D0554941

# SABISTON TEXTBOOK OF SURGERY

## 19TH EDITION

# SABISTON TEXTBOOK OF SURGERY:

## THE BIOLOGICAL BASIS OF MODERN SURGICAL PRACTICE

### 19TH EDITION


**COURTNEY M. TOWNSEND, JR., MD**
Professor and John Woods Harris Distinguished Chairman
Robertson-Poth Distinguished Chair in General Surgery
Department of Surgery
The University of Texas Medical Branch
Galveston, Texas

**R. DANIEL BEAUCHAMP, MD**
J.C. Foshee Distinguished Professor and Chairman, Section of Surgical Sciences
Professor of Surgery and Cell and Developmental Biology and Cancer Biology
Vanderbilt University School of Medicine
Surgeon-in-Chief, Vanderbilt University Hospital
Nashville, Tennessee

**B. MARK EVERS, MD**
Professor and Vice-Chair for Research, Department of Surgery
Director, Lucille P. Markey Cancer Center
Markey Cancer Foundation Endowed Chair
Physician-in-Chief, Oncology Service Line UK Healthcare
The University of Kentucky
Lexington, Kentucky

**KENNETH L. MATTOX, MD**
Professor and Vice Chairman
Michael E. DeBakey Department of Surgery
Baylor College of Medicine
Chief of Staff and Chief of Surgery
Ben Taub General Hospital
Houston, Texas


with 1645 illustrations


ELSEVIER
SAUNDERS

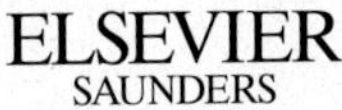

SAUNDERS

1600 John F. Kennedy Blvd.
Ste 1800
Philadelphia, PA 19103-2899

SABISTON TEXTBOOK OF SURGERY

ISBN: 978-1-4377-1560-6
International Edition ISBN: 978-1-4557-1146-8



## Notices

Knowledge and best practice in this field are constantly changing. As new research and experience broaden our understanding, changes in research methods, professional practices, or medical treatment may become necessary.

Practitioners and researchers must always rely on their own experience and knowledge in evaluating and using any information, methods, compounds, or experiments described herein. In using such information or methods they should be mindful of their own safety and the safety of others, including parties for whom they have a professional responsibility.

With respect to any drug or pharmaceutical products identified, readers are advised to check the most current information provided (i) on procedures featured or (ii) by the manufacturer of each product to be administered, to verify the recommended dose or formula, the method and duration of administration, and contraindications. It is the responsibility of practitioners, relying on their own experience and knowledge of their patients, to make diagnoses, to determine dosages and the best treatment for each individual patient, and to take all appropriate safety precautions.

To the fullest extent of the law, neither the Publisher nor the authors, contributors, or editors, assume any liability for any injury and/or damage to persons or property as a matter of products liability, negligence or otherwise, or from any use or operation of any methods, products, instructions, or ideas contained in the material herein.

**Library of Congress Cataloging-in-Publication Data or Control Number**
Sabiston textbook of surgery : the biological basis of modern surgical practice.—19th ed. / [edited by] Courtney M. Townsend Jr. … [et al.].
p. ; cm.
Textbook of surgery
Includes bibliographical references and index.
ISBN 978-1-4377-1560-6 (hardcover : alk. paper)
I. Sabiston, David C., 1924-2009. II. Townsend, Courtney M. III. Title: Textbook of surgery.
[DNLM: 1. Surgical Procedures, Operative. 2. General Surgery. 3. Perioperative Care. WO 500]
617—dc23

2011040621

*Global Content Development Director:* Judith Fletcher
*Content Developmental Manager:* Maureen Iannuzzi
*Publishing Services Manager:* Catherine Jackson
*Senior Project Manager:* Rachel E. McMullen
*Design Direction:* Louis Forgione

Printed in Canada

Last digit is the print number: 9 8 7 6 5 4 3 2 1

# DEDICATION

TO OUR PATIENTS, who grant us the privilege of practicing our craft; to our students, residents, and colleagues, from whom we learn; and to our wives—Mary, Shannon, Karen, and June—without whose support this would not have been possible.

# CONTRIBUTORS

**ANDREW B. ADAMS, MD, PHD**
Associate, Department of Surgery, Emory Transplant Center, Emory University School of Medicine, Atlanta, Georgia
*Transplantation Immunobiology and Immunosuppression*

**CHARLES A. ADAMS, JR., MD**
Chief of Trauma and Surgical Critical Care, Rhode Island Hospital; Assistant Professor of Surgery, Alpert Medical School of Brown University, Providence, Rhode Island
*Surgical Critical Care*

**AHMED AL-MOUSAWI, MD**
Clinical Fellow, Burns & Critical Care, Shriners Burns Hospital for Children, Department of Surgery, University of Texas Medical Branch, Galveston, Texas
*Metabolism in Surgical Patients*

**WADDAH B. AL-REFAIE, MD, FACS**
Co-Director, Minnesota Surgical Outcomes Workgroup, Associate Professor of Surgery and Staff Surgeon, Division of Surgical Oncology, Department of Surgery, University of Minnesota and Minneapolis VAMC, Minneapolis, Minnesota
*Exocrine Pancreas*

**NANCY L. ASCHER, MD, PHD**
Professor and Chair, Department of Surgery, University of California at San Francisco, San Francisco, California
*Liver Transplantation*

**STANLEY W. ASHLEY, MD**
Chief Medical Officer, Vice President for Medical Affairs, Brigham and Women's Hospital; Frank Sawyer Professor of Surgery, Harvard Medical School, Boston, Massachusetts
*Acute Gastrointestinal Hemorrhage*

**PAUL S. AUERBACH, MD, MS, FACEP**
Redlich Family Professor of Surgery, Department of Surgery, Division of Emergency Medicine, Stanford University School of Medicine, Stanford, California
*Bites and Stings*

**BRIAN BADGWELL, MD**
Assistant Professor, Department of Surgery, University of Arkansas for Medical Sciences, Little Rock, Arkansas
*Abdominal Wall, Umbilicus, Peritoneum, Mesenteries, Omentum, and Retroperitoneum*

**FAISAL G. BAKAEEN, MD, FACS**
Chief of Cardiothoracic Surgery, The Michael E. DeBakey VA Medical Center; Associate Professor, Cardiothoracic Surgery, Baylor College of Medicine, Houston, Texas
*Acquired Heart Disease: Coronary Insufficiency*

**PHILIP S. BARIE, MD, MBA, FIDSA, FCCM, FACS**
Professor of Surgery and Public Health, Weill Cornell Medical College; Chief, Preston A. (Pep) Wade Acute Care Surgery Service, New York–Presbyterian Hospital–Weill Cornell Medical Center, New York, New York
*Surgical Infections and Antibiotic Use*

**B. TIMOTHY BAXTER, MD**
Professor of Vascular Surgery, Department of Surgery, University of Nebraska Medical Center, Omaha, Nebraska
*The Lymphatics*

**R. DANIEL BEAUCHAMP, MD**
J.C. Foshee Distinguished Professor and Chairman, Section of Surgical Sciences, Professor of Surgery and Cell and Developmental Biology and Cancer Biology, Vanderbilt University School of Medicine; Surgeon-in-Chief, Vanderbilt University Hospital, Nashville, Tennessee
*Perioperative Patient Safety*

**YOLANDA BECKER, MD, FACS**
Professor of Surgery, Director, Kidney and Pancreas Program, Division of Transplant Surgery, University of Chicago, Chicago, Illinois
*Kidney and Pancreas Transplantation*

**PAUL R. BEERY, MD**
Clinical Assistant Professor, Department of Surgery, Ohio State University Grant Medical Center, Columbus, Ohio
*Surgery in the Pregnant Patient*

**DAVID H. BERGER, MD**
Professor of Surgery and Vice-Chair, Michael E. DeBakey Department of Surgery, Baylor College of Medicine; Operative Care Line Executive, Michael E. DeBakey VA Medical Center, Houston, Texas
*Surgery in the Geriatric Patient*

**JOSHUA I.S. BLEIER, MD, FACS, FASCRS**
Assistant Professor, Department of Surgery, University of Pennsylvania, Philadelphia, Pennsylvania
*Colon and Rectum*

**DANIEL BORJA-CACHO, MD**
HPB Fellow, Department of Surgery, University of Minnesota, Minneapolis, Minnesota
*Exocrine Pancreas*

**HOWARD BRODY, MD, PHD**
Director, Institute for the Medical Humanities; John P. McGovern Centennial Chair in Family Medicine, Family Medicine, University of Texas Medical Branch, Galveston, Texas
*Ethics and Professionalism in Surgery*

**BRUCE D. BROWNER, MD, MS, FACS**
Gray-Gossling Chair, Professor and Chairman Emeritus, Department of Orthopedic Surgery, New England Musculoskeletal Institute, University of Connecticut Health Center; Director of Orthopaedics, Hartford Hospital, Farmington, Connecticut
*Emergency Care of Musculoskeletal Injuries*

**THOMAS A. BUCHHOLZ, MD, FACR**
Head, Division of Radiation Oncology, The University of Texas M.D. Anderson Cancer Center, Houston, Texas
*Diseases of the Breast*

**BRIAN B. BURKEY, MD, FACS**
Vice-Chairman and Section Head, Head and Neck Surgery and Oncology, Head and Neck Institute, Cleveland Clinic Foundation; Adjunct Professor, Department of Otolaryngology, Vanderbilt University Medical Center, Nashville, Tennessee
*Head and Neck*

**KATHLEEN E. CARBERRY, BSN, RN, MPH**
Research Specialist–Clinical Outcomes, Center for Clinical Outcomes, Congenital Heart Surgery Service, Texas Children's Hospital, Houston, Texas
*Congenital Heart Disease*

**CHARLIE C. CHENG, MD**
Assistant Professor, Division of Vascular Surgery and Endovascular Therapy, University of Texas Medical Branch, Galveston, Texas
*Peripheral Arterial Occlusive Disease*

**KENNETH J. CHERRY, JR., MD**
Professor, Department of Surgery, School of Medicine, University of Virginia, Charlottesville, Virginia
*Aorta*

**LORI CHOI, MD**
Assistant Professor, Division of Vascular Surgery and Endovascular Therapy, University of Texas Medical Branch, Galveston, Texas
*Peripheral Arterial Occlusive Disease*

**DANNY CHU, MD**
Associate Chief of Cardiothoracic Surgery, Operative Care Line, Michael E. DeBakey VA Medical Center; Assistant Professor of Surgery, Michael E. DeBakey Department of Surgery, Texas Heart Institute/Baylor College of Medicine, Houston, Texas
*Acquired Heart Disease: Coronary Insufficiency*

**DAI H. CHUNG, MD**
Professor and Chairman, Janie Robinson and John Moore Lee Endowed Chair, Department of Pediatric Surgery, Vanderbilt University Medical Center, Nashville, Tennessee
*Pediatric Surgery*

**WILLIAM G. CIOFFI, MD**
Surgeon-in-Chief, Department of Surgery, Rhode Island Hospital; Professor and Chairman of Surgery, Alpert Medical School of Brown University, Providence, Rhode Island
*Surgical Critical Care*

**MICHAEL COBURN, MD**
Professor and Chair, Scott Department of Urology, Baylor College of Medicine; Carlton-Scott Chair in Urologic Education; Chief of Urology, Ben Taub General Hospital, Houston, Texas
*Urologic Surgery*

**MARION E. COUCH, MD, PHD**
Associate Professor, Department of Otolaryngology/Head and Neck Surgery, University of North Carolina School of Medicine, Chapel Hill, North Carolina
*Head and Neck*

**MICHAEL D'ANGELICA, MD**
Associate Member, Department of Surgery, Memorial Sloan-Kettering Cancer Center; Associate Attending Surgeon, Department of Surgery, Memorial Hospital for Cancer and Allied Diseases; Associate Professor, Department of Surgery, Cornell University, Weill Medical College, New York, New York
*The Liver*

**ALAN DARDIK, MD, PHD**
Associate Professor of Surgery, Yale University School of Medicine; Chief, Peripheral Vascular Surgery, VA Connecticut Healthcare System, West Haven, Connecticut
*Surgery in the Geriatric Patient*

**MERRIL T. DAYTON, MD**
Professor and Chairman, Department of Surgery, State University of New York–Buffalo; Chief of Surgery, Kaleida Health System, Buffalo General Hospital, Buffalo, New York
*Surgical Complications*

**JOSE J. DIAZ, MD, CNS, FACS, FCCM**
Professor of Surgery, Chief Acute Care Surgery, R. Adams Cowley Shock Trauma Center, University of Maryland Medical Center, Baltimore, Maryland
*Bedside Surgical Procedures; The Difficult Abdominal Wall*

**QUAN-YANG DUH, MD**
Professor of Surgery, University of California San Francisco; Surgical Service, San Francisco VA Medical Center, San Francisco, California
*The Adrenal Glands*

**WILLIAM D. DUTTON, MD, CDR, MC, USN**
Instructor of Surgery, Acute Care Surgery Fellow, Division of Trauma and Surgical Critical Care, Vanderbilt University Medical Center, Nashville, Tennessee
*The Difficult Abdominal Wall*

**TIMOTHY J. EBERLEIN, MD**
Bixby Professor and Chairman of the Department of Surgery, Spencer T. and Ann W. Olin Distinguished Professor and Director, The Alvin J. Siteman Cancer Center, Barnes-Jewish Hospital and Washington University School of Medicine; Surgeon-in-Chief, Barnes-Jewish Hospital, St. Louis, Missouri
*Tumor Biology and Tumor Markers*

**JAMES S. ECONOMOU, MD, PHD**
Beaumont Professor of Surgery, Chief of Division of Surgical Oncology, Professor of Microbiology, Immunology and Molecular Genetics, Professor of Molecular and Medical Pharmacology, UCLA School of Medicine; Vice Chancellor for Research, University of California, Los Angeles, California
*Tumor Immunology and Immunotherapy*

**E. CHRISTOPHER ELLISON, MD**
Robert M. Zollinger Professor and Chair, Department of Surgery, Ohio State University Medical Center, Columbus, Ohio
*Surgery in the Pregnant Patient*

**STEVEN R.T. EVANS, MD**
Professor of Surgery, Chief Medical Officer and Vice President for Medical Affairs, Georgetown University Hospital, Washington, DC
*Biliary System*

**B. MARK EVERS, MD**
Professor and Vice-Chair for Research, Department of Surgery, Director, Lucille P. Markey Cancer Center, Markey Cancer Foundation Endowed Chair, Physician-in-Chief, Oncology Service Line UK Healthcare, The University of Kentucky, Lexington, Kentucky
*Small Intestine*

**FARHOOD FARJAH, MD, MPH**
Department of Surgery, University of Washington, Seattle, Washington
*Evidence-Based Surgery: Critically Assessing Surgical Literature*

**MITCHELL P. FINK, MD**
Professor, Departments of Surgery and Anesthesiology, Vice-Chair of Department of Surgery, UCLA David Geffen School of Medicine, Los Angeles, California
*The Inflammatory Response*

**NICHOLAS A. FIORE, II, MD, FACS**
Cy-Fair Hand and Wrist, Houston, Texas
*Hand Surgery*

**DAVID R. FLUM, MD, MPH**
Professor of Surgery and Adjunct Professor of Health Services and Pharmacy, Director of the Surgical Outcomes Research Center, University of Washington, Seattle, Washington
*Evidence-Based Surgery: Critically Assessing Surgical Literature*

**YUMAN FONG, MD**
Murray F. Brennan Chair in Surgery, Department of Surgery, Division of Hepatopancreatobiliary Surgery, Memorial Sloan-Kettering Cancer Center; Professor of Surgery, Weill Cornell Medical Center, New York, New York
*The Liver*

**CHARLES D. FRASER, JR., MD**
Chief and The Donovan Chair in Congenital Health Surgery, Surgeon-in-Chief, Texas Children's Hospital; Professor of Surgery and Pediatrics, Susan V. Clayton Chair in Surgery, Baylor College of Medicine, Houston, Texas
*Congenital Heart Disease*

**JULIE A. FREISCHLAG, MD**
The William Steward Halsted Professor and Chair, Department of Surgery, Johns Hopkins University, Baltimore, Maryland
*Venous Disease*

**GERALD M. FRIED, MD, CM, FRCS(C), FACS, FCAHS**
Adair Family Professor and Chairman, Department of Surgery, McGill University; Surgeon-in-Chief, McGill University Health Centre, Montreal, Quebec, Canada
*Emerging Technology in Surgery: Informatics, Robotics, and Electronics*

**ROBERT D. FRY, MD**
Emilie and Roland deHellebranth Professor of Surgery, Chief of the Division of Colon and Rectal Surgery, University of Pennsylvania Health System; Chairman, Department of Surgery, Pennsylvania Hospital, Philadelphia, Pennsylvania
*Colon and Rectum*

**DAVID A. FULLERTON, MD**
Head, Division of Cardiothoracic Surgery, University of Colorado School of Medicine, Aurora, Colorado
*Acquired Heart Disease: Valvular*

**JAIME GASCO, MD**
Assistant Professor, Division of Neurological Surgery, University of Texas Medical Branch, Galveston, Texas
*Neurosurgery*

**GERD G. GAUGLITZ, MMS, MD**
Department of Dermatology and Allergy, Ludwig-Maximilian University, Munich, Germany
*Burns*

**JASON P. GLOTZBACH, MD**
Postdoctoral Research Fellow, Stanford University Department of Surgery, Stanford, California; General Surgery Resident, University of North Carolina Department of Surgery, Chapel Hill, North Carolina
*Regenerative Medicine*

**S. PETER GOEDEGEBUURE, PHD**
Research Associate Professor, Department of Surgery, Washington University School of Medicine, St. Louis, Missouri
*Tumor Biology and Tumor Markers*

**RAJA R. GOPALDAS, MD**
Assistant Professor of Cardiothoracic Surgery, Hugh E. Stephenson Department of Surgery, University of Missouri-Columbia School of Medicine, Columbia, Missouri
*Acquired Heart Disease: Coronary Insufficiency*

**MARJORIE C. GREEN, MD**
Associate Professor of Medicine and Internist, Department of Breast Medical Oncology, Division of Cancer Medicine, The University of Texas M.D. Anderson Cancer Center, Houston, Texas
*Diseases of the Breast*

**OLIVER L. GUNTER, MD**
Assistant Professor, Division of Trauma and Surgical Critical Care, Vanderbilt University School of Medicine, Nashville, Tennessee
*Bedside Surgical Procedures*

**GEOFFREY C. GURTNER, MD, FACS**
Professor and Associate Chair of Surgery, Stanford University Department of Surgery, Stanford, California
*Regenerative Medicine*

**FADI HANBALI, MD, FACS**
Assistant Professor of Neurosurgery, Texas Tech University Health Science Center, El Paso, Texas
*Neurosurgery*

**JOHN B. HANKS, MD**
C. Bruce Morton Professor and Chief, Division of General Surgery, Department of Surgery, University of Virginia, Charlottesville, Virginia
*Thyroid*

**ALDEN H. HARKEN, MD**
Chairman, Department of Surgery, University of California at San Francisco (East Bay), San Francisco, California
*Acquired Heart Disease: Valvular*

**JENNIFER A. HELLER, MD**
Assistant Professor of Surgery, Director of Johns Hopkins Vein Center, Johns Hopkins Bayview Medical Center, Baltimore, Maryland
*Venous Disease*

**DAVID N. HERNDON, MD, FACS**
Chief of Staff, Shriners Burns Hospital for Children; Professor of Surgery and Jesse H. Jones Distinguished Chair in Burn Surgery, The University of Texas Medical Branch, Galveston, Texas
*Burns; Metabolism in Surgical Patients*

**MICHAEL S. HIGGINS, MD, MPH**
Professor, Department of Anesthesiology, Surgery and Biomedical Informatics, Vanderbilt University School of Medicine, Nashville, Tennessee
*Perioperative Patient Safety*

**ASHER HIRSHBERG, MD, FACS**
Professor of Surgery, State University of New York Downstate College of Medicine; Director of Emergency Vascular Surgery, Kings County Hospital Center, Brooklyn, New York
*The Surgeon's Role in Mass Casualty Incidents*

**GINGER E. HOLT, MD**
Associate Professor, Department of Orthopaedic Surgery, Vanderbilt Orthopaedic Institute, Vanderbilt University Medical Center, Nashville, Tennessee
*Bone Tumors*

**MICHAEL D. HOLZMAN, MD, MPH**
Associate Professor of Surgery and Lester and Sara Jayne Williams Chair in Academic Surgery, General Surgery Division, Vanderbilt University Medical Center, Nashville, Tennessee
*The Spleen*

**KELLY K. HUNT, MD**
Hamill Foundation Distinguished Professor of Surgery, Chief of Surgical Breast Oncology, M.D. Anderson Cancer Center, Houston, Texas
*Diseases of the Breast*

**PATRICK G. JACKSON, MD**
Chief of Gastrointestinal Surgery, Department of Surgery, Georgetown University Hospital, Washington, DC
*Biliary System*

**ERIC H. JENSEN, MD**
Assistant Professor of Surgery, University of Minnesota, Minneapolis, Minnesota
*Exocrine Pancreas*

**MARC JESCHKE, MD, PHD, FACS, FRCSC**
Director, Ross Tilley Burn Centre, Sunnybrook Health Sciences Centre; Associate Professor, Department of Surgery, Division of Plastic Surgery, University of Toronto; Senior Scientist, Sunnybrook Research Institute, Toronto, Ontario, Canada
*Burns*

**HOWARD W. JONES, III, MD**
Professor and Chairman, Department of Obstetrics and Gynecology, Vanderbilt University School of Medicine, Nashville, Tennessee
*Gynecologic Surgery*

**ALLAN D. KIRK, MD, PHD**
Professor, Department of Surgery, Emory University School of Medicine, Atlanta, Georgia
*Transplantation Immunobiology and Immunosuppression*

**KIMBERLY S. KIRKWOOD, MD, FACS**
Professor of Surgery, Department of Surgery, University of California at San Francisco, San Francisco, California
*The Appendix*

**SAE HEE KO, MD**
Postdoctoral Research Fellow, Stanford University Department of Surgery, Stanford, California; General Surgery Resident, University of Pittsburgh Department of Surgery, Pittsburgh, Pennsylvania
*Regenerative Medicine*

**TIEN C. KO, MD**
Jack H. Mayfield, M.D. Distinguished Professor in Surgery; Vice Chairman for Harris County Hospital District, The University of Texas Health Science Center; Chief of Surgery, Lyndon B. Johnson General Hospital, Houston, Texas
*Molecular and Cell Biology*

**SETH B. KRANTZ, MD**
Research Fellow, Robert H. Lurie Comprehensive Cancer Center and the Department of Surgery, Northwestern University Feinberg School of Medicine, Chicago, Illinois
*Stomach*

**MAHMOUD N. KULAYLAT, MD**
Associate Professor of Surgery, Department of Surgery, State University of New York–Buffalo, Buffalo General Hospital, Buffalo, New York
*Surgical Complications*

**TERRY C. LAIRMORE, MD**
Professor of Surgery and Director, Division of Surgical Oncology, Scott and White Memorial Hospital and Clinic, Texas A&M University System Health Science Center College of Medicine, Temple, Texas
*The Multiple Endocrine Neoplasia Syndromes*

**CHRISTIAN P. LARSEN, MD, DPHIL**
Joseph B. Whitehead Professor and Chairman of Surgery; Associate Vice-President and Executive Director, Emory Transplant Center, Emory University School of Medicine, Atlanta, Georgia
*Transplantation Immunobiology and Immunosuppression*

**MIMI LEONG, MD, MS**
Assistant Professor, Plastic Surgery Division, Baylor College of Medicine; Staff Physician, Section of Plastic Surgery, Operative Care Line, Michael E. DeBakey Department of Surgery, Houston, Texas
*Wound Healing*

**MICHAEL T. LONGAKER, MD, MBA, FACS**
Deane P. and Louise Mitchell Professor and Vice-Chair in Department of Surgery, Co-Director of Stanford Institute for Stem Cell Biology and Regenerative Medicine, Director of Program in Regenerative Medicine, Stanford University School of Medicine, Palo Alto, California
*Regenerative Medicine*

**ROBERT R. LORENZ, MD, MBA**
Medical Director Payment Reform, Risk & Contracting; Head and Neck Surgery, Laryngotracheal Reconstruction and Oncology, Head and Neck Institute, Cleveland Clinic, Cleveland, Ohio
*Head and Neck*

**JOHN MAA, MD**
Assistant Professor, Department of Surgery, University of California at San Francisco, San Francisco, California
*The Appendix*

**NAJJIA N. MAHMOUD, MD**
Associate Professor of Surgery, Department of Surgery, University of Pennsylvania, Philadelphia, Pennsylvania
*Colon and Rectum*

**DAVID M. MAHVI, MD**
James R Hines Professor, Department of Surgery, Northwestern University Feinberg School of Medicine, Chicago, Illinois
*Stomach*

**MARY S. MAISH, MD, MPH**
Associate Professor of Surgery, Director of the UCLA Center for Esophageal Disorders, UCLA David Geffen School of Medicine, Los Angeles, California
*Esophagus*

**MARK A. MALANGONI, MD**
Associate Executive Director; American Board of Surgery, Philadelphia, Pennsylvania
*Hernias*

**DAVID J. MARON, MD, MBA**
Associate Director of Colorectal Surgery Residency Program, Staff Surgeon, Department of Colorectal Surgery, Cleveland Clinic Florida, Weston, Florida
*Colon and Rectum*

**SILAS T. MARSHALL, MD**
Resident, Department of Orthopaedic Surgery, University of Connecticut, Farmington, Connecticut
*Emergency Care of Musculoskeletal Injuries*

**ABIGAIL E. MARTIN, MD**
Assistant Professor of Surgery, Divisions of Pediatric General Surgery and Abdominal Transplant Surgery, Duke University Medical Center, Durham, North Carolina
*Small Bowel Transplantation*

**R. SHAYN MARTIN, MD**
Assistant Professor of Surgery, Department of Surgery, Wake Forest School of Medicine; Director, Surgical Critical Care, Wake Forest Baptist Medical Center, Winston-Salem, North Carolina
*Management of Acute Trauma*

**NADER MASSARWEH, MD, MPH**
Surgical Resident, Department of Surgery, University of Washington, Seattle, Washington
*Evidence-Based Surgery: Critically Assessing Surgical Literature*

**ADDISON K. MAY, MD**
Professor of Surgery and Anesthesiology, Division of Trauma and Surgical Critical Care, Vanderbilt University Medical Center, Nashville, Tennessee
*Bedside Surgical Procedures*

**MARY H. MCGRATH, MD, MPH, FACS**
Professor, Division of Plastic Surgery, Department of Surgery, University of California San Francisco, San Francisco, California
*Plastic Surgery*

**SHAUN MCKENZIE, MD**
Assistant Professor, University of Kentucky Department of Surgery, Markey Cancer Center, Lexington, Kentucky
*Small Intestine*

**KELLY M. MCMASTERS, MD, PHD**
Ben A. Reid, Sr. M.D. Professor and Chairman, Department of Surgery, University of Louisville School of Medicine, Louisville, Kentucky
*Melanoma and Cutaneous Malignancies*

**J. WAYNE MEREDITH, MD, FACS**
Richard T. Meyers Professor and Chair, Department of Surgery, Wake Forest University School of Medicine; Chief of Surgery, Wake Forest University Baptist Medical Center, Winston-Salem, North Carolina
*Management of Acute Trauma*

**DEAN J. MIKAMI, MD**
Assistant Professor of Surgery, Department of Surgery, Ohio State University Medical Center, Columbus, Ohio
*Surgery in the Pregnant Patient*

**RICHARD S. MILLER, MD, FACS**
Professor of Surgery, Chief of the Division of Trauma and Surgical Critical Care, Vanderbilt University Medical Center, Nashville, Tennessee
*The Difficult Abdominal Wall*

**AARON MOHANTY, MD**
Assistant Professor, Pediatric Neurosurgery, University of Texas Medical Branch, Galveston, Texas
*Neurosurgery*

**JEFFREY F. MOLEY, MD**
Professor of Surgery, Department of Surgery, Chief, Section of Endocrine and Oncologic Surgery, Washington University School of Medicine; Associate Director, Alvin Siteman Cancer Center; Attending Surgeon, Surgical Service, St. Louis VA Medical Center, St. Louis, Missouri
*The Multiple Endocrine Neoplasia Syndromes*

**KEVIN MURPHY, MD, MCH, FRCS(PLAST.)**
Hand Surgery Fellow, Division of Plastic Surgery, Baylor College of Medicine, Houston, Texas
*Hand Surgery*

**ELAINE E. NELSON, MD, FACEP**
Chairman, Department of Emergency Medicine, Regional Medical Center of San Jose, San Jose, California
*Bites and Stings*

**HEIDI NELSON, MD**
Fred C. Andersen Professor, Department of Surgery, Chair Division of Surgery Research, Mayo Clinic, Rochester, Minnesota
*Anus*

**DAVID NETSCHER, MD**
Clinical Professor, Division of Plastic Surgery; Professor, Department of Orthopedic Surgery, Baylor College of Medicine; Adjunct Professor of Clinical Surgery (Plastic Surgery), Weill Medical College, Cornell University; Chief of Hand Surgery, St. Luke's Episcopal Hospital; Chief of Plastic Surgery, VA Medical Center, Houston, Texas
*Hand Surgery*

**LEIGH NEUMAYER, MD**
Professor of Surgery, Department of Surgery, University of Utah; Jon and Karen Huntsman Presidential Professor in Cancer Research, Huntsman Cancer Institute; Co-Director, Multidisciplinary Breast Program, Huntsman Cancer Hospital, Salt Lake City, Utah
*Principles of Preoperative and Operative Surgery*

**ROBERT L. NORRIS, MD**
Professor, Department of Surgery and Chief, Division of Emergency Medicine, Stanford University School of Medicine, Stanford, California
*Bites and Stings*

**BRANT K. OELSCHLAGER, MD, FACS**
Byers Endowed Professor of Esophageal Research, Chief, Gastrointestinal and General Surgery and Center for Videoendoscopic Surgery, University of Washington, Seattle, Washington
*Hiatal Hernia and Gastroesophageal Reflux Disease*

**JOEL T. PATTERSON, MD**
Associate Professor of Neurosurgery and Otolaryngology, Samuel R. Snodgrass, MD Professorship in Neurosurgery, Chief and Program Director, Division of Neurosurgery, Department of Surgery, The University of Texas Medical Branch, Galveston, Texas
*Neurosurgery*

**CARLOS A. PELLEGRINI, MD, FACS, FRCSI(HON)**
The Henry N. Harkins Professor and Chairman, Department of Surgery, University of Washington Medical Center, Seattle, Washington
*Hiatal Hernia and Gastroesophageal Reflux Disease*

**REBECCA P. PETERSEN, MD, MSC**
Senior Fellow and Acting Instructor, Department of Surgery, University of Washington, Seattle, Washington
*Hiatal Hernia and Gastroesophageal Reflux Disease*

**LINDA G. PHILLIPS, MD**
Truman G. Blocker, Jr., MD, Distinguished Professor and Chief, Division of Plastic Surgery, Department of Surgery, The University of Texas Medical Branch, Galveston, Texas
*Wound Healing; Breast Reconstruction*

**IRAKLIS I. PIPINOS, MD**
Professor, Vascular Surgery, Department of Surgery, University of Nebraska Medical Center, Omaha, Nebraska
*The Lymphatics*

**JASON POMERANTZ, MD**
Assistant Professor, Department of Surgery, University of California San Francisco, San Francisco, California
*Plastic Surgery*

**RUSSELL G. POSTIER, MD**
John A. Schilling Professor and Chairman, Department of Surgery, University of Oklahoma Health Sciences Center, Oklahoma City, Oklahoma
*Acute Abdomen*

**DONALD S. PROUGH, MD**
Professor and Chair, Department of Anesthesiology, The University of Texas Medical Branch, Galveston, Texas
*Anesthesiology Principles, Pain Management, and Conscious Sedation*

**JOE B. PUTNAM, JR., MD**
Ingram Professor of Surgery, Chairman of Department of Thoracic Surgery, Professor of Biomedical Informatics, Vanderbilt University School of Medicine, Nashville, Tennessee
*Lung, Chest Wall, Pleura, and Mediastinum*

**PETER RHEE, MD, MPH, DMCC**
Professor of Surgery and Molecular Cellular Biology, Chief of Trauma, Critical Care and Emergency Surgery, University of Arizona, Tucson, Arizona
*Shock, Electrolytes, and Fluid*

**TAYLOR S. RIALL, MD, PHD**
Associate Professor, John Sealy Distinguished Chair in Clinical Research, Department of Surgery, University of Texas Medical Branch, Galveston, Texas
*Endocrine Pancreas*

**WILLIAM O. RICHARDS, MD**
Professor and Chair, Department of Surgery, University of South Alabama College of Medicine, Mobile, Alabama
*Morbid Obesity*

**NOE A. RODRIGUEZ, MD**
Post-Doctoral Fellow Burn Research, Department of Surgery, University of Texas Medical Branch, Galveston, Texas
*Metabolism in Surgical Patients*

**KENDALL R. ROEHL, MD**
Assistant Professor, Division of Plastic and Reconstructive Surgery, Texas A&M Health Sciences Center, Scott and White Hospital Clinics, Temple, Texas
*Breast Reconstruction*

**MICHAEL J. ROSEN, MD**
Chief of Gastrointestinal Surgery, Director Case Comprehensive Hernia Center Department of Surgery, University Hospitals Case Medical Center, Cleveland, Ohio
*Hernias*

**RONNIE A. ROSENTHAL, MD**
Professor of Surgery, Yale University School of Medicine, New Haven and Chief, Surgical Service, VA Connecticut Healthcare System, West Haven, Connecticut
*Surgery in the Geriatric Patient*

**IRA RUTKOW, MD, MPH, DRPH**
Clinical Professor of Surgery, University of Medicine and Dentistry of New Jersey, Newark, New Jersey
*History of Surgery*

**LESLIE J. SALOMONE, MD**
Clinical Endocrinologist, Jacksonville, Florida
*Thyroid*

**HERBERT S. SCHWARTZ, MD**
Professor and Chairman, Department of Orthopaedic Surgery, Vanderbilt Orthopaedic Institute, Vanderbilt University Medical Center, Nashville, Tennessee
*Bone Tumors*

**STEVEN R. SHACKFORD, MD, FACS**
Professor Emeritus, Department of Surgery, College of Medicine, University of Vermont, Burlington, Vermont
*Vascular Trauma*

**JULIA SHELTON, MD**
Resident, Department of General Surgery, Vanderbilt University Medical Center, Nashville, Tennessee
*The Spleen*

**EDWARD R. SHERWOOD, MD, PHD**
Professor, James F. Arens Endowed Chair, Vice Chair for Research, Department of Anesthesiology, The University of Texas Medical Branch, Galveston, Texas
*Anesthesiology Principles, Pain Management, and Conscious Sedation*

**JASON K. SICKLICK, MD**
Department of Surgery, Division of Surgical Oncology, Moores UCSD Cancer Center, University of California at San Diego, La Jolla, California
*The Liver*

**MICHAEL B. SILVA, JR., MD**
Fred J. and Dorothy E. Wolma Professor in Vascular Surgery, Professor of Radiology, Chief, Division of Vascular Surgery and Endovascular Therapy, Director, Texas Vascular Center, University of Texas Medical Branch, Galveston, Texas
*Peripheral Arterial Occlusive Disease*

**SAMUEL SINGER, MD**
Chief, Gastric and Mixed Tumor Service, Department of Surgery, Memorial Sloan-Kettering Cancer Center, New York, New York
*Soft Tissue Sarcomas*

**MICHAEL J. SISE, MD**
Clinical Professor of Surgery, University of California, San Diego School of Medicine; Medical Director, Division of Trauma, Scripps Mercy Hospital, San Diego, California
*Vascular Trauma*

**PHILIP W. SMITH, MD**
Assistant Professor of Surgery, Endocrine and General Surgery, Department of Surgery, University of Virginia, Charlottesville, Virginia
*Thyroid*

**JULIE ANN SOSA, MD, MA, FACS**
Associate Professor of Surgery and Medicine (Medical Oncology), Divisions of Endocrine Surgery and Surgical Oncology, Yale University School of Medicine, New Haven, Connecticut
*The Parathyroid Glands*

**RONALD A. SQUIRES, MD**
Professor, Department of Surgery, University of Oklahoma Health Sciences Center, Oklahoma City, Oklahoma
*Acute Abdomen*

**MICHAEL STEIN, MD**
Director of Trauma, Rabin Medical Center, Petach Tivka, Israel
*The Surgeon's Role in Mass Casualty Incidents*

**ANDREW STEPHEN, MD**
Staff, Division of Trauma and Surgical Critical Care, Rhode Island Hospital; Alpert Medical School of Brown University, Providence, Rhode Island
*Surgical Critical Care*

**RONALD M. STEWART, MD**
Professor and Chair, Jocelyn and Joe Straus Endowed Chair, Department of Surgery, University of Texas Health Science Center San Antonio, San Antonio, Texas
*Bites and Stings*

**DEBRA L. SUDAN, MD**
Professor of Surgery and Pediatrics, Division Chief Abdominal Transplant Surgery, Vice-Chair for Clinical Operations, Duke University School of Medicine, Durham, North Carolina
*Small Bowel Transplantation*

**MARCUS C.B. TAN, MBBS(HONS)**
Resident in General Surgery, Department of Surgery, Barnes-Jewish Hospital, Washington University in St. Louis, St. Louis, Missouri
*Tumor Biology and Tumor Markers*

**ALI TAVAKKOLIZADEH, MD**
Associate Surgeon, Brigham and Women's Hospital; Assistant Professor of Surgery, Harvard Medical School, Boston, Massachusetts
*Acute Gastrointestinal Hemorrhage*

**JAMES S. TOMLINSON, MD, PHD**
Assistant Professor of Surgery, Division of Surgical Oncology, University of California, Los Angeles, Los Angeles, California
*Tumor Immunology and Immunotherapy*

**COURTNEY M. TOWNSEND, JR., MD**
Professor and John Woods Harris Distinguished Chairman, Robertson-Poth Distinguished Chair in General Surgery, Department of Surgery, The University of Texas Medical Branch, Galveston, Texas
*Endocrine Pancreas*

**MARGARET C. TRACCI, MD, JD**
Assistant Professor, Division of Vascular and Endovascular Surgery, University of Virginia, Charlottesville, Virginia
*Aorta*

**RICHARD H. TURNAGE, MD**
Academic Affiliation; Professor and Chairman; University of Arkansas for Medical Sciences (UAMS); Little Rock, Arkansas
*Abdominal Wall, Umbilicus, Peritoneum, Mesenteries, Omentum, and Retroperitoneum*

**ROBERT UDELSMAN, MD, MBA**
William H. Carmalt Professor of Surgery and Oncology and Chairman, Department of Surgery, Yale University School of Medicine, New Haven, Connecticut
*The Parathyroid Glands*

**MARSHALL M. URIST, MD**
Champ Lyons Professor and Vice-Chairman, Department of Surgery, University of Alabama at Birmingham, Birmingham, Alabama
*Melanoma and Cutaneous Malignancies*

**CHERYL E. VAIANI, PHD**
Assistant Professor, Clinical Ethicist, Institute for the Medical Humanities, University of Texas Medical Branch, Galveston, Texas
*Ethics and Professionalism in Surgery*

**DANIEL VARGO, MD, FACS**
Associate Professor, Department of Surgery, University of Utah School of Medicine, Salt Lake City, Utah
*Principles of Preoperative and Operative Surgery*

**SELWYN M. VICKERS, MD, FACS**
Jay Phillips Professor and Chairman, Department Chair, Department of Surgery, University of Minnesota, Minneapolis, Minnesota
*Exocrine Pancreas*

**BRADON J. WILHELMI, MD**
Leonard Weiner Endowed Professor, Chief of Plastic Surgery, Residency Program Director, Division of Plastic and Reconstructive Surgery, University of Louisville, Louisville, Kentucky
*Breast Reconstruction*

**COURTNEY G. WILLIAMS, MD**
Associate Professor, Department of Anesthesiology, The University of Texas Medical Branch, Galveston, Texas
*Anesthesiology Principles, Pain Management, and Conscious Sedation*

**FELICIA N. WILLIAMS, MD**
Chief Resident, Department of Surgery, East Carolina University, Pitt County Memorial Hospital, Greenville, North Carolina
*Burns*

**JAMES C. YANG, MD**
Senior Investigator, Surgery Branch, Center for Cancer Research, National Cancer Institute, Bethesda, Maryland
*Tumor Immunology and Immunotherapy*

**MICHAEL W. YEH, MD, FACS**
Associate Professor of Surgery and Medicine (Endocrinology), Chief, Section of Endocrine Surgery, UCLA David Geffen School of Medicine, Los Angeles, California
*The Adrenal Glands*

# FOREWORD

"How many a man has dated a new era in his life from the reading of a book."

Henry David Thoreau (1817-1862)

This 19th edition of *Sabiston Textbook of Surgery,* the fourth edited by Dr. Townsend and his co-editors Drs. Maddox, Beauchamp, and Evers, extends the tradition of textbook excellence and leadership initiated 18 editions ago. The emphasis on clinical relevance and outcomes characteristic of earlier editions has been enhanced by the addition of three new chapters on organ transplantation, two new chapters in the vascular section: "The Aorta" and "Peripheral Arterial Occlusive Disease," and new chapters on the cutting edge topics of tumor immunology and immunotherapy and the "difficult abdominal wall." Other chapters have been embellished by inclusion of the latest information on biomaterials, organ procurement issues, specific gene therapy, biliary tumors, urinary system tumors, and simulation in surgery. Still other content has been revised to increase the focus on evidence-based practice by coverage of comparative effectiveness and patient-specific therapeutics.

The recruitment of more than 50 new authors and co-authors has guaranteed timeliness of the text, ensured full display of state of the art technology, and refreshed the trove of illustrations which by tradition have amplified and corroborated the text. The authors have also provided over 400 self-assessment questions which will assist the reader in preparing for and successfully achieving recertification.

As was true with the previous edition, ownership of the print text of this edition gives free access to the online product "Expert Consult," which includes full text and art, updates (journal articles selected by the editors and authors and keyed to chapter topics), board review questions, and videos on topics ranging from pleural effusion to hand transplantation and total aortic replacement. Expert Consult makes access to the text and all related material as convenient as the nearest computer.

This 19th edition of Sabiston successfully integrates print and electronic media to provide complete coverage of surgical practice. Full use of all features of this text will increase the reader's practice of evidence-based surgery, facilitate the reader's recertification activities, and promote the reader's acquisition and maintenance of the professional competencies. In short this is truly a text that as foretold by Thoreau will launch each reader on a new era in his or her surgical life.

BASIL A. PRUITT, JR., MD, FACS, FCCM

# PREFACE

SURGERY CONTINUES TO EVOLVE as new technology, techniques, and knowledge are incorporated into the care of surgical patients. The 19th edition of the *Sabiston Textbook of Surgery* reflects these exciting changes and new information. We have incorporated eight new chapters and more than 77 new authors to ensure that the most current information is presented. For example, safety is paramount in the care of our surgical patients; our chapter on safety describes the surgeon's roles and responsibilities to ensure safety. We have included a new chapter on management of the difficult abdominal wall, which can be a vexing problem for even the most experienced surgeon. Distant surgery, using robotic and telementoring technology, has become a reality, and minimally invasive techniques are being used in almost all invasive procedures. This new edition has revised and enhanced the current chapters to reflect these changes. Finally, we have extensively updated chapters dealing with basic science aspects that are important to surgeons and, in many cases, represent scientific advances in which surgeons are leading the charge. This is most evident in the chapters on tumor biology and tumor immunology, transplantation immunology, and the rapidly emerging field of regenerative medicine.

The primary goal of this new edition is to remain the most thorough, useful, readable, and understandable textbook presenting the principles and techniques of surgery. It is designed to be equally useful to students, trainees, and experts in the field. We are committed to maintaining this tradition of excellence, begun in 1936. Surgery, after all, remains a discipline in which the knowledge and skill of a surgeon combine for the welfare of all patients.

COURTNEY M. TOWNSEND, JR., MD

# ACKNOWLEDGMENTS

WE WOULD LIKE TO recognize the invaluable contributions of Karen Martin, Steve Schuenke, Eileen Figueroa, and administrator Barbara Petit. Their dedicated professionalism, tenacious efforts, and cheerful cooperation are without parallel. They accomplished whatever was necessary, often on short or immediate deadlines, and were vital for the successful completion of the endeavor.

Our authors, respected authorities in their fields, all busy physicians and surgeons, did an outstanding job in sharing their wealth of knowledge.

We would also like to acknowledge the professionalism of our colleagues at Elsevier: Maureen R. Iannuzzi, Content Developmental Manager; Louis Forgione, Senior Book Designer; Rachel E. McMullen, Senior Project Manager; Catherine Jackson, Publications Services Manager; and Judith Fletcher, Global Content Development Director.

# CONTENTS

# VIDEO CONTENTS

# SECTION I

# SURGICAL BASIC PRINCIPLES

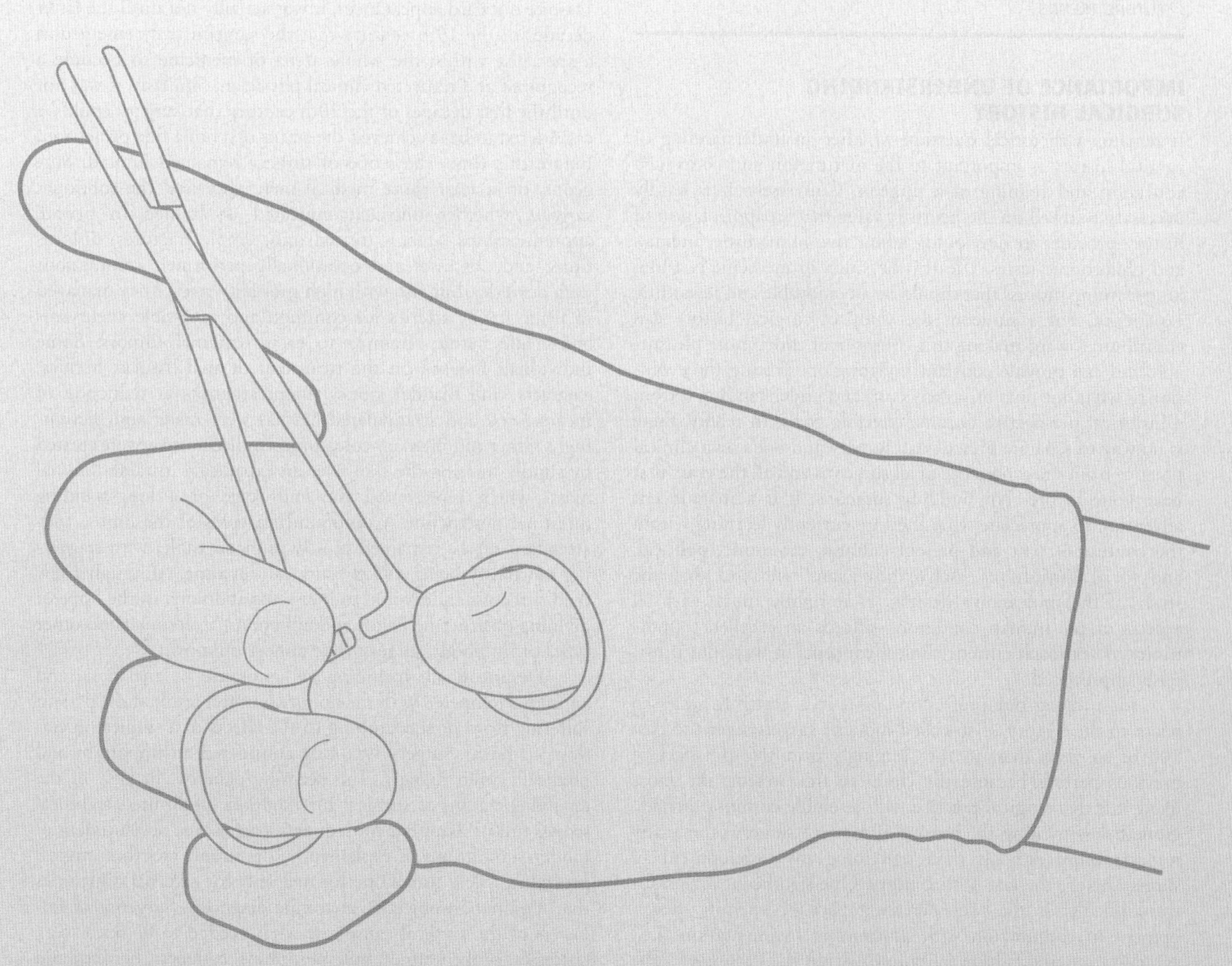

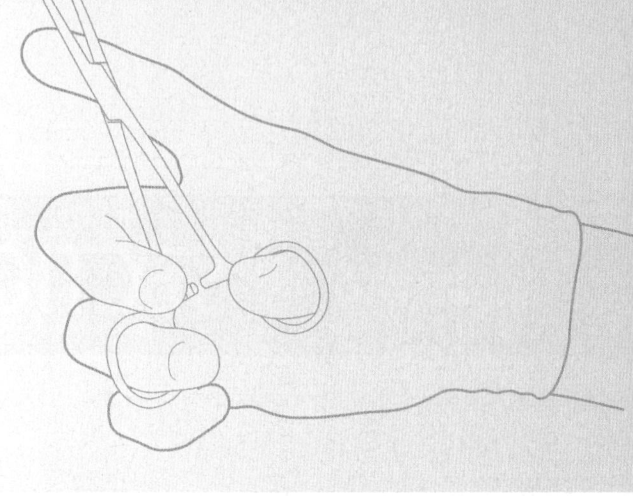

CHAPTER 1

# HISTORY OF SURGERY

Ira Rutkow



## IMPORTANCE OF UNDERSTANDING SURGICAL HISTORY

It remains a rhetorical question whether an understanding of surgical history is important to the maturation and continued education and training of a surgeon. Conversely, it is hardly necessary to dwell on the heuristic value that an appreciation of history provides in developing adjunctive humanistic, literary, and philosophic tastes. Clearly, the study of medicine is a lifelong learning process that should be an enjoyable and rewarding experience. For a surgeon, the study of surgical history can contribute toward making this educational effort more pleasurable and can provide constant invigoration. Tracing the evolution of what one does on a daily basis and understanding it from a historical perspective become enviable goals. In reality, there is no way to separate present-day surgery and one's own clinical practice from the experience of all surgeons and all the years that have gone before. For budding surgeons, it is a magnificent adventure to appreciate what they are currently learning within the context of past and present cultural, economic, political, and social institutions. Active physicians will find that the study of the profession—dealing, as it rightly must, with all aspects of the human condition—affords an excellent opportunity to approach current clinical concepts in ways not previously appreciated.

In studying our profession's past, it is certainly easier to relate to the history of so-called modern surgery over the past 100 or so years than to the seemingly primitive practices of previous periods because the closer to the present, the more likely it is that surgical practices will resemble current practices. Nonetheless, writing the history of modern surgery is in many respects more difficult than describing the development of surgery before the late 19th century. One significant reason for this difficulty is the ever-increasing pace of scientific development in conjunction with unrelenting fragmentation (i.e., specialization and subspecialization) within the profession. The craft of surgery is in constant flux and, the more rapid the change, the more difficult it is to obtain a satisfactory historical perspective. Only the lengthy passage of time permits a truly valid historical analysis.

### Historical Relationship Between Surgery and Medicine

Despite outward appearances, it was actually not until the latter decades of the 19th century that the surgeon truly emerged as a specialist within the whole arena of medicine to become a recognized and respected clinical physician. Similarly, it was not until the first decades of the 20th century that surgery could be considered to have achieved the status of a bona fide profession. Before this time, the scope of surgery remained limited. Surgeons, or at least those medical men who used the sobriquet *surgeon,* whether university-educated or trained in private apprenticeships, at best treated only simple fractures, dislocations, and abscesses and occasionally performed amputations with dexterity, but also with high mortality rates. They managed to ligate major arteries for common and accessible aneurysms and made heroic attempts to excise external tumors. Some individuals focused on the treatment of anal fistulas, hernias, cataracts, and bladder stones. Inept attempts at reduction of incarcerated and strangulated hernias were made and, hesitatingly, rather rudimentary colostomies or ileostomies were created by simply incising the skin over an expanding intra-abdominal mass, which represented the end stage of a long-standing intestinal obstruction. Compound fractures of the limbs, with attendant sepsis, remained mostly unmanageable, with staggering morbidity being a likely surgical outcome. Although a few bold surgeons endeavored to incise the abdomen in the hope of dividing obstructing bands and adhesions, abdominal and other types of intrabody surgery were almost unknown.

Despite it all, including an ignorance of anesthesia and antisepsis tempered with the not uncommon result of the patient suffering from or succumbing to the effects of a surgical operation (or both), surgery was long considered an important and medically valid therapy. This seeming paradox, in view of the terrifying nature of surgical intervention, its limited technical scope, and its damning consequences before the development of modern conditions, is explained by the simple fact that surgical procedures were usually performed only for external difficulties that required an objective anatomic diagnosis. Surgeons or followers of the surgical cause saw what needed to be fixed (e.g., abscesses, broken bones, bulging tumors, cataracts, hernias) and would treat the problem in as rational a manner as the times permitted. Conversely, the physician was forced to render subjective care for disease processes that were neither visible nor understood. After all, it is a difficult task to treat the symptoms of illnesses such as arthritis, asthma, heart failure, and diabetes, to name but a few, if there is no scientific understanding or internal knowledge of what constitutes their basic pathologic and physiologic underpinnings.

With the breathtaking advances made in pathologic anatomy and experimental physiology during the 18th and first part of the 19th centuries, physicians would soon adopt a therapeutic viewpoint that had long been prevalent among surgeons. It was no longer a question of just treating symptoms; the actual pathologic problem could ultimately be understood. Internal disease processes that manifested themselves through difficult to treat external signs and symptoms were finally described via physiology-based experimentation or viewed pathologically through the lens of a microscope. Because this reorientation of internal medicine occurred within a relatively short time and brought about such dramatic results in the classification, diagnosis, and treatment of disease, the rapid ascent of mid-19th century internal medicine might seem more impressive than the agonizingly slow, but steady, advance of surgery. In a seeming contradiction of mid-19th century scientific and social reality, medicine appeared as the more progressive branch, with surgery lagging behind. The art and craft of surgery, for all its practical possibilities, would be severely restricted until the discovery of anesthesia in 1846 and an understanding and acceptance of the need for surgical antisepsis and asepsis during the 1870s and 1880s. Still, surgeons never needed a diagnostic and pathologic revolution in the manner of the physician. Despite the imperfection of their scientific knowledge, the pre–modern era surgeon did cure with some technical confidence.

That the gradual evolution of surgery was superseded in the 1880s and 1890s by the rapid introduction of startling new technical advances was based on a simple culminating axiom—the four fundamental clinical prerequisites that were required before a surgical operation could ever be considered a truly viable therapeutic procedure had finally been identified and understood:

1. Knowledge of human anatomy
2. Method of controlling hemorrhage and maintaining intraoperative hemostasis
3. Anesthesia to permit the performance of pain-free procedures
4. Explanation of the nature of infection, along with the elaboration of methods necessary to achieve an antiseptic and aseptic operating room environment

The first two prerequisites were essentially solved in the 16th century, but the latter two would not be fully resolved until the ending decades of the 19th century. In turn, the ascent of 20th century scientific surgery would unify the profession and allow what had always been an art and craft to become a learned vocation. Standardized postgraduate surgical education and training programs could be established to help produce a cadre of scientifically knowledgeable physicians. Moreover, in a final snub to an unscientific past, newly established basic surgical research laboratories offered the means of proving or disproving the latest theories while providing a testing ground for bold and exciting clinical breakthroughs.

## Knowledge of Human Anatomy

Few individuals have had an influence on the history of surgery as overwhelmingly as that of the Brussels-born Andreas Vesalius (1514-1564; Fig. 1-1). As professor of anatomy and surgery in Padua, Italy, Vesalius taught that human anatomy could be learned only through the study of structures revealed by human dissection. In particular, his great anatomic treatise, *De Humani Corporis Fabrica Libri Septem* (1543), provided fuller and more detailed descriptions of human anatomy than any of his illustrious predecessors. Most importantly, Vesalius corrected errors in traditional anatomic teachings propagated 13 centuries earlier by Greek and Roman authorities, whose findings were based on animal rather than human dissection. Even more radical was Vesalius' blunt assertion that anatomic dissection must be completed by physician-surgeons themselves—a direct renunciation of the long-standing doctrine that dissection was a grisly and loathsome task to be performed by a diener-like individual while the perched physician-surgeon lectured by reading from an orthodox anatomic text from on high. This principle of hands-on education would remain Vesalius' most important and long-lasting contribution to the teaching of anatomy. Vesalius' Latin *literae scriptae* ensured its accessibility to the most well-known physicians and scientists of the day. Latin was the language of the intelligentsia and the *Fabrica* became instantly popular, so it was only natural that over the next 2 centuries, the work would go through numerous adaptations, editions, and revisions, although always remaining an authoritative anatomic text.

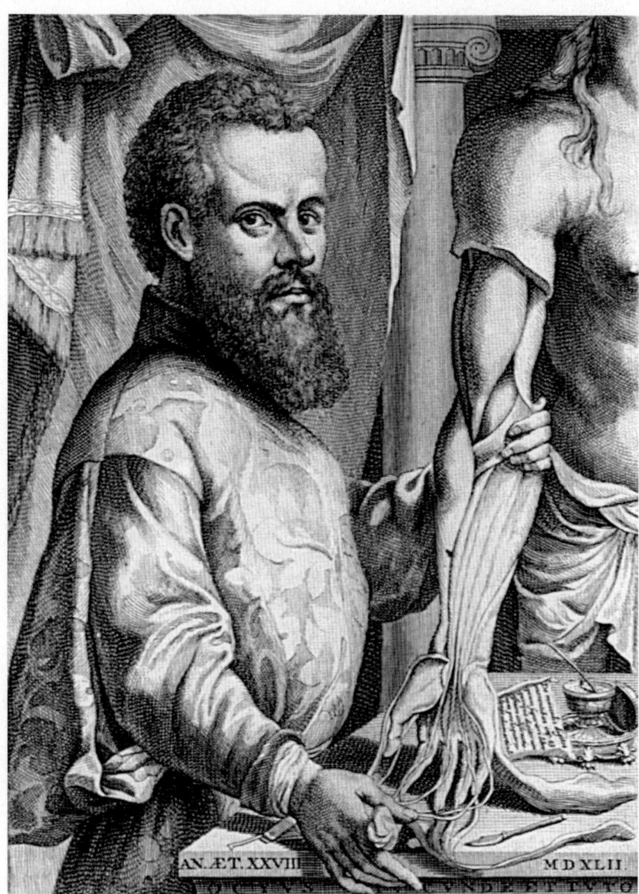


**FIGURE 1-1** Andreas Vesalius (1514-1564).

## Method of Controlling Hemorrhage

The position of Ambroise Paré (1510-1590) in the evolution of surgery remains of supreme importance (Fig. 1-2). He played

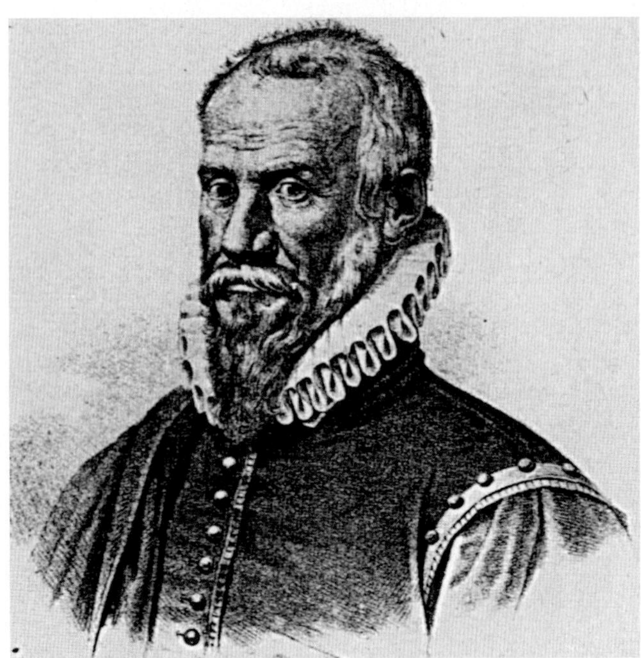

**FIGURE 1-2** Ambroise Paré (1510-1590).

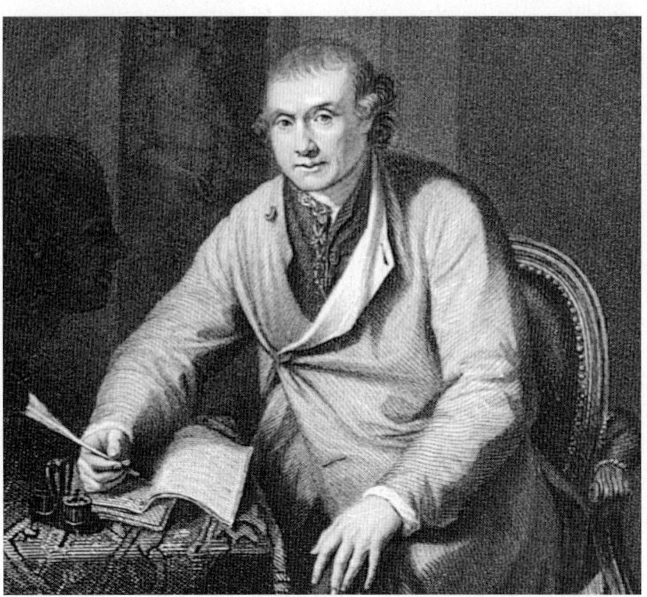

**FIGURE 1-3** John Hunter (1728-1793).

the major role in reinvigorating and updating Renaissance surgery and represents severing of the final link between surgical thought and techniques of the ancients and the push toward more modern eras. From 1536 until just before his death, Paré was engaged as an army surgeon, during which time he accompanied different French armies on their military expeditions, or was performing surgery in civilian practice in Paris. Although other surgeons made similar observations about the difficulties and nonsensical aspects of using boiling oil as a means of cauterizing fresh gunshot wounds, Paré's use of a less irritating emollient of egg yolk, rose oil, and turpentine brought him lasting fame and glory. His ability to articulate such a finding in a number of textbooks, all written in the vernacular, allowed his writings to reach more than just the educated elite. Among Paré's important corollary observations was that when performing an amputation, it was more efficacious to ligate individual blood vessels than to attempt to control hemorrhage by means of mass ligation of tissue or with hot oleum. Described in his *Dix Livres de la Chirurgie avec le Magasin des Instruments Necessaires à Icelle* (1564), the free or cut end of a blood vessel was doubly ligated and the ligature was allowed to remain undisturbed in situ until, as a result of local suppuration, it was cast off. Paré humbly attributed his success with patients to God, as noted in his famous motto, *"Je le pansay. Dieu le guérit,"*—that is, "I treated him. God cured him."

## Pathophysiologic Basis of Surgical Diseases

Although it would be another 3 centuries before the third desideratum, that of anesthesia, was discovered, much of the scientific understanding concerning efforts to relieve discomfort secondary to surgical operations was based on the 18th century work of England's premier surgical scientist, John Hunter (1728-1793; Fig. 1-3). Considered one of the most influential surgeons of all time, his endeavors stand out because of the prolificacy of his written word and the quality of his research, especially in using experimental animal surgery as a way to understand the pathophysiologic basis of surgical diseases. Most impressively, Hunter relied little on the theories of past authorities but rather on personal observations, with his fundamental pathologic studies first described in the renowned textbook *A Treatise on the Blood, Inflammation, and Gun-Shot Wounds* (1794). Ultimately, his voluminous research and clinical work resulted in a collection of more than 13,000 specimens, which became one of his most important legacies to the world of surgery. It represented a unique warehousing of separate organ systems, with comparisons of these systems—from the simplest animal or plant to humans—demonstrating the interaction of structure and function. For decades, Hunter's collection, housed in England's Royal College of Surgeons, remained the outstanding museum of comparative anatomy and pathology in the world, until a World War II Nazi bombing attack of London created a conflagration that destroyed most of Hunter's assemblage.

## Anesthesia

Since time immemorial, the inability of surgeons to complete pain-free operations had been among the most terrifying of medical problems. In the preanesthetic era, surgeons were forced to be more concerned about the speed with which an operation was completed than with the clinical efficacy of their dissection. In a similar vein, patients refused or delayed surgical procedures for as long as possible to avoid the personal horror of experiencing the surgeon's knife. Analgesic, narcotic, and soporific agents such as hashish, mandrake, and opium had been used for thousands of years. However, the systematic operative invasion of body cavities and the inevitable progression of surgical history could not occur until an effective means of rendering a patient insensitive to pain was developed.

As anatomic knowledge and surgical techniques improved, the search for safe methods to prevent pain became more pressing. By the early 1830s, chloroform, ether, and nitrous oxide had been discovered and so-called laughing gas parties and ether frolics were in vogue, especially in America. Young people were amusing themselves with the pleasant side effects of these compounds as itinerant so-called professors of chemistry traveled to hamlets, towns, and cities to lecture on and demonstrate the exhilarating effects of these new gases. It soon became evident to various physicians and dentists that the pain-relieving qualities of ether and nitrous oxide could be applicable to surgical operations and tooth extraction. On October 16, 1846, William T.G. Morton (1819-1868), a Boston dentist, persuaded John Collins Warren (1778-1856), professor of surgery at the Massachusetts General Hospital, to let him administer sulfuric ether to a surgical patient from whom Warren went on to remove a small, congenital vascular tumor of the neck painlessly. After the operation, Warren, greatly impressed with the new discovery, uttered his famous words, "Gentlemen, this is no humbug."

Few medical discoveries have been so readily accepted as inhalational anesthesia. News of the momentous event spread rapidly throughout the United States and Europe, and a new era in the history of surgery had begun. Within a few months after the first public demonstration in Boston, ether was used in hospitals throughout the world. Yet, no matter how much it contributed to the relief of pain during surgical operations and decreased the surgeon's angst, the discovery did not immediately further the scope of elective surgery. Such technical triumphs awaited the recognition and acceptance of antisepsis and asepsis. Anesthesia helped make the illusion of surgical cures more seductive, but it could not bring forth the final prerequisite—all-important hygienic reforms.

Still, by the mid-19th century, both physicians and patients were coming to hold surgery in relatively high regard for its pragmatic appeal, technologic virtuosity, and unambiguously measurable results. After all, surgery appeared a mystical craft to some. To be allowed to consensually cut into another human's body, to gaze at the depth of that person's suffering, and to excise the demon of disease seemed an awesome responsibility. It was this very mysticism, however, long associated with religious overtones, that so fascinated the public and their own feared but inevitable date with a surgeon's knife. Surgeons had finally begun to view themselves as combining art and nature, essentially assisting nature in its continual process of destruction and rebuilding. This regard for the natural would spring from the eventual, although preternaturally slow, understanding and use of Joseph Lister's (1827-1912) techniques (Fig. 1-4).

## Antisepsis, Asepsis, and Understanding the Nature of Infection

In many respects, the recognition of antisepsis and asepsis was a more important event in the evolution of surgical history than the advent of inhalational anesthesia. There was no arguing that the deadening of pain permitted a surgical operation to be conducted in a more efficacious manner. Haste was no longer of prime concern. However, if anesthesia had never been conceived, a surgical procedure could still be performed, albeit with much difficulty. Such was not the case with listerism. Without antisepsis and asepsis, major surgical operations more than likely ended in death rather than just pain. Clearly, surgery needed both anesthesia and antisepsis, but in terms of overall importance, antisepsis proved to be of greater singular impact.

In the long evolution of world surgery, the contributions of several individuals stand out as being preeminent. Lister, an English surgeon, can be placed on such a select list because of his monumental efforts to introduce systematic, scientifically based antisepsis in the treatment of wounds and the performance of surgical operations. He pragmatically applied others' research into fermentation and microorganisms to the world of surgery by devising a means of preventing surgical infection and securing its adoption by a skeptical profession.

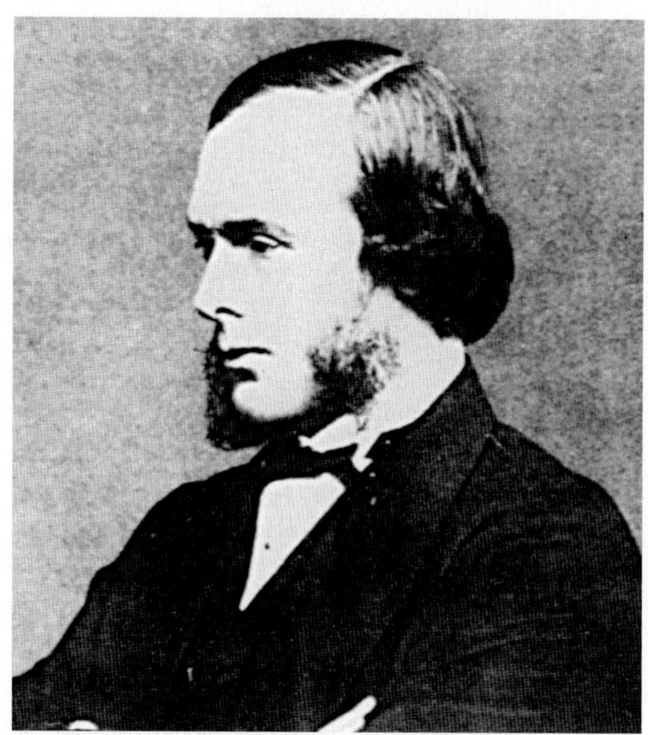

**FIGURE 1-4** Joseph Lister (1827-1912).

It was evident to Lister that a method of destroying bacteria by excessive heat could not be applied to a surgical patient. He turned, instead, to chemical antisepsis and, after experimenting with zinc chloride and the sulfites, decided on carbolic acid. By 1865, Lister was instilling pure carbolic acid into wounds and onto dressings. He would eventually make numerous modifications in the technique of dressings, manner of applying and retaining them, and choice of antiseptic solutions of varying concentrations. Although the carbolic acid spray remains the best remembered of his many contributions, it was eventually abandoned in favor of other germicidal substances. Lister not only used carbolic acid in the wound and on dressings but also went so far as to spray it into the atmosphere around the operative field and table. He did not emphasize hand scrubbing but merely dipped his fingers into a solution of phenol and corrosive sublimate. Lister was incorrectly convinced that scrubbing created crevices in the palms of the hands where bacteria would proliferate. A second important advance by Lister was the development of sterile absorbable sutures. He believed that much of the deep suppuration found in wounds was created by previously contaminated silk ligatures. Lister evolved a carbolized catgut suture that was better than any previously produced. He was able to cut the ends of the ligature short, thereby closing the wound tightly and eliminating the necessity of bringing the ends of the suture out through the incision, a surgical practice that had persisted since the days of Paré.

The acceptance of listerism was an uneven and distinctly slow process, for many reasons. First, the various procedural changes that Lister made during the evolution of his methodology created confusion. Second, listerism, as a technical exercise, was complicated by the use of carbolic acid, an unpleasant and time-consuming nuisance. Third, various early attempts to use antisepsis in surgery had proved abject failures, with many leading surgeons unable to replicate Lister's generally good results. Finally, and most importantly, acceptance of listerism depended entirely on an understanding and ultimate recognition of the veracity of the germ theory, a hypothesis that many practical-minded surgeons were loath to accept.

As a professional group, German-speaking surgeons would be the first to grasp the importance of bacteriology and the germ theory. Consequently, they were among the earliest to expand on Lister's message of antisepsis, with his spray being discarded in favor of boiling and use of the autoclave. The availability of heat sterilization led to the development of sterile aprons, drapes, instruments, and sutures. Similarly, the use of face masks, gloves, hats, and operating gowns also naturally evolved. By the mid-1890s, less clumsy aseptic techniques had found their way into most European surgical amphitheaters and were approaching total acceptance by American surgeons. Any lingering doubts about the validity and significance of the momentous concepts that Lister had put forth were eliminated on the battlefields of World War I. There, the importance of just plain antisepsis became an invaluable lesson for scalpel bearers, whereas the exigencies of the battlefield helped bring about the final maturation and equitable standing of surgery and surgeons within the worldwide medical community.

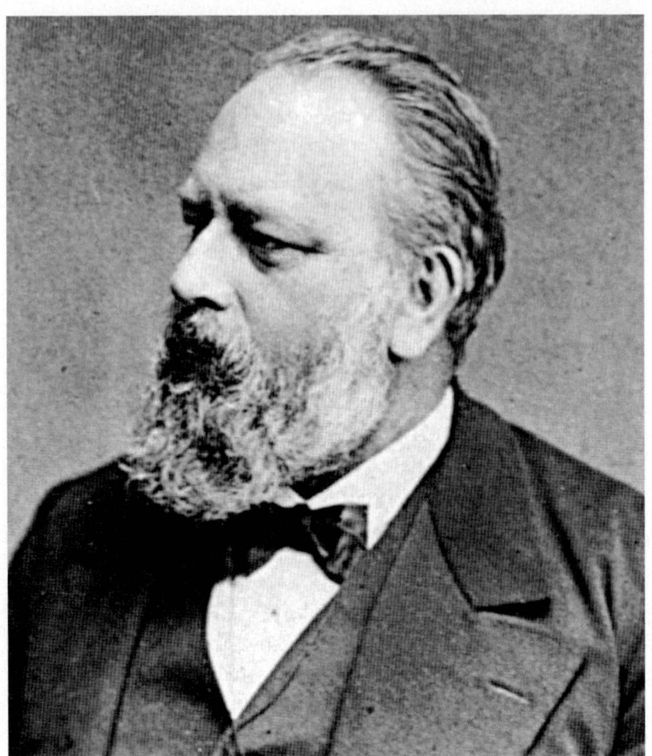

**FIGURE 1-5** Theodor Billroth (1829-1894).

## X-Rays

Especially prominent among other late 19th century discoveries that had an enormous impact on the evolution of surgery was research conducted by Wilhelm Roentgen (1845-1923), which led to his 1895 elucidation of x-rays. Having grown interested in the phosphorescence from metallic salts that were exposed to light, Roentgen made a chance observation when he passed a current through a vacuum tube and noticed a greenish glow coming from a screen on a shelf 9 feet away. This strange effect continued after the current was turned off. He found that the screen had been painted with a phosphorescent substance. Proceeding with full experimental vigor, Roentgen soon realized that there were invisible rays capable of passing through solid objects made of wood, metal, and other materials. Most significantly, these rays also penetrated the soft parts of the body in such a manner that the more dense bones of his hand were able to be revealed on a specially treated photographic plate. In a short time, numerous applications were developed as surgeons rapidly applied the new discovery to the diagnosis and location of fractures and dislocations and the removal of foreign bodies.

## EARLY 20TH CENTURY

By the late 1890s, the interactions of political, scientific, socioeconomic, and technical factors set the stage for what would become a spectacular showcasing of surgery's newfound prestige and accomplishments. Surgeons were finally wearing antiseptic-looking white coats. Patients and tables were draped in white, and basins for bathing instruments in bichloride solution abounded. Suddenly, all was clean and tidy, with conduct of the surgical operation no longer a haphazard affair. This reformation would be successful not because surgeons had fundamentally changed but because medicine and its relationship to scientific inquiry had been irrevocably altered. Sectarianism and quackery, the consequences of earlier medical dogmatism, would no longer be tenable within the confines of scientific truth.

With all four fundamental clinical prerequisites in place by the turn of the century, highlighted by the emerging clinical triumphs of various English surgeons, including Robert Tait (1845-1899), William Macewen (1848-1924), and Frederick Treves (1853-1923); German-speaking surgeons, including Theodor Billroth (1829-1894; Fig. 1-5), Theodor Kocher (1841-1917; Fig. 1-6), Friedrich Trendelenburg (1844-1924), and Johann von Mikulicz-Radecki (1850-1905); French surgeons, including Jules Peán (1830-1898), Just Lucas-Championière (1843-1913), and Marin-Theodore Tuffiér (1857-1929); Italian surgeons, most notably Eduardo Bassini (1844-1924) and Antonio Ceci (1852-1920); and several American surgeons, exemplified by William Williams Keen (1837-1932), Nicholas Senn (1844-1908), and John Benjamin Murphy (1857-1916), scalpel wielders had essentially explored all cavities of the human body. Nonetheless, surgeons retained a lingering sense of professional and social discomfort and continued to be pejoratively described by nouveau scientific physicians as nonthinkers who worked in little more than an inferior and crude manual craft.

It was becoming increasingly evident that research models, theoretical concepts, and valid clinical applications would be necessary to demonstrate the scientific basis of surgery to a wary public. The effort to devise new operative methods called for an even greater reliance on experimental surgery and its absolute encouragement by all concerned parties. Most importantly, a scientific basis for therapeutic surgical recommendations—consisting of empirical data, collected and analyzed according to nationally and internationally accepted rules and set apart from individual authoritative assumptions—would have to be

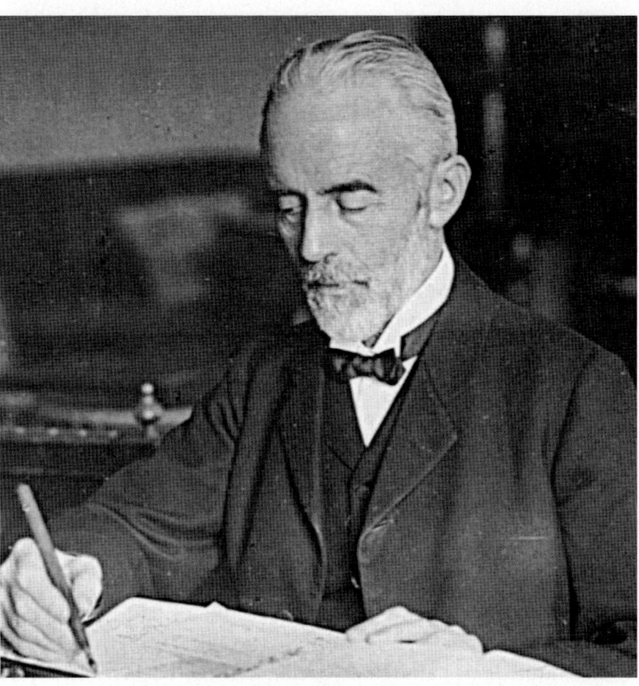

**FIGURE 1-6** Theodor Kocher (1841-1917).

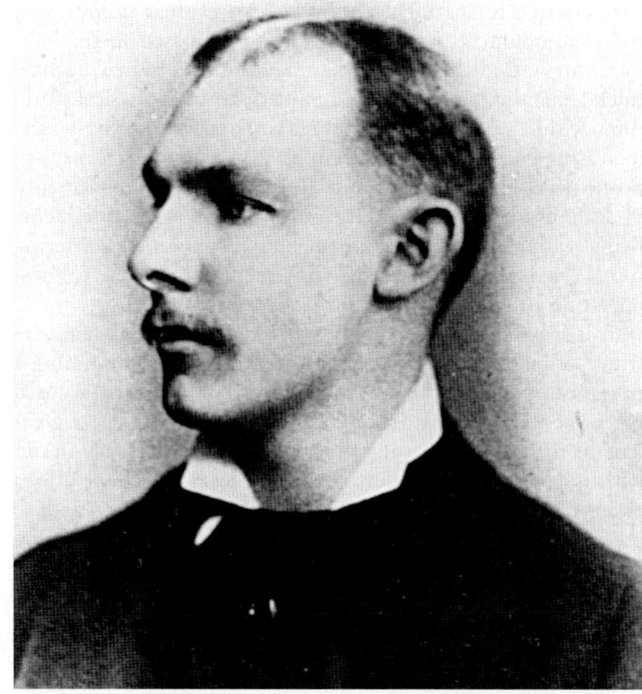

**FIGURE 1-7** William Halsted (1852-1922).

developed. In contrast to previously unexplainable doctrines, scientific research would triumph as the final arbiter between valid and invalid surgical therapies.

In turn, surgeons had no choice but to allay society's fear of the surgical unknown by presenting surgery as an accepted part of a newly established medical armamentarium. This would not be an easy task. The immediate consequences of surgical operations, such as discomfort and associated complications, were often of more concern to patients than the positive knowledge that an operation could eliminate potentially devastating disease processes. Accordingly, the most consequential achievement by surgeons during the early 20th century was ensuring the social acceptability of surgery as a legitimate scientific endeavor and the surgical operation as a therapeutic necessity.

## Ascent of Scientific Surgery

William Stewart Halsted (1852-1922), more than any other surgeon, set the scientific tone for this most important period in surgical history (Fig. 1-7). He moved surgery from the melodramatics of the 19th-century operating theater to the starkness and sterility of the modern operating room, commingled with the privacy and soberness of the research laboratory. As professor of surgery at the newly opened Johns Hopkins Hospital and School of Medicine, Halsted proved to be a complex personality, but the impact of this aloof and reticent man would become widespread. He introduced a new surgery and showed that research based on anatomic, pathologic, and physiologic principles and the use of animal experimentation made it possible to develop sophisticated operative procedures and perform them clinically with outstanding results. Halsted proved, to an often leery profession and public, that an unambiguous sequence could be constructed from the laboratory of basic surgical research to the clinical operating room. Most importantly, for surgery's own self-respect, he demonstrated during this turn of the century renaissance in medical education that departments of surgery could command a faculty whose stature was equal in importance and prestige to that of other more academic or research-oriented fields, such as anatomy, bacteriology, biochemistry, internal medicine, pathology, and physiology.

As a single individual, Halsted developed and disseminated a different system of surgery so characteristic that it was termed a *school of surgery*. More to the point, Halsted's methods revolutionized the world of surgery and earned his work the epithet "halstedian principles," which remains a widely acknowledged and accepted scientific imprimatur. Halsted subordinated technical brilliance and speed of dissection to a meticulous and safe, albeit sometimes slow performance. As a direct result, Halsted's effort did much to bring about surgery's self-sustaining transformation from therapeutic subservience to clinical necessity.

Despite his demeanor as a professional recluse, Halsted's clinical and research achievements were overwhelming in number and scope. His residency system of training surgeons was not merely the first such program of its type—it was unique in its primary purpose. Above all other concerns, Halsted desired to establish a school of surgery that would eventually disseminate throughout the surgical world the principles and attributes that he considered sound and proper. His aim was to train able surgical teachers, not merely competent operating surgeons. There is little doubt that Halsted achieved his stated goal of producing "not only surgeons but surgeons of the highest type, men who will stimulate the first youth of our country to study surgery and to devote their energies and their lives to raising the standards of surgical science." So fundamental were his contributions that without them, surgery might never have fully developed and could have remained mired in a quasiprofessional state.

The heroic and dangerous nature of surgery seemed appealing in less scientifically sophisticated times, but now surgeons were courted for personal attributes beyond their unmitigated technical boldness. A trend toward hospital-based surgery was increasingly evident, in equal parts resulting from new, technically demanding operations and modern hospital physical structures within which surgeons could work more effectively. The increasing complexity and effectiveness of aseptic surgery, diagnostic necessity of the x-ray and clinical laboratory, convenience of 24-hour nursing, and availability of capable surgical residents living within a hospital were making the hospital operating room the most plausible and convenient place for a surgical operation to be performed.

It was obvious to both hospital superintendents and the whole of medicine that acute care institutions were becoming a necessity, more for the surgeon than for the physician. As a consequence, increasing numbers of hospitals went to great lengths to supply their surgical staffs with the finest facilities in which to complete operations. For centuries, surgical operations had been performed under the illumination of sunlight, candles, or both. Now, however, electric lights installed in operating rooms offered a far more reliable and unwavering source of illumination. Surgery became a more proficient craft because surgical operations could be completed on stormy summer mornings, as well as on wet winter afternoons.

## Internationalization, Surgical Societies, and Journals

As the sophistication of surgery grew, internationalization became one of its underlying themes, with surgeons crossing the great oceans to visit and learn from one another. Halsted and Hermann Küttner (1870-1932), director of the surgical clinic in Breslau, Germany (now known as Wroclaw and located in southwestern Poland), instituted the first known official exchange of surgical residents in 1914. This experiment in surgical education was meant to underscore the true international spirit that had engulfed surgery. Halsted firmly believed that young surgeons achieved greater clinical maturity by observing the practice of surgery in other countries, as well as in their own.

An inevitable formation of national and international surgical societies and the emergence and development of periodicals devoted to surgical subjects proved to be important adjuncts to the professionalization process of surgery. For the most part, professional societies began as a means of providing mutual improvement via personal interaction with surgical peers and the publication of presented papers. Unlike surgeons of earlier centuries, who were known to guard so-called trade secrets closely, members of these new organizations were emphatic about publishing transactions of their meetings. In this way, not only would their surgical peers read of their clinical accomplishments, but a written record was also established for circulation throughout the world of medicine.

The first of these surgical societies was the Académie Royale de Chirurgie in Paris, with its *Mémoires* appearing sporadically from 1743 through 1838. Of 19th century associations, the most prominent published proceedings were the *Mémoires* and *Bulletins* of the Société de Chirurgie of Paris (1847), the *Verhandlungen* of the Deutsche Gesellschaft für Chirurgie (1872), and the *Transactions* of the American Surgical Association (1883). No surgical association that published professional reports existed in 19th century Great Britain, and the Royal Colleges of Surgeons of England, Ireland, and Scotland never undertook such projects. Although textbooks, monographs, and treatises had always been the mainstay of medical writing, the introduction of monthly journals, including August Richter's (1742-1812) *Chirurgische Bibliothek* (1771), Joseph Malgaigne's (1806-1865) *Journal de Chirurgie* (1843), Bernard Langenbeck's (1810-1887) *Archiv für Klinische Chirurgie* (1860), and Lewis Pilcher's (1844-1917) *Annals of Surgery* (1885), had a tremendous impact on updating and continuing the education of surgeons.

## World War I

Austria-Hungary and Germany continued as the dominant forces in world surgery until World War I. However, results of the conflict proved disastrous to the central powers (Austria-Hungary, Bulgaria, Germany, and the Ottoman Empire), especially to German-speaking surgeons. Europe took on a new social and political look, with the demise of Germany's status as the world leader in surgery a sad but foregone conclusion. As with most armed conflicts, because of the massive human toll, especially battlefield injuries, tremendous strides were made in multiple areas of surgery. Undoubtedly, the greatest surgical achievement was in the treatment of wound infection. Trench warfare in soil contaminated by decades of cultivation and animal manure made every wounded soldier a potential carrier of any number of pathogenic bacilli. On the battlefront, sepsis was inevitable. Most attempts to maintain aseptic technique proved inadequate, but the treatment of infected wounds by antisepsis was becoming a pragmatic reality.

Surgeons experimented with numerous antiseptic solutions and various types of surgical dressing. A principle of wound treatment entailing débridement and irrigation eventually evolved. Henry Dakin (1880-1952), an English chemist, and Alexis Carrel (1873-1944; Fig. 1-8), the Nobel prize–winning French American surgeon, were the principal protagonists in the development of this extensive system of wound management. In addition to successes in wound sterility, surgical advances were made in the use of x-rays in the diagnosis of battlefield injuries, and remarkable operative ingenuity was evident in

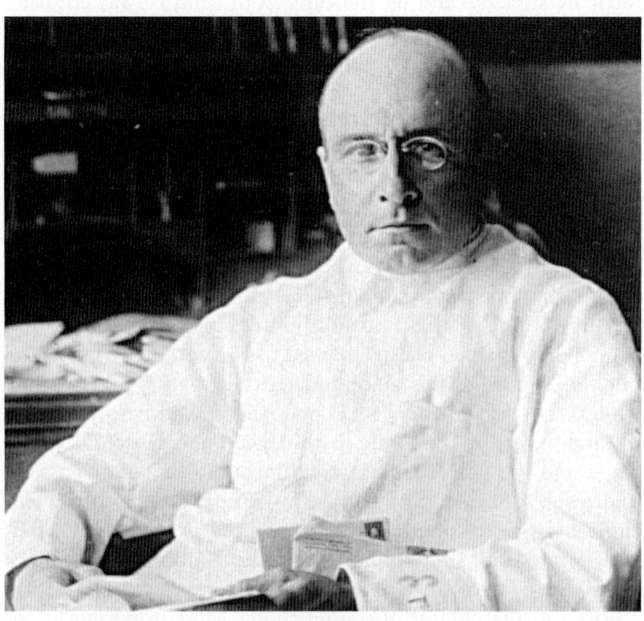

**FIGURE 1-8** Alexis Carrel (1873-1944).

reconstructive facial surgery and the treatment of fractures resulting from gunshot wounds.

## American College of Surgeons

For American surgeons, the years just before World War I were a time of active coalescence into various social and educational organizations. The most important and influential of these societies was the American College of Surgeons, founded in 1913 by Franklin Martin (1857-1935), a Chicago-based gynecologist. Patterned after the Royal Colleges of Surgeons of England, Ireland, and Scotland, the American College of Surgeons established professional, ethical, and moral standards for every graduate in medicine who practiced in surgery and conferred the designation Fellow of the American College of Surgeons (FACS) on its members. From the outset, its primary aim was the continuing education of surgical physicians. Accordingly, the requirements for fellowship were always related to the educational opportunities of the period. In 1914, an applicant had to be a licensed graduate of medicine, receive the backing of three fellows, and be endorsed by the local credentials committee.

In view of the stipulated peer recommendations, many physicians, realistically or not, viewed the American College of Surgeons as an elitist organization. With an obvious so-called blackball system built into the membership requirements, there was a difficult to deny belief that many surgeons who were immigrants, females, or members of particular religious and racial minorities were granted fellowships sparingly. Such inherent bias, in addition to questionable accusations of fee splitting along with unbridled contempt of certain surgeons' business practices, resulted in some very prominent American surgeons never being permitted the privilege of membership.

The 1920s and beyond proved to be a prosperous time for American society and its surgeons. After all, the history of world surgery in the 20th century is more a tale of American triumphs than it ever was in the 18th or 19th centuries. Physicians' incomes dramatically increased and surgeons' prestige, aided by the ever-mounting successes of medical science, became securely established in American culture. Still, a noticeable lack of standards and regulations in surgical specialty practice became a serious concern to leaders in the profession. The difficulties of World War I had greatly accentuated this realistic need for specialty standards, when many of the physicians who were self-proclaimed surgical specialists were found to be unqualified by military examining boards. In ophthalmology, for example, more than 50% of tested individuals were deemed unfit to treat diseases of the eye.

It was an unmistakable reality that there were no established criteria with which to distinguish a well-qualified ophthalmologist from an upstart optometrist or to clarify the differences in clinical expertise between a well-trained, full-time ophthalmologic specialist and an inadequately trained, part-time general physician–ophthalmologist. In recognition of the gravity of the situation, the self-patrolling concept of a professional examining board, sponsored by leading voluntary ophthalmologic organizations, was proposed as a mechanism for certifying competency. In 1916, uniform standards and regulations were set forth in the form of minimal educational requirements and written and oral examinations, and the American Board for Ophthalmic Examinations, the country's first, was formally incorporated. By 1940, six additional surgical specialty boards were established—orthopedic (1934), colon and rectal (1934), urologic (1935), plastic (1937), surgical (1937), and neurologic (1940).

As order was introduced into surgical specialty training and the process of certification matured, it was apparent that the continued growth of residency programs carried important implications for the future structure of medical practice and the social relationship of medicine to overall society. Professional power had been consolidated, and specialization, which had been evolving since the time of the Civil War, was now recognized as an essential, if not integral, part of modern medicine. Although the creation of surgical specialty boards was justified under the broad imprimatur of raising the educational status and evaluating the clinical competency of specialists, board certification undeniably began to restrict entry into the specialties.

As the specialties evolved, the political influence and cultural authority enjoyed by the profession of surgery were growing. This socioeconomic strength was most prominently expressed in reform efforts directed toward the modernization and standardization of America's hospital system. Any vestiges of so-called kitchen surgery had essentially disappeared, and other than numerous small private hospitals predominantly constructed by surgeons for their personal use, the only facilities in which major surgery could be adequately conducted and postoperative patients appropriately cared for were the well-equipped and physically impressive modern hospitals. Thus, the American College of Surgeons and its expanding list of fellows had a strong motive to ensure that America's hospital system was as up to date and efficient as possible.

On an international level, surgeons were confronted with the lack of any formal organizational body. Not until the International College of Surgeons was founded in 1935 in Geneva would such a society exist. At its inception, this organization was intended to serve as a liaison to the existing colleges and surgical societies in the various countries. However, its goals of elevating the art and science of surgery, creating greater understanding among the surgeons of the world, and affording a means of international postgraduate study never came to full fruition, in part because the American College of Surgeons adamantly opposed the establishment—and continues to do so—of a viable American chapter of the International College of Surgeons.

## Women Surgeons

One of the many overlooked areas of surgical history concerns the involvement of women. Until recent times, women's options for obtaining advanced surgical training were severely restricted. The major reason was that through the mid-20th century, only a handful of women had performed enough surgery to become skilled mentors. Without role models and with limited access to hospital positions, the ability of the few practicing female physicians to specialize in surgery seemed an impossibility. Consequently, women surgeons were forced to use different career strategies than men and to have more divergent goals of personal success to achieve professional satisfaction. Despite these difficulties, and through the determination and aid of several enlightened male surgeons, most notably William Byford (1817-1890) of Chicago and William Keen of Philadelphia, a small cadre of female surgeons did exist in late 19th century America. Mary Dixon Jones (1828-1908), Emmeline Horton Cleveland (1829-1878), Mary Harris Thompson (1829-1895), Anna Elizabeth Broomall (1847-1931), and Marie Mergler

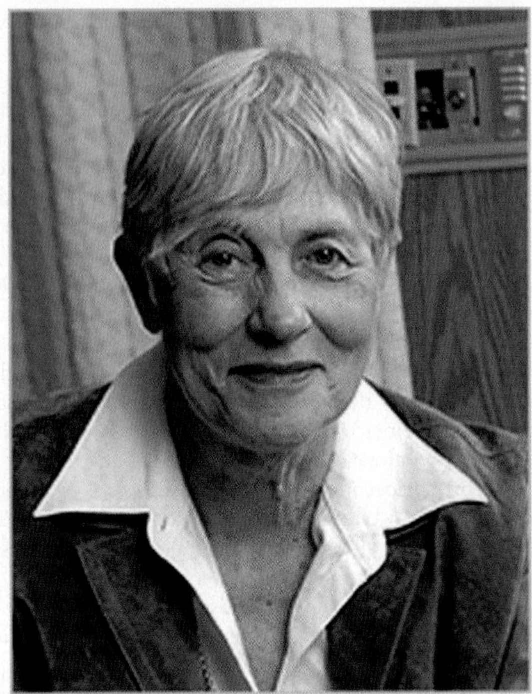

**FIGURE 1-9** Olga Jonasson (1934-2006). (Courtesy University of Illinois, Chicago.)

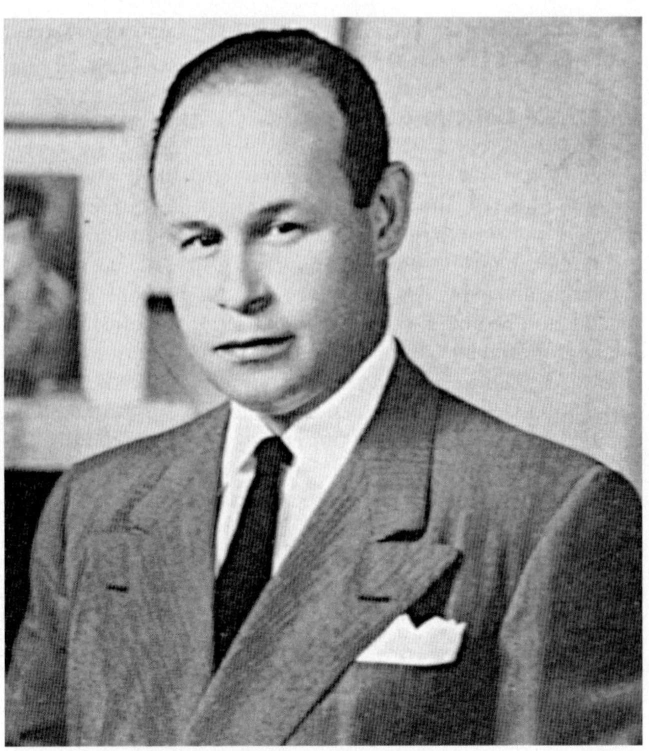

**FIGURE 1-10** Charles Drew (1904-1950).

(1851-1901) would act as a nidus toward greater gender equality in 20th century surgery. Olga Jonasson (1934-2006; Fig. 1-9), a pioneer in the field of clinical transplantation, played a leading role in encouraging women to enter the modern, male-dominated world of surgery. In 1987, when she was named chair of the department of surgery at Ohio State University College of Medicine, Jonasson became the first woman in the United States to head an academic surgery department at a coeducational medical school.

## African American Surgeons

There is little disputing the fact that both gender and racial bias have influenced the evolution of surgery. Every aspect of society is affected by such discrimination, and African Americans, like women, were innocent victims of injustices that forced them into never-ending struggles to attain competency in surgery. As early as 1868, a department of surgery was established at Howard University. However, the first three chairmen were all white Anglo-Saxon Protestants. Not until Austin Curtis was appointed professor of surgery in 1928 did the department have its first African American head. Like all black physicians of his era, he was forced to train at so-called Negro hospitals, in Curtis' case Provident Hospital in Chicago, where he came under the tutelage of Daniel Hale Williams (1858-1931), the most influential and highly regarded of early African American surgeons. In 1897, Williams received considerable notoriety when he reported successful suturing of the pericardium for a stab wound of the heart.

With little likelihood of obtaining membership in the American Medical Association or its related societies, African American physicians joined together in 1895 to form the National Medical Association. Black surgeons identified an even more specific need when the Surgical Section of the National Medical Association was opened in 1906. These National Medical Association surgical clinics, which preceded the Clinical Congress of Surgeons of North America, the forerunner to the annual congress of the American College of Surgeons by almost half a decade, represented the earliest examples of organized, so-called "show me" surgical education in the United States.

Admittance to surgical societies and attainment of specialty certification were important social and psychological accomplishments for early African American surgeons. When Daniel Williams was named a Fellow of the American College of Surgeons in 1913, the news spread rapidly throughout the African American surgical community. Still, African American surgeons' fellowship applications were often acted on rather slowly, which suggests that denials based on race were clandestinely conducted throughout much of the country. As late as the mid-1940s, Charles Drew (1904-1950; Fig. 1-10), chairman of the department of surgery at Howard University School of Medicine, acknowledged that he refused to accept membership in the American College of Surgeons because this so-called nationally representative surgical society had, in his opinion, not yet begun to accept capable and well-qualified African American surgeons freely. Claude H. Organ, Jr. (1926-2005; Fig. 1-11), was a distinguished editor, educator, and historian. Among his books, the two-volume *A Century of Black Surgeons: The U.S.A. Experience* and the authoritative *Noteworthy Publications by African-American Surgeons* underscored the numerous contributions made by African American surgeons to the nation's health care system. In addition, as the long-standing editor-in-chief of *Archives of Surgery*, as well as serving as president of the American College of Surgeons and chairman of the American Board of Surgery, Organ wielded enormous influence over the direction of American surgery.

FIGURE 1-11 Claude H. Organ, Jr. (1926-2005). (Courtesy the American College of Surgeons, Chicago, and Dr. James C. Thompson.)

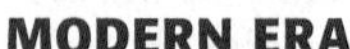

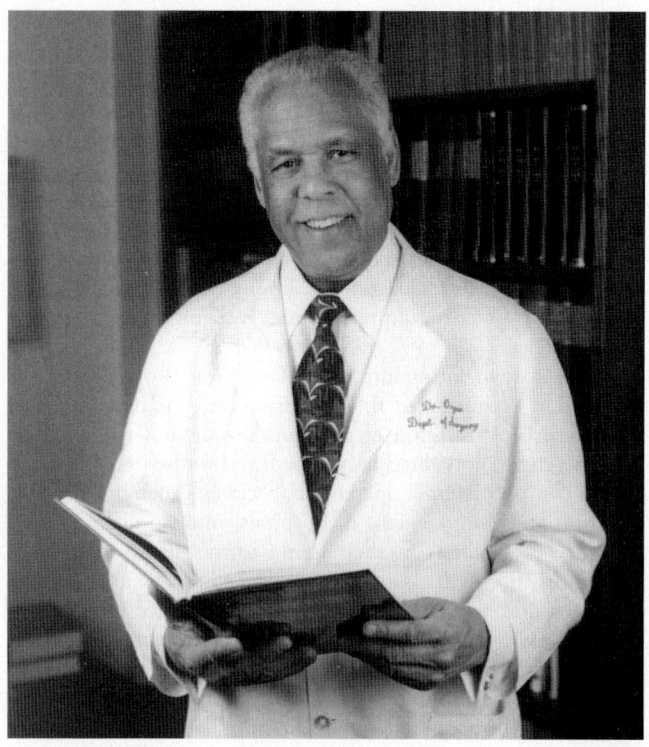

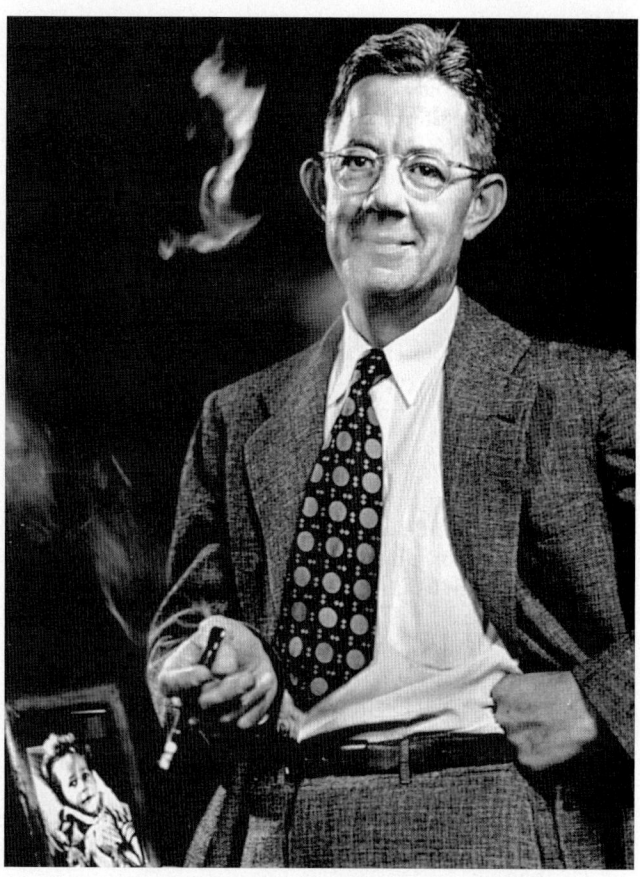

FIGURE 1-12 Alfred Blalock (1899-1964).

## MODERN ERA

Despite the global economic depression in the aftermath of World War I, the 1920s and 1930s signaled the ascent of American surgery to its current position of international leadership. Highlighted by educational reforms in its medical schools, Halsted's redefinition of surgical residency programs, and the growth of surgical specialties, the stage was set for the blossoming of scientific surgery. Basic surgical research became an established reality as George Crile (1864-1943), Alfred Blalock (1899-1964; Fig. 1-12), Dallas Phemister (1882-1951), and Charles Huggins (1901-1997) became world-renowned surgeon-scientists.

Much as the ascendancy of the surgeon-scientist brought about changes in the way in which the public and profession viewed surgical research, the introduction of increasingly sophisticated technologies had an enormous impact on the practice of surgery. Throughout the evolution of surgery, the practice of surgery—the art, the craft and, finally, the science of working with one's hands—had largely been defined by its tools. From the crude flint instruments of ancient peoples, through the simple tonsillotomes and lithotrites of the 19th century, up to the increasingly complex surgical instruments developed in the 20th century, new and improved instruments usually led to a better surgical result. Progress in surgical instrumentation and surgical techniques went hand in hand.

Surgical techniques would, of course, become more sophisticated with the passage of time but, by the conclusion of World War II, essentially all organs and areas of the body had been fully explored. In fact, within a short half-century, the domain of surgery had become so well established that the profession's foundation of basic operative procedures was already completed. As a consequence, there were few technical surgical mysteries left. What surgery now needed to sustain its continued growth was the ability to diagnose surgical diseases at an earlier stage, locate malignant growths while they remained small, and have more effective postoperative treatment so that patients could survive ever more technically complex operations. Such thinking was exemplified by the introduction of cholecystography in 1924 by Evarts Graham (1883-1957) and Warren Cole (1898-1990). In this case, an emerging scientific technology introduced new possibilities into surgical practice that were not necessarily related solely to improvements in technique. To the surgeon, the discovery and application of cholecystography proved most important, not only because it brought about more accurate diagnoses of cholecystitis but also because it created an influx of surgical patients where few had previously existed. If surgery was to grow, large numbers of individuals with surgical diseases were needed.

It was an exciting era for surgeons, with important clinical advances being made in the operating room and basic science laboratory. Among the most notable highlights were the introduction in 1935 of pancreaticoduodenectomy for cancer of the pancreas by Allen Oldfather Whipple (1881-1963) and a report in 1943 on vagotomy for the operative treatment of peptic ulcer disease by Lester Dragstedt (1893-1976). Other significant advances included the following:

- Frank Lahey (1880-1953) stressed the importance of identifying the recurrent laryngeal nerve during the course of thyroid surgery.
- Owen Wangensteen (1898-1981) successfully decompressed mechanical bowel obstructions by using a newly devised suction apparatus in 1932.
- George Vaughan (1859-1948) successfully ligated the abdominal aorta for aneurysmal disease in 1921.
- Max Peet (1885-1949) presented splanchnic resection for hypertension in 1935.
- Walter Dandy (1886-1946) performed intracranial section of various cranial nerves in the 1920s.
- Walter Freeman (1895-1972) described prefrontal lobotomy as a means of treating various mental illnesses in 1936.
- Harvey Cushing (1869-1939) introduced electrocoagulation in neurosurgery in 1928.
- Marius Smith-Petersen (1886-1953) described a flanged nail for pinning a fracture of the neck of the femur in 1931 and introduced Vitallium cup arthroplasty in 1939.
- Vilray Blair (1871-1955) and James Brown (1899-1971) popularized the use of split-skin grafts to cover large areas of granulating wounds.
- Earl Padgett (1893-1946) devised an operative dermatome that allowed calibration of the thickness of skin grafts in 1939.
- Elliott Cutler (1888-1947) performed a successful section of the mitral valve for relief of mitral stenosis in 1923.
- Evarts Graham completed the first successful removal of an entire lung for cancer in 1933.
- Claude Beck (1894-1971) implanted pectoral muscle into the pericardium and attached a pedicled omental graft to the surface of the heart, thus providing collateral circulation to that organ, in 1935.
- Robert Gross (1905-1988) reported the first successful ligation of a patent arterial duct in 1939 and resection for coarctation of the aorta with direct anastomosis of the remaining ends in 1945.
- John Alexander (1891-1954) resected a saccular aneurysm of the thoracic aorta in 1944.

With such a wide variety of technically complex surgical operations now possible, it had clearly become impossible for any single surgeon to master all the manual skills and pathophysiologic knowledge necessary to perform such cases. Therefore, by the middle of the century, a consolidation of professional power inherent in the movement toward specialization, with numerous individuals restricting their surgical practice to one highly structured field, had become among the most significant and dominating events in 20th century surgery. Ironically, the United States, which had been much slower than European countries to recognize surgeons as a distinct group of clinicians separate from physicians, would now spearhead this move toward surgical specialization with great alacrity. Clearly, the course of surgical fragmentation into specialties and subspecialties was gathering tremendous speed as the dark clouds of World War II settled over the world. The socioeconomic and political ramifications of this war would bring about a fundamental change in the way that surgeons viewed themselves and their interactions with the society in which they lived and worked.

## Last Half of the 20th Century

The decades of economic expansion after World War II had a dramatic impact on surgery's scale, particularly in the United States. It was as though being victorious in battle permitted medicine to become big business overnight, with the single-minded pursuit of health care rapidly transformed into society's largest growth industry. Spacious hospital complexes were built that not only represented the scientific advancement of the healing arts, but also vividly demonstrated the strength of American's postwar socioeconomic boom. Society was willing to give surgical science unprecedented recognition as a prized national asset.

The overwhelming impact of World War II on surgery was the sudden expansion of the profession and the beginnings of an extensive distribution of surgeons throughout the country. Many of these individuals, newly baptized to the rigors of technically complex trauma operations, became leaders in the construction and improvement of hospitals, multispecialty clinics, and surgical facilities in their home towns. Large urban and community hospitals established surgical education and training programs and found it relatively easy to attract interns and residents. For the first time, residency programs in general surgery were rivaled in growth and educational sophistication by those in all the special fields of surgery. These changes served as fodder for further increases in the number of students entering surgery. Not only would surgeons command the highest salaries, but society was also enamored of the drama of the operating room. Television series, movies, novels, and the more than occasional live performance of a heart operation broadcast on a network beckoned the lay individual.

Despite lay approval, success and acceptability in the biomedical sciences are sometimes difficult to determine, but one measure of both in recent times has been awarding of the Nobel Prize in medicine and physiology. Society's continued approbation of surgery's accomplishments can be seen in the naming of nine surgeons as Nobel laureates (Table 1-1).

## Cardiac Surgery and Organ Transplantation

Two clinical developments truly epitomized the magnificence of post–World War II surgery and concurrently fascinated the public—the maturation of cardiac surgery as a new surgical specialty and the emergence of organ transplantation. Together, they would stand as signposts along the new surgical highway. Fascination with the heart goes far beyond that of clinical medicine. From the historical perspective of art, customs, literature, philosophy, religion, and science, the heart has represented the seat of the soul and the wellspring of life itself. Such reverence also meant that this noble organ was long considered a surgical untouchable. The late 19th and 20th centuries witnessed a steady march of surgical triumphs in opening successive cavities of the body, but the final achievement awaited the perfection of methods for surgical operations in the thoracic space.

Such a scientific and technologic accomplishment can be traced back to the repair of cardiac stab wounds by direct suture and the earliest attempts at fixing faulty heart valves. As triumphant as Luther Hill's (1862-1946) first known successful suture of a wound that penetrated a cardiac chamber was in 1902, it would not be until the 1940s that the development of safe intrapleural surgery could be counted on as something other than an occasional event. During World War II, Dwight Harken (1910-1993) gained extensive battlefield experience in removing

**Table 1-1 Nobel Laureate Surgeons in Medicine and Physiology**

| SURGEON | COUNTRY | FIELD (YEAR OF AWARD) |
|---|---|---|
| Theodor Kocher (1841-1917) | Switzerland | Thyroid disease (1909) |
| Allvar Gullstrand (1862-1930) | Sweden | Ocular dioptrics (1911) |
| Alexis Carrel (1873-1944) | France and United States | Vascular surgery (1912) |
| Robert Bárány (1876-1936) | Austria | Vestibular disease (1914) |
| Frederick Banting (1891-1941) | Canada | Insulin (1922) |
| Walter Hess (1881-1973) | Switzerland | Midbrain physiology (1949) |
| Werner Forssmann (1904-1979) | Germany | Cardiac catheterization (1956) |
| Charles Huggins (1901-1997) | United States | Oncology (1966) |
| Joseph Murray (1919-) | United States | Organ transplantation (1990) |

bullets and shrapnel in or in relation to the heart and great vessels without a single fatality. Building on his wartime experience, Harken and other pioneering surgeons, including Charles Bailey (1910-1993) of Philadelphia and Russell Brock (1903-1980) of London, proceeded to expand intracardiac surgery by developing operations for the relief of mitral valve stenosis. The procedure was progressively refined and evolved into the open commissurotomy repair used today.

Despite mounting clinical successes, surgeons who operated on the heart had to contend not only with the quagmire of blood flowing through an area in which difficult dissection was taking place, but also with the unrelenting to and fro movement of a beating heart. Technically complex cardiac repair procedures could not be developed further until these problems were solved. John Gibbon (1903-1973; Fig. 1-13) addressed this enigma by devising a machine that would take on the work of the heart and lungs while the patient was under anesthesia, in essence pumping oxygen-rich blood through the circulatory system while bypassing the heart so that the organ could be operated on at leisure. The first successful open heart operation in 1953, conducted with the use of a heart-lung machine, was a momentous surgical contribution. Through single-mindedness of purpose, Gibbon's research paved the way for all future cardiac surgery, including procedures for correction of congenital heart defects, repair of heart valves, revascularization operations, and heart transplantation. David Sabiston (1924-2009; Fig. 1-14) was an inspirational surgical leader who served 30 years as chairman of the department of surgery at Duke University. Trained under Alfred Blalock at Johns Hopkins, Sabiston performed early and innovative coronary artery bypass operations that paved the way for more effective cardiac surgery procedures. Sabiston assumed numerous leadership roles throughout his career, including President of the American College of Surgeons, the American Surgical Association, and the American Association for Thoracic Surgery. As an eminent editor-in-chief, he guided the *Annals of Surgery* for 25 years and oversaw six previous editions of this text, the legendary *Sabiston Textbook of Surgery: The Biological Basis of Modern Surgical Practice.* Michael DeBakey (1908-2008; Fig. 1-15) was a renowned cardiac and vascular surgeon, clinical researcher, medical educator, and international medical statesman, who was the long-time Chancellor of Baylor College of Medicine and senior attending surgeon of the Methodist Hospital in Houston. He pioneered the use of Dacron grafts to replace or repair blood vessels, invented the roller pump, developed ventricular assist devices, was among the first to perform a coronary artery bypass and carotid endarterectomy, demonstrated the link between cigarette smoking and lung cancer, and created an early version of what became the mobile army surgical hospital or MASH unit. DeBakey was an influential advisor to the federal government about health care policy and served as chairman of the President's Commission on Heart Disease, Cancer, and Stroke during the Johnson administration. Among DeBakey's numerous honors were the Presidential Medal of Freedom, Congressional Gold Medal, and Lasker Clinical Medical Research Award.

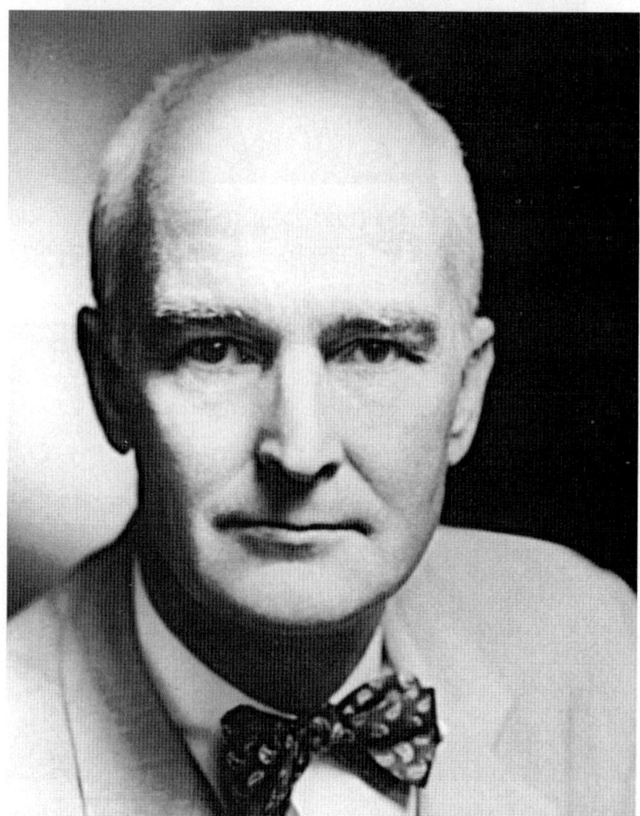

**FIGURE 1-13** John Gibbon (1903-1973).

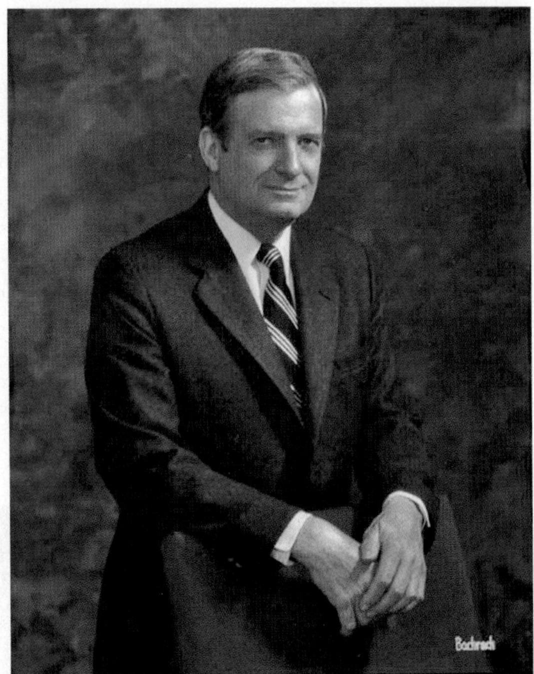

**FIGURE 1-14** David Sabiston (1924-2009). (From Anderson R: David C. Sabiston, Jr, MD. J Thorac Cardiovasc Surg 137:1307–1308, 2009.)

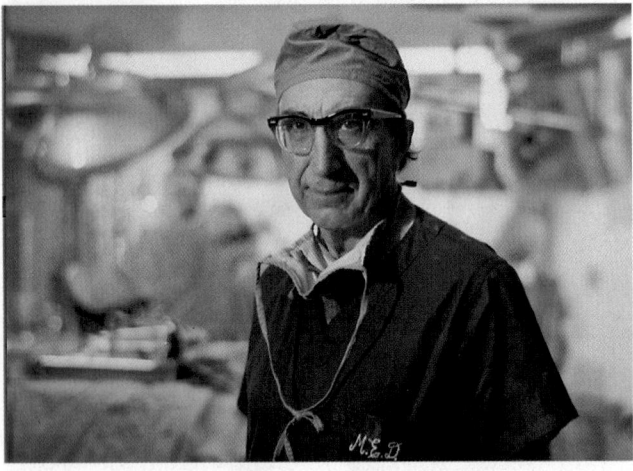

**FIGURE 1-15** Michael DeBakey (1908-2008). (Courtesy Baylor College of Medicine, Houston.)

Since time immemorial, the focus of surgery was mostly on excision and repair. However, beginning in the 20th century, the opposite end of the surgical spectrum—reconstruction and transplantation—became realities. Experience in the 19th century had shown that skin and bone tissues could be autotransplanted from one site to another in the same patient. It would take the horrendous and mutilating injuries of World War I to advance skin transplantation decisively and legitimize the concept of surgery as a method of reconstruction. With Harold Gillies (1882-1960) of England and Vilray Blair of the United States establishing military-based plastic surgery units to deal with complex maxillofacial injuries, a turning point in the way in which society viewed surgery's raison d'être occurred. Now, not only would surgeons enhance nature's healing powers, but they could also dramatically alter what had previously been little more than one's physical foregone conclusion. For example, Hippolyte Morestin (1869-1919) described a method of mammaplasty in 1902. John Staige Davis (1872-1946) of Baltimore popularized a manner of splinting skin grafts and later wrote the first comprehensive textbook on this new specialty, *Plastic Surgery: Its Principles and Practice* (1919). Immediately after the war, Blair would go on to establish the first separate plastic surgery service in a civilian institution at Barnes Hospital in St. Louis. Vladimir Filatov (1875-1956) of Odessa, Russia, used a tubed pedicle flap in 1916 and, in the following year, Gillies introduced a similar technique.

What about the replacement of damaged or diseased organs? After all, even in the mid-20th century, the very thought of successfully transplanting worn-out or unhealthy body parts verged on scientific fantasy. At the beginning of the 20th century, Alexis Carrel had developed revolutionary new suturing techniques to anastomose the smallest of blood vessels. Using his surgical élan on experimental animals, Carrel began to transplant kidneys, hearts, and spleens. Technically, his research was a success, but some unknown biologic process always led to rejection of the transplanted organ and death of the animal. By the middle of the century, medical researchers had begun to clarify the presence of underlying defensive immune reactions and the necessity of creating immunosuppression as a method to allow the host to accept the foreign transplant. Using high-powered immunosuppressant drugs and other modern modalities, kidney transplantation soon blazed the way, and it was not long before many organs and even hands and faces were being replaced.

### Political and Socioeconomic Influences

Despite the 1950s and 1960s witnessing some of the most magnificent advances in the history of surgery, political and socioeconomic influences were starting to overshadow many of the clinical triumphs by the 1970s. It was the beginning of a schizophrenic existence for surgeons in that complex and dramatic lifesaving operations were completed to innumerable accolades whereas concurrently public criticism of the economics of medicine, in particular, high-priced surgical practice, portrayed the scalpel holder as a greedy, financially driven, selfish individual. This was in stark contrast to the relatively selfless and sanctified image of the surgeon before the growth of specialty work and the introduction of government involvement in health care delivery.

Although they are philosophically inconsistent, the dramatic and theatrical features of surgery that make surgeons heroes from one perspective and symbols of corruption, mendacity, and greed from the opposite point of view are the very reasons why society demands so much of its them. There is the precise and definitive nature of surgical intervention, expectation of success that surrounds an operation, short time frame in which outcomes are realized, high income levels of most surgeons, and almost insatiable inquisitiveness of lay individuals about all aspects of the act of consensually cutting into another human's flesh. These phenomena, ever more sensitized in this age of mass media and instantaneous telecommunication, make surgeons seem more accountable than their medical colleagues and, simultaneously, symbolic of the best and worst in medicine. In ways that were previously unimaginable, this vast social transformation of surgery controls the fate of the individual physician in the present era to a much greater extent than surgeons as a collective force can control it by their attempts to direct their own profession.

## 20TH CENTURY SURGICAL HIGHLIGHTS

Among the difficulties in studying 20th century surgery is the abundance of famous names and important written contributions—so much so that it becomes a difficult and invidious task to attempt any rational selection of representative personalities along with their significant writings. Although many justly famous names might be missing, the following description of surgical advances is intended to highlight some of the stunning clinical achievements of the past century chronologically.

In 1900, the German surgeon Hermann Pfannenstiel (1862-1909) described his technique for a suprapubic surgical incision. That same year, William Mayo (1861-1939) presented his results on partial gastrectomy before the American Surgical Association. The treatment of breast cancer was radically altered when George Beatson (1848-1933), professor of surgery in Glasgow, proposed oophorectomy and the administration of thyroid extract as a possible cure (1901). John Finney (1863-1942) of the Johns Hopkins Hospital authored a paper on a new method of gastroduodenostomy, or widened pyloroplasty (1903). In Germany, Fedor Krause (1856-1937) was writing about total cystectomy and bilateral ureterosigmoidostomy. In 1905, Hugh Hampton Young (1870-1945) of Baltimore was presenting early studies of his radical prostatectomy for carcinoma. William Handley (1872-1962) was surgeon of the Middlesex Hospital in London when he authored *Cancer of the Breast and Its Treatment* (1906). In that work, he advanced the theory that in breast cancer, metastasis is caused by extension along lymphatic vessels and not by dissemination via the bloodstream. That same year, José Goyanes (1876-1964) of Madrid used vein grafts to restore arterial flow. William Miles (1869-1947) of England first wrote about his technique of abdominoperineal resection in 1908, the same year that Friedrich Trendelenburg (1844-1924) attempted pulmonary embolectomy. Martin Kirschner (1879-1942) of Germany described a wire for skeletal traction and for stabilization of bone fragments or joint immobilization 3 years later. Donald Balfour (1882-1963) of the Mayo Clinic provided the initial account of his important operation for resection of the sigmoid colon, as did William Mayo for his radical operation for carcinoma of the rectum in 1910.

In 1911, Fred Albee (1876-1945) of New York began to use living bone grafts as internal splints. Wilhelm Ramstedt (1867-1963), a German surgeon, described a pyloromyotomy (1912) at the same time that Pierre Fredet (1870-1946) was reporting a similar operation. In 1913, Henry Janeway (1873-1921) of New York developed a technique for gastrostomy in which he wrapped the anterior wall of the stomach around a catheter and sutured it in place, thereby establishing a permanent fistula. Hans Finsterer (1877-1955), professor of surgery in Vienna, improved on Franz von Hofmeister's (1867-1926) description of a partial gastrectomy with closure of a portion of the lesser curvature and retrocolic anastomosis of the remainder of the stomach to the jejunum (1918). Thomas Dunhill (1876-1957) of London was a pioneer in thyroid surgery, especially in his operation for exophthalmic goiter (1919). William Gallie (1882-1959) of Canada used sutures fashioned from the fascia lata in herniorrhaphy (1923). Barney Brooks (1884-1952), professor of surgery at Vanderbilt University in Nashville, Tennessee, initially introduced clinical angiography and femoral arteriography in 1924. Reynaldo dos Santos (1880-1970), a Portuguese urologist, reported the first translumbar aortogram 5 years later. Cecil Joll (1885-1945), professor of surgery in London, described the treatment of thyrotoxicosis by means of subtotal thyroidectomy in the 1930s.

In 1931, George Cheatle (1865-1951), professor of surgery in London, and Max Cutler (1899-1984), a surgeon from New York, published their important treatise, *Tumours of the Breast.* In that same year, Cutler detailed his systemic use of ovarian hormone for the treatment of chronic mastitis. Around the same time, Ernst Sauerbruch (1875-1951) of Germany completed the first successful surgical intervention for cardiac aneurysm and his countryman, Rudolph Nissen (1896-1981), removed an entire bronchiectatic lung. Geoffrey Keynes (1887-1982) of St. Bartholomew's Hospital in England articulated the basis for the opposition to radical mastectomy and his favoring of radium treatment for breast cancer (1932). The Irish surgeon Arnold Henry (1886-1962) devised an operative approach for femoral hernia in 1936. Earl Shouldice (1891-1965) of Toronto first began to experiment with a groin hernia repair based on overlapping layers brought together by a continuous wire suture during the 1930s. René Leriche (1879-1955) proposed an arteriectomy for arterial thrombosis in 1937 and, later, periarterial sympathectomy to improve arterial flow. Leriche also described a syndrome of aortoiliac occlusive disease in 1940. In 1939, Edward Churchill (1895-1972) of the Massachusetts General Hospital performed a segmental pneumonectomy for bronchiectasis. Charles Huggins (1901-1997; Fig. 1-16), a pioneer in endocrine therapy for cancer, found that antiandrogenic treatment consisting of orchiectomy or the administration of estrogens could produce long-term regression in patients with advanced prostatic cancer. These observations formed the basis for the current treatment of prostate and breast cancer by hormonal manipulation; Dr. Huggins was awarded the Nobel Prize in 1966 for these

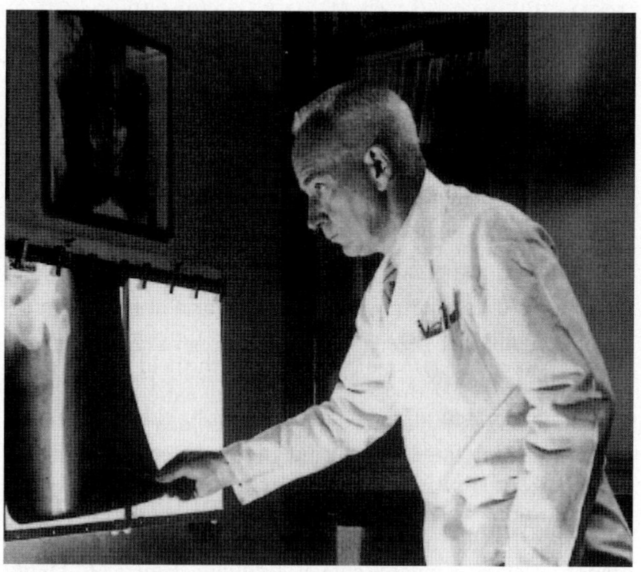

**FIGURE 1-16** Charles Huggins (1901-1997). (Used with permission from the University of Chicago Hospitals, Chicago.)

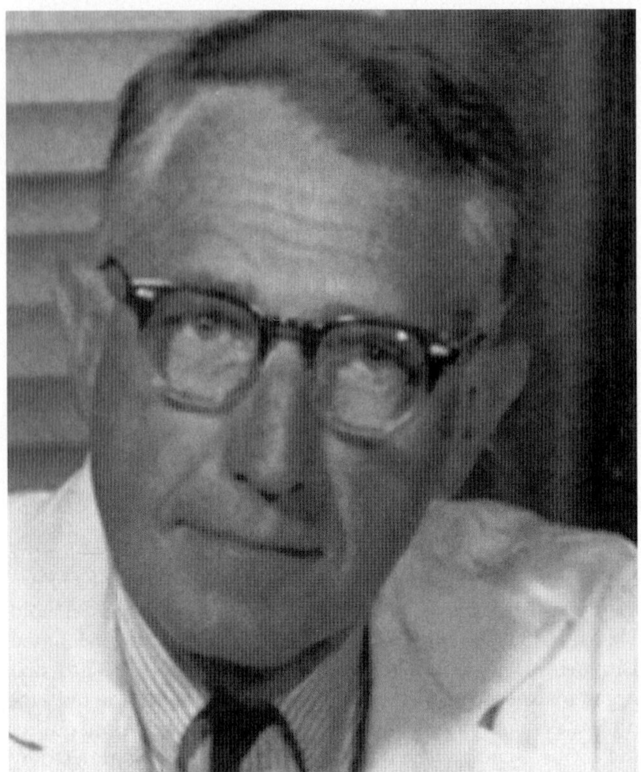

**FIGURE 1-17** Francis D. Moore (1913-2001).

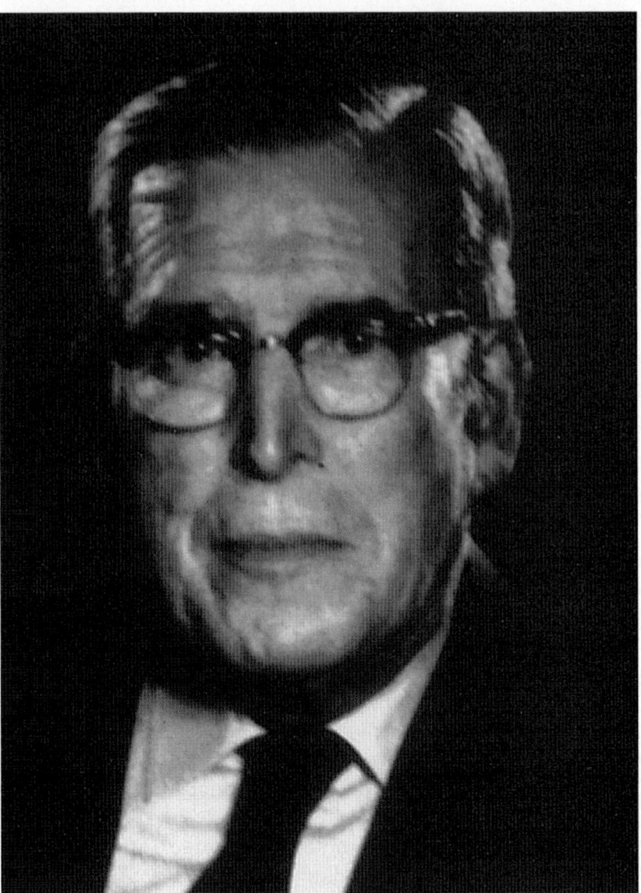

**FIGURE 1-18** Jonathan Rhoads (1907-2002). (Courtesy Dr. James C. Thompson.)

monumental discoveries. Clarence Crafoord (1899-1984) pioneered his surgical treatment of coarctation of the aorta in 1945. The following year, Willis Potts (1895-1968) completed an anastomosis of the aorta to a pulmonary vein for certain types of congenital heart disease. Chester McVay (1911-1987) popularized a repair of groin hernias based on the pectineal ligament in 1948.

Working at Georgetown University Medical Center in Washington, DC, Charles Hufnagel (1916-1989) designed and inserted the first workable prosthetic heart valve in a man (1951). That same year, Charles Dubost (1914-1991) of Paris performed the first successful resection of an abdominal aortic aneurysm and insertion of a homologous graft. Robert Zollinger (1903-1994) and Edwin Ellison (1918-1970) first described their eponymic polyendocrine adenomatosis in 1955. The following year, Donald Murray (1894-1976) completed the first successful aortic valve homograft. At the same time, John Merrill (1917-1986) was performing the world's first successful homotransplantation of the human kidney between identical twin brothers. Francis D. Moore (1913-2001; Fig. 1-17) defined objectives of metabolism in surgical patients and in 1959 published his widely quoted book, *Metabolic Care of the Surgical Patient.* Moore was also a driving force in the field of transplantation and pioneered the technique of using radioactive isotopes to locate abscesses and tumors. In the 1960s, Jonathan E. Rhoads (1907-2002; Fig. 1-18), in collaboration with colleagues Harry Vars and Stan Dudrick, described the technique of total parenteral nutrition, which has become an important and lifesaving treatment for the management of a critically ill patient who cannot tolerate standard enteral feedings. James D. Hardy (1918-2003), at the University of Mississippi, performed the first lung (1963) and heart (1964) transplants in a human. Judah

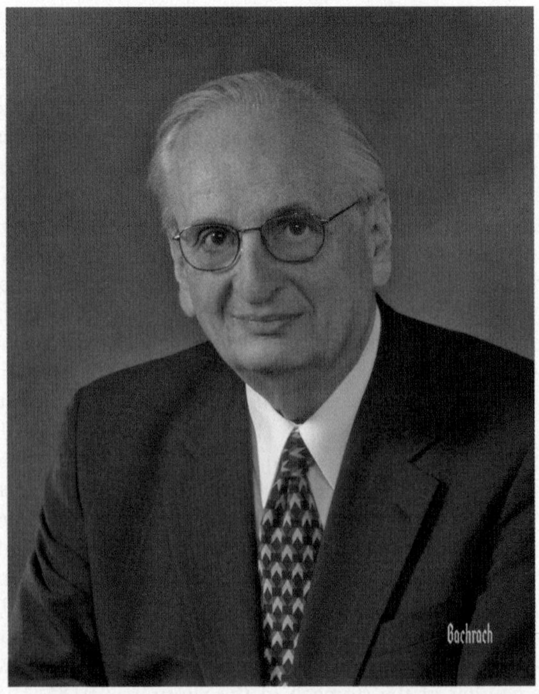


**FIGURE 1-19** Judah Folkman (1933-2008). (Courtesy Children's Hospital, Boston.)

Folkman (1933-2008; Fig. 1-19) was surgeon-in-chief at Children's Hospital in Boston, where he devoted much of his time to basic science research. He was best known for his studies on angiogenesis, the process whereby a tumor forms blood vessels to nourish itself and grow. Folkman's work led to antiangiogenesis therapy—the concept that cancers can be contained by using chemotherapeutic agents to inhibit their blood supply.

## FUTURE TRENDS

Throughout most of its evolution, the practice of surgery has been largely defined by its tools and the manual aspects of the craft. The last decades of the 20th century saw unprecedented progress in the development of new instrumentation and imaging techniques. These refinements have not come without noticeable social and economic cost. Advancement will assuredly continue because if the study of surgical history offers any lesson, it is that progress can always be expected, at least relative to technology. There will be more sophisticated surgical operations with better results. Eventually, automation may even robotize the surgeon's hand for certain procedures. Still, the surgical sciences will always retain their historical roots as fundamentally a manually based art and craft.

In many respects, the surgeon's most difficult future challenges are not in the clinical realm but instead in better understanding the socioeconomic forces that affect the practice of surgery and in learning how to manage them effectively. Many splendid schools of surgery now exist in almost every major industrialized city, but none can lay claim to dominance in all the disciplines that comprise surgery. Similarly, the presence of authoritative individual personalities who help guide surgery is more unusual today than in previous times. National aims and socioeconomic status have become overwhelming factors in securing and shepherding the future growth of surgery worldwide. In light of an understanding of the intricacies of surgical history, it seems an unenviable and obviously impossible task to predict what will happen in the future. In 1874, John Erichsen (1818-1896) of London wrote that "the abdomen, chest, and brain will forever be closed to operations by a wise and humane surgeon." A few years later, Theodor Billroth remarked that "A surgeon who tries to suture a heart wound deserves to lose the esteem of his colleagues." Obviously, the surgical crystal ball is a cloudy one at best.

To study the fascinating history of our profession, with its many magnificent personalities and outstanding scientific and social achievements, may not necessarily help us predict the future of surgery. However, it does shed much light on current clinical practices. To a certain extent, if surgeons in the future wish to be regarded as more than mere technicians, the profession needs to appreciate the value of its past experiences better. Surgery has a distinguished heritage that is in danger of being forgotten. Although the future of the art, craft, and science of surgery remains unknown, it assuredly rests on a glorious past.

## SELECTED REFERENCES

Allbutt TC: The Historical Relations of Medicine and Surgery to the End of the Sixteenth Century, London, 1905, Macmillan.

An incisive and provocative address by the Regius Professor of Physics in the University of Cambridge concerning the sometimes strained relationships between early medical and surgical physicians.

Billings JS: The history and literature of surgery. In Dennis FS, editor: System of Surgery, vol 1, Philadelphia, 1895, Lea Brothers, pp 17–144.

Surgeon, hospital architect, originator of *Index Medicus*, and director of the New York Public Library, Billings has written a comprehensive review of surgery, albeit based on a hagiographic theme.

Bishop WJ: The Early History of Surgery, London, 1960, Robert Hale.

This book by Bishop, a distinguished medical bibliophile, is best for its description of surgery in the Middle Ages, the Renaissance, and 17th and 18th centuries.

Bliss M: Harvey Cushing, A Life in Surgery, New York, 2005, Oxford.

Prized as a fascinating biography of one of America's most influential surgeons. Bliss is a wonderful writer who provides an incisive and colorful description of surgery during the late 19th and early 20th centuries.

Cartwright FF: The Development of Modern Surgery from 1830, London, 1967, Arthur Barker.

An anesthetist at King's College Hospital in London, Cartwright has produced a work rich in detail and interpretation.

Cope Z: A History of the Acute Abdomen, London, 1965, Oxford University Press.

Cope Z: Pioneers in Acute Abdominal Surgery, London, 1939, Oxford University Press.

These two works by the highly regarded English surgeon provide overall reviews of the evolution of surgical intervention for intra-abdominal pathology.

Earle AS: Surgery in America: From the Colonial Era to the Twentieth Century, New York, 1983, Praeger.

A fascinating compilation of journal articles by well-known surgeons that traces the development of the art and science of surgery in America.

Edmondson JM: American Surgical Instruments, San Francisco, 1997, Norman Publishing.

Although a wealth of information is available about the practice of surgery and the men who performed it in colonial and 19th-century America, this book details the lost story of the instrument makers and dealers who supplied the all-important tools for these physicians.

Gurlt EJ: Geschichte der Chirurgie und ihrer Ausübung, 3 vols 1–3, Berlin, 1898, A. Hirschwald.

A monumentally detailed history of surgery from the beginnings of recorded history to the end of the 16th century. Gurlt, a German surgeon, includes innumerable translations from ancient manuscripts. Unfortunately, this work has not been translated into English.

Hurwitz A, Degenshein GA: Milestones in Modern Surgery, New York, 1958, Hoeber-Harper.

The numerous chapters by these surgical attending physicians at Maimonides Hospital in Brooklyn contain prefatory information, including a short biography of various surgeons (with portrait) and a reprinted or translated excerpt of each one's most important surgical contribution.

Kirkup J: The Evolution of Surgical Instruments: An Illustrated History from Ancient Times to the Twentieth Century, Novato, Calif, 2006, Norman Publishing.

Surgeons are often defined by their surgical armamentarium, and this treatise provides detailed discussions on the evolution of all manner of surgical instruments and the materials from which they are constructed.

Leonardo RA: History of Surgery, New York, 1943, Froben.
Leonardo RA: Lives of Master Surgeons, New York, 1948, Froben.
Leonardo RA: Lives of Master Surgeons, Supplement 1, New York, 1949, Froben.

These texts by the eminent Rochester, New York, surgeon and historian together provide an in-depth description of the whole of surgery, from ancient times to the mid-20th century. Especially valuable are the countless biographies of famous and near-famous scalpel bearers.

Malgaigne JF: Histoire de la chirurgie en occident depuis de VIe jusqu'au XVIe siècle, et histoire de la vie et des travaux d'Ambroise Paré. In Malgaigne JF, editor: Ambroise Paré, oeuvres complètes, vol 1, introduction, Paris, 1840–1841, JB Baillière.

This history by Malgaigne, considered among the most brilliant French surgeons of the 19th century, is particularly noteworthy for its study of 15th and 16th century European surgery. This entire work was admirably translated into English by Wallace Hamby, an American neurosurgeon, in *Surgery and Ambrose Paré* by JF Malgaigne (Norman, Oklahoma, 1965, University of Oklahoma Press).

Meade RH: An Introduction to the History of General Surgery, Philadelphia, 1968, WB Saunders.
Meade RH: A History of Thoracic Surgery, Springfield, Ill, 1961, Charles C. Thomas.

Meade, an indefatigable researcher of historical topics, practiced surgery in Grand Rapids, Michigan. With extensive bibliographies, his two books are among the most ambitious of such systematic works.

Porter R: The Greatest Benefit to Mankind, a Medical History of Humanity, New York, 1997, WW Norton.

A wonderful literary tour de force by one of the most erudite and entertaining of modern medical historians. Although more a history of the whole of medicine than of surgery specifically, this text has become an instantaneous classic and should be required reading for all physicians and surgeons.

Ravitch MM: A Century of Surgery: 1880–1980, The History of the American Surgical Association, vols 1 and 2, Philadelphia, 1981, JB Lippincott.

Ravitch, among the first American surgeons to introduce mechanical stapling devices for use in the United States, was highly regarded as a medical historian. This text provides a year by year account of the meetings of the American Surgical Association, the most influential of America's numerous surgical organizations.

Richardson, R: The Story of Surgery: An Historical Commentary, Shrewsbury, England, 2004, Quiller Press.

An absorbing account of surgical triumphs written by a physician turned medical historian.

Rutkow IM: American Surgery, An Illustrated History, Philadelphia, 1998, Lippincott-Raven.
Rutkow IM: Bleeding Blue and Gray: Civil War Surgery and the Evolution of American Medicine, New York, 2005, Random House.
Rutkow IM: James A. Garfield, New York, 2006, Times Books/Henry Holt and Company.
Rutkow IM: Seeking the Cure: A History of Medicine in America, New York, 2010, Scribner.
Rutkow IM: Surgery, An Illustrated History, St. Louis, 1993, Mosby–Year Book.
Rutkow IM: The History of Surgery in the United States, 1775–1900, vols 1 and 2, San Francisco, 1988 and 1992, Norman Publishing.

Using biographic compilations, colored illustrations, and detailed narratives, these books explore the evolution of medicine and surgery, internationally and in the United States.

Schwartz S: Gifted Hands: America's Most Significant Contributions to Surgery, Amherst, NY, 2009, Prometheus Books.

A remarkably researched book that details the wide-ranging tale of American surgery's rise to world eminence.

Thorwald J: The Century of the Surgeon, New York, 1956, Pantheon.
Thorwald J: The Triumph of Surgery, New York, 1960, Pantheon.

In a most dramatic literary fashion, Thorwald uses a fictional eyewitness narrator to create continuity in the story of the development of surgery during its most important decades of growth, the late 19th and early 20th centuries. Imbued with a myriad of true historical facts, these books are among the most enjoyable to be found within the genre of surgical history.

Wangensteen OH, Wangensteen SD: The Rise of Surgery, from Empiric Craft to Scientific Discipline, Minneapolis, 1978, University of Minnesota Press.

Not a systematic history but an assessment of various operative techniques (e.g., gastric surgery, tracheostomy, ovariotomy, vascular surgery) and technical factors (e.g., débridement, phlebotomy, surgical amphitheater, preparations for surgery) that contributed to or retarded the evolution of surgery. Wangensteen was a noted teacher of experimental and clinical surgery at the University of Minnesota and his wife was an accomplished medical historian.

Zimmerman LM, Veith I: Great Ideas in the History of Surgery, Baltimore, 1961, Williams & Wilkins.

Zimmerman, late professor of surgery at the Chicago Medical School, and Veith, a masterful medical historian, provide well-written biographic narratives to accompany numerous readings and translations from the works of almost 50 renowned surgeons of varying eras.

CHAPTER 2

# ETHICS AND PROFESSIONALISM IN SURGERY

Cheryl E. Vaiani and Howard Brody

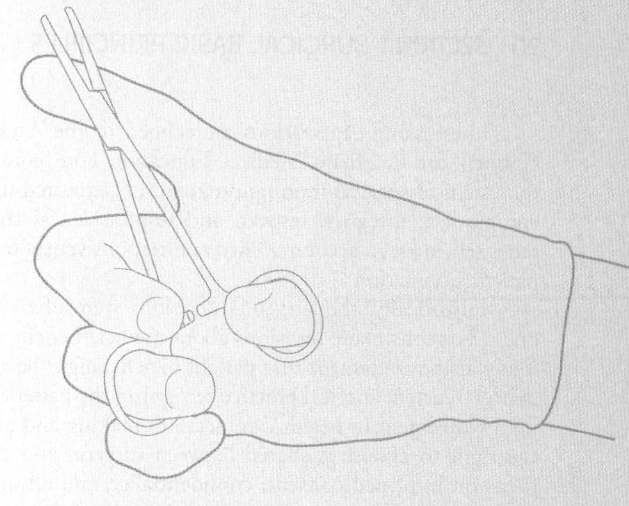



## THE IMPORTANCE OF ETHICS IN SURGERY

Although the ethical precepts of respect for persons, beneficence, nonmaleficence, and justice have been fundamental to the practice of medicine since ancient times, ethics has assumed an increasingly visible and codified position in health care over the past 50 years. The Joint Commission, the courts, presidential commissions, medical school and residency curriculum planners, professional organizations, the media, and the public have all grappled with determining the right course of action in health care matters. The explosion of medical technology and knowledge, changes in the organizational arrangement and financing of the health care system, and challenges to traditional precepts posed by the corporatization of medicine have all created new ethical questions.

The practice of medicine or surgery is, at its center, a moral enterprise. Although clinical proficiency and surgical skill are crucial, so are the moral dimensions of a surgeon's practice. According to sociologist Charles Bosk, the surgeon's actions and patient outcome are more closely linked in surgery than in medicine, and that linkage dramatically changes the relationship between surgeon and patient.[1] Surgeon and humanist Miles Little has suggested that there is a distinct moral domain within the surgeon-patient relationship. According to Little, "testing and negotiating the reality of the category of rescue, negotiating the inherent proximity of the relationship, revealing the nature of the ordeal, offering and providing support through its course, and being there for the other in the aftermath of the surgical encounter, are ideals on which to build a distinctively surgical ethics."[2] Because surgery is an extreme experience for the patient, surgeons have a unique opportunity to understand their patients' stories and provide support for them. The virtue and duty of engaged presence as described by Little extends beyond a warm, friendly personality and can be taught by both precept and example. Although Little does not specifically identify trust as a component of presence, it seems inherent to the moral depth of the surgeon-patient relationship. During surgery the patient is in a totally vulnerable position and a high level of trust is demanded for the patient to place his or her life directly in the surgeon's hands. Such trust, in turn, requires that the surgeon strive to act always in a trustworthy manner.

From the Hippocratic Oath to the 1847 American Medical Association statement of medical principles through the present, the traditional ethical precepts of the medical profession have included the primacy of patient welfare. The American College of Surgeons was founded in 1913 on the principles of high-quality care for the surgical patient and the ethical and competent practice of surgery. The preamble to its Statement on Principles states the following[3]:

> The American College of Surgeons has had a deep and effective concern for the improvement of patient care and for the ethical practice of medicine. The ethical practice of medicine establishes and ensures an environment in which all individuals are treated with respect and tolerance; discrimination or harassment on the basis of age, sexual preference, gender, race, disease, disability, or religion, are proscribed as being inconsistent with the ideals and principles of the American College of Surgeons.

The Code of Professional Conduct continues[4]:

> As Fellows of the American College of Surgeons, we treasure the trust that our patients have placed in us, because trust is integral to the practice of surgery. During the continuum of pre-, intra-, and post-operative care, we accept responsibilities to:
>
> - Serve as effective advocates of our patients' needs.
> - Disclose therapeutic options, including their risks and benefits.
> - Disclose and resolve any conflict of interest that might influence decisions regarding care.
> - Be sensitive and respectful of patients, understanding their vulnerability during the perioperative period.
> - Fully disclose adverse events and medical errors.
> - Acknowledge patients' psychological, social, cultural, and spiritual needs.
> - Encompass within our surgical care the special needs of terminally ill patients.
> - Acknowledge and support the needs of patients' families.
> - Respect the knowledge, dignity, and perspective of other health care professionals.

These same expectations are echoed in the Accreditation Council for Graduate Medical Education core competencies that medical-surgical training programs are expected to achieve: compassion, integrity, respect, and responsiveness that supersedes self-interest, accountability, and responsiveness to a diverse patient population.[5]

Historically, the surgeon's decisions were often unilateral ones. Surgeons made decisions about medical benefit with little if any acknowledgment that patient benefit might be a different matter. Current surgical practice recognizes the patient's increasing involvement in health care decision making and grants that the right to choose is shared between surgeon and patient. A focus on informed consent, confidentiality, and advance directives acknowledges this changed relationship of the surgeon and patient. However, the moral dimensions of a surgeon's practice extend beyond those issues to ask how the conscientious, competent, ethical surgeon should reveal damaging mistakes to a family when they have occurred, balance the role of patient advocate with that of being a gatekeeper, handle a colleague who is too old or too impaired to operate safely, or think about surgical innovation. Jones and colleagues,[6] in a helpful casebook of surgical ethics, have noted that even a matter as mundane as the order of patients in a surgical schedule may conceal important ethical decisions.

## END-OF-LIFE CARE

Care of patients at the end of life has garnered increasing attention in recent years. The decade of the 1990s was characterized by the expansion of efforts to educate physicians and inculcate palliative care practices into medical institutions. Surgeons who often are best known for their ability to be decisive—to do something—began to recognize their role in appropriate end-of-life care and to develop standards for palliative surgical care. In February 1998, The American College of Surgeons approved "The Statement of Principles of Care at the End of Life," which includes a responsibility to provide appropriate palliative and hospice care and respect a patient's right to refuse treatment and the physician's responsibility to forgo futile interventions.[7] A Surgeons Palliative Care Workgroup met in 2000 to foster awareness, education, and research in palliative care. In the first of a series of articles concerning palliative care by the surgeon in the *Journal of the American College of Surgeons*, Dunn and Milch[8] have explained that palliative care provides the surgeon with a "new opportunity to rebalance decisiveness with introspection, detachment with empathy." They also suggested that although surgeons might appreciate cognitively the need for palliative care, it also presents surgeons with difficult emotional challenges and ambiguities. In recognition of his leadership in the areas of hospice and palliative care, Robert A. Milch received the inaugural Hastings Center Cunniff-Dixon Physician Award in 2010 for leadership in care near the end of life. Dr. Milch said, in accepting the award, that "to the extent that we are able to play a part in that wonder, helping to heal even when we cannot cure, tending the wounds of body and spirit, we are ourselves elevated and transformed."[9]

### Resuscitation in the Operating Room

One of the most difficult issues in end-of-life care for the surgical patient concerns resuscitation. Informed decisions about cardiopulmonary resuscitation (CPR) require that patients have an accurate understanding of their diagnosis, prognosis, likelihood of CPR's success in their situation, and risks involved. Surgeons sometimes are reluctant to honor a patient's request not to be resuscitated when the patient is considering an operative procedure. Patients with terminal illness may desire surgery for palliation, pain relief, or vascular access yet not desire resuscitation if they experience cardiac arrest. Both the American College of Surgeons and American Society of Anesthesiologists have rejected the unilateral suspension of orders not to resuscitate in surgery without a discussion with the patient, but some physicians believe that patients cannot have surgery without being resuscitated and view a DNR order as "as an unreasonable demand to lower the standard of care."[10] Providers may worry that an order to forgo CPR may be extended inappropriately to withholding other critical interventions, such as measures required to control bleeding and maintain blood pressure. They may also fear being prevented from resuscitating patients for whom the arrest is the result of a medical error.

Discussions with the patient or surrogate about his or her goal for care and desires in various scenarios can help guide decision making. Such conversations allow a mutual decision that respects the patient's autonomy and physician's professional obligations. A patient who refuses resuscitation because the current health status is burdensome can clearly be harmed by intervening to resuscitate while in the operating room (OR). On the other hand, a patient who refuses because of the (presumed) low likelihood of success may change this decision once she or he understands the more favorable outcomes of intraoperative resuscitation.[11] A physician can certainly choose to transfer the care of the patient to another physician if he or she is uncomfortable with the patient's decision about interventions but should not impose this decision on the patient. CPR is not appropriate for every patient who has a cardiac or pulmonary arrest, even if that patient is in the operating room. Physicians need to develop skills in communicating accurate information about the risks and benefits of resuscitation with patients and families in light of the patient's condition and prognosis, make this discussion a routine part of the plan of care, and develop an appropriate team relationship between the surgeon and anesthesiologist to implement the decision.

## CULTURAL SENSITIVITY

Much has been said about the culture of surgery and the personality type of surgeons. The slogan "when in doubt, cut it out" is representative of the surgeon's imperative to act. Harsh generalizations of surgeons as egotistical, having a "God complex," and acting as playground bullies are frequent. As an often-stereotyped specialty, surgeons should have an astute appreciation for the impact of culture in the clinical encounter. The interaction between the surgeon who recommends operative treatment, and the patient who believes that the pain is from a spiritual source and cannot be treated by surgery, is unlikely to go well unless the surgeon has the tools to understand and respect the patient's cultural beliefs, values, and ways of doing things.

Training for cultural competence in health care is an essential clinical skill in the increasingly diverse U.S. population and has been recognized and integrated into the current education of medical professionals. Strong evidence of racial and ethnic disparities in health care supports the critical need for such training. Patient-centered care must recognize culture as a major force in shaping an individual's expectations of a physician, perceptions of good and bad health, understanding of a disease's cause, methods of preventive care, interpretation of symptoms, and recognition of appropriate treatment. Being a culturally competent surgeon is more than having knowledge about specific cultures; in fact, cultural knowledge must be carefully handled to avoid stereotyping or oversimplification. Instead, cultural competence involves the "exploration, empathy, and responsiveness to patients' needs, values, and preferences."[12] Self-assessment is often the first step to developing the attitude and skill of cultural competence. Honest and insightful inquiry into one's own feelings, beliefs, and values, including assumptions, biases, and stereotypes, is essential to awareness of the impact of culture on care.

The Association of American Medical Colleges' statement on education for cultural competence lists the following clinical skills as essential for medical students to acquire[13]:

1. Knowledge, respect, and validation of differing values, cultures, and beliefs, including sexual orientation, gender, age, race, ethnicity, and class
2. Dealing with hostility and discomfort as a result of cultural discord
3. Eliciting a culturally valid social and medical history
4. Communication, interaction, and interviewing skills
5. Understanding language barriers and working with interpreters
6. Negotiating and problem-solving skills
7. Diagnosis, management, and patient-adherent skills leading to patient compliance

Various models for effective cross-cultural communication and negotiation exist[14-21] to assist the physician in discovering and understanding the patient's cultural frame of reference. The BELIEF instrument by Dobbie and colleagues[22] is one such model:

**B**eliefs about health: What caused your illness/problem?
**E**xplanation: Why did it happen at this time?
**L**earn: Help me to understand your belief/opinion.
**I**mpact: How is this illness/problem impacting your life?
**E**mpathy: This must be very difficult for you.
**F**eelings: How are you feeling about it?

These models demand the skills of good listening, astute observation, and skillful communication used within the framework of respect and flexibility on the part of the physician. Bridging the cultural divide uses the same skills and traits that engender patient trust and satisfaction and improve quality of care. As Kleinman and associates[16] have explained in a classic paper, BELIEF types of questions are excellent to ask during every patient encounter, and not only those with patients from markedly different cultures. They stress the usefulness of regarding every patient interaction as a type of cross-cultural experience.

## SHARED DECISION MAKING

Ethically and legally, informed consent is at the heart of the relationship between the surgeon and patient. The term *informed consent* originated in the legal sphere and still conveys a sense of legalism and bureaucracy to many physicians. The term *shared decision making* has become more popular recently. It is, for all purposes, essentially synonymous with the idea of informed consent, but suggests a clinical and educational context that most physicians find more congenial.

Shared decision making is the process of educating the patient and assessing that he or she has understood and given permission for diagnostic or therapeutic interventions. The underlying ethical principle is respect for persons, or autonomy. Informed consent reflects the legal and ethical rights people have to make choices about what happens to their body in accordance with their values and goals and the ethical duty of the physician to enhance the patient's well-being.

There is no absolute formula for obtaining informed consent for a procedure, treatment plan, or therapy. A common error is to confuse the signing of a consent form with the process of informed consent. At best, the form is documentation that the process of shared decision making has occurred, not a substitute for that process. The process should include explanations from the physician in language the patient can understand and provide the opportunity for the patient to ask questions and consult with others, if necessary. Clarification of the patient's understanding is an important part of the decision making process. Asking patients to explain in their own words what they expect to happen and possible outcomes is much more indicative of their understanding than the ability merely to repeat what the physician has stated (What do you understand about the surgery that has been recommended to you?). Ideally, the process allows the physician and patient to work together to choose a course of treatment using the physician's expertise and the patient's values and goals.

Determining a patient's capacity to participate in decision making is an important role of the physician and inherent in the process of informed consent. Although capacity is generally assumed in adult patients, there are numerous occasions when the capacity for decision making is questionable or absent. Illness, medication, and altered mental status may result in an inability to participate independently in medical decision making. Capacity for decision making occurs along a continuum, and the more serious the consequences of the decision, the higher the level of capacity that it is prudent to require. Decisional capacity may also change over time; an individual may be capable of medical decisions one day or even at a particular time of day, but not at another. Probably the most common reason for questioning a patient's capacity is patient refusal of a treatment, procedure, or plan that the physician thinks is indicated. A patient's refusal certainly raises a red flag and may be an appropriate indicator for an evaluation of capacity, but it should not be the only one. Determination of capacity should be an essential part of the informed consent process for any decision.

How does a physician best evaluate a patient's capacity? There is no one definitive assessment tool for capacity. Although there are many guides and standards for evaluating capacity, it is most generally a common sense judgment that arises from a clinician's interaction with the patient. Mental status tests that assess orientation to person, place, and time are less useful than direct assessment of patient's ability to make a particular medical decision. Simple questions such as these assess the evaluation of capacity in the clinical setting more directly[23,24]:

- What do you understand about what is going on with your health right now?
- What treatment, diagnostic test, and/or procedure has been proposed to you?

- What are the benefits and risks?
- Why have you decided …?

## PROFESSIONALISM

Within medical ethics, the topic of professionalism has received increasing attention in the last decade or so. Although the more usual approaches to ethics focus on what decisions one ought to make in a particular situation, professionalism instead addresses questions of enduring moral character—what sort of physician one is, rather than only what one does or does not do.

A common way to address professionalism is to list a series of desirable character traits.[25] Almost all discussions of professionalism, however, ultimately rely heavily on two simple points. First, physicians are presumed, by virtue of entering into practice, to have made a moral commitment to place the interests of their patients above their own self-interests, at least to a considerable degree. Second, approaching medicine as a profession is commonly contrasted with viewing medical practice as merely a business.

Common challenges to surgeons' professionalism arise during interactions with the pharmaceutical and medical device industries, in which one may earn a substantial monetary reward for activities that promote the marketing interests of companies, even if those activities fail to promote better health for patients. If care is to remain affordable for most patients, the need to control U.S. health care costs represents another major challenge to professionalism. Will physicians and their professional societies act like special interest lobbies, mainly interested in maintaining generous reimbursements for their favored procedures, regardless of evidence about the procedures' efficacy? Or, will physicians rise to the challenge of supporting evidence-based medicine and take leadership in identifying low-efficacy procedures whose restricted use could conserve scarce health care resources?[26]

## CONCLUSION

The challenges of contemporary surgical practice necessitate attention not only to the lessons of the past but also contemplation of the future. Traditional codes and oaths provide guidance but reflection, self-assessment, and deliberation about what it means to be a good surgeon and how a good surgeon ought to act are essential. Educational efforts must inculcate the professional attitudes, values, and behaviors that recognize and support a culture of integrity and ethical accountability.

## SELECTED REFERENCES

Brody H: Hooked: Ethics, the Medical Profession, and the Pharmaceutical Industry, Lanham, Md, 2007, Rowman & Littlefield.

Examines the relationships between physicians and the pharmaceutical industry and how the integrity of the professional of medicine is threatened by those relationships.

Cassell EJ: The Nature of Suffering and the Goals of Medicine, New York, 1991, Oxford University Press.

Experienced internist's reflections on suffering and the relationship between patient and physician.

Chen PW: Final Exam: A Surgeon's Reflections on Mortality, New York, 2007, Alfred A. Knopf.

A transplant surgeon's narrative about her own fears and doubts about confronting death and how she helps her patients face the same issues.

Gawande A: Complications: A Surgeon's Notes on an Imperfect Science, New York, 2002, Metropolitan Books.

A young surgeon's thoughts on fallibility, mystery, and uncertainty in surgical practice.

Jonsen AR, Siegler M, Winslade WJ: Clinical Ethics: A Practical Approach to Ethical Decisions in Clinical Medicine, ed 7, New York, 2010, McGraw-Hill.

The standard physician's pocket guide to clinical and ethical decision making.

May WF: The Physician's Covenant: Images of the Healer in Medical Ethics, Philadelphia, 1983, Westminster John Knox Press.

Reflections on the physician as parent, fighter, technician, and teacher.

McCullough LB, Jones JW, Brody BA: Surgical Ethics, New York, 1998, Oxford University Press.

Nineteen chapters on surgical ethics, varying from principles and practice through research and innovation to finances and institutional relationships.

Nuland SB: How We Die: Reflections on Life's Final Chapter, New York, 1994, Vintage Books.

A national bestseller by a senior surgeon, writer, and historian of medicine.

Selzer R: Letters to a Young Doctor, New York, 1982, Simon & Schuster.

Sage advice for young surgeons from a seasoned surgeon-writer.

## REFERENCES

1. Bosk CL: Forgive and remember: managing medical failure, ed 2, Chicago, 2003, University of Chicago Press.
2. Little M: Invited commentary: Is there a distinctively surgical ethics? Surgery 129:668–671, 2001.
3. American College of Surgeons: Statements on principles, 2004 (http://www.facs.org/fellows_info/statements/stonprin.html).
4. American College of Surgeons: Code of professional conduct, 2003 (http://www.facs.org/memberservices/codeofconduct.html).
5. Accreditation Council for Graduate Medical Education (ACGME): Common program requirements: General competencies, 2007 (http://www.acgme.org/outcome/comp/GeneralCompetencies Standards21307.pdf).
6. Jones JW, McCullough LB, Richman BW: The Ethics of Surgical Practice: Cases, Dilemmas, and Resolutions, New York, 2008, Oxford University Press.
7. American College of Surgeons' Committee on Ethics: Statement on principles guiding care at the end of life. Bull Am Coll Surg 83:46, 1998.

8. Dunn GP, Milch RA: Introduction and historical background of palliative care: Where does the surgeon fit in? J Am Coll Surg 193:325–328, 2001.
9. Hastings Center: Surgeon and hospice founder accepts Hastings Center Cunniff-Dixon Physician Award, 2011 (http://www.thehastingscenter.org/News/Detail.aspx?id=4422).
10. Youngner SJ, Cascorbi HF, Shuck JM: DNR in the operating room. Not really a paradox. JAMA 266:2433–2434, 1991.
11. Girardi LN, Barie PS: Improved survival after intraoperative cardiac arrest in noncardiac surgical patients. Arch Surg 130:15–18, 1995.
12. Betancourt JR: Cultural competence—marginal or mainstream movement? N Engl J Med 351:953–955, 2004.
13. Association of American Medical Colleges: Cultural competence education, 2005 (https://www.aamc.org/download/54338/data/culturalcomped.pdf).
14. Stuart MR, Lieberman JA, III: The Fifteen-Minute Hour: Applied Psychotherapy for the Primary Care Physician, New York, 1993, Praeger.
15. Levin SJ, Like RC, Gottlieb JE: ETHNIC: A framework for culturally competent ethical practice. Patient Care 34:188–189, 2000.
16. Kleinman A, Eisenberg L, Good B: Culture, illness, and care: clinical lessons from anthropologic and cross-cultural research. Ann Intern Med 88:251–258, 1978.
17. Green AR, Betancourt JR, Carrillo JE: Integrating social factors into cross-cultural medical education. Acad Med 77:193–197, 2002.
18. Flores G: Culture and the patient-physician relationship: Achieving cultural competency in health care. J Pediatr 136:14–23, 2000.
19. Carrillo JE, Green AR, Betancourt JR: Cross-cultural primary care: A patient-based approach. Ann Intern Med 130:829–834, 1999.
20. Betancourt JR, Carrillo JE, Green AR: Hypertension in multicultural and minority populations: Linking communication to compliance. Curr Hypertens Rep 1:482–488, 1999.
21. Berlin EA, Fowkes WC, Jr: A teaching framework for cross-cultural health care. Application in family practice. West J Med 139:934–938, 1983.
22. Dobbie AE, Medrano M, Tysinger J, et al: The BELIEF Instrument: A preclinical teaching tool to elicit patients' health beliefs. Fam Med 35:316–319, 2003.
23. Boyle RJ: The process of informed consent. In Fletcher JC, Lombardo PA, Marshall MF, et al, editors: Introduction to Clinical Ethics, ed 2, Hagerstown, Md, 1997, University Publishing Group, pp 89–105.
24. Lo B: Resolving Ethical Dilemmas: A Guide for Clinicians, ed 3, New York, 2005, Lippincott Williams & Wilkins.
25. Medical Professionalism Project: Medical professionalism in the new millennium: A physician's charter. Lancet 359:520–522, 2002.
26. Brody H: Medicine's ethical responsibility for health care reform—the Top Five list. N Engl J Med 362:283–285, 2010.

CHAPTER 3

# MOLECULAR AND CELL BIOLOGY

Tien C. Ko

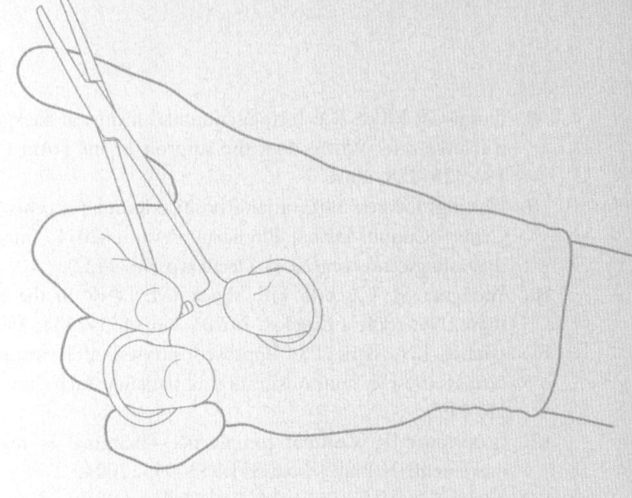

- HUMAN GENOME
- RECOMBINANT DNA TECHNOLOGY
- CELL SIGNALING
- CELL DIVISION CYCLE
- CELL DEATH
- HUMAN GENOME PROJECT
- NOVEL TREATMENT STRATEGIES
- ETHICAL, PSYCHOLOGICAL, AND LEGAL IMPLICATIONS

Since the 1980s, there has been an explosion in knowledge regarding molecular and cellular biology. These advances will transform the practice of surgery to one that is based on molecular techniques for the prevention, diagnosis, and treatment of many surgical diseases. This has been made possible by the achievements of the Human Genome Project, which is intended to reveal the complete genetic instruction of humans. The core knowledge of molecular and cellular biology has been presented in detail in several textbooks.[1,2] An overview of the field is presented here, with emphasis on basic concepts and techniques.

## HUMAN GENOME

Mendel first defined genes as information-containing elements that are distributed from parents to offspring. Genes contain the design that is essential for the development of each human. The field of molecular biology began in 1944, when Avery demonstrated that DNA was the hereditary material that made up genes. Translation of this genetic information into RNA and then protein leads to the expression of specific biologic characteristics or phenotypes. Major advances made in the field of molecular biology are listed in Table 3-1. In this section, the structures of genes and DNA are reviewed, as are the processes whereby genetic information is translated into biologic characteristics.

### Structure of Genes and DNA

DNA is composed of two antiparallel strands of unbranched polymer wrapped around each other to form a right-handed double helix (Fig. 3-1).[3] Each strand is composed of four types of deoxyribonucleotides containing the bases adenine (A), cytosine (C), guanine (G), and thymine (T). The nucleotides are joined together by phosphodiester bonds that join the 5′carbon of one deoxyribose group to the 3′ carbon of the next. Whereas the sugar-phosphate backbone remains constant, the attached bases can vary to encode different genetic information. The nucleotide sequences of the opposing strands of DNA are complementary to each other, thus allowing the formation of hydrogen bonds that stabilize the double-helix structure. Complementary base pairs require that A always pairs with T and C always pairs with G.

The entire human genetic information, or human genome, contains $3 \times 10^9$ nucleotide pairs. However, less than 10% of the DNA sequences are copied into messenger RNA (mRNA) molecules, which encode proteins, or structural RNA, such as transfer RNA (tRNA) or ribosomal RNA (rRNA) molecules. Each nucleotide sequence in a DNA molecule that directs the synthesis of a functional RNA molecule is called a gene (Fig. 3-2). DNA sequences that do not encode genetic information may have structural or other unknown functions. Human genes commonly contain more than 100,000 nucleotide pairs, yet most mRNA molecule–encoding proteins consist of only 1000 nucleotide pairs. Most of the extra nucleotides consist of long stretches of noncoding sequences, called introns, that interrupt the relatively short segments of coding sequences called exons. For example, the thyroglobulin gene has 300,000 nucleotide bases and 36 introns, whereas its mRNA has only 8700 nucleotide bases. The processes whereby genetic information encoded in DNA is transferred to RNA and protein molecules are discussed later.

The human genome contains 24 different DNA molecules; each DNA has $10^8$ bases and is packaged in a separate chromosome. Thus, the human genome is organized into 22 different autosomes and two different sex chromosomes. Because humans are diploid organisms, each somatic cell contains two copies of each different autosome and two sex chromosomes, for a total of 46 chromosomes. One copy of chromosomes is inherited from the mother and one is inherited from the father. Germ cells contain only 22 autosomes and one sex chromosome. Each chromosome contains three types of specialized DNA sequences that are important in the replication or segregation of chromosomes during cell division (Fig. 3-3). To replicate, each chromosome contains many short, specific DNA sequences that act as replication origins. A second sequence element, called a centromere, attaches DNA to the mitotic spindle during cell division. The third sequence element is a telomere, which contains G-rich repeats located at each end of the chromosome. During DNA replication, one strand of DNA becomes a few bases shorter at its 3′ end because of limitation in the replication machinery. If this is not remedied, DNA molecules will become progressively shorter in their telomere segments with each cell division. This problem is solved by an enzyme called telomerase, which periodically extends the telomerase sequence by several bases.

Each chromosome, when stretched out, would span the cell nucleus thousands of times. To facilitate DNA replication and segregation, each chromosome is packaged into a compact structure with the aid of special proteins, including histones. DNA and histones form a repeated array of particles called nucleosomes; each consists of an octomeric core of histone proteins around which the DNA is wrapped twice. The condensed complex of DNA and proteins is known as chromatin. Not only does chromosome packaging facilitate DNA replication and segregation, but it also influences the activity of genes (see later).

## DNA Replication and Repair

Before cell division, DNA must be duplicated precisely so that a complete set of chromosomes can be passed to each progeny. DNA replication must occur rapidly, yet with extremely high accuracy. In humans, DNA is replicated at the rate of approximately 50 nucleotides/second, with an error rate of one in every $10^9$ base pair replications. This efficient replication of genetic material requires an elaborate replication machinery consisting of several enzymes. Because each strand of DNA double helix encodes nucleotide sequences complementary to its partner strand, both strands contain identical genetic information and serve as templates for the formation of an entirely new strand.

Eventually, two complete DNA double helices are formed that contain identical genetic information. The fidelity of DNA replication is of critical importance because any mistake, called a mutation, will result in wrong DNA sequences being copied to daughter cells. Mistake in a single base pair is called a point mutation, which results in a missense mutation or nonsense mutation (Fig. 3-4). In a missense mutation, a single amino acid is changed, which can cause changes in the structure of the protein, leading to altered biologic activity. In a nonsense mutation, point mutation results in the replacement of an amino acid codon with a stop codon, leading to premature termination of translation and truncation of the encoded protein. If there is an addition or deletion of a few base pairs, it is called a frameshift mutation, which leads to the introduction of unrelated amino acids or a stop codon. Some mutations are silent and will not affect the function of the organism. Several proofreading mechanisms are used to eliminate mistakes during DNA replication.

**Table 3-1 Major Events in Molecular Biology**

| YEAR | EVENT |
|---|---|
| 1941 | Genes are found to encode proteins. |
| 1944 | DNA is determined to carry the genetic information. |
| 1953 | DNA structure is determined. |
| 1962 | Restriction endonucleases are discovered. |
| 1966 | Genetic code is deciphered. |
| 1973 | DNA cloning technique is established. |
| 1976 | First oncogene is discovered. |
| 1977 | Human growth hormone is produced in bacteria. |
| 1978 | Human insulin gene is cloned. |
| 1981 | First transgenic animal is produced. |
| 1985 | Polymerase chain reaction is invented. |
| | First tumor suppressor gene is discovered. |
| 1990 | Human Genome Project is created. |
| 1998 | First mammal is cloned. |

## RNA and Protein Synthesis

In the early 1940s, geneticists demonstrated that genes specify the structure of individual proteins. The transfer of information from DNA to protein proceeds through the synthesis of an intermediate molecule known as RNA. RNA, like DNA, is made up of a linear sequence of nucleotides composed of four complementary bases. RNA differs from DNA in two respects:

1. Its sugar-phosphate backbone contains ribose instead of deoxyribose sugar
2. Thymine (T) is replaced by uracil (U), a closely related base that pairs with adenine (A)

RNA molecules are synthesized from DNA by a process known as DNA transcription, which uses one strand of DNA as a template. DNA transcription differs from DNA replication in that RNA is synthesized as a single-stranded molecule and is

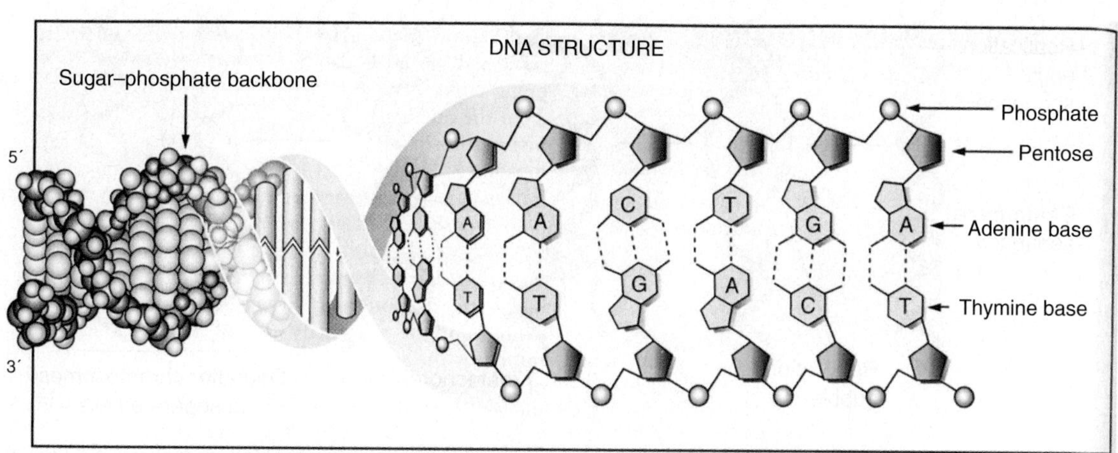


**FIGURE 3-1** DNA double-helix structure. The sequence of four bases (guanine, adenine, thymine, and cytosine) determines the specificity of genetic information. The bases face inward from the sugar-phosphate backbone and form pairs *(dashed lines)* with complementary bases on the opposing strand. (Adapted from Rosenthal N: DNA and the genetic code. N Engl J Med 331:39–41, 1994.)

relatively short in comparison to DNA. Several classes of RNA transcripts are made, including mRNA, tRNA, and rRNA. Even though all these RNA molecules are involved in the translation of information from RNA to protein, only mRNA serves as the template. RNA synthesis is a highly selective process, with only approximately 1% of the entire human DNA nucleotide sequence transcribed into functional RNA sequences. Although each cell contains the same genetic material, only specific genes are transcribed. RNA transcription is controlled by regulatory proteins that bind to specific sites on DNA, close to the coding sequence of a gene. The complex regulation of gene transcription occurs during development and tissue differentiation and allows differential patterns of gene expression.

After transcription, mRNA is processed for transport out of the nucleus (Fig. 3-5). One important step is RNA splicing, which removes noncoding sequences or introns. Once in the cytoplasm, RNA directs the synthesis of a particular protein through a process called RNA translation. The sequence of nucleotides in mRNA is translated into the amino acid sequence of a protein. Each triplet of nucleotides forms a codon that specifies one amino acid. Because RNA is composed of four types of nucleotides, there are 64 possible codon triplets ($4 \times 4 \times 4$). However, only 20 amino acids are commonly found in proteins, so most amino acids are specified by several codons. The rule whereby different codons are translated into amino acids is called the genetic code (Table 3-2).

Protein translation requires a ribosome, which is composed of more than 50 different proteins and several rRNA molecules. Ribosomes bind an mRNA molecule at the initiation codon (AUG) and begin translation in the 5′ to 3′ direction. Protein synthesis ceases once one of the three termination codons is encountered. The rate of protein synthesis is controlled by initiation factors that respond to the external environment, such as growth factor and nutrients. These regulatory factors help coordinate cell growth and proliferation.

## Control of Gene Expression

The human body is made up of millions of specialized cells, each performing predetermined functions. This is characteristic of all multicellular organisms. In general, different human cell types contain the same genetic material (i.e., DNA), yet they synthesize and accumulate different sets of RNA and protein molecules. This difference in gene expression determines whether a cell is a hepatocyte or a cholangiocyte. Gene expression can be controlled at six major steps in the synthetic pathway from DNA to RNA to protein.[4] The first control is at the level of gene transcription, which determines when and how often a given gene is transcribed into RNA molecules. The next step is RNA

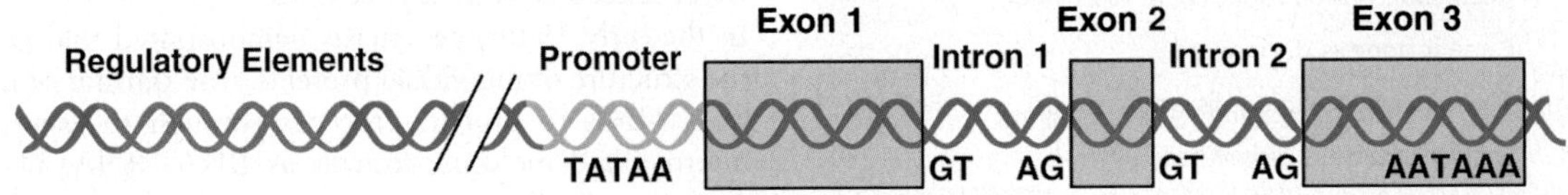


**FIGURE 3-2** Gene structure. The DNA sequences that are transcribed as RNA are collectively called the gene and include exons (expressed sequences) and introns (intervening sequences). Introns invariably begin with the nucleotide sequence GT and end with AG. An AT-rich sequence in the last exon forms a signal for processing the end of the RNA transcript. Regulatory sequences that make up the promoter and include the TATA box occur close to the site where transcription starts. Additional regulatory elements are located at variable distances from the gene. (Adapted from Rosenthal N: Regulation of gene expression. N Engl J Med 331:931–933, 1994.)

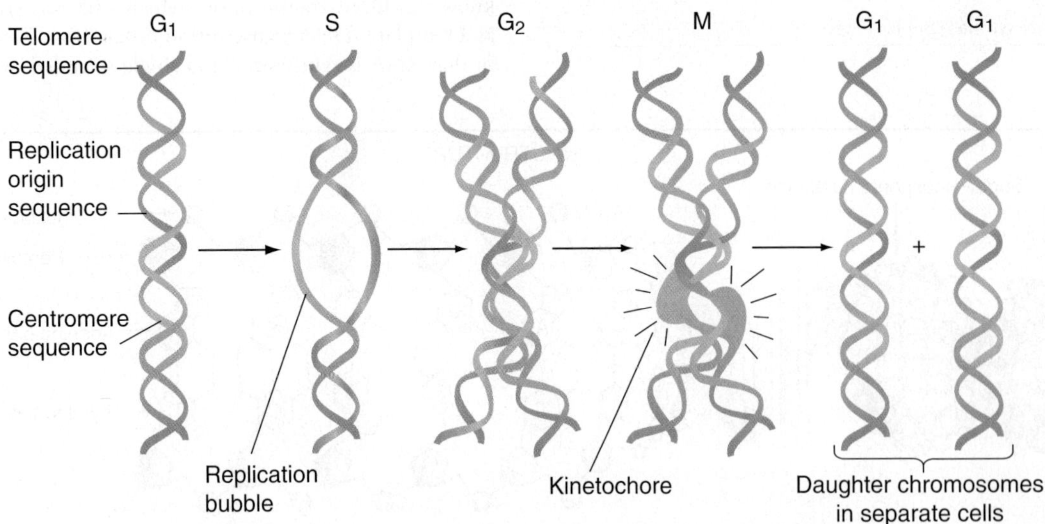


**FIGURE 3-3** Chromosome structure. Each chromosome has three types of specific sequences that facilitate its replication during the cell cycle. Origins of replication are located throughout each chromosome to facilitate DNA synthesis. The centromere holds the duplicated chromosome together and is attached to the mitotic spindle through a protein complex called a kinetochore. Telomere sequences are located at each end of the chromosome and are replicated in a special way to preserve chromosome integrity.

```
Wild-type sequences
  Amino acid  N-Phe  Arg  Trp  Ile  Ala  Asn-C
  mRNA        5'–UUU CGA  UGG  AUA  GCC  AAU–3'
  DNA         3'–AAA GCT  ACC  TAT  CGG  TTA–5'
              5'–TTT CGA  TGG  ATA  GCC  AAT–3'

Missense
              3'–AAT GCT  ACC  TAT  CGG  TTA–5'
              5'–TTA CGA  TGG  ATA  GCC  AAT–3'
              N-Leu  Arg  Trp  Ile  Ala  Asn-C

Nonsense
              3'–AAA GCT  ATC  TAT  CGG  TTA–5'
              5'–TTT CGA  TAG  ATA  GCC  AAT–3'
              N-Phe  Arg  Stop

Frameshift by addition
              3'–AAA GCT  ACC  ATA  TCG  GTT  A–5'
              5'–TTT CGA  TGG  TAT  AGC  CAA  T–3'
              N-Phe  Arg  Trp  Tyr  Ser  Gln

Frameshift by deletion
                 GCTA
                 CGAT
              3'–AAA CCT  ATC  GGT  TA–5'
              5'–TTT GGA  TAG  CCA  AT–3'
              N-Phe  Gly  Stop
```

**FIGURE 3-4** Different types of mutations. Point mutations involve alteration in a single base pair. Small additions or deletions of several base pairs directly affect the sequence of only one gene. A wild-type peptide sequence and the mRNA and DNA encoding it are shown at the top. Altered nucleotides and amino acid residues are enclosed in a box. Missense mutations lead to a change in a single amino acid in the encoding protein. In a nonsense mutation, a nucleotide base change leads to the formation of a stop codon that results in premature termination of translation, thereby generating a truncated protein. Frameshift mutations involve the addition or deletion of any number of nucleotides that is not a multiple of three, thus causing a change in the reading frame. (From Lodish HF, Baltimore D, Berk A, et al [eds]: Molecular cell biology, ed 3, New York, 1998, Scientific American, p 267.)

processing control, which regulates how many mature mRNA molecules are produced in the nucleus. The third step is RNA transport control, which determines which mature mRNA molecules are exported into the cytoplasm where protein synthesis occurs. The fourth step involves mRNA stability control, which determines the rate of mRNA degradation. The fifth step involves translational control, which determines how often mRNA is translated by ribosomes into proteins. The final step is post-translational control, which regulates the function and fate of protein molecules.

Control of gene transcription is the best studied step of regulation for most genes. RNA synthesis begins with assembly and binding of the general transcription machinery to the promoter region of a gene (see Fig. 3-5). The promoter is located upstream of the transcription initiation site at the 5′ end of the gene and consists of a stretch of DNA sequence primarily composed of T and A nucleotides (i.e., the TATA box). The general transcription machinery is composed of several proteins, including RNA polymerase II and general transcription proteins. These general transcription factors are abundantly expressed in all cells and are required for the transcription of most mammalian genes. The rate of assembly of the general transcription machinery to the promoter determines the rate of transcription, which is regulated by gene regulatory proteins. In contrast to the small number of general transcription proteins, there are thousands of different gene regulatory proteins. Most bind to specific DNA sequences, called regulatory elements, to activate or repress transcription.

Gene regulatory proteins are expressed in small amounts in a cell, and different selections of proteins are expressed in different cell types. Similarly, different combinations of regulatory elements are present in each gene to allow differential control of gene transcription. Many human genes have more than 20 regulatory elements; some bind transcriptional activators, whereas others bind transcriptional repressors. Ultimately, the balance between transcriptional activators and repressors determines the rate of transcription, which can vary by a factor of more than $10^6$ between genes that are expressed and those that are repressed. Most regulatory elements are located at a distance (i.e., thousands of nucleotide bases) away from the promoter. These distant regulatory elements are brought into the proximity of the promoter through DNA bending, thus enabling control of promoter activity. In summary, the combination of regulatory elements and the types of gene regulatory proteins expressed determines where and when a gene is transcribed.

Post-translational control is another important step in the regulation of gene expression because most proteins are modified in one form or another.[5] Modifications such as proteolytic cleavage, disulfide formation, glycosylation, lipidation, and biotinylation allow the protein to achieve the proper structural conformation essential for its biologic activity. The complexity of regulation is greatly increased by additional amino acid modifications that can occur at multiple sites of a protein. Examples of amino acid modification include phosphorylation, acetylation, methylation, ubiquitination, and sumoylation.

## RECOMBINANT DNA TECHNOLOGY

Advances in recombinant DNA technology, beginning in the 1970s, have greatly facilitated study of the human genome. It is now routine practice in molecular laboratories to excise a specific region of DNA, produce unlimited copies of it, and determine its nucleotide sequences. Furthermore, isolated genes can be altered (engineered) and transferred back into cells in culture or into the germline of an animal or plant so that the altered gene is inherited as part of the organism's genome. The most important recombinant DNA technology includes the ability to cut DNA at specific sites by restriction nucleases, rapidly amplify DNA sequences, quickly determine the nucleotide sequences, clone a DNA fragment, and create a DNA sequence.[6]

### Restriction Nucleases

Restriction nucleases are bacterial enzymes that cut the DNA double helix at specific sequences of four to eight nucleotides. More than 400 restriction nucleases have been isolated from different species of bacteria and they recognize over 100 different specific sequences. Commonly used restriction enzymes often recognize a six–base pair palindromic sequence, such as GAATTC. Each restriction nuclease will cut a DNA molecule into a series of specific fragments, which can be joined to other DNA fragments with compatible ends (Fig. 3-6*A*). By using a combination of different restriction enzymes, a restriction map of each DNA can be created, thus facilitating the isolation of individual genes.

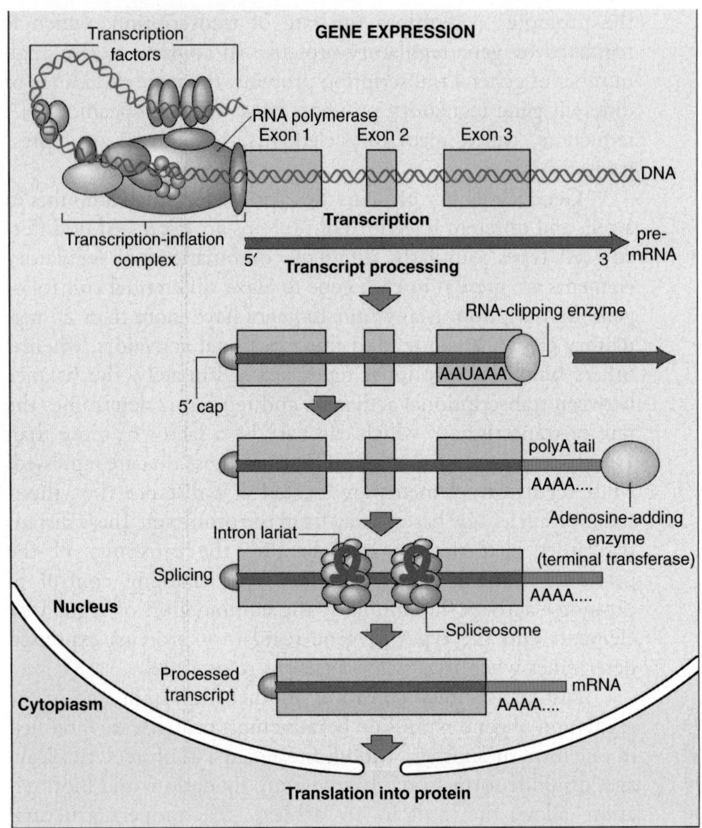


**FIGURE 3-5** Process of gene transcription. Gene expression begins with the binding of multiple protein factors to enhancer sequences and promoter sequences. These factors help form the transcription-initiation complex, which includes the enzyme RNA polymerase and multiple polymerase-associated proteins. The primary transcript (pre-mRNA) includes exon and intron sequences. Post-transcriptional processing begins with changes at both ends of the RNA transcript. At the 5′ end, enzymes add a special nucleotide cap; at the 3′ end, an enzyme clips the pre-mRNA approximately 30 base pairs after the AAUAAA sequence in the last exon. Another enzyme adds a polyadenylate (polyA) tail, which consists of as many as 200 adenine nucleotides. Next, spliceosomes remove the introns by cutting the RNA at the boundaries between exons and introns. The process of excision forms lariats of the intron sequences. The spliced mRNA is then mature and can leave the nucleus for protein translation in the cytoplasm. (Adapted from Rosenthal N: Regulation of gene expression. N Engl J Med 331:931–933, 1994.)

**Table 3-2 The Genetic Code**

| | Second Position | | | | |
|---|---|---|---|---|---|
| **FIRST POSITION (5′ END)** | **U** | **C** | **A** | **G** | **THIRD POSITION (3′ END)** |
| U (uracil) | Phe | Ser | Tyr | Cys | U |
| | Phe | Ser | Tyr | Cys | C |
| | Leu | Ser | Stop | Stop | A |
| | Leu | Ser | Stop | Trp | G |
| C (cytosine) | Leu | Pro | His | Arg | U |
| | Leu | Pro | His | Arg | C |
| | Leu | Pro | Gln | Arg | A |
| | Leu | Pro | Gln | Arg | G |
| A (adenine) | Ile | Thr | Asn | Ser | U |
| | Ile | Thr | Asn | Ser | C |
| | Ile | Thr | Lys | Arg | A |
| | Met | Thr | Lys | Arg | G |
| G (guanine) | Val | Ala | Asp | Gly | U |
| | Val | Ala | Asp | Gly | C |
| | Val | Ala | Glu | Gly | A |
| | Val | Ala | Glu | Gly | G |

## Polymerase Chain Reaction

An ingenious technique to amplify a segment of a DNA sequence in vitro rapidly was developed in 1985 by Saiki and coworkers.[7] This method, called the polymerase chain reaction (PCR), can enzymatically amplify a segment of DNA a billion-fold. The principle of the PCR technique is illustrated in Figure 3-6*B*.

To amplify a segment of DNA, two single-stranded oligonucleotides, or primers, must be synthesized, each designed to complement one strand of the DNA double helix and lying on opposite sides of the region to be amplified. The PCR reaction mixture consists of the double-stranded DNA sequence (the template), two DNA oligonucleotide primers (heat stable), DNA polymerase, and four types of deoxynucleotide triphosphate. Each round of amplification involves separation of the DNA template into two single strands, hybridization of the two DNA primers to complementary sequences on each strand of the DNA template, and DNA synthesis downstream of each primer. Each round of PCR requires only approximately 5 minutes and results in a doubling of the double-stranded DNA molecules, which serve as templates for subsequent reactions. After only 32 cycles, more than 1 billion copies of the desired DNA segment are produced. Not only is the PCR technique extremely powerful, but it is also the most sensitive technique to detect a single copy of a DNA or RNA molecule in a sample. To detect RNA molecules, they must first be transcribed into complementary DNA sequences with the enzyme reverse transcriptase. The number of research and clinical applications for PCR continues to grow. In molecular laboratories, PCR has been used for cloning of DNA, engineering of DNA, analysis of allelic sequence variations, and sequencing of DNA. PCR techniques have many clinical applications, including the

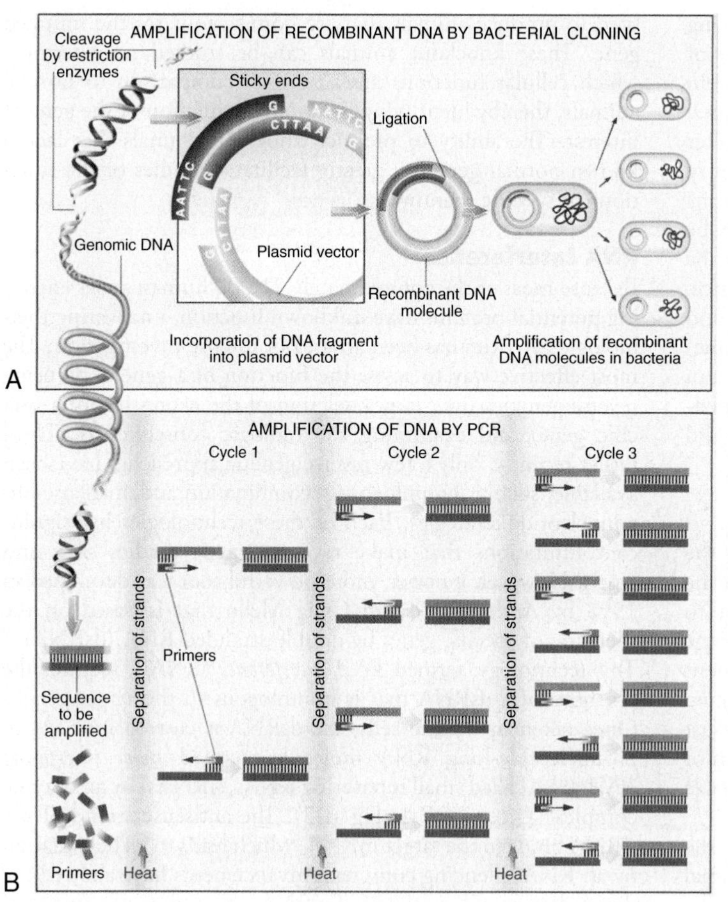


**FIGURE 3-6** Amplification of recombinant DNA and amplification by PCR. **A,** The DNA segment to be amplified is separated from surrounding genomic DNA by cleavage with a restriction enzyme. The enzymatic cuts often produce staggered, or sticky, ends. In the example shown, the restriction enzyme EcoRI recognizes the sequence GAATTC and cuts each strand between G and A; the two strands of genomic DNA are shown as *black*. The same restriction enzyme cuts the circular plasmid DNA (*gray*) at a single site, thereby generating sticky ends that are complementary to the sticky ends of the genomic DNA fragment. The cut genomic DNA and the remainder of the plasmid, when mixed together in the presence of a ligase enzyme, form smooth joints on each side of the plasmid–genomic DNA junction. This new molecule, recombinant DNA, is carried into bacteria, which replicate the plasmid as they grow in culture. **B,** The DNA sequence to be amplified is selected by primers, which are short synthetic oligonucleotides that correspond to sequences flanking the DNA to be amplified. After an excess of primers is added to the DNA, together with a heat-stable DNA polymerase, the strands of both the genomic DNA and primers are separated by heating and allowed to cool. A heat-stable polymerase elongates the primers on either strand, thus generating two new, identical, double-stranded DNA molecules and doubling the number of DNA fragments. Each cycle takes just a few minutes and doubles the number of copies of the original DNA fragment. (From Rosenthal N: Tools of the trade—recombinant DNA. N Engl J Med 331:315–317, 1994.)

diagnosis of genetic diseases, assay of infectious agents, and genetic fingerprinting for forensic samples.

## DNA Sequencing

DNA encodes information for proteins and, ultimately, the phenotype of a human being. Each gene may contain over 3000 nucleotide bases. Identification of the nucleotide sequences of a fragment of DNA has been made possible through the development of rapid techniques that take advantage of the ability to separate DNA molecules of different lengths, even those differing by only a single nucleotide. Currently, the standard method for sequencing DNA is based on an enzymatic method requiring in vitro DNA synthesis. This method is rapid and can be automated to allow sequencing of large segments of DNA. With these techniques, it is possible to determine the boundaries of a gene and the amino acid sequence of the protein that it codes. Sequencing techniques have enabled the identification and in vitro synthesis of important proteins such as insulin, interferon, hemoglobin, and growth hormones.

## DNA Cloning

DNA cloning techniques allow identification of a gene of interest from the human genome. First, the entire DNA content of a cell is cut with a restriction nuclease to generate DNA fragments, which are joined to a self-replicating genetic element (a virus or plasmid). Viruses or plasmids are small circular DNA molecules that occur naturally and can replicate rapidly when introduced into bacterial cells. They are extremely useful tools for amplifying a segment of unknown DNA. With this method, a collection of bacteria plasmids containing the entire human genome can be created. This human DNA library can then be used to identify genes of interest.

## DNA Engineering

One of the most important outcomes of recombinant DNA technologies is the ability to generate new DNA molecules of any sequence through DNA engineering. New DNA molecules can be synthesized by the PCR method or by using automated oligonucleotide synthesizers. The PCR method can be used to amplify any known segment of the human genome and to redesign its two ends. Automated oligonucleotide synthesizers enable the rapid production of DNA molecules, up to approximately 100 nucleotides in length. The sequence of such synthetic DNA molecules is entirely determined by the experimenter. Larger DNA molecules are formed by combining two or more DNA molecules that have complementary cohesive ends created by restriction enzyme digestion. One powerful application of DNA engineering is the synthesis of large quantities of cellular proteins for medical applications. Most cellular proteins are produced in small amounts in human cells, making it difficult to purify and study these proteins. However, with DNA engineering, it is possible to place a human gene into an expression vector that is introduced into bacterial, yeast, insect, or mammalian cells to produce a large quantity of protein. The protein can easily be purified and used for scientific studies or clinical applications. Medically useful proteins, such as human insulin, growth hormone, interferon, and viral antigens for vaccines, have been produced by engineering expression vectors containing these genes of interest.

DNA engineering techniques are also important for solving problems in cell biology. One of the fundamental challenges of cell biology is to identify the biologic functions of the protein product of a gene. With the use of DNA engineering techniques, it is now possible to alter the coding sequence of a gene to alter the functional properties of its protein product or the regulatory region of a gene and thus produce an altered pattern of its expression in the cell. The coding sequence of a gene can be changed in such subtle ways that the protein encoded by the gene has only one or a few alterations in its amino acid sequence. The modified gene is then inserted into an expression vector and transfected into the appropriate cell type to examine the function of the redesigned protein. With this strategy, one can analyze which parts of the protein are important for fundamental processes, such as protein folding, enzyme activity, and protein-ligand interactions.

## Transgenic Animals

The ultimate test of the function of a gene is to overexpress the gene in an organism and observe its effect or delete it from the genome and evaluate the consequences. It is much easier to overexpress a gene of interest than to delete it from the genome of an organism. To overexpress a gene, the DNA fragment encoding the gene of interest, the transgene, must be constructed with recombinant DNA techniques.[7,8] The DNA fragment must contain all the components necessary for efficient expression of the gene, including a promoter and regulatory region that drives transcription.

The type of promoter used can determine whether the transgene is expressed in many tissues of the transgenic animal or in a specific tissue. For example, selective expression in the acinar pancreas can be achieved by linking the amylase promoter to the coding sequence of the transgene. The transgene DNA fragments are introduced into the male pronucleus of a fertilized egg via microinjection techniques. Animals are then screened for the presence of the transgene. Analysis of these animals has provided important insight into the functions of many human genes, as well as animal models of human diseases. For example, transgenic animals engineered to overexpress a mutant form of the gene for the β-amyloid protein precursor (the *APP* gene) have neuropathologic changes similar to those in patients with Alzheimer's disease. This transgenic model not only supports the role of the *APP* gene in the development of Alzheimer's disease, but is also a model for testing methods of prevention or treatment of Alzheimer's disease.

A major disadvantage of using transgenic animals is that they will reveal only dominant effects of the transgene because these animals still retain two normal copies of the gene in their genome. Therefore, it is extremely useful to produce animals that do not express both copies of the gene of interest.[9] These knockout animals are much more difficult to develop than transgenic animals and require gene-targeting techniques. To knock out a gene, it is important to modify the gene of interest by DNA engineering to create a nonfunctioning gene. This altered gene is inserted into a vector and then inserted into germ cell lines. Although most mutated genes are inserted randomly into one of the chromosomes, a mutated gene will, rarely, replace one of the two copies of the normal gene by homologous recombination. Germ cells with one copy of the normal gene and one copy of the mutated gene will give rise to heterozygous animals. Heterozygous males and females are generated and can then be bred to produce animals that are homozygous for the mutated gene. These knockout animals can be studied to determine which cellular functions are altered in comparison to normal animals, thereby identifying the biologic function of the gene of interest. The ability to produce knockout animals that lack a known normal gene has greatly facilitated studies of the functions of specific mammalian genes.

## RNA Interference

Because most of the approximately 21,000 human genes encoding potential proteins have unknown function, uncovering their biologic activities has been an area of intense investigation. The most effective way to assess the function of a gene is by using reverse genetics (i.e., target deletion of the expression of a specific gene) and examining the biologic consequences. Until rather recently, only a few reverse genetic approaches have been available, such as homologous recombination and antisense oligonucleotide strategies. Each of these technologies has significant limitations that make reverse genetic studies slow and costly. However, a newer, more powerful tool was developed in 1998 by Andrew Fire and Craig Mello that is based on the silencing of specific genes by double-stranded RNA (dsRNA).[10] This technology, termed *RNA interference* (RNAi), requires the synthesis of a dsRNA that is homologous to the target gene.[11] Once taken up by the cells, the dsRNA is cleaved into 21- to 23-nucleotide-long RNA molecules termed *short interfering RNAs* (also called small interfering RNAs, siRNAs) by an enzyme complex (Dicer-RDE-1; Fig. 3-7). The antisense strand of the siRNA binds to the target mRNA, which leads to its degradation by an RNAi silencing complex. Advancements have allowed the direct design and synthesis of siRNAs, as well as placement of

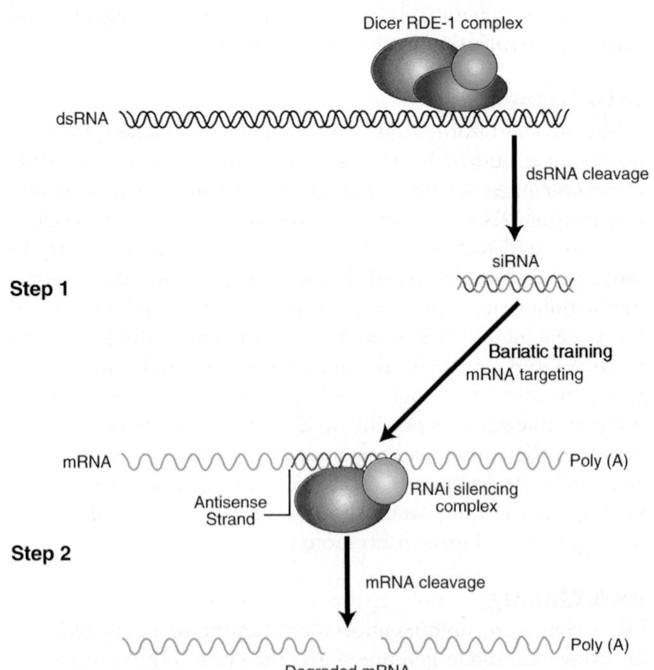


**FIGURE 3-7** RNA interference. Long double-stranded RNA (dsRNA) is processed by the Dicer-RDE-1 complex to form siRNA. The antisense strand of siRNA is used by an RNA interference (RNAi) silencing complex to guide specific mRNA cleavage, thus promoting mRNA degradation. *RDE-1,* RNAi deficient-1.

these siRNAs into viral vectors. Not only will this technology transform future studies in the analysis of gene function, but siRNAs might also be used as gene therapy to silence the function of specific genes.

## CELL SIGNALING

The human body is composed of billions of cells that must be coordinated to form specific tissues. Both neighboring and distant cells influence the behavior of cells through intercellular signaling mechanisms. Whereas normal cell signaling ensures the health of the human, abnormal cell signaling can lead to diseases such as cancer. Through powerful molecular techniques, the sophisticated signaling mechanisms used by mammalian cells have become better understood. This section reviews the general principles of intercellular signaling and examines the signaling mechanisms of the two main families of cell surface receptor proteins.[12]

### Ligands and Receptors

Cells communicate with one another by means of multiple signaling molecules, including proteins, small peptides, amino acids, nucleotides, steroids, fatty acid derivatives, and even dissolved gases, such as nitric oxide and carbon monoxide. Once these signaling molecules are synthesized and released by a cell, they may act on the signaling cell (autocrine signaling), affect adjacent cells (paracrine signaling), or enter the systemic circulation to act on distant target cells (endocrine signaling). These signaling molecules, also called ligands, bind to specific proteins, called receptors, expressed in the plasma membrane or the cytoplasm of the target cells. On ligand binding, the receptor becomes activated and generates a cascade of intracellular signals that alter the behavior of the cell. Each human cell is exposed to hundreds of different signals from its environment, but it is genetically programmed to respond only to specific sets of signals. Cells may respond to one set of signals by proliferating, to another set by differentiating, and to another by achieving cell death. Furthermore, different cells may respond to the same set of signals with different biologic activities.

Most extracellular signals are mediated by hydrophilic molecules that bind to receptors on the cell surface of the target cells. These cell surface receptors are divided into three classes based on the transduction mechanism used to propagate signals intracellularly. Ion channel–coupled receptors are involved in rapid synaptic signaling between electrically excitable cells. These receptors form gated ion channels that open or close rapidly in response to neurotransmitters. G protein–coupled receptors regulate the activity of other membrane proteins through a guanosine triphosphate–binding regulatory protein, called G protein.[13] Enzyme-coupled receptors act directly as enzymes or are associated with enzymes.[14] Most of these receptors are protein kinases or are associated with protein kinases that phosphorylate specific proteins in the cell.

Some extracellular signals are small hydrophobic molecules, such as steroid hormones, thyroid hormones, retinoids, and vitamin D. They communicate with target cells by diffusing across the plasma membrane and binding to intracellular receptor proteins. These cytoplasmic receptors are structurally related and constitute the intracellular receptor superfamily. On ligand activation, the intracellular receptors enter the nucleus, bind specific DNA sequences, and regulate transcription of the adjacent gene.

Some dissolved gases, such as nitric oxide and carbon monoxide, act as local signals by diffusing across the plasma membrane and activating intracellular enzymes in the target cells. In the case of nitric oxide, it binds and activates the enzyme guanylyl cyclase, which leads to the production of the intracellular mediator cyclic guanosine monophosphate (cGMP).

### G Protein–Coupled Receptors

G protein–coupled receptors are the largest family of cell surface receptors and mediate cellular responses to a broad range of signaling molecules, including hormones, neurotransmitters, and local mediators.[15] These receptors include β-adrenergic receptors, $\alpha_2$-adrenergic receptors, and glucagon receptors. They share a similar structure with an extracellular domain that binds ligand and an intracellular domain that binds to a specific trimeric G protein. There are at least six distinct trimeric G proteins based on their intracellular signaling mechanisms; each is composed of three different polypeptide chains, called α, β, and γ.[13] On ligand binding, the G protein–coupled receptor activates its trimeric G protein (Fig. 3-8). Activated trimeric G protein alters the concentration of one or more small intracellular signaling molecules, referred to as second messengers.

Two major second messengers regulated by G protein–coupled receptors are cyclic adenosine monophosphate

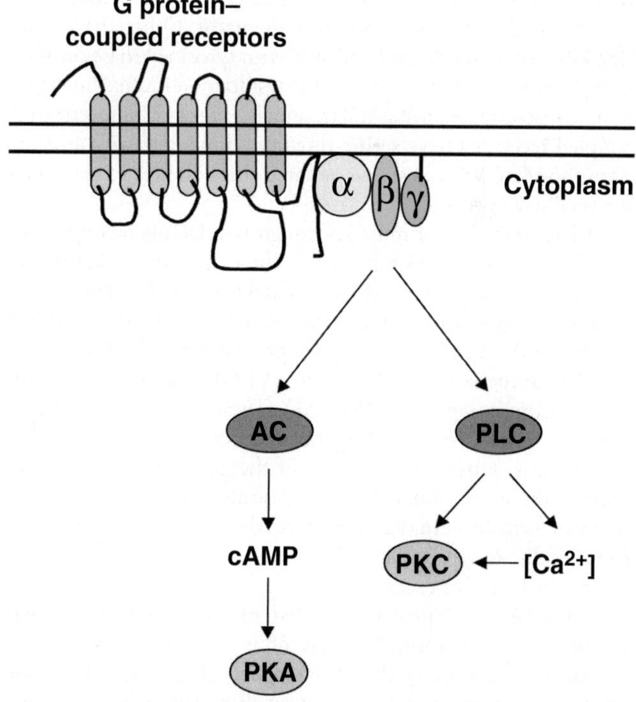


**FIGURE 3-8** G protein–coupled receptor signaling pathway. G protein–coupled receptors are seven-transmembrane domain proteins activated by the binding of ligands. Activated receptors initiate a cascade of events leading to amplification of the original signal. First, the receptor activates a trimer G protein consisting of α, β, and γ subunits. G proteins can activate adenylyl cyclase (AC) to generate cAMP or phospholipase C (PLC) to release intracellular calcium. cAMP can activate protein kinase A (PKA), whereas PLC or intracellular calcium can activate PKC.

(cAMP) and calcium. cAMP is synthesized by the enzyme adenylyl cyclase and can be rapidly degraded by cAMP phosphodiesterase.[16] Intracellular calcium is stored in the endoplasmic reticulum and released into the cytoplasm on proper signaling. Some trimeric G proteins can activate adenylyl cyclase, whereas others inhibit its activity. Trimeric G protein can also activate the enzyme phospholipase C, which produces the necessary signal molecules to activate release of calcium from the endoplasmic reticulum. Activation of phospholipase C can also lead to the activation of protein kinase C (PKC), which initiates a cascade of kinases. Changes in cAMP or calcium concentrations in the cell directly affect the activities of specific kinases that phosphorylate target proteins. The end result is altered biologic activity of these target proteins, which leads to a specific biologic response to the initial signal molecule. Despite the differences in signaling details, all G protein–coupled receptors use a complex cascade of intracellular mediators to amplify the biologic response to the initial extracellular signals greatly.

### Enzyme-Coupled Receptors

Enzyme-coupled receptors are a diverse family of transmembrane proteins with similar structures. Each receptor has an extracellular ligand-binding domain and a cytosolic domain that has intrinsic enzyme activity or is associated directly with an enzyme. Enzyme-coupled receptors are classified according to the type of enzymatic activity used for their intracellular signal transduction. Some receptors have guanylyl cyclase activity and generate cGMP as an intracellular mediator. Others have tyrosine kinase activity or are associated with tyrosine kinase proteins that phosphorylate specific tyrosine residues on intracellular proteins to propagate intracellular signals. Finally, some enzyme-coupled receptors have serine-threonine kinase activity and can phosphorylate specific serine or threonine residues to transduce intracellular signals.

The receptors for most known growth factors belong to the tyrosine kinase receptor family.[14] These include receptors for epidermal growth factor (EGF), platelet-derived growth factor (PDGF), fibroblast growth factor (FGF), hepatocyte growth factor (HGF), insulin, insulin-like growth factor I (IGF-I), vascular endothelial growth factor (VEGF), and macrophage colony-stimulating factor (M-CSF). These growth factor receptors play crucial roles during normal development and tissue homeostasis. Furthermore, many of the genes that encode proteins in the intracellular signaling cascades that are activated by receptor tyrosine kinases were first identified as oncogenes in cancer cells. Inappropriate activation of these proteins causes a cell to proliferative excessively.

Similar to G protein–coupled receptors, tyrosine kinase receptors use a complex cascade of intracellular mediators to propagate and amplify the initial signals (Fig. 3-9). On ligand binding, the tyrosine kinase receptor dimerizes, which activates the kinase. Activated receptor kinase initiates an intracellular relay system, first by cross-phosphorylation of tyrosine residues of the cytoplasmic domain of the receptor. Next, small intracellular signaling proteins bind to phosphotyrosine residues on the receptor and form a multiprotein signaling complex from which the signal propagates to the nucleus. The Ras proteins serve as crucial links in the signaling cascade.[17] On activation, Ras proteins initiate a cascade of serine-threonine phosphorylation that converges on mitogen-activated protein (MAP) kinases.

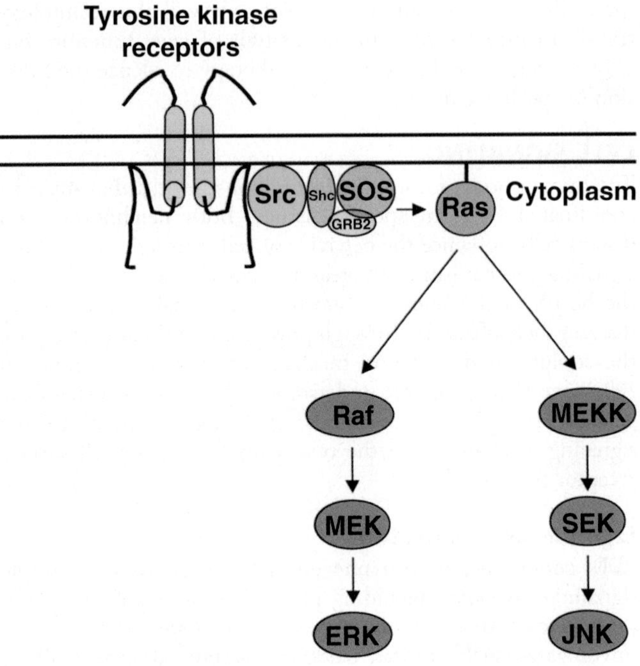


**FIGURE 3-9** Tyrosine kinase receptor signaling pathway. Tyrosine kinase receptors are single transmembrane proteins that form a dimer on ligand binding. The activated receptors bind to several proteins (Src, Shc, SOS, GRB2) to form a multiprotein signal complex. This protein complex can activate Ras, which can initiate several kinase cascades. One kinase cascade includes the Raf, MEK, and ERK members, whereas another includes the MEKK, SEK, and JNK proteins.

Activated MAP kinases relay signals downstream by phosphorylating transcription factors, thereby leading to the regulation of gene expression.

As noted, human cells integrate many different extracellular signals and respond with biologic behaviors such as proliferation, differentiation, and cell death. In the following sections, we review the mechanisms governing these important biologic processes.

## CELL DIVISION CYCLE

The cell division cycle is the fundamental means whereby organisms propagate and normal tissue homeostasis is maintained. The cell division cycle is an organized sequence of complex biologic processes that is traditionally divided into four distinct phases (Fig. 3-10). Replication of DNA occurs in the S phase (S = synthesis), whereas nuclear division and cell fission occur in the mitotic (M) phase. The intervals between these two phases are called the $G_1$ and $G_2$ phases (G = gap). After division, cells enter the $G_1$ phase, where they can receive extracellular signals and a determination is made whether to proceed with DNA replication or to exit the cell cycle. In this section, we review the proteins that regulate progression through each phase of the cell cycle and how they control key checkpoints of the cell cycle, followed by a discussion of how many cell cycle proteins are mutated or deleted in human cancers.

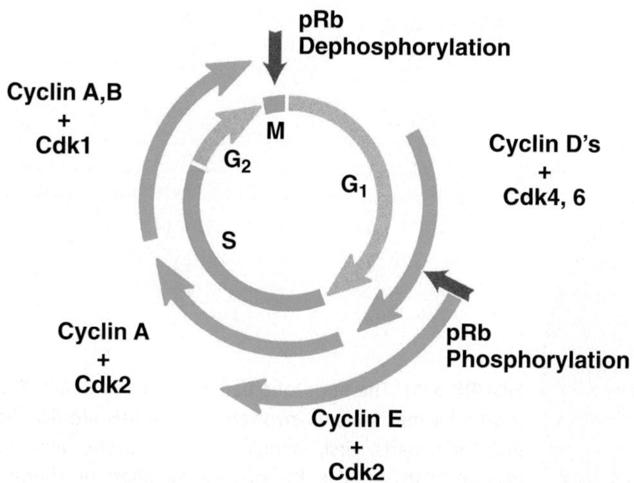


**FIGURE 3-10** Mechanisms regulating mammalian cell cycle progression. The cell cycle consists of four phases: Gl (first gap) phase, S (DNA synthetic) phase, G2 (second gap) phase, and M (mitotic) phase. Progression through the cell cycle is regulated by a highly conserved family of serine-threonine protein kinases composed of a regulatory subunit (the cyclins) and a catalytic subunit (the Cdks). Cell cycle progression can be inhibited by a class of regulators called the cyclin kinase inhibitors and by phosphorylation of the retinoblastoma (pRb) protein.

### Regulation of the Cell Division Cycle by Cyclin, Cyclin-Dependent Kinase, and Cdk Inhibitory Proteins

Progression of the mammalian cell cycle through these specific phases is governed by the sequential activation and inactivation of a highly conserved family of regulatory proteins, cyclin-dependent kinases (Cdks).[18] Cdk activation requires the binding of a regulatory protein (cyclin) and is controlled by positive and negative phosphorylation. Cdk activities are inhibited by Cdk inhibitory proteins (CKIs). The active cyclin-Cdk complex is involved in the phosphorylation of other cell cycle regulatory proteins. Cyclin proteins are classified according to their structural similarities. Each cyclin exhibits a cell cycle–phase-specific pattern of expression. In contrast, Cdk proteins are expressed throughout the cell cycle. The cyclins, Cdks, and CKIs form the fundamental regulatory units of the cell cycle machinery.

### Cell Cycle Checkpoints

In proliferating cells, cell cycle progression is regulated at two key checkpoints, the G1-S and the $G_2$-M transitions. Progression through early to mid-$G_1$ is dependent on Cdk4 and Cdk6, which are activated by association with one of the D-type cyclins, D1, D2, or D3.[18] Progression through the late $G_1$ phase and into the S phase requires the activation of Cdk2, which is sequentially regulated by cyclins E and A, respectively. The subsequent activation of Cdk1 (cdc2) by cyclin B is essential for the transition from the $G_2$ phase into the M phase. There are two families of CKIs, the CIP-KIP family and the INK family. The four known INK proteins (p15INK4B, p16INK4A, p18INK4C, and p19INK4D) selectively bind and inhibit Cdk4 and Cdk6 and are expressed in a tissue-specific pattern. The three members of the CIP-KIP family (p21CIP1, p27KIP1, and p57KIP2) share a conserved amino-terminal domain that is sufficient for binding to cyclin-Cdk complexes and inhibition of Cdk-associated kinase activity. Each CIP-KIP protein can inhibit all known Cdks. One of the key targets of the $G_1$ Cdks is the retinoblastoma tumor suppressor protein (pRb), which belongs to the Rb family of pocket proteins (pRb, p107, p130).[19] In their hypophosphorylated form, pocket proteins can sequester cell cycle regulatory transcription factors, including heterodimers of the E2F and DP families of proteins.[20] Phosphorylation of pRb, first by cyclin D–dependent kinases and then by cyclin E-Cdk2 during late $G_1$, leads to the release of E2F-DP and subsequent activation of genes that participate in the entry into the S phase.

### Oncogenes and Tumor Suppressor Genes

The genes encoding cell cycle regulatory proteins are often targets of mutation during neoplastic transformation. If the mutated gene is cancer-causing, it is referred to as an oncogene and its normal counterpart is called a proto-oncogene. Many proto-oncogenes have been identified and are typically involved in the relay of stimulatory signals from growth factor receptors to the nucleus. They include the intracellular signaling protein Ras and the cell cycle regulatory protein cyclin D1. Mutation of a single copy of a proto-oncogene is sufficient to bring about increased cellular proliferation, one of the hallmarks of cancer. Several antiproliferative gene–encoding proteins such as pRb, p15, and p16 also negatively control the cell division cycle. These genes are often referred to as tumor suppressor genes because they prevent excess and uncontrolled cellular proliferation. These genes are inactivated in some forms of cancer to bring about the loss of control of proliferation. However, unlike proto-oncogenes, both copies of a tumor suppressor gene must be deleted or inactivated during malignant transformation.

## CELL DEATH

Cell proliferation must be balanced by an appropriate process of cell death to maintain tissue homeostasis. There are three type of cell death based on the morphologic appearance of the dying cell.[21] Type 1 cell death, or apoptosis, has been best studied and is characterized by chromatin condensation, nuclear fragmentation, shrunken cytoplasm with intact cytoplasmic organelles, and eventual formation of plasma membrane–bound vesicles termed *apoptotic bodies,* which are then eliminated by neighboring phagocytic cells. Type 2 cell death, or autophagic cell death, is characterized by massive vacuolization of the cytoplasm without chromatin condensation. Type 3 cell death, or necrosis, is characterized by increased cell volume, swelling of cytoplasmic organelles, and rupture of plasma membrane.

Cell death has important physiologic functions, including the remodeling of tissues during development, removal of senescent cells and cells with genetic damage beyond repair, and maintenance of tissue homeostasis. In this section, we review the molecular machinery that controls apoptosis and autophagic cell death.

### Apoptosis

Two main pathways of apoptosis have been characterized, the extrinsic or death receptor pathway and intrinsic or stress pathway.[22] In the extrinsic pathway, cell surface death receptors bind to proapoptotic ligands, such as tumor necrosis factor (TNF), leading to the recruitment of a multiprotein complex called the death-inducing signaling complex (DISC) and an

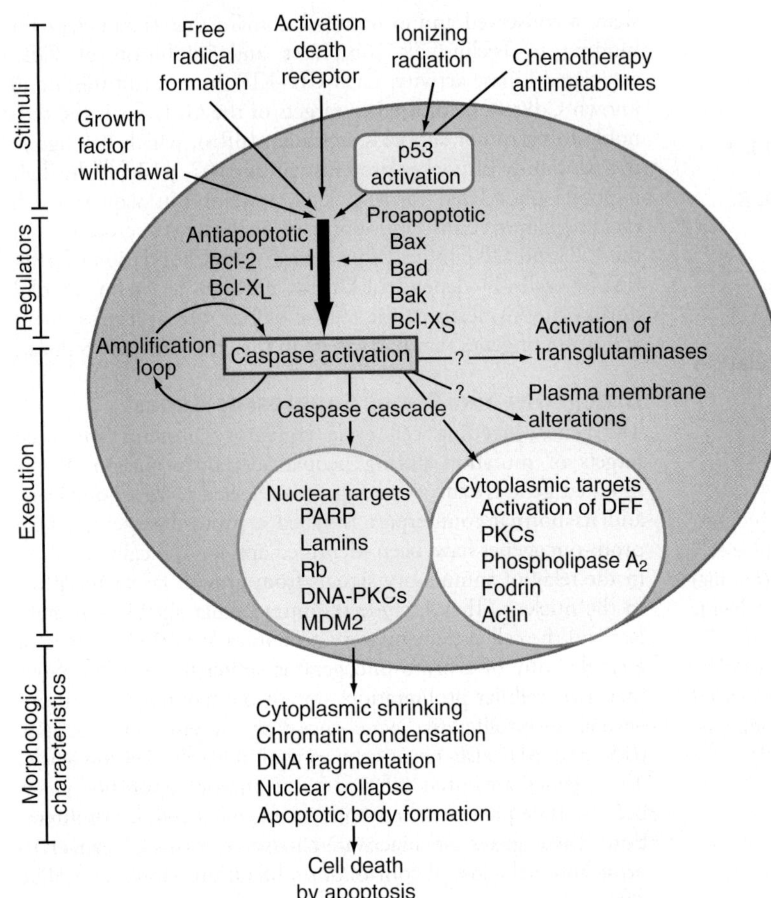


**FIGURE 3-11** The apoptotic pathways of cell death. The molecular mechanisms involved in apoptosis are divided into three parts. First, stimuli of the apoptotic pathway include DNA damage by ionizing radiation or chemotherapeutic agents (p53 activation), activation of death receptors, free radical formation, and loss of growth factor signaling. Second, progression of these stimuli to the central execution pathway is positively or negatively regulated by expression of the Bcl-2 family of proteins. Third, the execution phase of apoptosis involves the activation of a family of evolutionarily conserved proteases called caspases. Caspase activation targets various nuclear and cytoplasmic proteins for activation or destruction, thereby leading to the morphologic and biochemical characteristics of apoptosis. (From Papaconstantinou HT, Ko TC: Cell cycle and apoptosis regulation in GI cancers. In Evers BM [ed]: Molecular mechanisms in gastrointestinal cancer, Austin, Tex, 1999, RG Landes, p 59.)

adapter protein called Fas-associated death domain (FADD). By contrast, the intrinsic pathway is activated when intracellular sensors detect proapoptotic stimuli, such as genotoxic damage or growth factor and nutrient deprivation, leading to the activation of Bax and Bak, which are proapoptotic members of the Bcl-2 family of proteins (see Fig. 3-11).[23] Bax and Bak are inserted in and destabilize the mitochondrial membrane, resulting in cytochrome c leakage. Prosurvival members of the Bcl-2 family such as Bcl-2, Bcl-$x_L$ and Bcl-w associate with the mitochondrial membrane to maintain its integrity. An example of intracellular sensors is the p53 tumor suppressor gene, which recognizes DNA damage. Activation of p53 results in $G_1$ phase cell cycle arrest to allow DNA repair; however, irreparable damage commits the cell to death by apoptosis.[24] Regardless of the many different signals and signal sensors involved in the activation of apoptosis, both the extrinsic and intrinsic pathways activate downstream caspases, the executioner of apoptosis.

Caspases, or ***c**ysteine **asp**artate prote**ases***, are highly conserved proteins first recognized as the *ced-3* gene product from the nematode *Caenorhabditis elegans*[25] and are intimately involved in the conserved biochemical pathway that mediates apoptosis. These proteolytic enzymes are synthesized as inactive proenzymes that require cleavage for activation. The protein substrates cleaved by activated caspases play a functional role in the morphologic and biochemical features seen in apoptotic cells. As indicated in Figure 3-11, activated caspases result in the destruction of cytoskeletal and structural proteins (α-fodrin and actin), nuclear structural components (NuMA and lamins), and cell adhesion factors (FAK). They induce cell cycle arrest through Rb cleavage, cytoplasmic release of p53 by cleavage of the regulatory double minute 2 (MDM2) protein, and subsequent nuclear translocation and activation of PKC-δ. DNA repair enzymes, such as poly(adenosine diphosphate [ADP]-ribose) polymerase and the 140-kDa component of DNA replication complex C, are inactivated by caspase proteolysis. Finally, DNA fragmentation is induced by the activation and nuclear translocation of a 45-kDa cytoplasmic protein called DNA fragmentation factor (DFF). Overall, the net effect of caspase activation is to halt cell cycle progression, disable homeostatic and repair mechanisms, initiate detachment of the cell from its surrounding tissue structures, disassemble structural components, and mark the dying cell for engulfment by surrounding phagocytic cells.

The complex molecular machinery of apoptosis, involving signaling, regulation of activation, promotion (or inhibition), and then execution, is a carefully choreographed process. Perturbations in this process at any of these three phases can result in loss of the apoptotic cell elimination pathway. Because apoptosis is a key regulator of cell number and therefore tissue homeostasis, it is easy to see how dysregulation of apoptosis can result in diseases such as cancer or autoimmunity.

## Autophagy

Although apoptosis is a well-characterized process, less is known about the autophagic cell death process. Autophagic cell death is a degradative process characterized by the sequestering of

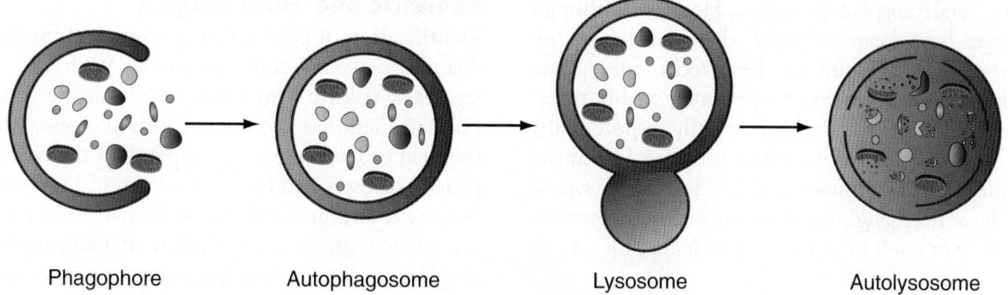


**FIGURE 3-12** The autophagy pathway. Autophagy proceeds through a series of regulated steps, including the formation of phagophores, leading to autophagosome. Autophagosomes fuse with lysosomes to form autolysosomes, in which cellular materials and organelles are degraded and building blocks are recycled.

organelles and portions of the cytoplasm in double-membrane vesicles known as autophagosomes.[22] Autophagosomes fuse with cytoplasmic lysosomes to form autolysosomes, enabling the lysosomal hydrolases to degrade engulfed cytoplasmic material and organelles (Fig. 3-12). This degradative process is genetically regulated and evolutionarily conserved, and is called autophagy. Autophagy plays an important role in protecting against infection, neurodegeneration, and tumor development. Autophagy is associated with cell death, but it is also associated with cell survival by sequestering and recycling damaged proteins and organelle during stress, or by regenerating building blocks for macromolecular synthesis during starvation. Autophagy is controlled by a group of genes (*ATG* genes) with at least 11 mammalian members. *ATG* genes control each step of autophagy, including the induction and formation of autophagic vesicles, fusion with lysosomes, and degradation of engulfed material. It is increasingly clear that dysregulation of autophagy contributes to the development of cancer, liver disease, aging, and inflammation.[26]

## HUMAN GENOME PROJECT

One of the most significant scientific undertakings of all times involved the identification and sequencing of the entire human genome, which was completed in the spring of 2003. The Human Genome Project has had a significant impact on the field of medicine by providing clinicians with an unprecedented arsenal of genetic information that will, it is hoped, lead to a better understanding and treatment of a variety of genetic diseases. For example, the Human Genome Project has been providing new information on the genetic variations in the human population by identifying DNA variants such as single nucleotide polymorphisms (SNPs), which occur approximately once every 300 to 500 bases along the 3 billion–base human genome.[27] SNPs are thought to serve as genetic markers for identifying disease genes by linkage studies in families or by the discovery of genes involved in human diseases. These findings may lead to better screening and help implement preventive medical therapy in the hope of reducing the development of certain diseases in patients found to have predisposing conditions. It is anticipated that knowing the sequence of human DNA will allow scientists to understand a host of diseases better. With new information and techniques to unravel the mysteries of human biology, this information will dramatically accelerate the development of new strategies for the diagnosis, prevention, and treatment of disease, not just for single-gene disorders, but for more common complex diseases, such as diabetes, heart disease, and cancer, for which genetic differences may contribute to the risk of contracting the disease and response to particular therapies.

The transition from genetics to genomics marks the evolution from an understanding of single genes and their individual functions to a more global understanding of the actions of multiple genes and their control of biologic systems. Technology emanating from the Human Genome Project is available to assess an array of genes that may change (increase or decrease) over time or with treatment. Such technology, using so-called DNA chips, provides one of the most promising approaches to large-scale studies of genetic variations, detection of heterogeneous gene mutations, and gene expression. DNA chips, which are also called microarrays, generally consist of a thin slice of glass or silicone approximately the size of a postage stamp on which threads of synthetic nucleic acids are arrayed.[28] Literally thousands of genes can be assessed on a single DNA chip. A clinical example of the use of microarrays includes the detection of human immunodeficiency virus (HIV) sequence variations, p53 gene mutations in breast tissue, and expression of cytochrome P-450 genes. In addition, microarray technology has been applied to genomic comparisons across species, genetic recombination, and large-scale analyses of gene copy number and expression, as well as protein expression in cancers.

As genome technology moves from the laboratory to the clinical setting, new methods will make it possible to read the instructions contained in an individual person's DNA. Such knowledge may predict future disease and alert patients and their health care providers to initiate preventive strategies. Individual DNA profiles, as well as the DNA profiles of tumors, may provide better stratification of patients for cancer therapies. The Human Genome Project is certain to have an important impact on all areas of clinical medicine. All surgical disciplines will be directly affected by this information. We focus on some specific examples here for which we foresee major developments that will greatly influence our clinical management.

### Transplantation

Despite the remarkable advances made in transplantation, organ procurement, and immunosuppression, a significant impediment remains the availability of suitable organs. The level of organ and tissue demand cannot be met by organ donation alone. Xenotransplantation has been proposed as a possible solution to the problem of organ availability and suitability for transplantation. A number of investigators have examined the possibility of using xenotransplanted organs. However, although short-term successes have been reported, there have been no long-term survivors with the use of these techniques. Data obtained from the Human Genome Project may enable transplant investigators to engineer animals genetically to potentially have more specific combinations of human antigens. It is anticipated that in the future, animals can be developed whose immune systems have been engineered to more closely resemble those of humans, thus eliminating dependence on organ donors.

Another possibility to address the organ donation problem is the potential for organ cloning. With the cloning of sheep and cattle, this topic has received a considerable amount of attention. Although the issue of whole-animal cloning is fascinating, the area that offers the greatest hope for transplant patients is the growing field of stem cell biology. By identifying stem cells of interest, the information gathered from the Human Genome Project could enable scientists to develop organ-cloning techniques that will revolutionize the field of transplantation. These pluripotent stem cells have the ability to divide without limit and give rise to many types of differentiated and specialized tissues with a specific purpose. It is anticipated that the identification of stem cells and the potential modification of these cells by gene therapy may allow investigators to engineer tissues of interest genetically.

### Oncology

The results of the Human Genome Project will have far-reaching effects on diagnostic studies, treatment, and counseling of cancer patients and family members.[28] Genetic testing is currently available for many disorders, including Tay-Sachs disease and cystic fibrosis. New tests have been developed to detect predispositions to Alzheimer's disease, colon cancer, breast cancer, and other conditions. Identification of the entire human genome will provide an unprecedented and powerful modality to increase our ability to screen high-risk groups and the general population.

With the identification of certain high-risk groups for the development of cancer, surgeons are playing an ever-increasing role in genetic assessment and ultimate therapy. Prophylactic surgery may soon become more prevalent as a first-line treatment in the fight against cancer. For example, discovery of the association between mutations of the *ret* proto-oncogene and hereditary medullary thyroid carcinoma has allowed surgeons to identify patients in whom medullary thyroid cancer will eventually develop. Genetic screening for mutations of the *ret* proto-oncogene in patients with multiple endocrine neoplasia type II allows prophylactic thyroidectomy to be performed at an earlier stage of the disease process than traditional biochemical screening. Other areas of active interest include testing of patients with familial adenomatous polyposis, in which the timing and extent of therapy may be based on the exact location of adenomatous polyposis coli (APC) mutations. Furthermore, additional testing will allow investigators to determine other genes that may contribute to this syndrome. Another area of controversy concerns the treatment of patients with mutations of the breast cancer susceptibility genes *BRCA1* and *BRCA2*. As more information becomes known regarding mutations of these genes and the clinical implications of these mutations, cancer treatment protocols will be altered accordingly.

### Pediatric and Fetal Surgery

Identification of the human genome will further aid in prenatal diagnostic testing and screening. With the identification of fetuses at risk for a number of identifiable genetic diseases, the Human Genome Project will increase research and activity in the field of fetal surgery by expanding the current knowledge of genetic diseases and rate of fetal surgical interventions involving current techniques and the combination or use of somatic gene therapy. In utero manipulation of identifiable genetic defects may, in the future, become a common intervention.

### Proteomics

An important offshoot of the Human Genome Project has been the realization for the need to examine the expression and function of the end product of the gene (i.e., the protein). This has led to the development of the field of proteomics, which is the study of the proteome. The term *proteome* was first coined by Marc Wilkins in 1995 to describe the entire collection of proteins of an organism.[29] The importance of proteomics is underscored by the fact that almost all cellular phenotypes and activities are directed by proteins.

Protein expression and modifications are regulated under normal physiologic conditions (e.g., differentiation, apoptosis, aging and are altered during pathophysiologic stresses, leading to the development and progression of disease). However, the human proteome is complex and dynamic, and its examination requires the development of new tools and technologies. The basic steps in proteomic studies consist of sample preparation, protein separation, protein imaging, and protein identification. Protein separation usually involves two-dimensional gel electrophoresis and protein identification by mass spectrometry (Fig. 3-13).[30] With the use of proteomic technologies, investigators have begun to elucidate patterns of protein changes between health and disease states by profiling complex biologic samples such as serum, urine, and tissues.[31,32] The field of proteomics has been advancing rapidly with the development of new and more powerful technologies to examine complex protein interactions and protein modifications. These advancements will lead to better detection and risk assessment, therapeutic targeting, and patient-tailored therapy for human diseases.

## NOVEL TREATMENT STRATEGIES

### Gene Therapy

The ability to alter specific genes of interest represents an exciting and powerful tool in the potential treatment of a wide array of diseases.[33-35] Instead of giving a patient a drug to treat or control the symptoms of a genetic disorder, physicians may be capable of treating the basic problem by altering the genetic makeup of the patient's cells. Several methods are available to introduce new genetic material into mammalian cells. Typically, two strategies have been considered, germline and somatic cell gene therapy. In the germline strategy, foreign DNA is introduced into the zygote or early embryo with the expectation that the newly introduced material will contribute to the germline of the recipient and therefore be passed to the next generation. In contrast, somatic cell gene therapy models represent the introduction of genetic material into somatic cells, which is then not transmitted to the germ cells.

A wide array of somatic cell gene therapy protocols designed to treat single-gene diseases, a variety of cancers, or HIV are

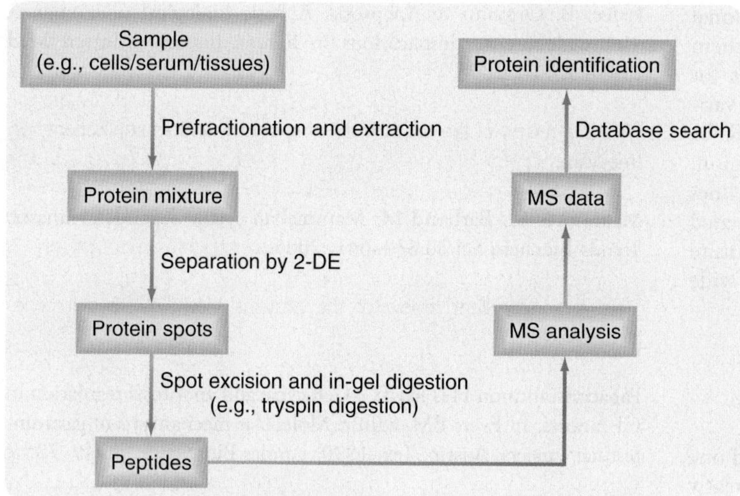


**FIGURE 3-13** Basic approach of proteomics-based research. *2-DE,* Two-dimensional gel electrophoresis; *MS,* mass spectrometry. (From Lam L, Lind J, Semsarian C: Application of proteomics in cardiovascular medicine. Int J Cardiol 108:12–19, 2006.)

under development, with some gene therapy protocols in clinical trials. The goals of human somatic gene therapy are generally one of the following: repair or compensate for a defective gene, enhance the immune response directed at a tumor or pathogen, protect vulnerable cell populations against treatments such as chemotherapy, or kill tumor cells directly.[36,37]

Several single-gene disorders are candidates for gene therapy and a number of protocols have been developed. In addition, current thinking has expanded from the treatment of single-gene disorders to include the treatment of acquired immunodeficiency syndrome (AIDS) and atherosclerosis with gene therapy techniques. Moreover, many protocols for the treatment of cancer are under evaluation, particularly for otherwise untreatable conditions. Strategies include the alteration of cancer cells or other host cells to produce cytokines or other molecules to alter the host response to the malignancy, expression of antigens on cancer cells to induce a host immune response, insertion of tumor suppressor genes or their sequences to slow cell growth, and introduction of drug-resistant genes into normal cells to facilitate more aggressive chemotherapy.

Although a number of in vitro experiments have shown great promise, in vivo trials have failed to match the in vitro results, partly as a result of the vehicles used for transfecting the DNA into cells. A repertoire of viral-based vectors have been analyzed, with each generation showing more promise than the previous modification.[38] Initially, retroviruses were used as vectors and are still used in certain cases. However, other potential vectors include adenovirus, herpesvirus, vaccinia, and other viruses. Nonviral systems, such as liposomes, DNA-protein conjugates, and DNA–protein-defective virus conjugates, also appear promising.[39] Safety issues, improvement of in vivo gene delivery, efficiency, and gene regulation after cellular transduction are the difficult issues that must be resolved in vector design. However, exciting and appealing the prospects of gene therapy may appear, this technique is still in the experimental stages.

## Short Interfering RNA

The discovery of siRNA as a method of gene silencing has provided another novel treatment strategy by targeting disease-causing genes. This powerful tool has already been tested in experimental conditions of viral infectious diseases and cancers. In infectious diseases, siRNAs against hepatitis B virus, HIV-1, and respiratory syncytial virus have been shown to inhibit viral replication.[40] Silencing of oncogenes such as K-*ras* and HER-2/*neu* has been shown to inhibit cancer cell growth. Although siRNA-based therapy holds great promise because of its potential for high selectivity and less toxicity, its clinical applications require overcoming the problem of the short half-life of siRNA and effective delivery to target tissues. Scientists are developing modifications of siRNA that will extend its half-life and improve cellular uptake.

## Drug Design

Based on information from the fields of genomics and structural biology, rational drug design can be devised to treat a host of diseases.[41] This technique has been used to generate potent drugs, many of which are currently in use or under study. For example, a rational design based on crystallographic data has led to the development of new classes of anti-HIV agents targeted against HIV protease. Once the critical proteins accounting for a disease are identified and their abnormal function understood, drugs can be designed to stimulate, inhibit, or substitute function.

Identification of human genetic variations will eventually allow clinicians to subclassify diseases and adapt therapies that are appropriate to the individual patient.[42] There may be differences in the effectiveness of medicines from one patient to the next. Furthermore, toxic reactions can occur that may be a consequence of genetically encoded host factors. These observations have spawned the field of pharmacogenomics, which attempts to use information on genetic variations in patients to predict responses to drug therapies. In addition to genetic tests that will predict responsiveness to therapies currently available, these genetic approaches to disease prevention and treatment should provide an expanding array of gene products that will be used in developing future drug therapies.

## Genetic Engineering of Antibodies

Monoclonal antibodies directed against specific antigens have been generated by using hybridoma techniques and are widely used in a number of fields of medicine, including oncology and transplantation. However, a major drawback is the fact that repeated treatment with murine antibodies results in an immune response directed against the antibody. Genetic engineering techniques have allowed the modification of mouse monoclonal antibodies to reduce the immune response directed against them by human recipients and to provide nonhuman resources for human antibodies.[43] This modification involves cloning the variable or hypervariable regions of the antibody from the mRNA of a hybridoma and fusing them with a human constant region, thus resulting in clones that can be expressed in human cell lines to produce large amounts of modified antibody. It is anticipated that such techniques will become more common in the future and provide a ready source of antibodies directed against a wide array of antigens.

## ETHICAL, PSYCHOLOGICAL, AND LEGAL IMPLICATIONS

The possibilities of genetic-based medicine are endless, and one can predict that in the next decade our lives will be greatly altered because of these rapid advances.[44] A number of ethical, psychological, and legal implications can be envisioned and will need to be addressed.[45,46] Such issues include ownership of the genetic information and who should have access to this information.[47] Another issue is how to counsel the patient and other family members correctly based on information obtained from genetic testing.

The surgeon of the future will need to participate actively and be knowledgeable in these emerging technologies because our management of specific problems will be greatly altered by the new knowledge gained from analysis of the human genome.[44,48,49] Most assuredly, these rapid advances will continue to alter current treatment strategies and challenge existing dogmas. Surgeons have the opportunity to be active participants and leaders in the research and complex decision making process that will affect the treatment of patients who require surgery. Surgeons, and all physicians, must rise to the occasion or otherwise be relegated to bystander status, with the possibility of these complex clinical and ethical decisions being made by nonclinicians.

## SELECTED REFERENCES

Alberts B, Johnson A, Lewis J, et al, editors: Molecular biology of the cell, ed 5, New York, 2008, Garland.

This textbook provides an excellent primer for the reader to understand the fundamental concepts of molecular biology.

Calvo KR, Liotta LA, Petricoin EF: Clinical proteomics: From biomarker discovery and cell signaling profiles to individualized personal therapy. Biosci Rep 25:107–125, 2005.

This is an extensive review of proteomics and its potential applications in clinical practice.

Collins FS: Shattuck Lecture—medical and societal consequences of the Human Genome Project. N Engl J Med 341:28–37, 1999.

This paper by the leader of the Human Genome Project provides an assessment of the progress toward completing this project, as well as future implications regarding human disease prevention and treatment.

Fadeel B, Orrenius S: Apoptosis: A basic biological phenomenon with wide-ranging implications in human disease. J Intern Med 258:479–517, 2005.

This is a review of the mechanism of apoptosis and its implications for medicine.

Malumbres M, Barbacid M: Mammalian cyclin-dependent kinases. Trends Biochem Sci 30:630–641, 2005.

This is an excellent review of the proteins that regulate cell cycle progression.

Papaconstantinou HT, Ko TC: Cell cycle and apoptosis regulation in GI cancers. In Evers BM, editor: Molecular mechanisms of gastrointestinal cancers, Austin, Tex, 1999, Landes Bioscience, pp 49–78.

This chapter provides an excellent review for the reader to understand regulation of the cell cycle and apoptosis.

Rychahou PG, Jackson LN, Farrow BJ, et al: RNA interference: Mechanisms of action and therapeutic consideration. Surgery 140: 719–725, 2006.

This is a review of progress in RNA interference technology and its potential clinical applications.

Sambrook J, Russell D, editors: Molecular cloning: A laboratory manual, ed 3, Plainview, NY, 2001, Cold Spring Harbor Laboratory Press.

This manual is a collection of laboratory protocols, including detailed discussion of DNA recombinant technology.

The Chipping Forecast. Nat Genet 21(Suppl):1–60, 1999.

This entire supplement provides an excellent primer for the reader to understand and appreciate the vast scientific potential and usefulness of microarray (i.e., gene chip) technology. A basic description of these techniques and possible limitations is presented.

## REFERENCES

1. Alberts B, Johnson A, Lewis J, et al: Molecular biology of the cell, ed 5, New York, 2008, Garland.
2. Lodish H, Berk A, Kaiser CA, et al: Molecular cell biology, ed 6, New York, 2008, WH Freeman.
3. Rosenthal N: DNA and the genetic code. N Engl J Med 331:39–41, 1994.
4. Mata J, Marguerat S, Bahler J: Post-transcriptional control of gene expression: A genome-wide perspective. Trends Biochem Sci 30: 506–514, 2005.
5. Yang XJ: Multisite protein modification and intramolecular signaling. Oncogene 24:1653–1662, 2005.
6. Rosenthal N: Tools of the trade—recombinant DNA. N Engl J Med 331:315–317, 1994.
7. Templeton NS: The polymerase chain reaction. History, methods, and applications. Diagn Mol Pathol 1:58–72, 1992.
8. Hofker MH, Breuer M: Generation of transgenic mice. Methods Mol Biol 110:63–78, 1998.

9. Majzoub JA, Muglia LJ: Knockout mice. N Engl J Med 334: 904–907, 1996.
10. Fire A, Xu S, Montgomery MK, et al: Potent and specific genetic interference by double-stranded RNA in Caenorhabditis elegans. Nature 391:806–811, 1998.
11. McManus MT, Sharp PA: Gene silencing in mammals by small interfering RNAs. Nat Rev Genet 3:737–747, 2002.
12. Signal transduction: Crosstalk. Trends Biochem Sci 17:367–443, 1992.
13. Wettschureck N, Offermanns S: Mammalian G proteins and their cell type specific functions. Physiol Rev 85:1159–1204, 2005.
14. Perona R: Cell signalling: Growth factors and tyrosine kinase receptors. Clin Transl Oncol 8:77–82, 2006.
15. Marinissen MJ, Gutkind JS: G-protein–coupled receptors and signaling networks: Emerging paradigms. Trends Pharmacol Sci 22:368–376, 2001.
16. Hurley JH: Structure, mechanism, and regulation of mammalian adenylyl cyclase. J Biol Chem 274:7599–7602, 1999.
17. Campbell SL, Khosravi-Far R, Rossman KL, et al: Increasing complexity of Ras signaling. Oncogene 17:1395–1413, 1998.
18. Malumbres M, Barbacid M: Mammalian cyclin-dependent kinases. Trends Biochem Sci 30:630–641, 2005.
19. Tonini T, Hillson C, Claudio PP: Interview with the retinoblastoma family members: Do they help each other? J Cell Physiol 192:138–150, 2002.
20. DeGregori J: The genetics of the E2F family of transcription factors: Shared functions and unique roles. Biochim Biophys Acta 1602:131–150, 2002.
21. Galluzzi L, Maiuri MC, Vitale I, et al: Cell death modalities: Classification and pathophysiological implications. Cell Death Differ 14:1237–1243, 2007.
22. Thorburn A: Apoptosis and autophagy: regulatory connections between two supposedly different processes. Apoptosis 13:1–9, 2008.
23. Cory S, Adams JM: The Bcl2 family: Regulators of the cellular life-or-death switch. Nat Rev Cancer 2:647–656, 2002.
24. Vousden KH, Lu X: Live or let die: The cell's response to p53. Nat Rev Cancer 2:594–604, 2002.
25. Lavrik IN, Golks A, Krammer PH: Caspases: Pharmacological manipulation of cell death. J Clin Invest 115:2665–2672, 2005.
26. Kroemer G, White E: Autophagy for the avoidance of degenerative, inflammatory, infectious, and neoplastic disease. Curr Opin Cell Biol 22:121–123, 2010.
27. Wang DG, Fan JB, Siao CJ, et al: Large-scale identification, mapping, and genotyping of single-nucleotide polymorphisms in the human genome. Science 280:1077–1082, 1998.
28. Khan J, Bittner ML, Chen Y, et al: DNA microarray technology: The anticipated impact on the study of human disease. Biochim Biophys Acta 1423:M17–M28, 1999.
29. Wilkins MR, Sanchez JC, Gooley AA, et al: Progress with proteome projects: Why all proteins expressed by a genome should be identified and how to do it. Biotechnol Genet Eng Rev 13: 19–50, 1996.
30. Lam L, Lind J, Semsarian C: Application of proteomics in cardiovascular medicine. Int J Cardiol 108:12–19, 2006.
31. Colantonio DA, Chan DW: The clinical application of proteomics. Clin Chim Acta 357:151–158, 2005.
32. Plebani M: Proteomics: The next revolution in laboratory medicine? Clin Chim Acta 357:113–122, 2005.
33. Prieto J, Herraiz M, Sangro B, et al: The promise of gene therapy in gastrointestinal and liver diseases. Gut 52(Suppl 2):49–54, 2003.
34. Meyerson SL, Schwartz LB: Gene therapy as a therapeutic intervention for vascular disease. J Cardiovasc Nurs 13:91–109, 1999.
35. Petrie NC, Yao F, Eriksson E: Gene therapy in wound healing. Surg Clin North Am 83:597–616, vii, 2003.
36. Lee JH, Klein HG: Cellular gene therapy. Hematol Oncol Clin North Am 9:91–113, 1995.
37. Crystal RG: In vivo and ex vivo gene therapy strategies to treat tumors using adenovirus gene transfer vectors. Cancer Chemother Pharmacol 43(Suppl):S90–S99, 1999.
38. Mah C, Byrne BJ, Flotte TR: Virus-based gene delivery systems. Clin Pharmacokinet 41:901–911, 2002.
39. Niidome T, Huang L: Gene therapy progress and prospects: Nonviral vectors. Gene Ther 9:1647–1652, 2002.
40. Rychahou PG, Jackson LN, Farrow BJ, et al: RNA interference: mechanisms of action and therapeutic consideration. Surgery 140:719–725, 2006.
41. Bailey DS, Bondar A, Furness LM: Pharmacogenomics—it's not just pharmacogenetics. Curr Opin Biotechnol 9:595–601, 1998.
42. Evans WE, McLeod HL: Pharmacogenomics—drug disposition, drug targets, and side effects. N Engl J Med 348:538–549, 2003.
43. Brekke OH, Sandlie I: Therapeutic antibodies for human diseases at the dawn of the twenty-first century. Nat Rev Drug Discov 2:52–62, 2003.
44. Hernandez A, Evers BM: Functional genomics: clinical effect and the evolving role of the surgeon. Arch Surg 134:1209–1215, 1999.
45. Vineis P: Ethical issues in genetic screening for cancer. Ann Oncol 8:945–949, 1997.
46. Grady C: Ethics and genetic testing. Adv Intern Med 44:389–411, 1999.
47. Nowlan W: Human genetics. A rational view of insurance and genetic discrimination. Science 297:195–196, 2002.
48. Vogelstein B: Genetic testings for cancer: The surgeon's critical role. Familial colon cancer. J Am Coll Surg 188:74–79, 1999.
49. Moulton G: Surgeons have critical role in genetic testing decisions, medical, legal experts say. J Natl Cancer Inst 90:804–805, 1998.

# CHAPTER 4

# THE INFLAMMATORY RESPONSE

Mitchell P. Fink

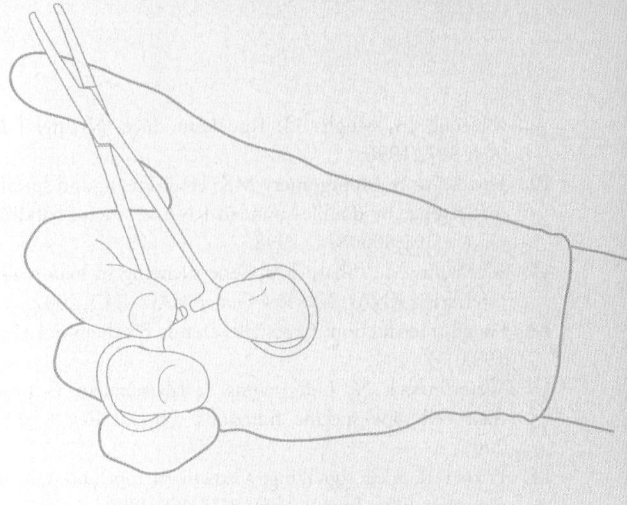



Celsus is credited with describing the cardinal clinical signs of inflammation—calor (warmth), dolor (pain), tumor (swelling), and rubor (redness). Classically, the term *inflammation* was used to denote the pathologic reaction whereby fluid and circulating leukocytes accumulate in extravascular tissue in response to injury or infection. Today, inflammation connotes not only localized effects, such as edema, hyperemia, and leukocytic infiltration, but also systemic phenomena—for example, fever and increased synthesis of certain acute-phase proteins and mediators of inflammation. The inflammatory response is closely interrelated with the processes of healing and repair. In fact, wound healing is impossible in the absence of inflammation. Accordingly, inflammation is involved in almost every aspect of surgery because proper healing of traumatic wounds, surgical incisions, and various types of anastomoses is entirely dependent on the expression of a tightly orchestrated and well-controlled inflammatory process.

Inflammation is fundamentally a protective response that has evolved to permit higher forms of life to rid themselves of injurious agents, remove necrotic cells and cellular debris, and repair damage to tissues and organs. However, the mechanisms used to kill invading microorganisms or to ingest and destroy devitalized cells as part of the inflammatory response can also be injurious to normal tissue. Thus, inflammation is a major pathogenic mechanism underlying numerous diseases and syndromes. Many of these pathologic conditions, such as inflammatory bowel disease (IBD), sepsis, and adult respiratory distress syndrome (ARDS), are of importance in the practice of surgery.

Initiation, maintenance, and termination of the inflammatory response are extremely complex processes involving numerous different cell types, as well as hundreds of different humoral mediators. A truly comprehensive account of the inflammatory response is beyond the scope of a single chapter in a text covering many other topics. Necessarily, therefore, this chapter will focus on the main initiators of inflammation and the most important cellular and humoral mediators of the inflammatory response.

For the purpose of describing the inflammatory process, this overview will make frequent mention of a common, but complicated, clinical entity—severe sepsis—as a paradigm of the inflammatory response. Severe sepsis is a syndrome caused by a systemic inflammatory response run amok. Sepsis is the most common cause of mortality in patients requiring care in an intensive care unit. Severe sepsis, which occurs in approximately 750,000 people in the United States every year, carries a mortality rate close to 30%. It is generally believed that the incidence of sepsis and septic shock is increasing, probably as a result of advances in many fields of medicine that have extended the use of complex invasive procedures and potent immunosuppressive agents. Given the importance of sepsis as a public health problem, efforts have been made to translate improvements in our understanding of inflammation and inflammatory mediators into the development of useful therapeutic agents. Some of these therapeutic agents are noted in the context of the overall discussion of inflammation.

## THE DANGER HYPOTHESIS: DANGER-ASSOCIATED MOLECULAR PATTERNS, PATHOGEN-ASSOCIATED MOLECULAR PATTERNS, AND ALARMINS

The immune system protects the host against disease caused by a wide range of exogenous pathogenic agents, such as viruses, bacteria, fungi, protozoa, and parasitic worms. The immune system, however, also plays a role in detecting and dealing with other threats to health, such as trauma, tissue necrosis, and malignant transformation, which typically are not caused by exogenous pathogens. To accomplish these goals, the immune system uses a layered strategy. The first layer consists of the innate responses, which occur early and are not antigen-specific. The innate responses depend largely on the proper functioning of natural killer (NK) cells and phagocytic cells, such as monocytes, macrophages, and neutrophils. The second layer is composed of adaptive responses, which develop later after the processing of antigen(s) by dendritic cells and the clonal expansion of T and B cell subsets. Adaptive responses are antigen-specific.

From an evolutionary standpoint, the innate immune system is truly ancient, whereas the adaptive immune system is a more recent biologic innovation. Aspects of the innate immune system can be found in primitive multicellular organisms, plants, insects, and other invertebrates. In contrast, an adaptive immune system is present only in vertebrate species. Key components of the innate immune system include the following: cells, such as macrophages, neutrophils, mast cells, and dendritic cells; the complement system; various secreted proteins, called cytokines and chemokines; and myriad small molecule mediators, such as prostaglandins, bradykinin, reactive oxygen species (ROS), and nitric oxide (NO·). The adaptive immune response is characterized by antigen specificity and memory (i.e., the ability to mount a more vigorous response to an antigen that has been encountered previously). T and B lymphocytes are the main cellular mediators of adaptive immune responses. B cells and their progeny, plasma cells, are responsible for the production of antibodies, which are the humoral mediators of the adaptive immune system.

T cells, which can be classified into various subtypes, play important roles in innate and adaptive immune responses. For example, natural killer T cells bridge the gap between the innate and adaptive immune systems because they are activated by glycolipid antigens presented by the glycoprotein, CD1d, on antigen-presenting cells.

T helper cells (Th), which express the surface protein, CD4, also play key roles in the orchestration of innate and adaptive immune responses. Naïve $CD4^+$ T cells (Th0 cells) can differentiate into at least four different Th subsets, called Th1, Th2, Th17, and T regulatory cells (Treg cells; Fig. 4-1). Th1 cells are responsible for directing the cell-mediated immune responses necessary for the eradication of intracellular pathogens, and favor macrophage activation. Th2 cells have been implicated in the pathogenesis of atopy and allergic inflammation and favor B cell growth and differentiation. Th1 cells produce the potent proinflammatory cytokines, interferon-γ (IFN-γ) and tumor necrosis factor-β (TNF-β; also called lymphotoxin). Th2 cells produce the cytokines interleukin-4 (IL-4), IL-5, IL-6, IL-10, and IL-13. The actions of IL-4, IL-10, and IL-13 are largely anti-inflammatory in nature. The actions of IL-6 can be both pro- and anti-inflammatory. Th17 cells produce several cytokines, notably IL-17A and IL-17F. Both IL-17A and IL-17F tend to be proinflammatory. The signature cytokines produced by Treg cells—namely transforming growth factor-β (TGF-β) and IL-10—are both anti-inflammatory. Thus, Th1 and Th17 lymphocytes are often viewed as being proinflammatory, whereas Th2 lymphocytes and Tregs are thought of as being anti-inflammatory. The cytokine, IL-12, drives Th1 differentiation, IL-4 induces Th2 differentiation, and TGF-β in combination with IL-6 promotes Th17 differentiation, but TGF-β in the absence of IL-6 promotes precursor cells to differentiate into Treg cells.[1]

Historically, activation of the immune system was thought to be triggered by the presence of antigens, which were recognized as being non-self in nature. However, the self-nonself model of immune surveillance and discrimination was burdened by the inability to account for numerous observations satisfactorily, such as the necessity for the presence of a tissue-damaging adjuvant to obtain a vigorous immune response to the nonself proteins present in vaccines. To address these concerns, the innovative immunologist, Polly Matzinger, formulated the danger model to explain immune system activation and discrimination.[2] According to this hypothesis, which is now widely accepted, activation of the innate immune system is triggered by a diverse set of molecules that indicate the presence of danger to the host (i.e., something that could threaten health and well-being). Danger might come in the form of an invasion of host tissues by a pathogenic microorganism, but danger also might

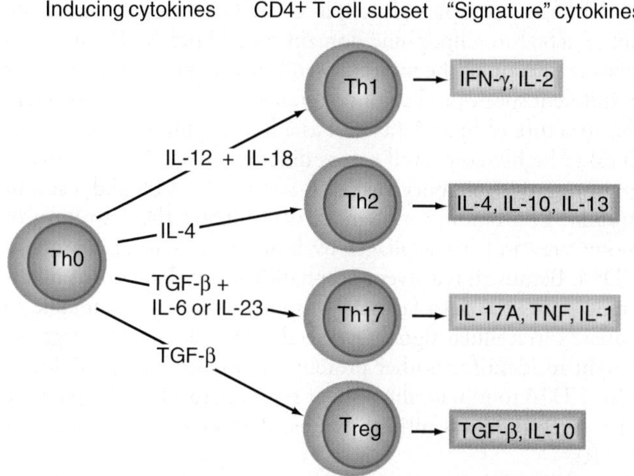


**FIGURE 4-1** Simplified representation of the differentiation of naïve helper T cells (Th0) into the four known $CD4^+$ helper T cell subtypes, which are called Th1, Th2, Th17, and Treg. A specific cytokine, secreted by the various helper T cell subtypes, constitutes a signature for that particular class of cells. Differentiation of Th0 cells into the various subtypes is driven by specific cytokines or, in some cases, a specific combination of two cytokines. For example, differentiation of Th0 cells along the Th1 pathway is driven by IL-12 in combination with IL-18, whereas differentiation of Th0 cells along the Th2 pathway is driven by IL-4.

come in the form of trauma or malignant transformation. The molecules that signal the presence of something dangerous share a number of recognizable biochemical features, and collectively are referred to as danger (or damage)-associated molecular patterns (DAMPs). Some DAMPs are host-derived; compounds in this class are called alarmins.[3] Other DAMPs are derived from pathogenic microorganisms and are called pathogen-associated molecular patterns (PAMPs).

Cells of the innate immune system recognize PAMPs and alarmins via a limited number of germline-encoded pattern recognition receptors (PRRs). The interaction between a DAMP and a PRR initiates intracellular signaling cascades that ultimately culminate in the expression of a broad range of molecules, including cytokines and chemokines, cell surface adhesion molecules, and enzymes, such as inducible nitric oxide synthase (iNOS) and cyclooxygenase-2 (COX-2), which underlie the development of the inflammatory response.

## Lipopolysaccharide

Much of our understanding of the innate immune system and the pathophysiology of inflammation has come from experimental studies with a compound called lipopolysaccharide (LPS) or endotoxin, which is a proinflammatory component of the cell wall of gram-negative bacteria. When experimental animals are injected with purified LPS, they manifest clinical and biochemical findings reminiscent of those observed in patients with severe sepsis or septic shock. Depending on myriad factors (e.g., the animal species being studied, the dose of LPS, its route of administration), the features of acute endotoxemia can include fever (or hypothermia), systemic arterial hypotension, leukocytosis or leukopenia, renal dysfunction, pulmonary dysfunction, hepatocellular damage, and metabolic acidosis.

LPS is a complex glycolipid composed of a polysaccharide tail attached to a lipophilic domain called lipid A. The polysaccharide portion of the molecule tends to be structurally different in different species and strains of gram-negative bacteria, whereas the structure of lipid A (as well as a few neighboring sugar residues) is highly conserved across different species and strains of gram-negative microorganisms. A complex of LPS and a serum protein, LPS-binding protein (LBP), initiates the activation of monocytes and macrophages by binding to a surface protein, CD14. Because it is a glycophosphatidylinositol-anchored membrane protein, CD14 lacks a cytosolic domain and is unable to initiate intracellular signaling directly. Accordingly, investigators sought to identify another protein that presumably participates with CD14 to initiate the cellular response to LPS. The putative LPS coreceptor was ultimately identified as a Toll-like receptor (TLR).[4]

### Toll-Like Receptors

TLR4, as well as other members of the TLR family of PRRs, is a homologue of a protein, Toll, which plays roles in embryogenesis as well as antifungal immunity in fruit flies. TLR4 was originally identified by studying an inbred strain of mice, C3H/HeJ, that is congenitally hyporesponsive to endotoxin. Subsequently, TLR4 knockout mice were generated and shown to be as hyporesponsive to LPS as C3H/HeJ mice, thus confirming the concept that expression of functional TLR4 is necessary for the activation of macrophages and monocytes by endotoxin. TLR4 mutations are also associated with endotoxin hyporesponsiveness in humans. MD-2, another protein associated with the extracellular domain of TLR4, is required for LPS responsiveness.

In addition to LPS, other PAMPs and alarmins are recognized by various TLRs (Table 4-1). For example, TLR2 recognizes various bacterial lipoproteins, as well as peptidoglycan derived from gram-positive bacteria. TLR5 recognizes flagellin, a 55-kDa protein found in the flagella of certain bacteria. TLR9 recognizes certain oligonucleotides containing unmethylated CpG motifs that are more common in bacterial DNA than in mammalian DNA.

Among the TLRs, TLR4 seems to be particularly important, because this receptor recognizes not only the PAMP, LPS, but several endogenous danger signals as well. These endogenous ligands for TLR4 include the following: heat shock protein (HSP) 70, an inducible cytosolic protein, which is important for the proper folding of nascent proteins; high-mobility group box-1(HMGB1), an abundant DNA-binding protein, which is important for transcription and repair of DNA; extra domain A of fibronectin, an abundant protein in the extracellular matrix; and fragments of hyaluronan, a glycosaminoglycan, which is one of the chief components of the extracellular matrix. Some of these alarmins, such as HMGB1, are actively secreted by immunostimulated macrophages or enterocytes, whereas others, such as hyaluronan fragments, are probably generated as a consequence of trauma to tissues. Accumulating evidence obtained by the Billiar group at the University of Pittsburgh has suggested that many of the deleterious host responses to severe trauma and/or hemorrhagic shock are mediated by the interaction of endogenous alarmins with TLR4.[4]

TLRs are glycoproteins. Their structure includes a ligand-binding domain, containing leucine-rich repeat (LRR) motifs, and a signaling domain, which is homologous to the signaling domain for the receptor for the cytokine IL-1 (see later). To date, 10 TLRs have been identified in humans, and these receptors can be divided into subfamilies based on the ligands they recognize. The receptors TLR3, TLR7, TLR8, and TLR9, are located intracellularly on membrane-bound endosomes, whereas the remaining members of the TLR family of receptors are situated so that they span the cytosolic membrane on the surface of cells.

### Other Families of Pattern Recognition Receptors

In addition to members of the TLR family, there are two other families of PRRs that are important for recognizing DAMPs and initiating innate immune responses. These two families are the retinoid acid-inducible gene I (RIG-I)–like receptors (RLRs) and the nucleotide-binding oligomerization domain (NOD)–like receptors (NLRs).[5] The two RIG-I–like receptors, RIG-I and melanoma differentiation-associated gene (MDA) 5, play a pivotal role in sensing the presence of viral double-stranded (ds) RNA in the cytoplasm. The interaction of ds-RNA with the C-terminal domains of RLRs initiates a signaling cascade, leading ultimately to the expression of cytokines important in antiviral immunity.

The two most extensively studied members of the NLR family of receptors are NOD1 and NOD2.[5] These PRRs sense PAMPs derived from the synthesis and degradation of bacterial peptidoglycan. NOD1 is activated by diaminopimelic acid produced by gram-negative bacteria, whereas NOD2 is activated by muramyl dipeptide (MDP), produced by gram-negative and gram-positive bacteria. As will be discussed in greater detail, NLRs are not only important for sensing certain intracellular pathogens, but these receptors also play a key role in the processing for secretion of two important proinflammatory cytokines, IL-1β and IL-18.

The receptor for advanced glycation end products (RAGE) is a receptor that has multiple potential ligands, including HMGB1, amyloid-β peptide, and certain members of the S100-calgranulin family of proteins.[6] Because RAGE-dependent signaling may be important for transducing some of the proinflammatory effects the alarmin, HMGB1, RAGE can be considered a PRR involved in innate immunity.

### High-Mobility Group Box 1

When mice are injected with a lethal bolus dose of LPS, circulating levels of TNF peak approximately 60 to 90 minutes later and are almost undetectable within 4 hours. Although mice show clinical signs of endotoxemia (e.g., decreased activity and ruffled fur) within a few hours after the injection of LPS, mortality typically does not occur until more than 24 hours later, long after circulating levels of the so-called alarm phase cytokines, TNF and IL-1β, have returned to normal. These observations suggested the possibility to Wang and colleagues that LPS-induced lethality might be mediated by a previously unidentified factor that is released much later than TNF or IL-1β.[6a] Prompted by this idea, these investigators carried out a prolonged search for the putative late-acting mediator. This research program ultimately resulted in the identification of HMGB1 (formerly called HMG-1) as a novel mediator of LPS-induced lethality.

HMGB1 was originally identified in 1973 as a nonhistone nuclear protein with high electrophoretic mobility. A characteristic feature of the protein is the presence of two folded DNA-binding motifs termed the *A domain* and the *B domain.* Both these domains contain a characteristic grouping of aromatic and

**Table 4-1 Recognition of Pathogen-Associated Molecular Patterns and Alarmins by Pattern Recognition Receptors**

| PRR[1] | PAMP[2] OR ALARMIN | COMPOUND | ORIGIN |
|---|---|---|---|
| **TLR[3]** | | | |
| TLR1/TLR2 | PAMP | Triacyl lipopeptides | Bacteria |
| TLR2/TLR6 | PAMP | Diacyl lipopeptides | Bacteria |
| TLR2/TLR6 | PAMP | Lipoteichoic acid | Gram-positive bacteria |
| TLR2 | PAMP | Lipoproteins | Bacteria |
| TLR2 | PAMP | Peptidoglycan | Bacteria |
| TLR2 | PAMP | Lipoarabinomannan | Mycobacteria |
| TLR2 | PAMP | Porins | *Neisseria* spp. |
| TLR2 | PAMP | Envelope glycoproteins | Viruses |
| TLR2 | PAMP | Glycoinositol-phospholipids | *Trypanosoma cruzi* |
| TLR2 | PAMP | Glycolipids | *Treponema maltophilum* |
| TLR2 | PAMP | Phospholipoprotein | *Candida* spp. |
| TLR2 | PAMP | Zymosan | Fungi |
| TLR2 | PAMP | β-Glycan | Fungi |
| TLR2 | Alarmin | HMGB1 | Host cells |
| TLR2 | Alarmin | EDN | Host hepatocytes, PMNs, macrophages |
| TLR3 | PAMP | ds-DNA4 | Viruses |
| TLR4 | PAMP | LPS5 | Gram-negative bacteria |
| TLR4 | PAMP | Envelope glycoproteins | Viruses |
| TLR4 | PAMP | Mannan | *Candida* spp. |
| TLR4 | Alarmin | HSP706 | Host cells |
| TLR4 | Alarmin | HMGB1 | Host cells |
| TLR4 | Alarmin | β-Defensin 2 | Host PMNs and epithelial cells |
| TLR4 | Alarmin | Hyaluronan oligomers | Host extracellular matrix |
| TLR4 | Alarmin | Heparan sulfate fragments | Host extracellular matrix |
| TLR4 | Alarmin | Extradomain A fragment of fibronectin | Host extracellular matrix |
| TLR5 | PAMP | Flagellin | Gram-negative bacteria with flagella |
| TLR7/8 | PAMP | ss-RNA7 | RNA viruses |
| TLR9 | PAMP | CpG DNA8 | Viruses, bacteria, protozoa |
| TLR10 | Unknown | Unknown | Unknown |
| TLR11 | PAMP | Profilin-like protein | *Toxoplasma gondii* |
| **NLR[9]** | | | |
| NOD1[10] | PAMP | Diaminopimelic acid | Gram-negative bacteria |
| NOD2 | PAMP | Muramyl dipeptide | Bacteria |
| NALP1[11] | PAMP | Muramyl dipeptide | Bacteria |
| NALP3 | Alarmin | ATP | Host cells |
| NALP3 | Alarmin | Uric acid crystals | Host cells |
| **RLR[12]** | | | |
| RIG-I[13] | PAMP | ds-RNA, short | Viruses |
| MDA5[14] | PAMP | ds-RNA, long | Viruses |
| **Miscellaneous** | | | |
| RAGE[15] | Alarmin | HMGB1 | Host cells |
| RAGE | Alarmin | S100A12 | Host phagocytic cells |
| PKR[16] | PAMP | ds-RNA | Viruses |

*EDN,* Eosinophil-derived neurotoxin; *PMN,* polymorphonuclear cell.

basic amino acids within a block of 75 residues termed the *HMG box*. HMGB1 has several functions within the nucleus, including facilitation of DNA repair and support of the transcriptional regulation of genes. When released by cells into the extracellular milieu, HMGB1 can interact with several different receptors, including TLR2, TLR4, and RAGE, on macrophages, endothelial cells, and enterocytes.[7] Activation of these receptors leads to the release of other proinflammatory mediators, such as TNF and NO·.

Although HMGB1 is normally not secreted by cells and levels of this protein are usually undetectable in plasma or serum, high circulating concentrations of HMGB1 can be detected in mice 16 to 32 hours after the onset of endotoxemia. Immunostimulated macrophages and enterocytes actively secrete HMGB1. Moreover, necrotic but not apoptotic cells release nuclear HMGB1. In this way, unexpected cell death, such as that secondary to trauma or infection, can act as a danger signal and lead to the induction of an inflammatory response.

Delayed passive immunization of mice with antibodies against HMGB1 confers significant protection against LPS-induced mortality. Furthermore, the administration of highly purified recombinant HMGB1 to mice is lethal. Thus, HMGB1 fulfills a modified version of Koch's criteria for being a mediator of LPS-induced lethality in mice. Direct application of HMGB1 into the airways of mice initiates an acute inflammatory response and lung injury that is reminiscent of ARDS in humans. In addition, HMGB1 (or a truncated form of the protein, including only the B box domain) increases the permeability of human enterocyte-like monolayers in culture and promotes intestinal barrier dysfunction when injected into mice.[8] Thus, it seems plausible that HMGB1 contributes to the development of organ dysfunction in human sepsis, a notion that is supported by the observation that circulating HMGB1 concentrations are significantly higher in patients with ultimately fatal sepsis than in patients with a less severe form of the syndrome.[9] Circulating levels of HMGB1 are also increased in victims of trauma[10] or burn injury.[11] Administration of a neutralizing anti-HMGB1 antibody improves survival in mice subjected to lethal hemorrhagic shock.[12] Ethyl pyruvate, a compound that blocks the release of HMGB1 from LPS-stimulated murine macrophage-like cells and inhibits release of the mediator in vivo, improves survival in mice with bacterial peritonitis, even when treatment with the compound is delayed for 24 hours after the onset of infection.[13]

### Heat Shock Proteins

The heat shock proteins were first identified as a family of molecules that are induced when cells or experimental animals are subjected to sublethal thermal stress. These proteins are also induced by many other stimuli, such as inflammation, oxidative stress, and infection. The primary role of HSPs is to serve as molecular chaperones to facilitate the proper folding of nascent proteins.

Like HMGB1, heat shock proteins are normally found inside cells but, under certain conditions, these proteins can be detected in the extracellular milieu. For example, elevated circulating levels of HSP70 have been found in trauma patients and patients in the immediate period after coronary artery bypass graft surgery. In addition, immunostimulated monocytes appear to be capable of actively secreting HSP70. Extracellular HSP70 (and the related protein, HSP60) can activate innate immune cells via a TLR4-dependent mechanism. Thus, like HMGB1, these proteins may serve as endogenous danger signals and trigger activation of the inflammatory response after damage to tissues.

## CYTOKINES AND CHEMOKINES

Cytokines are small proteins or glycoproteins secreted for the purpose of altering the function of target cells in an endocrine (uncommon), paracrine, or autocrine fashion. In contrast to classic hormones, such as insulin or thyroxine, cytokines are not secreted by specialized glands but, instead, are produced by cells individually (e.g., lymphocytes or macrophages) or as components of a tissue (e.g., the intestinal epithelium). Many cytokines are pleiotropic; these cytokines are capable of inducing many different biologic effects, depending on the target cell types involved and the presence or absence of other modulating factors. Redundancy is another characteristic feature of cytokines—that is, several different cytokines can exert very similar biologic effects.

Chemokines are a special family of cytokines that are small proteins with molecular weights in the range of 8 to 11 kDa. The chemokines have as their primary biologic activity the ability to act as chemoattractants for leukocytes or fibroblasts. Another cytokine subclass is a group of proteins that act primarily to stimulate the growth or differentiation (or both) of hematopoietic progenitor cells; these mediators are collectively referred to as colony-stimulating factors. Other growth and differentiation factors, including the various platelet-derived growth factors, epidermal growth factor, and keratinocyte growth factor, also fit into the broad category of cytokines.

Overall, hundreds of soluble proteins involved in cell to cell signaling, variously called cytokines, chemokines, interleukins, colony-stimulating factors, and growth factors, have been identified and characterized. Some pertinent facts about some of the most important cytokines are provided in Table 4-2 and some of these mediators are discussed in greater detail in the sections that follow.

### Interferon-γ and Granulocyte-Macrophage Colony-Stimulating Factor

The interferons, named for their ability to interfere with viral infection, were initially discovered in the 1950s as soluble factors secreted by leukocytes. The type 1 interferons, IFN-α and IFN-β, are primarily involved as mediators of innate (and acquired) immune responses to viral infection. IFN-γ, although also important in the immune response to viral infection, has much broader activity as a proinflammatory mediator.

For the most part, IFN-γ is produced by three types of cells—$CD4^+$ Th1 cells, $CD8^+$ Th1 cells, and natural killer (NK) cells. IFN-γ, along with IL-12, plays a critical role in promoting the differentiation of $CD4^+$ T cells into the Th1 phenotype. Because Th1 cells also produce IFN-γ, the potential exists for a positive feedback loop. IL-12, produced by monocytes and macrophages, stimulates the production of IFN-γ by Th1 and NK cells. In turn, IFN-γ further activates monocytes and macrophages, thereby creating another positive feedback loop.

In addition to promoting the differentiation of uncommitted $CD4^+$ T cells into Th1 cells, IFN-γ inhibits the differentiation of lymphocytes into cells with the Th2 phenotype. Because Th2 cells secrete the counterregulatory cytokines IL-4 and IL-10, the effect of IFN-γ to downregulate the production of these

**Table 4-2 Cellular Sources and Important Biologic Effects of Selected Cytokines**

| CYTOKINE | ABBREVIATION | MAIN SOURCES | IMPORTANT BIOLOGIC EFFECTS |
|---|---|---|---|
| Tumor necrosis factor | TNF | Mφ, others | See Table 4-3 |
| Lymphotoxin-α | LT-α | Th1, NK | Same as TNF |
| Interferon-α | IFN-α | Leukocytes | Increases expression of cell surface class I MHC molecules; inhibits viral replication |
| Interferon-β | IFN-β | Fibroblasts | Same as IFN-α |
| Interferon-γ | IFN-γ | Th1 | Activates Mφ; promotes differentiation of CD4⁺ T cells + cells into cells into Th1 cells; inhibits differentiation of CD4⁺ T cells into Th2 cells |
| Interleukin-1α | IL-1α | Keratinocytes, others | See Table 4-3 |
| Interleukin-1β | IL-1β | Mφ, NK, DC | See Table 4-3 |
| Interleukin-2 | IL-2 | Th1 | In combination with other stimuli, promotes proliferation of T cells; promotes proliferation of activated B cells; stimulates secretion of cytokines by T cells; increases cytotoxicity of NK cells |
| Interleukin-3 | IL-3 | T cells, NK | Stimulates pluripotent bone marrow stem cells to increase production of leukocytes, erythrocytes, and platelets |
| Interleukin-4 | IL-4 | Th2 | Promotes growth and differentiation of B cells; promotes differentiation of CD4⁺ T cells into Th2 cells; inhibits secretion of proinflammatory cytokines by Mφ |
| Interleukin-5 | IL-5 | T cells, mast cells, Mφ | Induces production of eosinophils from myeloid precursor cells |
| Interleukin-6 | IL-6 | Mφ, Th2, EC, enterocytes | Induces fever; promotes B cell maturation and differentiation; stimulates hypothalamic- pituitary-adrenal axis; induces hepatic synthesis of acute-phase proteins |
| Interleukin-8 | IL-8 | Mφ, EC, enterocytes | Stimulates chemotaxis by PMN; stimulates oxidative burst by PMN |
| Interleukin-9 | IL-9 | Th2 | Promotes proliferation of activated T cells; promotes immunoglobulin secretion by B cells |
| Interleukin-10 | IL-10 | Th2, Mφ | Inhibits secretion of proinflammatory cytokines by Mφ |
| Interleukin-11 | IL-11 | DC, bone marrow | Increases production of platelets; inhibits proliferation of fibroblasts |
| Interleukin-12 | IL-12 | Mφ, DC | Promotes differentiation of CD4⁺ T cells into Th1 cells; enhances IFN-γ secretion by $T_H1$ cells |
| Interleukin-13 | IL-13 | Th2, others | Inhibits secretion of proinflammatory cytokines by Mφ |
| Interleukin-17A | IL-17A | Th17 | Stimulates production of proinflammatory cytokines by Mφ and many other cell types |
| Interleukin-18 | IL-18 | Mφ, others | Costimulation with IL-12 of IFN-γ secretion by Th1 cells and NK cells |
| Interleukin-21 | IL-21 | Th2, Th17 | Modulation of B cell survival; inhibition of IgE synthesis; inhibition of proinflammatory cytokine production by Mφ |
| Interleukin-23 | IL-23 | Mφ, DC | In conjunction with TGF-β, promotes differentiation of naïve T cells into Th17 cells |
| Interleukin-27 | IL-27 | Mφ, DC | Suppresses effector functions of lymphocytes and Mφ |
| Monocyte chemotactic protein-1 | MCP-1 | EC, others | Stimulates chemotaxis by monocytes; stimulates oxidative burst by Mφ |
| Granulocyte-macrophage colony-stimulating factor | GM-CSF | T cells, Mφ, EC, others | Enhances production of granulocytes and monocytes by bone marrow; primes Mφ to produce proinflammatory mediators after activation by another stimulus |
| Granulocyte colony-stimulating factor | G-CSF | Mφ, fibroblasts | Enhances production of granulocytes by bone marrow |
| Erythropoietin | EPO | Kidney cells | Enhances production of erythrocytes by bone marrow |
| Transforming growth factor-β | TGF-β | T cells, Mφ, platelets, others | Stimulates chemotaxis by monocytes and induces synthesis of extracellular proteins by fibroblasts; promotes differentiation of naïve T cells into Treg cells; with IL-6 or IL-23, promotes differentiation of naïve T cells into $T_H17$ cells; inhibits immunoglobulin secretion by B cells; downregulates activation of NK cells |

*DC,* Dendritic cells; *EC,* endothelial cells; *Mφ,* cells of the monocyte-macrophage lineage; *MHC,* major histocompatibility complex; *NK,* natural killer cells; *PMN,* polymorphonuclear neutrophils; *Th1, Th2, Th17,* subsets of differentiated CD4⁺ T helper cells.

cytokines by Th2 cells further promotes the development of an inflammatory response to an invading pathogen. In target cells, such as macrophages or enterocytes, IFN-γ induces the expression or activation of a number of key proteins involved in the innate immune response to microbes. Among these proteins are other cytokines, such as TNF and IL-1, and enzymes, such as iNOS and the reduced form of nicotinamide adenine dinucleotide phosphate (NADPH) oxidase complex. Thus, IFN-γ stimulates the release of a number of other proinflammatory mediators, including cytokines, such as TNF, and small molecules, such as superoxide radical anion ($O_2^-\cdot$), an oxidant produced by NADPH oxidase, and NO·, produced by iNOS. Secretion of these inflammatory mediators by activated macrophages and other cell types is inhibited by IL-4 and IL-10. Accordingly, IFN-γ–mediated downregulation of the Th2 phenotype—and thereby production of IL-4 and IL-10—further promotes the development of an inflammatory response.

The crucial role of IFN-γ in the host's innate immune response to microbial invasion, particularly by intracellular pathogens, has been emphasized by experiments using transgenic mice with targeted disruption of the genes coding for IFN-γ or the ligand-binding subunit of the IFN-γ receptor (IFN-γR). These knockout mice manifest increased susceptibility to infections caused by *Listeria monocytogenes, Mycobacterium tuberculosis,* or bacille Calmette-Guérin.

When responsive target cells are exposed to IFN-γ, a number of genes are activated within minutes and without the synthesis of new copies of intermediate signaling proteins. IFN-γ–induced signal transduction occurs through the activation of a protein tyrosine phosphorylation cascade known as the JAK-STAT pathway (Fig. 4-2). JAK initially stood for "just another kinase" because the biologic role of these proteins was not established when they were initially discovered. Because these receptor-associated kinases look both outside and inside the cell, JAK has now come to stand for Janus kinases, after the two-faced Roman god. The moniker STAT, an acronym for ***s***ignal ***t***ransducers and ***a***ctivators of ***t***ranscription, was appropriately chosen because, in medical parlance, an action to be carried out immediately is a stat order and signaling involving these proteins similarly occurs without delay. In addition to IFN-γ, a large number of other cytokines, including IL-6 and IL-11 (see later), also use versions of the JAK-STAT signaling mechanism. In mammals, there are seven mammalian STAT proteins (STAT1, STAT2, STAT3, STAT4, STAT5A, STAT5B, and STAT6) and four JAK proteins (JAK1, JAK2, JAK3, and TYK2).

IFN-γR is a heterodimer that consists of a 90-kDa glycoprotein, the α chain, which is required for binding of the ligand, and a transmembrane protein, the β chain, which is required for signaling. Associated with the receptor are two members of the JAK family of kinases, JAK1 and JAK2. Interaction of IFN-γ with its receptor results in the dimerization of IFN-γR, which brings JAK1 and JAK2 into close association and leads to mutual phosphorylation and activation (see Fig. 4-2). The activated JAK kinases then catalyze the phosphorylation of tyrosine residues on the α chains of IFN-γR, which results in docking to the receptor complex by the transcription factor STAT1. After tyrosine phosphorylation, two copies of STAT1 form a homodimer (IFN-γ activation factor [GAF]) that subsequently dissociates from the receptor complex and translocates to the nucleus, where binding to the regulatory regions of target genes

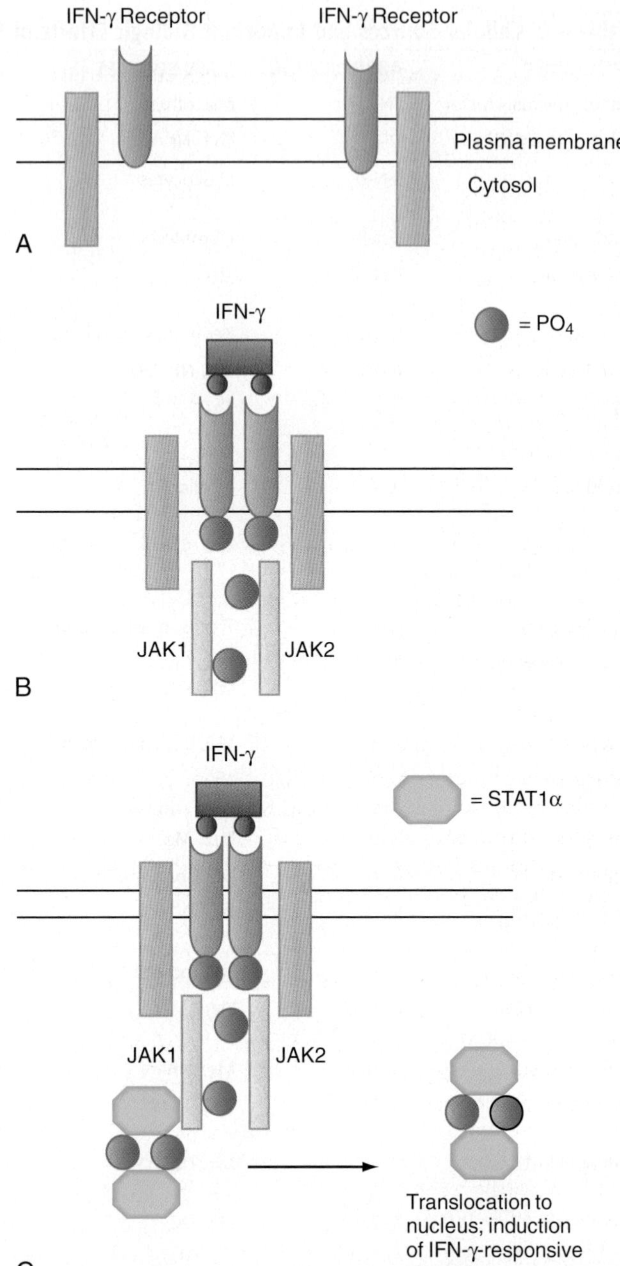


**FIGURE 4-2** Simplified representation of intracellular signaling mediated by binding of IFN-γ to its receptor (IFN-γR). **A,** IFN-γR is a dimer that consists of a ligand-binding α chain and a transmembrane signaling β chain. **B,** Binding of IFN-γ leads to dimerization of IFN-γR and brings two signaling proteins, JAK1 and JAK2, into association with the receptor complex. **C,** The association of JAK1 and JAK2 with the receptor leads to mutual tyrosine phosphorylation of these proteins, as well as phosphorylation of tyrosine residues on the ligand-binding chains of IFN-γR and docking of two copies of the preformed transcription factor STAT1α to the receptor complex. After tyrosine phosphorylation, STAT1α forms a homodimer. The homodimer dissociates from the receptor complex and translocates to the nucleus, where binding to the promoter regions of various IFN-γ–responsive genes leads to transcriptional activation.

containing the IFN-γ activation site (GAS) nucleotide sequence leads to transcriptional activation.

JAK-STAT–dependent signaling is regulated in cells by a variety of mechanisms. Because STATs are activated by tyrosine phosphorylation, phosphotyrosine phosphatases are implicated in the negative regulation of JAK-STAT signaling pathways. In this regard, the first to be described were Src homology 2 domain (SH2)–containing tyrosine phosphatases such as SHP1 and SHP2. The presence of a characteristic amino acid sequence, the SH2 domain, in these cytoplasmic enzymes promotes the association of these phosphatases with phosphotyrosines present on activated receptors or on signaling molecules, as well as on activated JAKs.[14] The transmembrane tyrosine phosphatase CD45, which is expressed on T and B cells, also downregulates JAK-STAT signaling. Two other important classes of proteins that regulate JAK-STAT signaling are the protein inhibitors of activated STAT (PIAS) and the inducible suppressors of cytokine signaling (SOCS).

The pivotal role played by IFN-γ in the regulation and expression of innate immunity to microbial pathogens led investigators to use this cytokine as a therapeutic agent to increase host resistance to infection, particularly for patients with congenital or acquired immunosuppression. For example, prophylactic treatment with recombinant IFN-γ has been shown to reduce the frequency of infections markedly in patients with chronic granulomatous disease, a life-threatening condition caused by an inherited defect in NADPH oxidase, the enzyme complex responsible for generating ROS in phagocytes. IFN-γ has been approved for this indication by the U.S. Food and Drug Administration (FDA). Severe trauma and burns are associated with defects in host antibacterial and antifungal defense and, in animal models of these conditions, treatment with IFN-γ has been found to increase resistance to infection. Three major clinical trials of prophylactic IFN-γ treatment were conducted in patients with multiple trauma or major thermal injury. Unfortunately, in all three studies, the incidence of infection and mortality was similar in cytokine- and placebo-treated patients.

It is unclear why treatment with IFN-γ failed to improve outcomes in these trials. However, treatment with IFN-γ was not individualized according to immunologic phenotype, and thus some of the deleterious effects of inflammation might have been fostered in certain subjects by administration of this potent proinflammatory cytokine. This concept is supported by results from an uncontrolled trial in which patients with sepsis and laboratory findings indicative of excessive immunosuppression (downregulation of human leukocyte antigen [HLA]-DR expression on circulating monocytes) were treated with IFN-γ. In this small study, administration of IFN-γ resulted in the resolution of sepsis in eight of nine patients. A small pilot study evaluated the use of prophylactic perioperative IFN-γ therapy to decrease the risk for infection in anergic high-risk patients undergoing major operations. Results from this study were inconclusive.

Another approach may be to substitute granulocyte-macrophage colony-stimulating factor (GM-CSF) for IFN-γ. GM-CSF is a hematopoietic growth factor and proinflammatory cytokine produced by multiple cell types, including bronchial epithelial cells, monocytes, and endothelial cells. As a growth factor, GM-CSF promotes an increase in the number of circulating polymorphonuclear nuclear cells (PMNs). However, in addition, GM-CSF has a number of IFN-γ–like features, including the use of JAK-STAT signaling pathways. In both in vitro and in vivo studies, treatment with GM-CSF primes monocytes to produce more proinflammatory cytokines, such as TNF, in response to LPS.

A randomized trial of adjuvant treatment with recombinant GM-CSF in neonates with sepsis and neutropenia has shown that survival is significantly improved in the group treated with the cytokine–growth factor.[15] Similarly, in a single-center randomized controlled trial (RCT), adjuvant treatment with recombinant GM-CSF significantly shortened hospital stay and decreased the number of infectious complications in patients with intra-abdominal sepsis.[16] A more recent multicentric RCT has suggested that adjuvant treatment with GM-CSF can improve outcome for selected patients with sepsis.[17] This study randomized 38 patients with severe sepsis and evidence of sepsis-induced immunosuppression to treatment with GM-CSF or placebo for 8 days. Although survival was similar in both groups, the GM-CSF–treated patients required mechanical ventilation and care in an ICU for a significantly shorter period of time

Crohn's disease is a chronic inflammatory disorder of the gastrointestinal (GI) tract. Treatment with corticosteroids often ameliorates symptoms of the disease, but chronic administration of corticosteroids is associated with many adverse side effects. Accordingly, clinicians and scientists are actively seeking better approaches to treat Crohn's disease. Because there is considerable evidence that Crohn's disease may result, at least in part, from impaired innate immunity (e.g., caused by a mutation in the NOD2 gene),[18] recombinant GM-CSF might be a therapeutic option for this condition. This hypothesis has been supported by the results from two RCTs, which showed that therapy with GM-CSF can induce remission in the absence of treatment with corticosteroids.[19,20]

## Interleukin-1 and Tumor Necrosis Factor

IL-1 and TNF are structurally dissimilar pluripotent cytokines. Although these compounds bind to different cellular receptors, their multiple biologic activities overlap considerably. For example, in vitro, both cytokines are capable of activating endothelial cells, leading to increased expression of cell surface adhesion molecules, such as intercellular adhesion molecule-1 (ICAM-1) and vascular cell adhesion molecule-1 (VCAM-1), which play important roles in the process whereby neutrophils extravasate from circulation into tissues at the site of infection and/or inflammation. Similarly, incubating cultured monocytes, neutrophils, endothelial cells, hepatocytes, mesangial cells, articular chondrocytes, or synovial fibroblasts with IL-1 or TNF leads to secretion of a chemokine, IL-8 (see later), which is important for recruiting neutrophils into inflammatory foci. Recombinant forms of IL-1β and TNF have been available for many years. Table 4-3 summarizes some of the biologic effects, which are observed when human subjects are injected with recombinant IL-1β or TNF. The information in this table should convince the reader that many of the features associated with the systemic inflammatory response syndrome (SIRS), such as increased circulating leukocyte count and fever, can be reproduced by injecting subjects with the alarm phase cytokines, IL-1β or TNF. Through their ability to potentiate the activation of helper T cells, IL-1 and TNF can promote almost all types of humoral and cellular immune responses. Furthermore, both these cytokines are capable of activating neutrophils and macrophages and inducing the expression of many other cytokines and inflammatory mediators. Many of the biologic effects of

**Table 4-3 Partial List of Physiologic Effects Induced by Infusing Interleukin-1 or Tumor Necrosis Factor Into Human Subjects**

| EFFECT | IL-1 | TNF |
|---|---|---|
| Fever | + | + |
| Headache | + | + |
| Anorexia | + | + |
| Increased plasma adrenocorticotropic hormone level | + | + |
| Hypercortisolemia | + | + |
| Increased plasma nitrite-nitrate levels | + | + |
| Systemic arterial hypotension | + | + |
| Neutrophilia | + | + |
| Transient neutropenia | + | + |
| Increased plasma acute-phase protein levels | + | + |
| Hypoferremia | + | + |
| Hypozincemia | | + |
| Increased plasma level of IL-1RA | + | + |
| Increased plasma level of TNF-R1and TNF-R2 | + | + |
| Increased plasma level of IL-6 | + | + |
| Increased plasma level of IL-8 | + | + |
| Activation of coagulation cascades | − | + |
| Increased platelet count | + | − |
| Pulmonary edema | − | + |
| Hepatocellular injury | − | + |

IL-1 or TNF are greatly potentiated by the presence of the other cytokine.

### Interleukin-1 and the Interleukin-1 Receptor

IL-1 was first described as a lymphocyte-activating factor produced by stimulated macrophages. IL-1 is not a single compound, but rather a family of three distinct proteins, IL-1α, IL-1β, and IL-1 receptor antagonist (IL-1RA), which are products of different genes located close to one another on the long arm of human chromosome 2. The genes for the two receptors for IL-1, IL-1RI and IL-1RII, are also located on chromosome 2. IL-1α and IL-1β are peptides composed of 159 and 153 amino acids, respectively. Although IL-1α and IL-1β are structurally distinct—only 26% of their amino acid sequences are homologous—the two compounds are almost identical from a functional standpoint. IL-1RA, the third member of the IL-1 family of proteins, is biologically inactive but competes with IL-1α and IL-1β for binding to IL-1 receptors on cells and thereby functions as a competitive inhibitor to limit IL-1–mediated effects.

IL-1 is synthesized by a wide variety of cell types, including monocytes, macrophages, B lymphocytes, T lymphocytes, NK cells, keratinocytes, dendritic cells, fibroblasts, neutrophils, endothelial cells, and enterocytes. Compounds that can trigger the production of IL-1 by monocytes, macrophages, or other cell types include PAMPs such as LPS (from gram-negative bacteria), lipoteichoic acid (from gram-positive bacteria), and zymosan (from yeast). Production of IL-1 can also be stimulated by other cytokines, including TNF, GM-CSF, and IL-1 itself.

Although many cell types express genes for both IL-1α and IL-1β, most cells produce predominantly one form of the cytokine. For example, human monocytes produce mostly IL-1β, whereas keratinocytes produce predominantly IL-1α. The two forms of IL-1 are both initially synthesized as 31-kDa precursors (pro–IL-1α and pro–IL-1β), which are then modified post-translationally to create the carboxyl terminal 17-kDa peptide forms of the mature cytokines. IL-1α is stored in the cytoplasm as pro–IL-1α or, after being phosphorylated or myristoylated, in a membrane-bound form. Whereas both pro–IL-1α and membrane-bound IL-1α are biologically active, pro–IL-1β is devoid of biologic activity. Pro–IL-1α is converted to the mature peptide by calpain and other nonspecific extracellular proteases. Pro–IL-1β is cleaved to its mature active form by a specific intracellular cysteine protease called IL-1β converting enzyme (ICE) or caspase-1. Like IL-1β, ICE–caspase-1 is stored in cells in an inactive form and must be proteolytically cleaved to become enzymatically active.

Transgenic mice deficient in ICE–caspase-1 are resistant to endotoxic shock and manifest an impaired ability to mount a local inflammatory response to intraperitoneal zymosan, a known inducer of sterile peritonitis. In contrast, ICE–caspase-1 knockout mice manifest increased susceptibility to infections caused by various pathogens, including *E. coli, Shigella flexneri, Salmonella typhimurium, Listeria monocytogenes,* and *Candida albicans.* Taken together, these data suggest that ICE-dependent processes, including secretion of the mature forms of IL-1β and the related cytokine, IL-18 (see later), are important for host defense against microbial infection but also are crucial for the pathologic manifestations of poorly controlled inflammation.[21] Various ICE-like enzymes, the caspases, have been identified as being important mediators of the process of programmed cell death, or apoptosis. A special form of apoptosis, called pyroptosis, can occur within minutes after macrophages are infected with certain intracellular pathogens. Pyroptosis is an ICE-dependent process.

The activation of ICE–caspase-1 can be triggered in cells by the formation of a molecular complex called the inflammasome.[21] Inflammasomes are oligomeric complexes, which are composed of ICE–caspase-1 as well as various members of the NLR family of PRRs called NALPs (***NA***CHT domain ***l***eucine-rich repeat and ***P***YD-containing protein) and an adapter protein called ASC (***a***poptosis-associated ***s***pecklike protein containing a ***C***ARD). Assembly of the inflammasome, which in many cases is triggered when an NLR family member senses the presence of PAMP molecules and ultimately leads to ICE–caspase-1 activation and secretion of IL-1β (and IL-18). Inflammasomes that contain a particular NALP (NALP3), can activate ICE–caspase-1 in response to a wide variety of unrelated compounds, including certain toxins, high concentrations of adenosine triphosphate (ATP), and crystals of monosodium urate (the mineral-like structures that are associated with gout). Alum, the adjuvant used in most vaccines to enhance immune responses to antigens, also has been shown to induce activation of the NALP3 inflammasome. All these compounds can lead to ICE–caspase-1 activation and secretion of IL-1β and the related cytokines, IL-18 and IL-33.

The mature 17-kDa form of IL-1β lacks a secretory signal peptide and is not secreted via the classic exocytic pathway used for the secretion of most proteins (including most other cytokines) from cells. ICE-dependent processing of pro–IL-1β and the secretory step appear to occur at the same time. Secretion of the leaderless mature peptide apparently occurs through the action of a specific transporter called ABC1, which can be inhibited by the oral hypoglycemic agent glyburide.

Similar to the other members of the IL-1 family, IL-1RA can be produced by a variety of cell types. However, unlike IL-1α and IL-1β, IL-1RA is synthesized with a leader peptide that allows normal secretion of the protein. A specialized form of IL-1RA, intracellular IL-1RA, is synthesized without a leader peptide sequence and therefore accumulates intracellularly in certain cell types. In some tissues, such as intestinal epithelium, the formation of intracellular IL-1RA may serve a counterregulatory function to limit inflammation and thereby confer mucosal protection. Moreover, an imbalance between the production of IL-1 and IL-1RA may promote the development of chronic inflammation in certain pathologic conditions, such as Crohn's disease. Cellular production of IL-1 and IL-1RA is differentially regulated. Certain cytokines, notably IL-4, IL-10, and IL-13, serve as anti-inflammatory mediators, in part by promoting the synthesis of IL-1RA. IL-6, although not usually considered an anti-inflammatory cytokine, is also capable of triggering the production of IL-1RA.

The importance of IL-1β as a proinflammatory cytokine and IL-1RA as an anti-inflammatory cytokine is emphasized by experiments using transgenic mouse strains deficient in IL-1RA, IL-1α, IL-1β, or both IL-1α and IL-1β (double knockout mice). In these studies, IL-1α knockout mice were able to mount a normal inflammatory response, whereas the IL-1β knockout animals manifested an impaired ability to mount a normal inflammatory response. In contrast, mice functionally deficient in IL-1RA manifested an exaggerated response to a systemic proinflammatory stimulus (intraperitoneal injection of turpentine).

There are two distinct IL-1 receptors, IL-1RI and IL-1RII. IL-1RI is an 80-kDa transmembrane protein with a long cytoplasmic tail. In contrast, IL-1RII, a 60-kDa protein, has only a very short cytoplasmic tail and is incapable of initiating intracellular signaling. As a consequence, IL-1RII is actually a decoy receptor that serves a counterregulatory role by competing with IL-1RI, the fully functional IL-1 receptor, for IL-1 in the extracellular space. IL-1RI is present on a wide variety of cell types, including T cells, endothelial cells, hepatocytes, and fibroblasts. IL-1RII is the predominant IL-1 receptor found on B cells, monocytes, and neutrophils. The extracellular domains of IL-1RI and IL-1RII are shed by activated neutrophils and monocytes. The shed receptors can act as a sink for secreted IL-1 and, thus, along with IL-1RA, represent an important counterregulatory component of the inflammatory response.

IL-1RI is a member of the IL-1R–TLR superfamily of receptors. The cytoplasmic portions of all the members of this superfamily of transmembrane proteins are homologous and are called Toll IL-1 receptor (TIR) domains. In contrast, the extracellular domains fall into two main subdivisions. In one subdivision, the extracellular portion of the molecule contains three immunoglobulin-like regions and is homologous to the structure of IL-1RI. In the other subdivision, which includes the TLRs, the extracellular domain contains leucine-rich repeats.

Because the cytoplasmic TIR domains of the TLRs are homologous to the cytoplasmic region of IL-1RI, it is not surprising that some shared mechanisms are responsible for downstream signaling (Figs. 4-3 and 4-4). In the MyD88-dependent

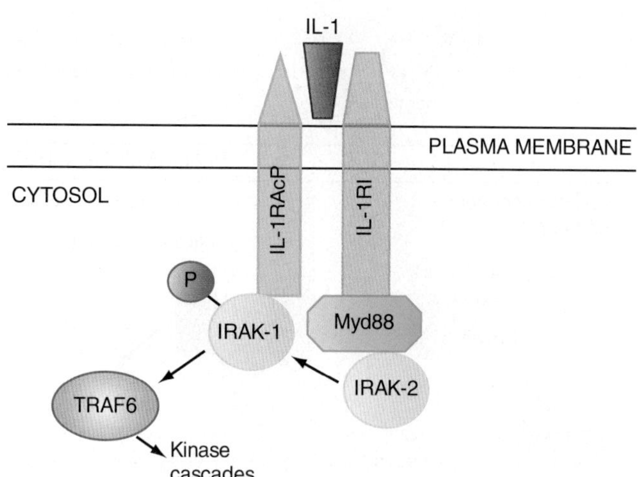


**FIGURE 4-3** Simplified representation of the intracellular signal transduction steps, which are initiated by the binding of IL-1 to its receptor. There are two IL-1 receptors, IL-1RI and IL-1RII. Only IL-1RI participates in signal transduction, and signaling via this receptor requires the participation of another transcytoplasmic protein, IL-1RAcP. The interaction of IL-1 with IL-1RI and IL-1RAcP leads to the formation of a trimolecular complex, which in turn results in the docking of yet another protein, IRAK-1. As a result of its interaction with MyD88, IRAK-1 is phosphorylated and activates another signaling protein, TRAF6. The IRAK-TRAF6 complex activates various downstream kinase cascades, ultimately leading to the activation of key transcription factors, such as NF-κB, and transcriptional activation of various IL-1–responsive genes.

pathway, an adapter protein, myeloid differentiation primary response factor 88 (MyD88), links the receptor to another protein called IL-1 receptor–associated kinase 1 (IRAK-1). On binding of the ligand to the TLR (or IL-1RI), IRAK-1 is phosphorylated and dissociates from the receptor complex, thereby allowing it to interact with another signaling protein, TNF receptor–activated factor 6 (TRAF6). This process results in the activation of nuclear factor κB (NF-κB), a pivotal proinflammatory transcription factor, as well as the phosphorylation signaling cascades involving mitogen-activated protein kinases (MAPKs).

In the case of activation of this signaling pathway by the binding of IL-1β to IL-1RI, the ligand-receptor interaction does not initiate signal transduction without the association of another transcytoplasmic protein called IL-1 receptor accessory protein (IL-1RAcP). Interestingly, the interaction of IL-18 (structurally related to IL-1) with IL-18R (another member of the IL-1R–TLR superfamily) does not trigger downstream signal transduction without the cooperation of a similar accessory protein called IL-18RAcP (or AcPL).

LPS can still activate MAPKs and NF-κB in macrophages derived from MyD88 knockout mice, although this activation occurs in a temporally delayed fashion.[22] This finding indicates that the interaction of LPS with TLR4 must be able to initiate MyD88-dependent and MyD88-independent signaling pathways. LPS-TLR4–induced signaling via the MyD88-independent pathway requires the adaptor proteins, TIR domain-containing adapter-inducing interferon-β (TRIF) and TRIF-related adaptor molecule (TRAM), and leads to the activation of the transcription factor, interferon regulatory factor 3 (IRF3). Translocation

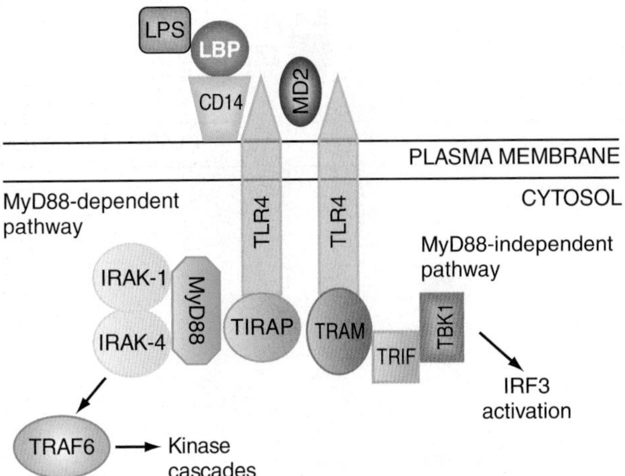


FIGURE 4-4 Simplified representation of the intracellular signal transduction steps, which are initiated by the binding of the microbial product, LPS, to TLR4. The interaction of LPS with TLR4 requires several extracellular accessory proteins–LBP, CD14 (a glycophosphoinositol-anchored cell surface receptor), and MD2. After assembly of the extracellular LPS-LBP-CD14-TLR4-MD2 complex, signaling can follow two different pathways. In the more immediate MyD88-dependent signaling pathway, an adapter protein, MyD88, links the intracellular portion of TLR4 to other adaptor proteins called IRAK-1 and IRAK-4. Phosphorylation of IRAK-1 allows it to dissociate from the receptor complex, thereby permitting it to interact with another signaling protein, TRAF6. This process results in the activation of NF-κB, a pivotal proinflammatory transcription factor, as well as signaling cascades involving MAPKs.6 In the more delayed MyD88-independent pathway, the adapter proteins, TRIF and TRAM, lead to the activation of the serine-threonine kinase, TANK-binding kinase (TBK) 1, which leads to the activation of the transcription factor, IRF3. After phosphorylation, IRF3 forms a complex with cyclic adenosine monophosphate (cAMP) response element-binding (CREB) protein-binding protein (CREBBP), and this complex translocates to the nucleus, leading to the transcription of the genes for IFN-α and IFN-β, as well as other interferon-induced genes. The association of TRIF with the TIR domain of TLR4 also leads to the activation of NF-κB via pathways, which involve TRAF6 as well as another adapter protein called RIP1 (not shown).

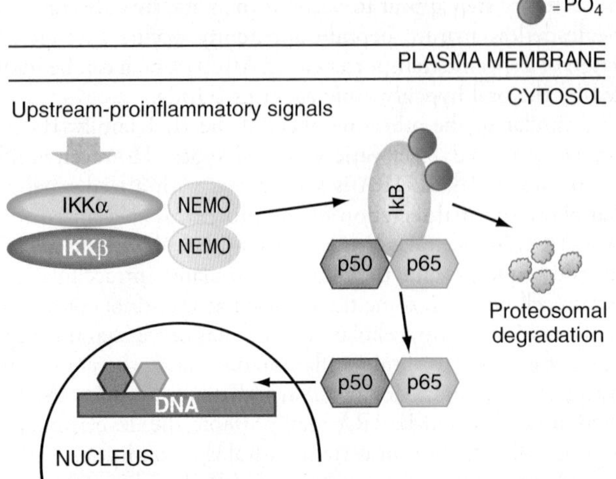


FIGURE 4-5 Simplified representation of the canonical pathway, leading to activation of the transcription factor NF-κB. In resting cells, the heterodimers, consisting of the NF-κB subunits p50 and p65, exist in the cytoplasm in an inactive form because of binding by a third inhibitory protein, IκB. On stimulation of the cell by a proinflammatory trigger (e.g., TNF, IL-1, or LPS), upstream signaling events lead to the phosphorylation of IκB on two key serine residues. Phosphorylation of IκB targets the molecule for ubiquitination and subsequent proteosomal degradation. Phosphorylation of IκB is mediated by an enzyme complex called IκB kinase (IKK), which contains two catalytic subunits, IKKα and IKKβ, as well as two copies of a regulatory scaffold protein called NF-κB essential modulator (NEMO). Phosphorylation and subsequent degradation of IκB permit translocation of transcriptionally active p50-p65 heterodimers into the nucleus. Binding of the transcription factor to *cis*-acting elements in the promoter regions of various NF-κB–responsive genes leads to transcription and ultimately translation of various proinflammatory proteins.

of activated IRF3 to the nucleus leads to transcription of the genes for IFN-α and IFN-β. The association of TRIF with the TIR domain of TLR4 also leads to the activation of NF-κB via pathways that involve TRAF6 and another adapter protein called RIP1.

The transcription factor, NF-κB, plays a central role in the orchestration of the inflammatory response. The Nobel Laureate, David Baltimore, originally identified NF-κB as a nuclear transcription factor involved in the activation of transcription of κ light chain immunoglobulin genes in B lymphocytes. Subsequently, NF-κB has been shown to regulate the transcription of more than 150 genes, particularly those related to inflammation, such as TNF, IL-6, IL-8, cyclooxygenase-2 (COX-2), inducible nitric oxide synthase (iNOS), and LBP. The transcriptionally active form of NF-κB is a homo- or heterodimer comprised of various proteins belonging to the NF-κB family. In mammals, these proteins include RelA–p65, c-Rel, NF-κB1 (p50-p105), NF-κB2 (p52-p100), and RelB. The most abundant form of NF-κB in many cell types is a heterodimer consisting of p65 and p50, and NF-κB is often loosely used to mean this particular entity.

In resting cells, the homo- or heterodimeric forms of NF-κB exist in the cytoplasm in an inactive form caused by binding by a third inhibitory protein, called IκB. In mammalian species, five IκB-like proteins have been identified—IκBα, IκBβ, IκBγ, IκBε, and Bcl-3. Several pathways exist for the activation of NF-κB–dependent signaling. Only the so-called canonical pathway will be described here (Fig. 4-5). On stimulation of the cell by a proinflammatory trigger (e.g., TNF, IL-1, or LPS), IκB is phosphorylated on two key serine residues (Ser32 and Ser36), which targets the molecule for ubiquitination and subsequent proteosomal degradation. Phosphorylation of IκB is mediated by an enzyme complex called IκB kinase (IKK) that contains two catalytic subunits, IKKα and IKKβ, as well as two copies of a regulatory scaffold protein called NF-κB essential modulator (NEMO) or, alternatively, IKKγ. Phosphorylation and subsequent degradation of IκB permit translocation of the transcriptionally active form of NF-κB into the nucleus and subsequent binding of the transcription factor to *cis*-acting elements in the promoter regions of various NF-κB-responsive genes.

IL-1 is an extremely potent mediator. Injecting healthy humans with as little as 1 ng/kg of recombinant IL-1β induces symptoms. Many IL-1–induced physiologic effects occur as a result of enhanced biosynthesis of other inflammatory mediators, including prostaglandin E2 (PGE2) and NO·. Thus, IL-1 increases the expression of the enzyme COX-2 in many cell types, thereby leading to increased production of PGE2. IL-1–induced hyperthermia is mediated by enhanced biosynthesis of PGE2 within the central nervous system (CNS) and can be blocked by the administration of COX inhibitors. IL-1 induces the enzyme iNOS in vascular smooth muscle cells and in other cell types. Induction of iNOS, which leads to increased production of the potent vasodilator NO· in the vascular wall, probably plays a key role in mediating hypotension triggered by the production of IL-1 and other cytokines released in response to LPS or other bacterial products.

Elevated circulating concentrations of IL-1β have been detected in normal human volunteers injected with tiny doses of LPS and in patients with septic shock. However, in subjects with acute endotoxemia or septic shock, circulating concentrations of IL-1β are relatively low in comparison to levels of other cytokines such as IL-6, IL-8, and TNF. In contrast, in normal subjects injected with LPS and in patients with sepsis or septic shock, circulating levels of IL-1RA increase substantially and, in some studies, have been shown to correlate with the severity of disease. Plasma levels of IL-1RII also increase dramatically in patients with serious infections. Although circulating concentrations of IL-1β tend to be relatively low in patients with sepsis, local concentrations of the cytokine can be elevated in patients with sepsis or related conditions, such as ARDS.

### Tumor Necrosis Factor

TNF was initially obtained from LPS-challenged animals and identified as a serum factor that was capable of killing tumor cells in vitro and causing necrosis of transplantable tumors in mice. The gene coding for the protein was sequenced and cloned shortly thereafter. At about the same time, another protein, cachectin, was identified in supernatants from LPS-stimulated macrophages on the basis of its ability to suppress the expression of lipoprotein lipase and other anabolic hormones in adipocytes. TNF and cachectin were later demonstrated to be the same protein. Administration of a large dose of TNF-cachectin to mice was shown to induce a lethal shocklike state remarkably similar to that induced by the injection of LPS, and passive immunization with antibodies to TNF-cachectin was shown to protect mice from endotoxin-induced mortality. Thus, a modern version of Koch's postulates was satisfied, and TNF-cachectin was identified as a pivotal mediator of endotoxic shock in animals. Gradually, the name cachectin was abandoned; the name TNF has survived. TNF is sometimes called TNF-α because it is structurally related to another cytokine that was originally called TNF-β but is now generally referred to as lymphotoxin α (LT-α). TNF and LT-α are both members of a large family of ligands that activate a corresponding family of structurally similar receptors. Other members of the TNF family include Fas ligand (FasL), receptor activator of NF-κB ligand (RANKL), CD40 ligand (CD40L) and TNF-related apoptosis-inducing ligand (TRAIL). Although cells of the monocyte-macrophage lineage are the major sources of TNF, other cell types, including mast cells, keratinocytes, T cells, and B cells, are also capable of releasing the cytokine. A wide variety of endogenous and exogenous stimuli (e.g., alarmins and PAMPs) can trigger induction of TNF expression. LT-α is produced by lymphocytes and NK cells.

TNF is initially synthesized as a 26-kDa cell surface–associated molecule anchored by an N-terminal hydrophobic domain. This membrane-bound form of TNF possesses biologic activity. The membrane-bound form of TNF is cleaved to form a soluble 17-kDa form by a specific TNF converting enzyme that is a member of the matrix metalloproteinase family of proteins. Like most of the other members of the TNF family of ligands, the soluble form of TNF exists as a homotrimer, a feature that is important for the cross linking and activation of TNF receptors.

TNF and LT-α are both capable of binding to two different receptors, TNFR1 (p55) and TNFR2 (p75). Both these receptors, like other receptors in the TNF receptor family, are transmembrane proteins that consist of two identical subunits. The extracellular domains of TNFR1 and TNFR2 are relatively homologous and manifest similar affinity for TNF, but the cytoplasmic regions of the two receptors are distinct. Accordingly, TNFR1 and TNFR2 signal through different pathways. Both receptors are present on most cell types except erythrocytes, but TNFR1 tends to be quantitatively dominant on cells of non-hematopoietic lineage.

The precise functions of the two TNF receptors remain to be elucidated. Nevertheless, considerable information about the roles of TNFR1 and TNFR2 has already been gleaned from experiments using genetically engineered strains of mice lacking one or the other or both of the TNF receptors. TNFR1 knockout mice are relatively resistant to LPS-induced lethality but manifest increased susceptibility to mortality caused by infection with the intracellular pathogens *L. monocytogenes* and *S. typhimurium.* TNFR2 knockout mice are relatively resistant to lethality induced by large doses of recombinant TNF but have an exaggerated circulating TNF response and manifest exacerbated pulmonary inflammation after intravenous (IV) challenge with LPS. Double knockout mice deficient in both TNFR1 and TNFR2 are phenotypically similar to mice lacking only TNFR1.

Most of the members of the TNF family of ligands are involved primarily in the regulation of cellular proliferation or the converse process, programmed cell death (apoptosis). For example, interaction of FasL with the Fas receptor is essential for the normal process of apoptosis in T lymphocytes. TNF itself is somewhat different from other members of the TNF family of ligands in that it is both an initiator of apoptosis and a potent proinflammatory mediator. Activation of inflammation by TNF depends, at least in part, on activation of the transcription factor NF-κB. Because activation of NF-κB tends to suppress apoptosis, it is generally necessary to suppress the synthesis of new proteins to observe TNF-mediated induction of apoptosis.

TNF-mediated signaling is initiated by trimerization of receptor subunits. The subsequent downstream events involved in TNF-mediated signaling are different for the two TNF receptors because the cytoplasmic domains for TNFR1 and TNFR2 are distinct. After ligand-induced trimerization of TNFR1, the first protein recruited to the receptor complex is TNFR1-associated death domain protein (TRADD). Subsequently, three more proteins are recruited to the receptor complex: receptor-interacting protein 1 (RIP1), Fas-associated death domain protein (FADD), and TNF receptor–associated factor 2 (TRAF2). When TNFR2 is trimerized after association of the ligand with the receptor, TRAF2 is recruited directly. TRAF1 then associates with TRAF2. The cytoplasmic domains of Fas, TNFRI, FADD, and TRADD all share a highly conserved sequence of appoximately 80 amino acids called the death domain, which seems to serve as a mediator of critical protein-protein interactions involved in Fas- and TNFR1-mediated signaling.

The downstream events leading to the activation of caspases (i.e., apoptosis) or gene transcription (i.e., inflammation) after recruitment of TRADD, TRAF2, or both are exceedingly complex. A deliberately oversimplified model is depicted in Figure 4-6. In the proapoptotic pathway, TRADD interacts with FADD, which in turn interacts with a protein called caspase-8 (also known as Fas-associated death domain–like IL-1β converting enzyme [FLICE]), the proximal element in the caspase cascade leading to programmed cell death. In the proinflammatory pathway induced by activation of TNFR1 or TNFR2, TRAF2 plays a central role in the early events that lead to activation of NF-κB and two important MAPK pathways—namely, those involving the proteins p38 MAPK and c-Jun N-terminal kinase (JNK). Overexpression of TRAF2 in engineered cells is sufficient to activate signaling pathways leading to the activation of NF-κB, as well as another proinflammatory transcription factor, activator protein-1 (AP-1). By triggering the association of FADD with the receptor complex, the interaction of FasL with Fas leads directly to the induction of apoptosis, whereas recruitment of FADD to the TNF-TNFR1 receptor complex requires an adaptor protein, TRADD, and thus initiates apoptotic processes less directly. Furthermore, the FasL-Fas interaction does not lead to activation of NF-κB, whereas signaling through NF-κB can apparently be initiated by TNF through more than one pathway (TRAF2 and RIP1).

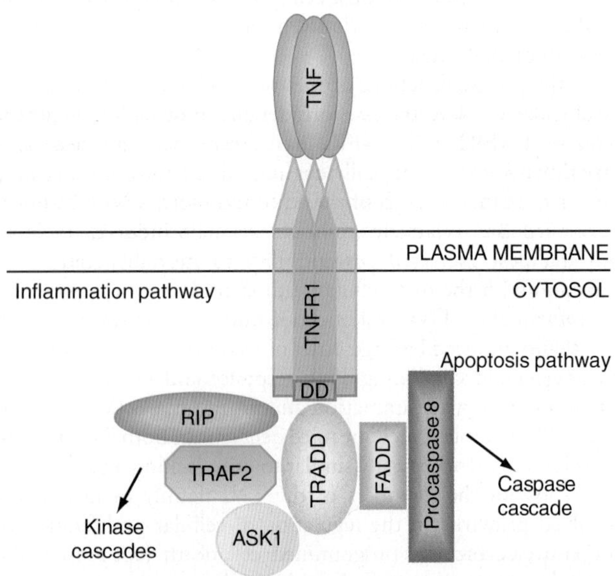


**FIGURE 4-6** Simplified view of intracellular signal transduction events initiated by TNF binding to its cellular receptors. There are two TNF receptors, TNFR1 and TNFR2. Both receptors are homodimeric transmembrane proteins. Although TNFR1 and TNFR2 are capable of initiating signal transduction, different pathways are involved. After TNF binds to TNFR1, a number of proteins, including RIP, FADD, and TRADD, associate with the receptor. The intracytoplasmic tail of TNFR1 and portions of these other signaling molecules share a highly conserved sequence of approximately 80 amino acids, called the death domain. Homotypic interactions among the death domains of these various proteins are essential for the formation of the functional signaling complex. After docking to the receptor complex, TRADD recruits other proteins (e.g., TRAF2 and MADD), which in turn initiate protein kinase pathways leading to the activation of the nuclear transcription factor NF-κB and the protein kinase JNK. TRAF2 can also interact with TNFR2. Association of FADD with the TNFR1 receptor complex leads to the activation of the proteolytic enzyme caspase-8, which is the proximal element in a signaling cascade leading to apoptosis (programmed cell death).

The extracellular domains of TNFR1 and TNFR2 are constitutively released by monocytes, and release of these soluble receptors is markedly increased when the cells are activated by LPS or phorbol ester. Both soluble TNFR1 (sTNFR1) and sTNFR2 are present at low concentrations in the circulation of normal subjects. In patients with sepsis or septic shock, circulating levels of sTNF-R1 and sTNF-R2 increase significantly. Higher concentrations portend a worse prognosis. When present in great molar excess, sTNF receptors can inhibit the biologic effects of TNF. However, when present at lower concentrations, sTNF receptors can stabilize the cytokine and potentially augment some of its actions.

The amount of TNF produced in response to a proinflammatory stimulus, such as exposure of cells to LPS, is determined, in part, by inherited differences (polymorphisms) in noncoding regions of the TNF gene. For example, if the base at position −308 in the TNF promoter is adenine (A), in vitro spontaneous and stimulated TNF production by monocytes is greater than if the base at this position is guanine (G). The more common allelic form of the TNF gene (TNF1) has guanine at position −308, whereas the less common allele (TNF2) has adenine at this position. Some studies have suggested that presence of the TNF2 allele markedly increases the risk for mortality in patients with septic shock, although other data dispute this notion. Interestingly, a G to A substitution at position +250 in the LT-α gene is similarly associated with increased production of TNF by stimulated mononuclear cells, and patients carrying this allele are also at higher risk for mortality from septic shock. In patients with community-acquired pneumonia (a relatively homogeneous population of patients with infection), the risk for development of septic shock is greatest for those who are homozygous for the so-called high TNF secretor genotype (i.e., AA) at position +250 in the LT-α gene.[23] Data such as these suggest that genotyping of patients may prove to be valuable in the coming years for tailoring anticytokine and other forms of adjuvant therapy for critically ill patients.

## Interleukin-1 and Tumor Necrosis Factor as Targets for Anti-Inflammatory Therapeutic Agents

In view of the central importance of IL-1 and TNF as mediators of the inflammatory response, investigators have regarded blocking the production or the actions of these cytokines as a reasonable strategy for treating a variety of conditions associated with excessive or poorly controlled inflammation. Although clearly different in many respects from sepsis in humans, the shocklike syndrome induced in rodents by injecting LPS IV or intraperitoneally has served as a useful paradigm for evaluating various anti-inflammatory strategies. In this model system, survival is improved when animals are treated with any one of a variety of different pharmacologic, immunologic, or genetic strategies that block the release of TNF or prevent this cytokine from interacting with its receptors after it is released. To a lesser extent, the same statement also applies to IL-1.

Glucocorticoids are a broad-spectrum and nonselective way to block IL-1– or TNF-mediated proinflammatory effects. As our understanding of the role of cytokines as mediators of inflammation has progressed, newer and more specific pharmacologic anti-inflammatory strategies have been developed and evaluated as adjunctive therapy for the treatment of sepsis in placebo-controlled prospective clinical trials. Unfortunately, results in these trials were disappointing. Positive results were obtained in only a single study, an open-label trial of recombinant IL-1RA that enrolled a relatively small number of patients. With the exception of this study, none of the agents tested significantly improved survival. In one trial, treatment of septic patients with a so-called fusion protein incorporating the extracellular domain of TNFR2 resulted in increased mortality, particularly in patients with gram-positive infection.

Despite the negative results obtained in sepsis trials, several agents designed to neutralize the effects of secreted TNF or IL-1β have significant clinical efficacy in other important inflammatory conditions such as Crohn's disease and rheumatoid arthritis. Infliximab, a monoclonal anti-TNF antibody, has been FDA-approved for administration to patients to provide long-term remission level control of the debilitating symptoms of Crohn's disease. Infliximab was approved for use, in combination with methotrexate, to reduce the signs and symptoms, inhibit the progression of structural damage, and improve physical function in patients with moderately to severely active rheumatoid arthritis who have had an inadequate response to methotrexate. Adalimumab, another monoclonal anti-TNF antibody, was FDA-approved for administration with or without methotrexate to patients with rheumatoid arthritis to ameliorate symptoms and disability. Etanercept, the TNFR2 fusion protein evaluated unsuccessfully for the treatment of sepsis, has been FDA-approved for the management of psoriatic arthritis. It can reduce the signs and symptoms and inhibit the progression of structural damage in patients with moderately to severely active rheumatoid arthritis, as well as reduce the signs and symptoms in patients 4 years of age and older with moderately to severely active polyarticular-course juvenile rheumatoid arthritis. Anakinra (recombinant human IL-1RA) was FDA-approved for administration alone or with other drugs (except TNF-modifying agents) to reduce the symptoms and modify the progression of structural damage in patients with moderate or severe rheumatoid arthritis who have failed one or more other disease-modifying antirheumatic drugs. TNF expression is upregulated in patients with severe asthma, and etanercept has been shown to decrease bronchial hyperreactivity in this condition.[24] Thus, cytokine-specific approaches to managing inflammatory conditions have moved from the research bench to the clinic and occupy an important role in the clinical management of common clinical conditions, even though this approach has not yet proven its efficacy for the treatment of sepsis and septic shock.

The network of cytokines associated with the inflammatory response interacts at multiple points with another component of the host's defense against injury and infection, the coagulation system. Thrombosis and coagulation help contain the invading organisms to a limited area. TNF, IL-1, and IL-6 (as well as some other proinflammatory cytokines) can activate the extrinsic pathway of coagulation, in part by promoting expression of tissue factor (TF), a transmembrane 45-kDa protein, on endothelial cells and monocytes. In addition, these cytokines also downregulate the expression of an important endogenous inhibitor of coagulation, thrombomodulin, on the surface of endothelial cells. Thus, TNF, IL-1, and IL-6 promote activation of the coagulation cascade. Numerous studies have documented that the extrinsic coagulation pathway is activated in patients with sepsis, even in the absence of frank, clinically evident disseminated intravascular coagulation (DIC).

Key components of the coagulation cascade are a group of proteins that function as endogenous anticoagulants and thus help provide counterregulatory balance to the system. It is therefore noteworthy that the inflammatory response leads not only to TF-mediated activation of coagulation but also to downregulation of these natural anticoagulant pathways. The result is a hypercoagulable state that in its most severe form is characterized by DIC.

Three major anticoagulant pathways exist and all can be inhibited by the inflammatory cascade—antithrombin, the protein C system, and tissue factor pathway inhibitor (TFPI). Antithrombin is a serine protease inhibitor that antagonizes thrombin and factor Xa. During severe inflammatory responses, antithrombin levels are markedly decreased as the result of consumption, impaired synthesis (negative acute phase response), and degradation by elastase from activated neutrophils.

Protein C is activated by thrombin bound to thrombomodulin. During systemic inflammation, protein C levels are reduced because of impaired synthesis and degradation by neutrophil elastase. Furthermore, the protein C system is inhibited by TNF- and IL-1β–mediated decreases in the expression of thrombomodulin. In addition to its role in regulating coagulation, the protein C system also modulates the inflammatory response. Activated protein C binds to the endothelial protein C receptor. Activation of this signaling pathway inhibits LPS-induced NF-κB nuclear translocation and thereby inhibits secretion of TNF, IL-1β, IL-6, and IL-8 by endothelial cells.

Circulating levels of protein C decrease in patients with severe sepsis or septic shock, and a marked deficiency of protein C in these patients is a prognostic indicator for an unfavorable outcome. Various strategies to inhibit excessive activation of the coagulation system have been extensively evaluated in animal models of endotoxemia and sepsis and in clinical trials. One of these approaches, the administration of recombinant human activated protein C, also called drotrecogin alfa (activated), was shown in a large multicentric randomized clinical trial to improve survival significantly in patients with severe sepsis[25]; it was FDA-approved for this indication. Because it is a protein, which inhibits coagulation, administration of drotrecogin alfa (activated) can be associated with bleeding complications.[26] Furthermore, its administration was not found to be beneficial for septic patients with an Acute Physiology and Chronic Health Evaluation II (APACHE II) score less than 25, postoperative patients with single-organ system dysfunction,[27] or pediatric patients with severe sepsis.[28] Prompted by concerns about the safety and efficacy of the recombinant protein, the European Medicines Agency (EMEA [European equivalent of the FDA]) threatened to withdraw its approval of drotrecogin alfa (activated) unless a second (postmarketing) pivotal trial yielded positive findings. This trial is currently in progress.

### Interleukin-6 and Interleukin-11

IL-6 and IL-11 warrant consideration together because along with several other proteins (e.g., oncostatin M), these cytokines use a specific transmembrane protein, gp130, for receptor function. IL-6 consists of 184 amino acids plus a 28–amino acid hydrophobic signal sequence. The protein is variably phosphorylated and glycosylated before secretion. IL-11 is translated as a precursor protein containing 199 amino acids, including a 21–amino acid leader sequence.

Like IL-1 and TNF, IL-6 is a pluripotent cytokine, which is intimately associated with the inflammatory response to injury or infection. IL-6 can be produced not only by immunocytes (e.g., monocytes, macrophages, lymphocytes) but also by many other cell types, including endothelial cells and intestinal epithelial cells. Factors known to induce the expression of IL-6 include IL-1, TNF, platelet-activating factor, LPS, and reactive oxygen metabolites. The promoter region of the IL-6 gene contains functional elements capable of binding NF-κB, as well as another important transcription factor, CCAAT (cytidine-cytidine-adenosine-adenosine-thymidine)/enhancer binding protein (C/EBP), previously called NF–IL-6. The cellular and physiologic effects of IL-6 are diverse and include induction of fever, promotion of B cell maturation and differentiation, stimulation of T cell proliferation and differentiation, promotion of differentiation of nerve cells, stimulation of the hypothalamic-pituitary-adrenal axis, and induction of the synthesis of acute-phase proteins (e.g., C-reactive protein) by hepatocytes. Plasmacytosis and hypergammaglobulinemia develop in transgenic mice that overexpress IL-6. Conversely, IL-6 knockout mice have an impaired acute-phase response to inflammatory stimuli, abnormal B cell maturation, deficient mucosal immunoglobulin A (IgA) production, and impaired host resistance to the intracellular pathogen *L. monocytogenes.* In other murine models of inflammation, the effects of genetic IL-6 deficiency have proven to be highly variable. For example, in a murine model of acute pancreatitis induced by repetitive injections of cerulein, inflammation was exacerbated in IL-6 knockout mice as compared with wild-type controls, a finding that emphasizes the anti-inflammatory effects of IL-6.[29] In contrast, in a murine model of hemorrhagic shock and resuscitation, IL-6 knockout mice exhibited less pulmonary inflammation and lung and gut mucosal injury than wild-type controls, findings that emphasize the proinflammatory effects of IL-6.[30] Although IL-6 knockout mice were not protected from the lethal effects of sepsis, treatment of septic wild-type mice with a carefully calibrated dose of an anti–IL-6 antibody improved survival.

IL-11 is expressed in a variety of cell types, including neurons, fibroblasts, and epithelial cells. Although constitutive expression of IL-11 can be detected in a range of normal adult tissues, expression of IL-11 can also be upregulated by IL-1, TGF-β, and other cytokines or growth factors. Regulation of IL-11 expression is under transcriptional and translational control. From a functional standpoint, IL-11 is a hematopoietic growth factor with particular activity as a stimulator of megakaryocytopoiesis and thrombopoiesis. IL-11 can also interact with epithelial cells in the gastrointestinal tract and inhibit the proliferation of enterocytic cell lines in vitro.

The mechanisms whereby IL-6– or IL-11–induced signals are transduced in target cells have been studied extensively. Activation of target cells via the IL-6 or IL-11 receptor complexes requires the cooperation of two distinct proteins. In the case of IL-6, the ligand-binding subunit is called IL-6R, whereas in the case of IL-11, the ligand-binding subunit is called IL-11R. For both receptors, a distinct protein called gp130 is required for signal transduction. Intracellular signal transduction involves association of the IL-6–IL-6R complex or the IL-11–IL-11R complex with gp130. Dimerization of gp130 leads to downstream signaling via members of the JAK family of protein tyrosine kinases. JAK kinase activation in turn leads to phosphorylation and activation of STAT3, a member of the STAT family of signaling proteins. Phosphorylation of STAT proteins leads to dimerization, translocation to the nucleus, binding to DNA, and transcriptional activation.

Circulating concentrations of IL-6 increase dramatically after tissue injury—for example, as a consequence of elective surgical procedures, accidental trauma, or burns. Elevated plasma levels of IL-6 are consistently observed in patients with sepsis or septic shock. The degree to which circulating IL-6 levels are elevated after tissue trauma or during sepsis has been shown to correlate with the risk for postinjury complications or death. Although it remains to be established whether high circulating IL-6 levels are directly or indirectly injurious to patients with sepsis or are simply a marker of the severity of illness, the observation that immunoneutralization of IL-6 improves outcome in experimental bacterial peritonitis suggests that elevated concentrations of this cytokine are deleterious.

Circulating levels of IL-11 increase in patients with DIC and sepsis. IV or oral administration of recombinant IL-11 improves survival in neutropenic rodents with sepsis, possibly by preserving the integrity of the intestinal mucosal barrier.[31] In a small phase 2 clinical study, treatment with recombinant IL-11 increased expression of von Willebrand factor in patients with mild von Willebrand disease.

### Interleukin-8 and Other Chemokines

*Chemotaxis* is the term used to denote the directed migration of cells toward increasing concentrations of an activating substance (chemotaxin). The ability to recruit leukocytes to an inflammatory focus by promoting chemotaxis is the primary biologic activity of a special group of cytokines called chemokines. More than 40 of these small proteins have been identified. Each contains approximately 70 to 80 amino acids, including three or four conserved cysteine residues. Four chemokine subgroups have been described. The subgroups are defined by the degree of separation of the first two $NH_2$-terminal cysteine residues. In the CXC or α-chemokines, the first two cysteine moieties are separated by a single nonconserved amino acid residue, whereas in the CC or β-chemokines, the $NH_2$-terminal cysteines are directly adjacent to each other. The C chemokine subgroup is characterized by the presence of only a single $NH_2$-terminal cysteine moiety. The $CX_3C$ subgroup has only one member (fractalkine); in this chemokine, the $NH_2$-terminal cysteine residues are separated by three intervening amino acids. A subclass of the CXC chemokines, exemplified by IL-8, contains a characteristic amino acid sequence (glutamate-leucine-arginine) near the $NH_2$-terminal end of the protein; these chemokines act primarily on PMNs. Other chemokines, including the CC chemokines and members of the CXC subgroup not containing the glutamate-leucine-arginine sequence, act, for the most part, on monocytes, macrophages, lymphocytes, or eosinophils. Many different cell types are capable of secreting chemokines; cells of the monocyte-macrophage lineage and endothelial cells are particularly important in this regard. Numerous proinflammatory stimuli, including cytokines, such as TNF and IL-1, and PAMPs, such as LPS, can stimulate the production of chemokines.

IL-8, the prototypical CXC chemokine, was first identified as a chemotactic protein by Yoshimura and associates in 1987.[31a] IL-8 is translated as a 99–amino acid precursor and is secreted after cleavage of a 20–amino acid leader sequence. In addition to attracting neutrophils along a chemotactic gradient, IL-8 also activates these cells by triggering degranulation, increased expression of surface adhesion molecules, and production of reactive oxygen metabolites. There are at least two distinct IL-8 receptors, CXCR1 (IL-8R1) and CXCR2 (IL-8R2). CXCR1 is predominantly expressed on neutrophils. Like other chemokine receptors, CXCR1 and CXCR2 are coupled to G proteins, and binding of ligand to these receptors leads to intracellular signal transduction via the generation of inositol triphosphate, activation of protein kinase C, and perturbations in intracellular ionized calcium concentrations.

Increased circulating concentrations of IL-8 were detected in experimental animal models of infection or endotoxemia and in patients with sepsis. Treatment of experimental animals with antibodies against IL-8 improves survival or prevents pulmonary injury in models of sepsis or ischemia-reperfusion injury. These observations support the concept that IL-8–mediated activation of neutrophils plays an important role in the pathogenesis of organ system damage in these syndromes.

Monocyte chemotactic protein-1 (MCP-1), the prototypical CC chemokine, was identified in the same year by two groups of investigators. MCP-1 is a chemotaxin for monocytes (but not neutrophils) and also activates monocytes by triggering the production of reactive oxygen metabolites and the expression of $\beta_2$ integrins (cell surface adhesion molecules). Elevated circulating concentrations of MCP-1 have been detected in endotoxemic mice and patients with sepsis. Pretreatment of mice with a polyclonal anti–MCP-1 antiserum ameliorates LPS-induced lung injury, thus suggesting an important role for this chemokine in the pathogenesis of sepsis-induced ARDS.

### Interleukin-12

IL-12, a cytokine produced primarily by antigen-presenting cells, is a heterodimeric protein composed of two disulfide-linked peptides (p35 and p40) encoded by distinct genes. Both subunits are required for biologic activity. The IL-12 receptor is expressed on T cells and NK cells. The most important biologic activity associated with IL-12 is to promote Th1 responses by helper T cells. In this regard, IL-12 promotes the differentiation of naive T cells into Th1 cells capable of producing IFN-γ after activation and serves to augment IFN-γ secretion by Th1 cells responding to an antigenic stimulus. Stimulation of IFN-γ production by IL-12 can be synergistically enhanced by the presence of other proinflammatory cytokines, notably TNF, IL-1, or IL-2. Conversely, counterregulatory cytokines, such as IL-4 and IL-10, are capable of inhibiting IL-12–induced IFN-γ secretion.

The immunologic responses governed by Th1 cells are central to the development of cell-mediated immunity necessary for appropriate host resistance to intracellular pathogens. It is not surprising, therefore, that transgenic mice deficient in IL-12 manifest increased susceptibility to infections caused by a number of intracellular pathogens, including *Mycobacterium avium* and *Cryptococcus neoformans.*

IL-12 may be a key factor in some of the deleterious inflammatory responses to LPS and gram-negative bacteria. Elevated circulating levels of IL-12 were measured in endotoxemic mice and baboons infused with viable *E. coli.* Elevated plasma levels of IL-12 were also detected in children with meningococcal septic shock and were correlated with outcome. However, in patients with postoperative sepsis, circulating IL-12 levels were lower than those in control subjects without sepsis and did not correlate with outcome.[32] Defective production of IL-12 by peripheral blood mononuclear cells after stimulation with IFN-γ and LPS is associated with an increased risk for the development of postoperative sepsis in preoperative patients.[33]

IL-12 has also been implicated in the pathogenesis of IBD. T cells eluted from the lamina propria of intestinal resection specimens from patients with Crohn's disease secrete cytokines consistent with a Th1-like profile. In addition, IL-12–secreting macrophages are present in large numbers in tissue specimens from patients with Crohn's disease but are rare in histologic sections from appropriate control subjects. Treatment with anti–IL-12 antibodies ameliorates the severity of disease in certain murine models of IBD. Treatment of patients with refractory IBD with thalidomide, a potent anti-inflammatory agent, decreases the production of TNF and IL-12 by mononuclear cells isolated from the lamina propria of gut mucosal biopsy samples and decreases disease activity.

Although excessive production of IL-12 has been implicated in the pathogenesis of acute inflammatory conditions such as septic shock and chronic inflammatory states, such as Crohn's disease, adequate production of IL-12 appears to be essential for orchestration of the normal host response to infection. When antibodies to IL-12 are administered to mice with fecal peritonitis induced by cecal ligation and perforation, mortality is increased and clearance of the bacterial load is impaired. Conversely, pretreatment or even post-treatment with recombinant IL-12 has been shown to improve survival in a murine model of bacterial peritonitis.

IL-12 is not the only member of the IL-12 family of cytokines. Two other cytokines, IL-23 and IL-27, are structurally related to IL-12. All three IL-12 family members are heterodimeric proteins, containing the IL-12p40 subunit or a homologue of IL-12p40 called Ebstein-Barr virus (EBV)-induced molecule 3 (EBI3). As noted, IL-12 is an IL-12p40–IL-12p35 heterodimer, IL-23 is an IL-12p40–IL-23p19 heterodimer, and IL-27 is a heterodimeric protein, consisting of EBI3 and IL-27p28. As will be discussed, IL-23 is clearly a proinflammatory cytokine, whereas IL-27 seems to be capable of exerting both proinflammatory and anti-inflammatory (or immunosuppressive) effects, depending on the experimental conditions being studied.[34]

### Interleukin-17 and Related Cytokines

IL-17, now sometimes called IL-17A, was discovered in 1995 by Yao and coworkers and shown to induce IL-6 and IL-8 production from human fibroblasts.[34a] Although it was not recognized at the time, IL-17 and other related cytokines were subsequently shown to play important and distinctive roles in host immunity and the development of various pathologic conditions.

In 1987, Mossman and Coffman proposed a model for adaptive immunity based on the concept that naïve precursor helper T cells can differentiate into one or the other of different classes of helper T cells (i.e., Th1 or Th2) characterized by different functions and different patterns of secreted cytokines.[34b] The Th1-Th2 paradigm proved to be robust and was accepted with little or no modification until approximately 2005, when a series of discoveries led to the recognition that a third, completely distinct subset of helper T cells, now called Th17, was important in the pathogenesis of inflammation associated with autoimmune conditions.

The discovery that IL-17 and related cytokines define a subset of helper T cells originally stemmed from studies of experimental autoimmune encephalomyelitis (EAE), a murine model of multiple sclerosis in humans.[35] According to the Th1-Th2 paradigm, autoimmunity was thought to be mediated by Th1 cells with specificity of self antigens. Unexpectedly, however, it was observed that IFN-γ and IFN-γR knockout mice, as well as mice deficient for other molecules (e.g., IL-12p35 or IL-18) involved in Th1 differentiation, were not protected from EAE but, on the contrary, developed a more severe form of the disease. These observations raised the possibility that a subset of T helper cells other than Th1 might be responsible for the induction of EAE or other organ-specific autoimmune conditions.

Meanwhile, in 2000, a novel cytokine chain, p19, was discovered in the process of screening for IL-6 homologues.[35] Whereas IL-12 is heterodimer, consisting of p35 and p40 chains, a newly discovered cytokine, IL-23, was shown to be a heterodimer made up of p40 and p19 chains. IL-23p19 knockout mice were shown to be protected from the development of EAE. Moreover, it was shown that IL-23 expands a population of T cells that produce IL-17 and, when adoptively transferred into naïve wild-type mice, induces EAE. These and other studies have established IL-17 as a key mediator of EAE and have also suggested that IL-23 is essential for the differentiation of the cells that produce IL-17. However, results from other studies called into question whether IL-23 is responsible for the differentiation of Th17 cells, and it is now established that a combination of TGF-β plus another cytokine (usually IL-6 but, under some conditions, also IL-23 or IL-21) is required to induce IL-17 production in a population of naïve T cells. It is noteworthy, therefore, that IL-6 knockout mice are resistant to the development of EAE, except under certain conditions.

Differentiation of naïve helper T cells into Th17 cells under the influence of TGF-β and IL-6 (or TGF-β plus IL-21) requires intracellular signaling mediated by a steroid receptor type of transcription factor, called RAR-related orphan receptor (ROR) γt. Cooperation with other transcription factors, such as interferon regulatory factor (IRF) 4, is probably also required.

There are six members of the IL-17 gene family named, in order of their discovery, IL-17A through IL-17F.[36] These molecules have a similar molecular weight (20 to 30 kDa), share sequence homology, and demonstrate overlapping, but not completely identical, biologic activities. The receptor for IL-17 is called IL-17R, and its structure is unlike that for any other cytokine receptor. In susceptible cells types, IL-17 activates signaling via multiple routes, including the MAPK pathways, various JAK-STAT pathways, and NF-κB. IL-17 or IL-17R knockout mice manifest increased susceptibility to selected pathogens, most notably *Klebsiella pneumoniae* and *C. albicans,* but are also partially protected from the development of EAE. Interestingly, in a murine model of IBD, IL-17A ameliorates the disease, whereas IL-17F exacerbates the disease.[35] Treatment with neutralizing anti–IL-17A antibodies improves survival in mice with sepsis induced by cecal ligation and puncture, even when therapy is instituted 12 hours after the onset of infection.[37]

### Interleukin-18

IL-18 is constitutively expressed by human peripheral blood mononuclear cells and murine intestinal epithelial cells, but IL-18 production can also be stimulated by a variety of proinflammatory microbial products. The main biologic activity of IL-18 is to induce production of IFN-γ by T cells and NK cells. In this regard, IL-18 acts most potently as a costimulant in combination with IL-12. IL-12–induced IFN-γ expression appears to depend on the presence of IL-18 inasmuch as transgenic mice (or cells from mice) deficient in IL-18 or ICE produce little IFN-γ in response to appropriate stimulation, even in the presence of ample IL-12. In addition to stimulating IFN-γ production, IL-18 induces the production of CC and CXC chemokines from human mononuclear cells and activates neutrophils, an effect that may contribute to organ injury and dysfunction in conditions such as sepsis and ARDS. Circulating concentrations of IL-18 are higher in patients with sepsis than in those only with injuries, and high levels of this cytokine are associated with a fatal outcome in patients with postoperative sepsis.

### Interleukin-4, Interleukin-10, and Interleukin-13

IL-4, IL-10, and IL-13 can be regarded as inhibitory, anti-inflammatory, or counterregulatory cytokines. All three of these cytokines are produced by Th2 cells and, among other roles, serve to modulate the production and effects of proinflammatory cytokines such as TNF and IL-1.

IL-4, originally described as a B cell growth factor, is a 15- to 20-kDa glycoprotein synthesized by Th2 cells, mast cells, basophils, and eosinophils. IL-4 has many biologic actions that promote the expression of the Th2 phenotype, characterized by downregulation of proinflammatory and cell-mediated immune responses and upregulation of humoral (B cell–mediated) immune responses. IL-4 induces differentiation of $CD4^+$ T cells into Th2 cells and, conversely, downregulates differentiation of $CD4^+$ T cells into Th1 cells. IL-4 inhibits the production of TNF, IL-1, IL-8, and PGE2 by stimulated monocytes or macrophages and downregulates endothelial cell activation induced by TNF. IL-4 acts as a comitogen for B cells and promotes expression of the class II major histocompatibility complex (MHC) on B cells.

IL-10, originally called cytokine synthesis inhibitory factor, was first isolated from supernatants of cultures of activated T cells. This cytokine is an 18-kDa protein produced primarily by Th2 cells but is also released by activated monocytes and other cell types. IL-10 acts to downregulate the inflammatory response through numerous mechanisms. For example, IL-10 inhibits the production of numerous proinflammatory cytokines, including IL-1, TNF, IL-6, IL-8, IL-12, and GM-CSF, by monocytes and macrophages; on the other hand, it increases synthesis of the counterregulatory cytokine IL-1RA by activated monocytes. In addition, IL-10 downregulates the proliferation and secretion of IFN-γ and IL-2 by activated Th1 cells, primarily by inhibiting the production of IL-12 by macrophages or other accessory cells. Conversely, IFN-γ downregulates IL-10 production by monocytes. At least some of the inhibitory effects of IL-10 are mediated by blocking IFN-γ–induced tyrosine phosphorylation of STAT1α, a key protein in the signal transduction pathway for IFN-γ.

The importance of IL-10 as a regulatory cytokine has been illustrated in experiments using transgenic mice deficient in IL-10. Such animals manifest increased resistance to the intracellular bacterial pathogen *L. monocytogenes*, thus suggesting that IL-10–mediated suppression of the Th1-type phenotype can impair the host's ability to eradicate certain types of infection. In contrast to these results, IL-10 knockout mice succumbed to the lethal effects of excessive inflammation when infected with another intracellular pathogen, the protozoan parasite *Toxoplasma gondii.* Results have been variable in mice with severe sepsis, but a genetic deficiency of IL-10 production alters the kinetics of the inflammatory process without affecting long-term survival. IL-10–deficient mice spontaneously develop a form of enterocolitis that is reminiscent of IBD in humans. Because the IBD-like syndrome in these animals can be suppressed by treating the animals with exogenous IL-10 or a neutralizing anti–IFN-γ antibody, the enterocolitis associated with IL-10 deficiency is thought to be caused by excessive expression of the Th1-type phenotype.

Production of IL-10 by peripheral blood mononuclear cells and $CD4^+$ T cells is increased in trauma patients, and elevated circulating concentrations of this cytokine have been measured in patients with trauma or sepsis. Moreover, in trauma and burn patients, increased production of IL-10 has been associated with a greater risk for serious infection and, in patients with sepsis, a greater risk for mortality or shock. These findings support the view that although excessive production of proinflammatory mediators may be deleterious in trauma and sepsis, development of the Th2 phenotype, characterized by increased production of IL-10 and IL-4 and decreased expression of the MHC type II antigen HLA-DR on monocytes, may lead to excessive immunosuppression and deleteriously affect the outcome on this basis. Evidence has been presented supporting the view that HLA-DR expression on monocytes is post-translationally downregulated by IL-10 in patients with sepsis.

Administering exogenous IL-10 in an effort to blunt excessive inflammation has led to mixed results in experimental models of sepsis or septic shock. In models in which experimental animals are challenged with IV LPS, treatment with recombinant IL-10 ameliorates fever and improves survival. In models such as cecal ligation and perforation, wherein the sepsis syndrome is induced by infection with viable bacteria, administration of exogenous IL-10 is beneficial or without effect. However, in mice with pneumonia caused by *Pseudomonas aeruginosa,* survival is improved when the animals are treated with an anti–IL-10 antibody to neutralize endogenous IL-10. Thus, although the use of recombinant IL-10 as an adjuvant treatment of sepsis is appealing, caution will need to be exercised in the design and conduct of clinical trials because excessive immunosuppression could adversely affect antibacterial defense mechanisms.

IL-13 is a 12-kDa protein closely related to IL-4. The two proteins have approximately 25% homology and share many structural characteristics. IL-13 is produced by Th2 cells and also undifferentiated $CD4^+$ T cells and $CD8^+$ T cells. The IL-13 receptor consists of two chains, one of which binds IL-4 but not IL-13, and another that binds IL-13 with high affinity. Binding of IL-4 or IL-13 to their respective receptors induces signaling by activating the same JAK kinases, JAK1 and Tyk2. IL-4, but not IL-13, also activates JAK3. The biologic activities of IL-13 are very similar to those of IL-4 with respect to B cell function although, unlike IL-4, IL-13 does not have any direct affects on T cells. IL-13 downregulates the production of proinflammatory cytokines (e.g., IL-1, TNF, IL-6, IL-8, IL-12, G-CSF, GM-CSF, MIP-1α) and PGE2 by activated monocytes and macrophages and, by the same token, increases the production of anti-inflammatory proteins, including IL-1RA and IL-1RII, from these cells. Additional anti-inflammatory properties of IL-13 include inhibition of induction of the enzyme COX-2, required for the production of prostaglandins, and induction of an enzyme, 15-lipoxygenase, that catalyzes the formation of a lipid mediator (lipoxin A4) with anti-inflammatory properties. Treatment of mice with recombinant IL-13 has been shown to prevent LPS-induced lethality and to decrease circulating levels of TNF and other proinflammatory cytokines. Conversely, treatment of septic mice with an anti–IL-13 antibody has been shown to increase mortality.

### Transforming Growth Factor-β

The TGF-β family of mediators exerts a number of effects on most cell types, including modulation of cell growth, inflammation, matrix synthesis, and apoptosis. Although more than 45 peptides in the TGF-β family have been isolated, TGF-β1 was the first identified and is the isoform most associated with modulation of immune function. The bioactive forms of the TGF-β proteins are produced from 50-kDa monomers that dimerize to form the 100-kDa TGF-β precursor. The TGF-β precursor undergoes intracellular cleavage by furin proteases to yield the active 25-kDa TGF-β homodimer. This active form of TGF-β remains associated with the remaining portion of its pro form, latency-associated peptide (LAP). This complex has been called latent TGF-β and is secreted in this inactive form into the extracellular matrix. This unusual mode of secretion allows the latent TGF-β complex to be considered to be an extracellular sensor. Latent TGF-β can be activated by the dissociation and degradation of LAP via proteolysis (catalyzed by plasmin or matrix metallopeptidases) or the nonenzymatic activity of integrins, thrombospondin-1, oxygen and nitrogen free radicals, or low pH. These activating factors are often perturbations of the extracellular matrix that are associated with phenomena such as angiogenesis, wound repair, inflammation, or cell growth. Thus, post-translational extracellular activation of TGF-β is the most important regulatory mechanism for this cytokine, a mode of activation that is unique among the cytokines.

Once activated, TGF-β–mediated signaling involves a cell surface heteromeric complex of transmembrane serine–threonine kinase receptors. Each receptor complex contains a pair of both TGF-β type I (TβRI) and type II (TβRII) receptors, which are activated by TGF-β binding and regulated by a number of intracellular proteins that interact directly with the receptor complex in a constitutive or ligand-induced manner. The intracellular signal transduction pathway responsible for gene induction or repression involves a family of structurally related proteins known as Smads. TGF-β receptor–activated Smads are phosphorylated by TβRI, form a heterotrimeric complex with the common partner Smad4, and translocate to the nucleus, where they can repress or activate transcription.

From a number of studies using transgenic and knockout mice, TGF-β1 was found to play an important role in leukocyte development and function, wound healing, inflammation, suppression of tumorigenesis, and organogenesis and homeostasis in tissues such as liver, kidney, pancreas, and lung. Furthermore, TGF-β1 administration reduces LPS-induced hypotension and mortality in a murine model of sepsis and, in trauma patients, lower circulating TGF-β1 levels are associated with the development of liver and kidney dysfunction, whereas higher TGF-β1 circulating levels 6 hours after admission to the intensive care unit are associated with an increased risk for sepsis.

TGF-β plays a dual role in the differentiation of naïve T helper cells. When present by itself, TGF-β promotes expression of the transcription factor, Foxp3, a differentiation of naïve helper T cells into Treg cells. However, when presented with IL-6 or IL-21, TGF-β abrogates Treg cell development and, instead, promotes differentiation of naïve helper T cells into Th17cells.[35] In the inactivated state, production of TGF-β fosters production of Treg cells, which tends to dampen immunologic or inflammatory responses. However, when IL-6 is produced in massive amounts as part of the acute-phase response to injury or infection, the balance is shifted to TGF-β–mediated induction of proinflammatory Th17 cells.[35]

### Macrophage Migration Inhibitory Factor

Macrophage migration inhibitory factor (MIF) was the first functional cytokine described. MIF is produced by monocytes and macrophages and acts in an autocrine and paracrine fashion to activate various cell types during inflammation. Immunostimulated macrophages secrete MIF. MIF appears to function proximally in the inflammatory cascade because MIF knockout mice exhibit a global reduction in the production of other inflammatory mediators such as TNF, IL-1β, and PGE2.

MIF is encoded by a unique gene that displays very high sequence conservation across species. MIF is constitutively expressed and, after translation, preformed MIF remains in cytoplasmic pools and is readily released from macrophages after inflammatory stimulation. The rapid release of preformed MIF is unlike most other cytokines, which are typically released after transcriptional activation and translation of new protein. The receptor for MIF, CD74, is also distinct from the other cytokine receptor superfamilies.

Apoptosis is an important mechanism for the resolution of the inflammatory response via the removal of activated monocytes and macrophages, and the proinflammatory action of MIF is caused, in part, by suppression of apoptosis. MIF also upregulates the expression of TLR4 on macrophages, thereby amplifying the response of the innate immune system to LPS (and possibly other proinflammatory substances such as HMGB1). Circulating MIF levels are increased in patients with sepsis and septic shock, but not in noninfected trauma patients. In mice with peritonitis, treatment with a neutralizing anti-MIF antibody improves survival.

### Complement

Complement was first identified as a heat-labile component in serum that complemented the function of humoral immunity in the killing of microorganisms. Rather than a single factor, complement is a complex system of more than 30 plasma and membrane-bound proteins. The nomenclature used to describe the multiple elements in the complement cascade follows their order of discovery rather than their sequential activation. Complement functions in consort with proteins of the coagulation, fibrinolysis, and kinin systems to augment the response to pathogenic stimuli via a series of catalytic reactions. The complement system is evolutionarily well preserved, thus suggesting that it represents a common ancestral host defense system. Although the complement system plays a key role in the host's defense against pathogenic microbes, dysregulated activation of the complement cascade can be deleterious and excessive complement activation has been implicated in the pathogenesis of a wide variety of immune and inflammatory conditions, ranging from ARDS and sepsis to asthma.[38]

Activation of complement occurs via three distinct pathways: the classical pathway is activated by antigen-antibody (IgG or IgM) complexes, the alternative pathway is initiated by recognition of certain bacterial cell surface markers, such as LPS, and the lectin-binding pathway is activated by detection of bacterial surface sugars, such as mannose (Fig. 4-7). Most of the complement proteins circulate in inactive form until they are cleaved by an upstream protease, which in turn activates their proteolytic activity. Thus, sequential activation of catalytically active proteins produces an escalating cascade of activity (similar to the coagulation system). Regardless of the activation pathway, the most important active products are the anaphylatoxins C3a and C5a and the membrane attack complex C5b-C9, which causes lysis of gram-negative bacteria. C3a induces the release of histamine from mast cells and causes smooth muscle cell contraction. C5a binds to its receptor (C5aR) on neutrophils and macrophages and triggers intracellular signaling, chemotaxis, enzyme release, and the generation of ROS, which participate in the killing of microorganisms.

Activation of the classical pathway is triggered by the interaction of antigen-antibody complexes with C1, which is a 790-kDa complex composed of a recognition protein C1q and a Ca2q-dependent tetramer consisting of two copies each of two proteases, C1r and C1s. Binding of C1 to a cellular or molecular target is mediated by C1q and results in the self-activation of C1r, which subsequently activates C1s. C1s then cleaves C4 and C2, thereby resulting in their activation. At this point, all pathways converge at C3 and lead to the activation of C3a and C5a and the terminal membrane attack complex C5b-C9, which creates pores in prokaryotic cell membranes that lead to bacterial cell lysis. Genetic defects in the classical pathway result in increased susceptibility to bacterial infections caused by organisms such as *Neisseria meningitidis, Haemophilus influenzae,* and *Streptococcus pneumoniae.*

The alternative pathway, triggered by bacterial products such as LPS, results in the sequential activation of C3a, C5a, and the membrane attack complex. The lectin-binding pathway, triggered by binding of bacterial sugars such as mannose to mannose-binding lectin protein, activates C4a and C5a and then joins the common pathway for activation of the membrane attack complex.

Activated complement products exert a number of biologic functions. C3b opsonizes pathogenic bacteria, which results in their enhanced phagocytosis by macrophages and neutrophils. Immune complexes bind to C3a and are then removed by binding with complement receptor 1 (CR1, discussed later). Clearance of necrotic and apoptotic cells may be facilitated by interaction with C1q. Complement factor deficiencies, which

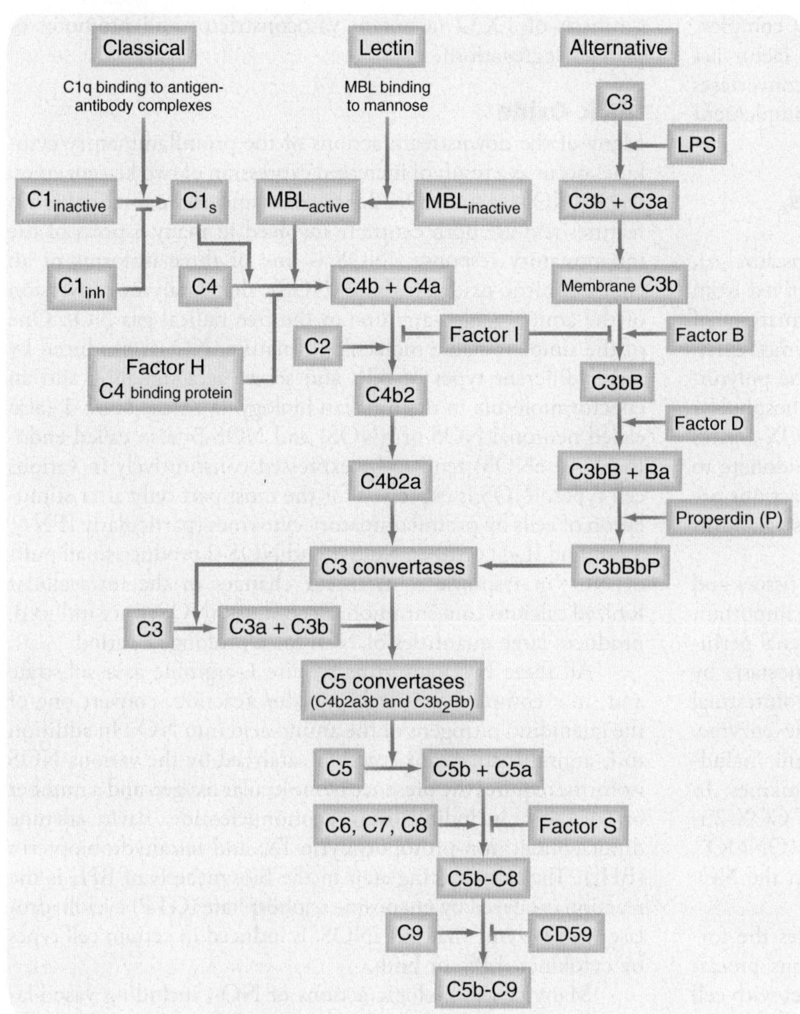


**FIGURE 4-7** Activation of the complement cascade via the classical, lectin, or alternative pathways leads to formation of the membrane attack complex (C5b-C9). Various complement inhibitors antagonize several steps in the cascade: C1 inhibitor ($C1_{inh}$), factor I, factor H, C4-binding protein, factor S, and CD59, among others not shown here. MBL, Mannose-binding lectin.

result in inadequate clearance of immune complexes and dead cells, may give rise to the development of autoimmunity.

Many of the effects of complement activation are mediated by the binding of activated complement products to specific receptors. Some receptors bind several different complement factors with varying affinity, thereby resulting in a variety of effects on different cells. Binding of C3b, C4b, and C1q by CR1, also known as CD35, results in the cleavage of C3 and C5 convertases, clearance of C3b-bound immune complexes, and activation of T lymphocytes. CR2, also known as CD21, is present on B and T lymphocytes and some endothelial cells. CR2 binds iC3b and C3d (C3b cleavage products) and causes stimulation of B lymphocytes and antibody production. EBV also binds to CR2. CR3 and CR4 are members of the integrin family and are expressed on myeloid cells. CR3 and CR4 bind iC3b, C3b, fibrinogen, ICAM-1, and other ligands. Binding of ligands to these receptors enhances antibody-mediated phagocytosis by neutrophils and macrophages. Although a number of different ligands bind to complement receptors 1 through 4, C3a and C5a bind to specific receptors (C3aR and C5aR, respectively). Both these receptors are present on a wide variety of cell types. Binding of C3a or C5a to their respective receptors activates intracellular signaling cascades involving MAPK pathways.

Detrimental actions of the complement system on the host are mediated by the overproduction of C3a and C5a during complement activation and the excessive formation of membrane attack complexes. In rodent models of sepsis, treatment with a neutralizing anti-C5a antibody improves survival and also decreases circulating levels of TNF and IL-6, thus suggesting that the activation of C5 receptors is associated with the release of these other mediators.[38]

Several inhibitors are present in plasma or are membrane-bound to prevent uncontrolled activation of the complement system. C1 inhibitor is present in plasma and prevents the activation of C1s and C1r, thereby antagonizing the classical pathway. In addition, C1 inhibitor also inhibits the lectin pathway. Heterozygous deficiency of C1 inhibitor results in life-threatening angioedema. Factor H and C4 binding protein are plasma proteins that inhibit C3 and C4 activation, thereby inhibiting all complement activation pathways. Factor I is a serine protease that inactivates C3b and C4b and therefore C3 and C5 convertases. C3a and C5a are also antagonized by carboxypeptidase N. S protein, fibronectin, and clusterin are plasma proteins that prevent insertion of C5b-C9 into cellular membranes. The membrane-bound complement inhibitors act at several points in the complement pathways. CD59 is a glycoprotein that prevents polymerization of C9 and blocks insertion of C9 into the membrane-bound C5b-C9 complex. Membrane cofactor protein and decay-accelerating factor act directly and with factor I to inhibit C3 and C5 convertases and cleave C3b and C4b, thereby inhibiting all complement pathways.

### Eicosanoids: Thromboxane, Prostaglandins, and Leukotrienes

The prostaglandins, including PGE2 and PGI2 (prostacyclin), and thromboxane A2 (TXA2) are lipid mediators derived from the unstable intermediate compound PGG2. Formation of PGG2 depends on the activity of two families of enzymes. First, isoforms of the enzyme phospholipase A2 liberate the polyunsaturated fatty acid arachidonate from membrane phospholipids. Second, the two cyclooxygenase isoforms COX-1 and COX-2 catalyze the stereospecific oxidation of arachidonate to form the cyclic endoperoxide PGG2. Both these reactions are major regulatory steps in the formation of prostaglandins and TXA2.

COX-1 is expressed constitutively in a variety of tissues and mediators produced by this isoform are thought to be important in various homeostatic processes, such as regulating renal perfusion and salt and water handling, maintaining hemostasis by modulating platelet aggregation, and preserving gastrointestinal mucosal integrity. COX-2, however, is an inducible enzyme. Expression of COX-2 is induced by a number of stimuli, including various growth factors and proinflammatory cytokines. In cells subjected to inflammatory stimuli, activation of COX-2 is thought to be mediated by the powerful oxidant $ONOO^-$, thereby providing a tight functional linkage between the NO· and prostaglandin mediator systems.

Once expressed and activated, COX-2 promotes the formation of PGG2 and PGH2 and, ultimately, various prostaglandins and TXA2. These mediators, in turn, interact with cell surface receptors belonging to the G protein–coupled receptor superfamily. Interaction of these receptors with cytosolic signaling pathways leads to rapid alterations in cell physiology manifested as physiologic or pathophysiologic phenomena such as vasodilation and increased microvascular permeability. Pharmacologic inhibition of cyclooxygenase activity is the basis for the anti-inflammatory actions of the class of compounds called nonsteroidal anti-inflammatory drugs (NSAIDs). Whereas the anti-inflammatory effects of NSAIDs are thought to be mediated by blocking the enzymatic activity of COX-2, some adverse side effects of these agents (e.g., gastric mucosal ulceration) are thought to be mediated by inhibition of COX-1. Accordingly, identification of COX-2 as the so-called inflammatory isoform of cyclooxygenase led to intense efforts to develop drugs selective for the inducible enzyme. Selective COX-2 inhibitors were initially widely prescribed by clinicians. However, data from large multicenter trials of rofecoxib, one of the compounds in this class, showed that treatment with this agent was associated with an increased risk for death from cardiovascular complications.[39,40] As a result of these findings, rofecoxib was withdrawn from the market. The increased risk for cardiovascular complications associated with rofecoxib, however, does not seem to be peculiar only to this specific agent but rather is thought to be a class effect associated with therapy with all isoform-selective COX-2 inhibitors, possibly as a result of greater inhibition of the synthesis of PGI2 (a vasodilator and inhibitor of platelet aggregation) relative to inhibition of the synthesis of TXA2 (a potent vasoconstrictor and promoter of platelet aggregation).

### Nitric Oxide

Many of the downstream actions of the proinflammatory cytokines occur as a result of increased expression of two key enzymes, iNOS (NOS-2) and COX-2. These enzymes share some common features and are both centrally involved in many aspects of the inflammatory response. iNOS is one of three isoforms of an enzyme, nitric oxide synthase (NOS), that catalyzes conversion of the amino acid L-arginine to the free radical gas NO·. One of the simplest stable molecules in nature, NO· is produced by many different types of cells and serves as a signaling and an effector molecule in mammalian biology. Whereas NOS-1 (also called neuronal NOS or nNOS) and NOS-3 (also called endothelial or eNOS) tend to be expressed constitutively in various cell types, iNOS is expressed for the most part only after stimulation of cells by proinflammatory cytokines (particularly IFN-γ, TNF, and IL-1) or LPS. NOS-1 and NOS-2 produce small puffs of NO· in response to transient changes in the intracellular ionized calcium concentration. In contrast, iNOS, once induced, produces large quantities of NO· for a prolonged period.

All three NOS isoforms require L-arginine as a substrate and, in a complex five-electron redox reaction, convert one of the guanidino nitrogens of the amino acid into NO·. In addition to L-arginine, the redox reaction catalyzed by the various NOS isoforms requires the presence of molecular oxygen and a number of cofactors, including flavin mononucleotide, flavin adenine dinucleotide, iron-protoporphyrin IX, and tetrahydrobiopterin ($BH_4$). The rate-limiting step in the biosynthesis of $BH_4$ is the reaction catalyzed by guanosine triphosphate (GTP) cyclohydrolase I, an enzyme that like iNOS, is induced in certain cell types by cytokines, LPS, or both.

Many of the biologic actions of NO·, including vasodilation, induction of vascular hyperpermeability, and inhibition of platelet aggregation, are mediated through the activation of the enzyme soluble guanylyl cyclase (sGC). Binding of NO· to the heme moiety of sGC activates the enzyme, thereby enabling it to catalyze the conversion of GTP to cyclic guanosine monophosphate (cGMP). NO· is not the only ligand that is capable of activating sGC; carbon monoxide (CO), another small gaseous molecule produced by mammalian cells, has also been shown to activate this enzyme. Signal transduction via the NO·-sGC (or the CO-sGC) pathway entails the activation of various cGMP-dependent protein kinase (PKG) isoforms. In vascular smooth muscle cells, NO·-induced vasodilation occurs as a result of PKG-mediated opening of high-conductance calcium and voltage-activated potassium channels. Excessive production of NO· as a result of iNOS induction in vascular smooth muscle cells is thought to be a major factor contributing to the loss of vasomotor tone and loss of responsiveness to vasopressor agents (vasoplegia) in patients with septic shock. Treatment with a drug that blocks production of NO·, such as $N^G$-monomethyl-L-arginine (L-NMMA), ameliorates hypotension in patients with septic shock. Unfortunately, treatment of septic patients with L-NMMA actually worsens survival, possibly because the drug does not selectively inhibit iNOS but also inhibits NOS-3 as well and therefore interferes with the normal regulation of microcirculatory perfusion. Some studies have suggested that iNOS knockout mice are partially resistant to the lethal effects of acute endotoxemia. In contrast, one study has shown that iNOS knockout mice are more susceptible than wild-type controls to lethality induced by bacterial peritonitis, possibly because enhanced NO· production is important for the host's defense against infection. In contrast, iNOS knockout mice are protected from sepsis-induced acute lung injury.[41]

Signaling via the sGC-PKG pathway is not the only way that NO· functions as an inflammatory mediator. In addition, NO· reacts rapidly with another free radical, superoxide anion ($O_2^-$·), to form peroxynitrite anion ($ONOO^-$), the conjugate base of the weak acid peroxynitrous acid (ONOOH). Being a potent oxidizing and nitrosating agent, $ONOO^-$-ONOOH is thought to be responsible for many of the toxic effects of NO·. For example, $ONOO^-$-ONOOH is capable of oxidizing sulfhydryl groups on various proteins at a rapid rate, peroxidizing membrane lipids, and inactivating mitochondrial aconitase. $ONOO^-$-ONOOH is also capable of damaging nuclear DNA, thus setting up a chain of events that ultimately leads to the activation of the enzyme poly(adenosine ribose diphosphate[ADP]) polymerase-1 (PARP-1). On activation, PARP-1 catalyzes the poly(ADP) ribosylation of proteins, a reaction that consumes oxidized nicotine adenine dinucleotide ($NAD^+$) and leads to energetic failure in cells.[42] Treatment with pharmacologic agents that do the following has been shown to improve organ system function, survival, or both in certain experimental models of inflammation, such as acute endotoxemia, mesenteric ischemia and reperfusion, hemorrhagic shock and resuscitation, and stroke:

1. Scavenge $ONOO^-$-ONOOH.
2. Selectively block iNOS (without blocking NOS-1 or NOS-3).
3. Block the activity of PARP-1.

### Carbon Monoxide

Although CO was identified as a poison in the mid-19th century, its role as an endogenous signaling molecule has been recognized only in the past few years. The toxicity of CO relates to its ability to impair the oxygen-carrying capacity of hemoglobin. Two mechanisms are involved. First, CO binds to hemoglobin with 250-fold greater affinity than $O_2$, thereby inhibiting $O_2$ binding and transport. Second, CO causes a conformational change in the hemoglobin molecule that impairs its ability to release bound $O_2$, thus shifting the oxyhemoglobin dissociation curve to the left. In addition, CO binds to and inactivates cytochrome $a_3$, thereby impairing mitochondrial respiration.

The concentrations of endogenously generated CO are far below the toxic level. Endogenously generated CO is a product of heme catabolism. The CO-generating reaction is catalyzed by a family of enzymes called heme oxygenases. There are three isoforms of heme oxygenase called HO-1, HO-2, and HO-3, although only HO-1 and HO-2 have been widely studied. HO-2 is constitutively expressed, whereas HO-1 is an inducible enzyme. HO-1 expression is induced by a wide variety of agents, including heme itself, heat shock stress, ROS, LPS, heavy metals, and ultraviolet radiation. HO-1 plays an important role in the defense of cells against oxidative stress, and both products of the degradation of heme by HO-1, bilirubin and CO, are important in this regard.

CO exerts a variety of physiologic effects. It causes relaxation of smooth muscle cells, which results in vasodilation and bronchodilation. CO inhibits the activation and aggregation of platelets. Like NO·, CO functions as a neurotransmitter. Finally, CO exerts a number of cytoprotective effects. Pretreatment of rodents with 250 ppm of inhaled CO ameliorates the development of acute lung injury after subsequent exposure to LPS or hyperoxia. CO also has antiproliferative effects on tumor cells and vascular endothelial and smooth muscle cells. Finally, CO has an anti-inflammatory role mediated via the MAPK pathway that results in suppression of TNF release and upregulation of IL-10 secretion.

Similar to NO·, CO mediates its effects by binding to the ferrous heme moieties of hemoproteins. Although the affinity of heme for NO· is higher than that for CO, the off rate for dissociation of CO from heme is much slower, so CO displaces NO· from heme over time. Thus, CO can modulate the effects of NO· in this manner. Binding of CO to the heme moiety of sGC results in the activation of sGC and is the primary mechanism responsible for many of the biologic effects of CO.

### Hydrogen Sulfide

In the past few years, it has become increasingly apparent that NO· and CO are not the only gaseous molecules used by mammalian species as signaling molecules. A third gas, hydrogen sulfide ($H_2S$), also seems to be important.[43] Long recognized as an environment pollutant, $H_2S$, a colorless gas with a characteristic odor of rotten eggs, is produced in mammalian cells from the amino acid, L-cysteine, via either of two enzymes, cystathionine γ-lyase or cystathione β-lyase. $H_2S$ is a potent vasodilator and produces this effect through a mechanism that is not dependent on the activation of sGC. In rodents with LPS-induced shock or septic shock, $H_2S$ levels are inversely correlated with arterial blood pressure, suggesting that it has a pathogenic role in the development of hypotension. Treatment of septic rats with propylargylglycine, a compound that blocks enzymatic $H_2S$ production, improves survival and decreases biochemical evidence of inflammation. These findings support the view that $H_2S$ is a proinflammatory mediator, although other findings have suggested that some of the effects of $H_2S$ are anti-inflammatory.

### Reactive Oxygen Species

ROS are reactive, partially reduced derivatives of molecular oxygen ($O_2$). Important ROS in biologic systems include superoxide radical anion ($O_2^-$·), hydrogen peroxide ($H_2O_2$), and hydroxyl radical (OH·). Closely related species include the hypohalous acids, particularly hypochlorous acid (HOCl), chloramine ($NH_2Cl$) and substituted chloramines (RNHCl or R′R″NCl), and singlet oxygen ($^1O_2$). Free radicals are atomic or molecular species with unpaired electrons. As a consequence of these unpaired electrons, free radicals are usually highly reactive and capable of modifying a wide range of cellular constituents, including lipids, proteins, and nucleic acids. ROS that are also free radicals include $O_2^-$·, OH·, peroxyl radical ($RO_2$·), and hydroxyperoxyl radical ($HO_2$·).

A variety of enzymatic and nonenzymatic processes can generate ROS in mammalian cells. Nevertheless, a few key reactions or processes constitute the main sources of these reactive species:

- NADPH oxidase catalyzes a one-electron reduction of $O_2$ to form $O_2^-$· according to the following equation: $2O_2 + NADPH \rightarrow 2O_2^-\cdot + NADP + 2H^+$. NADPH oxidase is an enzyme complex that is assembled and activated after the activation of phagocytes by microbes or microbial products (e.g., LPS) or various proinflammatory mediators such as leukotriene $B_4$, platelet activating factor, TNF, or IL-8. In resting cells, the components of NADPH oxidase are present in the cytosol and membranes of various intracellular organelles. When the cell is activated, the components are assembled on a membrane-bound vesicle, which then fuses with the plasma membrane, and $O_2^-\cdot$ is released outward into the extracellular milieu and inward into the phagocytic vesicle. The reaction catalyzed by NADPH oxidase is critical for the formation of ROS in phagocytic cells, such as macrophages and PMNs. NADPH oxidase, however, is also present in other cell types, including vascular smooth muscle cells and endothelial cells.

- Superoxide dismutase (SOD) catalyzes the conversion (dismutation) of two moles of $O_2^-$ to form one mole each of $O_2$ and $H_2O_2$. Two forms of SOD are present in cells. Copper-zinc SOD (CuZn-SOD) is a constitutive enzyme localized to the cytoplasm, whereas manganese SOD (Mn-SOD) is an inducible enzyme present in mitochondria. Increased expression of Mn-SOD is induced by oxidant stress or various proinflammatory cytokines.
- In the presence of free ionized iron or copper in a low oxidation state (i.e., $Fe^{2+}$ or $Cu^+$, respectively), $H_2O_2$ reacts nonenzymatically to form $OH\cdot$ and hydroxyl anion according to the following equation: $H_2O_2 + Fe^{2+} \rightarrow OH\cdot + OH^- + Fe^{3+}$. The lower oxidation state of the transition metal cation can then be regenerated by the action of any number of reducing agents within the cellular milieu (e.g., ascorbic acid) and the cycle then repeated. This cycle constitutes the so-called Fenton reaction.
- Myeloperoxidase (MPO) is an enzyme present in phagocytes that catalyzes oxidation of the halide ions chloride ($Cl^-$), bromide ($Br^-$), and iodide ($I^-$) by $H_2O_2$ to form the corresponding hypohalous acids (HOCl, HOBr, and HOI, respectively). MPO, a colored heme-containing enzyme, is responsible for the greenish tint that is sometimes noticeable in purulent exudates.
- Xanthine oxidase (XO) catalyzes the oxidation of xanthine (or hypoxanthine) by molecular oxygen to form uric acid and $O_2^-\cdot$ according to the following equation: $\text{xanthine} + H_2O + 2O_2 \rightarrow \text{uric acid} + 2O_2^- + 2H^+$. An enzyme related to XO, xanthine dehydrogenase (XDH), uses reduced nicotinamide adenine dinucleotide (NADH) as a cofactor and converts xanthine (or hypoxanthine) to uric acid without forming partially reduced forms of molecular oxygen. During episodes of tissue ischemia, XDH is proteolytically converted to XO, and adenosine triphosphate is degraded to xanthine and hypoxanthine. During reperfusion, $O_2$ is available and XO acts on the accumulated substrates (xanthine and hypoxanthine), which leads to a burst in the production of ROS.
- Although the various NOS isoforms ordinarily catalyze the formation of NO· and L-citrulline from L-arginine, these enzymes can generate $O_2^-\cdot$ if L-arginine availability is limiting.
- ROS are also produced as a byproduct of the normal metabolism of oxygen in mitochondria and have important roles in cell signaling. Leakage of electrons from the mitochondrial electron transport chain with resultant formation of $O_2^-\cdot$ is quantitatively the most important mechanism, leading to ROS production within cells. Somewhat paradoxically, tissue hypoxia, such as that occurring during hemorrhagic shock, can enhance mitochondrial ROS production. It is noteworthy, therefore, that administration of a synthetic ROS scavenger, which has been designed to be concentrated in mitochondria, can prolong survival of rats with lethal hemorrhagic shock.[44]

To counter the activity of ROS, cells are equipped with a number of antioxidant systems, including SOD, catalase, glutathione, glutathione peroxidase, ascorbic acid (vitamin C), α-tocopherol (vitamin E), and thioredoxin. Under normal circumstances, the reducing milieu in cells prevents ROS-induced cellular damage. However, during times of stress, ROS production can increase dramatically and overwhelm normal antioxidant defenses, thereby leading to so-called oxidative stress and damage to cells and tissues on this basis.

Sepsis is associated with oxidative stress. Low plasma ascorbate levels are predictive of the development of multiorgan dysfunction in septic patients, and some data have shown a reduction in the incidence of organ failure when antioxidants are administered to critically ill surgical patients.

## NEUROENDOCRINE CONTROL OF THE INFLAMMATORY RESPONSE

The neuroendocrine system plays an important role in regulating immune and inflammatory responses. From a teleologic standpoint, regulation of innate immune responses by the CNS makes good sense. Innate immune responses to danger signals, whether caused by infection or trauma, need to occur quickly, and the CNS is capable of responding to external stimuli within milliseconds to minutes. Additionally, the CNS recognizes and responds to painful stimuli, which are often associated with trauma of various sorts. The three main components of regulatory influence of the CNS are mediated by hormones secreted by the adrenal cortex, hormones secreted by the adrenal medulla, and a neurotransmitter, acetylcholine, released by terminals of the vagus nerve.

### Corticosteroids

The adrenal cortex synthesizes the mineralocorticoid, aldosterone, various weak androgens (e.g., dehydroepiandrosterone), and the glucocorticoid, cortisol (hydrocortisone). Because it is lipophilic, cortisol diffuses across the cytosolic membrane of cells and binds to a cytosolic receptor. The cortisol-receptor complex translocates into the nucleus, where it interacts with glucocorticoid responsive elements in the regulatory regions of hundreds of genes. The production of cortisol is regulated by the CNS via the hypothalamic-pituitary axis. In response to physiologic or psychological stress, secretion of adrenocorticotrophic hormone (ACTH) from the anterior pituitary gland increases, which leads to increased secretion of cortisol from the adrenal cortex.

Clinicians and scientists have long recognized that the natural and synthetic glucocorticoids, such as hydrocortisone and dexamethasone, are potent anti-inflammatory agents. Glucocorticoids modulate the secretion of cytokines and chemokines by lymphocytes, macrophages, and other cell types. The effects of glucocorticoids on the pattern of cytokine and chemokine secretion are myriad, but some of the most important, as summarized by Prigent and colleagues,[45] are as follows:

inhibition of IL-2 and IFN-γ secretion by T cells; inhibition of IL-1β, TNF, IL-6, IL-8 and IL-12 secretion by monocytes and macrophages; increased secretion of anti-inflammatory cytokines (IL-10, IL-1RA and TGF-β) secretion by various cell types; downregulation of COX-2 and iNOS expression; and inhibition of adhesion molecule expression on various cell types.

These anti-inflammatory actions of hydrocortisone and related compounds are mediated by more than one mechanism. One important action of glucocorticoids is to downregulate signaling mediated by a key transcription factor, NF-κB, known to activate many genes associated with the inflammatory response. Glucocorticoid-induced downregulation of NF-κB activation is a result of augmented expression of a protein, IκB, that is an inhibitory component of the NF-κB complex. An additional anti-inflammatory action of glucocorticoids is to inhibit the activation of another signaling pathway, the JNK-SAPK cascade, which leads to decreased translation of TNF mRNA and thus decreased production of TNF. Still another mechanism whereby glucocorticoids inhibit inflammation is through decreased expression of the enzyme ICE, required for post-translational processing of pro–IL-1β and thus decreased secretion of mature IL-1β.

In some experimental models of sepsis, early treatment with high doses of a potent synthetic glucocorticoid, such as methylprednisolone or dexamethasone, improves survival. Unfortunately, several large clinical trials have failed to confirm the benefit of high-dose glucocorticoid therapy for the adjuvant treatment of patients with septic shock or the related condition, ARDS. As a result, the notion of using glucocorticoids for these indications seemed to be a dead issue. However, the concept of using glucocorticoids as anti-inflammatory agents in the management of ARDS or septic shock has been resurrected, at least transiently. Several small studies have shown that prolonged therapy with relatively low doses of hydrocortisone or methylprednisolone improve systemic hemodynamics, pulmonary function, or both in patients with ARDS or septic shock. These findings were confirmed by the results obtained in a 300-patient, multicenter RCT carried out in one country (France).[46] Although somewhat controversial, the results of this study supported the view that administration of a relatively low dose of hydrocortisone could improve survival in patients with volume-unresponsive pressor-dependent septic shock and an inadequate circulating cortisol response to an injection of ACTH. Prompted by the results from this study, 499 patients with volume-unresponsive pressor-dependent septic shock were enrolled in a multicenter trial of IV hydrocortisone.[47] At 28 days, there was no difference in mortality between patients in the two study groups, although the corticosteroid-treated patients had more episodes of superinfection. Similarly disappointing results were obtained in a study of the administration of corticosteroids during the late (so-called fibroproliferative) phase of ARDS.[48] Although some experts still advocate treating selected patients with sepsis or septic shock with corticosteroids, the results of these most recent studies suggest that this practice should be abandoned.

## Catecholamines

The catecholamines, norepinephrine and epinephrine, are the principal neuroendocrine mediators of the sympathoadrenal axis. Norepinephrine is a neurotransmitter released by the terminals of postganglionic sympathetic neurons, whereas epinephrine is a hormone secreted by chromaffin cells in the adrenal medulla in response to stimulation via preganglionic sympathetic nerve fibers. To a lesser extent, the adrenal medulla also releases two other catecholamines, norepinephrine and dopamine. Epinephrine and norepinephrine released from nerve terminals or the adrenal gland can bind to and activate $\beta_2$-adrenergic receptors on macrophages and monocytes, upregulating secretion of IL-10 and downregulating secretion of TNF. Although $\alpha_2$-adrenergic stimulation can have the opposite effect and increase TNF secretion, activation of the sympathoadrenal axis has anti-inflammatory effects almost exclusively.[49]

## Cholinergic Anti-Inflammatory Pathway

In addition to the fight-or-flight responses of the sympathoadrenal axis, there is another neural pathway that clearly plays a role in modulating innate immune responses. This pathway, which has both afferent and efferent arms and uses the vagus nerve as a conduit, was identified in a series of ground-breaking studies carried out by the neurosurgeon and immunologist, Kevin Tracey.[50] It is now clear that macrophages express a receptor for the neurotransmitter, acetylcholine. This receptor, called the α7 acetylcholine receptor, belongs to the nicotinic subclass of cholinergic receptors. Occupation of this receptor by acetylcholine or a pharmacological nicotinic cholinergic agonist suppresses the secretion of proinflammatory cytokines by immunostimulated macrophages. In experimental animals, stimulating the vagus nerve with an electrode suppresses innate immune responses, whereas sectioning the vagus nerve leads to exacerbation of pathologic inflammatory responses. In extensive preclinical studies, using animal models of human diseases, activation of the cholinergic anti-inflammatory pathway via various means has been shown to ameliorate the manifestations of acute pancreatitis, visceral ischemia-reperfusion injury, hemorrhagic shock, arthritis, and severe sepsis. At present, it is not known whether manipulation of vagal tone or the cholinergic anti-inflammatory pathway can ameliorate human diseases associated with dysregulated inflammation, but is likely that studies to address this topic will be carried out within the next few years.

## SELECTED REFERENCES

Angus DC, Linde-Zwirble WT, Lidicker J, et al: Epidemiology of severe sepsis in the United States: Analysis of incidence, outcome, and associated costs of care. Crit Care Med 29:1303–1310, 2001.

A large observational cohort study that estimates that the incidence of severe sepsis is over 750,000 cases/year in the United States, with an expected growth rate of 1.5%/annum. It is also estimated that 215,000 patients with severe sepsis die annually, a number roughly equal to that associated with acute myocardial infarction.

Bernard GR, Vincent JL, Laterre PF, et al: Efficacy and safety of recombinant human activated protein C for severe sepsis. N Engl J Med 344:699–709, 2001.

Large, multicentric randomized trial demonstrating that treatment with recombinant human activated protein C (rhAPC) reduces mortality in patients with severe sepsis. The incidence of serious bleeding events was higher in the group that received rhAPC, but this did not reach statistical significance.

Bettelli E, Carrier Y, Gao W, et al: Reciprocal developmental pathways for the generation of pathogenic effector Th17 and regulatory T cells. Nature 441: 235–238, 2006.

A landmark paper that identified the key role of IL-6 in the determination of whether naïve T cell exposed to TGF-β will differentiate into Th17 or Treg cells.

Matzinger P: The danger model: A renewed sense of self. Science 296:301–305, 2002.

The classic view of the immune system proposed that an immunologic distinction is made between self and nonself. This article proposes a paradigm shift in this concept. In fact, the immune system may be more concerned with entities that do damage than with those that are foreign, and the release of so-called danger signals from dead or dying cells may alert the immune system to such substances.

Sprung CL, Annane D, Keh D, et al: Hydrocortisone therapy for patients with septic shock. N Engl J Med. 2008; 358:111–124.

Important contribution to the evidence-based critical care literature demonstrating that treatment with low doses of glucocorticosteroids significantly fails to reduce mortality in patients with septic shock.

## REFERENCES


1. Steinman L: A brief history of T(H)17, the first major revision in the T(H)1/T(H)2 hypothesis of T cell-mediated tissue damage. Nat Med 13:139–145, 2007.
2. Matzinger P: The danger model: A renewed sense of self. Science 296:301–305, 2002.
3. Bianchi ME: DAMPs, PAMPs and alarmins: All we need to know about danger. J Leukoc Biol 81:1–5, 2007.
4. Mollen KP, Anand RJ, Tsung A, et al: Emerging paradigm: Toll-like receptor 4-sentinel for the detection of tissue damage. Shock 26:430–437, 2006.
5. Mogensen TH: Pathogen recognition and inflammatory signaling in innate immune defenses. Clin Microbiol Rev 22:240–273, 2009.
6. Yan SF, Ramasamy R, Schmidt AM: Receptor for AGE (RAGE) and its ligands—cast into leading roles in diabetes and the inflammatory response. J Mol Med 87:235–247, 2009.

6a. Wang H, Bloom O, Zhang M, et al: HMG-1 as a late mediator of endotoxin lethality in mice. Science 285:248–251, 1999.

7. Lotze MT, Tracey KJ: High-mobility group box 1 protein (HMGB1): Nuclear weapon in the immune arsenal. Nat Rev Immunol 5:331–342, 2005.
8. Sappington PL, Yang R, Yang H, et al: HMGB1 B box increases the permeability of Caco-2 enterocytic monolayers and impairs intestinal barrier function in mice. Gastroenterology 123:790–802, 2002.
9. Fink MP: Bench-to-bedside review: High-mobility group box 1 and critical illness. Crit Care 11:229, 2007.
10. Peltz ED, Moore EE, Eckels PC, et al: HMGB1 is markedly elevated within 6 hours of mechanical trauma in humans. Shock 32:17–22, 2009.
11. Lantos J, Foldi V, Roth E, et al: Burn trauma induces early HMGB1 release in patients: Its correlation with cytokines. Shock 33:562–567, 2010.
12. Yang R, Harada T, Mollen KP, et al: Anti-HMGB1 neutralizing antibody ameliorates gut barrier dysfunction and improves survival after hemorrhagic shock. Mol Med 12:105–114, 2006.
13. Ulloa L, Ochani M, Yang H, et al: Ethyl pyruvate prevents lethality in mice with established lethal sepsis and systemic inflammation. Proc Natl Acad Sci U S A 99:12351–12356, 2002.
14. Valentino L, Pierre J: JAK-STAT signal transduction: Regulators and implication in hematological malignancies. Biochem Pharmacol 71:713–721, 2006.
15. Bilgin K, Yaramis A, Haspolat K, et al: A randomized trial of granulocyte-macrophage colony-stimulating factor in neonates with sepsis and neutropenia. Pediatrics 107:36–41, 2001.
16. Orozco H, Arch J, Medina-Franco H, et al: Molgramostim (GM-CSF) associated with antibiotic treatment in nontraumatic abdominal sepsis: A randomized, double-blind, placebo-controlled clinical trial. Arch Surg 141:150–153, 2006.
17. Meisel C, Schefold JC, Pschowski R, et al: Granulocyte-macrophage colony-stimulating factor to reverse sepsis-associated immunosuppression: A double-blind, randomized, placebo-controlled multicenter trial. Am J Respir Crit Care Med 180:640–648, 2009.
18. Ogura Y, Bonen DK, Inohara N, et al: A frameshift mutation in NOD2 associated with susceptibility to Crohn's disease. Nature 411:603–606, 2001.
19. Valentine JF, Fedorak RN, Feagan B, et al: Steroid-sparing properties of sargramostim in patients with corticosteroid-dependent Crohn's disease: A randomised, double-blind, placebo-controlled, phase 2 study. Gut 58:1354–1362, 2009.
20. Korzenik JR, Dieckgraefe BK, Valentine JF, et al: Sargramostim for active Crohn's disease. N Engl J Med 352:2193–2201, 2005.
21. McIntire CR, Yeretssian G, Saleh M: Inflammasomes in infection and inflammation. Apoptosis 14:522–535, 2009.
22. Kawai T, Akira S: TLR signaling. Semin Immunol 19:24–32, 2007.
23. Waterer GW, Quasney MW, Cantor RM, et al: Septic shock and respiratory failure in community-acquired pneumonia have different TNF polymorphism associations. Am J Respir Crit Care Med 163:1599–1604, 2001.
24. Berry MA, Hargadon B, Shelley M, et al: Evidence of a role of tumor necrosis factor alpha in refractory asthma. N Engl J Med 354:697–708, 2006.
25. Bernard GR, Vincent JL, Laterre PF, et al: Efficacy and safety of recombinant human activated protein C for severe sepsis. N Engl J Med 344:699–709, 2001.
26. Castelli EE, Culley CM, Fink MP: Challenge and rechallenge: Drotrecogin alfa (activated)-induced prolongation of activated partial thromboplastin time in a patient with severe sepsis. Pharmacotherapy 25:1147–1150, 2005.
27. Abraham E, Laterre PF, Garg R, et al: Drotrecogin alfa (activated) for adults with severe sepsis and a low risk of death. N Engl J Med 353:1332–1341, 2005.
28. Goldstein B, Nadel S, Peters M, et al: ENHANCE: Results of a global open-label trial of drotrecogin alfa (activated) in children with severe sepsis. Pediatr Crit Care Med 7:200–211, 2006.
29. Cuzzocrea S, Mazzon E, Dugo L, et al: Absence of endogenous interleukin-6 enhances the inflammatory response during acute pancreatitis induced by cerulein in mice. Cytokine 18:274–285, 2002.
30. Yang R, Han X, Uchiyama T, et al: IL-6 is essential for development of gut barrier dysfunction after hemorrhagic shock and

resuscitation in mice. Am J Physiol Gastrointest Liver Physiol 285:G621–629, 2003.

**31.** Opal SM, Keith JC Jr, Jhung J, et al: Orally administered recombinant human interleukin-11 is protective in experimental neutropenic sepsis. J Infect Dis 187:70–76, 2003.

**31a.** Yoshimura T, Matsushima K, Tanaka S, et al: Purification of a human monocyte-derived neutrophil chemotactic factor that has peptide sequence similarity to other host defense cytokines. Proc Natl Acad Sci U S A 84:9233–9237, 1987.

**32.** Emmanuilidis K, Weighardt H, Matevossian E, et al: Differential regulation of systemic IL-18 and IL-12 release during postoperative sepsis: high serum IL-18 as an early predictive indicator of lethal outcome. Shock 18:301–305, 2002.

**33.** Weighardt H, Heidecke CD, Westerholt A, et al: Impaired monocyte IL-12 production before surgery as a predictive factor for the lethal outcome of postoperative sepsis. Ann Surg 235:560–567, 2002.

**34.** Hunter CA: New IL-12-family members: IL-23 and IL-27, cytokines with divergent functions. Nat Rev Immunol 5:521–531, 2005.

**34a.** Yao Z, Painter SL, Fanslow WC, et al: Human IL-17: a novel cytokine derived from T cells. J Immunol 155:5483–5486, 1995.

**34b.** Mossmann TR, Coffman RL: Two types of mouse helper T-cell clone. Immunol Today 8:223–227, 1987.

**35.** Korn T, Bettelli E, Oukka M, et al: IL-17 and Th17 Cells. Annu Rev Immunol 27:485–517, 2009.

**36.** Kawaguchi M, Adachi M, Oda N, et al: IL-17 cytokine family. J Allergy Clin Immunol 114:1265–1273; quiz 1274, 2004.

**37.** Flierl MA, Rittirsch D, Gao H, et al: Adverse functions of IL-17A in experimental sepsis. FASEB J 22:2198–2205, 2008.

**38.** Guo RF, Ward PA: Role of C5a in inflammatory responses. Annu Rev Immunol 23:821–852, 2005.

**39.** Bresalier RS, Sandler RS, Quan H, et al: Cardiovascular events associated with rofecoxib in a colorectal adenoma chemoprevention trial. N Engl J Med 352:1092–1102, 2005.

**40.** Curfman GD, Morrissey S, Drazen JM: Expression of concern: Bombardier et al., "Comparison of upper gastrointestinal toxicity of rofecoxib and naproxen in patients with rheumatoid arthritis," N Engl J Med 2000;343:1520–1528. N Engl J Med 353:2813–2814, 2005.

**41.** Razavi HM, Werhun R, Scott JA, et al: Effects of inhaled nitric oxide in a mouse model of sepsis-induced acute lung injury. Crit Care Med 30:868–873, 2002.

**42.** Fink MP: Cytopathic hypoxia. Mitochondrial dysfunction as mechanism contributing to organ dysfunction in sepsis. Crit Care Clin 17:219–237, 2001.

**43.** Lowicka E, Beltowski J: Hydrogen sulfide ($H_2S$)—the third gas of interest for pharmacologists. Pharmacol Rep 59:4–24, 2007.

**44.** Macias CA, Chiao JW, Xiao J, et al: Treatment with a novel hemigramicidin-TEMPO conjugate prolongs survival in a rat model of lethal hemorrhagic shock. Ann Surg 245:305–314, 2007.

**45.** Prigent H, Maxime V, Annane D: Clinical review: Corticotherapy in sepsis. Crit Care 8:122–129, 2004.

**46.** Annane D, Sebille V, Charpentier C, et al: Effect of treatment with low doses of hydrocortisone and fludrocortisone on mortality in patients with septic shock. JAMA 288:862–871, 2002.

**47.** Sprung CL, Annane D, Keh D, et al: Hydrocortisone therapy for patients with septic shock. N Engl J Med 358:111–124, 2008.

**48.** Steinberg KP, Hudson LD, Goodman RB, et al: Efficacy and safety of corticosteroids for persistent acute respiratory distress syndrome. N Engl J Med 354:1671–1684, 2006.

**49.** Pavlov VA, Tracey KJ: Neural regulators of innate immune responses and inflammation. Cell Mol Life Sci 61:2322–2331, 2004.

**50.** Tracey KJ: Physiology and immunology of the cholinergic antiinflammatory pathway. J Clin Invest 117:289–296, 2007.

# CHAPTER 5

# SHOCK, ELECTROLYTES, AND FLUID

Peter Rhee

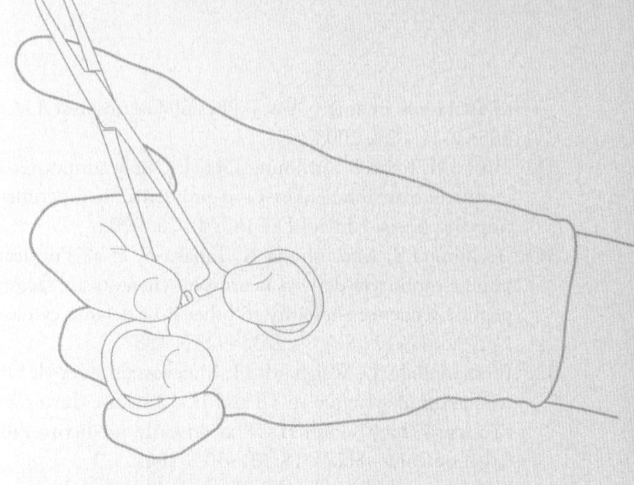



Surgeons are the masters of fluids because they need to be. They care for patients who cannot eat or drink for various reasons—for example, they have hemorrhaged, undergone surgery, or lost fluids from tubes, drains, or wounds. Surgeons are obligated to know how to care for these patients, as they have put their lives in our hands. This topic might appear simple only for those who do not understand the complexities of the human body and its ability to regulate and compensate fluids. In reality, the task of managing patients' blood volume is one of the most challenging burdens surgeons face, often requiring complete control of the intake and output of fluids and electrolytes, often in the presence of blood loss. Surgeons do not yet completely understand the physiology of shock and resuscitation, and our knowledge is superficial. Given the nature of our profession, we have studied fluids and electrolytes as we dealt with patients who have bled and even exsanguinate. Historically, wartime experience has always helped us move ahead in our knowledge of the management of fluids and resuscitation are no exceptions as we have learned much from them as well. The current wars in Iraq and Afghanistan.

Constant attention to, and titration of, fluid loss therapy is required, because the human body is dynamic. The key to treatment is to realize the patient's initial condition and understand that the fluid status is constantly changing. Bleeding, sepsis, neuroendocrine disturbances, and dysfunctional regulatory systems can all affect patients who are undergoing the dynamic changes of illness and healing. The correct management of blood volume is highly time-dependent. If managed well, surgeons are afforded the chance to deal with other aspects of surgery, such as nutrition, administration of antibiotics, drainage of abscesses, relief of obstruction and incarceration, treatment of ischemia, and resection of tumors. Knowing the difference among dehydration, anemia, hemorrhage, and overresuscitation is vital.

The human body is predominantly water, which resides in the intravascular, intracellular, and interstitial (or third) spaces. Water moves among these spaces and depends on many variables. Because surgeons can only control the intravascular space, this chapter will concentrate on the correct management of the intravascular space, because this is the only means to control the other two fluid compartments.

This chapter will also examine historical aspects of shock, fluids, and electrolytes—not just to note interesting facts or pay tribute to deserving physicians, but also to try to understand how this knowledge was gained. Doing so is vital to understanding past changes in management and to accept future changes. Surgeons are often awed at the discoveries made, yet also astounded by how often they were wrong, and why. Future surgeons will look back at the current body of knowledge and be amazed at how little was known. Recent changes in the management of shock, fluids, and electrolytes have been major ones. Knowledge of the history helps explain why these changes were required. As a consequence of not studying the past, we have often repeated history in many ways.

After the historical highlights, this chapter will discuss fluids that are now used, along with fluids under development. Finally, caring for perioperative patients will be explored from a daily needs perspective.

## HISTORY

History may be disliked by those who are in a hurry to learn only the basics. Learning from the past, however, is essential, to know treatments that have and have not worked. Dogma must always be challenged and questioned. Were the treatments based on science? To understand what to do, surgeons must know how the practice evolved to the current management methods. Studying the history of shock is important for at least three reasons:

1. Physicians and physiologists have been fascinated with blood loss out of necessity.
2. Experiments that have been carried out need to be reassessed.
3. It is necessary to know more, because the current understanding of shock is elementary.

### Resuscitation

One of the earliest authenticated resuscitations in the medical literature is the miraculous deliverance of Anne Green, who was executed by hanging on December 14, 1650. Green was executed in the customary way by being forced off a ladder to hang by the neck. She hung for 30 minutes, during which time some of her friends pulled "with all their weight upon her legs, sometimes lifting her up, and then pulling her down again with a sudden jerk, thereby the sooner to dispatch her out of her pain"[1]

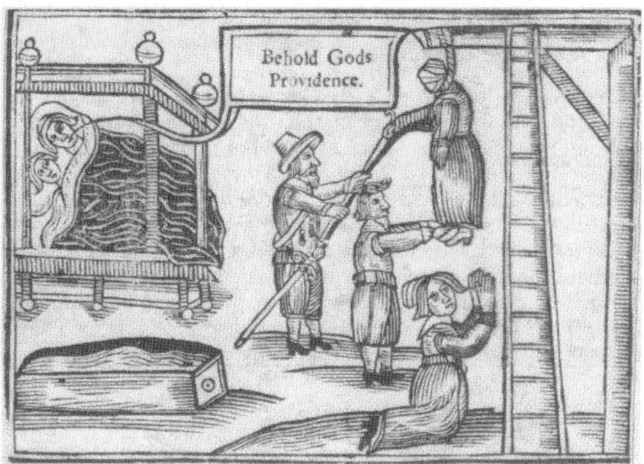


**FIGURE 5-1** Miraculous deliverance of Anne Green, who was executed in 1650. (From Hughes JT: Miraculous deliverance of Anne Green: an Oxford case of resuscitation in the seventeenth century. Br Med J [Clin Res Ed] 285:1792–1793, 1982; by kind permission of the Bodleian Library, Oxford.)

(Fig. 5-1). When everyone thought she was dead, the body was taken down, put in a coffin, and carried to the private house of Dr. William Petty—who, by the king's orders, was allowed to perform autopsies on the bodies of everyone who had been executed.

When the coffin was opened, Green was observed to take a breath and a rattle was heard in her throat. Petty and his colleague, Thomas Willis, abandoned all thoughts of a dissection and proceeded to revive their patient. They held her up in the coffin and then, by wrenching her teeth apart, poured hot cordial into her mouth, which caused her to cough. They rubbed and chafed her fingers, hands, arms, and feet; after 15 minutes of these efforts, they put more cordial into her mouth. Then, after tickling her throat with a feather, she opened her eyes momentarily.

At that stage, they opened a vein and bled 5 ounces of blood. They continued administering the cordial and rubbing her arms and legs. Next, they applied compression bandages to her arms and legs. Heating plasters were put to her chest, and another plaster was inserted as an enema "to give heat and warmth to her bowels." They then put her in a warm bed, with another woman to lie with her to keep her warm. After 12 hours, Green began to speak; 24 hours after her revival, she was answering questions freely. After 2 days, her memory was normal, apart from her recollection of her execution and the resuscitation.

## Shock

Hemorrhagic shock has been extensively studied and written about for many years. Injuries, whether intentional or not, have occurred so frequently that much of the understanding of shock has been learned by surgeons taking care of the injured.

What is shock? The current widely accepted definition is inadequate perfusion of tissue. However, many subtleties lie behind this statement. Nutrients for cells are required, but which nutrients are not well defined at this point. The most critical nutrient is oxygen, but concentrating on oxygenation alone probably represents elemental thinking. Blood is highly complex and carries countless nutrients, buffers, cells, antibodies, hormones, chemicals, electrolytes, and antitoxins. Even if we think in an elemental fashion and try to optimize the perfusion of tissue, the delivery side of the equation is affected by blood volume, anemia, and cardiac output. Moreover, the use of nutrients is affected by infection and drugs. The vascular tone plays a role as well; for example, in neurogenic shock, the sympathetic tone is lost and, in sepsis, systemic vascular resistance decreases, because of a broken homeostatic process or possibly because of evolutionary factors.

Many advances in medicine have been achieved by battlefield observations. Unfortunately, in military and civilian trauma, hemorrhagic shock is the leading cause of preventable death. Repeatedly, wounded patients have survived their initial injuries, with adequate control of the hemorrhage, only to undergo malaise and deterioration, resulting in death. Such cases led to many explanations; most observers theorized a circulating toxic agent, thought to be secondary to the initial insult. The first record available that shows an understanding of the need for fluid in injured patients was apparently from Ambroise Paré (1510-1590), who urged the use of clysters (enemas to administer fluid into the rectum) to prevent "noxious vapors from mounting to the brain." Yet, he also wrote that phlebotomy is "required in great wounds when there is fear of deflexion, pain, delirium, raving, and unquietness"; he and others practiced bloodletting during that era, because shock accompanying injury was thought to be from toxins.

The term *shock* appears to have been first used in 1743 in a translation of the French treatise of Henri Francois Le Dran regarding battlefield wounds. He used the term to designate the act of impact or collision, rather than the resulting functional and physiologic damage. However, the term can be found in the book *Gunshot Wounds of the Extremities*, published in 1815 by Guthrie, who used it to describe the physiologic instability.

Humoral theories persisted until the late 19th century but, in 1830, Herman provided one of the first clear descriptions of intravenous (IV) fluid therapy. In response to a cholera epidemic, he attempted to rehydrate patients by injecting 6 ounces of water into the vein. In 1831, O'Shaughnessy also treated cholera patients by administering large volumes of salt solutions intravenously and published his results in *Lancet*.[2] Those were the first documented attempts to replace and maintain the extracellular internal environment or the intravascular volume. Note, however, that the treatment of cholera and dehydration is not the ideal treatment of hemorrhagic shock.

In 1872, Gross defined shock as "a manifestation of the rude unhinging of the machinery of life." His definition, given its accuracy and descriptiveness, has been repeatedly quoted in the literature. Theories on the cause of shock persisted through the late 19th century; although it was unexplainable, it was often observed. George Washington Crile investigated it and concluded, at the beginning of his career, that the lowering of the central venous pressure in the shock state in animal experiments was caused by a failure of the autonomic nervous system.[3] Surgeons witnessed a marked change in ideas about shock between 1888 and 1918. In the late 1880s, there were no all-encompassing theories, but most surgeons accepted the generalization that shock resulted from a malfunctioning of some part of the nervous system. Such a malfunctioning has now been shown *not* to be the main reason—but surgeons are still perplexed by the mechanisms of hemorrhagic shock, especially regarding the complete breakdown of the circulatory system that occurs in the later stages of shock.

In 1899, using contemporary advances with sphygmomanometers, Crile proposed that a profound decline in blood pressure (BP) could account for all symptoms of shock. He also helped alter how physicians diagnosed shock and followed its course. Before Crile, most surgeons relied on respiration, pulse, or declining mental status when evaluating the condition of patients. After Crile's first books were published, many surgeons began measuring BP. In addition to changing how surgeons thought about shock, Crile was part of the therapeutic revolution. His theories remained generally accepted for almost 2 decades, predominantly in surgical circles. Crile's work persuaded Harvey Cushing to measure BP during all operations, which in part led to the general acceptance of BP measurement in clinical medicine. Crile also concluded that shock was not a process of dying, but rather a marshaling of the body's defenses in patients struggling to live. He later deduced that the reduced volume of circulating blood, rather than the diminished BP, was the most critical factor in shock.

Crile was instrumental in forming numerous theories of shock but was also known for the "anoci-association" theory of shock, which accounted for pain and its physiologic response during surgery. He realized that the constant administration of nitrous oxide during surgery was required, which necessitated having an additional professional at the operating table—the skilled nurse anesthetist. In 1908, he trained Agatha Hodgins, one of his nurses at Western Reserve, who later founded the American Association of Nurse Anesthetists.

Crile's theories evolved as he continued his experimentations; in 1913, he proposed the kinetic system theory. He was interested in thyroid hormone and its response to wounds, but realized that adrenalin was a key component of the response to shock. He relied on experiments by Walter B. Cannon, who found that adrenalin was released in response to pain or emotion, shifting blood from the intestines to the brain and extremities. Adrenalin release also stimulated the liver to convert glycogen to sugar for release into the circulation. Cannon argued that all the actions of adrenalin aided the animal in its effort to defend itself.[4]

Crile incorporated Cannon's study into his theory. He proposed that impulses from the brain after injury stimulated glands to secrete their hormones, which in turn resulted in sweeping changes throughout the body. Crile's kinetic system included a complex interrelationship among the brain, heart, lungs, blood vessels, muscles, thyroid gland, and liver. He also noted that if the body underwent too much stress, the adrenal glands would run out of adrenalin, the liver of glycogen, the thyroid of its hormone, and the brain itself of energy, accounting for autonomic changes. Once the kinetic system ran out of energy, BP would fall, and the animal would go into shock.

At the end of the 19th century, surgeons for the most part used a wide variety of tonics, stimulants, and drugs. Through careful testing, Crile demonstrated that most of those agents were ineffective, stressing that only saline solutions, adrenalin, blood transfusions, and safer forms of anesthesia were beneficial for treating shock. In addition, he vigorously campaigned against the customary approach of polypharmacy, instead promoting only drugs of proven value. He stated that stimulants, long a mainstay of treatment in shock, did not raise BP and should be discarded: "a surgeon should not stimulate an exhausted vasomotor center with strychnine. That would be as futile as flogging a dead horse."

**BOX 5-1 Causes of Shock (According to Blalock)**

- Hematogenic (oligemia)
- Neurogenic (caused primarily by nervous influences)
- Vasogenic (initially decreased vascular resistance and increased vascular capacity, as in sepsis)
- Cardiogenic (failure of the heart as a pump, as in cardiac tamponade or myocardial infarction)
- Large volume loss (extracellular fluid, as in patients with diarrhea, vomiting, and fistula drainage)

Data from Blalock A: Principles of surgical care: Shock and other problems, St Louis, 1940, CV Mosby.

Henderson recognized the importance of decreased venous return and its effect on cardiac output and arterial pressure. His work was aided by advances in techniques that allowed careful recording of the volume curves of the ventricles. Fat embolism also led to a shocklike state, but its possible contribution was questioned because study results were difficult to reproduce. The vasomotor center and its contributions in shock were heavily studied in the early 1900s. In 1914, Mann noted that unilaterally innervated vessels of the tongues of dogs, ears of rabbits, and paws of kittens appeared constricted during shock, as compared with contralaterally denervated vessels.

Battlefield experiences continued to intensify research on shock. During the World War I era, Cannon used clinical data from the war and data from animal experiments to examine the shock state carefully. He theorized that toxins and acidosis contributed to the previously described lowering of vascular tone. He and others then focused on acidosis and the role of alkali in preventing and prolonging shock. The adrenal gland and effect of cortical extracts on adrenalectomized animals were studied with fascination during this period.

Then, in the 1930s, a unique set of experiments by Blalock[5] determined that almost all acute injuries were associated with changes in fluid and electrolyte metabolism. Such changes were primarily the result of reductions in the effective circulating blood volume. Blalock showed that those reductions after injury could be the result of several mechanisms (Box 5-1). He clearly showed that fluid loss in injured tissues involved the loss of extracellular fluid (ECF) that was unavailable to the intravascular space for maintaining circulation. The original concept of a "third space," in which fluid is sequestered and therefore unavailable to the intravascular space, evolved from Blalock's studies.

Carl John Wiggers first described the concept of irreversible shock.[6] His 1950 textbook, *Physiology of Shock,* represented the attitudes toward shock at that time. In an exceptionally brilliant summation, Wiggers assembled the various signs and symptoms of shock from various authors in that textbook (Fig. 5-2), along with his own findings. His experiments used what is now known as the Wiggers prep. In his usual experiments, he used previously splenectomized dogs and cannulated their arterial systems. He took advantage of an evolving technology that allowed him to measure the pressure in the arterial system, and he studied the effects of lowering BP through blood withdrawal. After removing the dogs' blood to an arbitrary set point (typically, 40 mm Hg), he noted that their BP soon spontaneously rose as fluid was spontaneously recruited into the intravascular space.

SYMPTOM COMPLEX OF SHOCK

**General appearance and reactions**

*Mental state*
Apathy
Delayed responses
Depressed cerebration
Weak voice
Listless or restlessness

*Countenance*
Drawn–anxious
Lusterless eyes
Sunken eyeballs
Ptosis of upper lids (slight)
Upward rotation of eyeballs (slight)

*Neuromuscular state*
Hypotonia
Muscular weakness
Tremors and twitchings
Involuntary muscular movements
Difficulty in swallowing

*Neuromuscular tests*
Depressed tendon reflexes
Depressed sensibilities
Depressed visual and auditory reflexes

*General but variable symptoms*
Thirst
Vomiting
Diarrhea
Oliguria
Visible or occult blood in vomitus, and stools

**Skin and mucous membranes**

*Skin*
Pale, livid, ashen gray
Slightly cyanotic
Moist, clammy
Mottling of dependent parts
Loose, dry, inelastic, cold

*Mucous membranes*
Pale, livid, slightly cyanotic

*Conjunctiva*
Glazed, lusterless

*Tongue*
Dry, pale, parched, shriveled

**Respiration and metabolism**

*Respiration*
Variable but not dyspneic
Usually increased rate
Variable depth
Occasional deep sighs
Sometimes irregular or phasic

*Temperature*
Subnormal, normal, supernormal

*Basal metabolic rate*
reduced (?)

**Circulation and blood**

*Superficial veins*
Collapsed and invisible
Failure to fill on compression or massage
Inconspicuous jugular pulsations

*Heart*
Apex sounds feeble
Rate, usually rapid

*Radial pulse*
Usually rapid
Small volume "feeble," "thready"

*Brachial blood pressures*
Lowered
Pulse pressure small

*Retinal vessels*
Narrowed

*Blood volume*
Reduced

*Blood chemistry*
Hemoconcentration or hemodilution
Venous $O_2$ decreased
A-V $O_2$ difference increased
Arterial $CO_2$ reduced
Alkali reserve reduced

**FIGURE 5-2** Wiggers' description of symptom complex of shock. (From Wiggers CJ: Present status of shock problem. Physiol Rev 22:74, 1942.)

To keep the dogs' BP at 40 mm Hg, Wiggers had to continually withdraw additional blood during this compensated stage of shock. During compensated shock, the dogs could use their reserves to survive. Water was recruited from the intracellular compartment as well as the extracellular space. The body tried to maintain the vascular flow necessary to survive. However, after a certain period, he found that to keep the dogs' BP at the arbitrary set point of 40 mm Hg, he had to reinfuse shed blood; he termed this phase *uncompensated* or *irreversible shock.* Eventually, after a period of irreversible shock, the dogs died.

If the dogs had not yet gone into the uncompensated phase, any type of fluid used for resuscitation would have made survival likely. In fact, most dogs at that stage, even without resuscitation, would self-resuscitate by going to a water source. Once they entered the uncompensated phase of shock, however, their reserves were exhausted; even if blood were given back, survival rates were better if additional fluid of some sort was administered. Uncompensated shock is surely what Gross meant by "unhinging of the machinery of life." Currently, hemorrhagic shock models are classified as involving controlled or uncontrolled hemorrhage. The Wiggers prep is controlled hemorrhage and is referred to as pressure-controlled hemorrhage.

Another animal model that uses controlled hemorrhage is the volume-controlled model. Arguments against this model include the inconsistency of the blood volume from one animal to another and the variability in response. Calculating blood volume is usually based on a percentage of body weight (typically, 7% of body weight), but such percentages are not exact and result in variability from one animal to another. However, proponents of the volume model and critics of the pressure model argue that a certain pressure during hypotension elicits a different response from one animal to another. Even in the pressure-controlled hemorrhage model, animals vary highly in regard to when they go from compensated to uncompensated shock. The pressure typically used in the pressure-controlled model is 40 mm Hg; the volume used in the volume-controlled model is 40%. The variance in the volume-controlled model can be minimized by specifying a narrow weight range for the animals (e.g., rats within 10 g, large animals within 5 pounds). It is also important to have the same experimenters doing the exact same procedure at the same time of the day in animals that were prepared and hydrated in exactly the same way.

The ideal model is uncontrolled hemorrhage, but its main problem is that the volume of hemorrhage is uncontrolled by the nature of the experiment. Variability is the highest in this model, even though it is the most realistic. Computer-assisted pressure models can be used that mimic the pressures during uncontrolled shock to reduce the artificiality of the pressure-controlled model.

## Fluids

How did the commonly used IV fluids, such as normal saline, enter medical practice? It is often taken for granted, given the vast body of knowledge in medicine, that they were adopted through a rigorous scientific process but that was not actually the case.

Normal saline has been used for many years and is extremely beneficial, but we now know that it also can be harmful. Hartog Jakob Hamburger, in his in vitro studies of red cell lysis in 1882, incorrectly suggested that 0.9% saline was the concentration of salt in human blood. This fluid is often referred to as physiologic or normal saline, but it is neither physiologic nor normal. Supposedly, 0.9% normal saline originated during the cholera pandemic that afflicted Europe in 1831, but an examination of the composition of the fluids used by physicians of that era found no resemblance to normal saline. The origin of the concept of normal saline remains unclear.[7]

In 1831, O'Shaughnessy described his experience in the treatment of cholera[8]:

> Universal stagnation of the venous system, and rapid cessation of the arterialization of the blood, are the earliest, as well as the most characteristic effects. Hence the skin becomes blue—hence animal heat is no longer generated—hence the secretions are suspended; the arteries contain black blood, no carbonic acid is evolved from the lungs, and the returned air of expiration is cold as when it enters these organs.

O'Shaughnessy wrote those words at the age of 22, having just graduated from Edinburgh Medical School. He tested his new method of infusing intravenous saline on a dog and observed no ill effects. Eventually, he reported that the aim of his method was to restore blood to its natural specific gravity and to restore its deficient saline matters. His experience with human cholera patients taught him that the practice of bloodletting, then highly common, was good for "diminishing the venous congestion" and that nitrous oxide (laughing gas) was not useful for oxygenation.

In 1832, Robert Lewins reported that he witnessed Thomas Latta injecting extraordinary quantities of saline into veins, with the immediate effects of "restoring the natural current in the veins and arteries, of improving the color of the blood, and [of] recovering the functions of the lungs." Lewins described Latta's saline solution as consisting of "two drachms of muriate, and two scruples of carbonate, of soda, to sixty ounces of water." Later, however, Latta's solution was found to equate to having

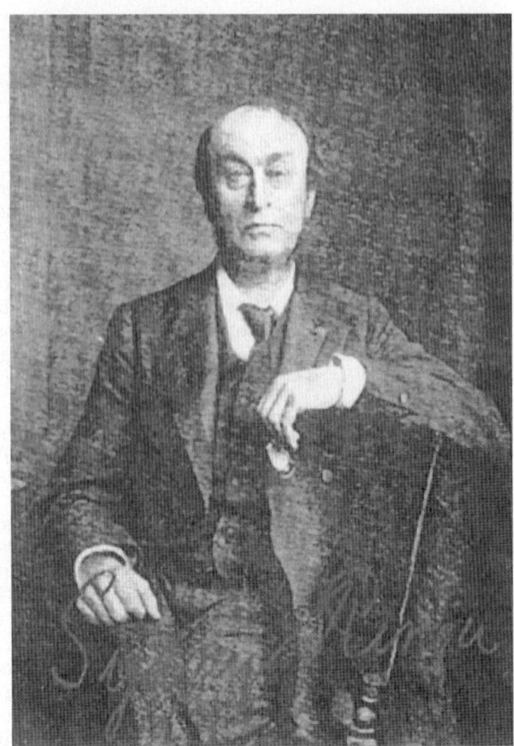

**FIGURE 5-3** Sydney Ringer, credited for the development of lactated Ringer's solution. (From Baskett TF: Sydney Ringer and lactated Ringers's solution. Resuscitation 58:5–7, 2003.)

134 mmol/liter of $Na^+$, 118 mmol/liter of $Cl^-$, and 16 mmol/liter of $HCO_3^-$.

Over the next 50 years, many reports cited various recipes to treat cholera, but none resembled 0.9% saline. In 1883, Sydney Ringer reported on the influence exerted by the constituents of the blood on the contractions of the ventricle (Fig. 5-3). Studying hearts cut out of frogs, he used 0.75% saline and a blood mixture made from dried bullocks' blood.[9] In his attempts to identify which aspect of blood caused better results, he found that a "small quantity of white of egg completely obviates the changes occurring with saline solution." He concluded that the benefit of white of egg was because of the albumin or potassium chloride. To show what worked and what did not, he described endless experiments, with alterations of multiple variables.

However, Ringer later published another article stating that his previously reported findings could not be repeated; through careful study, he realized that the water used in his first article was actually not distilled water, as reported, but rather tap water from the New River Water Company. It turned out that his laboratory technician, who was paid to distill the water, took shortcuts and used tap water instead. Ringer analyzed the water and found that it contained many trace minerals (Fig. 5-4). Through careful and diligent experimentation, he found that calcium bicarbonate or calcium chloride—in doses even smaller than those in blood—restored good contractions of the frog ventricles. The third component that he found essential to good contractions was sodium bicarbonate. He knew the importance of the trace elements. He also stated that fish could live for weeks unfed in tap water, but would die in distilled water in a few hours; minnows, for example, died in an average of 4.5 hours.

| They consist of: | | |
|---|---|---|
| Calcium | 38.3 | per million. |
| Magnesium | 4.5 | " |
| Sodium | 23.3 | " |
| Potassium | 7.1 | " |
| Combined carbonic acid | 78.2 | " |
| Sulphuric acid | 55.8 | " |
| Chlorine | 15 | " |
| Silicates | 7.1 | " |
| Free carbonic acid | 54.2 | " |

**FIGURE 5-4** Sidney Ringer's report of contents in water from the New River Water company. (From Baskett TF: Sydney Ringer and lactated Ringers's solution. Resuscitation 58:5–7, 2003.)

Thus, the three ingredients that he found essential were potassium, calcium, and bicarbonate. Ringer's solution soon became ubiquitous in physiologic laboratory experiments.

In the early 20th century, fluid therapy by injection under the skin (hypodermoclysis) and infusion into the rectum (proctoclysis) became routine. Hartwell and Hoguet reported its use in intestinal obstruction in dogs, laying the foundation for saline therapy in human patients with intestinal obstruction.

As IV crystalloid solutions were developed, Ringer's solution was modified, most notably by pediatrician Alexis Hartmann. In 1932, attempting to develop an alkalinizing solution to administer to his acidotic patients, Hartmann modified Ringer's solution by adding sodium lactate. The result was lactated Ringer's (LR), or Hartmann's solution. He used sodium lactate (instead of sodium bicarbonate)—the conversion of lactate into sodium bicarbonate was slow enough to lessen the danger posed by sodium bicarbonate, which could rapidly shift patients from compensated acidosis to uncompensated alkalosis.

In 1924, Rudolph Matas, regarded as the originator of modern fluid treatment, introduced the concept of the continued IV drip but also warned of the potential dangers of saline infusions. He stated that "Normal saline has continued to gain popularity but the problems with metabolic derangements have been repeatedly shown but seem to have fallen on deaf ears." In healthy volunteers, normal saline has been shown to cause abdominal discomfort and pain, nausea, drowsiness, and decreased mental capacity to perform complex tasks.

The point is that normal saline and LR solutions have been formulated for conditions other than the replacement of blood, and the reasons for the formulation are archaic. Such solutions have been useful for dehydration; when used in relatively small volumes (1 to 3 liters/day), they are well tolerated and relatively harmless, they provide water, and the human body can tolerate the amounts of electrolytes they contain. Over the years, LR has attained widespread use for the treatment of hemorrhagic shock. However, normal saline and LR are mostly permeable through the vascular membrane, but are poorly retained in the vascular space. After a few hours, only about 175 to 200 mL of a 1-liter infusion remains in the intravascular space. In countries other than the United States, LR is often referred to as Hartmann's solution, and normal saline is referred to as physiologic (sometimes even spelled "fisiologic") solution. With the advances in science in the last 50 years, it is hard to understand why more advances in resuscitation fluids have not been made.

## Blood Transfusions

Concerned about the blood that injured patients lost, Crile began to experiment with blood transfusions. As he stated, "After many accidents, profuse hemorrhage often led to shock before the patient reached the hospital. Saline solutions, adrenalin, and precise surgical technique could substitute only up to a point for the lost blood." At the turn of the 19th century, transfusions were seldom used. Their use waxed and waned in popularity because of transfusion reactions and difficulties in preventing clotting in donated blood. Through his experiments in dogs, Crile showed that blood was interchangeable: he transfused blood without blood group matching. Alexis Carrel was able to sew blood vessels together with his triangulation technique, using it to connect blood vessels from one person to another for the purpose of transfusions. However, Crile found Carrel's technique too slow and cumbersome in humans, so he developed a short cannula to facilitate transfusions.

By World War II, shock was recognized as the single most common cause of treatable morbidity and mortality. At the time of the Japanese attack on Pearl Harbor on December 7, 1941, no blood banks or effectual blood transfusion facilities were available. Most military locations had no stocks of dried pooled plasma. Although the wounded of that era were evacuated quickly to a hospital, the mortality rate was still high. IV fluids of any type were essentially unavailable, except for a few liters of saline manufactured by means of a still in the operating room. IV fluid was usually administered using an old Salvesen flask and reused rubber tubing. Often, a severe febrile reaction resulted from the use of that tubing.

The first written documentation of resuscitation in World War II patients was 1 year after Pearl Harbor, in December 1942, in notes from the 77th Evacuation Hospital in North Africa. Churchill stated that "The wounded in action had for the most part either succumbed or recovered from any existing shock before we saw them. However, later cases came to us in shock, and some of the early cases were found to be in need of whole blood transfusion. There was plenty of reconstituted blood plasma available. However, some cases were in dire need of whole blood. We had no transfusion sets, although such are available in the United States: no sodium citrate; no sterile distilled water; and no blood donors."

The initial decision to rely on plasma rather than blood appears to have been based in part on the view held by the Office of the Surgeon General of the Army, and in part on the opinion of the civilian investigators of the National Research Council. Those civilian investigators thought that in shock, the blood was thick and the hematocrit level high. On April 8, 1943, the Surgeon General stated that no blood would be sent to the combat zone. Seven months later, he again refused to send blood overseas because of the following: (1) his observations of overseas theaters had convinced him that plasma was adequate for the resuscitation of wounded men; (2) from a logistics standpoint, it was impractical to make locally collected blood more available than that from general hospitals in the combat zone; and (3) shipping space was too small. Vasoconstricting drugs such as adrenalin were condemned because they were thought to decrease blood flow and tissue perfusion as they dammed the blood in the arterial portion of the circulatory system.

**Table 5-1 Four Classes of Hemorrhagic Shock***

| | Class | | | |
|---|---|---|---|---|
| **PARAMETER** | **I** | **II** | **III** | **IV** |
| Blood loss (%) | 0-15 | 15-30 | 30-40 | >40 |
| Central nervous system | Slightly anxious | Mildly anxious | Anxious or confused | Confused or lethargic |
| Pulse (beats/min) | <100 | >100 | >120 | >140 |
| Blood pressure | Normal | Normal | Decreased | Decreased |
| Pulse pressure | Normal | Decreased | Decreased | Decreased |
| Respiratory rate | 14-20/min | 20-30/min | 30-40/min | >35/min |
| Urine (mL/hr) | >30 | 20-30 | 5-15 | Negligible |
| Fluid | Crystalloid | Crystalloid | Crystalloid + blood | Crystalloid + blood |

*According to the ATLS course.

During World War II, out of necessity, efforts to make blood transfusions available heightened and led to the institution of blood banking for transfusions. Better understanding of hypovolemia and inadequate circulation favored the use of plasma as a resuscitative solution, in addition to whole blood replacement. Thus, the treatment of traumatic shock greatly improved. The administration of whole blood was thought to be extremely effective, so it was widely used. Mixed with sodium citrate in a 6:1 ratio to bind the calcium in the blood, which prevented clotting, worked well.

However, no matter which solution was used—blood, colloids, or crystalloids—the blood volume seemed to increase by only a fraction of what was lost. In the Korean War era, it was recognized that more blood had to be infused to regain the blood volume that was lost adequately. The reason for the need for more blood was unclear, but was thought to be because of hemolysis, pooling of blood in certain capillary beds, and loss of fluid into tissues. Considerable attention was given to elevating the feet of patients in shock.

## PHYSIOLOGY OF SHOCK

### Bleeding

Research and experience have both taught us much about the physiologic responses to bleeding. The Advanced Trauma Life Support (ATLS) course defines four classes of shock (Table 5-1). In general, that categorization has helped point out the physiologic responses to hemorrhagic shock, emphasizing the identification of blood loss and guiding treatment. Shock can be thought of anatomically at three levels (Fig. 5-5). It can be cardiogenic, with extrinsic abnormalities (e.g., tamponade) or intrinsic abnormalities (e.g., pump failure caused by infarct, overall cardiac failure, or contusion). Large vessels can cause shock if they are injured and bleeding results. If the anatomic problem is at the small vessel level, neurogenic dysfunction or sepsis can be the culprit.

The four classes of shock as taught in the ATLS course are problematic because they were not rigorously tested and proven. The developers of the ATLS course have agreed that these classes were fairly arbitrary and not necessarily based on rigorous scientific data. Patients in shock do not always follow the physiology as taught in the ATLS course, and a high degree of variance exists among patients, particularly in children and older patients. Children, in general, seem to be able to compensate, even after large volumes of blood loss, because of the higher water composition of their bodies. However, when they decompensate, the process can be rapid. Older patients do not compensate well; when they start to collapse physiologically, the process can be devastating because their ability to recruit fluid is not as good and their cardiac reserves are less.

The problem with the signs and symptoms classically shown in the ATLS classes is that in reality, the manifestations of shock can be confusing and difficult to assess. For example, consider whether an individual patient's change in mental status is caused by factors such as blood loss, traumatic brain injury (TBI), pain, or illicit drugs. The same dilemma applies for respiratory rate and skin changes. Are alterations in a patient's respiratory rate or skin caused by factors such as pneumothorax, rib fractures, or inhalation injury?

To date, despite the many potential methods of monitoring shock, none has been found clinically reliable for replacing BP. Clinicians all know that there is a wide range of normal BPs. The question often is this: What is the baseline BP of the patient being treated? When a seemingly normal BP is treated, is that hypotension or hypertension compared with the patient's normal BP? How do we know how much blood has been lost? Even if blood volume is measured directly (rapid methods are now available), what was the patient's baseline blood volume? To what blood volume should the patient be resuscitated? The end point of resuscitation has been elusive. The variance in all the variables makes assessment and treatment a challenge.

One important factor to recognize is that clinical symptoms are relatively few in patients who are in class I shock. The only change in class I shock is anxiety, which is practically impossible to assess—is it the result of factors such as blood loss, pain, trauma, or drugs? A heart rate higher than 100 beats/min has been used as a physical sign of bleeding, but evidence of its significance is minimal. Brasel and colleagues[10] have shown that heart rate is neither sensitive nor specific in determining the need for emergent intervention, need for packed red blood cell (PRBC) transfusions in the first 2 hours after an injury, or severity of an injury. Heart rate was not altered by the presence of hypotension (systolic BP <90 mm Hg).

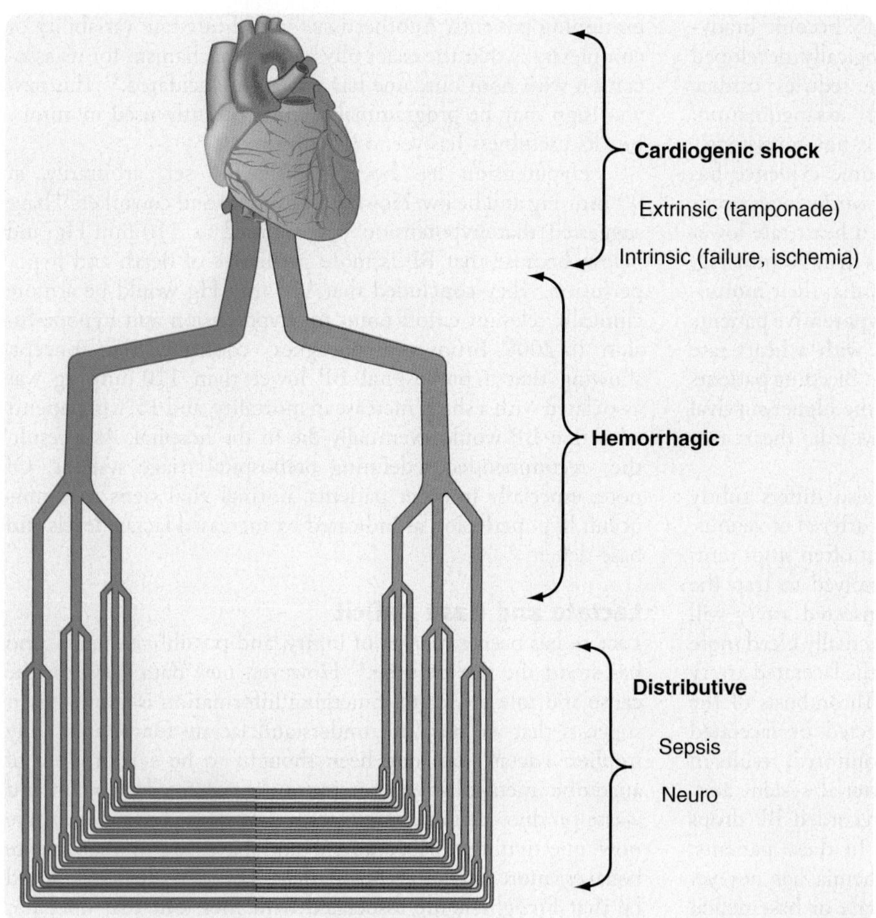


**FIGURE 5-5** Types of shock.

In patients who are in class II shock, we are taught that their heart rate is increased but, again, this is a highly unreliable marker; pain and mere nervousness can also increase heart rate. The change in pulse pressure—the difference between systolic and diastolic pressure—is also difficult to identify, because the baseline BP of patients is not always known. The change in pulse pressure is thought to be caused by an adrenalin response, which constricts vessels and results in higher diastolic pressures. It is important to recognize that the body compensates well.

Not until patients are in class III shock does BP supposedly decrease. At this stage, patients have lost 30% to 40% of their blood volume; for an average man weighing 75 kg/168 lbs, that can mean up to 2 liters of blood loss (Fig. 5-6). It is helpful to remember that a can of soda or beer is 355 mL; a six pack is 2130 mL. Theoretically, if a patient is hypotensive from blood loss, we are looking for a six pack of blood. Small amounts of blood should not result in hypotension. Although intracranial bleeding can cause hypotension in the last stages of herniation, it is almost impossible that it is the result of large volumes of blood loss intracranially because there is not enough room for that volume of blood. It is critical to recognize uncontrolled bleeding, and even more critical to stop bleeding before patients go into class III shock. It is more important to recognize blood loss than it is to replace blood loss. A common mistake is to think that trauma patients are often hypotensive; hypotension is rare in trauma patients (occurring less than 6% of the time).

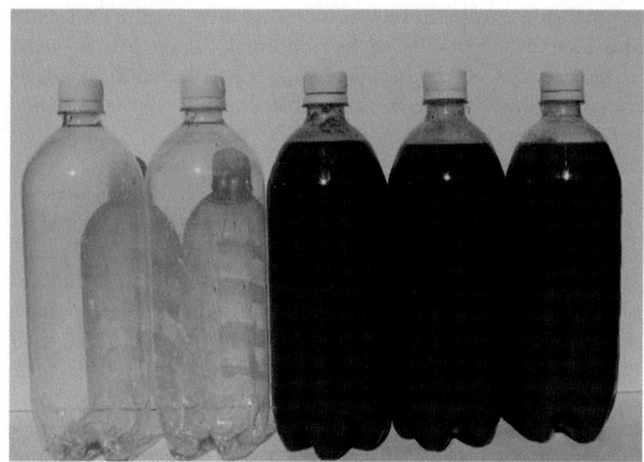

**FIGURE 5-6** Liters of blood lost for class III shock, or 40% of 5 liters, according to the ATLS.

In addition, the ATLS course, which was designed for physicians who are not surgeons, does not recognize many subtle but important aspects of bleeding. The concepts of the course are relatively basic. However, surgeons know that there are nuances of the varied responses to injuries in animals and humans. In the case of arterial hemorrhage, for example, we know that animals do not necessarily manifest tachycardia as their first response when bleeding, but actually become bradycardic. It is speculated that this is a teleologically developed mechanism because a bradycardic response reduces cardiac output and minimizes free uncontrolled exsanguination; however, a bradycardic response to bleeding is not consistently shown in all animals, including humans. Some evidence has shown that this response, termed *relative bradycardia,* does occur in humans. Relative bradycardia is defined as a heart rate lower than 100 beats/min when the systolic BP is less than 90 mm Hg. When bleeding patients have relative bradycardia, their mortality rate is lower. Interestingly, up to 44% of hypotensive patients have relative bradycardia. However, patients with a heart rate lower than 60 beats/min are usually moribund. Bleeding patients with a heart rate of 60 to 90 beats/min have the higher survival rate as compared with patients who are tachycardic (heart rate >90 beats/min).[11]

The physiologic response to bleeding also differs subtly according to whether the source of bleeding is arterial or venous. Arterial bleeding is obviously problematic, but often stops temporarily on its own; the human body has evolved to trap the blood loss in adventitial tissues, and the transected artery will spasm and thrombose. A lacerated artery can actually bleed more than a transected artery because the spasm of the lacerated artery can actually enlarge the hole in the vessel. Thrombosis of the artery sometimes does not occur in transected or lacerated vessels. Arterial bleeding, when constantly monitored, results in rapid hypotension: there is a leak in the arterial system and, because the arterial system is valveless, the recorded BP drops early, even before large-volume loss occurs. In these patients, hypotension ensues quickly but because ischemia has not yet had a chance to occur, measurements of lactate or base deficit often yield normal results.

Venous bleeding, however, is slower; the human body compensates, and sometimes large volumes of blood are lost before hypotension ensues. In venous bleeding, there is time for lactate and base deficit results to be abnormal. Blood loss is often slower, but can still be massive before it is reflected in hypotension. The slower nature of venous bleeding also allows for compensatory mechanisms to interact because water is recruited intravascularly from cells and the interstitial spaces.

It is generally taught that the hematocrit or hemoglobin level is not reliable for predicting blood loss. This is true for patients with a high hematocrit or hemoglobin level but in patients resuscitated with fluids, a rapid drop in the hematocrit and hemoglobin levels can occur immediately. Bruns and associates[12] have shown that the hemoglobin level can be low within the first 30 minutes after the patient arrives at a trauma center. Therefore, although patients with a high or normal hemoglobin level may have significant bleeding, a low hemoglobin level, because it occurs rapidly, usually reflects the actual hemoglobin level and extent of blood loss. Infusion of acellular fluids often will dilute the blood and decrease the hemoglobin levels even further.

The lack of good indicators to distinguish which patients are bleeding has led many investigators to examine heart rate variability or complexity as a potential new vital sign. Many clinical studies have shown that heart rate variability or complexity is associated with poor outcome, but this has yet to catch on, perhaps because of the difficulty of calculating it. Heart rate variability or complexity would have to be calculated using software, with a resulting index on which clinicians would have to rely; this information would not be available merely by examining patients. Another issue with heart rate variability or complexity is that the exact physiologic mechanism for its association with poor outcome has yet to be elucidated.[13] This new vital sign may be programmable into currently used monitors, but its usefulness has yet to be confirmed.

Hypotension has been traditionally set, arbitrarily, at 90 mm Hg and below. However, Eastridge and coworkers[14] have suggested that hypotension be redefined as 110 mm Hg and below, because that BP is more predictive of death and hypoperfusion. They concluded that 110 mm Hg would be a more clinically relevant cutoff point for hypotension and hypoperfusion. In 2008, Bruns and colleagues[15] confirmed that concept, showing that a prehospital BP lower than 110 mm Hg was associated with a sharp increase in mortality, and 15% of patients with that BP would eventually die in the hospital. As a result, they recommended redefining prehospital triage systems. Of note, especially in older patients, normal vital signs may miss occult hypoperfusion as indicated by increased lactate levels and base deficit.[16]

### Lactate and Base Deficit

Lactate has been a marker of injury, and possibly ischemia, and has stood the test of time.[16] However, new data question the cause and role of lactate. Emerging information is confusing; it suggests that we may not understand lactate for what it truly implies. Lactate has long been thought to be a byproduct of anaerobic metabolism and is routinely perceived to be an end waste product that is completely unfavorable. Physiologists are now questioning this paradigm and have found that lactate behaves more advantageously than not. An analogy would be that firefighters are associated with fires, but that does not mean that firefighters are bad, nor does it mean that they caused the fires.

Research has shown that lactate accumulates in muscle and blood during exercise; it is at its highest level at, or just after, exhaustion. Accordingly, it was assumed that lactate was a waste product. We also know that lactic acid appears in response to muscle contraction and continues in the absence of oxygen. In addition, accumulated lactate disappears when oxygen is present in tissues.

Recent evidence has indicated that lactate is an active metabolite, capable of moving among cells, tissues, and organs, where it may be oxidized as fuel or reconverted to form pyruvate or glucose. It now appears that increased lactate production and concentration, as a result of anoxia or dysoxia, are often the exception rather than the rule. Lactate seems to be a shuttle for energy; the lactate shuttle is now the subject of much debate. The end product of glycolysis is pyruvic acid. Lack of oxygen is thought to convert pyruvate into lactate. However, lactate formation may allow carbohydrate metabolism to continue through glycolysis. It is postulated that lactate is transferred from its site of production in the cytosol to neighboring cells and to various organs (e.g., heart, liver, kidney), where its oxidation and continued metabolism can occur.

Lactate is also being studied as a pseudohormone because it seems to regulate the cellular redox state through exchange and conversion into pyruvate and through its effects on the ratio of nicotinamide adenine dinucleotide to nicotinamide adenine dinucleotide (reduced)—the $NAD^+$/NADH ratio. It is released into the systemic circulation and taken up by distal tissues and organs, where it also affects the redox state in those cells. Further evidence has shown that it affects wound regeneration, with the promotion of increased collagen deposition and neovascularization. Lactate may also induce vasodilation and catecholamine release and stimulate fat and carbohydrate oxidation.

Lactate levels in blood are highly dependent on the equilibrium between production and elimination from the bloodstream. The liver is predominantly responsible for clearing lactate; acute or chronic liver disease affects lactate levels. Lactate was always thought to be produced from anaerobic tissues, but it now seems that various tissue beds that are not undergoing anaerobic metabolism produce lactate when signaled of distress.

In canine muscle, lactate is produced by moderate-intensity exercise when the oxygen supply is ample. A high adrenergic stimulus also causes a rise in lactate level as the body prepares or responds to stress. A study of climbers of Mount Everest has shown that the resting $Po_2$ on the summit was approximately 28 mm Hg and decreased even more during exercise.[17] The blood lactate level in those climbers was essentially the same as at sea level. These studies have allowed us to question lactate and its true role.

In humans, lactate may be the preferred fuel in the brain and heart; infused lactate is used before glucose at rest and during exercise. Because it is glucose sparing, lactate allows glucose and glycogen levels to be maintained. However, some data point to lactate's protective role in TBIs.[18] Lactate fuels the human brain during exercise. The level of lactate, whether it is a waste product or source of energy, seems to signify tissue distress, from anaerobic conditions or other factors.[19] Release of epinephrine and other catecholamines will result in higher lactate levels.

Base deficit, a measure of the number of millimoles of base required to correct the pH of 1 liter of whole blood to 7.4, seems to correlate well with lactate level, at least in the first 24 hours after an injury. Rutherford, in 1992, showed that a base deficit of 8 is associated with a 25% mortality rate in patients older than 55 years without a head injury or in patients younger than 55 with a head injury. When base deficit remains elevated, most clinicians believe that it is an indication of ongoing shock.

One of the problems with base deficit is that it is commonly influenced by the chloride from various resuscitation fluids, resulting in a hyperchloremic nongap acidosis. In patients with renal failure, base deficit can also be a poor predictor of outcome. In the acute stage of renal failure, a base deficit lower than 6 mmol/liter is associated with a poor outcome.[20] With the use of hypertonic saline (HTS), which has three to eight times the sodium chloride concentration as normal saline, depending on the concentration used, in trauma patients, the hyperchloremic acidosis has been shown to be relatively harmless. However, when HTS is used, the base deficit should be interpreted with caution.

## Compensatory Mechanisms

When needed, blood flow to less critical tissues is diverted to more critical tissues. The earliest compensatory mechanism in response to a decrease in intravascular volume is an increase in sympathetic activity. Such an increase is mediated by pressure receptors or baroreceptors in the aortic arch, atria, and carotid bodies. A decrease in pressure inhibits parasympathetic discharge while norepinephrine and epinephrine are liberated and causes adrenergic receptors in the myocardium and vascular smooth muscle to be activated. Heart rate and contractility are increased; peripheral vascular resistance is also increased, resulting in an increased BP. However, the various tissue beds are not affected equally; blood is shunted from less critical organs (e.g., skin, skeletal muscle, splanchnic circulation) to more critical organs (e.g., brain, liver, kidneys).

Then, the juxtaglomerular apparatus in the kidney—in response to the vasoconstriction and decrease in blood flow—produces the enzyme renin, which generates angiotensin I. The angiotensin-converting enzyme located on the endothelial cells of the pulmonary arteries converts angiotensin I to angiotensin II. In turn, angiotensin II stimulates an increased sympathetic drive, at the level of the nerve terminal, by releasing hormones from the adrenal medulla. In response, the adrenal medulla affects intravascular volume during shock by secreting catechol hormones—epinephrine, norepinephrine, and dopamine—which are all produced from phenylalanine and tyrosine. They are called *catecholamines* because they contain a catechol group derived from the amino acid tyrosine. The release of catecholamines is thought to be responsible for the elevated glucose level in hemorrhagic shock. Although the role of glucose elevation in hemorrhagic shock is not fully understood, it does not seem to affect outcome.[21]

Cortisol, also released from the adrenal cortex, plays a major role in that it controls fluid equilibrium. In the adrenal cortex, the zona glomerulosa produces aldosterone in response to stimulation by angiotensin II. Aldosterone is a mineralocorticoid that modulates renal function by increasing the recovery of sodium and excretion of potassium. Angiotensin II also has a direct action on the renal tubules, reabsorbing sodium. The control of sodium is a primary mechanism whereby the human body controls water absorption or secretion in the kidneys. One of the problems in shock is that the release of hormones is not infinite; the supply can be exhausted.

This regulation of intravascular fluid status is further affected by the carotid baroreceptors and atrial naturetic peptides. Signals are sent to the supraoptic and paraventricular nuclei in the brain. Antidiuretic hormone (ADH) is released from the pituitary, causing retention of free water at the level of the kidney. Simultaneously, volume is recruited from the extravascular and cellular spaces. A shift of water occurs as hydrostatic pressures fall in the intravascular compartment. At the capillary level, hydrostatic pressures are also reduced, because the precapillary sphincters are vasoconstricted more than the postcapillary sphincters.

## Lethal Triad

The triad of acidosis, hypothermia, and coagulopathy is common in resuscitated patients who are bleeding or in shock from various factors. Our basic understanding is that inadequate tissue perfusion results in acidosis caused by lactate production. In the shock state, the delivery of nutrients to the cells is thought to be inadequate, so adenosine triphosphate (ATP) production decreases. The human body relies on ATP production to maintain homeostatic temperatures; ATP is the source of heat in all homeothermic (warm-blooded) animals. Thus, if ATP production is inadequate to maintain body temperature, the body will trend toward the ambient temperature. For most patients, this is 22° C (72° F), the temperature inside typical hospitals. The resulting hypothermia then affects the efficiency of enzymes, which work best at 37° C. For surgeons, the critical problem with hypothermia is that the coagulation cascade depends on enzymes affected by hypothermia; if enzymes are not functioning optimally because of hypothermia, coagulopathy worsens, which in surgical patients can contribute to uncontrolled bleeding from injuries or the surgery itself. Further bleeding continues to fuel the triad. The optimal method to stop the vicious cycle of death is to stop the bleeding and the causes of hypothermia. In most typical scenarios, hypothermia is not spontaneous from ischemia but is induced because of using room temperature fluid or cold blood products.

### Acidosis

Bleeding causes a host of responses. During the resuscitative phase, the lethal triad (acidosis, hypothermia, and coagulopathy) is frequent, most likely because of two major factors. First, tissue ischemia from the lack of blood flow results in lactic acidosis. Some believe that the acidotic state is not necessarily undesirable, because the body tolerates acidosis better than alkalosis. Oxygen is more easily offloaded from the hemoglobin molecules in the acidotic environment; many who try to preserve tissue have found that cells live longer in an acidotic environment. Correcting acidosis with sodium bicarbonate has classically been avoided because it is treating a number or symptom when the cause needs to be addressed. Treating the pH alone has shown no benefit, but it can lead to complacency; patients appear to be better resuscitated, but the underlying cause of their acidosis has not been adequately addressed. It is also argued that rapidly injecting sodium bicarbonate can worsen intracellular acidosis because of the diffusion of the converted $CO_2$ into the cells.

The best fundamental approach to metabolic acidosis from shock is to treat the underlying cause of shock. However, some clinicians believe that treating the pH has advantages, because the enzymes necessary for the coagulation cascade work better at an optimal temperature and optimal pH. Coagulopathy can contribute to uncontrolled bleeding, so some have recommended treating acidosis for patients in dire scenarios. Treating acidosis with sodium bicarbonate may have a benefit in an unintended and unrecognized way. Rapid infusion is usually accompanied by a rise in BP in hypotensive patients, which is usually attributed to correcting the pH. However, sodium bicarbonate in most urgent situations is given in ampules. The 50-mL ampule of sodium bicarbonate has 1 mEq/mL—in essence, similar to giving a hypertonic concentration of sodium, which quickly draws fluid into the vascular space. Given its high sodium concentration, a 50-mL bolus of sodium bicarbonate has physiologic results similar to those of 325 mL of normal saline or 385 mL of LR. Essentially it is like giving small doses of HTS. Sodium bicarbonate quickly increases $CO_2$ levels by its conversion in the liver, so if the minute ventilation is not increased, respiratory acidosis can result.

THAM (tromethamine; tris[hydroxymethyl]aminomethane) is a biologically inert amino alcohol of low toxicity that buffers $CO_2$ and acids. It is sodium-free and limits the generation of $CO_2$ in the process of buffering. At 37° C, the $pK_a$ of THAM is 7.8, making it a more effective buffer than sodium bicarbonate in the physiologic range of blood pH. In vivo, THAM supplements the buffering capacity of the blood bicarbonate system by generating sodium bicarbonate and decreasing the partial pressure of $CO_2$. It rapidly distributes to the extracellular space and slowly penetrates the intracellular space, except in the case of erythrocytes and hepatocytes, and is excreted by the kidney. Unlike sodium bicarbonate, which requires an open system to eliminate $CO_2$ to exert its buffering effect, THAM is effective in a closed or semiclosed system and it maintains its buffering ability during hypothermia. THAM acetate (0.3 M; pH, 8.6) is well tolerated, does not cause tissue or venous irritation, and is the only formulation available in the United States. THAM may induce respiratory depression and hypoglycemia, which may require ventilatory assistance and the administration of glucose.

The initial loading dose of THAM acetate (0.3 M) for the treatment of acidemia may be estimated as follows:

$$\text{THAM (in mL of 0.3 M solution)} = \text{lean body weight (in kg)} \times \text{the base deficit (in mmol/liter)}$$

The maximal daily dose is 15 mmol/kg/day for an adult (3.5 liters of a 0.3-M solution in a patient weighing 70 kg). It is indicated in the treatment of respiratory failure (acute respiratory distress syndrome [ARDS ] and infant respiratory distress syndrome) and has been associated with the use of hypothermia and permissive hypercapnia (controlled hypoventilation). Other indications are diabetic and renal acidosis, salicylate and barbiturate intoxication, and increased intracranial pressure associated with brain trauma. It is used in cardioplegic solutions and during liver transplantation. Despite these features, THAM has not been documented clinically to be more efficacious than sodium bicarbonate.

### Hypothermia

Hypothermia can be beneficial and detrimental. A fundamental knowledge of hypothermia is of vital importance in the care of surgical patients. The beneficial aspects of hypothermia are mainly because of decreased metabolism. Injury sites are often iced, creating vasoconstriction and decreasing inflammation through decreased metabolism. This concept of cooling to slow metabolism is also the rationale behind using hypothermia to decrease ischemia during cardiac, transplantation, pediatric, and neurologic surgery. Also, amputated extremities are iced before reimplantation. Cold water near-drowning victims have higher survival rates thanks to the preservation of the brain and other vital organs. The Advanced Life Support Task Force of the International Liaison Committee of Resuscitation now recommends cooling (to 32° to 34° C) unconscious adults, who have spontaneous circulation after out of hospital cardiac arrest caused by ventricular fibrillation, for 12 to 24 hours. Induced hypothermia is vastly different from spontaneous hypothermia, which is typically from shock, inadequate tissue perfusion, or cold fluid infusion.

Medical or accidental hypothermia is also very different from trauma-associated hypothermia (Table 5-2). The survival rates after accidental hypothermia range from approximately 12% to 39%; the average temperature drop is to approximately 30° C (range, 13.7° to 35.0° C). The lowest recorded temperature in a survivor of accidental hypothermia (13.7° C [56.7° F]) was in an extreme skier in Norway; she was trapped under the ice and eventually fully recovered neurologically.

The data in patients with trauma-associated hypothermia differ. Their survival rate falls dramatically with their core temperature, reaching 100% mortality when it reaches 32° C at any point—whether in the emergency room, operating room, or

**Table 5-2 Classification of Hypothermia by Cause**

| | Cause | |
|---|---|---|
| **DEGREE** | **TRAUMA** | **ACCIDENT** |
| Mild | 36°-34° C | 35°-32° C |
| Moderate | 34°-32° C | 32°-28° C |
| Severe | <32° C (<90° F) | <28° C (<82° F) |

intensive care unit (ICU). In trauma patients, hypothermia is caused by shock and is thought to perpetuate uncontrolled bleeding because of the associated coagulopathy. Trauma patients with a postoperative core temperature lower than 35° C have a fourfold increase in mortality and lower than 33° C, a sevenfold increase in mortality. Hypothermic trauma patients tend to be more severely injured and older, with bleeding as indicated by blood loss and transfusions.[22]

Surprisingly, in a study using the National Trauma Data Bank, Shafi and associates have shown that hypothermia and its associated poor outcome are not related to the state of shock. It was previously thought that a core temperature lower than 32°C was uniformly fatal in trauma patients who have the additional insult of tissue injury and bleeding. However, a small number of trauma patients have now survived, despite a recorded core temperature lower than 32° C. In a multi-institutional trial, Beilman and coworkers[23] have recently demonstrated that hypothermia is associated with more severe injuries, bleeding, and a higher rate of multiorgan dysfunction in the ICU, but not with death.

To understand hypothermia, we have to remember that humans are homeothermic (warm-blooded) animals, in contrast to poikilothermic (cold-blooded) animals, such as snakes and fish. To maintain a body temperature of 37° C, our hypothalamus uses various mechanisms to control core body temperature tightly. We use oxygen as the key ingredient, or fuel, to generate heat in the mitochondria in the form of ATP. When ATP production is below its lowest threshold, one side effect is the lowering of body temperature to the ambient temperature, which typically is less than core body temperature. In contrast, during exercise, we use more oxygen, because more ATP is required and we produce excess heat. In an attempt to modulate core temperature, we start perspiring to use the cooling properties of evaporation.

Hypothermia, although potentially beneficial, is detrimental in trauma patients, mainly because it causes coagulopathy. Cold affects coagulopathy by decreasing enzyme activity, enhancing fibrinolytic activity, and causing platelet dysfunction. Platelets are affected by the inhibition of thromboxane B2 production, resulting in decreased aggregation. A heparin-like substance is released, causing a diffuse intravascular coagulation (DIC)–like syndrome. Hageman factor (factor XII ) and thromboplastin are some of the enzymes most affected. Even a drop in core temperature of only a few degrees results in 40% inefficiency in activity of some enzymes.

Heat affects the coagulation cascade so much that when blood is drawn from cold patients and sent to the laboratory, the sample is heated to 37° C, because even 1° or 2° C of cold delays clotting and renders test results inaccurate. Thus, in a cold and coagulopathic patient, if the coagulation profile obtained from the laboratory shows an abnormality, the result represents the same level of coagulopathy as if the patient (and not just the sample) had been warmed to 37° C. Therefore, a cold patient is always more coagulopathic than indicated by the coagulation profile. A normal coagulation profile does not necessarily represent what is occurring in the body.

Heat is measured in calories. One calorie is the amount of energy required to raise the temperature of 1 mL of water (which has, by definition, a specific heat of 1.0). It takes 1 kcal to raise the temperature of 1 liter of water by 1° C. If an average man (weight, 75 kg) consisted of pure water, then it would take 75 kcal to raise his temperature by 1° C. However, humans are not made of pure water and blood has a specific heat coefficient of 0.87. Thus, the human body has a specific heat of 0.83. Therefore, it actually takes 62.25 kcal (75 kg × 0.83) to raise the body temperature by 1° C. If a patient were to lose 62.25 kcal, the body temperature would decrease by 1° C. This basic science is important when choosing methods to retain heat or treat hypothermia or hyperthermia. It allows the efficacy of one method to be compared with another.

The normal basal metabolic heat generation is approximately 70 kcal/hr; shivering can increase this to 250 kcal/hr. Heat is transferred to and from the body by contact or conduction (as in a frying pan or Jacuzzi), air or convection (as in an oven or sauna), radiation, and evaporation. Convection is an extremely inefficient way to transfer heat because the air molecules are so far apart as compared with liquids and solids. Conduction and radiation are the most efficient ways to transfer heat. However, heating the patient with radiation is fraught with inconsistencies and technical challenges and is difficult to apply clinically, so we are left with conduction to transfer energy efficiently.

Warming or cooling through manipulation of the temperature of IV fluids is useful because it uses conduction to transfer heat. Although IV fluids can be warmed, the U.S. Food and Drug Administration (FDA) only allows fluid warmers to be set at a maximum of 40° C. Therefore, the differential between a cold trauma patient (34° C) and warmed fluid is only 6° C. Thus, 1 liter of warmed fluids can only transfer 6 kcal to the patient. As previously calculated, approximately 62 kcal is needed to raise the core temperature by 1° C. Therefore, 10.4 liters of warmed fluids are needed to raise the core temperature by 1° C, to 35° C. Once that has been achieved, the differential is now only 5° C between the patient and the warmed fluid, so it actually takes 12.5 liters of warmed fluids to raise the patient's temperature from 35° to 36° C. A cold patient at 32° C needs to be given 311 kcal (75 kg × 0.83) to warm him or her to 37° C. Note that 1 liter of fluid must be given at the highest rate possible, because if the infusion rate is slow the fluid cools to room temperature as the IV line is exposed to ambient room temperature. To avoid IV line cooling, devices that warm fluids up to the point of insertion into the body should be used.

Warming patients by infusing warmed fluids is difficult, but fluid warmers are still critically important; the main reason to warm fluids is so that patients are not cooled. Cold fluids can cool patients quickly. The fluids that are typically infused are at room temperature (22° C) or at 4° C, which is the temperature of a refrigerator in which blood products are stored. Therefore, it takes 5 liters of 22° C fluid or 2 liters of cold blood to cool a patient by 1° C. Again, the main reason for using fluid warmers is not necessarily to warm patients but to prevent their cooling during resuscitation.

**Table 5-3 Classification of Warming Techniques**

| | Active | |
|---|---|---|
| **PASSIVE** | **EXTERNAL** | **INTERNAL** |
| Drying the patient | Bair Hugger | Warmed fluids |
| Warm fluids | Heated warmers | Heat ventilator |
| Warm blankets, sheets | Lamps | Cavity lavage, chest tube, abdomen, bladder |
| Head covers | Radiant warmers | Continuous arterial or venous rewarming |
| Warming the room | Clinitron bed | Full or partial bypass |

**Table 5-4 Calories Delivered by Active Warming**

| METHOD | KCAL/HR |
|---|---|
| Airway from vent | 9 |
| Overhead radiant warmers | 17 |
| Heating blankets | 20 |
| Convective warmers | 15-26 |
| Body cavity lavages | 35 |
| CAVR | 92-140 |
| Cardiopulmonary bypass | 710 |

*CAVR*, Continuous arteriovenous rewarming.

Rewarming techniques are classified as passive or active. Active warming is further classified as external or internal (Table 5-3). Passive warming involves preventing heat loss. An example of passive warming is to dry the patient to minimize evaporative cooling, giving warm fluids to prevent cooling, or covering the patient so that the ambient air temperature immediately around the patient can be higher than the room temperature. Covering the patient's head helps reduce a tremendous amount of heat loss. Using aluminum-lined head covers is preferred; they reflect back the infrared radiation that is normally lost through the scalp. Warming the room technically helps reduce the heat loss gradient, but the surgical staff usually cannot work in a humidified room at 37° C. Passive warming also includes closing open body cavities, such as the chest or abdomen, to prevent evaporative heat loss. The most important way to prevent heat loss is to treat hemorrhagic shock by controlling bleeding. Once shock has been treated, the body's metabolism will heat the patient from his or her core. This point cannot be overemphasized.

Active warming actively transfers calories to the patient, externally through the skin or internally. Skin and fat are designed to be highly efficient in preventing heat transfer, so active external warming is inefficient as compared with internal warming. Forced-air heating, such as with Bair Hugger temperature management therapy (Arizant Healthcare, Eden Prairie, Minn), is technically classified as active warming, but air is a terribly inefficient medium and not many calories are provided to patients. Forced-air heating only increases the patient's ambient temperature but it can actually cool the patient initially because it increases evaporative heat loss if the patient is wet from blood, fluids, clothes, or sweat. Warming the skin may feel good to the patient and surgeon, but it actually decreases shivering, which is a highly efficient method of internal warming that tricks the thermoregulatory nerve input on the skin. Because forced-air heating uses convection, the actual amount of active warming is estimated to be only 10 kcal/hour.

Active external warming is better performed by placing patients on heating pads, which use conduction to transfer heat. Beds are available that can warm patients faster, such as the Clinitron bed (Hill-Rom, Batesville, Ind), which uses heated air fluidized beads. Such beds are not practical in the operating room, but are applicable in the ICU. Removing wet sheets and wet clothes remains an essential aspect of rewarming.

The best method to warm patients is to deliver the calories internally (Table 5-4). Heating the air used for ventilators is technically internal active warming, but is inefficient because, again, the heat transfer method is convection. The surface area of the lungs is massive, but the energy is mainly transferred through humidified water droplets, mostly using convection and not conduction. The amount of heat transferred through warmed humidified air is also minimal by comparison to methods that use conduction. Body cavities can be lavaged by infusing warmed fluids through chest tubes or merely by irrigating the abdominal cavity with hot fluids. Other methods, which have been written about but rarely used in practice, include gastric lavage and esophageal lavage with special tubes. If gastric lavage is desired, one method is to place two nasogastric tubes and infuse warm fluids in one while the other sucks the fluid back out. Bladder irrigation with an irrigation Foley catheter is useful. Instruments to warm the hand through conduction show much promise but are not yet readily available.

The best means to deliver heat is through countercurrent exchange of fluids, using conduction to transfer calories. Again, heating IV fluids is technically active internal warming but, because of the limitations of how much fluids can be heated, it is relatively inefficient. Heating fluids before infusion minimizes cooling rather than active warming. Full cardiopulmonary bypass is unmatched; it delivers more than 5 liters/min of heated blood to every part of the body that contains capillaries. If full cardiopulmonary bypass is not available or not desired, alternatives include continuous venous and arterial rewarming. Venous-venous rewarming is most easily accomplished using the roller pump of a dialysis machine, which is often more available to the average surgeon. A prospective study has shown arterial-venous rewarming to be highly effective. It can warm patients to 37° C in approximately 39 minutes, as compared with an average warming time of 3.2 hours using standard techniques. Special Gentilello arterial warming catheters are inserted into the femoral artery and a second line is inserted into the opposite femoral vein. The pressure from the artery produces flow, which is then directed to a fluid warmer and back into the vein. This method highly depends on the patient's BP because flow is directly related to BP.

Over the last several decades, with the changes in resuscitation methods, the incidence of hypothermia has decreased and is now less of a problem. Dilutional coagulopathy also occurs less frequently because the use of crystalloids has been minimized.

## Coagulopathy

Coagulopathy in surgical patients is multifactorial. In addition to acidosis and hypothermia, the other main cause of coagulopathy is usually decreased clotting factors. This decrease is caused by consumption (from the innate attempt to stop bleeding), dilution (from infused fluids devoid of factors), and genetic (hemophilia) factors.

The methods to define and treat coagulopathy are still varied; no standardization is apparent. Hypothermia has a vital role in coagulopathy because the coagulation cascade is dependent on enzymatic activities. Thus, coagulopathy is associated with shock and increased mortality. Bleeding from coagulopathy or any other cause perpetuates shock, which induces more acidosis, hypothermia, and consumption and use of fluids. The only way to break this vicious cycle is to stop the bleeding.

In recent years, interest in using drugs to stop bleeding and correct coagulopathy has increased. Recombinant factor VIIa (rFVIIa) was developed for use in hemophiliacs and works with tissue factor and activated platelets. Tissue factor is ubiquitous but, with tissue injury, is released at high levels at the site of injury, as are activated platelets. Theoretically, because rFVIIa targets sources of tissue injury, it is ideal in surgery. For example, if one were in a car accident and the spleen and femur were injured, the bleeding would stop at the spleen and other injured tissues with the aid of rFVIIa, but would not cause thrombotic or embolic problems elsewhere. It was used off-label in patients with massive bleeding with coagulopathy, and case reports started to appear in the literature. Then case series appeared and, eventually, reports with recommendations of how and when to use it were published.

Boffard and colleagues[24] have shown, in a randomized, double-blind, placebo-controlled trial, that blunt trauma patients who receive rFVIIa have a significantly lower blood transfusion requirement and a lower incidence of massive transfusion. The trial also showed similar trends in penetrating trauma patients, as well as improved early outcomes in blunt and penetrating trauma patients. However, the difference was not statistically significant. In addition, the trial showed a trend toward a lower incidence of multiorgan dysfunction syndrome (MODS) and ARDS. In a post hoc analysis, Rizoli and associates examined the efficacy of rFVIIa in coagulopathic patients, stating that it significantly reduces the need for blood transfusions and incidence of MODS and ARDS. Enthusiasm for its use has waned, however, because the relative cost of the drug is high and prospective trials did not show a survival advantage. The average cost for the drug is \$1/μg/kg; for a 75-kg person, that equates to \$7500/dose.

The military, which began using rFVIIa during the war in Iraq, reported a decreased 30-day mortality rate without an increased risk of severe thrombotic events, but eventually there were reports of complications. Caution started to emerge as the concerns about thromboembolic events were being reported. It seems that injured vessels were at risk for thrombosis. The correct dose of the drug is still unclear, as is the optimal timing of administration.

Selecting the correct patient population for rFVIIa is also a major factor. Some reports did not show a significant impact on mortality, but this could be a result of the drug only being used in moribund patients, for whom no medical therapy would have improved outcome. The reason for not using it early or on nonmoribund patients was because of the high cost of the drug. A large multicenter prospective trial of rFVIIa was initiated; it was difficult to implement and then was stopped early, given how difficult it was to enroll patients—for various reasons, including problems with informed consent. The main issue with the aborted trial was that the FDA required the primary outcome to be 30-day mortality and the overall mortality rate in this study was lower than expected; thus, continuing the study would have been futile and costly because the difference in mortality rate would have had less of a chance of reaching statistical significance. Although rFVIIa does decrease the need for blood transfusions, it may or may not save lives; mortality is often affected by more than blood transfusions.

Although the use of rFVIIa has not yet shown to be beneficial in traumatic shock, it may be particularly useful for patients with traumatic brain injuries (TBIs).[25] It may not be the ultimate solution to coagulopathy, but it has certainly garnered interest about using drugs to combat coagulopathy. Recently, there other drugs have started to emerge with a potential role in the treatment of coagulopathy. Factor IX, or prothrombin complex concentrate (PCC), has become popular for the treatment of surgical coagulopathy. For patients on warfarin, PCC is the option of choice when treatment with fresh- frozen plasma (FFP) is problematic because of time for preparation and the concern of worsening cardiac heart failure caused by the volume of plasma. PCC actually contains many factors (factors II, VII, IX, X), including variable amounts of factor VIIa, depending on the brand of PCC used. Recent experience with factor IX has shown that it is efficacious, at 10% of the cost of rFVIIa. The use of blood-based component therapy is paramount for treating coagulopathy (see later, "Evolution of Modern Resuscitation"). However, the concept of treating traumatic bleeding with a drug needs to be thoroughly tested and developed. If there were a drug that when administered, would stop or reduce bleeding, treat coagulopathy at a low cost, and not cause serious complications, it would be a real contribution to medicine. Again, the problem is that current modes are expensive and the adverse events from administering such a drug is still unknown.

## Oxygen Delivery

The definition of shock is inadequate tissue perfusion, but some believe that the fundamental problem is tissue oxygenation. Much of what we know about oxygen delivery and consumption has come from a physiologist named Archibald V. Hill. He was an avid runner who measured the oxygen consumption of four runners running around an 88-m grass track (Fig. 5-7). In the process of his work, Hill defined the terms *maximum $O_2$ intake, $O_2$ requirement,* and *$O_2$ debt.* He is mostly known for his work with Otto Meyerhof, who unraveled the distinction between aerobic and anaerobic metabolism, for which they were awarded the Nobel Prize in 1922.

Blood delivers oxygen by red cells, which contain hemoglobin. The simple calculation of oxygen delivery ($Do_2$) is the cardiac output (CO) multiplied by the content of oxygen carried by a volume of blood ($Cao_2$):

$$Do_2 = CO \times Cao_2$$

The average hemoglobin carries 1.34 mL of $O_2$/g, depending on the arterial hemoglobin (Hgb) saturation ($Sao_2$) of the red cell. In addition, a minor amount of oxygen is dissolved in plasma; this amount is calculated by multiplying the solubility constant by 0.003 times the content of oxygen in the arterial blood ($Pao_2$). The $Cao_2$ of arterial blood is calculated as follows:

$$Cao_2 = (1.34 \times Hgb \times Sao_2) + (0.003 \times Pao_2)$$

where is Hgb is in g/dL. Cardiac output is heart rate multiplied by the stroke volume. In a normal state, the stroke volume can be increased by shunting blood from one tissue bed to the central vasculature, but most of the change in cardiac output is determined by heart rate. In states of hemorrhage and resuscitation, the stroke volume is affected because it can be controlled by infusion of fluids. As blood volume is decreased, it will ultimately affect stroke volume, which is compensated by an increase in heart rate.

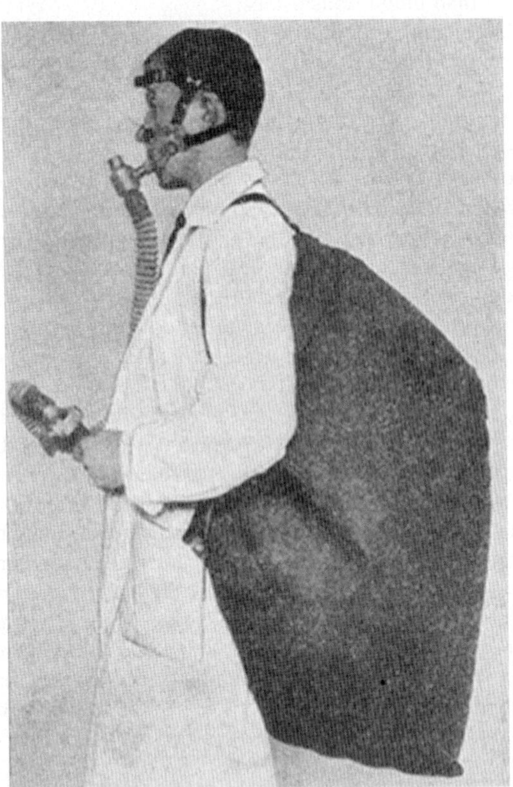

**FIGURE 5-7** Bag with side tube, low on the left-hand side, for use while running. The tap is carried in the left hand. (From Hill AV, Lupton H: Muscular exercise, lactic acid, and the supply and utilization of oxygen. Q J Med 16:135–171, 1923.)

Oxygen consumption by cells is calculated by subtracting the content of oxygen in the red cells in the venous system just before it is reoxygenated ($Cv_{O_2}$):

$$V_{O_2} = CO \times (Ca_{O_2}O_2 - Cv_{O_2})$$

After simplifying the terms and converting the units, the result is as follows:

$$V_{O_2} = CO \times 1.34 \times Hgb \times (Sa_{O_2} - Sv_{O_2})$$

The arterial oxygen content is measured by sampling the arterial blood with a blood gas. The venous oxygen content is measured by sampling the blood in the pulmonary artery just before it is reoxygenated. The most conventional method of sampling the venous oxygen content is by drawing back blood from the most distal port of a pulmonary artery catheter. The sample is taken from the pulmonary artery because venous blood is mixed there from all parts of the body. Oxygen content in the inferior vena cava is typically higher than in the superior vena cava, which this is higher than the blood in the coronary sinus. The average mixed venous sample is 75% saturated, so the oxygen consumption is thought to average 25% of the oxygen delivered (Fig. 5-8). This means that in general, an ample reserve of oxygen is delivered to tissues.

With advancements in technology, catheters are now available that can continuously measure the venous saturation in the pulmonary artery. These use technology similar to the pulse oximeter built into the tip of a pulmonary artery catheter, which uses near-infrared light waves to measure the saturation state of hemoglobin. Also because of new technology, cardiac output can be shown continuously. In the past, cardiac output was inferred by measuring the rate of change in temperature in the heart, at the distal aspect of a pulmonary artery catheter, by infusing a standard volume of iced or room temperature water into the proximal port and measuring the change in temperature.

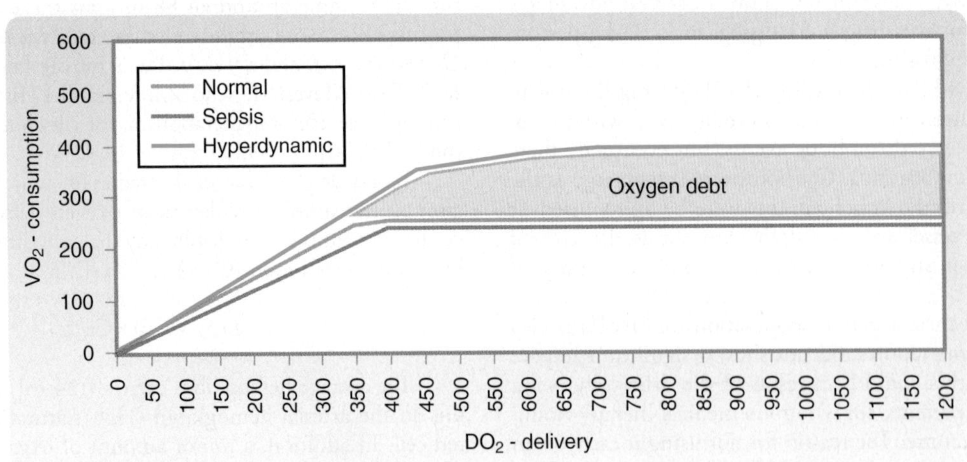


**FIGURE 5-8** Oxygen delivery and consumption. During normal states, oxygen delivery is approximately 1000 mL/min of $O_2$. The oxygen consumption in a normal state is 25% of delivery and is approximately 250 mL/min. At very low oxygen delivery, it is believed that consumption is delivery-dependent and occurs in shock. There is oxygen debt during shock and during recovery, and there is a hyperdynamic stage during which the circulatory system is paying back its oxygen debt.

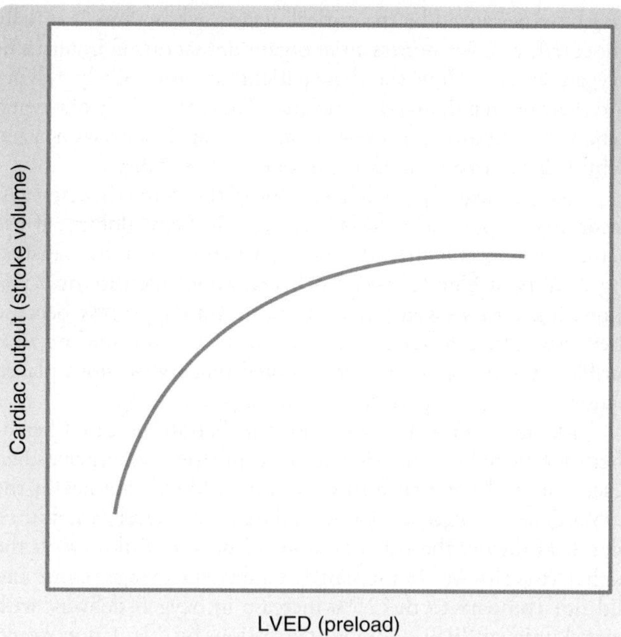


**FIGURE 5-9** Starling curve. As LEVD pressure is increased, the fibers of the heart muscles are lengthened, resulting in increased contraction resulting in increased cardiac output. This occurs to a certain point, at which increases in volume and length do not result in increases in cardiac output.

Cardiac output and oxygen delivery are also affected by the end-diastolic volume of the left ventricle. As described by Starling in 1915, cardiac output increases when the ventricular fibers increase in length, to a point (Fig. 5-9). Left ventricular end-diastolic (LVED) volume can be estimated by using a pulmonary artery catheter and measuring the wedge pressure; this reflects the pressure in the left ventricle, because the vessel from the pulmonary artery to the left ventricle has no valves. Alternative approaches can help optimize the filling volume in the left ventricle. Pulmonary artery catheters for calculating the right ventricular end-diastolic (RVED) volume are now available. Echocardiography using transthoracic or esophageal probes can directly estimate the filling volumes in the heart. However, variations in volume and heart size can distort results; heart size is also affected by medical conditions that can stress and dilate the heart. The interpretation of heart data is also subjective.

Such variables are considered important because it was assumed that lessons learned from physiology applied to patients in shock. During the late 1980s, surgical critical care evolved into a specialty, focusing heavily on optimizing oxygen delivery to tissues. One of the pioneers of modern surgical critical care, William Shoemaker, theorized that during shock, because of a lack of oxygen delivery, there was anaerobic metabolism and an oxygen debt that needed to be repaid. He showed that after volume loading, if oxygen delivery increased, consumption would also increase—until a certain point, when an additional increase in oxygen delivery did not result in consumption. This process was thought to be paying back the oxygen debt that occurred during ischemia throughout the body. Patients in shock were found to have a hyperdynamic stage, in which increased oxygen delivery resulted in increased consumption. The assumption was that increased consumption was caused by the oxygen debt that the body had incurred.

## Optimization (Supernormalization)

Shoemaker popularized the concept of optimization or supernormalization of oxygen delivery, which means that oxygen delivery is maximized or increased until its consumption no longer increases but, instead, levels off. The idea was to continue to increase the delivery of oxygen as long as consumption increased. If the body used more oxygen, the thought was that it was because it needed it. The optimization process involves administering a rapid bolus of fluid and confirming that it raises wedge pressure. Because the response to fluid infusion is dynamic, the infusion process much occur over a short period, such as 20 minutes. If it takes longer, determining whether changes in the vascular space, specifically the heart, may be caused by other variables in addition to the fluids used. Also, if not measured immediately after infusion, the effects of the infusion degraded quickly as fluids moved out of the vascular space.

Another rationale for rapidly infusing fluids as boluses and checking the results frequently is that any changes in preload and cardiac output may be short-lived with the shifts in fluid. Wedge pressure and cardiac output must be measured minutes before fluid infusion and immediately afterward to determine whether it is effective. If cardiac output increased with the wedge pressure increase, then it is assumed that oxygen delivery increases. By sampling the central venous oxygen content when measuring cardiac output, clinicians can determine whether oxygen consumption also increases. This process was originally repeated, over and over, until it was demonstrated that the fluid bolus does not increase cardiac output. The goal was to optimize oxygen delivery from the delivery-dependent portion of the curve to the portion that was not delivery-dependent (Fig. 5-8).

The preferred fluid during this optimization process was LR, for cost reasons, but colloid was also acceptable. Once the Starling curve was optimized, in that LVED volume could no longer be increased with increases in wedge pressure, wedge pressure would be kept at that maximal level. Further increases in wedge pressure, without increasing LVED volume, meant that patients might suffer from unnecessary pulmonary edema.

Once fluid infusion maximized cardiac output and oxygen delivery, if oxygen consumption continued to increase, it was concluded that patients needed further oxygen delivery to pay back the oxygen debt or meet the oxygen needs of the tissues. At that stage, an inotropic agent would be added to push cardiac output further to a higher level. The agent recommended at that time was dobutamine. The dose was increased and its effect on cardiac output was documented. With each maneuver, oxygen consumption was measured and cardiac output optimized to meet the consumption demands. This optimizing process maximized oxygen delivery to ensure that all tissue beds were being fed adequately. Shoemaker's earlier clinical trials had shown that patients resuscitated in this manner had a lower incidence of MODS and death. During this optimizing era, ARDS and MODS were the leading causes of late death in trauma patients.

However, subsequent clinical studies failed to repeat Shoemaker's success. Randomized prospective trials showed that the optimization of oxygen delivery and consumption did not improve outcome.[26] In general, patients who responded to the optimization process did well, but those who could not have their oxygen delivery augmented to a higher level did poorly.

Thus, although response to optimization was prognostic of outcome, the process itself did not seem to change outcome. One reason why the earlier studies succeeded might have been because the control patients were not adequately resuscitated. With the later trials, when patients were adequately resuscitated, the optimization process did not improve outcome. In fact, the aggressive use of fluids to achieve supranormal oxygen delivery could cause abdominal compartment syndrome.[27]

Moreover, oxygen delivery in hyperdynamic patients could not be driven to a point at which consumption seemed to level off. One theory was that as the heart was being pushed with the supernormalization process, its metabolism increased so that the heart was the major organ that seemed to consume all the excess oxygen being delivered. The harder the heart worked to deliver the oxygen, the more it had to use. It must be remembered that normal cardiac output for an average adult is approximately 5 liters/min, but patients were often driven to a cardiac output of 15 liters/min, or more, for days at a time.

The critics of the optimization process asserted that there was a point during oxygen delivery at which it was flow-dependent, but the coupling of consumption and delivery made it seem like increased delivery was the factor that increased consumption. Furthermore, optimization advocates neglected the fact that the body was usually already at the flat part of the oxygen consumption curve. Rarely was oxygen delivered when it was critical or when the body was consuming all that was being delivered. The result of the optimization process usually meant that patients were flooded with fluids. The hyperdynamic response and MODS may have been caused by the fluids used, which may have caused an inflammatory response at excessive volumes.

The concept of oxygen debt might have some vital flaws.[28] Hill's original work on aerobic and anaerobic metabolism in only four patients has now been propagated for a century. However, modern exercise physiology studies have shown that oxygen debt is repaid over a short period; it does not take days. In contrast, the optimization process showed oxygen debt for long periods.

During massive hemorrhage, some ischemia to some tissues is theoretically possible. In acute hemorrhage, however, when the BP falls to 40 mm Hg, cardiac output and thus oxygen delivery are typically only reduced by 50%. Before resuscitation with acellular fluids, the hemoglobin level does not fall significantly; in this state, oxygen delivery is cut by only 50% and the body is designed to have plenty of reserves (cells consume only 25% of the delivered oxygen in the normal state). Whether any ongoing anaerobic metabolism is actually occurring is questionable because, theoretically, the oxygen delivered has to decrease to 25% of baseline to be anaerobic. When resuscitation takes place without blood to restore the vascular volume to the original volume, the hemoglobin level theoretically may decrease by 25%, but cardiac output is usually restored to the original state. Again, oxygen delivery is only halved, with plenty of oxygen still being delivered to avoid ongoing anaerobic metabolism. It is difficult to calculate cardiac output and hemoglobin level that fall to a point at which oxygen delivery is reduced by 75%—that is, to below the anaerobic threshold.

In hypovolemic shock states, it was thought that even though global oxygen delivery might be adequate, regional hypoxia is ongoing. Different organs and tissue beds are not similar in their oxygen needs or consumption. Hypoxic insult may be experienced by the critical organs, whose flow is usually preserved, whereas nonessential organs are sacrificed in terms of oxygen delivery. However, these patients are not actively moving and their oxygen demand is minimal. Thus, the theory of oxygen debt is in question. In exercise states, even if there is oxygen debt, it is paid back quickly and does not take days.

To optimize oxygen delivery, one of the most efficient ways, according to past calculations, was to add hemoglobin . If the hemoglobin level increased from 8.0 to 10 dL/liter, by transfusing 2 units of blood, oxygen delivery would increase by 25%. Blood transfusions were part of the optimization process, because they also increased wedge pressure and LVED volume and thus cardiac output, but it was rarely noted that transfusions placed patients on the flat part of the consumption curve.

Decades ago, it was also thought that an increased hematocrit level would reduce flow to the capillaries, so clinicians had reservations about transfusing too much blood. Studies in the 1950s demonstrated better flow at the capillary level with diluted blood. However, the small amount of decreased flow with the higher viscosity was in the range of a few percentage points and did not compare to the 25% increase in oxygen delivery with several units of PRBCs. Blood transfusions by calculation would be the most efficient way of increasing oxygen delivery, if that were the goal.

Current exercise physiology studies have shown that professional athletes perform better when their hemoglobin levels are above normal. The athletes who blood dope, by undergoing blood transfusions or by taking red cell production enhancers, such as erythropoietin, are now banned for illegal performance enhancement. Such athletes have cardiac outputs of more than 20 to 50 liters/min; they do not seem to have any problem with sludging caused by the higher flow and thicker than normal blood. The argument against this analogy of athletes and their capability to deliver oxygen despite a high hematocrit level is that injured patients have capillaries that are not vasodilated and are often plugged with white and red cells.

## Global Perfusion Versus Regional Perfusion

Gaining the ability to measure BP was revolutionary. However, because the main functions of the vascular system are to deliver needed nutrients and carry excreted substances from the cells, clinicians constantly ask whether pressure or flow is more important. During sepsis, systemic vascular resistance is low. A malfunction somewhere in the regulatory system is assumed.

A teleologic explanation is also possible. Lower systemic vascular resistance could be a way that our body evolved so that cardiac output could be easily increased as afterload is reduced. Some shunting is believed to occur at the capillary level, however, so should BP be augmented with the exogenous administration of pressor agents, normalizing BP at the expense of capillary flow? High doses of pressor agents most likely worsen flow, because lactate levels increase if the pressor dose is too high. That rise could be the result of a stress response because catecholamines are known to increase lactate levels or decrease flow to the capillary beds.

Purists would prefer to have lower BP pressure, as long as flow is adequate, but some organs are somewhat sensitive to pressure. For example, the brain and kidneys are traditionally thought to be pressure-dependent; however, when early experiments were done, it was difficult to isolate flow from pressure, because those two values are interrelated. With the concept that flow might be more important than just pressure, technology has focused on measuring nutrient flow rather than pressure.

During hemorrhage or hypovolemia, blood is redirected to organs such as the brain, liver, and kidneys—at the expense of tissue beds such as the skin, muscle, and gut. Thus, the search ensued to find the reason for this. The gastrointestinal (GI) tract became the focus of much research. Two main methods were developed, gastric tonometry and near-infrared (NIR) technology.

Gastric tonometry measures the adequacy of blood flow in the GI tract through placement of a $CO_2$-permeable balloon, filled with saline, in the stomach of a patient after gastric acid suppression. The balloon is left intact with the mucosa of the stomach for 30 minutes, allowing the $CO_2$ of the gastric mucosa to pass into the balloon and equilibrate. The saline and gas are then withdrawn from the balloon; the partial pressure of the $CO_2$ is measured. That value, in conjunction with the arterial bicarbonate ($HCO_3^-$) level, is used in the Henderson-Hasselbalch equation to calculate the pH of the gastric mucosa and, by inference, to determine the adequacy of blood flow to the splanchnic circulation.

The logistic difficulties of gastric tonometry are concerning. Data on its use have suggested that even though it can help predict survival, resuscitating patients to a certain value has no benefit. Most clinicians have now abandoned gastric tonometry. A multicenter trial has shown that in patients with septic shock, gastric tonometry is predictive of outcome, but implementing it is no better than using the cardiac index as a resuscitation goal.[29] Regional variables of organ dysfunction are thought to be better monitoring variables than global pressure-related hemodynamic variables. However, the data seem to indicate consistently that initial resuscitation of critically ill patients with shock does not require monitoring of regional variables. After stabilization, regional variables are, at best, merely predictors of outcome.

The optimal device for monitoring the adequacy of resuscitation should be noninvasive, simple, cheap, and portable. NIR spectroscopy uses the NIR region of the electromagnetic spectrum from approximately 800 to 2500 nm. Typical applications are wide ranging and include the areas of physics, astronomy, chemistry, pharmaceuticals, medical diagnostics, and food and agrochemical quality control. The main attraction of NIR is that light, at those wavelengths, can penetrate skin and bone. This is why your hand looks red when placed over a flashlight as the other visible light waves are absorbed or reflected, but red and infrared light pass through easily.

A common device using NIR technology that has now become standard in the medical industry is the pulse oximeter. Using slightly different light waves, it correlates with such variables as cytochrome $aa_3$ status by adding a third light wave in the 800-nm region. When the oxygen supply is less than adequate, the rate of electron transport is reduced and oxidative phosphorylation decreases, leading ultimately to anaerobic metabolism. Optical devices that use NIR wavelengths can determine the redox potential of copper atoms on cytochrome aa3 and have been used to study intracellular oxidative processes noninvasively. Thus, with NIR technology, the question of oxygenation or perfusion is bypassed; the metabolic rate of tissue can be directly determined to assess whether it is being adequately oxygenated. Animal models of hemorrhagic shock have validated the potential use of NIR technology in that they showed changes in regional tissue beds (Fig. 5-10). The

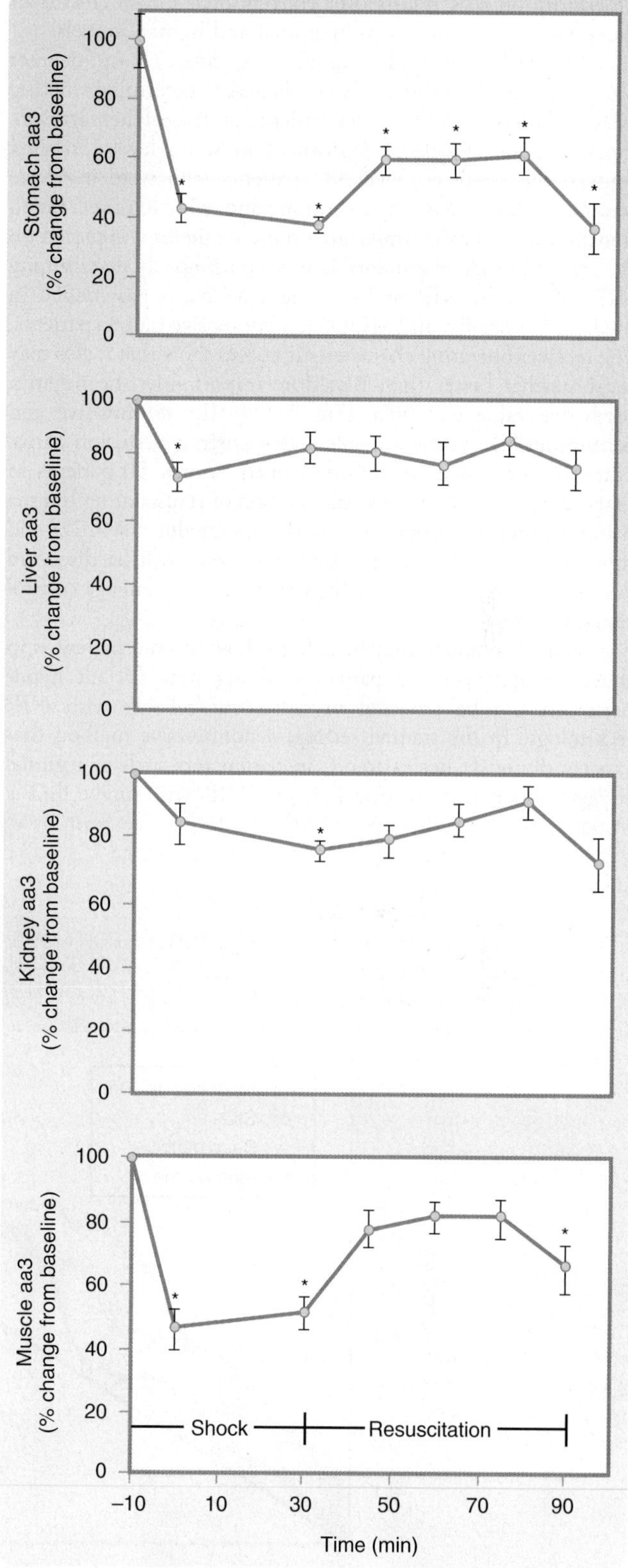


**FIGURE 5-10** Cytochrome aa3 measurements in rabbits during hemorrhagic shock. Shown are regional tissue beds and implied tissue oxygenation. Oxygenation at the mitochondrial level is preserved in kidney and liver compared with muscle and stomach. (From Rhee P, Langdale L, Mock C, et al: Near-infrared spectroscopy: Continuous measurement of cytochrome oxidation during hemorrhagic shock. Crit Care Med 25:166–170, 1997.)

superiority of NIR results over conventional measurements of shock have also been shown in animal and human models.

In search of the ideal monitoring device, a multicenter prospective study was recently conducted to determine whether NIR technology could detect patients at risk of hemorrhagic shock and its sequelae.[30] Performed in seven level I trauma centers, the study enrolled 383 patients who were in severe traumatic shock, with hypotension, and who required blood transfusions. A probe similar to a pulse oximeter was placed on the thenar muscle of patients' hands, continuously determining NIR values. The NIR probe was as sensitive as base deficit in predicting mortality and MODS in hypotensive trauma patients. The receiver operating characteristic curves show that it also may be somewhat better than BP. More importantly, the negative predictive value was 90% (Fig. 5-11). The noninvasive and continuous NIR probe was able to demonstrate perfusion status. Note, however, that MODS developed in only 50 patients in that study, probably because the method of resuscitating trauma patients changed during this period, which reduced MODS and mortality rates. The changes that took place will be discussed later in this chapter but, briefly, was because of damage control resuscitation.

NIR technology may be able to show when a patient is in shock or even when a patient is doing well. Occult hypoperfusion can be detected or ruled out reliably with NIR technology. In the trauma setting, a noninvasive method that can continuously detect trends in parameters such as regional oxygenation status, base deficit, and BP will surely find a role, but will this technology change how patients are treated? The debate now centers on this issue and raises some questions:

- Once a patient's hypoperfusion status has been determined, whether by BP, NIR technology, or some other modality, what do we do with that information?
- Is it necessary to increase oxygen delivery to regional tissue beds that are inadequately oxygenated?
- Previous studies have shown that optimizing global oxygen delivery is not useful and that regional tissue monitoring with gastric tonometry has also failed to show benefit, so will NIR technology be helpful or harmful?

An example of harm is overresuscitating a patient to fix an abnormal value that might not mean much clinically. The end point of resuscitation is constantly being debated. Because NIR results correlate well with base deficit, though, NIR technology may someday be used to monitor a surrogate marker indirectly, such as base deficit, even though it does not measure that value directly.

NIR technology has other promising uses in surgery, such as directly monitoring flow and tissue oxygenation in high-risk patients (e.g., those undergoing organ transplantation, free flap perfusion, classification of burn injuries, intraoperative assessment of bowel ischemia, with compartment syndrome or subdural and epidural hematomas). Perhaps the most useful application will be in the ICU in septic shock patients at risk for MODS.

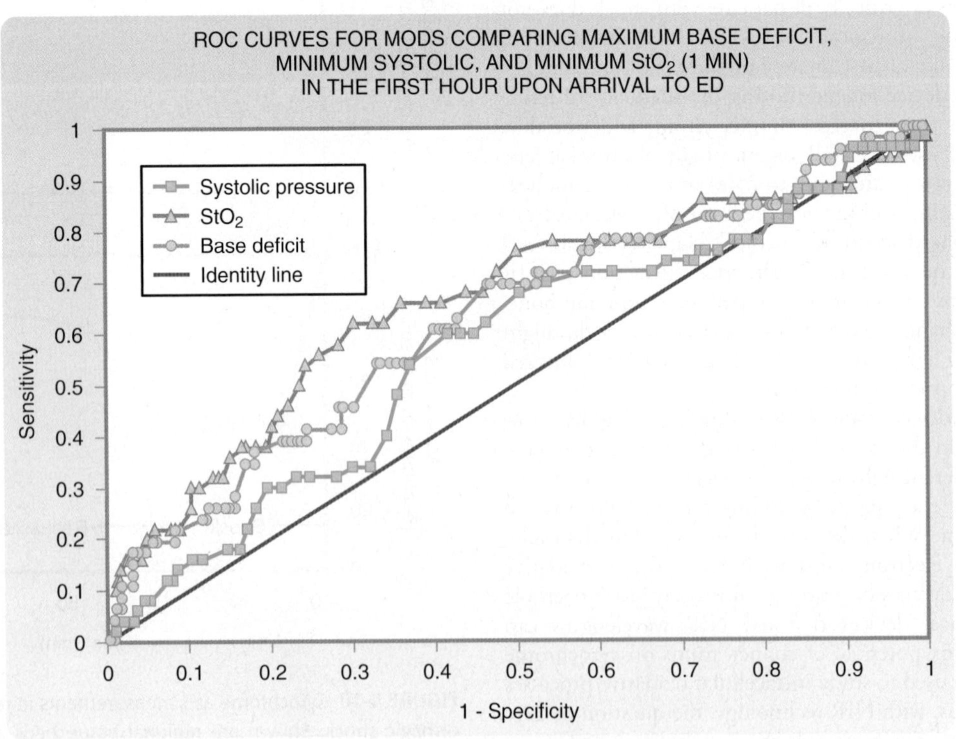


**FIGURE 5-11** NIR spectroscopy in 383 patients with traumatic hemorrhagic shock with hypotension who required blood transfusion. NIR measured tissue oxygenation levels in the thenar muscle noninvasively and was found to correlate well with arterial base deficit. (From Cohn SM, Nathens AB, Moore FA, et al: Tissue oxygen saturation predicts the development of organ dysfunction during traumatic shock resuscitation. J Trauma 62(1):44–55, 2007.)

## Septic Shock

International experts strongly agree on many recommendations for the best care of patients with severe sepsis. The Surviving Sepsis Campaign clinical guidelines were published in 2004.[31] These treatment methods were graded by a panel of 55 international experts, using grades ranging from high (A) to very low (D) to assess the quality of evidence. Strong recommendations (rated as a 1) indicated that an intervention's desirable effects clearly outweigh its undesirable effects (e.g., risk, burden, cost) or clearly do not. Weak recommendations (rated as a 2) indicated that the tradeoff between desirable and undesirable effects is less clear. The rating of strong or weak is considered of greater clinical importance than a difference in the letter grade for the quality of evidence. In areas without complete agreement, a formal process of resolution was developed and applied. Key recommendations, listed by category, are given in Box 5-2.

## Other Supportive Therapeutic Options for Severe Sepsis

Symbols are as shown in Box 5-2 (✓ indicates a strong recommendation, or "we recommend"; ◦ indicates a weak recommendation, or "we suggest"). Strength of recommendation and quality of evidence have been assessed using the GRADE (***g***rades of ***r***ecommendation, ***a***ssessment, ***d***evelopment, and ***e***valuation) criteria, presented in the parentheses after each recommendation.

### Blood Product Administration

✓Give red blood cells when hemoglobin level decreases to <7.0 g/liter (<70 g/liter) to target a hemoglobin level of 7.0 to 9.0 g/dL in adults (1B). A higher hemoglobin level may be required in special circumstances (e.g., myocardial ischemia, severe hypoxemia, acute hemorrhage, cyanotic heart disease, lactic acidosis).

### BOX 5-2 International Guidelines for Management of Severe Sepsis and Septic Shock: Hemodynamic Support and Adjunctive Therapy

Strength of recommendation and quality of evidence have been assessed using the GRADE criteria, presented in the parentheses after each guideline:

✓Indicates a strong recommendation, or "we recommend"

◦Indicates a weak recommendation, or "we suggest"

**Fluid Therapy**

✓Fluid-resuscitate using crystalloids or colloids (1B).

✓Target a CVP of ≥8 mm Hg (≥12 mm Hg if mechanically ventilated) (1C).

✓Use of fluid challenge technique while associated with a hemodynamic improvement (1D).

✓Give fluid challenges of 1000 mL of crystalloids or 300-500 mL or colloids over 30 min. More rapid and larger volumes may be required in sepsis-induced tissue hypoperfusion (1D).

✓Rate of fluid administration should be reduced if cardiac filling pressures increase without concurrent hemodynamic improvement (1D).

**Vasopressors**

✓Maintain MAP ≥ 65 mm Hg (1C).

✓Norepinephrine and dopamine centrally administered are the initial vasopressors of choice (1C).

◦Epinephrine, phenylephrine, or vasopressin should not be administered as the initial vasopressor in septic shock (2C). Vasopressin, 0.03 units/min, may be subsequently added to norepinephrine with anticipation of an effect equivalent to norepinephrine alone.

◦Use epinephrine as the first alternative agent in septic shock when blood pressure is poorly responsive to norepinephrine or dopamine. (2B).

✓Do not use low-dose dopamine for renal protection (1A).

✓In patients requiring vasopressors, insert an arterial catheter as soon as practical (1D).

**Inotropic Therapy**

✓Use dobutamine in patients with myocardial dysfunction as supported by elevated cardiac filling pressures and low cardiac outputs (1C).

✓Do not increase cardiac index to predetermined supranormal levels (1B).

**Steroids**

◦Consider IV hydrocortisone for adult septic shock when hypotension responds poorly to adequate fluid resuscitation and vasopressors (1C).

◦ACTH stimulation test is not recommended to identify the subset of adults with septic shock who should receive hydrocortisone (2B).

◦Hydrocortisone is preferred to dexamethasone (2B).

◦Fludrocortisone (50 μg PO, once daily) may be included if an alternative to hydrocortisone is being used that lacks significant mineralocorticoid activity. Fludrocortisone is optional if hydrocortisone is used (2C).

◦Steroid therapy may be weaned once vasopressors are no longer required (2D).

✓Hydrocortisone does should be ≤300mg/day (1A).

✓Do not use corticosteroids to treat sepsis in the absence of shock unless the patient's endocrine or corticosteroid history warrants it (1D).

**Recombinant Human Activated Protein C**

◦Consider rhAPC in adult patients with sepsis-induced organ dysfunction with clinical assessment of high risk of death (typically APCAHE II score ≥25 or multiorgan failure) if there are no contraindications (2B, 2C postoperative patients).

✓Adult patients with severe sepsis and low risk of death (typically, APACHE II score <20 or one organ failure) should not receive rhAPC (1A).

From Dellinger RP, Levy MM, Carlet JM, et al: Surviving Sepsis Campaign: International guidelines for management of severe sepsis and septic shock: 2008. Crit Care Med 36:296–327, 2008.

*ACTH,* Adrenocorticotropic hormone; *APACHE,* Acute Physiology and Chronic Health Evaluation; *CVP,* central venous pressure; *GRADE,* grades of recommendation, assessment, development and evaluation; *MAP,* mean arterial pressure; *rhAPC,* recombinant human activated protein C.

◦Do not use erythropoietin to treat sepsis-related anemia. Erythropoietin may be used for other accepted reasons (1B).
◦Do not use FFP to correct laboratory clotting abnormalities unless there is bleeding or planned invasive procedures (2D).
✓Do not use antithrombin therapy (1B).
◦Administer platelets when (2D):
Counts are <5,000 mm$^3$ (5 × 10$^9$/liter) regardless of bleeding
Counts are 5,000 to 30,000/mm$^3$ (5-30 × 10$^9$/liter) and there is significant bleeding risk
Higher platelet counts (≥50,000 mm$^3$ [5-50 × 10$^9$/liter]) are required for surgery or invasive procedures

### Mechanical Ventilation of Sepsis-Induced Acute Lung Injury or Acute Respiratory Distress Syndrome

✓Target a tidal volume of 6 mL/kg (predicted) body weight in patients with acute lung injury (ALI) or ARDS (1B).
✓Target an initial upper limit plateau pressure to ≤30 cm $H_2O$. Consider chest wall compliance when assessing plateau pressure (1C).
✓Allow $PaCO_2$ to increase above normal, if needed, to minimize plateau pressures and tidal volumes (1C).
✓Set positive end-expiratory pressure (PEEP) to avoid extensive lung collapse at end-expiration (1C)
◦Consider using the prone position for ARDS patients requiring potentially injurious levels of $FIO_2$ or plateau pressure, provided they are not put at risk from positional changes (2C).
✓Maintain mechanically ventilated patients in a semirecumbent position (head of the bed raised to 45 degrees) unless contraindicated (1B), between 30 and 45 degrees (2C).
◦Noninvasive ventilation should be considered in the minority of ALI or ARDS patients with mild to moderate hypoxemic respiratory failure. These patients need to be hemodynamically stable, comfortable, easily arousable, able to protect and clear their airway, and expected to recover rapidly (2B).
✓Use a weaning protocol and an spontaneous breathing trial (SBT) regularly to evaluate the potential for discontinuing mechanical ventilation (1A).
✓SBT options include a low level of pressure support with continuous positive airway pressure, 5 cm $H_2O$, or a T piece.
✓Before the SBT, patients should:
Be arousable.
Be hemodynamically stable without vasopressors.
Have no new potentially serious conditions.
Have low ventilatory and end-expiratory pressure requirements.
Require $FIO_2$ levels that can be safely delivered with a face mask or nasal cannula.
✓Do not use a pulmonary artery catheter for the routine monitoring of patients with ALI or ARDS (1A).
✓Use a conservative fluid strategy for patients with established ALI who do not have evidence of tissue hypoperfusion (1C).

### Sedation, Analgesia, and Neuromuscular Blockade

✓Use sedation protocols with a sedation goal for critically ill, mechanically ventilated patients (1B).
✓Use intermittent bolus sedation or continuous infusion sedation to predetermined end points (sedation scales), with daily interruption or lightening to produce awakening. Retitrate if necessary (1B).
✓Avoid neuromuscular blockers where possible. Monitor depth of block with train-of-four test when using continuous infusions (1B).

### Glucose Control

✓Use IV insulin to control hyperglycemia in patients with severe sepsis following stabilization in the ICU (1B).
✓Aim to keep blood glucose level <150 mg/dL (8.3 mmol/liter) using a validated protocol for insulin dose adjustment (2C).
✓Provide a glucose calorie source and monitor blood glucose levels every 1 to 2 hours (4 hours when stable) in patients receiving IV insulin (1C).
✓Interpret with caution low glucose levels obtained with point of care testing, because these techniques may overestimate arterial blood or plasma glucose levels (1B).

### Renal Replacement

◦Intermittent hemodialysis and continuous venovenous hemofiltration (CVVH) are considered equivalent (2B).
◦CVVH offers easier management in hemodynamically unstable patients (2D).

### Bicarbonate Therapy

✓Do not use bicarbonate therapy for improving hemodynamics or reducing vasopressor requirements when treating hypoperfusion-induced lactic acidemia with pH ≥7.15 (1B).

### Deep Vein Thrombosis Prophylaxis

✓Use low-dose unfractionated heparin (UFH) or low-molecular-weight heparin (LMWH), unless contraindicated (1A).
✓Use a mechanical prophylactic device, such as compression stockings or an intermittent compression device, when heparin is contraindicated (1A).
◦Use a combination of pharmacologic and mechanical therapy for patients who are at very high risk for deep vein thrombosis (2C).
◦In patients at very high risk, LMWH should be used rather than UFH (2C).

### Stress Ulcer Prophylaxis

✓Provide stress ulcer prophylaxis using an $H_2$ blocker (1A) or proton pump inhibitor (1B). Benefits of prevention of upper GI bleed must be weighed against the potential for development of ventilator-acquired pneumonia.

### Consideration for Limitation of Support

◦Discuss advance care planning with patients and families. Describe likely outcomes and set realistic expectations (1D).

Some of the most crucial recommendations are as follows: early goal-directed resuscitation of the septic patient during the first 6 hours after recognition of sepsis (1C); blood cultures before antibiotic therapy (1C); prompt performance of imaging studies to confirm potential source of infection (1C); administration of broad-spectrum antibiotic therapy within 1 hour after diagnosis of septic shock (1B) and of severe sepsis without septic shock (1D); reassessment of antibiotic therapy with microbiologic and clinical data to narrow coverage, when appropriate (1C); a usual 7 to 10 days of antibiotic therapy guided by the clinical response (1D); source control with attention to the balance of risks and benefits of the chosen method (1C); administration of crystalloid or colloid fluid resuscitation (1B); fluid challenge to restore mean circulating filling pressure (1C); reduction in rate of fluid administration with rising filling pressures if tissue perfusion is not improving (1D); vasopressor preference for norepinephrine or dopamine to maintain an initial target of mean arterial pressure (MAP) of at least 65 mm Hg (1C); dobutamine inotropic therapy when cardiac output remains low, despite fluid resuscitation and despite combined inotropic-vasopressor therapy (1C); stress dose steroid therapy only for septic shock patients whose BP responds poorly to fluid and vasopressor therapy (2C); and recombinant activated protein C in patients with severe sepsis who are clinically deemed at high risk of death (2B, but rated 2C in postoperative patients).

In patients without tissue hypoperfusion, coronary artery disease, or acute hemorrhage, major recommendations are as follows: target hemoglobin level of 7 to 9 g/dL (1B); low tidal volume (1B) and limitation of inspiratory plateau pressure strategy (1C) in patients with acute lung injury (ALI) or ARDS, application of at least a minimal amount of positive end-expiratory pressure in patients with ALI (1C); head of bed elevation for mechanically ventilated patients unless contraindicated (1B); avoidance of routine use of pulmonary artery catheters in patients with ALI or ARDS (1A); reduction in the number of days of mechanical ventilation and in ICU length of stay, as well as a conservative fluid strategy, in patients with established ALI and/or ARDS who are not in shock (1C); protocols for weaning and for sedation or analgesia (1B); intermittent bolus sedation or continuous infusion sedation with daily interruptions or lightening (1B); avoidance of neuromuscular blockers, if possible (1B); institution of glycemic control (1B); target blood glucose level lower than 150 mg/dL after initial stabilization (2C); equivalency of CVVH or intermittent hemodialysis (2B); prophylaxis for deep vein thrombosis (1A); use of stress ulcer prophylaxis to prevent upper GI bleeding by using histamine ($H_2$ blockers) (1A) or proton pump inhibitors (1B); and consideration of limiting support, when appropriate (1D).

Recommendations specific to pediatric patients with severe sepsis include greater use of physical examination therapeutic end points (2C), use of dopamine as the first drug of choice for hypotension (2C), use of steroids only in children with suspected or proven adrenal insufficiency (2C), and nonuse of recombinant activated protein C (1B).

## RESUSCITATION

### Problems With Resuscitation

Lessons learned from the Korean War showed that resuscitation with blood and blood products was useful. Throughout that war, the concept prevailed that a limited amount of salt and water should be given to patients after injuries. That derived, in part, from the work of Coller and Moyer in experiments done at the University of Michigan. By the time of the Vietnam War, volume resuscitation in excess of replacement of shed blood became an acceptable practice to maintain adequate homeostasis. The practice may have been induced by hemorrhagic shock experiments performed by Tom Shires. In his classic study, Shires used the Wiggers model and bled 30 dogs to a mean BP of 50 mm Hg for 90 minutes. He then infused LR (5% of body weight) followed by blood in 10 dogs, plasma (10 mL/kg) followed by blood in another 10 dogs, and shed blood alone in the remaining 10 dogs. The dogs that received LR had the best survival rates. Shires concluded that although the replacement of lost blood with whole blood remains the primary treatment of shock, adjunctive replacement of the coexisting functional volume deficit with a balanced salt solution appears to be of value.

Soon, the surgical community went from being judicious with crystalloid solutions to being aggressive. Surgeons returning from the Vietnam War advocated the use of crystalloids, a seemingly cheap and easy method of resuscitating patients. They touted the lives that were saved. However, what evolved from this method of resuscitation was the so-called *Da Nang lung*, eventually known as *ARDS*. (The U.S. Navy had its field hospital in Da Nang, Vietnam.) The explanation for the evolution of the new condition was that battlefield patients were now living long enough to develop it, because their lives were saved with aggressive resuscitation and better critical care, including a greater capability to treat renal failure. In contrast, in previous wars, it was thought that patients died early from inadequately treated shock.

However, that explanation had no supporting evidence. The killed in action (KIA) rate (the number of wounded patients who died before reaching a facility that had a physician present) had not changed for over a century (Table 5-5). The died of wounds (DOW) rate (the number of wounded patients who died after reaching a facility that had a physician present) had decreased during World War II because of the use of antibiotics, but it was slightly higher during the Vietnam War. The perceived reason for the slightly higher DOW rate was that patients in Vietnam were transported to medical facilities more quickly by helicopters. Transport times had decreased, from an average of 4 hours to 40 minutes, but if the sicker patients who would have normally died in the field were transported more quickly to die in the medical facility, the KIA rate should have fallen—and it did not.

Moreover, the renal failure rate and cause of renal failure did not significantly change between the Korean War and the Vietnam War. Another false argument was that the wounds seen during the Vietnam War were worse, because of the enemy's high-velocity AK-47 rifles. Actually, the rounds or bullets used by the AK-47 were similar to those used by the enemy in the Russo-Japanese War, World War I, and World War II. The 7.62-mm round used in the AK-47 rifle was invented by the Japanese in the 1890s.

In the early 1970s, the prehospital system in the United States started to evolve. Previously, ambulances were usually hearses driven by morticians, which is why early ambulances

**Table 5-5**

| WAR | KILLED IN ACTION (%) | DIED OF WOUNDS (%) |
|---|---|---|
| Civil War | 16.0 | 13.0 |
| Russo-Japanese War | 20.0 | 9.0 |
| WW I | 19.6 | 8.1 |
| WW II | 19.8 | 3.0 |
| Korean War | 19.5 | 2.4 |
| Vietnam | 20.2 | 3.5 |

**Table 5-6 Prehospital Fluid Studies in Trauma Patients**

| STUDY | STUDY SETTING |
|---|---|
| Aprahamian et al: The effect of a paramedic system on mortality of major open intra-abdominal vascular trauma. J Trauma 23:687–690, 1983. | Paramedic system<br>Open intra-abdominal vascular trauma |
| Kaweski SM et al: The effect of prehospital fluids on survival in trauma patients. J Trauma 30:1215–1218, 1990. | Prehospital fluids<br>Trauma patients |
| Bickell et al. Immediate versus delayed fluid resuscitation for hypotensive patients with penetrating torso injuries. N Engl J Med 331:1105–1109, 1994. | Presurgery fluids<br>Hypotensive penetrating torso injuries |
| Turner et al: A randomised controlled trial of prehospital intravenous fluid replacement therapy in serious trauma. Health Technol Assess 4:1–57, 2000. | Prehospital<br>1309 serious trauma patients |
| Kwan et al: Timing and volume of fluid administration for patients with bleeding following trauma. Cochrane Database Syst Rev (1):CD002245, 2001. | Prehospital<br>Bleeding trauma patients |
| Dula et al: Use of prehospital fluids in hypotensive blunt trauma patients. Prehosp Emerg Care 6:417–420, 2002. | Prehospital<br>Hypotensive blunt trauma patients |
| Greaves et al: Fluid resuscitation in pre-hospital trauma care: A consensus view. J R Coll Surg Edinb 47:451–457, 2002. | Prehospital<br>Consensus view |
| Dutton et al: Hypotensive resuscitation during active hemorrhage: Impact on in-hospital mortality. J Trauma 52:1141–1146, 2002. | Presurgery fluids<br>Hypotensive active hemorrhage |
| Dula et al: Use of prehospital fluids in hypotensive blunt trauma patients. Prehosp Emerg Care 6:417-420, 2002. | Prehospital fluids<br>Hypotensive patients |

were of the station wagon configuration. As the career paths of emergency medical technicians and paramedics grew, they began resuscitative efforts in the field and continued them to the trauma center. The ATLS course was created in the mid-1970s by an orthopedic surgeon who survived a small plane crash, but saw his family perish in a rural area with physicians unfamiliar with modern trauma management.

To prevent shock, the ATLS course recommended that all trauma patients have two large-bore IV lines placed and receive 2 liters of LR. The actual recommendation in the ATLS text specifically states that patients in class III shock should receive 2 liters of LR followed by blood products. However, clinicians though that crystalloid solutions seemed innocuous and definitely improved BP in hypotensive patients.

In the 1980s and early 1990s, aggressive resuscitation was taught and endorsed. The two large-bore IV lines started in the field were converted to larger IV lines through a wire-guided exchange system; central lines were placed for aggressive fluid resuscitation. Some trauma centers performed cutdowns on the saphenous vein at the ankle to place IV tubing directly into the vein and thereby maximize flow during resuscitation.

Technology soon caught up, and machines were built to infuse crystalloid solutions rapidly; however, studies showed that outcomes actually worsened. The literature was filled with data showing that ischemia to tissues resulted in disturbances of all types. Optimization of oxygen delivery was the goal. As a result, massive volumes of crystalloids were poured into patients. Residents were encouraged to "pound" patients with fluids. If trauma patients did not develop ARDS, it was taught that they were not adequately resuscitated, but many clinical trials showed that prehospital fluids did not improve outcome (Table 5-6).

### Bleeding

One of the most influential studies on hemorrhagic shock was performed by Ken Mattox and, in 1994, the results were reported by Bickell and coworkers.[32] The aim of Mattox's study, a prospective clinical trial, was to determine whether withholding prehospital fluids affected outcome in hypotensive patients after a penetrating torso injury. IV lines were started in patients with BP lower than 90 mm Hg. On alternating days, patients received standard fluid therapy in the field or had fluids withheld until they reached the hospital. Withholding prehospital fluids conferred a statistically significant survival advantage—a revolutionary counterintuitive finding that shocked surgeons. To reiterate, if no fluids were given in the prehospital setting to hypotensive patients with penetrating torso injuries, they would survive more often than if fluids were given in the field.

Critics of Mattox's study claimed that reanalysis of the data using the methodology of intention to treat made the statistical significance no longer valid because the $P$ value for survival was higher than 0.05. The authors of this study excluded patients who were dead in the field when paramedics arrived. It made sense that fluids would not help those who had already died in the field, and thus should not be counted, but purists asserted that those patients should have been included in the final analysis. Even if that assertion were accounted for, Mattox's study would still show that patients who did not receive fluids had a survival advantage, albeit the difference would no longer be statistically significant. Everything that surgeons had been taught before 1994 stressed that not treating hypotensive patients with fluids would surely lead to death, yet Mattox's study showed the opposite.

That 1994 article popularized the concept of permissive hypotension—that is, allowing hypotension during uncontrolled hemorrhage. The fundamental rationale for permissive hypotension was that restoration of BP with fluids would increase bleeding from uncontrolled sources. Cannon, in 1918, had stated that "inaccessible or uncontrolled sources of blood loss should not be treated with IV fluids until the time of surgical control."

Animal studies have validated the idea of permissive hypotension. Burris and colleagues have shown that moderate resuscitation results in the best outcome compared with no resuscitation or aggressive resuscitation. In a swine model of uncontrolled hemorrhage, Sondeen has shown that raising BP with fluids or pressors could lead to increased bleeding. The idea was that increasing BP would burst the clot that had formed. The study also found that the pressure that would cause rebleeding was a MAP of 64 ± 2 mm Hg, with a systolic pressure of 94 ± 3 mm Hg and diastolic pressure of 45 ± 2 mm Hg. Other animal studies have confirmed these hypotheses.

The next question was whether the continued strategy of permissive hypotension in the operating room would result in improved survival. Dutton and associates randomized one group of patients to a target systolic BP higher than 100 mm Hg and another group to a target systolic BP of 70 mm Hg. Fluid therapy was titrated until definitive hemorrhage control was achieved. However, despite attempts to maintain BP at 70 mm Hg, the average BP was 100 mm Hg in the low-pressure group and 114 mm Hg in the high-pressure group. Patients' BPs rose spontaneously. Titrating their BP to the low target was difficult, even with less use of fluids. The survival rate did not differ between the two groups.

The idea of permissive hypotension was slow to catch on. The arguments against allowing anything but aggressive resuscitation was dismissed. Critics continued to emphasize that the Mattox trial focused only on penetrating injuries and should not be extrapolated to blunt trauma. Clinicians feared that patients with traumatic blunt head injuries would be harmed without a normalized BP. However, Shafi and Gentilello examined the National Trauma Data Bank and found that hypotension was an independent risk factor for death, but did not increase the mortality rate in patients with TBIs any more than in patients without TBIs. The risk of death quadrupled in patients with hypotension in the TBI group (odds ratio [OR], 4.1; 95% confidence interval [CI], 3.5 to 4.9) and the non-TBI group (OR, 4.6; 95% CI, 3.4 to 6.0). Furthermore, in 2006, Plurad and coworkers[43] showed that emergency department hypotension is not an independent risk factor for acute renal dysfunction or failure.

### Trauma Immunology and Inflammation

The 1990s witnessed an explosion of information regarding alterations of homeostasis and cellular physiochemistry during shock. The scientific investigations of Shires, Carrico, Baue, and countless others shed light on the basic mechanisms underlying the resuscitation of patients in shock. The pathophysiology has been identified as having an aberrant inflammatory status, resulting in the body's own immune system damaging the endothelial tissues and ultimately the end organ. This inflammatory state leads to a spectrum of conditions ranging from sequestration of fluid leading to edema, progressing to Acute Lung Injury (ALI), Systemic Inflammatory Response Syndrome (SIRS), Acute Respiratory Distress Syndrome (ARDS) and the Multiple Organ Failure (MOF) which was later termed Multiple Organ Dysfunction Syndrome (MODS).[33] Such conditions were in every surgical ICU; attention focused on biochemical perturbations and altered mediators as sites for possible interventions. The fundamental cause was thought to be that ischemia and reperfusion, as shown in animal models, would create a state of damage to the capillary endothelium and subsequent changes to the end organ. It was generally accepted that the reason for the reperfusion injury was mediated by activated neutrophils that emitted deleterious cytokines and oxygen-free radicals, which was popular then because assays to study them had been developed. The animal model used to study this pathophysiology was often the gut mesentery ischemia and reperfusion model which entailed the clamping of the mesenteric artery for a time period (e.g., the superior mesenteric artery that fed the intestines) before the clamp was removed, thus reperfusing the organ. However, ischemia reperfusion injury is different than resuscitation injury as it was later discovered.

Death after traumatic injury was described as trimodal. Some patients died within a short time after injury, some died in the hospital within a few hours, and many died late in the hospital course. However, a study in trauma patients has shown that deaths occur in a logarithmic decay fashion and follow the rule of biology; no grouping of deaths can be seen, unless the data are represented or lumped together as immediate, early, or late. The only reason for the initial trimodal distribution was that patients who died after 24 hours were labeled under late deaths.[34]

According to the traditional (although now discredited) trimodal pattern, patients who typically died first could be aided by a better prehospital system and, more importantly, by injury prevention. For the second group of patients, better resuscitation was thought to be a potentially lifesaving intervention. For the third group (the late deaths), immunomodulation was considered to be key; given these patients' responses to SIRS, a sterile phenomenon, the cause was thought to be the inflammatory adaptive aberrancy after successful resuscitation. When there is prolonged end arteriole cessation of flow producing tissue ischemia for a period of time, followed by reperfusion, it is termed *reperfusion injury*. For example, with an injury to the femoral artery that requires 4 to 6 hours to restore circulation, muscle cells may have undergo reperfusion injury and will start to swell, causing a compartment syndrome in the lower leg. This reperfusion injury was thought to occur following hemorrhagic shock. However, the pathophysiology is more one of resuscitation injury rather than reperfusion injury.

With improved technology, the immunologic response after trauma was heavily researched; in the past, we were limited to studying physiology. A theory started to evolve that shock caused an aberrant inflammatory response, which then needed to be modulated and suppressed. Many literature reports showed that the inflammatory system was upregulated or activated after shock. The white cells in the blood became activated. Neutrophils were identified as the key mediators in the acute phase of shock, even though lymphocytes are typically have a major role in chronic diseases (e.g., cancer) and in viral infections. Shock, caused by various mechanisms, was thought to induce ischemia to tissues and, after reperfusion, to set off an inflammatory response, which primarily affected the microcirculation and caused leaks (Fig. 5-12).

Typically, neutrophils are rapidly transported through capillaries. When signaled by chemokines, however, neutrophils will start to roll, adhere firmly to the endothelium, and migrate out of the capillaries to find the body's foes and initiate healing. Early researchers thought that neutrophils would battle invaders (e.g., bacteria) through phagocytic activity and the release of oxygen free radicals; this was thought to be the reason for the leak in the capillary system (Fig. 5-13). Because neutrophils can be primed to have an enhanced response, a massive search took place to identify causes of neutrophil priming and downregulation. The many cytokines targeted included interleukin (IL), types 1 through 18, tumor necrosis factor (TNF), and adhesion molecules, such as intercellular adhesion molecules (ICAMs), vascular cell adhesion molecules (VCAMs), E-selectin, L-selectin, P-selectin, and platelet-activating factor (PAF).

That research had much overlap with the research being performed in the arenas of reimplantation, vascular ischemia, and reperfusion. Clinically, it was already known that the implantation of severed extremities would have pathophysiologic results, similar to those from ischemia, reperfusion, and swelling caused by leaky capillaries. The immune response was described as bimodal; if the body was first primed by trauma or shock, it would be set up for an exaggerated response when hit with a second insult (e.g., infection).

In the late 1990s, other researchers focused on the role of the alimentary tract. They knew that the splanchnic circulation was shunted of blood by vasoconstriction during hemorrhagic shock, so the gut suffers the most ischemia during shock and is the most susceptible to reperfusion injury. The animal model most often used to study the gut's role in inflammation was a rat model of superior mesenteric artery (SMA) occlusion and reperfusion. Because SIRS is a sterile phenomenon, the gut was implicated as a potential player in the development of MODS.

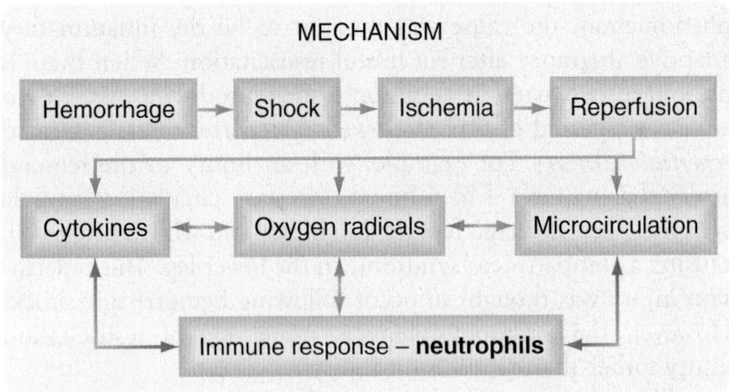


**FIGURE 5-12** Hemorrhage causing neutrophil activation.

Animals were shown to have a translocation of bacteria into the portal system; initiation of the inflammatory cascade was investigated as the source of MODS. Investigators also knew that the release of *Escherichia coli* bacteria in the blood released endotoxins, which further initiated the release of cytokines (e.g., TNF, cachectin). However, studies in humans failed to demonstrate translocation of bacteria in intraoperative samples of portal vein during resuscitation. Although complete occlusion of the SMA for hours, followed by reperfusion, does result in swollen necrotic injured bowel, the problem was that these findings were extrapolated to humans undergoing hemorrhagic shock. Again, during hemorrhagic shock, the SMA is not occluded and, even during severe states, there is a trickle flow of blood to the splanchnic organs.

Because patients in shock bleed and receive blood transfusions, transfusion of PRBCs was also implicated as the cause of MODS. Patients who required massive amounts of PRBCs were most likely to develop MODS. Researchers in this elucidating area found that the use of older PRBCs was an independent risk factor for the development of MODS. PRBCs have a shelf life of 42 days in the refrigerated state. As blood ages, changes occur in the fluid that have been shown to affect the immune response negatively.

In the past, when technology was limited, PRBCs were mainly tested for the red cells' capability to carry oxygen and their viability under the microscope and in the body. Most major trauma centers now have learned to use leukoreduced PRBCs—that is, the small number of white cells that can release oxygen free radicals and cytokines are now routinely filtered, before the PRBCs are stored. Leukoreduction removes 99.9% of donor white cells and, in one large Canadian study, reduced the mortality rate from 7.03% to 6.19%. Other trauma studies have shown no reduction in the mortality rate but still showed a decrease in rates of infection, infectious complications, and late ARDS. To date, the largest study of leukoreduction in trauma patients has not shown any reduction in the rates of infection, organ failure, or mortality.[35]

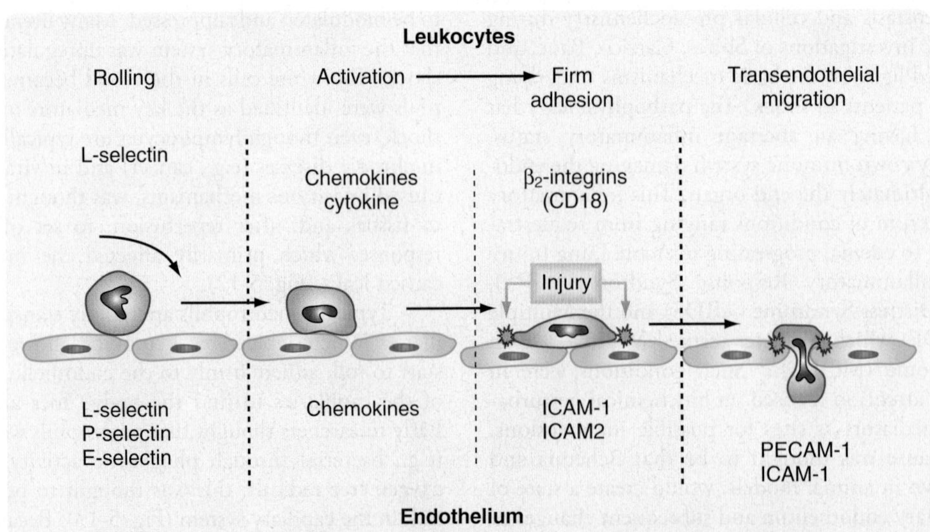


**FIGURE 5-13** Intravascular neutrophils that are activated will adhere and roll until another set of mechanisms causes firm adherence, and transendothelial migration out of the vascular system occurs. It is believed that this transmigration process injures the endothelium, with the release of an oxygen free radical. This could result in fluid leaks out of the vascular system.

Numerous trials have examined the blockage of cytokines to treat septic patients. Two prospective, randomized, multicentered, double-blinded trials—the North American Sepsis Trial (NORASEPT) and the International Sepsis Trial (INTERSEPT)—studied at the 28-day mortality rate of critically ill patients who received anti-TNF antibody. Neither trial showed any benefit. Other trials testing other potential cytokines were also disappointing. The cytokines tested included CD11/CD18,[36] anti–IL-1 receptor, antiendotoxin antibodies, bradykinin antagonists, and PAF receptor antagonists. The search continues for one key mediator that could be manipulated to solve the toxemia of shock.[37] However, such attempts to simplify the events and find one solution to the problem may be the main problem because there is no simple answer and no simple solution. The answer may lie in cocktails of substances; the humoral and endocrine systems, which are always mediated by blood, is exceedingly complex. Shock has many causes and mechanisms. Understanding this is crucial as we look for solutions.

## Evolution of Modern Resuscitation

### Detrimental Impact of Fluids

As early as the 1996, the U.S. Navy used a swine model to study the effects of fluids on neutrophil activation after hemorrhagic shock resuscitation. It was shown that neutrophils are activated after a 40% blood volume hemorrhage when followed by resuscitation with LR. That finding was not surprising; what was enlightening was that the level of neutrophil activation was similar in control animals that did not undergo hemorrhagic shock but merely received LR and in animals that were bled and resuscitated with LR (Fig. 5-14). In the other control animals, which did not receive LR but instead were resuscitated with shed blood or HTS, the neutrophils were activated significantly less after hemorrhagic shock. The implication was that the inflammatory process was not caused by shock and resuscitation, but by LR itself.

Those findings were repeated over several years in a series of experiments using human blood in small and large animal models of hemorrhagic shock. When the blood was diluted with various resuscitation fluids, the inflammatory changes depended on the fluid used; despite similar physiologic results in vivo, the immunologic results were different (Fig. 5-15). The response was ubiquitous throughout the entire inflammatory response system, including at the levels of DNA and RNA expression.

Ultimately, the cause of the enhanced inflammatory response to fluids was recognized. All the artificial fluids used to raise BP could cause the inflammatory sequelae of shock; the fluids themselves were responsible (Table 5-7). What might be obvious today was not obvious then, and was unrecognized for decades; it was not recognized that blood is extremely complex. It does so more than raise BP and carry red cells. In the past, we studied the complexity of the body's immune response, but failed to realize that fluids such as LR and normal saline that were developed more than 100 years ago were not a substitute for blood.

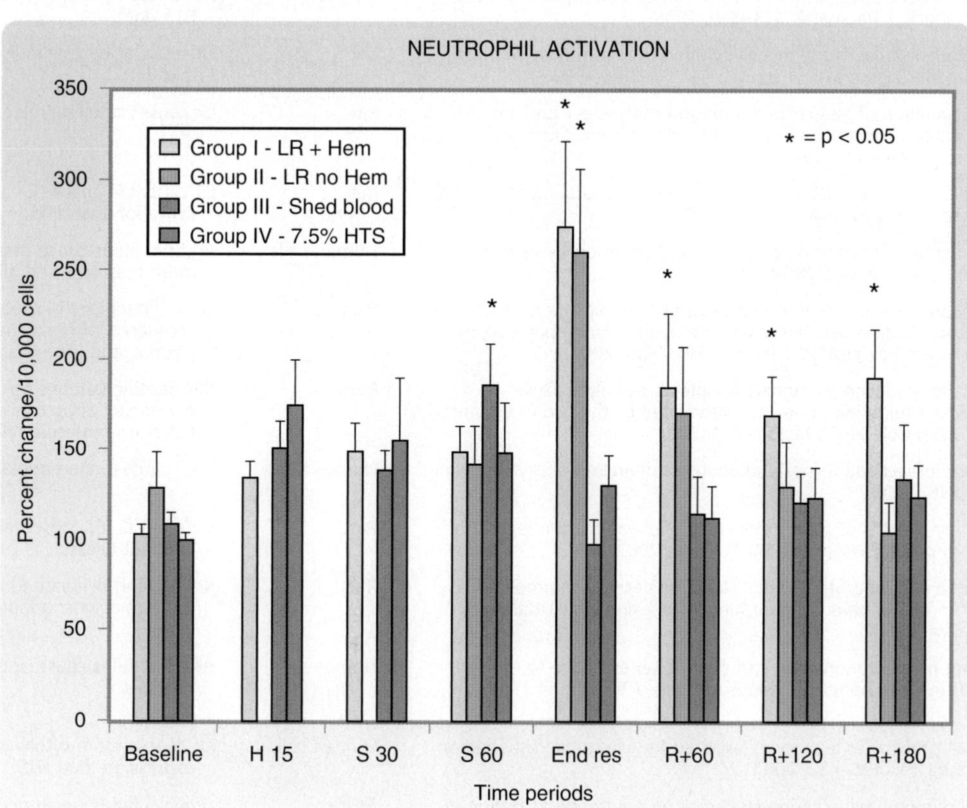


**FIGURE 5-14** Neutrophil activation in whole blood of swine measured by flow cytometry. The highest neutrophil activation occurred following hemorrhagic shock and resuscitation using LR. Similar neutrophil activation occurred when the animal was not resuscitated but was infused with LR. No activation occurred when shocked animals were resuscitated with whole blood or 7.5% HTS. (From Rhee P, Burris D, Kaufmann C, et al: Lactated Ringer's resuscitation causes neutrophil activation after hemorrhagic shock. J Trauma 44:313–319, 1998.)

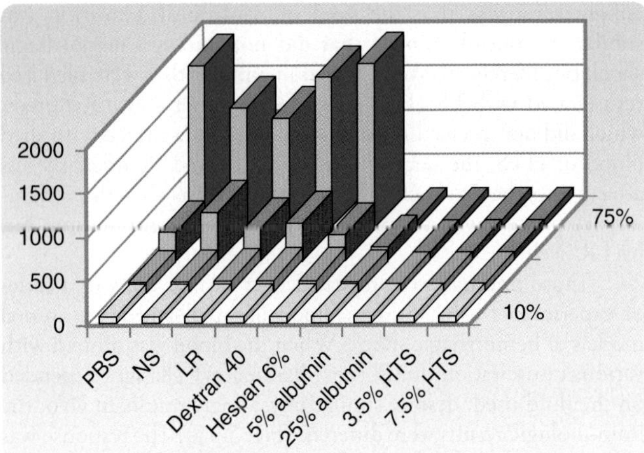


**FIGURE 5-15** Human neutrophil activation using whole blood diluted various resuscitation fluids, as measured by flow cytometry. Phosphate-buffered saline (PBS) was used because it has a pH of 7.4. (From Rhee P, Wang D, Ruff P, et al: Human neutrophil activation and increased adhesion by various resuscitation fluids. Crit Care Med 28:74–78, 2000.)

Further investigations showed that when the lactate in LR was replaced with other sources of energy that could be better used by the mitochondria, the inflammatory aspects were attenuated; one such novel fluid was ketone Ringer's solution (Table 5-8). Lactic acid occurs in two stereoisomeric forms, as well as in a racemic mixture of those isomers. In biologic systems, the true racemic mixture, or equal molarity of the isomers, rarely occurs. Usually, one or the other isomer predominates. The stereoisomers are named L(+) and D(−) lactic acid. L(+)-lactate is a normal intermediary of mammalian metabolism. The unnatural isomer, D(−)-lactate, is produced when tissue glyoxalase converts methylglyoxal into a lactic acid of the D form. L(+)-Lactate has low toxicity as a consequence of the rapid metabolism. D(−)-Lactate, however, has higher toxic potential. Psychoneurotic disturbances have been described with pure D(−)-lactate; increasing evidence has indicated a connection between high plasma concentration of racemic lactate and anxiety and panic disorders. Racemic dialysis fluids have reportedly been associated with clinical cases of D-lactate toxicity. Experiments with the isomers have shown that D(−)-lactate causes significant inflammatory changes in rats and swine as well as activation of human neutrophils.

**Table 5-7 Summary of Studies by U.S. Navy Demonstrating Fluids Causing Inflammation After Resuscitation**

| STUDY | MODEL | SUMMARY OF FINDINGS |
|---|---|---|
| Rhee et al: Lactated Ringer's solution resuscitation causes neutrophil activation after hemorrhagic shock. J Trauma 44:313–319, 1998. | Swine | LR causes neutrophils activation, blood; HTS does not. |
| Deb et al: Resuscitation with lactated Ringer's solution in rats with hemorrhagic shock induces immediate apoptosis. J Trauma 46:582–588, 1999. | Rat | LR cause apoptosis in liver and gut more than HTS. |
| Sun et al: Early up-regulation of intercellular adhesion molecule-1 and vascular cell adhesion molecule-1 expression in rats with hemorrhagic shock and resuscitation. Shock 11:416–422, 1999. | Rat | LR causes cytokine release more than HTS. |
| Alam et al: E- and P-selectin expression depends on the resuscitation fluid used in hemorrhaged rats. J Surg Res 94:145–152, 2000. | Rat | LR causes increased E- and P-selectin than activation than HTS. |
| Rhee et al: Human neutrophil activation and increased adhesion by various resuscitation fluids. Crit Care Med 28:74–78, 2000. | Human cells | Artificial fluids cause neutrophil activation more than HTS and albumin. |
| Deb et al: Lactated Ringer's solution and hetastarch but not plasma resuscitation after rat hemorrhagic shock is associated with immediate lung apoptosis by the up-regulation of the Bax protein. J Trauma 49:47–53, 2000. | Rats | LR and hetastarch increase lung apoptosis compared with plasma whole blood, plasma, and albumin. |
| Alam et al: Resuscitation-induced pulmonary apoptosis and intracellular adhesion molecule-1 expression in rats are attenuated by the use of ketone Ringer's solution. J Am Coll Surg 193:255–263, 2001. | Rats | Substituting ketones for lactate reduces pulmonary apoptosis and intracellular adhesion molecule release. |
| Koustova et al: Effects of lactated Ringer's solutions on human leukocytes. J Trauma 52:872–878, 2002. | Human cells | D-LR causes inflammation more than L-LR. |
| Alam et al: cDNA array analysis of gene expression following hemorrhagic shock and resuscitation in rats. Resuscitation 54:195–206, 2002. | Rats | Different fluids cause gene expression at different levels. |
| Koustova et al: Ketone and pyruvate Ringer's solutions decrease pulmonary apoptosis in a rat model of severe hemorrhagic shock and resuscitation. Surgery 134:267–274, 2003. | Rats | Ketone and pyruvate Ringer's solution protects against apoptosis compared with LR. |
| Stanton et al: Human polymorphonuclear cell death after exposure to resuscitation fluids in vitro: Apoptosis versus necrosis. J Trauma 54:1065–1074, 2003. | Human cells | Artificial fluids cause apoptosis and necrosis. |
| Gushchin et al: cDNA profiling in leukocytes exposed to hypertonic resuscitation fluids. J Am Coll Surg 197:426–432, 2003. | Human cells | LR causes more cytokines release via gene expression than HTS. |
| Alam et al: Effect of different resuscitation strategies on neutrophil activation in a swine model of hemorrhagic shock. Resuscitation 60:91–99, 2004. | Swine | Artificial fluids cause neutrophil activation despite resuscitation rates. |
| Jaskille et al: D-Lactate increases pulmonary apoptosis by restricting phosphorylation of bad and eNOS in a rat model of hemorrhagic shock. J Trauma 57:262–269, 2004. | Rats | D-Lactate in fluids causes more apoptosis than L-Lactate. |

**Table 5-8 Components of Ketone Ringer's Solution***

| COMPONENT | NORMAL SALINE (mEq/LITER) | D-LR (mEq/LITER) | L-LR (mEq/LITER) | KETONE RINGER'S SOLUTION (mEq/LITER) |
|---|---|---|---|---|
| D-Lactate | – | 14 | – | – |
| L-Lactate | – | 14 | 28 | – |
| 3-D-β-hydroxybutryate | – | – | – | 28 |
| Sodium | 154 | 130 | 130 | 130 |
| Potassium | – | 4 | 4 | 4 |
| Calcium | – | 3 | 3 | 3 |
| Chloride | 154 | 109 | 109 | 109 |

*Replacing lactate with an alternative fuel source such as ketone affected the immunologic response following resuscitation.

In 1999, with new evidence implicating LR as the cause of ARDS and MODS, the U.S. Navy contracted with the Institute of Medicine to review the topic of the optimal resuscitation fluid.[38] Their report made many recommendations; key recommendations were that LR be manufactured with only the L(+) isomer of lactate and that researchers continue to search for alternative resuscitation fluids that do not contain lactate but contain other nutrients, such as ketones. It stated that the optimal resuscitation fluid is 7.5% HTS because of the decreased inflammation associated with it and its logistic advantage in terms of weight and size. Although the Institute of Medicine had been asked to make recommendations for the military, the report's authors thought that the evidence was also applicable to civilian injuries as well.

HTS has a long record of research and development. It has been used in humans for decades and has been consistently shown to be less inflammatory than LR. This immunologic advantage had always been attributed to its own properties as compared with LR or normal saline. However, more recent evidence involving proper controls have shown that HTS is not necessarily better than LR, but that LR is worse than HTS. This is important because for the first time investigators started to recognize that LR and normal saline may be detrimental. Again, blood is complex, and the fluids used in the past were a poor replacement.

PRBCs, different from whole blood, were also a poor replacement—PRBCs are separated, washed, and then filtered. with much of the plasma stripped out. Clotting factors, glucose, hormones, and cytokines crucial for signaling were not in PRBCs or in most of the fluids formerly used for resuscitation. Evidence that the fluid type affects the inflammatory response is now growing and has been confirmed in a number of studies.[39]

Based on these findings, a national consensus panel of experts recommended a plasma volume expander, 6% hetastarch (Hespan), as the fluid of choice for the military.[40] The rationale was that even though the Institute of Medicine recommended 7.5% HTS, it was not commercially available was not approved by the FDA. In addition, the panel of experts convened by the U.S. military believed that a colloid offered the benefit of less weight and cube, meaning that the average medic could resuscitate patients with one third of the volume (as compared with HTS) and would not have to carry large bags of LR or normal saline in the field.

After this recommendation was presented, another workshop was convened and changed the recommendation to 6% hetastarch in LR (Hextend). The predominant rationale was that a single study had shown that in patients undergoing cardiac surgery, Hextend decreased transfusion requirements postoperatively (as compared with Hespan), possibly because the calcium in LR aided in coagulation, but this was not substantiated. Subsequent studies have shown no difference in coagulation properties between hetastarches, whether the carrier is saline or LR.

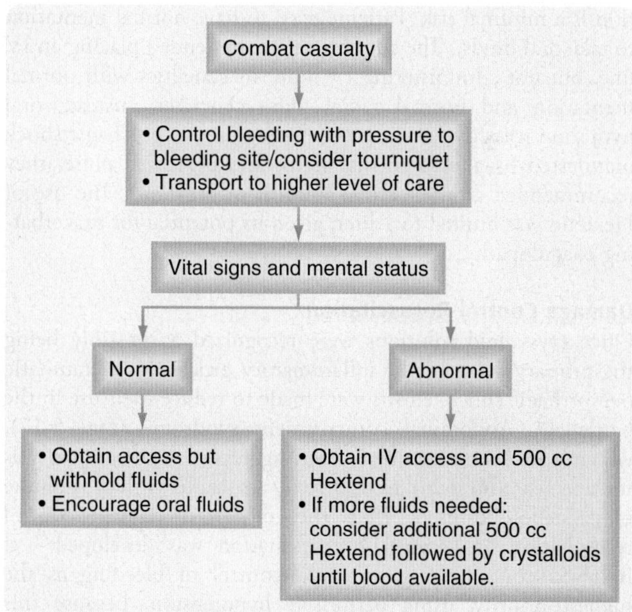


**FIGURE 5-16** New recommendation for fluid resuscitation for the U.S. Military by the Committee on Tactical Combat Casualty Care. (From Rhee P, Koustova E, Alam H: Searching for the optimal resuscitation method: Recommendations for the initial fluid resuscitation in combat casualties. J Trauma 54:S52–S62, 2003.)

The Committee on Tactical Combat Casualty Care was formed in 2000 by the U.S. Navy and now sets policy on the prehospital management of combat casualties. Their recommendations and algorithm for resuscitation were revolutionary compared with the civilian recommendations (Fig. 5-16). The algorithm was formed with the following points in mind:

1. Most combat casualties do not require fluid resuscitation.
2. Oral hydration is an underused option.

3. Aggressive resuscitation has not been shown to be beneficial in civilian victims of penetrating trauma.
4. Moderate resuscitation in animal models of uncontrolled hemorrhage offers the best outcome.
5. Large volumes of LR are not safe.
6. Colloid or HTS offers a significant advantage in terms of less weight and cube for the military medic.

The committee recommended Hextend, which seemed similar to Hespan but with the potential for benefit in terms of coagulopathy. It was recognized that the most casualties were not undergoing hemorrhagic shock and were not in any jeopardy of bleeding to death. Only a minority of patients required fluid resuscitation in the field. Surgeons and anesthesiologists generally would prefer all patients to be NPO to avoid aspiration during induction of anesthesia and surgery, but trauma patients are never NPO. With the rapid induction of anesthesia, aspiration is a minimal risk. Patients need to have normal mentation to take oral fluids,. The committee recommended placing an IV line, but not administering IV fluid, in casualties with normal mentation and normal radial pulse character; instead, oral hydration was advised. In those undergoing hemorrhagic shock manifested by altered mental status and decreased pulse, they recommended administering 500 mL of Hextend. The use of Hextend was limited to 1 liter, given its potential for exacerbating coagulopathy.

## Damage Control Resuscitation

Once crystalloid solutions were recognized as possibly being the primary cause of the inflammatory process after traumatic hemorrhagic shock, efforts were made to reduce their use in the battlefield. Abdominal compartment syndrome (Fig. 5-17), which had been described when aggressive resuscitation was routine, was also found to be directly associated with the volume of crystalloid infused. Thus, the concept of damage control resuscitation or hemostatic resuscitation was developed.[41] It involved concentrating on rapid control of bleeding as the highest priority, using permissive hypotension, because this would minimize the use of acellular fluids and not burst the clot, minimizing the use of crystalloid solutions, using HTS to reduce the total volume of crystalloid necessary, using blood products early, and considering the use of drugs such as rFVIIa or factor IX to stop bleeding and reduce coagulopathy (Box 5-3). The rationale for the early use of blood products was that large volumes of crystalloids were detrimental; because fresh whole blood was not available, component therapy with pRBCs, thawed plasma, and platelets would approximate whole blood and minimize the use of acellular fluids. Component therapy was not ideal compared with fresh whole blood but because of logistic problems, it was not available, and component therapy used empirically for some patients with ongoing uncontrolled hemorrhage would be better in the long term. Mental status was thought to be a useful to guide to determine who needed care; the use of the radial pulse was preferred over BP cuffs, which are not practical when personnel are under fire in the combat setting.

With the promotion of damage control resuscitation, clinical studies indicated that aggressive early use of blood products, such as PRBCs and FFP, reduce the total volume of PRBCs used by 25%.[42] These studies also used permissive hypotension and focused on surgical control of hemorrhage, rather than on resuscitation before surgical control of hemorrhage. Other studies have shown that with damage control resuscitation, the incidence of ARDS decreases, from 25% of ICU admissions to 9%.[43] ARDS now occurs in patients with pulmonary contusion, pneumonia, or sepsis, but is no longer a routine complication in trauma patients who undergo damage control resuscitation.

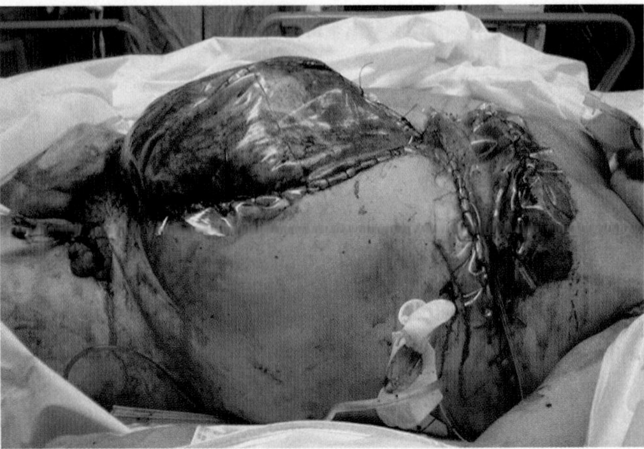

**FIGURE 5-17** Patient following damage control surgery with abdominal and thoracic compartment syndrome caused by massive fluid resuscitation. (Courtesy Dr. Demetri Demetriades, Trauma Recovery Surgical Critical Care Program, USC University Hospital, Los Angeles.)

**BOX 5-3 Components of Damage Control or Hemostatic Resuscitation**

- Initiate permissive hypotension until definitive surgical control is achieved.
- Minimize crystalloid use.
- Initially use 5% HTS.
- Use blood products early (PRBC, FFP, platelets, cryoprecipitates).
- Consider rFVIIa or factor IX.
- Avoid hypothermia.

## Whole Blood Resuscitation

Damage control resuscitation was developed because surgeons in the recent war in Iraq came back and stated that fresh whole blood was useful for massively bleeding soldiers. Although the surgeons early in this war were hesitant and reluctant to try the walking blood bank (see later) that was used to obtain fresh whole blood from noncombat soldiers, eventually it was tried and found to be highly successful and easy. Returning surgeons repeatedly noted that patients resuscitated with whole blood did not seem to have the coagulation or pulmonary problems seen previously. After operative procedures, even patients who underwent several blood volume replacement procedures were warm and not acidotic. Trauma surgeons were starting to recognize that crystalloid resuscitation should and could be avoided by using damage control resuscitation. Because they had only recently started to recognize that currently used fluids had an impact on outcome, they had not yet had a chance to develop the optimal resuscitation fluid to replace blood. As a result, military surgeons advocated the aggressive use of FFP, not because it was ideal, but because it was probably better than crystalloid or colloidal solutions.

The military has a logistic advantage that the civilian sector does not yet have. When casualties arrive, military surgeons can activate the walking blood bank—hundreds of noncombat soldiers on the base will come to the medical facility to donate their blood. Given the relative safety of these donors, because they were all prescreened for infectious agents and had been blood-typed, fresh whole blood was readily available. In the military, when surgical units are available, it is usually at a base where many do not go out on patrol and can donate blood. Obviously, those in combat roles are not eligible to donate because they would no longer be fit to be a combatant. Bleeding patients are transfused with PRBCs and given HTS and crystalloid solution until fresh whole blood is ready for infusion, usually within about 30 minutes after activation of the walking blood bank.

When military surgeons receive a warning about incoming casualties, they can activate the walking blood bank ahead of their arrival and make fresh whole blood available even sooner. The blood is withdrawn and mixed with 50 to 100 mL of citrate-phosphate-dextrose (CPD), which binds calcium and prevents clotting in the bag. The bag of fresh whole blood is then transfused within minutes after donation. The body usually has ample stores of calcium, which makes coagulopathy from CDP rare; calcium can also be injected IV with 10 mL of 10% calcium chloride.

When the military started its practice of using whole blood, no data supported it. Reports eventually emerged showing its safety and efficacy, even when PRBCs were readily available.[44] and now coalition forces have also started the practice of whole blood transfusions. The controversy over the use of fresh whole blood will continue, because randomized prospective studies are not logistically feasible in the war zone.

### Resuscitation With 1:1:1

As news of these successful battlefield practices spread, the civilian literature started to echo the benefits of surgical hemorrhage control before resuscitation and the aggressive use of PRBCs and FFP, summarized in Table 5-9. Because whole blood was not available in the civilian sector, efforts focused on trying to re-create whole blood by transfusing components of blood together. It had been though that component therapy needed to be directed by laboratory results. Surgeons could transfuse only patients with documented coagulopathy and could transfuse only the necessary components. Empirical use was discouraged.

Whole blood is separated into its various components by centrifugation. The plasma is drawn off and separated into fibrinogen and platelets. PRBCs, with a hematocrit level of 60 to 70, are washed, anticoagulants and preservatives are added, and they are then stored. Component separation has made the best use of whole blood, reducing waste. However, component therapy is analogous to eating coffee beans, sugar, cream, and hot water separately to make coffee internally.

The U.S. Army reported its success with the aggressive use of FFP, largely because of the efforts of Holcomb, who had access to the Military Trauma Registry. Registry data have consistently confirmed the benefits of transfusing blood components in a ratio of 1 unit of PRBCs to 1 unit of FFP to 1 unit of platelets, at ratio now termed *1:1:1*. In a civilian setting, Maegele and colleagues have reported that the aggressive use of FFP also resulted in improved outcome. Duchesne and associates wondered whether they might have been wrong for 60 years by not being aggressive with FFP, and showed in another study that it reduced mortality and coagulopathy.

Tiexaira and coworkers have shown that although it is better to be aggressive, the ratio of 1 unit of PRBCs to 2 units of FFP may be equivalent. The previous studies had a tendency to place patients with a 1:2 ratio into the aggressive group, and could not clearly distinguish among 1:1 versus 1:2 versus 1:3. Other studies also failed to find a survival benefit with FFP but showed that it reduces coagulopathy.

An ongoing multicenter, prospective, cohort study was designed to characterize the genomic and proteomic response in injured patients at risk for MODS after traumatic injury and hemorrhagic shock. So far, the data have shown a decreased mortality rate in patients transfused with a high ratio of FFP to PRBCs (i.e., a ratio >1:5).

Snyder and colleagues have show a higher survival rate if FFP use is more aggressive. However, their retrospective study could have had a selection bias toward less moribund patients being in the FFP group, because these patients obviously survived long enough to receive FFP transfusions. Other studies have tried to eliminate patients who die early from both groups (FFP versus no FFP), only including patients who lived at least 6 hours; the continuing trend seems to be that early and aggressive use of FFP is beneficial.

Aggressive use of platelets[45] and fibrinogen[46] has also been shown to improve outcome. In a six-center retrospective study, Zink and associates[47] have shown that the early administration of a high ratio of FFP and platelets improve survival and decrease overall need for PRBCs in massively transfused patients. The largest difference in mortality occurred during the first 6 hours after admission, suggesting that the early administration of FFP and platelets is critical. Most hospitals use apheresis platelets, which are pooled platelets; 1 unit is equivalent to what was previously called a *six pack of platelets*.

### Massive Transfusion Protocol

Studies have led to the development of the massive transfusion protocol (MTP), which calls for the aggressive use of component therapy. The protocol was designed to enable a hospital's blood bank to improve logistic systems for the empirical use of blood components. A number of studies have shown that implementing an MTP improves survival in trauma patients.[48] To qualify as a trauma center, the American College of Surgeons Verification Review Committee recommends that all trauma centers have their own MTP in place.

An example of an MTP directive is that for severely injured patients, the blood bank should bring a cooler with 2 units of unmatched O-negative blood that can be immediately used for resuscitation (Table 5-10). Most patients do not require massive transfusion, usually defined as a transfusion of more than 10 units of PRBCs in 24 hours. If possible, a patient's blood sample should be drawn before the uncrossmatched blood is transfused; even 1 unit of PRBCs can sometimes interfere with crossmatching. If a patient requires more PRBCs before crossmatched blood is available, an additional 4 units of O-negative blood should be made available. If crossmatched blood is available, the next 4 units transfused should be crossmatched blood.

Because most patients do not require more than 6 units of PRBCs, most do not receive FFP. For patients who require more PRBCs, 7 to 12 units of PRBCs should be delivered, along with 6 units of FFP and 1 unit of apheresis platelets. Preferably, the

**Table 5-9 Recent Retrospective Studies on the Use of Fresh-Frozen Plasma**

| STUDY | SUMMARY OF FINDINGS |
|---|---|
| Borgman et al: The ratio of blood products transfused affects mortality in patients receiving massive transfusions at a combat support hospital. J Trauma 63:805–813, 2007. | Retrospective study of 246 patients PRBC-to-FFP ratio group of 1 : 1.4 had better survival rates. |
| Gonzalez et al: Fresh-frozen plasma should be given earlier to patients requiring massive transfusion. J Trauma 62:112–119, 2007. | Retrospective study of 97 patients; they recommended early use of FFP before ICU admission. |
| Kashuk et al: Postinjury life threatening coagulopathy: Is 1 : 1 fresh-frozen plasma : packed red blood cells the answer? J Trauma 65:261–270, 2008. | Retrospective study on 133 patients and logistic regression showed improved coagulopathy but no improvement in survival. |
| Gunter et al: Optimizing outcomes in damage control resuscitation: Identifying blood product ratios associated with improved survival. J Trauma 65:527–534, 2008. | Retrospective study of 259 patients and increased use of FFP and platelets improved survival after major trauma. |
| Holcomb et al: Increased plasma and platelet to red blood cell ratios improves outcome in 466 massively transfused civilian trauma patients. Ann Surg 248:447–458, 2008. | Retrospective study of 467 patients undergoing transfusion of 10 units of PRBCs or more showed increased survival with use of FFP and platelets. |
| Spinella et al: Effect of plasma and red blood cell transfusions on survival in patients with combat related traumatic injuries. J Trauma 64:S69–S77, 2008. | 708 patients undergoing transfusion showed that FFP use was associated with improved survival. |
| Maegele et al: Red blood cell to plasma ratios transfused during massive transfusion are associated with mortality in severe multiple injury: A retrospective analysis from the Trauma Registry of the Deutsche Gesellschaft fur Unfallchirurgie. Vox Sang 95:112–119, 2008. | Retrospective study of 713 patients showed improved survival with increased aggressive use of FFP in patients undergoing massive transfusion. |
| Duchesne JC, Hunt JP, Wahl G, et al: Review of current blood transfusions strategies in a mature level I trauma center: Were we wrong for the last 60 years? J Trauma 65:272–276, 2008. | Retrospective study of 135 patients with massive transfusions who had better outcomes with 1 : 1. |
| Sperry et al: An FFP : PRBC transfusion ratio ≥1 : 1.5 is associated with a lower risk of mortality after massive transfusion. J Trauma 65:986–993, 2008. | Multicenter prospective cohort study with 415 patients showed that higher FFP use was associated with lower mortality. |
| Moore et al: Is there a role for aggressive use of fresh-frozen plasma in massive transfusion of civilian trauma patients? Am J Surg 196:948–958, 2008. | Retrospective study of 93 patients and concluded that damage control resuscitation with FFP may have a role in civilian trauma. |
| Teixeira et al: Impact of plasma transfusion in massively transfused trauma patients. J Trauma 66:693–697, 2009. | Retrospective study in 383 patients showing that more FFP use was associated with better survival. |
| Duchesne et al: Hemostatic resuscitation during surgery improves survival in patients with traumatic–induced coagulopathy. J Trauma 67:33–37, 2009. | Seven-year retrospective study with 435 patients showed survival advantage in patients receiving FFP-to-RBC ratio of 1 : 1 compared with 1 : 4. |
| Snyder et al: The relationship of blood product ratio to mortality: Survival benefit or survival bias? J Trauma 66:358–362, 2009. | Retrospective study of 134 patients showed improved survival with higher use of FFP, but the advantage was not persistent when adjusted for survival bias. |
| Watson et al: Fresh-frozen plasma is independently associated with a higher risk of multiple organ failure and acute respiratory distress syndrome. J Trauma 67:221–227, 2009. | Prospective multicenter cohort study of blunt trauma patients showed that FFP was associated with increased risk of MODS and ARDS. |
| Zink et al: A high ratio of plasma and platelets to packed red blood cells in the first 6 hours of massive transfusion improves outcomes in a large multicenter study. Am J Surg 197:565–570, 2009. | Retrospective 16-center study with 466 patients who had lower mortality if FFP and platelets were used early and as 1 : 1. |
| Riskin et al: Massive transfusion protocols: The role of aggressive resuscitation versus product ratio in mortality reduction. J Am Coll Surg 209:198–205, 2009. | Retrospective study of 77 patients; they concluded that massive transfusion protocol was associated with improved survival. |

FFP and platelets should be transfused first, before the next 6 units of PRBCs are transfused. Thus, for a severely injured patient who will require massive transfusion, the ratio now starts to approach the preferred 1 : 1 : 1 ratio. The "trick" that has gained popularity is to attach a large visible label on the back of all the blood products and to number them sequentially; thus, the emergency department, operating room, or ICU personnel can always quickly determine which unit of PRBCs, FFP, or platelets is being transfused (Fig. 5-18). The use of uncrossmatched blood is a predictor of the need for the MPT, but has also been associated with complications such as ARDS and sepsis.[49]

Our current approach—namely, allowing permissive hypotension, minimizing crystalloid resuscitation, using HTS, and aggressively using blood and blood products—may seem obvious now, but it is different than the approach used 15 years ago. It is now recognized that whole blood is highly complex and that crystalloids do not resemble blood in any way. Crystalloids are acceptable when used for rehydrating patients, providing daily water needs, and delivering medications into the veins but can be harmful when used to replace liters of lost blood in the massive quantities formerly used. Not that long ago, more than 30 liters of fluid might have been administered within a few hours after a trauma patient arrived at the trauma center.

### Current Status of Fluid Types

In January 2010, the U.S. Army had another consensus meeting to examine the different fluid types and make recommendations for future research. A summary of the results will soon be published.

### Crystalloids

The mechanism responsible for acidosis, after large volumes of normal saline are infused, is the dilution of serum bicarbonate ($HCO_3^-$) through the replacement of lost plasma with fluids that do not contain bicarbonate. Normally, chloride and bicarbonate ions are reciprocated up or down with each other. Often, the result of massive normal saline infusion is a hyperchloremic anion gap metabolic acidosis. At extreme levels, acidosis can impair cardiac performance and decrease responsiveness to cardiac inotropic drugs. Many would argue that for cellular protection, the human body offloads oxygen from hemoglobin in the acidotic state and that acidosis, at least to a degree, is actually better for a patient.

Regardless of the advantages and disadvantages of induced metabolic acidosis, no clinical evidence exists that it matters. A study of injured soldiers with hemorrhagic shock has found no significant difference in base deficit between a group of 26 men resuscitated perioperatively with blood and LR (mean, 6.4 liters) and a group of 27 men resuscitated with blood and normal saline (mean, 5.9 liters). Surgeons with experience using HTS encounter induced metabolic acidosis frequently and have found it to be of minimal clinical consequence. Induced metabolic hyperchloremic acidosis is different from spontaneous metabolic acidosis and from hypovolemic lactic acidosis. No evidence exists that induced it causes anything more than confusion in interpreting blood gas levels. Given the lack of any significant proven benefit of one crystalloid over another, many trauma systems use normal saline in the prehospital arena; stocking just one form of fluid is convenient. Another issue is that when blood is being transfused, LR would have to be switched to normal saline anyway. However, this is a regulatory matter because studies have shown that the use of LR as a carrier in the same IV line as blood has no relevant side effects.

Plasma-Lyte (Baxter, Deerfield, Ill), a balanced crystalloid solution, was developed more than 20 years ago and contains additional electrolytes, such as acetate and gluconate. The overall chloride level is also lower. Plasma-Lyte also contains potassium and magnesium, so one should be careful when infusing in patients with renal failure as they will not be able to clear these electrolytes. It is similar to other crystalloids in that it can cause lung edema and increase intracranial pressure (ICP) and generalized edema. The numerous reports of its use have addressed its safety during the priming of extracorporeal circulation pumps and its use in cold ischemia, circulatory arrest, organ transplantation, and organ preservation.

In a study examining the use of HTS with dextran (HTSD), patients were randomized to receive 7.5% HTSD or Plasma-Lyte A. The 2-hour sodium, bicarbonate, $CO_2$, and pH values were comparable. The HTSD group required less crystalloid. However, the volumes infused were also different. In a study by McFarlane, 30 patients undergoing hepatobiliary or pancreatic surgery were randomized to 0.9% normal saline or Plasma-Lyte 148 at 15 mL/kg/hr, which equates to approximately 1125 mL/75 kg. During surgery, Plasma-Lyte was found to be more efficacious; it was balanced, with less hyperchloremia and less base deficit. However, no significant difference in sodium, potassium, or blood lactate level was found in either group.

**Table 5-10 Massive Transfusion Protocol at the University of Arizona**

| | Cooler No. | | | | | |
|---|---|---|---|---|---|---|
| | 1 | 2 | 3 | 4 | 5 | 6 |
| Units of PRBCs | 2 | 4 | 6 | 6 | 6 | 6 |
| Units of FFP | | | 6 | 6 | 6 | 6 |
| Units of platelets | | | 1 | 1 | | 1 |
| Units of cryoprecipitate | | | | 20 | | 10 |

Platelets are pooled and are equivalent to a six-pack of platelets. The sample is immediately sent for type, crossmatching, and coagulation profile. Coolers 3 and higher have crossmatched PRBCs. Coolers 7, 9, 11, 13, and 15 have the same contents as cooler 5 and coolers 8, 10, 12, and 14 have the same contents as cooler 6. Each unit has a large label with a number on it.

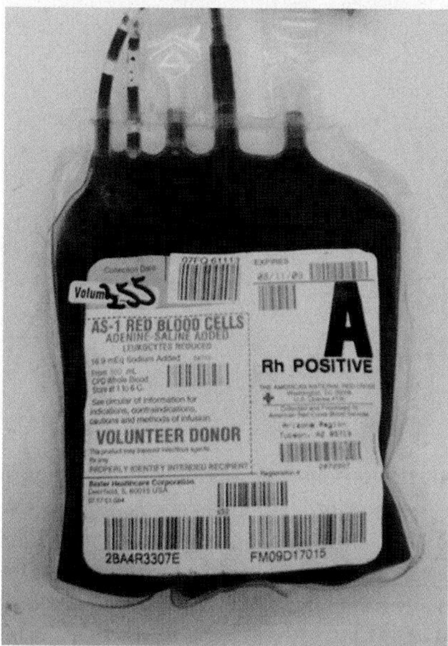


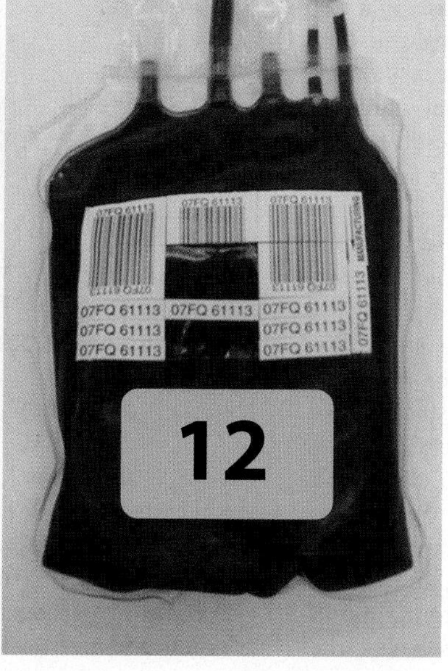


**FIGURE 5-18** Label on back of transfused unit.

**Table 5-11 Composition of Commercially Available Crystalloids**

| COMPONENT | NORMAL SALINE | LACTATED RINGER'S | PLASMALYTE-A | NORMOSOL-R | PLASMA |
|---|---|---|---|---|---|
| **Positive Ions** | | | | | |
| Sodium | 154 | 130 | 140 | 140 | 134-145 |
| Pottasium | | 4 | 5 | 5 | 3.4-5 |
| Calcium | | 3 | | | 2.25-2.65 |
| Magnesium | | | 3 | 3 | 0.7-1.1 |
| **Negative Ions** | | | | | |
| Chloride | 154 | 109 | 98 | 98 | 98-108 |
| Lactate | | 28 | 27 | 27 | |
| Bicarbonate | | | | | 22-32 |
| Gluconate | | | 23 | 23 | |
| pH | 5.4-7.0 | 6.5 | 7.4 | 7.4 | 7.4 |
| Osmolarity | 308 | 273 | 294 | 295 | 280-295 |

Compared with LR and normal saline, Plasma-Lyte may be a better balanced solution, but no studies exist that show its effects in large volumes. It may be an ideal solution for daily maintenance fluid, but does not offer a significant benefit for resuscitation more than other crystalloids. In a kidney transplantation study, Plasma-Lyte A did not increase lactate levels (like LR) and did not cause acidosis (like normal saline); the best metabolic profile was maintained in patients receiving Plasma-Lyte A. Plasma-Lyte is also favored in various cell preparations and as a storage medium for platelets. The components of the various crystalloids are shown in Table 5-11. The cost for LR and normal saline are typically less than $1.00; the costs of Plasma-Lyte and other balanced solutions is closer to $2.00.

### Hypertonic Saline

HTS has been extensively studied, with more than 6869 reports, and at least 1217 since 2005. In summary, the studies have shown that sodium is the main electrolyte that controls intravascular volume. Investigators who have worked with HTS in bleeding animals were surprised to learn, after infusing large volumes of crystalloids to obtain a physiologic response, that the same response can be achieved with a much smaller volume—as long as the salt load was the same. For example, in an animal model of hemorrhagic shock, if 1 liter of normal saline is required to achieve a BP of 120 mm Hg, the same result can be obtained with an infusion of 120 mL of 7.5% normal saline. For 5% HTS, only 182 mL would be needed. In a normal animal undergoing hemorrhage, HTS will pull water in from the cells and interstitial space, similar to the results of pouring in isotonic crystalloids.

Immunologically, HTS has consistently been shown to reduce the inflammatory response; thus, it is thought to be immunomodulatory (Fig. 5-19). Randomized prospective studies have been done with HTS alone or with a colloid such as hetastarch or dextran; results show that HTS is equivalent to crystalloid solutions. The concentration that has been studied the most is 7.5% HTS. Studies have not shown a survival advantage with HTS, but it has been conclusively shown to be safe, and hyperchloremic acidosis does not seem to be a problem. From 1995 to 2005, when inflammation was being extensively studied, the

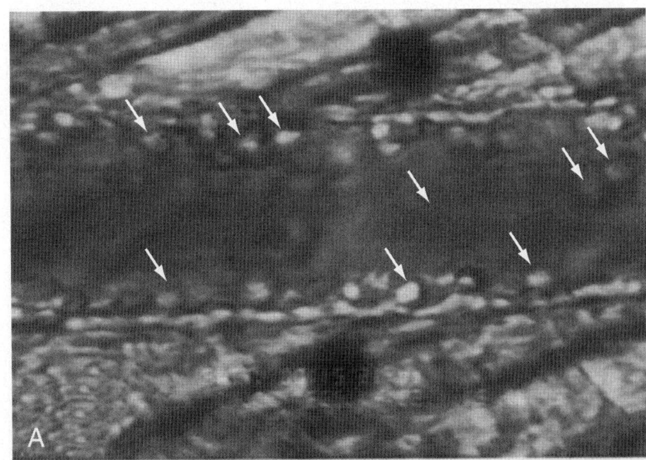


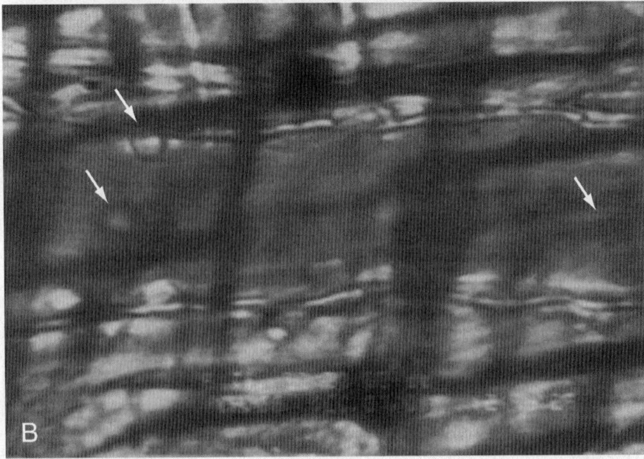


**FIGURE 5-19** Immunologic response from hypertonic resuscitation is less than that after LR has been given. (From Pascual JL, Khwaja KA, Ferri LE, et al: Hypertonic saline resuscitation attenuates neutrophil lung sequestration and transmigration by diminishing leukocyte-endothelial interactions in a two-hit model of hemorrhagic shock and infection. J Trauma 54:121–132, 2003.)

theoretical advantages of HTS—decreasing the inflammatory response and potentially reducing ARDS and MODS—made it the ideal fluid of choice in shock resuscitation.

One of the main problems with 7.5% HTS is that no manufacturer makes it; no profit can be gained by selling salt water. Currently, 7.5% HTS is not approved by the FDA. The process of obtaining approval for the indication of resuscitation is costly and no company has an interest in making that investment. In Europe, 7.5% HTS is manufactured and sold with dextran added; there is currently a market for that.

The Resuscitation Outcomes Consortium (ROC), which is comprised of ten trauma centers in the United States and Canada, has been funded to participate in trauma and emergency medicine trials. The funding comes, in part, from the National Institutes of Health. ROC is the first prehospital, federally funded organization to examine potential prehospital interventions.

The first trauma trial by ROC was the HTS trial, a prospective randomized trial that enrolled hypotensive patients (systolic BP <70 mm Hg) with blunt or penetrating trauma, with and without traumatic head injury. Patients were randomized into one of three arms by dose and fluid: (1) 250 mL bolus of normal saline; (2) 250 mL bolus of 7.5% HTS; and (3) 250 mL of 7.5% HTS with 6% dextran 70. The HTS trial enrolled 2221 patients, with the need for informed consent waived. Two other trials by ROC were the hemorrhagic shock trial (894 patients) and the TBI trial (1327 patients). The TBI trial enrolled patients with or without hypotension; the main enrollment criterion was a Glasgow Outcome Score (GCS) of 8 or less.

The HTS shock trial showed that patients' demographic and physiologic characteristics were similar, except that patients receiving HTS had a mild elevation in their sodium level (147 mEq/liter versus 140 mEq/liter in the normal saline group). The admission hemoglobin level was also significantly different; the patients who received HTS with or without dextran had a hemoglobin level of 10.2 g/dL. However, 11.1 g/dL in the normal saline group. The overall 28-day survival rates were almost identical: HTS patients, 73%; HTS with dextran patients, 74.5%; and normal saline patients, 74.4% ($P = .91$).

However, the HTS trial was stopped before the end of its planned enrollment by the Drug Safety and Monitoring Board (DSMB) for two main reasons. First, interim analysis showed futility as the mortality outcomes were so similar and the completion of the study would not have shown significant differences. Second, a detailed subgroup analysis found a potential for harm in patients who received no PRBC transfusion in the first 24 hours; for unexplained reasons, their mortality rate was significantly higher if they received HTS or HTS with dextran. HTS and HTS with dextran patients who received more than 10 units of PRBCs within the first 24 hours had a lower mortality rate, although the difference was not statistically significant.

The design of the HTS trial has been criticized. First, it allowed for only a small dose in the prehospital phase; HTS infusion did not continue in the hospital. Also, the sodium level was raised to only 147 mEq/liter; studies showing an immunomodulatory effect from HTS have suggested that the sodium level should be raised to approximately 155 mEq/liter. The second criticism was that the HTS trial essentially compared HTS with permissive hypotension (similar to the Bickell study[32]). In hypotensive patients, 250 mL of normal saline is clinically irrelevant but because 250 mL of HTS with dextran D or HTS is approximately equivalent to 2 liters of normal saline, the group of patients who received HTS were being resuscitated whereas the normal saline group was not. Thus, the trial seemed to compare 250 mL of normal saline to the equivalent of 2 liters of normal saline. Support for this theory is that the hemoglobin level was lower in the group of patients who received HTS. The trial of HTS in patients with TBI was also halted; the interim analysis also showed futility, meaning that the primary outcome was almost identical between the normal saline and HTS groups. Such an outcome can also be interpreted as showing that HTS is safe, but technically the trial was not powered to show noninferiority. HTS was studied in TBI, because preliminary studies had shown promise; HTS infusion is highly effective in decreasing intracranial pressure (ICP) and can do this while increasing blood volume, BP, and blood flow to the brain. Compared with mannitol, which is customarily used for lowering ICP, HTS might do this without dehydrating patients or putting them at further risk for secondary brain injury caused by hypotension or renal failure. Patients on high-dose mannitol drips are also susceptible to pulmonary insufficiency, causing longer ICU stays; infusing mannitol requires high daily volumes. Mannitol is safe if used carefully in patients with isolated TBIs, but in hypotensive multitrauma patients it can be detrimental and might cause hypotension.

HTS may still be beneficial, but this ROC study will probably stop further HTS trials for many years. The funding also came in part from the U.S. Army, which invested in the HTS trial hoping to determine noninferiority. Most studies are efficacy trials; the federal government currently endorses the concept that all future drug trials should show efficacy for the FDA to approve new drugs or treatment. This is an attempt to contain health care costs; if drug A is merely equivalent to drug B, the FDA should not approve it because it will result in uncontrolled health care costs. However, in the military combat casualty care setting, a fluid has less volume and weight but can do the same thing as standard crystalloids and would be logistically beneficial. Thus, one of the mandates of the ROC trial was to show safety, efficacy, and noninferiority. A much larger sample is needed to show that a drug or fluid is not inferior.

Finally, most animal and human studies have used 7.5% HTS, an arbitrary concentration; 10% HTS was found to be highly irritating to peripheral veins, so 7.5% HTS was developed. HTS injected rapidly into human volunteers causes pain at the infusion site. The preferred route is through the central vein. In animal studies, if 7.5% HTS is given through the interosseous route, osteomyonecrosis and compartment syndrome can ensue. Commercially, HTS comes in 23%, 5%, and 3% concentrations. Curiously, all the human studies used 7.5% HTS, which is not commercially available. This could be the main strategic mistake of the HTS studies. Some nontrauma studies have used 3% and 23% concentrations, but almost no clinical experience has been reported with 5%. Also, 23% HTS is primarily used for patients with hyponatremia and to reduce ICP in TBI patients.

However, one study has shown that the use of 5% HTS in trauma patients, with or without TBI, is safe.[50] This finding is logical, because the 7.5% HTS studies have shown it to be safe. Using 5% HTS may be the best strategy to recruit intravascular volume as compared with crystalloid resuscitation. The method used in trauma patients is to give 5% HTS in 250-mL infusions and, if more than 500 mL is needed, to check sodium levels.

The sodium content of 250 mL of 5% HTS is equivalent to 1645 mL of LR. Thus, a bolus can be given quickly, without having to use hypotonic solutions such as LR. If 500 mL of 5% HTS is used in acute trauma patients, some believe that this can resuscitate patients without having to give 3 liters of a crystalloid solution. This complies with the concept of damage control resuscitation, in which one of the goals is to minimize crystalloid use.

## Colloids

Extensive randomized control trials have examined the safety and efficacy of 5% albumin, 6% hetastarch, and 6% dextran. However, no evidence has shown that one colloid is superior to another, nor that colloids are better or worse than crystalloids. Colloids can have proinflammatory effects similar to those of crystalloids. In some cases, colloids will do more harm in large volumes than crystalloids, but all colloids should not be considered the same. The commonly used colloids are plasma, albumin, dextran, and starch-based colloids. It is well known that artificial colloids can perpetuate coagulopathy; dextran is used specifically to help prevent clotting after vascular surgery. The inflammatory system is tightly interwoven with the coagulation process; thus, we limit the use of Hextend to 1 liter in trauma patients, who are often harmed if they have coagulopathy from increased bleeding. In animal models, albumin seems to be better for preventing inflammation, whereas hetastarch and dextran, in high doses, appear to cause inflammation and coagulopathy.

Albumin has many theoretical advantages, especially in animal studies. clinically, though, it has not been shown to make a difference. Its main theoretical advantage is that compared with crystalloids, it is less inflammatory, probably because it is a natural molecule, and not artificial. Other than its dilutional effect, albumin is associated with minimal coagulopathy. No clinical evidence has shown that albumin is better than other colloids, but the SAFE study in Australia has shown 4% albumin to be safe, compared with normal saline, in ICU patients.[51] The SAFE study, whose main intent was to show equivalency, found no difference in the primary outcome (28-day mortality rate) or in any secondary outcome. The Tactical Combat Casualty Care Committee (TCCC) has recommended a low-volume resuscitation fluid—currently, for tactical reasons, 500 mL of Hextend. The reason for that choice was that 7.5% HTS is not commercially available. The military has adopted the idea of damage control or hemostatic resuscitation, which entails limited use of crystalloid fluids, one-time use of HTS, early use of blood and blood products, and other adjuncts, such as factor VIIa or IX. The result has been an improved outcome, decreased blood use, and decreased incidence of ARDS.[52] ARDS and MODS still occur, but at a much lower rate than previously seen; they usually occur in patients with a pulmonary contusion or an infectious process.

However, 25% albumin offers many advantages over artificial colloids. It has a proven immunologic anti-inflammatory effect and five times less volume than current artificial colloids; unlike artificial colloids, it does not potentially lead to coagulopathic side effects. It has been proven safe from infectious and clinical standpoints. The volume of fluid that has to be carried is obviously much less (Fig. 5-20). The cost of albumin is approximately 30 times more than crystalloids and three times more than dextran or Hextend, but those comparisons were made against 5% human albumin. The cost of 100 mL of 25% albumin, when compared with 500 mL of Hextend on a physiologic basis, is only approximately three times as much. During the Vietnam War, 25% albumin was first made available and worked well: it was packaged in a green can that could be transported without damage, had a long shelf life, and was easy to use.

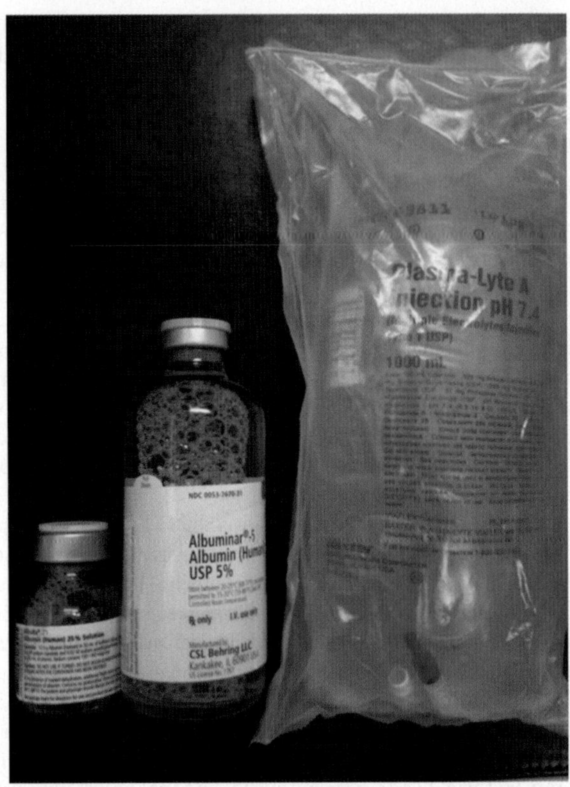


**FIGURE 5-20** Comparison of container sizes: 50 mL of 25% albumin, 500 mL of 5% albumin, and 1 liter of LR. 50 mL of 25% albumin is physiologically equivalent to approximately 2000 to 2500 mL of crystalloids.

## Future Resuscitation Research

### Blood Substitutes

In contrast to volume expanders, blood substitutes are fluids that can carry oxygen. In the United States, 15 million units of PRBCs are transfused annually. Methods to decrease the need for blood transfusions include preoperative autologous donation, intraoperative blood retrieval and reinfusion, and isovolemic hemodilutions. These allow for withdrawing a patient's blood at the start of surgery, replacing it with volume expanders and then, at the end of surgery, retransfusing with the patient's own donated blood. Because of blood supply limitations, infectious and transfusion complications, and storage limitations, the need for blood substitutes remains. The ideal blood substitute would do the following:

- Deliver oxygen
- Require no compatibility testing
- Have few side effects
- Have prolonged storage capabilities
- Persist in the circulation
- Be cost-effective

Currently, blood substitutes are hemoglobin- or nonhemoglobin-based. Research on hemoglobin-based fluids dates back to the 1920s, when the stroma of cells was lysed to obtain hemoglobin. Purification and sterilization were hurdles that took decades to overcome, but it was soon realized that free hemoglobin had toxic effects because of its breakdown products. Problems with free hemoglobin include osmotic diuretic effects, renal toxicity, coagulation abnormalities, short half-life, and vasoactive effect, which is known to be caused by hemoglobin solutions scavenging nitric oxide.

During the next 3 decades (1930s to 1950s), efforts concentrated on stabilizing the hemoglobin molecule to increase its persistence in the circulation and prevent toxic effects. Such strategies included crosslinking the molecule between the tetramer subunit, polymerizing it, encapsulating it in an artificial red cell or in liposomes, and using microsphere technology to form 1 million stable micromolecules. Development of some hemoglobin substitutes advanced to clinical trials.

Blood substitutes are referred to as *hemoglobin oxygen carriers* (HBOCs). Current second-generation HBOCs are pasteurized and free of communicable pathogens; they also have no ABO, Rh, or other blood antigens. They are universally compatible and require no blood banking and can be easily administered without special training or expertise. The problems of a short half-life and renal toxicity have now been overcome, but some troublesome side effects remain, including free radical generation and exacerbation of reperfusion injury, methemoglobin production, and immunologic effects (e.g., immunosuppression, potentiation of endotoxin-related pathogenicity).

The hemoglobin for blood substitutes comes from various sources, such as outdated donated human blood, bovine or swine blood, and transgenic *E. coli*. Each source has its benefits (e.g., availability, cost) and side effects (e.g., infections, other complications). Human hemoglobin has the advantage of being a naturally occurring product that has been extensively studied; its obvious disadvantage is lack of availability. About 2 units of discarded blood are required to make 1 unit of the HBOC. Even if all the discarded human blood were captured, the numbers of units made would only be 50% of what was discarded.

The potential advantages of animals as a source of hemoglobin are tremendous—they are a relatively cheap source, and their supply is ample. However, despite efforts at controlling a herd, problems such as bovine spongiform encephalitis will inevitably surface.

Recombinant hemoglobin has problems as well gigantic volumes of bacterial culture are needed and the stringent processing methods are costly. It is estimated that only 0.1 g of hemoglobin can be generated from 1 liter of *E. coli* culture (750 liters would make 1 unit). Production of 3 million units would require more than 1.125 billion liters of culture.

One of the first HBOC products tested was manufactured in 1999. Diaspirin cross-linked hemoglobin (DCLHb), known as HemAssist (Baxter), was tested. This chemically modified human hemoglobin solution was used in a highly publicized trial in patients with traumatic hemorrhagic shock, one of the first trials to use community consent instead of individual patient consent. Baxter terminated the trial early because patients who received the test product had a higher 28-day mortality rate (47%) than those who received normal saline (25%; $P < .015$). The trial brought disappointment to investigators anticipating the success of the first red cell substitute.

A recent analysis has compared data from the Baxter trial with 17 U.S. emergency departments and the parallel 27 European Union prehospital systems now using DCLHb but showed no difference in outcome. In this study, neither mean BP nor elevated BP readings correlated with DCLHb treatment of traumatic hemorrhagic shock patients. As such, no clinically demonstrable DCLHb pressor effect could be directly related to the adverse mortality outcome observed in the Baxter trial.

Two other products currently have potential for clinical use. Both are polymerized rather than tetramerized. Polymerization is thought to be more efficacious because the molecular weights are higher (130 kDa) than with tetramerization (65 kDa), resulting in a longer intravascular presence. Some investigators have proposed that polymerization avoids contact with nitric oxide, attenuating the vasoconstriction seen with previous products. One of those products is HBOC-201 (Hemopure, Biopure), made from bovine blood. It is universally compatible and stable at room temperature for up to 3 years. Animal studies showed great promise and human trials with orthopedic patients also showed promise, but safety issues were a concern. Patients who received Hemopure had an increased number of serious adverse events. The vasoconstrictive properties of Hemopure may have caused myocardial infarction in susceptible patients. Biopure went bankrupt in 2009 and was taken over by OPK Biotech (Cambridge, Mass), which manufactures a product called Oxyglobin (HBOC-301) for veterinary use. FDA approval for Hemopure is still pending. OPK Biotech has continued to develop Hemopure for human use; the U.S. Navy is supporting research for potential use in the military setting.

The company shut down its operations after it was informed by the FDA that the risks outweighed the benefits. The more promising hemoglobin-based product was PolyHeme (Northfield Laboratories, Evanston, Ill). The way it is produced removes almost all the cross-linked tetrameric hemoglobin (<1%). PolyHeme is made from outdated human donated blood and has a shelf life of approximately 1 year at room temperature. The most recent human trial was a multicenter study in trauma patients, with the need for informed consent waived.[53] Patients were randomized to receive PolyHeme or crystalloids and PRBCs. A total of 29 trauma centers enrolled 714 patients. It was reported that patients can be resuscitated with PolyHeme, without using stored blood, up to 6 units within 12 hours after injury. Outcomes between the two groups were comparable in regard to 30-day mortality rates, 13.4% in the PolyHeme group and 9.6% in the control group. However, the PolyHeme group had more serious adverse events—specifically, an increased number of myocardial infarctions. Nonetheless, the risk-benefit ratio of PolyHeme is favorable when blood is needed but unavailable.

A meta-analysis of 16 HBOC trials, including four trauma trials involving HemAssist or PolyHeme, has shown that HBOC patients have a significantly increased risk of myocardial infarction and death as compared with controls. The problem of vasoconstriction will have to be addressed further. Vasodilators can be added to mitigate vasoconstriction, but whether enthusiasm for HBOCs persists remains to be seen. However, they have a real potential benefit for patients who do not have access to PRBCs, such as in rural areas or the military.

Third-generation hemoglobin substitutes have begun to address the deficiencies of earlier formulations. The encapsulation of hemoglobin in liposomes is an innovation, but efforts to make it ideal continue. The mixing of phospholipids and cholesterol in the presence of free hemoglobin forms a sphere, with hemoglobin in the center. These liposomes have oxygen dissociation curves similar to those of red blood cells and administration can transiently achieve high circulating levels of hemoglobin and oxygen-carrying capacity. However, research is still in the preclinical testing stage; progress in prolonging the half-life and elucidating the effects on the immune system, particularly reticuloendothelial sequestration, are crucial before clinical testing can begin.

### Perfluorocarbons

Perfluorocarbons (PFCs) are completely inert biologically and are similar to Teflon and Gore-Tex. Altering the molecule by fluoridating the ring structure lowers the melting point and makes it a liquid at room temperature. in 1966, PFCs captured the imagination of many people when photographs were released of a mouse completely submerged in the liquid form but breathing and surviving in it (Fig. 5-21). PFCs dissolve larger quantities of oxygen and $CO_2$ than plasma. They have yet to find a purpose in liquid form, but enthusiasm has increased for their use in partial liquid ventilation (PLV). Trials in adults with ARDS have shown no benefit, but studies are still ongoing in children with hyaline membrane disease.

PFCs have two challenges to overcome for use as blood substitutes. The first is that the liquid form is immiscible in water; thus, PFCs must be suspended as microdroplets with the use of emulsifying agents. The second is that unlike hemoglobin, the oxygen dissolved in PFCs has a linear relationship to the partial pressure of oxygen, whereas hemoglobin has a sigmoidal disassociation curve favoring full loading at normal atmospheric oxygen levels. Thus, the $F_{IO_2}$ that has to be applied is too high.

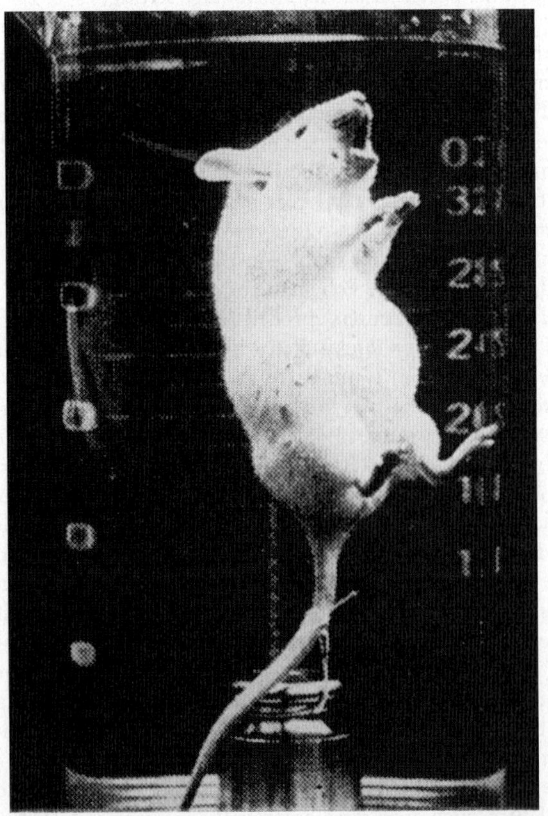

**FIGURE 5-21** Mouse surviving while submerged in perfluorocarbons. (From Shaffer TH, Wolfson MR: Liquid ventilation. In Polin RA, Fox WW, Abman SH [eds]: Fetal and neonatal physiology, ed 3, WB Saunders, 2003, Philadelphia.)

Second-generation PFCs have been formulated to allow more oxygen-carrying capacity, with alterations in their emulsion properties. These new compounds can also be stored at 4° C, whereas previous solutions had to be frozen. Oxygent (Alliance Pharmaceutical, San Diego) is a 60% perflubron emulsion with a median particle diameter less than 0.2 μm. The use of lecithin as an emulsifier eliminated the adverse effects of complement activation observed in earlier studies of PFCs. Possible current uses include cardiopulmonary bypass with normovolemic hemodilution and balloon angioplasty to provide oxygenated blood past the catheter while inflated. In a phase 3 study, Oxygent was shown to reduce the need for red blood cell (RBC) transfusion in patients undergoing noncardiac surgery (16%, Oxygent group; 26%, control group; $P < .05$). Oxygent patients, however, had more serious adverse events (32% in the Oxygent group versus 21% in the control group; $P < .05$). In another phase 3 study, in patients undergoing cardiac bypass, Oxygent possibly increased the incidence of strokes. All further studies were halted.

Two other PFC products have been introduced. In early-phase clinical trials, OxyFluor (Hemagen, Columbia, Md) produced mild thrombocytopenia and flulike symptoms in healthy volunteers. Baxter International has withdrawn support for further development. Phase 2 trials of Oxycyte were suspended; its manufacture was taken over by Oxygen Biotherapuetics (Morrisville, NC) and is being sold over the counter as a cosmetic product known as Dermacyte, an oxygen concentrate gel for wound healing. Dermacyte is also being investigated for the treatment of cancer during chemotherapy or radiation therapy because oxygen free radicals are thought to kill cancer cells. PFCs are not free of side effects and are not efficacious for oxygen delivery and use.

### Novel Fluids

The recognition that currently available fluids are not a replacement for blood and that they can be harmful if used in large amounts to expand blood volume has initiated exciting research for better fluids. Blood is so highly complex that the ultimate goal is to develop artificial whole blood; the ideal method would be to manufacture whole blood with a bioreactor using stem cells, but this development would take decades.

The permutations of future fluid development are endless. Novel crystalloids are being tested, as are hypertonic solutions with and without oxygen carriers, hypertonic colloids, FDPs, and drug therapy.

In 1999, the Institute of Medicine recommended research to eliminate lactate in LR and to investigate the use of alternative energy substrates in resuscitation fluids. It recognized that, although reperfusion injury can occur in shock resuscitation, a separate entity, called *resuscitation injury*, is a result of the method of resuscitation and the fluids used.

Two substances have since been identified that could alter the inflammatory response after resuscitation. In small and large animal models, studies have found that simply replacing the lactate in LR with ketones or pyruvate reduces the inflammatory response after hemorrhagic shock resuscitation. Other investigators have concentrated on various forms of pyruvate to minimize resuscitation injury; ethyl pyruvate seems promising.[54] From a cellular level, a combination of anti-inflammatory constituents in fluids seems more efficacious.

Studies of the mechanisms of these improved results have found that monocarboxylate-supplemented resuscitation provides energy substrates, with minimal alteration in the conventionally used fluids, such as LR. Replacing the lactate in LR with pyruvate or ketones protected the brain and other tissues after shock.[55] This finding led to research on causes of this protective effect and on the potential of using drugs alone to treat hemorrhagic shock.

### Freeze-Dried Plasma

Clinical studies showing better outcomes with minimizing crystalloids and aggressively using blood products led to the development of FDP, or lyophilized plasma. This approach was used in World War II and the Korean War, but became less popular over time (Fig. 5-22), partly because research showing that crystalloids and colloids might not make a difference, as well as concern about possible transmission of infection. However, the capability of removing potential infectious agents, along with improved technology for manufacturing lyophilized plasma, resurrected research in this field. The advantages of lyophilized plasma are that it avoids the difficult logistics of storing fresh-frozen products and the preparation time of thawing FFP.

Through funding by the U.S. Navy, plasma separated from fresh porcine blood was lyophilized to produce FDP and then compared with FFP. After a 60% blood volume hemorrhage, pigs were resuscitated with reconstituted FDP, which was just as efficacious as thawed plasma and had an identical coagulation profile. A multi-institutional polytrauma animal trial found that FDP was better than Hextend, which led to anemia and coagulopathy.[56] Currently, this is a promising area of research and development.

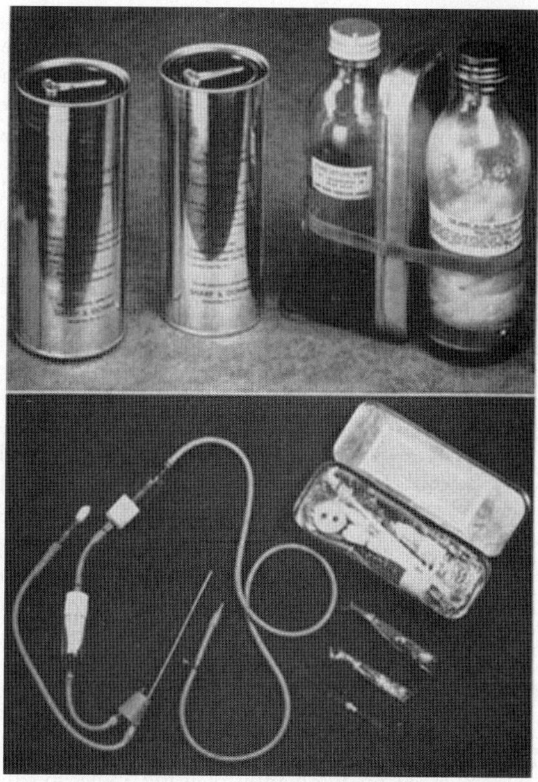

**FIGURE 5-22** Freeze-dried plasma used during World War II. (Courtesy Office of Medical History, U.S. Army Medical Department, Center of History and Heritage, Washington, DC.)

From the military perspective, a method of developing artificial whole blood was needed that was practical and not harmful. Again, fresh whole blood is so complex that simple fluids are not a replacement. The reality of artificial whole blood is many years away, but FDP is available much sooner in terms of being able to treat hemorrhagic shock without causing as much harm as currently available colloids and crystalloids do. FDP can also undo physiologic derangements by restoring intravascular volume and treating coagulopathy. The logistic advantages of a product that can be easily reconstituted would be a tremendous advance. There are many studies being undertaken of oxygen carriers and small volume resuscitation, so the concept that FDP can be reconstituted with less water—and initial resuscitation performed with a hypertonic, hyperoncotic resuscitation fluid—is exciting.

### Pharmacologic Agents

This area of work is an example of translational research that is novel and could be revolutionary. DNA transcription is regulated, in part, by the acetylation of nuclear histones that are controlled by two groups of enzymes, histone deacetylases (HDACs) and histone acetyltransferases (HATs). Animal experiments have shown that hemorrhagic shock and resuscitation are associated with HDAC-HAT activity misbalance, and that the acetylation status of cardiac histones is influenced by the choice of resuscitation strategy. Shock-induced changes can be reversed through the infusion of a pharmacologic HDAC inhibitor, even when it is administered for only a limited period after the insult. Animal experiments have shown promise in elucidating mechanisms behind the success of using an HDA inhibitor to prolong life after shock.[55]

Alam and colleagues[57] have been investigating the role of valproic acid (VPA, an anticonvulsant) in improving tolerance to shock by cells, in part because of the preservation of the Akt survival pathway. In their study, large swine subjected to trauma (femoral and liver injury) and to severe hemorrhage (60% blood loss) were randomized into one of three groups—no treatment (control group), treatment with fresh whole blood, or treatment with VPA (400 mg/kg) without resuscitation. The early survival rate was 100% in the fresh whole blood group, 86% in the VPA group, and 25% in the control group.

Given concerns that inflammation after trauma might be a pathologic event, another unique approach is to use estrogen and progesterone to treat patients after traumatic hemorrhagic shock. Independent laboratory studies have indicated that the use of estrogen and progesterone is a promising method to reduce secondary injury in hemorrhagic shock and other similar processes. These studies have shown that the early administration of estrogen (a strong antioxidant, anti-inflammatory, and mitochondrial stabilizer and antiapoptotic agent) significantly decreased the severity of injury caused by early, devastating cell death.

The use of estrogen has now been tested in 60 clinical trials, mostly in the fields of prostate cancer, uremic bleeding, liver transplantation, spine surgery, cardiology, cardiac surgery, and

TBI. Its safety record is good. Currently, the Resuscitations Outcome Consortium, made up of 10 trauma centers in Canada and the United States, has a study planned to investigate the efficacy of administering estrogen IV in the prehospital environment.

### Suspended Animation

The military has supported research to develop a technique to prevent patients from dying from exsanguination. Reparable torso hemorrhage is still a major cause of preventable death in the battlefield, so research is being conducted to identify a method of preserving a patient's life long enough to repair the sources of hemorrhage later. This concept is termed *suspended animation.* Rather than resuscitation, the goal is to stop cellular death with induced hypothermia or by chemical means.

Initially, animal studies focused on identifying hibernation inducers that signal cells chemically to decrease metabolism. Serum from hibernating squirrels can be injected into nonhibernating squirrels and induce hibernation. Metabolism slows, heart rate decreases, and life seems to be suspended. Many mammals are highly tolerant of ischemia, such as diving seals, which can remain underwater for 45 minutes at a time. Bears hibernate in the cold, and turtles can bury themselves in mud without dying. The search continues to determine how human life can persist at the normal metabolic rate without oxygenation. This fascinating area of research should help us understand the meaning of life at the cellular level, but the clinical use of hibernating inducers has not yet been elucidated.

Hypothermia or cooling reduces the metabolic needs of cells. Thus, as noted, the use of induced hypothermia has been studied to determine whether it can put life on hold. Once metabolic demands are decreased, life can be slowed or suspended. This metabolic suspension can be effectively achieved with hypothermia and with various chemical infusions. Interestingly, life or metabolism does not seem to end with the cessation of perfusion; rather, it actually ends during reperfusion, when irreversible cellular damage has occurred. Reperfusion of cells that have exhausted their supply of nutrients can damage cells and thus end life. The mechanisms are complex, but calcium exchange may be a key component.

Because exsanguination is a major cause of death, the suspension of life with hypothermia or chemical cellular arrest could buy time to transport patients to a hospital where their vascular injuries could be repaired and life restored. Animal studies have been performed to perfect a method of inducing suspended animation and then successfully restoring life without neurologic injury. Clinically, induced hypothermic arrest is already being used in cardiothoracic surgery and neurosurgery. However, the length of time that flow to the brain can be halted is only approximately 45 minutes. In cardiac surgery, the heart is arrested and cooled while the rest of the body is perfused with a pump. The idea is to take the methods used to preserve the heart and apply them to the whole body, including the brain but such methods are complex and require extensive preparation and immense teamwork. It is unknown whether they can be simplified for emergencies, such as unexpected exsanguination.

Animal work on this topic has been performed for 60 years. Dr. Peter Safar, often called the "father of CPR" (cardiopulmonary resuscitation), studied induced profound hypothermic arrest in dogs and rats under controlled conditions. Research was funded by the U.S. Navy that involved experiments showing that profound hypothermia to 10° C can be induced by infusing cold fluids containing massive doses of potassium. Essentially, the process is similar to achieving cardioplegia except that a solution is infused to arrest not only the heart but the entire body. The solution used to induce such massive hypothermic and chemical arrest is an organ preservation fluid (HypoThermosol, Sigma-Aldrich, St Louis,) that contains 70 mEq/liter of potassium.

Patients who have, in effect, died from exsanguinating traumatic hemorrhage typically undergo a resuscitative thoracotomy in the emergency department to stop their bleeding and attempts are made to resuscitate them. However, this is a desperate maneuver, with dismal results; only 7.4% of these patients survive. The U.S. Navy developed a new method—once the chest is opened, instead of trying to resuscitate patients, they are infused with cold HypoThermosol.

Large animal (swine) models have been used to develop the techniques that induce suspended animation in the emergent setting; studies have repeatedly shown that swine could be put into whole body arrest and then rapidly (within 20 to 30 minutes) made hypothermic to 10° C. During this process, all the blood is removed from the swine and they are left in that state for about 1 to 3 hours. This, by clinical definition, kills the swine: no metabolism occurs during that state, no brain or heart activity can be detected, and no blood is in the body.

Theoretically, this is the period during which human patients could be taken to the operating room for vascular repairs; these patients almost always have suffered major vascular injury causing exsanguination. Because the vascular repairs would be done in an asanguineous state, no blood loss would occur during the repairs. These repairs are accomplished using portable pumps smaller than a can of soda.[58] also, this is when human patients could be put on a standard bypass machine by a second team of surgeons; that machine would be used to revive patients by flushing out the potassium and warming them while infusing blood. In the swine model, this entire process has been shown to be feasible, even after extended periods of shock and with associated vascular, solid organ, and hollow viscous injuries.

Research on this concept by the military has advanced to where a multicenter clinical trial is now planned. The mechanisms and methods to suspend life and then restart it have clearly been identified. The traditional teaching was that hypothermia during trauma care is harmful, but the difference between spontaneous hypothermia and induced hypothermia is huge. Spontaneous hypothermia indicates hemorrhagic shock and is often associated with massive resuscitation with cold or room temperature fluids. Such severely injured patients will do poorly, given their blood loss and the dilutional coagulopathy, which is obviously detrimental when patients have uncontrolled bleeding. Appropriately induced hypothermia, however, can be beneficial.

## PERIOPERATIVE FLUID MANAGEMENT

### Body Water

Humans are made predominantly of water (50% to 70% of body weight). The precise percentage is affected by gender, body fat, and age. The body can do without many things for long periods, but water is essential. In the body, water resides in three compartments or spaces—intracellular, intravascular, and interstitial. The intracellular compartment has the largest volume of water, constituting about 30% to 40% of body weight (two thirds of the body's total water). The intravascular volume is usually calculated as 5% to 7% of body weight. Water shifts rapidly among the three compartments. Large resources of water can be pulled from the intracellular compartment into the intravascular compartment, and large volumes of water can be stored in the interstitial compartment. Water in the interstitial compartment is recirculated by the lymphatics and eventually returns to the intravascular compartment.

A fixed amount of water is in bones and dense connective tissue, but this water is relatively stable and not considered to be in circulation. Water is secreted by various cells in the skin, cerebrospinal fluid, and intraocular, synovial, renal, and gastrointestinal systems; this water is also not considered to be in circulation.

Clinical tools are available to measure the volume of water in the body accurately. One method is bioimpedance spectroscopy, which measures electrical current impedance that is imperceptible to a person, to estimate total body water. The method is best used to estimate body fat.

Methods to measure intravascular volume are also commercially available. They usually involve injecting a known concentration of tagged molecules (e.g., potassium-40 or albumin) that remain intravascular for a known period. Potassium is predominantly an intracellular solute and albumin is predominantly extracellular. Sampling the blood and calculating the volume based on the decreased concentration of the injected tracer is fairly accurate. This method is not widely used clinically because the baseline volume is unknown; even if it were known, the intravascular volume is contractible and expandable, so the desired target volume cannot yet be determined. During injuries and illnesses, when homeostasis has not been maintained, normal values may not be applicable or desirable during resuscitation. The practicality of measuring these spaces has not been identified; however, research has shown that a person's extracellular volume can be expanded even if he or she is dehydrated intracellularly.

The main intracellular electrolytes are potassium and magnesium. Intracellularly, they are the principal cations and phosphates and proteins are the principal anions. Extracellularly, in contrast, sodium is the predominant cation; chloride and bicarbonate are the predominant anions. In plasma, given its higher protein content, the result of organic anions, the total concentrations of cations are higher and the concentrations of inorganic anions are lower than in interstitial fluids. The Gibbs-Donnan equilibrium equation states that the product of the concentrations of any pair of diffusible cations and anions on one side of a semipermeable membrane will equal the product of the same pair of ions on the other side. Cell walls are semipermeable membranes; the flow of water is determined by the osmotically active particles (≈290 to 310 mOsm). The effective osmotic pressure depends on those substances that fail to pass through the pores of the semipermeable membrane.

The unit of mEq/liter refers to the number of electrical charges; the unit of mOsm/liter refers to the number of osmotically active particles, or ions. A milliequivalent in a solution must be precisely balanced by the same number of milliequivalents of a cation and anion. The balance affects the direction of water as it equilibrates. The osmotic pressure of a solution refers to the actual number of osmotically active particles present in the solution, but does not depend on the chemical combining capacities of the substances. For example, sodium chloride dissociates to 2 mOsm, whereas sodium sulfate ($Na_2SO_4$) dissociates into three particles, 2 mOsm of sodium and 1 mOsm of sulfate. However, 1 mOsm of an unionized substance such as glucose is equal to 1 mOsm of the substance.

Dissolved proteins in the plasma are responsible for the effective osmotic pressure between the plasma and interstitial fluid, frequently referred to as the *colloid osmotic pressure.* Sodium is pumped outside the cell and potassium inside the cell. Thus, sodium is the major electrolyte responsible for the osmotic pressure, but glucose and urea, which do not easily penetrate the cell membrane, also increase the effective osmotic pressure. Water passes across the cell membrane freely, so sodium has a highly important impact on the movement of water. However, the concentration of sodium is not necessarily related to the volume status of ECF. A severe extracellular volume deficit can occur with a low or high sodium concentration over time.

The osmotic gradient is also important when controlling water. The number of osmotic particles is the key, and the size of the osmotic particle does not matter. For example, transfusion of PRBCs will actually cause water to pass from the intravascular space to the interstitial space. Immediately after the transfusion of PRBCs, hydrostatic pressure increases inside the vascular space and water is pushed out. Although the hematocrit level of PRBCs is 60% to 70%, the red cells act as one osmotic particle. Because the size difference between red cells and proteins in the blood is so significant, fewer osmotic particles are in a given volume of blood as compared with normal whole blood. Therefore, the osmotic pressure intravascularly is actually reduced after transfusion of PRBCs. PRBCs are prepared by centrifuging the red cells and removing the plasma. Thus, the number of osmotic particles in PRBCs is markedly reduced.

The size difference between a red cell and albumin is huge (like a soccer ball versus a grain of sand), but each will act as one osmotic particle. The number of soccer balls that can fit into a stadium is limited, but the number of grains of sand that can fit is many orders of magnitude higher. Similarly, with a transfusion of PRBCs, water is pushed out of the intravascular space into the interstitial or intercellular space, because of the decrease in the number of osmotic particles or volume.

## Maintenance Fluids

In surgical patients, assessing the intravascular status is a pivotal task, but one of the most difficult. Surgical patients have blood loss from trauma, operations, and diseases. In addition, volume deficits occur from losses of gastrointestinal fluids because of vomiting, diarrhea, nasogastric suctioning, fistulas, and drains. Fluid also shifts out of the intravascular space because of burns, inflammation (as in pancreatitis), intestinal obstruction, infection, and sepsis.

Nonetheless, the main daily task of perioperative patient care is assessing the intravascular status. Is it where it needs to be? It is safer for surgeons to assume that a patient is hypovolemic or hypervolemic than normal; the normovolemic band is very small. Normovolemia occurs only as patients pass from hypervolemia to hypovolemia. The maintenance fluid should constantly be adjusted, depending on the patient's current status.

**BOX 5-4 Maintenance Fluid Calculation**

**IV Fluid Calculation**
- 4 mL/kg for first 10 kg
- 2 mL/kg for next 10 kg
- 1 mL/kg for every kg over 20 kg

*Sample calculation for 45-kg patient:*
- 10 kg × 4 mL / kg = 40 mL
- 10 kg × 2 mL / kg = 20 mL
- 25 kg × 1 mL / kg = 25 mL

Maintenance rate = 85 mL / hr

*Sample calculation for 73-kg patient:*
- 10 kg × 4 mL / kg = 40 mL
- 10 kg × 2 mL / kg = 20 mL
- 53 kg × 1 mL / kg = 53 mL

Maintenance rate = 113 mL / hr

Surgeons must pay attention to each patient's fluid status and bodily needs, rather than infusing maintenance fluid at the same rate.

For the routine preoperative care of patients about to undergo elective surgery, the customary approach is to start a maintenance drip of crystalloids. However, note that patients who undergo same day surgery have little need for preoperative fluids. All preoperative patients are asked not to take in any fluids by mouth starting the night before surgery, a directive that typically does not result in any problems. Remember that everyone is NPO when they sleep; people do not normally wake up hypotensive or in renal failure. Thus, for patients about to undergo major surgery requiring inpatient hospitalization after surgery, IV fluids the night before are not necessary: they typically will receive plenty of fluids from the anesthesiologist during surgery.

In patients who have undergone a colectomy, a small, prospective randomized study has shown that minimizing crystalloids during surgery leads to a better outcome; these patients have less nausea and vomiting, decreased hospital length of stay, and faster return of gastrointestinal function. However, starting these patients on a maintenance fluid is safe, mainly to provide water (Box 5-4). In adult patients weighing more than 40 kg, the simple rule for calculating the fluid rate is 40 plus their weight in kilograms; that is, a 73-kg patient's maintenance rate would be 113 kg/hr (73 + 40).

Maintenance fluids have not been rigorously tested, so the ideal fluid is unknown. The current standard is to use 5% dextrose in water ($D_5$) half-normal (0.45%) saline with 40 mEq/liter of potassium. The source of the standard's formulation remains unclear. For a 70-kg NPO man, it would provide sodium and potassium, but this is not what the average person requires (Table 5-12). The average 70-kg man's requirements are listed in Table 5-13.

The average daily salt intake in American men has been difficult to assess; the median is an estimated 7.8 to 11.8 g/day. Because that range does not include salt added at the table, it is probably an underestimate. The U.S. Department of Agriculture recommends a salt intake of less than 2.3g/day. Normal saline contains 9 g of sodium chloride in 1 liter of water. The amount of fluids and electrolytes infused into patients with the standard formulation is highly inaccurate. The decision to give $D_5$ in maintenance fluid is thought to derive from fasting studies of Harvard medical students in the 1920s. Those studies found that providing approximately 100 g of glucose decreased protein spillage in the urine. The rationale for the use of half-normal saline and 20 mEq/liter of potassium is unknown. A survey of critical care intensivists found that the vast majority did not know the daily recommended intake of sodium or potassium.

**Table 5-12 Contents of Maintenance Solution***

| COMPONENT | 24-HR TOTAL |
|---|---|
| Water | 2760 mL |
| Dextrose | 132 g |
| Sodium | 11.8 g (203 mEq) |
| Potassium | 1.9 g (53 mEq) |

*With $D_5$ half-normal saline with 40 mEq/liter of potassium in a 70-kg patient over 24 hours.

**Table 5-13 Normal Daily Needs for 70-kg Man/Day**

| COMPONENT | 24-HR TOTAL |
|---|---|
| Water | 2000 mL |
| Urine | 1500 mL |
| Sodium | 2-4 g |
| Potassium | 100 mEq |

Surgeons fear that an insufficient volume of fluid will lead to renal failure. Oliguria in a 70-kg man is defined as less than 400 mL of urine produced and excreted in a 24-hour period. This is the minimum volume required to maintain normal serum blood urea nitrogen (BUN) and creatinine levels so that the kidney can function maximally. This volume equates to 0.24 mL/kg/hr. Historically, surgical residents were mandated to give patients enough IV maintenance fluid to produce 0.5 mL/kg/hr, probably to build in a safety margin to ensure enough volume. Today, it is not uncommon for residents to give patients a 1-liter fluid bolus of crystalloids for urine output of less than 50 mL/kg/hr, a practice that will usually lead to overhydration, but the kidneys can compensate for this. In general, overhydration has not been typically seen as a problem, and anasarca has been seen as harmless; however, this view is accurate only for patients who are not on a ventilator. Studies have suggested that excess fluids may delay the return of bowel function.

Postoperatively, in general, patients are more often initially hypervolemic. Because of the bleeding from surgery and the need for IV infusion, anesthesiologists often give patients too much blood and fluids during surgery. Giving a few liters of blood and fluid is probably inconsequential, but for patients who have lost liters of blood, accurate measurement is impossible; their volume status has to be estimated. Patients who have lost a minimal amount of blood during elective surgery who have received liters of crystalloids and have adequate urine output do not necessarily need IV maintenance fluids. For typical patients on the surgical ward, normally functioning kidneys will generally make up for any errors in the amount of blood and fluid given. However, for ICU patients on a ventilator who have severe traumatic injuries, sepsis, or blood loss, there is less room for error.

For ICU patients, in general, too much intravascular volume is better than too little. Too much volume equates to increased time on the ventilator, according to practicing intensivists, but too little equates to renal insufficiency or renal failure. Pulmonary failure has an associated mortality rate of 20% to 25%, whereas renal failure has an associated mortality rate of 48%. Managing volume correctly could equate to a perfect number of days on the ventilator and to no days on dialysis.

Immediately after surgery, volume requirements are vastly different than the next day. Again, for ICU patients, it is generally better to err on the conservative side, with increased IV volume postoperatively for a predetermined period. Most surgeons have no problem with giving several 1-liter boluses of fluids, but are afraid of having an IV rate of 500 mL for 4 hours, even though the total volume of fluid may be the same. When fluids are given as a bolus, the body has a tendency to be confused; hormone release fluctuates wildly as the body tries to compensate for such wide swings in pressure and volume in the vascular system.

Surgical patients are often hypovolemic intravascularly, despite being overhydrated during the surgery. The body can be dramatically overloaded by many liters (at least according to calculations of how much fluid has been infused), but still be hypovolemic intravascularly. The total daily water input in these patients may be higher, but determining current intravascular volume is vital to try to predict the volume status over time as the water shifts from the interstitial to the intravascular space.

The same maintenance rate over days can be problematic, especially for ICU patients. Again, determining fluid status is difficult. Surgeons need to obtain as much information as possible to estimate the IV maintenance rate. Knowing the BUN-to-creatinine ratio is helpful; a ratio higher than 20 is generally thought to be on the dry side, and a ratio less than 10, on the wet side. Such generalizations are only true for patients with normal renal function. Urine output is an excellent way to determine kidney function. High output generally will mean that the body is trying to rid itself of water; surgeons should assist by decreasing the maintenance fluid rate. Anasarca is a helpful clue, as are the customary vital signs.

In older patients with heart failure or sepsis who are intravascularly hypovolemic, anasarca can be profound. Many of these patients will need more IV fluids, despite having anasarca. To help estimate vascular volume, central venous pressure and data from pulmonary artery catheters, if available, are useful. However, caution should be taken when interpreting heart rate. Central venous pressure, wedge pressure from pulmonary artery catheter, stroke volume, cardiac output, and volume status all roughly correlate, but heart rate and intravascular volume are difficult to correlate. Heart rate is affected by many variables, including pain, anxiety, hormone levels, and temperature.

For patients with arterial blood gases, the $PaO_2$-to-$FIO_2$ or the P/F ratio is extremely helpful. The P/F ratio is the ratio of arterial oxygen concentration to the fraction of inspired oxygen. In a healthy young patient without heart disease, the arterial oxygen content is approximately 100; because room air is 0.21% oxygen, the P/F ratio is approximately 500 (100/0.21). That same patient, if placed on 100% oxygen, would have an arterial oxygen content of 500 and a P/F ratio of 500. In a healthy patient who does not have pneumonia, sepsis, or pulmonary contusion, the P/F ratio can reflect interstitial or lung water status; it will help direct the maintenance rate. If patients have a calculated maintenance IV rate, the surgeon evidently believes that their intravascular volume rate is ideal and that the water shifts are not expected to be an issue (because the total water content is deemed ideal).

In surgical patients with low urine output, the most common error is to provide furosemide as an IV bolus. In most if not all these patients, low urine output postoperatively means that they have deceased renal blood flow because of insufficient intravascular volume. When blood flow to the kidneys is decreased, the kidneys sense inadequate intravascular volume; therefore, the renin-angiotensin system, ADH, atrial natriuretic peptide, carotid baroreceptors, and other mechanisms will be activated in an effort to preserve water. If furosemide is injected as a bolus, it poisons the distal Henle loop, rendering it unable to hold in water, thus increasing urine output. Increased urine output in patients with an intravascular volume deficit worsens the deficit. An entire set of compensatory mechanisms will again be activated in an effort to preserve more water.

Low urine output is a signal that the maintenance rate should be higher; high urine output is usually a signal that the maintenance rate should be lower. If surgeons are forced to pull water out of a patient's body because of life-threatening hypoxia, diuretics such as dopamine or furosemide can be used in a drip form, which does not result in the toxic side effects seen with a bolus of furosemide. Still, decreasing intravascular volume status will have a number of effects on many organs.

For resuscitation of patients, our knowledge of biochemistry and physiology might suggest that one particular fluid would make much more sense than another. For example, fluids such as Plasma-Lyte (Normosol-R, Hospira, Lake Forest, Ill) resemble the contents of the electrolytes in blood more than solutions such as LR or normal saline. Solutions resembling serum may be optimal in that they lessen the chance of hyperchloremic acidosis caused by the higher concentration of chloride in normal saline. In the body, $Cl^-$ and $HCO_3^-$ seem to be in equilibrium; in the presence of high levels of chloride, a nonanion gap acidosis will result. However, advocates of normal saline argue that even though acidosis caused by anaerobic metabolism is not generally desired, hyperchloremic acidosis is not necessarily bad. It may help offload oxygen at the tissue level from the hemoglobin molecule.

Despite all these arguments, no evidence shows any clinical benefit of one crystalloid solution over another. Using the cheapest and most readily available fluid may make the most sense. Hospital costs of LR and normal saline are currently approximately \$0.98 per liter; Plasma-Lyte and Normosol-R cost approximately \$1.49 per liter. Because the difference in cost is so small, the cost saving argument is probably invalid.

Fluids that are devoid of some elements and require later replacement of other—for example, potassium—raise a more pertinent issue. They may not be cost-effective in the long run, even if initially cheaper. The costs of monitoring and replacing electrolytes can add up to significant amounts. Because surgical patients often require blood transfusions, purists will urge the use of crystalloids as carriers without calcium, because it is feared that calcium will cause blood to clot in the IV lines. LR contains 3 mEq/liter of calcium, which will exceed the chelating capability of the citrate in the blood bag. However, whole blood or PRBCs mixed with an equal volume of LR have not increased clot formation in vitro as compared with saline reconstitution.

## Adrenal Gland

As noted, the adrenal medulla affects intravascular volume during shock by secreting catechol hormones. They are called *catecholamines* because they contain a catechol group derived from the amino acid tyrosine. The most abundant catecholamines are epinephrine, norepinephrine, and dopamine, all of which are produced from phenylalanine and tyrosine. Cortisol is also released from the adrenal cortex and plays a major role in that it controls fluid equilibrium. Aldosterone is produced from the adrenal cortex and zona glomerulosa in response to stimulation by angiotensin II. Aldosterone is a mineralocorticoid that modulates renal function by increasing the recovery of sodium and excretion of potassium. One of the problems in shock is that the release of all these hormones is not infinite; they can be exhausted.

Many other organs are involved in the control of hormones, including the hypothalamic-pituitary interface, which leads to the release of adrenocorticotropic hormone (ACTH) from the anterior pituitary gland. This system is affected by various factors, including intravascular pressure, intravascular volume, and electrolytes such as sodium. The juxtaglomerular apparatus of the kidneys produces the enzyme renin, which generates angiotensin I. Angiotensin I is then converted to angiotensin II by the angiotensin-converting enzyme located on the endothelial cells of the pulmonary arteries. This regulation of intravascular fluid status is further affected by the carotid baroreceptors and atrial natriuretic peptides. To infuse or block any of these hormones leads to compensatory mechanisms and perturbations within this complicated system.

The system is also affected by many other factors that we have recently found, and will be affected by others that have yet to be discovered. For example, TBI has shown us that the hypothalamic-pituitary interface can be directly affected by mechanical trauma or ICP. For these patients, treatment becomes difficult to control because they go through a wide range of physiologic responses. Patients undergoing brain herniation go from a bradycardic hypertensive state to a profoundly tachycardic and hypotensive state. During these widely varying states, urine output is also affected and diabetes insipidus (DI) can occur. Most likely, the human body has teleologically evolved to try to reduce brain edema at all costs and high-volume urine output often results, requiring vasopressin infusions. Patients whose regulating system is malfunctioning or whose adrenal glands have been exhausted also have a need for high-dose pressors. However, it has been shown that the infusion of cortisol and thyroid hormone in drip form can decrease such instability and minimize the need for fluid infusion and pressors. Patients undergoing brain herniation illustrate the complexity of the regulatory system; surgeons must be cognizant of the changes that can occur every minute.

Adrenal glucocorticoid insufficiency, but not complete failure, occurs in patients with impaired function of the hypothalamic-pituitary-adrenal axis. These patients produce limited amounts of corticosteroids. Clinical problems develop when patients are stressed by hypovolemia caused by hemorrhage, onset of an infection, fear, or hypothermia. When evaluating patients during a surgical emergency, chronic adrenal insufficiency may be initially diagnosed after intractable hypotension is found. Pathologic causes of chronic adrenal insufficiency include autoimmune destruction of the adrenal gland and adrenalitis, in which cytotoxic lymphocytes gradually destroy cortisol-synthesizing cells in the adrenal cortex. Patients with adrenalitis gradually develop symptoms of fatigue, inanition, weight loss, and postural dizziness. Their chief complaint may be vague cramping abdominal pain, nausea, and change in bowel habits. Laboratory findings suggesting adrenal insufficiency include hyperkalemia, acidemia, hyponatremia, and elevated serum creatinine levels. The diagnosis of adrenal insufficiency secondary to end-organ failure is established by disproportionately elevated ACTH levels, as compared with cortisol levels.

Clinical findings in patients with sudden acute adrenal insufficiency can be nonspecific. If plasma cortisol levels precipitously decline to nil, patients will have abdominal pain syndrome, vomiting, and tender abdomen and then will progress to prostration, coma, and hypotension unresponsive to catecholamine infusion. Signs and symptoms of a gradual reduction in cortisol function include malaise, fatigue, and hyponatremia with hyperkalemia. Patients with a complete loss of circulating glucocorticoids can die within hours after irreversible hypotension.

In critically ill patients, quickly establishing the diagnosis of adrenal insufficiency is difficult. Laboratory tests can confirm that plasma levels of the hormones are depressed, but test results take hours to obtain. Pending the laboratory test results, surgeons treat these patients with hormone replacement therapy. Treatment of glucocorticoid deficiency in adults consists of an IV infusion of 100 mg of hydrocortisone, which has an onset of action within 1 to 2 hours and a duration of action of 8 hours. Thus, the commonly recommended replacement dose in an adult is 100 mg of IV hydrocortisone, infused every 8 hours and then rapidly tapered over subsequent days as the patient's condition stabilizes and laboratory test results become available.

Other glucocorticoids used for IV replacement therapy include methylprednisolone and dexamethasone. Methylprednisolone has an anti-inflammatory milligram per milligram potency of 5 and dexamethasone, 25 (relative to 1.0 for hydrocortisone). Patients whose adrenal glands are destroyed may also require replacement of mineralocorticoids. Patients with primary adrenal failure should be treated with 50 to 200 μg/day of fludrocortisone.

## Antidiuretic Hormone and Water

ADH causes water to be reabsorbed and thus reduces urine output. The pituitary releases ADH or arginine vasopressin (AVP). Synthesized in the hypothalamic region, ADH is stored in the pituitary. Excess production or release of ADH causes overhydration: water is retained and thus sodium levels are lowered. Because serum osmolality is predominantly related to sodium, it will be lower than normal (285 mmol/kg) with excess ADH.

One example of overhydration is a syndrome called *SIADH* (syndrome of inappropriate ADH). Despite being overhydrated because of too much ADH production, the kidneys are signaled to hold onto water. Therefore, urine osmolality will be high (>300 mmol/kg), even though serum osmolality is low. However, if ADH is not synthesized or released (e.g., patients with TBI), the kidneys will start to release high volumes of water and urine osmolality will be as low as 100 mmol/kg. The resulting dehydration will lead to elevated serum sodium levels. In patients with TBI, the development of DI is associated with significant brain injury and poor prognosis. In patients with DI or SIADH, the body's thermostat or regulator is dysfunctional;

close attention needs to be paid to maintain volume control. Treatment of patients with DI should include desmopressin (DDAVP) and treatment of patients with SIADH includes water restriction.

## ELECTROLYTES

### Sodium

Sodium is vital for homeostasis and the action potential in the body. It is the predominant molecule that controls water movement in and out of the vascular system. Hyponatremia and hypernatremia, heavily controlled by ADH, are common problems in surgical patients. In general, mild forms of hyponatremia and hypernatremia are not problematic, but hyponatremia is more concerning than hypernatremia. Of the many signs and symptoms associated with each, they are nonspecific; none of the signs or symptoms alone would lead a clinician to diagnose a sodium abnormality. A blood test is always required.

#### Hyponatremia

Hyponatremia can be mild (130 to 138 mEq/liter), moderate (120 to 130 mEq/liter), or severe (<120 mEq/liter). Mild hyponatremia and moderate hyponatremia are common but only rarely symptomatic. Severe hyponatremia, however, can cause headaches and lethargy; patients can become comatose or have seizures, although chronic severe hyponatremia can often be asymptomatic. Hyponatremia is problematic when cells swell as a result of the body's decreased ability to maintain homeostatic osmolality outside the cells. Typically, hyponatremia is caused by pathologic processes in the brain or lungs.

Patients with hyponatremia are usually hypotonic; on occasion, they may be hypertonic, with high serum glucose or mannitol levels. In severe hyperglycemia, ECF osmolality rises and exceeds that of the intracellular fluid (ICF). The reason is that glucose penetrates cell membranes slowly when insulin is absent, so hyperglycemia pulls water out of the cells into the ECF. Serum sodium concentration falls in proportion to the dilution caused by the hyperglycemia; the measured sodium level is lowered by 1.6 mEq/liter for every additional 100 mg/dL of glucose. This phenomenon is referred to as *transitional hyponatremia*, because no net change in body water occurs. No specific therapy is required; artificially lowered sodium concentrations will return to normal once the plasma glucose level is normalized. The most common formulas for sodium for clinical use are shown in Box 5-5.

The patient's fluid volume status is critical when assessing hyponatremia. In general, hyponatremia is considered as renal or extrarenal. Excretion of sodium by the kidneys is caused by renal failure or problems with ADH or diuretics. Extrarenal causes include sodium loss caused by wounds, burns, sweating, congestive heart failure, cirrhosis, hypothyroidism, gastrointestinal losses, and cerebral salt wasting syndrome. Acute hyponatremia can also occur if dehydrated patients are infused with fluids containing no sodium. In patients who have bled or who are intravascularly depleted of water (e.g., because of vomiting, diarrhea, pancreatitis, or burns), IV infusion of $D_5$ can rapidly cause hyponatremia. The problem is exacerbated in hypovolemic patients because the hypothalamus is secreting ADH in an effort to preserve water. The normal response to hyponatremia is the suppression of ADH to secrete water to increase the sodium concentration in the serum. Thus, hyponatremic patients should have undetectable levels of ADH. However, ADH release can be stimulated by elevated ECF osmolality and by reduced ECF volume. In hypovolemic patients, baroreceptors also stimulate the hypothalamus to retain water through ADH release.

**BOX 5-5 Sodium Equations for Clinical Use**

**Sodium Deficit**
Sodium deficit (mEq) = ([Na] goal − [Na] plasma) × TBW
TBW = total body water = body weight × 60%

**Free Water Deficit**
Free water deficit = ([Na]/140) −1) × TBW

**Corrected Sodium**
Corrected sodium = ([Na] + 0.016) × (glucose − 100)

**Serum Osmolality (Calculated)**
(2 × [Na]) + (BUN/2.8) + (glucose/18)

**Fractional Excretion of Sodium ($Fr_{exc}$ Na)**
$Fr_{exc}$ Na = ([Na] urine) + (creatinine plasma/[Na] plasma) + (creatinine urine)
<1% = prerenal (hypovolemia)
>2% = intrinsic renal disorder

Diuresis with furosemide or mannitol can also cause hyponatremia in addition to causing intravascular fluid loss. In addition, it increases sodium loss by the kidneys and increases ADH release as the body tries to counteract the rapid fluid loss by preserving water. Hyperglycemia, if high enough for glucose to be spilled in the urine, will also induce an osmotic diuresis that depletes extracellular water and also leads to hyponatremia. Along with diuresis, hyperglycemia can lead to various electrolyte imbalances involving many regulatory mechanisms and can cause wild hormonal swings and imbalances.

Renal loss of sodium can lead to hyponatremia and excessive release of natriuretic peptides related to brain injury or disease. One particularly difficult condition to treat is cerebral salt wasting syndrome. Even when treating these patients with salt, the regulatory mechanisms cause a high urine output, up to 4 to 6 liters/day, with consequent urine sodium losses. Those losses correlate with elevated brain natriuretic peptide levels in plasma. The lost sodium must be replaced via an IV line or by enteral intake.

In patients with a brain injury, hyponatremia that is normally well tolerated may be devastating; it is thought to cause cerebral intracellular swelling as osmolality is reduced. In these patients, infusion of HTS may be needed. HTS is available commercially (in a 3%, 5%, or 23% concentration). A pharmacist can also formulate HTS at any desired concentration. Depending on the electrolyte imbalance, salt infusions can take various forms; sodium can be provided as sodium chloride, sodium acetate, sodium bicarbonate, or a combination of these.

If HTS is to be infused at concentrations higher than 5%, the preferred route is via central IV catheters; higher concentrations can be caustic to peripheral veins and can also cause pain. In general, no more than 10 mEq/day of sodium should be provided. The volume of fluids needed should be taken into consideration when choosing the concentration. If a patient requires a large volume of fluids in a 4-hour period, 0.9% normal saline will elevate the sodium level. However, in hypervolemic patients, the goal is to minimize the volume infused, so a higher concentration can be used, such as 5%. The reason for elevating the sodium level slowly is to avoid central pontine myelinolysis, which can occur 1 to 6 days later. This manifests as pseudobulbar palsy, quadriparesis, seizures, movement disorders, and decreased level of consciousness.

If urologic or gynecologic surgery is performed with hypo-osmotic irrigation, acute hyponatremia can occur. During endometrial resection and transurethral resection of the prostrate, acute water intoxication has been reported as a complication.

In surgical ICU patients, a frequent cause of hyponatremia is SIADH. This syndrome can be acute or chronic. In hypovolemic patients, the body's natural response is to release ADH. If the body is euvolemic and still releases ADH inappropriately, the patient has SIADH, so this diagnosis should only be made in euvolemic patients. Given the aberrant release of ADH, the serum osmolality is often lower than 270 mmol/kg, but the kidneys still excrete concentrated urine.

A hyponatremic patient with a urine osmolality of 350 mmol/kg is producing ADH and the kidneys are concentrating it as they should; the source of hyponatremia is usually extrarenal. ADH-secreting tumors (e.g., carcinoid tumors, small cell carcinomas of the lung) can cause chronic SIADH. Up to 35% of patients with active acquired immunodeficiency syndrome (AIDS) who are admitted for hospitalization have SIADH. Hyponatremia can also be caused by renal dysfunction in patients with conditions that impair the capability to retain sodium, such as medullary cystic disease, polycystic kidney disease, analgesic nephropathy, chronic pyelonephritis, and obstructive uropathy after decompression syndrome.

### Hypernatremia

Moderate hypernatremia (146 to 159 mEq/liter) is fairly well tolerated. Causes include endocrine syndromes, in which ADH synthesis or release fails, the failure of renal tubular cells to respond to ADH, increased salt intake or infusion, and loss of water. Hypernatremia can be problematic in that it pulls water out of the cells; the primary concern is that it is thought to contract the cerebral cells. However, my recent experience with HTS has shown that acutely elevated sodium levels are relatively safe. HTS is used to contract cerebral intracellular volume in patients with TBI to reduce the total brain volume when intracranial swelling or mass effect is a factor. The normal response to hypernatremia is for the kidneys to generate hyperosmolar urine and retain water. Renal correction of hypernatremia depends on the patient having access to water.

Pathologically, hypernatremia, like hyponatremia, is considered as renal or extrarenal. Renal fluid losses are caused by diuretics, the polyuric phase of acute tubular necrosis (ATN), or postobstructive diuresis of the kidney. After decompression of a chronically obstructed ureter, renal tubular cells seem to respond less to ADH. Nephrogenic DI is defined as an impaired capacity of the renal tubules to respond to ADH and concentrate urine. Moderate hypernatremia develops in patients with nephrogenic DI when they lose water in dilute urine, despite elevated plasma levels of ADH. If an infusion of ADH does not increase urine osmolality, DI is the likely diagnosis. Drugs such as lithium, glyburide, demeclocycline, and amphotericin B can cause DI. The treatment in patients with lithium-induced nephrogenic DI is amiloride (5 to 10 mg daily).

Hyperkalemia or severe hypokalemia also impairs the capacity of renal tubular cells to absorb sodium. Patients with end-stage renal dysfunction and low glomerular filtration rates may produce a fixed volume of 2 to 4 liters/day of iso-osmotic urine. In hot and arid environments, these patients are particularly susceptible to dehydration and hypernatremia.

The extrarenal causes of hypernatremia include loss of water from vomiting, diarrhea, nasogastric tube suctioning, burns, sweating, fever, and problems with insufficient ADH levels. Infusion of sodium, like HTS, can also cause hypernatremia; the duration depends on the amount of crystalloids infused for resuscitation over 24 hours. A recent study on the use of 5% HTS in trauma patients has shown that sodium levels rise above 150 mEq/liter and remain elevated for days. In contrast, previous studies on the use of 7.5% HTS infusions found that the duration of the hypernatremia was short. The transient hypernatremia was probably caused by aggressive use of other crystalloids for resuscitation after the HTS infusion, which quickly diluted the hypernatremia.

When dealing with hypernatremia, it is again important first to assess volume status; correcting the hypernatremia depends on volume status. In hypovolemic patients, offsetting the volume deficit with isotonic fluids is sufficient. However, nonhypovolemic patients need free water replacement with hypotonic solutions. In hypervolemic patients, diuretics may be used, but carefully. In general, in asymptomatic patients, sodium levels should not be corrected too rapidly; doing so could cause cerebral edema. In patients with acute hypernatremia, the rate is usually no more than 1 to 2 mEq/hr; with chronic hyponatremia, no more than 0.5 mEq/hr. Sodium levels should not be corrected at a rate higher than 8 mEq/day. Careful and frequent sodium monitoring is often required.

Patients with DI are producing dilute urine at a rate of hundreds of milliliters per hour. They should be treated with DDAVP, a synthetic analogue of ADH that has a half-life of several hours. DDAVP increases water movement out of the collecting duct but does not have the vasoconstrictive properties of ADH. Patients with mild DI can be treated with intranasal DDAVP and water. It can be administered orally, intranasally, SC, or IV. The intranasal dose is 10 μg once or twice daily. In ICU patients, IV administration is preferred for control and accuracy.

## Potassium

Potassium is the main intracellular ion and sodium is the main extracellular ion. The normal potassium concentration in serum is 4.5 mmol/liter. Small changes in serum reflect large intracellular changes. The daily average intake of potassium is 50 to 100 mmol/day. The kidneys control the daily excretion, which ranges widely, from 20 to 400 mmol/day. The renin-angiotensin-aldosterone hormone axis is the key regulator of potassium clearance. As the plasma aldosterone concentration increases, so does potassium excretion.

### Hypokalemia

Patients with hypokalemia have a potassium concentration $[K^+]$ lower than 3.5 mmol/liter. The result is hyperpolarization of the resting potential of the cell, which interferes with neuromuscular function. Generalized symptoms commonly associated with depressed serum levels include fatigue, weakness, and ileus. Occasionally, rhabdomyolysis occurs in patients whose $[K^+]$ drops below 2.5 mmol/liter. Flaccid paralysis with respiratory compromise can occur as $[K^+]$ decreases to lower than 2 mmol/liter.

Hypokalemia is caused by renal losses, extrarenal losses, or intracellular shifts from medications or hyperthyroidism. Extrarenal losses can be caused by persistent vomiting, gastric tubes, diarrhea, or high-output enteric or pancreatic fistulas. Hypokalemia is a common problem in patients with congestive heart failure who are on multiple drugs. It can also develop in patients treated with diuretics that force renal function to excrete urine with an elevated potassium concentration. Long-term diuretic therapy can produce a sustained negative potassium balance. Patients with a chronic potassium deficiency can develop a cardiac rhythm disturbance. The electrocardiogram (ECG) of patients with hypokalemia will show depressed T waves and U waves. Hypokalemia leads to cardiac arrhythmia, particularly atrial tachycardia with or without block, atrioventricular dissociation, ventricular tachycardia, and ventricular fibrillation. The risk for hypokalemia-associated arrhythmia is higher in patients treated with digoxin, even when potassium concentrations are in the low-normal range. Hypokalemia not caused by diuretics may be caused by a rare endocrine disorder, including primary hyperaldosteronism and renin-secreting tumors.

**Treatment of Acute Hypokalemia** Hypokalemic patients require potassium replacement by the oral or IV route. Oral supplementation is generally 40 to 100 mEq/day, in two to four doses. The IV rate is 10 to 20 mEq/hr; if potassium is infused at rates higher than10 mEq/hr, cardiac monitoring is required. In emergency situations, the rate can be as high as 40 mEq/hr, but a central vein should be used because high concentrations of potassium in IV fluids can be irritating to peripheral veins. In patients with renal dysfunction, whose potassium excretion is reduced, the IV rate of potassium replacement and total dose should be lower.

After treatment, frequent monitoring of potassium levels is necessary. Because hypokalemia represents large intracellular deficits, replenishing total body levels may take days. Potassium therapy is given as the chloride salt because hypokalemia is commonly associated with a contraction in the extracellular water, in which chloride is the predominant anion. Potassium in foods is linked to phosphate. Potassium phosphate salts may need to be given via the IV route, particularly when expansion of intracellular water is anticipated. To reduce the risk of serious cardiac arrhythmia in patients with cardiac disease or after cardiac surgery who have a serum level lower than 3.5 mmol/liter, serum [$K^+$] should be promptly corrected to a level higher than 4.0 mmol/liter. Patients with substantial and continuing gastrointestinal loss of potassium require extraordinary potassium replacement to correct the hypokalemia.

Magnesium levels should be monitored concomitantly; hypomagnesemia can produce refractory hypokalemia. Magnesium is an important cofactor for potassium uptake and for the maintenance of intracellular potassium levels. In addition, supplemental magnesium reduces the risk of arrhythmia.

Hypokalemic patients with concurrent acidemia are treated with potassium replacement, before their pH is corrected by bicarbonate administration. Diabetic patients with ketoacidosis may initially have a normal [$K^+$], but hypokalemia rapidly develops as insulin is administered and as glucose shifts into cells. For these patients, potassium supplements should be added to the resuscitation fluid once the physician is confident that renal function is adequate. If hypokalemia develops while patients are undergoing diuretic therapy, additional drugs can reduce the renal loss of potassium. For example, triamterene or spironolactone blocks the effect of aldosterone and reduces potassium loss in urine.

## Hyperkalemia

Hyperkalemia is defined as a [K+] higher than 5.0 mmol/liter. If levels exceed 6 mmol/liter, perturbations in the resting cell membrane potential occur and normal depolarization and repolarization are impaired. The most common cause of hyperkalemia is renal failure in hospitalized patients. The transport of potassium is passive, but the transport of sodium requires energy. This difference across the cell is maintained by $Na^+$,$K^+$-ATPase activity, which requires energy. The energy is in the form of cellular ATP; its levels are highly variable in different stages of shock when nutrients are not available (whether carbohydrates or oxygen). When cellular ATP levels fall, the sodium pump is impaired. If sodium or potassium levels are severely high or low, the membrane potential will be affected. Eventually, without energy, cell death occurs, and the $Na^+$-$K^+$ gradient cannot be maintained; the sodium gradient is needed to maintain the membrane potential.

The primary clinical problem is cardiac arrhythmia, which can be lethal. Hyperkalemia is associated with peaked T waves; dangerous hyperkalemia (6 to 7 mmol/liter) is indicated by T waves higher than R waves (Fig. 5-23).

The most common cause of hyperkalemia is acute onset of renal dysfunction or failure. Cellular injury (e.g., sepsis or ischemia reperfusion) can also release potassium from its intracellular source, which can overwhelm the kidneys' ability to clear potassium. At least 20% of normal renal function is required to respond to ADH and maintain normal potassium levels. The reperfusion of ischemic tissues resulting in rhabdomyolysis causes high potassium levels; to prevent cardiac arrest, a bolus of IV sodium bicarbonate may be of some benefit. The bicarbonate shifts potassium intracellularly. Note that impaired aldosterone levels (as with infarction of bilateral adrenal glands) can activate other renal mechanisms and stimulate potassium excretion, resulting in moderate levels of hyperkalemia.

Drugs can have a direct effect on the renal tubules and on potassium excretion, such as triamterene, spironolactone, beta

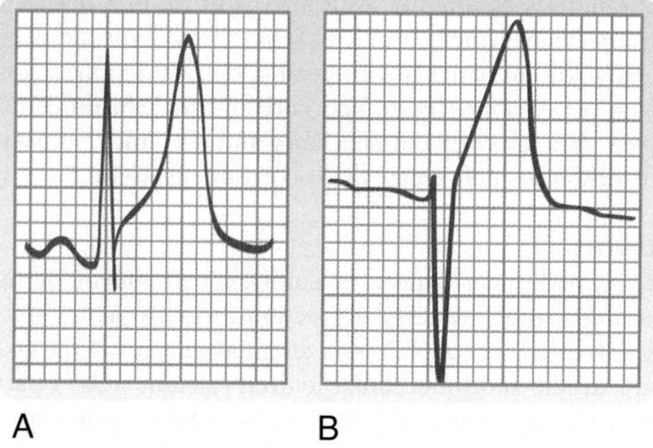


**FIGURE 5-23** Electrocardiographic changes. **A,** Indicating hyperkalemia. The T wave is tall, narrow, and symmetrical. **B,** Indicating acute myocardial infarction. The T wave is tall but broad-based and asymmetrical. (From Somers MP, Brady WJ, Perron AD, et al: The prominent T wave: Electrocardiographic differential diagnosis. Am J Emerg Med 20:243–251, 2002.)

blockers, cyclosporine, and tacrolimus. They are usually a contributing factor but not a primary cause. Succinylcholine, a depolarizing paralytic agent, is used in patients with muscle atrophy from disuse, prolonged bed rest, neurologic denervation syndromes, severe burns, direct muscle trauma, or rhabdomyolysis; it can cause severe hyperkalemia, resulting in cardiac arrest. When drawing blood samples from patients, clinicians must recognize that sample hemolysis can release potassium, so laboratory test results could be spurious. If the sample or test results are suspect, another sample should be taken before drastic efforts are made to treat hyperkalemia.

**Treatment of Hyperkalemia** In patients at risk of developing cardiac arrhythmia from hyperkalemia, several interventions are useful. IV calcium can immediately reduce the risk of arrhythmia by antagonizing the depolarization effect of elevated $[K^+]$. Sodium bicarbonate infusion buffers extracellular protons and allows for the net transfer of cytosolic protons across the cell membrane via carbonic acid. The shift of protons out of the cell is associated with a shift of potassium into the cells. Bicarbonate therapy is most effective in hyperkalemic patients with metabolic acidemia. Insulin and glucose infusions prompt an increase in $Na^+,K^+$-ATPase activity and decline in extracellular water potassium concentration as the extracellular water potassium is pumped into the cell.

In patients with aldosterone deficiency and hyperkalemia, a mineralocorticoid drug such as 9α-fludrocortisone will increase the renal excretion of potassium. In patients with acute renal failure, hemodialysis is the most reliable method to control hyperkalemia. Continuous filtration methods clear $K^+$ at a slower rate than hemodialysis. Chronic hyperkalemia associated with renal dysfunction can be managed by oral or rectal administration of sodium polystyrene sulfonate, a cation exchange resin that binds potassium in the gut lumen. Rectally administered binding resins are particularly effective because the colonic mucosa can excrete mucus with large amounts of potassium. Surgeons should clearly establish a process for managing hyperkalemia, because rapidly escalating potassium levels pose an immediate threat and require rapidly delivered effective therapy (Box 5-6). Dysfunctional renal handling of potassium from mineralocorticoid deficiency or resistance leads to hyperkalemia. Renal failure is commonly associated with tubular defects and potassium management problems, along with hyperaldosteronism. However, in patients with normal renal function, assessing levels of aldosterone, renin, and cortisol can help differentiate between mineralocorticoid deficiency and resistance. In patients with aldosterone deficiency, fludrocortisone is useful.

**BOX 5-6 Guidelines for Treatment of Adult Patients With Hyperkalemia**

First: Stop all infusion of potassium.

**Electrocardiographic Evidence of Pending Arrest**

Loss of P wave and broad slurring of QRS; immediate effective therapy indicated

1. IV infusion of calcium salts:
   10 mL of 10% calcium chloride over 10-minute period
   *or*
   10 mL of 10% calcium gluconate over 3- to 5-minute period
2. IV infusion of sodium bicarbonate: 50-100 mEq over 10- to 20-minute period; benefit proportional to extent of pretherapy acidemia

**Electrocardiographic Evidence of Potassium Effect**

Peaked T waves; prompt therapy needed

1. Glucose and insulin infusion: IV infusion of 50 mL of $D_{50}W$ and 10 units of regular insulin; monitor glucose
2. Immediate hemodialysis

**Biochemical Evidence of Hyperkalemia and No Electrocardiographic Changes**

Effective therapy needed within hours

1. Potassium-binding resins into the gastrointestinal tract, with 20% sorbitol
2. Promotion of renal kaliuresis by loop diuretic

*$D_{50}W$*, 50% dextrose in water.

## Calcium

Calcium, a divalent cation, is a critical component of many extracellular and intracellular reactions. For surgeons, it is of particular interest because it is an essential cofactor in the coagulation cascade, and intracellular ionized calcium ($iCa^{2+}$) participates in the regulation of neuronal, hormonal, muscular, and renal cellular function. Total serum calcium concentration, normally, 8.5 to 10.5 mg/dL, is present in three molecular forms—protein-bound calcium, diffusible calcium bound to anions (e.g., bicarbonate, phosphate, acetate), and freely diffusible calcium as $iCa^{2+}$.

The biochemically active species is $iCa^{2+}$, which constitutes about 45% of total serum calcium. More than 80% of protein-bound calcium is attached to albumin, so the total calcium concentration in serum will decrease in patients with hypoalbuminemia. Physiologically, the total plasma calcium level must be corrected relative to the albumin level. Normal calcium levels may range from 8.5 to 10.5 mg/day, assuming an albumin level of 4.5 g/dL. The calcium concentration [Ca] usually changes by 0.8 mg/dL for every change of 1.0 g/dL in plasma albumin concentration. This formula estimates the actual total plasma calcium level:

$$\text{Corrected } iCa^{2+} = \text{total } [Ca] + (0.8 \times [4.5 - \text{albumin level}])$$

Acidosis decreases the amount of calcium bound to albumin, whereas alkalosis increases the bound fraction of calcium. A small amount of calcium (≈6%) is bound to anions such as citrate and sulfate. The remainder is $iCa^{2+}$, which is biologically active.

The increase in $iCa^{2+}$ concentration $[iCa^{2+}]$ is controlled by cell membrane enzymes that transport calcium out of the cell. In muscle cells, $iCa^{2+}$ is stored in the sarcoplasmic reticulum and can be quickly released into ICF, where it has a key role in the molecular events that cause muscle contraction. Tight control of $[iCa^{2+}]$ in ECF is essential. The serum [Ca] is controlled by the interaction of parathyroid hormone (PTH), calcitonin, and vitamin D. PTH and calcitonin are hormones subject to regulatory release by endocrine cells, whereas vitamin D is consumed in the diet or formed in the skin as cholecalciferol in response to ultraviolet irradiation. Bone contains an enormous reservoir of calcium in the form of a matrix of calcium and other molecules. Turnover of calcium salts in bone is constant and integral to maintaining a stable $[iCa^{2+}]$ in ECF. Receptors in the membranes of parathyroid cells release PTH when [iCa$^{2+}$] in ECF declines. PTH activates osteoclasts in bones, which release calcium from the structural matrix of bone. PTH stimulates tubule cells in the proximal nephron to absorb calcium from the filtrate and excrete phosphates. PTH with vitamin D enhances calcium absorption from the lumen of the gut.

Calcitonin has the opposite effects on calcium metabolism compared with PTH. As calcitonin levels in ECF increase because of its excretion from type C cells of the thyroid, [iCa$^{2+}$] declines as more calcium is bound to bone matrix. Vitamin D circulating in the blood is converted in the liver to 25-hydroxycholecalciferol (25-D). Then, 25-D circulating in blood encounters kidney cells that further hydroxylate the sterol to 1,25-dihydroxycholecalciferol (1,25-D), which is the most potent calcium-modulating hormone. Next, 1,25-D increases the transport of calcium and phosphate from the lumen of the bowel into the ECF of the intestine. Furthermore, in conjunction with PTH, 1,25-D increases bone resorption, increasing the [Ca] in ECF. In summary, a number of hormonal mechanisms produce a balance of influences on the concentration of calcium in ECF.

### Hypocalcemia

Hypocalcemia varies from an asymptomatic biochemical abnormality to a life-threatening disorder, depending on its duration, severity, and rapidity of development. It is caused by the loss of calcium from the circulation or by insufficient entry of calcium into the circulation.

Acute hypocalcemia can be life-threatening. It impairs transmembrane depolarization; [iCa$^{2+}$] below 0.8 mEq/liter can lead to central nervous system dysfunction. Hypocalcemic patients can have paresthesias, muscle spasms (including tetany), and seizures. As [iCa$^{2+}$] declines, patients can notice numbness, paresthesias of the distal extremities, and painful muscle spasms. If patients hyperventilate, a respiratory alkalosis may exacerbate their condition and further reduce [iCa$^{2+}$]. Cardiac dysfunction is also common. Patients with a low [iCa$^{2+}$] may require IV infusion of calcium to restore cardiac function. Hypocalcemic patients have a prolonged QT interval on ECGs that may progress to complete heart block or ventricular fibrillation.

Hypoparathyroidism, the most common cause of hypocalcemia, often develops because of surgery in the central neck, such as radical resection of head and neck cancers. It develops in 1% to 2% of patients after a total thyroidectomy. The hypocalcemia may be transient, permanent, or intermittent, as with vitamin D deficiency during the winter. Autoimmune hypoparathyroidism can be an isolated defect or be part of polyglandular autoimmune syndrome type I in association with adrenal insufficiency and mucocutaneous candidiasis; most of these patients have autoantibodies directed against the calcium-sensing receptor. Congenital causes of hypocalcemia include activation of mutations of the calcium-sensing receptor, which resets the calcium–PTH relationship to a lower serum calcium level. Mutations affecting intracellular processing of the pre-pro-PTH molecule can lead to hypoparathyroidism, hypocalcemia, or both. Finally, some cases of hypoparathyroidism are associated with hypoplasia or aplasia of the parathyroid glands; the best known is DiGeorge syndrome.

Pseudohypoparathyroidism is a group of disorders characterized by postreceptor resistance to PTH. One classic variant is Albright's hereditary osteodystrophy, associated with low stature, round facies, short digits, and mental retardation. Hypomagnesemia induces PTH resistance and also affects PTH production. Severe hypermagnesemia (>6 mg/dL) can lead to hypocalcemia by inhibiting PTH secretion. When associated with decreased dietary calcium intake, vitamin D deficiency leads to hypocalcemia. The low calcium level stimulates PTH secretion (secondary hyperparathyroidism), leading to hypophosphatemia.

Rhabdomyolysis and tumor lysis syndrome cause loss of calcium from the circulation when large amounts of intracellular phosphate are released, thereby increasing calcium levels in bone and extraskeletal tissues. A similar mechanism causes hypocalcemia with phosphate administration.

Acute pancreatitis results in calcium sequestration in the abdomen, causing hypocalcemia. After surgery for hyperparathyroidism, patients with severe prolonged disease (e.g., those with secondary or tertiary hyperparathyroidism who are in renal failure) can develop a form of hypocalcemia known as *hungry bone syndrome*, in which serum calcium is rapidly deposited into the bone. The syndrome is rarely seen after the correction of long-standing metabolic acidosis or after thyroidectomy for hyperthyroidism.

Several medications (e.g., ethylenediaminetetraacetic acid [EDTA], citrate present in transfused blood, lactate, foscarnet) chelate calcium in the circulation, sometimes producing hypocalcemia in which [iCa$^{2+}$] is decreased, even though the total calcium level may be normal. Extensive osteoblastic skeletal metastases (e.g., from prostate and breast cancers) may also cause hypocalcemia. Chemotherapy, including cisplatin, 5-fluorouracil, and leucovorin, causes hypocalcemia mediated through hypomagnesemia. Hypocalcemia after surgery can be mediated by the citrate content of transfused blood or by large-volume fluid administration and hypoalbuminemia. In patients with sepsis, hypocalcemia is usually associated with hypoalbuminemia.

Tumor lysis syndrome is a constellation of electrolyte abnormalities that include hypocalcemia, hyperphosphatemia, hyperuricemia, and hyperkalemia. These occur when antineoplastic therapy causes a sudden surge in tumor cell death and release of cytosolic contents. Solid tumors and lymphomas have been implicated. Acute renal failure occurs in patients with tumor lysis syndrome and prevents spontaneous correction of the electrolyte abnormalities; emergency dialysis may be the only way to correct the abnormalities comprehensively.

Acute hypocalcemia is frequent after resuscitation from shock. In a study of patients in burn shock, Wray and colleagues hypothesized that a major factor contributing to the development of hypocalcemia was depressed levels of 1,25-D, perhaps caused by a sudden lack of vitamin D in the diet. In patients with severe pancreatitis, the decrease in calcium level is speculated to be the consequence of ionized extracellular calcium becoming linked to fats in the peripancreatic inflammatory phlegmon. Rapid infusion of a citrate load during the transfusion of blood products, particularly platelet concentrates and FFP, may also lead to acute severe hypocalcemia ([iCa$^{2+}$] <0.62 mmol/liter) and to hypotension. Rapid increases in the serum phosphate level can occur after improper administration or excessive dosing of phosphate-containing cathartics; as the phosphate concentration increases, severe hypocalcemia ensues.

**Treatment of Hypocalcemia** Patients with acute symptomatic hypocalcemia (calcium level <7.0 mg/dL; [iCa$^{2+}$] level <0.8 mmol/liter) should be treated promptly with IV calcium.

Calcium gluconate, preferred over calcium chloride, causes less tissue necrosis if extravasated, so it should be given through the central vein route. The first 100 to 200 mg of elemental calcium (1 to 2 g calcium gluconate) should be given over 10 to 20 minutes. Faster administration may result in cardiac dysfunction, even arrest. The first 100 to 200 mg should then be followed by a slow calcium infusion, at a rate of 0.5 to 1.5 mg/kg/hr. Calcium infusion should continue until the patient has received effective doses of oral calcium and vitamin D. Calcium for infusion should be diluted in saline or dextrose solution to avoid vein irritation. The infusion should not contain bicarbonate or phosphate, which can form an insoluble calcium salt. If bicarbonate or phosphate administration is necessary, a separate IV line should be used.

Coexisting hypomagnesemia should be corrected in every patient. Care should be taken in patients with renal insufficiency because they cannot excrete excess magnesium. Magnesium is given via infusion, initiated with 2 g magnesium sulfate over 10 to 15 minutes, followed by 1 g/hr. In patients with severe hyperphosphatemia (e.g., those with tumor lysis syndrome, rhabdomyolysis, or chronic renal failure), treatment is focused on correcting the hyperphosphatemia.

Acute hyperphosphatemia usually resolves in patients with intact renal function. Phosphate excretion may be aided by saline infusion but be cautious, because this can lead to worsening of hypocalcemia. In addition, acetazolamide, a carbonic anhydrase inhibitor, can be given at 10 to 15 mg/kg every 3 to 4 hours. Hemodialysis may be necessary for patients with symptomatic hypocalcemia and hyperphosphatemia, especially if renal function is impaired. Chronic hyperphosphatemia is managed by a low-phosphate diet and phosphate binders with meals.

Chronic hypocalcemia (hypoparathyroidism) is treated by oral calcium administration and, if that is insufficient, vitamin D supplementation. The serum calcium level should be targeted to approximately 8.0 mg/dL. Most patients will be entirely asymptomatic at that level. Further elevation will lead to hypercalciuria because of the lack of PTH effect on the renal tubules. Chronic hypercalciuria carries the risks of nephrocalcinosis, nephrolithiasis, and renal impairment.

Several oral calcium preparations are available. Calcium carbonate is the cheapest form, but may be poorly absorbed, especially in older patients and those with achlorhydria. Similarly, various forms of vitamin D are available. If oral calcium preparations cannot achieve adequate calcium repletion, vitamin D should be added. The usual initial daily dosage is 50,000 IU of 25-hydroxyvitamin D (or 0.25 to 0.5 mg of 1,25-hydroxyvitamin D). Calcium and vitamin D doses are established by gradual titration. When adequate calcemia is achieved, urinary calcium excretion is measured. If hypercalciuria is detected, a thiazide diuretic may be added to diminish calciuria and further increase the serum calcium level, which should be monitored. If the phosphorus level is higher than 6.0 mg/dL when the calcium level is satisfactory, an unabsorbable phosphate binder should be added. Once calcium and phosphorus levels are controlled, the patient should be monitored every 3 to 6 months for both levels and for urinary calcium excretion.

Special consideration is necessary for the treatment of women with hypoparathyroidism who are pregnant or nursing. During pregnancy, vitamin D requirements gradually increase, up to three times as high as the prepregnancy requirements. Supplementary doses of vitamin D should be titrated, using frequent serum calcium level measurements. After delivery, if the baby is to be bottle-fed, the dose should be decreased to the prepregnancy dose. If the baby is to be nursed, the dose of calcitriol should be decreased to 50% of the prepregnancy dose because endogenous calcitriol production is stimulated by prolactin and by the increased production of PTH-related peptide (PTHrP), which is also stimulated by prolactin.

Several reports have described successful control of hypocalcemia using synthetic PTH (1,34-PTH, teriparatide) via twice-daily SC administration, with a lower risk of hypercalciuria.

### Hypercalcemia

Mild hypercalcemia is suspected when the total serum calcium level is in the range of 10.5 to 12 mg/dL. Patients with a serum [Ca] of 12 to 14.5 mg/dL have moderate hypercalcemia. Patients with transient hypercalcemia are generally asymptomatic. Those with sustained elevations in renal calcium excretion are susceptible to the development of renal lithiasis. Patients have severe hypercalcemia when serum calcium levels exceed 15 mg/dL; these patients have symptoms of weakness, stupor, and central nervous system dysfunction. In hypercalcemic patients, a renal concentrating defect also occurs, leading to polyuria and loss of sodium and water; many hypercalcemic patients are dehydrated. Hypercalcemic crisis is a syndrome in which total serum calcium levels exceed 17 mg/dL; these patients are subject to life-threatening cardiac tachyarrhythmia, coma, acute renal failure, and ileus with abdominal distention.

The most common cause of hypercalcemia (in 90% of all patients) is primary hyperparathyroidism; other causes include unregulated PTH secretion and malignancy. Signs and symptoms of hypercalcemia are nonspecific. Usually, a patient's clinical presentation is recognized as related to hypercalcemia only after it has been diagnosed by blood test results. It is extremely difficult to diagnose hypercalcemia by a patient's history alone.

Bone demineralization is found in patients with severe and prolonged hyperparathyroidism. Most of these patients (85%) have a solitary hyperfunctioning adenoma in one parathyroid gland; the remaining 15% have excessive PTH release as a result of hyperplasia of all four glands. PTH induces phosphaturia and depresses serum phosphate concentration; this laboratory finding corroborates the diagnosis of primary hyperparathyroidism. Secondary hyperparathyroidism, an endocrine disease characterized by hyperplasia of the parathyroid glands, develops in patients with chronic renal failure. Decreased renal function results in impaired synthesis of 1,25-D. Although patients have low serum calcium levels, their osteomalacia indicates excessive PTH secretion. To control elevated PTH levels in patients with secondary hyperparathyroidism, surgical removal of most of the parathyroid tissue may be required.

Humoral hypercalcemia of malignancy (HHM) is a clinical syndrome in which elevated calcium levels are caused by synthesis of the humoral factor by the tumoral process. Usually, HHM is applied to patients with excessive tumoral production of PTHrP. However, rare cases characterized by excessive production of PTH and calcitriol have also been described. Patients with HHM constitute about 80% of all patients with hypercalcemia associated with malignancy. PTHrP and PTH share the same receptor, but the clinical presentation differs. HHM patients have a markedly larger degree of renal calcium excretion; PTH potently stimulates tubular calcium resorption, and hypercalciuria is less pronounced. HHM is usually associated with low serum calcitriol levels; PTH stimulates calcitriol production, and its level is usually elevated. PTHrP stimulates only bone resorption, with very low osteoblastic activity and therefore usually normal alkaline phosphatase levels; PTH stimulates bone resorption and formation.

HHM patients usually have a clinically obvious malignant disease and a poor prognosis. The only exceptions to this are patients with small, well-differentiated endocrine tumors (e.g., pheochromocytomas, islet cell tumors). However, these tumors constitute a minority of cases. HHM is most commonly seen with squamous cell carcinomas (e.g., of the lung, esophagus, cervix, or head and neck) and with renal, bladder, and ovarian cancers. Treatment of HHM patients is aimed at reducing the tumor burden, reducing osteoclastic resorption of the bone, and increasing calcium excretion through the urine.

Most cases of hypercalcemia are associated with Hodgkin's disease. The other third of cases are associated with non-Hodgkin's lymphoma and are caused by increased production of calcitriol by the malignant cells. Hypercalcemia usually responds well to treatment with corticosteroids. Multiple myeloma, lymphoma, and solid tumors metastatic to bone (particularly breast, lung, and prostate cancer) cause hypercalcemia by excessive osteoclastic activity. Drugs can also cause hypercalcemia, including theophylline, lithium, thiazide diuretics, and extraordinarily high doses of vitamin A and D. In addition, hypercalcemia can develop in young, normally active patients with high bone turnover rates who are suddenly forced into immobility, such as during forced bed rest after injury or major illness. This hypercalcemia of immobilization resolves with return to normal activity.

Another cause of hypercalcemia is milk-alkali syndrome, a rare condition caused by the ingestion of large amounts of calcium together with sodium bicarbonate. It is currently associated with the ingestion of calcium carbonate in over-the-counter antacid preparations and in drugs used to prevent and treat osteoporosis. Features of the syndrome include hypercalcemia, renal failure, and metabolic alkalosis. The exact pathophysiologic mechanism is unknown. In rare cases, the amount of calcium ingested may be as low as 2000 to 3000 mg/day, but in most patients, the amount is between 6000 and 15,000 mg/day. Treatment consists of rehydration, diuresis, and cessation of calcium and antacid ingestion. If diuresis is impossible because of renal failure, dialysis using a dialysate with a low [Ca] is effective. Renal failure usually resolves in patients with short-term hypercalcemia, but may persist in those with chronic hypercalcemia.

**Treatment** Definitive management of hypercalcemia depends on correction of the primary problem. Thus, patients with hyperparathyroidism secondary to a parathyroid adenoma or hyperplasia are cured by excision of the diseased parathyroid tissue. Hypercalcemic patients taking thiazide drugs should be converted to alternative therapies. Patients with a malignancy and hypercalcemia may respond to surgical excision, radiation therapy, or chemotherapy. Symptomatic patients with malignancy-related severe hypercalcemia can be quickly and effectively treated by saline infusion to expand intravascular volume, followed by the administration of a loop diuretic (i.e., furosemide) to induce saline diuresis, with associated urinary calcium clearance. Patients with severe hypercalcemia frequently have a contracted extracellular volume, so isotonic saline infusion is essential. Hypercalcemic patients in renal failure who cannot benefit from drug-induced diuresis can be treated by hemodialysis.

Severe hypercalcemia related to the release of calcium from bone by tumor can be managed by the administration of bisphosphonates. These drugs have a potent capacity to reduce osteoclast-mediated release of calcium from bone. Several formulations of bisphosphonates are available—in order of preference, zoledronic acid, pamidronate disodium, and etidronate disodium—all of which produce a slow decline in [$iCa^{2+}$] over several days. In patients with metastatic breast cancer, bisphosphonates given as long-term prophylactic agents at a regular dosage have been shown to prevent hypercalcemia effectively.

Administration of exogenous calcitonin is often initially effective in patients with hypercalcemia. Calcitonin, the calcium-lowering hormone produced by parafollicular cells of the thyroid gland, induces renal excretion of calcium and suppresses reabsorption of bone by osteoclasts. However, long-term treatment frequently leads to tachyphylaxis, possibly related to the development of antibodies to the exogenous calcitonin. Chelating agents (e.g., EDTA, phosphate salts) that bind and neutralize $iCa^{2+}$ are rarely indicated. They are associated with the complications of metastatic calcification and acute renal failure and the risk of depressing [$iCa^{2+}$] to hypocalcemic levels.

## Magnesium

Magnesium, an essential cation in the cell, is the second most prevalent anion. It is a critical cofactor in any reaction powered by ATP, so deficiencies can affect metabolism. It also acts as a calcium channel antagonist and plays a key role in the modulation of any activity involving calcium, such as muscle contraction and insulin release. The normal concentration of magnesium [$Mg^{2+}$] in plasma ranges between 1.5 and 2.0 mEq/liter. Like calcium, it exists in three states—protein-bound (30%, bound mostly to albumin), bound to anions (10%), and ionized (60%).

Less than 1% of the total body magnesium content is found in ECF. Measured plasma magnesium levels often do not reflect total body magnesium content. Clinical sequelae of altered magnesium content depend more on tissue magnesium levels than on the blood [$Mg^{2+}$]. Consequently, it is often difficult to consistently correlate symptoms to specific plasma magnesium levels. One method to estimate the tissue magnesium level is a physiologic test that measures the renal response to a magnesium load. Patients who retain more than 30% of an 800-mg load of IV magnesium are thought to be magnesium-depleted, whereas those who retain less than 20% are said to be magnesium-replete.

The kidneys are responsible for maintaining magnesium balance by excreting the absorbed magnesium. The ionized and bound forms of magnesium are freely filtered at the glomerulus. The distal tubule resorbs 10% of the filtered magnesium and plays an important role in calcium-independent magnesium homeostasis. The hormonal regulation of magnesium homeostasis has not been completely determined. PTH, glucagon, and ADH increase the resorption of magnesium in the Henle loop. In the distal convoluted tubule, aldosterone, ADH, and glucagon are thought to increase magnesium resorption. To maintain magnesium homeostasis, renal resorption of magnesium varies widely. Fractional resorption of filtered magnesium can decline to almost zero in the presence of hypermagnesemia or reduced glomerular filtration rate. In contrast, in response to magnesium depletion or decreased intake, the fractional resorption of $Mg^{2+}$ can increase to 99.5% to minimize urinary losses.

### Hypomagnesemia

In ICU patients, the prevalence of hypomagnesemia ranges from 11% to 65%, but it is usually asymptomatic. Some studies have shown little significance of hypomagnesemia; other studies have shown an association with mortality. Any association with mortality is not necessarily causal, obviously, and may merely reflect a patient's state of health. Symptoms from hypomagnesemia have been reported at modest degrees of depletion but, in general, symptoms become more common as the serum [$Mg^{2+}$] falls below 1.2 mg/dL. Associating specific symptoms with hypomagnesemia is difficult.

Hypokalemia is commonly associated with hypomagnesemia and reportedly occurs in 40% of patients with hypomagnesemia. The converse is also true; 60% of patients with hypokalemia are hypomagnesemic. There are a number of causes of hypomagnesemia, including renal, gastrointestinal, and skin losses, as well as hungry bone syndrome. Skin losses can be caused by burns or toxic epidermal necrolysis. Renal losses can be caused by many drugs, but the most common are diuretics.

Hypomagnesemia also causes a specific disorder of renal potassium wasting that is refractory to potassium supplementation until magnesium is adequately repleted. Recently, the mechanism whereby magnesium depletion results in renal potassium loss has been elucidated. Decreased intracellular magnesium slows ATP production. Throughout the body, such slowed ATP production has a negative effect on $Na^+$,$K^+$-ATPase activity. The result is loss of intracellular potassium, which flows down its concentration gradient into the tubule and is lost in the urine.

Hypocalcemia, hyponatremia, and hypophosphatemia are also common in patients with hypomagnesemia. Intracellular hypomagnesemia can develop in patients with chronic diarrhea syndrome or in those who undergo prolonged aggressive diuretic therapy. Magnesium deficiency is also common in patients with heavy alcohol intake. Diabetic patients with persistent osmotic diuresis from glycosuria commonly have hypomagnesemia.

**Treatment** Patients with symptomatic hypomagnesemia should be treated with IV magnesium. The most common formulation is $MgSO_4$; 1 g of magnesium sulfate contains 0.1 g of elemental magnesium. No trials have been done to determine the optimal regimen for magnesium replacement, but consensus statements have suggested 8 to 12 g of magnesium sulfate in the first 24 hours, followed by 4 to 6 g/day for 3 or 4 days to replete body stores. IV magnesium therapy is advocated for some acutely ill patients without documented magnesium depletion. The American College of Cardiology (ACC) and American Heart Association (AHA) recommend 1 to 2 g of magnesium sulfate as an IV bolus over 5 minutes for torsades de pointes therapy. Emerging data have suggested that magnesium may also play a role in reducing reperfusion injury and decreasing infarct size in patients with acute myocardial infarction. Currently, the AHA recommends 2 g of $MgSO_4$ over 15 minutes, followed by 18 g over 24 hours in patients with suspected myocardial infarction who have hypomagnesemia.

Magnesium replacement should be done cautiously in patients with renal insufficiency. Recommendations call for dose reductions of 50% to 75%. During infusions, patients should be monitored closely for decreased deep tendon reflexes. Magnesium levels should be checked at regular intervals. Oral supplementation has been shown to correct increased magnesium retention successfully. Potassium-sparing diuretics may be helpful in patients with chronic renal magnesium wasting. Diuretics that block the sodium channel in the distal convoluted tubule, such as amiloride and triamterene, reduce magnesium wasting in some patients. Severe hypomagnesemia (<1.0 mEq/liter) requires sustained therapy because of the slow equilibration of extracellular magnesium with intracellular stores. Correction of hypomagnesemia can also reduce the risk of cardiac arrhythmia. Frequently, the magnitude of magnesium deficiency parallels the magnitude of hypocalcemia. Hypocalcemia in patients with magnesium deficiency is resistant to calcium replacement alone, so these patients should receive magnesium concurrently.

### Hypermagnesemia

Hypermagnesemia is a common abnormality in patients with renal failure but is otherwise uncommon. Theophylline toxicity, now rare, was formerly associated with hypermagnesemia . Hypermagnesemia can be exacerbated by the ingestion of magnesium-containing drugs, particularly antacids; Epsom salts also contain magnesium, as does magnesium citrate, which is often used in surgical care. High levels of magnesium seem to be tolerated well and, in general, without sequelae. In one report, a patient in diabetic ketoacidosis with hypomagnesemia received 50 g of magnesium sulfate over 6 hours, rather than the intended 2 g. Despite a documented magnesium level of 24 mg/dL and significant short-term morbidity, the patient recovered completely.

IV magnesium overdoses may be better tolerated than oral overdoses. Hypermagnesemia caused by the oral ingestion of magnesium is unusual in the absence of renal insufficiency. A fatal case of hypermagnesemia was documented in a developmentally disabled child who was given magnesium to relieve constipation. Despite calcium infusions and dialysis, the child died. The chronic ingestion of magnesium likely made the child's condition refractory to treatment, perhaps because of a greater total body magnesium burden from chronic overload. Hypermagnesemia has also been repeatedly reported after the use of magnesium-containing enemas.

Magnesium can block synaptic transmission of nerve impulses. It also causes the initial loss of deep tendon reflexes and may lead to flaccid paralysis and apnea. Neuromuscular toxicity also affects smooth muscle, resulting in ileus and urinary retention. In cases of oral intoxication, the development of ileus can slow intestinal transit times, further increasing absorption of magnesium. Hypermagnesemia has also been reported to cause a parasympathetic blockade resulting in fixed and dilated pupils, mimicking brainstem herniation. Other neurologic signs include lethargy, confusion, and coma.

Magnesium blocks the shift of calcium into myocardial cells and can act as a calcium channel blocker. In cardiac tissue, it also blocks potassium channels needed for repolarization. Patients with severe hypermagnesemia can show evidence of heart failure. Other cardiac manifestations of hypermagnesemia, at least initially, include bradycardia and hypotension. Higher magnesium levels cause a prolonged PR interval, increased QRS duration, and a prolonged QT interval. Extreme cases can result in complete heart block or cardiac arrest.

Metabolic disturbances caused by hypermagnesemia have been recognized less than those caused by hypomagnesemia. Hypocalcemia can occur, although it is typically mild and asymptomatic. Symptomatic hypermagnesemia, despite normal renal function, has been reported with magnesium infusions, typically during treatment of patients who are in preterm labor or who have preeclampsia or eclampsia. Routine magnesium measurements are often not performed, although the infusion protocols (a load of 4 to 6 g, followed by 1 to 2 g/hr) result in serum magnesium levels of 4 to 8 mg/dL. Obstetric patients who experience accidental overdoses of magnesium usually have good outcomes, despite magnesium levels as high as 19 mg/dL.

**Treatment** In patients with hypermagnesemia and intact renal function, stopping the infusion or supply of magnesium will allow them to recover. Calcium salts can reverse hypotension and respiratory depression. Patients are typically given 100 to 200 mg of IV elemental calcium over 5 to 10 minutes. To speed the renal clearance of magnesium, loop diuretics and saline diuresis are intuitive options, but no literature explicitly supports its use.

In critically ill patients, disorders of magnesium homeostasis can have dramatic effects on physiology. However, such disorders often go unrecognized. In ICU patients, hypomagnesemia is common and associated with poor outcomes, so measurement of the serum magnesium level should be routine. Unlike magnesium depletion, hypermagnesemia is a rare but frequently iatrogenic and fatal problem.

In patients with renal insufficiency, dialysis rapidly corrects hypermagnesemia and is the only way to lower magnesium levels acutely. Aggressive use of dialysis may improve survival. In patients with severe renal dysfunction, dialysis offers a modality to clear magnesium rapidly. Both peritoneal dialysis and hemodialysis are effective for lowering magnesium levels. Intermittent hemodialysis corrects hypermagnesemia more rapidly than peritoneal dialysis or continuous renal replacement therapy.

## SELECTED REFERENCES

Awad S, Allison SP, Lobo DN: The history of 0.9% saline. Clin Nutr 27:179–188, 2008.

Summary of how saline was developed, noting that the science behind its development is lacking.

Bickell WH, Wall MJ, Jr, Pepe PE, et al: Immediate versus delayed fluid resuscitation for hypotensive patients with penetrating torso injuries. N Engl J Med 331:1105–1109, 1994.

Classic study, probably the most referenced paper in trauma, showing that despite being hypotensive in the field after penetrating torso injury, treating these patients with crystalloid solutions resulted in worse outcome and not infusing fluids improved outcome.

Cohn SM, Nathens AB, Moore FA, et al: Tissue oxygen saturation predicts the development of organ dysfunction during traumatic shock resuscitation. J Trauma 62:44–54, 2007.

Multicenter prospective study using seven busy level I trauma centers to determine usefulness of measuring tissue oxygenation. It showed that this noninvasive tool, which attaches to the thenar muscle, correlates well with base excess and can predict poor outcome. However, the study selected out the most severely injured patients with bleeding requiring transfusions and the ability to predict that these patients will do poorly was obvious. It also showed that the number of patients who developed multiple organ failure was small.

Committee on Fluid Resuscitation for Combat Casualties: Fluid resuscitation: State of the science for treating combat casualties and civilian injuries. Report of the Institute of Medicine, Washington, DC, 1999, National Academy Press.

Considered a white paper by the Institute of Medicine, it was considered radical in that it did not recommend lactated Ringer's as the fluid of choice for civilians and the military. It recommended hypertonic saline and additional research to eliminate d-isomer lactate from lactated Ringer's and to investigate other metabolites, such as ketones, as an alternative.

Finfer S, Bellomo R, Boyce N, et al: A comparison of albumin and saline for fluid resuscitation in the intensive care unit. N Engl J Med 350:2247–2256, 2004.

Prospective multicenter study designed to show that albumin is safe in the intensive care unit. However, it used 4% albumin and showed that the outcome was no different.

Fluid resuscitation of combat casualties. Conference proceedings. June 2001 and October 2001. J Trauma 54(Suppl):S1–S234, 2003.

This entire supplement summarizes the rationale for the changes recommended for the treatment of combat casualties.

Holcomb JB, Jenkins D, Rhee P, et al: Damage control resuscitation: Directly addressing the early coagulopathy of trauma. J Trauma 62:307–310, 2007.

This paper describes the evolution of damage control resuscitation and rationale behind the recommendation of permissive hypotension, reduction of crystalloid use, use of hypertonic saline, and aggressive use of blood products early and often for best results.

Moore EE, Moore FA, Fabian TC, et al: PolyHeme Study Group: Human polymerized hemoglobin for the treatment of hemorrhagic shock when blood is unavailable: The USA multicenter trial. J Am Coll Surg 208:1–13, 2009.

Study showing that artificial hemoglobin made from expired human blood could be used safely and as a replacement of blood in the field and in the hospital.

Plurad D, Martin M, Green D, et al: The decreasing incidence of late post-traumatic acute respiratory distress syndrome: The potential role of lung protective ventilation and conservative transfusion practice. J Trauma 63:1–7, 2007.

This paper shows that decreasing incidence of ARDS in trauma and its association with decreased crystalloid use.

Spinella PC, Perkins JG, Grathwohl KW, et al: Warm fresh whole blood is independently associated with improved survival for patients with combat-related traumatic injuries. J Trauma 66:S69–S76, 2009.

Describes the usefulness of whole blood transfusion practice found by the military.

Velmahos GC, Demetriades D, Shoemaker WC, et al: End points of resuscitation of critically injured patients: normal or supranormal? A prospective randomized trial. Ann Surg 232:409–418, 2000.

Excellent study showing in a prospective manner that increasing oxygen delivery through increasing content and cardiac output did not improve survival in trauma patients in the intensive care unit.

## REFERENCES

1. Hughes JT: Miraculous deliverance of Anne Green: An Oxford case of resuscitation in the seventeenth century. Br Med J (Clin Res Ed) 285:1792–1793, 1982.
2. O'Shaughnassy WB: Experiments on the blood in cholera. Lancet 32:490–495, 1831.
3. Crile GW: An experimental research into surgical shock, Philadelphia, 1899, JB Lippincott.
4. Cannon WB: The emergency function of the adrenal medulla in pain and the major emotions. Am J Physiol 33:356–372, 1914.
5. Blalock A: Experimental shock: The cause of low blood pressure caused by muscle injury. Arch Surg 20:959–996, 1930.
6. Wiggers CJ: The present status of shock problem. Physiol Rev 22:74–123, 1942.
7. Awad S, Allison SP, Lobo DN: The history of 0.9% saline. Clin Nutr 27:179–188, 2008.
8. O'Shaughnessy WB: Proposal of a new method of treating the blue epidemic cholera by the injection of highly-oxygenated salts into the venous system. Lancet 17:366–371, 1831.
9. Ringer S: Concerning the Influence exerted by each of the constituents of the blood on the contraction of the ventricle. J Physiol 3:380–393, 1882.
10. Brasel KJ, Guse C, Gentilello LM, et al: Heart rate: Is it truly a vital sign? J Trauma 62:812–817, 2007.
11. Ley EJ, Salim A, Kohanzadeh S, et al: Relative bradycardia in hypotensive trauma patients: A reappraisal. J Trauma 67:1051–1054, 2009.
12. Bruns B, Lindsey M, Rowe K, et al: Hemoglobin drops within minutes of injuries and predicts need for an intervention to stop hemorrhage. J Trauma 63:312–315, 2007.
13. Riordan WP, Jr, Norris PR, Jenkins JM, et al: Early loss of heart rate complexity predicts mortality regardless of mechanism, anatomic location, or severity of injury in 2178 trauma patients. J Surg Res 156:283–289, 2009.
14. Eastridge BJ, Salinas J, McManus JG, et al: Hypotension begins at 110 mm Hg: Redefining "hypotension" with data. J Trauma 63:291–297, 2007.
15. Bruns B, Gentillelo L, Elliot A, et al: Prehospital hypotension redefined. J Trauma 65(6):1217–1221, 2008.
16. Martin JT, Alkhoury F, O'Connor JA, et al: Normal vital signs belie occult hypoperfusion in geriatric trauma patients. Am Surg 76:65–69, 2010.
17. Grocott MP, Martin DS, Levett DZ, et al: Arterial blood gases and oxygen content in climbers on Mount Everest. N Engl J Med 360:140–149, 2009.
18. Cureton EL, Kwan RO, Dozier KC, et al: A different view of lactate in trauma patients: Protecting the injured brain. J Surg Res 159:468–473, 2010.
19. Reynolds PS, Barbee RW, Ward KR: Lactate profiles as a resuscitation assessment tool in a rat model of battlefield hemorrhage resuscitation. Shock 30:48–54, 2008.
20. Bilello JF, Davis JW, Lemaster D, et al: Prehospital hypotension in blunt trauma: Identifying the "crump factor." J Trauma 2009.
21. Sperry JL, Frankel HL, Nathens AB, et al: Characterization of persistent hyperglycemia: What does it mean postinjury? J Trauma 66:1076–1082, 2009.
22. Inaba K, Teixeira PG, Rhee P, et al: Mortality impact of hypothermia after cavitary explorations in trauma. World J Surg 33:864–869, 2009.
23. Beilman GJ, Blondet JJ, Nelson TR, et al: Early hypothermia in severely injured trauma patients is a significant risk factor for multiple organ dysfunction syndrome but not mortality. Ann Surg 249:845–850, 2009.
24. Boffard KD, Riou B, Warren B, et al: Recombinant factor VIIa as adjunctive therapy for bleeding control in severely injured trauma patients: Two parallel randomized, placebo-controlled, double-blind clinical trials. J Trauma 59:8–15, 2005.
25. Mayer SA, Brun NC, Begtrup K, et al: Recombinant activated factor VII for acute intracerebral hemorrhage. N Engl J Med 352:777–785, 2005.
26. Velmahos GC, Demetriades D, Shoemaker WC, et al: Endpoints of resuscitation of critically injured patients: normal or supranormal? A prospective randomized trial. Ann Surg 232:409–418, 2000.
27. Madigan MC, Kemp CD, Johnson JC, et al: Secondary abdominal compartment syndrome after severe extremity injury: Are early, aggressive fluid resuscitation strategies to blame? J Trauma 64:280–285, 2008.
28. Noakes TD: How did A V Hill understand the VO2max and the "plateau phenomenon?" Still no clarity? Br J Sports Med 42:574–580, 2008.
29. Palizas F, Dubin A, Regueira T, et al: Gastric tonometry versus cardiac index as resuscitation goals in septic shock: A multicenter, randomized, controlled trial. Crit Care 13:R44, 2009.
30. Cohn SM, Nathens AB, Moore FA, et al: Tissue oxygen saturation predicts the development of organ dysfunction during traumatic shock resuscitation. J Trauma 62:44–54, 2007.
31. Dellinger RP, Levy MM, Carlet JM, et al: Surviving Sepsis Campaign: International guidelines for management of severe sepsis and septic shock: 2008. Crit Care Med 36:296–327, 2008.
32. Bickell WH, Wall MJ, Jr, Pepe PE, et al: Immediate versus delayed fluid resuscitation for hypotensive patients with penetrating torso injuries. N Engl J Med 331:1105–1109, 1994.
33. Eiseman B, Beart R, Norton L: Multiple organ failure. Surg Gynecol Obstet 144:323–326, 1977.
34. Demetriades D, Kimbrell B, Salim A, et al: Trauma deaths in a mature urban trauma system: is "trimodal" distribution a valid concept? J Am Coll Surg 201:343–348, 2005.
35. Englehart MS, Cho SD, Morris MS, et al: Use of leukoreduced blood does not reduce infection, organ failure, or mortality following trauma. World J Surg 33:1626–1632, 2009.

36. Rhee P, Morris J, Durham R, et al: Recombinant humanized monoclonal antibody against CD18 (rhuMAb CD18) in traumatic hemorrhagic shock: Results of a phase II clinical trial. Traumatic Shock Group. J Trauma 49:611–619, 2000.
37. Todd SR, Kao LS, Catania A, et al: Alpha-melanocyte stimulating hormone in critically injured trauma patients. J Trauma 66:465–469, 2009.
38. Committee on Fluid Resuscitation for Combat Casualties: Fluid resuscitation: State of the science for treating combat casualties and civilian injuries. Report of the Institute of Medicine, Washington, DC, 1999, National Academy Press.
39. Gao J, Zhao WX, Xue FS, et al: Effects of different resuscitation fluids on acute lung injury in a rat model of uncontrolled hemorrhagic shock and infection. J Trauma 67:1213–1219, 2009.
40. Fluid resuscitation of combat casualties. Conference proceedings. June 2001 and October 2001. J Trauma 54(Suppl):S1–S234, 2003.
41. Holcomb JB, Jenkins D, Rhee P, et al: Damage control resuscitation: Directly addressing the early coagulopathy of trauma. J Trauma 62:307–310, 2007.
42. Teixeira PG, Oncel D, Demetriades D, et al: Blood transfusions in trauma: Six-year analysis of the transfusion practices at a Level I trauma center. Am Surg 74:953–957, 2008.
43. Plurad D, Martin M, Green D, et al: The decreasing incidence of late post-traumatic acute respiratory distress syndrome: The potential role of lung protective ventilation and conservative transfusion practice. J Trauma 63:1–7, 2007.
44. Spinella PC, Perkins JG, Grathwohl KW, et al: Warm fresh whole blood is independently associated with improved survival for patients with combat-related traumatic injuries. J Trauma 66:S69–S76, 2009.
45. Perkins JG, Cap AP, Spinella PC, et al: An evaluation of the impact of apheresis platelets used in the setting of massively transfused trauma patients. J Trauma 66:S77–S84, 2009.
46. Stinger HK, Spinella PC, Perkins JG, et al: The ratio of fibrinogen to red cells transfused affects survival in casualties receiving massive transfusions at an army combat support hospital. J Trauma 64:S79–S85, 2008.
47. Zink KA, Sambasivan CN, Holcomb JB, et al: A high ratio of plasma and platelets to packed red blood cells in the first 6 hours of massive transfusion improves outcomes in a large multicenter study. Am J Surg 197:565–570, 2009.
48. Dente CJ, Shaz BH, Nicholas JM, et al: Improvements in early mortality and coagulopathy are sustained better in patients with blunt trauma after institution of a massive transfusion protocol in a civilian level I trauma center. J Trauma 66:1616–1624, 2009.
49. Inaba K, Branco BC, Rhee P, et al: Impact of ABO-identical vs ABO-compatible nonidentical plasma transfusion in trauma patients. Arch Surg 145:899–906, 2010.
50. DuBose JJ, Kobayashi L, Lozornio A, et al: Clinical experience using 5% hypertonic saline as a safe alternative fluid for use in trauma. J Trauma 68:1172–1177, 2010.
51. Finfer S, Bellomo R, Boyce N, et al: A comparison of albumin and saline for fluid resuscitation in the intensive care unit. N Engl J Med 350:2247–2256, 2004.
52. Martin M, Salim A, Murray J, et al: The decreasing incidence and mortality of acute respiratory distress syndrome after injury: A 5-year observational study. J Trauma 59:1107–1113, 2005.
53. Moore EE, Moore FA, Fabian TC, et al: Human polymerized hemoglobin for the treatment of hemorrhagic shock when blood is unavailable: the USA multicenter trial. J Am Coll Surg 208:1–13, 2009.
54. Cruz, Jr, RJ, Harada T, Sasatomi E, et al: Effects of ethyl pyruvate and other α-keto carboxylic acid derivatives in a rat model of multivisceral ischemia and reperfusion. J Surg Res 165:151–157, 2011.
55. Lin T, Chen H, Koustova E, et al: Histone deacetylase as therapeutic target in a rodent model of hemorrhagic shock: Effect of different resuscitation strategies on lung and liver. Surgery 141:784–794, 2007.
56. Alam HB, Bice LM, Butt MU, et al: Testing of blood products in a polytrauma model: Results of a multi-institutional randomized preclinical trial. J Trauma 67:856–864, 2009.
57. Alam HB, Shuja F, Butt MU, et al: Surviving blood loss without blood transfusion in a swine poly-trauma model. Surgery 146:325–333, 2009.
58. Alam HB, Casas F, Chen Z, et al: Development and testing of portable pump for the induction of profound hypothermia in a swine model of lethal vascular injuries. J Trauma 61:1321–1329, 2006.

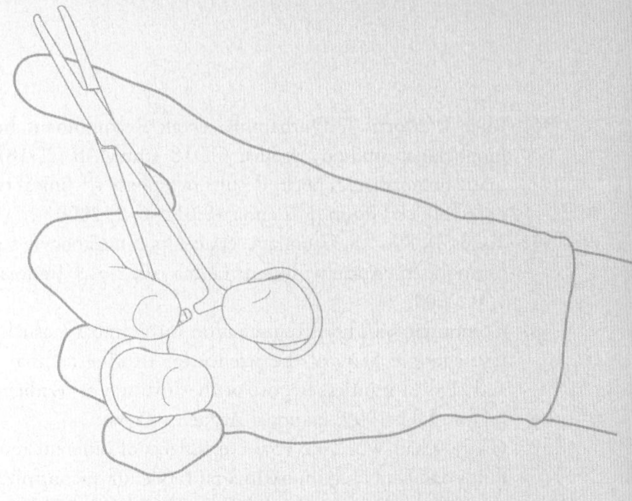

CHAPTER 6

# METABOLISM IN SURGICAL PATIENTS

Ahmed Al-Mousawi, Noe A. Rodriguez, and David N. Herndon



Metabolism involves a diverse range of chemical processes required to sustain life and enable growth, healing, development, reproduction, homeostasis, and adaptation and response to the environment. Through highly efficient metabolic pathways, nutrients are absorbed, transformed, and broken down to release energy. The nutritional status of an individual depends on an adequate diet, function of the alimentary tract, and physiologic condition. In surgical and critically ill patients, metabolic and nutritional processes may be impaired as a consequence of environmental, pathologic, or traumatic factors, leading to a need for nutritional supplementation to enable healing and recovery. Development and implementation of nutritional support represents one of the main advances of the last century that has led to improved patient care and surgical outcomes.

Over recent decades, major progress has occurred in our understanding of the physiologic response to injury, increasing focus on improved nutrition in surgical care. Catabolism of skeletal muscle protein has been recognized as a major factor contributing to adverse outcomes following major surgery and trauma. In 1905, Sneve[1] described the catabolic response as metabolic exhaustion and emaciation seen in burn patients. Cuthbertson[2] studied the effects of long bone fractures in animal models, characterizing physiologic and metabolic responses into two phases: the early ebb phase and the flow phase. The former occurs the first several hours after injury, typically lasts 2 to 3 days, and is distinguished by reduced oxygen consumption ($Vo_2$), glucose tolerance, cardiac output, and basal metabolic rate. The latter typically starts several days after injury, lasts days to weeks, and features catabolic breakdown of skeletal muscle, negative nitrogen balance, hyperglycemia, and increased cardiac output, $Vo_2$, and respiratory rate.

In 1953 Cope and colleagues[3] correlated muscle wasting following thermal injury with a measured rise in metabolic rate. Moore's book, in 1959,[4] proposed the use of continuous feeding to attenuate proteolysis and muscle catabolism observed following trauma. Establishing the feasibility of long-term parenteral nutrition (PN) in the late 1960s, Dudrick[5] recognized that malnourished surgical patients with a preexisting protein deficit were at increased risk of complications.

It was then shown that the hypermetabolic response seen in patients with major burns resulted in part from an increase in catecholamine serum levels and that the metabolic response could be attenuated by ambient temperature and pharmacologic means. Further studies showed that severe trauma and burns lead to a hypercatabolic response, with deleterious effects on various organs, and that the inflammatory response contributes to hypermetabolism and subsequent catabolism seen following severe injury (Fig. 6-1).[6] Modulation of this hypermetabolic response through pharmacologic and nutritional interventions, alteration of the environment, and improved surgical management are cornerstones of advancing surgical care.

Although widely quoted, the classic description of the ebb and flow response may not be apt for critically ill patients in a modern intensive care setting. A refined description has been proposed for these patients, who may suffer further insults from multiple operations or repeated bouts of sepsis (Fig. 6-2). The classic description may also oversimplify the array of responses that occur; these remain incompletely understood, particularly in the prolonged flow phase, which includes a short-term acute response and prolonged adaptive response.

The metabolic response to injury aims to restore homeostasis. It is characterized by changes in the flow of substrates among organs, increasing glucose and amino acid supply to the wound or site of injury to facilitate repair and healing. Neuroendocrine and inflammatory mediators of the stress response induce changes such as muscle proteolysis, leading to the release of amino acids, primarily alanine and glutamine. These are needed for protein synthesis at the site of injury and are also converted to glucose by hepatic gluconeogenesis. Glutamine serves as a fuel supply to the gut and is converted to alanine and ammonia, which are used by the liver or converted to urea. Hypermetabolism results in critically ill patients when the metabolic response is severe and prolonged, together with a hyperdynamic circulation, muscle catabolism, increased nitrogen loss, and glucose intolerance.

## NUTRITIONAL REQUIREMENTS

The primary goal of nutritional support is to provide an adequate energy supply and all the nutrients necessary to support life and function. Nutrients in the diet require ingestion, digestion, absorption, and regulation before the substrates released are used, stored, or expended for energy. The major components

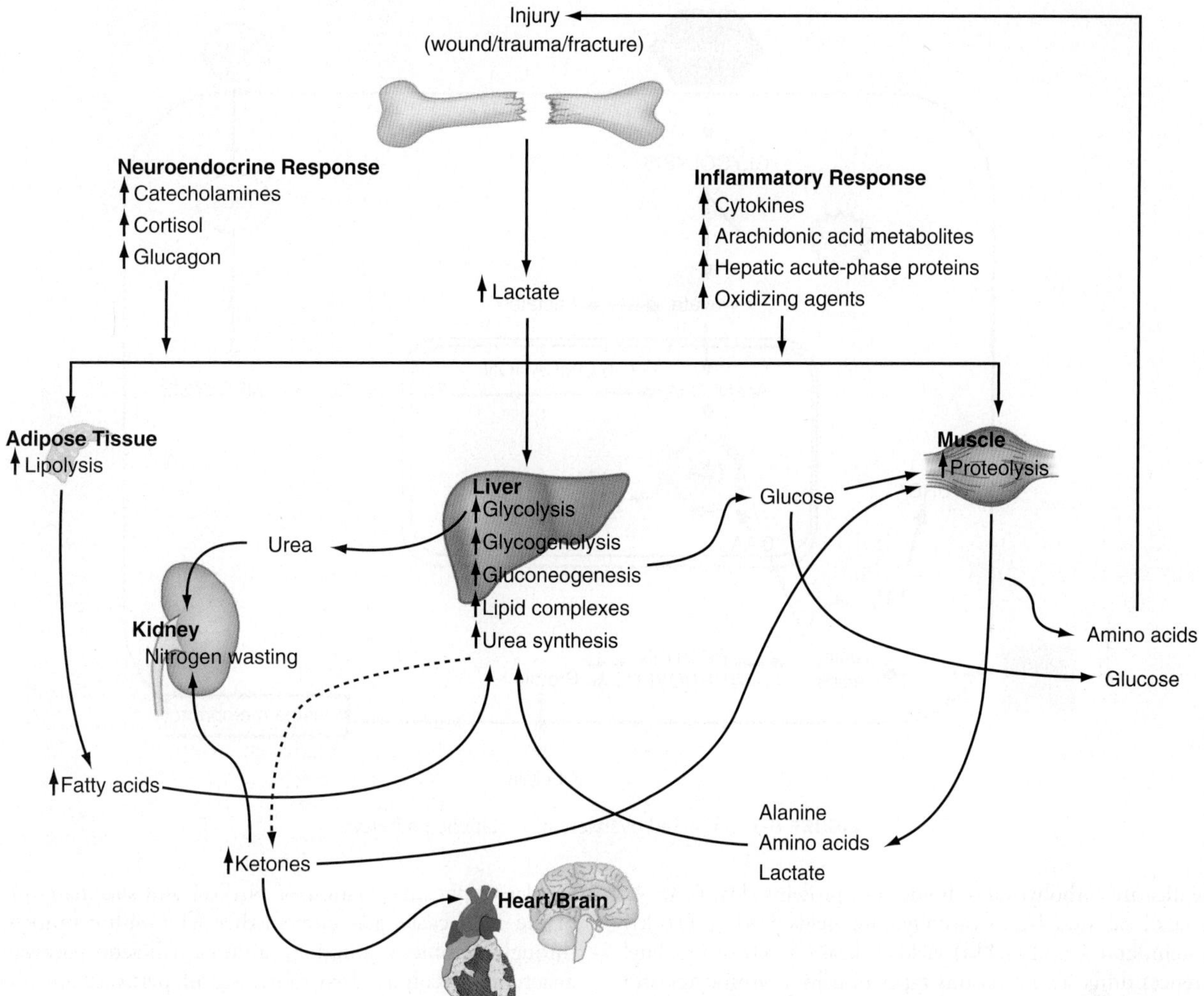

Injury
(wound/trauma/fracture)
Neuroendocrine Response
↑Catecholamines
↑Cortisol
↑Glucagon
Inflammatory Response
↑Cytokines
↑Arachidonic acid metabolites
↑Hepatic acute-phase proteins
↑Oxidizing agents
↑Lactate
Adipose Tissue
↑Lipolysis
Muscle
↑Proteolysis
Liver
↑Glycolysis
↑Glycogenolysis
↑Gluconeogenesis
↑Lipid complexes
↑Urea synthesis
Glucose
Urea
Kidney
Nitrogen wasting
Amino acids
Glucose
↑Fatty acids
Alanine
Amino acids
Lactate
↑Ketones
Heart/Brain

**FIGURE 6-1** Metabolic response to injury and trauma.

Increased metabolic rate
Decreased metabolic rate
Recovery phase
Initial injury
A
Time
Chronic phase
Initial injury
B
Time

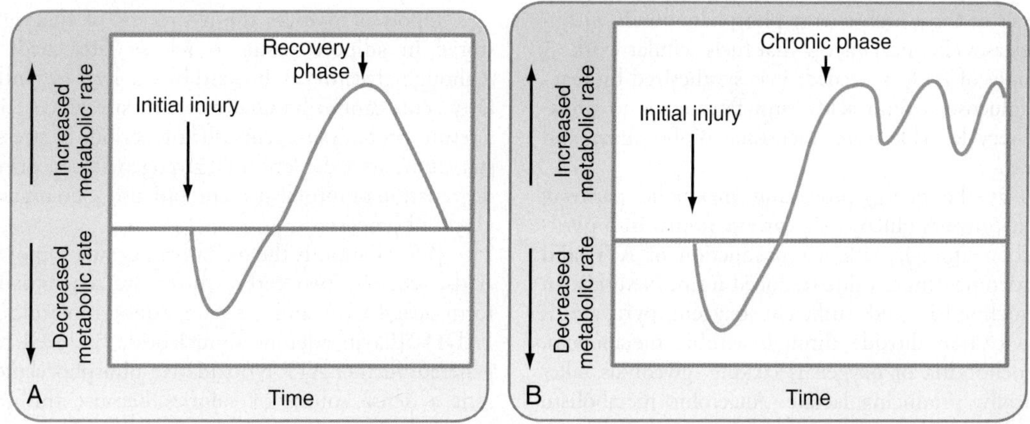

**FIGURE 6-2** **A,** Classic ebb and flow phases of the acute stress response. The metabolic rate initially falls below normal and then increases to supranormal levels before returning to normal. **B,** Ebb and flow revisited. In the population of chronically ill patients in critical care, the classic ebb and flow pattern is altered. Recurrent bouts of sepsis and other proinflammatory stimuli result in a fluctuating metabolic demand, which remains chronically elevated. (Adapted from Ball S, Baudouin SV: Endocrine disorders in the critically ill: The endocrine response to critical illness. In Hall GM, Hunter JM, Cooper MS [eds]: Core topics in endocrinology in anaesthesia and critical care, Cambridge, England, 2010, Cambridge University Press, pp 126–131.)

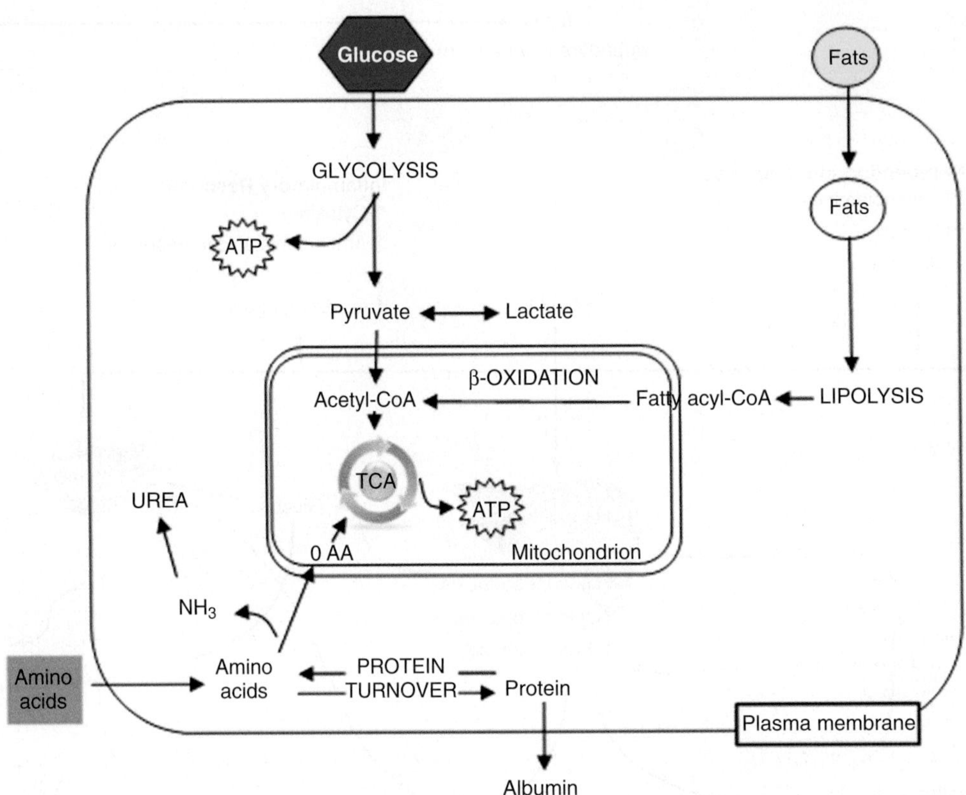


**FIGURE 6-3** Simplified overview of metabolic pathways.

of the diet are carbohydrates, lipids, and proteins (Fig. 6-3). As a source of calories, 1 g of carbohydrate yields 3.4 kcal (16 kJ) of protein, and 4 kcal (17 kJ) yields 9 kcal (37 kJ) of fat. Fuel preferences differ across various types of cells; erythrocytes and neurons use glucose preferentially, muscle and cardiac myocytes can also use fat, and enterocytes and lymphocytes can metabolize the amino acid glutamine. Adaptation to different fuels can occur under circumstances of starvation.

At the cellular level, adenosine triphosphate (ATP) is the main source of energy that drives reactions and metabolic processes. Hydrolysis of three high-energy phosphate bonds within the molecule releases chemical energy that fuels cellular work. A continuous supply of ATP is needed; it is synthesized by reactions that use glucose, amino acids, and fatty acids to phosphorylate and recycle ATP from adenosine diphosphate and monophosphate.

Glycolysis is the energy-producing metabolic pathway within cells that converts glucose (six carbon atoms) into pyruvate (three carbon atoms), with net production of ATP and nicotinamide adenine dinucleotide (reduced form, NADH). In cells with mitochondria and sufficient oxygen, pyruvate is metabolized to carbon dioxide through aerobic metabolism, whereas if mitochondria or oxygen is lacking, glycolysis takes place anaerobically, producing lactate. Anaerobic metabolism occurs in cells during states of hypoperfusion, in muscle cells during bursts of increased activity, and in cells without mitochondria such as red blood cells, in which anaerobic glycolysis is the only energy-producing pathway.

Phosphorylation of ATP occurs in the cell cytoplasm during glycolysis (anaerobic, substrate level phosphorylation) and in mitochondria in the tricarboxylic acid (TCA) cycle. Oxidative phosphorylation of NADH and succinate, products of the TCA cycle, generates further ATP within mitochondria through aerobic respiration, a more efficient pathway than anaerobic glycolysis. Two molecules of pyruvate are produced from each molecule of glucose that enters glycolysis, yielding two ATP molecules. In comparison, a single molecule of glucose yields approximately 32 molecules of ATP through glycolysis, subsequent oxidation of pyruvate to acetyl coenzyme A (acetyl-CoA), and progress into the TCA cycle, which ends with oxidative phosphorylation of the products.

Lipolysis involves the hydrolysis of triacylglycerol (TAG) stored in adipose tissue to release fatty acids and glycerol. Although glycerol can be used by the liver to synthesize glucose, fatty acids cannot be used to synthesize glucose in humans. As a result, proteolysis occurs during periods of stress or prolonged starvation after depletion of glycogen stores, primarily through degradation of muscle protein, but also solid organs, to maintain glucose homeostasis.

β-Oxidation is the oxidative degradation of saturated fatty acids, whereby two carbon units are sequentially removed to form acetyl-CoA and electron donor molecules (NADH and $FADH_2$ [flavin adenine dinucleotide, reduced form]) used to generate further ATP by oxidative phosphorylation. Fats represent a dense source of calories because this process has an extremely high energy yield, with 129 molecules of ATP being formed from one molecule of the typical fatty acid palmitate.

## Carbohydrate Metabolism

Carbohydrates are a primary source of calories and are divided into four groups: simple carbohydrates, which include monosaccharides (one sugar unit) and disaccharides (two sugar units);

and complex carbohydrates, which include oligosaccharides (three to ten sugar units) and polysaccharides (>ten sugar units).

Carbohydrate digestion begins in the mouth with the action of salivary amylase, which hydrolyzes polysaccharide bonds in the amylose and amylopectin molecules that constitute starch. Breakdown continues in the gut by the action of pancreatic amylase and of the enzymes sucrase, lactase, maltase, and isomaltase from intestinal epithelial cells to yield monosaccharides. Bacteria in normal gut flora enable the breakdown of certain polysaccharides and starches, which humans lack the enzymes to digest, and help prevent the invasion of pathogenic strains in the intestine.

The products of intestinal digestion yield the monosaccharides glucose, fructose, and galactose. These sugars are rapidly absorbed and transported to the liver. Approximately 90% of portal venous glucose is removed from the blood by hepatocytes through carrier-facilitated diffusion. Carrier molecules on the sinusoidal domain of hepatocytes are capable of binding and transferring the sugars into the cytoplasm.

Glycogen is the stored form of carbohydrate in the liver and skeletal muscle. The liver plays a key role in processes that synthesize and degrade glycogen (glycogenesis and glycogenolysis), and in the endogenous synthesis of glucose (gluconeogenesis). Glycogen can be stored in the liver, in up to 65 g/kg of tissue, and is stored in muscle for its exclusive use. Hepatic synthesis of glycogen begins with a core composed of a high-density protein (glycogenin) and the action of a rate-determining enzyme, glycogen synthase. This enzyme is activated by insulin and glucose, both of which are elevated in the postprandial state, leading to elongation of the glycogen chain by the addition of glucose units. Conversely, glycogen synthase is inhibited by glucagon and epinephrine. During fasting, glycogenolysis leads to the release of glucose, with the rate-limiting enzyme glycogen phosphorylase activated by glucagon and epinephrine and inhibited by insulin. Glycogen stores are exhausted within 48 hours of fasting, and body protein stores must be mobilized to maintain adequate glucose supply to the brain.

In addition to glycogenolysis, glucose levels are maintained through the conversion of noncarbohydrate substrates by gluconeogenesis, which occurs primarily in the liver and, to a lesser extent, in the renal cortex. Substrates for this pathway include all amino acids except lysine and leucine, derived from the proteolysis of skeletal muscle, glycerol derived from the degradation of triglycerides (TGs) in adipose tissue, and lactate produced from anaerobic glycolysis (see Fig. 6-1). The enzyme-catalyzed reactions of the gluconeogenic pathway include the reversal of several steps of glycolysis and four irreversible reactions.

## Lipid Metabolism

Lipids are hydrophobic molecules that include fatty acids, phospholipids, glycerolipids, sphingolipids, eicosanoids, and vitamins. They play key roles in cell structure and function, including energy storage and expenditure, formation of biologic membranes, and cell signaling. If lipids are not immediately used by cells, they can be stored in the form of TGs, the most potent caloric stores in the body, because 1 g of fat delivers 9 kcal (37.7 kJ).

Dietary TGs are unable to pass through the intestinal epithelial cells and must first be emulsified and hydrolyzed to monoacylglycerols or free fatty acids. This process is mediated by a mixture of lipases, biliary, pancreatic, and intestinal secretions from glands positioned along the gastrointestinal (GI) tract (tongue, stomach, pancreas, glycocalyx of intestinal wall). The stomach plays two important roles; it secretes gastric lipase, responsible for the digestion and absorption of up to 20% of total TGs, and it initiates the process of emulsification. Fat then enters the upper duodenum, 80% in the form of TGs and the rest in the form of partially hydrolyzed compounds. Emulsified TGs stimulate the contraction of the gallbladder and the release of bile and pancreatic fluid containing lipase, colipase, phospholipase A2, and cholesteryl esterase. Bile acids and colipase enable pancreatic lipase to act on TGs to produce diacylglycerols (DAGs), monoacylglycerols (MAGs), and free fatty acids.

Lipolysis occurs within the cytosolic lipid droplets of adipocytes, in which a series of lipases initiate the breakdown of TAG into free fatty acids and glycerol. Hormone-sensitive lipase (HSL) was until recently thought to be the only enzyme to hydrolyze TGs in adipose tissue. A second enzyme, adipose triglyceride lipase (ATGL), is now believed to catalyze the first step in the hydrolysis of TGs (Fig. 6-4).[7]

In the postabsorptive state, adipose tissue releases free fatty acids and glycerol to the circulation for use as energy. Hepatic β-oxidation of fatty acids produces ketone bodies, acetoacetate, and 3-hydroxybutyrate, which can be used directly as fuel sources by cardiac muscle, skeletal muscle, and the renal cortex as well as cerebral tissue after a week of fasting. This switch of the central nervous system (CNS) during starvation, away from the primary use of carbohydrates to the use of ketone bodies as a fuel, represents a critically important adaptive step that has a secondary sparing effect on body protein.

Desnutrin-ATGL initiates lipolysis by hydrolyzing TAG to diacylglycerol. HSL hydrolyzes DAG to MAG, which is subsequently hydrolyzed by MAG lipase (MGL) to generate glycerol and three fatty acids. Fatty acids generated during lipolysis can be released into the circulation for use by other organs or oxidized within adipocytes. During fasting, catecholamines, by binding to Gαs-coupled β-adrenergic receptors (β-ARs), activate adenylate cyclase (AC) to increase cyclic adenosine monophosphate (cAMP) and activate protein kinase A (PKA). PKA phosphorylates HSL, resulting in the translocation of HSL from the cytosol to the lipid droplet. PKA also phosphorylates the lipid droplet–associated protein perilipin. Also, during fasting, glucocorticoids increase the expression of desnutrin-ATGL.

## Protein Metabolism

Proteins are essential to the structure and function of every cell and participate in cell adhesion, signaling, and immunogenicity. The digestion of protein into peptides begins in the stomach through acid denaturation and the enzymatic action of pepsin. Digestion of peptides into tripeptides, dipeptides, and amino acids takes place at the level of the duodenum through proteases secreted from the pancreas and peptidases associated with the glycocalyx of the intestinal wall. Dipeptides, oligopeptides, and single amino acids are absorbed in the small intestine.

Human protein synthesis requires 20 amino acids; eight are termed *essential amino acids* because they cannot be synthesized de novo from other amino acids (10 if arginine and histidine are included as essential in infants) and must therefore be obtained in the diet. Six amino acids are termed *conditionally essential amino acids* because during childhood, illness, and other conditions, they may not be synthesized at rates that meet

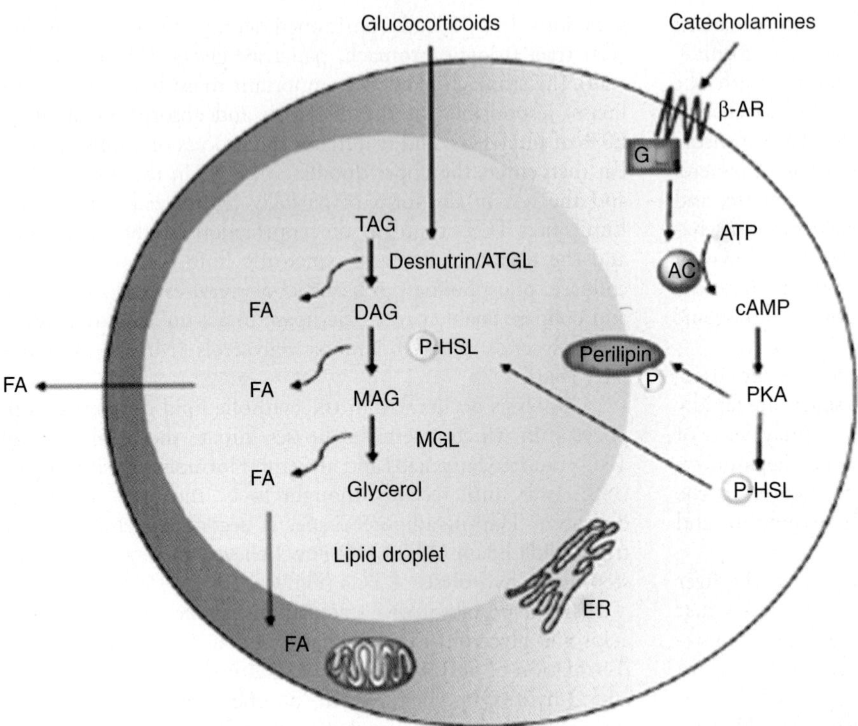


**FIGURE 6-4** Regulation of lipolysis within adipocytes. (Adapted from Ahmadian M, Wang Y, Sul HS: Lipolysis in adipocytes. Int J Biochem Cell Biol 42:555–559, 2010.)

requirements and may therefore need to be supplemented. The remaining six are termed *nonessential amino acids* because they can be synthesized internally (Table 6-1).

Various tissues, including liver, muscle, kidney, lung, and adipose tissue, share regulatory roles in amino acid metabolism, although the catabolism of most essential amino acids takes place in the liver. However, the three branched-chain amino acids (BCAAs)—leucine, isoleucine, and valine—are an exception, because these are poorly metabolized during first-pass metabolism in the liver and are degraded by skeletal muscle. The breakdown of BCAAs in muscle generates alanine and glutamine.

Alanine is released from skeletal muscle, in addition to lactate, during the anaerobic glycolysis of glucose, which releases ATP. In the Cori cycle, the liver converts lactate produced by muscle back to glucose for muscle fuel in an ATP-dependent manner. Similarly, alanine can be used by the liver and is a preferred precursor for hepatic gluconeogenesis as part of the glucose-alanine cycle (see Fig. 6-1). Alanine is provided by either muscle during protein turnover or amino acids in the diet.

Metabolism of nitrogen-containing compounds in the body, including amino acids, produces ammonia, which is converted to urea, a less toxic substance, by a series of reactions that comprise the urea cycle. The urea cycle generates urea from ammonia produced from amino acid oxidation, in which certain amino acids enter the urea cycle directly as intermediates, including arginine. Increased catabolism of protein and the release of amino acids for gluconeogenesis lead to excess nitrogen production, negative nitrogen balance, and increased excretion of urea by the kidneys (see Fig. 6-1). Liver failure can lead to hepatic encephalopathy because of the buildup of nitrogenous compounds, including ammonia; inborn errors of metabolism also give rise to disorders from dysfunction of the urea cycle.

## Regulation of the Amino Acid Pool

Anabolic or catabolic hormonal signaling, various pathophysiologic mechanisms, type and availability of nutrients, and their routes of administration are all factors that regulate the pool of free amino acids. During enteral nutrition (EN), the portal venous system delivers ingested amino acids to the liver; 25% of these reach the general circulation to supply the plasma pool of amino acids, 55% are converted to urea, 6% are used for the synthesis of constitutive plasma proteins (e.g., albumin, prealbumin), and 14% become liver protein. In a severe hypermetabolic response to surgery or trauma, there is a significant increase in demand for amino acids and proteins. Similarly, increase in demand is noted during growth, physical activity, pregnancy, and lactation.

### Glucose-Alanine and Glucose-Lactate Amino Acid Cycles

After severe injury or major surgery, the rates of glucose uptake, glycolysis, and oxidation of BCAAs in muscle are increased. Stimulated by glucagon, the liver transfers the amino group from alanine via the urea cycle to produce pyruvate.

Pyruvate enters the gluconeogenesis pathway via the mitochondrial enzyme pyruvate carboxylase. Glucose is then synthesized and released back to the circulation. Of the 20 amino acids, 18 are gluconeogenic, with alanine being the most frequent source. This amino acid pathway is referred to as the *glucose-alanine cycle.*

Lactate is a byproduct of the anaerobic metabolism of glucose. In physiologic states, it is produced by red blood cells (anaerobic cells) and skeletal muscle and taken up by the liver, where it is initially converted to pyruvate and subsequently to glucose via the gluconeogenic pathway. This is commonly known as the *glucose-lactate*, or Cori, cycle. The reactions that convert lactate back to glucose require a great deal of energy, which is supplied through lipolysis and β-oxidation of fat (see Fig. 6-1).

**Table 6-1 Amino Acids**

| AMINO ACID GROUP (ABBREVIATION) | FEATURES |
|---|---|
| **Essential Amino Acids** | Must be contained in diet because these cannot be synthesized |
| Valine (Val) | Branched-chain amino acid |
| Leucine (Leu) | Branched-chain amino acid |
| Isoleucine (Ile) | Branched-chain amino acid |
| Lysine (Lys) | |
| Methionine (Met) | |
| Threonine (Thr) | |
| Phenylalanine (Phe) | |
| Tryptophan (Trp) | |
| **Conditionally Essential** | Conditionally indispensable because low synthesis rates may exceed requirements under certain conditions, especially in infants |
| Arginine (Arg) | Essential depending on health status of individual and for infants because it cannot be synthesized quickly enough |
| Histidine (His) | Previously considered essential for infants; now also considered essential for adults |
| Tyrosine (Tyr) | Can be synthesized from phenylalanine |
| Cysteine (Cys) | Can be synthesized from methionine |
| Glutamine (Gln) | Major energy source for intestinal mucosa |
| Proline (Pro) | |
| **Nonessential Amino Acids** | Needs can be fully met by synthesis |
| Alanine (Ala) | |
| Asparagine (Asn) | |
| Aspartate (Asp) | |
| Glutamate (Glu) | |
| Glycine (Gly) | |
| Serine (Ser) | |

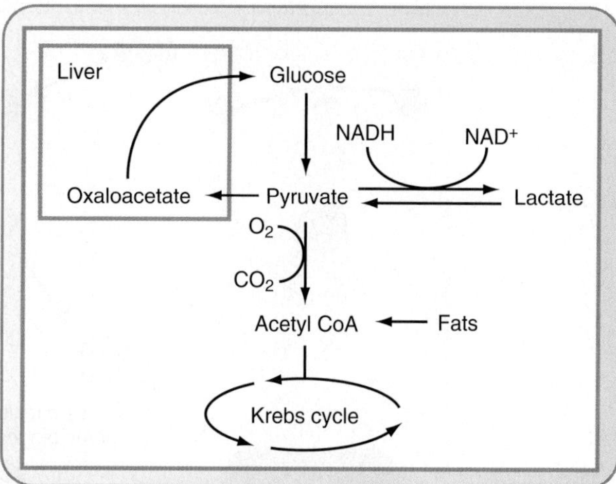


**FIGURE 6-5** Oxidative decarboxylation of pyruvate is a pivotal step in the overall oxidative metabolism of carbohydrates and fats. Overwhelmingly high levels of glucose may lead to lactate production, even in the presence of oxygen. (Adapted from Gore DC, Ferrando A, Barnett J, et al: Influence of glucose kinetics on plasma lactate concentration and energy expenditure in severely burned patients. J Trauma 49:673–677, 2000.)

In the critically ill patient, lactate serves as a global marker of tissue hypoperfusion and insufficient oxygen delivery. However, there are additional mechanisms to explain lactate accumulation in these patients; elevations in plasma lactate levels in severely injured patients may in part be related to increases in glucose flux and may not totally be a reflection of a deficit in oxygen availability (Fig. 6-5).[8]

## Intestinal Health

After dietary ingestion, polysaccharides such as fiber and starch undergo bacterial fermentation in the colonic lumen. Bacterial fermentation is essential for two major reasons: (1) support of the normal flora of the gut lumen, which in turn prevents colonization and subsequent infection (e.g., *Clostridium difficile*); and (2) production of acetoacetate, propionate, and butyrate (a short-chain fatty acid). Butyrate appears to be the preferred fuel of colonic mucosa cells, followed by acetoacetate, glutamine, and finally glucose, and butyrate is therefore essential for mucosal integrity. With the advent and prolonged use of elemental diets for the purpose of achieving total absorption within the small intestine, adequate delivery of fiber to the colonic mucosa is not ensured, bacterial fermentation does not take place, butyrate-producing bacteria are suppressed, and mucosal integrity may be consequently impaired.

Following critical injury, there is thinning of the gut mucosa and a decrease in gut mucosal weight, protein, and DNA content, which are indicative of decreased cellular mass and absorptive surface of the small bowel, changes that result from an increased rate of small bowel mucosal apoptosis, with a relative decrease in small bowel cell proliferation.[9] These changes have been associated with decreased absorption, deranged transportation, and increased gut permeability.

## Protein Turnover

Protein turnover is continuously altered by dietary intake, synthesis, and protein breakdown. Amino acids are removed from the free pool of amino acids by protein synthesis and conversion to urea in a dynamic balance referred to as *protein turnover*. Net synthesis of protein is indicative of an anabolic state, whereas degradation of protein is indicative of a catabolic state. During critical illness, sepsis, trauma, or severe burn injury, there is an increased rate of synthesis and breakdown of muscle protein, although the magnitude of the latter is more significant and leads to a catabolic state.[6] Increased proteolysis initiates an imbalance of the supply and demand of free amino acids; if protein breakdown persists, net protein catabolism leads to significant muscle wasting.

### Proteolysis

The triggers and cellular signaling pathways that induce proteolysis and muscle catabolism, along with therapeutic targets and therapies to prevent muscle wasting, are areas of intense research

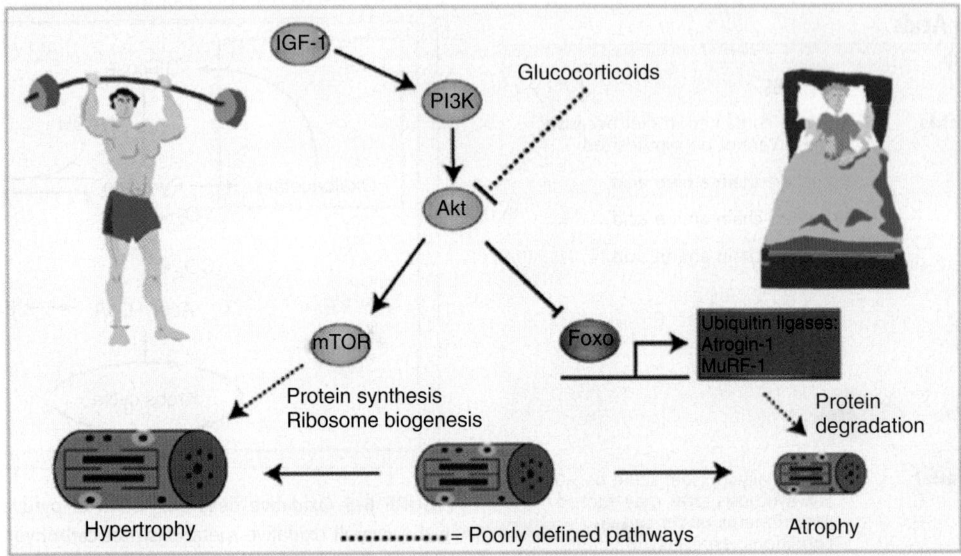


**FIGURE 6-6** The proteins Akt1 and Foxo at the decision point of atrophy versus hypertrophy. (From Hoffman EP, Nader GA: Balancing muscle hypertrophy and atrophy. Nat Med 10:584–585, 2004.)

interest but remain incompletely understood. Proteolysis may be induced to varying degrees by a range of conditions that include fasting, cancer, neurologic genetic disorders, disease, diabetes, sepsis, AIDS, burns, hyperthyroidism, and excess glucocorticoids. The terminal biochemical process involves conjugation of ubiquitin to the amino group of lysine residues in proteins through a series of enzyme: (1) E1 ubiquitin-activating enzyme; (2) E2 ubiquitin-conjugating enzyme; and (3) E3 ubiquitin ligases. The key enzymes in this process are the E3 ligases. Three E3 ubiquitin ligases are expressed in muscle: atrogin-1 (also known as *MAFbx*), muscle RING finger protein 1 (MuRF1), and E3α-I. Approximately 85 specialized proteases that act on ubiquitin are encoded in human genes. Nuclear factor-κB is a major transcription factor that triggers muscle protein degradation via ubiquitination.

Recent studies have proposed that Akt1 is the balancing force between muscle atrophy and hypertrophy. Insulin-like growth factor-1 (IGF-1) and other anabolic stimuli activate the PI3K-Akt1 pathway, leading to the activation of downstream targets (mTOR and S6K1) that stimulate muscle protein synthesis and hypertrophy (Fig. 6-6). Conversely, Akt1 is responsible for the phosphorylation status of the Foxo family of transcription factors. If Foxo is phosphorylated by Akt1, it leaves the nucleus and becomes inactive, thereby preventing the induction of atrophy. However, if Akt1 activity is suppressed, Foxo becomes dephosphorylated and transcriptionally active and directly binds the key atrogin-1 ubiquitination gene, among others, inducing increased protein degradation and muscle atrophy.

### Vitamins and Micronutrients

In addition to requiring macronutrients, proteins, carbohydrates, and fats, numerous cellular processes and enzymes require the provision of trace quantities of vitamins, minerals, and trace elements (Table 6-2).

Decreased levels of vitamins and trace elements have been implicated in impaired wound healing and immune dysfunction. Micronutrients and vitamin deficiencies are rarely seen in patients receiving EN but can occur more often in patients receiving parenteral nutrition (PN). Although deficiencies are avoidable with adequate supplementation, some vitamins and micronutrients require portal passage for conversion or activation, which is potentially bypassed with parenteral infusion. In patients with short bowel syndrome or extensive ileal resection, vitamins and micronutrients that normally require enterohepatic circulation are not adequately absorbed or activated. Patients with adult-onset pernicious anemia or atrophic gastritis with hypochlorhydria can have vitamin $B_{12}$ deficiency. Fat malabsorption induced by pancreatic insufficiency can lead to inadequate uptake of fat-soluble micronutrients. Extensive inflammatory bowel disease can result in iron and vitamin deficiencies. Plasma levels of trace elements are also significantly depressed for prolonged periods after injury because of increased urinary excretion and significant cutaneous losses.

## NUTRITIONAL ASSESSMENT AND MONITORING

Nutritional assessment of surgical patients includes evaluation of preexisting malnutrition or obesity, medical conditions and metabolic disorders, malabsorption, dental disease, drug dependency, and alcoholism. In addition to requiring a comprehensive medical history and physical examination, nutritional assessment may include relevant laboratory tests, anthropometric measurements, and other assessments of body composition and energy expenditure, combined with the serial evaluation of results and response to therapy (Box 6-1). Malnutrition may exist primarily because of underlying pathology or inadequate intake, secondary to disease, trauma, and inflammatory processes or as a consequence of surgical interventions and operative procedures.

Stress responses to trauma and critical illness lead to derangement of normal metabolic and physiologic processes, induction of inflammatory cascades, hepatic acute-phase protein responses, capillary leakage of plasma proteins and subsequent fluid compartment shifts, elevated basal energy expenditure, and

## Table 6-2 Vitamins and Micronutrients in Surgical Care

| MICRONUTRIENT | FUNCTION | DEFICIENCY | RELEVANCE |
|---|---|---|---|
| Vitamin A | Cofactor in collagen synthesis and cross linking; antioxidant; immune stimulation; macrophage extravasation; mucosal integrity; regulation of glycoprotein synthesis | Dermatitis, night blindness, xerophthalmia, respiratory ailments (pneumonia, bronchopulmonary dysplasia), impaired gut epithelial integrity | Wound healing and epithelial regeneration; deficiency can result in diminished activity of helper T cells, impaired mucous secretion; retinol-binding protein sensitive to nutritional status of individuals |
| Vitamin D | Promotes absorption of calcium and phosphorus (by intestine and kidney), bone growth, and bone remodeling (by osteoblasts and osteoclasts); regulates the synthesis of several structural proteins, including type I collagen | Bone demineralization | Deficiency and impairment, causing bone demineralization and osteopenia |
| Vitamin E | Antioxidant properties promote cell membrane integrity | Increased platelet aggregation, decreased red blood cell survival, hemolytic anemia, neurologic abnormalities, decreased serum creatinine level, excessive creatinuria | Prolonged steatorrhea and neuronal degeneration |
| Vitamin K | Essential for coagulation; prerequisite for wound healing | Bruising, hemorrhage | Deficiency reported in long-term antibiotic therapy, TPN lacking fat emulsions, malabsorption |
| Vitamin $B_1$ (Thiamin) | Cofactor in collagen cross linking; facilitates entry of glucose into the TCA cycle | Beriberi, lactic acidosis, anorexia, fatigue, peripheral neuropathy, Wernicke-Korsakoff syndrome, cardiomegaly | Deficiency reported in depleted patients who receive sudden load of carbohydrates; wound healing; treated with 25-100 mg thiamine/day |
| Vitamin $B_5$ (pantothenic acid) | Component of coenzymes involved in energy release from macronutrients and synthesis of heme and fat | Fatigue, sleep disturbances, nausea, abdominal cramps, vomiting, diarrhea, muscle cramps, mental depression, hypoglycemia | Deficiency leading to poor wound healing and skin graft take |
| Biotin | Coenzyme in carboxylation reactions (gluconeogenesis, fatty acid, propionate synthesis) | Glossitis, dermatitis, pallor, hair loss | Long-term TPN, alcoholism, postgastrectomy |
| Vitamin C | Antioxidant, protects against free radical damage; collagen cross linking and hydroxylation of lysine and proline during collagen formation; immune-mediated and antibacterial functions of white blood cells; DNA, RNA replication and lymphocyte function | Fatigue, anorexia, muscular pain, scurvy (anemia, hemorrhagic disorders, defective collagen in bone, cartilage, teeth, connective tissues, muscle degeneration, gingivitis, capillary weakness, impaired wound healing) | Crucial in wound healing; facilitates tissue regeneration, collagen formation in bone, teeth, connective tissue |
| Calcium | Remodeling and degradation of collagen rely on calcium-dependent collagenases | Osteoporosis | Important in reducing osteopenia and function of collagenases; deficiency leading to hypotension, cardiovascular collapse, unresponsiveness to fluids and pressors, PTH end-organ resistance, dysrhythmias |
| Copper | Promotes cross linking of collagen and elastin synthesis; scavenges free radicals | Skeletal demineralization, impaired glucose tolerance, anemia, neutropenia, leucopenia, changes in skin and hair pigmentation; linked to fatal arrhythmias and poorer outcomes | Significant wound exudate; losses of copper and zinc known to occur in pediatric burn patients[60] |
| Iron | Essential in heme-containing molecules for oxygen transport (hemoglobin) and storage (myoglobin), electron transport, and redox reactions (cytochromes) | Anemia, cheilosis, glossitis, hair loss, brittle finger nails, koilonychias, pallor, tissue hypoxia, exertional dyspnea, heart enlargement | Deficiency may occur because of anemia and blood loss; inadequacy leading to reduced resistance to infection and cold intolerance |
| Magnesium | Cofactor in protein and collagen synthesis | Nausea, muscle weakness, irritability, mental derangement | Deficiency can lead to cardiac arrhythmia, increased nervous system irritability, tetany |
| Selenium | Reduces intracellular hydroperoxides; protects membrane lipids from oxidative damage; may reduce mortality in critically ill patients | Growth retardation, muscle pain and weakness, myopathy, cardiomyopathy | Important in cell-mediated immune function; deficiency can lead to altered thyroid hormone metabolism, increased plasma glutathione levels |
| Zinc | Essential cofactor in a wide range of enzyme systems involved in protein synthesis, metalloenzymes, DNA replication, immune function, collagen formation, cross linking | Hair loss, dermatitis, growth retardation, delayed sexual maturation, testicular atrophy, decreased appetite, depressed smell and taste acuity, depression, diarrhea | Deficiency can cause impaired wound healing, may affect bone formation; wound exudate losses |

Adapted from Norbury WB, Situ E, Herndon DN: Nutritional support in the critically ill. In Cameron JL (ed): Current surgical therapy, ed 9, Philadelphia, 2007, Mosby Elsevier, pp 1234–1245.

*PTH,* Parathyroid hormone.

**BOX 6-1 Methods of Nutritional Assessment**

Clinical history
Body weight
Anthropomorphic measurements: IBW, BMI, skin fold thickness
Indirect calorimetry
Oxygen consumption, determination of respiratory quotient
Body composition analysis: Dual-energy X-ray absorptiometry
Biochemical measurements: albumin, transferrin, prealbumin
Measurement of nitrogen balance
Measurements of immunologic function

catabolism of muscle protein, which result in organ dysfunction and associated morbidity. The aim should be to assess and accurately meet nutritional demands while avoiding overfeeding.

Overfeeding is detrimental, leading to hypercapnia and metabolic acidosis, hyperglycemia, hypertriglyceridemia, hepatic dysfunction, and azotemia.[10] Goal-directed nutritional support is essential for improving outcomes following trauma and surgery and should be based on repeated assessment of response to feeding. Nutritional support should be started as soon as possible if circumstances indicate that adequate oral intake will be unlikely for a patient within 5 days or if a preexisting nutritional deficit is present.

## Malnutrition and Starvation

Up to 50% of patients admitted to the hospital may be malnourished[11] and an additional 25% to 30% become malnourished during their hospital stay. Malnutrition can occur as a result of protein-calorie deficiency, predominant protein deficiency, and deficiency of specific micronutrients. Malnutrition can also result from a hypermetabolic state following trauma, critical illness, sepsis, severe burns, or major surgery. It leads to impairment of multiple organ systems, including the immune system, leading to an increased incidence of infection and delayed wound healing. Severe malnutrition and prolonged starvation eventually lead to reduced GI barrier function, respiratory insufficiency, skeletal muscle wasting, decreased myocardial mass, renal atrophy, diastolic cardiac dysfunction, and decreased sensitivity to inotropic agents.

In the metabolic response to starvation, glycogen serves as the primary body fuel for the first 12 to 24 hours. Once glycogen stores are depleted, gluconeogenesis increases and amino acids begin to be degraded to fuel. Over time, ketone bodies from fat can serve as the primary oxidative fuel source. In hypercatabolic states, increases occur in catabolic hormones—cortisol, glucagon, catecholamines, and a number of inflammatory mediators. Hyperglycemia, elevated lactate levels, and increased urinary nitrogen excretion are characteristic features. The body uses fat and muscle as sources of energy. Muscle protein is used preferentially relative to visceral protein. Hence, the rate of loss of lean body mass exceeds that of overall weight loss.

Malnutrition caused by starvation responds to restoration of nutrition, whereas malnutrition secondary to the stress response and disease is often less responsive to nutritional support. Enteral feeding enhances the immune response, and increasing the protein content of the enteral diet has been shown to reduce immunosuppression.

## Physical Body Measurements

### Body Weight

Body weight reflects both fluid balance and nutritional status. Significant weight loss, particularly if rapid or unplanned, is a powerful predictor of mortality.[12] Patients should be weighed daily, and accurate intake and output records should be maintained:

$$\text{Weight loss (\%)} = ([\text{usual weight} - \text{present weight}]/\text{usual weight}) \times 100$$

In critically ill patients, daily changes in weight can be misleading when used for monitoring nutritional requirements and should be interpreted with some caution. Fluid retention and shifts can mask weight loss from skeletal muscle. It should be remembered that overprovision of calories and protein does not avert persistence of muscle protein breakdown, and weight gains may be caused by increases in body fat. Overweight and obese patients may be unable to use fat stores following injury and may not be as well nourished as is often assumed, with these patients having low muscle mass in relation to their weight.

### Anthropometric Measurements

Anthropometric measurements comprise a range of physical body measurements that are compared with standard values or used to evaluate individual changes in nutritional status over time. These also include estimation of ideal body weight (IBW) and body mass index (BMI).

**Ideal Body Weight** A practical anthropomorphic approach is the calculation of IBW, particularly when the usual body weight or weight of the patient before the onset of illness is unknown. Values for IBW can be found in standardized tables that relate height to expected weight, or IBW can be estimated by the following equations[13]:

- Men: 106 lb (48 kg) for the first k (152 cm) and 6 lb (2.7 kg) for each inch (2.54 cm) over k.
- Women: 100 lb (45 kg) for the first k (152 cm) and 5 lb (2.3 kg) for each inch (2.54 cm) over 5 ft.

**Body Mass Index** BMI is a statistical index that uses height and weight to provide an estimate of body fat in males and females of all ages. However, individual variation can occur, and it should not be used as the sole means of classifying a person as obese or malnourished. The U.S. National Health and Nutrition Examination Survey of 2007 indicates that 63% of Americans are overweight, with 26% in the obese category (a BMI of 30 or more). In children, BMI percentile allows comparison with children of the same sex and age. A BMI that is less than the fifth percentile is considered underweight and above the 95th percentile is considered obese.

$$\text{BMI} = \text{weight (in kg)}/\text{height}^2\ (\text{in m}^2)$$

***Interpretation of Body Mass Index***

Severely underweight: <16.5
Underweight: 16.5-18.4
Normal weight: 18.5 -24.9
Overweight: 25-29.9

Obesity grade I: 30-34.9
Obesity grade II: 35-39.9
Obesity grade III: ≥40

## Evaluating Caloric Requirements

Determining nutritional requirements of critically ill patients is essential because the provision of inadequate or excess calories can adversely affect outcome. Measuring the resting energy expenditure (REE) or basal metabolic rate can be extremely useful in the nutritional management of surgical patients under various types of stress who may experience significantly increased energy demands, which can be difficult to predict. Estimates of caloric requirements can be made using several different equations, calculated using blood gas measurements with the Fick equation, or measured by indirect calorimetry using bedside metabolic carts to determine REE.

### Energy Expenditure Equations

Several different equations are commonly used to estimate nutritional requirements. These formulas provide only an estimate because energy demands may vary considerably among patients and requirements will also depend on a patient's condition and activity level. These formulas are based on parameters including age, gender, height, and weight. Examples include the Harris-Benedict,[61] American College of Chest Physicians, Ireton-Jones (1997), Penn State (2003), and Swinamer (1990) equations. In severely burned patients, these and other equations can estimate nutritional requirements. Included in these other equations are the Curreri and Galveston formulas, which additionally take into consideration body surface area and burn percentage. It is important to select the appropriate equation based on age and correct estimate of degree of injury, because their inappropriate use can lead to significant overestimation of caloric needs and increased risk of overfeeding.

**Harris-Benedict Equation** Most patients can be fed adequately by supplying 100% to 120% of the predicted REE as calculated by the Harris-Benedict equation.[14] This equation estimates basal metabolic rate (BMR), assuming a normal resting physiologic state.

For men:

$$\text{BMR} = 66.5 + (13.75 \times \text{weight in kg}) + (5.003 \times \text{height in cm}) - (6.775 \times \text{age in years})$$

For women:

$$\text{BMR} = 655.1 + (9.563 \times \text{weight in kg}) + (1.850 \times \text{height in cm}) - (4.676 \times \text{age in years})$$

Therefore, multiplication by a stress factor is generally needed, usually ranging from 1.2 to 1.5 in ventilated patients with sepsis. A stress factor of 1.1 and 1.2 has been suggested for minor and major elective surgery, 1.35 and 1.6 for skeletal trauma and head injury, and 1.1, 1.5, and 1.8 for mild, moderate, and severe infection, respectively, has also been suggested.[15] This may rise to 1.2 to 1.95 in burn injuries of 40% to 100% of total body surface area (TBSA).

**Indirect Calorimetry** An evaluation of the metabolic status can be performed by indirect calorimetry using bedside metabolic carts, which measure REE using expired gas volumes; $\dot{V}O_2$ and carbon dioxide production ($\dot{V}CO_2$) are measured directly. A tight-fitting face mask or connection to a mechanical ventilator circuit is needed. The measured REE value may need to be increased approximately 10% to 20% if used to estimate caloric requirements in patients to allow for activity and fluctuations in their overall metabolic rate.

$$\text{REE (in kcal/day)} = 1.44\,(3.9\ \dot{V}O_2\ [\text{in mL/min}] + 1.1\ \dot{V}CO_2\ [\text{in mL/min}])$$

Measurements obtained are generally reliable and reproducible over a wide range of catabolic conditions, metabolic rates, and values of $FIO_2$.Indirect calorimetry may also be used to monitor the adequacy of feeding by calculating the respiratory quotient ($RQ = \dot{V}CO_2/\dot{V}O_2$) and evaluating substrate uptake. An RQ in the range of 0.7 to 1.0 is seen in the normal uptake of mixed substrates. An RQ of 0.7 or less is consistent with pure fat uptake and is indicative of underfeeding, whereas an RQ higher than 1.0 may indicate fat synthesis from carbohydrate and overfeeding. Overfeeding has been shown to be detrimental to critically ill patients and induces a rise in $\dot{V}CO_2$ because of increased lipogenesis.[16] Such a rise in $\dot{V}CO_2$ may also contribute to difficult weaning from ventilatory support.

Poor agreement between measured and predicted REEs has been reported in certain circumstances, being as high as 635 ± 526 kcal/day in severely burned children.[17] Bedside carts are therefore recommended to calculate optimal nutritional requirements in certain patient populations, including the following: (1) severely burned children; (2) ventilator-dependent patients; (3) patients with clinical signs of overfeeding or underfeeding; (4) patients with spinal cord injury or coma; (5) critically ill patients who are morbidly obese; and (6) those with failure to respond adequately to the use of diets determined according to equations, with failure determined by lack of improvement in clinical or biochemical nutritional measurements.

### Dual-Energy X-Ray Absorptiometry

Dual-energy x-ray absorptiometry is a useful technique for monitoring long-term nutritional progress. It is used to measure body composition changes, including lean body mass, fat mass, and bone density. It is a noninvasive investigation, with scans obtained with the patient lying supine on a table. It measures the attenuation of two x-ray beams, one high energy and the other low energy, and it delivers a low dose of radiation. These measurements are compared with standard models used for bone and soft tissue. Results are separated into lean body mass, fat mass, and bone mineral content. Maintaining and enhancing skeletal muscle as lean body mass is a principal objective of nutritional support; these measurements are therefore useful in nutritional assessment. Assessment of body composition when patients have been treated with surgical staples or are undergoing fluid shifts in cellular and whole-body water may confound the assessment of lean body mass.

## Monitoring Nutritional Status

Careful monitoring is necessary to ensure optimal feeding and prevent underfeeding or overfeeding, regardless of the method used to estimate nutritional needs. This involves regular clinical assessment of vital signs, respiratory status, functional improvement, and wound healing, all of which may present important clues about the true nutritional status. In addition to clinical assessment, monitoring trends in a range of parameters will serve to guide nutritional support and the need to enhance or adjust feeding regimens.

### Nitrogen Balance

Nitrogen balance can be calculated to monitor the adequacy of protein intake. A negative nitrogen balance occurs when the excretion of nitrogen exceeds the daily intake, an indication of muscle breakdown, whereas a positive nitrogen balance is associated with muscle gain.

Nitrogen balance can be estimated using equations based on common measurements, such as urine urea nitrogen (UUN), urine nonurea nitrogen (estimated as 20% of UUN), 24-hour urine output (UO), and an additional 2 g/day to account for nonurinary nitrogen losses (stool and skin).

$$\text{24-hour UUN (g/day)} = \text{UUN (mg/dL)} \times \text{UO (ml/day)} \times 1/1000\ \text{(g/mg)} \times 1/100\ \text{(dl/mL)}$$

$$\text{Total nitrogen loss (g/day)} = \text{24-hour UUN (g/day)} + (0.20 \times \text{24-hour UUN [g/day]}) + 2\ \text{(g/day)}$$

$$\text{Total nitrogen balance (g/day)} = \text{Total nitrogen intake (g/day)} - \text{total nitrogen loss (g/day)}$$

Serial monitoring of total nitrogen balance in patients permits one to evaluate the response to nutritional support and identify patients at risk of developing muscle protein loss. Persistent loss of nitrogen and protein catabolism leads to decreased muscle strength, altered body composition, increased infectious complications, and subsequent delayed rehabilitation.

### Pediatric Assessment

Nutritional assessment in children, in addition to clinical history, physical examination, and biochemical markers, also includes plotting their growth on percentile charts. The Centers for Disease Control and Prevention (CDC) has published revised, standard, gender-specific percentile charts for growth, including stature and weight for age and BMI. These charts are demographically representative of the U.S. population from 2 to 20 years, with charts also available for younger children (Fig. 6-7). These charts are used to monitor a patient's long-term nutritional progress. A patient's position on the growth chart is the best simple tool to evaluate overall nutritional status in the acute setting. A value below the fifth percentile or a trend line crossing two major percentile lines indicates a serious failure to thrive.

### Serum Proteins

A range of serum proteins are commonly used as indicators of nutritional status, with albumin being the most frequently used. Albumin accounts for more than 50% of the total protein in serum and is the major contributor to colloid osmotic pressure. An albumin level below 3 g/dL suggests suboptimal nutrition and has been used as the primary preoperative serum marker of malnutrition (Table 6-3). Albumin has a long half-life ($t_{1/2}$), approximately 20 days, and perioperative albumin levels have been found to be a better prognostic indicator than anthropomorphic measurements for morbidity and mortality in surgical patients.[18,19] Serum proteins with a shorter circulating duration are also used; these include transferrin ($t_{1/2}$ = 10 days), prealbumin ($t_{1/2}$ = 3 days), and retinol binding protein ($t_{1/2}$ = 12 to 24 hours), because these are more sensitive indicators of recent changes.

**Table 6-3 Surgical Risk by Serum Albumin Level**

| SERUM ALBUMIN (g/dL) | 30-DAY MORTALITY RATE (%) | 30-DAY MORBIDITY RATE (%) |
|---|---|---|
| >4.5 | ≤1 | ≤10 |
| 3.5 | 5 | 25 |
| 3.0 | 9 | 35 |
| 2.5 | 15 | 45 |
| <2.1 | ≈30 | 65 |

Adapted from Gibbs J, Cull W, Henderson W, et al: Preoperative serum albumin level as a predictor of operative mortality and morbidity: Results from the National VA Surgical Risk Study. Arch Surg 134:36–42, 1999.

Perioperative levels of serum albumin have been shown to be powerful predictors of morbidity and mortality.

During the acute stress response to injury, significant downregulation of 50% to 70% of proteins with a longer half-life, such as albumin and transferrin, occurs in parallel to the upregulation of hepatic acute-phase proteins. The degree of downregulation of constitutive proteins after trauma is used as a predictor of mortality and stress severity. Patients with albumin levels below 3 g/dL show an independently associated increased risk of developing serious complications within 30 days of surgery, including sepsis, acute renal failure, coma, failure to wean from ventilation, cardiac arrest, pneumonia, and wound infection.

Albumin levels are also useful in detecting protein-energy malnutrition, which is frequently difficult to recognize in patients not presenting with low body weight and results from increased demands associated with the stress of illness, injury, or infection. If these requirements are not met from dietary sources, body protein stores are depleted, leading to complications (e.g., malabsorption, impaired immunologic response, reduced production of other constitutive proteins). Counterintuitively, IV administration of albumin is usually ineffective because it degrades quickly after infusion and does not treat the underlying cause of malnutrition.

The use of serum protein levels as indicators of nutritional status may be limited in the acute phase following injury, inflammation, infection, and surgical stress. Fluid shifts and increased capillary permeability lead to protein leakage from the intravascular compartment, which results in hemodilution and false hypoproteinemia.

## NUTRITIONAL SUPPORT

Surgical patients with suboptimal nutritional support have impaired wound healing, altered immune responses, accelerated catabolism, increased organ dysfunction, delayed recovery, and increased morbidity and mortality.[20] Following surgery, patients who are inadequately fed become undernourished within 10 days and display a marked increase in mortality.[21] Feeding should therefore be initiated as early as possible,

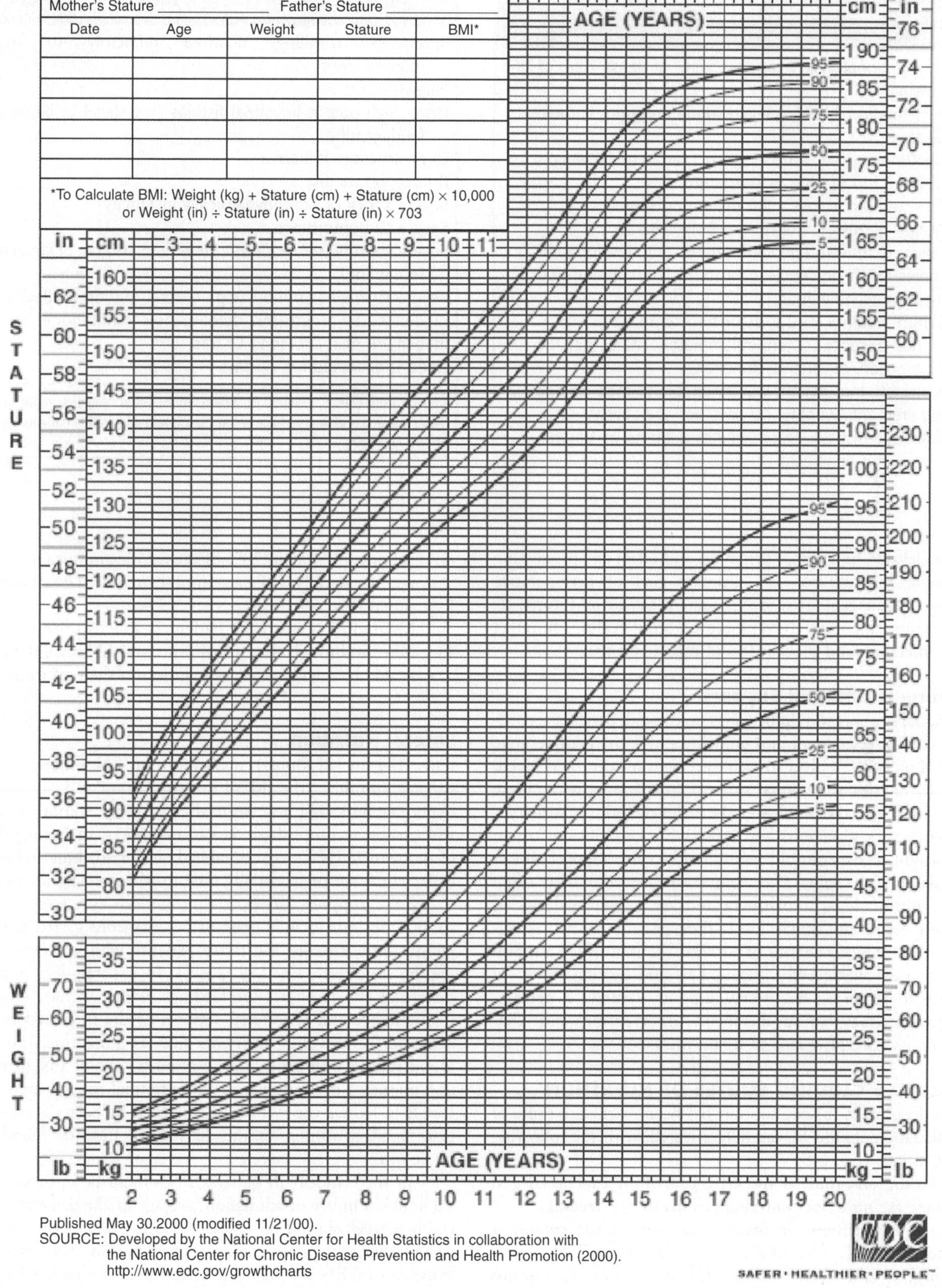


**FIGURE 6-7** Stature- and weight-for-age percentile charts for boys ages 2 to 20 years. (From Centers for Disease Control and Prevention: Growth charts, 2000, http://www.cdc.gov/growthcharts.)

**BOX 6-2 Criteria to Initiate Perioperative Nutritional Support[23-25]**

Severe nutritional risk expected with at least one of the following:
- Past medical history: Severe undernutrition, chronic disease.
- Involuntary loss >10%-15% of usual body weight within 6 mo or >5% within 1 mo
- Expected blood loss >500 mL during surgery
- Weight of 20% under IBW or BMI <18.5 kg/m$^2$
- Failure to thrive on pediatric growth and development curves (<5th percentile or a trend line crossing two major percentile lines)
- Serum albumin <3.0 g/dL or transferrin <200 mg/dL in the absence of an inflammatory state, hepatic dysfunction, or renal dysfunction
- Anticipate that patient will be unable to meet caloric requirements within 7-10 days perioperatively.
- Catabolic disease (e.g., significant burns or trauma, sepsis, and pancreatitis)

**BOX 6-3 Contraindications to Enteral Nutrition**

Intractable vomiting, diarrhea refractory to medical management
Paralytic ileus
Distal high-output intestinal fistulas (too distal to bypass with feeding tube)
GI obstruction, ischemia
Diffuse peritonitis
Severe shock or hemodynamically instability
Severe GI hemorrhage
Severe short bowel syndrome (less than 100 cm of small bowel remaining)
Severe GI malabsorption (e.g., enteral nutrition failed, as evidenced by progressive deterioration in nutritional status)
Inability to gain access to GI tract
Need is expected for <7 days

Adapted from Villet S, Chiolero RL, Bollmann MD, et al: Negative impact of hypocaloric feeding and energy balance on clinical outcome in ICU patients. Clin Nutr 24:502–509, 2005.

address elevated nutritional demands, and offset any preexisting nutritional impairment. The ultimate goal of perioperative nutritional management is to supplement caloric and nutrient-specific requirements safely to promote wound healing, diminish risk of infection, and prevent loss of muscle protein.

### Initiating Nutritional Support

Nutritional support should be considered for all patients according to clinical assessment and guidelines over the perioperative period (Box 6-2).[23-25] If a surgical intervention can be delayed, 10 to 14 days of nutritional support for patients with severe nutritional risk has been shown to be beneficial prior to surgery.[22] Obviously critical patients and those with a significant loss in body weight or a premorbid state should receive support almost immediately (<3 days) after admission, because they often exhibit immunologic impairment and are at increased risk of infection. Significant weight loss in these patients is often associated with a reduced chance of survival. Malnourished surgical patients also have severely impaired wound healing times. In addition to requiring nutritional support, severely hypercatabolic patients may require therapeutic interventions and rehabilitation exercise programs to regain muscle mass.

## PRINCIPLES GUIDING ROUTES OF NUTRITION

After a decision to initiate support has been reached, a route of administration should be carefully selected, with the following considerations (Fig. 6-8)[5,26,27]:

1. Use the oral route if the GI tract is fully functional and there are no other contraindications to oral feeding.[28]
2. Initiate nutrition via the enteral route if the patient is not expected to be on a full oral diet within 7 days postsurgery and there are no GI tract contraindications (Box 6-3).[28]
3. If the enteral route is contraindicated or not tolerated, use the parenteral route within 24 to 48 hours in patients who are not expected to be able to tolerate full enteral nutrition (EN) within 7 days.[21,27]
4. Administer at least 20% of the caloric and protein requirements enterally while reaching the required goal with additional PN.
5. Maintain PN until the patient is able to tolerate 75% of calories through the enteral route and EN until the patient is able to tolerate 75% of calories via the oral route.

### Enteral Nutrition

Early (24 to 48 hours) institution of EN following major surgery minimizes the risk of undernutrition and can abate the hypermetabolic response seen after surgery. Administration of EN can be accomplished via various routes, including the use of nasogastric (NG), nasoduodenal, and nasojejunal tubes (Fig. 6-9), which are preferentially used in patients who are expected to require support for short time periods (<4 weeks). Other surgical options include open or percutaneous gastrostomy and jejunostomy, usually for those patients who are expected to require long-term EN (>4 weeks). In general, EN offers the beneficial effects of trophic feedings, which include structural maintenance and functional support of the intestinal mucosa, achieved by providing nutrients such as glutamine, preserving blood supply, and promoting peristalsis. Use of EN to protect and maintain the integrity of the intestinal mucosa may therefore help reduce the risk of sepsis caused by bacterial translocation. Feeding routes for the delivery of EN are described in Table 6-4.

In the critically ill patient, EN should be initiated within 48 hours of injury or admission; average intake delivered within the first week should be at least 60% to 70% of the total estimated energy requirements, as determined by the assessment. Provision of EN in this time frame and at this level may be associated with decreased length of hospital stay, days on mechanical ventilation, and infectious complications.

Feeding through a NG tube is the most cost-effective method for EN support and perhaps the most helpful for preventing postoperative complications, such as gastroparesis. The

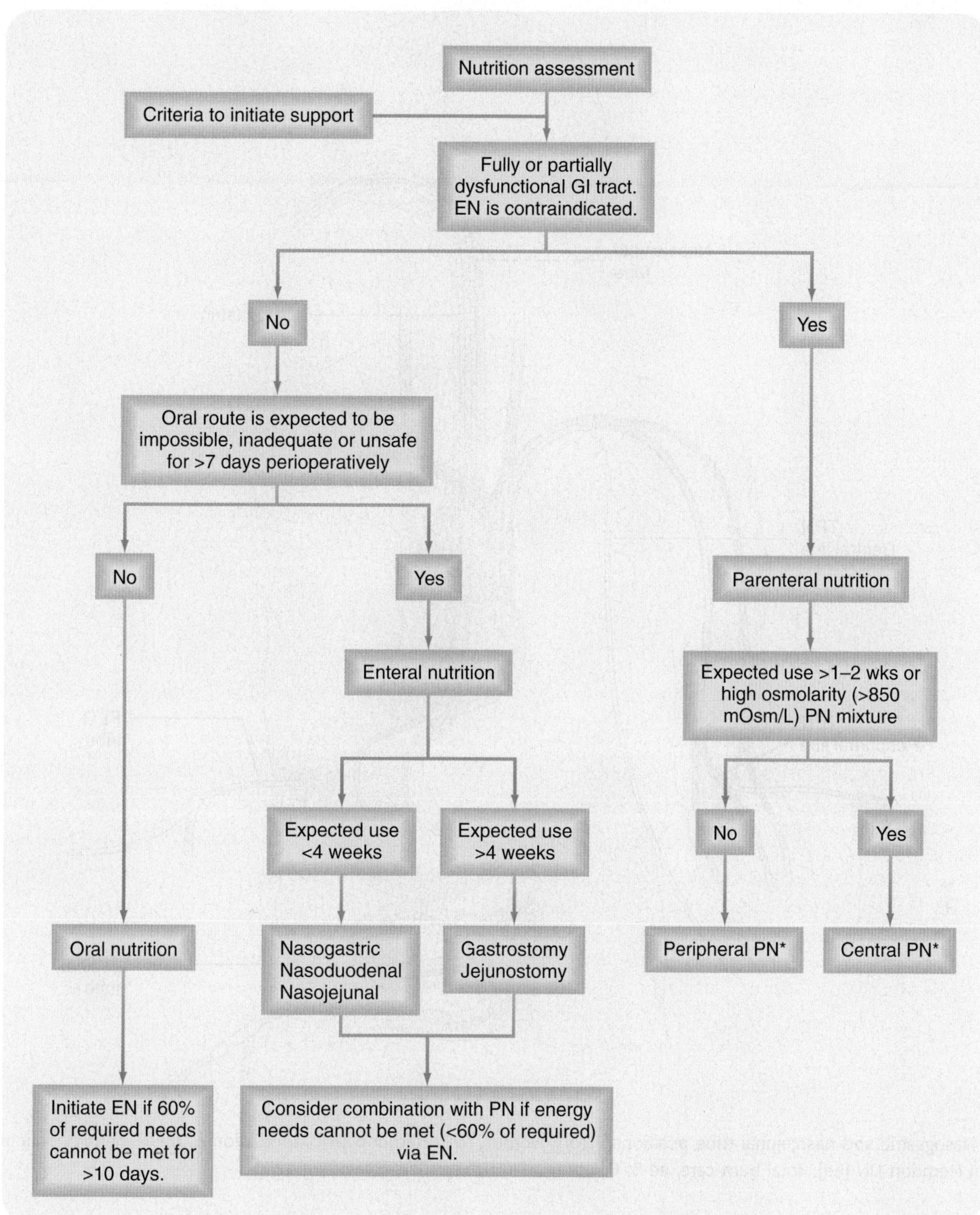


**FIGURE 6-8** Algorithm for route of nutritional support in surgical patients.

use of NG tubes conveniently facilitates the ability to supply caloric needs and to monitor the volume of gastric residuals. To decrease reflux and the risk of aspiration, it is recommended that the head of the bed be raised to 35 degrees and the volume of residuals not exceed 50 mL/hour. Although the residual volume should be rechecked after 1 hour from a single elevated value, feeding does not have to stop automatically.

GI ileus may reflect an underlying deterioration; therefore, monitoring gastric residual volumes serves as an indicator of intercurrent conditions, such as sepsis. In burn patients, residuals that increase above the amount of food delivered routinely every hour have been shown to correlate with the development of bacterial sepsis, and a full sepsis workup is indicated when gastric residuals exceed 200 mL.[30,31]

The practice of checking the positioning of tubes by X-ray prior to their use is a time-consuming process that has been motivated, in part, by the unintended placement of small-diameter tubes into lower airways. However, NG tubes may be placed with confidence by auscultation over the stomach while delivering 50 mL of air quickly with an irrigation syringe. Nasojejunal and duodenal tubes may be too small for this procedure. Contraindications to EN include prolonged ileus or gastroparesis, bowel obstruction, acute pseudo-obstruction, ischemic enterocolitis, and other causes of malabsorption.

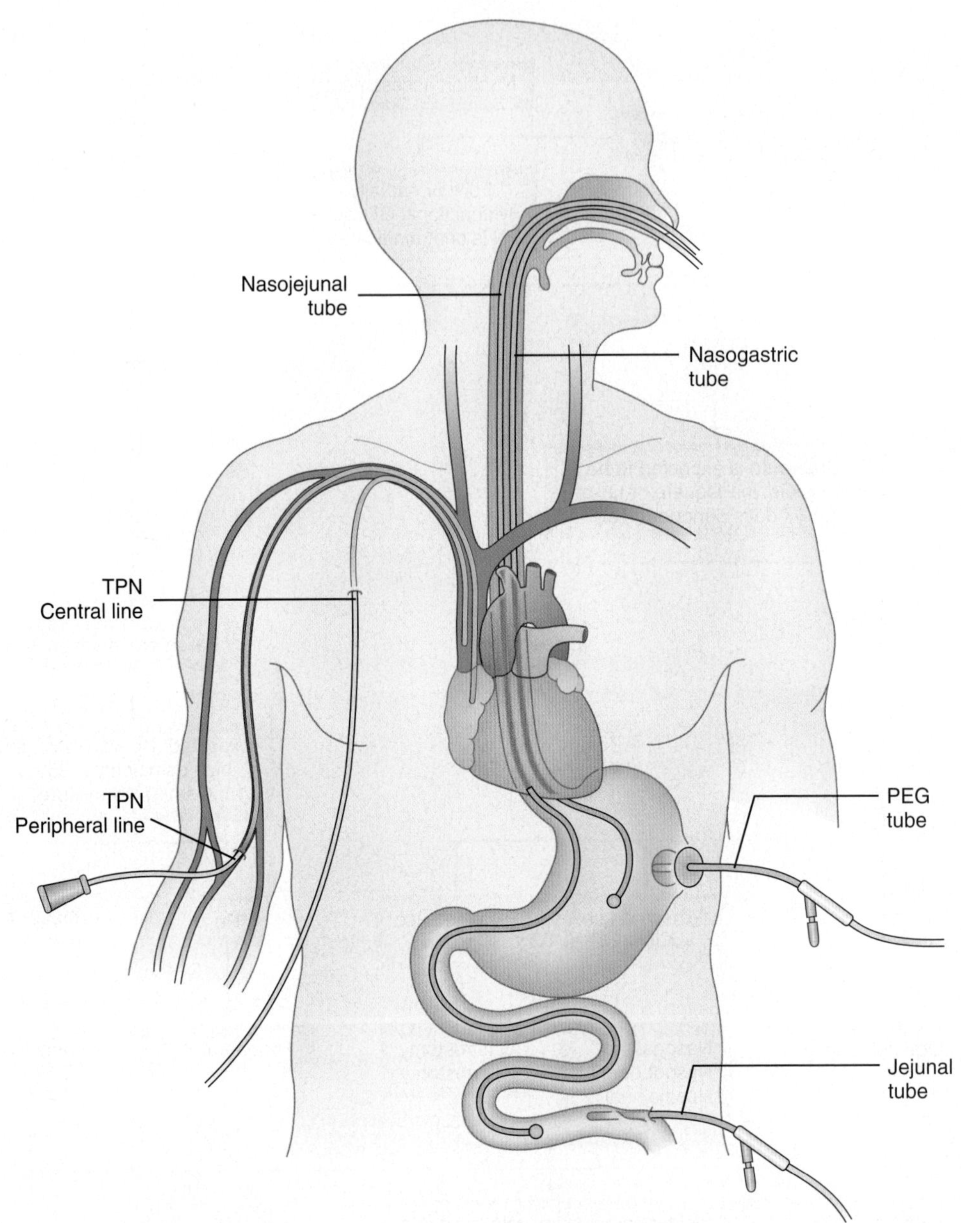


**FIGURE 6-9** Nasogastric and nasojejunal tube positions. (From Norbury WB, Herndon DN: Modulation of the hypermetabolic response after burn injury. In Herndon DN [ed]: Total burn care, ed 3, Edinburgh, 2007, Saunders Elsevier, p 423.)

With nasoenteric feeding beyond the stomach, the tube should be advanced through the duodenum, ideally past the ligament of Treitz to the proximal jejunum, because this reduces the risk of aspiration. Nasojejunal feeding may be preferable in some settings because it does not need to be stopped prior to surgery to prevent aspiration. However, nasojejunal feeding requires continuous infusion, and gastric residual volumes cannot be checked to confirm progress. Nasojejunal feeding should not be commenced until the patient is fully volume-resuscitated and hemodynamically stable. Percutaneous feeding options should be considered if a patient requires nasal tube feeding for a prolonged period beyond 2 or 3 weeks.

Ileus associated with severe injury is not as common as previously thought. Ileus derived from mesenteric hypoperfusion prior to adequate resuscitation is reversed once the patient has been resuscitated. Conversely, overresuscitation leads to GI edema and should also be avoided. Postinjury ileus does not affect the small bowel as profoundly as the stomach. Therefore, feeding using a nasoduodenal tube passed through the pylorus, or a nasojejunal tube advanced past the ligament of Treitz, can be initiated as soon as possible, preferably within 6 hours following injury. This approach also allows continuous feeding during surgeries and physical therapy sessions. The initiation of immediate enteral feeding allows the delivery of calculated caloric requirements by the third day postinjury. Reduction of hypermetabolism by initiating enteral feeding soon after injury is possible, with this reduction in metabolic rate associated with less intense elevations in glucagon, cortisol, and catecholamine levels.[32]

**Table 6-4 Enteral Nutrition Feeding Routes**

| ROUTE | SUITABILITY | INSERTION METHOD, CONFIRMATION | ADVANTAGES | DISADVANTAGES |
|---|---|---|---|---|
| Nasogastric | Short term—functional GI tract | Blind at bedside; fluoroscopy guided | Easy to insert, replace; can monitor gastric pH and residual volume; bolus feeding | Aspiration risk, misplacement complications, sinusitis, epistaxis, nasal necrosis, esophageal strictures, erosive esophagitis |
| Nasoduodenal, nasojejunal | Short term—functional GI tract but poor gastric emptying, reflux, aspiration risk; commence feed only when volume-resuscitated and hemodynamically stable | Blind at bedside; fluoroscopy guided, endoscopy guided | Reduced aspiration risk; some tubes enable decompression of stomach while feeding into jejunum | Easily clogged or displaced, aspiration risk, misplacement complications, displacement and reflux into stomach, sinusitis, epistaxis, nasal necrosis; requires continuous infusion; cannot check gastric residuals except with specialized gastric port |
| Gastrostomy | Long term—good gastric emptying; avoid if significant reflux or aspiration problem | Surgical, percutaneous, endoscopic, radiologic | Bolus feeding; large-bore tube less likely to block | Procedure risks include bleeding, perforation, aspiration risk, dislodgment with peritoneal contamination, wound site infection, granulation |
| Jejunostomy | Long term—functional GI tract but poor gastric emptying, reflux, aspiration risk, gastroparesis or gastric dysfunction | Surgical, percutaneous, endoscopic, radiologic | Reduced aspiration risk | Bleeding, infection, perforation, migration, aspiration, dislodgement and leakage into peritoneal cavity, occlusion, pneumatosis, intestinal ischemia or infarction, bowel obstruction; difficult to replace; cannot check residuals; requires continuous infusion |

Adapted from Al-Mousawi A, Branski LK, Andel HL, et al: Ernährungstherapie bei Brandverletzten. In Kamolz LP, Herndon DN, Jeschke MG (eds): Verbrennungen: Diagnose, Therapie und Rehabilitation des thermischen Traumas, German Edition, New York, 2009, Springer-Verlag, pp 183–194.

### Formulations

Numerous enteral formulations are available and can be classified according to their composition. Standard formulas are sterile, nutritionally complete, and intended for patients with a normal GI tract who cannot ingest adequate nutrients and calories by regular oral diets. Specialty formulations may be more efficiently absorbed in patients suffering from short gut syndrome, severe trauma, burn injury, and chronic malabsorptive diarrhea. Whole-protein formulations are appropriate for most patients. Peptide-based or free amino acid formulations may be considered for patients with a severely compromised GI tract or severe protein-fat malabsorption. Modular formulas consist of a singular macronutrient as a source of calories (e.g., fiber, protein) and are generally used by mixing with standard or specialty formulas. Immune-enhancing formulas consist of nutritional components enriched with arginine, glutamine, nucleotides, and omega-3 fatty acids. Although most formulations are hyperosmolar at full strength, dilution by 25% to 50% to make isotonic and hypotonic formulas is initially preferred to minimize the possibility of diarrhea from excess osmotic load and to facilitate absorption (Table 6-5). Continuous enteral feeding with milk or a soy-based milk substitute can maintain total body weight throughout the hospital course but may not be able to maintain lean body mass.

In patients undergoing a severe hypermetabolic response, peripheral breakdown of fat is increased. Fatty acids are delivered to the liver and undergo re-esterification; their accumulation leads to fatty liver changes. The use of high-fat diets such as milk, which consists of 44% fat, 42% carbohydrate, and 14% protein, needs to be carefully considered because additional fat may lead to increased levels fat in the liver. The use of high-sugar, high-protein diets consisting of 3% fat, 82% carbohydrate, and 15% protein stimulate protein synthesis, increase endogenous insulin production, and improve lean body mass accretion.[33]

Muscle protein degradation is markedly decreased with the administration of a high-carbohydrate diet compared with fat-containing diets. Endogenous insulin concentration is increased, improving the net balance of skeletal muscle protein caused by decreased protein breakdown.

### Complications

Complications of nasogastric and enteric feeding include nausea and vomiting, epistaxis, sinusitis, nasal necrosis, aspiration leading to pneumonia, tube malpositioning, dislodgment, and feeding-associated diarrhea. Fine-bore tubes are more comfortable but can become blocked easily. Auscultation examination of gastric fluid aspirate and pH testing can be used to confirm tube position, particularly for large-bore nasal tubes, although many units prefer radiologic confirmation. Tubes can also be inserted under endoscopic or fluoroscopic guidance. Monitoring guidelines and potential metabolic complications of EN are given in Tables 6-6 and 6-7.

Refeeding syndrome can be precipitated following prolonged fasting and IV fluid administration in chronically malnourished patients. The transition from metabolizing body fat to carbohydrate in the feed can cause an abrupt rise in insulin and disturbances of intracellular electrolytes. Electrolyte abnormalities can result in cardiac failure and dysrhythmias, respiratory failure, neurologic disturbances, and renal and hepatic dysfunction. With all nutritional support, the rate of feeding should commence slowly to prevent abrupt metabolic changes.

Aside from mechanical issues related to the feeding tube, the most common complications of enteral feedings result

**Table 6-5 Composition of Various Enteral Nutrition Formulations***

| | Composition | | | | | |
|---|---|---|---|---|---|---|
| FORMULA | kcal/mL | CHO, g/L (% CALORIES) | PRO, g/L (% CALORIES) | FAT, g/L (% CALORIES) | OSMOLALITY (mOsm/L) | COMMENTS |
| **Standard** | | | | | | |
| Similac | 0.67 | 72 (43) | 15 (8) | 36 (49) | | Infant nutrition |
| Enfamil | 0.67 | 73 (44) | 14 (8) | 35 (48) | | Infant nutrition |
| Isomil | 0.67 | 68 (41) | 18 (10) | 37 (49) | | Infant nutrition, lactose-free, used in cow protein allergy |
| Isosource HN | 1.2 | 160 (53) | 53 (18) | 39 (29) | 490 | High nitrogen |
| Ensure Plus | 1.5 | 208 (57) | 54 (15) | 46 (28) | 680 | Concentrated calories |
| Pediasure Enteral | 1.0 | 133 (53) | 30 (12) | 40 (35) | 335 | For ages 1-13 yr, with fiber, not easily digestible |
| Jevity 1 Cal | 1.06 | 155 (54) | 44 (17) | 35 (29) | 300 | Isotonic nutrition with fiber |
| Boost Kid Essential | 1.0 | 135 (54) | 30 (12) | 38 (34) | 550-600 | Oral or tube feeding |
| Boost HP | 1.0 | 137 (55) | 62 (24) | 25 (21) | 650 | Oral or tube feeding, high protein |
| Promote | 1.0 | 130 (52) | 62 (25) | 26 (23) | 340 | High protein, oral or tube feeding |
| Promote w/Fiber | 1.0 | 138 (50) | 62 (25) | 28 (25) | 380 | Very high protein, oral or tube feeding |
| Nutren 1.0 | 1.0 | 127 (51) | 40 (16) | 38 (33) | 370 | With fiber, decreases diarrhea |
| **Immune-Enhancing** | | | | | | |
| Crucial | 1.5 | 89 (36) | 63 (25) | 45 (39) | 490 | With ARG, critical illness, major surgery, transitional feedings, hydrolyzed protein |
| Impact | 1.0 | 130 (53) | 56 (22) | 28 (25) | 375 | With ARG, GLN, and fiber |
| Impact GLN | 1.3 | 150 (46) | 78 (24) | 43 (30) | 630 | Immunonutrition, GLN, ARG, omega-3 PUFA, nucleic acids |
| Oxepa | 1.5 | 105 (28) | 63 (17) | 94 (55) | 535 | ARDS, acute lung injury, sepsis; concentrated |
| **Specialty** | | | | | | |
| Glucerna | 1.0 | 96 (34) | 42 (17) | 54 (49) | 355 | For glucose-intolerant or diabetic patients, low CHO |
| Nepro | 1.8 | 167 (34) | 81 (18) | 96 (48) | 585 | For CKD and patients on dialysis; concentrated |
| Osmolite1Cal | 1.06 | 144 (54) | 44 (17) | 35 (29) | 300 | Isotonic, for use in those intolerant to hyperosmolar nutrition |
| Vivonex RTF | 1.0 | 175 (70) | 50 (20) | 12 (10) | 630 | Transitional feeding, low fat, easily digestible |
| Vivonex TEN | 1.0 | 210 (82%) | 38 (15%) | 2.8 (3%) | 630 | 100% free amino acids, very low fat, used for severe trauma (e.g., burns) or surgery, transitional feeding |
| Vivonex Plus | 1.0 | 190 (76%) | 45 (18%) | 6.7 (6%) | 650 | 100% free amino acids, very low fat, used for severe trauma (e.g., burns) or surgery, transitional feeding |
| Elecare | 0.67 | 72 (43%) | 20 (15%) | 32 (42%) | 350 | Prepared at 9.4 g/60 mL; amino acid–based nutrition |
| **Modular** | | | | | | |
| Resource Benefiber | 0.27 | 66 (100%) | 0% | 0% | – | Prepared at 4 g/60 mL; tasteless, odorless, soluble fiber, used for constipation |
| Resource Beneprotein | 0.83 | 0% | 200 (100%) | 0% | – | Prepared at 7 g/30 mL; whey protein, mixed in foods, protein-calorie malnutrition |

Adapted from Al-Mousawi A, Branski LK, Andel HL, et al: Ernährungstherapie bei Brandverletzten. In Kamolz LP, Herndon DN, Jeschke MG (eds): Verbrennungen: Diagnose, Therapie und Rehabilitation des thermischen Traumas, German edition, New York, Springer-Verlag, 2009, pp 183–194.

*ARDS,* Acute respiratory distress syndrome; *ARG,* arginine; *CHO,* carbohydrate; *CKD,* chronic kidney disease; *GLN,* glutamine; *PRO,* protein.

*Data extrapolated from Nestle Clinical Nutrition: Enteral product reference guide, Nestle, 2010, Minneapolis; and Abbott Laboratories: Abbott nutrition pocket guide, Abbott Park, Ill, 2009, Abbott Laboratories.

from solute overload. Inappropriately rapid administration of hyperosmolar solutions may result in diarrhea, dehydration, electrolyte imbalance, hyperglycemia, and loss of potassium, magnesium, and other ions through diarrhea. If aggressive administration of hyperosmolar solute continues, pneumatosis intestinalis with bowel necrosis and perforation can result. Hyperosmolar nonketotic coma can also occur with enteral feedings, as with PN.

**Table 6-6 Suggested Monitoring Schedule for Enteral Feeding**

| PARAMETER | ACUTE PATIENT | STABLE PATIENT |
|---|---|---|
| Electrolytes | Daily | 1-2×/week |
| Complete blood count | Daily | 1-2×/week |
| Glucose level | 3×/day; more often if poor control | 3×/day; less often if good control |
| Creatinine and urea levels | Daily | Weekly or twice weekly |
| Nitrogen balance | Daily | 2-3×/week |
| Input and output | Daily | 2-3×/week |
| Body weight | Daily | 2-3×/week |
| Urine output | Hourly | every 4 hours |
| Stool | Per motion | Daily |

## Parenteral Nutrition

PN developed during the 1960s and soon became a major advancement in the nutrition of patients with a nonfunctioning GI tract. It involves the IV infusion of nutrients in an elemental form, bypassing the usual processes of digestion. When long-term delivery of hyperosmolar regimens is required, total PN (TPN) is facilitated through a dedicated central line (Fig. 6-9). A peripheral line can be used to provide for lower osmolar solutions during shorter periods of time.

Since its early use, PN has benefited patients who meet the criteria for nutritional support because of temporary or permanent limitation of GI tract function. Because of lower costs and improved outcomes of patients administered EN, the use of PN has declined from its previous popularity and is now reserved for patients in whom contraindications to EN are present (see Box 6-2). To promote gut integrity and motility in patients on PN alone, small volumes of EN are encouraged, when possible. Prior to initiating PN, patients should be hemodynamically stable and able to tolerate the fluid volume and nutrient content of parenteral formulations; PN should be used with caution in patients with congestive heart failure, pulmonary disease, diabetes mellitus, and other metabolic disorders (Table 6-8).

**Table 6-7 Complications of Enteral Feeding**

| PROBLEM | COMMON CAUSES | MANAGEMENT |
|---|---|---|
| Diarrhea | Medications (e.g., antibiotics, $H_2$ blockers, laxatives, hyperosmotic, hypertonic solutions), feeding intolerance (osmolarity, fat), acquired lactase deficiency | Measure stool output.<br>Rule out infection (bacterial, viral, parasitic).<br>Supply fiber.<br>Change medication or formula.<br>Check osmolarity and infusion rate.<br>Administer antimotility medications (e.g., loperamide, codeine). |
| Nausea and vomiting | Delayed stomach emptying, constipation, abdominal distention, odor and appearance of formulations | Administer feedings at room temperature.<br>Use isotonic formulations.<br>Use a closed system when possible.<br>Reduce doses of narcotics.<br>Use gastroprokinetic agents (metoclopramide).<br>Monitor gastric residuals and stool output. |
| Constipation, fecal impaction | Dehydration, lack or excess of fiber | Monitor fluid balance daily.<br>Carry out rectal disimpaction.<br>Consider the use of cathartics, stool softeners, laxatives, or enemas. |
| Aspiration pneumonitis | Long-term supine position, delayed stomach emptying, altered mental status, malpositioned feeding tube, vomiting | Place head of bed at 45 degrees during feedings.<br>Stop EN if gastric residual volume exceeds 200 mL.<br>Use nasoduodenal or nasojejunal tubes in patients at risk. |
| Hyponatremia, overhydration | Excess fluid intake, refeeding syndrome, organ failure (e.g., liver, heart, kidney) | Monitor fluid balance and body weight daily.<br>Consider fluid restriction.<br>Change formula (avoid low- sodium intake).<br>Initiate diuretic therapy. |
| Hypernatremia | Dehydration, inadequate fluid intake | Increase free water. |
| Dehydration | Diarrhea, inadequate fluid intake | Determine cause.<br>Increase fluid intake. |
| Hyperglycemia | High content of carbohydrate in feedings, insulin resistance | Evaluate and adjust feeding formula.<br>Consider insulin regimen. |
| Hypokalemia, hypomagnesemia, hypophosphatemia | Diarrhea, refeeding syndrome | Correct electrolyte abnormalities.<br>Determine cause.<br>Reduce rate if refeeding syndrome is present and monitor patient. |
| Hyperkalemia | Excess potassium intake, renal impairment | Change feeding formula.<br>Reduce potassium intake.<br>Consider insulin regimen. |

**Table 6-8 Clinical Conditions Requiring Cautious Use of Parenteral Nutrition**

| CONDITION | SUGGESTED CRITERIA |
|---|---|
| Hyperglycemia | Glucose >300 mg/dL |
| Azotemia | BUN >100 mg/dL |
| Hyperosmolality | Serum osmolality >350 mOsm/kg |
| Hypernatremia | Na >150 mEq/L |
| Hypokalemia | K <3 mEq/L |
| Hyperchloremic metabolic acidosis | Cl >115 mEq/L |
| Hypophosphatemia | Phosphorus <2 mg/dL |
| Hypochloremic metabolic alkalosis | Cl <85 mEq/L |

From Mirtallo JM, In Gottschlich MM: The A.S.P.E.N. nutrition support core curriculum: a case-based approach: the adult patient, Silver Spring, Md, 2007, American Society for Parenteral and Enteral Nutrition, p 268.

*BUN,* Blood urea nitrogen.

**Table 6-9 Composition of Parenteral Nutrition Formulations**

| | Caloric Content | | | |
|---|---|---|---|---|
| SAMPLE NUTRITION* | g/dL | kcal/g | kcal/mL | mOsm/L |
| **2-in-1 Solutions** | | | | |
| Dextrose | | | | |
| DW 10% | 10 | 3.4 (CHO) | 0.34 | 505 |
| DW 30% | 30 | 3.4 (CHO) | 1.02 | 1510 |
| DW 70% | 70 | 3.4 (CHO) | 2.38 | 3530 |
| Amino acids | | | | |
| Aminosyn RF 5.2% | 5.2 | 4 (PRO) | 0.2 | 427 |
| Travasol 10% | 10 | 4 (PRO) | 0.4 | 998 |
| Prosol 20% | 20 | 4 (PRO) | 0.8 | 1835 |
| Lipid emulsion | | | | |
| Intralipid 10% | 10 | 11 (FAT)† | 1.1 | 300 |
| Intralipid 20% | 20 | 10 (FAT)† | 2 | 350 |
| Intralipid 30% | 30 | 10 (FAT)† | 3 | 310 |

*CHO,* Carbohydrate; *PRO,* protein.

*3-in-1 solutions: total nutrient admixture (TNA)

†Estimated at 9 kcal/g for fat plus additional calories from glycerol.

The use of PN is vital for patients with partial or complete GI dysfunction and who therefore are unable to digest and absorb sufficient nutrients, including patients with bowel obstruction, enteritis, fistulas or short bowel syndrome, and chemotherapy toxicity. Critically ill patients who are candidates for PN should be hemodynamically stable and have a clear contraindication to enteral feeding (e.g., ileus, acute GI bleeding, bowel obstruction), because in most other cases the efficacy of PN feeding remains controversial. The use of primary PN is uncertain in patients with Crohn's disease, ulcerative colitis, anorexia nervosa, scheduled cardiac surgery, or prolonged respiratory support. In patients undergoing chemotherapy, radiation, or marrow transplantation, the routine use of PN is associated with increased infectious complications, increased morbidity, and lack of survival improvement.[34]

### Formulations

PN includes all IV formulations, emulsions, or admixtures of nutrients that are administered in an elemental form. In the United States, PN formulations are traditionally composed of 60% to 70% dextrose and 10% to 20% amino acids, both administered daily and combined as 2-in-1 solutions. Formulations may also include 10% to 30% lipid emulsion, which may be combined together into a single formulation (3-in-1 solution) or supplemented separately, usually less often (once or twice weekly). Parenteral formulations can be ordered in solutions in a wide range of concentrations, including 10%-70% dextrose, 5.2%-20% amino acids, and 10%-30% lipid emulsions (Table 6-9).

In addition containing to sterile water, electrolytes, vitamins, and minerals, PN formulations can include medications, such as insulin and histamine 2 ($H_2$) blockers. Various combinations of these components are incorporated into the regimen for IV administration based on the patient's individual requirements.

### Ordering Parenteral Nutrition

In general, minimal fluid requirements in the absence of GI or other losses are 25 to 35 mL/kg/day (Fig. 6-10). Feeding volume is built up slowly over a few days. Using the example of a 70-kg person, one first calculates the overall caloric goal and the proportion contributed by protein, usually as follows:

$$\text{Total kilocalories } (25\text{–}35 \text{ kcal/kg/day}) = 30 \text{ kcal/kg/day} \times 70 \text{ kg} = 2100 \text{ kcal}$$

$$\text{Protein } (1.5 \text{ g/kg/day}) = 1.5 \text{ kcal/kg/day} \times 70 \text{ kg} = 105 \text{ g protein}$$

1. For TPN formulated without lipid (2-in-1 solution; in our practice, we recommend lipid infusion at least every 1 to 2 weeks for most patients to prevent essential fatty acid deficiency):

$$\text{Total kilocalories} = 2100 \text{ kcal}$$

$$\text{Calories from amino acids} = 105 \text{ g} \times 4 \text{ kcal/g} = 420 \text{ kcal}$$

$$\text{Remaining calories} = 2100 - 420 = 1680 \text{ kcal}$$

Then, make up the difference with dextrose:

$$1680 \text{ kcal}/(3.4 \text{ kcal/g}) = 494 \text{ g dextrose}$$

2. For TPN formulated with lipid (3-in-1 solution):

$$\text{Total kilocalories} = 2100 \text{ kcal}$$

Provide 20% of the total calories as lipid:

$$\text{Lipid} = 2100 \text{ kcal} \times 0.2 = 420 \text{ kcal}$$

$$420 \text{ kcal}/(9 \text{ kcal/g}) = 47 \text{ g lipid}$$

## Physician Orders
### PARENTERAL NUTRITION (PN) - ADULT

**Primary Diagnosis:** ______________ **Ht:** ______ cm **Dosing Wt:** ______ kg
**PN Indication:** ______________ **Allergies:** ______________

**Instructions:** This form must be completed for a new order or continuation of PN and faxed to the Pharmacy by **[Insert Time]** to receive same day preparation. PN administration begins at **[Insert Time]**. Contact the Nutrition Support Service at: (XXX)-XXX-XXXX for additional information.

**Administration Route:** ☐ CVC or PICC — *Note: Proper tip placement of the CVC or PICC must be confirmed prior to PN infusion*
☐ Peripheral IV (PIV) — *(Final PN Osmolarity ≤ ______ mOsm/L)*

**Monitoring:** Daily weights, strict input & output, bedside glucose monitoring every ______ hours
☐ Na, K, Cl, $CO_2$, glucose, BUN, Scr, Mg, $PO_4$, every ______________
☐ T. Bili, Alk Phos, AST, ALT, Albumin, Triglycerides, Calcium every ______________

**Base Solution:** *Select one* — *Parenteral nutrition **MUST** be administered through a dedicated infusion port and filtered with a 1.2-micron in-line filter at all times. Discard any unused volume after 24 hours.*

| ☐ **PERIPHERAL 2-in-1** | ☐ **CENTRAL 2-in-1** | ☐ **CENTRAL 3-in-1** |
|---|---|---|
| Dextrose ______ g | Dextrose ______ g | Dextrose ______ g |
| Amino Acids (*Brand* __________) ______ g | Amino Acids (*Brand* __________) ______ g | Amino Acids (*Brand* __________) ______ g |
| *For patients with PIV and established glucose tolerance: Provides _____ kcal; Maximum Rate not to exceed ______ mL/hour* | *For patients with CVC or PICC and established glucose tolerance: Provides _____ kcal; Maximum Rate not to exceed ______ mL/hour* | Fat Emulsion (*Brand* __________) ______ g |
| | | *For patients with CVC or PICC and established glucose/fat emulsion tolerance: Provides _____ kcal; Maximum Rate not to exceed ______ mL/hour* |
| | | *Use of additional fat emulsion not required with 3-in-1 base solution* |

**RATE & VOLUME:** ______ mL/hour for ______ hours = ______ mL/day
***Must specify***

*or* **CYCLIC INFUSION:** ______ mL/hour for ______ hours, then ______ mL/hour for ______ hours = ______ mL/day

**Fat Emulsion** (*Brand* __________) **- *via PIV or CVC with 2-in-1 base solutions*** *(Select caloric density & volume)*

☐ 10% ☐ 250 mL Infuse at ______ mL/hour over ______ hours Frequency __________
☐ 20% ☐ 500 mL *(Note: Infusions <4 or >12 hours not recommended)* *Discard any unused volume after 12 hours.*

| **Additives: (per day)** | | ***Normal Dosages*** |
|---|---|---|
| **Sodium** Chloride | ______ mEq | *1–2 mEq Sodium/kg/day* |
| as Acetate | ______ mEq | *pH or $CO_2$ dependent* |
| as Phosphate | ______ mmol of $PO_4$ | *Consider if hyperkalemic* |
| **Potassium** Chloride | ______ mEq | *1–2 mEq Potassium/kg/day* |
| as Acetate | ______ mEq | *pH or $CO_2$ dependent* |
| as Phosphate | ______ mmol of $PO_4$ | *20–40 mmol/day (1 mmol Phos = 1.5 mEq K)* |
| Calcium **Gluconate** | ______ mEq | *5–15 mEq/day* |
| Magnesium **Sulfate** | ______ mEq | *8–24 mEq/day* |
| Adult **Multivitamins** | ______ mL/day | *Contains Vitamin K 150 mcg* |
| Adult **Trace Elements** | ______ mL/day | *Zn ___ mg, Cu ___ mg, Mn ___ mg, Cr ___ mcg, Se ___ mcg (with normal hepatic function)* |
| **$H_2$ Antagonist** ______ | ______ mg | *___ mg/day with normal renal function* |
| **Other:** | | |

**Additives: (per day)**
**Regular Insulin** ______ units
*Recommend if hyperglycemic, start with 1 unit for every 10 g of dextrose*

***Pharmacy Use Only:* Ca/$PO_4$ Limit checked** ___
*(Note: Some brands of amino acids contain phosphate)*

**Physician's Signature:** ______________ **PagerNumber:** ______________ **Date/time:** __________
**Orders transcribed by:** __________ **Date/time:** __________ **Orders verified by:** __________ **Date/time:** __________
**SEND COMPLETED ORDERS TO PHARMACY**

**FIGURE 6-10** Adult PN order form. This template can serve as a guide to meet the criteria for mandatory and strongly recommended components of a PN order form. These components are not intended to be guidelines for formulas or monitoring. The PN order form content should be adapted to meet the needs of the individual institution based on patient population, prescribing patterns, and judgment by health care professionals. See text. (Adapted from Mirtallo J, Canada T, Johnson D, et al: Safe practices for parenteral nutrition. JPEN J Parenter Enteral Nutr 28[Suppl]:S39–S70, 2004.)

Calories from amino acids:

$$105\ g \times 4\ kcal/g = 420\ kcal$$

Remaining calories:

$$2100 - 420 - 420 = 1260\ kcal$$

Then, make up the difference with dextrose:

$$1260\ kcal/(3.4\ kcal/g) = 370\ g\ dextrose$$

Final volume (for 3-in-1, maximally concentrated):

$$\text{Amino acids (10\% stock solution)} = 105\ g = 1050\ mL$$

$$\text{Dextrose (70\% stock solution)} = 370\ g = 528\ mL$$

$$\text{Lipids (20\% stock solution)} = 47\ g = 235\ mL$$

$$\text{Total volume} = 1813\ mL/day$$

The final concentrations (wt/vol) are 5.8% amino acids, 20.4% dextrose, and 2.6% lipid.

### Complications

Parenteral feeding is associated with complications arising from line insertion and infection, which include pneumothorax, hematoma, bacteremia, endocarditis, damage to vessels and other structures, air embolism, and thrombosis. In contrast to EN, TPN has been associated with increased rates of bacterial translocation.[35] TPN has also been associated with increased proinflammatory cytokine levels and increased pulmonary dysfunction. The use of TPN, even as a simple supplement of maximally tolerated enteral feeding to reach nutritional requirements, has been associated with impairment of hepatic function and immune response.[36]

Overfeeding patients can lead to major complications. The overfeeding of carbohydrates results in elevated respiratory quotients, increased fat synthesis, and increased $CO_2$ elimination, leading to difficulty in weaning from ventilator support. Excess carbohydrate or fat can also lead to fat deposition in the liver. Excess protein replacement leads to elevations in blood urea nitrogen levels (Table 6-10).[10]

### Carbohydrate Content

Designated chemically as D-glucose, dextrose is the most commonly used carbohydrate substrate and provides 3.4 kcal/g (16 kJ). Dextrose solutions come in a wide range of concentrations and can be diluted as required to provide calories and adjust blood glucose levels. PN may contain dextrose or other carbohydrates as part of the formulation or be administered separately. Concentrated hypertonic dextrose solutions of 20% to 70% are usually administered via central lines, because these will cause irritation if administered into peripheral veins and can lead to thrombophlebitis. Contraindications to the use of concentrated dextrose solutions include alcohol withdrawal and delirium tremens in a dehydrated patient and suspected intracranial or intraspinal hemorrhage. Once metabolized, carbohydrates are ultimately oxidized to carbon dioxide and water,

**Table 6-10 Complications of Parenteral Nutrition**

| PROBLEM | COMMON CAUSES | MANAGEMENT |
|---|---|---|
| Hypoglycemia | Excess insulin administration, sudden cessation of PN infusion | Stop insulin.<br>Start 10% dextrose IV.<br>Give a 50% dextrose ampule before resuming central line feeding. |
| Hyperglycemia | Excess dextrose concentration, stress-associated (e.g., sepsis), chromium deficiency | 0.1-0.2 U insulin/g dextrose therapy, SQ or IV insulin sliding scale, limit dextrose content, consider discontinuing PN until improved blood glucose control |
| Hypertriglyceridemia (acceptable concentrations <400 mg/dL) | Dextrose overfeeding, rapid administration of intravenous fatty emulsion (>110 mg/kg/hr) | Infusion of IVFE should be restricted to less than 30% of total calories or 1g/kg/day, given slowly, over no less than 8 to 10 hr, if administered separately |
| Essential fatty acid deficiency (e.g., dermatitis, alopecia, hepatomegaly, thrombocytopenia, anemia) | 1- to 3-wk administration of PN lacking linoleic and alpha-linolenic fatty acid emulsions | 2%-4% daily energy requirements should be derived from linoleic acid, 0.5% from alpha-linolenic acid[43] (500 mL of 10% IVFE over 8 to 10 hr, twice weekly) |
| Electrolyte and mineral abnormalities | Inadequate monitoring | Modification of subsequent infusions<br>Parenteral iron uncommonly increases risk of anaphylactic reactions |
| Azotemia | Dehydration, excess protein, inadequate carbohydrate calories | Free water, 5% dextrose via a peripheral vein |
| Metabolic bone disease (osteoporosis in 41% of those on long- term home PN) | Unclear, multifactorial (e.g., postmenopausal, long-term PN, Cushing's syndrome, Crohn's disease, malabsorption, multiple myeloma, osteogenesis imperfect, corticosteroids, heparin, immobilization) | Early screening of risk factors, DEXA, management of premorbid conditions<br>Special PN considerations: Supplement calcium, P, Mg, Cu<br>Minimize aluminum contamination, treat metabolic acidosis, avoid heparin |
| Elevated liver function parameters (increased transaminase, bilirubin, alkaline phosphatase levels) | Common following initiation; usually temporary | If persistent, usually caused by amino acid load; reduce protein delivery. |

*DEXA,* Dual-energy x-ray absorptiometry.

so caution should be used to control infusion rates to avoid hyperglycemia and hypercapnia when weaning patients from ventilator support.

In the acute setting, supplying sufficient carbohydrate reduces liver glycogen breakdown; it may also exert a protein-sparing effect by supplying an alternate fuel to amino acids. Endogenous glucose production has been shown to be significantly suppressed when glucose is infused at a rate of 1 mg/kg/min and maximally suppressed at 4 mg/kg/min, with or without exogenous insulin infusion,[37] because infusion at a faster rate does not suppress gluconeogenesis further.

Glucose infusion rates require greater monitoring and caution in pediatric patients because of the increased risk of hyperglycemia and hypoglycemia. A suggested guideline maximum concentration is 25% dextrose at an infusion rate of up to 7 mg/kg/min.

When calculating TPN requirements, protein requirements are usually calculated first and subtracted from total calories, with remaining calorie requirements met with carbohydrate, with or without lipids. Formulations are often concentrated because patients in a critical care setting may often be at risk of volume overload.

### Lipid Content

IV fat emulsions (IVFEs) provide a dense source of calories and are particularly useful when carbohydrate administration approaches maximal limits or blood glucose control is an issue. They are also useful in preventing essential fatty acid deficiency. The optimal use of lipid emulsions during parenteral feeding remains controversial, however, especially with regard to critically ill surgical patients and patients under metabolic stress, because changes in fatty acid metabolism following severe injuries may predispose these particular patients to the adverse effects of lipid infusions. Delivery of lipid emulsion has been associated with immune suppression, modulation of the inflammatory response, and adverse clinical outcomes.[38] In polytrauma patients, infusion of IVFE in the early postinjury period has been associated with increased length of intensive care unit (ICU) and hospital stay, prolonged mechanical ventilation, and increased susceptibility to infection compared with patients not given IVFE until after 10 days.[39] However, it remains uncertain whether these differences are attributable to withholding lipid or provision of less total calories.

Commercially available parenteral regimens in the United States are composed of soybean oil rich in the omega-6 fatty acid linoleic acid, a precursor of arachidonic acid used in the synthesis pathway of prostaglandins, thromboxanes, and leukotrienes. Because of this proinflammatory potential, there is a trend to limiting omega-6 content and switching to lipids such as fish oil or to those rich in omega-3 fatty acids, such as eicosapentaenoic acid, which competes to reduce cell membrane availability of arachidonic acid and its products. Reduced prostaglandin and leukotriene levels lead to diminished chemotaxis and cytokine production and decreased platelet aggregation, coagulation, and smooth muscle contraction. Other potential effects of excessive levels of long-chain omega-6 fatty acids include depletion of available antioxidants in plasma lipoproteins.

Polyunsaturated omega-3 fatty acids found in fish oil have been shown to prevent the development of inflammatory conditions by modulating the synthesis of eicosanoids and other inflammatory mechanisms. A recent meta-analysis that examined the use of fish oil emulsions and included six non-U.S. randomized controlled trials in elective surgical patients has shown a significant reduction in infectious complications and shortened hospital stay, although it demonstrated no mortality benefit overall.[40] However, an earlier meta-analysis of the immunologic effects of lipid emulsions found no clear evidence that long-chain TGs detrimentally affect immune function.[41]

Potential deficiency of essential fatty acids may occur after the first week of parenteral feeding, although patients with large adipose stores can go for much longer without supplementation. In our practice, a minimum of 500 mL of lipid emulsion every 2 weeks is recommended to avoid essential fatty acid deficiency during parenteral feeding.

### Protein Content

The recommended daily amount of protein intake for most healthy adults is 0.8 g/kg body weight/day (46-56 g/day). Muscle protein degradation following severe injury leads to loss of lean mass, which persists for months after visible wound healing,[42] and approximately 20% of total energy requirements is needed in the form of protein intake to limit this loss, at least. This is equivalent to 1.5 to 2.0 g protein/kg IBW/day in fasted surgical patients and up to 3.0 g/kg/day in severely injured patients. Most standard enteral and parenteral feeding mixtures provide this increased quantity of protein if sufficient volume of formula is delivered to meet the patients increased caloric requirements. Traditionally, the nitrogen-to-calorie ratio for most feeding formulas prepared for surgical patients has been 1:150 (i.e., 1 g of nitrogen for every 150 kcal), and for PN a protein-fat-glucose caloric ratio has generally approximated 20:30:50. Patients with chronic renal failure and hepatic failure have conventionally been treated with low-protein diets.

### Fluid and Electrolytes

Patients with GI disorders, particularly those leading to extensive bowel resection, may experience demanding water and electrolyte imbalances. These patients require extra vigilance; monitoring is critical for the prevention, early diagnosis, and treatment of these imbalances. In adult patients with PN, at least 30 to 40 mL/kg of fluid, 1 to 2 mEq/kg of sodium and potassium, 10 to 15 mEq of calcium, 8 to 20 mEq of magnesium, and 20 to 40 mmol of phosphate should be administered daily.[43] Patients who are rapidly anabolic, including those previously malnourished, may require additional potassium, magnesium, and phosphorus, whereas those with renal impairment may require restriction.

## SPECIAL CONSIDERATIONS

This section considers nutritional support in relation to a number of surgical conditions and describes current metabolic and nutritional strategies.

### Burn Injury and the Metabolic Stress Response

Following all forms of major trauma, inflammatory and hormonal responses are activated and greatly influence metabolic pathways and mechanisms. Nutrient intake, absorption, and substrate uptake will be affected during the different stages of the stress response.

Elevated metabolic rate is a common feature of critical illness, arising in such conditions as trauma, major surgery, severe burns, and sepsis. The stress response leads to activation of an array of physiologic processes that respond to altered metabolic requirements and attempt to restore homeostasis. Although these changes may initially be beneficial, in critical illness and sepsis, inflammation and associated changes are often exaggerated and prolonged, leading to clinical complications, delayed recovery, and increased mortality. Nutrient requirements will increase but become more difficult to predict, and enteral or parenteral feeding will often be necessary to meet vastly increased nutritional requirements.

Severe burns affecting approximately 30% or more of the TBSA are associated with a major elevation in metabolic rate. The inflammatory and hormonal mechanisms underlying this response are complex but are known to include a prolonged rise in circulating catecholamine, glucocorticoid, and glucagon levels, leading to elevated rates of gluconeogenesis, glycogenolysis, and protein catabolism. Other features of metabolic dysfunction include insulin resistance and increased peripheral lipolysis.

Burns are classified according to their size, mechanism, and depth of injury. They range from superficial burns affecting the epidermis only to partial-thickness (second-degree) burns that involve the dermis and full-thickness (third-degree) burns extending through all layers of the skin. An estimate of the body surface burned can be obtained using the rule of nines (modified for pediatric use according to age) or a Lund-Browder chart.

Patients with severe burns need fluid resuscitation to prevent hypovolemic shock, guided by the percentage of body surface area burned and body weight. Several different formulas are used to calculate requirements over the first 24 hours (see Chapter 21). Urine output remains the best indicator of volume status, with minimum target values of 0.5 mL/kg/hr in adults and 1 mL/kg/hr in children. Overresuscitation should be avoided to prevent complications of fluid overload, including pulmonary edema and cardiac dysfunction.

Early resuscitation of severely burned patients is of primary importance. In circumstances in which medical care is not immediately available—for example, in isolated locations or in mass casualty situations—this may be possible through oral rehydration and basic electrolyte replacement, because most patients will initially be able to drink.

Nutritional support should be initiated as early as possible to supply vastly elevated caloric and protein demands. Patients will usually have a functioning GI tract but may be incapable of sufficient oral intake to meet requirements, particularly after larger burns, and enteral feeding is the route of choice to supplement or replace oral intake. Although nutritional support aims to offset losses and maintain energy requirements, nutritional supplementation alone has not been found to be completely effective for arresting loss of muscle mass. Strategies to counteract the features of hypermetabolism and catabolism include pharmacologic, surgical, and environmental interventions.

Early volume resuscitation and enteral feeding are important to preserve the integrity of the GI mucosa; otherwise, diminished splanchnic blood flow will increase the risk of mucosal atrophy, bacterial overgrowth, translocation, and sepsis. Early excision of deep burns and wound closure with a skin graft or skin substitute, maintaining environmental temperature to prevent excessive heat loss, and early use of nutritional feeding have all significantly improved outcomes after injury. For example, modulating the hormonal and inflammatory response, improving wound healing, and reducing muscle catabolism have led to great reductions in morbidity and mortality.

Caloric requirements in patients with severe burns can be difficult to predict accurately, because energy expenditure is drastically increased and varies with the condition of the patient, operative interventions, and septic episodes. A variety of formulas can be used to estimate caloric requirements in burn patients although, if available, indirect calorimetry provides a superior estimate of energy needs and can also be used to determine the respiratory quotient to detect overfeeding (Tables 6-11 and 6-12). Indirect calorimetry provides a value for REE, with the measurement typically increased by 10% to 20% to allow for variability and activity when used to guide feeding.

Severe burn injuries of 30% or more of the TBSA represent one of the most severe forms of trauma, with extreme and prolonged muscle wasting seen in these patients. Negative nitrogen balance, insulin resistance, lipolysis, and protein wasting may persist for up to 1 year following severe injuries, leading to a significant delay in rehabilitation.

Pharmacologic treatments have been investigated for their potential to counteract catabolic effects and attenuate the metabolic response in the acute and rehabilitation phases. These include anabolic agents such as recombinant human growth hormone (in children), oxandrolone, insulin, IGF-1, and β-adrenergic receptor (AR) blockers, such as propranolol. Nonpharmacologic strategies include early wound closure, prevention of infection, environmental thermoregulation, high-carbohydrate, high-protein continuous enteral feeding, and early institution of resistive exercise programs. Modulation of the stress response also includes pain and anxiety control through the administration of analgesia and anxiolytics and psychological therapy.

**Table 6-11 Formulas for Estimating Caloric Requirements in Adult Burn Patients**

| FORMULA | EQUATION | COMMENTS |
|---|---|---|
| **Harris-Benedict**[61] | | |
| Men | BEE (kcal/ day) = 66.5 + (13.75 × W ) + (5.00 × H ) − (6.76 × A) | Multiply BEE by stress factor of 1.2-2.0 (1.2-1.5 sufficient for most burns) to estimate caloric requirement. |
| Women | BEE (kcal/day) = 655 + (9.56 × W) + (1.85 × H) − (4.68 × A) | |
| **Curreri** | | |
| Age, 16-59 yr | Calories (kcal/day) = (25 × W) + (40 × % BSAB) | Specific for burns, may significantly overestimate energy requirements, maximum 50% BSAB |
| Age > 60 yr | Calories (kcal/day) = (20 × W) + (65 × % BSAB) | |

*A,* Age (yr); *BEE,* basal energy expenditure; *% BSAB,* percentage of total body surface area burned; *H,* height (cm); *W,* weight (kg).

**Table 6-12 Formulas for Estimating Caloric Requirements in Pediatric Burn Patients**

| FORMULA | SEX / AGE (YEARS) | EQUATION (DAILY REQUIREMENT IN KCAL) |
|---|---|---|
| WHO | Males 0-3 | $(60.9 \times W) - 54$ |
| | 3-10 | $(22.7 \times W) + 495$ |
| | 10-18 | $(17.5 \times W) + 651$ |
| | Females 0-3 | $(61.0 \times W) - 51$ |
| | 3-10 | $(22.5 \times W) + 499$ |
| | 10-18 | $(12.2 \times W) + 746$ |
| RDA | 0-6 months | $108 \times W$ |
| | 6 months-1 year | $98 \times W$ |
| | 1-3 | $102 \times W$ |
| | 4-10 | $90 \times W$ |
| | 11-14 | $55 \times W$ |
| Curreri junior | <1 | RDA + (15 × %BSAB) |
| | 1-3 | RDA + (25 × %BSAB) |
| | 4-15 | RDA + (40 × %BSAB) |
| Galveston infant | 0-1 | 2100 kcal/ $m^2$ BSA + 1000 kcal/$m^2$ BSAB |
| Galveston revised | 1-11 | 1800 kcal/ $m^2$ BSA+ 1300 kcal/$m^2$ BSAB |
| Galveston adolescent | 12+ | 1500 kcal/ $m^2$ BSA+ 1500 kcal/$m^2$ BSAB |

Adapted from Al-Mousawi A, Branski LK, Andel HL, et al: Ernährungstherapie bei Brandverletzten. In Kamolz LP, Herndon DN, Jeschke MG (eds): Verbrennungen: Diagnose, Therapie und Rehabilitation des thermischen Traumas, German Edition. New York: Springer-Verlag/Wien, 2009, pp 183–194.

*BSA,* Body surface area; *RDA,* recommended dietary allowance.

**Table 6-13 Effect of Omega-3 Polyunsaturated Fatty Acids on Eicosanoid Synthesis***

| METABOLITE | PHYSIOLOGIC ACTION | OMEGA-3 EFFECT |
|---|---|---|
| **AA Eicosanoid** | | |
| $PGE_2$ | Proinflammatory, vasodilator† | ↓ |
| $TXA_2$ | Potent platelet aggregation and vasoconstrictor | ↓ |
| $LTB_4$ | Proinflammatory, neutrophil chemotaxis | ↓ |
| **EPA Eisocanoid** | | |
| $TXA_3$ | Mild platelet aggregation | ↑ |
| $PGI_3$ | Mild platelet disaggregation | ↑ |
| RvE1 | Potent anti-inflammatory | ↑ |
| **DHA Docosanoid** | | |
| RvD1 | Potent anti-inflammatory | ↑ |
| NPD1 | Potent anti-inflammatory, neuroprotective bioactivity | ↑ |

*AA,* Arachidonic acid; *DHA,* docosahexaenoic acid; *EPA,* eicosapentaenoic acid; *LT,* leukotriene; *NP,* neuroprotectin; *PG,* prostaglandin; *PGI,* prostacyclin; *Rv,* resolvin; *TX,* thromboxane.

*Biochemical basis of a less inflammatory phenotype.

†Prostaglandin E2 has been reported to have dual activity as both a pro- and anti-inflammatory. The latter, although weak, has been reported to be the effect of the induced production of lipoxins.

Early excision of full-thickness burn wounds and application of skin grafts or substitutes is known to decrease metabolic rates greatly in these patients when compared with those whose surgery is delayed to 1 week after injury. By keeping ambient temperatures at 33° C, the metabolic rate in patients with large burns is also reduced.[44] Providing a structured exercise program in conjunction with occupational and physical therapy during rehabilitation improves passive and active range of motion, muscle strength, and lean body mass.[45] Propranolol is a nonselective β-AR antagonist that has been shown to reduce thermogenesis, tachycardia, and REE in burn patients. Catecholamines trigger increased peripheral lipolysis in injured patients; propranolol may help reduce the impact of excessive circulating catecholamines on lipolysis and substantially decrease fatty infiltration of the liver.

In severely burned children, recombinant human growth hormone and oxandrolone, a synthetic testosterone analogue and anabolic agent, have both shown promising results during hypermetabolic states, significantly improving growth and lean body mass. In adult patients, however, a European multicenter trial has reported significantly greater mortality in critical care patients administered growth hormone,[46] and its use is therefore only considered for children.

## Immunonutrition

Major injury, whether traumatic or induced by surgery, results in significant suppression of immune function, which may influence a patient's recovery. Specific nutrients, including arginine, omega-3 polyunsaturated fatty acids, glutamine, and nucleotides, have been shown to modulate the host response in animal and clinical experiments, with potential improvements in immune function but inconsistent clinical evidence. The working hypothesis is that the clinical use of a solution containing increased amounts of arginine stimulates T lymphocytes and provides a substrate for the generation of NO, whereas the inclusion of omega-3 fatty acids promotes the synthesis of more favorable prostaglandins, and inclusion of nucleotides nonspecifically enhances immune competence. Long-chain omega-3 fatty acids decrease the production of inflammatory eicosanoids, cytokines, and adhesion molecules. This occurs directly by replacing arachidonic acid as an eicosanoid substrate, inhibiting arachidonic acid metabolism, and giving rise to anti-inflammatory resolvins. The indirect effect occurs through the modulation of transcription factors that regulate the expression of inflammatory genes. Omega-3 polyunsaturated fatty acids are potentially useful anti-inflammatory agents and may be beneficial for patients at risk of acute and chronic inflammatory conditions (Table 6-13).[47]

A number of clinical trials have evaluated the efficacy of immune-enhancing enteral formulas and have shown superior outcomes compared with standard formulations in certain patient populations. Their use has been recommended from 7 days prior to 7 days after surgery in the following circumstances[25,28,48]:

- Major neck surgery for cancer (e.g., laryngectomy, pharyngectomy)
- Severely malnourished patients (serum albumin level <2.8 g/dL) or patients undergoing major oncologic GI surgery (e.g., esophagus, stomach, pancreas, duodenum, hepatobiliary tree)

- Patients with severe trauma to two or more body systems (e.g., abdomen, chest, head, spinal cord, extremities) and an injury severity score ≥18 or abdominal trauma index ≥20, which generally includes grade 3 pancreatoduodenal, grade 4 colonic, and grade 4 hepatic or gastric injuries
- Patients with mild sepsis (APACHE II score <15); although possibly harmful and not recommended for patients with severe sepsis
- Patients with acute respiratory distress syndrome (ARDS)

No sufficient data are available to support the use of immune-enhancing formulations in burned patients. However, reduced mortality, wound healing time, and length of hospital stay have been shown in burn patients receiving glutamine supplementation to standard EN formulations.[49,50]

### Omega-3 and Omega-6 Fatty Acids

These include linoleic acid (an omega-6 polyunsaturated fatty acid) and alpha-linolenic acid (an omega-3 polyunsaturated fatty acid). The omega number refers to the position of the first carbon-carbon double bond (unsaturated) relative to the omega end of the fatty acid. Rich sources of both fatty acids may be found in plants, whereas fish also contain high levels of omega-3. Linoleic and alpha-linolenic acids are essential fatty acids that the body cannot produce from alternative sources. These are important compounds in the production of highly unsaturated fatty acids and are critical for the growth of skin, blood, and neural cells as well as for the configuration of highly specialized lipid membranes, such as those of neural synapses, retinal pigment epithelium cells, and myocardial cells. By means of elongation, desaturation, and β-oxidation steps, these essential fatty acids also give rise to eicosanoids. These compounds are involved in cell signaling and contribute to the regulation of a number of responses, including arterial pressure, hemostasis, bronchoconstriction, vasoconstriction, platelet aggregation, and inflammatory and immune responses.

Linoleic acid is converted to arachidonic acid in the omega-6 pathway of essential fatty acids. Arachidonic acid, an omega-6 polyunsaturated fatty acid, is a precursor in the biosynthesis of eicosanoids such as prostaglandins, prostacyclins, lipoxins, thromboxanes, and leukotrienes. Alpha-linolenic acid is first converted to eicosapentaenoic acid and subsequently to docosahexaenoic acid in the omega-3 pathway. Regulation of these pathways involves multiple factors (e.g., diet, hormones, toxins), but the key regulating enzymes are Δ-6-desaturase and Δ-5-desaturase. Table 6-13 shows precursor fatty acids, their metabolites, respective physiologic actions, and theoretical effect of omega-3–enriched diets.

**Optimal Omega-6-to-Omega-3 Ratio in the Diet** Potential benefits of nutritional supplementation with fish oil–derived omega-3 fatty acids, compared with the more common omega-6 fatty acids from plant sources include improved immune responses and outcomes. These benefits may derive from a reduced incidence of hyperglycemia and decreased production of proinflammatory cytokines such as prostaglandin E2 and leukotrienes. These are derived from arachidonic acid metabolism, through which omega-6 fatty acids are also metabolized.

Various and controversial reports contrasting the effects of arachidonic (n-6), eicosapentaenoic (n-3), and docosahexaenoic (n-3) acid in particular (as it pertains to immunomodulation) have raised the issue of whether the n-6–to–n-3 polyunsaturated fatty acid (PUFA) ratio may need to be controlled in the administration of nutritional support. It is clear that n-3 fatty acids play important roles in prostaglandin metabolism, thrombosis, atherosclerosis, immunology and inflammation, and membrane function. There is evidence to support the use of n-3 fatty acids in inflammatory disorders such as Crohn's disease, ulcerative colitis, rheumatoid arthritis, and asthma.

## Organ Transplantation

In organ transplantation, consideration must be given to the assessment of the patient's nutritional status and preparation for metabolic disturbances in the postoperative period. Although organ recipients do not necessarily have a propensity to develop high metabolic rates unless secondary conditions are present (e.g., sepsis, other surgical complications), an elevated REE has been reported following surgery, by up to 42% above predicted values 10 days after liver transplantation,[51] and to be persistently increased up to 1 year post-transplantation. Therefore, 1.3 to 1.5 times the calculated basal energy expenditure, or 30 to 35 kcal/kg, are recommended for these patients to prevent loss of weight and lean body mass. A number of immunosuppressive medications are used to prevent and treat rejection of newly transplanted organs. The side effects of these drugs often have an impact on nutrient intake and digestion, most commonly in the form of GI disorders (e.g., constipation, diarrhea, nausea and vomiting, dyspepsia, pancreatitis). Malnutrition is therefore an important factor influencing outcome after organ transplantation, and optimization of overall nutritional status prior to and following surgery is critical for the living donor and the recipient.

## Inflammatory Bowel Disease

During the course of their disease, patients with inflammatory bowel disease often experience a range of complications that impair their nutritional status, including significant weight loss caused by sitophobia (aversion to food), diarrhea, protein-wasting enteropathy, GI bleeding, development of fistulas, and abdominal pain. Acute exacerbations may also cause increased energy demands and worsening of these complications. In Crohn's disease, criteria to initiate nutritional support are similar to those for other patients (see earlier). When EN is indicated, formulas low in fat content show improved efficacy compared with elemental or semielemental formulas. PN usually does not have a primary role unless EN is contraindicated. Additionally, PN may be used temporarily (<2 weeks) in combination with antibiotics with the intention of allow healing of the GI mucosa that would further facilitate surgery. In Crohn's patients with severe short bowel syndrome, home PN is particularly suitable.

## Short Bowel Syndrome

Short bowel syndrome results from resection of functioning gut to a length below that necessary for adequate digestion and absorption of nutrients. In adults, resection is most commonly performed because of Crohn's disease, mesenteric thrombosis, and volvulus, whereas in infants, necrotizing enterocolitis is the most common cause. Within 24 to 48 hours after resection, the intestinal adaptation process begins with epithelial hyperplasia in the intestinal crypts. If a patient is left with 1.5 feet of small bowel anastomosed to the left colon, hypertrophy of the remaining small bowel will, in most cases, enable survival while reducing the need of daily PN support to twice weekly. The goal of nutritional support in short bowel syndrome is to maximize intestinal adaptation through aggressive EN while limiting complications. EN has a potent trophic effect on the intestinal mucosa, resulting in lengthening of intestinal villi, increasing absorptive surface area, and improving digestive and absorptive function. Patients receiving home TPN commonly survive for 10 to 20 years or even longer, which was not possible prior to the development of TPN. Some patients undergo sufficient hypertrophy of the remaining small bowel that the need for home TPN is ultimately decreased or removed. Efforts to promote more rapid hypertrophy of the small bowel by using gut-specific hormones, fiber, fuels, and isotonic solutions have been reported. More randomized prospective trials are needed to determine the efficacy of nutrient and non-nutrient stimuli in maximizing intestinal adaptation and optimizing the management of short bowel syndrome.

## Malnutrition States

### Marasmus

Marasmus is caused by a deficiency in dietary calories. It is a serious worldwide problem, particularly affecting children in developing countries. In surgical patients, it is commonly associated with infections and GI tract disturbances. The changes in metabolism seen during marasmus are similar to those in starvation, discussed earlier. Marasmus can result from decreased energy intake, increased loss of ingested calories (diarrhea, emesis), or increased energy expenditure. The response to energy deficiency is a decrease in basal energy metabolism, slowing of growth, and loss of muscle mass and subcutaneous fat deposits. Management of marasmus involves cautious nutritional rehabilitation, correction of electrolyte imbalance, and aggressive treatment of complications such as infections, dehydration, anemia, and heart failure. During treatment, these patients are at significant risk of developing refeeding syndrome and potential death, particularly if weight loss more than 10% has recently been recorded. This is also true even in nonmarasmatic surgical patients with starvation periods of at least 7 to 10 days who are hypercatabolic or who have a history of anorexia nervosa, chronic alcoholism, or cancer.

### Kwashiorkor

Kwashiorkor is a condition caused by protein-energy malnutrition. In developing countries, kwashiorkor is more commonly caused by famine or an insufficient food supply. In the developed world, most cases are an indication of severe neglect or abuse. Secondary protein-energy malnutrition has been attributed to gastric surgery, anorexia nervosa, and diseases involving significant loss of ingested nutrients (e.g., pancreatic insufficiency, celiac disease, ulcerative colitis, cystic fibrosis, renal failure, malignancies). Features of kwashiorkor include pedal edema, apathy, hepatic enlargement, skin atrophy and depigmentation, and decreased muscle mass. The World Health Organization (WHO) has devised a three-phase management approach; the patient is first resuscitated and stabilized (phase 1), prior to starting nutritional rehabilitation (phase 2), and final follow-up and recurrence prevention (phase 3).[52]

## Sepsis

Sepsis is a major cause of death among hospitalized patients, causing over 200,000 deaths yearly in the United States and accounting for more than $10 billion spent on health care.[53] Following the onset of sepsis, proinflammatory cytokines stimulate the secretion of cortisol, glucagon, and catecholamines. These hormones promote glycogenolysis and gluconeogenesis. Once glycogen stores are exhausted, lipid and protein become the major sources of energy. Infection causes modifications in the production and uptake of glucose, resulting in hyperglycemia. As sepsis progresses, visceral blood flow is reduced, leading to the development of hypoglycemia. Metabolism during sepsis is associated with an increase in metabolic rate of up to 50% above basal energy expenditure.

Protein metabolism is also deranged during sepsis. There is increased synthesis of certain proteins, associated with a reprioritization of hepatic protein synthesis, and an increase in the synthesis of acute-phase proteins such as C-reactive protein, whereas synthesis of constitutive proteins such as albumin and prealbumin decreases. Increased synthesis of glutamine occurs during sepsis. Glutamine serves as a primary fuel for the immune system and gut epithelium, maintaining the protective barrier function of the gut mucosa and increasing blood flow to the intestine. The excretion of breakdown products of muscle such as urea, creatinine, uric acid, and ammonia is increased. The net protein loss in severe sepsis can exceed 2 g/kg/day. Studies have shown that despite receiving adequate nutritional support, septic patients can lose more than 10% of total body protein in 3 weeks.[54] If the catabolic state is not modified, tissue repair and immune response are impaired, with severe loss of skeletal and visceral proteins also occurring.

The catabolic hormones induce lipolysis of triacylglycerol (TAG) stored in adipose tissue to glycerol and free fatty acids. In severe sepsis, hyperlipidemia and hyperlactemia are present, with a discrepancy occurring between lactate production and lactate uptake, which results in increased plasma lactate concentrations; increasing levels are associated with severe sepsis.

Nutritional support helps combat the negative effects of sepsis and maintain immunity, reduce skeletal muscle breakdown, improve wound healing, and preserve gut mucosal barrier function. The beneficial effect of nutrition lies in providing additional substrate for acute-phase protein synthesis. Outcomes in critical care populations have improved with the initiation of early enteral feeding; improved nutrition supports a functional immune system and reduces septic morbidity and mortality.

## Hepatic Insufficiency

The liver has a remarkable ability to recover and compensate, with 80% to 90% impairment required for features of hepatic insufficiency to appear (e.g., decreased albumin, prolonged prothrombin time, mental confusion). Hepatic insufficiency results in a catabolic state similar to sepsis. Cytokines have been implicated in this catabolic state. Increased levels of tumor necrosis factor (TNF), interleukin-1 (IL-1), and IL-6 are seen, which have catabolic effects on muscle, adipose tissue, and liver. Lipids and proteins replace carbohydrates as primary sources of energy, resulting in depletion of lipid and protein reserves. There is a derangement of carbohydrate, lipid, and protein metabolism. Glucose intolerance occurs, along with decreased storage of glycogen in the liver and muscle. Fatty acid levels, ketone body levels, and ketone body production are increased. Inhibition of lipoprotein lipase affects lipid storage, resulting in an imbalance between fat synthesis and catabolism. There is an increase in urine nitrogen losses with normal renal function. The increased protein catabolism does not return to normal with feeding. The net effect of these metabolic abnormalities is protein-calorie malnutrition.

A serum amino acid imbalance is also seen with increased levels of phenylalanine, tyrosine, and tryptophan (aromatic amino acids) and decreased levels of the BCAAs leucine, valine, and isoleucine. This imbalance results in abnormal amine neurotransmitter products in which norepinephrine and dopamine are replaced by compounds such as octopamine and phenylethanolamine.[55] This imbalance is a possible basis for hepatic encephalopathy. Treatment involves monitoring protein intake. The quantity of amino acid in the diet is reduced to 20 to 40 g/day. If encephalopathy worsens or does not improve, formulations are administered with increased concentration of BCAAs and reduced aromatic amino acid concentration. In general, parenteral formulations are better tolerated than enteral formulations.

Most patients with hepatic failure have increased losses of potassium, magnesium, and zinc, so close attention to fluid and electrolyte management is necessary. Significant ascites can be treated with fluid restriction.

### Gastric Bypass Surgery

In a Roux-en-Y gastric bypass, the stomach volume is reduced by creating a small pouch at the top of the stomach using surgical staples or a plastic band. The stomach is then connected directly to the middle portion of the small intestine (jejunum), bypassing the rest of the stomach, duodenum, and proximal portion of jejunum. GLP-1, produced by L cells in the distal intestinal tract, is a powerful incretin. Patients who have a Roux-en-Y gastric bypass have increased levels of GLP-1 with improvement in diabetes, results not seen after restrictive bariatric procedures. Following gastric bypass and jejunointestinal bypass, a pleiotropic endocrine response may contribute to the improved glycemic control, appetite reduction, and long-term changes in body weight.[56]

### Intensive Insulin and Glycemic Control

In diabetic and nondiabetic surgical patients, hyperglycemia and hypoglycemia have been associated with increased morbidity and mortality. Hyperglycemia increases inflammation and has deleterious effects on the immune, respiratory, renal, and nervous systems. Hyperglycemia increases infection rates, length of hospital stay, ventilator dependence, and mortality and decreases the rate of wound healing.[57] Hypoglycemia results in detrimental effects, especially in the central and autonomic nervous systems and circulatory system. Clinically, it is manifested by dizziness, drowsiness, fatigue, tachycardia, seizures, and coma. Control of systemic and local glucose levels are critical to local wound healing and overall outcomes.

Using intensive insulin protocols to maintain tight glycemic control has emerged as an important therapy in improving outcomes and reducing complications in critical care patients.[57] The severe stress response of critical illness leads to insulin resistance and impaired uptake of glucose, and these protocols help reduce the incidence of hyperglycemic episodes by maintaining normoglycemia. Controversy persists regarding the blood glucose levels to target and indications for initiating intensive insulin therapy.

### Pancreatitis

The incidence of acute pancreatitis continues to rise worldwide, correlating with increasing alcohol consumption at a current rate of 35/100,000, with mortality reaching 40% in severe cases and up to 80% in septic patients with multiorgan failure. Severe cases of pancreatitis are associated with the development of sepsis and prolonged organ failure; however, patients have traditionally been kept NPO to minimize pancreatic stimulation and decrease its subsequent inflammation. Currently, this practice is known to lead to intestinal ischemia, bacterial translocation, and potential sepsis. A meta-analysis of 291 patients has revealed that patients with acute pancreatitis who received EN had significantly reduced infectious complications, although no significant differences were observed in mortality.[58] Presently, no evidence suggests a beneficial action of the addition of prokinetics in patients with severe acute pancreatitis.

In patients with acute pancreatitis, initial volume resuscitation and pain control should be followed by early postpyloric enteral feeding, commencing within 24 hours of admission; this has been shown to reduce complications, length of stay, and mortality.[59] Patients with mild acute pancreatitis may commence a low-fat oral diet.

The pancreas only manifests signs of endocrine or exocrine insufficiency after 90% of its cell mass has been destroyed. In chronic pancreatitis, pain and continued alcoholism are mainly associated with the development of early malnutrition before organ damage reaches criteria for insufficiency. It is essential, therefore, that nutritional management in these patients begin with abstinence from alcohol and relief from abdominal pain, with the addition of pancreatic enzymes as necessary, management of nutrient-specific deficiencies, and initiation of PN, when indicated.

### Obesity

The prevalence of obesity in the industrialized world is increasing and has resulted in a growing number of obese patients. Extensive research in humans and animals provides evidence that obesity is caused by dietary and genetic factors. Gene defects in the coding sequences for leptin and the melanocortin-4 receptor have been identified as being contributory to the occurrence of clinically severe obesity. These gene defects are very rare, however, and there are currently 600 candidate genes under investigation that are suspected to be involved in a polygenic manner in the development of obesity. However, genetic factors are only contributory and susceptibility factors in obesity, with dietary behavior identified as the main factor responsible for the huge increase.

Unbalanced caloric intake compared with energy needs is one of the leading factors leading to weight gain. Altered nutritional behaviors in the industrialized world over recent decades, with larger portions of processed high-calorie foods, sugar-sweetened drinks, and increasingly sedentary lifestyles, all have contributed significantly to the pandemic development of obesity. Even small, consistent, daily excesses in caloric intake have major long-term effects because this positive balance accumulates over time.

In addition to technical challenges in anesthesia and surgical procedures, obese patients can have additional needs in terms of nutrition because of metabolic alterations, requiring enhanced perioperative care. Obesity is associated with an increased incidence of preexisting comorbidities, including endocrine

**Table 6-14 Body Weight Classification***

| | | Waist Circumference | |
|---|---|---|---|
| CLASSIFICATION | BMI (kg/m²) | MEN, ≤40 INCH WOMEN, ≤35 INCH | MEN, >40 INCH WOMEN, >35 INCH |
| Underweight | <18.5 | | |
| Normal | 18.5-24.9 | | |
| Overweight | 25.0-29.9 | Increased | High |
| Obesity I | 30.0-34.9 | High | Very high |
| Obesity II | 35.0-39.9 | Very high | Very high |
| Obesity III | >39.9 | Extremely high | Extremely high |

Adapted from National Heart, Lung, and Blood Institute: The practical guide: Identification, evaluation, and treatment of overweight and obesity in adults, 2000 (http://www.nhlbi.nih.gov/guidelines/obesity/prctgd_c.pdf.)

*According to BMI and relative risk of type 2 diabetes, hypertension, and cardiovascular disease, compared with normal weight individuals, according to waist measurement.

disorders, cardiovascular disease and risk factors, GI conditions, and immune dysfunction. Consequently, obese patients are predisposed to a higher incidence of clinical complications, morbidity, and mortality; therefore, additional clinical care requirements need to be considered and addressed during their operative stay.

Assessment of the BMI was described earlier. The BMI has been shown to compare relatively accurately with the percentage of total body fat and morbidity. The classification of body weight with respect to underweight, normal weight, overweight, and obesity can be seen in Table 6-14. This classification is commonly applied to the whole population, although it does have some limitations. There are two exceptions; total body fat can be overestimated in trained athletes because they have a higher percentage of lean body mass, and total body fat may be underestimated in older individuals because of muscle loss. For children and adolescents, the BMI needs to be adjusted, because males and females have different growth characteristics, with the distribution of fat, muscle mass, and bone mineral content varying with growth. The body mass indices in this population are compared against growth charts considering their age and gender and expressed as a BMI for age percentile to make them analogous. Underweight is classified as lower than the 5th percentile, healthy weight from the 5th to 85th percentile, overweight 85th to the 95th percentile, and obese equal to the 95th percentile or higher. Evaluation of weight status according to a patient's BMI is important because this can provide information regarding the patient's potential comorbidities and risk for complications during hospitalization.

### Comorbidities and Preexisting Conditions

Patients with a BMI higher than 30 are considered especially at high risk and need special consideration during their hospital stay because of preexisting comorbidities and increased incidence of clinical complications. In most cases, more than one comorbidity in the obese patient is present. The most important related factors that need to be considered in surgical patients are presented here.

**Type 2 Diabetes Mellitus** Almost 80% of obese patients suffer from type 2 diabetes mellitus. A strong causality between obesity and diabetes mellitus type 2 has been shown. Type 2 diabetes can lead to obesity, and obesity can also induce diabetes. Type 2 diabetes is caused by insulin resistance in peripheral cells and a decreased production of insulin in the pancreas. Insulin resistance can lead to diminished liver function and impaired wound healing and healing, and it is molecularly linked with the inflammatory response.

**Cardiovascular Disease** Obesity is associated with an increased incidence of cardiovascular disease, including coronary heart disease, cardiomyopathy, congestive heart failure, sudden death, and stroke. These factors need to be considered when planning of surgical procedures requiring anesthesia and during the perioperative hospital stay.

**Deep Vein Thrombosis and Embolism** Hospitalized patients are at high risk for thromboses and consequently for embolic events. It has been shown that obesity independently increases the risk of these events. The major contributing factors are abdominal fat distribution, venous insufficiency, congestive heart failure, and systemic hyperlipidemia. Moreover, it has been suggested that obesity contributes to the development of thrombotic complications by an increase in prothrombotic factors. These factors need to be considered, especially in immobilized patients, along with close monitoring and prophylactic treatment.

**Hepatobiliary Disease** The metabolic state in obese patients has been shown to be associated with several conditions in the hepatobiliary tract. It is one of the most common causes of nonalcoholic liver disease. This can range from nonsymptomatic steatosis hepatis to an inflammatory steatosis, fatty infiltration, and liver cirrhosis. This liver damage results in altered metabolism and severe changes in the production of liver proteins. There is an association among the development of gallstones, cholelithiasis, and obesity. With these adverse changes in liver metabolism, there is a need to substitute essential proteins. Moreover, the dosages of these drugs need to be adjusted because of their altered rate of metabolism.

**Osteoarthritis** The incidence of osteoarthritis is increased in obesity because of functional effects on weight-bearing joints. Pain in weight-bearing joints can range from functional limitations to invalidism. These circumstances have to be considered in the differential diagnosis, especially in patients susceptible to trauma. Moreover, joint pain needs to be considered as a differential diagnosis in tumor patients, who are susceptible to bone metastases.

**Metabolic Syndrome** A special form of obesity is described by the metabolic syndrome. This is a combination of simultaneous risk factors associated with central obesity that lead to a greatly increased risk of coronary artery disease, stroke, and type 2 diabetes. Underlying causes are similar to those of regular obesity. Genetic factors, physical inactivity, and age are involved. Around 20% to 25% of the world's population is estimated to have the metabolic syndrome. This high incidence also needs to be addressed in the treatment of surgical patients.

A key feature of the syndrome includes body fat distribution in a central (abdominal) pattern. According to the International Diabetes Federation, a waist circumference more than 40 inches for men and 35 inches for women meets the criteria for the metabolic syndrome (see Table 6-14) when at least two of the following criteria are also met:

- Increased TG level: ≥150 mg/dL (>1.70 mmol/liter) (or receiving specific treatment)
- Decreased high-density lipoprotein cholesterol: <40 mg/dL (<1.03 mmol/liter) for men and <50 mg/dL (<1.29 mmol/liter) for women (or receiving specific treatment)
- Systolic blood pressure (BP) ≥130 mm Hg or diastolic BP ≥85 mm Hg (or hypertension previously diagnosed and treated)
- Fasting plasma glucose level ≥100 mg/dL (5.6 mmol/liter) or diagnosed type 2 diabetes mellitus

The metabolic syndrome has a high prevalence in middle-aged and older patients (30% to 40%). It is associated with increased cardiovascular morbidity and mortality, including arterial hypertonia, and in most cases is associated with subclinical organ damage, such as microalbuminuria, decreased glomerular filtration rate, left ventricular hypertrophy, diastolic dysfunction, and arterial thickening.

### The Surgical Obese Patient

The characteristics described need to be considered at admission and during the course of the hospital stay. Secondary metabolic changes only rarely require a special enteric or parenteral treatment regimen. During catabolic phases especially, hyperinsulinemia is normalized rapidly. In general, some weight loss should be considered before the admission of obese patients. Weight reduction by 10% of the total body weight should be considered prior to planned elective admissions, if feasible, as it can result in significant improvements in lung function parameters and a vast normalization of metabolism. Some recent studies have indicated that after operative procedures and during the hospital stay, a moderate, hypocaloric, protein-rich balanced diet should be given. This results in the mobilization of endogenous fat depots; the high protein content contributes to preserve lean body mass from catabolic breakdown.

Unfortunately, only a few studies and investigations about the high incidence of these problems have been conducted. Therefore, current knowledge and specialized treatment regimens are limited, although the overweight and obese patient needs special attention throughout her or his entire hospital stay.

## SUMMARY

Recognition of the importance of nutritional support for optimal outcomes in surgical patients and the critically ill has prompted research and development into a wide variety of regimens and strategies. Surgery, trauma, and sepsis lead to the release of inflammatory mediators and systemic hormonal and metabolic adaptations from the stress response. Nutritional support is a key component of modern surgical care and collaboration with nutrition specialists will assist in providing appropriate support while avoiding complications. When nutritional support is required and no contraindications are present, EN is the first choice for most patients, with calculations based on individual patient requirements. Various methods are available for the delivery of nutritional support; PN should be used, when necessary, in patients in whom EN is contraindicated. In addition to operative interventions to address underlying pathology, catabolism and hypermetabolism can be managed by prompt treatment of infection and by environmental and pharmacologic strategies to diminish these factors, and nutritional support begun as early as possible to meet elevated demands.

## SELECTED REFERENCES

Cuthbertson DP: Post-shock metabolic response (Arris-Gale Lecture to the Royal College of Surgeons of England). Lancet 239:433–437, 1942.

A landmark of the hypermetabolic response. Sir Cuthbertson characterized the metabolic response of surgical and trauma patients as observed during his experiments in animal models.

Fischer JE: Nutrition and metabolism in the surgical patient, ed 2, Boston, 1996, Little, Brown.

This work encompasses the background biochemistry and practical knowledge of surgical nutrition and metabolism.

Herndon DN: Total burn care, ed 3, Edinburgh, 2007, Saunders Elsevier.

This book represents the efforts of surgeons, anesthesiologists, residents, nurses, and allied health professionals dedicated to the management of the most severe hypermetabolic and hypercatabolic surgical patients—burn patients.

Moore FD: Metabolic care of the surgical patient, Philadelphia, 1959, WB Saunders.

This is a classic of surgical metabolism, with great contributions to the understanding of fluids and nutrition.

Wilmore DW, Long JM, Mason AD, Jr, et al: Catecholamines: Mediator of the hypermetabolic response to thermal injury. Ann Surg 180:653–669, 1974.

Classic work that introduced catecholamines as primary mediator of the hypermetabolic response and not thyroid hormones. This was among the first to suggest the possibility of a pharmacological intervention.

Gottschlich MM, DeLegge MH, Guenter P, editors: The A.S.P.E.N. nutrition support core curriculum, Silver Spring, Md, 2008, American Society for Parenteral and Enteral Nutrition.

Comprehensive text covering all aspects of nutritional support in depth. Numerous case studies and examples are provided.

## REFERENCES


1. Sneve H: The treatment of burns and skin grafting. JAMA 45:1–8, 1905.
2. Cuthbertson DP: Post-shock metabolic response (Arris-Gale Lecture to the Royal College of Surgeons of England). Lancet 239:433–437, 1942.
3. Cope O, Nardi GL, Quijano M, et al: Metabolic rate and thyroid function following acute thermal trauma in man. Ann Surg 137:165–174, 1953.
4. Moore FD: Metabolic care of the surgical patient, Philadelphia, 1959, WB Saunders.
5. Dudrick SJ: Early developments and clinical applications of total parenteral nutrition. JPEN J Parenter Enteral Nutr 27:291–299, 2003.
6. Jeschke MG, Chinkes DL, Finnerty CC, et al: Pathophysiologic response to severe burn injury. Ann Surg 248:387–401, 2008.
7. Ahmadian M, Wang Y, Sul HS: Lipolysis in adipocytes. Int J Biochem Cell Biol 42:555–559, 2010.
8. Gore DC, Ferrando A, Barnett J, et al: Influence of glucose kinetics on plasma lactate concentration and energy expenditure in severely burned patients. J Trauma 49:673–677, 2000.
9. Chung DH, Evers BM, Townsend CM, Jr, et al: Burn-induced transcriptional regulation of small intestinal ornithine decarboxylase. Am J Surg 163:157–162, 1992.
10. Klein CJ, Stanek GS, Wiles CE, 3rd: Overfeeding macronutrients to critically ill adults: Metabolic complications. J Am Diet Assoc 98:795–806, 1998.
11. Reilly JJ Jr, Hull SF, Albert N, et al: Economic impact of malnutrition: A model system for hospitalized patients. JPEN J Parenter Enteral Nutr 12:371–376, 1988.
12. Chang DW, DeSanti L, Demling RH: Anticatabolic and anabolic strategies in critical illness: A review of current treatment modalities. Shock 10:155–160, 1998.
13. Hamwi GJ: Changing dietary concepts. In Danowski TS, editor: Diabetes mellitus: Diagnosis and treatment, New York, 1964, American Diabetes Association, pp 73–78.
14. Miles JM: Energy expenditure in hospitalized patients: implications for nutritional support. Mayo Clin Proc 81:809–816, 2006.
15. Van Way CW: Nutrition secrets, Philadelphia, 1999, Hanley & Belfus.
16. Ireton-Jones C, Turner W: The use of respiratory quotient to determine the efficacy of nutrition support regimens. J Am Diet Assoc 87:1880–1883, 1987.
17. Suman OE, Mlcak RP, Chinkes DL, et al: Resting energy expenditure in severely burned children: Analysis of agreement between indirect calorimetry and prediction equations using the Bland-Altman method. Burns 32:335–342, 2006.
18. Gibbs J, Cull W, Henderson W, et al: Preoperative serum albumin level as a predictor of operative mortality and morbidity: results from the National VA Surgical Risk Study. Arch Surg 134:36–42, 1999.
19. Khuri SF, Daley J, Henderson W, et al: Risk adjustment of the postoperative mortality rate for the comparative assessment of the quality of surgical care: Results of the National Veterans Affairs Surgical Risk Study. J Am Coll Surg 185:315–327, 1997.
20. Hoffman EP, Nader GA: Balancing muscle hypertrophy and atrophy. Nat Med 10:584–585, 2004.
21. Sandstrom R, Drott C, Hyltander A, et al: The effect of postoperative intravenous feeding (TPN) on outcome following major surgery evaluated in a randomized study. Ann Surg 217:185–195, 1993.
22. Von Meyenfeldt MF, Meijerink WJ, Rouflart MM, et al: Perioperative nutritional support: A randomised clinical trial. Clin Nutr 11:180–186, 1992.
23. ASPEN Board of Directors and the Clinical Guidelines Task Force: Guidelines for the use of parenteral and enteral nutrition in adult and pediatric patients. JPEN J Parenter Enteral Nutr 26(Suppl):1SA–138SA, 2002.
24. Gottschlich MM, DeLegge Mark H, Guenter P, editors: The A.S.P.E.N. nutrition support core curriculum, Silver Spring, Md, 2007, American Society for Parenteral and Enteral Nutrition.
25. Weimann A, Braga M, Harsanyi L, et al: ESPEN Guidelines on Enteral Nutrition: Surgery including organ transplantation. Clin Nutr 25:224–244, 2006.
26. Dudrick SJ, Wilmore DW, Vars HM, et al: Long-term total parenteral nutrition with growth, development, and positive nitrogen balance. Surgery 64:134–142, 1968.
27. Singer P, Berger MM, Van den Berghe G, et al: ESPEN Guidelines on Parenteral Nutrition: Intensive care. Clin Nutr 28:387–400, 2009.
28. Kreymann KG, Berger MM, Deutz NE, et al: ESPEN Guidelines on Enteral Nutrition: Intensive care. Clin Nutr 25:210–223, 2006.
29. Villet S, Chiolero RL, Bollmann MD, et al: Negative impact of hypocaloric feeding and energy balance on clinical outcome in ICU patients. Clin Nutr 24:502–509, 2005.
30. Wolf SE, Jeschke MG, Rose JK, et al: Enteral feeding intolerance: An indicator of sepsis-associated mortality in burned children. Arch Surg 132:1310–1313, 1997.
31. Greenhalgh DG, Saffle JR, Holmes JHT, et al: American Burn Association consensus conference to define sepsis and infection in burns. J Burn Care Res 28:776–790, 2007.
32. Alexander JW, Gottschlich MM: Nutritional immunomodulation in burn patients. Crit Care Med 18:S149–S153, 1990.
33. Hart DW, Wolf SE, Zhang XJ, et al: Efficacy of a high-carbohydrate diet in catabolic illness. Crit Care Med 29:1318–1324, 2001.
34. Koretz RL, Lipman TO, Klein S: AGA technical review on parenteral nutrition. Gastroenterology 121:970–1001, 2001.
35. Alverdy J, Aoys E, Moss G: Total parenteral nutrition promotes bacterial translocation from the gut. Surgery 104:185–190, 1988.
36. Herndon DN, Barrow RE, Stein M, et al: Increased mortality with intravenous supplemental feeding in severely burned patients. J Burn Care Rehabil 10:309–313, 1989.
37. Wolfe RR, Allsop JR, Burke JF: Glucose metabolism in man: Responses to intravenous glucose infusion. Metabolism 28:210–220, 1979.
38. Wanten GJ, Calder PC: Immune modulation by parenteral lipid emulsions. Am J Clin Nutr 85:1171–1184, 2007.
39. Battistella FD, Widergren JT, Anderson JT, et al: A prospective, randomized trial of intravenous fat emulsion administration in trauma victims requiring total parenteral nutrition. J Trauma 43:52–58, 1997.
40. Wei C, Hua J, Bin C, et al: Impact of lipid emulsion containing fish oil on outcomes of surgical patients: Systematic review of randomized controlled trials from Europe and Asia. Nutrition 26:474–481, 2010.
41. Wirtitsch M, Wessner B, Spittler A, et al: Effect of different lipid emulsions on the immunological function in humans: A systematic review with meta-analysis. Clin Nutr 26:302–313, 2007.
42. Hart DW, Wolf SE, Mlcak R, et al: Persistence of muscle catabolism after severe burn. Surgery 128:312–319, 2000.

43. Mirtallo J, Canada T, Johnson D, et al: Safe practices for parenteral nutrition. JPEN J Parenter Enteral Nutr 28:S39–S70, 2004.
44. Wilmore DW, Long JM, Mason AD, Jr, et al: Catecholamines: Mediator of the hypermetabolic response to thermal injury. Ann Surg 180:653–669, 1974.
45. Neugebauer CT, Serghiou M, Herndon DN, et al: Effects of a 12-week rehabilitation program with music and exercise groups on range of motion in young children with severe burns. J Burn Care Res 29:939–948, 2008.
46. Takala J, Ruokonen E, Webster NR, et al: Increased mortality associated with growth hormone treatment in critically ill adults. N Engl J Med 341:785–792, 1999.
47. Calder PC: n-3 polyunsaturated fatty acids, inflammation, and inflammatory diseases. Am J Clin Nutr 83(Suppl):1505S–1519S, 2006.
48. Consensus recommendations from the US summit on immune-enhancing enteral therapy. JPEN J Parenter Enteral Nutr 25(Suppl):S61–S63, 2001.
49. Garrel D, Patenaude J, Nedelec B, et al: Decreased mortality and infectious morbidity in adult burn patients given enteral glutamine supplements: A prospective, controlled, randomized clinical trial. Crit Care Med 31:2444–2449, 2003.
50. Zhou YP, Jiang ZM, Sun YH, et al: The effect of supplemental enteral glutamine on plasma levels, gut function, and outcome in severe burns: A randomized, double-blind, controlled clinical trial. JPEN J Parenter Enteral Nutr 27:241–245, 2003.
51. Plank LD, Metzger DJ, McCall JL, et al: Sequential changes in the metabolic response to orthotopic liver transplantation during the first year after surgery. Ann Surg 234:245–255, 2001.
52. World Health Organization: Management of severe malnutrition: A manual for physicians and other senior health workers, 1999 (http://whqlibdoc.who.int/hq/1999/a57361.pdf).
53. Marshall JC: Sepsis: Current status, future prospects. Curr Opin Crit Care 10:250–264, 2004.
54. Plank LD, Hill GL: Sequential metabolic changes following induction of systemic inflammatory response in patients with severe sepsis or major blunt trauma. World J Surg 24:630–638, 2000.
55. Fischer JE, Baldessarini RJ: False neurotransmitters and hepatic failure. Lancet 2:75–80, 1971.
56. le Roux CW, Aylwin SJ, Batterham RL, et al: Gut hormone profiles following bariatric surgery favor an anorectic state, facilitate weight loss, and improve metabolic parameters. Ann Surg 243:108–114, 2006.
57. van den Berghe G, Wouters P, Weekers F, et al: Intensive insulin therapy in the critically ill patients. N Engl J Med 345:1359–1367, 2001.
58. McClave SA, Chang WK, Dhaliwal R, et al: Nutrition support in acute pancreatitis: A systematic review of the literature. JPEN J Parenter Enteral Nutr 30:143–156, 2006.
59. Marik PE: What is the best way to feed patients with pancreatitis? Curr Opin Crit Care 15:131–138, 2009.
60. Voruganti VS, Klein GL, Lu HX, et al: Impaired zinc and copper status in children with burn injuries: Need to reassess nutritional requirements. Burns 31:711–716, 2005.
61. Harris JA, Benedict VS: Biometric studies of basal metabolism in man, Washington, DC, 1919, Carnegie Institute of Washington.

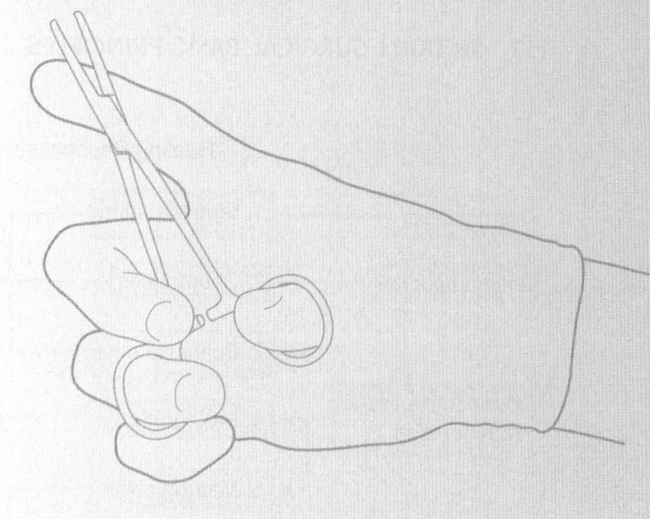

CHAPTER 7

# WOUND HEALING

Mimi Leong and Linda G. Phillips

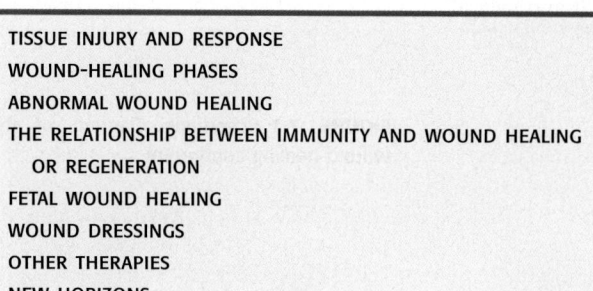

The treatment and healing of wounds are some of the oldest subjects discussed in the medical literature. Yet despite knowledge of the steps involved, the exact mechanisms underlying wound healing are not completely understood.

## TISSUE INJURY AND RESPONSE

Wound repair is the effort of injured tissues to restore their normal function and structural integrity after injury. During the effort to restore barriers to fluid loss and infection, reestablish normal blood and lymphatic flow patterns, and restore the mechanical integrity of the injured system, flawless repair is sacrificed because of the urgency to return to function. Regeneration, in contrast, is perfect restoration of the preexisting tissue architecture in the absence of scar formation. Although regeneration is the goal of wound healing, it is found only in embryonic development, in lower organisms such as the stone crab and salamander, or in certain tissue compartments such as bone and liver. In wound healing in adult humans, however, the accuracy of regeneration is sacrificed for the speed of repair.

All wounds undergo the same basic steps of repair. Acute wounds proceed in an orderly and timely reparative process to achieve sustained restoration of structure and function. A chronic wound, in contrast, does not proceed to restoration of functional integrity. It is stalled in the inflammatory phase as a result of a variety of causes and does not proceed to closure.

## WOUND-HEALING PHASES

The three phases of wound healing are inflammation, proliferation, and maturation. In a large wound such as a pressure sore, the eschar or fibrinous exudate reflects the inflammatory phase, the granulation tissue is part of the proliferative phase, and the contracting or advancing edge is part of the maturational phase. All three phases may occur simultaneously, and the phases may overlap with their individual processes (Fig. 7-1).

### Inflammatory Phase

During the immediate reaction of the tissue to injury, hemostasis and inflammation occur. This phase represents an attempt to limit damage by stopping the bleeding, sealing the surface of the wound, and removing any necrotic tissue, foreign debris, or bacteria present. The inflammatory phase is characterized by increased vascular permeability, migration of cells into the wound by chemotaxis, secretion of cytokines and growth factors into the wound, and activation of the migrating cells (Fig. 7-2).

#### Hemostasis and Inflammation

During an acute tissue injury, blood vessel damage results in initial intense local vasoconstriction of arterioles and capillaries followed by vasodilation and increased vascular permeability (Fig. 7-3). Erythrocytes and platelets adhere to the damaged capillary endothelium, resulting in plugging of capillaries and leading to cessation of hemorrhage. Activation of these platelets by binding to the exposed type IV and V collagen from the damaged endothelium results in platelet aggregation. The initial contact between platelets and collagen requires von Willebrand factor (vWF) VIII, a heterodimeric protein synthesized by megakaryocytes and endothelial cells. Platelet adhesion to the endothelium is primarily mediated through the interaction between high-affinity glycoprotein receptors and the integrin receptor GPIIb-IIIa ($\alpha_{IIb}\beta_3$). Platelets also express other integrin receptors that mediate direct binding to collagen ($\alpha_2\beta_1$) and laminin ($\alpha_6\beta_1$) or indirect binding by attaching to subendothelial matrix-bound fibronectin ($\alpha_5\beta_1$), vitronectin ($\alpha_v\beta_3$), and other ligands.

#### Increased Vascular Permeability

Platelet binding results in conformational changes in platelets that trigger intracellular signal transduction pathways that lead to platelet activation and the release of biologically active proteins. Platelet alpha granules are storage organelles that contain platelet-derived growth factor (PDGF), transforming growth factor-β (TGF-β), insulin-like growth factor type I (IGF-I), fibronectin, fibrinogen, thrombospondin, and vWF. The dense bodies contain vasoactive amines, such as serotonin, that cause vasodilation and increased vascular permeability. Mast cells adherent to the endothelial surface release histamine and serotonin, resulting in increased permeability of endothelial cells and causing leakage of plasma from the intravascular space to the

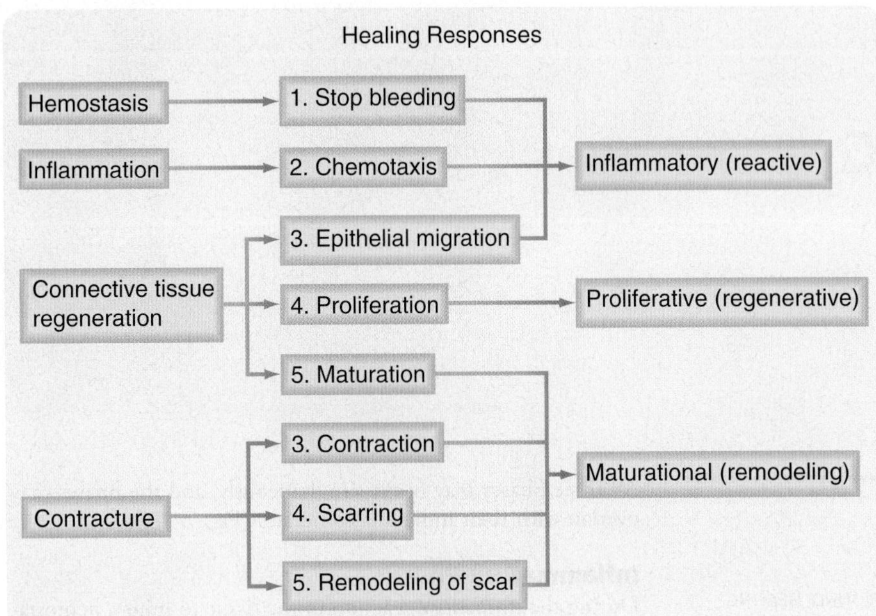


**FIGURE 7-1** Schematic diagram of the wound-healing continuum.

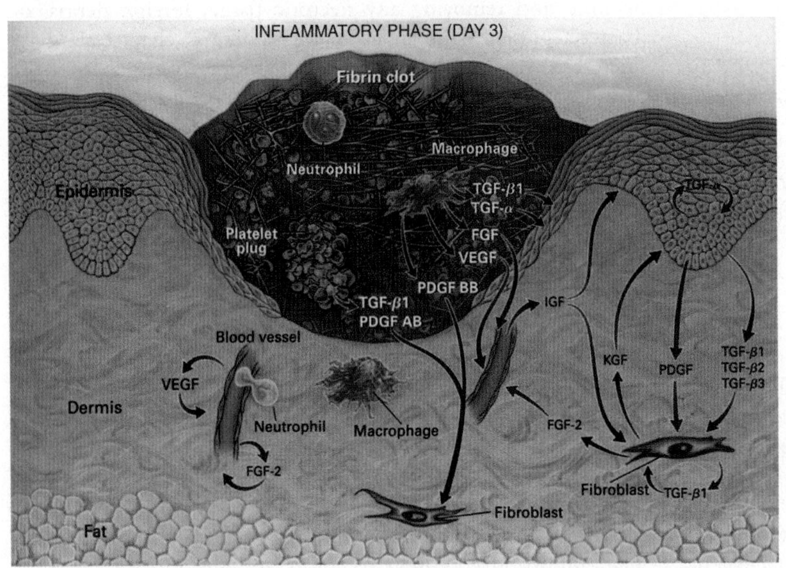


**FIGURE 7-2** Cutaneous wound 3 days after injury. The cells and growth factors necessary to facilitate cell migration into the wound are shown. (From Singer AJ, Clark RAF: Mechanisms of disease: Cutaneous wound healing. N Engl J Med 341:738–746, 1999.)

extracellular compartment. The clotting cascade is initiated through the intrinsic and extrinsic pathways. As the platelets become activated, the membrane phospholipids bind factor V, which allows interaction with factor X. Membrane-bound prothrombinase activity is generated and potentiates thrombin production exponentially. The thrombin itself activates platelets and catalyzes the conversion of fibrinogen to fibrin. The fibrin strands trap red blood cells to form the clot and seal the wound. The lattice framework that results will be the scaffold for endothelial cells, inflammatory cells, and fibroblasts. Thromboxane A2 and prostaglandin F2α, formed from the degradation of cell membranes in the arachidonic acid cascade, also assist in platelet aggregation and vasoconstriction. Although these activities serve to limit the amount of injury, they can also cause localized ischemia, resulting in further damage to cell membranes and the release of more prostaglandin F2α and thromboxane A2.

### Chemokines

Chemokines stimulate the migration of different cell types, particularly inflammatory cells, into the wound and are active participants in the regulation of the different phases of wound healing. The CXC, CC, and C ligand families bind to G protein–coupled surface receptors called CXC receptors and CC receptors.

Macrophage chemoattractant protein (MCP-1, or CCL2) is induced in keratinocytes after injury. It is a potent chemoattractant for monocytes/macrophages, T lymphocytes, and mast cells.[1] Expression of this chemokine is sustained in chronic wounds and results in the prolonged presence of polymorphonuclear cells (PMNs) and macrophages, leading to the prolonged inflammatory response.[2] CXCL1 (GRO-α) is a potent PMN chemotactic regulator and is increased in acute wounds. It is also involved in reepithelialization.[3] Interleukin-8 (IL-8,

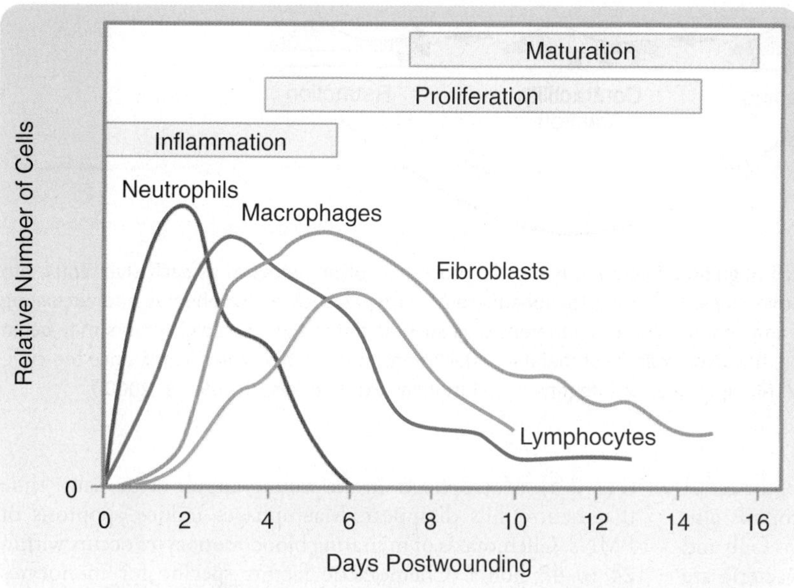


**FIGURE 7-3** Time course of the appearance of different cells in the wound during healing. Macrophages and neutrophils are predominant during the inflammatory phase (peak at days 3 and 2, respectively). Lymphocytes appear later and peak at day 7. Fibroblasts are the predominant cells during the proliferative phase. (Adapted from Witte MB, Barbul A: General principles of wound healing. Surg Clin North Am 77:509–528, 1997.)

or CXCL8) expression is increased in acute and chronic wounds.[4] It is involved in reepithelialization and induces the leukocyte expression of matrix metalloproteinases (MMPs), which stimulates remodeling. It is also a strong chemoattractant for PMNs and participates in inflammation.[4] Relatively low levels of IL-8 are found in fetal wounds and may be why fetal wounds have decreased inflammation and heal without scars.[5] Expression of the keratinocyte-produced chemokine interferon inducible protein 10 (IP-10 or CXCL10) is elevated in acute wounds as well as chronic inflammatory conditions.[6] It impairs wound healing by increasing inflammation and recruiting lymphocytes to the wound. It also inhibits proliferation by decreasing reepithelialization and angiogenesis and preventing fibroblast migration.[3] Stromal cell-derived factor-1 (SDF-1, or CXCL12) is expressed by endothelial cells, myofibroblasts, and keratinocytes and is involved in inflammation by recruiting lymphocytes to the wound and promoting angiogenesis. It is a potent chemoattractant for endothelial cells and bone marrow progenitors from the circulation to peripheral tissues.[7] It also enhances keratinocyte proliferation, resulting in reepithelialization.[8]

### Polymorphonuclear Cells

The release of histamine and serotonin leads to vascular permeability of the capillary bed. Complement factors such as C5a and leukotriene B4 promote neutrophil adherence and chemoattraction. In the presence of thrombin, endothelial cells exposed to leukotriene C4 and D4 release platelet-aggregating factor, which further enhances neutrophil adhesion. Monocytes and endothelial cells produce the inflammatory mediators IL-1 and tumor necrosis factor-α (TNF-α), and these mediators further promote endothelial-neutrophil adherence. The increased capillary permeability and the various chemotactic factors facilitate diapedesis of neutrophils into the inflammatory site. As the neutrophils begin their migration, they release the contents of their lysosomes and enzymes such as elastase and other proteases into the extracellular matrix (ECM), which further facilitates neutrophil migration. The combination of intense vasodilation and increased vascular permeability leads to clinical findings of inflammation, rubor (redness), tumor (swelling), calor (heat), and dolor (pain). Local tissue swelling is further promoted by the deposition of fibrin, a protein end product of coagulation, and the fibrin becomes entrapped in lymphatic vessels.

Evidence suggests that the migration of PMNs requires sequential adhesive and de-adhesive interactions between $\beta_1$ and $\beta_2$ integrins and ECM components. Integrin molecules are a family of cell surface receptors that are closely coupled with the cell's cytoskeleton. These molecules serve two major functions:

1. Interaction with components of the ECM, such as fibronectin, to provide adhesion
2. Signal transduction to the interior of the cell

Integrins are crucial for cell motility and are required in inflammation and normal wound healing, as well as in embryonic development and tumor metastases. After extravasation, PMNs, attracted by chemotaxins, migrate through the ECM by means of transient interactions between integrin receptors and their ligands. Four phases of integrin-mediated cell motility have been described: adhesion, spreading, contractility or traction, and retraction. Activation of specific integrins though ligand binding has been shown to increase cell adhesion and activate reorganization of the cell's actin cytoskeleton. Spreading is characterized by the development of lamellipodia and filopodia. Traction at the leading edge of the cell develops through binding of integrin, followed by translocation of the cell over the adherent segment of the plasma membrane. The integrin is shifted to the rear of the cell and releases its substrate, thereby permitting cell advancement (Fig. 7-4). Regulation of integrin function by adhesive substrates offers a mechanism for local control of migrant cells. Within the assembled framework of the ECM, binding sites for integrins have been identified on collagen, laminin, and fibronectin.

The chemotactic agent mediates the PMN response through signal transduction as the chemotaxin binds to receptors on the cell surface. Bacterial products such as *N*-formyl-methionyl-leucyl-phenylalanine bind to induce cyclic adenosine

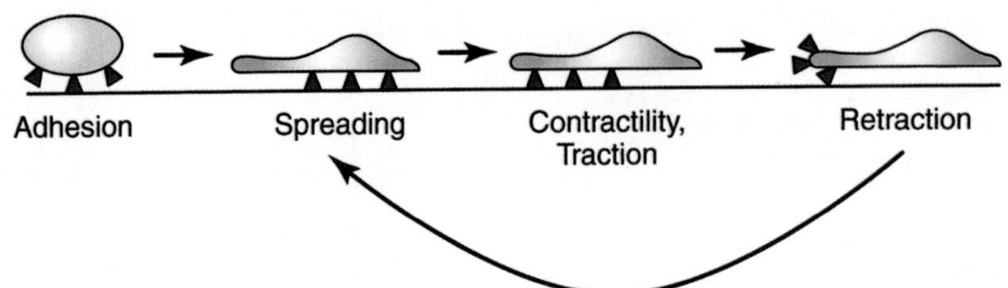


**FIGURE 7-4** Schematic of a cycle of integrin-mediated cell migration. Migration is a cyclic process involving integrins at each step. Entry into the migration cycle can take place at either of the first two steps. For example, nonadherent cell types such as lymphomas and circulating carcinomas begin the migration cycle at the first step of attachment, whereas adherent cells such as fibroblasts and solid tumors may begin the cycle at the spreading step. Regardless of the cell type, however, cells must maintain attachment to the extracellular matrix once the cycle has begun. (Adapted from Holly SP, Larson MK, Parise LV: Multiple roles of integrins in cell motility. Exp Cell Res 261:69–74, 2000.)

monophosphate (cAMP) but if there is maximal receptor occupancy, superoxide is produced at peak rates. Neutrophils also possess receptors for IgG and the complement proteins C3b and C3bi. As the complement cascade is released and bacteria are opsonized, binding of these proteins to cell receptors on neutrophils allows recognition by the neutrophils and phagocytosis of the bacteria. When neutrophils are stimulated, they express more CR1 and CR3 receptors, thereby permitting more efficient binding and phagocytosis of these bacteria.

Functional activation occurs after migration of PMNs into the wound site, which may induce new cell surface antigen expression, increased cytotoxicity, or enhanced production and release of cytokines. These activated neutrophils scavenge for necrotic debris, foreign material, and bacteria and generate free oxygen radicals, with electrons donated by the reduced form of nicotinamide adenine dinucleotide phosphate (NADPH). The electrons are transported across the membrane into lysosomes, where superoxide anion ($O_2^-$) is formed. Superoxide dismutase catalyzes the formation of hydrogen peroxide ($H_2O_2$), which is then degraded by myeloperoxidase in the azurophilic granules of neutrophils. This interaction oxidizes halides, with the formation of byproducts such as hypochlorous acid. The iron-catalyzed reaction between $H_2O_2$ and $O_2^-$ forms hydroxyl radicals (OH·). This potent free radical is bactericidal, but is also toxic to neutrophils and surrounding viable tissues.

Migration of PMNs stops when wound contamination has been controlled, usually within the first few days after injury. PMNs do not survive longer than 24 hours. After 24 to 48 hours, the predominance of cells in the wound cleft shifts to mononuclear cells. If wound contamination persists or secondary infection occurs, continuous activation of the complement system and other pathways provides a steady supply of chemotactic factors, resulting in a sustained influx of PMNs into the wound. In addition to the delay in healing, this prolonged inflammation can be deleterious in terms of destruction of normal tissue, with progression to tissue necrosis, abscess formation, and possibly systemic infection. PMNs are not essential for wound healing because their role in phagocytosis and antimicrobial defense may be taken over by macrophages. Sterile incisions will heal normally without the presence of PMNs.

### Macrophages

The macrophage is the one cell that is truly crucial to wound healing in that it serves to orchestrate the release of cytokines and stimulate many of the subsequent processes of wound healing (Fig. 7-5). Macrophages in the wound appear at the same time that neutrophils disappear. Macrophages induce apoptosis of PMNs. Chemotaxis of migrating blood monocytes occurs within 24 to 48 hours. Chemotactic factors specific for monocytes include bacterial products, complement degradation products (C5a), thrombin, fibronectin, collagen, TGF-β, and PDGF-BB. Monocyte chemotaxis is also facilitated by the interaction of integrin receptors on the monocyte surface with ECM proteins such as fibrin and fibronectin. The β integrin receptor also transduces the signal for macrophage phagocytic activity. Activated integrin expression promotes adhesion-mediated gene induction in monocytes that transforms them into wound macrophages; such transformation results in increased phagocytic activity and selective expression of cytokines and signal transduction elements by messenger RNA (mRNA), including the early growth response genes *EGR2* and c-*fos*. Macrophages have specific receptors for immunoglobulin G (IgG; Fc receptor), C3b (CR1 and CR3), and fibronectin (integrin receptors) that permit surface recognition of opsonized pathogens and facilitate phagocytosis.

Bacterial debris such as lipopolysaccharide can activate monocytes to release free radicals and cytokines that mediate angiogenesis and fibroplasia. The presence of IL-2 increases the release of free radicals and thus enhances bactericidal activity, and the activity of the free radicals is potentiated by IL-2. In addition, the free radicals generate bacterial debris, which further potentiates the activation of monocytes. Activated wound macrophages also produce nitric oxide (NO), a substance that has been demonstrated to have many functions other than antimicrobial properties.

As the monocyte or macrophage is activated, phospholipase is induced, cell membrane phospholipids are enzymatically degraded, and thromboxane A2 and prostaglandin F2α are released. The macrophage also releases leukotrienes B4 and C4 and 15- and 5-hydroxyeicosatetraenoic acid. Leukotriene B4 is a potent chemotaxin for neutrophils and increases their adherence to endothelial cells.

Wound macrophages release proteinases, including matrix metalloproteinases (MMP-1, MMP-2, MMP-3, and MMP-9; Fig. 7-6), that degrade the ECM and are crucial for removing foreign material, promoting cell movement through tissue spaces, and regulating ECM turnover. This activity is dependent on the cAMP pathway and thus can be blocked by nonsteroidal anti-inflammatory drtugs (NSAIDs) or glucocorticoid drugs. Colchicine and retinoic acid appear to decrease collagenase production as well.

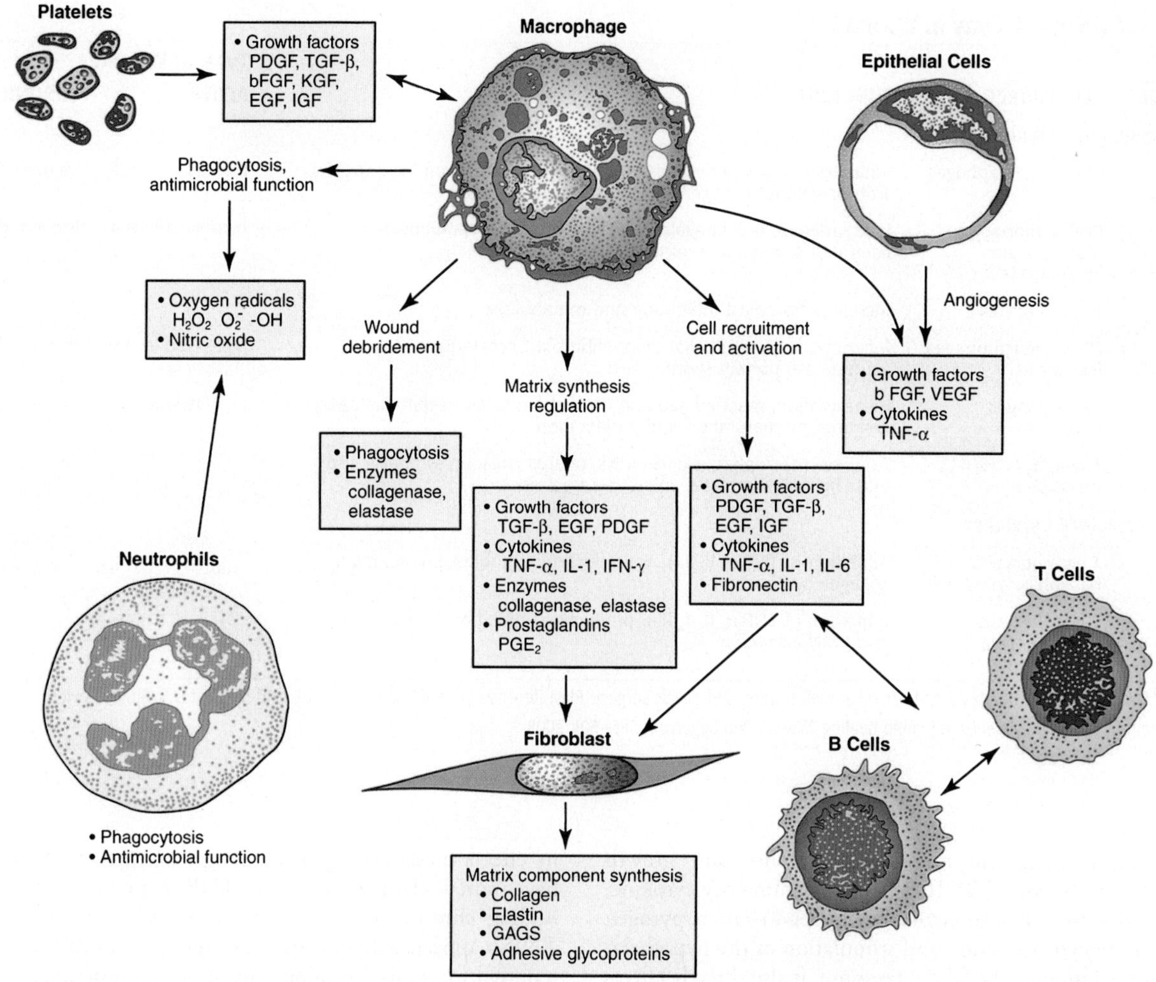

Platelets

• Growth factors PDGF, TGF-β, bFGF, KGF, EGF, IGF

Macrophage

Epithelial Cells

Phagocytosis, antimicrobial function

• Oxygen radicals $H_2O_2$ $O_2^-$ -OH
• Nitric oxide

Wound debridement

• Phagocytosis
• Enzymes collagenase, elastase

Matrix synthesis regulation

• Growth factors TGF-β, EGF, PDGF
• Cytokines TNF-α, IL-1, IFN-γ
• Enzymes collagenase, elastase
• Prostaglandins $PGE_2$

Cell recruitment and activation

• Growth factors PDGF, TGF-β, EGF, IGF
• Cytokines TNF-α, IL-1, IL-6
• Fibronectin

Angiogenesis

• Growth factors b FGF, VEGF
• Cytokines TNF-α

Neutrophils

• Phagocytosis
• Antimicrobial function

T Cells

B Cells

Fibroblast

Matrix component synthesis
• Collagen
• Elastin
• GAGS
• Adhesive glycoproteins

**FIGURE 7-5** Interaction of cellular and humoral factors in wound healing. Note the key role of the macrophage. *bFGF,* Basic fibroblast growth factor; *$H_2O_2$,* hydrogen peroxide; *$O_2^-$,* superoxide; *PGE2,* prostaglandin E2. (Adapted from Witte MB, Barbul A: General principles of wound healing. Surg Clin North Am 77: 509–528, 1997.)

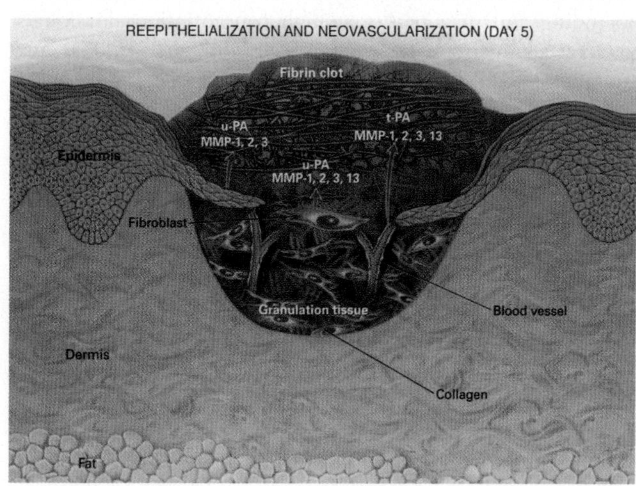


**FIGURE 7-6** Cutaneous wound 5 days after injury. Blood vessels are seen sprouting into the fibrin clot as epidermal cells resurface the wound. Some of the proteinases involved in cell movement at this time point are shown. *MMP-1, -2, -3, -13,* Matrix metalloproteinases 1, 2, 3, and 13 (collagenase 1, gelatinase A, stromelysin 1, and collagenase 3, respectively); *t-PA,* tissue plasminogen activator; *u-PA,* urokinase-type plasminogen activator. (Adapted from Singer AJ, Clark RAF: Mechanisms of disease: Cutaneous wound healing. N Engl J Med 341:738–746, 1999.)

**Table 7-1 Cytokine Activity in Wound Healing**

| | | | Type of Wound | |
|---|---|---|---|---|
| **CYTOKINE** | **CELL SOURCE** | **FUNCTION** | **ACUTE** | **CHRONIC** |
| **Proinflammatory Cytokines** | | | | |
| TNF-α | PMNs, macrophages | Inflammation, reepithelialization, PMN margination and cytotoxicity, with or without collagen synthesis; provides metabolic substrate | Increased levels | Increased levels |
| IL-1 | PMNs, monocytes, macrophages, keratinocytes | Inflammation, reepithelialization, fibroblast and keratinocyte chemotaxis, collagen synthesis | Increased levels | Increased levels |
| IL-2 | T lymphocytes | Increases fibroblast infiltration and metabolism | | |
| IL-6 | PMNs, macrophages, fibroblasts | Inflammation, reepithelialization, fibroblast proliferation, hepatic acute-phase protein synthesis | Increased levels | Increased levels |
| IL-8 | Macrophages, fibroblasts | Inflammation, macrophage and PMN chemotaxis; reepithelialization, keratinocyte maturation and proliferation | Increased levels | Increased levels |
| IFN- γ | T lymphocytes, macrophages | Activates macrophages and PMNs, retards collagen synthesis and cross-linking, stimulates collagenase activity | | |
| **Anti-Inflammatory Cytokines** | | | | |
| IL-4 | T lymphocytes, basophils, mast cells | Inhibition of TNF-α, IL-1, IL-6 production; fibroblast proliferation, collagen synthesis | | |
| IL-10 | T lymphocytes, macrophages, keratinocytes | Inhibition of TNF-α, IL-1, IL-6 production, inhibition of macrophage and PMN activation | | |

Adapted from Rumalla VK, Borah GL: Cytokines, growth factors, and plastic surgery. Plast Reconstr Surg 108:719–733, 2001; and Barrientos S, Stojadinovic O, Golinko MS, et al: Growth factors and cytokines in wound healing. Wound Rep Regen 16: 585–601, 2008.

Macrophages secrete numerous cytokines and growth factors (Tables 7-1 and 7-2). IL-1, a proinflammatory cytokine, is an acute-phase response cytokine. This endogenous pyrogen causes lymphocyte activation and stimulation of the hypothalamus, thereby inducing the febrile response. It also directly affects hemostasis by inducing the release of vasodilators and stimulating coagulation. Its effect is further amplified as endothelial cells produce it in the presence of TNF-α and endotoxin. IL-1 has numerous effects, such as enhancement of collagenase production, stimulation of cartilage degradation and bone reabsorption, activation of neutrophils, regulation of adhesion molecules, and promotion of chemotaxis. It stimulates other cells to secrete proinflammatory cytokines. Its effects also extend into the proliferative phase, during which it increases fibroblast and keratinocyte growth and collagen synthesis. Studies have demonstrated increased levels of IL-1 in chronic nonhealing wounds, thus suggesting its role in the pathogenesis of poor wound healing. The early beneficial responses of IL-1 in wound healing appear to be maladaptive if elevated levels last beyond the first week after injury.

Microbial byproducts induce macrophages to release TNF. TNF-α is crucial in initiating the response to injury or bacteria. It upregulates cell surface adhesion molecules that promote the interaction of immune cells and endothelium. TNF-α is detected in the wound within 12 hours and peaks after 72 hours. Its effects include hemostasis, increased vascular permeability, and enhanced endothelial proliferation. Like IL-1, TNF-α induces fever, increased collagenase production, reabsorption of cartilage and bone, and release of PDGF, as well as the production of more IL-1. Excessive production of TNF-α, however, has been associated with multisystem organ failure and increased morbidity and mortality in inflammatory disease states, partly through its effects on activating macrophages and neutrophils. Studies have noted elevated levels of TNF-α in nonhealing versus healing chronic venous ulcers. Thus, as in the case of IL-1, TNF-α appears to be essential in the early inflammatory response required for wound healing, but local and systemic persistence of this cytokine may lead to impaired wound maturation.

IL-6, which is produced by monocytes and macrophages, is involved in stem cell growth, activation of B and T cells, and regulation of the synthesis of hepatic acute-phase proteins. Within acute wounds, IL-6 is also secreted by PMNs and fibroblasts, and its increase parallels the increase in the PMN count locally. IL-6 is detectable within 12 hours of experimental wounding and may persist at high concentrations for longer than 1 week. It also works synergistically with IL-1, TNF-α, and endotoxins. It is a potent stimulator of fibroblast proliferation and is decreased in aging fibroblasts and fetal wounds.

IL-8 (also called CXCL8) is secreted primarily by macrophages and fibroblasts in the acute wound, with peak expression within the first 24 hours. Its major effects have been discussed but include increased PMN and monocyte chemotaxis, PMN degranulation, and expression of endothelial cell adhesion molecules.

Interferon-γ (IFN-γ), another proinflammatory cytokine, is secreted by T lymphocytes and macrophages. Its major effects are macrophage and PMN activation and increased cytotoxicity. It has also been shown to reduce local wound contraction and aid in tissue remodeling. IFN-γ has been used in the treatment of hypertrophic and keloid scars, possibly by its effect in slowing collagen production and cross linking, whereas collagenase (MMP-1) production increases. Experimentally, however, it has been shown to impair reepithelialization and wound strength in a dose-dependent manner when applied locally or systemically.

**Table 7-2 Growth Factors That Affect Wound Healing**

| GROWTH FACTOR | CELL SOURCE | FUNCTION | Type of Wound ACUTE | CHRONIC |
|---|---|---|---|---|
| PDGF | Platelets, macrophages, endothelial cells, keratinocytes, fibroblasts | Inflammation; granulation tissue formation; reepithelialization; matrix formation and remodeling; chemotactic for PMNs, macrophages, fibroblasts, and smooth muscle cells, activates PMNs, macrophages and fibroblasts; mitogenic for fibroblasts, endothelial cells; stimulates production of MMPs, fibronectin, and HA; stimulates angiogenesis and wound contraction | Increased levels | Decreased levels |
| TGF-β (including isoforms $\beta_1$, $\beta_2$, and $\beta_3$) | Platelets, T lymphocytes, macrophages, endothelial cells, keratinocytes, fibroblasts | Inflammation; granulation tissue formation; reepithelialization; matrix formation and remodeling; chemotactic for PMNs, macrophages, lymphocytes, fibroblasts; stimulates TIMP synthesis, keratinocyte migration, angiogenesis, and fibroplasia; inhibits production of MMPs and keratinocyte proliferation; induces TGF-β production | Increased levels | Decreased levels |
| EGF | Platelets, macrophages, fibroblasts | Mitogenic for keratinocytes and fibroblasts; stimulates keratinocyte migration | Increased levels | Decreased levels |
| FGF-1 and FGF-2 family | Macrophages, mast cells, T lymphocytes, endothelial cells, fibroblasts, keratinocytes, smooth muscle cells, chondrocytes | Granulation tissue formation; reepithelialization; matrix formation and remodeling; chemotactic for fibroblasts, mitogenic for fibroblasts and keratinocytes; stimulates keratinocyte migration; angiogenesis; wound contraction and matrix deposition | Increased levels | Decreased levels |
| KGF (also called FGF-7) | Fibroblasts, keratinocytes, smooth muscle cells, chondrocytes, endothelial cells, mast cells | Stimulate proliferation and migration of keratinocytes, increase transcription of factors involved in detoxification of ROS, potent mitogen for vascular endothelial cells; upregulates VEGF, stimulates endothelial cell production of UPA | Increased levels | Decreased levels |
| VEGF | Keratinocytes, platelets, PMNs, macrophages, endothelial cells, smooth muscle cells, fibroblasts | Granulation tissue formation; increases vasopermeability; mitogenic for endothelial cells | Increased levels | Decreased levels |
| TGF-α | Macrophages, T lymphocytes, keratinocytes, platelets, fibroblasts, lymphocytes | Reepithelialization; increase keratinocyte migration and proliferation | | |
| IGF-1 | Macrophages, fibroblasts | Stimulates elastin production and collagen synthesis, fibroblast proliferation | | |

Adapted from Schwartz SI (ed): Principles of surgery, ed 7, New York, 1999, McGraw-Hill, p 269; and Barrientos S, Stojadinovic O, Golinko MS, et al: Growth factors and cytokines in wound healing. Wound Rep Regen 16: 585–601, 2008.

*HA,* Hyaluronic acid.

These findings suggest that administration of IFN-γ may improve scar hypertrophy by decreasing the strength of the wound.

Macrophages also release growth factors that stimulate fibroblast, endothelial cell, and keratinocyte proliferation and are important in the proliferative phase (see Table 7-2). Macrophage-secreted PDGF stimulates collagen and proteoglycan synthesis. PDGF exists as three isomers—PDGF-AA, PDGF-AB, and PDGF-BB. However, the PDGF-BB isomer is the only growth factor preparation approved by the U.S. Food and Drug Administration and is the most widely studied clinically. Topical application of recombinant PDGF has improved wound-breaking strength and healing time in human and murine models of acute wounding. Administration of PDGF-BB has improved wound closure in chronic and diabetic nonhealing ulcers in humans and rodents but did not have the same effect in steroid-treated animals.

TGF-α and TGF-β are both released by activated monocytes. TGF-α stimulates epidermal growth and angiogenesis. TGF-β itself stimulates monocytes to express other peptides such as TGF-α, IL-1, and PDGF. TGF-β, which is also released by platelets and fibroblasts within wounds, exists as at least three isomers—$\beta_1$, $\beta_2$, and $\beta_3$—and its effects include fibroblast migration and maturation and ECM synthesis. TGF-$\beta_1$ has been shown to play an important role in collagen metabolism and healing of gastrointestinal injuries and anastomoses. In experimental models, TGF-$\beta_1$ accelerates wound healing in normal, steroid-impaired, and irradiated animals.

TGF-β is the most potent stimulant of fibroplasia, and its strong mitogenic effects have been implicated in the fibrogenesis seen in disease states such as scleroderma and interstitial pulmonary fibrosis. Enhanced expression of TGF-$\beta_1$ mRNA is found in keloid and hypertrophic scars. In contrast, fetal wounds have been demonstrated to have a paucity of TGF-β, thus suggesting that the scarless repair seen in utero occurs because of low or absent amounts of TGF-β. Studies of the three isomers have suggested that although TGF-$\beta_1$ and TGF-$\beta_2$ play an important role in tissue fibrosis and postinjury scarring, TGF-$\beta_3$ may limit scarring. As the concentration of TGF-β rises in the inflammatory site, fibroblasts are directly stimulated to produce collagen and fibronectin, thus leading to the proliferative phase.

### Lymphocytes

T lymphocytes appear in significant number in the wound at approximately the fifth day, with a peak occurring at approximately the seventh day. B lymphocytes do not appear to play a significant role in wound healing but seem to be involved in downregulating healing as the wound closes. Lymphocytes exert most of their effects on fibroblasts by producing stimulatory cytokines, such as IL-2 and fibroblast-activating factor, and inhibitory cytokines, such as TGF-β, TNF-α, and IFN-γ. Initially, lymphocytes were thought to play a minimal role in acute wound healing, particularly in the absence of excessive inflammation. The macrophage processes foreign debris such as bacteria or enzymatically degraded host proteins and serves as an antigen-presenting cell to lymphocytes. This interaction stimulates lymphocyte proliferation and release of cytokines. T cells produce IFN-γ, which stimulates the macrophage to release a cascade of cytokines, including TNF-α and IL-1. IFN-γ also causes decreased synthesis of prostaglandins, which enhances the effect of inflammatory mediators. In addition, IFN-γ suppresses collagen synthesis and inhibits macrophages from leaving the site of injury. Thus, IFN-γ appears to be an important mediator of chronic nonhealing wounds, and its presence suggests that T lymphocytes are primarily involved in chronic wound healing.

Some studies, however, have questioned the belief that lymphocytes are not essential for acute wound healing. Drugs that suppress T-lymphocyte function and proliferation, such as steroids and immunosuppressive agents (e.g., cyclosporine, tacrolimus), have been found to result in impaired wound healing in experimental wound models, possibly through decreased NO synthesis. In vivo lymphocyte depletion suggests the existence of an incompletely characterized T cell lymphocyte population that is neither $CD4^+$ nor $CD8^+$, and it is this subset that seems to be responsible for the promotion of wound healing.

## Proliferative Phase

As the acute responses of hemostasis and inflammation begin to resolve, the scaffolding is laid for repair of the wound through angiogenesis, fibroplasia, and epithelialization. This stage is characterized by the formation of granulation tissue, which consists of a capillary bed, fibroblasts, macrophages, and a loose arrangement of collagen, fibronectin, and hyaluronic acid.

A number of studies have used growth factors to modify granulation tissue, particularly fibroplasia. Adenoviral transfer, topical application, and subcutaneous injection of PDGF, TGF-β, keratinocyte growth factor (KGF), vascular endothelial growth factor (VEGF), and epidermal growth factor (EGF) have been tested to increase the proliferation of granulation tissue.

### Angiogenesis

Angiogenesis is the process of new blood vessel formation and is necessary to support a healing wound environment. After injury, activated endothelial cells degrade the basement membrane of postcapillary venules, thereby allowing the migration of cells through this gap. Division of these migrating endothelial cells results in tubule or lumen formation. Eventually, deposition of the basement membrane occurs and results in capillary maturation.

After injury, the endothelium is exposed to numerous soluble factors and comes in contact with adhering blood cells. These interactions result in upregulation of the expression of cell surface adhesion molecules, such as vascular cell surface adhesion molecule-1 (VCAM-1). Matrix-degrading enzymes, such as plasmin and the metalloproteinases, are released and activated, and degrade the endothelial basement membrane. Fragmentation of the basement membrane allows migration of endothelial cells into the wound, promoted by fibroblast growth factor (FGF), PDGF, and TGF-β. Injured endothelial cells express adhesion molecules, such as the integrin $\alpha_v\beta_3$, which facilitates attachment to fibrin, fibronectin, and fibrinogen and thus facilitates endothelial cell migration along the provisional matrix scaffold. Platelet endothelial cell adhesion molecule-1 (PECAM-1), also found on endothelial cells, modulates their interaction with each other as they migrate into the wound.

Capillary tube formation is a complex process that involves cell-cell and cell-matrix interactions, modulated by adhesion molecules on endothelial cell surfaces. PECAM-1 has been observed to mediate cell-cell contact, whereas $\beta_1$ integrin receptors may aid in stabilizing these contacts and forming tight junctions between endothelial cells. Some of the new capillaries differentiate into arterioles and venules, whereas others undergo involution and apoptosis, with subsequent ingestion by macrophages. Regulation of endothelial apoptosis is not well understood.

Angiogenesis appears to be stimulated and manipulated by a variety of cytokines predominantly produced by macrophages and platelets. As the macrophage produces TNF-α, it orchestrates angiogenesis during the inflammatory phase. Heparin, which can stimulate the migration of capillary endothelial cells, binds with high affinity to a group of angiogenic factors.

VEGF, a member of the PDGF family of growth factors, has potent angiogenic activity. It is produced in large amounts by keratinocytes, macrophages, endothelial cells, platelets, and fibroblasts during wound healing.[9-12] Cell disruption and hypoxia, hallmarks of tissue injury, appear to be strong initial inducers of potent angiogenic factors at the wound site, such as VEGF and its receptor. VEGF family members include VEGF-A, VEGF-B, VEGF-C, VEGF-D, VEGF-E, and placental growth factor (PLGF).[13] VEGF-A promotes early events in angiogenesis and subsequently is crucial to wound healing.[14] It binds to tyrosine kinase surface receptors Flt-1 (VEGF receptor-1, or VEGFR-1) and KDR (VEGF receptor-2, or VEGFR-2).[15] Flt-1 is required for blood vessel organization, whereas KDR is important for endothelial cell chemotaxis, proliferation, and differentiation.[16,17] Animal studies have shown that VEGF-A administration restores impaired angiogenesis found in diabetic ischemic limbs[18]; however, other studies have shown that exogenous VEGF results in vascular leakage and disorganized blood vessel formation.[19,20] VEGF-C, which is also elevated during wound healing, is primarily released by macrophages and is important during the inflammatory phase of wound healing.[21] Although it works primarily through VEGF receptor-3 (VEGFR-3), which is expressed in macrophages and lymphatic endothelium, it can also activate VEGFR-2, thereby increasing vascular permeability.[21] In vivo administration of VEGF-C in an animal model using an adenoviral vector to genetically diabetic mice resulted in accelerated healing.[13] PLGF is another proangiogenic factor that is elevated after wounding. It is involved in inflammation and expressed by keratinocytes and endothelial cells. It is believed to work synergistically with VEGF, thereby potentiating its proangiogenic function.[22]

Both acidic and basic FGFs (FGF-1 and FGF-2) are released from disrupted parenchymal cells and are early stimulants of angiogenesis. FGF-2 provides the initial angiogenic stimulus within the first 3 days of wound repair, followed by a subsequent prolonged stimulus mediated by VEGF from days 4 through 7. There is a dose-dependent effect of VEGF and FGF-2 on angiogenesis. Both TGF-α and EGF stimulate endothelial cell proliferation. TNF-α is chemotactic for endothelial cells; it promotes formation of the capillary tube and may mediate angiogenesis through its induction of hypoxia-inducible factor 1 (HIF-1). It regulates the expression of other hypoxia-responsive genes, including inducible NO synthase and VEGF. HIF-1α mRNA is prominently present in wound inflammatory cells during the initial 24 hours, and HIF-1α protein is present in cells isolated from the wound 1 and 5 days after injury in vitro. Data also suggest that there is a positive interaction between endogenous NO and VEGF, with endogenous NO enhancing VEGF synthesis. Similarly, VEGF has been shown to promote NO synthesis in angiogenesis, thus suggesting that NO mediates aspects of VEGF signaling required for endothelial cell proliferation and organization.

TGF-β is a chemoattractant for fibroblasts and probably assists in angiogenesis by signaling the fibroblast to produce FGFs. Other factors that have been shown to induce angiogenesis include angiogenin, IL-8, and lactic acid. Several of the matrix materials, such as fibronectin and hyaluronic acid from the wound site, are angiogenic. Fibronectin and fibrin are produced by macrophages and damaged endothelial cells. Collagen appears to interact by causing the tubular formation of endothelial cells in vitro. Angiogenesis thus results from the complex interaction of ECM material and cytokines.

### Fibroplasia

Fibroblasts are specialized cells that differentiate from resting mesenchymal cells in connective tissue; they do not arrive in the wound cleft by diapedesis from circulating cells. After injury, the normally quiescent and sparse fibroblasts are chemoattracted to the inflammatory site, where they divide and produce the components of the ECM. After stimulation by macrophage- and platelet-derived cytokines and growth factors, the fibroblast, which is normally arrested in the $G_0$ phase, undergoes replication and proliferation. Platelet-derived TGF-β stimulates fibroblast proliferation indirectly by releasing PDGF. The fibroblast can also stimulate replication in an autocrine manner by releasing FGF-2. To continue proliferating, fibroblasts require further stimulation by factors such as EGF or IGF-I. Although fibroblasts require growth factors for proliferation, they do not need growth factors to survive. Fibroblasts can live quiescently in growth factor–free media in monolayers or three-dimensional cultures.

The primary function of fibroblasts is to synthesize collagen, which they begin to produce during the cellular phase of inflammation. The time required for undifferentiated mesenchymal cells to differentiate into highly specialized fibroblasts accounts for the delay between injury and the appearance of collagen in a healing wound. This period, generally 3 to 5 days, depending on the type of tissue injured, is called the lag phase of wound healing. Fibroblasts begin to migrate in response to chemotactic substances such as growth factors (PDGF, TGF-β), C5 fragments, thrombin, TNF-α, eicosanoids, elastin fragments, leukotriene B4, and fragments of collagen and fibronectin.

The rate of collagen synthesis declines after 4 weeks and eventually balances the rate of collagen destruction by collagenase (MMP-1). At this point, the wound enters a phase of collagen maturation. The maturation phase continues for months or even years. Glycoprotein and mucopolysaccharide levels decrease during the maturation phase, and new capillaries regress and disappear. These changes alter the appearance of the wound and increase its strength.

### Epithelialization

The epidermis serves as a physical barrier to prevent fluid loss and bacterial invasion. Tight cell junctions within the epithelium contribute to its impermeability and the basement membrane zone gives structural support and provides attachment between the epidermis and the dermis. The basement membrane zone consists of several layers:

1. The lamina lucida (electron clear), consisting of laminin and heparan sulfate
2. The lamina densa (electron dense), containing type IV collagen
3. Anchoring fibrils, consisting of type IV collagen, which secure the epidermodermal interface and connect the lamina densa to the dermis

The basal layer of the epidermis attaches to the basement membrane zone by hemidesmosomes. Reepithelialization of wounds begins within hours after injury. Initially, the wound is rapidly sealed by clot formation and then by epithelial (epidermal) cell migration across the defect. Keratinocytes located at the basal layer of the residual epidermis or in the depths of epithelium-lined dermal appendages migrate to resurface the wound. Epithelialization involves a sequence of changes in wound keratinocytes—detachment, migration, proliferation, differentiation, and stratification. If the basement membrane zone is intact, epithelialization proceeds more rapidly. The cells are stimulated to migrate. Attachments to neighboring and adjoining cells and to the dermis are loosened, as demonstrated by intracellular tonofilament retraction, dissolution of intercellular desmosomes and hemidesmosomes linking the epidermis to the basement membrane, and formation of cytoplasmic actin filaments.

Epidermal cells express integrin receptors that allow them to interact with ECM proteins such as fibronectin. The migrating cells dissect the wound by separating the desiccated eschar from viable tissue. This path of dissection is determined by the integrins that the epidermal cells express on their cell membranes. Degradation of the ECM, required if epidermal cells are to migrate between the collagenous dermis and fibrin eschar, is driven by epidermal cell production of collagenase (MMP-1) and plasminogen activator, which activates collagenase and plasmin. The migrating cells are also phagocytic and remove debris in their path. Cells behind the leading edge of migrating cells begin to proliferate. The epithelial cells move in a leapfrog and tumbling fashion until the edges establish contact. If the basement membrane zone is not intact, it will be repaired first. The absence of neighboring cells at the wound margin may be a signal for the migration and proliferation of epidermal cells. Local release of EGF, TGF-α, and KGF and increased expression of their receptors may also stimulate these processes. Topical application of KGF-2 in young and aged animals accelerates reepithelialization. Basement membrane proteins, such as laminin, reappear in a highly ordered sequence from the margin of the wound inward. After the wound is completely reepithelialized, the cells become columnar and stratified again while firmly attaching to the reestablished basement membrane and underlying dermis.

### Extracellular Matrix

The ECM exists as a scaffold to stabilize the physical structure of tissues, but it also plays an active and complex role by regulating the behavior of cells that contact it. Cells within it produce the macromolecular constituents, including the following:

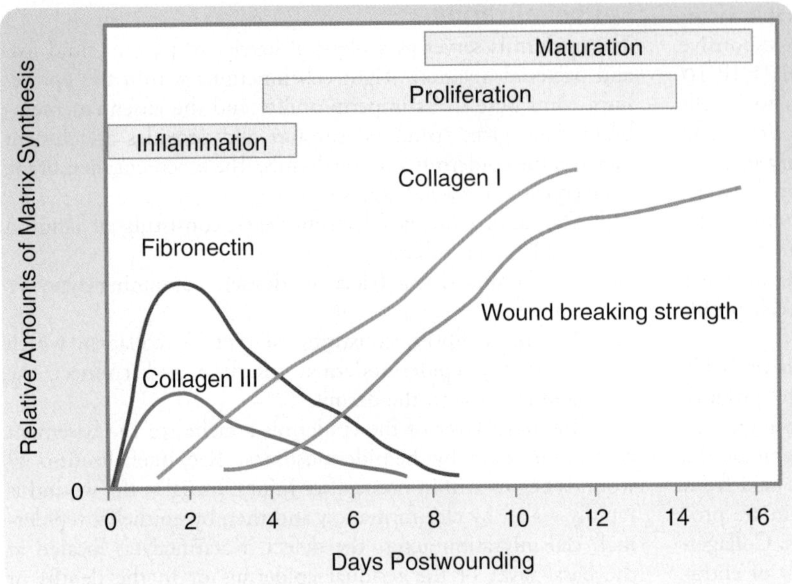


**FIGURE 7-7** Wound matrix deposition over time. Fibronectin and type III collagen constitute the early matrix. Type I collagen accumulates later and corresponds to the increase in wound-breaking strength. (Adapted from Witte MB, Barbul A: General principles of wound healing. Surg Clin North Am 77: 509–528, 1997.)

1. Glycosaminoglycans (GAGs), or polysaccharide chains, usually found covalently linked to protein in the form of proteoglycans
2. Fibrous proteins such as collagen, elastin, fibronectin, and laminin[23]

In connective tissue, proteoglycan molecules form a gel-like ground substance. This highly hydrated gel allows the matrix to withstand compressive force while permitting rapid diffusion of nutrients, metabolites, and hormones between blood and tissue cells. Collagen fibers within the matrix serve to organize and strengthen it, whereas elastin fibers give it resilience and matrix proteins have adhesive functions.[23]

The wound matrix accumulates and changes in composition as healing progresses, balanced between new deposition and degradation (Fig. 7-7). The provisional matrix is a scaffold for cellular migration and is composed of fibrin, fibrinogen, fibronectin, and vitronectin. GAGs and proteoglycans are synthesized next and support further matrix deposition and remodeling. Collagens, which are the predominant scar proteins, are the end result. Attachment proteins, such as fibrin and fibronectin, provide linkage to the ECM through binding to cell surface integrin receptors.

Stimulation of fibroblasts by growth factors induces upregulated expression of integrin receptors, thereby facilitating cell-matrix interactions. Ligand binding induces clustering of integrin into focal adhesion sites. Regulation of integrin-mediated cell signaling by the extracellular divalent cations $Mg^{2+}$, $Mn^{2+}$, and $Ca^{2+}$ is perhaps caused by induction of conformational changes in the integrins.

A dynamic and reciprocal relationship exists between fibroblasts and the ECM. Cytokine regulation of fibroblast responses is altered by variations in the composition of the ECM. For example, expression of matrix-degrading enzymes, such as the MMPs, is upregulated after cytokine stimulation of fibroblasts. Collagenolytic MMP-1 is induced by IL-1 and downregulated by TGF-β. Activation of plasminogen to plasmin by plasminogen activator and procollagenase to collagenase by plasmin results in matrix degradation and facilitates cell migration. Modulation of these processes provides additional mechanisms whereby the cell-matrix interaction can be regulated during wound healing. Matrix modulation is also seen in tumor metastasis. Neoplastic cells lose their dependence on anchorage, mediated mainly by integrins; this is probably caused by decreased production of fibronectin and subsequent decreased adhesion and, as a result, these cells can break away from the primary tumor and metastasize.

An example of the necessary dynamic interactions occurring in the provisional matrix during wound healing is the effect of TGF-β on incisional wounds sealed with fibrin sealant. Fibrin sealant is a derivative of plasma components that mimics the last step in the coagulation cascade. Commercially available fibrin sealant has an approximately 10-fold greater concentration of fibrin than plasma and consequently provides a more airtight, waterproof seal. Fibrin sealant may serve as a mechanical barrier to the early cell-mediated events occurring in wound healing. Supplementation of fibrin sealant with TGF-β has been demonstrated to reverse the inhibitory effects of fibrin sealant on wound healing and increase tensile strength as compared with sutured wounds. The increased tensile strength may be a result of improved cell migration into the wound site, more rapid clearance of fibrin sealant, suppression of gelatinase (MMP-9), and enhancement of ECM synthesis in TGF-β–supplemented wounds.

**Collagen Structure** Collagens are found in all multicellular animals and are secreted by a variety of cell types. They are a major component of skin and bone and constitute 25% of the total protein mass in mammals. The proline- and glycine-rich collagen molecule is a long, stiff, triple-stranded helical structure that consists of three collagen polypeptide α chains wound around one another in a ropelike superhelix. With its ringlike structure, proline provides stability to the helical conformation in each α chain, whereas glycine, because of its small size, allows tight packing of the three α chains to form the final superhelix. There are at least 20 types of collagen, the main constituents of connective tissue being types I, II, III, V, and XI. Type I is the principal collagen of skin and bone and is the most common.[23] In adults, the skin is approximately 80% type I and 20% type

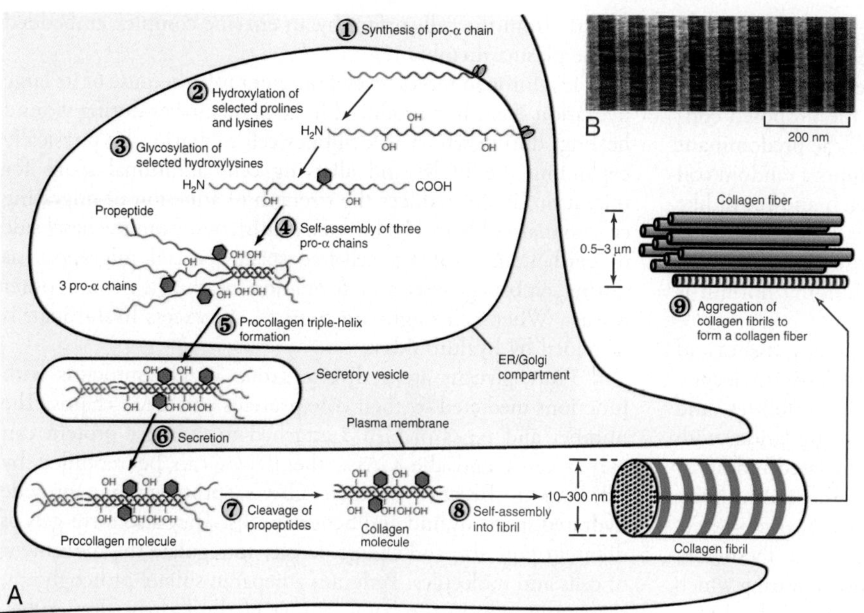


**FIGURE 7-8** Intracellular and extracellular events in the formation of a collagen fibril. **A,** Collagen fibrils are shown assembling in the extracellular space contained within a large infolding in the plasma membrane. As one example of how collagen fibrils can form ordered arrays in the extracellular space, they are shown further assembling into large collagen fibers, which are visible with a light microscope. The covalent cross links that stabilize the extracellular assemblies are not shown. **B,** Electron micrograph of a negatively stained collagen fibril revealing its typical striated appearance. *ER,* Endoplasmic reticulum. (**A,** From Alberts B, Johnson A, Lewis J, et al [eds]: Molecular biology of the cell, ed 4, New York, 2002, Garland, p 1100; **B,** Courtesy Robert Horne.)

III. In newborns, the content of type III collagen is greater than that found in adults. In early wound healing, there is also increased expression of type III collagen. Type I collagens are the fibrillar, or fibril-forming, collagens. They are secreted into the extracellular space, where they assemble into collagen fibrils (10 to 300 nm in diameter), which then aggregate into larger, cable-like bundles called collagen fibers (several micrometers in diameter).

Other types of collagens include types IX and XII (fibril-associated collagens) and types IV and VII (network-forming collagens). Types IX and XII are found on the surface of collagen fibrils and serve to link the fibrils to one another and to other components in the ECM. Type IV molecules assemble into a meshlike pattern and are a major part of the mature basal lamina. Dimers of type VII form anchoring fibrils that help attach the basal lamina to the underlying connective tissue and are especially abundant in the skin.

Type XVII and XVIII collagens are two of a number of collagen-like proteins. Type XVII has a transmembrane domain and is found in hemidesmosomes. Type XVIII is located in the basal laminae of blood vessels. The peptide endostatin, which inhibits angiogenesis and shows promise as an anticancer drug, is formed by cleavage of the C-terminal domain of type XVIII collagen.

**Collagen Synthesis** Collagen polypeptide chains are synthesized on membrane-bound ribosomes and enter the endoplasmic reticulum (ER) lumen as pro–α chains (Fig. 7-8). These precursors have amino-terminal signal peptides to direct them to the ER, as well as propeptides at both the N- and C-terminal ends. Within the lumen of the ER, some of the prolines and lysines undergo hydroxylation to form hydroxyproline and hydroxylysine. Hydroxylation results in the stable triple-stranded helix through the formation of interchain hydrogen bonds. The pro–α chain then combines with two others to form procollagen, a hydrogen-bonded, triple-stranded helical molecule. In conditions such as vitamin C (ascorbic acid) deficiency (scurvy), proline hydroxylation is prevented, thereby resulting in the formation of unstable triple helices secondary to the synthesis of defective pro–α chains. Vitamin C deficiency is characterized by the gradual loss of preexisting normal collagen, which leads to fragile blood vessels and loose teeth.

After secretion into the ECM, specific proteases cleave the propeptides of the procollagen molecules to form collagen monomers. These monomers assemble to form collagen fibrils in the ECM, driven by collagen's tendency to self-assemble. Covalent cross linking of the lysine residues provides tensile strength. The extent and type of cross linking vary from tissue to tissue. In tissues such as tendons, in which tensile strength is crucial, collagen cross linking is extremely high. In mammalian skin, the fibrils are organized in a basket weave pattern to resist multidirectional tensile stress. In tendons, on the other hand, fibrils are in parallel bundles aligned along the major axis of tension.[23]

A number of factors can affect collagen synthesis. Vitamin C (ascorbic acid), TGF-β, IGF-I, and IGF-II increase collagen synthesis. IFN-γ decreases type I procollagen mRNA synthesis and glucocorticoids inhibit procollagen gene transcription, thereby leading to decreased collagen synthesis.

Several genetic disorders are caused by abnormalities in collagen fibril formation. In osteogenesis imperfecta, deletion of one procollagen $\alpha_1$ allele results in weak and easily fractured bones. Ehlers-Danlos syndrome is a result of mutations affecting type III collagen and is characterized by fragile skin and blood vessels and hypermobile joints.

**Elastic Fibers** Tissues such as skin, blood vessels, and lungs require strength and elasticity to function. Elastic fibers in the ECM of these tissues provide the resilience to allow recoil after transient stretching.

Elastic fibers are predominantly composed of elastin, a highly hydrophobic protein (≈750 amino acids long). Soluble tropoelastin is secreted into the extracellular space, where it forms lysine cross links to other tropoelastin molecules to generate a large network of elastin fibers and sheets. Elastin is composed of hydrophobic and alanine- and lysine-rich α-helical segments that alternate along the polypeptide chain. The hydrophobic segments are responsible for the molecule's elastic properties. The alanine- and lysine-rich α-helical segments form cross links between adjacent molecules. Although the proposed conformation of elastin molecules is controversial, the predominant theory is that the elastin polypeptide chain adopts a random coil conformation that allows the network to stretch and recoil like a rubber band. Elastic fibers consist of an elastin core covered by a sheath of microfibrils, which are composed of several distinct glycoproteins such as fibrillin. Elastin-binding fibrillin is essential for integrity of the elastic fibers.

Microfibrils appear before elastin in developing tissues and seem to form a scaffold on which the secreted elastin molecules are deposited. Elastin is produced early in life, stabilizes, and does not undergo much further synthesis or degradation, with a turnover that approaches the life span. Age-related modification is a result of progressive degradation as the elastic fibers gradually become tortuous, frayed, and porous. Scanning electron microscopy shows that in humans, the elastic meshwork grows largely undistorted during postnatal growth, during which fibers seem to enlarge in synchrony with growth of the tissue. In nonwounded circumstances, there is little elastin degradation, probably because of elastin's hydrophobic nature, which makes the interior of this highly folded protein inaccessible. As a result of this high degree of three-dimensionality and extensive cross linking, cleavage must be considerable before there is much loss of elasticity. Both IGF-1 and TGF-β stimulate the production of elastin. Glucocorticoids and basic FGF reduce adult skin cell production of elastin.

Mutations causing a deficiency of elastin protein result in arterial narrowing as a consequence of excessive smooth muscle cell proliferation in the arterial wall (intimal hyperplasia). These findings suggest that the normal elasticity of an artery is needed to prevent proliferation of these cells. Gene mutations in fibrillin result in Marfan syndrome; severely affected individuals are prone to aortic rupture.

**Glycosaminoglycans and Proteoglycans** GAGs are unbranched polysaccharide chains composed of repeating disaccharide units, a sulfated amino sugar (*N*-acetylglucosamine or *N*-acetylgalactosamine) and uronic acid (glucuronic or iduronic). GAGs are highly negatively charged because of the sulfate or carboxyl groups on most of their sugars. Four types of GAGS exist[23]:

1. Hyaluronan
2. Chondroitin sulfate and dermatan sulfate
3. Heparan sulfate
4. Keratan sulfate

The GAGs in connective tissue usually constitute less than 10% of the weight of the fibrous proteins. Their highly negative charge attracts osmotically active cations, such as $Na^+$, which causes large amounts of water to be incorporated into the matrix. This results in porous hydrated gels and is responsible for the turgor that enables the matrix to withstand compressive force.[23]

Hyaluronan is the simplest of the GAGs. It is composed of repeating nonsulfated disaccharide units and is found in adult tissues, but is especially prevalent in fetal tissues. Its abundance in fetal wounds is believed to be a factor in the scarless wound healing seen in fetal tissues. Unlike the other GAGs, hyaluronan is not covalently attached to any protein and is synthesized directly from the cell surface by an enzyme complex embedded in the plasma membrane.

Hyaluronan serves several different roles because of its large hydration shell. It is produced in large quantities during wound healing, during which it facilitates cell migration by physically expanding the ECM and allowing cells additional space for migration; it also reduces the strength of adhesion of migrating cells to matrix fibers. Hyaluronan synthesized from the basal side of epithelium creates a cell-free space for cell migration, as during embryogenesis and formation of the heart and other organs. When cell migration finishes, the excess hyaluronan is degraded by hyaluronidase.

Proteoglycans are a diverse group of glycoproteins with functions mediated by their core proteins and GAG chains. The number and types of GAGs attached to the core protein can vary greatly, and the GAGs themselves can be modified by sulfonation. Because of their GAGs, proteoglycans provide hydrated space around and between cells. They also form gels of different pore size and charge density to regulate the movement of cells and molecules. Perlecan, a heparan sulfate proteoglycan, serves this role in the basal lamina of the kidney glomerulus. Decreased levels of perlecan are believed to play a role in diabetic albuminuria.

Proteoglycans function in chemical signaling by binding various secreted signal molecules, such as growth factors, and modulating their signaling activity. Proteoglycans can also bind other secreted proteins, such as proteases and protease inhibitors. Such binding allows proteoglycans to regulate proteins by the following:

1. Immobilizing the protein and restricting its range of action
2. Providing a reservoir of the protein for delayed release
3. Altering the protein to allow more effective presentation to cell surface receptors
4. Prolonging the protein's action by protecting it from degradation
5. Blocking the activity of the protein

Proteoglycans can be components of plasma membranes and have a transmembrane core protein or are attached to the lipid bilayer by a glycosylphosphatidylinositol anchor. These proteoglycans act as coreceptors that work with other cell surface receptor proteins in binding cells to the ECM and initiating the response of cells to extracellular signaling proteins. For example, the syndecans are transmembrane proteoglycans located on the surface of many cells, including fibroblasts and epithelial cells. In fibroblasts, syndecans are found in focal adhesions, where they interact with fibronectin on the cell surface and with cytoskeletal and signaling proteins inside the cell. Mutations leading to inactivation of these coreceptor proteoglycans result in severe developmental defects.[23]

The ECM has other noncollagen proteins, such as the fibronectins, that have multiple domains and can bind to other matrix macromolecules and cell surface receptors. These interactions help organize the matrix and facilitate cell attachment. Fibronectin is important in animal embryogenesis.

Fibronectin exists as soluble and fibrillar isoforms. Soluble plasma fibronectin circulates in various body fluids and enhances blood clotting, wound healing, and phagocytosis. The highly insoluble fibrillar forms assemble on cell surfaces and are deposited in the ECM. The fibronectin fibrils that form on the surface of fibroblasts are usually coupled with neighboring intracellular actin stress fibers. The actin filaments promote assembly of the fibronectin fibril and influence fibril orientation. Integrin transmembrane adhesion proteins mediate these interactions. The contractile actin and myosin cytoskeleton pulls on the fibronectin matrix and generates tension.[23]

**Basal Lamina** Basal laminae are flexible, thin (40- to 120-nm–thick) mats of specialized ECM that separate cells and epithelia from the underlying or surrounding connective tissue. In skin, the basal lamina is tethered to the underlying connective tissue by specialized anchoring fibrils. This composite of basal lamina and collagen is the basement membrane.

The basal lamina acts in numerous ways:

1. As a molecular filter to prevent the passage of macromolecules (i.e., in the kidney glomerulus)
2. As a selective barrier to certain cells (i.e., the lamina beneath the epithelium prevents fibroblasts from contacting epithelial cells, but does not stop macrophages or lymphocytes)
3. As a scaffold for regenerating cells to migrate
4. As an important element in tissue regeneration in locations where the basal lamina survives

Although its composition may vary from tissue to tissue, most mature basal laminae contain type IV collagen, perlecan, and the glycoproteins laminin and nidogen. Type IV collagen has a more flexible structure than the fibrillar collagens; its triple-stranded helix is interrupted, thereby allowing multiple bends.

Laminins, in general, consist of three long polypeptide chains ($\alpha$, $\beta$, and $\gamma$). Mice lacking the laminin $\gamma_1$ chain die during embryogenesis because they cannot make a basal lamina. The laminin in basement membranes consists of several domains that bind to perlecan, nidogen, and laminin receptor proteins found on cell surfaces. The type IV collagen and laminin networks are connected by nidogen and perlecan, which act as stabilizing bridges. Many of the cell surface receptors for type IV collagen and laminin are members of the integrin family. Another important type of laminin receptor is dystroglycan, a transmembrane protein that together with integrins may organize assembly of the basal lamina.

**Degradation of the Extracellular Matrix** Regulated turnover of the ECM is crucial to many biologic processes. ECM degradation occurs during metastasis when neoplastic cells migrate from their site of origin to distant organs via the bloodstream or lymphatics. In injury or infection, localized degradation of the ECM occurs so that cells can migrate across the basal lamina to reach the site of injury or infection. Locally secreted cellular proteases, such as MMPs or serine proteases, degrade the ECM components. Matrix proteolysis helps the cell migrate in the following ways:

1. Clearing a path through the matrix
2. Exposing binding sites, thereby promoting cell binding or migration
3. Facilitating cell detachment so that a cell can move forward
4. Releasing signal proteins that promote cell migration

Proteolysis is tightly regulated. Many proteases are secreted as inactive precursors that are activated when required. In addition, cell surface receptors bind these proteases to ensure that they act only on sites where they are needed. Finally, protease inhibitors, such as the tissue inhibitors of metalloproteinase (TIMPs), can bind these enzymes and block their activity.

## Maturational Phase

Wound contraction occurs by centripetal movement of the whole thickness of the surrounding skin and reduces the amount of disorganized scar. Wound contracture, in contrast, is a physical constriction or limitation of function and is a result of the process of wound contraction. Contractures occur when excessive scar exceeds normal wound contraction, and it results in a functional disability. Scars that traverse joints and prevent extension or scars that involve the eyelid or mouth and cause an ectropion are examples of contractures.

Wound contraction appears to take place as a result of a complex interaction of the extracellular materials and fibroblasts, which is not completely understood. Using a fibroblast-populated collagen lattice, Ehrlich demonstrated that aborted cell locomotion appears to cause bunching and contraction of the collagen fibers.[23a] In this in vitro model, trypsinized collagen is populated by fibroblasts that adhere to it in culture. If normal dermal fibroblasts are cultured, they attempt to move but are trapped by the collagen fibers. The tractional forces cause the lattice to bunch and contract.

Numerous studies have shown that fibroblasts in a contracting wound undergo change to stimulated cells, referred to as myofibroblasts. These cells have function and structure in common with fibroblasts and smooth muscle cells and express alpha smooth muscle actin in bundles called stress fibers. The actin appears at day 6 after wounding, persists at high levels for 15 days, and is gone by 4 weeks, when the cell undergoes apoptosis. It appears that a stimulated fibroblast develops contractile ability related to the formation of cytoplasmic actin-myosin complexes. When this stimulated cell is placed in the fibroblast-populated collagen lattice, contraction occurs even faster. The tension that is exerted by the fibroblasts' attempt at contraction appears to stimulate the actin-myosin structures in their cytoplasm. If colchicine, which inhibits microtubules, or cytochalasin D, which inhibits microfilaments, is added to the tissue culture, the result is minimal contraction of the collagen gels. Fibroblasts develop a linear arrangement in the line of tension that when removed, causes the cells to round up.

Stimulated fibroblasts, or myofibroblasts, are found to be a constant feature present in abundance in diseases involving excessive fibrosis. Such diseases include hepatic cirrhosis, renal and pulmonary fibrosis, Dupuytren's contracture, and desmoplastic reactions induced by neoplasia. The actin microfilaments are arranged linearly along the long axis of the fibroblast. They are associated with dense bodies that allow attachment to the surrounding ECM. Fibronexus is the attachment entity that connects the cytoskeleton to the ECM and spans the cell membrane in doing so.

MMPs also appear to be important for wound contraction. It has been demonstrated that stromelysin-1 (MMP-3) strongly affects wound contraction. MMPs may be necessary to allow cleavage of the attachment between the fibroblast and the collagen so that the lattice can be made to contract. Different populations of fibroblasts, from different organs, respond to the contraction stimulus in a heterogeneous fashion. It is likely that the stromelysin-1, with the participation of $\beta_1$ integrins, allows modification of attachment sites between fibroblasts and the

**BOX 7-1 Factors That Inhibit Wound Healing**

Infection
Ischemia
  Circulation
  Respiration
  Local tension
Diabetes mellitus
Ionizing radiation
Advanced age
Malnutrition
Vitamin deficiencies
  Vitamin C
  Vitamin A
Mineral deficiencies
  Zinc
  Iron
Exogenous drugs
  Doxorubicin (Adriamycin)
  Glucocorticosteroids

collagen fibrils. Similarly, cytokines such as TGF-$\beta_1$ affect contraction by increasing the expression of $\beta_1$ integrin.

### Remodeling

The fibroblast population decreases and the dense capillary network regresses. Wound strength increases rapidly within 1 to 6 weeks and then appears to plateau up to 1 year after the injury (see Fig. 7-8). When compared with nonwounded skin, tensile strength is only 30% in the scar. An increase in breaking strength occurs after approximately 21 days, mostly as a result of cross linking. Although collagen cross linking causes further wound contraction and an increase in strength, it also results in a scar that is more brittle and less elastic than normal skin. Unlike normal skin, the epidermodermal interface in a healed wound is devoid of rete pegs, the undulating projections of epidermis that penetrate into the papillary dermis. Loss of this anchorage results in increased fragility and predisposes the neoepidermis to avulsion after minor trauma.

## ABNORMAL WOUND HEALING

In such a complex series of interweaving events as wound healing, a number of factors can impede the outcome (Box 7-1). The amount of tissue lost or damaged, amount of foreign material or bacterial inoculation, and length of exposure to toxic factors affect the time to recovery. Intrinsic factors such as age, chemotherapeutic agents, atherosclerosis, cardiac or renal failure, and location on the body all affect wound healing.

Ultimately, the type of scar—whether it is adequate, inadequate, or proliferative—is dictated by the amount of collagen deposition and balanced by the amount of collagen degradation. If the balance is tipped in either direction, the result is poor.

### Hypertrophic Scars and Keloids

Keloids and hypertrophic scars are proliferative scars characterized by excessive collagen deposition versus collagen degradation (Fig. 7-9). Keloids are defined as scars that grow beyond the borders of the original wounds, and these scars rarely regress with time. Keloids are more prevalent in patients with more darkly pigmented skin; they develop in 15% to 20% of African

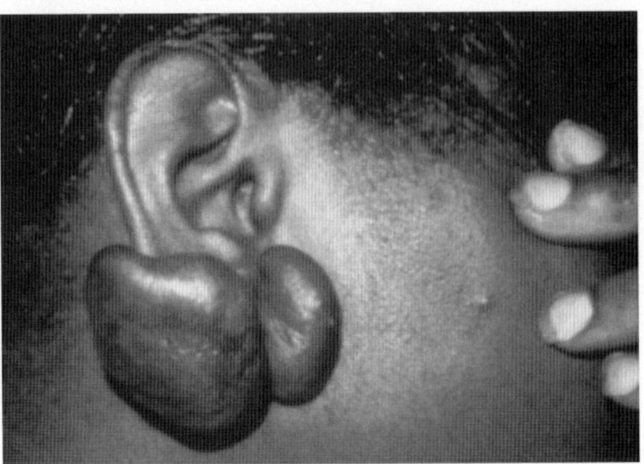

FIGURE 7-9 Keloids caused by ear piercing.

Americans, Asians, and Hispanics. Keloids appear to have a genetic predisposition. Keloid scars tend to occur above the clavicles, on the trunk, on the upper extremities, and on the face. They cannot be prevented at this time and are often refractory to medical and surgical intervention. Hypertrophic scars, in contrast, are raised scars that remain within the confines of the original wound and frequently regress spontaneously. These scars also differ histologically from normal scars. Keloids and hypertrophic scars have stretched collagen bundles aligned in the same plane as the epidermis, as opposed to normal scar tissue, in which the collagen bundles are randomly arrayed and relaxed. In addition, keloid scars have thicker, more abundant collagen bundles that form acellular nodelike structures in the deep dermal portion of the keloid lesion. The center of keloid lesions also contains a paucity of cells in comparison to hypertrophic scars, which have islands composed of aggregates of fibroblasts, small vessels, and collagen fibers throughout the dermis.

Hypertrophic scars are often preventable. Prolonged inflammation and insufficient resurfacing, such as can occur with a burn wound, lead to hypertrophic scars. It appears that the tension that signals the formation of activated fibroblasts also causes excessive collagen to be deposited. Scars perpendicular to the underlying muscle fibers tend to be flatter and narrower, with less collagen formation than when they are parallel to the underlying muscle fibers. The position of an elective scar can be chosen in such a way to make a narrower and less obvious scar in the distant future (Fig. 7-10). As muscle fibers contract, the wound edges become reapproximated if they are perpendicular to the underlying muscle. If, however, the scar is parallel to the underlying muscle, contraction of that muscle tends to cause gaping of the wound edges and leads to more tension and scar formation.

There is some indication of biochemical differences between proliferative scars and normal wound scars. Hypertrophic scars represent a hyperproliferative phenotype that develops after multiple stimulatory effects. This phenotype can be reversed once the stimulation, such as excessive skin tension or growth factors, is removed. Keloids, however, represent a unique phenotype that appears to be genetically predisposed to changes in ECM production and is switched on irreversibly by factors such as TGF-β. Expression of the isoforms TGF-$\beta_1$ and TGF-$\beta_2$ is increased in human keloid cells in comparison to normal human

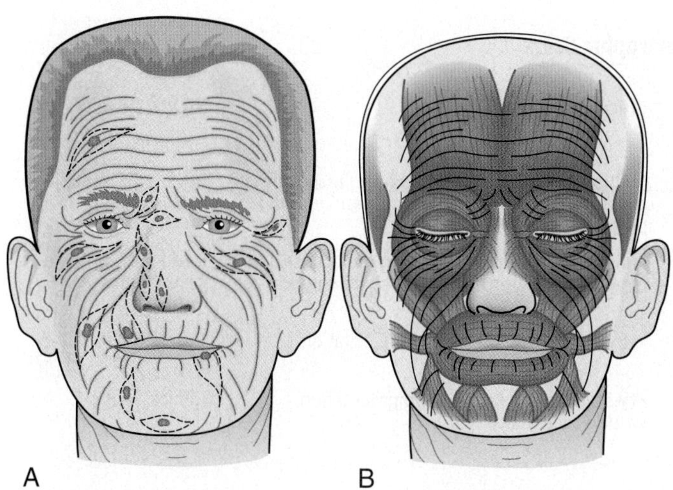


**FIGURE 7-10** The preferred orientation for elective skin incisions **(A)** is parallel to lines of facial expression **(B).** (From Kraissl CJ: The selection of appropriate lines for elective surgical incisions. Plast Reconstr Surg 8:1–28, 1951.)

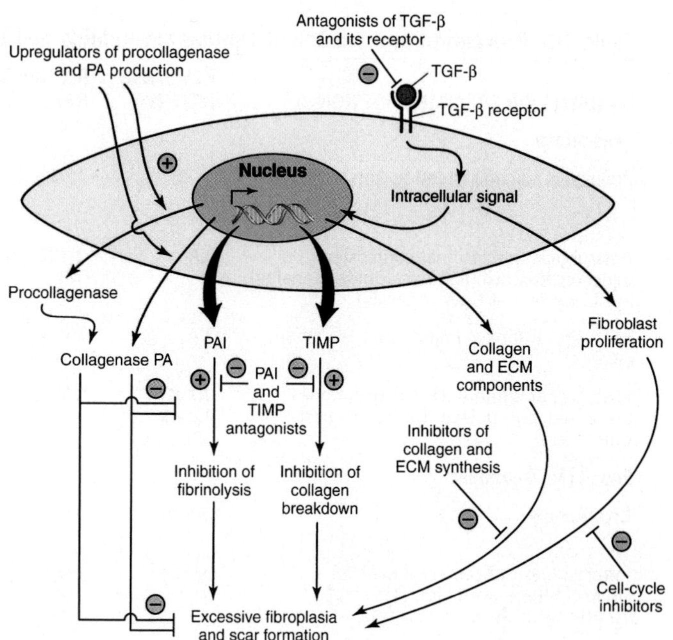


**FIGURE 7-11** Pathways in causing excessive fibroplasia by TGF-β and means for therapeutic intervention. TGF-β increases the cellular production of ECM proteins, such as fibronectin and collagen, and also increases the cellular expression of integrins (not shown). Furthermore, the synthesis of inhibitors of degrading enzymes of plasminogen activator inhibitor (PAI) and TIMPs is also increased by TGF-β, whereas expression of collagenase and plasminogen activator (PA) is decreased. This upregulation of inhibitor synthesis plus downregulation of protease synthesis further augments the accumulation of ECM proteins induced by TGF-β and is the basis for fibrotic tissue formation secondary to excessive action of TGF-β. Possible means of therapeutic intervention are highlighted. Antagonists of TGF-β and its receptor would shift the ECM equilibrium toward degradation, as would upregulators of PA production and PAI antagonists. Inhibitors of collagen and ECM synthesis would prevent excessive ECM deposition. Cell cycle inhibitors would prevent the proliferation of fibroblasts. (From Tuan TL, Nichter LS: The molecular basis of keloid and hypertrophic scar formation. Mol Med Today 41:19–24, 1998.)

dermal fibroblasts. Hypertrophic scar fibroblasts produce more TGF-$\beta_1$. In contrast to the elevated collagen synthesis seen in these scars, collagen degradation is low. Both MMP-1 (collagenase) and MMP-9 (gelatinase involved in early tissue repair) are decreased in hypertrophic scars and keloids. MMP-2 (gelatinase in late tissue remodeling) is significantly elevated in hypertrophic scars and keloids. Studies involving antibodies to TGF-β have shown that its activity can be blocked and fibrosis decreased. Growth factors have also been implicated in fibrosis and have been studied as targets for the blockade of fibrosis. IFN-γ, which suppresses collagen synthesis, has been tested clinically in keloid scars and has produced an average 30% reduction in scar thickness (Fig. 7-11).

Keloids and hypertrophic scars are challenging to manage and, although both respond to the same therapy, hypertrophic scars are easier to treat. However, there is no single proven best therapy and the large number of treatment options reflects the lack of quality research on this topic (Table 7-3).[24]

## Chronic Nonhealing Wounds

Chronic wounds, by definition, are wounds that have failed to proceed through an orderly and timely reparative process to produce anatomic and functional integrity over a period of 3 months. These wounds are a significant challenge to the health care system and its professionals, with a huge economic burden.

Chronic wounds, like other abnormal wounds, appear to have derangements in the various stages of wound healing and have unusually elevated or depressed levels of cytokines, growth factors, or proteinases. Chronic wound fluid, unlike acute wound fluid, has been demonstrated to have greater levels of IL-1, IL-6, and TNF-α; levels of these proinflammatory cytokines decreased as the wound healed. In addition, an inverse relationship between TNF-α and essential growth factors such as EGF and PDGF has been demonstrated.

The amount of normal wound ECM is determined by a dynamic balance among overall matrix synthesis, deposition, and degradation. Proteolytic degradation of ECM is an essential feature of repair and remodeling during cutaneous repair. Evidence suggests that proteolytic degradation in the wound environment is a major cause of failure to heal. MMPs are a family of structurally related enzymes that have the ability to degrade ECM components and are differentiated by their substrate specificity and inhibited by TIMPs. TNF-α has been shown to increase the production of MMPs while inhibiting the production of TIMPs. Conversely, inhibition of MMPs results in decreased levels of TNF-α in wound fluid and decreased inflammatory cell numbers while increasing wound tensile strength and levels of TGF-β.

Studies in chronic wounds, such as pressure ulcers in human and animal models, have demonstrated elevated levels of MMPs, particularly MMP-1, MMP-2, MMP-8, and MMP-9, and decreased levels of TIMPs. This finding has led many investigators to conclude that a chronic wound is a result of persistently elevated levels of MMPs and depressed levels of their inhibitors. These MMPs have been shown to degrade the adhesive substrates for cell migration and signaling molecules, such

**Table 7-3 Prevention and Treatment Options for Keloids and Hypertrophic Scars**

| MODALITY OR TREATMENT OPTION | RESPONSE RATE (%) | RECURRENCE RATE (%) | COMMENTS | STUDY DESIGN |
|---|---|---|---|---|
| **Prevention** | | | | |
| Preventive silicone sheeting (postsurgery) | 0-75 | 25-36 | Multiple preparations available; tolerated by children; expensive; avoid on open wounds; poor study design | Review of multiple case studies |
| Postsurgical intralesional corticosteroid injection (triamcinolone acetonide [Kenalog], 10-40 mg/mL at 6-wk intervals) | NA | 0-100 (mean, 50) | Patient acceptance and safety; may cause hypopigmentation, skin atrophy, telangiectasia | Review of multiple case studies |
| Postsurgical topical imiquimod, 5% cream (Aldara) | NA | 28 | May cause hyperpigmentation, irritation | Case study |
| Postsurgical fluorouracil, triamcinolone acetonide, and pulsed dye lasers (best outcomes) | 70 at 12 wk | NA | Effective; may cause hyperpigmentation, wound ulceration | Clinical trial |
| **First-Line Treatment** | | | | |
| Cryotherapy | 50-76 | NA | Useful on small lesions; easy to perform; may cause hypopigmentation, pain | Review of multiple case studies |
| Intralesional corticosteroid injection (triamcinolone acetonide [Kenalog], 10-40 mg/mL at 6-wk intervals) | 50-100 | 9-50 | Inexpensive, requires multiple injections; may cause discomfort, skin atrophy, telangiectasia | Review of multiple case studies |
| Silicone elastomer sheeting | 50-100 | NA | Multiple preparations available; tolerated by children; expensive; poor study design | Review of multiple case studies |
| Pressure dressing (24-30 mm Hg) worn for 6-12 mo | 90-100 | NA | Inexpensive; difficult schedule; poor adherence | Review of multiple case studies |
| Surgical excision | NA | 50-100 | Z-plasty option for burns; immediate postsurgical treatment needed to prevent regrowth | Review of multiple case studies |
| Combined cryotherapy and intralesional corticosteroid injection | 84 | NA | See benefits of individual treatments; may cause hypopigmentation | Case study |
| Triple-keloid therapy (surgery, corticosteroids, silicone sheeting) | 88 at 13 mo | 12.5 at 13 mo | Tedious; time-intensive; expensive | Case study |
| Pulsed dye laser | NA | NA | Specialist referral needed; expensive; variable results depending on trial (controversial) | Case studies |
| **Second-Line and Alternative Treatment** | | | | |
| Verapamil, 2.5 mg/mL, intralesional injection combined with perilesional excision and silicone sheeting | 54 at 18 months | NA | Repeated injections; limited experience; may cause discomfort | Clinical trial |
| Fluorouracil, 50 mg/mL, intralesional injection 2-3 times/wk | 88 | 0 | Effective; may cause hyperpigmentation, wound ulceration | Review of multiple case studies |
| Bleomycin tattooing, 1.5 IU/mL | 92, 88 | NA | Effective; may cause pulmonary fibrosis, cutaneous reactions | Review of case study<br>Control trial |
| Postsurgical interferon-a2b, 1.5 million IU, intralesional injection bid for 4 days | 30-50 | 8-19 | Expensive; may cause pruritus, altered pigmentation, pain | Review of multiple case studies |
| Radiation therapy alone | 56 (mean) | NA | Local growth inhibition; may cause cancer, hyperpigmentation, paresthesias | Review of multiple case studies |
| Postsurgical radiation therapy | 76 | NA | Local growth inhibition; may cause cancer | Review of multiple case studies |
| Onion extract topical gels (Mederma) | NA | NA | Limited effect alone, better in combination with silicone sheeting | Prospective case study |

Adapted from Juckett G, Hartman-Adams H: Management of keloids and hypertrophic scars. Am Fam Physician: 80:253–260, 2009.

*NA,* Not available.

as growth factors and cytokines. In addition, excessive proteolysis may cause the release of high levels of breakdown products of connective tissue that will activate inflammatory cell processes inappropriately. With increased inflammation of the wound, there is less likelihood that the wound will progress to healing. The balance is slanted in favor of collagen degradation rather than collagen synthesis.

Wounds that are chronically inflamed and do not proceed to closure are susceptible to the development of squamous cell carcinoma (Fig. 7-12). Originally reported in chronic burn scars

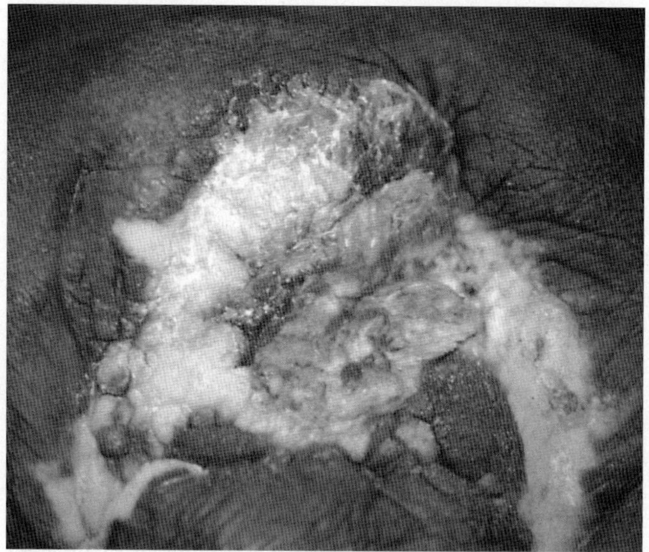

**FIGURE 7-12** Squamous cell carcinoma in a chronic pressure sore.

by Marjolin, other conditions have also been associated with this problem, including osteomyelitis, pressure sores, venous stasis ulcers, and hidradenitis.[24a] The wound appears irregular, raised above the surface, and has a white, pearly discoloration. The premalignant state is pseudoepitheliomatous hyperplasia. If this report is obtained on a biopsy specimen, the biopsy is repeated because squamous cell carcinoma may be present in other areas.

### Infection

Probably the most common cause of healing delays is wound infection. If the bacterial count in the wound exceeds $10^5$ organisms/g of tissue or if any beta-hemolytic streptococci are present, the wound will not heal by any means, including flap closure, skin graft placement, or primary suture. Bacteria prolong the inflammatory phase and interfere with epithelialization, contraction, and collagen deposition. The endotoxins themselves stimulate phagocytosis and release of collagenase, which contributes to collagen degradation and destruction of surrounding, previously normal tissue. Treatment to decrease the bacterial count, either mechanically or with the use of systemic antibiotics, therefore limits the amount of inflammation and allows closure of the wound. Bacteria may accelerate the expression or increase concentrations of MMPs, growth factors, and cytokines in chronic-type wounds; their role, as yet, has not been clearly defined.

## Other Causes of Abnormal Wound Healing

### Hypoxia

Molecular oxygen is essential for collagen formation. Ischemia can be caused by atherosclerosis, cardiac failure, or simple wound tension preventing localized perfusion. Under hypoxic conditions, energy derived from glycolysis may be sufficient to initiate collagen synthesis, but the presence of molecular oxygen is critical for post-translational hydroxylation of the prolyl and lysyl residues required for triple-helix formation and cross linking of collagen fibrils. Although hypoxia will stimulate angiogenesis, this essential step in collagen fibril assembly proceeds poorly when the $PO_2$ falls below 40 mm Hg. Optimal $PO_2$ for collagen synthesis is present at the periphery of the wound whereas the center remains hypoxic.

The role of anemia in wound healing has long been attributed to be predominantly secondary to hypoperfusion. However, studies evaluating colonic anastomoses in a crystalloid-resuscitated hemorrhagic shock model have demonstrated altered histologic parameters—decreased white blood cell infiltration, angiogenesis, fibroblast production, and collagen production. Use of tobacco products has a similar impact on wound healing because of both the vasoconstriction that occurs with smoking and elevated carbon monoxide serum levels, which can limit the oxygen-carrying capacity of blood.

### Diabetes

Diabetes mellitus impairs wound healing at all stages of the process. A diabetic patient with associated neuropathy and atherosclerosis is prone to tissue ischemia, repetitive trauma, and infection. Tissue hypoxia, as indicated by reduced dorsal foot transcutaneous oxygen tension ($TcO_2$), is a consequence of vascular disease and has been well demonstrated in diabetic patients. In addition to large-vessel disease, many diabetic patients have abnormalities at the microvascular level. The thickened basement membrane of the capillaries causes decreased perfusion in the microenvironment, and there is increased perivascular localization of albumin, which suggests that these capillaries are leaky.

VEGF upregulation in diabetic patients is also impaired.[25] Hypoxia is normally a potent upregulator of VEGF. However, a recent study has demonstrated that cells from diabetic patients do not upregulate VEGF expression in response to hypoxia and diabetic animals are unable to increase VEGF production following soft tissue ischemia.[25] This failure was attributed to a decrease in transactivation by the transcription factor HIF-1$\alpha$ as a result of high glucose levels. HIF-1$\alpha$ mediates hypoxia-stimulated VEGF expression. Decreased binding of HIF-1$\alpha$ to its coactivator p300 resulted in decreased HIF-1$\alpha$ functional activity. Covalent binding of the dicarbonyl metabolite methylglyoxal to p300 resulted in modification of the p300 and was responsible for the decreased association of HIF-1$\alpha$ and p300. Administration of deferoxamine, an inhibitor of methylglyoxal conjugation, to diabetic mice resulted in normalization of HIF-1$\alpha$–p300 interaction and transactivation of HIF-1$\alpha$, with increased neovascularization and enhanced wound healing.

Diabetic patients are prone to repeated trauma as a result of the diabetic neuropathy that affects sensory and motor function in the somatic and autonomic pathways. Furthermore, diabetics are susceptible to infection because of an attenuated inflammatory response, impaired chemotaxis, and inefficient bacterial killing. Infection also increases local tissue metabolism, thus further imposing a burden on an already tenuous blood supply and thereby amplifying the risk for tissue necrosis. Lymphocyte and leukocyte function are impaired, and there is increased collagen degradation and decreased collagen deposition. The collagen that is formed is more brittle than normal collagen, probably because of glycosylation from the increased levels of glucose present in the ECM. Glycation of collagen also affects focal adhesion formation, resulting in alteration of fibroblast and matrix interactions and decreased fibroblast migration.[26]

#### Ionizing Radiation

Ionizing radiation causes endothelial cell injury with endarteritis and results in atrophy, fibrosis, and delayed tissue repair. Unlike most hypoxic wound beds, angiogenesis is not initiated. Because its greatest effect is on cells in the $G_2$ through M phase, rapidly dividing cell populations are most sensitive to radiation. Such cells include keratinocytes and fibroblasts during wound healing, injury to which impairs epithelialization and the formation of granulation tissue.

#### Aging

Older patients are more likely to sustain surgical wound rupture and delayed healing than younger patients. With aging, collagen undergoes qualitative and quantitative changes. Dermal collagen content decreases with aging, and aging collagen fibers show distorted architecture and organization. Upregulation of MMP-2 and MMP-9 was enhanced in healthy older subjects after experimental wounding as compared with younger controls. Studies in aged animals have also demonstrated decreased reepithelialization, depressed collagen synthesis, and impaired angiogenesis, with decreased levels of growth factors, including the proangiogenic factors FGF-2 and VEGF. Other studies have suggested that the early inflammatory period of wound healing is altered in older adults, including impaired macrophage activity with reduced phagocytosis and delayed infiltration of macrophages and B lymphocytes into wounds. In addition, with aging, there is a decrease in response to hypoxia, as demonstrated by decreased MMP activation and TGF-$\beta_1$ receptor expression by keratinocytes isolated from aged donors.

#### Malnutrition

Malnutrition has an impact on wound healing. Protein catabolism can result in a delay in wound healing. A hypoalbuminemic patient can experience wound-healing delay or even dehiscence; although the albumin level must be lower than 2.0 g/dL to have an effect on wound healing. Protein supplements can reverse this deficiency.

Vitamin deficiencies affect wound healing primarily as a result of their effect as cofactors. Delayed healing can occur in as few as 3 months of vitamin C deprivation. This deficiency can be reversed by the administration of as little as 10 mg/day and no more than 2000 g/day.[26a] Deficiency of vitamin A impedes monocyte activation and deposition of fibronectin, thus further affecting cellular adhesion, and impairs TGF-β receptors. Vitamin A contributes to lysosomal membrane destabilization and directly counteracts the effect of glucocorticoids. The main effect of vitamin K deficiency is to limit the synthesis of prothrombin and factors VII, IX, and X. Vitamin K metabolism is impeded by antibiotics. Patients who have chronic or recurrent infections need to have their clotting parameters checked before surgical procedures.

A few minerals, if deficient in the diet, adversely affect wound healing. Zinc deficiency is rare, except in patients with conditions such as large burns, severe multiple trauma, and hepatic cirrhosis. Zinc is a necessary cofactor for RNA polymerase and DNA polymerase. Deficiency of zinc results in early wound healing delays. Iron deficiency anemia is a debatable cause of wound healing delay. Although the ferrous ion is a cofactor needed to convert proline to hydroxyproline, reports are conflicting regarding the effects that acute and chronic anemia have on wound healing. In general, patients benefit most by a well-rounded diet consisting of adequate protein intake and caloric value, plus vitamin and mineral supplementation.

#### Drugs

Some exogenous drugs directly inhibit wound healing. Doxorubicin (Adriamycin) is a potent inhibitor, particularly if administered preoperatively. Although clinical studies have shown little impairment, experimental models have indicated that nitrogen mustard, cyclophosphamide, methotrexate, bischloroethylnitrosourea (BCNU), and doxorubicin are the most potent wound inhibitors. These chemotherapeutic agents reduce mesenchymal cell proliferation and reduce the number of platelets, inflammatory cells, and growth factors available, especially if given preoperatively. Tamoxifen, an antiestrogen, is known to decrease cellular proliferation. In addition, there appears to be a dose-dependent decrease in wound-breaking strength associated with tamoxifen. This effect may be caused by decreased TGF-β production. Glucocorticosteroids impair fibroblast proliferation and collagen synthesis. The amount of granulation tissue formed is also decreased. Steroids stabilize the lysosomal membranes. This particular effect can be reversed by the administration of vitamin A. The decrease in breaking strength caused by the administration of exogenous steroids appears to be both time- and dose-related. High doses of NSAIDs have been reported to delay healing, but doses in the therapeutic range are unlikely to have an effect.

### Relationship Between Immunity and Wound Repair or Regeneration

There exists substantial evidence in different model organisms that the immune system is extremely important in shaping the quality of the repair, including the amount of scarring and restoration of the structure and function. Evidence suggests that as the immune system becomes more developed, the ability to regenerate is lost.[27] However, other studies have contradicted this and suggest that a functional immune response does not prevent regeneration; in fact, it may play a positive role in the capability to regenerate. Modulation of the local immune response, therefore, may prove to be effective therapeutic strategy in cases of impaired wound healing.

## FETAL WOUND HEALING

Fetal skin wounds heal rapidly and without the scarring and inflammation characteristic of adult skin wounds. It was thought that fetal wound healing represented ideal tissue repair and that understanding fetal wound healing would provide surgeons the tools to regulate and control the different steps in adult wound healing. In adult cutaneous healing, as opposed to fetal healing, dermal appendages such as hair follicles, sweat glands, and sebaceous glands fail to regenerate. Furthermore, there are changes in collagen in adult wounds, with the healed wound demonstrating densely packed collagen bundles oriented perpendicularly to the wound surface, unlike that of normal uninjured skin and fetal skin, both of which have a reticular pattern.

Fetal wounds reepithelialize faster, with less neovascularization and a faster increase in strength. Fetal wound research has demonstrated that fetal wounds differ from adult wounds in inflammatory responses, ECM components, and growth factor expression and responses.

Fetal repair is dependent on gestational age and wound size. There may be a wound size threshold (the diameter of excised skin at which 50% of wounds heal without scarring at a given gestational age). The wound size threshold for 60- and 70-day-gestation animals is 6 to 10 mm and 4 to 6 mm for 80- and 90-day-gestation animals. It has been suggested that larger wounds may extend the time of the healing response and expose wound tissue to a different ECM and growth factor profile. Larger excisional wounds may also stimulate the formation of myofibroblasts in the wound and thereby result in scar formation. The transition from scarless to scarring repair occurs near the end of the second trimester and the beginning of the third. Wounds heal faster in a fetus than in a neonate, and they heal slowest in adults. Normal development of skin appendages occurs when fibroblasts of the dermis induce the epithelium to form hair follicles or glands. Wounds created early in gestation heal without scarring and with dermal appendages, thus suggesting tissue regeneration versus repair. Late-gestation wounds, in contrast, heal with scarring and without dermal appendages. The transition from scarless healing to healing without dermal appendages suggests that the fetal fibroblast loses its ability to induce the epithelium to form dermal appendages with advancing gestational age.

Investigators have cited intrinsic (oxygen tension of the human fetus) and extrinsic (amniotic fluid environment) differences between fetal and adult wound healing, with most noting that the intrinsic differences are the key determinants in whether wounds will heal with scars.[28] Intrinsic differences include fetal oxygen tension, which is markedly decreased (fetal sheep, mean $PaO_2$ of 20 mm Hg) when compared with adult animals (adult sheep, mean $PaO_2$ of 116 mm Hg). This decrease in fetal oxygenation is partially compensated by the relative affinity of fetal hemoglobin for oxygen.

The fetal environment, an extrinsic difference between fetal and adult wounds, is characterized by a hyaluronic acid–rich amniotic fluid. Studies have suggested that the increased number of hyaluronic acid receptors and increased amount of hyaluronic acid may create a permissive environment in which fibroblast movement is facilitated, thereby resulting in the increased rate and efficiency of fetal healing.[28]

Much of fetal wound-healing research has focused on the role of fibroblasts. Fetal fibroblasts appear to have characteristics quite different from those of adult fibroblasts. Proline hydroxylation is a rate-limiting step in collagen synthesis by dermal cells; early-gestation fetal human fibroblasts have increased prolyl hydroxylase activity, which gradually decreases to adult levels after 20 weeks of gestation. Collagens I, III, V, and VI appear earlier and the ratio of type III to type I is greater in fetal wounds, which is consistent with the higher prevalence of type III collagen in normal fetal tissue. Fetal fibroblasts in vitro have higher collagen production than their adult counterparts. This may be secondary to the unique regulatory mechanism for prolyl hydroxylase and may explain why there is higher fibroblast activity in fetuses younger than 20 weeks' gestation.

Collagen synthesis falls to adult levels after 20 weeks' gestation. There appears to be an increase in collagen degradation as a function of gestational age. Studies have found marked increases in the gene expression of MMP-1, MMP-3, and MMP-9 that correlate with the onset of scar formation in nonwounded fetal skin. These findings suggest that late-gestation fetal rat skin undergoes an adult type of tissue remodeling after wounding that leads to the scarring seen in adult skin.

There are also differences in the components of the ECM of fetal and adult wounds. After injury, fibronectin levels are similar in adults and fetuses, but tenascin, an inhibitor of fibronectin, increases earlier and returns to normal more rapidly in the fetus. Larger amounts of fibronectin in fetal wounds stimulate immediate cell attachment, whereas the more rapid deposition of tenascin in the fetus allows cells to migrate and fully epithelialize the wound more rapidly and thus decrease wound-healing time.

Levels of hyaluronic acid are persistently elevated in fetal wounds. During gestation, decreasing levels of hyaluronic acid correlate with increasing scarring potential. The unique ECM composition of fetal tissues may influence collagen fibril deposition by facilitating cell mobility and migration, thereby leading to the loose collagen pattern seen in healed fetal wounds as opposed to the dense collagenous pattern seen in adult scars. However, few studies have examined the effect of modifying the ECM components.

Differences in fetal wound healing also occur in the inflammatory phase. The fetus exhibits a reduced inflammatory response with a lack of neutrophil infiltration and decreased infiltration of endogenous immunoglobulins. The paucity of macrophages and a difference in the temporal appearance of macrophages in a fetal wound may explain why there are differences in growth factor profiles between adult and fetal wounds and why there is a reduced inflammatory response.[28a] These studies cite a direct correlation between increased macrophage recruitment in older fetuses and the development of increased scarring.

Fetal wounds have been demonstrated to have minimal levels of TGF-β and FGF-2 by immunohistochemistry. Furthermore, PDGF in fetal wounds disappears more rapidly than in adult wounds. This lack of growth factors may be explained by the decreased inflammatory cell recruitment. Normal inflammatory (adult-type) wound healing may have evolved to reduce the risk of infection at the expense of healing quality.

TGF-β is the growth factor that has been most extensively studied in fetal wound repair. $TGF\text{-}\beta_1$ has been shown to induce rapid healing and scar formation when added to adult rat wounds and to induce inflammation and fibrosis when added to fetal rabbit wounds. TGF-β production may be blunted in hypoxemic conditions, which has led to the theory that the decreased oxygen tension in the fetal environment inhibits TGF-β production and results in decreased scar formation. More recent work has suggested that differential expression of the different TGF-β isoforms, rather than the mere presence of TGF-β, may be important in explaining the differences in repair.

Growth factor manipulation to make wounds more fetal-like with less angiogenesis, less fibrosis, and improved ECM migratory ability has not resulted in completely scarless healing, and there is still failure of regeneration of dermal appendages. Some inconsistencies in fetal wound healing are not clearly understood. It has been shown that there are differences in species with regard to scarless fetal wound healing and that not all fetal tissues are capable of scarless healing. For example, fetal lamb diaphragm and gastric wounds scar, whereas concurrent skin wounds heal without scarring.

Studies have demonstrated a correlation between the presence of myofibroblasts and scar formation; this suggests that a transition in fibroblast phenotype may contribute to the onset of scarring. Excisional wounds in 75-day-gestation fetal lambs have shown an absence of scar formation and alpha smooth muscle actin expression. Alpha smooth muscle actin appears after 100 days of gestation along with scar formation, which suggests that the mechanisms of scarless fetal wound healing have yet to be completely elucidated.

## WOUND DRESSINGS

Wound dressings have been used since the time of antiquity. Treatment of wounds originally consisted of homemade remedies and evolved very little for many years but, in 1867, Lister introduced antiseptic dressings by soaking lint and gauze in carbolic acid. Although there are currently many more sophisticated dressings, there are several points to consider.

Wound healing is most successful in a moist, clean, and warm environment. Subsequently, in treating a wound in a nonsurgical conservative manner, certain characteristics are important in the wound dressing (Box 7-2). It is important to note that not all dressings can provide all the aforementioned characteristics and not all wounds require all these functions. It is essential that the choice of dressing match the specific wound conditions.

Two concepts that are critical when selecting appropriate dressings for wounds are occlusion and absorption. Studies have demonstrated that the rate of epithelialization under an occlusive dressing is twice that of a wound that is left uncovered and allowed to dry. Placement of an occlusive dressing over the wound provides a mildly acidic pH and low oxygen tension on the wound surface; this is a good environment for the proliferation of fibroblasts and formation of granulation tissue. A relatively occlusive dressing is a good choice for many wounds. However, wounds that have a significant amount of exudate or wounds with high bacterial counts will require a dressing that is absorptive and prevents maceration of the surrounding skin. These wounds also require a dressing that reduces the bacterial load within the wound while removing the exudate produced. Placement of a pure occlusive dressing without bactericidal properties will allow bacterial overgrowth and worsen the infection.

An in-depth discussion on the types of wound dressings exceeds the scope of this text, but it is important to mention the various classes of dressings (Table 7-4).[29] Wound dressings can be categorized into four classes—nonadherent fabrics, absorptive dressings, occlusive dressings, and creams, ointments, and solutions. A brief discussion of these categories follows.

**BOX 7-2 Characteristics of Ideal Dressing**

Creates a moist environment
Removes excess exudate
Prevents dessication
Allows for gaseous exchange
Impermeable to microorganisms
Thermally insulating
Prevents particulate contamination
Nontoxic to beneficial host cells
Provides mechanical protection
Nontraumatic
Easy to use
Cost-effective

Adapted from Morin RJ, Tomaselli NL: Interactive dressings and topical agents. Clin Plast Surg 34:643–658, 2007.

Nonadherent fabrics are generally fine-mesh gauze supplemented with a substance to augment their occlusive properties or antibacterial abilities. An example of this type of dressing is Scarlet Red, a relatively nonocclusive dressing that is impregnated with *O*-tolylazo-*O*-tolylazo-β-naphthol, which has some antimicrobial abilities. Another example of this class is Xeroform, a relatively occlusive, hydrophobic dressing containing 3% bismuth tribromophenate in a petrolatum base, which helps mask wound odors and has some antimicrobial activity against *Staphylococcus aureus* and *Escherichia coli.*

The absorptive class is used mainly for wounds that produce a significant amount of exudate. Exudate production from leg ulcers can be as much as 12 g/10 $cm^2$/24 hours.[30] Wide-mesh gauze is the oldest of this type of dressing and is very absorbent, but it loses its effectiveness when saturated. Newer materials, such as foam dressings, provide the absorbent qualities for removing large quantities of exudate and have a nonadherent quality to prevent disruption of newly formed granulation tissue on removal. Examples of these foams are Lyofoam (ConvaTec, Skillman, NJ), Allevyn (Smith & Nephew, Largo, Fla), Curafoam (Kendall Company, Mansfield, Mass), Flexzan (Dow Hickam, Sugar Land, Tex), and VigiFOAM (Bard, Murray Hill, NJ). Wound healing beneath absorptive dressings appears to be slower than under occlusive dressings, possibly because of wicking of cytokines from the wound bed or decreased keratinocyte migration.

The occlusive dressing class provides moisture retention, mechanical protection, and a barrier to bacteria. The occlusive class can be divided into biologic and nonbiologic dressings. Examples of biologic dressings are allograft, xenograft, amnion, and skin substitutes. Homograft is a graft transplanted between genetically unique humans, whereas a xenograft is a graft transplanted between species. Pigskin is the most commonly used xenograft. Homografts and xenografts are temporary dressings in that both are rejected if left on a wound for an extended period. Amnion is derived from human placentas and is another effective biologic wound dressing. These dressings are often used in the treatment of burn wounds; however, they can be used as a temporary measure in other types of wounds as well.

The newest type of wound dressings are skin substitutes that can be used for structural support and scaffolding for regeneration.[31,32] Examples include Integra (Integra LifeSciences, Plainsboro, NJ), Apligraf (Novartis, Basel, Switzerland), and AlloDerm (LifeCell, Branchburg, NJ). Integra is a bilayer membrane system for skin replacement. The first layer is made of a porous matrix of cross-linked bovine tendon collagen and a GAG (chondroitin 6-sulfate). The second layer is made of synthetic polysiloxane polymer (silicone) and functions to control moisture loss from the wound. The first layer serves as a template for the infiltration of fibroblasts, macrophages, lymphocytes, and capillaries from the wound bed. During the healing process, a new collagen matrix is deposited by fibroblasts and the dermal layer of the template is degraded. Once vascularization of the dermal layer is complete, a thin autograft can be applied after removal of the silicone layer. AlloDerm is an acellular dermal matrix derived from donated human skin tissue. It provides the matrix for revascularization and incorporation into host tissue. It must be noted that although AlloDerm will incorporate and serves well to provide additional strength, it will not provide a

**Table 7-4 Types of Dressings**

| CATEGORY | COMPOSITION AND CHARACTERISTICS | FUNCTION | EXAMPLES | COMMENTS |
|---|---|---|---|---|
| Nonadherent fabrics | Fine-mesh gauze with supplement to augment occlusive and nonadherent properties, healing facilitating capabilities, and antibacterial characteristics | Protection, moist environment | Scarlet Red, Vaseline gauze, Xeroform, Xeroflo, Mepitel, Adaptic, Telfa | Scarlet Red, Xeroform, Telfa, Vaseline gauze– hydrophobic, more occlusive; Xeroflo, Mepitel, Adaptic–less occlusive, allow drainage of fluid into overlying dressing layers |
| **Absorptive** | | | | |
| Gauze | Wide mesh gauze | Removing exudates, prevents maceration | Wide-mesh gauze | Not effective when saturated; can be used for wound débridement if in contact with wound |
| Foams | Hydrophobic polyurethane sheets | Protection, absorption of exudate | Lyofoam, Allevyn, Curafoam, Flexzan, Vigifoam | Advantages—comfortable, can expand and conform to wound, easily removed for cleansing Disadvantages—need to be replaced as wounds heal, custom shapes are labor intensive to make, limited protection from bacteria, cannot be used while bathing |
| **Occlusive** | | | | |
| Nonbiologic | | Insulation, moisture retention, protective barrier acts against bacteria | | |
| Films | Clear polyurethane membranes with acrylic adhesive on one side | See above | Tegaderm, Mefilm, Carrafilm, Bioclusive, Transeal, Opsite | Waterproof; permeable to oxygen, carbon dioxide, and water vapor; do not interfere with patient function; allow visualization of wound; nonabsorptive, can leak; require intact skin around wound area; wound contraction may be slowed, removal may disrupt new epithelium |
| Hydrocolloids | Hydrocolloid matrix (gelatin, pectin, carboxymethyl cellulose) | As above; absorbs water from wound exudates, swells, liquefies to form moist gel | Duoderm, NuDerm, Comfeel, Hydrocol, Cutinova, Tegasorb | Available as adhesive wafers, paste, powders; similar features as films, but bulkier; more protection but may interfere more with function |
| Alginates | Cellulose-like polysaccharide fibers derived from calcium salt of alginate (seaweed) | As above; calcium alginate conversion to soluble sodium salt following contact with wound exudates results in hydrophilic gel | Algiderm, Algosteril, Kaltostat, Curasorb, Carasorb, Melgisorb, SeaSorb, Kalginate, Sorbsan | Occlusive environment; various forms—ropes, ribbons, pads |
| Hydrogels | Polyethylene oxide or carboxymethyl cellulose polymer and water (80%) | As above; rehydrating agents for dry wounds; little water absorption (high water content) | Vigilon, Nu-gel, Tegagel, FlexiGel, Curagel, Flexderm | Available as gels, sheets, impregnated gauze; occlusive environment |
| Biologic | | Similar to nonbiologics | | |
| Homograft | Derived from genetically unique humans | | Cadaver skin | Temporary dressing; is rejected if left on wound for extended period |
| Xenograft | Interspecies graft (e.g., pig) | | Pigskin | Same as above |
| Amnion | Human placenta | | | Good biologic dressing |
| Skin substitutes | Different compositions | | Integra, Alloderm, Apligraf, Biobrane, Transcyte | Integra—bilayered membrane skin substitute; AlloDerm—acellular cadaveric dermis; Apligraf—living, bilayered, biologic dressing composed of neonatal dermal fibroblasts on collagen matrix |

*Continued*

**Table 7-4 Types of Dressings—cont'd**

| CATEGORY | COMPOSITION AND CHARACTERISTICS | FUNCTION | EXAMPLES | COMMENTS |
|---|---|---|---|---|
| **Creams, Ointments, and Solutions** | | | | |
| Antibacterial | Different compositions | Used to treat infected wounds | Acetic acid (gram-negative, *Pseudomonas*); Dakin's solution (broad antibacterial spectrum); iodine-containing antibacterials (Iodosorb, Iodoflex, Betadine; broad antibacterial and antifungal spectrum); silver nitrate (broad antibacterial spectrum); mafenide acetate (Sulfamylon; broad antibacterial spectrum) silver sulfadiazine (Silvadene; broad antibacterial, antifungal, and antiviral spectrum); Acticoat (broad antibacterial spectrum) | Acetic acid— impairs wound healing; Dakin's— toxic to fibroblasts; iodine-containing solutions—toxic to fibroblasts, impairs wound healing; silver nitrate—treats burns, slows epithelialization, hyponatremia, stains clothes black; mafenide acetate— penetrates eschar, painful application, inhibits reepithelialization, carbonic anhydrase inhibitor; silver sulfadiazine—transient neutropenia, accelerates epithelialization of partial-thickness burns, neovascularization, commonly used for burns; Acticoat—silver-impregnated occlusive dressing, antibacterial activity lasts 3 days |
| Antibacterial Ointments | Different compositions | Used to treat infected wounds; soothing to apply; lubricates wound surface; occlusive; antibacterial activity lasts 12 hours | Bacitracin (gram-positive cocci and bacilli); neomycin (gram-negative) polymyxin B sulfate (gram-negative); polysporin (polymyxin B, bacitracin); neosporin (polymyxin B, bacitracin, neomycin); triple antibiotic ointment (polymyxin B, bacitracin, neomycin) | Neosporin—increased reepithelialization in experimental wounds by 25% compared with wounds with no dressing |
| Enzymatic | Different compositions; uses naturally occurring enzymes | Removal of necrotic tissue | Sutilains (derived from *Bacillus subtilis*); collagenase (Santyl; derived from *Clostridium histolyticum*); papain (derived from vegetable pepsin) | Sutilains—digests denatured collagen; collagenase—digests denatured and native collagen; papain—effective against collagen in presence of cofactor containing sulfhydryl group; addition of urea doubles enzymatic action of papain |
| Other | Normal saline wet to dry gauze dressing | Removal of necrotic tissue | | Nondiscriminating—both necrotic and newly formed granulation tissue and epithelium removed; can be painful |

Adapted from Lionelli GT, Lawrence WT: Wound dressings. Surg Clin North Am 2003; 83:617–638, 2003.

dermal matrix to support a skin graft as would Integra; therefore, AlloDerm is not frequently used as a skin substitute. Apligraf is a living, bilayered biologic dressing that has been designed to simulate normal skin. Initially, neonatal-derived dermal fibroblasts are cultured in a collagen matrix for 6 days. Human keratinocytes are then cultured on top of this neodermis. The dressing contains matrix proteins and expresses cytokines; however, it does not contain melanocytes, Langerhans cells, macrophages, lymphocytes, or the adnexal structures normally present in human skin. These are only three examples of the types of skin substitutes that are currently available. Many other substitutes are in development and will continue to provide options for the surgeon.

The final class of wound dressings consists of creams, ointments, and solutions. This is a broad category that extends from traditional materials, such as zinc oxide paste, to cutting edge preparations containing growth factors. The various categories include those with antibacterial properties such as acetic acid, Dakin's solution, silver nitrate, mafenide (Sulfamylon), silver sulfadiazine (Silvadene), iodine-containing ointments (Iodosorb), and bacitracin. Application of these products is indicated when clinical signs of infection, such as an increase in exudate or cellulitis, are present or if quantitative culture demonstrates more than $10^5$ organisms/g of tissue.

Many types of wound dressings are available to the surgeon and the number is increasing. The surgeon must have information about the available that allow effective wound management (Box 7-3).

## OTHER THERAPIES

### Hyperbaric Oxygen

Wound ischemia is believed to be the most common cause of wound healing failure. Hyperbaric oxygen (HBO) therapy uses oxygen as a drug and the hyperbaric chamber as the tool for elevating oxygen concentration at the target area.

Hyperbaric oxygen therapy was first used for treatment of bacterial infections and later for decompression sickness. Hyperbaric medicine has since been used for a myriad of disease processes, including improvement of split-thickness skin graft take, flap survival and salvage, treatment of acute thermal burns, necrotizing fasciitis, chronic wounds, hypoxic wounds, and radiation injuries.[33] The rationale for its use is that ischemia or tissue hypoxia (oxygen levels below 30 mm Hg) results in

**BOX 7-3 Dressing Options for Noninfected Clean Wounds**

- Incisional wound
  - Three-layer dressings
  - Ointments
  - Occlusive dressings
- Partial thickness wounds (e.g., abrasions, donor sites)
  - No dressing (scab)
  - Impregnated gauze
  - Creams, ointments
  - Occlusive dressings
- Full-thickness wounds (e.g., pressure sores)
  - Alginates or hydrogels—rarely applicable
  - Creams, gels (e.g., Silvadene)
  - Wet to dry dressing changes
  - Vacuum-assisted closure (VAC) device

significant impairment of normal metabolic activity and wound healing by impairing aspects of wound healing, such as fibroblast proliferation, collagen synthesis, and epithelialization.[34,35] In addition, because HBO therapy involves inhalation of 100% oxygen at pressures of 1.9 to 2.5 atm, tissue oxygen levels can be 10 times higher than usual.[35] The higher arterial partial pressure of oxygen is sufficient to supply the tissue with all its metabolic requirements, even in the absence of hemoglobin; this elevated level lasts for 2 to 4 hours after termination of HBO therapy and induces synthesis of endothelial cell nitric oxide synthase, as well as angiogenesis.[36]

Vascular evaluation and revascularization, if needed, is a prerequisite prior to HBO therapy. Patients who will benefit from HBO therapy as adjuvant therapy are patients with who have hypoxic wounds that show marked improvement in wound hypoxia during oxygen breathing at hyperbaric conditions.[33] Transcutaneous oxygen pressure ($TcPO_2$) is used to assess wound perfusion and oxygenation. A patient with a wound $TcPO_2$ lower than 35 mm Hg in room air has tissue hypoxia. A measurement of in-chamber $TcPO_2$ of 200 mm Hg or higher suggests that the patient would benefit from HBO therapy.[37]

HBO treatments for hypoxic wounds are usually delivered at 1.9 to 2.5 atm for sessions of 90 to 120 minutes each, with the patient breathing 100% oxygen during the treatment. Treatments are given once daily, five to six times/week, and should be given as an adjunct to surgical or medical therapies. Clinical evidence of wound improvement should be noted after 15 to 20 treatments.

Complications of HBO therapy are caused by atmospheric pressure changes or by the rise in oxygen partial pressure. Middle ear barotrauma, which ranges from hyperemia of the eardrum to ear drum perforation, is the most common complication caused by changes in atmospheric pressure. The most serious barotrauma side effect, although rare, is pneumothorax or tension pneumothorax. Complications associated with oxygen partial pressure increases are brain oxygen toxicity, manifested by convulsions resembling grand mal seizures, oxygen lung toxicity, resulting from damage from oxygen free radicals to lung parenchyma and airways and ranging from tracheobronchitis to full-blown respiratory distress syndrome, and transient myopia.

Absolute contraindications to HBO therapy are as follows: (1) uncontrolled pneumothorax; (2) current or recent treatment with doxorubicin, bleomycin, or doxorubicin

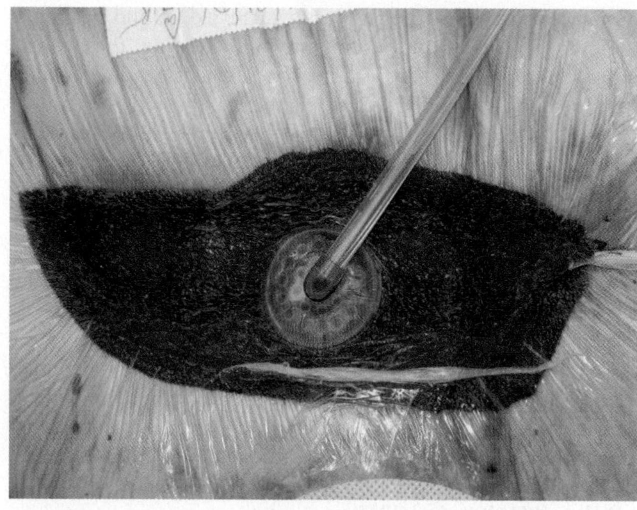

**FIGURE 7-13** Negative pressure–assisted wound closure sponge in place on a patient's abdomen.

(potential aggravation of cardiac and pulmonary toxicity); and (3) treatment with disulfiram (increases risk of developing oxygen toxicity).

Randomized, controlled clinical trials have demonstrated that HBO therapy is a useful adjunct therapy for diabetic ischemic foot ulcers and reduces the incidence of leg amputations.[38] These studies, however, like all human studies, are difficult to interpret because of the length of time chronic wounds take to heal and the variability among wounds that cannot be controlled. Interestingly, despite the obvious potential flaws in the scientific literature surrounding hyperbaric oxygen therapy, medical insurance companies have decided that there is enough evidence to support HBO therapy as an adjunct treatment for perfused, chronic, nonhealing lower extremity wounds, provided that the limbs have already undergone revascularization.[37]

## Negative Pressure–Assisted Wound Closure

In the past 15 years, there have been significant advances in complex acute and chronic wound management. One of the most significant discoveries was the improvement in wounds with negative pressure–assisted wound closure (Fig. 7-13). With this technology, the surgeon now has additional options in addition to immediate closure of wounds (i.e., adjunctive therapy before or after surgery, or an alternative to surgery in the extremely ill).

The original description of negative pressure–assisted wound closure was presented by Argenta and associates in 1997.[38a] By applying subatmospheric pressure to wounds, they demonstrated removal of chronic edema, an increase in local blood flow, and stimulation of granulation tissue. This technique may be used on acute, subacute, and chronic wounds. Additional studies have demonstrated significant improvement in wound depth in chronic wounds treated with negative-pressure therapy as compared with wounds treated with saline wet to moist dressings. In addition, treatment with negative pressure results in faster healing times, with fewer associated complications.

The exact mechanism of the improvement in healing with negative-pressure therapy has yet to be determined. Many initially believed that the reason for increased wound healing is the removal of wound exudates while keeping the wound moist.[38a] As originally hypothesized by Argenta and associates, with negative-pressure therapy, there is a fivefold increase in blood flow to cutaneous tissues. Further studies have shown an increase in capillary caliber and stimulated endothelial proliferation and angiogenesis. It is well known that increased bacterial loads result in slowed wound healing; however, despite increased wound healing with negative-pressure therapy, it has been shown to result in increased bacterial counts. Other studies have suggested that negative pressure therapy produces three-dimensional stress within the cells (microstrain) as well as across the whole area of the wound (macrostrain), resulting in changes such as increased cellular proliferation and higher microvessel density.[39] Evidence also suggests that negative pressure therapy alters wound fluid composition by removing potentially deleterious proteinases and inflammatory cytokines, such as MMP-1, MMP-2, MMP-9, and TNF-α.

Even though the mechanisms resposible for the improvement achieved with negative-pressure therapy have yet to be clearly elucidated, such treatment represents a significant improvement in cost-effectiveness and has decreased length of stay after acute and chronic wounds. There have been reports of a 78% decrease in hospital stay and a 76% decrease in cost with negative-pressure therapy. This cost decrease and effectiveness of wound treatment with negative-pressure therapy have translated to home health care treatment of Medicare patients.

Clinical benefits of negative pressure therapy have been demonstrated in randomized control trials and case-control studies. These benefits include decrease in wound volume or size, accelerated wound bed preparation, accelerated wound healing, improved rate of graft take, decreased drainage time for acute wounds, reduction of complications, enhancement of response to first-line treatment, increased patient survival, and decreased cost.

## NEW HORIZONS

### Tissue Engineering

In 1987, the National Science Foundation bioengineering panel defined that tissue engineering was "the application of the principles and methods of engineering and the life sciences toward the development of biologic substitutes to restore, maintain, or improve function."[39a] These principles and methods have been used toward the creation of skin products made of cells, ECM components, or combinations of the two. This tissue-engineered skin has developed and progressed rapidly over the past 20 years, mainly because of the limitations associated with autografts, and may function by providing the cellular or matrix components that could be necessary for wounds to heal. The use of biologic dressings (see earlier), as well as scaffolds, stem cell therapy, and gene therapy are a few examples of tissue engineering, in which new tissues are created rather than transferred.

### Scaffolds

When dressings alone fail to achieve healing, the clinician now has a variety of advanced therapeutics that can be used. Topical application of growth factors to chronic wounds has not been as beneficial as anticipated, presumably because they are degraded by proteases in the wound fluid. Researchers have been investigating whether localized gene therapy may be a better delivery system for providing growth factors to the wound bed. In addition, dressings that actively alter the wound matrix are being developed. One such device, oxidized regenerated cellulose-collagen, has been found to promote human dermal fibroblast proliferation and cell migration, accelerate wound closure in diabetic mice, and possibly sequester or inactivate proteases. Biodegradable scaffolds, natural or synthesized, may also alter the wound milieu so it is more favorable. Porcine small intestinal submucosa has been demonstrated in a number of applications to provide a scaffold for tissue repair and reconstruction. Although xenogeneic, this acellular scaffold is minimally immunogenic and has been shown to be completely degraded and replaced by host tissue. Hyaluronic acid conjugated with glycidyl methacrylate, chondroitin sulfate, or gelatin has been shown to have vulnerary effects on wound-healing parameters.

The addition of live cells to scaffolds is a promising therapy for chronic wounds that are difficult to heal. Whether using actual cultured skin with both fibroblasts and keratinocytes or fibroblasts integrated into a dermal matrix, the neonatal cells provide growth factors and matrix elements consistent with rapid healing. They are currently cost-prohibitive for large wounds and are primarily applicable only to shallow ulcerations.

### Gene and Stem Cell Therapy

Gene and stem cell therapy are emerging as promising approaches for the treatment of acute and chronic wounds. Although tissue-engineered biologic dressings such as Apligraf have had some success in the healing of diabetic ulcers, they are expensive, with low engraftment rates.

Embryonic stem cells (ESCs) were discovered in 1981 and it was quickly recognized that their regenerative properties could potentially be harnessed for treating chronic wounds.[40] Because of ethical issues, however, their use and research has been limited. This has led to the investigation and subsequent discovery of self-renewing multipotent adult progenitor cells (MAPCs),[41] which do not have the same ethical limitations.

Whole bone marrow was first investigated as a possible candidate for cellular therapy because of the ease of harvest and because it is a source of autologous MAPCs. Studies have demonstrated that bone marrow can increase vascularity and accelerate closure of chronic wounds.[42] However, because bone marrow is composed of different cell types, including MAPCs, which make up a very small portion of the bone marrow, it is unclear which cell populations are actually beneficial for wound healing. Isolation of mesenchymal stromal cells (MSC) from bone marrow. a heterogenous group of MAPCs, and their use in wound healing studies has demonstrated that MSCs result in improved granulation tissue formation and neovascularization compared with whole bone marrow.[43]

MSCs are self-renewing and can differentiate into different mesenchymal lineages, including adipocytes and chrondrocytes.[44] They have been isolated in vivo from many different tissues, including bone marrow, skeletal muscle, adipose, and blood. They have been shown to improve acute and chronic wound healing in human and animal models.[45] Although it was thought that the mechanism of action was totally understood, studies have suggested that MSCs act through a number of mechanisms, including cell differentiation, growth factor and cytokine production, immune system modulation, maintenance of the ECM, and wound contraction.[46]

Several methods of MSC delivery into the wound have been proposed, including direct injection of a single cell suspension, gel or matrix delivery systems, and synthetic bioinspired polymers. In addition, recruitment of endogenous MSCs is another method to deliver these cells to the wound.

Bone marrow or whole blood–derived endothelial progenitor cells (EPCs) are endothelial precursors and play a role in angiogenesis and vasculogenesis. These cells improve tissue perfusion by increasing neovascularization.[47] Subsequently, these cells, which can secrete angiogenic factors such as VEGF, are potentially important in the treatment of a number of disease processes, including wound healing, myocardial infarction, vascular disease, and cancer.

Skin has been also been shown to be a large repository of MAPCs. These MAPCs can arise from the epidermis, dermis, hair follicle bulge, dermal sheath, and dermal papillae. In particular, the hair follicle bulge area is considered an abundant, easily accessible source of actively growing MAPCs.[48] Hair follicle MAPCs have been shown to differentiate into neurons, glial cells, keratinocytes, and smooth muscle cells.[48] Because of their location, skin-derived MAPCs are present in the wound and are accessible for harvest.

Gene therapy, or the insertion of a gene into recipient cells, has the potential to affect wound healing by recruiting MAPCs to the wound in vivo or through ex vivo modification of MAPCs; that modified cell can then be used for cellular therapy. Gene therapy using vectors has been used experimentally to improve wound healing through overexpression of chemokine genes known to have effects on MAPC homing.[46] Gene therapy allows for the continuous production of the desired protein into the wound by the transduced cells. Direct administration of proteins into the wound, on the other hand, could potentially result in degradation of the proteins by wound proteases. Gene therapy–mediated overexpression of HIF-1α and SDF-1α have been used to improve wound healing in a diabetic mouse model.[49]

Although much is still not known about the use of gene therapy in wound healing, there is a great deal of research currently underway. As more is learned about the molecular biology of wound healing, there will likely be greater use of gene therapy to accelerate wound healing.

In summary, the therapy of choice needs to be based on the basics of wound bed preparation and modified according to the characteristics of the wound. Despite the availability of many dressings and alternative therapies, there have been no substantial studies showing a difference in healing between therapies of the same category. In fact, the cost-benefit ratio of some of the therapeutic modalities is still unclear. Thus, a systematic approach that addresses débridement, exudate management, and bacterial burden should be the standard of clinical practice and can be accomplished even in situations with limited resources.

## SELECTED REFERENCES

Alberts B, Johnson A, Lewis J, et al, editors: Cell junctions, cell adhesion, and the extracellular matrix. The Molecular Biology of the Cell, ed 4, New York, 2002, Garland, pp 1091–1114.

This chapter gives a comprehensive review of matrix and integrin biology and their critical role in biologic processes, including tissue repair.

Bello YM, Falabella AF, Eaglstein WH: Tissue-engineered skin. Current status in wound healing. Am J Clin Dermatol 2:305–313, 2001.

This article discusses the various skin substitutes available and their uses in wound healing.

Barrientos S, Stojadinovic O, Golinko MS, et al: Growth factors and cytokines in wound healing. Wound Repair Regen 16:585–601, 2008.

Review of cytokines, growth factors, and chemokines in wound healing.

Dang C, Ting K, Soo C, et al: Fetal wound healing current perspectives. Clin Plast Surg 30:13–23, 2003.

This review article discusses the morphologic, cellular, and molecular aspects of scarless fetal wound healing.

Eming SA, Hammerschmidt M, Krieg T, et al: Interrelation of immunity and tissue repair or regeneration. Semin Cell Dev Biol 20:517–527, 2009.

This article gives a review of the complex role of the immune system in tissue repair as well as in regeneration.

Herdrich BJ, Lind RC, Liechty KW: Multipotent adult progenitor cells: Their role in wound healing and the treatment of dermal wounds. Cytotherapy 10:543–550, 2008.

Comprehensive review of the current state of stem cell therapy in wound healing.

Hunter JE, Teot L, Horch R, et al: Evidence-based medicine: Vacuum-assisted closure in wound care management. Int Wound J 4:256–269, 2007.

Review of negative-pressure wound closure using evidence-based medicine.

Juckett G, Hartman-Adams H: Management of keloids and hypertrophic scars. Am Fam Physician 80:253–260, 2009.

This article discusses the current evidence-based treatment of keloids and hypertrophic scars.

Kulikovsky M, Gil T, Mettanes I, et al: Hyperbaric oxygen therapy for non-healing wounds. Isr Med Assoc J 11:480–485, 2009.

Review of negative-pressure wound closure topics and uses.

Lionelli GT, Lawrence WT: Wound dressings. Surg Clin North Am 83:617–638, 2003.

Thorough discussion of classes and uses of wound dressings.

Singer AJ, Clark RAF: Cutaneous wound healing. N Engl J Med 341:738–746, 1999.

Comprehensive review of the cellular and molecular aspects of wound healing.

## REFERENCES


1. Raja KS, Garcia MS, et al: Wound re-epithelialization: Modulating keratinocyte migration in wound healing. Front Biosci 12:2849–2868, 2007.
2. Wetzler C, Kampfer H, Stallmeyer B, et al: Large and sustained induction of chemokines during impaired wound healing in the genetically diabetic mouse: Prolonged persistence of neutrophils and macrophages during the late phase of repair. J Invest Dermatol 115:245–253, 2000.
3. Christopherson K II, Hromas R: Chemokine regulation of normal and pathologic immune responses. Stem Cells 19:388–396, 2001.
4. Rennekampff HO, Hansbrough JF, Kiessig V, et al: Bioactive interleukin-8 is expressed in wounds and enhances wound healing. J Surg Res 93:41–54, 2000.
5. Liechty KW, Crombleholme TM, Cass DL, et al: Diminished interleukin-8 (IL-8) production in the fetal wound healing response. J Surg Res 77:80–84, 1998.
6. Barrientos S, Stojadinovic O, Golinko MS, et al: Growth factors and cytokines in wound healing. Wound Repair Regen 16:585–601, 2008.
7. Grunewald M, Avraham I, Dor Y, et al: VEGF-induced adult neovascularization: Recruitment, retention, and role of accessory cells. Cell 124:175–189, 2006.
8. Florin L, Maas-Szabowski N, Werner S, et al: Increased keratinocyte proliferation by JUN-dependent expression of PTN and SDF-1 in fibroblasts. J Cell Sci 118:1981–1989, 2005.
9. Banks RE, Forbes MA, Kinsey SE, et al: Release of the angiogenic cytokine vascular endothelial growth factor (VEGF) from platelets: Significance for VEGF measurements and cancer biology. Br J Cancer 77:956–964, 1998.
10. Gaudry M, Bregerie O, Andrieu V, et al: Intracellular pool of vascular endothelial growth factor in human neutrophils. Blood 90:4153–4161, 1997.
11. Jazwa A, Loboda A, Golda S, et al: Effect of heme and heme oxygenase-1 on vascular endothelial growth factor synthesis and angiogenic potency of human keratinocytes. Free Radic Biol Med 40:1250–1263, 2006.
12. Nissen NN, Polverini PJ, Koch AE, et al: Vascular endothelial growth factor mediates angiogenic activity during the proliferative phase of wound healing. Am J Pathol 152:1445–1452, 1998.
13. Saaristo A, Tammela T, Farkkila A, et al: Vascular endothelial growth factor-C accelerates diabetic wound healing. Am J Pathol 169:1080–1087, 2006.
14. Suzuma K, Takagi H, Otani A, et al: Hypoxia and vascular endothelial growth factor stimulate angiogenic integrin expression in bovine retinal microvascular endothelial cells. Invest Ophthalmol Vis Sci 39:1028–1035, 1998.
15. Thomas KA: Vascular endothelial growth factor, a potent and selective angiogenic agent. J Biol Chem 271:603–606, 1996.
16. Shalaby F, Rossant J, Yamaguchi TP, et al: Failure of blood-island formation and vasculogenesis in Flk-1-deficient mice. Nature 376:62–66, 1995.
17. Waltenberger J, Claesson-Welsh L, Siegbahn A, et al: Different signal transduction properties of KDR and Flt1, two receptors for vascular endothelial growth factor. J Biol Chem 269:26988–26995, 1994.
18. Walder CE, Errett CJ, Bunting S, et al: Vascular endothelial growth factor augments muscle blood flow and function in a rabbit model of chronic hindlimb ischemia. J Cardiovasc Pharmacol 27:91–98, 1996.
19. Carmeliet P: VEGF gene therapy: Stimulating angiogenesis or angioma-genesis? Nat Med 6:1102–1103, 2000.
20. Nagy JA, Vasile E, Feng D, et al: Vascular permeability factor/vascular endothelial growth factor induces lymphangiogenesis as well as angiogenesis. J Exp Med 196:1497–1506, 2002.
21. Schoppmann SF, Birner P, Stockl J, et al: Tumor-associated macrophages express lymphatic endothelial growth factors and are related to peritumoral lymphangiogenesis. Am J Pathol 161:947–956, 2002.
22. Carmeliet P, Moons L, Luttun A, et al: Synergism between vascular endothelial growth factor and placental growth factor contributes to angiogenesis and plasma extravasation in pathological conditions. Nat Med 7:575–583, 2001.
23. Alberts B, Johnson A, Lewis J, et al, editors: Cell junctions, cell adhesion, and the extracellular matrix. The Molecular Biology of the Cell, ed 4, New York, 2002, Garland, pp 1091–1114.

23a. Ehrlich HP: Wound closure: Evidence of cooperation between fibroblasts and collagen matrix. Eye 2:149–157, 1988.

24. Juckett G, Hartman-Adams H: Management of keloids and hypertrophic scars. Am Fam Physician 80:253–260, 2009.

24a. Marjolin J-N: Ulcere. Dictionnaire de Medecine, vol 21, Pratique, 1828.

25. Thangarajah H, Yao D, Chang EI, et al: The molecular basis for impaired hypoxia-induced VEGF expression in diabetic tissues. Proc Natl Acad Sci U S A 106:13505–13510, 2009.
26. Loughlin DT, Artlett CM: 3-Deoxyglucosone-collagen alters human dermal fibroblast migration and adhesion: implications for impaired wound healing in patients with diabetes. Wound Repair Regen 17:739–749, 2009.

26a. http://ods.od.nih.gov/factsheets/vitaminc/accessed June 1, 2011.

27. Eming SA, Hammerschmidt M, Krieg T, et al: Interrelation of immunity and tissue repair or regeneration. Semin Cell Dev Biol 20:517–527, 2009.
28. Dang C, Ting K, Soo C, et al: Fetal wound healing current perspectives. Clin Plast Surg 30:13–23, 2003.

28a. Cowin AJ, Brosnan MP, Holmes TM, et al: Endogenous inflammatory response to dermal wound healing in the fetal and adult mouse. Dev Dyn 212:385–393, 1998.

29. Lionelli GT, Lawrence WT: Wound dressings. Surg Clin North Am 83:617–638, 2003.
30. Thomas S, Fear M, Humphreys J, et al: The effect of dressings on the production of exudates from venous leg ulcers. Wounds 18:145–150, 1996.
31. Bello YM, Falabella AF, Eaglstein WH: Tissue-engineered skin. Current status in wound healing. Am J Clin Dermatol 2:305–313, 2001.
32. Singer AJ, Clark RAF: Cutaneous wound healing. N Engl J Med 341:738–746, 1999.
33. Kulikovsky M, Gil T, Mettanes I, et al: Hyperbaric oxygen therapy for non-healing wounds. Isr Med Assoc J 11:480–485, 2009.
34. Hunt TK, Pai MP: The effect of varying ambient oxygen tensions on wound metabolism and collagen synthesis. Surg Gynecol Obstet 135:561–567, 1972.
35. Niinikoski J: Effect of oxygen supply on wound healing and formation of experimental granulation tissue. Acta Physiol Scand Suppl 334:1–72, 1969.
36. Boykin JV: Hyperbaric oxygen therapy: a physiological approach to selected problem wound healing. Wounds 8:183–198, 1996.

**37.** Fife CE: Hyperbaric oxygen therapy applications in wound care. In Sheffield PJ, Smith APS, Fife CE, editors: Wound Care Practice, Flagstaff, Ariz, 2004, Bet Publishing, pp 661–684.

**38.** Abidia A, Kuhan G, Laden G: Hyperbaric oxygen therapy for diabetic leg ulcers—a double-blind randomized controlled trial. Eur J Vas Endovasc Surg 25(6):513–518, 2003.

**38a.** Argenta LC, Morykwas MJ: Vacuum-assisted closure: A new method for wound control and treatment: Clinical experience. Ann Plast Surg 38:563–576; discussion 577, 1997.

**39.** Hunter JE, Teot L, Horch R, et al: Evidence-based medicine: Vacuum-assisted closure in wound care management. Int Wound J 4:256–269, 2007.

**39a.** Skalak R, Fox CF: Tissue engineering. Granlibakken, Lake Tahoe: Proc wrkshop; New York, 1988, Liss, pp 26–29.

**40.** Herdrich BJ, Lind RC, Liechty KW: Multipotent adult progenitor cells: Their role in wound healing and the treatment of dermal wounds. Cytotherapy 10:543–550, 2008.

**41.** Jiang Y, Jahagirdar BN, Reinhardt RL, et al: Pluripotency of mesenchymal stem cells derived from adult marrow. Nature 418:41–49, 2002.

**42.** Ichioka S, Kouraba S, Sekiya N, et al: Bone marrow-impregnated collagen matrix for wound healing: Experimental evaluation in a microcirculatory model of angiogenesis, and clinical experience. Br J Plast Surg 58:1124–1130, 2005.

**43.** Javazon EH, Keswani SG, Badillo AT, et al: Enhanced epithelial gap closure and increased angiogenesis in wounds of diabetic mice treated with adult murine bone marrow stromal progenitor cells. Wound Repair Regen 15:350–359, 2007.

**44.** Pittenger MF, Mackay AM, Beck SC, et al: Multilineage potential of adult human mesenchymal stem cells. Science 284:143–147, 1999.

**45.** Yoshikawa T, Mitsuno H, Nonaka I, et al: Wound therapy by marrow mesenchymal cell transplantation. Plast Reconstr Surg 121:860–877, 2008.

**46.** Badillo AT, Redden RA, Zhang L, et al: Treatment of diabetic wounds with fetal murine mesenchymal stromal cells enhances wound closure. Cell Tissue Res 329:301–311, 2007.

**47.** Asahara T, Takahashi T, Masuda H, et al: VEGF contributes to postnatal neovascularization by mobilizing bone marrow-derived endothelial progenitor cells. EMBO J 18:3964–3972, 1999.

**48.** Jensen TG: Cutaneous gene therapy. Ann Med 39:108–115, 2007.

**49.** Badillo AT, Chung S, Zhang L, et al: Lentiviral gene transfer of SDF-1alpha to wounds improves diabetic wound healing. J Surg Res 143:35–42, 2007.

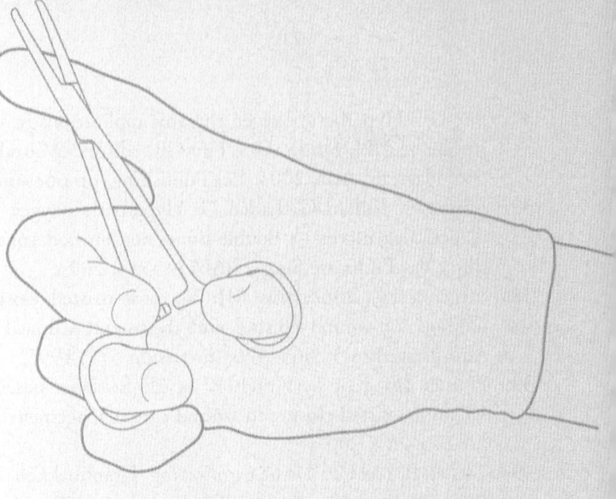

CHAPTER 8

# REGENERATIVE MEDICINE

JASON P. GLOTZBACH, SAE HEE KO, GEOFFREY C. GURTNER, AND MICHAEL T. LONGAKER



Regeneration refers to the restoration of normal tissue and organ architecture and function after injury or disease. Although numerous complex organisms retain impressive capacity to regenerate limbs and organs throughout adult life, humans have sacrificed regenerative ability for speed and strength of repair. This has allowed us to enjoy remarkable evolutionary success, but it also leads to significant scarring that causes significant loss of function and aesthetic consequences. It may be possible to improve on the normal recovery from injury and illness by promoting true tissue regeneration instead of repair through fibrosis and scarring. Surgeons have understood these dynamics for decades, but comprehensive tissue and organ regeneration have remained elusive in clinical practice. The field of regenerative medicine is largely focused on stem cells, which are powerful undifferentiated cells that have the ability to self-renew and give rise to one or more different cell types. As basic scientific research has uncovered the biology of stem cells, translational opportunities for stem cell–based therapies have become increasingly plausible. In addition to stem cell biology, the field of regenerative medicine includes the disciplines of tissue engineering and biomaterials, which aim to create molecular and structural niches to deliver regenerative therapies. This chapter provides an overview of the current status of stem cell biology and tissue engineering research and outlines the future steps required for regenerative medicine to become clinically useful.

## STEM CELL SOURCES

Stem cells are defined by their capacity to self-renew and differentiate into multiple functional cell types (Table 8-1). Traditionally, they have been divided into two main groups based on their potential to differentiate (Fig. 8-1). Pluripotent stem cells (embryonic) can differentiate into every cell of the body, whereas multipotent stem cells (adult) can differentiate into multiple, but not all, cell lineages. In addition to the traditional stem cell classification, a new class of stem cells has recently been described—induced pluripotent stem (iPS) cells—which are derived from genetically reprogrammed adult cells. These diverse cell populations hold much promise to provide researchers and clinicians with an expanded armamentarium to treat diseased and dysfunctional organs.

### Embryonic Stem Cells

During development, two distinct lineages emerge during the transition from morula to blastocyst, the trophoectoderm and the inner cell mass. Embryonic stem cells (ESCs) are immortal cell lines derived from the inner cell mass of the blastocyst. The two hallmark characteristics of ESCs are their unlimited in vitro self-renewal capacity and their ability to differentiate into all somatic cell types.[1] A number of transcription factors, most prominently Oct4, Sox2, and Nanog, are essential regulators that ensure the maintenance of pluripotency while suppressing differentiation.[2] The two glycolipid antigens SSEA3 and SSEA4 are operational cell surface markers used to identify human ESCs.[3] Since the successful isolation of mouse and human ESCs, their potential for cell replacement therapy and regenerative medicine has been widely acknowledged.[4] Both mouse and human ESCs have demonstrated an in vitro capacity to form cardiomyocytes, hematopoietic progenitors, neurons, skeletal myocytes, adipocytes, osteocytes, chondrocytes, and pancreatic islet cells when cultured under specific growth factor conditions.[5,6]

However, a number of limitations currently exist regarding the use of human ESCs in regenerative medicine. Although pluripotentiality and unlimited ability for self-renewal make ESCs attractive for cell replacement therapy, these same characteristics simultaneously translate into unregulated differentiation and formation of teratomas and teratocarcinomas. These tumors contain differentiated cells that contain all three primary germ layers, as well as undifferentiated pluripotent stem cells. This tendency to form tumors has been observed when ESCs are transplanted into mice, raising the concern that human ESC–based therapy may also lead to unwanted tumor formation.[1] Without the elimination of this possibility, the clinical use of ESC-derived tissue will remain limited.

In addition, any cell-based therapy must be free of animal contaminants that might contain pathogens or elicit an immune reaction after transfer to a host. Both mouse cell and human ESC lines are generally grown on a mouse-derived feeder layer of fibroblasts that provides additional factors that promote ESC proliferation as well as inhibit their differentiation. One example of possible animal product contamination is the demonstration that human ESCs grown on mouse feeder cells express a nonhuman sialic acid that could elicit a host's immune response.[7]

**Table 8-1 Definitions of Stem Cell-Related Terms**

| TERM | DEFINITION |
|---|---|
| Totipotent | Ability to form all cell types and lineages of organism (e.g., fertilized egg) |
| Pluripotent | Ability to form all lineages of the body (e.g., embryonic stem cells) |
| Multipotent | Ability of adult stem cells to form multiple cell types of one lineage (e.g., mesenchymal stem cells) |
| Unipotent | Cells form one cell type (e.g., follicular bulge skin stem cells) |
| Reprogramming | Dedifferentiation into an embryonic state; can be induced by nuclear transfer, genetic manipulation, viral transduction, and related methods |

Concerns have also been raised over the possible transfer of murine viruses from feeder layers to human ESCs. Many laboratories are working to solve this problem, with some studies demonstrating the ability to culture human ESCs under serum-free defined medium conditions on human cell-derived feeders or under feeder-free conditions.[8]

Furthermore, there are significant political and ethical hurdles that hinder further investigations of human ESCs. At this time, the limited number of ESC lines available and the restrictions placed on their use have precluded major progress in ESC-based applications. Although President Obama in recent months has largely reversed the restrictions put in place by President Bush, alternative solutions are needed to advance cell-based regenerative strategies.

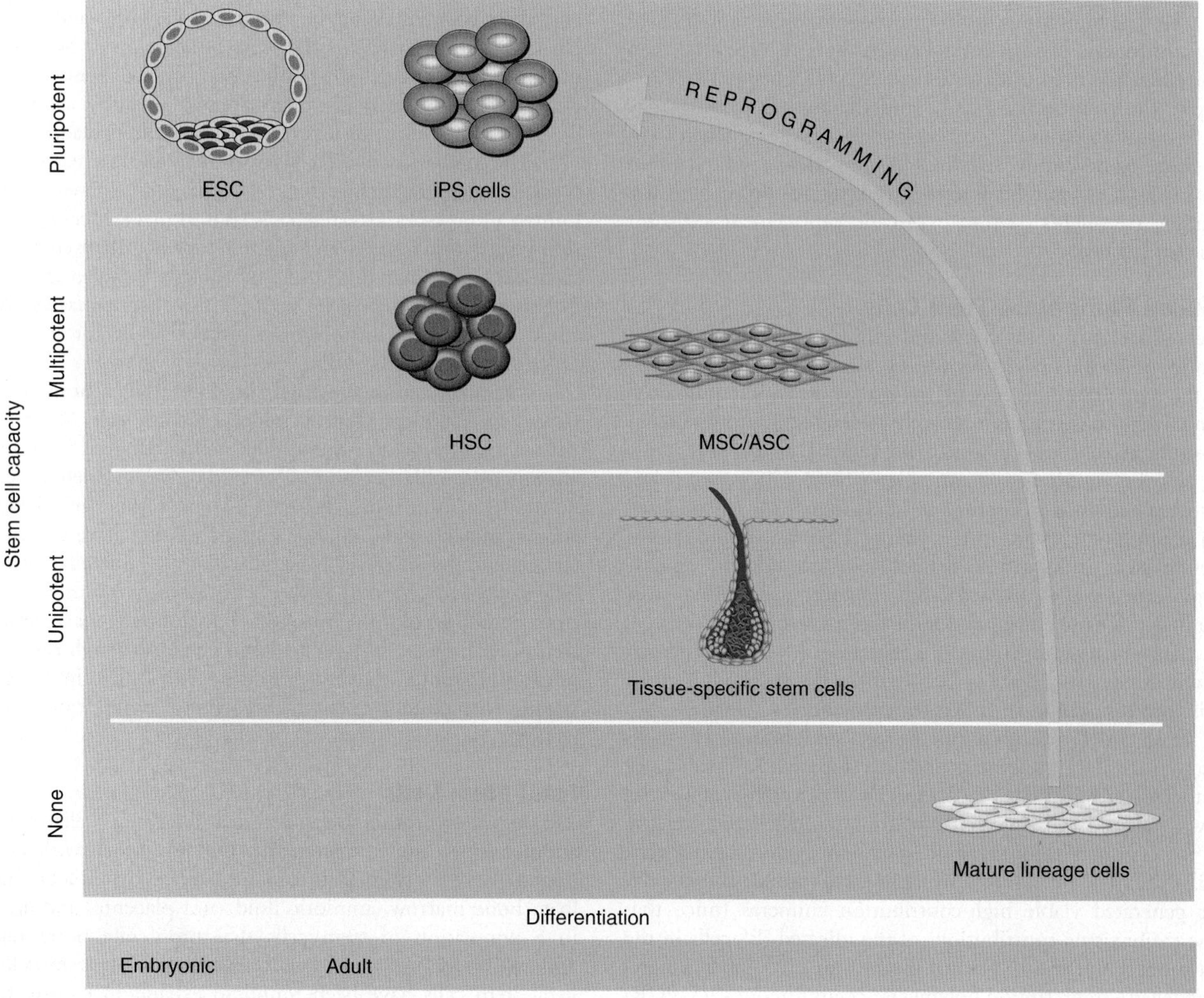


**FIGURE 8-1** Schematic of stem cell organization. ESCs, derived from the inner cell mass of the blastocyst, have the highest stem cell capacity (pluripotent) and are the least committed to any tissue lineage. Adult stem cells such as HSCs and MSCs are multipotent and are limited to certain tissue lineages, although they remain in a relatively undifferentiated state at rest. Tissue-specific stem cells, such as skin follicular bulge cells, are limited to producing a single cell and tissue type (unipotent), although they retain considerable proliferative capacity to regenerate their specific tissue. Mature lineage cells, such as mature epithelium, do not have regenerative potential. iPS cells are mature lineage cells or adult stem cells that have been reprogrammed to a state of relative pluripotency and have much of the same regenerative potential as ESCs.

### Somatic Cell Nuclear Transfer

Somatic cell nuclear transfer (SCNT), also referred to as reproductive cloning, involves the transfer of nuclei from postnatal somatic cells into an enucleated ovum. Mitotic divisions of this cell in culture lead to the generation of a blastocyst capable of yielding a whole new organism. Major advances in this field came in 1997 with the production of a normal sheep (Dolly),[9] and this procedure has been reproduced in other mammals, including mice, cattle, pigs, cats, and dogs.[10]

These experimental studies suggest that a similar approach using SCNT might work in humans for therapeutic cloning, whereby human ESCs produced by this approach could be subsequently differentiated into therapeutically useful cells and transplanted back into patients with degenerative diseases. A recent report on primate ESC lines, which were derived from rhesus macaque SCNT blastocysts using adult male skin fibroblasts as nuclear donors, is an important step in this direction.[11]

However, similar to human ESCs, SCNT is embroiled in an ethically complex debate about the moral status of created embryo and concerns about obtaining human unfertilized eggs. The technical limitations of this procedure have also dampened early enthusiasm, because several studies have reported less than 10% efficiency in the derivation of SCNT-generated ESCs.[12] Despite the controversy, SCNT and therapeutic cloning may still be a promising means to generate genetically matched stem cell lines. Long-lasting cell lines from patients with diseases created via SCNT can be used to screen potentially useful drugs or other treatments and may provide replacement cells for damaged organs.

### Induced Pluripotent Stem Cells

Given the complex logistical and ethical considerations surrounding donated oocytes for SCNT, alternatives that recapitulate the reprogramming process in vitro while avoiding the need for oocytes altogether are ultimately preferable. A groundbreaking study in 2006 by Takahashi and Yamanaka[13] defined a specific set of transcription factors, Oct4, Sox2, Klf4, and cMyc, that were sufficient to reprogram adult mouse fibroblasts back into a pluripotent state, thus creating ESC-like induced pluripotent stem (iPS) cells. Takahashi and coworkers[14] quickly demonstrated that the same combination of transcription factors is sufficient for the pluripotent induction of human cells as well. The ease and reproducibility of generating iPS cells compared with SCNT has raised the hope that iPS cells might fulfill much of the promise of human ESCs in regenerative medicine.

It is widely accepted that mouse and human iPS cells closely resemble molecular and developmental features of blastocyst-derived ESCs.[13,15] A number of research groups have shown that iPS cells injected into immunodeficient mice give rise to teratomas comprising all three embryonic germ layers, similar to ESCs. In addition, when injected into blastocysts, iPS cells generated viable high-contribution chimeras (mice that show major tissue contributions of the injected iPS cells in the host mouse) and contributed to the germline.[13,15] Furthermore, using reverse transcription polymerase chain reaction (RT-PCR) assays and immunocytochemistry, studies have shown that iPS cells express key markers of ESCs.

However, recent evidence has demonstrated that iPS cells are not identical to ESCs. Global gene expression analysis comparing iPS cells with human ESCs using microarrays has demonstrated that approximately 4% of the over 32,000 analyzed genes had more than a fivefold difference in expression.[16] Furthermore, chimeras and progeny mice derived from iPS cells had higher than normal rates of tumor formation than those derived from ESCs, which in some cases may have been caused by reactivation of the transfected *c-Myc* oncogene.[17] These key differences need to be elucidated further to define the safety of iPS cell use in regenerative medicine.

Another potential complication with the generation of iPS cells is the use of retroviral and lentiviral vectors to activate the necessary reprogramming transcription factors. Specifically, the viral genome could be inserted near endogenous genes, resulting in gene activation or silencing. This risk of insertional mutagenesis could lead to uncontrolled modification of the genome, with potential development of cancer. Much progress has been made in generating integration-free murine iPS cells, and various recent studies using adenoviral, plasmid-based, and recombinant protein-based strategies have reported that viral integration is not required for the reprogramming process.[18,19] Even without viral integration, the safety of iPS cells needs to be rigorously tested, because all essential reprogramming factors are oncogenes and their overexpression has been linked with cancers.[20] The characterization of iPS cells will be enhanced by ongoing improvements in the high-resolution analysis of genomic integrity via DNA sequencing technology to identify even minor deletions, inversions, or loss of individual alleles readily.

The generation of iPS cells is likely to create a major impact on regenerative medicine. These iPS cells can be generated from human adipose-derived stem cells (ASCs) in a feeder-free condition with a faster speed and higher efficiency than comparable strategies targeting adult human fibroblasts.[21] Given the ease of isolating a large quantity of ASCs from lipoaspirates, ASCs could be an ideal autologous source of cells for generating individual-specific iPS cells.

The therapeutic potential of iPS cells has been demonstrated in several preclinical models. For example, Wernig and colleagues have demonstrated that neurons derived from reprogrammed fibroblasts could alleviate the disease phenotype in a rat model of Parkinson's disease.[22] Using a humanized sickle cell anemia mouse model, Hanna and associates[23] have shown that the genetic defect could be corrected using transplantation of hematopoietic stem cells (HSCs) derived from iPS cells (derived from fibroblasts of those mice) that had homologous recombination of an intact wild-type β-globin gene. Although these early preclinical studies are very promising, iPS cell technology will require further refinement before clinical applications can be feasible.

### Fetal Stem Cells

Although less prominently discussed, fetal stem cells represent another source for a regenerative building block with clinical potential. Fetal stem cells can be derived from fetal blood, liver, bone marrow, amniotic fluid, and placenta, and are rich in a population of stem cells that proliferate more rapidly and exhibit greater multipotentiality than adult stem cells.[24,25] Fetal stem cells have been found to expand in culture for at least 20 passages, and their capacity for adipogenic, osteogenic, and chondrogenic differentiation has been demonstrated under appropriate culture conditions.[26] In addition, transplantation into a xenogeneic sheep model has shown the ability of these cells to engraft and undergo site-specific tissue differentiation.

Despite these promising findings, however, significant debate has been raised over the issue of using cells from fetuses and the attendant risks associated with intrauterine procedures. Nonetheless, fetal stem cells may still provide a novel means whereby future autogenous in utero cellular and genetic therapies can be devised.

### Adult Stem Cells

Once embryonic development has completed, humans and other complex organisms lose their cache of embryonic stem cells. During adult life, the regenerative capacity of tissues and organs is maintained by adult stem cells, which reside in mature tissues and in general repositories throughout bone marrow and adipose tissue. Unlike embryonic stem cells and induced pluripotent stem cells, adult stem cells are multipotent; they can differentiate into some but not all tissue lineages and are typically confined to a certain tissue type and microenvironment, usually termed a *stem cell niche*.[27] The most studied and best characterized adult stem cell types is the hematopoietic stem cell, which has served as the experimental paradigm for basic studies into the biology of adult stem cell biology.[28] Recently, much insight has been gained into the organization and function of mesenchymal stem cells and adipose stromal cells, which have shown considerable promise for the field of regenerative medicine.

### Tissue-Specific Stem Cells

Given the frequent cellular turnover and significant regenerative capacity of epithelial organs such as the cornea, small intestine, and skin,[29] it is not surprising that these tissues harbor robust resident stem cell populations. However, resident stem cells have also been isolated from organ systems that were thought to have little or no regenerative capacity, such as cardiac tissue[30] and neural tissue,[31] suggesting that most or all mature mammalian tissues and organs have corresponding stem cell populations that play some role in local tissue homeostasis and organ regeneration. These tissue-specific resident multipotent stem cells are characterized by profound self-renewal capacity, which allows them to maintain lifelong homeostasis of mature tissues in the absence of disease or injury.

Although a thorough discussion of each tissue-specific stem cell type is beyond the scope of this chapter, a limited description of a few cell types that are most relevant to surgeons is warranted. In the skin, stem cells reside in two general niches, along the hair follicles in the bulge region deep to the sebaceous glands and in the deep interfollicular epidermis.[32] The follicular bulge cells proliferate and form the hair shaft as it grows and may contribute to epidermal regeneration after trauma or injury. The deep interfollicular epidermal cells migrate upward to replenish the layers of the epidermis during normal homeostasis of the epidermis, a process that replaces all skin cells every 3 to 4 weeks. In the small intestine, a group of proliferative cells resides at the base of the crypts and send differentiating cells upward to repopulate the mature gut epithelium, with rapid turnover every 4 to 5 days. It is clear that intestine-specific stem cells exist, but the lack of specific antigens for cell isolation has made precise identification of the putative intestinal stem cell elusive, and the structure of the intestinal stem cell compartment remains controversial.[33] Interestingly, not all adult organs with regenerative potential depend on stem cell proliferation. The liver and pancreas appear to regenerate through proliferation of adult cells.[34,35] In the heart, resident stem cells have limited regenerative potential and have not been shown to engraft when administered exogenously after myocardial injury.[36] More experimental work is needed before these populations of tissue-specific resident stem cells can be effectively exploited for regenerative medicine applications.

### Adult Multipotent Stem Cells

Multipotent cells exist in several reservoirs in the adult and retain the ability to form many different cellular lineages (Fig. 8-2). Although the differentiation potential of these cells is not as complete as ESCs or induced pluripotent stem cells, their relative abundance and ease of isolation from adult patients establishes adult stem cells as a highly relevant cell type for regenerative medicine applications. Accordingly, adult multipotent stem cells have been a focus of intensive research efforts over the past several decades.

### Hematopoietic Stem Cells

HSCs have been the most studied and best characterized adult multipotent stem cell type after being definitively isolated in mice several decades ago.[37] These blood-forming cells reside in specialized niches within adult bone marrow and function to maintain homeostasis of all lineages of hematopoietic cells. HSCs have become the paradigm for the experimental investigation of adult stem cell biology. They form the basis of the most successful clinical application of stem cell–based therapy—bone marrow transplantation for hematologic malignancies and other disorders, through which HSCs repopulate all lineages of the hematopoietic system after bone marrow ablation.[28] Despite the enormous ability of HSCs to regenerate the hematopoietic system, the preponderance of evidence does not support the concept that HSCs can transdifferentiate into other tissue lineages, thus limiting their usefulness in cell-based therapeutic interventions outside of the hematopoietic system.[38] In addition, HSCs cannot readily be grown in cell or tissue culture conditions in vitro, further limiting their usefulness for regenerative medicine applications. Although direct transplantation of HSCs is not likely to be used for regenerative medicine (outside of hematopoietic deficiencies and malignancies), stem cell biologists have been investigating a possible role for HSCs in the induction of tolerance in preparation for organ transplantation.[39]

### Mesenchymal Stem Cells

The stromal fraction of adult bone marrow contains of heterogeneous population of cells that were originally described as supportive cells for hematopoietic cells and later termed mesenchymal stem cells (MSCs). This group of multipotent cells is derived from embryonic mesenchyme and can differentiate into mesenchymal-derived structures, such as bone, fat, cartilage, and muscle.[40] MSCs are rare in the bone marrow, because they only make up approximately 1 of 10,000 total bone marrow cells. They have traditionally been isolated in vitro through their ability to adhere to polystyrene tissue culture plastic; however, it is increasingly recognized that this isolation method produces a heterogeneous mix of cells, which has made comparison of experimental protocols and standardization of results difficult. Reports of human MSC surface antigen expression profiles vary widely; there is no one agreed on group of surface markers that can be used for prospective isolation protocols. A comprehensive

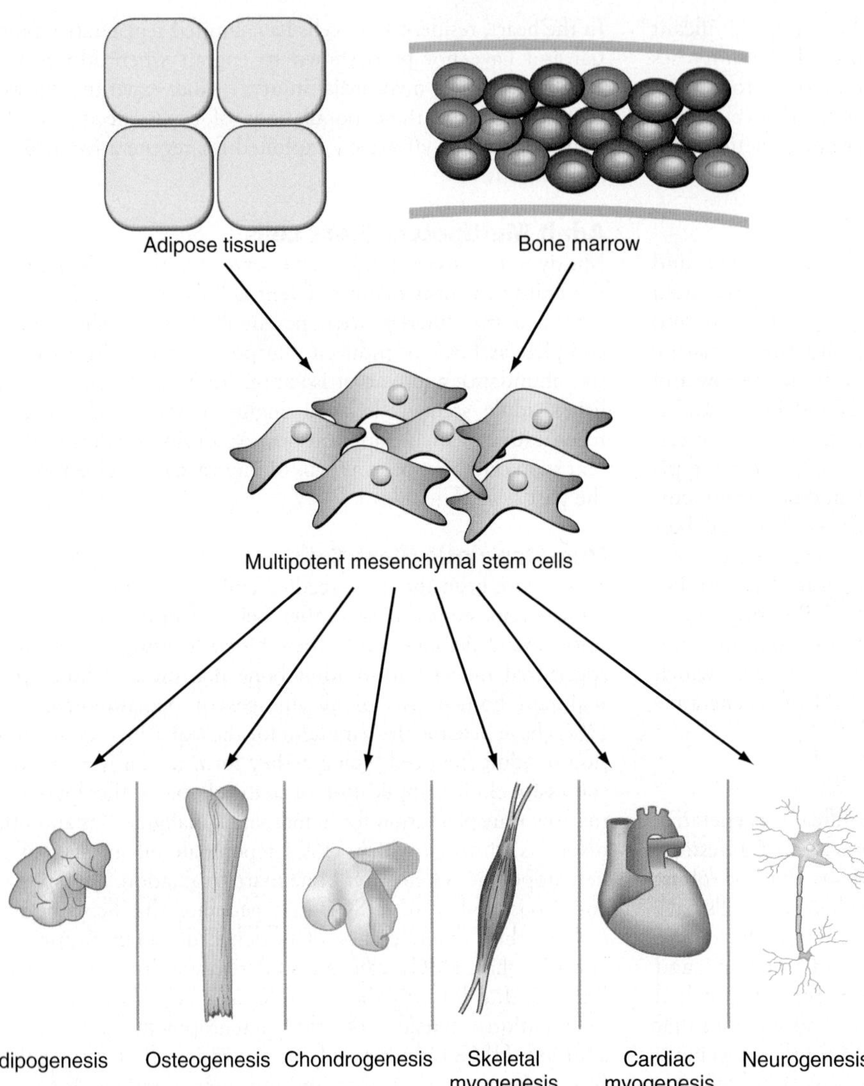


**FIGURE 8-2** Adult multipotent mesenchymal stem cells can be isolated from adipose tissue (ASCs) or from bone marrow (MSCs). These cells have been shown to differentiate into multiple tissue types in vitro, including adipose tissue (apidogenesis), bone (osteogenesis), cartilage (chondrogenesis), skeletal and cardiac muscle (skeletal and cardiac myogenesis), and nerve (neurogenesis) tissues. There has been varying success in differentiating these cells in these tissue types in vivo, which will be necessary before adult multipotent stem cells can be clinically useful for regenerative medicine applications.

review of the literature has documented that MSCs typically express the surface antigens CD13, CD29, CD44, CD73, CD90, CD105, CD146, CD166, CD271, and Stro-1, and typically do not express the hematopoietic markers CD11b, CD31, CD34, CD117, and CD45.[41] Development of a standardized isolation protocol for MSCs is an active area of ongoing research.

MSCs have shown significant promise for use in regenerative medicine applications, largely because of their ability to form multiple mature lineages. MSCs have been widely studied for use in the regeneration of cartilage and skeletal defects; results from animal models of both metabolic and traumatic skeletal injuries have been encouraging.[42] MSCs have also been shown to improve myocardial function after infarction in animal models,[43] although results in human trials using systemic injection of bone marrow cells after myocardial infarction have been mixed.[44,45] Another significant challenge that must be overcome is promoting MSC survival in infarcted myocardium and other damaged tissues, which often present a hostile environment to the engraftment and proliferation of stem cells.[46] Because of these local factors, it is possible that MSCs play a supportive role in tissue regeneration by creating a favorable local environment through secretion of growth factors and angiogenic signals. For example, MSCs have been shown to increase wound healing in chronic wounds, although the cells do not persist in the wounds over time.[47]

## Adipose-Derived Stromal Cells

There is growing excitement in the field of regenerative medicine concerning the usefulness of the stromal vascular fraction of subcutaneous adipose tissue, which contains a heterogeneous group of undifferentiated cells that are collectively referred to as ASCs. These cells have also been referred to as processed lipoaspirate (PLA) cells, adipose-derived stem cells (ADSCs), and adipose-derived mesenchymal cells (ADMCs). Although there are subtle differences among isolation protocols, a detailed discussion is out of the scope of this chapter. Zuk and coworkers have demonstrated that these cells can be coaxed to differentiate into bone, adipose tissue, cartilage, and muscle in vitro.[48] In addition, there have been several reports of limited differentiation of ASCs into neural tissue[49] and cardiac myocytes.[50] The major advantage of ASCs is their relative abundance and ease of isolation from subcutaneous adipose tissue through standard lipoaspirate techniques; approximately 1 billion cells/liter of lipoaspirate specimen can be isolated. More studies are ongoing to characterize thoroughly the heterogeneous mixture of cells that are present in adipose tissue, but unpublished data from our group has suggested that multiple subpopulations with differential abilities to produce specific tissue types may be present in ASCs. In addition, by applying different growth factors, such as bone morphogenic protein or fibroblast growth factor, ASCs can be induced to form a specific tissue.[51] Once characterized, appropriately selected ASC cells treated with specific growth factors could prove profoundly important for tissue-specific regenerative medicine applications.

### Endothelial Progenitor Cells

Circulating cells that concurrently express some hematopoietic antigens in addition to endothelial cell markers have been isolated from the peripheral blood in animals and humans. These cells have been termed *endothelial progenitor cells* (EPCs), because there is substantial evidence that they are recruited from the bone marrow and traffic to sites of vascular injury and ischemia to effect vasculogenesis, the growth of new blood vessels from circulating progenitors, in response to hypoxia and tissue ischemia.[52] Similar to MSCs and ASCs, these cells appear to be mesenchymal or stromal in origin, but there is no widely agreed on profile of surface antigen expression or isolation protocol for these cells. Furthermore, it is not clear whether these cells differentiate into mature endothelial cells or merely serve as supportive perivascular cells during the process of vasculogenesis.

### Stem Cells and Cancer

The tremendous self-renewal and regenerative potential of stem cells comes with a price. If the asymmetrical division and self-renewal process of stem cells become dysregulated, the risk of malignant transformation increases significantly.[53] Mutations and dysregulation of stem cell self-renewal underlie most hematopoietic malignancies, and also have been implicated in cancers of the breast, gastrointestinal system, and central nervous system and in many other solid tumors.[54] Oncologic surgeons know well that even microscopic disease left behind after resection of a cancerous lesion can cause recurrent disease; the corollary with stem cell–based therapy is that small numbers of dysregulated stem cells can, if implanted, become a clinically significant tumor. As stem cell–based therapy is adapted for clinical use, these lessons from cancer biology must be heeded, because the neoplastic potential of pluripotent and multipotent stem cells is not trivial.

## BIOENGINEERING FOR REGENERATIVE MEDICINE

### Research Applications

Stem cells are profoundly influenced by their surroundings, as evidenced by the importance of the niche for maintenance of stem cell populations in vivo. This aspect of stem cell physiology has prompted the field of regenerative medicine to expand from pure stem cell biology to include engineering of biomaterials and mechanical systems to create synthetic niches on which to grow stem cells to facilitate detailed experimental studies and provide therapeutic platforms on which to deliver stem cells to patients (Fig. 8-3).[55] Such biomaterials are referred to as biomimetic because they mimic the anatomic and/or physiologic environment necessary for cellular engraftment and proliferation. One of the most basic applications of this principle has been in designing complex culture systems to provide a more physiologic environment than standard two-dimensional rigid polystyrene plastic for studying stem cell growth in vitro. For example, by coating a culture dish with the ligand leukemia inhibitory factor bound to a thin polymer, Alberti and colleagues have demonstrated a significant increase in mouse ESC proliferation.[56] A group in Switzerland has demonstrated that ASCs expanded in a three-dimensional, ceramic, scaffold-based perfusion culture system had improved osteogenic capabilities as compared with traditional two-dimensional expansion in tissue culture dishes.[57] An additional offshoot of the incorporation of engineering concepts into the field of regenerative medicine has been an increasing awareness of the influence of mechanical forces on stem cell behavior and the importance of understanding and controlling the mechanical environment of engineered tissue grafts for use in regenerative therapies.

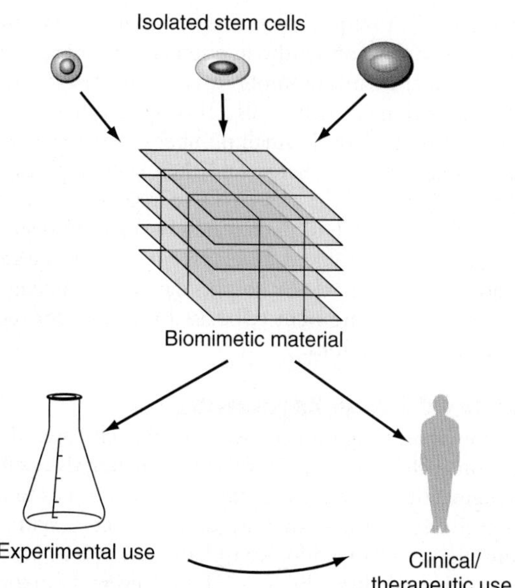


**FIGURE 8-3** Biomimetic materials are engineered to create favorable stem cell niches for both in vitro experimental stem cell biology studies and for clinical use in regenerative medicine applications. Because all stem cells are exquisitely sensitive to environmental cues, the bioengineering component of regenerative medicine will be crucial to modulate and control stem cell behavior to allow effective cell-based therapies to be used clinically.

### Biomaterials as Constructs for Cell Delivery and Directed Differentiation

In addition to experimental tools, bioengineered materials hold much promise as platforms for cell delivery in regenerative medicine applications. Up to this point, most efforts have centered on the use of biomaterials such as collagen polymers, polyglycolic acid (PGA), poly(lactic-co-glycolic acid) (PLGA), and polyethylene glycol (PEG) hydrogels, which are porous to allow cell ingress and can be easily molded and shaped to a desired configuration. Several groups have also used modified ink jet printers to create precisely patterned scaffolds and hydrogels to devise finely tuned systems for cellular support and growth factor delivery.[58] A frequently articulated goal of these biomaterial studies is to develop synthetic systems to mimic physiologic extracellular matrix and promote in vivo–directed proliferation and differentiation of stem cells. This approach would allow implantation of a relatively small number of stem cells within a bioengineered construct that would then encourage expansion and differentiation of the stem cells to regenerate the desired tissue.[59] Although much of the research in this field is still in the early stages of discovery and development, significant advances have moved us much closer to the day when bioengineered constructs will facilitate stem cell–based therapies for regenerative medicine applications.

### Organ-Level Tissue Engineering

In addition to creating mimetic scaffolds for cell-based therapies and custom culture systems, the fields of materials science and tissue engineering have recently expanded their focus to include organ-level engineering—that is, to construct a synthetic or partially engineered organ for transplantation into a patient with end-stage organ failure. Because of the severe limitations on donor organ availability, the prospect of engineering replacement organs from a patient's own cells is highly appealing to overcome the problem of organ scarcity. Urology has taken the lead in this field, because urologic structures such as the bladder and urethra lend themselves well to organ engineering. Atala and colleagues have demonstrated the clinical feasibility of urethral and bladder grafts engineered from collagen matrices and seeded cells.[58] Although organ engineering appears to be on the verge of clinical viability for hollow organs such as the bladder, ex vivo engineering of solid organs with complex physiology, such as the liver and kidney, represents a much more difficult challenge.

The kidney presents an enormous challenge because of its complex three-dimensional architecture and the diverse functional requirements of each cellular component. Nonetheless, several groups have reported limited success with a bioartificial kidney containing living tubule cells and connected through standard hemodialysis access lines.[60] Although this is a nonimplanted temporary ex vivo solution, these early studies suggest that an engineered cell-scaffold construct may be able to supplant long-term renal replacement therapy. Ongoing studies using collagen matrices and in vitro expansion of renal cells to create anatomically and physiologically appropriate glomerulotubular units have shown some promise in animal studies.[61] The liver also represents a significant clinical need for replacement organs, but organ-level engineering is difficult because of the inherent complexity of hepatic anatomy and physiology. Isolated hepatocyte transplantation has shown some short-term effectiveness in treating Crigler-Najjar syndrome and other metabolic disorders of the liver, but whole-organ replacement has not been achieved.[62] Several groups are working to seed expanded or immortalized human liver cells on biomimetic scaffolds, but these experiments are in the preliminary stages of development.[63] In total, although organ-level engineering has significant potential, much more work is required before this field will have clinical applicability.

## CLINICAL APPLICATIONS OF STEM CELLS

Stem cell therapies are setting a new paradigm for regenerative medicine, with tremendous potential to repair and regenerate tissue injury and diseases. Although there is considerable optimism for novel cell-based treatments, their use needs to be carefully evaluated by early clinical trials. Early clinical experience with stem cell therapies is summarized in Table 8-2. Many of these studies have attempted to expand on the success of bone marrow HSC transplantation in treating blood disorders and cancer to evaluate the safety and efficacy of stem cell–based therapies to treat a number of diseases.

### Embryonic Stem Cells

Clinical studies on the use of pluripotent stem cells have begun to take place. In 2009, the U.S. Food and Drug Administration (FDA) approved the first clinical trial using ESCs. The study, led by the biotechnology company Geron, will be evaluating the use of ESC in the treatment of complete spinal cord injury.[64] The company recently enrolled the first human patient into this Phase I trial to assess the safety and tolerability of hESC-derived oligodendrocyte progenitor cells. Many other applications using ESCs are expected to enter clinical trials. Regulatory approval is being sought for the use of ESCs to treat blindness associated with retinal loss based on encouraging in vitro and in vivo preclinical studies, and efforts are also underway to develop beta islet cells from ESCs for the correction of type 1 diabetes.[65]

### Fetal Stem Cells

Fetal neural stem cells are also being explored to address difficult genetic diseases. The biotechnology company, California Stem Cell, is evaluating the transplantation of fetal neural stem cells to treat children with lysosomal storage diseases.[65] Concerns were raised by the report of multifocal brain tumor development in a child with ataxia telangiectasia treated with intracerebellar and intrathecal injections of fetal neural stem cells in Russia.[66] The glioneuronal neoplasm was found to be derived from the transplanted neural stem cells. More research and ongoing clinical vigilance are needed to ensure safety in stem cell transplantation.

### Multipotent Adult Stem Cells

Because of the ethical and political concerns related to the use of embryonic and fetal cells and tissues as the basis of clinical treatments, the field of regenerative medicine has begun to emphasize the potential of adult multipotent stem cells as the foundation for stem cell–based therapies. MSCs and ASCs readily differentiate into the mesenchymal lineages of bone, cartilage, fat, and muscle, which make them ideal candidates for regeneration of those tissues in adult patients. There have been several case reports of ASCs and MSCs used to repair bone defects, but there have been no rigorous clinical trials performed as of this writing. Based on promising results in animal models, there has been considerable interest in the implantation of bone marrow cells in the setting of myocardial infarction and ischemic cardiomyopathy.[43] Several trials have been performed using intramyocardial or intracoronary injection of bone marrow–derived cells. These studies have generated mixed results, with modest increases in left ventricular ejection fraction but little evidence of long-term survival benefits. More studies are needed to determine the role of stem cell–based treatments in ischemic myocardial pathologies.

Overall, there is much promise for stem cell–based therapies, but this potential has been largely unrealized to date. Despite this, regenerative medicine seems poised to become clinically relevant in the near term, which likely will considerably expand the tools available to surgeons and their patients.

**Table 8-2 Reported Clinical Applications of Stem Cells**

| CLINICAL APPLICATION | CELL TYPE | DELIVERY METHOD |
|---|---|---|
| Inflammatory bowel disease (Crohn's)[a] | ASC | Surgical implantation into perianal fistulae |
| Muscular dystrophy[b] | Muscle-derived progenitors, $CD133^+$ | Local injection |
| Ischemic cardiomyopathy (MAGNUM Trial)[c] | Bone marrow (BM) MSC | Surgically implanted three-dimensional collagen matrix |
| Acute myocardial infarction (BOOST Trial)[d] | Total bone marrow | Intracoronary injection |
| Acute myocardial infarction (REPAIR-AMI Trial)[e] | Total bone marrow | Intracoronary injection |
| Acute myocardial infarction (ASTAMI Trial)[f] | BM MNC | Intracoronary injection |
| Ischemic cardiomyopathy[g] | Total bone marrow | Systemic injection |
| Tracheobronchomalacia[h] | BM MSC | Differentiated to chondrocytes and surgically implanted |
| Traumatic calvarial defect[i] | ASC | Surgical implantation in fibrin glue |
| Achondroplasia[j] | BM MSC | Transplantation concurrently with distraction osteogenesis |

[a]From Garcia-Olmo D, Herreros D, Pascual M, et al: Treatment of enterocutaneous fistula in Crohn's disease with adipose-derived stem cells: A comparison of protocols with and without cell expansion. Int J Colorectal Dis 24:27–30, 2009.

[b]From Torrente Y, Belicchi M, Marchesi C, et al: Autologous transplantation of muscle-derived $CD133^+$ stem cells in Duchenne muscle patients. Cell Transplant 16:563–577, 2007.

[c]From Chachques JC, Trainini JC, Lago N, et al: Myocardial assistance by grafting a new bioartificial upgraded myocardium (MAGNUM trial): Clinical feasibility study. Ann Thorac Surg 85:901–908, 2008.

[d]From Wollert KC, Meyer GP, Lotz J, et al: Intracoronary autologous bone-marrow cell transfer after myocardial infarction: the BOOST randomised controlled clinical trial. Lancet 364:141–148, 2004.

[e]From Schächinger V, Erbs S, Elsässer A, et al; REPAIR-AMI Investigators: Intracoronary bone marrow-derived progenitor cells in acute myocardial infarction. N Engl J Med 355:1210–1221, 2006.

[f]From Lunde K, Solheim S, Aakhus S, et al: Intracoronary injection of mononuclear bone marrow cells in acute myocardial infarction. N Engl J Med 355:1199–1209, 2006.

[g]From Meyer GP, Wollert KC, Lotz J, et al: Intracoronary bone marrow cell transfer after myocardial infarction: 5-year follow-up from the randomized-controlled BOOST trial. European heart journal 30:2978–2984, 2009.

[h]From Macchiarini P, Jungebluth P, Go T, et al: Clinical transplantation of a tissue-engineered airway. Lancet 372:2023–2030, 2008.

[i]From Lendeckel S, Jödicke A, Christophis P, et al: Autologous stem cells (adipose) and fibrin glue used to treat widespread traumatic calvarial defects: Case report. J Craniomaxillofac Surg 32:370–373, 2004.

[j]From Kitoh H, Kitakoji T, Tsuchiya H, et al: Transplantation of marrow-derived mesenchymal stem cells and platelet-rich plasma during distraction osteogenesis—a preliminary result of three cases. Bone 35:892–898, 2004.

## SELECTED REFERENCES

Atala A: Engineering organs. Curr Opin Biotechnol 20:575–592, 2009.

This excellent review from a leader in the field of regenerative medicine outlines the progress made and challenges faced by tissue and organ engineering as is relates to regenerative medicine.

Beltrami AP, Barlucchi L, Torella D, et al:Adult cardiac stem cells are multipotent and support myocardial regeneration. Cell 114:763–776, 2003.

This paper discusses the isolation of resident cardiac stem cells and their potential uses in myocardial regeneration. Resident cardiac stem cells are a prime example of the limits of tissue-specific stem cell populations for use in regenerative medicine.

Blanpain C, Horsley V, Fuchs E: Epithelial stem cells: Turning over new leaves. Cell 128:445–458, 2007.

This excellent review describes the current understanding of epithelial stem cells and discusses their potential applications for regenerative medicine.

Kiel MJ, He S, Ashkenazi R, et al: Haematopoietic stem cells do not asymmetrically segregate chromosomes or retain BrdU. Nature 449:238–242, 2007.

This important paper demonstrates that asymmetrical cell division does not occur in HSCs. This establishes the concept that not all adult stem cells are clonal populations and that heterogeneity of transcription is likely the normal state of a stem cell population.

Lutolf MP, Gilbert PM, Blau HM: Designing materials to direct stem cell fate. Nature 462:433–441, 2009.

This comprehensive review describes the role of bioengineering in stem cell biology research and regenerative medicine.

Pittenger MF, Mackay AM, Beck SC, et al: Multilineage potential of adult human mesenchymal stem cells. Science 284:143–147, 1999.

This paper was the first description of human mesenchymal stem cells. In this report, the authors demonstrated the existence of a nonhematopoietic cell population in the bone marrow with multipotent differentiation ability.

Spangrude GJ, Heimfeld S, Weissman IL: Purification and characterization of mouse hematopoietic stem cells. Science 241:58–62, 1988.

This was the original description of hematopoietic stem cell isolation, which established the paradigm for adult stem cell research.

Takahashi K, Yamanaka S: Induction of pluripotent stem cells from mouse embryonic and adult fibroblast cultures by defined factors. Cell 126:663–676, 2006.

This was the original description of the creation of induced pluripotent stem cells by viral transfection with four genes. Subsequent studies have generated iPS cells from human skin cells and ASCs. Because the original transfection methods involved genomic integration of viral particles, much work is ongoing to allow the safe induction of pluripotency in cells by using techniques that would allow these cells to be used clinically.

Thomson JA, Itskovitz-Eldor J, Shapiro SS, et al: Embryonic stem cell lines derived from human blastocysts. Science 282:1145–1147, 1998.

These authors were the first group to isolate and describe human embryonic stem cells. This paper created much interest in ESCs as potential sources of cell-based therapies for the field of regenerative medicine, but also raised several important ethical concerns that are the source of ongoing debate in the scientific and broader community.

Zuk PA, Zhu M, Ashjian P, et al: Human adipose tissue is a source of multipotent stem cells. Mol Biol Cell 13:4279–4295, 2002.

In this seminal description of adipose stromal cells, the authors demonstrated that multipotent mesenchymal stem cells could be isolated from the stromal vascular fraction of human adipose tissue. This was the first account of an adult stem cell population isolated from a tissue other than the bone marrow.

## REFERENCES


1. Thomson JA, Itskovitz-Eldor J, Shapiro SS, et al: Embryonic stem cell lines derived from human blastocysts. Science 282:1145–1147, 1998.
2. Boyer LA, Lee TI, Cole MF, et al: Core transcriptional regulatory circuitry in human embryonic stem cells. Cell 122:947–956, 2005.
3. International Stem Cell Initiative; Adewumi O, Aflatoonian B, Ahrlund-Richter L,et al: Characterization of human embryonic stem cell lines by the International Stem Cell Initiative. Nat Biotechnol 25:803–816, 2007.
4. Martin GR: Isolation of a pluripotent cell line from early mouse embryos cultured in medium conditioned by teratocarcinoma stem cells. Proc Natl Acad Sci U S A 78:7634–7638, 1981.
5. Poliard A, Nifuji A, Lamblin D, et al: Controlled conversion of an immortalized mesodermal progenitor cell towards osteogenic, chondrogenic, or adipogenic pathways. J Cell Biol 130:1461–1472, 1995.
6. Wu DC, Boyd AS, Wood KJ: Embryonic stem cell transplantation: potential applicability in cell replacement therapy and regenerative medicine. Front Biosci 12:4525–4535, 2007.
7. Martin MJ, Muotri A, Gage F, Varki A: Human embryonic stem cells express an immunogenic nonhuman sialic acid. Nat Med 11:228–232, 2005.
8. Amit M, Shariki C, Margulets V, Itskovitz-Eldor J: Feeder layer- and serum-free culture of human embryonic stem cells. Biol Reprod 70:837–845, 2004.
9. Wilmut I, Schnieke AE, McWhir J, et al: Viable offspring derived from fetal and adult mammalian cells. Nature 385:810–813, 1997.
10. Lee BC, Kim MK, Jang G, et al: Dogs cloned from adult somatic cells. Nature 436:641, 2005.
11. Byrne JA, Pedersen DA, Clepper LL, et al: Producing primate embryonic stem cells by somatic cell nuclear transfer. Nature 450:497–502, 2007.
12. Perry AC: Progress in human somatic-cell nuclear transfer. N Engl J Med 353:87–88, 2005.
13. Takahashi K, Yamanaka S: Induction of pluripotent stem cells from mouse embryonic and adult fibroblast cultures by defined factors. Cell 126:663–676, 2006.
14. Takahashi K, Tanabe K, Ohnuki M, et al: Induction of pluripotent stem cells from adult human fibroblasts by defined factors. Cell 131:861–872, 2007.
15. Wernig M, Meissner A, Foreman R, et al: In vitro reprogramming of fibroblasts into a pluripotent ES-cell-like state. Nature 448: 319–324, 2007.
16. Chin MH, Mason MJ, Xie W, et al: Induced pluripotent stem cells and embryonic stem cells are distinguished by gene expression signatures. Cell Stem Cell 5:111–123, 2009.
17. Okita K, Ichisaka T, Yamanaka S: Generation of germline-competent induced pluripotent stem cells. Nature 448:313–317, 2007.
18. Stadtfeld M, Nagaya M, Utikal J, et al: Induced pluripotent stem cells generated without viral integration. Science 322:945–949, 2008.
19. Zhou H, Wu S, Joo JY, et al: Generation of induced pluripotent stem cells using recombinant proteins. Cell Stem Cell 4:381–384, 2009.
20. Liu SV: iPS cells: A more critical review. Stem Cells Dev 17:391–397, 2008.
21. Sun N, Panetta NJ, Gupta DM, et al: Feeder-free derivation of induced pluripotent stem cells from adult human adipose stem cells. Proc Natl Acad Sci U S A 106:15720–15725, 2009.
22. Wernig M, Zhao JP, Pruszak J, et al: Neurons derived from reprogrammed fibroblasts functionally integrate into the fetal brain and improve symptoms of rats with Parkinson's disease. Proc Natl Acad Sci U S A 105:5856–5861, 2008.
23. Hanna J, Wernig M, Markoulaki S, et al: Treatment of sickle cell anemia mouse model with iPS cells generated from autologous skin. Science 318:1920–1923, 2007.
24. Guillot PV, O'Donoghue K, Kurata H, Fisk NM: Fetal stem cells: Betwixt and between. Semin Reprod Med 24:340–347, 2006.
25 De Coppi P, Bartsch G, Jr, Siddiqui MM, et al: Isolation of amniotic stem cell lines with potential for therapy. Nat Biotechnol 25:100–106, 2007.
26. Götherström C, Ringdén O, Tammik C, et al: Immunologic properties of human fetal mesenchymal stem cells. Am J Obstet Gynecol 190:239–245, 2004.
27. Moore KA, Lemischka IR: Stem cells and their niches. Science 311:1880–1885, 2006.
28. Orkin SH, Zon LI: Hematopoiesis: An evolving paradigm for stem cell biology. Cell 132:631–644, 2008.
29. Blanpain C, Horsley V, Fuchs E: Epithelial stem cells: Turning over new leaves. Cell 128:445–458, 2007.
30. Beltrami AP, Barlucchi L, Torella D, et al: Adult cardiac stem cells are multipotent and support myocardial regeneration. Cell 114:763–776, 2003.

**31.** Gross CG: Neurogenesis in the adult brain: Death of a dogma. Nat Rev Neurosci 1:67–73, 2000.

**32.** Gurtner GC, Werner S, Barrandon Y, Longaker MT: Wound repair and regeneration. Nature 453:314–321, 2008.

**33.** Garrison AP, Helmrath MA, Dekaney CM: Intestinal stem cells. J Pediatr Gastroenterol Nutr 49:2–7, 2009.

**34.** Cantz T, Manns MP, Ott M: Stem cells in liver regeneration and therapy. Cell Tissue Res 331:271–282, 2008.

**35.** Dor Y, Brown J, Martinez OI, Melton DA: Adult pancreatic beta-cells are formed by self-duplication rather than stem-cell differentiation. Nature 429:41–46, 2004.

**36.** Li Z, Lee A, Huang M, et al: Imaging survival and function of transplanted cardiac resident stem cells. J Am Coll Cardiol 53:1229–1240, 2009.

**37.** Spangrude GJ, Heimfeld S, Weissman IL: Purification and characterization of mouse hematopoietic stem cells. Science 241:58–62, 1988.

**38.** Balsam LB, Wagers AJ, Christensen JL, et al: Haematopoietic stem cells adopt mature haematopoietic fates in ischaemic myocardium. Nature 428:668–673, 2004.

**39.** Weissman IL, Shizuru JA: The origins of the identification and isolation of hematopoietic stem cells, and their capability to induce donor-specific transplantation tolerance and treat autoimmune diseases. Blood 112:3543–3553, 2008.

**40.** Pittenger MF, Mackay AM, Beck SC, et al: Multilineage potential of adult human mesenchymal stem cells. Science 284:143–147, 1999.

**41.** Kolf CM, Cho E, Tuan RS: Mesenchymal stromal cells. Biology of adult mesenchymal stem cells: Regulation of niche, self-renewal and differentiation. Arthritis Res Ther 9:204, 2007.

**42.** El Tamer MK, Reis RL: Progenitor and stem cells for bone and cartilage regeneration. J Tissue Eng Regen Med 3:327–337, 2009.

**43.** Orlic D, Kajstura J, Chimenti S, et al: Bone marrow cells regenerate infarcted myocardium. Nature 410:701–705, 2001.

**44.** Rosenzweig A: Cardiac cell therapy—mixed results from mixed cells. N Engl J Med 355:1274–1277, 2006.

**45.** Gersh BJ, Simari RD, Behfar A., et al: Cardiac cell repair therapy: A clinical perspective. Mayo Clin Proc 84:876–892, 2009.

**46.** Hosoda T, Kajstura J, Leri A, Anversa P: Mechanisms of myocardial regeneration. Circ J 74:13–17, 2010.

**47.** Falanga V, Iwamoto S, Chartier M, et al: Autologous bone marrow-derived cultured mesenchymal stem cells delivered in a fibrin spray accelerate healing in murine and human cutaneous wounds. Tissue Eng 13:1299–1312, 2007.

**48.** Zuk PA, Zhu M, Ashjian P, et al: Human adipose tissue is a source of multipotent stem cells. Mol Biol Cell 13:4279–4295, 2002.

**49.** Ashjian PH, Elbarbary AS, Edmonds B, et al: In vitro differentiation of human processed lipoaspirate cells into early neural progenitors. Plast Reconstr Surg 111:1922–1931, 2003.

**50.** Léobon B, Roncalli J, Joffre C, et al: Adipose-derived cardiomyogenic cells: In vitro expansion and functional improvement in a mouse model of myocardial infarction. Cardiovasc Res 83:757–767, 2009.

**51.** An C, Cheng Y, Yuan Q, Li J: IGF-1 and BMP-2 induces differentiation of adipose-derived mesenchymal stem cells into chondrocyte-like cells. Ann Biomed Eng 38:1647–1654, 2010.

**52.** Asahara T, Murohara T, Sullivan A, et al: Isolation of putative progenitor endothelial cells for angiogenesis. Science 275:964–967, 1997.

**53.** Morrison SJ, Kimble J: Asymmetric and symmetric stem-cell divisions in development and cancer. Nature 441:1068–1074, 2006.

**54.** Rossi DJ, Jamieson CH, Weissman IL: Stems cells and the pathways to aging and cancer. Cell 132:681–696, 2008.

**55.** Lutolf MP, Gilbert PM, Blau HM: Designing materials to direct stem-cell fate. Nature 462:433–441, 2009.

**56.** Alberti K, Davey RE, Onishi K, et al: Functional immobilization of signaling proteins enables control of stem cell fate. Nat Methods 5:645–650, 2008.

**57.** Scherberich A, Galli R, Jaquiery C, et al: Three-dimensional perfusion culture of human adipose tissue-derived endothelial and osteoblastic progenitors generates osteogenic constructs with intrinsic vascularization capacity. Stem Cells 25:1823–1829, 2007.

**58.** Atala A: Engineering organs. Curr Opin Biotechnol 20:575–592, 2009.

**59.** Xu Y, Shi Y, Ding S: A chemical approach to stem-cell biology and regenerative medicine. Nature 453:338–344, 2008.

**60.** Song JH, Humes HD: The bioartificial kidney in the treatment of acute kidney injury. Curr Drug Targets 10:1227–1234, 2009.

**61.** Humes HD, Buffington DA, MacKay SM, et al: Replacement of renal function in uremic animals with a tissue-engineered kidney. Nat Biotechnol 17:451–455, 1999.

**62.** Dalgetty DM, Medine CN, Iredale JP, Hay DC: Progress and future challenges in stem cell-derived liver technologies. Am J Physiol Gastrointest Liver Physiol 297:G241–G248, 2009.

**63.** Kobayashi N: Life support of artificial liver: Development of a bioartificial liver to treat liver failure. J Hepatobiliary Pancreat Surg 16:113–117, 2009.

**64.** Couzin J: Biotechnology. Celebration and concern over U.S. trial of embryonic stem cells. Science 323:568, 2009.

**65.** Trounson A: New perspectives in human stem cell therapeutic research. BMC Med 7:29, 2009.

**66.** Amariglio N, Hirshberg A, Scheithauer BW, et al: Donor-derived brain tumor following neural stem cell transplantation in an ataxia telangiectasia patient. PLoS Med 6:e1000029, 2009.

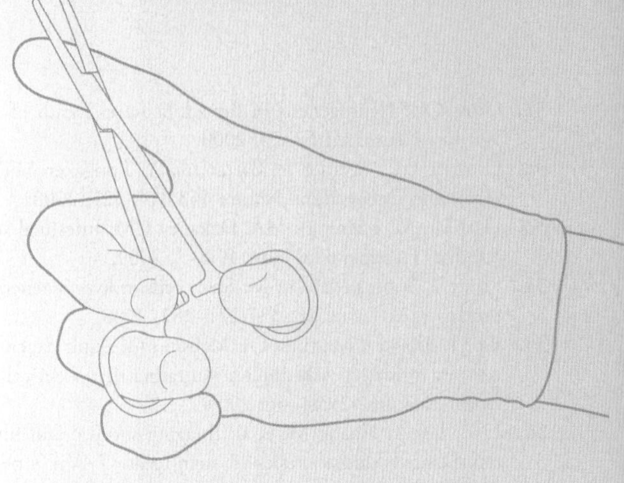

CHAPTER 9

# EVIDENCE-BASED SURGERY: CRITICALLY ASSESSING SURGICAL LITERATURE

David R. Flum, Farhood Farjah, and Nader Massarweh



Not long ago, case series published by a single surgeon or group of surgeons reporting the results of a novel management strategy or new technique were the mainstay of communication in the surgical community. These reports highlighted surgical advances that could be applied to patients, but often reflected the best surgeons reporting their best results. Such reports represented much of the evidence base that guided surgical practice. However, with growing recognition that almost everyone will require surgery at some point in their lives, surgical disease is being increasingly considered in the context of the public's health. From this perspective, the published experience of one surgeon becomes less relevant than evidence that describes how surgical procedures actually work in the general community, how their effectiveness compares with other strategies, and the full spectrum of outcomes needed to assess a procedure's impact on patients and the health care system. Over the last decade, surgical health services and outcomes research has emerged as an essential approach for informing the modern surgical era with evidence. Surgical investigators apply a range of research methods to draw truths from the collective surgical experience, with the goal of integrating the best available evidence into what surgeons do in general practice. Distinct from the past era of surgical research, current efforts aim to move beyond reporting what can be done to patients to establishing what should be done for patients.

Outcomes and health services research are broad terms for scientific inquiries evaluating health care outcomes, care delivery, and the systems delivering that care. This enterprise does not focus on outcomes alone, but also considers the daily actions performed by health care teams and surgeons (processes of care) as well as the environment in which services are delivered (structures of care). With the medical community facing increasing regulatory oversight and a drive for more accountable care, it is essential that surgeons understand and embrace the approach of evidence-based surgery so they can improve the care of their patients and maintain a leadership role in health policy and quality improvement activities. The goal of this chapter is to help the reader become a more critical evaluator of the surgical literature and advance the use of better evidence in surgical practice. To that end, this chapter is framed through questions that a critical reader should ask when reading a research study.

## WHAT IS THE PURPOSE OF THE STUDY?

Assessing the value of a study requires an understanding of the investigator's intended purpose. Most studies can be placed into one of two general categories, descriptive (or exploratory) and analytic (Fig. 9-1). Most descriptive studies should be considered hypothesis-generating rather than causality-focused whereas analytic studies test a prespecified hypothesis. A study's purpose should drive the selection of study groups, outcomes of interest, data sources, study design, and analytic plan. Unfortunately, many studies fall short in linking study purpose and methodology; investigators may sometimes try to establish causality from descriptive studies. For example, in a study describing trends in the misdiagnosis of appendicitis during a time when there was increased use of diagnostic testing, an attempt to establish a causal link between these two findings (i.e., the trend in misdiagnosis was caused by the trend in diagnostic testing) would be overreaching the descriptive nature of the study.[1] The intent of descriptive studies should be identifying possible associations and serving as an impetus for future investigations using more rigorous analytic approaches.

## WHAT IS BEING COMPARED?

Many surgical studies evaluate outcomes (e.g., complications, cost, efficacy, effectiveness, quality of life, functional status, patient satisfaction) of one intervention or strategy compared with another. The method of classifying subjects into one group or another and the fact that some exposures vary with time pose important methodologic challenges to be considered when evaluating the strength of evidence provided by a study.

### Misclassification

Misclassification is the incorrect categorization of a subject into a study group. This issue is important because in the context of misclassification, even a properly performed analysis with an appropriate study design will yield biased results. There are two

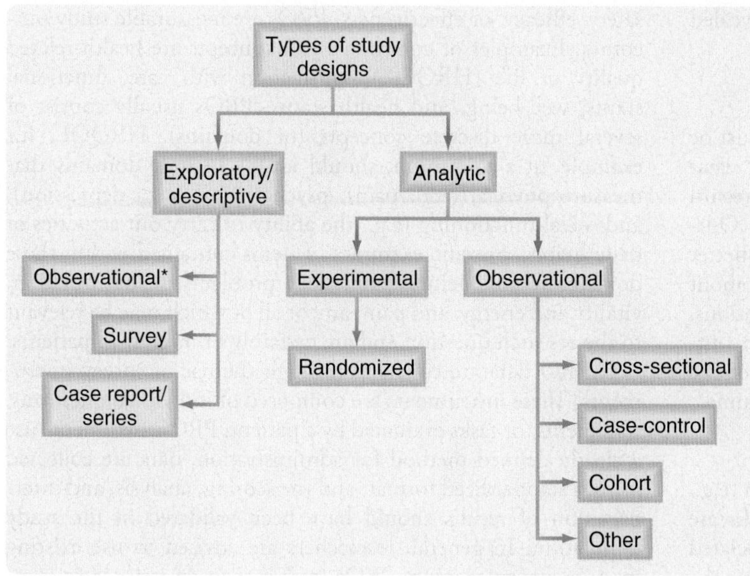


**FIGURE 9-1** Hierarchy of study designs. The asterisk means that the same study designs found in the other branch apply.

types of misclassification, nondifferential and differential. Nondifferential misclassification indicates an equal and random chance that any one subject will be misclassified (or included as part of the wrong study group). With differential misclassification, the chance a subject is misclassified is nonrandom.

Stage migration, also known as the Will Rogers phenomenon, is a classic example of misclassification.[2] Cancer stage has a well-defined relationship with long-term survival. Patients may be staged through clinical examination, radiographic assessment, invasive procedures, or pathologic tissue examination (the gold standard). Staging techniques other than pathology-based approaches may be inaccurate. It is not uncommon for higher accuracy staging modalities to be associated with higher observed survival rates when compared with lower accuracy methods (e.g., a clinical examination). Patients only assessed clinically might be understaged—categorized as early-stage cancer but actually with late-stage cancer. Survival rates for early- stage patients would then be worse than they really were because misclassified late-stage patients lower the group average. Similarly, if overstaged patients were considered with truly late-stage patients, survival would be better than in actuality. This phenomenon has been demonstrated in a study of lung cancer patients in which those who underwent pathologic staging had better 5-year survival rates compared with those who underwent clinical staging.[3]

If a difference in outcome truly exists between two groups, nondifferential misclassification will bias the results toward the null hypothesis, a conservative bias. With differential misclassification, the bias may be conservative or anticonservative, depending on the manner in which patients were misclassified and the true relationship between group assignment and outcome. Because nondifferential error leads to a conservative bias, preferable to nonconservative, which could lead to false-positive findings, differential misclassification is the more serious concern. Consider a hypothetical study of a surgical intervention for cancer involving two groups of patients, one classified based on clinical staging and the other on pathologic staging. In this case, incorrectly assuming that both groups have been equally classified would be a mistake. If the study demonstrated a significant benefit for the surgical intervention in the pathologically staged group, the reader would have to wonder whether the observed difference in survival was attributable to the intervention or to differential misclassification (understaging) of patients in the clinically staged group. By comparison, if staging in both study groups were based on a radiographic evaluation, each patient would have an equal chance of being overstaged or understaged. Failure to demonstrate a difference in outcome between the two interventions might be a false-negative finding attributable to nondifferential misclassification.

## Time-Varying Exposures

Time-varying (or time-dependent) exposures refer to predictors whose value may vary with time (e.g., smoking status, transplantation status). Failure to account for time-varying exposures in the analysis of an observational study may lead to biased results and incorrect conclusions. An example of potential bias arising from time-varying covariates is an analysis of heart transplantation survival data.[4] The impact of heart transplantation on survival was assessed by comparing patients who received a transplant with those who did not. Although the initial analysis revealed a survival benefit associated with transplantation, the manner in which patients were grouped (treating transplantation as a fixed variable) led to bias in favor of transplanted patients.

Transplantation wait times are often long and many patients die while awaiting a donor organ; therefore, patients on the transplantation wait list, but who died a short time after being listed, did not have a chance to undergo transplantation. When the investigators retrospectively assigned patients to these two study groups (transplanted versus not transplanted), the patients who survived long enough to receive a new heart introduced selection bias in favor of transplantation, because their survival times were on average longer than in the nontransplantation group. In actuality, each subject's exposure status (transplanted versus not transplanted) was time-dependent. While on the wait list and prior to transplantation, a subject could contribute survival time to the nontransplantation group; subsequent to transplantation, the same subject could then contribute survival time to the transplantation group. Reanalysis of the data evaluating exposure status in a time-dependent fashion revealed no association between transplantation and survival.[5]

## WHAT IS THE OUTCOME OF INTEREST?

Concluding that operation A is better than operation B must be supported by evidence of a difference in outcomes. But what does "better" mean? What if operation A is better with regard to one type of outcome but worse in terms of another? Outcomes assessment cannot determine which procedure is better for the patient, but it can inform patients and providers about differences between two or more competing therapeutic options. Readers judging a study's value should determine which outcomes were assessed, from what perspective, and whether the chosen outcomes were consistent with the study's stated aims.

### Safety

Safety end points capture the inherent risks of an operation (e.g., surgical site infection), natural history of the underlying disease process in the context of therapy (e.g., malignancy-associated deep venous thrombosis in a postoperative patient), and/or the safety of health care delivery (e.g., wrong-site surgery). Operative mortality and postoperative complications (morbidity) are the most commonly measured markers of safety. Safety end points are often used in studies because they are relatively easy to measure and only require a short follow-up period to determine whether the event occurred. However, these are generally rare events, so large numbers of patients are usually necessary to characterize the association between a given intervention and the chosen safety outcome appropriately.

### Effectiveness and Efficacy

Efficacy refers to the extent to which a treatment intervention achieves its purported benefit and the durability of that result. Efficacy is usually determined in a controlled research environment, requires comparison of the selected intervention to a control group, may include randomization, and usually necessitates longer follow-up. For all these reasons, efficacy studies are more challenging to execute and more expensive to fund than simple descriptive studies. A related outcome often confused with efficacy is effectiveness. Whereas efficacy usually relates to outcomes in the context of research studies (e.g., randomized trials) and ideal patient care conditions, effectiveness relates to outcomes in real-world practice.

The distinction, although subtle, is an important one because much of the surgical literature is written by experts at academic centers and/or centers of excellence that more closely approximate ideal patient care conditions. They may fail to capture variability in the quality of care provided by the average physician at an average medical center in an average community. It is exactly for this reason that studies of comparative effectiveness, comparing the benefits and harms of different interventions in real-world settings, have gained increased attention because they are believed to provide the health care community with information on outcomes that more closely approximates actual practice in the general community.

### Patient-Reported Outcomes

Patient-reported outcomes (PROs) measure subjective outcomes (termed *concepts* in the PRO literature) of care reported by the patient directly, without further interpretation of this response by a provider or researcher. Similar to outcomes informing safety, efficacy, or effectiveness, PROs are measurable study outcomes. Examples of common PRO concepts are health-related quality of life (HRQOL), satisfaction with care, functional status, well-being, and health status. PROs usually consist of several more discrete concepts (or domains). HRQOL, for example, at a minimum, should ideally include domains that measure physical (e.g., pain), psychological (e.g., depression), and social functioning (e.g., the ability to carry out activities of daily living). Specific examples of items contained within these domains might include pain, sleep problems, sexual function, vitality and energy, and pain, any or all of which may be relevant to the research question and are certainly of interest to patients.

PRO data are collected through the use of survey instruments. These instruments are composed of individual questions, statements, or tasks evaluated by a patient. PRO instruments use a clearly defined method for administration, data are collected using a standardized format, and the scoring, analysis, and interpretation of results should have been validated in the study population. In general, researchers are advised to use existing instruments to measure PROs (rather than creating their own) because the appropriate development of an instrument requires significant time, resources, testing, and validation before application.[6] Knowing whether the chosen instrument has been validated in the population of interest is also essential when interpreting the results and should be questioned when reading a study reporting PROs.

Although PROs represent a useful, informative, and important outcome, they are difficult to measure accurately and can be controversial. For example, there is often a disconnect between what clinicians and patient believe to be a low HRQOL associated with a chronic condition. When patients actually experience a chronic health condition that seems intolerable, they may shift their frame of reference, and there is also a degree of patient adaptation that is difficult to quantify. For instance, the quality of life reported by a newly wheelchair-bound patient compared with one who has been in a wheelchair for a number of years could be drastically different—the former might be quite low, whereas the latter might be higher than anticipated. Part of the difficulty is that PROs are a more subjective, less tangible outcome than mortality or readmission. However, incorporating these measures into outcomes assessment is paramount in counseling future patients.

### Resource Utilization

Resource utilization refers to the use of health services related to an intervention. In the context of surgical care, this includes utilization of hospital resources—length of stay, hospital readmission, use of outpatient, pharmacy, and durable medical equipment (e.g., wheelchairs and oxygen) services, and emergency room use. Defining criteria for expected utilization is challenging and average use is often considered as a benchmark. Excess resource utilization, as compared with the average, is considered an inferior outcome and is often associated with some form of complication. It can be challenging to determine how much resource utilization is related to the intervention or procedure under study and how much is attributable to a patient's baseline clinical conditions (e.g., chronic disease, adverse events) and nonclinical factors (e.g., patient-level social support, patient preference for in-hospital versus out of hospital care, insurance status precluding use of home nursing). For example, an investigator might use Medicare data to study readmission after pancreatic resection for cancer. Although readmission events are readily identified, it is not possible to know whether the readmission was planned (for chemotherapy administration) or unplanned (because of a complication).

The chosen timeline for assessing health care utilization is also critical. Only measuring immediate health care utilization associated with a diagnostic test would miss the potential downstream impact on future diagnostic and therapeutic care. Limiting assessment to brief periods might miss potentially important future implications over a patient's life. For example, although the quality and use of high-resolution imaging studies (e.g., computed tomography [CT] scan) has risen, the number of incidentalomas identified (e.g., adrenal, lung, or liver lesions too small to be diagnosed accurately on imaging) has concurrently increased. If an investigator hoped to describe the impact of CT scanning as a cancer screening modality, only measuring the individual screening study would fail to capture the downstream effect in the form of multiple, costly follow-up studies and/or biopsies to evaluate an incidentaloma further.

## Costs

Charges are the amount of money requested for health services and supplies. By comparison, costs are the actual amount of money required to deliver care. Differentiating the two is critical because health economic studies should aim to characterize the costs of care. Most data used for health economic analyses provide information on health care charges. If charges are evaluated instead of costs, an intervention or management strategy would appear more expensive than it actually is. When reading the methods section of such a study, the critical reader must look for several important points. First, the investigators should describe if and how they converted charges to costs, generally through the use of a charge-to-cost ratio. Second, costs should be discounted (typically, 3% to 5%) to account for the fact that a dollar today will be worth less than a dollar in the future. Finally, studies spanning several years should adjust for inflation.

The perceived relationship between health care utilization and costs depends on the perspective (e.g., patient, provider, hospital, payer, or societal) taken by the investigator. A hospital may be reimbursed a prespecified amount for performing a procedure and all patient care associated with that operation for the subsequent 90 days. If the patient experiences a complication and requires multiple clinic visits to deal with that complication, this health care utilization may be viewed as a poor outcome from the perspective of the patient, surgeon, and hospital or clinic. However, in this scenario, from the payer's perspective, the cost of all complications-related care within 90 days of the operation would be irrelevant because they do not have to pay more for it. Alternatively, some types of hospitals (critical access) can receive greater reimbursement for greater care delivery; therefore, increased utilization may not be an adverse outcome for a given hospital or surgeon, even though it may be for the health care system as a whole. The perspective of the study will define which costs are necessary to ascertain and include in the analysis. For example, whereas a societal perspective would include the costs of care as well as the direct and indirect monetary costs associated with care (e.g., travel and boarding expenses, lost productivity at work, caretaker expenses), a hospital's perspective would be more selective, not considering the patient's out of pocket expenses, but certainly including whether delivered care is covered by a global payment to the hospital.

There are several different methods for comparative health economic analyses. All methods consider the costs of care in terms of dollars, but differ in terms of how they quantify health benefit. A cost-benefit analysis quantifies health benefit in terms of dollars. Although easy to compare and interpret such results, the great challenge with this approach is assigning a dollar value to a life or a specific health outcome. A cost-utility analysis quantifies health benefits in terms of quality-adjusted life-years (QALYs). Utilities are a measure of overall quality of life, usually scaled between 0 and 1, with 1 being perfect health, and are ascertained using a visual analogue scale, the time trade-off, or standard gamble techniques.[7] Utilities are multiplied by survival time to determine QALYs. When this outcome metric is evaluated as a cost/QALY, it is readily comparable between interventions. An intervention with an associated cost/QALY of $50,000 or less has typically been considered cost-effective. In the original Medicare law that included dialysis as a publicly funded treatment, $50,000 was determined to be the cost of dialysis. However, there is ongoing debate about the validity of this metric and a range of costs/QALY of $20,000 to $100,000 has been proposed as more reasonable.[8] Cost-effectiveness analyses measure health benefit in terms of an outcome metric called the incremental cost-effectiveness ratio (ICER), which is the difference in costs between two competing therapeutic options divided by the difference in health outcome. If the ICER comparing a treatment with a standard reveals that it is more expensive and less efficacious, it is considered to be dominated by the standard and not favored, whereas a less expensive and more efficacious treatment dominates the standard and is favored. Circumstances in which an intervention is more expensive and efficacious or less expensive and efficacious represent a trade-off.

## Surrogate End Points

Interest in surrogate end points has emerged because definitive clinical outcomes may be difficult to assess secondary to the infrequency of a chosen clinical end point, the cost of ascertainment, or a long lag time to development. Surrogate end points are commonly used in studies of new pharmaceutical interventions when efficient data gathering about treatment effect is essential to move a product to the marketplace rapidly.[9] The true clinical benefits of an intervention may take years to recognize, and it may be desirable to identify an intermediate outcome that could serve as a surrogate for the actual clinical effect. Unfortunately, the problem with using surrogate end points is that an intervention may influence an outcome through various, and potentially unintended or unanticipated, pathways.

A classic example illustrating the dangers of using surrogate end points was the Cardiac Arrhythmia Suppression Trial.[10] This study hypothesized that the incidence of sudden cardiac death could be reduced through the administration of flecainide or encainide. These drugs became popular because they had been designed to reduce the rate of ventricular ectopy, a common rhythm aberrancy thought to cause sudden cardiac death. Although these drugs had been shown to reduce ventricular ectopy, when mortality (a clinical, nonsurrogate end point) was measured in this trial, administration of these drugs was found to result in a threefold increase in the rate of death. Suppression of ventricular ectopy was therefore a poor surrogate for the intended clinical impact (improved survival) of these agents.

When evaluating a study, the reader must not only ask whether the selected outcome can answer the research question, but also whether that outcome is a meaningful clinical end point or simply a more easily measured surrogate. Criteria for validating a surrogate end point have been proposed—the surrogate end point should be correlated with the clinical end point of interest and fully capture the net effect of the intervention on the end point of interest.[9] For example, with stage III colon cancer, there was interest in using adjuvant chemotherapy to improve survival. Disease-free survival was proposed as a surrogate for overall survival. Clearly, these two end points are correlated, satisfying the first criterion. Using meta-analysis, adjuvant chemotherapy was shown to result in similar relative improvement in both disease-free and overall survival.[9] In other words, disease-free survival fully captured the net effect of adjuvant chemotherapy for stage III colon cancer, suggesting that it might be a valid surrogate for assessing overall survival benefit. Unless a chosen surrogate outcome has been validated and vetted in other surgical studies, the results and conclusions should be interpreted with caution.

## WHAT IS THE STUDY DESIGN?

Several study designs are commonly used in surgical research. Appropriate study design selection depends on the study question or aim and the availability of resources to conduct the research. The informed reader should make sure that the investigators have used an acceptable study design to address the research question.

### Randomized Controlled Trials

Randomized controlled trials (RCTs) provide the highest level of evidence supporting causality—one intervention leads to better outcomes when compared with another—or noninferiority (see later). If randomization is performed properly, variables that might bias results or act as confounding agents should be distributed equally between groups, resulting in the main advantages of an RCT. That is, outcomes between two or more groups can be compared without the influence of these measured and unmeasured confounding factors and causality can be more definitively established. However, conducting an RCT is challenging because of issues associated with subject accrual and retention, the sometimes complex nature of surgical interventions, significant research costs, and problems relating to the unique environments in which RCTs are usually performed. The effect of the latter influences how much the trial outcomes can be generalized to routine clinical practice environments. To increase the quality and transparency of RCTs, many journals now require online study registration with the International Standard Randomized Controlled Trial Number (ISRCTN) registry so that the research questions, study population, and analytic plan are detailed before the study begins, as well as requiring minimum reporting standards based on the Consolidated Standards of Reporting Trials (CONSORT) guidelines.[11-13] The CONSORT guidelines require that details about various methodologic issues pertinent to the conduct of RCTs (e.g., randomization, blinding, intent to treat) be included in the final manuscript.

In an RCT, subjects are randomly assigned to an intervention group, where they receive an experimental intervention (a given trial may randomize to one or more interventions), or to a control group, where they receive a controlled measurable alternative (placebo or a standard form of existing therapy). Subjects are then followed to measure the occurrence of the outcome(s) of interest. Successful randomization eliminates systematic differences in potential confounding variables between the study groups. Subjects (single-blind) and, in some cases the investigators (double-blind), may be blinded to which study intervention individual subjects are assigned. Blinding of study subjects is intended to mitigate the influence of a placebo effect, whereas blinding the investigators reduces bias from differential delivery of care and outcomes assessment between study groups.

An important analytic issue with RCTs is intent-to-treat (ITT). When an analysis is conducted following the ITT principle, outcome comparisons between control and treatment groups are based on the initial randomization and disregard any crossover—that is, subjects who were randomized to control but received the study intervention, or those assigned to an intervention but received the control. If analytic approaches other than ITT are used, the benefits of randomization will be lost. Without performing the analysis based on the initial randomization, the absence of systematic differences in patient characteristics (confounders) cannot be guaranteed. For example, an investigator who is an advocate of an intervention might prefer that only those patients in an RCT who actually underwent that procedure be included in the analysis (known as a per-protocol analysis), excluding those randomized to the treatment but who crossed over to the control group. However, ITT analysis is essential because it allows surgeons and patients to discuss whether choosing that intervention is best for that particular patient. At the point of a care decision (should the patient agree to undergo a procedure or not), neither the patient nor the surgeon knows whether the patient will be able to complete the intervention or strategy or will require a more conventional approach, perhaps because of the patient's inability to tolerate the procedure. ITT creates an evidence-based approach to inform patients about how the intervention compares at the moment the decision is being made, because ITT incorporates all the factors affecting that decision.

If two interventions are compared using a superiority design, in which the hypothesis is that one therapy is better than the other, and a statistically significant difference is not identified, the reader may be tempted to conclude that the two therapies are equivalent in terms of that outcome. However, it is important to understand that the absence of evidence is not the same as having evidence of absence. In other words, not finding a statistically significant difference (the absence of evidence) does not exclude the possibility that one intervention is clinically and/or meaningfully worse than another (evidence of absence). Noninferiority RCTs are a special case in which the hypothesis is that competing interventions have equivalent outcomes (i.e., no difference in outcome between therapies). It is mathematically impossible to design a study with sufficient power to prove no difference in outcomes. Instead, investigators specify a priori the minimum difference in outcome that would be clinically important. The analysis is then designed to determine whether differences in outcomes are greater than this minimally important difference. Although noninferiority designs have clear value in surgical research, they are uncommon. As compared with superiority designs, in which the hypothesized difference in outcome is relatively large, vast patient enrollment is required to power noninferiority trials adequately to test what is usually a much smaller hypothesized difference.

One example of a noninferiority RCT was a study conducted by the Clinical Outcomes Surgical Therapy Study

Group evaluating whether minimally invasive colon resection provided equivalent oncologic outcomes compared with conventional resection.[14] Prior to the study, the investigators determined that a 23% higher risk of tumor recurrence in the laparoscopic group would be clinically important. The results of the trial showed no statistically significant difference between recurrence rates for laparoscopic and open colon resection and also found that laparoscopic resection had a risk of recurrence no higher than 17%, representing the upper bound of the confidence interval. Because the 95% confidence interval did not include what was determined to be a clinically meaningful difference (23%), the investigators safely concluded equivalence for these two interventions.

RCTs are not ideal for all research questions. For example, an RCT would be suboptimal for assessing rare safety events or for addressing questions about the effectiveness of an intervention across broad populations of patients and practice environments. The pragmatic RCT is an emerging methodology that capitalizes on the benefits of randomization, but also accounts for variable practice environments and settings.

## Meta-Analysis

Any one study may be underpowered to answer a given research question. Meta-analysis is a technique that pools available published data in an effort to increase the statistical power of an analysis. Meta-analysis is not only applicable to RCT data, but can also be used to pool results from observational studies. Similar to the CONSORT criteria for randomized trials, the QUOROM (Quality of Reporting of Meta-Analyses)[15] and MOOSE (Meta-Analysis of Observational Studies in Epidemiology)[16] guidelines have been developed to ensure the quality and validity of results obtained through meta-analysis. These should be considered when evaluating the quality of evidence provided by a pooled analysis.

Regardless of the type of pooled data, in all cases, an important consideration in appraising a meta-analysis is the homogeneity of the pooled studies. If the included studies evaluated similar end points, patient populations, and comparison groups, using similar definitions of variables and methods of outcome ascertainment, then the pooled results may be informative. Significant heterogeneity indicates more variation in study outcomes than chance alone can explain, a sign that the designs or results of the included studies may not be compatible and should not be pooled. This is particularly a concern when observational data have been aggregated, because these studies tend to have less control of variability and minimal control of confounding and bias.

As an example, several randomized trials have been conducted to determine whether goal-directed therapy aimed at optimizing gut perfusion and oxygen delivery decreases the incidence of gastrointestinal complications after noncardiac surgery. Most individual studies favored goal-directed therapy but, possibly because of low sample size ($N = 33$ to 138 subjects in the published studies), most were unable to demonstrate a statistically significant benefit. A meta-analysis including 16 of these studies ($N = 1079$) demonstrated a statistically significant 58% decrease in the odds of gastrointestinal complications as a result of goal-directed therapy.[17] And, as important, there was no statistical heterogeneity or inconsistency detected in any of the analyses.

## Cohort Study

Cohort studies follow, prospectively or retrospectively, nonrandomized groups of patients over time to determine whether a clinical event or outcome occurs with greater or less frequency. If the study aim is descriptive in nature, it is reasonable to describe unadjusted outcomes or results adjusted for potential confounding factors. However, unadjusted comparisons are likely to be biased if there are nonrandom reasons why patients are in one group versus the other, a common problem. The advantages of cohort studies are the ability to estimate the incidence (or rate) of both exposures and outcomes, simultaneously assess multiple outcomes, and study rare exposures. Cohort studies are inefficient for evaluating outcomes that are rare or occur a long time after exposure.

For example, in a secondary analysis of the PREVENTION VI trial data, outcome differences between patients who underwent endoscopic versus open saphenous vein harvesting during coronary artery bypass grafting were evaluated.[18] After adjusting for potential confounding factors, the authors found that rates of death and the two composite end points were statistically higher among the endoscopic harvesting group. This study highlights two advantages of the cohort design—it allowed an estimation of the rate of adverse events associated with competing interventions and the simultaneous assessment of multiple outcomes.

## Case-Control

Case-control studies compare the frequency of exposures between patients who have and have not experienced an outcome of interest. These studies begin by enrolling subjects with and without the outcome of interest and then look back in time to search for differences in subject exposure to potential risk factors. Case-control designs are infrequently used in the surgical literature. However, one example involved an evaluation of risk factors associated with retained foreign bodies after surgery.[19] The researchers reviewed the medical records of all patients who made claims or provided incident reports to a large, statewide malpractice insurer ($N = 54$). Each case was matched to four control patients ($N = 235$) who did not make such claims. Risk factors for retained foreign bodies included emergency surgery, unplanned change in the operation, and body mass index. This study highlighted two advantages of the case-control design, the ability to evaluate risk factors for a rare outcome and to assess multiple risk factors simultaneously.

Case-control studies are sometimes confused with cohort studies, perhaps because of difficulty regarding the meaning of case and control in the research context. In health services and epidemiologic research, a case refers to a subject who has experienced an outcome of interest whereas a control refers to a patient who has not experienced that outcome. All patients experiencing the outcome should be included in a case-control study, particularly when that outcome is rare. It is unnecessary to sample all those without the outcome because there is no statistical benefit for including more than four controls for each case. Because of the manner in which subjects are sampled in a case-control study, it is not possible to estimate the frequency of the exposure in the population at large from case-control studies. Advantages of the case-control design include efficiency in evaluating rare outcomes or outcomes occurring a long time after exposure and the ability to evaluate multiple exposures simultaneously. When measurement of an exposure is expensive or time-consuming (e.g., costly laboratory assays, detailed interviews), this can be a much more efficient way to use resources.

### Case Reports and Case Series

Case reports and case series report on one or more patients treated by a single surgeon or group of surgeons at a single institution. A case report aims to highlight an unusual or unexpected procedure or event, whereas a case series demonstrates that such events can happen more than once. A benefit of these studies is that they can reveal a potentially unrecognized benefit or adverse effect of surgical therapy and may generate new hypotheses, prompting more rigorous scientific evaluation. Laparoscopic radical prostatectomy is an established approach for treating localized prostate cancer and reportedly offers equivalent oncologic benefit to open resection. However, since 1994, surgeons have reported 14 total cases of port site metastasis, highlighting a rare but potentially serious risk of a minimally invasive approach to prostatectomy.[20] These studies are distinct from cohort investigations because there is no comparison made between competing strategies or interventions.

## WHAT IS THE SOURCE OF DATA?

Data can be collected prospectively or retrospectively. Prospective data are advantageous because investigators can collect information about variables of interest as they relate to the research question. Retrospective data are advantageous because they are readily available and generally inexpensive, although they are more likely to include a limited number of variables that may or may not be pertinent to the study question. Data are available from a variety of sources. A synopsis of the main advantages, limitations, and examples of each of these data sources is presented in Table 9-1.

## ARE THERE NONANALYTIC ISSUES WORTHY OF CONSIDERATION?

### Confounding

One of the most important issues to consider in the evaluation and conduct of outcomes research using observational data is confounding. A confounder is a measured or unmeasured variable associated with the exposure of interest and associated with the outcome. This dual relationship can influence the degree and direction of, or even completely mitigate, an observed association between exposure and outcome. As an example, consider a hypothetical study aiming to determine whether there is an association between insurance status and long-term survival among resected colon cancer patients. The results demonstrate a significantly lower survival rate among uninsured compared with insured patients. However, the authors did not measure and therefore adjust for cancer stage, a well-known and strong determinant of long-term survival. Also, patients without insurance may present with later stage cancer because of limited access to care. Without controlling for the higher proportion of patients with higher stage cancer in the uninsured groups, the results are biased, so that the uninsured would appear to have worse outcomes than they actually have, because of the higher proportion of late-stage patients in that group. A comprehensive report about the direction of bias resulting from confounding is available.[21]

Authors of observational studies should ideally address confounding in two ways, analytically and in their discussion of the study's limitations. Multivariate regression, propensity score, and instrumental variable analysis are all analytic methods of addressing confounding using measured variables. For variables that were not measured or cannot be measured, the authors of a study should itemize these variables and discuss the potential direction and magnitude of bias that could result from them.

### Generalizability

Generalizability refers to the ability to take the information from research studies and apply them reproducibly in the community at large. For example, RCTs are conducted in a highly controlled setting, with strict inclusion and exclusion criteria, staff dedicated to follow-up and protocol adherence, and usually at academic or tertiary care centers. Although RCTs provide the highest level of evidence about the efficacy of competing interventions, the environment in which they take place may limit other providers' ability to reproduce the delivery of care and outcomes in a nonresearch setting. However, generalizability can also be a problem with observational studies. For example, Medicare data are limited to older and disabled patients. As

**Table 9-1 Data Sources for Outcomes and Health Services Research**

| DATA SOURCE | ADVANTAGES | DISADVANTAGES | EXAMPLE |
|---|---|---|---|
| Medical records | Easy to do; useful as hypothesis-generating exercise | Missing data; time-consuming; inability to measure certain information (e.g., intent); limited scientific value | Case reports, case series |
| Administrative | Large numbers; real-world data; often generalizable; easy to obtain; affordable | Limited clinical variables; data collected for billing, not research | Medicare; state discharge data sets |
| Registry | Often contains clinical data; population-based real-world data not restricted to tertiary or referral centers | Missing data; only cross-sectional data on interventions | SEER, National Cancer Database |
| Linked data sets | Same as registry; richer source of data than either registry or administrative alone; allows longitudinal assessment of episodes of care | Missing data; inability to capture intent of therapy | SEER-Medicare |
| Quality improvement | Prospectively collected data; rich in clinical, laboratory, and demographic patient data | Overrepresentation of tertiary or referral centers; only a random sample of patients, not comprehensive | National Surgical Quality Improvement Project; Society of Thoracic Surgeons database |
| National surveys | National sample; 2.5 yr of longitudinal diagnoses and health care claims data | May overrepresent certain racial groups in survey sample | Medical expenditure panel survey |

such, practice patterns and outcomes among Medicare patients may or may not be generalizable to non-Medicare patients. Critical readers should consider why care patterns and outcomes described in research studies might not be reproducible in the broader scope of community medical practice.

### Determining Causality Using Observational Data

Observational data may reveal associations between exposures (i.e., competing therapies) and outcomes. Investigators hope to infer a causal relationship between exposures and outcomes based on such associations. One criterion for inferring causality is that the exposure must happen before the outcome. Otherwise, the exposure cannot plausibly lead to the outcome. The association and hypothesized causal relationship must also be biologically (clinically) plausible. Finally, the magnitude of association between the exposure and outcome must be large and, if there are varying degrees of exposure, there should also be varying magnitudes of association between exposure and outcome (e.g., dose-response relationship). Beware of observational studies in which the conclusion is that A causes B. As noted, such studies can be hypothesis-generating and may show clear associations, but A causes B cannot be proven without a properly performed prospective trial.

## HOW WERE THE DATA ANALYZED?

The statistical analysis of any study should stem from the study aims, design, and data sources. An understanding of several methodologic concepts will serve as a foundation for reviewing the literature critically.

### Variable Types and Descriptive Statistics

Defining the type of variable used in a study is the first step in evaluating descriptive and comparative statistics. Table 9-2 provides a summary of commonly used descriptive and comparative statistics. A continuous variable is one that can take on an infinite number of values. Age and length of stay are examples of a continuous variable. Descriptive statistics are used to describe the central tendency of continuous variables. The arithmetic mean provides a good estimate of central tendency for normally distributed (gaussian, or bell-shaped) data. If the data are skewed (not normally distributed), the mean will be a biased estimator of the central tendency. In these cases, the median or geometric mean provides a better estimate.

Categorical variables have discrete values. The simplest categorical variable is a binary variable that can only take on one of two values, such as sex (man, woman [male, female]). Ordinal variables are ordered categorical variables. Cancer stage is a classic example of an ordinal categorical variable. Nominal variables are unordered categorical variables, such as race. Categorical variables may be described in terms of proportions.

Time to event variables consist of two variables, a continuous variables that measures the time interval from an established start point (e.g., date of diagnosis or therapy) to a failure event (e.g., death or disease recurrence) or the end of the observation period and a binary variable, which indicates whether the failure event occurred. Long-term survival is a classic example of a time to event variable. The Kaplan-Meier method is the most common way to provide a description of the probability of an event occurring at a certain point in time (e.g., survival at 5 years). This method takes into consideration that over time, the number of patients at risk for an event decreases; as patients drop out of a study or experience the outcome event, there will be progressively fewer patients at risk for having the outcome (a patient who dies cannot die again). The Kaplan-Meier method may overestimate risk in the setting of competing risks. For example, time to re-intervention has competing risks—the disease process may evolve prompting re-intervention; over time a contraindication to re-intervention may develop, or death may occur, in which case a patient is no longer at risk. However, methods exist for handling time to event variables in the setting of competing risks.[22]

**Table 9-2 Commonly Used Parameters in Surgical Outcomes and Health Services Research**

| TYPE OF VARIABLE | MEASUREMENT | DESCRIPTIVE STATISTIC | MULTIVARIATE REGRESSION MODEL |
|---|---|---|---|
| Continuous | Mean, median | Unpaired t-test; paired t-test for repeated measures, or ANOVA for two or more groups | Linear |
| Categorical | Proportion | $\chi^2$ (chi-squared) | Logistic |
| Time to event | Kaplan-Meier | Log-rank | Cox hazard |

### Hypothesis Testing

Hypothesis testing uses comparative or analytic statistics to determine whether observed differences between two or more groups are real or are attributable to chance. The *P* value is a statistical summary measure for hypothesis testing. A significance level of 5% ($P = .05$) is widely used to indicate a statistically significant finding, although this value is arbitrary. A *P* value is interpreted as the probability that the observed difference in outcomes between groups is the result of chance (i.e., the difference is not actually based on the effect of the intervention). The smaller the *P* value, the less likely the difference could represent a false-positive finding. As a general rule, the larger the difference being compared and the larger the sample size for a given comparison, the lower the *P* value, and the less likely that the finding is the result of chance alone).

Two types of errors can occur with hypothesis testing. An alpha (or type I) error occurs when one observes a difference in outcomes when one does not actually exist. Readers should be particularly cognizant of the potential for this type of error in studies that use a large database (e.g., Medicare or National Inpatient Sample data). In these cases, if the research question and analysis have not been specified a priori and numerous statistical tests are performed on many and varied subgroups (sometimes known as mining the data), the chance of finding a *P* value that achieves the threshold of significance is increased. For example, if a threshold of 5% were considered statistically significant, 5 of 100 statistical tests could potentially demonstrate a statistically significant finding that is attributable to chance alone (a false-positive finding). This exemplifies the problem with multiple comparisons—performing multiple post hoc (or nonprespecified) analyses, looking for differences in one or more outcomes among subgroups of study subjects. If multiple comparisons are anticipated, the Bonferroni correction (the *P* value [at the set significance level, such as .05] divided by the number of planned post hoc comparisons) is a simple and highly conservative way to guard against type I errors. A beta (or type II) error occurs when no difference in outcomes is observed when a difference truly exists (a false-negative finding). This type of error occurs when a study has insufficient power to detect true differences in outcomes between groups. Power is directly related to sample size and the size of the observed difference.

For smaller studies, there may be situations in which zero outcome events are observed in one of the study groups. In this case, the "rule of 3s" is useful for obtaining the upper bound of the 95% confidence interval: if $N$ patients are observed, none of whom have the outcome, the upper bound of the 95% confidence interval (CI) for the probability of the outcome goes from 0 to $3/N$. Hypothesis testing is also possible by examining CIs. Summary measures of the difference between groups are provided as an estimated ratio (outcomes in the study group divided by outcomes in the standard or control group) or as an absolute difference, with a 95% CI. The CI provides an estimate of the uncertainty around a given value; a wide CI indicates a lack of precision, whereas a tight (small) interval would be indicative of minimal uncertainty. When the summary measure is a ratio, a CI inclusive of 1.0 indicates no statistical difference in outcomes. Put another way, the CI demonstrates that the group difference could actually have a value of 1.0, indicating that outcomes in both groups might be similar. If the summary measure is the absolute difference, a CI inclusive of 0 indicates no statistically significant difference.

Table 9-2 provides a summary of statistical tests that are often used for hypothesis testing by variable type. The unpaired t-test is used to compare two independent groups that have continuous outcome variables. A paired t-test is used to compare two dependent groups that have continuous outcome variables. An example of a dependent group comparison is serial blood pressure measurements on the same person. An analysis of variance (ANOVA) is used when comparing more than two groups with a continuous outcome variable. The chi-square statistic is often used to compare the distributions of two or more groups with categorical outcome variables. Fisher's exact test is more appropriate for such comparisons when the sample size is small. A log-rank test is used to compare two groups with time to event outcome variables.

## Multivariable Analysis

Multivariate regression models are among the most commonly used methods to evaluate the relationship between variables and outcomes in the absence of the influence of other measured variables. Linear regression is used to evaluate the relationship between factors potentially associated with a continuous outcome variable, such as length of stay. This model assumes the outcome variable in normally distributed. Unfortunately, in the case of most health services end points, such as length of stay, that assumption is often violated. To deal with non-normal outcomes, a "transformation" might be used to create a new variable that more closely approximates a normal distribution—for example, taking the logarithm of the length of stay. The summary measure provided by a linear regression is a risk difference.

Logistic regression is used when the outcome variable is binary (e.g., operative mortality). Probabilities and odds, although calculated differently, are both measures of risk and are usually presented in the form of a ratio (the odds or risk in the study group divided by the control group). Understanding the difference between these measures is important because the odds will overestimate the probability if the outcome occurs frequently in the population. When the outcome is rare, the odds generally provide a good approximation of the probability.

Cox proportional hazard regression is used for the evaluation of time to event outcomes. The summary measure of risk provided by this model is also in the form of a ratio. A hazard simply refers to the instantaneous risk of an event at any time. The proportional hazards assumption must be valid to interpret the results of this type of regression and requires that the differences in risks of an event between groups remain constant over time.

## Propensity Score Analysis

Propensity score analysis is an alternative method of risk adjustment. When two groups are being compared, logistic regression is used to calculate a given subject's risk or probability (or propensity) of having an exposure of interest (e.g., minimally invasive as compared with open surgery). The subject's calculated probability of receiving that therapy is the propensity score. The outcomes of interest for patients with a similar propensity score can then be compared without having to adjust for other variables. Study subjects can be matched based on their propensity score or can be grouped based on tertiles, quartiles, or quintiles of the score. Stratifying subjects into discrete groups based on their propensity score is a form of risk adjusting. As an alternative to stratification, the propensity score can be used as an adjustment variable in regression models.

Propensity score analyses appeal to some because they seem intuitive; they compare outcomes across groups who have a similar probability of receiving the therapy of interest. This analysis is often described as being similar to an RCT in the sense that it compares outcomes between groups at equal propensity for receiving the therapy of interest. Unfortunately this analogy often leads people to believe that propensity score analyses provide advantages in risk adjustment over multivariate regression techniques. However, this is generally unsubstantiated because the analytic approach has no bearing on a key measurement issue, the ability to measure all confounders, including unknown, using observational data. The reader should really be aware of three circumstances in which the use of propensity scores may be more appropriate than multivariate regression: (1) there are many confounders requiring adjustment, and using traditional regression techniques could underpower the analysis; (2) there is no interest in the association between the adjustment factors and outcome; and (3) the relationship between the exposure and propensity for treatment can be estimated more accurately than the relationship between the exposure and outcome.[23,24] Otherwise, propensity scores are not superior to multivariate techniques, but are simply an adequate alternative.

## Instrumental Variable Analysis

Instrumental variable analysis is another method of accounting for unmeasured confounding and controlling bias. The principle underlying this type of analysis is that there are unmeasured, or immeasurable, confounders that might bias the study's results. Because these confounders cannot be determined, they cannot be controlled for. Selecting a variable exogenous to the study subject, one that the study subject has no control over, that is strongly associated with the exposure but not associated with the outcome (except possibly through the causal pathway involving the exposure) will control for any and all confounding factors associated with the outcome and exposure of interest.

Although the use of instrumental variables can be extremely useful for decreasing confounding, there are several notable limitations of which the reader must be aware. The best example of an instrumental variable is randomization. In an RCT, randomization is strongly associated with the exposure under study, but is not in any way associated with the measured outcome, except through the randomization assignment. The best instruments are those that act as a surrogate for randomization. However, well-selected instrumental variables are very rare in surgical research. As a result, if a poorly selected instrument (one that has weak correlation with the exposure) is used, bias can actually be accentuated. Also, there are no statistical methods that allow the investigator to demonstrate clearly whether the chosen instrument is a good one. It is how strong an argument that the investigator makes in favor of the chosen instrument that validates the choice. Therefore, readers must decide whether they agree with the choice of the instrumental variable and whether they will believe the results. A publication evaluating the association between cardiac catheterization and mortality provides a good demonstration of the use of an instrumental variable as compared with other common risk adjustment techniques.[25]

### Missing Data

Missing data is a common problem in all types of studies. If the study is small and the investigator ignores (throws out) subjects with missing data, the power of the study is compromised. More importantly, if data are missing in a systematic way (e.g., related to the exposure and outcome), excluding subjects with missing data will likely bias the analysis. Missing data can fall into one of three categories with unfortunate names—missing completely at random (MCAR), missing at random (MAR), and missing not at random (MNAR).

Data that are MCAR are missing for random reasons unrelated to the exposure, covariate, or outcome. A good example of how MCAR may occur is when a research assistant accidentally drops a test tube of blood from a study subject. The reason for the lost data has nothing to do with the treatment that the patient received, outcome that they may experience, or the patient's gender, race, or social status. When data are MAR, the data are missing conditional on some other measured value. For example, women may be less willing to give information about their weight. As such, one could predict the likelihood of missing weight data based on gender. When data are MNAR, the data is missing conditional on an unmeasured value. For example, a patient may be unwilling to offer information about their income, perhaps because she or he considers it to be too high or too low. In this case, the reason for missing information about income is the level of the income itself.

Unfortunately, it is difficult to establish whether missing data are MCAR, MAR, or MNAR, and thus investigators must make informed assumptions. If missing data do not vary across factors associated with an outcome, and the authors are unaware of any systematic reason for missing data, it would be reasonable to assume MCAR. If missing data occur more frequently across certain groups of patients, then one might assume MAR, although the possibility of MNAR cannot be excluded. If the investigator is aware of MNAR, there is no good solution for handling missing data. With MCAR and MAR, there are a number of methods for handling missing data, including the missing data indicator method (in which missing data points are coded as a separate category instead of missing), as well as various methods of imputation. However, multiple imputation appears to introduce the least bias.[26] Finally, with MCAR, one could conduct a case-complete analysis (i.e., throw out subjects with missing data), but at the expense of the study's power.

### Correlated Data

Correlated data has implications for statistical inference in studies that make repeated measures of an outcome over time (longitudinal study), and/or examine subjects that cluster within groups. Several investigators were interested in examining differences over time in HRQOL between men and women who underwent coronary artery bypass grafting (CABG).[27] Self-administered questionnaires were collected at 6 weeks, 6 months, and 1 year after CABG. Women had lower scores than men at 1 year, but both groups improved over time and the rate of recovery was similar for men and women. The authors used generalized linear models to account for baseline and follow-up correlations. In general, methods used to handle correlated data in the context of repeated outcome measures take into account variability in outcome within a subject and between subjects.

For example, clustering refers to the notion that patients treated by the same surgeons and/or at the same medical center are likely to be more similar to each other than patients treated by a different surgeon. Similarly, surgeons working at a particular type of hospital are more likely to be similar to each other than surgeons/institution working at a different hospital. Under such circumstances, the outcomes of a patients under the care of a particular surgeon, and a surgeon working at a particular hospital, are more likely to be similar (or correlated). For example, investigators examined the relationship between surgeon volume and operative mortality for several different procedures, after adjusting for patient characteristics and hospital volume.[28] Their analysis involved three levels of variables—those pertaining to patients (age, gender, comorbidity), surgeons (procedural volume), and hospitals (procedural volume). For most procedures, higher surgeon volume was associated with lower adjusted operative mortality rates. The authors used a special statistical model (binary mixed effects) to account for clustering of patients within surgeons and clustering of surgeons within hospitals.

Failure to account for correlated data in the analysis can result in a conservative (inappropriately accepting the null hypothesis) or anticonservative (inappropriately rejecting the null hypothesis) inference. For example, it has been shown that adjusting for correlated data attenuates the significance of the volume-outcome relationship.[29] Stated differently, failure to account for clustering might result in an anticonservative inference (e.g., concluding that a volume-outcome relationship exists when it does not). Statistical methods accounting for correlated data may include hierarchical regression models, Bayesian analysis, or clustering adjustment. A further discussion of correlated data and the use of associated statistical methods is beyond the scope of this chapter. Surgeons reading the scientific literature should be aware of situations in which correlated data may exist and look for how the authors chose to handle the correlation.

## ARE THERE ETHICAL CONSIDERATIONS?

There are two main ethical issues worthy of consideration when evaluating a surgical study. It is not uncommon for surgeons and investigators to serve in advisory roles for pharmaceutical companies or device manufacturers. Such associations may affect a

**Table 9-3 IDEAL Model for Evaluation of New Surgical Innovations**

| PARAMETER | 1: IDEA | 2A: DEVELOPMENT | 2B: EXPLORATION | 3: ASSESSMENT | 4: LONG-TERM STUDY |
|---|---|---|---|---|---|
| Purpose | Proof of concept | Development | Learning | Assessment | Surveillance |
| Number and types of patients | Single digit; highly selected | Few; selected | Many; may expand to mixed; broadening indication | Many; expanded indications (well defined) | All eligible |
| Number and types of surgeons | Very few; innovators | Few; innovators and some early adopters | Many; innovators, early adopters, early majority | Many; early majority | All eligible |
| Output | Description | Description | Measurement; comparison | Comparison; complete information for non-RCT participants | Description; audit, regional variation: quality assurance, risk adjustment |
| Intervention | Evolving; procedure inception | Evolving; procedure development | Evolving; procedure refinement; community learning | Stable | Stable |
| Method | Structured case reports | Prospective development studies | Research database; explanatory or feasibility RCT (efficacy trial); diseased-based (diagnostic) | RCT with or without additions, modifications; alternative designs | Registry; routine database (e.g., SCOAP, STS, NSQIP); rare case reports |
| Outcomes | Proof of concept; technical achievement; disasters, dramatic successes | Mainly safety; technical and procedural success | Safety; clinical outcomes (specific and graded); short-term outcomes; patient-centered (reported outcomes; feasibility outcome | Clinical outcomes (specific and graded); middle-term and long-term outcomes; patient-centered (reported) outcomes; cost-effectiveness | Rare events long-term outcomes; quality assurance |
| Ethical approval | Sometimes | Yes | Yes | Yes | No |

Adapted from McCulloch P, Altman DG, Campbell WB, et al: No surgical innovation without evaluation: The IDEAL recommendations. Lancet 374:1105–1112, 2009.

*IDEAL, I*dea, *d*evelopment, *e*xploration, *a*ssessment, *l*ong-term study; *NSQIP,* National Surgical Quality Improvement Project; *SCOAP,* Surgical Care and Outcomes Assessment Program; *STS,* Society of Thoracic Surgeons.

researcher's objectivity if, for example, a study's hypothesis addresses the effect of that company's product, constituting a conflict of interest. These considerations loom largest over industry-sponsored trials. When reading an RCT supported by the corporation that makes a given drug or device, it is crucial to read the methods, results, and conclusions with a critical eye to ensure that any potential influence from the sponsor has not affected study validity. Similarly, when reading the conclusion, the reader must make certain the investigators' claims have not overstepped the results. Claims and conclusions should be substantiated by the results obtained from the study and not simply be based on what the investigator or sponsor believes. Furthermore, it is the responsibility of all investigators to disclose all associations fully (for themselves or their families) that could conceivably be construed as a conflict of interest. Without such disclosures, the objectivity and validity of a given study must be even more closely scrutinized.

The second ethical issue deals with the importance of new technology assessment. As health care innovation continues to move forward, these evaluations will increasingly become a necessary focus of surgical studies. Investigators must always consider how best to conduct such studies ethically and safely. Unfortunately, in the current health care environment, rapid adoption of novel diagnostic and surgical procedures often precedes scientific evidence that demonstrates the safety and efficacy (or lack thereof) of the innovation. There are two main reasons why innovations reach the health care market prior to the availability of confirmatory evidence:

1. RCTs (the gold standard for demonstrating the efficacy of an intervention) suffer from low patient accrual, expense, and time.
2. There is a lack of formalized registries or secondary data sources to track use and outcomes, which at least allow preliminary safety and effectiveness assessments.

Although administrative data (e.g., Medicare) or established registries (e.g., Surveillance, Epidemiology, and End Results [SEER] program) can provide data for such assessments, there is often a significant lag between when the innovation becomes widely available and when the data are accessible.

Recently, the Balliol Collaboration of research methodologists and surgical trial experts developed a framework for assessing surgical research and innovation.[30] The IDEAL (Innovation, Development, Exploration, Assessment, and Long-term study) model has been proposed as a means of guiding the ethical, regulatory, methodologic, and funding issues associated with each stage of surgical innovation (Table 9-3). This model may be considered as a framework and set of standards for future evidence-based surgical care.

## CONCLUSIONS

The practice of surgery using the best available evidence is the responsibility of all surgeons. Navigating the complex issues underlying the evidence requires an understanding of the components of outcomes and health services research. The questions posed in this chapter should serve as a guide for critically examining of the surgical literature. Only by becoming more critical evaluators of the surgical literature will the next generation of surgeons be able to embrace fully the promise of evidence-based surgery.

## SELECTED REFERENCES

Bridges JF, Onukwugha E, Mullins CD: Health care rationing by proxy: Cost-effectiveness analysis and the misuse of the $50,000 threshold in the US. Pharmacoeconomics 28:175–184, 2010.

The benchmark of $50,000 per QALY is often used in cost-effective assessments. This article provides an excellent review of the accuracy and appropriateness of this cost per QALY metric and includes a timely discussion regarding health care cost-effectiveness research.

Donders AR, van der Heijden GJ, Stijnen T, et al: Review: A gentle introduction to imputation of missing values. J Clin Epidemiol 59:1087–1091, 2006.

Most surgical studies use data sets that contain missing data points, often for potentially important variables. Therefore, understanding how missing values can bias study results and knowing how to deal with missing values are important for being able to appraise a surgical study critically.

Fleming TR: Surrogate end points and FDA's accelerated approval process. Health Aff (Millwood) 24:67–78, 2005.

The selection of appropriate end points is perhaps the most important issue in the design of any research study, in particular, RCTs. This article provides a thorough discussion of surrogate end points, studies that have used surrogate end points, and how such end points can influence study results.

McCulloch P, Altman DG, Campbell WB, et al: No surgical innovation without evaluation: The IDEAL recommendations. Lancet 374:1105–1112, 2009.

This article, as well as its two companion pieces, discuss the importance and limitations of evaluating new surgical technology and provides a framework that can and should be used for new and timely technology assessment.

Stukel TA, Fisher ES, Wennberg DE, et al: Analysis of observational studies in the presence of treatment selection bias: Effects of invasive cardiac management on AMI survival using propensity score and instrumental variable methods. JAMA 297:278–285, 2007.

This study provides a good example, comparison, and discussion of several commonly used methodologic techniques in the surgical literature.

## REFERENCES

1. Flum DR, Morris A, Koepsell T, et al: Has misdiagnosis of appendicitis decreased over time? A population-based analysis. JAMA 286:1748–1753, 2001.
2. Feinstein AR, Sosin DM, Wells CK: The Will Rogers phenomenon. Stage migration and new diagnostic techniques as a source of misleading statistics for survival in cancer. N Engl J Med 312:1604–1608, 1985.
3. Mountain CF: Revisions in the International System for Staging Lung Cancer. Chest 111:1710–1717, 1997.
4. Clark DA, Stinson EB, Griepp RB, et al: Cardiac transplantation in man. VI. Prognosis of patients selected for cardiac transplantation. Ann Intern Med 75:15–21, 1971.
5. Crowley J, Hu M: Covariance analysis of heart transplant survival data. JASA 72:27–36, 1977.
6. Patrick DL, Erickson P: Health status and health policy: quality of life in health care evaluation and resource allocation, Oxford, Oxford University Press, 1993.
7. Neumann PJ, Goldie SJ, Weinstein MC: Preference-based measures in economic evaluation in health care. Annu Rev Public Health 21:587–611, 2000.
8. Bridges JF, Onukwugha E, Mullins CD: Health care rationing by proxy: Cost-effectiveness analysis and the misuse of the $50,000 threshold in the US. Pharmacoeconomics 28:175–184, 2010.
9. Fleming TR: Surrogate end points and FDA's accelerated approval process. Health Aff (Millwood) 24:67–78, 2005.
10. Echt DS, Liebson PR, Mitchell LB, et al: Mortality and morbidity in patients receiving encainide, flecainide, or placebo. The Cardiac Arrhythmia Suppression Trial. N Engl J Med 324:781–788, 1991.
11. Moher D, Jones A, Lepage L: Use of the CONSORT statement and quality of reports of randomized trials: A comparative before-and-after evaluation. JAMA 285:1992–1995, 2001.
12. Moher D, Schulz KF, Altman D: The CONSORT statement: Revised recommendations for improving the quality of reports of parallel-group randomized trials. JAMA 285:1987–1991, 2001.
13. Moher D: CONSORT: An evolving tool to help improve the quality of reports of randomized controlled trials. Consolidated Standards of Reporting Trials. JAMA 279:1489–1491, 1998.
14. Clinical Outcomes of Surgical Therapy Study Group: A comparison of laparoscopically assisted and open colectomy for colon cancer. N Engl J Med 350:2050–2059, 2004.
15. Moher D, Cook DJ, Eastwood S, et al: Improving the quality of reports of meta-analyses of randomised controlled trials: The QUOROM statement. Quality of Reporting of Meta-analyses. Lancet 354:1896–1900, 1999.
16. Stroup DF, Berlin JA, Morton SC, et al: Meta-analysis of observational studies in epidemiology: A proposal for reporting. Meta-analysis Of Observational Studies in Epidemiology (MOOSE) group. JAMA 283:2008–2012, 2000.
17. Giglio MT, Marucci M, Testini M, et al: Goal-directed haemodynamic therapy and gastrointestinal complications in major surgery: A meta-analysis of randomized controlled trials. Br J Anaesth 103:637–646, 2009.
18. Lopes RD, Hafley GE, Allen KB, et al: Endoscopic versus open vein-graft harvesting in coronary-artery bypass surgery. N Engl J Med 361:235–244, 2009.
19. Gawande AA, Studdert DM, Orav EJ, et al: Risk factors for retained instruments and sponges after surgery. N Engl J Med 348:229–235, 2003.
20. Savage SJ, Wingo MS, Hooper HB, et al: Pathologically confirmed port site metastasis after laparoscopic radical prostatectomy: Case report and literature review. Urology 70:1222, e1229–e1211, 2007.
21. Mehio-Sibai A, Feinleib M, Sibai TA, et al: A positive or a negative confounding variable? A simple teaching aid for clinicians and students. Ann Epidemiol 15:421–423, 2005.

**22.** Blackstone EH, Lytle BW: Competing risks after coronary bypass surgery: The influence of death on reintervention. J Thorac Cardiovasc Surg 119:1221–1230, 2000.

**23.** Joffe MM, Rosenbaum PR: Invited commentary: propensity scores. Am J Epidemiol 150:327–333, 1999.

**24.** D'Agostino RB, Jr: Propensity score methods for bias reduction in the comparison of a treatment to a non-randomized control group. Stat Med 17:2265–2281, 1998.

**25.** Stukel TA, Fisher ES, Wennberg DE, et al: Analysis of observational studies in the presence of treatment selection bias: Effects of invasive cardiac management on AMI survival using propensity score and instrumental variable methods. JAMA 297:278–285, 2007.

**26.** Donders AR, van der Heijden GJ, Stijnen T, et al: Review: A gentle introduction to imputation of missing values. J Clin Epidemiol 59:1087–1091, 2006.

**27.** Lindquist R, Dupuis G, Terrin ML, et al: Comparison of health-related quality-of-life outcomes of men and women after coronary artery bypass surgery through 1 year: Findings from the POST CABG Biobehavioral Study. Am Heart J 146:1038–1044, 2003.

**28.** Birkmeyer JD, Stukel TA, Siewers AE, et al: Surgeon volume and operative mortality in the United States. N Engl J Med 349:2117–2127, 2003.

**29.** Panageas KS, Schrag D, Riedel E, et al: The effect of clustering of outcomes on the association of procedure volume and surgical outcomes. Ann Intern Med 139:658–665, 2003.

**30.** McCulloch P, Altman DG, Campbell WB, et al: No surgical innovation without evaluation: the IDEAL recommendations. Lancet 374:1105–1112, 2009.

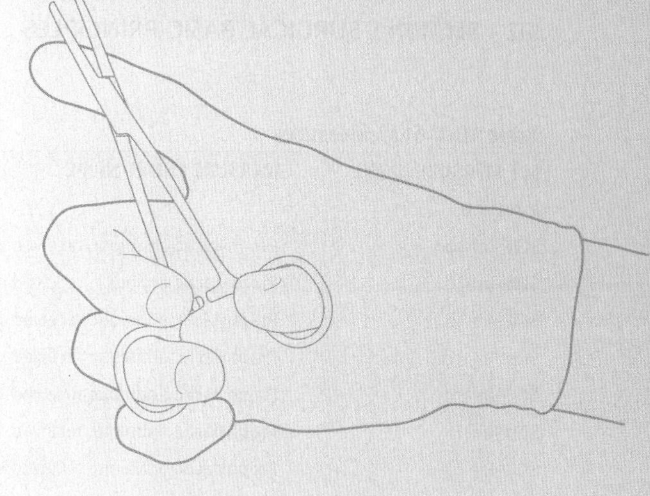

CHAPTER 10

# PERIOPERATIVE PATIENT SAFETY

R. Daniel Beauchamp and Michael S. Higgins



## HISTORY AND PERSPECTIVE

Patient safety in the health care environment is recognized as less than optimal or desirable. A series of eye-opening reports were published in the 1990s and provided clear evidence of high rates of serious adverse events that resulted in serious harm to hospitalized patients. The Institute of Medicine (IOM), in its landmark report, *To Err is Human,* published in 1999, estimated that as many as 1 million people/year were injured and up to 98,000 died annually because of medical errors.[1] When the focus was specifically turned to surgical patients, surgical care accounted for between 48% and 66% of adverse events among nonpsychiatric hospital discharges.[2] In regard to operative procedures and deliveries, 3% resulted in adverse events, and surgical adverse events were associated with a 5.6% mortality rate, accounting for 12.2% of hospital deaths. Furthermore, 54% of surgical adverse events were judged to be preventable.

Adverse events in surgical patients encompass those common to all hospitalized patients, such as adverse drug events, falls, missed diagnoses, deep venous thrombosis, pulmonary embolism, aspiration events, respiratory failure, nosocomial pneumonia, myocardial infarction, and cardiac arrhythmias. In addition, surgical specific adverse events include technique-related complications, wound infections, and postoperative bleeding.

In 2000, the IOM called for a national effort to reduce medical errors by 50% within 5 years; however, progress has fallen far short of that goal, despite numerous private and public initiatives aimed at finding solutions. Leape and colleagues[3] have proposed that these efforts fell short because health care organizations did not undertake the major cultural changes required to accomplish true and lasting improvements in performance. They proposed that health care entities must become "high-reliability organizations" that hold themselves accountable to offer safe andeffective patient-centered care consistently. They proposed five transforming concepts for adoption by health care organizations seeking such cultural transformative changes:

1. Transparency must be a practiced value in everything we do.
2. Care must be delivered by multidisciplinary teams working in integrated care platforms.
3. Patients must become full partners in all aspects of health care.
4. Health care workers need to find joy and meaning in their work.
5. Medical education must be redesigned to prepare new physicians to function in this new environment.

## SURGICAL INFECTION PREVENTION AND SURGICAL CARE IMPROVEMENT PROJECT

Because surgical site infections (SSIs) were recognized as the second most common site of nosocomial infections and a major cause of morbidity, readmissions, excessive costs, and death, the Centers for Medicare and Medicaid Services (CMS) and the Centers for Disease Control and Prevention (CDC) initiated the National Surgical Care Improvement Project (SCIP) in 2002.[4] The goal of surgical infection prevention (SIP) was to reduce the incidence and impact of SSIs in surgical populations, particularly in high-volume procedures. In 2003, the national SIP project convened a meeting of the Surgical Infection Prevention Guideline Writers Workgroup of experts and representatives from several surgical specialty societies to develop evidence-based and consensus guidelines for antimicrobial prophylaxis for abdominal and vaginal hysterectomy, hip or knee arthroplasty, and cardiothoracic, vascular, and colon surgery.

The SIP project focused on three primary quality performance measures. The first SIP measure was that prophylactic antibiotics should be given within the 60-minute interval immediately preceding the surgical skin incision (within 2 hours for vancomycin, with appropriate documentation of the reason). The second measure was that the appropriate prophylactic antibiotic for the scheduled procedure should be selected based on consensus recommendations. The third SIP measure was that the prophylactic antibiotic should be discontinued within 24 hours of the end of the procedure.

The SIP project has transitioned into the SCIP, and includes additional process performance measures aimed at reducing SSIs. Three additional measures to reduce SSIs have been added to the original SIP measures: (1) glucose control in cardiac surgical patients; (2) appropriate hair removal at the surgical site (using clippers, not razors); and (3) maintenance of normothermia in patients undergoing colorectal operations. In addition to

**Table 10-1 SCIP Measures**

| SET MEASURE ID NO. | MEASURE SHORT NAME |
|---|---|
| **Infection** | |
| SCIP-Inf-1a | Prophylactic antibiotic received within 1 hr prior to surgical incision, overall rate |
| SCIP-Inf-1b | Prophylactic antibiotic received within 1 hr prior to surgical incision, CABG |
| SCIP-Inf-1c | Prophylactic antibiotic received within 1 hr prior to surgical incision, other cardiac surgery |
| SCIP-Inf-1d | Prophylactic antibiotic received within 1 hr prior to surgical incision, hip arthroplasty |
| SCIP-Inf-1e | Prophylactic antibiotic received within 1 hr prior to surgical incision, knee arthroplasty |
| SCIP-Inf-1f | Prophylactic antibiotic received within 1 hr prior to surgical incision, colon surgery |
| SCIP-Inf-1g | Prophylactic antibiotic received within 1 hr prior to surgical incision, hysterectomy |
| SCIP-Inf-1h | Prophylactic antibiotic received within 1 hr prior to surgical incision, vascular surgery |
| SCIP-Inf-2a | Prophylactic antibiotic selection for surgical patients, overall rate |
| SCIP-Inf-2b | Prophylactic antibiotic selection for surgical patients, CABG |
| SCIP-Inf-2c | Prophylactic antibiotic selection for surgical patients, other cardiac surgery |
| SCIP-Inf-2d | Prophylactic antibiotic selection for surgical patients, hip arthroplasty |
| SCIP-Inf-2e | Prophylactic antibiotic selection for surgical patients, knee arthroplasty |
| SCIP-Inf-2f | Prophylactic antibiotic selection for surgical patients, colon surgery |
| SCIP-Inf-2g | Prophylactic antibiotic selection for surgical patients, hysterectomy |
| SCIP-Inf-2h | Prophylactic antibiotic selection for surgical patients, vascular surgery |
| SCIP-Inf-3a | Prophylactic antibiotics discontinued within 24 hr after surgery end time, overall rate |
| SCIP-Inf-3b | Prophylactic antibiotics discontinued within 48 hr after surgery end time, CABG |
| SCIP-Inf-3c | Prophylactic antibiotics discontinued within 48 hr after surgery end time, other cardiac surgery |
| SCIP-Inf-3d | Prophylactic antibiotics discontinued within 24 hr after surgery end time, hip arthroplasty |
| SCIP-Inf-3e | Prophylactic antibiotics discontinued within 24 hr after surgery end time, knee arthroplasty |
| SCIP-Inf-3f | Prophylactic antibiotics discontinued within 24 hr after surgery end time, colon surgery |
| SCIP-Inf-3g | Prophylactic antibiotics discontinued within 24 hr after surgery end time, hysterectomy |
| SCIP-Inf-3h | Prophylactic antibiotics discontinued within 24 hr after surgery end time, vascular surgery |
| SCIP-Inf-4 | Cardiac surgery patients with controlled 6 am postoperative blood glucose level |
| SCIP-Inf-6 | Surgery patients with appropriate hair removal |
| SCIP-Inf-9 | Urinary catheter removed on postoperative day 1 or 2, with day of surgery being day 0 |
| SCIP-Inf-10 | Surgery patients with perioperative temperature management |
| **Cardiac** | |
| SCIP-Card-2 | Surgery patients on beta blocker therapy prior to arrival who received a beta blocker during the perioperative period |
| **VTE** | |
| SCIP-VTE-1 | Surgery patients with recommended VTE prophylaxis ordered |
| SCIP-VTE-2 | Surgery patients who received appropriate VTE prophylaxis within 24 hr prior to surgery to 24 hr after surgery |

From Centers for Medicare and Medicaid Services, The Joint Commission: National Hospital Inpatient Quality Measures: Specifications Manual, Version 3.1, June, 2010 (http://www.qualitynet.org/dcs/ContentServer?c=Page&pagename=QnetPublic%2FPage%2FQnetTier4&cid=1228749003528).
*VTE,* Venous thromboembolism.

the six performance measures aimed at reducing SSIs, measures aimed at preventing cardiovascular complications and venous thromboembolism after major surgical procedures were proposed (Table 10-1).[5] To reduce perioperative ischemic heart complications, patients who have been on β-adrenergic blocking medications prior to operation, should be maintained on beta blockade in the perioperative period and during hospitalization. The final SCIP measures are for the use of appropriate venous thromboembolism prophylaxis in surgical patients at risk for deep venous thrombosis and pulmonary embolism.

## Use of Quality Data to Improve Outcomes of Surgical Patients

How do we know which interventions work and which fail to improve outcomes? Despite the intuitive appeal of quality- and safety-motivated process improvements, it is challenging to generate accurate data in a timely manner to support the effectiveness of the safety measures that have been undertaken. The rise of health services research programs and rigorous population-based research in academic medical centers and the involvement of surgeons in these programs have led to several landmark

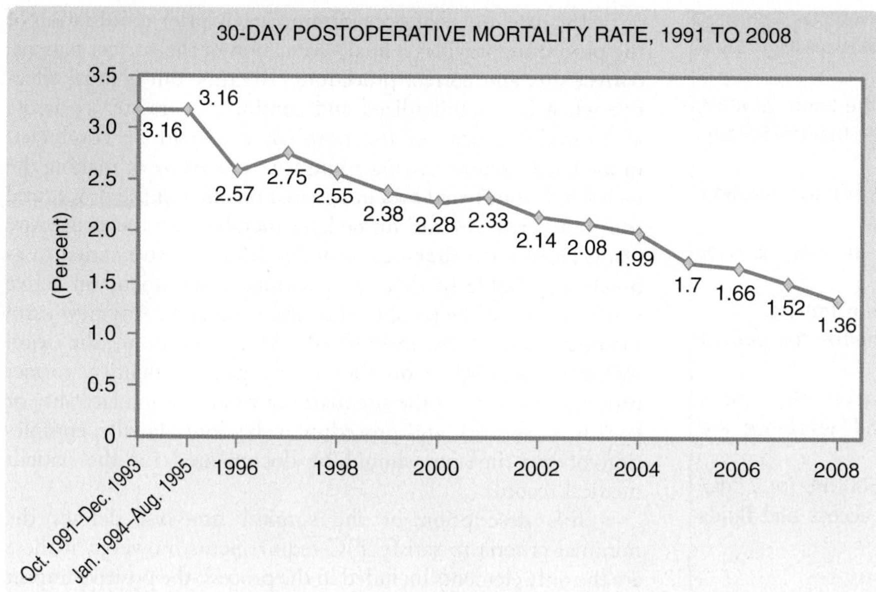


**FIGURE 10-1** Actual mortality trend for the National Surgery Quality Improvement Program (15 years from inception through fiscal year 2008). (From the Congressional Budget Office: Quality initiatives undertaken by the Veterans Health Administration, August 2009 [http://www.cbo.gov/ftpdocs/104xx/doc10453/08-13-VHA.pdf].)

studies that have helped identify some risk factors that affect morbidity and mortality in surgical populations. The development of broad-based prospective databases, such as the American College of Surgeons–National Surgical Quality Improvement Program (ACS-NSQIP) database, the Society of Thoracic Surgeons (STS) national database, and the American College of Surgeons National Trauma Data Bank (NTDB) are all examples of the development of critical tools necessary for such important population-based outcomes research to be completed.

The National Veterans Affairs Surgical Quality Improvement Program was initiated in 1991 to improve surgical outcomes in Veterans Administration (VA) hospitals.[6] The NSQIP is a risk-adjusted outcomes database comprised of over 90 data elements gathered by specially trained nurses who review the preoperative, intraoperative, and postoperative periods. This database was validated in the VA system, in which the data are provided back to hospitals and providers and used to inform strategies aimed at reducing morbidity and mortality, with considerable success (Fig. 10-1).[7]

The ACS-NSQIP is a national civilian database launched in 2004 as an outgrowth of the VA NSQIP. The ACS-NSQIP is a prospectively collected, multi-institution clinical registry database of general and vascular surgery patients that provides feedback on risk-adjusted outcomes to member hospitals across the United States for quality improvement purposes; however, the data are also available for population-based research. A recent examination of the ACS-NSQIP data reviewed the overall and major complication rates and risk-adjusted death rates of 84,730 patients who underwent inpatient general or vascular surgical procedures from 2005 through 2007.[8] Interestingly, the death rates in these surgical patients ranged from 3.5% in the quintile of very low-mortality hospitals to 6.9% in the quintile of very high-mortality hospitals (double the rate of the low mortality hospitals), whereas the rates of overall and major complications were not significantly different when comparing these two groups of hospitals. The difference in overall risk-adjusted mortality was almost twice as high after a major complication in the very high-mortality hospitals (21.4%) as compared with the very low-mortality hospitals (12.5%). Although processes and systems aimed at the avoidance of complications seem intuitively important, it is not always possible in the performance of complex procedures, particularly in populations at high risk. This report demonstrated that failure to rescue patients after a serious complication was associated with an increased death rate in the high-mortality hospitals as compared with the low-mortality hospitals. The same authors found similar results when analyzing patient outcomes from a Medicare database.[9]

## Effective Teams and Communication

Perioperative team building has parallels in the aviation industry in that teams intermittently come together for relatively short, defined periods of time to accomplish a complex task, requiring the specialized skills of each team member, under potentially stressful conditions in which there is inherent danger. A recent investigation of the impact of implementing a standardized surgical safety checklist (Box 10-1) has demonstrated that complication rates ranged from 6.1% to 21% (total of 11%) of 3733 surgical patients across eight major hospitals in eight cities worldwide and the rate of postoperative death ranged from 0.8% to 3.7% (total of 1.5%) prior to implementation of the checklist.[10] After implementation of the surgical checklist with preoperative sign-in, time-out and postprocedural sign-out elements the overall rate of complications decreased to 7% (range, 3.6% to 9.7%) and the rate of death declined to 0.8% (range, 0% to 1.7%).[10]

The Joint Commission (TJC) has made the implementation of the Universal Protocol for the prevention of wrong site, wrong-patient, and wrong-procedure surgery, including the preprocedural time-out, accreditation requirements.[11,12] The Universal Protocol includes the following elements: preprocedural verification, site marking, and final verification during the preprocedural time-out. The preprocedural verification includes verification of the appropriate history and physical examination in the medical record, presence of a signed consent form, nursing assessment, and preanesthesia assessment (when

**BOX 10-1 Elements of the Surgical Safety Checklist**

**Sign In**

Before induction of anesthesia, members of the team (at least the nurse and an anesthesia professional) state that the following have been done:

- The patient has verified his or her identity, surgical site and procedure, and consent.
- The surgical site is marked or site marking is not applicable.
- The pulse oximeter is on the patient and functioning.
- All members of the team are aware of whether the patient has a known allergy.
- The patient's airway and risk of aspiration have been evaluated and appropriate equipment and assistance are available.
- If there is a risk of blood loss of at least 500 mL (or 7 mL/kg body weight in children), appropriate access and fluids are available.

**Time-Out**

Before skin incision, the entire team (nurses, surgeons, anesthesia professionals, and any others participating in the care of the patient) states aloud the following:

- Confirms that all team members have been introduced by name and role
- Confirms the patients identity, surgical site, and procedure
- Reviews the anticipated critical events
    - Surgeon reviews critical and unexpected steps, operative duration, anticipated blood loss
    - Anesthesia staff review concerns specific to patient
    - Nursing staff reviews confirmation of sterility, equipment availability, other concerns
- Confirms that prophylactic antibiotics have been administered ≤60 min before incision is made or that antibiotics are not indicated
- Confirms that all essential imaging results for correct patient are displayed in OR

**Sign Out**

Before the patient leaves the operating room, the following are done:

- Nurse reviews the following aloud with the team:
    - Name of procedure, as recorded
    - That needle, sponge, and instrument counts are complete (or not applicable)
    - That specimen (if any) is correctly labelled, including patient's name
    - Whether there are any issues with equipment that need to be addressed
- The surgeon, nurse, and anesthesia professional review aloud the key concerns for the recovery and care of the patient.

Adapted from Haynes AB, Weiser TG, Berry WR, et al: A surgical safety checklist to reduce morbidity and mortality in a global population. N Engl J Med 360:491–499, 2009.

applicable). It also includes verification that the necessary diagnostic laboratory, radiology, and other test results are present and properly displayed. The requirement for and presence of blood products, implants, devices, and/or special equipment is also confirmed in the preprocedural verification process.

The time-out that occurs immediately prior to initiation of the procedure provides a final verification of the correct patient, correct site, and correct procedure. The time-out is most effective when it is standardized and conducted consistently across all procedural areas of the hospital; it should be conducted immediately before starting an invasive procedure or making the incision. It is initiated by a designated member of the procedural team and involves the immediate members of the procedure team. During the time-out, other activities are suspended to as much as possible so that team members may focus on active confirmation of the patient, site, and procedure. Any new team members should be introduced. At a minimum, the team members must agree on the correct patient identity, correct procedural site (with the site marking verified when laterality or level is a concern), and procedure to be done. Finally, completion of the time-out should be documented for the patient medical record.

This description of the surgical time-out defines the minimal criteria to satisfy TJC requirements; however, if these are the only elements included in the process, the positive impact will be limited. The Crew Resource Management (CRM) training and discipline around the Universal Protocol enables organizations to enhance communication between health care professionals in the perioperative management teams and to incorporate process improvement measures, such as those defined by the SCIP, into the checklists. These evidence-based interventions include timely administration of perioperative antibiotics, administration of beta blockers in patients at risk of ischemic heart disease, venous thromboembolism prophylaxis, and intraoperative normothermia. The time-out checklist may also include availability and sterility of instrumentation and implantable devices. The conclusion of the optimal surgical time-out should include an open invitation for any member of the team to speak up at any time during the procedure if she or he recognizes a problem that poses risk to the patient or health care team.

### Handoffs and Surgical Safety

During the surgical experience, patients are managed by teams of physicians and nurses that commonly transfer primary responsibility for patient care between one another. Unfortunately, transfers of care have been demonstrated to be associated with an increase in medical errors.[13,14] In a recent review of 258 surgical errors from closed malpractice claims, breakdowns in communication were determined to be a factor in almost 25%.[15] Another study examined the handover of patients in the intensive care unit (ICU) and noted that significant degradation of important patient information occurred frequently during these transfers of care.[16] Medication discrepancies have also shown to be common in resident sign-out lists.

To address these communications challenges, experts have turned to other high-risk industries, such as nuclear power and the space program, to understand their strategies better and apply useful practices to health care. There are unique differences between the work environments in these industries and health care, which can present challenges to the direct transfer of approaches. However, the use of checklists and structured communication procedures such as SBAR (situation-background-assessment-recommendation) have been advocated almost universally.[17] As a result of this emerging evidence of the importance of communication in medical errors, TJC made the standardization of hand-off communications a national patient safety goal and an area of focus for institutional reviews. Also, the use of simulation has been advocated to improve the effectiveness of teaching hand-off procedures and for use in the assessment of performance. As reviewed elsewhere in this chapter, the use of information technology has been demonstrated to improve patient hand-offs and has been leading to the implementation of new tools in large health care systems, such as the Veterans Administration.

### Phases in Perioperative Care

**Preoperative Phase** Preoperative preparation, review of the clinical history, relevant radiologic images, pathology, relevant anatomy, and anticipation of potential problems that may be encountered during the course of the operative procedure are essential components of the surgeon's preparation. Communication with the patient and/or family members is critical to ensure that all are in agreement regarding the operation, site of procedure, risks, benefits, and possible alternative approaches. Documentation of a discussion of these should be included as part of the consent for operation. Comorbidities and their possible impact on outcome should be assessed and understood by the surgeon, the anesthesiologist, and the patient and family.

**Intraoperative Phase** The operating room is a complex and often high-stress environment in which there are multiple opportunities for the occurrence of errors or events that could adversely affect patient outcomes. As noted, the Universal Protocol initiated in the preoperative holding area is continued and completed in the operating room to minimize the risk of wrong surgery. We believe that the time of anesthetic induction, patient positioning, and performance of the time-out are critical portions of any surgical procedure that requires the presence and collaborative involvement of the attending surgeon, the anesthesiologist and/or anesthetist, scrub nurse, and circulating nurse to achieve the maximum safety and quality of care. This is a critical time for the surgeon and anesthesiologist to communicate regarding the anticipated intraoperative course, anticipated problems, including blood loss, anticipated case length, and any special requests. Special requests may include avoidance of excessive crystalloid in an older patient with a history of heart failure or chronic obstructive pulmonary disease. It may also include the avoidance of long-acting muscle relaxants in patients undergoing resections that are near important motor nerve structures, such as in the face, neck, or axilla. This early phase of the operation is also an excellent opportunity to put all in the room at ease, introduce any new team members and, as noted earlier, invite participants to speak up at any time during the procedure if there are questions or concerns. To enhance the safe conduct of the operation, a neutral zone between the surgeon and scrub nurse should be defined and agreed on for sharp instruments.

The surgeon's responsibility is to perform the operative procedure with the utmost skill, efficiency, and safety. During the surgical procedure, the surgeon should continually communicate with the anesthesiologist and the rest of the team regarding the progress of the operation, any unexpected findings, hemorrhage, or technical complications. Similarly, the anesthesia team should communicate any significant changes in the physiologic status of the patient, especially those related to hypotension, $O_2$ desaturation events, and critical laboratory values. Such communications should be verified in both directions by verbal acknowledgment, and a plan of management should be agreed on. In addition, the surgeon and operating room (OR) team must communicate regarding the instrument, needle, and sponge counts and requirement, if any, for intraoperative imaging to confirm the absence of unplanned retained foreign bodies. Confirmation of the disposition of pathologic specimens should also occur between the surgeon and circulating nurse prior to the surgeon and patient leaving the operating room. In addition, the checkout procedure should include discussion between the surgeon and anesthesiologist regarding postoperative disposition of the patient. This should include agreement about the need for special postoperative care, such as intensive care, anticipated prolonged recovery room stay, and need for telemetry.

**Postoperative Phase** For most patients, the immediate postoperative period consists of a monitored period of transition to normal neurophysiologic function, with some treatment of pain, nausea, and body temperature being relatively common. Although relatively rare, catastrophic complications such as myocardial ischemia or infarction, stroke, airway obstruction, and acute hemorrhage may occur. In addition, there is occasionally the need for continued pharmacologic and fluid therapy management during the early postoperative phase. Early recognition and effective intervention to correct physiologic derangements associated with impending crisis are key to rescuing patients at risk. This requires an efficient and collaborative team of caregivers who have instituted a system of excellent communication. Effective intervention also requires multidisciplinary collaborative teams of providers—often including specialty consultative services—appropriate escalation of care, timely implementation of antibiotic therapy for sepsis, effective critical care teams, and appropriate interventions aimed at the source of the complication. Ghaferi and colleagues[9] have pointed out that effective recognition and communication regarding patient status requires a high-quality nursing staff, with staffing ratios sufficient to enable nurses to perform regular patient assessments. For example, studies have demonstrated an association between a high nurse-to-bed ratio and decreased perioperative mortality.[18] The higher nurse-to-patient ratios are also associated with greater job satisfaction and reduced rates of burnout among nurses. As noted, appropriate and timely escalation of care is crucial for patients who have become ill from a serious complication. This often involves transfer of a patient to an ICU, in which an increased nurse-to-patient ratio is associated with reduced resource use and daily rounds by a dedicated intensive care physician is associated with reduction in inpatient mortality.[19]

## Physician Fatigue and Surgical Safety

There has been increased focus on the relationship of physician fatigue and patient safety that gained prominence with the publication of *To Err Is Human*.[1] Based in part on emerging data regarding physician fatigue and performance, including in the procedural environment,[20] the Accreditation Council for Graduate Medical Education (ACGME) mandated duty hour restrictions for physician in training in 2003, with recent recommendations by an IOM committee to extend those restrictions.[21]

Some studies have demonstrated variable results regarding the impact of these changes on patient safety. A study of interns working in ICUs has shown that the medical error rate is reduced with work hour restrictions.[22] However, another study has shown higher error rates after the implementation of work hour restrictions in New York.[23] Larger scale studies have demonstrated similar variability. Investigations of all Medicare beneficiaries and VA hospitals[24] have failed to demonstrate a change in mortality for surgical patients. However, a more recent investigation has noted a reduction in the percentage of surgical complications attributed to providers, from 48.3% to 38.6%, and a reduction in mortality rate, from 1.9% to1.1%, after the restrictions, with the improvement attributed to the increased participation of attending surgeons in clinical care and possibly to other concurrent improvement initiatives.[25]

Various hypotheses have been advanced to explain the variable results of duty hour restrictions. One argument is that the initial restriction of duty hours did not limit prolonged shifts that were thought to have the greatest impact on performance. In addition, the resulting increase in patient hand-offs, which are known to increase the risk of errors, may offset the improved safety from reduced fatigue. Duty hour restrictions may not necessarily translate into reduced fatigue. It has also been suggested that shift length has a greater impact on patient safety than overall hours.[26] Hour restrictions may also interfere with physician education, which can negatively affect clinical performance and patient safety. These effects are certainly reinforced by surgical resident perceptions.

Several recent surveys have shown a negative impact of resident duty hour restrictions on attending surgeon job satisfaction, time for teaching, and overall workload.[27,28] An early investigation after the duty hour restrictions showed that general surgeons worked a mean (standard deviation [SD]) of 73.8 (14.1) hours/week and only 44% reported 1 day/week away from clinical duties.[29] In a study of surgical errors, fatigue was self-reported by attending physicians as a contributing factor in 16% of adverse events.[30] Although a retrospective review of cardiac procedures performed by sleep-deprived surgeons has shown no difference in complication rates,[31] more recent work has shown an association between limited sleep opportunity, increased work duration, and complication rates.[32] As a result of these emerging data, some have argued that attending surgeon duty hours should be limited as well, and a variety of strategies have been proposed, such as implementing a surgical hospitalist service.

Despite the conflicting data, it seems logical that rested physicians make better decisions that should improve patient safety. For these reasons, work week and shift length limitations, napping, and other validated strategies to reduce fatigue may have beneficial effects on surgical patient safety. However, the resulting expansion of the labor pool is estimated to cost as much as $3.4 million/life saved, making this a substantial economic issue for the health care system, especially for academic medical centers.[33] Moreover, the known safety risks that result from the increased number of lesser trained providers and the increased frequency of hand-offs must be considered. These concerns may be addressed by strategies to improve competency through the use of communication tools, such as checklists, and structured communications at critical events, such as transitions in care. There is also a significant need for additional research to understand the complex association between interventions designed to improve physician fatigue and their relationship to the safety of surgical patients in complex health care delivery systems better.

## Use of Information Technology to Enhance Surgical Patient Safety

The IOM's seminal report, *Crossing the Quality Chasm: A New Health System for the 21st Century*, called for a radical redesign of the health care system, with a focus on the use of information technology as a means to improve the quality and safety of health care and reduce cost.[33a] Since then, the federal government has made significant investments to improve the development and deployment of health care information technology (HCIT), including the establishment of a federal executive position of National Coordinator for Health Information Technology and financial incentives in efforts to promote widespread adoption of HCIT.

### Computerized Order Entry

Computerized provider order entry (CPOE) is recommended by the Agency for Healthcare Research and Quality and the National Quality Forum as one of the 30 safe practices for better health care. The Leapfrog group has also recommended CPOE implementation as one of its first three recommended leaps for improving patient safety. These positions are informed by the evidence that 90% of medication errors occur at the ordering or prescribing step and that clinical decision support systems (CDSSs), which are the engines for CPOEs, have been demonstrated to reduce drug administration errors significantly.[34]

Despite these strong recommendations, hospitals have been slow to implement CPOE. A 2009 study found that only 17% of U.S. hospitals had implemented a CPOE system, and the proportion of outpatient practices using CPOE is even smaller.[35] Cost is likely a major factor, as is the resistance to change at the organizational and individual provider levels coupled with a lack of systems that have been implemented successfully in a variety of clinical settings.

CPOE and computerized prescription writing already have shown the ability to reduce medical errors and variability in surgical patient care. A large study in Texas has demonstrated an improvement in mortality for patients undergoing coronary artery bypass grafting (CABG).[36] Vikoren and colleagues[37] have demonstrated the ability of a CPOE to reduce variability in patient care for patients undergoing total joint surgery. Compliance with medication and care protocols related to national quality initiatives, such as SCIP, are improved with the use of CPOE systems, as demonstrated for perioperative blood glucose control,[38] prophylactic antibiotic administration,[39] and other quality initiatives.

Other work, however, has shown no change in medication errors for surgical patients after CPOE implementation.[40] One study has shown a reduction in medication errors but an overall increase in mortality, thought to have resulted from other effects on patient care work flow.[41] These results have prompted investigations of all the factors related to CPOE implementations that could affect patient care (Box 10-2).[42-44] There are also issues related to the underlying clinical decision support systems that may affect outcomes. Specifically, the guidelines may not be applicable to all clinical environments and may not be current.

Consequently, Weir and associates have recommended the implementation of a set of safety indicators that should be tracked during CPOE implementation to ensure that any risks are mitigated.[45] Also, clinicians must ensure that the decision support algorithms are reviewed and validated prior to implementation to benefit from drug interaction alerts and other

**BOX 10-2 Types of Unintended Consequences of Computerized Provider Order Entry Systems**

- More or new work for clinicians
- Unfavorable work flow issues
- Never-ending system demands
- Problems related to persistence of paper orders
- Unfavorable changes in communication patterns and practices
- Negative feelings toward the new technology
- Generation of new types of errors
- Unexpected changes in an institution's power structure, organizational culture, or professional roles
- Overdependence on the technology

From Campbell EM, Sittig DF, Ash JS, et al: Types of unintended consequences related to computerized provider order entry. J Am Med Inform Assoc 13:547–556, 2006.[44]

critically important decision support measures.[46] Similarly, a system was developed to test CPOE systems against the criteria established by the Leapfrog group that CPOEs should detect at least 50% of common prescribing errors.[47]

### Other Applications for Information Technology in Surgical Patient Safety

There is evidence to suggest that a significant number of surgical errors occur because of poor communication and lack of access to critical patient information. In a root cause analysis of operative and postoperative events from 1995 to 2002, TJC found that almost 70% of events were associated with communication failures. Other studies have shown that transitions of care are associated with higher risk for errors, as well as demonstrating an increase in medical errors with an increase in the number of patient transfers.[14] Various strategies have been successfully used to improve surgical safety, including the use of standardized communication events and checklists. Several information technology solutions have been suggested to enhance these and other strategies to improve surgical patient safety. The use of computer checklists has been demonstrated as a means to transfer patient information more effectively and efficiently. Similarly, a computerized medication reconciliation process can improve continuation of medications postoperatively.[48] The use of information management systems for the documentation of perioperative care also provides the opportunity for the use of clinical decision support algorithms and care alerts to improve antibiotic redosing[49] and compliance with surgical time-out elements.

Emerging technologies may also prove to be beneficial, including the use of bar code and radiofrequency tracking systems as a means to eliminate "never events," such as wrong-patient and wrong-site surgery and retained foreign objects. Intraoperative video systems may also allow the opportunity to record and debrief procedures during patient care, as they have in emergency departments, or potentially to monitor and intercede to provide enhanced patient support.

## CREATING AN ORGANIZATIONAL STRUCTURE TO PROMOTE PATIENT SAFETY AND QUALITY CARE

The health care culture must be changed to focus on quality care and patient safety. As noted earlier, Leape and coworkers[3] have proposed five transforming concepts for adoption by health care organizations that seek such transformative changes (see earlier).

How do we change the culture to incorporate these concepts? At our institution (Vanderbilt University Medical Center, Nashville, Tenn), the commitment has been made to change the culture from the top of the organization. Of the five pillars of excellence that form the framework for setting organizational goals and direction, quality is the central pillar. The other four pillars include people, service, growth and finance, and innovation. Under the quality pillar, institutional goals are set on an annual basis and the entire medical center is managed and operated within a framework to accomplish the goals that have been set. Each year, the goals become more challenging to continue to drive improvements.

Institutionally, there is a chief quality officer who works with clinical leadership, nursing, and administration within the patient care areas to identify priorities and identify necessary resources to support quality improvement and address safety issues promptly. Our Center for Clinical Improvement provides assistance with resources to support root cause analyses of patient deaths, adverse outcomes, and near-misses. Reporting adverse outcomes and near-misses is encouraged in a blame-free environment. Within the Perioperative Enterprise, there is a Surgical Site Infection Collaborative and Perioperative Quality and Safety Committee that collaborate with each another and that receive input from the various surgical services, perioperative nursing services, and infection control services. Each surgical service conducts weekly to biweekly morbidity, mortality, and improvement (MM&I) conferences. Cases identified in these service-level MM&I conferences that exemplify systems concerns or issues are referred to a multidisciplinary MM&I committee, which selects cases for presentation at an institution-wide MM&I conference that is held on a quarterly basis.

Organizational transparency is achieved through the sharing of performance data across the institution. Quality and safety performance data are fed back to the clinicians and staff on a monthly basis, with benchmark comparators when available. Multidisciplinary teams are central to how we are organized around patient care, quality, and safety. The patient is central to all we do in the clinical care setting and, within our service pillar goals, are patient satisfaction targets dependent on provider or physician-patient communication. Under our people pillar goals are faculty and staff satisfaction goals, because we believe that health care workers who are happy in their roles and feel fulfilled provide better quality care. We reward such behaviors financially and symbolically. We teach the students in our medical center, at all levels, how each member of the team contributes to quality care and safety, and this is incorporated into the medical and nursing curriculum.

## SELECTED REFERENCES

Aiken LH, Clarke SP, Sloane DM, et al: Hospital nurse staffing and patient mortality, nurse burnout, and job dissatisfaction. JAMA 288:1987–1993, 2002.

The objective of this study was to determine the association between the patient-to-nurse ratio and patient mortality, failure-to-rescue (deaths following complications) among surgical patients, and factors related to nurse retention.

Fry DE: Surgical site infections and the surgical care improvement project (SCIP): Evolution of national quality measures. Surg Infect (Larchmt) 9:579–584, 2008.

This is a recent comprehensive review of the national SCIP effort to reduce SSI. The National SIP Project was an initiative sponsored jointly by the Centers for Medicare and Medicaid Services and the U.S. Centers for Disease Control and Prevention to decrease the incidence of SSI in major surgical procedures.

Ghaferi AA, Birkmeyer JD, Dimick JB: Variation in hospital mortality associated with inpatient surgery. N Engl J Med 361:1368–1375, 2009.

This was a landmark study of 84,730 patients who had undergone inpatient general and vascular surgery from 2005 through 2007, using data from the American College of Surgeons National Surgical Quality Improvement Program.

Haynes AB, Weiser TG, Berry WR, et al: A surgical safety checklist to reduce morbidity and mortality in a global population. N Engl J Med 360:491–499, 2009.

Surgery has become an integral part of global health care, with an estimated 234 million operations performed yearly. This study demonstrates the efficacy of the surgical safety checklist in diverse settings.

Khuri SF, Daley J, Henderson W, et al: The Department of Veterans Affairs' NSQIP: The first national, validated, outcome-based, risk-adjusted, and peer-controlled program for the measurement and enhancement of the quality of surgical care. National VA Surgical Quality Improvement Program. Ann Surg 228:491–507, 1998.

This study was designed to provide reliable risk-adjusted morbidity and mortality rates after major surgery to the 123 Veterans Affairs Medical Centers (VAMCs) performing major surgery, and to use risk-adjusted outcomes in the monitoring and improvement of the quality of surgical care to all veterans.

Veasey S, Rosen R, Barzansky B, et al: Sleep loss and fatigue in residency training: A reappraisal. JAMA 288:1116–1124, 2002.

The authors reviewed studies addressing the effects of sleep loss on cognition, performance, and health in surgical and nonsurgical residents.

## REFERENCES


1. Kohn LT, Corrigan JM, Donaldson MS, editors: To err is human: Building a safer health system, Washington, DC, 1999, National Academy Press.
2. Gawande AA, Thomas EJ, Zinner MJ, et al: The incidence and nature of surgical adverse events in Colorado and Utah in 1992. Surgery 126:66–75, 1999.
3. Leape L, Berwick D, Clancy C, et al: Transforming health care: A safety imperative. Qual Saf Health Care 18:424–428, 2009.
4. Bratzler DW, Houck PM: Antimicrobial prophylaxis for surgery: An advisory statement from the National Surgical Infection Prevention Project. Am J Surg 189:395–404, 2005.
5. Fry DE: Surgical site infections and the surgical care improvement project (SCIP): Evolution of national quality measures. Surg Infect (Larchmt) 9:579–584, 2008.
6. Khuri SF, Daley J, Henderson W, et al: The Department of Veterans Affairs' NSQIP: The first national, validated, outcome-based, risk-adjusted, and peer-controlled program for the measurement and enhancement of the quality of surgical care. National VA Surgical Quality Improvement Program. Ann Surg 228: 491–507, 1998.
7. DePalma RG: Surgical quality programs in the Veterans Health Administration. Am Surg 72:999–1004 1133–1048, 2006.
8. Ghaferi AA, Birkmeyer JD, Dimick JB: Variation in hospital mortality associated with inpatient surgery. N Engl J Med 361: 1368–1375, 2009.
9. Ghaferi AA, Birkmeyer JD, Dimick JB: Complications, failure to rescue, and mortality with major inpatient surgery in medicare patients. Ann Surg 250:1029–1034, 2009.
10. Haynes AB, Weiser TG, Berry WR, et al: A surgical safety checklist to reduce morbidity and mortality in a global population. N Engl J Med 360:491–499, 2009.
11. The Joint Commission: National patient safety goals, 2010 (http://www.jointcommission.org/PatientSafety/NationalPatientSafetyGoals).
12. Traynor K: Joint Commission updates National Patient Safety Goals for 2010. Am J Health Syst Pharm 66:2062–2064, 2009.
13. Horwitz LI, Moin T, Krumholz HM, et al: Consequences of inadequate sign-out for patient care. Arch Intern Med 168: 1755–1760, 2008.
14. Kitch BT, Cooper JB, Zapol WM, et al: Handoffs causing patient harm: A survey of medical and surgical house staff. Jt Comm J Qual Patient Saf 34:563–570, 2008.
15. Greenberg CC, Regenbogen SE, Studdert DM, et al: Patterns of communication breakdowns resulting in injury to surgical patients. J Am Coll Surg 204:533–540, 2007.
16. Pickering BW, Hurley K, Marsh B: Identification of patient information corruption in the intensive care unit: Using a scoring tool to direct quality improvements in handover. Crit Care Med 37:2905–2912, 2009.
17. Haig KM, Sutton S, Whittington J: SBAR: A shared mental model for improving communication between clinicians. Jt Comm J Qual Patient Saf 32:167–175, 2006.
18. Aiken LH, Clarke SP, Sloane DM, et al: Hospital nurse staffing and patient mortality, nurse burnout, and job dissatisfaction. JAMA 288:1987–1993, 2002.
19. Pronovost PJ, Jenckes MW, Dorman T, et al: Organizational characteristics of intensive care units related to outcomes of abdominal aortic surgery. JAMA 281:1310–1317, 1999.
20. Weinger MB, Ancoli-Israel S: Sleep deprivation and clinical performance. JAMA 287:955–957, 2002.
21. Ulmer C, Wolman DM, Johns MME, editors: Resident duty hours: Enhancing sleep, supervision, and safety, Washington, DC, 2008, National Academies Press.
22. Landrigan CP, Rothschild JM, Cronin JW, et al: Effect of reducing interns' work hours on serious medical errors in intensive care units. N Engl J Med 351:1838–1848, 2004.
23. Poulose BK, Ray WA, Arbogast PG, et al: Resident work hour limits and patient safety. Ann Surg 241:847–856, 2005.
24. Volpp KG, Rosen AK, Rosenbaum PR, et al: Mortality among patients in VA hospitals in the first 2 years following ACGME resident duty hour reform. JAMA 298:984–992, 2007.
25. Privette AR, Shackford SR, Osler T, et al: Implementation of resident work hour restrictions is associated with a reduction in

mortality and provider-related complications on the surgical service: A concurrent analysis of 14,610 patients. Ann Surg 250:316–321, 2009.

**26.** Barger LK, Ayas NT, Cade BE, et al: Impact of extended-duration shifts on medical errors, adverse events, and attentional failures. PLoS Med 3:e487, 2006.

**27.** Coverdill JE, Finlay W, Adrales GL, et al: Duty-hour restrictions and the work of surgical faculty: Results of a multi-institutional study. Acad Med 81:50–56, 2006.

**28.** Vanderveen K, Chen M, Scherer L: Effects of resident duty-hours restrictions on surgical and nonsurgical teaching faculty. Arch Surg 142:759–764; discussion 764–756, 2007.

**29.** Winslow ER, Bowman MC, Klingensmith ME: Surgeon work hours in the era of limited resident work hours. J Am Coll Surg 198:111–117, 2004.

**30.** Gawande AA, Zinner MJ, Studdert DM, et al: Analysis of errors reported by surgeons at three teaching hospitals. Surgery 133:614–621, 2003.

**31.** Ellman PI, Law MG, Tache-Leon C, et al: Sleep deprivation does not affect operative results in cardiac surgery. Ann Thorac Surg 78:906–911, 2004.

**32.** Rothschild JM, Keohane CA, Rogers S, et al: Risks of complications by attending physicians after performing nighttime procedures. JAMA 302:1565–1572, 2009.

**33.** Nuckols TK, Bhattacharya J, Wolman DM, et al: Cost implications of reduced work hours and workloads for resident physicians. N Engl J Med 360:2202–2215, 2009.

**33a.** Committee on Quality of Health Care in America, Institute of Medicine: Crossing the quality chasm: a new health system for the 21st century, 2001.

**34.** Bates DW, Leape LL, Cullen DJ, et al: Effect of computerized physician order entry and a team intervention on prevention of serious medication errors. JAMA 280:1311–1316, 1998.

**35.** Jha AK, DesRoches CM, Campbell EG, et al: Use of electronic health records in U.S. hospitals. N Engl J Med 360:1628–1638, 2009.

**36.** Amarasingham R, Plantinga L, Diener-West M, et al: Clinical information technologies and inpatient outcomes: A multiple hospital study. Arch Intern Med 169:108–114, 2009.

**37.** Vikoren TH, Musser RC, Tcheng JE, et al: From clinical pathways to CPOE: Challenges and opportunities in standardization and computerization of postoperative orders for total joint replacement. J Surg Orthop Adv 15:195–200, 2006.

**38.** Donaldson S, Villanuueva G, Rondinelli L, et al: Rush University guidelines and protocols for the management of hyperglycemia in hospitalized patients: Elimination of the sliding scale and improvement of glycemic control throughout the hospital. Diabetes Educ 32:954–962, 2006.

**39.** Kanter G, Connelly NR, Fitzgerald J: A system and process redesign to improve perioperative antibiotic administration. Anesth Analg 103:1517–1521, 2006.

**40.** Stone WM, Smith BE, Shaft JD, et al: Impact of a computerized physician order-entry system. J Am Coll Surg 208:960–967; discussion 967–969, 2009.

**41.** Han YY, Carcillo JA, Venkataraman ST, et al: Unexpected increased mortality after implementation of a commercially sold computerized physician order entry system. Pediatrics 116: 1506–1512, 2005.

**42.** Khajouei R, de Jongh D, Jaspers MW: Usability evaluation of a computerized physician order entry for medication ordering. Stud Health Technol Inform 150:532–536, 2009.

**43.** Rahimi B, Timpka T, Vimarlund V, et al: Organization-wide adoption of computerized provider order entry systems: A study based on diffusion of innovations theory. BMC Med Inform Decis Mak 9:52, 2009.

**44.** Campbell EM, Sittig DF, Ash JS, et al: Types of unintended consequences related to computerized provider order entry. J Am Med Inform Assoc 13:547–556, 2006.

**45.** Weir CR, McCarthy CA: Using implementation safety indicators for CPOE implementation. Jt Comm J Qual Patient Saf 35:21–28, 2009.

**46.** Bradley VM, Steltenkamp CL, Hite KB: Evaluation of reported medication errors before and after implementation of computerized practitioner order entry. J Healthc Inf Manag 20:46–53, 2006.

**47.** Kilbridge PM, Welebob EM, Classen DC: Development of the Leapfrog methodology for evaluating hospital implemented inpatient computerized physician order entry systems. Qual Saf Health Care 15:81–84, 2006.

**48.** Murphy EM, Oxencis CJ, Klauck JA, et al: Medication reconciliation at an academic medical center: Implementation of a comprehensive program from admission to discharge. Am J Health Syst Pharm 66:2126–2131, 2009.

**49.** St Jacques P, Sanders N, Patel N, et al: Improving timely surgical antibiotic prophylaxis redosing administration using computerized record prompts. Surg Infect (Larchmt) 6:215–221, 2005.

# SECTION II

# PERIOPERATIVE MANAGEMENT

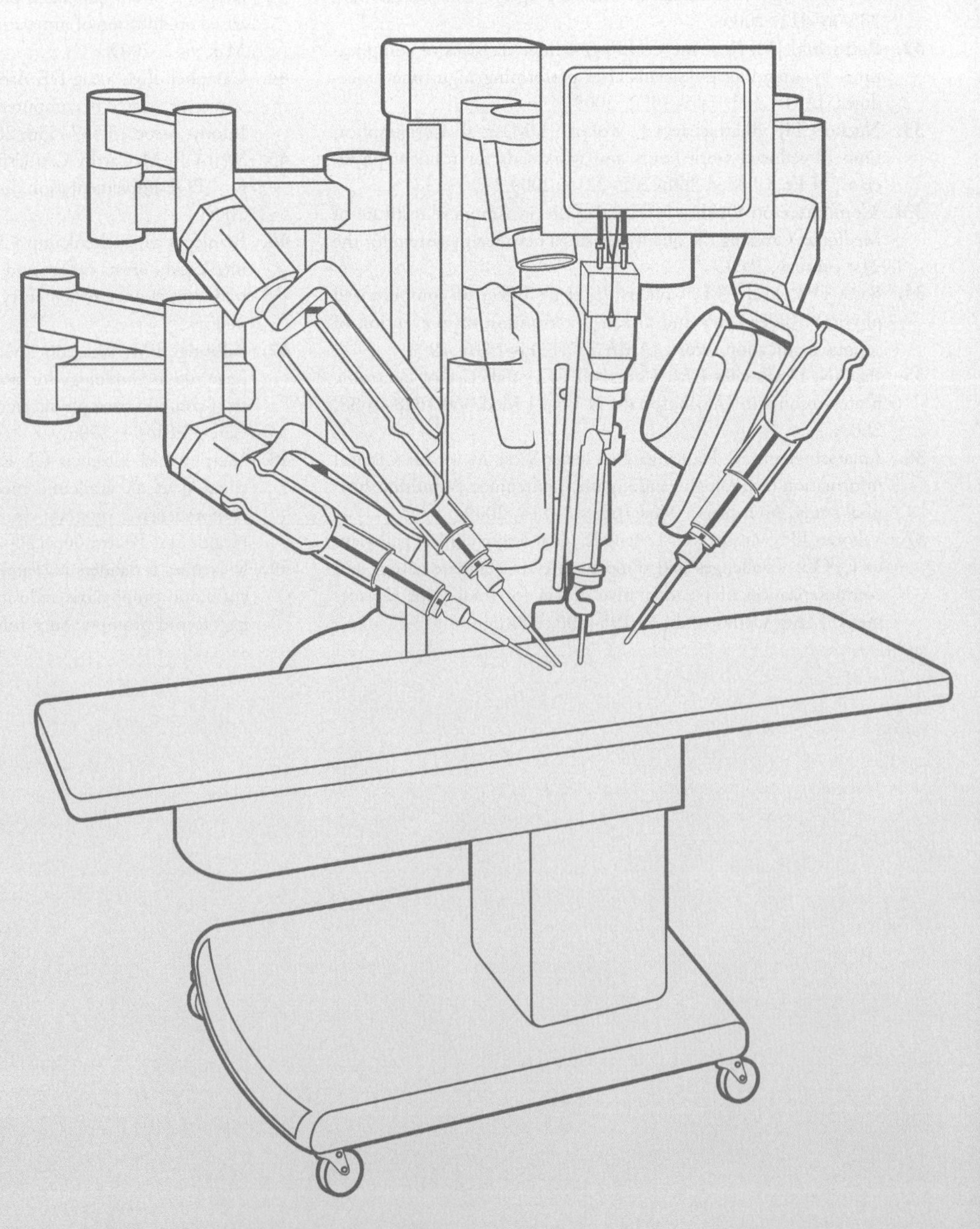

CHAPTER 11

# PRINCIPLES OF PREOPERATIVE AND OPERATIVE SURGERY

LEIGH NEUMAYER AND DANIEL VARGO

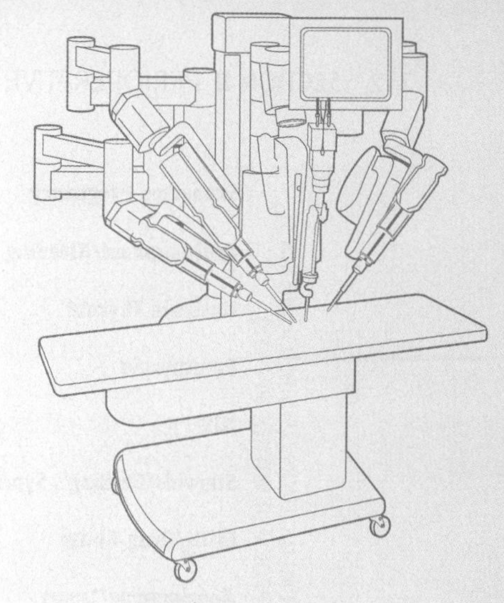



## PREOPERATIVE PREPARATION OF THE PATIENT

The modern preparation of a patient for surgery is epitomized by the convergence of the art and science of the surgical discipline. The context in which preoperative preparation is conducted ranges from an outpatient office visit to hospital inpatient consultation to emergency department evaluation of a patient. Approaches to preoperative evaluation differ significantly, depending on the nature of the complaint and the proposed surgical intervention, patient health and assessment of risk factors, and results of directed investigation and interventions to optimize the patient's overall status and readiness for surgery. This chapter reviews the components of risk assessment applicable to the evaluation of any patient for surgery and attempts to provide some basic algorithms to aid in the preparation of patients for surgery.

## PRINCIPLES OF, AND PREPARATION FOR, OPERATIVE SURGERY

Proper operative technique is of paramount importance for optimizing outcome and enhancing the wound healing process. There is no substitute for a well-planned and conducted operation to provide the best possible surgical outcome. One of the most reliable means of ensuring that surgeons provide quality care in the operating room is through participation in high-quality surgical training programs, which provide opportunities for repetitive observation and performance of surgical procedures in a well-structured environment. With their participation, young surgeons in training can progressively develop the technical skills necessary to perform the most demanding and complex operative procedures.

### Determining the Need for Surgery

Patients are often referred to surgeons with a suspected surgical diagnosis and the results of supporting investigations in hand. In this context, the surgeon's initial encounter with the patient may be largely directed toward confirmation of relevant physical findings and review of the clinical history and laboratory and investigative tests that support the diagnosis. A recommendation regarding the need for operative intervention can then be made by the surgeon and discussed with the patient and family members. A decision to perform additional investigative tests or consideration of alternative therapeutic options may postpone the decision for surgical intervention from this initial encounter to a later time. It is important for the surgeon to explain the context of the illness and the benefit of different surgical interventions, further investigation, possible nonsurgical alternatives, when appropriate, as well as what would happen if no intervention were undertaken.

The surgeon's approach to the patient and family during the initial encounter should be one that fosters a bond of trust and opens a line of communication among all participants. A professional and unhurried approach is mandatory, with time taken to listen to concerns and answer questions posed by the patient and family members. The surgeon's initial encounter with a patient should result in the patient being able to express a basic understanding of the disease process and the need for further investigation and possible surgical management. A well-articulated follow-up plan is essential.

### Perioperative Decision Making

Once the decision has been made to proceed with operative management, a number of considerations must be addressed regarding the timing and site of surgery, type of anesthesia, and preoperative preparation necessary to understand the patient's risk and optimize the outcome. These components of risk assessment take into account the perioperative (intraoperative period through 48 hours postoperatively) and later postoperative (up to 30 days) period and seek to identify factors that may contribute to patient morbidity during these periods.

### Preoperative Evaluation

The aim of preoperative evaluation is not to screen broadly for undiagnosed disease, but to identify and quantify any comorbidity that may affect the operative outcome. This evaluation is driven by findings on the history and physical examination suggestive of organ system dysfunction or by epidemiologic data suggesting the benefit of evaluation based on age, gender, or patterns of disease progression. The goal is to uncover problem areas that may require further investigation or be amenable to preoperative optimization (Table 11-1).[1] Routine preoperative

**Table 11-1 Suggestions for Adult Preoperative Testing**

| TEST | BASIC: MINOR SURGERY IN HEALTHY PATIENT (WITHIN 90 DAYS) | | | | Additive Surgical and Medical Factors — SURGICAL PROCEDURES (WITHIN 90 DAYS) | | | | | | | CLINICALLY SIGNIFICANT AND CHANGING DISORDERS AND/OR MEDICATIONS (SHADED = WITHIN 90 DAYS; LIGHT = TEST FOR DISORDER PROBABLY SHOULD BE PERFORMED WITHIN 30 DAYS) | | | | | | | | | | | | | | | | | | | |
|---|---|---|---|---|---|---|---|---|---|---|---|---|---|---|---|---|---|---|---|---|---|---|---|---|---|---|---|---|---|---|---|
| | **Healthy Adult <45 y/o** | **H45-54 y/o** | **55-69 y/o** | **>70 y/o** | **Cardiac/Thoracic** | **Vascular** | **Major Intraperitoneal/Abdominal** | **Anticipated >2 U EBL** | **Intracranial** | **Orthopedic Prosthesis** | **TURP, Hysterostomy** | **Hypertension** | **Smoking** | **Morbid Obesity** | **h/o Stroke** | **Cancer (?Metastatic)** | **Seizure Medications** | **Cardiovascular** | **Respiratory** | **Diabetes** | **Hepatic** | **Renal** | **Fluid or Electrolyte Loss** | **Autoimmune/Lupus** | **EtOH/Drug Abuse** | **Steroids/Cushing's Syndrome** | **HIV** | **Parathyroid** | **Unstable Thyroid** | **Anticoagulant/Bleeding** | **Suspected Pregnancy** |
| ECG | | M | Y | Y | Y | Y | Y | Y | Y | | | Y | Y | Y | Y | Y | | Y | Y | Y | Y | Y | ± | Y | Y | Y | Y | Y | Y | | |
| CBC + platelets | | | Y | Y | Y | Y | Y | Y | Y | Y | Y | | | Y | Y | Y | Y | Y | Y | Y | Y | Y | Y | Y | Y | Y | Y | Y | Y | Y | |
| Electrolytes | | | | Y | Y | Y | Y | Y | Y | Y | Y | Y | | Y | Y | Y | | Y | Y | Y | Y | Y | Y | Y | Y | Y | Y | Y | Y | | |
| BUN/creatinine | | | | Y | Y | Y | Y | Y | Y | Y | Y | Y | | | Y | Y | | Y | Y | Y | Y | Y | | Y | Y | Y | Y | Y | Y | | |
| Glucose | | | | Y | Y | Y | Y | Y | Y | Y | Y | | | Y | Y | Y | | Y | | Y | Y | Y | | | Y | Y | Y | Y | Y | | |
| LFTs | | | | | | | ± | | | | | | | | | Y | Y | | | | Y | | | | Y | | Y | | | | |
| Calcium | | | | | | | | | | | | | | | | | | | | | | | | | | | | Y | | | |
| PT/PTT | | | | | Y | | | Y | Y | | | | | | | | | | | | Y | Y | | Y | Y | | | | | Y | |
| U/A, culture | | | | | | | | | | S | | | | | | | | | | | | | | | | | | | | | |
| CXR | | | | | Y | | | | | | | | | | | S | | | Y | | | | | | | | S | | | | |
| Hormone levels | | | | | | | | | | | | | | | | | | | | | | | | | | | | | Y | | |
| Bleeding time | | | | | | | | | S | | | | | | | | | | | | | | | | | | | | | ± | |
| Pregnancy | | | | | | | | | | | | | | | | | | | | | | | | | | | | | | | Y* |
| Drug levels | | | | | | | | | S | | | | | | | | S | | | | | | | | ± | | | | | | |
| Tumor markers | | | | | | | | | | | | | | | | S | | | | | | | | | | | | | | | |
| Clot | Depends primarily on extensiveness of proposed surgery, as per Blood Bank MSBOS guidelines | | | | | | | | | | | | | | | | | | | | | | | | | | | | | | |

Adapted from Halaszynski TM, Juda R, Silverman DG: Optimizing postoperative outcomes with efficient preoperative assessment and management. Crit Care Med 32:S76–S86, 2004.

*BUN,* Blood urea nitrogen; *CXR,* chest x-ray; *EBL,* estimated blood loss; *EtOH,* ethanol; *HIV,* human immunodeficiency virus; *h/o,* history of; *LFTs,* liver function tests; *M,* usually indicated for male; *MSBOS*, maximum surgical blood order schedule; *PT/PTT,* prothrombin time/partial thromboplastin time; *S,* may be requested (and reviewed) by the surgeon as part of surgical workup; *TURP,* transurethral resection of the prostate; *U/A,* urinalysis; *Y,* usually indicated; ±, if situation acute or severe.

*At a minimum, a urine pregnancy test should be performed on the morning of surgery in any woman of childbearing age, unless the uterus or ovaries are surgically absent.

*Shaded area,* Timing of test is not typically critical; results from 90 days (and possibly 180 days) may be acceptable; *light area,* typically best to obtain within 30 days of surgery.

**Note:** (1) Times and test listings are suggestions; they are not absolute and should not preclude other testing in given settings, nor should they prevent a case from proceeding if the anesthesiologist and surgeon deem it to be appropriate. (2) Testing for a given disorder depends on the severity of the disorder in the context of the planned surgery; that is, are the tests likely to generate potentially clinically significant information and provide information that would be an important component of the history and physical examination?

testing is not cost-effective and, even in older adults, is less predictive of perioperative morbidity than the American Society of Anesthesiologists (ASA) status or American Heart Association (AHA)/American College of Cardiology (ACC) guidelines for surgical risk.

The preoperative evaluation is determined in light of the risk of the planned procedure (low, medium, or high), planned anesthetic technique, and postoperative disposition of the patient (outpatient or inpatient, ward bed, or intensive care). In addition, the preoperative evaluation is used to identify patient risk factors for postoperative morbidity and mortality. Along with being a generally accepted program for risk adjustment to monitor and improve surgical outcomes, The National Surgical Quality Improvement Program (NSQIP) has been used to develop predictive models for postoperative morbidity and mortality, and several factors have consistently been found to be independent predictors of postoperative events (Table 11-2), both in the Department of Veterans Affairs (VA) and in a more recent comparison between the VA and private sector hospitals.[2] It is important to understand that the NSQIP has been validated as an excellent quality improvement tool by accounting for the influence of patient risk on outcomes from surgery and allowing hospitals to compare their outcomes to that of their peers. Although risk prediction models have been developed and are available to use in the VA, they have yet to be validated prospectively as they might apply to individual patients. The potential ability to predict an individual patient's risk may have its biggest impact in allowing the surgeon to intervene with measures shown to decrease that risk.

If preoperative evaluation uncovers significant comorbidity or evidence of poor control of an underlying disease process, consultation with an internist or medical subspecialist may be required to facilitate the workup and direct management. In this process, communication between the surgeon and consultants is essential to define realistic goals for this optimization process and to expedite surgical management.

For all patients, their general risk should be categorized using the American Society of Anesthesiologist classification. The ASA classification was one of the first risk categorization systems. It has five stratifications:

I. Normal healthy patient
II. Patient with mild systemic disease
III. Patient with severe systemic disease that limits activity but is not incapacitating
IV. Patient who has incapacitating disease that is a constant threat to life
V. Moribund patient not expected to survive 24 hours with or without an operation

The letter "E" is added to any of these for an emergency operation. Even though the system seems subjective, it continues to be a significant independent predictor of mortality.[2] Although the ASA class should be determined for each patient, a more in-depth assessment of risk is indicated for procedures more involved than a skin biopsy.

**Table 11-2 Top Patient Risk Factors Most Predictive of Post-Operative Mortality***

| VARIABLE | ODDS RATIO | 95% CI |
|---|---|---|
| **14 Private Sector Hospitals (*N* = 54,450; C-index = 0.934)** | | |
| ASA 4/5 | 8.1 | 6.0-11.0 |
| ASA 3 | 3.5 | 2.7-4.7 |
| Albumin g/dL | 0.62 | 0.56-0.69 |
| Emergency operation | 2.6 | 2.2-3.1 |
| Age/yr | 1.04 | 1.03-1.04 |
| Platelet count <150,000 | 1.9 | 1.6-2.2 |
| Disseminated cancer | 2.9 | 2.3-3.7 |
| Dyspnea at rest | 1.6 | 1.3-2.0 |
| Dyspnea with minimal exertion | 1.3 | 1.0-1.5 |
| DNR | 3.9 | 2.6-5.8 |
| BUN >40mg/dL | 1.3 | 1.0-1.6 |
| Work RVU/unit | 1.02 | 1.01-1.03 |
| **128 VA Hospitals (*N* = 129,546; C-index = 0.900)** | | |
| ASA 4/5 | 5.3 | 4.3-6.6 |
| ASA 3 | 2.6 | 2.2-3.2 |
| Albumin g/dL | 0.6 | 0.57-0.63 |
| Emergency operation | 2.0 | 1.9-2.2 |
| Disseminated cancer | 3.3 | 2.9-3.8 |
| Age/yr | 1.04 | 1.03-1.04 |
| Work RVU/unit | 1.05 | 1.04-1.05 |
| Dyspnea at rest | 1.4 | 1.2-1.6 |
| Dyspnea with minimal exertion | 1.3 | 1.2-1.5 |
| DNR | 2.8 | 2.4-3.3 |
| Ascites | 2.3 | 1.9-2.7 |
| BUN >40mg/dL | 1.4 | 1.2-1.6 |

Adapted from Khuri SF, Henderson WG, Daley J, et al: Successful implementation of the Department of Veterans Affairs' National Surgical Quality Improvement Program in the private sector: The Patient Safety in Surgery study. Ann Surg 248:329-336, 2008.

*ASA,* American Society of Anesthesiologist's Patient Severity Score; *BUN,* blood urea nitrogen; *CI,* confidence index; *DNR,* do not resuscitate; *RVU,* relative value units.

*NSQIP comparison of private sector hospitals to VA hospitals.

## SYSTEMS APPROACH TO PREOPERATIVE EVALUATION

### Cardiovascular System

Cardiovascular disease is the leading cause of death in the industrialized world and its contribution to perioperative mortality during noncardiac surgery is significant. Of the 27 million patients undergoing surgery in the United States every year, 8 million, or almost 30%, have significant coronary artery disease or other cardiac comorbid conditions. One million of these patients will experience perioperative cardiac complications, with substantial morbidity, mortality, and cost. Consequently, much of the preoperative risk assessment and patient preparation centers on the cardiovascular system.

Assessment tools for stratification of the cardiovascular portion of anesthetic risk have been available for some time. The premiere example is Goldman's criteria of cardiac risk for noncardiac surgery (Table 11-3).[3] This strategy, designed by multivariate analysis, assigns points to easily reproducible characteristics. The points are then added to yield a total, which has been correlated with perioperative cardiac risk. One of the more

**Table 11-3 Cardiac Risk Indices**

| CARDIAC RISK INDEX WITH VARIABLES | POINTS | COMMENTS |
|---|---|---|
| **Goldman Cardiac Risk Index, 1977** | | **Cardiac complication rate** |
| 1. Third heart sound or jugular venous distention | 11 | 0-5 points = 1% |
| 2. Recent myocardial infarction | 10 | 6-12 points = 7% |
| 3. Nonsinus rhythm or premature atrial contraction on ECG | 7 | 13-25 points = 14% |
| 4. >5 premature ventricular contractions | 7 | >26 points = 78% |
| 5. Age >70 yr | 5 | |
| 6. Emergency operations | 4 | |
| 7. Poor general medical condition | 3 | |
| 8. Intrathoracic, intraperitoneal, or aortic surgery | 3 | |
| 9. Important valvular aortic stenosis | 3 | |
| **Detsky Modified Multifactorial Index, 1986** | | **Cardiac complication rate** |
| 1. Class 4 angina | 20 | >15 = high risk |
| 2. Suspected critical aortic stenosis | 20 | |
| 3. Myocardial infarction within 6 mo | 10 | |
| 4. Alveolar pulmonary edema within 1 wk | 10 | |
| 5. Unstable angina within 3 mo | 10 | |
| 6. Class 3 angina | 10 | |
| 7. Emergency surgery | 10 | |
| 8. Myocardial infarction >6 mo ago | 5 | |
| 9. Alveolar pulmonary edema resolved >1 wk ago | 5 | |
| 10. Rhythm other than sinus or PACs on ECG | 5 | |
| 11. >5 PVCs any time before surgery | 5 | |
| 12. Poor general medical status | 5 | |
| 13. Age >70 yr | 5 | |
| **Eagle's Criteria for Cardiac Risk Assessment, 1989** | | |
| 1. Age >70 yr | 1 | <1, no testing |
| 2. Diabetes | 1 | 1-2, send for noninvasive test |
| 3. Angina | 1 | ≥3, send for angiography |
| 4. Q waves on ECG | 1 | |
| 5. Ventricular arrhythmias | 1 | |
| **Revised Cardiac Risk Index** | | |
| 1. Ischemic heart disease | 1 | Each increment in points increases risk for postoperative myocardial morbidity |
| 2. Congestive heart failure | 1 | |
| 3. Cerebral vascular disease | 1 | |
| 4. High-risk surgery | 1 | |
| 5. Preoperative insulin treatment of diabetes | 1 | |
| 6. Preoperative creatinine level >2 mg/dL | 1 | |

Adapted from Akhtar S, Silverman DG: Assessment and management of patients with ischemic heart disease. Crit Care Med 32(Suppl):S126–S136, 2004.

*PAC,* Premature atrial contraction; *PVC,* premature ventricular contraction.

important contributions of this work was the inclusion of functional capacity, clinical signs and symptoms, and operative risk assessment to estimate the patient's overall risk and plan preoperative interventions. This concept has been further refined in the Revised Cardiac Risk Index, which uses six predictors of complications to estimate cardiac risk in noncardiac surgical patients, and is also shown in Table 11-3. In addition, several other investigators have proposed cardiac risk indices; however, many were found to be expensive and time-consuming.

In an attempt to assess and optimize the cardiac status of patients undergoing noncardiac surgery, a joint committee

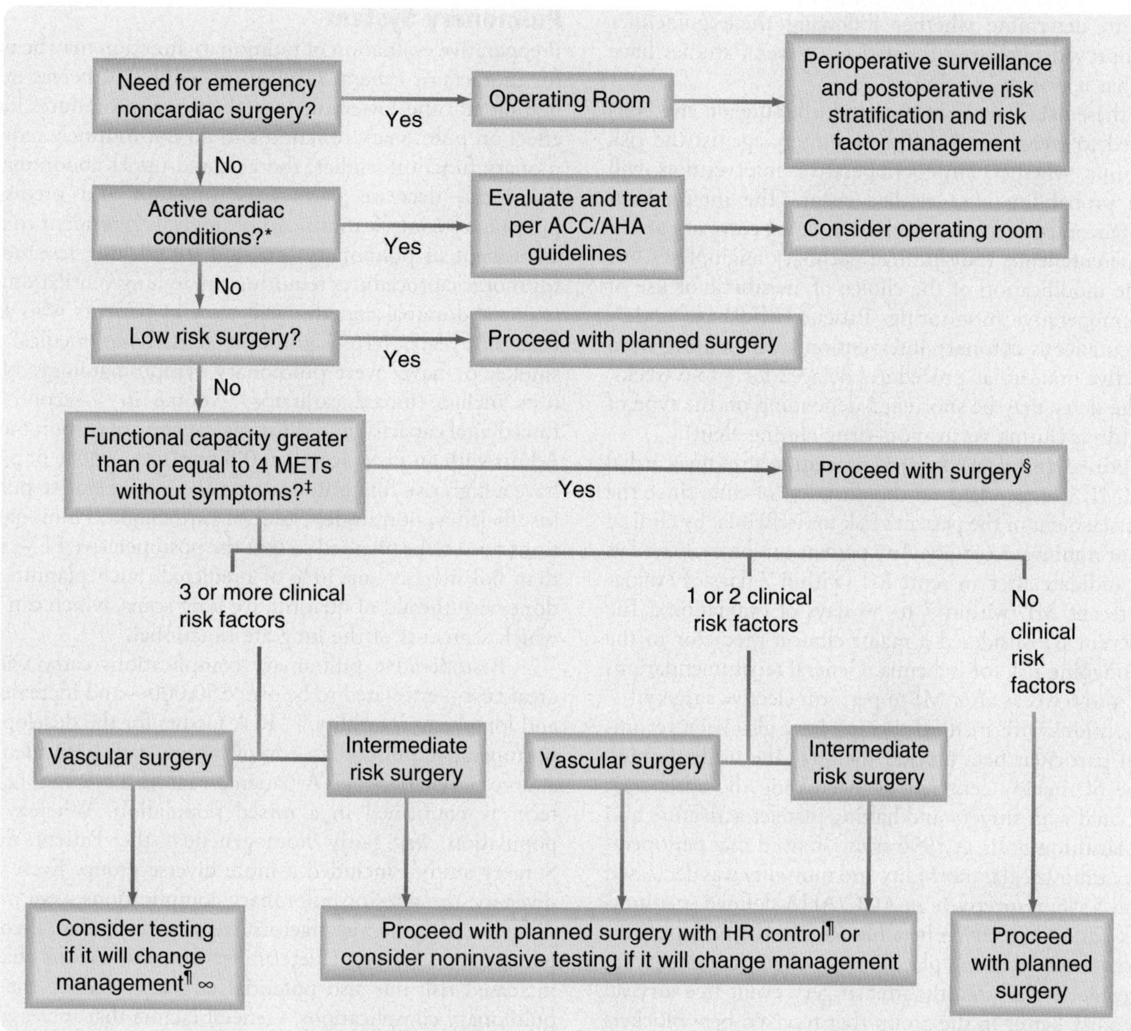


**FIGURE 11-1** Stepwise approach to preoperative cardiac assessment for non-cardiac surgery. *HR,* Heart rate; *MET,* metabolic equivalent. Adapted from Fleisher LA, Beckman JA, Brown KA, et al. ACC/AHA 2007 Guidelines on Perioperative Cardiovascular Evaluation and Care for Noncardiac Surgery: Executive Summary: A Report of the American College of Cardiology/American Heart Association Task Force on Practice Guidelines (Writing Committee to Revise the 2002 Guidelines on Perioperative Cardiovascular Evaluation for Noncardiac Surgery). Circulation 116:1971–1996, 2007.

*Active cardiac conditions include unstable coronary syndromes, decompensated heart failure (New York Heart Association functional class IV, worsening or new-onset heart failure), significant arrhythmias (high grade atrioventricular block, Mobitz type II block, third degree block, symptomatic ventricular arrhythmias, supraventricular arrhythmias with uncontrolled ventricular rate, symptomatic bradycardia, newly recognized ventricular tachycardia), severe valvular disease (severe aortic stenosis, symptomatic mitral stenosis).

‡An abbreviated list of METs includes the following: activities such as taking care of yourself, eating, getting dressed, 1 MET; light housework, 4 METs; climbing a flight of stairs or walking up a hill, 5 METs; engaging in strenuous sports, 10 METs.

§Noninvasive testing may be considered before surgery in specific patients with risk factors if it will change management. Clinical risk factors include ischemic heart disease, compensated or prior heart failure, diabetes mellitus, renal insufficiency, and cerebrovascular disease.

¶Consider perioperative beta blockade for patient populations in whom this has been shown to reduce morbidity and mortality.

of the ACC and AHA has developed an easily used tool (Fig. 11-1).[4] This methodology takes into account previous coronary revascularization and evaluation and clinical risk assessment, divided into major, intermediate, and minor clinical predictors. The next factor taken into account is the patient's functional capacity, which is estimated by obtaining a history of the patient's daily activities. The earlier mentioned variables and type of surgery are then used to determine whether the pretest probability can be altered by noninvasive testing.

The standard exercise stress test, with or without thallium for perfusion imaging, can be limited by the functional capacity of the patient. Patients not able to exercise to an acceptable stress level may require pharmacologic stress testing with dipyridamole; thereafter, perfusion defects can be assessed via thallium or a dobutamine-induced stress, followed by functional evaluation with echocardiography. Angiography can then be used to define the anatomic abnormalities contributing to the ischemia exactly. Although no large prospective randomized trial has been conducted to determine whether following these guidelines result in improved outcomes for patients, several studies have suggested that it is useful to do so.[3]

Once these data have been obtained, the surgeon and consultants need to weigh the benefits of surgery against the risk and determine whether any perioperative intervention will reduce the probability of a cardiac event. The intervention usually centers on coronary revascularization via coronary artery bypass or percutaneous transluminal coronary angioplasty but may include modification of the choice of anesthetic or use of invasive intraoperative monitoring. Patients who have undergone a percutaneous coronary intervention with stenting need to have elective noncardiac procedures delayed for 4 to 6 weeks, although the delay may be shortened depending on the type of stent used (drug-eluting versus non–drug-eluting stent).[3]

The optimal timing of a surgical procedure after myocardial infarction (MI) is dependent on the duration of time since the event and assessment of the patient's risk for ischemia, by clinical symptoms or noninvasive study. Any patient can be evaluated as a surgical candidate after an acute MI (within 7 days of evaluation) or a recent MI (within 7 to 30 days of evaluation). The infarction event is considered a major clinical predictor in the context of ongoing risk for ischemia. General recommendations are to wait 4 to 6 weeks after MI to perform elective surgery.[3]

Interventions with medical therapy have also been recommended, in particular beta blocker therapy. The underpinning of this type of therapy centered on decreasing the adrenergic surge associated with surgery and halting platelet activation and microvascular thrombosis. A 1996 study showed that perioperative risk for cardiovascular morbidity and mortality was decreased by 67% and 55%, respectively in ACC/AHA-defined medium- to high-risk patients receiving beta blockers in the perioperative period versus those receiving placebo. Although the benefit was most noticeable in the 6 months after surgery, event-free survival was significantly better in the group that received beta blockers up to 2 years after surgery.[5] In 2007, the results of another large randomized trial (***P***eri***O***perative ***IS***chemic ***E***valuation—POISE) showed the potential harm of perioperative beta blocker therapy.[6] The POISE trial enrolled over 8000 patients undergoing noncardiac surgery. Although the results confirmed the reduction in perioperative cardiac events such as myocardial infarction, cardiovascular death, and cardiac arrest, this benefit was offset by an increased rate of stroke and total mortality with perioperative beta blocker therapy. Unlike the prior study, this study started high-dose, extended-release metoprolol on the day of surgery. The results were important enough to stimulate the ACC/AHA to modify their recommendations (Table 11-4).[7] The current recommendations are to continue beta blockers for those who are on them preoperatively, consider them for high-risk patients (more than one risk factor), titrating to heart rate and blood pressure, and not to give them to low-risk patients.

An easy and inexpensive method to determine cardiopulmonary functional status for noncardiac surgery is the patient's ability or inability to climb two flights of stairs. Two flights of stairs are needed because it demands more than 4 metabolic equivalents (METs). In a review of all studies of stair climbing as preoperative assessment, prospective studies have shown it to be a good predictor of mortality associated with thoracic surgery.[8] In major noncardiac surgery, an inability to climb two flights of stairs is an independent predictor of perioperative morbidity, but not mortality.

## Pulmonary System

Preoperative evaluation of pulmonary function may be necessary for thoracic or general surgical procedures. Whereas extremity, neurologic, and lower abdominal surgical procedures have little effect on pulmonary function and do not routinely require pulmonary function studies, thoracic and upper abdominal procedures can decrease pulmonary function and predispose to pulmonary complications. Accordingly, it is prudent to consider assessment of pulmonary function for all lung resection cases, for thoracic procedures requiring single-lung ventilation, and for major abdominal and thoracic cases in patients who are older than 60 years, have significant underlying medical disease, smoke, or have overt pulmonary symptomatology. Necessary tests include forced expiratory volume in 1 second ($FEV_1$), forced vital capacity, and diffusing capacity of carbon monoxide. Adults with an $FEV_1$ less than 0.8 liter/sec, or 30% of predicted, have a high risk for complications and postoperative pulmonary insufficiency; nonsurgical solutions are sought. Pulmonary resections need to be planned so that the postoperative $FEV_1$ is higher than 0.8 liter/sec, or 30% of predicted. Such planning can be done with the aid of quantitative lung scans, which can indicate which segments of the lung are functional.

Postoperative pulmonary complications carry with them great cost—estimated to be over $50,000—and increased short- and long-term mortality.[9,10] Risk factors for the development of postoperative pulmonary complications have been identified in a large population of VA patients (Tables 11-5 and 11-6), and recently confirmed in a mixed population. Whereas the VA population was fairly homogeneous, the Patient Safety in Surgery study[11] included a more diverse group. Even with the diversity, the rates of pulmonary complications were not much different and the risk factors were very similar. Preoperative pulmonary assessment determines not only factors that confer increased risk but also potential targets to reduce the risk for pulmonary complications. General factors that increase risk for postoperative pulmonary complications include increasing age, lower albumin level, dependent functional status, weight loss, and possibly obesity. Concurrent comorbid conditions such as impaired sensorium, previous stroke, congestive heart failure, acute renal failure, chronic steroid use, and blood transfusion are also associated with increased risk for postoperative pulmonary complications. Specific pulmonary risk factors include chronic obstructive pulmonary disease, smoking, preoperative sputum production, pneumonia, dyspnea, and obstructive sleep apnea.

Preoperative interventions that may decrease postoperative pulmonary complications include smoking cessation (within 2 months before the planned procedure), bronchodilator therapy, antibiotic therapy for preexisting infection, and pretreatment of asthmatic patients with steroids. In addition, encouraging exercise preoperatively may improve a patient's recovery postoperatively. A reasonable recommendation would be to encourage the patients to walk 3 miles in less than 1 hour several times weekly. Perioperative strategies include the use of epidural anesthesia, vigorous pulmonary toilet and rehabilitation, and continued bronchodilator therapy.

## Renal System

Approximately 5% of the adult population has some degree of renal dysfunction that can affect the physiology of multiple organ systems and cause additional morbidity in the

**Table 11-4 American Heart Association/American College of Cardiology Perioperative Focused Update Recommendations**

| CURRENT RECOMMENDATION | CHANGE FROM PREVIOUS RECOMMENDATION |
|---|---|
| **Class I*** | |
| Beta blockers should be continued in patients undergoing surgery who are receiving beta blockers for treatment of conditions with ACCF/AHA class I guideline indications for the drugs. | Revised wording; recommendation of giving beta blockers to high cardiac risk vascular patients with findings of ischemia on preoperative testing moved down in class of recommendation (see class IIa) |
| **Class IIa** | |
| 1. Beta blockers titrated to heart rate and blood pressure are probably recommended for patients undergoing vascular surgery who are at high cardiac risk because of coronary artery disease or the finding of cardiac ischemia on preoperative testing. | Modified or combined recommendation, moved down in classification |
| 2. Beta blockers titrated to heart rate and blood pressure are reasonable for patients in whom preoperative assessment for vascular surgery identifies high cardiac risk, as defined by the presence of more than one clinical risk factor. | Modified recommendation (added "titrated to heart rate and blood pressure" and changed "are probably recommended" to "are reasonable") |
| 3. Beta blockers titrated to heart rate and blood pressure are reasonable for patients in whom preoperative assessment identifies coronary artery disease or high cardiac risk, as defined by the presence of more than one clinical risk factor, who are undergoing intermediate-risk surgery. | Revised wording |
| **Class IIb** | |
| 1. The usefulness of beta blockers is uncertain for patients who are undergoing intermediate-risk procedures or vascular surgery in whom preoperative assessment identifies a single clinical risk factor in the absence of coronary artery disease. | Revised wording |
| 2. The usefulness of beta blockers is uncertain in patient undergoing vascular surgery with no clinical risk factors who are not currently taking beta blockers. | No change from 2007 recommendations |
| **Class III** | |
| 1. Beta blockers should not be given to patients undergoing surgery who have absolute contraindications to beta blockade. | No changes from 2007 recommendations |
| 2. Routing administration of high-dose beta blockers in the absence of dose titration is not useful and may be harmful to patients not currently taking beta blockers who are undergoing noncardiac surgery. | New recommendation |

Adapted from Fleischmann KE, Beckman JA, Buller CE, et al: 2009 ACCF/AHA focused update on perioperative beta blockade. J Am Coll Cardiol 54:2102–2128, 2009.

*Class of recommendation is based on the size of the treatment effect combined with an estimate of certainty (precision) of the treatment effect. Clinical risk factors include history of ischemic heart disease, history of compensated or prior heart failure, history of cerebrovascular disease, diabetes mellitus, and renal insufficiency (defined in the revised cardiac risk index as a preoperative serum creatinine level >2 mg/dL).

perioperative period. In fact, a preoperative creatinine level of 2.0 mg/dL or higher is an independent risk factor for cardiac complications. Identification of coexisting cardiovascular, circulatory, hematologic, and metabolic derangements secondary to renal dysfunction are the goals of preoperative evaluation in these patients.

A patient with known renal insufficiency undergoes a thorough history and physical examination, with particular questioning about previous MI and symptoms consistent with ischemic heart disease. The cardiovascular examination seeks to document signs of fluid overload. The patient's functional status and exercise tolerance are carefully elicited. Diagnostic testing for the patient with renal dysfunction includes an electrocardiogram (ECG), serum chemistry panel, and complete blood count (CBC). If physical examination findings are suggestive of heart failure, a chest radiograph may be helpful. Urinalysis and urinary electrolyte studies are not often helpful in the setting of established renal insufficiency, although they may be diagnostic in patients with new-onset renal dysfunction.

Laboratory abnormalities are often seen in a patient with advanced renal insufficiency. Some metabolic derangements in a patient with advanced renal failure may be mild and asymptomatic and are revealed by electrolyte or blood gas analysis. Anemia, when present in these patients, may range from mild and asymptomatic to that associated with fatigue, low exercise tolerance, and exertional angina. Such anemia can be treated with erythropoietin or darbepoietin preoperatively or perioperatively. Because the platelet dysfunction associated with uremia is often a qualitative one, platelet counts are usually normal. A safe course is to communicate with the anesthesiologist about the potential need for agents to be available in the operating room to assist in improving platelet function. A patient with end-stage renal disease frequently requires additional attention in the perioperative period. Pharmacologic manipulation of hyperkalemia, replacement of calcium for symptomatic hypocalcemia, and use of phosphate-binding antacids for hyperphosphatemia are often required. Sodium bicarbonate is used in the setting of metabolic acidosis not caused by hypoperfusion when serum bicarbonate levels are below 15 mEq/liter. It can be administered in intravenous (IV) fluid as one to two ampules in one liter of a 5% dextrose solution. Hyponatremia is treated by volume restriction, although dialysis is commonly required within the perioperative period for control of volume and electrolyte abnormalities.

**Table 11-5 Risk Factors for Development of Postoperative Pneumonia and Respiratory Failure***

| RISK FACTOR | POSTOPERATIVE PNEUMONIA RISK INDEX (OR 95% CI) | POINT VALUE | RESPIRATORY FAILURE RISK INDEX (OR 95% CI) | POINT VALUE |
|---|---|---|---|---|
| **Type of Surgery** | | | | |
| AAA repair | 4.29 (3.34-5.50) | 15 | 14.3 (12.0-16.9) | 27 |
| Thoracic | 3.92 (3.36-4.57) | 14 | 8.14 (7.17-9.25) | 21 |
| Upper abdominal | 2.68 (2.38-3.03) | 10 | 4.21 (3.80-4.67) | 14 |
| Neck | 2.30 (1.73-3.05) | 8 | 3.10 (2.40-4.01) | 11 |
| Neurosurgical | 2.14 (1.66-2.75) | 8 | 4.21 (3.80-4.67) | 14 |
| Vascular | 1.29 (1.10-1.52) | 3 | 4.21 (3.80-4.67) | 14 |
| Emergency surgery | 1.33 (1.16-1.54) | 3 | 3.12 (2.83-3.43) | 11 |
| General anesthesia | 1.56 (1.36-1.80) | 4 | 1.91 (1.64-2.21) | – |
| **Age** | | | | |
| >80 yr | 5.63 (4.62-6.84) | 17 | – | – |
| 70-79 yr | 3.58 (2.97-4.33) | 13 | – | – |
| 60-69 yr | 2.38 (1.98-2.87) | 9 | – | – |
| 50-59 yr | 1.49 (1.23-1.81) | 4 | – | – |
| <50 yr | 1.00 (referent) | – | – | – |
| 60-69 yr | – | – | 1.51 (1.36-1.69) | 4 |
| <60 yr | – | – | 1.00 (referent) | – |
| ≥70 yr | – | – | 1.91 (1.71-2.13) | 6 |
| **Functional Status** | | | | |
| Totally dependent | 3.83 (2.33-3.43) | 10 | 1.92 (1.74-2.11) | 7 |
| Partially dependent | 1.83 (1.63-2.06) | 6 | 1.92 (1.74-2.11) | 7 |
| Independent | 1.00 (referent) | – | 1.00 (referent) | – |
| **Albumin Level** | | | | |
| <3.0 g/dL | – | – | 2.53 (2.28-2.80) | 9 |
| >3.0 g/dL | – | – | 1.00 (referent) | – |
| Weight loss >10% (within 6 mo) | 1.92 (1.68-2.18) | 7 | 1.37 (1.19-1.57)* | – |
| Chronic steroid use | 1.33 (1.12-1.58) | 3 | – | – |
| Alcohol, >two drinks/day (within 2 wk) | 1.24 (1.08-1.42) | 2 | 1.19 (1.07-1.33)* | – |
| Diabetes, insulin-treated | – | – | 1.15 (1.00-1.33)* | – |
| History of COPD | 1.72 (1.55-1.91) | 5 | 1.81 (1.66-1.98) | 6 |
| **Current Smoker** | | | | |
| Within 1 yr | 1.28 (1.17-1.42) | 3 | – | – |
| Within 2 wk | – | – | 1.24 (1.14-1.36)* | – |
| Preoperative pneumonia | – | – | 1.70 (1.24-2.13)* | – |
| **Dyspnea** | | | | |
| At rest | – | – | 1.69 (1.36-2.09)* | – |
| With minimal exertion | – | – | 1.21 (1.09-1.34)* | – |
| | – | – | 1.00 (referent) | – |
| **No Dyspnea** | | | | |
| Impaired sensorium | 1.51 (1.26-1.82) | 4 | 1.22 (1.04-1.43)* | – |
| History of CVA | 1.47 (1.28-1.68) | 4 | 1.20 (1.05-1.38)* | – |
| History of CHF | – | – | 1.25 (1.07-1.47)* | – |

*Continued*

**Table 11-5 Risk Factors for Development of Postoperative Pneumonia and Respiratory Failure—cont'd**

| RISK FACTOR | POSTOPERATIVE PNEUMONIA RISK INDEX (OR 95% CI) | POINT VALUE | RESPIRATORY FAILURE RISK INDEX (OR 95% CI) | POINT VALUE |
|---|---|---|---|---|
| **Blood Urea Nitrogen Level** | | | | |
| <8 mg/dL | 1.47 (1.26-1.72) | 4 | 1.00 (referent) | – |
| 8-21 mg/dL | 1.00 (referent) | – | 1.00 (referent) | – |
| 22-30 mg/dL | 1.24 (1.11-1.39) | 2 | 1.00 (referent) | – |
| >30 mg/dL | 1.41 (1.22-1.64) | 3 | 2.29 (2.04-2.56) | 8 |
| Preoperative renal failure | – | – | 1.67 (1.23-2.27)* | – |
| Preoperative transfusion (>4 units) | 1.35 (1.07-1.72) | 3 | 1.56 (1.28-1.91) * | – |

Adapted from Arozullah AM, Khuri SF, Henderson WG, et al: Development and validation of a multifactorial risk index for predicting postoperative pneumonia after major noncardiac surgery. Ann Intern Med 135:847–857, 2001; and Arozullah AM, Daley J, Henderson WG, Khuri SF: Multifactorial risk index for predicting postoperative respiratory failure in men after major noncardiac surgery. Ann Surg 232:242–253, 2000.

*AAA,* Abdominal aortic aneurysm; *CHF,* congestive heart failure; *CI,* confidence interval; *COPD,* chronic obstructive pulmonary disease; *CVA,* cerebrovascular accident; *OR,* odds ratio.

*The risk factor was statistically significant in multivariable analysis but was not included in the respiratory failure risk index.

**Table 11-6 Pulmonary Risk Class Assignment**

| RISK CLASS | POSTOPERATIVE PNEUMONIA RISK INDEX (POINT TOTAL) | PREDICTED PROBABILITY OF PNEUMONIA (%) | RESPIRATORY FAILURE RISK INDEX (POINT TOTAL) | PREDICTED PROBABILITY OF RESPIRATORY FAILURE (%) |
|---|---|---|---|---|
| 1 | 0-15 | 0.2 | 0-10 | 0.5 |
| 2 | 16-25 | 1.2 | 11-19 | 2.2 |
| 3 | 26-40 | 4.0 | 20-27 | 5.0 |
| 4 | 41-55 | 9.4 | 28-40 | 11.6 |
| 5 | >55 | 15.3 | >40 | 30.5 |

Adapted from Arozullah AM, Khuri SF, Henderson WG, et al: Development and validation of a multifactorial risk index for predicting postoperative pneumonia after major noncardiac surgery. Ann Intern Med 135:847–857, 2001; and Arozullah AM, Daley J, Henderson WG, Khuri SF: Multifactorial risk index for predicting postoperative respiratory failure in men after major noncardiac surgery. Ann Surg 232:242–253, 2000.

Patients with chronic end-stage renal disease undergo dialysis before surgery to optimize their volume status and control the potassium level. Intraoperative hyperkalemia can result from surgical manipulation of tissue or transfusion of blood. Such patients are often dialyzed on the day after surgery as well. In the acute setting, patients who have a stable volume status can undergo surgery without preoperative dialysis, provided that no other indication exists for emergency dialysis.[12] Prevention of secondary renal insults in the perioperative period include the avoidance of nephrotoxic agents and maintenance of adequate intravascular volume throughout this period. In the postoperative period, the pharmacokinetics of many drugs may be unpredictable, and adjustments in dosage need to be made according to pharmacy recommendation. Notably, narcotics used for postoperative pain control may have prolonged effects despite hepatic clearance, and nonsteroidal agents are avoided in patients with renal insufficiency.

## Hepatobiliary System

Hepatic dysfunction may reflect the common pathway of a number of insults to the liver, including viral-, drug-, and toxin-mediated disease. A patient with liver dysfunction requires careful assessment of the degree of functional impairment, as well as a coordinated effort to avoid additional insult in the perioperative period (Fig. 11-2).[13]

A history of any exposure to blood and blood products or exposure to hepatotoxic agents is obtained. Patients frequently know whether hepatitis has been diagnosed and need to be questioned about when the diagnosis was made and what activity led to the infection. Although such a history may not affect further patient evaluation, it is important to obtain in case an operative team member is injured during the planned surgical procedure. A review of systems specifically inquires about symptoms such as pruritus, fatigability, excessive bleeding, abdominal distention, and weight gain. Evidence of hepatic dysfunction may be seen on physical examination. Jaundice and scleral icterus may be evident with serum bilirubin levels higher than 3 mg/dL. Skin changes include spider angiomas, caput medusae, palmar erythema, and clubbing of the fingertips. Abdominal examination may reveal distention, evidence of fluid shift, and hepatomegaly. Encephalopathy or asterixis may be evident. Muscle wasting or cachexia can be prominent.

A patient with liver dysfunction should undergo standard liver function tests. Elevations in hepatocellular enzyme levels

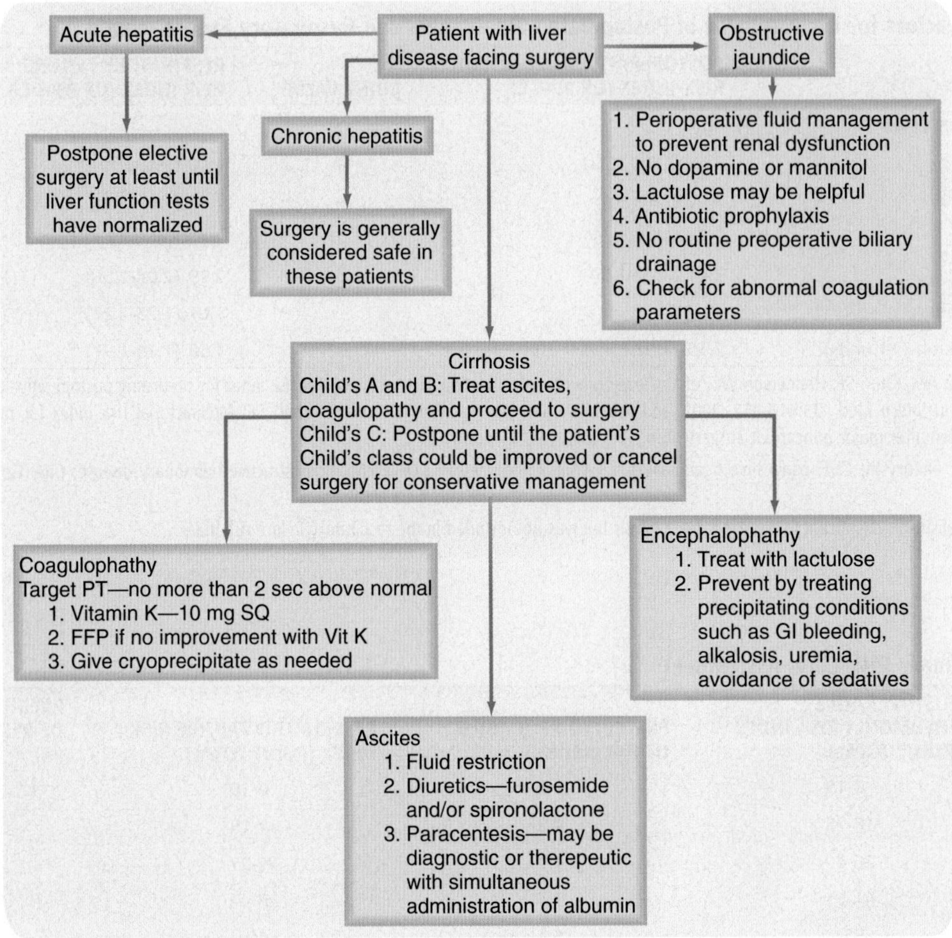


**FIGURE 11-2** Approach to a patient with liver disease. *FFP*, fresh-frozen plasma; *GI*, Gastrointestinal; *SQ*, subcutaneous. (Adapted from Rizvon MK, Chou CL: Surgery in the patient with liver disease. Med Clin North Am 87:211–227, 2003.)

may suggest a diagnosis of acute or chronic hepatitis, which can be investigated by serologic testing for hepatitis A, B, and C. Alcoholic hepatitis is suggested by lower transaminase levels and an aspartate aminotransferase-to-alanine transaminase ratio (AST/ALT) higher than 2. Laboratory evidence of chronic hepatitis or clinical findings consistent with cirrhosis is investigated with tests of hepatic synthetic function, notably serum albumin, prothrombin, and fibrinogen levels. Patients with evidence of impaired hepatic synthetic function also have a CBC and serum electrolyte analysis. Type and screen are indicated for any procedure in which blood loss could be more than minimal.

In the event of an emergency situation requiring surgery, such an investigation may not be possible. A patient with acute hepatitis and elevated transaminase levels is managed nonoperatively, when feasible, until several weeks beyond normalization of laboratory values. Urgent or emergency procedures in these patients are associated with increased morbidity and mortality. A patient with evidence of chronic hepatitis may often safely undergo surgery. A patient with cirrhosis may be assessed with the Child-Pugh classification, which stratifies operative risk according to a score based on abnormal albumin and bilirubin levels, prolongation of the prothrombin time (PT), and degree of ascites and encephalopathy (Table 11-7). This scoring system was initially used to predict mortality in cirrhotic patients undergoing portacaval shunt procedures, although it has been shown to correlate with mortality in cirrhotic patients undergoing a wider spectrum of procedures as well. Data generated more than 25 years ago showed that patients with Child class A, B, and C cirrhosis had mortality rates of 10%, 31%, and 76%, respectively, during abdominal operations; these figures have been validated more recently.[8] Although the figures may not represent current risk for all types of abdominal operations, little doubt exists that the presence of cirrhosis confers additional risk for abdominal surgery, proportional to the severity of disease. Other factors that affect outcomes in these patients are the emergency nature of a procedure, prolongation of the PT more than 3 seconds above normal and refractory to correction with vitamin K, and presence of infection.

Two common problems requiring surgical evaluation in a cirrhotic patient are hernia (umbilical and groin) and cholecystitis. An umbilical hernia in the presence of ascites is a difficult management problem because spontaneous rupture is associated with increased mortality rates. Elective repair is best after the ascites has been reduced to a minimum preoperatively, although the procedure is still associated with mortality rates as high as 14%. Repair of groin hernias in the presence of ascites is less risky in terms of recurrence and mortality.

**Table 11-7 Child-Pugh Scoring System**

| PARAMETER | Points 1 | 2 | 3 |
|---|---|---|---|
| Encephalopathy | None | Stage I or II | Stage III or IV |
| Ascites | Absent | Slight (controlled with diuretics) | Moderate despite diuretic treatment |
| Bilirubin (mg/dL) | <2 | 2-3 | >3 |
| Albumin (g/liter) | >3.5 | 2.8-3.5 | <2.8 |
| PT (prolonged seconds) | <4 | 4-6 | >6 |
| INR | <1.7 | 1.7-2.3 | >2.3 |

Class A, 5-6 points; class B, 7-9 points; class C, 10-15 points.
*INR*, International normalized ratio; *PT*, prothrombin time.

**Table 11-8 Insulin Types**

| TYPE OF INSULIN | ONSET OF ACTION | PEAK EFFECT | DURATION OF ACTION |
|---|---|---|---|
| Rapid acting (Lispro, NovoLog, Apidra) | 10-30 min | 30-90 min | 3-4 hr |
| Short-acting (Regular, Humulin, Novolin) | 30-60 min | 2-5 hr | 6-10 hr |
| Intermediate-acting (NPH, Lente) | 1-4 hr | 4-12 hr | 12-24 hr |
| Long-acting (Glargine [Lantus]) | 1-2 hr | 3-20 hr | 24-30 hr |

Adapted from Ahmed Z, Lockhart CH, Weiner M, et al: Advances in diabetic management: Implications for anesthesia. Anesth Analg 100:666–669, 2005.

Several reports have shown decreased rates of complication with laparoscopic procedures performed in cirrhotic patients. Among the best-described procedures is laparoscopic cholecystectomy performed in patients with Child class A through C. When compared with open cholecystectomy, lower morbidity in terms of blood loss and wound infection has been observed.[13a]

Malnutrition is common in cirrhotic patients and is associated with a reduction in hepatic glycogen stores and reduced hepatic protein synthesis. Patients with advanced liver disease often have a poor appetite, tense ascites, and abdominal pain. Attention must be given to appropriate enteral supplementation, as for all patients at significant nutritional risk.

## Endocrine System

A patient with an endocrine condition such as diabetes mellitus, hyperthyroidism or hypothyroidism, or adrenal insufficiency is subject to additional physiologic stress during surgery. The preoperative evaluation identifies the type and degree of endocrine dysfunction to permit preoperative optimization. Careful monitoring identifies signs of metabolic stress related to inadequate endocrine control during surgery and throughout the postoperative course.

### Perioperative Diabetic Management

The evaluation of a diabetic patient for surgery assesses the adequacy of glycemic control and identifies the presence of diabetic complications, which may have an impact on the patient's perioperative course. The patient's history and physical examination document evidence of diabetic complications, including cardiac disease, circulatory abnormalities, and presence of retinopathy, neuropathy, or nephropathy. Preoperative testing may include fasting and postprandial glucose and hemoglobin A1C levels. Serum electrolyte, blood urea nitrogen, and creatinine levels are determined to identify metabolic disturbances and renal involvement. Urinalysis may reveal proteinuria as evidence of diabetic nephropathy. An ECG is considered for patients with long-standing disease. The existence of neuropathy in diabetics may be accompanied by cardiac autonomic neuropathy, which increases the risk for cardiorespiratory instability in the perioperative period.

Management of diabetic patients has evolved in the last decade. The introduction of new drugs for non–insulin-dependent diabetics, in addition to new types of insulin and new insulin delivery systems in insulin-dependent diabetics, has changed how these patients are approached in the perioperative period.

Insulin is available in several types and is typically classified by its length of action (Table 11-8). Rapid- and short-acting insulin preparations are usually withheld when the patient stops oral intake and are used for acute management of hyperglycemia during the NPO period. Intermediate- and long-acting insulin preparations are administered at two thirds the normal evening dose the night before surgery and half the normal morning dose the day of surgery, with frequent bedside glucose determinations and treatment with short-acting insulin, as needed. An infusion of 5% dextrose is initiated the morning of surgery.

Insulin pumps are used by some patients as their method of glucose management. These pumps use short-acting insulin (Velosulin) and have a variable delivery rate that can be programmed to simulate endogenous insulin production more closely. On the day of surgery, the patient continues with the basal insulin infusion. The pump is then used to correct the glucose level as it is measured. Patients generally have a correction or sensitivity factor that will decrease their glucose by 50 mg/dL. It is important to know this factor before the planned surgical procedure so that glucose can be managed in the operating room.[14]

Patients who take oral hypoglycemic agents (sulfonylureas, such as chlorpropamide and glyburide) typically withhold their normal dose the day of surgery. Patients can resume their oral agent once diet is resumed. An exception is metformin. If the patient has altered renal function, this agent needs to be discontinued until renal function normalizes or stabilizes to avoid potential lactic acidosis.[15] Coverage for hyperglycemia is with a short-acting insulin preparation based on blood glucose monitoring.

### Management of Other Endocrinopathies

A patient with known or suspected thyroid disease is evaluated with a thyroid function panel, in particular the thyroid-stimulating hormone (TSH) level. Evidence of hyperthyroidism (very low TSH level) is addressed preoperatively and surgery is deferred until a euthyroid state has been achieved, when feasible. These patients need to have their electrolyte levels determined and an ECG performed as part of their preoperative evaluation. In addition, if the physical examination suggests signs of airway compromise from a large goiter, further imaging may be warranted. A patient with hyperthyroidism who takes antithyroid medication such as propylthiouracil or methimazole is instructed to continue this regimen on the day of surgery. The patient's usual doses of beta blockers or digoxin are also continued. In the event of urgent surgery in a thyrotoxic patient at risk for thyroid storm, a combination of adrenergic blockers and glucocorticoids may be required; these are administered in consultation with an endocrinologist. Patients with newly diagnosed hypothyroidism generally do not require preoperative treatment, although they may be subject to increased sensitivity to medications, including anesthetic agents and narcotics. Severe hypothyroidism (high TSH level) can be associated with myocardial dysfunction, coagulation abnormality, and electrolyte imbalance, notably hypoglycemia. Severe hypothyroidism needs to be corrected before elective operations. It should also be considered for a severely ill patient who is not recovering from surgery in a normal fashion.

A patient with a history of steroid use may require supplementation for a presumed abnormal adrenal response to perioperative stress (Box 11-1). Patients who have taken more than 5 mg of prednisone (or equivalent)/day for more than 3 weeks within the past year are considered at risk when undergoing major surgery. Lower doses of steroid or minor procedures are not generally associated with adrenal suppression.

The adequacy of the hypothalamic-pituitary response to adrenocorticotropic hormone (ACTH) can be tested in any patient who may have some degree of suppression secondary to chronic or intermittent steroid use. A low-dose (1 μg) ACTH stimulation test may demonstrate abnormal response to adrenal stimulation and suggest the need for perioperative steroid supplementation. Recent guidelines suggest titrating the dosage of glucocorticoid replacement to the degree of surgical stress (see Box 11-1). Minor operations such as hernia repair under local anesthesia may not require any additional steroid. Moderate operations such as open cholecystectomy or lower extremity revascularization require 50 to 75 mg/day of hydrocortisone equivalent for 1 or 2 days. Major operations such as colectomy or cardiac surgery are covered with 100 to 150 mg/day of hydrocortisone equivalent for 2 to 3 days. Inadequacy of the hypothalamic-pituitary-adrenal axis (HPAA) in the perioperative period can lead to unexplained hypotension.

Patients with pheochromocytoma require preoperative pharmacologic management to prevent intraoperative hypertensive crises or hypotension leading to cardiovascular collapse. The state of catecholamine excess associated with pheochromocytoma is controlled by a combination of α-adrenergic and β-adrenergic blockade before surgery. One to 2 weeks is generally required to achieve adequate therapeutic effect by alpha blockade; this can be accomplished with a nonselective agent such as phenoxybenzamine or a selective $\alpha_1$-adrenergic agent such as prazosin. Alpha blockade usually uncovers a vascular volume deficit that is not apparent clinically. In addition, patients have generally been placed on a sodium-restricted diet as part of their hypertension management. Liberalization of sodium in the diet may aid in replenishing plasma volume. Beta blockade is initiated several days after the α-adrenergic agent is begun and serves to inhibit the tachycardia that accompanies nonselective alpha blockade and to control arrhythmia. Patients with pheochromocytoma may undergo surgery when pharmacologic blood pressure control is achieved.

**BOX 11-1 Perioperative Supplemental Glucocorticoid Regimens**

**No HPAA Suppression**

Less than 5 mg of prednisone or equivalent/day for any duration

Alternate-day single morning dose of short-acting glucocorticoid of any dose or duration

Any dose of glucocorticoid for less than 3 wk

- Rx: Give the usual daily glucocorticoid dose during the perioperative period.

**HPAA Suppression Documented or Presumed**

More than 20 mg of prednisone or equivalent/day for 3 wk or longer

Cushingoid appearance

Biochemical adrenal insufficiency on a low-dose ACTH stimulation test

Minor procedures or local anesthesia

- Rx: Give the usual glucocorticoid dose before surgery.
- No supplementation unless signs or symptoms of adrenal insufficiency, then 25 mg hydrocortisone IV

Moderate surgical stress

- Rx: 50 mg hydrocortisone IV before induction of anesthesia, 25 mg hydrocortisone every 8 hr thereafter for 24-48 hr, then resume usual dose
- Major surgical stress
- Rx: 100 mg hydrocortisone IV before induction of anesthesia, 50 mg hydrocortisone every 8 hr thereafter for 48-72 hr, then resume usual dose

**HPAA Suppression Uncertain**

5-20 mg of prednisone or its equivalent for 3 wk or longer

5 mg or more of prednisone or its equivalent for 3 wk or more in the year before surgery

Minor procedures or local anesthesia

- Rx: Give the usual glucocorticoid dose before surgery.
- No supplementation

Moderate or major surgical stress

- Check the low-dose ACTH stimulation test to determine HPA axis suppression, or
- Give supplemental glucocorticoids as though suppressed.

Adapted from Schiff RL, Welsh GA: Perioperative evaluation and management of the patient with endocrine dysfunction. Med Clin North Am 87:175–192, 2003; and Kohl, BA, Schwartz S: Surgery in the patient with endocrine dysfunction. Med Clin North Am 93:1031–1047, 2009.

## Immune System

The approach to a patient with suspected immunosuppression is the same, regardless of whether this state results from antineoplastic drugs in a cancer patient or immunosuppressive therapy in a transplant patient, or is the result of advanced disease in patients with acquired immunodeficiency syndrome. The goal is to optimize immunologic function before surgery and to minimize the risk for infection and wound breakdown.

Preoperative assessment includes the following: a thorough history of the patient's underlying disease and current functional status; a history of immunosuppressive treatment, including names of medications and duration of treatment; and a history of recent changes in weight. The physical examination seeks to document any signs of organ dysfunction that may underlie progression of the disease or be related to its treatment. Laboratory assessment includes a CBC with differential and platelet count, electrolyte determination, and liver function tests; an ECG and chest radiograph are obtained when age or physical findings suggest risk. Possible sites of infection must be investigated, including examination of any indwelling catheters, and a complete workup of any suspected infectious focus may be warranted. Additional studies of T cell, B cell, polymorphonuclear, or complement function may be helpful to delineate the degree of immune system compromise. Neutropenia, anemia, or thrombocytopenia may accompany the underlying disease process or result from treatment of the condition with immunosuppressive medication. Decisions regarding red blood cell transfusion or the use of synthetic erythropoietin or colony-stimulating factors are often based on the degree of dysfunction and other patient risk factors. Careful attention is paid to nutritional deficiency in this patient population, with supplementation indicated in the perioperative period. Appropriate antibiotic prophylaxis is critical.

Immunocompromised patients may be at risk for wound complications, especially if they are receiving exogenous steroid therapy. When taken within 3 days of surgery, steroids reduce the degree of wound inflammation, epithelialization, and collagen synthesis, which can lead to wound breakdown and infection. In addition, patients receiving sirolimus as part of their antirejection protocol can have difficulties with wound healing, so this drug should be discontinued if possible prior to operation.

### Human Immunodeficiency Virus–Infected Patients and Surgery

As morbidity and mortality continue to decrease with improved medical management of human immunodeficiency virus (HIV) infection, more HIV-infected patients are requiring surgery. It is important to understand how the agents used to treat HIV will affect the patient during surgery.

HIV treatment involves antiretroviral drugs from one of four classes: protease inhibitors, fusion inhibitors, nucleoside-nucleotide reverse transcriptase inhibitors (NRTIs), and non-nucleoside reverse transcriptase inhibitors (NNRTIs). It is important to note that these agents are not immunosuppressive agents but work directly on the pathway of HIV cell integration and reproduction. For this reason, they do not have a significant effect on wound healing or infection rates. The patient's white blood cell count or, more specifically, the absolute neutrophil count, in addition to the direct HIV titer, is more predictive of postoperative complications. One specific finding with NRTIs is that of lactic acidosis as a result of mitochondrial toxicity.[16] This condition needs to be added to the differential diagnosis of a critically ill patient with known HIV infection who has a persistently elevated lactate concentration. Hypoperfusion is ruled out initially, but drug complication needs to be investigated. Treatment is discontinuation of the agent.

## Hematologic System

Hematologic assessment may lead to the identification of disorders such as anemia, inherited or acquired coagulopathy, or a hypercoagulable state. Substantial morbidity may result from failure to identify these abnormalities preoperatively. The need for perioperative prophylaxis for venous thromboembolism must be carefully reviewed in every surgical patient.

Anemia is the most common laboratory abnormality encountered in preoperative patients. It is often asymptomatic and can require further investigation to understand its cause. The history and physical examination may uncover subjective complaints of energy loss, dyspnea, or palpitations, and pallor or cyanosis may be evident. Patients are evaluated for lymphadenopathy, hepatomegaly, or splenomegaly, and pelvic and rectal examinations are performed. A CBC, reticulocyte count, and serum iron, total iron-binding capacity, ferritin, vitamin $B_{12}$, and folate levels are obtained to investigate the cause of anemia. Preoperative treatment and optimization are appropriate for an anemic patient. The decision to transfuse a patient perioperatively is made with consideration of the patient's underlying risk factors for ischemic heart disease, estimated magnitude of blood loss during surgery, and potential for improving or worsening outcomes after surgery with a preoperative transfusion. Generally, patients with normovolemic anemia without significant cardiac risk or anticipated blood loss can be managed safely without transfusion, with most healthy patients tolerating hemoglobin levels of 6 or 7 g/dL (Box 11-2).[17]

All patients undergoing surgery are questioned to assess their bleeding risk. Coagulopathy may result from inherited or acquired platelet or factor disorders or may be associated with organ dysfunction or medications. The inquiry begins with direct questioning about a personal or family history of abnormal bleeding. Supporting information includes a history of easy bruising or abnormal bleeding associated with minor procedures or injury. A history of liver or kidney dysfunction or recent common bile duct obstruction needs to be elicited, as well as an assessment of nutritional status. Medications are carefully reviewed, and the use of anticoagulants, salicylates, nonsteroidal anti-inflammatory drugs (NSAIDs), and antiplatelet drugs are noted. Physical examination may reveal bruising, petechiae, or signs of liver dysfunction. Patients with thrombocytopenia may have qualitative or quantitative defects as a result of immune-related disease, infection, drugs, or liver or kidney dysfunction. Qualitative defects may respond to medical management of the underlying disease process, whereas quantitative defects may

**BOX 11-2 Guidelines for Red Blood Cell Transfusion for Acute Blood Loss**

- Evaluate the risk for ischemia.
- Estimate or anticipate the degree of blood loss. Less than 30% rapid volume loss probably does not require transfusion in a previously healthy individual.
- Measure the hemoglobin concentration: <6 g/dL, transfusion usually required; 6-10 g/dL, transfusion dictated by clinical circumstance; >10 g/dL, transfusion rarely required.
- Measure vital signs and tissue oxygenation when hemoglobin is 6-10 g/dL and the extent of blood loss is unknown. Tachycardia and hypotension refractory to volume suggest the need for transfusion; $O_2$ extraction ratio <50% and decreased $V_{O_2}$ suggest that transfusion is usually needed.

Adapted from Simon TL, Alverson DC, AuBuchon J, et al: Practice parameters for the use of red blood cell transfusions: Developed by the Red Blood Cell Administration Practice Guideline Development Task Force of the College of American Pathologists. Arch Pathol Lab Med 122:130–138, 1998.

**Table 11-9 Recommendations for Perioperative Management of Patients Taking Chronic Anticoagulation**

| INDICATION FOR CHRONIC ANTICOAGULATION | PATIENT CHARACTERISTICS | PERIOPERATIVE MANAGEMENT |
|---|---|---|
| Prosthetic heart valves | High risk<br>Recent (<1 mo) stroke or transient ischemic attack (TIA)<br>Any mitral valve<br>Caged ball or tilting disc aortic valve | Strongly recommend bridging |
| | Moderate risk—bileaflet aortic valve with two or more risk factors for stroke* | Consider bridging |
| | Low risk—bileaflet aortic valve with fewer than two risk factors for stroke* | Bridging optional |
| Chronic atrial fibrillation | High risk<br>Recent stroke or TIA<br>Rheumatic mitral valve disease | Strongly recommend bridging |
| | Moderate risk—chronic atrial fibrillation with two or more risk factors for stroke* | Consider bridging |
| | Low risk—chronic atrial fibrillation with fewer than two risk factors for stroke* | Bridging optional |
| Venous thromboembolism | High risk<br>Recent (≤3 wk) VTE<br>Active (<6 mo or palliative) cancer<br>Antiphospholipid antibody†<br>Major comorbid disease (cardiac or pulmonary) | Strongly recommend bridging |
| | Moderate risk<br>VTE in last 6 mo<br>VTE with interruption of anticoagulation | Consider bridging |
| | Low risk—none of the above | Bridging optional |

Adapted from Douketis JD, Berger PB, Dunn AS, et al: The perioperative management of antithrombotic therapy: American College of Chest Physicians Evidence-Based Clinical Practice Guidelines (8th Edition). Chest 133:299S–339S, 2008.

*Risk factors for stroke: atrial fibrillation, previous stroke, TIA, or systemic embolism; age >75 yr; hypertension, diabetes mellitus, left ventricular dysfunction.

†Antiphospholipid antibodies—anticardiolipin antibody, lupus anticoagulant.

require platelet transfusion when counts are lower than 50,000/mL in a patient at risk for bleeding. Coagulation studies are not routinely ordered, but patients with a history suggestive of coagulopathy should undergo coagulation studies before surgery. Coagulation studies are also carried out before the procedure if considerable bleeding is anticipated or any significant bleeding would be catastrophic. Patients with documented disorders of coagulation may require perioperative management of factor deficiencies, often in consultation with a hematologist.

Patients receiving anticoagulation therapy usually require preoperative reversal of the anticoagulant effect, most times bridging the patient with low-molecular-weight heparin (LMWH). In patients taking warfarin, the drug is withheld for five scheduled doses preoperatively to allow the international normalized ratio (INR) to fall to the range of 1.5 or less, assuming that the patient is maintained at an INR of 2.0 to 3.0. For all but those procedures that carry a high risk of postoperative bleeding, warfarin can be restarted the day of or day after surgery because it will take up to five doses to become therapeutic. Additional recommendations for specific diagnoses requiring chronic anticoagulation are based on risk-benefit analysis. Patients at high risk for a thromboembolic event while off chronic anticoagulation (e.g., recent venous thromboembolism, stroke or transient ischemic attack; valvular heart disease with risk of stroke; or acute arterial embolism) are strongly recommended to have full bridging while off their warfarin. This may be therapeutic dose LMWH or perioperative IV heparinization. For those on LMWH, it is recommended to give the last dose 20 to 24 hours prior to surgery, restarted approximately 12 to 24 hours postoperatively. For those requiring systemic heparinization, it should be stopped within 6 hours of surgery and restarted within 12 to 24 hours postoperatively. For procedures with a high risk of postoperative bleeding, or in which large surfaces have been dissected, consider using prophylactic-dose LMWH for the dosing regimen for several days and then switch back to therapeutic dosing. When possible, surgery is postponed in the first month after an episode of venous or arterial thromboembolism. Patients taking anticoagulants for less than 2 weeks for pulmonary embolism (PE) or proximal deep venous thrombosis (DVT), or those for whom the risk of perioperative bleeding is high, should be considered for retrievable inferior vena cava filter placement before surgery (Table 11-9).[18,19]

All surgical patients are assessed for their risk for venous thromboembolism and receive adequate prophylaxis according to current guidelines (Table 11-10).[20,21] Patients are questioned to elicit any personal or family history suggestive of a hypercoagulable state. Levels of protein C, protein S, antithrombin III, and antiphospholipid antibody can be determined. Risk factor stratification is achieved by considering a number of factors, including age, type of surgical procedure, previous thromboembolism, cancer, obesity, varicose veins, cardiac dysfunction, indwelling central venous catheters, inflammatory bowel disease, nephrotic syndrome, pregnancy, and estrogen or tamoxifen use. A number of regimens may be appropriate for the prophylaxis of venous thromboembolism, depending on assessed risk coupled with the perceived risk of perioperative bleeding. These include the use of unfractionated heparin, LMWH, intermittent compression devices, and early ambulation. Initial prophylactic doses of heparin can be given preoperatively, within 2 hours of surgery, and with compression devices in place before induction of anesthesia. For very high-risk patients (orthopedic procedures, multiple risk factors),

**Table 11-10 Levels of Risk for Thromboembolism in Surgical Patients Without Prophylaxis and Successful Prevention Strategies**

| LEVEL OF RISK | DEFINITION OF RISK LEVEL | CALF DVT (%) | PROXIMAL DVT (%) | CLINICAL PE (%) | FATAL PE (%) | PREVENTION STRATEGY |
|---|---|---|---|---|---|---|
| Low | Minor surgery in patients <40 yr with no additional risk factors | 2 | 0.4 | 0.2 | 0.002 | Aggressive, early mobilization |
| Moderate | Minor surgery in patients with additional risk factors; nonmajor surgery in patients 40-60 yr with no additional risk factors; major surgery in patients <40 yr with no additional risk factors | 10-20 | 2-4 | 1-2 | 0.1-0.4 | Graded compression stockings; IPC; LDUH, 5000 U q12h; LMWH—enoxaparin, 40 mg/day SC; daltaparin, 5000 IU/day SC; factor Xa inhibitor (Fondaparinux, 2.5 mg/day SC) |
| High | Nonmajor surgery in patients >60 yr or with additional risk factors; major surgery in patients >40 yr or with additional risk factors | 20-40 | 4-8 | 2-4 | 0.4-1.0 | LDUH 5000 U q8h; LMWH—enoxaparin 40 mg/day SC; daltaparin, 5000 IU/day SC; factor Xa inhibitor (Fondaparinux, 2.5 mg/day SC); combined IPC plus anticoagulant strategy above |
| For moderate- and high-risk patients, initiate pharmacologic prophylaxis within 12-24 hr after procedure for 7-10 days | | | | | | |
| Very high risk | Major surgery in patients >40 yr plus previous VTE, cancer, or molecular hypercoagulable state; hip or knee arthroplasty, hip fracture surgery, major trauma, spinal cord injury | 40-80 | 10-20 | 4-10 | 0.2-5 | LDUH, 5000 U q8h; LMWH—enoxaparin, 40 mg/d SC; daltaparin, 5000 IU/day SC; tinzaparin, 3500 IU/day SC); factor Xa inhibitor (Fondaparinux, 2.5 mg/day SC); combined IPC plus anticoagulant strategy above |
| For very high-risk patients, initiate pharmacologic prophylaxis 2-12 hr before or 12-24 hr after procedure. Continue for at least 7-10 days. Consideration should be given to continuing for 4 wk postoperatively in those not requiring chronic anticoagulation. If the bleeding risk posed by the operation is high, consider placement of a removable IVC filter preoperatively for patients with current DVT. | | | | | | |

Adapted from Geerts WH, Heit JA, Clagett GP, et al: Prevention of venous thromboembolism. Chest 119:132S–175S, 2001. and Muntz JE and Michota FA: Prevention and management of venous thromboembolism in the surgical patient: Options by surgery type and individual patient risk factors. Am J Surg 1991A:S11–S20, 2010.

*ES*, Elastic stockings; *IPC*, intermittent pneumatic compression; *LDUH*, low-dose unfractionated heparin.

continuation of venous thromboembolism (VTE) prophylaxis may be considered after discharge from the hospital.

## ADDITIONAL PREOPERATIVE CONSIDERATIONS

### Age

Older adults account for a disproportionate percentage of surgical patients. Risk assessment must carefully consider the effect of comorbid illness in this population. Although age has been reported as an independent risk factor for postoperative mortality, this observation may represent the unmeasured aspects of comorbid disease, the severity of illness and, perhaps, limited reserve.

In an older adult patient, the preoperative evaluation seeks to identify and quantify the magnitude of comorbid disease and optimize the patient's condition before surgery, when possible. Preoperative testing is based on findings suggested in the history and physical examination. Generally, older patients have an ECG, chest radiograph, CBC, and determination of glucose, creatinine, blood urea nitrogen, and albumin levels. Additional preoperative studies are based on the criteria discussed earlier for the evaluation of patient and procedural risk.

Predicting and preventing postoperative delirium are important aspects of the perioperative care of older adults. Patients with three or more of the following factors have a 50% risk for postoperative delirium: 70 years or older; self-reported alcohol abuse; poor cognitive status; poor functional status; markedly abnormal preoperative serum sodium, potassium, and/or glucose level; noncardiac thoracic surgery; and aortic aneurysm surgery.[22] This risk is explained to the patient and family, along with the symptoms of postoperative delirium. If delirium does occur, metabolic and infectious causes need to be investigated before labeling the event as sundowning.

### Nutritional Status

Evaluation of the patient's nutritional status is part of the preoperative evaluation. A history of weight loss greater than 10% of body weight over a 6-month period or 5% over a 1-month period is significant. Albumin or prealbumin levels may help identify patients with some degree of malnutrition, and physical findings of temporal wasting, cachexia, poor dentition, ascites, or peripheral edema may be corroborative. The degree of malnutrition is estimated on the basis of weight loss, physical findings, and plasma protein level assessment. The adequacy of a nutritional regimen can be confirmed with a number of serum markers. Albumin (half-life, 14 to 18 days), transferrin (half-life, 7 days), and prealbumin (half-life, 3 to 5 days) levels can be determined on a regular basis in hospitalized patients. These proteins are responsive to stress conditions, however, and their synthesis may be inhibited in the immediate perioperative period. Once a patient is on a stable regimen and in the anabolic phase of recovery, these markers reflect the adequacy of nutritional efforts.

The effect of perioperative nutritional support on outcomes has been studied in a number of trials. Patients with severe malnutrition—as defined by a combination of weight loss, visceral protein indicators, and prognostic indices—appear to benefit most from preoperative nutrition (enteral, if possible). Well-nourished patients undergoing surgery do not appear to

**Table 11-11 National Research Council Classification of Operative Wounds and Rates of Wound Infection**

| CLASSIFICATION | FEATURES | RATE OF INFECTION (%) |
|---|---|---|
| Clean (class I) | Nontraumatic<br>No inflammation<br>No break in technique<br>Respiratory, alimentary, or genitourinary tract not entered | 2.1 |
| Clean-contaminated (class II) | Gastrointestinal or respiratory tract entered without significant spillage | 3.3 |
| Contaminated (class III) | Major break in technique<br>Gross spillage from the gastrointestinal tract<br>Traumatic wound, fresh<br>Entrance into the genitourinary or biliary tracts in the presence of infected urine or bile | 6.4 |
| Dirty and infected (class IV) | Acute bacterial inflammation encountered, without pus<br>Transection of "clean" tissue for the purpose of surgical access to a collection of pus<br>Traumatic wound with retained devitalized tissue, foreign bodies, fecal contamination, or delayed treatment, or all of these, or from a dirty source | 7.1 |

Adapted from Kumar S, Leaper DJ: Classification and management of acute wounds. Surgery (Oxford) 23(2):47–51, 2005.

benefit from aggressive perioperative nutritional support. Generally, nutritional support begins within 5 to 10 days after surgery in patients unable to resume their normal diet. The exception to this is trauma victims (including those with burns) who, because of their general catabolic state, benefit from much earlier commencement of nutritional support if it is anticipated that they will not be able to manage oral intake within a few days. For all patients, an enteral route of feeding is preferred; however, in circumstances in which the patient cannot tolerate enteral feeds or they are contraindicated, the parenteral route is used.

### Obesity

The perioperative mortality rate is significantly increased in patients with clinically severe obesity (body mass index [BMI] <40 kg/m$^2$, or BMI <35 kg/m$^2$ with significant comorbid conditions). The goal of preoperative evaluation of an obese patient is to identify risk factors that might modify perioperative care of the patient. Clinically severe obesity is associated with a higher frequency of essential hypertension, pulmonary hypertension, left ventricular hypertrophy, congestive heart failure, and ischemic heart disease. Patients with none or one of these risk factors receive a beta blocker preoperatively for cardioprotection. Patients with two or more risk factors undergo noninvasive cardiac testing preoperatively.[23]

Obesity is also a risk factor for postoperative wound infection. The rate of wound infections is much lower with laparoscopic surgery in this group, which could have a bearing on selection of the operative approach. Obesity is an independent risk factor for DVT and PE; therefore, appropriate prophylaxis is instituted in these patients.

## PREOPERATIVE CHECKLIST

The preoperative evaluation concludes with a review of all pertinent studies and information obtained from investigative tests. This review is documented in the chart, which represents an opportunity to ensure that all necessary and pertinent data have been obtained and appropriately interpreted. Informed consent after discussion with the patient and family members regarding the indication for the anticipated surgical procedure, as well as its risks and proposed benefits, are documented in the chart. The preoperative checklist also gives the surgeon an opportunity to review the need for beta blockade, DVT prophylaxis, and prophylactic antibiotics.

Preoperative orders are written and reviewed. The patient receives written instructions regarding the time of surgery and management of special perioperative issues such as fasting, bowel preparation, and medication use.

### Antibiotic Prophylaxis

Appropriate antibiotic prophylaxis in surgery depends on the most likely pathogens encountered during the surgical procedure. The type of operative procedure (Table 11-11) is helpful for deciding the appropriate antibiotic spectrum and is considered before ordering or administering any preoperative medication. Prophylactic antibiotics are not generally required for clean (class I) cases, except in the setting of indwelling prosthesis placement, or when bone is incised. Patients who undergo class II procedures benefit from a single dose of an appropriate antibiotic administered before the skin incision. For abdominal (hepatobiliary, pancreatic, gastroduodenal) cases, cefazolin is generally used. Contaminated (class III) cases require mechanical preparation or parenteral antibiotics with aerobic and anaerobic activity. Such an approach is taken in the setting of emergency abdominal surgery, as for suspected appendicitis, and in trauma cases. Dirty or infected cases often require the same antibiotic spectrum, which can be continued into the postoperative period in the setting of ongoing infection or delayed treatment.

The appropriate antibiotic is chosen before surgery and administered before the skin incision is made (Table 11-12).[24] Repeat dosing occurs at an appropriate interval, usually 3 hours for abdominal cases or twice the half-life of the antibiotic, although the patient's renal function may alter the timing (Table 11-13).[25] Perioperative antibiotic prophylaxis generally is not continued beyond the day of surgery. With the advent of minimal access surgery, the use of antibiotics seems less justified because the risk for wound infection is extremely low. For example, routine antibiotic prophylaxis in patients undergoing laparoscopic cholecystectomy for uncomplicated symptomatic cholelithiasis is of questionable value. It may have a role, however, in cases that result in prosthetic graft (i.e., mesh) placement, such as laparoscopic hernia repair.

**Table 11-12 Antimicrobial Prophylaxis for Surgery**

| NATURE OF OPERATION | COMMON PATHOGENS | RECOMMENDED ANTIMICROBIALS | ADULT DOSAGE BEFORE SURGERY[a] |
|---|---|---|---|
| Cardiac | *Staphylococcus aureus, S. epidermidis* | Cefazolin *or*<br>Vancomycin[c] | 1-2 g IV[b]<br>1 g IV |
| **Gastrointestinal** | | | |
| Esophageal, gastroduodenal | Enteric gram-negative bacilli, gram-positive cocci | *High risk*[d] *only:* Cefazolin[g] | 1-2 g IV |
| Biliary tract | Enteric gram-negative bacilli, enterococci, clostridia | *High risk*[e] *only:* Cefazolin[g] | 1-2 g IV |
| Colorectal | Enteric gram-negative bacilli, anaerobes, enterococci | *Oral:* Neomycin + erythromycin base[f] *or*<br>Metronidazole[f]<br>*Parenteral:* Cefoxitin[g] *or*<br>Cefazolin *plus*<br>Metronidazole[g] *or*<br>Ampicillin-sulbactam | <br><br>1-2 g IV<br>1-2 g IV<br>0.5 g IV<br>3 g IV |
| Appendectomy, nonperforated[h] | Enteric gram-negative bacilli, anaerobes, enterococci | Cefoxitin[g] *or*<br>Cefazolin plus<br>Metronidazole[g] *or*<br>Ampicillin-sulbactam | 1-2 g IV<br>1-2 g IV<br>0.5 g IV<br>3 g IV |
| Genitourinary | Enteric gram-negative bacilli, enterococci | *High risk*[i] *only:* Ciprofloxacin | 500 mg PO or 400 mg IV |
| **Gynecologic and Obstetric** | | | |
| Vaginal, abdominal, or laparoscopic hysterectomy | Enteric gram-negative bacilli, anaerobes, group B streptocci, enterococci | Cefoxitin[g] *or* cefazolin[g] *or*<br>Ampicillin-sulbactam[g] | 1-2 g IV<br>3 g IV |
| Cesarean section | Same as for hysterectomy | Cefazolin[g] | 1-2 g IV after cord clamping |
| Abortion | Same as for hysterectomy | *First trimester, high risk*[j]: Aqueous penicillin G *or*<br>Doxycycline<br>*Second trimester:* Cefazolin[g] | 2 million U IV<br>300 mg PO[k]<br>1-2 g IV |
| **Head and Neck Surgery** | | | |
| Incisions through oral or pharyngeal mucosa | Anaerobes, enteric gram-negative bacilli, *S. aureus* | Clindamycin<br><br>Cefazolin + metronidazole | 600-900 mg IV<br>1-2 mg IV<br>0.5 g IV |
| **Neurosurgery** | *S. aureus, S. epidermidis* | Cefazolin *or*<br>Vancomycin[c] | 1-2 g IV<br>1 g IV |
| **Ophthalmic** | *S. epidermidis, S. aureus,* streptococci, enteric gram-negative bacilli, *Pseudomonas* spp. | Gentamicin, tobramycin, ciprofloxacin, gatifloxacin, levofloxacin, moxifloxacin, ofloxacin, or neomycin-gramicidin-polymyxin B<br>Cefazolin | Multiple drops topically over 2 to 24 hr<br><br>100 mg subconjunctivally |
| **Orthopedic** | *S. aureus, S. epidermidis* | Cefazolin[l] or<br>Cefuroxime[l] *or*<br>Vancomycin[c,l] | 1-2 g IV<br>1.5 g IV<br>1 g IV |
| **Thoracic (noncardiac)** | *S. aureus, S. epidermidis,* streptococci, enteric gram-negative bacilli | Cefazolin *or*<br>Cefuroxime *or*<br>Vancomycin[c] | 1-2 g IV<br>1.5 g IV<br>1 g IV |
| **Vascular** | | | |
| Arterial surgery involving prosthesis, abdominal aorta, or groin incision | *S. aureus, S. epidermidis,* enteric gram-negative bacilli | Cefazolin *or*<br>Vancomycin[c] | 1-2 g IV<br>1 g IV |
| Lower extremity amputation for ischemia | *S. aureus, S. epidermidis,* enteric gram-negative bacilli, clostridia | Cefazolin *or*<br>Vancomycin[c] | 1-2 g IV<br>1 g IV |

Treatment guidelines from the Medical Letter 7(82):47–52, 2009.

[a]Parenteral prophylactic antimicrobials can be given as a single IV dose begun 60 min or less before the operation. For prolonged operations (>4 hr) or those with major blood loss, additional intraoperative doses should be given at intervals one to two times the half-life of the drug for the duration of the procedure in patients with normal renal function. If vancomycin or a fluoroquinolone is used, the infusion should be started 60-120 min before the initial incision to minimize the possibility of an infusion reaction close to the time of induction of anesthesia and to have adequate tissue levels at the time of incision.

[b]Some consultants recommend an additional dose when patients are removed from bypass during open heart surgery.

[c]Vancomycin is used in hospitals in which methicillin-resistant *S. aureus* (MRSA) and *S. epidermidis* are frequent causes of postoperative wound infection, for patients previously colonized with MRSA, or for those who are allergic to penicillins or cephalosporins. Rapid IV administration may cause hypotension, which could be especially dangerous during induction of anesthesia. Even when the drug is given over 50 min, hypotension may occur; treatment with diphenhydramine (e.g., Benadryl) and further slowing of the infusion rate may be helpful. Some experts would give 15 mg/kg of vancomycin to patients weighing more than 75 kg, up to a maximum of 1.5 g, with a slower infusion rate (90 min for 1.5 g). To provide coverage against gram-negative bacteria, most *Medical Letter* consultants would also include cefazolin or cefuroxime in the prophylaxis regimen for patients not allergic to cephalosporins, ciprofloxacin, levofloxacin, gentamicin, or aztreonam, each one in combination with vancomycin, which can be used in patients who cannot tolerate a cephalosporin.

[d]Morbid obesity, esophageal obstruction, decreased gastric acidity, or gastrointestinal motility.

[e]Age >70 yr, acute cholecystitis, nonfunctioning gallbladder, obstructive jaundice, or common duct stones.

[f]After appropriate diet and catharsis, 1 g of neomycin plus 1 g of erythromycin at 1 PM, 2 PM, and 11 PM or 2 g of neomycin plus 2 g of metronidazole at 7 PM and 11 PM the day before an 8 AM operation.

[g]For patients allergic to penicillins and cephalosporins, clindamycin with gentamicin, ciprofloxacin, levofloxacin, or aztreonam is a reasonable alternative.

[h]For a ruptured viscus, therapy is often continued for approximately 5 days. Ruptured viscus in a postoperative setting (dehiscence) requires antibacterials to include coverage of nosocomial pathogens.

[i]Urine culture positive or unavailable, preoperative catheter, transrectal prostatic biopsy, placement of prosthetic material.

[j]Patients with previous pelvic inflammatory disease, previous gonorrhea, or multiple sex partners.

[k]Divided into 100 mg 1 hr before the abortion and 200 mg ½ hour after the abortion.

[l]If a tourniquet is to be used in the procedure, the entire dose of antibiotic must be infused prior to its inflation.

**Table 11-13 Suggested Initial Dose and Time Until Redosing of Antimicrobial Drugs Commonly Used for Surgical Prophylaxis**

| | Renal Half-Life (HR) | | | | | |
|---|---|---|---|---|---|---|
| **ANTIMICROBIAL** | **PATIENTS WITH NORMAL RENAL FUNCTION** | **PATIENTS WITH END-STAGE RENAL DISEASE** | **RECOMMENDED INFUSION DURATION** | **STANDARD DOSE** | **WEIGHT-BASED DOSE RECOMMENDATION**[a] | **RECOMMENDED REDOSING INTERVAL**[b] **(hr)** |
| Aztreonam | 1.5-2 | 6 | 3-5 min,[c] 20-60 min[d] | 1-2 g IV | 2 g maximum (adults) | 3-5 |
| Ciprofloxacin | 3.5-5 | 5-9 | 60 min | 400 mg IV | 400 mg | 4-10 |
| Cefazolin | 1.2-2.5 | 40-70 | 3-5 min,[c] 15-60 min[d] | 1-2 g IV | 20-30 mg/kg (if <80 kg, use 1 g; if >80 kg, use 2 g) | 2-5 |
| Cefuroxime | 1-2 | 15-22 | 3-5 min,[c] 15-60 min[d] | 1.5 g IV | 50 mg/kg | 3-4 |
| Cefamandole | 0.5-2.1 | 12.3-18[e] | 3-5 min,[c] 15-60 min[d] | 1 g IV | | 3-4 |
| Cefoxitin | 0.5-1.1 | 6.5-23 | 3-5 min,[c] 15-60 min[d] | 1-2 g IV | 20-40 mg/kg | 2-3 |
| Cefotetan | 2.8-4.6 | 13-25 | 3-5 min,[c] 20-60 min[d] | 1-2 g IV | 20-40 mg/kg | 3-6 |
| Clindamycin | 2-5.1 | 3.5-5.0[f] | 10-60 min (do not exceed 30 mg/min) | 600-900 mg IV | If <10 kg, use at least 37.5 mg; if >10 kg, use 3-6 mg/kg | 3-6 |
| Erythromycin base[h] | 0.8-3 | 5-6 | NA | 1 g PO 19, 18, and 9 hr before surgery | 9-13 mg/kg | NA |
| Gentamicin | 2-3 | 50-70 | 30-60 min | 1.5 mg/kg IV[g] | —[g] | 3-6 |
| Neomycin[h] | 2-3 (3% absorbed under normal gastrointestinal conditions) | 12-24 or longer | NA | 1 g PO 19, 18, and 9 hr before surgery | 20 mg/kg | NA |
| Metronidazole | 6-14 | 7-21; no change | 30-60 min | 0.5-1 g IV | 15-mg/kg initial dose (adult); 7.5 mg/kg on subsequent doses | 6-8 |
| Vancomycin | 4-6 | 44.1-406.4 ($C_{Cr}$ <10 mL/min) | 1 g over 60-min period (use longer infusion time if dose >1 g) | 1 g IV | 10-15 mg/kg (adult) | 6-12 |

Adapted from Bratzler DW, Honck PM: Antimicrobial prophlyaxis for surgery: An advisory statement from the National Surgical Infection Prevention Project. Clin Inf Dis 38:1706–1715, 2004.

$C_{Cr}$, Creatinine clearance rate.

[a]Data are primarily from published pediatric recommendations.

[b]For procedures of long duration, antimicrobials should be readministered at intervals of one to two times the half-life of the drug. The intervals in the table were calculated for patients with normal renal function.

[c]Dose injected directly into a vein or via running intravenous fluids.

[d]Intermittent intravenous infusion.

[e]In patients with a serum creatinine level of 5 to 9 mg/dL.

[f]The half-life of clindamycin is the same or slightly increased in patients with end-stage renal disease as in those with normal renal function.

[g]If a patient's body weight is more than 30% higher than ideal body weight (IBW), the dosing weight (DW) can be determined as follows: DW = IBW = 0.4 × (*IBW*, total body weight).

[h]Routine oral antibiotic preparation can be omitted in most operations on the colon if IV antibiotics are used.

## Review of Medications

Careful review of the patient's home medications is part of the preoperative evaluation before any operation; the goal is to use medications that control the patient's medical illnesses appropriately while minimizing the risk associated with anesthetic-drug interactions or the hematologic or metabolic effects of some commonly used medications and therapies. The patient is asked to name all medications, including psychiatric drugs, hormones, and alternative or herbal medications, and to provide dosages and frequency.

In general, patients taking cardiac drugs, including beta blockers and antiarrhythmics, pulmonary drugs such as inhaled or nebulized medications, or anticonvulsants, antihypertensives, or psychiatric drugs are advised to take their medications with a sip of water on the morning of surgery. Parenteral forms or substitutes are available for many drugs and may be used if the patient remains NPO for any significant period postoperatively. It is important to return patients to their normal medication regimen as soon as possible. Two notable examples are the additional cardiovascular morbidity associated with the perioperative discontinuation of beta blockers and rebound hypertension with abrupt cessation of the antihypertensive clonidine. Medications such as lipid-lowering agents or vitamins can be omitted on the day of surgery.

Some drugs are associated with an increased risk for perioperative bleeding and are withheld before surgery. Drugs that affect platelet function are withheld for variable periods; aspirin and clopidogrel (Plavix) are withheld for 7 to 10 days, whereas NSAIDs are withheld between 1 day (ibuprofen and indomethacin) and 3 days (naproxen and sulindac), depending on the drug's half-life. Because the use of estrogen and tamoxifen has been associated with an increased risk for thromboembolism, they probably need to be withheld for a period of 4 weeks preoperatively.[26]

The widespread use of herbal medications has prompted review of the effects of some commonly used preparations and their potential adverse outcomes during the perioperative period. These substances may fail to be recorded in the preoperative evaluation, although important metabolic and hematologic effects can result from their regular use (Table 11-14).[27] Generally, the use of herbal medications is stopped preoperatively, but this needs to be done with caution in patients who report the use of valerian, which may be associated with a benzodiazepine-like withdrawal syndrome.

## Preoperative Fasting

The standard order of "NPO past midnight" for preoperative patients is based on the theory of reduction of volume and acidity of the stomach contents during surgery. Guidelines have recommended a shift to allow a period of restricted fluid intake for up to a few hours before surgery. The ASA recommends that adults stop intake of solids for at least 6 hours and clear fluids for 2 hours. When the literature was reviewed by the Cochrane group, they found 22 trials in healthy adults that provided 38 controlled comparisons.[28] There was no evidence that the volume or pH of gastric contents differed with the length and type of fasting. Although not reported in all the trials, there appeared to be no increased risk for aspiration or regurgitation with a shortened period of fasting. Very few trials have investigated the fasting routine in patients at higher risk for regurgitation or aspiration (pregnant, older age, obese, or with stomach disorders). There has also been increasing evidence that preoperative carbohydrate supplementation is safe and may improve a patient's response to perioperative stress.[29,30] Surgeons and anesthesiologists should evaluate the evidence and consider adjusting their standard fasting policies.

**Table 11-14 Perioperative Concerns and Recommendations for Herbal Medicines**

| COMMON NAME OF HERB | PERIOPERATIVE CONCERNS | PREOPERATIVE RECOMMENDATIONS |
|---|---|---|
| Echinacea | Allergic reactions; decreased effectiveness of immunosuppressants; potential for immunosuppression with long-term use | No data |
| Ephedra | Risk for myocardial ischemia and stroke from tachycardia and hypertension; ventricular arrhythmias with halothane; long-term use depletes endogenous catecholamines and may cause intraoperative hemodynamic instability; life-threatening interaction with monoamine oxidase inhibitors | Discontinue at least 24 hr before surgery |
| Garlic | Potential to increase risk for bleeding, especially when combined with other medications that inhibit platelet aggregation | Discontinue at least 7 days before surgery |
| Ginkgo | Potential to increase risk for bleeding, especially when combined with other medications that inhibit platelet aggregation | Discontinue at least 36 hr before surgery |
| Ginseng | Hypoglycemia; potential to increase risk for bleeding; potential to decrease anticoagulative effect of warfarin | Discontinue at least 7 days before surgery |
| Kava | Potential to increase sedative effect of anesthetics; potential for addiction, tolerance, and withdrawal after abstinence unstudied | Discontinue at least 24 hr before surgery |
| St. John's wort | Induction of cytochrome P-450 enzymes, with effect on cyclosporine, warfarin, steroids, protease inhibitors, and possibly benzodiazepines, calcium channel blockers, and many other drugs; decreased serum digoxin levels | Discontinue at least 5 days before surgery |
| Valerian | Potential to increase sedative effect of anesthetics; benzodiazepine-like acute withdrawal; potential to increase anesthetic requirements with long-term use | No data |

Adapted from Ang-Lee MK, Moss J, Yuan CS: Herbal medicines and perioperative care. JAMA 286:208–216, 2001.

## POTENTIAL CAUSES OF INTRAOPERATIVE INSTABILITY

A patient who is under anesthesia can have physiologic derangements that need to be addressed. Some can be dramatic and require immediate attention; others allow for investigation before introduction of therapy. These derangements are usually of a cardiac or pulmonary nature, or are related to the administration of anesthesia.

### Myocardial Infarction

It has been estimated that 1.5% of patients who undergo noncardiac surgery will suffer a perioperative MI.[31] Some of these events will occur in the operating room. The typical presentation is that of new-onset electrocardiographic changes, dysrhythmias, and/or hypotension. If the patient has reasonable hemodynamics and no evidence of decreased perfusion, the procedure can usually be completed. Any evidence of instability, however, should lead to termination of the procedure and cardiac evaluation. Temporary abdominal closure techniques can be used, if needed. Intervention decisions for MI should be made in conjunction with cardiology.

### Pulmonary Embolism

Depending on the procedure, PE can be a significant source of intraoperative instability. It has been estimated that up to 2% of patients undergoing hip surgery will have a PE during the procedure. Signs of intraoperative PE include new tachycardia, evidence of right heart strain, hypotension, and complete cardiovascular collapse. The onset is sudden and rapid diagnosis and treatment are paramount.

Intraoperative transesophageal echocardiography (TEE) is a modality that is now commonly used in the operating room. TEE can be used to identify the PE directly or to show the physiologic effects on cardiac function and allow for an inferred diagnosis.[32] Right ventricular dysfunction, tricuspid regurgitation, and leftward bowing of the interatrial septum are the typical findings. If an embolism is suspected, management will depend on the stability of the patient. If unstable, the procedure should be aborted and efforts to address the PE instituted. This includes cardiovascular support, thrombolytics and, in severe cases, pulmonary embolectomy.

### Pneumothorax

Pneumothorax is a known complication of laparoscopy. As more procedures are approached with minimally invasive techniques, especially esophageal procedures, the risk of pneumothorax increases. The main risk of pneumothorax with laparoscopy is development of a tension pneumothorax and associated cardiovascular collapse. Clinically, ballooning of the diaphragm can be seen. Physiologic changes include deoxygenation, hypercarbia, and hypotension. Electrocardiographic changes can also be noted.

Diagnosis and treatment are straightforward. If the patient is decompensating and there are decreased breath sounds in one hemithorax, abdominal insufflation should be released. Needle decompression or tube thoracostomy should be performed. Chest radiographic confirmation is not necessary and can delay treatment, leading to further instability. Once a chest tube has been placed, pneumoperitoneum can be reintroduced and patient physiology followed. If no derangements are noted, the procedure can be completed.

### Anaphylaxis and Latex Allergy

Intraoperative anaphylactic reactions may occur as frequently as 1 in 4500 surgical procedures and carry a 3% to 6% risk for mortality.[33] Causative agents are most often muscle relaxants, latex, anesthetic induction agents such as etomidate and propofol, and narcotic drugs. Additional agents administered while patients are under anesthesia that may be associated with anaphylaxis include dyes (e.g., isosulfan blue dye for sentinel node procedures), colloid solutions, antibiotics, blood products, protamine, and mannitol.

The manifestations of anaphylactic reactions occurring under anesthesia may range from mild cutaneous eruptions to hypotension, cardiovascular collapse, bronchospasm, and death. When suspected, use of the offending agent is discontinued and the patient is given epinephrine, 0.3 to 0.5 mL of a 1 : 1000 solution subcutaneously; with severe anaphylaxis, it is given IV and repeated at 5- to 10-minute intervals as needed. Histamine 1 ($H_1$) blockade with diphenhydramine, 50 mg IV or IM, plus $H_2$ blockade with ranitidine, 50 mg IV, as well as hydrocortisone, 100 to 250 mg IV every 6 hours, is usually required. Additional supportive measures in the setting of hemodynamic or respiratory collapse may include fluid boluses, pressors, orotracheal intubation, and nebulized $\beta_2$-adrenergic agonists or racemic epinephrine. Postoperative monitoring in the intensive care unit is generally required for a patient who has had a severe intraoperative anaphylactic reaction.

Latex sensitivity is the second most common cause of anaphylactic reactions (after muscle relaxants) and must be screened for in the medical history. Although the incidence of such sensitivity may be less than 5% in the general population, higher risk groups, including those with a genetic predisposition (atopic conditions) or chronic exposure to latex and individuals with spina bifida, may have rates as high as 72%. Those who give a history consistent with possible latex sensitivity undergo skin testing before anticipated operative procedures. Appropriate intraoperative measures to ensure a latex-free environment obviates most perioperative risk in a patient with latex allergy.

### Malignant Hyperthermia

The incidence of malignant hyperthermia (MH) is higher in children and young adults than in adults; a rate of 1 in 15,000 has been estimated in the group at highest risk, boys younger than 15 years.[34] MH represents an acute episode of hypermetabolism and muscle injury related to the administration of halogenated anesthetic agents or succinylcholine. Susceptibility to MH is inherited according to an autosomal dominant pattern, with apparent incomplete penetrance. The patient may therefore fail to reveal familial knowledge of the trait and a personal history of muscle disorder may not be evident.

An acute episode of MH may be recognized by increased sympathetic nervous system activity, muscle rigidity, and high fever. Associated derangements include hypercapnia, arrhythmia, acidosis, hypoxemia, and rhabdomyolysis. When suspected, MH is treated by discontinuing inhalational anesthetic agents and succinylcholine, completely changing the anesthesia circuit, and administering dantrolene sodium at doses of 2 to 3 mg/kg IV. This drug may be titrated to the abatement of symptoms. Additional supportive measures include active or passive cooling and pharmacologic treatment of the arrhythmia, hyperkalemia, and acidosis.

### Wrong-Site Surgery and Universal Protocol

In 2004, the Joint Commission (TJC) adopted, as a national patient safety goal, the elimination of wrong-site, wrong-procedure, wrong-patient procedures.[35,36] A Universal Protocol was developed and the concept of the time-out was instituted. The protocol includes preoperative marking of the surgical site, confirmation of the site by comparing physician notes, consent, mark, and patient identification, and ensuring that the proper implants or devices are available for the procedure. Many institutions add other pieces of information to their time-out, such as antibiotic and venous thromboembolism prophylaxis. An example of such a time-out process is shown in Figure 11-3. Although the problem of wrong-site surgery has now been well defined and systems have been put into place to try to prevent it, there are no data currently available to show its effectiveness.[36]

## THE OPERATING ROOM

Preparation for surgery does not end with evaluation of the patient and selection of the operative procedure. It is the responsibility of the surgeon to ensure that everything needed for the procedure is available on the day of surgery, including any special equipment required to carry out the operation and the availability of any implants, blood, blood products, or special medications.

To run an operating room efficiently requires well-trained surgeons, anesthesiologists, and operating room staff, as well as an operating room equipped with an easily maneuverable operating table, good lighting, and ample space for personnel and equipment. The room is cleaned and the table checked for malfunction before and after each case. It is extremely costly and stressful to replace the operating table or other equipment with the patient already in the operating room. Preoperative

SURGICAL SAFETY CHECKLIST

Prior to procedure

- Patient **identification** confirmed with TWO identifiers (per policy)
- **Site/side/procedure** confirmed
- Site **marked** by physician or appropriate designee (per policy)
- Signed **consent** with correct procedure, patient, and site/side
- **History and physical** completed
- **NPO** status documented
- Patient **allergies** documented
- **Anesthesia** assessment completed
- **Special requirements:**
  - **Anesthesia issues** identified (e.g., difficult airway, aspiration risk)
  - Patient and family **education** completed and understanding evaluated
  - When applicable:
    - Availability of **special equipment**
    - Availability of **implants or devices**
    - Availability of **imaging films and results**
    - Availability of **blood products**

In operative suite

- All team members verbally **introduced** and **sign in** on white board
- **Pulse oximeter** on patient and functioning
- **TIME-OUT** procedure prior to surgical incision (surgeon, anesthesia provider, nurse, and scrub tech verbally confirm):
  - **Correct patient** identity
  - Signed **consent** with correct procedure, patient, side/site
  - **Correct procedure and position** identified
  - **Side and site marked**
  - **Special requirements** have been verifed (see above)
  - Any **inconsistencies** have been resolved (e.g., questions, concerns)
  - **Safety precautions** addressed based on patient history/medication use (e.g., allergies)
  - **Antibiotic** administration (prophylaxis and irrigation fluids)
  - Relevant **imaging and results** labeled and displayed, if applicable

At completion of procedure

- **Procedure confirmed** by attending surgeon or designee and documented
- Instrument, sponge, and needle **counts** are correct (or corrective action taken)
- **Specimens** reviewed, labeled, and destination confirmed
- **Equipment or other problems** addressed
- **Major medical conditions** summarized
- **Recovery location** stated

**FIGURE 11-3** Example of perioperative time-out process.

communication among surgeons, anesthesiologists, and operating room staff is vitally important. Such communication helps save time, prevents confusion and undue frustration in the management of equipment use, accounts for patient needs and personnel requirements, and makes planned procedures progress safely and efficiently. The modern operating room for a trauma service has a temperature control panel that allows the room temperature to be modified rapidly to avoid hypothermia. Patients are positioned and secured on the table. Position-related neuromuscular and/or orthopedic injury can be prevented with careful positioning and padding. Barriers consisting of sterile drapes and gowns are established between the surgeon, patient, and other operating room staff. The barriers need to be impermeable to water and other body fluids. Finally, a hands-free communication system (e.g., intercom, voice-activated speaker phone) must be functioning in the room to facilitate communication among surgeons and pathologists, radiologists, blood bank, pharmacy, and the patient's family members. Most importantly, if an unexpected situation arises, help can be summoned immediately.

### Maintenance of Normothermia

Hypothermia averaging only 1.5° C below normal is associated with adverse outcomes that add hospitalization costs of $2500 to $7000 for each surgical patient. Many factors increase the risk for perioperative hypothermia—extremes of age, female gender, ambient room temperature, length and type of surgical procedure, cachexia, preexisting conditions, significant fluid shifts, use of cold irrigants, and use of general or regional anesthesia. The term *normothermia* is defined as a core temperature between 36° and 38° C. Preventive warming measures are used to avoid hypothermia. Passive insulation includes warmed cotton blankets, socks, head covering, limited skin exposure, circulating water mattresses, and increase in ambient room temperature (68° to 75° F). Some patients may require active warming, which includes use of a forced air convection warming system, humidified and warmed anesthetic gases, and warmed IV fluids. The greatest temperature decline occurs during the first hour of surgery. Therefore, even in short procedures, temperature monitoring is indicated.[37]

### Preoperative Skin Preparation

Preoperative skin preparation of the patient and surgeon is important in preventing surgical site infection. The effectiveness of the preparation is dependent on the type of antiseptic used and the method of application. The Centers for Disease Control and Prevention (CDC) recommends that the size of the area prepared be sufficient, the solution applied in concentric circles, the applicator discarded once the periphery has been reached, and time allowed for the solution to dry, especially when alcoholic solutions are used, because they are flammable. The Association of Operating Room Nurses has added that the applicator needs to be sterile and the solution needs to be applied with the use of friction and extend from the incision site to the periphery. A review of this subject has revealed six evaluable studies; however, all described a unique comparison and thus could not be combined for meta-analysis.[38] It was concluded at that time that there was insufficient evidence to recommend one skin preparation antiseptic over another. A more recent randomized, controlled study investigated chlorhexidine-alcohol versus povidone iodine for the prevention of surgical site infections.[39] In this study, 849 patients were randomized and, at 30 days, there were significantly fewer wound infections in the chlorhexidine-alcohol group. The results were significant for superficial and deep surgical site infections. There were no differences in adverse events related to the solution used. Hair removal, if needed, is accomplished by clipping with electric clippers rather than shaving with a razor.

### Hemostasis

Minimizing blood loss is an important technical aspect of surgery. Increased blood loss exacerbates the stress of surgery and resuscitation; less blood loss allows the performance of a technically superior operation. In the presence of adequate hemostasis, one can conduct a more precise dissection and shorten operating and recovery times for the patient. Avoidance of blood transfusion obviates the risk for transfusion-related complications and the transmission of bloodborne diseases.[40]

Essential operative technique dictates that larger vessels (smaller than 1 mm in diameter) be tied, clipped, or sealed with monopolar or bipolar electrocautery or high-frequency ultrasonic devices. Major named vessels, in particular, are not only tied but also undergo suture ligation. Hemoclip application is acceptable, especially in an operating field with an extremely confined space or when dealing with delicate vessels, such as portal vein branches. With limited access procedures, such as those performed with minimal access techniques, clip application seems to be a better choice than knot tying. At times, it is necessary to use hemoclips, such as when performing an oncologic procedure in which outlining of the margins provides a radiopaque marker for postoperative irradiation.

In the event of catastrophic bleeding, such as when confronted with an unexpected intraoperative major vessel injury, intraperitoneal rupture of an aortic aneurysm, or bleeding from major intra-abdominal trauma, temporary occlusion of the aorta at the esophageal hiatus with a compression device such as a sponge on a stick or vascular clamp or manual compression is considered. Such a maneuver may be lifesaving by allowing the anesthesia staff to catch up with blood loss by aggressive resuscitation. It also allows the surgeon to remove intraperitoneal blood and clots with lap sponges or suction devices until the exact bleeding site can be identified, controlled, and repaired primarily or with an interposition graft. Occasionally, a partial vascular injury may need to be extended or converted to a complete transection to allow a better repair. This approach is particularly applicable to injury of the aorta and vena cava.

Bleeding that occurs from multiple sites in a trauma patient, such as liver laceration, pelvic fracture, or both, especially in a hypothermic patient, may best be treated with packing alone or in conjunction with angiographic embolization to achieve temporary control followed by a second-look operation. This maneuver of damage control is of paramount importance. It may be the only way that a patient's life can be saved. In fact, this principle of damage control can and should be applied beyond the trauma patient to all surgical procedures when unexpected bleeding is encountered or a second-look laparotomy will be necessary. Other adjunctive measures that may be helpful in dealing with wide areas of surface tissue oozing include microwave coagulation, laser coagulation, and the application of topical hemostatic agents (e.g., Surgicel, thrombin, Gelfoam, and fibrin glue).

**Table 11-15 Comparison of Absorbable Sutures**

| SUTURE | TYPES | RAW MATERIAL | TENSILE STRENGTH RETENTION IN VIVO | TISSUE REACTION |
|---|---|---|---|---|
| Surgical gut | Chromic | Collagen derived from healthy beef and sheep | Individual patient characteristics can affect rate of tensile strength loss | Moderate reaction |
| Monocryl (poliglecaprone 25) | Monofilament | Copolymer of glycolide and epsilon-caprolactone | ≈50%-60% (violet, 60%-70%) remains at 1 wk<br>≈20%-30% (violet, 30%-40%) remains at 2 wk<br>Lost within 3 wk (violet, 4 wk) | Minimal acute inflammatory reaction |
| Coated Vicryl (polyglactin 910) | Braided, Monofilament | Glycolide and L-Lactide coated with a copolymer of lactide and calcium stearate | ≈75% remains at 2 wk<br>≈50% remains at 3 wk<br>25% remains at 4 wk | Minimal acute inflammatory reaction |
| PDS II (polydioxanone) | Monofilament | Polyester polymer | ≈70% remains at 2 wk<br>≈50% remains at 4 wk<br>≈25% remains at 6 wk | Slight reaction |

Adapted from Ethicon: Wound closure manual, Somerville, NJ, 2007, Ethicon.

**Table 11-16 Comparison of Nonabsorbable Sutures**

| SUTURE | TYPES | RAW MATERIAL | TENSILE STRENGTH RETENTION IN VIVO | TISSUE REACTION |
|---|---|---|---|---|
| Perma-Hand–silk suture | Braided | Organic protein called fibroin | Progressive degradation of fiber may result in gradual loss of tensile strength over time | Acute inflammatory reaction |
| Ethilon–nylon suture | Monofilament | Long-chain aliphatic polymers nylon 6 or nylon 6,6 | Progressive hydrolysis may result in gradual loss of tensile strength over time | Minimal acute inflammatory reaction |
| Nurolon–nylon suture | Braided | Long-chain aliphatic polymers nylon 6 or nylon 6,6 | Progressive hydrolysis may result in gradual loss of tensile strength over time | Minimal acute inflammatory reaction |
| Mersilene–polyester fiber suture | Braided Monofilament | Poly(ethylene terephthalate) | No significant change known to occur in vivo | Minimal acute inflammatory reaction |
| Ethibond Excel–polyester fiber suture | Braided | Poly(ethylene terephthalate) coated with polybutilate | No significant change known to occur in vivo | Minimal acute inflammatory reaction |
| Prolene–polypropylene suture | Monofilament | Isotactic crystalline stereoisomer of polypropylene | Not subject to degradation or weakening by action of tissue enzymes | Minimal acute inflammatory reaction |
| Pronova–poly (hexafluoropropylene-VDF suture) | Monofilament | Polymer blend of poly (vinylidene fluoride) and poly(vinylidene fluoride-cohexafluoropropylene) | Not subject to degradation or weakening by action of tissue enzymes | Minimal acute inflammatory reaction |

Adapted from Ethicon: Wound closure manual, Somerville, NJ, 2007, Ethicon.

## Wound Closure

Wound closure can be temporary or permanent; the latter can be primary or secondary. Critical factors in making this decision are the patient's condition, clinical setting, area of the body involved, condition of the wound itself, and disease process or injury that led to surgical intervention.

Various methods can be chosen to close wounds in different parts of the body, depending on the clinical circumstance. In general, clean noncontaminated wounds with healthy local tissue conditions are best closed by primary permanent closure. In a patient with a condition requiring reexploration or one suffering from abdominal compartment syndrome, temporary closure is preferable. Heavily contaminated extremity or trunk wounds are left open with packing. Heavily contaminated abdominal wounds are best served by fascial closure alone, with the skin left open and packed. The principle of eliminating dead space to reduce the risk for seroma and hematoma formation is important and can be achieved internally with sutures or a suction device or externally with a compression appliance.

Permanent closure can be achieved with running or interrupted sutures. Suture can be monofilament or multifilament, braided or nonbraided, and dissolvable or nondissolvable (Tables 11-15 and 11-16). In general, when proven infection or contamination is a concern, monofilament nonbraided suture is preferred. For abdominal wall closure in a debilitated, malnourished cancer patient, permanent closure with nondissolvable suture seems prudent. In a cirrhotic patient with established ascites or a patient with potential for the development of postoperative ascites, the abdomen is closed with running suture and a multilayer watertight closure must be achieved.

Temporary closure of the abdominal wall may be appropriate in the setting of a multiply injured patient or one with intra-abdominal hypertension. This can be achieved with a vacuum suction device or a prosthesis bridging technique using a sterile IV bag or polypropylene mesh (Table 11-17). The vacuum suction technique (Vac-Pac) involves using a two-sided temporary closing material made of a Ioban over a blue towel. The Ioban faces the intestine and prevents adhesion to the

**Table 11-17 Types of Synthetic Mesh and Their Uses**

| TYPE OF MESH | TRADE NAME | TYPE | COMMENTS |
|---|---|---|---|
| **Nonabsorbable** | | | |
| Polypropylene | Marlex, Prolene, Atrium | Monofilament | Highly elastic, withstands infection well; widely used for abdominal wall reconstruction, hernia repair |
| Polytetrafluoroethylene (PTFE) | Teflon | Multifilament | Nonexpanded mesh; associated with a large number of complications; limited usefulness |
| Expanded PTFE | Gore-Tex | Multifilament | Greatest elongation in comparison to other nonabsorbable meshes; minimal tissue incorporation; multiple uses in abdominal, vascular reconstruction |
| Polyethylene terephthalate | Mersilene, Dacron | Multifilament | Polyester fiber mesh with broad usefulness in abdominal wall, hernia repair; less extensively used than polypropylene |
| **Absorbable** | | | |
| Polyglycolic acid | Dexon | Multifilament | Useful for temporary abdominal closure; resists infection |
| Polyglactin 910 | Vicryl | Multifilament | Useful for temporary abdominal closure; resists infection |

Adapted from Fenner DE: New surgical mesh. Clin Obstet Gynecol 43:650–658, 2000.

blue towel. The membrane is tucked beneath the abdominal wall, with the blue towel side facing up to provide retention and prevent potential loss of domain. The central portion of the drape is fenestrated before placement. Suction catheters and gauze dressings are placed beneath a second Biodrape that covers the entire abdominal wall and seals the closure (Fig. 11-4). This technique has a number of advantages; it is quick and easy to use, the temporary closure can be constructed from materials that are readily available in the operating room, no suturing is required; and therefore the integrity of the abdominal fascia is maintained for later permanent closure, and the applied suction prohibits fluid from accumulating in the abdominal cavity. Disadvantages include an inability to inspect the intestine (as with an IV bag) at the bedside and increased complexity of fluid and electrolyte balance because of potentially large fluid losses. It has been our practice to return these patients to the operating room every 3 to 4 days for replacement of the temporary closure. If possible, interrupted permanent fascial closure sutures are placed at the superior and inferior ends of the fascia to close the fascia gradually, over the course of up to four trips to the operating room.

Two rather recent concepts in abdominal surgery include the use of adhesion reduction barriers and synthetic biomembranes for abdominal wall closure. Two types of adhesion reduction barriers are available, hyaluronic acid–carboxymethylcellulose and oxidized regenerated cellulose. Both these materials are applied to the raw surface of the bowel before abdominal closure and within 1 hour they turn to a gelatinous substance.[41] Although the use of these membranes does not obviate adhesions totally, they have been demonstrated in clinical trials to decrease their severity.[42] The second innovation is that of using engineered tissue matrices for abdominal wall closure. These materials are constructed from donor integumentary tissue and processed to remove the epidermal and dermal cellular portions, and thus the antigenic component of the allograft. The resulting product is a collagen-based matrix with its native tensile strength intact but its capacity to generate an immune response abrogated. The interstices of the allograft are then colonized by cellular populations from the recipient.[43] This material promises to yield an adjunct to closure of a complex abdominal wall defect that has good strength and is more resistant to infection than with the use of synthetic materials such as polypropylene mesh.

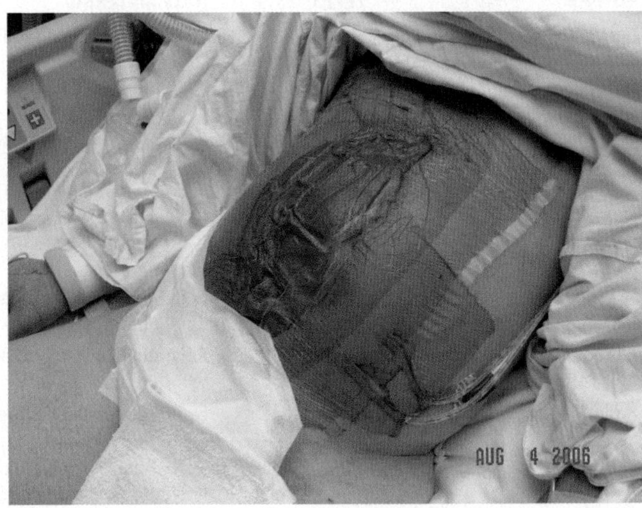


**FIGURE 11-4** Vac-Pac temporary abdominal wound closure. This closure method allows easy reentry into the abdomen and does not compromise the fascia. To fashion, place a surgical towel between two medium sticky drapes. Then place it in the abdomen and tuck the edges underneath the fascia with an overlap of several centimeters. Closed suction drains are placed along the edges and brought out through the skin. Another surgical towel is then placed over the open portion of the wound and a large sticky drape is used to cover the entire abdomen. The drains are immediately connected to wall suction to provide adequate compression of the dressing.

## Staplers

Surgical staplers have changed the practice of surgery in a profound way, most notably within the field of minimally invasive technology. Several different devices are available for stapling:

1. Skin staplers
2. Ligating and dividing staplers (LDSs)
3. Gastrointestinal anastomosis (GIA) staplers
4. Thoracoabdominal (TA) staplers

5. End-to-end anastomosis (EEA) staplers
6. Laparoscopic hernia mesh tackers
7. Open hernia mesh staplers
8. Endo-GIA staplers

A modification of the GIA stapler for laparoscopic use, the endo-GIA, has particularly broad usefulness. It can facilitate the ligation and transection of major vascular pedicles in laparoscopy, as in the performance of splenectomy, nephrectomy, or hepatectomy, or facilitate GIA or transection of solid organs such as the pancreas. In a video-assisted thoracoscopic surgical procedure, it can aid in wedge resection of an injured or diseased lung. The GIA (endo-GIA or standard version) stapler may aid in the transection of thick or indurated mesentery during intestinal resection in patients with inflammatory bowel disease.

### Surgical Adhesives

Surgical adhesives have been widely used in modern surgery. They can be used for a simple task such as skin closure or for more complex wound problems. Many agents are clinically available and are used for a variety of purposes. Fibrin seal adhesive has been used to close fistulas, prevent lymphatic leakage after complete lymphadenectomy in the axilla or groin, and prevent leakage from tissue surfaces that have been newly transected, such as staple lines of the lung or pancreatic resection. It also has been adapted to seal the terminal bronchus via bronchoscopy as a noninvasive means for treating a small subset of patients with pneumothorax. Fibrin seal adhesive has become the preferred way to treat pseudoaneurysms in the groin or axilla that result from arterial puncture. Ultrasound-guided direct injection into such lesions has been reported to be successful, with low complication rates.[44] Adhesives can also be used as an adjunct to reinforce and provide a watertight seal to a delicate gastrointestinal anastomosis, such as one involving the biliary tract or pancreas.

Surgical adhesives work by admixing a two-component agent derived from whole blood; each is secured in separate containers for shipping and storage. When mixed, the components form a viscous semiliquid tissue glue that can be applied onto a suture line, fistula tract or cavity, or other raw tissue surface or potential small dead space. When set, it becomes a solid adhesive biomembrane, sealant, or plug that will be self-retained. Major obstacles to its widespread use are cost and the potential for complications related to disease transmission with the use of blood products.

Two other commonly used agents are 2-octylcyanoacrylate (Dermabond) and butyl-2-cyanoacrylate (Histoacryl). Cyanoacrylate has been used for repair of organs and as an adhesive in many orthopedic procedures. Dermabond has been demonstrated to be an adequate replacement for the traditional suture closure of simple skin lacerations. Dermabond also allows the patient to resume showering within a few hours of wound closure.

## SURGICAL DEVICES AND ENERGY SOURCES

### Electrosurgery and Electrocautery

In 1928, Cushing first published a series of 500 neurosurgical procedures performed with an electrocautery device that was developed by Bovie. Since then, electrocautery and electrosurgery have become the most important and basic surgical tools in the operating room.

High-frequency alternating current can be delivered in unipolar or bipolar fashion. The unipolar (or monopolar) device is composed of a generator, electrode for application, and electrode for the returning current to complete the circuit. The patient's body becomes part of the circuit when the system is activated. Because the effectiveness of energy conversion into heat is inversely related to the area of contact, the application electrode is designed to be small to generate heat efficiently and the returning electrode is designed to be large to disperse energy and prevent burn injury. The heat generated is dependent on three other factors in addition to the size of the contact area: (1) the power setting or frequency of the current; (2) the length of activation time; and (3) whether the waveform released from the generator is continuous or intermittent. Unipolar devices can be used to incise tissue when activated with a constant waveform and to coagulate when activated with an intermittent waveform. In the cutting mode, much heat is generated relatively quickly over the target, with minimal lateral thermal spread. As a result, the device cuts through tissue without coagulating any underlying vessels. In contrast, in the coagulation mode, electrocautery generates less heat on a slower frequency, with the potential for large lateral thermal spread. Such spread results in tissue dehydration and vessel thrombosis. A blended waveform can be chosen that will be able to take advantage of the cutting and coagulation modes. A large grounding pad must be placed securely on the patient for the unipolar electrosurgical or electrocautery device to function properly and prevent thermal burn injury at the current reentry electrode site.

Bipolar electrocautery establishes a short circuit between the tips of the instrument, whether a tissue grasper or forceps, without the requirement for a grounding pad. The tissue grasped between the tips of the instrument completes the circuit. In generating heat that affects only the tissue within the short circuit, it provides precise thermal coagulation. Bipolar electrocautery is more effective than the monopolar instrument in coagulating vessels because it adds the mechanical advantage of compression of tissue between the tips of the instrument to the thermal coagulation. Bipolar electrocautery is particularly useful when conducting a procedure in which lateral thermal injury or an arcing phenomenon needs to be avoided.

### Lasers

Lasers use photons to excite the chromophore molecules within target tissue and generate kinetic energy that is released as heat, which causes protein denaturation and coagulation necrosis. This effect occurs without much collateral damage to surrounding tissue. It can be applied to the surface of target tissue or interstitially with a fiberoptic probe placed under precision image guidance. The energy generated and the depth of tissue penetration can be varied with the power setting selected and the photon chosen for the particular task. The laser effect can be enhanced by photosensitizing agents. The most common types of laser currently in use are the argon, carbon dioxide, and neodymium:yttrium-aluminum-garnet (Nd-YAG) lasers. The depth of energy penetration within the target organ is least with the argon laser, moderate with the carbon dioxide laser, and deepest with the Nd-YAG laser.

Interstitial laser photocoagulation is a fairly recently adopted laser treatment technology. With a precisely placed optic fiber (or fibers) inside the target tissue, laser light is delivered and absorbed by the surrounding structure and tissue. The degree of absorption within and around the target tissue depends on the wavelength of the laser chosen and specific optical properties of the tissue. The optical properties of different tumors or tissues are markedly different and depend on their tissue composition and density, degree of parenchymal fibrosis, vascularity, and presence or absence of necrosis.

## Argon Beam Coagulator

The argon beam coagulator creates a monopolar electric circuit between a hand-held probe and the target tissue by establishing a steady flow of electrons through a channel of electrically activated and ionized argon gas. This high-flow argon gas conducts electrical current to the target tissue and generates thermal coagulation of this tissue. The depth of the thermal penetration of tissue varies from fractions of a millimeter to a maximum of 6 mm, depending on three factors:

1. Power setting
2. Distance between the probe and the target
3. Length of its application

The hand-held control is usually combined with the regular Bovie, which can provide much more focused tissue coagulation for any identifiable vessels. The argon gas blows blood away from the surface of the target argon beam coagulation is more effective for the bleeding parenchyma of an organ. Visibility is also improved by the same mechanism. It is most commonly used to treat parenchymal hemorrhage of an organ, particularly the liver, but can be used on the spleen, kidney, or any other solid organ with surface oozing.

## Photodynamic Therapy

Photodynamic therapy is a rather recently developed treatment that allows destruction of cancer cells and has been expanded to the eradication of metaplastic cells. It begins with the administration of a target-specific photosensitizer that is eventually concentrated in the target tissue. The photosensitizing agent is then activated with a wavelength-specific light energy source, which leads to the generation of free radicals cytotoxic to the target tissue. Photodynamic therapy has been used to treat different types of late-stage cancers, mainly in a palliative setting, but has also been used for the treatment of some chemoresistant tumors. Applications reported in the literature include treating early radiographically detected non–small cell lung cancer, pancreatic cancer, squamous cell and basal cell carcinoma of the skin, recurrent superficial bladder cancer, chest wall involvement from breast cancer, and even chest wall recurrence of breast cancer. Its usefulness has been expanded to include the treatment of noncancer conditions, such as Barrett's esophagus and psoriasis.[45]

## High-Frequency Sound Wave Techniques

Ultrasound has had a strong impact on the practice of modern medicine. It has different functions, depending on the frequency of ultrasound generated by the machine. At a low power level, it causes no tissue damage and is mainly used for diagnostic purposes. With a high-frequency setting, ultrasound can be used to dissect, cut, and coagulate. Several high-frequency ultrasonic devices are available for use in surgical practice.

Another beneficial manipulation of acoustic wave technology is that of extracorporeal shock wave lithotripsy. It has been used in treating cholelithiasis and nephrolithiasis. In this modality, the patient is placed in a water bath and a high-energy acoustic shock wave is generated by piezoelectric or electromagnetic technology and focused. The water-tissue interface allows the wave to pass through normal tissue without injuring it. The energy of the shock wave is focused on the offending stone by ultrasound and causes disruption and fragmentation of the calculus, which is then passed via the ureter.

### Harmonic Scalpel

The harmonic scalpel is an instrument that uses ultrasound technology to dissect tissue in bipolar fashion with only minimal collateral tissue damage. The device vibrates at a high frequency, approximately 55,000 times/second, to cut tissue. The high-frequency vibration of tissue molecules generates stress and friction in the tissue, which in turn generates heat and denaturation of protein. Because of this unique capability to dissect tissue and coagulate small blood vessels all at once, with minimal energy transfer to surrounding tissue, the device has gained recognition among surgeons. It has been used in many different types of minimally invasive surgery and its application has also been extended to many open procedures.

### Ultrasonic Cavitation Devices

The Cavitron ultrasonic surgical aspirator uses lower frequency ultrasound energy to fragment and dissect tissue of low fiber content. It is basically an ultrasound probe combined with an aspirator, so it functions as an acoustic vibrator and suction device at the same time. The Cavitron has a variety of applications. Because the instrument fragments and aspirates tissue of low collagen and high water content, it can be effective surgically for liver and pancreatic procedures without causing damage to surrounding tissue. When compared with the dissection technique of other instruments, such as the scalpel or cautery, the advantages of using this device are less blood loss, improved visibility, and reduced collateral tissue injury. It has been used for resecting lesions in noncirrhotic liver and pancreatic tumors, especially small endocrine tumors within a soft normal pancreas, without fibrosis. It has also been used for partial nephrectomy, salvage splenectomy, head and neck procedures, and treatment of many gynecologic tumors.

## Radiofrequency Ablation

Radiofrequency energy can be used for tissue ablation in a curative or a palliative attempt to treat different cancers. It is also effective for treating benign conditions such as neuralgia, bone pain, and cardiac arrhythmias (e.g., atrial fibrillation). The basic method of radiofrequency application is to place an electrode (or electrodes) into or over the target tissue to transmit a high-frequency alternating current to the tissue in the range of 350 to 500 kHz. Rapid alternating directional movement of ions results in the release of kinetic energy. It can raise the temperature of the target tissue to higher than 100° C and cause protein denaturation, desiccation, and coagulation necrosis; it has a built-in sensor for automatically terminating transmission of the current at a particular set point to prevent overheating and unwanted collateral damage. The main use of this modality is for tumors in the liver parenchyma. Its applications have been expanded to tumors in the lung, kidney, adrenal gland, breast, thyroid, pancreas, and bone. The indications for radiofrequency ablation are continuing to grow because it is inexpensive and can be reliably used to destroy a larger tumor mass.

### Cryoablation

Cryotherapy can be applied topically to treat skin conditions or tumors or interstitially for the ablation of liver lesions. It destroys cells by freezing and thawing. With liquid nitrogen or argon circulating through a probe placed over or within the target lesion, the tissue can be frozen to a temperature of −35° C or lower. Cell damage occurs as a result of disruption of subcellular structures, with ice crystal formation in the freezing phase and degradation during the thawing process. Ischemia of the tissue from focal disruption of the circulation, shifting of water and electrolyte content in situ, and protein denaturation also contribute to the tissue damage induced by cryotherapy. Lesions that contact major vessels can be difficult to treat with this modality, however, because of the heat sink effect introduced by circulating blood. Nonetheless, it has been reported to be effective in treating primary and secondary lesions of the liver that are unresectable. The major disadvantage of interstitial cryotherapy is its cost. Patients usually need general anesthesia for the procedure, the equipment is more expensive than a radiofrequency system, and the process itself is time-consuming. Complications such as hemorrhage from tissue fracture are a concern. Cryoablation is currently used to treat solid tumors in the lung, liver, breast, kidney, and prostate.

### Microwave Ablation and Radiosurgery

Microwave coagulation is achieved by using a generator to transmit microwave energy at a frequency of 2450 MHz via a probe placed under image guidance within target organs or tissue. A rapidly alternating electrical field is created in the target tissue to induce motion of polar molecules in the tissue, such as water. Kinetic energy is dissipated as heat, which causes coagulation necrosis. It was initially used for lesions in the liver; however, its applications have been expanded to the treatment of cardiac rhythm disturbances, prostatic hyperplasia, endometrial bleeding, sterilization of bony margins, and partial nephrectomy. The major limiting factor is that the area that can be ablated with the current equipment is very small, thus necessitating multiple insertions of the microwave probe to treat a single lesion.[37]

The premiere tool in radiosurgery is the gamma knife; its principal area of use is in neurosurgery. This tool allows more than 200 separate sources of high-energy gamma radiation, arranged in a circular fashion, to be focused stereotactically onto a minute area in the brain. Avoiding injury to normal brain tissue requires that the head be held motionless by an external fixation device. This ability to destroy finite areas within the brain has been applied to the treatment of benign and malignant brain neoplasms, arteriovenous malformations, and epilepsy.

## OUTPATIENT SURGERY

Over the past 25 years, outpatient surgery has become more commonplace. It is estimated that up to 75% of elective surgical procedures are now performed in an outpatient setting, which means that patients do not experience an overnight stay around the time of the procedure. Even patients who will need a postoperative inpatient stay after the procedure are usually admitted to the hospital after the surgery. Outpatient surgery can take place in an operating room associated with a large hospital, in a freestanding outpatient surgery center, or even in a physician's office. Preoperative evaluation of the patient usually takes place on an ambulatory basis, and more coordination is required by the surgeon to ensure that the evaluation is completed and acted on in a timely fashion. Patients with significant comorbid conditions are evaluated by the anesthesia staff at least 1 day before the planned procedure (Box 11-3).[46] The standards for perioperative monitoring are similar regardless of the setting and are tailored to the complexity of the procedure and comorbid condition(s) of the patient. In addition, the patient's postoperative disposition takes into account the distance from the

**BOX 11-3 Conditions for Which Preoperative Evaluation May Be Recommended Before Day of Surgery**

**General**
- Medical condition inhibiting the patient's ability to engage in normal daily activity
- Medical condition necessitating continual assistance or monitoring at home within past 6 mo
- Admission within past 2 mo for acute condition or exacerbation of a chronic condition

**Cardiocirculatory**
- History of angina, coronary artery disease, myocardial infarction
- Symptomatic arrhythmias
- Poorly controlled hypertension (diastolic <110 mm Hg, systolic <160 mm Hg)
- History of congestive heart failure

**Respiratory**
- Asthma, chronic obstructive pulmonary disease requiring chronic medication or with acute exacerbation and progression within the past 6 mo
- History of major airway surgery or unusual airway anatomy
- Upper or lower airway tumor or obstruction
- History of chronic respiratory distress requiring home ventilatory assistance or monitoring

**Endocrine**
- Insulin-dependent diabetes mellitus
- Adrenal disorders
- Active thyroid disease

**Neuromuscular**
- History of seizure disorder or other significant central nervous system disease (e.g., multiple sclerosis)
- History of myopathy or other muscle disorder

**Hepatic**
- Any active hepatobiliary disease or compromise

**Musculoskeletal**
- Kyphosis or scoliosis causing functional compromise
- Temporomandibular joint disorder
- Cervical or thoracic spine injury

**Oncology**
- Patients receiving chemotherapy
- Other oncology process with significant physiologic residual or compromise

**Gastrointestinal**
- Massive obesity (<140% of ideal body weight)
- Hiatal hernia
- Symptomatic gastroesophageal reflux

place of surgery, as well as who will be around to monitor the patient.

In general, procedures performed under local anesthesia without sedation are such that patients can be discharged home under their own recognizance. The need for postoperative pain control with narcotic-based agents may alter patients' suitability for transporting themselves and thus is considered when making decisions about disposition. Any patient who receives sedation, general anesthetic, or both at a minimum needs to have a ride home. Ideally, the patient will have a responsible individual staying overnight in the same residence. Again, the patient's ability to perform tasks at home will be influenced by the need for narcotics, as well as any restrictions or limitations dictated by the procedure. Patients who will be unable to maintain oral intake after surgery, because of the operation itself or the need for postoperative ventilatory support, or who will need IV or other nonoral pain medication, will require postoperative hospitalization. The need for postoperative care will have a bearing on the type of facility in which the surgeon chooses to carry out the procedure.

## SELECTED REFERENCES

Caprini JA: Venous thromboembolism in surgery—a preventable complication. Introduction. Am J Surg 199:S1–S2, 2010.

A comprehensive overview of venous thromboembolism and its prevention and treatment in surgical populations.

Eagle KA, Berger PB, Calkins H, et al: ACC/AHA guideline update on perioperative cardiovascular evaluation for noncardiac surgery: A report of the American College of Cardiology/American Heart Association Task Force on Practice Guidelines (Committee to Update the 1996 Guidelines on Perioperative Cardiovascular Evaluation for Noncardiac Surgery). Circulation 105:1257–1267, 2002.

Evidence-based guidelines for perioperative cardiovascular evaluation for noncardiac surgery, updated in 2002 by the American College of Cardiology/American Heart Association Task Force on Practice Guidelines.

Fleisher LA, Rosenbaum SH: Perioperative patient care. Med Clin North Am 93:xiii–xiv, 2009.

An overview of the components of a medical consultation of the potential operative candidate.

Gould JC, Melvin WS: Advances and controversies in minimally invasive surgery. Surg Clin North Am 88:xv–xvi, 2008.

An overview of the basic principles behind the technology commonly used in the operating room and for diagnostic purposes.

Khuri SF, Henderson WG, Daley J, et al: The patient safety in surgery study: Background, study design, and patient populations. J Am Coll Surg 204:1089–1102, 2007.

This volume of the *Journal of the American College of Surgeons* is comprised of many articles presenting the results of this important study, which tested the applicability and validity of the National Surgical Quality Improvement Program (NSQIP) outside the VA.

Napolitano LM, Bass BC: Risk-adjusted outcomes and perioperative care. Surg Clin North Am 85(6):1341–1346, 2005.

Overview of the perioperative concerns of patients, surgeons, and anesthesiologists, including topics addressing risk adjustment, hospital systems, and patient safety.

## REFERENCES

**1.** Halaszynski TM, Juda R, Silverman DG: Optimizing postoperative outcomes with efficient preoperative assessment and management. Crit Care Med 32:S76–86, 2004.

**2.** Khuri SF, Henderson WG, Daley J, et al: Successful implementation of the Department of Veterans Affairs' National Surgical Quality Improvement Program in the private sector: The Patient Safety in Surgery study. Ann Surg 248:329–336, 2008.

**3.** Akhtar S, Silverman DG: Assessment and management of patients with ischemic heart disease. Crit Care Med 32:S126–136, 2004.

**4.** Eagle KA, Berger PB, Calkins H, et al: ACC/AHA guideline update for perioperative cardiovascular evaluation for noncardiac surgery—executive summary: A report of the American College of Cardiology/American Heart Association Task Force on Practice Guidelines (Committee to Update the 1996 Guidelines on Perioperative Cardiovascular Evaluation for Noncardiac Surgery). J Am Coll Cardiol 39:542–553, 2002.

**5.** Mangano DT, Layug EL, Wallace A, et al: Effect of atenolol on mortality and cardiovascular morbidity after noncardiac surgery. Multicenter Study of Perioperative Ischemia Research Group. N Engl J Med 335:1713–1720, 1996.

**6.** Devereaux PJ, Yang H, Yusuf S, et al: Effects of extended-release metoprolol succinate in patients undergoing non-cardiac surgery (POISE trial): A randomised controlled trial. Lancet 371:1839–1847, 2008.

**7.** Fleischmann KE, Beckman JA, Buller CE, et al: 2009 ACCF/AHA focused update on perioperative beta blockade. J Am Coll Cardiol 54:2102–2128, 2009.

**8.** Biccard BM: Relationship between the inability to climb two flights of stairs and outcome after major non-cardiac surgery: Implications for the pre-operative assessment of functional capacity. Anaesthesia 60:588–593, 2005.

**9.** Dimick JB, Chen SL, Taheri PA, et al: Hospital costs associated with surgical complications: A report from the private-sector National Surgical Quality Improvement Program. J Am Coll Surg 199:531–537, 2004.

**10.** Khuri SF, Henderson WG, DePalma RG, et al: Determinants of long-term survival after major surgery and the adverse effect of postoperative complications. Ann Surg 242:326–341, 2005.

**11.** Johnson RG, Arozullah AM, Neumayer L, et al: Multivariable predictors of postoperative respiratory failure after general and vascular surgery: Results from the Patient Safety in Surgery study. J Am Coll Surg 204:1188–1198, 2007.

**12.** Joseph AJ, Cohn SL: Perioperative care of the patient with renal failure. Med Clin North Am 87:193–210, 2003.

**13.** Rizvon MK, Chou CL: Surgery in the patient with liver disease. Med Clin North Am 87:211–227, 2003.

**13a.** Yerdel MA, Koksoy C, Aras N, et al: Laparoscopic versus open cholecystectomy in cirrhotic patients: A prospective study. Surg Laparosc Endosc 7:483–486, 1997.

**14.** Ahmed Z, Lockhart CH, Weiner M, et al: Advances in diabetic management: Implications for anesthesia. Anesth Analg 100: 666–669, 2005.

15. Turina M, Christ-Crain M, Polk HC, Jr: Impact of diabetes mellitus and metabolic disorders. Surg Clin North Am 85:1153–1161, ix, 2005.
16. Carr A, Cooper DA: Adverse effects of antiretroviral therapy. Lancet 356:1423–1430, 2000.
17. Simon TL, Alverson DC, AuBuchon J, et al: Practice parameter for the use of red blood cell transfusions: Developed by the Red Blood Cell Administration Practice Guideline Development Task Force of the College of American Pathologists. Arch Pathol Lab Med 122:130–138, 1998.
18. Kearon C, Hirsh J: Management of anticoagulation before and after elective surgery. N Engl J Med 336:1506–1511, 1997.
19. Douketis JD, Berger PB, Dunn AS, et al: The perioperative management of antithrombotic therapy: American College of Chest Physicians Evidence-Based Clinical Practice Guidelines (8th Edition). Chest 133:299S–339S, 2008.
20. Geerts WH, Heit JA, Clagett GP, et al: Prevention of venous thromboembolism. Chest 119:132S–175S, 2001.
21. Muntz JE, Michota FA: Prevention and management of venous thromboembolism in the surgical patient: options by surgery type and individual patient risk factors. Am J Surg 199:S11–20, 2010.
22. Marcantonio ER, Goldman L, Mangione CM, et al: A clinical prediction rule for delirium after elective noncardiac surgery. JAMA 271:134–139, 1994.
23. Abir F, Bell R: Assessment and management of the obese patient. Crit Care Med 32:S87–S91, 2004.
24. Bratzler DW, Houck PM, Richards C, et al: Use of antimicrobial prophylaxis for major surgery: Baseline results from the National Surgical Infection Prevention Project. Arch Surg 140:174–182, 2005.
25. Weed HG: Antimicrobial prophylaxis in the surgical patient. Med Clin North Am 87:59–75, 2003.
26. Mercado DL, Petty BG: Perioperative medication management. Med Clin North Am 87:41–57, 2003.
27. Ang-Lee MK, Moss J, Yuan CS: Herbal medicines and perioperative care. JAMA 286:208–216, 2001.
28. Brady M, Kinn S, Stuart P: Preoperative fasting for adults to prevent perioperative complications. Cochrane Database Syst Rev (4):CD004423, 2003.
29. Diks J, van Hoorn DE, Nijveldt RJ, et al: Preoperative fasting: An outdated concept? JPEN J Parenter Enteral Nutr 29:298–304, 2005.
30. Melis GC, van Leeuwen PA, von Blomberg-van der Flier BM, et al: A carbohydrate-rich beverage prior to surgery prevents surgery-induced immunodepression: A randomized, controlled, clinical trial. JPEN J Parenter Enteral Nutr 30:21–26, 2006.
31. Wijeysundera DN, Bender JS, Beattie WS: Alpha-2 adrenergic agonists for the prevention of cardiac complications among patients undergoing surgery. Cochrane Database Syst Rev (4):CD004126, 2009.
32. Rosenberger P, Shernan SK, Body SC, et al: Utility of intraoperative transesophageal echocardiography for diagnosis of pulmonary embolism. Anesth Analg 99:12–16, 2004.
33. Lieberman P: Anaphylactic reactions during surgical and medical procedures. J Allergy Clin Immunol 110:S64–69, 2002.
34. Rosenbaum HK, Miller JD: Malignant hyperthermia and myotonic disorders. Anesthesiol Clin North America 20:623–664, 2002.
35. Makary MA, Sexton JB, Freischlag JA, et al: Patient safety in surgery. Ann Surg 243:628–632, 2006.
36. Michaels RK, Makary MA, Dahab Y, et al: Achieving the National Quality Forum's "Never Events": Prevention of wrong site, wrong procedure, and wrong patient operations. Ann Surg 245:526–532, 2007.
37. Jeran L: Patient temperature: An introduction to the clinical guideline for the prevention of unplanned perioperative hypothermia. J Perianesth Nurs 16:303–304, 2001.
38. Edwards PS, Lipp A, Holmes A: Preoperative skin antiseptics for preventing surgical wound infections after clean surgery. Cochrane Database Syst Rev (3):CD003949, 2004.
39. Darouiche RO, Wall MJ, Jr, Itani KM, et al: Chlorhexidine-alcohol versus povidone-iodine for surgical site antisepsis. N Engl J Med 362:18–26, 2010.
40. Hebert PC, Wells G, Tweeddale M, et al: Does transfusion practice affect mortality in critically ill patients? Transfusion Requirements in Critical Care (TRICC) Investigators and the Canadian Critical Care Trials Group. Am J Respir Crit Care Med 155: 1618–1623, 1997.
41. DeCherney AH, diZerega GS: Clinical problem of intraperitoneal postsurgical adhesion formation following general surgery and the use of adhesion prevention barriers. Surg Clin North Am 77: 671–688, 1997.
42. Vrijland WW, Tseng LN, Eijkman HJ, et al: Fewer intraperitoneal adhesions with use of hyaluronic acid–carboxymethylcellulose membrane: A randomized clinical trial. Ann Surg 235:193–199, 2002.
43. Mizuno H, Takeda A, Uchinuma E: Creation of an acellular dermal matrix from frozen skin. Aesthetic Plast Surg 23:316–322, 1999.
44. Friedman SG, Pellerito JS, Scher L, et al: Ultrasound-guided thrombin injection is the treatment of choice for femoral pseudoaneurysms. Arch Surg 137:462–464, 2002.
45. Salo JA, Salminen JT, Kiviluoto TA, et al: Treatment of Barrett's esophagus by endoscopic laser ablation and antireflux surgery. Ann Surg 227:40–44, 1998.
46. Pasternak LR: Preoperative screening for ambulatory patients. Anesthesiol Clin North America 21:229–242, 2003.

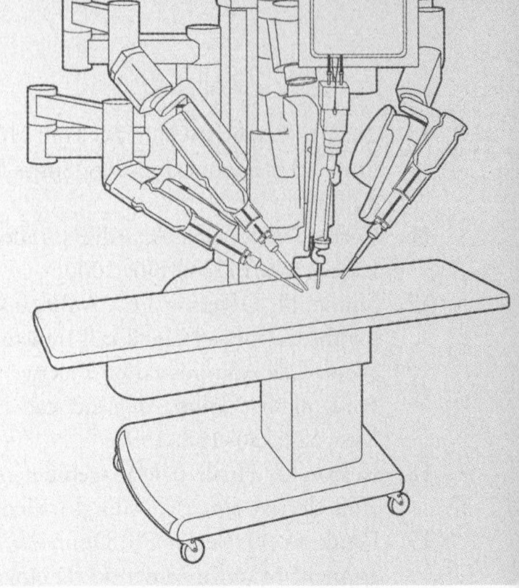

CHAPTER 12

# SURGICAL INFECTIONS AND ANTIBIOTIC USE

Philip S. Barie



Traditionally, surgical infections have been considered to be those that require surgical therapy (e.g., complicated intra-abdominal infections [cIAIs] and skin or soft tissue infections [cSSTIs]). However, surgical patients are particularly vulnerable to nosocomial infections, so a more expansive definition includes any infection that affects surgical patients. Examples of infections that may complicate perioperative care include surgical site infections (SSIs), central line–associated bloodstream infections (CLABSIs), urinary tract infections (UTIs), and hospital- or ventilator-associated pneumonia (HAP, VAP). This chapter takes the more encompassing view, recognizing that the surgical patient is at particular risk for nosocomial infections for numerous reasons.

Surgery's inherent invasiveness creates portals of entry for pathogens to invade the host through natural epithelial barriers. Surgical illness is immunosuppressive (e.g., trauma, burns, malignant tumors), as is therapeutic immunosuppression following solid organ transplantation. General anesthesia almost always means a period of endotracheal intubation and mechanical ventilation, and a period of reduced consciousness during emergence that poses a risk of pulmonary aspiration of gastric contents; both increase the risk of pneumonia. Considering that the development of a postoperative infection has a negative impact on surgical outcomes, recognizing and minimizing risk and an aggressive approach to the diagnosis and treatment of these infections are crucial.

Although morbid and costly, infection is preventable to some degree, and every physician who has patient contact must do his or her utmost to prevent infection. An ensemble of prevention methods is required, because no single method is universally effective. Infection control is paramount. Surgical incisions and traumatic wounds must be handled gently, inspected daily, and dressed if necessary using strict asepsis. Drains and catheters must be avoided, if possible, and removed as soon as practicable. Prophylactic and therapeutic antibiotics, whether empirical or directed against a known infection, should be used sparingly to minimize antibiotic selection pressure on the development of multidrug-resistant (MDR) pathogens. Each of these aspects is discussed in detail.

## RISK FACTORS FOR INFECTION

### Host Factors

The host is defined by genotype, expressed phenotypically as characteristic traits. Innate immunity provides continuous surveillance against tissue invasion by foreign antigens in the interstitial spaces just beneath epithelial barriers. Potential pathogens are ubiquitous in the environment, but although colonization of epithelia occurs even in healthy hosts, invasion generally requires a portal of entry, which for surgical patients might include injured tissue, incision, puncture site for vascular access, or indwelling catheter. Injury also stimulates a repair response (inflammation), which may cause a wide-ranging autodestructive augmentation of the inflammatory response.

The phenotypic stress response augments cardiovascular function through the autonomic nervous system, promotes glycogenolysis, catabolizes peripheral lean tissue and fat for gluconeogenesis, enhances coagulation to stanch hemorrhage, and stimulates a proinflammatory cytokine response to begin the tissue repair process (Box 12-1).[1] Innate and adaptive immunity are depressed in large part by the actions of cortisol (Table 12-1 and Box 12-2).[2]

Older age (generally, age ≥65 years) is a definite risk factor for adverse outcomes from infection,[3] related to immune senescence and an increased incidence of nosocomial infection. Hyperglycemia induces immune cell dysfunction (Box 12-3) and is a recognized risk factor for infection (Box 12-4). Even transitory hyperglycemia is associated with an increased risk of SSIs[4-7] and other nosocomial infections, and translates into increased mortality after trauma[8,9] and critical surgical illness[10,11] for diabetic and nondiabetic patients.

### Genetics and Genomics of Trauma and Sepsis

It is controversial as to whether gender makes a difference in outcome following infection and sepsis. Androgens are immunosuppressive in vitro and in animal studies, and male animals have higher mortality after trauma and sepsis,[12,13] but human data are conflicting. Population-based studies have cast doubt on the clinical importance of the laboratory observations of

**BOX 12-1 Overview of the Stress Response to Injury**

Activation of the autonomic nervous system
Activation of hypophyseal-pituitary-adrenal axis (HPAA)
Peripheral insulin resistance
Production of pro-inflammatory and anti-inflammatory cytokines and lipid mediators
Production of reactive oxygen and nitrogen intermediates
Acute-phase changes of hepatic protein synthesis
Recruitment and activation of neutrophils, monocytes-macrophages, and lymphocytes
Upregulation of procoagulant activity

**BOX 12-2 Immune Dysfunction After Injury**

**Lymphopenia**
Helper-to-suppressor T cell ratio <1
Downregulated:
- T, B cell proliferation
- NK cell activity
- IL-2 receptor expression
- IL-4, IL-10 production
- HLA-DR expression
- DTH skin test response

**Nonspecific Immunity**
Monocytosis
Upregulated:
- Acute-phase proteins
- Inflammatory cytokine production
- Eicosanoid production

Downregulated:
- Neutrophil function

*DTH,* Delayed-type hypersensitivity; *HLA,* human leukocyte antigen; *NK,* natural killer cell.

**Table 12-1 Principal Hormonal Responses to Surgical Stress**

| ENDOCRINE GLAND | HORMONES | CHANGE IN SECRETION |
|---|---|---|
| Anterior pituitary | Corticotropin | Increased |
| | Growth hormone | Increased |
| | Thyrotropin | Variable |
| | Follicle-stimulating hormone, luteinizing hormone | Variable |
| Posterior pituitary | Arginine vasopressin | Increased |
| Adrenal cortex | Cortisol | Increased |
| | Aldosterone | Increased |
| Pancreas | Insulin | Decreased |
| | Glucagon | Increased |
| Thyroid | Thyroxine | Decreased |
| | Triiodothyronine | Decreased |

**BOX 12-3 Glucose Dyshomeostasis During Stress and Effects on Cellular Immunity**

**Effects of Hyperglycemia Upon Immune Cell Function**
- Decreased respiratory burst of alveolar macrophages
- Decreased insulin-stimulated chemokinesis
- Glucose-induced protein kinase C activation
- Increased adherence
- Increased adhesion molecule generation
- Spontaneous activation of neutrophils

**Effects of Stress Response on Carbohydrate Metabolism**
- Enhanced peripheral glucose uptake
- Hyperlactatemia
- Increased gluconeogenesis
- Depressed glycogenolysis
- Peripheral insulin resistance

**BOX 12-4 Medical Conditions Known to Increase Risk of Postoperative Infection**

- Extremes of age (neonates, very old adults)
- Malnutrition
- Obesity
- Diabetes mellitus
- Prior site irradiation
- Hypothermia
- Hypoxemia
- Coexisting infection remote to surgical site
- Corticosteroid therapy
- Recent operation, especially of chest or abdomen
- Chronic inflammation
- Hypocholesterolemia

gender-based differences. Gannon and colleagues[14] have found no gender-based difference of mortality among 18,892 trauma patients; of interest, males were more likely to develop pneumonia, but females were more likely to succumb. Angus and associates[15] were unable to detect any adverse outcomes from sepsis among females in a nationwide U.S. population-based study.

Modern high-throughput, multiplexed assays allow the molecular characterization of pathologic conditions. Most genes have hundreds or thousands of nucleotides, but only a relatively short sequence is needed for the precise identification of each. The DNA microarray, minute quantities of vast numbers (i.e., many thousands) of short, gene-specific probe nucleotides affixed to a slide chip can be used to identify messenger RNA that can be isolated from cells or tissues and labeled to produce complimentary nucleotides (cDNA or cRNA). When incubated with the microarray, the cDNA or cRNA will bind by conventional base pairing. With a scanner and the aid of computational biomedicine, the label signal intensity (mRNA abundance) may be calculated and compared, generating an expression profile called the *transcriptome* for the cell or tissue of interest. Such techniques have furthered the understanding of host predisposition and response to sepsis[16,17]; application of related techniques of cell separation, genome-wide expression, and cell-specific pathway analyses may be useful to characterize alterations in human disease or the presence of specific microbes. However, their presence does not distinguish whether the microbe is a colonist or a pathogen.

In infection, genomic variability may correlate with disease susceptibility. Single nucleotide polymorphisms (SNPs), single point mutations in the nucleotide structures of genes related to inflammation (e.g., tumor necrosis factor-α [TNF-α], interleukin [IL]-1, -6, and -8), the anti-inflammatory response (e.g., IL-10, IL-1 receptor antagonist), the innate immune response (e.g., Toll-like receptor 4), and the coagulation system (e.g., factor V, plasminogen activator inhibitor-1) have been associated with a predisposition to sepsis.[18] However, heterogeneity in the immune response and predisposition to infection, as well as the severity of infections and resultant mortality, make conclusions difficult to determine, which makes it unlikely that a single SNP will be identifiable in an individual patient to characterize risk.

## Interactions Between the Host and Therapy

The risk of infection may exist as the result of injury itself, impairment of host defenses, resuscitation, or definitive care. Hypothermia may occur as the result of exposure, large-volume infusion of unwarmed fluids or blood products, or evaporative losses during intracavitary surgery, especially if the chest and abdomen are opened. Peripheral and cutaneous vasoconstriction occur to preserve core heat, but vasoconstriction decreases microcirculatory blood flow, which may also be disrupted by hypovolemia, inflammatory response, activation of coagulation, and decreased deformability of transfused red blood cells (see below).[19] Hypothermia is immunosuppressive, affects cardiovascular performance adversely, and increases mortality after trauma and surgery.[20,21]

Tissue hypoxia after trauma may result from injury to the face, airways, lungs, or chest wall, inability to secure the airway, massive blood loss, cardiovascular instability, disruption of the microcirculation, or acute respiratory distress syndrome (ARDS). Tissue hypoxia appears to predispose to SSI.[22] Administration of supplemental oxygen ($FiO_2 = 0.8$) reduces the risk of SSI after elective surgery (meta-analysis).[21]

The manner of resuscitation may influence outcome. Fluids are necessary to restore hemodynamics and microcirculatory perfusion, but the quantity and type of fluid that should be administered is still debated. Historically, crystalloid fluids were preferred to colloids, being less expensive and with results that were at least equivalent.[23] Although some trials, such as that of the SAFE investigators,[24] have led to a reappraisal, the question remains controversial. Delaney and coworkers[25] have conducted a meta-analysis of 17 trials (1977 subjects); eight trials were specifically of colloid versus crystalloid for resuscitation of patients with sepsis. Using a fixed effects model, colloid resuscitation was associated with reduced mortality (odds ratio [OR], 0.82; 95% confidence interval [CI], 0.67 to 1.0; $P = 0.047$), but not when a more robust random effects model was used for the meta-analysis (OR, 0.84; 95% CI, 0.69 to 1.02; $P = 0.08$). However, six of the trials included, by a single investigator, have been called into question for scientific misconduct[26]; omission of those results from the meta-analysis still produced a significant result by fixed effects meta-analysis (OR, 0.76; 95% CI, 0.62 to 0.95; $P = 0.015$). Functionally, resuscitation of the immune system may be the crucial determinant, as evidenced by observations that a persistent systemic inflammatory response after injury is associated with an increased risk of nosocomial infection and death.[27]

### Blood Transfusion

Blood transfusion can be lifesaving after trauma or hemorrhage, but increased risk of infection is the consequence. Transfusions express immunosuppression through altered leukocyte antigen presentation and a shift to the T helper 2 phenotype.[28] Claridge and colleagues[29] have identified an exponential relationship between transfusion and infection risk among trauma patients, detectable after even 1 unit of transfusion, and becoming a near-certainty after more than 15 units of transfused blood (relative risk [RR], 1.084; 95% CI, 1.028 to 1.142). Hill and associates[30] have estimated by meta-analysis that the risk of infection related to blood transfusion is increased for trauma patients by more than fivefold (OR, 5.26; 95% CI, 5.03 to 5.43) and, for surgical patients, by more than threefold. This increased risk for infection by transfusion has also been identified for critically ill patients in general[31] and for CLABSI[32] and VAP[33] specifically. Loss of membrane high-energy phosphates associated with prolonged storage of banked blood leads to impaired erythrocyte deformability, disruption of the microcirculation, and impaired oxygen offloading.[34] Consequently, blood transfusion does not increase oxygen consumption in severe sepsis[35] and may actually increase organ dysfunction.[36] It is safe to be conservative in the administration of red blood cell concentrates to stable patients in the ICU.[37]

### Control of Blood Sugar

Not only does hyperglycemia impair host immune function, it also reflects the catabolism and insulin resistance associated with surgical stress. Poor perioperative glycemic control increases the risk of infection and worsens outcomes from sepsis for diabetic and nondiabetic patients. Cardiac surgery patients have a higher risk of infection of sternal incision and lower extremity donor sites. Moderate hyperglycemia (>200 mg/dL) at any time on the first postoperative day increases the risk of SSI fourfold after cardiac[6] and noncardiac surgery.[7] Insulin infusion to keep the blood glucose level less than 110 mg/dL was associated with a 40% decrease in mortality among critically ill postoperative patients (≈70% of whom had undergone cardiac surgery), and also fewer nosocomial infections and less organ dysfunction.[38] However, glycemic control has become somewhat controversial because of nonconfirmation of a salutary effect in critically ill medical patients. Moreover, concern regarding an increased incidence of hypoglycemia (≈6%, <60 mg/dL) in patients treated with intensive insulin therapy, and resultant increased mortality, has led to relaxation of glycemic control targets to approximately 140 to 180 mg/dL.[39] Nonetheless, a meta-analysis of recent trials by Greisdale and associates[10] has indicated that the risk of mortality is decreased significantly for patients treated with intensive insulin therapy in dedicated surgical intensive care units (ICUs; RR, 0.63; 95% CI, 0.44 to 0.91), regardless of whether the patients had diabetes mellitus. However, countervailing opinion as to the usefulness and safety of intensive insulin therapy is prevalent.[21]

Nutritional support is crucial, considering that restoration of anabolism requires calories and nitrogen in excess of basal requirements of 25 to 30 kcal and 1 g nitrogen/kg/day. It is challenging to provide adequate calories and protein while simultaneously avoiding hyperglycemia. Parenteral nutrition may convey no advantage over not feeding the patient at all,[40] perhaps because of the inherent morbidity of central IV feeding (i.e., the risks of CLABSI and hyperglycemia). By contrast, early enteral feeding within the first 48 hours, perhaps immediately if the gut is functional, is clearly beneficial, with the possible exceptions of intestinal ischemia and pneumonia prevention (see later). The risk of infection was reduced by 55% (OR, 0.45; 95% CI, 0.30 to 0.66) in a meta-analysis of 15 randomized trials of early enteral feeding following surgery, trauma, or burns.[41]

## INFECTION CONTROL

General principles of surgical care, critical care, and infection control must be adhered to at all times. Resuscitation must be rapid, yet precise; overresuscitation and underresuscitation increase the risk of infection. Pathology must be identified and treated as soon as possible. Central venous catheters inserted under suboptimal barrier precautions (e.g., lack of cap, mask, sterile gown, and sterile gloves for the operator and a full bed drape for the patient) must be removed and replaced, if necessary, by a new puncture at a new site as soon as the patient's condition permits. Drains should be avoided and removed as soon as possible, if required.[42] Detailed evidence-based guidelines for the general prevention of SSIs,[43] CLABSIs,[44,45] and VAP have been published.[46,47]

Infection control is a individual and collective responsibility. Hand hygiene is the most effective means to reduce the spread of infection, but compliance is a continual challenge.[48] Alcohol gel hand cleansers are effective,[49] except against the spores of *Clostridium difficile*, which requires cleansing with soap and water.[50] Universal precautions—cap, mask, gown, gloves, and protective eyewear—must be observed whenever there is a risk of splashing of body fluids.

Endogenous flora are the source of most bacterial pathogens, Skin surfaces, artificial airways, gut lumen, wounds, catheters, and inanimate surfaces (e.g., bed rails, computer terminals)[51] may become colonized. Any break in natural epithelial barriers (e.g., incisions, percutaneous catheters, airway or urinary catheters) creates a portal of entry for invasion of pathogens. The fecal-oral route is the most common manner whereby pathogens reach the portal, but health care workers facilitate the transmission of pathogens on their hands.

Contact isolation is an important part of infection control and should be used selectively to prevent the spread of pathogens such as methicillin-resistant *Staphylococcus aureus* (MRSA), vancomycin-resistant enterococci (VRE), or MDR gram-negative bacilli. However, contact isolation may decrease the amount of direct patient contact.[52] An appropriate balance must be struck, because reduced nurse staffing of ICUs has been independently associated with an increased risk of a number of nosocomial infections.[53]

### Catheter Care

Optimal catheter care includes avoidance when unnecessary, appropriate skin preparation and barrier protection during insertion, proper catheter selection (e.g., antimicrobial- or antiseptic-coated), proper dressing of indwelling catheters, and removal as soon as no longer needed, or as is practicable, but no longer than 24 hours, after insertion under less than ideal circumstances (e.g., trauma bay, cardiac resuscitation).

Risks and benefits must be weighed when deciding to place any catheter, including the risk of infection. Almost all indwelling catheters carry such a risk, but nontunneled central venous catheters and pulmonary artery catheters pose the highest risk, including local site infections and CLABSIs. Other catheters that pose increased infection risk include endotracheal tubes, intercostal thoracostomy catheters (inserted as an emergency), ventriculostomy catheters for intracranial pressure monitoring, and urinary bladder catheters. Each day of endotracheal intubation and mechanical ventilation increases the risk of pneumonia by 1% to 3%[54]; it is controversial whether tracheostomy decreases that risk.[55]

Chlorhexidine gluconate, a phenolic biguanidine derivative, is used in concentrations of 0.5% to 4.0% alone or in lower concentrations in combination with an alcohol as a skin antiseptic. The microbicidal action, which is bactericidal, viricidal, and fungicidal, is somewhat slow, but persistent. Chlorhexidine should be used preferentially for skin preparation for vascular catheter insertion; it is superior to povidone-iodine solution[56] and is also recommended for surgical skin preparation,[57] topical bathing of critically ill patients,[58,59] and as an antiseptic coating for indwelling central vascular catheters.[60] If povidone-iodine solution is used for surgical site preparation, it must be allowed to dry for microbicidal effect. Note that its use is discouraged unless a mucous membrane is to be prepped. Full barrier precautions are mandatory for all bedside catheterization procedures, except arterial and urinary bladder catheterization, for which sterile gloves and a sterile field suffice if maintained meticulously. Whenever a central venous catheter is inserted under suboptimal conditions, it must be removed—and replaced at a different site if still needed—as soon as permitted by the patient's hemodynamic status, but no longer than 24 hours after insertion. A single dose of a first-generation cephalosporin (e.g., cefazolin) may prevent some infections following emergency tube thoracostomy or ventriculostomy, but is not indicated for vascular or bladder catheterizations.

It is crucial to maintain dressings carefully, which can be challenging if the patient is agitated or the body surface is irregular (e.g., the neck [internal jugular vein catheterization] as opposed to the chest wall [subclavian vein catheterization]). Marking the dressing clearly with the date and time of each change is simple and effective. Dressing carts or similar equipment should not be brought from patient to patient; instead, sufficient supplies should be kept in each patient's room. The potential for transmission of pathogens on inanimate fomites (e.g., scissors) must be borne in mind. Implementation of care bundles and dedicated catheter care teams substantially reduces the risk of CLABSIs and UTIs.[61,62]

The choice of catheter may play a role in decreasing the risk of infection related to endotracheal tubes, central venous catheters, and urinary catheters. Continuous aspiration of subglottic secretions (CASS) via an endotracheal tube with an extra lumen that opens to the airway just above the balloon facilitates the removal of secretions that accumulate below the vocal cords but above the endotracheal tube balloon, an area that cannot be reached by routine suctioning. The incidence of VAP is decreased by 50% by CASS.[63] Silver-impregnated endotracheal tubes are effective in reducing airway colonization[64] and may reduce the incidences of VAP and mortality.[65] Antibiotic-coated (e.g., minocycline/rifampin) or antiseptic-coated central venous catheters (e.g., chlorhexidine, silver sulfadiazine) can reduce the incidence of catheter-related bloodstream infections (CRBSIs),[44,66] especially in high-prevalence units; minocycline- or rifampin-coated catheters may be more effective. Urinary bladder catheters coated with ionic silver reduce the incidence of catheter-related bacterial cystitis by a similar amount.[67,68]

Ventilator weaning by protocol, including daily sedation holidays and spontaneous breathing trials, allows endotracheal extubation sooner and decreases the risk of VAP (see later).[69] An even better strategy may be avoidance of endotracheal intubation entirely. Respiratory failure can sometimes be managed with noninvasive positive-pressure ventilation delivered by mask (e.g., continuous positive airway pressure [CPAP]).[70] Improved resuscitation and noninvasive monitoring techniques have decreased the utilization of pulmonary artery catheters, which pose a particularly high risk of infection.[71] Most drains do not decrease the risk of infection; in fact, the risk is probably increased[72] because the catheters hold open a portal for invasion by bacteria.

## SPECIFIC INFECTIONS

### Surgical Site Infection

The spectrum of bacterial contamination of the surgical site is well described.[72] Clean surgical procedures affect only skin structures and other soft tissues. Clean-contaminated procedures open a hollow viscus under controlled circumstances (e.g., elective aerodigestive or genitourinary tract surgery). Contaminated procedures introduce a large inoculum of bacteria into a normally sterile body cavity, but too briefly for infection to become established during surgery (e.g., penetrating abdominal trauma, enterotomy during adhesiolysis for mechanical bowel obstruction). Dirty procedures are those performed to control established infection (e.g., colon resection for perforated diverticulitis).

The microbiology of SSI depends on the nature of the procedure, location of the incision, and whether a body cavity or hollow viscus is entered during surgery. Most SSIs are caused by skin flora that are inoculated into the incision during surgery, therefore, the most common SSI pathogens are all gram-positive cocci—*Staphylococcus epidermidis, S. aureus,* and *Enterococcus* spp. For infrainguinal incisions and intracavitary surgery, gram-negative bacilli such as *Escherichia coli* and *Klebsiella* spp. are potential pathogens. When surgery is performed on the pharynx, lower gastrointestinal tract, or female genital tract, anaerobic bacteria become potential SSI pathogens. Antibiotic prophylaxis should be suitably directed against likely pathogens (see later).

The incidence of SSIs has been estimated to be about 3% in the United States, although the incidence varies greatly from less than 5% for clean surgery to more than 20% for emergency colon surgery, which is often performed in a dirty field. Moreover, the overall estimate is almost certainly an underestimate, considering that SSI following ambulatory surgery, which now represents more than 70% of all operations in the United States, is seldom reported. Numerous factors determine whether a patient will develop an SSI, including those related to the patient, environment, and treatment (Box 12-5).[72] As incorporated in the National Nosocomial Infections Surveillance System (NNIS) and its successor program, the National Healthcare Safety Network (NHSN),[73-75] the most recognized factors are wound classification, American Society of Anesthesiologists class 3 or higher (class 3 is chronic active medical illness), and prolonged operative time, where time is longer than the 75th percentile for the given procedure. According to the NNIS-NHSN, the risk of SSI increases as the number of risk factors present increases, irrespective of the type of operation.[76] Laparoscopic surgery is associated with a decreased incidence of SSI under most circumstances. There are several possible reasons why laparoscopic surgery decreases the risk of SSI, including decreased wound size, limited use of cautery in the abdominal wall, and a diminished stress response to tissue injury.

**BOX 12-5 Risk Factors for the Development of Surgical Site Infections**

**Patient Factors**
Ascites (for abdominal surgery)
Chronic inflammation
Corticosteroid therapy (controversial)
Obesity
Diabetes
Extremes of age
Hypocholsterolemia
Hypoxemia
Peripheral vascular disease (for lower extremity surgery)
Postoperative anemia
Prior site irradiation
Recent operation
Remote infection
Skin or nasal carriage of staphylococci
Skin disease in the area of infection (e.g., psoriasis)
Undernutrition

**Environmental Factors**
Contaminated medications
Inadequate disinfection/sterilization
Inadequate skin antisepsis
Inadequate ventilation

**Treatment Factors**
Drains
Emergency procedure
Hypothermia
Inadequate antibiotic prophylaxis
Oxygenation (controversial)
Prolonged preoperative hospitalization
Prolonged operative time

Host-derived factors contribute importantly to the risk of SSI, including increased age,[77] obesity, malnutrition, diabetes mellitus,[7] hypocholesterolemia,[78] and several other factors not accounted for specifically by the NNIS-NHSN (see Box 12-5). In a study of 5031 noncardiac surgical patients, the incidence of SSI was 3.2%.[79] Independent risk factors for the development of SSI included ascites, diabetes mellitus, postoperative anemia, and recent weight loss, but not chronic obstructive pulmonary disease, tobacco use, or corticosteroid use. In another prospective study of 9016 patients, 12.5% of patients developed an infection of some type within 28 days after surgery.[80] Multivariable analysis revealed that decreased serum albumin concentration, increased age, tracheostomy, and amputations were associated with an early infection, whereas a dialysis shunt, vascular repair, and early infection were associated with hospital readmission. Factors associated with 28-day mortality included increased age, low serum albumin concentration, increased serum creatinine concentration, and an early infection.

Hypothermia during surgery is common if patients are not warmed actively because of evaporative water loss, administration of room temperature fluids, and other factors.[81]

Maintenance of normal core body temperature is unequivocally important for decreasing the incidence of SSIs. Mild intraoperative hypothermia is associated with an increased incidence of SSIs following elective colon surgery[82] and diverse operations[83]

It is controversial whether perioperative oxygen administration is beneficial for the prevention of infection.[84] The ischemic milieu of the fresh surgical incision is vulnerable to bacterial invasion. Moreover, oxygen has been postulated to have a direct antibacterial effect.[85,86] Although clinical trials have had conflicting results,[87,88] one recent meta-analysis has suggested a benefit of supplemental oxygen administration specifically to reduce the incidence of SSIs,[21] but further studies may be needed before the practice becomes routine.

Skin closure of a contaminated or dirty incision is believed to increase the risk of SSIs, but few good studies exist to evaluate the multiplicity of wound closure techniques available to surgeons. Open abdomen techniques of temporary abdominal closure for management of trauma or severe peritonitis are increasingly being used. Retrospective data have indicated that antibiotics are not indicated for prophylaxis of the open abdomen,[89] although an inability to achieve primary abdominal closure is associated with several infectious complications (e.g., pneumonia, bloodstream infection, SSIs). Infectious complications, in turn, significantly increase costs from prolonged length of stay, but not mortality.[90]

Drains placed in incisions probably cause more infections than they prevent. Epithelialization of the wound is prevented and the drain becomes a conduit, holding open a portal for invasion by pathogens colonizing the skin. Several studies of drains placed into clean or clean-contaminated incisions have shown that the rate of SSI is not reduced[91,92]; in fact, the rate is increased.[93-96] Considering that drains pose this risk, they should be used as little as possible and removed as soon as possible.[97] Under no circumstances should prolonged antibiotic prophylaxis be administered to cover indwelling drains (see later).

Wound irrigation is a controversial means to reduce the risk of SSIs. Routine low-pressure saline irrigation is ineffective,[98] but high-pressure (i.e., pulsed) irrigation may be beneficial.[99] Intraoperative topical antibiotics can minimize the risk of SSIs,[100-102] but the use of antiseptics rather than antibiotics might minimize the development of resistance.

Surgical site infection remains a clinical diagnosis. Presenting signs and symptoms depend on the depth of infection, typically as early as postoperative day 4 or 5, although rare necrotizing SSIs caused by *Streptococcus pyogenes* or *Clostridium perfringens* may develop within 24 hours after surgery. Clinical signs range from local induration only to the hallmarks of infection (e.g., erythema, edema, tenderness, warmth, pain-related immobility), which may manifest before wound drainage. In cases of deep incisional SSIs, tenderness may extend beyond the margin of erythema, and crepitus, cutaneous vesicles, or bullae may be present. With ongoing infection, signs of systemic inflammatory response syndrome (SIRS; two or more of fever, leukocytosis, tachycardia, or tachypnea) herald the development of sepsis. In intracavitary (organ, space) SSIs, symptoms specific to the involved organ system will usually predominate, such as ileus, respiratory distress or failure, or altered sensorium.

Cultures are not mandatory for the management of superficial incisional SSIs, particularly if drainage and wound care alone will suffice without antibiotics and if superficial swab cultures are collected, which are susceptible to contamination by nearby skin colonists. In cases of deeper infection or hospital-acquired infection, exudates or drainage specimens should be sent for analysis from the surgically opened wound—as opposed to the already opened wound, which becomes colonized.

More severe SSIs, especially the dangerous forms of necrotizing soft tissue infection (NSTI), are true emergencies that need immediate surgical attention. Even modest delays can increase mortality substantially. Freischlag and coworkers[103] have shown that mortality increases from 32% to 70% when therapy is delayed longer than 24 hours. Immediate widespread débridement is indicated for established NSTIs without waiting for identification of the causative pathogen or development of a specific symptom. Sequential surgical débridements may be needed to control the infection.

The first steps in the treatment of SSIs are to open and examine the suspicious portion of the incision and decide about further surgical treatment.[104] If the infection is confined to the skin and superficial underlying subcutaneous tissue, opening the incision and providing local wound care may be all the treatment that is necessary. Antibiotic therapy of superficial incisional SSIs is indicated only for erythema extending beyond the wound margin or for systemic signs of infection. Deeper SSIs may require formal surgical exploration and débridement to obtain local control of the infection. Surgical site infection must also be considered as a cause of delayed or failed wound healing and prompt the same decisions as described earlier.

Organ or space SSIs occur within a body cavity (e.g., intra-abdominal, intrapleural, intracranial) and are directly related to a surgical procedure. These deep infections may remain occult or present with few symptoms, mimicking incisional SSIs and leading to inadequate initial treatment; they become apparent only when a major complication ensues. The diagnosis of organ or space SSIs usually requires some form of imaging to confirm the site and extent of infection. Adequate source control requires a drainage procedure, whether open or percutaneous.

Experimentally, vacuum-assisted wound closure (VAC) was first appraised by Morykwas and colleagues[105] in a porcine model in 1997. Therapy by VAC optimizes blood flow, decreases edema, and aspirates accumulated fluid, thereby facilitating bacterial clearance. Negative pressure promotes wound contraction to cover the defect and may trigger intracellular signaling that increases cellular proliferation.[106] The clinical usefulness of VAC has been described only anecdotally, mostly for sternal infections following cardiac surgery, abdominal wall dehiscence, management of complex perineal wounds, or securing skin grafts.[107,108]

Many general and specific tactics for the prevention of SSIs have been brought together in a bundle known as the Surgical Care Improvement Project (SCIP), the effectiveness of which has been called into question.[109,110] A predecessor program, the National Surgical Infection Prevention Project (SIP), focused primarily on the quality of antibiotic prophylaxis, including choice of agent, timing of administration, and duration of prophylaxis. A national audit found that the agents being prescribed for prophylaxis were often inappropriate, the effectiveness of prophylaxis was decreased because the timing of administration was suboptimal, and only 40% of patients administered surgical antibiotic prophylaxis had the antibiotic discontinued within 24 hours, risking adverse events (e.g., superinfection, development of bacterial resistance).[111] It was advised that antibiotic administration should occur within 60 minutes before incision and

**BOX 12-6 Surgical Care Improvement Project Performance Measures***

**Antibiotic Prophylaxis**

Proportion of patients who have their antibiotic dose initiated within 1 hour before surgical incision (2 hours for vancomycin or a fluoroquinolone)

Proportion of patients who receive an approved antibiotic agent for prophylaxis consistent with current recommendations (published guidelines; see Table 12-2)

Proportion of patients whose prophylactic antibiotics were discontinued within 24 hours of the surgery end time (48 hours for cardiac surgery)

Clindamycin use is preferred for patients allergic to β-lactam antibiotics.

Vancomycin is allowed for prophylaxis of cardiac, vascular, and orthopedic surgery if there is a physician-documented reason in the medical record or documented β-lactam allergy.

**Glucose Control (Cardiac Surgery Patients)**

Blood glucose concentration must be maintained <200 mg/dL for the first 2 days after surgery.

Blood glucose determination closest to 6 am on postoperative days 1 and 2 (surgery end date is postoperative day 0) is monitored.

**Hair Removal**

- No hair removal should be performed; if hair is removed, clippers or a depilatory agent should be used immediately prior to surgery. Razors are not to be used.

**Normothermia (Colorectal Surgery Patients)**

- Core body temperature should be between 96.8° to 100.4° F within the first hour after leaving the operating room.

*Relevant to prevention of surgical site infection.

**Table 12-2 Surgical Care Improvement Program: Approved Antibiotic Prophylactic Regimens for Elective Surgery**

| TYPE OF OPERATION | ANTIBIOTIC(S) |
|---|---|
| Cardiac (including CABG),[a] vascular[b] | Cefazolin or cefuroxime or vancomycin[c] |
| Hip, knee arthroplasty[b] | Cefazolin or cefuroxime or vancomycin[c] |
| Colon[d,e] | Oral: Neomycin sulfate plus erythromycin base or metronidazole, administered for 18 hr before surgery<br>Parenteral: Cefoxitin or cefotetan or ertapenem or cefazolin plus metronidazole or ampicillin-sulbactam |
| Hysterectomy[f] | Cefazolin or cefoxitin or cefotetan or cefuroxime or ampicillin-sulbactam |

*CABG,* Coronary artery bypass grafting.

[a]Prophylaxis may be administered for up to 48 hr for cardiac surgery; for all other cases, the limit is 24 hr.

[b]For β-lactam allergy, clindamycin or vancomycin are acceptable substitutes for cardiac, vascular, and orthopedic surgery.

[c]Vancomycin is acceptable with a physician-documented justification for use in the patient's medical record.

[d]For β-lactam allergy, clindamycin plus gentamicin, a fluoroquinolone, or aztreonam, or metronidazole plus gentamicin or a fluoroquinolone are acceptable choices.

[e]For colon surgery, oral or parenteral prophylaxis alone, or both combined, are acceptable.

[f]For β-lactam allergy, clindamycin plus gentamicin, a fluoroquinolone, or aztreonam, or metronidazole plus gentamicin or a fluoroquinolone or clindamycin monotherapy, are acceptable choices.

that prophylaxis should continue for no longer than 24 hours.[112] Implementation demonstrated improved adherence to process measures.[113]

The SIP was incorporated into SCIP, with additional process measures added (Box 12-6), including recommendations for agents to be used for prophylaxis in specific circumstances (Table 12-2). As a U.S. federal program, SCIP includes reporting mandates, with financial incentives for compliance that will eventually become penalties for noncompliance.[114] Perhaps not unexpectedly, several studies have reported that the incidence of SSIs has not decreased under SCIP,[109,110] possibly for several reasons.[115] Baseline infection rates may have increased as a result of improved reporting, masking any decrease from process improvement. The inherent assumption, that a focus on process improvement will result in an improved outcome, may be flawed. Causes and prevention of SSIs are complex and multifactorial and compartmentalization by SCIP may be an oversimplification. Moreover, SCIP is not a smorgasbord of tactics from which the clinician may pick and choose; prevention of SSIs requires the flawless execution of an ensemble of prevention tactics,[116] not all of which are included in SCIP. For example, correction of patient factors is notably missing. Nonetheless, all the SCIP measures are supported by ample, good-quality evidence, and the search for processes that lead to meaningful improvements in outcome must continue.

## Postoperative Pneumonia

Surgical patients are particularly susceptible to pneumonia, particularly if they require mechanical ventilation (Table 12-3). VAP, defined as pneumonia occurring 48 to 72 hours after endotracheal intubation, is the most common ICU infection among surgical and trauma patients. The incidence appears to be decreasing but, unfortunately, VAP is partially iatrogenic, and sometimes associated with difficult to treat MDR pathogens. Increasingly ill patients, nonspecific diagnostic criteria, indiscriminate antibiotic use, and unclear therapeutic end points have all contributed to the increased prevalence of VAP caused by MDR pathogens. In turn, MDR pathogens increase the likelihood of inadequate initial antimicrobial therapy, which exerts further selection pressure for these pathogens and results in higher mortality.

Distinction is sometimes made between early-onset VAP (occurring <5 days after intubation) and late-onset VAP (occurring ≥5 days after intubation). Early-onset VAP, to which trauma patients are particularly prone, is often a result of aspiration of gastric contents and is usually caused by antibiotic-sensitive bacteria such as methicillin-sensitive *S. aureus, Streptococcus pneumoniae,* and *Haemophilus influenzae.*[46,117,118] Conversely, patients with late-onset VAP are at increased risk for infection with MDR pathogens (e.g., MRSA, *Pseudomonas aeruginosa, Acinetobacter* spp.).

The incidence of VAP depends on the diagnostic criteria used and therefore varies in published reports. Clinical criteria

**Table 12-3 Rates of Health Care–Associated Pneumonia Among Various ICU Types***

| | TT Use | | VAP Rate (Mean/Median) | |
|---|---|---|---|---|
| ICU TYPE | 1992-2004 | 2006-2008 | 1992-2004 | 2006-2008 |
| Medical | 0.46 | 0.48 | 4.9/3.7 | 2.4/2.2 |
| Pediatric | 0.39 | 0.42 | 2.9/2.3 | 1.8/0.7 |
| Surgical | 0.44 | 0.39 | 9.3/8.3 | 4.9/3.8 |
| Cardiovascular | 0.43 | 0.39 | 7.2/6.3 | 3.9/2.6 |
| Neurosurgical | 0.39 | 0.36 | 11.2/6.2 | 5.3/4.0 |
| Trauma | 0.56 | 0.57 | 15.2/11.4 | 8.1/5.2 |

From National Nosocomial Infections Surveillance (NNIS) System Report, data summary from January 1992 through June 2004, issued October 2004. Am J Infect Control 32:470–485, 2004; and Edwards JR, Peterson KD, Mu Y, et al: National Healthcare Safety Network (NHSN) report: Data summary for 2006 through 2008, issued December 2009. Am J Infect Control 37:783–805, 2009.

*TT use,* Number of days of indwelling endotracheal tube or tracheostomy/1000 patient-days in ICU; *VAP,* ventilator-associated pneumonia.
*Infection rates are indexed per 1000 patient-days.

**BOX 12-7 Risk Factors for the Development of Ventilator-Associated Pneumonia**

Age ≥60 yr
Acute respiratory distress syndrome
Chronic obstructive pulmonary disease or other underlying pulmonary disease
Coma or impaired consciousness
Serum albumin level <2.2 g/dL
Burns, trauma
Blood transfusion
Organ failure
Supine position
Large-volume gastric aspiration
Sinusitis
Immunosuppression
Prolonged mechanical ventilation

**Table 12-4 Strategies to Prevent Ventilator-Associated Pneumonia**

| STRATEGY | RECOMMENDED | INSUFFICIENT EVIDENCE |
|---|---|---|
| Universal infection control precautions | + | |
| Orotracheal intubation (versus nasotracheal) | + | |
| Maintenance of endotracheal cuff pressure >20 cm $H_2O$ | + | |
| Continuous aspiration of subglottic secretions | + | |
| Semirecumbent positioning | + | |
| Modified cuff technology | + | |
| Sliver-impregnated endotracheal tube | + | |
| Postpyloric feeding | | + |
| Postponement of enteral feeding for at least 48 hr following intubation | + | |
| Selective decontamination of the digestive tract | | ? |
| Topical chlorhexidine (pharynx or bathing) | + | |
| Transfusion restriction | + | |
| Antibiotic cycling | | + |

alone (e.g., those of the Centers for Disease Control and Prevention [CDC]), which do not require the identification of a pathogen) underestimate the incidence of VAP as compared with microbiologic or histologic data.[119,120] A systematic review of 89 studies of mechanically ventilated patients with VAP[121] has reported a pooled incidence of VAP of 22.8% (95% CI, 18.8 to 26.9). The risk for trauma patients, especially those with traumatic brain injury, is especially high. The incidence of VAP increases with the duration of mechanical ventilation at a rate of 3%/day during the first 5 days, 2%/day during days 5 to 10, and 1%/day after that.[54]

Risk factors for VAP are summarized in Box 12-7. Perhaps most important is airway intubation itself. The risk of HAP increases 6- to 20-fold in mechanically ventilated patients[121,122]; VAP is especially common in patients with ARDS because of prolonged mechanical ventilation and devastated local airway host defenses.[123]

Several evidence-based strategies can prevent VAP but, to be used effectively, a thorough understanding of modifiable risk factors is required (Table 12-4).[124] Prevention of VAP begins with the minimization of endotracheal intubation and duration of mechanical ventilation. Noninvasive positive-pressure ventilation (NIPPV) should be used when possible (e.g., awake patient with intact airway reflexes), because it is associated with a lower incidence of VAP.[125] When the airway must be secure, orotracheal intubation is preferred to the nasotracheal route; the former decreases the risk of VAP by 50%[126] by decreasing the risk of nosocomial sinusitis, a known antecedent of VAP. Evidence-based strategies to decrease the duration of mechanical ventilation include daily assessment for readiness to extubate by interruption of sedation and spontaneous breathing trials,[127] standardized weaning protocols, and adequate ICU staffing.[128]

After intubation, most VAP preventive measures aim to decrease the risk of aspiration. Maintenance of endotracheal cuff pressure more than 20 cm $H_2O$, new balloon cuff materials and technology that facilitate a better seal between balloon and tracheal side wall,[129] and continuous aspiration of subglottic secretions (CASS)[63] reduce the incidence of VAP significantly. Semirecumbent positioning (30 to 45 degrees, head up) is also protective as compared with supine positioning, especially during enteral feeding.[130] Postpyloric feeding may decrease the risks of gastroesophageal reflux and aspiration. A meta-analysis of 11 randomized trials has reported a RR of 0.77 (95% CI, 0.60 to 1.00; $P = .05$) for VAP with postpyloric as compared with gastric feedings,[131] but promotility agents such as erythromycin facilitate safe intragastric feeding.[132] However, early enteral feedings may increase the risk of VAP. Shorr and colleagues[33] have reported that enteral nutrition begun 48 hours or less after the initiation of mechanical ventilation is independently associated with the development of VAP (OR, 2.65; 95% CI, 1.93 to 3.63; $P < .0001$).

Pharmacologic strategies to minimize the risk of VAP include stress ulcer prophylaxis and selective decontamination of the digestive tract (SDD) with topical or systemic antibiotics or antiseptics. Many clinical trials have examined the effect of SDD on the incidence of VAP, but the literature is limited by questionable study methodology,[133] study in ICUs in which MDR pathogens were rare, and an increased number of infections caused by MDR bacteria observed in the SSD groups,[134,135] especially gram-positive cocci. For these reasons, the use of SDD remains controversial for the routine prevention of VAP. However, a meta-analysis of studies of oropharyngeal decontamination with topical chlorhexidine has provided sufficient evidence to recommend the practice,[136] especially for cardiac surgical patients.

Ample data document the relationship between blood transfusion and infection risk in surgical, trauma, and critically ill patients.[28-32] Shorr and associates[33] have found red blood cell transfusion to be an independent risk factor for VAP (OR, 1.89; 95% CI, 1.33 to 2.68; $P = .0004$). Earley and coworkers[137] have documented a 90% decreased incidence of VAP in a surgical ICUs following implementation of an anemia management protocol that resulted in fewer blood transfusions.

The diagnosis of VAP is challenging to make accurately, because noninfectious processes that produce abnormal chest radiographs (CXRs) and gas exchange (e.g., congestive heart failure, atelectasis, ARDS, pulmonary embolism, pulmonary hemorrhage) may coexist. Intubated sedated patients cannot mobilize respiratory secretions without assistance. Moreover, immunocompromised patients, such as solid organ transplant recipients, may have pneumonia without fever, cough, sputum production, or leukocytosis.[138] The diagnosis of VAP requires not only determination if the patient has pneumonia, but also determination of the causative agent. Poor specificity (false-positive results) is problematic because it exposes patients to risk from overtreatment with antibiotics and also increases the risk of emergence of MDR bacteria.[139,140] Conversely, inadequate initial therapy is associated with increased mortality that cannot be reduced by subsequent modification of the antibiotic regimen.[141]

According to CDC criteria, the diagnosis of VAP requires one or more of the following: fever, leukocytosis or leukopenia, purulent sputum, hypoxemia, or a new or evolving CXR infiltrate. No pathogen need be identified. However, noninfectious processes mimic these nonspecific signs, so clinical criteria alone are unreliable. A new CXR infiltrate, along with two of the criteria mentioned, is only 69% sensitive and 75% specific for VAP as compared with postmortem histology.[142] Subsequent reports have confirmed the low specificity of the clinical diagnosis of VAP[143]; microbiologic confirmation occurs in fewer than 50% of cases.[144] Computed tomography (CT) has only a fair correlation with the diagnosis of pneumonia in complex patients.[145]

The clinical pulmonary infection score (CPIS) incorporates clinical, radiographic, and microbiologic criteria (e.g., temperature, leukocyte count, CXR infiltrates, appearance and volume of tracheal secretions, $PaO_2$, $FIO_2$, culture and Gram stain of tracheal aspirate—0 to 2 points each) to yield a maximum score of 12 points.[146] A CPIS higher than 6 points indicates a high probability of VAP. However, the specificity of CPIS is no better than clinical acumen alone when compared with lower respiratory tract cultures obtained via bronchoscopic bronchoalveolar lavage (BAL) or protected specimen brush (PSB),[147,148] and is inaccurate for use on trauma patients.[149] However, the negative predictive value of a negative Gram stain from a stable patient is almost 100%.[150]

Because of the low specificity of traditional diagnostic criteria, culture of lower respiratory tract samples is mandatory for nosocomial pneumonia prior to the administration of antibiotics to minimize false-negative results. The methods of specimen collection (invasive versus noninvasive) and specimen analysis (semiquantitative versus quantitative) have been debated. Noninvasive techniques include endotracheal suction aspiration (EA), blinded plugged telescoping catheter (PTC), blinded PSB, and mini-BAL. Endotracheal aspirates are less specific because of an increased likelihood of contamination by oropharyngeal flora reflecting colonization rather than infection, which is the crucial issue in diagnosis.

Invasive techniques (BAL or PSB) collect samples by fiberoptic bronchoscopy and allow direct inspection of the airways, but are more expensive and resource-intensive. Whereas semiquantitative microbiology reports growth in ordinal categories (e.g., light, moderate, heavy), quantitative microbiology reports growth in terms of colony forming units (CFU) per milliliter of aliquot; a threshold value is assigned to distinguish colonization from infection. Commonly used thresholds are $10^3$ CFU/mL for PSB, $10^4$ CFU/mL for BAL, and $10^5$ CFU/mL for EA. Any threshold should be lowered by one order of magnitude for antibiotic therapy prior to sample acquisition.[151]

Bronchoscopic specimen techniques are more specific than blinded techniques and both techniques are superior to EA, although it is unclear whether this makes a difference clinically. Shorr and colleagues[152] have performed a meta-analysis of randomized trials that compared outcomes of patients with VAP managed with invasive versus noninvasive sampling when both samples were cultured quantitatively. Although the pooled OR suggested a survival advantage to the invasive approach (OR, 0.62), the result was not significant. However, patients in the invasive group were significantly more likely to undergo changes in the antimicrobial regimen, whether narrowing of therapy or cessation.

Organisms that may be pathogens in VAP or contaminants when recovered from the airway include *P. aeruginosa*, *Enterobacteriaceae*, *S. pneumoniae*, *S. aureus*, and *H. influenzae*. Conversely, isolation of enterococci, viridans streptococci, coagulase-negative staphylococci, and *Candida* spp. are rarely, if ever, a cause of respiratory dysfunction.

**Table 12-5 Rates of Central Venous Catheter Use and Central Line-Associated Bloodstream Infection Among Various ICU Types**

| | CVC Use | | CLABSI Rate (Mean/Median) | |
|---|---|---|---|---|
| ICU TYPE | 1992-2004 | 2006-2008 | 1992-2004 | 2006-2008 |
| Medical | 0.52 | 0.45 | 5.0/3.9 | 1.9/1.0 |
| Pediatric | 0.46 | 0.48 | 6.6/5.2 | 3.0/2.5 |
| Surgical | 0.61 | 0.59 | 4.6/3.4 | 2.3/1.7 |
| Cardiovascular | 0.79 | 0.71 | 2.7/1.8 | 1.4/0.8 |
| Neurosurgical | 0.48 | 0.44 | 4.6/3.1 | 2.5/1.9 |
| Trauma | 0.61 | 0.63 | 7.4/5.2 | 3.6/3.0 |

From National Nosocomial Infections Surveillance (NNIS) System Report, data summary from January 1992 through June 2004, issued October 2004. Am J Infect Control 32:470–485, 2004; and Edwards JR, Peterson KD, Mu Y, et al: National Healthcare Safety Network (NHSN) report: Data summary for 2006 through 2008, issued December 2009. Am J Infect Control 37:783–805, 2009.

*CVC use,* Number of days of central venous catheter placement/1000 patient-days in ICU.

Infection rates are indexed per 1000 patient-days.

## Central Line–Associated Bloodstream Infection

Critically ill patients often require reliable large-bore central venous access (e.g., femoral, internal jugular, subclavian vein), but the catheters are prone to infection. Strict adherence to infection control, proper insertion technique, and catheter care are crucial for prevention (see earlier) because surgical and trauma patients are at high risk (Table 12-5). When placed under elective (controlled) circumstances, optimal technique includes chlorhexidine skin preparation (not povidone-iodine), maximum barrier precautions (i.e., draping the entire bed into the sterile field; donning a cap, mask, and sterile gown and gloves), and implementing a formal catheter care protocol. If insertion technique is breached, the risk of infection increases exponentially, and the catheter should be removed and replaced (if still needed) at a different site using strict asepsis and antisepsis as soon as the patient's condition permits, but certainly within 24 hours. Infection risk is highest for femoral vein catheters and lowest for catheters placed via the subclavian route.[153] Peripheral vein catheters, peripherally placed central catheters (PICCs), and tunneled central venous catheters (e.g., Hickman, Broviac) pose less risk of infection than percutaneous central venous catheters. Implementation of bundles and checklists are effective measures to decrease the risk of CLABSIs when implemented and adhered to rigorously.[154-157] Antibiotic- and antiseptic-coated catheters are controversial, but may help decrease the risk of infection in units that have a high rate of infection.[44]

All intravascular devices and insertion sites must be assessed daily to determine ongoing need and whether signs of local infection are present (e.g., inflammation or purulence at the exit site or along the tunnel). Contaminated catheter hubs are common portals of entry for organisms colonizing the endoluminal surface of the catheter. Infusate (e.g., fluid, blood products, IV medications) can become contaminated and cause bacteremia or fungemia, which is likely to result in septic shock. Abrupt onset of signs and symptoms of sepsis or shock in patients with an indwelling vascular catheter should prompt suspicion of catheter infection. Positive blood cultures for staphylococci or *Candida* spp. strongly suggest infection of a vascular catheter, which should prompt removal and culture of the catheter. Studies have demonstrated the reliability of semiquantitative or quantitative catheter tip culture methods for the diagnosis of a colonized catheter.[158] The predictive value of a positive catheter culture is low when there is a low pretest probability of catheter-related line sepsis, and catheters removed from ICU patients should only be cultured if there is strong clinical suspicion of CLABSI. For patients undergoing evaluation for fever who do not have SIRS, there is usually no need to remove or change all indwelling catheters immediately; however, this would be prudent in a patient with a prosthetic heart valve or fresh arterial graft and is strongly recommended for severe sepsis or septic shock, peripheral embolization, disseminated intravascular coagulation, or ARDS.

Suppurative phlebitis of a central vein caused by a centrally placed catheter is unusual. With suppurative phlebitis, bloodstream infection characteristically originates from a peripheral vein catheter site with an infected intravascular thrombus, producing a picture of overwhelming sepsis with high-grade bacteremia or fungemia. This syndrome is encountered most often in burn patients or other ICU patients who develop catheter-related infection that goes unrecognized, permitting microbes to proliferate. In patients with persistent *S. aureus* bacteremia or fungemia, echocardiography is appropriate to assess for endocarditis and guide further therapy.[159]

## Urinary Tract Infection

Catheter-associated bacteriuria or candiduria usually represents colonization, is rarely symptomatic, and is an unlikely cause of fever or secondary bloodstream infection,[160,161] even in immunocompromised patients,[162] unless there is urinary tract obstruction, history of recent urologic manipulation, injury, or surgery, or neutropenia.[163,164] As such, there has been relatively little emphasis until recently on the prevention of nosocomial UTIs compared with VAP or CLABSIs.[165] As effective prevention tactics, emphasis is now being placed on avoidance or brief duration of catheterization (e.g., <48 hours for elective surgery patients)[157,165] and on the use of silver alloy–coated catheters[67,68] when instrumentation is required.

Traditional signs and symptoms (e.g., dysuria, urgency, pelvic or flank pain, fever or chills) that correlate with bacteriuria in noncatheterized patients are rarely reported in ICU patients with documented catheter-associated bacteriuria or candiduria (>$10^5$ CFU/mL).[166,167] In the ICU, most urinary tract infections are related to urinary catheters and are caused by multiresistant, nosocomial, gram-negative bacilli other than *E. coli, Enterococcus* spp., and yeasts.[165]

When clinical evaluation suggests the urinary tract as a possible source of fever, a urine specimen should be evaluated by direct microscopy, Gram stain, and quantitative culture.[161] The specimen should be aspirated from the catheter sampling port after disinfecting the port with 70% to 90% alcohol, not collected from the drainage bag. Urine collected for culture should reach the laboratory promptly to prevent multiplication of bacteria within the receptacle, which might lead to the misdiagnosis of infection; any delay should prompt refrigeration of the specimen.

In contrast to community-acquired urinary tract infections, in which pyuria is highly predictive of important bacteriuria, pyuria may be absent with catheter-associated urinary tract infection. Even if present, pyuria is not a reliable predictor of UTI in the presence of a catheter.[167] The concentration of urinary bacteria or yeast needed to cause symptomatic urinary tract infection or fever is unclear. Whereas it is clear that counts higher than $10^3$ CFU/mL represent true bacteriuria or candiduria in catheterized patients,[168] no evidence has shown that higher counts are more likely to represent symptomatic infection.

Whereas it is appropriate to collect urine specimens in the investigation of fever (see later), routine monitoring or surveillance cultures of urine contribute little to patient management. Rapid dipstick tests, which detect leukocyte esterase and nitrite, are unreliable in the setting of a catheter-related UTI. The leukocyte esterase test correlates with the degree of pyuria, which may or may not be present in a catheter-related UTI. The nitrite test reflects *Enterobacteriaceae*, which convert nitrate to nitrite, and is therefore unreliable to screen for *Enterococcus, Candida,* and *Staphylococcus* spp.

### Intra-Abdominal Infection

Intra-abdominal infections (IAIs) represent a diverse group of diseases commonly encountered in surgical practice. Such infections are dichotomized traditionally and for clinical research purposes into uncomplicated (uIAI) and complicated (cIAI)[169] and, more recently, as to whether they arose in the community-associated (CA-IAI) or hospital-associated (HA-IAI) setting (e.g., associated with a colon anastomotic dehiscence), and whether they are low, moderate, or high risk for clinical failure, morbidity, or death. In uIAIs, infection is contained within a single organ and there may be no perforation of the gastrointestinal (GI) tract. Uncomplicated IAIs almost never cause serious illness and will not considered further here, although a complicating nosocomial infection could make matters worse.[170]

By contrast, cIAIs extend beyond the source organ and into the peritoneal cavity through a perforated viscus, thereby stimulating a greater SIRS response. The extent of infection depends on containment by local intraperitoneal host defenses. Contained infection results in the formation of an abscess, which is facilitated by foreign bodies to lower the inoculum size and microbial synergy, and creates a low pH environment that impairs phagocyte function and impedes permeation of immune cells and antibiotics. Uncontained spread of infection leads to diffuse peritonitis, a condition characterized by higher mortality that necessitates urgent celiotomy.[171]

Most IAIs may be controlled effectively, with low associated morbidity, through removal or repair of the infected focus, treatment with narrow-spectrum, pathogen-specific antimicrobial therapy (if indicated), and restoration of anatomy if resection is performed for definitive source control. However, in cases of high-risk or hospital-acquired cIAI, broad-spectrum empirical antimicrobial therapy is indicated because of an increased risk of causative MDR pathogens.[172,173] Inappropriate initial antimicrobial therapy of high-risk patients with cIAIs leads to increased rates of clinical failure and death,[174,175] often caused by multiorgan dysfunction syndrome (MODS). In cases of severe sepsis or septic shock secondary to IAI, termed *abdominal sepsis,* mortality is approximately 25% to 35%,[176,177] but may exceed 70%.[178,179] Treatment of abdominal sepsis is predicated on adequate physical drainage or resection of the infected focus (termed *source control*), which may range from percutaneous drainage to serial laparotomies and open abdominal wound management in severe cases.[180]

Mortality from HA-IAIs is higher than from CA-IAIs.[181,182] Health care–associated nonpostoperative IAIs, which arise in patients hospitalized for reasons unrelated to abdominal pathology, portend a particularly poor prognosis.[183] In these cases, diagnosis is often delayed because of a low index of suspicion, poor underlying health status, and altered sensorium. Health care–associated IAIs are significantly more likely to involve pathogens that are resistant to narrow-spectrum agents[173] and therefore are more likely to be treated inadequately as compared with patients with CA-IAIs, contributing to treatment failures and a higher incidence of morbidity and mortality.[175]

## ANTIBIOTIC USE

### Pharmacokinetic and Pharmacodynamic Principles

Pharmacokinetics (PK) involves the principles of drug absorption, distribution, and metabolism.[184] Dose-response relationships are influenced by dose, dosing interval, and route of administration. Plasma and tissue drug concentrations are influenced by absorption, distribution, and elimination, which in turn depend on drug metabolism and excretion. Serum drug concentrations may be correlated, depending on tissue penetration but, to the extent that they are correlated, relationships between local drug concentration and effect are defined by pharmacodynamic (PD) principles (see later).

Basic concepts of PK include *bioavailability*, the percentage of drug dose that reaches the systemic circulation. Bioavailability is 100% after IV administration but is affected by absorption, intestinal transit time, and degree of hepatic metabolism after oral administration. The *half-life* ($t_{1/2}$), the time required for the serum drug concentration to reduce by one half, reflects *clearance* and *volume of distribution* ($V_D$)[184] and is useful to estimate for the interpretation of drug concentration data. $V_D$, a derived proportionality constant of no particular physiologic significance that is independent of a drug's clearance or $t_{1/2}$, is useful for estimating the plasma drug concentration achievable from a given dose. $V_D$ varies substantially because of pathophysiology; a reduced $V_D$ causes a higher plasma drug concentration for a given dose, whereas fluid overload and hypoalbuminemia, which decrease drug binding, increase $V_D$, making dosing more complex.

Clearance refers to the volume of liquid from which a drug is eliminated completely per unit of time, whether by tissue distribution, metabolism, or elimination. Knowledge of drug clearance is important for determining the dose of drug necessary to maintain a steady-state concentration. Drug elimination may be by metabolism, excretion, or dialysis. Most drugs are metabolized by the liver to polar compounds for eventual renal excretion, which may occur by filtration or active or passive transport. The degree of filtration is determined by molecular size and charge and by the number of functional nephrons. In general, if 40% or more of administered drug or its active metabolites is eliminated unchanged in the urine, decreased renal function will require a dosage adjustment.

PD is unique for antibiotic therapy because drug-patient, drug-microbe, and microbe-patient interactions must be accounted for.[184] In contrast to most drug treatment, the key drug interaction is not with the host, but with the microbe. Microbial physiology, inoculum size, microbial growth phase, mechanisms of resistance, microenvironment (e.g., local pH), and host response are important factors to consider. Because of microbial resistance, the mere administration of a drug may not be microbicidal if an adequate concentration is not achieved.

Antibiotic PD parameters determined by laboratory analysis include the minimal inhibitory concentration (MIC), the lowest serum drug concentration that inhibits bacterial growth ($MIC_{90}$ refers to 90% inhibition). However, some antibiotics may suppress bacterial growth at subinhibitory concentrations (*postantibiotic effect,* PAE). Appreciable PAE can be observed with aminoglycosides and fluoroquinolones for gram-negative bacteria, and with some β-lactam drugs (notably carbapenems) against *S. aureus*. However, MIC testing may not detect resistant bacterial subpopulations within the inoculum (e.g., heteroresistance of *S. aureus*).[185] Moreover, in vitro results may be irrelevant if bacteria are inhibited only by drug concentrations that cannot be achieved clinically.

Sophisticated analytic strategies use both PK and PD—for example, by determination of the peak serum concentration–to–MIC ratio, duration of time (T) that plasma concentration remains above the MIC (T > MIC), and area of the plasma concentration–time curve above the MIC (area under the curve, AUC). Accordingly, aminoglycosides exhibit concentration-dependent killing,[186] whereas β-lactam agents exhibit efficacy determined by time above the MIC.[187] For β-lactam antibiotics with a short $t_{1/2}$, it may be efficacious to administer by continuous infusion.[188,189] Some agents (e.g., fluoroquinolones) exhibit both properties; bacterial killing increases as drug concentration increases up to a saturation point, after which the effect becomes concentration-independent.

## Antibiotic Prophylaxis

Prophylactic antibiotics are used most often to prevent infection of a surgical incision. Preoperative antibiotic prophylaxis is proved to reduce the risk of postoperative SSIs in many circumstances. However, only the incision itself is protected, and only while it is open and thus vulnerable to inoculation. If not administered properly, antibiotic prophylaxis is ineffective and may be harmful. Antibiotic prophylaxis of surgery does not prevent postoperative nosocomial infections, which actually occur at an increased rate after prolonged prophylaxis,[190] selecting for more resistant pathogens when infection does develop.[42]

Antibiotic prophylaxis is indicated for most clean-contaminated and contaminated (or potentially contaminated) operations. An example of a clean-contaminated operation in which antibiotic prophylaxis is usually not indicated is elective laparoscopic cholecystectomy.[191] A meta-analysis of five trials (899 patients) revealed no benefit compared with placebo for prevention of SSIs (OR, 0.68; 95% CI, 0.24 to 1.91), major infection, or distant infection. Antibiotic prophylaxis is indicated for high-risk biliary surgery; high-risk is conferred by age older than 70 years, diabetes mellitus, or a recently instrumented biliary tract (e.g., biliary stent).

Elective colon surgery is a clean-contaminated procedure in which preparatory practices are in evolution,[192,193] although the evidence of benefit of systemic antibiotic prophylaxis is unequivocal. Antibiotic bowel preparation, standardized in the 1970s by the oral administration of nonabsorbable neomycin and erythromycin base in addition to mechanical cleansing, reduced the risk of SSIs to the present rate of approximately 15%. However, mechanical bowel preparation and preoperative oral antibiotics are omitted increasingly according to the belief that there is no additive benefit beyond parenteral antibiotic prophylaxis, and that the risk of anastomotic dehiscence and *Clostridium difficile*–associated disease (CDAD) may be increased. Current SCIP guidelines for antibiotic prophylaxis of elective colon surgery give equal weighting to oral prophylaxis alone, parenteral prophylaxis alone, or the combination (see Table 12-2), despite the fact that two meta-analyses (that asked different questions) are in conflict about the efficacy of oral prophylaxis for colorectal surgery. Song and Glenny[194] have compared oral antibiotics alone with oral or systemic antibiotic prophylaxis (five trials), and found a higher SSI rate with oral prophylaxis alone (OR, 3.34; 95% CI, 1.66 to 6.72). In contrast, Lewis[192] performed a meta-analysis of 13 randomized trials of systemic versus combined oral and systemic prophylaxis and showed significant benefit for the combined approach (RR, 0.51; 95% CI, 0.24 to 0.78).

Antibiotic prophylaxis of clean surgery is controversial. When bone is incised (e.g., craniotomy, sternotomy) or a prosthesis is inserted, antibiotic prophylaxis is generally indicated. Some controversy persists with clean surgery of soft tissues (e.g., breast, hernia). Meta-analysis of randomized controlled trials has shown some benefit of antibiotic prophylaxis of breast cancer surgery without immediate reconstruction,[195,196] but no decrease of SSI rate for groin hernia surgery,[197,198] even when nonabsorbable mesh is implanted.

Arterial reconstruction with a prosthetic graft is an example of clean surgery in which the risk of infection is high, especially infra-inguinal. In a meta-analysis[199] of 23 randomized controlled trials of prophylactic systemic antibiotics for peripheral arterial reconstruction (Table 12-6), it was found that prophylactic systemic antibiotics reduced the risk of SSI by approximately 75%, and early graft infection by about 69%. There was no benefit to prophylaxis for longer than 24 hours, of antibiotic bonding to the graft material itself, or preoperative bathing with an antiseptic agent compared with unmedicated bathing.

Four principles guide the administration of antimicrobial agent for prophylaxis[112]:

1. Safety
2. An appropriate narrow spectrum of coverage of relevant pathogens
3. Little or no reliance on the agent for therapy of infection (because of the possible induction of resistance with heavy usage)
4. Administration within 1 hour before surgery and for a defined brief period thereafter (no longer than

**Table 12-6 Meta-Analysis of Measures to Prevent Infection Following Arterial Reconstruction**

| INTERVENTION | NO. OF TRIALS | ODDS RATIO | 95% CI |
|---|---|---|---|
| Systemic antibiotic prophylaxis | | | |
| Surgical site infection | 10 | 0.25 | 0.17-0.38 |
| >24 hours prophylaxis | 3 | 1.28 | 0.82-1.98 |
| Early graft infection | 5 | 0.31 | 0.11-0.85 |
| Rifampicin bonding of polyester grafts | | | |
| Graft infection (1 mo) | 3 | 0.63 | 0.27-1.49 |
| Graft infection (2 yr) | 2 | 1.05 | 0.46-2.40 |
| Suction wound drainage, groin | | | |
| Surgical site infection | 2 | 0.96 | 0.50-1.86 |
| Preoperative antiseptic bath | | | |
| Surgical site infection | 3 | 0.97 | 0.70-1.36 |
| In situ surgical technique | | | |
| Surgical site infection | 2 | 0.48 | 0.31-0.74 |

From Stewart A, Eyers PS, Earnshaw JJ: Prevention of infection in arterial reconstruction. Cochrane Database Syst Rev (3):CD003073, 2006.

24 hours, 48 hours for cardiac surgery, and ideally, a single dose)

According to these principles, quinolones or carbapenems are undesirable agents for surgical prophylaxis, although ertapenem and quinolone prophylaxis have been endorsed by SCIP for the prophylaxis of colon surgery (the latter with metronidazole for penicillin-allergic patients; see Table-12-2).

Most SSIs are caused by gram-positive cocci, so prophylaxis should be directed primarily against staphylococci for clean cases and for high-risk, clean-contaminated, elective biliary and gastric surgery. A first-generation cephalosporin is preferred in almost all circumstances (Table 12-7), with clindamycin used for penicillin-allergic patients.[112] If gram-negative or anaerobic coverage is required, a second-generation cephalosporin or the combination of a first-generation agent plus metronidazole are most experts' first-choice regimens. Vancomycin prophylaxis is generally appropriate only in institutions in which the incidence of MRSA infection is high (>20% of all SSIs caused by MRSA).

The optimal time to give parenteral antibiotic prophylaxis is within 1 hour prior to incision.[200] Antibiotics given sooner are ineffective, as are agents given after the incision is closed. A 2001 audit of prescribing practices in the United States indicated that only 56% of patients who received prophylactic antibiotics did so within 1 hour prior to the skin incision; timeliness was documented in only 76% of cases in a 2005 audit in Department of Veterans Affairs hospitals.[201] Most inappropriately timed first doses of prophylactic antibiotic occur too early; changing institutional processes to administer the drug in the operating room can improve compliance with best practices. Antibiotics with short half-lives ($t_{1/2} < 2$ hours; e.g., cefazolin or cefoxitin) should be redosed every 3 to 4 hours during surgery if the operation is prolonged or bloody.[202] Even though SCIP specifies a 24-hour limit for prophylaxis, single-dose prophylaxis (with intraoperative redosing, if indicated) is equivalent to multiple doses for the prevention of SSI.[203] Unfortunately, excessively prolonged antibiotic prophylaxis is pervasive and potentially harmful. Prolonged prophylaxis increases the risk of nosocomial infections unrelated to the surgical site and of the emergence of MDR pathogens. Pneumonia and vascular catheter-related infections have been associated with prolonged prophylaxis,[204,205] as has the emergence of SSI caused by MRSA.[42]

Evidence has shown that only 40% of patients who receive antibiotic prophylaxis do so for less than 24 hours.[111] As a result of ischemia caused by surgical hemostasis, antibiotic penetration into the incision immediately after surgery is questionable until neovascularization occurs (24 to 48 hours). Antibiotics should not be given to cover indwelling drains or catheters, in lavage or irrigation fluid, or as a substitute for poor surgical technique.

## Principles of Antibiotic Therapy

Antimicrobial therapy is a mainstay of the treatment of infections, but widespread overuse and misuse of antibiotics have led to an alarming increase in MDR pathogens. New agents may allow shorter courses of therapy and prophylaxis, which are desirable for cost savings and control of microbial flora. Effective therapy with no toxicity requires a careful but expeditious search for the source of infection and an understanding of the principles of PK (see earlier).

### Evaluation of Possible Infection

Absent a fever, any hypotension, tachycardia, tachypnea, confusion, rigors, skin lesions, respiratory manifestations, oliguria, lactic acidosis, leukocytosis, leukopenia, immature neutrophils (i.e., bands >10%), or thrombocytopenia may indicate a workup for infection and immediate empirical therapy. Although the initial manifestation may be the development of organ dysfunction in some cases, new temperature elevation is usually the trigger for an evaluation for the presence of infection (fever workup). However, some infected patients do not become febrile and may be even be hypothermic. Hypothermic or euthermic patients may have a life-threatening infection. These include older patients, those with open abdominal wounds, or with end-stage liver disease or chronic renal failure, and patients taking anti-inflammatory or antipyretic drugs. Moreover, fever, especially in the postoperative period, may have an noninfectious cause; therefore, fever does not equate with infection (Box 12-8).[206]

The definition of fever is arbitrary, and depends on how and when temperature was measured. In addition to host biology, a variety of environmental forces in an ICU can also alter body temperature, such as specialized mattresses, lighting, heating or air conditioning, peritoneal lavage, and renal replacement therapy.[207] Thermoregulatory mechanisms can be disrupted by drugs or by injury to the central nervous system. Thus, it is often difficult to determine whether an abnormal temperature is a reflection of a physiologic process, drug, or environmental influence. Moreover, in surgical patients, the substantial possibility (≈50%) that a fever has a noninfectious cause must be considered.[206]

Many ICUs consider any patient with a core temperature 38.3° C or higher (≥101° F) to be febrile and to warrant evaluation for possible infection. However, a lower threshold may be decided on for immunocompromised patients. Laboratory tests

**Table 12-7 Appropriate Cephalosporin Prophylaxis for Selected Types of Surgery**

| PROCEDURE | ALTERNATIVE PROPHYLAXIS IN SERIOUS PENICILLIN ALLERGY |
|---|---|
| **First-Generation Cephalosporin** | |
| **Cardiovascular and thoracic** | |
| Median sternotomy | Clindamycin (for all cardiovascular and thoracic cases except amputation) |
| Pacemaker insertion | |
| Vascular reconstruction involving abdominal aorta, insertion of prosthesis, or groin incision (except carotid endarterectomy, which requires no prophylaxis) | |
| Implantable defibrillator | |
| Pulmonary resection | |
| Lower limb amputation | Gentamicin and metronidazole |
| **General** | |
| Cholecystectomy (high risk only) | Gentamicin |
| Gastrectomy (high risk only; not uncomplicated chronic duodenal ulcer) | Gentamicin and metronidazole |
| Hepatobiliary | Gentamicin and metronidazole |
| Major débridement of traumatic wound | Gentamicin |
| Genitourinary (ampicillin plus gentamicin is a reasonable alternative) | Ciprofloxacin |
| **Gynecologic** | |
| Cesarean section (STAT) | Metronidazole or doxycycline, after cord clamping |
| Hysterectomy (cefoxitin is a reasonable alternative) | Doxycycline |
| **Head and neck, oral cavity** | |
| Major procedures entering oral cavity or pharynx | Gentamicin and clindamycin or metronidazole |
| **Neurosurgery** | |
| Craniotomy | Clindamycin, vancomycin |
| **Orthopedics** | |
| Major joint arthroplasty | Vancomycin[†] |
| Open reduction of closed fracture | Vancomycin[†] |
| **Second-Generation Cephalosporin**[‡] | |
| Appendectomy | Metronidazole plus gentamicin |
| Colon surgery[§] | |
| Surgery for penetrating abdominal trauma | |

*STAT,* Emergency.

*Should be given as a single IV dose just before the operation. Consider an additional dose if the operation is prolonged longer than 3-4 hr.

[†]Primary prophylaxis with vancomycin (i.e., for the non–penicillin-allergic patient) may be appropriate for cardiac valve replacement, placement of a nontissue peripheral vascular prosthesis, or total joint replacement in institutions in which a high rate of infections with MRSA or MRSE has occurred. The precise definition of high rate is debated. A single dose administered immediately before surgery is sufficient unless the procedure lasts for more than 6 hr, in which case the dose should be repeated. Prophylaxis should be discontinued after a maximum of two doses, but may be continued for up to 48 hr.

[‡]An intraoperative dose should be given if cefoxitin is used and the duration of surgery exceeds 3-4 hr, because of the short half-life of the drug. A postoperative dose is not necessary, but is permissible for up to 24 hr.

[§]Benefit beyond that provided by bowel preparation with mechanical cleansing and oral neomycin and erythromycin base is debatable.

or imaging studies should be performed only after a clinical assessment (history and physical examination) indicates that infection may be present. Fever is common during the initial 72 hours following surgery and is usually noninfectious in origin.[207] Muscle compression injury (direct trauma or as a result of compartment syndrome) and tetanus are two rare complications of traumatic wounds that may cause fever. Other potentially serious noninfectious causes of postoperative fever include deep venous thrombosis, tissue ischemia or necrosis, pulmonary embolism, adrenal insufficiency, drug-induced fever, anesthesia-induced malignant hyperthermia, and acute allograft rejection. However, once a patient is more than 96 hours postoperative, fever is more likely to represent infection.

Drug fever is decidedly unusual in surgical patients and must be considered as a diagnosis of exclusion. Some drugs cause fever by producing local infusion site inflammation (e.g., phlebitis, sterile abscesses, soft tissue reaction), such as amphotericin B, erythromycin, and potassium chloride. Some drugs may also

**BOX 12-8 Miscellaneous Causes of Fever Related to Noninfectious States**

Acalculous cholecystitis
Acute myocardial infarction
Acute respiratory distress syndrome (fibroproliferative phase)
Adrenal insufficiency
Cytokine release syndrome
Fat embolism
Gout
Hematoma
Heterotopic ossification
Immune reconstitution inflammatory syndrome (IRIS)
Infarction of any tissue
Intracranial hemorrhage (trauma or vascular cause)
Myocardial infarction
Pancreatitis
Pericarditis
Pulmonary infarction
Stroke
Thyroid storm
Transfusion of blood or blood products
Transplant rejection
Tumor lysis syndrome
Venous thromboembolic disease
Withdrawal syndromes (e.g., drug, alcohol)

stimulate heat production (e.g., thyroxine), limit heat dissipation (e.g., atropine, epinephrine), or alter thermoregulation (e.g., butyrophenone tranquilizers, phenothiazines, antihistamines, antiparkinson drugs). Drug fever in surgical ICUs is most often attributed to antimicrobial agents (e.g., vancomycin, β-lactams), and anticonvulsants (especially phenytoin). Malignant hyperthermia and neuroleptic malignant syndrome deserve consideration when fever is especially high because the results can be devastating if left untreated.[208] Malignant hyperthermia can be delayed in onset for as long as 24 hours, especially if the patient is on corticosteroids. Malignant hyperthermia is a genetically determined response mediated by a dysregulation of cytoplasmic calcium flux in skeletal muscle, resulting in intense muscle contraction, fever, and increased creatinine phosphokinase (CPK) concentration. It can be caused by succinylcholine and inhalational anesthetics. The neuroleptic malignant syndrome is slightly more common and more often identified in the ICU than malignant hyperthermia. It has been associated with phenothiazines, thioxanthines, and butyrophenones. It also manifests as muscle rigidity, fever, and increasing CPK concentration. However, unlike malignant hyperthermia, the initiator of muscle contraction is central, the syndrome is often less intense, and mortality is lower.

Drug withdrawal syndromes may be associated with fever, tachycardia, diaphoresis, and hyperreflexia, including those caused by alcohol, opioids, barbiturates, and benzodiazepines. It is important to recognize that a history of use of these drugs may not be available when the patient is admitted to the ICU. Withdrawal and related fever may therefore occur several hours or days after admission.

Fever can be related to hematoma or SSI. Surgical site infection is rare in the first few days after operation, except for group A streptococcal infections and clostridial infections that can develop within hours to 1 to 3 days after surgery. These causes should be suspected on the basis of inspection of the incision. Thus, it is mandatory to remove the surgical dressing to inspect the incision as part of any fever evaluation. However, if an incision is opened and cultured, a deep culture specimen should be collected; swabbing an open wound superficially or collecting fluid from drains (if present) for culture is unhelpful because the likelihood of colonization is high.

A CXR is optional for evaluation of postoperative fever unless long-term mechanical ventilation, respiratory rate, auscultation, abnormal blood gas levels, or pulmonary secretions suggest a high yield. The clinician must be alert to the possibility that the patient could have aspirated during the perioperative period, or the uncommon event that the patient was incubating a community-acquired pneumonia prior to the operation caused, for example, by pneumococci or influenza A. A urinalysis or culture is not mandatory to evaluate fever during the initial 3 days postoperatively unless there is reason, by history or examination, to suspect a UTI. After trauma, UTI is common only after injury to the urinary tract.

### Blood Cultures

Blood cultures should be obtained from patients with a new fever when clinical evaluation does not suggest strongly a noninfectious cause. The site of venipuncture should be cleaned with 2% chlorhexidine gluconate in 70% isopropyl alcohol or 1% to 2% tincture of iodine. Povidone-iodine (10%), although acceptable, is not bactericidal until dry; some false-positive blood cultures may be caused by premature specimen collection.[209] One blood culture is defined as a 20- to 30-mL sample of blood drawn at a single time from a single site, regardless of how many bottles or tubes are filled for processing; the minimum inoculum for an adult blood culture should be 10 mL/bottle. The sensitivity of blood culturing for detection of true bacteremia or fungemia is related to many factors, most importantly the volume of blood drawn and obtaining the cultures before the initiation of anti-infective therapy.[210]

Evidence has suggested that the cumulative yield of pathogens is optimized when three blood cultures with adequate volume (20 to 30 mL each) are drawn.[210] Each culture should ideally be drawn by separate venipuncture or through a separate intravascular device, but not through multiple ports of the same intravascular catheter. There is no evidence that the yield of cultures drawn from an artery or vein is different. Drawing two to three blood cultures with appropriate volume from separate sites of access at the onset of fever is the most effective way to discern whether an organism found in blood culture represents a true pathogen (multiple cultures are often positive), a contaminant (only one of multiple blood cultures is positive for an organism commonly found on skin and clinical correlation does not support infection), or a bacteremia or fungemia from an infected catheter (one culture from the source catheter is positive, often with a positive catheter tip, and other cultures are not).[211]

### Empirical Antibiotic Therapy

Empirical antibiotic therapy must be administered judiciously. Injudicious therapy could result in undertreatment of established infection or unnecessary therapy when the patient has only inflammation or bacterial colonization; either may be deleterious. Inappropriate treatment (e.g., delay,[212,213] therapy misdirected against usual pathogens, failure to treat MDR pathogens) leads unequivocally to increased mortality.[141,214,215]

Strategies have been promulgated to optimize antibiotic administration, including reliance on physician prescribing patterns, computerized decision support, administration by protocol, and formulary restriction programs. These are considered under the general framework of antibiotic stewardship.[216] Because of the increasing prevalence of MDR pathogens, it is crucial for initial empirical antibiotic therapy to be targeted appropriately, administered in a sufficient dosage to ensure bacterial killing, narrowed in spectrum (de-escalation)[217] as soon as possible based on microbiology data and clinical response, and continued only as long as necessary.[218] Appropriate antibiotic prescribing not only optimizes patient care, but supports infection control practices and preserves microbial ecology.

### Choice of Antibiotic

Antibiotic choice is based on several interrelated factors (Box 12-9). Paramount is activity against identified or likely (for empirical therapy) pathogens, presuming that infecting and colonizing organisms can be distinguished and narrow-spectrum coverage is always desired. Estimation of likely pathogens depends on the disease process believed responsible, whether the infection is community-, health care–, or hospital-acquired, and whether MDR organisms are present, or likely to be. Local knowledge of antimicrobial resistance patterns is essential, even at the unit-specific level. Patient-specific factors of importance include age, debility, immunosuppression, intrinsic organ function, prior allergy or other adverse reaction, and recent antibiotic therapy. Institutional factors of importance include guidelines that could specify a particular therapy, formulary availability of specific agents, outbreaks of infections caused by MDR pathogens, and antibiotic control programs.

A number of agents are available for therapy (Box 12-10).[219] Agents may be chosen based on spectrum, whether broad or targeted (e.g., antipseudomonal, antianaerobic), in addition to the factors noted. If a nosocomial gram-positive pathogen is suspected (e.g., wound infection, SSI, CLABSI, HAP, VAP) or MRSA is endemic, empirical vancomycin (or linezolid) is appropriate. Some authorities recommend dual-agent therapy for serious *Pseudomonas* infections (an antipseudomonal β-lactam drug plus an aminoglycoside), but evidence of efficacy is mixed.[220-222] Combination therapy of a specific pathogen (e.g., double coverage of *Pseudomonas*) may, in fact, worsen outcomes. A meta-analysis of β-lactam monotherapy versus β-lactam–aminoglycoside combination therapy for immunocompetent patients with sepsis (64 trials, 7586 patients) found no difference in mortality (RR, 0.90; 95% CI, 0.77 to 1.06) or development of resistance.[221] In fact, clinical failure was more common with combination therapy, as was the incidence of acute kidney injury. However, it is important for empirical therapy of any infection that might be caused by a gram-positive or gram-negative organism (e.g., HAP-VAP, HA-IAI) to include activity against all likely pathogens.[47,223]

### Duration of Therapy

The end point of antibiotic therapy is largely undefined, in part because quality data are few. If cultures are negative, empirical antibiotic therapy should usually be stopped after no more than 48 to 72 hours. Unnecessary antibiotic therapy increases the risk of MDR infection, so prolonged therapy with negative cultures

**BOX 12-9 Factors Influencing Antibiotic Choice**

Activity against known/suspected pathogens
Disease believed responsible
Distinguish infection from colonization
Narrow-spectrum coverage most desirable
Antimicrobial resistance patterns
Patient-specific factors
- Severity of illness (?)
- Age (?)
- Immunosuppression
- Organ dysfunction
- Allergy

Institutional guidelines/restrictions

**BOX 12-10 Antibacterial Agents for Empirical Use**

**Antipseudomonal**
Piperacillin-tazobactam
Cefepime, ceftazidime
Imipenem-cilastatin, meropenem, doripenem
? Ciprofloxacin, levofloxacin (depending on local susceptibility patterns)
Aminoglycosides
Polymyxins (polymyxin B, colistin [polymyxin E])

**Targeted-spectrum**
**Gram-positive**
Glycopeptide (e.g., vancomycin, telavancin)
Lipopeptide (e.g., daptomycin; not for known/suspected pneumonia)
Oxazolidinone (e.g., linezolid)
**Gram-negative**
Third-generation cephalosporin (not ceftriaxone)
Monobactam
Polymyxins (polymyxin B, colistin [polymyxin E])
**Antianaerobic**
Metronidazole

**Broad-Spectrum**
Piperacillin-tazobactam
Carbapenems
Fluoroquinolones (depending on local susceptibility patterns)
Tigecycline (plus an antipseudomonal agent)

**Antianaerobic**
Metronidazole
Carbapenems
β-lactam and β-lactamase combination agents
Tigecycline

**Anti-MRSA**
Ceftaroline
Daptomycin (not for use against pneumonia)
Minocycline (oral only)
Linezolid
Telavancin
Tigecycline (not in pregnancy or for children under the age of eight years)
Vancomycin

is usually unjustifiable. The morbidity of antibiotic therapy also includes allergic reactions, development of nosocomial superinfections, (e.g., fungal, enterococcal, and *C. difficile*–related infections), organ toxicity, reduced yield from subsequent cultures, and vitamin K deficiency with coagulopathy or accentuation of warfarin effect.

If infection is evident, treatment is continued as indicated clinically. Some infections can be treated for 5 days or less. Every decision to start antibiotics must be accompanied by an a priori decision regarding the duration of therapy. A reason to continue therapy beyond the predetermined end point must be compelling. Bacterial killing is rapid in response to effective agents, but the host response may not subside immediately. Therefore, the clinical response of the patient should not be the sole determinant. If a patient still has SIRS at the predetermined end point, it is more useful to stop therapy and reevaluate for persistent or new infection, MDR pathogens, and noninfectious causes of SIRS than to continue therapy uninformed.

## DISEASE-, PATHOGEN-, AND ANTIBIOTIC-SPECIFIC CONSIDERATIONS

### Pneumonia

Following initiation of therapy for suspected VAP, lower respiratory tract cultures may reveal no growth or growth below the predetermined threshold value, substantial (above threshold) growth of a susceptible pathogen, or growth of a MDR pathogen. Under the first scenario, antimicrobial therapy may be discontinued if the patient has not deteriorated.[224] Under the second scenario, therapy is de-escalated[225] to a narrow-spectrum agent active against the pathogen. In the third scenario, the initial broad-spectrum agent active against the pathogen is continued or therapy is escalated to target the MDR pathogen.

Once pathogen-specific therapy has been initiated, its duration must be determined, with the goal of avoiding prolonged unnecessary administration. Resolution of clinical and radiographic parameters typically lags the eradication of infection.[47] Dennesen and colleagues[226] have noted a clinical response to therapy (e.g., normalization of temperature, white blood cell count, and arterial oxygen saturation and decreased bacterial count in sputum) within 6 days of therapy of VAP. A randomized multicenter trial of 401 patients (VAP proved by bronchoscopy and quantitative microbiology)[227] showed an 8-day course (versus 15 days) of initially appropriate antimicrobial therapy to be effective, provided that the patient was stable and the pathogen was not a nonfermenting gram-negative bacillus. In select patients (i.e., those unlikely to have VAP based on a CPIS $\leq 6$), a 3-day course of therapy may be sufficient.[228]

Nonresponders to therapy for VAP pose a dilemma.[47] Inadequate therapy, misdiagnosis, or a pneumonia-related complication (e.g., empyema, lung abscess) must be considered. The evaluation should be repeated, including quantitative sputum cultures using a quantitative diagnostic threshold one log lower, given recent antibiotic exposure. Broadened empirical antibiotic coverage should be reinstituted thereafter until new data become available.

### Central Line–Associated Bloodstream Infection

The pathogens of CLABSI are predominantly gram-positive cocci, most commonly methicillin-related *S. epidermidis* (MRSE), MRSA, and enterococci. Unfortunately, MRSE is the most common cause of CRBSIs and of false-positive blood cultures because of contamination during the collection process. Most authorities consider the isolation of MRSE from a single blood culture to be a contaminant and do not treat, especially if the patient has no indwelling hardware that might become infected secondarily (e.g., prosthetic joint, heart valve). Gram-negative bacillary pathogens are less common, but are seldom contaminants. Fungal CLABSIs are less common in surgical patients than medical patients, but must be treated empirically in critically ill patients at risk.

Treatment is by catheter removal (for peripheral or percutaneous central venous catheters) and parenteral antibiotics, at least initially.[3,229] It is unclear whether a positive catheter culture requires therapy beyond catheter removal without local signs of infection or a true-positive blood culture. Bloodstream infections caused by *S. aureus* probably require at least 2 weeks of therapy regardless of cause, although some argue for a longer course (4 to 6 weeks) because of the risk of metastatic infection (e.g., pneumonia, endocarditis). Vancomycin or linezolid may be chosen for MRSA CLABSIs (or MRSE when treatment is indicated), with daptomycin as an alternative. Therapy for enterococcal or gram-negative CLABSIs is dictated by bacterial susceptibility, with no clear consensus about the duration of therapy. Beyond removal of the catheter, treatment of fungal CLABSIs is controversial; some recommend at least 2 weeks of systemic antifungal therapy. Multidrug-resistant fungal pathogens are less common in surgical patients. except for solid organ transplant recipients, so initial empirical therapy with a echinocandin is often de-escalated to fluconazole after susceptibility is reported.[229a]

### Intra-Abdominal Infection

Only approximately 15% of patients with secondary peritonitis are ill enough to require ICU care. Severe secondary peritonitis may follow penetrating intestinal injury that is not recognized or treated promptly (>12-hour delay). Other causes include dehiscence of a bowel anastomosis with leakage or development of an intra-abdominal abscess. Secondary peritonitis is polymicrobial, with anaerobic gram-negative bacilli (e.g., *B. fragilis*) predominating and *E. coli* and *Klebsiella* spp. commonly isolated from community-onset infections. Various antibiotic regimens of an appropriate spectrum may be prescribed.[223] Enterococci, *Pseudomonas,* and other bacteria may be isolated, but do not require specific therapy if the patient is otherwise healthy (e.g., not immunocompromised) and responding to therapy as prescribed.

When HA-IAI is a complication of disease or therapy, the flora are more likely to reflect MDR pathogens[173,175] and outcomes are worsened if empirical therapy is not appropriate. For example, enterococci, *Enterobacter,* and *Pseudomonas* are more prevalent, whereas *E. coli* and *Klebsiella* are less common.[230] Antibiotic therapy must be adjusted accordingly and surgical source control must be achieved. Failure of two source control procedures with persistent intra-abdominal collections is referred to as *tertiary peritonitis.* Tertiary peritonitis is also characterized by complete failure of intra-abdominal host defenses.[231] There is debate regarding whether tertiary peritonitis is a true invasive infection or is peritoneal colonization with incompetent local host defenses, so whether antibiotic therapy is indicated is controversial. Bacteria isolated in tertiary peritonitis are avirulent opportunists, such as MRSE, enterococci, *Pseudomonas,* and

*C. albicans,* supporting the incompetent host defense hypothesis. Some authorities recommend management with an open abdomen technique, so that peritoneal toilet can be provided manually—at the bedside in some cases—under sedation or anesthesia, until local host defenses recover. There may be no alternative to open abdomen management if the infection extends to involve the abdominal wall, and extensive débridement is required.

### *Clostridium difficile*–Associated Disease

CDAD, or *C. difficile* infection (CDI), develops because antibiotic therapy disrupts the balance of colonic flora, allowing the overgrowth of *C. difficile,* which is present in the fecal flora of approximately 3% of normal hosts. Any antibiotic can induce this selection pressure, even when given appropriately as surgical prophylaxis, although clindamycin, third-generation cephalosporins, and fluoroquinolones have a predilection.[232] Paradoxically, even antibiotics used to treat CDAD (e.g., metronidazole) have been associated with CDAD. Restriction of cephalosporin and fluoroquinolone prescribing can reduce the rate of infection.[233]

CDAD is unquestionably a nosocomial infection. Spores persist on inanimate surfaces for prolonged periods, and can be transmitted patient to patient by contaminated equipment (e.g., bedpans, rectal thermometers) or by health care workers as fomites. Alcohol gel hand disinfection is not active against spores of *C. difficile,* so hand washing with soap and water is necessary when caring for an infected patient, or generally during outbreaks.

The clinical spectrum of CDAD is wide, ranging from asymptomatic (8% of affected patients do not have diarrhea) to life-threatening transmural pancolitis with perforation and severe sepsis or septic shock. The typical patient will have fever, abdominal distention with or without tenderness, copious diarrhea, and leukocytosis. Colon hemorrhage is rare and, if observed, should prompt consideration of an alternative diagnosis.

Treatment of mild cases consists of withdrawal of the putative offending antibiotic; oral antibiotic therapy is often prescribed but may not be necessary. More severe cases may require parenteral metronidazole or oral or enteral vancomycin (by gavage or enema, if ileus precludes oral therapy); parenteral vancomycin is ineffective. The new oral macrolide fidaxomicin is noninferior to vancomycin and may reduce the risk of relapsed disease, a major clinical problem.[234] Some patients with severe or fulminating disease may require a colectomy, usually a total abdominal colectomy.[235] The prevalence of severe disease has increased markedly with the emergence of a new strain of *C. difficile.* The new strain has undergone mutation of a gene that suppresses toxin production so that far more toxin is elaborated, resulting in clinically severe disease.[236] More of these patients will require surgery, but it remains to be determined whether or how antibiotic therapy should be modified to combat this dangerous bacterium.

### Complicated Skin and Soft Tissue Infections

Complicated SSTIs involve deeper tissues or require major surgical intervention. Infection in the presence of medical comorbidities, particularly chronic kidney disease, diabetes mellitus, or peripheral arterial disease, also defines a cSSTI. Examples include major abscesses, deep space infections, diabetic foot infections, some postoperative SSIs (those with systemic signs of infection), infected decubitus ulcers, and NSTIs. In randomized controlled trials, comparable outcomes of antibiotic therapy for cSSTIs (except NSTIs, which are usually [≈80%] polymicrobial), are achieved by agents that treat only gram-positive cocci (e.g., vancomycin, linezolid, daptomycin, telavancin). Because of the heterogeneity of these infections, the reader is referred to comprehensive treatment guidelines for the management of cSSTI (Box 12-11).[237]

Patients with diabetes mellitus are at risk for considerable morbidity as a result of chronic foot ulceration and foot infection, including limb loss. Diabetic foot infections (DFIs) are usually a consequence of skin ulceration from ischemia or trauma to a neuropathic foot. The compartmentalized anatomy of the foot, with its various spaces, tendon sheaths, and neurovascular bundles, allows ischemic necrosis to affect tissues within a compartment or spread along anatomic tissue planes. Recurrent infections are common, and 10% to 30% of affected patients eventually require amputation. Diabetic patients are predisposed to foot infections, not only because of the portal of entry and poor blood supply, but also because of defects in humoral immunity (e.g., impaired neutrophil chemotaxis, phagocytosis, intracellular killing) and impaired monocyte-macrophage function, which correlate with the adequacy of glycemic control. Cell-mediated immunity and complement function may also be impaired.

Acute infections are usually caused by gram-positive cocci. *S. aureus* is the most important pathogen in DFIs. It is often present as a monomicrobial infection, but usually it is also an important pathogen in polymicrobial infections. Chronic wounds, recurrent infections, and infections in hospitalized patients are more likely to harbor complex flora, including aerobic and anaerobic flora. Among gram-negative bacilli, bacteria of the family Enterobacteriaceae are common, and *Pseudomonas aeruginosa* may be isolated from wounds that have been treated with hydrotherapy or wet dressings. Enterococci may be recovered from patients treated previously with a cephalosporin. Anaerobic bacteria seldom cause DFIs as the sole pathogen, but may be isolated from deep infections or necrotic tissue. Antibiotic-resistant bacteria, especially MRSA, may be isolated from patients who have received antibiotics previously or who have been hospitalized or reside in long-term care facilities. Agents that have been shown to be effective for therapy of DFIs in clinical trials include cephalosporins, β-lactamase inhibitor combination antibiotics, fluoroquinolones, clindamycin, carbapenems, vancomycin, and linezolid. The optimal duration of therapy for DFIs has not been determined; common practice is to treat mild infections for 1 week, whereas serious infections may require up to a 2-week course of therapy. Adequate débridement, resection, or amputation can shorten the necessary duration of therapy.

### Antibiotic Activity Spectra

Susceptibility testing of specific organisms is necessary for the treatment of serious infections, including all nosocomial infections. Recommendations will focus on agents useful for the treatment of nosocomial infections. Recommended agents for specific organisms are guidelines only, because in vitro susceptibilities may not correlate with clinical efficacy. Exposure to certain agents has been associated with the emergence of specific MDR bacteria, which require a different empirical antibiotic choice or modification of a regimen if identified or suspected (Table 12-8).

**BOX 12-11 Recommendations from Guidelines for Treatment of Complicated Skin and Soft Tissue Infections**

**Non-Necrotizing Cellulitis**

Most frequent causative agent is *Streptococcus pyogenes;* other agents include *Haemophilus influenzae* and pneumococcus.

Parenteral penicillin is TOC; treatment failures may occur in severe disease.

Protein synthesis inhibitory agents alone or in combination with cell wall active agents should be given in severe cases, but macrolide resistance is increasing.

Other regimens may include antistaphylococcal penicillins, cefazolin, ceftaroline, and ceftriaxone.

**Complicated Skin and Soft Tissue Infections**

Involve a broad variety of pathogens; frequently polymicrobial

*S. aureus* is most common isolate; community-acquired (CA) MRSA increasingly common

Simple abscesses may respond to incision and drainage alone.

Complex abscesses and abscesses with cellulitis require adjuvant antibiotics.

Empirical antibiotic therapy should be directed toward the most likely pathogens, including CA-MRSA in most settings.

Suspected polymicrobial infections should be managed with coverage of enteric gram-negative and anaerobic pathogens.

**Necrotizing Soft Tissue Infections**

Delays in diagnosis increase morbidity and mortality.

Presence of gas in soft tissue is specific for necrotizing infections, but insensitive.

CT and magnetic resonance imaging (MRI) improve detection of soft tissue gas, but radiographic findings of tissue fluid and edema are neither sensitive nor specific.

Clinical features suggestive of NSTIs are:

- Pain disproportionate to physical examination findings
- Tense edema
- Bullae
- Skin ecchymosis, necrosis
- Cutaneous anesthesia
- Systemic toxicity
- Progression despite antibiotic therapy

Predictive laboratory values:

- White blood cell count $>14 \times 10^9$/L
- Serum sodium level <135 mmol/L
- Blood urea nitrogen level >15 mg/dL

Early antibiotic coverage of likely pathogens is indicated; this depends on the clinical setting, inciting pathophysiology, and previous antibiotic exposure.

Timely, wide surgical débridement of involved tissue improves outcome.

Frequent reevaluation or return to the operating room within 24 hours ensures adequacy of débridement and lack of progression.

Necrotizing infections are usually polymicrobial; they may involve anaerobic and aerobic gram-positive and gram-negative pathogens.

Possible single-agent regimens include imipenem-cilastatin, meropenem, ertapenem, piperacillin-tazobactam, ticarcillin–clavulanic acid, and tigecycline.

**Diabetic Foot Infections**

These may involve a wide variety of pathogens; separating colonizing bacteria from pathogens may be difficult.

Gram-positive cocci are most common, but gram-negative bacilli and anaerobes may be involved. Chronic wounds may have resistant pathogens.

Empirical therapy should take local susceptibility patterns, previous antibiotic exposure, and prior pathogens into considerations.

Adequate tissue cultures should be obtained.

Possible antibiotic regimens include cefazolin, ceftriaxone, cefoxitin, ceftaroline, ampicillin-sulbactam, piperacillin-tazobactam, and a carbapenem; daptomycin and linezolid can be used with the addition of gram-negative coverage.

For MRSA infections, vancomycin, telavancin, ceftaroline, daptomycin, tigecycline, and linezolid can be considered.

Modified from May AK, Stafford RE, Bulger EM, et al: Treatment of complicated skin and soft tissue infections. Surg Infect (Larchmt) 10:467–499, 2009.

**Table 12-8 Causes and Consequences of Bacterial Resistance as Related to Empirical Antibiotic Choices**

| INITIAL THERAPEUTIC AGENT | EMERGENT RESISTANT BACTERIA | TREATMENT OF RESISTANT BACTERIA |
|---|---|---|
| Fluoroquinolones | MRSA<br>MDR gram-negative bacilli*<br>*Clostridium difficile* infection | Vancomycin, others (see Box 12-11)<br>Carbapenem or polymyxin or tygecycline (not for *Pseudomonas*)<br>Vancomycin or metronidazole or fidaxomycin |
| Vancomycin | VRE<br>VISA | Tigecycline, linezolid, daptomycin<br>Ceftaroline, tigecycline, linezolid, daptomycin |
| Cephalosporins | VRE<br>MDR gram-negative bacilli<br>*Clostridium difficile* infection | Tigecycline, linezolid, daptomycin<br>Carbapenem or polymyxin or tigecycline (not for *Pseudomonas*)<br>Vancomycin or metronidazole or fidaxomycin |
| Carbapenems | MDR gram-negative bacilli<br>*Stenotrophomonas maltophilia*<br>*Clostridium difficile* infection | Carbapenem or polymyxin or tigecycline (not for *Pseudomonas*)<br>Trimethoprim/sulfamethoxazole<br>Vancomycin or metronidazole or fidaxomycin |

*VISA,* Vancomycin intermediate-resistant *Staphylococcus aureus.*

*MDR, gram-negative bacilli include producers of extended-spectrum β-lactamases, metallo-β-lactamases, and carbapenemases.

## Cell Wall Active Agents

**β-Lactam Antibiotics** The β-lactam antibiotic group consists of penicillins, cephalosporins, monobactams, and carbapenems. Within this group, several agents have been combined with β-lactamase inhibitors to broaden the spectrum of activity. Several subgroups of antibiotics are recognized within the group, notably several generations of cephalosporins and penicillinase-resistant penicillins.

***Penicillins*** Penicillinase-resistant semisynthetic penicillins include methicillin, nafcillin, oxacillin, cloxacillin, and dicloxacillin. These agents are used primarily as therapy for sensitive strains of staphylococci. Hospitalized patients should not be treated empirically with these agents because of high rates of MRSA, and almost all enterococcal strains are resistant. However, if the *S. aureus* isolate is susceptible, these drugs are the treatment of choice (TOC).

With the exception of carboxy penicillins and ureidopenicillins, penicillins retain little or no activity against most gram-negative bacilli. Carboxypenicillins (ticarcillin and carbenicillin) and ureidopenicillins (azlocillin, mezlocillin, and piperacillin; sometimes referred to as *acylampicillins*) have some activity against gram-negative bacteria and *P. aeruginosa.* Ureidopenicillins have greater intrinsic activity against *Pseudomonas,* but none are used widely any more without a β-lactamase inhibitor in combination (BLIC). Combination with a β-lactamase inhibitor (e.g., sulbactam, tazobactam, clavulanic acid) enhances the effectiveness of the parent β-lactam agent (piperacillin > ticarcillin > ampicillin) and, to a lesser extent, the inhibitor (tazobactam > sulbactam ~ clavulanic acid). The spectrum of activity varies within the class, so the treating clinician needs to be familiar with each of the drugs. All the BLIC drugs are effective against streptococci and MRSA, and highly effective against anaerobes (except for *C. difficile*). Piperacillin-tazobactam has the widest spectrum of activity against gram-negative bacteria and the most potency among β-lactam drugs against *P. aeruginosa*. Ampicillin-sulbactam is unreliable against *E. coli* and *Klebsiella* (resistance rate ≅ 50%), but it has useful activity against *Acinetobacter* spp. because of the sulbactam moiety.

***Cephalosporins*** More than 20 cephalosporins comprise the class; the characteristics of the drugs vary widely, but are similar within four broad generations. First- and second-generation agents are useful only for prophylaxis, uncomplicated infections, or de-escalation therapy when results of susceptibility testing are known. Third-generation agents have enhanced activity against gram-negative bacilli (some have specific antipseudomonal activity), but most are ineffective against gram-positive cocci and none against anaerobes. Cefepime, the fourth-generation cephalosporin available in the United States, has enhanced antipseudomonal activity and has regained activity against most gram-positive cocci, but not MRSA. Ceftaroline (usual dose, 600 mg IV, every 12 hours) has not been classified, but has anti-MRSA activity unique among the cephalosporins while retaining modest activity comparable to first-generation agents against gram-negative bacilli.[238] None of the cephalosporins are active against enterococci. The heterogeneity of spectra, especially among third-generation agents, requires broad familiarity with all these drugs.

**Third-Generation Cephalosporins.** Third-generation cephalosporins include cefoperazone, cefotaxime, cefpodoxime, cefprozil, ceftazidime, ceftibuten, ceftizoxime, ceftriaxone, and lorcarbicef. They possess a modestly extended spectrum of activity against gram-negative bacilli but not against gram-positive bacteria (except for ceftriaxone) or anaerobic bacteria. Third-generation cephalosporins, particularly ceftazidime, have been associated with the induction of extended-spectrum β-lactamase (ESBL) production among many of the Enterobacteriaceae (see Table 12-8). Their activity is only reliable against non-ESBL–producing species of Enterobacteriaceae, including *Enterobacter, Citrobacter, Providencia,* and *Morganella* but no longer reliable for empirical use as monotherapy against nonfermenting gram-negative bacilli (e.g., *Acinetobacter* spp., *P. aeruginosa, Stenotrophomonas maltophilia*).

**Fourth-Generation Cephalosporins.** The gram-negative spectrum of cefepime is broader than that of the third-generation cephalosporins (the antipseudomonal activity exceeds that of ceftazidime), whereas the anti–gram-positive activity is comparable to that of a first-generation cephalosporin. The safety profile is excellent and the potential for induction of ESBL production is less. There is no activity against enterococci or enteric anaerobes. Similar to the carbapenems, cefepime appears to be intrinsically more resistant to hydrolysis by β-lactamases, but not enough for its activity to be reliable against ESBL-producing bacteria.

***Monobactams*** The single available agent of this class, aztreonam, has a spectrum of activity against gram-negative bacilli similar that of to the third-generation cephalosporins, with no activity against gram-positive organisms or anaerobes. Aztreonam is not a potent inducer of β-lactamases. Resistance to aztreonam is widespread, but the drug may be useful for directed therapy against known susceptible strains and may be used safely for penicillin-allergic patients because the incidence of cross-reactivity is low (see later).

***Carbapenems*** Carbapenems have a five-carbon ring attached to the β-lactam nucleus. The alkyl groups are oriented in a *trans* configuration rather than the *cis* configuration characteristic of other β-lactam agents, making these drugs resistant to β-lactamases. Four drugs, imipenem-cilastatin, meropenem, doripenem, and ertapenem, are available in the United States. Imipenem-cilastatin, meropenem, and doripenem have the widest (and generally comparable) antibacterial spectrum of any antibiotics, with excellent activity against aerobic and anaerobic streptococci, methicillin- sensitive staphylococci, and almost all gram-negative bacilli except *Acinetobacter, Legionella, P. cepacia,* and *S. maltophilia*.[239] Activity against the Enterobacteriaceae exceeds that of all antibiotics, with the possible exceptions of piperacillin-tazobactam and cefepime, and activities of meropenem and doripenem against *P. aeruginosa* are approached only by that of amikacin. All carbapenems are superlative antianaerobic agents, so there is no reason to combine a carbapenem with metronidazole except, for example, to treat concurrent mild *C. difficile* colitis in a patient with a life-threatening infection that mandates carbapenem therapy.

Meropenem and doripenem have less potential for neurotoxicity than imipenem-cilastatin, which is contraindicated in patients with active central nervous system disease or injury (except the spinal cord), because of the rare (≈0.5%) appearance of myoclonus or generalized seizures in patients who have received high doses (with normal renal function) or inadequate dosage reductions with renal insufficiency. With all carbapenems, widespread disruption of host microbial flora may lead to superinfections (e.g., fungi, *C. difficile*, *Stenotrophomonas*, resistant enterococci).

Ertapenem is not useful against *Pseudomonas*, *Acinetobacter*, *Enterobacter* spp., or MRSA, but its long half-life permits once-daily dosing.[240] Ertapenem is highly active against ESBL-producing Enterobacteriaceae and also has less potential for neurotoxicity.

**Lipoglycopeptides**

Vancomycin, a soluble lipoglycopeptide, is bactericidal, but only on dividing organisms. Unfortunately, tissue penetration of vancomycin is universally poor, which limits its effectiveness. Both *S. aureus* and *S. epidermidis* are usually susceptible to vancomycin, although MICs for *S. aureus* are increasing, requiring higher doses for effect,[241,242] and leading to rates of clinical failure that have exceeded 50% in some reports (Table 12-9).[243] *Streptococcus pyogenes*, group B streptococci, *S. pneumoniae* (including penicillin-resistant *S. pneumoniae* [PRSP]), and *C. difficile* are also susceptible. Most strains of *Enterococcus faecalis* are inhibited (but not killed) by attainable concentrations, but *Enterococcus faecium* is increasingly VRE.

It is important for public health that widespread inappropriate use of vancomycin be curtailed. Actual indications include serious infections caused by MRSA or MRSE, gram-positive infections in patients with serious penicillin allergy, and oral therapy (or by enema in patients with ileus) for serious cases of CDI. Parenteral vancomycin (a starting dose of 15 mg/kg is now recommended for patients with normal renal function to achieve a minimum trough concentration of 15 to 20 µg/mL)[241,242] must be infused over at least 1 hour to avoid toxicity (e.g., red man syndrome). Despite concern about MRSA as a causative pathogen for SSIs, properly designed randomized trials are lacking and routine vancomycin prophylaxis is not recommended.[244]

Telavancin, a synthetic derivative of vancomycin, has been approved for the treatment of cSSTIs.[245] The drug is active against MRSA, pneumococci, including PRSP, and vancomycin-susceptible enterococci, with MICs generally lower than 1 µg/mL. There appears to be a dual mechanism of action, including cell membrane disruption and inhibition of cell wall synthesis. The most common side effects are taste disturbance, nausea, vomiting, and headache. There may be a small increased risk of acute kidney injury. The usual dose is 10 mg/kg, infused IV over 60 minutes, every 24 hours for 7 to 14 days; dosages reductions are necessary in renal insufficiency. No information is available regarding dosing during renal replacement therapy.

**Table 12-9 Causes of Vancomycin Failure***

| PARAMETER PREDICTING FAILURE | ADJUSTED ODDS RATIO | 95% CI |
|---|---|---|
| Infective endocarditis | 4.55 | 2.26-9.15 |
| Nosocomial acquisition of infection | 2.19 | 1.21-3.97 |
| Initial vancomycin trough concentration <15 µg/mL | 2.00 | 1.25-3.22 |
| Vancomycin MIC >1 µg/mL | 1.52 | 1.09-2.49 |

From reference 245.

*In a single-venter cohort of 320 patients with documented MRSA bacteremia, using logistic regression analysis.

**Cyclic Lipopeptides**

Daptomycin has potent, rapid bactericidal activity against most gram-positive organisms. The mechanism of action is via rapid membrane depolarization, potassium efflux, arrest of DNA, RNA, and protein synthesis, and cell death. Daptomycin exhibits concentration-dependent killing and has a long half-life (8 hours). A dose of 4 mg/kg once daily is recommended for cSSTIs, versus 6 mg/kg/day for bacteremia. Daptomycin is excreted in the urine, so the dosing interval should be increased to 48 hours when creatinine clearance is lower than 30 mL/min. No antagonistic drug interactions have been observed.

Daptomycin is active against many aerobic and anaerobic gram-positive bacteria, including MDR strains such as MRSA, MRSE, and VRE. Furthermore, daptomycin is also effective against a variety of anaerobes, including *Peptostreptococcus* spp., *C. perfringens*, and *C. difficile.* Resistance to daptomycin has been reported for MRSA and VRE.

Importantly, daptomycin must not be used for the treatment of pneumonia or as empirical therapy when pneumonia is in the differential diagnosis, even when caused by a susceptible organism, because daptomycin penetrates lung tissue poorly and is also inactivated by pulmonary surfactant.[246]

**Polymyxins**

Polymyxins are cyclic, cationic peptide antibiotics that have fatty acid residues[247]; of the five polymyxins described originally (polymyxins A to E), two (B and E) have been used clinically. Polymyxin B and polymyxin E (colistin) differ by a single amino acid. Polymyxins bind to the anionic bacterial outer membrane, leading to a deterrent effect that disrupts membrane integrity. High-affinity binding to the lipid of a moiety of lipopolysaccharide may have an endotoxin-neutralizing effect. Commercial preparations of polymyxin B are standardized, but those of colistimethate (a less toxic prodrug of colistin that is administered clinically) are not, so dosing depends on which preparation is being supplied. Most recent reports have described colistimethate use, but the drugs are therapeutically equivalent.

Dosing of polymyxin B is 1.5 to 2.5 mg/kg (15,000 to 25,000 U/kg) daily in divided doses, whereas dosing of colistimethate ranges from 2.5 to 6 mg/kg/day, also in divided doses. The diluent is voluminous, adding substantially to daily fluid intake. Data on PK are scant, but the drugs exhibit rapid concentration-dependent bacterial killing against a wide variety of gram-negative bacilli, including most isolates of *E. coli*, *P. aeruginosa*, *S. maltophilia*, and *Klebsiella*, *Enterobacter*, and *Acinetobacter* spp. Activity has remained generally excellent despite the widespread emergence of MDR pathogens. Combinations of polymyxin B or colistimethate and rifampin exhibit synergistic activity in vitro. Uptake into tissue is poor, but intrathecal and inhalational administration have been described. Clinical response rates for respiratory tract infections appear to be lower than for other sites of infection.

Polymyxins had fallen out of favor because of nephrotoxicity and neurotoxicity issues, but the emergence of MDR pathogens has returned them to clinical use. Up to 40% of colistimethate-treated patients (5% to 15% for polymyxin B) will have an increase of serum creatinine levels, but renal replacement therapy is seldom required. Neurotoxicity (5% to 7%

for both) usually becomes manifest as muscle weakness or polyneuropathy.

## Protein Synthesis Inhibitors

Several classes of antibiotics, although dissimilar structurally and having divergent spectra of activity, exert their antibacterial effects via binding to bacterial ribosomes and inhibition of protein synthesis. This classification is valuable mechanistically, linking several classes of antibiotics conceptually that have few clinically useful members.

### Aminoglycosides

Once disdained for its toxicity, a resurgence of aminoglycoside use has occurred as resistance to newer antibiotics (especially third-generation cephalosporins and fluoroquinolones) has developed. Gentamicin, tobramycin, and amikacin are still used frequently. Aminoglycosides bind to the bacterial 30S ribosomal subunit, inhibiting protein synthesis. With the exception of gentamicin's modest activity against gram-positive cocci, the spectrum of activity for the various agents is almost identical. Prescribing decisions should be based on toxicity and local resistance patterns.

Nevertheless, the potential toxicity is real, and aminoglycosides are now seldom used as first-line therapy, except in a synergistic combination to treat a serious *Pseudomonas* infection, enterococcal endocarditis, or an infection caused by an MDR gram-negative bacillus. As second-line therapy, these drugs are highly efficacious against the Enterobacteriaceae, but there is less activity against *Acinetobacter*, and limited activity against *P. cepacia, Aeromonas* spp., and *S. maltophilia.*

Aminoglycosides kill bacteria most effectively with a concentration peak–to–MIC ratio higher than 12, so a loading dose is necessary and serum drug concentration must be monitored. Synergistic therapy with a β-lactam agent is theoretically effective because bacterial cell wall damage caused by the β-lactam drug enhances intracellular penetration of the aminoglycoside; however, evidence of improved clinical outcomes is controversial,[220-222,248] especially with conventional dosing. Conventional dosing for serious infections requires 5 mg/kg/day of gentamicin or tobramycin after a 2-mg/kg loading dose, or 15 mg/kg day of amikacin after a loading dose of 7.5 mg/kg. PK is variable and unpredictable in critically ill patients, and higher doses are sometimes necessary (e.g., for burn patients). High doses (e.g., gentamicin, 7 mg/kg/day; amikacin, 20 mg/kg/day) given once daily can obviate these problems in many patients. Marked dosage reductions are necessary in renal insufficiency, but the drugs are dialyzed and a maintenance dose should be given after each hemodialysis treatment.

### Tetracyclines

Tetracyclines bind irreversibly to the 30S ribosomal subunit but, unlike aminoglycosides, they are bacteriostatic. Widespread resistance limits their usefulness in the hospital setting (with two exceptions, doxycycline and tigecycline). Tetracyclines are active against anaerobes; *Actinomyces* can be treated successfully. Doxycycline is active against *B. fragilis*, but is seldom used for this purpose. All tetracyclines are contraindicated in pregnancy and for children younger than 8 years because of dental toxicity.

Tigecycline is a rather new glycylcycline derived from minocycline.[249] With the major exceptions of *Pseudomonas* spp. and *P. mirabilis*, the spectrum of activity is broad, including many MDR gram-positive and gram-negative bacteria, including MRSA, VRE, and *Acinetobacter* spp. Tigecycline overcomes typical bacterial resistance to tetracyclines because of a modification at position 9 of its core structure, which enables high-affinity binding to the 30S ribosomal unit. Tigecycline is active against aerobic and anaerobic streptococci, staphylococci, MRSA, MRSE, and enterococci, including VRE. Activity against gram-negative bacilli is directed against Enterobacteriaceae, including ESBL-producing strains, *P. multocida, A. hydrophila, S. maltophilia, E. aerogenes,* and *Acinetobacter* spp. Antianaerobic activity is excellent. The drug is approved for therapy of cIAIs and cSSTIs.

Concern has been raised recently by a post hoc analysis indicating that the mortality of tigecycline-treated patients is higher in pooled phase 3 and 4 clinical trials, including unpublished registration trials.[250] The adjusted risk difference for all-cause mortality based on a random effects model stratified by trial weight was 0.6% (95% CI, 0.1 to 1.2) between tigecycline and comparator agents. However, an independent meta-analysis has found no such survival disadvantage in an analysis of eight published randomized controlled trials (4651 patients).[251] Overall, no difference was identified for the pooled clinically (OR, 0.92; 95% CI, 0.76 to 1.12) or microbiologically evaluable populations (OR, 0.86; 95% CI, 0.69 to 1.07) from these trials.

### Oxazolidinones

Oxazolidinones bind to the ribosomal 50S subunit, preventing complexing with the 30S subunit. Assembly of a functional initiation complex for protein synthesis is blocked, preventing translation of mRNA. This mode of action is novel compared with that of other protein synthesis inhibitors that permit mRNA translation but then inhibit peptide elongation. Preventing the initiation of protein synthesis is inherently no more lethal than prevention of peptide elongation; therefore, linezolid is bacteriostatic against most susceptible organisms. The ribosomes of *E. coli* are as susceptible to linezolid as those of gram-positive cocci but, with minor exceptions, gram-negative bacteria are oxazolidinone-resistant because oxazolidinones are excreted by efflux pumps.

Linezolid is equally active against MSSA and MRSA, vancomycin-susceptible enterococci, and VRE, and against susceptible and PRSP pneumococci. Most gram-negative bacteria are resistant, but *Bacteroides* spp. are susceptible. Linezolid requires no dosage reduction in renal insufficiency and exhibits excellent tissue penetration, but it is uncertain whether this provides clinical benefit in the treatment of cSSTIs or HAP-VAP.[252] A meta-analysis has suggested that linezolid is equivalent to vancomycin for HAP-VAP,[253] but some clinicians believe that linezolid should supplant vancomycin as first-line therapy for serious infections caused by gram-positive cocci.

### Macrolide-Lincosamide-Streptogramin Family

**Clindamycin** The only lincosamide in active clinical use is clindamycin, which also binds to the 50S ribosome. Clindamycin has good antianaerobic activity (although *B. fragilis* resistance is increasing), and reasonably good activity against susceptible gram-positive cocci, not MRSA or VRE. Clindamycin is used occasionally for anaerobic infections and is preferred over vancomycin for prophylaxis of clean surgical cases in penicillin-allergic patients (see Box 12-6).[112] Because clindamycin inhibits exotoxin production in vitro, it has been advocated in preference to penicillin as first-line therapy for invasive *S. pyogenes* infections. The use of clindamycin has been associated with the development of CDI.

## Drugs That Disrupt Nucleic Acids

### Fluoroquinolones

Fluoroquinolones inhibit bacterial DNA synthesis by inhibiting DNA gyrase, which folds DNA into a superhelix in preparation for replication. The fluoroquinolones exhibit a broad spectrum of activity, excellent oral absorption and bioavailability, and are generally well tolerated (except for photosensitivity and cartilage [especially in children] and tendon damage). These are potent agents with an unfortunate propensity to develop (and induce) resistance rapidly (see Table 12-9). Agents with parenteral and oral formulations include ciprofloxacin, levofloxacin, and moxifloxacin, which has some antianaerobic activity. Several others have been withdrawn from the market or have never been approved because of toxicity.

Fluoroquinolones are most active against enteric gram-negative bacteria, particularly the Enterobacteriaceae and *Haemophilus* spp. There is some activity against *P. aeruginosa, S. maltophilia,* and gram-negative cocci. Activity against gram-positive cocci is variable; it is least for ciprofloxacin and best for the so-called *respiratory quinolone* (e.g., moxifloxacin). Ciprofloxacin is most active against *P. aeruginosa.* However, rampant overuse of fluoroquinolones is rapidly causing resistance that might limit severely the future usefulness of these agents.[254] Fluoroquinolone use has been associated with the emergence of resistant *E. coli, Klebsiella* spp., *P. aeruginosa,* and MRSA.[255,256] Fluoroquinolones prolong the QTc interval and may precipitate the ventricular dysrhythmia torsades de pointes, so electrocardiographic measurement of the QTc interval before and during fluoroquinolone therapy is important. Also, fluoroquinolones interact with warfarin to cause a rapid marked prolongation of the international normalized ratio (INR), so anticoagulation must be monitored closely during therapy.

### Cytotoxic Antibiotics

**Metronidazole** Metronidazole is active against almost all anaerobes and against many protozoa that parasitize human beings. Metronidazole has potent bactericidal activity, including activity against *B. fragilis, Prevotella* spp., *Clostridium* spp. (including *C. difficile*), and anaerobic cocci, although it is ineffective against actinomycosis. Resistance remains rare and is of negligible clinical significance.

Metronidazole causes DNA damage after intracellular reduction of the nitro group of the drug. Acting as a preferential electron acceptor, it is reduced by low redox potential electron transport proteins, decreasing the intracellular concentration of the unchanged drug and maintaining a transmembrane gradient that favors uptake of additional drug. The drug therefore penetrates well into almost all tissues, including neural tissue, making it effective for deep-seated infections and bacteria that are not multiplying rapidly. Absorption after oral or rectal administration is rapid and almost complete. The $t_{1/2}$ of metronidazole is 8 hours because of an active hydroxy metabolite. Increasingly, IV metronidazole is administered every 8 to 12 hours in recognition of the active metabolite, but once-daily dosing is possible.[257] No dosage reduction is required for renal insufficiency, but the drug is dialyzed effectively and administration should be timed to follow dialysis if twice-daily dosing is used. PK in patients with hepatic insufficiency suggests a dosage reduction of 50% with marked impairment.

**Trimethoprim-Sulfamethoxazole** Sulfonamides exert bacteriostatic activity by interfering with bacterial folic acid synthesis, a necessary step in DNA synthesis. Resistance is widespread, thus limiting its use. The addition of sulfamethoxazole to trimethoprim, which prevents the conversion of dihydrofolic acid to tetrahydrofolic acid by the action of dihydrofolate reductase (downstream from the action of sulfonamides) accentuates the bactericidal activity of trimethoprim.

The combination of trimethoprim-sulfamethoxazole (TMP-SMX) is active against S. *aureus, S. pyogenes, S. pneumoniae, E. coli, P. mirabilis, Salmonella* and *Shigella* spp., *Yersinia enterocolitica, S. maltophilia, L. monocytogenes,* and *Pneumocystis jirovici.* Used for urinary tract infections, acute exacerbations of chronic bronchitis, and *Pneumocystis* infections, TMP-SMX is a treatment of choice for infections caused by *S. maltophilia* and outpatient and sometimes inpatient treatment of infections caused by community-acquired MRSA.

A fixed-dose combination of TMP-SMX (1 : 5) is available for parenteral administration. The standard oral formulation is TMP, 80 mg, and SMX, 400 mg, but lesser and greater strength tablets are available. Oral absorption is rapid and bioavailability is almost 100%. Tissue penetration is excellent. The parenteral formulation, 10 mL, contains TMP, 160 mg, and SMX, 800 mg. Full doses (150 to 300 mg TMP in three or four divided doses) may be given if creatinine clearance is higher than 30 mL/min, but the drug is not recommended when the creatinine clearance is less than 15 mL/min.

## ANTIBIOTIC TOXICITIES

### β-Lactam Allergy

Allergic reaction is the most common toxicity of β-lactam antibiotics. The incidence is approximately 7 to 40/1000 treatment courses of penicillin.[258] Parenteral therapy is more likely to provoke an allergic reaction. Most serious reactions occur in patients with no history of penicillin allergy, simply because a history of penicillin allergy is commonly sought and is reported by 5% to 20% of patients, far in excess of the true incidence. Patients with a prior reaction have a four- to sixfold increased risk of another reaction compared with the general population. However, this risk decreases with time, from 80% to 90% skin test reactivity at 2 months to 20% reactivity at 10 years. The risk of cross-reactivity between penicillins and carbapenems and cephalosporins is approximately 5%, being highest for first-generation cephalosporins. There is negligible cross-reactivity to monobactams.

### Red Man Syndrome

Tingling and flushing of the face, neck, or thorax may occur with parenteral vancomycin therapy, but is less common than fever, rigors, or local phlebitis. Although a hypersensitivity reaction, it is not an allergic phenomenon because of the clear association with too rapid infusion of the drug (<1 hour, which can also cause hypotension). The cause is believed to be histamine release caused by local hyperosmolality. A maculopapular rash caused by hypersensitivity occurs in approximately 5% of patients.

## Nephrotoxicity

There is little difference among aminoglycosides in terms of nephrotoxic potential. Aminoglycosides do not provoke inflammation; thus, there are no allergic components to any manifestation of aminoglycoside toxicity. The mechanisms of clinical toxicity relate to ischemia and toxicity to the renal proximal tubular cell.[258] Ultimately, injury is manifested by necrosis of the proximal tubular cell, reduction of the glomerular filtration rate, and decreased creatinine clearance but is usually reversible, and progression to dialysis dependence is rare. Aminoglycoside nephrotoxicity is accentuated by several cofactors, including frequent dosing, older age, sodium and volume depletion, acidemia, hypokalemia, hypomagnesemia, and coexistent liver disease. The risk of injury is ameliorated by single daily dose therapy. If renal function deteriorates, it is advisable to discontinue therapy unless treatment is for a life-threatening infection.

Vancomycin nephrotoxicity is increasing because of higher dosing and concurrent administration of other nephrotoxins. Nephrotoxicity of polymyxins may be an unavoidable consequence of the need to use an agent with known nephrotoxic potential to treat serious infections cause by MDR gram-negative bacilli when there are few alternative, if any.

## Ototoxicity

Aminoglycosides cause cochlear or vestibular toxicity that is usually irreversible, and may develop after the cessation of therapy.[259] Repeated exposures create cumulative risk. Most patients develop cochlear toxicity or a vestibular lesion; rarely are both organs injured. Cochlear toxicity can be subtle, because few patients have baseline audiograms and formal screening programs are seldom undertaken. Few patients complain of hearing loss but, when sought, the incidence of cochlear toxicity may be more than 60%. Clinical hearing loss may occur in 5% to 15% of patients.

Ototoxicity caused directly by vancomycin is accepted as fact, but has been poorly documented in the literature. Hearing loss attributed to vancomycin is better described as neurotoxicity, manifesting as auditory nerve damage, tinnitus, and loss of acuity for high-frequency tones. Synergistic injury is possible with coadministration of other ototoxic drugs, especially aminoglycosides and furosemide. There is no correlation between ototoxicity and nephrotoxicity for drugs that cause both (e.g., aminoglycosides, vancomycin).

## Avoiding Toxicity: Adjustment of Antibiotic Dosage

### Hepatic Insufficiency

The liver metabolizes and eliminates drugs that are too lipophilic for renal excretion. The cytochromes P450 (a gene superfamily consisting of >300 different enzymes) oxidize lipophilic compounds to water-soluble products. Other enzymes convert drugs or metabolites by conjugating them with sugars, amino acids, sulfate, or acetate to facilitate biliary or renal excretion, whereas enzymes such as esterases and hydrolases act by other distinct mechanisms. Oxidation, in particular, is disrupted when liver function is impaired.

Drug dosing in hepatic insufficiency is complicated by insensitivity of clinical assessments to quantify liver function and changing metabolism as the degree of impairment fluctuates (e.g., resolving cholestasis). Changes in renal function with progressive hepatic impairment add considerable complexity. Renal blood flow is decreased in cirrhosis and glomerular filtration is decreased in cirrhosis with ascites. Adverse drug reactions are more frequent with cirrhosis than with other forms of liver disease.

The effect of liver disease on drug disposition is difficult to predict in individual patients; none of the usual tests of liver function can be used to guide dosage.[260] Generally, a dosage reduction of up to 25% of the usual dose is considered if hepatic metabolism is 40% or lower and renal function is normal (Box 12-12). Greater dosage reductions (up to 50%) are advisable if the drug is administered chronically, there is a narrow therapeutic index, protein binding is significantly reduced, or the drug is excreted renally and renal function is severely impaired.

### Renal Insufficiency

Renal drug elimination depends on glomerular filtration, tubular secretion, and reabsorption, any of which may be altered with renal dysfunction. Renal failure may affect hepatic and renal drug metabolic pathways. Drugs whose hepatic metabolism is likely to be disrupted in renal failure include aztreonam, several cephalosporins, macrolides, and carbapenems.

Accurate estimates of renal function are important in patients with mild to moderate renal dysfunction, because the clearance of many drugs by dialysis actually makes management easier. Factors influencing drug clearance by hemofiltration include molecular size, aqueous solubility, plasma protein binding, equilibration kinetics between plasma and tissue, and

**BOX 12-12 Antibiotics Requiring Dosage Reduction for Hepatic and Renal Insufficiency**

**Hepatic**

Aztreonam
Cefoperazone
Chloramphenicol
Clindamycin
Erythromycin
Isoniazid
Linezolid
Metronidazole
Nafcillin
Quinupristin-dalfopristin
Rifampin
Tigecycline

**Renal**

Aminoglycosides
Aztreonam
Carbapenems
Cephalosporins (most)
Chloramphenicol
Fluoroquinolones
Macrolides (except erythromycin and fidoxamycin)
Penicillins
Polymyxins
Sulfonamides
Trimethoprim/sulfamethoxazole
Vancomycin

the apparent $V_D$. New high-flux polysulfone dialysis membranes can clear molecules up to 5 kDa efficiently (the molecular weight of vancomycin is 1.486 kDa). The need to dose patients during or after a renal replacement therapy treatment must be borne in mind; during continuous renal replacement therapy, the estimated creatinine clearance is approximately15 to 25 mL/min in addition to the patient's intrinsic clearance.[261] Cefaclor, cefoperazone, ceftriaxone, chloramphenicol, clindamycin, cloxacillin, dicloxacillin, doxycycline, erythromycin, linezolid, methicillin, nafcillin, oxacillin, metronidazole, rifampin, and tigecycline do not require dosage reductions in renal failure (see Box 12-12).

## IMPORTANT PATHOGENS OF CRITICALLY ILL PATIENTS

### Vancomycin-Resistant Enterococci

Vancomycin-resistant enterococci are predominantly *E. faecium* and thus usually manifest high-level resistance to ampicillin as well, which limits therapeutic options. Patients at risk include those with prolonged hospitalizations, multiple ICU admissions, and multiple or prolonged courses of antibiotics, especially cephalosporins and vancomycin (see Table 12-8). Although many isolates of VRE reflect colonization rather than invasive infection, isolation of VRE from the bloodstream or purulent closed space collections in symptomatic patients merits antimicrobial treatment. At present, there are four approved agents for VRE infection—daptomycin, linezolid, quinupristin-dalfopristin (Q-D), and tigecycline—although chloramphenicol also has activity. Although there are no direct comparative trials of these agents, the side effect profiles of the other three agents appear favorable compared with Q-D. Linezolid-resistant VRE strains are being reported, particularly in patients with inadequately drained or nonremovable foci of infection who receive protracted therapy.

### *Staphylococcus aureus*

With the advent of effective infection control procedures, the incidence of MRSA infections may be decreasing.[262,263] Nonetheless, MRSA remains a formidable and dangerous pathogen. Vancomycin has been the traditional first-line therapy of choice for most serious MRSA infections; however, there is increasing awareness of its limitations.[242,264] Vancomycin achieves only slow bactericidal activity, has poor lung and central nervous system penetration, and poor activity in prosthetic biofilms. Heteroresistance to vancomycin has been detected in high-inoculum infections, and intermediate and complete vancomycin resistance has been described recently, although it remains rare. Combination therapy with gentamicin may enhance its bactericidal activity; however, this use does not alter clinical cure rates. In vancomycin-intolerant patients or vancomycin-refractory MRSA infections (i.e., vancomycin failures),[243] linezolid or Q-D, have shown modest efficacy as a salvage option.[265] Daptomycin is bactericidal rapidly against *S. aureus* (including MRSA), but whether rapid bacterial killing confers a clinical advantage for therapy of most infections is debatable. Tigecycline is active (bacteriostatic) against MRSA, which does not confer a clinical disadvantage in most therapeutic situations. Ceftaroline is the newest option for the treatment of MRSA infections.

### *Pseudomonas aeruginosa*

*Pseudomonas aeruginosa* is a ubiquitous, avirulent opportunist whose virulence is enhanced in critically ill patients.[266] It is the second most common isolate from ICU infections, and infections caused by *P. aeruginosa* are the leading cause of death from nosocomial infection in the ICU, with infection-associated mortality as high as 70% in patients with pneumonia or bacteremia. Therapy is complex because of intrinsic and acquired resistance to a diverse spectrum of antimicrobial agents. Resistance is mediated via chromosomal-mediated β-lactamases, aminoglycoside-modifying enzymes, and mutations of outer membrane porin channels, which impede entry of carbapenems into the periplasmic space. A prominent characteristic is a high rate (20% to 40%) of de novo resistance developing during antipseudomonal therapy, a major cause of failed therapy.[267] Meropenem and doripenem may provide slightly higher activity than imipenem-cilastatin, with a lower propensity for central nervous system toxicity.

### Multidrug-Resistant Enterobacteriaceae, Including *Klebsiella* Species

Resistance to β-lactams and other antibiotics in the Enterobacteriaceae family is increasingly associated with plasmid-mediated resistance determinants that are transferred easily among species, including ESBLs and carbapenemases, specifically the CTX-M family of ESBLs, KPC family of serine carbapenemases, and VIM, IMP, and NDM-1 metallo–β-lactamases.[268-270] These enzymes are now appearing worldwide in multiple combinations of ESBLs and carbapenemases, thereby conferring resistance to almost all β-lactam antibiotics. The increasing prevalence of carbapenem-resistant gram-negative bacteria is particularly disconcerting.

*Klebsiella* spp. and other Enterobacteriaceae are notable for exhibiting chromosome-mediated inducible β-lactamases, which deactivate antipseudomonal penicillins (e.g., ticarcillin, piperacillin), aztreonam, and cephalosporins. Ceftazidime is a potent inducer of chromosomal β-lactamase expression and is increasingly avoided as monotherapy or combination therapy of infections caused by even susceptible organisms. Cefepime does not appear to induce this type of chromosome-mediated resistance to the same degree, but itself is susceptible to the action of ESBLs. Because most ESBL-producing strains also coexpress resistance to other agents (e.g., aminoglycosides, fluoroquinolones), there are few antimicrobials available to treat infections with these organisms and data regarding agents in development are limited to in vitro studies. Therapeutic options are limited to carbapenems (the mainstay of therapy for ESBL producers) and tigecycline.

### *Stenotrophomonas maltophilia*

At present, there are no clinical laboratory standards for the interpretation of disk diffusion susceptibilities for *S. maltophilia*. In the absence of broth dilution testing results, the most reliable agents have been TMP-SMX alone or TMP-SMX and ticarcillin–clavulanic acid in combination. The use of other agents has been associated with high rates of clinical failure despite in vitro susceptibility.

### *Acinetobacter baumannii* Complex

*Acinetobacter baumannii* is a pleomorphic, aerobic, gram-negative bacillus (referred to sometimes as a *coccobacillus*) that is isolated commonly from the hospital environment and hospitalized patients. *A. baumannii* colonizes aquatic environments preferentially, and is not part of normal fecal flora. This organism is often cultured from hospitalized patients' respiratory secretions, wounds or surgical sites, and urine. Historically, most *Acinetobacter* isolates recovered from hospitalized patients represented colonization rather than infection, especially in the ICU setting, being particularly common with endotracheal intubation, multiple IV catheters, monitoring devices, surgical drains, urinary catheters, or prior antimicrobial therapy with agents that have little or no activity against *Acinetobacter*. Colonization of the gastrointestinal tract by *Acinetobacter* is uncommon.

Although *A. baumannii* is avirulent, it is capable of causing infection of the seriously ill host.[271,272] *Acinetobacter* infections are increasingly common; when they occur, they usually involve organ systems with a high fluid content (e.g., sputum, cerebrospinal fluid, peritoneal fluid, urine), manifesting most commonly as pneumonia, catheter-associated bacteriuria, or bloodstream infection. *Acinetobacter* pneumonias have a predilection to occur in outbreaks. Nosocomial meningitis may occur in colonized neurosurgical patients with externalized ventricular drains (i.e., ventriculostomy). *Acinetobacter* is rarely associated with meningitis, endocarditis (native and prosthetic valve infections), peritonitis, urinary tract infections, community-acquired pneumonia, or cholangitis.

*A. baumannii* is inherently resistant to several antibiotics, but MDR strains have emerged that are susceptible to relatively few antibiotics. Antibiotics to which MDR *Acinetobacter* is usually susceptible include meropenem, doripenem, amikacin, tigecycline, colistin, and polymyxin B, with one of the latter two agents increasingly being used. There are no clinical laboratory standards for the interpretation of disk diffusion susceptibilities for tigecycline against *A. baumannii.* Mortality and morbidity resulting from *A. baumannii* infection relate to the underlying immune status of the host rather than the inherent virulence of the organism.

## FUNGAL INFECTIONS

Fungi are ubiquitous heterotrophic eukaryotes, resilient to environmental stress and adaptable to diverse environments. The most important human pathogens are the yeasts and molds. Invasive mycoses have emerged as a major cause of morbidity and mortality in hospitalized surgical patients. The U.S. incidence of nosocomial candidemia is approximately 8/100,000 population, at a cost of approximately $1 billion/year. Fungemia is the fourth most common type of bloodstream infection in the United States, but many surgical patients develop invasive infections without positive blood cultures. Host or therapeutic immunosuppression, organ transplantation, implantable devices, and human immunodeficiency virus (HIV) infection have all changed the landscape of fungal pathogenicity.

### Risk Factors

Whereas the incidence of hospital-acquired fungal infections almost doubled in the past decade, the greatest increase occurred in critically ill surgical patients, making the surgical ICU population an extremely high-risk group.[273] Several conditions (patient-dependent and disease-specific) are independent predictors for invasive fungal infection, including ICU length of stay, extent of medical comorbidity, host immune suppression, and number of medical devices present. Neutropenia, diabetes mellitus, new-onset renal replacement therapy, total parenteral nutrition, broad-spectrum antibiotic administration, bladder catheterization, azotemia, diarrhea, and corticosteroid therapy have also been associated with candidemia.[274,275]

#### Diabetes Mellitus

Diabetes mellitus is an independent predictor for mucosal candidiasis, invasive candidiasis, and aspergillosis. Diabetic ketoacidosis has a strong association with rhinocerebral *Mucor* (produced by Zygomycetes) and other atypical fungal infections, with hyperglycemia being the strongest predictor of candidemia after liver transplantation and cardiopulmonary bypass. Glycosylation of cell surface receptors facilitates fungal binding and subsequent internalization and apoptosis of targeted cells. Glycosylation of opsonins disables fungal antigen recognition. The serum of diabetic patients has diminished capacity to bind iron, therefore making it available to the pathogen. Altered Th1 (helper phenotype) lymphocyte recognition of fungal targets impairs the production of interferon-$\gamma$ (IFN-$\gamma$). *Candida* spp. overexpress a $C_3$ receptor–like protein that facilitates adhesion to endothelium and mucosal surfaces.

#### Neutropenia

There is a direct correlation between the degree of neutropenia and risk of invasive fungal infection.[277a] Although a recent meta-analysis has concluded that there is little benefit from prophylaxis in neutropenic cancer patients, empirical antifungal therapy is standard for febrile neutropenia patients after chemotherapy or bone marrow transplantation. When profound neutropenia exists, the risk for breakthrough candidemia during antifungal therapy is significantly higher.

#### Organ Transplantation and Immunosuppression

The two most common opportunistic fungal pathogens of transplant patients are *Candida* and *Aspergillus* spp. The risk of fungal infection decreases 6 months after transplantation, unless a rejection episode requires intensification of the immunosuppression. In the solid organ transplant recipient, the graft itself is often affected. In liver transplantation, the risk of fungemia increases with the duration of the operation and number of transfusions. Other risk factors include the type of bile duct anastomosis (Roux-en-Y), tissue ischemia, cytomegalovirus (CMV) infection, and graft-versus-host disease. *Aspergillus* tracheobronchitis in lung transplant patients is most likely to occur at the bronchial anastomosis. Surveillance bronchoscopy is recommended in this setting. *Aspergillus* is also the main organism responsible for fungemia after heart transplantation, and is second only to CMV as the cause of pneumonia in the first month after surgery.

Infectious complications are the primary cause of morbidity and mortality after pancreas and kidney-pancreas transplantation. The most common pathogens are gram-positive cocci, followed by gram-negative bacilli and *Candida.* Risk factors for fungal infections in this setting include bladder rather than enteric drainage (in cases of pancreas transplantation) and the use of muromonab-CD3 for antirejection therapy. Kidney recipients have the lowest incidence of infectious complications of all solid organ transplants, but the risk is sufficiently high that all solid organ transplant recipients (kidney recipients included) receive fungal prophylaxis with fluconazole (see later).

#### Malignant Disease

Cancer and chemotherapy produce three types of immune dysfunction that render the patient vulnerable to opportunistic infections: neutropenia (see earlier), deficits in lymphocyte-mediated innate immunity (e.g., lymphoma and during corticosteroid treatment), and adaptive immunodeficiency (e.g., multiple myeloma, Waldenström macroglobulinemia, and after splenectomy). As many as one third of cases of febrile neutropenia after chemotherapy for malignant disease are caused by invasive fungemia (see later). The type of lymphopenia is as important as the nadir of the lymphocyte count. Whereas Th1-type responses (TNF-α, IFN-γ, and IL-12) confer protection, Th2 (IL-4 and IL-10) suppressor phenotype responses are associated with progression of disease. Corticosteroids have anti-inflammatory properties related to their inhibitory effects on the activation of various transcription factors, in particular NF-κB. In murine models, steroid treatment increases the production of IL-10 and decreases the recruitment of mononuclear cells in response to a fungal challenge. However, IL-8–mediated neutrophil is unaffected.

#### Central Venous Catheters

Many episodes of candidemia represent a CLABSI. Isolation of *C. parapsilosis* from blood is strongly associated with CLABSI, parenteral nutrition, and prosthetic devices. In non-neutropenic subjects, the most common portals of entry for catheter contamination and subsequent infection are the skin during catheter placement, manipulation of an indwelling catheter, and cross-infection among ICU patients attributed to health care workers. Other possible sources for primary catheter colonization include contaminated parenteral nutrition solution, multidrug administration with repetitive violation of the sterile fluid path, and presence of other medical devices. The secondary route of contamination for devices in direct contact with the bloodstream (e.g., pacemakers, cardiac valves, joint prostheses) is candidemia originating from the gastrointestinal tract. Endogenous flora are also the most common source in neutropenic and other immunosuppressed patients. Once the catheter is contaminated, a stereotypical series of events occurs. Yeast adhere to the catheter surface and develop hyphae that integrate into a biofilm that increases in size and tridimensional complexity. A biofilm is the main reservoir for candidemia secondary to contaminated medical devices, because it induces stasis and sequesters the fungi from antimycotic medication and the immune response.

In general, catheter removal is indicated following the diagnosis of systemic fungal infections and fungemia. Antifungal agents are usually continued after the catheter is removed, and *Candida* endophthalmitis should be ruled out (see later).

### Prediction of Invasive *Candida* Infection

Overgrowth and recovery of *Candida* spp. from multiple sites, even from asymptomatic patients, carries a high likelihood of invasive candidiasis. Risk factors for the development of *Candida* colonization include female gender, antibiotic therapy prior to an ICU admission, prolonged stay in the ICU, and multiple gastrointestinal operations.[276] The source of the pathogen in the surgical context of is usually the gastrointestinal tract.

Because colonization with *Candida* spp. presages invasive disease, it is desirable to identify and characterize patients further in terms of risk. Surveillance cultures may be used to screen ICU patients. Several scoring systems have been proposed to quantify the risk of invasive fungal infection (Box 12-13). Pittet and colleagues[277] have proposed the colonization index, which has been validated in surgical patients. A threshold index of 0.5 or higher has been proposed for the initiation of empirical antifungal therapy in critically ill patients (see later). The *Candida* score, developed by Leon and associates,[278] considers dynamic patient factors that are present before the fact of colonization is identified, and thus may be an earlier indicator. A threshold score of 2.5 points is indicative of high risk. Comparisons between the two are few, but the *Candida* score may perform better.[279,280] The colonization index developed[281] and modified[282] by Ostrosky-Zeichner and coworkers suggests that high-risk patients are those who remain in the ICU for 4 days or longer, have a central venous catheter in place or are treated with antibiotics, and two of the following: use of total parenteral nutrition, need for dialysis, recent major surgery, diagnosis of pancreatitis, and treatment with systemic corticosteroids or other immunosuppressive agents.

Shorr and colleagues[283] have described a score to predict candidemia specifically, using data present on hospital admission (not specifically for surgical patients). This simple model assesses six factors (see Box 12-13), including age, absence of fever, recent hospitalization, admission from another health care facility, and need for mechanical ventilation; it differentiates patients' risk for candidemia in a graded fashion (e.g., no risk factors, 0.4%, three risk factors, 3.2%; six risk factors, 27.3%; $P <$ .0001) on presentation to the hospital.

The use of broad-spectrum antibiotics is a well-documented risk factor for fungal colonization and subsequent infection. Interrelations between bacteria and fungi in human disease are complex. Antibiotics that have some antianaerobic therapy are associated with substantial increases in colony counts of yeast flora of the gut, whereas antibiotics with poor anaerobic activity are less likely to produce this effect. Sawyer and associates[284] have demonstrated that *C. albicans i*nduces bacterial translocation into abscesses, but the relationship is one of direct competency, rather than synergy or cooperation. The precise mechanism of action for this observation is unknown, but is probably related to fungi to microbe competence and growth suppression. *Candida* may enhance the pathogenicity of certain bacteria but not others; this interaction remains to be elucidated.

#### Intensive Care Unit and Invasive Mechanical Ventilation

Epidemiologic observations have correlated the duration of mechanical ventilation and amount of intensive care required with the occurrence of fungal colonization and invasive infections. Other factors related to susceptibility for systemic candidiasis are total parenteral nutrition, prophylaxis of stress-related gastric mucosal hemorrhage, radiation therapy, previous bacteremia, abdominal surgery, renal replacement therapy, extremes of age, recurrent mucocutaneous candidiasis, and duration of cardiopulmonary bypass longer than 120 minutes.

### Fungal Pathogens

#### *Candida albicans*

*C. albicans* is a common cause of human disease, which can be focal or disseminated.[285] *C. albicans* accounts for about 60% of *C.* isolates, followed by *Candida glabrata* (15% to 25% of all *Candida* infections). The incidence of candidemia has increased

**BOX 12-13 Scoring Systems for Risk Stratification for Invasive Candidiasis**

***Candida* Colonization Index**[277]

This is the number of cultures sites positive for the identical yeast isolate, divided by the number of sites cultured. At least three sites should be cultured (oral mucosa, axillae, rectum, gastric contents, urine). A score ≧0.5 points is considered high risk for subsequent infection. Discrimination statistics were not reported.

***Candida* Score**[278]

Five dichotomous variables are awarded points. A summed total score ≥2.5 points is strongly predictive of invasive fungal infection (sensitivity, %; specificity, %; C statistic = 0.847).

Total parenteral nutrition: 1 point
Surgery on ICU admission: 1 point
Multifocal *Candida* species colonization: 1 point
Severe sepsis: 2 points

**Ostrosky-Zeichner Score (2007)**[280]

This is a prediction rule that provides a dichotomous risk assessment based on the presence of at least three risk factors: relative risk, 5; sensitivity, 0.27, specificity; 0.93, positive predictive value; 0.13, negative predictive value; 0.97, accuracy, 0.90.

Any systemic antibiotic (days 1-3 of the ICU stay) *or*
Central venous catheter (days 1-3) *and*
At least two of the following:

- Total parenteral nutrition (days 1-3)
- Any renal replacement therapy (days 1-3)
- Any major surgery (days –7 to 0)
- Pancreatitis (days –7 to 0)
- Any steroid use (days –7 to –3)

Any other immunosuppression (days –7 to 0)

**Ostrosky-Zeichner Modified Score (2011)**[279]

This is a prediction rule that provides a dichotomous risk assessment based on the presence of at least three risk factors: relative risk, 4; sensitivity, 0.50; specificity, 0.83; positive predictive value, 0.10; negative predictive value, 0.97; accuracy, 0.81.

Mechanical ventilation >48 hr (days 1-4) *and*
Any systemic antibiotic (days 1-3 of the ICU stay) *and*
Central venous catheter (days 1-3) *and*
At least one of the following:

- Total parenteral nutrition (days 1-3)
- Any renal replacement therapy (days 1-3)
- Any major surgery (days –7 to 0)
- Pancreatitis (days –7 to 0)
- Any steroid or other immunosuppression (days –7 to 0)

**Shorr Candidemia Score**[282]

A simple, equal-weight score (1 point each) differentiated reasonably well among patients admitted with a bloodstream infection, with a C statistic of 0.70.

Age <65 yr
Temperature ≦98° F or severe altered mental status
Cachexia
Hospitalization within the previous 30 days
Admission from another health care facility
Need for mechanical ventilation

over the past 30 years, representing 8% to 15% of all nosocomial bloodstream infections, with mortality rates reported in some series to be as high as 80%. *Candida* bloodstream infection carries an independent increased risk of death in adult ICU patients.[286]

A morphologic transition from yeast to hyphal forms is the most important determinant of dissemination of *C. albicans,* because the mycelial phase is invasive[287] because of upregulated elaboration of proteinases. Host and pathogen play a role in this dimorphism. Phenotypic switching accompanied by changes in antigen expression, colony morphology, and tissue affinities are recognized, but the inducer mechanisms and triggering stimuli are unknown.

Multifocal candidiasis is the simultaneous isolation of *Candida* from two or more of the following normally sterile locations: respiratory, digestive, and urinary tracts, wounds, or drainage. Disseminated candidiasis requires microbiologic evidence of yeast in fluids from normally sterile sites such as cerebrospinal, pleural, pericardial, or peritoneal fluid, histologic samples from viscera, or a diagnosis of endophthalmitis or candidemia with negative catheter tip cultures. Disseminated candidiasis and true fungemia can lead to septic shock, similar to that seen with bacterial pathogens. The dimorphic transition results in shock and end-organ failure in susceptible individuals, mechanistically independent of TNF-α.

The diagnosis of fungemia as the cause of a patient's sepsis depends on a strong clinical suspicion, because fungemia and bacteremia are indistinguishable based on clinical criteria.[288] Blood cultures for *Candida* are false-negative more than 50% of the time; moreover, bacterial pathogens may interfere with the recovery of *Candida.* Biomarkers including the fungal cell wall component (1 → 3)-β-D-glucan,[289] anti-*Candida* immunoglobulin G (IgG) antibodies,[290] and procalcitonin[291] are suggestive but not sufficiently accurate for diagnosis. There are no reliable laboratory tests to identify the presence of *Candida* or to differentiate between *Candida* colonization and invasive candidiasis. No single site of isolation is superior to others in predicting which patients have systemic infection. Purpura fulminans and unexplained myalgias are suggestive of candidiasis in the appropriate clinical context. The presence of three or more colonized sites or two positive blood cultures at least 24 hours apart, with one obtained after the removal of any central venous catheter, are strong indicators of fungemia.[292] Whereas asymptomatic recovery of *Candida* in urine rarely requires therapy, candiduria should be treated if symptomatic, after instrumentation or renal transplantation, or if the patient is neutropenic. Removing or changing the bladder drainage catheter is required.

Fungal endophthalmitis usually occurs as a result of hematogenous spread from systemic fungemia.[293] *Candida* spp. are the most common offenders, although *Aspergillus, Cryptococcus, Fusarium, Scedosporium,* and others are known causes of endophthalmitis. Retinal involvement has been diagnosed in 28% to 45% of all patients with known candidemia and may be the first sign of hitherto undetected fungemia. Early treatment of invasive fungal infection decreases the incidence of endophthalmitis, All patients with invasive candidiasis or fungemia must undergo a formal ophthalmologic assessment to rule out eye involvement. The observation of a classic three-dimensional, retina-based, cotton wool vitreal inflammatory process is diagnostic of *Candida* endophthalmitis.

Treatment of endophthalmitis consists of IV antifungal therapy and may require intraocular injections of amphotericin B, caspofungin, or voriconazole. In patients in whom extension to the vitreous or pars anterior is evident, surgical débridement or vitrectomy may be required. Delay in treatment frequently leads to blindness.

#### Non–*albicans Candida*

The incidence of non-*Candida* fungemia and sepsis is increasing, accounting for up to 50% of non–*albicans Candida* adult ICU infections. Undoubtedly, the pressure of antifungal therapy is an explanation for the emergence of *C. glabrata* and *C. krusei* as pathogens.[294] Other species of yeast are related to specific events, such as *C. parapsilosis* in the presence of an indwelling central venous catheter. An increased incidence of *C. tropicalis* in oncology patients is secondary to the inherent invasiveness of the organism, especially through damaged gastrointestinal mucosa. Clinically, the features of these infections are indistinguishable from those of *C. albicans.*

#### *Aspergillus*

Noninvasive types of aspergillosis include allergic bronchopulmonary aspergillosis, a form of hypersensitivity reaction in asthmatics, and aspergilloma. These entities, without tissue invasion, usually do not require antifungal therapy. However, invasive aspergillosis is increasing in incidence and has become a major cause of death among patients with liquid tumors. Although invasive *Aspergillus* infections usually occur via inhalation of conidia, the fungus may also be ingested on food (e.g., pepper, regular and herbal teas, fruits, corn, rice). Spores of *Aspergillus* and other filamentous fungi are thermotolerant, difficult to eradicate, and threaten the immunocompromised host. Conidia that are not cleared by alveolar macrophages germinate in the alveoli; hyphal forms invade the pulmonary parenchyma, with prominent vascular invasion and early dissemination.[295]

#### Other Emerging Fungal Pathogens

Zygomycetes (*Mucor*) are becoming increasingly important in ICU patients. The portal of entry in the immunocompromised host is usually inhalation of aerosolized thermotolerant spores, although percutaneous exposure (surgical or traumatic wounds and burns) has been reported. The source of these spores is usually decaying organic matter in soil, but they can be found in hospital food, including fruit, bread, cookies, crackers, regular and herbal tea, and pepper. The major risk factors for mucormycosis are diabetic ketoacidosis, neutropenia, iron overload, deferoxamine therapy, and protein-calorie malnutrition. Infection may cause extensive tissue necrosis; treatment includes surgical débridement, depending on the extent of the disease.

### Prophylaxis

The substantial morbidity and mortality of invasive fungal infections has led to the practice of administering prophylactic antifungal agents, usually fluconazole, to critically ill patients. Early on, concern was raised that increasing the use of azole antifungals would lead to increased resistance to the agents.[296,297] A prospective, randomized, placebo-controlled trial of enteral fluconazole, 400 mg/day, was conducted among 260 critically ill surgical patients with a length of stay of 3 days or longer in a tertiary-care surgical ICU.[298] After adjusting for potentially confounding effects of the Acute Physiology and Chronic Health Evaluation (APACHE) III score, days to first dose, and fungal colonization at enrollment, the risk of fungal infection was reduced by 55% in the fluconazole group, but no difference in mortality was observed. In a follow-up prospective, observational study,[299] subjects admitted for 3 days or longer to the surgical ICU underwent surveillance fungal cultures of rectal-fecal swabs, urine, and endotracheal aspirates on admission, once weekly thereafter, and on ICU discharge while fluconazole prophylaxis of high-risk surgical patients continued as usually carried out. *C. glabrata* colonization was not more common among patients in the later cohort as compared with earlier (adjusted odds ratio [AOR], 0.90; 95% CI, 0.57 to 1.41). Patients with invasive candidiasis in the latter cohort were not more likely than those in the earlier trial to have infection caused by *C. glabrata* (AOR, 1.93; 95% CI, 0.20 to 18.98), whereas patients with invasive candidiasis in the 2003 cohort were less likely than patients in the 1998 trial to have acquired invasive candidiasis in the ICU (AOR, 0.08; 95% CI, 0.01 to 0.82).

Four randomized studies comparing fluconazole to placebo for the prevention of fungal infections in the surgical ICU were subjected to meta-analysis.[300] The studies enrolled 626 patients but used differing dosing regimens of fluconazole. All trials were double-blinded and two were multicenter studies. Fluconazole prophylaxis significantly reduced the incidence of fungal infections (pooled OR, 0.44; 95% CI, 0.27 to 0.72; $P < .001$). However, fluconazole prophylaxis was not associated with a survival advantage (pooled OR for mortality, 0.87; 95% CI, 0.59 to 1.28). Fluconazole did not alter the rate of candidemia, perhaps because it developed in only 2.2% of all participants. Data were insufficient to allow comment on the impact of fluconazole prophylaxis on resource use, distribution of non-*albicans* species of *Candida*, or emergence of resistance.

Prophylactic fluconazole administration in general surgical ICU patients appears to decrease the incidence of mycotic infections, but does not improve survival. The absence of a survival advantage may reflect the paucity of data in this area and the possibility that this issue requires further study. Current guidelines recommend fluconazole prophylaxis for high-risk patients (Box 12-14).[301]

#### Antifungal Prophylaxis of Solid Organ Transplant Recipients

Solid organ transplantation is lifesaving for end-stage organ failure, but post-transplantation invasive fungal infections remain a major cause of morbidity and mortality. To improve outcomes, various prevention strategies been tested, including antifungal prophylaxis with systemic and topical nonabsorbable agents. Currently, data support the use of antifungal prophylaxis in liver, lung, small bowel, and pancreas transplant recipients (see Box 12-14).[301]

In a meta-analysis of randomized placebo-controlled trials with fluconazole prophylaxis, the incidence of fungal infections was significantly reduced; however, there was no survival advantage, similar to antifungal prophylaxis of critically ill general surgical patients.[302] For liver transplant patients, the number needed to treat (NNT) to prevent one infection is 14, given an incidence of 10%. The meta-analysis also concluded that for lower risk recipients (i.e., renal homograft recipients), the NNT increases to 28.

**BOX 12-14 Synopsis of Clinical Practice Guidelines for the Management of Candidiasis***

**Antifungal Prophylaxis for Solid-Organ Transplant Recipients and ICU Patients**

- Solid-organ transplant recipients:
  Postoperative antifungal prophylaxis for liver (A-I), pancreas (B-II), and small bowel (B-III) transplant recipients at high risk of candidiasis, daily for 7-14 days.
  - Fluconazole (200-400 mg [3-6 mg/kg] daily)
  - Liposomal amphotericin B (L-AmB) (1-2 mg/kg)
- Patients hospitalized in the ICU:
  Fluconazole (400 mg [6 mg/kg] daily) is recommended for high-risk patients in adult units that have a high incidence of invasive candidiasis (B-I).

**Treatment of identified Candidemia in Non-Neutropenic Patients**

- Initial therapy for most adult patients (A-I):
  Fluconazole (loading dose of 800 mg [12 mg/kg], then 400 mg [6 mg/kg] daily) *or*
  Echinocandin
  - Caspofungin: Loading dose of 70 mg, then 50 mg daily, *or*
  - Micafungin: 100 mg daily, *or*
  - Anidulafungin: Loading dose of 200 mg, then 100 mg daily is recommended
- An echinocandin for is favored for patients with moderate to severe illness or for patients who have had recent azole exposure (A-III). Fluconazole is recommended for patients who are less critically ill and who have had no recent azole exposure (A-III). The same therapeutic approach is advised for children, with attention to differences in dosing.
- Transition from an echinocandin to fluconazole is recommended for patients who have isolates likely to be susceptible to fluconazole (e.g., *C. albicans*) and who are clinically stable (A-II).
- For infection caused by *C. glabrata,* an echinocandin is preferred (B-III). Transition to fluconazole or voriconazole therapy is not recommended without confirmation of isolate susceptibility (B-III). For patients who received fluconazole or voriconazole initially, have improved clinically, and have negative follow-up cultures, continuation of the azole to completion of therapy is reasonable (B-III).
- For infection caused by *C. parapsilosis,* treatment with fluconazole is recommended (B-III). Patients who have received an echinocandin initially, have improved clinically, and have negative follow-up cultures, continuation of the ehinocandin to completion of therapy is reasonable (B-III).
- Amphotericin B deoxycholate (AmB-d), 0.5-1.0 mg/kg daily, or a lipid formulation of AmB (LFAmB), 3-5 mg/kg daily, are alternatives if there is intolerance to or limited availability of other antifungal agentss (A-I). Transition from AmB-d or LFAmB to fluconazole is recommended if isolates are likely to be susceptible to fluconazole (e.g., *C. albicans*) and the patient is stable clinically (A-I).
- Voriconazole, 400 mg (6 mg/kg) twice daily for two doses, and then 200 mg (3 mg/kg) twice daily thereafter is effective for candidemia (A-I), but there is little advantage over fluconazole, and is recommended as step-down oral therapy for selected cases of candidiasis caused by *C. krusei* or voriconazole-susceptible *C. glabrata* (B-III).
- The recommended duration of therapy for candidemia without obvious metastatic complications is for 2 weeks after documented clearance of *Candida* from the bloodstream and resolution of symptoms attributable to candidemia (A-III).
- IV catheter removal is strongly recommended (A-II).

**Empirical Treatment for Suspected Invasive Candidiasis in Non-Neutropenic Patients**

- Empirical therapy for suspected candidiasis in nonneutropenic patients is similar to that for proven candidiasis (B-III):
  - Fluconazole (loading dose of 800 mg [12 mg/kg], then 400 mg [6 mg/kg] daily)
  - Caspofungin (loading dose of 70 mg, then 50 mg daily)
  - Anidulafungin (loading dose of 200 mg, then 100 mg daily)
  - Micafungin (100 mg daily)

An echinocandin is preferred for patients who have had recent azole exposure, whose illness is moderately severe or severe, or who are at high risk of infection caused by *C. glabrata* or *C. krusei* (B-III).

- AmB-d (0.5-1.0 mg/kg daily) or LFAmB (3-5 mg/kg daily) are alternatives if there is intolerance to or limited availability of other antifungals (B-III).
- Empirical antifungal therapy should be considered for critically ill patients with risk factors for invasive candidiasis and no other known cause of fever, based on clinical assessment of risk, serologic markers for invasive candidiasis, or culture data from nonsterile sites (B-III).

Adapted from Playford EG, Webster AC, Sorrell TC, et al: Systematic review and meta-analysis of antifungal agents for preventing fungal infections in liver transplant recipients. Eur J Clin Microbiol Infect Dis 25:549–561, 2006.
*Infectious Diseases Society of America, 2009; strength of evidence-based recommendations is shown in parentheses.

A systematic review and meta-analysis of antifungal prophylaxis in liver transplant recipients evaluated ten randomized trials (1106 patients) of any prophylactic antifungal regimen versus no antifungal agent or another antifungal regimen.[303] In general, results were consistent across trials, despite clinical and methodological heterogeneity. Antifungal prophylaxis did not reduce mortality (RR, 0.84; 95% CI, 0.54 to 1.30), but fluconazole prophylaxis reduced invasive fungal infections (RR, 0.28; 95% CI: 0.13 to 0.57). Fluconazole prophylaxis did not significantly increase colonization or infection with azole-resistant fungi, although data were limited.

## Antifungal Therapy

Candidemia is defined as the following: (1) one blood culture that grows *Candida* spp. and histologically documented invasive candidiasis or an ophthalmic examination consistent with candidal endophthalmitis; (2) at least two blood cultures obtained at different times from a peripheral vein that grow the same *Candida* spp; or (3) one blood culture obtained peripherally and one blood culture obtained through an indwelling central line, both of which grow identical *Candida* spp. Patients with one positive blood culture drawn through an IV line and a positive semiquantitative catheter tip culture

**Table 12-10 Antifungal Agents**

| ANTIFUNGAL AGENT | INDICATIONS | ROUTE AND DOSAGE |
|---|---|---|
| Amphotericin B | *Candida albicans* (>95%), *C. glabrata* (95%), *C. parapsilosis* (>95%), *C. krusei* (>95%), *C. tropicalis* (99%), *C. guillermondi, C. lusitaniae*<br>Variable activity: *Aspergillus* spp., ferrous *Trichosporon beigelii, Fusarium* spp., *Blastomyces dermatidis* | IV: 0.5-1.0 mg/kg/day over 2-4 hr<br>Oral: 1 mL oral suspension, swish and swallow 4× daily, ×2 wk |
| Amphotericin B liposomal (less nephrotoxicity) | *C. albicans* (>95%), *C. glabrata* (>95%), *C. parapsilosis* (>95%), *C. krusei* (>95%), *C. tropicalis* (99%), *C. guillermondi, C. lusitaniae*<br>Variable activity: *Aspergillus* spp. | IV: 3-5 mg/kg/day |
| Amphotericin B colloidal dispersion | *C. albicans* (>95%), *C. glabrata* (>95%), *C. parapsilosis* (>95%), *C. krusei* (>95%), *C. tropicalis* (99%), C. guillermondi, *C. lusitaniae*<br>Variable activity: *Aspergillus* spp. | IV: 3-5 mg/kg/day |
| Amphotericin B lipid complex | *C. albicans* (>95%), *C. glabrata* (>95%), *C. parapsilosis* (>95%), *C. krusei* (>95%), *C. tropicalis* (99%), *C. guillermondi, C. lusitaniae*<br>Variable activity: *Aspergillus* spp. | IV: 5 mg/kg/day |
| Ketoconazole | *C. albicans* | PO: 200-400 mg/daily |
| Voriconazole | *Aspergillus* spp., *Fusarium* spp., *C. albicans* (99%), *C. glabrata* (99%), *C. parapsilosis* (99%), *C. tropicalis* (99%), *C. krusei* (99%), *C. guillermondi* (>95%), *C. lusitaniae* (95%) | IV: 6 mg/kg q12h ×2, then 4 mg/kg IV every 12 hr<br>PO: >40 kg, 200 mg every 12 hr; <40 kg, 100 mg every 12 hr |
| Fluconazole | *C. albicans* (97%), *C. glabrata* (85%–90% resistant, intermediate), *C. parapsilosis* (99%) *C. tropicalis* (98%), *C. krusei* (5%)<br>Fungistatic against *Aspergillus* spp. | Candidiasis—prophylaxis (IV or oral), 100-400 mg/day; invasive, 400-800 mg/day<br>Oropharyngeal: 200 mg day 1, then 100 daily for 2 wk |
| Itraconazole | Fungicidal to *Aspergillus* spp., *C. albicans* (93%), *C. glabrata* (50%), *C. parapsilosis* (45%), *C. tropicalis* (58%), *C. krusei* (69%), *C. guillermondi, C. lusitaniae*<br>Blastomycoses, histoplasmosis, chromomycosis | IV: Load 200 mg IV 2× daily ×4 doses, then 200 mg 4× daily maximum 14 days<br>Oral: 200 mg daily or 2× daily<br>Life-threatening: Load 600-800/day ×3-5/days, then 400-600 mg/day |
| Caspofungin | *C. albicans, C. glabrata, C. parapsilosis, C. tropicalis, C. krusei, C. guillermondi, C. lusitaniae* | IV: 70 mg IV, then 50 mg IV every day |
| Micafungin | *C. albicans, C. glabrata, C. parapsilosis, C. tropicalis, C. krusei, C. guillermondi, C. lusitaniae* | IV: 100-200 mg IV daily |
| Anidulafungin | *C. albicans, C. glabrata, C. parapsilosis, C. tropicalis, C. krusei, C. guillermondi, C. lusitaniae* | Esophageal candidiasis: 100 mg IV day 1, 50 mg/day thereafter.<br>Candidemia: 200 mg IV day 1, 100 mg/day thereafter |
| Flucytosine | Not effective for *C. krusei*<br>Effective for *C. albicans, C. tropicalis, C. parapsilosis, C. lusitaniae* | PO: 50-150 mg/kg/day divided qid |
| Nystatin | *C. albicans* | 100,000 U swish and swallow qid |
| Clotrimazole | Thrush (usually not cultured) | Oral troches daily for 14 days |

are not considered infected unless they satisfy one of these criteria.

Severe non-bloodstream candidal infections are defined as *Candida* spp. isolated from a normally sterile body site and the presence of at least one of the following: fever (>38.5° C [101.3° F]) or hypothermia (<36° C [96.8° F]); unexplained prolonged hypotension (systolic blood pressure <80 mm Hg for >2 hours, unresponsive to volume challenge); absence of response to adequate antibiotic treatment for a suspected bacterial infection. *Candida* spp. Pneumonia, which some authorities believe does not exist in immunocompetent hosts, requires the recovery of $>10^5$ CFU/mL of *Candida* spp. in BAL fluid, in addition to the appearance of a new infiltrate on CXR. Invasive fungal infections in non-neutropenic ICU patients are treated if histology or cytopathology shows yeast cells or pseudohyphae from a needle aspiration or biopsy (excluding mucous membranes), a positive culture obtained aseptically from a normally sterile and clinically or radiologically abnormal site consistent with infection (excluding urine, sinuses, and mucous membranes), or a positive percutaneous blood culture in patients with temporally related clinical signs and symptoms compatible with the relevant organism. Survival is more likely from candidemia than from other forms of invasive candidiasis, and is strongly influenced negatively by critical illness.[304]

The repertoire of antifungal agents has expanded with the introduction of less toxic formulations of amphotericin B, improved triazoles, echinocandins, and other agents that target the fungal cell wall.[305] Table 12-10 lists available antifungal agents. Amphotericin B is a natural polyene macrolide that binds primarily to ergosterol, the principal sterol in the fungal cell membrane, leading to disruption of ion channels, production of oxygen free radicals, and apoptosis. It is active against most fungi, including in cerebrospinal fluid. Because of its high level of protein binding, tissue concentrations are not usually affected by hemodialysis. Infusion-related reactions can occur in up to 73% of patients with the first dose and often diminish

**Table 12-11 Usual Susceptibilities of *Candida* Species to Selected Antifungal Agents**

| *CANDIDA* SPP. | FLUCONAZOLE | ITRACONAZOLE | VORICONAZOLE (NOT STANDARDIZED) | AMPHOTERICIN B | CASPOFUNGIN (NOT STANDARDIZED) |
|---|---|---|---|---|---|
| *C. albicans* | S | S | S | S | S |
| *C. tropicalis* | S | S | S | S | S |
| *C. parapsilosis* | S | S | S | S | S to I (?R) |
| *C. glabrata* | S-DD to R | S-DD to R | S to I | S to I | S |
| *C. krusei* | R | S-DD to R | S to I | S to I | S |
| *C. lusitaniae* | S | S | S | S to R | S |

*I,* Intermediate; *R,* resistant; *S,* susceptible; *S-DD,* susceptible dose-dependent (increased MIC may be overcome by higher dosing, such as 12 mg/kg/day fluconazole).

during continued therapy. Amphotericin B–associated nephrotoxicity can lead to azotemia and hypokalemia, although acute potassium release with rapid infusion can occur and lead to cardiac arrest. Amphotericin B lipid formulations allow for higher dose administration with lessened nephrotoxicity, but whether outcomes are enhanced is unproved. Nystatin is a polyene similar in structure to amphotericin B, and is currently used topically for *C. albicans.* Flucytosine is a fluorinated pyrimidine analogue that is converted to 5-fluorouracil, which causes RNA miscoding and inhibits DNA synthesis. It is available in the United States in oral form only and has been used with amphotericin B for synergism against *Candida* spp. But, in general, there is scant evidence that dual-agent therapy for fungal infections is beneficial.[306]

The azoles inhibit the cytochrome P450–dependent enzyme, 14-alpha reductase, altering fungal cell membranes through the accumulation of abnormal 14-alpha-methyl sterols. Ketoconazole is available only in tablet form and is indicated for candidiasis and candiduria. Fluconazole and itraconazole are available in oral and parenteral formulations and are active against *Candida* spp., except *C. krusei,* and *Fusarium* spp. Itraconazole is active against *Aspergillus* spp. As noted, *C. glabrata* and *C. krusei* resistance has been observed with fluconazole. The tissue concentration of both drugs is influenced by many agents such as antacids, $H_2$ antagonists, isoniazid, phenytoin, and phenobarbital. Biofilms produced by *Candida* spp. are penetrated by fluconazole and most other antifungal agents.[307,308]

Second-generation antifungal triazoles include posaconazole, ravuconazole, and voriconazole. They are active against *Candida* spp., including fluconazole-resistant strains, and *Aspergillus* spp. For the latter, voriconazole is emerging as the treatment of choice.[309,310]

The echinocandins include caspofungin, micafungin, and anidulafungin, each of which is approved therapy for candidiasis and candidemia but is third-line treatment for invasive aspergillosis.[311] Because of their distinct mechanism of action, disrupting the fungal cell wall by inhibiting (1 → 3)-β-D-glucan synthesis, the echinocandins can theoretically be used in combination with other standard antifungal agents.[306] The echinocandins have activity against *Candida* and *Aspergillus* spp., but are not reliably active against other fungi. Echinocandin activity is excellent against most *Candida* spp., but moderate against *C. parapsilosis, C. guillermondi,* and *C. lusitaniae.* Echinocandins exhibit no cross-resistance with azoles or polyenes.[312] Prospective randomized trials have demonstrated that micafungin is noninferior to caspofungin for therapy of invasive candidiasis[313] and as effective as liposomal amphotericin B.[314] Micafungin may be cost-effective in comparison to fluconazole therapy.

With the proliferation of non-*albicans Candida* infections caused by the widespread use of fluconazole, empirical therapy regimens recommend an echinocandin or lipid formulation of amphotericin B as the first-line agent for therapy of seriously or critically ill patients (see Box 12-14 and Table 12-10).[303,315] Once the pathogen has been identified as *Candida,* therapy may be de-escalated to fluconazole, except for *C. glabrata* and *C. krusei,* for which continuation therapy with an echinocandin may be indicated (Table 12-11).

## REFERENCES


1. Desborough JP: The stress response to trauma and surgery. Br J Anaesth 85:109–117, 2000.
2. Napolitano LM, Faist E, Wichmann MW, et al: Immune dysfunction in trauma. Surg Clin North Am 79:1385–1416, 1999.
3. Gardner EM, Murasko DM: Age-related changes in Type 1 and Type 2 cytokine production in humans. Biogerontology 3:271–290, 2002.
4. Latham R, Lancaster AD, Covington JF, et al: The association of diabetes and glucose control with surgical-site infections among cardiothoracic surgery patients. Infect Control Hosp Epidemiol 22:607–612, 2001.
5. Cheadle WG: Risk factors for surgical site infection. Surg Infect (Larchmt) 7(Suppl 1):S7–11, 2006.
6. Zerr KJ, Furnary AP, Grunkemeier GL, et al: Glucose control lowers the risk of wound infection in diabetics after open heart operations. Ann Thorac Surg 63:356–361, 1997.
7. Pomposelli JJ, Baxter JK, 3rd, Babineau TJ, et al: Early postoperative glucose control predicts nosocomial infection rate in diabetic patients. JPEN J Parenter Enteral Nutr 22:77–81, 1998.
8. Yendamuri S, Fulda GJ, Tinkoff GH: Admission hyperglycemia as a prognostic indicator in trauma. J Trauma 55:33–38, 2003.
9. Bochicchio GV, Bochicchio KM, Joshi M, et al: Acute glucose elevation is highly predictive of infection and outcome in critically injured trauma patients. Ann Surg 252:597–602, 2010.
10. Griesdale DE, de Souza RJ, van Dam RM, et al: Intensive insulin therapy and mortality among critically ill patients: A meta-analysis including NICE-SUGAR study data. CMAJ 180:821–827, 2009.
11. Eachempati SR, Hydo LJ, Shou J, et al: Implementation of tight glucose control for critically ill surgical patients: A process improvement analysis. Surg Infect (Larchmt) 10:523–531, 2009.

12. Wichmann MW, Zellweger R, DeMaso CM, et al: Enhanced immune responses in females, as opposed to decreased responses in males following haemorrhagic shock and resuscitation. Cytokine 8:853–863, 1996.
13. Diodato MD, Knoferl MW, Schwacha MG, et al: Gender differences in the inflammatory response and survival following haemorrhage and subsequent sepsis. Cytokine 14:162–169, 2001.
14. Gannon CJ, Napolitano LM, Pasquale M, et al: A statewide population-based study of gender differences in trauma: Validation of a prior single-institution study. J Am Coll Surg 195:11–18, 2002.
15. Angus DC, Linde-Zwirble WT, Lidicker J, et al: Epidemiology of severe sepsis in the United States: Analysis of incidence, outcome, and associated costs of care. Crit Care Med 29:1303–1310, 2001.
16. Laudanski K, Miller-Graziano C, Xiao W, et al: Cell-specific expression and pathway analyses reveal alterations in trauma-related human T cell and monocyte pathways. Proc Natl Acad Sci U S A 103:15564–15569, 2006.
17. Arcaroli J, Fessler MB, Abraham E: Genetic polymorphisms and sepsis. Shock 24:300–312, 2005.
18. Gunderson KL, Steemers FJ, Lee G, et al: A genome-wide scalable SNP genotyping assay using microarray technology. Nat Genet 37:549–554, 2005.
19. Machiedo GW, Powell RJ, Rush BF, Jr, et al: The incidence of decreased red blood cell deformability in sepsis and the association with oxygen free radical damage and multiple-system organ failure. Arch Surg 124:1386–1389, 1989.
20. Danks RR: Triangle of death. How hypothermia acidosis and coagulopathy can adversely impact trauma patients. JEMS 27:61–66, 68–70, 2002.
21. Dickinson A, Qadan M, Polk HC, Jr: Optimizing surgical care: A contemporary assessment of temperature, oxygen, and glucose. Am Surg 76:571–577, 2010.
22. Ives CL, Harrison DK, Stansby GS: Tissue oxygen saturation, measured by near-infrared spectroscopy, and its relationship to surgical-site infections. Br J Surg 94:87–91, 2007.
23. Cochrane Injuries Group Albumin Reviewers: Human albumin administration in critically ill patients: Systematic review of randomised controlled trials. BMJ 317:235–240, 1998.
24. Finfer S, Bellomo R, Boyce N, et al: A comparison of albumin and saline for fluid resuscitation in the intensive care unit. N Engl J Med 350:2247–2256, 2004.
25. Delaney AP, Dan A, McCaffrey J, et al: The role of albumin as a resuscitation fluid for patients with sepsis: A systematic review and meta-analysis. Crit Care Med 39:386–391, 2011.
26. Shafer SL: Notice of retraction. Anesth Analg 111:1567, 2010.
27. Bochicchio GV, Napolitano LM, Joshi M, et al: Persistent systemic inflammatory response syndrome is predictive of nosocomial infection in trauma. J Trauma 53:245–250, 2002.
28. Nathens AB, Nester TA, Rubenfeld GD, et al: The effects of leukoreduced blood transfusion on infection risk following injury: a randomized controlled trial. Shock 26:342–347, 2006.
29. Claridge JA, Sawyer RG, Schulman AM, et al: Blood transfusions correlate with infections in trauma patients in a dose-dependent manner. Am Surg 68:566–572, 2002.
30. Hill GE, Frawley WH, Griffith KE, et al: Allogeneic blood transfusion increases the risk of postoperative bacterial infection: a meta-analysis. J Trauma 54:908–914, 2003.
31. Taylor RW, O'Brien J, Trottier SJ, et al: Red blood cell transfusions and nosocomial infections in critically ill patients. Crit Care Med 34:2302–2308; quiz 2309, 2006.
32. Shorr AF, Jackson WL, Kelly KM, et al: Transfusion practice and bloodstream infections in critically ill patients. Chest 127:1722–1728, 2005.
33. Shorr AF, Duh MS, Kelly KM, et al: Red blood cell transfusion and ventilator-associated pneumonia: A potential link? Crit Care Med 32:666–674, 2004.
34. Scharte M, Fink MP: Red blood cell physiology in critical illness. Crit Care Med 31:S651–S657, 2003.
35. Fernandes CJ, Jr, Akamine N, De Marco FV, et al: Red blood cell transfusion does not increase oxygen consumption in critically ill septic patients. Crit Care 5:362–367, 2001.
36. Moore FA, Moore EE, Sauaia A: Blood transfusion. An independent risk factor for postinjury multiple organ failure. Arch Surg 132:620–624, 1997.
37. Offner PJ, Moore EE, Biffl WL, et al: Increased rate of infection associated with transfusion of old blood after severe injury. Arch Surg 137:711–716, 2002.
38. van den Berghe G, Wouters P, Weekers F, et al: Intensive insulin therapy in the critically ill patients. N Engl J Med 345:1359–1367, 2001.
39. Krinsley JS: Understanding glycemic control in the critically ill: 2011 update. Hosp Pract (Minneapolis) 39:47–55, 2011.
40. Heyland DK, MacDonald S, Keefe L, et al: Total parenteral nutrition in the critically ill patient: a meta-analysis. JAMA 280:2013–2019, 1998.
41. Marik PE, Zaloga GP: Early enteral nutrition in acutely ill patients: A systematic review. Crit Care Med 29:2264–2270, 2001.
42. Manian FA, Meyer PL, Setzer J, et al: Surgical site infections associated with methicillin-resistant Staphylococcus aureus: Do postoperative factors play a role? Clin Infect Dis 36:863–868, 2003.
43. Mangram AJ, Horan TC, Pearson ML, et al: Guideline for prevention of surgical site infection, 1999. Hospital Infection Control Practices Advisory Committee. Infect Control Hosp Epidemiol 20:250–278, 1999.
44. O'Grady NP, Alexander M, Burns LA, et al: Guidelines for the prevention of intravascular catheter-related infections. Clin Infect Dis 52:e162–e193, 2011.
45. Mermel LA, Allon M, Bouza E, et al: Clinical practice guidelines for the diagnosis and management of intravascular catheter-related infection: 2009 update by the Infectious Diseases Society of America. Clin Infect Dis 49:1–45, 2009.
46. Minei JP, Nathens AB, West M, et al: Inflammation and the host response to injury, a large-scale collaborative project: Patient-oriented research core–standard operating procedures for clinical care. II. Guidelines for prevention, diagnosis and treatment of ventilator-associated pneumonia (VAP) in the trauma patient. J Trauma 60:1106–1113, 2006.
47. American Thoracic Society; Infectious Diseases Society of America: Guidelines for the management of adults with hospital-acquired, ventilator-associated, and healthcare-associated pneumonia. Am J Respir Crit Care Med 171:388–416, 2005.
48. Erasmus V, Daha TJ, Brug H, et al: Systematic review of studies on compliance with hand hygiene guidelines in hospital care. Infect Control Hosp Epidemiol 31:283–294, 2010.
49. Prospero E, Barbadoro P, Esposto E, et al: Extended-spectrum beta-lactamases Klebsiella pneumoniae: Multimodal infection

control program in intensive care units. J Prev Med Hyg 51:110–115, 2010.

50. Oughton MT, Loo VG, Dendukuri N, et al: Hand hygiene with soap and water is superior to alcohol rub and antiseptic wipes for removal of Clostridium difficile. Infect Control Hosp Epidemiol 30:939–944, 2009.

51. Dancer SJ: The role of environmental cleaning in the control of hospital-acquired infection. J Hosp Infect 73:378–385, 2009.

52. Evans HL, Shaffer MM, Hughes MG, et al: Contact isolation in surgical patients: A barrier to care? Surgery 134:180–188, 2003.

53. Stone PW, Pogorzelska M, Kunches L, et al: Hospital staffing and health care–associated infections: A systematic review of the literature. Clin Infect Dis 47:937–944, 2008.

54. Cook DJ, Walter SD, Cook RJ, et al: Incidence of and risk factors for ventilator-associated pneumonia in critically ill patients. Ann Intern Med 129:433–440, 1998.

55. Harrington DT, Phillips B, Machan J, et al: Factors associated with survival following blunt chest trauma in older patients: Results from a large regional trauma cooperative. Arch Surg 145:432–437, 2010.

56. Milstone AM, Passaretti CL, Perl TM: Chlorhexidine: Expanding the armamentarium for infection control and prevention. Clin Infect Dis 46:274–281, 2008.

57. Darouiche RO, Wall MJ, Jr, Itani KM, et al: Chlorhexidine-alcohol versus povidone-iodine for surgical-site antisepsis. N Engl J Med 362:18–26, 2010.

58. Evans HL, Dellit TH, Chan J, et al: Effect of chlorhexidine whole-body bathing on hospital-acquired infections among trauma patients. Arch Surg 145:240–246, 2010.

59. Dixon JM, Carver RL: Daily chlorohexidine gluconate bathing with impregnated cloths results in statistically significant reduction in central line–associated bloodstream infections. Am J Infect Control 38:817–821, 2010.

60. Weber DJ, Rutala WA: Central line-associated bloodstream infections: Prevention and management. Infect Dis Clin North Am 25:77–102, 2011.

61. Bonello RS, Fletcher CE, Becker WK, et al: An intensive care unit quality improvement collaborative in nine Department of Veterans Affairs hospitals: Reducing ventilator-associated pneumonia and catheter-related bloodstream infection rates. Jt Comm J Qual Patient Saf 34:639–645, 2008.

62. Jain M, Miller L, Belt D, et al: Decline in ICU adverse events, nosocomial infections and cost through a quality improvement initiative focusing on teamwork and culture change. Qual Saf Health Care 15:235–239, 2006.

63. Muscedere J, Rewa O, McKechnie K, et al: Subglottic secretion drainage for the prevention of ventilator-associated pneumonia: A systematic review and meta-analysis. Crit Care Med 39:1985–1991, 2011.

64. Rello J, Kollef M, Diaz E, et al: Reduced burden of bacterial airway colonization with a novel silver-coated endotracheal tube in a randomized multiple-center feasibility study. Crit Care Med 34:2766–2772, 2006.

65. Afessa B, Shorr AF, Anzueto AR, et al: Association between a silver-coated endotracheal tube and reduced mortality in patients with ventilator-associated pneumonia. Chest 137:1015–1021, 2010.

66. Hanna HA, Raad II, Hackett B, et al: Antibiotic-impregnated catheters associated with significant decrease in nosocomial and multidrug-resistant bacteremias in critically ill patients. Chest 124:1030–1038, 2003.

67. Beattie M, Taylor J: Silver alloy versusuncoated urinary catheters: A systematic review of the literature. J Clin Nurs 2011.

68. Johnson JR, Kuskowski MA, Wilt TJ: Systematic review: Antimicrobial urinary catheters to prevent catheter-associated urinary tract infection in hospitalized patients. Ann Intern Med 144:116–126, 2006.

69. Ely EW, Baker AM, Dunagan DP, et al: Effect on the duration of mechanical ventilation of identifying patients capable of breathing spontaneously. N Engl J Med 335:1864–1869, 1996.

70. Esteban A, Frutos-Vivar F, Ferguson ND, et al: Noninvasive positive-pressure ventilation for respiratory failure after extubation. N Engl J Med 350:2452–2460, 2004.

71. Shah MR, Hasselblad V, Stevenson LW, et al: Impact of the pulmonary artery catheter in critically ill patients: Meta-analysis of randomized clinical trials. JAMA 294:1664–1670, 2005.

72. Barie PS: Surgical site infections: Epidemiology and prevention. Surg Infect (Larchmt) 3(Suppl 1):S9–21, 2002.

73. National Nosocomial Infections Surveillance (NNIS) System Report, Data Summary from January 1992-June 2001, issued August 2001. Am J Infect Control 29:404–421, 2001.

74. National Nosocomial Infections Surveillance (NNIS) System Report, data summary from January 1992 through June 2004, issued October 2004. Am J Infect Control 32:470–485, 2004.

75. Edwards JR, Peterson KD, Mu Y, et al: National Healthcare Safety Network (NHSN) report: Data summary for 2006 through 2008, issued December 2009. Am J Infect Control 37:783–805, 2009.

76. Garibaldi RA, Cushing D, Lerer T: Risk factors for postoperative infection. Am J Med 91:158S–163S, 1991.

77. Raymond DP, Pelletier SJ, Crabtree TD, et al: Surgical infection and the aging population. Am Surg 67:827–832, 2001.

78. Delgado-Rodriguez M, Medina-Cuadros M, Martinez-Gallego G, et al: Total cholesterol, HDL-cholesterol, and risk of nosocomial infection: A prospective study in surgical patients. Infect Control Hosp Epidemiol 18:9–18, 1997.

79. Malone DL, Genuit T, Tracy JK, et al: Surgical site infections: Reanalysis of risk factors. J Surg Res 103:89–95, 2002.

80. Scott JD, Forrest A, Feuerstein S, et al: Factors associated with postoperative infection. Infect Control Hosp Epidemiol 22:347–351, 2001.

81. Hedrick TL, Heckman JA, Smith RL, et al: Efficacy of protocol implementation on incidence of wound infection in colorectal operations. J Am Coll Surg 205:432–438, 2007.

82. Kurz A, Sessler DI, Lenhardt R: Perioperative normothermia to reduce the incidence of surgical-wound infection and shorten hospitalization. Study of Wound Infection and Temperature Group. N Engl J Med 334:1209–1215, 1996.

83. Flores-Maldonado A, Medina-Escobedo CE, Rios-Rodriguez HM, et al: Mild perioperative hypothermia and the risk of wound infection. Arch Med Res 32:227–231, 2001.

84. Brar MS, Brar SS, Dixon E: Perioperative supplemental oxygen in colorectal patients: A meta-analysis. J Surg Res 166:227–235, 2011.

85. Knighton DR, Halliday B, Hunt TK: Oxygen as an antibiotic. A comparison of the effects of inspired oxygen concentration and antibiotic administration on in vivo bacterial clearance. Arch Surg 121:191–195, 1986.

86. Gottrup F: Oxygen in wound healing and infection. World J Surg 28:312–315, 2004.

87. Greif R, Akca O, Horn EP, et al: Supplemental perioperative oxygen to reduce the incidence of surgical-wound infection. N Engl J Med 342:161–167, 2000.
88. Pryor KO, Fahey TJ, 3rd, Lien CA, et al: Surgical site infection and the routine use of perioperative hyperoxia in a general surgical population: A randomized controlled trial. JAMA 291:79–87, 2004.
89. Miller RS, Morris JA, Jr, Diaz JJ, Jr, et al: Complications after 344 damage-control open celiotomies. J Trauma 59:1365–1371, 2005.
90. Vogel TR, Diaz JJ, Miller RS, et al: The open abdomen in trauma: Do infectious complications affect primary abdominal closure? Surg Infect (Larchmt) 7:433–441, 2006.
91. Al-Inany H, Youssef G, Abd ElMaguid A, et al: Value of subcutaneous drainage system in obese females undergoing cesarean section using Pfannenstiel incision. Gynecol Obstet Invest 53:75–78, 2002.
92. Magann EF, Chauhan SP, Rodts-Palenik S, et al: Subcutaneous stitch closure versus subcutaneous drain to prevent wound disruption after cesarean delivery: A randomized clinical trial. Am J Obstet Gynecol 186:1119–1123, 2002.
93. Siegman-Igra Y, Rozin R, Simchen E: Determinants of wound infection in gastrointestinal operations: The Israeli study of surgical infections. J Clin Epidemiol 46:133–140, 1993.
94. Noyes LD, Doyle DJ, McSwain NE, Jr: Septic complications associated with the use of peritoneal drains in liver trauma. J Trauma 28:337–346, 1988.
95. Magee C, Rodeheaver GT, Golden GT, et al: Potentiation of wound infection by surgical drains. Am J Surg 131:547–549, 1976.
96. Vilar-Compte D, Mohar A, Sandoval S, et al: Surgical site infections at the National Cancer Institute in Mexico: A case-control study. Am J Infect Control 28:14–20, 2000.
97. Barie PS: Are we draining the life from our patients? Surg Infect (Larchmt) 3:159–160, 2002.
98. Platell C, Papadimitriou JM, Hall JC: The influence of lavage on peritonitis. J Am Coll Surg 191:672–680, 2000.
99. Cervantes-Sanchez CR, Gutierrez-Vega R, Vazquez-Carpizo JA, et al: Syringe pressure irrigation of subdermic tissue after appendectomy to decrease the incidence of postoperative wound infection. World J Surg 24:38–41, 2000.
100. Andersen B, Bendtsen A, Holbraad L, et al: Wound infections after appendicectomy. I. A controlled trial on the prophylactic efficacy of topical ampicillin in non-perforated appendicitis. II. A controlled trial on the prophylactic efficacy of delayed primary suture and topical ampicillin in perforated appendicitis. Acta Chir Scand 138:531–536, 1972.
101. Yoshii S, Hosaka S, Suzuki S, et al: Prevention of surgical site infection by antibiotic spraying in the operative field during cardiac surgery. Jpn J Thorac Cardiovasc Surg 49:279–281, 2001.
102. O'Connor LT, Jr, Goldstein M: Topical perioperative antibiotic prophylaxis for minor clean inguinal surgery. J Am Coll Surg 194:407–410, 2002.
103. Freischlag JA, Ajalat G, Busuttil RW: Treatment of necrotizing soft tissue infections. The need for a new approach. Am J Surg 149:751–755, 1985.
104. Turina M, Cheadle WG: Management of established surgical site infections. Surg Infect (Larchmt) 7:S33–S41, 2006.
105. Morykwas MJ, Argenta LC, Shelton-Brown EI, et al: Vacuum-assisted closure: A new method for wound control and treatment: animal studies and basic foundation. Ann Plast Surg 38:553–562, 1997.
106. Venturi ML, Attinger CE, Mesbahi AN, et al: Mechanisms and clinical applications of the vacuum-assisted closure (VAC) Device: a review. Am J Clin Dermatol 6:185–194, 2005.
107. Heller L, Levin SL, Butler CE: Management of abdominal wound dehiscence using vacuum-assisted closure in patients with compromised healing. Am J Surg 191:165–172, 2006.
108. Schaffzin DM, Douglas JM, Stahl TJ, et al: Vacuum-assisted closure of complex perineal wounds. Dis Colon Rectum 47:1745–1748, 2004.
109. Stulberg JJ, Delaney CP, Neuhauser DV, et al: Adherence to surgical care improvement project measures and the association with postoperative infections. JAMA 303:2479–2485, 2010.
110. Ingraham AM, Cohen ME, Bilimoria KY, et al: Association of surgical care improvement project infection-related process measure compliance with risk-adjusted outcomes: Implications for quality measurement. J Am Coll Surg 211:705–714, 2010.
111. Bratzler DW, Houck PM, Richards C, et al: Use of antimicrobial prophylaxis for major surgery: Baseline results from the National Surgical Infection Prevention Project. Arch Surg 140:174–182, 2005.
112. Bratzler DW, Houck PM: Antimicrobial prophylaxis for surgery: An advisory statement from the National Surgical Infection Prevention Project. Am J Surg 189:395–404, 2005.
113. Dellinger EP, Hausmann SM, Bratzler DW, et al: Hospitals collaborate to decrease surgical site infections. Am J Surg 190:9–15, 2005.
114. Barie PS: No pay for no performance. Surg Infect (Larchmt) 8:421–433, 2007.
115. Dellinger EP: Adherence to Surgical Care Improvement Project measures: The whole is greater than the parts. Future Microbiol 5:1781–1785, 2010.
116. Lee JT: Nonmagical tools. Infect Control Hosp Epidemiol 24:769–771, 2003.
117. Kollef MH, Shorr A, Tabak YP, et al: Epidemiology and outcomes of health-care-associated pneumonia: Results from a large US database of culture-positive pneumonia. Chest 128:3854–3862, 2005.
118. Rello J, Ollendorf DA, Oster G, et al: Epidemiology and outcomes of ventilator-associated pneumonia in a large U.S. database. Chest 122:2115–2121, 2002.
119. Fagon JY, Chastre J, Wolff M, et al: Invasive and noninvasive strategies for management of suspected ventilator-associated pneumonia. A randomized trial. Ann Intern Med 132:621–630, 2000.
120. Safdar N, Dezfulian C, Collard HR, et al: Clinical and economic consequences of ventilator-associated pneumonia: a systematic review. Crit Care Med 33:2184–2193, 2005.
121. Celis R, Torres A, Gatell JM, et al: Nosocomial pneumonia. A multivariate analysis of risk and prognosis. Chest 93:318–324, 1988.
122. Torres A, Aznar R, Gatell JM, et al: Incidence, risk, and prognosis factors of nosocomial pneumonia in mechanically ventilated patients. Am Rev Respir Dis 142:523–528, 1990.
123. Markowicz P, Wolff M, Djedaini K, et al: Multicenter prospective study of ventilator-associated pneumonia during acute respiratory distress syndrome. Incidence, prognosis, and risk factors. ARDS Study Group. Am J Respir Crit Care Med 161:1942–1948, 2000.

124. Pieracci FM, Barie PS: Strategies in the prevention and management of ventilator-associated pneumonia. Am Surg 73:419–432, 2007.
125. Antonelli M, Conti G, Rocco M, et al: A comparison of noninvasive positive-pressure ventilation and conventional mechanical ventilation in patients with acute respiratory failure. N Engl J Med 339:429–435, 1998.
126. Holzapfel L, Chevret S, Madinier G, et al: Influence of long-term oro- or nasotracheal intubation on nosocomial maxillary sinusitis and pneumonia: Results of a prospective, randomized, clinical trial. Crit Care Med 21:1132–1138, 1993.
127. Kress JP, Pohlman AS, O'Connor MF, et al: Daily interruption of sedative infusions in critically ill patients undergoing mechanical ventilation. N Engl J Med 342:1471–1477, 2000.
128. Marelich GP, Murin S, Battistella F, et al: Protocol weaning of mechanical ventilation in medical and surgical patients by respiratory care practitioners and nurses: Effect on weaning time and incidence of ventilator-associated pneumonia. Chest 118:459–467, 2000.
129. Zanella A, Scaravilli V, Isgro S, et al: Fluid leakage across tracheal tube cuff, effect of different cuff material, shape, and positive expiratory pressure: A bench-top study. Intensive Care Med 37:343–347, 2011.
130. Drakulovic MB, Torres A, Bauer TT, et al: Supine body position as a risk factor for nosocomial pneumonia in mechanically ventilated patients: A randomised trial. Lancet 354:1851–1858, 1999.
131. Heyland DK, Dhaliwal R, Drover JW, et al: Canadian clinical practice guidelines for nutrition support in mechanically ventilated, critically ill adult patients. JPEN J Parenter Enteral Nutr 27:355–373, 2003.
132. Berne JD, Norwood SH, McAuley CE, et al: Erythromycin reduces delayed gastric emptying in critically ill trauma patients: A randomized, controlled trial. J Trauma 53:422–425, 2002.
133. van Nieuwenhoven CA, Buskens E, van Tiel FH, et al: Relationship between methodological trial quality and the effects of selective digestive decontamination on pneumonia and mortality in critically ill patients. JAMA 286:335–340, 2001.
134. Verwaest C, Verhaegen J, Ferdinande P, et al: Randomized, controlled trial of selective digestive decontamination in 600 mechanically ventilated patients in a multidisciplinary intensive care unit. Crit Care Med 25:63–71, 1997.
135. Lingnau W, Berger J, Javorsky F, et al: Changing bacterial ecology during a five-year period of selective intestinal decontamination. J Hosp Infect 39:195–206, 1998.
136. Chlebicki MP, Safdar N: Topical chlorhexidine for prevention of ventilator-associated pneumonia: A meta-analysis. Crit Care Med 35:595–602, 2007.
137. Earley AS, Gracias VH, Haut E, et al: Anemia management program reduces transfusion volumes, incidence of ventilator-associated pneumonia, and cost in trauma patients. J Trauma 61:1–5, 2006.
138. Sawyer RG, Crabtree TD, Gleason TG, et al: Impact of solid organ transplantation and immunosuppression on fever, leukocytosis, and physiologic response during bacterial and fungal infections. Clin Transplant 13:260–265, 1999.
139. Neuhauser MM, Weinstein RA, Rydman R, et al: Antibiotic resistance among gram-negative bacilli in US intensive care units: Implications for fluoroquinolone use. JAMA 289:885–888, 2003.
140. Niederman MS: Appropriate use of antimicrobial agents: Challenges and strategies for improvement. Crit Care Med 31:608–616, 2003.
141. Alvarez-Lerma F: Modification of empirical antibiotic treatment in patients with pneumonia acquired in the intensive care unit. ICU-Acquired Pneumonia Study Group. Intensive Care Med 22:387–394, 1996.
142. Fabregas N, Ewig S, Torres A, et al: Clinical diagnosis of ventilator associated pneumonia revisited: Comparative validation using immediate post-mortem lung biopsies. Thorax 54:867–873, 1999.
143. Mabie M, Wunderink RG: Use and limitations of clinical and radiologic diagnosis of pneumonia. Semin Respir Infect 18:72–79, 2003.
144. Fagon JY, Chastre J, Domart Y, et al: Nosocomial pneumonia in patients receiving continuous mechanical ventilation. Prospective analysis of 52 episodes with use of a protected specimen brush and quantitative culture techniques. Am Rev Respir Dis 139:877–884, 1989.
145. Winer-Muram HT, Steiner RM, Gurney JW, et al: Ventilator-associated pneumonia in patients with adult respiratory distress syndrome: CT evaluation. Radiology 208:193–199, 1998.
146. Fartoukh M, Maitre B, Honore S, et al: Diagnosing pneumonia during mechanical ventilation: The clinical pulmonary infection score revisited. Am J Respir Crit Care Med 168:173–179, 2003.
147. Luyt CE, Chastre J, Fagon JY: Value of the clinical pulmonary infection score for the identification and management of ventilator-associated pneumonia. Intensive Care Med 30:844–852, 2004.
148. Veinstein A, Brun-Buisson C, Derrode N, et al: Validation of an algorithm based on direct examination of specimens in suspected ventilator-associated pneumonia. Intensive Care Med 32:676–683, 2006.
149. Croce MA, Swanson JM, Magnotti LJ, et al: The futility of the clinical pulmonary infection score in trauma patients. J Trauma 60:523–527, 2006.
150. Blot F, Raynard B, Chachaty E, et al: Value of gram stain examination of lower respiratory tract secretions for early diagnosis of nosocomial pneumonia. Am J Respir Crit Care Med 162:1731–1737, 2000.
151. Torres A, El-Ebiary M: Bronchoscopic BAL in the diagnosis of ventilator-associated pneumonia. Chest 117:198S-202S, 2000.
152. Shorr AF, Sherner JH, Jackson WL, et al: Invasive approaches to the diagnosis of ventilator-associated pneumonia: a meta-analysis. Crit Care Med 33:46–53, 2005.
153. McGee DC, Gould MK: Preventing complications of central venous catheterization. N Engl J Med 348:1123–1133, 2003.
154. Pronovost P: Interventions to decrease catheter-related bloodstream infections in the ICU: The Keystone Intensive Care Unit Project. Am J Infect Control 36:S171 e171–e175, 2008.
155. Pronovost PJ, Goeschel CA, Colantuoni E, et al: Sustaining reductions in catheter related bloodstream infections in Michigan intensive care units: Observational study. BMJ 340:c309, 2010.
156. Furuya EY, Dick A, Perencevich EN, et al: Central line bundle implementation in US intensive care units and impact on bloodstream infections. PLoS One 6:e15452, 2011.
157. Miller RS, Norris PR, Jenkins JM, et al: Systems initiatives reduce healthcare-associated infections: A study of 22,928 device days in a single trauma unit. J Trauma 68:23–31, 2010.

158. Clinical and Laboratory Standards Institute: Principles and procedures for blood cultures; approved guideline, 2007 (http://www.clsi.org/source/orders/free/m47-a.pdf).
159. Mermel LA, Farr BM, Sherertz RJ, et al: Guidelines for the management of intravascular catheter-related infections. Clin Infect Dis 32:1249–1272, 2001.
160. Tambyah PA, Maki DG: Catheter-associated urinary tract infection is rarely symptomatic: A prospective study of 1,497 catheterized patients. Arch Intern Med 160:678–682, 2000.
161. Golob JF, Jr, Claridge JA, Sando MJ, et al: Fever and leukocytosis in critically ill trauma patients: It's not the urine. Surg Infect (Larchmt) 9:49–56, 2008.
162. Safdar N, Slattery WR, Knasinski V, et al: Predictors and outcomes of candiduria in renal transplant recipients. Clin Infect Dis 40:1413–1421, 2005.
163. Bryan CS, Reynolds KL: Hospital-acquired bacteremic urinary tract infection: Epidemiology and outcome. J Urol 132:494–498, 1984.
164. Quintiliani R, Klimek J, Cunha BA, et al: Bacteraemia after manipulation of the urinary tract. The importance of pre-existing urinary tract disease and compromised host defences. Postgrad Med J 54:668–671, 1978.
165. Ksycki MF, Namias N: Nosocomial urinary tract infection. Surg Clin North Am 89:475–481, ix–x, 2009.
166. Laupland KB, Bagshaw SM, Gregson DB, et al: Intensive care unit-acquired urinary tract infections in a regional critical care system. Crit Care 9:R60–65, 2005.
167. Schwartz DS, Barone JE: Correlation of urinalysis and dipstick results with catheter-associated urinary tract infections in surgical ICU patients. Intensive Care Med 32:1797–1801, 2006.
168. Schiotz HA: The value of leucocyte stix results in predicting bacteriuria and urinary tract infection after gynaecological surgery. J Obstet Gynaecol 19:396–398, 1999.
169. Solomkin JS, Hemsell DL, Sweet R, et al: Evaluation of new anti-infective drugs for the treatment of intra-abdominal infections. Infectious Diseases Society of America and the Food and Drug Administration. Clin Infect Dis 15(Suppl 1):S33–S42, 1992.
170. Merlino JI, Yowler CJ, Malangoni MA: Nosocomial infections adversely affect the outcomes of patients with serious intraabdominal infections. Surg Infect (Larchmt) 5:21–27, 2004.
171. Nathens AB, Rotstein OD, Marshall JC: Tertiary peritonitis: Clinical features of a complex nosocomial infection. World J Surg 22:158–163, 1998.
172. Pacelli F, Doglietto GB, Alfieri S, et al: Prognosis in intra-abdominal infections. Multivariate analysis on 604 patients. Arch Surg 131:641–645, 1996.
173. Roehrborn A, Thomas L, Potreck O, et al: The microbiology of postoperative peritonitis. Clin Infect Dis 33:1513–1519, 2001.
174. Sturkenboom MC, Goettsch WG, Picelli G, et al: Inappropriate initial treatment of secondary intra-abdominal infections leads to increased risk of clinical failure and costs. Br J Clin Pharmacol 60:438–443, 2005.
175. Montravers P, Gauzit R, Muller C, et al: Emergence of antibiotic-resistant bacteria in cases of peritonitis after intra-abdominal surgery affects the efficacy of empirical antimicrobial therapy. Clin Infect Dis 23:486–494, 1996.
176. Barie PS, Hydo LJ, Shou J, et al: Efficacy and safety of drotrecogin alfa (activated) for the therapy of surgical patients with severe sepsis. Surg Infect (Larchmt) 7(Suppl 2):S77–S80, 2006.
177. Barie PS, Vogel SB, Dellinger EP, et al: A randomized, double-blind clinical trial comparing cefepime plus metronidazole with imipenem-cilastatin in the treatment of complicated intra-abdominal infections. Cefepime Intra-abdominal Infection Study Group. Arch Surg 132:1294–1302, 1997.
178. Farthmann EH, Schoffel U: Principles and limitations of operative management of intraabdominal infections. World J Surg 14:210–217, 1990.
179. Garcia-Sabrido JL, Tallado JM, Christou NV, et al: Treatment of severe intra-abdominal sepsis and/or necrotic foci by an 'open-abdomen' approach. Zipper and zipper-mesh techniques. Arch Surg 123:152–156, 1988.
180. Marshall JC, Maier RV, Jimenez M, et al: Source control in the management of severe sepsis and septic shock: an evidence-based review. Crit Care Med 32:S513–S526, 2004.
181. Wittmann DH, Aprahamian C, Bergstein JM: Etappenlavage: Advanced diffuse peritonitis managed by planned multiple laparotomies utilizing zippers, slide fastener, and Velcro analogue for temporary abdominal closure. World J Surg 14:218–226, 1990.
182. Ohmann C, Wittmann DH, Wacha H: Prospective evaluation of prognostic scoring systems in peritonitis. Peritonitis Study Group. Eur J Surg 159:267–274, 1993.
183. Gajic O, Urrutia LE, Sewani H, et al: Acute abdomen in the medical intensive care unit. Crit Care Med 30:1187–1190, 2002.
184. DiPiro JT, Edmiston CE, Jr, Bohnen JM: Pharmacodynamics of antimicrobial therapy in surgery. Am J Surg 171:615–622, 1996.
185. Anstead GM, Owens AD: Recent advances in the treatment of infections due to resistant Staphylococcus aureus. Curr Opin Infect Dis 17:549–555, 2004.
186. Kashuba AD, Bertino JS, Jr, Nafziger AN: Dosing of aminoglycosides to rapidly attain pharmacodynamic goals and hasten therapeutic response by using individualized pharmacokinetic monitoring of patients with pneumonia caused by gram-negative organisms. Antimicrob Agents Chemother 42:1842–1844, 1998.
187. Thomas JK, Forrest A, Bhavnani SM, et al: Pharmacodynamic evaluation of factors associated with the development of bacterial resistance in acutely ill patients during therapy. Antimicrob Agents Chemother 42:521–527, 1998.
188. Benko AS, Cappelletty DM, Kruse JA, et al: Continuous infusion versus intermittent administration of ceftazidime in critically ill patients with suspected gram-negative infections. Antimicrob Agents Chemother 40:691–695, 1996.
189. Lau WK, Mercer D, Itani KM, et al: Randomized, open-label, comparative study of piperacillin-tazobactam administered by continuous infusion versus intermittent infusion for treatment of hospitalized patients with complicated intra-abdominal infection. Antimicrob Agents Chemother 50:3556–3561, 2006.
190. Velmahos GC, Toutouzas KG, Sarkisyan G, et al: Severe trauma is not an excuse for prolonged antibiotic prophylaxis. Arch Surg 137:537–541, 2002.
191. Al-Ghnaniem R, Benjamin IS, Patel AG: Meta-analysis suggests antibiotic prophylaxis is not warranted in low-risk patients undergoing laparoscopic cholecystectomy. Br J Surg 90:365–366, 2003.
192. Lewis RT: Oral versus systemic antibiotic prophylaxis in elective colon surgery: A randomized study and meta-analysis send a message from the 1990s. Can J Surg 45:173–180, 2002.
193. Centers for Medicare & Medicaid Services: Anticipated public reporting of National Hospital Quality Measure SIP-2 (SCIP

Infection 2), appropriate antibiotic selection for surgical prophylaxis, 2006, (http://www.cms.hhs.gov/HospitalQualityInits/Downloads/HospitalSDPSMemoRandum.pdf).

194. Song F, Glenny AM: Antimicrobial prophylaxis in colorectal surgery: A systematic review of randomized controlled trials. Br J Surg 85:1232–1241, 1998.

195. Tejirian T, DiFronzo LA, Haigh PI: Antibiotic prophylaxis for preventing wound infection after breast surgery: A systematic review and meta-analysis. J Am Coll Surg 203:729–734, 2006.

196. Cunningham M, Bunn F, Handscomb K: Prophylactic antibiotics to prevent surgical site infection after breast cancer surgery. Cochrane Database Syst Rev (2):CD005360, 2006.

197. Aufenacker TJ, Koelemay MJ, Gouma DJ, et al: Systematic review and meta-analysis of the effectiveness of antibiotic prophylaxis in prevention of wound infection after mesh repair of abdominal wall hernia. Br J Surg 93:5–10, 2006.

198. Sanchez-Manuel FJ, Seco-Gil JL: Antibiotic prophylaxis for hernia repair. Cochrane Database Syst Rev (4):CD003769, 2004.

199. Stewart A, Eyers PS, Earnshaw JJ: Prevention of infection in arterial reconstruction. Cochrane Database Syst Rev (3): CD003073, 2006.

200. Classen DC, Evans RS, Pestotnik SL, et al: The timing of prophylactic administration of antibiotics and the risk of surgical-wound infection. N Engl J Med 326:281–286, 1992.

201. Hawn MT, Gray SH, Vick CC, et al: Timely administration of prophylactic antibiotics for major surgical procedures. J Am Coll Surg 203:803–811, 2006.

202. Zanetti G, Giardina R, Platt R: Intraoperative redosing of cefazolin and risk for surgical site infection in cardiac surgery. Emerg Infect Dis 7:828–831, 2001.

203. McDonald M, Grabsch E, Marshall C, et al: Single- versus multiple-dose antimicrobial prophylaxis for major surgery: A systematic review. Aust N Z J Surg 68:388–396, 1998.

204. Namias N, Harvill S, Ball S, et al: Cost and morbidity associated with antibiotic prophylaxis in the ICU. J Am Coll Surg 188:225–230, 1999.

205. Fukatsu K, Saito H, Matsuda T, et al: Influences of type and duration of antimicrobial prophylaxis on an outbreak of methicillin-resistant Staphylococcus aureus and on the incidence of wound infection. Arch Surg 132:1320–1325, 1997.

206. Barie PS, Hydo LJ, Eachempati SR: Causes and consequences of fever complicating critical surgical illness. Surg Infect (Larchmt) 5:145–159, 2004.

207. O'Grady NP, Barie PS, Bartlett JG, et al: Guidelines for evaluation of new fever in critically ill adult patients: 2008 update from the American College of Critical Care Medicine and the Infectious Diseases Society of America. Crit Care Med 36:1330–1349, 2008.

208. Caroff SN, Mann SC: Neuroleptic malignant syndrome and malignant hyperthermia. Anaesth Intensive Care 21:477–478, 1993.

209. Trautner BW, Clarridge JE, Darouiche RO: Skin antisepsis kits containing alcohol and chlorhexidine gluconate or tincture of iodine are associated with low rates of blood culture contamination. Infect Control Hosp Epidemiol 23:397–401, 2002.

210. Cockerill FR, 3rd, Wilson JW, Vetter EA, et al: Optimal testing parameters for blood cultures. Clin Infect Dis 38:1724–1730, 2004.

211. Mermel LA, Maki DG: Detection of bacteremia in adults: Consequences of culturing an inadequate volume of blood. Ann Intern Med 119:270–272, 1993.

212. Kumar A, Roberts D, Wood KE, et al: Duration of hypotension before initiation of effective antimicrobial therapy is the critical determinant of survival in human septic shock. Crit Care Med 34:1589–1596, 2006.

213. Barie PS, Hydo LJ, Shou J, et al: Influence of antibiotic therapy on mortality of critical surgical illness caused or complicated by infection. Surg Infect (Larchmt) 6:41–54, 2005.

214. Kollef MH, Ward S, Sherman G, et al: Inadequate treatment of nosocomial infections is associated with certain empirical antibiotic choices. Crit Care Med 28:3456–3464, 2000.

215. Garnacho-Montero J, Garcia-Garmendia JL, Barrero-Almodovar A, et al: Impact of adequate empirical antibiotic therapy on the outcome of patients admitted to the intensive care unit with sepsis. Crit Care Med 31:2742–2751, 2003.

216. Dellit TH, Owens RC, McGowan JE, Jr, et al: Infectious Diseases Society of America and the Society for Healthcare Epidemiology of America guidelines for developing an institutional program to enhance antimicrobial stewardship. Clin Infect Dis 44:159–177, 2007.

217. Kollef MH, Micek ST: Strategies to prevent antimicrobial resistance in the intensive care unit. Crit Care Med 33:1845–1853, 2005.

218. Hayashi Y, Paterson DL: Strategies for reduction in duration of antibiotic use in hospitalized patients. Clin Infect Dis 52:1232–1240, 2011.

219. Giamarellou H: Treatment options for multidrug-resistant bacteria. Expert Rev Anti Infect Ther 4:601–618, 2006.

220. Aarts MA, Hancock JN, Heyland D, et al: Empiric antibiotic therapy for suspected ventilator-associated pneumonia: A systematic review and meta-analysis of randomized trials. Crit Care Med 36:108–117, 2008.

221. Paul M, Benuri-Silbiger I, Soares-Weiser K, et al: Beta lactam monotherapy versus beta lactam-aminoglycoside combination therapy for sepsis in immunocompetent patients: Systematic review and meta-analysis of randomised trials. BMJ 328:668, 2004.

222. Kumar A, Zarychanski R, Light B, et al: Early combination antibiotic therapy yields improved survival compared with monotherapy in septic shock: A propensity-matched analysis. Crit Care Med 38:1773–1785, 2010.

223. Solomkin JS, Mazuski JE, Bradley JS, et al: Diagnosis and management of complicated intra-abdominal infection in adults and children: Guidelines by the Surgical Infection Society and the Infectious Diseases Society of America. Surg Infect (Larchmt) 11:79–109, 2010.

224. Kollef MH, Kollef KE: Antibiotic utilization and outcomes for patients with clinically suspected ventilator-associated pneumonia and negative quantitative BAL culture results. Chest 128:2706–2713, 2005.

225. Eachempati SR, Hydo LJ, Shou J, et al: The pathogen of ventilator-associated pneumonia does not influence the mortality rate of surgical intensive care unit patients treated with a rotational antibiotic system. Surg Infect (Larchmt) 11:13–20, 2010.

226. Dennesen PJ, van der Ven AJ, Kessels AG, et al: Resolution of infectious parameters after antimicrobial therapy in patients with ventilator-associated pneumonia. Am J Respir Crit Care Med 163:1371–1375, 2001.

**227.** Chastre J, Wolff M, Fagon JY, et al: Comparison of 8 vs 15 days of antibiotic therapy for ventilator-associated pneumonia in adults: a randomized trial. JAMA 290:2588–2598, 2003.

**228.** Singh N, Rogers P, Atwood CW, et al: Short-course empirical antibiotic therapy for patients with pulmonary infiltrates in the intensive care unit. A proposed solution for indiscriminate antibiotic prescription. Am J Respir Crit Care Med 162:505–511, 2000.

**229.** Pappas PG, Rex JH, Sobel JD, et al: Guidelines for treatment of candidiasis. Clin Infect Dis 38:161–189, 2004.

**229a.** O'Grady NP, Chertow DS: Managing bloodstream infections in patients who have short-term central venous catheters. Cleve Clin J Med 78(1):10–17, 2011.

**230.** Pieracci FM, Barie PS: Intra-abdominal infections. Curr Opin Crit Care 13:440–449, 2007.

**231.** Buijk SE, Bruining HA: Future directions in the management of tertiary peritonitis. Intensive Care Med 28:1024–1029, 2002.

**232.** Pepin J, Saheb N, Coulombe MA, et al: Emergence of fluoroquinolones as the predominant risk factor for Clostridium difficile-associated diarrhea: A cohort study during an epidemic in Quebec. Clin Infect Dis 41:1254–1260, 2005.

**233.** Price J, Cheek E, Lippett S, et al: Impact of an intervention to control Clostridium difficile infection on hospital- and community-onset disease: An interrupted time series analysis. Clin Microbiol Infect 16:1297–1302, 2010.

**234.** Louie TJ, Miller MA, Mullane KM, et al: Fidaxomicin versus vancomycin for Clostridium difficile infection. N Engl J Med 364:422–431, 2011.

**235.** Lamontagne F, Labbe AC, Haeck O, et al: Impact of emergency colectomy on survival of patients with fulminant Clostridium difficile colitis during an epidemic caused by a hypervirulent strain. Ann Surg 245:267–272, 2007.

**236.** McDonald LC, Killgore GE, Thompson A, et al: An epidemic, toxin gene-variant strain of Clostridium difficile. N Engl J Med 353:2433–2441, 2005.

**237.** May AK, Stafford RE, Bulger EM, et al: Treatment of complicated skin and soft tissue infections. Surg Infect (Larchmt) 10:467–499, 2009.

**238.** Kaushik D, Rathi S, Jain A: Ceftaroline: a comprehensive update. Int J Antimicrob Agents 37:389–395, 2011.

**239.** Rodloff AC, Goldstein EJ, Torres A: Two decades of imipenem therapy. J Antimicrob Chemother 58:916–929, 2006.

**240.** Zhanel GG, Johanson C, Embil JM, et al: Ertapenem: Review of a new carbapenem. Expert Rev Anti Infect Ther 3:23–39, 2005.

**241.** Liu C, Bayer A, Cosgrove SE, et al: Clinical practice guidelines by the Infectious Diseases Society of America for the treatment of methicillin-resistant Staphylococcus aureus infections in adults and children: Executive summary. Clin Infect Dis 52:285–292, 2011.

**242.** Rybak MJ, Lomaestro BM, Rotschafer JC, et al: Vancomycin therapeutic guidelines: A summary of consensus recommendations from the infectious diseases Society of America, the American Society of Health-System Pharmacists, and the Society of Infectious Diseases Pharmacists. Clin Infect Dis 49:325–327, 2009.

**243.** Kullar R, Davis SL, Levine DP, et al: Impact of vancomycin exposure on outcomes in patients with methicillin-resistant Staphylococcus aureus bacteremia: Support for consensus guidelines suggested targets. Clin Infect Dis 52:975–981, 2011.

**244.** Falagas ME, Alexiou VG, Peppas G, et al: Do changes in antimicrobial resistance necessitate reconsideration of surgical antimicrobial prophylaxis strategies? Surg Infect (Larchmt) 10: 557–562, 2009.

**245.** Chang MH, Kish TD, Fung HB: Telavancin: A lipoglycopeptide antimicrobial for the treatment of complicated skin and skin structure infections caused by gram-positive bacteria in adults. Clin Ther 32:2160–2185, 2010.

**246.** Silverman JA, Mortin LI, Vanpraagh AD, et al: Inhibition of daptomycin by pulmonary surfactant: In vitro modeling and clinical impact. J Infect Dis 191:2149–2152, 2005.

**247.** Landman D, Georgescu C, Martin DA, et al: Polymyxins revisited. Clin Microbiol Rev 21:449–465, 2008.

**248.** Bailey JA, Virgo KS, DiPiro JT, et al: Aminoglycosides for intra-abdominal infection: equal to the challenge? Surg Infect (Larchmt) 3:315–335, 2002.

**249.** Stein GE, Craig WA: Tigecycline: A critical analysis. Clin Infect Dis 43:518–524, 2006.

**250.** U.S. Food and Drug Administration: FDA drug safety communication: Increased risk of death with Tygacil (tigecycline) compared with other antibiotics used to treat similar infections, 2010 (www.fda.gov/Drugs/DrugSafety/ucm224370.htm).

**251.** Cai Y, Wang R, Liang B, et al: Systematic review and meta-analysis of the effectiveness and safety of tigecycline for treatment of infectious disease. Antimicrob Agents Chemother 55:1162–1172, 2011.

**252.** Eckmann C, Dryden M: Treatment of complicated skin and soft-tissue infections caused by resistant bacteria: value of linezolid, tigecycline, daptomycin and vancomycin. Eur J Med Res 15:554–563, 2010.

**253.** Walkey AJ, O'Donnell MR, Wiener RS: Linezolid vs glycopeptide antibiotics for the treatment of suspected methicillin-resistant Staphylococcus aureus nosocomial pneumonia: A meta-analysis of randomized controlled trials. Chest 139:1148–1155, 2011.

**254.** Nseir S, Di Pompeo C, Soubrier S, et al: First-generation fluoroquinolone use and subsequent emergence of multiple drug-resistant bacteria in the intensive care unit. Crit Care Med 33:283–289, 2005.

**255.** Livermore DM, Woodford N: The beta-lactamase threat in Enterobacteriaceae, Pseudomonas and Acinetobacter. Trends Microbiol 14:413–420, 2006.

**256.** Charbonneau P, Parienti JJ, Thibon P, et al: Fluoroquinolone use and methicillin-resistant Staphylococcus aureus isolation rates in hospitalized patients: A quasi experimental study. Clin Infect Dis 42:778–784, 2006.

**257.** Sprandel KA, Drusano GL, Hecht DW, et al: Population pharmacokinetic modeling and Monte Carlo simulation of varying doses of intravenous metronidazole. Diagn Microbiol Infect Dis 55:303–309, 2006.

**258.** De Broe ME, Giuliano RA, Verpooten GA: Aminoglycoside nephrotoxicity: Mechanism and prevention. Adv Exp Med Biol 252:233–245, 1989.

**259.** Bates DE: Aminoglycoside ototoxicity. Drugs Today (Barc) 39:277–285, 2003.

**260.** Roberts JA, Lipman J: Antibacterial dosing in intensive care: Pharmacokinetics, degree of disease and pharmacodynamics of sepsis. Clin Pharmacokinet 45:755–773, 2006.

**261.** Trotman RL, Williamson JC, Shoemaker DM, et al: Antibiotic dosing in critically ill adult patients receiving continuous renal replacement therapy. Clin Infect Dis 41:1159–1166, 2005.

**262.** Centers for Disease Control and Prevention (CDC): Vital signs: central line-associated bloodstream infections—United States, 2001, 2008, and 2009. MMWR Morb Mortal Wkly Rep 60: 243–248, 2011.

**263.** Burton DC, Edwards JR, Horan TC, et al: Methicillin-resistant Staphylococcus aureus central line-associated bloodstream infections in US intensive care units, 1997–2007. JAMA 301:727–736, 2009.

**264.** Moellering RC, Jr.: Vancomycin: a 50-year reassessment. Clin Infect Dis 42(Suppl 1):S3-S4, 2006.

**265.** Tverdek FP, Crank CW, Segreti J: Antibiotic therapy of methicillin-resistant Staphylococcus aureus in critical care. Crit Care Clin 24:249–260, vii-viii, 2008.

**266.** Wu LR, Zaborina O, Zaborin A, et al: Surgical injury and metabolic stress enhance the virulence of the human opportunistic pathogen Pseudomonas aeruginosa. Surg Infect (Larchmt) 6:185–195, 2005.

**267.** Driscoll JA, Brody SL, Kollef MH: The epidemiology, pathogenesis and treatment of Pseudomonas aeruginosa infections. Drugs 67:351–368, 2007.

**268.** Tenover FC: Mechanisms of antimicrobial resistance in bacteria. Am J Med 119:S3–10, 2006.

**269.** Bush K: Bench-to-bedside review: The role of beta-lactamases in antibiotic-resistant gram-negative infections. Crit Care 14:224, 2010.

**270.** Patel G, Bonomo RA: Status report on carbapenemases: challenges and prospects. Expert Rev Anti Infect Ther 9:555–570, 2011.

**271.** Bonomo RA, Szabo D: Mechanisms of multidrug resistance in Acinetobacter species and Pseudomonas aeruginosa. Clin Infect Dis 43(Suppl 2):S49–S56, 2006.

**272.** Grupper M, Sprecher H, Mashiach T, et al: Attributable mortality of nosocomial Acinetobacter bacteremia. Infect Control Hosp Epidemiol 28:293–298, 2007.

**273.** Vincent JL, Anaissie E, Bruining H, et al: Epidemiology, diagnosis and treatment of systemic Candida infection in surgical patients under intensive care. Intensive Care Med 24:206–216, 1998.

**274.** Blumberg HM, Jarvis WR, Soucie JM, et al: Risk factors for candidal bloodstream infections in surgical intensive care unit patients: The NEMIS prospective multicenter study. The National Epidemiology of Mycosis Survey. Clin Infect Dis 33:177–186, 2001.

**275.** Paphitou NI, Ostrosky-Zeichner L, Rex JH: Rules for identifying patients at increased risk for candidal infections in the surgical intensive care unit: Approach to developing practical criteria for systematic use in antifungal prophylaxis trials. Med Mycol 43:235–243, 2005.

**276.** Chow JK, Golan Y, Ruthazer R, et al: Risk factors for albicans and non-albicans candidemia in the intensive care unit. Crit Care Med 36:1993–1998, 2008.

**277.** Pittet D, Monod M, Suter PM, et al: Candida colonization and subsequent infections in critically ill surgical patients. Ann Surg 220:751–758, 1994.

**277a.** Ziakas PD, Kourbeti IS, Voulgarelis M, et al: Effectiveness of systemic antifungal prophylaxis in patients with neutropenia after chemotherapy: a meta-analysis of randomized controlled trials. Clin Ther 32(14):2316–2336, 2010.

**278.** Leon C, Ruiz-Santana S, Saavedra P, et al: A bedside scoring system ("Candida score") for early antifungal treatment in non-neutropenic critically ill patients with Candida colonization. Crit Care Med 34:730–737, 2006.

**279.** Leon C, Ruiz-Santana S, Saavedra P, et al: Usefulness of the "Candida score" for discriminating between Candida colonization and invasive candidiasis in non-neutropenic critically ill patients: A prospective multicenter study. Crit Care Med 37:1624–1633, 2009.

**280.** Kratzer C, Graninger W, Lassnigg A, et al: Design and use of Candida scores at the intensive care unit. Mycoses 2011 May 3 [Epub ahead of print].

**281.** Ostrosky-Zeichner L, Sable C, Sobel J, et al: Multicenter retrospective development and validation of a clinical prediction rule for nosocomial invasive candidiasis in the intensive care setting. Eur J Clin Microbiol Infect Dis 26:271–276, 2007.

**282.** Ostrosky-Zeichner L, Pappas PG, Shoham S, et al: Improvement of a clinical prediction rule for clinical trials on prophylaxis for invasive candidiasis in the intensive care unit. Mycoses 54:46–51, 2011.

**283.** Shorr AF, Tabak YP, Johannes RS, et al: Candidemia on presentation to the hospital: development and validation of a risk score. Crit Care 13:R156, 2009.

**284.** Sawyer RG, Adams RB, May AK, et al: Development of Candida albicans and C. albicans/Escherichia coli/Bacteroides fragilis intraperitoneal abscess models with demonstration of fungus-induced bacterial translocation. J Med Vet Mycol 33:49–52, 1995.

**285.** Eggimann P, Garbino J, Pittet D: Epidemiology of Candida species infections in critically ill non-immunosuppressed patients. Lancet Infect Dis 3:685–702, 2003.

**286.** Felk A, Kretschmar M, Albrecht A, et al: Candida albicans hyphal formation and the expression of the Efg1-regulated proteinases Sap4 to Sap6 are required for the invasion of parenchymal organs. Infect Immun 70:3689–3700, 2002.

**287.** Prowle JR, Echeverri JE, Ligabo EV, et al: Acquired bloodstream infection in the intensive care unit: Incidence and attributable mortality. Crit Care 15:R100, 2011.

**288.** Shorr AF, Lazarus DR, Sherner JH, et al: Do clinical features allow for accurate prediction of fungal pathogenesis in bloodstream infections? Potential implications of the increasing prevalence of non-albicans candidemia. Crit Care Med 35:1077–1083, 2007.

**289.** Mohr JF, Sims C, Paetznick V, et al: Prospective survey of (1→3)-beta-D-glucan and its relationship to invasive candidiasis in the surgical intensive care unit setting. J Clin Microbiol 49:58–61, 2011.

**290.** Pitarch A, Nombela C, Gil C: Prediction of the clinical outcome in invasive candidiasis patients based on molecular fingerprints of five anti-Candida antibodies in serum. Mol Cell Proteomics 10:M110 004010, 2011.

**291.** Charles PE, Castro C, Ruiz-Santana S, et al: Serum procalcitonin levels in critically ill patients colonized with Candida spp: New clues for the early recognition of invasive candidiasis? Intensive Care Med 35:2146–2150, 2009.

**292.** Dean DA, Burchard KW: Surgical perspective on invasive Candida infections. World J Surg 22:127–134, 1998.

**293.** Riddell JT, Comer GM, Kauffman CA: Treatment of endogenous fungal endophthalmitis: focus on new antifungal agents. Clin Infect Dis 52:648–653, 2011.

**294.** Meersseman W, Vandecasteele SJ, Wilmer A, et al: Invasive aspergillosis in critically ill patients without malignancy. Am J Respir Crit Care Med 170:621–625, 2004.

**295.** Eggimann P, Pittet D: Postoperative fungal infections. Surg Infect (Larchmt) 7(Suppl 2):S53–S56, 2006.

**296.** Rocco TR, Reinert SE, Simms HH: Effects of fluconazole administration in critically ill patients: Analysis of bacterial and fungal resistance. Arch Surg 135:160–165, 2000.

**297.** Gleason TG, May AK, Caparelli D, et al: Emerging evidence of selection of fluconazole-tolerant fungi in surgical intensive care units. Arch Surg 132:1197–1201, 1997.

**298.** Pelz RK, Hendrix CW, Swoboda SM, et al: Double-blind placebo-controlled trial of fluconazole to prevent candidal infections in critically ill surgical patients. Ann Surg 233:542–548, 2001.

**299.** Magill SS, Swoboda SM, Shields CE, et al: The epidemiology of Candida colonization and invasive candidiasis in a surgical intensive care unit where fluconazole prophylaxis is utilized: Follow-up to a randomized clinical trial. Ann Surg 249:657–665, 2009.

**300.** Shorr AF, Chung K, Jackson WL, et al: Fluconazole prophylaxis in critically ill surgical patients: A meta-analysis. Crit Care Med 33:1928–1935; quiz 1936, 2005.

**301.** Pappas PG, Kauffman CA, Andes D, et al: Clinical practice guidelines for the management of candidiasis: 2009 update by the Infectious Diseases Society of America. Clin Infect Dis 48:503–535, 2009.

**302.** Brizendine KD, Vishin S, Baddley JW: Antifungal prophylaxis in solid organ transplant recipients. Expert Rev Anti Infect Ther 9:571–581, 2011.

**303.** Playford EG, Webster AC, Sorrell TC, et al: Systematic review and meta-analysis of antifungal agents for preventing fungal infections in liver transplant recipients. Eur J Clin Microbiol Infect Dis 25:549–561, 2006.

**304.** Horn DL, Ostrosky-Zeichner L, Morris MI, et al: Factors related to survival and treatment success in invasive candidiasis or candidemia: A pooled analysis of two large, prospective, micafungin trials. Eur J Clin Microbiol Infect Dis 29:223–229, 2010.

**305.** Chen SC, Playford EG, Sorrell TC: Antifungal therapy in invasive fungal infections. Curr Opin Pharmacol 10:522–530, 2010.

**306.** Ostrosky-Zeichner L: Combination antifungal therapy: A critical review of the evidence. Clin Microbiol Infect 14(Suppl 4):65–70, 2008.

**307.** Mukherjee PK, Zhou G, Munyon R, et al: Candida biofilm: A well-designed protected environment. Med Mycol 43:191–208, 2005.

**308.** Al-Fattani MA, Douglas LJ: Penetration of Candida biofilms by antifungal agents. Antimicrob Agents Chemother 48:3291–3297, 2004.

**309.** Herbrecht R, Denning DW, Patterson TF, et al: Voriconazole versus amphotericin B for primary therapy of invasive aspergillosis. N Engl J Med 347:408–415, 2002.

**310.** Kullberg BJ, Sobel JD, Ruhnke M, et al: Voriconazole versus a regimen of amphotericin B followed by fluconazole for candidaemia in non-neutropenic patients: A randomised non-inferiority trial. Lancet 366:1435–1442, 2005.

**311.** Glöckner A: Treatment and prophylaxis of invasive candidiasis with anidulafungin, caspofungin and micafungin: Review of the literature. Eur J Med Res 16:167–179, 2011.

**312.** Anidulafungin (Eraxis) for Candida infections. Med Lett Drugs Ther 48:43–44, 2006.

**313.** Pappas PG, Rotstein CM, Betts RF, et al: Micafungin versus caspofungin for treatment of candidemia and other forms of invasive candidiasis. Clin Infect Dis 45:883–893, 2007.

**314.** Kuse ER, Chetchotisakd P, da Cunha CA, et al: Micafungin versus liposomal amphotericin B for candidaemia and invasive candidosis: A phase III randomised double-blind trial. Lancet 369:1519–1527, 2007.

**315.** Zilberberg MD, Kothari S, Shorr AF: Cost-effectiveness of micafungin as an alternative to fluconazole empirical treatment of suspected ICU-acquired candidemia among patients with sepsis: A model simulation. Crit Care 13:R94, 2009.

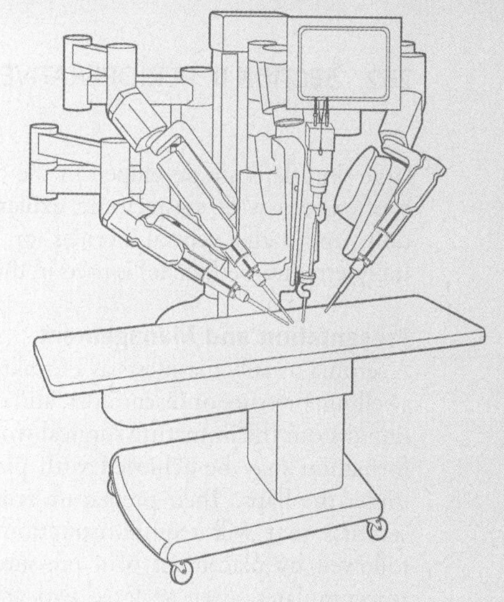

CHAPTER 13

# SURGICAL COMPLICATIONS

Mahmoud N. Kulaylat and Merril T. Dayton



Surgical complications remain a frustrating and difficult aspect of the operative treatment of patients. Regardless of how technically gifted and capable surgeons are, all will have to deal with complications that occur after operative procedures. The cost of surgical complications in the United States runs into millions of dollars; in addition, such complications are associated with lost work productivity, disruption of family life, and stress to employers and society in general. Frequently, the functional results of the operation are compromised by complications; in some cases the patient never recovers to the preoperative level of function. The most significant and difficult part of complications is the suffering borne by a patient who enters the hospital anticipating an uneventful operation but is left suffering and compromised by the complication.

Complications can occur for a variety of reasons. A surgeon can perform a technically sound operation in a patient who is severely compromised by the disease process and still have a complication. Similarly, a surgeon who is sloppy or careless or hurries through an operation can make technical errors that account for the operative complications. Finally, the patient can be healthy nutritionally, have an operation performed meticulously, and yet suffer a complication because of the nature of the disease. The possibility of postoperative complications remains part of every surgeon's mental preparation for a difficult operation.

Surgeons can do much to avoid complications by careful preoperative screening. When the surgeon sees the surgical candidate for the first time, a host of questions come to mind, such as the nutritional status of the patient and the health of the heart and lungs. The surgeon will make a decision regarding performing the appropriate operation for the known disease. Similarly, the timing of the operation is often an important issue. Some operations can be performed in a purely elective fashion, whereas others must be done in an urgent fashion. Occasionally, the surgeon will require that the patient lose weight before the operation to enhance the likelihood of a successful outcome. At times, a wise surgeon will request preoperative consultation from a cardiologist or pulmonary specialist to make certain that the patient will be able to tolerate the stress of a particular procedure.

Once the operation has begun, the surgeon can do much to influence the postoperative outcome. Surgeons must handle tissues gently, dissect meticulously, and honor tissue planes. Performing the technical portions of the operation carefully will lower the risk for a significant complication. At all costs, surgeons must avoid the temptation to rush, cut corners, or accept marginal technical results. Similarly, the judicious use of antibiotics and other preoperative medications can influence the outcome. For a seriously ill patient, adequate resuscitation may be necessary to optimize the patient before giving a general anesthetic.

Once the operation is completed, compulsive postoperative surveillance is mandatory. Thorough and careful rounding on patients on a regular basis postoperatively gives the operating surgeon an opportunity to be vigilant and seek postoperative complications at an early stage, when they can be most effectively addressed. During this process, the surgeon will carefully check all wounds, evaluate intake and output, check temperature profiles, ascertain what the patient's activity levels have been, evaluate nutritional status, and check pain levels. Over years of experience, the clinician can begin to assess these parameters and detect deviations from the normal postoperative course. Expeditious response to a complication makes the difference between a brief, inconvenient complication and a devastating, disabling one. In summary, a wise surgeon will deal with complications quickly, thoroughly, and appropriately.

## SURGICAL WOUND COMPLICATIONS

### Seroma

#### Causes

A seroma is a collection of liquefied fat, serum, and lymphatic fluid under the incision. The fluid is usually clear, yellow, and somewhat viscous and is found in the subcutaneous layer of the skin. Seromas represent the most benign complication after an operative procedure and are particularly likely to occur when large skin flaps are developed in the course of the operation, as is often seen with mastectomy, axillary dissection, groin dissection, and large ventral hernias or when a prosthetic mesh (polytetrafluoroethylene) is used in the repair of a ventral hernia.

#### Presentation and Management

A seroma usually manifests as a localized and well-circumscribed swelling, pressure or discomfort, and occasional drainage of clear liquid from the immature surgical wound. Prevention of seroma formation may be achieved with placement of suction drains under the flaps. Their premature removal often results in large seromas that will require aspiration under sterile conditions, followed by placement of a pressure dressing. A seroma that reaccumulates after at least two aspirations is evacuated by opening the incision and packing the wound with saline-moistened gauze to allow healing by secondary intention. In the presence of synthetic mesh, open drainage is best performed in the operating room, the incision is best closed to avoid exposure and infection of the mesh, and suction drains are placed. An infected seroma is also treated with open drainage. The presence of synthetic mesh in these cases will prevent the wound from healing. Management of the mesh depends on the severity and extent of infection. In the absence of severe sepsis and spreading cellulitis and the presence of localized infection, the mesh can be left in situ and removed at a later date when the acute infectious process has resolved. Otherwise, the mesh must be removed and the wound managed with open wound care.

### Hematoma

#### Causes

A hematoma is an abnormal collection of blood, usually in the subcutaneous layer of a recent incision or in a potential space in the abdominal cavity after extirpation of an organ (e.g., splenic fossa hematoma after splenectomy or pelvic hematoma after proctectomy). Hematomas are more worrisome than seromas because of the potential for secondary infection. Hematoma formation is related to inadequate hemostasis, depletion of clotting factors, or the presence of coagulopathy. A host of disease processes can contribute to coagulopathy, including myeloproliferative disorders, liver disease, renal failure, sepsis, clotting factor deficiencies, and medications. Medications most commonly associated with coagulopathy are antiplatelet drugs, such as acetylsalicylic acid (ASA, aspirin), clopidogrel, ticlopidine, eptifibatide, and abciximab, and anticoagulants, such as unfractionated heparin (UFH), low-molecular-weight heparin (LMWH [e.g., enoxaparin, dalteparin sodium, tinzaparin]), and vitamin K antagonist (VKA [e.g., warfarin sodium]).

#### Presentation and Management

The clinical manifestations of a hematoma may vary with its size, location, and presence of infection. A hematoma may manifest as an expanding, unsightly swelling and/or pain in the area of a surgical incision. In the neck, a large hematoma may cause compromise of the airway; in the retroperitoneum, it may cause a paralytic ileus, anemia, and ongoing bleeding caused by local consumptive coagulopathy; and, in the extremity and abdominal cavity, it may result in compartment syndrome. On physical examination, the hematoma appears as a localized soft swelling with purplish blue discoloration of the overlying skin. The swelling varies from small to large and may be tender to palpation or associated with drainage of dark red fluid out of the fresh wound.

Hematoma formation is prevented preoperatively by correcting any clotting abnormalities and discontinuing medications that alter coagulation. Antiplatelet medications and anticoagulants may be given to patients undergoing procedures for a variety of reasons. Clopidogrel is given after implantation of a coronary stent, ASA is given for the treatment of coronary artery disease (CAD) and stroke, and VKA is given after implantation of a mechanical mitral valve for atrial fibrillation, venous thromboembolism, and hypercoagulable states. These medications must be temporarily discontinued before surgery. There are no specific studies that have addressed the issue of timing of discontinuation of such medications.

One must balance the risk of significant bleeding caused by uncorrected medication-induced coagulopathy and the risk of thromboembolic events after discontinuation of therapy. The risk of bleeding varies with the type of surgery or procedure and adequacy of hemostasis; the risk of thromboembolism depends on the indication for antithrombotic therapy and presence of comorbid conditions.[1] In patients at high risk for thromboembolism (e.g., those with a mechanical mitral valve or older generation aortic valve prosthesis, venous thromboembolism within 3 months, severe thrombophilia, recent atrial fibrillation [within 6 months], stroke or transient ischemic attack who are scheduled to undergo an elective major surgical procedure involving a body cavity), the VKA must be discontinued 4 to 5 days before surgery to allow the international normalized ratio (INR) to be lower than 1.5. In patients whose INR is still elevated (>1.5), low-dose vitamin K (1 to 2 mg) is given orally. Patients are then given bridging anticoagulation—that is, a therapeutic dose of rapidly acting anticoagulant, intravenous (IV) UFH or to LMWH. Those receiving IV UFH (half-life, 45 minutes) can have the medication discontinued 4 hours before surgery and those receiving therapeutic dose LMWH SC (variable half-life) 16 to 24 hours before surgery. VKA is then resumed 12 to 24 hours after surgery (takes 2 to 3 days for anticoagulant effect to begin after start of VKA) and when there is adequate hemostasis. In patients at high risk of bleeding (major surgery or high bleeding risk surgery) for whom postoperative therapeutic LMWH or UFH is planned, initiation of therapy is delayed for 48 to 72 hours, low-dose LMWH or UFH is administered, or the therapy is completely avoided. Patients at low risk for thromboembolism do not require heparin therapy after discontinuation of the VKA. Patients on ASA or clopidogrel must have the medication withheld 6 to 7 days before surgery; otherwise, the surgery must be delayed until the patient has completed the course of treatment. Antiplatelet therapy is resumed approximately 24 hours after surgery. In patients with a bare metal coronary stent who require surgery within 6 weeks of stent placement, ASA and clopidogrel are continued in the perioperative period. In patients who are receiving VKAs and require urgent surgery, immediate reversal of anticoagulant effect requires transfusion with fresh-frozen plasma or other prothrombin concentrate and low-dose IV or oral vitamin K. During surgery, adequate hemostasis must be achieved with ligature, electrocautery, fibrin glue, or topical bovine thrombin before closure. Closed suction drainage systems are placed in large potential spaces and removed postoperatively when the output is not bloody and scant.

Evaluation of a patient with a hematoma, especially one that is large and expanding, includes assessment of preexisting risk factors and coagulation parameters (e.g., prothrombin time [PT], activated partial prothrombin time [aPTT], INR, platelet count, bleeding time) and appropriate treatment. A small hematoma does not require any intervention and will eventually resorb. Most retroperitoneal hematomas can be managed by expectant waiting after correction of associated coagulopathy (platelet transfusion if bleeding time is prolonged, desmopressin in patients who have renal failure, and fresh-frozen plasma in patients who have an increased INR). A large or expanding hematoma in the neck is managed in a similar fashion and best evacuated in the operating room urgently after securing the airway if there is any respiratory compromise. Similarly, hematomas detected soon after surgery, especially those developing under skin flaps, are best evacuated in the operating room.

## Acute Wound Failure (Dehiscence)

### Causes

Acute wound failure (wound dehiscence or a burst abdomen) refers to postoperative separation of the abdominal musculoaponeurotic layers. It is among the most dreaded complications faced by surgeons and is of great concern because of the risk of evisceration, the need for some form of intervention, and the possibility of repeat dehiscence, surgical wound infection, and incisional hernia formation.

Acute wound failure occurs in approximately 1% to 3% of patients who undergo an abdominal operation. Dehiscence most often develops 7 to 10 days postoperatively but may occur anytime after surgery, from 1 to more than 20 days. A multitude of factors may contribute to wound dehiscence (Box 13-1). Acute wound failure is often related to technical errors in placing sutures too close to the edge, too far apart, or under too much tension. Local wound complications such as hematoma and infection can also predispose to localized dehiscence. In fact, a deep wound infection is one of the most common causes of localized wound separation. Increased intra-abdominal pressure (IAP) is often blamed for wound disruption and factors that adversely affect wound healing are cited as contributing to the complication. In healthy patients, the rate of wound failure is similar whether closure is accomplished with a continuous or interrupted technique. In high-risk patients, however, continuous closure is worrisome because suture breakage in one place weakens the entire closure.

**BOX 13-1 Factors Associated With Wound Dehiscence**

Technical error in fascial closure
Emergency surgery
Intra-abdominal infection
Advanced age
Wound infection, hematoma, and seroma
Elevated intra-abdominal pressure
Obesity
Chronic corticosteroid use
Previous wound dehiscence
Malnutrition
Radiation therapy and chemotherapy
Systemic disease (uremia, diabetes mellitus)

### Presentation and Management

Acute wound failure may occur without warning and evisceration makes the diagnosis obvious. A sudden, dramatic drainage of a relatively large volume of a clear, salmon-colored fluid precedes dehiscence in 25% of patients. More often, patients report a ripping sensation. Probing the wound with a sterile, cotton-tipped applicator or gloved finger may detect a partial dehiscence.

Prevention of acute wound failure is largely a function of careful attention to technical detail during fascial closure, such as proper spacing of the suture, adequate depth of bite of the fascia, relaxation of the patient during closure, and achieving a tension-free closure. For very high-risk patients, interrupted closure is often the wisest choice. Alternative methods of closure must be selected when primary closure is not possible without undue tension. Although retention sutures were used extensively in the past, their use is less common today, with many surgeons opting to use a synthetic mesh or bioabsorbable tissue scaffold.

Treatment of dehiscence depends on the extent of fascial separation and the presence of evisceration and/or significant intra-abdominal pathology (e.g., intestinal leak, peritonitis). A small dehiscence, especially in the proximal aspect of an upper midline incision 10 to 12 days postoperatively, can be managed conservatively with saline-moistened gauze packing of the wound and use of an abdominal binder. In the event of evisceration, the eviscerated intestines must be covered with a sterile, saline-moistened towel and preparations made to return to the operating room after a very short period of fluid resuscitation. Similarly, if probing of the wound reveals a large segment of the wound that is open to the omentum and intestines, or if there is peritonitis or suspicion of intestinal leak, plans to take the patient back to the operating room are made.

Once in the operating room, thorough exploration of the abdominal cavity is performed to rule out the presence of a septic focus or an anastomotic leak that may have predisposed to the dehiscence. Management of that infection is of critical importance before attempting to close. Management of the incision is a function of the condition of the fascia. When technical mistakes are made and the fascia is strong and intact, primary closure is warranted. If the fascia is infected or necrotic, débridement is performed. The incision can then be closed with retention sutures; however, to avoid tension, use of a prosthetic material may be preferred. Closure with an absorbable mesh (polyglactin or polyglycolic acid) may be preferable because the mesh is well tolerated in septic wounds and allows bridging the gap between the edges of the fascia without tension, prevents evisceration, and allows the underlying cause of the patient's dehiscence to resolve. Once the wound has granulated, a skin graft is applied and wound closure is achieved by advancing local tissue. This approach uniformly results in the development of a hernia, the repair of which requires the subsequent removal of the skin graft and use of a permanent prosthesis. An alternative method of closure is dermabrasion of the skin graft followed by fascial closure using the component separation technique. Attempts to close the fascia under tension guarantee a repeat dehiscence and, in some cases, result in intra-abdominal hypertension (IAH). The incision is left open (laparotomy), closed with a temporary closure device (open abdomen technique), closed with synthetic mesh or biologic graft (acellular dermal matrix), or closed by using negative-pressure wound therapy.

The open abdomen technique avoids IAH, preserves the fascia, and facilitates reaccess of the abdominal cavity. With laparotomy, the wound is allowed to heal with secondary intention and/or subsequently closed with a skin graft or local or regional tissue. This approach is associated with prolonged healing time, fluid loss, and risk of complex enterocutaneous fistula formation as a result of bowel exposure, desiccation, and traumatic injury. Furthermore, definitive surgical repair to restore the integrity of the abdominal wall will eventually be required. A temporary closure device (vacuum pack closure) protects abdominal contents, keeps patients dry, can be quickly removed with increased IAP, and avoids secondary complications seen with laparotomy. A fenestrated, nonadherent, polyethylene sheet is applied on the bowel omentum, moist surgical towels or gauze with drains are placed on top, and an iodophore-impregnated adhesive dressing is placed. Continuous suction is then applied. If the fascia cannot be closed in 7 to 10 days, the wound is allowed to granulate and then covered with a skin graft.

Absorbable synthetic mesh provides wound stability and is resistant to infection. It is associated with fistula and hernia formation repair, which is difficult and may require reconstruction of the abdominal wall. Repair with nonabsorbable synthetic mesh such as polypropylene, polyester, or polytetrafluoroethylene (PTFE) is associated with complications that will require removal of the mesh (e.g., abscess formation, dehiscence, wound sepsis, mesh extrusion, bowel fistulization). Although PTFE is more desirable because it is nonadherent to underlying bowel, it is expensive, does not allow skin grafting, and is associated with chronic infections. An acellular dermal matrix (bioprosthesis) has the mechanical properties of a mesh for abdominal wall reconstruction and physiologic properties that make it resistant to contamination and/or infection. The bioprosthesis provides immediate coverage of the wound and serves as mechanical support in a single-stage reconstruction of compromised surgical wounds. It is bioactive because it functions as tissue replacement or scaffold for new tissue growth; it stimulates cellular attachment, migration, neovascularization, and repopulation of the implanted graft. A bioprosthesis also reduces long-term complications (e.g., erosion, infection, chronic pain). Available acellular materials are animal-derived (e.g., porcine intestinal submucosa, porcine dermis, cross-linked porcine dermal collagen) or human-derived (e.g., cadaveric human dermis). However, the rate of wound complications (e.g., superficial wound or graft infection, graft dehiscence, fistula formation, bleeding) and hernia formation or laxity of the abdominal wall is 25% to 50%.[2]

Negative-pressure wound therapy is based on the concept of wound suction. A vacuum-assisted closure device is most commonly used. The device consists of a vacuum pump, canister with connecting tubing, open-pore foam (e.g., polyurethane ether, polyvinyl alcohol foam) or gauze, and semiocclusive dressing. The device provides immediate coverage of the abdominal wound, acts as a temporary dressing, does not require suturing to the fascia, minimizes IAH, and prevents loss of domain. Applying suction of 125 mm Hg, the open-pore foam decreases in size and transmits the negative pressure to surrounding tissue, leading to contraction of the wound (macrodeformation) and removal of extracellular fluid (via decrease in bowel edema, evacuation of excess abdominal fluid, decrease in wound size), stabilization of the wound environment, and microdeformation of the foam-wound interface, which induces cellular proliferation and angiogenesis. The secondary effects of the vacuum-assisted closure device include acceleration of wound healing, reduction and changes in bacterial burden, changes in biochemistry and systemic responses, and improvement in wound bed preparation—increase in local blood perfusion and induction healing response through microchemical forces.[3] This approach results in successful closure of the fascia in 85% of cases. However, the device is expensive and cumbersome to wear and may cause significant pain, cause bleeding (especially in patients on anticoagulant therapy), be associated with increased levels of certain bacteria, and be associated with evisceration and hernia formation. There is also an increased incidence of intestinal fistulization at enterotomy sites and enteric anastomoses, and in the absence of anastomoses.

## Surgical Site Infection (Wound Infection)

### Causes

Surgical site infections (SSIs) still continue to be a significant problem for surgeons. Despite major improvements in antibiotics, better anesthesia, superior instruments, earlier diagnosis of surgical problems, and improved techniques for postoperative vigilance, wound infections continue to occur. Although some may view the problem as merely cosmetic, that view represents a shallow understanding of this problem, which causes significant patient suffering, morbidity, and even mortality, and is a financial burden to the health care system. Furthermore, SSIs represent a risk factor for the development of incisional hernia, which requires surgical repair. Currently, in the United States, SSIs account for almost 40% of hospital-acquired infections among surgical patients.

The surgical wound encompasses the area of the body, internally and externally, that involves the entire operative site. Wounds are thus categorized into three general categories:

1. Superficial, which includes the skin and subcutaneous tissue
2. Deep, which includes the fascia and muscle
3. Organ space, which includes the internal organs of the body if the operation includes that area

The Centers for Disease Control and Prevention has proposed specific criteria for the diagnosis of surgical site infections (Box 13-2).[4]

Surgical site infections develop as a result of contamination of the surgical site with microorganisms. The source of these microorganisms is mostly patients' flora (endogenous source) when integrity of the skin and/or wall of a hollow viscus is violated. Occasionally, the source is exogenous when a break in the surgical sterile technique occurs, thus allowing contamination from the surgical team, equipment, implant or gloves, or surrounding environment. The pathogens associated with a surgical site infections reflect the area that provided the inoculum for the infection to develop. The microbiology, however, varies, depending on the types of procedures performed in individual practices. Gram-positive cocci account for half of the infections (Table 13-1)—*Staphylococcus aureus* (most common), coagulase-negative *Staphylococcus,* and *Enterococcus* spp. *S. aureus* infections

**BOX 13-2 Centers for Disease Control and Prevention Criteria for Defining a Surgical Site Infection**

**Superficial Incisional**

Infection less than 30 days after surgery

Involves skin and subcutaneous tissue only, *plus* one of the following:

- Purulent drainage
- Diagnosis of superficial surgical site infection by a surgeon
- Symptoms of erythema, pain, local edema

**Deep Incisional**

Less than 30 days after surgery with no implant and soft tissue involvement

Infection less than 1 year after surgery with an implant; involves deep soft tissues (fascia and muscle), *plus* one of the following:

- Purulent drainage from the deep space but no extension into the organ space
- Abscess found in the deep space on direct or radiologic examination or on reoperation
- Diagnosis of a deep space surgical site infection by the surgeon
- Symptoms of fever, pain, and tenderness leading to wound dehiscence or opening by a surgeon

**Organ Space**

Infection less than 30 days after surgery with no implant

Infection less than 1 year after surgery with an implant and infection; involves any part of the operation opened or manipulated, *plus* one of the following:

- Purulent drainage from a drain placed in the organ space
- Cultured organisms from material aspirated from the organ space
- Abscess found on direct or radiologic examination or during reoperation
- Diagnosis of organ space infection by a surgeon

Adapted from Mangram AJ, Horan TC, Pearson ML, et al: Guideline for prevention of surgical site infection. Infect Control Hosp Epidemiol 20:252, 1999.

**Table 13-1 Pathogens Isolated from Postoperative Surgical Site Infections at a University Hospital**

| PATHOGEN | PERCENTAGE OF ISOLATES |
|---|---|
| *Staphylococcus* (coagulase-negative) | 25.6 |
| *Enterococcus* (group D) | 11.5 |
| *Staphylococcus aureus* | 8.7 |
| *Candida albicans* | 6.5 |
| *Escherichia coli* | 6.3 |
| *Pseudomonas aeruginosa* | 6.0 |
| *Corynebacterium* | 4.0 |
| *Candida* (non-*albicans*) | 3.4 |
| Alpha-hemolytic *Streptococcus* | 3.0 |
| *Klebsiella pneumoniae* | 2.8 |
| Vancomycin-resistant *Enterococcus* | 2.4 |
| *Enterobacter cloacae* | 2.2 |
| *Citrobacter* spp. | 2.0 |

From Weiss CA, Statz CI, Dahms RA, et al: Six years of surgical wound surveillance at a tertiary care center. Arch Surg 134:1041–1048, 1999.

normally occur in the nasal passages, mucous membranes, and skin of carriers. The organism that has acquired resistance to methicillin (methicillin-resistant *S. aureus* [MRSA]) consists of two subtypes, hospital- and community-acquired MRSA. Hospital-acquired MRSA is associated with nosocomial infections and affects immunocompromised individuals. It also occurs in patients with chronic wounds, those subjected to invasive procedures, and those with prior antibiotic treatment. Community-acquired MRSA is associated with a variety of skin and soft tissue infections in patients with and without risk factors for MRSA. Community-acquired MRSA (e.g., the USA300 clone) has also been noted to affect SSIs. Hospital-acquired MRSA isolates have a different antibiotic susceptibility profile—they are usually resistant to at least three β-lactam antibiotics and are usually susceptible to vancomycin, teicoplanin, and sulfamethoxazole. Community-acquired MRSA is usually susceptible to clindamycin, with variable susceptibility to erythromycin, vancomycin, and tetracycline. There is evidence to indicate that hospital-acquired MRSA is developing resistance to vancomycin (vancomycin intermediate-resistant *S. aureus* [VISA] and vancomycin-resistant *S. aureus* [VRSA]).[5] *Enterococcus* spp. are commensals in the adult gastrointestinal (GI) tract, have intrinsic resistance to a variety of antibiotics (e.g., cephalosporins, clindamycin, aminoglycoside), and are the first to exhibit resistance to vancomycin.

In approximately one third of SSI cases, gram-negative bacilli (*Escherichia coli, Pseudomonas aeruginosa,* and *Enterobacter* spp.) are isolated. However, at locations at which high volumes of GI operations are performed, the predominant bacterial species are the gram-negative bacilli. Infrequent pathogens are group A beta-hemolytic streptococci and *Clostridium perfringens.* In recent years, the involvement of resistant organisms in the genesis of SSIs has increased, most notable in MRSA.

A host of patient- and operative procedure–related factors may contribute to the development of SSIs (Box 13-3).[6] The risk of infection is related to the specific surgical procedure performed and, hence, surgical wounds are classified according to the relative risk of surgical site infections occurring—clean, clean-contaminated, contaminated, and dirty (Table 13-2). In the National Nosocomial Infections Surveillance System, the risk of patients is stratified according to three important factors: (1) wound classification (contaminated or dirty); (2) longer duration operation, defined as one that exceeds the 75th percentile for a given procedure; and (3) medical characteristics of the patients as determined by the American Society of Anesthesiology score of III, IV, or V (presence of severe systemic disease that results in functional limitations, is life-threatening, or is expected to preclude survival from the operation) at the time of operation.[7]

### Presentation

SSIs most commonly occur 5 to 6 days postoperatively but may develop sooner or later than that. Approximately 80% to 90%

of all postoperative infections occur within 30 days after the operative procedure. With the increased use of outpatient surgery and decreased length of stay in hospitals, 30% to 40% of all wound infections have been shown to occur after hospital discharge. Nevertheless, although less than 10% of surgical patients are hospitalized for 6 days or less, 70% of postdischarge infections occur in that group.

**BOX 13-3 Risk Factors for Postoperative Wound Infection**

| Patient Factors | Environmental Factors | Treatment Factors |
|---|---|---|
| Ascites | Contaminated medications | Drains |
| Chronic inflammation | Inadequate disinfection/ sterilization | Emergency procedure |
| Undernutrition<br>Obesity | Inadequate skin antisepsis | Inadequate antibiotic coverage |
| Diabetes | Inadequate ventilation | Preoperative hospitalization |
| Extremes of age | Presence of a foreign body | Prolonged operation |
| Hypercholesterolemia | | |
| Hypoxemia | | |
| Peripheral vascular disease | | |
| Postoperative anemia | | |
| Previous site of irradiation | | |
| Recent operation | | |
| Remote infection | | |
| Skin carriage of staphylococci | | |
| Skin disease in the area of infection | | |
| Immunosuppression | | |

Data from National Nosocomial Infections Surveillance Systems (NNIS) System Report: Data summary from January 1992–June 2001, issued August 2001. Am J Infect Control 29:404–421, 2001.

**Table 13-2 Classification of Surgical Wounds**

| CATEGORY | CRITERIA | INFECTION RATE (%) |
|---|---|---|
| Clean | No hollow viscus entered<br>Primary wound closure<br>No inflammation<br>No breaks in aseptic technique<br>Elective procedure | 1-3 |
| Clean-contaminated | Hollow viscus entered but controlled<br>No inflammation<br>Primary wound closure<br>Minor break in aseptic technique<br>Mechanical drain used<br>Bowel preparation preoperatively | 5-8 |
| Contaminated | Uncontrolled spillage from viscus<br>Inflammation apparent<br>Open, traumatic wound<br>Major break in aseptic technique | 20-25 |
| Dirty | Untreated, uncontrolled spillage from viscus<br>Pus in operative wound<br>Open suppurative wound<br>Severe inflammation | 30-40 |

Superficial and deep SSIs are accompanied by erythema, tenderness, edema, and occasionally drainage. The wound is often soft or fluctuant at the site of infection, which is a departure from the firmness of the healing ridge present elsewhere in the wound. The patient may have leukocytosis and a low-grade fever. According to the Joint Commission (TJC), a surgical wound is considered infected if (1) there is drainage of grossly purulent material drains from the wound, (2) the wound spontaneously opens and drains purulent fluid, (3) the wound drains fluid that is culture-positive or Gram stain–positive for bacteria, and (4) the surgeon notes erythema or drainage and opens the wound after determining it to be infected.

### Treatment

Prevention of surgical site infections relies on changing or dealing with modifiable risk factors that predispose to surgical site infections. However, many of these factors cannot be changed, such as age, complexity of the surgical procedure, and morbid obesity. Patients who are heavy smokers are encouraged to stop smoking at least 30 days before surgery, glucose levels in diabetics must be treated appropriately, and severely malnourished patients should be given nutritional supplements for 7 to 14 days before surgery.[8] Obese patients must be encouraged to lose weight if the procedure is elective and there is time to achieve significant weight loss. Similarly, patients who are taking high doses of corticosteroids will have lower infection rates if they are weaned off corticosteroids or are at least taking a lower dose. Patients undergoing major intra-abdominal surgery are administered a bowel preparation in the form of a lavage solution or strong cathartic, followed by oral nonabsorbable antibiotic(s), particularly for surgery of the colon and small bowel. Bowel preparation lowers the patient's risk for infection from that of a contaminated case (25%) to a clean-contaminated case (5%). Hair is removed by clipping immediately before surgery and the skin is prepped at the time of operation with an antiseptic agent (e.g., alcohol, chlorhexidine, iodine).

The role of preoperative decolonization in carriers of *S. aureus* undergoing general surgery is questionable, and the routine use of prophylactic vancomycin or teicoplanin (effective against MRSA) is not recommended. Although perioperative antibiotics are widely used, prophylaxis is generally recommended for clean-contaminated or contaminated procedures in which the risk of SSIs is high or in procedures in which vascular or orthopedics prostheses are used because the development of SSIs will have grave consequences (Table 13-3). For dirty or contaminated wounds, the use of antibiotics is for therapeutic purposes rather than for prophylaxis. For clean cases, prophylaxis is controversial. For some surgical procedures, a first- or second-generation cephalosporin is the accepted agent of choice. A small but significant benefit may be achieved with the prophylactic administration of a first-generation cephalosporin for certain types of clean surgery (e.g., mastectomy, herniorrhaphy). For clean-contaminated procedures, administration of preoperative antibiotics is indicated. The appropriate preoperative antibiotic is a function of the most likely inoculum based on the area being operated. For example, when a prosthesis may be placed in a clean wound, preoperative antibiotics would include something to protect against *S. aureus* and streptococcal species.

**Table 13-3 Prophylactic Antimicrobial Agent for Selected Surgical Procedures**

| PROCEDURE | RECOMMENDED AGENT | POTENTIAL ALTERNATIVE |
|---|---|---|
| Cardiothoracic | Cefazolin or cefuroxime | Vancomycin, clindamycin |
| Vascular | Cefazolin or cefuroxime | Vancomycin, clindamycin |
| Gastroduodenal | Cefazolin | Cefoxitin, cefotetan, aminoglycoside, or fluoroquinolone + antianaerobe |
| Open biliary | Cefazolin | Cefoxitin, cefotetan, or fluoroquinolone + antianaerobe |
| Laparoscopic cholecystectomy | None | – |
| Nonperforated appendicitis | Cefoxitin, cefotetan, cefazolin + metronidazole | Ertapenem, aminoglycoside, or fluoroquinolone + antianaerobe |
| Colorectal | Cefoxitin, cefotetan, ampicillin-sulbactam, ertapenem, cefazolin + metronidazole | Aminoglycoside, or fluoroquinolone + antianaerobe, aztreonam + clindamycin |
| Hysterectomy | Cefazolin, cefuroxime, cefoxitin, cefotetan, ampicillin-sulbactam | Aminoglycoside, or fluoroquinolone + antianaerobe, aztreonam + clindamycin |
| Orthopedic implantation | Cefazolin, cefuroxime | Vancomycin, clindamycin |
| Head and neck | Cefazolin, clindamycin | – |

From Kirby JP, Mazuski JE: Prevention of surgical site infection. Surg Clin North Am 89:365–389, 2009.

A first-generation cephalosporin, such as cefazolin, would be appropriate in this setting. For patients undergoing upper GI tract surgery, complex biliary tract operations, or elective colonic resection, administration of a second-generation cephalosporin such as cefoxitin or a penicillin derivative with a β-lactamase inhibitor is more suitable. Alternatively, ertapenem can be used for operations involving the lower GI tract. The surgeon will give a preoperative dose, intraoperative doses approximately 4 hours apart, and two postoperative doses appropriately spaced. The timing of administration of prophylactic antibiotics is critical. To be most effective, the antibiotic is administered IV within 30 minutes before the incision so that therapeutic tissue levels have developed when the wound is created and exposed to bacterial contamination. Usually, a period of anesthesia induction, preparation, and draping takes place that is adequate to allow tissue levels to build up to therapeutic levels before the incision is made. Of equal importance is making certain that the prophylactic antibiotic is not administered for extended periods postoperatively. To do so in the prophylactic setting is to invite the development of drug-resistant organisms, as well as serious complications, such as *Clostridium difficile*–associated colitis.

At the time of surgery, the operating surgeon plays a major role in reducing or minimizing the presence of postoperative wound infections. The surgeon must be attentive to personal hygiene (hand scrubbing) and that of the entire team. In addition, the surgeon must make certain that the patient undergoes a thorough skin preparation with appropriate antiseptic solutions and is draped in a sterile, careful fashion. During the operation, steps that have a positive impact on outcome are followed:

1. Careful handling of tissues
2. Meticulous dissection, hemostasis, and débridement of devitalized tissue
3. Compulsive control of all intraluminal contents
4. Preservation of blood supply of the operated organs
5. Elimination of any foreign body from the wound
6. Maintenance of strict asepsis by the operating team (e.g., no holes in gloves, avoidance of the use of contaminated instruments, avoidance of environmental contamination, such as debris falling from overhead)
7. Thorough drainage and irrigation of any pockets of purulence in the wound with warm saline
8. Ensuring that the patient is kept in a euthermic state, well-monitored, and fluid-resuscitated
9. Expressing a decision about closing the skin or packing the wound at the end of the procedure

The use of drains remains somewhat controversial in preventing postoperative wound infections. In general, there is almost no indication for drains in this setting. However, placing closed suction drains in very deep, large wounds and wounds with large wound flaps to prevent the development of a seroma or hematoma is a worthwhile practice.

Treatment of SSIs depends on the depth of the infection. For both superficial and deep SSIs, skin staples are removed over the area of the infection and a cotton-tipped applicator may be easily passed into the wound, with efflux of purulent material and pus. The wound is gently explored with the cotton-tipped applicator or a finger to determine whether the fascia or muscle tissue is involved. If the fascia is intact, débridement of any nonviable tissue is performed; the wound is irrigated with normal saline solution and packed to its base with saline-moistened gauze to allow healing of the wound from the base anteriorly, thus preventing premature skin closure. If widespread cellulitis or significant signs of infection (e.g., fever, tachycardia), are noted, administration of IV antibiotics must be considered. Empirical therapy is started and tailored according to culture and sensitivity data. The choice of empirical antibiotics is based on the most likely culprit, including the possibility of MRSA. MRSA is treated with vancomycin, linezolid, or clindamycin. Cultures are not routinely performed, except for patients who will be treated with antibiotics so that resistant organisms can be treated adequately. However, if the fascia has separated or purulent material appears to be coming from deep to the fascia, there is obvious concern about dehiscence or an intra-abdominal abscess that may require drainage or possibly a reoperation.

Wound cultures are controversial. If the wound is small, superficial, and not associated with cellulitis or tissue necrosis, cultures may not be necessary. However, if fascial dehiscence and a more complex infection are present, a culture is sent. A deep SSI associated with grayish, dishwater-colored fluid, as well as frank necrosis of the fascial layer, raises suspicion for the presence of a necrotizing type of infection. The presence of crepitus in any surgical wound or gram-positive rods (or both) suggests the possibility of infection with *C. perfringens.* Rapid and expeditious surgical débridement is indicated in these settings.

Most postoperative infections are treated with healing by secondary intention, allowing the wound to heal from the base anteriorly, with epithelialization being the final event. In some cases, when there is a question about the amount of contamination, delayed primary closure may be considered. In this setting, close observation of the wound for 5 days may be followed by closure of the skin or negative-pressure wound therapy if the wound looks clean and the patient is otherwise doing well.

## COMPLICATIONS OF THERMAL REGULATION

### Hypothermia

#### Causes

Optimal function of physiologic systems in the body occurs within a narrow range of core temperatures. A 2° C drop in body temperature or a 3° C increase signifies a health emergency that is life-threatening and requires immediate intervention. Hypothermia can result from a number of mechanisms preoperatively, intraoperatively, or postoperatively. A trauma patient with injuries in a cold environment can suffer significant hypothermia, and paralysis can lead to hypothermia because of loss of the shiver mechanism.

Hypothermia develops in patients undergoing rapid resuscitation with cool IV fluids, transfusions, or intracavitary irrigation with cold irrigant, and in patients undergoing a prolonged surgical procedure with low ambient room temperature and a large, exposed operative area subjected to significant evaporative cooling. Almost all anesthetics impair thermoregulation and render the patient susceptible to hypothermia in the typically cool operating room environment.[9] Advanced age and opioid analgesia also reduce perioperative shivering. Propofol causes vasodilation and significant redistribution hypothermia. Postoperatively, hypothermia can result from cool ambient room temperature, rapid administration of IV fluids or blood, and failure to keep patients covered when they are only partially responsive. More than 80% of elective operative procedures are associated with a drop in body temperature, and 50% of trauma patients are hypothermic on arrival in the operating suite.

#### Presentation

Hypothermia is uncomfortable because of the intense cold sensation and shivering. It may also be associated with profound effects on the cardiovascular system, coagulation, wound healing, and infection. A core temperature lower than 35° C after surgery triggers a significant peripheral sympathetic nervous system response, consisting of an increased norepinephrine level, vasoconstriction, and elevated arterial blood pressure. Patients in shock or with a severe illness often have associated vasoconstriction that results in poor perfusion of peripheral organs and tissues, an effect accentuated by hypothermia. In a high-risk patient, a core temperature lower than 35° C is associated with a twofold to threefold increase in the incidence of early postoperative ischemia and a similar increase in the incidence of ventricular tachyarrhythmia. Hypothermia also impairs platelet function and reduces the activity of coagulation factors, thereby resulting in an increased risk for bleeding. Hypothermia results in impaired macrophage function, reduced tissue oxygen tension, and impaired collagen deposition, which predisposes wounds to poor healing and infection. Other complications of hypothermia include a relative diuresis, compromised hepatic function, and some neurologic manifestations. Similarly, the patient's ability to manage acid-base abnormalities is impaired. In severe cases, the patient can have significant cardiac slowing and may be comatose, with low blood pressure, bradycardia, and a very low respiratory rate.

#### Treatment

Prevention of hypothermia entails monitoring core temperature, especially in patients undergoing body cavity surgery or surgery lasting longer than 1 hour, children and older adults, and patients in whom general epidural anesthesia is being conducted.[9] Sites of monitoring include pulmonary artery blood, tympanic membrane, esophagus and pharynx, rectum, and urinary bladder. While the patient is being anesthetized, and during skin preparation, significant evaporative cooling can take place; the patient is kept warm by increasing the ambient temperature and using heated humidifiers and warmed IV fluid. After the patient is draped, the room temperature can be lowered to a more comfortable setting. A forced-air warming device that provides active cutaneous warming is placed on the patient. Passive surface warming is not effective in conserving heat. There is some evidence that a considerable amount of heat is lost through the head of the patient, so simply covering the patient's head during surgery may prevent significant heat loss.

In the perioperative period, mild hypothermia is commonplace and patients usually shiver because the anesthesia impairs thermoregulation. Many patients who shiver after anesthesia, however, are hypothermic. Treatment of the hypothermia with forced-air warming systems and radiant heaters will also reduce the shivering.[9] In a severely hypothermic patient who does not require immediate operative intervention, attention must be directed toward rewarming by the following methods:

1. Immediate placement of warm blankets, as well as currently available forced-air warming devices
2. Infusion of blood and IV fluids through a warming device
3. Heating and humidifying inhalational gases
4. Peritoneal lavage with warmed fluids
5. Rewarming infusion devices with an arteriovenous system
6. In rare cases, cardiopulmonary bypass

Special attention must be paid to cardiac monitoring during the rewarming process because cardiac irritability may be a significant problem. Similarly, acid-base disturbances must be aggressively corrected while the patient is being rewarmed. Once in the operating room, measures noted earlier to keep the patient warm are applied.

## Malignant Hyperthermia

### Causes

Malignant hyperthermia (MH) is a life-threatening hypermetabolic crisis manifested during or after exposure to a triggering general anesthetic in susceptible individuals. It is estimated that MH occurs in 1 in 30,000 to 50,000 adults. Mortality from MH has decreased to less than 10% in the last 15 years as a result of improved monitoring standards that allow early detection of MH, availability of dantrolene, and increased use of susceptibility testing.

Susceptibility to MH is inherited as an autosomal dominant disease with variable penetrance. To date, two MH susceptibility genes have been identified in humans and four mapped to specific chromosomes but not definitely identified. The mutation results in altered calcium regulation in skeletal muscle in the form of enhanced efflux of calcium from the sarcoplasmic reticulum into the myoplasm. Halogenated inhalational anesthetic agents (e.g., halothane, enflurane, isoflurane, desflurane, and sevoflurane) and depolarizing muscle relaxants (e.g., succinylcholine, suxamethonium) cause a rise in the myoplasmic $Ca^{2+}$ concentration. When an MH-susceptible individual is exposed to a triggering anesthetic, there is abnormal release of $Ca^{2+}$, which leads to prolonged activation of muscle filaments, culminating in rigidity and hypermetabolism. Uncontrolled glycolysis and aerobic metabolism give rise to cellular hypoxia, progressive lactic acidosis, and hypercapnia. The continuous muscle activation with adenosine triphosphate breakdown results in excessive generation of heat. If untreated, myocyte death and rhabdomyolysis result in hyperkalemia and myoglobulinuria. Eventually, disseminated coagulopathy, congestive heart failure (CHF), bowel ischemia, and compartment syndrome develop.

### Presentation and Management

MH can be prevented by identifying at-risk individuals before surgery. MH susceptibility is suspected preoperatively in a patient with a family history of MH or a personal history of myalgia after exercise, a tendency for the development of fever, muscular disease, and intolerance to caffeine. In these cases, the creatine kinase level is checked, and a caffeine and halothane contraction test (or an in vitro contracture test developed in Europe) may be performed on a muscle biopsy specimen from the thigh.[10] MH-susceptible individuals confirmed by abnormal skeletal muscle biopsy findings or those with suspected MH susceptibility who decline a contracture test are given a trigger-free anesthetic (e.g., barbiturate, benzodiazepine, opioid, propofol, etomidate, ketamine, nitrous oxide, nondepolarizing neuromuscular blocker).

Unsuspected MH-susceptible individuals may manifest MH for the first time during or immediately after the administration of a triggering general anesthetic. The clinical manifestations of MH are not uniform and vary in onset and severity. Some patients manifest the abortive form of MH (e.g., tachycardia, arrhythmia, raised temperature, acidosis). Others, after intubation with succinylcholine, demonstrate loss of twitches on neuromuscular stimulation and develop muscle rigidity. An inability to open the mouth as a result of masseter muscle spasm is a pathognomonic early sign and indicates susceptibility to MH. Other manifestations include tachypnea, hypercapnia, skin flushing, hypoxemia, hypotension, electrolyte abnormalities, rhabdomyolysis, and hyperthermia.

**BOX 13-4 Management of Malignant Hyperthermia**

Discontinue the triggering anesthetic.
Hyperventilate the patient with 100% oxygen.
Administer alternative anesthesia.
Terminate surgery.
Give dantrolene, 2.5 mg/kg, as a bolus and repeat every 5 min, then 1 to 2 mg/kg/hr until normalization or disappearance of symptoms.
Check and monitor arterial blood gas and creatine kinase, electrolyte, lactate, and myoglobin levels.
Monitor the electrocardiogram, vital signs, and urine output.
Adjunctive and supportive measures are carried out:

- Volatile vaporizers are removed from the anesthesia machine.
- Carbon dioxide canisters, bellows, and gas hoses are changed.
- Surface cooling is achieved with ice packs and core cooling with cool parenteral fluids.
- Acidosis is monitored and treated with sodium bicarbonate.
- Arrhythmias are controlled with beta blockers or lidocaine.
- Urine output more than 2 mL/kg/hr is promoted; furosemide (Lasix) or mannitol and a glucose-insulin infusion (0.2 U/kg in a 50% glucose solution) are given for hyperkalemia, hypercalcemia, and myoglobulinuria.

The patient is transferred to the intensive care unit to monitor for recurrence.

Once MH is suspected or diagnosed, the steps outlined in Box 13-4 are followed. Dantrolene is a muscle relaxant. In the solution form, it is highly irritating to the vein and must be administered in a large vein. When given intravenously, it blocks up to 75% of skeletal muscle contraction and never causes paralysis. The plasma elimination half-life is 12 hours. Dantrolene is metabolized in the liver to 5-hydroxydantrolene, which also acts as a muscle relaxant. Side effects reported with dantrolene therapy include muscle weakness, phlebitis, respiratory failure, GI discomfort, hepatotoxicity, dizziness, confusion, and drowsiness. Another agent, azumolene, is 30 times more water-soluble than and equipotent to dantrolene in the treatment of MH; like dantrolene, it does not affect the heart. Its main side effect is marked pulmonary hypertension. However, azumolene is not in clinical use at this time.

## Postoperative Fever

### Causes

One of the most concerning clinical findings in a patient postoperatively is the development of fever. Fever describes a rise in core temperature, modulation of which is managed by the anterior hypothalamus. Fever may result from bacterial invasion or their toxins, which stimulate the production of cytokines. Trauma (including surgery) and critical illness also invoke a cytokine response. Cytokines are low-molecular-weight proteins that act in an autocrine, paracrine, and/or endocrine fashion to influence a broad range of cellular functions and exhibit proinflammatory and anti-inflammatory effects. The inflammatory

**BOX 13-5 Causes of Postoperative Fever**

| Infectious | Noninfectious |
|---|---|
| Abscess | Acute hepatic necrosis |
| Acalculous cholecystitis | Adrenal insufficiency |
| Bacteremia | Allergic reaction |
| Decubitus ulcers | Atelectasis |
| Device-related infections | Dehydration |
| Empyema | Drug reaction |
| Endocarditis | Head injury |
| Fungal sepsis | Hepatoma |
| Hepatitis | Hyperthyroidism |
| Meningitis | Lymphoma |
| Osteomyelitis | Myocardial infarction |
| Pseudomembranous colitis | Pancreatitis |
| Parotitis | Pheochromocytoma |
| Perineal infections | Pulmonary embolus |
| Peritonitis | Retroperitoneal hematoma |
| Pharyngitis | Solid organ hematoma |
| Pneumonia | Subarachnoid hemorrhage |
| Retained foreign body | Systemic inflammatory response syndrome |
| Sinusitis | Thrombophlebitis |
| Soft tissue infection | Transfusion reaction |
| Tracheobronchitis | Withdrawal syndromes |
| Urinary tract infection | Wound infection |

response results in the production of a variety of mediators that induce a febrile inflammatory response, also known as systemic inflammatory response syndrome.[11] Hence, fever in the postoperative period may be the result of an infection or caused by systemic inflammatory response syndrome. Fever after surgery is reported to occur in up to two thirds of patients, and infection is the cause of fever in approximately one third of cases. Numerous disease states can cause fever in the postoperative period (Box 13-5).

The most common infections, however, are health care–associated infections—SSI, urinary tract infection (UTI), intravascular catheter–related bloodstream infection (CR-BSI), and pneumonia. Urinary tract infection is a common postoperative event and a significant source of morbidity in postsurgical patients. A major predisposing factor is the presence of a urinary catheter; the risk increases with increased duration of catheterization (>2 days). Endogenous bacteria (colonic flora, most common *E. coli*) are the most common source of catheter-related urinary tract infection in patients with short-term catheterization. With prolonged catheterization, additional bacteria are found. In the critically ill surgical patient, candiduria accounts for approximately 10% of nosocomial urinary tract infections. The presence of an indwelling catheter, diabetes mellitus, use of antibiotics, advanced age, and underlying anatomic urologic abnormalities are risk factors for candiduria.[12]

The use of central venous catheters carries a risk of CR-BSI that increases hospital stay and morbidity and mortality. The infections are preventable and are considered a "never" complication by the Centers of Medicare and Medicaid Services.[13] CR-BSI results from microorganisms that colonize the hubs or from contamination of the injection site of the central venous catheter (intraluminal source) or skin surrounding the insertion site (extraluminal source). Coagulase-negative staphylococci, hospital-acquired bacteria (e.g., MRSA, multidrug-resistant gram-negative bacilli, fungal species [*Candida albicans*]) are the most common organisms responsible for CR-BSI. *S. aureus* bacteremia is associated with higher mortality and venous thrombosis. Metastatic infections (endocarditis) are uncommon but represent a serious complication of CR-BSI. The duration of central venous catheter placement, patient location (outpatient versus inpatient), type of catheter, number of lumens and manipulations daily, emergent placement, need for total parenteral nutrition (TPN), presence of unnecessary connectors, and whether best care practices are followed are risk factors for BSI.[14]

### Presentation and Management

In evaluating a patient with fever, one has to take into consideration the type of surgery performed, patient's immune status, underlying primary disease process, duration of hospital stay, and epidemiology of hospital infections.

High fever that fluctuates or is sustained and that occurs 5 to 8 days after surgery is more worrisome than fever that occurs early postoperatively. In the first 48 to 72 hours after abdominal surgery, atelectasis is often believed to be the cause of the fever. Occasionally, clostridial or streptococcal SSIs can manifest as fever within the first 72 hours of surgery. Temperatures that are elevated 5 to 8 days postoperatively demand immediate attention and, at times, intervention. Evaluation involves studying the six Ws: wind (lungs), wound, water (urinary tract), waste (lower GI tract), wonder drug (e.g., antibiotics), and walker (e.g., thrombosis). The patient's symptoms usually indicate the organ system involved with infection; cough and productive sputum suggest pneumonia, dysuria and frequency indicate a UTI, watery foul-smelling diarrhea develops as a result of infection with *C. difficile,* pain in the calf may be caused by deep venous thrombosis (DVT), and flank pain may be caused by pyelonephritis. Physical examination may show an SSI, phlebitis, tenderness on palpation of the abdomen, flank, or calf, or cellulitis at the site of a central venous catheter.

A complete blood count, urinalysis and culture, radiograph of the chest, and blood culture are essential initial tests. A chest radiograph may show a progressive infiltrate suggestive of the presence of pneumonia. Urinalysis showing more than $10^5$ colony-forming units/milliliter (CFU/mL) in a noncatheterized patient and more than $10^3$ CFU/mL in a catheterized patient indicates a urinary tract infection. The diagnosis of CR-BSI rests on culture data because physical examination is usually unrevealing. There is no gold standard for how to use blood cultures. Two simultaneous blood cultures or paired blood cultures (i.e., simultaneous peripheral and central blood cultures) are commonly used. Peripheral blood cultures showing bacteremia and isolation of 15 CFUs or $10^2$ CFUs from an IV catheter indicate the presence of a CR-BSI. In tunneled catheters, a quantitative colony count that is 5- to 10-fold higher in cultures drawn through the central venous catheter is predictive of CRC-BSI. If paired cultures are obtained, positive culture more than 2 hours before peripheral culture indicates the presence of CR-BSI. After removal of the catheter, the tip may be sent for quantitative culture. Serial blood cultures and a transesophageal echocardiogram are obtained in patients with *S. aureus* bacteremia and valvular heart disease, prosthetic valve, or new onset of murmur. Patients who continue to have fever, slow clinical progress, and no discernible external source may require computed tomography (CT) of the abdomen to look for an intra-abdominal source of infection.

Prevention of urinary tract infection starts with minimizing the duration of catheterization and maintenance of a closed drainage system. When prolonged catheterization is required, changing the catheter before blockage occurs is recommended because the catheter serves as a site for pathogens to create a biofilm. The efficacy of strategies to prevent or delay the formation of a biofilm, such as the use of silver alloy or impregnated catheters and the use of protamine sulfate and chlorhexidine in reducing catheter-related UTIs has yet to be established.[15]

On the other hand, most if not all CR-BSIs are preventable by adopting maximal barrier precautions and infection control practice during insertion. Educational programs that stress best practice that targets those placing the catheter and those responsible for maintenance of the catheter are important. Removal of catheters when they are not needed is paramount. On placing the catheter, there must be strict adherence to aseptic technique, the same as in the operating room—hand hygiene, skin antisepsis, full barrier precaution and stopping insertion when breaks in sterile technique occur. The subclavian vein is preferable to jugular and femoral vein. Involvement of a catheter care team for proper catheter care after insertion has proven effective in reducing the incidence of CR-BSIs. Antiseptic- and antibiotic-impregnated catheters decrease catheter colonization and CR-BSIs but their routine use is not recommended.

#### Treatment

Management of postoperative fevers is dictated by the results of a careful workup. Management of the elevated temperature itself is controversial. Although the fever may not be life-threatening, the patient is usually uncomfortable. Attempts to bring the temperature down with antipyretics are recommended. If pneumonia is suspected, empirical broad-spectrum antibiotic therapy is started and then altered according to culture results.

A UTI is treated with removal or replacement of the catheter with a new one. In systemically ill patients, broad-spectrum antibiotics are started, because most offending organisms exhibit resistance to several antibiotics, and then tailored according to culture and susceptibility results. In patients with asymptomatic bacteruria, antibiotics are recommended for immunocompromised patient, patients undergoing urologic surgery, implantation of a prosthesis, or patients with infections caused by strains with a high incidence of bacteremia. Patients with candiduria are managed in a similar fashion. The availability of fluconazole, a less toxic antifungal than amphotericin B, however, has encouraged clinicians to use it more frequently.

The treatment of CR-BSI entails removal of the catheter, with adjunctive antibiotic therapy. A nontunneled catheter can be easily removed after establishing an alternative venous access. Single-agent therapy is sufficient and usually involves vancomycin, linezolid, or empirical coverage of gram-negative bacilli and *Candida* spp. in patients with severe sepsis or immunosuppression. Treatment is continued for 10 to 14 days. For patients with septic thrombosis or endocarditis, treatment is continued for 4 to 6 weeks. Catheter salvage is indicated in patients with tunneled catheters that are risky to remove or replace, or in patients with coagulase-negative staphylococci who have no evidence of metastatic disease or severe sepsis, do not have tunnel infection, or do not have persistent bacteremia. Catheter salvage is achieved by antibiotic lock therapy whereby the catheter is filled with antibiotic solution for several hours.

## RESPIRATORY COMPLICATIONS

### General Considerations

A host of factors contribute to abnormal pulmonary physiology after an operative procedure. First, loss of functional residual capacity is present in almost all patients. This loss may be the result of a multitude of problems, including abdominal distention, painful upper abdominal incision, obesity, strong smoking history with associated chronic obstructive pulmonary disease, prolonged supine positioning, and fluid overload leading to pulmonary edema. Almost all patients who undergo an abdominal or thoracic incision have a significant alteration in their breathing pattern. Vital capacity may be reduced up to 50% of normal for the first 2 days after surgery for reasons that are not completely clear. The use of narcotics substantially inhibits the respiratory drive, and anesthetics may take some time to wear off. Most patients who have respiratory problems postoperatively have mild to moderate problems that can be managed with aggressive pulmonary toilet. However, in some patients, severe postoperative respiratory failure develops; this may require intubation and ultimately may be life-threatening.

Two types of respiratory failure are commonly described. Type I, or hypoxic, failure results from abnormal gas exchange at the alveolar level. This type is characterized by a low $Pa{O_2}$ with a normal $Pa{CO_2}$. Such hypoxemia is associated with ventilation-perfusion ($\dot{V}/\dot{Q}$) mismatching and shunting. Clinical conditions associated with type I failure include pulmonary edema and sepsis. Type II respiratory failure is associated with hypercapnia and is characterized by a low $Pa{O_2}$ and high $Pa{CO_2}$. These patients are unable to eliminate $CO_2$ adequately. This condition is often associated with excessive narcotic use, increased $CO_2$ production, altered respiratory dynamics, and adult respiratory distress syndrome (ARDS). The overall incidence of pulmonary complications exceeds 25% in surgical patients. Of all postoperative deaths, 25% are caused by pulmonary complications, and pulmonary complications are associated with 25% of the other lethal complications. Thus, it is of critical importance that the surgeon anticipate and prevent the occurrence of serious respiratory complications.

One of the most important elements of prophylaxis is careful preoperative screening of patients. Most patients have no pulmonary history and need no formal preoperative evaluation. However, all patients with a history of heavy smoking, maintained on home oxygen, unable to walk one flight of stairs without severe respiratory compromise, previous history of major lung resection, and older patients who are malnourished must be carefully screened with pulmonary function tests. Similarly, patients managed by chronic bronchodilator therapy for asthma or other pulmonary conditions also need to be assessed carefully. Although there is some controversy about the value of perioperative assessment, most careful clinicians will study a high-risk pulmonary patient before making an operative decision. The assessment may start with posteroanterior and lateral chest radiographs to evaluate the appearance of the lungs. It serves as a baseline if the patient should have problems postoperatively.

Similarly, a patient with polycythemia or chronic respiratory acidosis warrants careful assessment. A room temperature arterial blood gas analysis is carried out in high-risk patients. Any patient with a $PaO_2$ lower than 60 mm Hg is at increased risk. If the $PaCO_2$ is more than 45 to 50 mm Hg, perioperative morbidity might be anticipated. Spirometry is a simple test that high-risk patients undergo before surgery. Probably the most important parameter in spirometry is the forced expiratory volume in 1 second ($FEV_1$). Studies have demonstrated that any patient with an $FEV_1$ higher than 2 liters will probably not have serious pulmonary problems. Conversely, patients with an $FEV_1$ lower than 50% of the predicted value will probably have exertional dyspnea. If bronchodilator therapy demonstrates an improvement in breathing patterns by 15% or more, bronchodilation is considered. Consultation with the patient includes a discussion about cessation of cigarette smoking 48 hours before the operative procedure, as well as a careful discussion about the importance of pulmonary toilet after the operative procedure.

## Atelectasis and Pneumonia

The most common postoperative respiratory complication is atelectasis. As a result of the anesthetic, abdominal incision, and postoperative narcotics, the alveoli in the periphery collapse and a pulmonary shunt may occur. If appropriate attention is not directed to aggressive pulmonary toilet with the initial symptoms, the alveoli remain collapsed and a buildup of secretions occurs and becomes secondarily infected with bacteria, resulting in pneumonia. The risk appears to be particularly high in patients who are heavy smokers, are obese, and have copious pulmonary secretions.

Pneumonia is the most common nosocomial infection occurring in hospitalized patients. Pneumonia occurring more than 48 hours after admission and without antecedent signs of infection is referred to as hospital-acquired pneumonia. Aspiration of oropharyngeal secretion is a significant contributing factor in its development. Extended intubation results in another subset of hospital-acquired pneumonia, ventilator-associated pneumonia—pneumonia occurring 48 hours after but within 72 hours of the initiation of ventilation. Health care–associated pneumonia refers to pneumonia occurring in patients who had been hospitalized in the last 90 days, patients in nursing facilities or frequenting a hemodialysis unit, and those who have received recent antibiotics, chemotherapy, or wound care. Although some consider hospital-acquired pneumonia and health care–associated pneumonia to be the same disease process, because both have the same prevalent organisms, the prognosis is different. Hospital-acquired pneumonia arising early (<5 days) has better prognosis than that arising late (>5 days). Numerous factors are associated with increased risk for pneumonia: depressed immune status, concomitant disease, poor nutritional status, increased length of hospital stay, smoking, increasing age, uremia, alcohol consumption, prior antibiotic therapy, presence of an endotracheal, nasogastric (NG), or enteric tube, and therapeutic proton pump inhibitor (PPI). Used to prevent stress ulceration, PPI increases colonization of the stomach with pathogenic bacteria that can increase the risk of ventilator-associated pneumonia. Tubes traversing the aerodigestive tract serve as conduits for bacteria to migrate to the lower respiratory tract.[16] The most common pathogens encountered in patients with hospital-acquired pneumonia depend on prior antibiotic therapy. In patients with early hospital-acquired pneumonia and no prior antibiotic therapy, the most common organisms are *Streptococcus pneumoniae* (colonizes upper airway), *Haemophilus influenzae, Enterobacteriaceae* spp. (*E. coli, Klebsiella* spp., and *Enterobacter* spp.), and *S. aureus* (mostly MRSA). Patients with early hospital-acquired pneumonia and recent antibiotic therapy and those with late hospital-acquired pneumonia also have gram-negative bacilli involved. The bacteria are occasionally resistant to first-generation cephalosporins. The organisms in patients with late-onset hospital-acquired pneumonia and prior history of antibiotics exhibit multidrug resistance (*P. aeruginosa, Acinetobacter baumannii,* and MRSA).

### Diagnosis

The most common cause of a postoperative fever in the first 48 hours after the procedure is atelectasis. Patients present with a low-grade fever, malaise, and diminished breath sounds in the lower lung fields. Frequently, the patient is uncomfortable from the fever but has no other overt pulmonary symptoms. Atelectasis is so common postoperatively that a formal workup is not usually required. With the use of incentive spirometry, deep breathing, and coughing, most cases of atelectasis will resolve without any difficulty. However, if aggressive pulmonary toilet is not instituted or the patient refuses to participate, frank development of pneumonia is likely. The patient with pneumonia will have a high fever and occasional mental confusion, and produces a thick secretion with coughing, leukocytosis, and chest radiograph that reveals infiltrates. If the patient is not expeditiously diagnosed and treated, this condition may rapidly progress to respiratory failure and require intubation. Concurrently with the initiation of aggressive pulmonary toilet, induced sputum for culture and sensitivity should be sent immediately to the laboratory. Quantitative cultures of the lower airways obtained by blind tracheobronchial aspiration, bronchoscopically guided sampling (bronchoalveolar lavage [BAL]), or protected specimen brush allow more targeted antibiotic therapy and, most importantly, decrease antibiotic use. Although pneumonia acquired in the hospital accounts for only 5% of all patients, particularly in older patients, the process may rapidly progress to frank respiratory failure requiring intubation.

### Treatment

To prevent atelectasis and pneumonia, smokers are encouraged to stop smoking for at least 1 week before surgery and the treatment of patients with chronic obstructive pulmonary disease, asthma, and CHF is optimized. Adequate pain control and proper pulmonary hygiene are important in the postoperative period. A patient-controlled analgesia device seems to be associated with better pulmonary toilet, as does the use of an epidural infusion catheter, particularly in patients with epigastric incisions. Encouraging the patient to use the incentive spirometer and cough while applying counterpressure with a pillow on the abdominal incision site is most helpful. Rarely, other modalities such as intermittent positive-pressure breathing and chest physiotherapy may be required. Patients on the ventilator are best kept in a semirecumbent position and subjected to proper oral hygiene. Chlorhexidine rinse or nasal gel has been shown to lower the rate of ventilator-associated pneumonia. Treatment with sucralfate as compared with a PPI for stress ulcer prophylaxis may be considered for patients not at high risk for GI bleeding. Proper endotracheal tube care, elimination of secretions pooling around the endotracheal cuff, frequent suctioning with a closed suction technique, and use of protocols designed to minimize mechanical ventilation can lead to decreased ventilator-associated pneumonia. Once the diagnosis is made, and while awaiting culture results, treatment with empirical antibiotic therapy is associated with decreased mortality. The choice of antimicrobial agent depends on the patient's risk factors, length of hospital stay, duration of mechanical ventilation, prior antibiotic therapy and culture results, and immunosuppression.

## Aspiration Pneumonitis and Aspiration Pneumonia

### Causes

Aspiration of oropharyngeal or gastric contents into the respiratory tract is a serious complication of surgery. Aspiration pneumonitis (Mendelson's syndrome) describes acute lung injury that results from the inhalation of regurgitated gastric contents, whereas aspiration pneumonia results from the inhalation of oropharyngeal secretions that are colonized by pathogenic bacteria. Although there is some overlap between the two disease entities with regard to predisposing factors, their clinicopathologic features are distinct.

Factors that predispose patients to regurgitation and aspiration include impairment of the esophageal sphincters (upper and lower) and laryngeal reflexes, altered GI motility, and absence of preoperative fasting. A number of iatrogenic maneuvers place the patient at increased risk for aspiration in a hospital setting. In the perioperative period, aspiration is more likely with urgent surgery, in patients with altered levels of consciousness, and in patients with GI and airway problems. Trauma patients and patients with peritonitis and bowel obstruction may have a depressed level of consciousness and airway reflexes, a full stomach as a result of a recent meal or gastric stasis, or GI pathology that predisposes to retrograde emptying of intestinal contents into the stomach. Patients with depressed levels of consciousness as a result of high doses of narcotics and patients who have suffered cerebrovascular accidents are obtunded and have neurologic dysphagia and dysfunction of the gastroesophageal junction. Anesthetic drugs lower esophageal sphincter tone and depress the patient's level of consciousness. Diabetics have gastroparesis and gastric stasis. Patients with an increased bacterial load in the oropharynx and depressed defense mechanisms as a result of an altered level of consciousness are at risk for aspiration pneumonia.

Older adults are particularly susceptible to oropharyngeal aspiration because of an increased incidence of dysphagia and poor oral hygiene. Patients with a NG tube or who are debilitated are also at risk for aspiration because they have difficulty swallowing and clearing their airway. The risk for aspiration pneumonia is similar in patients receiving feeding via an NG, nasoenteric, or gastrostomy tube; patients receiving nutrition via a gastrostomy tube frequently have scintigraphic evidence of aspiration of gastric contents. The critically ill are at an increased risk for aspiration and aspiration pneumonia because they are in a supine position, have an NG tube in place, exhibit gastroesophageal reflux, even with the absence of an NG tube, and have altered GI motility. Prophylactic histamine 2 ($H_2$) receptor antagonists or PPIs that increase gastric pH and allow the gastric contents to become colonized by pathogenic organisms, tracheostomy, reintubation, and previous antibiotic exposure are other factors associated with an increased risk for health care–related pneumonia. The risk of aspiration is high after extubation because of the residual effect of sedation, the NG tube, and oropharyngeal dysfunction.

The pathophysiology of aspiration pneumonitis is related to the pulmonary intake of gastric contents at a low pH associated with particulate matter. The severity of lung injury increases as the volume of aspirate increases and its pH decreases. The process often progresses rapidly, may require intubation soon after the injury occurs, and later sets the stage for bacterial infection. The infection is refractory to management because of the combination of infection occurring in an injured field. The pathophysiology of aspiration pneumonia is related to bacteria gaining access to the lungs.

### Presentation and Diagnosis

A patient with aspiration pneumonitis often has associated vomiting and may have received general anesthesia or had an NG tube placed. The patient may be obtunded or have altered levels of consciousness. Initially, the patient may have associated wheezing and labored respiration. Many patients who aspirate gastric contents have a cough or a wheeze. Some patients, however, have silent aspiration suggested by an infiltrate on a chest radiograph (CXR) or decreased $PaO_2$. Others have cough, shortness of breath, and wheezing that progress to pulmonary edema and ARDS. In the great majority of patients with aspiration pneumonia, on the other hand, in a susceptible patient, the condition is diagnosed after a chest radiograph shows an infiltrate in the posterior segments of the upper lobes and the apical segments of the lower lobes.

### Treatment

Prevention of aspiration in patients undergoing surgery is achieved by instituting measures that reduce gastric contents, minimize regurgitation, and protect the airway. For adults, a period of no oral intake, usually 6 hours after a night meal, 4 hours after clear liquids, and a longer period for diabetics, is necessary to reduce gastric contents before elective surgery.[17] Routine use of $H_2$ antagonists or PPIs to reduce gastric acidity and volume has not been shown to be effective in reducing the mortality and morbidity associated with aspiration and hence is not recommended. When a difficult airway is encountered, awake fiberoptic intubation is performed. In emergency situations in patients with a potentially full stomach, preoxygenation is accomplished without lung inflation, and intubation is performed after applying cricoid pressure during rapid-sequence induction. In the postoperative period, identification of an older or overly sedated patient, or a patient whose condition is deteriorating, mandates instituting maneuvers to protect the patient's airway. Postoperatively, it is important to avoid the overuse of narcotics, encourage the patient to ambulate, and cautiously feed a patient who is obtunded, older, or debilitated.

A patient who sustains aspiration of gastric contents needs to be placed on oxygen immediately and have a chest radiograph to confirm the clinical suspicions. A diffuse interstitial pattern is usually seen bilaterally and is often described as bilateral, fluffy infiltrates. Close surveillance of the patient is absolutely essential. If the patient is maintaining oxygen saturation via a face mask without excessively high work of breathing, intubation may not be required. However, if the patient's oxygenation deteriorates or the patient is obtunded, the work of breathing increases, as manifested by an increased respiratory rate, and prompt intubation must be accomplished. After intubation for suspected aspiration, suctioning the bronchopulmonary tree will confirm the diagnosis and remove any particulate matter. Administration of antibiotics shortly after aspiration is controversial, except in patients with bowel obstruction or other conditions associated with colonization of gastric contents. Administration of empirical antibiotics is also indicated for a patient with aspiration pneumonitis that does not resolve or improve within 48 hours of aspiration. Corticosteroid administration does not provide any beneficial effects to patients with aspiration pneumonitis. Antibiotic therapy with activity against gram-negative organisms is indicated for patients with aspiration pneumonia.

## Pulmonary Edema, Acute Lung Injury, and Adult Respiratory Distress Syndrome

### Causes

A wide variety of injuries to the lungs or cardiovascular system, or both, may result in acute respiratory failure. Three of the most common manifestations of such injury are pulmonary edema, acute lung injury, and ARDS. The clinician's ability to recognize and distinguish among these conditions is of critical importance because clinical management of these three entities varies considerably.

Pulmonary edema is a condition associated with accumulation of fluid in the alveoli. As a result of the fluid in the lumen of the alveoli, oxygenation cannot take place and hypoxemia occurs. As a consequence, the patient must increase the work of breathing, including an increased respiratory rate and exaggerated use of the muscles of breathing. Pulmonary edema is usually caused by increased vascular hydrostatic pressure associated with CHF and acute myocardial infarction (MI). It is also commonly associated with fluid overload as a result of overly aggressive resuscitation (Box 13-6).

A consensus conference has identified acute lung injury and ARDS as two separate grades of respiratory failure secondary to injury. In contrast to pulmonary edema, which is associated with increased wedge and right-sided heart pressure, acute lung injury and ARDS are associated with hypo-oxygenation because of a pathophysiologic inflammatory response that leads to the accumulation of fluid in the alveoli, as well as thickening in the space between the capillaries and the alveoli. Acute lung injury is associated with a $PaO_2/FIO_2$ (fraction of inspired oxygen) ratio of less than 300, bilateral infiltrates on chest radiography, and a wedge pressure less than 18 mm Hg. It tends to be shorter in duration and not as severe. On the other hand, ARDS is associated with a $PaO_2/FIO_2$ ratio of less than 200 and also has bilateral infiltrates and a wedge pressure less than 18 mm Hg.

**BOX 13-6 Conditions Leading to Pulmonary Edema, Acute Lung Injury, and Adult Respiratory Distress Syndrome**

**Increased Hydrostatic Pressure**
Acute left ventricular failure
Chronic congestive heart failure
Obstruction of the left ventricular outflow tract
Thoracic lymphatic insufficiency
Volume overload

**Altered Permeability State**
Acute radiation pneumonitis
Aspiration of gastric contents
Drug overdose
Near-drowning
Pancreatitis
Pneumonia
Pulmonary embolus
Shock states
Systemic inflammatory response syndrome and multiple organ failure
Sepsis
Transfusion
Trauma and burns

**Mixed or Incompletely Understood Pathogenesis**
Hanging injuries
High-altitude pulmonary edema
Narcotic overdose
Neurogenic pulmonary edema
Postextubation obstructive pulmonary edema
Reexpansion pulmonary edema
Tocolytic therapy
Uremia

### Presentation and Management

Patients with pulmonary edema often have a corresponding cardiac history, recent history of massive fluid administration, or both. In the presence of a frankly abnormal chest radiograph, invasive monitoring in the form of a Swan-Ganz catheter for evaluation of pulmonary capillary wedge pressure may be indicated. Patients with an elevated wedge pressure are managed by fluid restriction and aggressive diuresis. Administration of oxygen via face mask in mild cases and intubation in more severe cases is also clinically indicated. In most cases, the pulmonary edema resolves quickly after diuresis and fluid restriction.

Patients with acute lung injury and ARDS generally have tachypnea, dyspnea, and increased work of breathing, as manifested by exaggerated use of the muscles of breathing. Cyanosis is associated with advanced hypoxia and is an emergency. Auscultation of the lung fields reveals poor breath sounds associated with crackles and, occasionally, with rales. Arterial blood gas analysis will reveal the presence of a low $PaO_2$ and high $PaCO_2$. Administration of oxygen alone does not usually result in improvement in the hypoxia.

In patients with impending respiratory failure, including tachypnea, dyspnea, and air hunger, management of acute lung injury and ARDS is initiated by immediate intubation plus careful administration of fluids; invasive monitoring with a Swan-Ganz catheter to assess wedge pressure and right-sided heart pressure is occasionally helpful. The strategy involves maintaining the patient on the ventilator with assisted breathing while the injured lung heals. A patient with severe acute lung injury or ARDS is initially placed on an $FIO_2$ of 100% and then weaned to 60% as healing takes place. Positive end-expiratory pressure is a valuable addition to ventilator management of

**Table 13-4 Criteria for Weaning from the Ventilator**

| PARAMETER | WEANING CRITERIA |
|---|---|
| Respiratory rate | <25 breaths/min |
| $Pa_{O_2}$ | >70 mm Hg ($F_{IO_2}$ of 40%) |
| $Pa_{CO_2}$ | <45 mm Hg |
| Minute ventilation | 8-9 liters/min |
| Tidal volume | 5-6 mL/kg |
| Negative inspiratory force | −25 cm $H_2O$ |

patients with this injury. Similarly, tidal volume needs to be 6 to 8 mL/kg, with peak pressure kept at 35 cm $H_2O$. Tidal volume is set at 10 to 12 mL/kg of body weight and the respiratory rate is chosen to produce a $Pa_{CO_2}$ near 40 mm Hg. In addition, the inspiratory-to-expiratory ratio is set at 1 : 2. Most patients will require heavy sedation and pharmacologic paralysis during the early phases of recuperation.

Careful monitoring of oxygenation, improvement of the respiratory rate with intermittent mandatory ventilation, and general alertness will suggest when the patient is ready to be extubated. Criteria for extubation are listed in Table 13-4.

## Pulmonary Embolism and Venous Thromboembolism

### Causes

Venous thromboembolism describes DVT and pulmonary embolism (PE). PE is a serious postoperative complication that represents a source of preventable morbidity and mortality in the United States and is responsible for 5% to 10% of all in-hospital deaths. Undiagnosed PE has a hospital mortality rate as high as 30%, which falls to 8% if diagnosed and treated appropriately.

Venous thromboembolism (VTE) is caused by a perturbation of the homeostatic coagulation system induced by intimal injury, stasis of blood flow, and a hypercoagulable state. Risk factors for the development of VTE are listed in Table 13-5.[18]

Thrombophilia describes hereditary and acquired biochemical states that predispose to VTE. One in four fatal PE cases occurs in surgical patients. Survivors of VTE are at increased risk for recurrence. The highest risk of VTE occurs in patients hospitalized for surgery. The prevalence of PE in patients with malignancy is 11%. The incidence of relative risk of DVT and PE in patients with inflammatory bowel disease is approximately 5% and 3%, respectively. In major trauma victims, the incidence of DVT exceeds 50%, with fatal emboli occurring in 0.4% to 2% of cases. Critically ill and intensive care unit patients have multiple risk factors and are also at higher risk for VTE. Central venous catheter–related thromboses are more common with femoral placement. Thrombosis ranges from 4% to 28% after subclavian vein cannulation and 4% to 33% after internal jugular catheterization. In patients with subclavian or axillary vein thrombosis, PE is reported in 9.4%.

Most PEs originate from an existing DVT in the legs, and the iliofemoral venous system represents the site from which most clinically significant pulmonary emboli arise. Approximately 50% of patients with proximal DVT develop a PE. Rare causes of PE include a fat embolus associated with fractures of long bones and air embolism, often related to operative procedures and the presence of central lines.

**Table 13-5 Risk Factors for Venous Thromboembolism**

| CATEGORY | FACTORS |
|---|---|
| General factors | Advancing age<br>Hospitalization or nursing home (with or without surgery)<br>Indwelling venous catheters<br>Neurologic disease (plegia and paresis)<br>Cardiomyopathy, myocardial infarction, or heart failure secondary to valve disease<br>Acute pulmonary disease (adult respiratory distress syndrome and pneumonia)<br>Chronic obstructive lung disease<br>Varicose veins |
| Inherited thrombophilia | Protein C deficiency<br>Protein S deficiency<br>Antithrombin III deficiency<br>Dysfibrinogenemia<br>Factor V Leiden mutation<br>Prothrombin gene mutation<br>Hyperhomocysteinemia<br>Anticardiolipin antibody<br>Paroxysmal nocturnal hemoglobinemia |
| Acquired thrombophilia | Malignancy<br>Inflammatory bowel disease<br>Heparin-induced thrombocytopenia<br>Trauma<br>Major surgery<br>Pregnancy/postpartum<br>Nephrotic syndrome<br>Behçet's syndrome<br>Systemic lupus erythematosus<br>History of venous thromboembolism |

**BOX 13-7 Symptoms and Signs of Pulmonary Embolism**

Pleuritic chest pain*
Sudden dyspnea*
Tachypnea
Hemoptysis*
Tachycardia*
Leg swelling*
Pain on palpation of the leg*
Acute right ventricular dysfunction
Hypoxia
Fourth heart sound*
Loud second pulmonary sound*
Inspiratory crackles*

*More common with pulmonary embolism.

### Presentation and Diagnosis

The physiologic response to PE depends on the size of the thrombus, coexisting cardiopulmonary disease, and various neurohormonal effects. More than 50% of DVTs are silent and PE may be the first manifestation of the disease. Most symptoms and signs associated with symptomatic PE are nonspecific and may be encountered with other disease states, such as MI, pneumothorax, and pneumonia (Box 13-7). CXR has limited value in the diagnosis of PE and is mainly used to rule out other causes of a patient's symptoms. Approximately 5% to 10% of patients develop a massive PE that results in hemodynamic instability (hypotension, with or without shock) and death. The probability of an individual having PE (pretest probability) is assessed by the sum of points given to VTE risk factors: the patient's symptoms, signs, and laboratory results (e.g., electrocardiogram [ECG], CXR, and arterial blood gas) most likely to be associated with PE. Using various scoring systems, patients are stratified into low-, moderate-, and high-probability categories.

Establishing the diagnosis of PE requires confirmatory tests (helical CT scan and/or a pulmonary angiogram) and ancillary tests (venous duplex ultrasound [VUS] and a D-dimer assay). Helical CT, also known as spiral CT or CT pulmonary angiography, has high specificity (92%) and sensitivity (86%), especially for central PE (main pulmonary artery or subsegmental branches) and has replaced the $\dot{V}/\dot{Q}$ scan as the initial test of choice. In addition to the findings listed in Box 13-7, spiral CT also allows diagnosis of other pulmonary causes of a patient's symptoms. The test, however, requires IV contrast, may not be available after normal working hours, requires a cooperative patient to avoid artifacts, may miss emboli in subsegmental arteries, which account for 20% of all pulmonary emboli, and may be inconclusive in approximately 10% of cases. Pulmonary angiogram is the gold standard test because it visualizes the arterial tree directly and detects intravascular filling defects. It is used less commonly, however, because it is invasive, requires expertise, and after-hours availability is limited.

Echocardiography is a rapid, noninvasive, available bedside test that provides quick results in a critically ill or hemodynamically unstable patient. Transthoracic echocardiography (TTE) shows the hemodynamic consequences of acute ventricular pressure overload—namely, right ventricle dysfunction (hypokinesia and dilation), interventricular septal flattening and paradoxical motion, elevated tricuspid gradient, pulmonary hypertension, and a patent foramen ovale.[19] Dysfunction of the right ventricle (RV) occurs in 30% to 50% of patients with PE who undergo echocardiography. The transesophageal echocardiogram also shows secondary changes in cardiac chamber size and functions caused by hemodynamic effects of the PE and may reveal a proximal intrapulmonary or free-floating intracardiac clot. Echocardiography also rules out other causes of shock such as a pericardial tamponade. Transesophageal echocardiography is not always available and requires specialty training.

VUS of the extremities is used as an indirect test for diagnosing PE. Approximately one third of patients with PE will demonstrate lower extremity findings consistent with DVT, and 80% of PE patients have a DVT on the venogram. D-dimer is a degradation product of a cross-linked fibrin blood clot. Levels are typically elevated in patients with acute thromboembolism. Of the many D-dimer tests, enzyme-linked immunosorbent assay (ELISA) is the most sensitive, with quick results. A negative test excludes the diagnosis, but a positive test does not rule in the diagnosis.

Based on the pretest clinical probability, a patient suspected of having PE requires a CXR, ECG, arterial blood gas (ABG) analysis, and D-dimer assay. If leg symptoms are present, VUS is performed and, if positive, the patient is considered to have PE and receives anticoagulant medication because treatment is similar to that for PE. If leg symptoms are absent, the spiral CT approach may be used. If the findings on spiral CT are suboptimal or negative and there is a high clinical probability of PE, an angiogram is obtained. This approach is not appropriate for patients with iodinated dye allergy.

In critically ill patients with high suspicion for PE and patients with suspected massive PE, the workup depends on their hemodynamic stability. In stable patients, anticoagulation is started if there are no contraindications, VUS is performed, and a spiral CT scan is obtained urgently. In unstable patients, anticoagulation is started and VUS and echocardiography are performed. If the echocardiographic results are positive, thrombolytic therapy is started and, if negative, a pulmonary angiogram is obtained.

### Treatment

Medications used in the treatment of venous thromboembolism are the heparins, fondaparinux, VKAs, and thrombolytic agents. Heparin prevents the thrombin-mediated conversion of fibrinogen to fibrin and stops propagation of the thrombus. UFH is inexpensive and highly effective, enhances antithrombotic activity of antithrombin III and factor Xa, and has a short plasma half-life. LMWH primarily inactivates factor Xa and has a longer half-life and more predictable anticoagulant property. VKAs (e.g., warfarin) have a delayed onset of action and the potential to interact with other medications. Fondaparinux is a synthetic pentasaccharide that selectively inhibits factor Xa. Thrombolytic agents (e.g., streptokinase, urokinase, recombinant tissue plasminogen activator) are used in the treatment of massive PE.

Treatment of PE starts with prevention. Because the great majority of PEs originates from existing clots in the deep venous system of the legs in at-risk patients, identifying patients at risk for DVT plus applying preventive measures is the only way to decrease VTE-related morbidity and mortality. The intensity of prophylaxis must match the risk for VTE and potential complications of the medication (e.g., bleeding, heparin-induced thrombocytopenia [HITT]). According to the American College of Clinical Pharmacy (ACCP), assessment of patients into low-, moderate- and high-risk categories for VTE is based on the type of surgery performed, patient mobility, risk of bleeding, and VTE risk based on the presence of additional risk factors.[20] Age is a significant risk factor, with the risk doubling with each decade beyond the age of 40 years. Most hospitalized patients have at least one risk factor for VTE and approximately 50% of them have more than three risk factors. Pharmacologic prophylaxis is an accepted and effective strategy.[21] In the critically ill, heparin is first-line prophylaxis. Prophylaxis is achieved with the administration of low-dose UFH given SC every 8 hours or LMWH given as a daily dose. Recent studies have suggested that LMWH is more effective prophylaxis than low-dose UFH (LDUF) in the critically ill and is associated a with reduced risk of major hemorrhage. Overt bleeding and thrombocytopenia are contraindications to chemical prophylaxis. In patients undergoing surgery, LDUF is administered (5000 U, 3 to 4 hours preoperatively and then every 8 hours). Fondaparinux has emerged as an alternative prophylactic after major orthopedic surgery. Nonpharmacologic prophylaxis can be achieved with elastic stockings, graduated compression stockings, intermittent pneumatic compression devices, or venous foot pumps. Compression devices are not associated with bleeding. They produce a satisfactory reduction in risk for DVT in high-risk surgical patients. However, little is known about their efficacy as sole prophylaxis in the critically ill and they may be most beneficial in combination with pharmacologic prophylaxis in the subset of high-risk patients or solely in patients for whom the risk of bleeding is high. The presence of leg ulcers and peripheral vascular disease precludes the use of mechanical devices.

Anticoagulation is the standard of care treatment for VTE. It prevents clot propagation and allows endogenous fibrinolytic activity to dissolve existing thrombi, a process that occurs over weeks and months. Incomplete resolution is not uncommon and predisposes to recurrent VTE. The initial treatment is with LMWH, UFH, or fondaparinux, followed by VKA, which is administered on the same day as LMWH or UFH, with overlap for 5 days or longer until the target INR is achieved. In patients with VTE and active cancer, anticoagulation is continued indefinitely. Surgical patients within 24 hours of surgery may be considered for a retrievable inferior vena cava filter until anticoagulation is initiated. In patients with a contraindication to anticoagulation, placement of an inferior vena cava filter protects against PE.

UFH is given intravenously (a weight-adjusted bolus of 70 U/kg is followed by 1000 U/hr) to achieve a partial thromboplastin time 1.5 to 2 times the control value. aPTT is determined 6 hours after the loading dose and then on a daily basis, and the dose of heparin is adjusted accordingly. UFH is easily reversible and hence the agent of choice. LMWH is given SC once or twice daily (enoxaparin, 1.5 mg/kg/day, or dalteparin, 10,000 to 18,000 U/day, depending on weight). Monitoring of LMWH is not necessary. Both UFH and LMWH may be associated with HITT, and therefore the platelet count is monitored between days 3 and 5. Warfarin is given orally and this therapy is allowed to overlap with heparin therapy until the INR is therapeutic for 2 consecutive days before heparin is discontinued. Therapy is continued for more than 3 months, with the goal to reach an INR of 2.5.

In massive PE, the goal of therapy is to maintain hemodynamic stability, enhance coronary flow, and minimize right ventricular ischemia. Once suspected, resuscitation is initiated, oxygen administered, and IV UFH therapy started. In the hemodynamically unstable, IV vasoactive medications are required. Thrombolytic therapy, if not contraindicated, has the advantage of dissolving the clot rapidly, with rapid improvement in pulmonary perfusion, hemodynamic alterations, gas exchange, and right ventricular function. The role of surgical embolectomy is controversial. The transcatheter technique (with or without low-dose thrombolytic therapy) is another therapeutic approach. Placement of an inferior vena cava filter reduces the risk for recurrence of PE.

Novel anticoagulants under investigation include factor Xa inhibitors (direct inhibitor [hypermethylated derivative of fondaparinux with a long half-life given IV or SC] or indirect inhibitor mediated by antithrombin [given orally or parenterally]) and direct thrombin inhibitors.

## CARDIAC COMPLICATIONS

### Postoperative Hypertension

#### Causes

Hypertension is a serious problem that can cause devastating complications in the preoperative, intraoperative, and postoperative periods. Perioperative hypertension (or hypotension) occurs in 25% of patients undergoing surgery. The risk of hypertension is related to the type of surgery performed and the presence of perioperative hypertension. Cardiovascular, thoracic, and intra-abdominal procedures are most commonly associated with hypertensive events. Preoperatively, most hypertension is essential hypertension; much less common are cases associated with renovascular causes and, even rarer, vasoactive tumors. Intraoperatively, fluid overload and pharmacologic agents may cause hypertension. Postoperatively, a host of causative factors are associated with hypertension, including pain, hypothermia, hypoxia, fluid overload in the postanesthesia period caused by fluid mobilization from the extravascular compartment, and discontinuation of chronic antihypertensive therapy before surgery. Other causes of postoperative hypertension include intra-abdominal bleeding, head trauma, clonidine withdrawal syndrome, and pheochromocytoma crisis.

#### Presentation and Management

Most cases of hypertension are detected during the routine preoperative workup. The observant surgeon will consider hypertension in the preoperative screening of patients, recognizing that failure to detect significant problems with hypertension can lead to needless hypertension-related complications. By definition, any patient who has a diastolic blood pressure higher than 110 mm Hg must be assessed and treated preoperatively if elective surgery is being contemplated. Patients taking chronic antihypertensive medications who are undergoing elective surgery are instructed to continue taking the medication up to the day of surgery. Patients receiving oral clonidine can be switched to a clonidine patch for at least 3 days before surgery. In emergency cases, the medications administered during induction and maintenance of anesthesia will assist in bringing the blood pressure down. Intraoperatively, the anesthesiologist must carefully monitor blood pressure, make certain that it stays within acceptable limits, and avoid fluid overload, hypoxia, and hypothermia. In the postoperative period, the patient is given adequate analgesia for pain control and long-term antihypertensive medications are resumed. In patients who are not able to take oral medications, beta blockers, angiotensin-converting enzyme (ACE) inhibitors, calcium channel antagonists, or diuretics are given parenterally or clonidine is administered as a transdermal patch.

Although hypertension in the postoperative period is common, a hypertensive crisis is uncommon, especially after noncardiac surgery. A hypertensive crisis is characterized by severe elevation of blood pressure associated with organ dysfunction—cerebral and subarachnoid hemorrhage and stroke, acute cardiac events, renal dysfunction, and bleeding from the operative wound. This particularly appears to be the case in carotid endarterectomy, aortic aneurysm surgery, and many head and neck procedures. Diastolic hypertension (>110 mm Hg) is significantly associated with cardiac complications and systolic hypertension (>160 mm Hg) is associated with an increased risk for stroke and death. In patients with new-onset or severe perioperative hypertension and patients with a hypertensive emergency, treatment with agents that have a rapid onset of action, short half-life, and few autonomic side effects to lower blood pressure is essential. Medications most commonly used in this setting include nitroprusside and nitroglycerin (vasodilators), labetalol and esmolol (beta blockers), enalaprilat (useful for patients receiving long-term ACE inhibitors), and nicardipine (calcium channel blocker). It is crucial in the acute setting not to decrease blood pressure more than 25% to avoid ischemic strokes and hypoperfusion injury to other organs.

## Perioperative Ischemia and Infarction

### Cause

Approximately 30% of all patients taken to the operating room have some degree of CAD. Older patients, patients with peripheral artery disease, and those undergoing vascular, thoracic, major orthopedic, or upper abdominal procedures are at high risk for an acute coronary syndrome in the postoperative period. Major risk factors for developing CAD are smoking, family history, adverse lipid profiles, diabetes mellitus, and elevated blood pressure.[22] Although management of nonoperative MI has improved, the mortality associated with perioperative MI remains approximately 30%. Perioperative myocardial complications result in at least 10% of all perioperative deaths. In the 1970s, the risk for recurrence of MI within 3 months of an MI was reported to be 30% and, if a patient underwent surgery within 3 to 6 months of infarction, the reinfarction rate was 15%; 6 months postoperatively the reinfarction rate was only 5%. However, improved preoperative assessment, advances in anesthesia and intraoperative monitoring, and the availability of more sophisticated intensive care unit monitoring have resulted in improvement in the outcome of patients at risk for an acute cardiac event. Individuals undergoing an operation within 3 months of an infarction have an 8% to 15% reinfarction rate; between 3 and 6 months postoperatively, the reinfarction rate is only 3.5%. The general mortality associated with MI in patients without a surgical procedure is 12%.

Myocardial ischemia and MI result from the imbalance between myocardial oxygen supply and demand. Primary causes that reduce myocardial perfusion and therefore oxygen supply include coronary artery narrowing caused by a thrombus that develops on a disrupted atherosclerotic plaque, dynamic obstruction caused by spasm of an epicardial coronary artery or diseased blood vessel, and severe narrowing caused by progressive atherosclerosis. Secondary causes that increase myocardial oxygen requirements, usually in the presence of a fixed restricted oxygen supply (limited myocardial perfusion), are extrinsic cardiac factors that include fever and tachycardia (increased myocardial oxygen demand), hypotension (reduced coronary blood flow), and anemia and hypoxemia (reduced myocardial oxygen delivery). The increased circulating catecholamines associated with surgical stress further increase myocardial oxygen demand.

### Presentation and Diagnosis

Acute coronary syndrome refers to a constellation of clinical symptoms that are compatible with myocardial ischemia and encompasses MI: ST-segment elevation myocardial infarction (STEMI) and depression (Q wave and non–Q wave), and unstable angina (UA)/non–ST-segment elevation myocardial infarction (NSTEMI). UA/NSTEMI is defined as ST-segment depression or prominent T wave inversion and/or positive biomarkers of myonecrosis in the absence of ST-segment elevation and in an appropriate clinical setting. The risk for myocardial ischemia and MI is greatest in the first 48 hours after surgery, and it may be difficult to make the diagnosis. The classic manifestation, chest pain radiating into the jaw and left arm region, is often not present. Patients may have shortness of breath, increased heart rate, hypotension, or respiratory failure. Perioperative myocardial ischemia and MI are often silent and, when they occur, are marked by shortness of breath (heart failure, respiratory failure), increased heart rate (arrhythmias), change in mental status, or excessive hyperglycemia in diabetics. Many perioperative MIs are non–Q wave NSTEMI. Periprocedural MI is associated with the release of biomarkers of necrosis, such as MB isoenzymes of creatinine kinase (CK-MB) and troponins, into the circulation. The troponin complex consists of three subunits, T (TnT), I (TnI), and C (TnC). TnT and TnI are derived from heart-specific genes and are referred to as cardiac troponins (cTns). cTns are not present in healthy individuals; their early release is attributable to the cytosolic pool and late release to the structural pool.

Patients considered to have acute coronary syndrome should have a 12-lead ECG and placed in an environment with continuous electrocardiographic monitoring and defibrillator capability. Biomarkers of myocardial necrosis are measured. CK-MB has a short half-life and is less sensitive and less specific than cTns. Troponins can be detected in blood as early as 2 to 4 hours but elevation may be delayed for up to 8 to 12 hours. The timing of elevation of cTns is similar to CK-MB but cTns persist longer, for up to 5 to 14 days. Elevated cTn levels above the 99th percentile of normal in two or more blood samples collected at least 6 hours apart indicates the presence of myocardial necrosis. Equivalent information is obtained with cTnI and cTnT, except in patients with renal dysfunction, in whom cTnI has a specific role. Each patient should have a provisional diagnosis of acute coronary syndrome with UA (electrocardiographic changes of ischemia and no biomarkers in the circulation), STEMI, or NSTEMI. The distinction has therapeutic implications because patients with STEMI may be considered for immediate reperfusion therapy (fibrinolysis or percutaneous intervention).[22]

### Treatment

Preventing coronary ischemia is a function of identifying patients prospectively at risk for a perioperative cardiac complication. This will allow improvement of the condition of the patient, possibly lowering the risk, selection of patients for invasive or noninvasive cardiac testing, and identifying patients who will benefit from more intensive perioperative monitoring. Preoperative cardiac risk assessment includes adequate history taking, physical examination, and basic diagnostic tests. The history is important to identify patients with cardiac disease or those at risk for cardiac disease, including previous cardiac revascularization, history of MI or stroke, and presence of valvular heart disease, heart failure, arrhythmia, hypertension, diabetes, lung disease, and renal disease. Unstable chest pain, especially crescendo angina, warrants careful evaluation and probable postponing of an elective operation. Physical examination may reveal uncontrolled hypertension, evidence of peripheral artery disease, arrhythmia, or clinical stigmata of heart failure (HF). The CXR may show pulmonary edema, ECG may show an arrhythmia, blood gas analysis may reveal hypercapnia or a low $PaO_2$, and blood tests may show abnormal kidney function. The patient who is found to have HF on physical examination or by history must have the problem treated before consideration for an elective operative procedure. *Guidelines for Perioperative Cardiovascular Evaluation for Noncardiac Surgery,* published by the American College of Cardiology (ACA) and American Heart Association (AHA), have stratified clinical predictors of increased perioperative cardiovascular risk leading to MI, CHF, or death into major, intermediate, and minor risks (Table 13-6) and

**Table 13-6 Clinical Predictors of Increased Perioperative Cardiovascular Risk Leading to Myocardial Infarction, Heart Failure, or Death**

| LEVEL OF RISK | RISK FACTOR |
|---|---|
| Major | Unstable coronary syndromes<br>Acute or recent MI with evidence of considerable ischemic risk as noted by clinical symptoms or noninvasive studies<br>Unstable or severe angina (Canadian class III or IV)<br>Decompensated heart failure<br>Significant arrhythmias<br>High-grade atrioventricular block<br>Symptomatic ventricular arrhythmias in the presence of underlying heart disease<br>Supraventricular arrhythmias with an uncontrolled ventricular rate<br>Severe valve disease |
| Intermediate | Mild angina pectoris (Canadian class I or II)<br>Previous MI identified by history or pathologic evidence<br>Q waves<br>Compensated or previous heart failure<br>Diabetes mellitus (particularly insulin dependent)<br>Renal insufficiency |
| Minor | Advanced age<br>Abnormal electrocardiogram (e.g., left ventricular hypertrophy, left bundle branch block, ST-T abnormalities)<br>Rhythm other than sinus (e.g., atrial fibrillation)<br>Low functional capacity (e.g., inability to climb one flight of stairs with a bag of groceries)<br>History of stroke<br>Uncontrolled systemic hypertension |

**Table 13-7 Cardiac Risk Stratification for Noncardiac Surgical Procedures**

| LEVEL OF RISK | RISK FACTOR |
|---|---|
| High (cardiac risk often >5%) | Emergency major operations, particularly in the elderly<br>Aortic and other major vascular surgery<br>Peripheral vascular surgery<br>Anticipated prolonged surgical procedures associated with large fluid shifts and blood loss |
| Intermediate (cardiac risk generally <5%) | Carotid endarterectomy<br>Intraperitoneal and intrathoracic surgery<br>Orthopedic surgery<br>Prostate surgery |
| Low (cardiac risk generally <1%) | Endoscopic procedures<br>Superficial procedures<br>Cataract surgery<br>Breast surgery |

From Eagle KA, Berger PB, Calkins H, et al: ACC/AHA Guideline Update for Perioperative Cardiovascular Evaluation for Noncardiac Surgery—Executive Summary. A report of the American College of Cardiology/American Heart Association Task Force on Practice Guidelines (Committee to Update the 1996 Guidelines on Perioperative Cardiovascular Evaluation for Noncardiac Surgery). Anesth Analg 94:1052–1064, 2002.

stratified cardiac risk into high, intermediate, and low (Table 13-7).[21]

The ACC/AHA guidelines permit more appropriate use of preoperative testing (echocardiography, dipyridamole myocardial stress perfusion imaging, traditional exercise stress test, or angiography) and beta blocker therapy, with probable cancellation of the elective operative procedure.[23] An algorithm for perioperative cardiovascular evaluation is presented in Figure 13-1. The role of preoperative coronary artery revascularization has yet to be determined. Percutaneous transluminal coronary angioplasty may be beneficial in reducing perioperative cardiac morbidity in a select group of patients.

Patients identified as being at high risk for myocardial events in the perioperative period are managed with beta blockers, careful intraoperative monitoring, maintenance of perioperative normothermia and vital signs, and continued postoperative pharmacologic management, including the administration of adequate pain medication. Given several days before surgery and continued for several days afterward, beta blockers (e.g., atenolol) have been shown to reduce perioperative myocardial ischemia by 50% in patients with CAD or CAD risk factors.[24] Patients with chronic stable angina continue with their antianginal medications, and beta blockers are continued to the time of surgery and thereafter. An ECG is obtained before, immediately after, and for 2 days after surgery. Patients are monitored for 48 hours, and in high-risk patients for 5 days, after surgery and cardiac enzyme levels are also checked. Invasive hemodynamic monitoring is appropriate for patients with left ventricular dysfunction, fixed cardiac output, and unstable angina or recent MI.

Shortness of breath and chest pain remain the two postoperative symptoms that must always be carefully evaluated and never written off as postoperative discomfort. Subtle changes in the ST segment and T wave hint of possible ischemia or MI. Evaluation of a patient suspected of having an intraoperative or postoperative MI includes immediate assessment by electrocardiography and measurement of biomarkers of myocardial necrosis. Constant electrocardiographic monitoring is required so that the development of any potentially lethal arrhythmia can immediately be treated. If the level of cardiac function is a concern, echocardiography is considered. Cardiac troponin levels identify patients with myocardial necrosis but do not identify the cause of necrosis. Cardiac-specific troponin levels begin to rise by 3 hours after myocardial injury. A troponin I level more than 1 ng/mL is specific, and elevations persist for 7 to 10 days. Troponin T elevations persist for 10 to 14 days after MI. Medical management of myocardial ischemia and MI includes immediate administration of high-flow oxygen, transfer to the intensive care unit, and early involvement of a cardiologist.

The goal of management of myocardial ischemia is to preserve the maximal amount of myocardial muscle possible, as well as improve coronary blood flow and decrease myocardial work. Immediate administration of beta blockers (oral or IV, dose-titrated to decrease heart rate to less than 70 beats/min) and aspirin (160 to 325 mg) is essential. Beta blockers are not indicated for patients with bradycardia, hypotension, severe left ventricular dysfunction, heart block, or severe bronchospastic disease. Nitroglycerin (given as a continuous IV infusion after a loading dose) alleviates pain and is beneficial for patients with MI complicated by HF or pulmonary edema. Systemic heparinization (or SC LMWH), if not contraindicated, is administered. In most cases, thrombolytic therapy is contraindicated in the postoperative period and can be used only in the situation in which minor surgery is performed. Studies have shown that emergency stricture dilation and coronary artery stenting may be more effective than thrombolytic therapy. ACE inhibitors may be given early after MI, especially anterior MI or with a

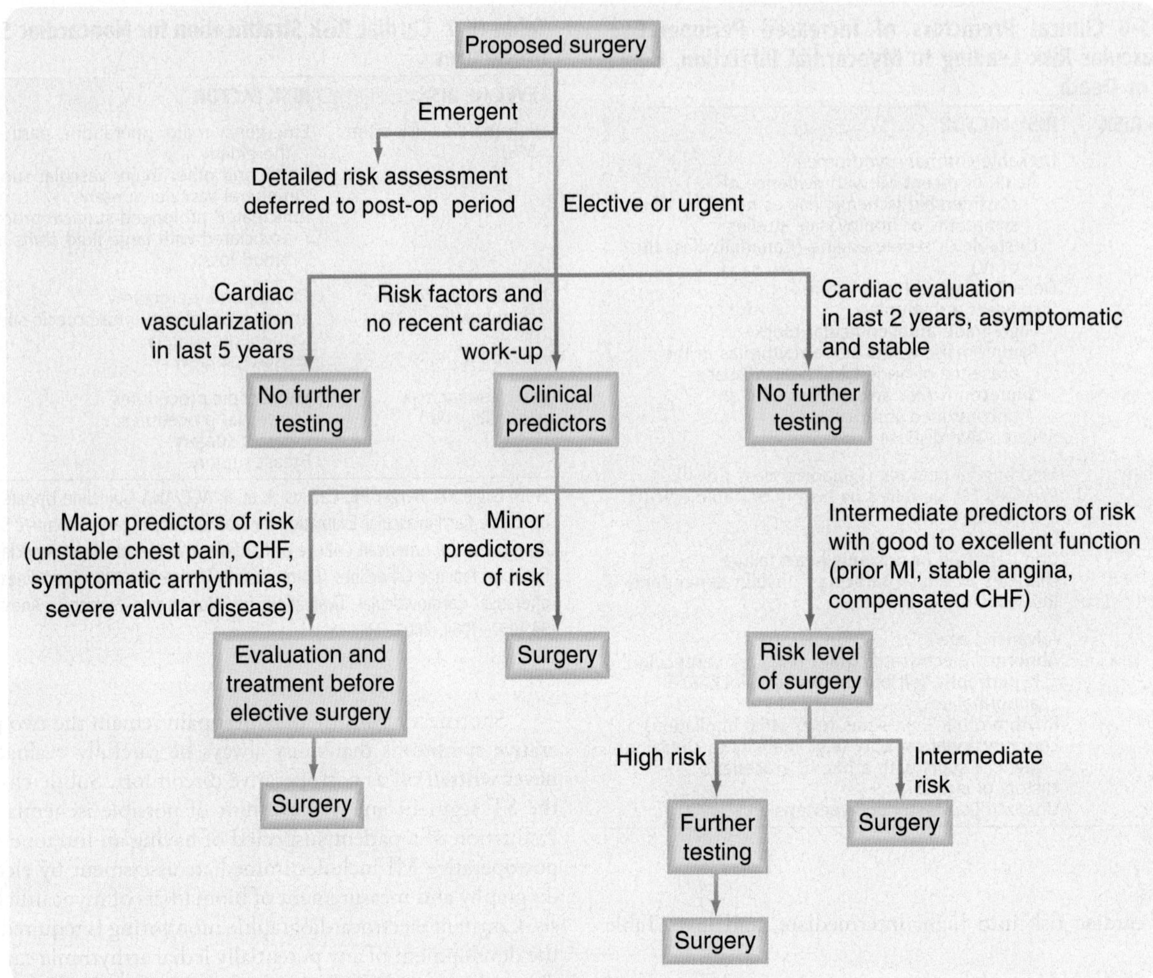


**FIGURE 13-1** Algorithm for perioperative cardiovascular evaluation for noncardiac surgery. Patients with major predictors of risk and patients with intermediate predictors of risk and a planned high-risk procedure undergo additional testing and resultant indicated treatment before elective surgery. *CHF,* Congestive heart failure; *MI,* myocardial infarction. (Adapted from Eagle KA, Brundage BH, Chaitman BR, et al: Guidelines for perioperative cardiovascular evaluation for noncardiac surgery. Report of the American College of Cardiology/American Heart Association Task Force on Practice Guidelines. J Am Coll Cardiol 27: 910–945, 1996.)

low left ventricular ejection fraction, and probably continued as a long-term therapy. Angiography must be strongly considered if the patient has ongoing myocardial ischemia that does not respond to pharmacologic therapy.

## Cardiogenic Shock

### Causes

Cardiogenic shock is one of the most serious sequelae of acute MI. Presumably, 50% or more of left ventricular muscle mass is irreversibly damaged, leading to a substantial reduction in cardiac output and resulting hypoperfusion. Other possible, less frequent causes of cardiogenic shock include ruptured papillary muscle or ventricular wall, aortic valvular insufficiency, mitral regurgitation, and ventricular septal defect. Cardiogenic shock is a highly lethal condition that results in the death of up to 75% of patients unless immediate management is instituted. Other serious sequelae from acute MI include CHF, arrhythmias, and thromboembolic complications.

### Presentation and Management

Observant physicians will watch a patient with an acute MI closely for evidence of the aforementioned complications. Cardiogenic shock usually develops rapidly over a short period and is marked by hypotension and respiratory failure. Aggressive management is required to save the life of a patient with this devastating condition. Immediate institution of mechanical ventilation with a high $FIO_2$, and occasional monitoring with a Swan-Ganz catheter, is important. For patients who do not respond to pharmacologic and conservative management, intra-aortic balloon pumps and ventricular assist devices may be lifesaving. For patients who have adequate myocardial reserve, coronary artery bypass may occasionally be indicated. Cardiac transplantation remains the gold standard treatment of end-stage HF.

## Postoperative Cardiac Arrhythmias

### Causes

Cardiac arrhythmias are common in the postoperative period and are more likely to occur in patients with structural heart disease. Cardiac arrhythmias are classified into tachyarrhythmia, bradyarrhythmia, and heart block. Tachyarrhythmia is further subdivided into supraventricular (sinus, atrial, nodal) and ventricular (premature ventricular contraction [PVC], ventricular tachycardia, ventricular fibrillation). Sustained supraventricular arrhythmia in patients undergoing major noncardiac surgery may be associated with an increased risk for a cardiac event (e.g., heart failure, MI, unstable angina) and cerebrovascular event.[24] Factors associated with increased risk for supraventricular arrhythmias are increasing age, history of heart failure, and type of surgery performed. Sinus tachycardia and atrial flutter or fibrillation are the most common types of tachyarrhythmia. Sinus tachycardia is caused by pain, fever, hypovolemia, anemia, anxiety and, less commonly, heart failure, MI, thyrotoxicosis, and pheochromocytoma. Atrial flutter or fibrillation occurs commonly in patients with electrolyte imbalance, history of atrial fibrillation, and chronic obstructive lung disease.

Ventricular ectopy occurs in one third of patients after major noncardiac surgery and risk factors associated with an increased risk for PVCs include the presence of preoperative PVCs, history of CHF, and cigarette smoking. Postoperative risk factors include hypoxia, acute hypokalemia, and hypercapnia. Ventricular arrhythmias consist of largely benign and sustained ventricular tachycardia and fibrillation. Nonsustained ventricular tachycardia commonly occurs during or after major vascular procedures.

### Presentation

The physiologic impact of an arrhythmia depends on its type and duration and the patient's underlying cardiac status and ventricular response. Most arrhythmias are transient and benign and are not associated with symptoms or physiologic changes. Occasionally, sinus tachycardia may precipitate ischemia and PVCs, and unsustained ventricular tachycardia may precipitate ventricular tachycardia. Arrhythmias may also represent a prelude to hemodynamic compromise, especially in patients with severe heart disease or a history of MI or cardiomyopathy. Both bradyarrhythmia and tachyarrhythmia may decrease cardiac output. Symptoms associated with arrhythmias include palpitations, chest pain, shortness of breath, dizziness, loss of consciousness, cardiac ischemia, and hypotension.

### Treatment

The patient's underlying cardiac status is the key to management of arrhythmias. Arrhythmias may signal the presence of reversible causes or precipitating factors that must be sought and dealt with, and treatment is based on the presence of adverse hemodynamic effects of the arrhythmia, not its mere presence. In tachyarrhythmia, control of the ventricular response is essential, and distinction between arrhythmias that traverse the atrioventricular node (atrial fibrillation, ectopic atrial tachycardia) from those that do not (ventricular tachycardia, fibrillation) is paramount. Antiarrhythmics that alter atrioventricular node conduction and control the ventricular rate are indicated in the treatment of arrhythmias that traverse the node and dangerous in those that do not. Beta blockers are avoided in patients with a low ejection fraction and bronchospastic lung disease. The ultimate goal of therapy is to achieve sinus rhythm and, if not possible, prevention of complications associated with arrhythmias must be addressed (e.g., anticoagulants given to patients with atrial fibrillation for more than 48 hours). The management of postoperative arrhythmias is outlined in Box 13-8.

**BOX 13-8 Management of Postoperative Cardiac Arrhythmias**

Cardiology consultation
Monitoring of the patient on a telemetry floor or in the intensive care unit
12-lead ECG and long strip to differentiate between atrial and ventricular arrhythmia
Clinical assessment
- Vital signs
- Peripheral perfusion
- Cardiac ischemia and congestive heart failure
- Level of consciousness

Treatment of arrhythmia
- Tachyarrhythmia
  - Unstable: Cardioversion
  - Stable
    Supraventricular tachyarrhythmia: Beta blockers (esmolol), ibutilide, or alternatives (e.g., digoxin, calcium channel blockers, amiodarone)
    Paroxysmal supraventricular tachyarrhythmia: vagal stimulation or adenosine. Digoxin, amiodarone, or calcium channel blocker if adenosine fails
    Multifocal atrial tachycardia: Beta blocker, calcium channel blocker, or amiodarone
    Ventricular tachycardia: Lidocaine, procainamide, or amiodarone
- Bradyarrhythmia
  - Sustained: Atropine or β-adrenergic agonist
  - Transient: No therapy
- Heart block: Persistent high-grade second- or third-degree block; insertion of a permanent pacemaker

## Postoperative Heart Failure

### Causes

Heart failure is a clinical syndrome characterized by any structural or functional cardiac disorder that impairs the ability of the ventricle to fill with or eject blood.[25] Several risk factors predispose to the development of heart failure, the most significant of which are CAD, hypertension, and increasing age. Poorly controlled heart failure represents one of the most serious cardiac risk factors for a preoperative patient, whereas patients with well-managed heart failure generally do well during an operation. Many factors can lead to new-onset heart failure or decompensation of preexisting heart failure in the perioperative period, including perioperative myocardial ischemia or MI, volume overload, hypertension, sepsis, occult cardiac valvular disease, PE, and new-onset atrial fibrillation. The risk for heart failure is greatest immediately after surgery and in the first 24 to 48 hours after surgery.

#### Presentation

Patients with poorly controlled heart failure or new-onset heart failure suffer from shortness of breath and wheezing. Physical examination often reveals tachycardia, a narrow pulse pressure, low pressure or orthostatic hypotension, jugular venous distention, peripheral edema, rales, and general evidence of poor peripheral perfusion. The ECG may reveal an MI, ventricular hypertrophy, atrial enlargement, or arrhythmias. A CXR may indicate cardiomegaly, pulmonary edema, and pleural effusion. Echocardiography assesses ventricular function and provides information about regional wall motion and valve function.

#### Treatment

Management of patients with heart failure is directed at optimizing preload, afterload, and myocardial contractility. Afterload reduction is accomplished by lowering the vascular resistance against which the heart must contract, and ACE inhibitors are a cornerstone of therapy for heart failure. Nitrates (venodilator) and hydralazine (vasodilator) reduce excessive preload and are used as an alternative in patients who cannot tolerate ACE inhibitors. β-Adrenergic blockade (selective or nonselective) for heart failure has proved effective in reducing mortality in patients with ischemic and nonischemic heart failure.[26] Digoxin (a sympatholytic agent) has traditionally been used for patients with heart failure in sinus rhythm. Its use has decreased given the superior and definitive beneficial effects of ACE inhibitors and beta blockers. Diuretics are necessary in all patients with heart failure for the management of volume overload and relief of symptoms of congestion. Calcium channel blockers are used only for the treatment of hypertension or angina not adequately controlled with other agents, such as ACE inhibitors or beta blockers. Inotropes increase cardiac contractility and are used in the critically ill and patients with end-stage heart failure.

## RENAL AND URINARY TRACT COMPLICATIONS

### Urinary Retention

#### Causes

The inability to evacuate a urine-filled bladder is referred to as urinary retention. This is a common postoperative complication seen with particularly high frequency in patients undergoing perianal operations and hernia repair. Urinary retention may also occur after surgery for low rectal cancer when an injury to the nervous system affects bladder function. Most commonly, however, the complication is a reversible abnormality resulting from discoordination of the trigone and detrusor muscles as a result of increased pain and postoperative discomfort. Urinary retention is also occasionally seen after spinal procedures and may occur after overly vigorous IV administration of fluid. Benign prostatic hypertrophy and, rarely, a urethral stricture may also be the cause of urinary retention.

#### Presentation and Management

Patients with postoperative urinary retention will complain of a dull constant discomfort in the hypogastrium. Urgency and actual pain in this area occur as the retention worsens. Percussion just above the pubis reveals fullness and tenderness.

To prevent urinary retention, the population at greatest concern, older adults and patients who have undergone low anterior resection, must be watched carefully. Adequate management of pain, including operative injection of local anesthetics, may also diminish the incidence of urinary retention. Judicious administration of IV fluids during the procedure and in the immediate postoperative period, especially in patients who have undergone anorectal surgery for benign disease, may similarly diminish the likelihood of postoperative urinary retention. Furthermore, awareness of how much time has passed since the last voiding to the present time is crucial in preventing acute retention. Most patients should not go more than 6 to 7 hours without passing some urine, and an observant clinician will make certain that no patient goes longer than that before undergoing straight catheterization.

General management principles for acute urinary retention include initial straight catheterization or placement of a Foley catheter, especially in older patients and patients who have undergone anterior resection because they may be unable to sense the fullness associated with retention. In high-risk patients, cystoscopy and cystometry may be required.

### Acute Renal Failure

#### Causes

Acute renal failure (ARF) is characterized by a sudden reduction in renal output that results in the systemic accumulation of nitrogenous wastes. This hospital-acquired renal insufficiency is more prevalent after major vascular procedures (ruptured aneurysm), renal transplantation, cardiopulmonary bypass procedures, major abdominal cases associated with septic shock, and major urologic operations. It may also occur in procedures in which there is major blood loss, with transfusion reactions, in serious diabetics undergoing operations, in life-threatening trauma, with major burn injuries, and in multiple organ system failure. Hospital-acquired renal insufficiency adversely affects surgical outcomes and is associated with significant mortality, especially when dialysis is required. Two types of ARF have been identified, oliguric and nonoliguric. Oliguric renal failure refers to urine in which volumes less than 480 mL are seen in a day. Nonoliguric renal failure involves output exceeding 2 liters/day and is associated with large amounts of isosthenuric urine that clears no toxins from the bloodstream. Factors leading to ARF can be inflow, parenchymal, or outflow, historically referred to as prerenal, renal, or postrenal, respectively (Table 13-8).

In normal kidneys, effective perfusion of the glomeruli is maintained by an autoregulatory mechanism involving the afferent and efferent arterioles. Any factor that interferes with or disrupts this mechanism results in ARF. Afferent constriction or efferent dilation decreases the glomerular filtration rate. Inflow, or prerenal, failure is secondary to hypotension, which causes afferent arteriolar constriction and efferent dilation, nonsteroidal anti-inflammatory drugs (NSAIDs), which inhibit afferent vasodilation, and gram-negative sepsis, which causes decreased peripheral vascular resistance while increasing renal vasoconstriction. Renal vascular stenosis and thrombosis can also be causes, although these are much less common. Outflow, or postrenal, ARF is caused by tubular obstruction from debris, crystals, or pigments, ureteric obstruction, or urinary bladder outflow obstruction. Ischemia, toxins, or nephritis cause parenchymal ARF.

The incidence of contrast-induced nephropathy has been increasing. Tubular damage can occur within 48 hours of dye

**Table 13-8 Causes of Postoperative Acute Renal Failure**

| INFLOW OR PRERENAL | PARENCHYMAL OR RENAL | OUTFLOW OR POSTRENAL |
|---|---|---|
| Sepsis<br>Medications<br>  Nonsteroidal anti-inflammatory drugs<br>  Angiotensin-converting enzyme inhibitors<br>Intravascular volume contraction<br>  Hypovolemia<br>  Hemorrhage<br>  Dehydration<br>  Atherosclerotic emboli<br>  Third spacing<br>  Cardiac failure | Renal ischemia<br>Drugs (aminoglycosides, amphotericin)<br>Iodinated contrast media<br>Interstitial nephritis | Cellular debris (acute tubular necrosis)<br>Crystals<br>  Uric acid<br>  Oxylate<br>Pigment<br>  Myoglobin<br>  Hemoglobin |

administration. Diabetic patients with vascular disease are at risk for major renal injury when contrast agents are administered. Administration of contrast to hypovolemic patients and those with preexisting renal dysfunction guarantees some degree of renal injury. The tubular injury is generally self-limited and reversible. Diabetic patients with creatinine clearance lower than 50 mL/min who receive 100 mL of contrast dye, however, can sustain severe tubular damage and may require dialysis. Blunt trauma with associated crush injuries places the patient at risk for ARF because of high serum levels of hematin and myoglobin, both of which are injurious to the renal tubules. ARF is a prominent feature in patients with acute compartment syndrome.[27] Growing awareness of this problem has led surgeons to intervene surgically, often resulting in dramatic improvement in renal function and preservation of renal filtering capacity.

### Presentation and Management

Prevention of hospital-acquired renal insufficiency requires the following: identification of patients with preexisting renal dysfunction; avoidance of hypovolemia, hypotension, and medications that depress renal function; and judicious use of nephrotoxic drugs. In the presence of renal impairment, the dose of antibiotics given for serious infections must be adjusted. The risk for contrast-induced nephropathy is reduced by adequate hydration and premedication with a free radical scavenger (e.g., *N*-acetylcysteine) or the use of alternative contrast (e.g., gadolinium). Renal hypoperfusion is avoided by optimizing cardiac output and volume expansion. Administration of fluid must be particularly judicious in patients with a history of heart failure. Monitoring renal function in all surgical patients, at times including creatinine clearance, is a sound clinical practice. Early intervention in cases of postrenal obstruction and abdominal compartment syndrome can obviate the development of renal injury.

Anuria that suddenly develops postoperatively in an otherwise healthy individual with no preexisting renal disease is postrenal in nature until proven otherwise. A kink in the Foley catheter or obstruction must be cleared. In patients who have undergone major pelvic surgery, ligation of the ureters is suspect. If renal ultrasound or a CT scan shows hydronephrosis, immediate surgical treatment is indicated. Postrenal causes of ARF are the most dramatic and straightforward to diagnose and treat, with significant immediate improvement after treatment.

ARF is otherwise diagnosed when there is a rise in the serum creatinine level, decrease in creatinine clearance, and urine output less than 400 mL/day (<20 mL/hr). Distinguishing between prerenal and renal azotemia, however, is complicated. Careful history taking may identify patients with preexisting renal dysfunction. Patients with large fluid losses from the GI tract (e.g., diarrhea, vomiting, fistula, high ileostomy output) often have associated profound dehydration. In such cases, the rise in the blood urea nitrogen (BUN) level is usually more than the rise in the creatinine level and the ratio of BUN to creatinine is more than 20. On the other hand, examination of the patient may reveal distended neck veins, rales in the lungs, and a cardiac gallop—all signs that a failing heart may be underperfusing the kidneys as the cause of the oliguria. Brown urine in the Foley bag in a trauma patient raises suspicion of myoglobinuria and requires rapid hydration, diuresis, and alkalinization of the urine. Evaluation of spun urine is helpful. The presence of hyaline casts indicates hypoperfusion and the presence of coarse granular casts indicates acute tubular necrosis. Lipoid casts are found with NSAID- and contrast-induced nephropathy and white and red cell casts are found with pyelonephritis. In patients with prerenal azotemia, the concentrating ability of the nephrons is normal, thereby resulting in normal urine osmolality and fractional excretion of sodium (>500 mOsm/liter and $FE_{Na}$ <1%, respectively). Conversely, with acute tubular necrosis, the concentrating ability of the kidney is lost and the patient produces urine with an osmolality equal to that of serum and high urine sodium levels (350 mOsm and >50 mg/L, respectively; Table 13-9). The best laboratory test for discriminating prerenal from renal azotemia is probably $FE_{Na}$. In prerenal patients, $FE_{Na}$ is 1% or less, whereas in renal azotemia patients it often exceeds 3%.

Once ARF is diagnosed, one has to ascertain whether the hypoperfusion of the kidney is caused by hypovolemia or cardiac failure. Distinguishing the two is critical because giving heart failure patients more fluid exacerbates an already failing system. Similarly, giving diuretics to a hypovolemic patient can worsen the renal failure. If the prerenal patient has no history of cardiac disease, administration of isosmotic fluid (normal saline or lactated Ringer's solution, or blood in patients who have hemorrhaged) is indicated. The IV fluid can be given rapidly (1 liter over a 20- to 30-minute period) in young patients with healthy hearts and a Foley catheter in place to measure hourly urine output, and must be administered until the patient is producing a minimum of 30 to 40 mL/hr of urine. If fluid administration does not result in improvement of the oliguria, placement of a central venous pressure or Swan-Ganz catheter is indicated to measure left- or right-sided heart filling pressure. In the presence of CHF, diuretics, fluid restriction, and appropriate cardiac medications are indicated. Ultrasound may show renal atrophy, reflecting the presence of chronic metabolic disease.

**Table 13-9 Diagnostic Evaluation of Acute Renal Failure**

| PARAMETER | PRERENAL | RENAL | POSTRENAL |
|---|---|---|---|
| Urine osmolality | >500 mOsm/liter | = Plasma | Variable |
| Urinary sodium | <20 mOsm/liter | >50 mOsm/liter | >50 mOsm/liter |
| Fractional excretion of sodium | <1% | >3% | Variable |
| Urine, plasma creatinine leve | >40 | <20 | <20 |
| Urine, plasma urea level | >8 | <3 | Variable |
| Urine, plasma osmolality | <1.5 | >1.5 | Variable |

Treatment of ARF includes the management of fluid and electrolyte imbalance, careful monitoring of fluid administration, avoidance of nephrotoxic agents, provision of adequate nutrition, and adjustment of doses of renally excreted medications until recovery of renal function. Most urgent in management of ARF is treating hyperkalemia and fluid overload. Hyperkalemia can be managed with a sodium-potassium exchange resin, insulin plus glucose, an aerosolized $\beta_2$-adrenergic agonist, and calcium gluconate. Insulin and $\beta_2$-adrenergic agonists shift potassium intracellularly. Hyperkalemia-associated cardiac irritability (prolonged PR interval or peaked T waves) is urgently treated with the administration of a 10% calcium gluconate solution over a 15-minute period, as well as simultaneous IV administration of insulin and glucose (10-U IV bolus with 50 mL of a 50% dextrose solution, followed by continuation of glucose to prevent hypoglycemia). A $\beta_2$-adrenergic agonist is given as a nebulizer containing 10 to 20 mg in 4 mL of saline over a period of 10 minutes or as an IV infusion containing 0.5 mg. Calcium gluconate is given as 10 mL of a 10% solution over a 5-minute period to reduce arrhythmias. Refractory hyperkalemia associated with metabolic acidosis and rhabdomyolysis requires hemodialysis. In less severe hyperkalemia, an ion exchange resin (sodium polystyrene [Kayexalate]) in enema form will help lower potassium levels. Phosphate levels also require careful monitoring. Hypophosphatemia can induce rhabdomyolysis and respiratory failure and is treated with the oral administration of Fleet Phospho-Soda. Hyperphosphatemia with hypercalcemia increases the risk for calciphylaxis and is treated with the administration of phosphorus binders (calcium carbonate) or dialysis. IV fluids are monitored with an emphasis on fluid restriction and occasional use of catheters to measure right- and left-sided heart filling pressure to avoid fluid overload.

When supportive measures fail, consideration must be given to hemodialysis.[28] Indications for hemodialysis are listed in Box 13-9. Although some hemodynamic instability may occur during dialysis, it is usually transient and may be treated with fluids. Dialysis may be continued on an intermittent basis until renal function has returned, which occurs in most cases.

**BOX 13-9 Indications for Hemodialysis**

Serum potassium > 5.5 mEq/liter
Blood urea nitrogen > 80-90 mg/dL
Persistent metabolic acidosis
Acute fluid overload
Uremic symptoms (pericarditis, encephalopathy, anorexia)
Removal of toxins
Platelet dysfunction causing bleeding
Hyperphosphatemia with hypercalcemia

## ENDOCRINE GLAND DYSFUNCTION

### Adrenal Insufficiency

#### Causes

Adrenal insufficiency is an uncommon but potentially lethal condition associated with failure of the adrenal glands to produce adequate glucocorticoids. Cortisol, the predominant corticosteroid secreted from the adrenal cortex, is under the influence of adrenocorticotropic hormone (ACTH) released from the pituitary gland, which in turn is under the influence of hypothalamic corticotropin-releasing hormone; both hormones are subject to negative feedback by cortisol itself. Cortisol is a stress hormone.

Chronic adrenal insufficiency may result from primary destruction of the adrenal gland or be secondary to a disease state or disorder involving the hypothalamus or anterior pituitary gland. Primary adrenal insufficiency is most frequently caused by autoimmune adrenalitis (Addison's disease), in which the adrenal cortex is destroyed by cytotoxic lymphocytes. Secondary adrenal insufficiency is most commonly caused by long-term administration of pharmacologic doses of glucocorticoids. Chronic use of glucocorticoids causes suppression of the hypothalamic-pituitary-adrenal axis, induces adrenal atrophy, and results in isolated adrenal insufficiency.

Acute adrenal insufficiency may occur as a result of abrupt cessation of pharmacologic doses of chronic glucocorticoid therapy, surgical excision or destruction of the adrenal gland (adrenal hemorrhage, necrosis, or thrombosis in patients with sepsis or antiphospholipid syndrome), or surgical excision or destruction (postpartum necrosis) of the pituitary gland. In addition, so-called functional or relative acute adrenal insufficiency may develop in critically ill and septic patients.

#### Presentation and Diagnosis

The clinical manifestations of adrenal insufficiency depend on the cause of the disease and associated endocrinopathies.[29] Symptoms and signs of chronic primary and secondary adrenal insufficiency are similar and nonspecific—fatigue, weakness, anorexia, weight loss, orthostatic dizziness, abdominal pain, diarrhea, depression, hyponatremia, hypoglycemia, eosinophilia,

**BOX 13-10 Rapid Adrenocorticotropic Hormone Stimulation Test in Patients With Adrenal Insufficiency**

- Determine baseline serum cortisol level.
  - Give 250 μg cosyntropin IV (or IM).
  - Measure serum cortisol levels 30 to 60 min after cosyntropin is given.
- Results
  - Normal adrenal function: Basal or postcorticotropin plasma cortisol concentration is at least 18 μg/dL (500 nmol/liter) or preferably 20 μg/dL (550 nmol/liter).
  - Primary adrenal insufficiency: Cortisol secretion is not increased.
  - Severe secondary adrenal insufficiency: Cortisol levels increase a little or not at all because of adrenocortical atrophy.

**Table 13-10 Relative Corticosteroid Potency Compared With Hydrocortisone**

| | GLUCOCORTICOID ACTIVITY | MINERALOCORTICOID ACTIVITY |
|---|---|---|
| **Short-Acting** | | |
| Hydrocortisone | 1 | 1 |
| Cortisone | 0.8 | 0.8 |
| **Intermediate-Acting** | | |
| Prednisone | 4 | 0.25 |
| Prednisolone | 4 | 0.25 |
| Methylprednisolone | 5 | Trace |
| Triamcinolone | 5 | Trace |
| **Long-Acting** | | |
| Dexamethasone | 20 | Trace |

Adapted from Druck P, Andersen DK: Diabetes mellitus and other endocrine problems. In Stillman RM (ed): Surgery: Diagnosis and therapy, New York, 1989, Lange, p 205.

decreased libido and potency. Patients with primary hypoadrenalism also show manifestations of elevated plasma levels of corticotropin and hyperpigmentation of the skin and mucous membranes. Patients with secondary disease, in contrast, initially have neurologic or ophthalmologic symptoms (headaches, visual disturbances) before showing signs of hypothalamic-pituitary-adrenal axis disease (hypopituitarism). Manifestations of hypothalamic-pituitary-adrenal axis suppression include hypoadrenalism, decreased levels of corticotropin, and manifestations of other hormone deficiencies (e.g., pallor, loss of hair in androgen-dependent areas, oligomenorrhea, diabetes insipidus, hypothyroidism).

Laboratory test abnormalities, including hyponatremia, hyperkalemia, acidosis, hypoglycemia or hyperglycemia, normocytic anemia, eosinophilia, and lymphocytosis, are present to a variable extent. The diagnosis, however, is established by measuring the morning plasma cortisol concentration. A level higher than 19 μg/dL (525 nmol/liter) rules out adrenal insufficiency and less than 3 μg/dL (83 nmol/liter) indicates its presence. A basal plasma corticotropin level exceeding 100 pg/mL (22 nmol/liter), low or low-normal basal aldosterone level, and increased renin concentration are indicative of primary hypoadrenalism. The rapid corticotropin stimulation test to determine adrenal responsiveness is the diagnostic procedure of choice when testing for primary adrenal insufficiency (Box 13-10).

To confirm the diagnosis of secondary adrenal insufficiency, the metyrapone test is performed. An insufficient increase in plasma 11-deoxycortisol and a low plasma cortisol concentration (<8 μg/dL) after the oral administration of metyrapone indicate the presence of secondary adrenal insufficiency. Magnetic resonance imaging (MRI) allows evaluation of the pituitary-hypothalamic region in patients with neurologic and ophthalmologic symptoms and CT is used to evaluate the adrenal glands in patients with primary hypoadrenalism.

The diagnosis of acute adrenal insufficiency can be especially difficult to make in the critically ill. The condition is suspected in patients exhibiting manifestations of preexisting or undiagnosed chronic adrenal insufficiency in whom unexplained hypotension or hemodynamic instability develops despite fluid resuscitation, as well as ongoing evidence of inflammation without an obvious source of infection. Hyponatremia is usually present and does not respond to saline infusion. A sodium level less than 120 mmol/liter is dangerous and may lead to delirium, coma, and seizures. Hypoglycemia and azotemia may also be present. An ECG will occasionally reveal low voltage and peaked T waves. To diagnose the condition, cortisol and corticotropin concentrations are checked and the short corticotropin stimulation test performed.

#### Treatment

Prevention and avoidance of adrenal insufficiency are achieved by a thorough preoperative history, detailed instruction of patients receiving chronic corticosteroid therapy regarding the dangers of abrupt termination of the medication, and adequate perioperative corticosteroid administration. Specific patients with rheumatoid arthritis, inflammatory bowel disease, or autoimmune disease and recipients of organ transplants are targeted. In the critically ill, a high index of suspicion can prevent a fatal outcome. A stress dose of hydrocortisone (100 mg) may be given with induction of anesthesia. For minor surgical procedures, the usual maintenance dose is continued postoperatively. For major surgical procedures, a stress dose (100 mg) is continued every 8 hours until the patient is stable or free of complications and then tapered to the usual maintenance dose.

Symptomatic patients are treated with hydrocortisone or cortisone. Fludrocortisone (substitute for aldosterone) is also administered to patients with primary disease. Patients who have received more than 20 mg of prednisone daily (or equivalent dose of another corticosteroid; Table 13-10) for more than 3 weeks within the previous year and patients with Cushing's syndrome who are undergoing surgery are presumed to have hypothalamic-pituitary-adrenal axis suppression and must be treated in a similar fashion.

Treatment of functional acute adrenal insufficiency involves immediate, rapid administration of high-dose hydrocortisone or methylprednisolone, with appropriate monitoring until clinical improvement is seen. Hypovolemia and hyponatremia are corrected with saline infusion.

## Hyperthyroid Crisis

### Causes

Hyperthyroidism refers to a sustained increase in the synthesis of thyroid hormones, and thyrotoxicosis is a clinical syndrome that results from an abnormal elevation of circulating levels of thyroid hormone, regardless of cause. Thyroid hormones are under the influence of pituitary gland thyroid-releasing hormone, which in turn is under the influence of hypothalamic thyrotropin-releasing hormone; both are subject to negative feedback by the thyroid hormones. Thyroid hormones have physiologic effects on many organ systems, but the greatest effect is on the cardiovascular system.

Thyroid crisis is a medical emergency that occurs in thyrotoxic patients with toxic adenoma or toxic multinodular goiter, but most often in patients with Graves' disease. The crisis is frequently precipitated by a stressful event and characterized by exacerbation of hyperthyroidism and decompensation of one or more organ systems. Mortality is high, ranging from 20% to 50% if the crisis is unrecognized and left untreated.

### Presentation and Diagnosis

Clinical manifestations of hyperthyroidism include nervousness, fatigue, palpitations, heat intolerance, weight loss, atrial fibrillation (in older patients), and ophthalmopathy characterized by eyelid retraction or lag, periorbital edema, and proptosis. The onset of thyroid crisis is sudden and manifested by accentuation of the symptoms and signs of thyrotoxicosis and organ system dysfunction, including hyperpyrexia, tachycardia out of proportion to fever, dehydration and collapse, central nervous system dysfunction (delirium, psychosis, seizure, coma), cardiac manifestations, GI symptoms, and liver dysfunction.

The diagnosis of thyrotoxicosis requires demonstration of elevated levels of circulating thyroid hormone and suppressed thyroid-stimulating hormone (TSH) levels and identification of the cause of the thyrotoxicosis. Free thyroxine ($T_4$) and triiodothyronine ($T_3$) represent the small unbound fraction of total thyroxine that is biologically active and correlate directly with the presence and severity of thyroid dysfunction. Thyroid scintigraphy with technetium pertechnetate ($^{99m}TcO_4^-$) or iodine 123 ($^{123}I$) provides information about the functional anatomy of the gland. In Graves' disease, there is diffuse uptake; in Plummer's disease (toxic multinodular goiter), there is an inhomogeneous pattern with hot, cold, and warm areas, and with Goetsch's disease (toxic solitary nodule), there is intense activity in the area of the nodule, with suppression of paranodular tissue.

### Treatment

In addition to the identification and treatment of the precipitating factor(s) and supportive care, specific medications (e.g., iodine, propylthiouracil, β-adrenergic blockers, dexamethasone) that target hormonal synthesis and release and block peripheral effects of the hormone are administered (Box 13-11).[30] Steroids are required to block the peripheral conversion of $T_4$ to $T_3$ and as a supplement because there is increased steroid demand and turnover and decreased physiologic effectiveness. Cardioversion for supraventricular tachyarrhythmia is ineffective during the thyrotoxic storm.

**BOX 13-11 Management of Thyroid Crisis**

Identification and treatment of the precipitating factor
Supportive care
- Oxygen
- IV fluid therapy
- Sedation (chlorpromazine)
- Venous thromboembolism prophylaxis with heparin
- Dexamethasone

Fever: antipyretics and cooling
Heart failure: Digoxin and diuretics
Atrial fibrillation: IV heparin
Beta blockers: Oral propranolol, 60-80 mg/4 hr (or diltiazem), to reduce the heart rate below 100 beats/min. In very sick patients, esmolol is given IV and reserpine is given to patients refractory to large doses of propranolol.
Propylthiouracil or methimazole
Lugol's solution given 4 hr after propylthiouracil
Plasmapheresis and charcoal plasma perfusion or exchange transfusion reserved for recalcitrant cases if no response in 24-48 hr
Once euthyroidism achieved, definitive therapy must be considered to prevent a second crisis

Definitive therapy for Graves' disease is accomplished with radioactive iodine or surgery. Radioactive iodine has obvious advantages in older, high-risk patients but needs to be avoided in children, pregnant women, and patients with large toxic adenomas. By using doses of $^{123}I$ in the range of 10 mCi (5 to 15 mCi) and subsequent levothyroxine, thyrotoxicosis can be successfully managed in 85% to 90% of patients. The main side effect of radioactive iodine is hypothyroidism. Surgery usually includes one of two operations, total thyroidectomy or a lobectomy on one side with a subtotal lobectomy on the other side. Total thyroidectomy is associated with a lower recurrence rate than subtotal thyroidectomy is (4% to 15%) but requires lifelong $T_4$ replacement postoperatively. Excision of the lesion is indicated for toxic adenoma, whereas total thyroidectomy is indicated for toxic multinodular goiter. Before surgery, patients must be made euthyroid with antithyroid drugs, and iodine is given for 7 days before surgery.

## Hypothyroidism

### Causes

Hypothyroidism is characterized by low systemic levels of thyroid hormone and may be exacerbated in the postoperative period in patients with preexisting chronic hypothyroidism or as a result of severe stress. Severe illness, physiologic stress, and drugs may inhibit the peripheral conversion of $T_4$ to $T_3$ and induce a hypothyroid-like state. Hypothyroidism may be primary (e.g., surgical removal, ablation, disease of the thyroid gland), secondary (e.g., hypopituitarism), or tertiary (e.g., hypothalamic disease).

### Presentation and Diagnosis

Patients with chronic hypothyroidism may be asymptomatic or, rarely, have the severe form (myxedema coma) characterized by coma, loss of deep tendon reflexes, cardiopulmonary collapse, and high mortality(≈40% to 50%). Most, however, demonstrate cold intolerance, constipation, brittle hair, dry skin, sluggishness, weight gain, and fatigue. The impact of hypothyroidism is greatest on the cardiovascular system, with effects such as bradycardia, hypotension, impaired cardiac function, conduction abnormalities, pericardial effusion, and increased risk for CAD. In the critically ill (e.g., those with trauma or sepsis), hypothyroidism is associated with worsening of pulmonary function, a predisposition to pleural effusion, and susceptibility to hypothermia.

The ECG usually shows bradycardia, low voltage, and prolonged PR, QRS, and QT intervals. In patients with primary hypothyroidism, serum total $T_4$, free $T_4$, and free $T_3$ levels are low, whereas the TSH level is elevated. In secondary disease, the TSH level, free $T_4$ index, and free $T_3$ are low. Distinguishing the two is important because adrenal insufficiency is present in secondary disease and administration of levothyroxine must be accompanied by cortisol or the disease could be exacerbated.

#### Treatment

Patients with known hypothyroidism who are receiving replacement hormonal therapy and are in the euthyroid state do not require any special treatment before surgery but are instructed to continue taking their medications. In patients with symptomatic chronic hypothyroidism, surgery is postponed until a euthyroid state has been achieved.

Patients with myxedema coma or those showing clinical signs of significant hypothyroidism (e.g., severe postoperative hypothermia, hypotension, hypoventilation, psychosis, obtundation) are immediately treated with thyroid hormone, concomitant with the IV administration of hydrocortisone, to avoid an addisonian crisis. IV levothyroxine or $T_3$ may be given until oral ingestion is possible.

### Syndrome of Inappropriate Antidiuretic Hormone Secretion

#### Causes

The syndrome of inappropriate antidiuretic hormone secretion (SIADH) is the most common cause of chronic normovolemic hyponatremia. Hyponatremia is defined as a serum sodium concentration lower than 135 mmol/liter. SIADH is diagnosed in any patient who remains hyponatremic despite all attempts to correct the imbalance in the presence of persistent antidiuretic activity from elevated arginine vasopressin levels. Vasopressin is a naturally occurring antidiuretic hormone that regulates free water excretion. It is synthesized in the hypothalamus, transported to the posterior pituitary, and stored until specific stimuli cause it to be secreted into the bloodstream. Thirst, hypovolemia, nausea, hypoglycemia, and drugs are among the many stimuli for vasopressin. Disorders and conditions that predispose to this relatively rare condition include trauma, stroke, antidiuretic hormone–producing tumors, drugs (ACE inhibitors, dopamine, NSAIDs), and pulmonary conditions.

#### Presentation

The clinical features of SIADH include anorexia, nausea, vomiting, obtundation, and lethargy. With more rapid onset, seizures, coma, and death can result. Clinical expression of the syndrome is caused by hyponatremia and is a function of the degree of hyponatremia, as well as the rapidity of its onset. The cardinal criteria of SIADH include hyponatremia with hypotonicity of plasma, urine osmolality in excess of plasma osmolality, increased renal sodium excretion, absence of edema or volume depletion, and normal renal function.

#### Treatment

Management of SIADH includes treatment of the underlying disease process and removal of excess water (i.e., treatment of the hyponatremia). Fluid restriction is the mainstay of management of chronic SIADH. IV administration of normal saline is used only in significantly symptomatic patients with chronic SIADH or those with symptomatic acute SIADH, with a duration of less than 3 days. Correction must occur at a rate of 0.5 mmol/liter/hr until the serum sodium concentration is 125 mg/dL or higher. Rapid correction leads to serious permanent neurologic damage. Diuretics such as furosemide occasionally help correct the imbalance. In some cases, IV administration of 3% saline solution may be required, but correction must be done in a constant, sustained fashion because overly rapid correction can result in seizure activity.

## GASTROINTESTINAL COMPLICATIONS

### Ileus and Early Postoperative Bowel Obstruction

#### Causes

Early postoperative bowel obstruction denotes obstruction occurring within 30 days after surgery. The obstruction may be functional (i.e., ileus), caused by inhibition of propulsive bowel activity, or mechanical as a result of a barrier. Ileus that occurs immediately after surgery in the absence of precipitating factors and resolves within 2 to 4 days is termed *primary* or *postoperative ileus.* On the other hand, ileus that occurs as a result of a precipitating factor and is associated with a delay in return of bowel function is termed *secondary, adynamic,* or *paralytic ileus.*[31] Mechanical bowel obstruction may be caused by a luminal, mural, or extraintestinal barrier.

The precise mechanism and cause of postoperative ileus are not completely understood. Several events that occur during an abdominal surgical procedure and in the perioperative period may interfere with or alter the contractile activity of the small bowel, which is governed by a complex interaction among the enteric nervous system, central nervous system, hormones, and local molecular and cellular inflammatory factors. Surgical stress and manipulation of the bowel result in sustained inhibitory sympathetic activity and release of hormones and neurotransmitters, as well as activation of a local molecular inflammatory response that results in suppression of the neuromuscular apparatus.[32] In the immediate postoperative period, restricted oral intake and postoperative narcotic analgesia also contribute to altered small bowel motility. Opiates and opioid peptides in the enteric nervous system suppress neuronal excitability. After transection and reanastomosis of the small bowel, the distal part of the bowel does not react to the pacemaker (found in the duodenum), and the frequency of contractions decreases. Other conditions listed in Box 13-12 are associated with or result in adynamic ileus.

Mechanical early postoperative small bowel obstruction is commonly caused by adhesions (92%), a phlegmon or abscess, internal hernia, intestinal ischemia, or intussusception. Intussusception occurring in the postoperative period is

**BOX 13-12 Causes of Intestinal Paralytic Ileus**

Pancreatitis
Intra-abdominal infection (peritonitis or abscess)
Retroperitoneal hemorrhage and inflammation
Electrolyte abnormalities
Lengthy surgical procedure and prolonged exposure of abdominal contents
Medications (e.g., narcotics, psychotropic agents)
Pneumonia
Inflamed viscera

relatively uncommon and is a rare occurrence after colorectal surgery. A phlegmon or abscess may be caused by leakage of intestinal contents from a disrupted anastomosis or by iatrogenic injury to the bowel during enterolysis or closure of laparotomy incision. With mechanical obstruction, there is an increased incidence of discrete, clustered contractions proximal to the obstruction that propel the intestinal contents past the point of obstruction (in cases of partial obstruction) and result in cramps. In high-grade or complete obstruction, the contents do not move distally, but accumulate in the proximal part of the bowel and initiate retrograde contractions that empty the small bowel contents into the stomach in preparation for expulsion during vomiting.

### Presentation

Postoperative ileus affects the stomach and colon primarily. After laparotomy, small bowel motility returns within several hours, gastric motility within 24 to 48 hours, and colonic motility in 48 to 72 hours. Secretions and swallowed air are not emptied from the stomach, and gastric dilation and vomiting may occur. The return of bowel activity is heralded by the presence of bowel sounds, flatus, and bowel movements.

Patients with early postoperative small bowel obstruction do not show manifestations of bowel activity or have temporary return of bowel function. In adynamic ileus, the stomach, small bowel, and colon are affected. In mechanical obstruction, the obstruction may be partial or complete, may occur in the proximal part of the small bowel (high obstruction) or in the distal part of the small bowel (low obstruction), and may be a closed-loop or open-ended obstruction.[33] There is stasis and progressive accumulation of gastric and intestinal secretions and gas; the bowel may lose its tone and dilate, thereby resulting in abdominal distention, pain, nausea and vomiting, and obstipation. The extent of the clinical manifestations varies with the cause, degree, and level of obstruction. Patients with high mechanical small bowel obstruction vomit early in the course and usually have no or minimal distention. The vomitus is generally bilious. Patients with distal obstruction, on the other hand, vomit later in the course and have more pronounced abdominal distention. The vomitus may initially be bilious and then becomes more feculent. Differentiation between adynamic ileus and mechanical obstruction can be difficult. With adynamic ileus, patients have diffuse discomfort but no sharp colicky pain and a distended abdomen. They often have a quiet abdomen, with few bowel sounds detected on auscultation with a stethoscope. With mechanical obstruction, high-pitched, tinkling sounds may be detected. Fever, tachycardia, manifestations of hypovolemia, and sepsis may also develop.

The diagnosis of bowel obstruction is usually based on clinical findings and plain radiographs of the abdomen.[33] However, in the postoperative period, differentiation between adynamic ileus and mechanical obstruction is imperative because the treatment is completely different. A CT scan, abdominal radiographs, and small bowel follow-through are variably used to establish the diagnosis and assist in treatment decision making. In adynamic ileus, abdominal radiographs reveal diffusely dilated bowel throughout the intestinal tract, with air in the colon and rectum. Air-fluid levels may be present, and the amount of dilated bowel varies greatly. With mechanical bowel obstruction, there is small bowel dilation with air-fluid levels and thickened valvulae conniventes in the bowel proximal to the point of obstruction and little or no gas in the bowel distal to the obstruction. A CT scan is more accurate for differentiating functional from mechanical obstruction by identifying the so-called transition point or cutoff at the obstruction site in cases of mechanical obstruction. It also determines the level (high or low) and degree of obstruction (partial versus high-grade or complete), differentiates between uncomplicated and complicated (compromised bowel, perforation) obstruction, and identifies specific types of obstruction (closed-loop obstruction, intussusception). In addition, CT may identify other associated disease states (e.g., bowel ischemia, phlegmon, abscess, pancreatitis). Small bowel follow-through is indicated if the clinical picture of postoperative small bowel obstruction is confusing, radiographs of the abdomen are not diagnostic, or the response to expectant management is inadequate. A standard battery of laboratory tests is also obtained, including a complete blood cell count with differential, determination of amylase, lipase, electrolyte, magnesium, and calcium levels, and urinalysis.

### Treatment

Preventive measures must be started intraoperatively and continued in the immediate postoperative period. A concerted effort must be made during any abdominal operation to minimize injury to the bowel and other peritoneal surfaces, the recognized source of adhesion formation. During the operation, the surgeon must handle the tissues gently and limit peritoneal dissection to only what is essential. The bowel must not be allowed to desiccate by prolonged exposure to air without protection. Moist laparotomy pads must be used to cover the bowel and must be moistened frequently if contact with the bowel is prolonged. Instrument injury to the bowel must be avoided. Given the importance of adhesion formation and the large magnitude of serious problems related to adhesions, adjunctive measures, such as antiadhesion barriers, may be considered. A number of antiadhesion barriers are available, including an oxidized cellulose product and a product that is a combination of sodium hyaluronate and carboxymethyl cellulose. These agents may inhibit adhesions wherever they are placed. However, a decrease in the number of adhesions at the site of application does not necessarily translate into a decrease in the rate of small bowel obstruction.

In the postoperative period, electrolyte levels are monitored and any imbalance corrected. Alternative analgesia to narcotics, such as NSAIDs and placement of a thoracic epidural with local anesthetic, may be used when possible. Intubation of the stomach with an NG tube needs to be applied selectively. Routine intubation does not confer any appreciable effect and is associated with discomfort, inhibits ambulation, and predisposes to aspiration, sinusitis, otitis, esophageal injury, and electrolyte imbalance. The use of prokinetic agents does not alter the outcome after colorectal surgery and other pharmacologic manipulations, such as parasympathetic agents, adrenergic blocking agents, and metoclopramide, also have no impact on resolving postoperative ileus.[32] The role of early postoperative feeding remains unclear.

Once early postoperative obstruction is suspected or diagnosed, a three-step approach is essential to guarantee a favorable outcome—resuscitation, investigation, and surgical intervention.[33] Emergency relaparotomy is performed if there is a closed-loop, high-grade, or complicated small bowel obstruction, intussusception, or peritonitis. Adynamic ileus is treated by resolving some of the abnormalities listed in Box 13-12 and waiting expectantly for resolution, with surgery not usually being required. Partial mechanical small bowel obstruction is also initially managed expectantly and for a longer period, 7 to 14 days, if the patient is stable and clinical and radiologic improvement continues. During this time, nutritional support is initiated and surgical intervention is performed if there are signs of deterioration or no improvement.

## Acute Abdominal Compartment Syndrome

### Cause

Abdominal compartment syndrome (ACS) describes increasing organ dysfunction or failure as a result of IAH. IAH is present when there is a consistent increased IAP value higher than 12 mm Hg, determined by a minimum of three measurements conducted 4 to 6 hours apart, measured at the end of expiration in a relaxed patient. ACS may be primary or secondary and develops when IAP is 20 mm Hg or higher, with or without abdominal perfusion pressure (APP) less than 50 mm Hg (at least three measurements performed 1 to 3 hours apart); it is associated with failure of one or more organ systems that was not present previously.

Primary ACS develops as a result of pathologic IAH caused by intra-abdominal pathology and secondary ACS develops in the absence of intra-abdominal primary pathology, injury, or intervention. Primary ACS is most commonly encountered in victims of multiple trauma, especially after damage control surgery, and develops as a result of ileus caused by bowel edema and contamination, continued bleeding, coagulopathy, packing used to control bleeding, capillary leak, and massive fluid resuscitation and transfusion. Closure of a noncompliant abdominal wall under tension in these situations is associated with IAH in 100% of cases. In nontrauma patients, IAH and possibly primary ACS have been reported to occur in patients with ascites, retroperitoneal hemorrhage, pancreatitis, or pneumoperitoneum and after reduction of chronic hernias that have lost their domain, repair of ruptured abdominal aortic aneurysm, complex abdominal procedures, and liver transplantation. Secondary ACS is in part iatrogenic and commonly encountered in patients with shock requiring aggressive fluid resuscitation with crystalloids, thermally injured and shock trauma victims, critically ill hypothermic and septic patients, and those who have sustained cardiac arrest. Shock and ischemia increase capillary permeability; combined with excessive crystalloid resuscitation (leading to dilution of plasma) and gut reperfusion, which further increase microvascular permeability, exudation of fluid with resultant interstitial edema, bowel wall edema and ascites occurs.

In healthy individuals, IAP ranges from subatmospheric to 5 mm Hg and fluctuates with respiration, body mass index, and activity. Following uncomplicated abdominal surgery, IAP ranges from 3 to 15 mm Hg. IAP reflects intra-abdominal volume and abdominal wall compliance. With increased volume, there is a decrease in compliance and any further change in volume results in an increase in pressure, leading to IAH. In the early stages of IAH, changes in organ function are not detectable and of questionable clinical significance. With further increase in IAP, deleterious effects are observed in the intra- and extra-abdominal organs and abdominal wall.[27] Upward displacement of the diaphragm results in decreased thoracic volume and compliance and increased intrapleural pressure. This results in an increase in peak airway pressure (PAP), ventilation-perfusion (V-P) mismatch, hypoxia, hypercapnia, and acidosis. When IAP reaches 25 mm Hg, there is an increase in end-respiratory pressure to achieve a fixed tidal volume. However, modest IAH can exacerbate acute lung injury, inhalation injury, or respiratory distress syndrome. Compression of the inferior vena cava and portal vein occurs and results in decreased venous return, and therefore a decrease in preload and pooling of blood in the splanchnic and lower extremity vascular beds, and increased peripheral vascular resistance. Venous return decreases with IAP higher than 20 mm Hg. As a result, cardiac output (CO), cardiac index, and right atrial and pulmonary artery occlusion pressures decrease. Increased intrathoracic pressure also decreases left ventricular compliance, thus reducing contractility and further decreasing the CO. Ventricular compliance is reduced when IAP is higher than 30 mm Hg. Cardiac output decreases, despite normovolemia or apparent high filling pressures and a normal ejection when the IAP is 20 to 25 mmHg. Systemic delivery of oxygen ($O_2$) decreases and whole body oxygen consumption is significantly reduced at an IAP higher than 25 mmHg.

Direct compression of the kidneys and obstruction of venous outflow, with resultant increase in prerenal vascular resistance and shunting of blood from the cortex to the medulla, results in a decrease in the glomerular filtration rate, renal plasma flow, glucose reabsorption, and urine output. In the postoperative patient admitted to the intensive care unit with an IAP higher than 18 mm Hg, renal function is impaired by 30%, independent of prerenal circulation. With an IAP higher than 25 mm Hg, renal output decreases in 65% of patients and in 100% of patients with an IAP higher than 35 mm Hg. Compression of the mesenteric vasculature leads to a decrease in splanchnic perfusion, mesenteric venous hypertension, and decreased hepatic arterial flow. This results in severe intramucosal acidosis, intestinal edema, and visceral swelling, increased intestinal permeability, and possible bacterial translocation. Gastric intramucosal acidosis develops with IAP higher than 20 to 25 cm $H_2O$ or 15 mm Hg. Elevated central venous pressure interferes with venous cerebral outflow, with consequent cerebral pooling and increase in intracerebral pressure. Also, with diminished CO and increasing intracerebral pressure, cerebral perfusion pressure decreases. Interleukin 6 (IL-6) and IL-1B levels increase in response to increased IAP. Blood flow to the abdominal wall decreases with a progressive increase in IAP. This may result in an increased rate of abdominal wound complications.

### Diagnosis

The clinical manifestations of primary and secondary ACS are similar. However, the effects of secondary ACS are more subtle, so the diagnosis may be missed and the clinical deterioration of the patient is usually attributed to severity of the primary illness or occurrence of irreversible shock. Secondary ACS often occurs during aggressive fluid resuscitation in patients with burns, extra-abdominal injury, or sepsis. Patients with ACS have difficulty breathing or are difficult to ventilate and exhibit rising PAP, decreased volumes, hypoxia, worsening hypercapnia, and deteriorating compliance. Oliguria rarely occurs in the absence of respiratory dysfunction or failure. The CO is reduced, despite apparent high filling pressures, and vasopressor therapy is required. The abdomen becomes distended and tense and neurologic deterioration may occur. The central venous pressure, pulmonary capillary wedge pressure (PCWP), and PAP become elevated and acidosis develops. Anuria, exacerbation of pulmonary failure, cardiac decompensation, and death ultimately occur.

Use of the urinary bladder catheter has been the gold standard and is the indirect method used to measure IAP.[28] IAP is measured in the following ways: (1) using a regular Foley catheter, disconnect from drainage tubing, directly inject 50 mL, clamp, insert needle, and measure; (2) a three-way Foley catheter with saline is injected into one port and IAP is measured through the other; or (3) a regular Foley catheter is serially connected to a three-way stopcock and a transducer. Other measurement kits have now become commercially available. Once measured, the pressure is graded: GI (IAP < 10 to 15 cm $H_2O$), GII (IAP < 16 to 25 cm $H_2O$), GIII (IAP < 26 to 35 cm $H_2O$), and GIV (IAP > 36 cm $H_2O$).

### Treatment

The prevention of primary ACS entails leaving the peritoneal cavity open in patients at risk for IAH and after high-risk surgical procedures. Patients at risk for secondary ACS receiving crystalloid resuscitation must be monitored closely and, when given more than 6 liters of crystalloid in a 6-hour period, IAP must be measured. In addition to blood pressure and urine output, monitoring APP (APP = mean arterial pressure − IAP) by continuously measuring IAP throughout resuscitation is a helpful indicator of the resuscitation end point. Routine measurement of IAP must also be considered in critically ill patients because IAH is the leading cause of chest wall impairment in ARDS. Monitoring gastric pH can detect cases of secondary ACS early after admission to the intensive care unit. A high incidence of suspicion is paramount, especially in cases of secondary ACS in which the onset is insidious and manifestations are subtle. Patients exhibiting the prodromal phase of ACS benefit from timely intervention to relieve the IAH and prevent progression to ACS (Box 13-13). Conservative fluid resuscitation, administration of analgesia, sedatives and pharmacologic paralysis, patient positioning, drainage of intra-abdominal fluid, escharotomy, renal placement therapy, and diuretics are measures that may prevent progression to ACS.

Optimizing treatment and identifying patients with IAH-ACS likely to benefit from decompression is a challenging task. The decision to intervene surgically is not based on IAH alone but rather on the presence of organ dysfunction in association with IAH. Few patients with a pressure of 12 mm Hg have any organ dysfunction, whereas IAP higher than 15 to 20 mmHg is significant in every patient. With grade III IAH, decompression may be considered when the abdomen is tense and signs of extreme ventilatory dysfunction and oliguria develop. In grade IV IAH, with signs of ventilator and renal failure, decompression is indicated. In patients with severe head injury and IAP higher than 20 mm Hg, even without overt ACS, or intractable intracranial hypertension without obvious head injury, abdominal decompression must be considered. Unlike primary ACS, in which reopening of the preexisting laparotomy incision for decompression can be easily done, there is usually reluctance to perform a formal laparotomy for decompression in cases of secondary ACS, especially in the absence of primary intra-abdominal pathology. If nonoperative measures (see earlier) prove ineffective, fascial release without exposing the peritoneal cavity using minimally invasive techniques has proven effective in lowering IAP in experimental animals.[34] Decompression (formal laparotomy) is an emergency and is performed in the operating room. Decompression leads to reduction of IAH, severe hypotension as a result of sudden decrease in systemic vascular resistance, and abrupt increase in the true tidal volume delivered to the patient, with washout of the byproducts of anaerobic metabolism from below the diaphragm. This results in respiratory alkalosis, decrease in effective preload, and a bolus of acid, potassium, and other

**BOX 13-13 Prevention of Abdominal Compartment Syndrome**

Patients at risk for IAH and abdominal compartment syndrome are identified (e.g., major trauma, complex abdominal procedure).

Organ function is monitored and assessed:

- Lungs: Hypercapnia, hypoxia, difficult ventilation, elevated pulmonary artery pressure, drop in $Pao_2/Fio_2$ ratio, decreased compliance, intrapulmonary shunt, increased dead space
- Heart: Decreased cardiac output and cardiac index and need for vasopressors
- Kidneys: Oliguria unresponsive to fluid therapy
- Central nervous system: Glasgow coma scale score <10 or neurologic deterioration in the absence of neurotrauma
- Abdomen: Distention; CT scan to check for fluid collections, narrowing of inferior vena cava, compression of the kidneys, and rounding of abdomen

Intra-abdominal pressure is measured and monitored with a urinary bladder or gastric catheter.

Other tests to check organ dysfunction:

- Gastric mucosal pH
- Near-infrared spectroscopy to measure muscle and gastric tissue oxygenation
- Abdominal perfusion pressure = mean arterial pressure − intra-abdominal pressure
- Renal filtration gradient = mean arterial pressure − 2× intra-abdominal pressure
- CT scan

Measures to lower IAH:

- Drainage of intra-abdominal fluid collections
- Muscle relaxation

Avoid primary closure of the incision—laparotomy or mesh, Bogota bag, biomesh, or vacuum-assisted closure.

byproducts delivered to the heart, where they cause arrhythmia or asystolic arrest. Hence, decompression is performed after adequate preload with volume has been established. Most patients respond to decompression and survive. Once stable, the patient may be returned to the operating room for definitive closure. If primary closure is not possible, closure may be effected with skin flaps only, composite mesh, bioprosthesis, bilateral medial advancement of rectus muscle and its fascia with lateral skin relaxation incisions, or tissue expanders and myocutaneous flaps.

## Postoperative Gastrointestinal Bleeding

### Causes

Postoperative GI bleeding is one of the most worrisome complications encountered by general surgeons. Possible sources in the stomach include peptic ulcer disease, stress erosion, a Mallory-Weiss tear, and gastric varices; possible causes include in the small intestine, arteriovenous malformations and bleeding from an anastomosis and, in the large intestine, anastomotic hemorrhage, diverticulosis, arteriovenous malformations, and varices.

In the critically ill, GI bleeding caused by stress ulceration is a serious complication. The incidence of bleeding from stress ulceration has decreased in the past 15 years, mainly because of improved supportive care, superior acid suppression, and enhanced resuscitative measures. Clinically significant bleeding that leads to hemodynamic instability, the need for transfusion of blood products, and occasionally operative intervention occurs in less than 5% of cases and is associated with significant mortality. Risk factors for stress ulceration are listed in Box 13-14.

### Presentation and Diagnosis

When considering the source of the hemorrhage, a previous history is important when assessing the patient. A history of peptic ulcer disease and previous upper GI bleeding lead one to consider a duodenal ulcer. Severe trauma, major abdominal surgery, central nervous system injury, sepsis, or MI may be associated with stress ulceration. An antecedent history of violent emesis leads to consideration of a Mallory-Weiss tear, and a history of portal hypertension or variceal bleeding is a clue regarding the presence of esophageal varices. A previous history of diverticulosis may indicate that the hemorrhage is diverticular in nature. With a recent surgical history of intestinal anastomosis, oozing from the suture or staple line may be the source of GI bleeding. In distal colorectal anastomoses, bleeding may be the first sign of anastomotic breakdown. A previous history of aortic aneurysm repair may indicate the presence of an aortoduodenal fistula. A history of intake of NSAIDs or anticoagulant or platelet inhibitor therapy will identify patients at high risk for postoperative bleeding.

**BOX 13-14 Risk Factors for Development of Stress Erosions**

Multiple trauma
Head trauma
Major burns
Clotting abnormalities
Severe sepsis
Systemic inflammatory response syndrome
Cardiac bypass
Intracranial operations

In general, bright red blood is considered to come from a colonic or distal small bowel source. Melanotic stools suggest a gastric cause of the bleeding. However, rapid bleeding at any site may result in bright red blood. Bleeding from the anastomosis may be a slow ooze or a rapid hemorrhage that can lead to hypotension. Patients who appear to have lost a significant amount of blood have associated tachycardia or hypotension or have a significant decrease in hematocrit level.

### Treatment

To prevent stress ulceration and decrease the risk for bleeding, patients at risk must receive aggressive fluid resuscitation to improve oxygen delivery and prophylaxis that neutralizes or reduces gastric acid. Patients with respiratory failure and coagulopathy benefit the most from prophylaxis. Maintaining the gastric pH above 4 is essential to minimize gastric mucosal injury and propagation of injury by acid. This can be achieved with antacids, $H_2$ blockers, $M_1$ cholinoreceptor antagonists, sucralfate, or PPIs.

The basic principles of management of postoperative GI bleeding include the following:

1. Fluid resuscitation and restoration of intravascular volume
2. Checking and monitoring clotting parameters and correcting abnormalities, as needed
3. Identification and treatment of aggravating factors
4. Transfusion of blood products
5. Identification and treatment of the source of the bleeding

In general, management of GI bleeding is best conducted in the intensive care unit setting. Fluid resuscitation with isosmotic crystalloids is begun after securing venous access. Blood samples are sent to assess the hematocrit, platelet count, prothrombin time, partial thromboplastin time, and INR. If the INR is elevated, vitamin K and fresh-frozen plasma are administered. Platelet transfusion is administered to patients with a prolonged bleeding time or to those who have been taking antiplatelet drugs; desmopressin acetate may also be given to patients in renal failure. Hypothermia, if present, is corrected.

Blood transfusion is recommended when tachycardia and hypotension refractory to volume expansion are present, with a hemoglobin concentration in the 6- to 10-g/dL range and the extent of blood loss is unknown, a hemoglobin concentration less than 6 g/dL, and rapid blood loss more than 30%, as well as in patients at risk for ischemia or those with an oxygen extraction ratio more than 50%, with a decrease in $V\text{O}_2$.[35] An NG tube is placed and the effluent checked for the presence of blood. Nonbloody bilious drainage almost rules out a gastroduodenal source of the bleeding. If blood is present, lavage with saline at room temperature is performed.

Identification and treatment of the source of bleeding can be achieved with endoscopy, angiography or, occasionally, laparotomy. Endoscopic control of bleeding can be achieved with an injection of epinephrine, electrocoagulation, laser coagulation, heater probe, argon plasma coagulator, clip application, banding, or any combination of these modalities, depending on the source of bleeding. Visceral angiography is indicated for patients who are actively bleeding or when endoscopy fails to control the bleeding. Once an actively bleeding vessel is identified, embolization (e.g., with Gelfoam, autologous blood clot, coils) often controls the bleeding. Infusion of vasopressin may be used in patients with severe stress ulceration, diverticulosis, and ongoing bleeding. Bleeding from an intestinal anastomosis and stress ulceration usually cease with expectant management. Rarely, a patient with an anastomosis may require a reoperation to resect the anastomosis and reconnect the bowel. Similarly, surgery for stress ulceration is reserved for patients who fail medical management. Usually, a generous gastrotomy is performed to evacuate the blood clots and oversew sites of active bleeding; uncommonly, total or subtotal gastrectomy, with or without vagotomy, is performed. Recurrence with both approaches is prevented in 50% to 80% of cases.

## Stomal Complications

### Causes

Stomas are widely used in the treatment of colorectal, intestinal, and urologic diseases. An intestinal stoma can be an ileostomy, colostomy, or urostomy, end, loop, or end-loop, temporary or permanent, diverting or decompressing, or continent or incontinent. A tube cecostomy and a blowhole are considered temporary decompressing colostomies performed in emergencies. Stomal complications are the result of several causative factors. Technical factors are most important in minimizing the complication rate of stoma construction and are largely preventable. Stomal complications are numerous (Table 13-11) and range from a bothersome problem with fit of the stomal appliance to major skin erosion and bleeding. Early complications are considered those that occur within 30 days after surgery.

### Presentation and Diagnosis

Ischemic necrosis results from impaired perfusion to the terminal portion of the bowel as a result of a tight aperture, overzealous trimming of mesentery, or mesenteric tension. Stomal retraction occurs early as a result of tension on the bowel or ischemic necrosis of the stoma. Late retraction is caused by increased thickness of the abdominal wall with weight gain. Stenosis occurs as a result of a small aperture, so-called natural maturation, ischemia, recurrence of Crohn's disease, or development of carcinoma. Mucocutaneous separation develops as a result of ischemia, inadequate approximation of mucosa to the dermal layer of skin, excessive bowel tension, or peristomal infection.

Stomal prolapse is most alarming to the patient and can result in incomplete diversion of stool, interfere with the stoma appliance, lead to leakage of stool, or become associated with obstructive symptoms and incarceration. Parastomal hernia formation occurs to some degree in most patients. A peristomal fistula is often a sign of Crohn's disease, may result from a deep suture used to mature the stoma, or may be caused by trauma from an appliance.

Chemical dermatitis is caused by contact of the stoma effluent with peristomal skin as a result of a large opening in the faceplate or leakage from an ill-fitted faceplate. Chemical dermatitis is initially manifested as erythema, ulceration (ileostomy effluent), encrustation (urostomy effluent), or pseudoepitheliomatous hyperplasia. Infectious dermatitis may be caused by fungus, bacteria, tinea corporis, or *C. albicans.* Allergic dermatitis may be related to any of the stomal equipment (e.g., faceplate, tape, belt), with skin manifestations appearing at the site of contact. Traumatic dermatitis occurs during change of the stomal device, from stripping of adhesive, or as a result of friction or pressure from the stomal device or supportive belt. Traumatic dermatitis is manifested as erythema, erosion, and ulceration.

Stoma patients are at risk for diarrhea and dehydration. The risk for dehydration depends on the type of stoma, underlying primary disease process, and any concomitant bowel resection; it commonly occurs in older patients, in hot weather, during strenuous exercise, and in association with short bowel syndrome.

Cutaneous manifestations of the disease may develop in the damaged peristomal skin in patients afflicted with certain skin conditions, such as psoriasis. Pyoderma gangrenosa may develop in patients with inflammatory bowel disease, and parastomal varices may develop in patients with liver disease.

### Treatment

To prevent most stomal complications, adherence to sound surgical technique is imperative. Application of the technical points shown in Box 13-15 ensures the construction of a healthy and well-positioned stoma in patients undergoing surgery. In emergencies and difficult cases such as the obese, distended bowel, and shortened mesentery, to ensure delivery of a viable stoma free of tension, the fascial aperture may be made larger, the bowel may have to be extensively mobilized, the ileocolic artery and inferior mesenteric artery may have to be divided at their origin, windows may need to be created in the mesentery, the stoma may be brought out at a site with less subcutaneous fat (above the umbilicus), or alternative stomas may be selected.

After construction of a stoma, a dusky appearance indicates some degree of ischemia. The ischemia may be mucosal or full thickness, and the extent and depth of ischemia dictate the need for immediate revision of the stoma. Viability of the stoma is checked with a test tube and a flashlight or endoscopy. Necrosis extending to and beyond the fascia requires immediate reoperation. Ischemia limited to a few millimeters is observed and may not result in any long-term sequelae. Repair of stomal retraction often requires laparotomy.

Skin-level stenosis can be repaired locally and stenoses from other causes can be repaired via laparotomy. Complete separation or detachment usually requires revision. Repair of end

**Table 13-11 Stomal Complications**

| | Complication | |
|---|---|---|
| **CATEGORY** | **EARLY** | **LATE** |
| Stoma | Poor location<br>Retraction*<br>Ischemic necrosis<br>Detachment<br>Abscess formation*<br>Opening wrong end | Prolapse<br>Stenosis<br>Parastomal hernia<br>Fistula formation<br>Gas<br>Odor |
| Peristomal skin | Excoriation<br>Dermatitis* | Parastomal varices<br>Dermatoses<br>Cancer<br>Skin manifestations of inflammatory bowel disease |
| Systemic | High output* | Bowel obstruction<br>Nonclosure |

*May also develop as a late complication.

**BOX 13-15 Technical Aspects of Stoma Construction**

**Abdominal Wall Aperture**
Excision of circular piece of skin approximately 2 cm in size
Preservation of subcutaneous fat to provide support for the stoma
Transrectus muscle placement of the stoma
Fascial aperture to admit two fingers

**Stoma**
Selection of normal bowel for the stoma
Adequate mobilization of bowel to avoid tension on the stoma
Preservation of blood supply to end of bowel (marginal artery of the colon and last vascular arcade of small bowel mesentery must be preserved)
Small bowel serosa must not be denuded of >5 cm of mesentery

**Maturation**
Primary maturation of end stoma or afferent limb of loop ileostomy
Avoidance of traversing skin with sutures during maturation

**Other Maneuvers***
Tunneling of bowel through extraperitoneal space of abdominal wall
Mesenteric-peritoneal closure
Fixation of mesentery or bowel to fascial ring
Use of supportive rod with loop stomas

*May be performed but have not been proved to be effective in preventing postoperative complications.

stomal prolapse can be achieved locally by making a circumferential incision at the mucocutaneous junction, excision of redundant bowel, and rematuration. Repair of loop stomal prolapse is achieved by local revision to an end stoma. Laparotomy may be required for the treatment of recurrent prolapse and prolapse associated with a parastomal hernia. Large permanent or complicated parastomal hernias are treated by relocating the stoma or reinforcing the fascia ring with mesh (synthetic or biomaterial). Treatment of a peristomal fistula entails resection of the diseased or involved segment of bowel and relocation of the stoma. Treatment of mucosal islands ranges from ablation with electrocautery to relocation of the stoma.

Treatment of chemical dermatitis entails cleaning the damaged skin, the use of barriers, and a properly fitting stomal management system. *Candida* dermatitis is best treated with nystatin powder. Allergic dermatitis is treated by removal of the offending item and symptomatic relief is produced by oral antihistamine or topical or oral steroid therapy. Traumatic dermatitis is treated by patient education and application of a skin barrier under the tape is used to secure the faceplate in place. Occasionally, in cases of severe dermatitis, the patient will have to be admitted to the hospital and placed on TPN while the skin around the stoma heals enough to allow subsequent placement of an appliance.

## *Clostridium difficile* Colitis

### Causes

*C. difficile* colitis (CDC) is an inflammatory bowel disease caused by toxins produced by unopposed proliferation of the bacterium *C. difficile*. Several factors are associated with increased risk for CDC (Table 13-12). There has been an increased incidence and diagnosis rate of *C. difficile* infection (CDI) in hospitalized patients, as well as an increase in severity, requiring admission to the intensive care unit, treatment failure of the disease, colectomies, and 30-day mortality (4.7% in 1992 to 13.8% in 2003).[36,37] These changes are caused by increased awareness of the disease, advanced age of inpatients, with numerous comorbidities, ubiquitous use of antibiotics, and emergence and spread of a hypervirulent strain. Historically, cephalosporins, clindamycin, and ampicillin-amoxicillin were most commonly associated with CDI. Fluoroquinolones, as a class of antibiotics, have emerged as the most prone and at increased risk to cause CDI, and the increased use of newer generation fluoroquinolones is implicated in outbreaks of a fluoroquinolone-resistant strain. Since 2000, a hypervirulent toxinotype III strain of *C. difficile* (designated BI/NAP1/027 strain) has been identified in Canada, the United States, and England. Virulence of the wild-type *C. difficile* bacteria is related to enterotoxin A and cytotoxin B encoded by the genes *tcdA* and *tcdB*. Polymorphisms or partial deletions (18-base pair deletion) in *tcdC* may lead to increased production of toxins A and B at levels 16 and 23 times higher than the wild type.

**Table 13-12 Factors Associated With Increased Risk for *Clostridium difficile* Colitis**

| CATEGORY | RISK FACTORS |
|---|---|
| Patient-related factors | Increasing age<br>Preexisting renal disease<br>Preexisting chronic obstructive lung disease<br>Impaired immune defense<br>Underlying malignancy<br>Underlying gastrointestinal disease |
| Treatment-related factors | Preoperative bowel cleansing<br>Antibiotic use<br>Immunosuppressive therapy<br>Surgery<br>Prolonged hospital stay |
| Facility-related factors | Intensive care units<br>Caregivers<br>Long-term facilities |

Antibiotic use continues to precede almost all cases of infection. Of patients contracting CDC, 90% have received antibiotic therapy and 70% have been treated with multiple antibiotics. Patients receiving prolonged courses of antibiotic therapy are particularly susceptible, and those receiving prophylaxis are also at risk. Prolonged hospital stay allows exposure to contaminated environmental surfaces by more susceptible people. Intensive care and long-term facility units are not only sites of heavy environmental contamination, but also house critically ill and vulnerable patients. Impaired host immune defense as a result of advanced age, surgery, immunosuppressive medications, HIV, and chemotherapy are major risk factors. The proportion of immunocompromised patients infected with *C. difficile* has increased from 20% to 30% in the past decade. Surgical patients account for 45% to 55% of CDC, and the highest rates of infection are noted in patients undergoing general and vascular surgery. *C. difficile* is a gram-positive anaerobic spore-forming bacillus; approximately 5% to 35% of bacteria do not produce toxins and thus do not cause colitis. The organism produces a capsule that resists degradation by phagocytes. The spore is heat-resistant, persists in the environment for months and years in a dormant phase, and survives on inanimate objects. Approximately 3% to 5% of the general population has the organism in their stool. This increases to 8.6% of patients with hematologic malignancies and 10% to 25% of adults during hospitalization.

Antibiotic use leads to a disturbance in the microflora of the colon and allows the nosocomial organism to grow, proliferate, and produce toxins. Toxin A, an enterotoxin, causes cell rounding, mucosal damage and inflammation, and release of inflammatory mediators. Toxin B is a potent cytotoxin that causes identical cell rounding and activates the release of cytokines from human monocytes. The toxins translocate to the portal circulation. Phagocytosis of toxins by macrophages in the liver results in the elaboration of several cytokines that act in the propagation of the systemic septic response.

### Presentation and Diagnosis

Overgrowth of the toxigenic strain of *C. difficile* results in a variety of disease states, with varied clinical courses. Watery diarrhea is the hallmark symptom and usually starts during or shortly after antibiotic use. One dose of antibiotic can result in the disease, but the incidence with prophylactic antibiotics increases with extended use of antibiotics beyond the recommended period. Approximately 25% to 40% of patients become symptomatic 10 weeks after completion of antibiotic therapy. The stools are foul-smelling and may be positive for the presence of occult blood. In mild to moderate cases, systemic signs of infection are absent or present to a mild degree. In severe colitis, the diarrhea becomes associated with abdominal cramps and anorexia, abdominal tenderness, dehydration, tachycardia, a raised leukocyte (white blood cell [WBC]) count, and bandemia (>10%). Pseudomembranous colitis is the more dramatic form of the disease and develops in 40% of patients who are significantly symptomatic.

Cell cytotoxin assay in tissue culture is a highly sensitive and specific test for the detection of toxin B (rounding effect) and is the gold standard diagnostic test for CDC. ELISA that detects toxin A or B in stool is highly sensitive and specific. Unlike the stool cytotoxic test, which requires 24 to 48 hours, results with ELISA are obtained within hours, the test is less expensive, and does not require specific training. Endoscopy reveals nonspecific colitis in moderate disease (mucosal edema and patchy erythema) or pseudomembranes in severe disease. The presence of pseudomembranes may be limited to the proximal colon in 10% of cases and the rectum may be spared in 60% of cases. Radiographs of the abdomen may be normal or show adynamic ileus, colonic dilation, thumb printing, or haustral thickening. CT scans may show a thickened and edematous colon wall and free peritoneal fluid.

Approximately 2% to 5% of patients develop fulminant colitis, despite timely medical therapy, and may succumb to cytokine-mediated cardiovascular collapse and death. This frequently develops in hospitalized and postoperative patients but may occur in the out of hospital setting. At-risk patients are the immunocompromised or those taking multiple antibiotics, patients with a previous diagnosis of *C. difficile* infection, those with vasculopathy, older adults, those with chronic obstructive pulmonary disease, and those in renal failure. In fulminant colitis, abdominal cramps, distention, and tenderness become more prominent and are associated with systemic signs of toxicity. Diarrhea may be absent in 5% to 12% of cases; the WBC count may be depressed but is most commonly increased with a rapid elevation (>20,000 cells/mm$^3$) and bandemia (>30%). A leukemoid reaction is a prominent feature that may suggest CDC or herald the onset of fulminant disease. Frank peritoneal signs and toxic megacolon may develop and rapidly progress to shock. Toxic megacolon usually develops slowly and is characterized by obstipation, a dilated colon, and systemic toxicity. In fulminant disease, the toxin assay is negative in 12.5% of cases. CT scanning is diagnostic and typically shows a boggy, edematous, and thickened colon wall (>3 mm) in 88%, pancolitis in 50%, serous ascites in 35%, pericolic inflammation in 35%, a clover leaf or accordion sign in 20%, and megacolon (transverse colon >8 cm) in 25% of cases. Sigmoidoscopy shows pseudomembranes in 90% of cases versus 23% in mild cases.

### Treatment

Treatment of CDC starts with prevention. However, this is difficult because disinfectants may eliminate *C.* difficile but not the highly resistant spores, antibiotics are ineffective in clearing stools of carriers and although effective, steam sterilization is expensive. Judicious use of antibiotics, application of standard hygiene measures to hospital staff, use of disposable gloves and single-use disposable thermometers, and ward closure and decontamination in case of outbreaks are important for decreasing the mortality and morbidity associated with CDC.

Once a diagnosis of CDC is made, medical therapy and timely surgical intervention improve recovery and lower the mortality rate. Death is related to delay in diagnosis, reliance on negative toxin assay, less than total abdominal colectomy, and additional patient-related factors. Infections with *C. difficile* usually follow a benign course. Although some patients respond to discontinuation of antibiotic therapy, others require treatment and respond within 3 to 4 days, and symptoms resolve in 95% to 98% within 10 days. Vancomycin (125 mg, four times/day) is given orally, down the NG tube or given or as an enema, or metronidazole (Flagyl) is given orally (250 mg, four times/day) or IV (500 mg, three times/day) for 2 weeks. Antimotility agents and narcotics are avoided. IV fluid therapy is instituted to correct dehydration. In the absence of ileus, oral intake is allowed. Approximately 25% to 30% of patients develop recurrent disease as a result of reinfection with a second strain or reactivation of toxigenic spores that persist in the colon. Treatment of relapse is similar to that of the primary infection. In patients with recurrent attacks, pulsed vancomycin therapy, combination therapy with vancomycin and rifampicin, or the administration of competitive organisms (e.g., *Lactobacillus acidophilus* and *Saccharomyces cerevisiae*) may be tried.

Most patients with CDI respond to medical treatment but, occasionally, the disease progresses to a more severe form, such as fulminant colitis, despite appropriate and timely medical treatment. Fulminant colitis is characterized by severe systemic inflammatory response (fever, hypotension, tachycardia, leucocytosis, and/or requirement for volume resuscitation), shock, multiple organ failure, and death caused by toxin-induced inflammatory mediators (e.g., IL-8, macrophage inflammatory protein-2, substance P, tumor necrosis factor-$\alpha$ [TNF-$\alpha$]) released locally in the colon. Hypotension that requires vasopressor support despite adequate volume resuscitation, lactate level 5 mmol/liter or higher, respiratory failure and ventilator support, and an increase in organ dysfunction are alarming premortem signs.[36,38]

Colectomy is indicated when medical treatment fails or when the patient develops hemodynamic instability, fulminant disease, toxic megacolon, or peritonitis. The timing of intervention is not well established. Although the end point of failure of medical therapy is not known, a 24- to 48-hour trial is considered minimal. Early intervention commits the patient to a major surgical procedure and an ileostomy, and a delayed intervention is associated with high mortality (35% to 75%).[36-38]

Once the patient develops fulminant CDC, multiple organ failure, and hypotension, surgical intervention is less likely to be beneficial. Mortality is also increased with advanced age (>65 years), prolonged duration of CDI, length of medical treatment, and elevated serum lactate levels.[36-38] Consequently, to lower mortality of severe CDI, patients at risk for fulminant disease are identified and the clinical features of the disease must be recognized. Most importantly, surgical intervention must be considered during a critical window that precedes the onset of multiple organ failure and hemodynamic collapse from prolonged septic shock. Early surgical intervention noted in recent years (2000-2006 versus 1995-1996) has changed the outcome, with a decrease in mortality from 65% to 32%.[36,37] The procedure of choice is total abdominal colectomy and ileostomy. Lesser procedures are less effective and associated with high mortality (70%) compared with 11% with abdominal colectomy.

## Anastomotic Leak

### Causes

Numerous factors can cause or are associated with an increased risk for anastomotic leak (Table 13-13). Mechanical bowel preparation has long been considered a critical factor in preventing infectious complications after elective colorectal surgery. In emergencies, surgeons have resorted to on-table colonic lavage to cleanse the colon and primary anastomosis, with good results. With decreased morbidity rates as a result of effective antibiotic prophylaxis, modern surgical techniques, and advances in patient care, the need for mechanical bowel preparation has been questioned. Studies have shown that mechanical bowel preparation results in adverse physiologic changes and structural alterations in the colonic mucosa and inflammatory changes in the bowel wall. Furthermore, some studies have suggested that its use in elective cases is not only unnecessary but also associated with increased anastomotic leaks, intra-abdominal and wound infections, and reoperation.[39] Proponents of intraoperative lavage have also become content with simply decompressing the dilated colon and milking away fecal matter in the area of the anastomosis instead of aggressive cleansing. Although there is a trend toward elimination of cleansing of the colon in elective and emergent colon resection, one must be cautioned against abandoning the practice completely, especially for anterior resections, in which the presence of stool in the rectum poses a problem with the use of staplers.

The level of the anastomosis in the GI tract is important. Although small bowel, ileocolic, and ileorectal anastomoses are considered safe, esophageal, pancreaticoenteric, and colorectal anastomoses are considered high risk for leakage. In the esophagus, lack of serosa appears to be a significant contributing factor. In the pancreas, the texture of the gland and size of the pancreatic duct, presence of pancreatic duct obstructive lesions, experience of the operating surgeon, and probably the type of enteric anastomosis are implicated (see later). In the rectum, the highest leak rate is found in anastomoses in the distal rectum, 6 to 8 cm from the anal verge.

Adequate microcirculation at the resection margins is crucial for the healing of any anastomosis. Factors interfering with the perianastomotic microcirculation include smoking, hypertension, locally enhanced coagulation activity as a result of surgical trauma, perianastomotic hematoma, and presence of macrovascular disease. In colorectal anastomoses, relative ischemia in the rectal remnant is a factor because its blood supply is derived from the internal iliac artery via the inferior hemorrhoidal vessels, contribution from the middle hemorrhoidal artery is minimal and, at best, variable because the vessels are mostly absent and, when present, are unilateral. Total mesorectal excision, neoadjuvant therapy, and extended lymphadenectomy with high ligation of the inferior mesenteric artery are additional contributing factors.

Intraluminal distention is believed to be responsible for rupture of an anastomosis. The mechanical strength of the anastomosis is important and, in the early period, is dependent on sutures or staples, with endothelial cells and fibrin-fibrinonectin complex additionally contributing to the tension force. Construction of a watertight and airtight anastomosis is therefore essential. Antiadhesive agents may predispose to leaks because they isolate the anastomosis from the peritoneum and omentum and, as found in animal studies, decrease anastomotic bursting pressure and hydroxyproline levels.[40]

Intra-abdominally placed open rubber drains are not helpful and, if left for more than 24 to 48 hours, are associated with an increased risk of infection. In the pelvis, drains have been shown in some studies to be associated with a higher leak rate. Conversely, drains may remove blood, cellular debris, and serum that act as good culture media for perianastomotic sepsis or abscess formation. Local sepsis affects the integrity of the anastomosis negatively as it reduces collagen synthesis and increases collagenase activity, which results in increased lysis of

**Table 13-13 Risk Factors Associated With Anastomotic Leak**

| DEFINITIVE FACTORS | IMPLICATED FACTORS |
|---|---|
| Technical aspects:<br>Blood supply<br>Tension on the suture line<br>Airtight and watertight anastomosis | Mechanical bowel preparation<br>Drains<br>Advanced malignancy<br>Shock and coagulopathy |
| Location in the GI tract:<br>Pancreaticoenteric<br>Colorectal<br>Above the peritoneal reflection<br>Below the peritoneal reflection | Emergency surgery<br>Blood transfusion<br>Malnutrition<br>Obesity<br>Gender |
| Local factors:<br>Septic environment<br>Fluid collection | Smoking<br>Steroid therapy<br>Neoadjuvant therapy |
| Bowel-related factors:<br>Radiotherapy<br>Compromised distal lumen<br>Crohn's disease | Vitamin C, iron, zinc, and cysteine deficiency<br>Stapler-related factors:<br>Forceful extraction of the stapler<br>Tears caused by anvil or gun insertion<br>Failure of the stapler to close |

collagen at the anastomosis. Defunctioning or protective stomas do not decrease the overall leak rate but rather minimize the severity and sequelae of perianastomotic contamination and decrease the reoperation rate. Defunctioning stomas, however, deprive the colon of short-chain fatty acids, resulting in exclusion colitis and delay in epithelialization of the anastomosis, and are associated with altered collagen metabolism observed in left-sided anastomoses.

Bevacizumab, an angiogenesis inhibitor, is associated with increased risk for surgical site complications. It is a humanized monoclonal antibody that targets vascular endothelial growth factor (VEGF). VEGF is a critical factor for the survival of endothelial cells and is selectively present in the neovasculature of growing tumors. Bevacizumab binds with high specificity and affinity to VEGF, inhibiting the binding of VEGF to its receptors and negatively affecting angiogenesis and/or the remodeling of the existing network of blood vessels. Bevacizumab is used in combination with standard chemotherapy IFL (irinotecan, 5-fluorouracil [FU], and leucovorin) in the treatment of patients with metastatic colorectal cancer. In animal studies, antiangiogenic cancer therapy inhibits dermal wound healing in a dose-related fashion and compromises healing of colonic anastomoses. In patients with metastatic colorectal cancer, it increases the risk of surgical site complications—spontaneous dehiscence of primary anastomosis and colocutaneous fistula formation from an anastomosis. Such complications may occur up to 2 years after surgery.[41] The mechanism is probably related to microthromboembolic disease leading to bowel ischemia, inhibition of angiogenesis in the microvascular bed of the new anastomosis, inhibition of neoangiogenesis in postradiated tissue, and reduction in the number of newly formed vessels in granulation tissue surrounding anastomotic sites. Risk factors for delayed anastomotic complications include a history of anastomotic complications, radiotherapy, and rectal location of anastomoses.

Emergency bowel surgery is associated with high morbidity and mortality, in part because of sepsis and anastomotic leakage. This is related to the poor nutritional status of the patient, presence of underlying malignancy, immunocompromised state, presence of intra-abdominal contamination or sepsis, and hemodynamic instability. Transfusion, on the one hand, causes impaired cell-mediated immunity and predisposes to infection and, on the other hand, alleviates anemia and improves the oxygen-carrying capacity of red blood cells that may have a positive impact on healing. Obesity increases the difficulty and complexity of the surgery, has been shown to be associated with increased postoperative complications, and is an independent risk factor for an increasing leakage rate, especially after a low colorectal anastomosis. Steroids affect healing by decreasing collagen synthesis, delaying the appearance of the inflammatory reaction, and reducing the production of transforming growth factor-β and insulin-like growth factor in wounds, which are essential for wound healing.

### Presentation and Diagnosis

Anastomotic leak is a dreadful complication to encounter. It results in sepsis and enteric fistula formation, leads to reoperation and a possible permanent stoma, and is associated with decreased survival and increased local recurrence rate after curative resection of cancer, and possibly leads to death.[42]

The clinical manifestations are the result of a cascade of events that start with loss of integrity of the anastomosis and leakage of intestinal contents. The leakage may be diffuse throughout the peritoneal cavity (uncontrolled leak) or become walled off by omentum, abdominal wall, and contiguous loops of bowel, pelvic wall or adhesions from prior operations. If a surgical drain is present, intestinal contents are discharged onto the skin. Intra-abdominal fluid collections may contain intestinal contents, frank pus, or pus mixed with intestinal contents. If the fluid collection is drained surgically or percutaneously, there is an initial discharge of purulent material followed by feculent material heralding the formation of an enterocutaneous fistula (controlled fistula). If allowed to drain through the surgical incision or abdominal wall, surgical wound infection and dehiscence with evisceration or an abdominal wall abscess may occur. If the fluid collection burrows into a contiguous structure such as the urinary bladder or vagina, spontaneous drainage occurs, with the formation of an enterovesical or enterovaginal fistula.

Hence, after the index surgery, a patient may have an initial normal postoperative course or may not have been progressing as expected. The early warning signs of anastomotic leak are malaise, fever, abdominal pain, ileus, localized erythema around the surgical incision, and leukocytosis. Patients may also develop bowel obstruction, induration, and erythema in the abdominal wall, rectal bleeding, or suprapubic pain. There may be an initial excessive drainage from the surgical wound or surgical wound dehiscence and/or evisceration. An intra-abdominal fluid collection or abdominal wall abscess may be identified and drained surgically or percutaneously. Patients may also experience pneumaturia, fecaluria, and pyuria. Once a fistulous communication is established, problems related to the loss of intestinal contents, perifistula skin, surgical wound, and malnutrition soon ensue.

Sepsis is a prominent feature of anastomotic leakage and results from diffuse peritonitis or localized abscess, abdominal wall infection, or contamination of a sterile site with intestinal contents. Abdominal wall infection develops as a result of contact of purulent material with the muscle and subcutaneous tissue, tissue necrosis associated with fascial sutures, and/or contact of corrosive intestinal juices with the abdominal wall, resulting in chemical erosion and extension of the infectious process. Nonclostridial necrotizing infections of the abdominal wall occur, particularly with fistulas of the lower GI tract that contain high concentrations of *Enterobacteriaceae*, nongroup A beta-hemolytic streptococci, and anaerobic cocci or penicillin-sensitive *Bacteroides* spp. Contamination of the urinary bladder with intestinal contents (enterovesical fistula) results in urosepsis.

### Treatment

Treatment of anastomotic leakage starts with prevention. In elective cases, nutritional support for 5 to 7 days is appropriate for patients who are malnourished or have lost significant amounts of weight. Mechanical and chemical bowel preparations are still recommended by many surgeons prior to colorectal resection. In patients receiving or who have received bevacizumab, the appropriate interval between the last dose administered and the surgery is not known. The terminal half-life of the medication is long—20 days—so wound healing complications are documented up to 56 days after treatment. It is advisable to delay elective surgery for at least 4 to 8 weeks or, preferably, three half-lives (60 days) after treatment. In patients with newly constructed anastomoses who are candidates for bevacizumab therapy, evaluation of the anastomosis prior to initiation of therapy with fine-cut CT scanning, barium enema, and colonoscopy allows identification of patients at risk for anastomotic complications. In emergencies, especially in hemodynamically unstable, immunocompromised, and nutritionally depleted patients, in the presence of fecal peritonitis, significant bowel dilation, and edema, an anastomosis is best avoided because a leak may prove fatal.

Construction of an anastomosis that is at low risk for disruption requires the following:

1. Adequate exposure, gentle handling of tissues, aseptic precaution, and meticulous, careful dissection
2. Adequate mobilization so that the two attached organs have a tension-free anastomosis
3. Correct technical placement of sutures or staples with little variance
4. Matching of the lumina of the two organs to be connected, which can be done by various techniques
5. Preservation of the blood supply to the ends of structures to be anastomosed

Sufficient microcirculation is essential for healing of the anastomosis. In intestinal anastomoses, the marginal artery of the colon and last vascular arcade of small bowel mesentery must be preserved. The small bowel serosa must not be denuded of mesentery more than 3 to 4 cm for hand-sewn anastomoses. In the distal colon, to ensure a tension-free anastomosis, the following maneuvers may be required: inferior mesenteric artery may be divided at its origin, windows created in the mesentery of the small bowel up to the third portion of the duodenum, and small branches interrupted between the arcades, creating mesenteric windows and dividing the ileocolic vessels at their origin. For intestinal and colorectal anastomoses, there is no difference in the rate of anastomotic leakage between hand-sewn and stapled anastomoses and among various stapling techniques, provided that sound surgical technique is followed. The decision to construct a one- or two-layer intestinal anastomosis is a matter of preference. A colorectal anastomosis is easier to perform in one layer. However, since the advent of stapling devices, an anastomosis deep in the pelvis has most commonly been stapled. The technique is not only faster but also improves asepsis because the anastomosis is performed in a closed fashion compared with a hand-sewn anastomosis, which is considered an "open anastomosis" and allows for more contamination. In low anterior resection, the omentum may be advanced to the pelvis and placed around the colorectal anastomosis. This maneuver may lower the rate of anastomotic leak or disruption but mostly appears to decrease the severity of the complication. Drainage of a colorectal anastomosis is advisable in difficult cases and when technical problems are encountered, or when neoadjuvant therapy has been used. Defunctioning stomas are used for extraperitoneal anastomoses, when technical difficulties are encountered, or after neoadjuvant therapy.

When constructing a pancreaticoenteric anastomosis, a pancreaticojejunostomy is equivalent to pancreaticogastrostomy. An end to side–duct to mucosa pancreaticojejunostomy is associated with a lower leak rate compared with an end-to-end invaginating pancreaticojejunostomy; obliteration of the main pancreatic duct with protamine gel or human fibrin sealant, or suture closure of the remnant pancreas without an anastomosis, is associated with the highest leak rate.[43] The routine placement of drains in proximity to pancreatic anastomoses is controversial. Drains and octreotide can be used when an anastomosis is performed to a soft pancreas with a small duct and in lower surgical volume centers or centers with a high leak rate (>10%). Pancreatic duct stents (placed intraoperatively) continue to be used, despite the lack of data to suggest that they decrease the leak rate.[43] A pancreatic stent placed prior to a distal pancreatectomy decompresses the pancreatic duct by abolishing the pressure gradient between the pancreatic duct and duodenum and may decrease the risk of fistula formation, thus allowing the site of a leak to seal.

Once an anastomotic leak is suspected or diagnosed, resuscitation is started immediately because patients are in the postoperative period and have been without nutrition. Furthermore, they have a contracted intravascular volume because of third spacing and lost intestinal contents, and may have an electrolyte imbalance. Intravascular volume is restored with crystalloid fluids and a blood transfusion if anemia is present and electrolyte imbalances are corrected. Oral intake is stopped and the bowel is put at rest to decrease luminal contents and GI stimulation and secretion. A NG tube is placed if obstructive symptoms are present. Infected surgical wounds are opened, and any abdominal wall abscesses are incised and drained. Reoperation is indicated if there is diffuse peritonitis, intra-abdominal hemorrhage, suspected intestinal ischemia, major wound disruption, or evisceration. Reoperation is a major undertaking and is associated with significant mortality and morbidity. The procedure is bloody and carries the risk of bowel injury. Primary closure of the leaking point only is avoided because failure is certain.

The management of duodenal and proximal jejunal leaks is a challenging task. In these situations, transgastric placement of a jejunal tube helps divert gastric and biliopancreatic secretions and placement of drains in close proximity to the leak allows external drainage of the intestinal contents. Pyloric exclusion and gastrojejunostomy should be used judiciously in these situations. Management of jejunal, ileal, and colorectal leaking anastomoses depends on the severity and duration of contamination, condition of the bowel, and hemodynamic stability of the patient. In a critically ill and unstable patient, especially one with fecal peritonitis, a damage control type of procedure is performed—the anastomosis is taken down, the ends of the bowel are stapled, peritoneal lavage is performed, and the incision is left open. A second-look laparotomy with stomal formation is performed in 24 to 48 hours or once the patient is more stable. Otherwise, in the small bowel, an anastomosis may be performed or the ends of the bowel are delivered as stomas; in the colon, the proximal end of the colon is brought out as a colostomy and the distal end closed or brought out as a mucous fistula; and, in the rectum, the distal end is closed and the proximal end of the colon delivered as a stoma. A proximal diverting stoma with drainage of the pelvis is not adequate treatment of leaking colorectal anastomoses associated with diffuse peritonitis. If the abdomen is left open, covering the bowel with the greater omentum (if available) or a biologic implant protects the bowel and prevents desiccation and spontaneous fistula formation. Negative-pressure wound therapy is best avoided when bowel is exposed, especially in the presence of unprotected suture or staple line.[44]

In the absence of diffuse peritonitis and evisceration, a CT scan may identify single or multiple abscesses, pneumoperitoneum, ascites and, at times, extravasation of oral contrast into the peritoneal cavity. Multiple abscesses require open drainage, a single intra-abdominal abscess can be drained percutaneously, and a pelvic abscess can be drained transrectally or transvaginally. Following drainage, an external fistula may develop. The management of a controlled fistula is outlined in the next section. If percutaneous drainage fails to control sepsis, reoperation is indicated. At the time of open drainage of a pelvic abscess, if there is any doubt about the origin of the abscess (de novo abscess versus abscess secondary to a small anastomotic leak that has sealed), a defunctioning stoma is constructed unless there is complete disruption of the anastomosis. In that case, the ends of the bowel are exteriorized as a stoma. A pancreaticojejunostomy leak, if small, can be treated by placing a drain next to the leak. However, for an anastomosis that has almost fallen apart, the patient will probably require completion pancreatectomy. A patient who has a bile duct leak will require drainage of the infection and placement of a drain next to the leak or, in the case of a large leak, may require bile duct reconstruction.

## Intestinal Fistulas

### Causes

A fistula represents an abnormal communication between two epithelialized surfaces, one of which is a hollow organ. In the GI tract, a fistula may develop between any two digestive organs or between a hollow organ and the skin and may be developmental or acquired. Acquired fistulas account for most GI fistulas and can be traumatic, spontaneous, or postoperative in nature.

GI fistulas are most commonly iatrogenic, develop after an operation, and may occur anywhere in the GI tract. Esophageal, aortoenteric, and rectal fistulas are not discussed in this section. In the past, acquired GI fistulas most commonly developed as a result of a difficult appendectomy. At present, they commonly occur as the result of anastomotic breakdown, dehiscence of a surgically closed segment of stomach or bowel, unrecognized iatrogenic bowel injury following adhesiolysis, or during closure of a laparotomy incision. Occasionally, they develop after instrumentation or drainage of a pancreatic, appendiceal, or diverticular fluid collection or abscess. The presence of intrinsic intestinal disease, such as Crohn's disease, radiation enteritis, distal obstruction, or a hostile abdominal environment, such as an abscess or peritonitis, are predisposing factors for fistula formation. The risk is also higher in emergencies when the patient may be malnourished or poorly prepped.

Gastric fistulas are uncommon and frequently occur after resection for cancer and less frequently after resection for peptic ulcer disease, necrotizing pancreatitis, an antireflux procedure, or bariatric surgery. Pancreatic fistulas develop as a result of disruption of the main pancreatic duct or its branches secondary to trauma or postoperatively following pancreatic biopsy, distal pancreatectomy, pancreaticoduodenectomy, pancreatic necrosectomy, and surgery on the stomach, biliary tree, or spleen. Intestinal fistulas develop after resection for cancer, diverticular disease, inflammatory bowel disease, or closure of a stoma.

### Presentation and Diagnosis

Enterocutaneous fistulas are usually associated with a triad of sepsis, fluid and electrolyte imbalance, and malnutrition. Patients are usually in the postoperative period and may not be progressing as expected or may have an initial normal postoperative course. They then start showing the manifestations of leakage of intestinal contents (see earlier). The seriousness and severity of these manifestations depend on the surgical anatomy and physiology of the fistula. Anatomically, the fistula may originate from the stomach, duodenum, small bowel (proximal or distal), or large bowel. The tract of the fistula may erode into another portion of the intestines (enteroenteric fistula) or another hollow organ (enterovesical), thus forming an internal fistula, or into the body surface (enterocutaneous and pancreatic fistula) or vagina (enterovaginal fistula), thus forming an external fistula. A mixed fistula describes an internal fistula associated with an external fistula. A superficial fistula drains on top of an open or granulating wound; in a deep fistula, the tract traverses the abdominal cavity and drains onto the skin. Physiologically, the fistula is classified as high or low output on the basis of the volume of discharge in 24 hours. The exact definition of low and high output varies from 200 to 500 mL/24 hr. However, three different categories are recognized—low output (<200 mL/24 hr), moderate output (200 to 500 mL/24 hr), and high output (>500 mL/24 hr). The ileum is the site of the fistula in 50% of high-output fistulas. The discussion in this section focuses mainly on external fistulas.

Sepsis is a prominent feature of postoperative intestinal fistulas and is present in 25% to 75% of cases. As noted earlier, sepsis is the result of diffuse peritonitis or localized abscess, abdominal wall or necrotizing infection, or contamination of a sterile hollow organ with intestinal contents.

Loss of intestinal contents through the fistula results in hypovolemia and dehydration, electrolyte and acid-base imbalance, loss of protein and trace elements, and malnutrition. In a high intestinal fistula, it also results in loss of the normal inhibitory effect on gastric secretion, thus resulting in a gastric hypersecretory state. With high-output enterocutaneous fistulas, there is also intrahepatic cholestasis related to the loss of bile salts, disruption of enterohepatic circulation, and bacterial overgrowth in the defunctionalized intestine. Malnutrition results from loss of protein-rich secretions, lack of nutrient intake, loss of absorption caused by bypass of the gut (e.g., gastrocolic, duodenocolic, high enterocutaneous fistulas), and sepsis that sets the stage for nutritional deficiency and rapid breakdown of body muscle mass. In gastroduodenal and proximal small bowel fistulas, the output is high and the fluid loss, electrolyte imbalance, and malabsorption are profound. In distal small bowel and colonic fistulas, the output is low and dehydration, acid-base imbalance, and malnutrition are uncommon. Significant electrolyte imbalance occurs in 45% of patients and malnutrition occurs in 55% to 90%.

Skin and surgical wound complications develop as a result of contact of GI effluent with skin or the wound. Effluent dermatitis results from the corrosive effect of intestinal contents, which cause irritation, maceration, excoriation, ulceration, and infection of the skin. Fecal dermatitis is marked by erythema and desquamation and may encourage skin sepsis. Superficial and deep surgical wound and necrotizing infections also develop. Pain and itching by contact of effluent with unprotected skin is intolerable and affects the morale of the patient.

### Treatment

Postoperative intestinal fistulas are not a new problem but rather continue to be a challenging clinical scenario. Their etiogenesis has changed and their management continues to evolve. In the past, the main focus of management involved suctioning of the

**Table 13-14 Factors Affecting Healing of External Intestinal Fistulas**

| FACTORS | FAVORABLE | UNFAVORABLE |
|---|---|---|
| Surgical anatomy of the fistula | Long tract, >2 cm<br>Single tract<br>No other fistulas<br>Lateral fistula<br>Nonepithelialized tract<br>Origin (jejunum, colon, duodenal stump, and pancreaticobiliary)<br>No adjacent large abscess | Short tract, <2 cm<br>Multiple tracts<br>Associated internal fistulas<br>End fistula<br>Epithelialized tract<br>Origin (lateral duodenum, stomach, and ileum)<br>Adjacent large abscess |
| Status of the bowel | No intestinal disease<br>No distal bowel obstruction<br>Small enteral defect, <1 cm | Intrinsic intestinal disease (Crohn's disease, radiation enteritis, recurrent or incompletely resected cancer)<br>Distal bowel obstruction<br>Large enteral defect, >1 cm |
| Condition of the abdominal wall | Intact<br>Not diseased<br>No foreign body | Disrupted (fistula opens into the base of the disrupted incision)<br>Infiltrated with malignancy or intestinal disease<br>Foreign body (mesh) |
| Physiology of the patient | No malnutrition<br>No sepsis | Malnutrition<br>Sepsis |
| Output of the fistula | No influence | Influence |

intestinal effluent and early surgical intervention. This approach has proven ineffective and is associated with significant patient morbidity and mortality and a high reoperation rate. At present, management requires the involvement of a surgeon, nutritionist, enterostomal therapist, interventional radiologist, and gastroenterologist; it entails initial medical treatment to allow spontaneous healing of the fistula, early surgical intervention in a select group of patients, and planned definitive surgery for patients whose fistulas have failed to heal. External intestinal fistulas result in prolonged hospital stays and enormous cost to the hospital and are associated with significant patient disability, morbidity, and mortality (6% to 30%). Although spontaneous closure occurs in 40% to 80% of cases, operative intervention may be required in 30% to 60% of cases.

The first step in the management of a GI fistula is to prevent its occurrence. Reducing the likelihood of an anastomotic leak requires adherence to sound surgical principles and proper techniques (see earlier). Should a fistula form, management involves several phases that are applied systematically and simultaneously (Table 13-14).

Once a leak is diagnosed or suspected, management involves resuscitation, TPN, correction of electrolyte imbalances, and transfusions, as appropriate. Oral intake is stopped and the bowel is put at rest, thus decreasing luminal contents and reducing GI stimulation and secretion. An NG tube is placed if obstructive symptoms are present. Routine NG placement is not helpful and subjects the patient to complications, such as sinusitis and aspiration. Broad-spectrum IV antibiotic therapy is started and later adjusted according to cultures.

The indications for early surgical intervention have been discussed earlier. Otherwise, resuscitation is continued. Treatment with $H_2$ antagonists or PPI helps decrease peptic ulceration and may decrease fistula output but does not aid in the closure of the fistula. Accurate measurement of output from all orifices and the fistula is paramount in maintaining fluid balance. Effective control of all sources of sepsis is important because continued sepsis is a major source of mortality that results in a state of hypercatabolism and the failure of exogenous nutritional support to restore and maintain body mass and immune function; it is also associated with a decreased rate of healing of GI fistulas. Infected surgical wounds are opened and drained, abdominal wall abscesses are incised and drained, and intra-abdominal fluid collections are drained percutaneously or surgically. Percutaneous drainage is tolerated better and allows changing a complex fistula (fistula associated with an abscess) to a simple fistula that has a better chance of spontaneous closure. A small pigtail catheter may be changed to a larger catheter that allows irrigation of the abscess cavity, later injection of contrast to assess resolution of the abscess, and study of the anatomy of the fistula.

Nutrition is one of the most important factors contributing to a successful outcome in the management of intestinal fistulas. TPN must be started early after the correction of electrolyte imbalance and repletion of volume. TPN allows bowel rest, which decreases output, eliminates negative nitrogen balance, improves the patient's nutritional status, allows better timing of the operation when needed, increases the rate of recovery, and may slightly improve the closure rate once sepsis is controlled. Trace elements, multivitamins, vitamin K, and medications such as octreotide may be added to the TPN. TPN is the initial nutritional support for any patient with a fistula and is continued in patients with high-output fistulas or patients who cannot tolerate oral intake. Somatostatin (SMS) analogues (e.g., octreotide, with a long half-life) help in management of the fistula by reducing GI secretions and inhibiting GI motility, thus controlling and reducing its output. Their value in healing intestinal fistulas is yet to be proven and routine use is limited because they are not without side effects. Somatostatin leads to cellular apoptosis, villous atrophy, and interruption of intestinal adaptation, and may be associated with acute cholecystitis. Enteral nutrition (low-residue diet, elemental diet, liquid whole protein diet) is administered to patients with low-output small bowel and colonic external fistulas. Fistuloclysis (i.e., infusion of nutrition directly through the fistula into the bowel distal to the fistula) is another option to deliver enteral nutrition to patients whose fistula has not healed spontaneously, provided there is more than 75 cm of healthy bowel distal that is in continuity with the fistula.[45] Fistuloclysis is safer and less expensive than TPN and prevents atrophy of the bowel distal to the fistula.

Early control of fistula output is essential to protect the perifistula skin from the corrosive effects of intestinal effluent, promote healing of damaged skin and surgical wounds, and facilitate nursing care of the patient. Early involvement by an enterostomal therapist and wound care team cannot be overemphasized. Protection of the skin is achieved with barriers, sealants, adhesives, and pouches. Negative-pressure wound therapy is another treatment strategy whereby the continuous suction of fistula output minimizes contact between intestinal contents and surrounding tissue. Hence, it protects perifistula skin, reduces the need for dressing changes, promotes wound healing, and even accelerates fistula closure, especially in deep fistulas. Closure has been reported to occur in 46% to 84% of cases.[46]

Once initial sepsis is controlled, nutrition provided, and wound and fistula care provided, studies are performed to define the surgical pathology of the fistula (origin, course, length of the fistula) and condition of the bowel (presence of intrinsic intestinal disease, presence of distal obstruction, continuity of the bowel) and to evaluate resolution of the intra-abdominal abscess. A fistulogram is performed by injecting a water-soluble contrast medium or barium through an existing drain or by inserting a 5 Fr pediatric feeding tube or a Foley catheter into the external opening of the fistula. A fistulogram delineates the anatomy of the fistula and identifies associated cavities, other fistulas, and distal obstructions. A contrast enema demonstrates the presence of a colocutaneous fistula in 90%, a colovesical fistula in 34%, and a coloenteric fistula in most cases. Enteroclysis allows evaluation for intrinsic intestinal disease. Cystoscopy identifies the fistula opening in 40% of enterovesical fistulas but the findings of localized bullous edema, with erythema and possible ulceration, are suggestive of the diagnosis in most patients. GI endoscopy allows direct visualization of colonic, intestinal, and gastroduodenal mucosa. A CT scan allows evaluation for the resolution of intra-abdominal abscesses and presence of intrinsic intestinal disease.

With such an orchestrated approach, most external fistulas heal spontaneously. Factors associated with spontaneous healing or failure to close are listed in Table 13-14. After control of sepsis, approximately 60% to 90% of external intestinal fistulas with favorable factors will close spontaneously with medical management, 90% will close within 4 to 6 weeks, and less than 10% in months 2 and 3. There are limited therapeutic options for enterocutaneous fistulas (ECFs) that fail to close—accept the fistula as a stoma awaiting optimal time for definitive closure or attempt direct closure.

Direct repair is applicable to a superficial bud fistula whereby limited dissection is performed to identify and close the edges of the fistula extraperitoneally and protect the suture line with a biologic dressing, with or without tissue adhesive. Although several attempts may be required to achieve successful closure of the fistula, the surgery is a local low-risk procedure and can be repeated. Definitive repair requires careful planning and may be a daunting task. Definitive closure requires a waiting period of 8 to 12 weeks, and requires that sepsis be controlled, nutrition provided, and skin is protected. The waiting period is crucial to allow recovery of immunologic competence, improvement of nutritional status, and resolution of the period of dense inflammatory reaction. There are no well-established guidelines to help in determining the timing of surgery. However, the experience of the surgeon, general condition of the patient, softness of the abdominal wall and abdominal cavity, and surgical anatomy of the fistula must be taken into consideration. A dense intra-abdominal inflammatory reaction occurs 10 to 21 days after surgery and lasts for 6 to 8 weeks before starting to resolve. A 6-month period is required for a neoperitoneal cavity to develop in fistulas within a laparoscopy wound. A simple fistula—single fistula with direct communication between the bowel and skin, a short tract and small enteral opening, and associated with other favorable factors—can be closed 12 weeks after the index surgery. A complex fistula—a fistula with a long tract and associated with other internal fistulas, large abscess cavity, fistula that opens into the base of a disrupted wound, or other unfavorable factors—is closed 6 to 12 months after the index surgery. Complex fistulas associated with intrinsic intestinal disease require definitive surgical intervention once the initial sepsis is controlled because spontaneous closure is highly unlikely and extirpation of the diseased bowel is essential. In patients with Crohn's disease, infliximab (Remicade) may also be used to aid in closure of the fistula in a select group of patients.

A controlled ECF that opens into the base of an interrupted wound requires abdominal wall construction at the time of definitive repair of the fistula. The fistulizing segment must not be excluded or bypassed to avoid the risk of blind loop syndrome. The fistula is excised, continuity of the GI tract reestablished, and the freshly constructed anastomosis wrapped with omentum, if available. Gastric, duodenal, and proximal jejunal fistulas that cannot be resected without a major surgical procedure are best managed with a Roux-en-Y intestinal anastomosis. The laparotomy incision is closed primarily or with durable well-vascularized coverage. Autogenous tissue reduces the risk of infection. Pedicle or free flaps with microvascular reconstruction may be considered; however, component separation when the rectus muscle is intact, with or without augmentation with acellular dermal matrix or synthetic mesh, is the preferred procedure.[47] Postoperative morbidity, ventral hernia formation, and recurrent ECFs develop in approximately 20% to 25% of cases. Biologic material (e.g., acellular human or porcine dermal matrix, porcine submucosa) used for visceral overlay protection or reconstruction is another viable option in this setting of compromised operative field because the implant resists infection and, when postoperative infection occurs, removal of the implant is not necessary. However, the product is expensive and the procedure is associated with a high rate of hernia formation and abdominal wall laxity.[48] Occasionally the incision is closed in stages. The incision may be left open (laparotomy), an absorbable mesh (polyglactin or polyglycolic acid) may be used to bridge the fascial defect, or negative-pressure wound therapy can be instituted. Once granulation tissue is formed, a split-thickness skin graft is applied.

New innovative approaches, such as transcatheter injection of diluted thrombin, endoscopic tissue sealant or clip application, and porcine small intestinal submucosa have been used in recalcitrant cases or as adjunctive therapy to hasten healing of the intestinal fistula, with some success.

## Pancreatic Fistulas

Overall, the physiologic classification, diagnosis, management, and outcome of postoperative external pancreatic fistulas are similar to that for external intestinal fistulas. However, pancreatic fistulas have additional distinctive features. Following pancreaticoduodenectomy, texture of the pancreas, size of the pancreatic duct, blood supply to the stump, and volume of pancreatic juice produced are the most significant risk factors for fistula formation. Pulmonary problems, autodigestion, and erosion into adjacent organs are additional significant morbidities associated with pancreatic fistulas. Sepsis and hemorrhage are associated with significant mortality (20% to 40%) and result in prolonged hospitalization and increased hospital expense. Postoperative pancreatic fistula is diagnosed when there is drain output of any measurable volume of fluid after postoperative day 3 with an amylase content more than three times the serum amylase activity. More often, the fluid amylase content is in the tens of thousands units/L. The fistula is demonstrated on a fistulogram or CT scan.

Efforts to decrease the morbidity and mortality of pancreatic fistulas after pancreaticoduodenectomy focus on preventing, decreasing, and controlling pancreatic leaks at the pancreatic-enteric reconstruction (see earlier, "Anastomotic Leak"). The benefit of perioperative somatostatin or its analogue has been evaluated in a meta-analysis study.[49] One study noted that somatostatin and octreotide reduce the rate of biochemical fistula but not the incidence of clinical anastomotic dehiscence, whereas the other noted a significant reduction in pancreatic fistula rate but no significant difference in postoperative mortality. Intraoperatively, a modified side to end pancreaticojejunal anastomosis provides a tension-free anastomosis to a pancreatic stump, with adequate blood supply and unobstructed flow of pancreatic juice is optimal. Common to this modified pancreaticojejunostomy is mobilization of the pancreatic stump to allow invagination of 3 to 4 cm of pancreatic stump into the jejunum, ablation of the jejuna mucosa in the area of the jejunum-pancreas interface, suturing the capsular edge of the pancreatic stump to mucosa of the everted jejunum, or the use of traction sutures between the capsular edge and jejunum proximal edge to avoid slippage of the stump out of the jejunum.

Once a pancreatic fistula has formed, medical treatment results in spontaneous closure in almost all fistulas after a pancreaticoduodenectomy and in up to 80% of all other cases of pancreatic fistulas. Octreotide therapy is beneficial because it significantly reduces fistula output and decreases the time to fistula closure. Endoscopic retrograde cholangiopancreatography (ERCP) is valuable because it defines the pancreatic duct anatomy and ductal obstruction and allows the placement of a stent that bypasses the high-resistance areas of the sphincter of Oddi, ductal strictures, and calculi, thus allowing pancreatic secretions to follow the path of least resistance. The stent may also block the ductal opening of the fistula. Operative treatment of a benign pancreaticocutaneous fistula depends on the location of the fistula (proximal versus distal portion of the pancreas) and status of the pancreatic duct (dilated versus stenotic duct). High excision of the fistula with fistuloenterostomy has been associated with the best results. Pseudocyst enterostomy is associated with an unacceptable recurrence and failure rate.

## HEPATOBILIARY COMPLICATIONS

### Bile Duct Injuries

#### Causes

The most dreaded complication of gallbladder surgery is injury to the extrahepatic bile duct system. Cholecystectomy accounts for most postoperative biliary injuries and strictures. The rate of major bile duct injury after laparoscopic cholecystectomy ranges from 0.4% to 0.7%, as opposed to 0.2% after open cholecystectomy.[50] Bile leak may be caused by a bile duct injury, cystic duct stump leak, divided accessory duct, or injury to the intestine. Acute cholecystitis, a foreshortened cystic duct, anomalies of the biliary tree, hemorrhage from injury to the cystic or hepatic artery, dissection with thermal instruments in the triangle of Calot, and failure to define the anatomy in the triangle of Calot clearly are among the most important factors associated with a higher frequency of duct injury after laparoscopic cholecystectomy.

The most common injury sustained during the laparoscopic procedure is complete transection at or below the hepatic duct bifurcation. Other less complex injuries include occlusion of the duct with a clip, thermal injury, avulsion of the cystic duct, and partial laceration.

### Presentation and Diagnosis

Most bile duct injuries are not identified at the time of surgery. Early in the postoperative period, patients may have manifestations related to a bile leak or have signs of a bile duct stricture later. Bile leaking from a lacerated divided duct may accumulate in the subhepatic space and form a biloma or seep into the peritoneal cavity and result in bile ascites. Patients in this situation have right upper quadrant pain, fever, nausea, abdominal distention, and malaise. The bile, on the other hand, may drain through an intraoperatively placed drain and be manifested as a bile leak. In this setting patients, may have leukocytosis and a slightly elevated bilirubin level. Patients with a clipped bile duct do not usually have symptoms but do have elevated liver enzyme levels. Bile duct strictures are usually accompanied by cholangitis, pain, fever, chills, and jaundice.

Diagnosis of bile duct injury requires the use of nuclear medicine imaging to demonstrate the presence of a leak or obstruction, a CT scan to identify bile collections or ascites, and ERCP to define the type and level of injury accurately. Percutaneous transhepatic cholangiography is indicated in cases of complete transection to define the proximal anatomy and site of injury. Magnetic resonance cholangiopancreatography is becoming the test of choice to diagnose late strictures and define the bile duct anatomy.

#### Treatment

Prevention of bile duct injury starts with proper surgical technique and adequate identification of the anatomy. The anatomic variability associated with severe inflammation creates a low threshold for converting a laparoscopic to an open cholecystectomy. During laparoscopic cholecystectomy, the infundibulum of the gallbladder must be retracted laterally and inferiorly to expose the triangle and widen the cystic–common bile duct angle. Dissection of the cystic duct and artery must commence close to the infundibulum of the gallbladder. The cystic duct and artery are divided once the anatomy is clearly delineated. Excessive traction on the gallbladder must be avoided because it will result in tenting of the common duct. If there is bleeding in the area of the cystic duct, blind clipping and cautery must be avoided and adequate exposure must be achieved, even if placement of another port is required. If there is an unexpected bile leak, unusual anatomy, or a second bile duct identified, or when technical difficulties and excessive bleeding are encountered, intraoperative cholangiography helps identify the anatomy and any injuries. Early conversion to an open procedure must also be considered.

Once a leak is diagnosed intraoperatively, immediate repair must be performed. The procedure is converted to an open one and the extent of duct injury is assessed. An accessory duct can be ligated, partial transection of the common duct can be repaired over a T tube, a divided duct or almost circumferential transection of the common duct can be repaired with an end-to-end anastomosis over a T tube, and a high injury can be repaired with a Roux-en-Y biliary enteric anastomosis. If repair of a high duct injury is difficult, drains are placed in the subhepatic space and the patient is referred to a tertiary center.

A leak or injury identified early in the postoperative period is treated as follows. The biloma is drained percutaneously, and a sphincterotomy is performed, a stent is placed, or both can be done if ERCP demonstrates a leak or partial narrowing. Surgical intervention is indicated for patients with major obstruction of the bile duct, major injury, or suspicion of a bowel injury. After adequate resuscitation, administration of antibiotics, and adequate drainage, patients are watched for a few days to make certain that they are not septic at the time of the operation. If there is evidence of adequate control of the leak, the surgeon may wait up to 5 to 7 days for inflammation in the area to subside before undertaking operative repair. Meticulous and careful dissection is required in this area because there is usually loss of common bile duct substance. After identifying the source of the bile extravasation, dissection plus débridement of nonviable common bile duct is prudent. Once it has been ascertained that there is tissue with good integrity, a Roux-en-Y limb can be anastomosed to the common bile duct. Multiple drains are left around the site of the repair.

**BOX 13-16 Causes of Acute Delirium**

Advanced age
Alcohol intoxication and withdrawal
Drugs (overdose or withdrawal)
- Anticholinergic drugs (tricyclic antidepressants, antihistamine)
- Oral hypoglycemic agents
- Antibiotics (cephalosporins)
- Histamine receptor blocking agents
- Anti-inflammatory drugs (e.g., steroidal, nonsteroidal)
- Anticonvulsant medications
- Anxiolytics (diazepam)
- Narcotics
- Cardiac medications (beta blockers, digoxin)

Structural brain abnormalities (e.g., edema, transient ischemic attack, neoplasm)
Metabolic and hemodynamic disturbances
- Electrolyte imbalance
- Hypoglycemia
- Hypoxemia
- Hypovolemia

Endocrine dysfunction
- Thyrotoxicosis
- Hypothyroidism
- Adrenocortical insufficiency

Sepsis and infections
Respiratory dysfunction (e.g., respiratory failure, pulmonary embolism, chronic obstructive pulmonary disease)
Liver, renal, cardiac disease (e.g., congestive heart failure, renal failure)
Trauma (surgical or otherwise)
Critical illness and intensive care unit stay

## NEUROLOGIC COMPLICATIONS

### Delirium, Cognitive Disorder, and Psychosis

#### Cause

Delirium refers to a state of acute confusion and is a common complication of surgery. Numerous factors are implicated in causing delirium (Box 13-16). The presence of a structural brain disorder (infarct) increases the individual's susceptibility to delirium. Anticholinergic medications and conditions that decrease the production of acetylcholine can precipitate delirium. In addition, a planned operation with loss of the patient's routine schedule, stress of the disease process, fear of the operation, loss of personal control, placement in an unfamiliar environment, addition of mind-altering pain medications, and pain can lead to dramatic alterations in behavior in postoperative patients. At particularly high risk for behavioral disorders in the postoperative period are older patients, patients with a previous history of substance abuse or psychiatric disorders, and children.

#### Presentation and Diagnosis

Early in the postoperative period, a patient may become acutely agitated, uncooperative, and confused. Patients with a previous psychiatric disorder may, however, become more withdrawn and depressed. Some patients may become noncommunicative and emotionally flat and may withdraw from any emotional exchange. Patients may also show an altered level of consciousness and changes in cognition. They may have reduced ability to focus, decreased levels of awareness, and difficulty with attention. In addition, they may have hallucinations and altered psychomotor activity and sleep-wake cycle. These changes have a tendency to fluctuate during the course of the day and are worse at night (sundowning). The severity of these manifestations depends on the underlying cause.

The incidence of postoperative delirium and cognitive disorders in geriatric patients varies with the type of surgery performed and preexisting dementia. Postoperative anemia (secondary to acute blood loss), electrolyte imbalance, sepsis, malnutrition, bladder catheterization, physical restraints, extended duration of anesthesia, infection, and respiratory complications are significant precipitating factors.

The most immediately threatening disorder encountered by physicians is delirium tremens, which may occur 48 hours to 14 days after acute alcohol withdrawal. In addition, delirium tremens is associated with extreme autonomic hyperactivity. Early signs of delirium tremens include fever, tremor, and tachycardia, and late signs include confusion, psychosis, agitation, and seizures. Because of the serious underlying nutritional and medical deficiencies, these patients have s moderately high mortality, which approaches 20% in some series.

#### Treatment

Management of delirium and cognitive disorders in a postoperative patient is a frustrating and challenging clinical scenario. Prevention starts with the identification of high-risk individuals before surgery and careful follow-up thereafter. Minimizing the dose or eliminating medications that interrupt mental function must be considered. Optimizing fluid status, providing nutrition and adequate pain control, and removing restraints early, including the Foley catheter, are essential. Early ambulation and transfer from the intensive care unit are encouraged.

Treatment of patients with acute confusion or a sudden change in behavior after surgery requires the following:

1. Recognition of the disorder
2. Close observation and monitoring
3. Identification and elimination of the precipitating factor
4. Treatment of any associated laboratory abnormalities
5. Selective use of imaging or other studies to rule out an organic brain lesion
6. Application of measures to protect the patient and staff
7. Treatment

A history of drug or alcohol abuse and of cardiac, pulmonary, renal, or liver disease or psychiatric illness must be sought. A list of medications used in the perioperative period must be checked. Clinical evaluation is performed to look for evidence of sepsis or a recent neurologic event. A thorough neurologic examination is performed while focusing on the level of consciousness and presence of focal neurologic deficits, ataxia, paresis, or paralysis. Cognitive tests are conducted. Blood samples are sent to check for evidence of infection and to identify metabolic, electrolyte, nutritional, and blood gas abnormalities. A CXR and urinalysis are performed to look for a source of infection. An ECG is obtained to look for evidence of MI. CT or MRI, and occasionally a spinal tap, may be helpful in select cases.

Measures to protect the patient and staff may include the occasional use of physical restraints, reassurance by speaking to the patient, and allowing family members to be involved in patient care. Medical therapy includes haloperidol, a neuroleptic (0.5 to 2 mg, given IV or IM to achieve a rapid effect and then PO for maintenance therapy). Benzodiazepines are the drug of choice for acute alcohol withdrawal. Other medications, including haloperidol (to control psychosis), beta blockers (to control autonomic manifestations), and clonidine (to control hypertension) are given in addition to benzodiazepine to patients with acute alcohol withdrawal.

### Seizure Disorders

#### Causes

Seizures are caused by paroxysmal electrical discharges from the cerebral cortex and may be primary or secondary. Primary causes include intracranial tumor, hemorrhage, trauma, and idiopathic seizure activity. Secondary causes include metabolic derangement, sepsis, systemic disease processes, and pharmacologic agents. Patients at particularly high risk for postoperative seizure include those with a previous history of epilepsy and patients acutely withdrawing from alcohol or medications or receiving other pharmacologic agents, including antidepressants, hypoglycemic agents, and lidocaine.

#### Presentation and Management

Seizures characterized by convulsions, rhythmic myoclonic activity, loss of consciousness, and change in mental status are often associated with fecal and urinary incontinence, lack of neurologic responsiveness, and postevent amnesia. On recognizing evidence of seizure activity, the patient must be carefully restrained so that injury is not sustained during convulsions and is carefully observed. Administration of IV benzodiazepines is essential to stop the seizure activity and is the standard for immediate care. Phenytoin (Dilantin) is the most commonly used anticonvulsant for new-onset generalized or focal seizures. It may be administered IV during acute convulsions or PO for maintenance. Phenytoin has several side effects, including rash and liver dysfunction. Occasionally, phenobarbital may be used but, because of sedation, is not an agent of choice. The two most commonly used agents for maintenance after seizures or for someone with status epilepticus are carbamazepine (Tegretol) and valproic acid. Neither of these agents can be given IV and thus are used for maintenance only. Gabapentin can be administered when the patient's condition is refractory to other agents. After adequate control of the seizure, a diagnostic workup for its cause is initiated. This includes a detailed history and physical examination, history of previous medication and drug use, WBC count to rule out occult infection, and electrolyte and metabolic assessment. CT or MRI is indicated for a patient with new-onset seizure activity because tumors are often the cause. Similarly, an electroencephalogram is obtained at some point to look for abnormal waveform activity.

### Stroke and Transient Ischemic Attacks

#### Causes

A stroke in the perioperative period is devastating and correlates with the type of operative procedure performed, age of the patient, and presence of risk factors for cardiovascular disease. Strokes are more commonly associated with cardiovascular procedures. Although older adults with cardiovascular disease are at a higher risk for a stroke, younger individuals are not exempt, especially those with an underlying inherited thrombophilia.

Postoperative strokes may be ischemic or hemorrhagic in nature. Ischemic strokes most commonly result from perioperative hypotension or overzealous control of hypertension, or from cardioemboli in patients with atrial fibrillation. Other sources of cardioemboli include MI and bacterial endocarditis. An embolus arising from DVT and traversing a patent foramen ovale (i.e., paradoxical embolization) may be responsible for strokes of unknown cause. Hemorrhagic strokes are less common and are mostly related to therapy with anticoagulants. Factors related to coagulation disorders, such as chronic abuse of alcohol, acquired immunodeficiency syndrome (AIDS), cocaine use, bleeding diathesis, and preexisting cerebrovascular anomalies, are associated with an increased risk for hemorrhagic stroke.

#### Presentation and Management

In all cases of stroke, the neurologic changes represent a dramatic departure from normal patient function. A focal alteration in motor function, alteration in mental status, aphasia, or occasionally unresponsiveness may be noted. Hemorrhagic strokes are uncommon, and their effect can be more devastating than ischemic strokes that are transient (occurring for seconds to minutes) or reversible (occurring for minutes to hours). In truly irreversible injury, the impact on the patient's overall health is immeasurable, and the patient's ability to function and enjoy a good quality of life is severely compromised.

Prevention of a perioperative stroke starts with the identification of at-risk patients. Patients with hypertension must receive adequate treatment, and overzealous correction must be avoided. Patients with atrial fibrillation benefit from prophylaxis with anticoagulants. Patients with a carotid bruit must be evaluated with noninvasive vascular studies and treated accordingly. Patients undergoing a high-risk surgical procedure (e.g., carotid endarterectomy) may be monitored intraoperatively with transcranial Doppler and electroencephalography. Adequate hydration and monitoring in the perioperative period to avoid hypotension and fluctuations in blood pressure are essential to avoid ischemic strokes.

On recognizing the clinical signs and symptoms of a stroke, the patient must have an IV line placed and be monitored for cardiac arrhythmias. Coagulation parameters are assessed for the presence of a coagulopathy, and blood is sent for culture and determination of the sedimentation rate to check for bacteremia and bacterial endocarditis. A diagnostic workup is started immediately to distinguish between hemorrhagic and ischemic stroke with a CT scan or MRI of the brain. Further tests depend on the clinical scenario, such as echocardiography to assess the heart for structural disease, carotid duplex scanning to assess patency of the carotid artery, and cerebral angiography to evaluate for vascular anomalies. Therapy is dictated by the underling mechanism of the stroke. A hypertensive hemorrhagic stroke is treated by aggressive control of the hypertension, an embolic stroke (cardiogenic or secondary to inherited thrombophilia) is treated by anticoagulation (in the absence of a contraindication) to prevent recurrence, and a hemorrhagic stroke is treated by reversal of the coagulopathy with protamine, if secondary to heparin, or platelet transfusion, if secondary to antiplatelet therapy. Mannitol and dexamethasone are given to reduce cerebral swelling. Treatment of any underlying cardiac arrhythmia is imperative to prevent recurrent embolization. Surgical intervention is indicated for patients with a localized hematoma or vascular anomaly, depending on the location and size of the hematoma, status of the patient, and accessibility of the aneurysm. Thrombolytic therapy (recombinant tissue plasminogen activator) is effective in restoring cerebral blood flow and minimizing brain injury if instituted early after the onset of an embolic event. Otherwise, low-dose aspirin therapy is the standard for acute ischemic infarction and, in patients who continue to have symptoms, antiplatelet agents (e.g., clopidogrel bisulfate, ticlopidine hydrochloride) are added.

## EAR, NOSE, AND THROAT COMPLICATIONS

### Epistaxis

Epistaxis may be associated with primary blood dyscrasias such as leukemia and hemophilia, excessive anticoagulation, and hypertension. Epistaxis is divided into two general categories, anterior and posterior. Anterior trauma is often caused by contusion or laceration of the nasal septum or turbinates during insertion of an NG or endotracheal tube. Firm pressure applied between the thumb and index finger to the nasal ala and held for 3 to 5 minutes is generally successful in stopping most cases of anterior epistaxis. Occasionally, packing with strip gauze for 10 to 15 minutes will aid in a particularly refractory case. If the bleeding fails to stop, packing for an extended period with petroleum jelly–covered strip gauze may be required. Removal of the packing in 1 to 3 days is usually associated with successful treatment of refractory epistaxis, along with treatment of the underlying condition or reversal of anticoagulation.

A more serious scenario is posterior nasal septal bleeding, which on occasion can be life-threatening. If all attempts to stop anterior nasal septal bleeding are unsuccessful, one may infer the probability of a posterior nasal hemorrhage, which may necessitate placement of a posterior pack of strip gauze covered in petroleum jelly ointment. For particularly refractory cases, a Foley catheter with a 30-mL balloon can be passed through the nasal passages and, after the pack is placed, pressure can be applied to it by pulling on the Foley catheter. This type of epistaxis may require concomitant anterior nasal packing to be successful. The packs on a difficult hemorrhage such as this may need to be left in place for 2 to 3 days. For epistaxis that defies all attempts at conservative management, ligation of the sphenopalatine artery or anterior ethmoidal artery may be required.

### Acute Hearing Loss

Abrupt loss of hearing in the postoperative period is an uncommon event. An immediate physical examination is performed to ascertain the degree of hearing loss. Unilateral hearing loss is generally associated with obstruction or edema related to an NG or feeding tube. Bilateral hearing loss is more often neural in nature and is usually associated with pharmacologic agents, such as aminoglycosides and diuretics. Examination with an otoscope will often reveal the presence of cerumen impaction or edema from a middle ear infection. If the otologic examination is completely normal, neural injury related to the agents just mentioned should be suspected. These drugs need to be discontinued immediately and hearing monitored over the ensuing 2 to 3 days to see whether recovery occurs. For cerumen impaction, use of a delicate speculum under direct vision is indicated. If the hearing loss is associated with edema related to an NG tube, merely removing the NG tube will result in resolution of the edema.

### Nosocomial Sinusitis

Nosocomial sinusitis is a recognized complication in the critically ill. Left untreated, sinusitis may be complicated by brain abscess formation, postorbital cellulitis, and nosocomial pneumonia. Patients at high risk for sinusitis are those receiving ventilatory support via a nasotracheal tube and those with nasal colonization with gram-negative bacteria. Also at risk are patients with facial trauma, those with an NG or feeding tube, and patients who have received antibiotic therapy.

Most nosocomial sinusitis occurs in the second week of hospitalization, and the maxillary sinuses are the most commonly affected. The classic signs encountered with community-acquired sinusitis (e.g., facial pain, malaise, fever, and purulent nasal discharge) may not be present because the patient is usually unconscious and intubated, has other sources of infection, and is receiving analgesics and antipyretics. The diagnosis is often made when CT is performed to look for a source of fever and the sinuses are included in the cuts. The CT scan generally shows thickened mucosa and the presence of an air-fluid level or opacification of the sinus.

Once diagnosed or suspected, nasal tubes are removed, decongestant is administered, and antibiotic therapy targeting the two most common organisms, *S. aureus* and *Pseudomonas* spp., is given. Other organisms that play a major role in nosocomial infections, such as MRSA and vancomycin-resistant *Enterococcus* and *Acinetobacter* spp., are also included in the coverage. With such treatment, clinical response occurs in 48 hours and a clinical and radiologic cure occurs in two thirds of patients. Failure of medical therapy leads to surgical drainage of the sinus involved. In rare cases, severe intractable sinusitis may require a drainage procedure via an operative technique.

### Parotitis

Parotitis most commonly occurs in an older man with poor oral hygiene and poor oral intake, with an associated decrease in saliva production. The pathophysiology involves obstruction of the salivary ducts or an infection in a diabetic or immunocompromised patient. The patient is noted to have significant edema and focal tenderness surrounding the parotid gland, which eventually progresses to involve edema of the floor of the mouth. If left undiagnosed and untreated, the parotitis can cause life-threatening sepsis. In the worst case scenario, the infection can dissect into the mediastinum and cause stridor from partial airway obstruction. Patients with advanced parotitis will have dysphagia and some respiratory occlusion. If the diagnosis of parotitis is being entertained, the patient receives IV, high-dose, broad-spectrum antibiotics with good coverage of *Staphylococcus,* the most common agent cultured from this disease. In the presence of a fluctuant area, incision plus drainage is indicated, with care taken to avoid the facial nerve. Rarely, advanced disease may even require emergency tracheostomy. Most patients with parotitis will have the condition arise 4 to 12 days after an initial operation. Because of the rapid progression of this disease, one must be aware of the diagnosis and, when present, institute immediate therapy, including occasional emergency surgery for patients with an obvious fluctuant area.

## SELECTED REFERENCES

Almanaseer Y, Mukherjee D, Kline-Rogers EM, et al: Implementation of the ACC/AHA guidelines for preoperative risk assessment in a general medicine preoperative clinic: Improving efficiency and preserving outcomes. Cardiology 103:24–29, 2005.

This paper describes the clinical predictors of increased cardiovascular risk leading to acute cardiac events in surgical patients. Implementation of these predictors may also allow better selection of patients who require more specific preoperative cardiac evaluation and beta blocker therapy.

Anderson JL, Adams CD, Antman EM, et al: ACC/AHA 2007 guidelines for the management of patients with unstable angina/non-ST-Elevation myocardial infarction: A report of the American College of Cardiology/American Heart Association Task Force on Practice Guidelines (Writing Committee to Revise the 2002 Guidelines for the Management of Patients With Unstable Angina/Non-ST-Elevation Myocardial Infarction) developed in collaboration with the American College of Emergency Physicians, the Society for Cardiovascular Angiography and Interventions, and the Society of Thoracic Surgeons endorsed by the American Association of Cardiovascular and Pulmonary Rehabilitation and the Society for Academic Emergency Medicine. J Am Coll Cardiol 50:e1–e157, 2007.

Patients with angina, particularly unstable angina, represent a high-risk group for surgery. The paper provides practical guidelines for the management of this challenging group of patients.

Anderson DJ, Kaye KS, Classen D, et al: Strategies to prevent surgical site infections in acute care hospitals. Infect Control Hosp Epidemiol 29(Suppl 1):S51–S61, 2008.

Surgical site infections (SSIs) remain a serious cause of significant postoperative morbidity, increased cost, and poor outcomes. This paper provides a realistic strategy for lowering or preventing SSIs in the acute care hospital setting.

Cooper MS, Stewart PM: Corticosteroid insufficiency in acutely ill patients. N Engl J Med 348:727–734, 2003.

This paper discusses the topic of functional adrenal insufficiency in critically ill patients and outlines the workup and treatment strategies.

Dronge AS, Perkal MF, Kancir S, et al: Long-term glycemic control and postoperative infectious complications. Arch Surg 141:375–380, 2006.

This paper addresses the importance of glycemic control as it relates to postoperative infections.

Eagle KA, Berger PB, Calkins H, et al: ACC/AHA Guideline Update for Perioperative Cardiovascular Evaluations for Noncardiac Surgery—Executive Summary. A report of the American College of Cardiology/American Heart Association Task Force on Practice Guidelines. (Committee to Update the 1996 Guidelines on Perioperative Cardiovascular Evaluation for Noncardiac Surgery). Anesth Analg 94:1052–1064, 2002.

This important report from the ACC and AHA carefully outlines the management of patients with cardiac risk factors who will undergo a noncardiac operation.

Geerts WH, Bergqvist D, Pineo GF, et al: Prevention of venous thromboembolism: American College of Chest Physicians Evidence-Based Clinical Practice Guidelines (8th Edition). Chest 133:381S–453S, 2008.

The ACCP offers evidence-based guidelines for preventing deep vein thrombosis in postoperative patients.

Heller L, Levin SL, Butler CE: Management of abdominal wound dehiscence using vacuum-assisted closure in patients with compromised healing. Am J Surg 191:165–172, 2006.

This paper deals with the concept of integration of vacuum-assisted closure systems in the management of wound dehiscence.

Lin HJ, Spoerke N, Deveney C, et al: Reconstruction of complex abdominal wall hernias using acellular human dermal matrix: A single institution experience. Am J Surg 197:599–603, 2009.

The development of a biologic prosthesis that can be placed in a contaminated field during hernia repair has provided a relatively new treatment paradigm for the management of these complex patients. This paper is a retrospective review of a single institute's experience with one type of biologic prosthesis.

Migneco A, Ojetti V, Testa A, et al: Management of thyrotoxic crisis. Eur Rev Med Pharmacol Sci 9:69–74, 2005.

This paper outlines the manifestations and treatment of an uncommon but potentially devastating complication of thyrotoxicosis.

Moore AFK, Hargest R, Martin M, et al: Intra-abdominal hypertension and the abdominal compartment syndrome. Br J Surg 91: 1102–1110, 2004.

This paper is important because it details the pathophysiology of intra-abdominal hypertension and abdominal compartment syndrome and attempts to provide guidelines for medical and surgical management of patients in whom these complications develop.

Perry SL, Ortel TL: Clinical and laboratory evaluation of thrombophilia. Clin Chest Med 24:153–170, 2003.

This review outlines the causes and workup of patients with a hypercoagulable state and provides recommendations for testing this high-risk group of patients.

Sailhamer EA, Carson K, Chang Y, et al: Fulminant Clostridium difficile colitis: Patterns of care and predictors of mortality. Arch Surg 144:433–439, 2009.

This recent description of a more virulent, resistant, and aggressive form of *C. dificile* makes this paper highly relevant.

Simon TL, Alverson DC, AuBuchon J, et al: Practice parameter for the use of red blood cell transfusions: Developed by the Red Blood Cell Administration Practice Guideline Development Task Force of the College of American Pathologists. Arch Pathol Lab Med 122: 130–138, 1998.

This paper is the result of a consensus conference held by the College of American Pathologists regarding blood transfusion and its usefulness for the treatment of surgical patients.

Slim K, Vicaut E, Panis Y, et al: Meta-analysis of randomized clinical trials of colorectal surgery with or without mechanical bowel preparation. Br J Surg 91:1125–1130, 2004.

This paper sheds light on the usefulness of mechanical bowel preparation before colorectal surgery.

## REFERENCES

1. Douketis JD, Berger PB, Dunn AS, et al: The perioperative management of antithrombotic therapy: American College of Chest Physicians Evidence-Based Clinical Practice Guidelines (8th Edition). Chest 133:299S–339S, 2008.
2. Diaz JJ, Jr, Conquest AM, Ferzoco SJ, et al: Multi-institutional experience using human acellular dermal matrix for ventral hernia repair in a compromised surgical field. Arch Surg 144:209–215, 2009.
3. Heller L, Levin SL, Butler CE: Management of abdominal wound dehiscence using vacuum- assisted closure in patients with compromised healing. Am J Surg 191:165–172, 2006.
4. Mangram AJ, Horan TC, Pearson ML, et al: Guideline for prevention of surgical site infection, 1999. Hospital Infection Control Practices Advisory Committee. Infect Control Hosp Epidemiol 20:250–278, 1999.
5. Awad SS, Elhabash SI, Lee L, et al: Increasing incidence of methicillin-resistant Staphylococcus aureus skin and soft-tissue infections: Reconsideration of empiric antimicrobial therapy. Am J Surg 194:606–610, 2007.
6. National Nosocomial Infections Surveillance (NNIS): System Report, Data Summary from January 1992–June 2001, issued August 2001. Am J Infect Control 29:404–421, 2001.
7. Culver DH, Horan TC, Gaynes RP, et al: Surgical wound infection rates by wound class, operative procedure, and patient risk index. National Nosocomial Infections Surveillance System. Am J Med 91:152S–157S, 1991.
8. Anderson DJ, Kaye KS, Classen D, et al: Strategies to prevent surgical site infections in acute care hospitals. Infect Control Hosp Epidemiol 29(Suppl 1):S51–S61, 2008.
9. Buggy DJ, Crossley AW: Thermoregulation, mild perioperative hypothermia and postanaesthetic shivering. Br J Anaesth 84:615–628, 2000.
10. Rosenberg H, Antognini JF, Muldoon S: Testing for malignant hyperthermia. Anesthesiology 96:232–237, 2002.
11. Jawa RS, Kulaylat MN, Baumann H, et al: What is new in cytokine research related to trauma/critical care? J Intensive Care Med 21:63–85, 2006.
12. Bukhary ZA: Candiduria: A review of clinical significance and management. Saudi J Kidney Dis Transpl 19:350–360, 2008.
13. Centers for Medicare and Medicaid Services (CMS), HHS: Medicare program; changes to the hospital inpatient prospective payment systems and fiscal year 2008 rates. Fed Regist 72: 47129–48175, 2007.
14. Edwards JR, Peterson KD, Andrus ML, et al: National Healthcare Safety Network (NHSN) Report, data summary for 2006, issued June 2007. Am J Infect Control 35:290–301, 2007.
15. Ksycki MF, Namias N: Nosocomial urinary tract infection. Surg Clin North Am 89:475–481, ix–x, 2009.
16. American Thoracic Society; Infectious Diseases Society of America: Guidelines for the management of adults with hospital-acquired, ventilator-associated, and healthcare-associated pneumonia. Am J Respir Crit Care Med 171:388–416, 2005.
17. Practice guidelines for preoperative fasting and the use of pharmacologic agents to reduce the risk of pulmonary aspiration: application to healthy patients undergoing elective procedures: A report by the American Society of Anesthesiologist Task Force on Preoperative Fasting. Anesthesiology 90:896–905, 1999.
18. Heit JA, Silverstein MD, Mohr DN, et al: Risk factors for deep vein thrombosis and pulmonary embolism: a population-based case-control study. Arch Intern Med 160:809–815, 2000.
19. Goldhaber SZ: Echocardiography in the management of pulmonary embolism. Ann Intern Med 136:691–700, 2002.
20. Geerts WH, Bergqvist D, Pineo GF, et al: Prevention of venous thromboembolism: American College of Chest Physicians Evidence-Based Clinical Practice Guidelines (8th Edition). Chest 133:381S–453S, 2008.

21. Eagle KA, Berger PB, Calkins H, et al: ACC/AHA Guideline Update for Perioperative Cardiovascular Evaluation for Noncardiac Surgery—Executive Summary. A report of the American College of Cardiology/American Heart Association Task Force on Practice Guidelines (Committee to Update the 1996 Guidelines on Perioperative Cardiovascular Evaluation for Noncardiac Surgery). Anesth Analg 94:1052–1064, 2002.
22. Anderson JL, Adams CD, Antman EM, et al: ACC/AHA 2007 guidelines for the management of patients with unstable angina/non-ST-Elevation myocardial infarction: A report of the American College of Cardiology/American Heart Association Task Force on Practice Guidelines (Writing Committee to Revise the 2002 Guidelines for the Management of Patients With Unstable Angina/Non-ST-Elevation Myocardial Infarction) developed in collaboration with the American College of Emergency Physicians, the Society for Cardiovascular Angiography and Interventions, and the Society of Thoracic Surgeons endorsed by the American Association of Cardiovascular and Pulmonary Rehabilitation and the Society for Academic Emergency Medicine. J Am Coll Cardiol 50:e1–e157, 2007.
23. Almanaseer Y, Mukherjee D, Kline-Rogers EM, et al: Implementation of the ACC/AHA guidelines for preoperative cardiac risk assessment in a general medicine preoperative clinic: improving efficiency and preserving outcomes. Cardiology 103:24–29, 2005.
24. Polanczyk CA, Goldman L, Marcantonio ER, et al: Supraventricular arrhythmia in patients having noncardiac surgery: clinical correlates and effect on length of stay. Ann Intern Med 129: 279–285, 1998.
25. Hunt SA, Baker DW, Chin MH, et al: ACC/AHA guidelines for the evaluation and management of chronic heart failure in the adult: Executive summary. J Heart Lung Transplant 21:189–203, 2002.
26. Bonet S, Agusti A, Arnau JM, et al: Beta-adrenergic blocking agents in heart failure: benefits of vasodilating and non-vasodilating agents according to patients' characteristics: A meta-analysis of clinical trials. Arch Intern Med 160:621–627, 2000.
27. Moore AF, Hargest R, Martin M, et al: Intra-abdominal hypertension and the abdominal compartment syndrome. Br J Surg 91:1102–1110, 2004.
28. Karsou SA, Jaber BL, Pereira BJ: Impact of intermittent hemodialysis variables on clinical outcomes in acute renal failure. Am J Kidney Dis 35:980–991, 2000.
29. Cooper MS, Stewart PM: Corticosteroid insufficiency in acutely ill patients. N Engl J Med 348:727–734, 2003.
30. Migneco A, Ojetti V, Testa A, et al: Management of thyrotoxic crisis. Eur Rev Med Pharmacol Sci 9:69–74, 2005.
31. Postoperative Ileus Management Council: Proceedings of Consensus Panel to Define Postoperative Ileus. Colorectal surgery consensus report, Atlanta, 2006, Thomson American Health Consultants.
32. Schwarz NT, Kalff JC, Turler A, et al: Selective jejunal manipulation causes postoperative pan-enteric inflammation and dysmotility. Gastroenterology 126:159–169, 2004.
33. Kulaylat MN, Doerr RJ: Small bowel obstruction. In Holzheimer RG, Mannick JA, editors: Surgical treatment—evidence-based and problem-oriented, New York, 2001, Zuckschwerdt, pp 102–113.
34. Kirkpatrick AW, Balogh Z, Ball CG, et al: The secondary abdominal compartment syndrome: Iatrogenic or unavoidable? J Am Coll Surg 202:668–679, 2006.
35. Simon TL, Alverson DC, AuBuchon J, et al: Practice parameter for the use of red blood cell transfusions: Developed by the Red Blood Cell Administration Practice Guideline Development Task Force of the College of American Pathologists. Arch Pathol Lab Med 122:130–138, 1998.
36. Seder CW, Villalba MR, Jr, Robbins J, et al: Early colectomy may be associated with improved survival in fulminant Clostridium difficile colitis: An 8-year experience. Am J Surg 197:302–307, 2009.
37. Sailhamer EA, Carson K, Chang Y, et al: Fulminant Clostridium difficile colitis: Patterns of care and predictors of mortality. Arch Surg 144:433–439; discussion 439–440, 2009.
38. Pepin J, Vo TT, Boutros M, et al: Risk factors for mortality following emergency colectomy for fulminant Clostridium difficile infection. Dis Colon Rectum 52:400–405, 2009.
39. Slim K, Vicaut E, Panis Y, et al: Meta-analysis of randomized clinical trials of colorectal surgery with or without mechanical bowel preparation. Br J Surg 91:1125–1130, 2004.
40. Uzunkoy A, Akinci OF, Coskun A, et al: Effects of antiadhesive agents on the healing of intestinal anastomosis. Dis Colon Rectum 43:370–375, 2000.
41. August DA, Serrano D, Poplin E: "Spontaneous," delayed colon and rectal anastomotic complications associated with bevacizumab therapy. J Surg Oncol 97:180–185, 2008.
42. Branagan G, Finnis D: Prognosis after anastomotic leakage in colorectal surgery. Dis Colon Rectum 48:1021–1026, 2005.
43. Stojadinovic A, Brooks A, Hoos A, et al: An evidence-based approach to the surgical management of resectable pancreatic adenocarcinoma. J Am Coll Surg 196:954–964, 2003.
44. Orgill DP, Manders EK, Sumpio BE, et al: The mechanisms of action of vacuum-assisted closure: More to learn. Surgery 146: 40–51, 2009.
45. Teubner A, Morrison K, Ravishankar HR, et al: Fistuloclysis can successfully replace parenteral feeding in the nutritional support of patients with enterocutaneous fistula. Br J Surg 91:625–631, 2004.
46. Wainstein DE, Fernandez E, Gonzalez D, et al: Treatment of high-output enterocutaneous fistulas with a vacuum-compaction device. A ten-year experience. World J Surg 32:430–435, 2008.
47. Wind J, van Koperen PJ, Slors JF, et al: Single-stage closure of enterocutaneous fistula and stomas in the presence of large abdominal wall defects using the components separation technique. Am J Surg 197:24–29, 2009.
48. Lin HJ, Spoerke N, Deveney C, et al: Reconstruction of complex abdominal wall hernias using acellular human dermal matrix: A single institution experience. Am J Surg 197:599–603, 2009.
49. Alghamdi A, Jawas A, Hart R: Use of octreotide for the prevention of pancreatic fistula after elective pancreatic surgery: a systematic review and meta-analysis. Canadian J Surg 50(6):459–466, 2007.
50. Krahenbuhl L, Sclabas G, Wente MN, et al: Incidence, risk factors, and prevention of biliary tract injuries during laparoscopic cholecystectomy in Switzerland. World J Surg 25:1325–1330, 2001.

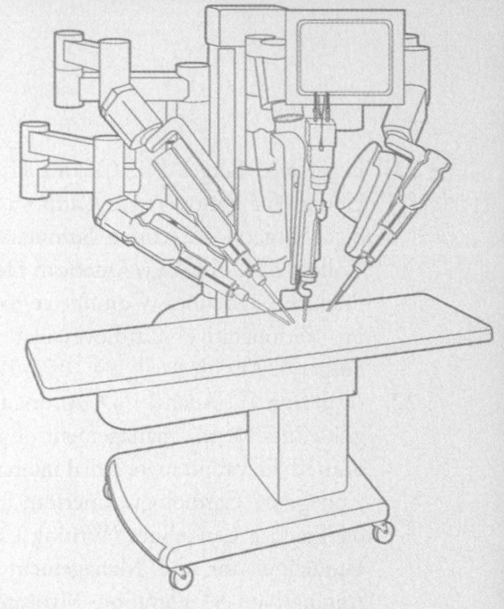

CHAPTER 14

# SURGERY IN THE GERIATRIC PATIENT

Alan Dardik, David H. Berger, and Ronnie A. Rosenthal



Over the past several generations, life expectancy in the United States has increased significantly. This is primarily the result of the implementation of public health and medical interventions such as improved sanitation, vaccinations, nutrition and lifestyle modifications, and antibiotics. From 1900 to the present, life expectancy at birth has increased almost 30 years (49.2 to 77.8 years), and the average 65-year-woman today can expect to live almost twice as long as her counterpart in 1900, or almost 20 years more (Table 14-1).[1]

With this increase in life expectancy comes an increase in the number of people living into old age with diseases and chronic conditions that would have caused death in earlier years. At present, more than 75% of those older than 65 years have at least one chronic condition and 20% of the Medicare population have 5 or more.[2] Many of these diseases and chronic conditions, such as cancer, degenerative joint disease, coronary artery disease, and visual impairment, have a surgical option as part of the treatment algorithm.

Over the next few decades, as the 78 million people in the Baby Boomer generation (born from 1946 to 1964) begin to reach age 65, there will be a rapid aging of the U.S. population (Fig. 14-1).[3] It is expected that by 2030, one in five people will be older than 65 years and, by 2050, almost 20 million people will be older than 85 years. Currently, Social Security, Medicare, and Medicaid benefits to older adults account for more than one third of U.S. spending and have the potential to consume the entire federal budget in the near future. Over the next decade, Medicare costs alone are expected to increase by 7%/year (Fig. 14-2).[4] The demand for health care services is likely to overwhelm the system if new ways to increase supply and delivery are not developed.

In April 2008, in response to the impending crisis in providing health services to older citizens, the Institute of Medicine (IOM) issued a report, in which the IOM "charged the Committee on the Future Health Care Workforce for Older Americans with determining the health care needs of Americans over 65 years of age and analyzing the forces that shape the health care workforce for these individuals."[2] The committee determined that to meet these needs, a three-pronged approach was necessary:

1. Enhancing the geriatric competence of the entire health care work force
2. Increasing the recruitment and retention of geriatrics specialists
3. Improving the way health care is delivered

The goal of this chapter is to help enhance the geriatric competence of surgeons and surgical trainees.

## AGING AND SURGERY

As the number of persons reaching old age continues to grow, there will be a concomitant need to provide surgical care to an increasing number of older patients. Over the past 2 decades alone, the percentage of surgeries in which the patient was older than 65 increased from 19% to 35% of all operations. When obstetric procedures are excluded, this portion rises to 43%. The proportion of the surgical workload across age groups in the specialties in non–federally funded hospitals is shown in Table 14-2.[5]

This increase in the percentage of operations in which the patient is older than 65 years is not entirely the result of the increase in the number of older patients; it is also a reflection of a greater willingness to offer surgical treatment to them and an increased expectation of older patients to remain active for as long as possible. Over the past several decades, advances in surgical and anesthetic techniques have allowed us to operate with much greater control and safety. Operative mortality in older patients has declined sharply. As a result, the risk associated with surgery has become somewhat less of a concern than the need to provide maximal medical management of disease.

The pattern of surgical management of malignant disease in older adults is an example of the changing views on surgery in this age group. Data from the National Cancer Institute's Surveillance, Epidemiology and End Results (SEER) program have indicated a decrease in the gap between the percentage of younger and older patients treated surgically for certain cancers. For early-stage breast, colon, and rectal cancers, in which the chance of surgical cure is high, the percentage of older patients receiving surgical treatment has approached that of younger patients. For localized gastric, pancreatic, lung, and liver cancers, operative percentages still decline sharply with age (Fig. 14-3).[6] At present, it is still unclear whether this decline is the result of appropriate decision making based on the overall health of the patient and patient treatment preference, or whether it is a

**Table 14-1 Life Expectancy of Older Persons**

| | White | | African American | |
|---|---|---|---|---|
| **AGE (YR)** | **MEN** | **WOMEN** | **MEN** | **WOMEN** |
| 65 | 17.1 | 19.8 | 15.1 | 18.6 |
| 70 | 13.6 | 15.9 | 12.3 | 15.1 |
| 75 | 10.5 | 12.3 | 9.8 | 12.0 |
| 80 | 7.8 | 9.3 | 7.7 | 9.3 |
| 85 | 5.7 | 6.7 | 5.9 | 7.1 |
| 90 | 4.0 | 4.7 | 4.5 | 5.3 |
| 95 | 2.8 | 3.3 | 3.5 | 3.9 |
| 100 | 2.0 | 2.3 | 2.6 | 2.8 |

Data from Arias E: United States life tables, 2006. Natl Vital Stat Rep 58:1–40, 2010.

**Table 14-2 Distribution of Procedure Types (by Age Group) Performed in Non–Federally Funded Hospitals (%)**

| | Age (yr) | | | |
|---|---|---|---|---|
| **TYPE OF PROCEDURE** | **<15** | **15-44** | **45-65** | **>65** |
| Ophthalmologic | 11 | 23 | 25 | 41 |
| Otolaryngologic | 26 | 34 | 20 | 20 |
| Thoracic | 5 | 14 | 33 | 48 |
| Cardiovascular | 3 | 10 | 36 | 51 |
| Gastrointestinal | 4 | 23 | 32 | 41 |
| Urologic | 3 | 21 | 35 | 41 |
| Gynecologic | 1 | 57 | 31 | 11 |
| Neurosurgical | 16 | 30 | 27 | 29 |
| Orthopedic | 3 | 21 | 36 | 39 |
| All | 4 | 33 | 28 | 36 |

Data from Hall, MJ, DeFrances CJ, Podgornik MN: 2007 National Hospital Discharge Survey. Adv Data 29:1–21, 2010.

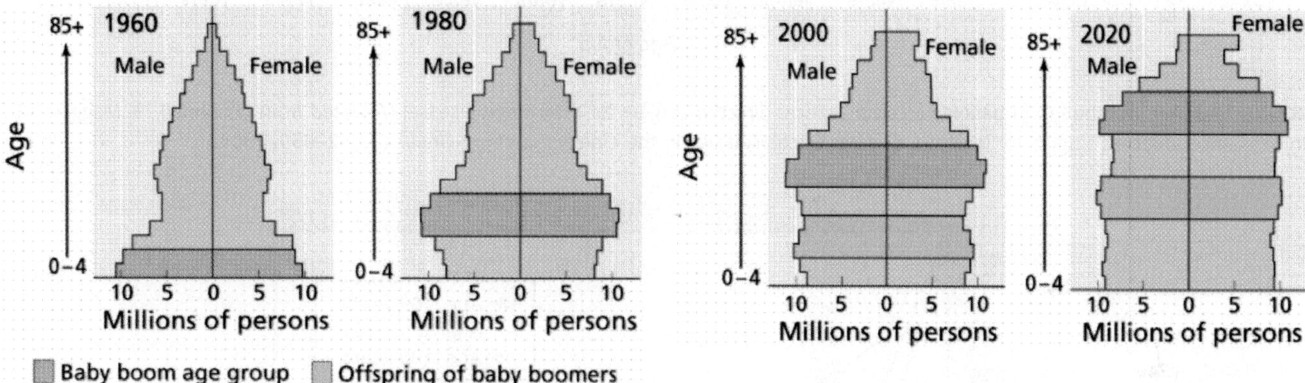


**FIGURE 14-1** Aging of the Baby Boom generation and offspring. (From Purves WK, Orians GH, Heller HC: Life: The science of biology, ed 4, New York, 1994, WH Freeman.)

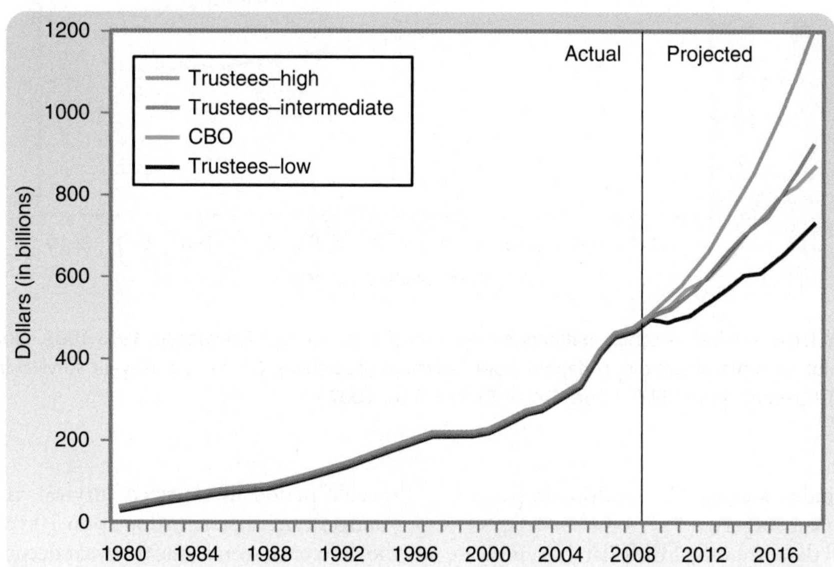


**FIGURE 14-2** Expected growth in Medicare spending over the next decade. (From Medicare Payment Advisory Commission: A data book: Healthcare spending and the Medicare program, MedPAC, 2009, Washington DC.)

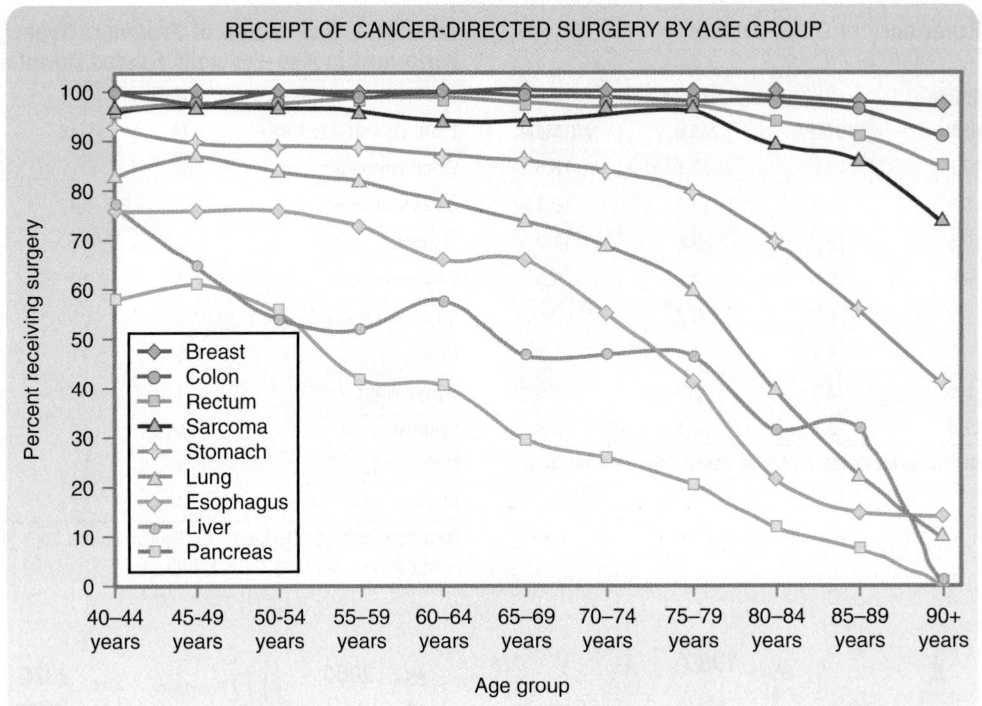


**FIGURE 14-3** Age distribution of patients receiving cancer-directed surgery for local stage disease. (Adapted from O'Connell JB, Maggard MA, Ko CY: Cancer-directed surgery for localized disease: Decreased use in the elderly. Ann Surg Oncol 11:962–969, 2004.)

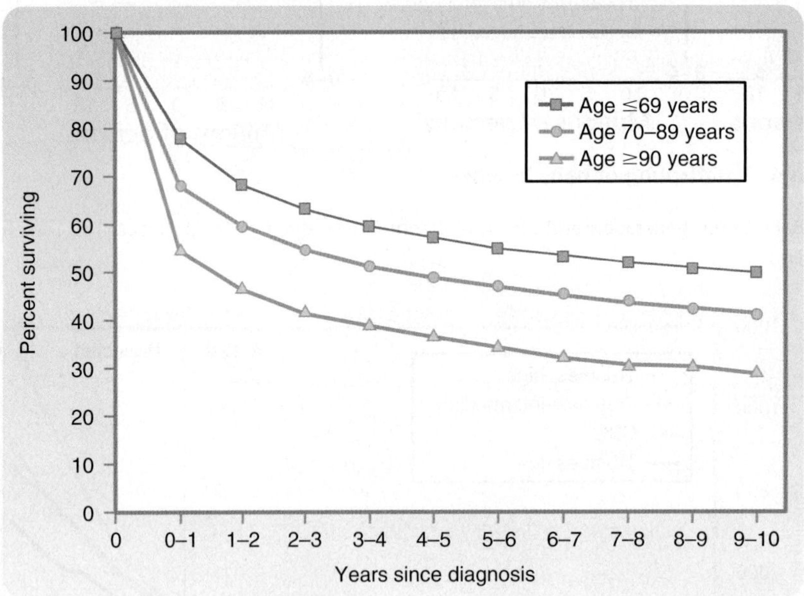


**FIGURE 14-4** Cumulative relative survival of cancer patients by age group from the SEER database, 1973-1998. Note that after the first year, survival curves are parallel for even the oldest old. (Adapted from Saltzstein SL, Behling CA: 5- and 10-year survival in cancer patients aged 90 and older: A study of 37,318 patients from SEER. J Surg Oncol 81:113–116, 2002.)

reflection of vestigial prejudice and age bias resulting in patients not being referred for cancer surgery.

However, additional data from the SEER database indicate that even in the oldest patients, those 90 years and older, cancer treatment is worthwhile. After the first year from diagnosis, relative survival, defined as the ratio of observed survival over a specific period to expected survival, is identical for older and younger cancer patients for up to 10 years (Fig. 14-4).[7] Most of the difference seen in the first year occurs in the first few months, and the only factor that positively influences first-year survival is whether the patient underwent surgical treatment of the cancer or other major surgery. This finding may be the result of selection bias, inasmuch as only the healthiest 90-year-olds may have been offered surgery. However, this serves to emphasize that age alone should not be the sole reason to deny surgical treatment of cancer.

There is no doubt that increasing age appears to have a negative effect on the outcome of surgery. However, most studies have indicated that chronologic age alone has little effect on outcome. Rather, it is the age-related decline in physiologic reserves and increase in comorbidity that is responsible for this observation. Even a compromised older patient can tolerate a surgical experience well if the procedure is carefully conducted and the postoperative course is uncomplicated. However, if even one complication occurs, mortality increases significantly. In a study of more than 26,000 patients older than 80 years undergoing major noncardiac surgery in Veterans Affairs Hospitals, mortality rose from 3.7% in patients with no complications to 26.1% in patients in whom one or more complication occurred.[8]

It is also most important to remember that the pattern of symptoms and natural history of the surgical disease in older patients may not be identical to that seen in their younger counterparts. The absence of typical signs and symptoms often leads to errors in diagnosis and delays in treatment. As a result, it is not unusual for an acute complication to be the first indication of disease. For example, acute cholecystitis and common bile duct (CBD) stones are more common indications for cholecystectomy in patients older than 65 years and biliary colic is more common in those younger than 65 years. This is unfortunate, because emergency surgery carries a 3- to 10-fold higher risk of operative mortality than comparable elective surgery. In addition, the extent of disease found at the time of surgery is often far more advanced in older patients when compared with younger patients; over 50% of appendices are perforated at the time of appendectomy in patients older than 65 years compared with less than 25% in those younger than 65 years. Therefore, a high index of suspicion is necessary to identify surgical disease early in older patients presenting with vague complaints or unexplained changes in mental status.

## SETTING GOALS FOR TREATMENT

Traditionally, surgeons have measured surgical success in terms of 30-day mortality and morbidity. For older patients, however, the definition of success is more complex. Although we are now able to perform even the most major surgery on our oldest patients with traditional surgical success, the quality of the outcome in the patient's view is more likely to depend on whether he or she can continue to function as before surgery. For some older patients, losing functional independence as a result of a major surgical intervention may be a far worse outcome than living with, or even dying of, the disease for which surgery is offered.

In a study of older patients with limited life expectancy because of serious chronic disease, Fried and colleagues[9] examined the impact of treatment burden (low, minor interventions, such as IV antibiotics; high, major interventions, such as surgery) and expected outcome (desirable versus undesirable) on patient preferences for treatment. Results indicated that more than 70% of older patients would not want even a low burden treatment if severe functional impairment or cognitive impairment was the expected outcome. The concern for functional and cognitive impairment was more dramatic than the concern for death (Fig. 14-5).

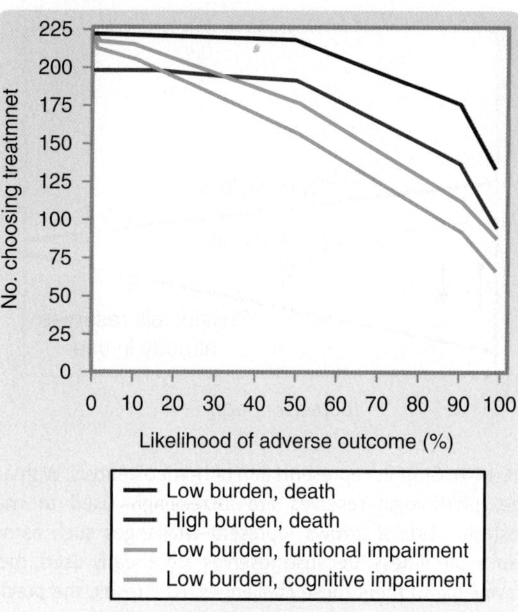


**FIGURE 14-5** Many patients are willing to undertake high- or low-burden treatments, even if the risk of death is high (up to 50%). However, when there is even a small risk of cognitive or functional decline, the number of patients willing to undergo even a low-burden treatment sharply declines. (Adapted from Fried TR, Bradley EH, Towle VR, et al: Understanding the treatment preferences of seriously ill patients. N Engl J Med 346:1061–1066, 2002.)

In another study of preferences for permanent nursing home placement in seriously ill hospitalized patients, 56% of patients were very unwilling or would rather die than live permanently in a nursing home. Correlation between the patient's wishes and both the surrogate's and physician's opinion of the patient's wishes was poor.[10]

Therefore, it is essential that the older patient be given a realistic estimate of the overall functional outcome of the proposed surgical treatment, in addition to the likelihood of control or cure of the particular disease. It is also essential that the surgeon understands the patient's preferences in the context of this broader view of surgical success.

## PHYSIOLOGIC DECLINE

With aging, there is a decline in physiologic function in all organ systems, but the magnitude of this decline is variable among organs and individuals. In the resting state, this decline usually has minimal functional consequence, although physiologic reserves may be used just to maintain homeostasis. However, when physiologic reserves are required to meet the additional challenges of surgery or acute illness, overall performance may deteriorate. This progressive age-related decline in organ system homeostatic reserves, termed *homeostenosis,* was first described by the physiologist Walter Cannon in the 1940s. Figure 14-6 is a graphic representation of the present concepts of homeostenosis.[11] With older age, there is increased use of physiologic reserves just to maintain normal homeostasis. Therefore, when stressed, fewer reserves are available to meet the challenge, and overall function may be pushed over the precipice of organ failure or death.

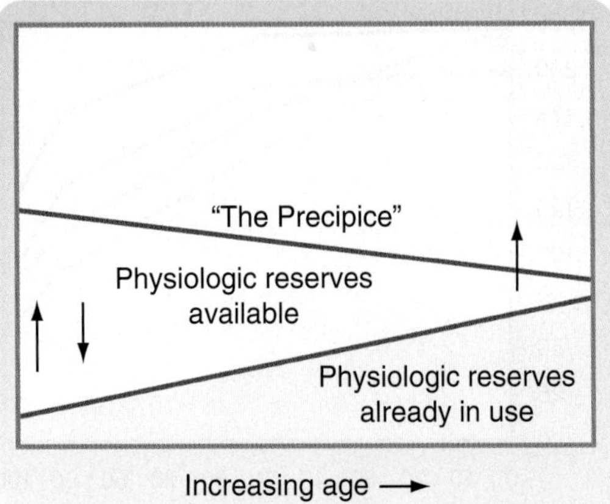


**FIGURE 14-6** Graphic representation of homeostenosis. With advancing age, physiologic reserves are increasingly used to maintain homeostasis. *Vertical arrows* represent challenges such as surgical stress or acute illness. Because reserves are already used, there are fewer available to meet these challenges. As a result, the precipice is crossed by a stress that would be easily tolerated in younger age. This precipice may be any relevant clinical marker, such as organ dysfunction or failure or death. (Adapted from Taffett GE: Physiology of aging. In Cassel CK, Leipzig RM, Cohen HJ, et al. [eds]: Geriatric medicine: An evidence-based approach, ed 4, New York, 2003, Springer-Verlag, pp 27–35.)

**BOX 14-1 Major Cardiovascular Changes With Age**

- Decreased number of myocytes
- Fibrosis of conducting pathways with increased arrhythmias
- Decrease ventricular and arterial compliance (increased afterload)
- Decreased β-adrenergic responsiveness
- Increased dependence on preload (including atrial kick)
- Increased diastolic dysfunction
- Increased silent ischemia

Over the past several decades, an enormous amount of research has been conducted to define the specific changes in organ function that are directly attributable to aging. This task is inherently difficult because aging is also accompanied by increased vulnerability to disease. It is often difficult to determine whether an observed decline in function is secondary to aging per se or to disease associated with aging. The overall effect, however, is still the same—a much smaller margin for error in the care of older patients. Understanding the changes in organ function can help minimize these errors.

## Cardiovascular System

Cardiovascular disease is the leading cause of death in the United States in men and women. Of these deaths, 83% occur in persons older than 65 years (Box 14-1). The prevalence of heart failure approaches 10 in 1000 persons in this age group. Congestive heart failure is a risk factor for several postoperative complications, including surgical site infections. Cardiac events are common in the postoperative period in older patients and are attributable to disease and to changes in the structure and function of the heart that accompany aging.

Morphologic changes are found in the myocardium, conducting pathways, valves, and vasculature of the heart and great vessels with increasing age. The number of myocytes declines as the collagen and elastin content increases, thereby resulting in fibrotic areas throughout the myocardium and an overall decline in ventricular compliance. Almost 90% of the autonomic tissue in the sinus node is replaced by fat and connective tissue, and fibrosis interferes with conduction in the intranodal tracts and bundle of His. These changes contribute to the high incidence of sick sinus syndrome, atrial arrhythmia, and bundle branch block. Sclerosis and calcification of the aortic valve are common but are usually of no functional significance. Progressive dilation of all four valvular annuli is probably responsible for the multivalvular regurgitation demonstrated in healthy older persons. Finally, there is a progressive increase in rigidity and decrease in distensibility of the coronary arteries and great vessels. Changes in the peripheral vasculature contribute to increased systolic blood pressure, increased resistance to ventricular emptying, and compensatory loss of myocytes, with ventricular hypertrophy.

The direct functional implications of these changes are difficult to assess accurately because age-related changes in body composition, metabolic rate, general state of fitness, and underlying disease all influence cardiac performance. It is now generally accepted that systolic function is well preserved with increasing age. Cardiac output and ejection fraction are maintained, despite the increase in afterload imposed by stiffening of the outflow tract. The mechanism whereby cardiac output is maintained during exercise, however, is somewhat different. In younger persons, output is maintained by increasing the heart rate in response to β-adrenergic stimulation. With aging, there is a relative hyposympathetic state in which the heart becomes less responsive to catecholamines, possible secondary to declining receptor function. The aging heart therefore maintains cardiac output not by increasing its rate, but by increasing ventricular filling (preload). Because of the dependence on preload, even minor hypovolemia can result in significant compromise in cardiac function.

Diastolic function, however, which depends on relaxation rather than contraction, is affected by aging.[12] Diastolic dysfunction is responsible for up to 50% of cases of heart failure in patients older than 80 years. Myocardial relaxation is more energy-dependent and therefore requires more oxygen than contraction. With aging, there is a progressive decrease in the partial pressure of oxygen. Consequently, even mild hypoxemia can result in prolonged relaxation, higher diastolic pressure, and pulmonary congestion. Because early diastolic filling is impaired, maintenance of preload becomes even more reliant on atrial kick. Loss of the atrial contribution to preload can result in further impairment of cardiac function.

It is also important to remember that the manifestation of cardiac disease in older adults may be nonspecific and atypical. Although chest pain is still the most common symptom of myocardial infarction, atypical symptoms such as shortness of breath, syncope, acute confusion, or stroke will occur in as many as 40% of older patients.

## Respiratory System

Chronic lower respiratory disease is the fourth leading cause of death after heart disease, cancer, and stroke. Respiratory problems are the most common postoperative complications in older

**BOX 14-2 Major Respiratory Changes With Age**

Decrease chest wall compliance
Decline in maximum inspiratory and expiratory force
Decrease in lung elasticity (small airway collapse)
Ventilation-perfusion mismatch
Decrease in $Pa_{O_2}$, no change in $Pa_{CO_2}$
Decreased FVC and $FEV_1$
Decline in ventilator responses to hypoxemia and hypercapnia
Decline in normal airway protective mechanisms (increased risk for aspiration)

**BOX 14-3 Major Renal Changes With Age**

Decrease in the number of functional nephrons
Decrease in the number of tubular cells
Decreased renal blood flow
Decreased GFR
Decline in creatinine clearance despite normal serum creatinine level
Decline in tubular function (loss of concentrating ability)
Increase susceptibility to dehydration
Decrease clearance of certain drugs
Increase in lower urinary track dysfunction and infection

patients (Box 14-2). Both disease- and age-related changes in lung structure and function contribute to this vulnerability.[13]

With aging there is a decline in respiratory function that is attributable to changes in the chest wall and lungs. Chest wall compliance decreases secondary to changes in structure caused by kyphosis and is exaggerated by vertebral collapse. Calcification of the costal cartilage and contractures of the intercostal muscles result in a decline in rib mobility. Maximum inspiratory and expiratory forces decrease by as much as 50% as a result of a progressive decrease in the strength of the respiratory muscles.

In the lung, there is loss of elasticity, which leads to increased alveolar compliance with collapse of the small airways and subsequent uneven alveolar ventilation with air trapping. Uneven alveolar ventilation leads to ventilation-perfusion mismatches, which in turn causes a decline in arterial oxygen tension of approximately 0.3 or 0.4 mm Hg/ year. The partial pressure of $CO_2$ does not change, despite an increase in dead space. This may be caused, in part, by the decline in production of $CO_2$ that accompanies the falling basal metabolic rates. Air trapping is also responsible for an increase in residual volume, or the volume remaining after maximal expiration.

Loss of support of the small airways also leads to collapse during forced expiration, which limits dynamic lung volumes and flow rates. Forced vital capacity decreases by 14 to 30 mL/year and forced expiratory volume in 1 second ($FEV_1$) decreases by 23 to 32 mL/year (in males). The overall effect of loss of elastic inward recoil of the lung is balanced somewhat by the decline in chest wall outward force. Total lung capacity therefore remains unchanged, and there is only a mild increase in resting lung volume, or functional residual capacity. Because total lung capacity remains unchanged, the increase in residual volume results in a decrease in vital capacity.

Control of ventilation is also affected by aging. Ventilatory responses to hypoxia and hypercapnia fall by 50% and 40%, respectively. The exact mechanism of this decline has not been well defined but it may be caused by declining chemoreceptor function at the peripheral or central nervous system level.

In addition to these intrinsic changes, pulmonary function is affected by alterations in the ability of the respiratory system to protect against environmental injury and infection. There is a progressive decrease in T cell function (see later), decline in mucociliary clearance, and decrease in several components of swallowing function. Loss of the cough reflex secondary to neurologic disorders, combined with swallowing dysfunction, may predispose to aspiration. The increased frequency and severity of pneumonia in older persons have been attributed to these factors and to an increased incidence of oropharyngeal colonization with gram-negative organisms. This colonization correlates closely with comorbidity and with the ability of older patients to perform activities of daily living (ADLs). This fact lends support to the idea that functional capacity is a crucial factor in assessing the risk for pneumonia in older patients.

## Renal System

Approximately 25% of all Americans 70 years and older have moderately or severely decreased kidney function (Box 14-3). Between the ages of 25 and 85, there is a progressive decrease in the renal cortex. Over time, approximately 40% of the nephrons become sclerotic. The remaining functional units hypertrophy in a compensatory manner. Sclerosis of the glomeruli is accompanied by atrophy of the afferent and efferent arterioles and by a decrease in renal tubular cell number. Renal blood flow also falls by approximately 50%. Functionally, there is a decline in the glomerular filtration rate (GFR) of approximately 45% by age 80 years.

Renal tubular function also declines with advancing age. The ability to conserve sodium and excrete hydrogen ion decreases, resulting in a diminished capacity to regulate fluid and acid-base balance. Dehydration becomes a particular problem because losses of sodium and water from nonrenal causes are not compensated for by the usual mechanisms. The inability to retain sodium is believed to be caused by a decline in the activity of the renin-angiotensin system. The increasing inability to concentrate the urine is related to a decline in end-organ responsiveness to antidiuretic hormone. The marked decline in the subjective feeling of thirst is also well documented but not well understood. Alterations of osmoreceptor function in the hypothalamus may be responsible for the failure to recognize thirst in spite of significant elevations in serum osmolality.[14]

Because of the decline in renal function with aging, it is often important to measure GFR in older patients as part of preoperative risk assessment and in hospital to provide accurate medication dosing. In older hospital patients, direct measurement of creatinine clearance (CrCl) is difficult because incontinence and cognitive impairment make 24-hour urine collection unreliable. Serum creatinine level measurement may be an unreliable indicator of renal function status because this value may remain unchanged as a result of a concomitant decrease in lean body mass and thus a decrease in creatinine production. A serum creatinine level of 1.0 mg/dL may represent a CrCl of over 100 mL/min in a 30-year old, but less than 60 mL/min in an 85-year old.[15]

To overcome these problems, formulas have been developed to estimate CrCl from plasma creatinine and patient characteristics. The most commonly used formulas are the

**Cockroft-Gault equation**

$C_{cr}$ = [(140 − Age in years) × Weight in kilograms]/(72 × Serum creatinine in mg/dL)

**MDRD study equation**

GFR = 175 × (Standardized serum creatinine in mg/dL)$^{-1.154}$ × (Age in years)$^{-0.203}$

**FIGURE 14-7** Equations for calculating creatinine clearance.

Cockcroft-Gault equation and the Modification of Diet in Renal Disease (MDRD) equation (Fig. 14-7). In a large study of older hospitalized patients, the Cockcroft-Gault equation has been shown to correlate more closely with directly measured CrCl.[16]

Acute kidney injury (AKI) is defined as a 0.3-mg/dL or 50% or higher change in the serum creatinine level from baseline or a reduction in urine output of less than 0.5 mL/kg/hr over a 6-hour interval, within a 48-hour period, following adequate volume resuscitation. AKI is a frequent occurrence after major surgery. Up to 7.5% of patients with a normal preoperative serum creatinine level will develop AKI. AKI is associated with increased short-term morbidity and mortality, as well as increased long-term mortality. Age, in addition, to emergency surgery, ischemic heart disease, and congestive heart failure, are risk factors for the development of postoperative AKI. Furthermore, older patients with already compromised renal function are at increased risk of postoperative AKI. The keys to avoiding postoperative AKI is to understand that older patients are at increased risk and to take steps to avoid unnecessary hypovolemia and ensure proper dosing of drugs that are cleared by the kidney and of drugs that are nephrotoxic.

The lower urinary tract also changes with increasing age. In the bladder, increased collagen content leads to limited distensibility and impaired emptying. Overactivity of the detrusor muscle secondary to neurologic disorders or idiopathic causes has also been identified. In women, decreased circulating levels of estrogen and decreased tissue responsiveness to this hormone cause changes in the urethral sphincter that predispose to urinary incontinence. In men, prostatic hypertrophy impairs bladder emptying. Together, these factors lead to urinary incontinence in 10% to 15% of older persons living in the community and 50% of those in nursing homes. There is also an increased prevalence of asymptomatic bacteruria with age, which varies from 10% to 50% depending on gender, level of activity, underlying disorders, and place of residence. Urinary tract infections alone are responsible for 30% to 50% of all cases of bacteremia in older patients. Alterations in the local environment and declining host defenses are thought to be responsible. Because of the lack of symptoms in older patients with bacteruria, preoperative urinalysis is important.

## Hepatobiliary System

Overall, hepatic function is well preserved with aging. However, there is as much as a fourfold increase in liver disease–related mortality in persons between the ages of 45 and 85 years.[17] Morphologic changes include a decrease in the number of hepatocytes and a reduction in overall weight, size, and volume. There is, however, a compensatory increase in cell size and proliferation of bile ducts. Functionally, hepatic blood flow decreases by approximately 0.3% to 1.5%/year to 40% to 45% of earlier values after 65 years of age.

**BOX 14-4 Major Hepatobiliary Changes With Age**

- Decrease in the number of hepatocytes
- Decline in hepatic blood flow
- Synthetic capacity remains unchanged
- Increased sensitivity to and decreased clearance of certain drugs
- Increased incidence of gallstones and gallstones related diseases

**BOX 14-5 Major Changes in Immune Function With Age**

- Decrease production and differentiation of naïve T cells
- Decrease in T cell mitogenic activity
- Increase in inflammatory cytokines
- Increased autoantibodies

The synthetic capacity of the liver, as measured by standard tests of liver function, remains unchanged (Box 14-4). However, the metabolism of and sensitivity to certain types of drugs is altered. Drugs requiring microsomal oxidation (phase I reactions) before conjugation (phase II reactions) may be metabolized more slowly, whereas those requiring only conjugation may be cleared at a normal rate. Drugs that act directly on hepatocytes, such as warfarin (Coumadin), may produce the desired therapeutic effects at lower doses in older adults because of an increased sensitivity of cells to these agents. Some recent evidence has also suggested that aging may be associated with a decline in the ability of the liver to protect against the effects of oxidative stress.

The most significant correlate of altered hepatobiliary function in older adults is the increased incidence of gallstones and gallstone-related complications. Gallstone prevalence rises steadily with age, although there is variability in the absolute percentages, depending on the population. Stones have been demonstrated in as many as 80% of nursing home residents older than 90 years. Biliary tract disease is the single most common indication for abdominal surgery in older adults (see later).

## Immune Function

Immune competence, like other physiologic parameters, declines with advancing age (Box 14-5). This immunosenescence is characterized by enhanced susceptibility to infections, an increase in

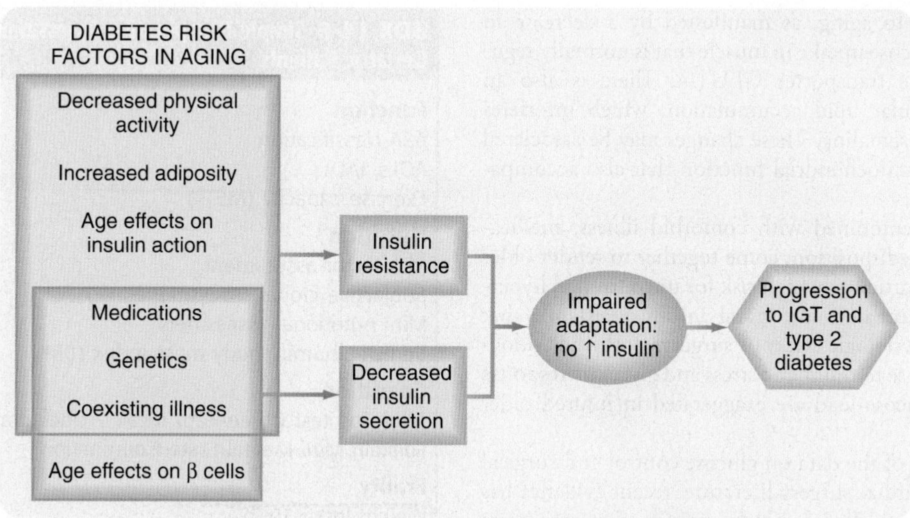


**FIGURE 14-8** The normal response to hyperglycemia is for the beta cell to adapt and secrete sufficient insulin to restore euglycemia. In aging, there is a decrease in insulin secretion and a probable increase in insulin resistance, which, when combined with comorbid illness, genetic factors, and medications, leads to a failure of this glucoregulatory process. *IGT,* Impaired glucose tolerance. (From Chang AM, Halter JB: Aging and insulin secretion. Am J Physiol Endocrinol Metab 284:E7–E12, 2003.)

autoantibodies and monoclonal immunoglobulins, and an increase in tumorigenesis. In addition, like other physiologic systems, this decline may not be apparent in the unchallenged state. For example, there is no decline in neutrophil count with age, but the ability of the bone marrow to increase neutrophil production in response to infection may be impaired. Older patients with major infections frequently have normal white blood cell (WBC) counts, but the differential count will show a profound shift to the left, with a large proportion of immature forms.

With aging, there is a decline in the hematopoietic stem cell pool in the bone marrow that leads to decreased production of naïve T cells from the thymus and of B cells from the bone marrow. Moreover, involution of the thymus gland, with a decline in thymic hormone levels, further impairs the production and differentiation of naïve T cells and leads to an increased proportion of memory T cells. This change in the population of T cells leaves older adult hosts less able to respond to new antigens. Furthermore, recent data have suggested that chronic infection with viruses such as cytomegalovirus produces nonfunctional T cell clonal expansions that may limit the space available for proliferating T cells.[18]

Some B cell defects have recently been identified, although it is thought that the functional deficits in antibody production are related to altered T cell regulation rather than intrinsic B cell changes. In vitro, there is increased helper T cell activity for nonspecific antibody production, as well as a decreased ability of suppressor T cells from old mice to recognize and suppress specific antigens from self. This is reflected in an increase in the prevalence of autoantibodies to more than 10% by 80 years of age. The mix of immunoglobulins also changes; immunoglobulin M (IgM) levels decrease, whereas IgG and IgA levels increase slightly.

Changes in the immune system with aging are similar those seen in chronic inflammation and cancer. In addition to the reduced mitogenic responses of T cells, there is an increase in the levels of acute-phase proteins. It is hypothesized that persistently elevated levels of inflammatory cytokines may be responsible for the downregulation of interleukin-2 production by chronically stimulated T cells. Markers of inflammation such as interleukin-6 have recently been shown to be increased in older patients. Chronic inflammation has been implicated in the syndrome of frailty, which is characterized by loss of muscle mass (sarcopenia), undernutrition, and impaired mobility. Inflammatory cytokines are also implicated in the normocytic anemia that is common in frail older adults.

The clinical implications of these changes are difficult to determine. When superimposed on the known immunosuppression caused by the physical and psychological stresses of surgery, insufficient immunologic responses are to be expected in older adults. The increased susceptibility to many infectious agents in the postoperative period, however, is more likely the result of a combination of stress and comorbid disease rather than physiologic decline alone.

## Glucose Homeostasis

Data from the National Health and Nutrition Examination Survey have shown a clear increase in the prevalence of disorders of glucose homeostasis with age; more than 20% of persons older than 60 years have type 2 diabetes. An additional 20% have glucose intolerance characterized by normal fasting glucose and a postchallenge glucose level higher than 140 mg/dL but less than 200 mg/dL. This glucose intolerance may be the result of a decrease in insulin secretion, increase in insulin resistance, or both (Fig. 14-8).[19]

There is now general consensus that beta cell function declines with age. This change is manifested by failure of the beta cell to adapt to the hyperglycemic milieu with an appropriate increase in insulin response. The question of insulin resistance is more controversial. Although insulin action has been shown to decrease in older adults, this change is thought to be more a function of changing body composition, with increased adipose tissue and decreased lean body mass, rather than age per se. Others believe that there is an increase in insulin resistance directly attributable to aging, as manifested by a decrease in insulin-mediated glucose uptake in muscle that is normally regulated by the glucose transporter GLUT-4. There is also an increase in intracellular lipid accumulation, which interferes with normal insulin signaling. These changes may be associated with the decline in mitochondrial function that also accompanies aging.[19]

These factors, combined with comorbid illness, medications, and genetic predisposition, come together to render older surgical patients at particularly high risk for uncontrolled hyperglycemia when subjected to the usual insulin resistance that accompanies the physiologic stress of surgery. Both the endogenous glucose response to traumatic stress and glycemic response to an exogenous glucose load are exaggerated in injured older patients.

Although most of the data on glucose control and surgical outcomes is in the cardiac surgery literature, recent evidence has confirmed that uncontrolled hyperglycemia in the immediate perioperative period is associated with an increase in infections in almost all types of surgery. The optimum level of glucose control, however, is still controversial. Earlier prospective studies indicated that tight control of blood sugar (80 to 110 mg/dL) achieved by continuous infusion of insulin improved some outcomes, including mortality in critically ill patients in the surgical intensive care unit, but more recent data have cast some doubt on the benefits of such strict control. In general, maintenance of the blood glucose level below 180 mg/dL in the perioperative period is now widely accepted as an appropriate target, even in older patients.

## PREOPERATIVE ASSESSMENT

The goals of preoperative assessment of an older patient are to define the extent of physiologic decline, characterize and optimize comorbid diseases, and determine how the stress of the surgical treatment will affect the patient's postoperative function and overall quality of life. Extensive testing for disease in every organ system is neither cost-effective, practical, nor necessary for most patients. A thorough history and physical examination will provide information to direct further workup, if necessary. It is important, however, to adjust the history and physical examination to look carefully for the risk factors, signs, and symptoms of the more common comorbid conditions. The addition of simple tools for the assessment of functional, cognitive, nutritional status and overall frailty will significantly enhance understanding of the individual patient's true operative risk (Box 14-6). When initial evaluation identifies specific disease or risk factors for disease, further workup may be indicated.

### BOX 14-6 Simple Preoperative Assessment Tools for Geriatric Patients

**Function**
ASA classification
ADLs, IADLs
Exercise capacity (METs)

**Nutrition**
Risk factor assessment
Subjective global assessment
Mini nutritional assessment
Serum albumin–body mass index (BMI)

**Cognition**
Mini-Cog test (three-item recall + clock drawing)
Folstein Mini-Mental State Examination

**Frailty**
Weight loss >10 lb
Weak grip strength
Low energy expenditure
Self-reported exhaustion
Slow walking speed

### Comorbidity

Like the surgical disease itself, the manifestations of comorbid illnesses in older adults are frequently less typical than in younger patients. For example, more than 40% of myocardial infarctions in patients older than 75 to 84 years are silent or unrecognized, as opposed to less than 20% in patients between the ages of 45 and 54. Cognitive and nutritional deficits occur frequently in the aged, but as many as two thirds and one half, respectively, are overlooked unless a specific assessment is undertaken. Swallowing disorders are also common but are often unrecognized.

In addition, comorbidity influences the overall life expectancy of the individual, irrespective of the surgical illness. For example, the mean life expectancy of cognitively intact persons aged 65 to 69 years is approximately 18 years, whereas the life expectancy for similarly aged patients with dementia is closer to 10 years. In older persons with congestive heart failure, 20% die within 1 year and 75% within 5 years of initial hospitalization. Understanding the impact of comorbidity on life expectancy is therefore essential in risk-benefit determinations.

Of all comorbid conditions, cardiovascular disease is the most prevalent, and cardiovascular events are a leading cause of severe perioperative complications and death. Therefore, the main thrust of preoperative evaluation in most patients, regardless of age, has focused on identifying patients at risk for cardiac complications. The American College of Cardiology (ACC) and American Heart Association (AHA) Task Force on Practice Guidelines first published an in-depth set of guidelines for preoperative cardiac evaluation in 1996, with updates in 2002 and 2007.[20] These guidelines provide a stepwise Bayesian strategy for determining which patients will need further testing to clarify risk or further treatment to minimize risk. Stratification is based on factors related to the patient and type of surgery. For older patients with known cardiac disease, rigorous workup may be necessary. For most patients, assessment of exercise tolerance and functional capacity is an accurate method of predicting the adequacy of cardiac and pulmonary reserves (see later).

Although the main focus of preoperative evaluation has been cardiac status, pulmonary complications in older patients are at least as common as cardiac complication, if not more so. Risk factors for pulmonary complications are not as well studied as those for cardiac complications, although many of the same issues apply to both. Poor exercise capacity and poor general health predict pulmonary and cardiac complications. In a systematic review of the literature for risk factor for pulmonary complications after noncardiac surgery (not limited to older adults) both patient and procedural factors were identified (Table 14-3).[21] Age older than 80 years was associated with the highest odds ratio (OR) of a pulmonary complication, even after adjusting for comorbidity. Indicators of impaired function, nutrition, and cognition, among others, were also important.

**Table 14-3 Potential Risk Factors for Postoperative Pulmonary Complications**

| PATIENT-RELATED FACTORS | ODDS RATIO | PROCEDURE-RELATED FACTORS | ODDS RATIO |
|---|---|---|---|
| Age (years) | | Aortic aneurysm repair | 6.90 |
| 70-79 | 3.90 | Thoracic surgery | 4.24 |
| ≥80 | 5.63 | Abdominal surgery | 3.01 |
| ASA class ≥ II | 3.12-4.87 | Upper abdominal surgery | 2.91 |
| Abnormal CXR | 4.81 | Neurosurgery | 2.53 |
| CHF | 2.93 | Prolonged surgery | 2.26 |
| Functionally dependent | 1.62-2.51 | Head and neck surgery | 2.21 |
| COPD | 2.36 | Emergency surgery | 2.21 |
| Weight loss | 1.62 | Vascular surgery | 2.10 |
| Medical Comorbidity | 1.48 | General anesthesia | 1.83 |
| Cigarette use | 1.40 | Perioperative transfusion | 1.47 |
| Impaired sensorium | 1.39 | | |
| Alcohol use | 1.21 | | |

Adapted from Smetana GW, Lawrence VA, Cornell JE: Preoperative pulmonary risk stratification for noncardiothoracic surgery: Systematic review for the American College of Physicians. Ann Intern Med 144:581–595, 2006.

Aortic aneurysm and thoracic and abdominal operations were the strongest procedure-related factors, but others, such as abdominal surgery, prolonged surgery, and emergency surgery, were also important.

Additional comorbid conditions, such as prior stroke, gastroesophageal reflux disease (GERD), and poor dentition, also place older patients at increased risk of aspiration. Subtle changes in cognitive and swallowing function are similarly common in older adults and are associated with aspiration pneumonia and other negative outcomes. Initial screening for aspiration risk can be accomplished easily with a simple 3-ounce water swallow test, which has been shown to have high sensitivity and negative predictive value. This test is accomplished by asking the patient to swallow 90 mL of water without stopping. Choking, coughing, wet quality to the voice after swallowing, or failure to complete the test indicates that a more thorough swallowing examination may be in order. Passing this test indicates a low risk for aspiration; however, the false-positive rate is high. Aspiration precautions, however, should be instituted for all older patients with any risk factors for aspiration

In a recent review of strategies to reduce postoperative pulmonary complications, only lung expansion interventions, such as incentive spirometry, were shown by good evidence to have an effect.[22] The selective use of nasogastric decompression (rather than routine use) and short-acting (as opposed to long-acting) intraoperative neuromuscular blockade was supported by fair evidence. Evidence supporting smoking cessation, epidural anesthesia and analgesia, laparoscopic versus open approaches, and nutritional supplementation was insufficient or conflicting.

## Function

Postoperative outcome in the geriatric surgical patient is largely determined by the impact of physiologic decline and comorbidity on an individual's functional reserves. Limited preoperative functional reserves also contribute to postoperative immobility, which in turn leads to complications such as atelectasis and pneumonia, venous stasis and pulmonary embolism, and multisystem deconditioning (see later). Function can be assessed in many ways.

### American Society of Anesthesiologists Classification

For decades, the physical status classification of the American Society of Anesthesiologists (ASA) has been used successfully to stratify operative risk. This simple classification ranks patients according to the functional limitations imposed by coexisting disease. When curves for mortality versus ASA class are examined with regard to age, there is little difference between younger and older patients, which indicates that mortality is a function of coexisting disease rather than chronologic age. ASA classification has been shown to predict postoperative mortality accurately, even in patients older than 80 years. In a large multicenter Department of Veterans Affairs study (National Surgical Quality Improvement Program [NSQIP]), surgical patients were assessed prospectively for operative risk and risk-adjusted models were then created to allow comparison of the quality of surgical care among different institutions. Of the 68 variables studied, the ASA functional classification was the factor most predictive of postoperative morbidity and the second most predictive of mortality.[23]

### Activities of Daily Living

The ability to perform ADLs (e.g., feeding, continence, transferring, toileting, dressing, bathing) and instrumental ADLs (IADLs; e.g., telephone use, transportation, meal preparation, shopping, housework, medication management, managing finances) have also been shown to correlate with postoperative mortality and morbidity.[24] Inactivity, defined as the inability to leave the home on one's own at least twice per week, has been associated with a higher incidence of all major surgical complications. Postoperative mortality in severely limited patients has been reported to be almost 10 times higher than mortality in active patients. In another study of functional recovery after major elective open abdominal operations, better recovery and shorter time to recovery of ADLs and IADLs were almost always predicted by a better preoperative physical performance status, as measured by three simple tests of strength and mobility.[25]

### Exercise Tolerance

Of all the methods of assessing overall functional capacity, exercise tolerance is the most sensitive predictor of postoperative cardiac and pulmonary complications in older adults. In an older but frequently quoted study comparing exercise tolerance and other assessment techniques, Gerson and associates demonstrated that an inability to raise the heart rate to 99 beats/min while performing 2 minutes of supine bicycle exercise was the most sensitive predictor of postoperative cardiac and pulmonary complications and death.[26]

ESTIMATED ENERGY REQUIREMENTS FOR VARIOUS ACTIVITIES*

| | | | |
|---|---|---|---|
| 1 MET ↓ 4 METs | Can you take care of yourself? Eat, dress, or use the toilet? Walk indoors around the house? Walk a block or two on level ground at 2–3 mph or 3.2–4.8 km/h? Do light work around the house like dusting or washing dishes? | 4 METs ↓ 10 METs | Climb a flight of stairs or walk up hill? Walk on level ground at 4 mph or 6.4 km/h? Run a short distance? Do heavy work around the house like scrubbing floors or lifting or moving heavy furniture? Participate in moderate recreational activities like golf, bowling, dancing, doubles tennis, or throwing a baseball or football? Participate in strenuous sports like swimming, singles tennis, football, basketball, or skiing? |

*MET, metabolic equivalent (see text).

**FIGURE 14-9** Estimated energy requirements for various activities. With increasing activity, the number of METs increases. An inability to function above 4 METs has been associated with increased perioperative cardiac events and long-term risk. (From Eagle KA, Berger PB, Calkins H, et al; American College of Cardiology/American Heart Association Task Force on Practice Guidelines [Committee to Update the 1996 Guidelines on Perioperative Cardiovascular Evaluation for Noncardiac Surgery]: ACC/AHA guideline update for perioperative cardiovascular evaluation for noncardiac surgery—executive summary. A report of the American College of Cardiology/American Heart Association Task Force on Practice Guidelines [Committee to Update the 1996 Guidelines on Perioperative Cardiovascular Evaluation for Noncardiac Surgery]. Circulation 105:1257–1267, 2002.)

Formal exercise testing, however, is not necessary in every older patient. The metabolic requirements for many routine activities have already been determined and are quantitated as metabolic equivalents (MET). One MET, defined as 3.5 mL/kg/min, represents the basal oxygen consumption of a 70-kg, 40-year-old man at rest. Estimated energy requirements for various activities are shown in Figure 14-9. An inability to function above 4 METs has been associated with increased perioperative cardiac events and long-term risk. By asking appropriate questions about the level of activity, functional capacity can be accurately determined without the need for additional testing.

## Cognition

Many people experience healthy aging without significant impairments, but a number of sensory, cognitive, and functional declines can occur with age, threatening independence. In cases of extreme sensory or cognitive loss, as seen with vascular and Alzheimer's dementia, the capacity to perform ADLs can be compromised. These age-associated changes in cognitive function may have profound effects on postsurgical recovery and outcome. Additionally, worse biologic functioning is often associated with lower cognitive performance.

The importance of preoperative cognitive status as a risk factor for negative postoperative outcomes in older patients is often overlooked. Cognitive assessment is rarely a part of the preoperative history and physical examination, and there are no widely accepted guidelines for such evaluation in surgical patients. However, preoperative cognitive deficits can have significant short- and long-term consequences in the postoperative period; preoperative cognitive deficits are the greatest risk factor for postoperative delirium and cognitive changes discovered postoperatively can persist for as long as 6 months after surgery.

It is most important to recognize that a change in mental status in older patients following surgery is often the earliest sign of a postoperative complication. Therefore, some form of assessment for mental status should be part of the routine postoperative evaluation. If an adequate preoperative cognitive evaluation has been conducted, postoperative assessment only requires brief observations of behavior and a comparison to baseline.

There are several methods for evaluating baseline cognitive function. The Folstein Mini- Mental State Examination (MMSE) has traditionally been used because of its ease of administration and reliability. It has been suggested that the Mini-Cog test detects clinically significant cognitive impairment as well as, if not better than, the MMSE in multiethnic older individuals.[27] It is easier to administer to non–English-speaking patients and is less biased by low education and literacy levels. The Mini-Cog test combines a three-item word learning and recall task (0 to 3 points; each correctly recalled word, 1 point), with a simple clock-drawing task (abnormal clock, 0 points; normal clock, 2 points) used as a distraction before word recall. Total possible Mini-Cog scores range from 0 to 5 points, with 0 to 2 suggesting high and 3 to 5 suggesting a low likelihood of cognitive impairment.

## Nutritional Status

Surgeons recognize the value of optimal nutritional status to minimize perioperative mortality and morbidity. However, older patients are at particular risk for malnutrition and therefore at increased risk for adverse perioperative events. It remains imperative for surgeons to continue to assess nutritional status and attempt to correct malnutrition to achieve optimal results. Although this may be difficult in any patient, detection plus correction of malnutrition in older patients is crucial.

The impact of poor nutrition as a risk factor for perioperative mortality and morbidity such as pneumonia and poor wound healing has long been appreciated. A variety of

**BOX 14-7 Factors Associated With Increased Risk of Malnutrition**

**Recent Weight Loss**

**Limited Ability to Get Food**
Immobility
Poverty

**Disinterest in Eating**
Depression
Isolation
Cognitive impairment
Decreased appetite
Decreased taste

**Difficulty Eating**
Poor dentition
Swallowing disorder
GERD

**Increased Gastrointestinal Losses**
Diarrhea
Malabsorption

**Systemic Diseases**
Chronic lung
Liver
Cardiac
Renal
Cancer

**Drugs and Medications**
EtOH
Suppressed appetite
Block nutrient metabolism

psychosocial issues and comorbid conditions common to older adults place this population at high risk for nutritional deficits. Malnutrition is estimated to occur in approximately 0% to 15% of community-dwelling older persons, 35% to 65% of older patients in acute care hospitals, and 25% to 60% of institutionalized older adults. Factors that lead to inadequate intake and uptake of nutrients in this population include the ability to obtain food (e.g., financial constraints, availability of food, limited mobility), desire to eat food (e.g., living situation, mental status, chronic illness), ability to eat and absorb food (e.g., poor dentition, chronic gastrointestinal disorders such as GERD or diarrhea), and medications that interfere with appetite or nutrient metabolism (Box 14-7).

In the frail older adult, a number of factors contribute to neuroendocrine dysregulation of the signals that control appetite and satiety and lead to what is termed *the anorexia of aging*. Although the anorexia of aging is a complex interaction of many interrelated events and systems, the result is chronic undernutrition and loss of muscle mass (sarcopenia). Malnutrition has also been associated with increased risk of falls and hospital admission.

Measurement of nutritional status in older adults, however, is difficult. Standard anthropomorphic measures do not take into account the changes in body composition and structure that accompany aging. Immune measures of nutrition are influenced by age-related changes in the immune system in general. Furthermore, criteria for the interpretation of biochemical markers in this age group have not been well established. Complicated markers and indices of malnutrition exist but are not necessary in the routine surgical setting. Subjective assessment by history and physical examination, in which risk factors and physical evidence of malnutrition are evaluated, has been shown to be as effective as objective measures of nutritional status. Several screening tools may be used, including the Subjective Global Assessment (SGA), Mini Nutritional Assessment (MNA), and Malnutrition Screening Tool (MST). The SGA is a relatively simple, reproducible tool for assessing nutritional status from the history and physical examination. SGA ratings are most strongly influenced by loss of subcutaneous tissue, muscle wasting, and weight loss. The SGA has been validated in older and critically ill patients, and has been related to the development of postoperative complications.[28] The MNA, which measures 18 factors, including body mass index (BMI), weight history, cognition, mobility, dietary history, and self-assessment, is also a reliable method for assessing nutritional status. Nutritional status, as determined by the SGA and MNA, has been shown to predict outcome in outpatient and hospitalized geriatric medical patients. The MST is also a simple screening tool and has been validated in older patients in hospital and residential settings.[29] Maintenance of adequate nutritional status in older residents of chronic residential facilities is improved with a nutritional coordinator program.

The serum albumin level has been implicated as a strong predictor of outcome, both perioperative mortality and morbidity, in surgical patients. Recent evidence has demonstrated that low serum albumin levels in older patients correlate with increased length of stay, increased rates of readmission, unfavorable disposition, and increased all-cause mortality. In the Veterans Affairs NSQIP study (see earlier),[23] a low serum albumin level was the most important predictive factor for mortality. This suggests that a low serum albumin level is a sensitive marker of outcome, regardless of whether it is directly related to poor nutritional status or to unidentified complex chronic illness; effects on outcome may correlate to a better extent with inflammation, at least in dialysis patients. More recently, albumin also has been shown to correlate with infection and in-hospital death.

Although there is no definitive evidence from large randomized trials on preoperative nutritional restoration, amelioration of malnutrition with protein or immune-enhancing supplementation may improve outcome in some groups of older patients.

## Frailty

Although recognizing an individual who is frail may seem easy, defining the physiologic components that describe the frail phenotype has proven more difficult. Frailty is primarily a geriatric syndrome in which declines in reserves across many organ systems leave the individual with a decreased ability to respond to many stressors. The frail individual typically has loss of muscle mass (sarcopenia), chronic undernutrition, weakness, and decreased exercise tolerance. For study purposes, the frail phenotype is currently defined by five characteristics: weight loss, weak grip strength, self-reported exhaustion, slow walking speed, and low energy expenditure.[30]

The presence of frailty is associated with many poor health outcomes, such as falls, disability, hospitalization, and death. Recent evidence has also suggested that frailty in surgical patients independently predicts higher postoperative complication rates, longer lengths of stay, and more frequent discharges to nursing facilities. The degree of frailty also predicts the magnitude of the increased risk with those classified as frail (four or five characteristics) having worse outcomes than those classified as intermediately frail (two or three characteristics).[31]

## SPECIFIC POSTOPERATIVE COMPLICATIONS

Although older surgical patients with comorbid disease are at higher risk for many of the same surgical complications that occur in patients of all ages, several serious complications are more specific to this age group. These likely reflect an overall decline in physiologic capacity and reserve.

### Delirium

Delirium, a disturbance of consciousness and cognition that presents over a short period of time, with a fluctuating course, is among the most common and potentially devastating postoperative complication seen in older patients. Postoperative delirium is associated with higher rates of morbidity (30 days) and mortality (6 months), longer intensive care unit (ICU) length of stay, longer hospital length of stay, higher rates of institutionalization after discharge, and higher overall hospital costs.[32] The incidence of postoperative delirium in older patients varies with the type of procedure: less than 5% after cataract surgery, 35% after vascular surgery, and 40% to 60% after hip fracture repair. The incidence in older patients requiring treatment in an ICU is over 50%.

Postoperative delirium is usually the result of an interaction between preexisting conditions (risk factors) and postoperative events or complications (precipitating factors). The onset of delirium maybe the first indication of a serious postoperative complication. Identifying risk factors preoperatively, and minimizing precipitating factors intraoperatively and postoperatively, is currently the best strategy to prevent delirium (Table 14-4).

**Table 14-4 Risk Factors and Precipitating Factors for Delirium**

| RISK FACTORS | PRECIPITATING FACTORS |
|---|---|
| Advanced age | Infection |
| Cognitive impairment | Medications |
| Functional impairment | Hypoxemia |
| Poor nutrition | Electrolyte abnormalities |
| Comorbidity | Under treated pain |
| Alcohol abuse | Neurologic events |
| Psychotropic medications | Dehydration |
| Sensory impairment | Sensory deprivation |
| Type of surgery | Sleep disruption |
| Severe illness | Use of bladder catheters<br>Unfamiliar environment<br>Use of physical restraints |

Adapted from Lagoo-Deenadayalan SA, Newell MA, Pofahl WE: Common perioperative complications in older patients. In Rosenthal RA, Zenilman ME, Katlic MR (eds): Principles and practice of geriatric surgery, ed 2, New York, 2011, Springer, pp 361–376.

#### Risk Factors

The most important risk factor for postoperative delirium in older patients is a preexisting cognitive deficit, so some form of cognitive assessment is an essential part of the preoperative workup. Other risk factors include poor functional status, undernutrition or malnutrition, serious coexisting illness, sensory deficits, depression, alcohol consumption, preoperative psychotropic drug use, severity of illness, and magnitude of surgical stress. In a large prospective study of patients older than 50 years undergoing elective, noncardiac surgery, Marcantonio and coworkers[33] have determined the relative importance of some of these factors in predicting delirium and developed a quantitative predictive rule to identify patients at risk.

#### Precipitating Factors

Precipitating factors for delirium in the postoperative setting include common postoperative complications (e.g., hypoxia, sepsis, metabolic disturbances), untreated or undertreated pain, medications (e.g., certain antibiotics, analgesics, antihypertensives, beta blockers, benzodiazepines), situational issues (e.g., unfamiliar environment, immobility, loss of sensory assist devices such as glasses and hearing aids), use of bladder catheters and other indwelling devices or restraints, and disruption of the normal sleep-wake cycle (e.g., medications and treatments given during usual sleep hours). No association has been found with the route of anesthesia (epidural versus general) or the occurrence of intraoperative hemodynamic complications. However, intraoperative blood loss, need for blood transfusion, and postoperative hematocrit level lower than 30% are associated with a significantly increased risk for postoperative delirium.

Although delirium is common in older patients following surgery, the diagnosis is frequently not appreciated. Agitation and confusion are usually recognized but depressed levels of consciousness may also be present. The Confusion Assessment Model (CAM) developed by Wei and colleagues[34] is a simple, well-validated tool to diagnose delirium. A positive CAM requires the following: (1) acute onset with waxing and waning course and (2) inattention, with (3) disordered thinking or (4) altered level of consciousness.

The best treatment for delirium is prevention. Strategies that focus on maintaining orientation (e.g., family at the bedside, sensory devices available), encouraging mobility, maintaining normal sleep-wake cycles (no medications during sleep hours), and avoiding dehydration and inappropriate medications have been shown to decrease the number and duration of episodes of delirium in hospitalized patients.[35] Pharmacologic prevention trials have not yet shown consistently positive results.

Once delirium is diagnosed, a thorough search for precipitating factors such as infections, hypoxia, metabolic disturbances, inappropriate medications, and undertreated pain should be conducted. Invasive devices and catheters should be removed as soon as possible and restraints should be avoided. A thorough review of the history should also be conducted and the family queried about possible predisposing factors, such as unrecognized alcohol consumption.

### Aspiration

Aspiration is a common cause of morbidity and mortality in older patients in the postoperative period. The incidence of

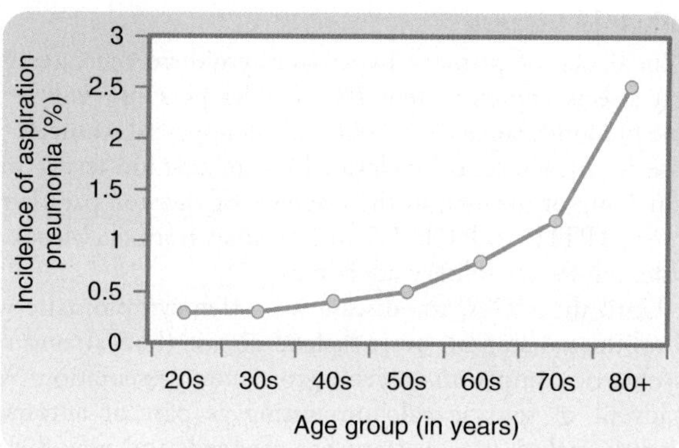


**FIGURE 14-10** There is almost an exponential increase in postoperative aspiration pneumonia with increasing age. (From Kozlow JH, Berenholtz SM, Garrett E, et al: Epidemiology and impact of aspiration pneumonia in patients undergoing surgery in Maryland, 1999-2000. Crit Care Med 31:1930–1937, 2003.)

**Table 14-5 Organ System Effects of Bed Rest**

| SYSTEM | EFFECT |
|---|---|
| Cardiovascular | ↓ Stroke volume, ↓ cardiac output, orthostatic hypotension |
| Respiratory | ↓ Respiratory excursion, ↓ oxygen uptake, ↑ potential for atelectasis |
| Muscles | ↓ Muscle strength, ↓ muscle blood flow |
| Bone | ↑ Bone loss, ↓ bone density |
| Gastrointestinal | Malnutrition, anorexia, constipation |
| Genitourinary | Incontinence |
| Skin | Sheering force, potential for skin break down |
| Psychological | Social isolation, anxiety, depression, disorientation |

From Kleinpell RM, Fletcher K, Jennings BM: Reducing functional decline in hospitalized elderly. In Hughes RG (ed): Patient safety and quality: An evidence-based handbook for nurses, AHRQ Publ No. 08-0043, Rockville, MD, 2008, Agency for Healthcare Research and Quality, pp 251–265.

postoperative aspiration pneumonia increases almost exponentially with increasing age, with patients older than 80 years having a 9- to 10-fold greater risk than those 18 to 29 years of age (Fig. 14-10).[36]

Swallowing is a complex, coordinated interaction of many neuromuscular events. As many as one third of independent functioning older persons report some difficulty with swallowing. With age, there is a decline in several of the elements of normal swallowing that predispose to aspiration. These include loss of teeth, decrease in the strength of the muscles of mastication, slowing of the swallow time, decreased laryngopharyngeal sensation, and decreased cough strength. Poor oral hygiene and the edentulous state are also associated with an overgrowth of pathologic organisms, which predispose to pneumonia following aspiration.

In general, other risk factors for aspiration in older patients can be categorized as disease- related (e.g., stroke, dementia, neuromuscular disorders such as Parkinson's disease, GERD), medication-related (e.g., drugs that cause dry mouth or altered mental status), and iatrogenic factors. The last of these is particularly relevant to surgical patients. The presence of devices crossing the oropharynx (e.g., nasogastric tubes [NG], endotracheal tubes [ET], esophageal thermometers, transesophageal echocardiographic [TEE] probes), has been shown to disrupt the swallowing mechanism further. The need for prolonged intubation is associated with swallowing dysfunction and aspiration, as is the use of enteral feeding tubes. The routine use of NG tubes in patients undergoing colon resection has been correlated with an increased risk of aspiration pneumonia, as has the use of TEEs in patients undergoing cardiac surgery. The occurrence of postoperative ileus also predisposes to aspiration.

Aspiration risk should be assessed preoperatively in all older patients with risk factors for aspiration and in those with any report of a swallowing abnormality (see earlier, "Preoperative Assessment"). Aspiration precautions should be ordered for any patient thought to be at risk. These include 30- to 45-degree upright positioning, careful evaluation of gastrointestinal function prior to starting feeding and frequently thereafter, careful monitoring of gastric residuals in patients with feeding tubes, and upright position during meals and for 30 to 45 minutes after meals in those on an oral diet.

## Deconditioning

In older patients, the prolonged period of immobility that follows hospitalization for a major surgical procedure often results in functional decline and overall deconditioning. Functional decline has been observed after as little as 2 days of immobility. Deconditioning is a distinct clinical entity, characterized by specific changes in function of many organ systems (Table 14-5).[37] Deconditioned individuals have ongoing functional limitations, despite improvement in the original acute illness. The period for functional recovery may be as much as three times longer than the period of immobility. Prolonged bed rest also leads to other postoperative complications, such as pressures ulcers and falls.

A major risk factor for deconditioning during hospitalization is a preexisting functional limitation. For example, patients requiring ambulation assist devices such as canes or walkers prior to hospitalization are more likely to suffer significant further functional decline. Other less obvious functional limitations, such as the inability to perform activities such as walking up a flight of steps carrying a bag of groceries (4 METs), are also associated with higher rates of postoperative complications and greater chances of functional decline. Other risk factors include two or more comorbidities, five or more medications, and a hospitalization or emergency room visit in the preceding year.[37] Patients who develop delirium while in the hospital are also at greater risk of developing serious functional decline and of requiring placement in short-term rehabilitation or long-term care facilities.

Assessment of functional capacity is an essential part of the preoperative assessment (see earlier). In patients identified at risk for functional decline, a plan for early directed methods to promote mobility, including early physical therapy consultation, should be establish prior to surgery. The "out of bed" order may be the most important of all routine postoperative orders for older patients.

Structured models for the in-hospital care of geriatric patients have been developed for patients hospitalized for medical illnesses. Adaptation of these models for surgery patients could promote improvements in functional and cognitive status. Preoperative conditioning to improve function prior to surgery, termed *prehabilitation* or *prehab,* has theoretical merit, although evidence to support its usefulness is still lacking.

## SURGERY OF MAJOR ORGAN SYSTEMS

### Endocrine Surgery

#### Thyroid Disease

Hypothyroidism occurs in 10% of women and 2% of men older than 60 years; hyperthyroidism occurs in 0.5% to 6% of persons older than 55. Hypothyroidism is caused by autoimmune disease, previous radioablation or surgery, and drugs that interfere with the synthesis of thyroid hormone, such as amiodarone. Hyperthyroidism is usually caused by toxic multinodular goiter, with Graves' disease being less common than in younger persons. Medical treatment of hypothyroidism in older adults is similar to that in younger patients. Surgical treatment of hyperthyroidism may be necessary for large goiters compressing the trachea. It is most important to remember that as with disorders of many other organ systems, symptoms of hypothyroidism and hyperthyroidism in this age group are easily overlooked or attributed to other causes. Failure to recognize the presence of either can result in serious perioperative problems.

The incidence of thyroid nodules increases throughout life, whether detected by physical examination, ultrasound, or autopsy, although physical examination is less sensitive because of fibrosis of the soft tissues of the neck and the gland. The incidence of nodules in autopsy series is 50%. Thyroid nodules are four times more common in females, but the risk for cancer in a nodule is higher in males. Most thyroid nodules are single when detected. Thyroid nodules change slowly over the short term. Prospective studies have shown, however, that up to 25% of colloid nodules can shrink over a period of 2 to 3 years and may disappear.

Well-differentiated thyroid cancer is divided into papillary and follicular subtypes. Sporadic papillary thyroid cancer has an almost bell-shaped distribution of age at diagnosis, with a decreasing trend in patients older than 60 years. Age is a negative prognostic factor for survival and other outcomes; patients older than 60 years have an increased risk for local recurrence, and patients younger than 20 and older than 60 have a higher risk for the development of distant metastasis. Similar results have been noted for follicular cancer. Increasing patient age correlates with increased risk for death by approximately twofold over a span of 20 years. Guidelines for the management of thyroid nodules and well-differentiated cancers can be found in the 2006 report of the American Thyroid Associations Guidelines Task Force.[38]

When thyroidectomy is indicated, it can usually be performed safely, even in patients much older than 80 years. However, older age does confer a higher risk of complications, longer hospital stays, more likely discharge to a location other than home, and higher rate of perioperative mortality. Surgical outcomes in older patients with multiple comorbidities have been shown to be better when the operative volume of the surgeon is more than 30 thyroidectomies/year.

#### Parathyroid Disease

The incidence of primary hyperparathyroidism increases with age; it affects approximately 2% of older persons, with a 3:1 female preponderance (1 in 1000 postmenopausal women). The disease is characterized by elevated serum calcium levels, often within 1 mg of normal, in the presence of elevated parathyroid hormone (PTH) to levels 1.5 to 2.0 times normal. Most cases in older adults are solitary adenomas.

Until the 1970s, the disease was often symptomatic with nephrolithiasis (stones), overt skeletal disease (bones), and neuropsychiatric complaints (psychic groans) on presentation. With the advent of routine calcium testing as part of automated chemistry analysis, this pattern has changed, and now 80% of cases are asymptomatic. A careful history, however, will frequently reveal the presence of less obvious psychological and emotional symptoms. Other subtle symptoms in older persons include memory loss, personality changes, inability to concentrate, exercise fatigue, and back pain. Several studies have shown that only 5% to 8% of patients are truly asymptomatic.

In response to the controversy regarding treatment of asymptomatic hyperparathyroidism, the National Institutes of Health (NIH) consensus conference in 1990 offered parameters for care. Participants agreed that truly asymptomatic patients, with serum calcium levels only mildly elevated, no previous history of life-threatening hypercalcemia, and normal renal, bone, and mental status, can be safely observed without surgery. Patients with CrCl decreased by 30% over age-matched controls, 24-hour urinary calcium excretion of more than 400 mg, and decreased bone mass more than 2 standard deviations (SDs) from age- and race-matched controls are offered surgical treatment.

Further indications for surgery include primary hyperparathyroidism in patients younger than 50 years and hyperparathyroidism in patients for whom close follow-up would be difficult or for whom significant concomitant illness complicates management. At a more recent NIH workshop in 2002, a panel reconsidered therapy for asymptomatic primary hyperparathyroidism. The threshold for parathyroidectomy was reduced to include patients with a serum calcium level more than 1 mg/dL above the upper limits of normal. This definition still leaves uncertain whether weakness and depression indicate symptomatic disease, although approximately 40% of patients with hyperparathyroidism have one or both complaints. Because the risk for morbidity and mortality associated with surgery is low, even in older patients, parathyroidectomy remains the treatment of choice unless other comorbid conditions preclude surgery.

Minimally invasive parathyroid surgery has gained acceptance with the adoption of sestamibi-directed surgery, intraoperative parathyroid hormone (PTH) assay, and videoscopic surgery. Cure rates in patients older than 70 years at one center have risen from 84% in the pre–minimally invasive era (before 2001) to 98% after the introduction of radioguided minimally invasive surgery under regional anesthesia.[39]

#### Breast Disease

**Epidemiology** Increasing age is a major risk factor for developing breast cancer. Worldwide, almost one third of breast cancer cases occur in patients older than 65 years. In the United States, more than 50% of new cases of breast cancer and approximately two thirds of breast cancer–related deaths occur in patients older than 65 years. Breast cancer incidence increases with age, peaking at age 75 and declining slightly thereafter. It is expected that as life expectancy continues to improve in Western countries, the proportion and absolute numbers of women with breast cancer will rise dramatically.[40]

**Presentation and Screening** The presentation of breast cancer is similar in older and younger populations. The painless mass represents the most common symptom of breast cancer. In older women, a new breast lump is likely to represent a malignancy. Breast pain, skin thickening, breast swelling, or nipple discharge or retraction should be vigorously pursued with biopsy in older women. Breasts become less dense with aging, making the clinical examination easier in older women. This difference also translates into an improved positive predictive value of an abnormal mammogram in women older than 65 years. The American Cancer Society recommends monthly breast self-examination, annual clinical breast examination, and annual mammography beginning at age 40, with no upper age limit as long as a woman remains in good health. If a woman's life expectancy is estimated to be less than 3 to 5 years, has severe functional limitations, or has multiple comorbidities that are likely to impair survival, discontinuation of screening is appropriate. The American Geriatrics Society Position Statement recommends annual or at least biennial mammography to age 75 years. Beyond the age of 75, mammography should be biennial or at least every 3 years if life expectancy is more than 4 years.[41]

**Pathology and Treatment Overview** Overall, breast cancers in older patients tend to be associated with more favorable pathologic prognostic factors. As patients' ages increase, their breast tumors are associated with more favorable tumor biology, as indicated by increased hormone sensitivity, attenuated epidermal growth factor receptor 2 (erb-b2) overexpression, and lower grades and proliferative indices. However, older patients are more likely to present with larger and more advanced tumors, and recent reports have suggested that the involvement of lymph nodes increases with age. Despite these differences, stage per stage, survival for older women with breast cancer is similar to that seen in younger women. Older women are less likely to receive definitive surgery, breast-conserving surgery, postlumpectomy radiotherapy, adjuvant hormonal therapy, and adjuvant chemotherapy.

Breast cancer trials in the United States have a disproportionately low enrollment of older women. Women 65 years and older are less likely than stage- and physician-matched younger women to be offered participation in breast cancer trials. Therefore, most recommendations for the treatment of older women with breast cancer have been derived from studies done in women younger than 70 years. Unlike the treatment of younger women with breast cancer, a central concept in decision making in older patients with breast cancer is that of life expectancy. Accurate predictions and knowledge of life expectancy are inherently important in decisions regarding screening older populations using mammography, treatment of the primary lesion, and use of systemic adjuvant therapy. Currently available treatment options often carry short-term risks and toxicities in older women that are not mitigated by long-term survival gains.

***Surgery*** Surgical resection of the primary tumor is recommended for all older patients unless they are poor surgical candidates, and breast-conserving therapy should be recommended when possible. Despite evidence that age is not a contraindication to breast-conserving surgery, older women have historically had lower rates of breast-conserving cancer surgery than younger women. Recent studies have indicated that the proportion of older women undergoing breast-conserving therapy is increasing. Omitting surgery exposes patients to a higher risk of local relapse and therefore is considered a suboptimal option, even for unfit older women. Tamoxifen alone had been previously recommended for the treatment of patients unfit for surgery and with short life expectancies, because tamoxifen antagonizes the estrogen receptor; in contrast to premenopausal women in whom the ovaries are responsible for estrogen production, the adrenal gland produces estrogen in postmenopausal women. Recent evidence[42] has indicated that the response to aromatase inhibitors, which block the synthesis of estrogen, is higher than tamoxifen in the neoadjuvant setting. Therefore, these agents may be more effective primary treatment for unfit older patients. Aromatase inhibitors are also associated with less thromboembolic complications than tamoxifen; however, the use of aromatase inhibitors in patients with severe osteoporosis is cautioned.

The role of axillary lymph node dissection (ALND) in the management of women with breast cancer has evolved over the last 10 to 15 years. ALND should be used when there is clinical suspicion of axillary lymph node involvement or a high-risk tumor. Biopsy of sentinel lymph nodes is a safe alternative to ALND in patients with clinically node-negative tumors. Older patients with tumor size smaller than 2 to 3 cm and no clinical evidence of axillary involvement should be offered a sentinel lymph node biopsy.[40]

***Radiation Therapy*** For women 70 years of age or older who have early, estrogen-receptor–positive breast cancer, the addition of adjuvant radiation therapy to tamoxifen does not significantly decrease the rate of mastectomy for local recurrence, increase the survival rate, or increase the rate of freedom from distant metastases. Therefore, tamoxifen alone is a reasonable choice for adjuvant treatment in such women. For older women with small, node-negative tumors, the decision to include breast irradiation after lumpectomy should be made on a case-by-case basis after careful discussion of the risks of locoregional recurrence and the side effects of radiation therapy. Alternatively, partial-breast irradiation with multicatheter interstitial brachytherapy, balloon catheter brachytherapy, three dimensional conformal external-beam radiotherapy, and intraoperative radiotherapy can be an option in selected older patients. Older women treated with mastectomy should be offered chest wall irradiation if they have tumors greater that 5 cm or more than four involved axillary lymph nodes.[40]

***Chemotherapy*** Tamoxifen and aromatase inhibitors, such as anastrozole, improve overall survival, reduce local recurrence, and reduce the risk of contralateral breast cancer for hormone-sensitive tumors in older women. Tamoxifen and anastrozole have side effects that can reduce their tolerance. Tamoxifen is associated with deep vein thrombosis, pulmonary emboli, cerebrovascular events, endometrial carcinoma, vaginal discharge and bleeding, and hot flashes. There are considerably more musculoskeletal complaints, including arthralgias and fractures, with anastrozole. The added value of chemotherapy in older women who receive endocrine therapy is influenced greatly by comorbidity and life expectancy. Models for estimating the benefits of chemotherapy in hormone receptor–positive older women have been developed, which demonstrate that a high risk of recurrence is needed to achieve a small survival benefit with adjuvant chemotherapy. For example, to reduce mortality risk at 10 years by 1% with chemotherapy, the risk of breast recurrence at 10 years has to be at least 25% for a 75-year-old woman in average health. These data suggest that chemotherapy for older women with hormone receptor–positive breast cancer should be offered only to node-positive patients who are in reasonable health, with a high risk of recurrence, and a life expectancy of more than 5 years. Older node-negative patients are unlikely to benefit from chemotherapy unless they have large hormone receptor–positive tumors with adverse pathologic characteristics or hormone receptor–negative tumors larger than 2 cm. An Internet based tool that incorporates age, health status, and tumor characteristics can help determine the potential benefit of adjuvant chemotherapy for breast cancer patients (http://www.adjuvantonline.com).[40,41]

## Gastrointestinal Surgery

### Esophagus

The esophagus undergoes characteristic changes with aging. Dysfunction of the proximal aspects of swallowing is noted during normal aging. Resting upper esophageal sphincter pressure and relaxation are decreased in the older normal population compared with a younger control population. The duration of oropharyngeal swallowing and sensory threshold for initiating a swallow are increased with advancing age. These factors increase the risk of pharyngeal stasis and potential for aspiration. Dysmotility of the cricopharyngeus (upper esophageal sphincter) with increasing age can result in Zenker's diverticulum (see Chapter 43). It appears that in normal healthy individuals, the physiologic function of the esophagus is preserved with increasing age, except for those older than 80 years. In the very old, the amplitude of esophageal contractions is decreased. It has been suggested that there is an association with GERD with the peristaltic dysfunction that occurs with aging. Although the lower esophageal sphincter resting pressure is normal and relaxes appropriately after deglutition, the sphincter fails to contract rapidly back to baseline, resulting in prolonged decreased tone. There is also an increased incidence of sliding hiatal hernia with aging, likely caused by laxity at the gastroesophageal junction. These conditions, in addition to delayed gastric emptying in older patients, predispose them to GERD. It is also important to remember that many medications prescribed for older patients increase the relaxation of the lower esophageal sphincter.[43]

The complications of GERD, including erosive esophagitis, Barrett's esophagus, and esophageal adenocarcinoma, are seen with an increased frequency in older patients. However, recent studies have demonstrated that symptoms may be attenuated in older adults. Specifically, older patients with severe esophagitis are least likely to have severe heartburn. Instead, they present with more nonspecific symptoms, such as dysphagia, anorexia, anemia, weight loss, and vomiting.[32] This absence of classic symptoms may be the result of an age-related decreased esophageal sensitivity to pain. Therefore, more aggressive diagnosis and/or treatment of GERD may be warranted for older patients, regardless of their presenting symptoms. The success of laparoscopic Nissen fundoplication for the correction of GERD in older patients provides a viable alternative to lifelong medications, which may also be less effective in older patients. As many as 90% of older patients report relief of symptoms, particularly vomiting and aspiration, after a Nissen procedure.

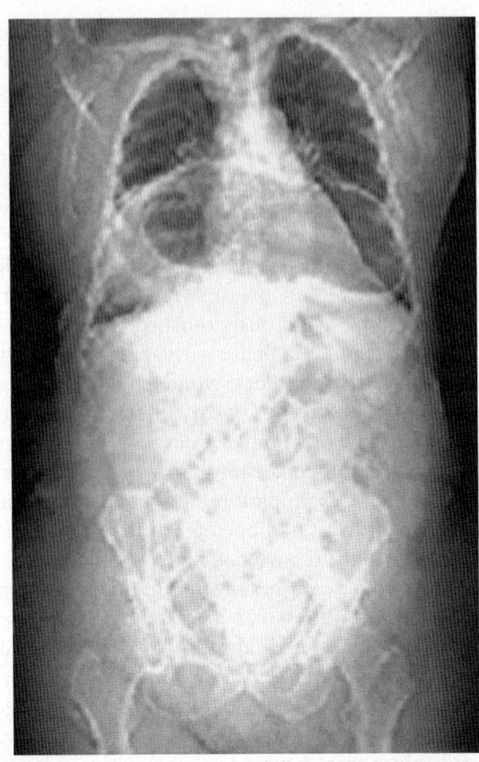

**FIGURE 14-11** Scout film for a CT scan showing a giant paraesophageal hernia with the entire stomach in the chest, rotated in an organoaxial direction.

Paraesophageal hernias also increase with advancing age and can reach enormous size without symptoms (Fig. 14-11). In the past, the fear of gastric volvulus, with subsequent strangulation, mandated immediate repair of paraesophageal hernias, even in the absence of symptoms. Watchful waiting is recommended, rather than immediate surgery for asymptomatic hernias, with a 1.1% annual probability of requiring an emergency operation.

Dysphagia is a frequent symptom in the older population that can cause significant problems in the perioperative period. Dysphagia in older adults can be divided into two categories—abnormalities affecting the neuromuscular mechanisms controlling movement of the tongue, pharynx, and upper esophageal sphincter (oropharyngeal dysphagia), and disorders affecting the esophagus itself (esophageal dysphagia). Causes of oropharyngeal dysphagia include stroke, Parkinson's disease, myasthenia gravis, diabetes, carcinomas, Zenker's diverticulum, and osteophytes. Causes of esophageal dysphasia can be divided into problems with motility, such as achalasia, diffuse esophageal spasm, and scleroderma, and structural problems, such as carcinoma, benign stricture, webs, and vascular compression.

Esophageal resection remains the only established curative treatment for cancer of the esophagus and gastric cardia. A major problem is that the surgery required is extensive, with a considerable risk of complications. Although the short-term mortality has decreased in recent years, the complication rate remains high. Recent studies have suggested that survival after resection of esophageal cancer is improving; however, this is may be partly the result of detection and treatment of earlier stage tumors. It appears that there is no difference in surgical complication rates between younger and older esophagectomy patients; however, overall morbidity and mortality rates are higher in older patients. This is most likely because of an increase in cardiopulmonary complications seen in the older age group undergoing esophageal resection.[44]

### Stomach

A progressive cephalad migration of the antral-fundic junction occurs with age. Studies have shown that between 25% and 80% of older persons have fasting achlorhydria. This is caused by progressive loss of parietal cells and decreased antral and serum concentrations of gastrin. Achlorhydria results in derangements in folate, iron, and vitamin $B_{12}$ absorption.[43]

The incidence of peptic ulcer disease increases with age. Up to 80% of peptic ulcer–related deaths occur in patients older than 65 years. Other factors that increase the risk of peptic ulcer disease in older adults are the use of nonsteroidal anti-inflammatory drugs (NSAIDs) and infection with *Helicobacter pylori*. NSAID use has increased markedly over the past few years, especially in older adults. The use of NSAIDs increases the risk of developing complicated peptic ulcer disease in older when compared with younger patients. Actual NSAID use is also a useful prognostic indicator; the mortality rate from peptic ulcer disease in older patients who take NSAIDs is twice that of those who do not. Similarly, 80% of all ulcer-related deaths are in patients taking NSAIDs. Despite this finding, NSAIDs are frequently prescribed to older patients, even those with previous gastrointestinal problems. *H. pylori* infections are believed to occur at a rate of 1%/year, yielding a substantial percentage of older adults harboring infections.

Older patients typically present for surgical correction of peptic ulcer disease in a delayed fashion and with more advanced disease. This translates to statistically significant increases in operative mortality for older patients undergoing surgery for complicated peptic ulcer disease. Age alone has not been shown to be an independent predictor of surgical risk. Multivariate analysis reveals three risk factors for operative mortality in perforated ulcer—the presence of concomitant disease, preoperative shock, and more than 48 hours of perforation. Age, amount of peritoneal soilage, and length of history of ulcer disease do not appear to be significant risks.

The incidence of gastric cancer rises progressively with age, with most patients between the ages of 50 and 70 years at presentation. Risks include dietary (e.g., pickled vegetables, salted fish, nitrates, nitrites), occupational (e.g., metal, asbestos, rubber workers), and geographic (Asia versus Western Hemisphere) factors. Chronic atrophic gastritis, previous gastric surgery, and chronic *H. pylori* infection, more frequently found in older patients, are associated with an increased risk of gastric cancer. Chronic atrophic gastritis and *H. pylori* infection are also risk factors for gastric lymphoma and its precursor, mucosal-associated lymphoid tissue. These patients typically present in the sixth decade of life. The presentation of gastric cancer is changing in older persons, leading to the need for more aggressive surgery. Older patients present with a predominance of intestinal type tumors rather than the more aggressive diffuse type. There is also a progression of the location of the tumor to more proximal areas of the stomach. As a result, total gastrectomy for cure in this population is now required in 13% to 34% of cases. No difference in resectability or the rate of positive lymph nodes found at surgery (60% to 70%) has been noted between younger and older patients.[45]

### Biliary Tract Disease

In almost all populations, and both genders, the prevalence of gallstones increases with increasing age, although the magnitude of this increase varies with the population. It is not surprising, therefore that biliary tract disease is the single most common cause of acute abdominal complaints in patients older than 65 years in the United States and accounts for approximately one third of all abdominal surgeries in this age group. In 2006, persons older than 65 years accounted for 50% of the hospital discharges for primary diagnosis cholelithiasis and one third of the over 400,000 inpatient cholecystectomies performed that year.

The increased frequency of gallstones in older adults is thought to result from changes in the composition of bile and impaired biliary motility. Alterations in the composition of bile with advancing age include an increase in the activity of 3-hydroxy-3-methylglutaryl coenzyme A (HMG-CoA, the rate-limiting enzyme in the synthesis of cholesterol) and a decrease in the activity of 7$\alpha$-hydroxylase (the rate-limiting enzyme in the synthesis of bile salts from cholesterol). This results in the supersaturation of bile with cholesterol and a decrease in the primary bile salt pool. The ratio of secondary to primary bile salts also increases. It is postulated that these secondary bile salts promote cholesterol gallstone formation by enhancing cholesterol synthesis, increasing the protein content of bile, decreasing nucleation time, and increasing the production of specific phospholipids that are thought to affect the production of mucin. It has also been suggested that the increase in secondary bile salts in older adults may promote the recycling of bilirubin, which in turn leads to the unconjugated bilirubin supersaturation necessary for pigment stone formation.

Alterations in gallbladder motility and bile duct motility are thought to be central to the development of cholesterol and brown pigment stones, respectively. The role of motility in black pigment stone formation, however, is less clear. Biliary motility is a complex interaction of hormonal and neural factors, but the major stimulus for gallbladder emptying is cholecystokinin (CCK). The sensitivity of the gallbladder wall to CCK has been shown to decrease with increasing age in animal models. In humans, gallbladder sensitivity to CCK is also decreased. However, there is a compensatory increase in the production of CCK in response to a stimulus that results in normal gallbladder contraction. The significance of this observation with regard to gallstone formation, however, is undetermined.

The indications for treatment of gallstone disease in older persons are the same as in younger patients, although complications of the disease, rather than biliary colic, are more common in those of advanced age. Older patients admitted to the hospital for cholecystectomy are more likely to have multiple biliary diagnoses, carry a concomitant diagnosis of cholangitis, undergo open operation, and require additional procedures such as endoscopic retrograde cholangiopancreatography (ERCP) or CBD exploration. The increased rate of complicated disease seen in older patients may be attributable to the increased severity of the disease, an increased prevalence of comorbid illnesses, or both. However, it is more likely to be a combination of factors, including delays in diagnosis and treatment caused by the frequent absence of typical biliary tract symptoms. Biliary colic, or episodic right upper quadrant pain radiating to the back, precedes the development of a complication only half as often in older as in younger patients. Even in the presence of acute cholecystitis, as many as 25% of older patients may have no abdominal tenderness, one third have no elevation in temperature or WBC count, and up to 59% have no peritoneal signs in the right upper quadrant.

Unfortunately, the outcome of biliary tract surgery in older patients hospitalized for treatment has not improved much over the past several decades. Older patients still have more complicated disease at the time of surgery, longer lengths of stay, higher rates of in-hospital mortality, and much higher rates of discharge to sites other than home (Fig. 14-12).[46] Until predictors of impending complications other than symptoms are identified, improving the outcome of biliary tract disease in older adults will be difficult. Increased awareness of the atypical manifestations of gallstone-related illness in this age group is essential.

Treatment of acute cholecystitis in older adults is somewhat controversial. Whereas considerable evidence supports the safety and efficacy of early laparoscopic cholecystectomy for acute cholecystitis in general, some authors favor percutaneous drainage, followed by delayed cholecystectomy, in older adults. Recent evidence has suggested that as many as 25% of older patients admitted to the hospital with a diagnosis of acute cholecystitis do not undergo cholecystectomy on the initial admission. However, readmission rates in this group are high, and 2-year survival is worse, even after adjustment for comorbidities and other patient risk factors.[47] The presence of CBD stones increases the likelihood of postoperative complications and death. In the prelaparoscopic era, bile duct stones were addressed at the time of cholecystectomy. Although open CBD exploration was extremely successful in clearing the bile duct of stones, it was associated with a significant increase in operative mortality and morbidity over simple cholecystectomy alone. Most clinicians now agree that if CBD stones are suspected from a dilated duct on ultrasound or from abnormal liver or pancreatic test results, a preoperative attempt at sphincterotomy and extraction via endoscopic retrograde cholangiopancreatography should be carried out. Successful duct clearance by this approach is reported in more than 90% of cases. Recurrence of CBD stones after sphincterotomy, however, even with antecedent or subsequent cholecystectomy, is higher in older than in younger patients (20% versus 4%). Risk factors for recurrence include a dilated CBD, duodenal diverticulum, angulation of the CBD, and previous cholecystectomy.

Management of the gallbladder after successful endoscopic treatment of CBD stones in patients without coincident acute cholecystitis is still controversial. Several studies have indicated that a complication related to the gallbladder will eventually develop in 4% to 24% of patients managed by endoscopic sphincterotomy alone and that 5.8% to 18% will require subsequent cholecystectomy. Unfortunately, because patients managed in this fashion are frequently the oldest and frailest patients, the mortality related to subsequent acute cholecystitis in these patients can be as high as 25%.

Special consideration must be given to the treatment of gallstones found at the time of laparotomy for an unrelated condition. The addition of cholecystectomy to the primary procedure usually adds little increased morbidity or mortality. Although some controversy still exists, many surgeons would proceed with incidental cholecystectomy if the patient were stable, exposure was appropriate, and the cholecystectomy added

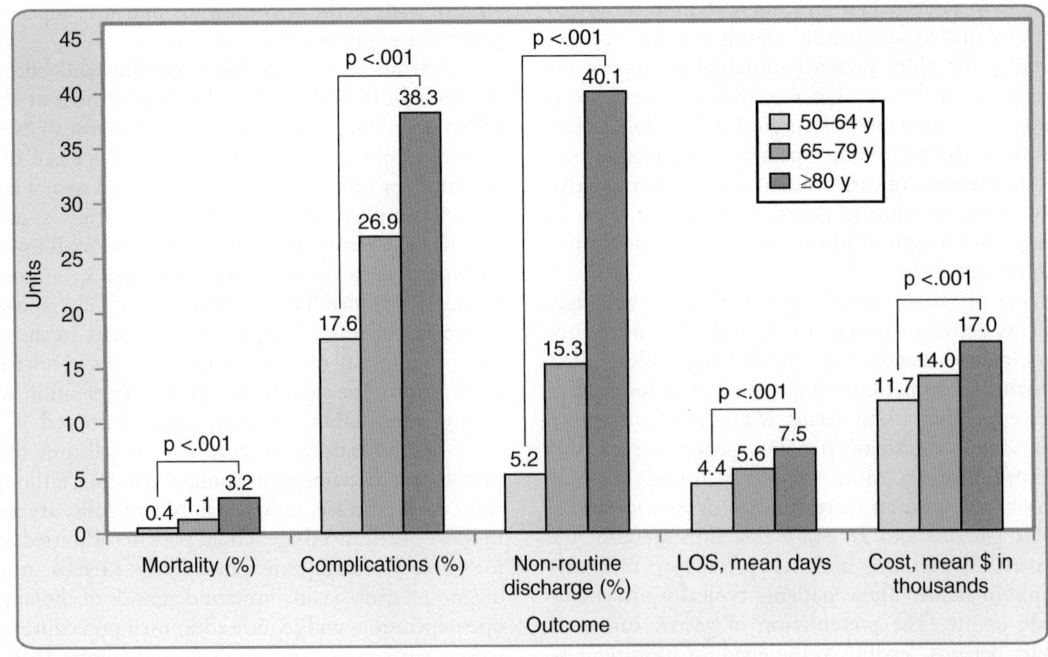


**FIGURE 14-12** Outcomes of inpatient cholecystectomy with age. (From Kuy S, Sosa JA, Roman SA, et al: Age matters: A study of clinical and economic outcomes following cholecystectomy in elderly Americans. Am J Surg 201(6):789–796, 2011.)

little additional operative time. In the past, stronger arguments for incidental cholecystectomy were based on concerns that the symptoms of acute postoperative cholecystitis might be unrecognized in the setting of a recent laparotomy incision. With better postoperative monitoring, more accurate imaging techniques, and percutaneous methods for decompressing the gallbladder should postoperative cholecystitis occur, these concerns have diminished.

### Liver

Tumors of the liver are 20 times more likely to arise from metastatic disease than from primary cancer. Metastatic tumors from gastrointestinal tract primaries are the most common type referred for resection. Patients with colon cancer have a 35% risk for recurrence in the liver, but only 10% to 20% of those identified have resectable disease. Patients resected have more than a 30% 5-year survival rate versus 0% if not resected.

Over the past 20 years the mortality associated with liver resection in patients older than 65 years has decreased. Today, the rates in younger and older patients are comparable.[48] Results are so similar that age alone is not necessarily a contraindication to simultaneous resection of colorectal malignancy and liver metastases.

In addition to surgical resection, treatments of hepatic cancer include radiologic embolization, cryotherapy and radiofrequency ablation therapy, which can be performed operatively or transcutaneously.

### Small Bowel Obstruction

Small bowel obstruction (SBO) is the most common and surgically relevant disorder of small intestinal function encountered in older persons. Although the exact incidence of SBO in older adults is difficult to ascertain, lysis of adhesions is the third most common gastrointestinal procedure after cholecystectomy and partial excision of the large bowel. Of the deaths associated with SBO, 50% occur in patients older than 70 years.

In Western countries, adhesions are responsible for a substantial majority of SBOs, followed by incarcerated hernias, neoplasms, and inflammatory bowel disease. It has been noted that patients with incarcerated hernias are slightly older than patients with adhesive obstruction. In addition, certain types of hernias, such as those that occur through the obturator foramen, are found almost exclusively in older adults and are particularly difficult to diagnose. Luminal obstruction, other than from deliberately ingested objects, accounts for less than 5% of cases. However, most cases of this type of obstruction occur in older adults . The two most common objects obstructing the lumen in adults are phytobezoars and gallstones. Phytobezoars, or large concretions of poorly digested fruit and vegetable matter, form with increased frequency in the stomach of older patients with poor dentition, decreased gastric acid, impaired gastric motility, and previous gastrectomy. In the stomach, these masses can become enormous without any symptoms. However, when a portion breaks free and migrates into the small bowel, obstruction ensues. Gallstones enter the small bowel usually through a fistula between the gallbladder and duodenum. Obturation of the small bowel lumen by an aberrantly located gallstone, incorrectly termed *gallstone ileus,* accounts for 1% to 3% of all SBOs but has been implicated in as many as 25% of obstructions in patients older than 65 with no abdominal wall hernia or history of previous surgery.

The pathophysiology, diagnosis, and treatment of SBO are discussed elsewhere in the text. It is important to note, however, that two important issues that determine management strategy—distinguishing functional (ileus) from mechanical obstruction and distinguishing simple from strangulated obstruction—are even more complex in older patients.

Many of the factors associated with ileus, such as systemic infections, intra-abdominal infections, metabolic abnormalities, and medications that affect motility, are more common in older persons. The relevance of these factors to the finding of abdominal distention is not always appreciated. Signs and symptoms of underlying infections such as pneumonia, urinary tract infection, or appendicitis may be subtle. Bowel distention may be erroneously considered the primary problem rather than a secondary event. Vomiting from a variety of nonobstructive causes can rapidly lead to dehydration and subsequent electrolyte abnormalities in older adults . The constellation of vomiting and bowel distention can easily be mistaken for obstruction.

In patients of all ages suspected of having adhesive SBO, initial nonoperative management with nasogastric decompression and IV hydration is standard. Although rates vary, only approximately 30% of patients with adhesive SBO will require surgery, usually for failure to progress or fear of strangulation. However, an accurate distinction between strangulated and simple mechanical SBO is difficult to make, particularly in older adults , because there are no objective markers that consistently identify which patient will require small bowel resection for ischemia at the time of surgery for SBO. Clinical findings of fever, tachycardia, elevated WBC count, and focal tenderness are notoriously misleading, particularly in older adults, in whom the risk for strangulation is the highest.

Several additional considerations are important in older adults. Although the natural reflex is to avoid unnecessary operations in sick older patients, prolonged conservative management can present new problems. Prolonged bed rest is associated with an increased incidence of venous stasis, pulmonary complications, and deconditioning. Prolonged nasogastric intubation is associated with an increased incidence of aspiration and pneumonia. Even a short period of nutritional deprivation may present a significant risk to an older patient with a baseline nutritional deficit. These factors together may result in a poor outcome if surgery becomes necessary after a prolonged attempt to avoid it.

In a review of more than 32,000 patients treated for SBO in California, 24% required surgery on the index admission.[49] Although length of stay was longer for those who had surgery, mortality was lower, readmissions for SBO were fewer, and the time interval to readmission for SBO was longer. The authors specifically stated that further research is needed to determine the importance of time to surgery on outcomes for the oldest and sickest patients.

In older patients who have undergone previous abdominal operations for malignant disease, the decision about when to operate is even more difficult. Metastatic obstruction presents several technical and ethical problems. Obstructing lesions are frequently found at a number of points in the bowel and resection may not be possible. Bypass of long, partially obstructed segments may be technically feasible but can leave the patient with a functionally short gut. Thirty-day operative mortality rates for this form of obstruction in older patients exceed 35%, and most patients die within 6 months. This discouraging outcome has led some to advocate prolonged periods of nonoperative decompression. Unfortunately, this approach produces only transient relief of obstructive symptoms. Furthermore, a previous history of malignancy is not an absolute indication that the obstruction is caused by metastatic disease. In 10% to 38% of patients with suspected malignant obstruction, a benign cause is found at the time of surgery.

Over the past decade, there has been increasing interest in using minimally invasive techniques to diagnose and treat SBO. At first glance, the laparoscopic approach in older adults has considerable appeal. Early intervention with minimal surgical stress would seem ideal. There are now numerous relatively small series by experienced laparoscopic surgeons that show diagnostic success in more than 90% of cases and total therapeutic success rates of 50% to 90%. However, laparoscopy in this setting can be technically challenging and not without complications. It is unclear at present how widely this option will be adopted as more surgeons become skilled in these advanced laparoscopic techniques.

### Appendicitis

Although appendicitis typically occurs in the second and third decades of life, 5% to 10% of cases present in old age. Appendicitis in older adults has increased in recent decades whereas the incidence in younger patients is declining. Inflammation of the appendix now accounts for 2.5% to 5% of acute abdominal disease in patients older than age 60 to 70 years. The overall mortality from appendicitis is only 0.8%, but the vast majority of deaths occur in the very young and the very old. In adults, the mortality rate after appendectomy is strongly related to age, ranging from a minimum of 0.07/1000 appendectomies in patients ages 20 to 29 years to a maximum of 164/1000 in nonagenarians.

The classic presentation of appendicitis—periumbilical pain that localizes over a period of several hours to the right lower quadrant, fever, anorexia, and leukocytosis—is present in less than 20% of older patients with appendicitis Although almost all older patients with acute appendicitis will present with abdominal pain, only 50% to 75% will have pain localized to the right lower quadrant. Almost one third of patients will have diffuse nonlocalizable abdominal pain. Because vague abdominal pain is a common complaint in older persons, its significance may be overlooked, leading to delays in treatment. Other signs of acute appendicitis are also unreliable in older adults. The WBC count and temperature are normal in 20% to 50% of older patients with appendicitis. Nausea, vomiting, and anorexia are also found less frequently in older patients.[50]

The indolent and nonspecific nature of the initial symptoms of appendicitis in older adults usually leads to delays of 48 to 72 hours before medical attention is sought. These delays are compounded by a delay in diagnosis once the patient reaches the hospital. Delays to operation longer than 24 hours are three times as likely to occur in older than in younger patients. As a result of these delays, over 50% of older patients will have perforated appendicitis identified at operation.[50] Older patients undergoing appendectomy for perforated appendicitis have a higher risk of complications and death than those undergoing simple appendectomy for appendicitis without peritonitis.

The use of laparoscopic surgery for the treatment of acute appendicitis has increased dramatically over the past decade. At laparoscopy, a significantly higher incidence of complicated appendicitis and other pathology is observed in older adults. These factors lead to a higher conversion rate to open surgery in older patients. There is no difference in infectious related morbidity between younger and older patients undergoing laparoscopic appendectomy (LA); however, older patients do experience a higher rate of cardiopulmonary complications. Older patients may benefit from a laparoscopic approach for the treatment of acute appendicitis. In a retrospective study of 2722 older patients,[51] significant reductions in length of stay were seen in the LA group compared with the open appendectomy (OA) group. Although LA did not result in statistically fewer complications than OA in older patients with perforated appendicitis, LA resulted in statistically fewer complications in the nonperforated appendicitis group. Importantly, there is a higher likelihood of discharge home compared with discharge to a skilled or nonskilled nursing facility and reduced mortality rates in LA patients.

The use of computed tomography (CT) scanning in the management of acute appendicitis has increased dramatically. Prior to urgent appendectomy, fewer than 20% of patients underwent preoperative CT in 1998 compared with over 90% of patients in 2007. It is important to note that the negative appendectomy rate in older adults has not changed during this same time period. Because of the atypical presentation of appendicitis in older adults and the expanded differential diagnosis, CT scanning has been advocated. If there is a suspicion of perforation and periappendiceal abscess, a CT scan should be obtained before operation. Percutaneous drainage and IV antibiotics are often preferable to exploration in the presence of a large abscess. In younger patients, this approach is followed by interval appendectomy approximately 6 weeks after the abscess has resolved. In older adults, recurrent appendicitis after resolution of the abscess is uncommon and interval appendectomy is therefore, not necessary in all cases. However, the possibility of perforated cancer in this age group does mandate a thorough evaluation of the colon when the acute process is controlled. Older patients presenting with signs and symptoms of acute appendicitis, but with longer duration of symptoms and a lower hematocrit than expected, should raise the concern for colon or appendiceal cancer.

### Carcinoma of the Colon and Rectum

Colorectal cancer is the third most common type of cancer and second most common cause of cancer-related deaths in the United States. Colorectal cancer is predominantly a disease of aging and is a major cause of morbidity and mortality in the older population. Colorectal cancer incidence is directly associated with increasing age, with most cases affecting older adults; 71% of new cases occur in patients 65 years and older and 42% occur in those 75 years and older. The annual incidence of colon cancer is almost 40 times higher for those older than 85 years compared with individuals 40 to 44 years of age. With the aging of the United States population, it is projected that the incidence of colorectal cancer will continue to increase.[52]

Increasing age is a poor prognostic factor in colorectal cancer. Patients older than 75 years have a significantly decreased 5-year disease-free survival compared with younger patients (Fig. 14-13). Although differences in colorectal cancer survival could be attributed in part to cancer biology and physiologic function specific to older adults, explicit differences in processes of care

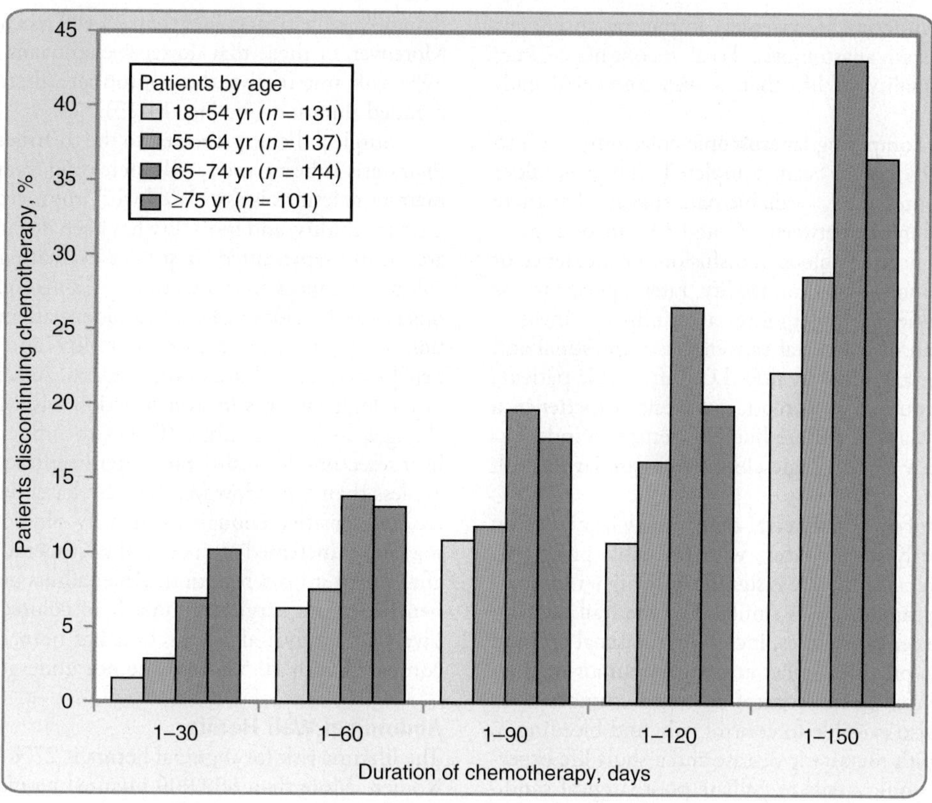


**FIGURE 14-13** Cumulative proportion of patients discontinuing chemotherapy by age. (From Kahn KL, Adams JL, Weeks JC, et al: Adjuvant chemotherapy use and adverse events among older patients with stage III colon cancer. JAMA 303:1037–1045, 2010.)

have been shown to be responsible for these outcome differences. Specifically, treatment disparities related to diagnosis, surgical care, and adjuvant and neoadjuvant therapies have been identified when comparing younger and older patients.[53]

The presenting signs and symptoms of colorectal cancer depend on the location of the tumor and do not vary substantially with age. Those with right-sided lesions tend to cause microcytic anemia from occult bleeding and present with fatigue, weakness, syncope, or a fall, and those with left-sided tumors tend to present with constipation, diarrhea, or a change in stool caliber. However, because fatigue, falls, constipation, and bowel dysfunction are accepted as common sequelae of aging, these symptoms are frequently ignored by the patient and physician. The diagnosis, therefore, is often not made until a complication occurs.

Older patients, regardless of the number of comorbidities they have, are less likely to receive screening for colorectal cancer. As a result, older adults are more likely to present with more advanced disease than younger patients. In addition, the proportion of unstaged cancers increases with advancing age. Screening for colorectal cancer in average risk individuals should begin at age 50; however, no upper age limit for colorectal cancer screening has been determined. Recommendations for screening include annual fecal occult blood testing and flexible sigmoidoscopy every 5 years, with full colonoscopy for positive occult blood or adenomatous polyps on flexible sigmoidoscopy, or colonoscopy every 5 to 10 years. Because older patients have an increased incidence of right-sided cancers and because more than 50% of patients with right-sided cancers have no lesions within reach of the flexible sigmoidoscope, colonoscopy may be a more effective screening tool in older patients. Colorectal cancer screening for older adults is not advised for individuals unlikely to live 5 years or for those who have significant comorbid medical conditions precluding treatment. Screening trials indicate that a difference in colorectal cancer mortality between screened and unscreened persons does not become noticeable until at least 5 years after screening. Therefore, persons with a life expectancy of 5 years or less are not likely to benefit from screening but are at risk for complications from procedures and the treatment of clinically unimportant disease.

Surgical resection is the only curative treatment for resectable colorectal cancer, regardless of the patient's age. For tumors of the abdominal colon, prohibitive anesthetic risk secondary to severe comorbidity and the presence of advanced metastatic disease are the only factors that should negatively influence the decision for surgery. There has been some concern about the ability of older patients to tolerate resectional procedures for low rectal cancers. This includes abdominoperineal resection, low anterior resection, and sphincter-saving coloanal anastomosis. Although technically more demanding than the traditional abdominoperineal resection, coloanal anastomosis provides a sphincter-saving alternative that is well tolerated by older adults in terms of operative mortality and postoperative complications. Both are equally effective for cure provided there is at least a 2-cm distal resection margin. Coloanal reconstruction can achieve continence in almost 80% of older individuals.

Assessment of anal function is extremely important in patient selection for low rectal anastomosis. Fecal incontinence may result in a worse quality of life than a well-controlled end-sigmoid colostomy.

Several studies comparing laparoscopic colectomy (LC) to open colectomy (OC) have been completed; however, older patients are underrepresented. Available data suggest that there is no significant difference between LC and OC in perioperative mortality rates, need for blood transfusion, or incidence of reoperation. Cardiopulmonary morbidity rates appear to be lower in older patients undergoing a minimally invasive approach to resection of colorectal cancer. Gastrointestinal and respiratory recovery are quicker after LC. After LC, patients report less pain, require less narcotic analgesia, experience a shorter hospital stay, and are more likely to return to independent status. Adequacy of oncologic clearance is similar in both treatment groups.

Local excision of low-lying rectal cancers may be an option for patients with early-stage cancers with favorable prognosis. Although the local recurrence rate is significantly higher for local excision, overall 5-year survival is similar. For the frail older or high-risk patient, lesser procedures, including transanal excision and fulguration, can provide local control of the tumor without disrupting continence. Local control of rectal tumors with chemoradiation is also possible to control pain and bleeding in poor-risk patients with metastatic disease and a short life expectancy. The use of colonic stents to palliate poor surgical candidates with impending obstruction should be considered.

Operative mortality for colorectal cancer in older patients is determined by the same two factors that influence operative mortality in older adults in general—the presence of coexisting disease and the need for emergency surgery. In patients with little or no comorbidity, operative mortality is similar, regardless of age. Even in patients older than 80 years, elective operative mortality rates are only approximately 2%. Unfortunately, because of the issues described, older patients are more likely to require emergency surgery than younger patients; colorectal cancer patients 85 years of age are twice as likely to need emergency surgery as those 65 years of age. In addition, with advancing age, a decreasing proportion of patients undergo curative resection at the time of surgery. When surgery is performed as an emergency, mortality increases threefold to fourfold over elective mortality for similar procedures. Length of hospital stays and hospital costs also increase. In addition, survivors of elective operations are twice as likely to return to independent living as are those surviving emergency surgery.

Survival after a diagnosis of colorectal cancer in older adults is disproportionately poor compared with that in younger patients. Methodology taking into account competing causes of death has established that older patients die more frequently from colorectal cancer, over and above expected age-related rates of death. In older patients with both colon and rectal cancers, the 5-year mortality following surgical resection is 1.5 to 2.5 times greater than for younger patients. The poorer survival seen in older patients with colorectal cancer may be a result of the reduced use of adjuvant therapy in this group. Despite the fact that most patients with colorectal cancer are older than 70 years, only 20% of patients in randomized trials are older than 70 years. The efficacy and tolerance of adjuvant chemotherapy for colon cancer and neoadjuvant chemoradiotherapy for rectal cancer in older patients have been demonstrated; however, less than 30% of patients older than 75 will receive adjuvant therapy. Moreover, of those that do receive adjuvant therapy, more than 50% will not receive the appropriate therapy for the recommended duration (see Fig. 14-13).[52]

Surgical therapy directed to the treatment of colorectal liver metastasis is being used with increasing frequency. Resection of metastatic lesions is associated with improved survival and operative morbidity, and mortality has been declining. Older patients are poorly represented in studies evaluating liver resection for colorectal cancer liver metastasis. As a result, surgery for liver metastases is seldom offered to older patients. Provider perception of high postoperative mortality and lack of oncologic benefit may contribute to this pattern. Although there are some physiologic changes in liver function with increasing age, these changes are not usually sufficient to influence the outcome of liver resection. Mortality rates after liver resection in older adults are less than 5%. However, because baseline liver function tests are not sensitive enough to identify physiologic decline, there may be an increased incidence of postoperative liver dysfunction after major impact resection. Older adults do derive a significant benefit from a surgical approach to colorectal liver metastases. Five-year survival after resection has been reported to be 32% compared with 10.5% in those not undergoing hepatectomy.

### Abdominal Wall Hernia

The lifetime risk for inguinal hernia is 27% for men and 3% for women. More than 600,000 inguinal hernias are repaired every year in the United States. There is a bimodal distribution for the development of inguinal hernia. Most develop for the first time in patients younger than 1 year and in those aged 55 to 85 years. The estimated incidence of abdominal wall hernia in persons older than 65 years is 13/1000, with a fourfold to eightfold higher incidence in men than in women. In patients older than 70 years, 65% of all hernias are inguinal, 20% are femoral, 10% are ventral, 3% are umbilical, and 1% are esophageal hiatal. Whereas the overwhelming majority of all groin hernias occur in men, 80% of femoral hernias occur in women. Older adults are also at risk for the more occult types of hernias, such as paraesophageal hernias and obturator hernias that do not become apparent until a complication has occurred.

It is clear that symptomatic groin and umbilical hernias in older adults should preferentially be repaired electively. Open, tension-free mesh repair of inguinal, femoral, and umbilical hernias can be performed as an outpatient procedure under epidural or local anesthesia with IV sedation. Mortality rates are low, even in patients with concomitant medical disease, and many reports have demonstrated mortality rates of 0%. Laparoscopic repair requires a general anesthetic in most cases, takes more operative time to complete, and incurs greater hospital costs. In older adults, the decreased economic benefit to society of an earlier return to normal activities and work seems to obviate the overall cost benefit of the laparoscopic operation. The trend in most centers is for laparoscopic repair to be restricted to bilateral and recurrent inguinal hernias, for which the results are excellent.

The issue of watchful waiting instead of immediate repair of asymptomatic and mildly symptomatic hernia in older adults remains controversial. Although some randomized studies have favored watchful waiting, others have suggested that repair may improve general health and decrease possible serious morbidity. Most studies agree that the risk of incarceration of asymptomatic hernias is small. One consideration that is most important in the decision to choose watchful waiting over repair is how the presence of the hernia might limit the activities of the aging individual. Maintenance of function and mobility is an important predictor of long-term survival and quality of life in older persons. In a recent follow-up to one randomized trial that initially showed that watchful waiting was safe, family members were surveyed about the ability of the hernia patient to perform four activities—normal activities around the home, normal work, social activities and recreational activities.[54] Of family members in the watchful waiting group, 25% to 30% reported some level of concern about the patient's ability to perform these activities. It was suggested these results favor repair.

Although the risk of incarceration of an asymptomatic hernia may be small, if it does occur, the results can be catastrophic, particular for the frail older person. This is mainly the result of the high incidence of strangulation found at the time of surgery. Intestinal resection is required in up to 12% to 20% of incarcerated inguinal hernias and as many as 40% of incarcerated femoral hernias. The decision to operate for asymptomatic or mildly symptomatic hernias is made on an individual basis by balancing the possible consequences of watchful waiting with the risks of the surgery. Care should be taken to determine whether the patient has limited his or her activities to avoid mild discomfort by seeking input from the family. Decreased activity presents more of a risk to the overall health of most older persons than the operative risk associated with inguinal hernia repair.

## Vascular Surgery

The most frequent peripheral vascular diseases seen in older patients are abdominal aortic aneurysms (AAAs), carotid artery disease, and peripheral arterial occlusive disease. Under elective conditions and in patients with well-managed concomitant disease, vascular surgery remains safe and effective; in many cases, endovascular technology is changing patterns of intervention.

### Abdominal Aortic Aneurysm

Mortality from elective AAA repair is generally considered to be less than 5% in patients 65 years and older, despite the high incidence of comorbidities in this age group. However, more recent evidence has called into question the effects of age on the outcome of AAA repair. On the basis of several studies, it has now been shown that there is a strong effect of age on mortality; males 85 years and older have almost five times the perioperative mortality rate of younger men, and females 85 years and older have over 10 times the mortality rate of younger women. Similarly, 5-year mortality after AAA repair in male and female older patients is approximately 80% to 90% compared with 25% to 30% in younger patients. As endovascular aneurysm repair (EVAR) has become more prevalent, experience with open AAA repair is diminishing, with concomitant increased mortality and morbidity associated with open surgery. In older patients, complications occur in approximately one third of open AAA repairs with infrarenal clamping and in over 50% of those with suprarenal clamping. Also, suprarenal clamping continues to be associated with increases in 30-day mortality, renal insufficiency, intraoperative blood loss, hospital length of stay, and rate of discharge to a nursing home. These results suggest that open AAA repair is becoming even less appropriate for most older patients, especially as the mean age of "older" patients increases. Fortunately, the increased availability of minimally invasive techniques, such as EVAR, may be associated with reduced mortality; many older and high-risk patients are receiving EVAR, with a mortality rate of approximately 2%, although complications continue to occur in about one third of cases. The true usefulness of EVAR may be with the repair of ruptured AAA. Emergency open repair for rupture is still associated with an operative mortality rate higher than 50% and an extremely high morbidity rate in those who do survive. However, reports of EVAR for ruptured aneurysms are encouraging, with reduced mortality; a recent collective review of worldwide experience with more than 1700 patients with ruptured aneurysms has shown, in experienced centers, a 30-day mortality rate of 19.7% in patients treated with EVAR compared with 36.3% in patients treated with open repair.[55] It is probable that the durability of stent grafts will increase over time, suggesting that EVAR is likely to be appropriate for older patients with suitable anatomy for repair.

### Carotid Artery Disease

Treatment of carotid disease for the prevention of stroke remains a common issue for older patients. In patients older than 65 to 80 years, the stroke rate from surgery is approximately 2.8% and the mortality rate is 2.4%. Survival of patients older than 80 years after carotid endarterectomy is similar to that in the general population. The incidence of neurologic symptoms after endarterectomy is lower than in an unoperated patient (13% versus 33%), and the incidence of late stroke is much lower as well (2% versus 17%), thus confirming the efficacy of endarterectomy in older patients. Suitable indications in octogenarians are similar to those in younger patients and include high-grade carotid lesions and hemispheric symptoms, with well-controlled concomitant disease. The development of carotid artery angioplasty and stenting (CAS) was originally thought to be a breakthrough, minimally invasive treatment for carotid disease, with wide applicability. However, patients older than 80 years old had an eightfold higher stroke rate (12.1% versus 1.7%) in the early report from the Carotid Revascularization Endarterectomy Versus Stenting Trial, the only randomized trial of carotid treatment sponsored by the NIH.[56] Recent European trials have confirmed the increased stroke rate with CAS. Patients older than 75 years have increased arch calcium deposits and increased arch tortuosity compared with younger patients, suggesting that increased stroke risk is inherent to standard femoral approaches generally used for CAS.

### Peripheral Vascular Disease

Peripheral vascular surgery for limb salvage is indicated for ischemic pain at rest, nonhealing ulcers, or frank gangrene. Although reports continue to show that age older than 80 years is a relative risk factor for increased perioperative mortality, surgery can generally be safely performed in older patients, especially when performed electively. In patients older than 80 years, the mortality rate associated with surgery is less than 5% and limb salvage rates over a period of 3 to 5 years are 50% to almost 90%. Five-year graft patency rates have been reported to be better in older than in younger patients with both prosthetic and autologous graft materials, although the small numbers of patients that have been studied suggests that larger series are still needed to validate these single center reports. Nevertheless, it is clear that older patients certainly do no worse than younger patients after infrageniculate bypass surgery. Treatment of graft infections in older patients is morbid, although aggressive wound care and muscle flap coverage is an option with good results (>50% graft salvage and 90% limb salvage). Endovascular approaches can also be used in the periphery in older patients, with reasonable durability in those with limited life expectancy. Angioplasty of the superficial femoral artery has a 5-year cumulative primary patency rate higher than 50% and a secondary patency rate of up to 70% in older patients. It is unclear whether these results will lead to increased treatment of older claudicant patients, as it has in younger patients.

Quality of life and preservation or restoration of functional independence are most important considerations in older patients. Amputation can be performed safely in older patients, with rates of perioperative mortality less than 10%. However, long-term survival after amputation is poor, with 1-year survival rates of approximately 50%; independent risk factors for mortality include high-level amputation, congestive heart failure, and inability to ambulate in the community. These functionally poor results of amputation lead many surgeons to continue to offer an aggressive approach to limb salvage in older patients.

## Cardiothoracic Disease

Cardiovascular disease has been the leading cause of death in the United States for almost 100 years. In the new millennium, cardiovascular disease is still present in approximately 64 million Americans, or 23% of the population. Most deaths attributable to cardiovascular disease occur in older patients.

Cardiac surgery is usually a dramatic event for patients and, accordingly, is one of the most frequently studied surgical procedures. Older patients have excellent results after cardiac surgery; as minimally invasive treatment of cardiac atherosclerosis changes patterns of referral to cardiac surgeons, patients are becoming older, with more frequent and severe comorbid conditions. Nevertheless, the uniformly good results with coronary artery bypass and valve replacement have encouraged continued performance of cardiac surgery, even in marginal candidates. Mortality in nonagenarians is approximately 14% but 5-year survival is approximately 59%.[57] Factors associated with excellent outcome in older patients include technically flawless surgery, meticulous hemostasis, excellent myocardial protection, and perfect anesthesia management.

### Coronary Artery Disease

The number of coronary artery bypass grafting (CABG) procedures performed on patients older than 65 years rose from 2.6 operations/1000 in 1980 to 13.0 operations/1000 in 1993. However, over the last decade, with the increasing use and success of percutaneous coronary artery interventions, the rate of CABG in persons older than 65 has fallen to 8.9/1000. This pattern is reflective of the performance of CABG in the general population, increasing from 7.2 cases/1000 discharges in 1988 to 12.2 cases in 1997, decreasing to 9.1 cases in 2003; nevertheless, overall mortality after CABG decreased from 5.4% in 1988 to approximately 3.3% in 2003.

Patients who are now referred for bypass usually have more complex disease or have failed alternative procedures. More than 50% of CABG procedures are now performed on patients older than 65 years. As the mortality and morbidity associated with cardiac surgical procedures have decreased, there has been a growing willingness to offer surgical therapy to older patients with reconstructible coronary artery disease. Unfortunately, older patients referred for cardiac surgery have a higher incidence of advanced disease (e.g., triple-vessel disease, left main or main equivalent disease, poor left ventricular function) and more symptomatic disease (90% of octogenarians are preoperatively classified as New York Heart Association [NYHA] functional class III or IV) and require emergency or urgent procedures more often.

Comorbid disease must be considered in older patients and may be extensive in some. Several preoperative risk factors for mortality after coronary bypass surgery have been identified, including an emergency procedure, severe left ventricular dysfunction, mitral insufficiency requiring a combined procedure, NYHA functional class IV, elevated preoperative creatinine level, chronic pulmonary disease, anemia (hematocrit <34%), and previous vascular surgery. Further risk factors for morbidity include obesity, diabetes mellitus, aortic stenosis, and cerebrovascular disease. These risk factors must be taken in the context of global patient comorbidity and considered as part of informed decision making for an individual patient. Risks attributable to patient age of 70 to 79 years are not significantly differently from those in patients younger than 60 years; however, patients older than 80 years have increased age-associated risk, equivalent to the presence of shock or acute (<6 hours) myocardial infarction.

In individuals older than 80 years, coronary artery bypass surgery is associated with an acceptable overall mortality of 7% to 12%, with mortality after elective procedures being lower than 3%. Nonagenarians have a perioperative mortality of approximately 15% to 20%, but a 5-year postoperative survival of approximately 50%, which represents a significant survival benefit associated with surgery. Early elective surgery is clearly preferable to emergency surgery, which is associated with two to ten times higher mortality. Unfortunately, with persistent reluctance to offer elective operations to many older patients, some series continue to report a significant percentage, as many as 40%, of older patients requiring urgent or emergency operations.

Morbidity after coronary surgery in older adults is high in many series. Pulmonary failure requiring prolonged intubation, neurologic events such as cerebrovascular accidents and delirium, and sternal wound infections increase with age and are associated with postoperative mortality. Other complications, including reoperation for bleeding, need for pacemaker insertion, perioperative myocardial infarction, and superficial wound infections, occur with equal frequency in both younger and older patients, although some studies have noted a slightly higher incidence of sternal wound infection in older patients.

The effectiveness of coronary artery bypass surgery versus medical management in octogenarians has been assessed in terms of cost per quality life year survival, and good late functional results have been demonstrated in elderly patients.[58] The cost per quality-adjusted life-year (QALY) saved was approximately $10,400, less than the cost for many common procedures, such as screening mammography. The survival rate in the surgery group was 80% and 69% at 3 and 4 years respectively, whereas, in the medical group, comparable survival rates were 64% and 32%. Using a validated health status assessment tool, the EurQol Questionnaire, the authors assessed quality of life in five domains: pain, activity, mobility, self-care, and depression and anxiety. In all areas, quality of life was better in the surgically treated than in the medically treated groups. Quality of life in the group of octogenarians who selected CABG was found to be equal to that of an average 55-year-old in the general population.

Older patients with end-stage heart failure have traditionally been excluded from the option of cardiac transplantation because of the scarcity of donor hearts and an inability to tolerate pharmacologic immunosuppression easily. Recent reports of partial left ventriculectomy are encouraging, with mortality and functional outcome in patients older than 65 years similar to that in younger patients.

### Valve Replacement

Since 1975, much data have accumulated that support the safety and efficacy of aortic valve replacement in older adults. Operative mortality is 3% to 10% and the long-term survival rate is approximately 75% to 80%. Although mortality in older patients is slightly higher than that in younger patients, most differences were not statistically significant. In addition, the vast majority of older patients receiving new aortic valves have great improvement in their quality of life. As many as 90% of older patients who were classified as NYHA functional class III or IV preoperatively and survive are reclassified postoperatively as class I or II. Because the average life expectancy for a healthy 70-year-old is approximately 13 years and that for an 80-year-old is approximately 8 years, safe aortic valve replacement surgery is preferable to the approximately 80% 4-year mortality associated with untreated symptomatic aortic stenosis.

Mitral valve disease in older adults has been less well investigated, partly because it is less common but also because the natural history is less well defined and the outcome of surgical therapy is less favorable, with slightly higher operative mortality after mitral valve replacement compared with aortic valve replacement in octogenarians. Left ventricular reserve is often compromised in older adults with mitral insufficiency because of the frequently associated ischemic disease. Low cardiac output is a particular problem after mitral valve replacement. Frequently, both aortic and mitral valve replacement are accompanied by additional procedures. There is some debate about whether valve replacement plus CABG or multiple valve replacement in the very old is too risky to justify the combined procedures. Many believe that with appropriate patient selection, even multiple procedures can be performed with relative safety, but the number of patients who meet the selection criteria is small. In centers that perform mitral valvuloplasty to repair the valve in patients with low ejection fractions, results in older patients are similar to those in younger patients.

The choice of valve material is also an important consideration in older patients. Mechanical valves are extremely durable but require lifelong anticoagulation. In patients older than 75 years, the mortality from long-term anticoagulation alone is almost 10%/year. Bioprosthetic valves do not require anticoagulation and are somewhat less durable, but may suffice for patients with a life expectancy of less than 10 years.

As experience with minimally invasive procedures become more common, it is likely that these procedures will become safer and will be used with increased frequency in older patients. Endovascular placement of valves, however, is likely to supersede additional advances in surgical therapy and become the procedure of choice in all patients, not just those unfit for open procedures. Endovascular valve replacement for degenerated porcine aortic valves is now being offered to some older patients.

### Lung Cancer

Lung cancer, usually adenocarcinoma or squamous cell carcinoma, remains a leading cause of death in industrialized countries; more than 150,000 deaths are still caused by lung cancer in the United States annually. Smoking remains the most important risk factor for lung cancer, and smoking cessation is an appropriate preventive measure for all patients. Appropriate therapy is critically dependent on accurate staging, and CT and $^{18}$F-fluorodeoxyglucose positron emission tomography are currently playing increasing diagnostic roles.

The incidence of non–small cell lung cancer (NSCLC) increases with age. There is still bias that older patients with early-stage (I to III) NSCLC do poorly with surgical resection, and thus these patients are often referred for limited resection or radiation therapy. Aggressive chemotherapy, particularly platinum-based adjuvant therapy, is often poorly tolerated by older patients. As such, many older patients have less than a full staging workup, incomplete histologic diagnoses, or undocumented performance status. Stage IV disease is initially diagnosed in most patients with NSCLC and they may be treated with combined chemotherapy and radiation therapy. However, older patients are not often considered candidates for this therapy. Some recent studies have shown that lower dose chemotherapy might be safe in older patients with limited comorbid illnesses, but well-performed controlled trials await publication. Neoadjuvant therapy is generally prescribed in older patients who are borderline candidates for surgery, would benefit from tumor downstaging, or would best be treated definitively by radiation therapy.

Recent evidence has suggested improved outcomes in older patients after surgical treatment of lung cancer.[59] Surgical resection for lung cancer is associated with an operative mortality rate of approximately 6%, although approximately 50% of patients still suffer some postoperative morbidity, such as atrial fibrillation, pneumonia, or retained secretions requiring bronchoscopy. Five-year survival in older patients after pulmonary resection for cancer is approximately 35%, with up to 40% survival in patients undergoing just lobectomy. Video-assisted thoracic surgery (VATS) is finding increased application, with some surgeons performing VATS for lung cancer resection. The potential for less operating time and blood loss, as well as short hospital length of stay and improved recovery time, holds great promise for all patients, especially older adults. Perioperative mortality rate for octogenarians treated with VATS is as low as 2%. VATS is associated with a similar 5-year survival rate compared with conventional open surgery. Increased age remains associated with more complications but only marginally worse survival. Results such as these suggest that VATS may increase the number of older patients who will be candidates for surgical therapy.

It is likely that future reports will define combinations of adjuvant and neoadjuvant therapy that will increase the number of older patients who will be surgical candidates and achieve disease-free survival. However, the outlook for older patients with preexisting pulmonary disease or other severe comorbid conditions remains poor.

## Trauma

Trauma is currently the fifth leading cause of death in older adults. Persons older than 65 years account for up to one third of trauma cases and 30% to 40% of trauma deaths, with more recent rates being the highest. Older patients have increased mortality, longer hospital stays, increased morbidity, and worse functional outcomes than younger patients. Motor vehicle accidents are the most common form of fatal injury in patients younger than 80 years and falls are the most frequent fatal injury after the age of 80. Interestingly, the incidence of death from motor vehicle accidents in older adults is the same whether they are passengers or pedestrians.

Older persons are at increased risk for blunt trauma and its complications. Age-associated central nervous system changes decrease coordination and mobility and increase the risk for accidents. Cerebral atrophy and decreased viscoelastic properties within the cranial vault make the brain more susceptible to blunt injury. Increased bone fragility results in an increased tendency for fracture. Decreased cardiac reserve and inability to increase cardiac output prevent avoidance of accidents. Concomitant use of drugs such as anticoagulants and antiplatelet agents increases the morbidity associated with traumatic events in older patients.

Significant injury can result from even simple falls from a level surface to the ground. The incidence of fracture or serious injury from such a fall is as high as 40% in an older person. After a fall with injury, there is significant morbidity. Of those hospitalized after a fall, up to 50% of patients need to be discharged from the hospital to a nursing facility, and only 50% are alive 1 year later. Elevator injuries in older patients are most commonly a slip, trip, or fall, but are associated with 15% hospital admission; 40% of these admissions are for a fractured hip.

Older patients have increased morbidity and mortality after head trauma, particularly when taking anticoagulant medications. Older people have increased rates of traumatic brain injury after head trauma and have longer disability. They take much longer to recover from head trauma than younger people and require more intensive rehabilitation. Blunt head trauma in an older person carries a particularly high mortality. Mortality in older patients with a Glasgow Coma Scale score of 5 is more than twice that of patients aged 20 to 40 years, and only 2% of older patients have a favorable recovery as compared with 38% of younger patients.

Injury from burns accounts for 8% of trauma in older patients. Older adults are at particular risk for burns because of impaired vision, decreased reaction time, depressed alertness, and decreased sensation of pain. In most older burn victims, injuries occur as a result of actions during ADLs—scalding, cooking accidents with flame, and electrical burns. In all patients, survival from burns is directly related to the total body surface area (TBSA) affected, but this association is more pronounced in older adults. In general, burns involving more than 40% of the TBSA in older persons have a poor prognosis. Reasons for the increased mortality are concomitant medical disease, burn wound sepsis, and multisystem failure, including pneumonia. For survivors of serious burns aged 59 years or older, fewer than 50% are discharged to independent living, one third to assisted living at home, and 20% to nursing facilities.

Older patients, whether they live with relatives or are institutionalized, are at risk for trauma as a result of elder abuse. It is estimated that 5% of older adults living in the community are subject to this type of maltreatment. It has also been shown that only one in 13 or 14 cases of elder abuse is reported. Maltreatment of older people can take one or more of six basic forms: physical abuse, sexual abuse, neglect, psychological abuse, financial exploitation, and violation of rights. As the older adult population increases, surgeons treating older trauma victims must learn to detect and report signs of physical and sexual abuse in addition to providing physical care of the patient's injuries, much as they have been mandated to do with children.

## Transplantation

In 1946, the first successful renal transplantation was performed. Early results with cadaveric renal transplants in patients older than 45 years were poor. The introduction of cyclosporine in the 1980s led to dramatic improvements, particularly in high-risk patients. As experience at transplantation centers has grown and the population of those older than 60 years has increased, the number of older patients who could potentially benefit from transplantation has also increased. Over the past 2 decades, the rate of persons older than 65 requiring renal replacement therapy in the United States has doubled and the rate in those older than 75 years has tripled.

The results of renal transplantation in older adults in terms of survival and quality of life justify extension of the age limit for this procedure. In one recent study of renal transplantation, patients older than 60 years had more delayed graft function and a longer initial hospital stay, but the incidence of acute rejection episodes was lower.[60] Patient survival, graft survival, and death-censored graft survival did not differ between older and younger patients, although follow-up of older patients was shorter (4.1 versus 6.7 years). The main cause of organ loss in older patients was death with a functioning kidney. Other have studies shown that 10-year allograft survival is higher in older patients than in patients younger than 60 years. However, the survival rate at 10 years in those older than 60 is 44% versus 81% for younger patients. Given the shortage of organ donors, the ethics of transplantation in older individuals with a higher likelihood of dying with a functioning allograft is questioned, although many believe that the evidence does not justify denying transplantation on the basis of age alone.

The number of older persons requiring liver transplantation has also increased. The percentage of liver recipients older than 65 years has increased from 4.9% in 1991 to 6.8% in 2002. Although age has been identified as a risk factor for a poorer outcome after liver transplantation, when patients are in better health (e.g., living at home at the time of transplantation), age is not a factor. Many studies have supported liver transplantation in low-risk, properly evaluated older adults.[61]

As the number of older transplant patients has increased, one important factor has emerged. The rate of acute and chronic rejection is clearly lower in older patients. This has been attributed to the overall decline in immunocompetence with age. However, this decline also renders older patients more susceptible to infection and malignancy. The high incidence of lymphoproliferative disorders in older transplant patients in general and the high rate of recurrent hepatitis C in older liver transplant patients in particular may be the result of excessive immunosuppression in this already compromised population. Decreasing immunosuppression in older patients may, in fact, improve both long- and short-term survival.

## SELECTED REFERENCES

Gerson MC, Hurst JM, Hertzberg VS, et al: Prediction of cardiac and pulmonary complications related to elective abdominal and non-cardiac thoracic surgery in geriatric patients. Am J Med 88:101–107, 1990.

An older but frequently quoted study comparing exercise tolerance and a variety of other assessment techniques demonstrating that an inability to raise the heart rate to 99 beats/min while performing 2 minutes of supine bicycle exercise was the most sensitive predictor of postoperative cardiac and pulmonary complications and death.

Hamel MB, Henderson WG, Khuri SF, et al: Surgical outcomes for patients aged 80 and older: morbidity and mortality from major noncardiac surgery. J Am Geriatr Soc 53:424–429, 2005.

A study of more than 26,000 patients older than 80 years undergoing major noncardiac surgery in Veterans Affairs Hospitals, showing the significance of complications on outcome in older patients. Mortality rose from 3.7% in patients with no complications to 26.1% in patients in whom one or more complication occurred.

Makary MA, Segev DL, Pronovost PJ, et al: Frailty as a predictor of surgical outcomes in older patients. J Am Coll Surg 210:901–908, 2010.

Frailty, a geriatric syndrome, independently predicts higher postoperative complication rates, longer lengths of stay, and more frequent discharges to nursing facilities in surgical patients.

Smetana GW, Lawrence VA, Cornell JE: Preoperative pulmonary risk stratification for noncardiothoracic surgery: systematic review for the American College of Physicians. Ann Intern Med 144:581–595, 2006.

A systematic review of the literature examining risk factor for pulmonary complications after noncardiac surgery, examining patient and procedural factors. This study showed that age older than 80 years was associated with the highest odds ratio of a pulmonary complication, even after adjusting for comorbidity.

Sollano JA, Rose EA, Williams DL, et al: Cost-effectiveness of coronary artery bypass surgery in octogenarians. Ann Surg 228:297–306, 1998.

Even in octogenarians, performing CABG is highly cost-effective. The quality of life of older adults who elect to undergo CABG is greater than that of their cohorts and equal to that of an average 55-year-old person in the general population.

## REFERENCES

1. Arias E: United States life tables, 2006. Natl Vital Stat Rep 58:1–40, 2010.
2. Rowe JW: Preface. In Committee on the Future Health Care Workforce for Older Americans Board on Health Care Services: Retooling for an aging america: Building the health care workforce, Washington DC, 2008, National Academy of Sciences, pp xi-xii.
3. Purves WK, Orians GH, Heller HC: Life: The science of biology, ed 4, New York, 1994, WH Freeman.
4. Medicare Payment Advisory Commission: A data book: Healthcare spending and the Medicare program, Washington DC, 2009, MedPAC.
5. Hall MJ, DeFrances CJ, Williams SN, et al: National Hospital Discharge Survey: 2007 summary. Natl Health Stat Report 24:1–20, 2010.
6. O'Connell JB, Maggard MA, Ko CY: Cancer-directed surgery for localized disease: Decreased use in the elderly. Ann Surg Oncol 11:962–969, 2004.
7. Saltzstein SL, Behling CA: 5- and 10-year survival in cancer patients aged 90 and older: A study of 37,318 patients from SEER. J Surg Oncol 81:113–116; discussion 117, 2002.
8. Hamel MB, Henderson WG, Khuri SF, et al: Surgical outcomes for patients aged 80 and older: Morbidity and mortality from major noncardiac surgery. J Am Geriatr Soc 53:424–429, 2005.
9. Fried TR, Bradley EH, Towle VR, et al: Understanding the treatment preferences of seriously ill patients. N Engl J Med 346: 1061–1066, 2002.
10. Mattimore TJ, Wenger NS, Desbiens NA, et al: Surrogate and physician understanding of patients' preferences for living permanently in a nursing home. J Am Geriatr Soc 45:818–824, 1997.
11. Taffett GE: Physiology of aging. In Cassel CK, Leipzig RM, Cohen HJ, et al., editors: Geriatric medicine: An evidence-based approach, ed 4, New York: 2003, Springer-Verlag, pp 27–35.
12. Sanders D, Dudley M, Groban L: Diastolic dysfunction, cardiovascular aging, and the anesthesiologist. Anesthesiol Clin 27:497–517, 2009.
13. Sharma G, Goodwin J: Effect of aging on respiratory system physiology and immunology. Clin Interv Aging 1:253–260, 2006.
14. Martin JE, Sheaff MT: Renal aging. J Pathol 211:198–205, 2007.
15. Luckey AE, Parsa CJ: Fluid and electrolytes in the aged. Arch Surg 138:1055–1060, 2003.
16. Pequignot R, Belmin J, Chauvelier S, et al: Renal function in older hospital patients is more accurately estimated using the Cockcroft-Gault formula than the modification diet in renal disease formula. J Am Geriatr Soc 57:1638–1643, 2009.
17. Schmucker DL: Age-related changes in liver structure and function: Implications for disease? Exp Gerontol 40:650–659, 2005.
18. Pawelec G, Koch S, Franceschi C, et al: Human immunosenescence: Does it have an infectious component? Ann N Y Acad Sci 1067:56–65, 2006.
19. Chang AM, Halter JB: Aging and insulin secretion. Am J Physiol Endocrinol Metab 284:E7–E12, 2003.
20. Freeman WK, Gibbons RJ: Perioperative cardiovascular assessment of patients undergoing noncardiac surgery. Mayo Clin Proc 84:79–90, 2009.
21. Smetana GW, Lawrence VA, Cornell JE: Preoperative pulmonary risk stratification for noncardiothoracic surgery: Systematic review for the American College of Physicians. Ann Intern Med 144:581–595, 2006.
22. Lawrence VA, Cornell JE, Smetana GW: Strategies to reduce postoperative pulmonary complications after noncardiothoracic surgery: Systematic review for the American College of Physicians. Ann Intern Med 144:596–608, 2006.

23. Khuri SF, Daley J, Henderson W, et al: Risk adjustment of the postoperative mortality rate for the comparative assessment of the quality of surgical care: Results of the National Veterans Affairs Surgical Risk Study. J Am Coll Surg 185:315–327, 1997.
24. Audisio RA, Pope D, Ramesh HS, et al: Shall we operate? Preoperative assessment in elderly cancer patients (PACE) can help. A SIOG surgical task force prospective study. Crit Rev Oncol Hematol 65:156–163, 2008.
25. Lawrence VA, Hazuda HP, Cornell JE, et al: Functional independence after major abdominal surgery in the elderly. J Am Coll Surg 199:762–772, 2004.
26. Gerson MC, Hurst JM, Hertzberg VS, et al: Prediction of cardiac and pulmonary complications related to elective abdominal and noncardiac thoracic surgery in geriatric patients. Am J Med 88:101–107, 1990.
27. Borson S, Scanlan JM, Watanabe J, et al: Simplifying detection of cognitive impairment: Comparison of the Mini-Cog and Mini-Mental State Examination in a multiethnic sample. J Am Geriatr Soc 53:871–874, 2005.
28. D'Alegria B, Cohen C, Medeiros F, et al: Nutritional diagnosis obtained by subjective global assessment in surgical patients and occurrence of post operative complications. Nutr Hosp 23:621, 2008.
29. Isenring EA, Bauer JD, Banks M, et al: The Malnutrition Screening Tool is a useful tool for identifying malnutrition risk in residential aged care. J Hum Nutr Diet 22:545–550, 2009.
30. Bandeen-Roche K, Xue QL, Ferrucci L, et al: Phenotype of frailty: Characterization in the women's health and aging studies. J Gerontol A Biol Sci Med Sci 61:262–266, 2006.
31. Makary MA, Segev DL, Pronovost PJ, et al: Frailty as a predictor of surgical outcomes in older patients. J Am Coll Surg 210:901–908, 2010.
32. Robinson TN, Raeburn CD, Tran ZV, et al: Postoperative delirium in the elderly: Risk factors and outcomes. Ann Surg 249:173–178, 2009.
33. Marcantonio ER, Goldman L, Mangione CM, et al: A clinical prediction rule for delirium after elective noncardiac surgery. JAMA 271:134–139, 1994.
34. Wei LA, Fearing MA, Sternberg EJ, et al: The Confusion Assessment Method: A systematic review of current usage. J Am Geriatr Soc 56:823–830, 2008.
35. Inouye SK, Bogardus ST, Jr, Charpentier PA, et al: A multicomponent intervention to prevent delirium in hospitalized older patients. N Engl J Med 340:669–676, 1999.
36. Kozlow JH, Berenholtz SM, Garrett E, et al: Epidemiology and impact of aspiration pneumonia in patients undergoing surgery in Maryland, 1999–2000. Crit Care Med 31:1930–1937, 2003.
37. Kleinpell RM, Fletcher K, Jennings BM: Reducing functional decline in hospitalized elderly. In Hughes RG, editor: Patient safety and quality: An evidence-based handbook for nurses, AHRQ Publ No. 08–0043, Rockville, MD, 2008, Agency for Healthcare Research and Quality, pp 251–265.
38. Cooper DS, Doherty GM, Haugen BR, et al: Revised American Thyroid Association management guidelines for patients with thyroid nodules and differentiated thyroid cancer. Thyroid 19: 1167–1214, 2009.
39. Pruhs ZM, Starling JR, Mack E, et al: Changing trends for surgery in elderly patients with hyperparathyroidism at a single institution. J Surg Res 127:58–62, 2005.
40. Wildiers H, Kunkler I, Biganzoli L, et al: Management of breast cancer in elderly individuals: Recommendations of the International Society of Geriatric Oncology. Lancet Oncol 8:1101–1115, 2007.
41. American Geriatrics Society Clinical Practice Committee: Breast cancer screening in older women. J Am Geriatr Soc 48:842–844, 2000.
42. Aapro M, Monfardini S, Jirillo A, et al: Management of primary and advanced breast cancer in older unfit patients (medical treatment). Cancer Treat Rev 35:503–508, 2009.
43. Salles N: Basic mechanisms of the aging gastrointestinal tract. Dig Dis 25:112–117, 2007.
44. Braiteh F, Correa AM, Hofstetter WL, et al: Association of age and survival in patients with gastroesophageal cancer undergoing surgery with or without preoperative therapy. Cancer 115:4450–4458, 2009.
45. Saif MW, Makrilia N, Zalonis A, et al: Gastric cancer in the elderly: An overview. Eur J Surg Oncol 36:709–717, 2010.
46. Kuy S, Sosa JA, Roman SA, et al: Age matters: An study of clinical and economic outcomes following cholecystectomy in elderly Americans. Am J Surg 201(6):789–796, 2011.
47. Riall TS, Zhang D, Townsend CM, Jr, et al: Failure to perform cholecystectomy for acute cholecystitis in elderly patients is associated with increased morbidity, mortality, and cost. J Am Coll Surg 210:668–677, 2010.
48. Lagoo-Deenadayalan SA, Newell MA, Pofahl WE: Common perioperative complications in older patients. In Rosenthal RA, Zenilman ME, Katlic MR, editors: Principles and practice of geriatric surgery, ed 2, New York, 2011, Springer, pp 361–376.
49. Foster NM, McGory ML, Zingmond DS, et al: Small bowel obstruction: A population-based appraisal. J Am Coll Surg 203:170–176, 2006.
50. Sheu BF, Chiu TF, Chen JC, et al: Risk factors associated with perforated appendicitis in elderly patients presenting with signs and symptoms of acute appendicitis. ANZ J Surg 77:662–666, 2007.
51. Harrell AG, Lincourt AE, Novitsky YW, et al: Advantages of laparoscopic appendectomy in the elderly. Am Surg 72:474–480, 2006.
52. Kahn KL, Adams JL, Weeks JC, et al: Adjuvant chemotherapy use and adverse events among older patients with stage III colon cancer. JAMA 303:1037–1045, 2010.
53. Anaya DA, Becker NS, Abraham NS: Global graying, colorectal cancer and liver metastasis: New implications for surgical management. Crit Rev Oncol Hematol 2010.
54. Gibbs JO, Giobbie-Hurder A, Edelman P, et al: Does delay of hernia repair in minimally symptomatic men burden the patient's family? J Am Coll Surg 205:409–412, 2007.
55. Veith FJ, Lachat M, Mayer D, et al: Collected world and single center experience with endovascular treatment of ruptured abdominal aortic aneurysms. Ann Surg 250:818–824, 2009.
56. Hobson RW, 2nd, Howard VJ, Roubin GS, et al: Carotid artery stenting is associated with increased complications in octogenarians: 30-day stroke and death rates in the CREST lead-in phase. J Vasc Surg 40:1106–1111, 2004.
57. Speziale G, Nasso G, Barattoni MC, et al: Operative and middle-term results of cardiac surgery in nonagenarians: A bridge toward routine practice. Circulation 121:208–213, 2010.

**58.** Sollano JA, Rose EA, Williams DL, et al: Cost-effectiveness of coronary artery bypass surgery in octogenarians. Ann Surg 228:297–306, 1998.

**59.** Dominguez-Ventura A, Allen MS, Cassivi SD, et al: Lung cancer in octogenarians: Factors affecting morbidity and mortality after pulmonary resection. Ann Thorac Surg 82:1175–1179, 2006.

**60.** Pedroso S, Martins L, Fonseca I, et al: Renal transplantation in patients over 60 years of age: A single-center experience. Transplant Proc 38:1885–1889, 2006.

**61.** Keswani RN, Ahmed A, Keeffe EB: Older age and liver transplantation: A review. Liver Transpl 10:957–967, 2004.

CHAPTER 15

# MORBID OBESITY

William O. Richards

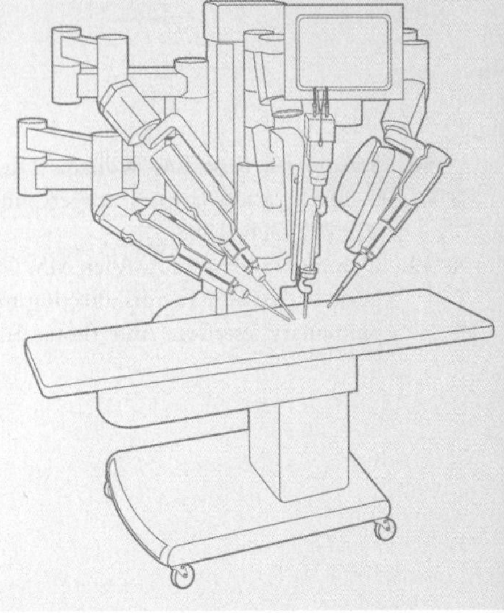



The surgical treatment of morbid obesity is termed *bariatric surgery.* It had its origin in the 1950s, when malabsorptive operations were first performed for severe hyperlipidemia syndromes. Subsequently, jejunoileal bypass to produce weight loss began to be performed sporadically during the 1960s and then more frequently in the 1970s. This operation, however, produced unacceptable metabolic complications and has been completely abandoned; other effective, low-morbidity operations have been developed.

This process has clearly pointed out two unique aspects of the field of bariatric surgery. The first is that this surgery involves the alteration of metabolic processes through fundamental changes in appetite, energy regulation, satiety, and metabolism, not just simply weight loss. The second is that long-term follow-up is essential to gauge the effect of these operations on a patient's overall health. Recent studies have all confirmed that operations such as the Roux-en-Y gastric bypass (RYGB), laparoscopic adjustable gastric banding (AGB), duodenal switch (DS), and laparoscopic sleeve gastrectomy result in sustained long-term weight loss, alterations in the metabolic consequences of morbid obesity, and a substantial reduction in mortality related to the improvement in lipid levels, diabetes, hypertension, obstructive sleep apnea, and cardiovascular events such as myocardial infarction. There is perhaps no other field in surgery that has accumulated more level 1 data and long-term comparative studies of medical and surgical treatment than bariatric surgery during the last decade. Moreover, the evidence conclusively shows that bariatric surgery is superior to medical therapy for weight loss, survival, and treatment of comorbidities, which are detailed in the chapter.

## OBESITY: MAGNITUDE OF THE PROBLEM

Morbid obesity is defined as being 100 lb above ideal body weight, twice ideal body weight, or a body mass index (BMI, which is weight [in kg]/height [in $m^2$]) of 40 $kg/m^2$. The latter definition is more accepted internationally and has essentially replaced the former ones for all practical and scientific purposes. A consensus conference by the National Institutes of Health (NIH) in 1991 suggested that the term *severe obesity* is more appropriate for defining people of this size.[1] This term shall be used interchangeably with morbid obesity in the remainder of this chapter.

It is estimated that more than one third of the U.S. adult population is obese; the prevalence of morbidly obese adults with a BMI of 40 or higher has gone from 2.9% in 1994 to 5.9% of the adult U.S. population in the National Health and Nutrition Examination Survey (NHANES) in 2006.[2] Patients undergoing bariatric surgery in the United States have average BMIs that are significantly higher than those reported in Europe. Australia, however, is not far behind, according to Australian bariatric surgeons. Even Europe, where severely obese individuals are not common in crowds, is now experiencing an overall enlargement of its population. Studies of adolescent obesity have estimated the incidence of obesity (40% above ideal body weight) as being in the 35% range for adolescents in the United States but more than 20% in most European countries. The problem is also growing at an alarmingly rapid rate in the United States. In 1985, when statistics of national obesity were first measured by the Centers for Disease Control and Prevention according to individual states, many states had no such data available. Of the approximately 50% that has these data, more than 50% reported a less than 10% incidence of people with a BMI higher than 30 $kg/m^2$. By 2008, every state except Colorado had reported that the incidence had risen to higher than 20% and 6 states reported that more than 30% of their population had a BMI of 30.0%.

Obesity is estimated to cause 300,000 deaths annually in the United States, whereas the total number of deaths annually from breast and colon cancers is only approximately 90,000/year.[3] After tobacco use, obesity is the second leading cause of preventable death in the United States and is second to smoking on the list of preventable factors responsible for increased health care costs. It is a sobering thought to realize that a 25-year-old morbidly obese man has a 22% reduction in life expectancy, or 12 years of life lost, when compared with a normal-sized man.[3] There is speculation that within the next decade, obesity may overtake tobacco as the leading cause of preventable death in the United States.

## PATHOPHYSIOLOGY AND ASSOCIATED MEDICAL PROBLEMS

The pathophysiology of severe obesity is poorly understood. Debate is ongoing regarding the relative genetic versus environmental components of the disease. There is a clear familial predisposition; it is rare for a single family member to have severe obesity and there is increasing evidence of specific genes, including *FTO* (fat mass and obesity-related) and *MC4R* (melanocortin 4 receptor) associated with obesity, increased fat mass, and insulin resistance.[4,5] The rapid increase in obesity from 1980 to 2010 emphasizes the considerable influence of environmental factors, such as easily available, cheap, high-density, caloric-rich foods and physical inactivity promoted by widespread ownership of cars, which also contributes to the problem.

Although there is no definitive answer to the pathophysiology of severe obesity, it is clear that a severely obese individual has, in general, persistent hunger that is not satiated by amounts of food that satisfy the nonobese. This lack of satiety or maintenance of hunger, with corresponding increases in caloric intake, may be the single most important factor in the process. Some studies have suggested that there are fundamental differences in the satiety and appetite hormonal control of eating that have created the current epidemic. This is hypothesized to occur when the brain's energy set point rises to increase energy intake through modulation of a person's appetite.

Another explanation of the obesity epidemic is that during human development, for thousands of years, the so-called *thrifty gene* marked those who could survive the periods of extreme protein calorie deprivation that marked early human development.[6] Because this thrifty gene allowed more efficient absorption and use of the calories ingested, the humans who had the thrifty gene had a distinct survival or fertility advantage. However, in modern society, in which we can drive through a fast food restaurant, drink high-fructose corn syrup soda, and eat a fat-laden, super-sized hamburger without getting out of the car, the thrifty gene does not convey a survival advantage. Instead, it helps increase the intake of calories in excess of metabolic needs.

We know that hormones, peptides, and vagal afferents to the brain have a major influence on satiety, appetite, and energy intake. The appetite hormone ghrelin, produced largely in the proximal part of the stomach by the presence of food, is involved in appetite and satiety.[7] Increased levels of ghrelin lead to increased food intake and increased ghrelin levels develop in individuals who are on low-calorie diets. This suggests one possible mechanism for the failure of most diets after 6 months—the increase in ghrelin. Interestingly, patients have normal to elevated ghrelin levels after laparoscopic AGB. Most studies have suggested that patients undergoing gastric bypass have suppressed postoperative levels of ghrelin, and appetite is dramatically reduced after gastric bypass, which leads to the incredible decrease in caloric intake that also leads to massive weight loss in the first 12 to 18 months after RYGB.[8]

Morbid obesity is a metabolic disease associated with numerous medical problems, some of which are almost unknown in the absence of obesity (Box 15-1). These problems must be carefully considered when one is contemplating offering weight reduction surgery to a patient. The most frequent problem is the combination of arthritis and degenerative joint disease, present in at least 50% of patients seeking surgery for severe obesity. The incidence of sleep apnea is high. Asthma is present in more than 25%, hypertension in more than 30%, diabetes in more than

**BOX 15-1 Medical Conditions Associated With Severe Obesity**

**Cardiovascular**
Hypertension
Sudden cardiac death myocardial infarction
Cardiomyopathy
Venous stasis disease
Deep venous thrombosis
Pulmonary hypertension
Right-sided heart failure

**Pulmonary**
Obstructive sleep apnea
Hypoventilation syndrome of obesity
Asthma

**Metabolic**
Metabolic syndrome (abdominal obesity, hypertension, dyslipidemia, insulin resistance)
Type 2 diabetes
Hyperlipidemia
Hypercholesterolemia
Nonalcoholic steatotic hepatitis (NASH) or nonalcoholic fatty liver disease (NAFLD)

**Gastrointestinal**
Gastroesophageal reflux disease
Cholelithiasis

**Musculoskeletal**
Degenerative joint disease
Lumbar disc disease
Osteoarthritis
Ventral hernias

**Genitourinary**
Stress urinary incontinence
End-stage renal disease (secondary to diabetes and hypertension)

**Gynecologic**
Menstrual irregularities

**Skin, Integumentary System**
Fungal infections
Boils, abscesses

**Oncologic**
Cancer of the uterus, breast, colon, kidney, prostate

**Neurologic, Psychiatric**
Pseudotumor cerebri
Depression
Low self-esteem
Stroke

**Social, Societal**
History of physical abuse
History of sexual abuse
Discrimination for employment
Social discrimination

20%, and gastroesophageal reflux in 20% to 30% of patients. The incidence of these conditions increases with age and with the severity and duration of the severe obesity.

The metabolic syndrome includes type 2 diabetes mellitus caused by insulin resistance, dyslipidemia, and hypertension. Patients with this constellation of problems are obese, with central body obesity being the primary essential feature (in women, waist circumference >35 inches; in men, >40 inches). The syndrome is characterized by impaired hepatic uptake of insulin, systemic hyperinsulinemia, and tissue resistance to insulin. Patients with metabolic syndrome are at high risk for early cardiovascular death.

Not listed in Box 15-1 are the associated societal discriminatory problems faced by severely obese individuals. Public facilities in terms of seating, doorways, and restroom facilities often make access to events held in these settings unavailable to a severely obese person. Travel on public transportation is sometimes difficult, if not impossible, especially in regard to air travel. Employment discrimination clearly exists for these individuals. Finally, the combination of low self-esteem, frequently a history of sexual or physical abuse, and these social difficulties coalesce to create a high incidence of depression in the morbidly obese patient population.

## MEDICAL VERSUS SURGICAL THERAPY

Medical therapy for severe obesity has limited short-term success and almost nonexistent long-term success. Once severely obese, the likelihood that a person will lose enough weight by dietary means alone and remain at a BMI below 35 kg/m$^2$ is estimated at 3% or less. The NIH consensus conference recognized that for this patient population, medical therapy has been uniformly unsuccessful in treating the problem.[1] A more recent review of the clinical trials of lifestyle interventions for the prevention of obesity in children has demonstrated that most were completely ineffective and the few that were marginally effective had an extremely small impact on BMI.[9] Despite massive efforts health care providers to influence weight through diet, physical activity, and lifestyle changes, the only effective long-term method for weight loss has been shown to be bariatric surgery. In a head to head trial, O'Brien and colleagues[10] randomized obese adolescents to lap band or to diet and lifestyle changes. Patients randomized to lap band lost 34.6 kg compared with the diet group, who lost 3.0 kg at the end of the 2-year trial. In another trial of obese adults, the surgical group achieved a 21.6% initial body weight loss whereas the medical group had a paltry 5.5% of initial body weight loss.[11]

Despite this limited success, it is generally agreed that a severely obese patient needs to be given the chance to comply with a medically supervised diet program to see whether any success can be achieved. A 10% weight loss attained over a period of months at a rate of 0.5 to 2 lb/week is the initial goal of medical therapy. Maintenance of the weight loss for 6 months defines the initial medical success with medical therapy, and further weight loss through a reduction in calories and increase in physical activity is encouraged. Insurance funding for surgery has traditionally been linked to such an attempt or, for some insurance companies, a well-documented history of several of these attempts. However, data showing any efficacy of the need for a prolonged diet attempt as positively influencing outcomes after bariatric surgery are lacking.

Very low-calorie diets fall into two categories, those that primarily restrict fat intake and those that primarily restrict carbohydrate intake. Both diets produce weight loss that is insufficient to affect any major change in health status.

In 2010, pharmacologic therapy focused on two medications. Sibutramine blocks presynaptic receptor uptake of norepinephrine and serotonin, thereby potentiating their anorexic effect in the central nervous system. Orlistat inhibits pancreatic lipase and thereby reduces absorption of up to 30% of ingested dietary fat. A maximum weight loss of up to 10% of body weight has been noted in unselected individuals taking either or both drugs; however, weight is regained within 12 to 18 months. For the severely obese individual, neither drug alone has proved to be effective therapy.

The Swedish Obesity Study (SOS) is our best evidence of the profound salutary effects of bariatric surgery on morbidity and mortality.[12] The study followed 98.9% of subjects undergoing bariatric surgery—gastric bypass, vertical banded gastroplasty, or nonadjustable silicone gastric banding—compared with a group of age-, gender-, and BMI-matched control subjects undergoing standard medical treatment. There was a significant long-term reduction in weight and in comorbid conditions, which resulted in a significant reduction in mortality in the bariatric surgery patients. Other excellent long-term studies have confirmed the benefits of bariatric surgery and have indicated a significant reduction in weight and long-term mortality in patients undergoing gastric bypass.[13]

Recently, experts from around the world met in Rome as part of the Diabetes Surgery Summit and put forth a position statement on recommendations for clinical and research issues related to the development of diabetes surgery.[14] During this extraordinary meeting, medical and surgical experts on bariatric surgery, obesity, and type 2 diabetes crafted a statement to develop methods for diabetes surgery to help improve access to proven surgical options while also suggesting research avenues to be pursued. Some of the recommendations included investigation of surgery on patients who have a BMI lower than 35, the previously defined cutoff for weight loss surgery.

## PREOPERATIVE CONSIDERATIONS

### Evaluation and Selection

#### Eligibility

Selection of patients for bariatric surgery is based strictly on currently accepted NIH guidelines. Patients must have a BMI higher than 40 kg/m$^2$ without associated comorbid medical conditions or a BMI higher than 35 kg/m$^2$ with an associated comorbid medical problem. They must have also failed dietary therapy. Beyond this, the NIH guidelines are not specific. However, it has been my experience that several practical criteria must also be used as guidelines for indications for surgery, including psychiatric stability, motivated attitude, and the ability to comprehend the nature of the operation and resultant changes in eating behavior and lifestyle. Criteria for eligibility for bariatric surgery are given in Box 15-2. An inability to fulfill these criteria is a contraindication to bariatric surgery.

One criterion not listed in Box 15-2 that unfortunately is often a significant issue for a severely obese patient is insurance coverage for the operation. Although bariatric surgery has been one of the most commonly studied operative procedures, with

**BOX 15-2 Indications for Bariatric Surgery**

Patients must meet the following criteria for consideration for bariatric surgery:

- BMI >40 kg/m$^2$ or BMI >35 kg/m$^2$ with an associated medical comorbidity worsened by obesity
- Failed dietary therapy
- Psychiatrically stable without alcohol dependence or illegal drug use
- Knowledgeable about the operation and its sequelae
- Motivated individual
- Medical problems not precluding probable survival from surgery

abundant information from controlled studies showing a significant survival advantage to the patient undergoing surgery, many insurance companies refuse to cover the procedure or establish multiple barriers to coverage for the individual patient. The Centers for Medicare and Medicaid Services (CMS), the federal agency that sets Medicare guidelines, established criteria for the coverage of open and laparoscopic gastric bypass, laparoscopic AGB, and DS operations in 2006. A controversial aspect of the ruling is the requirement that bariatric surgery be performed only by surgeons in hospitals that are designated as Centers of Excellence by the American Society of Bariatric Surgeons or level I centers by the American College of Surgeons. These unique requirements for Medicare beneficiaries were at least partly the results of concern by policymakers that the morbidity and mortality associated with bariatric surgery were high and that the explosive growth in the number of hospitals and surgeons performing the procedures did not correlate with hospital oversight of these procedures and resulting complications. Nevertheless, this marks a watershed moment in surgery in which, increasingly, payers are demanding that surgeons and hospitals meet stringent requirements for infrastructure, training of personnel, and ultimately, results of the procedures. Bariatric surgeons have risen to the occasion, as evidenced by the most recent data from National Surgical Quality Improvement Program (NSQIP)[15] and the Longitudinal Assessment of Bariatric Surgery (LABS) consortium[16] of the extremely low morbidity and mortality for laparoscopic bariatric surgery across the United States. These recent studies suggest that the imposition of the Center of Excellence standard has been at least partially responsible of the decline in operative morbidity and mortality.

Medical contraindications to bariatric surgery are not clear. All patients with comorbid conditions are at greater risk. The surgeon must ensure that these risks are well understood by all patients before bariatric surgery, especially those at high risk. Ideally, several family members are included in these discussions. Some individuals have end-stage organ dysfunction of the heart, lungs, or both; they are unlikely to gain the benefit of longevity and improved health.

Patients who cannot walk have greater risk than those who can ambulate, and surgery is contraindicated in patients who are unable to ambulate. Prader-Willi syndrome is another absolute contraindication because no surgical therapy affects the constant need to eat by these patients.

Patients who weigh more than 500 lb are at increased risk for mortality and have more complications. Many options for diagnostic testing, such as computed tomography (CT), are exceeded by this weight limit. At this weight, operating room tables, moving and lift equipment and teams, blood pressure cuffs, sequential compression device (SCD) boots, and any sort of invasive bedside procedures such as central venous catheters become extraordinarily difficult or problematic. It has been my practice to encourage strongly patients weighing more than 500 lb to lose weight down to that level by nonoperative methods, even if it means enforced hospitalization.

Age is a controversial contraindication to bariatric surgery. For adolescents, most pediatric bariatric surgeons recommend that the operation be performed after the major growth spurt (mid to late teens), thus allowing increased maturity on the part of the patient. Simple restrictive operations are thought to be most appropriate for patients in this age group. In the United States, although the laparoscopic AGB procedure (LAP-BAND) has been approved by the U.S. Food and Drug Administration (FDA) only for patients 18 years or older, several groups have modest experiences using this device under FDA guidelines.[10] Increasing experience will be required to determine which operation is most effective in adolescents.

Although I have generally set the age of 65 years as an approximate cutoff for performing gastric bypass, patients older than 65 have been individually evaluated. Such evaluations focus on the patient's relative physiologic age and potential for longevity rather than chronologic age. The duration and degree of obesity are the most important factors when evaluating an older patient. In general, the duration and severity of obesity and the number of comorbid medical problems that exist lower the potential for such individuals to benefit from bariatric surgery.

## Evaluation

Preoperative assessment of a bariatric surgical patient involves two distinct areas. One is a specific preoperative assessment of candidacy for bariatric surgery and evaluation for comorbid conditions. The second is a general assessment and preoperative preparation, as for any major abdominal surgery, which is discussed in depth in Chapter 11.

**General Measures** A team approach is required for the optimal care of a morbidly obese patient (Box 15-3). Box 15-4 summarizes the steps and tests routinely performed for the preoperative evaluation of bariatric patients in the my clinics.

Proper preoperative patient education is essential and attendance at educational sessions is mandatory. After preoperative testing is completed, a final counseling session with the surgeon and an education session with the nurse educator and nutritionist are held.

A first-generation cephalosporin, in a dose appropriate for weight, is given preoperatively, and antibiotics are continued for less than 24 hours. Data support the use of preoperative antibiotics, but no data have established the optimal regimen for deep venous thrombosis (DVT) prophylaxis. In the era of open surgery, pulmonary embolism (PE) was one of the most common causes of death after bariatric surgery. However, recent data have shown that pulmonary embolism is uncommon after laparoscopic RYGB and that measures such as early ambulation and sequential compression devices, without pharmacologic agents, such as heparin, can be used successfully to prevent DVT and PE in many patients undergoing laparoscopic gastric bypass or laparoscopic AGB.[17] High-risk patients (e.g., those with history of DVT, venous stasis ulcers, known or highly suspected

**BOX 15-3 Bariatric Multidisciplinary Team**

Surgeon
Assisting surgeon
Nutritionist
Anesthesiologist
Operating room nurse
Operating room scrub technician, nurse
Nurse care coordinator, educator
Secretary, administrator
Psychiatrist, psychologist
Primary care physician
Medical specialists for cardiac, pulmonary, gastrointestinal, endocrine, musculoskeletal, and neurologic conditions, as indicated

**BOX 15-4 Preoperative Evaluation**

**Before the Clinic Visit**
Documented, medically supervised diet
Counseling and referral from the primary care physician
Reading a comprehensive written brochure and/or attendance at a seminar regarding operative procedures, expected results, and potential complications

**Initial Clinic Visit**
Group presentation on information in the booklet
Group presentation on preoperative and postoperative nutritional issues by the nutritionist
Individual assessment by the surgeon's team
Individual counseling session with the surgeon
Individual counseling session with the nutritionist
Screening blood tests

**Subsequent Events and Evaluations**
Full psychological assessment and evaluation, as indicated
Medical specialist evaluations, as indicated
Insurance approval for coverage of the procedure
Screening flexible upper endoscopy, as indicated
Screening ultrasound of the gallbladder (if present)
Arterial blood gas analysis, as indicated

**Subsequent Clinic Visits**
Counseling session with the surgeon (including selection of the date for surgery)
Education session with the nurse educator
Preoperative evaluation by the anesthesiologist
Final paperwork by the preadmissions center

pulmonary hypertension, hypoventilation syndrome of obesity, or need for reoperation during the initial hospitalization) are given SC injections of heparin or low-molecular-weight heparin (LMWH) on call in the operating room and then twice daily until discharge at home, for a full 2-week course. Prophylactic vena cava filters are inserted, if possible on a temporary basis, in patients at extremely high risk for DVT and PE.

**Specific Comorbid Conditions** Cardiovascular evaluation of a bariatric patient must include a history of recent chest pain and functional assessment of activity in relation to cardiac function. Patients with a history of recent chest pain or a change in exercise tolerance need to undergo a formal cardiology assessment, including stress testing, as indicated. I almost never resort to invasive central monitoring with a Swan-Ganz catheter because central venous and pulmonary hypertension are the norm and must not be interpreted as volume overload. The use of intraoperative transesophageal echocardiography is occasionally helpful for patients with cardiomyopathy.

Pulmonary assessment includes a search for obstructive sleep apnea because a significant number of patients undergoing bariatric surgery will have undiagnosed obstructive sleep apnea.[16] A history of falling asleep while driving or at work or a history of feeling tired after a night's sleep, coupled with a history of snoring or even witnessed apnea, is strongly suggestive of the condition. Patients with suggestive histories of clinically significant sleep apnea need to undergo preoperative sleep study testing. If found to have the condition, use of a continuous or bilevel positive airway pressure apparatus postoperatively while sleeping can eliminate the stressful periods of hypoxia that would otherwise result in these patients. Although tolerated under normal circumstances, these hypoxic episodes in the immediate postoperative period are more dangerous because of the enhanced effect of narcotic pain medications and postoperative fluid shifts, which affect hemodynamic stability.

Reactive asthma is another common problem of the severely obese that is underrecognized. It requires less preoperative preparation in terms of testing than sleep apnea and is less dangerous.

Hypoventilation syndrome of obesity (pickwickian syndrome) is a diagnosis that should be suspected in the superobese (BMI >60 kg/m$^2$) by the patient's clinical appearance. Individuals with this diagnosis have plethoric faces, may appear clinically cyanotic, and clearly exhibit difficulty in normal respiratory efforts at baseline or with mild exertion. Arterial blood gas analysis reveals $Paco_2$ higher than $Pao_2$ and an elevated hematocrit. Pulmonary artery pressure is greatly elevated. These patients have extremely high cardiopulmonary morbidity and mortality and require significant preoperative weight loss and optimization of the patient's cardiopulmonary physiology prior to the operative procedure. A planned intensive care unit admission postoperatively is usually needed. Prolonged ventilator support is often required, and management of intravascular volume is based on the patient's baseline status.

Because there is a considerable incidence of hypertension or diabetes in patients with concomitant renal disease, the serum creatinine level is an excellent preoperative screening test for baseline renal function.

Musculoskeletal conditions, especially arthritis and degenerative joint disease, are the most common group of comorbid diseases found in severely obese patients. Over 50% of patients have some form of these conditions, often to an advanced degree. Limited ambulation, joint replacement, severe back pain, and other sequelae are not uncommon. Before surgery, it is important for patients to understand that any preexisting structural damage cannot be reversed by weight loss. Fortunately, significant weight loss often alleviates or even reverses the chronic pain or disability from such conditions. Significant weight loss after bariatric surgery will make subsequent knee and hip replacement surgery more effective and safer.

Metabolic problems are common in severely obese patients, particularly hyperlipidemia, hypercholesterolemia, and type 2 diabetes mellitus. All are easily determined by simple blood tests.

Of severely obese patients, 20% to 30% undergoing bariatric surgery have clinically significant type 2 diabetes. Diabetes needs to be controlled preoperatively to reduce the incidence of perioperative morbidity.

Skin must be examined for fungal infection and venous stasis changes, which are associated with a greatly increased incidence of postoperative DVT.

Umbilical or ventral hernias may be present. It has been my practice to postpone repair of ventral and incisional hernias until after significant weight loss. This has the advantage of performing the operation when intra-abdominal pressure is greatly reduced and after ongoing weight loss so that the patient is in positive nitrogen balance rather than actively losing weight. Repair of the hernias at the time of abdominoplasty enables the bariatric surgeon to complete physical reconstruction of the abdominal wall and place prosthetic mesh to reinforce the abdominal wall, which often cannot be accomplished during the initial bariatric procedure.

Cholelithiasis is the most prevalent of the several gastrointestinal conditions and, if gallstones are present, most surgeons agree that cholecystectomy needs to be performed simultaneously with the bariatric surgery. The incidence of gallstone or sludge formation after gastric bypass is approximately 30%. For patients undergoing malabsorptive operations, gallstone formation is so frequent that prophylactic cholecystectomy is a standard part of these procedures. However, for restrictive operations, screening ultrasound is recommended, particularly in patients undergoing RYGB, because endoscopic retrograde cholangiopancreatography (ERCP) is not possible. Ursodeoxycholic acid (ursodiol), 300 mg twice daily for 6 months postoperatively, reduces the incidence of gallstone formation to 3% in patients who follow this treatment plan. My current recommendations for patients undergoing laparoscopic bariatric surgery are simultaneous cholecystectomy if gallstones are present and ursodiol therapy for 6 months after surgery if the gallbladder is normal.

Gastroesophageal reflux disease (GERD) is common in severely obese patients because of the increased abdominal pressure and shortened lower esophageal sphincter. Preoperative upper endoscopy is indicated in all patients who have GERD to detect Barrett's esophagus and the presence of hiatal hernias and to evaluate the lower part of the stomach in patients undergoing RYGB.

A patient with nonalcoholic steatotic hepatitis (NASH) presents a potential problem. The size of the left lobe of the liver often inhibits the surgeon's ability to complete an operation laparoscopically. Patients with a known enlarged fatty liver may benefit from caloric restriction, especially carbohydrate restriction, for a period of several weeks preoperatively. Bariatric surgery is beneficial for NASH; weight loss improves the prognosis. NASH is not a contraindication to bariatric surgery if there is no cirrhosis and portal hypertension or hepatocellular decompensation. Liver biopsy should be performed at the time of bariatric surgery in any patient whose liver appears abnormal.

## Special Equipment

### Clinic

The clinic for evaluating bariatric patients must be constructed with the needs of the patient in mind. The waiting area must contain comfortable benches with backs, not standard-sized chairs. Doorways must be extra wide to accommodate wheelchairs. This is true for bathrooms as well, which must be equipped with toilets on the floor, not mounted on the wall. A scale that can weigh up to 1000 lb is necessary. Large-sized gowns, wide examining tables stable enough for large patients, and wide blood pressure cuffs are needed. A large room with appropriate seating is needed for the patient group education session.

### Operating Room

The operating room needs to contain a hydraulically operated operating room table that can accommodate up to 800 lb. Side attachments to widen the table are required, as needed. Foam cushioning, extra large SCD stockings, wide and secure padded straps for the abdomen and legs, and a footboard for the operating room table are all essential to secure the patient safely for placement in a steep reverse Trendelenburg position during surgery.

Videotelescopic equipment, as used for any laparoscopic abdominal procedure, is necessary. Two monitors, one near each shoulder, and high-flow insufflators able to maintain pneumoperitoneum are essential.

I have found a 45-degree telescope, extra-long staplers, atraumatic graspers, and other instruments to be most useful. Extra-long trocars may be needed. An ultrasonic scalpel is most helpful in all aspects of the dissection.

A fixed retractor device secured to the operating room table for clamping and holding the liver retractor is also essential. This can pose one of the most difficult technical challenges in patients with a large thick liver. Sometimes, two retractors may be necessary for a large liver.

## OPERATIVE PROCEDURES

Primary laparoscopic bariatric operations are preferred over the open procedures because of the increased availability of the laparoscopic approach and overwhelming advantages of the laparoscopic approach. These include reduced mortality, wound infections, pulmonary complications, thromboembolic complications, reduced rate of incisional hernias, and decreased hospitalization.[15,16]

We are only just now starting to recognize the many reasons why bariatric operations produce weight loss. The primary pathway to weight loss is the profound and long-lasting reduction of oral intake induced by changes in the gut-brain axis.[18] The other is malabsorption of ingested food. Box 15-5 lists the major procedures to be described.

**BOX 15-5 Bariatric Operations: Mechanism of Action**

**Restrictive**

Vertical banded gastroplasty (VBG; historic purposes only)
Laparoscopic adjustable gastric banding (AGB)
Laparoscopic sleeve gastrectomy (LSG)

**Largely Restrictive, Mildly Malabsorptive**

Roux-en-Y gastric bypass (RYGB)

**Largely Malabsorptive, Mildly Restrictive**

Biliopancreatic diversion (BPD)
Duodenal switch (DS)

### Vertical Banded Gastroplasty

This procedure has now largely been abandoned in favor of others because of poor long-term weight loss, high rate of late stenosis of the gastric outlet, and tendency for patients to adopt a high-calorie liquid diet, thereby leading to regain of weight.

### Laparoscopic Adjustable Gastric Banding

The AGB procedure may be performed with any of various types of adjustable bands. The two bands approved for use by the FDA in the United States are the LAP-BAND (INAMED Health, Santa Barbara, Calif) and the Realize band (Ethicon Endo-Surgery, Cincinnati, Ohio). The Swedish Adjustable Gastric Band (Obtech Medical, Baar, Switzerland), the MIDBAND (Medical Innovation Development, Villeurbanne, France), and the Heliogast band (Helioscopie, Vienne, France) are other banding systems used in Europe, Asia, the Middle East, and South America. The techniques of placement of the bands are similar; only the locking mechanisms, band shape and configuration, and adjustment schedules vary somewhat for the different types of bands. They all work on the principle of reduction of oral intake by augmenting the early satiety and decrease in appetite triggered by distention of the proximal part of the stomach and feedback to the brain eating center via the vagal nerves.[18] Their advantage over other bariatric procedures is adjustability and a markedly lower initial operative morbidity and mortality.

Trocar placement for AGB is shown in Figure 15-1. The surgeon stands to the patient's right, the assistant is to the patient's left, and the camera operator is adjacent to the surgeon. Most surgeons place the patient in the supine position, but some prefer to have the patient's legs spread so that the surgeon can stand between his or her legs. The peritoneum at the angle of His is divided to create an opening in the peritoneum between the angle of His and the top of the spleen (Fig. 15-2*A*). The telescope is placed through the left upper quadrant port for this part of the operation to maximally view the angle of His area.

The pars flaccida technique has become the approach of choice for placing the adjustable band. It begins by dividing the gastrohepatic ligament in its thin area, just over the caudate lobe of the liver. The anterior branch of the vagus nerve is spared, and any aberrant left hepatic artery is preserved. The base of the right crus of the diaphragm is identified. Care must be taken to identify the crus clearly because occasionally the vena cava can lie close to the caudate lobe. The surgeon gently follows the surface of the right crus posterior and inferior to the esophagus while aiming for the angle of His (see Fig. 15-2*B*). A gentle spreading and pushing technique is used to create an avascular tunnel along this plane. Once the tip of the tunneling instrument is seen near the top of the spleen, it is gently pushed through any remaining peritoneal layers to complete the tunnel (see Fig. 15-2*C*). The adjustable band has already been placed in the peritoneal cavity through the large 15-mm trocar located in the right upper quadrant before dissection of the pars flaccida. The narrow end of the band itself is grasped by the tunneling instrument and pulled through the tunnel from the greater to the lesser side of the stomach (Fig. 15-3). That end is then threaded through the locking mechanism of the band, after which the band is locked. Once the band has been locked in place, the buckle is adjusted to lie on the lesser curvature side of the stomach (Fig. 15-4). A 5-mm grasper inserted between the band and stomach ensures that the band is not too tight.

The anterior gastric wall is plicated over the band with three or four interrupted nonabsorbable sutures (Fig. 15-5). There needs to be just enough stomach above the level of the band for incorporating that tissue into the suture. Suturing is carried as far posterolaterally as possible because this region has been the most frequent area of fundus herniation through the band. The band is thus ideally secured approximately 1 cm below the gastroesophageal junction with this technique.

The Silastic tubing leading from the band is pulled through the 15-mm trocar site in the right upper quadrant paramedian area to complete the laparoscopic portion of the operation. The

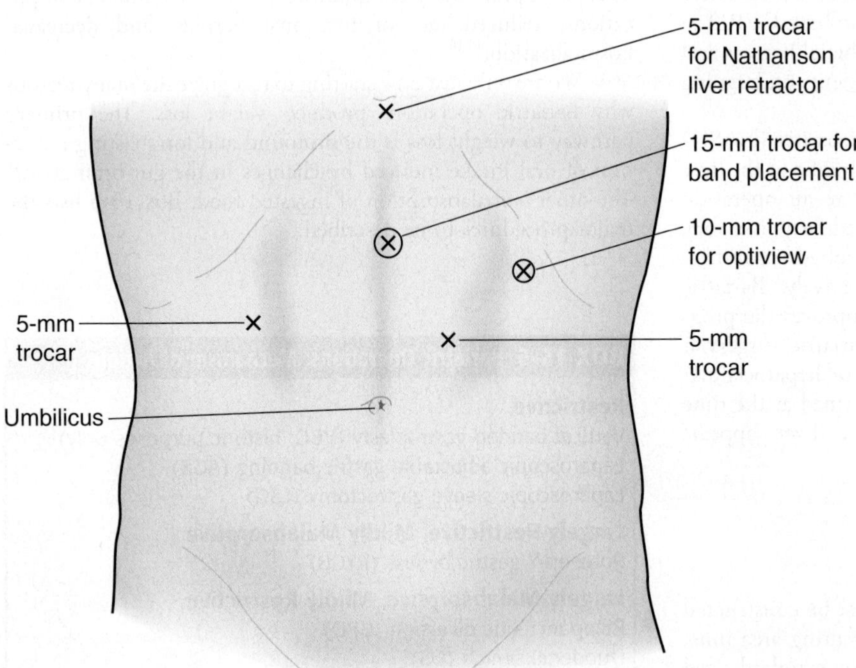


**FIGURE 15-1** Trocar location for adjustable gastric banding.

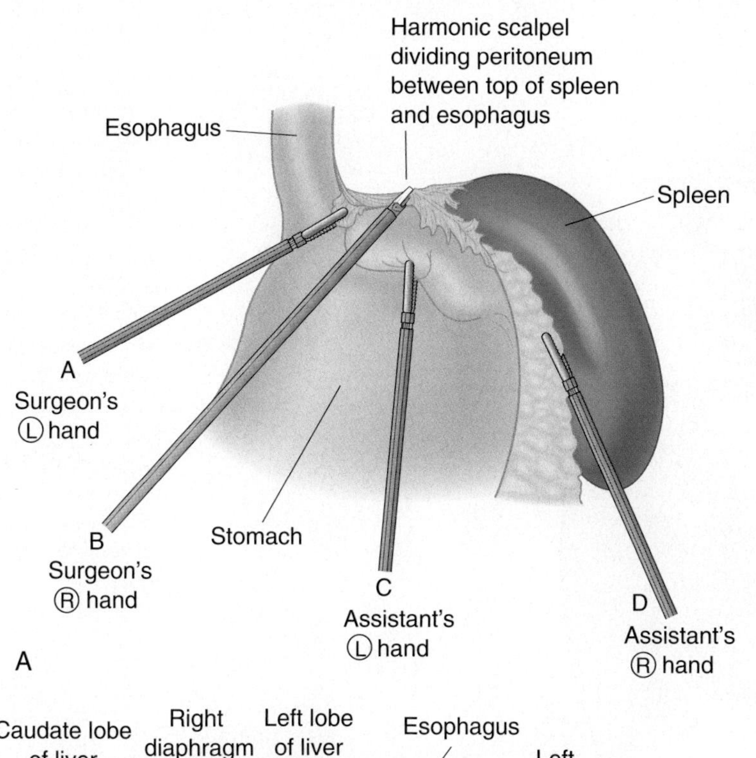


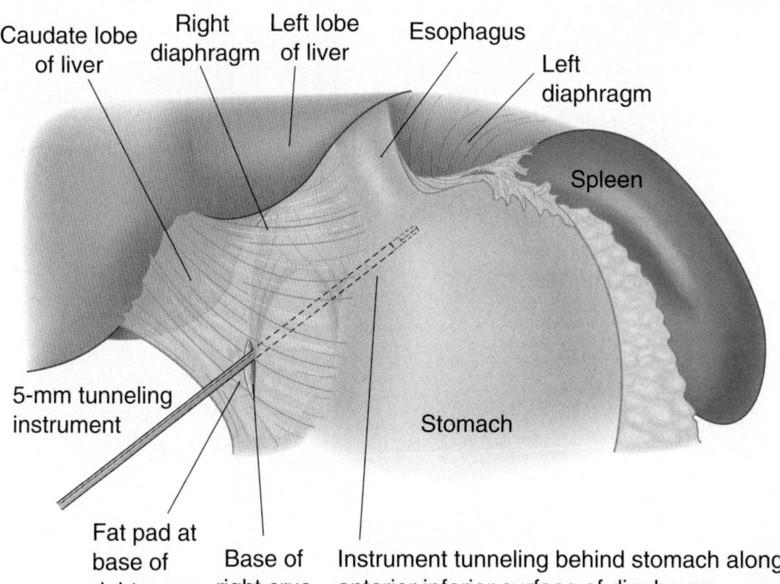


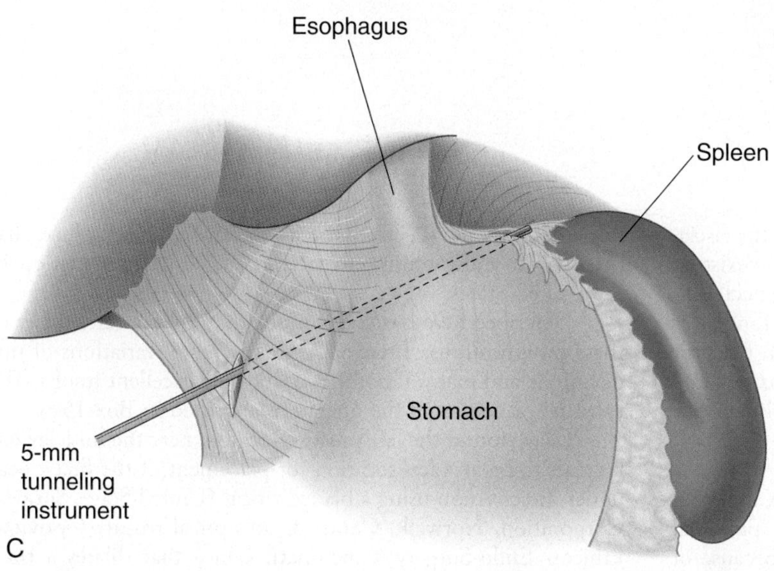


**FIGURE 15-2** **A,** Dividing the peritoneum at the angle of His. **B,** Pars flaccida technique in which the fat pad is divided at the base of the right crus. **C,** Tunnel posterior to the stomach completed.

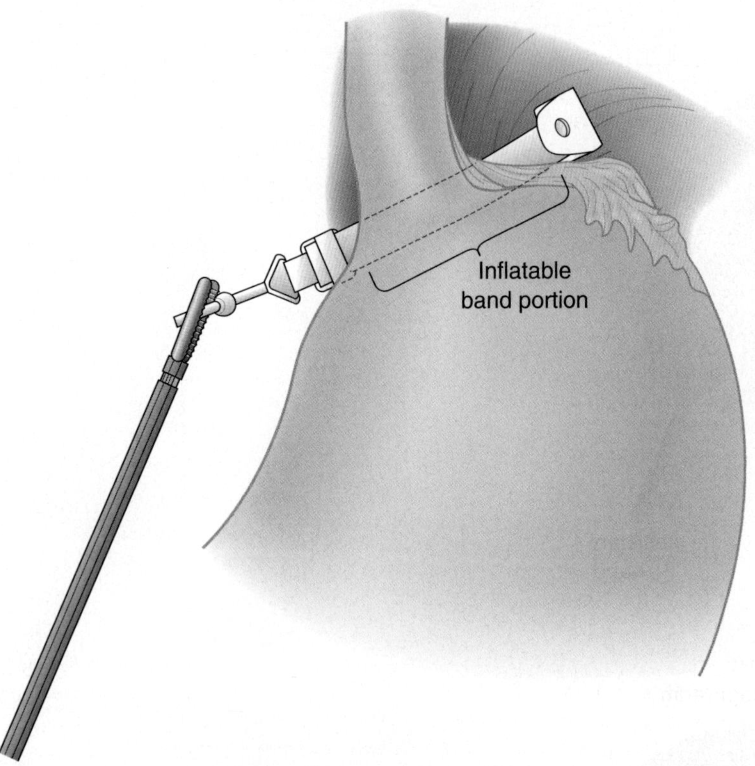


FIGURE 15-3 Pulling the LAP-BAND through the tunnel.

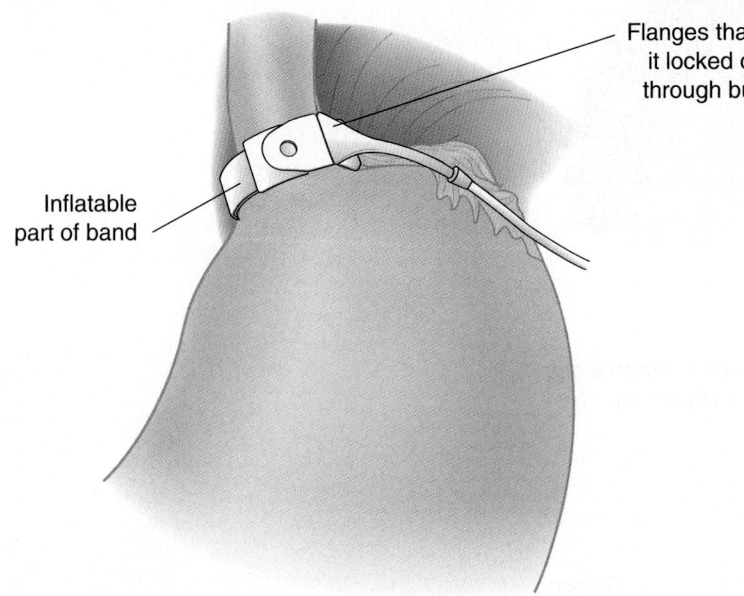


FIGURE 15-4 Locking the LAP-BAND.

trocar site incision is enlarged to reveal the anterior rectus fascia, which is exposed approximately 2 to 4 cm lateral to the existing fascial defect for the trocar, and the access port is connected to the inflation tubing. Four sutures inserted through the four holes on the access port are placed in the fascia, after which the port is tied to the fascia (Fig. 15-6). The redundant tubing is replaced in the abdominal cavity, with care taken to avoid kinking.

## Roux-en-Y Gastric Bypass

The gastric bypass, first described by Mason and Ito in 1969, incorporated a loop of jejunum anastomosed to a proximal gastric pouch. This operation proved unacceptable because of bile reflux, and RYGB, which eliminates bile reflux, has become the most commonly performed bariatric operation in the United States.

Described here is one technique that incorporates many of these modifications. There are certainly many variations of this technique and many, if not most, will yield excellent results. The essential principles of the operation are listed in Box 15-6.

I have found the left subcostal region, near the midclavicular line, to be an ideal location for placement of the first trocar under direct vision using a bladed trocar (United States Surgical Corporation, Norwalk, Conn) or an optical trocar (Optiview, Ethicon Endo-Surgery, Cincinnati, Ohio) that dilates a tract

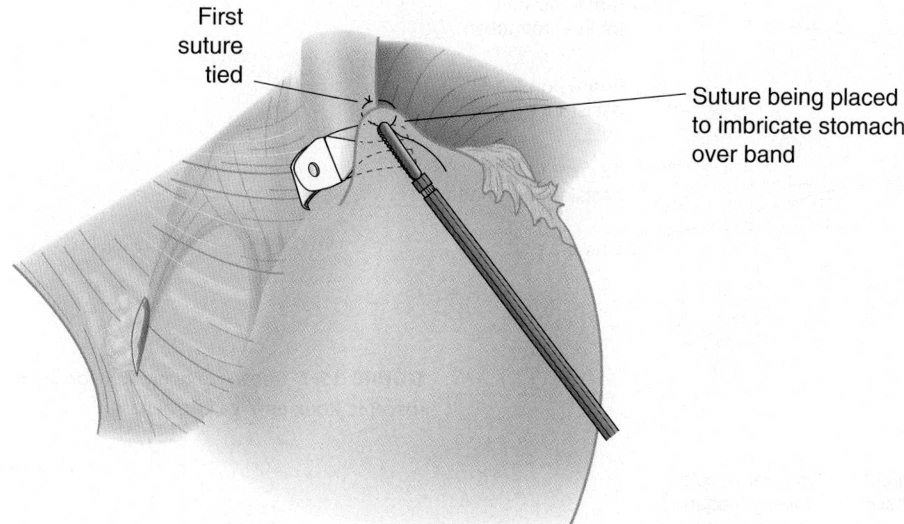


**FIGURE 15-5** Imbricating the anterior aspect of the stomach over the LAP-BAND.

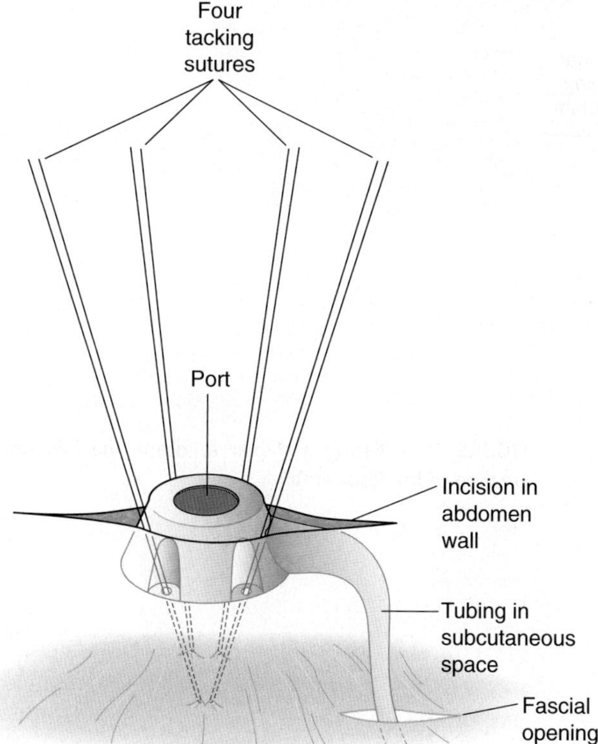


**FIGURE 15-6** Passing the inflation tubing through the abdominal wall sufficiently far from the port site to prevent acute kinking of the tubing.

under direct vision can be used. Subsequent trocars are placed under laparoscopic vision to achieve the configuration shown in Figure 15-7.

Once the omentum is mobilized, the ligament of Treitz is identified. A location approximately 30 to 40 cm distal to the ligament is chosen for division of the jejunum with an endoscopic stapler (Fig. 15-8). The mesentery is then further divided with staples or a harmonic scalpel.

**BOX 15-6 Essential Components of Roux-en-Y Gastric Bypass**

- Small proximal gastric pouch
- Gastric pouch constructed from the cardia of the stomach to prevent dilation and minimize acid production
- Gastric pouch divided from the distal part of the stomach
- Roux limb at least 75 cm in length
- Enteroenterostomy constructed to avoid stenosis or obstruction
- Closure of all potential spaces for internal hernias

The length of the Roux limb is influenced in my practice by patient weight. Patients with a BMI in the 40s will be well served with a Roux limb of 80 to 120 cm, whereas patients with a BMI significantly in excess of 50 are usually given a Roux limb of approximately 150 cm. The proximal jejunum is left to remain at the patient's right side and the Roux limb is lifted cephalad and coiled in the curve of the transverse colon mesentery (Fig. 15-9). This technique allows the proximal jejunum to be aligned directly alongside the designated point on the Roux limb for the distal anastomosis. The stapler is placed through the surgeon's right-hand port because the bowel segments are easily aligned to facilitate placement of the stapler into enterotomies created in each segment of bowel at the desired location of the anastomosis (Fig. 15-10). Another firing of the stapler, this time from the left side of the patient, creates a large side-to-side anastomosis. Once the anastomosis is created, the stapler defect is closed with the stapler. The mesenteric defect between the loops of small bowel is now closed with running permanent sutures (Fig. 15-11).

The Roux limb may be passed toward the proximal gastric pouch through a retrocolic or antecolic pathway. The retrocolic route may then take a retrogastric or antegastric pathway, whereas the antecolic route always takes an antegastric pathway. All routes seem to work well. I use the antecolic antegastric approach because there appears to be no difference in leak rates and the passage of the Roux limb through the transverse colon mesentery to a retrogastric position can be challenging (see Fig. 15-11). Care must be taken to ensure that the Roux limb is passed with the mesentery downward, and not twisted.

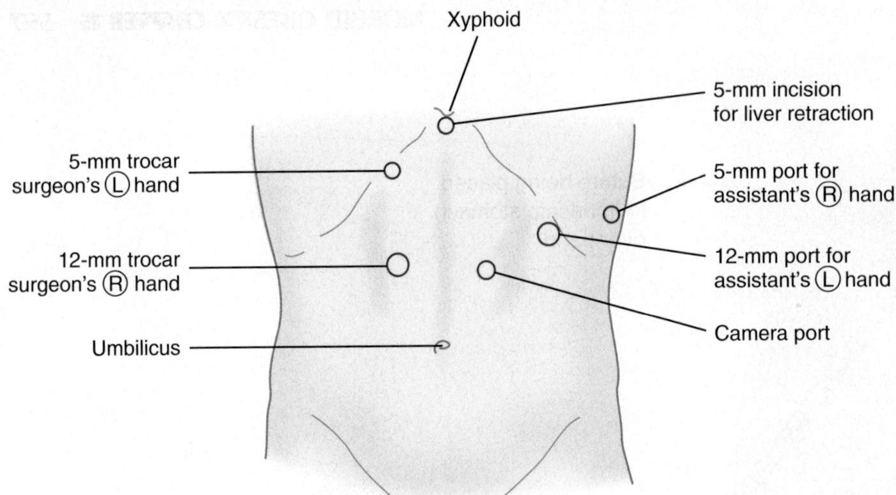


**FIGURE 15-7** Trocar configuration for laparoscopic Roux-en-Y gastric bypass.

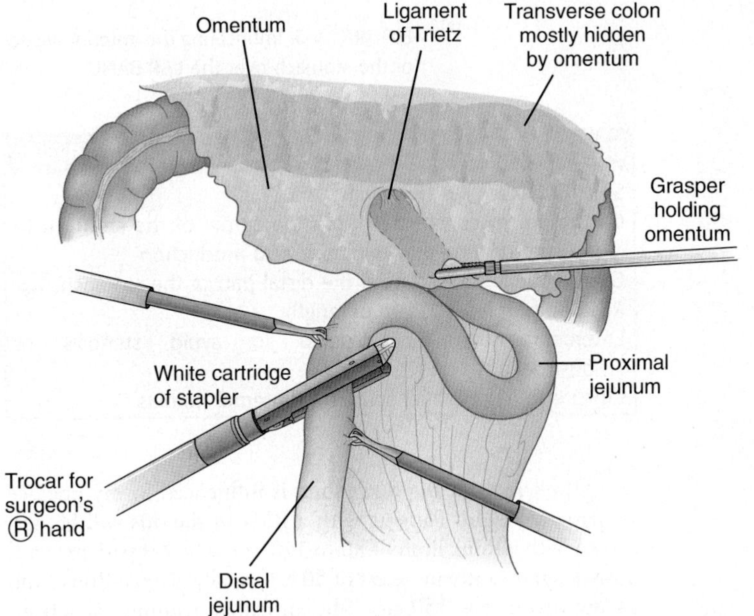


**FIGURE 15-8** Placing a stapler to divide the jejunum for creation of the Roux limb.

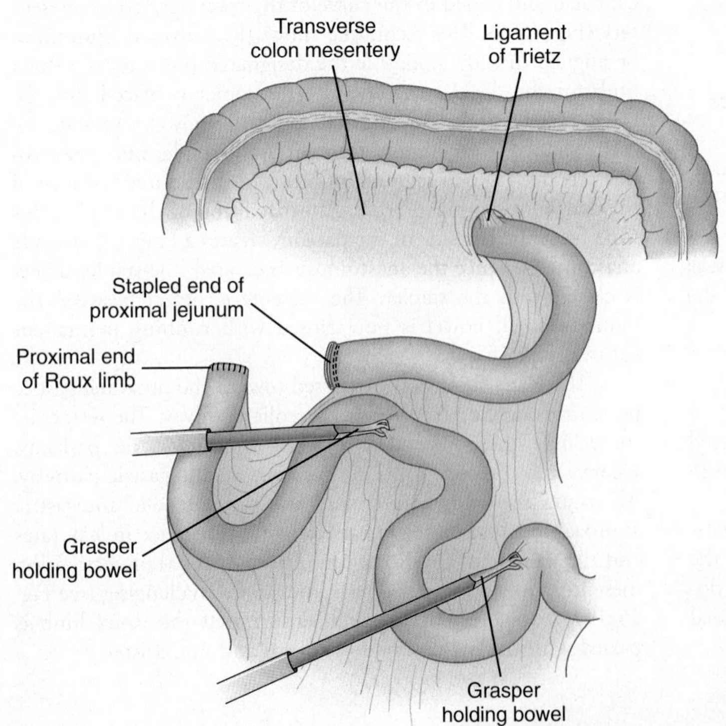


**FIGURE 15-9** Measuring and laying out the jejunum to set up a distal anastomosis for the length of the Roux-en-Y gastric bypass.

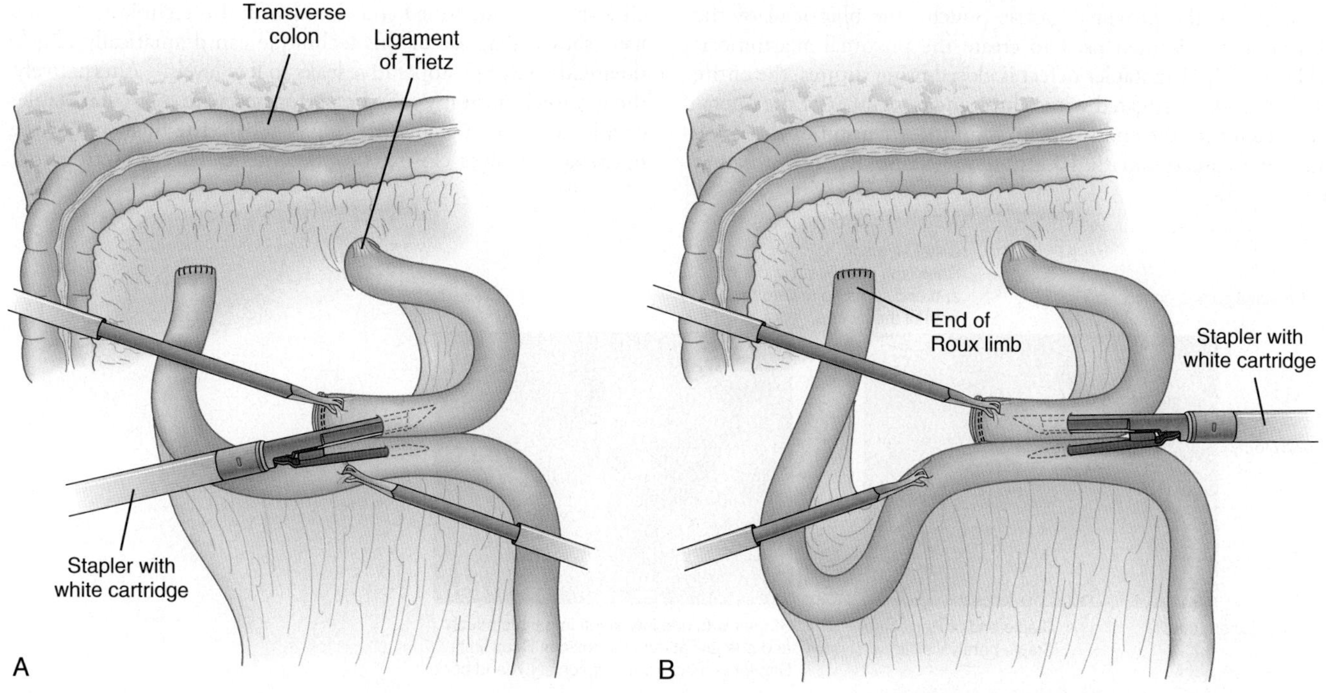


**FIGURE 15-10** Placing the stapler to create an enteroenterostomy.

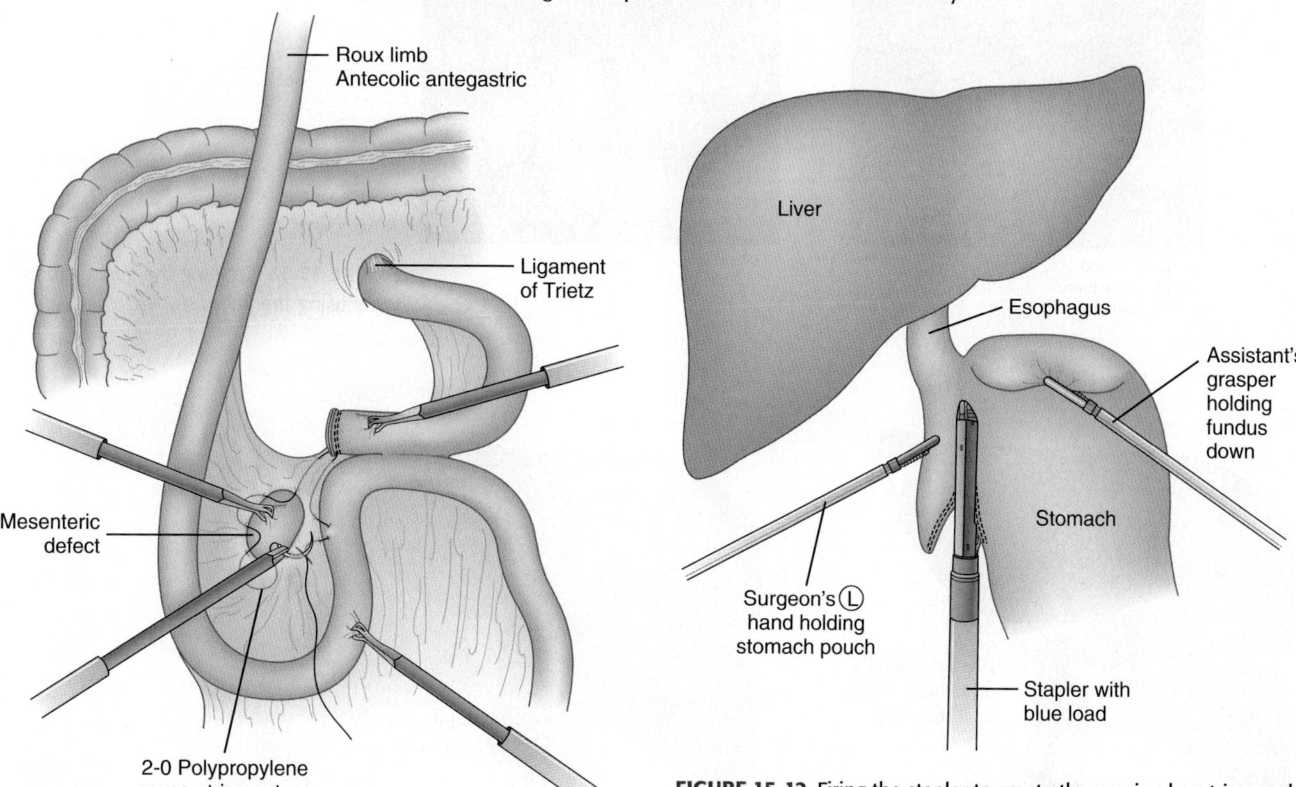


**FIGURE 15-11** Sewing the mesenteric defect and placing an antiobstruction stitch.

**FIGURE 15-12** Firing the stapler to create the proximal gastric pouch.

The left lobe liver retractor is now placed and the patient placed in the reverse Trendelenburg position. Exposure of the angle of His allows division of the peritoneum between the top of the spleen and gastroesophageal junction with the ultrasonic scalpel. The lesser sac is entered through the gastrohepatic ligament, 3 to 4 cm below the gastroesophageal junction. The blue load of the linear stapler is now fired multiple times to create a 10- to 15-mL proximal gastric pouch, based on the upper lesser curvature of the stomach Fig. 15-12. Once the gastric pouch is created, the Roux limb is placed in a position adjacent to the proximal gastric pouch. The blue load of the linear stapler is then used to create the proximal anastomosis (Fig. 15-13). The stapler defect is closed using sutures, the entire anastomosis is irrigated with saline, and a member of the operative team uses the endoscope to monitor occlusion of the Roux limb with an atraumatic 10-mm bowel clamp. Even the smallest air leak can be identified and closed with this technique. Studies have shown that use of this technique can dramatically reduce the incidence of postoperative leaks to low levels.[19] Alternatively, the gastrojejunostomy may be performed with a circular stapler or a hand-sutured technique (Fig. 15-14). The final step of the operation involves closing the mesenteric defects. Retrogastric

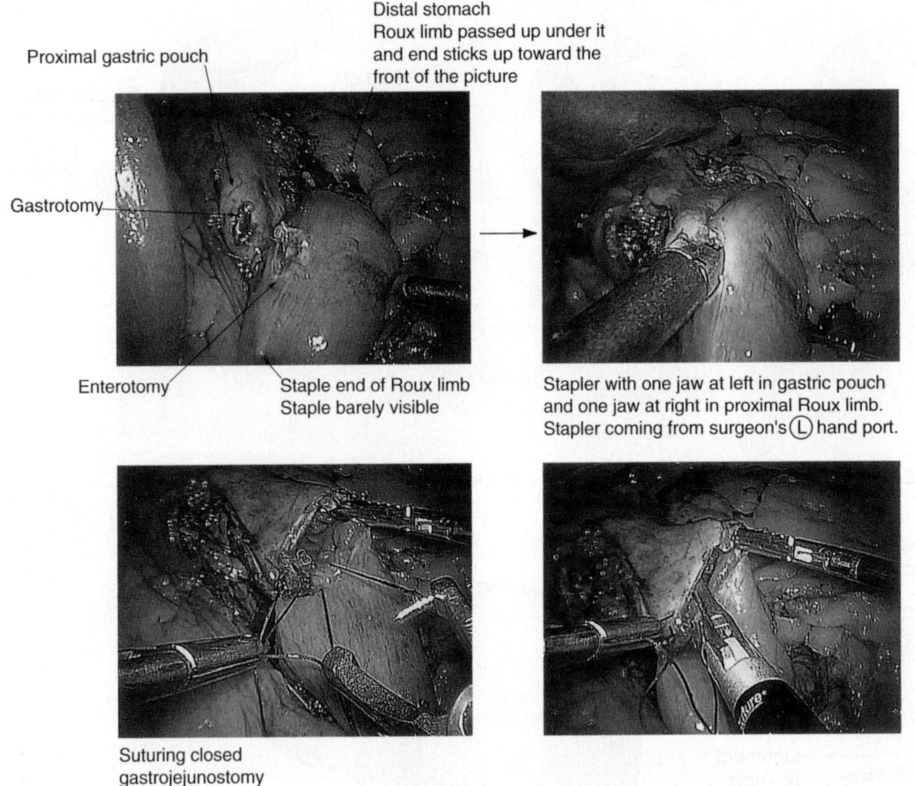


**FIGURE 15-13** Creating the gastrojejunostomy using the linear stapler.

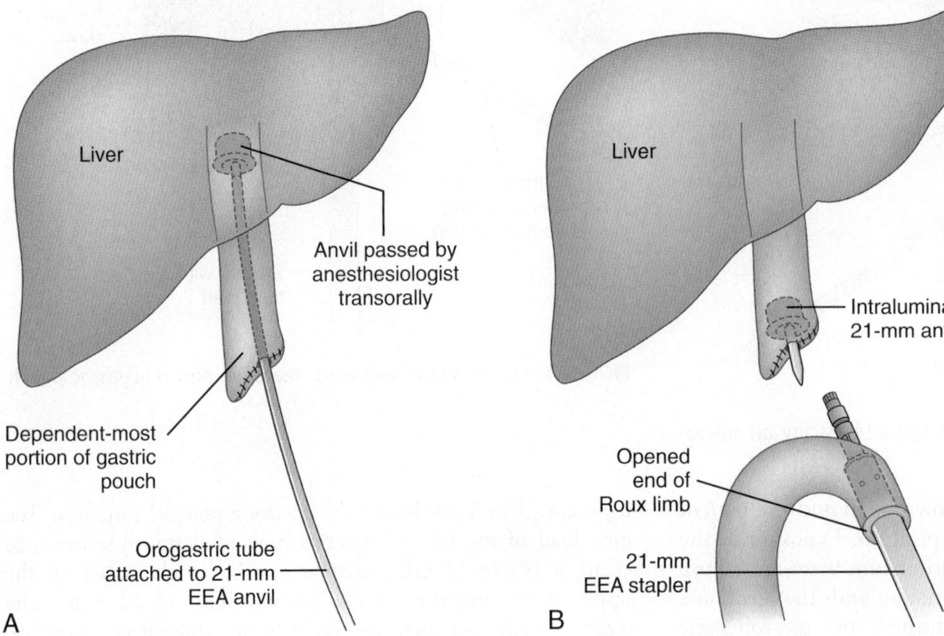


**FIGURE 15-14** Creating the gastrojejunostomy using a circular stapler.

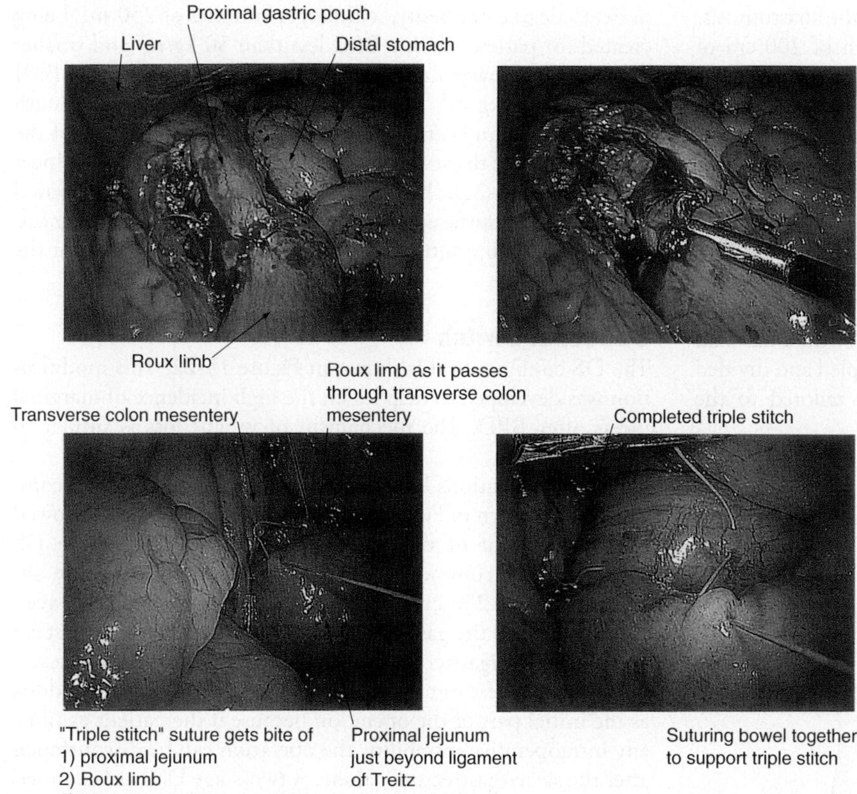


**FIGURE 15-15** Placing the triple stitch to close the mesenteric defects.

herniation of the Roux limb was a problem because sutures often pulled through the fatty mesentery of the transverse colon and allowed subsequent bowel herniation and obstruction. I have solved this problem by performing an antecolic roux limb or by attaching the Roux limb to the proximal jejunum near the ligament of Treitz with permanent sutures to fix a segment of the two pieces of bowel together (Fig. 15-15). This technique also closes Petersen's hernia defect.

## Biliopancreatic Diversion

Biliopancreatic diversion (BPD), like most bariatric operations that had been performed through an open approach, can now be performed through a laparoscopic approach. BPD produces weight loss based primarily on malabsorption, but it also has a restrictive component.

The anatomic configuration of BPD is shown in Figure 15-16. The intestinal tract is reconstructed to allow only a short so-called *common channel* of the distal 50 cm of terminal ileum for absorption of fat and protein. The alimentary tract beyond the proximal part of the stomach is rearranged to include only the distal 200 cm of ileum, including the common channel. The proximal end of this ileum is anastomosed to the proximal end of the stomach after performing a distal hemigastrectomy. The ileum proximal to the end that is anastomosed to the stomach is in turn anastomosed to the terminal ileum within the 50- to 100-cm distance from the ileocecal valve, depending on the surgeon's preference and the patient's size.

The laparoscopic procedure is performed with a trocar alignment (Fig. 15-17). The initial portion of the operation involves exposing the terminal ileum and cecum. Appendectomy is optional. The terminal ileum is measured to a length of 50 cm

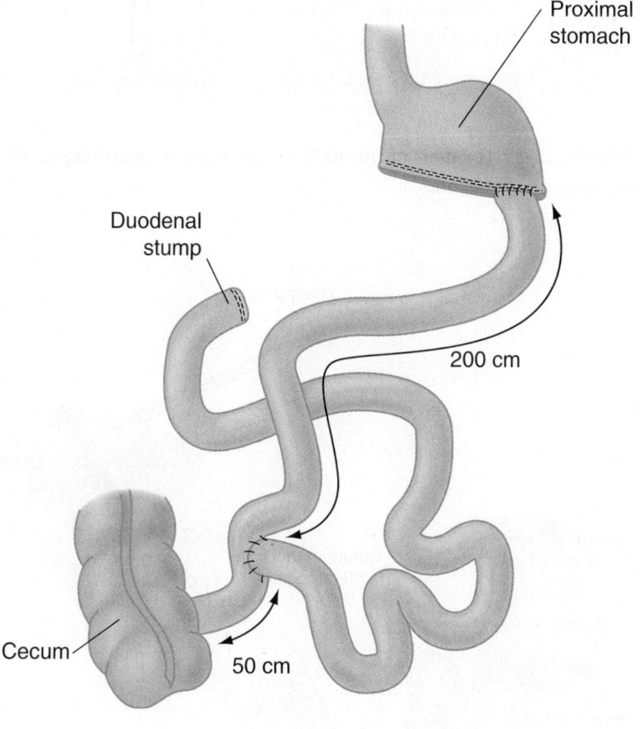


**FIGURE 15-16** Anatomic configuration of biliopancreatic diversion.

with a marking suture placed for the location of the anastomosis. After placing the marking suture, a total length of 200 cm of ileum is measured and, at this point, the ileum is divided with the vascular staple load (Fig. 15-18). The proximal end of the bowel is then anastomosed to the terminal ileum at the site of the marking suture with a standard linear stapling technique and the mesenteric defects are closed with sutures (Fig. 15-19). The alimentary tract limb can be extended beyond a 200-cm total length if there is concern that the patient may not eat a protein-rich diet.

Attention is now turned toward the stomach. A distal gastrectomy is performed with serial applications of the blue load of the stapler (Fig. 15-20). The duodenum is stapled and divided distal to the pylorus. Gastric volume may be tailored to the patient's degree of obesity, with larger volumes of 250 mL being created for patients with a BMI less than 50 kg/m$^2$ and smaller pouches to a lower limit of 150 mL for patients with a BMI more than 50 kg/m$^2$. The proximal end of the 200-cm length of terminal ileum is anastomosed to the posterior surface of the proximal end of the stomach with the blue cartridge of the linear stapler (Fig. 15-21). The stapler defect is closed and the bowel secured to the surface of the stomach beyond the anastomosis with an anchoring suture to prevent kinking of the bowel at the gastroileostomy.

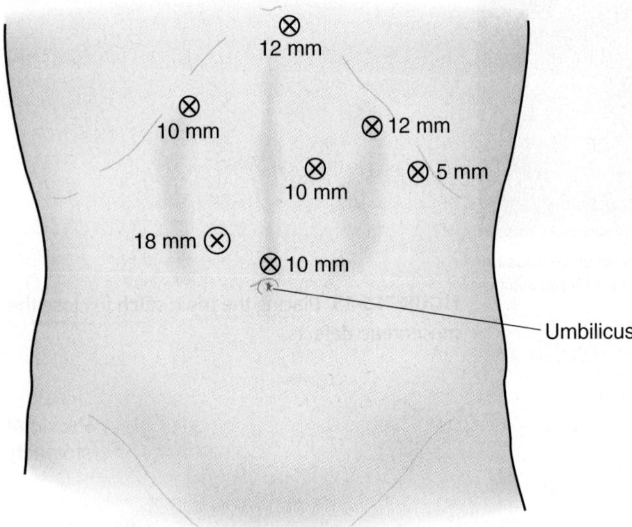


**FIGURE 15-17** Location of trocars for performing a laparoscopic biliopancreatic diversion.

## Duodenal Switch

The DS configuration is shown in Figure 15-22. This modification was developed to help lessen the high incidence of marginal ulcers after BPD. The mechanism of weight loss is similar to that of BPD.

Trocar locations for performing the operation laparoscopically are as shown in Figure 15-17. An appendectomy is followed by measurement of the terminal ileum. Notably, in the DS procedure, the common channel is 100 cm and the entire alimentary tract is 250 cm. However, the major difference between DS and BPD is the gastrectomy and proximal anatomy. Instead of a distal hemigastrectomy, a sleeve gastrectomy of the greater curvature of the stomach is performed. This procedure is done as the initial part of the operation because if the patient exhibits any intraoperative instability, the operation can be discontinued after the sleeve gastrectomy alone. A two-stage DS has been used in patients who have an extremely high BMI and are high operative risks.[20] The sleeve gastrectomy alone usually produces enough weight loss to make the second stage of the operation technically easier. This approach lowers the mortality rate, despite the need to undergo two operative procedures. Others have found weight loss after the initial sleeve gastrectomy to be sufficient to preclude subsequent conversion to a DS.[21,22]

The first step of a laparoscopic DS is to perform the sleeve gastrectomy with a stapling technique that begins at the mid-antrum; a staple line is created parallel to the lesser curvature of

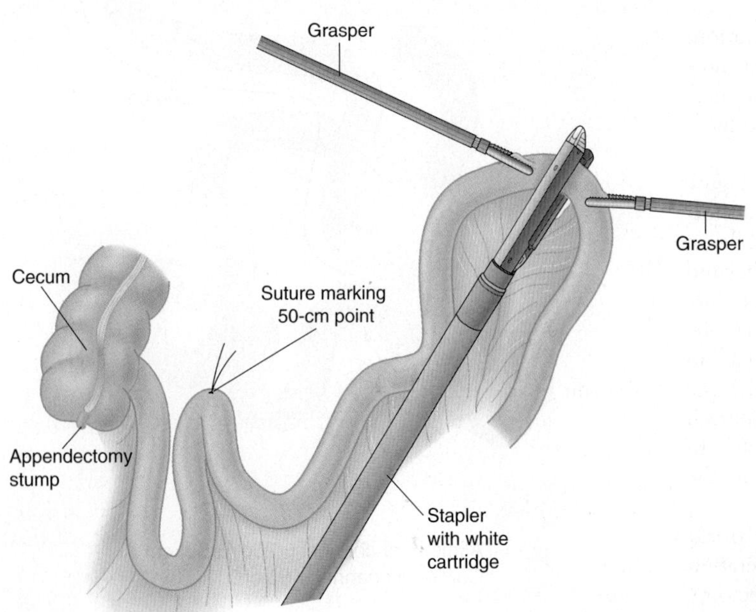


**FIGURE 15-18** Dividing the ileum at the 200-cm location proximal to the ileocecal valve after having already marked the 50-cm location.

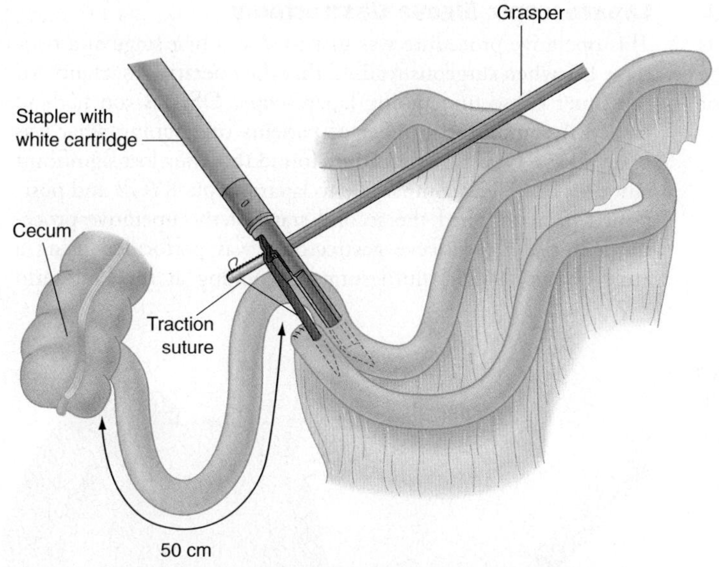


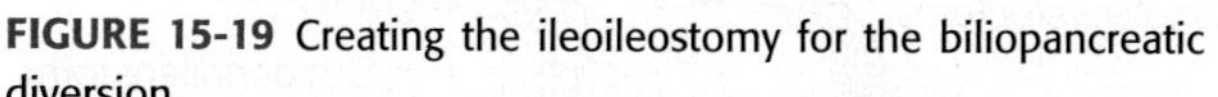

**FIGURE 15-19** Creating the ileoileostomy for the biliopancreatic diversion.

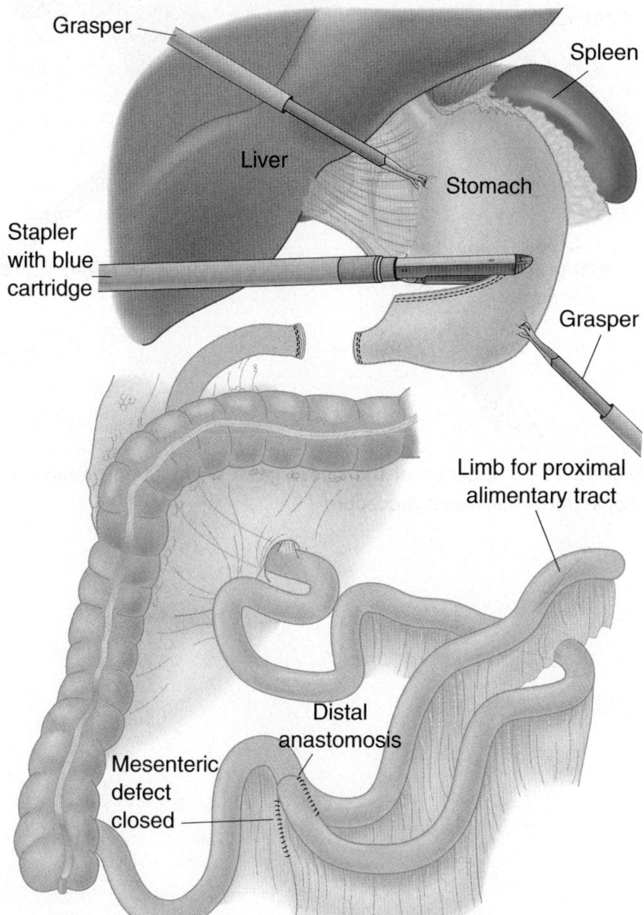


**FIGURE 15-20** Performing the distal gastrectomy.

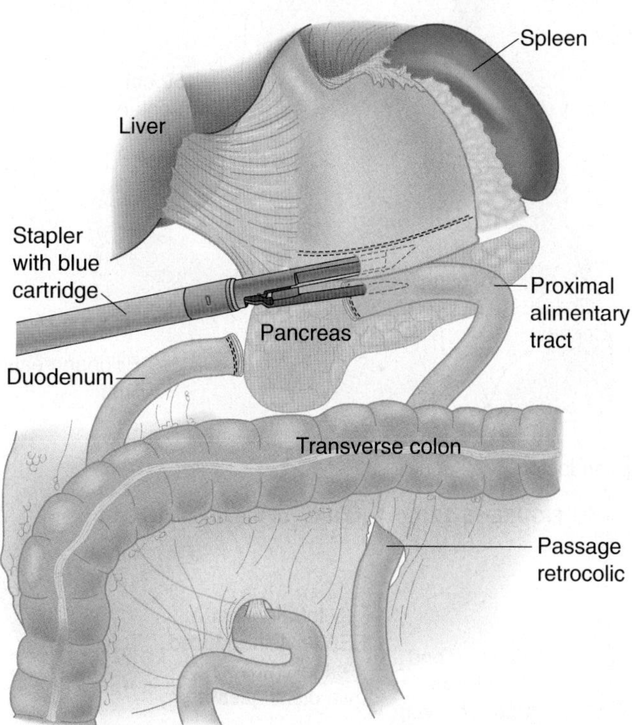


**FIGURE 15-21** Creation of the gastrojejunostomy between the ileum and proximal part of the stomach.

the stomach, with a 40 to 60 Fr Maloney dilator placed along the lesser curve to prevent narrowing. The staple line is created with multiple firings of the stapler until the angle of His is reached (Fig. 15-23). The goal is to produce a lesser curvature gastric sleeve with a volume of 150 to 200 mL.

After sleeve gastrectomy, or preceding it in smaller patients, the duodenum is divided with the stapler approximately 2 cm beyond the pylorus. The distal connections are performed as for BPD. The distal anastomosis is created at the 100-cm point proximal to the ileocecal valve. The proximal anastomosis is created between the proximal end of the 250 cm of terminal ileum and the first portion of the duodenum. The duodenoileostomy is an antecolic end-to-side anastomosis. This anastomosis is the one of the most critical parts of the operation and can be performed with a circular stapler (Fig. 15-24) or using a hand-sewn technique. If the end-to-end anastomosis (EEA) stapler is used, the anvil is directly inserted through the staple line of the duodenal stump via a gastrotomy under suture guidance or through an oral approach with a nasogastric tube.

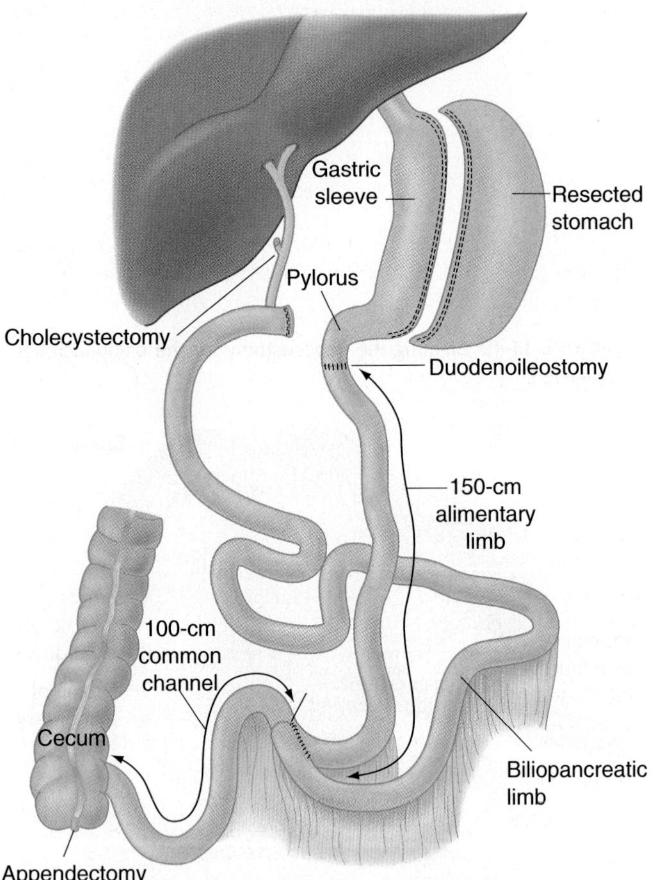


**FIGURE 15-22** Configuration of the duodenal switch.

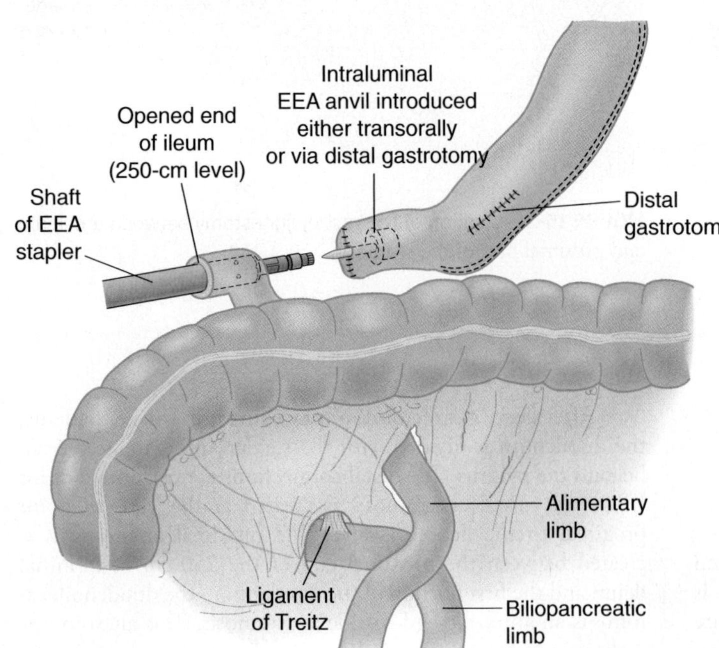


**FIGURE 15-24** Creation of the duodenoenterostomy. *EEA*, End-to-end anastomosis.

## Laparoscopic Sleeve Gastrectomy

This operative procedure was first used as a first stage of a two-stage DS when surgeons realized that the operative mortality for the super obese undergoing laparoscopic DS was too high to justify. A significant number of patients undergoing what was planned as a two-stage procedure found that they lost significant amounts of weight comparable to laparoscopic RYGB and post-poned or abandoned the second stage of the operative procedure. Initially, the sleeve gastrectomy was performed using a large bougie (60 Fr) until surgeons looking at the long-term

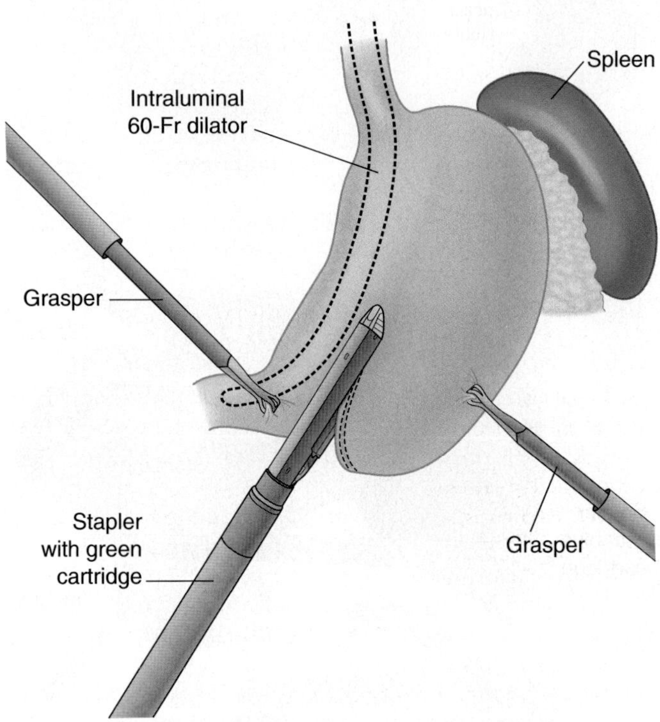


**FIGURE 15-23** Creation of the sleeve gastrectomy during a laparoscopic duodenal switch procedure.

results found that a smaller sized gastric pouch and extension into the antrum of the stomach were found to enhance the results of the procedure enough to consider its use as a primary stand-alone procedure.

As a primary procedure, the surgeon takes down the entire greater curvature, leaving intact the tissue within 4 to 6 cm of the pylorus, up to the angle of His, and exposing the left crus of the diaphragm. Then, using a 32 to 40 Fr bougie, the stomach is divided from the antrum to the angle of His using sequential firings of the stapler. It is vitally important to preserve the left gastric vessels and lesser curve blood supply and to prevent twisting or spiraling of the gastric tube. Some surgeons routinely suture the staple line to reinforce its integrity or use some form of staple line reinforcement to prevent it from bleeding or leaking.

This procedure has proven value as the first stage of a two-stage procedure to reduce mortality in the superobese. As more surgeons developed this procedure as an effective two-stage procedure, it became clear that this was also an effective primary procedure. Several longer term studies have shown long-term weight loss to be equal to laparoscopic RYGB. In one randomized study, laparoscopic sleeve gastrectomy was found to result in superior weight loss and better appetite control 3 years post-surgery compared with laparoscopic AGB.[23] Another randomized trial has shown the laparoscopic sleeve gastrectomy to be more effective in weight loss and induction of satiety than laparoscopic RYGB.[24] Increasingly, I and other surgeons have promoted the laparoscopic sleeve gastrectomy as a primary procedure. Recognizing its usefulness, a current procedural terminology (CPT) code was given to the procedure in 2010 by the AMA (American Medical Association).

Advantages of the laparoscopic sleeve gastrectomy include its technical simplicity, preservation of the pylorus (avoidance of dumping), metabolic reduction of ghrelin levels,[24] lack of need for serial adjustments (like the laparoscopic AGB), reduction in internal hernias (seen after laparoscopic RYGB), reduction in malabsorption (seen with laparoscopic RYGB), and ability to modify the gastric sleeve later to a laparoscopic RYGB or laparoscopic DS configuration in a second stage of the operation. Advantages and specific clinical scenarios for the use of the laparoscopic sleeve gastrectomy are listed in Table 15-1.

Disadvantages of the procedure seem to focus on the Achilles heel of the operation, which is leakage along the long gastric staple line. Although leakage after gastric bypass is one of the most feared complications, those following laparoscopic sleeve gastrectomy appear to be slightly more common than in laparoscopic RYGB and more difficult to treat.[25] Leaks tend to be accompanied by long-term fistula formation. Other concerns are the long-term outcomes of the procedure, which are not as well characterized as for other bariatric procedures.

## POSTOPERATIVE CARE AND FOLLOW-UP

Excellent surgical outcomes require the appropriate selection of patients, thorough preoperative preparation, technically well-performed operations, and attentive postoperative care. A bariatric patient requires particularly attentive and special postoperative care in several areas above and beyond those for the average surgical patient.

The most dreaded complication after bariatric surgery is a leak from the gastrointestinal tract. Tachycardia, at times accompanied by tachypnea or agitation, is often the only manifestation of this severe intra-abdominal problem. A severely obese patient might not be subject to the development of fever or signs of peritonitis, as would a patient with a normal body habitus. A high index of suspicion for a leak must be present for the patient who has sustained postoperative tachycardia, fever, or increased pain. The surgeon must use further diagnostic studies, including gastrografin esophageal swallow studies and oral contrast CT scans, and even be prepared to reexplore the patient before overwhelming sepsis from the leak of gastric contents induces multisystem organ failure.

Appropriate fluid resuscitation is essential. A 200-kg patient who undergoes open gastric bypass can easily require 6 to 10 liters of fluid for replacement of maintenance, third-space, and operative fluid or blood losses. My postoperative protocol after open surgery calls for 400 mL/hr of a balanced salt solution (usually lactated Ringer's), with boluses given as needed for low urine output. A Foley catheter is used intraoperatively and urine output is monitored carefully. Patients undergoing laparoscopic surgery usually have much less third-space and operative blood loss than patients undergoing open surgery and can be managed with 125 mL/hr of IV fluids. Urine output intraoperatively is

**Table 15-1 Potential Role of Laparoscopic Sleeve Gastrectomy (LSG) in Bariatric Surgery**

| CONDITION | PROCEDURES CONTRAINDICATED | POTENTIAL ADVANTAGES OF LSG |
|---|---|---|
| Iron deficiency anemia | RYGB, BPD | Preservation of duodenum |
| Crohn's small bowel disease | RYGB, DS, BPD, laparoscopic AGB if on steroids | Preservation of small bowel |
| Transplant patients on immunosuppressive meds | Laparoscopic AGB if on steroids; relative contraindications for RYGB, DS, BPD | More stable absorption of antirejection medications |
| Cardiac failure patients | Malabsorption of medications by RYGB, DS, BPD a relative contraindication | More stable absorption of critically needed medications |
| Severe arthritis requiring NSAID use | RYGB and BPD contraindicated because of ulcer risk | Preservation of stomach allows continued use of NSAIDs |
| Patients who may not be able to comply with frequent follow-up | Laparoscopic AGB, RYGB, DS, BPD | Less risk of malabsorption and reduced need for laparoscopic AGB adjustments |
| Patients with preexisting vitamin deficiencies, vitamin D, iron ect | RYGB, DS, BPD | Preservation of entire small bowel reduces risk of vitamin deficiencies |
| Autoimmune connective tissue disorder | Laparoscopic AGB contraindicated | Laparoscopic SG may be good option |

*NSAID,* Nonsteroidal anti-inflammatory drug.

normally low because of the pneumoperitoneum and usually improves in the recovery room setting. Some patients who have been taking diuretics for many years will not have adequate urine output without diuretic use, but the surgeon must ensure that the patient is adequately volume-resuscitated before giving diuretics. Higher than expected fluid requirements, oliguria, and tachycardia are a constellation of postoperative findings suggesting intra-abdominal problems.

Adequate pain control is essential. Narcotic requirements are decreased with a laparoscopic approach. A patient-controlled analgesia (PCA) pump is appropriate and helpful. The value of an epidural catheter for pain relief is controversial. It has been my experience that these catheters are often difficult to place and easy to dislodge in the severely obese population. In addition, the use of LMWH for DVT prophylaxis may preclude safe placement.

DVT prophylaxis is important. Pulmonary embolism is one of the leading causes of death after open bariatric surgery. No data have substantiated one regimen of prophylaxis to be better than another. I use a combination of early ambulation (the same day as surgery, generally within 4 to 6 hours) and the use of SCDs for most patients who have a BMI less than 60, are ambulatory, and have undergone an uncomplicated laparoscopic operation.[17] For patients with higher BMIs, who are restricted in their ambulation, or have a history of venous stasis or DVT, SC administration of LMWH (e.g., enoxaparin) is used.

My standard practice procedure is to obtain a radiographic study of the gastrointestinal tract on the first postoperative day only if there are clinical signs of a leak, which include a temperature higher than 100° C or a heart rate higher than 100 beats/min. If neither is present, I start a water trial and progress the diet to liquids. Using this approach has led to excellent clinical results, but the surgeon must investigate persistent tachycardia or fever, which can be the only signs of a clinically significant leak. Failure to diagnose and promptly treat a leak after bariatric surgery often leads to catastrophic outcomes, and early intervention uniformly results in survival.

Discharge, regardless of the bariatric operation, occurs when the patient is mobile, is tolerating an oral liquid diet, has adequate pain control with oral analgesics, and exhibits no signs of problems (e.g., fever or wound cellulitis). The timing of discharge, once these criteria are met, is often influenced by cultural issues, patient expectation, or distance between the home and hospital. Thus, the duration of hospitalization is not always an accurate reflection of optimal outcomes when comparing published studies in the literature.

Although the schedule of postoperative visits varies, all patients must undergo long-term follow-up. This guarantees that the surgeon will obtain feedback on the operative results and helps ensure that any preventable long-term metabolic or other procedure-related complications will be avoided. The potential for such metabolic complications is inherently present for all the malabsorptive procedures. The restrictive procedures have minimal health risks from metabolic complications but, instead, have their own potential problems, such as band slippage or erosion in patients undergoing AGB. Moreover, improved weight loss occurs in patients who see their surgeon for adjustments to the band.[26]

A typical regimen for monitoring a patient after AGB would be to have the initial visit take place within the first month postoperatively to evaluate oral intake, food tolerance, and wound healing and to determine whether appropriate restriction has resulted from placement of the noninflated band. Subsequent visits, usually scheduled monthly to bimonthly in the beginning and then less frequently, involve counseling with a nutritionist and evaluation of weight loss and the need for band adjustment. A goal of 1 to 2 lb/week of weight loss is adjusted for initial body weight. Less weight loss is an indication for the instillation of additional saline into the band system via the port. This is initially done under fluoroscopic control until the surgeon has sufficient experience and confidence to perform these adjustments in the office or clinic without fluoroscopic guidance. Blood tests are performed periodically throughout the patient's follow-up, depending on metabolic indications, patient's underlying medical illnesses, and other indications.

After RYGB, a typical postoperative checkup regimen would include a visit within the first 2 to 3 weeks postoperatively to assess wound healing, advance from a liquid diet to solid food, and check overall recovery. Subsequent visits are scheduled at 6 weeks, 3 months, 6 months, and 1 year after surgery and then annually. Visits during the first year are for monitoring weight loss; those after the first year are for checking maintenance of weight loss and nutritional competence. The risk for iron, folate, vitamin A, vitamin D, and vitamin $B_{12}$ deficiency is lifelong.

Patients undergoing malabsorptive operations must understand the necessity of meticulous compliance with a strict follow-up plan. After BPD or DS, a patient is seen within the first 2 weeks to be certain that diarrhea is not too prolific and dehydration has not resulted. The patient must be taught the signs of dehydration and plans for its treatment. Replacement of fat-soluble vitamins is mandatory, and patient compliance must be documented. Initial visits after the first month take place monthly for the first several months until the risks of dehydration, poor protein intake, and significant metabolic consequences of rapid weight loss have lessened. The potential for protein-calorie malnutrition exists after these procedures and it will usually be manifested during this time. Thereafter, as weight loss slows, periodic visits separated by 3-month intervals are indicated for the first year and semiannually thereafter. Weight loss will taper after the first 12 to 18 months. Lifelong follow-up to assess fat-soluble vitamin deficiencies and protein levels, liver function, and metabolic stability is indicated after BPD or DS.

Most bariatric practices use patient support groups as a component of their postoperative support system. These groups are variously organized and managed but usually consist of patients who have undergone weight reduction surgery or are contemplating it. They meet to discuss personal experiences with respect to their surgery, recovery, experience of losing weight, and maintenance of lost weight. Although no data exist regarding their medical benefit, groups that are vigorous and successful seem to provide an excellent forum for patients to exchange information; they provide psychological and emotional support and encouragement to patients before and after surgery.

## OUTCOMES

There is no consensus on the definition of success for any of these operations in terms of percentage of weight loss or extent of reversal of comorbid conditions, but there is much evidence demonstrating that bariatric procedures are effective in achieving long-term weight loss and improvement in comorbid diseases. Several studies have shown improved survival or improvement in cardiovascular risk in patients undergoing bariatric surgery as compared with a matched set of individuals who did not undergo this surgery.[27,28] Resolution and improvement of comorbid conditions after all types of bariatric surgery have been confirmed in two meta-analyses (Table 15-2).[29,30]

The most striking evidence of efficacy has come from trials comparing morbidly obese diabetics who underwent bariatric surgery with those who did not and were treated medically. A Swedish study[12] has shown an 80% decrease in the annual mortality of diabetic individuals in the surgical weight loss group versus a group of control patients not undergoing surgery (9% mortality at 9 years versus 28% mortality in the control group). The decrease in mortality is not limited to diabetics undergoing bariatric surgery. In a study comparing matched control subjects with those who underwent bariatric surgery in Canada, Christou and colleagues[28] have demonstrated that weight loss surgery reduces the relative risk of mortality by 89% (95% confidence interval [CI], 73% to 96%) 5 years later. Adams and associates[13] have matched patients undergoing gastric bypass (GBP) to obese subjects applying for a Utah driver's license and found substantial reduction in long-term mortality for the patients who underwent GBP. I believe it to be self-evident that the continued reports of improvement in cardiovascular risk factors seen after bariatric surgery, such as diabetes, hypertension, and dyslipidemia, will lead to a reduction in cardiovascular mortality.

Results can be determined only after adequate long-term follow-up and with procedures done in adequate numbers by a variety of surgeons. The applicability of some operations may vary depending on patient factors, such as size or previous abdominal surgery; however, there is considerable variation in the use of bariatric surgery that does not appear to be related to the prevalence of morbid obesity in that region.[31]

**Table 15-2 Results of Two Major Bariatric Procedures**

| | Study (Year) | |
|---|---|---|
| PARAMETER | BUCHWALD ET AL (2004)[30] | MAGGARD ET AL (2005)[29] |
| AGB weight loss, range (kg) | 39.7 (42.2-37.2) | 34.8 (29.5-40.1) |
| AGB EWL, range (%) | 61.2 (64.4-58.1) | |
| AGB mortality | 0.1% (2297 patients) | 0.02% (9222 patients) |
| RYGB weight loss, range (kg) | 43.5 (48.1-38.8) | 41.5 (37.4-45.6) |
| RYGB EWL, range (%) | 61.6 (66.5-56.7) | |
| RYGB mortality | 0.5% (5644 patients) | 0.3% (11,290 patients) |
| BPD-DS weight loss, range (kg) | 46.4 (51.6-41.2) | 53.1 (47.4-58.8) |
| BPD-DS EWL, range (%) | 70.1 (73.9-66.3) | |
| BPD/DS mortality | 1.1% (3030 patients) | 0.9% (2808 patients) |

## Adjustable Gastric Banding

Patients undergoing AGB experience an operation that may last as little as 1 hour in experienced hands. Discharge from the hospital after an overnight stay is the norm, with a few reports of same-day discharge but more frequent reports of longer time to discharge based on cultural norms and acceptance. Table 15-3 gives the results of laparoscopic AGB in several large reported series in the literature with long-term follow-up.

The band is initially placed without adding any saline to distend it. Saline is added in 1.0- to 1.5-mL increments to produce a desired weight loss of 1 to 2 kg/wk. Excess weight loss may lead to actual removal of a small amount of saline, whereas inadequate weight loss is an indication for the addition of more saline to the system to increase restriction of the band. The incidence of metabolic problems is low after AGB because there is no disruption of the normal gastrointestinal tract. One potential problem is esophageal dilation from chronic obstruction secondary to band slippage.

Weight loss after AGB has averaged 39.7 kg (61.2% excess weight loss [EWL]) and 34.8 kg in two meta-analyses of bariatric surgery (see Table 15-2).[29,30] The pattern of weight loss is such that weight loss continues after the first year, up to a maximal amount that is usually achieved by the third year. Series with a 5-year follow-up have confirmed that the weight loss may even

**Table 15-3 Results of Laparoscopic Adjustable Gastric Banding Procedures**

| | Study (Year) | | | |
|---|---|---|---|---|
| PARAMETER | O'BRIEN ET AL* | BUCHWALD ET AL (2004)[30] | MAGGARD ET AL (2005)[29] | PONCE ET AL (2005)[32] |
| No. of patients | 709 | 1848 | 5562 (1 yr) | 1014 |
| Age (yr) | 41 | NR | NR | NR |
| Body mass index (kg/m$^2$) | 45 | NR | NR | NR |
| Operating room time (min) | 56 | NR | NR | NR |
| Conversion (%) | 1.0 | NR | NR | NR |
| Follow-up (yr) | 0.25-6 | NR | 1/>3 | 1/4 |
| EWL/yr (%) | 54/5 | 47.5/NR | NR | 41/1, 64/4 |
| Weight loss, kg (yr) | NR | 28.6/NR | 30 (1)/35 (>3) | NR |

*From O'Brien PE, Dixon JB, Brown W, et al: The laparoscopic adjustable gastric band (Lap Band): a prospective study of medium-term effects on weight, health and quality of life. Obes Surg 12:652–660, 2002.

*NR*, Not reported.

improve slightly more after 3 years. In series with longer than a 5-year follow-up, baseline BMI decreased from an average of 42 to 46 kg/m$^2$ to 30 to 36 kg/m$^2$ at 5 years.[32]

The LAP-BAND has been shown to resolve type 2 diabetes in 47.9% and improve the condition in 80.8% of patients in the meta-analyses published.[30] The laparoscopic AGB was compared with medical treatment in a prospective randomized trial in Australia. This study demonstrated substantial weight loss in the surgical group associated with remission of the type 2 diabetes in 73%; the medically treated patients had insignificant weight loss and only 13% achieved remission of their diabetes.[33] Hypertension was resolved in 42% and improved in 70.8% of patients after this procedure. Improvement in dyslipidemia was also noted in 58.9% of patients. Other comorbid conditions such as obstructive sleep apnea, GERD, and venous stasis improved or resolved after weight loss with AGB.[32] Another randomized trial compared weight loss after laparoscopic AGB with medically treated patients and found that the laparoscopic AGB group had significantly better weight loss than the medical group. Even in adolescents, the laparoscopic AGB group had much greater weight loss compared with patients randomized to medical treatment.[10] The results of these three trials support the use of the laparoscopic AGB over medical therapy for weight loss, remission of diabetes, improvement in quality of life, and resolution of obesity-related comorbidites.[11,34]

Quality of life has been shown to improve for the domains of physical activity, self-esteem, and general health in adolescents 2 years after laparoscopic AGB compared with no improvement in the group randomized to medical therapy.[10] In another randomized trial of adults undergoing laparoscopic AGB, quality of life improved in eight of eight subscores of the Short Form-36, whereas the medically treated patients had only three of eight subscores improve.[11]

### Roux-en-Y Gastric Bypass

RYGB has an established track record, longer than that of any other operation. Its performance has been modified over the years, and the results presented in Table 15-4 reflect data in series from the era of its performance as both an open and laparoscopic procedure. Recovery after RYGB is improved after a laparoscopic approach, as has been demonstrated for several other abdominal operations. This improvement is largely related to the decrease in postoperative pain experienced by patients after laparoscopic RYGB versus open RYGB. One prospective randomized study has compared open and laparoscopic RYGB. In that study, patients were monitored for 1 year, at which time weight loss with both approaches was comparable (68% loss of excess weight for laparoscopic RYGB versus 62% loss of excess weight for open RYGB). Nguyen and associates[35] have reported a shorter length of hospitalization and more rapid return to activities of daily living with laparoscopic RYGB. Although the early improvement in quality of life reported after laparoscopic RYGB (3 months postoperatively) was better than with open RYGB, the data were comparable for the two groups at 6 months after surgery, thus suggesting that the major recovery benefit with a laparoscopic approach is limited to the first 3 months postoperatively.

Another important advantage of the laparoscopic approach for RYGB is a decrease in the incidence of wound complications and incisional hernia seen after the procedure. A long-term follow-up of a prospective randomized trial comparing laparoscopic and open gastric bypass found a much higher rate of incisional hernias in the open surgery group.[36] There was, however, no difference in the rate resolution of comorbid conditions or weight loss between the two procedures. Maggard and coworkers[29] have also found laparoscopic RYGB to be superior to the open procedure in regard to a decreased incidence of incisional hernias and respiratory and wound complications.

The duration of hospitalization has been found to decrease in all patients undergoing RYGB. Patients undergoing laparoscopic RYGB are usually hospitalized for approximately 2 days. Since the advent of laparoscopic RYGB, I have seen patients who undergo open RYGB or require conversion to open RYGB discharged within 1 day of patients after laparoscopic RYGB, probably because of protocols in place that encourage early ambulation and oral intake after RYGB that did not exist before the era of laparoscopic RYGB.

Two meta-analyses of long-term follow-up studies have shown that RYGB results in weight loss of 43.5 and 41.5 kg (see

**Table 15-4 Results of Roux-en-Y Gastric Bypass**

| | Study (Year) | | |
|---|---|---|---|
| **PARAMETER** | **BUCHWALD ET AL (2004)[30]** | **MAGGARD ET AL (2005)[29]** | **SUGERMAN (2003)*** |
| Number of patients | 4204 | 1281 | 1025 |
| Age (yr) | NR | NR | 39 |
| Body mass index (kg/m$^2$) | NR | NR | 51 |
| Follow-up (yr) | NR | 1/>3 | 10-12 |
| EWL (%) | 62 | NR | 52 |
| Weight loss (kg) | 43 | 43/41 | NR |
| Resolution, improvement (%) | NR | NR | NR |
| Diabetes mellitus type 2 | 93 | NR | 83 |
| Hypertension | 87 | NR | 69 |
| Obstructive sleep apnea | 95 | NR | NR |
| Osteoarthritis | NR | NR | 18 |

*Sugerman HJ, Wolfe LG, Sica DA, et al: Diabetes and hypertension in severe obesity and effects of gastric bypass-induced weight loss. Ann Surg 237:751–758, 2003.

Table 15-2).[29,30] Long-term follow-up studies have shown 58% loss of excess weight at 5 years and 49% at 14 years after RYGB.

Resolution of comorbid conditions after open and laparoscopic RYGB has generally been excellent. A meta-analysis of the effects of RYGB on diabetes has shown resolution in 83.7% and improvement in 93.2% of patients.[30] Torquati and colleagues[37] have found a substantial reduction in hemoglobin A1c levels and resolution of diabetes in 74% of diabetics undergoing laparoscopic RYGB. Preoperative factors that predicted failure of diabetes to resolve were need for insulin preoperatively or waist circumference more than 50 inches in men and more than 40 inches in women. All series demonstrated that resolution of diabetes begins immediately after surgery and may be partially related to enteric factors regulating glucose metabolism. Rubino and associates[38] have been proponents of intestinal factors, particularly in the case of RYGB, especially in regard to the effect of duodenal bypass on the improvement in diabetes unrelated to weight loss.[14] Long-term follow-up after RYGB shows that most patients who resolve their diabetes maintain good control of the diabetes unless they regain substantial amounts of weight.[39] Thus, although there may be a benefit to bypassing the duodenum, sustained long-term weight loss appears to be an essential element of the salutatory effects of RYGB on type 2 diabetes.

Metabolic syndrome is cured or ameliorated with gastric bypass.[40] Mattar and coworkers[41] have shown that gastric bypass is also effective in improving NASH.

The meta-analysis of the effect of RYGB on comorbid conditions has indicated remarkable improvement in every disease studied.[30] Hypertension resolved in 67.5% and improved in 87.2%; obstructive sleep apnea resolved in 80.4% and improved in 94.8% of patients. Hyperlipidemia, hypercholesterolemia, and hypertriglyceridemia improved in 96.9%, 94.9%, and 91.2%, respectively, of patients undergoing RYGB.

RYGB has also been shown to resolve the symptoms of pseudotumor cerebri and cure the difficult problem of venous stasis ulcers. Immediate resolution of the symptoms of GERD occurs in more than 90% of cases. The extremely small gastric pouch has a limited reservoir for holding gastric juice, and the cardia is a low acid-producing area of the stomach.

## Biliopancreatic Diversion and Duodenal Switch

Most malabsorptive procedures performed in the United States are the DS modification of BPD, so this section will discuss the results of both operations. The EWL after BPD-DS is the highest of the bariatric operations discussed in this chapter, with a mean weight loss of 46.4 and 53.1 kg found by two meta-analyses (see Table 15-2).[29,30] The percentage EWL for BPD-DS was 70.1%, also the highest for any of the procedures discussed in this chapter.

In a recent study comparing morbidly obese patients with a BMI higher than 50 kg/m$^2$, there was significantly more EWL at 12, 18, and 24 months postoperatively after DS than after RYGB. Twelve months postoperatively, EWL was 65% in the DS group and 57% in the RYGB group.[42] Thus, some surgeons have argued that superobese patients fare better and maintain weight loss better in the long term after undergoing DS than after other bariatric procedures. Others have noted that side effects, mortality, and morbidity are much higher with DS and therefore the incremental improvements in EWL are not justified.

BPD-DS has also been highly effective in treating comorbid conditions, including hypertension, diabetes, lipid disorders, and obstructive sleep apnea. Lipid disorders and type 2 diabetes are almost uniformly resolved after BPD-DS (Table 15-5). Hypertension is cured in 83.4% and obstructive sleep apnea resolves in 91.9% of patients.[30]

**Table 15-5 Results of Malabsorptive Operations***

| | Study (Year) | | |
|---|---|---|---|
| PARAMETER | SCOPINARO† | BUCHWALD ET AL (2004)[30] | MAGGARD ET AL (2005)[29] |
| No. of patients (BPD-DS) | 1356 | 2480 | 735 |
| Age (yr) | 37 | NR | NR |
| Body mass index (kg/m$^2$) | 47 | NR | NR |
| Follow-up (yr) | 12 | NR | 1/>3 |
| Loss of excess weight (%) | 78 | 70 | NR |
| No. of bowel movements/day | 2-4 | NR | NR |
| Weight loss (kg) | NR | 46 | 52/53 |
| Resolution, improvement (%) | NR | NR | NR |
| Diabetes mellitus type 2 | 100 | 98.9 | NR |
| Hypertension | 87 | 83.4 | NR |
| Cholesterol | 100 | 87 | NR |

*BPD-DS.

†Scopinaro N, Gianetta E, Adami GF, et al: Biliopancreatic diversion for obesity at eighteen years. Surgery 119:261–268, 1996.

After BPD, patients typically have between two and four daily bowel movements. Excessive flatulence and foul-smelling stools are the rule. Relatively selective malabsorption of starch and fat provides the major mechanism of weight loss, although the partial gastric resection does contribute a restrictive component to the operation.

Surgeons caring for these patients must be alert to measure protein levels for confirmation of adequate absorption. When protein malnutrition does occur, the common channel may need to be lengthened with a reoperation. Patients must also be aware that their ability to absorb simple sugars, alcohol, and short-chain triglycerides is good and that overindulgence of sweets, milk products, soft drinks, alcohol, and fruit may produce excess weight gain.

Major considerations for achieving excellent results in patients offered BPD-DS include the ability to monitor these patients reliably and confirm that they are being compliant with the recommendations to take appropriate vitamin supplements. Supplements include multivitamins, and at least 1800 mg of oral calcium/day. Supplemental fat-soluble vitamins, including vitamins D, K, and A, are indicated monthly as well.

The reported experience with laparoscopic DS is still somewhat limited. Prachand and colleagues[42] have reported the results of 185 DS procedures, most which were performed laparoscopically. The patients in this series, having been chosen because they had a BMI higher than 50 kg/m$^2$, were larger than

**Table 15-6 Outcomes of Sleeve Gastrectomy**

| VARIABLE | HIGH-RISK PATIENTS, STAGED APPROACH | PRIMARY PROCEDURE | ALL PATIENTS |
|---|---|---|---|
| No. of studies* (no. of patients) | 13 (821) | 24 (1749) | 36 (2570) |
| Preoperative BMI (kg/m$^2$) | | | |
| Range | 49.1-69.0 | 37.2-54.5 | 37.2-69.0 |
| Mean | 60.0 | 46.6 | 51.2 |
| Postoperative BMI (kg/m$^2$) | | | |
| Range | 36.4-53.0 | 26.0-39.8 | 26.0-53.0 |
| Mean | 44.9 | 32.2 | 37.1 |
| Follow-up (mo) | 4-60 | 3-36 | 3-60 |
| Excess weight loss (%) | | | |
| Range | 33.0-61.4 | 36.0-85.0 | 33.0-85.0 |
| Mean | 46.6 | 60.7 | 55.4 |
| Complication rate (%) | | | |
| Range | 0-23.8 | 0-21.7 | 0-23.8 |
| Mean | 9.4 | 6.2 | |
| Studies with >100 patients (%) | 3.3-15.3 | 0-14.1 | 0-14.1 |
| Leaks† | 8/686 (1.2) | 45/1681 (2.7)‡ | 53/2367 (2.2) |
| Bleeding† | 11/686 (1.6) | 7/1681 (1.0)§ | 28/2367 (1.2) |
| Strictures† | 6/686 (0.9) | 9/1681 (0.5)§ | 15/2367 (0.6) |
| Mortality¶ | 2/821 (0.24) | 3/1749 (0.17)§ | 5/2570 (0.19) |

From Clinical Issues Committee of the American Society for Metabolic and Bariatric Surgeons: Updated position statement on sleeve gastrectomy as a bariatric procedure. Surg Obes Relat Dis 6:1–5, 2010.

*One study included clearly defined patients in both groups.

†Included studies with detailed complication data only.

‡$P = .02$ compared with high-risk group.

§$P$ not significant compared with high-risk group.

¶Thirty-day postoperative mortality; ( ) reflect %.

patients in most selected series. A median loss of 73% of excess weight was noted at 18 months after surgery. There was a 0.5% mortality rate (one patient), which is the lowest ever reported for BPD-DS.

Because of a high incidence of morbidity and mortality (23% and 6.5%) in patients with a BMI higher than 60 kg/m$^2$ undergoing laparoscopic DS, surgeons developed the two-stage DS, with sleeve gastrectomy alone performed as the first stage to decrease morbidity in this superobese patient population. The Clinical Issues Committee of the American Society for Metabolic and Bariatric Surgery (ASBMS) comprehensively reviewed 13 studies of 821 high-risk patients who underwent a staged approach with laparoscopic sleeve gastrectomy. On average, the preoperative BMI was 60.0; after 4- to 60-month follow-ups, the postoperative BMI was 44.9. The complications in this high-risk patients population showed a leak rate of 1.2%, bleeding rate of 1.6%, and mortality of 0.24%. The ASMBS committee concluded that laparoscopic sleeve gastrectomy has value as the initial stage of a bariatric surgery in high-risk patients.[25]

## Laparoscopic Sleeve Gastrectomy

The initial reports of laparoscopic sleeve gastrectomy were part of the first stage of a two-stage bariatric procedure, although some patients never reached the second stage. A few surgeons, after seeing these patients lose prodigious amounts of weight, suggested that laparoscopic sleeve gastrectomy be used as a primary procedure. Some surgeons have suggested that the percentage of EWL 1 year after laparoscopic sleeve gastrectomy (36% to 85%) is sufficient to preclude conversion to laparoscopic RYGB or laparoscopic DS.[25] The weight loss resulting from LSG was comparable to that in patients undergoing DS or RYGB; they conclude that LSG produces adequate weight loss, with morbidity comparable to that after AGB and emphasized the use of a 32–40 Fr sizing tube for the operation.[25] The ASMBS position paper regarding laparoscopic sleeve gastrectomy as a primary bariatric procedure reviewed 24 studies of 1749 patients who underwent laparoscopic sleeve gastrectomy as a primary procedure.[25] The results shown in Table 15-6 demonstrate a mean EWL of 60.7% and a low rate of complications. Although the ASMBS views these early results as promising, it was suggested that long-term weight loss data will be essential in confirming the efficacy of this procedure. Level 1 data about laparoscopic sleeve gastrectomy is available from France from a randomized trial comparing laparoscopic sleeve gastrectomy to laparoscopic AGB after 3 years.[23] Weight loss and loss of feelings of hunger were better in the laparoscopic sleeve gastrectomy patients compared with laparoscopic AGB patients at 1 and 3 years after surgery.

**Table 15-7 Comparison of Complications After Laparoscopic and Open Roux-en-Y Gastric Bypass**

| ADVERSE EVENT AND TYPE OF PROCEDURE | ADVERSE EVENT RATE (%) | ODDS RATIO (95% CI) | NO. OF PATIENTS |
|---|---|---|---|
| Respiratory (including pneumonia, atelectasis, and respiratory insufficiency) | | | |
| Open vs. laparoscopic (range) | 3.0 vs. 1.9 | 1.54 (0.17-19.42) | 101 vs. 104 |
| Surgical, preventable and not preventable (including wound, hernia, splenic injury, repeated operation, anastomotic events) | | | |
| Open vs. laparoscopic | 31.1 vs. 26.1 | 1.32 (0.72-2.43) | 122 vs. 134 |
| Wound, all | | | |
| Open vs. laparoscopic | 13.1 vs. 0.0 | Not estimable | 122 vs. 134 |
| Wound infection, major | | | |
| Open vs. laparoscopic | 3.0 vs. 0.0 | Not estimable | 101 vs. 104 |
| Wound infection, minor | | | |
| Open vs. laparoscopic | 14.3 vs. 0.0 | Not estimable | 21 vs. 30 |
| Incisional hernia | | | |
| Open vs. laparoscopic | 8.2 vs. 0.0 | Not estimable | 122 vs. 134 |
| Internal hernia | | | |
| Open vs. laparoscopic | 0.0 vs. 1.3 | 0.00 (0.00-40.40) | 76 vs. 79 |
| Reoperation | | | |
| Open vs. laparoscopic | 0.0 vs. 4.0 | 0.00 (0.00-38.94) | 25 vs. 25 |
| Deep venous thrombosis, pulmonary embolism, or both | | | |
| Open vs. laparoscopic | 1.0 vs. 0.9 | 1.22 (0.02-96.69) | 97 vs. 109 |

From Maggard MA, Shugarman LR, Suttorp M, et al: Meta-analysis: Surgical treatment of obesity. Ann Intern Med 142:547–559, 2005.

Potential advantages of the laparoscopic sleeve gastrectomy are the technical ease of the procedure, induction of satiety through reduction in ghrelin levels, reduced need for postoperative adjustments as opposed to laparoscopic AGB, preservation of the pylorus, avoidance of dumping, reduced risk of malabsorption, and apparent safety of the procedure in high-risk individuals. Use of the laparoscopic sleeve gastrectomy may be advantageous for some patient populations (see Table 15-1). I believe that it is clear that the fastest rising procedure is the laparoscopic sleeve gastrectomy; it will probably be used by bariatric surgeons more frequently in the future.

## COMPLICATIONS

The procedures described are associated with complications that can occur with any intra-abdominal operation, such as pulmonary embolism. However, each operation has unique complications and different rates of occurrence of some common complications seen after any abdominal operation.

A number of reports have shown laparoscopic procedures to be associated with less respiratory, surgical wound, and thrombotic complications (Table 15-7).[16,29,43] The benefits promoted for laparoscopic surgery go beyond the cosmetic effects and actually influence postoperative complication rates, which makes the laparoscopic technique my preferred approach for almost every patient, including remedial operations.

### Adjustable Gastric Banding

The mortality associated with AGB (0.02% to 0.1%) has been significantly lower than that for RYGB (0.3% to 0.5%) or either of the malabsorptive operations (0.9% to 1.1%).[16,29,30] Complications for the procedure are described in this section and summarized in Table 15-8. A major complication of RYGB or BPD-DS is the risk of leakage from the anastomosis, which does not occur with AGB; however, from the meta-analysis, it appears that the need for reoperation and complications related to surgery occur in all types of bariatric procedures.

A common complication that plagued AGB in the mid to late 1990s was the high incidence of band slippage, which was reported in 15% of patients in one series, a figure that was comparable to other reports for the initial perigastric band placement. Before the pars flaccida technique, the band was placed around the proximal part of the stomach, with the posterior portion of the band free within the lesser sac, a technique termed the *perigastric approach.* This allowed much more movement of the stomach and, despite the anterior imbricating sutures, the fundus of the stomach herniated up through the band in a significant percentage of cases. In a randomized trial of the two techniques, O'Brien and coworkers[34] have shown that use of the pars flaccida technique is associated with a much lower rate of slippage than was seen with use of the perigastric technique (4% versus 15%). The pars flaccida technique has subsequently become the preferred approach.

This so-called *slippage* is usually manifested as the sudden development of food intolerance or, occasionally, gastroesophageal reflux. The latter symptom is also indicative of any form of obstruction at the site of the band. Slippage is the most common cause of obstruction but, on occasion, erosion and fibrosis can also cause similar symptoms. A patient with obstructive symptoms or food intolerance has a plain radiograph of the abdomen taken. In its appropriate position, the band is oriented in a diagonal direction, along the 1- to 7-o'clock or 2- to 8-o'clock axis in the epigastric region. A plain film showing the band in a horizontal or 10- to 4-o'clock position is diagnostic of slippage and altered band position. Slippage or any other obstructive process at the band site will cause functional stenosis of the gastrointestinal tract at the proximal end of the stomach. As a result, esophageal dilation can occur if this situation is not corrected.

**Table 15-8 Complications After Laparoscopic Adjustable Gastric Banding**

| | Study (Year)* | | | | |
|---|---|---|---|---|---|
| **PARAMETER** | **FLUM ET AL (2009)†** | **O'BRIEN ET AL (2002)[10]** | **BUCHWALD ET AL (2004)[30]** | **MAGGARD ET AL (2005)[29]** | **PONCE ET AL (2005)[32]** |
| No. of patients | 1198 | 1120 | 2297 | 9222 | 1014 |
| Mortality | 0 | 0 | 0.1% | 0.04 | 0 |
| Postoperative complications | 1.0 | 1.5 | | 13.2 | |
| Slippage | | 13.9 | | | 21 (PG)/1.4 (PF) |
| Erosions | | 3 | | | 0.2 |
| Port complications | | 5.4 | | | 1.2 |
| Reoperations | | 25.3 | | 7.7 | |
| DVT-PE | 0.3% | 0 | | | |
| Wound infection | | 0.9 | | | |

*PF,* Pars flaccida; *PG,* perigastric.

*All numbers, except number of patients, represent percentages.

†O'Brien PE, Dixon JB, Laurie C, et al: Weight loss and early and late complications–the international experience. Am J Surg 184:42S–45S, 2002.

Erosion of the band into the lumen of the stomach is a less frequent complication but requires reoperation. The incidence of erosion may increase in the future but currently, however, the incidence remains below 1% for many large series and up to 3%, as noted earlier in the Australian studies. Erosion may be manifested as abdominal pain or as a port access site infection. In cases in which the band does erode into the stomach, it is presumed that the band is too tight or the stomach was imbricated too close to the buckle of the band, which causes erosion over time. Surprisingly, this complication is rarely life-threatening and many reports have described removal of the eroded band, repair of the stomach, and replacement of a new band at the same operative setting.

Port access site problems are the most numerous of the complications that occur after AGB. These problems also require reoperative therapy in most cases, but the procedure can often be performed under local anesthesia and does not involve the peritoneal cavity. Leakage of the access tubing is a common problem that occurs in up to 11% of cases. In addition, kinking of the tubing as it passes through the fascia is another relatively common reason for port access difficulties. Port site infection is the least common port access problem (<1%), but needs to be evaluated with upper endoscopy to be certain that band erosion has not occurred.

## Roux-en-Y Gastric Bypass

Mortality rates after RYGB have generally been in the 0.3% to 1.0% range for large reported series. Meta-analyses have shown a 30-day mortality rate of 0.3% to 0.5% for RYGB (see Table 15-2).[16,29,30]

Causes of mortality have varied but include pulmonary embolism, anastomotic leak, cardiac events, intra-abdominal abscess, and multiorgan failure. Mortality rates are obviously influenced heavily by patient selection. Male gender is also associated with an increased risk for morbidity and mortality in some series[44] but not in the most recent LABS experience. The LABS study identified BMI and a history of venous thromboembolism as independent predictors of complications.[16] As noted, the use of a laparoscopic approach has greatly lessened the incisional hernia and wound complication rates.[35] Anastomotic leaks or complications occurred in 2.2%, and the reoperation rate was 1.6% in the meta-analysis.[29] Table 15-9 summarizes data regarding complications after RYGB.

**Table 15-9 Complications After Roux-en-Y Gastric Bypass**

| | Study (Year) | | |
|---|---|---|---|
| **PARAMETER** | **SUGERMAN (2003)*** | **MAGGARD ET AL (2005)[29]** | **BUCHWALD ET AL (2004)[30]** |
| No. of patients | 1025 | 11,290 | 5644 |
| Mortality (%) | 0.9 | 0.3 | 0.5 |
| Gastrointestinal bleeding (%) | | 2.0 | |
| Leak, major wound complications (%) | 3 | 2.2 | |

*Sugerman HJ, Wolfe LG, Sica DA, et al: Diabetes and hypertension in severe obesity and effects of gastric bypass-induced weight loss. Ann Surg 237:751–758, 2003.

Pulmonary embolism is one of the most feared complications after any form of bariatric surgery; its incidence in large reported series of open RYGB sometimes exceeds 1%. Thrombotic complications such as DVT and pulmonary embolism appear to be less frequently associated with laparoscopic surgery than with open gastric bypass.

Improvement in postoperative morbidity after laparoscopic procedures is not limited to incisional hernia, as detailed in Table 15-7. Specifically, postoperative atelectasis, pneumonia, and respiratory insufficiency are 1.54 times more common after open bariatric than after laparoscopic procedures.

Although nausea and vomiting are not unusual in isolated circumstances after RYGB, especially in relation to a patient's adaptation to food restriction, these symptoms, if persistent, can lead to the obvious problem of dehydration. This must be aggressively treated in the postoperative period or when associated with a viral or other gastrointestinal illness compounding the problem and further limiting oral intake. IV fluids are indicated when in doubt. This is the case for all bariatric operations, not just RYGB.

One specific problem that may arise with persistent vomiting after any of the bariatric operations and that is *imperative* for the surgeon to remember and treat is Wernicke's encephalopathy from prolonged vomiting. This neurologic deficit is preventable with appropriate administration of parenteral thiamine (vitamin $B_1$) when the patient has persistent and severe vomiting. If the neurologic symptoms become significant, they may often not be fully reversed, despite thiamine therapy.

Because depression is so frequent in the patient population undergoing bariatric surgery, severe postoperative depression may also develop after any bariatric operation. When it occurs, the patient may totally stop eating, thereby producing what at first seems like wonderful weight loss, but soon, when gone beyond its desired end point, it progresses to a loss of critical visceral and musculoskeletal protein mass, which can be life-threatening.

Complications specific to RYGB include anastomotic leaks from the proximal or distal anastomosis. Leaks from the gastrojejunostomy are more common and are generally the cause of a significant percentage of the life-threatening complications and deaths. Evidence has suggested that a surgeon's experience will influence the leak rate, especially early in the laparoscopic experience with RYGB. Most large series of open RYGB procedures reported a leak rate of 1% to 2%, whereas some laparoscopic surgeons, early in their experience, were observing a leak rate approaching 5%. Maggard and colleagues[29] found a leak rate of 2.2% in open and laparoscopic RYGB. Fortunately, this appears to be a transient phenomenon on the learning curve of some surgeons; most large series of laparoscopic RYGB have reported anastomotic leak rates of 1% to 2%, and some have treated large series without a leak.[19]

Another specific life-threatening complication that may result after RYGB is bowel obstruction. Patients who have a clinical or radiographic picture of small bowel obstruction after RYGB need a reoperation. The potential for internal hernias after this operation makes strangulation obstruction a frequent type of bowel obstruction. Patients with bowel obstruction and not ileus in the immediate postoperative period—I perform CT with contrast or an upper gastrointestinal series to confirm or rule out obstruction—must be promptly operated on before retrograde distention of the biliopancreatic limb and distal part of the stomach results in rupture of the distal gastric staple line, with subsequent peritonitis.

Stenosis of the gastrojejunostomy may occur after RYGB and has been reported in 2% to 14% of patients in various series. The higher incidence seems to be associated with circular stapler versus sutured-type anastomoses. Postoperative anastomotic stenosis is usually manifested at 4 to 6 weeks postoperatively as progressive intolerance to solids and then to liquids in a setting in which they were previously tolerated. The problem is successfully treated with endoscopic or fluoroscopic balloon dilation. Unless a marginal ulcer is associated with the stenosis, the problem does not require a reoperation.

A marginal ulcer occurs after 2% to 10% of RYGB procedures. The incidence can be decreased by preoperative treatment of patients for *Helicobacter pylori* colonization of the stomach. Patients with a marginal ulcer typically have continuous, boring epigastric pain. Treatment consists of medical therapy with proton pump inhibitors. Medical treatment resolves all marginal ulcers unless the ulcer has fistulized to the lower part of the stomach and created an ongoing source of acid to exacerbate the ulcer.

Iron and vitamin $B_{12}$ deficiencies are the two most common long-term metabolic complications of RYGB. The incidence of iron insufficiency varies in reported series. Iron is preferentially absorbed in the duodenum and proximal jejunum. Hence, RYGB bypasses the area of maximal iron absorption in the gut. The iron deficiency, based on serum values, is between 15% and 40%, whereas actual iron deficiency anemia occurs in as many as 20% of patients after RYGB. In most cases, this problem is easily treated with oral iron supplements. The gluconate form of iron is best absorbed in a nonacid environment.

The incidence of vitamin $B_{12}$ deficiency after RYGB is reported as 15% to 20%, although it rarely causes anemia. Peripheral neural complications from low vitamin $B_{12}$ levels after RYGB are almost unknown. Vitamin $B_{12}$ deficiency is caused by inefficient absorption because of delayed mixing with intrinsic factor. Several preparations include intrinsic factor and will maximize absorption in the terminal ileum. Other routes of vitamin $B_{12}$ administration include sublingual medication, nasal spray, and parenteral injections.

Analysis of the NSQIP database has shown the operative mortality and complication rate for the laparoscopic approach to be significantly lower than the open approach (odds ratio, 2.08; 95% CI, 1.33 to 3.25).[43]

The incidence of associated splenectomy, wound infection, incisional hernia, respiratory complications, and DVT-PE was lower with laparoscopic RYGB than with open RYGB.[29] In contrast, the incidence of bowel obstruction, especially early bowel obstruction, appears to be higher in patients undergoing laparoscopic RYGB.

## Biliopancreatic Diversion

Mortality rates after BPD-DS were reported to be 1.1% in the meta-analysis of Buchwald and colleagues and 0.9% in Maggard and associates' study.[29] Surgical wound complications occurred in 5.9% of patients, leaks developed in 1.8%, and reoperations occurred 4.2% of the time, as summarized in Table 15-10.[30]

The most significant and specific long-term complication seen after BPD is protein malnutrition, which occurs in 11.9% of patients. Treatment is hospitalization, with 2 to 3 weeks of parenteral nutrition. This particular problem is usually manifested within the first few months after surgery, but it can occur sporadically, although less frequently, after surgery. In the collected series, 4% of patients eventually required a reoperation to reverse the BPD completely or lengthen the common channel.[29,30] The revision rate was approximately 0.1% annually for the first 6 years, and the rehospitalization rate for malabsorption or diarrhea was 0.93% annually during the same period. The percentage of patients averaging more than three daily bowel movements was 7%, and 34% believed that the unpleasant odor of stools and flatus was a problem. Abdominal bloating was experienced in one third of patients more than once weekly. Bone pain was reported in 29% of patients. Metabolic complications and side effects included iron deficiency in 9%, low ferritin level in 25%, low calcium concentration in 8%, and low level of vitamin A in 5% of patients; elevated parathyroid hormone levels were present in 17%.

Malabsorption of fat-soluble vitamins is one of the major problems associated with BPD-DS. Slater and coworkers[45] have

**Table 15-10 Complications After Malabsorptive Operations (Biliopancreatic Diversion and Duodenal Switch)**

| | Study (Year) | | | |
|---|---|---|---|---|
| PARAMETER | SCOPINARO (1998)* | BUCHWALD ET AL (2004)[30] | MAGGARD ET AL (2005)[29] | REN (2004)[26] |
| Number of patients | 2241 | 3030 | 2808 | 170 |
| Mortality | 0.5 | 1.1 | 0.9 | |
| Leak | 0.1 | | 1.8 | |
| DVT-PE | 0.06 | | | |
| Medical problems, malnutrition | 3† | | | |
| Iron deficiency anemia | 40 | | | |
| Vitamin A deficiency | 2.9%‡ | | | 69 |
| Vitamin K deficiency | | | | 68 |
| Vitamin D deficiency | | | | 63 |

All numbers except number of patients represent percentages.

*Scopinaro N, Adami GF, Marinari GM, et al: Biliopancreatic diversion. World J Surg 22:936–946, 1998.

†Severe protein/calorie malnutrition.

‡Night blindness caused by Vitamin A deficiency.

shown that vitamin D and A levels 2 years after BPD are significantly depressed, with vitamin D deficiency in 63%, vitamin A deficiency in 69%, evidence of bone resorption in 3%, and all patients having essential fatty acid deficiency. Lack of clinical correlation with these levels suggests that the problem may be more prevalent than originally reported or suspected from past series.

Although the complication of protein malnutrition and poor intake is theoretically most likely to occur soon after BPD-DS, the fact that late deaths occur from protein malnutrition and Wernicke's encephalopathy suggests that these patients may always be at risk for these problems. Marginal ulcers are a distinct problem of BPD, which has been solved with the DS modification preserving the pylorus. Perhaps it is the overall difficulty of the operation, as well as the potential dangers of the operation, that has left BPD as the least popular operation performed in the United States. Even the DS modification does not represent more than 10% of bariatric operations. Further studies are needed to evaluate the long-term consequences of BPD and DS to justify their performance as a primary procedure.

## REOPERATIVE SURGERY

A controversial topic is the appropriateness of performing repeat bariatric operations for failed previous procedures. There are no specific rules to govern the appropriateness of repeat bariatric surgery. The absolute definition of a failed operation is unclear, but most surgeons would accept returning to the criteria listed in Box 15-2 as appropriate when considering reoperation. If a patient has undergone an operation that has been proven by mass experience to be ineffective, a repeat operation for failure of that procedure is appropriate. Complications of procedures, such as stenosis causing gastric outlet obstruction after vertical banded gastroplasty or metabolic complications after jejunoileal bypass, are obvious indications for revisional surgery. One mistake frequently made by a nonbariatric surgeon when correcting a complication of a bariatric operation is simply to perform a procedure that corrects the complication but does not provide for continued weight restriction. In these circumstances, a typical long-term course is for patients to slowly regain weight to the same degree of obesity as before the initial bariatric procedure and then seek further surgical assistance.

In assessing a patient for the appropriateness of reoperative surgery, the surgeon must determine whether the original bariatric operation is intact and still appropriate anatomically for maintaining weight loss. If not, consideration for reoperation is appropriate. However, a patient who has failed an anatomically intact and well-constructed bariatric operation is, in my opinion, at high risk to fail a second or revisional bariatric operation. Although little has been reported, there are no reports contradicting this. It is known that the incidence of infection, organ ischemia, anastomotic leakage, blood transfusion, and other severe intra-abdominal complications is increased in revisional surgery.

All bariatric operations have some degree of failure. A figure of approximately 10% is often used in discussions regarding the failure rate of various well-established operations considered effective, including all those described in this chapter. The definition of failure is varied; it may include inadequate weight loss, inadequate resolution of medical comorbid conditions, development of side effects negatively influencing lifestyle and satisfaction, and development of complications requiring medical or surgical intervention or those requiring alteration or reversal of the operation.

Jejunoileal bypass, a relic of history, still exists in a small number of patients, who need to have it reversed to prevent progression to cirrhosis, liver failure, and other severe metabolic consequences. Any reversal should include a replacement weight reduction operation.

Failed RYGB secondary to a dilated gastric pouch or dilated gastrojejunostomy has been treated with laparoscopic placement of an AGB has been successful in several centers, including mine. Failed RYGB has been treated by adding a malabsorptive component to the original procedure by reconnecting the efferent end of the RYGB halfway down the length of the alimentary bowel and thereby decreasing the alimentary tract by 50%.

Although patients experience a decrease in BMI, protein malnutrition can develop in a significant number. Conversion of patients after failed open or laparoscopic gastroplasty to RYGB has been shown to decrease BMI. Other sporadic reports of small case series in the literature have suggested that even reoperations can, under appropriate circumstances, be performed laparoscopically and have relatively good results, although not with as low a complication rate as the initial surgery.

## ADDITIONAL CONSIDERATIONS

### Controversies in Bariatric Surgery

Flum and colleagues[46] have suggested that morbidity and mortality after bariatric surgery in routine practice is much higher than published results reported by experienced surgeons. They accessed the Medicare database for all bariatric surgical procedures from 1997 to 2002 and found that the 30-day mortality rate was 2.0%—much higher than the rate reported in two meta-analyses. They found high mortality within the first 30 days, but also a surprisingly high death rate (4.6%) within the first year after surgery. Their conclusion was that mortality rates were much higher in real-life practice than those reported in retrospective case reviews or prospective studies. Nguyen and associates[47] have shown that high-volume academic hospitals have a lower mortality rate, length of hospital stay, complication rate, and cost. In patients older than 55 years, mortality was 3.1% at low-volume hospitals and 0.9% at high-volume centers.

These reports of high morbidity and mortality after bariatric surgery and the reduction in rates in high-volume centers have led to a spate of editorials and policy changes aimed at reducing the risks associated with bariatric surgery. One of the most important developments was the medical policy decision handed down by CMS for Medicare beneficiaries in February 2006, which is notable for the dramatic step of requiring that surgery be performed only in Centers of Excellence as certified by the American College of Surgeons or ASBMS. The requirement for surgeons and the hospitals in which the surgery is performed to go through a significant vetting process, demonstration of surgical results, and demonstration of the processes and readiness of the facilities to take care of the needs of morbidly obese patients is a seminal event in the practice of surgery in this country. Recent studies from the NSQIP[15] have demonstrated that laparoscopic bariatric surgery complication rates across the United States are much lower than those reported during the 1997 to 2002 era. A combination of improved laparoscopic techniques, surgeon experience, institution of the Center of Excellence concept, and better patient preparation and postoperative care have led to the dramatic lowering of operative complications and death after bariatric surgery.

### Investigational Bariatric Procedures

A number of procedures have been investigated for weight loss surgery but have not been totally accepted by the surgical community. Gastric pacing has been performed in several trials but has not been shown to have any long-term effect and has been abandoned. Others have investigated vagal blocking with implantable electrodes placed laparoscopically around the abdominal vagal trunks. Early clinical trials of this technique are promising but the FDA has not yet released the device for sale in the United States. Endoscopic incisionless surgery has focused on patients after RYGB who have inadequate weight loss or significant weight regain and who have a dilated gastrojejunostomy. It is thought that these patients lose restriction because of the dilated gastrojejunostomy and thus overeat. Surgeons have tried endoscopic injection of sclerosing agents to create scar and a smaller anastomosis, with variable effects. There are a number of ongoing studies to demonstrate and evaluate the effectiveness of various endoscopic suturing devices and/or injection therapies designed to reduce the anastomosis size and thus impose more restrictions on food intake.[48] These have been met with variable success and, in some cases, are not paid for by the insurance company, leaving patients to pay out of pocket for the procedure.

Another endoscopic and laparoscopic procedure that has some scientific merit is the concept that duodenal bypass improves type 2 diabetes independent of weight loss through a poorly defined mechanism of action. Rubino and colleagues[38] have been the major proponent of the theory that duodenal bypass improves glucose control in diabetics through reduction of the anti-incretin effect, thus improving the diabetes. Because the action of incretins in the distal small bowel is to increase insulin secretion and cause beta cell proliferation, increasing either the secretion or effect of the incretins should help patients with diabetes.

Increasingly, surgeons are observing the effects of bariatric operations on more than the physical reduction of caloric intake or malabsorption. Alteration in comorbid conditions caused by metabolic processes may prove equally as important. For example, bariatric operations may have important metabolic components that alter the hormonal, cytokine, and/or metabolic rate of patients.[18,49]

### The Bariatric Revolution and Counterrevolution

Bariatric surgery could still be considered as being in the midst of a revolution. In many U.S. hospitals, bariatric surgical procedures are the most commonly performed operation on the general surgical service.[50] There are several reasons for this. The most important one, which temporally corresponds with the rapid rise in patient demand for bariatric surgery, is the use of a laparoscopic approach for operations. Although a laparoscopic approach was more commonplace in Europe and Australia in the mid-1990s with the advent of the popularity of laparoscopic AGB, use of the laparoscopic approach for RYGB in the United States actually only began in 1999. Before then, only a few medical centers were offering that approach. Laparoscopic AGB was not performed in the United States until 2001, but has become the most common bariatric procedure performed in some U.S. centers.

Mass media and the rapid dissemination of information are also a major factor in the bariatric revolution. Patients may now access many sites on the Internet to obtain information about bariatric surgery. Television stations show videos of actual operations. Internet chat groups and blogs, in which former and prospective patients discuss bariatric surgery, are common, and many patients participate before and after surgery. Media and television personalities have undergone bariatric surgery, with superb results that they have been willing to share with the public. The combination of all these factors has led to a patient population that is more informed and aware of the potential of this surgery to treat their morbid obesity.

Finally, the surgical community itself has adjusted its perception of bariatric surgery. It is now a desirable area of specialization for graduating residents, who enjoy the technical challenge of advanced laparoscopic surgery combined with the rewards of performing a life-altering and usually highly successful operation for their patients.

## CONCLUSION

Surgical treatment of morbid obesity is no longer considered out of the mainstream of general surgery. It is now a component of most surgical residents' training programs and currently represents the fastest growing area of general surgery. Patient demand for the procedure has vastly increased; at present, surgeons operate annually on less than 2% of eligible patients who would benefit from bariatric surgery. This chapter has discussed all aspects of the performance of bariatric surgery in current surgical practice, including the most commonly performed current procedures. The disease process of morbid obesity is, unfortunately, incompletely understood but rapidly increasing in prevalence. At present, surgical therapy is the only effective treatment of morbid obesity.

## SELECTED REFERENCES

Ashrafian H, le Roux CW: Metabolic surgery and gut hormones—a review of bariatric entero-humoral modulation. Physiol Behav 97: 620–631, 2009.

A superb review article of the gut hormone changes associated with metabolic operations known as bariatric surgery. The article also summarizes the effects of these hormones on appetite and energy regulation in an attempt to explain the differential effects of bariatric surgical procedures on eating behavior and weight loss.

Buchwald H, Avidor Y, Braunwald E, et al: Bariatric surgery: A systematic review and meta-analysis. JAMA 292:1724–1737, 2004.

The authors reviewed the literature and selected 136 studies (22,094 patients) that they reviewed and subjected to meta-analysis. Bariatric surgery was found to be effective for weight loss and resulted in improvement or cure of serious comorbid conditions (diabetes, dyslipidemia, hypertension, and sleep apnea) in most patients. This comprehensive meta-analysis provides compelling data on the effectiveness and beneficial results of bariatric surgery.

Christou NV, Sampalis JS, Liberman M, et al: Surgery decreases long-term mortality, morbidity, and health care use in morbidly obese patients. Ann Surg 240:416–423, 2004.

In a study comparing matched control subjects with subjects who underwent bariatric surgery in Canada, it was demonstrated that weight loss surgery reduces the relative risk for mortality by 89% (95% CI, 73% to 96%) 5 years after surgery. This is a substantial argument for the effectiveness of bariatric surgery, not only to reduce weight but to also ameliorate or cure the comorbid conditions, which increases survival.

Maggard MA, Shugarman LR, Suttorp M, et al: Meta-analysis: Surgical treatment of obesity. Ann Intern Med 142:547–559, 2005.

The authors assessed 147 studies on bariatric surgery to analyze weight loss, mortality, and complications. They found that laparoscopic gastric bypass resulted in fewer wound complications, incisional hernias, and respiratory complications than the open approach. They concluded from the analysis of weight loss and resolution of comorbid conditions that bariatric surgery was more effective than medical treatment in patients with a BMI of 40 kg/m2 or higher. This study supports the use of bariatric surgery as being safe and effective.

Nguyen NT, Goldman C, Rosenquist CJ, et al: Laparoscopic versus open gastric bypass: A randomized study of outcomes, quality of life, and costs. Ann Surg 234:279–289, 2001.

The first prospective randomized trial comparing laparoscopic with open gastric bypass. Patients were monitored for 1 year, at which time weight loss with both approaches was comparable (68% loss of excess weight for laparoscopic RYGB versus 62% loss of excess weight for open RYGB), but the laparoscopic approach had a shorter length of hospitalization and more rapid return to activities of daily living than the open procedure.

Rubino F, Kaplan LM, Schauer PR, et al: The Diabetes Surgery Summit consensus conference: Recommendations for the evaluation and use of gastrointestinal surgery to treat type 2 diabetes mellitus. Ann Surg 251:399–405, 2010.

A greater understanding of bariatric surgery has concluded that these operations provide benefits for patients with type 2 diabetes above and beyond the weight loss associated with surgery. This led to the world conference of experts who defined the problem and submitted recommendations for future research into surgical treatments for type 2 diabetes.

Sjostrom L, Narbro K, Sjostrom CD, et al: Effects of bariatric surgery on mortality in Swedish obese subjects. N Engl J Med 357:741–752, 2007.

This study compared a group of patients undergoing bariatric surgery with a group of matched control subjects and monitored them for 10.9 years. They had an unparalleled follow-up rate of 99.9% of the subjects in the study. A significant decrease in the weight and risk of death in individuals in the surgical weight loss group was found, as compared with control patients not undergoing surgery (unadjusted overall hazard ratio was 0.76 in the surgery group [$P = .4$] compared with the control group). This is excellent long-term study indicated that bariatric surgery results in sustained weight loss, resolution of comorbid conditions, and increased survival in comparison to standard medical treatment.

Dixon JB, O'Brien PE, Playfair J, et al: Adjustable gastric banding and conventional therapy for type 2 diabetes: A randomized controlled trial. JAMA 299:316–323, 2008.

O'Brien PE, Dixon JB, Laurie C, et al: Treatment of mild to moderate obesity with laparoscopic adjustable gastric banding or an intensive medical program: A randomized trial. Ann Intern Med 144:625–633, 2006.

O'Brien PE, Sawyer SM, Laurie C, et al: Laparoscopic adjustable gastric banding in severely obese adolescents: A randomized trial. JAMA 303:519–526, 2010.

These three studies by an Australian group has provided level I evidence of the superiority of bariatric surgery compared with medical treatment in three distinct scenarios. One study demonstrated that laparoscopic AGB is superior in adolescents and another showed that laparoscopic AGB is superior in adult patients compared with medical therapy. Dixon and colleagues' study showed a significantly improved weight loss and resolution of diabetes 2 years after laparoscopic AGB surgery compared with a group of diabetics who were treated medically. The evidence is mounting that bariatric surgery provides better weight loss and resolution of comorbidities than medical therapy in severely obese patients.

## REFERENCES


1. Gastrointestinal surgery for severe obesity: National Institutes of Health Consensus Development Conference Statement. Am J Clin Nutr 55(Suppl):615S–619S, 1992.
2. Ogden CL, Carroll MD, Curtin LR, et al: Prevalence of overweight and obesity in the United States, 1999–2004. JAMA 295:1549–1555, 2006.
3. Mokdad AH, Marks JS, Stroup DF, et al: Actual causes of death in the United States, 2000. JAMA 291:1238–1245, 2004.
4. Frayling TM, Timpson NJ, Weedon MN, et al: A common variant in the FTO gene is associated with body mass index and predisposes to childhood and adult obesity. Science 316:889–894, 2007.
5. Eric Hu X, Wos JA, Dowty ME, et al: Small-molecule melanin-concentrating hormone-1 receptor antagonists require brain penetration for inhibition of food intake and reduction in body weight. J Pharmacol Exp Ther 324:206–213, 2008.
6. Prentice AM, Hennig BJ, Fulford AJ: Evolutionary origins of the obesity epidemic: Natural selection of thrifty genes or genetic drift following predation release? Int J Obes (Lond) 32:1607–1610, 2008.
7. Cummings DE: Ghrelin and the short- and long-term regulation of appetite and body weight. Physiol Behav 89:71–84, 2006.
8. Cummings DE, Weigle DS, Frayo RS, et al: Plasma ghrelin levels after diet-induced weight loss or gastric bypass surgery. N Engl J Med 346:1623–1630, 2002.
9. Summerbell CD, Waters E, Edmunds LD, et al: Interventions for preventing obesity in children. Cochrane Database Syst Rev (3):CD001871, 2005.
10. O'Brien PE, Sawyer SM, Laurie C, et al: Laparoscopic adjustable gastric banding in severely obese adolescents: A randomized trial. JAMA 303:519–526, 2010.
11. O'Brien PE, Dixon JB, Laurie C, et al: Treatment of mild to moderate obesity with laparoscopic adjustable gastric banding or an intensive medical program: A randomized trial. Ann Intern Med 144:625–633, 2006.
12. Sjostrom L, Narbro K, Sjostrom CD, et al: Effects of bariatric surgery on mortality in Swedish obese subjects. N Engl J Med 357:741–752, 2007.
13. Adams TD, Gress RE, Smith SC, et al: Long-term mortality after gastric bypass surgery. N Engl J Med 357:753–761, 2007.
14. Rubino F, Kaplan LM, Schauer PR, et al: The Diabetes Surgery Summit consensus conference: Recommendations for the evaluation and use of gastrointestinal surgery to treat type 2 diabetes mellitus. Ann Surg 251:399–405, 2010.
15. Lancaster RT, Hutter MM: Bands and bypasses: 30-day morbidity and mortality of bariatric surgical procedures as assessed by prospective, multi-center, risk-adjusted ACS-NSQIP data. Surg Endosc 22:2554–2563, 2008.
16. Flum DR, Belle SH, King WC, et al: Perioperative safety in the longitudinal assessment of bariatric surgery. N Engl J Med 361:445–454, 2009.
17. Clements RH, Yellumahanthi K, Ballem N, et al: Pharmacologic prophylaxis against venous thromboembolic complications is not mandatory for all laparoscopic Roux-en-Y gastric bypass procedures. J Am Coll Surg 208:917–921, 2009.
18. Ashrafian H, le Roux CW: Metabolic surgery and gut hormones—a review of bariatric entero-humoral modulation. Physiol Behav 97:620–631, 2009.
19. Sekhar N, Torquati A, Lutfi R, et al: Endoscopic evaluation of the gastrojejunostomy in laparoscopic gastric bypass. A series of 340 patients without postoperative leak. Surg Endosc 20:199–201, 2006.
20. Cottam D, Qureshi FG, Mattar SG, et al: Laparoscopic sleeve gastrectomy as an initial weight-loss procedure for high-risk patients with morbid obesity. Surg Endosc 20:859–863, 2006.
21. Armstrong J, O'Malley SP: Outcomes of sleeve gastrectomy for morbid obesity: A safe and effective procedure? Int J Surg 8:69–71, 2010.
22. Bohdjalian A, Langer FB, Shakeri-Leidenmuhler S, et al: Sleeve gastrectomy as sole and definitive bariatric procedure: 5-year results for weight loss and ghrelin. Obes Surg 20:535–540, 2010.
23. Himpens J, Dapri G, Cadiere GB: A prospective randomized study between laparoscopic gastric banding and laparoscopic isolated sleeve gastrectomy: Results after 1 and 3 years. Obes Surg 16:1450–1456, 2006.
24. Karamanakos SN, Vagenas K, Kalfarentzos F, et al: Weight loss, appetite suppression, and changes in fasting and postprandial ghrelin and peptide-YY levels after Roux-en-Y gastric bypass and sleeve gastrectomy: A prospective, double-blind study. Ann Surg 247:401–407, 2008.
25. Clinical Issues Committee of the American Society for Metabolic and Bariatric Surgery: Updated position statement on sleeve gastrectomy as a bariatric procedure. Surg Obes Relat Dis 6:1–5, 2010.
26. Ren CJ: Controversies in bariatric surgery: Evidence-based discussions on laparoscopic adjustable gastric banding. J Gastrointest Surg 8:396–397, 2004.
27. Sjostrom L, Lindroos AK, Peltonen M, et al: Lifestyle, diabetes, and cardiovascular risk factors 10 years after bariatric surgery. N Engl J Med 351:2683–2693, 2004.
28. Christou NV, Sampalis JS, Liberman M, et al: Surgery decreases long-term mortality, morbidity, and health care use in morbidly obese patients. Ann Surg 240:416–423, 2004.
29. Maggard MA, Shugarman LR, Suttorp M, et al: Meta-analysis: Surgical treatment of obesity. Ann Intern Med 142:547–559, 2005.
30. Buchwald H, Avidor Y, Braunwald E, et al: Bariatric surgery: A systematic review and meta-analysis. JAMA 292:1724–1737, 2004.
31. Poulose BK, Holzman MD, Zhu Y, et al: National variations in morbid obesity and bariatric surgery use. J Am Coll Surg 201:77–84, 2005.
32. Ponce J, Paynter S, Fromm R: Laparoscopic adjustable gastric banding: 1,014 consecutive cases. J Am Coll Surg 201:529–535, 2005.
33. Dixon JB, O'Brien PE, Playfair J, et al: Adjustable gastric banding and conventional therapy for type 2 diabetes: A randomized controlled trial. JAMA 299:316–323, 2008.
34. O'Brien PE, Dixon JB, Laurie C, et al: A prospective randomized trial of placement of the laparoscopic adjustable gastric band: comparison of the perigastric and pars flaccida pathways. Obes Surg 15:820–826, 2005.
35. Nguyen NT, Goldman C, Rosenquist CJ, et al: Laparoscopic versus open gastric bypass: a randomized study of outcomes, quality of life, and costs. Ann Surg 234:279–289, 2001.

**36.** Puzziferri N, Austrheim-Smith IT, Wolfe BM, et al: Three-year follow-up of a prospective randomized trial comparing laparoscopic versus open gastric bypass. Ann Surg 243:181–188, 2006.

**37.** Torquati A, Lutfi R, Abumrad N, et al: Is Roux-en-Y gastric bypass surgery the most effective treatment for type 2 diabetes mellitus in morbidly obese patients? J Gastrointest Surg 9:1112–1116, 2005.

**38.** Rubino F, Schauer PR, Kaplan LM, et al: Metabolic surgery to treat type 2 diabetes: Clinical outcomes and mechanisms of action. Annu Rev Med 61:393–411, 2010.

**39.** Kim S, Richards WO: Long-term follow-up of the metabolic profiles in obese patients with type 2 diabetes mellitus after Roux-en-Y gastric bypass. Ann Surg 251:1049–1055, 2010.

**40.** Madan AK, Orth W, Ternovits CA, et al: Metabolic syndrome: Yet another comorbidity gastric bypass helps cure. Surg Obes Relat Dis 2:48–51, 2006.

**41.** Mattar SG, Velcu LM, Rabinovitz M, et al: Surgically-induced weight loss significantly improves nonalcoholic fatty liver disease and the metabolic syndrome. Ann Surg 242:610–617, 2005.

**42.** Prachand VN, Davee RT, Alverdy JC: Duodenal switch provides superior weight loss in the super-obese (BMI > or = 50 kg/m2) compared with gastric bypass. Ann Surg 244:611–619, 2006.

**43.** Hutter MM, Randall S, Khuri SF, et al: Laparoscopic versus open gastric bypass for morbid obesity: A multicenter, prospective, risk-adjusted analysis from the National Surgical Quality Improvement Program. Ann Surg 243:657–662, 2006.

**44.** Poulose BK, Griffin MR, Moore DE, et al: Risk factors for post-operative mortality in bariatric surgery. J Surg Res 127:1–7, 2005.

**45.** Slater GH, Ren CJ, Siegel N, et al: Serum fat-soluble vitamin deficiency and abnormal calcium metabolism after malabsorptive bariatric surgery. J Gastrointest Surg 8:48–55, 2004.

**46.** Flum DR, Salem L, Elrod JA, et al: Early mortality among Medicare beneficiaries undergoing bariatric surgical procedures. JAMA 294:1903–1908, 2005.

**47.** Nguyen NT, Paya M, Stevens CM, et al: The relationship between hospital volume and outcome in bariatric surgery at academic medical centers. Ann Surg 240:586–593, 2004.

**48.** Herron DM, Birkett DH, Thompson CC, et al: Gastric bypass pouch and stoma reduction using a transoral endoscopic anchor placement system: A feasibility study. Surg Endosc 22:1093–1099, 2008.

**49.** le Roux CW, Aylwin SJ, Batterham RL, et al: Gut hormone profiles following bariatric surgery favor an anorectic state, facilitate weight loss, and improve metabolic parameters. Ann Surg 243:108–114, 2006.

**50.** Nguyen NT, Root J, Zainabadi K, et al: Accelerated growth of bariatric surgery with the introduction of minimally invasive surgery. Arch Surg 140:1198–1202, 2005.

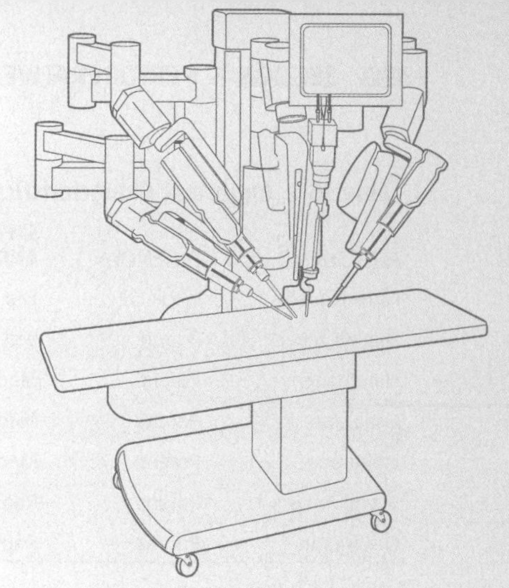

CHAPTER 16

# ANESTHESIOLOGY PRINCIPLES, PAIN MANAGEMENT, AND CONSCIOUS SEDATION

Edward R. Sherwood, Courtney G. Williams, and Donald S. Prough



The relatively brief history of anesthesiology began more than 150 years ago with the administration of the first ether anesthetic. Throughout much of its subsequent history, the risk of anesthesia-related mortality and morbidity was unacceptably high because of primitive equipment, complication-prone drugs, and lack of adequate monitors. However, during the past 5 decades, rapid technologic and pharmacologic progress have resulted in the ability to provide anesthesia safely for complex surgical procedures, even in patients with severe underlying disease.

The most notable advances in anesthesia equipment have been the development of anesthetic machines that reduce the possibility of providing hypoxic gas mixtures, vaporizers that provide accurate doses of potent inhalational agents, and intraoperative anesthesia ventilators that provide more precise and sophisticated respiratory support. Pharmacologic advances have generally consisted of shorter acting drugs, with fewer significant side effects. However, the greatest advances have been in monitoring devices. These include in-circuit oxygen analyzers, capnometers, pulse oximeters, and anesthetic vapor–specific analyzers. Although these monitors do not guarantee a successful outcome, they markedly increase its probability. This chapter will review the major principles defining the modern practice of anesthesiology.

## PHARMACOLOGIC PRINCIPLES

The initial practice of anesthesiology used single drugs such as ether or chloroform to abolish consciousness, prevent movement during surgery, ensure amnesia, and provide analgesia. In contrast, current anesthesia practice combines a number of agents, often including regional techniques, to achieve specific end points. Although inhalational agents remain the core of modern anesthetic combinations, most anesthesiologists initiate anesthesia with intravenous (IV) induction agents and then maintain anesthesia with inhalational agents supplemented by IV opioids and muscle relaxants. Benzodiazepines are often added to induce anxiolysis and amnesia.

### Inhalational Agents

The original inhalational anesthetics—ether, nitrous oxide, and chloroform—had important limitations. Subsequent drug development has emphasized inhalational agents that facilitate rapid induction and emergence and are nontoxic; these include isoflurane, sevoflurane, and desflurane. Although halothane and enflurane were also commonly used in the past, the use of both agents has decreased dramatically during the last 5 to 10 years. The important aspects of each volatile anesthetic can be summarized in terms of their key clinical attributes (Table 16-1). Two of the most important characteristics of inhalational anesthetics are the blood-gas (B-G) solubility (partition) coefficient and the minimum alveolar concentration (MAC). The B-G solubility coefficient is a measure of the uptake of an agent by blood. In general, less soluble agents (lower B-G solubility coefficients), such as nitrous oxide and desflurane, are associated with more rapid induction of and emergence from anesthesia, whereas induction and emergence are slower with agents having high solubility in blood, such as halothane. MAC is a measure of potency and is defined as the concentration of an agent required to prevent movement in response to a skin incision in 50% of patients. A higher MAC represents a less potent volatile anesthetic. Among volatile agents, halothane is the most potent, with a MAC of 0.75%, whereas desflurane has a MAC of 6% and is the least potent of the hydrocarbon-based volatile agents. Nitrous oxide has a MAC of 104% at sea level, meaning that nitrous oxide alone is generally not suitable for the maintenance of general anesthesia. The pungency of anesthetic agents also has practical implications. Agents with low pungency, such as halothane and sevoflurane, do not cause significant airway irritation when delivered at commonly used concentrations and are useful for inhalation induction of anesthesia. Desflurane is highly irritating to the airways and is not useful for inhalation induction under most conditions.

**Table 16-1 Important Characteristics of Inhalational Agents**

| ANESTHETIC | POTENCY | SPEED OF INDUCTION AND EMERGENCE | SUITABILITY FOR INHALATIONAL INDUCTION | SENSITIZATION TO CATECHOLAMINES | METABOLIZED (%) |
|---|---|---|---|---|---|
| Nitrous oxide | Weak | Fast | Insufficient alone | None | Minimal |
| Diethyl ether | Potent | Very slow | Suitable | None | 10 |
| Halothane | Potent | Medium | Suitable | High | 20+ |
| Enflurane | Potent | Medium | Not suitable | Medium | <10 |
| Isoflurane | Potent | Medium | Not suitable | Minimal | <2 |
| Sevoflurane | Potent | Rapid | Suitable | Minimal | <5 |
| Desflurane | Potent | Rapid | Not suitable | Minimal | 0.02 |

### Nitrous Oxide

Nitrous oxide provides only partial anesthesia at atmospheric pressure because its MAC is 104% of inspired gas at sea level. Nitrous oxide minimally influences respiration and hemodynamics. In addition, it has low solubility in blood. Therefore, it is often combined with one of the potent volatile agents to permit a lower dose of the potent volatile agent, thus limiting side effects, reducing cost, and facilitating rapid induction and emergence. The most important clinical problem with nitrous oxide is that it is 30 times more soluble than nitrogen and diffuses into closed gas spaces faster than nitrogen diffuses out. Because nitrous oxide increases the volume or pressure of these spaces, it is contraindicated in the presence of closed gas spaces such as pneumothorax, small bowel obstruction, and middle ear surgery, as well as in retinal surgery, in which an intraocular gas bubble is created. Because nitrous oxide gradually accumulates in the pneumoperitoneum, some clinicians prefer to avoid its use during laparoscopic procedures. However, periodic venting can prevent buildup, and some investigators have suggested that nitrous oxide might be preferable to carbon dioxide as the insufflated gas.[1]

### Isoflurane

Approved by the U.S. Food and Drug Administration (FDA) in 1979, isoflurane has rapidly replaced halothane as the most commonly used potent inhalational agent. Despite the release of sevoflurane and desflurane, isoflurane is commonly used in modern operating rooms, at least in part because the cost of the now-generic compound is well below that of the newer agents. Isoflurane has several advantages over halothane, including less reduction in cardiac output, less sensitization to the arrhythmogenic effects of catecholamines, and minimal metabolic effects. However, isoflurane-induced tachycardia, a variable response, can increase myocardial oxygen consumption. Careful observation of the heart rate is necessary when used in patients with coronary artery disease (CAD). In concentrations of 1.0 MAC or less, isoflurane causes little increase in cerebral blood flow and intracranial pressure (ICP) and depresses cerebral metabolic activity more than halothane or enflurane. Its pungent odor almost precludes its use for inhalational induction.

### Sevoflurane

Sevoflurane's relatively low solubility facilitates rapid induction and emergence. Sevoflurane is associated with faster emergence than isoflurane, especially in longer cases, although its slightly faster emergence does not result in earlier discharge after outpatient surgery. Sevoflurane is associated with a lower incidence of postoperative somnolence and nausea in the post-anesthesia care unit (PACU) and in the first 24 hours after discharge than isoflurane. Unlike isoflurane, sevoflurane is pleasant to inhale, thus making it suitable for inhalational induction in children. Sevoflurane is clinically suitable for outpatient surgery, mask induction of patients with potentially difficult airways, and maintenance of patients with bronchospastic disease. When sevoflurane, halothane, and isoflurane were compared, all these potent agents decreased respiratory resistance in endotracheally intubated nonasthmatics. However, sevoflurane reduced airway resistance more than halothane or isoflurane.[2]

Considerable metabolic transformation of sevoflurane takes place and results in increases in the serum fluoride ion concentration and, in the presence of soda lime, production of compound A, a metabolite that is nephrotoxic in experimental animals. However, β-lyase, the enzyme responsible for the formation of compound A,[3] has 8 to 30 times greater activity in rat kidneys than in human kidney tissue. Therefore, the nephrotoxicity of compound A in humans appears to be theoretical and not clinically important.

### Desflurane

Desflurane is rapidly taken up and eliminated. After anesthesia lasting more than 3 hours, desflurane was associated with more rapid recovery than isoflurane.[4] Its pungent odor precludes inhalational induction. In addition, desflurane is associated with tachycardia and hypertension if the concentration is increased too rapidly. When exposed to dry carbon dioxide absorbent, volatile anesthetics are partially converted to carbon monoxide. Desflurane, enflurane, and isoflurane produce more carbon monoxide than halothane or sevoflurane does. Carbon monoxide production is greater with dry $CO_2$ absorbent, with Baralyme more than with soda lime, at higher temperatures, and at higher anesthetic concentrations.[5] Because continued gas flow in an unused machine will desiccate the $CO_2$ absorbent, turning gas flow off in anesthesia machines when they are not in use can reduce carbon monoxide production. It is also prudent to run fresh gas through an anesthesia machine that has not been used for 1 or 2 days to wash out any carbon monoxide that might be present prior to patient contact.

## Intravenous Agents

IV agents are an indispensable component of modern anesthetic practice. They are used primarily for induction of

**Table 16-2 Clinical Characteristics of Intravenous Induction Agents**

| IV INDUCTION AGENT | DOSE (MG/KG) | COMMENTS | SIDE EFFECTS | SITUATIONS REQUIRING CAUTION | RELATIVE INDICATIONS |
|---|---|---|---|---|---|
| Thiopental | 2-5 | Inexpensive; slow emergence after high doses | Hypotension | Hypovolemia; compromised cardiac function | Suitable for induction in many patients |
| Ketamine | 1-2 | Psychotropic side effects controllable with benzodiazepines; good bronchodilator; potent analgesic at subinduction doses | Hypertension; tachycardia | Coronary disease; severe hypovolemia | Rapid-sequence induction of asthmatics, patients in shock (reduced doses) |
| Propofol | 1-2 | Burns on injection; good bronchodilator; associated with low incidence of postoperative nausea and vomiting | Hypotension | Coronary artery disease; hypovolemia | Induction of outpatients; induction of asthmatics |
| Etomidate | 0.1-0.3 | Cardiovascularly stable; burns on injection; spontaneous movement during induction | Adrenal suppression (with continuous infusion) | Hypovolemia | Induction of patients with cardiac contractile dysfunction; induction of patients in shock (reduced doses) |
| Midazolam | 0.15-0.3 | Relatively stable hemodynamics; potent amnesia | Synergistic ventilatory depression with opioids | Hypovolemia | Induction of patients with cardiac contractile dysfunction (usually in combination with opioids) |

anesthesia and as part of a multidrug combination to produce balanced anesthesia.

## Induction Agents

Induction with thiopental, the oldest IV induction agent, is rapid and pleasant. Although the drug is remarkably well tolerated by a wide variety of patients, several clinical situations necessitate caution (Table 16-2). In hypovolemic patients and those with congestive heart failure, thiopental-induced vasodilation and cardiac depression can lead to severe hypotension unless doses are markedly reduced. In these patients, etomidate or ketamine is an alternative agent. Although thiopental does not directly precipitate bronchospasm, it does not blunt airway reactivity in response to the intense airway stimulation produced by endotracheal intubation as effectively as propofol or ketamine, which are attractive alternatives for patients with reactive airway disease.

In the usual doses used for induction of anesthesia, thiopental is associated with rapid emergence because of redistribution of the agent from the brain to peripheral tissues, particularly fat. In higher doses or after prolonged infusion, circulating blood levels increase and the action of thiopental must be terminated by hepatic metabolism, which eliminates only approximately 10%/hr. Therefore, prolonged sedation may exist under those conditions.

Ketamine, which produces a dissociative state of anesthesia, is the only IV induction agent that increases blood pressure and heart rate and decreases bronchomotor tone. Usually associated with increased sympathetic tone, ketamine causes direct cardiac depression that may become evident if given to patients with high preanesthetic sympathetic tone, as in patients in hemorrhagic shock. In markedly reduced doses (15% to 20% of the usual induction dose), ketamine is an appropriate choice for IV induction of severely hypovolemic patients, in whom it causes the least fall in blood pressure of any of the induction agents. Ketamine is an appropriate agent for IV induction of asthmatic patients because it reduces bronchomotor tone and decreases the airway reactivity associated with endotracheal intubation. Among the IV induction agents, ketamine also causes the least amount of ventilatory depression and loss of airway reflexes. However, because of the induction of copious oropharyngeal secretions, an antisialogogue such as glycopyrrolate is generally administered with ketamine. Ketamine can be used as the sole anesthetic for brief superficial procedures because it produces profound amnesia and somatic analgesia. It is less useful, however, for abdominal cases or delicate surgery because it produces no muscular relaxation, does not control visceral pain, and may not completely control patient movement. The potent pain-relieving effects of ketamine have been exploited for preemptive analgesia. In patients in whom ketamine was infused continuously before incision and continued through wound closure, postoperative morphine consumption was significantly lower on postoperative days 1 and 2 than in patients who did not receive ketamine.[6]

In patients with CAD, ketamine is usually avoided because tachycardia and hypertension may cause myocardial ischemia. In patients with increased ICP (e.g., after traumatic brain injury), ketamine may further increase ICP because it is the only IV agent that increases cerebral blood flow. Another clinically important side effect of ketamine is emergence delirium. In adults and older children, supplemental benzodiazepines or volatile agents are generally effective in preventing emergence delirium.

Propofol, commonly used as an induction agent for ambulatory surgery, is a short-acting induction agent associated with smooth, nausea-free emergence. Small doses are also useful for short-term sedation during brief procedures such as retrobulbar or peribulbar eye blocks. The primary limitations of propofol are pain on injection and blood pressure reduction. The latter precludes use in patients who may be hypovolemic and prompts caution in patients who may tolerate hypotension poorly, such as those with severe CAD.

Propofol also produces excellent bronchodilation. In asthmatic patients, 0% of those who received propofol wheezed at

2 or 5 minutes after intubation versus 45% of those who received a thiobarbiturate and 26% of those who received an oxybarbiturate.[7] In nonasthmatic patients, 75% of whom smoked, airway resistance was less after induction with propofol than after induction with thiopental or etomidate. Brown and Wagner[8] have demonstrated that the bronchodilatory effects of propofol and ketamine are mediated through the blockade of vagus nerve–mediated cholinergic bronchoconstriction.

Etomidate is an imidazole compound that produces minimal hemodynamic changes. Because it preserves blood pressure in most patients, etomidate is often chosen as an alternative for induction of patients with cardiovascular disease. Major drawbacks include burning pain on injection, abnormal muscular movements (myoclonus), and adrenal suppression when given as a prolonged infusion for sedation of critically ill patients.

Although not used as an induction agent, dexmedetomidine has gained increased value as a sedative agent in anesthetic care.[9] Dexmedetomidine is a selective $\alpha_2$-adrenergic receptor agonist that has sedative, amnestic, and analgesic properties. It has value as a preoperative sedative, anesthetic adjunct and sedative-hypnotic for the management of sedation in critically ill patients. It causes minimal respiratory depression but can have significant cardiovascular effects, including bradycardia and hypotension, if given too rapidly or used for patients with significant hypovolemia.[9]

### Opioids

Opioids are used in most patients undergoing general anesthesia and are given as adjuncts to patients receiving regional or local anesthesia. As a component of a multifaceted anesthetic, opioids produce profound analgesia and minimal cardiac depression. Their disadvantages include ventilatory depression and inconsistent hypnosis and amnesia, which must usually be provided by other agents.

Several reasons explain the universal popularity of opioids in anesthetic management. First, they reduce the MAC of potent inhalational agents. For example, fentanyl (3 ng/mL plasma concentration) decreased the MAC of sevoflurane by 59% and reduced $MAC_{awake}$ (the alveolar concentration at which an emerging patient responds to commands) by 24%.[10] Second, they blunt the hypertension and tachycardia associated with manipulations such as endotracheal intubation and surgical incision. Third, they provide analgesia that extends throughout the early postemergence interval and facilitates smoother awakening from anesthesia. Fourth, in doses 10 to 20 times the analgesic dose, opioids act as complete anesthetics in a high proportion of patients by providing not only analgesia but also hypnosis and amnesia. This characteristic has prompted their use for cardiac surgery patients, sometimes as sole anesthetic agents and more often as a major component of the anesthetic. Finally, they are now often added to local anesthetic solutions in epidural and intrathecal blocks to improve the quality of analgesia.

Morphine, hydromorphone, and meperidine are inexpensive, intermediate-acting agents that are less commonly used for maintenance of anesthesia than for postoperative analgesia. Fentanyl, a synthetic opioid that is 100 to 150 times more potent than morphine, is commonly used for maintenance of anesthesia because of its shorter duration of action and rapid onset. Newer synthetic, short-acting opioids, including sufentanil and alfentanil, are also used during anesthesia because they are quickly metabolized and excreted. Remifentanil, an opioid metabolized by serum esterases, is particularly short-acting. Remifentanil does not accumulate during prolonged infusions and is therefore often used as part of IV anesthetics. It is also useful as part of the anesthesia induction sequence because of its rapid onset and short duration of action.

### Neuromuscular Blockers

Decades ago, anesthesia was typically conducted with single, potent, inhalational agents that produced all the components of general anesthesia, including whatever degree of muscle relaxation was necessary for the conduct of surgery. Among the drawbacks of this approach was the fact that the depth of anesthesia necessary to produce profound muscle relaxation was much deeper than that necessary to provide hypnosis and amnesia, which caused prolonged emergence times and, possibly, undesirable hemodynamic alterations. The addition of muscle relaxants afforded the opportunity to deliver only enough of the inhalational and IV agents to achieve hypnosis, amnesia, and analgesia while still providing satisfactory operating conditions.

The two categories of neuromuscular blockers in clinical use are depolarizing (noncompetitive) and nondepolarizing (competitive) agents. The depolarizing agents exert agonistic effects at the cholinergic receptors of the neuromuscular junction, initially causing contractions evident as fasciculations, followed by an interval of profound relaxation. The nondepolarizing neuromuscular blockers compete for receptor sites with acetylcholine, with the magnitude of block dependent on the availability of acetylcholine and affinity of the agent for the receptor.

Succinylcholine, the only depolarizing agent still in clinical use, continues to be useful for endotracheal intubation because of its rapid onset and short duration of action. However, it is associated with serious hazards, including hyperkalemia and malignant hyperthermia, in a small proportion of patients. The drug can be administered in a relatively high dose for intubation because it is rapidly metabolized by plasma pseudocholinesterase, except in a small fraction of patients with atypical or absent pseudocholinesterase. Because its duration of action is only 5 minutes, a patient who cannot be successfully intubated can be ventilated by mask for a short time until spontaneous respiration resumes. However, a patient who cannot be ventilated by mask will not resume spontaneous breathing after an intubating dose of succinylcholine before the onset of life-threatening hypoxemia.[11]

Side effects of succinylcholine include bradycardia, especially in children, and severe, life-threatening hyperkalemia in patients with burns, paraplegia, quadriplegia, and massive trauma. Succinylcholine, when combined with a volatile agent, is also implicated in triggering malignant hyperthermia in susceptible individuals. Therefore, it is best avoided in patients at risk for malignant hyperthermia, including those with muscular dystrophy or a family history of malignant hyperthermia. Some anesthesiologists avoid succinylcholine in children, especially boys, because of the possibility of an undiagnosed myopathology that could predispose the patient to severe hyperkalemia or malignant hyperthermia. Masseter spasm is also a common occurrence that may presage malignant hyperthermia in children, but it is usually a benign effect. Because succinylcholine is a depolarizing agent that causes visible muscle fasciculations, it has been implicated in causing postoperative muscle pain, which can be reduced by pretreatment with a small dose of a nondepolarizing agent. As a result of the many sporadic

**Table 16-3 Dose-Response Relationships of Nondepolarizing Neuromuscular Blocking Drugs in Humans**

| DRUG | DURATION | $ED_{50}$ (MG/KG) | $ED_{95}$ (MG/KG) | INTUBATING DOSE (MG/KG) |
|---|---|---|---|---|
| Pancuronium | Long | 0.036 (0.022-0.042) | 0.067 (0.059-0.080) | 0.08-0.12 |
| Vecuronium | Intermediate | 0.027 (0.015-0.031) | 0.043 (0.037-0.059) | 0.1-0.2 |
| Cisatracurium | Intermediate | 0.026 (0.15-0.31) | 0.04 (0.32-0.55) | 0.15-0.2 |
| Mivacurium | Short | 0.039 (0.027-0.052) | 0.067 (0.045-0.081) | 0.15-0.2 |
| Rocuronium | Intermediate | 0.147 (0.069-0.220) | 0.305 (0.257-0.521) | 0.6-1.0 |

Adapted from Naguib M, Lien CA: Pharmacology of muscle relaxants and their antagonists. In Miller RD, Fleisher LA, Johns RA, et al (eds): Miller's anesthesia, ed 6, Philadelphia, 2005, Churchill Livingstone, pp 481–572.

*$ED_{50}$*, Dose effective for surgical relaxation in 50% of patients; *$ED_{95}$*, dose effective for surgical relaxation in 95% of patients; values expressed as mean (95% confidence limits). Somewhat larger doses are required to facilitate endotracheal intubation.

problems associated with the use of succinylcholine, some anesthesiologists now reserve its use only for situations in which an airway must be rapidly secured (i.e., rapid-sequence induction). In other situations, nondepolarizing agents, chosen largely on the basis of their mode of excretion and duration of action, are preferable.

Nondepolarizing relaxants are used when succinylcholine is contraindicated, as an alternative to succinylcholine for patients in whom easy endotracheal intubation is anticipated, and when prolonged intraoperative relaxation is required to facilitate surgical exposure. Knowledge of the side effects of individual agents, often related to vagolysis or release of histamine, and routes of metabolism plays a major role in the selection of specific agents for individual cases. Doses required to provide satisfactory operating conditions are summarized in Table 16-3. Dosing of nondepolarizing agents requires knowledge of several important characteristics. First, the use of neuromuscular blockers prevents movement in response to noxious stimuli. Therefore, chemical paralysis can mask the signs of inadequate anesthesia, or sedation or analgesia in postoperative patients. Medicolegal claims of intraoperative awareness during general anesthesia were more than twice as frequent in patients receiving intraoperative muscle relaxants.[12] Second, higher doses are required to provide satisfactory conditions for intubation than for surgical relaxation. Therefore, if a nondepolarizer is used only after intubation, smaller doses are required. Third, other anesthetic drugs potentiate the actions of nondepolarizing agents. Potent inhalational agents potentiate the effects of competitive neuromuscular blockers in a dose-dependent fashion. The newer inhalational agent desflurane potentiates the effects of vecuronium approximately 20% more than isoflurane.[13] Fourth, individual responses to muscle relaxants vary widely, with patients demonstrating markedly increased and decreased neuromuscular blockade in comparison to expected levels.

Fifth, and most important, subtle blockade can be difficult to detect and can be associated with postoperative weakness. The importance of subtle residual paralysis has been quantified by using the train-of-four (TOF) fade ratio, a semiquantitative monitoring technique used to assess the adequacy of neuromuscular blockade and the adequacy of pharmacologic reversal. A 1997 report characterized the symptoms of volunteers receiving graded doses of muscle relaxants at various TOF ratios.[14] A sustained 5-second head lift, a commonly used clinical index of adequate reversal, was achieved if the TOF ratio was higher than 0.60. At TOF ratios higher than 0.70, all subjects maintained patent airways and oxygen saturation higher than 96%. However, in a 2003 study, at TOF ratios less than 0.90, subjects had diplopia and difficulty tracking objects in all directions. The ability to oppose the incisors strongly did not return until the TOF ratio was higher than 0.90. It was concluded that satisfactory return of neuromuscular function requires return of the TOF ratio to higher than 0.90 and, ideally, to 1.0.[15] In patients who received the intermediate-acting neuromuscular blockers atracurium, vecuronium, or rocuronium only for endotracheal intubation, the TOF ratio was lower than 0.9 in 37% of patients 2 hours after receiving the muscle relaxant.[15]

The use of neuromuscular blocking agents in general, and nondepolarizing agents in particular, necessitates a strategy to ensure adequate muscular function at the conclusion of anesthesia. Many of the complications associated with neuromuscular blockers relate to inadequate reversal at the conclusion of cases or inadequate assessment of reversal. Nondepolarizing relaxants are generally pharmacologically reversed with an anticholinesterase (neostigmine or edrophonium), accompanied by atropine or glycopyrrolate to counteract the muscarinic effects of the anticholinesterase. However, recovery depends on the intensity of neuromuscular blockade at the time that reversal is attempted and on the effects of the reversal agent. At the end of anesthesia, profound neuromuscular blockade may preclude reliable antagonism by an anticholinesterase.

With the longer acting muscle relaxants, such as pancuronium, residual blockade can potentially complicate postoperative recovery. In a clinical trial, 691 patients undergoing abdominal, gynecologic, or orthopedic surgery under general anesthesia were randomized to receive pancuronium, vecuronium, or atracurium. After reversal with neostigmine, a higher proportion (26%) of patients who had received pancuronium had residual neuromuscular blockade (TOF $< 0.70$) than patients who had received vecuronium or atracurium (5.3% combined).[16] Patients who received pancuronium and had a TOF ratio less than 0.70 had a higher incidence of atelectasis or pneumonia on postoperative chest radiographs (16.9% of 59 patients in that category). There was no association between postoperative pulmonary complications and residual blockade with the other two muscle relaxants, with intermediate durations of action.

One key factor determining recovery from neuromuscular blockade is the ability to metabolize and excrete the drugs. In patients with renal disease, the half-lives of rocuronium,

**BOX 16-1 Electronic Monitors Used for Anesthesia and Their Indications**

**Routine Monitors**

Pulse oximetry
- Blood oxygen saturation
- Heart rate
- Tissue perfusion (via plethysmography)

Automated blood pressure cuff
- Blood pressure

Electrocardiography
- Heart rhythm
- Heart rate
- Monitor of myocardial ischemia

Capnography
- Adequacy of ventilation
- Intratracheal placement of endotracheal tube

Pulmonary perfusion

Oxygen analyzer
- Monitoring of delivered oxygen concentration

Ventilator pressure monitor
- Ventilator disconnection during general anesthesia
- Monitoring of airway pressure

Temperature monitoring

**Specialized Monitors**

Monitoring of urine output (Foley catheter)
- Gross indicator of intravascular volume status and renal perfusion

Arterial catheter
- Continuous measurement of arterial blood pressure
- Sampling of arterial blood

Central venous catheter
- Continuous measurement of central venous pressure
- Delivery of centrally acting drugs
- Rapid administration of fluids and blood

Pulmonary artery catheter
- Measurement of pulmonary artery pressure
- Measurement of left ventricular pressure
- Measurement of cardiac output
- Measurement of mixed venous oxygenation

Precordial Doppler
- Detection of air embolism

Transesophageal echocardiography
- Evaluation of myocardial performance
- Assessment of heart valve function
- Assessment of intravascular volume
- Detection of air embolism

Esophageal Doppler
- Assessment of descending aortic blood flow
- Assessment of cardiac preload

Transpulmonary indicator dilution
- Measurement of cardiac output
- Measurement of preload

Esophageal and precordial stethoscope
- Auscultation of breathing and heart sounds

Electroencephalography, bispectral array

Depth of anesthesia

vecuronium, and pancuronium are prolonged. In such patients, alternative drugs include atracurium or cisatracurium, which are metabolized by Hofman degradation and thus do not have prolonged half-lives in patients with renal dysfunction.

## ANESTHESIA EQUIPMENT

Anesthesia equipment has undergone rapid development over the past several decades. The central piece of equipment for delivery of anesthesia is the modern anesthesia machine, which functions primarily to deliver oxygen and volatile anesthetics to the patient. In addition, modern anesthetic machines have sophisticated ventilators that allow for effective respiratory support and integrated monitors that accurately measure oxygen delivery, inspired and end-tidal gas concentrations, airway pressures, minute ventilation, and fresh gas flows. Despite many years of improving design, the hazards of gas delivery systems must still be considered. The primary concern is inadvertent delivery of a hypoxic gas mixture. Adverse anesthetic outcomes were associated with gas delivery equipment in 72 of 3791 cases in the American Society of Anesthesiologists (ASA) closed claims database. Misuse of equipment occurred in 75% of incidents, and 78% could have been detected with monitoring of pulse oximetry or capnography.[17]

In addition to the anesthesia machine, the other major components of anesthesia equipment are monitors. The use of monitors to assess changes in respiratory and cardiovascular function during anesthesia and surgery has been instrumental in improving overall safety.

## PATIENT MONITORING DURING AND AFTER ANESTHESIA

Effective monitoring is a critical aspect of anesthesia care. The essential components of monitoring include observation and vigilance, instrumentation, data analysis, and institution of corrective measures, if indicated. The goal of patient monitoring is to provide optimal anesthetic management and detect abnormalities early in their course so that corrective measures can be instituted before serious or irreversible injury occurs. Although it is difficult to relate improved patient outcomes with specific monitors directly, the reduction in anesthesia-related morbidity and mortality has paralleled the institution of current monitoring practices.

The indications, risks, and benefits associated with the use of noninvasive and invasive electronic monitors must be assessed for each individual patient (Box 16-1). These decisions are guided by the patient's medical condition, type of surgery, and potential complications associated with invasive monitoring. However, the proliferation of electronic monitoring devices does not circumvent the need for clinical skills such as observation, inspection, auscultation, and palpation. The ASA has established standards for basic anesthetic monitoring.[18] These have been designed to integrate clinical skills and electronic monitoring with the goal of enhancing patient safety.

Standard I asserts that a qualified anesthesia care provider must be continuously present in the operating room during the administration of anesthesia. The physician must continuously monitor the status of the patient and alter anesthesia care based on the patient's response to the dynamic changes associated with anesthesia and surgery.

Standard II mandates continuous assessment of ventilation, oxygenation, circulation, and temperature during all anesthetics. Specific requirements include the following:

1. The use of an oxygen analyzer with a low–oxygen concentration alarm during general anesthesia.
2. Quantitative assessment of blood oxygenation such as by pulse oximetry.
3. The adequacy of ventilation must be continuously ensured by clinical evaluation. Quantitative monitoring of the $CO_2$ content in expired gas and volume of expired gas is strongly recommended.
4. Clinical assessment and monitors to determine the presence of $CO_2$ in expired gases to ensure correct endotracheal tube placement after intubation. A device capable of detecting disconnection of breathing system components during mechanical ventilation must be in continuous use. This device must give an audible signal when its alarm threshold is exceeded.
5. The electrocardiogram (ECG) must be continuously monitored during anesthesia, and blood pressure and heart rate must be evaluated at least every 5 minutes. In patients undergoing general anesthesia, adequacy of circulatory function must be continuously monitored by electronic means, palpation, or auscultation.
6. A means of temperature evaluation must be readily available in the operating room; it is used during periods of intended or expected changes in body temperature.

## Blood Pressure Monitoring

Blood pressure monitoring is required during the administration of all anesthetics. Noninvasive blood pressure monitoring is appropriate for most surgical cases, and most modern operating rooms are equipped with automated oscillometric blood pressure analyzers. Indications for invasive blood pressure monitoring include intraoperative use of deliberate hypotension, continuous blood pressure assessment in patients with significant end-organ damage or during high-risk surgical procedures, anticipation of wide perioperative blood pressure swings, need for multiple blood gas analyses, and inadequacy of noninvasive blood pressure measurements, such as in morbidly obese patients. Several sites for arterial cannulation are available, each with inherent advantages and potential for complications. The radial artery is most commonly cannulated because of its superficial location, relative ease of cannulation and, in most patients, adequate collateral flow from the ulnar artery. Other potential sites for percutaneous arterial cannulation include the femoral, brachial, axillary, ulnar, dorsalis pedis, and posterior tibial arteries. Possible complications of intra-arterial monitoring include hematoma, neurologic injury, arterial embolization, limb ischemia, infection, and inadvertent intra-arterial injection of drugs. Intra-arterial catheters are not placed in extremities with potential vascular insufficiency. However, with proper patient selection, the complication rate associated with intra-arterial cannulation is low and its benefits can be important.

## Electrocardiography

Electrocardiographic monitoring is a standard of care during the administration of anesthesia. Information regarding dysrhythmias and cardiac ischemia can be readily obtained from these data. Analysis of electrocardiographic tracings is the cornerstone of cardiopulmonary resuscitation protocols.

## Ventilation Monitoring

Sedation and opioid administration and induction of general or regional anesthesia can depress or abolish spontaneous ventilation and thus necessitate intraoperative ventilatory support. Several means are available to assess the adequacy of ventilation, including physical assessment of chest expansion, auscultation of breath sounds, and evaluation for evidence of upper airway obstruction and stridor. Precordial and esophageal stethoscopes provide continuous input regarding air movement and the development of wheezing. During mechanical ventilation, monitors of airway pressure and minute ventilation alert the anesthesiologist to conditions that can impair ventilation, such as disconnection of the ventilatory circuit, dislodgment of the endotracheal tube, obstruction of the gas delivery system, and changes in airway resistance or compliance, or both.

The advent of end-tidal carbon dioxide ($ETCO_2$) monitoring has greatly enhanced the monitoring of ventilation and detection of esophageal intubation. In normal individuals, the difference between $ETCO_2$ and $PaCO_2$ is 2 to 5 mm Hg. The gradient between end-tidal and arterial $CO_2$ reflects dead space ventilation, which is increased in cases of decreased pulmonary blood flow, such as pulmonary air embolism or thromboembolism and decreased cardiac output. Therefore, $ETCO_2$ monitoring can also provide important information regarding pulmonary perfusion.

## Oxygenation Monitoring

Monitoring of $FIO_2$ and hemoglobin oxygen saturation is a standard of care during all general anesthetics. Modern anesthesia machines are equipped with oxygen analyzers that detect the delivered oxygen concentration ($FIO_2$). This monitor, in combination with fail-safe devices, low–oxygen delivery alarms, and oxygen ratio monitors, greatly decreases the chance of delivering a hypoxic gas mixture during anesthesia.

## Temperature Monitoring

Temperature is monitored in all patients undergoing general anesthesia. The site of measurement is dependent on the surgical procedure and physical characteristics of the patient. Esophageal temperature is most commonly measured during general anesthesia. Other sites of temperature monitoring include rectal, cutaneous, tympanic membrane, bladder, and nasopharyngeal sites and, in patients with pulmonary artery catheters, the pulmonary artery. Because of the potential morbidity associated with hypothermia and hyperthermia, it is important to monitor body temperature and institute measures to maintain temperature as close to normal as possible.

## Neuromuscular Blockade Monitoring

Because of variability in sensitivity to neuromuscular blockers among patients, it is essential to monitor neuromuscular function in patients receiving intermediate- and long-acting muscle relaxants. The most common sites of monitoring are at the ulnar or orbicularis oculi muscles. The basis of neuromuscular monitoring is assessment of muscle activity after proximal nerve stimulation (Box 16-2). This evaluation indicates acetylcholine receptor blockade at the neuromuscular junction. The degree of

**BOX 16-2 Techniques for Assessing Neuromuscular Blockade**

**Train-of-Four Fade Ratio (Four Successive 200-μsec Stimuli Over 2-Sec Period)**

Twitch height progressively fades with increasing blockade:

- Loss of fourth twitch indicates 75% receptor blockade
- Loss of third twitch indicates 80% blockade
- Loss of second twitch indicates 90% blockade
- Loss of first twitch indicates 100% blockade
- Clinical relaxation requires 75% to 95% blockade

Presence of four twitches without fade suggests adequate reversal of neuromuscular blockade.

**Double-Burst Stimulation: Two Successive Sets of 50-Hz Bursts (Three Stimuli/Burst) Separated by 750 μsec (Appears as Two Twitches)**

Easier to detect fade visually with this technique than with train-of-four fade ratio

Loss of second twitch indicates 80% receptor blockade

Presence of twitches without fade suggests adequate reversal of neuromuscular blockade

**Tetany: Sustained 50- or 100-Hz Burst**

Duration of sustained contraction fades with increasing blockade

Sustained contraction for 5 sec suggests adequate reversal of neuromuscular blockade

neuromuscular blockade is indicated by a decreased evoked response to twitch stimulation.

### Central Nervous System Monitoring

Awareness during anesthesia is an uncommon but disturbing complication. Many years of experience with intraoperative electroencephalographic signal processing has resulted in development of the bispectral array (BIS), which is thought to monitor awareness during anesthesia. The monitor is essentially a modified electroencephalogram (EEG) that assesses brain wave activity and reports numbers from 0 to 100, which correlate with the level of awareness. A value of 100 represents complete awareness and 0 represents complete suppression of brain wave activity. Evidence has suggested that BIS is an accurate indicator of the depth of anesthesia.[19] Monitoring the depth of anesthesia may improve time to awakening and discharge in the outpatient setting. Furthermore, some reports have indicated that BIS values lower than 40 for more than 5 minutes during general anesthesia may be associated with increased perioperative morbidity, including myocardial infarction (MI) and stroke in high-risk patients.[20] In addition, BIS monitors are gaining acceptance as a means of assessing awareness in locations such as emergency departments and intensive care units.

## PREOPERATIVE EVALUATION

The ASA has established basic standards for preanesthetic care in which an anesthesiologist is required to evaluate the medical status of the patient, derive a plan for anesthetic care, and discuss the plan with the patient.[21] The Joint Commission (TJC) requires that all patients receiving anesthesia undergo a preanesthetic evaluation. Because a decreasing percentage of patients are admitted to the hospital on the day before surgery, preoperative testing clinics have been developed to facilitate preoperative evaluation. The advent of preoperative clinics has facilitated the efficient use of operating room resources. Ferschel and colleagues[22] have reported that development of an anesthesia preoperative evaluation clinic in a teaching hospital reduced day of surgery cancellations and delays. Optimally, preoperative clinics need to be efficient, predictable, and thorough. In modern practice, many patients without complicated medical problems who are scheduled for elective, low-risk procedures can be interviewed by telephone or online teleconference prior to surgery and given preoperative instructions.

A well-focused history will allow the physician to perform targeted physical and laboratory examinations. Laboratory tests performed within 6 months of surgery generally do not need to be repeated unless a significant change in the patient's medical status has occurred. Healthy patients undergoing elective procedures may not need any preoperative laboratory testing. In the current climate of cost containment, preoperative testing must be minimized but effective. The use of routine preoperative testing is associated with significant costs, both in dollars and potential harm. False-positive test results can cause needless delays in surgery and could require follow-up, which will increase costs and could lead to harm or injury associated with further tests and procedures. Studies have shown that routine testing adds to costs but has little impact on patient care. However, targeted testing based on results of the history and physical examination can significantly improve overall patient care. Investigation of conditions associated with increased perioperative morbidity is important for reducing the risks related to anesthesia and surgery. Coexisting conditions that must be carefully evaluated include intravascular volume status, airway abnormalities, cardiovascular disease, pulmonary disease, neurologic disease, renal and hepatic disease, and disorders of nutrition, endocrinology, and metabolism. Preoperative pregnancy testing is controversial. The rationale for performing preoperative pregnancy testing is the potential for spontaneous abortion and birth anomalies associated with surgery and anesthesia. There is no clear evidence to demonstrate an association of anesthetic drugs with the development of fetal anomalies in humans, but animal studies have shown that some anesthetics, such as nitrous oxide, may cause developmental abnormalities. A clear sexual history and documentation of the last menstrual cycle is obtained from women of childbearing age. In ambiguous situations, a preoperative pregnancy test is indicated.

### Airway Examination

Assessing the airway is a crucial step in developing an anesthetic plan. Even if regional anesthesia is planned, general anesthesia and the need to maintain a patent airway might be necessary. The goal of the airway examination is to identify characteristics that could hinder assisted mask ventilation or tracheal intubation. A history of diseases or conditions that are associated with airway closure or difficult laryngoscopy will alert the physician to potential airway difficulties. Review of previous anesthetic records can provide invaluable information regarding previous airway management. The airway examination is completed by systematic inspection of the mouth opening, thyromental distance, neck mobility, and size of the tongue in relation to the oral cavity (Box 16-3). The patient is observed in frontal and profile views because many airway abnormalities, such as a receding mandible, will not be evident from a frontal view. The size of the tongue in relation to the oral cavity can be graded by

**BOX 16-3 Important Factors When Performing an Airway Examination**

**Patient History**
Previous anesthetic history
Medical history (e.g., history of oropharyngeal mass, pharyngeal disease)
Review of chart to assess prior airway management during previous anesthesia

**Physical Examination**
Mouth opening (should be 6-8 cm [three to four fingerbreadths])
Cervical spine mobility
Mallampati classification
Thyromental distance (should be 6-8 cm [three to four fingerbreadths])
Frontal and profile view
Assessment for disease-associated airway abnormalities
Presence of facial hair

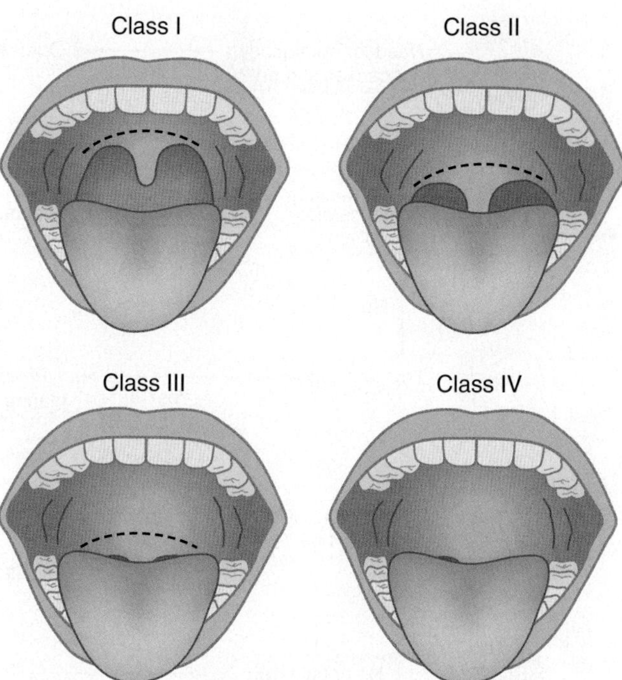


**FIGURE 16-1** The Mallampati classification relates tongue size to pharyngeal size. This test is performed with the patient in the sitting position, the head held in a neutral position, the mouth wide open, and the tongue protruding to the maximum. The subsequent classification is assigned according to the pharyngeal structures that are visible: class I, visualization of the soft palate, fauces, uvula, and anterior and posterior pillars; class II, visualization of the soft palate, fauces, and uvula; class III, visualization of the soft palate and the base of the uvula; and class IV, soft palate not visible at all. (From Mallampati SR, Gatt SP, Gugino LD, et al: A clinical sign to predict difficult tracheal intubation: A prospective study. Can Anaesth Soc J 32:429–434, 1985.)

using the Mallampati classification (Fig. 16-1). The Mallampati examination is performed with the patient sitting and the head in a neutral position, mouth opened as wide as possible, and tongue protruded maximally. The observer views the oral and pharyngeal structures that are evident. In general, a patient in whom the uvula, tonsillar pillars, and soft palate are visible (class I) will be easy to mask ventilate and intubate. Patients in whom only the hard palate is visible, a class IV airway, have a higher likelihood of being difficult to mask-ventilate and intubate. However, the Mallampati classification is only one component of the airway examination; it must be used in conjunction with other aspects of the airway examination and the patient's history to provide a complete airway assessment. Other physical factors associated with uncomplicated airway management are adequate mouth opening, neck extension, and thyromental distance. In a meta-analysis examining more than 50,000 patients, Shiga and associates[23] have reported that individual physical characteristics, by themselves, have poor predictive value for identifying airway difficulties. However, the combined presence of two or more physical end points that predict difficult airway management increasingly improves sensitivity and specificity.

## Cardiovascular Disease

The risk for perioperative myocardial ischemia and infarction and the risk for cardiac death have become important issues as progressively more complex surgery has been offered to patients with increasingly severe systemic disease. The apparent incidence of perioperative myocardial ischemia depends on the perspective of the study, prospective or retrospective, sensitivity of the markers used, and type of surgical procedure. Based on review of the available literature, the American College of Cardiology (ACC) and the American Heart Association (AHA) have published guidelines for the evaluation and treatment of CAD in noncardiac surgical patients.[24] These guidelines focus on the patient's history of CAD, exercise tolerance and type of surgery proposed. A detailed history and physical examination are required to assess the presence of underlying cardiovascular disease. Assessment of functional status and the ability to perform common daily tasks is a critical part of the assessment. Patients with active major cardiovascular conditions require evaluation and treatment before undergoing noncardiac surgery. The following are considered active cardiac conditions:

1. Unstable coronary syndromes
2. Decompensated congestive heart failure
3. Significant arrhythmias
4. Severe valvular disease

In the 2007 revision of the ACC/AHA guidelines, the previously used intermediate-risk category was replaced with clinical risk factors from the Revised Cardiac Risk Index, with the exclusion of the type of surgery, which is included elsewhere in the approach to the patient.[24] These clinical risk factors are incorporated into the overall evaluation of the patient (Fig. 16-2). The clinical risk factors that are part of the Revised Cardiac Risk Index include the following:

1. History of ischemic heart disease
2. History of compensated or prior heart failure
3. History of cerebrovascular disease
4. Diabetes mellitus
5. Renal insufficiency

Distinguishing unstable coronary syndromes from a history of ischemic heart disease can be difficult in some situations.

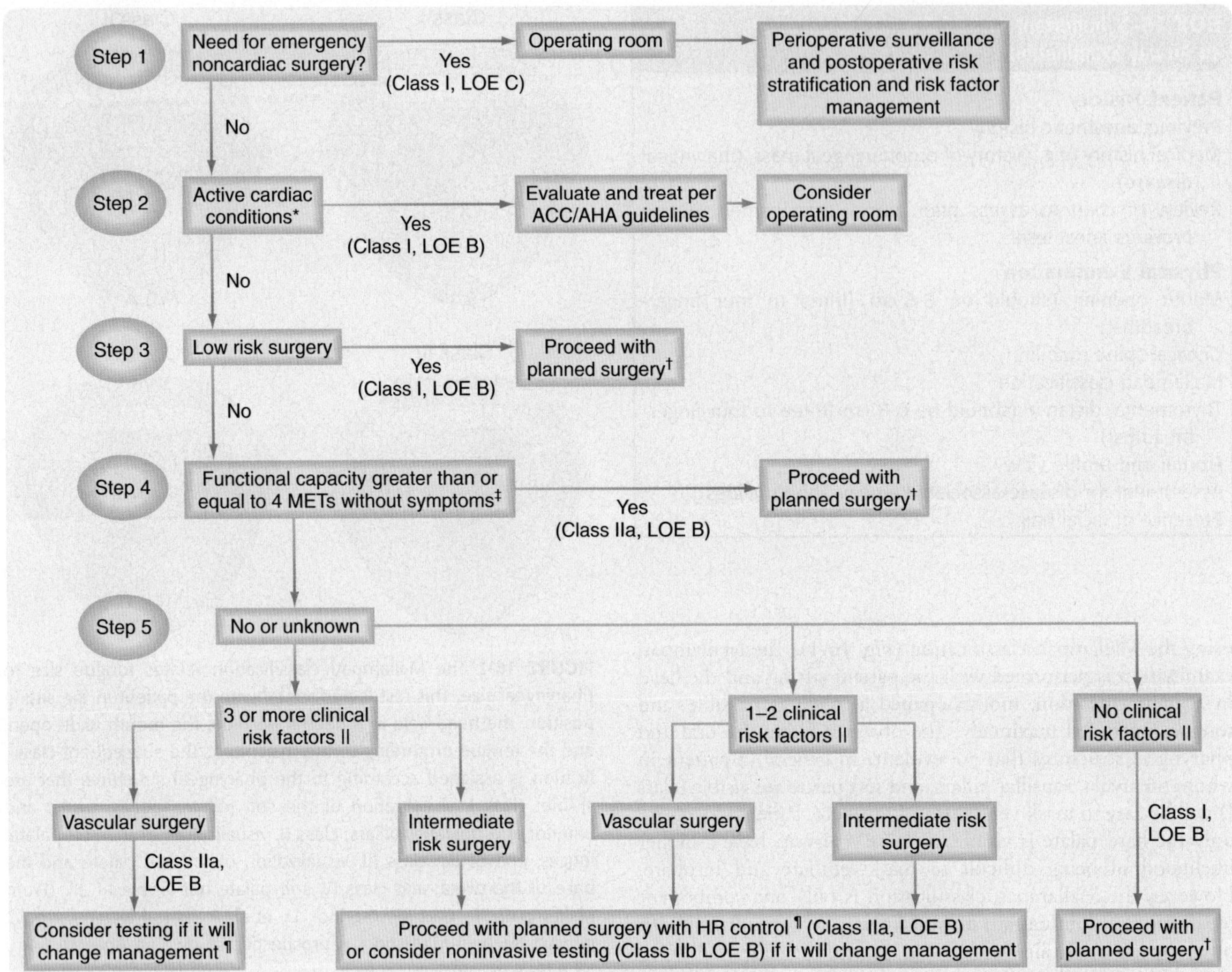


**FIGURE 16-2** Cardiac evaluation and care algorithm for noncardiac surgery based on active clinical conditions, known cardiovascular disease, or cardiac risk for patients 50 years of age or older. *Class I, LOE* (level of evidence) *C* indicates benefit much greater than risk based on expert opinion or standard of care; *Class I, LOE B* indicates benefit much greater than risk based on single randomized trial or nonrandomized studies; *Class IIa, LOE B* indicates benefit greater than risk based on single randomized trial or nonrandomized studies; *Class IIb, LOE B* indicates benefit greater than or equal to risk based on single randomized trial or nonrandomized studies. (From Fleisher LA, Beckman JA, Brown KA, et al: 2009 ACCF/AHA focused update on perioperative beta blockade incorporated into the ACC/AHA 2007 guidelines on perioperative cardiovascular evaluation and care for noncardiac surgery. Circulation 120:e169–e276, 2009.)

Overall, a history of MI or abnormal Q waves determined by electrocardiography is listed as a clinical risk factor, whereas an acute MI (at least one documented MI 7 days or less before the examination) or recent MI (more than 7 days but 1 month or less before the examination), with evidence of important ischemic risk by clinical symptoms or noninvasive study, is an active cardiac condition that requires further evaluation. Thus, the separation of MI into the traditional 3- and 6-month intervals has been altered. Current management of MI provides for risk stratification during convalescence. If a recent stress test does not indicate residual myocardium at risk, the likelihood of reinfarction after noncardiac surgery is low. Although there are no adequate clinical trials on which to base firm recommendations, it appears reasonable to wait 4 to 6 weeks after MI to perform elective surgery, assuming that adequate medical management and/or revascularization has been instituted.

Minor predictors are recognized markers for cardiovascular disease that have not been proven to increase perioperative risk independently. These include advanced age (>70 years), abnormal ECG (left ventricular [LV] hypertrophy, left bundle branch block, ST-T abnormalities), rhythm other than sinus, and uncontrolled systemic hypertension. The presence of a number of minor predictors might lead to a higher suspicion of CAD but is not incorporated into the recommendations for treatment.

Figure 16-2 presents a framework for determining which patients are candidates for preoperative cardiac testing. The clinician must consider several interacting variables and give them appropriate weight. Since publication of the perioperative cardiovascular evaluation guidelines in 2002, several new randomized trials and cohort studies have led to modification of the original algorithm. The following stepwise approach is recommended[24]:

**Step 1:** The urgency of noncardiac surgery must be considered. In many cases, patient- or surgery-specific factors dictate an obvious strategy (e.g., emergency surgery) that may not allow for further cardiac assessment or treatment. In such cases, the consultant may function best by providing recommendations for perioperative medical management and surveillance. Selected postoperative risk stratification is often appropriate for patients with elevated risk for long-term coronary events who have never had such an assessment previously. This is usually initiated after the patient has recovered from the surgical stress.

**Step 2:** Does the patient have an active cardiac condition? If not, proceed to step 3. In patients being considered for elective noncardiac surgery, the presence of unstable coronary disease, decompensated heart failure, or severe arrhythmia or valvular heart disease usually leads to cancellation or delay of surgery until the cardiac problem has been clarified and treated appropriately. Examples of unstable coronary syndromes include previous MI with evidence of important ischemic risk by clinical symptoms or noninvasive study, unstable or severe angina, and new or poorly controlled ischemia-mediated heart failure. Many patients in these circumstances are referred for coronary angiography to assess further therapeutic options. Depending on the results of the test or interventions and the risk of delaying surgery, it may be appropriate to proceed to the planned surgery with maximal medical therapy.

**Step 3:** Is the patient undergoing low-risk surgery? Many procedures are associated with a combined morbidity and mortality rate less than 1%, even in high-risk patients. Additionally, mortality on the day of surgery, for most ambulatory surgical procedures, is actually lower than mortality on day 30, which suggests that the incremental risk of ambulatory surgery is negligible or may be protective. Therefore, interventions based on cardiovascular testing in stable patients would rarely result in a change in management, and it would be appropriate to proceed with the planned surgical procedure.

**Step 4:** Does the patient have a functional capacity of 4 metabolic equivalents (METs) or more, without symptoms? Functional status has been shown to be reliable for perioperative and long-term prediction of cardiac events. In highly functional asymptomatic patients, management will rarely be changed based on the results of any further cardiovascular testing. It is therefore appropriate to proceed with the planned surgery. In patients with known cardiovascular disease or at least one clinical risk factor, perioperative heart rate control with beta blockade may be appropriate.

If the patient has not had a recent exercise test, functional status can usually be estimated from the ability to perform activities of daily living. Functional capacity can be expressed as METs; the resting or basal oxygen consumption ($\dot{V}O_2$) of a 70-kg, 40-year-old man in a resting state is 3.5 mL/kg/min, or 1 MET. For this purpose, functional capacity has been classified as excellent (>10 METs), good (7 to 10 METs), moderate (4 to 6 METs), poor (<4 METs), or unknown. The predicted MET level for a certain activity is influenced by the degree of conditioning and genetic predisposition. Perioperative cardiac and long-term risks are increased in patients unable to meet a 4-MET demand during most normal daily activities. Examples of leisure activities associated with less than 4 METs are slow ballroom dancing, golfing with a cart, playing a musical instrument, and walking at a speed of approximately 2 to 3 mph. Activities that require more than 4 METs include moderate cycling, climbing hills, ice skating, roller blading, skiing, singles tennis, and jogging.

**Step 5:** If the patient has poor functional capacity, is symptomatic, or has unknown functional capacity, the presence of clinical risk factors will determine the need for further evaluation. If the patient has no clinical risk factors, it is appropriate to proceed with the planned surgery, and no further change in management is indicated.

If the patient has one or two clinical risk factors, it is reasonable to proceed with the planned surgery and initiate heart rate control with beta blockade, or consider testing if it will change management. Two studies in vascular surgery patients with one or two clinical risk factors were unable to demonstrate any difference in outcome in the group who proceeded with the planned surgery with good medical management or tight heart rate control, but there are circumstances in which the clinician may change aspects of care based on the results of the test.[24]

In patients with three or more clinical risk factors, the surgery-specific cardiac risk is important. The surgery-specific cardiac risk (Table 16-4) of noncardiac surgery is related to two important factors. First, the type of surgery itself may identify a patient with a greater likelihood of underlying heart disease and higher perioperative morbidity and mortality. Perhaps the most extensively studied example is vascular surgery, in which underlying CAD is present in a substantial portion of patients. If the patient is undergoing vascular surgery, testing should only be considered if it will change management. Other types of surgery may be associated with similar risk to vascular surgery but have not been studied extensively. For nonvascular surgery, the degree of hemodynamic cardiac stress dictates the surgery-specific risk. Depending on the noncardiac surgical procedure, it may be associated with profound alterations in heart rate, blood pressure, vascular volume, pain, bleeding, clotting tendencies, oxygenation, neurohumoral activation, and other perturbations. The intensity of these coronary and myocardial stressors helps determine the likelihood of perioperative cardiac events.

**Table 16-4 Cardiac Risk* Stratification for Noncardiac Surgical Procedures**

| RISK STRATIFICATION | PROCEDURE EXAMPLES |
|---|---|
| Vascular (reported cardiac risk often more than 5%) | Aortic and other major vascular surgery; peripheral vascular surgery |
| Intermediate (reported cardiac risk generally 1% to 5%) | Intraperitoneal and intrathoracic surgery; carotid endarterectomy; head and neck surgery; orthopedic surgery; prostate surgery |
| Low (reported cardiac risk generally less than 1%)† | Endoscopic procedures; superficial procedure; cataract surgery; breast surgery; ambulatory surgery |

*Combined incidence of cardiac death and nonfatal myocardial infarction.
†These procedures do not generally require further preoperative cardiac testing.

The perioperative morbidity related to the procedures ranges from 1% to 5%. In these patients, who are considered ready to undergo intermediate-risk surgery, there are insufficient data to determine the best strategy—proceeding with the planned surgery with tight heart rate control with beta blockade or further cardiovascular testing if it will change management.

Hypertension is a common disorder that can be associated with end-organ damage, relative hypovolemia and, if inadequately treated, intraoperative blood pressure lability. In hypertensive patients, assessment of cardiovascular, neurologic, and renal function is necessary to quantify the extent of end-organ impairment. The preoperative antihypertensive regimen and compliance with that regimen should be reviewed preoperatively. In general, antihypertensive medications are continued throughout the perioperative period.

Numerous investigators have assessed the efficacy and safety of beta blockers in the management of cardiovascular disease during the perioperative period. Current studies have suggested that beta blockers reduce perioperative myocardial ischemia and may reduce the risk of MI and cardiovascular death in high-risk patients. However, recent results reported in the POISE trial have shown that the routine administration of higher dose, long-acting metoprolol on the day of surgery in patients who have previously not received beta blocker therapy, and in the absence of dose titration, is associated with an overall increase in mortality related to hypotension and stroke.[25] However, the POISE results do not address continuation of beta blockers in patients undergoing surgery who are receiving beta blockers for ACCF/AHA class I guideline indications. Currently, the ACC Foundation (ACCF)/AHA recommends continuation of beta blocker therapy in those patients. In addition, available evidence suggests, but does not definitively prove that when possible, and where indicated, beta blockers should be started days to weeks before elective surgery. The dose should be titrated perioperatively to achieve adequate heart rate control to increase the likelihood that the patient will receive the benefit of ACCF/AHA blockade while seeking to minimize the considerable risks of hypotension and bradycardia seen in POISE. Titrated rate control with ACCF/AHA blockers should continue during the intraoperative and postoperative periods. These assertions have been supported by a recent prospective trial, which reported that perioperative administration of ACCF/AHA blockers according to the Perioperative Cardiac Risk Reduction protocol was associated with decreased 30-day and 1-year mortality, whereas perioperative withdrawal of ACCF/AHA blockers was associated with increased mortality.[26] However, routine administration of high-dose ACCF/AHA blockers in the absence of dose titration for patients undergoing noncardiac surgery is not useful, may be harmful, and cannot be advocated, according to ACCF/AHA recommendations.[24]

### Endocarditis Prophylaxis

Some patients with congenital or valvular heart disease are at increased risk for the development of infective endocarditis (IE). The AHA previously proposed long-standing guidelines that recommended antibiotic prophylaxis for patients at risk for the development of IE who underwent dental, urinary, gastrointestinal, or respiratory surgical procedures. However, the AHA guidelines for endocarditis prophylaxis were changed significantly in 2007.[27] The new recommendations are based on more recent research indicating that the chance of developing IE is much more likely to result from random bacteremias caused by daily activities such as chewing and tooth brushing, rather than as a result of bacteremia generated by dental and surgical procedures. Therefore, antibiotic prophylaxis is not recommended based solely on an increased lifetime risk of developing IE and should be reserved for patients at highest risk (Box 16-4). The AHA panel has recommended that antibiotic prophylaxis is reasonable for dental procedures that involve manipulation of gingival tissues, periapical region of teeth or perforation of oral mucosa, and respiratory tract procedures or procedures that manipulate infected skin or musculoskeletal structures in patients at highest risk. Antibiotic prophylaxis solely to prevent IE is not recommended for genitourinary (GU) or gastrointestinal (GI) tract procedures. For recommended procedures and indications, oral amoxicillin is the drug of choice. Alternative drugs and routes are recommended for patients unable to take oral medications or those with penicillin allergy (Table 16-5).

**BOX 16-4 Cardiac Conditions Associated With Highest Risk of Adverse Outcome from Endocarditis for Which Prophylaxis with Dental Procedures Is Reasonable**

Prosthetic cardiac valve or prosthetic material used for cardiac valve repair
Previous infective endocarditis
CHD*
- Unrepaired cyanotic CHD, including palliative shunts and conduits
- Completely repaired congenital heart defect with prosthetic material or device, whether placed by surgery or catheter intervention, during first 6 mo after procedure†
- Repaired CHD with residual defects at site or adjacent to site of prosthetic patch or prosthetic device, which inhibit endothelialization

Cardiac transplantation recipients who develop cardiac valvulopathy

*Except for the conditions listed, antibiotic prophylaxis is no longer recommended for any other form of CHD.
†Prophylaxis is reasonable because endothelialization of prosthetic material occurs within 6 months after the procedure.

### Pulmonary Disease

Surgical patients often have obstructive or restrictive pulmonary disease. The preoperative history focuses on functional status, exercise tolerance, severity of the disease, and current medications. Recent worsening of symptoms needs to be closely evaluated. A thorough chest physical examination must be performed. Findings on the history and physical examination, as well as an understanding of the planned surgical procedure, suggest appropriate preoperative testing, which may include chest radiography, arterial blood gas analysis, and pulmonary function testing. The goal of preoperative evaluation is to detect and treat reversible pulmonary pathology, optimize medical management, and allow planning for postoperative ventilatory support, if indicated.

The perioperative risk associated with preexisting pulmonary disease has been extensively studied. Qaseem and coworkers,[28] reviewing the topic of preoperative pulmonary evaluation, identified patient-related risk factors, factors related to the

**Table 16-5 Regimens for a Dental Procedure**

| SITUATION | AGENT | Regimen (Single Dose 30-60 min Before Procedure) ADULTS | CHILDREN (MG/KG) |
|---|---|---|---|
| Oral | Amoxicillin | 2 g | 50 |
| Unable to take oral medication | Ampicillin *or* cefazolin or ceftriaxone | 2 g IM or IV<br>1 g IM or IV | 50 IM or IV<br>50 IM or IV |
| Allergic to penicillins or ampicillin, oral | Cephalexin*† *or*<br>Clindamycin *or*<br>Azithromycin or clarithromycin | 2 g<br>600 mg<br>500 mg | 50<br>20<br>15 |
| Allergic to penicillins or ampicillin and unable to take oral medication | Cefazolin or ceftriaxone† *or*<br>Clindamycin | 1 g IM or IV<br>600 mg IM or IV | 50 IM or IV<br>20 IM or IV |

*Or other first- or second-generation oral cephalosporin in equivalent adult or pediatric dosage.

†Cephalosporins should not be used in an individual with a history of anaphylaxis, angioedema, or urticaria with penicillins or ampicillin.

**Table 16-6 Risk Factors Associated With Postoperative Pulmonary Complications**

| PATIENT-ASSOCIATED RISK FACTORS | RELATIVE RISK ASSOCIATED WITH FACTOR | PROCEDURE-ASSOCIATED RISK FACTORS | RELATIVE RISK ASSOCIATED WITH FACTOR |
|---|---|---|---|
| Age > 60 yr | 2.1-3.0 | Surgery > 3 hr | 2.1 |
| Functional dependence | 2.5 | | |
| ASA class > II | 4.9 | General anesthesia | 1.8 |
| Congestive heart failure | 2.9 | | |
| Smoking | 1.3 | Emergency surgery | 2.2 |
| Obesity | 1.3 | | |
| COPD | 1.8 | | |

Modified from Qaseem A, Snow V, Fitterman N, et al: Risk assessment for strategies to reduce perioperative pulmonary complications for patients undergoing non-cardiovascular surgery: A guideline from the American College of Physicians. Ann Intern Med 144:575–580, 2006.

surgical site, and other factors related to surgery, such as the duration of surgery, the choice of general anesthesia, and intraoperative use of pancuronium (Table 16-6). Major patient-associated risk factors are ASA class higher than II, age older than 60 years, functional dependence, and presence of chronic obstructive pulmonary disease (COPD) or congestive heart failure. A serum albumin concentration less than 3.5 g/dL was also a strong predictor of pulmonary complications. Unadjusted rates of pulmonary complications were 27% and 7% in patients with low or normal serum albumin concentrations, respectively.[29] Current smoking was a minor predictor of pulmonary complications. The presence of obesity or mild to moderate asthma was not significantly associated with perioperative pulmonary complications.

In a cohort of patients in whom asthma was diagnosed and who subsequently required surgery at the Mayo Clinic (general or regional anesthesia), perioperative bronchospasm was documented in 1.7% (confidence interval [CI] 95%, 0.9% to 3%).[30] All attacks were treated successfully, and there were no episodes of pneumothorax, pneumonia, or death. The risk was highest in patients who were older, had recently used antiasthmatic medications, had recent asthma symptoms, and had recently required physician attention for bronchospasm or required hospitalization.[31]

The other major factors predicting perioperative pulmonary complications are related to surgical and anesthetic interventions and include surgery lasting longer than 3 hours, emergency surgery, and use of general anesthesia. Procedures with an increased risk for pulmonary complications include abdominal surgery, thoracic surgery, neurosurgery, head and neck surgery, and vascular surgery.

Pulmonary function testing remains controversial, in part because of changing expectations regarding the ability of patients with chronic pulmonary disease to tolerate extensive surgery. Pulmonary function testing has variable predictive value, cannot define a threshold above which the risk associated with surgery is prohibitive, and identifies no group at high risk but without clinical evidence of pulmonary disease. Arterial blood gas analysis also does not identify a group for whom the risk of surgery is prohibitive. Spirometry may be helpful for a patient who has unexplained cough, dyspnea, or exercise intolerance or if there is a question regarding optimal improvement of airflow obstruction. Warner and colleagues[30] have compared 135 patients who had undergone spirometry, were undergoing abdominal surgery, and met objective criteria for obstructive pulmonary disease (mean forced expiratory volume in 1 second, 0.9 ± 0.2 liters) with 135 patients matched for gender, surgical site, smoking history, and age. Although there was a significantly greater incidence of bronchospasm, the incidence of prolonged endotracheal intubation, prolonged intensive care unit admission, or readmission was no different. These results have been reiterated in the meta-analysis performed by Qaseem and associates.[28]

## Renal and Hepatic Disease

Renal and hepatic dysfunctions alter the metabolism and disposition of many anesthetic agents, as well as impair many systemic functions. Patients with acute renal or hepatic insufficiency do no undergo elective surgery until these conditions can be adequately stabilized. Chronic renal insufficiency (CRI) provides many perioperative management challenges, including acid-base abnormalities, electrolyte disturbances, and coagulation disorders. A thorough history must include the cause of CRI, presence of systemic complications related to CRI, and other systemic diseases. Current daily urinary output, type and frequency of dialysis, and dialysis-related complications must also be evaluated. The physical examination focuses on identifying systemic complications of CRI, including evidence of altered volume status, coagulopathy, anemia, pericardial effusion, and encephalopathy. Laboratory evaluation includes assessment of anemia, electrolyte abnormalities, coagulopathy, and cardiovascular disease. Dialysis is performed 18 to 24 hours before surgery to avoid the fluid and electrolyte shifts that occur immediately after dialysis.

A patient with chronic liver disease poses many perioperative challenges. The presence of liver disease alters anesthetic drug metabolism and hypoalbuminemia increases the free fraction of many drugs, thus making these patients sensitive to the acute and long-term effects of many anesthetics. The perioperative risks associated with anesthesia and surgery are dependent on the severity of hepatic dysfunction. The preoperative evaluation focuses on hepatic synthetic and metabolic function and presence of coagulopathy, encephalopathy, and ascites, as well as nutritional status of the patient.

## Nutrition, Endocrinology, and Metabolism

Diabetes mellitus warrants discussion because of its high prevalence and potential for comorbidity. Preanesthetic evaluation focuses on the duration and type of diabetes, as well as the current medical regimen. Review of end-organ function with emphasis on autonomic dysfunction, cardiovascular disease, renal insufficiency, retinopathy, and neurologic complications is mandatory. Patients with diabetes are considered to have delayed gastric emptying and to be at risk for gastroesophageal reflux. Perioperative plasma glucose levels need to be well controlled, yet hypoglycemia must be prevented. Appropriate control of perioperative blood sugar in diabetics is difficult to define. Over the long term, there is compelling evidence of a correlation between hyperglycemia and long-term diabetic complications. It is much less clear whether blood sugar must be tightly controlled during the acute stress of surgery. However, there is a strong correlation between mortality and tight control of glucose in critically ill patients, including surgical patients.[32]

In diabetic patients undergoing surgery, several principles of management are generally accepted:

1. Substitute shorter acting for longer acting insulin.
2. Provide a reduced dose of insulin on the morning of surgery.
3. Once a diabetic who is receiving nothing by mouth (NPO) is given insulin, provide glucose in IV fluids.
4. In patients with type 2 diabetes, long-acting sulfonylurea drugs such as chlorpropamide are stopped and shorter acting agents are substituted.
5. Metformin is always stopped because of a slight risk for perioperative drug-induced lactic acidosis. Perioperative insulin requirements vary, depending on body weight, liver disease, steroid therapy, infection, and whether cardiopulmonary bypass surgery has been performed.

Patients who have received systemic glucocorticoids during the year before surgery may not be able to respond to surgical stress adequately. Because of the remote risk for adrenal insufficiency during anesthesia, patients who receive chronic glucocorticoids generally receive perioperative glucocorticoid coverage. Recommendations regarding identification of patients at risk and appropriate dosing were formerly based on anecdote. Newer recommendations are based on the preoperative dosage of glucocorticoid, duration of therapy, and type of surgery. For minor surgical stress, the equivalent of 25 mg of hydrocortisone on the operative day is recommended; for moderate surgical stress, 50 to 75 mg equivalent for 1 to 2 days; and, for major surgical stress, 100 to 150 mg/day for 2 to 3 days.

## Fasting Before Surgery

Pulmonary aspiration of gastric contents during anesthesia is an uncommon, but serious complication. To prevent aspiration, NPO guidelines have been developed for patients scheduled for anesthesia and surgery. Traditionally, orders for "NPO after midnight" forbade any intake of liquids and solids. However, applying the same guidelines for clear liquids (gastric emptying time, 1 to 2 hours) and solids (gastric emptying time, 6 hours) has been questioned. The ASA adopted guidelines in 1998 that recommended a minimum fasting period of 2 hours after the ingestion of clear liquids and 6 hours for solids and nonclear liquids, such as milk or orange juice (Box 16-5). Clear liquids are defined as liquids that can be seen through and do not contain solids or particulates. The routine use of GI stimulants, gastric acid secretion blockers, antacids, and antiemetics is not recommended. However, many patients have medical conditions that cause decreased gastric emptying. In these patients, the use of agents to improve gastric emptying and neutralize gastric acid may be warranted. In addition, precautions are instituted to decrease the risk for aspiration during anesthesia in patients undergoing emergency procedures.

The reported incidence of aspiration during anesthesia in various studies has varied from 1.4 to 11/10,000 anesthetic procedures. A higher incidence has been noted during emergency surgery and in patients with underlying disease processes that cause decreased gastric emptying. Interestingly, some reports have suggested that aspiration is at least as common during emergence from anesthesia as during the induction phase. Of patients in whom aspiration is suspected, less than 50% exhibit

**BOX 16-5 Summary of Preoperative Fasting Recommendations***

| Ingested Material (Minimum Fasting Period) |
|---|
| Clear liquids† (2 hr) |
| Breast milk (4 hr) |
| Infant formula (6 hr) |
| Nonhuman milk (6 hr) |
| Solid food (6 hr) |

Adapted from Practice guidelines for preoperative fasting and the use of pharmacologic agents to reduce the risk of pulmonary aspiration: Application to healthy patients undergoing elective procedures: A report by the American Society of Anesthesiologist Task Force on Preoperative Fasting. Anesthesiology 90:896–905, 1999.

*To reduce the risk of pulmonary aspiration; applies to healthy patients undergoing elective procedures.

†Examples of clear liquids are water, fruit juices without pulp, black coffee, clear tea, carbonated beverages.

evidence of pulmonary injury and approximately one third of patients require postoperative intubation and ventilation. Most of these patients were extubated within 6 hours of surgery. Approximately 10% of patients required intubation and ventilation for 24 hours or longer. Approximately 50% of patients requiring ventilation for longer than 24 hours after aspiration of gastric contents died of pulmonary complications.

### Assessment of Physical Status

The ASA has developed a graded descriptive scale to categorize preoperative comorbidity. The classification is independent of operative procedure and serves as a standardized method of communicating patient physical status to anesthesiologists and other health care providers. Patients are categorized as follows:

ASA I—No organic, physiologic, biochemical, or psychiatric disturbance.

ASA II—A patient with mild systemic disease that results in no functional limitation. Examples are well-controlled hypertension and uncomplicated diabetes mellitus.

ASA III—A patient with severe systemic disease that results in functional impairment. Examples are diabetes mellitus with vascular complications, previous MI, and uncontrolled hypertension.

ASA IV—A patient with severe systemic disease that is a constant threat to life. Examples are congestive heart failure and unstable angina pectoris.

ASA V—A moribund patient who is not expected to survive, with or without the surgery. Examples are ruptured aortic aneurysm and intracranial hemorrhage with elevated ICP.

ASA VI—A declared brain-dead patient whose organs are being harvested for transplantation.

E—Emergency surgery is required. For example, ASA IE represents an otherwise healthy patient undergoing emergency appendectomy.

## SELECTION OF ANESTHETIC TECHNIQUES AND DRUGS

Selection of anesthetic techniques and drugs begins with the preoperative anesthetic evaluation. Recognition of important preexisting conditions and chronic medication use may suggest that certain approaches are preferable. The requirements of the surgical procedure and surgeon are then considered:

- What is the operative site?
- How will the patient be positioned?
- What is the expected duration of surgery?
- Is the patient expected to return home after an ambulatory procedure or is hospital admission anticipated?
- Finally, in this era of cost constraints, are the costs of newer drugs justified by probable clinical benefit?

Evidence of the increasing safety of anesthesia is the fact that multiple options can often be used safely and effectively for the same procedure and the same patient.

After completing the preanesthetic evaluation, the anesthesiologist discusses various options regarding anesthetic care with the patient. Together, sometimes with input from the patient's surgeon, the anesthesiologist and patient choose an anesthetic technique. Continued progress in the pharmacology of anesthetic drugs, improvements in the accuracy and applicability of monitoring devices, and parallel improvements in the management of chronic disease processes have resulted in the ability to customize the anesthetic management of individual patients extensively.

### Risk of Anesthesia

Patients often desire information regarding the risk of death or major complications associated with anesthesia. However, because perioperative death and major complications have become so uncommon, the risk associated with anesthesia is difficult to quantify. The risk for cardiac arrest attributable to anesthesia appears to be less than 1/10,000 cases.[33,34] Schwilk and coworkers[35] have prospectively studied preoperative risk factors as predictors of perioperative adverse events in 26,907 patients undergoing noncardiac surgery. In this study, 14 variables proved to be independent risk factors, including gender, age, ASA status, general condition, nutritional state, coronary disease, airway and lung pathology, Mallampati classification, fluid and electrolyte balance, metabolic state, grade of urgency, operative site, duration of surgery, and anesthetic technique (lower risk with regional than with general anesthesia). With the use of a point system, patients could be reliably separated into low- and high-risk groups.

Because so many surgical procedures are now performed without admission to the hospital, the risk associated with ambulatory anesthesia is particularly important. To assess this risk, 38,598 patients who had undergone 45,090 consecutive ambulatory surgical procedures were contacted within 72 hours and 30 days of surgery (99.94% and 95.9% of patients, respectively). No patient died of a medical complication within 1 week of surgery.[36] The total death rate was 1/11,273 (four deaths), and the total complication rate was 1/1366.

### Selection of a Specific Technique

The first step in selecting a specific anesthetic technique for an individual patient is to consider whether the procedure can be appropriately performed with monitored anesthesia care (also sometimes abbreviated as MAC, but which must be distinguished from the identical abbreviation for minimum alveolar concentration), regional anesthesia (including regional upper and lower extremity blocks, subarachnoid blocks, and epidural anesthesia), or general anesthesia. Monitored anesthesia care supplements local anesthesia performed by surgeons. Anesthesiologists usually participate because an individual patient or procedure requires higher doses of potent sedatives or opioids or because an acutely or chronically ill patient requires close monitoring and hemodynamic or respiratory support. Regional anesthesia (see later) is useful for operations on the upper and lower extremities, pelvis, and lower part of the abdomen. Other procedures, such as carotid endarterectomy and so-called awake craniotomy, can also be successfully performed under a regional or field block. Patients receiving regional anesthesia can generally remain awake and, if needed, can receive IV sedation or analgesics. Although regional anesthesia avoids general anesthesia and intuitively appears to be safer, hazards specific to regional anesthesia must be considered. Such hazards include, among others, post–dural puncture headache, local anesthetic toxicity, and peripheral nerve injury. In addition, an inadequate regional anesthetic may require rapid transition to heavy sedation or general anesthesia.

General anesthesia is a reversible state of unconsciousness. Although the mechanism of general anesthetics remains speculative and controversial, the four components of general anesthesia—amnesia, analgesia, inhibition of noxious reflexes, and skeletal muscle relaxation—are usually achieved in modern anesthesia by a combination of IV anesthetics and analgesics, inhalational anesthetics and, frequently, muscle relaxants. Because the drugs that produce these components cause desirable and undesirable physiologic changes, the pharmacologic effects of these agents must be matched to the pathophysiology of the patient's medical problems. The major adverse changes associated with anesthetic drugs are respiratory depression, cardiovascular depression, and loss of airway maintenance and protection. Important complications of general anesthesia include hypoxemia (with possible central nervous system [CNS] damage), hypotension, cardiac arrest, and aspiration of acidic gastric contents, which can lead to severe pulmonary damage. Dental damage is more frequent but not life-threatening.

Regardless of the suitability of a particular technique for a specific surgical procedure, other factors, including the patient's preferences, must be considered. For example, regional anesthesia might not be chosen if a patient were extremely anxious or could not communicate effectively because of a language barrier. Monitored anesthesia care might be inappropriate if a patient were unlikely to lie quietly during delicate or prolonged surgery. Any procedure planned under regional anesthesia or monitored anesthesia care can require conversion to general anesthesia if the original choice proves unsatisfactory.

## AIRWAY MANAGEMENT

Airway management is perhaps the most critical skill in anesthesiology. As noted, the preoperative evaluation focuses on recognition of patients who may be difficult to mask-ventilate or intubate. Knowledge of and skill with various techniques for establishment of a patent airway constitutes the central group of skills critical for the safe practice of anesthesiology. Fortunately, the incidence of difficult intubations is low. Difficult direct laryngoscopy occurs in 1.5% to 8.5% and failed intubation occurs in 0.13% to 0.3% of general anesthetic procedures. The laryngeal mask airway, Combitube, lighted stylet, Bullard laryngoscope, and GlideScope are developments that have made ventilation and intubation possible for many patients who have failed intubation with a conventional laryngoscope. The fiberoptic bronchoscope is an additional tool for the management of a difficult airway.

Because of the importance of a prompt effective response to difficult intubation, the ASA has developed guidelines for managing difficult airways (Fig. 16-3). A key factor is the initial airway examination and recognition of patients with potentially difficult airways. If the physician suspects that mask ventilation and tracheal intubation will be difficult, it is recommended that spontaneous ventilation be preserved. Approaches to these patients include awake intubation or use of anesthetic techniques that preserve spontaneous ventilation. In some cases, establishment of a surgical airway in an awake patient under local anesthesia may be indicated. However, some patients are found to have a difficult airway only after anesthesia and muscle relaxation have been induced. This is an emergency situation that must be rectified quickly to avoid hypoxemia, brain injury, and/or death. A variety of airway adjuncts are available to preserve ventilation and facilitate tracheal intubation under emergency conditions. The physician always must call for assistance in these situations to optimize patient care and consider reestablishment of spontaneous ventilation. It is essential to have alternate means for securing the airway available for all patients in the event of an unanticipated difficult airway.

## REGIONAL ANESTHESIA

Regional anesthesia is an attractive anesthetic option for many types of operative procedures and can provide excellent postoperative pain management in select patients. However, like any anesthetic technique, the risks and benefits associated with regional anesthesia must be assessed for each individual. Several regional techniques are in common use, including spinal, epidural, and peripheral nerve blocks. Each technique has specific benefits and risks, which depend in part on the choice of local anesthetic drugs.

### Local Anesthetic Drugs

Local anesthetics have played a critical role in intraoperative anesthesia, almost since they were first described. The two classes of local anesthetic drugs in common use are amino esters and amino amides, often referred to as esters and amides. The mechanism of action of local anesthetics is dose-dependent blockade of sodium currents in nerve fibers. Local anesthetic drugs differ in terms of their physicochemical characteristics. Of these characteristics, the most important are $pK_a$, protein binding, and degree of hydrophobicity. $pK_a$ refers to the pH at which half the drug exists in the basic uncharged form and half exists in the cationic form. In general, agents with a lower $pK_a$ have a faster onset than agents with a higher $pK_a$, although some agents, such as chloroprocaine, can be given at much higher concentrations, thereby offsetting the effects of a high $pK_a$. Because all commonly used local anesthetics have relatively high $pK_a$ values, they are largely ineffective in acidotic (inflamed) environments, in which local anesthetics exist primarily in the ionized form, which does not penetrate nerves. In general, greater hydrophobicity is associated with greater potency, and increased protein binding correlates with a longer duration of action. The speed of onset, duration of action, and typical doses of agents commonly used for regional anesthesia or local anesthesia are summarized in Table 16-7.

**FIGURE 16-3** ASA difficult airway algorithm. The likelihood and clinical impact of basic management problems such as difficult intubation, difficult mask ventilation, and difficulty with patient cooperation or consent should be assessed in all patients for whom airway management is being contemplated. The clinician should consider the relative merits and feasibility of basic management choices, including the use of awake intubation techniques, preservation of spontaneous ventilation, and use of surgical approaches to establish a secure airway. (From American Society of Anesthesiologists Task Force on Management of the Difficult Airway: Practice guidelines for management of the difficult airway: An updated report by the American Society of Anesthesiologists Task Force on Management of the Difficult Airway. Anesthesiology 98:1269–1277, 2003.)

DIFFICULT AIRWAY ALGORITHM

1. Access the likelihood and clinical impact of basic management problems:
   A. Difficult ventilation
   B. Difficult intubation
   C. Difficulty with patient cooperation or consent
   D. Difficult tracheostomy
2. Actively pursue opportunities to deliver supplemental oxygen throughout the process of difficult airway management
3. Consider the relative merits and feasibility of basic management choices:

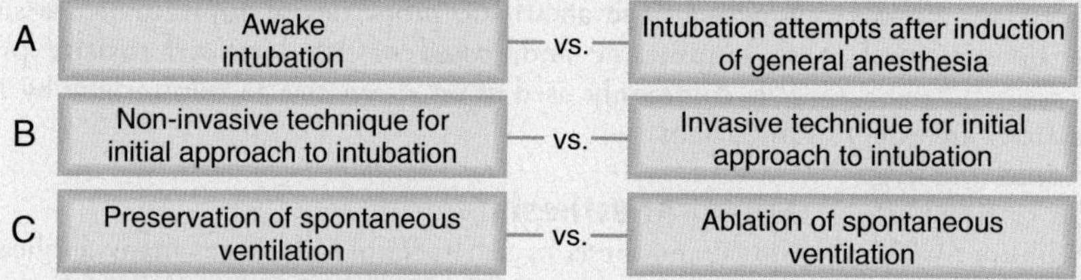

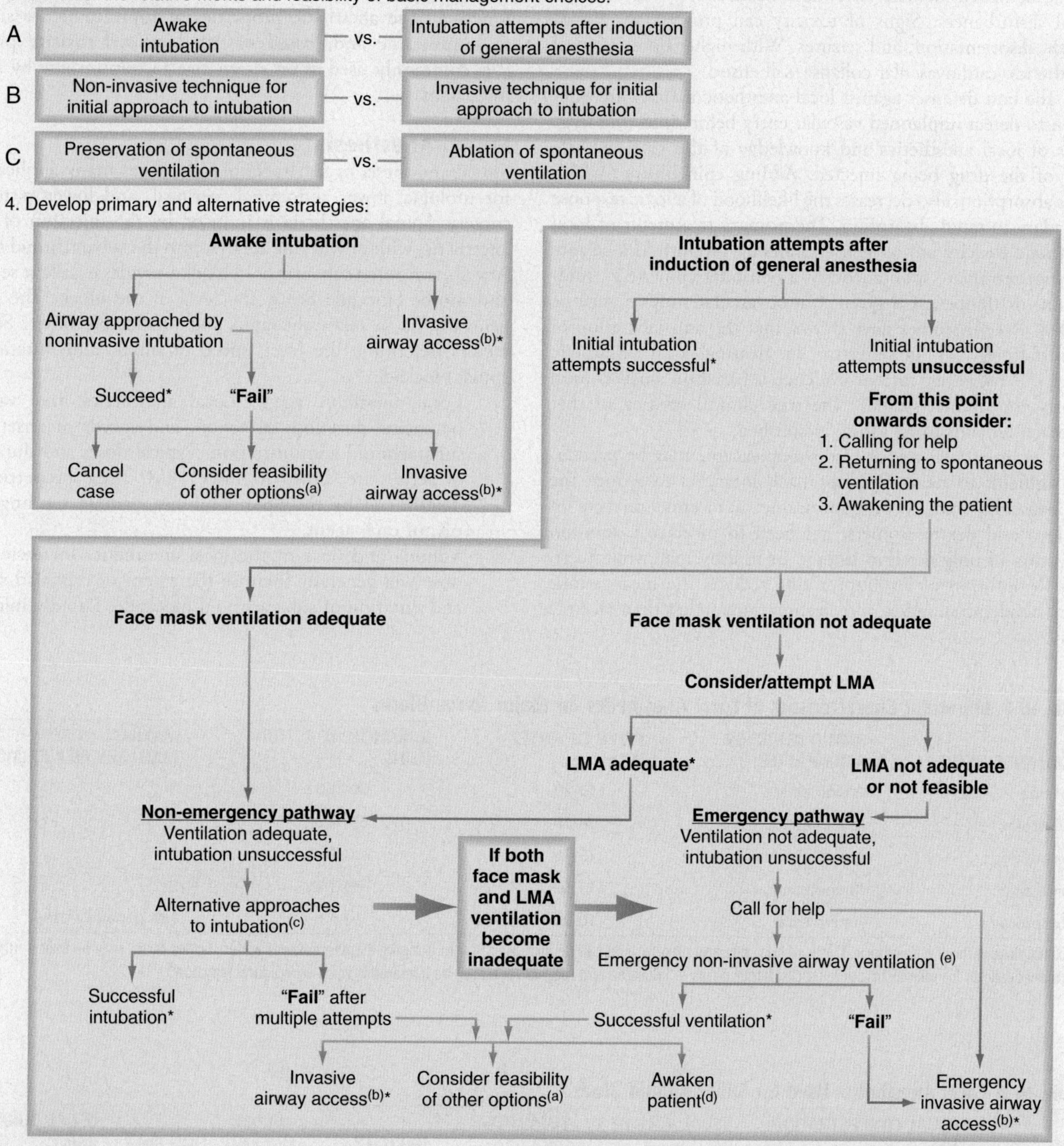

4. Develop primary and alternative strategies:

**Awake intubation**

Airway approached by noninvasive intubation

Invasive airway access(b)*

Succeed*

**"Fail"**

Cancel case

Consider feasibility of other options(a)

Invasive airway access(b)*

**Intubation attempts after induction of general anesthesia**

Initial intubation attempts successful*

Initial intubation attempts **unsuccessful**

**From this point onwards consider:**
1. Calling for help
2. Returning to spontaneous ventilation
3. Awakening the patient

**Face mask ventilation adequate**

**Face mask ventilation not adequate**

**Consider/attempt LMA**

**LMA adequate***

**LMA not adequate or not feasible**

**Non-emergency pathway**
Ventilation adequate, intubation unsuccessful

Alternative approaches to intubation(c)

**If both face mask and LMA ventilation become inadequate**

**Emergency pathway**
Ventilation not adequate, intubation unsuccessful

Call for help

Emergency non-invasive airway ventilation (e)

Successful intubation*

**"Fail"** after multiple attempts

Successful ventilation*

**"Fail"**

Invasive airway access(b)*

Consider feasibility of other options(a)

Awaken patient(d)

Emergency invasive airway access(b)*

***Confirm ventilation, tracheal intubation, or LMA placement with exhaled $CO_2$**

a. Other options include (but are not limited to): surgery utilizing face mask or LMA anesthesia, local anesthesia infiltration or regional nerve blockade. Pursuit of these options usually implies that mask ventilation will not be problematic. Therefore, these options may be of limited value if this step in the algorithm has been reached via the Emergency Pathway.

b. Invasive airway access includes surgical or percutaneous tracheostomy or cricothyrotomy.

c. Alternative noninvasive approaches to difficult intubation include (but are not limited to): use of different laryngoscope blades, LMA as an intubation conduit (with or without fiberoptic guidance), fiberoptic intubation, intubating stylet or tube changer, light wand, retrograde intubation, and blind oral or nasal intubation.

d. Consider repreparation of the patient for awake intubation or canceling surgery.

e. Options for emergency non-invasive airway ventilation include (but are not limited to): rigid bronchoscope, esophageal-tracheal combitube ventilation, or transtracheal jet ventilation.

When used for regional anesthesia, the toxicity of local anesthetics is dependent on the site of injection and speed of absorption. Inadvertent intravascular injection of local anesthetics will produce toxicity with much smaller doses. The main symptoms of local anesthetic toxicity involve the CNS and cardiovascular system. The earliest signs of an overdose or inadvertent intravascular injection are numbness or tingling of the tongue or lips, a metallic taste, light-headedness, tinnitus, and visual disturbances. Signs of toxicity can progress to slurred speech, disorientation, and seizures. With higher doses of local anesthetics, cardiovascular collapse will ensue.

The best defenses against local anesthetic toxicity are aspiration to detect unplanned vascular entry before injecting large doses of local anesthetics and knowledge of the maximal safe dose of the drug being injected. Adding epinephrine, which slows absorption, also decreases the likelihood of a toxic response secondary to rapid absorption. The primary treatments of local anesthetic toxicity are oxygen and airway support. If a seizure does not terminate spontaneously, a benzodiazepine (e.g., midazolam) or thiopental is given. Cardiovascular support may be needed. Recent studies have shown that the administration of an intralipid may be effective in treating local anesthetic toxicity.[36a] However, current evidence is based on small clinical reports and animal studies. The true clinical efficacy of that approach remains to be firmly established.

Cardiovascular toxicity from bupivacaine may be particularly difficult to treat. One approach intended to reduce the cardiovascular toxicity of bupivacaine, a racemic mixture of the levo and dextro isomers, has been to produce a solution consisting of only the levo isomer. In healthy male volunteers, slow IV infusion of levobupivacaine reduces the mean stroke index, acceleration index, and ejection fraction less than racemic bupivacaine. Ropivacaine, a newer potent amide local anesthetic, was compared with bupivacaine and lidocaine in volunteers receiving a slow IV infusion until CNS symptoms first occurred. Echocardiography and electrocardiography were used to quantify systolic, diastolic, and electrophysiologic effects. Bupivacaine increased QRS width during sinus rhythm as compared with the other two treatments and reduced systolic and diastolic function, whereas ropivacaine reduced only systolic function. The anesthetic properties of ropivacaine are similar to bupivacaine and, based on its decreased toxicity profile, it is commonly used as an alternative to bupivacaine by many physicians.

## Spinal Anesthesia

Spinal anesthesia or subarachnoid block has many applications for urologic, lower abdominal, perineal, and lower extremity surgery. Spinal anesthesia is induced by the injection of local anesthetic, with or without opiates, into the subarachnoid space. A well-performed subarachnoid block provides excellent sensory and motor blockade below the level of the block. The block generally has a relatively rapid and predictable onset. Several factors determine the level, speed of onset, and duration of spinal blockade.

1. Local anesthetic agent. Local anesthetics have varying potencies, durations of action, and speeds of onset after subarachnoid administration. Typical doses and durations of action are shown in Table 16-8. These properties are determined by the lipid solubility, protein binding, and $pK_a$ of each agent.
2. Volume and dose of the local anesthetic. Increasing the dose will generally increase the extent of cephalad spread and duration of subarachnoid blockade. Rapidly injecting

**Table 16-7 Important Characteristics of Local Anesthetics for Major Nerve Blocks**

| LOCAL ANESTHETIC | AMINO AMIDE OR AMINO ESTER | SPEED OF ONSET (MIN) | DURATION OF ACTION (MIN) | MAXIMAL DOSE* (AXILLARY BLOCK) (MG/KG) |
|---|---|---|---|---|
| Lidocaine | Amino amide | 10-20 | 60-180 | 5 |
| Mepivacaine | Amino amide | 10-20 | 60-180 | 5 |
| Bupivacaine | Amino amide | 15-30 | 180-360 | 3 |
| Ropivacaine | Amino amide | 15-30 | 180-360 | 3 |
| Chloroprocaine | Amino ester | 10-20 | 30-50 | Not generally used |

*Maximal dose without epinephrine. Doses of lidocaine and mepivacaine can be increased to 7 to 8 mg/kg if epinephrine is added. Lower doses may be toxic if infiltrated subcutaneously, as for intercostal nerve blocks; larger doses of lidocaine and mepivacaine may be tolerated if given by epidural injection.

**Table 16-8 Local Anesthetics Used for Subarachnoid Block**

| DRUG | USUAL CONCENTRATION (%) | USUAL VOLUME (ML) | TOTAL DOSE (MG) | BARICITY | GLUCOSE CONCENTRATION (%) | USUAL DURATION (MIN) |
|---|---|---|---|---|---|---|
| Lidocaine | 1.5, 5.0 | 1-2 | 30-100 | Hyperbaric | 7.5 | 30-60 |
| Tetracaine | 0.25-1.0 | 1-4 | 5-20 | Hyperbaric | 5.0 | 75-200 |
| | 0.25 | 2-6 | 5-20 | Hypobaric | 0 | 75-200 |
| | 1.0 | 1-2 | 5-20 | Isobaric | 0 | 75-200 |
| Bupivacaine | 0.5 | 2-4 | 10-20 | Isobaric | 0 | 75-200 |
| | 0.75 | 1-3 | 7.5-22.5 | Hyperbaric | 8.25 | 75-200 |

From Berde CB, Strichartz GR: Local anesthetics. In Miller RD (ed): Anesthesia, ed 5, Philadelphia, 2000, Churchill Livingstone, pp 491–522.

local anesthetic solutions leads to turbulent flow and unpredictable spread.

3. Patient position and local anesthetic baricity. Local anesthetic solutions can be prepared as hypobaric, isobaric, or hyperbaric solutions. Cerebrospinal fluid (CSF) has low specific gravity (i.e., only slightly higher than that of water). Local anesthetic solutions prepared in water have a slightly lower specific gravity than CSF and will therefore ascend within CSF. Plain local anesthetic solutions are isobaric, and local anesthetics mixed in 5% dextrose are hyperbaric relative to CSF. The baricity of the local anesthetic solution and position of the patient at the time of injection and until the local anesthetic firmly binds to nervous tissue will determine the level of block. For example, administration of hyperbaric bupivacaine at the low lumbar level to a patient in the sitting position will result in intense lumbosacral blockade. The longer the patient remains in the sitting position, the less the cephalad spread of the block.
4. Vasoconstrictors. The addition of epinephrine, particularly to short-acting local anesthetics, will increase the duration of action.
5. Addition of opioids. The addition of small doses of fentanyl (e.g., 20 μg) or morphine (e.g., 0.25 mg) will prolong the duration of analgesia and increase the duration of analgesia and tolerance for tourniquet pain.
6. Anatomic and physiologic factors. A higher than expected level of spinal anesthesia can result from anatomic factors that decrease the relative volume of the subarachnoid space, such as obesity, pregnancy, increased intra-abdominal pressure, previous spine surgery, and abnormal spinal curvature. Older patients tend to be more sensitive to intrathecally injected local anesthetics.

Spinal anesthesia provides the advantage of avoiding manipulation of the airway and potential complication of tracheal intubation, as well as the potential side effects of general anesthetics such as nausea, vomiting, and prolonged emergence or drowsiness. Spinal anesthesia also provides advantages for several types of surgery, including endoscopic urologic procedures, particularly transurethral resection of the prostate, in which an awake patient provides a valuable monitor for assessment of hyponatremia or bladder perforation. Less confusion and postoperative delirium have been reported in older patients after repair of hip fractures under spinal anesthesia. Intrathecal opiate administration can provide high-quality postoperative analgesia for patients undergoing abdominal, lower extremity, urologic, and gynecologic procedures.

In most cases, spinal anesthesia is administered as a single bolus injection. Therefore, the block is of limited duration and is not suitable for prolonged procedures. The practice of continuous spinal anesthesia with the use of small-bore catheters has largely been abandoned because of neurologic complications associated with local anesthetic toxicity. However, continuous spinal anesthesia with relatively large-bore epidural catheters can provide the advantages of incremental titration and the ability to administer additional doses in select older patients. Unfortunately, this technique has a high likelihood of inducing a post–dural puncture headache in young patients.

Complications of subarachnoid block include hypotension (sometimes refractory), bradycardia, post–dural puncture headache, transient radicular neuropathy, backache, urinary retention, infection, epidural hematoma, and excessive cephalad spread, resulting in cardiorespiratory compromise. Frank neurologic injury, although described with continuous techniques using small-bore catheters, is rare. Hypotension, which occurs as a consequence of sympathectomy, usually responds readily to fluids and small doses of pressors such as ephedrine. The efficacy of fluid preloading in providing prophylaxis against hypotension is controversial.

Post–dural puncture headache occurs after a small proportion of subarachnoid blocks. Factors that increase its incidence include female gender, younger age, and larger needles. Epidural analgesia would appear to avoid the complication but, if the dura is inadvertently punctured, leaves a much larger dural rent. When compared with epidural anesthesia, spinal anesthesia has a quicker onset, is more predictably satisfactory for surgery, and is less frequently associated with backache. Transient radicular neuropathy, a painful but usually self-limited condition, has become evident in association with an increase in enthusiasm for the use of lidocaine for subarachnoid block.

When cardiac arrest results from excessive cephalad spread of subarachnoid block or protracted hypotension, cardiopulmonary resuscitation is notoriously difficult. Patients who suffer cardiac arrest during subarachnoid block have poor survival, possibly because the profound sympathectomy causes difficulty in generating adequate coronary perfusion pressure. Relatively large doses of epinephrine may be necessary to achieve adequate perfusion pressure during cardiopulmonary resuscitation after spinal anesthesia. Absolute contraindications to spinal anesthesia include sepsis, bacteremia, and infection at the site of injection, severe hypovolemia, coagulopathy, therapeutic anticoagulation, increased ICP, and patient refusal.

## Epidural Anesthesia

Epidural block, another form of neuraxial regional block, has application in a wide variety of abdominal, thoracic, and lower extremity procedures. Induction of epidural anesthesia or analgesia results from the injection of local anesthetics, with or without opiates, into the lumbar or thoracic epidural space. Generally, a catheter is inserted after the epidural space has been located with a needle. The presence of the catheter provides several advantages. First, local anesthetic can be added in a controlled fashion so that the time to onset of the block can be well controlled. Second, the catheter can be use for repeated dosing so that anesthesia can be provided for the duration of lengthy procedures. Third, local anesthetics or opiates can be administered for several days to provide postoperative analgesia.

Epidural anesthesia has specific advantages for thoracic surgery, peripheral vascular surgery, and gastrointestinal surgery. Epidural anesthesia has also been shown to decrease blood loss and deep venous thrombosis during total joint arthroplasty. Postoperative epidural analgesia for thoracic surgery provides superior pain control, less sedation, and better pulmonary function than parenteral opiates.

Christopherson and colleagues[37] have randomized 100 patients undergoing major elective vascular reconstruction to receive epidural anesthesia followed by postoperative epidural analgesia or general anesthesia followed by patient-controlled analgesia (PCA). Epidural anesthesia was associated with a lower rate of reoperation for vascular insufficiency (2 versus 11 in the general anesthesia group). Other morbidity and mortality rates were similar. However, the choice of anesthesia apparently does not influence overall morbidity in patients undergoing peripheral vascular surgery.

The use of low concentrations of local anesthetics in conjunction with epidural opiates has been associated with earlier ambulation and less postoperative ileus after abdominal surgery. Thoracic epidural anesthesia, but not lumbar epidural anesthesia, appears to be associated with more rapid recovery of GI function after major abdominal surgery. However, IV lidocaine also results in more rapid return of bowel function, flatus and bowel movement. Therefore, circulating lidocaine may account for at least some of the effects of epidural anesthesia on postoperative bowel function. A continuing controversy relates to whether epidural or subarachnoid analgesia reduces subsequent analgesic requirements after the block has resolved, so-called preemptive analgesia.

The complications and contraindications associated with epidural anesthesia are similar to those for spinal anesthesia. However, a special cautionary note is indicated regarding epidural anesthesia and anticoagulation. Because of the risk of spinal hematoma, placement and removal of epidural catheters in patients receiving oral or parenteral anticoagulation is performed in conjunction with an anesthesiologist. The advent of low-molecular-weight heparin (LMWH) for prophylaxis of deep venous thrombosis has resulted in an increase in the incidence of epidural hematomas associated with the removal or placement of epidural catheters. Although LMWH is effective as prophylaxis against venous thromboembolism, spinal hematomas have occurred in association with perioperative use of LMWH in patients given neuraxial analgesia. The timing of catheter placement and removal in the setting of LMWH use is critical for avoiding this rare but catastrophic complication. Although many of the guidelines are based on evidence provided by small clinical studies and case reports, a general consensus exists regarding the placement and removal of epidural catheters in patients receiving LMWH.[38] In general, an epidural catheter should not be placed earlier than 24 hours after treatment with LMWH, and LMWH should not be started before 6 hours after epidural catheter placement. An epidural catheter should not be removed earlier than 12 hours after the last dose of LMWH, and LMWH should not be restarted earlier than 2 hours after catheter removal. A high index of suspicion of epidural hematoma must be maintained for patients undergoing neuraxial blockade who have received or will receive LMWH. All persons involved in the care of patients receiving continuous epidural analgesia need to be aware of the signs of epidural hematoma, including back pain, lower extremity sensory and motor dysfunction, and bladder and bowel abnormalities. To reduce the risk, needle placement is not done less than 10 to 12 hours after the last dose, and subsequent dosing is delayed at least 2 hours. Epidural catheters are withdrawn at least 10 to 12 hours after the last dose of LMWH.

A final rare complication, epidural abscess, is considered for patients in whom back pain develops after epidural injection; magnetic resonance imaging (MRI) is an effective diagnostic tool for such patients.

### Peripheral Nerve Blocks

Blockade of the brachial plexus, lumbar plexus, and specific peripheral nerves is an effective means of providing surgical anesthesia and postoperative analgesia for many surgical procedures involving the upper and lower extremities. The advantage of peripheral nerve blocks is reduced physiologic stress in comparison to spinal or epidural anesthesia, avoidance of airway manipulation and potential complications associated with endotracheal intubation, and avoidance of the potential side effects associated with general anesthesia. However, successful nerve block anesthesia requires a cooperative patient, an anesthesiologist skilled in peripheral nerve blocks, and a surgeon accustomed to operating on awake patients. All patients undergoing peripheral nerve block receive full preoperative evaluation under the assumption that general anesthesia could be used if the block is inadequate.

Improvements in nerve block equipment and methodology, as well as the availability of a wide range of local anesthetics, have greatly improved the effectiveness and safety of peripheral nerve blocks. In addition to providing surgical anesthesia, peripheral nerve blocks and placement of indwelling catheters for a prolonged nerve block provide excellent analgesia for many types of upper extremity surgery and trauma. An additional application of indwelling catheters is enhancement of blood flow after reattachment of amputated limbs and for patients with peripheral vascular disease. Each particular block has specific associated risks and benefits. However, general complications of peripheral nerve blocks include local anesthetic toxicity, neurologic injury, inadvertent neuraxial block, and intravascular injection of local anesthetics.

## CONSCIOUS SEDATION

When anesthesiologists participate in the sedation of patients undergoing surgical procedures, the procedure is termed *monitored anesthesia care.* Monitored anesthesia care encompasses a wide range of depths of sedation, ranging from minimal sedation to brief intervals of complete unconsciousness (e.g., during placement of a retrobulbar block by an ophthalmologist). When nonanesthesia personnel administer sedation for surgical procedures, the process is generally termed *conscious sedation,* although the term *moderate sedation* is preferable. Moderate sedation implies that the patient can respond purposefully to verbal or tactile stimulation, has a patent airway requiring no intervention, demonstrates adequate spontaneous ventilation, and has maintained cardiovascular function. There is a narrow margin between minimal sedation, which may be inadequate for surgery to continue, and deep sedation, which may result in airway compromise and cardiovascular and respiratory depression. Although relatively rare in this setting, a closed claims analysis has shown that hypoventilation and hypoxemia are the most common major complications.[39] Because of the risks associated with moderate sedation, TJC requires that patients be managed with precautions similar to what they would receive if an anesthesiologist were managing the sedation. Important factors include the necessity for preprocedure evaluation, continuous presence of a trained monitoring assistant who has no other responsibilities throughout the procedure, immediate availability of airway and resuscitation equipment, monitoring after the procedure until the effects of sedation have resolved, and specific written postoperative instructions. Physicians who perform procedures under conscious sedation are granted privileges in line with their training and experience in the appropriate resuscitative procedures.

Drugs used for moderate sedation usually consist of opioids such as fentanyl or morphine, often combined with an anxiolytic such as midazolam. Titration of these agents requires careful assessment of a patient's level of pain or anxiety and the requirements for the surgical procedure. Induction agents such as propofol are becoming increasingly popular for the induction of moderate sedation outside of the operating room. Although generally safe when used under the proper conditions, those agents introduce an added element of risk and increase the need for caution because of potentially rapid progression to deep sedation or even general anesthesia. Most hospitals now have specific policies and procedures governing moderate sedation. Those who use moderate sedation outside hospitals (e.g., in office-based surgical practices) need to follow the same precautions as those practiced in the hospital environment.

## POSTANESTHESIA CARE

The PACU is the area designated for the care of patients recovering from the immediate physiologic and pharmacologic consequences associated with anesthesia and surgery. The PACU ideally is located close to the operating rooms. Monitors for the assessment of ventilation, oxygenation, and circulation must be available for all recovering patients. The extent of monitoring depends on the condition of the patient. The ASA has established standards of postanesthesia care,[40] which mandate the following:

1. All patients undergoing general, regional, or monitored anesthesia care will receive appropriate postanesthesia care as dictated by the responsible anesthesiologist and/or policies and procedures that have been approved by the Department of Anesthesiology.
2. An anesthesia provider who is knowledgeable of the patient's condition will accompany the patient to the PACU.
3. On arrival in the PACU, the patient's condition will be reassessed and a report given to the care provider assuming responsibility for care.
4. The patient's condition will be evaluated continually in the PACU.
5. A physician is responsible for discharge of the patient from the PACU.

Recovery from anesthesia is usually uneventful and routine. Most patients stay in the PACU for 30 to 60 minutes until they are fully reactive and can be moved to a second-stage recovery area—for ambulatory patients who are returning home that day—or to a bed on a surgical floor. However, several criteria need to be met before the patient can be safely discharged from the PACU. All patients must be awake and oriented and have stable vital signs. Patients must be breathing without difficulty, able to protect their airways, and oxygenating appropriately. Pain, shivering, nausea, and vomiting must be adequately controlled. Patients receiving regional anesthesia must be observed for resolution of the block. There can be no evidence of surgical complications such as postoperative bleeding.

Several types of anesthesia-related complications can be encountered in the PACU and must be promptly recognized and treated to prevent serious injury.

### Postoperative Agitation and Delirium

Pain and anxiety are often manifested as postoperative agitation. However, agitation may also signal serious physiologic disturbances such as hypoxemia, hypercapnia, acidosis, hypotension, hypoglycemia, surgical complications, and adverse drug reactions. Serious underlying conditions must be excluded as the cause of agitation before treating patients empirically with pain medications, sedatives, or physical restraints.

### Respiratory Complications

Respiratory problems are the most frequently occurring major complications in the PACU. Airway obstruction is most commonly caused by obstruction of the oropharynx by the tongue or oropharyngeal soft tissues as a result of the residual effects of general anesthetics, pain medications, or muscle relaxants. Other causes of airway obstruction include laryngospasm, blood, vomitus, or debris in the airway, glottic edema, vocal cord paralysis, and external compression of the airway by a hematoma, dressing, or cervical collar. Oxygen must be administered to a patient with airway obstruction while measures are taken to relieve the obstruction. The characteristic physical signs of airway obstruction are sonorous respiratory sounds and paradoxical chest movement.

Many obstructions can be relieved by applying a head tilt and jaw thrust maneuver, with or without placement of an oral or nasopharyngeal airway. Suctioning the airway may also be beneficial, and the patient needs to be examined for evidence of external airway compression. In cases of laryngospasm, continuous positive airway pressure (CPAP) is applied, followed by the administration of 10 to 20 mg of succinylcholine if CPAP is ineffective. Patients may require mask ventilation and endotracheal intubation if the laryngospasm does not resolve promptly. In children, glottic edema or postextubation croup can result in airway obstruction. Mild cases are treated with humidified oxygen. Refractory obstruction may require the administration of systemic steroids and racemic epinephrine by nebulization. Reintubation may also be required.

Hypoxemia is a surprisingly common problem. The incidence of mild hypoxemia ($Spo_2$ = 86% to 90%) and severe hypoxemia ($Spo_2 \leq 85\%$) was found to be 7% and 0.7%, respectively, in the PACU for patients undergoing superficial elective plastic surgery, 38% and 3%, respectively, for patients undergoing upper abdominal surgery, and 52% and 20%, respectively, for patients undergoing thoracoabdominal surgery.[41] Hypoxemia can result from hypoventilation, ventilation-perfusion mismatching, or right-to-left intrapulmonary shunting. Reluctance to inspire deeply after abdominal or thoracic surgery may also result in hypoxemia. Clinically, hypoxemia must be suspected as an underlying problem in patients exhibiting restlessness, tachycardia, or cardiac irritability. Bradycardia, hypotension, and cardiac arrest are late signs. Hypoxemia in the PACU may be secondary to atelectasis, which may respond to incentive spirometry or vigorous encouragement to inspire deeply and cough. Treatment of hypoxemia requires the administration of oxygen, assurance of adequate ventilation, and treatment of the underlying causes.

Hypoventilation (synonymous with hypercapnia) can result from airway obstruction, central respiratory depression caused by the residual effects of anesthetic agents, hypothermia, CNS injury, or restriction of ventilation secondary to muscle relaxants, abdominal distention, and/or electrolyte abnormalities. Signs can include prolonged somnolence, a slow (or rapid) respiratory rate, airway obstruction, shallow breathing, tachycardia, and arrhythmias. Severe hypoventilation can result in hypoxemia, although augmented inspired oxygen will limit the severity of hypoventilation-induced hypoxemia. Treatment is aimed at identification and treatment of the underlying problem. In all cases, ventilation must be supported until corrective measures are instituted. Obtundation, circulatory depression, and severe respiratory acidosis are indications for endotracheal intubation and ventilatory support.

## Postoperative Nausea and Vomiting

Perhaps one of the most annoying problems for patients and staff in the PACU is postoperative nausea and vomiting. A wide variety of agents have varying degrees of effectiveness for prevention or treatment postoperative nausea and vomiting (Table 16-9). No single technique has yet proven to be uniformly therapeutic and cost-effective. The use of propofol for induction of anesthesia has also been shown to be effective in decreasing the incidence of postoperative nausea and vomiting. One important complication related to the IV coadministration of ondansetron and metoclopramide has been the production of bradyarrhythmias, including a slow junctional escape rhythm and ventricular bigeminy. The FDA has placed a so-called black box warning on the use of droperidol, in which additional electrocardiographic monitoring is required before and after administration of the drug because of an alleged increase in serious cardiac arrhythmias caused by QT prolongation. This FDA warning has been controversial because of the good safety profile of droperidol during the past 35 years and relative lack of scientific evidence to support the recommendation.[42] A study comparing droperidol and saline did not show a significant effect of either intervention on the QT interval during or after anesthesia.[43] Nevertheless, the FDA recommendation has caused a significant reduction in the use of droperidol for the treatment of postoperative nausea and vomiting.

The approach to the prophylaxis and treatment of postoperative nausea and vomiting are guided by an understanding of the mechanisms causing nausea and vomiting. Areas in the brainstem that control nausea and vomiting reflexes, such as the chemoreceptor trigger zone, contain receptors for dopamine, acetylcholine, histamine, and serotonin. Binding of all these receptors may precipitate nausea, vomiting, or both. Effective pharmacologic approaches to the treatment of postoperative nausea and vomiting include the use of anticholinergics, serotonin receptor antagonists, antidopaminergics, and antihistamines (Table 16-9). The use of any particular agent is based on its efficacy, potential side effects, and cost.

**Table 16-9 Commonly Used Antiemetic Agents**

| DRUG CLASS | COMMON SIDE EFFECTS |
|---|---|
| **Dopamine Receptor Antagonists (DA-2)** | |
| Phenothiazines | |
| Fluphenazine | |
| Chlorpromazine | |
| Prochlorperazine | Sedation |
| Butyrophenones | Dissociation |
| Droperidol | Extrapyramidal effects |
| Haloperidol | |
| Substituted benzamide | |
| Metoclopramide | |
| **Antihistamines ($H_1$)** | |
| Diphenhydramine | Sedation |
| Promethazine | Dry mouth |
| **Anticholinergics** | |
| Scopolamine | Sedation |
| Atropine | Dry mouth |
| | Tachycardia |
| **Serotonin Receptor Antagonists** | |
| Ondansetron | Headache |
| Dolasetron | |
| **Corticosteroids** | |
| Dexamethasone | Glucose intolerance |
| Methylprednisolone | Altered wound healing |
| Hydrocortisone | Immunosuppression |
| | Renal effects |

## Hypothermia

Hypothermia has been extensively studied as a perioperative complication. The most important issues related to perioperative hypothermia include the risk of increased oxygen consumption postoperatively because of shivering, alterations in drug metabolism, effects on blood coagulation and the possibility that hypothermia could increase the rate of surgical infections. Increased oxygen consumption could be a particular problem in patients with CAD, in whom shivering could trigger myocardial ischemia. However, the risk associated with mild hypothermia has not been well defined in otherwise healthy patients. Nevertheless, the Center for Medicare and Medicaid Services has designated perioperative normothermia as a pay for performance issue. This means that hospitals and medical centers that report on and achieve perioperative normothermia (36° C within 30 minutes of arrival in the PACU for procedures lasting longer than 1 hour) receive financial incentives.

General anesthesia has profound effects on thermoregulatory mechanisms and active intraoperative warming is required to maintain normothermia under most conditions. Forced-air and circulating water warmers are the most effective techniques for providing active intraoperative warming, each having advantages under different conditions. IV fluid warmers and airway warming devices can also be useful for minimizing heat loss but do not allow for active warming. Because of the effects of anesthesia on heat redistribution to the skin and peripheral tissues, preoperative warming is required to minimize core hypothermia in patients undergoing procedures lasting less than 1 hour. In most cases, prophylactic warming will decrease the incidence of postoperative hypothermia and need for intervention in the outpatient surgical setting. However, time to PACU discharge and patient satisfaction are not affected. The use of prophylactic warming is associated with a significant increase in cost. Therefore, guidelines for temperature management during short outpatient surgical procedures remain to be fully implemented.

## Circulatory Complications

Hypotension in the PACU is most commonly caused by hypovolemia, left ventricular dysfunction, or arrhythmias. Other causes include anaphylaxis, transfusion reactions, cardiac tamponade, pulmonary emboli, adverse drug reactions, adrenal insufficiency, and hypoxemia. Treatment involves support of the circulation with fluids, administration of inotropic agents, use of the Trendelenburg position, and delivery of oxygen until the underlying cause is diagnosed and treated.

Hypertension is a common finding in the PACU. Common causes include pain, anxiety, and inadequately managed essential hypertension. Hypoxemia and hypercapnia always need to be ruled out. Other less common causes include hypoglycemia, drug reactions, diseases such as hyperthyroidism, pheochromocytoma, or malignant hyperthermia, and bladder distention. The fundamental goal in control of postoperative hypertension is to identify and correct the underlying cause.

## ACUTE PAIN MANAGEMENT

Pain, one of the most common symptoms experienced by surgical patients, has historically been poorly evaluated and frequently undertreated. There have been important changes in medical care with respect to pain management, with inclusion of pain management in medical school curricula, establishment of institutional protocols and procedures for pain management, development of the subspecialty of pain medicine, creation of organizations focused on pain, and increased interest on the part of governmental and third-party payers. These changes will continue and medical personnel must continue to increase their knowledge of pain control and commitment to provide optimal analgesia as a key component of patient care. Surveys have shown that continued improvement is necessary to reduce the high incidence of moderate to severe acute postoperative pain further.

Acute pain occurs frequently in the setting of surgery and trauma. The pain experience may be part of the symptom complex that prompts the patient to seek medical care or may be caused by tissue injury sustained as a result of surgery or trauma. The term *acute* refers to pain that is expected to be of relatively short duration and that should resolve with tissue healing or withdrawal of the noxious stimulus. Acute pain generally resolves within minutes, hours, or days. Chronic pain, which can persist for years, is defined as pain that persists for at least 1 month beyond the usual course of an acute disease or beyond a reasonable time in which an injury would be expected to heal. The acute stress response associated with acute pain serves a useful function, although undertreatment may result in harmful pathophysiologic changes. Chronic pain serves no useful function and is now recognized not only as a part of certain disease processes, such as cancer, but also often as a disease itself.

### Mechanisms of Acute Pain

The International Association for the Study of Pain defines pain as "an unpleasant sensory and emotional experience associated with actual or potential tissue damage or described in terms of such damage."[43a] This definition emphasizes not only the sensory experience but also the affective component of pain. The tissue injury that leads to the complaint of pain results in a process called nociception, which has four steps: transduction, transmission, modulation, and perception (Fig. 16-4). With transduction, the noxious stimulus is converted into an electrical signal at free nerve endings, also known as nociceptors. Nociceptors are widely distributed throughout the body in somatic and visceral tissues.

With transmission, the electrical signal is sent via nerve pathways toward the CNS. Nerve pathways include primary sensory afferents, primarily A delta and C fibers, that project to the spinal cord, ascending tracts (including the spinothalamic tract) to the brainstem and thalamus, and thalamocortical pathways to the cortex. Modulation, the process that enhances or suppresses the pain signal, occurs primarily in the dorsal horn of the spinal cord—in particular, the substantia gelatinosa. Perception, the final step in the nociceptive process, occurs when the pain signal reaches the cerebral cortex. The first three steps in nociception are important for the sensory and discriminative aspects of pain. The fourth step, perception, is integral to the subjective and emotional experience.

### Methods of Analgesia

A number of agents, routes of administration, and modalities are available for effective management of acute pain. Analgesic agents include opioids, nonsteroidal anti-inflammatory drugs (NSAIDs), acetaminophen, and local anesthetics. Less traditional agents that may be used more frequently include clonidine, dexmedetomidine, dextromethorphan, and gabapentin. Routes of administration include the oral, parenteral, epidural, and intrathecal routes. The oral route is the preferred route for analgesic delivery. Patients experiencing mild to moderate acute pain and who can receive agents orally can obtain effective analgesia. Parenteral administration is preferred for patients experiencing moderate to severe pain, who require rapid control of pain, and who cannot receive agents through the GI tract. The IV route is preferred over IM and SC injections when the parenteral route is indicated. IM injections are painful, result in erratic absorption, and lead to variable blood levels of the administered agent.

#### Opioids

Opioids are potent analgesic agents that are effective but frequently underused. By binding to opioid receptors in the CNS and probably also in peripheral tissues, opioids modulate the nociceptive process. The best-characterized opioid receptors are $\mu_1$, $\mu_2$, $\delta$, $\kappa$, $\varepsilon$, and $\sigma$ receptors. The $\mu_1$ receptors are involved in supraspinal analgesia. The $\delta$ and $\kappa$ receptors are involved in spinal analgesia. Opioids can be administered by a number of routes, including oral, parenteral, neuraxial, rectal, and transdermal.

Opioids have varying degrees of potency. Strong opioids are ideal for moderate to severe pain and for pain that is constant in frequency. Weak opioid agents are suitable for mild to moderate pain that is intermittent in frequency. Morphine, the prototype strong opioid, can be delivered by a variety of routes and techniques. Other strong opioids include hydromorphone, fentanyl, and meperidine. Morphine is metabolized to morphine-3-glucuronide and morphine-6-glucuronide, which can accumulate in patients with renal impairment. For moderate to severe pain in patients with renal dysfunction, fentanyl and hydromorphone are more suitable agents. Historically, meperidine has frequently been the preferred strong opioid. This practice has declined because meperidine is metabolized to normeperidine, a unique toxic metabolite that can accumulate and cause seizure-like activity. Patients who are particularly vulnerable to this side effect include older patients, patients who are dehydrated, and those with renal impairment. Fentanyl is

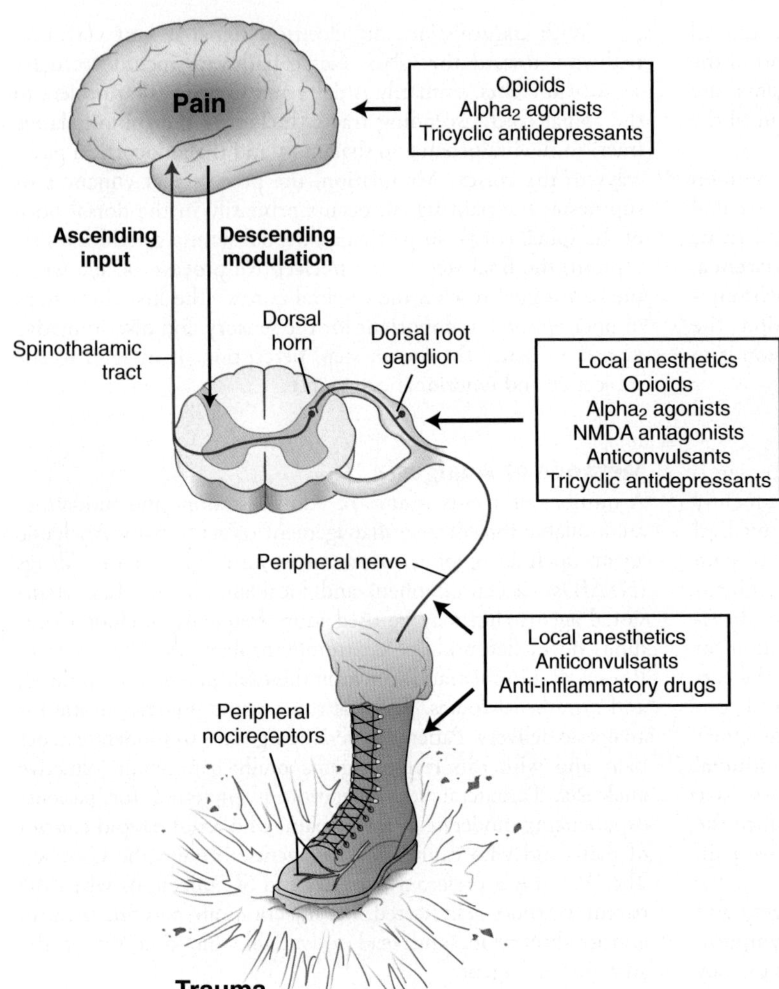


**FIGURE 16-4** Schematic diagram outlining the nociceptive pathway for the transmission of painful stimuli. Interventions that prevent nociceptive transmission are shown at the points in the pathway that are thought to be their sites of action. (From Buckenmaier CC III, Bleckner LL [eds]: Military advanced regional anesthesia and analgesia handbook, Washington DC, 2008, Borden Institute, Walter Reed Army Medical Center.)

available in a transdermal preparation, but this route is not recommended for acute pain management.

Weak opioid agents, such as hydrocodone and codeine, are commonly combined with aspirin or acetaminophen. Tramadol is an analgesic that is a nonopioid but has some opioid-like effects. It is a centrally acting agent that is administered orally and can be used for mild to moderate pain. Common opioid-related side effects include nausea, pruritus, sedation, mental clouding, decreased gastric motility, urinary retention, and respiratory depression. Appropriate selection of agents, monitoring, and treatment can prevent or ameliorate these side effects.

One major barrier to the effective use of opioid agents by patients, physicians, and other health care providers is the fear of addiction, which can be manifested as underdosing, use of excessively wide dosing intervals, administration of weak opioids for moderate to severe pain, and underreporting of pain. In the setting of acute postoperative pain, the use of opioids has not been shown to be a risk factor for the development of an addiction disorder. Key terms to understand include the terms *tolerance, addiction* (psychological dependence), and *physical dependence.* Tolerance occurs when a previously effective opioid dose fails to provide adequate analgesia. It is a normal physiologic effect and should not be confused with addiction. Tolerance develops not only to the analgesic effect of opioids but also to most opioid-related side effects. The duration of opioid exposure also plays a role in the development of tolerance. In patients manifesting tolerance, an increased dose is required to achieve effective analgesia. Addiction or psychological dependence is a compulsive disorder manifested by preoccupation with obtaining and inappropriate use of a substance, continued use despite harm, decreased quality of life, and denial. Psychological dependence should not be confused with physical dependence, which is a normal physiologic process. Physical dependence is manifested by the occurrence of a withdrawal syndrome when use of a drug is stopped suddenly or when an antagonist is given. The duration of opioid treatment is a factor in the development of physical dependence. The short-term use of opioids in the perioperative period rarely results in physical dependence. Slow tapering of opioids generally prevents withdrawal symptoms.

### Nonsteroidal Anti-Inflammatory Agents

NSAIDs are an important component of perioperative analgesia that when used as a part of the analgesic regimen, reduce pain and can decrease opioid consumption. Their mechanism of action is achieved through the inhibition of cyclooxygenase (COX) enzyme activity, which results in decreased production of prostaglandins. Prostaglandins are potent mediators of pain that act directly at nociceptors and also increase nociceptor sensitivity. Inhibition of prostaglandin production results in analgesia but can also lead to side effects such as gastric ulceration, bleeding, and renal injury. These side effects have limited the used of NSAIDs in the perioperative period. Contrary to previous evidence that NSAIDs act mainly in peripheral tissues, there is now evidence that NSAIDs also work in the CNS.

There is a wide range of compounds in this analgesic class, with differing chemical structures. Most of these agents are intended for oral administration, which limits their use perioperatively. Ketorolac is available for parenteral administration and has been shown to be effective for analgesia and safe with appropriate patient selection. Ketorolac is avoided in patients with a history of gastropathy, platelet dysfunction, or thrombocytopenia, in those with a history of allergy to the agent, and in patients with renal impairment or hypovolemia. It is used with caution in older patients. A loading dose of 30 mg IV, followed by 15 mg IV every 6 hours for a short course, can provide effective analgesia for mild to moderate pain or can be a useful adjunct for moderate to severe pain when combined with opioids or other analgesic techniques.

Rather recent advances in this analgesic category involve the introduction of agents that are selective in their inhibition of subtypes of the COX enzyme. There are at least two subtypes of this enzyme, COX-1 (constitutive) and COX-2 (inducible). Traditional NSAIDs are nonselective inhibitors of COX. Newer agents (e.g., celecoxib, rofecoxib, valdecoxib) are selective COX-2 inhibitors. COX-2 inhibitors appear to offer similar analgesia with a somewhat reduced risk of causing GI bleeding, bleeding diathesis, and renal compromise.[44] They have mostly been studied and used clinically in the management of arthritis-related pain but have become more frequently used in the perioperative period. Currently available COX-2 inhibitors are for oral administration. Parecoxib is being studied for parenteral use. There are indications that COX-2 inhibitors are associated with a lower incidence of gastropathy. Concerns about the use of these selective NSAIDs include the risk for cardiovascular events and their effects on bone healing. Some of these agents (e.g., rofecoxib, valdecoxib) have been removed from the market because of the risk for cardiovascular complications. Valdecoxib was removed from commercial distribution because of the risk for severe skin reaction and cardiovascular complications.

### Local Anesthetics for the Management of Acute Pain

Local anesthetics work by blocking conduction in nerve fibers, the second step in the process of nociception. These agents are used to provide regional anesthesia for surgery, but their effects last into the postoperative period and contribute to preemptive analgesia. Local anesthetics used in doses lower than those required for anesthesia can also provide analgesia by a variety of application techniques, including local infiltration, topical application, epidural infusion, and peripheral nerve infusion. Local infiltration of local anesthetic before the surgical incision may reduce the sensitization of nociceptors and thereby result in reduced conduction of pain signals to the CNS. This may be manifested as decreased postoperative pain and analgesic requirements. Local infiltration on wound closure may also be helpful. Topical application of local anesthetic includes the use of agents such as a eutectic mixture of local anesthetics (e.g., EMLA cream), which contains prilocaine and lidocaine. This agent can be used for superficial procedures and can be placed before the surgical incision. Placement of peripheral nerve catheters for local anesthetic infusion has become a frequently used technique for postoperative pain management. The development of disposable and lightweight infusion pumps has led to the increased use of peripheral nerve infusion in the ambulatory setting. Peripheral nerve infusion analgesia has been shown to provide improved postoperative pain control when compared with opioid administration.[45]

### Combination Analgesic Therapy

By combining agents from different analgesic classes, synergy may be obtained. Synergy results in the potentiation of effect and reduced dosage of each individual agent, with fewer and less severe side effects from each agent. Common combinations include opioids and NSAIDs in an analgesic regimen or epidural administration of a local anesthetic with an opioid. The choice of agent and technique depends on factors such as the patient's medical history, patient preference, extent of surgery, expected degree of postoperative pain, experience of the staff providing care for the patient, and postoperative setting in which the patient will recover. Gabapentin, an anticonvulsant used for the management of chronic neuropathic pain, has shown efficacy for analgesia in the acute postoperative period, including improved pain control and reduced opioid-related side effects.[46]

The concept of preemptive analgesia is being actively explored and used in the perioperative period. Induced by a variety of agents and techniques, the goal of preemptive analgesia is to influence the analgesic process before initiation of the noxious stimulus (e.g., surgical incision). This minimizes sensitization of the nervous system and moderates the process of nociception described previously. Effective preemptive analgesia results in decreased postoperative pain, reduced postoperative analgesic requirement, decreased side effects from analgesics, increased compliance with postoperative rehabilitation, and decreased incidence of chronic postsurgical pain syndromes.

### Neuraxial Analgesia

Neuraxial routes of administration include the epidural and intrathecal (subarachnoid) routes. These modes of administration require consultation from acute pain specialists, usually anesthesiologists who have received specialized training in use of the neuraxial route for the administration of anesthesia and analgesia. Neuraxial agents are delivered by a single injection into the epidural or subarachnoid space, intermittent injections through an indwelling epidural catheter, by continuous infusion through an indwelling epidural catheter, or patient-controlled epidural analgesia through an indwelling catheter. Indwelling subarachnoid catheters are rarely used for acute pain. An important consideration when selecting patients for neuraxial analgesia is the presence of abnormal coagulation, including concurrent use of antiplatelet and anticoagulant agents. Knowledge of such coagulation issues is important to minimize the risk for intraspinal bleeding and spinal hematoma formation, which can lead to severe neurologic injury. The neuraxial route requires education of the medical and nursing staff and use of protocols and guidelines. In general, patients can be managed on surgical floors with these analgesic techniques. However, monitoring procedures need to be in place to minimize the development of side effects and enhance patient safety.

Agents such as opioids and local anesthetics are given via the neuraxial route to achieve analgesia. Other agents that have been used neuraxially include clonidine, neostigmine, and acetaminophen. Opioids, when delivered by the neuraxial route, provide analgesia by their action at opioid receptors located in the dorsal horn of the spinal cord. An important determinant of opioid action when delivered by the neuraxial route is the drug's degree of lipid solubility. Morphine is hydrophilic, which accounts for its slow onset of analgesia, long duration of action, ability to provide analgesia over a wide dermatomal distribution, and risk for late respiratory depression. Fentanyl is lipophilic, which accounts for its fast onset and short duration of action, ability to provide segmental analgesia, and limited risk for late respiratory depression. A hydrophilic opioid such as morphine, when delivered into the epidural or subarachnoid space, remains in the CSF longer than a lipophilic opioid. The drug can travel rostrally to the brain and influence the respiratory centers hours after initial delivery.

Local anesthetics, when used for neuraxial analgesia, provide analgesia by blocking nerve conduction. To achieve neuraxial analgesia, local anesthetics are delivered in smaller doses and weaker concentrations than those required to achieve surgical anesthesia. This resulting sensory blockade is sufficient to provide analgesia but is not sufficiently profound to interfere with motor function and mask complications. Analgesic concentrations of local anesthetics also cause less impairment of sympathetic tone. Bupivacaine and ropivacaine are the most commonly used local anesthetics for epidural analgesia and peripheral nerve infusion analgesia. They affect sensory fibers more than motor fibers (differential blockade) and have a lower incidence of tachyphylaxis (tolerance to local anesthetic action). Neuraxial analgesia for acute pain commonly combines opioids and local anesthetics. Each agent has a different mechanism of action; combining these agents produces synergistic analgesia and thereby results in reduced doses of each agent and a decreased incidence and severity of side effects. A meta-analysis of the efficacy of postoperative epidural analgesia has concluded that epidural analgesia, regardless of agent, location of catheter placement, and type of pain assessment, provides analgesia superior to that of parenteral opioids.[47]

### Intravenous Patient-Controlled Analgesia

An increasingly popular and effective modality using the parenteral route of administration is IV PCA. This modality minimizes the steps involved in the delivery of analgesia and increases patient autonomy and control. Opioids are the agents of choice for IV PCA. In comparing IV PCA with conventional, intermittent, nurse-administered opioid delivery, patients obtain prompt analgesia, receive smaller doses of opioids at more frequent intervals, can maintain blood concentration of drug in the analgesic range, and have a lower incidence of drug-related side effects. Candidates for IV PCA are patients who can understand the basic steps involved in use of the device, who are willing to assume control of their analgesia, and who are physically capable of activating the device. Such patients include children as young as 4 years of age and most adults, including geriatric patients.

The preferred agents for IV PCA are opioids, with morphine sulfate most commonly chosen. Other opioids used for IV PCA include hydromorphone, fentanyl, and meperidine. Methadone IV PCA has been described. Physicians' orders for IV PCA must specify the drug, drug concentration, loading dose, bolus dose, continuous infusion rate (basal rate), lockout interval, and dose limits. Selection of these parameters is based on the patient's age, medical status, and level of pain. The routine use of a continuous basal infusion rate with IV PCA remains controversial. With a continuous infusion, drug is delivered to the patient regardless of demand, thus resulting in the potential for a higher incidence of drug-related side effects, including respiratory depression. It is safest to restrict the use of basal infusions to patients in special categories, including those with severe pain from extensive surgery or trauma and patients who are tolerant because of chronic opioid use.

The use of structured protocols and guidelines is encouraged for facilities using IV PCA. The medical and nursing staffs need to receive training in the care of patients using this modality. There is an increased risk for complications if staff members are not trained in the following: to understand the concept of IV PCA; to perform appropriate patient selection, education, and assessment; to use appropriate drug and dose selection; and to establish appropriate monitoring requirements and protocols for management of side effects.

## Chronic Pain

In a subset of patients, pain persists after the expected healing time despite the lack of sufficient pathology to account for the pain. Pain that persists for 1 month beyond the expected time for recovery or initial onset is considered evidence of a chronic pain syndrome. Such patients with persistent pain frequently use terms such as *burning, shooting,* and *shocklike* to describe their pain, which is generally associated with a neuropathic pain syndrome. Neuropathic pain syndromes occur when there has been injury to the nervous system (central, peripheral, or both). Central sensitization is believed to underlie the development of neuropathic pain. Examples include patients with persistent pain after head and neck surgery, thoracotomy, mastectomy, hernia repair, and amputation. Certain factors that may increase the risk for chronic pain include infection at the surgical site, intraoperative trauma to nerves, diabetes mellitus, and nerve entrapment by cancer. There is some evidence that preemptive analgesia may help minimize the occurrence of these syndromes.

Because chronic pain syndromes can be difficult to diagnose in the early postoperative period, it is important for physicians to perform appropriate pain assessment during postoperative follow-up. For example, after amputation, patients might consider it strange to continue to feel sensation and pain in the location of an amputated limb and might be reluctant to volunteer information that they believe could suggest psychological instability. In such circumstances, appropriate questioning may elicit the complaint and result in patient reassurance and appropriate treatment. Referral to a pain medicine consultant is appropriate when the diagnosis of a chronic postoperative pain syndrome is made. Treatment modalities include the use of adjuvant medications such as antidepressants and anticonvulsants, nerve blocks, physical therapy, and psychological techniques.

## Specific Types of Acute Pain Patients

### Patients With a History of Chronic Pain

Patients who have a history of chronic pain may experience acute pain as a result of surgery or trauma differently from patients who have no history of chronic pain. Their experience of pain is affected by their experience with chronic pain. Some of these patients may be receiving chronic opioid therapy as part of their chronic pain management. It is likely that these patients will manifest tolerance to opioid therapy and have a decreased pain threshold, which may result in the patient reporting higher levels of pain and the physician increasing the opioid dose. Obtaining a pain history preoperatively, choosing anesthetic and surgical techniques to minimize tissue trauma and the response to trauma, and appropriate planning for postoperative analgesia can assist in achieving effective analgesia.

### Patients With a History of Substance Abuse

Patients with a history of substance abuse are frequently undertreated for acute pain complaints. The stigma associated with drug abuse, misunderstanding on the part of health care providers, and inappropriate pain behavior contribute to undertreatment for this patient population. Effective analgesia can be obtained with strict guidelines, patient education, and appropriate use of consultants and modalities such as regional analgesia.

### Pediatric Patients

Pediatric patients experience a similar severity of acute postoperative and post-traumatic pain as adults. A major historical myth that has been refuted is the belief that neonates, infants, and children do not perceive pain in the same way as adults. Effective analgesia for a pediatric patient experiencing acute pain can be achieved with pain assessment tools that are tailored for this population and the use of modalities and agents similar to those used for adults. Dosage selection in a pediatric patient must be guided by calculations based on patient weight. With neonates, nurse-controlled analgesia is standard. Older children can effectively use PCA. Regional anesthesia is increasingly being used for pediatric surgery, with the benefits of analgesia extending into the postoperative period and reduced opioid requirements. Epidural analgesia, usually via a caudally placed catheter or a single injection into the caudal canal, can provide effective analgesia. Placement of a peripheral catheter for infusion of local anesthetics can also be used. Topical anesthesia with local anesthetics such as the application of EMLA cream can similarly minimize pain from IV catheter placement and superficial procedures.

### Older Patients

As the proportion of older adults in the general population increases, a growing percentage of geriatric patients are undergoing surgery or being treated for trauma. These patients will require pain assessment and evaluation tailored to their mental status and cognitive abilities. The modalities and agents used to manage acute pain in this population must take into consideration underlying disease states and decreased organ function.

## CONCLUSION

Modern anesthesia is safe and effective for the vast majority of patients, in large part because of important advances in anesthesia equipment, monitors, and drugs. With a wide variety of specific techniques to choose from, selection of anesthetic and postoperative pain regimens for each patient can be based on the requirements of the surgical procedure, patient preferences, and experience and expertise of the anesthesiologist.

## SELECTED REFERENCES

Benumof JL, Dagg R, Benumof R: Critical hemoglobin desaturation will occur before return to an unparalyzed state following 1 mg/kg intravenous succinylcholine. Anesthesiology 87:979–982, 1997.

Using a combination of pharmacologic and physiologic information from the literature, the authors provide a detailed discussion of factors that influence the rate at which clinically important hypoxemia occurs in relation to the expected duration of succinylcholine. This contributes an important counterargument to the common misconception that succinylcholine will be metabolized before hypoxemia-induced harm occurs.

Debaene B, Plaud B, Dilly MP, et al: Residual paralysis in the PACU after a single intubating dose of nondepolarizing muscle relaxant with an intermediate duration of action. Anesthesiology 98:1042–1048, 2003.

In a study of 526 patients who received a single dose of vecuronium, rocuronium, or atracurium to facilitate tracheal intubation, received no more relaxant thereafter, and did not undergo reversal of neuromuscular blockade, residual paralysis was present in 45% overall and 37% after 2 hours. The authors emphasize the importance of quantitative measurement of neuromuscular transmission.

Devereaux PJ, Yang H, Yusuf S, et al: Effects of extended-release metoprolol succinate in patients undergoing non-cardiac surgery (POISE trial): A randomised controlled trial. Lancet 371:1839–1847, 2008.

This widely publicized study reported that beta blocker–naïve patients receiving perioperative treatment with high-dose, extended-release metoprolol had a decreased incidence of perioperative myocardial ischemia but increased hypotension, stroke, and death.

Fleisher LA, Beckman JA, Brown KA, et al: 2009 ACCF/AHA focused update on perioperative beta blockade incorporated into the ACC/AHA 2007 guidelines on perioperative cardiovascular evaluation and care for noncardiac surgery. J Am Coll Cardiol 54:e13–e118, 2009.

In this extensive review, a joint task force of the American College of Cardiology and American Heart Association reports guidelines for evaluation of patients with cardiovascular disease who are scheduled for noncardiac surgery. They thoroughly examine the importance of the history, physical findings, available tests, and influence of various types of surgery, as well current recommendations on the perioperative use of beta blockers. This is a valuable update of a consensus approach to this difficult topic.

Qaseem A, Snow V, Fitterman N, et al: Risk assessment for strategies to reduce perioperative pulmonary complications for patients undergoing non-cardiovascular surgery: A guideline from the American College of Physicians. Ann Intern Med 144:575–580, 2006.

Report of a consensus conference that reviewed the topic of preoperative pulmonary evaluation. This group identified patient-related risk factors, factors related to the surgical site, and other factors related to surgery, such as the duration of surgery, choice of general anesthesia, and intraoperative use of pancuronium. Major patient-associated risk factors were ASA class greater than 2, age older than 60 years, functional dependence, and presence of COPD or congestive heart failure. A serum albumin concentration lower than 3.5 g/dL was also a strong predictor of pulmonary complications.

Sprung J, Warner ME, Contreras MG, et al: Predictors of survival following cardiac arrest in patients undergoing noncardiac surgery—a study of 518,294 patients at a tertiary referral center. Anesthesiology 99:259–269, 2003.

Cardiac arrest occurred in 223 of 518,294 patients (4.3/10,000) undergoing noncardiac surgery between January 1, 1990, and December 31, 2000. The frequency of arrest in patients receiving general anesthesia decreased over time (7.8/10,000 during 1990-1992; 3.2/10,000 during 1998-2000). The immediate survival rate after arrest was 46.6%, and the hospital survival rate was 34.5%. Twenty-four patients (0.5/10,000) had cardiac arrest related primarily to anesthesia.

Wallace AW, Au S, Cason BA: Association of the pattern of use of perioperative beta-blockade and postoperative mortality. Anesthesiology 113:794–805, 2010.

This study retrospectively analyzed a large cohort of surgical patients from 1996-2008. The authors report that perioperative withdrawal of beta blockers resulted in increased morbidity and mortality and that use of perioperative beta blockers and that overall use of beta blockers reduces perioperative mortality.

White PF, Song D, Abrao J, et al: Effect of low-dose droperidol on the QT interval during and after general anesthesia: A placebo-controlled study. Anesthesiology 102:1101–1105, 2005.

The FDA has issued a black box warning concerning the use of droperidol for the treatment of postoperative nausea and vomiting because of reported prolongation of the QT interval and potential development of ventricular arrhythmias. This study showed that the use of droperidol (0.625–1.25 mg IV) for antiemetic prophylaxis during general anesthesia was not associated with a statistically significant increase in the QTc interval when compared with saline.

## REFERENCES


1. Diemunsch PA, Van Dorsselaer T, Torp KD, et al: Calibrated pneumoperitoneal venting to prevent $N_2O$ accumulation in the $CO_2$ pneumoperitoneum during laparoscopy with inhaled anesthesia: an experimental study in pigs. Anesth Analg 94:1014–1018, 2002.
2. Rooke GA, Choi JH, Bishop MJ: The effect of isoflurane, halothane, sevoflurane, and thiopental/nitrous oxide on respiratory system resistance after tracheal intubation. Anesthesiology 86: 1294–1299, 1997.
3. Spracklin DK, Kharasch ED: Evidence for metabolism of fluoromethyl 2,2-difluoro-1-(trifluoromethyl)vinyl ether (compound A), a sevoflurane degradation product, by cysteine conjugate beta-lyase. Chem Res Toxicol 9:696–702, 1996.
4. Beaussier M, Deriaz H, Abdelahim Z, et al: Comparative effects of desflurane and isoflurane on recovery after long-lasting anaesthesia. Can J Anaesth 45:429–434, 1998.
5. Fang ZX, Eger EI, 2nd, Laster MJ, et al: Carbon monoxide production from degradation of desflurane, enflurane, isoflurane, halothane, and sevoflurane by soda lime and Baralyme. Anesth Analg 80:1187–1193, 1995.
6. Fu ES, Miguel R, Scharf JE: Preemptive ketamine decreases postoperative narcotic requirements in patients undergoing abdominal surgery. Anesth Analg 84:1086–1090, 1997.
7. Eames WO, Rooke GA, Wu RS, et al: Comparison of the effects of etomidate, propofol, and thiopental on respiratory resistance after tracheal intubation. Anesthesiology 84:1307–1311, 1996.
8. Brown RH, Wagner EM: Mechanisms of bronchoprotection by anesthetic induction agents: Propofol versus ketamine. Anesthesiology 90:822–828, 1999.
9. Tan JA, Ho KM: Use of dexmedetomidine as a sedative and analgesic agent in critically ill adult patients: A meta-analysis. Intensive Care Med 36:926–939, 2010.
10. Katoh T, Ikeda K: The effects of fentanyl on sevoflurane requirements for loss of consciousness and skin incision. Anesthesiology 88:18–24, 1998.
11. Benumof JL, Dagg R, Benumof R: Critical hemoglobin desaturation will occur before return to an unparalyzed state following 1 mg/kg intravenous succinylcholine. Anesthesiology 87:979–982, 1997.
12. Domino KB, Posner KL, Caplan RA, et al: Awareness during anesthesia: A closed claims analysis. Anesthesiology 90:1053–1061, 1999.
13. Wright PM, Hart P, Lau M, et al: The magnitude and time course of vecuronium potentiation by desflurane versus isoflurane. Anesthesiology 82:404–411, 1995.
14. Kopman AF, Yee PS, Neuman GG: Relationship of the train-of-four fade ratio to clinical signs and symptoms of residual paralysis in awake volunteers. Anesthesiology 86:765–771, 1997.
15. Debaene B, Plaud B, Dilly MP, et al: Residual paralysis in the PACU after a single intubating dose of nondepolarizing muscle relaxant with an intermediate duration of action. Anesthesiology 98:1042–1048, 2003.
16. Berg H, Roed J, Viby-Mogensen J, et al: Residual neuromuscular block is a risk factor for postoperative pulmonary complications. A prospective, randomised, and blinded study of postoperative pulmonary complications after atracurium, vecuronium and pancuronium. Acta Anaesthesiol Scand 41:1095–1103, 1997.
17. Caplan RA, Vistica MF, Posner KL, et al: Adverse anesthetic outcomes arising from gas delivery equipment: A closed claims analysis. Anesthesiology 87:741–748, 1997.
18. American Society of Anesthesiologists: Standards guidelines and statements. Standards for basic anesthetic monitoring. Committee of Origin: Standards and Practice Parameters (Approved by the ASA House of Delegates on October 21, 1986, and last amended on October 20, 2010 with an effective date of July 1, 2011) (http://www.asahq.org/publicationsAndServices/sgstoc.htm).
19. Kreuer S, Bruhn J, Larsen R, et al: A-line, bispectral index, and estimated effect-site concentrations: A prediction of clinical end-points of anesthesia. Anesth Analg 102:1141–1146, 2006.
20. Leslie K, Myles PS, Forbes A, et al: The effect of bispectral index monitoring on long-term survival in the B-aware trial. Anesth Analg 110:816–822, 2010.

**21.** American Society of Anesthesiologists: Standards, guidelines, and statements. Basic standards of preanesthesia care. (Approved by the ASA House of Delegates Oct 14, 1987 and last affirmed on October 20, 2010) (www.asahq.org/For-Members/Clinical-Information/~/media/For%2520Members/documents/Standards%2520Guidelines%2520Stmts/Preanesthesia%2520Care%2520Basic%2520Standards%2520for.ashx).

**22.** Ferschl MB, Tung A, Sweitzer B, et al: Preoperative clinic visits reduce operating room cancellations and delays. Anesthesiology 103:855–859, 2005.

**23.** Shiga T, Wajima Z, Inoue T, et al: Predicting difficult intubation in apparently normal patients: a meta-analysis of bedside screening test performance. Anesthesiology 103:429–437, 2005.

**24.** Fleisher LA, Beckman JA, Brown KA, et al: 2009 ACCF/AHA focused update on perioperative beta blockade incorporated into the ACC/AHA 2007 guidelines on perioperative cardiovascular evaluation and care for noncardiac surgery. J Am Coll Cardiol 54:e13–e118, 2009.

**25.** Devereaux PJ, Yang H, Yusuf S, et al: Effects of extended-release metoprolol succinate in patients undergoing non-cardiac surgery (POISE trial): A randomised controlled trial. Lancet 371: 1839–1847, 2008.

**26.** Wallace AW, Au S, Cason BA: Association of the pattern of use of perioperative beta-blockade and postoperative mortality. Anesthesiology 113:794–805, 2010.

**27.** Wilson W, Taubert KA, Gewitz M, et al: Prevention of infective endocarditis: Guidelines from the American Heart Association: A guideline from the American Heart Association Rheumatic Fever, Endocarditis, and Kawasaki Disease Committee, Council on Cardiovascular Disease in the Young, and the Council on Clinical Cardiology, Council on Cardiovascular Surgery and Anesthesia, and the Quality of Care and Outcomes Research Interdisciplinary Working Group. Circulation 116:1736–1754, 2007.

**28.** Qaseem A, Snow V, Fitterman N, et al: Risk assessment for and strategies to reduce perioperative pulmonary complications for patients undergoing noncardiothoracic surgery: A guideline from the American College of Physicians. Ann Intern Med 144:575–580, 2006.

**29.** Smetana GW: Preoperative pulmonary evaluation. N Engl J Med 340:937–944, 1999.

**30.** Warner DO, Warner MA, Barnes RD, et al: Perioperative respiratory complications in patients with asthma. Anesthesiology 85:460–467, 1996.

**31.** Warner DO, Warner MA, Offord KP, et al: Airway obstruction and perioperative complications in smokers undergoing abdominal surgery. Anesthesiology 90:372–379, 1999.

**32.** van den Berghe G, Wouters P, Weekers F, et al: Intensive insulin therapy in the critically ill patients. N Engl J Med 345:1359–1367, 2001.

**33.** Newland MC, Ellis SJ, Lydiatt CA, et al: Anesthetic-related cardiac arrest and its mortality: A report covering 72,959 anesthetics over 10 years from a US teaching hospital. Anesthesiology 97:108–115, 2002.

**34.** Sprung J, Warner ME, Contreras MG, et al: Predictors of survival following cardiac arrest in patients undergoing noncardiac surgery: A study of 518,294 patients at a tertiary referral center. Anesthesiology 99:259–269, 2003.

**35.** Schwilk B, Muche R, Treiber H, et al: A cross-validated multifactorial index of perioperative risks in adults undergoing anaesthesia for non-cardiac surgery. Analysis of perioperative events in 26907 anaesthetic procedures. J Clin Monit Comput 14:283–294, 1998.

**36.** Warner MA, Shields SE, Chute CG: Major morbidity and mortality within 1 month of ambulatory surgery and anesthesia. JAMA 270:1437–1441, 1993.

**36a.** Corman SL, Skledar SJ: Use of lipid emulsion to reverse local anesthetic toxicity. Ann Pharmacother 41:1873–1877, 2007.

**37.** Christopherson R, Beattie C, Frank SM, et al: Perioperative morbidity in patients randomized to epidural or general anesthesia for lower extremity vascular surgery. Perioperative Ischemia Randomized Anesthesia Trial Study Group. Anesthesiology 79:422–434, 1993.

**38.** Horlocker TT, Wedel DJ, Benzon H, et al: Regional anesthesia in the anticoagulated patient: defining the risks (the second ASRA Consensus Conference on Neuraxial Anesthesia and Anticoagulation). Reg Anesth Pain Med 28:172–197, 2003.

**39.** Metzner J, Domino KB: Risks of anesthesia or sedation outside the operating room: The role of the anesthesia care provider. Curr Opin Anaesthesiol 23:523–531, 2010.

**40.** American Society of Anesthesiologists Task Force on Postanesthetic Care: Practice guidelines for postanesthetic care: A report by the American Society of Anesthesiologists Task Force on Postanesthetic Care. Anesthesiology 96:742–752, 2002.

**41.** Xue FS, Li BW, Zhang GS, et al: The influence of surgical sites on early postoperative hypoxemia in adults undergoing elective surgery. Anesth Analg 88:213–219, 1999.

**42.** White PF, Abrao J: Drug-induced prolongation of the QT interval: What's the point? Anesthesiology 104:386–387, 2006.

**43.** White PF, Song D, Abrao J, et al: Effect of low-dose droperidol on the QT interval during and after general anesthesia: A placebo-controlled study. Anesthesiology 102:1101–1105, 2005.

**43a.** IASP Task Force on Taxonomy, Part III: Pain terms, a current list with definitions and notes on usage. In Merskey H, Bogduk N, editors: Classification of chronic pain, ed 2, Seattle, 1994, IASP Press, pp 209–214.

**44.** Buvanendran A, Kroin JS, Tuman KJ, et al: Effects of perioperative administration of a selective cyclooxygenase 2 inhibitor on pain management and recovery of function after knee replacement: A randomized controlled trial. JAMA 290:2411–2418, 2003.

**45.** Richman JM, Liu SS, Courpas G, et al: Does continuous peripheral nerve block provide superior pain control to opioids? A meta-analysis. Anesth Analg 102:248–257, 2006.

**46.** Turan A, White PF, Karamanlioglu B, et al: Gabapentin: An alternative to the cyclooxygenase-2 inhibitors for perioperative pain management. Anesth Analg 102:175–181, 2006.

**47.** Block BM, Liu SS, Rowlingson AJ, et al: Efficacy of postoperative epidural analgesia: A meta-analysis. JAMA 290:2455–2463, 2003.

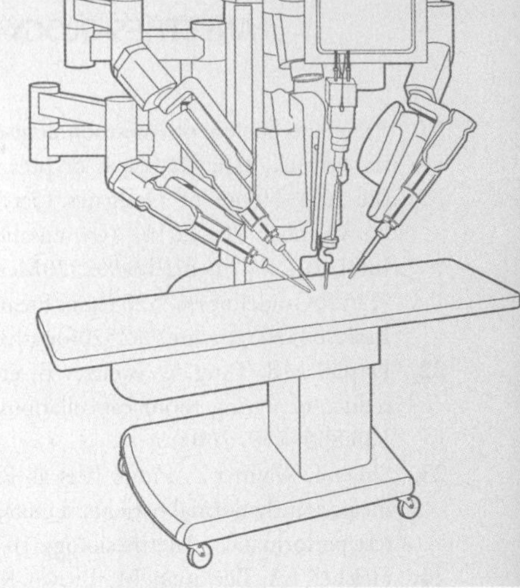

CHAPTER 17

# EMERGING TECHNOLOGY IN SURGERY: INFORMATICS, ROBOTICS, AND ELECTRONICS

GERALD M. FRIED



There has been a dramatic change in surgical care over the past 20 years with the introduction of digitization, miniaturization, improved optics, novel imaging techniques, and computerized information systems in the operating room (Fig. 17-1). Whereas surgery has traditionally required large incisions large enough to allow the surgeon to introduce his or her hands into the patient's body and allow sufficient light to see the structures being operated on, innovations have stimulated a radical change in how surgical procedures are performed. Many surgical procedures have become image-guided. These can be done by manipulating instruments from outside the patient while directing them by looking at displays of direct images of the target tissues (e.g., endoscopic or laparoscopic surgery) or at indirect images of the region of interest (e.g., endovascular catheter-based treatments, energy-focused ablation of tumors). Image-guided surgery has enabled the use of very small incisions or punctures to introduce surgical instruments. In other cases, the surgical instruments can be passed to the target tissue through anatomic conduits (e.g., arteries, veins) or natural orifices (e.g., mouth, anus, vagina, urethra) without the need for any visible incision. Other innovations to minimize the damage of access to the patient include single-incision laparoscopic surgery and minilaparoscopy.

Although the patient may benefit substantially in terms of the pain and complications that occur as a result of the access to the organ being operated on, the techniques require an entirely novel skill set for the surgeons. The concept of the procedure may be familiar to the surgeon from open surgical experience, but the skills required to perform the surgery are different and must be learned and practiced to avoid the risk of complications during this learning or transition phase. This chapter will introduce the concepts of innovative image-guided surgical techniques, including minimal access concepts and robotics, address the approaches to training and establishing proficiency, and provide some thoughts on the potential for simulation in training surgeons and planning surgery.

## MINIMALLY INVASIVE SURGERY

Accessing internal body cavities, such as the chest, abdomen, and pelvis, requires an incision. The size of the incision is determined by the need of the surgeon to see and manipulate the target tissues. If resection is required, the incision size must take into account the dimensions of the tissues to be removed. In some cases, thorough histologic examination of the removed tissue is not critical (e.g., splenectomy for idiopathic thrombocytopenic purpura [ITP], hysterectomy for fibroids) and the resected organ may be pulverized or morcellated to ease its removal through a small incision. In other cases, such as colectomy for cancer, it is important to examine the removed tissues accurately for staging and grading purposes and to ensure that the resection margins are free of disease. In the latter cases, the incision must be sufficient to avoid compromising the accuracy of the pathologic examination. The goal of minimal access surgery is to diminish the trauma of access without compromising the overall goal of the surgical procedure (Fig. 17-2).

The cost to the patient of this access incision is multifactorial. Generally, larger incisions are associated with more postoperative pain, longer recovery periods, a period of physical disability, greater morbidity in cases of wound infection, more risk of incisional hernias, and a higher rate of symptomatic adhesive bowel obstruction in the future. It is estimated that approximately 20% to 30% of laparotomies result in incisional hernias. Because the success of incisional hernia repair is poor (approximately 30% of repairs fail), a large laparotomy incision in itself may result in up to 30% patients requiring a second operation and another 9% or more requiring a third operation to deal with complications of access.

Image-guided surgery greatly diminishes the postoperative pain and morbidity of wound infection and the longer term problems related to hernias and adhesions. However, the smaller incisions present some real challenges to the operating surgeon.[1]

Laparoscopic surgery involves the placement of a small telescope into the body cavity. The telescope illuminates the target tissues and conveys a bright magnified, high-definition image to the surgeon through an attached or incorporated camera system. The view is startling in its clarity (Fig. 17-3). It eliminates shadows and affords all members of the operating team the identical view of the surgery. An important limitation of laparoscopic imaging is that it is generally monocular compared with the binocular view in open surgery, because traditional telescopes have a single-lens system. With a monocular optical system, the surgeon obtains a two-dimensional view of the body displayed on a video monitor. Other cues must be developed to appreciate the relative positions of the instruments and visualized tissues in three dimensions. This is a learned skill, and most surgeons are able to adjust to laparoscopic imaging with a little practice. The currently available robotic platform uses binocular imaging, providing the surgeon with a truly immersive three-dimensional view (Fig. 17-4).

Most telescope-camera systems can be zoomed electronically and adjusted for light sensitivity. These systems are also ideal for recording static images or videos for documentation of findings or for teaching purposes. These images can be attached to the medical record and stored with radiologic picture archiving and communication system (PACS) images. In this way, they are available for the radiologist, pathologist, and other consultants for patient care or quality improvement initiatives. A drawback of laparoscopy is the limited field of view; the laparoscope must be moved to maintain an ideal image. The closer the laparoscope image is to the target, the better the illumination, magnification, and image detail, but the field of view is more limited. Constant communication between the surgeon performing the operation and the assistant managing the telescope is essential for safe surgery.

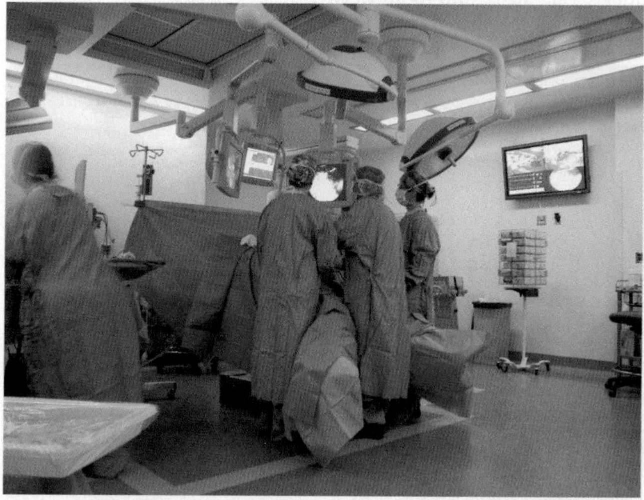

**FIGURE 17-1** Integrated OR. This provides digital information on multiple displays, controlled by the surgical team. The large flat panel displays four images on the screen—endoscopic view, patient's vital signs, image of the abdomen captured by a camera in the OR light, and a room view. The central display in the surgical field is a touch screen, allowing the surgeon to control the operating room environment. The green lighting allows the surgical team to see well and do their work, while avoiding glare on the surgical displays.

Laparoscopic images give the surgeon a view of the surface of tissues. In open surgery, the surgeon can palpate and compress tissues to gain a sense of the presence of the pathology that lies deep to the surface. Because direct manual evaluation is not available during laparoscopy, the surgeon must adopt other methods to evaluate the tissues beneath the surface. Some of this information can be acquired before surgery by assessing the patient with cross-sectional imaging, such as ultrasound, computed tomography (CT), and magnetic resonance imaging (MRI). Digital CT and MR images can be displayed in the operating room using surface markers to help the surgeon consolidate these findings with the visual display of the tissue surface during surgery. An advantage of ultrasound (Fig. 17-5) is that it is easy to use intraoperatively and can be positioned to provide real-time information of the tissue being viewed through the laparoscope. A surgeon proficient in intraoperative ultrasound can incorporate the surface and cross-sectional information to evaluate the target tissues carefully.

During minimally invasive surgery the surgeon's eye is on the display monitor.[2] One opportunity presented by laparoscopy is the display of multiple pieces of information on the imaging screen. Most data required by the surgical team are available digitally and can be routed to any display device. Because the anesthesiologist acquires important hemodynamic data on the patient, this information can be displayed on the surgeon's monitor. When operating on an unstable patient, this provides valuable real-time data to the surgeon. Similarly, the surgeon can display real-time imaging information provided by intraoperative ultrasound, flexible endoscopy or fluoroscopy, or preoperatively acquired images (e.g., CT or MRI scans) simultaneously with the laparoscopic images using picture-in-picture, split screen, or quad split screen displays (Fig. 17-6). The surgeon can use telestration techniques (e.g., used to outline plays on TV sports broadcasts) to communicate with the assistant or point out findings to students (Fig. 17-7).

Videoconferencing is readily available, bringing consultant pathologists and radiologists right into the operating room environment. This provides useful context for their interpretation of findings. The surgeon can have access to a whole dashboard of information and select the relevant data for heads-up display

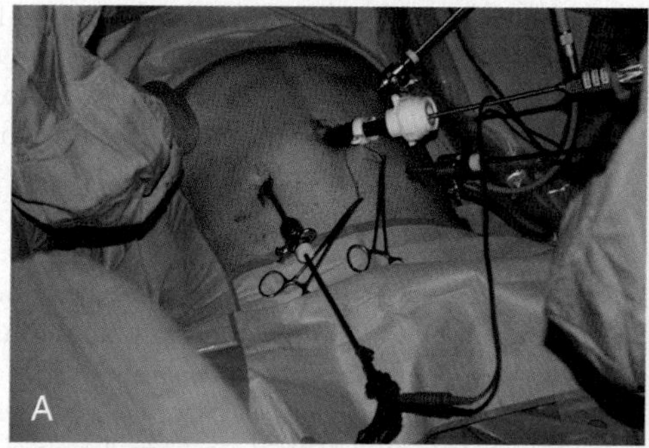

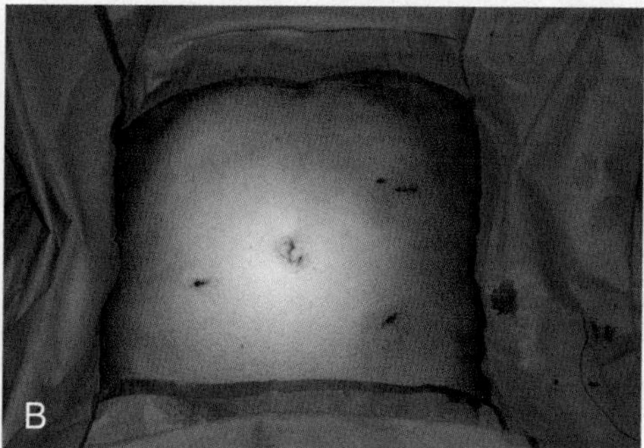

**FIGURE 17-2** Surgical field for laparoscopic colectomy. **A,** The instruments are passed through trocars in the abdominal wall. **B,** The small incisions at the completion of the surgery. The largest incision at the umbilicus was to extract the specimen.

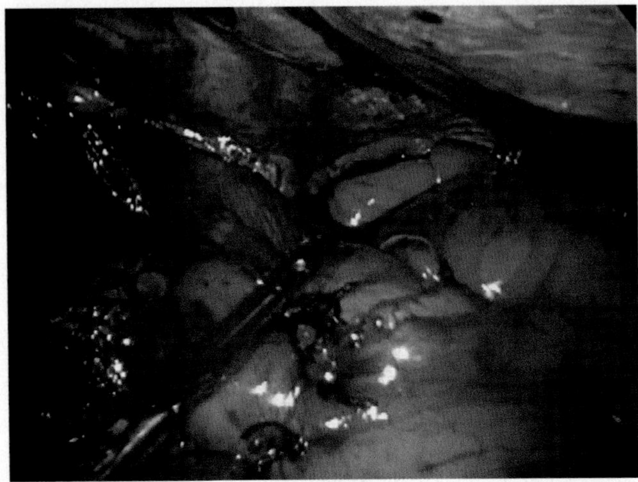

**FIGURE 17-3** Laparoscopic image, which provides a magnified, high-resolution, and well-illuminated view for the entire surgical team.

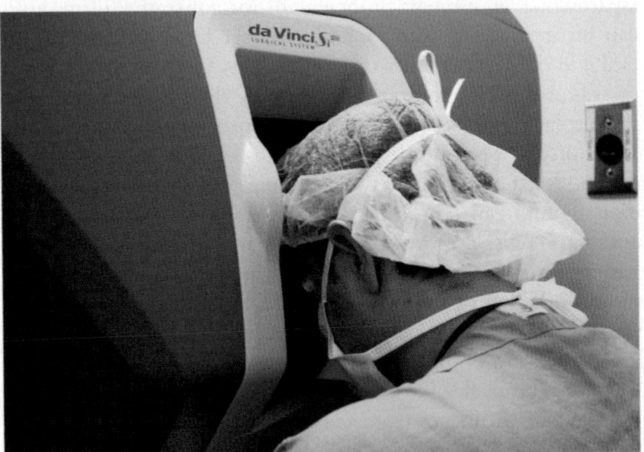


**FIGURE 17-4** Surgeon is working in three-dimensional immersive visualization environment while doing robotic surgery.

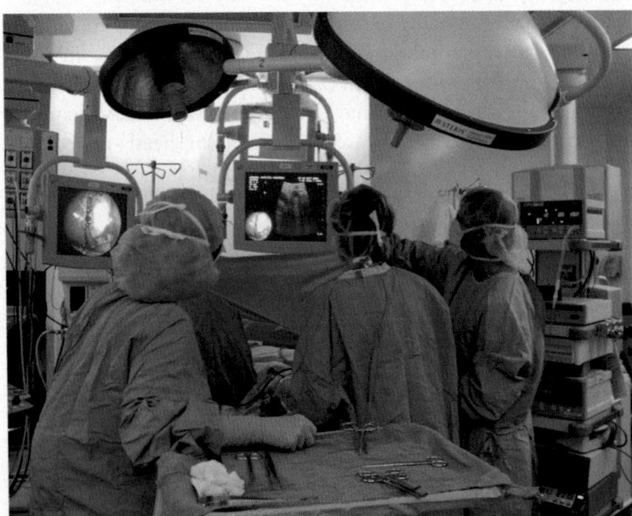

**FIGURE 17-5** Laparoscopic ultrasound. The combination of surface imaging by laparoscopy and cross-sectional imaging with ultrasound are complementary.

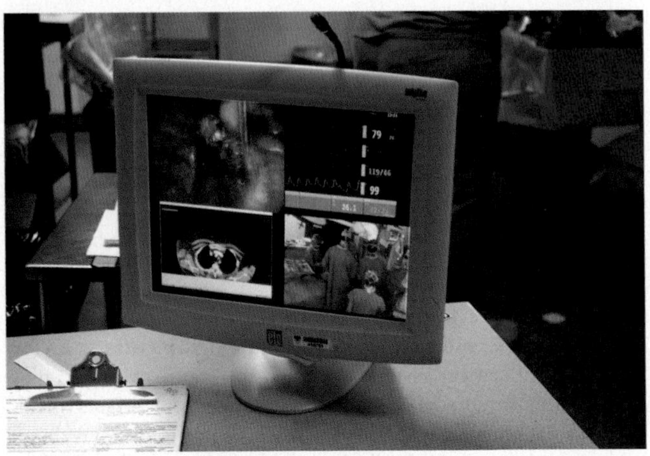

**FIGURE 17-6** Quad screen display. The surgeon can select up to four images to be displayed simultaneously on a monitor. This display at the nursing station shows the endoscopic image, preoperative CT image, vital signs, and room view.

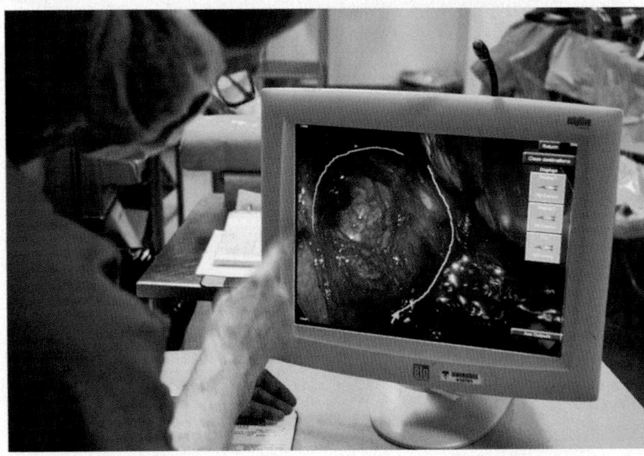

**FIGURE 17-7** Telestration allows the surgeon to use the touch screen to annotate the image for documentation or teaching.

during the procedure. The routing of digital information to display(s) can be carried out using voice controls or touch screens in the surgical field. The operating room images can also be accessed remotely in real time with appropriate security and privileges (Fig. 17-8).

The operating room environment has been completely redesigned to provide an optimal setting for image-guided surgery.[3] Ambient tinted room lighting provides the surgeon with a glare-free view of the display monitors while allowing others in the operating room (OR) sufficient illumination to move around the room and carry out their work safely. The surgical team has access to multiple monitors to display the surgical images and other digital information. It is not unusual to have six or seven monitors in an image-guided surgical suite. Each monitor can be moved into an ergonomically comfortable viewing position, and it has been shown that the monitor position has an impact on the precision and efficiency of the surgical procedure. Integrated ORs have been designed so that all devices, lighting, and image routing can be controlled from the surgical field or a control station. The surgeon can have access to multiple

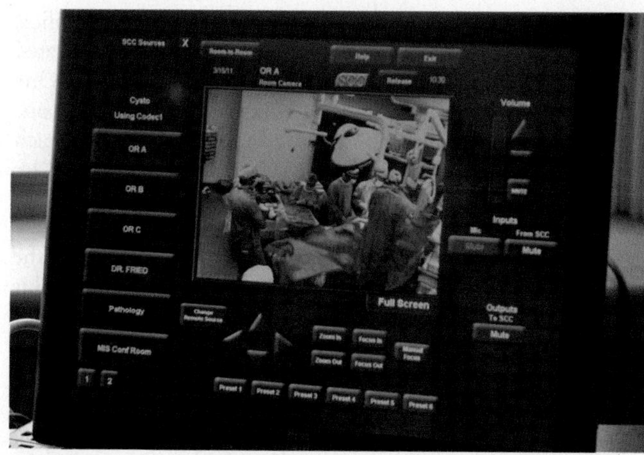


**FIGURE 17-8** The touch interface in the surgeon's office allows the image source to be selected and displayed remotely.

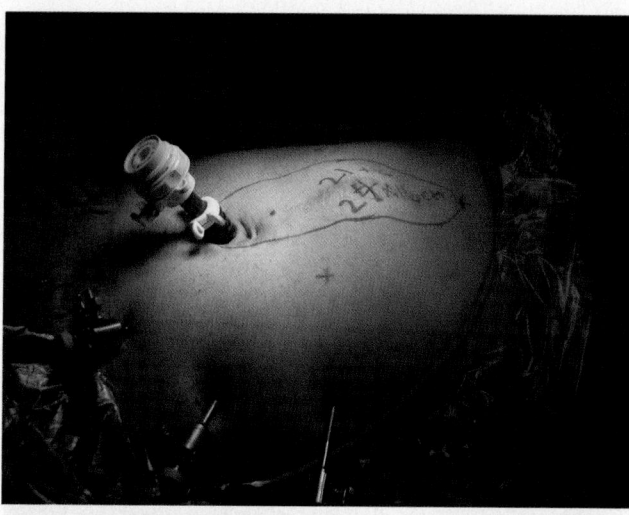

**FIGURE 17-9** Surgeon working through trocars during incisional hernia repair.

images simultaneously (e.g., laparoscope, flexible endoscope, ultrasound, fluoroscopy, preoperative CT and MRI images). By controlling the interface, any digital image or combination of images can be routed to any monitor. Any image can be recorded to document the surgical findings. The images or video clips can be annotated by verbal recordings or by textual description. This provides valuable documentation of the surgical findings for the medical record. Prompts can be embedded into the system so that a visual or auditory reminder can alert the surgical team when it is time for the next dose of antibiotics.

Despite the many advantages, image-guided surgery includes some unique challenges. When operating through a large incision, there are relatively few constraints on the range of motion of surgical instruments. If a surgeon wants to move the instrument tip upward, he or she can move the whole hand and instrument upward. In laparoscopy, the abdomen is insufflated with gas to create a working space. Generally, 5 to 6 liters of carbon dioxide is pumped into the abdominal cavity, separating structures and allowing the lens to focus on the target tissue from a suitable distance. To avoid loss of this working space, instruments must be passed through trocars or ports placed through the abdominal wall. These ports have gaskets that seal around the instruments, maintaining the positive pressure and working space. The design of these ports poses some limitations on instrument design. such as the geometry and curvature of the instrument shafts (Fig. 17-9). Because the handles of the instruments are outside the patient, the shafts are generally long. Interposing the laparoscopic instrument between the surgeon's hands and the target tissue dampens tactile feedback. Surgeons rely on their determination of texture and compressibility to evaluate tissue characteristics and pathology. In laparoscopic surgery, the surgeon must learn how to interpret these characteristics through the instrument. In robotic laparoscopic surgery, the surgeon operates a device at a console outside the patient, which then controls instruments inside the patient. This results in complete loss of the sense of touch to evaluate tissues. Prototype instruments are being developed to display force feedback (tissue resistance) optically or by sound feedback. They have not yet been widely incorporated into clinical care.

Because laparoscopic instruments are placed through trocars that are fixed in the abdominal wall, this creates a lever or fulcrum effect. Range of motion is limited to six directions—up, down, right, left, clockwise, or counterclockwise rotation. As a result, if the surgeon wishes to deflect the instrument tip upward, she or he must angle the handle downward. This reciprocal movement takes some time to become natural. Furthermore, depending on the proportion of the total length of the instrument outside compared with inside the patient, there may be amplification of the movement of the instrument tip compared with the hand. Working with long instruments across a fulcrum may amplify any existing tremor, making it difficult to carry out procedures that require fine movements. Many of these limitations and challenges presented by laparoscopy can be addressed by better education, practice using simulators, and further development of enabling technologies, such as robotics.

As surgeons have become more skilled in laparoscopy, the variety of surgical procedures to which minimally invasive surgery techniques have been applied has continued to grow, bolstered by evidence of effectiveness and safety, patient demand, and better instrumentation. Relative contraindications have continued to diminish. Currently, most elective abdominal surgical procedures are being done laparoscopically.

## Beyond Laparoscopic Surgery

Having realized the tremendous benefit to the patients of laparoscopy, there is a desire for further improvements by diminishing the injury of access to internal body cavities. Several approaches have been developed and are being evaluated to assess potential benefit over traditional laparoscopic surgery. The goals are to diminish postoperative pain, accelerate surgical recovery, and improve cosmetic outcome while maintaining the safety and effectiveness of the surgery.

One approach is to miniaturize the diameter of the surgical instruments and telescopes further (minilaparoscopy; Fig. 17-10). As camera light sensitivity and image quality improve, high-quality images can be obtained through progressively smaller laparoscopes. Whereas a 10- mm diameter telescope was once needed to provide sufficient light and image quality to perform surgery, current 5-mm telescopes can provide images

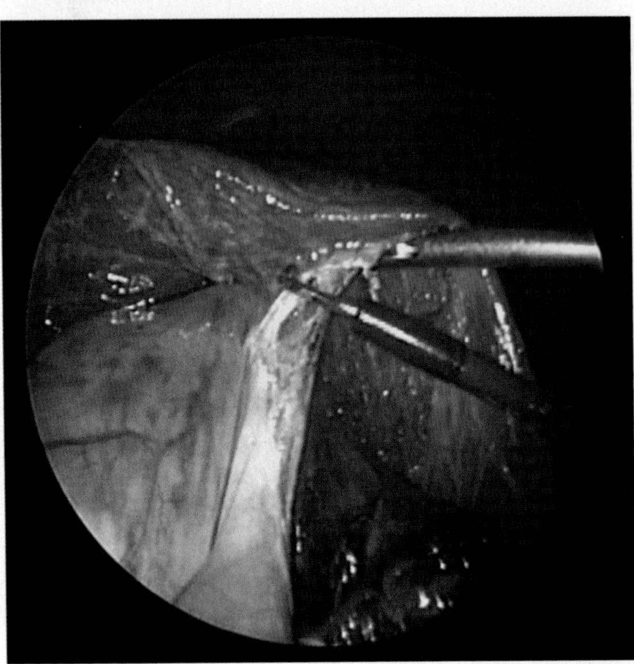

FIGURE 17-10 Laparoscopic cholecystectomy using 3-mm instruments and laparoscope.

that are hard to distinguish from those of 10-mm telescopes. Progressive reduction in their diameter allows the surgeon to move the telescope easily from port to port to provide different views of the surgical target and minimize the cosmetic and functional problems related to these incisions. In minilaparoscopy, surgeons can insert instruments as small as 2 mm into the body cavity through needle-sized incisions, leaving almost no scar. Other than the modification of instruments, there is no real difference in the conduct of the surgery, nor is further training required. The step from laparoscopy to minilaparoscopy is natural. Unfortunately, the reduced access size further constrains instrument design. Minilaparoscopy instruments are less robust and more limited in curvature than 5- or 10-mm instruments.[4]

Another approach has been to put the laparoscope and all instruments through a single port (usually placed at the depth of the umbilical dimple). This single incision is usually approximately 2 to 3 cm in length and can be placed in many patients so that the scar is almost invisible once healed. Placing all instruments through a single port creates further challenges because of instruments colliding with each other and creates a laparoscopic view that is parallel to the instruments, further impeding the surgeon's depth perception. This has been addressed by designing deflectable tip laparoscopes and instruments with wristlike flexibility to help surgeons accommodate to these new challenges. Although there is clearly a learning curve for acquiring skills in single-incision laparoscopy, even for proficient laparoscopic surgeons, this learning curve can be overcome to a great extent by deliberate practice in the simulation environment.[5]

Natural orifice transluminal endoscopic surgery (NOTES) is a novel approach whereby access to the abdominal cavity is achieved without any incision in the abdominal wall.[6] This is truly scarless surgery, conducted by accessing the abdominal cavity through a natural orifice (mouth, rectum, vagina). After placing a flexible or rigid endoscope through a natural orifice, an organ (stomach, colon, or vagina) is intentionally perforated and the endoscope is advanced into the peritoneal cavity. One way this is accomplished is by passing a flexible endoscope through the mouth into the stomach and through the stomach wall into the abdominal cavity. Other surgical instruments are advanced through or around the gastroscope and then out through this opening into the abdominal cavity. After the procedure is completed, the resected tissue is retrieved through the mouth and the gastrotomy is closed. As might be imagined, this technique is fraught with challenges. Very long instruments are required that need to be directed by manipulating the visualization platform (endoscope) using specially designed elevators at its distal end. This makes it difficult to move the instruments without moving the view. The operating platform is flexible and is unstable for the surgeon to work with. It also requires an iatrogenic perforation of a viscus to obtain access. Any failure of healing can result in peritonitis. Although access through the vagina is less risky than the stomach or colon, its potential use is limited to women, and the risk of postoperative dyspareunia remains to be determined. Currently, prospective trials are being conducted to compare NOTES with laparoscopic cholecystectomy. NOTES techniques may be more applicable to procedures other than cholecystectomy, such as those that already require an opening in the digestive tract.[7]

## CATHETER-BASED THERAPIES

Vascular surgery has traditionally involved replacing or bypassing occluded or aneurysmal vessels. Endovascular procedures have revolutionized vascular surgery in much the same way as laparoscopy has affected general surgery. Imaging is provided by fluoroscopy and contrast solution is injected to outline the vascular anatomy. By accessing the vascular system by puncture or cut-down, instruments can be threaded along the vessel, narrowings can be dilated with balloons, and intraluminal stents can be threaded into position, guided by real-time fluoroscopic imaging. Large incisions required for access in patients with serious comorbidity can be avoided entirely. Results of endovascular procedures are excellent, recovery is hastened, and the requirements for prolonged hospitalization and intensive care unit (ICU) care are reduced.[8,9]

In cardiac surgery, similar transcatheter endovascular approaches have been used to treat coronary artery disease, close septal defects, dilate stenotic valves, and even replace cardiac valves. The idea of avoiding the stress and morbidity of a major incision is particularly appealing in those patients with serious underlying disease. Despite this, the effectiveness and durability of these less invasive therapies must be compared with traditional surgical approaches.

## IMAGE-GUIDED ABLATIVE THERAPIES

High-intensity focused ultrasound (HIFU) is a technique whereby ultrasound or MRI can be used to direct focused ultrasound energy to pathologic tissues. The acoustic energy absorbed by the targeted tissue causes rapid heating and destruction of the tissue. Currently, applications are mostly for the ablation of uterine fibroids and benign prostatic hyperplasia. This is an exciting example of image-guided surgery without any incision. The application of HIFU is growing and it is being evaluated for destruction of metastatic disease and treatment of arrhythmias.[10-12]

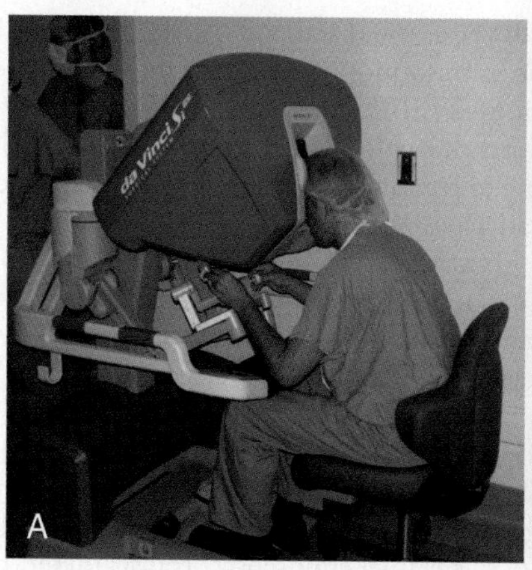


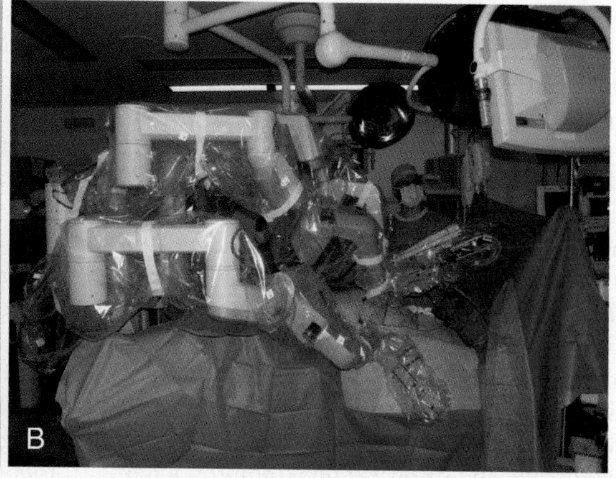


**FIGURE 17-11** Robotic surgery. **A,** Surgeon at console using hands and feet to control robot arms. **B,** Robotic setup at patient.

An analogous image-guided therapy is radiofrequency ablation (RFA). Using any of a number of imaging techniques (e.g., laparoscopy, ultrasound, CT scan, MRI), RFA energy is used to destroy pathologic tissues. Whereas HIFU can be delivered transcutaneously, RFA requires direct access to the target tissue for its effect. It has been shown to be an effective modality to treat tumors of the lung, liver, bone, and kidney.

## MINIMALLY INVASIVE ROBOTIC SURGERY

The concept of robotic surgery is to use the enabling characteristics of robots to improve the capabilities of the surgeon compared with working freehand.[13] Unlike the use of robotics in industry, the robot does not work autonomously in most surgical applications, but acts as an interface between the operating surgeon and patient. In this master-slave relationship, the master (surgeon) sits at a console, in an ergonomic and comfortable position, and uses movements of both hands and feet to control movement of the laparoscope and instruments (slave) in the patient. The commercially available robotic system uses a proprietary laparoscope with two optical systems providing binocular (three-dimensional) vision. The surgical instruments are wristed near their distal tips, so the movements of the surgeon's hands can be reproduced by the instruments without the usual limitations of the fulcrum effect seen with traditional laparoscopic instruments. The degrees of freedom of the instrument are increased, making it easier to carry out fine maneuvers than with traditional laparoscopic surgery. The surgeon can work from within the operating room or even remotely because there is no direct contact between the surgeon at the console and the instruments (Fig. 17-11). One consequence of this interface is that the surgeon has no tactile sense of the tissues, but must adapt by using visual information.

Robotic surgery has opened up the concept of telesurgery. Theoretically, the surgeon can operate on patients at great distance.[14] Before this can be applied practically, issues of licensing and liability must be addressed, and latent delays between motion of the surgeon and movement of the instrument must be resolved. The longer the distance that the data needs to be transmitted from the console to the patient, the greater the latent delay. Delays of more than 250 milliseconds can have a significant impact on the quality of the surgery. Robotic surgical platforms are appealing for support of the injured soldier and of

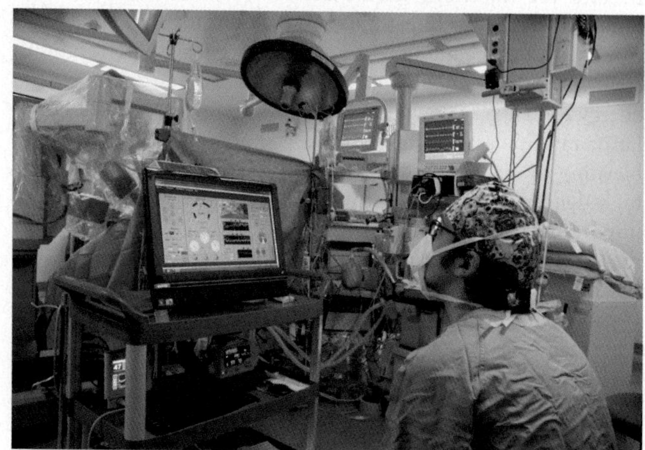

**FIGURE 17-12** In this operation, robotic prostatectomy is being done with robotic-controlled anesthesia.

patients in hostile environments, such as outer space missions, deep sea exploration, and polar expeditions.

Robotic surgery provides other exciting opportunities to enhance surgical performance. Because there is an interface between the surgeon and effector instruments, it is possible to modulate the relationship between the surgeon's movement and that of the instrument electronically. The robot can adjust the gain or the scale of movement. In this way, the surgeon can make larger movements to affect very fine movements of the instrument tip. This can be helpful for surgery that requires fine and precise movements, such as suturing small vessels together. Algorithms can also be incorporated to dampen tremor using embedded filters.

Currently, minimally invasive surgery robotic systems are widely used in urologic surgery and gynecology and, to a lesser extent in cardiac surgery, otolaryngology, and general surgery.[15-24] The main drawbacks are the costs, bulkiness, setup time for the equipment, and absence of compelling data to show superiority of robotic operations over those done by well-trained laparoscopic surgeons. Recently, robotic surgery has been carried out in conjunction with robotic-assisted anesthesia (Fig. 17-12).

This is an automated platform on which anesthesia agents are controlled using computer-assisted devices that calculate moment to moment anesthesia doses in a closed-loop system to provide optimal dosing.[25]

## FLEXIBLE ENDOSCOPE AS A SURGICAL PLATFORM

The development of the flexible endoscope has opened up a whole field of diagnostic and therapeutic opportunities. With only topical anesthesia or IV sedation, it is easy to pass a flexible endoscope through the mouth or nose into the upper gastrointestinal (GI) tract or respiratory tree, or a colonoscope up through the rectum (Fig. 17-13). The endoscope is advanced by deflecting its tip using wheels at the handle, guided by the image provided by the miniature charge coupled-device (CCD) chip at the end of the endoscope and displayed on a monitor. Channels in the endoscope provide access for instruments, and the lens can be irrigated and the field suctioned through the endoscope. Instruments have been developed for pinch biopsy, needles for injection, needle-knives for incisions, snares for removing polyps or foreign bodies, balloons for stretching strictures, clips for occluding bleeding vessels or sealing perforations, stents for deployment across strictures or perforations, and energy for delivery down the endoscope in the form of monopolar or multipolar electrocautery, lasers, or heater probes to stop bleeding or ablate tumors. The flexible endoscope can provide high-definition images of the interior of the body and is an important diagnostic modality. It is increasingly being used for therapeutic purposes and is an important tool for the GI and thoracic surgeon. As surgeons have become increasingly comfortable with the flexible endoscope as a surgical platform, they have sought some of these capabilities for use in laparoscopic surgery. This has led to the development of flexible tip laparoscopes, which can provide effective visualization of hard to reach areas in the chest, abdomen, and pelvis.

Like other image-guided therapies, the flexible endoscope demands the surgeon be comfortable operating while viewing a monitor with a monocular optical system, and carry out therapies using long instruments interposed between the hands and target tissue. Recent advances have combined the outstanding imaging capability of the flexible endoscope with an ultrasound transducer at the distal end. Applications in the GI tract (endoscopic ultrasound [EUS]) and bronchial tree (endobronchial ultrasound [EBUS]) extend the capability of the endoscope to visualize the complete thickness of the wall of the organ for staging of tumors, adjacent lymph nodes, which can be biopsied, and adjacent structures (e.g., evaluation of the common bile duct or pancreas through the duodenum or stomach during EUS). Surgical procedures can now be performed using EUS guidance, such as pancreatic pseudocyst drainage into the stomach.

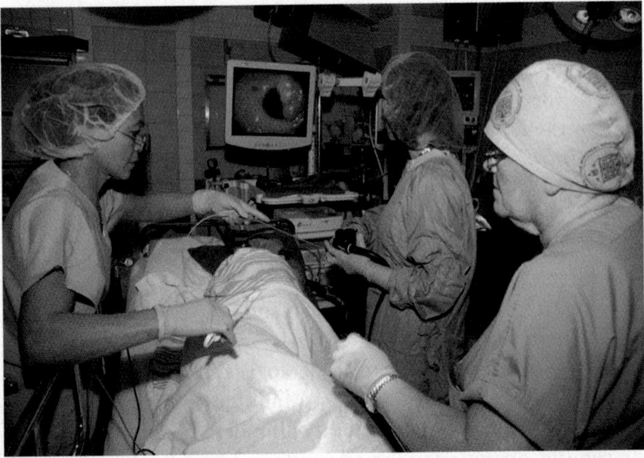

**FIGURE 17-13** Flexible endoscopy is a platform for surgical therapy or an adjunct to open or laparoscopic surgery.

## SIMULATION FOR SURGICAL TRAINING AND OPERATIVE PLANNING

Image-guided surgery, whether performed by laparoscopy, robotics, flexible endoscopy, transcatheter methods, or other techniques generally requires a set of specific technical skills distinct from those required for traditional open surgical procedures. Each technique makes specific demands on the surgeon, requiring specific training programs. It cannot be assumed that a surgeon who is proficient at performing a splenectomy by laparotomy can smoothly adopt the laparoscopic technique for this operation without further training.

There is a concept of the learning curve during which the surgeon acquires proficiency with a technique in the course of applying the technique in surgical practice. It has never been clear when the learning curve has been completed. Furthermore, the evaluation of a new technology or technique can be biased by evaluating the outcome of the procedure in the hands of a surgeon in the learning curve. The outcome measured may be more reflective of the surgeon's experience or proficiency with the technique than with the outcome of the procedure itself.

Learning a surgical technique in a simulation environment has many practical advantages. The specific learning objectives can be defined and modeled for learning. In this way, the surgeon can repeatedly practice the specific skills required to make the transition. Practice on a simulator focuses the experience on the learner, not on the patient. The learner can be allowed to progress at his or her own pace, go beyond the comfort level, and experiment with different techniques or approaches. The surgeon can be allowed to make errors and be required to correct them. Performance can be measured in a standardized and objective way and compared with an accepted performance standard (proficiency level).[26-28]

Here, we will explore the role of simulation-based education for training surgeons to perform laparoscopic surgery. Many of the principles learned through this process can provide educational paradigms for teaching other innovative surgical techniques

### Simulation Training for Minimally Invasive Surgery

The advent of the laparoscopic era, with the shift to image-based surgical technologies, has required abdominal surgeons to learn new skills. This was not a seamless transition, as evidenced by the increase in common bile duct injuries associated with the introduction of laparoscopic cholecystectomy in the early 1990s. Weekend courses simply did not prepare experienced open surgeons adequately to be proficient in the new image-based, two-dimensional environment, with the reduction in tactile feedback and increased hand-eye coordination required. Similarly, training programs struggled with how best to prepare residents for laparoscopic surgery. Coincident with the need to teach image-based surgery, other factors challenged the traditional apprenticeship model of surgical training, including an increased focus on patient safety, rising operating room costs, and limitations in resident work hours. These needs led to the development of models to allow the acquisition and assessment of fundamental laparoscopic skills outside the operating room, through simulation.[29,30] This training paradigm shift was also occurring for open surgical skills[26,27] and in other technical specialties such as anesthesia, similar to the use of flight simulators in the aviation industry.

Simulation allows for the acquisition of skills through learner-centered, deliberate practice in a safe environment, analogous to practicing an instrument. For example, instead of learning how to dissect the gallbladder from the liver bed during laparoscopic cholecystectomy in the operating room, trainees acquire the fundamental psychomotor skills in a simulation center (Fig. 17-14), allowing them to focus on operative strategy, anatomy, and judgment with their clinical proctor in the OR. As such, simulation is best seen as a potentially important adjunct to clinical experience, especially during early training for a particular skill or procedure and, ideally, within a developed curriculum. In laparoscopy, simulations include the use of live animals, human cadavers, box trainers, and virtual reality trainers. Simulations may teach and assess fundamental skills (part task trainers [PTTs]), or entire procedures, teamwork, and professional skills. However, these technologies do not exist in isolation, and innovations such as the integration of trainers with actors to create human-simulator hybrids may enhance effectiveness. Simulation is often costly in terms of technologic and human resources. Objective assessment of performance is an important component of simulation-based training to set practice goals, guide remediation, and judge the effectiveness of these new educational interventions.

In this section, an overview of the role of simulation in surgical education will be presented, focusing on its role in training and assessment for image-based interventions, and high-level evidence supporting the transferability of skills from the simulated to clinical environment. Extensive reviews of this subject are available.[9]

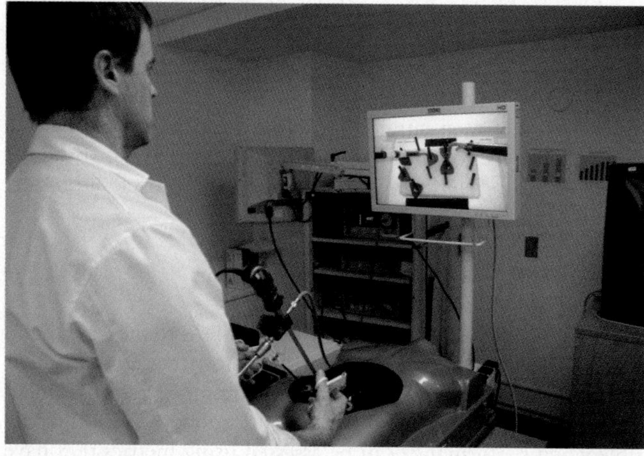

**FIGURE 17-14** Students practicing fundamental laparoscopic skills in the simulation center.

### Teaching Fundamental Skills With Partial Task Trainers

Partial task simulators are used to teach and assess the component skills required to perform procedures, but do not model entire operations. In laparoscopic surgery, these include box trainers and virtual reality systems, with tasks that develop depth perception, hand-eye coordination, and bimanual dexterity. These are accomplished using drills requiring the coordinated use of both hands in a two-dimensional space and more complex tasks (e.g., suturing). The primary role is to enable novice surgeons to acquire baseline psychomotor skills through deliberate practice outside the OR.

A widely available part-task box-trainer system is the Fundamentals of Laparoscopic Surgery (FLS) program.[30] FLS incorporated the McGill Inanimate System for Training and Evaluation of Laparoscopic Skills (MISTELS) box trainer to teach and certify fundamental technical skills in laparoscopy. Like other box trainers, FLS consists of a box covered with an opaque membrane through which trocars for instruments and a camera are placed. The trainee visualizes the interior of the box on a monitor, modeling intra-abdominal laparoscopy. Standard laparoscopic instruments, including curved dissectors, scissors, and needle drivers are used. FLS currently includes five tasks scored for efficiency and accuracy in a standardized fashion, with error scores applied to penalize specific actions that should be discouraged. There is ample published evidence to support the validity and reliability of the performance metrics[29]; FLS performance correlates with intraoperative performance as measured during gallbladder dissection from the liver bed in laparoscopic cholecystectomy. A proficiency-based curriculum has been developed based on FLS training to a specific performance goal. FLS training to proficiency results in greater improvements in OR performance compared with standard clinical training.[31] In other words, these fundamental psychomotor skills, acquired in a low-fidelity PTT, such as FLS transfer to the OR environment. Simulation-based training is efficient and effective. The FLS program has established minimal standards of knowledge about laparoscopic surgery and the technical skills that must be demonstrated as the basis for practicing laparoscopy; the American Board of Surgery now requires FLS certification for general surgeons to qualify for the board examination. The requisite skills may be developed by practicing using simple box trainer simulations or more complex virtual reality systems.

After acquiring proficiency using PTT simulations, these skills can be applied to the performance of laparoscopic procedures. Using virtual reality and physical training systems, entire procedures can be learned and performance assessed in the safety of a simulation environment. The advantage of this approach is that the learner can acquire skills rapidly, explore different approaches to performing an operation, assess specific enabling devices and instrumentation, and practice dealing with complications that could occur in practice. Simulation is oriented around the learner, whereas patient safety is paramount in the clinical learning environment. When the procedure evolves (e.g., from multiport laparoscopy to single-port laparoscopy), the learner can upgrade her or his skills using simulation to decrease the learning curve (Fig. 17-15).

Reliable and valid rating scales have recently been developed for assessment of clinical performance during laparoscopic surgery. These metrics provide specific assessment of performance during each critical phase of an operation and reflect

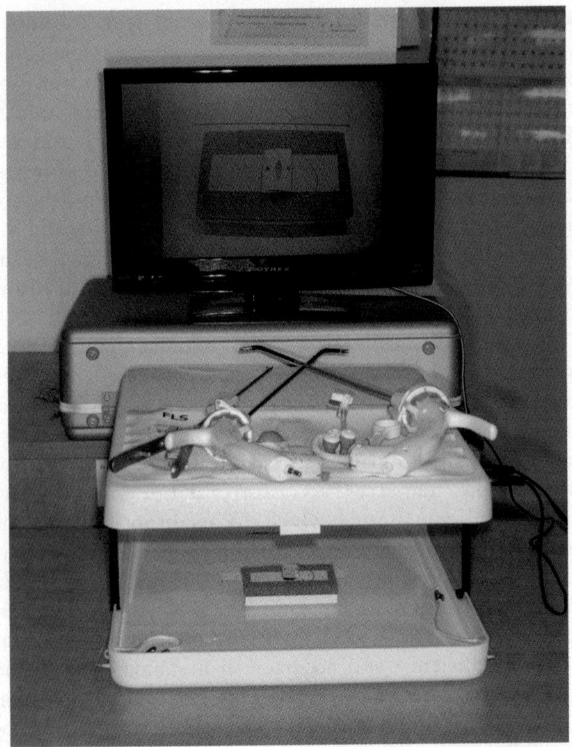

**FIGURE 17-15** Part task trainer box used for the FLS. This can be readily modified to practice skills required for single-port laparoscopy.

specific skills fundamental to performance of that operation. Using this information as a needs assessment, a specific curriculum can be developed for each individual learner, creating a highly efficient and effective personal learning program.

## Types of Simulations

### Simulation for Endovascular Procedures

Endovascular procedures are ideally suited for simulation training. A number of high-fidelity simulators are available to learn these procedures. Virtual reality displays provide images of the clinical problem and wires, balloons, and stents can be deployed to treat various pathologies in almost any anatomic location. This is an effective platform for training in endovascular procedures for the vascular surgeon, cardiac surgeon, radiologist, or cardiologist. A single simulator can provide educational opportunities to practice interventions on the carotids, cerebral aneurysms, coronary arteries, and iliofemoral vessels and for aortic valve replacement.

### Urology Simulators

Urology has been a specialty that has a long history of application of image-guided or minimally invasive therapies. Transurethral approaches to the prostate, bladder, and urinary tract are well established. Recent advances in tissue ablation, such as the holmium laser, have enabled prostatectomy for benign disease to be done with low morbidity. Most urinary stone diseases can be treated by endoscopic or percutaneous methods and/or lithotripsy on an ambulatory basis, without the need for general anesthesia. Because many of these procedures require specific skills unique to the procedure, simulation has proven to be a useful platform to develop and practice these skills. Similar to endovascular procedures, commercially available virtual reality systems are excellent platforms to practice a large variety of urologic procedures. Scenarios are available to challenge the learner with cases of varying difficulty, and performance can be easily evaluated.

### Flexible Gastrointestinal and Respiratory Endoscopy Simulators

Although the flexible endoscope is an exciting platform for diagnosis and therapy, it requires substantial experience before its use can be fully mastered. A number of simulators have been developed for teaching GI and respiratory endoscopy, including endoscopic therapeutic procedures, EUS, and endoscopic retrograde cholangiopancreatography (ERCP). These devices come with a variety of clinical scenarios of different degrees of difficulty and complexity. The learner can become comfortable with the endoscope interface, practice manipulating the endoscope to navigate the appropriate anatomic channel, test his or her diagnostic acumen, and experience various endoscopic therapies delivered through the endoscope. Metrics imbedded in the simulator allows the learner to track performance over time and to compare performance with that of a peer group or a proficiency standard.

### Simulation for Surgical Planning

The great promise of surgical simulation is the concept of preoperative surgical rehearsal based on the anatomy and pathology of the specific patient being operated on. Sophisticated imaging techniques provide anatomic and functional information in a digital format, so this approach is now possible for neurosurgery procedures with a novel surgical simulator. Prototype systems have been developed whereby patient-specific imaging data can be modeled into a virtual reality model with realistic haptic (tactile) properties, and with deformation with pressure and traction mimicking human tissue characteristics. The surgeon can then explore different approaches for performing a complex or high-risk surgical procedure. The virtual environment allows the surgeon to interact with the patient's unique anatomy and pathology. The computerized platform can convey tactile sensation and simulate bleeding. It allows evaluation of the completeness of resection and helps to predict probable functional deficits from injury to normal tissue. A prototype of this system, developed by the National Research Council of Canada, is currently being assessed for neurosurgery.[32] The application for neurosurgery is particularly attractive, because the skull forms a rigid framework to the brain, allowing accurate stereotactic representation. In theory, a surgical procedure can be created like a movie, with editing parts of the procedure that can be done better, recording all the movements, and playing back the perfect operation in the OR.

## Measuring Surgical Performance During Simulation

The best incentive to improve technical skills is to measure them. Having a measure of performance skill allows the establishment of norms, proficiency target goals for training, comparison to peers, and objective standards for certification. This is only possible when performance can be assessed using metrics that have passed the tests of reliability and validity required to use them in a high-stakes environment. The parameters measured must reflect and predict clinical performance and be practical to apply, meaningful to the learner, and generalizable to different learning environments. The attraction of measuring performance in a simulated environment is that the context for testing can be standardized, unaffected by patient differences in body habitus, anatomy, and pathology. The level of difficulty can be altered. By providing a standardized test environment, the metrics can be evaluated scientifically.

- *Reliability:* Any test measurement must be reliable, inferring that the measurements are consistent between evaluators (interrater reliability), when an individual is assessed on different days or in different places (test-retest reliability), and that there is internal consistency among the results of the different items on the test when these are used to generate a total score reflective of performance.
- *Validity:* Any test provides an inference regarding an attribute (e.g., knowledge, judgment, skills). The accuracy with which the test, conducted in an artificial or simulated environment, evaluates the attributes or constructs (e.g., technical skill in the operating room) is a measure of the validity of the test.

  For a test to be valid, it must meet several standards:
  - Face validity reflects the expert opinion regarding whether the metrics used for evaluation make sense. Are they logical values reflective of the quality of performance in the context of the surgical skills being assessed?
  - Content validity is the measure of how well the test reflects the breadth of the content being assessed. If a test of laparoscopic skills only measures whether a surgeon could move her or his instrument to touch a specific target, it would not show good content validity. It would not reflect the other requirements of bimanual dexterity, such as the ability to transfer objects by coapting the instruments in a single point in space.
  - Criterion validity (e.g., predictive validity) is a test whereby the measurements in the test are compared with a measure of the same skill in the actual clinical environment. Because valid measures are not often available for evaluating clinical performance, indirect measures are often used to test construct validity. Such evidence would be based on an assumption—for example, surgeons with more clinical experience would perform better on the simulated test than those with less experience (known group differences), or that surgical residents with superior in-training evaluation scores for technical skills would perform better than those receiving average or below-average scores (concurrent validity).

A summary of the process used to test the reliability and validity of the FLS program can serve as a useful example of the methodology involved in establishing useful simulation metrics.

## CONCLUSION

Surgery has been going through a rapid growth spurt as the advancements in technology, digitization, and optics have been adapted to the operating room. This is a stimulating time in the field of surgery. The rate of growth and the potential for merging many of these technologies holds great promise for patient safety and for delivering surgical care, with its values of effective and durable treatment, at a much lower cost to the patient in terms of pain and suffering.

## SELECTED REFERENCES

Bitterman N: Technologies and solutions for data display in the operating room. J Clin Monit Comput 20:165–173, 2006.

The operating room is becoming a complex environment. In the digital era, information can be brought to the surgeon at the point of care and displayed in real time to direct surgical care.

Dillon M, Cardwell C, Blair PH, et al: Endovascular treatment for ruptured abdominal aortic aneurysm. Cochrane Database Syst Rev (1):CD005261, 2007.

The use of endovascular techniques for treatment of abdominal aortic aneurysm has been studied rigorously. These trials are an example of high-quality studies of innovative techniques in surgery.

DiRaddo R, Tomanek B, Laroche D, et al: Patient-specific virtual reality systems for brain tumor surgery. Neuro-Oncology 11:698–698, 2009.

This is an intriguing description of the development of a simulation, based on point of care clinical imaging, that allows the surgeon to rehearse an operation using the anatomy and pathology of the patient to be operated on.

Faulkner H, Regehr G, Martin J, et al: Validation of an objective structured assessment of technical skill for surgical residents. Acad Med 71:1363–1365, 1996.

This manuscript describes OSATS (objective structured assessment of technical skill) developed to evaluate surgical skill. The paper also provides good validation data in support of its use. OSATS is one of the most widely used metrics for technical skill evaluation.

Fried GM, Feldman LS, Vassiliou MC, et al: Proving the value of simulation in laparoscopic surgery. Ann Surg 240:518–525, 2004.

This paper provides an excellent summary of the process of validation of simulation as a useful and effective way to assess technical skill in surgery. Using the hands-on component of the FLS program as an example, the authors describe how the metrics were validated and how the educational effectiveness was measured.

Gurusamy KS, Samraj K, Ramamoorthy R, et al: Miniport versus standard ports for laparoscopic cholecystectomy. Cochrane Database Syst Rev (3):CD006804, 2010.

Once laparoscopy became firmly entrenched as a means of providing effective surgical care with less injury of access, efforts have increased to add further benefit by using NOTES or by reducing the size of the abdominal wall incisions used. This review summarizes and analyzes the current evidence in support of the use of reduced size laparoscopy (minilaparoscopy), in comparison to traditional laparoscopy.

Swanstrom LL, Fried GM, Hoffman KI, et al: Beta test results of a new system assessing competence in laparoscopic surgery. J Am Coll Surg 202:62–69, 2006.

The FLS program has been developed to teach the fundamental knowledge, judgment, and technical skills that form the foundation for laparoscopic surgery. It is currently mandatory to pass the FLS certification test to be eligible for certification by the American Board of Surgery. This paper describes the science that underlies the use of this program as a high-stakes assessment.

Tsuda S, Scott D, Doyle J, et al: Surgical skills training and simulation. Curr Probl Surg 46:271–370, 2009.

This is a comprehensive and current review of surgical simulation, with an excellent bibliography.

## REFERENCES


1. Keus F, de Jong JA, Gooszen HG, et al: Laparoscopic versus open cholecystectomy for patients with symptomatic cholecystolithiasis. Cochrane Database Syst Rev (4):CD006231, 2006.
2. Bitterman N: Technologies and solutions for data display in the operating room. J Clin Monit Comput 20:165–173, 2006.
3. Computer-aided surgery. A GPS for the OR. Health Devices 38:206–218, 2009.
4. Gurusamy KS, Samraj K, Ramamoorthy R, et al: Miniport versus standard ports for laparoscopic cholecystectomy. Cochrane Database Syst Rev (3):CD006804, 2010.
5. Edwards C, Bradshaw A, Ahearne P, et al: Single-incision laparoscopic cholecystectomy is feasible: Initial experience with 80 cases. Surg Endosc 24:2241–2247, 2010.
6. Chukwumah C, Zorron R, Marks JM, et al: Current status of natural orifice translumenal endoscopic surgery (NOTES). Curr Probl Surg 47:630–668, 2010.
7. Navarra G, Curro G: SILS and NOTES cholecystectomy: A tailored approach. ANZ J Surg 80:769–770, 2010.
8. Dillon M, Cardwell C, Blair PH, et al: Endovascular treatment for ruptured abdominal aortic aneurysm. Cochrane Database Syst Rev (1):CD005261, 2007.
9. Malas MB, Freischlag JA: Interpretation of the results of OVER in the context of EVAR trial, DREAM, and the EUROSTAR registry. Semin Vasc Surg 23:165–169, 2010.
10. Wikimedia Foundation: Wikipedia: High-intensity focused ultrasound, 2011 (http://en. wikipedia.org/wiki/High-intensity_focused_ultrasound).
11. Coussios CC, Farny CH, Haar GT, et al: Role of acoustic cavitation in the delivery and monitoring of cancer treatment by high-intensity focused ultrasound (HIFU). Int J Hyperthermia 23:105–120, 2007.
12. Hwang JH, Crum LA: Current status of clinical high-intensity focused ultrasound. Conf Proc IEEE Eng Med Biol Soc 2009:130–133, 2009.
13. Maeso S, Reza M, Mayol JA, et al: Efficacy of the Da Vinci surgical system in abdominal surgery compared with that of laparoscopy: A systematic review and meta-analysis. Ann Surg 252:254–262, 2010.
14. Anvari M: Remote telepresence surgery: The Canadian experience. Surg Endosc 21:537–541, 2007.
15. Ballantyne GH: Telerobotic gastrointestinal surgery: Phase 2—safety and efficacy. Surg Endosc 21:1054–1062, 2007.
16. Braga LH, Pace K, DeMaria J, et al: Systematic review and meta-analysis of robotic-assisted versus conventional laparoscopic pyeloplasty for patients with ureteropelvic junction obstruction: Effect on operative time, length of hospital stay, postoperative complications, and success rate. Eur Urol 56:848–857, 2009.
17. Davis JW, Castle EP, Pruthi RS, et al: Robot-assisted radical cystectomy: An expert panel review of the current status and future direction. Urol Oncol 28:480–486, 2010.
18. Desai PH, Tran R, Steinwagner T, et al: Challenges of telerobotics in coronary bypass surgery. Expert Rev Med Devices 7:165–168, 2010.
19. Idrees K, Bartlett DL: Robotic liver surgery. Surg Clin North Am 90:761–774, 2010.
20. Kang DC, Hardee MJ, Fesperman SF, et al: Low quality of evidence for robot-assisted laparoscopic prostatectomy: Results of a systematic review of the published literature. Eur Urol 57:930–937, 2010.
21. Li M, Mazilu D, Horvath KA: Computer aided minimally invasive cardiac procedures. Minerva Chir 65:439–450, 2010.
22. Lum MJ, Rosen J, Lendvay TS, et al: TeleRobotic fundamentals of laparoscopic surgery (FLS): Effects of time delay—pilot study. Conf Proc IEEE Eng Med Biol Soc 2008:5597–5600, 2008.
23. Moses GR, Doarn CR: Barriers to wider adoption of mobile telerobotic surgery: Engineering, clinical and business challenges. Stud Health Technol Inform 132:308–312, 2008.
24. Reza M, Maeso S, Blasco JA, et al: Meta-analysis of observational studies on the safety and effectiveness of robotic gynaecological surgery. Br J Surg 97:1772–1783, 2010.
25. Hemmerling TM: Automated anesthesia. Curr Opin Anaesthesiol 22:757–763, 2009.
26. Faulkner H, Regehr G, Martin J, et al: Validation of an objective structured assessment of technical skill for surgical residents. Acad Med 71:1363–1365, 1996.
27. Grantcharov TP, Reznick RK: Teaching procedural skills. BMJ 336:1129–1131, 2008.
28. Tsuda S, Scott D, Doyle J, et al: Surgical skills training and simulation. Curr Probl Surg 46:271–370, 2009.
29. Fried GM, Feldman LS, Vassiliou MC, et al: Proving the value of simulation in laparoscopic surgery. Ann Surg 240:518–525, 2004.
30. Swanstrom LL, Fried GM, Hoffman KI, et al: Beta test results of a new system assessing competence in laparoscopic surgery. J Am Coll Surg 202:62–69, 2006.
31. Sroka G, Feldman LS, Vassiliou MC, et al: Fundamentals of laparoscopic surgery simulator training to proficiency improves laparoscopic performance in the operating room—a randomized controlled trial. Am J Surg 199:115–120, 2010.
32. DiRaddo R, Tomanek B, Laroche D, et al: Patient-specific virtual reality systems for brain tumor surgery. Neuro-Oncology 11:698–698, 2009.

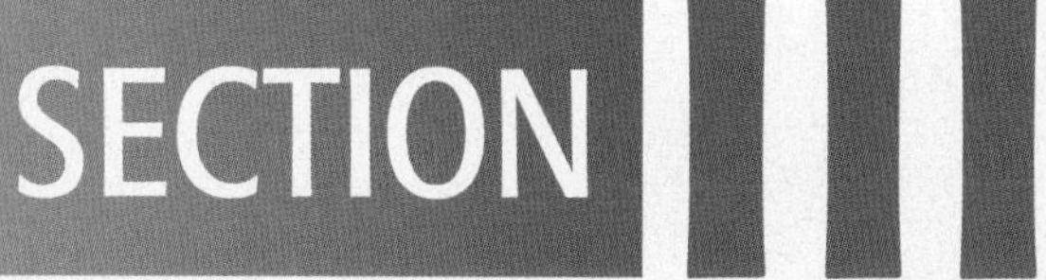

# SECTION III

# TRAUMA AND CRITICAL CARE

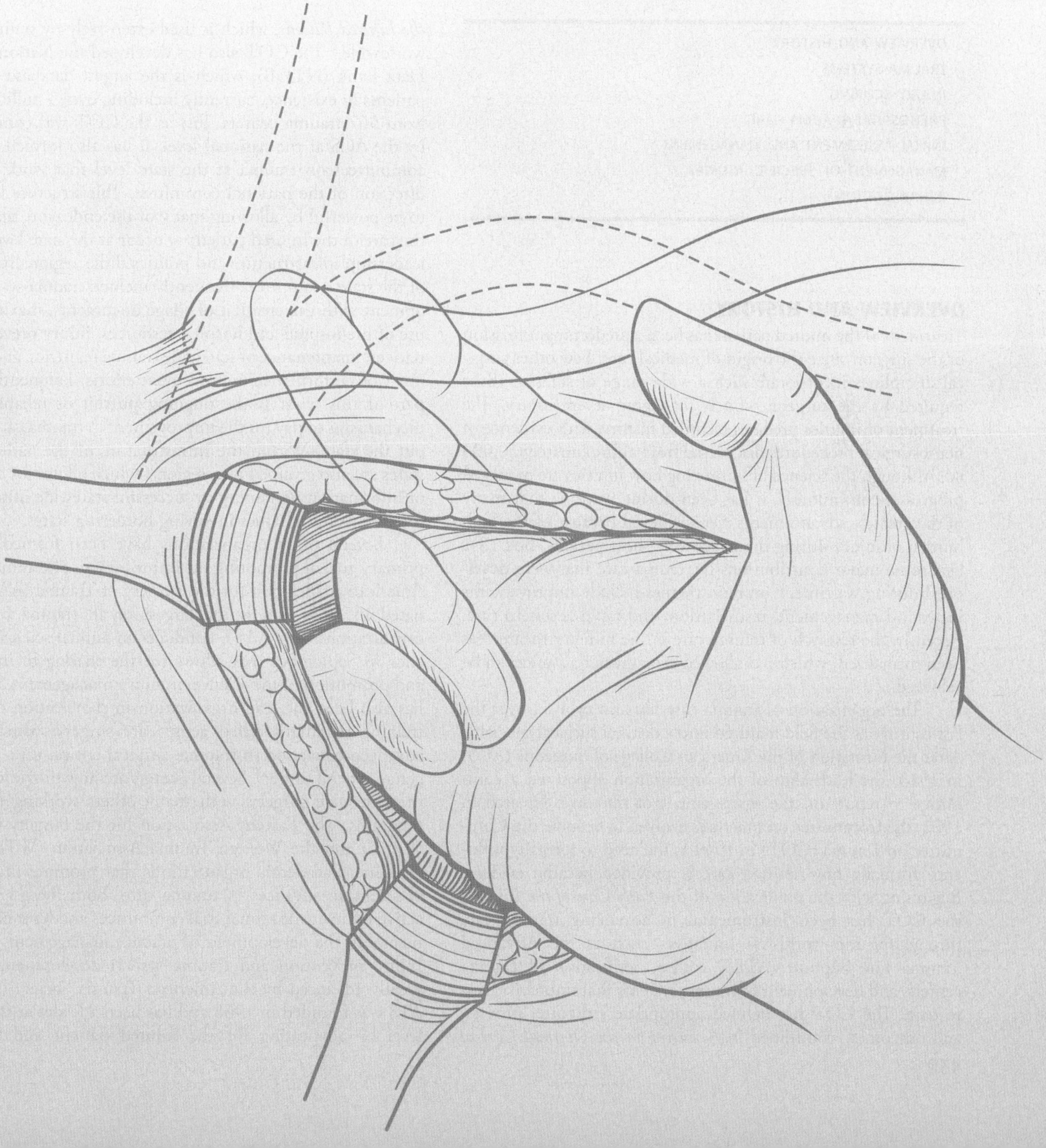

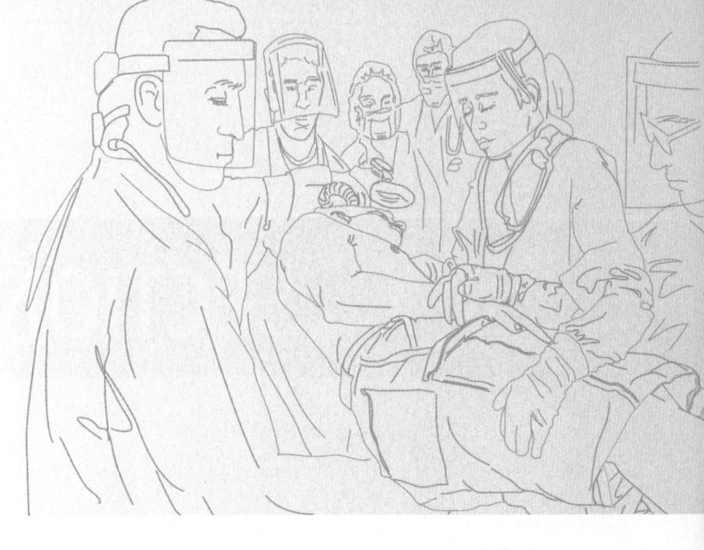

CHAPTER 18

# MANAGEMENT OF ACUTE TRAUMA

R. Shayn Martin and J. Wayne Meredith



## OVERVIEW AND HISTORY

Treatment of the injured patient has been a predominant mission of the surgeon since the origin of medical care. Few other surgical disciplines incorporate such a wide range of skills as those required by the surgeon who is managing severe injury. The treatment of injuries predates recorded history, with evidence of neurosurgical procedures discovered from approximately 10,000 BC. Although the science of improving how injuries are managed progresses continuously, it has been during wartime that many of the greatest advancements were achieved because of the high burden of injury during these relatively short periods. Box 18-1 lists some major contributions to trauma care that were developed during wartime. Common themes include improvements in wound management, resuscitation, and rapid access to care. Recently, the research of trauma care in the military theater has been formalized, which has allowed even greater advances to be achieved.

The organization of trauma care has also evolved over the last century as the field matured into a distinct surgical specialty. After the formation of the American College of Surgeons (ACS) in 1913, the leadership of the organization appointed a committee to report on the management of fractures. Created in 1922, the Committee on Fractures evolved to become the Committee on Trauma (COT) in 1949 as the need to formally influence formally how trauma care is provided became evident. Beginning with the publication of the *Early Care of the Injured,* the COT has been instrumental in advancing trauma care throughout the world via initiatives such as the Advanced Trauma Life Support (ATLS) course, verification of trauma centers, and development of trauma systems that improve access to care. The COT has defined appropriate structure, process, and outcomes, as outlined in *Resources for the Optimal Care of the Injured Patient,* which is used extensively by trauma centers worldwide.[1] The COT also has developed the National Trauma Data Bank (NTDB), which is the largest database of trauma patients in existence, currently including over 3 million patients from 567 trauma centers. Just as the COT was commissioned by the ACS at the national level, it has also formed individual committees on trauma at the state level that work under the direction of the national committee. This structure has proven to be powerful by allowing many of the endeavors that advance the care of the injured patient to occur at the state level, because leadership infrastructure and politics differ regionally. Activities of the state committees frequently include trauma system development with the creation of triage documents, maximizing the use of prehospital and hospital resources, injury prevention initiatives, maintenance of statewide trauma registries, and advancement of performance improvement efforts. Frequently, a major part of this work is the ongoing pursuit of reliable funding mechanisms to pay for the improvement in trauma care throughout the state. Within the infrastructure of the national COT, states are also grouped into regions, which allows for the sharing of information pertaining to successful statewide initiatives and the discussion of issues involving bordering states.

Several other organizations have been formed, with the primary goal of promoting the improvement of trauma care. The American Association for the Surgery of Trauma (AAST) originated in 1938 and is the largest of all trauma professional organizations. The AAST conducts an annual scientific conference in September that allows for the sharing of information and promotion of the science of injury management. The AAST has also been the lead organization in the creation of the new training paradigm called acute care surgery, which includes advanced education in trauma, surgical critical care, and emergency general surgery. Several centers are now providing training in acute care surgery, with many others working to develop programs. The Eastern Association for the Surgery of Trauma (EAST) and the Western Trauma Association (WTA) are also prominent academic organizations that promote the exchange of scientific advances in trauma care. Both these groups have active multi-institutional trial committees and have been instrumental in the development of practice management guidelines. Injury prevention and trauma system development has been greatly advanced by the American Trauma Society (ATS). The ATS was founded in 1968 and has been a leader at the national level by advocating for the injured patient and promoting

**BOX 18-1 Advances and Discoveries in Trauma Care During War**

French and Indian War (1754-1763)
- Wound contraction during healing
- Primary and secondary healing
- Description of granulation tissue and epithelialization

American Revolutionary War (1775-1783)
- Exhaustive therapy (bleeding, diarrhea, vomiting, salivation, sweating)
- Centralization of medical care
- Establishment of first medical school

American Civil War (1861-1865)
- Primary amputation (versus secondary)
- Use of topical antiseptic agents
- Whole blood infusion
- Development of specialty hospitals (eye-ear, orthopedics, hernia)
- Extremity traction splinting

World War I (1914-1918)
- Laparotomy for penetrating abdominal trauma
- Wound débridement and delayed closure
- Early use of plasma and crystalloid
- First blood bank

World War II (1939-1945)
- Guillotine amputation and delayed primary closure
- Exteriorization of colon injuries
- Mobile surgical teams
- Organ dysfunction after injury described

Korean War (1950-1953)
- Vascular surgery for limb salvage
- Hypovolemic shock recognition
- Mobile surgical hospital units (MASH units)

Vietnam War (1955-1964)
- Aeromedical transfer (helicopter)
- Sulfamylon for burn care
- Recognition of acute respiratory distress syndrome (Da Nang lung)

Iraq wars (Iraq, 2003 to present)
- Damage control resuscitation
- Highly efficient trauma systems
- Reemergence of tourniquet use

trauma-related legislation. Finally, the care of the injured patient is a multidisciplinary process, which has accordingly driven the formation of organizations in many other fields that play a role in trauma care. The Orthopedic Trauma Association (OTA), American Association of Neurological Surgeons (AANS), and Society of Trauma Nurses (STN) represent three organizations whose members are part of the multidisciplinary team dedicated to improving the care of the injured patient.

## TRAUMA SYSTEMS

Interstate 40 runs 2550 miles from Wilmington, on the coast of North Carolina, to Barstow, California. If a car crash were to occur along I-40, the unfortunate reality is that the outcome after a given severity of injury is dependent on where along the highway the crash occurs. This illogical finding is a reflection of the variability in a patient's access to care that is provided throughout the United States and the rest of the world. Regions that are better able to respond to injury have developed an organized approach to providing all the elements that maximize the potential for meaningful recovery, called a trauma system. Trauma systems encompass the entire care continuum, starting at the time of the injury, with a patient's access to care, through the rehabilitation process. At the most basic level, one might think of the goal of a trauma system as getting the right patient to the right place at the right time.

**BOX 18-2 Components of Comprehensive Inclusive Trauma System**

Injury prevention efforts
Prehospital care
Tachypnea
Triage
Communication
Transportation
Acute care facilities
Trauma center designation, verification
Post–acute care, rehabilitation
Performance improvement
Education and outreach
Legislation

Historically, the provision of trauma care was centered around the large academic hospitals that provided the vast majority of injury management. Prehospital efforts focused on getting all patients to the trauma center, regardless of the degree of injury. Although initially found to be beneficial to those patients who were transported to the trauma center, this exclusive type of system failed to address the needs of patients who were geographically distant from the trauma center. Furthermore, this type of system did not capitalize on the resources that could be provided in non–trauma center hospitals. The solution was the development of inclusive trauma systems designed to address the needs of all injured patients, regardless of their severity of injury or geographic location. Inclusive trauma systems capitalize on the resources of all hospitals from critical access facilities to the large levels I and II trauma centers. Guided by predeveloped triage protocols, injured patients are transported to facilities that can provide the level of care necessary to manage injuries of varying severity. At times, this requires transferring patients from smaller hospitals to larger hospitals or trauma centers. Box 18-2 lists the common components of an inclusive trauma system that must be coordinated to maximize the efficiency of getting the injured patient to the care location that he or she needs most. The benefits of this approach include the efficient use of all available resources, reduction in potentially overwhelming trauma centers with patients of lower acuity, and allowing most patients to receive appropriate care within their own community. Finally, it is essential to recognize that legislation plays a large role in the establishment and maintenance of trauma systems. Only through ongoing legislative support can the systematic approach to trauma care grow to eliminate the possibility of a patient lacking access to appropriate, high-quality care for his or her injuries.

The establishment of trauma systems is a relatively new development, with Illinois and Maryland first creating a system for addressing injuries in the early 1970s. Congress recognized the need for a coordinated approach to the management of injuries and passed the Trauma Care Systems Planning and Development Act of 1990, which formally addressed the need for trauma systems. The development of trauma systems was further advanced with the release of the Model Trauma Care System Plan by the Health Resources and Services Administration (HRSA).[2] Originally released in 1992 and then revised in 2006, the newly titled *Model Trauma System Planning and Evaluation* document applied a public health approach to trauma and provided valuable direction for developing and evaluating trauma systems. This public health approach identified trauma as a disease, the impact of which can be prevented or decreased by applying already established systems that address other health-related issues, such as infectious diseases. Finally, the American College of Surgeons' COT established the Trauma Systems Consultation Program in 1996 to guide states or regions in the process of developing a systematic approach to trauma care.

The impact of trauma systems on the care people receive after injury has been well studied and provides support for ongoing societal investment in this approach. In 2000, Nathens and colleagues published their evaluation of more than 400,000 patients treated over a 17-year period.[3] During the study period, trauma systems were established and developed in many of the regions evaluated. After correcting for all identifiable injury prevention and management improvements, the development of a trauma system over an approximately 10-year period resulted in a reduction in mortality by 8%.[3] Several others have also reported this effect, demonstrating an improvement in outcomes in areas that establish a systematic approach to injury management. Most recently, the National Study on Costs and Outcomes of Trauma (NSCOT) was performed to evaluate variations in injury care and outcomes between trauma centers and non–trauma centers. Supported by the National Center for Injury Prevention and Control of the Centers for Disease Control and Prevention (CDC), NSCOT represents one of the largest epidemiologic studies ever to evaluate trauma care; it included more than 5000 patients from 69 hospitals. NSCOT established that injured patients treated at a trauma center experienced improved outcomes over those treated at non–trauma centers. After correction for injury severity, care at a trauma center was associated with a reduction in mortality of 20% in-hospital and 25% at 1 year.[4]

Trauma system development and maintenance benefit from the contributions of physicians of all different types who work at locations ranging from the smallest rural hospital to the largest academic medical center. Even in areas in which definitive trauma care is not provided, health care personnel play a vital role by establishing triage plans and providing initial stabilization and patient transfer. Highly functional trauma systems require the involvement of local leaders from hospitals, government, and prehospital agencies to develop the regional trauma system and work with surrounding trauma centers to ensure appropriate care for patients with all levels of injury severity.

## INJURY SCORING

To characterize injuries accurately for the purposes of clinical management, benchmarking, and research, several injury scoring systems have been developed. These typically are based on the anatomy of the injury or the resulting physiology, with several types systems created and evaluated over the last 40 years. One of the first anatomy-based scoring systems was the Abbreviated Injury Scale (AIS), initially published in 1971. The AIS characterizes injuries using a six-digit taxonomy that describes the body region, type of anatomic structure, and specific anatomic detail of the injury. As seen in Table 18-1, the first digit of the AIS score defines the affected body region, allowing clinicians and researchers to identify the location of described injuries quickly. The AIS also assigns a severity code to the injury as a seventh digit, which ranges between 1 (minimal severity) and 6 (presumably fatal). The AIS has been updated six times since the original publication and remains one of the most commonly used injury coding systems.

**Table 18-1 Abbreviated Injury Scale (AIS) Body Regions**

| AIS FIRST DIGIT | BODY REGION |
|---|---|
| 1 | Head |
| 2 | Face |
| 3 | Neck |
| 4 | Thorax |
| 5 | Abdomen |
| 6 | Spine |
| 7 | Upper extremity |
| 8 | Lower extremity |
| 9 | Unspecified |

Although the AIS successfully describes individual injuries, it fails to reflect the impact of multiple injuries sustained by the same patient. In 1974, Baker and colleagues[5] presented the Injury Severity Score (ISS), calculated by summing the squares of the AIS severity codes for the three most severely injured body regions. Minor injury has been defined as an ISS less than 9, whereas moderate injury is between 9 and 16, serious injury is between 16 and 25, and severe injury is suggested by a score more than 25. The ISS has been used extensively since its development as a way of quantifying the overall injury burden sustained by a given patient. Many other anatomic injury coding systems have since been developed, each with their own merits, although a comprehensive discussion of these exceeds the scope of this chapter. One of the most recent advances in injury coding has been the development of the Organ Injury Scales (OIS) by the American Association for the Surgery of Trauma (AAST), which have been incorporated into the most recent update of the AIS.[6] The OIS provides greater anatomic detail to specific organs that was lacking in the AIS. They also have introduced the concept of injury grades, which provide a standard way of describing organ injury severity and the associated risk of morbidity and mortality. Another attribute of the OIS taxonomy is that the severity suggested by the injury grade has been validated using the NTDB.[6]

Although anatomic scoring methods are more readily used to compare groups of like injuries, physiologic scoring systems may have more real-time clinical value. Physiologic scores provide a better indication of the injured patient's condition and can therefore be used to make treatment decisions or develop a prognosis. Probably the most commonly used is the Glasgow Coma Scale (GCS), which reflects a patient's level of consciousness. With scores ranging from 3 to 15, the GCS is composed of a measure of eye opening, verbal response, and motor function. The GCS and more specifically the motor score alone have

**Table 18-2 Glasgow Coma Scale**

| PARAMETER | SCORE |
|---|---|
| **Eye Opening** | |
| Spontaneous | 4 |
| To voice | 3 |
| To pain | 2 |
| None | 1 |
| **Verbal Response** | |
| Oriented | 5 |
| Confused | 4 |
| Inappropriate | 3 |
| Incomprehensible | 2 |
| None | 1 |
| **Motor Response** | |
| Obeys commands | 6 |
| Localizes pain | 5 |
| Withdraws to pain | 4 |
| Flexion | 3 |
| Extension | 2 |
| None | 1 |
| **Total Glasgow Coma Score** | 3-15 |

**Table 18-3 Revised Trauma Score**

| GLASGOW COMA SCORE | SYSTOLIC BLOOD PRESSURE (mm Hg) | RESPIRATORY RATE (breaths/min) | CODED VALUE |
|---|---|---|---|
| 13-15 | >89 | 10-29 | 4 |
| 9-12 | 76-89 | >29 | 3 |
| 6-8 | 50-75 | 6-9 | 2 |
| 4-5 | 1-49 | 1-5 | 1 |
| 3 | 0 | 0 | 0 |
| **Total Revised Trauma Score** | | | 0-12 |

been found to be reflective of patient outcome after traumatic brain injury.[7] Other examples of physiologic scores commonly used are the Trauma Score (TS) and the Revised Trauma Score (RTS), which are composed of the GCS as well as physiologic variables, such as systolic blood pressure, respiratory rate, and capillary refill time to quantify the injured patient's condition. The GCS and the RTS are depicted in Tables 18-2 and 18-3. These scores have been of value for research purposes and have been used for making triage decisions with some success.

## PREHOSPITAL TRAUMA CARE

Immediately after a patient is injured, the prehospital phase of care begins with the goal of moving a patient to a location capable of providing definitive injury management as quickly as possible. Because of the time-dependent nature of many severe injuries, prehospital personnel play an integral role in the ultimate outcome of the trauma patient. The initial approach to prehospital injury care can be summarized into four priorities:

1. Evaluate the scene.
2. Perform an initial assessment.
3. Make critical interventions and triage-transport decision.
4. Transport the patient.

This list of priorities is intentionally brief because the outcome for each patient depends greatly on how quickly definitive hemorrhage control is obtained. For that reason, only critical interventions should occur prior to initiating transportation to the definitive care facility.

Prehospital providers must begin by evaluating the scene first to ensure his or her safety. The remaining scene assessment should be rapid and completed as the patient is approached. The initial assessment consists of a systematic approach to identify life-threatening conditions immediately that require urgent intervention. This assessment follows the well known ABC mnemonic, in which ***a***irway, ***b***reathing, and ***c***irculation are sequentially addressed. During this time, an airway is established and assisted ventilation is provided if necessary. Spinal immobilization is provided with a hard collar and long spine board. Assessment and support of circulation includes immediate control of external hemorrhage and initiation of fluid resuscitation.

The success of the prehospital trauma management hinges on immediately making a triage and transport decision. Severely injured patients should be immediately transported to an appropriate hospital for definitive care using the "Load and go" philosophy, with all remaining care provided en route. Valuable prehospital care including a head to toe examination, continuous monitoring, placement of subsequent intravenous access, and environmental control can be provided while the patient is being transported. Although the decision to depart the scene rapidly is often simple, where to go and how to get there can be much more challenging. These decisions should be made well in advance and then implemented in the form of well-outlined protocols and agreements that were developed during trauma system planning endeavors. To guide this process, the COT and the CDC have developed a Field Triage Decision Scheme, which is included in the updated COT document[1] (Fig. 18-1). This systematic approach to triage uses physiologic status, mechanism of injury, and identification of high-risk patients to assist in deciding who might benefit from immediate transfer to a trauma center. Finally, the value of rapidly making a triage and transport decision within minutes of patient arrival and then quickly departing to keep scene times less than 10 minutes cannot be overemphasized.

One of the primary goals of prehospital trauma care is maintaining control of the injured patient's airway. The gold standard for airway maintenance in severely injured patients remains oral endotracheal intubation, typically using a rapid-sequence technique with spine stabilization. There has been some controversy recently that has questioned whether advanced airway management in the prehospital setting is more harmful than basic airway support with a bag valve mask and basic airway adjuncts. The existing literature has been unable to address this question adequately. For example, Eckstein and colleagues[8] have retrospectively evaluated 496 injured patients and found that endotracheal intubation was associated with a greater mortality compared with bag valve mask support. Studies such as these are limited by selection bias and at best can suggest that this

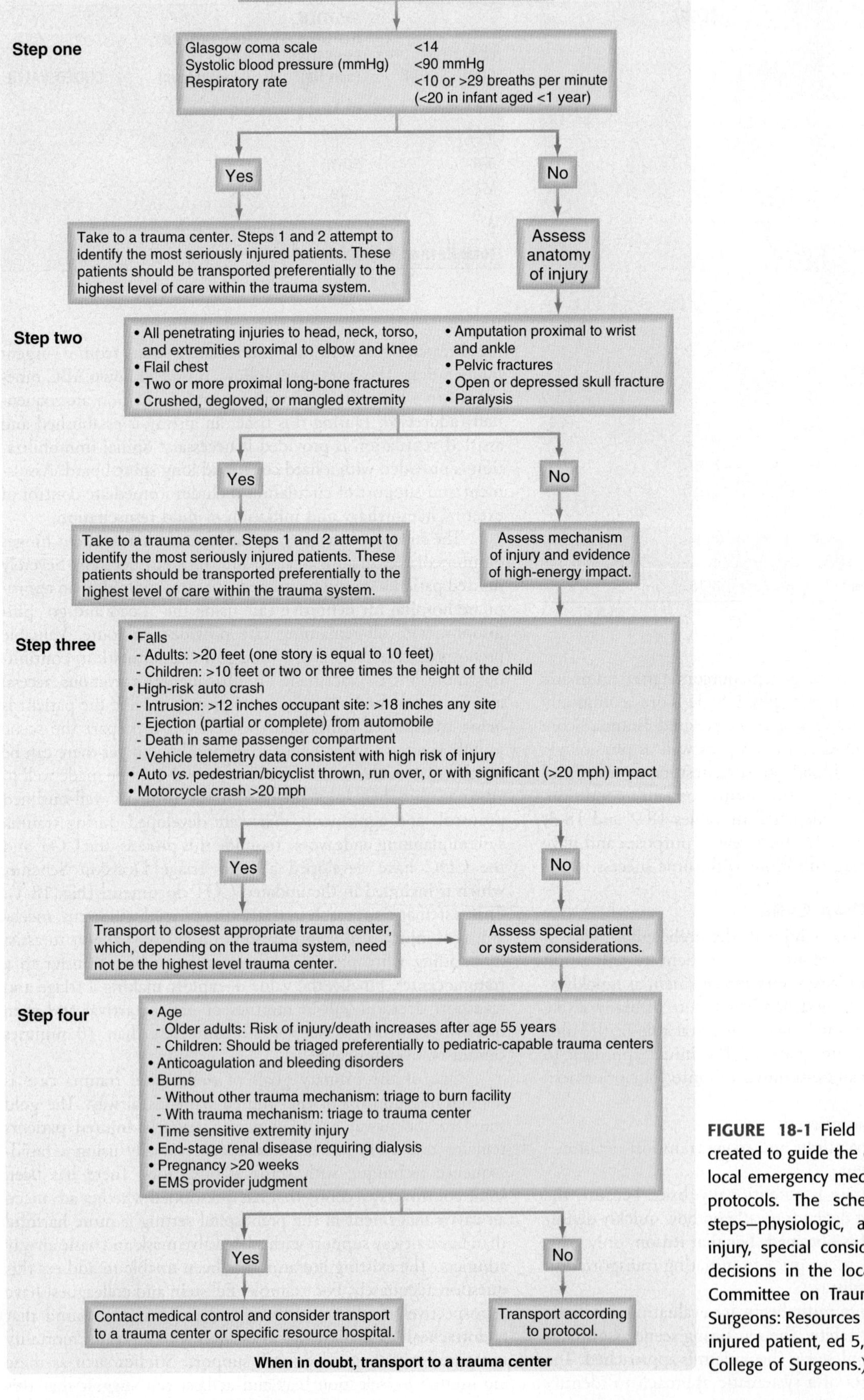

Measure vital signs and level of consciousness
Step one
Glasgow coma scale <14
Systolic blood pressure (mmHg) <90 mmHg
Respiratory rate <10 or >29 breaths per minute (<20 in infant aged <1 year)
Yes
No
Take to a trauma center. Steps 1 and 2 attempt to identify the most seriously injured patients. These patients should be transported preferentially to the highest level of care within the trauma system.
Assess anatomy of injury
Step two
• All penetrating injuries to head, neck, torso, and extremities proximal to elbow and knee
• Flail chest
• Two or more proximal long-bone fractures
• Crushed, degloved, or mangled extremity
• Amputation proximal to wrist and ankle
• Pelvic fractures
• Open or depressed skull fracture
• Paralysis
Yes
No
Take to a trauma center. Steps 1 and 2 attempt to identify the most seriously injured patients. These patients should be transported preferentially to the highest level of care within the trauma system.
Assess mechanism of injury and evidence of high-energy impact.
Step three
• Falls
- Adults: >20 feet (one story is equal to 10 feet)
- Children: >10 feet or two or three times the height of the child
• High-risk auto crash
- Intrusion: >12 inches occupant site: >18 inches any site
- Ejection (partial or complete) from automobile
- Death in same passenger compartment
- Vehicle telemetry data consistent with high risk of injury
• Auto vs. pedestrian/bicyclist thrown, run over, or with significant (>20 mph) impact
• Motorcycle crash >20 mph
Yes
No
Transport to closest appropriate trauma center, which, depending on the trauma system, need not be the highest level trauma center.
Assess special patient or system considerations.
Step four
• Age
- Older adults: Risk of injury/death increases after age 55 years
- Children: Should be triaged preferentially to pediatric-capable trauma centers
• Anticoagulation and bleeding disorders
• Burns
- Without other trauma mechanism: triage to burn facility
- With trauma mechanism: triage to trauma center
• Time sensitive extremity injury
• End-stage renal disease requiring dialysis
• Pregnancy >20 weeks
• EMS provider judgment
Yes
No
Contact medical control and consider transport to a trauma center or specific resource hospital.
Transport according to protocol.
When in doubt, transport to a trauma center


**FIGURE 18-1** Field triage decision scheme created to guide the development of state and local emergency medical services (EMS) triage protocols. The scheme uses four decision steps—physiologic, anatomic, mechanism of injury, special considerations—to guide triage decisions in the local trauma system. (From Committee on Trauma, American College of Surgeons: Resources for the optimal care of the injured patient, ed 5, Chicago, 2006, American College of Surgeons.)

question be studied prospectively. There has also been work specifically in brain-injured patients that argues the converse and thus supports the use of prehospital endotracheal intubation.[9] Finally, it is of value to have several airway rescue techniques and methods available because many have been found to facilitate intubation or provide a bridge to a definitive airway. Two examples that are well studied are the gum elastic bougie and blind insertion airway devices.

Resuscitation with isotonic crystalloid solution is initiated in the prehospital phase of care for patients in shock. Although this principle remains well accepted, the need for intravenous (IV) fluid resuscitation in some patient groups has been questioned and the concept of hypotensive resuscitation has been introduced. The rationale is that overresuscitation before management of bleeding could potentially increase the rate of blood loss by disrupting areas that had become hemostatic. Bickell and associates[10] have performed a prospective trial that compared standard crystalloid administration with the concept of withholding prehospital fluid resuscitation in patients with penetrating torso trauma. The group of patients who had resuscitation withheld until reaching the hospital had a lower mortality than the immediate resuscitation group. These results are intriguing, but the study represented a unique cohort of penetrating trauma patients in an urban setting, with short transport times to definitive care. Nevertheless, it suggests that prehospital fluid resuscitation be judiciously administered to support some minimal level of perfusion to support the maintenance of hemostasis.

Finally, recent military experience has reintroduced the use of tourniquets for prehospital extremity hemorrhage control. For some time, tourniquets were infrequently used because of concern about muscle and nerve injury. Recent advances in device development and provider education have lessened the associated risk and have again demonstrated the potential benefit of tourniquets in certain situations. Several series now have demonstrated improved outcomes related to the use of tourniquets in the military theater.[11] Many prehospital agencies are now including tourniquets on standard equipment lists so that they may be used when confronted with a patient with devastating extremity injuries with uncontrolled arterial hemorrhage. Although many commercial devices are now available, Figure 18-2 illustrates a tourniquet that can be used in the prehospital setting.

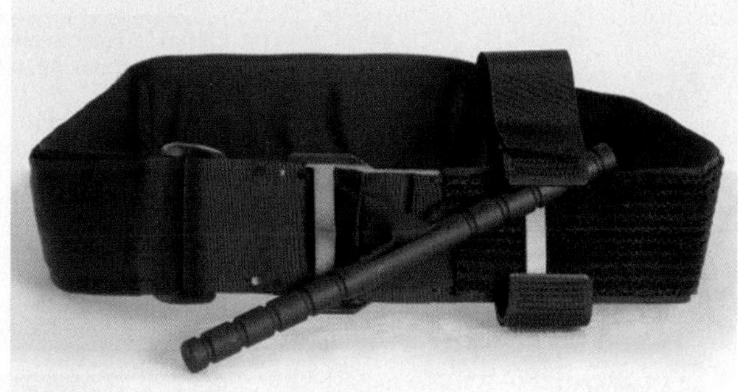

**FIGURE 18-2** Example of a tourniquet. Tourniquets are now more commonly being used to prevent extremity exsanguination in military and civilian prehospital environments.

## INITIAL ASSESSMENT AND MANAGEMENT

Since its inception over 30 years ago, the Advanced Trauma Life Support (ATLS) course has presented a safe approach to the initial assessment and management of the injured patient.[12] ATLS has been widely adopted as the standard approach in most trauma centers. All physicians who provide initial care to trauma patients should complete the ATLS course to become familiar with the concept of rapidly identifying and addressing life-threatening conditions during the initial patient assessment. Furthermore, ATLS teaches three important concepts that greatly enhance the ability to manage injured patients, regardless of where care is provided:

1. Treat the greatest threat to life first.
2. The lack of a definitive diagnosis should not delay the application of an indicated urgent treatment.
3. An initial, detailed history is not essential to begin the evaluation of a patient with acute injuries.

The initial assessment follows a well-defined order that is based on the patient's risk of death. At this time, the identification of life-threatening conditions requires immediate intervention. This initial assessment and management, also termed the *primary survey*, follows the mnemonic ABCDE (Fig. 18-3):

**A**irway and cervical spine protection
**B**reathing
**C**irculation
**D**isability or neurologic condition
**E**xposure and Environmental control

Finally, the safety of the health care team is of upmost importance. Therefore, prior to any patient contact, personal protective equipment must be donned to reduce the risk of infectious disease transmission.

### Airway

On receiving an injured patient in the emergency department, the status of the patient's airway should be immediately assessed. This is best achieved by eliciting a verbal response, because speaking patients are typically able to protect their airway. The inability to speak indicates severe mental status depression or some obstruction to air flow through the upper airway. In either of these situations, however, the patient is frequently unable to maintain an adequate airway to support acceptable oxygenation and ventilation. Further indicators of airway compromise include noisy breathing, severe facial trauma, specifically with oropharyngeal blood or foreign body, and patient agitation. A determination of the adequacy of the airway should be completed within seconds of the patient's arrival, as well as a decision to obtain better airway control if necessary. Even if an airway is thought to be secure, frequent reassessment for decompensation and the development of airway compromise is paramount.

Also of importance during this time is protecting the cervical spine. Injured patients should be suspected of having a cervical spine injury until a thorough evaluation can be completed to eliminate this possibility. Cervical spine protection includes the use of a hard cervical collar and the maintenance of the log roll technique for all patient movement. Spine protection during patient transportation can be augmented by the use of a long spine board but patients should be removed from these devices shortly after emergency department arrival to prevent the development of pressure sores, which can occur within a short period

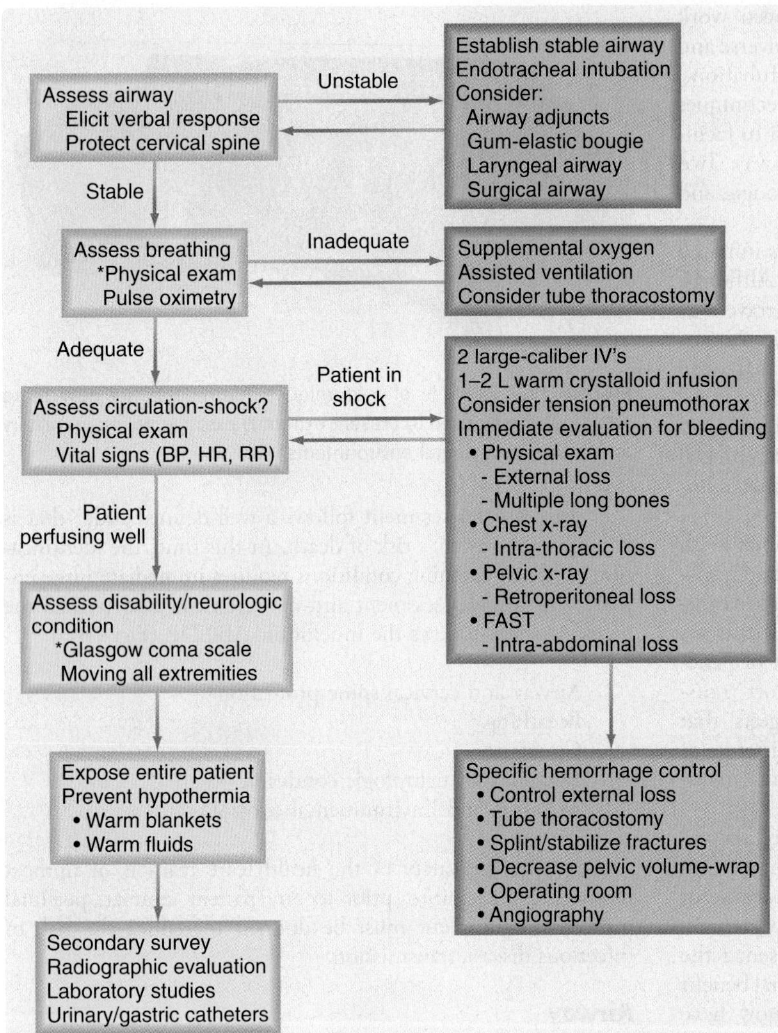


**FIGURE 18-3** Algorithm for the initial assessment of the injured patient. *BP,* Blood pressure; *HR,* heart rate; *RR,* respiratory rate.

of time. During airway assessment and intervention, the anterior portion of the collar can be removed to facilitate exposure and airway manipulation but manual stabilization should be provided by an assistant throughout this period.

Immediate airway adjuncts include supplemental oxygen, oropharyngeal and nasopharyngeal airways, and bag valve mask ventilation. These can be applied quickly to support the failing patient while preparing to secure a more definitive airway. The definitive airway of choice for most injured patients is oral endotracheal intubation provided using a rapid-sequence technique. With cricoid pressure applied, the patient is provided a sedative and fast-acting neuromuscular blocker such as succinylcholine to maximally enhance glottic visualization. Direct laryngoscopy and intubation are performed, with care taken to avoid cervical spine motion. Endotracheal tube position must be confirmed using chest and abdomen auscultation, end-tidal carbon dioxide measurement, and ultimately a chest radiograph. The presence of highly experienced airway personnel can be extremely advantageous and may be an important component of the trauma alert system.

Several recent developments have broadened the capabilities of airway physicians when challenged with a difficult airway. The gum elastic bougie has been shown to improve the rate of successful intubation, especially in the setting of a challenging airway. For injured patients who cannot undergo cervical extension, require cricoid pressure, or have upper airway injuries, the normal view of the glottis may be obscured. In this setting, the bougie can be placed with a limited view of the vocal cords, resulting in an improved rate of appropriately placing an endotracheal tube. Another rescue technique that should be remembered in the setting of an inability to intubate successfully is the use of a blind insertion airway device. Some commonly used devices include the laryngeal mask airway (LMA), multilumen esophageal airway (Combitube), and laryngeal tube airway (King LT-D). These are typically placed blindly and function essentially by occluding the esophagus and the posterior pharynx, allowing assisted ventilation to pass selectively down the trachea. These have been found to be easy to place and are valuable tools in a rescue situation.[13]

If a difficult airway requires the intubating physician to progress to a backup plan, preparation for a surgical airway should begin. A cricothyroidotomy can be performed with limited equipment and should commence prior to cardiovascular collapse. The inability to maintain oxygenation with a bag valve mask between intubation attempts is a reasonable indication for establishment of a surgical airway. To perform a

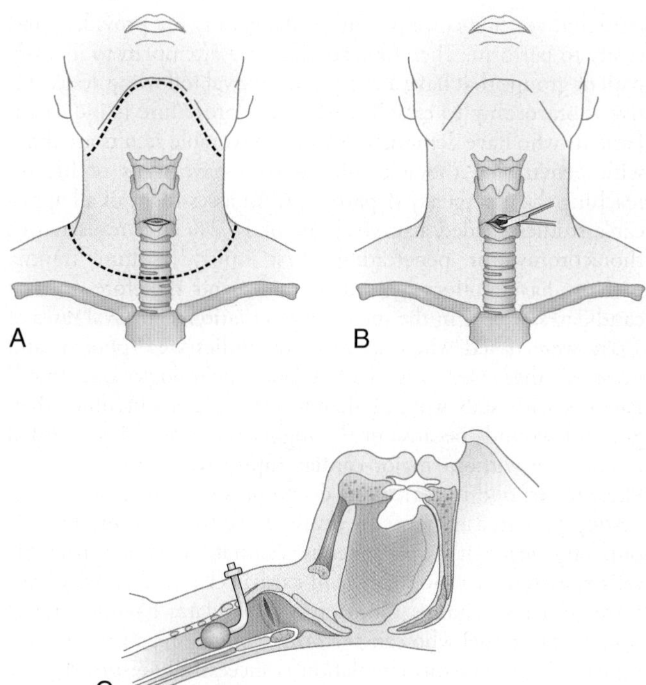


**FIGURE 18-4** Technique of cricothyroidotomy. The cricothyroid membrane is identified by palpation **(A)** and a transverse incision is made over the membrane **(B)**. The incision and dissection are continued through the cricothyroid membrane and the cricothyroidotomy is spread, allowing the passage of a tracheal tube.

cricothyroidotomy (Fig. 18-4), the front portion of the cervical collar is removed and in-line stabilization of the cervical spine is maintained. After preparation, a transverse incision is made over the cricothyroid membrane, which can be palpated between the thyroid cartilage and cricoid ring. Spreading the overlying soft tissue reveals the cricothyroid membrane. The membrane is transversely incised and the cricothyroidotomy is spread longitudinally. A tracheostomy or endotracheal tube is then advanced through the incised membrane and down the trachea. After balloon inflation, tube position is immediately confirmed with lung auscultation and end-tidal carbon dioxide determination. Finally, patients suspected of having a laryngeal injury might have involvement of the airway in the vicinity of the cricothyroid membrane and therefore could benefit from a tracheostomy instead of a cricothyroidotomy.

## Breathing

Breathing is rapidly assessed by visualizing or palpating the chest, auscultating breath sounds, and measuring oxygen saturation. Limited respiratory effort or dyspnea are indicative of the need for airway stabilization and ventilatory support. Inability to ventilate the patient adequately could be secondary to tension pneumothorax, massive hemothorax, or flail chest with pulmonary contusion. Tension pneumothorax should be recognized on the primary survey and radiographic confirmation is not required prior to treatment. Deviation of the trachea in the sternal notch, in combination with unilaterally absent or diminished breath sounds and cardiopulmonary compromise, is diagnostic of a tension pneumothorax. Thoracic decompression should immediately be performed with a large-bore needle–angiocatheter or a tube thoracostomy, depending on the availability of equipment and supplies. Massive hemothorax may also require urgent placement of a tube thoracostomy and severe pulmonary contusion can only be managed with aggressive mechanical ventilation, often with elevated levels of positive end-expiratory pressure (PEEP). With severe pulmonary contusion one should resist continuously disconnecting the ventilator to suction or bag the patient when oxygenation will only improve with uninterrupted PEEP.

**BOX 18-3 Indicators of Shock in the Injured Patient**

Agitation, confusion
Tachycardia
Tachypnea
Diaphoresis
Cool, mottled extremities
Weak distal pulses
Decreased pulse pressure
Decreased urine output
Hypotension

## Circulation

After respiratory stabilization, an immediate assessment for cardiovascular compromise is completed. Simply, the physician must determine whether the injured patient is in shock. Box 18-3 lists the most common immediate indicators of shock. It is important to recognize that a patient can be in shock before developing hypotension because this is one of the last findings before complete cardiovascular collapse. Cardiovascular dysfunction in injured patients is secondary to hemorrhage in most patients. In less common situations, a spinal cord injury (neurogenic shock), or preinjury heart failure or sepsis could be the cause. On recognition of shock, resuscitation is immediately initiated with 1 to 2 liters of warm crystalloid solution infused through two large-bore, short, peripheral IV catheters. A rapid assessment for the source(s) of blood loss is then completed. It may be valuable to approach this assessment by recognizing the five major locations for exsanguinating blood loss: chest, abdomen, retroperitoneum (often a pelvic fracture), multiple long bone fractures, and external sites. Immediately, a brief physical examination will identify long bone fractures and sources of external hemorrhage. A chest radiograph will evaluate for thoracic blood loss and a pelvic radiograph will identify a pelvic fracture. The focused abdominal sonography in trauma (FAST) scan or diagnostic peritoneal lavage (DPL) for gross blood can be obtained to evaluate for intra-abdominal bleeding. The FAST scan is a rapidly obtainable ultrasound that assesses for fluid within the abdomen. The FAST scan assesses the hepatorenal, splenorenal, and pelvic spaces for fluid which in the setting of trauma most likely represents blood. A FAST scan can be performed quickly in the trauma bay by the surgeon and can be rapidly repeated if necessary. Figure 18-5 demonstrates blood in the hepatorenal space on FAST scan.

After the initial 1- to 2-liter crystalloid bolus is infused, patients are reassessed for response by determining whether the indicators of shock have improved. Patients who respond favorably can then continue to undergo a standard evaluation to identify their injuries. It is important to decrease the administered IV fluid to a maintenance rate so that signs of ongoing

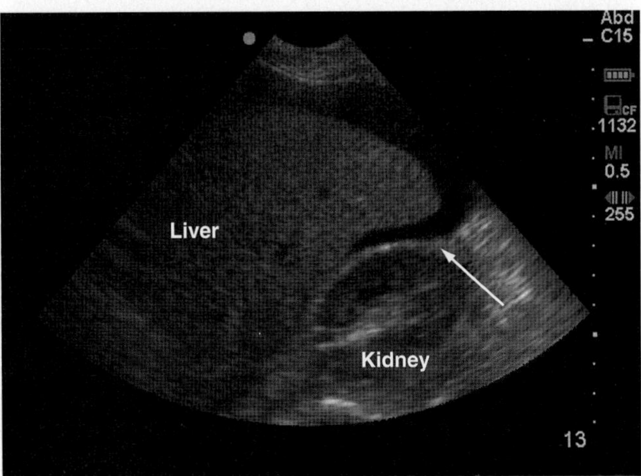


**FIGURE 18-5** FAST scan demonstrating fluid in the hepatorenal space (Morrison's pouch). The *arrow* identifies fluid (blood) between the liver and right kidney.

blood loss will not be masked by continuous fluid infusion. Those that fail to respond to the IV fluid bolus need immediate intervention based on the assessment for bleeding. External bleeding should be managed and fractures splinted. A tube thoracostomy may be required for thoracic blood loss, with subsequent thoracotomy as needed. Intra-abdominal bleeding in the hemodynamically unstable patient warrants emergent laparotomy. Finally, bleeding from pelvic fractures may require a pelvic binder followed by pelvic angiography with embolization for arterial hemorrhage. While the management of hemorrhage is occurring, ongoing resuscitation with blood products should be provided commensurate with the estimated blood loss.

### Disability and Exposure

A rapid determination of neurologic function can be achieved by quickly calculating the GCS. This will reflect the patient's eye opening, verbal, and motor responses and potentially reflect the degree of neurologic injury. If possible, this should be assessed prior to administering sedating or paralyzing medications. Also, the ability to move the extremities should be determined because this may be indicative of a spinal cord injury, especially in the setting of shock without an identified source of blood loss. The evaluation described during the primary survey requires complete exposure of the patient to ensure that important findings are not obscured by clothing. Despite this, maintaining body temperature is of upmost priority. A core body temperature should be obtained and documented. Warm blankets should be applied whenever an examination is not being performed and the trauma resuscitation room should be kept warm. All fluids provided to the trauma patient must be warm and body warmers should be considered as needed.

### Resuscitative Thoracotomy

Rarely, select patients who experience cardiac arrest in the emergency department may be candidates for a resuscitative thoracotomy. There are four main goals of a thoracotomy in the emergency department: opening of the pericardium to relieve cardiac tamponade, internal cardiac massage, cross-clamping of the distal thoracic aorta, and management of intra-thoracic bleeding. Although potentially lifesaving for some patients, a resuscitative thoracotomy can be dangerous for providers and costly to perform. Therefore, studies have attempted to identify patient groups that have a chance of survival following resuscitative thoracotomy to establish when the procedure is indicated. Patients who have demonstrated more favorable results are those with penetrating thoracic injuries who have signs of life on reaching the emergency department. An assessment of all applicable studies yielded a survival rate of 11.2% after resuscitative thoracotomy for penetrating chest injury.[14] Blunt trauma patients have uniformly dismal results and therefore are not candidates, except in the most select situations. Survival rates of 1.6% were noted when appropriate studies were pooled, and most of these survivors had a poor neurologic outcome.[14] Patients with stab wounds demonstrate better outcomes than gunshot wounds because of the higher incidence of pericardial tamponade without major cardiac injury which may be more likely to respond to pericardial decompression. Signs of life suggesting potential response to resuscitative thoracotomy include pupillary reactivity, spontaneous respiratory effort, palpable pulses, extremity movement, and cardiac electrical activity. Performing a resuscitative thoracotomy mandates having surgical support personnel who can perform definitive repair of thoracic injuries if spontaneous circulation is successfully resumed.

### Secondary Survey

A head to toe evaluation is completed on all stable patients after the primary survey. All body regions are thoroughly examined to identify injuries or the need for further evaluation. At this time, a more detailed neurologic evaluation can be completed and abnormalities of the face and neck identified. This includes posterior surfaces that are more difficult to visualize and may be obscured by the cervical collar. The torso is examined, especially with respect to pulmonary dysfunction and abdominal tenderness. Seatbelt or other superficial injury to the neck and abdomen may prompt further evaluation. The pelvis is assessed for tenderness, with care taken to avoid excessive compression because this technique to identify stability may only disrupt hemostasis. A rectal examination with a nonbloody glove to assess the prostate and the presence of gross gastrointestinal (GI) blood should be included. The extremities are evaluated for closed or open deformities and each joint should be manipulated to identify abnormalities. Careful assessment of distal perfusion is extremely important, especially in the presence of an associated extremity injury. This frequently includes an evaluation of pulse quality and blood pressure comparison between extremities. The patient should be rolled to assess the spine for deformity or tenderness and the long spine board can be removed at this time. Penetrating mechanisms require meticulous surveillance for all penetrating injuries, especially those that may be difficult to identify in areas such as the scalp, mouth, axilla, perineum, and throughout the back. On identification of these injuries, labeling with a radiopaque marker may allow localization on imaging studies.

## MANAGEMENT OF SPECIFIC INJURIES

### Damage Control Principles

Historically, in many centers, trauma patients who required immediate operation for life-threatening injuries would undergo surgery until all injuries were definitively repaired. Some patients would experience progressive physiologic derangement during these operations, often developing hypothermia, coagulopathy, and metabolic acidosis, a combination that has become labeled as the deadly triad or the bloody vicious cycle. To avoid certain death, this cycle must be halted by quickly managing bleeding and providing aggressive resuscitation. In 1993, Rotondo and associates[15] coined the term *damage control* to describe an approach to managing patients who were progressing rapidly toward death as their injuries were being definitively repaired. Damage control includes immediate surgical control of hemorrhage and contamination without immediate definitive reconstruction. All surgical bleeding is controlled and intra-abdominal or intrathoracic packing is frequently required to achieve hemostasis. Hollow visceral resection with temporary GI discontinuity is also commonly used. The chest or abdomen is then temporarily closed, frequently using a vacuum-type closure method. The patient is aggressively resuscitated in the intensive care unit with the goal of achieving adequate cardiopulmonary function and metabolic hemostasis. On improvement in body temperature, coagulopathy, and acidosis, definitive reconstruction of injuries can occur, followed by chest or abdominal closure when feasible. Initially, the concept of damage control was used for severe abdominal injuries but the principles have been applied to injuries of the chest, pelvis, and extremities. Using a similar approach, some have even advocated damage control orthopedics, which is based on the theory that rapid fracture stabilization may reduce the inflammatory response to injury and result in fewer long-term sequelae.

Recently, traditional methods of resuscitation immediately after injury have been questioned. Born out of military experience, an approach now called damage control resuscitation has evolved, with promising early results. In damage control resuscitation, replacement of lost blood is provided as a more equivalent distribution of all blood components. The military experience found that resuscitating with equal amounts of packed red blood cells, plasma, platelets, and cryoprecipitate resulted in preventing severe coagulopathy, which was associated with less physiologic derangement after severe injury.[16] Although some studies have reported improved outcomes with this approach, others have questioned the validity of these findings when applied to civilian patient populations. Nevertheless, many trauma centers have implemented this approach. Prospective trials are greatly needed to definitively evaluate this practice.

## Injuries to the Brain

Traumatic brain injuries (TBIs) remain one of the greatest causes of death and disability despite significant improvements in the care of these injuries over the last several decades. Injuries to the brain are common with a substantial percentage resulting in death or permanent disability. Commonly, the outcome of a patient with multiple injuries is dictated by the impact of the brain injury. According to data from the CDC, 1.4 million brain injuries are sustained each year, with 1.1 million evaluated in U.S. emergency departments.[17] Falls are the most common cause of brain injuries, with those at the extremes of age being the most vulnerable to this mechanism. The mortality rate for the 235,000 patients with TBI that require hospitalization is 21.3% and the number of people experiencing permanent TBI-related disability exceeds 80,000 each year.

### Mechanism and Pathophysiology

Injuries to the brain result from direct transmission of energy to the cranium and the underlying brain tissue, as well as damage resulting from movement of the brain within the rigid cranial vault. Compression of brain tissue can also result from tearing of intracranial blood vessels, which causes accumulation of blood. Secondary brain injury can occur following the initial insult and results from ischemia and compression by adjacent tissue edema. Because of the rigidity of the bony cranium, the volume within the skull remains constant. The Monro-Kellie doctrine states that any increase in the volume of intracranial contents results in an elevation of intracranial pressure with an associated decrease in the volume of other tissues, such as the brain parenchyma and cerebrospinal fluid. Figure 18-6 depicts the relationship between intracranial volume and pressure, which explains why injury resulting in increased intracranial blood and edema can have such a detrimental effect on the surrounding brain tissue. Epidural hematomas (Fig. 18-7) typically result from a lateral fracture of the cranium causing bleeding from the middle meningeal artery or a nearby vessel. The classic clinical course includes a brief loss of consciousness followed by a lucid interval, during which time the hematoma is expanding. Ultimately, symptoms again develop and can be profound without intervention. When identified and treated early, patients with epidural hematomas can have favorable outcomes because the hematoma itself is usually not associated with underlying brain parenchymal injury. This is in distinction to subdural hematomas, which commonly are associated with severe underlying brain tissue injury (Fig. 18-8). Subdural hematomas are believed to result from tearing of the bridging veins between the dura and cerebral cortex. The hematoma can be compressive but it is frequently the underlying brain contusion and axonal injury that dictate the outcome after these injuries. Subarachnoid hemorrhage after TBI is common and in itself has little deleterious effect. The presence of blood in the subarachnoid space likely is a reflection of the presence of a TBI, which should prompt surveillance. Parenchymal contusions of brain tissue result from a direct blow to the cranium or from movement of the brain within the rigid cranial vault, resulting in injury on the opposite side, also described as a contra-coup injury. Typically, the blood and hematoma associated with these contusions are not overly

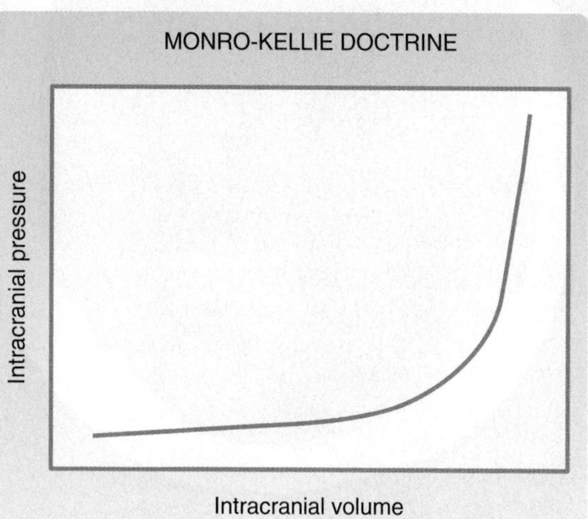


**FIGURE 18-6** The Monro-Kellie doctrine describes the increase in intracranial pressure as intracranial volume increase secondary to hemorrhage or edema. This relationship of pressure to volume is a result of the rigid cranial vault, which exhibits a fixed volume.

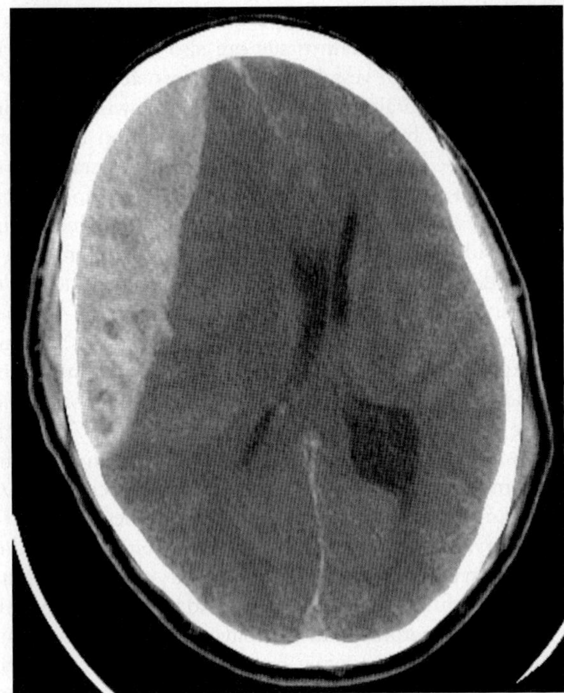

**FIGURE 18-7** Cranial CT scan demonstrating an epidural hematoma. Blood appears as high-density fluid *(white)* identified in the right parietal region. Note the associated midline shift.

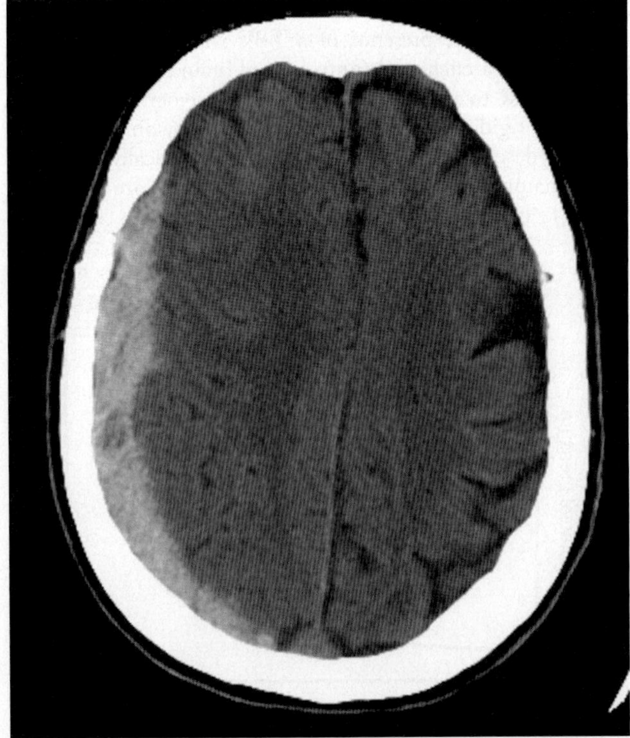

**FIGURE 18-8** Cranial CT scan demonstrating a subdural hematoma. Blood appears as high-density fluid *(white)* identified in the right posterior parietal region. Note how the blood follows the contour of the underlying brain.

large but the edema that develops over the subsequent days can be profound and a major source of secondary brain injury. Finally, diffuse axonal injury describes the phenomenon of disruption of the axon from the neuronal body secondary to severe rotational forces that are believed to create a shearing effect. Frequently, the magnitude of this type of injury cannot be appreciated on imaging and the ultimate severity is determined clinically during the weeks that follow. Diffuse axonal injury may be suggested on imaging by the presence of scattered punctuate hemorrhages within the parenchyma and, at times, a loss of the differentiation of gray and white mater.

### Immediate Management

Prevention of secondary brain injury is of highest priority as soon as a patient with a TBI is encountered. Given our current capabilities, little can be done to reverse the effects of the primary brain-injuring process, but intervention can be provided to prevent secondary insult. At the most basic level, this includes ensuring that the injured brain receives adequate blood flow to supply necessary quantities of oxygen. Therefore, emphasis must be placed on maintaining the ABCs throughout all prehospital and hospital phases of care. This includes early recognition of severe TBI, with immediate establishment of an acceptable airway and initiation of physiologic ventilatory support. Hemorrhage control and resuscitation should be initiated to prevent hypoperfusion, which can be highly detrimental to the injured brain. Determination of the GCS can be valuable to compare the patient's neurologic condition throughout the continuum of care. Patients known to be on antithrombotic therapy urgently need reversal of the anticoagulant effects, which may worsen intracranial hemorrhage. Because of the time-dependent nature of certain intracranial injuries, decreasing the time from injury to the operating room can be lifesaving for some patients. Therefore, hospitals without neurosurgical support should quickly assess whether they have the capability to care for a patient with a presumed TBI and then make the appropriate transfer arrangements. This should be a high priority and should not be delayed to obtain studies that will have no immediate impact on the care of the patient.

### Evaluation

The evaluation of TBI begins during the primary survey, when a brief assessment of neurologic function is completed. Typically, this includes determination of the GCS, with emphasis on elucidating the best motor function, because this can be most predictive of neurologic function. The inability to follow commands is a valuable indicator of a severe brain injury. An assessment of the character of the pupils is also included because this can be indicative of progressive compression within the cranium that is impinging on the cranial nerves. If possible, a neurological examination should be performed before it is obscured by sedating or paralyzing agents such as those used for intubation.

Although the management of airway compromise and shock are of highest priority, patients with a TBI benefit from early imaging of the cranium after stabilization. Computed tomography (CT) of the head without IV contrast is the most important diagnostic study during the initial evaluation of TBI because it provides a highly sensitive determination of acute intracranial pathology. When reviewing a CT scan of the head, acute blood appears as high-density fluid that can be further characterized by location within the cranium. Intraparenchymal contusion as well as edema with mass effect can also be identified by cranial CT. Because the presence of certain hematomas on CT scans may prompt emergent craniotomy, it is important to expedite imaging as soon as stability is ensured in all patients with a suspected TBI. Imaging of the cranium with magnetic resonance imaging (MRI) may be able to provide better anatomic detail, especially in the setting of ischemia, but has no role in the initial evaluation of the brain injured patient.

### Management

Early cranial CT will identify patients who might benefit from operative intervention. Neurosurgical consultation should be obtained early to allow for rapid transfer to the operating room when necessary. Findings on cranial CT that may benefit from urgent surgery include epidural and subdural hematomas, especially in the setting of an associated mass effect. Severely depressed skull fractures may also benefit from early operation to manage hemorrhage and elevate the depressed bone. Epidural and subdural hematomas are managed with craniotomy, followed by evacuation of hematoma and cessation of intracranial bleeding. Because of the underlying parenchymal injury, significant edema can often develop after hematoma evacuation, especially in the setting of a subdural hematoma. Following surgery, patients will frequently require ongoing surveillance of neurologic function and management of intracranial hypertension. Occasionally, patients with intracranial hypertension refractory to all nonoperative interventions are considered for decompressive craniectomy, which includes removal of a portion of the cranium and may include parenchymal resection in severe cases.

Most patients with intracranial hemorrhage require close monitoring of neurologic function and vital signs, which is usually best performed in a higher level of care setting, such as the intensive care unit. Guidelines published by the Brain Trauma Foundation provide an excellent assessment of the literature and represent the most comprehensive, evidence-based recommendations available.[18] Secondary brain injury should be prevented by ensuring adequate cardiovascular and pulmonary function. Many patients with severe TBI require measurement of the intracranial pressure (ICP) to guide management, which is aimed at reducing associated brain tissue edema. Cerebral perfusion pressure (CPP), which is the difference between the mean arterial pressure and the ICP, is also commonly used to guide severe TBI management. Although many physicians preferentially use ICP or CPP to direct management, it has been determined that neither one is superior to the other. It has been recognized that the overaggressive treatment of CPP may be deleterious. Figure 18-9 demonstrates an approach to the management of the patient with a severe TBI.

To manage elevations in ICP, several interventions have been suggested. Placement of a ventriculostomy allows both the measurement of ICP and the drainage of cerebrospinal fluid, which may assist with intracranial hypertension. Head of bed elevation is a simple technique that can provide gravity-assisted reduction in ICP but requires sufficient stability of the thoracolumbar spine. Ventilated patients benefit from mild hyperventilation, with the goal being maintenance of the $P_{CO_2}$ between 30 and 35 mm Hg because the use of more profound hyperventilation has been found to be deleterious. Hypoventilation must be avoided. Sedation aimed at reducing ICP is a valuable tool, although the depth of suppression should be kept at a minimum to ensure a productive neurologic examination. Hyperosmolar therapy with mannitol or, more recently, hypertonic saline that functions by reducing brain tissue edema is frequently useful. Administration of these agents requires monitoring of serum osmolarity to prevent severe electrolyte derangement. Occasionally, paralysis and barbiturate coma induction are implemented but should be used only in cases refractory to other interventions. Finally, it has been well established that corticosteroid administration has no role in the management of TBI.

## Injuries to the Spinal Cord and Vertebral Column

Spinal cord injuries (SCIs) have profound immediate and long-term effects on patients often resulting in years of disability. Except for high cervical spine injuries, mortality directly related to SCIs is low, although the associated morbidity is substantial and irreversible. Many patients sustaining SCIs are young and therefore experience many years of debilitation. In the NTDB, approximately 1% of blunt and penetrating trauma patients sustained a SCI, with an associated mortality of 13.3% and 15.1%, respectively. Motor vehicle crashes (MVCs) remain the leading cause of SCIs whereas in penetrating injuries, gunshot wounds cause the vast majority. Vertebral column fractures without SCI are 10-fold more common than those that occur with a SCI. Again, most commonly caused by MVCs, vertebral column fractures are present in 11.8% of all blunt trauma patients in the NTDB and are associated with a mortality rate of 6.3%. Approximately one third of these fractures involve the cervical spine.

Injuries to the spinal cord can occur after blunt or penetrating mechanisms. Blunt trauma to the spine can result in cord injury through direct impingement or indirect manipulation. Fractures and dislocations can reduce the size of the spinal canal and cause direct tissue damage or secondary injury through ischemia, bleeding, or edema. The spinal cord can also sustain injury through mechanisms that distract or severely rotate the cord, causing neuronal damage. Penetrating mechanisms directly lacerate the spinal cord tissue or cause adjacent injury and indirect damage. Occasionally, injury to the spinal cord can occur without abnormality of the vertebral column identified on imaging. The phenomenon known as spinal cord injury without radiographic abnormality (SCIWORA) can be extremely frustrating because the lack of bony injury can result in missed opportunities to prevent neurologic injury. Fractures of the vertebral column can occur after almost any form of physical force. Common mechanisms include flexion and extension, especially in the cervical spine, as well as compressive forces that commonly affect the lumbar spine. A Chance fracture is a well-described pattern with transverse disruption through all vertebral elements that occurs most commonly during an MVC. During a high-speed frontal crash, an occupant wearing a seatbelt above the iliac crest experiences flexion and distraction of a lumbar vertebrae, resulting in this fracture pattern (Fig. 18-10).

### Immediate Management

Management of injuries involving the spine begins immediately on prehospital personnel arrival. Spinal immobilization with a rigid cervical collar and a long spine board should be performed immediately and should include manual assistance throughout all patient transfers. All blunt and select penetrating trauma patients are assumed to have an injury to the spine until a proper

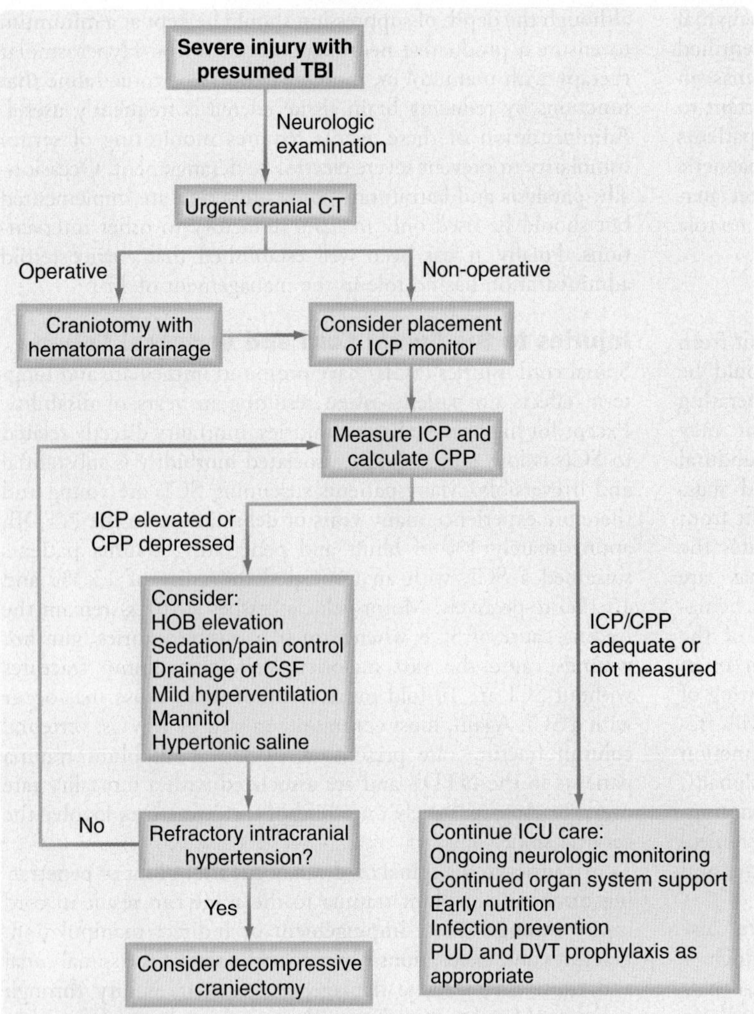


**FIGURE 18-9** Algorithm for the management of traumatic brain injury. *CSF,* Cerebrospinal fluid; *DVT,* deep venous thrombosis; *HOB,* head of bed; *PUD,* peptic ulcer disease.

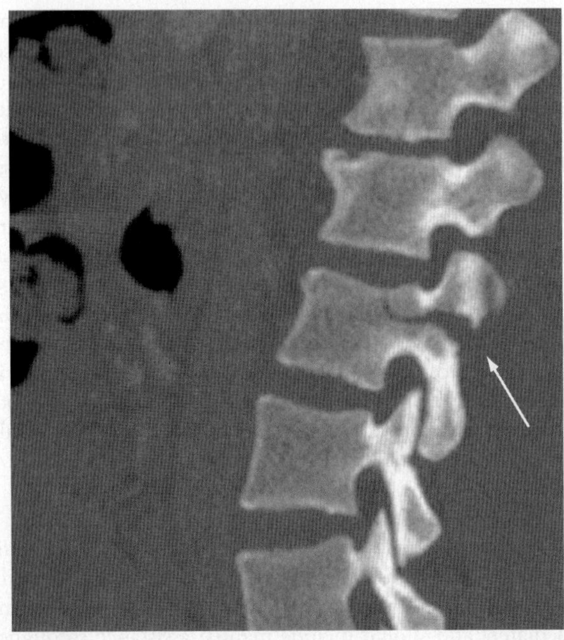

**FIGURE 18-10** Chance fracture on lumbar spine CT scan, sagittal view. Note the fracture involvement of all posterior elements *(arrow).*

evaluation can exclude the diagnosis. Management of the airway with support of ventilation may be required in the setting of high cervical spine injuries. Injuries to the spine superior to C5 may have varying degrees of respiratory depression because of paresis of the phrenic nerves. Patients with neurogenic shock caused by a loss of sympathetic tone require intravascular volume expansion and, at times, initiation of vasopressors early in the course of treatment. Typically, this is indicated by the presence of hypotension in a patient with warm, well-perfused extremities that also demonstrate decreased motor function. Finally, depending on spine surgeon preference, corticosteroid therapy may be initiated during the initial time period in the emergency department, although this practice remains extremely controversial.

## Evaluation

During the primary survey, an assessment of extremity movement can evaluate for a SCI grossly. A more comprehensive assessment should occur during the secondary survey, with a detailed determination of neurologic function obtained in those patients who demonstrate a deficit. The level of sensory loss should be determined, as well as the muscle groups that exhibit weakness or paralysis. This information may serve to assist in identifying the location of the injury but also to track progression of symptoms, which may affect therapeutic decisions. SCIs are deemed complete if all neurologic function below a specific cord level is absent or incomplete if there is motor or sensory function identified below this level. Spine surgeons' consultation should be done early so that they are actively involved in this evaluation. Examination may also reveal tenderness over the injured vertebrae or the presence of a deformity consistent with disruption of the vertebral column. Patients who have no findings on examination, demonstrate no decreased level of consciousness, and have no distracting injuries can undergo clearance of the spine by clinical means alone.

Further evaluation of the spine typically involves CT of the cervical, thoracic, and lumbar vertebral bodies. Although plain radiographs of the spine are acceptable, the high-quality images and rapid availability associated with CT have made this the modality of choice in most emergency departments. Visualization of the cervicothoracic junction on plain radiographs can be extremely challenging, especially in larger patients, and can often require numerous repeat studies. For this reason, many have transitioned to obtaining a dedicated cervical spine CT during the initial imaging of the patient. CT also provides the ability to reconstruct the images into sagittal and coronal planes to provide even better anatomic visualization. SCIs are less well delineated on CT than bony injuries but are suggested by the presence of spinal canal compromise and soft tissue edema identified adjacent to the spinal cord. Figure 18-11 demonstrates a severe cervical spine fracture with subluxation and anterior displacement.

The thoracic and lumbar vertebral columns are more conducive to imaging with plain radiography than the cervical spine. Identification of the alignment of the vertebral bodies as well as an assessment of the vertebral height are the main features evaluated on plain radiography. Many centers obtain CT scans

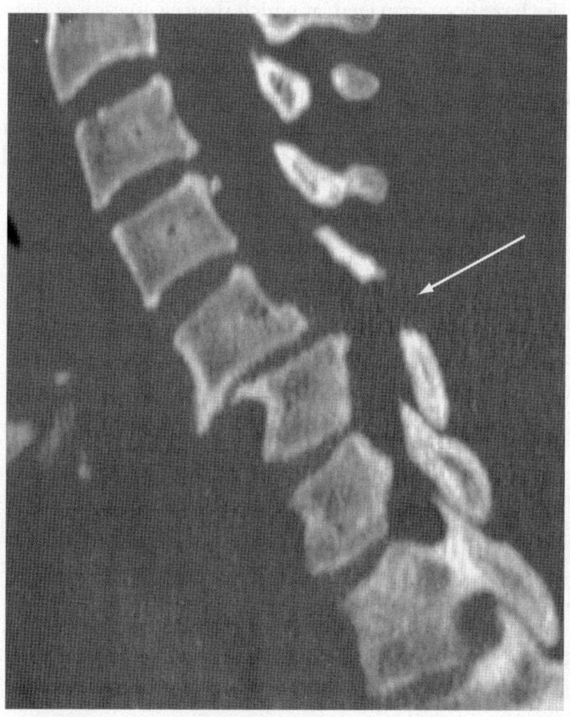

**FIGURE 18-11** Cervical spine fracture with severe anterior subluxation and compromise of the spinal canal. The *arrow* identifies the severe narrowing of the spinal canal.

of the chest, abdomen, and pelvis during the radiographic evaluation for truncal injuries. These images can be reformatted to focus on the thoracic and lumbar spines in the sagittal and coronal planes. The anatomic detail provided by these images is excellent and has been shown to be more sensitive for bony injury than plain radiographs. Because these studies require no further imaging and provide superior visualization, many centers have now abandoned plain radiographs in exchange for reformatted thoracic and lumbar spine CT scans. The presence of a significant injury identified on reformatted imaging may require a dedicated study to formulate an operative plan better. Although CT is the study of choice for evaluating the bony structures, assessment of the spinal cord frequently requires MRI to visualize injured soft tissue better. Obtaining these images, especially in the acute setting, must be carefully considered with respect to the patient's overall level of stability.

#### Management

As noted, the spine requires protection with strict immobilization throughout the entire evaluation until injuries can be ruled out. Typically, this includes the use of a hard collar and maintenance of the log roll technique when movement is required. Although a long spine board is generally used during the transport of patients in an ambulance, it is important to remove it as soon as possible to prevent the development of pressure wounds, which can develop quickly when a patient is lying on a rigid device. On recognizing the presence of a SCI, a spine surgeon consultation should be obtained promptly. In facilities that have no spine surgery services available, arrangements for transfer should begin immediately. Further studies and interventions should only occur if the results will have an immediate impact on the care provided. For example, imaging to identify an associated vertebral column fracture will have no effect on care if a spine surgeon is not available and therefore transfer should not be delayed. SCIs with neurogenic shock, occurring most commonly with cervical injuries, require resuscitation because of a loss of sympathetic tone. Neurogenic shock frequently responds to volume expansion with crystalloid solution but occasionally requires vasopressor agents such as dopamine or epinephrine. Hypotension should be avoided because it may contribute to cord ischemia and progression of the SCI. The value of corticosteroid administration has been extensively studied but remains controversial. Several large randomized trials have demonstrated small improvements in recovery after methylprednisolone administration, especially when initiated early after injury.[19] Others investigators have been unable to reproduce these results and have found an increased incidence of steroid-related complications with methylprednisolone therapy. Therefore, most authors agree that steroids remain an option that should be considered after consultation with the spine surgeon. When administered, methylprednisolone is provided as a bolus of 30 mg/kg body weight followed by an infusion of 5.4 mg/kg/hr for 23 hours if the bolus was given within 3 hours of injury. The infusion duration is extended to 48 hours if the bolus was administered between 3 and 8 hours after injury whereas SCIs that occurred more than 8 hours prior should not be treated.

Cervical fracture-dislocation injuries may benefit from the application of traction in the emergency department to restore vertebral column alignment. Based on the injury pattern and associated injuries, some SCIs benefit from early operative decompression to reduce cord impingement, as determined by the spine surgeon. Other injuries may require fixation because of instability on a semielective basis after immediate patient care needs are addressed. Fractures without instability may require only immobilization with a hard collar or brace over a several-week time period. Table 18-4 lists commonly encountered vertebral column fractures with management options. It is important that any patient with an SCI or significant vertebral column injury be monitored closely for changes in neurologic examination that might prompt urgent intervention.

## Injury to the Maxillofacial Region

Facial injuries are common but rarely life-threatening. The main concern during the initial evaluation and management of facial trauma is airway maintenance and bleeding. Injuries to the face were identified in 24.8% of NTDB cases, with an associated mortality of 4.7%. It is likely that a significant majority of these deaths were caused by associated TBIs because their simultaneous presence is high. Facial injuries can result from direct impact during a blunt mechanism, such as an MVA or fall. Fractures of the facial bones and soft tissue injuries predominate. Lefort fractures represent a specific pattern of facial bone injuries that consist of three variations of midface disruption from the surrounding facial bones. Despite their frequent description, Lefort fractures are uncommonly identified. Penetrating mechanisms such as gunshot and knife-related wounds are not uncommon and can result in large soft tissue injuries, especially with the passage of a bullet through the face. Injuries to the face can also result in disruption of sensory function when associated with eye, nose, ear, or mouth involvement.

### Immediate Management

Establishment of a secure airway is the greatest concern with facial injuries, especially those with severe lower face soft tissue and bony involvement. Early intubation prior to the development of significant edema may be lifesaving. Securing the airway may be complicated by distortion of the anatomy and by presence of blood and debris in the mouth and posterior pharynx. The application of multiple airway options, including a surgical approach, may be necessary. Control of bleeding is also of great importance given the extensive vascularity of the face. Bleeding can be from soft tissue or exposed bone edges and should be initially treated with direct pressure and resuscitation. Suture ligation of identified bleeding vessels or rapid closure of wounds with suture or staples can be highly effective. Frequently, bleeding from the face is exacerbated by hypothermia and coagulopathy, which should be aggressively prevented or treated.

### Evaluation

Most facial injuries are evident on physical examination. Soft tissue injuries can be characterized and the involvement of facial organs assessed. The eyes should be examined for changes in visual acuity and the presence of diplopia. The condition of the globe and the surrounding orbit requires careful evaluation for rupture or extraocular muscle entrapment, which would require urgent treatment. Injury to the external ears and nose are also identified on physical examination. The stability of the midface and jaw should be assessed, as well as the condition and proper occlusion of the dentition and alveolar ridge. Deformities of the forehead and cheeks indicate underlying frontal bone and maxillary fractures, respectively. If possible, function of the facial nerve should be assessed by testing the motor groups of the face.

CT performed with thin cuts provides excellent visualization of the facial bones and is the most common modality used in the evaluation of the face. Sagittal and coronal, as well as three-dimensional reconstructions, can aid in the thorough assessment of the bones and deep soft tissue. Severe external injury to the face should prompt obtaining a facial CT scan. Patients who undergo head CT can have the facial bones assessed for obvious fracture or fluid within the sinuses, which should suggest the need for facial CT. Critically injured patients might have facial injury suggested by physical examination after severe injuries have been managed, at which time evaluation with facial CT can be performed.

### Management

Severe soft tissue injuries and fractures to the face frequently benefit from the assistance of maxillofacial surgery specialists

**Table 18-4 Fractures of the Vertebral Column**

| FRACTURE | DESCRIPTION | TYPICAL MANAGEMENT |
|---|---|---|
| C1 Jefferson fracture | Disruption of C1 ring in multiple locations; blow-out of ring | Stable transverse ligament: Hard collar<br>Unstable transverse ligament: Traction or surgery |
| Odontoid fractures | Type I: Tip of odontoid<br>Type II: Through base<br>Type III: Involves C2 body | Type I: Hard collar<br>Type II: Halo vest or surgery<br>Type III: Halo vest |
| C2 hangman fracture | Bilateral C2 pedicles with spondylolisthesis | Halo vest or surgery if displacement severe |
| Cervical vertebral body fractures | Compression or burst of vertebral body, with or without retropulsion into canal | Mild loss of height: Hard collar<br>Involvement of multiple columns or presence of retropulsion into canal: Surgical stabilization |
| Thoracic vertebral body fractures | Compression or burst of vertebral body, with or without retropulsion into canal | Anterior column only: TLSO<br>Anterior and posterior columns: Surgical stabilization |
| Lumbar vertebral body fractures | Compression or burst of vertebral body, with or without retropulsion into canal | Anterior column only: TLSO<br>Anterior and posterior columns: Surgical stabilization |
| Chance fracture | Avulsion of posterior elements of lumbar vertebrae seen with high seatbelt use | Surgical stabilization |

*TLSO,* Thoracolumbosacral orthosis.

to assist in management. As noted, airway management and bleeding are the greatest priority. Bleeding frequently responds to direct pressure or suture closure of the wound although, in severe cases, angiography with embolization of bleeding facial blood vessels may be necessary. Lacerations can frequently be closed with local anesthesia using deep absorbable sutures followed by closure of the epidermis with 5-0 or 6-0 interrupted or running sutures. Prior to closure, wounds should be débrided to remove all jagged or nonviable skin edges, as well as irrigated with sterile fluid. Closure of lacerations to the lip, nose, ear, and orbit require special consideration to facilitate optimal wound healing.

Management of facial fractures is almost never required acutely. Severely depressed facial bone fractures are the exception because these may involve the underlying brain and require urgent reduction. Large facial wounds may necessitate multiple washouts but the formal reconstruction is still usually delayed. Most maxillofacial fractures are intentionally repaired in a delayed fashion to allow reduction in the associated edema that almost uniformly develops. Large open wounds and fractures involving sinuses or the aerodigestive tract require antibiotics shortly after admission but overextending this course should be avoided. Most fractures benefit from open reduction and internal fixation, typically using screws and plates. The goal of reconstruction is to restore optimal functional and cosmetic results. Orbital fractures with rectus muscle injuries require reconstruction to preserve normal ocular movements. Mandibular fractures are commonly encountered and can be characterized by the anatomic location of the fracture. Minimally displaced fractures can be treated with maxillary-mandibular fixation using wires or bars whereas plating may be necessary for fractures with significant displacement.

## Injuries to the Neck

The neck can be one of the more overwhelming regions when confronted with severe injury, likely because of the presence of multiple vital structures in close proximity to one another. Nevertheless, as with other areas of the body, addressing neck injuries can be manageable by implementing an organized approach. Although only 1% of all injuries in the NTDB involve the neck, the associated mortality rate is the highest of all regions, reaching 9.7%. Penetrating mechanisms are the most common ,with gunshot and stab wounds accounting for most neck injuries. Penetrating injuries can result in direct laceration of vascular and aerodigestive structures, resulting in substantial bleeding or contamination, respectively. Blunt injuries to the neck can cause compression, with fracture of the larynx or trachea. Blunt pharyngeal or esophageal injuries are extremely rare but can result in leakage into the surrounding soft tissue with sepsis if not adequately addressed. Blunt cerebrovascular injuries (BCVIs) involving the carotid arteries commonly result from compression by a seatbelt; the vertebral arteries are vulnerable to severe flexion and extension mechanisms. Injury severity ranges from intimal tears, with or without thrombosis, to full-thickness injury with pseudoaneurysm formation. One of the greatest concerns after BCVIs is stroke secondary to thromboembolism developing from the disrupted vessel wall.

### Immediate Management

Much of the trepidation related to neck injuries is the urgency commonly related to the initial management. Of greatest primary concern is establishment of a secure airway, especially given the rapidity with which deterioration can occur in the setting of a neck injury. Airway compromise can occur secondary to direct injury to the larynx or trachea, as well as blood or debris within the upper airway. Expanding neck hematomas can quickly compress the upper airway, leading to cessation of adequate ventilation. The presence of an expanding neck hematoma mandates immediate intubation by experienced personnel before complete airway obstruction occurs. Great care should be taken in managing the airway in the setting of a suspected laryngotracheal injury. Patients who are maintaining their own airway should undergo planning that might include intubation or awake tracheostomy in the operating room. Attempted intubation could worsen a tenuous situation and should not be performed without a backup plan, unless in an emergent situation. The surgical airway of choice for an upper airway injury is a tracheostomy because injury to the larynx could make cricothyroidotomy ineffective.

Hemorrhage is the other major concern in the immediate period after neck injuries. Most bleeding can be controlled with direct pressure, at least during transport to the operating room and initiation of neck exploration. Hemorrhage through a penetrating wound should be immediately treated with digital pressure in the wound until operative exposure can be achieved. Resuscitation with blood products should be initiated in the setting of substantial bleeding from the neck because large quantities of blood can be lost quickly. It is of great importance that patients suspected of having a vascular injury be rapidly transferred to the operating room for surgical management of ongoing bleeding.

### Evaluation

Unstable patients should be taken immediately to the operating room and will therefore undergo the entire evaluation of the neck under direct visualization. Those who are stable on initial evaluation require further assessment for suspected injuries. In the setting of penetrating trauma, evaluation and management of the neck have typically depended on the anatomic location of the injury. For descriptive purposes, the neck can be divided into three zones (Fig. 18-12). Zone I extends from the thoracic inlet to the cricoid cartilage and contains large vascular structures, as well as the trachea and esophagus. Zone II is bordered inferiorly by the cricoid cartilage and superiorly by the angle of the mandible. Zone II is the most accessible surgically and contains the carotid and vertebral arteries, jugular veins, and structures of the aerodigestive tract. Zone III includes the neck between the angle of the mandible and the base of the skull. This zone includes vascular structures that are difficult to expose surgically. Traditionally, injuries to zone II mandated operative exploration whereas zones I and III were evaluated with diagnostic studies to determine the presence of injury. It has since been recognized that only patients with evidence of active bleeding or an obvious aerodigestive injury require mandatory neck exploration. Others, regardless of anatomic location, can be evaluated with diagnostic studies.[20]

In patients undergoing evaluation of penetrating neck trauma, an assessment of the vasculature is required. Frequently, this can be achieved with CT angiography, which can delineate the vascular anatomy of the neck with great accuracy. CT angiography can be performed quickly in the emergency department and is effective at revealing vascular injuries to the neck.

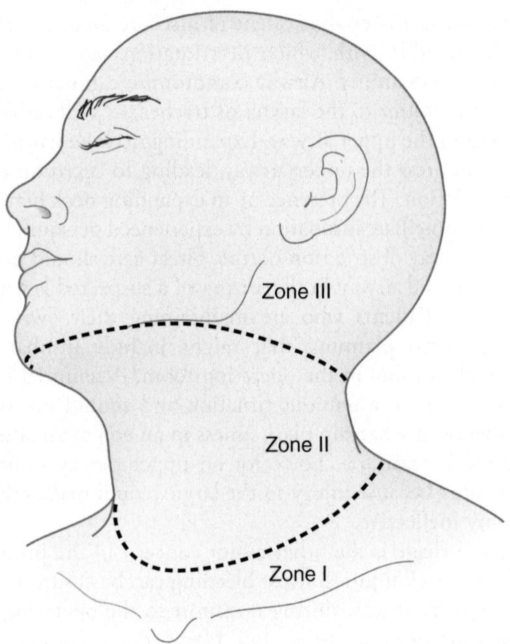


**FIGURE 18-12** Zones of the neck. Zone 1 extends from the thoracic inlet to the cricoid cartilage. Zone 2 is between the cricoid cartilage and the angle of the mandible. Zone 3 extends from the angle of the mandible to the skull base.

Furthermore, the tract of the penetrating object can frequently be identified on advanced-generation scanners, which often allows selective evaluation of other structures of the neck. CT angiography can be limited by the presence of metallic missile debris, which results in image scatter. In this situation, or when further evaluation is required, standard digital subtraction angiography can be valuable. Duplex ultrasonography is also an option for evaluation of the carotid and vertebral arteries after penetrating neck trauma.

Evaluation for BCVIs has evolved substantially over the last decade. Although initially thought to be extremely rare, the emergence of high-risk screening criteria and improved imaging technology has led to a significant increase in the diagnosis of BCVIs. In 1999, Biffl and coworkers published a set of criteria that accurately identified a group of patients at high risk for BCVIs.[21] Digital subtraction angiography of the carotid and vertebral arteries was then more readily applied to these high-risk patients, resulting in the identification of BCVIs in over 30% of this cohort. This work led to the establishment of the Denver criteria, which suggests which patients require evaluation for BCVIs. Box 18-4 lists the findings most commonly used to prompt further evaluation.[21] Although originally these injuries were all identified using standard angiography, recent advances in CT angiography have changed how many of these injuries are diagnosed. It appears that the skill of the radiologist is of great importance, but CT angiography has demonstrated a sensitivity and specificity comparable to that of standard angiography.[22] Other studies have questioned the usefulness of CT angiography in this setting, citing a significantly worse ability to detect these injuries. Nevertheless, with the improved logistics of obtaining a CT scan and the more favorable associated risk profile, most centers now rely heavily on CT imaging for BCVI evaluation.

**BOX 18-4 Indicators of High Risk for Blunt Cerebrovascular Injury**

**Signs and Symptoms**

Expanding neck hematoma
Arterial hemorrhage from neck, nose, mouth
Focal neurologic deficit
Cervical bruit (patient age <50 yr)
Stroke on CT or MRI
Neurologic deficit unexplained by CT findings

**Risk Factors**

Severe midface fracture, Lefort II or III
Basilar skull fracture involving the carotid canal
Diffuse axonal injury and GCS ≤6
Significant cervical spine fracture or ligamentous injury
Significant soft tissue injury to anterior neck (e.g., seatbelt mark)
Near-hanging with anoxia

Neck injuries also require an assessment of the aerodigestive tract. This can be achieved by performing bronchoscopy to assess the trachea. Evaluation of the larynx can be challenging and is best accomplished with laryngoscopy. Finally, the esophagus requires evaluation, which is best done by performing contrast esophagraphy and esophagoscopy. Separately, these two studies may miss up to 20% of esophageal injuries, but together almost all injuries will be identified. At times, more severe injuries cannot safely be evaluated with a contrast study and therefore require a thorough endoscopic evaluation. Frequently, information obtained from the neck CT scan will allow the clinician to perform these diagnostic studies selectively when the involvement of a given structure has clearly been avoided.

### Management

Shock, active bleeding, expanding neck hematoma, and/or obvious aerodigestive injuries require immediate neck exploration. Neck exploration is most commonly performed using an incision along the anterior border of the sternocleidomastoid muscle on the side of the injury. Occasionally, a collar incision is more versatile, especially if both sides of the neck need exploration. The platysma is divided and the anterior border of the sternocleidomastoid muscle is identified and dissected from the underlying tissue. The internal jugular vein is next identified and exposed. The internal jugular vein is commonly injured and requires direct repair or ligation if closure is not possible. Along the anterior border of the internal jugular vein, the facial vein is identified and exposed. Ligation of the facial vein will allow the deep structures of the neck to be approached. With the internal jugular vein retracted laterally, the carotid sheath is exposed. If necessary, proximal and distal carotid control are obtained and the artery is exposed. Care should be taken to avoid injuring the adjacent vagus nerve and the hypoglossal nerve, which crosses the internal carotid artery superiorly. Injuries to the carotid artery require repair with simple closure or end-to-end anastomosis. Frequently, reconstruction of the carotid artery with a synthetic graft or autologous vein is necessary. In damage control situations, the carotid artery can be ligated if no other options exist.

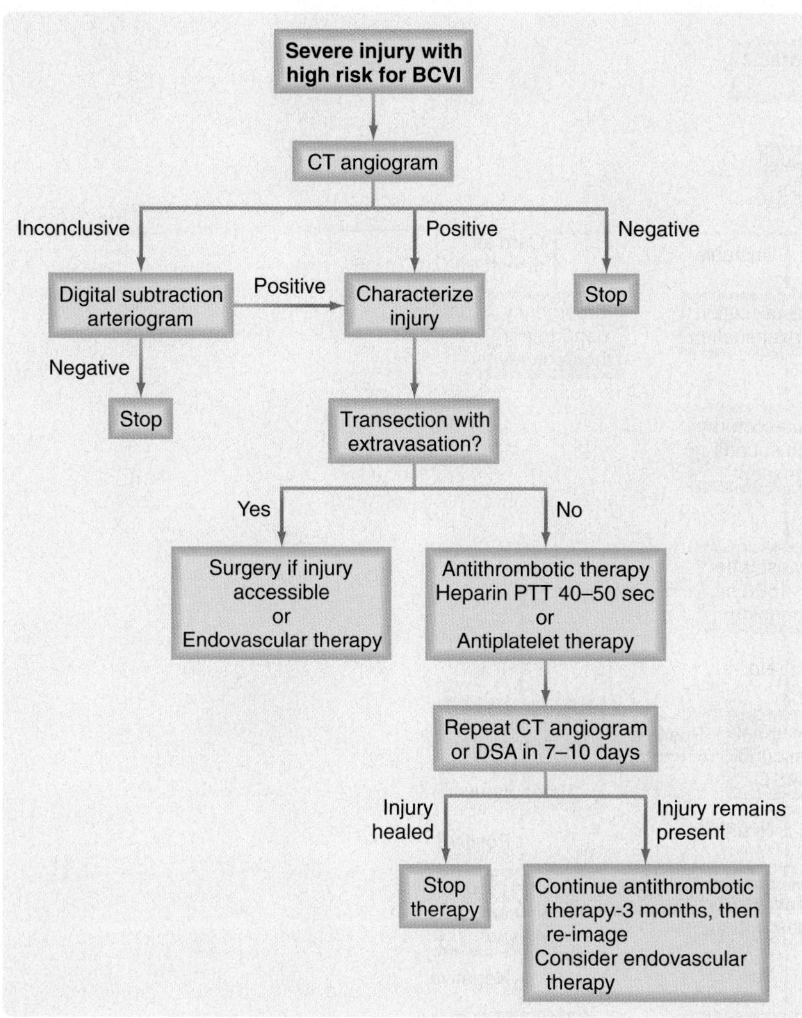


**FIGURE 18-13** Algorithm for the management of blunt cerebrovascular injury. *DSA,* Digital subtraction angiography. (Adapted from Biffl WL, Cothren CC, Moore EE, et al: Western Trauma Association critical decisions in trauma: Screening for and treatment of blunt cerebrovascular injuries. J Trauma 67:1150–1153, 2009.)

To explore the trachea or esophagus, the carotid artery is retracted laterally and dissection is continued medially. This exploration may be greatly aided by the placement of a nasogastric tube to allow palpation of the esophagus. Injuries to the esophagus should be débrided to expose the entirety of the perforation. Closure can be with one or two layers and meticulous drainage is important. Covering the esophageal repair with viable muscle may be highly beneficial, especially in the setting of adjacent tracheal or vascular repair. In the setting of massive tissue loss or delayed presentation, esophageal diversion with the creation of an esophagostomy may be necessary. Simple tracheal lacerations can be primarily closed with absorbable suture if the injury is small and will approximate in a tension-free fashion. Larger defects require resection and reanastomosis although some anterior tracheal injuries are amenable to tracheostomy creation through the injury. After maturation of the tracheostomy tract, the tube can be removed and closure usually occurs spontaneously.

The treatment of BCVIs has evolved significantly over the last decade. Following the increased recognition of these injuries, it was determined that anticoagulation and antiplatelet therapy substantially reduced the risk of stroke. Typically, patients who are identified as high risk undergo CT angiography or digital subtraction angiography shortly after admission to evaluate for a BCVI. Many patients have a contraindication to immediate anticoagulation and antiplatelet therapy but treatment should be initiated as soon as safely possible, because a significant percentage of strokes occur days to weeks after injury. An approach to the diagnosis and management of BCVIs was recently published by the Western Trauma Association (Fig. 18-13).[23] The suggested treatment includes initiation of anticoagulation, with heparin aimed at achieving a partial thromboplastin time between 40 and 50 seconds. Antiplatelet therapy is another option for those who cannot receive full anticoagulation. After 7 days, a repeat CT angiogram can be obtained and those patients who demonstrate complete healing no longer require therapy. Others require ongoing treatment for 3 months, followed by reevaluation. The presence of a pseudoaneurysm may benefit from endovascular management with stent placement or embolization for vertebral artery injuries.

## Injuries to the Chest

Thoracic injuries are common, with up to one of five patients presenting with trauma involving the chest. Given that the chest contains the most vital cardiopulmonary structures, these injuries have the potential of being severe. In the NTDB, chest injuries are present in 13.8% of all blunt and 12.2% of all penetrating trauma patients, associated with an overall mortality

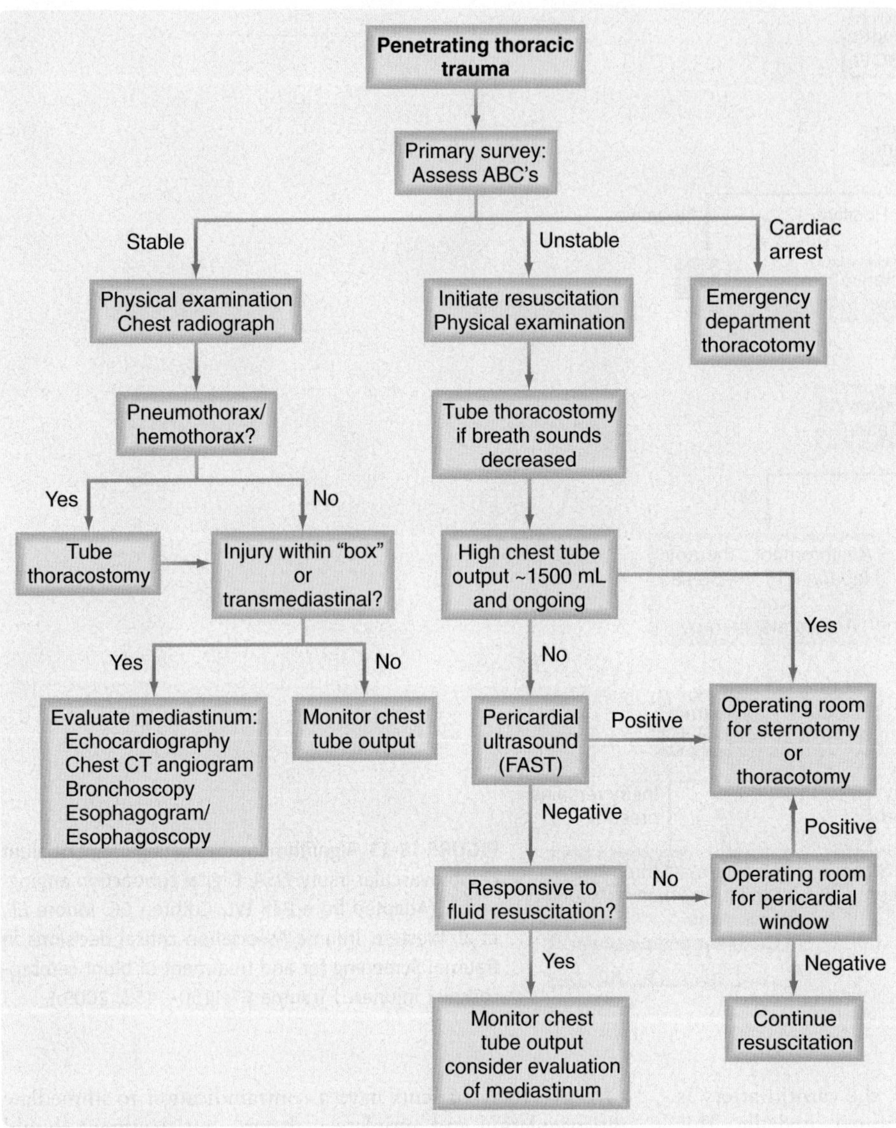


**FIGURE 18-14** Algorithm for the management of penetrating thoracic injuries.

rate of 8.4%.[24] Among patients sustaining blunt thoracic trauma, the mortality is significantly greater, ranging from 9.5% to 47.5%, depending on injury severity. Despite the seriousness of these injuries, most can be treated effectively by basic maneuvers that can be provided in the emergency department. MVAs are the most common cause of blunt thoracic injuries, followed by falls, with injury resulting from the transmission of energy to the chest wall and underlying structures. Direct compression, as well as deceleration and rotational physical mechanisms, contribute to the incidence of thoracic injury. The size and location of the chest make it vulnerable to penetrating mechanisms, such as gunshot and stab wounds. The lungs and mediastinal structures are susceptible to lacerations and perforations when exposed to penetrating trauma.

### Immediate Management

Many injuries to the thorax require immediate intervention during the primary survey to support cardiopulmonary function. As noted earlier, establishment of a secure airway and ventilatory assistance should occur immediately in patients with respiratory compromise. Poor compliance on ventilation with decreased breath sounds may indicate a tension pneumothorax, which requires urgent placement of a tube thoracostomy. External bleeding should be controlled with direct pressure while resuscitation with crystalloid solution and blood products is initiated. Hemodynamic instability may indicate a tension pneumothorax requiring decompression, hypovolemia requiring hemorrhage control and resuscitation, or cardiac dysfunction secondary to pericardial tamponade, cardiac contusion or myocardial infarction, or coronary air embolism. Evaluation for sources of bleeding should commence and an assessment for pericardial fluid with ultrasound or pericardial window be completed, especially in the setting of penetrating trauma. Based on these initial interventions, decisions regarding subsequent management such as immediate operation can be determined. Cardiac arrest, especially in the setting of penetrating mechanisms, requires resuscitative thoracotomy (see earlier). An approach to the initial evaluation and management of penetrating chest injuries is presented in Figure 18-14.

### Evaluation

Most thoracic injuries can be identified with a physical examination and plain chest radiography. Physical examination will reveal superficial injuries, including chest wall defects and penetrating wounds. Overall respiratory effort and chest wall movement can be visualized to reflect injuries to the ribs and sternum. Deviation of the trachea at the sternal notch may reveal intrathoracic tension on the side opposite the trachea. Distended neck veins indicate cardiac failure, which requires further evaluation. Chest radiography is performed on all significantly injured patients at risk for thoracic injuries. This study can be obtained rapidly in the trauma bay, with the results quickly revealed. The chest radiograph easily identifies the presence of a pneumothorax or hemothorax, as well as rib and sternal fractures. The appearance of the mediastinum may suggest a thoracic aortic injury. An ultrasound of the pericardium is a component of the FAST examination, which may reveal pericardial blood. In recent years, thoracic CT angiography has emerged as a valuable tool in the evaluation of blunt thoracic trauma. CT provides visualization of the chest wall and hemithoraces, allowing determination of rib fractures, pneumothoraces and hemothoraces, and pulmonary contusion. Of great value has been the ability to evaluate the thoracic aorta for injury that historically required standard angiography when suggested by a chest radiograph. Chest CT angiography is able to identify transection of the aortic wall, as well as lower grade injuries that involve only the aortic intima. Many thoracic surgeons have even evolved their technique and proceed with operative intervention based on the chest CT alone, without formal angiography. Some injuries continue to require standard thoracic angiography to characterize anatomy better that is indeterminate on CT imaging.

Penetrating injuries to the chest that cross the mediastinum or are in the vicinity of the heart and mediastinal structures require a methodical evaluation. Penetrating wounds in an area defined by the sternal notch superiorly, the costal margin inferiorly, and the nipples laterally are in this group requiring further evaluation. This includes an assessment of the cardiovascular and aerodigestive structures of the mediastinum. Immediate ultrasound is performed to evaluate the pericardium for effusion. If the pericardium is communicating with one of the hemithoraces, ultrasound may yield false-negative results. Further evaluation has historically included an angiogram of the chest, which has now been replaced by CT angiography in most situations. The heart and great vessels are evaluated for injury, although this can be impeded by the presence of retained missile fragments that cause scatter on CT. Standard angiography can be valuable in this setting. Depending on the trajectory of the penetrating object, the trachea and proximal airways may require evaluation with bronchoscopy. If injury is suspected, the esophagus should be assessed with a combination of esophagoscopy and contrast esophagography. In isolation, these studies have an approximate 20% false-negative rate, although their combined sensitivity approaches 100%. Frequently, thoracic CT will accurately identify the trajectory of the wound and thus guide the need for further evaluation.

### Management

Up to 85% of all thoracic injuries can be managed with nothing more than a tube thoracostomy. In most cases, the placement of a chest tube is urgent but may still be performed in a controlled manner that includes strict sterile preparation and excellent surgical technique. This of great importance given the morbidity associated with an empyema that can result from improper chest tube placement. The chest should be prepared appropriately using more than just a splash of povidone-iodine (Betadine) as well as wide draping to maintain the sterility of the field and the tube to be placed. The skin incision should be at the level of the nipple to stay superior enough to avoid the highest reach of the diaphragm. A tunnel is created in a superior direction and the chest is entered bluntly in an interspace above the skin incision. The lung is palpated to confirm chest entry and evaluate for intrathoracic adhesions. A tube large enough to drain blood (typically 32 to 36 Fr) is then advanced superiorly through the incision and posterior to the lung. Chest tubes that are being placed only for a pneumothorax can be positioned in the anterior hemithorax. A valuable maneuver is to spin the tube to confirm that it is not kinked, which would result in poor drainage. The thoracostomy is then connected to an underwater drainage device providing 20 cm $H_2O$ suction.

Tube thoracostomies that drain large amounts of blood on initial placement or demonstrate ongoing output may indicate active intrathoracic bleeding that requires thoracotomy. Typically, immediate thoracotomy is indicated for more than 1500 mL of blood drained on chest tube insertion or more than 300 mL/hr for 3 hours. Although these values clearly may be associated with intrathoracic bleeding, the decision to operate should be carefully considered, especially with regard to the immediate output. Occasionally, chest tubes that initially drain 1500 mL but then have little ongoing output in the setting of hemodynamic stability indicate bleeding from a lung laceration, which ceases with lung reexpansion and may not require or benefit from thoracotomy. Other indications for immediate thoracotomy include a massive air leak with associated pneumothorax or drainage of esophageal or gastric contents from the chest tube. The choice of thoracic approach depends on the presumed injured structures. Access to the lungs, pulmonary vasculature, and hemidiaphragm is through a posterolateral thoracotomy that is best performed through the fifth interspace, with or without removal of the fifth rib. On the right, this incision also exposes the proximal and midesophagus, as well as the trachea and bilateral mainstem bronchi. A left thoracotomy is valuable for approaching the distal esophagus, the left lung, the left ventricle, the descending aorta, and the left subclavian artery. A median sternotomy can be a highly versatile approach, allowing exposure of the right heart, ascending aorta, aortic arch with right-sided arch vessels, and pulmonary vasculature.

**Chest Wall and Pleural Space Injuries** Fractures of the ribs are the most common thoracic injury following blunt trauma, with almost 80% of patients with chest injuries sustaining one or more fractures. The chest wall is also commonly involved during penetrating mechanisms, present in 25% of penetrating chest trauma cases. The mortality rate associated with chest wall injuries following blunt trauma is approximately 10%; it exceeds 20% for penetrating injuries. Rib fractures typically occur secondary to compression of the thoracic cage in an anteroposterior or lateral direction that often will dictate the location of the cortical disruption along the rib. Steering wheels and seatbelts are commonly identified as the impinging structure resulting in a fracture. In its most severe form, large amounts of energy transferred to the chest wall can result in the creation of a flail segment, defined as two or more adjacent ribs that are each

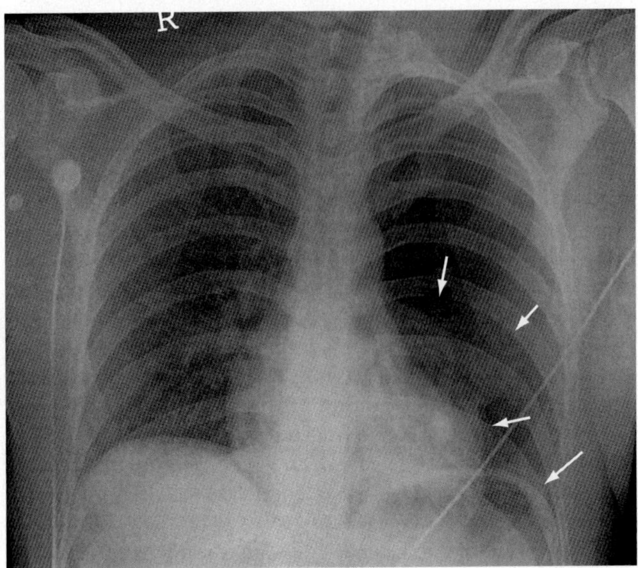


**FIGURE 18-15** Large left-sided pneumothorax on plain chest radiograph. *Arrows* identify the lateral border of the collapsed lung.

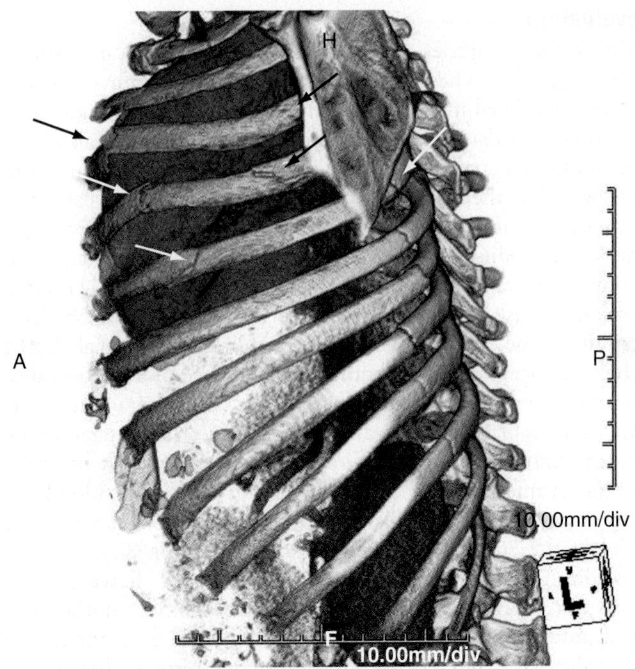


**FIGURE 18-16** Multiple rib fractures with flail segment on three-dimensional CT reconstruction. *Arrows* identify the multiple adjacent rib fractures. Note the underlying pulmonary contusion, which appears as a blue color.

fractured in two or more locations. This results in a separation of a segment of the chest wall. Although pulmonary mechanics can be disrupted in the setting of a flail segment, the greatest physiologic insult is caused by the underlying pulmonary contusion that almost invariably occurs. A pneumothorax occurs with compression of the chest that tears the surface of the lung through a blow-out type mechanism or via laceration from a fractured rib, causing the accumulation of air in the pleural space. Similarly, bleeding from the injured chest wall or lacerated lung can result in a hemothorax as blood accumulates in the pleural space.

During the primary or secondary survey, chest wall injuries are commonly recognized. Chest wall tenderness and changes in chest wall motion are suggestive. Some patients require immediate intervention for chest injuries, but most will subsequently undergo further evaluation. Injuries involving the chest wall or pleural space can frequently be identified on chest radiographs. Figure 18-15 demonstrates a large left pneumothorax on chest radiograph. Chest CT is a common part of the evaluation for thoracic injuries at many centers. CT identifies rib and sternal fractures, as well as pleural air and blood with a great degree of sensitivity. At times, a so-called occult pneumothorax that was not identified on a chest radiograph can be visualized by CT, especially when it only occupies the anterior hemithorax. Figure 18-16 demonstrates a flail segment on chest CT with three-dimensional reconstruction.

Pneumothorax or a large hemothorax on a chest radiograph requires placement of a tube thoracostomy. Chest tube drainage should continue until any pulmonary air leak has resolved and drainage is not excessive. Hemothoraces should be drained if it is thought that the quantity of blood in the pleural space could result in lung entrapment as the hematoma matures. Occasionally, hemothoraces that do not resolve after insertion of a tube thoracostomy benefit from thoracoscopic drainage and tube placement. Patients who demonstrate an occult pneumothorax by chest CT and have no respiratory compromise can be managed with observation and a repeat chest radiograph the following day. Enlargement of the pneumothorax on follow-up imaging necessitates a chest tube. Patients who demonstrate a large amount of subcutaneous air without significant pneumothorax should be followed closely, with a low threshold for placing a chest tube, because a pulmonary air leak may still be present.

Rib fractures can vary greatly in severity, depending on the number present and patient characteristics. Associated pain can be severe and a great concern is the development of respiratory infections. Aggressive analgesia should be provided to allow adequate pulmonary toilet and promote comfort. Adequate analgesia can be achieved with IV narcotics in mild cases but, in more severe cases, patients benefit greatly from the provision of epidural analgesia. Epidural analgesia after chest wall injuries has been associated with fewer ventilator days, shorter intensive care unit length of stay, and fewer hospital days. Furthermore, Bulger and coworkers[25] have demonstrated fewer pulmonary infections and decreased duration of mechanical ventilation with the use of epidural analgesia in patients with three or more rib fractures. Nonsteroidal anti-inflammatory drugs (NDAIDs) are also beneficial in conjunction with narcotics. Aggressive pulmonary toilet, including deep breathing, frequent coughing, and incentive spirometry, should be highly encouraged. Chest physical therapy and positive expiratory pressure exercises may also be beneficial. Severe chest wall injuries with pulmonary failure may require mechanical ventilation. There has been renewed interest in the operative fixation of rib fractures, although the optimal indications to perform these procedures and their associated benefit remains incompletely defined. Sternal fractures are managed similar to rib fractures requiring analgesia and pulmonary toilet. Occasionally, sternal fractures result in the development of a mediastinal hematoma. Although these typically do not require specific treatment, the presence of active bleeding from the adjacent internal mammary artery may require angioembolization or open ligation in the setting of hemodynamic instability.

**Pulmonary Injuries** The lungs are susceptible to injury during blunt and penetrating mechanisms. Although reported in up to 15% of cases in some series, pulmonary contusion after blunt trauma is present in 5.5% of patients in the NTDB. Among patients with blunt chest trauma, pulmonary contusion is common, being identified in 40% of cases. Mortality can be severe, ranging from 10% to 25%, and respiratory failure with the acute respiratory distress syndrome, as well as pneumonia, are frequently encountered. Pulmonary contusion results from energy transfer through the chest wall to the pulmonary parenchyma, resulting in tissue damage, as well as hemorrhage into the alveolar and interstitial spaces. The result is the development of physiologic shunt with hypoxemia. These injuries are also associated with a profound inflammatory response that can lead to further respiratory dysfunction and systemic inflammation. Frequently, pulmonary contusion is identified in the presence of a flail segment and is the major cause of associated morbidity and mortality. Penetrating mechanisms can result in lung contusions or laceration of the pulmonary parenchyma. In one larger multicenter series, 24% of patients with thoracic trauma sustained a penetrating mechanism, of which 2.8% required an urgent thoracotomy for management of pulmonary bleeding.[26]

Pulmonary injuries might first be identified on examination or through the drainage of large amounts of blood or air from a tube thoracostomy. Chest radiographs obtained shortly after patient arrival may demonstrate pneumothorax or hemothorax indicative of an underlying pulmonary injury. Lung contusions may be present on the initial chest radiograph but typically require time to become evident on plain film. Pulmonary contusions identified early on chest film are frequently severe and rapidly progressive to respiratory failure. A pulmonary contusion is easily identified by thoracic CT, although at times it can be challenging to differentiate contusion from atelectasis. A basic rule of thumb is that atelectasis does not cross pulmonary fissures, whereas contusions are not limited by ventilatory segments. Also, higher density pulmonary tissue in the vicinity of chest wall injuries, especially when not in dependent areas, is highly suggestive of pulmonary contusion. Figure 18-17 demonstrates a pulmonary contusion on a thoracic CT scan.

Chest tube drainage of large quantities of blood or air may require thoracotomy. The classic guidelines have been described earlier, and the surgeon must make a determination regarding the likelihood of ongoing bleeding that would benefit from operative management. In most cases, tube thoracostomy alone with lung expansion adequately manages low-pressure lung bleeding and small air leaks. Ongoing blood loss indicates a more central, high-pressure source, which should prompt thoracotomy. Bleeding vessels within the parenchyma of the lung should be identified and controlled with suture ligatures. Missile tracts can be opened by passing a GIA stapler through the wound and performing a tractotomy that then exposes injured vessels so they can be controlled. Occasionally, pulmonary resection is required in anatomic or nonanatomic patterns to manage larger segments of injured lung tissue. In the setting of damage control, surgical bleeding can be controlled with sutures or staplers, followed by packing the chest with laparotomy sponges and temporary closure with a sponge and suction dressing. Unlike abdominal packing, the packs should occupy minimal space and be constructed to allow maximal lung expansion.

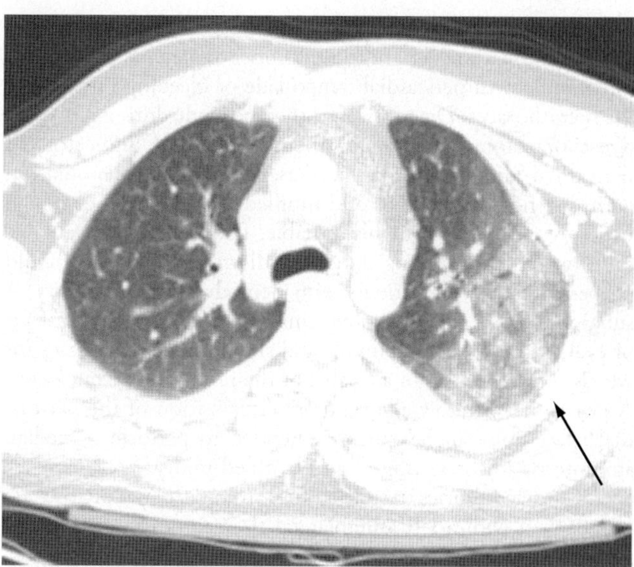

**FIGURE 18-17** Left pulmonary contusion on thoracic CT. The *arrow* identifies contused lung, which appears as higher density tissue because of air space hemorrhage and associated edema.

The management of pulmonary contusion is largely supportive. Patients should be monitored for indications of respiratory decompensation such as hypoxemia, increased work of breathing, and agitation, which mandate intubation and mechanical ventilation. Pulmonary function is supported until the physiologic insult related to the contusion resolves. Efforts to prevent ventilator-associated pneumonia are valuable because of a significantly increased risk. Intubation should be guided by the patient's observed respiratory function and should not be performed prophylactically simply on recognition of pulmonary contusion. Similarly, the presence of a pulmonary contusion or flail chest does not require mandatory chest tube placement in the absence of a pneumothorax or hemothorax. Patients with pulmonary contusion should not be managed with fluid restriction, which is a common misconception.[27] Appropriate resuscitation to maintain acceptable whole-body perfusion should be provided as for other severely injured patients. Excessive volume expansion should be avoided and might benefit from placement of a pulmonary artery catheter to guide fluid administration, especially when significant ventilatory support is required. Aggressive pulmonary toilet can be beneficial, as well as adequate pain control, when concomitant chest wall injuries are present.

**Cardiac Injuries** For obvious reasons, cardiac injuries represent some of the most severe problems experienced by patients after penetrating and blunt trauma. Penetrating injury to the heart occurred in 2% of patients with penetrating trauma in the NTDB and 16% in the subset of penetrating chest trauma alone. These numbers likely underestimate the true incidence of penetrating cardiac injuries because many are immediately lethal and never present to a hospital. In those that do survive to emergency department arrival, the mortality rate is 62%.

Penetrating cardiac injuries will frequently be evident on initial examination. A significant number of patients will present in extremis with pericardial tamponade or bleeding into one of the hemithoraces. Diagnosis may then be made during resuscitative thoracotomy in agonal patients. In others, indicators of pericardial tamponade may be present, including hypotension with distended neck veins and muffled heart sounds, although their presence can be highly variable. Ultrasound is a valuable tool for quickly assessing the pericardium for fluid and should be performed in all patients with hemodynamic instability. A subxiphoid pericardial window remains the most valuable means of evaluating for cardiac injury and should be used in cases for which ultrasound is not available or the results are inconclusive. A pericardial window allows direct visualization of the pericardial space and can be quickly extended to perform a median sternotomy in the setting of an identified injury.

Cardiac injuries resulting in cardiovascular collapse are approached with a left anterolateral thoracotomy in the emergency department. Injuries that are identified and allow transport to the operating room are best exposed through a median sternotomy. Injuries to the atria can be grasped in a side-biting fashion with a Satinsky clamp and then closed with running or interrupted permanent monofilament sutures. Ventricular injures can be more challenging and usually are associated with significant bleeding. The laceration can be held closed manually while the defect is closed with horizontal mattress sutures, which are reinforced with pledgets. To gain temporary control, one option is to close the laceration using skin staples; this allows resuscitation and transport to the operating room. Another option is the passage of a Foley catheter through the wound, followed by inflation of the balloon and maintenance of outward tension to occlude the opening until definitive closure can be done.

Blunt cardiac injury resulting in cardiac contusion or more severe structural abnormalities such as septal defects or valvular failure result less frequently, identified in only 3.8% of cases of blunt chest trauma. Most of these represent a contusion of the myocardium that results in arrhythmias and that are frequently self-limiting. In rare cases, blunt cardiac injury results in heart failure, with cardiogenic shock.

The diagnosis of cardiac contusion has been studied extensively but remains somewhat controversial. Although several laboratory and radiographic studies have been found to be associated with cardiac contusion, in practical terms it is only the presence of clinical sequelae that needs to be considered. The presence of an arrhythmia on an electrocardiogram (ECG), most commonly tachyarrhythmias, or cardiogenic shock is the pertinent clinical sequela that requires intervention and therefore is diagnostic in itself. Clinical findings of cardiac contusion that are absent on admission are highly unlikely to develop and, in their continued absence, require no further evaluation. Positive cardiac enzyme levels or radiographic studies have no impact on therapy that is not dictated by clinical and electrocardiographic findings. The presence of hemodynamic instability with evidence of heart failure should prompt an echocardiogram to assess cardiac wall and septal motion, as well as valvular function, which in rare cases can be injured during blunt thoracic trauma.

Blunt cardiac injuries require an ECG at the time of initial evaluation. Patients with mild electrocardiographic changes that do not require treatment should be monitored for 12 hours with telemetry. No further intervention is required if telemetry has revealed no arrhythmias and a follow-up ECG is normal. Those with more severe electrocardiographic changes or arrhythmias on admission require telemetry for 24 to 48 hours and therapy initiated for the specific electrical abnormality. Most patients demonstrate arrhythmias on initial assessment that do not require medical treatment and resolve quickly during the course of monitoring. Heart failure may require treatment with inotropic support and right ventricular afterload reduction, given the frequent involvement of the right heart. Patients who demonstrate structural abnormalities on echocardiography may require urgent operation to repair cardiac injuries.

**Thoracic Aortic Injuries** Injuries to the thoracic aorta are also highly severe but fortunately not common. Only 0.3% of patients sustaining blunt trauma in the NTDB sustained an aortic injury, although the associated mortality rate exceeded 47%. As with cardiac injuries, this likely underestimates the true incidence because aortic transection is a common cause of immediate death in blunt trauma patients who never present to the emergency department. In 3.8% of cases, the aorta is involved in penetrating thoracic trauma; almost all these injuries are fatal (mortality = 86.1%). The cause of blunt aortic injuries had traditionally been believed to be a result of rapid deceleration, which tears the aortic wall in the vicinity of the ligamentum arteriosum, where it is fixed to the thorax. Lateral mechanisms may also contribute, during which the aortic arch acts as a lever and causes torque to develop at the aortic isthmus. The result of these mechanisms can range from a tear in the aortic intima to full-thickness transection of the wall. Only patients who experience containment of the rupture by the surrounding mediastinal tissue present to the hospital.

Penetrating aortic injury may be discovered at the time of thoracotomy or sternotomy, often in the setting of patient extremis. Blunt aortic injury may be suggested by a chest radiograph that demonstrates findings such as a widened mediastinum, apical capping, loss of the aortic knob, or deviation of the left mainstem bronchus. Because of a high rate of missed injuries by plain radiograph, most patients involved in high-energy injury mechanisms undergo helical CT angiography of the chest to evaluate for aortic injury. Injuries to the thoracic aorta can be identified on CT as a disruption in the intima or as a pseudoaneurysm with a mediastinal hematoma, which appears as contrast contained outside the aortic lumen. Usually, this study alone is sufficient to plan operative repair, although standard angiography is necessary in some cases, usually at the discretion of the thoracic surgeon. A contained pseudoaneurysm from an aortic transection is depicted on a chest CT scan in Figure 18-18.

Patients who present with a blunt thoracic aortic rupture that is contained will require operative repair. The natural history of these injuries is slow expansion, which ultimately culminates with free aortic rupture. It has been recognized that there is usually a delay in this progression that allows other more urgent issues, such as acute hemorrhage, to be addressed. In the interim, medical therapy with beta antagonists aimed at controlling aortic wall stress is absolutely essential and should be instituted early. Open surgical therapy to repair the aorta is accomplished through a left thoracotomy. Small penetrating injuries to the aorta can be closed primarily if exposed prior to exsanguination. Larger penetrating injuries

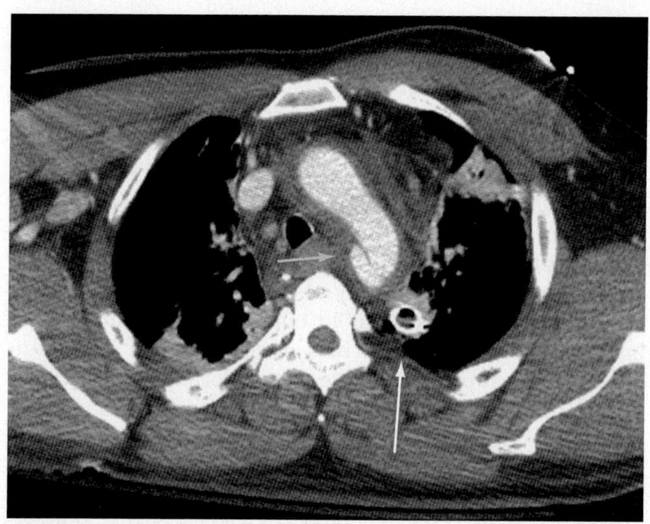

**FIGURE 18-18** Aortic transection with pseudoaneurysm and associated hematoma on a thoracic CT scan. This injury occurred at the typical location, just distal to the left subclavian artery at the aortic isthmus. The *yellow arrow* identifies a pseudoaneurysm; the *white arrow* identifies a left-sided tube thoracostomy.

and blunt transection require replacement of a segment of the aorta with a prosthetic graft. This is most commonly performed with the assistance of cardiopulmonary bypass, with full bypass through a femoral-femoral approach or with a centrifugal pump and left heart bypass. The use of cardiopulmonary bypass has been associated with a decreased incidence of paraplegia, which can result from cessation of aortic blood flow during the clamp and sew technique. Proximal and distal aortic control, as well as control of the left subclavian artery, are achieved and the injured segment replaced. This occasionally requires reimplantation of the left subclavian artery, depending on the proximal extent of the injury.

More recently, there has been a great deal of interest in the use of endovascular stent grafts to repair the injured thoracic aorta. This is particularly appealing for those patients at high operative risk and with favorable vascular anatomy, but further study is required to establish the role of this modality confidently. In many centers, this approach is becoming a mainstay of treatment for managing these injuries. Described advantages associated with the endovascular repair of aortic injury include a reduction in the incidence of paraplegia and a potential improvement in mortality. Although rare, patients with an intimal tear only may be candidates for nonoperative management because many of these injuries will heal without intervention. Patients should be treated with beta blocker therapy and undergo follow-up imaging to ensure the absence of expansion and ultimately the resolution of the injury.

**Tracheobronchial Injuries** Injuries to the tracheobronchial tree are uncommon but are associated with significant morbidity and mortality. In the NTDB, there are a total of only 275 tracheobronchial injuries, representing 0.02% of all patients injured by a blunt mechanism and 0.05% of all patients injured by a penetrating mechanism. Based on a literature survey, Kiser and colleagues[28] have reported on 265 blunt tracheobronchial injuries from a period of 123 years, in which 59% were caused by MVAs. The mortality from these injuries since 1970 was only 9% but it is believed that many patients with these injuries succumb prior to the arrival of prehospital personnel. Approximately 50% of these injuries involved the right mainstem bronchus within 2 cm of the carina. It is though that these injuries result from the application of a large amount of energy to the anterior chest, which pulls the lungs laterally and avulses the bronchi from the fixed carina. Another proposed mechanism is a rupture caused by rapid compression of the lungs and airways against a closed glottis, which perforates the trachea along the membranous portion. Penetrating injuries, mainly secondary to gunshot wounds, can also result in injuries to the tracheobronchial tree.

Identification of tracheobronchial injuries depends somewhat on the location of airway disruption. Significant subcutaneous air may be present on physical examination. Injuries that involve the thoracic trachea and proximal bronchi may result in large amounts of pneumomediastinum identified by chest radiography or chest CT. More distal airway injuries will typically cause a pneumothorax requiring insertion of a tube thoracostomy. A continuous air leak with persistent pneumothorax is highly suggestive of an injury to a bronchus or large bronchiole. Diagnosis is made with bronchoscopy, which most commonly is performed with a flexible bronchoscope because the use of a rigid bronchoscope requires neck extension, which is usually not feasible prior to excluding a cervical spine injury. Bronchoscopy allows for the identification of the injury and a detailed characterization, such as the location and severity of the disruption.

Initial management of tracheobronchial injuries includes careful airway management. With the placement of any airway, avoiding any further disruption is vital and may benefit from bronchoscopic guidance under direct visualization. Injuries that occupy less than one third of the luminal circumference may be considered for nonoperative management if any pneumothorax and associated air leak that were present resolve after insertion of a chest tube and the lung expands completely. Management includes antibiotics, humidified oxygen, careful suctioning, and close observation to be sure that infectious sequelae do not develop. Operative management of the trachea, right-sided airways, and proximal left mainstem bronchus is best approached through a right posterolateral thoracotomy. Distal left-sided injuries are repaired through a left thoracotomy. A vascularized intercostal muscle flap should be mobilized and preserved on opening the chest because placement of a retractor will prevent harvest of this potential tissue coverage. Repair includes débridement of devitalized tissue or segmental resection with closure, using absorbable sutures. The repair then benefits from coverage with a tissue pedicle, such as a previously preserved intercostal muscle flap. Patients requiring ongoing ventilation may benefit from passage of the endotracheal tube distal to the repair to provide protection. Other options include dual-lung ventilation and extracorporeal life support during the immediate postoperative time period.

**Esophageal Injuries** Injuries to the thoracic esophagus occur predominantly after penetrating trauma but remain uncommon by any cause. Only 2% of all patients in the NTDB with penetrating chest trauma sustained an injury to the esophagus. Most of these are caused by gunshot wounds, followed by stab wounds in fewer than 20% of cases. The mortality associated with these injuries is significant (39%) because of the severe nature of esophageal perforation and because the adjacent vital structures can also be injured along with the esophagus. Blunt esophageal injury is exceedingly rare, identified in only 0.02% of blunt trauma patients in the NTDB. Of these patients, 25% die because of the significant energy required to rupture the thoracic esophagus. Blunt esophageal injury is believed to be caused by a rapid elevation in intraluminal pressure during compression of the chest or abdomen. An impact to the upper abdomen can compress the distended stomach, leading to transmission of air and fluid up the esophagus and resulting in a perforation of the wall, usually in the distal segment.

Penetrating esophageal injuries may be suggested by the trajectory of a missile or weapon. Injuries in the vicinity of the mediastinum require consideration of possible esophageal injury. The esophagus is best evaluated through a combination of contrast esophagography and esophagoscopy. The combination of these two modalities results in a sensitivity of almost 100% for esophageal injury. Findings include extravasation of contrast from the esophageal lumen or a disruption of the mucosa visualized on endoscopy. These studies should also be used to determine the location of the injury along the esophagus to assist in operative planning. Blunt trauma patients may demonstrate large amounts of pneumomediastinum, which prompts a further workup with esophagography and esophagoscopy. Chest CT may reveal air adjacent to the esophagus but outside the lumen, as well as surrounding soft tissue inflammation. At times, the defect itself can be visualized on CT. Esophageal injuries at the gastroesophageal junction may result in abdominal pain and tenderness.

The rapid identification and management of esophageal injuries are paramount because delays are associated with worse outcomes. Clinical evaluation and studies that reveal an esophageal injury should prompt immediate operative repair. The upper and midthoracic esophagus are best approached through a right posterolateral thoracotomy through the fourth or fifth interspace, whereas the lower esophagus is exposed from the left through the sixth or seventh interspace. Contrast studies that demonstrate the injury within the abdomen benefit from a laparotomy to repair the esophagus from an abdominal approach. Again, maintenance of a vascularized intercostal muscle flap is of great value for coverage of the repair. The injury should be entirely exposed, which usually requires opening the muscular layer superiorly and inferiorly to reveal the extent of the mucosal defect, which is commonly larger than the muscular disruption. The esophagus is then closed in one or two layers, frequently using an absorbable mucosal suture followed by interrupted muscular sutures using a permanent material. The repair is covered with the muscle flap or another adjacent tissue to provide protection, given the high rate of leak and fistula formation. Esophageal repairs at the gastroesophageal junction can be covered with a fundoplication of gastric tissue. Chest and mediastinal drains should be placed in the vicinity of the repair to control any leak that may develop. A gastrostomy and feeding jejunostomy are frequently advisable to allow gastric decompression and early nutritional support. Esophageal injuries that are identified late may not allow primary repair because of the massive amounts of inflammation that can develop. In some situations, esophagectomy is the only option to allow recovery from the associated inflammatory insult, followed by planned elective reconstruction, when feasible.

**Diaphragmatic Injuries** Injuries to the diaphragm can be a diagnostic challenge. They are often first identified at the time of laparotomy for penetrating injury or late following blunt trauma. Approximately 3% of patients with trauma to the torso have a diaphragmatic injury identified, with approximately two thirds of them secondary to penetrating trauma. In the NTDB, 26.6% of penetrating chest injuries included a diaphragmatic injury, which was associated with a 22.5% mortality. This is secondary to injuries involving adjacent vital organs because diaphragmatic injuries themselves are usually of limited threat to life. Blunt diaphragmatic injuries occur in only 1.8% of blunt thoracic injuries and are believed to be a result of a rapid increase in intra-abdominal pressure during an anterior impact that causes a blowout of the diaphragmatic tissue. Injuries are most commonly recognized on the left side, with only 25% occurring adjacent to the liver or in the central portion of the diaphragm. Because of the high energy required to create a blunt diaphragmatic rupture, there is a significant associated mortality, approximately 29%. The morbidity related to diaphragmatic injuries is occasionally identified months to years later when the perforation was not initially recognized and repaired. The natural history of these injuries includes progressive enlargement with herniation of abdominal viscera into the chest, which is commonly the identified abnormality on radiographic evaluation.

Diagnosis requires a high index of suspicion when confronted with even the most subtle indicators of injury to the diaphragm. Frequently, penetrating diaphragmatic injuries are discovered on operative exploration of the chest or abdomen. Identifying the trajectory of the injury will usually allow recognition of the diaphragmatic defect. Blunt injuries can be more elusive. The chest radiograph may identify injuries to the diaphragm by demonstrating the presence of abdominal viscera, most commonly the stomach, within the chest, although this finding may be absent in a significant number of injuries. Figure 18-19 illustrates a left diaphragmatic injury on a plain chest radiograph. Passage of a nasogastric tube can be of assistance if

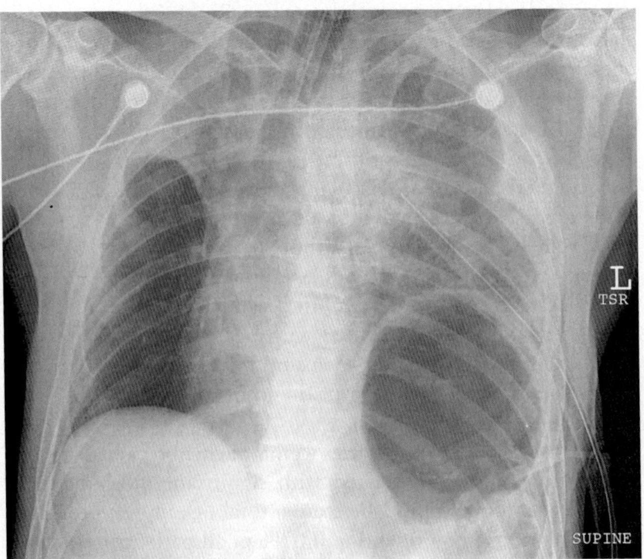


**FIGURE 18-19** Left-sided diaphragmatic injury on a plain chest radiograph. The gas-filled stomach can be visualized in the left chest; this was caused by herniation through a large diaphragmatic laceration.

the tube is identified in the lower left hemithorax; the administration of gastric contrast may add to the detection. Chest and abdominal CT scans may demonstrate the presence of abdominal viscera in the chest or an abnormality of the diaphragm itself, such as discontinuity, thickening, or elevation. At times, three-dimensional reconstruction of the CT developed from newer generation scanners can demonstrate the diaphragmatic defect with high sensitivity. Given the challenge of diagnosis, operative exploration may be required when imaging is suggestive. In patients who have no other indication for laparotomy, video-assisted thoracoscopy or cautious laparoscopy conducted to avoid tension pneumothorax may offer less invasive means to visualize the diaphragm.

Repair of diaphragmatic injuries includes débridement of nonviable tissue and closure of the defect. Typically, the diaphragm exhibits enough redundancy to close all but the largest defects primarily. Closure is commonly performed with a nonabsorbable suture in a single layer, incorporating large full-thickness bites of healthy diaphragmatic tissue. Hemostasis in this layer is important because branches of the phrenic artery may be exposed at the edges of the tear. When the repair involves mostly muscle, horizontal mattress sutures may reinforce the suture line. Large areas of tissue loss are rare in traumatic rupture but, when present, may require reconstruction with a prosthetic. Nonabsorbable synthetic materials are reasonable in noncontaminated fields although they should not be placed when the GI tract has been injured. When the diaphragm has been traumatically detached from the periphery, it may be reinserted to the chest wall one or two interspaces superior.

## Injuries to the Abdomen

Abdominal injuries are frequently encountered in the management of trauma patients. Of all patients in the 2009 NTDB, 13% sustained abdominal injuries, associated with an overall mortality rate of 7.7%.[24] During the evaluation of the injured patient, the abdomen is of high priority because the vital nature of the contained organs and structures. Blunt trauma can result in the laceration of solid organs usually causing bleeding, which in its most severe form manifests as hemorrhagic shock or as visceral perforation of the GI tract. Penetrating trauma to the abdomen can result in laceration of solid organs and perforation of hollow organs, which must be discovered and repaired at the time of laparotomy.

### Immediate Management

Immediate management of abdominal injuries consists of resuscitation and evaluation (see earlier). Patients in shock require initiation of resuscitation with crystalloid solutions and blood products, as well as a rapid assessment for the source of bleeding. Retained foreign bodies traversing the abdominal wall should be maintained throughout the initial evaluation and protected from excessive movement. These should then be removed only after defining a definitive plan, which almost always includes abdominal operation.

### Blunt Abdominal Trauma Evaluation

Patients who present with blunt versus penetrating mechanisms of injury frequently require varying approaches to evaluation. Blunt trauma patients who are unstable and have intra-abdominal fluid identified on FAST require an emergent laparotomy to manage bleeding.[29] Surgeons can quickly become skilled at performing the FAST examination and should be actively involved in obtaining and interpreting the study. If FAST is unavailable, aspiration of 10 mL or more of gross blood on DPL also suggests an intra-abdominal source of hemorrhage requiring emergent operation. Furthermore, patients with peritonitis require abdominal exploration to evaluate for hollow visceral injury. Other patients will undergo further workup of the abdomen to evaluate for intra-abdominal injury. Figure 18-20 presents an approach to evaluating the blunt trauma patient with possible abdominal injury.

Abdominal CT has become the mainstay of imaging for the stable blunt trauma patient and has led to the emergence of nonoperative management of many solid abdominal organ injuries. Abdominal CT is typically performed with IV contrast timed to capture the portal venous phase, which best demonstrates the vasculature and visceral perfusion of the solid abdominal organs. CT provides excellent visualization of the solid organs, allowing the characterization of injury severity (injury grade) and the recognition of active bleeding, which appears as contrast extravasation. Imaging findings assist in making management decisions regarding the need for operative, nonoperative, or angiographic therapy. The retroperitoneal structures are also well visualized on CT, identifying injuries that are difficult to evaluate with FAST or DPL. DPL demonstrating more than 100,000 red blood cells/mm$^3$ is indicative of intra-abdominal injury and historically mandated a laparotomy. The high nontherapeutic laparotomy rate associated with this practice has led to the nonoperative principles commonly used today because a large percentage of abdominal structures that had bled were no longer bleeding at the time of abdominal exploration. The frequent lack of bleeding at laparotomy suggested that the patient's physiologic condition was more important than the presence of intra-abdominal blood when making treatment decisions.

Abdominal CT is less sensitive for detecting hollow visceral injury, although this has improved as imaging technology has progressed from the older 4- and 16-slice CT scanners to the newer 64- and 128-channel machines. Hollow viscous injury is suggested by the recognition of bowel wall thickening, inflammation in the surrounding adipose tissue seen as stranding, or presence of free intraperitoneal fluid. Administration of oral contrast is not necessary and might increase the risk of vomiting with aspiration.[30] It is paramount that the presence of unexplained free fluid on imaging be carefully evaluated and a high index of suspicion for bowel injury be maintained. Frequently, a combination of these radiographic findings, with clinical signs and symptoms such as an abdominal seatbelt mark or tenderness on examination, are suggestive and may require exploration. A challenging scenario is the identification of intra-abdominal fluid on imaging without the presence of solid organ injury to explain its presence. In a significant percentage of cases, this fluid represents blood from a mesenteric tear that is no longer bleeding, but being confident that a bowel injury is not present can be difficult. The amount of fluid identified may be helpful, with fluid visualized in more than one abdominal quadrant suggestive of a bowel injury requiring laparotomy. In many cases, patients can provide an adequate abdominal examination to follow for symptoms indicative of a hollow viscous injury. In patients for whom mental status or concomitant injuries compromise the abdominal examination, DPL may provide valuable information. Findings on lavage fluid evaluation, including more than 500 white blood cells/mm$^3$, amylase, bilirubin, or particulate

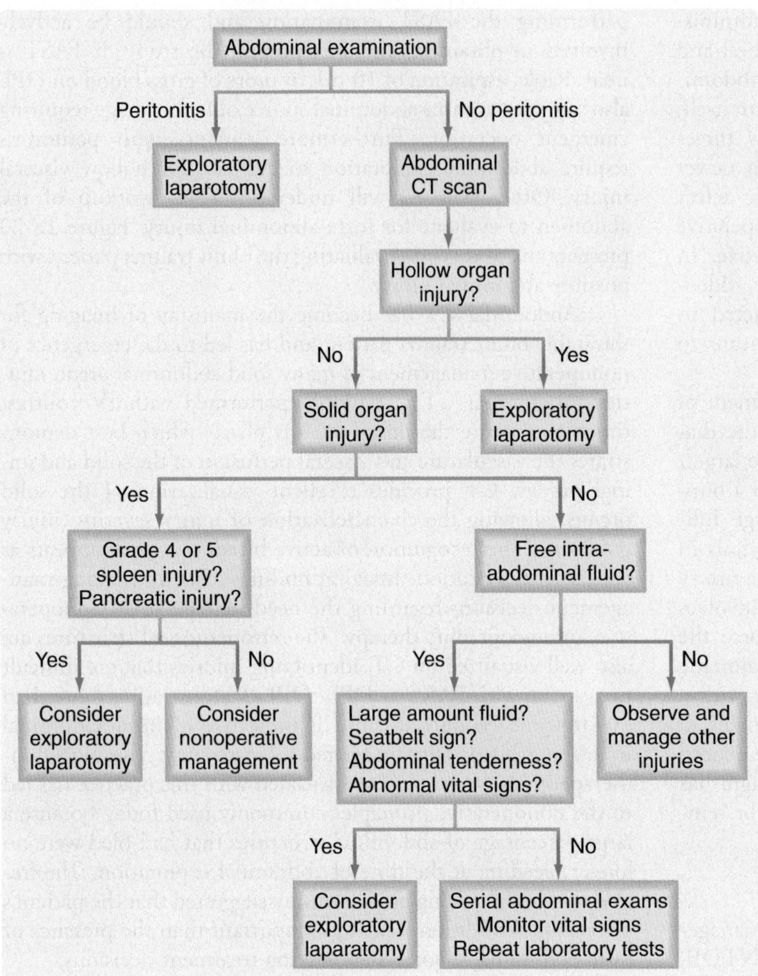


**FIGURE 18-20** Algorithm for the evaluation and management of blunt abdominal trauma.

matter, have been found to be indicative of a hollow visceral injury.

### Penetrating Abdominal Trauma Evaluation

Penetrating abdominal trauma is typically evaluated differently than blunt mechanisms. Because of the high rate of intra-abdominal injury, patients sustaining anterior abdominal gunshot wounds are frequently transferred quickly to the operating room for laparotomy. Depending on the location of the penetrating wound, the chest may require evaluation for mediastinal, pleural, or pulmonary injuries. It may be valuable to attempt to determine the trajectory of the missiles while preparing for surgery because this may assist in directing the exploration. Penetrating wounds of the skin should be identified with radiopaque markers and plain radiographs obtained to determine their location and relation to missile position. The number of missiles and skin wounds should add up to an even number, or a more intense search for injuries is required. This evaluation should be brief and not delay operation, especially in the hemodynamically unstable patient.

Abdominal stab wounds can be managed somewhat differently. Figure 18-21 presents one approach that was recently developed after a multicenter trial facilitated by the Western Trauma Association.[31] Patients with hemodynamic instability, peritonitis, or evisceration require immediate laparotomy with repair of injuries. Others can have the penetrating wound explored locally to determine whether the anterior or posterior abdominal fascia was violated. Those without fascial penetration can be discharged to home. In the setting of a positive or equivocal local wound exploration, patients should be monitored with serial abdominal examinations and determinations of hemoglobin levels every 8 hours. Throughout this evaluation, the development of peritonitis, hemodynamic instability, significant decreases in hemoglobin level, or development of leukocytosis should prompt further evaluation, usually with laparotomy. Patients without clinical change after 24 hours can have a diet instituted and be discharged to home. The important principle determined by the group was that many stab wounds failed to result in intra-abdominal injury that required repair, even in the setting of peritoneal violation. This approach requires the presence of an infrastructure that allows close surveillance of these patients, although this may not be possible in all facilities. Others believe that penetration of the abdominal fascia warrants exploration to identify any possible injury immediately, with the understanding that this will result in a higher nontherapeutic laparotomy rate.

An additional tool that has been used more recently is laparoscopy, mainly to establish or exclude the presence of peritoneal penetration. It remains fairly well accepted that laparoscopy in most hands is not sufficient to explore the entire abdomen but it can be used to identify violation of the parietal peritoneum, which can then prompt laparotomy to

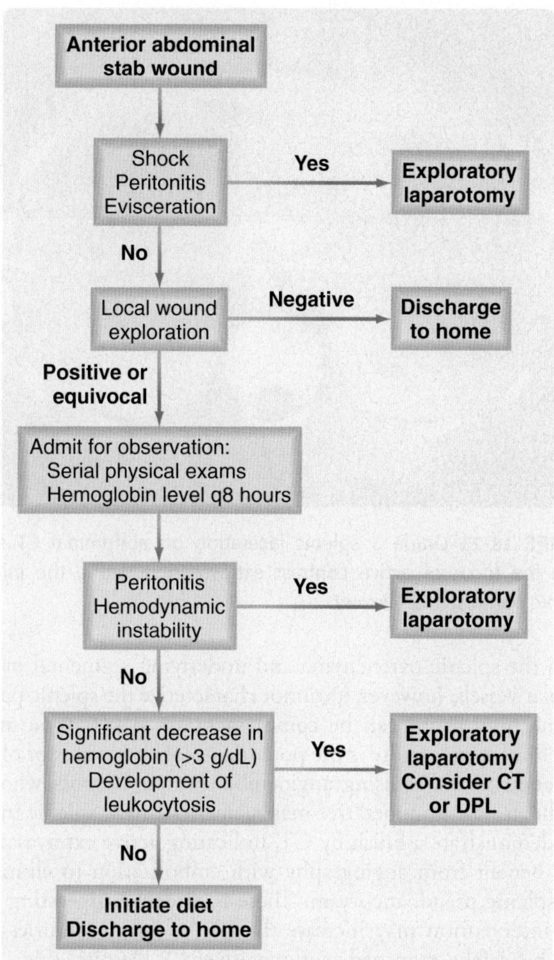


**FIGURE 18-21** Algorithm for the evaluation and management of anterior abdominal stab wounds. (Adapted from Biffl WL, Kaups KL, Cothren CC, et al: Management of patients with anterior abdominal stab wounds: A Western Trauma Association multicenter trial. J Trauma 66:1294–1301, 2009.)

address injuries. Patients without peritoneal penetration can be discharged to home after recovery from anesthesia in the absence of other injury or illness.

Penetrating wounds from both high- and low-energy mechanisms that occur posterior to the midaxillary lines and throughout the back may benefit from three-dimensional imaging with CT. Patients with abdominal symptoms or a track that clearly enters the abdomen require abdominal exploration. Otherwise, the thickness and density of the retroperitoneum often result in penetrating injuries avoiding significant structures, therefore requiring no operative intervention. CT can often determine the track of the penetrating injury by lining up external markers with internal missiles and locules of air within the tissues. Establishment of the injury track often allows decisions to be made regarding further evaluation or necessary injury management. Information regarding vertebral column, spinal cord, pelvic, and vascular injuries within the retroperitoneum can also be obtained by CT. Injury tracks identified by CT that are within close proximity to intra-abdominal organs typically require abdominal exploration. One limitation of this approach is the presence of radiographic scatter caused by retained missiles, which may obscure findings on CT scans.

#### Management

Patients who require laparotomy should undergo a systematic exploration so that all areas of the abdomen are assessed and injuries are not missed. As noted earlier, this approach may require abbreviation in the setting of deteriorating physiologic condition. As a standard technique, the abdomen is opened from the xiphoid process to pubic symphysis to provide adequate exposure of all abdominal structures. The falciform ligament is divided, separating the liver from the abdominal wall to improve retraction and perihepatic packing. Using a hand-held retractor, blood is quickly evacuated from all four quadrants of the abdomen and laparotomy sponges are placed to provide temporary hemostasis. Many surgeons then prefer to place a fixed retractor to provide necessary exposure. Packed sponges are removed to address bleeding structures and hemostasis is achieved, or the packs are replaced in the damage control setting. The entire GI tract is carefully evaluated, from the gastroesophageal junction to the rectum at the peritoneal reflection. This includes entering the lesser sac to evaluate the posterior stomach and the pancreas. Areas stained with blood that are of concern for injury should be explored further with careful dissection. The required management of specific injuries is detailed later. Developing physiologic compromise should be promptly recognized; this requires open lines of communication with anesthesia providers throughout the operation. In this setting, the operation should be abbreviated, with the only goals becoming hemorrhage and contamination control with temporary abdominal closure. Otherwise, the abdominal fascia can be closed in a single layer and the subcutaneous wound addressed as dictated by the level of intra-abdominal contamination.

**Splenic Injuries** The spleen is the most commonly injured abdominal organ in the NTDB, with 3.2% of all injured patients and 50.7% of patients with blunt abdominal trauma demonstrating splenic injuries. This is similar to a large multicenter series that included data from 1993 to 1997 in which 2.6% of injured patients sustained splenic trauma.[32] The ability to manage splenic injuries is required for anyone who definitively treats patients with blunt abdominal trauma. A significant mortality of 10.8% is associated with blunt splenic injury among centers who contribute to the NTDB. Many of these deaths are caused by associated injuries and prehospital delays; it would be hoped that few patients should succumb to an injury that can be rapidly addressed. The pathophysiology of blunt splenic injury can include direct compression of the organ in the left upper quadrant of the abdomen or a deceleration mechanism that tears the splenic capsule or parenchyma, mainly at areas fixed or tethered to the retroperitoneum. A subcapsular hematoma of the spleen is demonstrated in Figure 18-22 at the time of splenectomy. Bleeding from a ruptured spleen can be ongoing at the time of presentation or frequently will have stopped. This cessation of bleeding allows many of these injuries to be managed without splenectomy, although reinitiation of bleeding from a splenic injury can be delayed. This is of obvious concern for patients who undergo nonoperative management and many studies have been devoted to identifying which patient populations are at greatest risk of delayed hemorrhage. The rate of late bleeding was determined to be 10.6% in a large series, although

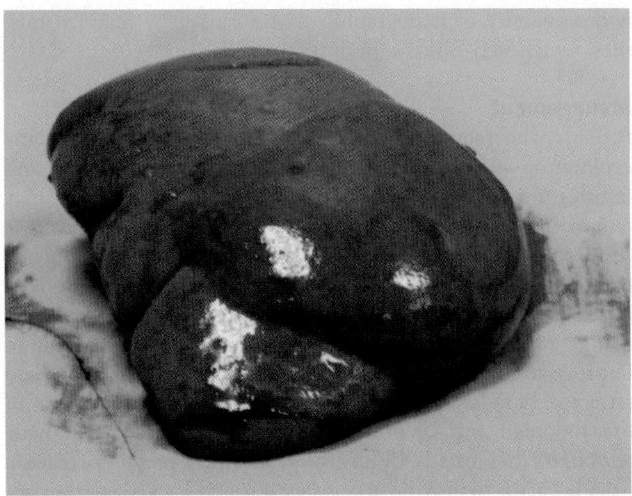

**FIGURE 18-22** Splenic injury with subcapsular hematoma. Despite only a 1-cm capsular tear, this injury demonstrated ongoing hemorrhage.

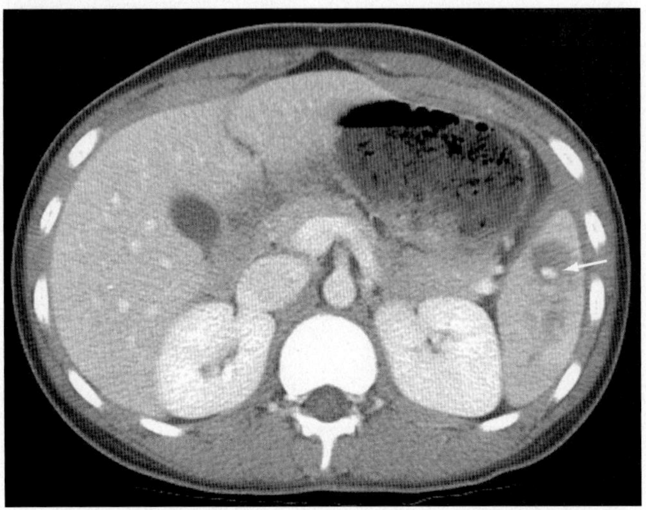

**FIGURE 18-23** Grade 3 splenic laceration on abdominal CT scan. Note the focus of active contrast extravasation within the injured splenic parenchyma *(arrow).*

this rate varies greatly with the grade of splenic injury.[32] Penetrating splenic trauma is less common but is still present in 14.5% of all penetrating abdominal injuries in the NTDB. This is somewhat higher than reported in a large series from Grady Memorial and Ben Taub General Hospitals during the 1980s and 1990s, in which 9.2% and 7.6%, respectively, of penetrating abdominal injuries involved the spleen.[33]

Identification of splenic injuries may occur during laparotomy in patients who are unstable and taken emergently to the operating room. As noted, unstable patients with intra-abdominal fluid on FAST require exploration, with the spleen commonly being the bleeding intra-abdominal organ. In stable patients, abdominal CT performed with IV contrast is the mainstay for diagnosing and characterizing splenic injuries. Images are typically obtained with the contrast in the portal venous phase to enhance the splenic parenchyma maximally while still being able to visualize the vasculature. Splenic injuries appear as disruptions in the normal splenic parenchyma, frequently with surrounding hematoma and free intra-abdominal blood. Occasionally, active extravasation of contrast, identified as a high-density blush, can be identified, contained within a pseudoaneurysm or bleeding into the peritoneal space. Figure 18-23 illustrates a splenic injury with active extravasation on an abdominal CT scan. Other findings can include a hematoma confined to the subcapsular space or even complete devascularization of the organ caused by injury of the hilar vessels. Table 18-5 demonstrates the AAST Organ Injury Scaling system of grading spleen injuries by anatomic characteristics. Spleen injury grading relies on describing parenchymal or subcapsular characteristics and the presence of vascular involvement.

A more recent advance in the management of splenic injury has been the use of angiography to evaluate further and, at times, treat these injuries. Usually, this modality has been used for injuries that demonstrate active extravasation by CT, although a well-defined indication for these studies is still being elucidated. Some centers have a lower threshold for angiography and use it in the setting of all high-grade injuries because of the greater risk of delayed bleeding during nonoperative management. Angiography can identify specific sites of bleeding from the splenic parenchyma and underlying segmental or trabecular vessels; however, it cannot characterize the splenic parenchymal injury but can be complementary to CT. One major benefit of angiography is the potential to obstruct sites of bleeding endovascularly using angioembolization. Patients who are candidates for nonoperative management of their splenic injury but demonstrate a blush by CT, indicating active extravasation, may benefit from angiography with embolization to eliminate the splenic pseudoaneurysm. There is evidence suggesting that this intervention may increase the rate of splenic injuries that can be safely managed nonoperatively.[34] Despite this, only patients not in shock who demonstrate hemodynamically stability should be considered for angiographic evaluation and possible angioembolic treatment.

With appropriate patient selection, many patients with blunt splenic trauma can be managed without splenectomy. The value of careful patient selection for nonoperative management cannot be overstated. It should not be overlooked that a definitive treatment for splenic bleeding exists in splenectomy, which does not have an overly great risk profile, especially in comparison to the adverse implications of ongoing hemorrhage. Therefore, no bleeding patient should go without splenectomy or splenic repair, especially in an attempt to push the figurative nonoperative envelope. Nevertheless, there are many patients who, at presentation, are no longer bleeding from a splenic injury and do benefit from avoiding an unnecessary operation. Fortunately, based on the patient's physiology, it is usually possible to elucidate those that have a hemostatic splenic injury and are appropriate candidates for nonoperative management. Another important point is that nonoperative management does not mean lack of intervention or care provided. Nonoperative management of splenic injury, done properly, is much more labor-intensive than operative therapy and requires greater resources over a longer period. Having the infrastructure in place is mandatory to provide the ongoing surveillance required to manage a spleen injury without surgery. To be a candidate for nonoperative management, there can be no physiologic indication of ongoing bleeding. Therefore, hemodynamic stability is a prerequisite and must be present without

**Table 18-5 American Association for the Surgery of Trauma: Spleen Organ Injury Scale**

| INJURY GRADE | INJURY TYPE | DESCRIPTION OF INJURY |
|---|---|---|
| I | Hematoma<br>Laceration | Subcapsular tear <10% surface area<br>Capsular tear <1 cm parenchymal depth |
| II | Hematoma<br>Laceration | Subcapsular tear, 10%-50% surface area; intraparenchymal, <5 cm in diameter<br>Capsular tear, 1-3 cm parenchymal depth that does not involve a trabecular vessel |
| III | Hematoma<br><br>Laceration | Subcapsular tear >50% surface area or expanding; ruptured subcapsular or parenchymal hematoma; intraparenchymal hematoma ≥5 cm or expanding<br>>3 cm parenchymal depth or involving trabecular vessels |
| IV | Laceration | Laceration involving segmental or hilar vessels producing major devascularization (>25% of spleen) |
| V | Hematoma<br>Laceration | Completely shattered spleen<br>Hilar vascular injury devascularizes spleen |

ongoing intravascular volume support. Hemodynamic stability is indicated by a normal blood pressure and lack of tachycardia, no physical examination findings indicating shock, and absence of metabolic acidosis. The initial hemoglobin level may not be reflective of actual blood loss until intravascular equilibration occurs. Patients who have experienced transient hemodynamic instability that responded to crystalloid infusion may be considered but a lower threshold for operation should be maintained.

Although the patient's physiologic condition is the most important factor when considering nonoperative management, there are other factors that may have an impact on this decision. Some controversy exists about whether older patients are at greater risk of failing nonoperative management. Two retrospective studies have compared failure rates between groups older and younger than 55 years of age and reached opposite conclusions.[35,36] The larger of these studies demonstrated a significantly greater rate (19% versus 10%) of failure of nonoperative management in patients older than 55 years.[36] Despite this, over 80% of older patients who underwent attempted nonoperative management still succeeded, so most would agree that age alone is not a contraindication to management without surgery, but that these patients require a greater degree of scrutiny. Another consideration that may affect decision making is the grade of splenic injury identified on imaging at admission. There are no prospective data to provide guidelines so this also has created a great deal of controversy. One multi-institutional retrospective study conducted by EAST identified failure rates of 33.3% in grade IV and 75% of grade V injuries, with 8% of failures occurring more than 9 days after injury.[32] Another multicenter study had few of these high-grade injuries but all of them failed nonoperative management.[37] Varying conclusions have resulted from these data. Some believe that failure rates after high-grade splenic injuries are unacceptably high, especially given that almost one in ten may occur after hospital discharge and that splenectomy does not carry a markedly high morbidity. Others think that a significant number can still be managed nonoperatively, despite the higher failure rate. The result is that this decision remains personal preference and is often guided by surgical intuition. Our preference is to reserve nonoperative management for grades I and II injuries, as well as grade III injuries that are isolated.

Operative management of splenic trauma may be in the setting of instability at admission, when the exact location of bleeding is unknown or after failed nonoperative management, when the spleen is suspected to be the culprit preoperatively. In either setting, the best approach is through a midline incision with packing of all four quadrants when instability is present. A fixed retractor facilitates exposure of the left upper quadrant. Splenectomy begins with division of the peritoneum laterally, which is facilitated by retracting the spleen posteromedially to expose these attachments. The dissection begins at the splenocolic ligament by dividing the peritoneum at the white line of Toldt and then continuing superiorly until the short gastric vessels are encountered. After the peritoneum is taken down, a blunt plane is created posterior to the spleen in a medial direction, extending behind the tail of the pancreas. This maneuver mobilizes the entire spleen and distal pancreas, which allows the spleen to be delivered into the visualized wound. The short gastric vessels are then identified and ligated, with care taken to avoid injuring the greater curve of the stomach. All that remains are the hilar vessels, which are clamped and ligated, being sure not to involve the tail of the pancreas in this division. Drains should not be placed unless there is concern that the tail of the pancreas was also injured. Postsplenectomy vaccines must be provided to ensure protection from encapsulated bacteria, including *Streptococcus pneumoniae, Neisseria meningitidis,* and *Haemophilus influenzae.* Several splenic salvage options exist, although these are becoming less commonly used because more patients who would commonly benefit from these techniques are managed nonoperatively. Splenic injury secondary to penetrating abdominal trauma is usually identified during laparotomy and should be addressed based on the presence or absence of ongoing bleeding. In the setting of damage control, the splenic injury can be packed but, more commonly, splenectomy is performed because of the rapidity at which the spleen can be removed and managed definitively.

**Hepatic Injuries** Second only to the spleen, injury to the liver is extremely common after blunt abdominal trauma. Overall, liver injuries occurred in 2.9% of all patients included in the NTDB, with 39.8% of those with blunt abdominal trauma sustaining injury to the liver. The mortality associated with these blunt hepatic injuries was 14.9%. Richardson and associates[38] have reported on their 25-year experience with hepatic trauma, during which the incidence of major liver injuries remained stable, ranging from 12% to 15%. Mechanisms of blunt hepatic trauma include compression with direct parenchymal damage and shearing forces, which tear hepatic tissue and disrupt vascular and ligamentous attachments. The liver is partially protected by the thoracic cage, although even the rigid ribs provide little support during high-energy mechanisms. Liver injury secondary to penetrating abdominal trauma is also common, given the sizable volume occupied by the liver in the abdomen. Nicholas and coworkers[33] have described the presence of liver injury in 34.4% of cases of penetrating abdominal trauma, which was similar to a comparison group that demonstrated an incidence of 29.3%. In the NTDB, the liver is the most commonly injured abdominal organ after penetrating trauma, present in 42.3% of cases. An associated mortality of 19.1% demonstrates the danger of these injuries. Penetrating mechanisms can cause variable degrees of tissue destruction, depending on the associated energy of the missile. Furthermore, penetrating injuries can cause significantly greater morbidity when vascular or biliary tree structures are involved.

As with splenic injuries, liver injuries are often first diagnosed on entering the abdomen in the unstable patient explored for the finding of free fluid on FAST examination. Stable patients with suspected hepatic trauma should undergo abdominal CT with IV contrast. Current CT modalities are excellent at providing significant anatomic detail that allows highly accurate characterization of injures. Findings on CT associated with liver injury include disruption of the hepatic parenchyma with perihepatic blood or hematoma, as well as hemoperitoneum. Occasionally, contrast extravasation visualized as a high-density blush is identified indicating the presence of a pseudoaneurysm or active bleeding external to the liver capsule. Figure 18-24 demonstrates a CT scan of a grade III liver laceration with extravasation of contrast. Findings on CT can be used to characterize the injury according to the AAST Organ Injury Scale for liver injuries. Liver injury grading involves the extent of parenchymal involvement and presence of vascular injury (Table 18-6).

Patients who are unstable during emergency department evaluation and are found to have intra-abdominal fluid require immediate laparotomy. Despite all that has evolved in the management of liver injuries, it should not be overlooked that unstable patients require operative management of bleeding. Patients who are stable benefit from a more conservative approach. As with spleen injuries, most injuries to the liver have stopped bleeding by the time of evaluation, which is usually reflected by the patient's physiologic condition. Hemostatic injuries benefit little from operative intervention but instead require close surveillance for indicators of rebleeding or associated complications. This approach has been shown to achieve excellent results in multiple series, with successful nonoperative management in 85% to 97% of cases.[39,40] Despite avoiding unnecessary operation in a significant number of patients, the application of a nonoperative approach for select patients has actually resulted in a decrease in mortality for liver injuries, despite an increase in overall injury severity over the last 3 decades.[38] To qualify for attempted nonoperative management, patients must demonstrate evidence that hepatic bleeding has stopped. This is typically indicated by the absence of tachycardia, hypotension, metabolic acidosis, and physical examination evidence of shock, being sure that the patient is not receiving ongoing fluid resuscitation that might mask cardiovascular compromise. Even more than in the setting of splenic injuries, physiologic stability is the major predictor of successful nonoperative management of hepatic trauma. This is true independently of injury severity, in that even high- grade liver injuries should be considered for nonoperative management as long as the patient remains hemodynamically stable, without evidence of bleeding.[40]

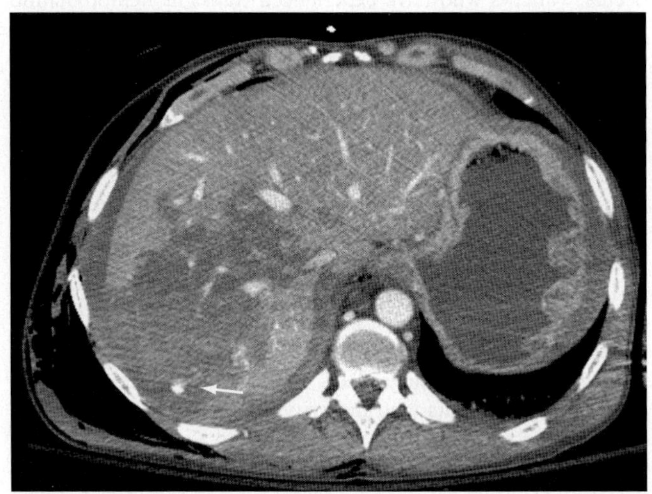

**FIGURE 18-24** Grade 4 liver laceration involving the right hepatic lobe on abdominal CT scan. Note the focus of active contrast extravasation within the injured liver parenchyma at the periphery of the injury *(arrow)*.

**Table 18-6 American Association for the Surgery of Trauma: Liver Organ Injury Scale**

| INJURY GRADE | INJURY TYPE | DESCRIPTION OF INJURY |
|---|---|---|
| I | Hematoma | Subcapsular tear <10% surface area |
| | Laceration | Capsular tear <1 cm parenchymal depth |
| II | Hematoma | Subcapsular tear, 10% to 50% surface area; intraparenchymal <10 cm in diameter |
| | Laceration | Capsular tear, 1-3 cm parenchymal depth, <10 cm in length |
| III | Hematoma | Subcapsular tear >50% surface area of ruptured subcapsular or parenchymal hematoma; intraparenchymal hematoma >10 cm or expanding |
| | Laceration | >3 cm parenchymal depth |
| IV | Laceration | Parenchymal disruption involving 25%-75% hepatic lobe or one to three Couinaud segments |
| V | Laceration | Parenchymal disruption involving >75% of hepatic lobe or more than one Couinaud segment within a single lobe |
| | Vascular | Juxtahepatic venous injuries (e.g., retrohepatic vena cava,central major hepatic veins) |
| VI | Vascular | Hepatic avulsion |

In contradistinction to spleen injuries, the operative intervention for liver trauma is less definitive and can be challenging. Therefore, hemodynamic decline requires operation but slow decreases in hemoglobin levels are at times tolerated and even occasionally treated with transfusion. This is especially true when there are other injuries that may account for some blood loss, and the decline in hemoglobin level may not be reflective of ongoing hepatic bleeding. Because many liver injuries are associated with some degree of hemoperitoneum, it is possible that a hollow visceral injury could be present but overlooked if the intra-abdominal fluid is attributed solely to the liver injury. Therefore, serial abdominal examinations to detect evidence of intestinal injury are an important part of nonoperative management of any solid abdominal organ.

In some cases, CT reveals a liver injury that demonstrates the extravasation of IV contrast from a disrupted vascular structure. These appear as a blush of high-density contrast, often within the injured-appearing hepatic parenchyma. In the setting of hemodynamic stability, this extravasation is usually contained within a pseudoaneurysm. The natural history of hepatic pseudoaneurysms is not exactly known but it is believed that they may be associated with an increased risk of delayed bleeding, especially when caused by hepatic arterial branches. A more recent advance in the management of hepatic pseudoaneurysms is the use of hepatic angiography, with embolization of blood vessels that demonstrate extravasation. Even with successful embolization, patients need standard surveillance, which is required for all hepatic injuries managed nonoperatively. When selected appropriately, the use of angioembolization has improved the rate of successful nonoperative management by reducing the number of conversions to operative therapy.[41,42] This has also allowed many higher grade injuries that historically might have required operation to be managed without surgery.

The evolution of nonoperative approaches to liver trauma has required advances in evaluating and managing complications that arise. In addition to delayed rebleeding, these include bile leaks with biloma formation, hemobilia, and development of liver abscesses. Frequently, these are suggested by the development of abdominal symptoms. with or without evidence of systemic infection or inflammation. CT or, at times, ultrasound will identify the liver injury–related pathology. Percutaneous drainage guided by CT or ultrasound is usually successful in managing abscess or biloma. Endoscopic retrograde cholangiopancreatography (ERCP) with stent placement is occasionally required to decompress the biliary tree and promote healing of a bile leak. Occasionally, a laparoscopy or laparotomy is necessary to manage biliary ascites not amenable to percutaneous drainage.

Operative management begins in the same fashion as with other abdominal injuries. A midline laparotomy is the most versatile approach for managing any liver injury that might be encountered. The falciform ligament is divided and perihepatic sponges are placed to manage bleeding from the liver temporarily. A fixed retractor is placed to expose the right upper quadrant structures. With perihepatic packing and manual compression, bleeding can be temporarily controlled and resuscitation provided. On patient stabilization, the packs are removed and the hepatic lacerations evaluated. Mild injuries with little or no ongoing bleeding may be managed with further compression, topical hemostatic agents, or suture hepatorrhaphy. Addressing these injuries may sometimes be facilitated by mobilizing the right or left hepatic lobes by dividing the triangular ligaments. This will allow injuries to be better exposed for interventions but may also allow better packing by optimizing anterior to posterior compression. Occasionally, however, when the risks of mobilization should be carefully considered if there is the possibility that the attachments of the liver are providing lifesaving tamponade of retrohepatic bleeding. This combination of superficial techniques will successfully manage most liver injuries encountered.

In the setting of more severe bleeding, a Pringle maneuver is a valuable adjunct. The hepatoduodenal ligament is encircled with a vessel loop or vascular clamp to occlude hepatic blood flow from the hepatic artery and portal vein. This maneuver helps distinguish hepatic venous bleeding, which persists from a portal vein, and hepatic artery bleeding that slows, allowing identification of sources of hemorrhage. The hepatic laceration can then be explored and any actively bleeding vessels controlled with suture ligation. Grossly devitalized hepatic parenchyma should be débrided when accessible and drains should be placed when injuries appear to be at risk for a bile leak. When feasible, a vascularized pedicle of omentum may be packed within the liver injury to reduce parenchymal bleeding and promote healing of the laceration.

Liver injuries in the vicinity of the retrohepatic vena cava that are not actively bleeding may benefit most from packing alone, without operative exploration. There are many heroic techniques seen in the literature that describe methods of repairing retrohepatic vena cava injuries, but it is likely that the approach with the greatest likelihood of success is maintaining the body's natural tamponade of this low-pressure region when feasible. An atriocaval shunt (Shrock shunt) is one method that entails isolation of the retrohepatic vena cava by placing an intracaval shunt between the right atrium and infrahepatic vena cava. Isolation of the liver with an atriocaval shunt with the addition of a Pringle maneuver allows repair of the vena cava or hepatic veins without ongoing associated blood loss. Damage control techniques are often of great value because many patients who require operative intervention for liver injuries have already deteriorated physiologically. This approach includes control of surgical bleeding followed by aggressive perihepatic packing and temporary abdominal closure. It is fruitless to leave surgical bleeding and hope that packing alone will provide control. Similarly, it is futile to continue surgical attempts with sutures to control diffuse liver bleeding from coagulopathy. Patients are then resuscitated in the intensive care unit until hypothermia, coagulopathy, and acidosis resolve, at which time the abdomen is reexplored and the packs removed. Angiography with embolization after damage control may provide additional assistance with managing ongoing bleeding from hepatic artery branches, although the mortality in this patient cohort remains high.[41]

**Gastric Injuries** Gastric injuries most commonly occur after penetrating abdominal trauma, with the stomach being the injured organ in approximately 17% of cases identified in two separate series from busy urban trauma centers.[33] This is similar to contemporary data obtained from the NTDB in which 18.1% of penetrating abdominal trauma involved the stomach were associated with a mortality of 19.7%. Penetrating injuries are frequently full-thickness perforations resulting in the spillage of gastric contents. Conversely, blunt gastric injuries are rare, occurring in 0.05% of all blunt trauma patients and 4.3% of patients with a blunt hollow visceral injury.[43] These injuries are associated with a significant mortality, reaching 28.2% in an EAST multi-institutional trial. In this series, gastric injury was independently associated with death when analyzed by regression analysis (relative risk [RR], 2.8; 95% confidence interval [CI], 1.8 to 4.4).[43] Blunt gastric injuries are equally as rare in the NTDB and are associated with a mortality rate of 28.3%. The proposed mechanism of blunt gastric rupture is an acute increase in intraluminal pressure from external forces that results in bursting of the gastric wall. Because of the high-energy nature of this mechanism, associated injuries are common and often include the liver, spleen, pancreas, and small bowel. Mortality is frequently attributed to these associated injuries.

Gastric injuries will often be identified on physical examination by the presence of peritonitis. Some gastric injuries are identified by CT or DPL but the value of these modalities is limited. The evaluation of gastric injuries follows the approach to tat for other hollow abdominal viscera (see earlier).

Repair of gastric injuries is based on severity and injury location. Large intramural hematomas should be evacuated to ensure the absence of perforation, followed by control of bleeding and closure of the seromusculature with nonabsorbable suture. Full-thickness perforations should be débrided to remove nonviable gastric tissue and then closed with one or two layers. The perforation is generally closed with an absorbable suture. followed by inversion of the suture line with nonabsorbable seromuscular stitches. Because of the size and redundancy of the stomach, this can also be repaired with a stapling device. Perforations involving the gastroesophageal junction, lesser curve, fundus, and posterior wall may be more challenging to approach and require better exposure of the upper abdomen. Rarely, destructive injuries to the stomach involving large portions of the gastric wall require a partial or even total gastrectomy. Reconstruction options include a Billroth I or II gastroenterostomy or creation of a Roux-en-Y esophagojejunostomy.

**Duodenal Injuries** Duodenal injuries are uncommon after blunt and penetrating trauma but can be challenging to diagnose and manage. Most are caused by penetrating mechanisms occurring in 6.7% of penetrating abdominal cases, most of which the result of to gunshot wounds. The associated mortality is significant, 22.1% in the NTDB. Only 0.1% of patients experiencing blunt trauma sustain a duodenal injury. In those that present with a blunt hollow visceral injury, 12% are located in the duodenum.[43] The mortality after blunt duodenal injury ranges from 11.4% to 14.8%. Blunt injuries are presumably caused by a blow to the epigastrium by a narrow object, resulting in contusion of the wall or a blowout secondary to acute elevation of intraluminal pressure. The classic description is the abdomen being struck by a steering wheel or, in children, a bicycle handlebar.

Although duodenal injuries after penetrating trauma are found at laparotomy, their identification after a blunt mechanism can be challenging and therefore require a high index of suspicion to avoid missed injuries. Because of the retroperitoneal location of a significant portion of the duodenum, physical examination findings may be limited. Even full-thickness perforations of the duodenum may not demonstrate peritoneal signs unless the perforation involves an intraperitoneal segment. The mainstay of evaluation for duodenal injury has become abdominal CT, with a low threshold for operative exploration. Findings on CT that reflect possible duodenal injury include thickened duodenal wall, air or fluid outside the bowel lumen, and contrast extravasation if oral contrast was administered. Some authors advocate the administration of oral contrast whereas others have found that it is not necessary with current imaging capabilities.[30] Low-grade injuries resulting in a duodenal hematoma can be identified by CT, although it is important also to evaluate the pancreas because of a high rate of concomitant injury. Any indication of duodenal perforation on examination or imaging should prompt operative exploration. At times, the findings are subtle but a low threshold for exploration should be maintained because of the potential for false-negative interpretations of the CT scan. Upper GI contrast studies, DPL, and laboratory studies such as serum amylase level determination, have at most a limited role in the evaluation of duodenal injuries.

Management of duodenal injuries depends on the severity and location of the injury. Hematomas of the duodenal wall typically require no treatment unless they are large and result in a gastric outlet obstruction. Treatment of obstructing hematomas consists of gastric decompression and initiation of total parenteral nutrition, with reevaluation of gastric emptying with a contrast study after 5 to 7 days. If after 2 weeks of upper GI bowel rest the obstruction persists, exploration is warranted to evaluate for perforation, stricture, or associated pancreatic injury. Duodenal hematomas identified at the time of laparotomy for another indication require careful evaluation for perforation. Frequently, they decompress during duodenal mobilization, although intentionally opening the serosa to drain an incidentally identified hematoma should generally be avoided in the absence of a full-thickness injury.

Most full-thickness injuries of the duodenal wall can be repaired primarily using a single- or double-layer approach, depending on the amount of tissue available. Adequate mobilization of the duodenum with a wide Kocher maneuver is required to provide necessary exposure and ensure a tension-free repair. Duodenal transection can be managed with primary anastomosis as long as the ampulla is not involved and the segment is short. Larger segments of duodenal destruction may require more complex reconstruction, frequently using bypass around the injured duodenum. Any repair can be protected from the enteric contents by performing a pyloric exclusion and creating a gastroenterostomy. In the damage control setting, the use of a duodenostomy tube or resection leaving the GI tract in discontinuity is highly effective for controlling contamination temporarily.

**Pancreatic Injuries** Because of their adjacent location, injuries to the duodenum are frequently associated with pancreatic injuries. These are rare in blunt and penetrating mechanisms, occurring in only 0.09% of the patients in the NTDB. Of those that sustain penetrating injuries to the abdomen, the pancreas is involved in 6.6% of the cases. Despite the infrequency of these injuries, they remain a serious problem, resulting in mortality rates of 23.4% and 30.2% for blunt and penetrating mechanisms, respectively. These high mortality rates can frequently be attributed to delays in diagnosis and treatment. Because of the caustic nature of pancreatic enzymes, delays in managing pancreatic injuries result in massive systemic inflammation, with subsequent poor outcomes. Pancreatic injuries can result from direct penetration of the organ or through the transmission of blunt force energy to the retroperitoneum. A commonly identified mechanism involves the crushing of the body of the pancreas between a rigid structure such as a steering wheel or seatbelt and the vertebral column. This can cause injury to the gland, ranging from mild contusion to complete transection with ductal disruption.

The diagnosis of pancreatic injuries can be extremely challenging and no single imaging modality has been found to be highly effective. As with the duodenum, the retroperitoneal location of the pancreas makes physical examination less helpful for diagnosis. Abdominal imaging with IV-enhanced CT can indicate the pancreatic injury but the sensitivity is limited for parenchymal injury and pancreatic duct disruption, as identified recently in a large multicenter trial.[44] Depending on the generation of scanner used, the sensitivity for detecting parenchymal or ductal injury did not surpass 60%. Peitzman and colleagues[45] have evaluated the usefulness of CT prospectively and found a somewhat better sensitivity, approximately 80%, likely reflecting the variations in radiologic interpretation among centers. Nevertheless, CT alone may not be satisfactory to rule out a pancreatic injury and a high index of suspicion must be maintained. Findings on CT that suggest pancreatic injury include malperfusion of the pancreatic parenchyma indicating disruption, surrounding fluid, or hematoma and stranding in the adjacent soft tissue. Figure 18-25 demonstrates an injury at the neck of the pancreas on an abdominal CT scan.

Given the limitations of imaging pancreatic trauma, the detection of injuries may require the use of other modalities. Although these injuries are uncommon, there is great value in minimizing the time to diagnosis because any delays could be associated with worse outcomes. Patients who are not responding appropriately to their known injuries require further evaluation for missed injuries. In this setting, repeat CT scanning may suggest a pancreatic injury that required time to develop radiographically evident pancreatic inflammation. Although not predictive as a screening tool, elevated serum amylase levels may reflect pancreatic trauma when obtained more than 3 hours after admission. Serum amylase levels may be sensitive but little is known about their specificity; therefore, the use of this indicator is limited and should not be routinely used. Imaging of the pancreatic ducts with ERCP and magnetic resonance cholangiopancreatography (MRCP) may be helpful, especially for those patients who have a suggestion of pancreatic injury but a lack of supporting studies. These modalities continue to be evaluated, but they may occasionally be of assistance in planning therapy and determining an operative approach.

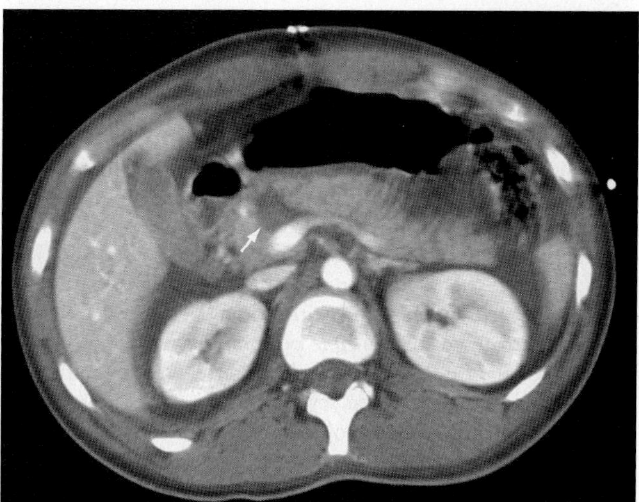

**FIGURE 18-25** Pancreatic injury on abdominal CT scan. The injury involves the pancreatic neck and appears as a 2-cm segment of nonperfused pancreas tissue, with surrounding edema *(arrow)*.

The mainstay of therapy for pancreatic injuries is surgical. Exposure of the entire gland to evaluate the pancreas comprehensively is required to exclude injury or select appropriate management. This exposure includes mobilization of the hepatic flexure of the colon and division of the gastrocolic ligament to retract the transverse colon and mesocolon inferiorly. A wide Kocher maneuver will mobilize the pancreatic head and facilitate evaluation. Assessment of the injury includes determining the degree of parenchymal involvement, location of the injury within the gland, and presence of pancreatic ductal involvement. The management of pancreatic injuries with ductal involvement depends on the location of the injury. Injuries to the left of the superior mesenteric vessels are managed with a distal pancreatectomy. The proximal stump can be managed by individually ligating the duct and oversewing the parenchyma or using a stapling device. Covering the stump with omentum may be advantageous and a closed suction drain should be placed. Managing injuries of the ductal system within the head of the pancreas can be more challenging. Although some advocate resection in this setting, the associated morbidity can be great, often necessitating a more conservative approach. Managing these injuries with drainage alone often successfully diverts the leakage of pancreatic fluid externally, creating a controlled fistula that frequently will close spontaneously. This healing may also be promoted with biliary decompression through the placement of stents via ERCP. Massive destruction of the pancreatic head with devitalized parenchyma or combined pancreatic and duodenal injuries may require a pancreaticoduodenectomy (Whipple procedure). This can be extremely challenging in this setting and is associated with a high postoperative complication rate. Performing a Whipple procedure in the setting of trauma requires ongoing patient stability or the operation should be abbreviated, with later reconstruction after the physiologic condition improves. Damage control for pancreatic injury includes hemorrhage control, external drainage, and temporary abdominal closure with plans for reexploration.

Adequate external drainage is an important principle in the management of most pancreatic injuries. The diversion of leaking pancreatic enzymes is required to prevent the devastating effects of uncontrolled accumulation of highly caustic digestive fluid, which will provoke a massive inflammatory response and progressive organ dysfunction. Pancreatic injuries not involving the pancreatic duct, including hematomas, parenchymal contusions, and lacerations of the capsule or superficial parenchyma, should be managed with external drainage alone. External drainage should be with a closed suction system because these are associated with a reduced rate of abscess development.[46] Distal feeding access should be considered based on the overall clinical picture. Figure 18-26 depicts an approach to the operative management of pancreatic injuries.

**Small Bowel Injuries** Depending on the series reviewed, the small intestine is one of the most frequently injured organs after penetrating abdominal trauma, likely secondary to the large percentage of the abdomen it occupies. Although the incidence of small

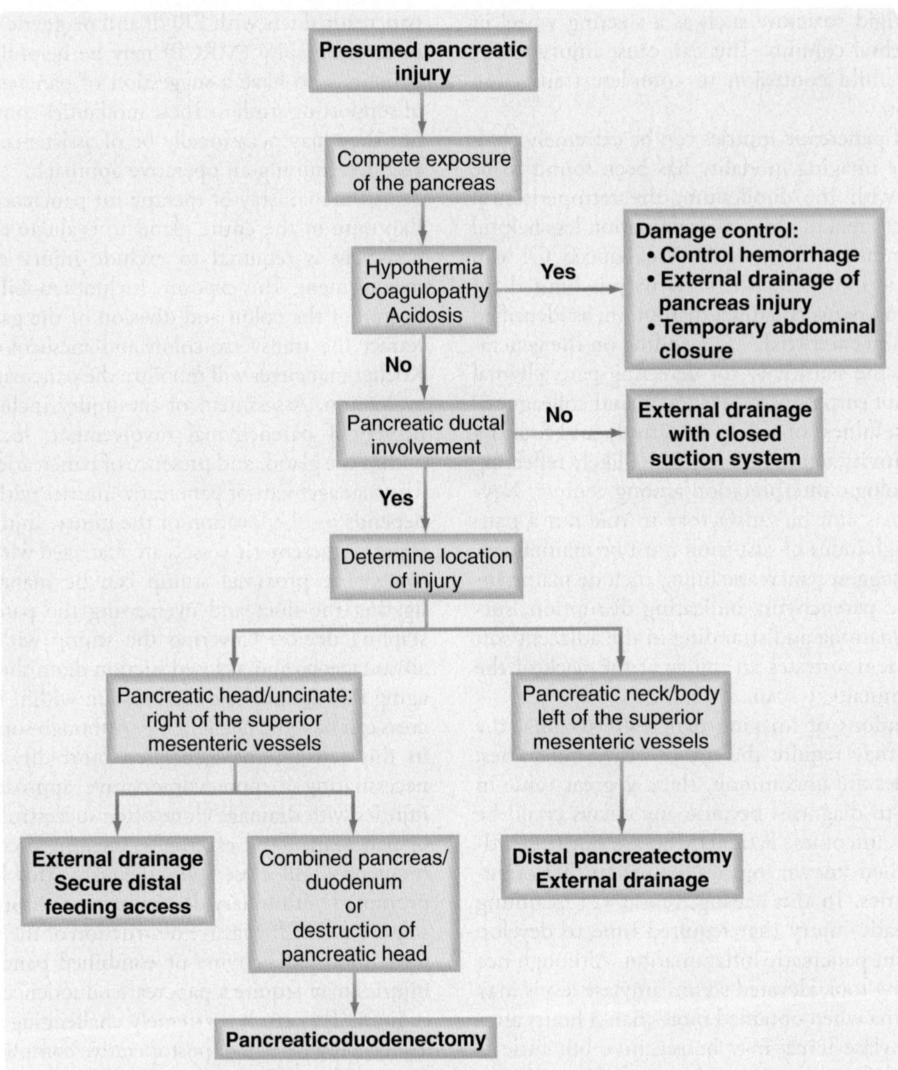


**FIGURE 18-26** Algorithm for the operative management of pancreatic injury.

bowel injury after penetrating abdominal trauma has been described as high as 60%, these injuries are less common in the NTDB, identified in 21.8% of cases. Mortality rates range from 10% to 25%, with most caused by associated vascular injuries. Penetrating injuries can vary from tiny perforations to large destructive injuries that destroy circumferential segments of small bowel. Blunt, small intestinal injuries are less common, present in 2.7% of all blunt abdominal injuries in the NTDB, although these injuries are associated with a significant mortality rate of 16.3%. Mechanisms of blunt small bowel injury include crushing, rupture, and shearing types of patterns. The small bowel can be crushed between the steering wheel or seatbelt and a rigid structure such as the vertebral column, resulting in direct tissue injury. Similar forces can result in a rupture-type injury during which the intraluminal pressure rapidly increases, causing a blowout along the antimesenteric border. Finally, deceleration mechanisms can result in a shearing of the serosa or muscularis throughout a segment of small bowel. Mesenteric injuries can cause devascularization of sections of small bowel without direct tissue injury.

Small intestinal injuries are often identified at the time of laparotomy. Otherwise, the evaluation can be challenging and is similar to the approach to other hollow abdominal viscera. The use of imaging and other modalities has been described earlier.

The repair of small bowel injuries depends on the extent of intestinal wall destruction in relation to the luminal circumference. Serosal tears can be reinforced with interrupted nonabsorbable suture, which imbricates the injury. Small perforations that can be closed without compromising the intestinal lumen can be débrided and repaired with one or two layers. This can safely be performed for multiple perforations as long as closure will not result in obstruction of the enteric contents, although many choose resection when several injuries are close together. Injuries occupying over 50% of the intestinal wall circumference should be addressed with resection and anastomosis. There has been no difference demonstrated between stapled and hand-sewn anastomoses for intestinal resections. Selection of the anastomosis technique should be based on the experience of the surgeon, with the method of greatest comfort used. Hand-sewn anastomoses are frequently constructed in two layers but single-layer methods are equally efficacious. The damage control approach to small bowel injuries includes rapid closure of perforations to control contamination and/or stapled resection of injured segments. Patients in shock may benefit from resection without immediate anastomosis because of related delays and a higher risk of anastomotic dehiscence. The abdomen is temporarily closed and the patient is resuscitated to correct physiologic derangements. Intestinal continuity can then reestablished on return to the operating room, following resuscitation.

**Colon Injuries** Similar to other hollow viscera, colon and rectal injuries occur most commonly after penetrating abdominal trauma and rarely after blunt mechanisms. The colon is one of the most frequently involved organs after penetrating abdominal trauma, occurring in 36% to 40% of patients in a series of 250 cases.[33] This incidence is similar to data from the NTDB, in which 34.3% of all cases of penetrating abdominal trauma involved the colon or rectum. The associated mortality for colon and rectal injuries is the lowest of all the abdominal viscera. Penetrating injuries can range in the degree of colonic wall destruction, depending on the level of energy associated with the mechanism. Penetrating injuries can also be obscured by the retroperitoneal location of some segments of colon. Blunt colon and rectal injury occur in less than 1% of all blunt trauma patients but, in those patients with blunt hollow visceral injury, the colon or rectum is involved in 30.2% of cases.[43] Mortality after blunt colon or rectal injury equals 16.3%, with much of this caused by associated injuries. Injuries to the colon can result from similar biomechanical mechanisms as those that occur in the small bowel. The colonic wall can be crushed by physical forces or rupture when the impact results in a rapid elevation in intraluminal pressure. Depending on the colonic segment involved, this perforation can occur into the retroperitoneum. The colon is also vulnerable to shearing forces, which can cause a separation of the serosa or muscularis over a long segment. Figure 18-27 demonstrates a segment of colon that was injured secondary to a shearing-type mechanism. Injury to the rectum can also occur when severe pelvic fractures result in a laceration by sharp bone fragments.

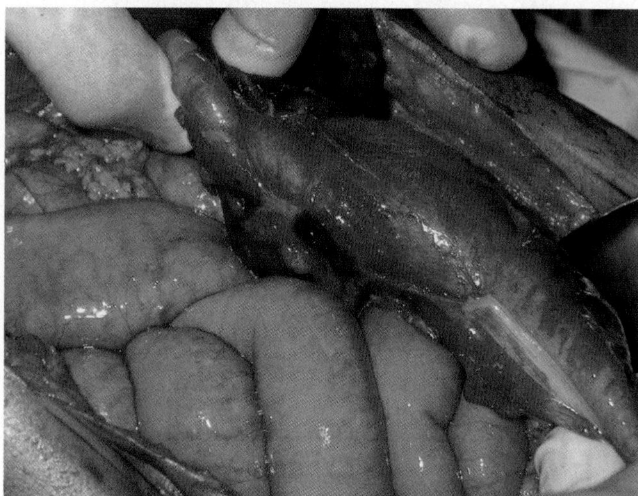

**FIGURE 18-27** Blunt left-sided colon injury at the time of laparotomy. The injury mechanism resulted in a deserosalizing-type injury that involved a several-centimeter-long segment of colon.

As with other hollow organ injuries, colonic injuries may be identified first at the time of laparotomy that was prompted by hemodynamic instability or the appropriate penetrating mechanism. Otherwise, evaluation is as described earlier for other hollow abdominal viscera. Care must be taken to assess segments of the colon that are retroperitoneal in location adequately.

Blood identified on rectal examination or a penetrating trajectory that suggests rectal involvement requires further evaluation. Rigid proctosigmoidoscopy can visualize the rectum and distal sigmoid colon to assist in determining the presence or absence of a rectal injury. This can be performed prior to laparotomy in hemodynamically stable patients to help plan the operative approach. Endoscopy may clearly reveal an injury to the rectum or only demonstrate hematoma in the rectal wall or a large amount of blood in the rectal vault. When possible, determining the size of the injury and location on the rectal wall may be valuable when planning the necessary management. Upper rectal injuries, especially those on the anterior or lateral surfaces, may be identified during examination of the pelvis during laparotomy.

Operative repair of colon injuries depends on the severity of the colonic wall injury and the patient's overall condition. Historically. it was believed that all colon injuries required resection with the creation of a colostomy because of a high risk of anastomotic dehiscence. A substantial amount of work has been dedicated to determining whether proximal fecal diversion was necessary to manage colonic perforation. Several randomized prospective trials have concluded that primary repair or resection with primary anastomosis is safe in select patients, resulting in a leak rate that was not significantly greater than that for colonic diversion.[47,48] Therefore, injuries that involve less than 50% of the colonic wall circumference can be repaired with one or two layers, being sure to imbricate the mucosal edge. Usually, compromising the colonic lumen is not as common a concern as in the small bowel. Destructive colon injuries that involve more than 50% of the colonic wall should be resected; many can then be anastomosed immediately. Injuries proximal to the middle colic artery are managed with a right hemicolectomy with creation of ileocolostomy, because this has been found to be a durable anastomosis. Distal injuries require segmental resection with colocolostomy anastomosis. In the setting of shock, immediate anastomosis may be associated with an unacceptably high leak rate and should be carefully considered.

There are two other options in the setting of hemodynamic instability to manage colon injuries. First, the injured segment can be resected and a diverting colostomy created. The second option is to resect the injured segment of colon and leave the GI tract in discontinuity until after the patient has been adequately resuscitated. On return visit to the operating room, delayed primary anastomosis or creation of a colostomy can be completed. Leak rates after delayed primary anastomosis have been found to be equivalent to immediate anastomosis performed in the setting of hemodynamic stability.[49] Other concerns that may suggest colostomy instead of primary repair or anastomosis include significant associated injuries, underlying medical disease, and delayed injury recognition with the development of severe peritoneal inflammation.

Rectal injuries that result in perforation present a significant risk of developing pelvic sepsis and thus require operative management. The mainstays of treatment for rectal injuries are fecal diversion and presacral drainage until healing has occurred, at which time the colostomy is reversed. This can be achieved with an end colostomy or a loop configuration as long as complete fecal diversion can be achieved. Historically, drainage of the presacral space has been considered an important part of managing rectal perforations because of data generated in the military theater. More recently, some have countered this edict, concluding that presacral drainage is an unnecessary component, especially in the setting of low-energy, nonmilitary types of penetrating rectal trauma.[50] Without definitive studies, one approach is to drain injuries that occur posteriorly or laterally, if in the lower third of the rectum, because these have likely entered the presacral space and are at greater risk of abscess formation. Other injuries to the extraperitoneal rectum can be managed with fecal diversion alone. Destructive rectal injuries that involve more than 50% of the rectal wall circumference may require resection of the rectum above the injury with the creation of an end colostomy.

**Abdominal Great Vessel Injuries** The great vessels of the abdomen are located within the retroperitoneum and abdominal mesenteries. Injuries to these vessels can be challenging to manage given the amount of blood loss that can be present when these structures are injured. Although these injuries frequently occur after blunt trauma, it is most commonly during penetrating injury that exploration of this region is required. Often, hematoma within the retroperitoneum is secondary to a pelvic fracture because hemorrhage from the pelvic vessels can dissect superiorly through the surrounding tissue. Abdominal vascular injuries are further addressed elsewhere in this text (Section 12, "Vascular Surgery") so only those concepts related to initial assessment and management will be presented here.

Vascular injuries in the abdomen are often first recognized at the time of laparotomy for penetrating abdominal trauma. Frequently, these injuries are associated with significant ongoing blood loss and hemodynamic instability. Exploration of penetrating injuries to the retroperitoneum results in a definitive diagnosis. Penetrating injuries to the back frequently benefit from three-dimensional imaging, given that most do not enter the peritoneal cavity. Current CT can often identify the path of the injury and therefore suggest possible injury to adjacent structures. After blunt trauma, injuries to the abdominal vasculature with associated hematoma are often identified via contrast-enhanced CT. Occasionally, blunt trauma to the retroperitoneum with vascular injury is identified during urgently performed laparotomy, although further identification of specific injury depends on the location of the hematoma.

Usually, penetrating injuries to the retroperitoneum identified during laparotomy require exploration. Injuries to the abdominal vasculature are detailed in the vascular surgery section of this text, but a knowledge of the basic approach to and exposure of these structures is important. Hematomas in the vicinity of the right renal hilum or infrarenal vasculature benefit from a right medial visceral mobilization, also known as the Cattel-Brasch maneuver. A wide Kocher maneuver is performed and the peritoneal dissection is continued inferiorly to mobilize the right colon. The dissection is continue around the cecum and then superiorly up the mesenteric root, allowing all the abdominal viscera to be retracted to the left, thus exposing the midline vascular structures. Basic tenets of vascular repair are paramount, including proximal and distal control of the injured vessel, when feasible. Injuries to the left renal hilum or the suprarenal vessels can be exposed by performing a left medial visceral mobilization (the Mattox maneuver). This is performed by dividing the left lateral peritoneum from above the spleen to the distal left colon. The plane posterior to the colonic mesentery and e pancreas is developed and the abdominal viscera are retracted to the right to expose the superior retroperitoneal vasculature.

Blunt abdominal vascular injuries that are not actively bleeding may require operation to repair or, as more recently found, may be considered for endovascular therapy. When confronted with a retroperitoneal hematoma during laparotomy for blunt trauma, the location of the hematoma suggests the appropriate treatment. Figure 18-28 depicts three zones used to classify these hematomas. Zone 1 hematomas require exploration because these frequently involve the aorta, proximal visceral vessels, or inferior vena cava. An exception may be the dark hematoma behind the liver, which suggests a retrohepatic vena cava injury. These injuries may be best served by not exposing the contained low-pressure injury or by gently packing the surrounding area; heroic management techniques can be extremely challenging. A hematoma in the region of zone 2 should only be explored if it appears that the hematoma is expanding and continuing to lose blood. Finally, a hematoma in zone 3 is usually secondary to pelvic fracture bleeding and should not be explored unless exsanguinating hemorrhage is present.

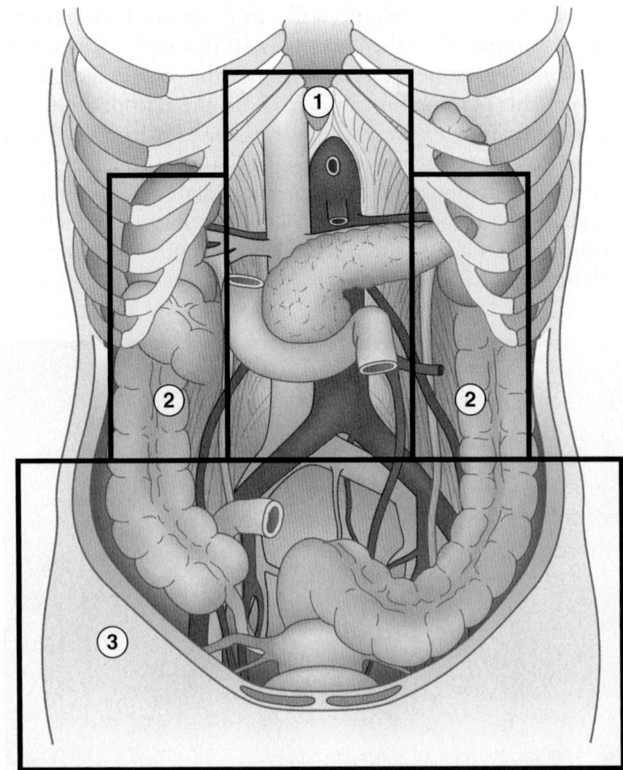


**FIGURE 18-28** Zones of the retroperitoneum visualized at the time of laparotomy. Zone 1 includes the central vascular structures, such as the aorta and vena cava. Zone 2 includes the kidneys and adjacent adrenal glands; zone 3 describes the retroperitoneum associated with the pelvic vasculature.

**Genitourinary Injuries** The genitourinary organs include the kidneys, ureters, bladder, and urethra, all contained within the retroperitoneum. Injury to these structures results in bleeding or urine extravasation. Blunt mechanisms can result in renal laceration and bladder rupture, which can occur intraperitoneally or extraperitoneally. Commonly, bladder injuries are associated with pelvic fractures when significant energy is transmitted to the urine-filled bladder, resulting in wall rupture. All genitourinary structures are vulnerable to penetrating mechanisms, many of which cause urine extravasation.

The evaluation and management of genitourinary injuries are described elsewhere in this text (see Chapter 73) and therefore will be only briefly outlined. The presence of gross or microscopic hematuria is the most valuable screen for injuries to the genitourinary organs and should prompt further evaluation. Imaging with IV contrast-enhanced CT frequently identifies injuries to the genitourinary organs. Renal trauma, as well as injury to the adrenal glands, are easily identified on CT; imaging also allows an assessment for urine extravasation from the collecting system. Injury to the bladder can be evaluated by obtaining a cystogram, which is now most easily achieved with CT. In males specifically, blood at the urethral meatus and prostatic abnormality on rectal examination are suggestive of a urethral injury and require evaluation. This is best achieved by performing retrograde urethrography, especially prior to placement of a urinary catheter. Penetrating genitourinary injuries may be identified at the time of laparotomy or suggested by imaging. Penetrating injuries to the back benefit from CT, which can characterize the injury tract and delineate adjacent organs.

During laparotomy for penetrating trauma, injuries to the kidney should be explored to ensure hemostasis but also to assess for a urine leak. Obtaining proximal control at the renal hilum is ideal and should be performed whenever possible. Many renal injuries are hemostatic at the time of exploration whereas others respond favorably to simple techniques. Devastating renal injuries, especially in the setting of shock with ongoing bleeding. may require nephrectomy after assessing the contralateral side for a kidney. Ureteral injuries require repair for which there are many described techniques, ranging from primary repair to nephrectomy. Intraperitoneal bladder injuries can be repaired in two layers of absorbable suture and the bladder drained with a Foley catheter or suprapubic cystostomy tube. Extraperitoneal bladder ruptures require only catheter drainage, with a follow-up cystogram to confirm healing.

Blunt retroperitoneal injury is most commonly identified on imaging and can be managed nonoperatively in most cases. Bleeding from the kidneys and adrenal glands is commonly self-limiting and requires no specific intervention. Nonoperative management requires clinical stability, which indicates the lack of ongoing blood loss. Deterioration mandates laparotomy, with management of uncontrolled bleeding. Patients with hemodynamic stability but pseudoaneurysm from a renal laceration on imaging may benefit from angioembolization. Renal hematomas after blunt trauma identified at laparotomy for other injuries should only be explored if it appears that the hematoma is expanding because this likely indicates ongoing hemorrhage.

### Injuries to the Pelvis and Lower Extremities

Orthopedic injuries to the pelvis and extremities are extremely common and are covered in depth elsewhere in this text. An approach to management as it relates to the general or trauma surgeon is presented here. Orthopedic injuries constituted the greatest number of cases in the 2009 NTDB, with 27.5% of patients having upper extremity and 35.1% having lower extremity trauma. Fortunately, the mortality is low for each group, just below 4%, but the long-term morbidity can be high. Pelvic fractures alone were seen in 6.4% of cases and had a substantially greater mortality, approximately 9%. A variety of physical mechanisms are responsible for orthopedic injuries, with MVAs and falls being the most common causes.

Open fractures are frequently easy to identify on initial examination, as are those with severe deformity. Plain radiography remained highly effective for diagnosis but CT has attained a greater role, especially with complex fracture patterns. Pelvic fractures are typically identified on initial pelvic radiography and then better characterized if an abdominal or pelvic CT is obtained. Although CT demonstrates the bony injury accurately, it also can identify an associated hematoma and the presence or absence of active contrast extravasation, which appears as high- density material, frequently within the hematoma. Extremity examination must include a thorough vascular assessment and evaluation for compartment syndrome. Evidence of vascular insufficiency or bleeding may require angiography to localize and characterize the injury. The role of CT angiography of the extremities remains to be elucidated.

The diagnosis and management of hemorrhage from pelvic fractures represents a unique challenge that requires a standardized approach involving a number of disciplines. Figure 18-29 presents an approach to these injuries. Unstable patients should have a pelvic radiograph quickly obtained and interpreted for pelvic fracture. An important point is that although some pelvic fracture patterns are more likely to bleed, any fracture is capable of bleeding and should not be disregarded in the unstable patient. Pelvic fractures that demonstrate an increase in pelvic volume should be compressed with a pelvic binder or sheet wrapped around the hips to reduce the space available for hematoma formation. This will frequently manage venous bleeding. Ongoing instability suggests an arterial source, which should be addressed with angiography and embolization if these resources are available. Embolization may also be warranted in those patients, with active contrast extravasation identified by pelvic CT. Some recent work has suggested that packing of the pelvis may be an alternative to embolization, especially when endovascular therapy is not immediately available. Stabilization of the pelvic ring with external fixation is then performed to maintain reduction of the pelvic volume and reduce ongoing venous bleeding.

## REHABILITATION

Although the acute management of injuries plays the greatest role in the reduction of mortality, it is the process of rehabilitation that functions to reduce the morbidity of injury. The rehabilitation process can be substantially longer than the hospital phase of care and is indispensible in restoring functionality and allowing patients to return to productive lives after severe injury. Much emphasis is placed on trauma-related fatalities, but there were approximately 30 million nonfatal injuries in 2008, many of which were severe and required some form of rehabilitation.

The rehabilitation process begins soon after the acute needs of the injured patient have been met. Hospital physical and occupational therapists frequently begin the process by initiating therapy and assessing which resources may be required when the

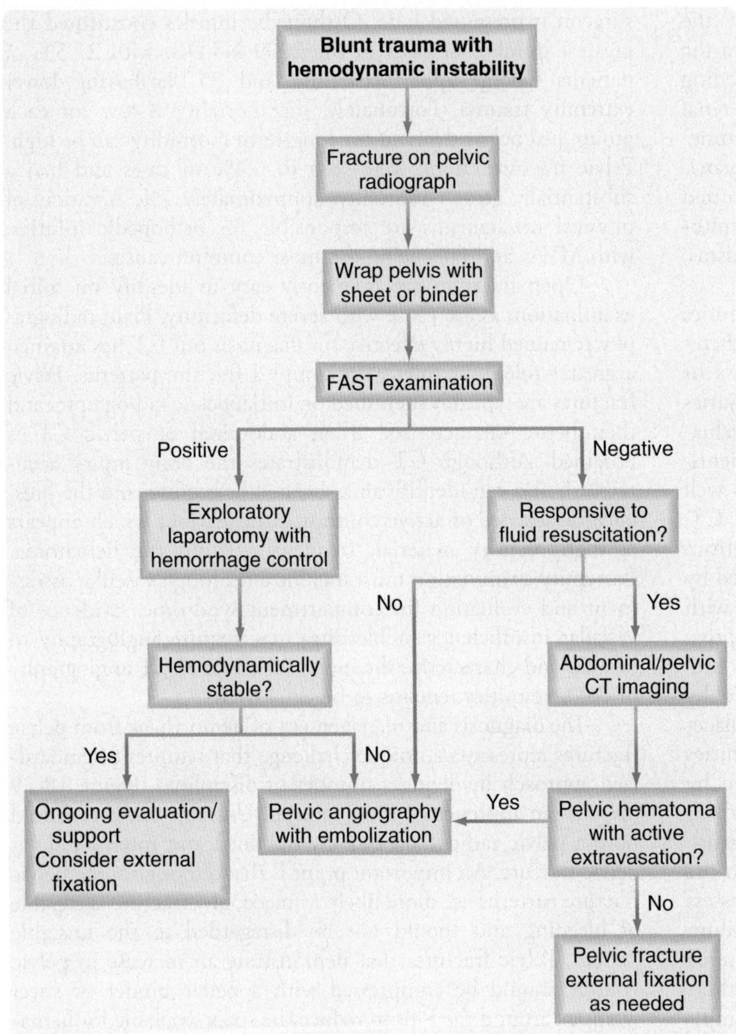


**FIGURE 18-29** Algorithm for the evaluation and management of pelvic fractures with associated hemorrhage.

patient leaves the hospital. With these recommendations available, case managers and social workers can begin the process of identifying available resources in the inpatient or outpatient setting to address the unique rehabilitation needs of the patient. More robust systems have regular input from the rehabilitation team to assist in expediting referrals and transfer to appropriate facilities. Many patients benefit from generic rehabilitation services, but some patient groups have unique needs, such as rehabilitation centers that focus on the recovery from traumatic brain and spinal cord injuries. These two patient cohorts have specific needs that are best addressed at centers with specialized expertise. Hospitals committed to the care of the injured patient must be sure to place adequate priority on reinforcing the rehabilitation process, because this clearly is one of the most important aspects of a patient's long-term recovery.

## SELECTED REFERENCES

American College of Surgeons: Advanced trauma life support for doctors, ed 8, Chicago, 2008, American College of Surgeons.

First released over 25 years ago, this ATLS course revolutionized the initial approach to the injured patient. The eighth edition contains the same systematic approach that has been taught since the initiation of the course, as well as a greater emphasis on the underlying support from the literature. This edition is the first to be released as a textbook rather than as a course manual and contains significantly revised text, tables, and figures.

Brain Trauma Foundation, American Association of Neurological Surgeons, Congress of Neurological Surgeons: Guidelines for the management of severe traumatic brain injury. J Neurotrauma 24(Suppl 1):S1–S106, 2007.

These guidelines represent the most comprehensive compilation of all literature related to traumatic brain injury. It is organized into evidence-based guidelines based on the strength of the associated studies. This document has been revised three times and therefore includes the most current published guidelines. Application of the guidelines has been associated with improved outcomes after traumatic brain injury.

Committee on Trauma, American College of Surgeons: Resources for the optimal care of the injured patient, ed 5, Chicago, 2006, American College of Surgeons.

This document outlines the necessary components for the optimal management of injured patients in a trauma center. Known as the *Green*

*Book*, this resource was developed by the Committee on Trauma and is frequently updated to remain current. The requirements to become verified as a trauma center and then maintain verification are contained within this document.

Feliciano DV, Mattox KL, Moore EE: Trauma, ed 6, New York, 2008, McGraw-Hill.

This textbook is the comprehensive resource for all injury specific information. Chapters incorporate all recent literature and provides an excellent presentation of all injuries sustained by the trauma patient. The text is frequently revised and chapters are written by world leaders in each specific subject matter.

MacKenzie EJ, Rivara FP, Jurkovich GJ, et al: A national evaluation of the effect of trauma-center care on mortality. N Engl J Med 354:366–378, 2006.

The National Study on Costs and Outcomes of Trauma (NSCOT), a large multicenter project supported by the Centers for Disease Control and Prevention, was initiated to define variations in injury care and outcomes between trauma and nontrauma centers. The project included over 5000 patients from 69 hospitals, spanning 12 states. This study demonstrated the benefit of care provided at a trauma center versus a nontrauma center. After correction for injury severity, trauma center care was associated with a reduction of in-hospital mortality (7.6% versus 9.5%; relative risk, 0.80; 95% confidence interval, 0.66 to 0.98), as well as 1-year mortality (10.4% versus 13.8%; relative risk, 0.75; 95% confidence interval, 0.60 to 0.95).

Nathens AB, Jurkovich GJ, Cummings P, et al: The effect of organized systems of trauma care on motor vehicle crash mortality. JAMA 283:1990–1994, 2000.

This study demonstrated the benefit of establishing a systematic method of managing trauma from the time of injury through the rehabilitation process. During a 17-year period, over 400,000 vehicle-related fatalities throughout the United States were evaluated to help establish a trauma system. The study identified a mortality benefit of 8% from trauma system development.

National Research Council: Accidental death and disability: The neglected disease of modern society, Washington, DC, 1966, National Academy of Sciences.

This landmark publication revealed the substandard way in, which injury and other emergency medical care was being provided in the United States. This document prompted the development of and improvement in emergency medical systems. Considered to be the white paper of emergency care, it provides valuable perspective regarding the maturation of modern emergency medical services.

Rotondo MF, Schwab CW, McGonigal MD, et al: "Damage control": An approach for improved survival in exsanguinating penetrating abdominal injury. J Trauma 35:375–383, 1993.

This article was the first to present the concept of damage control,, which has become the standard of care in managing multiple severe injuries. It was not until the development of this approach did surgeons use the abbreviation of abdominal surgery to prevent the deadly cycle of worsening hypothermia, coagulopathy, and acidosis. Based on the success of this methodology, other areas of trauma management, such as orthopedics and resuscitation, have developed similar approaches.

U.S. Department of Health and Human Services, Health Resources and Services Administration: Trauma-EMS systems program. Model trauma systems planning and evaluation. 2006. (www.ncdhhs.gov/dhsr/EMS/trauma/pdf/hrsatraumamodel.pdf).

In response to studies that demonstrated a paucity of trauma systems in the United States, the Health Resources and Services Administration released this document which outlines how systems for the management of injuries are developed and evaluated. It emphasizes the value of a public health approach to trauma care. It has also been valuable in securing governmental funding for trauma system development.

## REFERENCES


1. Committee on Trauma, American College of Surgeons: Resources for the optimal care of the injured patient, ed 5, Chicago, 2006, American College of Surgeons.
2. U.S. Department of Health and Human Services, Health Resources and Services Administration: Trauma–EMS systems program. Model trauma systems planning and evaluation. 2006. (www.ncdhhs.gov/dhsr/EMS/trauma/pdf/hrsatraumamodel.pdf).
3. Nathens AB, Jurkovich GJ, Cummings P, et al: The effect of organized systems of trauma care on motor vehicle crash mortality. JAMA 283:1990–1994, 2000.
4. MacKenzie EJ, Rivara FP, Jurkovich GJ, et al: A national evaluation of the effect of trauma-center care on mortality. N Engl J Med 354:366–378, 2006.
5. Baker SP, O'Neill B, Haddon W, et al: The injury severity score: A method for describing patients with multiple injuries and evaluating emergency care. J Trauma 14:187–196, 1974.
6. Tinkoff G, Esposito T, Reed J, et al: American Association for the Surgery of Trauma Organ Injury Scale I: Spleen, liver, and kidney, validation based on the National Trauma Data Bank. J Am Coll Surg 207:646–655, 2008.
7. Healey C, Osler TM, Rogers FB, et al: Improving the Glasgow coma scale: Motor score alone is a better predictor. J Trauma 54:671–680, 2003.
8. Eckstein M, Chan L, Schneir A, et al: Effect of prehospital advanced life support on outcomes of major trauma patients. J Trauma 48:643–648, 2000.
9. Winchell RJ, Hoyt DB: Endotracheal intubation in the field improves survival in patients with severe head injury. Arch Surg 132:592–597, 1997.
10. Bickell WH, Wall MJ, Jr, Pepe PE, et al: Immediate versus delayed fluid resuscitation for hypotensive patients with penetrating torso injuries. N Eng J Med 331:1105–1109, 1994.
11. Kragh JF, Jr, Walters TJ, Baer DG, et al: Survival with emergency tourniquet use to stop bleeding in major limb trauma. Ann Surg 249:1–7, 2009.
12. American College of Surgeons: Advanced trauma life support for doctors, ed 8, Chicago, 2008, American College of Surgeons.
13. Parmet JL, Colonna-Romano P, Horrow JC, et al: The laryngeal mask airway reliably provides rescue ventilation in cases of unanticipated difficult tracheal intubation along with difficult mask ventilation. Anesth Analg 87:661–665, 1998.
14. Asensio JA, Wall M, Minei J, et al; Working Group, Ad Hoc Subcommittee on Outcomes, American College of Surgeons

Committee on Trauma: Practice management guidelines for emergency department thoracotomy. J Am Coll Surg 193:303–309, 2001.

15. Rotondo MF, Schwab CW, McGonigal MD, et al: "Damage control": An approach for improved survival in exsanguinating penetrating abdominal injury. J Trauma 35:375–383, 1993.
16. Fox CJ, Gillespie DL, Cox ED: The effectiveness of a damage control resuscitation strategy for vascular injury in a combat support hospital: Results of a case control study. J Trauma 64:S99–S107, 2008.
17. Langlois JA, Rutland-Brown W, Thomas KE: Traumatic brain injury in the United States: emergency department visits, hospitalizations, and deaths, Atlanta, 2004, Centers for Disease Control and Prevention, National Center for Injury Prevention and Control.
18. Brain Trauma Foundation, American Association of Neurological Surgeons, Congress of Neurological Surgeons: Guidelines for the management of severe traumatic brain injury. J Neurotrauma 24(Suppl 1):S1–S106, 2007.
19. Bracken MB, Holford TR: Neurological and functional status 1 year after acute spinal cord injury: Estimates of functional recovery in National Acute Spinal Cord Injury Study II from results modeled in National Acute Spinal Cord Injury Study III. J Neurosurg 96:259–266, 2002.
20. Golueke PJ, Goldstein AS, Sclafani SJ, et al: Routine versus selective exploration of penetrating neck injuries: A randomized prospective study. J Trauma 24:1010–1014, 1984.
21. Biffl WL, Moore EE, Offner PJ, et al: Optimizing screening for blunt cerebrovascular injuries. Am J Surg 178:517–522, 1999.
22. Eastman AL, Chason DP, Perez CL, et al: Computed tomographic angiography for the diagnosis of blunt cervical vascular injury: Is it ready for prime time? J Trauma 60:925–929, 2006.
23. Biffl WL, Cothren CC, Moore EE, et al: Western Trauma Association critical decisions in trauma: Screening for and treatment of blunt cerebrovascular injuries. J Trauma 67:1150–1153, 2009.
24. Committee on Trauma, American College of Surgeons: National Trauma Data Bank annual report 2009, Chicago, 2009, American College of Surgeons.
25. Bulger EM, Edwards T, Klotz P, et al: Epidural analgesia improves outcome after multiple rib fractures. Surgery 136:426–430, 2004.
26. Karmy-Jones R, Jurkovich GJ, Shatz DV, et al: Management of traumatic lung injury: A Western Trauma Association multicenter review. J Trauma 51:1049–1053, 2001.
27. Richardson JD, Franz JL: Pulmonary contusion and hemorrhage—crystalloid versus colloid replacement. J Surg Res 16:330–336, 1974.
28. Kiser AC, O'Brien SM, Detterbeck FC: Blunt tracheobronchial injuries: Treatment and outcomes. Ann Thorac Surg 71:2059–2065, 2001.
29. McKenney M, Lentz K, Nunez D, et al: Can ultrasound replace diagnostic peritoneal lavage in the assessment of blunt trauma? J Trauma 37:439–441, 1994.
30. Holmes JF, Offerman SR, Chang CH, et al: Performance of helical computed tomography without oral contrast for the detection of GI injuries. Ann Emerg Med 43:120–128, 2004.
31. Biffl WL, Kaups KL, Cothren CC, et al: Management of patients with anterior abdominal stab wounds: A Western Trauma Association multicenter trial. J Trauma 66:1294–1301, 2009.
32. Peitzman AB, Heil B, Rivera L, et al: Blunt splenic injury in adults: Multi-institutional study of the Eastern Association for the Surgery of Trauma. J Trauma 49:177–189, 2000.
33. Nicholas JM, Parker Rix E, Easley KA, et al: Changing patterns in the management of penetrating abdominal trauma: The more things change, the more they stay the same. J Trauma 55:1095–1110, 2003.
34. Haan JM, Bochicchio GV, Kramer N, et al: Nonoperative management of blunt splenic injury: A 5-year experience. J Trauma 58:492–498, 2005.
35. Cocanour CS, Moore FA, Ware DN, et al: Age should not be a consideration for nonoperative management of blunt splenic injury. J Trauma 48:606–612, 2000.
36. Harbrecht BG, Peitzman AB, Rivera L, et al: Contribution of age and gender to outcome of blunt splenic injury in adults: Multicenter study of the Eastern Association for the Surgery of Trauma. J Trauma 51:887–895, 2001.
37. Cogbill TH, Moore EE, Jurkovich GJ, et al: Nonoperative management of blunt splenic trauma: A multicenter experience. J Trauma 29:1312–1317, 1989.
38. Richardson JD, Franklin GA, Lukan JK, et al: Evolution in the management of hepatic trauma: A 25-year perspective. Ann Surg 232:324–330, 2000.
39. Meredith JW, Young JS, Bowling J, et al: Nonoperative management of blunt hepatic trauma: The exception or the rule. J Trauma 36:529–535, 1994.
40. Croce MA, Fabian TC, Menke PG, et al: Nonoperative management of blunt hepatic trauma is the treatment of choice for hemodynamically stable patients. The results of a prospective trial. Ann Surg 221:744–753, 1995.
41. Duane TM, Como JJ, Bochicchio GV, et al: Reevaluating the management and outcomes of severe blunt liver injury. J Trauma 57:494–500, 2004.
42. Asensio JA, Roldàn G, Petrone P, et al: Operative management and outcomes in 103 AAST-OIS grades IV and V complex hepatic injuries: Trauma surgeons still need to operate, but angioembolization helps. J Trauma 54:647–654, 2003.
43. Watts DD, Fakry SM; EAST Multi-Institutional Hollow Viscus Injury Research Group: Incidence of hollow viscus injury in blunt trauma: An analysis from 276,557 trauma admissions from the EAST multi-institutional trial. J Trauma 54:289–294, 2003.
44. Phelan HA, Velmahos GC, Jurkovich GJ, et al: An evaluation of multidetector computed tomography in detecting pancreatic injury: results of a multicenter AAST study. J Trauma 66:641–647, 2009.
45. Peitzman AB, Makaroun MS, Slasky BS, et al: Prospective study of computed tomography in the initial management of blunt abdominal trauma. J Trauma 26:585–592, 1986.
46. Fabian TC, Kudsk KA, Croce MA, et al: Superiority of closed suction drainage for pancreatic trauma. A randomized, prospective study. Ann Surg 211:724–728, 1990.
47. Stone HH, Fabian TC: Management of perforating colon trauma: Randomization between primary closure and exteriorization. Ann Surg 190:430–436, 1979.
48. Demetriades D, Murray JA, Chan L, et al: Penetrating colon injuries requiring resection: Diversion or primary anastomosis? An AAST prospective multicenter study. J Trauma 50:765–775, 2001.
49. Miller PR, Chang MC, Hoth JJ, et al: Colonic resection in the setting of damage control laparotomy: Is delayed anastomosis safe? Am Surg 73:606–610, 2007.
50. Gonzalez RP, Falimirski ME, Holevar MR: The role of presacral drainage in the management of penetrating rectal injuries. J Trauma 45:656–661, 1998.

CHAPTER 19

# THE DIFFICULT ABDOMINAL WALL

Jose J. Diaz, William D. Dutton, and Richard S. Miller

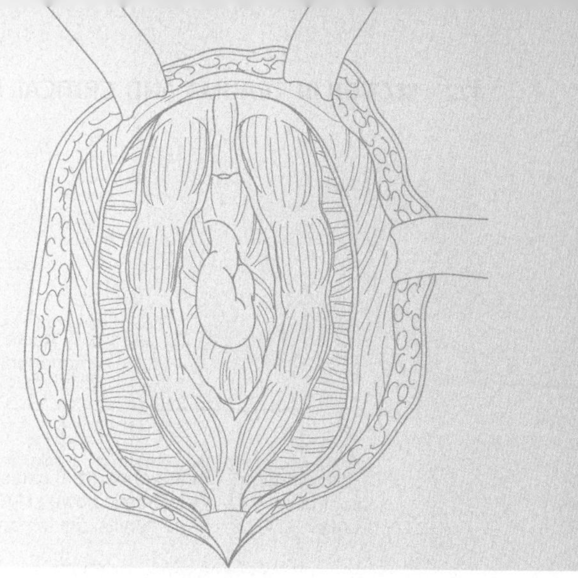



## ACUTE PRESENTATION

### Definitions and Management

The final step in a laparotomy is abdominal facial closure. Usually, the fascia and the skin are closed primarily. However, as medicine has advanced, surgeons have had to treat sicker patients with a higher burden of advanced comorbid disease. In the trauma setting, the clinical success of nonoperative management of solid organ injuries has reduced the total number of operative cases. However, trauma patients requiring operation are often at their physiologic limits. Techniques in damage control have become essential adjuncts in trauma, general, and vascular surgery.

Stone and Lucas and colleagues[1,2] in the 1980s and Rotondo and Morris[3,4] and associates in the 1990s defined the primary goals of damage control surgery in the trauma patient, which included the initial three phases we know today. Fabian and coworkers[5] have described the five phases of damage control surgery, from the initial operation to restoration of abdominal wall integrity:

Phase 1: Emergent laparotomy with control of bleeding and contamination, abdominal packing of medical bleeding, and abbreviated abdominal wound closure
Phase 2: Resuscitation: Correction of end points of resuscitation—hypothermia, coagulopathy, and acidosis
Phase 3: Reexploration, staged abdominal repair, and delayed primary fascial closure[4]
Phase 4: Planned ventral hernia
Phase 5: Abdominal wall reconstruction (Fig. 19-1)

During phase 3, the abdominal fascia is closed more than 65% of the time. All intra-abdominal injuries are repaired, peritonitis controlled, and other disease states corrected. However, there may still be unresolved visceral edema and/or loss of domain with retraction of the abdominal wall. This is the most common scenario giving rise to the difficult abdominal wall. The goal of delayed primary fascial closure is to have the fascia closed within 8 days. Complications increase exponentially after this point, including intra-abdominal abscess and formation of intestinal fistulas, which can increase to 25% to 45%.[6] However, the risk of developing intra-abdominal hypertension or abdominal compartment syndrome, ongoing inflammatory response syndrome, lack of source control, and/or intra-abdominal abscess or intestinal fistula may be reason enough to delay primary closure of the abdominal fascia (Box 19-1).

### Intra-Abdominal Hypertension or Abdominal Compartment Syndrome Complicating the Difficult Abdominal Wall

Once reexploration and staged abdominal reconstruction have been completed, the next goal is to close the abdomen with the least amount of physiologic stress. Intra-abdominal hypertension is known to cause ischemia to the viscera and abdominal wall, which can progress to abdominal compartment syndrome with organ dysfunction. In 2004, the World Congress of Abdominal Compartment Syndrome met to develop consensus definitions for intra-abdominal hypertension and abdominal compartment syndrome.[7,8] These consensus definitions are used to define intra-abdominal hypertension and primary, secondary, and recurrent abdominal compartment syndrome. The World Congress of Abdominal Compartment Syndrome definitions have helped further define the disease processes of intra-abdominal hypertension and abdominal compartment syndrome (Boxes 19-2 and 19-3). Abdominal compartment syndrome is not necessarily an end stage process but a continuum of disease, which might be amenable to medical management at an earlier stage. Grade III intra-abdominal hypertension (intra-abdominal pressure >20 mm Hg) should be further monitored with intravesicular pressure monitoring. Medical therapies should be instituted at this point—supine positioning, judicious crystalloid resuscitation, and drainage of intra-abdominal fluid collections.[9] If these fail to improve intra-abdominal hypertension or organ dysfunction develops, serious consideration must be given to decompressive laparotomy. Other therapies to decrease intra-abdominal hypertension may include neuromuscular blockade, increased sedation, diuresis, evacuation of intra-luminal contents, and hemodialysis or hemofiltration.

Abdominal decompression lowers intra-abdominal hypertension and results in improvement in lung dynamic compliance.[10] Bladder pressures higher than 25 mm Hg have been

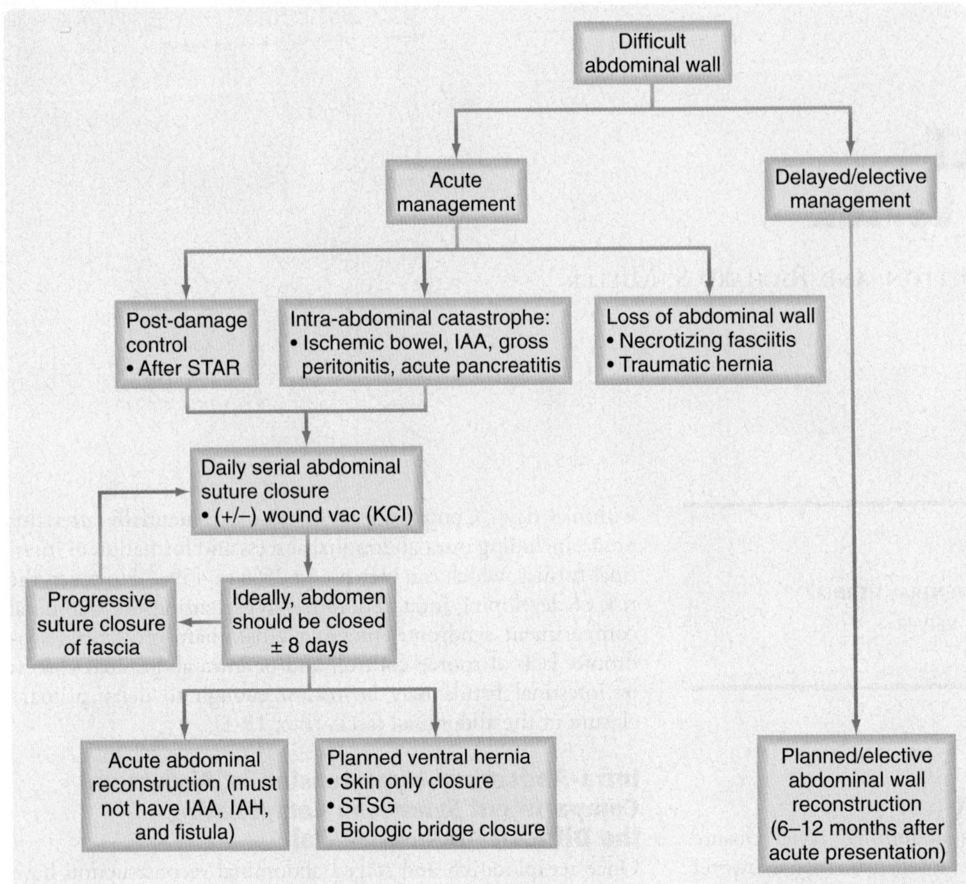


**FIGURE 19-1** Flow diagram of the difficult abdominal wall.

**BOX 19-1 Causative Factors Leading to Open Abdomen**

- Abdominal compartment syndrome
- Trauma—damage control
- Acute pancreatitis
- Emergency general surgery or abdominal sepsis
- Vascular emergencies

**BOX 19-2 World Congress Abdominal Compartment Syndrome Definitions: Intra-Abdominal Hypertension and Abdominal Compartment Syndrome**

Normal intra-abdominal pressure is ≈5-7 mm Hg in critically ill adults.

Intra-abdominal hypertension is defined by a sustained or repeated pathologic elevation in intra-abdominal pressure ≥12 mm Hg.

Intra-abdominal hypertension is graded as follows (in mm Hg):

- Grade I: Intra-abdominal pressure, 12-15
- Grade II: Intra-abdominal pressure, 16-20
- Grade III: Intra-abdominal pressure, 21-25
- Grade IV: Intra-abdominal pressure, >25

Abdominal compartment syndrome is defined as a sustained intra-abdominal pressure >20 mm Hg (with or without abdominal perfusion pressure <60 mm Hg) associated with new organ dysfunction or failure.

**BOX 19-3 Types of Abdominal Compartment Syndrome**

- Primary abdominal compartment syndrome is a condition associated with injury or disease in the abdominopelvic region that frequently requires early surgical or interventional radiologic intervention.
- Secondary abdominal compartment syndrome refers to conditions that do not originate from the abdominopelvic region.
- Recurrent abdominal compartment syndrome refers to the condition in which abdominal compartment syndrome redevelops following previous surgical or medical treatment of primary or secondary abdominal compartment syndrome.

suggested to indicate abdominal compartment syndrome.[11] Using the definition of abdominal compartment syndrome—the development of significant respiratory compromise, including elevated inspiratory pressure (≈35 cm $H_2O$), renal dysfunction (urine <30 mL/hr), hemodynamic instability requiring catecholamines, and a rigid or tense abdomen, it has been found that in these patients, emergency abdominal decompression results in a significant increase in the cardiac index, tidal volume, and urine output, with a resultant decrease in bladder pressure, heart rate, central venous pressure, pulmonary artery occlusion pressure, peak airway pressure, partial pressure of arterial carbon dioxide, and lactate level. Abdominal decompression may also be of benefit in the setting of increased intracranial pressure.

Secondary abdominal compartment syndrome may occur after exsanguination from an extremity injury and/or when massive volume resuscitation is required. Recurrent abdominal compartment syndrome occurs after damage control in a patient with an open abdomen with ongoing hemorrhage or massive volume resuscitation. In all scenarios, intra-abdominal pressure should be monitored.[12,13]

### Abdominal Catastrophe Complicating the Difficult Abdominal Wall

Tissue loss of the abdominal wall posses a uniquely difficult problem. Blast, shear, and penetrating traumatic injuries and necrotizing skin and soft tissue infections can all result in significant tissue loss. Loss of abdominal wall tissue will require creative temporary abdominal closure, with the goal of maintaining integrity of the bowel. In these clinical scenarios, a definitive repair of the abdominal wall defect may require the use of autologous tissue or biologic or synthetic mesh. In severe cases, acute primary repair of the ventral hernia is not recommended because of the high incidence of gastrointestinal contamination, resolving source control of infection, and continued risk of wound infection. In these cases, synthetic mesh is contraindicated because of the high risk of mesh infection.[14]

### Other Conditions Complicating the Difficult Abdominal Wall

After the abdomen has been opened, adhesions develop and the viscera will become cocooned. This makes reexploration of the bowel for fistula repair or bowel obstructions almost impossible without causing further injury. The development of bowel fistula will commonly occur at the site of an anastomosis, but may be in exposed small bowel not previously injured.[6,15]

After any traumatic or emergency laparotomy in which bleeding and gastrointestinal injury occurred, the risk of an intra-abdominal abscess can be as high as 25% to 35%.[6] Most intra-abdominal abscesses can be percutaneously drained, but may still require open drainage. In the setting of intra-abdominal abscess, enteroatmospheric fistula, tissue loss, loss of abdominal domain, and massive visceral edema, the safest course in an open abdomen is to proceed with a planned ventral hernia.

## TEMPORARY ABDOMINAL CLOSURE

### Techniques

The development of the open abdomen technique has posed a new problem—how to close the abdomen temporarily in a way that is easy to apply, tension-free, atraumatic, and inexpensive, and allows for a high rate of delayed primary fascial closure. The options for temporary abdominal closure can be broadly classified as dynamic (securing a device to the fascial edges for serial approximation to achieve delayed primary fascial closure) or tension-free (atraumatic abdominal visceral coverage). Current and historical techniques are presented in Table 19-1. The most widely used delayed primary fascial closure techniques now used in the United States are the artificial burr, vacuum pack, and commercially available vacuum pack device.

**Table 19-1 Current and Historical* Techniques for Temporary Abdominal Closure**

| TECHNIQUE | DESCRIPTION | MECHANISM |
|---|---|---|
| Vacuum-assisted closure (VAC) | A perforated plastic sheet covers the viscera and a sponge is placed between the fascial edges. The wound is covered by an airtight seal, which is pierced by a suction drain connected to a suction pump and fluid collection system. | The (active and adjustable) negative pressure supplied by the pump keeps constant tension on the fascial edges while it collects excess abdominal fluid and helps resolve edema. |
| Vacuum pack | A perforated plastic sheet covers the viscera, damp surgical towels are placed in the wound, and a surgical drain is placed on the towels. An airtight seal covers the wound and negative pressure is applied through the drain. | The negative pressure keeps constant tension on the fascial edges and excess fluid is collected. |
| Artificial burr (Wittmann patch) | Two opposite Velcro sheets (hooks and loops, one on each side) are sutured to the fascial edges. The Velcro sheets connect in the middle. | This technique allows for easy access and stepwise reapproximation of the fascial edges. |
| Dynamic retention sutures | The viscera are covered with a sheet (e.g., ISODrape, Microtek [Microban], Huntersville, NC). Horizontal sutures are placed through a large-diameter catheter and through the entire abdominal wall on both sides. | The sutures keep tension on the fascia and may be tightened to allow staged reapproximation of the fascial edges. This may be combined with a vacuum system. |
| Plastic silo (Bogota bag) | A sterile x-ray film cassette bag or sterile 3-liter urology irrigation bag is sutured between the fascial edges or the skin and opened in the middle. | This is an easy technique that allows for easy access. The bag may be reduced in size to approximate the fascial edges. |
| Mesh, sheet | An absorbable or nonabsorbable mesh or sheet is sutured between the fascial edges. Examples are Dexon, Marlex, or Vicryl mesh. Examples of sheets are Silastic or silicone sheets. | The mesh or sheet may be reduced in size to allow for reapproximation. Nonresorbable meshes may be removed or left in place at the end of the open abdominal period. |
| Loose packing* | The fascial defect is covered by standard wound dressing only. | This technique is simple but does not prevent fascial retraction. |
| Skin approximation | The skin is closed over the fascial defect with towel clips or a running suture. | Skin provides a natural cover for the viscera, but the towel clips obstruct radiologic imaging and do not prevent fascial retraction. |
| Zipper* | A mesh or sheet with a sterilized zipper is sutured between the fascial edges. | This technique is comparable to the mesh/sheet and allows for easy access. |

*Denotes a historical technique.

The artificial burr consists of two sheets of hook and burr material, similar to Velcro, that is sewn to the fascial edges after a plastic drape is placed over the viscera. The hook and burr is then overlapped with limited tension to provide a secure temporary abdominal closure. Gauze is used to pack the subcutaneous tissue.[16] Pulling the Velcro-like material apart easily allows reexploration of the abdomen. At the completion of the subsequent operations, the patch can be tightened to keep fascial tension. Repeated tightening allows for a sequential approximation of the fascia until it can be closed without undue tension. In 2009, Van Hensbroek and colleagues[17] have suggested that the artificial burr, along with dynamic retention sutures paired with a commercially available vacuum pack device, have the highest success in fascial closure rates.

In 1995, Brock and associates[18] first described the vacuum pack, which is a three-layer temporary abdominal closure. A fenestrated polyvinyl sheet is draped over the exposed viscera and tucked under the fascial edges. A surgical towel is placed under the fascia, followed by two silicone drains, which are placed on top of the towel. An adhesive, iodophor-impregnated polyester drape is placed over the skin laterally to the anterior axillary lines to seal the wound. The surgical drains are connected to a wall suction, creating a negative-pressure dressing. The vacuum pack–negative-pressure temporary abdominal closure has gained wide acceptance because it can be applied quickly, is inexpensive and atraumatic, and allows for control of abdominal fluids. It is cost-effective. approximately $50/application.[17] In most of this trauma population, delayed primary fascial closure was possible at the second laparotomy. Although delayed primary fascial closure is less common in the emergent surgery population, combined fascial closure rates as high as 68% have been demonstrated.[19] Fistula and leak rates are no different than with other types of temporary abdominal closure (TAC), with reported fistula rates of 3% to 5%.[19,20]

A commercial version of the vacuum pack is available. Results have been similar to primary fascial closure and complication rates comparable to the vacuum pack. A modification of the technique, incorporating dynamic serial fascial closure in conjunction with a commercial vacuum pack, has demonstrated 90% delayed primary fascial closure rates. This technique extends beyond the 8-day benchmark, with low complication rates in some series.[19,21] A recent review has suggested that the vacuum pack and artificial burr are associated with the highest closure rates as well as the lowest mortality rates.[17]

### Assessing Readiness for Abdominal Closure

Patients are prepared to return for reconstruction of internal injuries[22] once they have been adequately resuscitated.[4] The goal of resuscitation is correction of hypothermia, coagulopathy, and acidosis. For the trauma patient, this can usually be accomplished within 36 hours. Recent clinical advances in the care for the critically ill and trauma patient have decreased the time to adequate resuscitation. Transfusion exsanguination protocols[23,24] have minimized the use of excessive crystalloid fluids.[25] Injured devitalized tissue is resected and gastrointestinal injuries can be anastomosed safely, mitigating the need for enterostomy. However, for high-risk patients (e.g., those with sepsis related to gastrointestinal perforation, severe postoperative bleeding, intraoperative hypotension), enterostomy remains the most conservative approach.[26]

Staging abdominal reconstruction serves three main functions—reduction of contamination and control of intra-abdominal sepsis, débridement of devitalized or contaminated tissue, and reconstruction. These techniques have been shown to improve outcomes in severely injured trauma patients.[27] Relaparotomy with routinely scheduled abdominal washout has been used as a means to manage the patient with severe intra-abdominal sepsis effectively. It has been well tolerated, with few gastrointestinal complications and lower mortality.[28,29] Use of this technique in severe necrotizing pancreatitis, in general, has correlated with improved mortality, although there have been mixed results in less severe cases.[14-16]

Source control remains the priority in most patients managed with an open abdomen. Clinical parameters such as renal dysfunction values, Acute Physiology and Chronic Health Evaluation score II (APACHE II), and multiorgan dysfunction score may be predictive of ongoing intra-abdominal sepsis[30,31] and can be used as indications for relaparotomy.[22,28] Patients who tolerate fascial closure had significantly lower scores than those with ongoing sepsis.

It is important to assess bladder pressure prior to closure of the abdomen.[32] Sustained intra-abdominal hypertension (15 to 20 mm Hg) and a rise of peak inspiratory pressure of 10 cm $H_2O$ during attempts at fascial closure are warning signs of high fascial tension, with the potential for vascular compromise to the abdominal wall and viscera. Closure of the fascia at a later date or a planned ventral hernia may be prudent for this subgroup of critically ill patients with an open abdomen.[7,9]

## ABDOMINAL CLOSURE OR PLANNED VENTRAL HERNIA?

After damage control surgery, patients commonly may leave the operating room with an open abdomen. Several key steps are advisable at reexploration:

1. Place a postligament of Treitz nasoenteral feeding access.
2. Preserve viable omentum; this will help protect the bowel.[33]
3. Place ostomies laterally to the rectus to preserve the rectus fascia for subsequent closure.
4. Leave the fascia open if there is more than a 10-cm $H_2O$ increase in peak airway pressures during attempted fascial closure.[34]

The complication rate with an open abdomen can be as high as 50%, with three clinical scenarios: (1) attempts at closing the fascia primarily under too much tension; (2) awaiting the formation of granulation tissue; and (3) using synthetic material for bridge closure.[35] The most serious and labor-intensive complication related to the open abdomen is the development of an enteroatmospheric fistula. This is defined as an intestinal fistula with bowel mucosa at the level of an open abdominal wound. It can occur at an anastomotic site or at the injured bowel; even uninjured exposed bowel can become traumatized to the point of developing a fistula in the absence of any overlying soft tissue coverage.[34] Once a fistula forms, the adjacent viscera must be protected and the effluent controlled.

Several novel techniques for enteroatmospheric fistula wound management have been described using stoma material and commercially available vacuum systems.[36-39] It is inadvisable to repair this type of fistula acutely in the inflamed surgical field and in a malnourished patient. A planned ventral hernia with control of the effluent is usually the safest option. Intubation of the fistula in the middle of a fixed visceral block is not recommended. Elective repair of the fistula should be delayed for several months when the fistula can be resected in conjunction with a delayed abdominal wall reconstruction. Closure of an enteroatmospheric fistula and/or stoma in the presence of a large abdominal wall defect is a challenging problem and is associated with a high complication rate. Several authors have suggested that this subgroup of patients can be managed in specialized units with added expertise in complex reconstruction.[36,40]

If the fascia cannot be approximated within the first 36 to 48 hours, dynamic serial partial closure is an option. Interrupted absorbable sutures are placed at the upper and lower portions of the abdominal wound; this can assist in maintaining the abdominal domain. Additionally, early enteral feeding (less than 4 days) has been associated with successful abdominal fascia closure and decreased fistula formation.[34] If the fascia cannot be primarily closed by day 8, decisions about abdominal visceral coverage must be considered. This can be achieved with two options, skin closure only or application of a skin graft. Prior to placing a skin graft, the fascial defect must be closed with an absorbable or biologic mesh. A granulation bed will develop that can accept a skin graft.

Creation of large skin flaps for skin only closure or performing acute component separation for a definitive repair of the abdominal wall defect is not recommended. These patients have significant soft tissue edema, may have unresolved infectious complications, and are commonly severely malnourished. Attempted early definitive closure may lead to major wound complications, including wound infection, skin flap necrosis, and loss of tissue options for definitive hernia repair.

The use of nonabsorbable synthetic mesh material in an open abdominal wound is not recommended because of the high rate of mesh infections, fibrosis, and fistula formation. Recently, biologic dermal matrix meshes have been commercially developed from human or animal sources. The primary use is for the surgical repair of complex abdominal wall defects. Although significantly more expensive than absorbable synthetic mesh, there are theoretical advantages for the use of biologic meshes over other techniques for bridging a fascial gap during the initial open abdomen phase. These include prevention of bowel desiccation and fistula formation, providing better integrity of the abdominal wall, accelerating angiogenesis and wound repair, achieving a biologic barrier to bacterial invasion, and allowing easier access to the peritoneal cavity for tentative abdominal wall reconstruction at a later time.[41,42]

In the acute setting, a bridge fascial repair with a biologic mesh will commonly result in bulging and laxity of the repair, which has been defined as a recurrence of the fascial defect. Several authors have demonstrated development of a bulge and hernia recurrence.[43,44] However, this technique may reduce the incidence of an enteroatmospheric fistula. If the skin cannot be closed over a biologic mesh, it is essential to keep it moist to promote granulation tissue formation and prevent desiccation. Silver topical antimicrobial dressings are effective for reducing the microbial burden and can improve the take of a split-thickness skin graft.[43,44]

## ELECTIVE PLANNED VENTRAL HERNIA REPAIR

### Dynamic Abdominal Wall Reconstruction

Once the patient has recovered from all the injuries and malnutrition has been corrected, a definitive abdominal wall reconstruction can be performed. Autologous tissue is the ideal choice for repairing this type of fascia defect, especially in a setting in which a bowel procedure would be performed. Preoperative computed tomography scanning is essential to obtain a complete picture of the abdominal wall and intra-abdominal anatomy and determine which tissue components are missing or inadequate and which can be used for reconstruction. The primary goal for this procedure is to reapproximate the rectus fascia and achieve a functional, dynamic abdominal wall. This is now accomplished using the Ramirez technique for the separation of myocutaneous flaps.[45] This allows the rectus muscle to be mobilized medially while releasing the external oblique, which will limit the mobilization. This technique can close defects up to 10 cm in the upper abdomen, 20 cm in the midabdomen, and 6 to 8 cm in the lower abdomen. Several modifications of the component separation technique have been described.[5]

### Component Separation

Component separation is classically described as separation of parts of the anterior abdominal wall. This is accomplished by division of the rectus, separation of the anterior rectus sheath and muscle from the posterior rectus sheath, and complete mobilization, ending with three suture lines. A single, lateral, relaxing incision anterior to the external oblique may be added to gain additional mobilization. The open book modification includes rotation of the anterior or posterior rectus fascia to increase the distance covered in the midabdomen.

The procedure is generally divided into the following critical steps:

1. The skin graft is removed over the abdominal viscera.
2. The viscera is freed from the abdominal wall to allow the abdominal wall to be mobilized medially. This may include extensive enterolysis and/or reversal of skin level ostomy.
3. Skin flaps are raised to expose the rectus and external oblique junction.
4. Relaxing incision are made in the external oblique from the anterior superior iliac spine to above the costal margin (Fig. 19-2).
5. The rectus is closed in the midline.
6. Biologic mesh can be used as an underlay (Fig. 19-3) and/or onlay (Fig. 19-4) to buttress the repair.

The hernia recurrence rate of a component separation repair alone is 22% to 32%. Reinforcing this closure using biologic mesh material has reduced hernia recurrence rates. It is important to achieve a wide underlay of the biologic matrix at least 3 to 5 cm lateral to the edge of the rectus fascia. This wide underlay is performed concurrently with the primary fascial closure, grasping a midline portion of the biologic material with a large absorbable suture so that it directly abuts the undersurface of the primary fascial repair.[46,47]

An overlay of biologic material can also be performed (sandwich technique) to reinforce the weakness in the lateral abdominal wall created by the component separation. One study using this multilayer reconstruction of the abdominal wall has found no recurrence rates at 16-month follow-up, with minimal complications.[48] The use of multiple closed suction drains under the skin flaps is necessary during these complex reconstructions to reduce seroma formation.[48]

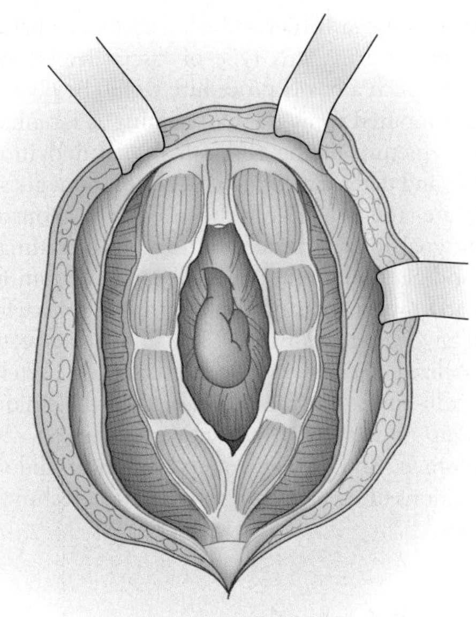

**FIGURE 19-2** Component separation, external oblique relaxing incision.

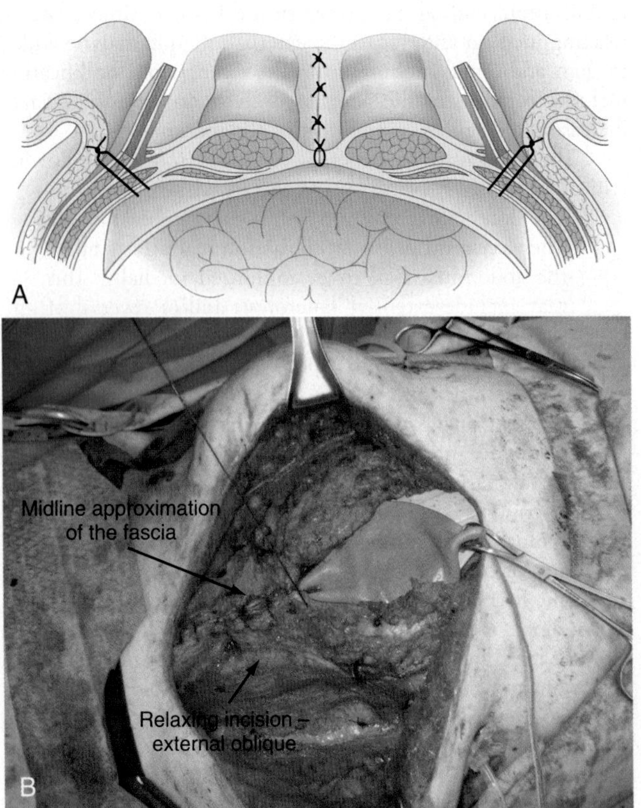


**FIGURE 19-3** Component separation with underlay technique **(A)** and underlay with biologic mesh **(B)**.

The Rives-Stoppa repair is another option for the complicated ventral hernia in a clean sterile surgical field.[49] This technique uses prosthetic mesh in a plane developed between the posterior rectus fascia and rectus muscle. An underlay of at least 5 to 10 cm from the lateral edge of the hernia defect and lateral

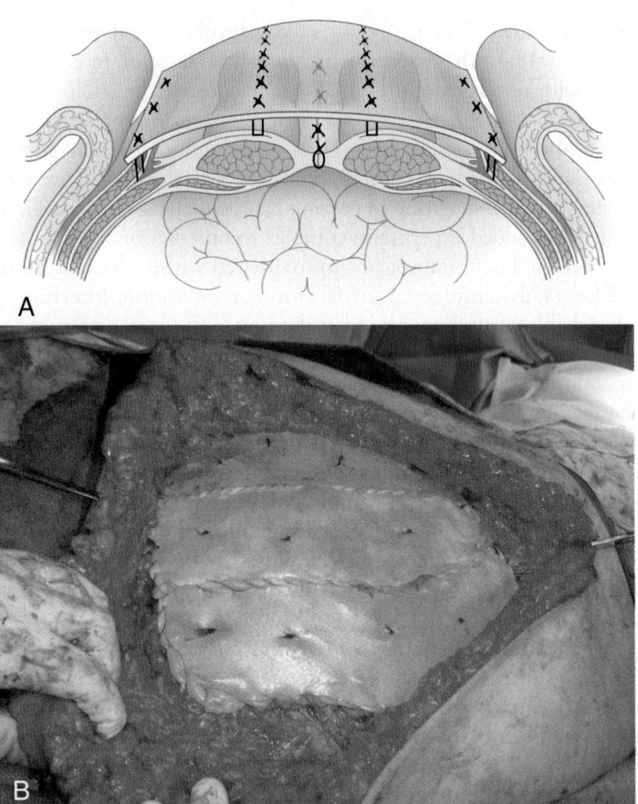


**FIGURE 19-4** Component separation with onlay technique **(A)** and onlay with biologic mesh **(B)**.

border of the prosthesis is necessary for adequate support. This procedure can be done extraperitoneally, thereby avoiding contact of the prosthetic mesh and viscera.

## SUMMARY

In most damage control laparotomies for trauma, vascular surgery, and/or emergency general surgery, primary fascial closure can be achieved in 60% to 90% of the cases. Patients for whom the abdomen cannot be closed make up the category of those with a difficult abdominal wall. This can then give rise to the complex ventral hernia. The causes of the difficult abdominal wall share features in common—loss of abdominal domain, risk of the development of intra-abdominal hypertension and/or abdominal compartment syndrome, development of intra-abdominal abscess or fistula, systemic inflammatory response syndrome, and a higher than 50% risk of hernia formation. When temporary coverage of the abdomen is necessary, the technique should be easy to apply, tension-free, atraumatic, and inexpensive and allow for a high rate of delayed primary fascial closure.

Following normalization of physiology, reexploration and a staged repair may be performed. It is not advisable to attempt delayed primary fascial closure if there is undue tension on the fascia or the peak inspiratory pressure rises more that 10 cm $H_2O$. However, the inability to close the open abdomen by 8 days is associated with a significant increase in complications, including enteroatmospheric fistulas. For this reason, some surgeons have bridged an abdominal wall defect with biologic mesh to protect the abdominal visceral. However, this repair should be considered as a temporizing measure because most bridging repairs will develop bulging and/or laxity within 1 year of closure. Delayed ventral hernia repair using component separation reinforced with biologic mesh has produced excellent results and is recommended for the closure of the complicated abdominal wall.

## SELECTED REFERENCES


Barker DE, Green JM, Maxwell RA, et al: Experience with vacuum-pack temporary abdominal wound closure in 258 trauma and general and vascular surgical patients. J Am Coll Surg 204:784–792, 2007.

This study describes 717 vacuum-pack closures that were performed in 258 surgical patients. Abdominal complications are described in detail.

Boele van Hensbroek P, Wind J, Dijkgraaf MG, et al: Temporary closure of the open abdomen: A systematic review on delayed primary fascial closure in patients with an open abdomen. World J Surg 33:199–207, 2009.

This study was designed to review the literature systematically to assess which TAC technique is associated with the highest delayed primary fascial closure (FC) rate. The techniques described were vacuum-assisted closure, vacuum pack, artificial burr, mesh or sheet, zipper, silo, skin closure, dynamic retention sutures, and loose packing.

Connolly PT, Teubner A, Lees NP, et al: Outcome of reconstructive surgery for intestinal fistula in the open abdomen. Ann Surg 247:440–444, 2008.

This is a discussion of the factors that influence the outcome of surgical techniques to close enterocutaneous fistulas within the open abdomen. Simultaneous reconstruction of the intestinal tract and abdominal wall remains associated with a high complication rate, justifying the management of such patients in specialized units.

Diaz JJ, Jr, Conquest AM, Ferzoco SJ, et al: Multi-institutional experience using human acellular dermal matrix for ventral hernia repair in a compromised surgical field. Arch Surg 144:209–215, 2009.

Four academic medical centers evaluate human acellular dermal matrix suitability for complex ventral hernia repair (CVHR). The hernia recurrence rate with human acellular dermal matrix in a compromised surgical field is less than that seen with primary repair, offering additional and improved surgical options for CVHR in this group of patients. Stoma or fistula takedown at the time of CVHR continues to be associated with significant complications.

de Vries Reilingh TS, van Goor H, Rosman C, et al: "Components separation technique" for the repair of large abdominal wall hernias. J Am Coll Surg 196:32–37, 2003.

This study evaluates the use of the component separation technique as a method for abdominal wall reconstruction. Special attention is dedicated to the reconstruction of large abdominal wall hernias, especially under contaminated conditions, in which the use of prosthetic material is contraindicated.

Fabian TC, Croce MA, Pritchard FE, et al: Planned ventral hernia. Staged management for acute abdominal wall defects. Ann Surg 219:643–650, 1994.

An analysis of a staged management scheme for the initial and definitive management of acute abdominal wall defects is provided. A four-stage scheme for managing acute abdominal wall defects is described: stage I—prosthetic insertion; stage II—2 to 3 weeks after prosthetic insertion and wound granulation, remal of prosthesis; stage III—2 to 3 days later, planned ventral hernia (split-thickness skin graft or full-thickness skin and subcutaneous fat graft); stage IV—6 to 12 months later, definitive reconstruction. Cases were evaluated retrospectively for the benefits and risks of the techniques used.

Miller RS, Morris JA, Jr, Diaz JJ, Jr, et al: Complications after 344 damage-control open celiotomies. J Trauma 59:1365–1371, 2005.

This study evaluated a large number of damage control abdomens. Morbidity is associated with the timing and method of wound closure and transfusion volume, but is independent of injury severity. Best outcomes with delayed primary fascial closure before 8 days.

Morris JA, Jr, Eddy VA, Blinman TA, et al: The staged celiotomy for trauma. Issues in unpacking and reconstruction. Ann Surg 217:576–584, 1993.

This article describes the important clinical events and decisions surrounding the reconstruction/unpacking portion of the staged celiotomy for trauma. The authors examined medical records to identify and characterize indications and timing of reconstruction, criteria for emergency return to the operating room, complications after reconstruction, and abdominal compartment syndrome (ACS).

Ramirez OM, Ruas E, Dellon AL: "Components separation" method for closure of abdominal-wall defects: An anatomic and clinical study. Plast Reconstr Surg 86:519–526, 1990.

This study suggests that large abdominal wall defects can be reconstructed with functional transfer of abdominal wall components without the need for the distant transposition of free muscle flaps. This demonstrated that the external oblique muscle can be separated from the internal oblique in a relatively avascular plane. The rectus muscle, with its overlying rectus fascia, can be elevated from the posterior rectus sheath. The compound flap of the rectus muscle, with its attached internal oblique transversus abdominis muscle, can be advanced 10 cm around the waistline.

Schecter WP, Hirshberg A, Chang DS, et al: Enteric fistulas: Principles of management. J Am Coll Surg 209:484–491, 2009.

The aim of this review is to present current principles in the management of enteric fistulas. Traditional management principles are evaluated to improve management and better understand the physiology and natural history of enteric fistulas.

Stone HH, Strom PR, Mullins RJ: Management of the major coagulopathy with onset during laparotomy. Annals of Surgery 197:532–535, 1983.

This is a classic description of the technique of abreviated laparotomy, abdominal packing, and correction of coagulopathy in 31 patients with an acceptable level of survival in previously nonsalvageable situations.

## REFERENCES


1. Lucas CE, Ledgerwood AM: Prospective evaluation of hemostatic techniques for liver injuries. J Trauma 16:442–451, 1976.
2. Stone HH, Strom PR, Mullins RJ: Management of the major coagulopathy with onset during laparotomy. Ann Surg 197:532–535, 1983.
3. Rotondo MF, Schwab CW, McGonigal MD, et al: "Damage control": An approach for improved survival in exsanguinating penetrating abdominal injury. J Trauma 35:375–382, 1993.
4. Morris JA, Jr, Eddy VA, Blinman TA, et al: The staged celiotomy for trauma. Issues in unpacking and reconstruction. Ann Surg 217:576–584, 1993.
5. Fabian TC, Croce MA, Pritchard FE, et al: Planned ventral hernia. Staged management for acute abdominal wall defects. Ann Surg 219:643–650, 1994.
6. Miller RS, Morris JA, Jr, Diaz JJ, Jr, et al: Complications after 344 damage-control open celiotomies. J Trauma 59:1365–1371, 2005.
7. Malbrain ML, Cheatham ML, Kirkpatrick A, et al: Results from the International Conference of Experts on Intra-abdominal Hypertension and Abdominal Compartment Syndrome. I. Definitions Intens Care Med 32:1722–1732, 2006.
8. Cheatham ML, Malbrain ML, Kirkpatrick A, et al: Results from the International Conference of Experts on Intra-abdominal Hypertension and Abdominal Compartment Syndrome. II. Recommendations. Intensive Care Med 33:951–962, 2007.
9. Cheatham ML: Nonoperative management of intra-abdominal hypertension and abdominal compartment syndrome. World J Surg 33:1116–1122, 2009.
10. Sugrue M, Jones F, Janjua KJ, et al: Temporary abdominal closure: A prospective evaluation of its effects on renal and respiratory physiology. J Trauma 45:914–921, 1998.
11. Ertel W, Oberholzer A, Platz A, et al: Incidence and clinical pattern of the abdominal compartment syndrome after "damage-control" laparotomy in 311 patients with severe abdominal and/or pelvic trauma. Crit Care Med 28:1747–1753, 2000.
12. Balogh Z, McKinley BA, Holcomb JB, et al: Both primary and secondary abdominal compartment syndrome can be predicted early and are harbingers of multiple organ failure. J Trauma 54:848–859, 2003.
13. Gracias VH, Braslow B, Johnson J, et al: Abdominal compartment syndrome in the open abdomen. Arch Surg 137:1298–1300, 2002.
14. Mayberry JC, Burgess EA, Goldman RK, et al: Enterocutaneous fistula and ventral hernia after absorbable mesh prosthesis closure for trauma: The plain truth. J Trauma 57:157–162, 2004.
15. Diaz JJ, Jr, Mejia V, Subhawong AP, et al: Protocol for bedside laparotomy in trauma and emergency general surgery: A low return to the operating room. Am Surg 71:986–991, 2005.
16. Wittmann DH, Aprahamian C, Bergstein JM, et al: A burr-like device to facilitate temporary abdominal closure in planned multiple laparotomies. Eur J Surg 159:75–79, 1993.
17. Boele van Hensbroek P, Wind J, Dijkgraaf MG, et al: Temporary closure of the open abdomen: A systematic review on delayed primary fascial closure in patients with an open abdomen. World J Surg 33:199–207, 2009.
18. Brock WB, Barker DE, Burns RP: Temporary closure of open abdominal wounds: The vacuum pack. Am Surg 61:30–35, 1995.
19. Barker DE, Green JM, Maxwell RA, et al: Experience with vacuum-pack temporary abdominal wound closure in 258 trauma and general and vascular surgical patients. J Am Coll Surg 204:784–792, 2007.
20. Navsaria PH, Bunting M, Omoshoro-Jones J, et al: Temporary closure of open abdominal wounds by the modified sandwich-vacuum pack technique. Br J Surg 90:718–722, 2003.
21. Cipolla J, Stawicki SP, Hoff WS, et al: A proposed algorithm for managing the open abdomen. Am Surg 71:202–207, 2005.
22. Holzheimer RG, Gathof B: Re-operation for complicated secondary peritonitis—how to identify patients at risk for persistent sepsis. Eur J Med Res 8:125–134, 2003.
23. Cotton BA, Gunter OL, Isbell J, et al: Damage control hematology: The impact of a trauma exsanguination protocol on survival and blood product utilization. J Trauma 64:1177–1182, 2008.
24. Duchesne JC, Hunt JP, Wahl G, et al: Review of current blood transfusions strategies in a mature level I trauma center: Were we wrong for the last 60 years? J Trauma 65:272–276, 2008.
25. Cotton BA, Au BK, Nunez TC, et al: Predefined massive transfusion protocols are associated with a reduction in organ failure and postinjury complications. J Trauma 66:41–48, 2009.
26. Weinberg JA, Griffin RL, Vandromme MJ, et al: Management of colon wounds in the setting of damage control laparotomy: A cautionary tale. J Trauma 67:929–935, 2009.
27. Hirshberg A, Wall MJ, Jr, Mattox KL: Planned reoperation for trauma: A two-year experience with 124 consecutive patients. J Trauma 37:365–369, 1994.
28. Stawicki SP, Brooks A, Bilski T, et al: The concept of damage control: Extending the paradigm to emergency general surgery. Injury 39:93–101, 2008.
29. Wittmann DH, Aprahamian C, Bergstein JM: Etappenlavage: Advanced diffuse peritonitis managed by planned multiple laparotomies utilizing zippers, slide fastener, and Velcro analogue for temporary abdominal closure. World J Surg 14:218–226, 1990.
30. Marshall JC: SIRS and MODS: What is their relevance to the science and practice of intensive care? Shock 14:586–589, 2000.
31. Goris RJ: Mediators of multiple organ failure. Intensive Care Med 16(Suppl 3):S192–S196, 1990.
32. Malbrain ML, De laet IE, De Waele JJ: IAH/ACS: The rationale for surveillance. World J Surg 33:1110–1115, 2009.
33. Brandt CP, McHenry CR, Jacobs DG, et al: Polypropylene mesh closure after emergency laparotomy: Morbidity and outcome. Surgery 118:736–740, 1995.
34. Miller RS, Morris JA, Jr: Current therapy of trauma and surgical critical care, St. Louis, 2008, Mosby-Elsevier.
35. Miller RS, Norris PR, Jenkins JM, et al: Systems initiatives reduce health care-associated infections: A study of 22,928 device days in a single trauma unit. J Trauma 68:23–31, 2010.
36. Schecter WP, Hirshberg A, Chang DS, et al: Enteric fistulas: Principles of management. J Am Coll Surg 209:484–491, 2009.
37. Fischer PE, Fabian TC, Magnotti LJ, et al: A ten-year review of enterocutaneous fistulas after laparotomy for trauma. J Trauma 67:924–928, 2009.
38. Scaff DW, Brooks AJ, Bilski T, et al: A technique for the management of the open abdomen in the presence of a fistula. Injury Extra 38:43–48, 2007.
39. Woodfield JC, Parry BR, Bissett IP, et al: Experience with the use of vacuum dressings in the management of acute enterocutaneous fistulas. ANZ J Surg 76:1085–1087, 2006.
40. Connolly PT, Teubner A, Lees NP, et al: Outcome of reconstructive surgery for intestinal fistula in the open abdomen. Ann Surg 247:440–444, 2008.

41. Diaz JJ, Jr, Conquest AM, Ferzoco SJ, et al: Multi-institutional experience using human acellular dermal matrix for ventral hernia repair in a compromised surgical field. Arch Surg 144:209–215, 2009.
42. Lee EI, Chike-Obi CJ, Gonzalez P, et al: Abdominal wall repair using human acellular dermal matrix: A follow-up study. Am J Surg 198:650–657, 2009.
43. Bluebond-Langner R, Keifa ES, Mithani S, et al: Recurrent abdominal laxity following interpositional human acellular dermal matrix. Ann Plast Surg 60:76–80, 2008.
44. de Moya MA, Dunham M, Inaba K, et al: Long-term outcome of acellular dermal matrix when used for large traumatic open abdomen. J Trauma 65:349–353, 2008.
45. Ramirez OM, Ruas E, Dellon AL: "Components separation" method for closure of abdominal-wall defects: an anatomic and clinical study. Plast Reconstr Surg 86:519–526, 1990.
46. de Vries Reilingh TS, van Goor H, Rosman C, et al: "Components separation technique" for the repair of large abdominal wall hernias. J Am Coll Surg 196:32–37, 2003.
47. de Vries Reilingh TS, van Goor H, Charbon JA, et al: Repair of giant midline abdominal wall hernias: "Components separation technique" versus prosthetic repair : Interim analysis of a randomized controlled trial. World J Surg 31:756–763, 2007.
48. Kolker AR, Brown DJ, Redstone JS, et al: Multilayer reconstruction of abdominal wall defects with acellular dermal allograft (AlloDerm) and component separation. Ann Plast Surg 55:36–41, 2005.
49. Williams RF, Martin DF, Mulrooney MT, et al: Intraperitoneal modification of the Rives-Stoppa repair for large incisional hernias. Hernia 12:141–145, 2008.

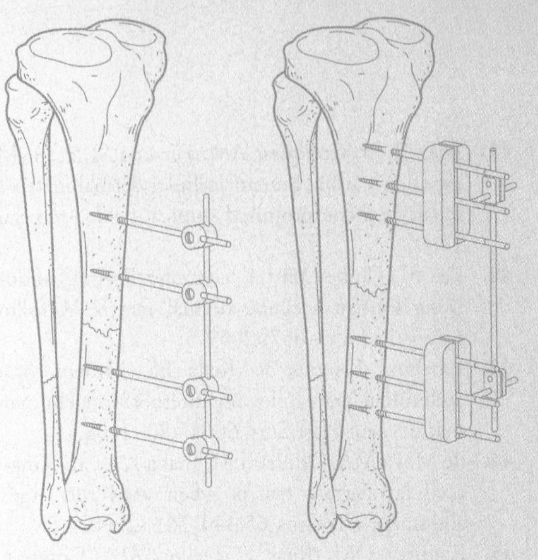

CHAPTER 20

# EMERGENCY CARE OF MUSCULOSKELETAL INJURIES

Silas T. Marshall and Bruce D. Browner



## EPIDEMIOLOGY OF ORTHOPEDIC INJURIES

Accidents continue to be a prominent cause of death and disability throughout the world. In the first 5 decades of life, trauma accounts for more deaths than any other cause. In all age groups, accidents are the fifth leading cause of death in the United States. In general, the amount of energy absorbed by a multiply injured patient corresponds to the extent of the musculoskeletal injuries. Because high energy is frequently involved, fractures and soft tissue injuries are common. Campbell et al found a 49% incidence of musculoskeletal injury among 5900 trauma patients seen at a level on trauma center from 2004–2006.[1] When the disability associated with musculoskeletal injuries is tabulated, the ensuing costs are staggering; hundreds of billions of dollars are consumed by medical expenses, lost productivity, and property damage annually.

At the national and global levels, substantial improvements in transportation safety and delivery of medical care have helped address this growing pandemic. Seatbelt and helmet laws, enforcement of drunk driving laws, mandates for improved safety features in automobiles, rapid deployment of emergency medical teams, and establishment of trauma centers have decreased the number of accident scene fatalities. With more victims now likely to survive accidents that might have been fatal in the past, caregivers will be challenged with managing more complex fractures and soft tissue wounds. These realities demand that trauma teams be aware of the frequency and consequences of musculoskeletal injuries in every trauma patient. An appreciation for the unique features of skeletal injury in patients who may also have severe head, thoracic, or intra-abdominal trauma is essential. In this way, a cohesive, integrated approach to the diagnosis and treatment of musculoskeletal injuries may be used in the care of the multiply injured patient.

## TERMINOLOGY

Communication among collaborating specialists is central to patient care. Trauma and emergency department findings need to be relayed precisely to consulting specialists. This task is particularly challenging in view of the variety of anatomic locations, fracture patterns, and associated soft tissue injuries encountered in orthopedics. Although many injuries are identified by eponyms within the orthopedic community, the most practical and universally understood characterizations of injuries are those that adhere to basic anatomic and mechanical principles.

### Fracture Types

A fracture is a disruption of the normal architecture of bone. Fractures can be acute, subacute, or chronic. Acute fractures have sharp, well-defined edges of the fragments. Subacute fractures have signs of healing present on x-ray. The edges become blunted and less well defined as bony resorption and new bone formation occur. Chronic fractures have a rounded and sclerotic appearance after resorption and remodeling of bone has occurred at the fracture ends (Fig. 20-1). This distinction can usually be made on clinical examination. Chronic fractures are often termed *delayed unions* or *nonunions.* A delayed union is defined as a fracture that is taking longer to show progression toward healing than would normally be expected. The expected healing time varies, depending on the age of the patient and anatomic location of the fracture. For example, long bones in adults typically take 6 to 8 weeks to achieve full bony union, whereas pediatric fractures and metaphyseal fractures take less time. A nonunion is a fracture that has lost the potential to progress with healing. Generally, nonunion of a long bone is a fracture that has failed to show evidence of healing over a 4- to 6-month period.[2] Chronic repetitive trauma can also cause microscopic disruptions when bone is stressed beyond its failure point. These injuries are termed *stress fractures* and are considered overuse injuries.

Because of increased plasticity, a more substantial periosteum, and the presence of growth plates, children's bones are at risk for a different set of fractures (Fig. 20-2). Plastic deformity of a long bone in a pediatric patient is deformation of the bone without actual disruption of the bony cortex. Diagnosis of the deformity often necessitates radiography of the contralateral

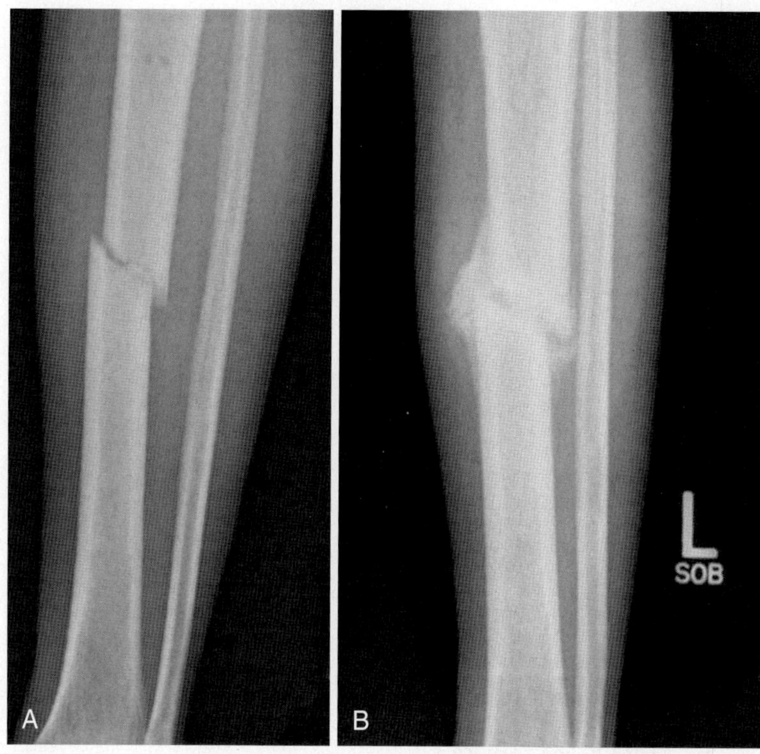


**FIGURE 20-1 A,** Acute fracture. Note the sharp, well-defined edges. **B,** Nonunion; 6 months later, the fracture line is still clearly visible, the edges of this fracture are blunted, and the bone ends are sclerotic. Clinically, there was still motion at the fracture site. The patient had significant chronic pain.

extremity to confirm asymmetry. Axial loads of long bones in children can lead to buckling of the cortex without a visible fracture line, appropriately termed a *buckle fracture.* Incomplete disruptions of the cortex are termed *greenstick fractures* in children or *infractions* in adults. A greenstick fracture consists of a cortical disruption on one side of the bone, with a buckle fracture or plastic deformation on the opposite side. The dense periosteal layer in children can contribute stability to many of these fractures if the layer remains intact. A fracture through the cartilaginous growth plate (physis) is another fracture type unique to children. A pure physeal fracture may not be radiographically apparent. These fractures are diagnosed clinically by the presence of pain over the growth plate.

When a bone fails through an area weakened by preexisting disease, it is termed a *pathologic fracture.* Causes may include weakness from primary bone tumors, metastatic lesions, infection, metabolic disease, and injury to an old fracture site. Although not commonly referred to in this way, fractures in osteoporotic bone are technically pathologic. However, the term *insufficiency* or *fragility fracture* is most frequently used to describe these injuries. In distinction to acute fractures in healthy bone, fragility fractures normally result from accidents with much lower energy, such as a fall from standing height. Hip fractures, compression fractures of the vertebral bodies, and distal radius fractures in older adults are common examples.

A fracture is considered open when an overlying wound produces communication between the fracture site and the outside environment. These fractures can range from an inside to outside poke hole in the skin to severe crush injuries. High-energy fracture patterns indicate that the soft tissues, as well as the bones, have absorbed large forces. Although the skin laceration is the most obvious component, the energy of the fracture, degree of contamination, and soft tissue injury must all be taken into account when grading the severity of the injury. Final grading of open fractures cannot be accomplished until all necrotic or contaminated tissue has been removed. Contamination of bone can lead to the development of osteomyelitis and all its catastrophic consequences, and thus necessitates emergency treatment.

An intra-articular fracture extends into a joint. When there is significant cartilage damage, late degenerative changes are likely. These injuries are normally caused by a compressive, or axial, load across the joint. Displaced intra-articular fractures require urgent anatomic reduction and rigid fixation to minimize the risk of post-traumatic arthritis. Anatomic reduction can be achieved directly with open arthrotomy or by arthroscopic means. It can also be achieved indirectly with fluoroscopic guidance.

Long bone fractures are characterized by anatomic location (Fig. 20-3). The epiphysis includes the area between the physis, or physeal scar, and articular surface. The metaphysis is located between the epiphysis and shaft and includes the growth plate. The diaphysis encompasses the shaft of the bone between the proximal and distal metaphyses. The diaphysis is made up of mostly dense cortical bone, which has less vascularity than the soft cancellous bone of the metaphysis. This difference in vascularity affects the rate at which the bone heals. Fractures can be described according to location within these three sections or according to the location in the bone—proximal, middle, and distal. In addition, fractures within the diaphysis are usually divided into thirds (i.e., proximal, middle and distal thirds). Distally, the humerus and femur flare to form their articular surfaces. These flares are termed the *epicondyles,* and fractures in these areas are referred to as supracondylar or intracondylar. The articular surfaces distal to the epicondyles are known as condyles. Intracondylar fractures are intra-articular and may extend proximally. Such distinctions are important because these injuries present difficult treatment challenges.

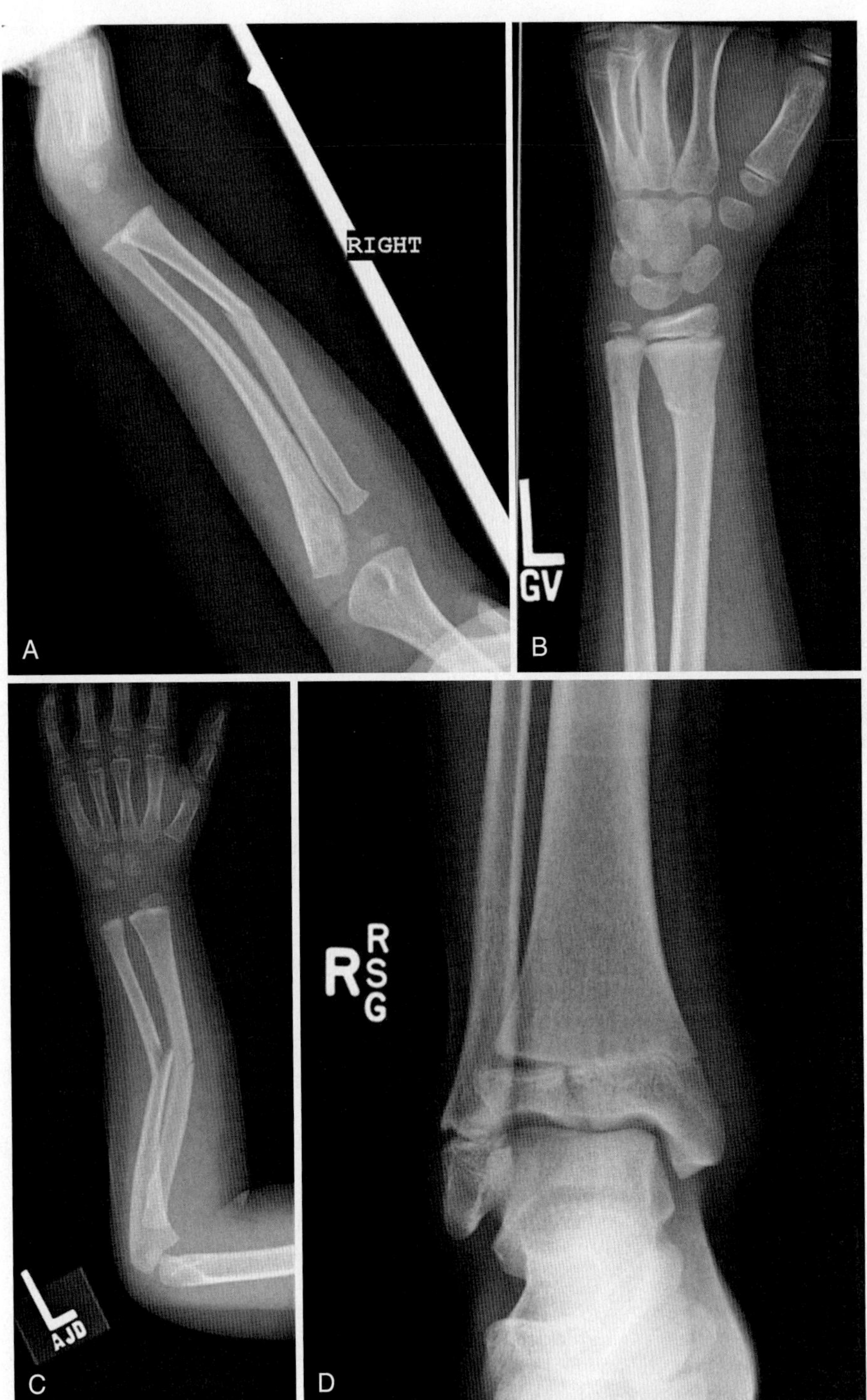


**FIGURE 20-2 A,** Plastic deformity. Note the bowing of the ulna. **B,** Buckle fracture. The cortex of the distal radius is deformed, but intact. **C,** Greenstick fracture; disruption of radial cortices, without disruption of the ulnar cortices in this forearm fracture in both bones. **D,** Physeal fracture. Note the gapping of the lateral tibial physis.

A fracture may also be described by the pattern of cortical disruption (Fig. 20-4). The orientation of the primary fracture line may be transverse, oblique, or spiral. Transverse and oblique fractures occur when a bending moment is applied. Oblique fractures can be further characterized as long or short oblique. Spiral fractures generally result from a rotational force about the long axis of the bone. Comminution is the presence of multiple fragments within an individual fracture site and usually indicates a higher-energy injury or weakened bone in an older patient. A butterfly fragment is an area of comminution in one of the simple fracture patterns described earlier. Segmental fractures are fractures that occur at multiple levels in the same bone.

Displacement, if present, is described from a combination of principles. These deformities may occur in any plane. When viewed on plain radiographs, all injuries will be resolved into pure coronal or sagittal displacement. However, it is important to realize that the true displacement usually occurs in a plane that is somewhere in between. Translation, angulation, rotation, and shortening are all components of fracture displacement. Translation is the relationship of the proximal fracture fragment

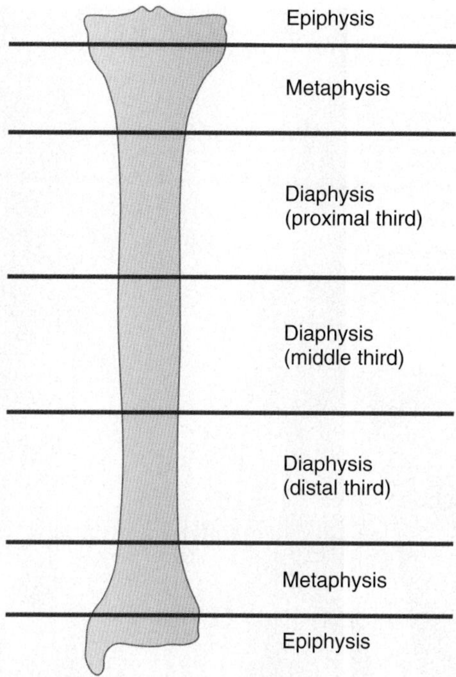


**FIGURE 20-3** Anatomic regions of the tibia.

to the distal one. It is described in terms of percentage of overlap. A fracture with 100% translation in any plane is completely displaced. Angulation is simply the angle created by the displaced fracture fragments. It is described by the direction of the apex formed by the fracture fragments (i.e., 20-degree apex lateral). The final component is rotation. To describe rotation exactly, a full-length film of the limb segment involved, including the joints above and below, must be examined. Alternatively, rotational deformity may be assessed clinically by comparing the injured limb with the contralateral side.

Once a fracture has been identified, it must be described in a consistent, systematic manner. All descriptions begin with whether the fracture is open or closed. The amount of soft tissue involvement is described. A closed fracture is assumed if, after careful evaluation, there is no observed communication between the fracture and outside world. The presence of an intra-articular fracture is then communicated. The side of the body and injured bone are stated next. A description of the pattern, followed by its location in the bone, is indicated. The displacement of the fracture fragments is related. Finally, it is important to indicate any associated, nonorthopedic injuries that may alter the timing and type of initial orthopedic management. Adherence to this scheme allows complete understanding of the fracture.

### Other Injuries

Ligamentous injuries are commonly encountered in association with traumatic injuries to bones and joints. When a ligament is damaged but is still in continuity, it is termed a *sprain.* Sprains can range in severity from minor injuries to significant instability about a joint. Grade I ligamentous injuries are caused by stretching of a ligament or ligament complex. They do not normally result in instability. A simple ankle sprain is a typical example of this type of injury. Partial ruptures of ligaments can result in minor instability and are considered grade II injuries. Complete ruptures, or grade III injuries, lead to significant instability at the associated joint. Avulsion fractures at the insertion of ligamentous structures also fall into this category. Ligamentous injuries cannot be overlooked because they can produce significant joint instability and endanger the surrounding soft tissue and neurovascular structures. This detail is critical when evaluating musculoskeletal injuries. A full neurovascular examination should be performed whenever there is suspicion of joint instability. Although most ligamentous injuries do not require urgent orthopedic management, stabilization or immobilization of the joint with a splint or brace is usually advisable.

A strain is an injury to a muscle or tendon. These injuries are most commonly of an overuse nature. Further loading of the already weakened structure can compound these injuries and lead to muscle or tendon rupture. Rest, ice, compression, and elevation are the mainstays of treatment for a strain; however, more urgent orthopedic management is necessary for a rupture. Although many tendon ruptures can be treated nonoperatively, proper positioning of the joint is important to ensure that the tendon scars down in a functional position. If operative management is pursued, it should occur fairly urgently. Scarring of the tendon tract and contracture of the muscle significantly complicate the operative procedure.

Joint injury without fracture is common in axial load injuries. Articular contusions, or bone bruises, usually heal with a period of rest and restricted weight bearing, but can lead to late degenerative changes in the joint. A more significant osteochondral defect (OCD) occurs when a piece of articular cartilage, along with its underlying subchondral bone, is separated from the surrounding joint surface. Small OCD lesions can be asymptomatic; however, many of these lesions can lead to chronic pain and joint degeneration. In some cases, the osteochondral fragment is large enough to see on plain radiographs. In these cases, it is important to immobilize the joint to minimize joint damage from the free-floating bony fragment. Other commonly injured joints are the intervertebral discs in the spine. These discs are made up of a viscoelastic nucleus pulposus surrounded by a dense, fibrous, annulus fibrosis. With a great enough axial load, the nucleus pulposus can herniate through the annulus, resulting in a disc herniation. This disc bulge can impinge on nerve roots, causing back and radicular pain. Disc herniations rarely need surgical intervention and often resolve with a course of physical therapy. Very rarely, severe disc bulge in the lumbar spine can cause significant impingement on the cauda equina, resulting in cauda equina syndrome. This is a surgical emergency and will be discussed in more detail later in the chapter.

## FIXATION PRINCIPLES

### External Fixation

External fixation provides stabilization of an injured limb segment through the use of pins or wires embedded in the bone. These pins are then connected to rods or rings via clamps. With the exception of the pins or wires, the rigid construct is external to the body, as the name implies. Newer designs are more complex, but easier to apply and more stable than previous designs. The addition of modularity has added to their prospective uses and has led to more adaptable and adjustable constructs.

External fixation is used for the treatment of open fractures, fractures in unstable patients who cannot tolerate significant anesthesia times or blood loss, complex fractures in which open

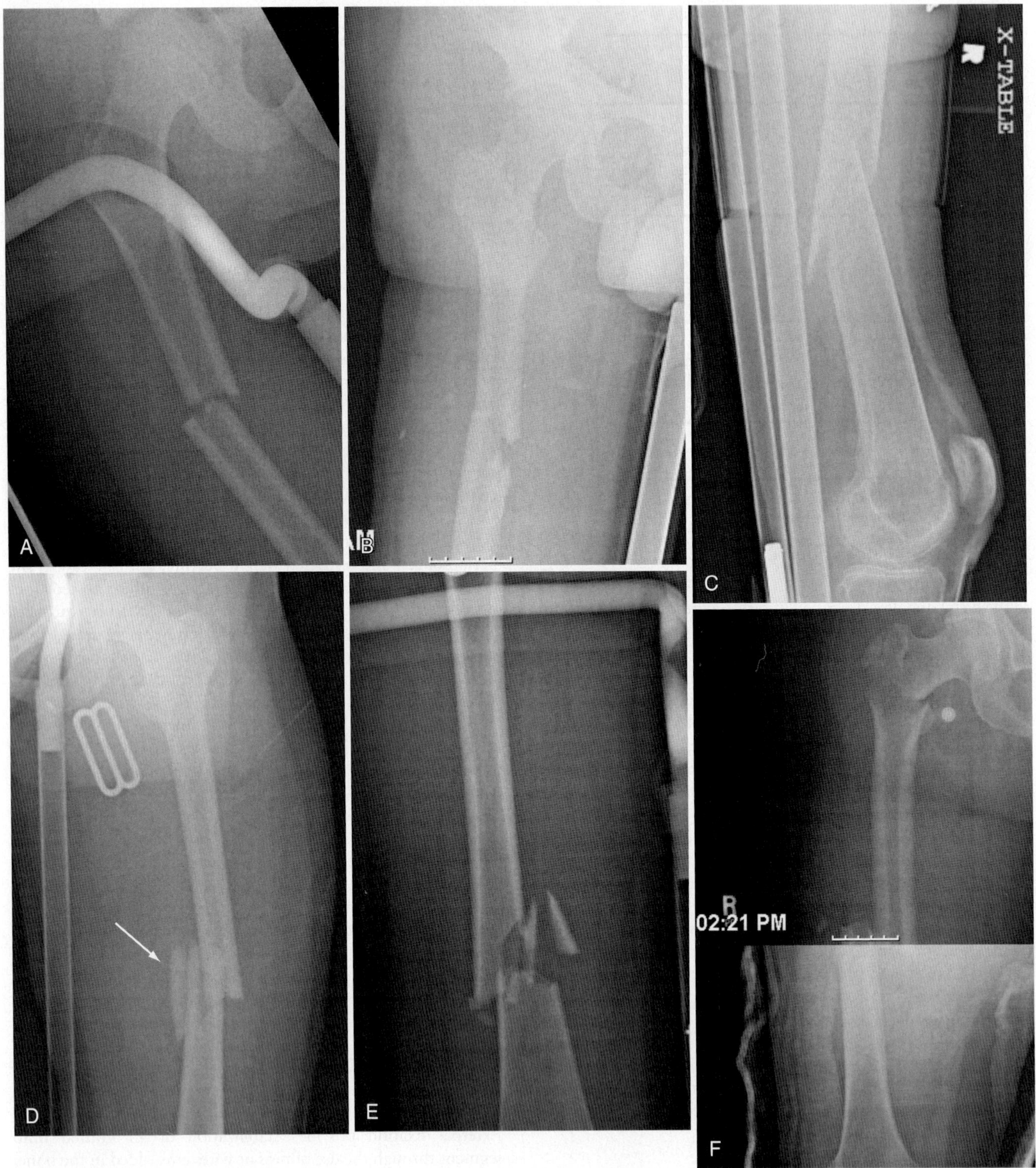


**FIGURE 20-4** Femur fracture patterns. **A,** Transverse. **B,** Oblique. **C,** Spiral. **D,** Butterfly fragment *(arrow)*. **E,** Comminuted. **F,** Segmental.

reduction and internal fixation (ORIF) is not warranted, and fractures with associated vascular injuries requiring stabilization and urgent vascular repair. Specialized external fixation devices are also used in limb reconstruction surgery. In fractures with soft tissue injuries, placement of percutaneously inserted pins that minimize further soft tissue damage and avoid the area of contamination helps decrease the incidence of infection and delayed union. External fixators may be used for temporary stabilization or for definitive treatment in select cases. In complex fractures around joints, fixation with implanted plates or screws

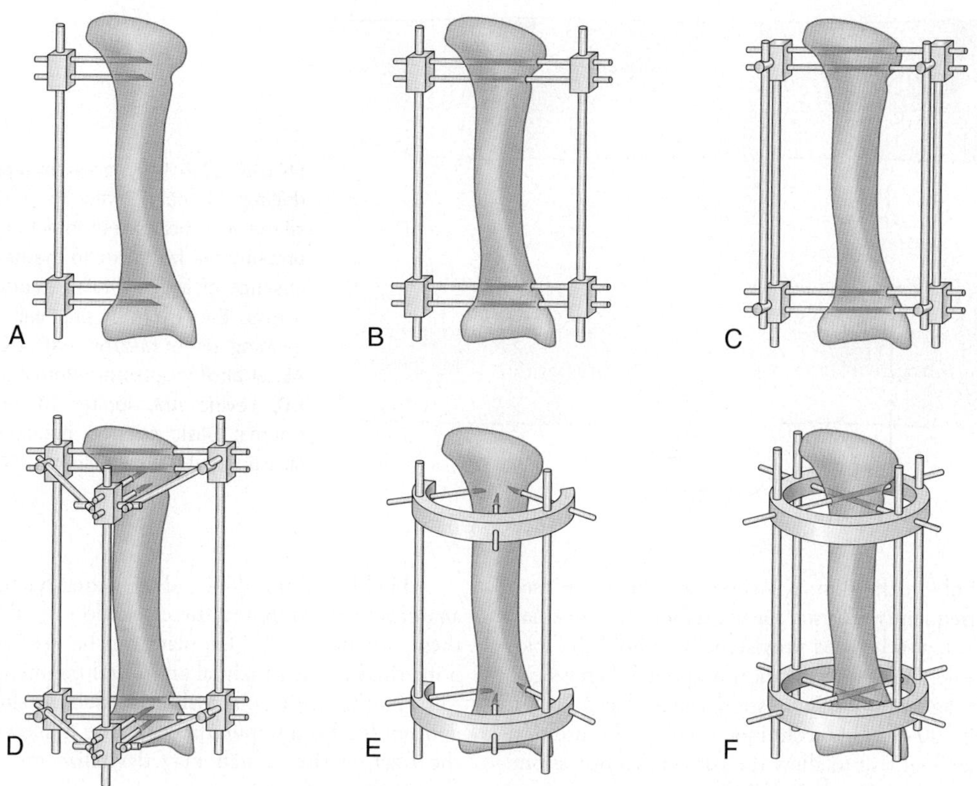


**FIGURE 20-5** Basic fixator configurations. **A,** Unilateral. **B,** Bilateral. **C,** Multiplanar (quadrilateral). **D,** Multiplanar (delta configuration). **E,** Hybrid fixator. **F,** Ring fixator. (From Green SA: Principles and complications of external fixation. In Browner, BD, Levine AM, Jupiter JB, et al [eds]: Skeletal trauma: Basic science, management, and reconstruction, ed 4, Philadelphia, 2008, WB Saunders.)

may not provide adequate stability. Additionally, overlying soft tissue damage makes operative exposure dangerous. In these cases, an external fixator, with the pins placed at a distance from the fracture and injured soft tissues, can provide the osseous stability necessary for fracture healing.

External frames are constructed from three components, pins, connectors, and rods or rings (Fig. 20-5). Pins are threaded or smooth and vary in length and diameter. They serve to connect the bone to the rest of the device. Pin placement is chosen to stabilize the fracture best while not compromising the viability of the fragments. Pins are never placed through compromised or infected skin. A variety of different clamps serves as connectors and secure pins to the rods that form the external frames. Most are universal joints that allow multiple degrees of freedom. Connecting clamps have advanced to the point that they now snap in place onto the pins and rods. They may be combined with rings or hinged rods and allow infinite permutations of frame constructs. Stabilizing rods are almost universally radiolucent to allow radiographic examination after application. Threaded rods, bone transport rails, motorized lengthening devices, and dynamic struts represent a small sample of the types of rods that can be used to achieve specific results.

There are a number of factors affecting the stiffness of the fixation construct. The stiffness of the pin material (usually stainless steel) and connecting bar material (titanium, stainless steel, or carbon fiber), as well as the diameter of the pins and bars, contributes to the stiffness of the frame. However, the loss of stiffness seen with more flexible materials, such as carbon fiber, or smaller diameter pins can easily be overcome by the frame configuration chosen. Increasing stiffness is seen with an increasing number of pins, increasing pin spread (distance between pins), decreasing distance between the bar and bone, increasing number of bars, and use of multiplanar constructs.

Once applied, external fixators require regular care and monitoring. Pin care is begun immediately and consists of cleansing with normal saline or half-strength peroxide solution. Drainage from pin sites must be addressed with local care, antibiotics, pin removal and replacement, or a combination of these measures. Pins are checked regularly to ensure that they have not loosened. Depending on the fracture pattern, fixator construct, and goals of treatment, the weight-bearing status is adjusted.

## Internal Fixation

ORIF implies that an incision is made at or near the site of injury to facilitate reduction of the fracture under direct vision (open reduction) and rigid stabilization with plates, screws, wires, rods, or combinations thereof (internal fixation). This technique allows anatomic reduction and the creation of constructs of varying levels of stability. Different types of implants can be used to achieve these results.

### Pins and Screws

Pins and screws are the simplest implants. They can be introduced in a variety of areas and are often placed percutaneously

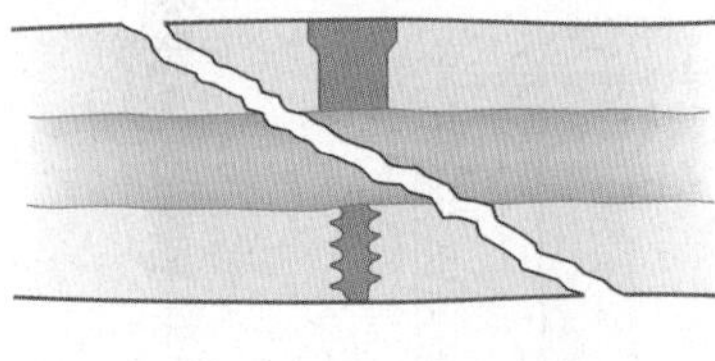
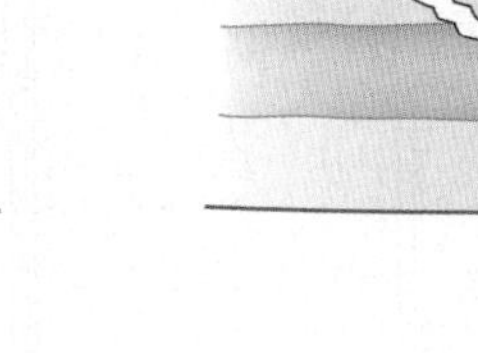
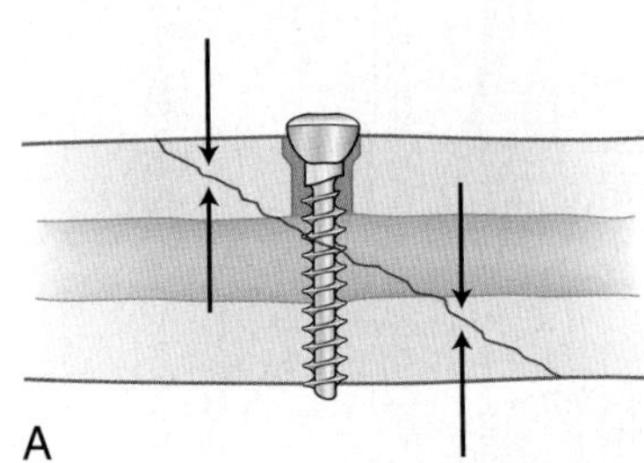

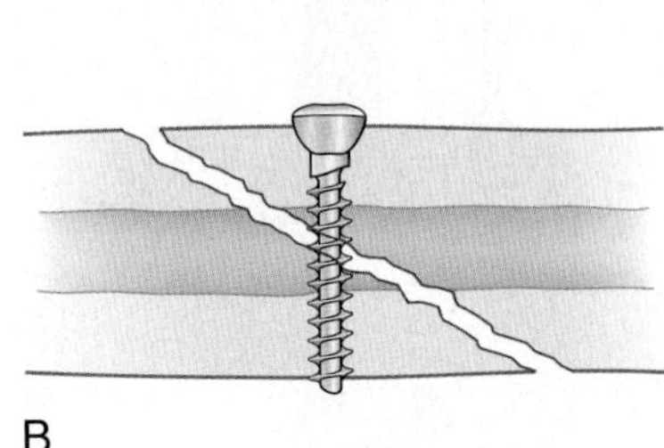


**FIGURE 20-6** Lag screws by application. **A,** Overdrilling the near cortex to produce a glide hole allows a cortical screw to act as a lag screw, compressing the far cortex to the near cortex. **B,** In the absence of a glide hole, a cortical screw inserted across the fracture site will maintain fracture gapping. (From Mazzocca AD, DeAngelis JD, Caputo AE, et al: Principles of internal fixation In Browner, BD, Levine AM, Jupiter JB, et al [eds]: Skeletal trauma: Basic science, management, and reconstruction, ed 4, Philadelphia, 2008, WB Saunders.)

through a poke hole in the skin. Kirschner wires may be used temporarily and frequently are used for the stabilization of small fragments. They can also be used provisionally to hold the fracture reduction while more stable fixation is applied. Screws can be used for interfragmentary compression when placed with a lag technique (Fig. 20-6). This technique involves the use of a gliding hole in one fragment to allow the screw to compress one fragment against another. Figure 20-6B shows a position screw. Without a gliding hole, a fully threaded screw will capture both fragments without compressing the far fragment to the near one, thus holding the position of the fragments.

### Plates

Plates are used frequently for the internal fixation of fractures. They allow even distribution of force across their length and can serve various biomechanical functions. The biomechanical properties of a plate depend on the material used, usually titanium or stainless steel, dimensions of the plate (thickness, width, and length), and technique with which it is applied (Fig. 20-7).

A neutralization plate is used to protect another form of fixation from excessive force. Often used in combination with a lag screw, these plates add stability by preventing torsion and bending. The addition of a neutralization plate allows mobilization earlier than would have been possible with less stable fixation.

Buttress plates are used to counteract forces that occur with axial loading. Longitudinal and oblique fractures near joints tend to displace along the line of the fracture when subjected to axial loads. Plates placed in a longitudinal fashion can form an axilla with the intact cortex that prevents axial displacement. Some plates are specifically designed for buttressing; however, any plate can be applied in a buttress mode.

Compression plating is used to increase the stability of fixation when the two major fracture fragments can be brought into contact. This technique allows direct compression of the fracture ends. Compression plates have oval screw holes with oblique edges that allow eccentric placement of screws. When a screw is applied eccentrically, the plate (and bone fragment fixed to it) translates as the screw tightens down against the plate to create compression at the fracture. Additionally, compression can also be achieved by overbending a plate or by introducing a tensioning device.

Highly comminuted and segmental fractures may not allow anatomic reduction and direct fixation of all the fragments. In these situations, a bridge plate can be used to stabilize a long bone rigidly. The proximal and distal fragments are rigidly fixed to each other with a plate while the fracture site is bypassed. This concept has been popularized because it allows less dissection at the fracture site, which may devitalize the comminuted and segmental fragments.

Special plates have been designed for certain fracture patterns and anatomic locations. Blade plates, dynamic condylar screws, and pelvic reconstruction plates are examples of these specialized plates.

### Tension Bands

When the forces across a fracture site tend to displace the fractured pieces in tension, the tension band technique can be applied to convert the displacing tensile forces on one side of a fracture into a compressive force across the entire contact area (Fig. 20-8). Traditionally, wires or cables are used to create tension bands. However, nonabsorbable suture and plates can also be used. Tension bands are used most frequently for fractures of the olecranon, where the pull of the triceps tends to distract the proximal fragment, and fractures of the patella, where the pull of the quadriceps tends to distract the superior pole. They are also commonly used for the femoral greater trochanter, humeral greater tuberosity, and medial malleolus.

### Intramedullary Nails

In contrast to wires, plates, and screws, intramedullary (IM) nails are placed in the medullary canal of long bones. They are used to splint or bridge a fracture and to control axial, bending, and rotational forces. IM nailing also permits fixation of a fracture through an incision distant from the fracture site. In this way, the periosteal blood supply at the fracture site is left undisturbed. Nails are made of various materials and can be fluted, smooth, solid, or cannulated (Fig. 20-9). When transverse screws are placed through the proximal and distal ends of the nail, the nail is said to be locked. Locked nails control rotation better and maintain bone length in the presence of comminution or bone loss. The locking holes in nails may be round or oval. Using a nail with an oval hole or leaving the nail unlocked at one end allows the bone fragment to slide axially along the nail and

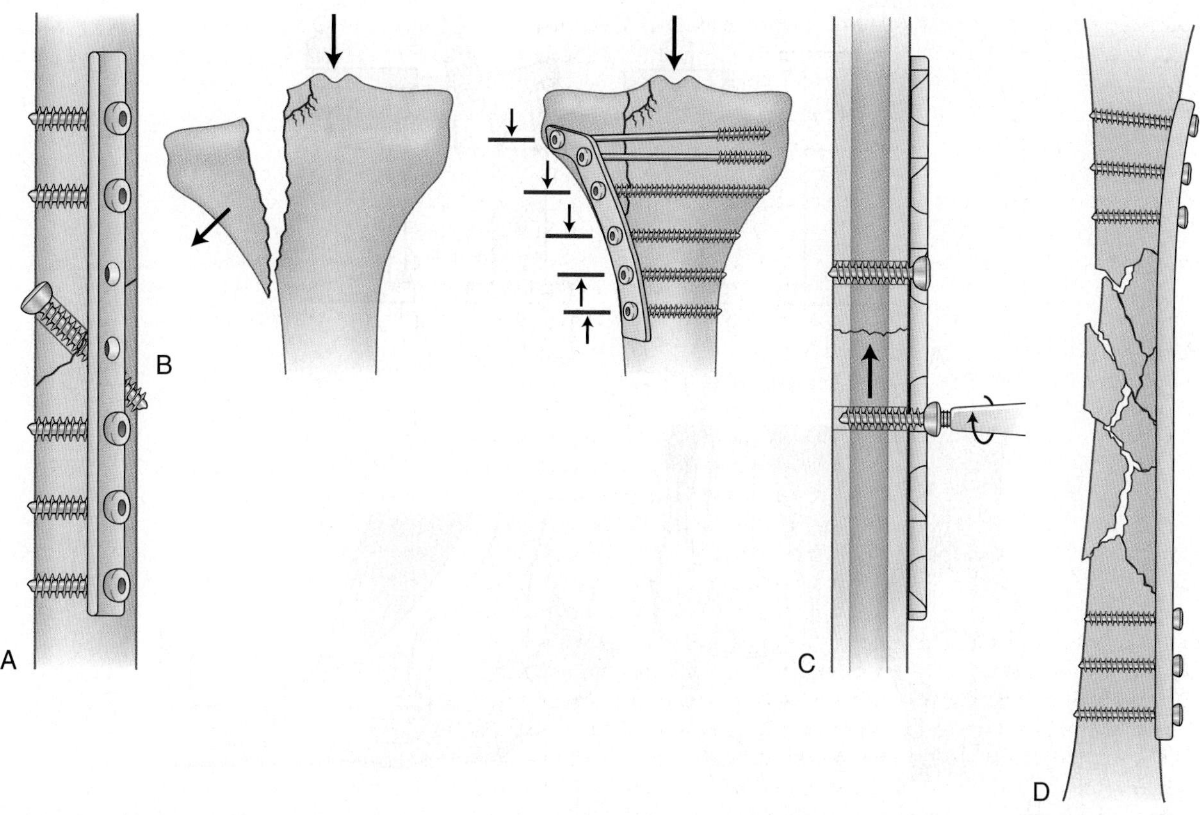


**FIGURE 20-7 A,** Interfragmentary screw fixation with a neutralization plate effectively resisting an external load. **B,** Buttress plate supporting the underlying cortex, effectively resisting displacement, which otherwise would result in angular deformity of the joint. The plate acts as a buttress or retaining wall. **C,** In the compression mode, the screw is inserted 1.0 mm eccentric to its final position in the hole on the side away from the fracture site. When the screw is tightened, its head slides down along the inclined plane, merging the eccentric circles and causing horizontal movement of the plate (1.0 mm). This results in fracture compression. **D,** The bridge plate maintains length and alignment by fixing to bone away from the comminution and preserving critical blood supply to that area by limiting surgical dissection. (From Mazzocca AD, DeAngelis JD, Caputo AE, et al: Principles of internal fixation. In Browner, BD, Levine AM, Jupiter JB, et al [eds]: Skeletal trauma: Basic science, management, and reconstruction, ed 4, Philadelphia, 2008, WB Saunders.)

produces compression at the fracture site. Nails locked in this fashion are dynamically locked. When screws are inserted through round holes in both ends of the nail, no motion is allowed within the construct; they are statically locked (Fig. 20-10).

IM nails can be introduced in a proximal to distal or distal to proximal direction and are termed *antegrade* and *retrograde,* respectively. Nails may be inserted with or without canal preparation by reaming. Reaming involves passing a large drill down the medullary canal to remove the cancellous bone and effectively widen the canal. This increased width allows the insertion of a larger diameter nail to increase the strength and stiffness of the construct. At the same time, reaming morcellizes the cancellous and cortical bone in the canal and deposits this exceptional autogenous bone graft at the fracture site. However, reaming leads to increased pressure in the medullary canal, increased temperature in the cortical bone, and embolization of marrow contents into the vascular system. In patients with severe derangement of pulmonary function or hemodynamic instability, embolization is not well tolerated.

Unreamed nails are inserted without reaming of the canal, and destruction of the cortical blood supply from the medullary system is largely avoided. In fractures in which there is a large degree of soft tissue loss or periosteal stripping, an unreamed nail is generally used.

## PATIENT EVALUATION

### History

Obtaining a detailed history of a skeletally injured patient is essential for accurate diagnosis and treatment. This can be challenging with multiply injured and older patients in the trauma setting; however, it is important to gather as much information as possible regarding the mechanism of injury. Often, trauma patients are unable to give accurate histories because of unconsciousness, intoxication, dementia, or delirium. In these cases, an account of the mechanism of injury and patient history should be obtained from family members, emergency medical response crew members, or other witnesses to the accident. Descriptions from the injury scene can be helpful because common patterns of injury follow from specific mechanisms (Table 20-1).

A general history that includes demographic information, past medical history, past surgical history, and social history are obtained. Knowledge of allergies, current medications, and time

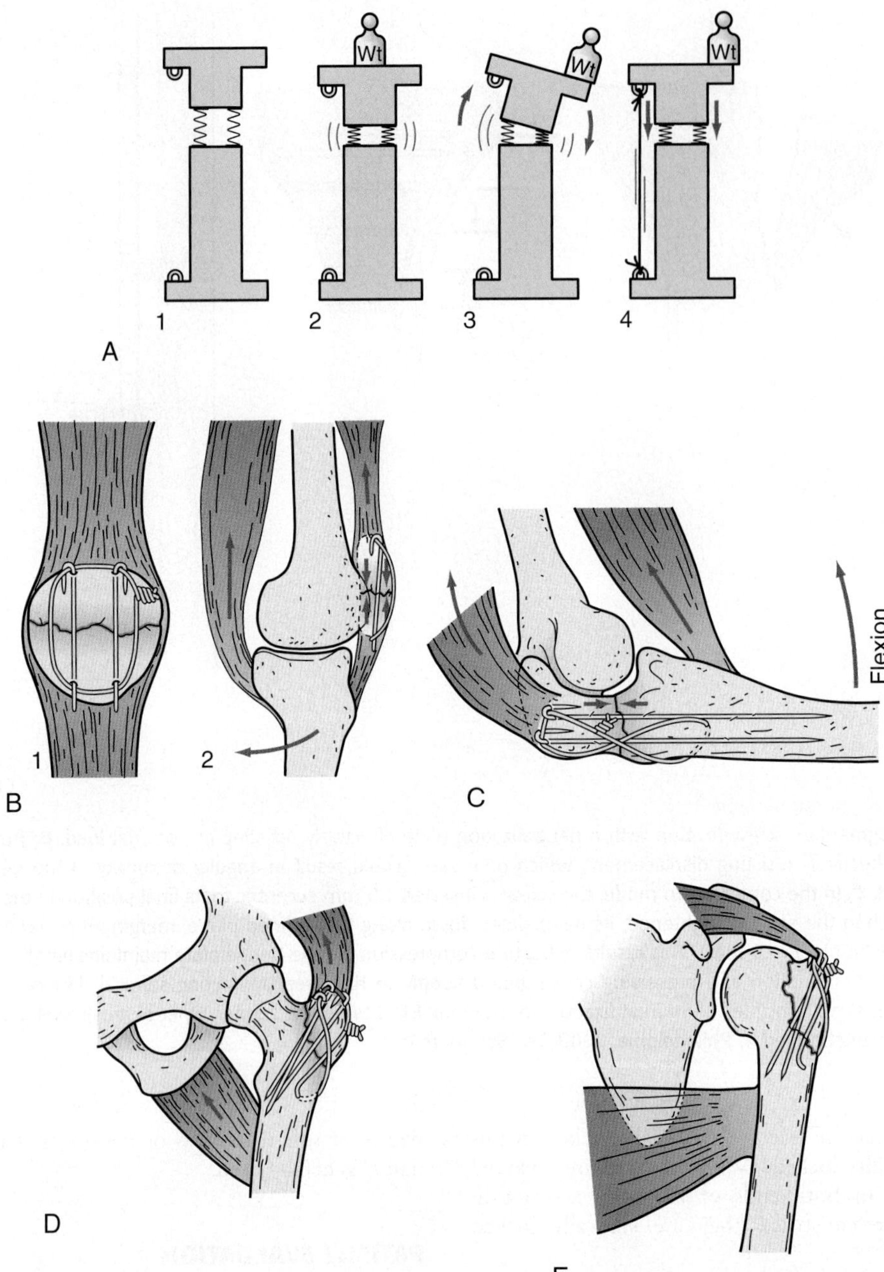


**FIGURE 20-8** Tension band principles. **A,** (1) An interrupted I-beam connected by two springs. (2) The I beam is loaded with a weight (Wt) placed over the central axis of the beam; there is uniform compression of both springs at the interruption. (3) When the I beam is loaded eccentrically by placing the weight at a distance from the central axis of the beam, the spring on the same side compresses, whereas the spring on the opposite side is placed in tension and stretches. (4) If a tension band is applied prior to the eccentric loading, it resists the tension that would otherwise stretch the opposite spring, thus causing uniform compression of both springs. **B,** The tension band principle applied to fixation of a transverse patellar fracture. (1) The AP view shows placement of the parallel Kirschner wires and anterior tension band. (2) The lateral view demonstrates antagonistic pull of the hamstrings and quadriceps, causing a bending moment of the patella over the femoral trochlea. An anterior tension band transforms this eccentric loading into compression at the fracture site. **C,** The tension band principle applied to fixation of a fracture of the ulna. The antagonistic pull of the triceps and brachialis causes a bending moment of the ulna over the humeral trochlea. The dorsal tension band transforms this eccentric load into compression at the fracture site. **D,** The tension band principle applied to fixation of a fracture of the greater trochanter. With the hip as a fulcrum, the antagonistic pull of the adductors and abductors causes a bending moment in the femur. The lateral tension band transforms this eccentric load into compression at the greater trochanteric fracture site. **E,** The tension band principle applied to fixation of a fracture of the greater tuberosity of the humerus. Using the glenoid as a fulcrum, the antagonistic pull of the pectoralis major and supraspinatus causes a bending moment of the humerus. The lateral tension band transforms this eccentric load into compression at the greater tuberosity fracture site. (From Mazzocca AD, DeAngelis JD, Caputo AE, et al: Principles of internal fixation. In Browner, BD, Levine AM, Jupiter JB, et al [eds]: Skeletal trauma: Basic science, management, and reconstruction, ed 4, Philadelphia, 2008, WB Saunders.)

since last oral intake is useful in guiding treatment. Information about the position of the limb before and after the injury, as well as the direction of the deforming force, can help predict the resulting injuries. Ambulatory status before the injury helps determine realistic goals for functional recovery. Any transient neurologic symptoms, such as loss of consciousness, numbness, parenthesis, and spasm, must be documented. Loss of bowel or bladder control in patients with back or neck pain must also be noted. The time elapsed since injury becomes critical information in a patient with a vascular injury, open wound, or dislocation.

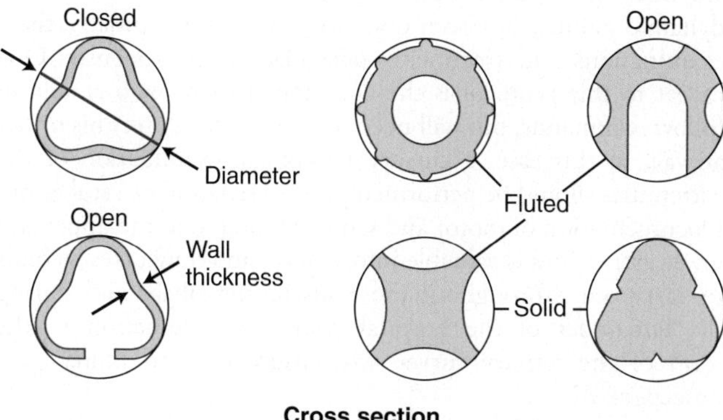


**FIGURE 20-9** Geometric features of an intramedullary nail that influence its performance. Note the cloverleaf, fluted, solid, and open designs. All these have the same diameter but different wall thicknesses. (From Mazzocca AD, DeAngelis JD, Caputo AE, et al: Principles of internal fixation. In Browner, BD, Levine AM, Jupiter JB, et al [eds]: Skeletal trauma: Basic science, management, and reconstruction, ed 4, Philadelphia, 2008, WB Saunders.)

**Table 20-1 Common Patterns and Associated Injuries**

| INJURY PATTERN OR MECHANISM | ASSOCIATED INJURIES |
|---|---|
| Fall from a height | Calcaneus fracture<br>Tibial plateau fracture<br>Fractures around the hip (proximal femur, acetabulum)<br>Vertebral burst fracture |
| Fall on outstretched hand (FOOSH) | Distal radius fracture<br>Posterior elbow dislocation<br>Pediatric<br>Both bones forearm fracture<br>Supracondylar humerus fracture |
| Ejection from a vehicle | Closed head injury<br>Spine fractures |
| T-bone motor vehicle accident | Lateral compression-type pelvic fracture<br>Closed head injury<br>Thoracic injury |
| Head-on motor vehicle accident | Abdominal visceral injury<br>Open-book pelvic fracture<br>Retroperitoneal bleeding<br>Injuries caused by floor board intrusion<br>Calcaneal fracture<br>Tibial plateau fracture<br>Posterior hip dislocation |
| Posterior knee dislocation | Popliteal artery injury |
| Supracondylar humerus fracture | Brachial artery injury<br>Nerve injury (median or radial) |
| Anterior shoulder dislocation | Axillary nerve injury |
| Posterior hip dislocation | Sciatic (peroneal division) nerve injury |

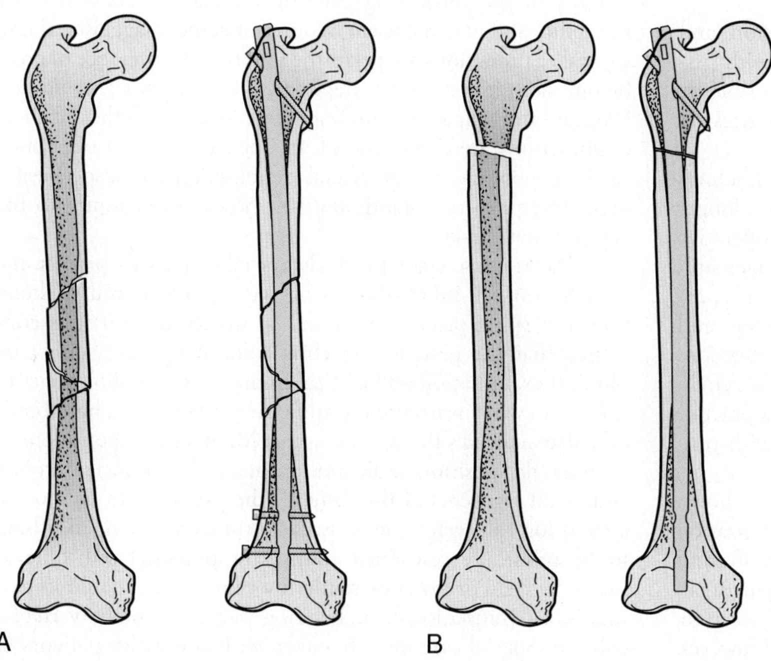


**FIGURE 20-10 A,** Static locked intramedullary nail fixed to both the proximal and distal fragments. **B,** Dynamic locked intramedullary nail fixed to the proximal (as shown) or distal fragment, but not to both.

## Trauma Room Evaluation

Examination of a multiply injured patient must first follow advanced trauma life support (ATLS) protocols in a systematic fashion and must be accompanied by appropriate treatment. The concept of life before limb demands that the ABCs (***a***irway, ***b***reathing, and ***c***irculation) be addressed prior to evaluating for any orthopedic injuries. Hemodynamically unstable patients are assumed to be in hemorrhagic shock until proven otherwise. A search for occult hemorrhage is undertaken and may include the pleural cavities, abdomen, retroperitoneum, and pelvis. A plain chest radiograph may quickly reveal a hemothorax. Chest tubes are placed, if necessary. Pelvic instability and the need for rapid external pelvic fixation are addressed. There is debate over whether the anteroposterior (AP) pelvic film, which has traditionally been considered part of the standard trauma radiographic series, is justified with the advent of newer, ultrafast computed tomography (CT) scanners. Recent data have shown that in a stable awake patient who has no evidence of pelvic injury on physical examination, routine use of this study may not be cost-effective.[3] However, in a patient with signs of pelvic injury on examination, hemodynamically unstable patient, or obtunded patient, the pelvic radiograph is essential for identifying unstable pelvic injury requiring immediate intervention in the trauma bay.[4] In addition, the pelvic radiograph is necessary for preoperative planning in operative fractures and as a comparison film when following fracture healing over time. A FAST (***f***ocused ***a***ssessment with ***s***onography in ***t***rauma) scan has been shown to be a rapid and effective technique for assessing for free fluid in the abdomen.[5] Positive scans have been shown to be strongly predictive of the need for laparotomy in hypotensive trauma patients. However, Gaarder and colleagues[6] have found that even in the hands of experienced radiologists, the FAST scan is a relatively unreliable technique for detecting intra-abdominal bleeding in the hemodynamically unstable patient. Cha and associates[7] have agreed with this conclusion and suggest that diagnostic peritoneal lavage and/or CT of the chest, abdomen, and pelvis be considered in hemodynamically unstable patients with suspected intra-abdominal injuries.

The patient's neurologic status is noted on admission, and the Glasgow Coma Scale score is calculated. Patients with suspected head injury need to be evaluated as soon as possible by CT. Peripheral vascular injuries and musculoskeletal injuries are next in priority, followed by maxillofacial injuries.

Although the previous dictum of addressing open fractures in the operating room within 6 hours of injury may no longer hold true, open fractures still require relatively urgent operative care. More importantly, emergent trauma room management, including administration of appropriate antibiotics, tetanus prophylaxis, gross débridement, copious irrigation, splinting, and wound coverage, is imperative for preventing future infection. Sterile dressings placed in the trauma room need to be left in place until the patient reaches the operating room. This practice has led to decreased infection rates when compared with routinely redressing wounds in the trauma area.

In their landmark article, Bone and coworkers[8] have shown that urgent (within the first 24 hours) versus late stabilization in the multiply injured patient reduces the incidence of adult respiratory distress syndrome (ARDS) and multisystem organ failure. In addition, with adequate stabilization of the fracture, the patient can be mobilized, avoiding convalescence. However, more recently, Morshed and colleagues[9] have shown that emergent fixation—within 12 hours—of femoral shaft fractures in polytrauma leads to an increased mortality rate. They suggest that this finding is likely caused by inadequate time for patient resuscitation in those taken to surgery in the first 12 hours from the time of injury. In isolated or less severe injuries, once the patient is stabilized, the timing of repair is less significant. Operative delay allows for resolution of the soft tissue swelling that may compromise soft tissue closure.

Unstable pelvic fractures are addressed in the primary survey because of the possibility of exsanguination. Traumatic spine injuries with associated neurologic compromise also deserve immediate attention. These exceptions aside, examination and management of the extremities are deferred to the secondary survey after the airway has been controlled and hemodynamic stability has been obtained. In a team approach, these examinations and treatments take place simultaneously. One caveat to this protocol is the conscious patient who is able to follow commands, but will need intubation to protect his or her airway. In this case, a cursory neurologic examination of the extremities should be performed prior to sedation or intubation. Documentation of motor and sensory function in the upper and lower extremities is valuable information and only takes seconds to carry out. Throughout the resuscitation phase and during the remainder of the hospital course, reexamination in the form of the tertiary survey will ensure that no injury goes unrecognized.

Evidence of pelvic fractures is assessed early in the resuscitative effort. Massive flank or buttock contusions and swelling are indicative of significant bleeding. The Morel-Lavallée lesion is an ecchymotic lesion over the greater trochanter that represents a subcutaneous degloving injury. This lesion is frequently associated with acetabular fractures. Blood at the urethral meatus, signifying injury to the genitourinary tract, may be a sign of an underlying pelvic fracture. Palpation of the symphysis pubis and the sacroiliac joints can help determine the presence of disruption of these joints. Gentle rocking and lateral compression through the anterior iliac crests can provide helpful clues to the stability of the pelvic ring. Any opening or looseness signifies instability and may represent a source of hemorrhage. Rectal and vaginal examinations are performed, noting the presence of gross blood, lacerations, bony fragments, hematomas, or masses. Wounds and palpable bony fragments found on either of these examinations are diagnostic of an open pelvic fracture, which carries a poor prognosis. Rectal examination can also reveal a high-riding prostate gland, another indication of injury to the genitourinary tract.

The trauma team must always take steps to protect the patient from self-inflicted or iatrogenic spinal cord injury. Therefore, full spine precautions must be observed until it is confirmed that the patient's vertebral column is intact, either by physical examination and clinical findings or by radiologic confirmation, when warranted. Fitting the patient with a hard cervical collar stabilizes the cervical spine. Maintaining the patient in a supine flat position at all times protects the thoracic, lumbar, and sacral segments of the spine. If the patient is to be moved, a strict log roll technique is used. At times, a patient may have to be physically restrained to prevent potential self-inflicted injury by head or lower extremity movements that could impart rotational, translational, or bending moments to the vertebral column. Special care must be taken with combative patients or those with altered mental status who may have lost the ability to protect themselves from further injury. On examination of the back, the examiner notes the presence of deformity, edema, or ecchymosis. Tenderness elicited on palpation of the spine is recorded for each level at which the patient complains of pain. Distinction is made regarding whether the pain is midline or paraspinal. Perianal sensation and rectal sphincter tone should be evaluated to test sacral nerve root function. Deep tendon reflexes and pathologic reflexes, such as the bulbocavernosus and Babinski reflexes, are tested.

Plain radiographs of the cervical spine, including AP, lateral, and open-mouth odontoid views were previously considered part of the standard trauma series of radiographs. Recently, however, Mathen and associates have shown that the standard plain films fail to identify 55.5% of clinically relevant fractures identified by multislice CT and add no clinically relevant data.[10] Similarly, a CT of the thoracic, lumbar, and sacral spine is faster and more accurate than radiography at identifying traumatic injury. With most trauma patients undergoing a CT of the chest, abdomen, and pelvis, reformatting the data into spinal reconstructions adds neither time nor radiation exposure. With this data, plain films are no longer indicated.

Examination of the extremities in a patient with isolated injuries or a multitrauma patient follows a simple, systematic, and reproducible pattern. Even when an isolated extremity injury is the primary reason for evaluation, the entire skeleton must be examined. The examiner must not be distracted from the task by obvious or severe injuries. Deformity, edema, ecchymosis, crepitus, tenderness, and pain with motion are the cardinal signs of an acute fracture. Each limb segment needs to be examined for lacerations and the signs of trauma described earlier. All joints are put through passive range of motion, at a minimum. Active range of motion is tested whenever possible. Joint effusions are evidence of intra-articular pathology (e.g., ligament or cartilage damage, or an intra-articular fracture). The joints are then manually stressed to assess the integrity of the ligamentous structures. A neurovascular examination is performed and documented. Pulses are recorded and compared with the opposite uninvolved extremity when possible. Doppler signals are obtained when palpable pulses are not present or are weak. Measuring the ankle-brachial index (ABI) is important when vascular injury is suspected. Motor function and sensation must be documented for the extremity dermatomes as well as the trunk in a patient with thoracic spine pain. To avoid the complications of a missed compartment syndrome, palpation of the involved compartments is performed. Any firm or tense compartments are checked for increased pressure if time and the patient's condition allow. Fasciotomies are performed urgently if pressures are elevated. Gross alignment and interim immobilization of long bone fractures are achieved before transportation of the patient from the trauma room. This helps prevent further damage to underlying soft tissues, reduces patient discomfort, facilitates transportation, and may help prevent further embolization of IM contents.[11] Traction splints or skeletal traction are applied when indicated.

## Diagnostic Imaging

Radiographic examination is used to supplement and enhance the information gathered during the primary survey, history, and physical examination. In a multiply injured patient, the ATLS protocol calls for a lateral cervical spine film and AP views of the pelvis and chest. However, as noted earlier for a stable, conscious patient with no physical examination findings of pelvic trauma, the pelvic film may be deferred for the pelvic CT. Cervical spine x-rays should be deferred for a CT of the cervical spine (if available). The secondary survey then dictates which extremity radiographs are necessary. When filming long bone injuries, it is important to verify the integrity of adjacent limb segments. Therefore, the joints above and below the level of injury are always included in the films. They are filmed separately if the cassette is not large enough to accommodate the entire view. Similarly, when pathology is suspected in a joint, the long bones above and below are also imaged. This practice helps identify commonly associated injuries to the adjacent limb segments that might otherwise be missed.

Because bone is a three-dimensional object, a single two-dimensional radiograph cannot describe a fracture. To understand the position and direction of the fracture fragments, orthogonal views (images taken at 90 degrees to one another) must be obtained. A bone may appear minimally displaced in one plane, but in another view may be significantly displaced (Fig. 20-11). All extremities with deformity need to be rotated to the anatomic position before taking radiographs to help decrease confusion when describing the fracture. When finer detail is necessary to evaluate a fracture pattern better or confirm the findings of an equivocal x-ray, a CT scan should be ordered. Magnetic resonance imaging (MRI) has become a particularly useful imaging modality. It is used to evaluate soft tissue, acute fractures, stress fractures, spinal cord injuries, and intra-articular pathology. Its role in the trauma setting has expanded as well, and it is particularly helpful in the setting of spinal cord injury. More frequently, MRI is used in the outpatient setting to evaluate soft tissue injuries and pathologic lesions. MRI is now commonly used for the diagnosis of acute fractures when plain films are negative.

Although AP and lateral views are generally adequate for most long bone fractures, there are a number of osseous structures that necessitate specific radiographs or routinely require more specialized studies, such as CT or MRI.

### Shoulder

True AP and lateral views of the shoulder must be taken in relation to the scapula because of the orientation of the joint. The most useful lateral view is an axillary radiograph. The tube is angled cephalad, with the plate on the superior aspect of the abducted shoulder. This view is often difficult to obtain because of pain or instability at the proximal end of the humerus. The Velpeau view is a modified axillary view, which provides orthogonally equivalent images. While wearing a sling, the patient leans backward 30 degrees over the cassette on the table. The x-ray tube is placed above the shoulder and the beam is projected vertically down through the shoulder onto the cassette (Fig. 20-12). This allows the x-ray to be taken with the shoulder adducted and in a sling, allowing acquisition of the axillary images without the pain of shoulder abduction.

### Elbow

AP and lateral views of the elbow provide visualization of most of the bony anatomy. Internal and external obliques are included in a complete elbow series and allow for better visualization of the medial and lateral epicondyles. On the lateral view, look for the fat pad sign or the sail sign for evidence of an occult fracture.

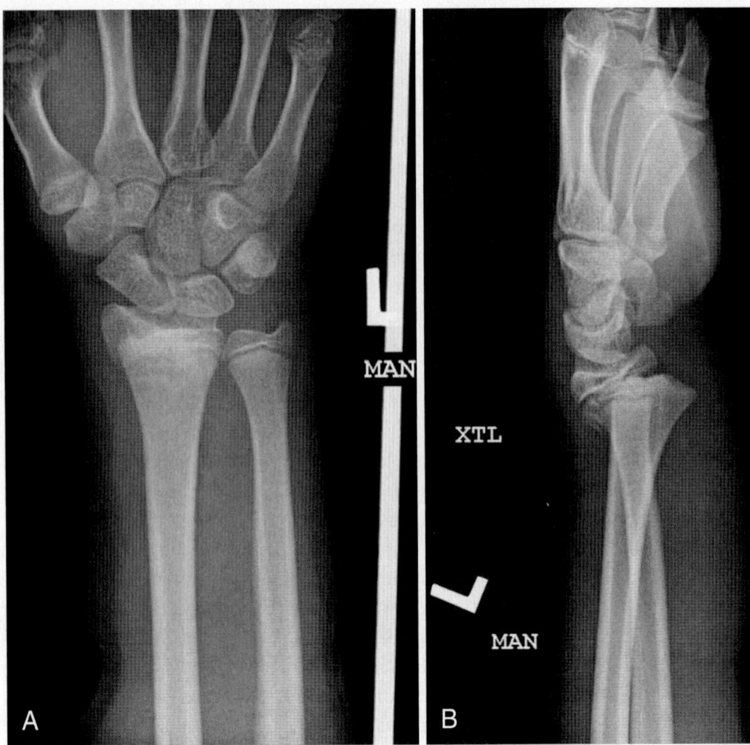


**FIGURE 20-11 A,** AP radiograph of the wrist showing disruption of the distal radial physis, but adequate alignment. **B,** Lateral view showing complete physeal separation, with 50% dorsal displacement and significant angulation.

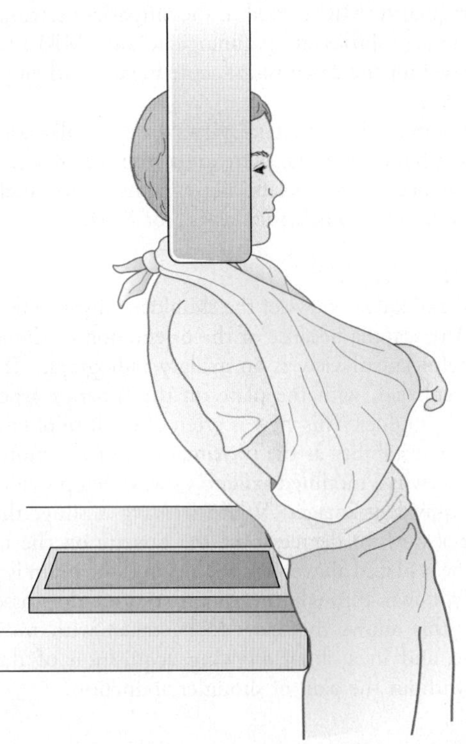

**FIGURE 20-12** Velpeau or Bloom-Obata modified axillary view. (From Green A, Norris TR: Proximal humeral fractures and glenohumeral dislocations. In Browner, BD, Levine AM, Jupiter JB, et al [eds]: Skeletal trauma: Basic science, management, and reconstruction, ed 4, Philadelphia, 2008, WB Saunders.)

The sail sign can be noted when hemiarthrosis from an intra-articular fracture forces the anterior and posterior fat pads out of the coronoid and olecranon fossae, respectively. On x-ray, the visualized fat pads resemble a sail (Fig. 20-13). Although the anterior fat pad can be visualized in a normal elbow, the presence of a posterior fat pad sign is strongly suggestive of occult fracture and, if clinically appropriate, warrants a CT scan.

### Pelvis and Acetabulum

The standard AP radiograph of the pelvis provides an overview to the structural integrity of the hips and pelvic ring. If pelvic pathology is noted on this film or suspected from physical examination, further views are necessary. Judet views, or 45-degree oblique views of the pelvis, are used to evaluate the acetabuli (Fig. 20-14). Because of the spatial orientation of the acetabulum, these views represent orthogonal projections when the x-ray tube is canted toward or away from the affected side. Similarly, inlet and outlet views of the pelvis allow closer examination of the sacroiliac joints and the sacrum itself, as well as identifying AP disruption in the pelvic ring. The inlet view is taken with the beam angled 60 degrees caudad, thus making the beam perpendicular to the pelvic brim. The sacral ala, displacement of the sacroiliac joints, and displacement of the pubic symphysis in the AP plane are easily seen. The outlet view is a 30-degree oblique view, with the tube angled cephalad. The sacrum is pictured en fosse, and the neural foraminae are easily evaluated. If not already obtained as part of the trauma workup, a pelvic CT should be ordered to evaluate fractures of the acetabuli and sacrum. This allows detailed evaluation of the amount of articular involvement, displacement, and presence of bony fragments within the joint. It also provides information regarding sacral displacement or neural foraminal involvement. Finally, it allows evaluation for intrapelvic hematoma. MRI has little role in acute, traumatic pelvic ring injury; however, it is the imaging modality of choice for suspected osteomyelitis or pelvic abscess.

### Hip

A hip series consists of AP and cross-table lateral x-rays. In an adult patient with acute groin pain and inability to bear weight, an occult hip fracture should be ruled out with an MRI or bone scan. In older patients with occult osteopenic hip fractures, bone scans, although accurate, are unreliable within 48 hours after injury. MRI has been shown to be at least as accurate as bone scans in the diagnosis of acute fractures. Additionally, the sensitivity and specificity of MRI were the same within 24 hours of admission as later. Earlier diagnosis can potentially lead to shorter hospital stays and, therefore, in theory offset the additional cost of MRI. In patients with femoral shaft fractures, the incidence of ipsilateral femoral neck fracture is as high as 9%. A protocol of AP internal rotation views of the hip, as well as thin cut CT (2-mm cuts) through the femoral neck in the emergency department (ED), has been shown to decrease the incidence of delayed diagnosis of this injury.[12]

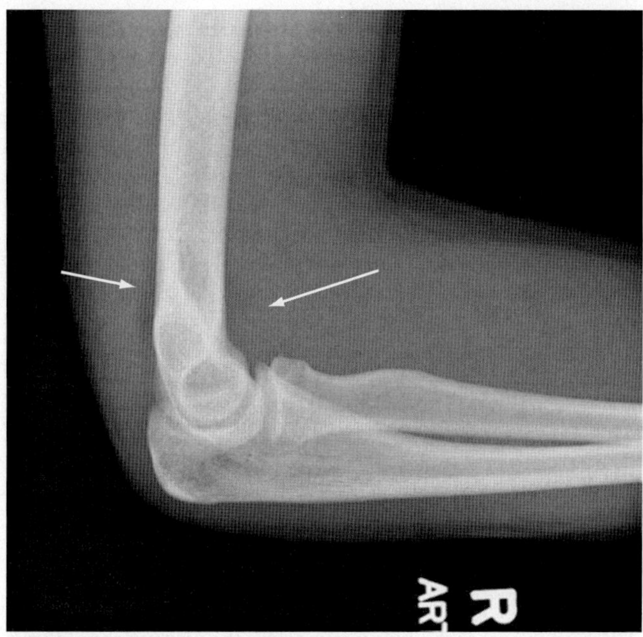


**FIGURE 20-13** Positive fat pad or sail sign in a patient with a nondisplaced radial neck fracture. Note the anterior and posterior areas of radiolucency *(arrows)* representing the extruded fat pads.

### Knee

AP, lateral, and internal or external oblique plain films allow visualization of most traumatic osseous abnormalities of the knee. If possible, standing films are useful for evaluating knee alignment and joint space narrowing. The lateral film can show an effusion, patellar fracture, posterior tibial plateau fracture, or tibial tubercle injury. If there is any doubt as to the degree of articular involvement, displacement, or depression, a CT scan should be ordered (Fig. 20-15). Although an MRI can be helpful in the acute setting, evaluation of ligamentous derangement is not urgent and can be deferred to the outpatient setting. In the setting of a knee dislocation, vascular injury should be assumed until proven otherwise. Serial measurements of the ABI are useful to monitor for vascular compromise, but vascular imaging in the form of CT angiography (CTA) or MR angiography (MRA) should be strongly considered in the setting of an acute knee dislocation.

### Ankle

In the ankle, it is important to confirm maintenance of the mortise. The stability of the mortise depends on bony and ligamentous support. With AP, mortise, and lateral x-rays, disruptions in the bony anatomy can be visualized directly. Although the ligamentous structures cannot be visualized directly, assumptions about their continuity can be made by evaluating the spaces between the bones. Three main parameters are commonly used are the tibia-fibula overlap, tibia-fibula clear space, and medial clear space (Fig. 20-16). All three parameters should be measured on the AP radiograph. The medial clear space is the distance between the medial border of the talus and lateral border of the medial malleolus. A normal value is less than 4 mm. The tibia-fibula clear space is the distance between the medial border of the fibula and floor of the incisura fibularis. A normal value is less than 5 mm. The tibia-fibula overlap is the amount of the lateral tibia overlapping the medial fibula. A

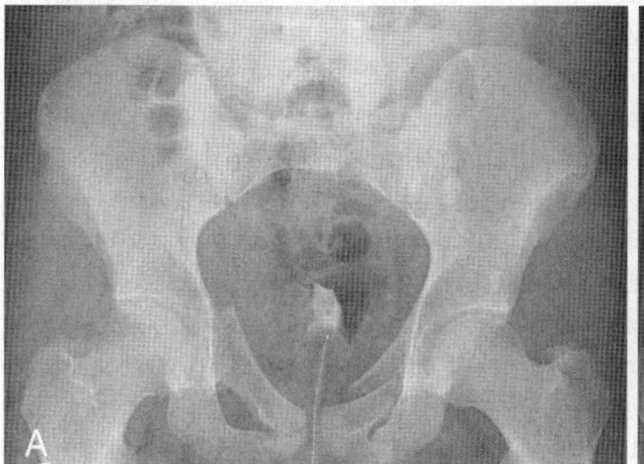

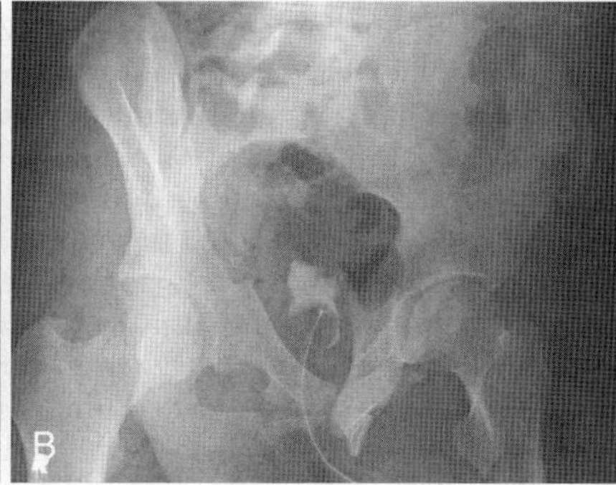

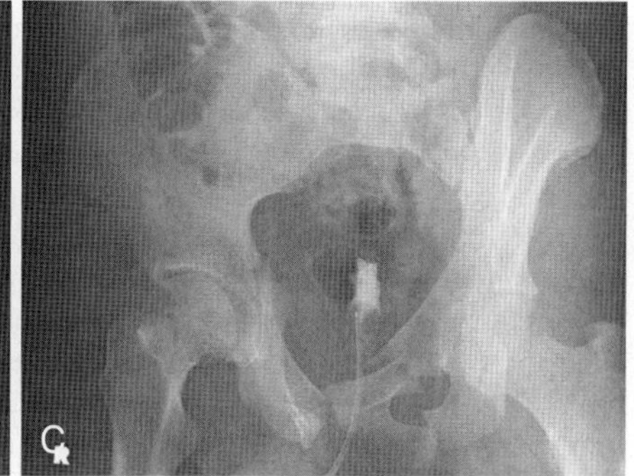


**FIGURE 20-14** AP and Judet pelvic radiographs clearly show the anterior and posterior walls and columns of both acetabuli. **A,** AP view showing bilateral inferior and superior pubic ramus fractures as well as a right acetabular fracture. **B,** Right obturator oblique view shows disruption of the anterior column and posterior wall of the right acetabulum. **C,** Right iliac oblique view shows disruption of the posterior column and anterior wall of the right acetabulum.

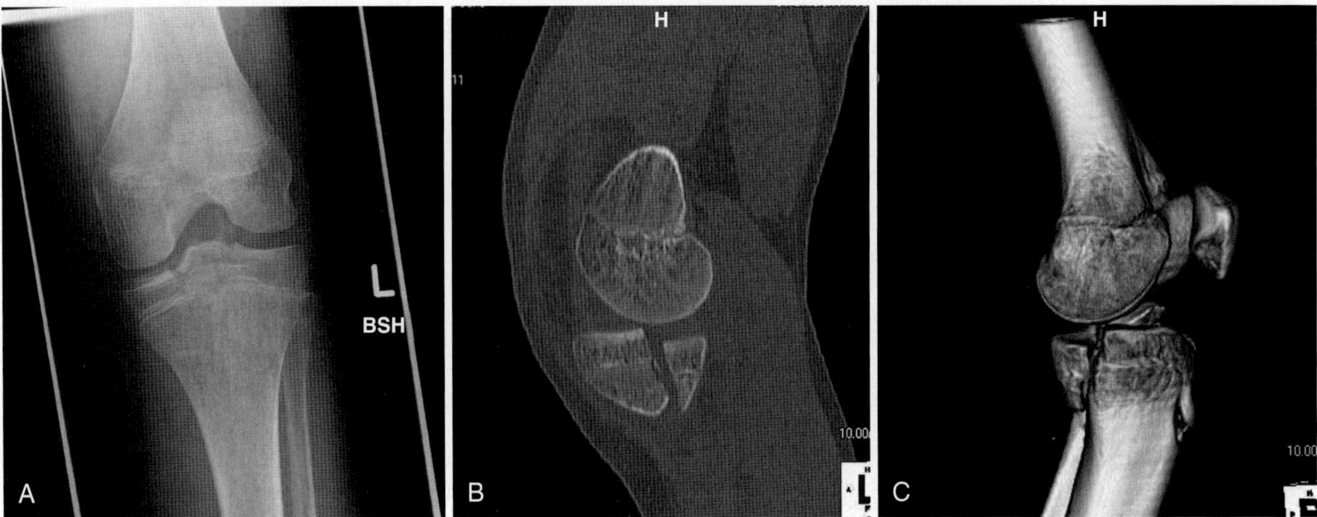


FIGURE 20-15 **A,** Minimally displaced fracture of the tibial eminence. **B,** CT scan of the knee shows a significant stepoff of the posterior medial tibial plateau. **C,** Three-dimensional reconstruction.

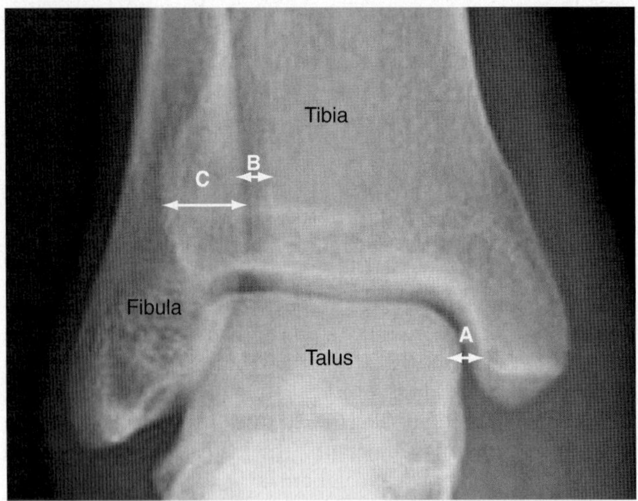


FIGURE 20-16 AP radiograph of the ankle showing medial clear space **(A)**, tibia-fibula clear space **(B)**, and tibia-fibula overlap **(C)**.

normal value is more than 10 mm. In an adult ankle, there should be some degree of tibia-fibula overlap in all views. Both the tibia-fibula clear space and overlap are measured 10 mm proximally to the tibial plafond. Excluding a direct blow injury, sustaining an isolated medial malleolar fracture is exceedingly rare. Most ankle injuries are caused by a twisting moment imparted to the ankle. The energy that enters through the medial malleolus must exit at some point on the lateral ankle. This may result in a lateral collateral ligament tear (rare), lateral malleolar fracture, or a more proximal fibula fracture. In some cases, the energy passes through the syndesmosis and exits at the proximal fibula. This is known as a Maisonneuve fracture. The disruption results in an unstable ankle mortise, which influences the treatment plan. Because of this, any isolated medial malleolar fracture should always get full-length AP and lateral tibia-fibula x-rays. In the case of an intra-articular fracture of the weight-bearing surface of the tibia (pilon fracture), a CT can be useful to evaluate the joint surface.

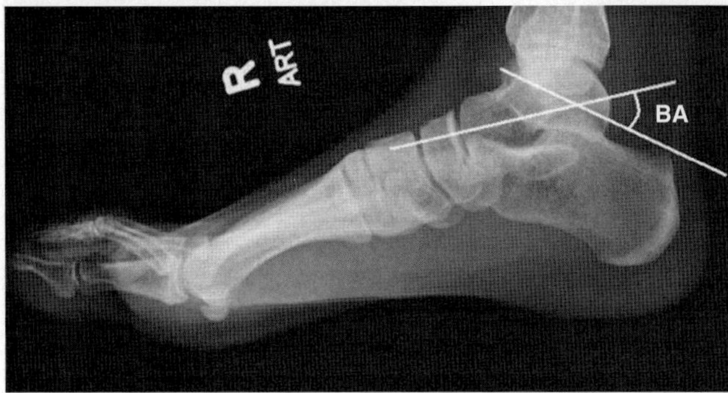


FIGURE 20-17 Lateral radiograph of the foot showing Bohler's angle (BA).

### Foot

When an injury of the foot is suspected, the workup should start with a standard series of AP, lateral, and oblique x-rays. However, because of the complex three-dimensional structure of the foot, this standard series of films may not be adequate to visualize certain bones. In the case of a calcaneus fracture, a Harris axial view should be added to evaluate the varus-valgus alignment of the tuberosity, as well as any sagittal splits in the bone. Bohler's angle—an angle formed by the bisection of a line drawn from the superior aspect of the calcaneal tuberosity to the superior aspect of the posterior facet and a line drawn from the tip of the anterior process to the superior aspect of the posterior facet—should be evaluated in the lateral view (Fig. 20-17). A normal Bohler's angle is between 20 and 40 degrees. A decrease in this angle usually indicates fracture, with depression of the posterior facet. When in doubt, films of the uninjured foot should be taken for comparison. For fractures of the talus, the AP and lateral films should be evaluated for articular congruence at the tibiotalar, subtalar, and talonavicular joints. There are specialized views of the bone (e.g., Canale view for the talar neck and Broden's view for evaluation of the subtalar joint); however, these views are radiology technician–dependent. In many cases, if a fracture is seen on the AP or lateral views, a CT scan is a

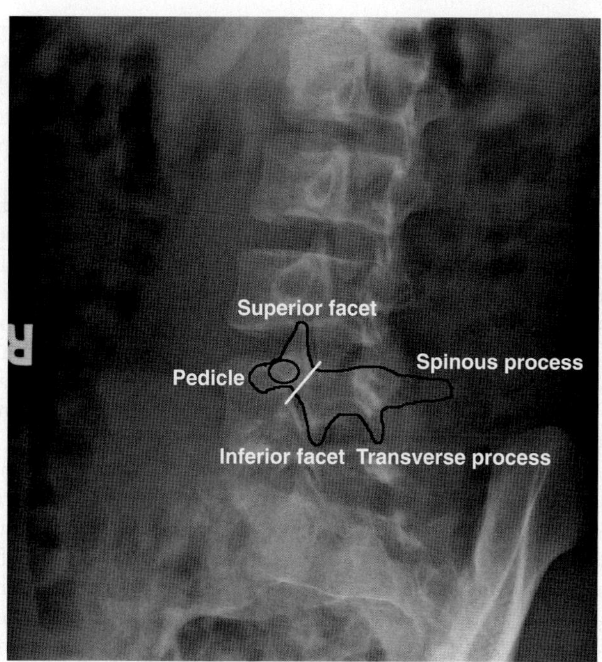


**FIGURE 20-18** Oblique radiograph of the lumbar spine with the Scotty dog outlined. Back leg, transverse process; ear, superior articular facet; eye, pedicle; front leg, inferior articular facet; neck, pars interarticularis; tail, spinous process (*white line* [the collar] represents a fracture).

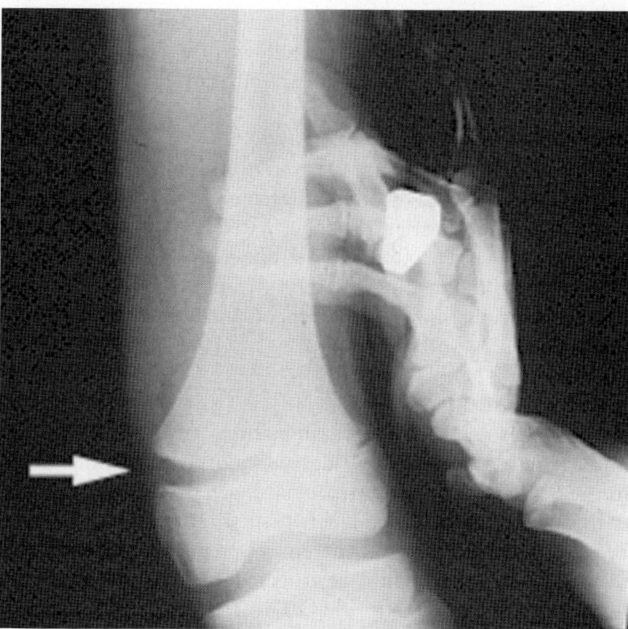

**FIGURE 20-19** Stress radiograph of a physeal injury of the distal femur. An AP radiograph with valgus stress applied reveals unstable physeal disruption.

faster and more cost-effective way to evaluate the displacement pattern. If x-rays are negative or equivocal and the patient has evidence of fracture—ecchymosis, pain out of proportion to plain film findings, significant soft tissue swelling—then a CT scan should be ordered. All but the most minimally displaced intra-articular fractures of the talus and calcaneus warrant a CT scan to define the fracture pattern and extent of articular displacement better. Except in the case of suspected osteomyelitis, MRI of the foot is of little use in the emergency setting.

## Spine

In patients with acute back pain, AP and lateral x-rays of the spine can be useful to look for fractures, spondylolisthesis, malalignment, or congenital anomalies. Oblique views are sometimes necessary to evaluate the bony anatomy of the spine more completely. Figure 20-18 shows the outline of the so-called Scotty dog. Each body part of the "dog" represents a portion of the vertebral body anatomy. The bony link between the superior and inferior facets, the pars interarticularis, is visualized as the neck of the dog. A "collar" around the dog's neck represents disruption of this bony link, fracture or spondylolysis, which can represent an unstable injury. In most cases of traumatic injury presenting with a complaint of back pain, suspicious findings on plain films, back pain out of proportion to x-ray findings, or neurologic deficit, further imaging is needed. CT is useful for defining bony anatomy. If ligamentous injury or neurologic compromise is suspected, MRI should be performed. In patients for whom MRI is contraindicated, a bone scan can be considered if occult fracture is suspected and CT myelography can be used to look for compromise of the spinal canal or intervertebral foraminae.

## Intra-Articular Fractures

The goal of radiographic assessment of intra-articular fractures is quantitation of articular incongruity and degree of malalignment. Orthogonal views of the joint and adjacent long bones are obtained. Radiographs made parallel to the articular surface best display any step-off that might be present. In complex intra-articular fractures, a CT scan is usually necessary to understand the position and displacement of all articular fragments fully. CT scans provide fine detail, help locate small fragments in the joint, and can further describe the extension of intra-articular fracture lines. They must not be used in lieu of acceptable plain radiographs, however. Plain radiographs are better suited to describe overall fracture characteristics and limb alignment accurately.

## Stress Radiographs

Stress radiographs are taken when ligamentous or growth plate injuries are suspected after clinical examination but are not evident on plain films. Gapping of the joint or physis while stressing the structure in question is diagnostic (Fig. 20-19). Cervical spine ligamentous injuries are often diagnosed this way with active flexion-extension radiographs. Passive flexion-extension must not be attempted.

## Vascular Injuries

Angiography is another important modality used for the evaluation of extremity and pelvic injuries. It is indicated whenever signs of distal ischemia are noted in an extremity. In addition, it should be considered for a patient with pelvic fractures who is hemodynamically unstable. Knee dislocations are concerning because of the high incidence of associated vascular injury. There is up to a 30% reported incidence of injury to the popliteal artery in patients with traumatic knee dislocation.[11] Current recommendations for evaluation of the leg following a knee injury include serial vascular examinations, using both manual palpation of pulses and the ABI, followed by selective arteriography of patients with abnormal examination findings.[13]

## INITIAL MANAGEMENT

Care of musculoskeletal injuries often begins in the field. The extent of fracture and wound management differs with the level of training and experience of the first responders—laypeople, police, and emergency medical personnel. Therefore, it is essential that the initial treating physician performs a thorough assessment and begins initial management, including splinting and wound care.

### Wound Management

After a thorough physical examination, treatment is begun immediately. All wound dressings and nontraction splints placed in the field should be removed by a single examiner to evaluate the degree of deformity and soft tissue injury. Superficial contamination by dirt, gravel, or grass is removed. Using sterile technique, wounds should be irrigated with sterile saline and mechanically débrided in the ED. If a significant delay is expected between presentation and formal operative irrigation and débridement, or if there is significant gross contamination, pulsatile lavage in the ED should be considered. Sterile saline solution or povidone-iodine–soaked dressings are then applied. After sterile dressings are placed over the wounds in the ED, they should remain in place until the time of operative irrigation and débridement (I&D). Careless wound management in the ED has been shown to increase the ultimate infection rate by 300% to 400%.[14] Tetanus prophylaxis and broad-spectrum intravenous (IV) antibiotics are administered. Immobilization is then undertaken in the same manner as for a closed injury. External bleeding in the extremities is controlled by direct manual pressure.

### Reduction and Immobilization

All displaced fractures and dislocations are gently reduced to reestablish limb alignment provisionally. If the patient's condition allows, precise reductions are performed and the extremities are splinted formally to maintain the fracture reduction. With time, the difficulty of reduction increases because of edema and muscle spasm. Therefore, reduction needs to be attempted as soon as possible and with the patient as relaxed as possible. Often, narcotic analgesics and sedatives are necessary, particularly with large joint dislocations. Muscle spasm can obstruct atraumatic reduction of these injuries. If a joint is still dislocated after adequate sedation and relaxation, general anesthesia may be necessary.

Reduction maneuvers follow the same principles for all fracture and dislocation types. First, in-line traction is applied to the limb. If the soft tissue envelope surrounding the fracture fragments is intact, in-line traction alone may produce satisfactory alignment via ligamentotaxis. In most cases, the deformity must be re-created and exaggerated to unhook the fractured ends. While still pulling traction, the mechanism of injury is reversed and the fracture reduced. Neurovascular status is documented before and after any reduction maneuver or splint application. Once satisfactory reduction or alignment is achieved, it must be maintained by immobilization through casting, splinting, or continuous traction. The joints above and below the fracture must be included to prevent displacement. Postreduction radiographs are required to confirm alignment and rotation. Nondisplaced fractures are treated like displaced fractures, without reduction. Most nondisplaced fractures do not require surgical treatment. Splints are placed initially and then changed to circumferential casts after the swelling subsides.

Ligamentous injuries may also require immobilization. The joint is fully evaluated as described earlier, and a thorough neurovascular examination is performed on the limb. Frequently, pain, effusions, or hemarthroses occur; these represent intra-articular pathology. Therapeutic aspiration of a traumatic hemiarthrosis is not recommended because this can lead to iatrogenic infection. In addition, release of the pressure of the effusion can precipitate more bleeding. The limb is then immobilized and reevaluated after the acute pain and swelling decrease.

The rationale for immobilization is threefold. First, splinting, particularly with traction or compression devices, reduces bleeding by reducing the volume of the muscular compartments. Second, additional soft tissue injury may be averted, and the chance of converting a closed to an open fracture by sharp bony fragments is reduced. Third, immobilization of the fracture reduces patient discomfort and facilitates transportation and radiographic evaluation of the patient. All fractures and dislocations are splinted or immobilized in the ED. Usually, splints are fashioned from padded plaster or fiberglass. Different splinting techniques are used to immobilize each type of fracture. A volar or ulnar gutter splint is used for fractures of the hand. A sugar tong splint (Figs. 20-20*A* to *D*) is used for wrist or forearm fractures. This splint prevents flexion and extension at the wrist and elbow, as well as pronation and supination of the forearm. A posterior elbow splint is applied for fractures or dislocations of this joint. For humeral shaft fractures, a coaptation or posterior splint is used. When there is minimal swelling present with a humeral shaft fracture, a functional fracture brace may be applied in the emergency room. A short-leg splint consisting of a posterior slab and a U or stirrup component (see Figs. 20-20*E* to *H*) is used for pathology of the foot and ankle. With the addition of side slabs crossing the knee, this splint can be extended into a long-leg splint for tibial fractures or knee dislocations (see Figs. 20-20*I* and *J*). Splints can be secured with a bias-cut stockinette, elastic wraps, or gauze bandage, provided that they are wrapped in a nonconstrictive fashion.

The role of circumferential casting in the acute setting is questionable. Because swelling of the injured extremity increases for 48 to 72 hours, a circular cast can be too constrictive and may lead to pressure necrosis or compartment syndrome. In select cases, in which a cast will be the definitive treatment (pediatric fractures or select nondisplaced fractures in adults), the initial circumferential cast can be applied and then cut longitudinally on two sides to allow swelling without splitting of the padding. This technique is called bivalving the cast; it maintains a reduction more effectively than an open splint while still allowing for soft tissue swelling.

### Traction

Traction is used to immobilize fractures or dislocations displaced by muscle forces that cannot be adequately controlled with simple splints. The most common indications are vertical shear injuries of the pelvis, hip dislocations, acetabular fractures, and fractures of the proximal femur or femoral shaft. Traction may be applied through the skin using a Buck's traction boot or

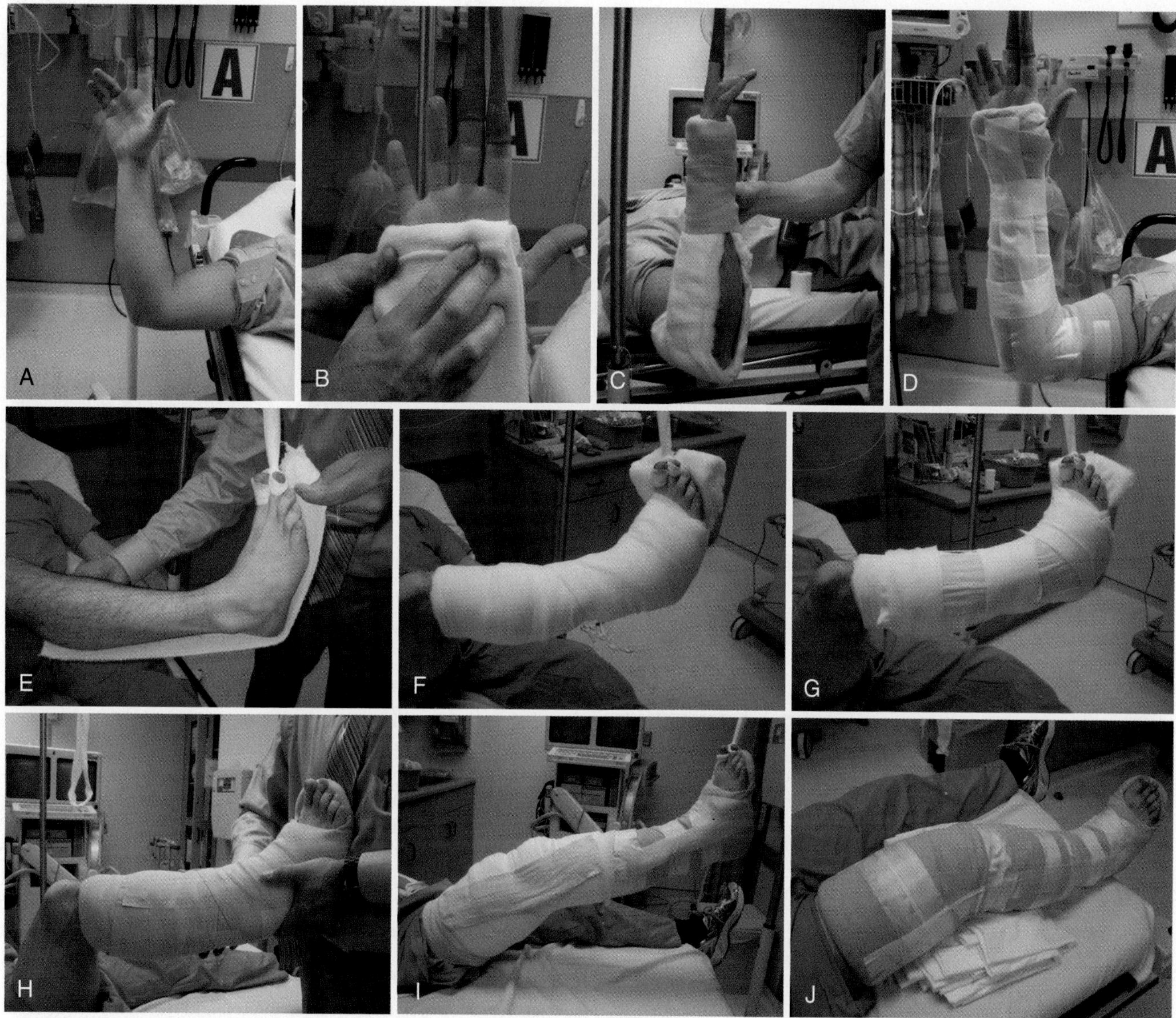


**FIGURE 20-20** Application of sugar tong **(A-D)**, short-leg **(E-H)**, and long-leg **(I-J)** splints. **A,** Finger traps are used to apply gravity traction. **B, C,** A well-padded splint (plaster or fiberglass) is measured and applied to the limb. The splint should extend from the distal palmer crease volarly **(B)** to the metacarpophalangeal (MCP) joints dorsally. This allows motion of the MCP joints. **D,** The compressive wrap (bias bandage or ace wrap) is applied and secured with tape. **E,** Gravity traction is applied by hanging the limb by the toes in a figure-4 position across the bed. This serves two functions. First, flexion at the knee relaxes the pull of the gastrocnemius muscle across the ankle; second, the inversion produced by this position helps maintain fibular length and the reduction of the medial malleolus. Both a posterior slab and U or stirrup component (plaster or fiberglass) are measured. **F,** The limb is protected with a soft dressing (circumferential Robert Jones cotton). **G,** The posterior followed by the stirrup splints are applied to the injured extremity and held in place with cast padding. **H,** The compressive wrap (bias bandage or Ace wrap) is applied and secured with tape. When possible, the knee is flexed and the ankle is placed in neutral position to prevent equinus contracture. **I,** The short-leg splint may be extended into a long-leg splint by protecting the remainder of the limb with a soft dressing and then applying medial and lateral side slabs overlapping the short-leg splint and extending to the proximal thigh. **J,** Again, the compressive wrap (bias bandage or Ace wrap) is applied and secured with tape.

through the bone using a skeletal traction pin placed through the bone distal to the fracture (Fig. 20-21). Traction of more than 8 pounds through the skin for any extended period causes skin damage. Therefore, skin traction is practical only for geriatric hip fractures and pediatric injuries requiring limited distraction force. The Hare traction splint applies a distraction force through an ankle stirrup and can provide effective immobilization for femoral shaft fractures (Fig. 20-22). It can be applied in the field and helps facilitate transport and mobilization, but should be used only temporarily due to the risk of skin breakdown from the stirrup.

Skeletal traction may be maintained for longer periods with more weight than that possible with skin traction. Up to 10% of body weight may be applied to a lower extremity skeletal traction pin. Neurovascular structures must be avoided during placement of the pins. As a rule of thumb, pins should be placed

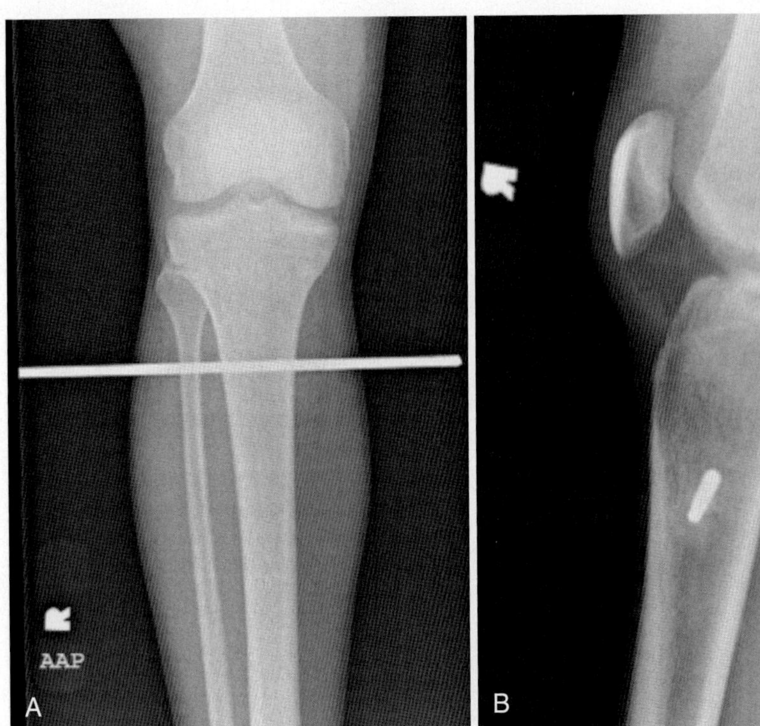


**FIGURE 20-21** **A, B,** Proximal tibial traction pin.

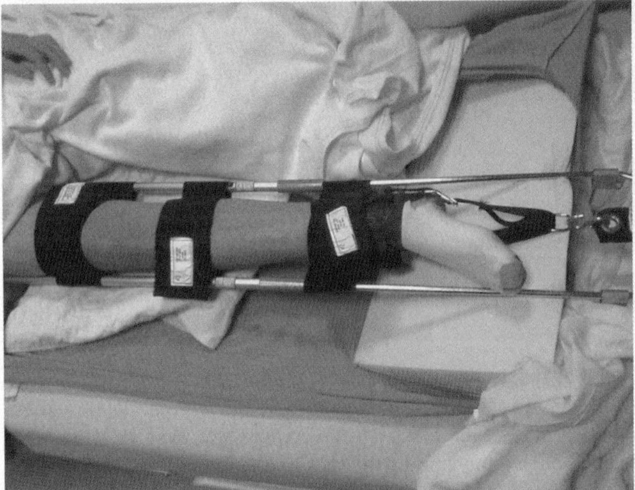

**FIGURE 20-22** Hare traction splint placed at the scene of the accident to stabilize a femoral shaft fracture.

from the side of the extremity containing the known structure at risk. This allows control over where the pin enters in relation to these structures. In the distal femur, the pin should be passed from medial to lateral to avoid the adductor hiatus containing the femoral artery and nerve. The pin should be placed parallel to the knee joint at the level of the superior pole of the patella and in the midpoint of the bone on the lateral x-ray. In the proximal tibia, the pin should be passed from lateral to medial to avoid the common peroneal nerve passing around the fibular head. The ideal pin placement is parallel to the joint, approximately 2 cm distal and 2 cm posterior to the top of the tibial tubercle. In the calcaneus, the pin should be passed medial to lateral to avoid the neurovascular bundle passing around the medial malleolus. The pin should be placed in the tuberosity, parallel to the ankle joint, as far posterior and inferior as possible while still passing through good bone. Once the pins are placed, the skin is checked for tension and relieved with incisions if necessary. The wounds are then dressed with povidone-iodine–soaked sponges. Pin tract infections are a common complication and can lead to osteomyelitis in the worst cases. For this reason, all pin sites are cleaned with a half-strength hydrogen peroxide solution and a sterile dressing applied at least twice daily.

## Prioritization of Surgical Care

After the secondary survey is completed and necessary diagnostic studies are obtained, a multiply injured patient may be moved to the operating room. Because operative decisions are made on a continuous basis as the patient's condition evolves, the trauma surgeon serves as the coordinator of care and prioritizes all surgical procedures after consulting with the anesthesiologist, neurosurgeon, and orthopedic surgeon. Critical procedures are carried out first, and each additional intervention is reviewed as the patient's status evolves. Intra-abdominal, intrapelvic, thoracic, retroperitoneal, and intracranial hemorrhages are immediate surgical priorities. These injuries include acute visceral hemorrhage, aortic or caval injuries, injuries to the heart and pulmonary vessels, intracranial mass lesions, depressed skull fractures, and pelvic fractures with associated instability. In addition to hemorrhage, immediate surgery is indicated for the prevention of local and systemic infections from open or devitalized wounds and limb salvage.

Stabilization of severe open and femoral shaft fractures may be performed simultaneously or after hemodynamic stabilization of the surgical patient. Limb-threatening vascular injuries are managed on an emergency basis because limiting the warm ischemia time to 6 hours is essential for optimal recovery.[15] Decisions regarding limb viability, compartment syndrome, and the need for amputation of a mangled extremity are made in concert with all services involved. Consideration must also be given to emergency capsulotomy and ORIF of femoral head fractures, as well as reduction of posterior hip dislocations, to prevent avascular necrosis. Definitive care of complex upper extremity fractures or intra-articular fractures is undertaken if the patient's condition permits. Spine, acetabular, and upper extremity injuries are addressed next. The operative repair of maxillofacial injuries can usually be delayed for several days, depending on the status of the patient.

## ORTHOPEDIC EMERGENCIES

### Open Fractures

Until recently, open fractures were considered surgical emergencies. The 6-hour rule dictated that open fractures require immediate operative management, within 6 hours of injury. It was believed that delay beyond the 6-hour window significantly increased the risk of deep infection in this patient population. A number of studies in the last 10 years have shown that there is little correlation between infection rate and time to surgery.[16,17] These studies have shown no difference in infection rate in patients washed out within 6 hours and those washed out within 12 or even 24 hours. These findings are important because they allow for more complete resuscitation of the patient and negate the need for after-hours surgery by a tired surgeon or a general operating room staff who may be less comfortable with orthopedic cases. The current belief is that open fractures warrant emergent ED management (antibiotics, tetanus, irrigation, and débridement) followed by urgent operative débridement, within 12 to 24 hours, because the long-term complications of infection or nonunion may threaten the patient's limb and can, with systemic sepsis, threaten the patient's life. The difficulty of open fracture management has been recognized for centuries. Amputation was the mainstay of treatment until the mid-1800s, when antiseptic technique came into use. Antisepsis, combined with débridement of all contaminated and devitalized tissue, provided the first reduction in open fracture–related mortality. Contemporaneous advances in antibiotic prophylaxis, aggressive débridement, open wound management, rotational muscle flaps, free tissue transfer, and bone grafting techniques have dramatically enhanced our capacity to treat severe open fractures resulting from high-energy trauma.

### Classification

A fracture is considered open when the fracture site communicates with the environment. Although the laceration or skin avulsion is the most obvious component, the entire zone of injury must be fully appreciated at the time of surgical exploration to assign an adequate severity grade (Fig. 20-23). Gustilo and Anderson have devised the most commonly cited classification of fractures with soft tissue injury.[18] They divided fractures into three grades based on the length of the skin opening, degree of comminution, soft tissue injury, and contamination (Table 20-2). Grade III fractures are further divided into three subtypes, depending on the degree of soft tissue stripping and presence or absence of vascular injury. This classification scheme represents a continuum. Sharp divisions between groups are difficult to discern, particularly among the intermediate grades; thus, interobserver variation occurs.

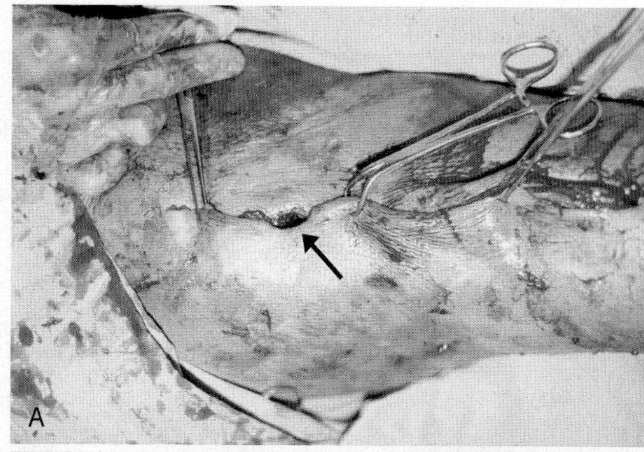


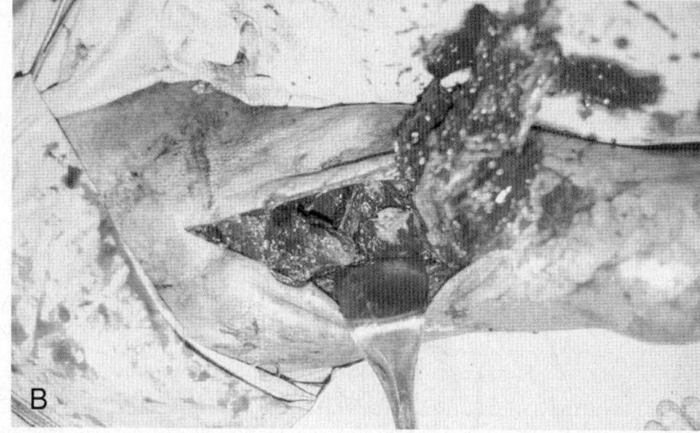


**FIGURE 20-23** Débridement of an open wound. **A,** The small original skin wound *(arrow)* is shown in the center of a surgical incision. **B,** The full extent of underlying soft tissue damage cannot be appreciated until after exploration.

The Gustilo-Andersen classification provides useful information regarding the prognosis and treatment of the injured extremity. Infection rates tend to increase from grades I through III. Infection rates range from 0% to 2% for grade I fractures, from 2% to 10% in grade II fractures, and from 10% to 50% for grade III fractures, with grade IIIc fractures exhibiting the highest rates of infection.[19] The predictive value of cultures prior to formal débridement is low. Therefore, the recommendation is to treat presumed bacterial contamination by a standard protocol rather than attempting to identify potential pathogens. Regardless of fracture grade, antimicrobials and tetanus prophylaxis are administered in the trauma room for any open fracture. In all open fractures and in closed fractures with soft tissue injuries, a first-generation cephalosporin is preferred. Most authors recommend addition of an aminoglycoside for grades II and III fractures. For any fracture with suspected soil contamination ("barnyard" injuries), high-dose penicillin is added to the regimen to cover *Clostridium* spp. (see Table 20-2). Current recommendations for duration of antibiotic therapy include 48 to72 hours of treatment initially and another 48 to 72 hours of therapy following each trip to the operating room for surgical débridement or closure.

The soft tissue destruction in a closed injury can be worse than that in comparable open injuries. Tscherne and Gotzen have classified closed fractures by creating a spectrum similar to what was recognized in open fractures (Table 20-3).[14] Although

**Table 20-2 Gustilo-Anderson Classification of Open Fractures**

| FRACTURE TYPE | DESCRIPTION | ANTIBIOTICS |
|---|---|---|
| I | Skin opening <1 cm, clean; most likely inside-to-outside lesion; minimal muscle contusion; simple transverse or oblique fracture | First-generation cephalosporin |
| II | Laceration >1 cm with extensive soft tissue damage, flaps, or avulsion; minimal to moderate crushing; simple transverse or short oblique fracture with minimal comminution | First-generation cephalosporin ± aminoglycoside |
| III | Extensive soft tissue damage, including muscle, skin, and neurovascular structures; often a high-velocity injury with a severe crushing component (barnyard injuries) | First-generation cephalosporin + aminoglycoside + penicillin G |
| IIIA | Extensive laceration, adequate bone coverage; segmental fracture; gunshot injuries | |
| IIIB | Extensive soft tissue damage with periosteal stripping and bone exposure necessitating formal soft tissue coverage; usually associated with massive contamination | |
| IIIC | Any open fracture with a vascular injury requiring repair | |

From Gustilo R, Mendoza R, Williams DN: Problems in the management of type III (severe) open fractures. J Trauma 24:742–746, 1984.

**Table 20-3 Tscherne Classification of Fractures with Soft Tissue Injuries**

| FRACTURE TYPE | DESCRIPTION |
|---|---|
| 0 | Minimal soft tissue damage; indirect violence; simple fracture patterns (e.g., torsion fracture of the tibia in skiers) |
| I | Superficial abrasion or contusion caused by pressure from within; mild to moderately severe fracture configuration (e.g., pronation fracture-dislocation of the ankle joint with a soft tissue lesion over the medial malleolus) |
| II | Deep contaminated abrasion associated with localized skin or muscle contusion; impending compartment syndrome; severe fracture configuration (e.g., segmental bumper fracture of the tibia) |
| III | Extensive skin contusion or crushing injury; underlying muscle damage may be severe; subcutaneous avulsion; decompensated compartment syndrome; associated major vascular injury; severe or comminuted fracture configuration |

From Tscherne H, Oestern H: Die Klassifizierung des Weichteilschadens bei offenen und geschlossenen Frakturen. Unfallheikunde 85:111–115, 1982.

this system has not been critically validated with outcome measures, it provides a means to gauge the significance of associated soft tissue injury. When these tissues become necrotic or if a surgical approach is carried out through them, infection rates could potentially increase.

## Initial Management

Early irrigation and débridement are the mainstays of treatment. Once the patient is in the operating room, dressings can be removed, along with all loose debris. Débridement requires meticulous removal and resection of all foreign and nonviable material from the wound. The goal is reduction of the bacterial count by leaving only clearly viable tissue behind. The wound is aggressively explored because the zone of injury is always larger than initially evident. Areas in which the extent of injury is commonly misjudged include the thigh and posterior leg because of their considerable muscle bulk. The fascial compartments are not completely decompressed by open fractures, and therefore fasciotomies are liberally performed during débridement to prevent compartment syndrome. Irrigation with copious amounts of sterile saline solution is then done. Many additives, including antibiotics, antiseptics, and surfactants, have been studied in an effort to increase the efficacy of wound irrigation. Of these three, only surfactants have shown promise for reducing infection rate. However, further studies are needed before surfactant solutions are recommended for routine use. Repeat débridement is performed 48 to 72 hours later because the tissue may demarcate and necrose. Surgical incisions used to enlarge the wound for exploration are closed primarily. The original wound created by the injury is usually left open. Dressings moistened with saline solution are applied and changed once or twice daily. In contrast to temporary dressings applied for transport from the emergency department, definitive wound management dressings should not be soaked in povidone-iodine because it causes tissue destruction.

Planning for wound coverage begins with the initial débridement. Early plastic surgery consultation may be helpful. If skin grafting or muscle flap coverage is necessary, it should be performed within the first 72 hours before secondary colonization and wound fibrosis develop. The desire to avoid nosocomial infection has promoted a trend toward immediate coverage of open fracture wounds. If there is a large soft tissue or bony void present following débridement, local antibiotic delivery may be beneficial while waiting for definitive soft tissue coverage. By using an antibiotic bead pouch (antibiotic-impregnated polymethylmethacrylate beads under an impermeable surgical dressing), high levels of local antibiotics can be delivered without the toxic effects that the same systemic dose would have on the patient.

### Limb Salvage Versus Primary Amputation

The choice between primary amputation and salvage of a severely injured extremity is a difficult one. Successful salvage depends on a number of factors, including vascular status, extent of soft tissue injury, degree of comminution, bone loss, and neurologic function. In addition to these local factors, ultimate success depends on systemic and psychological elements. Patients with poor nutrition, multisystem injuries, or psychoses and those unable to cooperate with a lengthy reconstructive process may not be candidates for limb salvage. Several scoring systems have been devised to help assess the need for primary amputation objectively. These systems were developed retrospectively in reference to injuries involving the lower part of the leg. Severely injured upper extremities have a far greater impact on the overall functioning status of the patient, and thus indications for upper extremity amputation are significantly more limited.

Absolute indications for primary amputation are an anatomically complete disruption of the tibial nerve in an adult and warm ischemia time longer than 6 hours. Relative indications are serious associated polytrauma, severe ipsilateral foot trauma, and an anticipated protracted course to achieve soft tissue coverage and bony reconstruction. If either of the absolute indications or two of the three relative indications are met, amputation is indicated. Although few studies have been performed to validate this scheme, these guidelines have been adopted widely and are considered the standard of care.

The mangled extremity severity score (MESS) is the most widely validated classification system. It is the product of a retrospective review of 25 charts of patients with severe open fractures of the lower extremity (Table 20-4).[15] Investigators found that limb salvage was related to vascular status, patient age, duration of ischemia, and absorbed energy. A score of 7 or higher consistently predicted the need for amputation, whereas all limbs with initial scores of 6 or less remained viable in the long term. This system has been validated prospectively and subsequent studies have almost uniformly supported the specificity of MESS in evaluating a severely injured lower leg. Subsequent studies have confirmed the high specificity (i.e., a low score reliability predicts limb salvage); however, these studies have also shown the sensitivity of the MESS to be low (i.e., a high score does not necessarily predict the need for amputation).[20] Other scoring systems have been shown to be equally poor predictors of the need for amputation.

**Table 20-4 Mangled Extremity Severity Score (MESS)**

| COMPONENT | POINTS |
|---|---|
| **Skeletal and Soft Tissue Injury** | |
| Low energy (stab, simple fracture, civilian gunshot wound) | 1 |
| Medium energy (open or multiplex fractures, dislocation) | 2 |
| High energy (close-range shotgun or military gunshot wound; crush injury) | 3 |
| Very high energy (same as above plus gross contamination, soft tissue avulsion) | 4 |
| **Limb Ischemia (Doubled if >6 hr)** | |
| Pulse reduced or absent but perfusion normal | 1 |
| Pulseless, paresthesias, diminished capillary refill | 2 |
| Cool, paralyzed, insensate, numb | 3 |
| **Shock** | |
| Systolic blood pressure always >90 mm Hg | 0 |
| Hypotensive transiently | 1 |
| Persistent hypotension | 2 |
| **Age (yr)** | |
| <30 | 0 |
| 30-50 | 1 |
| >50 | 2 |

From Johansen K, Daines M, Howey T, et al: Objective criteria accurately predict amputation following lower extremity trauma. J Trauma 30:568–573, 1990.

Few studies have compared the functional outcome of below-knee amputation (BKA) with that of salvaged limbs. A meta-analysis of studies comparing the two has shown that functional outcome up to 7 years out from the initial injury was no different between the two groups of patients.[21] Both groups had equal length of initial hospital stay, but the patients who underwent limb salvage had increase length of rehabilitation, a greater number of additional surgeries, greater likelihood of rehospitalization, and likely higher total cost. In contrast however, the BKA group required multiple prostheses and prosthesis modifications over their lifetime, with significant associated costs. Rates of return to work and self-reported disability were equal between the groups. Psychologically, most patients would prefer salvage to amputation initially; however, all patients who experienced failed limb salvage stated that they would have chosen primary amputation if given the choice again. This study outlines the importance of avoiding a failed salvage attempt and emphasizes the need for better scoring systems to determine the success of salvage.

When presented with a severely mangled extremity, it is important to document all pertinent local and systemic factors accurately. A MESS should be calculated for each patient but should be used with caution as a guideline to supplement the clinical findings. Whenever possible, pictures should be taken and added to the permanent medical record. Primary amputation should be performed when injuries include complete tibial or sciatic nerve injury in an adult or irreparable osseous or arterial injury. When the indications are not absolute, it is essential that several surgeons evaluate the patient independently and document their opinion in the medical record.

### Skeletal Stabilization

Skeletal stabilization has been shown to be crucial for soft tissue healing. When compared with cast and splints, internal or external fixation permits greater access for wound care and is more effective in controlling pain during mobilization. At the cellular level, the inflammatory response is shortened and the spread of bacteria is diminished. The decision to use one mode of fixation over another is dependent on the fracture pattern, degree of contamination, and surgeon preference.

One of the most widely accepted methods of fixation has been external fixation. In unstable patients or grossly contaminated wounds, standard or ringed external fixation can be used for temporary stabilization or for definitive fixation. External fixation minimizes dissection and avoids the insertion of large metallic implants. It is easily removed, replaced, and adjusted and can be combined with other means of fixation. However, external fixators are not without their problems. Although pin tract osteomyelitis has become rare with changes in design and the technique of pin insertion, superficial infection with drainage occurs in approximately 30% of all patients. Because of their size and location, further débridement and coverage can be cumbersome. In the tibia, for example, pin insertion through the subcutaneous anteromedial border reduces pin tract infection but often results in obstructed access for plastic and reconstructive surgery. In other cases, more extensive fracture patterns may require more complex frame constructs that further limit access. Although effective in providing skeletal stabilization during soft tissue reconstruction, external fixation is not ideal for achieving fracture union. Additional surgery, including bone grafting or conversion to internal fixation, is often necessary.

For these reasons, IM nailing appears to be an attractive option. Definitive fracture care can usually be accomplished in a single operation. Without bulky exposed hardware, mobilization and daily wound care are facilitated. However, several early series have reported an unacceptably high incidence of infection when reamed IM nails were used for type III open tibial fractures.[22] Originally, the increased infection rate was believed to be caused by destruction of cortical blood flow by reaming. The injury itself causes periosteal stripping and significant soft tissue loss. The loss of the medullary blood supply potentially further weakens the bone's healing potential and resistance to infection. However, studies in animals have shown that the endosteal blood supply reconstitutes over a relatively short period of time.[22a] Reaming the IM canal prior to insertion of the nail allows for placement of a larger diameter nail and forces bone marrow in between the fractured bone ends, which facilitates healing. In a subsequent meta-analysis of management of open tibial fractures, Bhandari and coworkers[22] have shown reduced risk of reoperation, malunion, and infection when comparing unreamed intramedullary nailing with external fixation; they also shown no difference in infection rate between reamed and unreamed nails. Although there is still controversy regarding reamed versus unreamed nailing, the general consensus is that in a stable patient, intramedullary nailing is the fixation of choice for open tibial fractures. High rates of infection have been shown when delayed conversion from external fixation to intramedullary nailing is performed; however, the infection rate is significantly reduced when the conversion happens within 2 weeks. Open periarticular fractures and fractures of the upper extremity should be treated with plate fixation if the patient's condition warrants.

## Acute Compartment Syndrome

Compartment syndrome can occur in any closed facial space. Usually, this occurs in a myofascial space secondary to trauma. The causes of compartment syndrome are numerous and include, but are not limited to, open and closed fractures, arterial injury, gunshot wounds, snake bites, extravasation at venous and arterial access sites, limb crush injuries, burns, constrictive dressings, and tight casts. Rapid diagnosis plus management of compartment syndrome is paramount to achieve a successful clinical outcome. This section addresses the pathogenesis, diagnosis, and management of acute compartment syndrome, specifically in the forearm and lower part of the leg.

Early recognition and treatment of compartment syndrome are critical in a trauma patient to avoid limb dysfunction, limb amputation, and even death. Volkmann was the first to describe the sequelae of postischemic contracture more than a century ago. He attributed permanent muscle contracture to trauma, swelling, and tight bandaging. As the late complications of compartment syndrome of the upper and lower extremities have been elucidated, the importance of early recognition and fasciotomy have become apparent. Failure to diagnose and treat this complication has resulted in numerous cases of preventable morbidity, rare cases of mortality, and many cases of litigation, often resulting in settlements in favor of the plaintiff.

### Pathogenesis

Compartment syndrome occurs secondary to increased pressure in the enclosed fascial space. The most common cause of compartment syndrome in an orthopedic patient is muscle edema from direct trauma to the extremity or reperfusion after vascular injury. This edema causes an increase in compartment pressure, which prevents venous outflow from the affected extremity. The backflow congestion furthers the cycle of increasing pressure and muscle ischemia. In the case of an orthopedic trauma patient with a long bone fracture, bleeding from the fracture produces a space-occupying hematoma that exacerbates the situation. On reduction of the fracture, compartment pressures increase secondary to a decrease in the compartmental volume. External compressive casts or bandages further reduce the ability of the compartment to expand.

Controversy exists regarding the level of compartment pressure for which surgical intervention is required. Mubarak and Hargens[23] have determined that an absolute tissue pressure of 30 mm Hg is the critical value at which fasciotomy should be performed. They concluded that because normal capillary pressure is 30 mm Hg, higher pressure would result in tissue necrosis. However, more recent studies have shown that the absolute pressure may be less important than the pressure in relation to the diastolic pressure ($\Delta P$). Whitesides and Heckman[24] have recommended a fasciotomy when intracompartmental $\Delta P$ approaches 20 mm Hg in the presence of documented rising tissue pressure, significant tissue injury, or a history of 6 hours of total ischemia time of an extremity. McQueen and Court-Brown[25] have shown that in patients who had a sustained intracompartmental pressure difference of 30 mm Hg or more relative to the diastolic blood pressure, there was no residual muscle damage at follow-up. They recommended this $\Delta P$ as an indication for fasciotomy. Current recommendations vary, but most authors agree that a $\Delta P$ of 30 mm Hg or less is an absolute indication for compartment release.[26]

Although there is controversy regarding when a fasciotomy should be performed, there is little debate regarding the effect of prolonged ischemia on skeletal muscle and nerve tissue. Investigators have determined that peripheral nerves and muscles can survive for as long as 4 hours under ischemic conditions without irreversible damage. An ischemic time of 6 hours results in a variable return of function in muscle and nerve tissue, and a total ischemic time longer than 8 hours leads to irreversible nerve and muscle injury.[24]

### Diagnosis

The diagnosis of acute compartment syndrome requires a high degree of clinical suspicion, a full understanding of the mechanism of injury, and careful serial physical examinations (Fig. 20-24). Tscherne and Gotzen[14] have stated that the more severe the initial soft tissue injury, the greater the probability that soft tissue complications, including compartment syndrome, will develop. The diagnosis of compartment syndrome relies on an understanding of high-risk injury patterns, subjective complaints of the patients, and an appreciation of early and late physical and clinical findings.

The presence of distal pulses and the absence of pallor cannot exclude the diagnosis of compartment syndrome because tissue perfusion in a compartment is dependent on arterial and capillary perfusion gradients. Paralysis and paresthesias are unreliable because studies have shown that peripheral nerves can

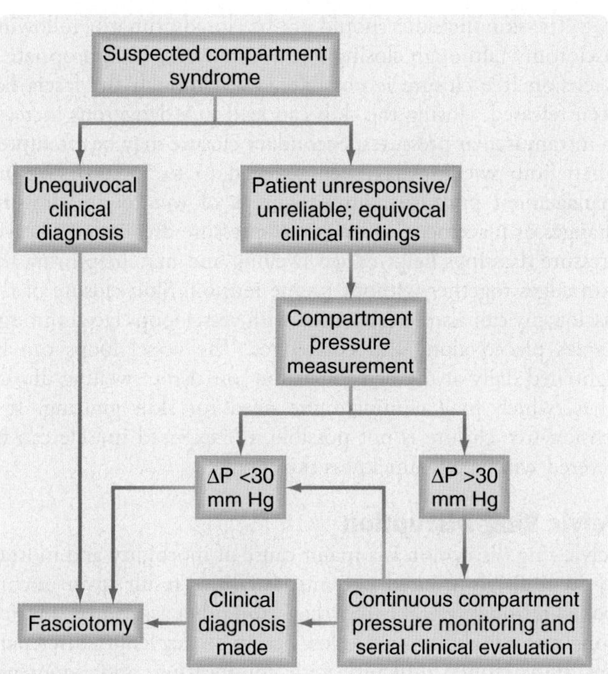


**FIGURE 20-24** Algorithm for the management of a patient with suspected compartment syndrome.

conduct impulses after 1 hour or more of total ischemic time. Because muscle ischemia causes pain, pain out of proportion to the injury is one of the most reliable symptoms in diagnosing acute compartment syndrome. Unusual requests for frequent narcotic analgesics can be reflective of ischemic pain. Passive stretching of the ischemic muscle of the compartment in question causes exquisite pain and is the most sensitive clinical finding in a developing compartment syndrome. Clinical palpation of the compartment in question plus comparison with the contralateral limb is useful for evaluating a compartment at risk, and any evidence of increased tension or fullness of the compartment should raise clinical suspicion. However, this diagnostic sign should only be used in combination with other concerning signs and symptoms because the ability to detect a rise in compartment pressure manually has been shown to be relatively unreliable.[27]

Although pain out of proportion to the injury is a cardinal clinical finding of an impending compartment syndrome, it must be emphasized that this pain will diminish as further ischemia occurs. In addition, the clinical findings may be obscured in patients medicated with narcotics; therefore, narcotic administration should be closely monitored. Systemic hypotension, vascular injury, external limb compression, coagulopathy, and deep venous thrombosis (DVT) predispose trauma patients to the development of compartment syndrome.

### Tissue Pressure Measurements

An unequivocal physical examination necessitates fasciotomy; however, if the examination is equivocal or the patient is uncooperative, intoxicated, intubated, or neurologically impaired, the diagnosis of compartment syndrome may depend more on the measurement of compartment pressures. Many methods have been described for evaluation of compartment pressures. The two most common techniques include the wick catheter and

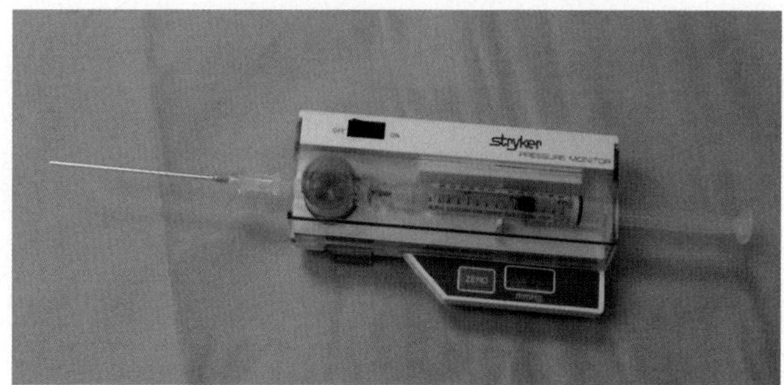


**FIGURE 20-25** Stryker STIC catheter.

side port needle. The wick catheter has the benefit of continuous pressure monitoring by using a continuous, low-volume infusion technique. This may be used as an indwelling device for recording compartment pressures at multiple time points. The most common method of measurement is the Stryker Intra-Compartmental Pressure Monitor System (STIC; Stryker, Mahwah, NJ), which uses the side port needle technique (Fig. 20-25). This hand-held electronic device is easily calibrated and used. Pressures are obtained by inserting the needle into each compartment and infusing a low volume of fluid until pressure equilibrium is reached. It is generally used to make measurements at one point in time and is not an indwelling device.

In place of invasive methods of measuring compartment pressure, fiberoptic devices are available in which near-infrared spectroscopy is used to measure tissue perfusion as a function of hemoglobin saturation. These devices allow continuous transcutaneous monitoring and are becoming more widely available. By using the absorptive wavelength of venous muscle oxyhemoglobin, near-infrared spectroscopy can be used to evaluate the viability of a compartment at risk. Increased application of this technology in the diagnosis of chronic compartment syndrome has led to its more routine use in the acute and subacute setting.

### Surgical Treatment

The two-incision approach to fasciotomy (Fig. 20-26) of the lower part of the leg is a reliable and straightforward procedure, given that the anatomy is well understood (Table 20-5). This approach involves making an anterolateral incision over the anterior and lateral compartments and a medial incision just posterior to the medial aspect of the tibia. The anterolateral incision is centered halfway between the fibular shaft and tibia. Once the fascia is identified, a small transverse incision is made to identify the anterior and lateral compartments, as well as the superficial peroneal nerve traveling in the lateral compartment. It is important to release the entire compartment, including the most proximal and distal aspects. The posteromedial incision is used to decompress the superficial and deep posterior compartments. The incision is made approximately 2 cm posterior to the tibial shaft. Care must be taken to preserve the saphenous nerve and vein. Once the fascia is identified, a transverse incision is made to delineate the superficial and deep compartments. The superficial posterior compartment is released first, proximally and distally to the medial malleolus. In similar fashion, the deep posterior compartment is released. To decompress the deep compartment completely, the soleus muscle must be taken down off the medial side of the tibia.

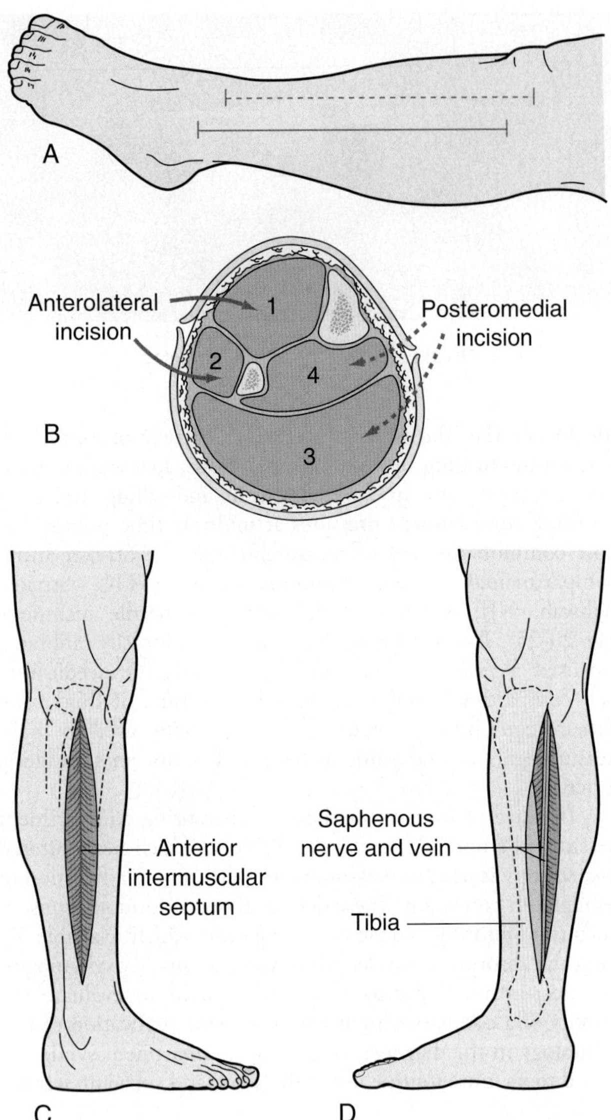


**FIGURE 20-26 A,** Double-incision technique for performing fasciotomies of all four compartments of the lower extremity. **B,** Cross section of the lower extremity showing positions of anterolateral and posteromedial incisions that allow access to the anterior and lateral compartments (*1* and *2*) and the superficial and deep posterior compartments (*3* and *4*).

The skin incisions should not be closed primarily following fasciotomy (although closing one incision may be appropriate if a tension free closure is possible). Even though the fascia has been released, closing the skin can lead to a dangerous increase in intramuscular pressures. Secondary closure may be attempted when limb swelling has been reduced (3 to 5 days). Wound management prior to closure consists of wet to dry dressing changes or placement of a negative-pressure dressing. Negative-pressure dressings help reduce swelling and may help bring the skin edges together without undue tension. Skin closure of the fasciotomy can also be facilitated with vessel loops laced through staples placed along the skin edges. The vessel loops can be tightened daily at the bedside as the soft tissue swelling diminishes, which may eliminate the need for skin grafting. If a tension-free closure is not possible, the exposed muscle can be covered with a split-thickness skin graft.

## Pelvic Ring Disruption

Pelvic ring disruption is a major cause of morbidity and mortality in multiply injured patients. Fatalities result from uncontrolled retroperitoneal hemorrhage and other associated injuries. Long-term disability such as low back pain, leg length discrepancies, dyspareunia, difficulty with childbearing, and impotence are caused by anatomic disruption of the pelvic ring. Pelvic fractures can be particularly lethal when they occur in conjunction with significant injuries to other major organ systems.[28] Because of the high force necessary to disrupt the pelvic ring in young patients, it is not surprising that up to 80% of these patients have additional musculoskeletal injuries. Mortality rates in patients with high-energy pelvic ring injuries are approximately 15% to 25%. Mortality increases almost 13-fold when the patient is hypotensive. When combined with a head or abdominal injury that requires surgical intervention, mortality increases to 50%. When both procedures are necessary, mortality approaches 90%.[11]

### Classification

Pelvic ring disruption can be broadly classified into two major groups, stable and unstable. A stable pelvis is defined as one that can withstand normal physiologic forces without being displaced. This stability depends on the integrity of the osseous and ligamentous structures (Fig. 20-27). Instability can be divided into rotational and vertical components (Fig. 20-28). Stable injuries include nondisplaced fractures of the pelvic ring and fractures resulting in less than 2.5 cm of displacement of anterior structures, the pubic rami or pubic symphysis. Rotational

**Table 20-5 Contents of Fascial Compartments in the Leg**

| COMPARTMENT | MUSCLES | VESSELS | NERVES |
|---|---|---|---|
| Anterior | Tibialis anterior<br>Extensor hallucis longus<br>Extensor digitorum communis | Anterior tibial | Deep peroneal |
| Deep posterior | Tibialis posterior<br>Flexor hallucis longus<br>Flexor digitorum longus | Posterior tibial | Tibial<br>Peroneal |
| Superficial posterior | Gastrocnemius<br>Soleus<br>Plantaris | | |
| Lateral | | | Superficial peroneal |

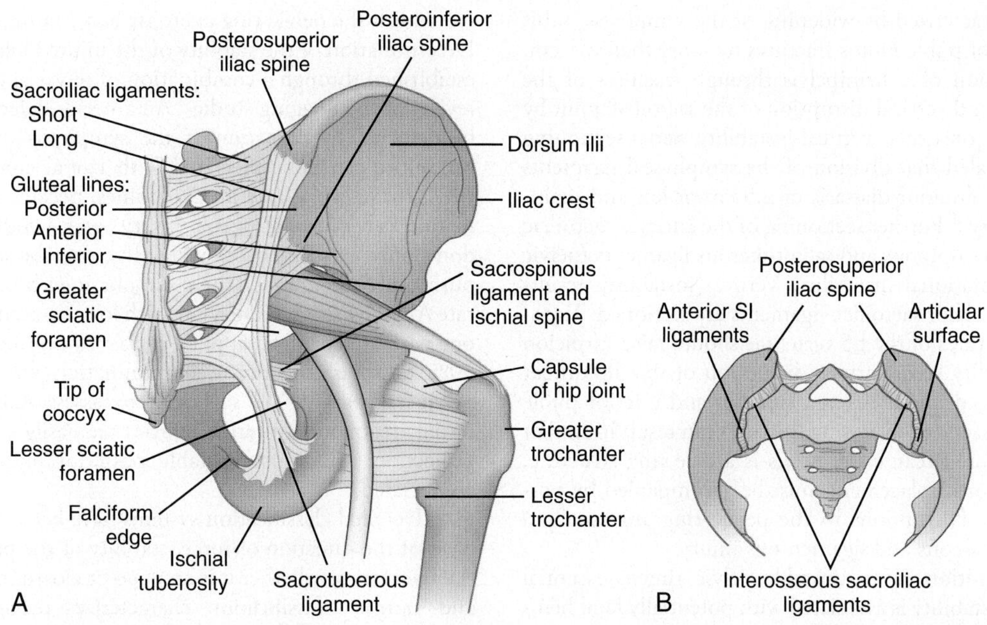


**FIGURE 20-27** Ligamentous complexes of the pelvis. **A,** Posteriorly, the major ligaments noted in the region of the SI joint are the posterior SI ligaments, both long and short. The long ligaments blend with the sacrospinous and sacrotuberous ligaments. **B,** In cross section, the orientation of the very thick posterior interosseous sacroiliac ligaments is noted. (From Stover MD, Mayo KA, Kellam JF: Pelvic ring disruptions. In Browner, BD, Levine AM, Jupiter JB, et al [eds]: Skeletal trauma: Basic science, management, and reconstruction, ed 4, Philadelphia, 2008, WB Saunders.)

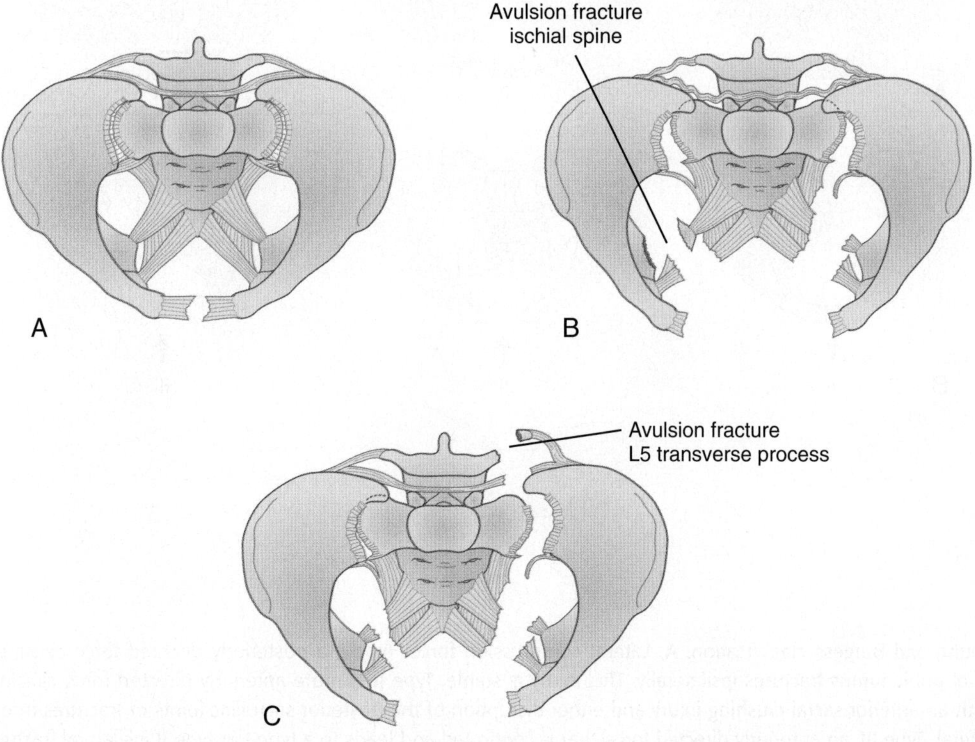


**FIGURE 20-28 A,** Division of the symphysis pubis allows the pelvis to open to approximately 2.5 cm with no damage to any posterior ligamentous structures. **B,** Division of the anterior SI and sacrospinous ligaments, either by direct division of their fibers (right) or by avulsion of the tip of the ischial spine (left), allows the pelvis to rotate externally until the posterior superior iliac spines about the sacrum. Note, however, that the posterior ligamentous structures (e.g., the posterior SI and iliolumbar ligaments) remain intact. Therefore, no displacement in the vertical plane is possible. **C,** Division of the posterior band ligaments—that is, the posterior SI, as well as the iliolumbar, causes complete instability of the hemipelvis. Note that global displacement is now possible. (From Stover MD, Mayo KA, Kellam JF: Pelvic ring disruptions. In Browner, BD, Levine AM, Jupiter JB, et al [eds]: Skeletal trauma: Basic science, management, and reconstruction, ed 4, Philadelphia, 2008, WB Saunders.)

instability is characterized by widening of the symphysis pubis or displacement of pubic ramus fractures by more than 2.5 cm. Superior translation of a hemipelvis through fractures of the sacrum or ilium and vertical disruption of the sacroiliac joint by more than 1 cm constitutes vertical instability. Serial sectioning studies have revealed that division of the symphyseal ligaments alone leads to an anterior diastasis of 2.5 cm or less and maintenance of stability.[29] Further sectioning of the anterior sacroiliac ligaments and sacrospinous and sacrotuberous ligaments (pelvic floor) imparts rotational instability. Vertical instability results only after the posterior sacroiliac ligaments are sectioned. Transverse process fractures of the L5 vertebrae should raise suspicion for pelvic instability secondary to disruption of the iliolumbar ligament. Displaced fractures (e.g., superior and inferior pubic ramus fractures, sacral or iliac wing fracture) can result in similar instability patterns. Because the pelvis is a true ring structure, significant anterior displacement must be accompanied by posterior disruption. Disruptions in the pelvic ring are usually a combination of osseous and ligamentous injury.

Early recognition of an unstable pelvic ring is essential because pelvic instability is associated with potentially fatal hemorrhage. Additionally, these injuries require intervention to reestablish the pelvic ring anatomy and minimize late disability. Determination of the stability of the injured hemipelvis must be established through a combination of physical examination and review of the imaging studies. An anterior defect can sometimes be detected by palpation at the symphysis pubis. Rotational instability can be appreciated with lateral compression of the pelvis through the anterior iliac spines. Because repeated manipulation can cause iatrogenic injury, such handling needs to be done only once. Vertical instability may be appreciated with push-pull radiographs. These are obtained by taking two separate AP pelvic x-rays, one view with lower extremity traction and one with an axial load applied to the leg on the affected side. In 90% of cases, the physical examination and anteroposterior pelvic radiograph are sufficient to assess stability and guide initial treatment. Anterior injuries are easily identified on this projection, and most unstable posterior injuries can also be appreciated.

Detailed classification systems have been developed on the basis of the direction of force, stability of the pelvis, location of the fracture, or whether it is an open or closed injury. The Young and Burgess classification characterizes pelvic ring fractures based on the mechanism of injury (Fig. 20-29).[11] Fracture

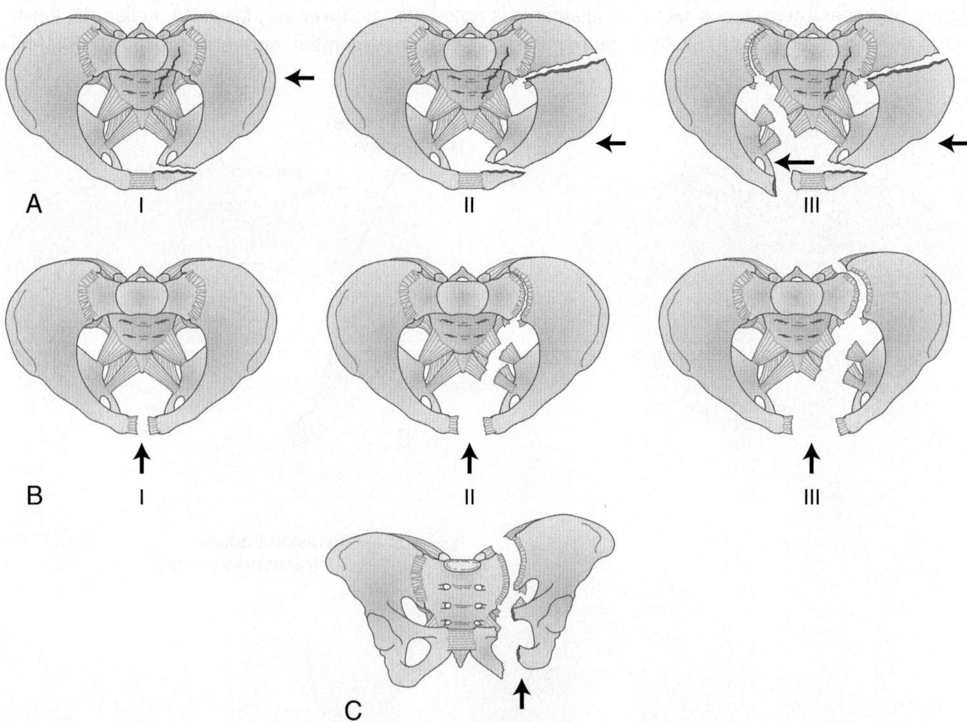


**FIGURE 20-29.** Young and Burgess classification. **A,** Lateral compression force. Type I, a posteriorly directed force causing a sacral crushing injury and horizontal pubic ramus fractures ipsilaterally. This injury is stable. Type II, a more anteriorly directed force causing horizontal pubic ramus fractures with an anterior sacral crushing injury and either disruption of the posterior sacroiliac joints or fractures through the iliac wing. This injury is ipsilateral. Type III, an anteriorly directed force that is continued and leads to a type I or type II ipsilateral fracture with an external rotation component to the contralateral side; the sacroiliac joint is opened posteriorly, and the sacrotuberous and spinous ligaments are disrupted. **B,** AP compression fractures. Type I, an AP-directed force opening the pelvis but with the posterior ligamentous structures intact. This injury is stable. Type II, continuation of a type I fracture with disruption of the sacrospinous and potentially the sacrotuberous ligaments and an anterior sacroiliac joint opening. This fracture is rotationally unstable. Type III, a completely unstable or vertical instability pattern with complete disruption of all ligamentous supporting structures. **C,** A vertically directed force(s) at right angles to the supporting structures of the pelvis leading to vertical fractures in the rami and disruption of all the ligamentous structures. This injury is equivalent to an AP type III or a completely unstable and rotationally unstable fracture. (Adapted from Young JWR, Burgess AR: Radiologic management of pelvic ring fractures, Baltimore, 1987, Urban and Schwarzenberg.)

patterns are divided into three types (A, B, C), depending on the direction of the deforming force. Type A results from a lateral compression (LC) force, type B results from an AP compression force (APC), and type C results from a vertical shear (VS) force. Types A and B fractures are further subdivided into types I, II, and III patterns, depending on the amount of ligamentous or osseous disruption. In both cases, type I fractures are stable, type II are rotationally unstable, and type III are rotationally and vertically unstable. APC-type injuries have the greatest risk for retroperitoneal hemorrhage. The APC III, also known as an open book pelvis, significantly increases the volume of the pelvis, allowing for massive blood loss in a short period of time (Fig. 20-30). Intrapelvic visceral injuries are also more common with the AP patterns. Mortality in AP compression–type injuries is related to a combination of retroperitoneal bleeding and visceral injuries. Lateral compression and vertical shear type fractures are associated with intra-abdominal and head injuries. Whereas intrapelvic hemorrhage occurs in LC-type fractures, the most common cause of death in a patient with this injury pattern is associated closed head trauma.[11]

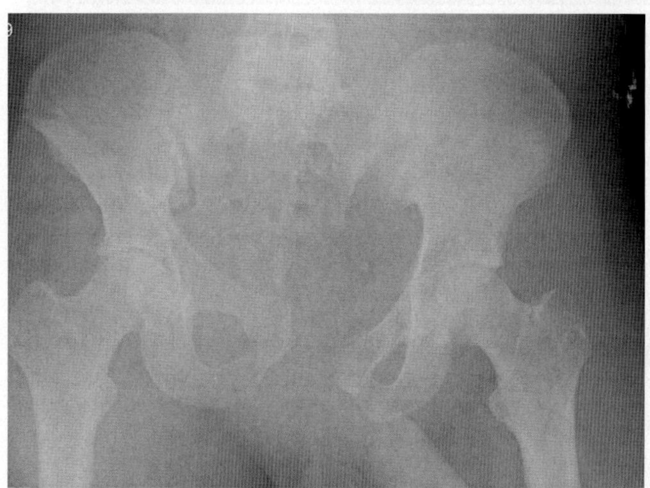

**FIGURE 20-30** AP pelvic radiograph showing the so-called open book pelvis. Complete disruption of the anterior and posterior ligamentous structures leaves this pelvis rotationally and vertically unstable.

### Hemorrhage in Pelvic Fracture

In most pelvic fractures, hemorrhage results from disruption of the pelvic venous plexus posteriorly and bleeding cancellous bone. Pelvic bleeding from a named artery occurs in less than 10% of cases.[30] Most bleeding resulting from pelvic fracture comes from the presacral venous plexus (Fig. 20-31). As a result, initial treatment of hemorrhage must focus on control of venous bleeding via reduction and stabilization of the pelvic ring. Reduction leads to a decrease in pelvic volume and tamponade of the bleeding vessels through compression of the viscera and pelvic hematoma. Stabilization maintains the reduction and avoids movement of the hemipelvis, thereby reducing pain and limiting disruption of any organizing thrombus. Because reduction and stabilization alone usually control venous bleeding, patients who do not respond to these maneuvers are more likely to have arterial bleeding.

### Stabilization

Reduction and stabilization of the pelvis can be achieved by various mechanical means. When field personnel detect unstable pelvic ring disruptions on physical examination, they can begin treatment by binding the pelvis with a rolled sheet or applying pneumatic antishock garments (PASGs). Like air splints applied to the extremities, the garment functions by compressing the pelvis. If applied in the field, PASGs should not be deflated until the patient is being resuscitated in the trauma room. A PASG has the advantage of ease of use, application in the field, and reusability. However, it blocks access to the patient and restricts excursion of the diaphragm, and there have been reports of gluteal and thigh compartment syndromes developing after extended use of PASGs in hypotensive patients. Because of this, the use of the pelvic binder has become more common. The binder can be applied quickly and easily. It effectively reduces pelvic volume, which can help control venous bleeding.[31]

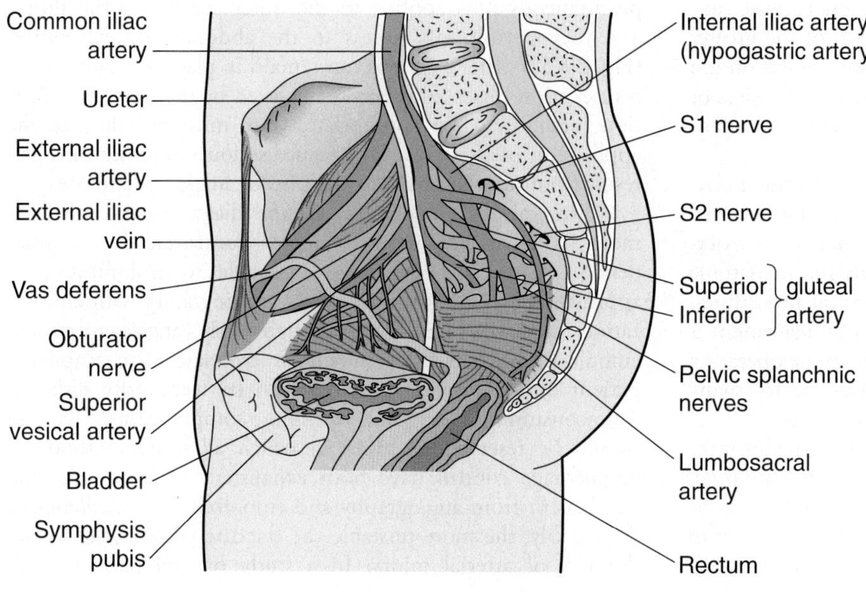


**FIGURE 20-31** Internal aspect of the pelvis showing the great vessels and lumbosacral plexus, as well as the pelvic floor, bladder, and rectum. The anterior column consists of the anterior two thirds of the vertebral body and the anterior longitudinal ligament. The middle column includes the posterior third of the vertebral body and the PLL. The posterior column includes all bony and ligamentous structures posterior to the PLL. (From Stover MD, Mayo KA, Kellam JF: Pelvic ring disruptions. In Browner, BD, Levine AM, Jupiter JB, et al [eds]: Skeletal trauma: Basic science, management, and reconstruction, ed 4, Philadelphia, 2008, WB Saunders.)

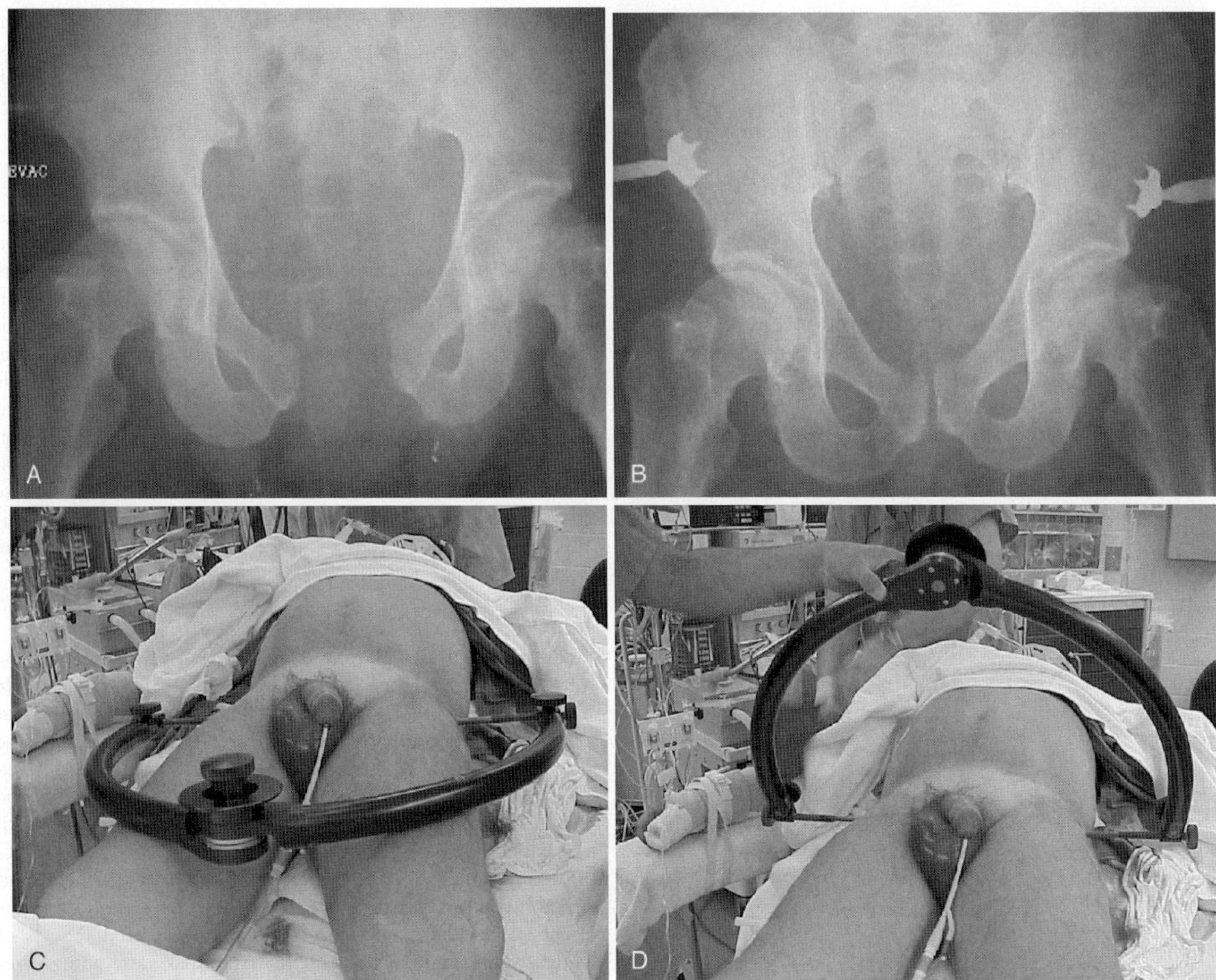

**FIGURE 20-32** Pelvic ring disruption with massive hemorrhage. **A,** AP radiograph of the pelvis showing disruption of the symphysis pubis and SI joint. **B,** AP view of the pelvis after reduction by the application of a pelvic stabilizer. **C, D,** Patient with the pelvic stabilizer in the standard position and elevated to allow access to the perineum or permit flexion of the hips for change to the lithotomy position.

However, caution must be used with these devices because they can exert dangerously high pressures at the level of the greater trochanter and iliac wing, leading to pressure sores if left on too long.[32] In addition, in the case of LC-type fractures, binders or sheets can overreduce the fracture, putting intrapelvic organs at risk.[31]

Historically, the standard method for controlling pelvic hemorrhage has been the application of an anterior external fixation frame. When applied properly, an anterior pelvic external fixator should provide stability to the pelvis and hematoma while allowing access to the abdomen for surgical procedures. Although these devices can be applied in the ED, placement is frequently deferred until the patient is brought to the operating suite. In these cases, the pelvis can remain displaced for many hours, with venous bleeding continuing uncontrolled.

If an external fixator cannot be applied expeditiously, another method of provisional stabilization must be used. Devices called pelvic C-clamps have been developed that can be applied rapidly to reduce and provisionally stabilize the pelvis in the ED. Their design allows compression of the pelvis through percutaneous pins applied to the outer surface of the ilium, and they permit easy access to the abdomen or extremities (Fig. 20-32). The C-clamps can remain in place throughout the resuscitation phase and then be replaced by definitive stabilization methods, when appropriate. Care must be taken in the application of these clamps because serious complications can result from misplacement of the pins or inappropriate use.

The role of angiography in the diagnosis and management of pelvic hemorrhage remains controversial. The incidence of arterial hemorrhage amenable to embolization is approximately 10%. In these cases, arteriography with embolization can be lifesaving. Although early angiography and embolization have been shown to correlate with improved patient outcomes, the procedure can be technically difficult, time-consuming and not without complications. Its use should be reserved for cases in which all other methods of hemorrhage control have been exhausted. Determining who will benefit from angiography and embolization is challenging. Predictably, the more unstable the fracture pattern, the higher the risk of arterial injury. In a study of 603 patients with

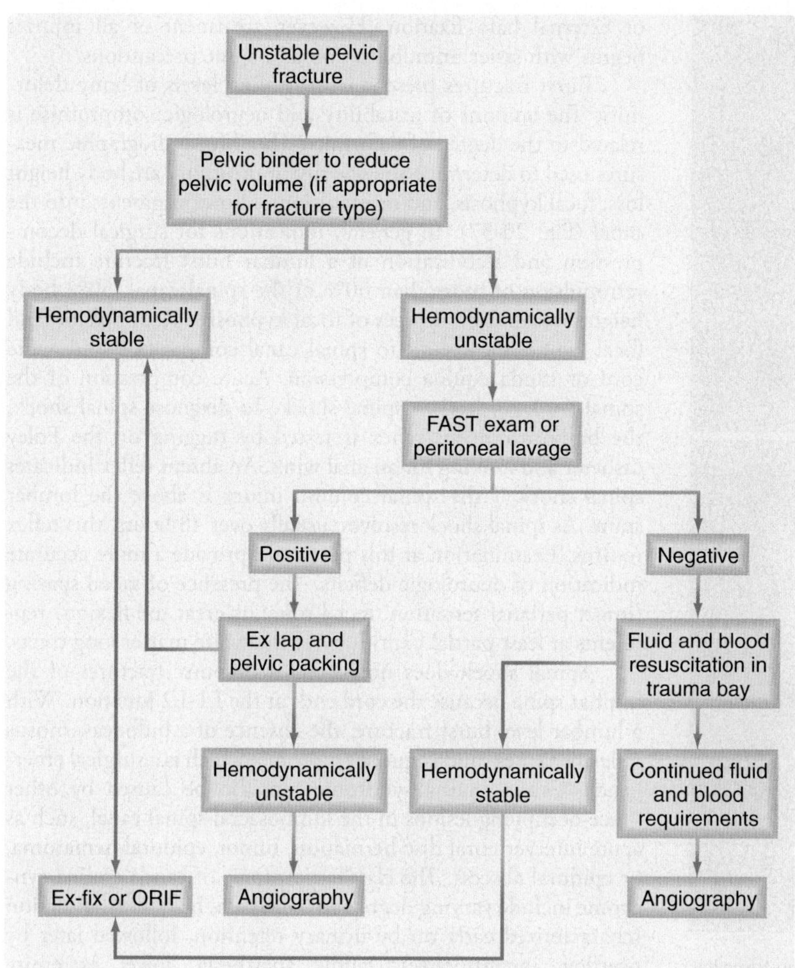


**FIGURE 20-33** Treatment algorithm for management of a patient with an unstable pelvic fracture. (Data from Hak DJ, Smith WR, Suzuki T: Management of hemorrhage in life-threatening pelvic fracture. J Am Acad Orthop Surg 17:447-457, 2009; Browner BD, DeAngelis JD: Emergency care of musculoskeletal injuries. In Townsend C, Beauchamp R, Evers B, Mattox K [eds]: Sabiston textbook of surgery, ed 18, Philadelphia, 2008, Saunders Elsevier; and Totterman A, Dormagen JB, Madsen JE, et al: A protocol for angiographic embolization in exsanguinating pelvic trauma: A report on 31 patients. Acta Orthop 77:462–468, 2006.)

pelvic fractures caused by blunt trauma, Salim and colleagues[33] have shown that disruption of the sacroiliac (SI) joint, female gender, and duration of hypotension were all predictors of a positive angiogram. Pelvic packing has long been used as a way to stop pelvic bleeding. More recently, a modified form of pelvic packing, retroperitoneal packing, has been shown to be as effective as embolization in controlling intrapelvic hemorrhage following pelvic fractures.[34] Many protocols and algorithms have been proposed for the management of pelvic fracture with hemodynamic instability.[30,35] A modified algorithm, taking into account the current data available in the literature, is presented in Figure 20-33.

### Management

Initial management of a patient with a pelvic ring injury was discussed earlier. Long-term definitive care of pelvic ring disruption is dependent on the pattern of injury and its severity. Stable fracture patterns usually require no more than restricted weight bearing. Frequently, an external fixator can provide definitive stabilization of unstable injuries if applied effectively and reduction is maintained. In cases in which the fixator may be obstructing access to the abdomen or an interim C-clamp has been applied, ORIF or closed reduction and percutaneous fixation may be indicated. When rotational or vertical instability is present, the anterior and posterior pelvis must be stabilized. Anteriorly, the symphysis is often secured with a plate and screws. Posteriorly, more options exist. The SI joint or sacral fractures can be secured with plates, bars, or percutaneously inserted cannulated screws (Fig. 20-34). When only rotational instability is present, the posterior ligaments are usually only partially disrupted. After the anterior pelvis is secured, pelvic ring stability should be reexamined. Often, no posterior fixation is necessary.

## Spinal Injuries

Cervical spine (C-spine) injuries can occur by several mechanisms, which can be divided into three main categories. The first involves direct trauma to the neck itself. The second mechanism involves motion of the head relative to the axial skeleton. This injury can occur by direct trauma to the head or continued movement of the head relative to the fixed body (whiplash), as often occurs in blunt trauma such as motor vehicle accidents, when the body is restrained. In attempting to tether the head against motion, the cervical spine endures a large bending or twisting moment that results in flexion-extension injuries or rotational injuries, respectively. A third mechanism of cervical spine injury involves a direct axial load imparted on the cranium that causes axial compression forces across the cervical vertebrae. This may result in a burst fracture and potential spinal cord injury. This pattern of injury is more commonly seen in the lumbar spine. An algorithm for diagnosing C-spine injuries is presented in Figure 20-35.

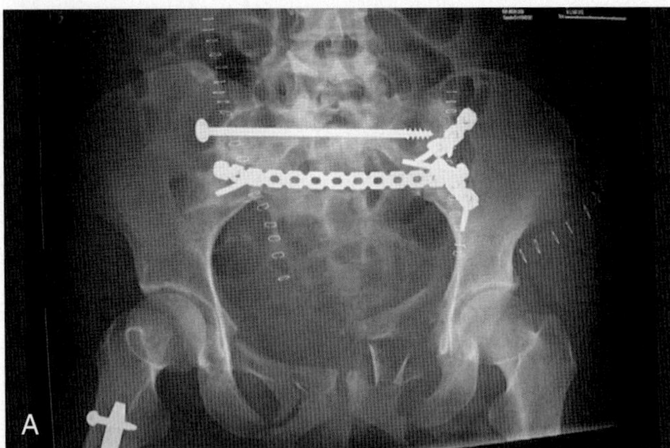

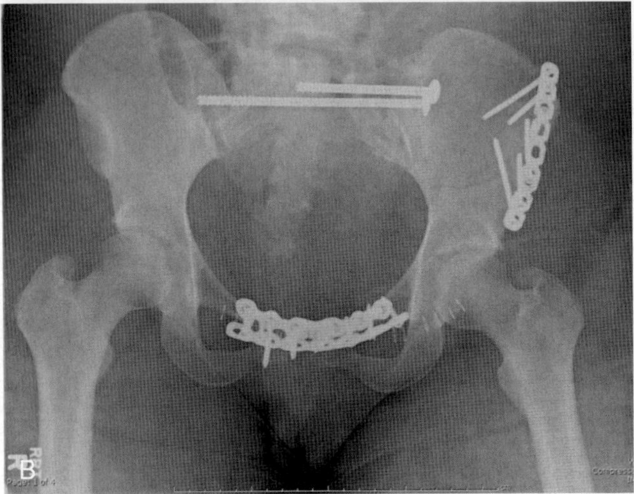

**FIGURE 20-34** Fixation of unstable pelvic fractures. **A,** One transiliac screw, one transiliac plate and two left SI plates were used to stabilize the posterior elements in this fracture. **B,** One transiliac screw and one SI screw were used to stabilize the posterior elements of this fracture. Plates were used to stabilize the pubic symphysis. An iliac crest plate was used to fix the left iliac wing fracture.

The spinal cord is divided into three columns (Fig. 20-36). The anterior column consists of the anterior two thirds of the vertebral body as well as the anterior longitudinal ligament. The middle column includes the posterior third of the vertebral body and the posterior longitudinal ligament (PLL). The posterior column includes all bony and ligamentous structures posterior to the PLL. In general, injury to one column results in a stable injury. Injury to two or three columns results in an unstable spinal segment. Instability in the spinal column puts the spinal cord at risk. Burst fractures, by definition, involve injury to the anterior and middle columns. These fractures are to be differentiated from compression fractures, which involve the anterior column only and are rarely associated with spinal cord injury. Burst fractures commonly occur after a fall from a height in which an axial load is transmitted to the upper axial skeleton when the feet strike the ground first. This mechanism results in a common pattern of fractures, including calcaneus, tibial plateau, proximal femur and lumbar burst fractures (see Table 20-1). Depending on the fracture pattern, treatment of spine injuries may range from observation to bracing, surgical fixation, or external halo fixation. However, treatment of all injuries begins with strict immobilization and spine precautions.

Burst fractures present with varying levels of bony deformity. The amount of instability and neurologic compromise is related to the degree of deformity. The three radiographic measures used to determine the severity of the injury are body height loss, focal kyphosis, and retropulsion of bony fragments into the canal (Fig. 20-37). In general, indications for surgical decompression and stabilization of a lumbar burst fracture include retropulsion of more than 50% of the spinal canal, 50% body height loss, and 25 degrees of focal kyphosis.[2] Retropulsion and focal kyphosis can lead to spinal canal compromise and acute cord or cauda equina compression. Acute compression of the spinal cord can lead to spinal shock. To diagnose spinal shock, the bulbocavernosus reflex is tested by tugging on the Foley catheter and looking for an anal wink. An absent reflex indicates spinal shock if the spinal column injury is above the lumbar spine. As spinal shock resolves, usually over 48 hours, this reflex returns. Examination at this point will provide a more accurate indication of neurologic deficits. The presence of sacral sparing (intact perianal sensation, rectal tone, or great toe flexion) represents at least partial continuity of the white matter long tracts.

Spinal shock does not occur with burst fractures of the lumbar spine because the cord ends at the L1-L2 junction. With a lumbar level burst fracture, the absence of a bulbocavernosus reflex indicates cauda equina syndrome, which is a surgical emergency. Cauda equina syndrome can also be caused by other space-occupying lesions in the lumbosacral spinal canal, such as acute intervertebral disc herniation, tumor, epidural hematoma, or epidural abscess. The classic symptoms of cauda equina syndrome include varying degrees of back pain, bladder dysfunction (characterized early on by urinary retention, followed later by overflow incontinence), saddle anesthesia, lower extremity numbness, and/or weakness and reduced rectal tone (a late finding). If cauda equina syndrome is suspected, a MRI should be ordered immediately to look for canal compromise. If MRI is not available or the patient cannot undergo an MRI, CT myelography can be performed. When a diagnosis of cauda equina syndrome is confirmed, surgical exploration and decompression should be performed within 24 to 48 hours.[36]

## Dislocations

Dislocation of any joint is considered an orthopedic emergency. Prolonged dislocation can lead to cartilage cell death, posttraumatic arthritis, ankylosis, and avascular necrosis. Dislocations of major joints (e.g., the shoulder, elbow, hip, knee, or ankle) are particularly concerning because of the high risk of neurovascular injury. These injuries, which are more likely to occur in young active patients, can have devastating consequences.

### Patient Evaluation

Most dislocations have characteristic physical findings. After a dislocation, muscles around the joint typically become spasmodic, thereby limiting range of motion as the limb assumes a distinctive position. In posterior hip dislocations, the thigh is held flexed and internally rotated. The affected limb is often shortened and cannot be passively extended. An anterior shoulder dislocation causes an externally rotated and adducted arm position. Elbow and knee dislocations (most commonly posterior) result in an extremity locked in extension (Fig. 20-38). As

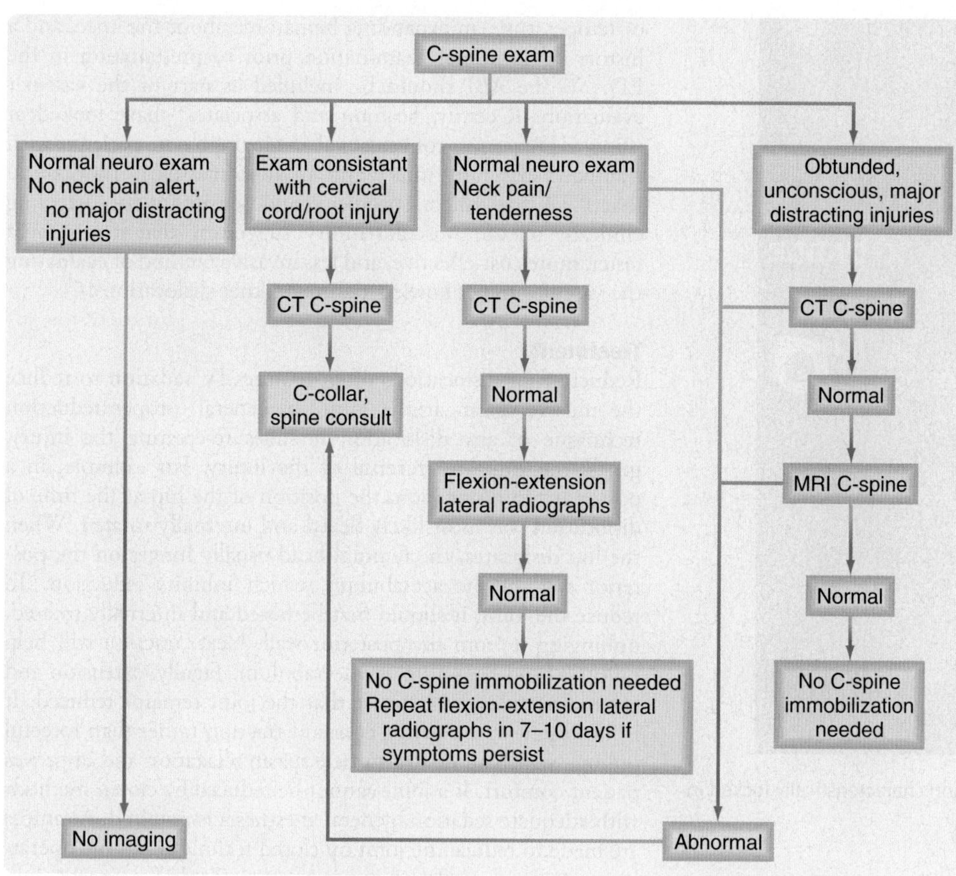


**FIGURE 20-35** Algorithm for imaging diagnosis of cervical spine injury. (Adapted from Lee Y, Templin C, Eismont F, et al: Thoracic and upper lumbar spine injuries. In Browner, BD, Levine AM, Jupiter JB, et al [eds]: Skeletal trauma: Basic science, management, and reconstruction, ed 4, Philadelphia, 2008, WB Saunders.)

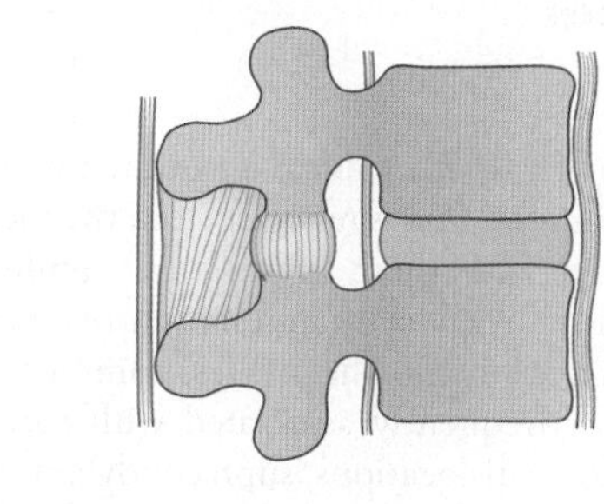

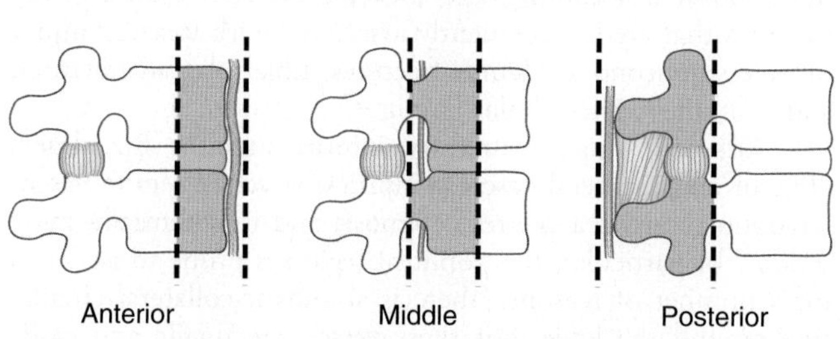


**FIGURE 20-36** Denis' three-column model of the spine. The anterior column consists of the anterior two thirds of the vertebral body and anterior longitudinal ligament. The middle column includes the posterior third of the vertebral body and PLL. The posterior column includes all bony and ligamentous structures posterior to the PLL. (From Lee Y, Templin C, Eismont F, et al: Thoracic and upper lumbar spine injuries. In Browner, BD, Levine AM, Jupiter JB, et al [eds]: Skeletal trauma: Basic science, management, and reconstruction, ed 4, Philadelphia, 2008, WB Saunders.)

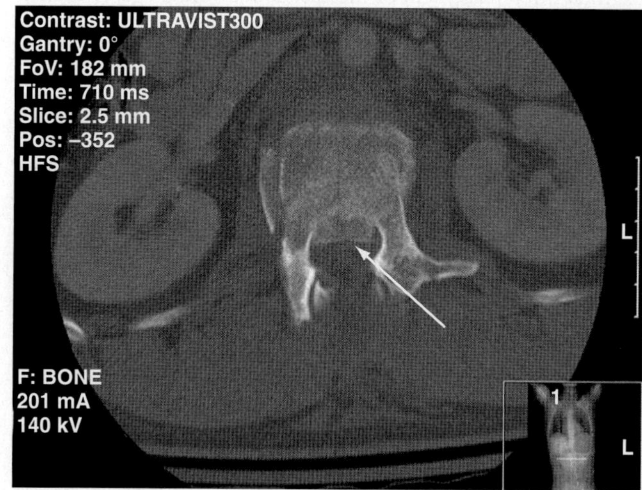


**FIGURE 20-37** Lumbar level burst fracture showing 50% retropulsion of bony fragments into the canal.

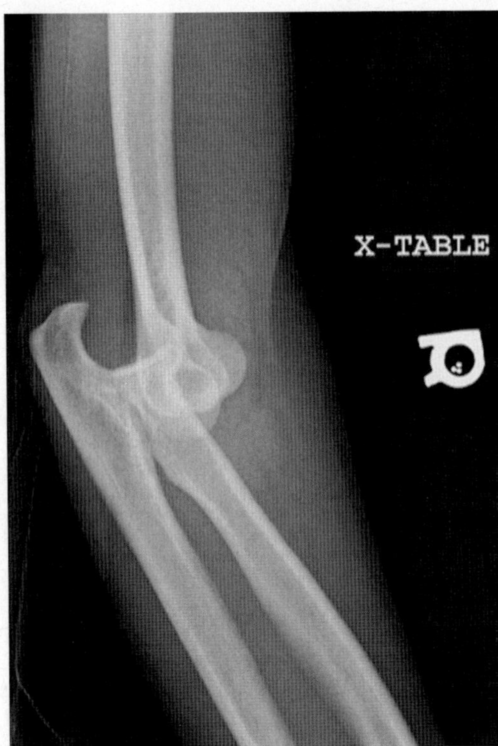


FIGURE 20-38 Posterior elbow dislocation characteristically locked in extension.

with all extremity injuries, a meticulous neurovascular examination must be performed and documented before and after manipulation.

Hip and knee dislocations require special discussion because of the extreme consequences of failure to recognize and address them in timely fashion. In the case of a hip dislocation, sciatic nerve injury, cartilage cell death, and avascular necrosis can result from delay in treatment. Of these complications, avascular necrosis is the most devastating because of its propensity to cause collapse of the femoral head and the subsequent development of degenerative joint disease. This problem can lead to the need for total hip replacement or hip fusion at a young age. Avascular necrosis usually develops in a time-dependent fashion. In the dislocated position, tension on the capsular blood vessels restricts blood flow to the femoral head. If the hip remains dislocated for 24 hours, avascular necrosis will ensue in 100% of cases. Although irreversible damage to the blood supply may occur at the time of injury, reduction within 6 hours is generally believed to reduce the incidence of ischemic changes.

Knee dislocations are a common cause of arterial injury secondary to the proximity of the popliteal vessels. Prompt reduction of these injuries is mandatory, followed by reevaluation of vascular status. Some authors have suggested that any patient with an acute knee dislocation should have angiography. However, this study is a costly procedure, with potential complications. Therefore, there has been a shift toward selective angiography. Recent data have shown that serial vascular examinations over a course of 24 to 48 hours can detect clinically relevant vascular injury.[37] Many have suggested that arteriography should be performed only in patients with abnormal vascular examination results, including decrease in pedal pulses, color, or temperature, an expanding hematoma about the knee, and a history of abnormal examination prior to presentation in the ED.[13,37] The ABI should be included as part of the vascular evaluation. Recently, Seamon and associates[38] have looked at using CTA versus conventional angiography in patients with traumatic extremity injury and an abnormal ABI. They found that CTA has 100% specificity and sensitivity for detecting clinically relevant vascular injury, suggesting that it may be a faster, more cost-effective, and less invasive method of evaluating the vascular tree following traumatic knee dislocations.

#### Treatment

Reduction of dislocations often requires IV sedation to reduce the muscle spasm at the joint. In general, proper reduction technique of any dislocation includes re-creating the injury, gentle traction, and reversal of the injury. For example, in a posterior hip dislocation, the position of the hip at the time of dislocation was most likely flexed and internally rotated. When the hip dislocates, the femoral head usually hinges on the posterior wall of the acetabulum, which inhibits reduction. To reduce the joint, it should first be flexed and internally rotated, unhinging it from the posterior wall. Next, traction will help pull the head back into the acetabulum. Finally, extension and external rotation will ensure that the joint remains reduced. It is important to use gentle constant traction rather than forceful pulling, which allows for muscle spasm relaxation and improves patient comfort. If a joint cannot be reduced by closed methods with adequate sedation, general anesthesia is required. Attempts are made to reduce the joint by closed techniques in the operating room, with staff and instruments available for open reduction if this fails.

### Vascular Injuries

#### Incidence

Although the rate of vascular injuries associated with blunt and penetrating extremity trauma is relatively low, the morbidity and limb loss associated with these injuries are significant. Distal ischemia is the most frequent manifestation of vascular injury in this setting and overt hemorrhage is less common. The orthopedic injuries most frequently associated with vascular insults include posterior knee dislocations, supracondylar humerus fractures, elbow dislocations, and unstable pelvic fractures. Other fractures that are less frequently associated with vascular injury include supracondylar femur fractures, tibial plateau fractures, and combined tibial-fibular fractures.

Although upper extremity injuries account for almost 30% of all peripheral vascular injuries, lower extremity vascular trauma carries a poorer prognosis and is potentially more serious. In particular, the popliteal region is prone to ischemia for a number of reasons. There is abundant collateral circulation around the knee, but these vessels are fragile and easily damaged by direct trauma or adjacent swelling. The popliteal artery begins at the adductor hiatus, which tethers it to the muscular fascia and restricts its movement. The soleus muscles also prevents excursion of the popliteal artery, thus making it prone to injury with knee dislocation. In the setting of popliteal artery thrombosis, lack of high-flow collaterals may lead to end-vessel thrombosis in situ secondary to low flow. Patency of these vessels is critical in limb salvage. Injuries to the superficial femoral artery rarely result in amputation because of the rich collateral circulation with the profunda femoris artery. Although rarely injured, injury to the profunda femoris may be clinically silent and the diagnosis must be made by angiography.

#### Management

Optimal results in treating combined vascular and orthopedic injuries depend on a high index of suspicion and expeditious intervention. A thorough vascular examination is performed in the trauma room, and all upper and lower extremity pulses are evaluated. Color, temperature, and the presence of pain or paresis are noted. Systolic pressure in the arm and at the ankle is recorded, and the ABI is calculated by dividing ankle pressure by brachial pressure. In the absence of chronic peripheral vascular disease, the index should be higher than 0.90. Usually, ABIs and pulses are symmetrical bilaterally. Audible bruits over blood vessels at affected areas may signify arterial injury or a traumatic fistula. Abnormal swelling may indicate deep vessel injury or rupture. Any pulse deficit or ABI less than 0.90 warrants formal arteriography. Prolonged or severe ischemia mandates immediate operative exploration. Intraoperative arteriography may be useful in planning vascular reconstruction if a vascular injury is present without critical ischemia. Direct arterial exploration of suspected injuries is warranted for open fractures.

Staging of skeletal stabilization and vascular repair should be individualized. When treating a fracture with an associated vascular injury, the order of fracture fixation and vascular repair is controversial. If the vessel is repaired first, the repair may be stretched or even damaged when the bones are pulled out to length. If the bone is fixed first, the extremity may suffer the effects of prolonged ischemia. Generally, vascular reconstruction precedes fracture fixation to restore limb perfusion. Disruption of the vascular repair after orthopedic fixation is rare, provided that the repair is performed with limb length restored. If there is significant shortening accompanying the fracture, placement of a temporary external fixator or femoral distracter is a fast and effective way to obtain appropriate limb length during vascular repair. The ipsilateral and contralateral limbs are prepared widely to allow access to the distal vessels and contralateral saphenous vein. Fasciotomy is performed before vascular repair if compartment syndrome is suspected. In knee dislocations, it is advisable to release the compartments of the lower part of the leg because of the chance of reperfusion injury and the development of compartment syndrome. Proximal and distal control is obtained before exploration of the hematoma. The artery and vein are carefully inspected and the injury is assessed.

In unstable fractures, the use of indwelling intraoperative shunts allows for stabilization of the fracture before definitive vascular repair. Studies have shown that this technique is effective for restoring limb perfusion, with relatively low complication rates.[39] Standard carotid endarterectomy shunts are often used in this setting. Proximal and distal thrombectomy is performed before shunt placement or repair. Frequently, arterial resection is necessary to obtain acceptable margins, and a saphenous vein graft is used if primary repair without tension is not possible. A completion arteriogram is routinely obtained because limb salvage depends on arterial patency. All major vein injuries are repaired to increase the patency rate of the arterial repair and prevent the sequelae of chronic venous congestion.

## COMMON LONG BONE FRACTURES

### Femur Fractures

#### Epidemiology and Significance

Femur fractures occur at a rate of 1/10,000 people/year. A closed femoral shaft fracture is considered a major injury when calculating the injury severity score (ISS). Therefore, another major injury in any other organ system qualifies the patient as multiply injured. With the exception of pathologic or insufficiency fractures in older patients, these fractures are the result of a high-energy injury. Frequently, these injuries lead to significant bleeding. Because of the geometry of the thigh, several units of blood can be lost into the tissues, with little external evidence of bleeding. Transfusion with packed red blood cells is often necessary. In addition to concerns about bleeding, the treating team should have a high suspicion of concomitant femoral neck fractures for all patients with femoral shaft fractures. As noted, there is almost a 10% incidence of these associated injuries.

#### Initial Management

All femur fractures must be immobilized before the patient is transported from the scene of the accident. Without immobilization, displaced femoral shaft fractures can cause increased edema, bleeding, and further damage to the surrounding soft tissues. Continued motion at the fracture site also results in increased fat embolization and contributes to the development of ARDS. Proper immobilization begins with in-line traction, which decreases the diameter of the thigh compartment, reducing its volume. The soft tissues are then under tension and can tamponade bleeding at the fracture site. As noted earlier, in-line traction in the field can be accomplished with a hare traction splint (see Fig. 20-22).[12] For patients in extremis, a posterior splint alone will suffice until formal traction or immobilization can be achieved. If time allows, a traction pin can be placed through the proximal tibia to provide skeletal traction and allow access to the distal femur (see Fig. 20-21). Up to 10% of a patient's body weight can be applied to properly placed skeletal traction.

#### Definitive Stabilization

Timing of definitive fixation of femoral shaft fractures is controversial. Until the end of the 20th century, delayed fixation of femoral fractures, sometimes up to 2 weeks after the initial injury, was the standard of care. However, in the early 1990s, thanks in large part to the work of Bone and coworkers,[8] there was a paradigm shift toward early fixation of these fractures. This prospective randomized trial of 178 patients with femur fractures showed a decreased rate of ARDS, fat embolism, and pneumonia, as well as shorter hospital stays, decreased days in the intensive care unit (ICU), and decreased cost of hospitalization for patients with femur fractures who were fixed within 24 hours of the injury, as opposed to those fixed after 48 hours. Immediate fixation leads to earlier mobilization, prevention of DVT and decubitus ulcers, easier nursing care, and decreased need for analgesia. Furthermore, the magnitude of fat embolized is also decreased.[8] Taken together, these factors can significantly improve pulmonary status and decrease the incidence of ARDS. This benefit is magnified as the ISS increases. In patients with severe trauma (ISS > 40), delayed fixation of femoral shaft fractures leads to a fivefold increase in the incidence of ARDS.

More recent studies, however, have suggested that immediate definitive fixation of femoral fractures in the multiply injured patient may not allow time for adequate resuscitation, leading to higher mortality rates. In a retrospective analysis of 3069 patients with multisystem trauma who underwent internal fixation of femoral shaft fractures, Morshed and colleagues[9] found a significantly increased mortality rate in patients fixed within 12 hours when compared with those fixed between 12 and 24 hours, between 48 and 120 hours, and more than 120 hours from the time of injury. This increase in mortality has been attributed to the so-called second hit phenomenon.[40] The initial trauma leads to an inflammatory response. The trauma of the surgery further increases this response, increasing levels of proinflammatory cytokines, which have been implicated in the development of ARDS. Morshed's paper suggested that patients with severe abdominal injury show the greatest benefit from delayed fixation; however, current recommendations also include hypothermia, coagulopathy, excessive intracranial pressure, and high pulmonary shunting as contraindications to immediate stabilization.[41] The findings in femoral fracture studies have been broadened to support immediate fixation of all long bone fractures, but definitive studies have not yet been carried out.

The fixation of femoral shaft fractures has become fairly uniform. The treatment of choice for closed fractures and types I through IIIA open fractures is closed, locked IM nailing. In contrast to open reduction methods, closed IM nailing reduces bleeding and soft tissue disruption at the fracture site. These minimally invasive techniques reduce perioperative stress and decrease the incidence of infection and nonunion. Treatment of types IIIB and IIIC open femoral shaft fractures is usually staged, with immediate I&D and external fixation followed by IM nailing or plating when there is sufficient soft tissue coverage of the bone.

## Tibial Shaft Fractures

### Epidemiology and Significance

Almost 26 tibia fractures occur per 100,000 people/year. The incidence has increased to approximately 500,000 cases in the United States annually. Fractures of the diaphysis of the tibia occur by direct and indirect mechanisms. Common mechanisms are bumper injuries, gunshot wounds, and bending or torsional injuries with a firmly planted foot. Because of the anatomy of the blood supply in the lower leg and the high energy involved in these injuries, treatment of tibial shaft fractures can present many difficulties. Further complicating matters, approximately 24% of all tibial shaft fractures are open injuries.[11]

### Blood Supply

Tibial shaft fractures tend to be slow healing as a result of their tenuous blood supply and limited soft tissue envelope. A single nutrient artery that branches from the posterior tibial artery serves the entire diaphysis. It enters the medullary canal and travels proximally and distally to anastomose with metaphyseal endosteal vessels. Although there is some contribution from the penetrating branches of the periosteal arteries that supply the outer third of the cortex, a diaphyseal fracture can easily compromise the nutrient arterial blood supply. Concomitant soft tissue stripping may leave an entire segment of tibia devascularized. This fragile environment predisposes tibial shaft fractures to impaired healing and, with open fractures, to osteomyelitis.

**Table 20-6 Nerves to the Foot**

| NERVE | SENSORY | MOTOR |
|---|---|---|
| Deep peroneal | First dorsal web space | Great toe dorsiflexion (extensor hallucis longus) |
| Superficial peroneal | Dorsum of foot | Eversion (peroneals) |
| Tibial | Plantar surface of foot | Great toe plantar flexion (flexor hallucis longus) |
| Sural | Lateral heel | None |
| Saphenous | Medial malleolus | None |

### Associated Soft Tissue Injuries

Aside from injuries to the overlying skin and muscle, tibial shaft fractures often have other associated soft tissue injuries. Ligamentous injuries causing knee instability are not uncommon and are often identified later as a source of continued morbidity. The incidence of compartment syndrome in tibial shaft fractures is as high as 9%, so close monitoring of patient symptoms and, if necessary, compartment pressures, is important.

Neurovascular injury should always be suspected and a careful examination must always be performed. The dorsalis pedis and posterior tibial arterial pulses should be palpated and capillary refill assessed. If injury is suspected, a Doppler probe can be used to assess arterial blood flow further. ABIs should also be calculated.

Neurologic examination includes assessment of all five major nerves that travel distally in the leg (Table 20-6). The deep peroneal nerve, traveling in the anterior compartment, can be evaluated by testing first dorsal web space sensation and foot and toe dorsiflexion. Testing sensation along the dorsum of the foot and eversion strength can assess the superficial peroneal nerve, which travels in the lateral compartment. The tibial nerve travels in the deep posterior compartment and provides sensation to the sole of the foot and motor function to the foot and toe plantar flexors. The sural and saphenous nerves travel superficially to the muscular compartments. They are both pure sensory nerves. The sural nerve supplies sensation to the lateral aspect of the heel and the saphenous nerve supplies sensation to the medial malleolus.

### Management and Treatment

Management and treatment of tibial shaft fractures have evolved over the years. A closed fracture with minimal displacement can be treated by cast immobilization and functional bracing. However, almost all moderate and severe fractures benefit from surgical stabilization. Reamed IM nailing is the technique of choice, when appropriate.

Plate fixation has fallen out of favor for diaphyseal fractures because of the high risk for wound-healing complications. However, it remains a valuable treatment option for diaphyseal fractures that extend proximally or distally into the metaphysis, which are less amenable to IM stabilization. Newer percutaneous plating techniques have improved the results of plate fixation by limiting surgical dissection in the zone of injury. When the patient's condition or the condition of the soft tissues about the leg preclude definitive fixation, external fixation continues to be a viable temporizing option for the treatment of tibial shaft fractures. Although it is generally reserved for temporary stabilization, with a good reduction, an external fixator can be used as definitive fixation. For complex fractures, a ringed external fixator is a powerful tool for correcting significant deformity or bony defects.

## Humeral Shaft Fractures

### Epidemiology and Significance

Humeral shaft fractures represent 3% to 5% of all fractures in adults. There is a bimodal distribution of incidence, with a small peak in the third decade for young men and a larger peak in the seventh decade for women. In younger patients, the injury is the result of high-energy trauma, whereas in older patients these fractures tend to be the result of osteoporosis. Most humeral shaft fractures can be treated nonoperatively. Studies have shown more than 95% union in those fractures treated without surgery.[42] In addition, the mobility of the shoulder and elbow joints will tolerate up to 15 degrees of malrotation, 20 degrees of flexion-extension deformity, 30 degrees of varus-valgus deformity, and 3 cm of shortening, without significant compromise in function or appearance.

A thorough neurovascular examination is imperative for patients with humeral fractures. There is up to an 18% incidence of radial nerve injury in humeral shaft fractures. With distal third spiral fractures (the so-called Holstein-Lewis fracture), the incidence is even higher because the radial nerve is at risk as it courses distally in the spiral groove (Fig. 20-39). In the trauma setting, right-sided humeral shaft fractures can be predictive of concomitant injury to the liver and other intra-abdominal organs.

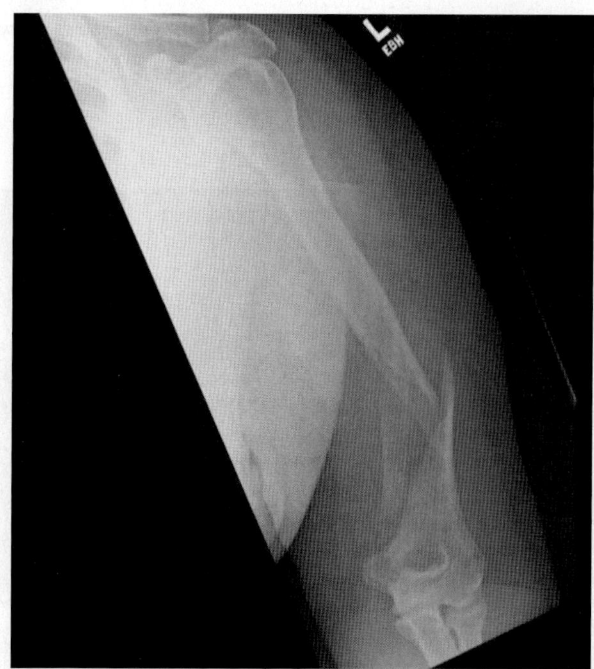


**FIGURE 20-39** Holstein-Lewis fracture of the humeral shaft. This patient had no radial nerve function at presentation. At the time of surgery, the nerve was found to be intact, but interposed between two fracture fragments. Full radial nerve function returned by 6 months.

### Treatment

Various nonoperative options exist for treating humeral shaft fractures—hanging arm casts, coaptation splints, sling and swathe, and functional bracing are all still used in the treatment of these fractures. Typically, a coaptation splint is applied in the acute setting and subsequently replaced by a functional fracture brace after the initial painful fracture period has passed (3 to 7 days). Patients are then allowed free elbow flexion-extension and arm abduction to 60 degrees. Gravity serves to correct alignment and to pull the bones out to length. Motion is encouraged to stimulate fracture healing because the hydraulic compression created by muscle contraction helps achieve fracture union.[42]

In certain circumstances, operative intervention is indicated. Failed closed reduction, intra-articular fractures, ipsilateral forearm or elbow fractures (floating elbow), segmental fractures, open fractures, and polytrauma patients all benefit from surgical management. Morbid obesity is a relative indication for operative treatment of these fractures. Obesity reduces the effectiveness of a functional fracture brace and the relatively abducted resting position of the arm in an obese patient leads to a high incidence of varus malunion. Of patients with radial nerve palsies, 70% to 90% are neurapraxias and recover spontaneously over 3 to 6 months. Surgical intervention for patients with radial nerve palsy following humeral shaft fractures is controversial. An algorithm for treatment of this problem is presented in Figure 20-40. Operative options include IM nailing, plate and screw fixation, and external fixation.

## CHALLENGES AND COMPLICATIONS

### Missed Injuries

Missed musculoskeletal injuries account for a large proportion of delays in diagnosis within the first few days of care of a critically injured patient. Clinical reassessment of trauma patients within 24 hours has reduced the incidence of missed injuries by almost 40%. Patients should be reexamined as they regain consciousness and resume activity. Repeat assessments should be routinely performed in all patients, especially unstable and neurologically impaired patients. The tertiary trauma survey includes a comprehensive examination and review of laboratory results and radiographs within 24 hours of initial evaluation. Specific injury patterns should be reviewed closely, especially in patients with multiple injuries and severe disability. External soft tissue trauma may be indicative of a more severe underlying injury. Missed cervical spine trauma occurs in 5% of all spine injuries and can potentially lead to paralysis and death.[43] Formal radiology rounds can facilitate increased recognition of occult injuries.

### Drug and Alcohol Use

The incidence of drug and alcohol use in patients with musculoskeletal injuries has been reported to be as high as 50%. Almost 25% of all patients test positive for two or more drugs.[44] Alcohol and drug use result in more severe orthopedic injuries and more frequent injuries requiring longer hospitalization. Associated complications include those from cocaine use, such as fever, hypertension, acute myocardial ischemia, arrhythmias, and stroke. Cocaine can also facilitate cardiac arrhythmias when combined with halothane, nitrous oxide, and/or ketamine. Furthermore, the use of alcohol or drugs can adversely affect the administration of premedicating drugs. Prophylaxis for delirium

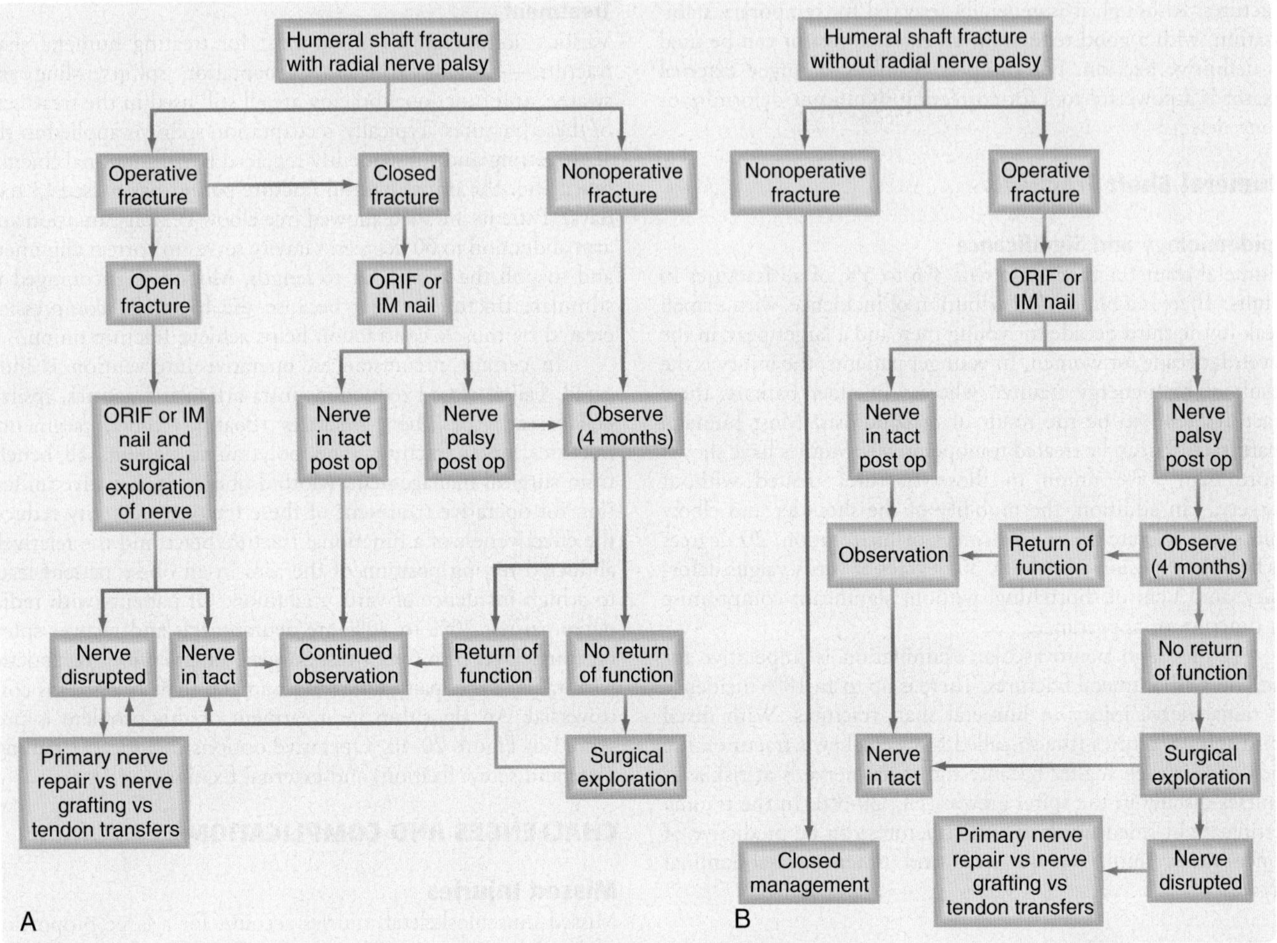

A

Humeral shaft fracture with radial nerve palsy

Operative fracture → Closed fracture

Nonoperative fracture

Open fracture

ORIF or IM nail

ORIF or IM nail and surgical exploration of nerve

Nerve in tact post op

Nerve palsy post op → Observe (4 months)

Nerve disrupted

Nerve in tact → Continued observation ← Return of function

No return of function

Surgical exploration

Primary nerve repair vs nerve grafting vs tendon transfers

B

Humeral shaft fracture without radial nerve palsy

Nonoperative fracture

Operative fracture

ORIF or IM nail

Nerve in tact post op

Nerve palsy post op

Observation ← Return of function ← Observe (4 months)

No return of function

Nerve in tact ← Surgical exploration

Closed management

Primary nerve repair vs nerve grafting vs tendon transfers ← Nerve disrupted

**FIGURE 20-40** Algorithms for management of a patient presenting with a humeral shaft fracture with **(A)** and without **(B)** radial nerve palsy.

tremens in postoperative patients should be performed when indicated. Inpatient detoxification consultation should be obtained before discharge.

## Thromboembolic Complications

When compared with patients with isolated injuries, multiply injured patients have an increased incidence of thromboembolic complications, including DVT and pulmonary embolism (PE; Fig. 20-41). In their study of venous thromboembolism (VTE) in trauma patients, Geerts and associates[45] have shown an overall incidence of 58%, with an 18% incidence of proximal clots. The incidence of pulmonary embolism in major trauma patients ranges from 2% to 22% and it is the third leading cause of death in these patients.[46] In addition to multiply injured trauma patients, patients undergoing elective neurosurgical, orthopedic, and oncologic surgery are also at increased risk for VTE. Long bone fractures, pelvic fractures, advanced age, spinal cord injuries, and surgical procedures are associated with an increased risk for VTE in trauma patients. The most common forms of pharmacologic prophylaxis include adjusted-dose unfractionated heparin, low-molecular-weight heparin (LMWH), warfarin, and aspirin. In addition, hirudin, a selective thrombin inhibitor and fondaparinux, an inhibitor of factor Xa, have been used for prophylaxis in elective hip and arthroplasty. Other forms of prophylaxis include mechanical devices, such as foot pumps and

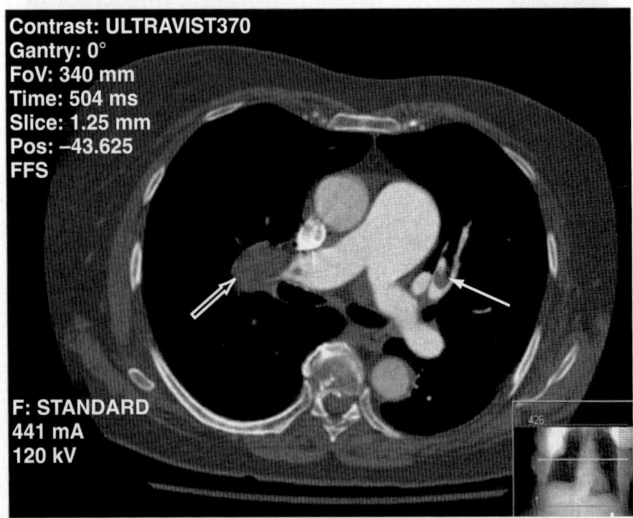


**FIGURE 20-41** CT angiogram showing a large PE completely occluding the right pulmonary artery *(solid arrowhead)* and a smaller PE occluding one of the segmental branches of the left pulmonary artery *(open arrowhead).*

sequential calf compression pumps, and barrier devices, such as inferior vena cava (IVC) filters.

It is generally agreed that prophylaxis is critical for a high-risk trauma patient. Two controversial issues in the prevention of VTE in a trauma patient are currently being debated. The first is the role of venous surveillance. Some physicians recommend routine duplex surveillance to detect thromboembolic events because the incidence of proximal DVT reported in some studies is higher than previously suspected. More recent literature, however, suggests that this is not necessary and that routine screening should be performed only for patients who are at high risk for VTE (e.g., in the presence of a spinal cord injury, lower extremity or pelvic fracture, or major head injury) and who have not received adequate thromboprophylaxis.[46] The second issue is appropriate prophylaxis. Adjusted-dose heparin and LMWH are currently the most common forms of prophylaxis. However, in a randomized study comparing low-dose unfractionated heparin with LMWH, Geerts and coworkers[45] documented an overall 44% incidence of DVT in trauma patients receiving low-dose unfractionated heparin versus 31% in those receiving enoxaparin. There was a slight increase in major bleeding in the enoxaparin-treated group; however, in none of the patients did the hemoglobin level drop by more than 2 g/dL.

In the most recent edition of the evidence-based recommendations for prevention of VTE, the American College of Chest Surgeons (ACCS) recommended the use of routine prophylaxis with LMWH while the patient is in the hospital. In patients with impaired mobility or those going to an inpatient rehabilitation facility, they recommended discharge on LMWH or warfarin (with an international normalized ratio [INR] goal of 2.0 to 3.0). In patients with a contraindication to anticoagulation, they recommended the use of intermittent pneumatic compression devices. These devices deliver sequential rhythmic compression to the calf and/or thigh and can help reduce the rate of DVT in trauma patients. In patients with lower extremity fractures or wounds, foot pumps should be used. Finally, the ACCS recommended against the routine use of IVC filters for patients at high risk of VTE. Because of the potential complications of filter placement, including migration of the filter, bleeding during or after placement, or filter thrombosis, these devices should be reserved for patients with known proximal DVT and either an absolute contraindication to chemical anticoagulation or impending major surgery. In either case, they recommended starting therapeutic anticoagulation as soon as the contraindication resolves.[46] Further research in this area is needed to determine the efficacy and safety of some of the newer agents for trauma patients with orthopedic injuries.

### Pulmonary Failure: Fat Emboli Syndrome and Adult Respiratory Distress Syndrome

Fat emboli syndrome (FES) is a condition characterized by respiratory distress, altered mental status, and skin petechiae. First described in humans in 1862, it occurs in multiply injured patients, especially those with orthopedic injuries. Clinical signs are evident hours to days after an injury involving long bone or pelvic fractures. Although fat embolization may occur in as many as 95% of traumatized patients, the incidence of FES ranges from 1% to 19%.[47] In patients with isolated long bone fractures, the incidence is between 2% and 5%. In a multiply injured patient with long bone or pelvic fractures, the incidence of FES is as high as 19%. Marrow fat from the fracture site is believed to enter the pulmonary circulation, where it causes activation of the coagulation cascade, platelet dysfunction, release of vasoactive substances and inflammatory cytokines, and subsequent neutrophil infiltration.[48] The treatment of FES is mostly supportive, but a recent meta-analysis by Bederman and colleagues[49] has shown that the use of corticosteroids in patients with multiple long bone fractures reduces the rate of FES by 78% without significantly increasing the risk of complications related to treatment of the fractures. Before the advent of modern ICU care, mortality rates in patients with FES were reported to be as high as 20%. Although that rate has dropped because of more modern resuscitative and supportive treatments (7% to 10%), mortality from FES is still a significant concern.[47]

FES may represent a subset of ARDS. ARDS is a pulmonary failure state defined as a $PaO_2/FIO_2$ ratio lower than 200 regardless of the level of positive end-expiratory pressure (PEEP), a pulmonary artery occlusion pressure of 18 mm Hg or less, or bilateral diffuse infiltrates on chest radiographs in the absence of congestive heart failure.[50] Early fixation of fractures has been shown to reduce the incidence of FES and ARDS in trauma patients; however, there has been some debate over whether the method of fixation affects the incidence of FES. In theory, IM nailing causes an increased embolic load, which could lead to an increased incidence of FES, but clinical and experimental studies have suggested that the presence of chest injury, not the method of fracture fixation, is responsible for ARDS.[41] Therefore, in patients with an acute chest injury with concomitant long bone fractures, it may be advisable to delay definitive fixation of the fracture until the patient's pulmonary status has stabilized.

## POSTOPERATIVE MOBILIZATION

The benefits of early fixation and mobilization of multiply injured patients have been discussed. However, a distinction between mobilization and weight bearing is essential. Mobilization is transfer of the patient from the supine position, either under the patient's own power or with the help of nurses and/or therapists. This includes turning the patient every shift by the nurse, sitting up in bed, or transferring the patient to a chair. All patients should be mobilized by the first or second postoperative day if their general condition permits. Mobilization helps prevent the development of pulmonary and septic complications.

Weight bearing, in contrast, is transmission of a load through an extremity. For a patient to be allowed to bear weight on an injured extremity, the following three conditions must be met:

1. There must be bone to bone contact at the fracture site as demonstrated intraoperatively or on postreduction radiographs. Without contact of the fracture ends, the fixation devices will be subjected to all the stresses applied to the extremity, which will frequently result in failure of the fixation.
2. Stable fixation of the fracture must be achieved. By definition, stable fixation is not disrupted when subjected to normal physiologic loads. Stable fixation is dependent on a number of factors. Fixation may be less than ideal in patients with osteopenic bone or severely comminuted fractures. When excessive loads

are anticipated, such as with heavy or obese patients, the typical fixation may not be adequate.

3. The patient must be able to comply with the weight-bearing status. Frequently, reliability of the patient is a significant consideration in the determination of weight-bearing status. Social, psychological, or emotional circumstances can affect a patient's ability to comply with weight-bearing restrictions.

Unless all three criteria are met, the fixation will need to be protected with restricted weight-bearing status. Touch-down weight bearing (TDWB) allows the patient to place the foot of his or her affected extremity flat on the floor, without bearing any of the patient's body weight. TDWB is often permitted in patients with injuries around the hip and allows extension of the hip and knee and dorsiflexion at the ankle. This natural position relaxes the hip musculature and minimizes joint reactive forces. Crutch walking with the foot off the floor (non–weight bearing [NWB]) leads to a significant increase in force across the hip joint because of contraction of the muscles about the hip. Toe-touch weight bearing (TTWB), a phrase often used synonymously with TDWB, is an unfortunate use of terminology. Most patients attempt to walk while touching only the toe of the injured extremity to the ground. In this position, the hip and knee are flexed and the ankle is held in equinus. When this status is maintained for any significant amount of time, contractures at the hip, knee, and ankle are common. For this reason, use of this terminology is discouraged.

Partial weight bearing (PWB) is defined in terms of the percentage of body weight applied to an injured extremity. It is gradually increased as the fracture gains stability through healing. With the use of a scale, the patient can learn what different amounts of body weight feel like. When a fracture and the patient are stable enough to withstand normal loads, weight bearing as tolerated (WBAT) is instituted. It is believed that reliable patients limit their own weight bearing according to their pain.

Even when weight bearing is not allowed, mobilization of affected and adjacent joints is typically performed within a few days. After surgical treatment, joints are typically immobilized briefly and then allowed passive or active range of motion in bed if weight bearing is not prudent. Early joint mobilization decreases the likelihood of fibrosis and therefore increases early mobility. Furthermore, joint motion is necessary for the good health of articular cartilage. Cartilage is nourished from synovial fluid most efficiently when the joint is moving. Early joint mobilization has become a basic tenet of orthopedic care and has led to a decrease in the morbidity associated with musculoskeletal injuries.

## SUMMARY

In the setting of acute trauma, preservation of a patient's life takes precedence over preservation of a limb. However, injuries to the extremities and axial skeleton may be life-threatening in rare circumstances (e.g., hemorrhage secondary to vascular injury from pelvic or long bone fractures). These must be recognized early and managed appropriately. Once the critical period has passed, musculoskeletal injuries are a major cause of post-traumatic morbidity, as demonstrated by increased health care costs, lost work days, physical disability, emotional distress, and diminished quality of life. Accordingly, it is essential that a detailed and complete extremity and axial musculoskeletal survey be performed on every patient, injuries be identified early, and the consulting orthopedic surgical team be notified of the specifics of these injuries in a timely fashion. It is essential that the trauma team have a high index of suspicion for the orthopedic emergencies discussed for any patient who has experienced high-energy trauma. Moreover, the patient should not be transported from the trauma room, unless necessary for lifesaving interventions, until the orthopedic team has evaluated and stabilized the involved extremity to protect it against further injury and morbidity. Finally, appropriate treatment of musculoskeletal injuries is a multidisciplinary undertaking. With cooperation and collaboration of all treating teams—general surgery, vascular surgery, neurosurgery, plastic surgery, internal medicine, and physical therapy—we will be able to ensure the best possible outcome for our patients.

## SELECTED REFERENCES

Bone LB, Johnson KD, Weigelt J, et al: Early versus delayed stabilization of femoral shaft fractures: A prospective randomized study. J Bone Joint Surg Am 71:336–340, 1989.

This classic article has shaped the treatment of multiply injured patients. It was the first clearly to define the benefits of early stabilization of femoral shaft fractures prospectively.

Browner BD, Levine AM, Jupiter JB, et al, editors: Skeletal trauma: Basic science, management and reconstruction, ed 4, Philadelphia, 2008, WB Saunders.

This is one of the premiere comprehensive texts covering traumatic musculoskeletal injuries, and this two-volume set is now in its fourth edition It is clearly written and visually appealing. The chapter authors are the elite orthopedic trauma surgeons in the world. It is an excellent reference for any physician dealing with a multiply injured patient.

Egol KA, Koval KJ, Zuckerma JD: Handbook of fractures, ed 4, Philadelphia, 2010, Lippincott Williams & Wilkins,.

This conveniently sized handbook is the ideal reference for physicians managing musculoskeletal injuries in the emergency setting. Comprehensive but concise, this guide discusses epidemiology, anatomy, mechanism of injury, clinical evaluation, radiologic evaluation, classification, treatment, and management of complications of most acute musculoskeletal injuries.

Gustilo R, Anderson J: Prevention of infection in the treatment of 1025 open fractures of long bones: Retrospective and prospective analyses. J Bone Joint Surg Am 58:453–458, 1976.

This classic article defined the classification and proposed management guidelines in patients with open fractures. It includes more than 300 cases reviewed retrospectively and another 600 prospective cases in which the new classification was applied.

Lieberman J: AAOS comprehensive orthopaedic review, Rosemont, Ill, 2009, American Academy of Orthopaedic Surgeons.

This text is a comprehensive review of all orthopedic subspecialties. Its bulleted format and well-organized layout allow for convienient referencing of a multitude of topics. It is an excellent reference for managing orthopedic patients.

Tscherne H, Gotzen L: Fractures with soft tissue injuries, Berlin, 1984, Springer-Verlag.

This fracture textbook is comprehensive in its coverage of open and closed fractures with soft tissue injuries. It covers all classifications, immediate management, fracture care, and wound care of these injuries. It uses the team approach to dealing with these complicated injuries.

## REFERENCES


1. Campbell BT, Saleheen H, Borrup K, et al: Epidemiology of trauma at a level 1 trauma center. Conn Med 73(7):389–394, 2009.
2. Lieberman J: AAOS comprehensive orthopaedic review, Rosemont, Ill, 2009, American Academy of Orthopaedic Surgeons.
3. Kessel B, Sevi R, Jeroukhimov I, et al: Is routine portable pelvic X-ray in stable multiple trauma patients always justified in a high technology era? Injury 38:559–563, 2007.
4. Fu CY, Wu SC, Chen RJ, et al: Evaluation of pelvic fracture stability and the need for angioembolization: Pelvic instabilities on plain film have an increased probability of requiring angioembolization. Am J Emerg Med 27:792–796, 2009.
5. Deunk J, Brink M, Dekker HM, et al: Predictors for the selection of patients for abdominal CT after blunt trauma: A proposal for a diagnostic algorithm. Ann Surg 251:512–520, 2010.
6. Gaarder C, Kroepelien CF, Loekke R, et al: Ultrasound performed by radiologists—confirming the truth about FAST in trauma. J Trauma 67:323–327, 2009.
7. Cha JY, Kashuk JL, Sarin EL, et al: Diagnostic peritoneal lavage remains a valuable adjunct to modern imaging techniques. J Trauma 67:330–334, 2009.
8. Bone LB, Johnson KD, Weigelt J, et al: Early versus delayed stabilization of femoral fractures. A prospective randomized study. J Bone Joint Surg Am 71:336–340, 1989.
9. Morshed S, Miclau T, 3rd, Bembom O, et al: Delayed internal fixation of femoral shaft fracture reduces mortality among patients with multisystem trauma. J Bone Joint Surg Am 91:3–13, 2009.
10. Mathen R, Inaba K, Munera F, et al: Prospective evaluation of multislice computed tomography versus plain radiographic cervical spine clearance in trauma patients. J Trauma 62:1427–1431, 2007.
11. Browner, BD, Levine AM, Jupiter JB, et al, editors: Skeletal trauma: Basic science, management, and reconstruction, ed 4, Philadelphia, 2008, WB Saunders.
12. Tornetta P, 3rd, Kain MS, Creevy WR: Diagnosis of femoral neck fractures in patients with a femoral shaft fracture. Improvement with a standard protocol. J Bone Joint Surg Am 89:39–43, 2007.
13. Levy BA, Fanelli GC, Whelan DB, et al: Controversies in the treatment of knee dislocations and multiligament reconstruction. J Am Acad Orthop Surg 17:197–206, 2009.
14. Tscherne H, Gotzen L: Fractures with soft tissue injuries, Berlin, 1984, Springer-Verlag.
15. Johansen K, Daines M, Howey T, et al: Objective criteria accurately predict amputation following lower extremity trauma. J Trauma 30:568–572, 1990.
16. Pollak AN, Jones AL, Castillo RC, et al: The relationship between time to surgical débridement and incidence of infection after open high-energy lower extremity trauma. J Bone Joint Surg Am 92: 7–15, 2010.
17. Ashford RU, Mehta JA, Cripps R: Delayed presentation is no barrier to satisfactory outcome in the management of open tibial fractures. Injury 35:411–416, 2004.
18. Gustilo RB, Anderson JT: Prevention of infection in the treatment of one thousand and twenty-five open fractures of long bones: Retrospective and prospective analyses. J Bone Joint Surg Am 58:453–458, 1976.
19. Zalavras CG, Marcus RE, Levin LS, et al: Management of open fractures and subsequent complications. J Bone Joint Surg Am 89:884–895, 2007.
20. Ly TV, Travison TG, Castillo RC, et al: Ability of lower-extremity injury severity scores to predict functional outcome after limb salvage. J Bone Joint Surg Am 90:1738–1743, 2008.
21. Busse JW, Jacobs CL, Swiontkowski MF, et al: Complex limb salvage or early amputation for severe lower-limb injury: A meta-analysis of observational studies. J Orthop Trauma 21:70–76, 2007.
22. Bhandari M, Guyatt GH, Swiontkowski MF, et al: Treatment of open fractures of the shaft of the tibia. J Bone Joint Surg Br 83: 62–68, 2001.

**22a.** Rudloff MI, Smith WR: Intramedullary reaming of the femur: current concepts concerning reaming. J Orthop Trauma 23:S12–S17, 2009.

23. Mubarak S, Hargens A: Compartment syndromes and Volkmann's contracture, Philadelphia, 1981, WB Saunders.
24. Whitesides TE, Heckman MM: Acute compartment syndrome: Update on diagnosis and treatment. J Am Acad Orthop Surg 4:209–218, 1996.
25. McQueen MM, Court-Brown CM: Compartment monitoring in tibial fractures. The pressure threshold for decompression. J Bone Joint Surg Br 78:99–104, 1996.
26. Olson SA, Glasgow RR: Acute compartment syndrome in lower extremity musculoskeletal trauma. J Am Acad Orthop Surg 13:436–444, 2005.
27. Shuler FD, Dietz MJ: Physicians' ability to manually detect isolated elevations in leg intracompartmental pressure. J Bone Joint Surg Am 92:361–367, 2010.
28. Lunsjo K, Tadros A, Hauggaard A, et al: Associated injuries and not fracture instability predict mortality in pelvic fractures: A prospective study of 100 patients. J Trauma 62:687–691, 2007.
29. Tile M: Pelvic ring fractures: should they be fixed? J Bone Joint Surg Br 70:1–12, 1988.
30. Hak DJ, Smith WR, Suzuki T: Management of hemorrhage in life-threatening pelvic fracture. J Am Acad Orthop Surg 17:447–457, 2009.
31. Krieg JC, Mohr M, Ellis TJ, et al: Emergent stabilization of pelvic ring injuries by controlled circumferential compression: A clinical trial. J Trauma 59:659–664, 2005.
32. Jowett AJ, Bowyer GW: Pressure characteristics of pelvic binders. Injury 38:118–121, 2007.
33. Salim A, Teixeira PG, DuBose J, et al: Predictors of positive angiography in pelvic fractures: A prospective study. J Am Coll Surg 207:656–662, 2008.
34. Osborn PM, Smith WR, Moore EE, et al: Direct retroperitoneal pelvic packing versus pelvic angiography: A comparison of two management protocols for haemodynamically unstable pelvic fractures. Injury 40:54–60, 2009.
35. Croce MA, Magnotti LJ, Savage SA, et al: Emergent pelvic fixation in patients with exsanguinating pelvic fractures. J Am Coll Surg 204:935–939, 2007.

**36.** Spector LR, Madigan L, Rhyne A, et al: Cauda equina syndrome. J Am Acad Orthop Surg 16:471–479, 2008.

**37.** Hollis JD, Daley BJ: 10-year review of knee dislocations: Is arteriography always necessary? J Trauma 59:672–675; discussion 675–676, 2005.

**38.** Seamon MJ, Smoger D, Torres DM, et al: A prospective validation of a current practice: The detection of extremity vascular injury with CT angiography. J Trauma 67:238–243, 2009.

**39.** Subramanian A, Vercruysse G, Dente C, et al: A decade's experience with temporary intravascular shunts at a civilian level I trauma center. J Trauma 65:316–324, 2008.

**40.** Morley JR, Smith RM, Pape HC, et al: Stimulation of the local femoral inflammatory response to fracture and intramedullary reaming: A preliminary study of the source of the second hit phenomenon. J Bone Joint Surg Br 90:393–399, 2008.

**41.** Pape HC, Tornetta P, 3rd, Tarkin I, et al: Timing of fracture fixation in multitrauma patients: the role of early total care and damage control surgery. J Am Acad Orthop Surg 17:541–549, 2009.

**42.** Sarmiento A, Zagorski JB, Zych GA, et al: Functional bracing for the treatment of fractures of the humeral diaphysis. J Bone Joint Surg Am 82:478–486, 2000.

**43.** Platzer P, Hauswirth N, Jaindl M, et al: Delayed or missed diagnosis of cervical spine injuries. J Trauma 61:150–155, 2006.

**44.** Levy RS, Hebert CK, Munn BG, et al: Drug and alcohol use in orthopedic trauma patients: A prospective study. J Orthop Trauma 10:21–27, 1996.

**45.** Geerts WH, Code KI, Jay RM, et al: A prospective study of venous thromboembolism after major trauma. N Engl J Med 331:1601–1606, 1994.

**46.** Geerts WH, Bergqvist D, Pineo GF, et al: Prevention of venous thromboembolism: American College of Chest Physicians Evidence-Based Clinical Practice Guidelines (8th Edition). Chest 133:381S–453S, 2008.

**47.** Talbot M, Schemitsch EH: Fat embolism syndrome: History, definition, epidemiology. Injury 37(Suppl 4):S3–7, 2006.

**48.** Blankstein M, Byrick RJ, Nakane M, et al: Amplified inflammatory response to sequential hemorrhage, resuscitation, and pulmonary fat embolism: An animal study. J Bone Joint Surg Am 92:149–161, 2010.

**49.** Bederman SS, Bhandari M, McKee MD, et al: Do corticosteroids reduce the risk of fat embolism syndrome in patients with long-bone fractures? A meta-analysis. Can J Surg 52:386–393, 2009.

**50.** Irwin R, Rippe J: Manual of intensive care medicine, ed 5, Philadelphia, 2010, Lippincott, Williams & Wilkins.

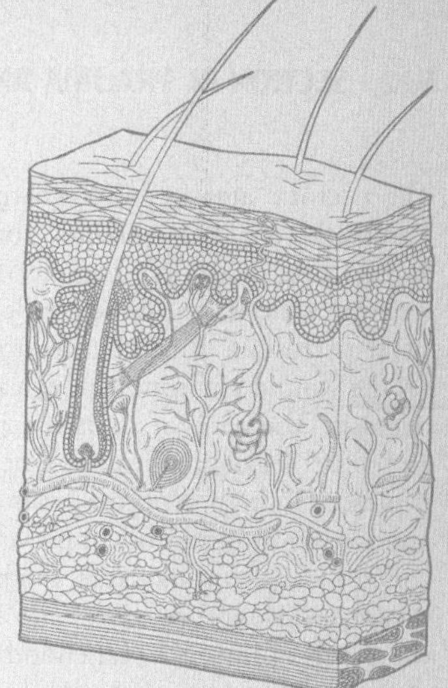

# CHAPTER 21

# BURNS

Marc Jeschke, Felicia N. Williams, Gerd G. Gauglitz, and David N. Herndon

CAUSES
PATHOPHYSIOLOGY OF BURN INJURIES
MANAGEMENT
WOUND CARE
SPECIAL CONSIDERATIONS: ELECTRICAL AND CHEMICAL BURNS
OUTCOMES
BURN UNITS
SUMMARY

More than 500,000 burn injuries occur annually in the United States.[1] Although most of these burn injuries are minor, approximately 40,000 to 60,000 burn patients require admission to a hospital or major burn center for appropriate treatment. The devastating consequences of burns have been recognized by the medical community and significant amounts of resources and research have successfully improved these dismal statistics.[2] Specialized burn centers (Box 21-1) and advances in therapy strategies, based on improved understanding of resuscitation, enhanced wound coverage, more appropriate infection control, improved treatment of inhalation injury, and better support of the hypermetabolic response to injury have further improved the clinical outcome of this unique patient population.[3] However, severe burns remain a devastating injury, affecting almost every organ system and leading to significant morbidity and mortality.[4,5]

## CAUSES

There is no greater trauma than a major burn injury, which can be classified according to different burn causes and different depths (Box 21-2). Of all cases, almost 4000 people die of complications related to thermal injury.[6] As in all trauma-related deaths, burn deaths generally occur immediately after the injury or weeks later as a result of multisystem organ failure. Of all burns, 66% occur at home and fatalities are predominant in the extremes of age, the very young and older adults. The most common causes are flame and scald burns.[7] Scald burns are most common in victims up to 5 years of age. There is a significant percentage of burns in children that are caused by child abuse. There are a number of risk factors that have been linked to burn injury—specifically age, location, demographics, and low economic status.[8] These risk factors underscore the fact that most burn injuries and fatalities are preventable and mandate intervention and prevention strategies. Overall, no single group is immune to the public health debt caused by burns.

Location plays a major role in the risk and treatment of burn. The available resources in a given community greatly influence morbidity and mortality. A lack of adequate resources affects the education, rehabilitation, and survival rates of burn victims. Someone with a severe burn in a resource-rich environment can receive care within minutes, whereas a burned individual in an austere environment may suffer for an extended period waiting for care. The ideal treatment of burns requires the collaboration of surgeons, anesthesiologists, occupational therapists, physiotherapists, nurses, nutritionists, rehabilitation therapists, and social workers just to accommodate the basic needs of a major burn survivor.[9] Any delay in reaching these resources compounds a delay in resuscitation and thus adds to the mortality risk.[10] For those who have access to adequate burn care, survival from a major burn is the rule, no longer the exception. The survival rate for all burns is 94.6%, but for at-risk populations, in communities lacking medical, legal, and public health resources, survival can be almost impossible.[7]

## PATHOPHYSIOLOGY OF BURN INJURIES

### Local Changes

Locally, thermal injury causes coagulative necrosis of the epidermis and underlying tissues, with the depth of injury dependent on the temperature to which the skin is exposed, the specific heat of the causative agent, and the duration of exposure. Burns are classified into five different categories of cause and depth of injury. The causes include injury from flame (fire), hot liquids (scald), contact with hot or cold objects, chemical exposure, and/or conduction of electricity (Box 21-2). The first three induce cellular damage by the transfer of energy, which induces coagulation necrosis. Chemical burns and electrical burns cause direct injury to cellular membranes in addition to the transfer of heat and can cause a coagulation or colliquation necrosis.

The skin, which is the largest organ on the human body, provides a staunch barrier in the transfer of energy to deeper tissues, thus confining much of the injury to this layer. Once the inciting focus is removed, however, the response of local tissues can lead to injury in the deeper layers. The area of cutaneous or superficial injury has been divided into three zones—zone of coagulation, zone of stasis, and zone of hyperemia (Fig. 21-1).

The necrotic area of burn where cells have been disrupted is termed the *zone of coagulation.* This tissue is irreversibly damaged at the time of injury. The area immediately surrounding the necrotic zone has a moderate degree of insult, with decreased tissue perfusion. This is termed the *zone of stasis* and, depending on the wound environment, can survive or go on to coagulative necrosis. The zone of stasis is associated with vascular damage and vessel leakage. Thromboxane A2, a potent vasoconstrictor, is present in high concentrations in burn wounds, and the local application of inhibitors improves blood flow and decreases the zone of stasis. Antioxidants, bradykinin antagonists, and subatmospheric wound pressures also improve blood flow and affect the depth of injury. Local endothelial interactions with neutrophils mediate some of the local inflammatory responses associated with the zone of stasis. Treatment directed at the control of local inflammation immediately after injury may spare the zone of stasis, indicated by studies demonstrating the blockage of leukocyte adherence with anti-CD18 or anti-intercellular adhesion molecules; monoclonal antibodies improve tissue perfusion and tissue survival in animal models. The last area is termed the *zone of hyperemia,* which is characterized by vasodilation from inflammation surrounding the burn wound. This region contains the clearly viable tissue from which the healing process begins and is generally not at risk for further necrosis.

### Burn Depth

The depth of burn varies, depending on the degree of tissue damage. Burn depth is classified into degree of injury in the epidermis, dermis, subcutaneous fat, and underlying structures (Fig. 21-2). First-degree burns are, by definition, injuries confined to the epidermis. First-degree burns are painful, erythematous, and blanch to the touch, with an intact epidermal barrier. Examples include sunburn or a minor scald from a kitchen accident. These burns do not result in scarring, and treatment is aimed at comfort with the use of topical soothing salves, with or without aloe, and oral nonsteroidal anti-inflammatory drugs (NSAIDs).

Second-degree burns are divided into two types, superficial and deep. All second-degree burns have some degree of dermal damage, by definition, and the division is based on the depth of injury into the dermis. Superficial dermal burns are erythematous, painful, blanch to touch, and often blister. Examples include scald injuries from overheated bathtub water and flash flame burns. These wounds spontaneously reepithelialize from retained epidermal structures in the rete ridges, hair follicles, and sweat glands in 1 to 2 weeks. After healing, these burns may have some slight skin discoloration over the long term. Deep dermal burns into the reticular dermis appear more pale and mottled, do not blanch to touch, but remain painful to pinprick. These burns heal in 2 to 5 weeks by reepithelialization from hair follicles and sweat gland keratinocytes, often with severe scarring as a result of the loss of dermis.

**BOX 21-1 Burn Unit Organization and Personnel**

Experienced burn surgeons (burn unit director and qualified surgeons)
Dedicated nursing personnel
Physical and occupational therapists
Social workers
Dietitians
Pharmacists
Respiratory therapists
Psychiatrists and clinical psychologists
Prosthetists

**BOX 21-2 Burn Classifications**

**Causes**
Flame—damage from superheated oxidized air
Scald—damage from contact with hot liquids
Contact—damage from contact with hot or cold solid materials
Chemicals—contact with noxious chemicals
Electricity—conduction of electrical current through tissues

**Depths**
First degree—injury localized to the epidermis
Superficial second degree—injury to the epidermis and superficial dermis
Deep second degree—injury through the epidermis and deep into the dermis
Third degree—full-thickness injury through the epidermis and dermis into subcutaneous fat
Fourth degree—injury through the skin and subcutaneous fat into underlying muscle or bone

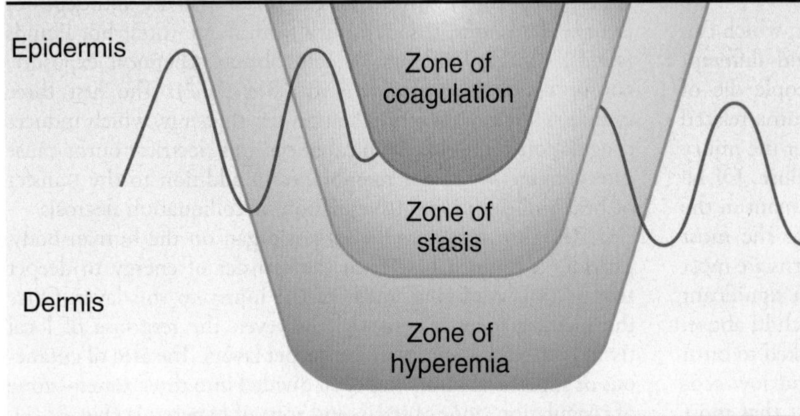


**FIGURE 21-1** Zones of injury after a burn. The zone of coagulation is the portion irreversibly injured. The zones of stasis and hyperemia are defined in response to the injury.

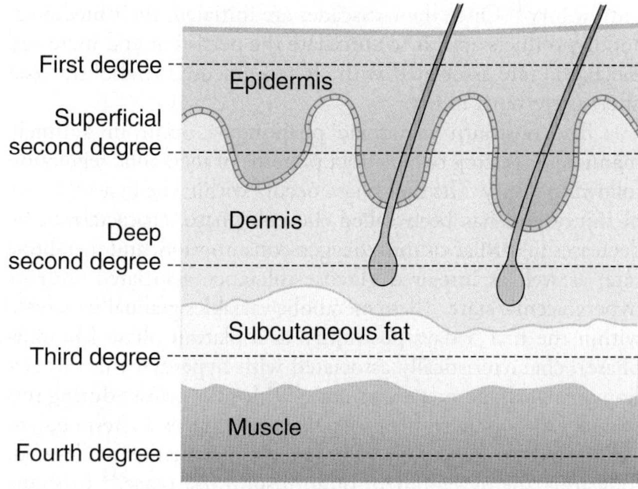


**FIGURE 21-2** Depths of a burn. First-degree burns are confined to the epidermis. Second-degree burns extend into the dermis (dermal burns). Third-degree burns are full thickness through the epidermis and dermis. Fourth-degree burns involve injury to underlying tissue structures such as muscle, tendons, and bone.

Third-degree burns are full-thickness burns through the epidermis and dermis and are characterized by a hard, leathery eschar that is painless and black, white, or cherry red. No epidermal or dermal appendages remain; thus, these wounds must heal by reepithelialization from the wound edges. Deep dermal and full-thickness burns require excision with skin grafting from the patient to heal the wounds in a timely fashion.

Fourth-degree burns involve other organs beneath the skin, such as muscle, bone, and brain.

Currently, burn depth is most accurately assessed by the judgment of experienced physicians. Accurate depth determination is critical to wound healing because wounds that will heal with local treatment are treated differently than those requiring operative intervention. Examination of the entire wound by the physicians ultimately responsible for their management is the gold standard used to guide further treatment decisions. Newer technologies, such as the multisensor laser Doppler flowmeter, hold promise for determining burn depth quantitatively. Several studies have claimed superiority of this method over clinical judgment in the determination of wounds requiring skin grafting for timely healing, which may lead to a change in the standard of care in the future.

## Burn Size

Determination of burn size estimates the extent of injury. Burn size is generally assessed by the rule of nines (Fig. 21-3). In adults, each upper extremity and the head and neck are 9% of the total body surface area (TBSA), the lower extremities and the anterior and posterior trunk are 18% each, and the perineum and genitalia are assumed to be 1% of the TBSA. Another method of estimating smaller burns is to equate the area of the open hand (including the palm and extended fingers) of the patient to be approximately 1% of the TBSA and then to transpose that measurement visually onto the wound for a determination of its size. This method is crucial when evaluating burns of mixed distribution.

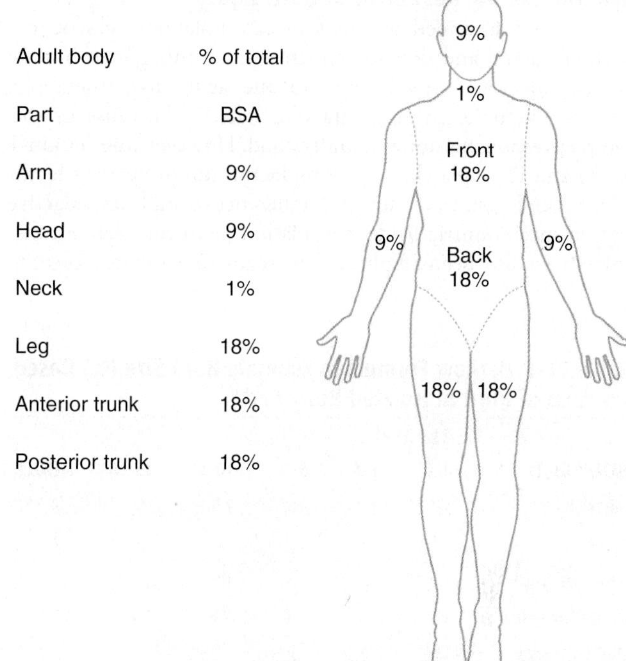


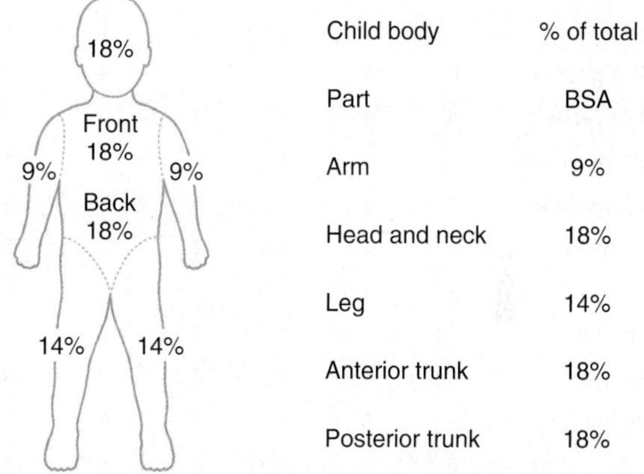


**FIGURE 21-3** Estimation of burn size using the rule of nines. (From American Burn Association: Advanced burn life support providers manual, Chicago, 2005, American Burn Association.)

Children have a relatively larger portion of the body surface area in the head and neck, which is compensated for by a relatively smaller surface area in the lower extremities. Infants have 21% of the TBSA in the head and neck and 13% in each leg, which incrementally approaches the adult proportions with increasing age. The Berkow formula is used to determine burn size accurately in children (Table 21-1).

## Systemic Changes

Severe burns covering more than 40% of the TBSA are typically followed by a period of stress, inflammation, and hypermetabolism, characterized by a hyperdynamic circulatory response with increased body temperature, glycolysis, proteolysis, lipolysis, and futile substrate cycling (Fig. 21-4). These responses are present in all trauma, surgical, and critically ill patients, but their severity, length, and magnitude are unique for burn patients.[4]

### Hypermetabolic Response to Burn Injury

Marked and sustained increases in catecholamine, glucocorticoid, glucagon, and dopamine secretion are thought to initiate the cascade of events leading to the acute hypermetabolic response, with its ensuing catabolic state.[11] The cause of this complex response is not well understood. However, interleukin-1 (IL-1) and IL-6, platelet-activating factor, tumor necrosis factor (TNF), endotoxins, neutrophil-adherence complexes, reactive oxygen species, nitric oxide, coagulation , and complement cascades have also been implicated in regulating this response to burn injury.[12] Once these cascades are initiated, their mediators and byproducts appear to stimulate the persistent and increased metabolic rate associated with altered glucose metabolism seen after severe burn injury.

**Table 21-1 Berkow Formula to Estimate Burn Size (%) Based on Area of Burn in Isolated Body Part***

| | Age (yr) | | | | | |
|---|---|---|---|---|---|---|
| **BODY PART** | **0-1** | **1-4** | **5-9** | **10-14** | **15-18** | **ADULT** |
| Head | 19 | 17 | 13 | 11 | 9 | 7 |
| Neck | 2 | 2 | 2 | 2 | 2 | 2 |
| Anterior trunk | 13 | 13 | 13 | 13 | 13 | 13 |
| Posterior trunk | 13 | 13 | 13 | 13 | 13 | 13 |
| Right buttock | 2.5 | 2.5 | 2.5 | 2.5 | 2.5 | 2.5 |
| Left buttock | 2.5 | 2.5 | 2.5 | 2.5 | 2.5 | 2.5 |
| Genitalia | 1 | 1 | 1 | 1 | 1 | 1 |
| Right upper arm | 4 | 4 | 4 | 4 | 4 | 4 |
| Left upper arm | 4 | 4 | 4 | 4 | 4 | 4 |
| Right lower arm | 3 | 3 | 3 | 3 | 3 | 3 |
| Left lower arm | 3 | 3 | 3 | 3 | 3 | 3 |
| Right hand | 2.5 | 2.5 | 2.5 | 2.5 | 2.5 | 2.5 |
| Left hand | 2.5 | 2.5 | 2.5 | 2.5 | 2.5 | 2.5 |
| Right thigh | 5.5 | 6.5 | 8 | 8.5 | 9 | 9.5 |
| Left thigh | 5.5 | 6.5 | 8 | 8.5 | 9 | 9.5 |
| Right leg | 5 | 5 | 5.5 | 6 | 6.5 | 7 |
| Left leg | 5 | 5 | 5.5 | 6 | 6.5 | 7 |
| Right foot | 3.5 | 3.5 | 3.5 | 3.5 | 3.5 | 3.5 |
| Left foot | 3.5 | 3.5 | 3.5 | 3.5 | 3.5 | 3.5 |

*Estimates are made, recorded, and then summed to gain an accurate estimate of the body surface area burned.

The postburn metabolic phenomena occur in a timely manner, suggesting two distinct patterns of metabolic regulation following injury. The first phase occurs within the first 48 hours of injury and has been called the ebb phase, characterized by decreases in cardiac output, oxygen consumption, and metabolic rate, as well as impaired glucose tolerance associated with its hyperglycemic state. These metabolic variables gradually increase within the first 5 days postinjury to a plateau phase (the flow phase), characteristically associated with hyperdynamic circulation and the hypermetabolic state.[11,13] Insulin release during this period was found to be twice that of controls in response to glucose load and plasma glucose levels are markedly elevated, indicating the development of an insulin resistance.[14] It is currently thought that these metabolic alterations resolve soon after complete wound closure. We have found that the hypermetabolic response to burn injury may last for more than 12 months after the initial event; in our recent studies,[15] we noted that sustained hypermetabolic postburn alterations, as shown by persistent elevations of total urine cortisol, serum cytokine, and catecholamine levels, and basal energy requirements, were accompanied by impaired glucose metabolism and insulin sensitivity that persisted for up to 3 years after the initial burn injury.

A 10- to 50-fold elevation of plasma catecholamine and corticosteroid levels occurs in major burns, which persist up to 3 years post-injury.[4,13,15] Cytokine levels peak immediately after the burn injury, approaching normal levels only after 1-month postinjury. Constitutive and acute-phase proteins are altered beginning 5 to 7 days postburn and remain abnormal throughout the acute hospital stay. Serum insulin-like growth factor I (IGF-I), IGF-binding protein 3 (IGFBP3), parathyroid hormone, and osteocalcin levels decrease immediately after the injury 10 fold, and remain significantly decreased up to 6 months postburn compared with normal levels. Sex hormone and endogenous growth hormone levels decrease at approximately 3 weeks postburn (Fig. 21-5).

For severely burned patients, the resting metabolic rate at a thermal neutral temperature (30° C) exceeds 140% of normal at admission, reduces to 130% once the wounds are fully healed, and then to 120% at 6 months after injury and 110% at 12

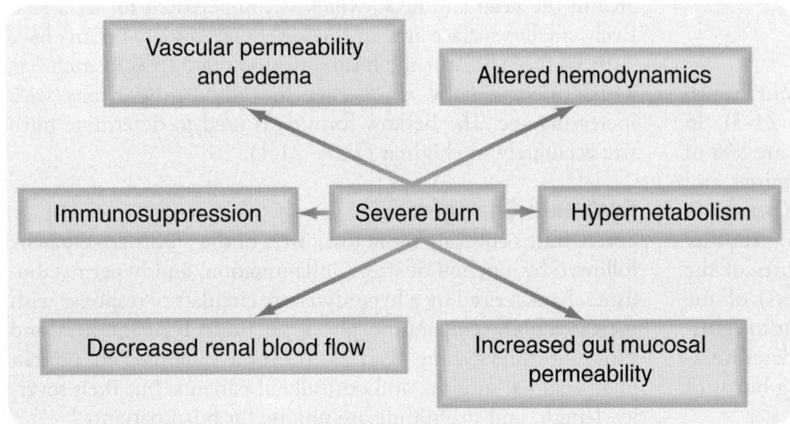


**FIGURE 21-4** Systemic effects of a severe burn.

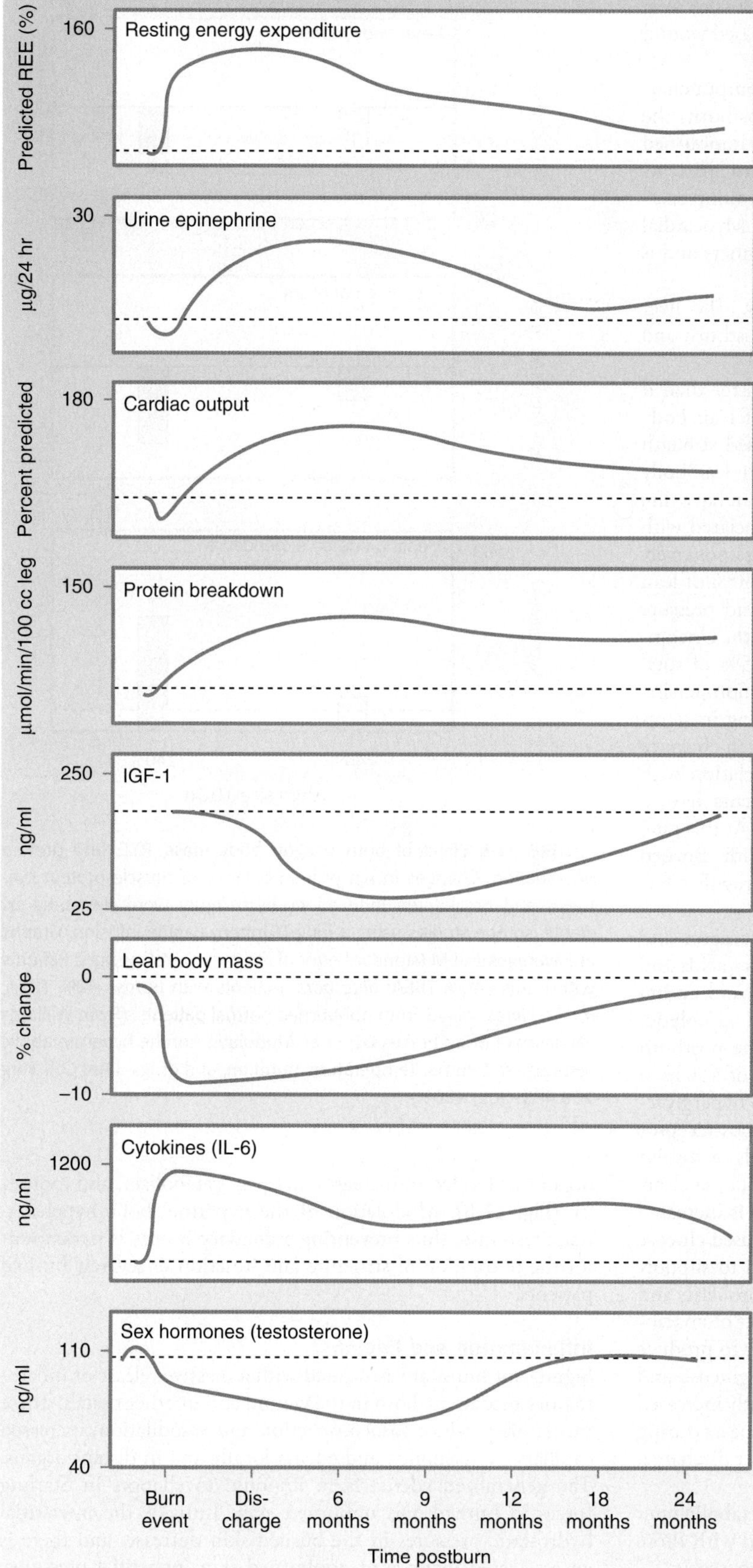


**FIGURE 21-5** Physiologic and metabolic changes after severe burn injury. This demonstrates changes in REE, stress hormones cardiac function, gender hormones, cytokines, and changes in body composition. Solid curves, A verages for burn patients; dashed lines, values from nonburned normal patients. (Data from Williams FN, Jeschke MG, Chinkes DL, et al: Modulation of the hypermetabolic response to trauma: Temperature, nutrition, and drugs. J Am Coll Surg 208:489–502, 2009.)

months postburn.[13] Increases in catabolism result in loss of total body protein, decreased immune defenses, and decreased wound healing.[4]

Immediate postburn patients have low cardiac output characteristic of early shock. However, 3 to 4 days postburn, the cardiac output is more than 1.5 times that of a nonburned healthy volunteer.[13] Heart rates of pediatric burn patients approach 1.6 times those of nonburned, healthy volunteers.[11] Postburn patients have increased cardiac work.[4] Myocardial oxygen consumption surpasses that of marathon runners and is sustained well into the rehabilitative period.

There is profound hepatomegaly after injury. The liver increases its size by 225% of normal by 2 weeks postburn and remains enlarged at discharge at 200% of normal.[13]

Postburn, muscle protein is degraded much faster than it is synthesized.[16] The net protein loss causes loss of lean body mass and severe muscle wasting, leading to decreased strength and failure to rehabilitate fully. Significant decreases in lean body mass related to chronic illness or hypermetabolism can have dire consequences. A 10% loss of lean body mass is associated with immune dysfunction. A 20% loss of lean body mass positively correlates with decreased wound healing. A loss of 30% of lean body mass leads to increased risk for pneumonia and pressure sores. A 40% loss of lean body mass can lead to death. Uncomplicated severely burned patients can lose up to 25% of total body mass after acute burn injury.[13] Protein degradation persists up to almost 1 year after severe burn injury, resulting in significant negative whole-body and cross-leg nitrogen balance (Fig. 21-6).[4] Protein catabolism has a positive correlation with increases in metabolic rates. Severely burned patients have a daily nitrogen loss of 20 to 25 g/m$^2$ of burned skin.[4] At this rate, a lethal cachexia can be reached in less than 1 month. Burned pediatric patients' protein loss leads to significant growth retardation for up to 24 months postinjury.[15]

Elevated circulating levels of catecholamines, glucagon, and cortisol after severe thermal injury stimulate free fatty acids and glycerol from fat, glucose production by the liver, and amino acids from muscle (Fig. 21-7).[4,11] Specifically, glycolytic-gluconeogenic cycling is increased 250% during the postburn hypermetabolic response, coupled with an increase of 450% in triglyceride fatty acid cycling. These changes lead to hyperglycemia and impaired insulin sensitivity related to postreceptor insulin resistance, as demonstrated by elevated levels of insulin and fasting glucose, and significant reductions in glucose clearance. Whereas glucose delivery to peripheral tissues is increased up to threefold, glucose oxidation is restricted. Increased glucose production is directed, in part, to the burn wound to support the relatively inefficient anaerobic metabolism of fibroblasts and endothelial and inflammatory cells. The end product of anaerobic glucose oxidation, lactate, is recycled to the liver to produce more glucose via gluconeogenic pathways. Serum glucose and insulin levels increase postburn and remain significantly increased through the acute hospital stay. Insulin resistance appears during the first week postburn and persists significantly after discharge, up to 3 years postburn.[13,15]

Septic patients have a profound increase in metabolic rates and protein catabolism, up to 40% more compared with those with burns of a similar size who do not develop sepsis.[17,18] A vicious cycle develops, because catabolic patients are more susceptible to sepsis caused by changes in immune function and immune response. The emergence of multidrug resistant organisms has led to increases in sepsis, catabolism, and mortality (Fig. 21-8). Modulation of the hypermetabolic hypercatabolic response, thus preventing secondary injury, is paramount for the restoration of structure and function of severely burned patients.

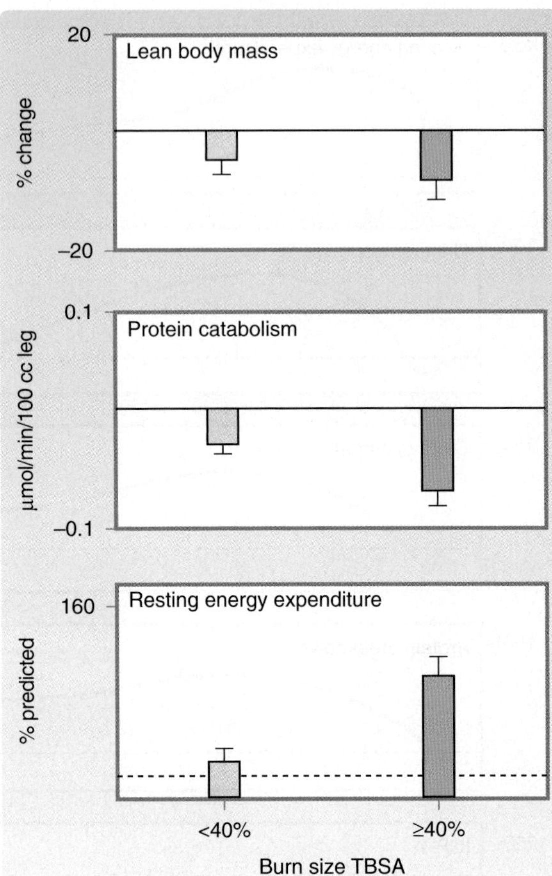


**FIGURE 21-6** Effect of burn size on body mass, REE, and protein degradation. Changes in net protein balance of muscle protein synthesis and breakdown induced by burn injury were measured by stable isotope studies using a [ring-D$_5$]phenyalanine infusion. Graphs are averages ± SEM (standard error of the mean). *Yellow bars,* Patients with burns <40% TBSA; *blue bars,* patients with burns >40% TBSA; *dashed lines,* values from nonburned normal patients. (From Williams FN, Jeschke MG, Chinkes DL, et al: Modulation of the hypermetabolic response to trauma: Temperature, nutrition, and drugs. J Am Coll Surg 208:489–502, 2009.)

## Inflammation and Edema

Significant burns are associated with a massive release of inflammatory mediators, both in the wound and in other tissues. These mediators produce vasoconstriction and vasodilation, increased capillary permeability, and edema locally and in distant organs. The generalized edema is in response to changes in Starling forces in burned and unburned skin. Initially, the interstitial hydrostatic pressures in the burned skin decrease, and there is an associated increase in nonburned skin interstitial pressures. As the plasma oncotic pressures decrease and interstitial oncotic pressures increase because of increased capillary permeability-induced protein loss, edema forms in the burned and nonburned

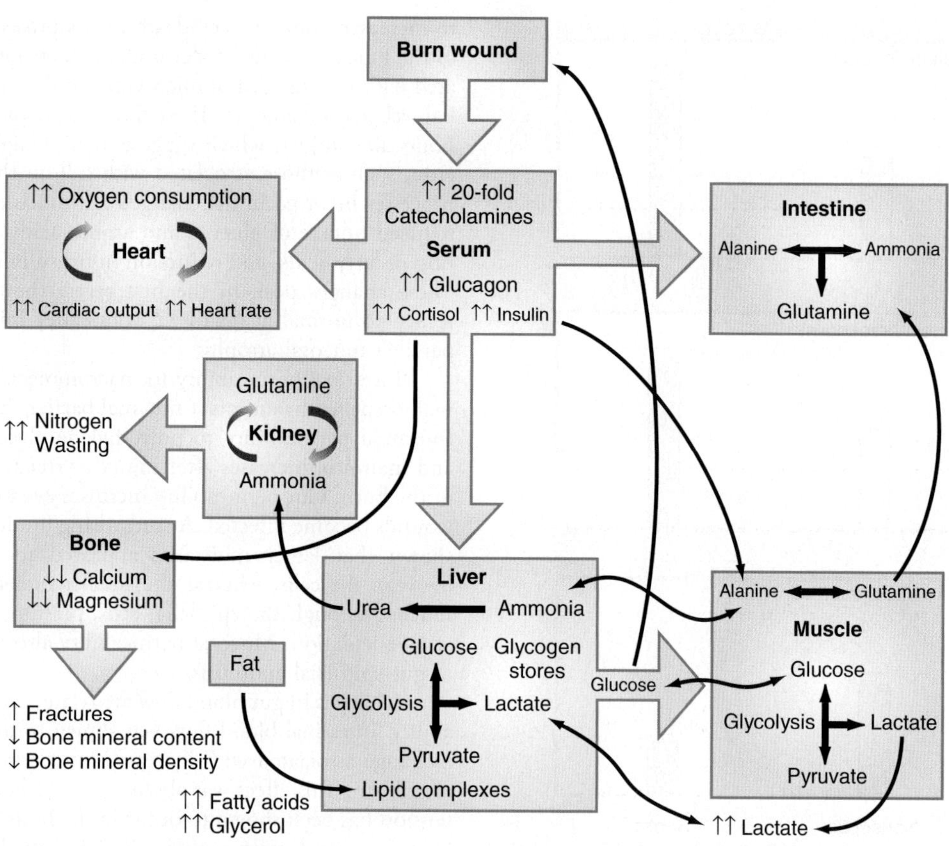


**FIGURE 21-7** Effects of metabolic dysfunction postburn. (From Williams FN, Jeschke MG, Chinkes DL, et al: Modulation of the hypermetabolic response to trauma: Temperature, nutrition, and drugs. J Am Coll Surg 208:489–502, 2009.)

tissues. The edema is greater in the burned tissues because of lower interstitial pressures.

Many mediators have been proposed to account for the changes in permeability after burns, including histamine, bradykinin, vasoactive amines, prostaglandins, leukotrienes, activated complement, and catecholamines. Mast cells in the burned skin release histamine in large quantities immediately after injury, which elicits a characteristic response in venules by increasing intercellular junction space formation. The use of antihistamines for the treatment of burn edema, however, has had limited success. In addition, aggregated platelets release serotonin, which plays a major role in edema formation. This agent acts directly to increase pulmonary vascular resistance and indirectly aggravates the vasoconstrictive effects of various vasoactive amines. Serotonin blockade improves the cardiac index, decreases pulmonary artery pressure, and decreases oxygen consumption after burn. When the antiserotonin methysergide was given to animals after scald injury, wound edema formation decreased as a result of local effects.

Another mediator likely to play a role in changes in permeability and fluid shifts is thromboxane A2; its level increases dramatically in the plasma and wounds of burn patients. This potent vasoconstrictor leads to vasoconstriction and platelet aggregation in the wound, contributing to expansion of the zone of stasis. It has also caused prominent mesenteric vasoconstriction and decreased gut blood flow in animal models, which compromised gut mucosal integrity and decreased gut immune function.

## Effects on the Cardiovascular System

Microvascular changes induce cardiopulmonary alterations characterized by loss of plasma volume, increased peripheral vascular resistance, and subsequent decreased cardiac output immediately after injury. Cardiac output remains depressed because of decreased blood volume and increased blood viscosity, as well as decreased cardiac contractility. Ventricular dysfunction during this period is attributed to a circulating myocardial depressant factor present in lymphatic fluid, although the specific factor has never been isolated. Burn patients with burns over 40% of their TBSA demonstrate an increased cardiac output, which significantly decreases over time. This is accompanied by an increase in heart rate. Severely burned pediatric patients have a marked tachycardia, with 160% to 170% predicted, which remains high at intensive care unit (ICU) discharge at (≈150%). Cardiac output at admission is 150% and remains high at discharge (≈130% predicted). There is some evidence that the heart rate remains elevated up to 2 years postburn.[13] Increased cardiac stress postburn is associated with myocardial depression. which has been shown in several studies.[19] The hypothesis that cardiac stress and myocardial dysfunction may be one of the main contributors to mortality in large burns was confirmed in a retrospective autopsy study, indicating the therapeutic need to improve cardiac stress and function.[20]

## Effects on the Renal System

Diminished blood volume and cardiac output result in decreased renal blood flow and glomerular filtration rate. Other

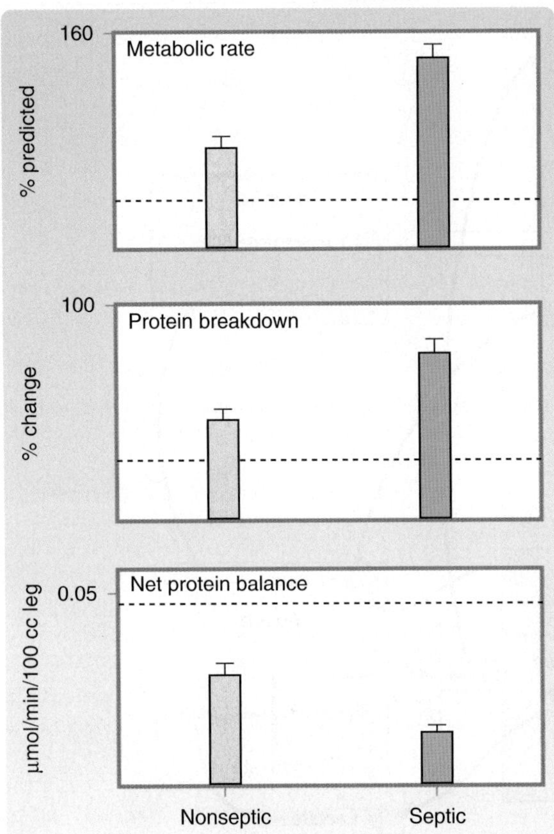


**FIGURE 21-8** Effect of sepsis on REE, muscle protein breakdown, and fractional synthetic rate of muscle protein synthesis compared with burns of similar size. Changes in net protein balance of muscle protein synthesis and breakdown induced by burn injury was measured by stable isotope studies using a [ring-$D_5$]phenyalanine infusion. Graphs are averages ± SEM. *Yellow bars,* Nonseptic patients with burns ≥40% TBSA; *blue bars,* septic patients with burns ≥40% TBSA; *dashed lines,* values from nonburned, normal patients. (From Williams FN, Jeschke MG, Chinkes DL, et al: Modulation of the hypermetabolic response to trauma: Temperature, nutrition, and drugs. J Am Coll Surg 208:489–502, 2009.)

stress-induced hormones and mediators, such as angiotensin, aldosterone, and vasopressin, reduce renal blood flow further immediately after the injury. These effects result in oliguria, which, if left untreated, will cause acute tubular necrosis and renal failure. Twenty years ago, acute renal failure in burn injuries was almost always fatal. Today, however, newer techniques in dialysis have become widely used to support the kidneys during recovery. The latest reports indicate an 88% mortality rate for severely burned adults and a 56% mortality rate for severely burned children in whom renal failure develops in the postburn period. Early resuscitation decreases the risks of renal failure and improves the associated morbidity and mortality rates.[10]

### Effects on the Gastrointestinal System

The gastrointestinal response to burn is highlighted by mucosal atrophy, changes in digestive absorption, and increased intestinal permeability. Atrophy of the small bowel mucosa occurs within 12 hours of injury in proportion to the burn size and is related to increased epithelial cell death by apoptosis. The cytoskeleton of the mucosal brush border undergoes atrophic changes associated with vesiculation of microvilli and disruption of the terminal web actin filaments. These findings are most pronounced 18 hours after injury, which suggests that changes in the cytoskeleton, such as those associated with cell death by apoptosis, are processes involved in the changed gut mucosa. Burn also causes reduced uptake of glucose and amino acids, decreased absorption of fatty acids, and reduction in brush border lipase activity. These changes peak in the first several hours after burn and return to normal at 48 to 72 hours after injury, a timing that parallels mucosal atrophy.

Intestinal permeability to macromolecules, which are normally repelled by an intact mucosal barrier, increases after burn. Intestinal permeability to polyethylene glycol 3350, lactulose, and mannitol increases after injury, correlating with the extent of the burn. Gut permeability increases even further when burn wounds become infected. A study using fluorescent dextrans has shown that larger molecules appeared to cross the mucosa between the cells, whereas the smaller molecules traversed the mucosa through the epithelial cells, presumably by pinocytosis and vesiculation. Mucosal permeability also paralleled increases in gut epithelial apoptosis.

Changes in gut blood flow are related to changes in permeability. Intestinal blood flow was shown to decrease in animals, a change associated with increased gut permeability at 5 hours after burn. This effect was abolished at 24 hours. Systolic hypotension has been shown to occur in the hours immediately after burn in animals with a 40% TBSA full-thickness injury. These animals showed an inverse correlation between blood flow and permeability to intact *Candida* spp.

### Effects on the Immune System

Burns cause a global depression in immune function, which is shown by prolonged allograft skin survival on burn wounds. Burn patients are then at great risk for a number of infectious complications, including bacterial wound infection, pneumonia, and fungal and viral infections. These susceptibilities and conditions are based on depressed cellular function in all parts of the immune system, including activation and activity of neutrophils, macrophages, T lymphocytes, and B lymphocytes. With burns of more than 20% TBSA, impairment of these immune functions is proportional to burn size.

Macrophage production after burn is diminished, which is related to the spontaneous elaboration of negative regulators of myeloid growth. This effect is enhanced by the presence of endotoxin and can be partially reversed with granulocyte colony-stimulating factor (G-CSF) treatment or inhibition of prostaglandin E2. Investigators have shown that G-CSF levels actually increase after severe burn. However, bone marrow G-CSF receptor expression is decreased, which may in part account for the immunodeficiency seen in burns. Total neutrophil counts are initially increased after burn, a phenomenon related to a decrease in cell death by apoptosis. However, neutrophils that are present are dysfunctional in terms of diapedesis, chemotaxis, and phagocytosis. These effects are explained, in part, by a deficiency in CD11b/CD18 expression after inflammatory stimuli, decreased respiratory burst activity associated with a deficiency in p47-phox activity, and impaired actin mechanics related to neutrophil motile responses. After 48 to 72 hours, neutrophil counts decrease, similar to macrophages with similar causes.

Helper T cell (Th cell) function is depressed after a severe burn associated with polarization from the IL-2 and interferon-γ (IFN-γ) cytokine-based Th1 response toward the Th2 response. The Th2 response is characterized by the production of IL-4 and IL-10. The Th1 response is important in cell-mediated immune defense, whereas the Th2 response is important in antibody responses to infection. As this polarization increases, so does the mortality rate. Administration of IL-10 antibodies and growth hormone has partially reversed this response and improved mortality rate after burn in animals. Burn also impairs cytotoxic T lymphocyte activity as a function of burn size, thus increasing the risk of infection, particularly from fungi and viruses. Early burn wound excision improves cytotoxic T cell activity.

## MANAGEMENT

### Basic Treatment

#### Prehospital Management

Before undergoing any specific treatment, burn patients must be removed from the source of injury and the burning process stopped. Inhalation injury should always be suspected and 100% oxygen should be given by face mask. While removing the patient from the source of injury, care must be taken so that the rescuer does not become another victim. All health care personnel and caregivers should be aware that they might be injured by contact with the patient or the patient's clothing. Universal precautions, including wearing gloves, gowns, mask, and protective eyewear, should be used whenever there is likely contact with blood or body fluids. Burning clothing should be extinguished and removed as soon as possible to prevent further injury. All rings, watches, jewelry, and belts should be removed because they retain heat and can produce a tourniquet-like effect. Room temperature water can be poured on the wound within 15 minutes of injury to decrease the depth of the wound, but any subsequent measures to cool the wound should be avoided to prevent hypothermia during resuscitation.

#### Initial Assessment

As with any trauma patient, the initial assessment of a burn patient is done by primary and secondary surveys. In the primary survey, immediate life-threatening conditions are quickly identified and treated. In the secondary survey, a more thorough head to toe evaluation of the patient is undertaken.

Exposure to heated gases and smoke results in damage to the upper respiratory tract. Direct injury to the upper airway results in edema, which, in combination with generalized whole-body edema associated with severe burn, may obstruct the airway. Airway injury must be suspected with facial burns, singed nasal hairs, carbonaceous sputum, and tachypnea. Upper airway obstruction may develop rapidly, and respiratory status must be continually monitored to assess the need for airway control and ventilatory support. Progressive hoarseness is a sign of impending airway obstruction, and endotracheal intubation should be instituted early, before edema distorts the upper airway anatomy. This is especially important in patients with massive burns, who may appear to breathe without problems early in the resuscitation period until several liters of volume have been given to maintain homeostasis, resulting in significant airway edema.

The chest should be exposed to assess breathing; airway patency alone does not ensure adequate ventilation. Chest expansion and equal breath sounds with $CO_2$ return from the endotracheal tube ensure adequate air exchange.

Blood pressure may be difficult to determine in burn patients with edematous or charred extremities. The pulse rate can be used as an indirect measure of circulation; however, most burn patients remain tachycardic, even with adequate resuscitation. For the primary survey of burn patients, the presence of pulses or Doppler signals in the distal extremities may be adequate to determine adequate circulation of blood until more effective monitoring modalities, such as arterial pressure measurements and urine output, can be established.

In patients who have been in an explosion or deceleration accident, a possibility exists for spinal cord injury. Appropriate cervical spine stabilization must be accomplished by whatever means necessary, including using cervical collars to keep the head immobilized until the condition can be evaluated.

#### Initial Wound Care

Prehospital care of the burn wound is basic and simple because it only requires protection from the environment, with application of a clean dry dressing or sheet to cover the involved part. Damp dressings should not be used. The patient should be wrapped in a blanket to minimize heat loss and for temperature control during transport. The first step in diminishing pain is to cover the wounds to prevent contact to exposed nerve endings. Intramuscular or subcutaneous narcotic injections for pain should never be used because drug absorption is decreased as a result of the peripheral vasoconstriction. This might become a problem later, when the patient is resuscitated, and vasodilation increases absorption of the narcotic depot with resulting apnea. Small doses of IV morphine may be given after complete assessment of the patient and after this has been determined to be safe by an experienced physician.

Although prehospital management is simple, it is often difficult to enact, particularly in at-risk populations. A recent study in New Zealand[21] has shown that initial first aid treatment of burns is inadequate in 60% of patients interviewed. This report also showed that inadequate first aid care is clearly associated with poorer outcomes. It was suggested that specific educational programs targeting at-risk populations might improve these outcomes.

#### Transport

Rapid uncontrolled transport of the burn victim is not a priority, except when other life-threatening conditions coexist. In most incidents involving major burns, ground transportation of victims to the receiving hospital is appropriate. Helicopter transport is of greatest use when the distance between the accident and hospital is 30 to 150 miles. For distances more than 150 miles, transport by fixed-wing aircraft is most appropriate. Whatever the mode of transport, it should be of appropriate size and have emergency equipment available, with trained personnel on board, such as nurses, physicians, paramedics, and/or respiratory therapists who are familiar with multiply injured trauma patients.

#### Resuscitation

Adequate resuscitation of the burn patient depends on the establishment and maintenance of reliable IV access. Increased times to beginning resuscitation of burn patients result in poorer outcomes and delays should be minimized. Venous access is best attained through short peripheral catheters in unburned skin; however, veins in burned skin can be used and are preferable to no IV access. Superficial veins are often thrombosed in full-thickness injuries and therefore are not suitable for cannulation. Saphenous vein cutdowns are useful in cases of difficult access and are used in preference to central vein cannulation because of lower complication rates. In children younger than 6 years, experienced physicians can use intraosseous access in the proximal tibia until IV access is accomplished. Lactated Ringer's solution without dextrose is the fluid of choice, except in children younger than 2 years, who should receive 5% dextrose Ringer's lactate. The initial rate can be rapidly estimated by multiplying the TBSA burned by the patient's weight in kilograms and then dividing by 8. The rate of infusion for an 80-kg man with a 40% TBSA burn can be calculated by the following formula:

$$80 \text{ kg} \times 40\% \text{ TBSA}/8 = 400 \text{ mL/hr}$$

This rate should be continued until a formal calculation of resuscitation needs is performed.

Many formulas have been devised to determine the proper amount of fluid to give a burn patient, all originating from experimental studies on the pathophysiology of burn shock. These experimental studies established the basis for modern fluid resuscitation protocols. It was shown that edema fluid in burn wounds is isotonic and contains the same amount of protein as plasma, and that the greatest loss of fluid is into the interstitium.[22] Various volumes of intravascular fluid were used to determine the optimal amount in terms of cardiac output and extracellular volume in a canine burn model; this was applied to the clinical setting by the Parkland formula (Table 21-2). Plasma volume changes were not related to the type of resuscitation fluid in the first 24 hours, but thereafter colloid solutions could increase plasma volume by the amount infused. From these findings, it was concluded that colloid solutions should not be used in the first 24 hours until capillary permeability returns closer to normal. Others have argued that normal capillary permeability is restored somewhat earlier after burn (6 to 8 hours), and therefore colloids could be used earlier.

Concurrently, researchers have shown the hemodynamic effects of fluid resuscitation in burns, which culminated in the Brooke formula (see Table 21-2). It was found that fluid resuscitation causes an obligatory 20% decrease in extracellular fluid and plasma volume that concludes after 24 hours. In the second 24 hours, plasma volume returns to normal with the administration of colloid. Cardiac output is low in the first day despite resuscitation, but it subsequently increases to supernormal levels as the flow phase of hypermetabolism is established. Since these studies, it has been found that much of the fluid needs are caused by leaky capillaries that permit passage of large molecules into the interstitial space to increase the extravascular colloid osmotic pressure. Intravascular volume follows the gradient to tissues, both into the burn wound and nonburned tissues. Approximately 50% of fluid resuscitation needs are sequestered in nonburned tissues in 50% TBSA burns.

Hypertonic saline solutions have theoretical advantages in burn resuscitation. These solutions decrease net fluid intake, decrease edema, and increase lymph flow, probably by the transfer of volume from the intracellular space to the interstitium. When using these solutions, hypernatremia must be avoided, and it is recommended that serum sodium concentrations should not exceed 160 mEq/dL. However, it must be noted that for patients with more than 20% TBSA burns who are randomized to hypertonic saline or lactated Ringer's solution, resuscitation does not have significant differences in volume requirements or changes in percentage of weight gain. Other investigators have found an increase in renal failure with hypertonic solutions that has tempered further efforts in this area of investigation. Some burn units successfully use a modified hypertonic solution of one ampule of sodium bicarbonate (50 mEq) in 1 liter of lactated Ringer's solution. Further research should be done to determine the optimal formula to reduce edema formation and maintain adequate cellular function.

Most burn units use something similar to the Parkland or Brooke formula, which calls for administering varying amounts of crystalloid and colloid for the first 24 hours. The fluids are generally changed in the second 24 hours, with an increase in colloid use. These are guidelines to direct resuscitation of the amount of fluid necessary to maintain adequate perfusion. Studies have shown that the Parkland formula often underestimates the volume of crystalloid received in the first 24 hours after severe burn, a phenomenon termed *fluid creep*. No single cause has clearly been identified. More liberal use of opioid analgesic and positive pressure ventilation has been suggested.[23] The increased fluid volumes are not without consequence; increased compartment pressures in the extremities, abdomen and, most recently, the orbit[24] have been suggested as requiring monitoring and possible release to prevent increased morbidity and mortality. The abdominal compartment is clinically monitored via the Foley catheter. When the pressure increases toward and above 30 mm Hg, complete abdominal escharotomy is ensured and paralytics are considered. If the increased abdominal pressure persists (>30 mm Hg), an improved outcome is based on the performance of a decompressive laparotomy. However, patients who require this procedure have mortality rates of 60% to almost 100%, depending on the series. Therefore, monitoring of the resuscitation is crucial to ensure an acceptable outcome. This is easily done in burn patients with normal renal function by following the volume of urine output, which should be 0.5 mL/hr in adults and 1.0 mL/kg/hr in children. Changes in IV fluid infusion rates should be made on an hourly basis, determined by the response of the patient to the

**Table 21-2 Resuscitation Formulas***

| | Volume | | |
|---|---|---|---|
| **FORMULA** | **CRYSTALLOID** | **COLLOID** | **FREE WATER** |
| Parkland | 4 mL/kg per % TBSA burn | None | None |
| Brooke | 1.5 mL/kg/% TBSA burn | 0.5 mL/kg per % TBSA burn | 2.0 liters |
| Galveston (pediatric) | 5000 mL/m² burned area + 1500 mL/m² total area | None | None |

*These guidelines are used for the initial fluid management after a burn injury. The response to fluid resuscitation should be continuously monitored, and adjustments in the rate of fluid administration should be made accordingly.

particular fluid volume administered. The exact formulas are shown in Table 21-2.

For burned children, formulas are commonly used that are modified to account for changes in surface area–to–mass ratios. These changes are necessary because a child with a comparable burn to that of an adult requires more resuscitation fluid per kilogram. The Galveston formula uses 5000 mL/TBSA burned (in $m^2$) + 2000 mL/$m^2$ total for maintenance in the first 24 hours. This formula accounts for maintenance needs and the increased fluid requirements of a child with a burn. All the formulas listed in Table 21-2 calculate the amount of volume given in the first 24 hours, with half is given in the first 8 hours.

The use of albumin during IV resuscitation has been debated. In a meta-analysis of 31 trials, it was shown that the risk of death is higher in burn patients receiving albumin compared with those receiving crystalloid, with a relative risk of death of 2.40 (95% confidence interval [CI], 1.11 to 5.19). Another meta-analysis of all critically ill patients refuted this finding, showing no differences in relative risk between albumin-treated and crystalloid-treated groups. As quality of the trials improved, the relative risks were reduced. Additional evidence has suggested that albumin supplementation, even after resuscitation, does not affect the distribution of fluid among the intracellular and extracellular compartments. What we can conclude from these trials and meta-analyses is that albumin used during resuscitation is at best equal to crystalloid and at worst detrimental to the outcome of burn patients. Thus, we cannot recommend the use of albumin during resuscitation.

To combat any regurgitation with an intestinal ileus, a nasogastric tube should be inserted in all patients with major burns to decompress the stomach. This is especially important for patients being transported in an aircraft at high altitudes. Also, all patients should be restricted from taking anything by mouth until the transfer has been completed. Decompression of the stomach is usually necessary because the apprehensive patient will swallow considerable amounts of air and distend the stomach. Additionally, a Dobhoff tube should be placed into the first (superior) part of the duodenum to feed the severely burned patient continuously.

Recommendations for tetanus prophylaxis are based on the condition of the wound and the patient's immunization history. All patients with burns of more than 10% of the TBSA should receive 0.5 mL of tetanus toxoid. If prior immunization is absent or unclear, or the last booster dose was more than 10 years ago, 250 U of tetanus immunoglobulin is also given.

### Escharotomies

When deep second- and third-degree burn wounds encompass the circumference of an extremity, peripheral circulation to the limb can be compromised. The development of generalized edema beneath a nonyielding eschar impedes venous outflow and eventually affects arterial inflow to the distal beds. This can be recognized by numbness and tingling in the limb and increased pain in the digits. Arterial flow can be assessed by the determination of Doppler signals in the digital arteries and the palmar and plantar arches in affected extremities. Capillary refill can also be assessed. Extremities at risk are identified on clinical examination or on measurement of tissue pressures higher than 40 mm Hg. These extremities require escharotomies, which are releases of the burn eschar performed at the bedside by incising the lateral and medial aspects of the extremity with a scalpel or

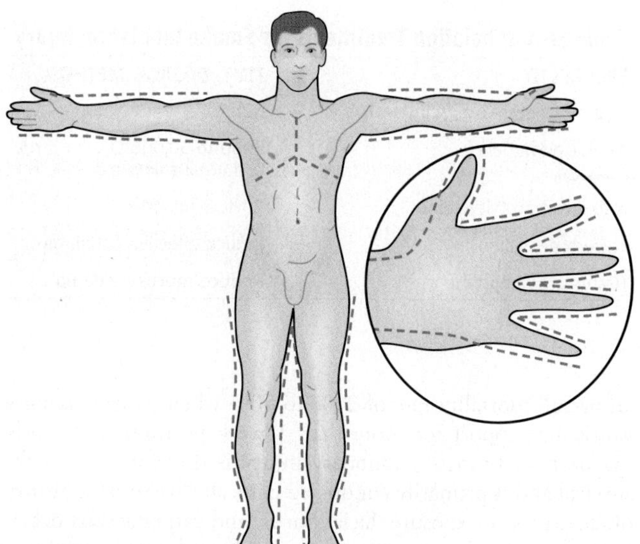

**FIGURE 21-9** Recommended escharotomies. In limbs requiring escharotomies, the incisions are made on the medial and lateral sides of the extremity through the eschar. In the case of the hand, incisions are made on the medial and lateral digits and on the dorsum of the hand.

electrocautery unit. The entire constricting eschar must be incised longitudinally to relieve the impediment to blood flow completely (Fig. 21-9). The incisions are carried down onto the thenar and hypothenar eminences and along the dorsolateral sides of the digits to open the hand completely, if it is involved. If it is clear that the wound will require excision and grafting because of its depth, escharotomies are safest to restore perfusion to the underlying nonburned tissues until formal excision. If vascular compromise has been prolonged, reperfusion after an escharotomy may cause reactive hyperemia and further edema formation in the muscle, making continued surveillance of the distal extremities necessary. Increased muscle compartment pressures may necessitate fasciotomies. The most common complications associated with these procedures are blood loss and the release of anaerobic metabolites, causing transient hypotension. If distal perfusion does not improve with these measures, central hypotension because hypovolemia should be suspected and treated.

A constricting truncal eschar can cause a similar phenomenon, except that the effect is to decrease ventilation by limiting chest excursion. Any decrease in ventilation of a burn patient requires inspection of the chest, with appropriate escharotomies to relieve the constriction and allow adequate tidal volumes. This need becomes evident in a patient on a volume control ventilator whose peak airway pressures increase.

## Specific Treatment

### Inhalation Injury

Even though mortality from major burns has significantly decreased during the past 20 years, inhalation injury still constitutes one of the most critical concomitant injuries following thermal insult. Approximately 80% of fire-related deaths result not from burns, but from inhalation of the toxic products of combustion, and inhalation injury has remained associated with

**Table 21-3 Inhalation Treatments for Smoke Inhalation Injury**

| TREATMENT | TIME, DOSAGE, METHOD |
|---|---|
| Bronchodilator (e.g., Albuterol) | q2h |
| Nebulized heparin | 5000 to 10,000 U with 3 mL normal saline q4h |
| Nebulized acetylcysteine | 20%, 3 mL q4h |
| Hypertonic saline | Induce effective coughing |
| Racemic epinephrine | Reduce mucosal edema |

**Table 21-4 Clinical Indications for Intubation**

| CRITERIA | VALUE |
|---|---|
| $Pao_2$ (mm Hg) | <60 |
| $Paco_2$ (mm Hg) | >50 (acutely) |
| $Pao_2/Fio_2$ ratio | <200 |
| Respiratory, ventilatory failure | Impending |
| Upper airway edema | Severe |

an overall mortality rate of 25% to 50% when patients require ventilator support for more than 1 week postinjury.[10,25] Early diagnosis of bronchopulmonary injury is therefore critical for survival and is primarily conducted clinically, based on a history of closed space exposure, facial burns, and carbonaceous debris in the mouth, pharynx or sputum. Evidenced-based experience on the diagnosis of inhalation injury, however, is rare. Chest x-rays are routinely normal until complications such as infections have developed. The standard diagnostic method should therefore be bronchoscopy of the upper airway of every burn patient. Endorf and Gamelli[26] have established a grading system of inhalation injury (0, 1, 2, 3, 4) derived from findings at initial bronchoscopy and based on the Abbreviated Injury Scale (AIS) criteria. Bronchoscopic findings consistent with inhalation injury include airway edema, inflammation, mucosal necrosis, presence of soot and charring in the airway, tissue sloughing, and carbonaceous material in the airway. The treatment of inhalation injury should start immediately with the administration of 100% oxygen via face mask or nasal cannula. Maintenance of the airway is critical. As noted, if early evidence of upper airway edema is present, early intubation is required because the upper airway edema normally increases over 9 to 12 hours. Prophylactic intubation without proper indications, however, should not be performed.

Advances in ventilator technology and treatment of inhalation injury have resulted in some improvement in mortality rates. Mechanical ventilation with a lower tidal volume than traditionally used has resulted in decreased mortality and increased the number of days without ventilator use. In addition, high-frequency ventilation decreased mortality to 29% from 41%. The management of inhalation injury consists of ventilatory support, aggressive pulmonary toilet (Table 21-3), bronchoscopic removal of casts, and nebulization therapy. Nebulization therapy can consist of heparin, alpha mimetics, or polymyxin B and is applied from two to six times daily. Pressure control ventilation with permissive hypercapnia is a useful strategy in the management of these patients, and $Paco_2$ levels as high as 60 mm Hg can be well tolerated if arrived at gradually. Prophylactic antibiotics are not indicated, but are imperative with documented lung infections. Clinical diagnosis of pneumonia includes two of the following[17]:

- Chest x-ray revealing a new and persistent infiltrate, consolidation, or cavitation
- Sepsis (as defined in Table 21-4)
- Recent change in sputum or purulence in the sputum, as well as quantitative culture

The clinical diagnosis can be made after using microbiologic data according to the American Burn Association Consensus Conference to Define Sepsis and Infection in Burns.[17] Empirical choices for the treatment of pneumonia, prior to culture results, should include coverage of methicillin-resistant *Staphylococcus aureus* (MRSA) and gram-negative organisms such as *Pseudomonas* and *Klebsiella* spp.[27]

## WOUND CARE

After the airway has been assessed and resuscitation is underway, attention must be turned to the burn wound. Treatment depends on the characteristics and size of the wound. All treatments are aimed at rapid and painless healing. Current therapy directed specifically toward burn wounds can be divided into three stages—assessment, management, and rehabilitation. Once the extent and depth of the wounds have been assessed and the wounds have been thoroughly cleaned and débrided, the management phase begins. Each wound should be dressed with an appropriate covering that serves several functions. First, it should protect the damaged epithelium, minimize bacterial and fungal colonization, and provide splinting action to maintain the desired position of function. Second, the dressing should be occlusive to reduce evaporative heat loss and minimize cold stress. Third, the dressing should provide comfort over the painful wound.

The choice of dressing is based on the characteristics of the treated wound (Table 21-5). First-degree wounds are minor, with minimal loss of barrier function. These wounds require no dressing and are treated with topical salves to decrease pain and keep the skin moist. Systemic NSAIDs given by mouth help with pain control. Second-degree wounds can be treated with daily dressing changes with topical antibiotics, cotton gauze, and elastic wraps. Alternatively, the wounds can be treated with a temporary biologic or synthetic covering to close the wound. Deep second- and third-degree wounds require excision and grafting for sizable burns; the choice of initial dressing should aim at holding bacterial proliferation in check and providing occlusion until the operation is performed.

### Antimicrobials

The timely and effective use of antimicrobials has revolutionized burn care by decreasing invasive wound infections. The untreated burn wound rapidly becomes colonized with bacteria and fungi because of the loss of normal skin barrier mechanisms. As the organisms proliferate to high wound counts (>$10^5$ organisms/g of tissue), they may penetrate into viable tissue. Organisms then invade blood vessels, causing a systemic infection that often leads to the death of the patient. This scenario has become uncommon in most burn units because of the effective use of antibiotics and

**Table 21-5 Burn Wound Dressings**

| DRESSINGS | ADVANTAGES AND DISADVANTAGES |
|---|---|
| **Antimicrobial Salves** | |
| Silver sulfadiazine (Silvadene) | Broad-spectrum antimicrobial; painless and easy to use; does not penetrate eschar; may leave black tattoos from silver ion; mild inhibition of epithelialization |
| Mafenide acetate (Sulfamylon) | Broad-spectrum antimicrobial; penetrates eschar; may cause pain in sensate skin; wide application may cause metabolic acidosis; mild inhibition of epithelialization |
| Bacitracin | Ease of application; painless; antimicrobial spectrum not as wide as above agents |
| Neomycin | Ease of application; painless; antimicrobial spectrum not as wide |
| Polymyxin B | Ease of application; painless; antimicrobial spectrum not as wide |
| Nystatin (Mycostatin) | Effective in inhibiting most fungal growth; cannot be used in combination with mafenide acetate |
| Mupirocin (Bactroban) | More effective staphylococcal coverage; does not inhibit epithelialization; expensive |
| **Antimicrobial Soaks** | |
| Silver nitrate 0.5% | Effective against all microorganisms; stains contacted areas; leaches sodium from wounds; may cause methemoglobinemia |
| Mafenide acetate 5% | Wide antibacterial coverage; no fungal coverage; painful on application to sensate wound; wide application associated with metabolic acidosis |
| Sodium hypochlorite 0.025% (Dakins solution) | Effective against almost all microbes, particularly gram-positive organisms; mildly inhibits epithelialization |
| Acetic acid 0.25% | Effective against most organisms, particularly gram-negative ones; mildly inhibits epithelialization |
| **Synthetic Coverings** | |
| OpSite | Provides a moisture barrier; inexpensive; decreased wound pain; use complicated by accumulation of transudate and exudate, requiring removal; no antimicrobial properties |
| Biobrane | Provides a wound barrier; associated with decreased pain; use complicated by accumulation of exudate, risking invasive wound infection; no antimicrobial properties |
| Transcyte | Provides a wound barrier; decreased pain; accelerated wound healing; use complicated by accumulation of exudate; no antimicrobial properties |
| Integra | Provides complete wound closure and leaves a dermal equivalent; sporadic take rates; no antimicrobial properties |
| **Biologic Coverings** | |
| Xenograft (pig skin) | Completely closes the wound; provides some immunologic benefits; must be removed or allowed to slough |
| Allograft (homograft, cadaver skin) | Provides all the normal functions of skin; can leave a dermal equivalent; epithelium must be removed or allowed to slough |

wound care techniques. The antimicrobials used can be divided into those given topically and those given systemically.

## Topical Antibiotics

Available topical antibiotics can be divided into two classes, salves and soaks. Salves are generally applied directly to the wound with cotton dressings placed over them, and soaks are generally poured into cotton dressings on the wound. Each of these classes of antimicrobials has advantages and disadvantages. Salves may be applied once or twice daily but may lose their effectiveness between dressing changes. Frequent dressing changes can result in shearing, with loss of grafts or underlying healing cells. Soaks remain effective because an antibiotic solution can be added without removing the dressing; however, the underlying skin can become macerated.

Topical antibiotic salves include 11% mafenide acetate (Sulfamylon), 1% silver sulfadiazine (Silvadene), polymyxin B, neomycin, bacitracin, mupirocin, and the antifungal agent nystatin. No single agent is completely effective, and each has advantages and disadvantages. Silver sulfadiazine is the most commonly used. It has a broad spectrum of activity because its silver and sulfa moieties cover gram-positive, most gram-negative, and some fungal forms. Some *Pseudomonas* spp. possess plasmid-mediated resistance. Silver sulfadiazine is relatively painless on application, has a high patient acceptance, and is easy to use. Occasionally, patients complain of a burning sensation after it is applied and, in a few patients, a transient leukopenia develops 3 to 5 days following its continued use. This leukopenia is generally harmless and resolves with or without treatment cessation.

Mafenide acetate is another topical agent with a broad spectrum of activity because of its sulfa moiety. It is particularly useful against resistant *Pseudomonas* and *Enterococcus* spp. It also can penetrate eschar, which silver sulfadiazine cannot. Disadvantages include painful application on skin, such as in second-degree wounds. It also can cause an allergic skin rash and has carbonic anhydrase inhibitory characteristics that can result in a metabolic acidosis when applied over large surfaces. Therefore, mafenide sulfate is typically reserved for small full-thickness injuries.

Petroleum-based antimicrobial ointments with polymyxin B, neomycin, and bacitracin are clear on application, painless, and allow for easy wound observation. These agents are commonly used for the treatment of facial burns, graft sites, healing donor sites, and small partial-thickness burns. Mupirocin is a relatively new petroleum-based ointment that has improved activity against gram-positive bacteria, particularly MRSA and select gram-negative bacteria. Nystatin in a salve or powder form can be applied to wounds to control fungal growth. Nystatin-containing ointments can be combined with other topical agents to decrease colonization of bacteria and fungus. The exception is the combination of nystatin and mafenide acetate; each inactivates the other.

Available agents for application as a soak include 0.5% silver nitrate solution, 0.025% sodium hypochlorite (Dakin's solution), 0.25% acetic acid, and mafenide acetate as a 5% solution. Silver nitrate has the advantage of being painless on application and having complete antimicrobial effectiveness. The disadvantages include its staining of surfaces to a dull gray or black when the solution dries. This can become problematic in determining wound depth during burn excisions and in keeping the patient and his or her surroundings clean of the black staining. The solution is also hypotonic, and continuous use can cause electrolyte leaching, with rare methemoglobinemia as another complication. A new commercial dressing containing biologically potent silver ions (Acticoat) that are activated in the presence of moisture is available. This dressing holds the promise to retain the effectiveness of silver nitrate without the problems of silver nitrate soaks.

Dakin's solution is effective against most microbes; however, it also has cytotoxic effects on the healing cells of patients' wounds. Low concentrations of sodium hypochlorite (0.025%) have less cytotoxic effects while maintaining most of the antimicrobial effects. Hypochlorite ion is inactivated by contact with protein, so the solution must be continually changed. The same is true for acetic acid solutions, which may be more effective against *Pseudomonas* spp. Mafenide acetate soaks have the same characteristics as the mafenide acetate salve, except in liquid form.

#### Systemic Antimicrobials

The use of perioperative systemic antimicrobials also has a role in decreasing burn wound sepsis until the burn wound is closed. Common organisms that must be considered when choosing a perioperative regimen include *S. aureus* and *Pseudomonas* spp., which are prevalent in burn wounds.

### Burn Wound Excision

Methods for handling burn wounds have changed and are similar for adults and children. Increasingly aggressive early tangential excision of the burn tissue and early wound closure, primarily by skin grafts, has led to significant improvement of mortality rates and substantially lower costs in this particular patient population. Furthermore, early wound closure has been found to be associated with decreased severity of hypertrophic scarring and joint contractures and stiffness, and promotes quicker rehabilitation. Techniques of burn wound excision have evolved substantially over the past decade. In general, most areas are excised with a hand skin graft knife or powered dermatome. Sharp excision with a knife or electrocautery is reserved for areas of functional cosmetic importance, such as the hand and face. In partial-thickness wounds, an attempt is being made to preserve viable dermis, whereas in full-thickness injuries, all necrotic and infected tissue must be removed, leaving a viable wound bed of fascia, fat, or muscle. The following techniques are generally used.

#### Tangential Excision

This technique, first described by Janzekovic in the 1970s, requires repeated shaving of deep, dermal, partial-thickness burns using a Braithwaite, Watson, or Goulian or dermatome, set at a depth of 0.005 to 0.010 inch until a viable dermal bed is reached. This is manifested clinically by punctuate bleeding from the dermal wound bed.

#### Full-Thickness Excision

A hand knife such as a Watson or powered dermatome is set at 0.015 to 0.030 inch and serial passes are made to excise the full-thickness wound. Excision is aided by traction on the excised eschar as it passes through the knife or dermatome. Adequate excision is signaled by a viable bleeding wound bed, which is usually fat.

#### Fascial Excision

This technique is reserved for burns extending down through the fat into muscle, where the patient presents late with large infected wounds and life-threatening invasive fungal infections. It involves surgical excision of the full thickness of the integument, including the subcutaneous fat down to the fascia, using a Goulian knife with a no. 11 blade. Unfortunately, fascial excision is mutilating and leaves a permanent contour defect, which is almost impossible to reconstruct. Lymphatic channels can be excised with this technique; peripheral lymphedema may develop.

Most patients can be managed with layered excisions, which optimize later appearance and function. Published estimates of the amount of bleeding associated with these operations range from 3.5% to 5% of the blood volume for every 1% of the body surface excised. The control of blood loss is one of the main determinants for outcome.[28] Therefore, several techniques should be used to control blood loss. Local application of fibrin or thrombin spray, topical application of epinephrine, 1/10,000 to 1/20,000, epinephrine-soaked laboratory pads (1/40,000), and immediate electrocautery of the blood vessel can control blood loss.[29] The use of a sterilized tourniquet can also limit blood loss. Finally, preexcisional tumescence with epinephrine saline can be used on the trunk, back, and extremities, but not the fingers.

### Burn Wound Coverage

Following burn wound excision, it is vital to obtain wound closure. Various biologic and synthetic substrates have been used to replace the injured skin postburn. Autografts from uninjured skin remains the mainstay of treatment for many patients. Because early wound closure using an autograft may be difficult when full-thickness burns exceed 40% of the TBSA, allografts (cadaver skin) frequently serve as skin substitute for severely burned patients (Fig. 21-10). Although this approach is still commonly used in burn centers throughout the world, it bears considerable risks, including antigenicity, cross infection, and limited availability. Xenografts have been used for hundreds of years as a temporary replacement for skin loss. Even though these grafts provide a biologically active dermal matrix, immunologic disparities prevent engraftment and predetermine rejection over time.

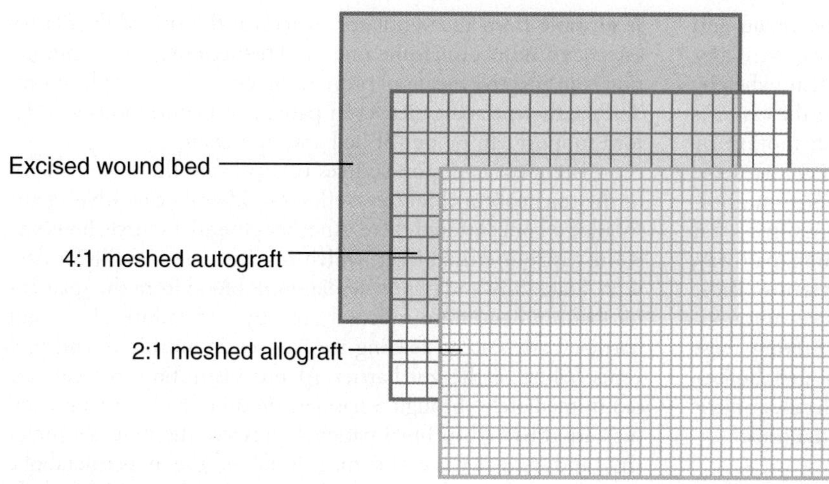


**FIGURE 21-10** Diagram of skin closure using widely meshed autografts. A widely meshed autograft is placed on a freshly excised viable wound bed. The remaining open wound between the interstices of the autograft is closed with an overlying layer of allograft, which can also be meshed to allow transudate, exudate, and hematoma to escape.

However, xenografts and allografts are only a temporary means of burn wound cover. True closure can only be achieved with living autografts or isografts. Autologous epithelial cells grown from a single full-thickness skin biopsy have been available for almost 2 decades. These cultured epithelial autografts (CEAs) have been shown to decrease mortality in massively burned patients in a prospective controlled trial. At our institution, we have found that CEAs used in combination with wide mesh autograft and allograft overlay in a pediatric patient population with burns of 90% or more of the TBSA to be associated with improved cosmetic results. However, widespread use of cultured autografts has been primarily hampered by poor long-term clinical results, exorbitant costs, and fragility and difficult handling of these grafts; these problems have been consistently reported by different burn units treating deep burns, even when cells were applied on properly prepared wound beds. Alternatively, dermal analogues have been made available for clinical use in recent years. Integra, an artificial dermal matrix (Integra LifeSciences, Plainsboro, NJ) has been approved by the U.S. Food and Drug Administration (FDA) for use in life-threatening burns. It has been successfully used for the immediate and delayed closure of full-thickness burns, leading to a reduction in length of hospital stay, favorable cosmetics, and improved functional outcome in a prospective and controlled clinical study. Our group recently conducted a randomized clinical trial using Integra in the management of severe full-thickness burns of 50% or more of the TBSA in a pediatric patient population, comparing it with a standard autograft-allograft technique, and found Integra to be associated with attenuated hepatic dysfunction, improved resting energy expenditure, and improved aesthetic outcome postburn.[30] Alloderm, an acellular human dermal allograft, has been advocated for the management of acute burns. Small clinical series and case reports have suggested that Alloderm may be useful in the treatment of acute burns. Tissue engineering technology is advancing rapidly. Fetal constructs have been successfully studied by Hohlfeld and associates[31]; the bilaminar skin substitute of Supp and Boyce (cultured skin substitute, CSS)[32] has been in clinical use and is promising.[29] Advances in stem cell culture technology may represent another promising therapeutic approach to deliver cosmetic restoration for burn patients.

## Multiorgan Failure

Early aggressive resuscitation regimens have improved survival rates dramatically. With the advent of vigorous fluid resuscitation, irreversible burn shock has been replaced by sepsis and subsequent multiorgan failure as the leading causes of death associated with burns. In our pediatric burn population, with burns of more than 80% of the TBSA, sepsis defined by bacteremia developed in 17.5% of [patients.[10] The mortality rate in the entire group was 33%; most of these deaths were attributable to multiorgan failure. Some of the patients who died were bacteremic and septic, but most were not. These findings highlight the observation that the development of multiorgan failure is often associated with infectious sepsis, but infection is by no means required to develop multiorgan failure. What is required is an inflammatory focus, which in severe burns is the massive skin injury that requires inflammation to heal. It has been postulated that the progression to multiorgan failure exists in a continuum with the systemic inflammatory response syndrome. Almost all burn patients meet the criteria for the systemic inflammatory response syndrome, as defined by the Consensus Conference of the American College of Chest Physicians.[17] It is therefore not surprising that multiorgan failure is common in burn patients.

### Causative Factors and Pathophysiology

The progression from the systemic inflammatory response syndrome to multiorgan failure is not well explained, although some of the mechanisms responsible are recognized. Most of these are found in patients with inflammation from infectious sources. In the burn patient, these infectious sources most likely emanate from invasive wound infection or from lung infection (e.g., pneumonia). As organisms proliferate out of control, endotoxins are liberated from gram-negative bacterial walls and exotoxins from gram-positive and gram-negative bacteria. Their release causes the initiation of a cascade of inflammatory mediators that can result, if unchecked, in organ damage and progression to organ failure. Occasionally, failure of the gut barrier with penetration of organisms into the systemic circulation may incite a similar reaction. However, this phenomenon has only been demonstrated in animal models and it remains to be seen whether this is a cause of human disease.

Inflammation from the presence of necrotic tissue and open wounds can incite a similar inflammatory mediator response as that seen with endotoxins. The mechanism whereby this occurs, however, is not well understood. Nevertheless, it is known that a cascade of systemic events is set in motion by invasive organisms or from open wounds, which initiates the systemic inflammatory syndrome and may progress to multiorgan failure. Evidence from animal studies and clinical trials has suggested that these events converge to a common pathway, which results in the activation of several cascade systems. Those circulating mediators can, if secreted in excessive amounts, damage organs distal from their site of origin. Among these mediators are endotoxins, the arachidonic acid metabolites, cytokines, neutrophils and their adherence molecules, nitric oxide, complement components, and oxygen free radicals.

#### Prevention

Because different cascade systems are involved in the pathogenesis of burn-induced multiorgan failure, it is impossible as of yet to pinpoint a single mediator that initiates the event. Thus, because the mechanisms of progression are not well known, prevention is the best solution. The current recommendations are to prevent the development of organ dysfunction and provide optimal support to avoid conditions that promote the onset.

The great reduction of mortality from large burns was observed with early excision and an aggressive surgical approach to deep wounds. Early removal of devitalized tissue prevents wound infections and decreases the inflammation associated with the wound. In addition, it eliminates small colonized foci, which are a frequent source of transient bacteremia. Those transient bacteremias during surgical manipulations may prime immune cells to react in an exaggerated fashion to subsequent insults, leading to whole-body inflammation and remote organ damage. We recommend complete early excision of clearly full-thickness wounds within 48 hours of the injury, or as early as possible.

Oxidative damage from reperfusion after low-flow states makes early aggressive fluid resuscitation imperative. This is particularly important during the initial phases of treatment and operative excision, with its attendant blood losses. Furthermore, the volume of fluid may not be as important as the timeliness with which it is given. In the study of children with more than 80% TBSA burns, it was found that one of the most important contributors to survival was the time required to start IV resuscitation, regardless of the initial volume given.

Topical and systemic antimicrobial therapy has significantly diminished the incidence of invasive burn wound sepsis. Perioperative antibiotics clearly benefit patients with burn injuries more than 30% of the TBSA. Vigilant and scheduled replacement of intravascular devices minimizes the incidence of catheter-related sepsis. We recommend changes of indwelling catheters every 5 days. The first can be done over a wire using the sterile Seldinger technique, but the second change requires a new site. This protocol should be followed as long as IV access is required. When possible, peripheral veins should be used for cannulation, even through burned tissue. The saphenous vein, however, should be avoided because of the high risk of thrombophlebitis.

Pneumonia, which contributes significantly to death in burn patients, should be vigilantly anticipated and aggressively treated. Every attempt should be made to wean patients as early as possible from the ventilator to reduce the risk of ventilator-associated nosocomial pneumonia. Furthermore, early ambulation is an effective means of preventing respiratory complications. With sufficient analgesics, even patients on continuous ventilatory support can be out of bed and in a chair.

The most common sources of sepsis are the wounds and/or the tracheobronchial trees; efforts to identify causative agents should be concentrated there. Another potential source, however, is the gastrointestinal tract, which is a natural reservoir for bacteria. Starvation and hypovolemia shunt blood from the splanchnic bed and promote mucosal atrophy and failure of the gut barrier. Early enteral feeding reduces septic morbidity and prevents failure of the gut barrier. At our institution, patients are fed immediately through a nasogastric tube. Early enteral feedings are tolerated in burn patients, preserve the mucosal integrity, and may reduce the magnitude of the hypermetabolic response to injury. Support of the gut goes along with carefully monitored hemodynamics.

### Organ Failure

Even with the best efforts at prevention, the presence of the systemic inflammatory syndrome that is ubiquitous in burn patients may progress to organ failure. It has been found that approximately 28% of patients with more than 30% TBSA burns will develop severe multiorgan dysfunction, of which 14% will also develop severe sepsis and septic shock. It generally begins to develop in the renal or pulmonary system and can progress through the liver, gut, hematologic system, and central nervous system. Although the development of multiorgan failure does not predict mortality, a recent study found a greater than 50% prevalence of multiorgan failure among nonsurvivors of burn injury.[18]

#### Renal Failure

With the advent of early aggressive resuscitation, the incidence of renal failure coincident with the initial phases of recovery has diminished significantly in severely burned patients. However, a second period of risk for the development of renal failure, 2 to 14 days after resuscitation, is still present. Renal failure is marked by decreasing urine output, fluid overload, electrolyte abnormalities, including metabolic acidosis and hyperkalemia, the development of azotemia, and increased serum creatinine levels. Treatment is aimed at averting complications associated with these conditions.

Urine output of more than 1 mL/kg is an adequate measure of renal perfusion in the absence of underlying renal disease. Decreasing the volume of fluid being given can alleviate volume overload in burn patients. These patients have increased insensible losses from the wounds, which can be roughly calculated at 1500 mL/m$^2$ TBSA + 3750 mL/m$^2$ TBSA burned. Further losses are accrued on air beds (1 liter/day in an adult). Decreasing the infused volume of IV fluids and enteral feedings to less than the expected insensate losses alleviates fluid overload problems. Electrolyte abnormalities can be minimized by decreasing potassium administration in the enteral feedings and giving oral bicarbonate solutions. Almost invariably, severely burned patients require exogenous potassium because of the heightened aldosterone response that results in potassium wasting.

If the problems listed overwhelm the conservative measures being used, some form of dialysis may be necessary. The indications for dialysis are volume overload or electrolyte abnormalities not amenable to other treatments. Peritoneal dialysis is effective for pediatric burn patients to remove volume and correct electrolyte abnormalities. In adults, hemofiltration is an effective approach. Continuous venous-venous hemodialysis is sometimes indicated because of the fluid shifts that occur. All hemodialysis techniques should be done in conjunction with experienced nephrologists who are experienced in these techniques.

After beginning dialysis, renal function may return, especially in pediatric and adult patients who maintain some urine output. Therefore, patients requiring such treatment may not require lifelong dialysis. It has been observed clinically that whatever urine output was present will decrease once dialysis is begun, but it may return in several days to weeks once the acute process of closing the burn wound nears completion.

#### Pulmonary Failure

Many burn patients require mechanical ventilation to protect the airway in the initial phases of their injury. We recommend that these patients be extubated as soon as possible after the risk is diminished. A trial of extubation is often warranted in the first few days after injury, and reintubation in this setting is not a failure. To perform this technique safely, however, requires the involvement of experts in obtaining an airway. The goal is extubation as soon as possible to allow patients to clear their airway, because they can perform their own pulmonary toilet better than through an endotracheal tube or tracheostomy. The first sign of impending pulmonary failure is a decline in oxygenation. This is best followed up with continuous oximetry and a decrease in saturation to less than 92% is indicative of failure. Increasing concentrations of inspired oxygen are necessary and, when ventilation begins to fail, denoted by increasing respiratory rate and hypercarbia, intubation is needed.

Some have stated that early tracheostomy (within the first week) might be indicated for those with significant burn injuries who are likely to require long-term ventilation. In one study, it was found that in severely burned children who underwent early tracheostomy that peak inspiratory pressures were lower after tracheostomy, with higher ventilatory volumes and pulmonary compliance, and higher $PaO_2/FIO_2$ ratios. No cases of tracheostomy site infections or tracheal stenoses were identified in the 28 patients studied. Another randomized study comparing those severely burned patients who underwent early tracheostomy with those who did not found similar improvements in oxygenation; however, no significant differences could be found in outcome measures, such as ventilator days, length of stay, incidence of pneumonia, or survival. In fact, 26% of those not undergoing tracheostomy were successfully extubated within 2 weeks of admission, implying that they would not have required tracheostomy at all. It seems that although tracheostomy may be required for some severely burned patients on ventilatory support, the advantages of early tracheostomy do not outweigh the disadvantages. Further studies from other centers may change this conclusion in the future.

#### Hepatic Failure

The development of hepatic failure in burn patients is a challenging problem without many solutions. The liver synthesizes circulating proteins, detoxifies the plasma, produces bile, and provides immunologic support. After severe burn injury, the liver increases in size to more than 200% of normal.[13] When the liver begins to fail, protein concentrations of the coagulation cascade decrease to critical levels and the patient becomes coagulopathic. Toxins are not cleared from the bloodstream and bilirubin concentrations increase. Complete hepatic failure is not compatible with life, but a gradation of liver failure with some decline of function is common. Efforts to prevent hepatic failure are the only effective methods of treatment.

With the development of coagulopathies, treatment should be directed at replacement of factors II, VII, IX, and X until the liver recovers. Albumin replacement may also be required. Attention to obstructive causes of hyperbilirubinemia, such as acalculous cholecystitis, should be considered as well. Initial treatment of this condition should be gallbladder drainage, which can be done percutaneously.

#### Hematologic Failure

Burn patients may become coagulopathic through two mechanisms, depletion and impaired synthesis of coagulation factors or thrombocytopenia. Factors associated with factor depletion are through disseminated intravascular coagulation associated with sepsis. This process is also common with coincident head injury. With breakdown of the blood-brain barrier, brain lipids are exposed to the plasma, which activates the coagulation cascade. Varying penetrance of this problem results in differing degrees of coagulopathy. Treatment of disseminated intravascular coagulation should include the infusion of fresh-frozen plasma and cryoprecipitate to maintain plasma levels of coagulation factors. For disseminated intravascular coagulation induced by brain injury, following the concentration of fibrinogen and levels with cryoprecipitate are the most specific indicators. Impaired synthesis of factors from liver failure is treated as noted earlier.

Thrombocytopenia is common in severe burns from depletion during burn wound excision. Platelet counts lower than 50,000/μL are common and do not require treatment. Only when the bleeding is diffuse and is noted to occur from IV sites should the administration of exogenous platelets be considered.

Paradoxically, it was found that severely burned patients are also at risk for thrombotic and embolic complications likely related to immobilization. It was found that complications of deep venous thrombosis were associated with increasing age, weight, and TBSA burned. These data indicate that deep venous thrombosis prophylaxis would be prudent for adult patients in the absence of bleeding complications.

#### Central Nervous System Failure

Obtundation is one of the hallmarks of sepsis, and burn patients are no exception. A new onset of mental status changes not attributed to sedative medications in a severely burned patient should incite a search for a septic source. Treatment is supportive.

## ATTENUATION OF THE HYPERMETABOLIC RESPONSE

### Nonpharmacologic Modalities

#### Nutritional Support

The response to injury known as hypermetabolism occurs dramatically after a severe burn. Increases in oxygen consumption, metabolic rate, urinary nitrogen excretion, lipolysis, and weight loss are directly proportional to the size of the burn. This response can be as high as 200% of the normal metabolic rate and returns to normal only with complete closure of the wound. Because the metabolic rate is so high, energy requirements are immense. These requirements are met by mobilization of carbohydrate, fat, and protein stores. Because the demands are prolonged, these energy stores are quickly depleted, leading to loss of active muscle tissue and malnutrition. This malnutrition is associated with functional impairment of many organs, delayed and abnormal wound healing, decreased immunocompetence, and altered cellular membrane active transport functions. Malnutrition in burns can be subverted to some extent by the delivery of adequate exogenous nutritional support. The goals of nutrition support are to maintain and improve organ function and prevent protein-calorie malnutrition.

Several formulas are used to calculate caloric requirements in burn patients. One formula multiplies the basal energy expenditure determined by the Harris-Benedict formula by 2 in burns of 40% of the TBSA, assuming a 100% increase in total energy expenditure. When total energy expenditure was measured by the doubly labeled water method, actual expenditures were found to be 1.33 times the predicted basal energy expenditure for pediatric patients with burns more than 40% of the TBSA. To meet the minimal needs of all the patients in this study, 1.55 times the predicted basal energy expenditure would be required; however, giving caloric loads in excess of this probably leads to fat accumulation without affecting lean mass accretion. This correlates to 1.4 times the measured resting energy expenditure by indirect calorimetry. Therefore, the calculation of twice the predicted basal energy expenditure might be too high.

Other commonly used calculations include the Curreri formula, which calls for 25 kcal/kg/day plus 40 kcal/% TBSA burned/day. This formula provides for maintenance needs plus the additional caloric needs related to the burn wounds. It was devised as a regression from nitrogen balance data in severely burned adults. In children, formulas based on body surface area are more appropriate because of the greater body surface area per kilogram of body weight. We recommend that the formula used should depend on the child's age (Table 21-6). These formulas were determined to maintain body weight in severely burned children; they change with age based on the body surface area alterations that occur with growth.

The composition of the nutritional supplement is also important. The optimal dietary composition contains 1 to 2 g/kg/day of protein, which provides a calorie-to-nitrogen ratio of approximately 100 : 1 with the caloric intakes suggested earlier.

**Table 21-6 Formulas to Predict Caloric Needs in Severely Burned Children**

| AGE GROUP | MAINTENANCE NEEDS | BURN WOUND NEEDS |
|---|---|---|
| Infants (0-12 mo) | 2100 kcal/% TBSA burned/24 hr | 1000 kcal/% TBSA burned/24 hr |
| Children (1-12 yr) | 1800 kcal/% TBSA burned/24 hr | 1300 kcal/% TBSA burned/24 hr |
| Adolescents (12-18 yr) | 1500 kcal/% TBSA burned/24 hr | 1500 kcal/% TBSA burned/24 hr |

This amount of protein provides for the synthetic needs of the patient, thus sparing the proteolysis occurring in the active muscle tissue to some extent. Nonprotein calories can be given as carbohydrate or as fat. Carbohydrates have the advantage of stimulating endogenous insulin production, which may have the same beneficial effects on muscle and burn wounds as an anabolic hormone. In addition, it has been shown that almost all the fat transported in very low-density lipoprotein after a severe burn is derived from peripheral lipolysis and not from de novo synthesis of fatty acids in the liver from dietary carbohydrates. As fat transporters are markedly decreased, we suggest a low-fat diet because additional fat to deliver noncarbohydrate calories has little support.

The diet may be delivered in two forms, either enterally through enteric tubes or parenterally through IV catheters. Parenteral nutrition may be given by isotonic solutions through peripheral catheters or by hypertonic solutions in central catheters. In general, the caloric demands of burn patients prohibit the use of peripheral parenteral nutrition. Total parenteral nutrition delivered centrally in burn patients has been associated with increased complications and mortality rates compared with enteral feedings. Total parenteral nutrition is reserved only for those patients who cannot tolerate enteral feedings. Enteral feeding has been associated with some complications, which include mechanical complications, enteral feeding intolerance, and diarrhea.

Interest in nutritional adjunctive treatment with anabolic agents has received attention as a means to decrease lean mass losses after severe injury. Agents used include growth hormone, IGF, insulin, oxandrolone, testosterone, and propranolol. Each of these agents has different actions to stimulate protein synthesis through an increase in protein synthetic efficiency. Simply put, the free amino acids available in the cytoplasm from stimulated protein breakdown with severe injury or illness are preferentially shunted toward protein synthesis rather than exported out of the cell. Some of these agents, such as insulin and oxandrolone, have shown efficacy, not only in improving protein kinetics but also in improving lean mass after severe burn. Further research will reveal whether these biochemical and physiologic measures translate to improved function.

### Environmental Support

Burn patients can lose as much as 4000 mL/m$^2$ burned/day of body water through evaporative loss from extensive burn wounds that have not definitive healed. The altered physiologic state resulting from the hypermetabolic response attempts to generate, at least partly, sufficient energy to offset heat losses associated with this inevitable water loss. The body attempts to raise skin and core temperatures to 2° C higher than normal. Raising the ambient temperature from 25° to 33° C can diminish the magnitude of this obligatory response from 2.0 to 1.4 resting energy expenditure (REE) units in patients with burns exceeding 40% of the TBSA (Fig. 21-11).[11] This simple environmental modulation is an important primary treatment goal that frequently is not realized.

### Exercise and Adjunctive Measures

A balanced physical therapy program is essential to restore metabolic variables and prevent burn wound contracture. Progressive resistance exercises in convalescent burn patients can maintain and improve body mass, augment incorporation of amino acids

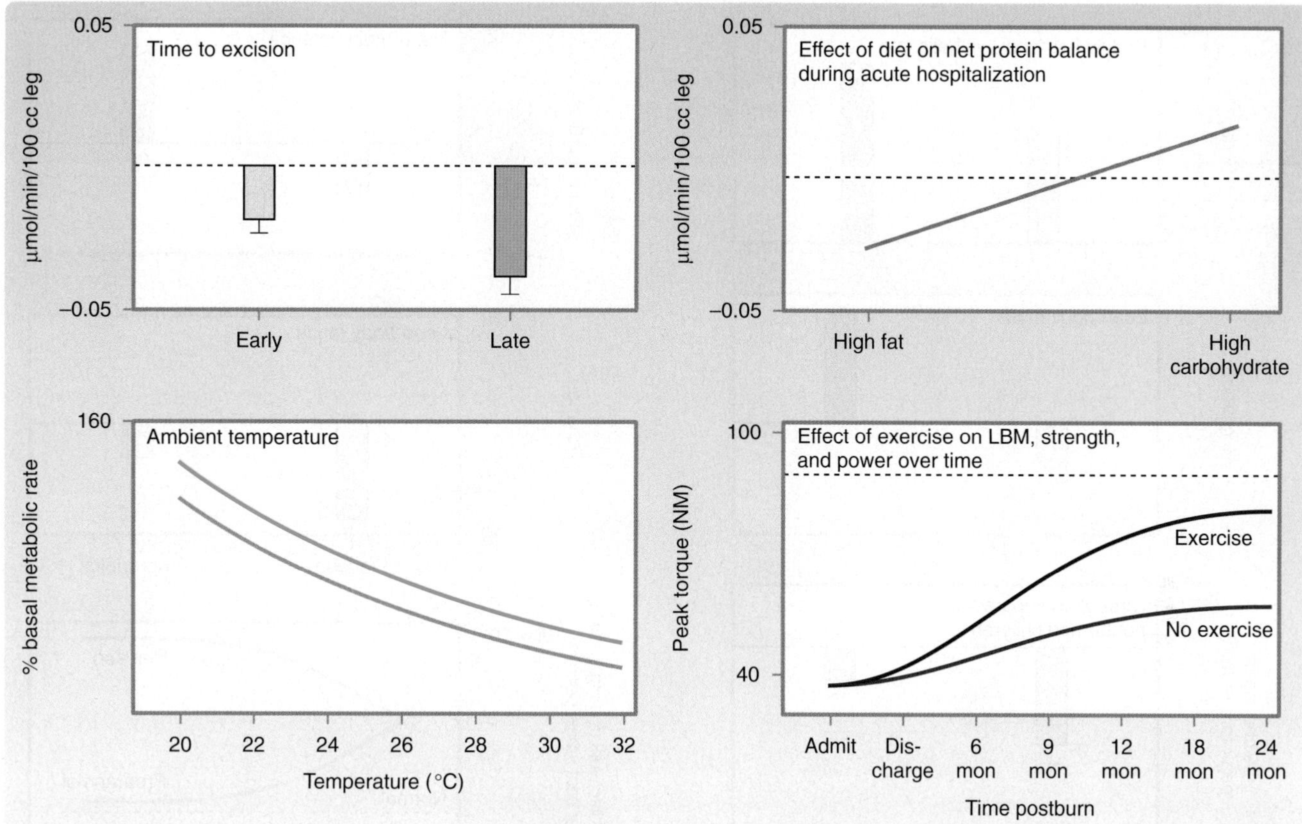


**FIGURE 21-11** Nonpharmacologic modulations of the hypermetabolic response postburn. This demonstrates the effect of early excision and grafting, environmental thermoregulation, high-carbohydrate diet, and exercise on physiologic derangements postburn. Graphs are averages ± SEM. *Yellow bar,* Patients with burns ≥40% TBSA who had early excision of burn eschar; *blue bar,* patients with burns ≥40% TBSA who had late excision of burn eschar; *solid curves,* averages for burn patients; *dashed lines,* values from nonburned normal patients. (From Williams FN, Jeschke MG, Chinkes DL, et al: Modulation of the hypermetabolic response to trauma: Temperature, nutrition, and drugs. J Am Coll Surg 208:489–502, 2009.)

into muscle proteins, and increase muscle strength and the ability to walk distances by approximately 50%. It has been demonstrated that resistance exercising can be safely accomplished in pediatric burn patients without exercise- related hyperpyrexia as the result of an inability to dissipate the heat generated. Although the initial burn injury and sepsis-related complications principally determine the extent of the metabolic response in burn victims, obligatory activity, background- and procedure-related pain, and anxiety also greatly increase the metabolic rate. Judicious maximal narcotic support, appropriate sedation, and supportive psychotherapy are mandatory to minimize their effects.

## Pharmacologic Modalities

### Recombinant Human Growth Hormone

The intramuscular administration of recombinant human growth hormone (rhGH) at doses of 0.2 mg/kg as a daily injection during acute burn care can favorably influence the hepatic acute-phase response, increased serum concentrations of its secondary mediator, IGF-I, improve muscle protein kinetics, maintain muscular growth, decrease donor site healing time by 1.5 days, improve REE, and decrease cardiac output.[33] These beneficial effects of rhGH are mediated by IGF-I and patients receiving this treatment have demonstrated a 100% increase in serum IGF-I and IGFBP3 levels compared with healthy individuals. However, in a prospective, multicenter, double-blind, randomized, placebo-controlled trial of 247 patients and 285 critically ill nonburned patients, Branski and coworkers[33] found that high doses of rhGH (0.10 ± 0.02 mg/kg body weight) were associated with increased morbidity and mortality. Others have found growth hormone treatment to be associated with hyperglycemia and insulin resistance. However, neither short- nor long-term administration of rhGH was associated with an increase in mortality in severely burned children.

### Insulin-Like Growth Factor

Because IGF-I mediates the effects of growth hormone (GH), the infusion of equimolar doses of recombinant human IGF-1 and IGFBP3 to burn patients has been demonstrated to improve protein metabolism effectively in catabolic pediatric subjects and adults, with significantly less hypoglycemia than rhGH itself. IGF-1 attenuates muscle catabolism and improves gut mucosal integrity in children with serious burns. Immune function is effectively improved by the attenuation of types 1 and 2 hepatic acute-phase responses, increased serum concentrations of constitutive proteins, and vulnerary modulation of the hypercatabolic use of body protein.[11] However, a study by Langouche and

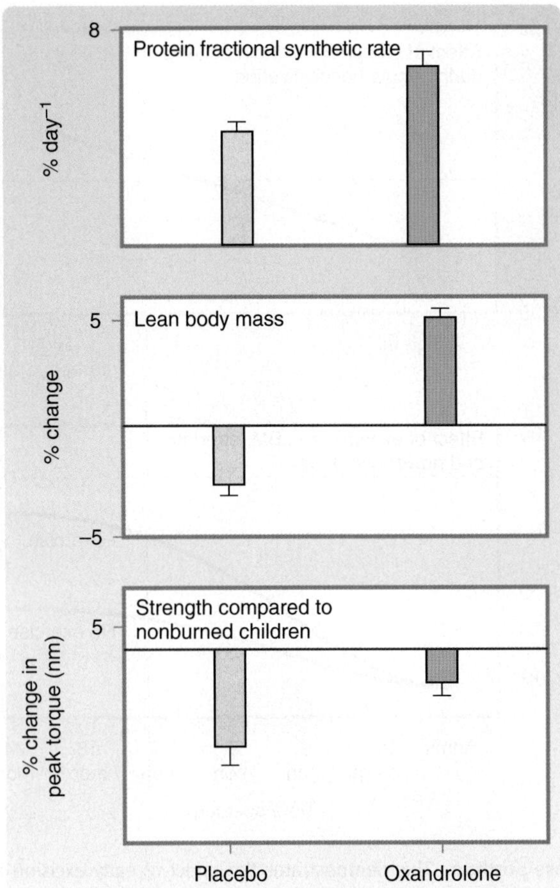


**FIGURE 21-12** Effects of oxandrolone treatment on the fractional synthetic rate of muscle protein synthesis, LBM, and strength. Changes in net protein balance of muscle protein synthesis and breakdown induced by burn injury were measured by stable isotope studies using [ring-$D_5$]phenyalanine infusion. Graphs are averages ± SEM. *Yellow bars,* Patients with burns ≥40% TBSA who received no anabolic agents; *blue bars,* patients with burns ≥40% TBSA randomized to receive oxandrolone. (From Williams FN, Jeschke MG, Chinkes DL, et al: Modulation of the hypermetabolic response to trauma: Temperature, nutrition, and drugs. J Am Coll Surg 208:489–502, 2009.)

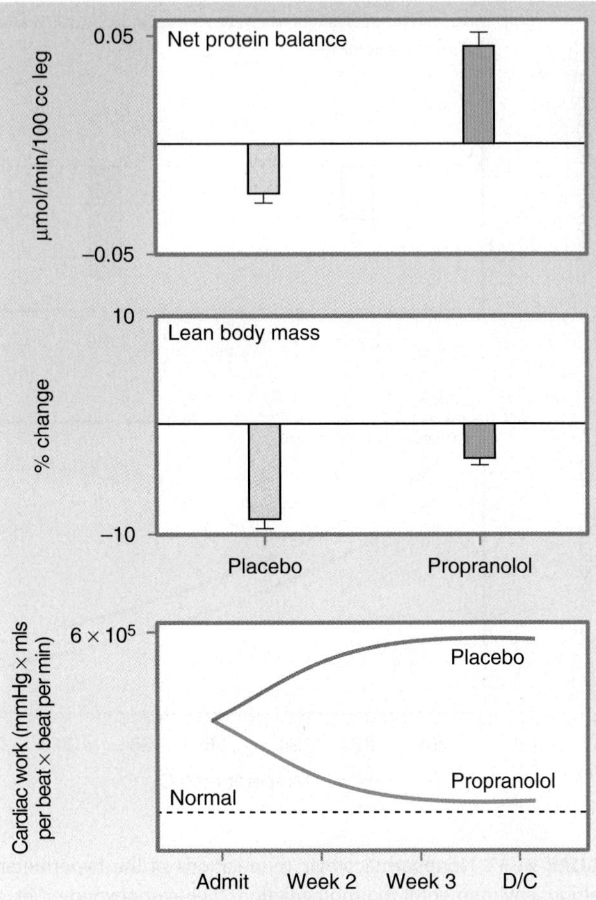


**FIGURE 21-13** Effect of propranolol treatment on the fractional synthetic rate of muscle protein synthesis, LBM, and cardiac work. Changes in net protein balance of muscle protein synthesis and breakdown induced by burn injury were measured by stable isotope studies using [ring-$D_5$]phenyalanine infusion. Graphs are averages ± SEM. *Yellow bars,* Patients with burns ≥40% TBSA who received no anabolic agents; *blue bars,* patients with burns ≥40% TBSA randomized to receive propranolol; *dashed lines,* values from nonburned normal patients. (From Williams FN, Jeschke MG, Chinkes DL, et al: Modulation of the hypermetabolic response to trauma: Temperature, nutrition, and drugs. J Am Coll Surg 208:489–502, 2009.)

van den Berghe[34] has indicated that the use of IGF-1 alone is not effective for critically ill patients without burns.

## Oxandrolone

Treatment with anabolic agents such as oxandralone, a testosterone analogue that possesses only 5% of the virilizing androgenic effects of testosterone, improves muscle protein catabolism via enhanced protein synthesis efficiency, reduces weight loss, and increases donor site wound healing. In a prospective randomized study, Wolf and associates[35] have demonstrated that the administration of 10 mg of oxandralone every 12 hours decreases hospital stay. In a large prospective, double-blinded, randomized single-center study, oxandrolone given at a dose of 0.1 mg/kg every 12 hours the shortened length of acute hospital stay, maintained lean body mass (LBM,) and improved body composition and hepatic protein synthesis (Fig. 21-12).[36] The effects were independent of age. Long-term treatment with this oral anabolic during rehabilitation in the outpatient setting is more favorably regarded by pediatric subjects then parenteral anabolic agents. Oxandrolone successfully abates the effects of burn-associated hypermetabolism on body tissues and significantly increases body mass over time, LBM at 6, 9, and 12 months after burn, and bone mineral content by 12 months after injury versus unburned controls.[37] Patients treated with oxandrolone show few complications relative to those treated with rhGH. However, it must be noted that although anabolic agents can increase LBM, exercise is essential to developing strength.

## Propranolol

β-Adrenergic blockade with propranolol probably represents the most efficacious anticatabolic therapy for the treatment of burns. The use of propranolol during acute care in burn patients, at a dose titrated to reduce the heart rate by 15% to 20%, has been found to diminish cardiac work[11] (Fig. 21-13). It also reduces fatty infiltration of the liver, which typically occurs in these patients as the result of enhanced peripheral lipolysis and altered substrate handling. Reduction of hepatic fat results from decreased peripheral lipolysis and reduced palmitate delivery and uptake by the liver, producing smaller livers, which adversely affect diaphragmatic function less frequently. Stable isotope and serial body composition studies have shown that the administration of propranolol reduces skeletal muscle wasting and increases lean body mass postburn.[11] The underlying mechanism of action of propranolol is still unclear; however, its effect appears to be caused by increased protein synthesis in the present of persistent protein breakdown and reduced peripheral lipolysis.[38] Studies now underway[39] suggest that the administration of propranolol, 4 mg/kg body weight/24 hr, also markedly decreases the amount of insulin necessary to decrease postburn elevated glucose levels. Propranolol may thus constitute a promising approach to overcome postburn insulin resistance.

## Attenuation of Postburn Hyperglycemia

### Insulin

Insulin represents probably one of the most extensively studied therapeutic agents, and novel therapeutic applications are constantly being found. In addition to its ability to decrease blood glucose levels by mediating peripheral glucose uptake into skeletal muscle and adipose tissue and suppressing hepatic gluconeogenesis, insulin is known to increase DNA replication and protein synthesis via control of amino acid uptake, increased fatty acid synthesis, and decreased proteinolysis.[12] The latter makes insulin particular attractive for the treatment of hyperglycemia in severely burned patients because insulin given during acute hospitalization has been shown to improve muscle protein synthesis, accelerate donor site healing time, and attenuate LBM loss and the acute-phase response (Fig. 21-14). In addition to its anabolic actions, insulin has been shown to exert totally unexpected anti-inflammatory effects, potentially neutralizing the proinflammatory actions of glucose.[40,41] These results suggest a dual benefit of insulin administration—reduction of the proinflammatory effects of glucose by restoration of euglycemia and a proposed, additional, insulin-mediated anti-inflammatory effect.[42]

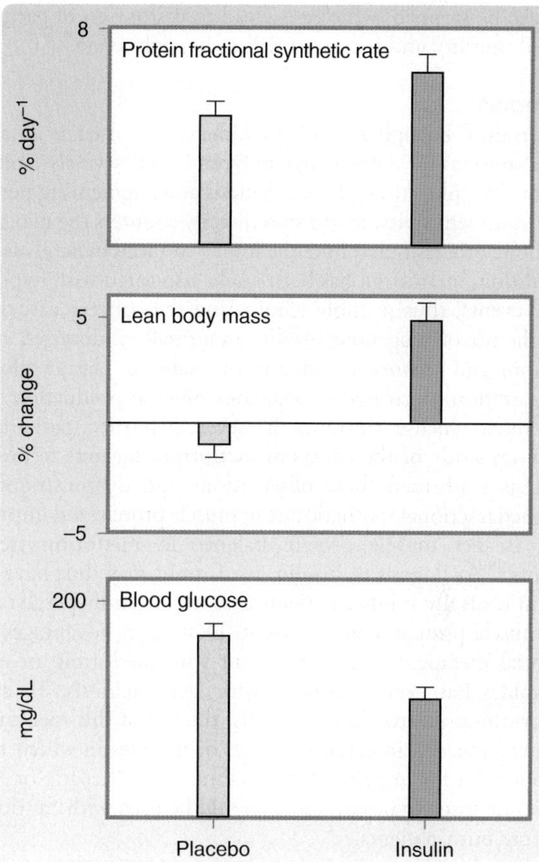


**FIGURE 21-14** Effect of insulin therapy on the fractional synthetic rate of muscle protein synthesis, LBM, and average blood glucose levels. Changes in net protein balance of muscle protein synthesis and breakdown induced by burn injury were measured by stable isotope studies using [ring-$D_5$]phenyalanine. Graphs are averages ± SEM. *Yellow bars,* Patients with burns ≥40% TBSA who received no anabolic agents or insulin; *blue bars,* patients with burns ≥40% TBSA randomized to receive insulin. (From Williams FN, Jeschke MG, Chinkes DL, et al: Modulation of the hypermetabolic response to trauma: Temperature, nutrition, and drugs. J Am Coll Surg 208:489–502, 2009.)

Insulin administered to maintain glucose at levels below 110 mg/dL decreases mortality, incidence of infections, sepsis, and sepsis-associated multiorgan failure in surgically critically ill patients. It has also been found to reduce newly acquired kidney injury significantly, accelerating weaning from mechanical ventilation and hastening discharge from the ICU and hospital.[43] When given during the acute phase, it not only improves acute hospital outcomes but also improves long-term rehabilitation and social reintegration of critically ill patients over a period of 1 year, indicating the advantage of insulin therapy.[44,45] However, because strict blood glucose control to maintain normoglycemia was required to obtain the most clinical benefit, a dialogue has emerged between those who believe that tight glucose control is beneficial for patient outcome and others who fear that high doses of insulin may lead to increased risks for hypoglycemic events and its associated consequences in these patients. A recent multicenter trial in Europe (Efficacy of Volume Substitution and Insulin Therapy in Severe Sepsis [VISEP] trial) has investigated the effects of insulin administration on morbidity and mortality in patients with severe infections and sepsis.[46] It was found that insulin administration does not affect mortality but the rate of severe hypoglycemia is fourfold higher in patients receiving intensive insulin therapy when compared with the conventional therapy group. Another large multicenter study has examined the use of a continuous, hyperinsulinemic, euglycemic clamp throughout the ICU stay and found a dramatic increase in serious hypoglycemic episodes.[47] Therefore, the ideal target glucose range has not been found, and several groups are currently undertaking clinical trials to define ideal glucose levels for the treatment of ICU and burn patients. Currently, the Surviving Sepsis Campaign recommendation is to maintain glucose levels below 150 mg/dL.[48] However, maintaining a continuous, hyperinsulinemic, euglycemic clamp in burn patients is particularly difficult because these patients are being continuously fed large caloric loads via enteral feeding tubes in an attempt to maintain euglycemia. Burn patients require weekly operations and daily dressing changes, so enteral nutrition occasionally needs to be stopped, which may lead to disruption of gastrointestinal motility and increased risk of hypoglycemia.[4]

### Metformin

Metformin (Glucophage), a biguanide, can be used as an alternative means to correct hyperglycemia in severely injured patients. By inhibiting gluconeogenesis and augmenting peripheral insulin sensitivity, metformin directly counters the two main metabolic processes that underlie injury-induced hyperglycemia. In addition, metformin has been rarely associated with hypoglycemic events, thus possibly eliminating the concern associated with the use of exogenous insulin. In a small randomized study by Gore and coworkers, metformin reduced plasma glucose concentration, decreased endogenous glucose production, and accelerated glucose clearance in severely burned patients. A follow-up study of the effects of metformin on muscle protein synthesis confirmed these observations and demonstrated an increased fractional synthetic rate of muscle protein and improvement in net muscle protein balance in metformin-treated patients.[49] Analogous to insulin, metformin may thus have efficacy in critically injured patients as both an antihyperglycemic and muscle protein anabolic agent. Despite its advantages and potential therapeutic uses, treatment with metformin or other biguanides has been associated with lactic acidosis. To avoid metformin-associated lactic acidosis, the use of this medication is contraindicated in certain diseases or illnesses in which there is a potential for impaired lactate elimination (hepatic or renal failure) or tissue hypoxia; it and should be used with caution in subacute burn patients.

### Novel Therapeutic Options

Other ongoing trials to decrease postburn hyperglycemia include the use of glucagon-like peptide 1 (GLP-1), peroxisome proliferator-activated receptor gamma (PPAR-γ) agonists (e.g., pioglitazone, thioglitazones), and a combination of various antidiabetic drugs. PPAR-γ agonists, such as fenofibrate, have been shown to improve insulin sensitivity in patients with diabetes. In a recent double-blind, prospective, placebo-controlled randomized trial, Cree and colleagues[50] have found that fenofibrate treatment significantly decreases plasma glucose levels and plasma glucose concentrations by improving insulin sensitivity and mitochondrial glucose oxidation. Fenofibrate also led to significantly increased tyrosine phosphorylation of the insulin receptor (IR) and IRS-1 in muscle tissue after hyperinsulinemic euglycemic clamp when compared with placebo-treated patients, indicating improved IR signaling.

## SPECIAL CONSIDERATIONS: ELECTRICAL AND CHEMICAL BURNS

## Electrical Burns

### Initial Treatment

Of all burn patients admitted, 3% to 5% are injured from electrical contact. Electrical injury is unlike other burn injuries in that the visible areas of tissue necrosis represent only a small portion of the destroyed tissue. Electrical current enters a part of the body, such as the fingers or hand, and proceeds through tissues with the lowest resistance to current, generally the nerves, blood vessels, and muscles. The skin has a relatively high resistance to electrical current and is therefore mostly spared. The current then leaves the body at a grounded area, typically the foot. Heat generated by the transfer of electrical current and passage of the current itself then injures the tissues. During this exchange, the muscle is the major tissue through which the current flows, and thus it sustains the most damage. Most muscle is in close proximity to bones. Blood vessels transmitting much of the electricity initially remain patent, but may proceed to progressive thrombosis as the cells die or repair themselves, thus resulting in further tissue loss from ischemia.

Injuries are divided into high- and low-voltage injuries. Low-voltage injury is similar to thermal burns without transmission to the deeper tissues; zones of injury from the surface extend into the tissue. Most household currents (110 to 220 V) produce this type of injury, which causes only local damage. The worst of these injuries are those involving the edge of the mouth (oral commissure), sustained when children gnaw on household electrical cords.

The syndrome of high-voltage injury consists of varying degrees of cutaneous burn at the entry and exit sites, combined with hidden destruction of deep tissue. Often, these patients also have cutaneous burns associated with the ignition of clothing from the discharge of electrical current. Initial evaluation consists of cardiopulmonary resuscitation if ventricular fibrillation is induced. Thereafter, if the initial electrocardiographic findings are abnormal or there is a history of cardiac arrest associated with the injury, continued cardiac monitoring is necessary, along with pharmacologic treatment for any dysrhythmias. The most serious derangements occur during the first 24 hours after injury. If patients with electrical injuries have no cardiac dysrhythmias on the initial electrocardiogram or recent history of cardiac arrest, no further monitoring is necessary.

Patients with electrical injuries are at risk for other injuries, such as being thrown from the electrical jolt or falling from heights after disengaging from the electrical current. In addition, the violent tetanic muscular contractions that result from alternating current sources may cause a variety of fractures and dislocations. These patients should be assessed in the same manner as any other patient with blunt traumatic injuries.

The key to managing patients with an electrical injury lies in the treatment of the wound. The most significant injury is within the deep tissue, and subsequent edema formation can cause vascular compromise to any area distal to the injury. Assessment should include circulation to distal vascular beds, because immediate escharotomy and fasciotomy may be required. If the muscle compartment is extensively injured and necrotic, so that the prospects for eventual function are dismal, early amputation may be necessary. We advocate early exploration of affected muscle beds and débridement of devitalized tissues, with attention given to the deeper periosteous planes, because this is the area with the most muscle tissue. Fasciotomies should be complete and may require nerve decompressions, such as carpal tunnel and Guyon canal releases. Tissue that has questionable viability should be left in place, with planned reexploration in 48 hours. Many such reexplorations may be required until the wound has been completely débrided. Electrical damage to vessels may be delayed and the extent of necrosis may extend after the initial débridements. After the devitalized tissues are removed, closure of the wound becomes paramount. Although skin grafts suffice as closure for most wounds, flaps may offer a better alternative, particularly with exposed bones and tendons. Even exposed and superficially infected bones and tendons can be salvaged with coverage by vascularized tissue. Early involvement by reconstructive surgeons experienced in the various methods of wound closure is optimal.

Muscle damage results in the release of hemochromogens (myoglobin), which are filtered in the glomeruli and may result in obstructive nephropathy. Therefore, vigorous hydration and infusion of IV sodium bicarbonate (5% continuous infusion) and mannitol (25 g every 6 hours for adults) are indicated to solubilize the hemochromogens and maintain urine output if significant amounts are found in the serum. These patients also require additional IV volumes over predicted amounts based on the wound area because most of the wound is deep and cannot be assessed by standard physical examination. In this situation, urine output should be maintained at 2 mL/kg/hr.

### Delayed Effects

Neurologic deficits may occur. Serial neurologic evaluations should be performed as part of the routine examination to detect any early or late neuropathology. Central nervous system effects such as cortical encephalopathy, hemiplegia, aphasia, and brainstem dysfunction injury have been reported up to 9 months after injury; delayed peripheral nerve lesions, characterized by demyelination with vacuolization and reactive gliosis, have also been seen. Another devastating long-term effect is the development of cataracts, which can be delayed for several years. These complications may occur in up to 30% of patients with significant high-voltage injury, and patients should be made aware of this possibility, even with the best treatment.

## Chemical Burns

Most chemical burns are accidental and caused by mishandling of household cleaners, although some of the most dramatic presentations involve industrial exposures. Thermal burns are, in general, short-term exposures to heat, but chemical injuries may be of longer duration, even hours, in the absence of appropriate treatment. The degree of tissue damage, as well as the level of toxicity, are determined by the chemical nature of the agent, its concentration, and duration of skin contact. Chemicals cause injury by protein destruction, with denaturation, oxidation, formation of protein esters, and/or desiccation of the tissue. In the United States, the composition of most household and industrial chemicals can be obtained from the Poison Control Center in the local area, which can provide suggestions for treatment.

Speed is essential for the management of chemical burns. For all chemicals, lavage with copious quantities of clean water should be done immediately after removing all clothing. Dry powders should be brushed from the affected areas before irrigation. Early irrigation dilutes the chemical, which is already in contact with the skin, and timeliness increases effectiveness. Several liters of irrigant may be required. For example, 10 mL of 98% sulfuric acid dissolved in 12 liters of water decreases its pH to 5.0, a range that can still cause injury. If the chemical composition is known (acid or base), monitoring of the pH of the spent lavage solution provides a good indication of lavage effectiveness and completion. A good rule of thumb is to lavage with 15 to 20 liters or more of tap water for significant chemical injuries. The lavage site should be kept drained to remove the earlier, more concentrated effluent. Care should be taken to drain away from uninjured areas to avoid further exposure.

All patients must be monitored according to the severity of their injuries. They may have metabolic disturbances, usually from pH abnormalities, because of exposure to strong acids or caustics. If respiratory difficulty is apparent, oxygen therapy and mechanical ventilation must be instituted. Resuscitation should be guided by the TBSA involved (burn formulas); however, the total fluid needs may be dramatically different from the calculated volumes. Some of these injuries may be more superficial than they appear, particularly in the case of acids, and therefore require less resuscitation volume. Injuries from bases, however, may penetrate beyond that which is apparent on examination and therefore require greater volume of water. Thus, patients with chemical injuries should be observed closely for signs of adequate perfusion, such as urine output. All patients with significant chemical injuries should be monitored with indwelling bladder catheters to measure outputs accurately.

Operative débridement, if indicated, should take place as soon as a patient is stable and resuscitated (Fig. 21-15). Following adequate lavage and débridement, burn wounds are covered with antimicrobial agents or skin substitutes. Once the wounds have stabilized with the indicated treatment, they are treated as with any loss of soft tissue. Skin grafting or flap coverage is performed, as needed.

### Alkali

Alkalis, such as lime, potassium hydroxide, bleach, and sodium hydroxide, are among the most common agents involved in chemical injury. Accidental injury frequently occurs in infants and toddlers who are exploring cabinets in which cleaning products are stored. There are three factors involved in the mechanism of alkali burns: (1) saponification of fat causes the loss of insulation of heat formed in the chemical reaction with tissue; (2) massive extraction of water from cells causes damage because of the hygroscopic nature of alkali; and (3) alkalis dissolve and unite with tissue proteins to form alkaline proteinates, which are soluble and contain hydroxide ions. These ions induce further chemical reactions, penetrating deeper into the tissue. Treatment involves immediate removal of the causative agent with lavage of large volumes of fluid, usually water. Attempts to neutralize alkali agents with weak acids are not recommended, because the heat released by neutralization reactions induces further injury. Particularly strong bases should be treated with lavage and consideration for the addition of wound débridement in the operating room. Tangential removal of affected areas is performed until the tissues removed are at a normal pH.

Cement (calcium oxide) burns are alkali in nature, occur commonly, and are usually work-related injuries. The critical substance responsible for the skin damage is the hydroxyl ion. Often, the agent has been in contact with the skin for prolonged periods, such as underneath the boots of a cement worker who seeks treatment hours after the exposure, or after the cement penetrates clothing and, when combined with perspiration, induces an exothermic reaction. Treatment consists of removing all clothing and irrigating the affected area with water and soap until all the cement is removed and the effluent has a pH lower than 8. Injuries tend to be deep because of exposure times, and surgical excision and grafting of the resultant eschar may be required.

### Acids

Acid injuries are treated initially like any other chemical injury, with removal of all chemicals by disrobing the affected area and copious irrigation. Acids induce protein breakdown by

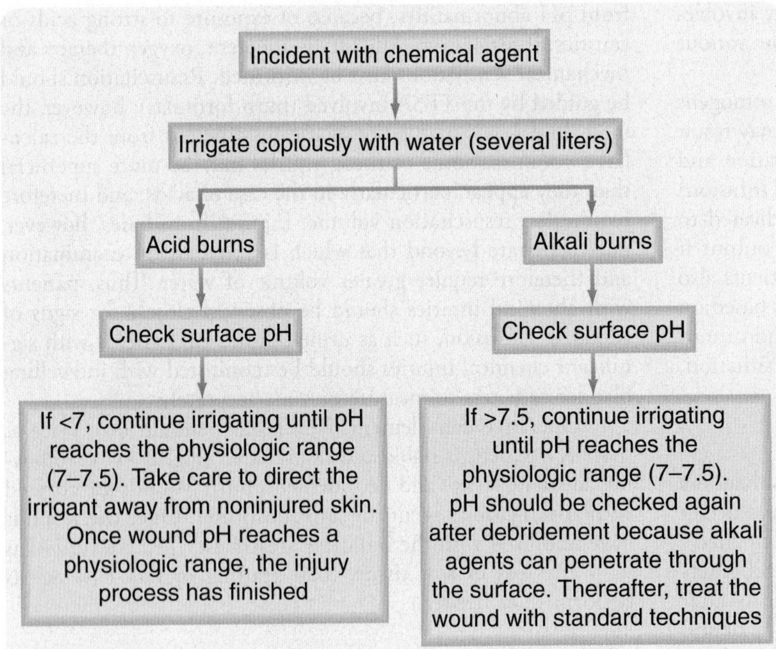


**FIGURE 21-15** Algorithm showing treatment of acid and alkali burns.

hydrolysis, which results in a hard eschar that does not penetrate as deeply as that caused by alkalis. These agents also induce thermal injury by heat generation with contact of the skin, causing further soft tissue damage. Some acids have added effects, discussed here.

Formic acid injuries are relatively rare, usually involving an organic acid used for industrial descaling and as a hay preservative. Electrolyte abnormalities are of great concern for patients who have sustained extensive formic acid injuries, with metabolic acidosis, renal failure, intravascular hemolysis, and pulmonary complications (acute respiratory distress syndrome) being common. Acidemia detected by a metabolic acidosis on arterial blood gas analysis should be corrected with IV sodium bicarbonate. Hemodialysis may be required when extensive absorption of formic acid has occurred. Mannitol diuresis is required if severe hemolysis occurs after deep injury. A formic acid wound typically has a greenish appearance and is deeper than what it initially appears to be; it is best treated by surgical excision.

Hydrofluoric acid is a toxic substance used widely in industrial and domestic settings and is the strongest inorganic acid known. Management of these burns differs from that for other acid burns in general. Hydrofluoric acid produces dehydration and corrosion of tissue with free hydrogen ions. In addition, the fluoride ion complexes with bivalent cations such as calcium and magnesium to form insoluble salts. Systemic absorption of the fluoride ion can then induce intravascular calcium chelation and hypocalcemia, which causes life-threatening arrhythmias. Beyond initial copious irrigation with clean water, the burned area should be treated immediately with copious amounts of 2% calcium gluconate gel. For example, 3.0 g of 2.5% calcium gluconate is mixed with 5 oz of water-soluable lubricant and applied to the wounds five times a day up to four times daily. Generally, these wounds are extremely painful because of the calcium chelation and associated potassium release. This finding can be used to determine the effectiveness of treatment. The gel should be changed at 15-minute intervals until the pain subsides, an indication of active fluoride ion removal. If pain relief is incomplete after several applications, or if symptoms recur, intradermal injections of 10% calcium gluconate (0.5 mL/cm$^2$ affected), intra-arterial calcium gluconate into the affected extremity, or both may be required to alleviate symptoms. If the burn is not treated in this way, decalcification of the bone underlying the injury and extension of the soft tissue injury may occur.

All patients with hydrofluoric acid burns should be admitted for cardiac monitoring, with particular attention paid to prolongation of the QT interval. To treat hypocalcemia, a total of 2 to 3 ampules of 10% calcium gluconate solution should be added to a liter of resuscitation fluid, and serum electrolyte levels closely monitored. Any electrocardiographic changes require a rapid response by the treatment team with IV calcium chloride to maintain heart function. Several grams of calcium may be required to fully abate the hydrofluoric acid burn. Speed in treatment of hydrofluoric burn is the key to effective treatment.

### Hydrocarbons

The organic solvent properties of hydrocarbons promote cell membrane dissolution and skin necrosis. Symptoms include erythema and blistering, and the burns are typically superficial and heal spontaneously. If absorbed systemically, toxicity can produce respiratory depression and eventual hepatic injury, thought to be associated with benzenes. Ignition of the hydrocarbons on the skin induces a deep full-thickness injury.

## OUTCOMES

Many of the treatments for burns are directed at improving functional psychological and work outcomes, which are only now being systematically studied. Authors are now reporting new methods to evaluate outcomes through Burn-Specific Health Scales and measures of adjustment. It has been found that severely burned adult patients adjust relatively well, although some develop clinically significant psychological disturbances, such as somatization and phobic anxiety. Children with severe burns were found to have similar somatization problems and sleep disturbances, but in general were well adjusted. Time off work in adult patients was found to be associated with increasing percentage of the TBSA burned, psychiatric history, and extremity burns, with considerable job disruption. In general, major burns can lead to significant disturbances in psychiatric health and outcomes, but these effects can be overcome.

## BURN UNITS

Improvements in burn care originated in specialized units specifically dedicated to the care of burn patients. These units consist of experienced personnel with resources to maximize outcome after these devastating injuries. Because of their specialized resources, burn patients are best treated in these facilities. Patients with the following criteria should be referred to a designated burn center:

1. Partial-thickness burns more than 10% of the TBSA
2. Burns involving the face, hands, feet, genitalia, perineum, and/or major joints
3. Any full-thickness burn
4. Electrical burns, including lightning injury
5. Chemical burns
6. Inhalation injury
7. Burns in patients with preexisting medical disorders that could complicate management, prolong recovery, or affect outcome
8. Any patient with burns and concomitant trauma (e.g., fractures) in which the burn injury poses the greater immediate risk of morbidity and mortality. In these cases, if the trauma poses the greater immediate risk, the patient may be initially stabilized in a trauma center before being transferred to a burn unit. Physician judgment is necessary in these cases and should be in conjunction with the regional medical control plan and triage protocols.
9. Burned children in hospitals without qualified personnel or equipment to care for children
10. Burns in patients who will require special social, emotional, or long-term rehabilitative intervention.

Specialized care for severely burned patients in burn centers has contributed to significant improvements in morbidity and mortality. The overall $LD_{50}$ for all burns is 70% of the TBSA, meaning that a 70% TBSA burn now has a 50% mortality rate for all ages[7]; 20 years ago, the $LD_{50}$ was a 50% TBSA.

## SUMMARY

The treatment of burns is complex. Minor injuries can be treated in the community by knowledgeable physicians. Moderate and severe injuries, however, require treatment in dedicated facilities with resources to maximize the outcomes from these often devastating events.

Novel concepts and techniques have been proposed and significantly improved over the past 30 years, resulting in a considerable decline in burn-related deaths and hospital admissions in the United States. Early excision and closure of the burn wound have probably been the single greatest advancement in treating patients with severe thermal injuries during the last 20 years, leading to substantially reduced REEs and subsequent improvement of mortality rates in this patient population. The adequate and rapid institution of fluid resuscitation maintains tissue perfusion and prevents organ system failure. Sepsis is successfully controlled by early excision of burn wounds and topical antimicrobial agents. Patients suffering from sustained inhalation injury require additional fluid resuscitation, humidified oxygen and, occasionally, ventilatory support. Enteral tube feeding is commenced early to control stress ulceration, maintain intestinal mucosal integrity, and provide fuel for the resulting hypermetabolic state. Therapeutic approaches to overcome this persistent hypermetabolism and associated hyperglycemia have remained challenging. At present, β-adrenergic blockade with propranolol represents probably the most efficacious anticatabolic therapy for the treatment of burns. Other pharmacologic strategies that have been successfully to attenuate the hypermetabolic response to burn injury include GH, IGF, and oxandrolone (Fig. 21-16). Maintaining blood glucose levels below 110 mg/dL using intensive insulin therapy has been shown to reduce mortality and morbidity in critically ill patients. However, associated hypoglycemic events have led to the investigation of other strategies, including the use of metformin and the PPAR-γ agonist fenofibrate.

Further studies are needed to address the primary determinants of death, inhalation injury complications, and pneumonia, as well as to ameliorate pain and scar formation, which are the persistent sequelae of this thermal injury. Better understanding of the basic mechanisms underlying the metabolic postburn alterations may lead to the development of novel therapeutic options. Centralized care in burn units and multidisciplinary team approaches will advance and extend current therapeutic strategies, further improving the prognosis for this unique patient population.

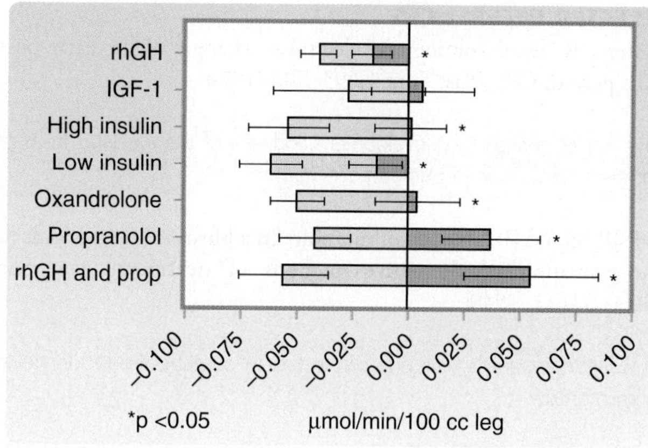


**FIGURE 21-16** Relative efficacy of the different anabolic agents to improve muscle protein synthesis compared with standard of care alone. Changes in net protein balance of muscle protein synthesis and breakdown induced by burn injury was measured by stable isotope studies using d5-phenyalanine infusion studies published previously. *p < 0.05. Graphs are averages ± SEM. Yellow bars represent patients with burns ≥40% total body surface area (TBSA) that received no anabolic agents. Blue bars represent patients with burns ≥40% TBSA that were randomized to receive drug. (From Williams FN, Jeschke MG, Chinkes DL, et al: Modulation of the hypermetabolic response to trauma: Temperature, nutrition, and drugs. J Am Coll Surg 208:489–502, 2009.)

## SELECTED REFERENCES

Baxter CR: Fluid volume and electrolyte changes of the early post-burn period. Clin Plast Surg 1:693–703, 1974.

This article defines the development and use of the Parkland formula for the resuscitation of burned patients.

Bull JP, Squire JR: A study of mortality in a burns unit; standards for the evaluation of alternative methods of treatment. Ann Surg 130:160–173, 1949.

This landmark article was one of the first to describe the incidence of burn mortality.

Herndon DN, Hart DW, Wolf SE, et al: Reversal of catabolism by beta-blockade after severe burns. N Engl J Med 345:1223–1229, 2001.

This landmark clinical trial shows that the efficacy of propranolol, a non-selective beta receptor antagonist, attenuates the profound hypermetabolic response and muscle-protein catabolism after severe burn injury.

Herndon DN, Tompkins RG: Support of the metabolic response to burn injury. Lancet 363:1895–1902, 2004.

This review is one of the premier articles to highlight the many methods for attenuating the hypermetabolic response and describe postburn physiologic and metabolic derangements.

Jeschke MG, Chinkes DL, Finnerty CC, et al: Pathophysiologic response to severe burn injury. Ann Surg 248:387–401, 2008.

This landmark clinical trial delineates the complexity of the hypermetabolic hypercatabolic response to severe burn injury.

Williams FN, Jeschke MG, Chinkes DL, et al: Modulation of the hypermetabolic response to trauma: Temperature, nutrition, and drugs. J Am Coll Surg 208:489–502, 2009.

This review highlights the significant pharmacologic and nonpharmacologic modulators of the postburn hypermetabolic response that have been shown to improve morbidity and mortality.

Wolf SE, Rose JK, Desai MH, et al: Mortality determinants in massive pediatric burns. An analysis of 103 children with > or = 80% TBSA burns (> or = 70% full-thickness). Ann Surg 225:554–565, 1997.

The treatment of very severely burned pediatric patients and the major determinants of mortality are described in this article. A formula was also devised to predict those who will survive or succumb to their injuries.

## REFERENCES

1. American Burn Association/American College of Surgeons: Guidelines for the operation of burn centers. J Burn Care Res 28:134–141, 2007.
2. Wolf SE: Critical Care in the severely burned: organ support and management of complications. In Herndon DN editor: Total burn care, ed 3, London, 2007, Saunders Elsevier, pp 454–476.
3. Herndon DN: Total burn care, ed 3, Philadelphia, 2007, Saunders Elsevier.
4. Herndon DN, Tompkins RG: Support of the metabolic response to burn injury. Lancet 363:1895–1902, 2004.
5. Bull JP, Squire JR: A study of mortality in a burns unit; standards for the evaluation of alternative methods of treatment. Ann Surg 130:160–173, 1949.
6. Flynn JD: Children playing with fire, National Fire Protection Association, 2009 (http://www.nfpa.org/assets/files/PDF/AnalysisChildrenPlaying.pdf).
7. American Burn Association: National Burn Repository: Report of data from 1999–2008, 2009 (http://www.ameriburn.org/2009NBRAnnualReport.pdf?PHPSESSID=12571a86a2cf103467eced2e6e290504). 7a-e
8. Centers for Disease Control and Prevention: Fire deaths and injuries: Fact sheet, 2009 (http://www.cdc.gov/HomeandRecreationalSafety/Fire-Prevention/fires-factsheet.html).
9. Herndon DN, Blakeney PE: Teamwork for total burn care: Achievements, directions, and hopes. In Herndon DN editor: Total burn care, ed 3, Philadelphia, 2007, WB Saunders, pp 9–13.
10. Wolf SE, Rose JK, Desai MH, et al: Mortality determinants in massive pediatric burns. An analysis of 103 children with > or = 80% TBSA burns (> or = 70% full-thickness). Ann Surg 225:554–565, 1997.
11. Williams FN, Jeschke MG, Chinkes DL, et al: Modulation of the hypermetabolic response to trauma: Temperature, nutrition, and drugs. J Am Coll Surg 208:489–502, 2009.
12. Gauglitz GG, Herndon DN, Jeschke MG: Insulin resistance postburn: Underlying mechanisms and current therapeutic strategies. J Burn Care Res 29:683–694, 2008.
13. Jeschke MG, Chinkes DL, Finnerty CC, et al: Pathophysiologic response to severe burn injury. Ann Surg 248:387–401, 2008.
14. Cree MG, Aarsland A, Herndon DN, et al: Role of fat metabolism in burn trauma–induced skeletal muscle insulin resistance. Crit Care Med 35:S476–483, 2007.
15. Gauglitz GG, Herndon DN, Kulp GA, et al: Abnormal insulin sensitivity persists up to three years in pediatric patients post-burn. J Clin Endocrinol Metab 94:1656–1664, 2009.
16. Herndon DN, Hart DW, Wolf SE, et al: Reversal of catabolism by beta-blockade after severe burns. N Engl J Med 345:1223–1229, 2001.
17. Greenhalgh DG, Saffle JR, Holmes JHt, et al; American Burn Association Consensus Conference on Burn Sepsis and Infection Group: American Burn Association consensus conference to define sepsis and infection in burns. J Burn Care Res 28:776–790, 2007.
18. Williams FN, Herndon DN, Hawkins HK, et al: The leading causes of death after burn injury in a single pediatric burn center. Crit Care 13:R183, 2009.
19. Willis MS, Carlson DL, Dimaio JM, et al: Macrophage migration inhibitory factor mediates late cardiac dysfunction after burn injury. Am J Physiol Heart Circ Physiol 288:H795–H804, 2005.
20. Pereira C, Murphy K, Herndon D: Outcome measures in burn care. Is mortality dead? Burns 30:761–771, 2004.
21. Sagraves SG, Phade SV, Spain T, et al: A collaborative systems approach to rural burn care. J Burn Care Res 28:111–114, 2007.
22. Baxter CR: Fluid volume and electrolyte changes of the early postburn period. Clin Plast Surg 1:693–703, 1974.
23. Sullivan SR, Friedrich JB, Engrav LH, et al: "Opioid creep" is real and may be the cause of "fluid creep." Burns 30:583–590, 2004.

24. Sullivan SR, Ahmadi AJ, Singh CN, et al: Elevated orbital pressure: Another untoward effect of massive resuscitation after burn injury. J Trauma 60:72–76, 2006.
25. Finnerty CC, Herndon DN, Jeschke MG: Inhalation injury in severely burned children does not augment the systemic inflammatory response. Crit Care 11:R22, 2007.
26. Endorf FW, Gamelli RL: Inhalation injury, pulmonary perturbations, and fluid resuscitation. J Burn Care Res 28:80–83, 2007.
27. Nugent N, Herndon DN: Diagnosis and treatment of inhalation injury. In Herndon DN editors: Total burn care, ed 3, Philadelphia, 2007, WB Saunders, pp 262–272.
28. Jeschke MG, Chinkes DL, Finnerty CC, et al: Blood transfusions are associated with increased risk for development of sepsis in severely burned pediatric patients. Crit Care Med 35:579–583, 2007.
29. Muller M, Gahankari D, Herndon, DN: Operative wound management. In Herndon DN, editor: Total burn care, ed 3, Philadelphia, 2007, WB Saunders, pp 177–195.
30. Branski LK, Herndon DN, Pereira C, et al: Longitudinal assessment of Integra in primary burn management: A randomized pediatric clinical trial. Crit Care Med 35:2615–2623, 2007.
31. Hohlfeld J, de Buys Roessingh A, Hirt-Burri N, et al: Tissue-engineered fetal skin constructs for paediatric burns. Lancet 366:840–842, 2005.
32. Supp DM, Boyce ST: Engineered skin substitutes: Practices and potentials. Clin Dermatol 23:403–412, 2005.
33. Branski LK, Herndon DN, Barrow RE, et al: Randomized controlled trial to determine the efficacy of long-term growth hormone treatment in severely burned children. Ann Surg 250:514–523. 2009.
34. Langouche L, Van den Berghe G: Glucose metabolism and insulin therapy. Crit Care Clin 22:119–129, 2006.
35. Wolf SE, Edelman LS, Kemalyan N, et al: Effects of oxandrolone on outcome measures in the severely burned: A multicenter prospective randomized double-blind trial. J Burn Care Res 27: 131–139, 2006.
36. Jeschke MG, Finnerty CC, Suman OE, et al: The effect of oxandrolone on the endocrinologic, inflammatory, and hypermetabolic responses during the acute phase postburn. Ann Surg 246:351–360, 2007.
37. Murphy KD, Thomas S, Mlcak RP, et al: Effects of long-term oxandrolone administration in severely burned children. Surgery 136:219–224, 2004.
38. Pereira CT, Jeschke MG, Herndon DN: Beta-blockade in burns. Novartis Found Symp 280:238–251, 2007.
39. Advanced Burn Life Support Providers Manual data.
40. Jeschke MG, Klein D, Bolder U, et al: Insulin attenuates the systemic inflammatory response in endotoxemic rats. Endocrinology 145:4084–4093, 2004.
41. Jeschke MG, Klein D, Herndon DN: Insulin treatment improves the systemic inflammatory reaction to severe trauma. Ann Surg 239:553–560, 2004.
42. Dandona P, Chaudhuri A, Mohanty P, et al: Anti-inflammatory effects of insulin. Curr Opin Clin Nutr Metab Care 10:511–517, 2007.
43. Van den Berghe G, Wilmer A, Hermans G, et al: Intensive insulin therapy in the medical ICU. N Engl J Med 354:449–461, 2006.
44. Ellger B, Debaveye Y, Vanhorebeek I, et al: Survival benefits of intensive insulin therapy in critical illness: Impact of maintaining normoglycemia versus glycemia-independent actions of insulin. Diabetes 55:1096–1105, 2006.
45. Ingels C, Debaveye Y, Milants I, et al: Strict blood glucose control with insulin during intensive care after cardiac surgery: Impact on 4-years' survival, dependency on medical care, and quality-of-life. Eur Heart J 27:2716–2724, 2006.
46. Brunkhorst FM, Engel C, Bloos F, et al: Intensive insulin therapy and pentastarch resuscitation in severe sepsis. N Engl J Med 358:125–139, 2008.
47. Langouche L, Vanhorebeek I, Van den Berghe G: Therapy insight: The effect of tight glycemic control in acute illness. Nat Clin Pract Endocrinol Metab 3:270–278, 2007.
48. Dellinger RP, Levy MM, Carlet JM, et al: Surviving Sepsis Campaign: International guidelines for management of severe sepsis and septic shock: 2008. Crit Care Med 36:296–327, 2008.
49. Gore DC, Herndon DN, Wolfe RR: Comparison of peripheral metabolic effects of insulin and metformin following severe burn injury. J Trauma 59:316–323, 2005.
50. Cree MG, Zwetsloot JJ, Herndon DN, et al: Insulin sensitivity and mitochondrial function are improved in children with burn injury during a randomized controlled trial of fenofibrate. Ann Surg 245:214–221, 2007.

# CHAPTER 22

# BITES AND STINGS

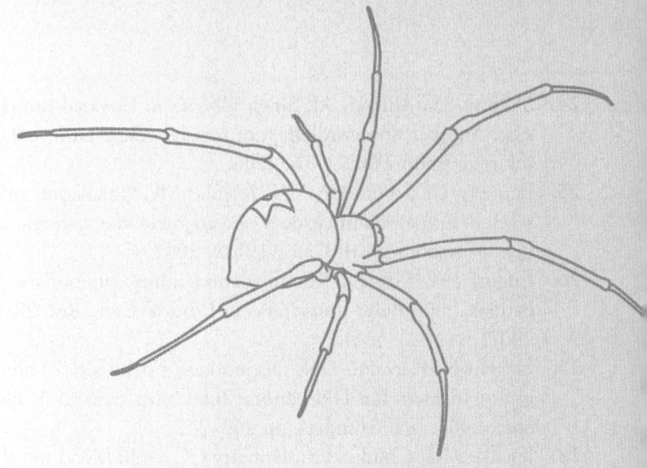

ROBERT L. NORRIS, PAUL S. AUERBACH, ELAINE E. NELSON, AND RONALD M. STEWART



## SNAKEBITES

### Epidemiology

An estimated 50,000 to 100,000 individuals worldwide die each year of venomous snakebites. Those at greatest risk include agricultural workers and hunters living in tropical countries.[1] In the United States, approximately 8000 bites by venomous snakes occur each year,[2] with approximately six deaths. Venomous species indigenous to the United States can be found in all states except Alaska, Maine, and Hawaii. The typical victim is a young male with a bite on an extremity. Lower extremity bites tend to result from stepping near a snake, whereas purposeful handling of a snake is more likely to produce a bite on the upper extremity. Those who are purposefully handling the snake are often intoxicated. Snakes are poikilothermic, which accounts for the higher incidence of bites during warmer months.

### Species

In the United States, snakes of the subfamily Crotalinae (pit vipers), which includes the rattlesnakes (Fig. 22-1), copperheads, and cottonmouths, are responsible for 99% of medically significant bites. Only 1% of bites are attributable to the other family of venomous snakes indigenous to the United States, the Elapidae (coral snakes).

Several characteristics distinguish pit vipers from nonvenomous snakes. Pit vipers tend to have relatively triangular heads, elliptical pupils, heat-sensing facial pits, large retractable anterior fangs, and a single row of subcaudal scales. Nonvenomous snakes often have more rounded heads, circular pupils, no fangs, and a double row of subcaudal scales (Fig. 22-2). Coral snakes possess a red, black, and yellow-banded pattern. In the United States, the alignment of red bands next to yellow reliably differentiates coral snakes from nonvenomous mimics. The old folk rhyme, "Red on yellow, kill a fellow, red on black, venom lack," may overstate the problem, but is a convenient way to remember the phenotypic appearance of coral snakes in North America. There are three species of coral snakes in the United States—the eastern and Texas coral snakes (*Micrurus fulvius* and *Micrurus tener*, respectively) and the Sonoran or Arizona coral snake (*Micruroides euryxanthus*).

### Toxicology

Snake venoms are complex and possess many peptides and enzymes. Peptides can damage vascular endothelium, thereby increasing permeability and leading to edema and hypovolemic shock. Enzymes include proteases and L-amino acid oxidase, which cause tissue necrosis, hyaluronidase, which facilitates the spread of venom through tissues, and phospholipase A2, which damages erythrocytes and muscle cells. Other enzymes include endonucleases, alkaline phosphatase, acid phosphatase, and cholinesterase.[3] In addition to causing local injury, these components also have deleterious effects on the cardiovascular, pulmonary, renal, and neurologic systems. Other components of the venom profoundly affect coagulation, fibrinolysis, platelet function, and vascular integrity, sometimes producing hemorrhagic or thrombotic sequelae.[4]

### Clinical Manifestations

#### Local

Approximately 20% of bites by pit vipers lack any venom injection (dry bites).[5] The only findings in such cases are puncture wounds or lacerations and minimal pain. Actual envenomation produces burning pain within minutes, followed by edema and erythema. Swelling progresses over the next few hours, and ecchymoses and hemorrhagic bullae may appear (Fig. 22-3). Involvement of the lymphatic system is common and heralded by lymphangitis and lymphadenopathy. With delayed or inadequate treatment, severe tissue necrosis can occur.

#### Systemic

Patients may complain of weakness, nausea, vomiting, perioral paresthesias, a metallic taste, and muscle twitching, although these systemic complaints are uncommon.[6] Diffuse capillary leakage leads to pulmonary edema, hypotension, and eventually shock. In victims of severe bites, a consumptive coagulopathy can develop within 1 hour.[4] Such patients can bleed spontaneously from almost any anatomic site, although clinically significant bleeding is uncommon, even in the face of significantly abnormal coagulation test results. Multifactorial acute renal

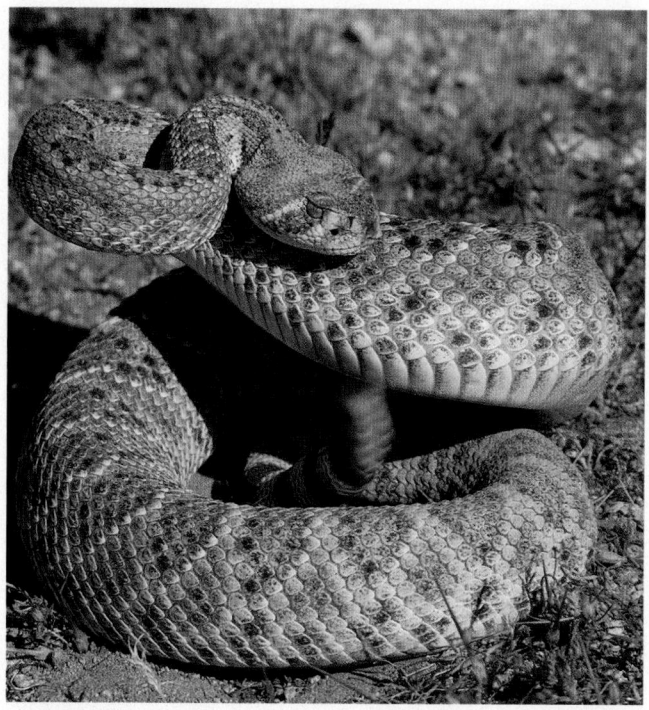

**FIGURE 22-1** A typical North American pit viper, the western diamondback rattlesnake, *Crotalus atrox.* (Courtesy Michael Cardwell.)

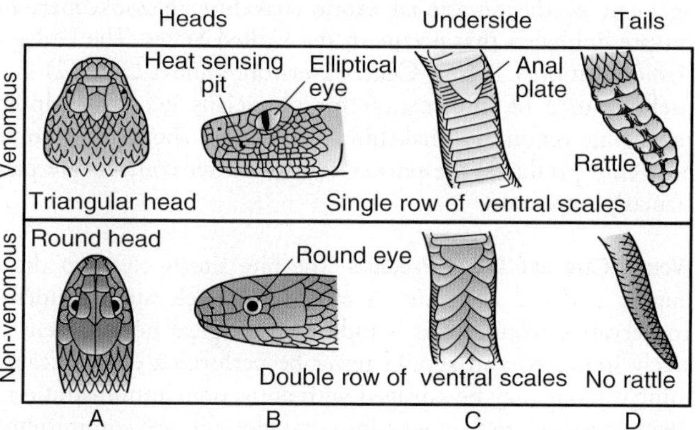


**FIGURE 22-2** Comparison of pit vipers and nonvenomous snakes. The rattle *(D, top panel)* applies to rattlesnakes only. (From Sullivan JB, Wingert WA, Norris RL: North American venomous reptile bites. In Auerbach PS [ed]: Wilderness medicine: Management of wilderness and environmental emergencies, ed 3, St Louis, Mosby–Year Book, 1995, p 684.)

failure resulting from direct nephrotoxins, circulatory collapse, myoglobinuria, and consumptive coagulopathy is possible. Laboratory abnormalities may include hypofibrinogenemia, thrombocytopenia, prolonged prothrombin and partial thromboplastin times, increased fibrin split products, elevated creatinine and creatine phosphokinase levels, proteinuria, hematuria, and anemia or hemoconcentration.[4, 6]

Unlike pit viper venoms, which tend to affect multiple organ systems, coral snake venom is primarily neurotoxic. Local injury is generally minimal or absent. Systemic signs of coral snake bites, including cranial nerve dysfunction and loss of deep tendon reflexes, may progress to respiratory depression and paralysis over a period of several hours. Differences in therapy make it important to distinguish between coral snake and pit viper bites.

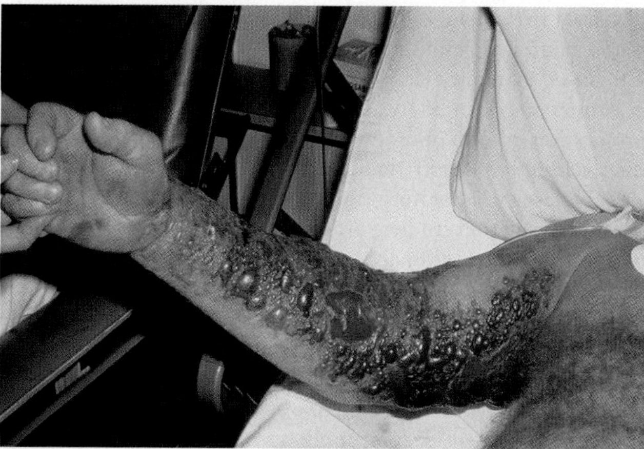

**FIGURE 22-3** A case of severe envenomation by a western diamondback rattlesnake *(Crotalus atrox)* 4 days after the bite. Note the soft tissue swelling and hemorrhagic and serum-filled vesicles. (Courtesy Dr. David Hardy.)

## Management

### Field Treatment

"Do no harm" first aid, consisting of rapid evacuation and proceeding to definitive care and immobilization, is the mainstay of first aid therapy. Removing the victim from the snake and placing him or her at rest is the first step. The wound is cleansed and immobilized at approximately heart level, if possible. Cryotherapy, suction, tourniquets, and electric shock therapy are harmful and ineffective. Therefore, these measures are not recommended. Most pit viper bites in the United States pose more of a threat to local tissues than to the life of the victim, and the use of any method to restrict venom to the bite site may be ill advised. The Australian pressure immobilization technique, in which the entire bitten extremity is snugly wrapped with a bandage, beginning at the bite site, and splinted, has been demonstrated in small studies to significantly limit the systemic spread of various snake venoms. This technique is the field treatment of choice for a non-necrotizing bite, such as from a coral snake,[7] but may make the local necrosis worse after a pit viper bite. Field measures must not delay transport to the nearest hospital appropriately equipped to handle a venomous snakebite. At least experimentally, antivenom (antivenin) reduces soft tissue loss and improves function,[8] and is probably time-dependent. In serious envenomations, delay in antivenin administration leads to greater tissue injury.

### Hospital Management

Caution must be exercised when handling any snake brought in with the patient for identification. Even dead snakes and severed heads can still have a bite reflex for as long as 1 hour. Handling of these animals by untrained healthcare personnel, even when the animal is dead, is not recommended.

A rapid, detailed history of the incident, type of snake, field management, and previous antivenom exposure is important.

Physical assessment emphasizes vital signs, cardiopulmonary status, neurologic examination, and wound appearance and size. The bitten extremity is marked at two or three locations so that circumferences can be measured every 15 minutes to judge the progression of local findings. Such measurements continue until the swelling has clearly stabilized.

Necessary laboratory analyses include a complete blood count, coagulation studies (prothrombin time, partial thromboplastin time, international normalized ratio [INR], fibrin degradation products, fibrinogen level), electrolyte, blood urea nitrogen, creatinine, and creatine phosphokinase levels, and urinalysis. No laboratory studies are necessary for a coral snake bite. A chest radiograph and electrocardiogram are obtained in older patients and anyone with systemic symptoms.

If the patient is completely asymptomatic 6 hours after a pit viper bite or 24 hours after a coral snake bite and all laboratory results are normal, it is unlikely that envenomation has occurred, and discharge is acceptable. All envenomated patients are best observed for at least 24 hours in the hospital.

**Antivenom Therapy** Deciding when to administer antivenom to a victim of a venomous snakebite requires significant clinical judgment, and consultation with an experienced clinician or toxicologist is prudent. The treating physician must quickly weigh the potential benefits of giving heterologous antiserum to the victim in an effort to halt the progression of envenomation against the risks inherent in the administration of such a product, such as an anaphylactoid reaction or serum sickness. Furthermore, because snake envenomation is a dynamic process, the decision for or against antivenom must be reevaluated as the syndrome manifests its severity over time. Currently, antivenom is administered to any patient with evidence of envenomation and clear progression in severity after arrival at the hospital or without delay in any patient with clearly serious poisoning (e.g., severe swelling, hypotension, respiratory distress).

Wyeth Polyvalent (Crotalidae) Antivenom is no longer manufactured. In 2000, the U.S. Food and Drug Administration (FDA) approved a second pit viper antivenom for use in the United States, CroFab (Protherics, Brentwood, Tenn). This product, produced in sheep and modified by Fab technology, appears to be more effective and safer to use than the previous polyvalent antivenin.[9-11] No skin testing is recommended, and no pretreatment in an effort to reduce the risk for an acute adverse reaction to the product is needed with CroFab.

Because antivenin works by neutralizing the antigens in the venom, its dose is based on the amount of venom injected, not the size of the patient. In the clinical setting, the exact amount of venom injected is impossible to determine; therefore, the dosing of antivenin requires significant experience and clinical judgment. For major envenomations, CroFab is given as six vials intravenously (IV) in 250 mL of diluent over a period of approximately 1 hour. If, after the initial dose, the severity of venom toxicity progresses over the next hour, an additional 4 to 6 vials are administered. This sequence is repeated as needed until the victim has stabilized. After stabilization, to prevent recurrence of the effects of the venom, two vials of CroFab are administered IV every 6 hours for three additional doses.[10] The same dosing regimen is used for children, and pregnancy is not a contraindication to antivenom therapy. Although expensive, postmarketing experience with CroFab has been favorable. Allergic reactions and side effects have been much less than with the previous Wyeth Polyvalent Antivenin.[12]

A separate antivenom, North American Coral Snake Antivenin, was also produced by Pfizer (formerly Wyeth-Ayerst) and is available for eastern and Texas coral snake bites, but this product is also not currently being manufactured. Current lot numbers have been extended until October 31, 2011, but these will then expire. No U.S. alternative for this antivenom exists. We recommend contacting your local poison control center for further information on coral snake envenomations. Administration is similar to that for CroFab, except that therapy is initiated in all patients in whom a positively identified coral snake bite has occurred, even in the absence of local or systemic symptoms, because such symptoms may be delayed many hours in onset. Once established, envenomation can be hard to reverse, even with the use of antivenom. There is no antivenom produced to treat Sonoran coral snake bites, but there have been no reported fatalities after bites by this small animal. Any currently available snakebite antivenom carries some risk for an acute anaphylactoid reaction and delayed serum sickness. Informed consent is obtained for its use whenever possible, and treatment of anaphylaxis with epinephrine and possible airway control must always be immediately available during administration. Patients should be warned of the symptoms of serum sickness before discharge from the hospital. Generally, serum sickness is easily treated with steroids and antihistamines.

Poison control centers and zoos can provide important information regarding the procurement of antivenom and management of the occasional exotic snakebite in zookeepers or private hobbyists that occurs in the United States. The University of National Poison Center Network (800-222-1222) is a useful source of information for physicians needing help in managing venomous snakebites. Given the shortage of some antivenin products, the poison control center contacts are particularly important.

**Wound Care and Blood Products** The bite site is cleansed thoroughly and the extremity is splinted and elevated. Prudent, conservative wound care is indicated. Surgical débridement is rarely indicated and should never be performed early, because injured tissue may be salvaged with antivenom administration.[8] Tetanus toxoid and tetanus immune globulin are administered as needed according to the patient's immunization history. Prophylactic antibiotics are reserved for cases in which misdirected first aid included incisions into the bite site or mouth suction. Otherwise, antibiotics are needed solely for the rare wound in which secondary infection develops.[13,14]

Blood products are needed only in the rare setting of clinically significant bleeding that is not reversed with antivenom. Patients with serious bleeding (e.g., gastrointestinal bleeding, intracranial bleeding, hemoptysis) may need packed red cells, platelets, fresh-frozen plasma, or cryoprecipitate, depending on the scenario and the results of serial complete blood counts and coagulation studies. Antivenom must be started before these second-line agents are infused, however.[13] Patients in whom coagulopathy has developed while in the hospital after a pit viper bite must be warned that coagulation abnormalities can recur for up to 2 weeks after the bite, even after antivenom therapy. They need to be advised to look for signs of bleeding and to avoid any elective surgery or activities, with an inherent high risk of injury during this period.

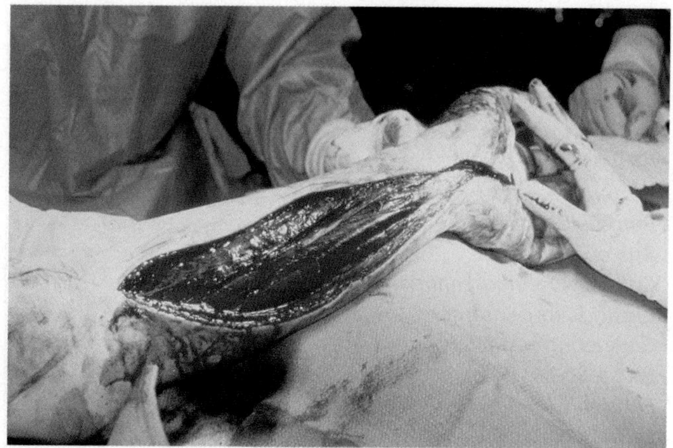

**FIGURE 22-4** Fasciotomy of the forearm compartments in a victim of a severe rattlesnake bite on the hand. Intracompartmental pressures were documented to be exceedingly elevated in this patient, despite limb elevation and large doses of antivenom. (Courtesy Dr. Robert Norris.)

**Fasciotomy** The great majority of snakebites result in the subcutaneous deposition of venom. Venom that is deposited by larger snakes into muscle compartments, however, can result in an increase in intracompartmental pressure. Subfascial deposition of venom is more likely in areas with less subcutaneous tissue (e.g., fingers, toes, anterior lower leg). Clinically differentiating a true compartment syndrome from the typical swollen, painful extremity seen after subcutaneous envenomation is difficult and may require measurement of compartment pressure. Fasciotomies are considered only if pressures are documented to exceed 30 to 40 mm Hg despite antivenom treatment and elevation (Fig. 22-4). There is no role for routine or prophylactic fasciotomy in venomous snakebites.[15] Preliminary animal evidence has suggested that fasciotomy may actually increase the severity of local myonecrosis in snake venom–induced compartment syndrome.[16] When a fasciotomy is required for treatment of compartment syndrome, antivenom should be aggressively administered and no débridement of injured tissue should be performed, because this tissue may be viable with antivenin therapy.[8] Negative-pressure wound therapy would seem a logical choice in the postoperative care of the patient following fasciotomy for intramuscular envenomation.

## MAMMALIAN BITES

### Epidemiology

The incidence of mammalian bite injuries is unknown because most patients with minor wounds never seek medical care. Although death from animal bites is uncommon in the United States, thousands of people are killed around the world each year, primarily by large animals such as lions and tigers. Dogs are responsible for 80% to 90% of animal bites in the United States, followed by cats and humans; an estimated 4.7 million dog bites occur annually in the United States and account for 1% of emergency department visits.[17] Most of these bites are from a family pet or a neighborhood dog. Pit bulls and Rottweilers account for most fatal dog bites in the United States.[18]Animal bites occur most frequently on the extremities of adults and on the head, face, and neck of children. More than 60% of reported bites occur in children, especially boys 5 to 9 years of age.

### Treatment

#### Evaluation

Humans attacked by animals are at risk for blunt and penetrating trauma. Animals produce blunt injuries by striking with their extremities, biting with their powerful jaws, and crushing with their body weight. Teeth and claws can puncture body cavities, including the cranium, and amputate extremities. Patients with serious injuries are managed in a similar fashion as other potential polytrauma victims, with special attention given to wound management. Useful laboratory tests include a hematocrit when blood loss is of concern and cultures when an infection is present. Radiographs are obtained to diagnose potential fractures, joint penetration, severe infections, and retained foreign bodies, such as teeth. The patient's tetanus status needs to be updated, as necessary.

#### Wound Care

Local wound management reduces the risk for infection and maximizes functional and aesthetic outcomes. Early wound cleansing is the most important therapy for preventing infection and zoonotic diseases such as rabies. Intact skin surrounding dirty wounds is scrubbed with a sponge and 1% povidone-iodine or 4% chlorhexidine gluconate solution. Alternatively, a 1% povidone-iodine solution can be used for irrigation, as long as the wound is flushed afterward with normal saline or water. Scrubbing the wound surface itself can increase tissue damage and infection and thus needs to be avoided. Wounds that are dirty or contain devitalized tissue are cleansed lightly with gauze or a porous sponge and sharply débrided.[17]

Options for wound repair include primary, delayed primary, and secondary closure. The anatomic location of the bite, source of the bite, and type of injury determine the most appropriate method. Primary closure is appropriate for head and neck wounds that are initially seen within 24 hours of the bite and for which aesthetic results are important and infection rates are low.[17,19,20] Primary closure can also be used for low-risk wounds to the arms, legs, and trunk if seen within 6 to 12 hours of the bite. Severe human bites and avulsion injuries of the face that require flaps have been successfully repaired by primary closure; however, this technique remains controversial. Wounds prone to the development of infection (Box 22-1), such as those initially seen longer than 24 hours after the bite (or longer than 6 hours if ear or nose cartilage is involved), are covered with moist dressings and undergo delayed primary closure after 3 to 5 days. Puncture wounds have an increased incidence of infection and are not sutured. Deep irrigation of small puncture wounds and wide excision have not proved beneficial. Larger puncture wounds, however, usually benefit from irrigation and débridement.[21] Healing by secondary intention generally produces unacceptable scars in cosmetic areas. The clinician should be alert to the fact that significant dog bites may have extensive undermined areas created by the large canine teeth. These wounds require operative intervention under general or regional anesthesia.

Bites involving the hands or feet have a much greater chance of becoming infected and are left open.[17] The primary goal in repairing bite wounds on the hand is to maximize functional

**BOX 22-1 Animal Bite Risk Factors for Infection**

**High Risk**

- Location
  - Hand, wrist, or foot
  - Scalp or face in infants (high risk of cranial perforation)
  - Over a major joint (possible perforation)
  - Through and through bite of a cheek
- Type of wound
  - Puncture (difficult to irrigate)
  - Tissue crushing that cannot be débrided
  - Carnivore bite over a vital structure (artery, nerve, joint)
- Patient
  - Older than 50 years
  - Asplenic
  - Chronic alcoholic
  - Altered immune status
  - Diabetic
  - Peripheral vascular insufficiency
  - Chronic corticosteroid therapy
  - Prosthetic or diseased heart valve or joint
- Species
  - Domestic cat
  - Large cat (deep punctures)
  - Human (hand bites)
  - Primates
  - Pigs

**Low Risk**

- Location
  - Face, scalp, or mouth
- Type of wound
  - Large, clean lacerations that can be thoroughly irrigated

Adapted from Keogh S, Callaham ML: Bites and injuries inflicted by domestic animals. In Auerbach PS (ed): Wilderness medicine: Management of wilderness and environmental emergencies, ed 4, St Louis, 2001, CV Mosby, pp 961–978.

**BOX 22-2 Common Bacteria Found in Animals, Mouths**

*Acinetobacter* spp.
*Actinobacillus* spp.
*Aeromonas hydrophila*
*Bacillus* spp.
*Bacteroides* spp.
*Bordetella* spp.
*Brucella canis*
*Capnocytophaga canimorsus*
*Clostridium perfringens*
*Corynebacterium* spp.
*Eikenella corrodens*
*Enterobacter* spp.
*Escherichia coli*
*Eubacterium* spp.
*Fusobacterium* spp.
*Haemophilus aphrophilus*
*Haemophilus haemolyticus*
*Klebsiella* spp.
*Leptotrichia buccalis*
*Micrococcus* spp.
*Moraxella* spp.
*Neisseria* spp.
*Pasteurella aerogenes*
*Pasteurella canis*
*Pasteurella dagmatis*
*Pasteurella multocida*
*Peptococcus* spp.
*Peptostreptococcus* spp.
*Propionibacterium* spp.
*Proteus mirabilis*
*Pseudomonas* spp.
*Serratia marcescens*
*Staphylococcus aureus*
*Staphylococcus epidermidis*
*Streptococcus* spp.
*Veillonella parvula*

Adapted from Keogh S, Callaham ML: Bites and injuries inflicted by domestic animals. In Auerbach PS (ed): Wilderness medicine: Management of wilderness and environmental emergencies, ed 4, St Louis, 2001, CV Mosby, pp 961–978.

outcome. Approximately one third of dog bites on the hand become infected, even with adequate therapy.[21] Healing by secondary intention is recommended for most hand lacerations. After thorough exploration, irrigation, and débridement, the hand is immobilized, wrapped in a bulky dressing, and elevated.

A common human bite wound associated with high morbidity is a clenched fist injury (fight bite) resulting from striking another person's mouth. Regardless of the history obtained, injuries over the dorsum of the metacarpophalangeal joints are treated as clenched fist injuries. These minor appearing wounds often result in serious injury to the extensor tendon or joint capsule and have significant oral bacterial contamination. The extensor tendon retracts when the hand is opened, so evaluation needs to be carried out with the hand in the open and clenched positions. Minor injuries are irrigated, débrided, and left open. Potentially deeper injuries and infected bites require exploration and débridement in the operating room and administration of IV antibiotics.[22]

All bite injuries are reevaluated in 1 or 2 days to rule out secondary infection.

### Microbiology

Given the large variety and concentration of bacteria in mouths, it is not surprising that wound infection is the main complication of bites, with 3% to 18% of dog bite wounds approximately 50% of cat bite wounds becoming infected. Infected wounds contain aerobic and anaerobic bacteria and yield an average of five isolates/culture (Box 22-2). Although many wounds are infected by *Staphylococcus* and *Streptococcus* spp. and anaerobes, *Pasteurella* spp. are the most common bacterial pathogen, found in 50% of dog bites and 75% of cat bites. Human bite wounds are frequently contaminated with *Eikenella corrodens* in addition to the microorganisms found after dog and cat bites.[22,23]

Systemic diseases such as rabies, cat scratch disease, cowpox, tularemia, leptospirosis, and brucellosis can be acquired through animal bites. Human bites can transmit hepatitis B and C, tuberculosis, syphilis, and human immunodeficiency virus (HIV).[20] Although HIV transmission from human bites is rare, seroconversion is possible when a person with an open wound, either from a bite or a preexisting injury, is exposed to saliva containing HIV-positive blood.[24] In this scenario, baseline and 6-month postexposure HIV testing is performed and prophylactic treatment with anti-HIV drugs is considered.

### Antibiotics

Although data are limited, preventive antibiotics are recommended for patients with high-risk bites.[17,21] The initial antibiotic choice and route are based on the type of animal and severity and location of the bite. Cat bites often cause puncture wounds that require antibiotics. Patients with low-risk dog and human bites do not benefit from prophylactic antibiotics unless the hand or foot is involved.[23] Patients seen 24 hours after a bite without signs of infection do not usually need prophylactic antibiotics. Routine cultures of uninfected wounds have not proved useful and are reserved for infected wounds.

Initial antibiotic selection needs to cover *Staphylococcus* and *Streptococcus* spp., anaerobes, *Pasteurella* spp. for dog and cat bites, and *E. corrodens* for human bites. Amoxicillin-clavulanate is an acceptable first-line antibiotic for most bites. Alternatives include second-generation cephalosporins, such as cefoxitin, or a combination of penicillin and a first-generation cephalosporin. Penicillin-allergic patients can receive clindamycin combined with ciprofloxacin (or combined with trimethoprim-sulfamethoxazole if the patient is pregnant or a child).[17, 20] Moxifloxacin has also been suggested as monotherapy. Infections developing within 24 hours of the bite are generally caused by *Pasteurella* spp. and are treated by antibiotics with appropriate coverage. Patients with serious infections require hospital admission and parenteral antibiotics such as ampicillin-sulbactam, piperacillin-tazobactam, cefoxitin, ticarcillin-clavulanate or clindamycin combined with a fluoroquinolone, or trimethoprim-sulfamethoxazole.

### Rabies

Annually, thousands of people die of rabies worldwide, with dog bites or scratches being the major source.[25] In the United States, rabies is primarily found in wildlife, with raccoons being the primary source, followed by skunks, bats, and foxes.[26] Cats and dogs account for less than 5% of cases since the establishment of rabies control programs. Although the number of infected animals in the United States continues to increase, with the total approaching 8000/year, human infection rates remain constant at one to three cases annually. Bats have been the main source of human rabies reported in this country during the past 20 years, although a history of bat contact is absent in most victims.

Rabies is caused by a rhabdovirus found in the saliva of animals and is transmitted through bites or scratches. Acute encephalitis develops and patients almost invariably die. The disease usually begins with a prodromal phase of nonspecific complaints and paresthesias, with itching or burning at the bite site spreading to the entire bitten extremity.[27] The disease then progresses to an acute neurologic phase. This phase generally takes one of two forms. The more common encephalitic or furious form is typified by fever and hyperactivity that can be stimulated by internal or external factors such as thirst, fear, light, or noise, followed by fluctuating levels of consciousness, aerophobia or hydrophobia, inspiratory spasm, and abnormalities of the autonomic nervous system. The paralytic form of rabies is manifested by fever, progressive weakness, loss of deep tendon reflexes, and urinary incontinence. Both forms progress to paralysis, coma, circulatory collapse, and death.

Adequate wound care and postexposure prophylaxis can prevent the development of rabies. Wounds are washed with soap and water and irrigated with a virucidal agent such as povidone-iodine solution. If rabies exposure is strongly suspected, consider leaving the wound open. The decision to administer rabies prophylaxis after an animal bite or scratch depends on the offending species and nature of the event. Guidelines for administering rabies prophylaxis can be obtained from local public health agencies or from the Advisory Committee on Immunization Practices. Research indicates that rabies prophylaxis is not being administered according to guidelines, which results in costly overtreatment or potentially life-threatening undertreatment.

Worldwide, almost 1 million people receive rabies prophylaxis each year, 40,000 from the United States.[25] Unprovoked attacks are more likely to occur by rabid animals. All wild carnivores must be considered rabid, but birds and reptiles do not contract or transmit rabies. In cases of bites by domestic animals, rodents, or lagomorphs, the local health department needs to be consulted before beginning rabies prophylaxis. A bite from a healthy-appearing domestic animal does not require prophylaxis if the animal can be observed for 10 days.

Rabies prophylaxis involves passive and active immunization. Passive immunization consists of administering 20 IU/kg body weight of rabies immune globulin. As much of the dose as possible is infiltrated into and around the wound. The rest can be given intramuscularly at a site remote from where the vaccine was administered. For healthy, immunocompromised patients, an active immunization consists of administering 1 mL of human diploid cell vaccine, purified chick embryo cell vaccine, or rabies vaccine absorbed intramuscularly into the deltoid in adults and into the anterolateral aspect of the thigh in children on days 0, 3, 7, and 14. For immunocompromised patients a five-dose schedule is recommended on days 0, 3, 7, 14, and 28. Patients with preexposure immunization do not require passive immunization and need active immunization only on days 0 and 3.[27]

## ARTHROPOD BITES AND STINGS

Although mammalian and reptilian bites inflict more serious injuries and are generally more dramatic in their presentations, many more people in the United States die from insect bites and stings, most often caused by anaphylaxis. Also, even more contract vector-related infectious diseases from the bites of insects.

### Black Widow Spiders

Widow spiders (genus *Latrodectus*) are found throughout the world. At least one of five species inhabits all areas of the United States except Alaska. The best-known widow spider is the black widow *(Latrodectus mactans)*. The female has a leg span of 1 to 4 cm and a shiny black body with a distinctive red ventral marking (often hourglass-shaped; Fig. 22-5). Variations in color occur among other species, with some appearing brown or red and some without the ventral marking. The nonaggressive female widow spider bites in defense. Males are too small to bite through human skin.

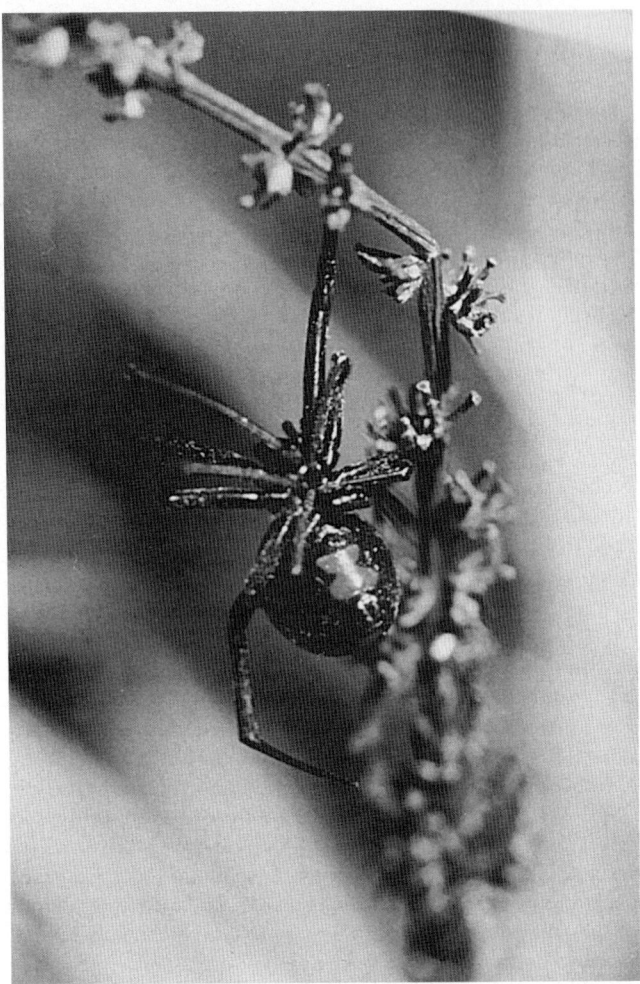

**FIGURE 22-5** Female black widow spider *(Latrodectus mactans)* with the characteristic hourglass marking. (Courtesy Dr. Paul Auerbach.)

#### Toxicology

Widow spiders produce neurotoxic venom with minimal local effects. The major component is α-latrotoxin, which acts at presynaptic terminals by enhancing the release of neurotransmitters. The ensuing clinical picture results from excess stimulation of neuromuscular junctions, as well as the sympathetic and parasympathetic nervous systems.

#### Clinical Manifestations

The bite itself may be painless or felt as a pinprick. Local findings are minimal. The patient may have systemic complaints and no history of a spider bite, thus making the diagnosis challenging. Neuromuscular symptoms may occur as early as 30 minutes after the bite and include severe pain and spasms of large muscle groups. Abdominal cramps and rigidity could mimic a surgical abdomen, but rebound is absent. Dyspnea can result from chest wall muscle tightness. Autonomic stimulation produces hypertension, diaphoresis, and tachycardia. Other symptoms include muscle twitching, nausea and vomiting, headache, paresthesias, fatigue, and salivation. Symptoms typically peak at several hours and resolve in 1 to 2 days. Mild pain and nonspecific symptoms, primarily neurologic, can persist for several weeks. Death is an unusual result of widow spider bites.

#### Treatment

Mild bites are managed with local wound care—cleansing, intermittent application of ice, and tetanus prophylaxis as needed. The possibility of delayed severe symptoms makes an observation period of several hours prudent. The optimal therapy for severe envenomation is controversial. IV calcium gluconate, previously recommended as a first-line drug to relieve muscle spasms after widow spider bites, has no significant efficacy. Narcotics and benzodiazepines are more effective agents to relieve muscular pain.

In the United States, antivenom derived from horse serum is available (Black Widow Spider Antivenin, Merck, West Point, Pa). Because this antivenom can cause anaphylactoid reactions or serum sickness, however, it must be reserved for serious cases. Antivenom is currently recommended for pregnant women, children younger than 16 years, individuals older than 60 years, and patients with severe envenomation and uncontrolled hypertension or respiratory distress. Skin testing for possible allergy to the U.S. antivenom is recommended by the manufacturer and is outlined in the package insert, although the reliability of such testing is low. Patients about to receive antivenom may be pretreated with antihistamines to reduce the likelihood or severity of a systemic reaction to the serum. The initial recommended dose is one vial IV or intramuscularly, repeated as necessary, although it is exceedingly rare for more than two vials to be required. Studies have demonstrated that antivenom can decrease a patient's hospital stay, with discharge occurring as early as several hours after administration. A high-quality antivenom is also available in Australia for *Latrodectus* bites. It appears that any widow spider antivenom is effective, regardless of which species inflicted the bite.[28]

### Brown Recluse Spiders

Envenomation by brown spiders of the genus *Loxosceles* is termed *necrotic arachnidism* or *loxoscelism*. These arthropods primarily inhabit North and South America, Africa, and Europe. Several species of *Loxosceles* are found throughout the United States, with the greatest concentration in the Midwest. Most significant bites in the United States are by *Loxosceles reclusa*, the brown recluse. The brown spiders are varying shades of brownish gray, with a characteristic dark brown, violin-shaped marking over the cephalothorax—hence, the name violin spider (Fig. 22-6). Whereas most spiders have four pairs of eyes, brown spiders have only three pairs. Both male and female specimens can bite and may do so when threatened.

#### Toxicology

Although several enzymes have been isolated from the venom, the major deleterious factor is sphingomyelinase D, which causes dermonecrosis and hemolysis. It is a phospholipase that interacts with the cell membranes of erythrocytes, platelets, and endothelial cells and causes hemolysis, coagulation, and platelet aggregation. Host responses have some significance in determining the severity of envenomation because functioning polymorphonuclear leukocytes and complement are necessary for the venom to have maximal effect.

#### Clinical Manifestations

Local findings at the bite site range from mild irritation to severe necrosis with ulceration.[29] The patient is often completely unaware of the bite or may have felt a slight stinging.

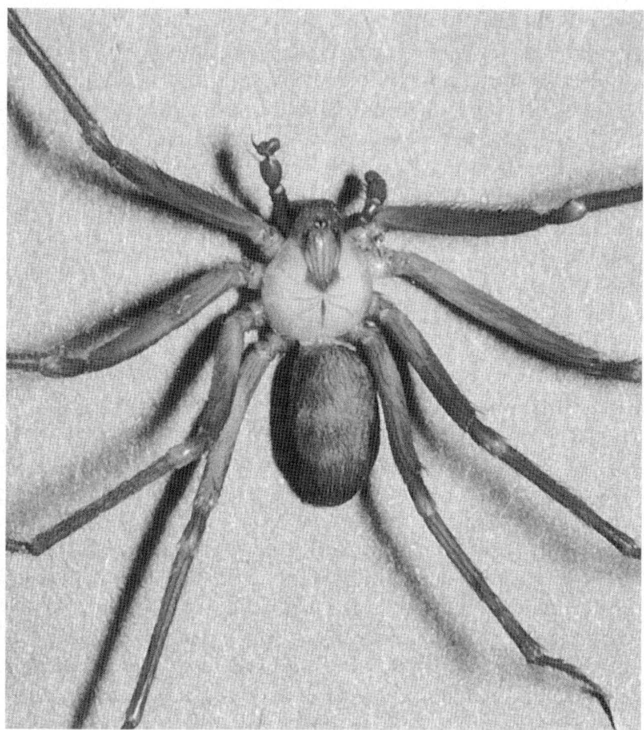

**FIGURE 22-6** Brown recluse spider *(Loxosceles reclusa)* with a violin-shaped marking on the cephalothorax. (Courtesy Dr. Sherman Minton.)

It is unusual for the victim to actually see or capture the spider. This can make the diagnosis very challenging because similar skin lesions can represent bites by other arthropods, skin infections (including methicillin-resistant *Staphylococcus aureus*), herpes zoster, dermatologic manifestation of a systemic illness, or other causes of dermatitis and vasculitis.[30] Within several hours of a *Loxosceles* bite, local tissue ischemia will develop in some patients, with resulting pain, itching, swelling, and erythema. A blister may form at the site. In more severe bites, the central area turns purple as a result of microvascular thrombosis. Peripheral vasoconstriction can also create a pale border surrounding the central region of necrosis. Over the next several days, an eschar develops over the widening necrotic area. The eschar separates and leaves an ulcer that usually heals over a period of many weeks to months, but occasionally skin grafting is required. Necrosis is most severe in fatty areas such as the abdomen and thigh.

Systemic features can include headache, nausea and vomiting, fever, malaise, arthralgias, and maculopapular rash. Additional findings may include thrombocytopenia, disseminated intravascular coagulation, hemolytic anemia, coma, and possibly death. Renal failure can result from intravascular hemolysis.

In patients with lesions consistent with brown spider bites, a search for evidence of systemic involvement (viscerocutaneous or systemic loxoscelism) is initiated, particularly if the victim has any systemic complaints. Appropriate laboratory tests include a complete blood count, with platelet count, and a bedside urine test for blood. If the results of any of these tests are abnormal, electrolyte, liver function, and coagulation studies are in order, but there are no truly diagnostic studies available. Systemic loxoscelism is more common in children and can occur with minimal local findings.

### Treatment

Recommended management remains controversial. The bite site is splinted, elevated, and treated with cold compresses. Cold therapy inhibits venom activity and reduces inflammation and necrosis. Heat application, in contrast, enhances tissue damage and ulcer development. Although controversial, a lipophilic prophylactic antibiotic such as erythromycin or cephalexin can be administered in standard doses for a few days. Tetanus status is updated as needed. Brown spider bites in which necrosis does not develop within 72 hours generally heal well and require no additional therapy. There is no commercial antivenom available in the United States.

Some research has suggested that more severe lesions may benefit from dapsone if administered within the first few days after the bite, even though the drug is not approved for this indication.[31] Dapsone may reduce local inflammation and necrosis by inhibiting neutrophil function. The suggested adult dosage is 100 mg/day. Dapsone can cause methemoglobinemia and is contraindicated in patients with glucose-6-phosphate dehydrogenase deficiency. Thus, levels of this enzyme are checked as therapy begins and dapsone is discontinued if the enzyme level is found to be deficient. Dapsone is not approved for use in children.

Early surgical intervention, other than simple conservative débridement of obviously necrotic tissue, is avoided. It is difficult or impossible to predict with any certainty the extent of eventual necrosis, and early surgery is apt to be overaggressive and needlessly disfiguring. Pyoderma gangrenosum, manifested as nonhealing ulcers and failure of skin grafts, occurs more often in patients undergoing early excision and débridement, possibly as a result of the rapid spread of venom.[28] After 1 to 2 weeks, when eschar margins are defined, débridement can be performed as necessary. In severe cases, wide excision and split-thickness skin grafting are necessary while dapsone therapy is continued.

The efficacy of using hyperbaric oxygen therapy for *Loxosceles* bites remains controversial.[32] Steroid administration, by any route, has never been proved to be beneficial in limiting dermonecrosis. A short course (a few days) of oral steroids can help stabilize red blood cell membranes and reduce hemolysis in the setting of systemic loxoscelism.

Patients with rapidly expanding necrotic lesions or a clinical picture suggesting systemic loxoscelism are admitted for close observation and management. Alternative diagnoses that may cause rapid expanding tissue necrosis should also be strongly considered in this situation, including serious soft tissue infection. Patients with less serious lesions can be monitored on an outpatient basis with frequent wound checks. Visits during the first 72 hours include reassessment for any evidence of systemic involvement based on symptoms and signs, and possibly a bedside urine test for blood.

## Scorpions

Significant scorpion envenomation occurs worldwide by species belonging to the family Buthidae. In this group, the bark scorpion *(Centruroides exilicauda)* is the only potentially dangerous species in the United States. It is found throughout Arizona and, occasionally, in immediately contiguous areas of surrounding states. It is a yellow to brown crablike arthropod up to 5 cm in length. Approximately 15,000 scorpion stings were reported during 2004 in the United States, and this is probably a significant underestimate of the total number of stings that occurred. Scorpions tend to be nocturnal and sting when threatened.

### Toxicology

Neurotoxic scorpion venoms, such as that produced by the bark scorpion, contain multiple low-molecular-weight basic proteins but possess very little enzymatic activity. The neurotoxins target excitable tissues and work primarily on ion channels, particularly sodium and potassium channels. They cause massive release of multiple neurotransmitters throughout the autonomic nervous system and the adrenal medulla.[33] Almost any organ system can be adversely affected, either by direct toxin effects or by the flood of autonomic neurotransmitters. Because of the speed of their systemic absorption, these neurotoxic scorpion venoms can cause rapid systemic toxicity and potentially death.

### Clinical Manifestations

Most scorpion stings in the United States cause short-lived, searing pain and mild, local irritation with slight swelling. Stings by the bark scorpion typically produce local paresthesias and burning pain. Systemic manifestations may include cranial nerve and neuromuscular hyperactivity and respiratory distress.[34] Signs of adrenergic stimulation, accompanied by nausea and vomiting, may also develop. Young children are at greatest risk for severe stings from the bark scorpion. Death can occur from bark scorpion stings but is rare.

### Treatment

All patients receive tetanus prophylaxis, if indicated, application of cold compresses to the sting site, and analgesics for pain. Victims of bark scorpion stings with signs of systemic envenomation require supportive care, with close monitoring of cardiovascular and respiratory status in an intensive care setting. Although an antivenom for this arthropod has been available in the past, production has currently ceased. The product was derived from goats, with a resultant risk for allergic sequelae, lacked FDA approval, and was available for use only in Arizona. Its use was highly controversial. There is an antivenom produced for related scorpions in Mexico that is currently being evaluated for possible use in the United States.

## Ticks

Several potentially serious diseases occur from tick bites, including Rocky Mountain spotted fever, ehrlichiosis, tularemia, babesiosis, Colorado tick fever, relapsing fever, and Lyme disease. Timely and adequate removal of the tick is important to prevent disease. Common lay recommendations for tick removal, such as the application of local heat, gasoline, methylated spirits, and fingernail polish, are ineffective. Proper removal involves grasping the tick by the body as close to the skin surface as possible with an instrument and applying gradual, gentle axial traction, without twisting. Commercial tick removal devices are superior to standard tweezers for this purpose.[35] An alternative removal method involves looping a length of suture material in a simple overhand knot around the body of the tick. The loop is slipped down as close to the patient's skin surface as possible. The knot is then tightened and the tick is pulled backward and out, over its head in a somersault action. Crushing the tick is avoided because potentially infectious secretions may be squeezed into the wound. After extraction, the wound is cleansed with alcohol or povidone-iodine. Any retained mouth parts of the tick are removed with the tip of a needle. If the tick was embedded for less than 24 hours, the risk of transmitting infection is very low. Tetanus immunization needs to be current. Occasionally, a granulomatous lesion requiring steroid injection or surgical excision may develop at the tick bite site a few weeks after the incident.[36] Patients in whom a local rash or systemic symptoms develop within 4 weeks of exposure to tick-infested areas, even in the absence of a known bite, need to be evaluated for infectious complications such as Lyme disease, the most common vector-borne disease in the United States.

Lyme disease is caused by the spirochete *Borrelia burgdorferi* and may initially be seen in any of three stages—early localized (stage 1), early disseminated (stage 2), or late-persistent (stage 3). Stage 1 findings of limited infection include a rash in at least 80% of patients that develops after an incubation period of approximately 3 to 30 days.[37,38] The rash, termed *erythema migrans*, is typically a round or oval erythematous lesion that begins at the bite site and expands at a relatively rapid rate, up to 1 cm/day, to a median size of 15 cm in diameter.[39] As the rash expands, there may be evidence of central clearing and, less commonly, a central vesicle or necrotic eschar. The rash may be accompanied by fatigue, myalgias, headache, fever, nausea, vomiting, regional lymphadenopathy, sore throat, photophobia, anorexia, and arthralgias. Without treatment, the rash fades in approximately 4 weeks. If untreated, the infection may disseminate and, between 30 and 120 days later, multiple erythema migrans lesions (generally smaller than the primary lesion) and neurologic, cardiac, or joint abnormalities may develop. Neuroborreliosis occurs in approximately 15% of untreated patients and is characterized by central or peripheral findings such as lymphocytic meningitis, subtle encephalitis, cranial neuritis (especially facial nerve palsy, which may be unilateral or bilateral), cerebellar ataxia, and motor neuropathies.[40] Cardiac findings occur in approximately 5% of untreated patients and are usually manifested as atrioventricular nodal block or myocarditis. Oligoarticular arthritis is a common finding in early disseminated Lyme disease and occurs in approximately 60% of untreated victims. There is a particular propensity for larger joints such as the knee, which becomes recurrently and intermittently swollen and painful. Findings of early disseminated Lyme disease eventually disappear with or without treatment. Over time, as much as 1 year after the initial tick bite, Lyme disease can progress to its chronic form, manifested by chronic arthritis, chronic synovitis, neurocognitive disorders, chronic fatigue, or any combination of these findings.

The diagnosis of Lyme disease is based largely on the presence of classic erythema migrans in a patient with a history of possible tick exposure in an endemic area or the presence of one or more findings of disseminated infection (e.g., nervous system, cardiovascular system, or joint involvement) and positive serology. Serologic testing is done in two stages. The first test to perform is an enzyme-linked immunosorbent assay (ELISA) for IgM and IgG antibodies to *B. burgdorferi*. If this test is reactive or indeterminate, it needs to be confirmed with a second test, a Western blot. If the patient has been ill for longer than 1 month, only IgG is assayed because an isolated positive IgM antibody level is probably a false-positive finding at this stage. Patients from highly endemic areas with the classic findings of stage 1 disease, including erythema migrans, can be treated without serologic confirmation because testing may be falsely negative at this early stage.[41]

First-line treatment of early or disseminated Lyme disease, in the absence of neurologic involvement, is oral doxycycline for 14 to 21 days. The second-line agent for use in children 8 years of age or younger and pregnant women is amoxicillin. An equally effective third choice is cefuroxime axetil. Each of these oral agents provides a cure in more than 90% of patients.[38] If the patient has any evidence of neuroborreliosis, treatment consists of daily IV ceftriaxone for 14 to 28 days. Similarly, patients with cardiac manifestations are treated via the IV route for at least part of their course and undergo cardiac monitoring if atrioventricular nodal block is significant (i.e., PR interval > 0.3 second). Oral antibiotics for 30 to 60 days or IV therapy for 30 days is usually effective for Lyme arthritis, although approximately 10% of patients will have persistent joint complaints after treatment.[39] Persistent arthritis in these nonresponders after antibiotic therapy is thought to be autoimmune-mediated because the spirochete has been eradicated.[42] Treatment of persistent arthritis after antibiotic therapy consists of anti-inflammatory agents or arthroscopic synovectomy.

Decisions to treat a victim of a tick bite prophylactically to prevent Lyme disease are controversial. Some authors condemn such an approach given the low (~1.4%) risk for transmission after a tick bite, even in an endemic area.[39] Research has shown, however, that a single dose of doxycycline, 200 mg orally given within 72 hours of a tick bite, can further reduce the already low risk of disease transmission.[38,43] A recent vaccine against Lyme disease has been withdrawn from the market because of adverse drug reactions. The best prevention for tick-borne diseases such as Lyme disease is the use of insect repellent and frequent body checks for ticks when traveling through their habitat.

## Hymenoptera

Most arthropod envenomation occurs by species belonging to the order Hymenoptera, which includes bees, wasps, yellow jackets, hornets, and stinging ants. In the United States, the order Hymenoptera accounts for most human fatalities, more than snake and mammalian bites combined. The winged Hymenoptera are located throughout the United States, whereas the so-called fire ants are currently limited to the southeastern and southwestern regions. The Africanized honeybee, which characteristically attacks in massive numbers, has recently migrated into the southwestern United States.

### Toxicology

Hymenopterans sting humans defensively, especially if their nests are disturbed. The stingers of most hymenopterans are attached to venom sacs located on the abdomen and can be used repeatedly. Some bees, however, have barb-shaped stingers that prevent detachment from the victim and thus render the bees capable of only a single sting. Hymenoptera venom contains vasoactive compounds such as histamine and serotonin, which are responsible for the local reaction and pain. The venom also contain peptides, such as melitin, and enzymes, primarily phospholipases and hyaluronidases, which are highly allergenic and elicit an IgE-mediated response in some victims.[44] Fire ant venom consists primarily of nonallergenic alkaloids that release histamine and cause a mild local necrosis. Allergenic proteins constitute only 0.1% of fire ant venom.

### Clinical Reactions

A Hymenoptera sting in a nonallergic individual produces immediate pain followed by a wheal and flare reaction. Fire ants characteristically produce multiple pustules from repetitive stings at the same site. Multiple Hymenoptera stings can produce a toxic reaction characterized by vomiting, diarrhea, generalized edema, cardiovascular collapse, and hemolysis, which can be difficult to distinguish from an acute anaphylactic reaction.

Large exaggerated local reactions develop in approximately 17% of envenomed subjects.[44] These reactions are manifested as erythematous, edematous, painful, and pruritic areas larger than 10 cm in diameter and may last 2 to 5 days. The precise pathophysiology of such reactions remains unclear, although they may partly be IgE-mediated.[45] Patients in whom large local reactions develop are at risk for similar episodes with future stings, but do not appear to be at increased risk for systemic allergic reactions.

Bee sting anaphylaxis develops in 0.3% to 3% of the general population and is responsible for approximately 40 reported deaths annually in the United States.[44] Fatalities occur most often in adults, usually within 1 hour of the sting. Symptoms generally occur within minutes and range from mild urticaria and angioedema to respiratory arrest secondary to airway edema and bronchospasm, and finally cardiovascular collapse. A positive IgE-mediated skin test to Hymenoptera extract helps predict an allergic sting reaction.

Unusual reactions to Hymenoptera stings include late-onset allergic reactions (>5 hours after the sting), serum sickness, renal disease, neurologic disorders such as Guillain-Barré syndrome, and vasculitis. The cause of these reactions is thought to be immune-mediated.

### Treatment

If a stinger has been left behind by an offending bee, it is removed as quickly as possible to prevent continued injection of venom.[46] The sting site is cleansed and locally cooled. Topical or injected lidocaine can help decrease pain from the sting. Antihistamines administered orally or topically can decrease pruritus. Blisters and pustules (typically sterile) from fire ant stings are left intact. Tetanus status is updated as needed.

Treatment of an exaggerated, local envenomation includes the aforementioned therapy in addition to elevation of the extremity and analgesics. A 5-day course of oral prednisone (1 mg/kg/day) is also recommended.[44] Isolated local reactions, typical or exaggerated, do not require epinephrine or referral for immunotherapy.

Mild anaphylaxis can be treated with 0.01 mg/kg (up to 0.5 mg) of 1:1000 (1 mg/mL, or 0.1%) intramuscular (mid-anterolateral thigh) epinephrine and an oral or parenteral antihistamine. More severe cases are also treated with steroids and may require oxygen, endotracheal intubation, IV epinephrine infusion, bronchodilators, IV fluids, or vasopressors. These patients are observed for approximately 24 hours in a monitored environment for any recurrence of severe symptoms.

Venom immunotherapy effectively prevents recurrent anaphylaxis from subsequent stings in patients with positive skin tests.[47] Those with previous severe, systemic, allergic reactions to Hymenoptera stings or in whom serum sickness develops are referred for possible immunotherapy. Referral is also recommended for adults with purely generalized dermal reactions, such as diffuse hives. Children with skin manifestations alone appear to be at relatively low risk for more serious anaphylaxis after subsequent stings and do not need referral. Patients with a history of systemic reactions resulting from Hymenoptera stings need to carry injectable epinephrine with them at all times; they also need to wear an identification medallion identifying their medical condition.

## MARINE BITES AND STINGS

Of all living creatures, 80% reside underwater. Hazardous marine animals are encountered by humans primarily in temperate or tropical seas. Exposure to marine life through recreation, research, and industry leads to frequent encounters with aquatic organisms. Injuries generally occur through bites, stings, or punctures and infrequently through electrical shock from creatures such as the torpedo ray.

### Initial Assessment

Injuries from marine organisms can range from mild local irritant skin reactions to systemic collapse from major trauma or severe envenomation. Several environmental aspects unique to marine trauma may make treatment of these patients challenging. Immersion in cold water predisposes patients to hypothermia and near-drowning. Rapid ascent after an encounter with a marine organism can cause air embolism or decompression illness in a scuba diver. Anaphylactic reaction to venom may further complicate an envenomation. Late complications include unique infections caused by a wide variety of aquatic microorganisms, as well as immune-mediated phenomena.

### Microbiology

Most marine isolates are gram-negative rods.[48] *Vibrio* spp. are of primary concern, particularly in immunocompromised hosts. In fresh water, *Aeromonas* spp. can be particularly aggressive pathogens. *Staphylococcus* and *Streptococcus* spp. are also frequently cultured from infections. The laboratory is notified that cultures are being requested for aquatic-acquired infections to alert them of the need for appropriate culture media and conditions.

### General Management

Initial management is focused on the airway, breathing, and circulation. Anaphylaxis needs to be anticipated and the victim treated accordingly. Patients with extensive blunt and penetrating injuries are managed as major trauma victims. Patients who have been envenomed receive specific intervention directed against a toxin (discussed separately, according to the marine animal), in addition to general supportive care. Antivenom can be administered, if available. Antitetanus immunization is updated after a bite, cut, or sting. Radiographs are obtained to locate foreign bodies and fractures. Magnetic resonance imaging is more useful than ultrasound or computed tomography to identify small spine fragments.

Selection of antibiotics is tailored to marine bacteriology. Third-generation cephalosporins provide adequate coverage for the gram-positive and gram-negative microorganisms found in ocean water, including *Vibrio* spp.[48] Ciprofloxacin, cefoperazone, gentamicin, and trimethoprim-sulfamethoxazole are acceptable antibiotics. Norfloxacin may be less efficacious against certain *Vibrio* spp. Other quinolones (e.g., ofloxacin, enoxacin, pefloxacin, fleroxacin, lomefloxacin, moxifloxacin) have not been extensively tested against *Vibrio* spp.; they may be useful alternatives, but this awaits definitive evaluation. Outpatient regimens include ciprofloxacin, trimethoprim-sulfamethoxazole, or doxycycline. Patients with large abrasions, lacerations, puncture wounds, or hand injuries, as well as immunocompromised patients, receive prophylactic antibiotics. Infected wounds are cultured. If a wound, commonly on the hand after a minor scrape or puncture, appears erysipeloid in nature, infection by *Erysipelothrix rhusiopathiae* is suspected. A suitable initial antibiotic based on this presumptive diagnosis would be penicillin, cephalexin, or ciprofloxacin.

### Wound Care

Meticulous wound care is necessary to reduce the risk for infection and optimize the aesthetic and functional outcomes.[49] Wounds are irrigated with normal saline. Débridement of devitalized tissue can decrease infection and promote healing. Large wounds are explored in the operating room. The decision to close a wound primarily must balance the cosmetic result against the risk for infection. Wounds are loosely closed and drainage allowed. Primary closure is avoided with distal extremity wounds, punctures, and crush injuries. For shark wounds, postoperative management may be prolonged and complicated by acute renal failure attributed to hypovolemia and shock, massive blood transfusion, myoglobinuria, and administration of nephrotoxic antibiotics. Rehabilitation may include the creation of prosthetic devices.

### Antivenom

Antivenom is available for several types of envenomation, including those from the box jellyfish, sea snake, and stonefish.[50] Patients demonstrating severe reactions to such envenomation benefit from antivenom. Skin testing to determine which patients might benefit from pretreatment with diphenhydramine or epinephrine can be performed before antivenom is administered, but it is not an absolute predictor of severe reactions. Ovine-derived antivenom (Commonwealth Serum Laboratories, King of Prussia, Pa) to treat severe *Chironex fleckeri* (box jellyfish) envenomation has been administered intramuscularly by field rescuers for many years without reports of a serious adverse reaction. Serum sickness is a complication of antivenom therapy and can be treated with corticosteroids. Regional poison control centers or major marine aquariums can sometimes assist in locating antivenom.

### Injuries from Nonvenomous Aquatic Animals

#### Sharks

Approximately 50 to 100 shark attacks are reported annually. However, these attacks cause fewer than 10 deaths/year.[49,51] Tiger, great white, gray reef, and bull sharks are responsible for most attacks. Most incidents occur at the surface of shallow water within 100 feet of the shore.[40] Sharks locate prey by detecting motion, electrical fields, and sounds and by sensing body fluids through smell and taste. Most sharks bite the victim once and then leave. Most injuries occur to the lower extremities.

Powerful jaws and sharp teeth produce crushing, tearing injuries. Hypovolemic shock and near-drowning are life-threatening consequences of an attack.[49] Other complications include soft tissue and neurovascular damage, bone fractures, and infection.[51] Most wounds require exploration and repair in the operating room (see the section on wound care). Radiographs may reveal one or more shark teeth in the wound.

Occasionally, bumping by sharks can produce abrasions, which are treated as second-degree burns.

### Moray Eels

Morays are bottom dwellers that reside in holes or crevices. Eels bite defensively and produce multiple small puncture wounds and, rarely, gaping lacerations. The hand is most frequently bitten. Occasionally, the eel remains attached to the victim, with decapitation of the animal required for release. Puncture wounds and bites on the hand from all animals, including eels, are at high risk for infection and must not be closed primarily if the capability exists for delayed primary closure.

### Alligators and Crocodiles

Crocodiles can attain a length of more than 20 feet and travel at speeds of 20 mph in water and on land. Like sharks, alligators and crocodiles attack primarily in shallow water. These animals can produce severe injuries by grasping victims with their powerful jaws and dragging them underwater, where they roll while crushing their prey. Injuries from alligator and crocodile attacks are treated like shark bites.

### Miscellaneous

Other nonvenomous animals capable of attacking include the barracuda, giant grouper, sea lion, mantis shrimp, triggerfish, needlefish, and freshwater piranha. Except for the needlefish, which spears a human victim with its elongated snout, these animals bite. Barracuda are attracted to shiny objects and have bitten fingers, wrists, scalps, or dangling legs adorned with reflective jewelry.

## Envenomation by Invertebrates

### Coelenterates

The phylum Coelenterata consists of hydrozoans, which include fire coral, hydroids, and Portuguese man-of-war, scyphozoans, which include jellyfish and sea nettles, and anthozoans, which include sea anemones. Coelenterates carry specialized living stinging cells called cnidocytes that encapsulate intracytoplasmic stinging organelles called cnidae, which include nematocysts.[52]

Mild envenomation, typically inflicted by fire coral, hydroids, and anemones, produces skin irritation.[50] The victim notices immediate stinging followed by pruritus, paresthesias, and throbbing pain with proximal radiation. Edema and erythema develop in the involved area, followed by blisters and petechiae. This can progress to local infection and ulceration.

Severe envenomation is caused by anemones, sea nettles, and jellyfish.[50] Patients have systemic symptoms in addition to the local manifestations. An anaphylactic reaction to the venom may contribute to the pathophysiology of envenomation. Fever, nausea, vomiting, and malaise can develop. Any organ system can be involved, and death is attributed to hypotension and cardiorespiratory arrest. One of the most venomous sea creatures, found primarily off the coast of northern Australia, is the box jellyfish *C. fleckeri*. In the United States, *Physalia physalis*, *Chiropsalmus quadrigatus*, and *Cyanea capillata* are substantial stingers.

Therapy consists of detoxification of nematocysts and systemic support. Dilute (5%) acetic acid (vinegar) can inactivate most coelenterate toxins and is applied for 30 minutes or until the pain is relieved.[50] This is critical with the box jellyfish. If a detoxicant is not available, the wound may be rinsed in seawater and gently dried.[50] Fresh water and vigorous rubbing can cause nematocysts to discharge. For a sting from the box jellyfish, Australian authorities previously recommended the pressure immobilization technique. This is no longer recommended. Instead, the envenomed limb is kept as motionless as possible and the victim is promptly taken to a setting in which antivenom and advanced life support are available.

To decontaminate other jellyfish stings, isopropyl alcohol is used only if vinegar is ineffective. Baking soda may be more effective than acetic acid for inactivating the toxin of U.S. eastern coastal Chesapeake Bay sea nettles.[50] Baking soda must not be applied after vinegar without a brisk saline or water rinse in between application of the two substances to avoid an exothermic reaction. Powdered or solubilized papain (meat tenderizer) may be more effective than other remedies for sea bather's eruption (often misnamed sea lice) caused by thimble jellyfishes or larval forms of certain sea anemones. Fresh lime or lemon juice, household ammonia, olive oil, or sugar may be effective, depending on the species of stinging creature.

After the skin surface has been treated, any remaining nematocysts must be removed. One method is to apply shaving cream or a flour paste and shave the area with a razor. The affected area again is irrigated, dressed, and elevated. Medical care providers need to wear gloves for self-protection. Cryotherapy, local anesthetics, antihistamines, and steroids can relieve pain after the toxin is inactivated. Prophylactic antibiotics are not usually necessary. Ocean bathers can be advised to apply Safe Sea jellyfish-safe sun block (Nidaria Technology, Jordan Valley, Israel) as a preventive measure before entering the water.

### Sponges

Two syndromes occur after contact with sponges.[50] The first is an allergic plant-like contact dermatitis characterized by itching and burning within hours of contact. This dermatitis can progress to soft tissue edema, vesicle development, and joint swelling. Large areas of involvement can cause systemic toxicity with fever, nausea, and muscle cramps. The second syndrome is an irritant dermatitis after penetration of the skin with small spicules. Sponge diver's disease is actually caused by anemones that colonize the sponges rather than by the sponges themselves.

Treatment consists of washing and drying gently the affected area. Dilute (5%) acetic acid (vinegar) is applied for 30 minutes three times daily.[50] Any remaining spicules can be removed with adhesive tape. A steroid cream can be applied to the skin after decontamination. Occasionally, a systemic glucocorticoid and an antihistamine are required.

### Echinodermata

Starfish, sea urchins, and sea cucumbers are members of the phylum Echinodermata. Starfish and sea cucumbers produce venom that can cause contact dermatitis.[52] Sea cucumbers occasionally feed on coelenterates and secrete nematocysts; therefore, local therapy for coelenterates also needs to be considered. Sea urchins are covered with venomous spines capable of causing local and systemic reactions similar to those from coelenterates. First aid consists of soaking the wound in hot, but tolerable water. Residual spines can be located with soft tissue radiographs or magnetic resonance imaging. Purple skin discoloration at the site of entrance wounds may be indicative of dye leached from the surface of an extracted urchin spine. This temporary tattoo disappears in 48 hours, which often confirms the absence of a retained foreign body. A spine is removed only if it is easily accessible or closely aligned to a joint or critical neurovascular structure. Reactive fusiform digit swelling attributed to a spine near a metacarpal bone or flexor tendon sheath may be alleviated by a high-dose glucocorticoid administered in an oral 14-day tapering schedule. Retained spines may cause the formation of granulomas that are amenable to excision or intralesional injection with triamcinolone hexacetonide, 5 mg/mL.

### Mollusks

Octopuses and cone snails are the primary envenoming species in the phylum Mollusca. Most harmful cone snails are found in Indo-Pacific waters. Envenomation occurs from a detachable harpoon-like dart injected via an extensible proboscis into the victim.[50,52] Blue-ringed octopuses can bite and inject tetrodotoxin, a paralytic agent. Both species can produce local symptoms such as burning and paresthesias. Systemic manifestations are primarily neurologic and include bulbar dysfunction and systemic muscular paralysis. Management of the bite site is best achieved by pressure and immobilization to contain the venom. This is accomplished by applying a 15-cm-wide circumferential wrap over a gauze pad or cloth that has been placed directly over the wound. The dressing is applied at venous-lymphatic pressure, with preservation of distal arterial pulses. Once the victim has been transported to a medical facility, the bandage can be released. Treatment of systemic complications is supportive.

### Annelid Worms (Bristleworms)

Annelid worms (bristleworms) carry rows of soft, easily detached fiberglass-like spines capable of inflicting painful stings and irritant dermatitis. Inflammation may persist for up to 1 week. Visible bristles are removed with forceps and adhesive tape or a commercial facial peel. Alternatively, a thin layer of rubber cement may be used to trap the spines and then peel them away. Household vinegar, rubbing alcohol, or dilute household ammonia may provide additional relief. Local inflammation is treated with a topical or systemic glucocorticoid.

## Envenomation by Vertebrates

### Stingrays

Rays are bottom dwellers ranging from a few inches to 12 feet long (tip to tail). Venom is stored in whiplike caudal appendages. Stingrays react defensively by thrusting their spines into a victim, causing puncture wounds and lacerations. The most common site of injury is the lower part of the leg and top of the foot. Local damage can be severe, with occasional penetration of body cavities. This is worsened by the vasoconstrictive properties of the venom, which produce cyanotic-appearing wounds. The venom is often myonecrotic. Systemic complaints include weakness, nausea, diarrhea, headache, and muscle cramps. The venom can cause vasoconstriction, cardiac dysrhythmias, respiratory arrest, and seizures.[53]

The wound is irrigated and then soaked in nonscalding hot water (up to 45° C) for 1 hour.[53] Débridement, exploration, and removal of spines are carried out during or after hot water soaking. Immersion cryotherapy is detrimental. The wound is not closed primarily. Lacerations heal by secondary intention or are repaired by delayed closure. The wound is dressed and elevated. Pain is relieved locally or systemically. Radiography is performed to locate any remaining spines. Acute infection with aggressive pathogens is anticipated.[50] In the event of a nonhealing draining wound, retention of a foreign body is suspected.

### Miscellaneous Fish

Other fish with spines that can produce injuries similar to those of stingrays include lionfish, scorpionfish, stonefish, catfish, and weeverfish. Each can cause envenomation, puncture wounds, and lacerations, with spines transmitting venom. Clinical manifestations and therapy are similar to those pertaining to stingrays. In the case of lionfish, vesiculations are sometimes noted. An equine-derived antivenom (Commonwealth Serum Laboratories) is available for administration in case of significant stonefish envenomation.

### Sea Snakes

Sea snakes of the family Hydrophiidae appear similar to land snakes. They inhabit the Pacific and Indian Oceans. Venom produces neurologic signs and symptoms, with possible death from paralysis and respiratory arrest. Local manifestations can be minimal or absent. Therapy is similar to that for coral snake (Elapidae) bites. The pressure immobilization technique is recommended in the field. Polyvalent sea snake antivenom is administered if any signs of envenomation develop.[53] The initial dose is one ampule, repeated as needed. Consultation with an experienced clinician, toxicologist or poison control center is recommended.

## SELECTED REFERENCES

Auerbach PS, editor: Wilderness medicine, ed 3, St Louis, 2007, CV Mosby.

This textbook is an in-depth review of wilderness medicine. Bites and stings by many organisms are discussed in detail by experts from each field. Many pertinent studies are reviewed.

Freeman TM: Clinical practice. Hypersensitivity to Hymenoptera stings. N Engl J Med 351:1978–1984, 2004.

The reactions to Hymenoptera stings are well organized in this practical monograph. The natural history of stinging insect allergy is reviewed and therapeutic considerations are discussed.

Gold BS, Dart RC, Barish RA: Bites of venomous snakes. N Engl J Med 347:347–356, 2002.

This article is a concise, practical review of snake venom poisoning in the United States. Proper use of the new North American antivenom is well summarized.

Isbister GK, Graudins A, White J, Warrell D: Antivenom treatment in arachnidism. J Toxicol Clin Toxicol 41:291–300, 2003.

This piece is an excellent review of the use of antivenom in spider bites around the world.

Mebs D: Venomous and poisonous animals, Boca Raton, Fla, 2002, CRC Press.

This book is a superbly illustrated collection of fascinating, detailed information about venoms and poisons in the animal kingdom, including marine and terrestrial animals.

Steere AC: Medical progress: Lyme disease. N Engl J Med 345:115–125, 2001.

This manuscript is a thorough review of the current understanding of Lyme borreliosis and clearly outlines diagnosis and treatment.

Swanson DL, Vetter RS: Bites of brown recluse spiders and suspected necrotic arachnidism. N Engl J Med 352:700–707, 2005.

This article is an excellent review of necrotic arachnidism, including the approach to diagnosis and management.

Williamson JA, Fenner PJ, Burnett JW, editors: Venomous and poisonous marine animals, Sydney, Australia, 1996, University of New South Wales Press.

This book is a superb reference, with a complete discussion of all common and uncommon toxic marine animals.

## REFERENCES


1. Warrell DA, Fenner PJ: Venomous bites and stings. Br Med Bull 49:423–439, 1993.
2. Parrish HM: Incidence of treated snakebites in the United States. Public Health Rep 81:269–276, 1966.
3. Ownby CL: Pathology of rattlesnake envenomation. In Tu AT, editor: Rattlesnake venoms, New York, 1982, Marcel Dekker, pp 164–169.
4. Hutton RA, Warrell DA: Action of snake venom components on the haemostatic system. Blood Rev 7:176–189, 1993.
5. Russell FE, Carlson RW, Wainschel J, et al: Snake venom poisoning in the United States. Experiences with 550 cases. JAMA 233:341–344, 1975.
6. Wingert WA, Chan L: Rattlesnake bites in southern California and rationale for recommended treatment. West J Med 148:37–44, 1988.
7. German BT, Hack JB, Brewer K, et al: Pressure-immobilization bandages delay toxicity in a porcine model of eastern coral snake (Micrurus fulvius fulvius) envenomation. Ann Emerg Med 45:603–608, 2005.
8. Stewart RM, Page CP, Schwesinger WH, et al: Antivenin and fasciotomy/debridement in the treatment of the severe rattlesnake bite. Am J Surg 158:543–547, 1989.
9. Consroe P, Egen NB, Russell FE, et al: Comparison of a new ovine antigen binding fragment (Fab) antivenin for United States Crotalidae with the commercial antivenin for protection against venom-induced lethality in mice. Am J Trop Med Hyg 53: 507–510, 1995.
10. Dart RC, Seifert SA, Carroll L, et al: Affinity-purified, mixed monospecific crotalid antivenom ovine Fab for the treatment of crotalid venom poisoning. Ann Emerg Med 30:33–39, 1997.
11. Gold BS, Dart RC, Barish RA: Bites of venomous snakes. N Engl J Med 347:347–356, 2002.
12. Corneille MG, Larson S, Stewart RM, et al: A large single-center experience with treatment of patients with crotalid envenomations: Outcomes with and evolution of antivenin therapy. Am J Surg 192:848–852, 2006.
13. Clark RF, Selden BS, Furbee B: The incidence of wound infection following crotalid envenomation. J Emerg Med 11:583–586, 1993.
14. Kerrigan KR, Mertz BL, Nelson SJ, et al: Antibiotic prophylaxis for pit viper envenomation: Prospective, controlled trial. World J Surg 21:369–372; discussion 372–363, 1997.
15. Bogdan GM, Dart RC, Falbo SC, et al: Recurrent coagulopathy after antivenom treatment of crotalid snakebite. South Med J 93:562–566, 2000.
16. Garfin SR, Castilonia RR, Mubarak SJ, et al: Role of surgical decompression in treatment of rattlesnake bites. Surg Forum 30:502–504, 1979.
17. Tanen DA, Danish DC, Grice GA, et al: Fasciotomy worsens the amount of myonecrosis in a porcine model of crotaline envenomation. Ann Emerg Med 44:99–104, 2004.
18. Centers for Disease Control and Prevention (CDC): Nonfatal dog bite-related injuries treated in hospital emergency departments—United States, 2001. MMWR Morb Mortal Wkly Rep 52:605–610, 2003.
19. Chen E, Hornig S, Shepherd SM, et al: Primary closure of mammalian bites. Acad Emerg Med 7:157–161, 2000.
20. Stefanopoulos PK, Tarantzopoulou AD: Facial bite wounds: Management update. Int J Oral Maxillofac Surg 34:464–472, 2005.
21. Callaham M: Prophylactic antibiotics in common dog bite wounds: A controlled study. Ann Emerg Med 9:410–414, 1980.
22. Perron AD, Miller MD, Brady WJ: Orthopedic pitfalls in the ED: Fight bite. Am J Emerg Med 20:114–117, 2002.
23. Broder J, Jerrard D, Olshaker J, et al: Low risk of infection in selected human bites treated without antibiotics. Am J Emerg Med 22:10–13, 2004.
24. Vidmar L, Poljak M, Tomazic J, et al: Transmission of HIV-1 by human bite. Lancet 347:1762, 1996.
25. World Health Organization: Rabies surveillance and control: The world survey of rabies. No. 35 for the year 1999, 2002 (http://www.who.int/rabies/resources/wsr1999/en).
26. Krebs JW, Wheeling JT, Childs JE: Rabies surveillance in the United States during 2002. J Am Vet Med Assoc 223:1736–1748, 2003.
27. Use of a reduced (4-dose) vaccine schedule for postexposure prophylaxis to prevent human rabies: recommendations of the advisory committee on immunization practices. Morbidity and Mortality Weekly Report. 59:RR-2. March 19, 2010.
28. Isbister GK, Graudins A, White J, et al: Antivenom treatment in arachnidism. J Toxicol Clin Toxicol 41:291–300, 2003.
29. Sams HH, Dunnick CA, Smith ML, et al: Necrotic arachnidism. J Am Acad Dermatol 44:561–573, 2001.
30. Swanson DL, Vetter RS: Bites of brown recluse spiders and suspected necrotic arachnidism. N Engl J Med 352:700–707, 2005.
31. King LE, Jr, Rees RS: Dapsone treatment of a brown recluse bite. JAMA 250:648, 1983.
32. Tutrone WD, Green KM, Norris T, et al: Brown recluse spider envenomation: Dermatologic application of hyperbaric oxygen therapy. J Drugs Dermatol 4:424–428, 2005.
33. LoVecchio F, McBride C: Scorpion envenomations in young children in central Arizona. J Toxicol Clin Toxicol 41:937–940, 2003.
34. Gateau T, Bloom M, Clark R: Response to specific Centruroides sculpturatus antivenom in 151 cases of scorpion stings. J Toxicol Clin Toxicol 32:165–171, 1994.
35. Stewart RL, Burgdorfer W, Needham GR: Evaluation of three commercial tick removal tools. Wilderness Environ Med 9:137–142, 1998.

**36.** Metry DW, Hebert AA: Insect and arachnid stings, bites, infestations, and repellents. Pediatr Ann 29:39–48, 2000.

**37.** Montiel NJ, Baumgarten JM, Sinha AA: Lyme disease—part II: Clinical features and treatment. Cutis 69:443–448, 2002.

**38.** Steere AC: Lyme disease. N Engl J Med 345:115–125, 2001.

**39.** Shapiro ED, Gerber MA: Lyme disease. Clin Infect Dis 31:533–542, 2000.

**40.** Steere AC: A 58-year-old man with a diagnosis of chronic lyme disease. JAMA 288:1002–1010, 2002.

**41.** DePietropaolo DL, Powers JH, Gill JM, et al: Diagnosis of lyme disease. Am Fam Physician 72:297–304, 2005.

**42.** Dinser R, Jendro MC, Schnarr S, et al: Antibiotic treatment of Lyme borreliosis: What is the evidence? Ann Rheum Dis 64:519–523, 2005.

**43.** Nadelman RB, Nowakowski J, Fish D, et al: Prophylaxis with single-dose doxycycline for the prevention of Lyme disease after an Ixodes scapularis tick bite. N Engl J Med 345:79–84, 2001.

**44.** Wright DN, Lockey RF: Local reactions to stinging insects (Hymenoptera). Allergy Proc 11:23–28, 1990.

**45.** Reisman RE: Insect stings. N Engl J Med 331:523–527, 1994.

**46.** Visscher PK, Vetter RS, Camazine S: Removing bee stings. Lancet 348:301–302, 1996.

**47.** Freeman TM: Clinical practice. Hypersensitivity to hymenoptera stings. N Engl J Med 351:1978–1984, 2004.

**48.** Williamson JA, Fenner PJ, Burnett JW, editors: Venomous and poisonous marine animals, Sydney, 1996, University of New South Wales Press.

**49.** Howard RJ, Burgess GH: Surgical hazards posed by marine and freshwater animals in Florida. Am J Surg 166:563–567, 1993.

**50.** Barber GR, Swygert JS: Necrotizing fasciitis due to Photobacterium damsela in a man lashed by a stingray. N Engl J Med 342:824, 2000.

**51.** Guidera KJ, Ogden JA, Highhouse K, et al: Shark attack. J Orthop Trauma 5:204–208, 1991.

**52.** McGoldrick J, Marx JA: Marine envenomations. Part 2: Invertebrates. J Emerg Med 10:71–77, 1992.

**53.** McGoldrick J, Marx JA: Marine envenomations: Part 1: Vertebrates. J Emerg Med 9:497–502, 1991.

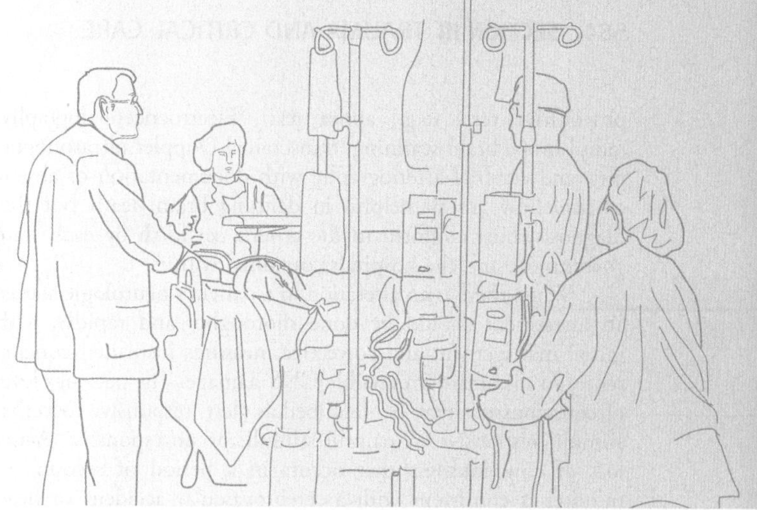

CHAPTER 23

# SURGICAL CRITICAL CARE

CHARLES A. ADAMS, JR., ANDREW STEPHEN, AND WILLIAM G. CIOFFI



The goal of surgical therapy, elective or urgent, is to enable patients to return to their preoperative state of health and functional status. However, some patients have surgical processes or injuries that are so severe that they would either not survive or would suffer significant long-term morbidity without specialized supportive care. These types of patients require multisystem surgical critical care delivered by specialized teams of trained health care providers in an intensive care unit (ICU). Although many of these ICUs are closed units or structured so that patient management decisions are made solely by the critical care team, it is important that surgeons remain current and acquainted with the ever-changing field of surgical critical care so that they can remain a vital part of the patient's health care team, especially in systems or institutions in which critical care of surgical patients is being delivered by nonsurgical specialists. In this chapter, we will approach the vast topic of surgical critical care in a system-based fashion and highlight recent developments and concepts.

## CENTRAL NERVOUS SYSTEM

### Neurologic Dysfunction

The central nervous system (CNS) is the most complex organ system in the body and is vulnerable to disturbances by a host of conditions and factors. The causes of an altered consciousness are so broad that a clouded sensorium is the norm in the ICU rather than the exception. This list of conscious-altering causes includes endogenous and exogenous factors. Some endogenous causes include sepsis, CNS infections, hypoxic-ischemic encephalopathy, tumors, trauma, electrolyte derangements, and metabolic conditions, whereas exogenous causes can include medications, environmental settings, and toxins. Any unexplained changes in a surgical patient's level of consciousness or sensorium should be worked up thoroughly. Ascribing such changes to ICU psychosis should be considered strictly a diagnosis of exclusion.[1] The term *altered mental status* is nonspecific and more descriptive definitions were offered by Plum and Posner almost 30 years ago in their text on stupor and coma and still apply today. The term *confusion* encompasses bewilderment, difficulty following commands, disturbed memory, and drowsiness or nighttime agitation, whereas delirium is a floridly abnormal mental state characterized by disorientation, fear, irritability, misperception of sensory stimuli and, often, visual hallucinations.

The presence of delirium can have far-reaching consequences and is associated with increased hospital length of stay and mortality.[2] Obtundation is defined as mental blunting associated with slowed psychological responses to stimulation. Stupor is described as a condition of deep sleep or behaviorally similar unresponsiveness in which the patient can be aroused only by vigorous and repeated stimuli. Coma is a state of unarousable psychological unresponsiveness in which the subject lies with eyes closed and shows no psychologically understandable response to external stimuli or inner need. A vegetative state is a state of wakefulness but with apparent complete lack of cognitive function. Death in the presence of cardiopulmonary function (brain death) refers to the absence of function of the brain and brainstem; there are specific criteria for this, but the absence of cerebral function is paramount. Cortical nonfunction must be accompanied by the loss of reflexes to pupillary light and corneal stimulation, loss of the vestibulo-ocular and oropharyngeal reflexes, and apnea in the presence of adequate stimulation ($Paco_2 > 60$ mm Hg for 30 seconds). Generally, two clinical examinations must be documented, separated by a defined time interval (e.g., 6 hours) and confirmed by independent physicians; however, there is no nationally accepted definition of brain death. It is important that there be a reason or physiologic insult sufficient to cause death and there are no complicating or reversible conditions (e.g., recent administration of sedative or anesthetic agents, hypothermia, hypo- or hyperglycemia, or severe hypo- or hypernatremia, or other significant metabolic derangements) that could interfere with brain death determination. If such complicating conditions preclude the completion of a clinical examination, additional tests are required, including provocative tests (e.g., apnea test). Electroencephalography, radioisotope brain scanning, transcranial Doppler ultrasonography, and cerebral arteriography with documentation of absent cortical flow are all helpful in defining brain death but this diagnosis must conform to the criteria set forth by each state government and the hospitals contained within.

When there is an alteration in a patient's neurologic status, an assessment should be done thoroughly and rapidly, with initial management and corrective measures instituted concurrently to minimize irreversible CNS damage. The patient's level of consciousness may be described as alert, responsive to verbal stimuli, responsive to painful stimuli, or unresponsive. Acute loss of consciousness that occurs in a period of seconds to minutes is consistent with a cerebrovascular accident or head trauma. A subacute course that occurs in many minutes to hours may suggest intoxication, infection, or a metabolic disturbance, whereas a more prolonged course of neurologic decline may suggest a CNS tumor. The pupillary examination can be particularly informative. Damage to the midbrain affects the reticular activating system, and thus consciousness, as well as pupil reactivity, whereas metabolic disease may produce coma but usually leaves the light reflex intact. Small reactive pupils are the hallmark of drug intoxication (particularly opiate) and metabolic disease, whereas large unreactive pupils may be associated with anticholinergic drugs, glutethimide, anoxia, or intracranial hypertension. A unilateral fixed and dilated pupil suggests third nerve dysfunction or uncal herniation. In the absence of purposeful eye movements, spontaneous roving eye movements imply intact cortical control of the brainstem. If no spontaneous eye movement is found, the vestibulo-ocular reflex (doll's eye maneuver) should be tested after excluding a cervical cord or spine lesion. This reflex is tested by turning the head rapidly from midline to one side. Contralateral conjugate eye movement, keeping the eyes seemingly fixed on a point in space, suggests an intact brainstem. The head should be turned in the opposite direction to check for symmetry. Failure of this reflex in either direction implies brainstem dysfunction. If this maneuver cannot be done, the vestibulo-ocular reflex may be assessed by a cold caloric testing technique instead. This is done by elevating the head to 30 degrees and rapidly instilling 50 mL of ice water into the external auditory canal, which results in reflex slow eye movement toward the stimulus. In an intact brain, the frontal eye fields attempt to override this stimulus, producing rapid saccades away from the stimulus (nystagmus). Conversely, if there is cortical damage, the eyes will maintain a fixed deviation, which implies a hemispheric lesion on the side toward which the eyes deviate. Assessment of motor function helps identify the location and severity of deficits. The motor component of the Glasgow Coma Scale is the most predictive portion of the scale following head trauma. Asymmetry of motor function suggests a focal cerebral lesion contralateral to the deficit. Decorticate (flexion of arms and extension of legs) and decerebrate (extension of both arms and legs) posturing are very poor prognostic signs.

Although it is important for staff physicians and surgical house personnel to become comfortable and proficient with the neurologic examination of critically ill and ventilated patients, it is tremendously beneficial when nurses provide frequent objective evaluations and can relay any significant changes to the surgical team, especially regarding states of delirium or confusion. ICU nurses generally care for limited numbers of patients simultaneously and thus are able to perform these evaluations on a frequent basis. The confusion assessment method for identifying ICU delirium (CAM-ICU) is a rapid, objective measuring tool to determine the presence of delirium and can be performed serially with relative ease.[2] CAM-ICU is straightforward and addresses whether there is an acute or fluctuating onset of a patient's mental status change or delirium, general inattention, disorganized thought, or altered level of consciousness. The mean time required for each CAM-ICU assessment is less than 1 minute and can be performed by any trained health care provider (e.g., physician, nurse, respiratory therapist); its reliability and accuracy has been validated in prospective cohort studies weighed against the standard of evaluations of delirium experts using criteria from the *Diagnostic and Statistical Manual of Mental Disorders*. The importance of a tool such as CAM-ICU lies in its ability to identify delirium quickly, accurately, and easily so that appropriate drug therapy may be instituted.

Laboratory studies also can help identify metabolic derangements such as hypothyroidism, electrolyte abnormalities, infections, and toxic ingestions. Urine toxicology screening is mandatory because drug intoxication is one of the most common initial causes of coma of unknown cause. Arterial blood gas (ABG) analysis should be performed to rule out hypoxia, hypercarbia, or acidosis as a cause of an altered mental state. Computed tomography (CT) is indicated for any patient with coma and focal neurologic findings or in patients with a depressed level of consciousness that prevents an adequate physical examination from being carried out. A lumbar puncture should be performed on any patient for whom the cause of coma is still unknown, especially patients in whom meningitis, encephalitis, or occult subarachnoid hemorrhage is suspected. In the post–head injury or neurosurgical postoperative patient, clinical deterioration in the absence of a new structural lesion (i.e., CT scan finding) coupled with signs of infection (e.g., fever, leukocytosis) may be a sign of CNS infection and a lumbar puncture is warranted.

Initial management begins with assurance of a patent ***a***irway and adequate ***b***reathing and ***c***irculation (the ABCs, as taught by the Advance Trauma Life Support program). Comatose patients should be intubated for airway protection; however, stability of the cervical spine must be ensured in trauma patients. If there is a possibility of increased intracranial pressure (ICP), lidocaine (1.5 mg/kg) or thiopental (3 to 5 mg/kg) should be administered to blunt sudden rises in ICP associated with intubation. Hypotension should be corrected promptly and aggressively with fluids and/or vasopressors to maintain an adequate cerebral perfusion pressure (CPP) of at least 55 to 60 mm Hg. CPP is calculated as the difference between a patient's mean arterial pressure (MAP) and intracranial pressure (CPP = MAP − ICP). A dose of 50 mL of 50% dextrose should be given immediately to any patient with coma of unknown cause . This will produce no detrimental effect on any causes of coma except Wernicke's encephalopathy (see later) and will correct the underlying problem if it is secondary to hypoglycemia. Even in those patients with hyperglycemia producing the coma, a marginal increase in the glucose concentration will not adversely affect the patient; however, the effects of any significant period of marked hypoglycemia may result in irreversible neurologic damage. In alcoholic patients or others with poor general nutrition, thiamine (1 mg/kg) should be administered before glucose. This may avoid acute Wernicke's encephalopathy (confusion, ataxia, ophthalmoplegia) and its associated necrosis of midline gray matter.

Narcotic overdose is a common cause of coma and is marked by shallow respirations, small reactive pupils, and hypotension. Naloxone (Narcan; 0.4 to 2 mg) is an opioid antagonist and should be given to patients with suspected opiate-induced coma. Flumazenil (0.2 mg) may be administered for suspected benzodiazepine intoxication, but care should be exercised in patients taking benzodiazepines on a chronic basis or suspected mixed ingestions because other agents may lower the seizure threshold, leading to severe seizures following flumazenil administration. Activated charcoal (25 to 50 mg) should be given for the ingestion of most drugs and toxins, but its effectiveness diminishes as the interval from ingestion to administration increases. Empirical antibiotic therapy directed at suspected demographic-associated pathogens is warranted if bacterial meningitis is suspected.

If increased ICP is assumed to be the cause of coma, treatment should be initiated immediately with elevation of the head of the bed to 30 to 45 degrees. Hyperventilation is effective in lowering the ICP, but prolonged or extreme hyperventilation can lead to cerebral vasoconstriction and detrimental regional ischemia. Also, it is likely that the vasoconstricting effects of hyperventilation to decrease ICP are lost within 24 hours as the cerebral circulation reflexively normalizes with the new lower $Paco_2$. Thus, a target $Paco_2$ of 35 to 40 mmHg is considered optimal and there is unlikely benefit of lower levels of $Paco_2$. Vasogenic cerebral edema leads to increased ICP according to the Monro-Kellie hypothesis, which states that the pressure inside the head must rise if any intracranial component increases (e.g., blood, brain, cerebrospinal fluid) because the cranial vault is a rigid, nonexpansive structure. Accordingly, the osmotic diuretic mannitol (0.5 to 1 g/kg) should be administered; this may be repeated every 4 to 6 hours as long as the serum sodium level and osmolarity remain less than 155 and 320 mmol/liter, respectively. However, mannitol should be avoided in situations in which such diuresis may compromise hemodynamics by decreasing the MAP and, in turn, the patient's CPP. Hypertonic saline 3% and, more recently, saline 23.4% have also been shown to be effective and safe therapies for managing intracranial hypertension via osmotic mechanisms without compromising the MAP as the way diuretics tend to do. Currently, most studies comparing hypertonic saline to mannitol are retrospective; thus, more randomized prospective investigation is warranted. Other factors involved in managing ICP include adequate sedation and suppression of fever and seizures. If the patient has refractory intracranial hypertension, second-tier therapies should be used, including ventriculostomy drainage, neuromuscular blockade, vasopressors to increase CPP, barbiturate coma, and decompressive craniectomy.

Seizure activity is often the first sign of a CNS complication. Because most seizures terminate rapidly, the most important initial intervention is protecting the patient from harm, most notably failure to protect the airway and self-injury. The cause of the seizures should be investigated and treated. CT scanning or magnetic resonance imaging (MRI) of the brain is indicated for new-onset seizures, and electroencephalograms should be obtained to exclude status epilepticus in patients who have persistent or recurrent seizures or who do not awaken after seizure activity. Status epilepticus should be treated with benzodiazepines, such as lorazepam (0.1 mg/kg), followed by phenytoin (1 g). If this regimen is unsuccessful in breaking the seizure activity, second-tier therapies should be administered, such as high-dose benzodiazepines, barbiturates, or propofol. The major systemic complications of seizures are rhabdomyolysis, hyperthermia, and cerebral edema.

## Analgesia, Sedation, and Neuromuscular Blockade

Pain and anxiety are common in ICU patients. Pain may be caused by an underlying disease state, trauma, invasive procedures, or surgical wounds. Pain is exacerbated by nursing interventions, invasive monitoring, therapeutic devices, immobility, and mechanical ventilation. Unrelieved pain can provoke a sympathetic stress response, as well as contribute to agitation and metabolic stress. Unfortunately, the severity of pain is often underappreciated in the ICU and consequently may be treated suboptimally. A universal goal for physicians is ensuring an optimal level of comfort and safety for all patients.

### Pain Assessment and Management

Perception of pain is influenced by prior experiences, negative expectations, and the cognitive capacity of the patient. The patient and family should be advised of the potential for pain and strategies to communicate pain. Patient self-reporting is the gold standard for the assessment of pain and the adequacy of analgesia. Pain assessment tools such as the visual analogue scale or numeric rating scale are most useful. In noncommunicative patients, assessment of behavioral (e.g., movements, facial expressions, posturing) and physiologic (e.g., heart rate, blood pressure, respiratory rate) indicators are necessary. It is paramount that the surgical staff and house officers communicate effectively with ICU nurses because their frequent assessments of pain consistently seem to lead to earlier and timelier administration of pain medications. Nurse-driven protocols for pain assessment and management have been shown to reduce ventilator days and ICU length of stay while at the same time providing patients with good pain relief.[3] The key concepts of nurse-driven protocols in the ICU are that they not only allow for but encourage nursing staff to use and hone their clinical assessment skills, especially useful because they have almost continuous interaction with their patients.

Opiates are the mainstay of pain management in the ICU. Nonpharmacologic interventions such as a comfortable environment, paying attention to positioning, arrangement of tubing and drains, and avoiding unnecessary noise, should be used as adjuncts to pain management. Opiates are particularly useful in the ICU because most have a rapid onset of action, are easily titrated, lack an accumulation of parent drug or active metabolites, and are relatively inexpensive. The most commonly prescribed opiates are morphine, fentanyl, and hydromorphone. Fentanyl has a rapid onset of action, a short half-life, and generates no active metabolites. It is ideal for use in hemodynamically unstable patients because it does not cause histamine release and its resultant vasodilatation, which can worsen hypotension. Continuous infusions of fentanyl have been associated with accumulation in lipid stores, resulting in a prolonged effect, and high doses have been associated with muscle rigidity syndromes. Morphine has a slower onset of action and longer half-life and may not be suitable for hemodynamically unstable patients because of its potential to cause histamine release and hypotension. This histaminergic effect is also responsible for morphine's propensity to cause pruritus. An active metabolite of morphine,

morphine-6-glucuronide, can accumulate in patients with renal insufficiency and lead to undesirable, continued sedating effects. Morphine also causes spasm of the sphincter of Oddi, which may be detrimental in patients with biliary tract disease or pancreatitis. Hydromorphone has a half-life similar to that of morphine, but generates no active metabolites and does not cause histamine release. It is typically used when high-dose morphine or fentanyl is ineffective or for patients in whom a large fluid volume is undesirable. To some extent, all opioid analgesics are associated with varying degrees of respiratory depression, hypotension, and ileus.

Preventing pain is more effective than treating established pain. Accordingly, continuous or scheduled intermittent dosing is preferable to as-needed (PRN) administration because ICU patients are often unable to express or advocate for their pain medication requirements. Patient-controlled analgesia (PCA) via specialized infusion pumps offers superior pain control but requires a patient to be an active participant in her or his care, which may not always be possible in the ICU setting. PCA can decrease opioid consumption, oversedation, and other adverse effects while providing good pain control. To avoid variable absorption, analgesics should be given IV to critically ill patients unless the patient is transitioning to a lower level of care. Alternatives to opioids include acetaminophen and nonsteroidal anti-inflammatory drugs (NSAIDs). Ketorolac is the prototypical IV NSAID and is an effective analgesic agent used alone or in combination with opiates. It is primarily eliminated by renal excretion, so it is relatively contraindicated for patients with renal failure, and it has been associated with bleeding complications, so its use in peptic ulcer disease or for fresh postoperative patients must be carefully weighed.

Epidural anesthesia is achieved by delivering drugs via a catheter placed in the extradural or epidural space. Many benefits of epidural anesthesia have been reported, including better suppression of surgical stress and pain, reductions in circulating levels of proinflammatory mediators, minimized hemodynamic effects, improved peripheral circulation, and reduced blood loss. A recent meta-analysis of 58 trials of thoracic and abdominal surgery in almost 6000 patients has also demonstrated that epidural opioid analgesia is associated with a decreased risk of postoperative pneumonia when compared with systemic opioid regimens; the report also cited a decreased need for prolonged mechanical ventilation and reintubation, along with improved oxygenation.[4] Patient-controlled epidural anesthesia is also possible and combines many of the benefits of PCA and epidural anesthesia.

**Table 23-1 Richmond Agitation Sedation Scale**

| SCORE | TERM | DESCRIPTION |
|---|---|---|
| +4 | Combative | Overly combative or violent; immediate danger to staff |
| +3 | Very agitated | Pulls or removes tubes or catheters; has aggressive behavior toward staff |
| +2 | Agitated | Frequent nonpurposeful movement; patient-ventilator dyssynchrony |
| +1 | Restless | Anxious or apprehensive but movements not aggressive or vigorous |
| 0 | Alert and calm | |
| −1 | Drowsy | Not fully alert, but has sustained (>10 sec) awakening with eye contact to voice |
| −2 | Light sedation | Briefly (<10 sec) awakens with eye contact to voice |
| −3 | Moderate sedation | Any movement (but no eye contact) to voice |
| −4 | Deep sedation | No response to voice, but any movement to physical stimulation |
| −5 | Unarousable | No response to voice or physical stimulation |

Adapted from Ely EW, Truman B, Shintani A, et al: Monitoring sedation status over time in ICU patients: Reliability and validity of the Richmond Agitation Sedation Scale (RASS). JAMA 289:2983–2991, 2003.

### Sedation

Inability to communicate, constant noise and light, disrupted sleep-wake cycles, various other stimuli common to the ICU setting, and immobility contribute to increased anxiety among ICU patients, which may be compounded further by mechanical ventilation. Sedation is necessary to alleviate anxiety and provide comfort, and prevent the patient from removing lines, catheters, and other necessary equipment. A predetermined sedation goal should be established and the level of sedation should be documented objectively based on a sedation scale such as the Richmond Agitation and Sedation Scale (RASS; Table 23-1). RASS is a rapid, simple construct that has been shown to detect changes in sedation in ICU patients over several days and facilitates the proper administration of analgesic and sedative medications. The nurse-driven protocols described earlier for managing pain and analgesic administration also apply to managing sedation. Much of the recent literature regarding pain and sedation protocols overlaps and also supports nurses implementing such protocols to assess and manage their patients' sedation needs actively when they are properly trained and educated about their use.[5]

The ideal level of sedation depends on the clinical situation, but a patient who is calm and easily arousable is generally considered as being appropriately sedated. Benzodiazepines have sedative and hypnotic effects, and some possess partial anterograde amnestic effects. They may potentiate opiates and moderate the pain response when used in combination with them; however, they are devoid of any analgesic properties. Diazepam, lorazepam, and midazolam are the most frequently used agents in the ICU. Diazepam has a short onset of action and short half-life, but its long-acting metabolite may accumulate following repetitive dosing. Lorazepam has a slow onset and intermediate half-life, making it most useful for medium- to long-term sedation. Lorazepam can accumulate in older patients with hepatic and renal dysfunction, resulting in prolonged sedation. Midazolam is a rapid-onset, short-acting drug with amnestic properties that can be used as an infusion or dosed intermittently; thus, it is the agent of choice for acutely agitated patients. Prolonged sedation with midazolam results in its accumulation and erratic effects and metabolism.

Propofol is a general anesthetic agent with significant sedative and hypnotic properties, but no analgesic effect. Propofol has rapid onset and an ultrashort duration of action. Its phospholipid vehicle can cause hypertriglyceridemia and pancreatitis, as well as pain, on injection. Propofol is most often used for sedation of neurosurgical patients, because it allows rapid awakening for

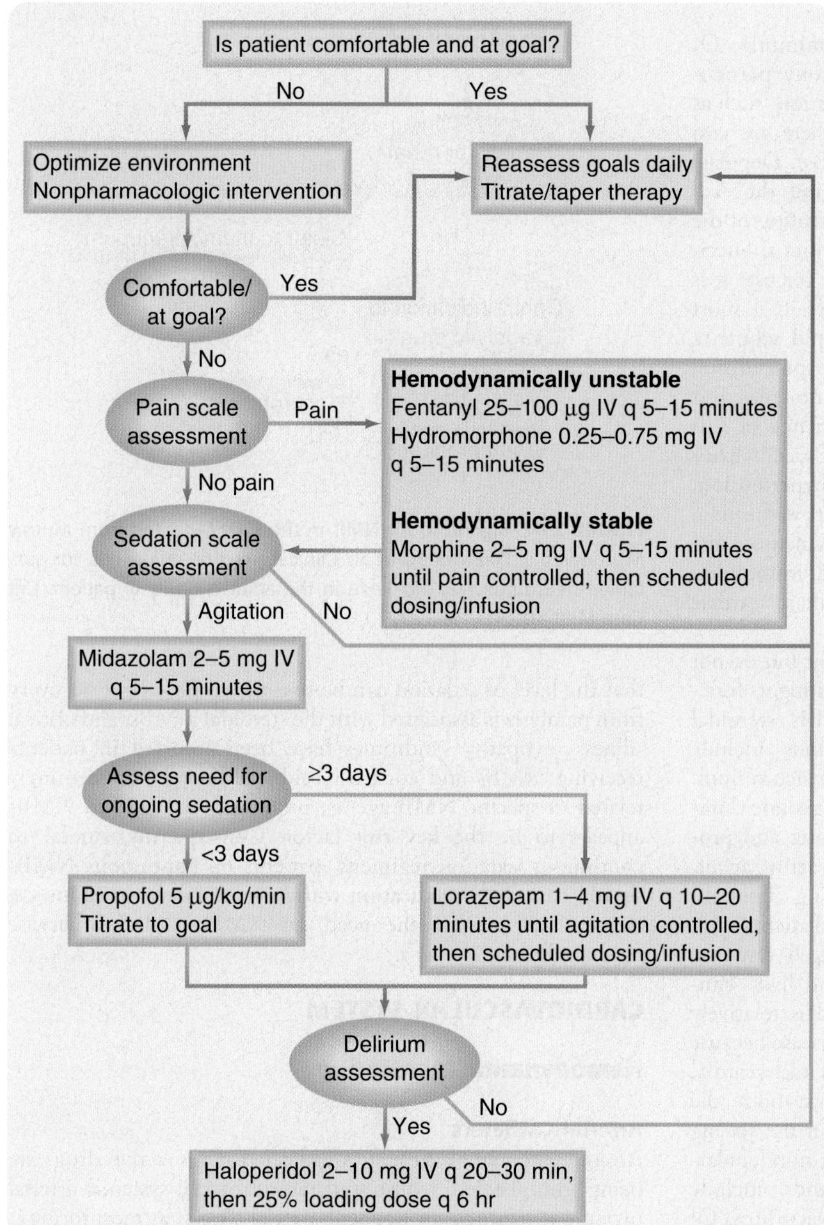


**FIGURE 23-1** Algorithm for analgesia and sedation in the ICU. (Adapted from Jacobi J, Fraser GL, Coursin DB, et al: Clinical practice guidelines for the sustained use of sedatives and analgesics in the critically ill adult. Crit Care Med 30:119–141, 2002.)

neurologic assessments and may decrease cerebral metabolism and reduce ICP. The main disadvantages of its prolonged use are its relative high cost and dose-related hypotension.

Figure 23-1 is an algorithm for the provision of analgesia and sedation in the ICU. It is important to be aware of the somewhat poorly understood propofol infusion syndrome, which manifests as rhabdomyolysis, lactic acidosis, and circulatory collapse. It is postulated that the likelihood of developing propofol infusion syndrome is increased if the patient is receiving concurrent vasopressors or steroids. The mechanism of this syndrome probably centers on decreased fatty acid metabolism coupled with damage to mitochondria, resulting in cardiac and peripheral myocyte dysfunction.

Dexmetomidine, a highly specific $\alpha_2$-adrenergic receptor agonist, has been increasingly used, especially in intubated patients, because it has been shown to decrease the amount of narcotic analgesics and sedatives that patients require while also providing a beneficial reduction in myocardial oxygen demands. Its main advantage over other agents is that it provides adequate sedation without significantly limiting a patient's respiratory drive so it can be used more easily and result in extubation.[6] Propofol and benzodiazepines are difficult to titrate to desired effect. Typically, when they are stopped in anticipation of extubation, patients become agitated to the point of requiring remedication, which may delay extubation and ventilator weaning. Recently, randomized data have shown decreased times of mechanical ventilation and ICU length of stay for patients placed on dexmedetomidine infusions for weaning from mechanical ventilation. The most significant disadvantages of using dexmedetomidine are its potential for creating hypotension and its cost, because it may be almost ten times more expensive than midazolam or propofol.

### Neuromuscular Blockade

Skeletal muscle relaxation may be warranted to minimize $O_2$ consumption or facilitate patient-ventilator synchrony, particularly when using nonconventional modes of ventilation, such as inverse ratio ventilation or prone positioning. There are two major categories of neuromuscular blockers (NMBs). Depolarizing NMBs mimic acetylcholine (Ach); they bind the Ach receptors of the motor end plate and cause depolarization of the muscle, which is clinically seen as muscle fasciculations. Succinylcholine is the only depolarizing NMB available for use. It is characterized by a rapid onset and a short half-life. It is most commonly used as the paralytic of choice for rapid sequence intubation and may be useful for short invasive procedures. Succinylcholine is degraded by plasma pseudocholinesterase and has a short half-life but in patients with a deficiency of this enzyme, prolonged effects can occur. Side effects of succinylcholine include muscle pain, rhabdomyolysis, ocular hypertension, malignant hyperthermia, and hyperkalemia. Patients with spinal cord injuries, large burns, upper and lower motor neuron diseases, renal failure, crush injury, and prolonged immobility are at particular risk for hyperkalemia and resultant cardiac dysrhythmias.

The nondepolarizing NMBs bind Ach receptors but do not activate them, thus blocking the receptor and inhibiting its function. There are two types of nondepolarizing NMBs, steroidal and nonsteroidal. The aminosteroidal compounds include agents such as rocuronium, vecuronium, and pancuronium. Rocuronium has a rapid onset of action and intermediate duration of action, making it useful for short procedures and prolonged relaxation. Vecuronium is an intermediate- acting agent, achieving NMB within 1 to 2 minutes and lasting about 30 minutes, but it can also be infused continuously. Patients with renal or hepatic dysfunction may have a prolonged response because vecuronium is cleared by the kidneys and liver. Pancuronium is long-acting (up to 90 minutes) and is relatively contraindicated in patients with coronary artery disease because its associated vagolytic effect causes pronounced tachycardia. Like vecuronium, pancuronium is eliminated via both the kidneys and liver and requires dose adjustments in the setting of renal or hepatic dysfunction. The nonsteroidal, nondepolarizing NMBs, or benzylisoquinolonium compounds, include atracurium, cisatracurium, tubocurarine, and mivacurium. Of these, atracurium and cisatracurium are the two agents most commonly used in the ICU. Atracurium is intermediate-acting with minimal cardiovascular effects but does have the tendency to promote histamine release. It is metabolized by plasma ester hydrolysis and spontaneous degradation; thus, it is most useful for patients with hepatic and renal dysfunction. A metabolite of atracurium may precipitate seizure activity if used at extremely high doses. Cisatracurium is an isomer of atracurium, with fewer tendencies to produce histamine release. Like atracurium, elimination is by ester hydrolysis and Hofmann elimination. An algorithm for the provision of NMB in the ICU is outlined in Figure 23-2.

Monitoring of NMB is accomplished by train-of-four testing, with one or two twitches considered to be the optimal depth. It is important to remember that in paralyzed patients, assessment of adequate analgesia and sedation is extremely difficult and patients must be presumptively medicated. Bispectral index monitoring is a form of electroencephalomyography that helps determine the level of awareness in a paralyzed patient so

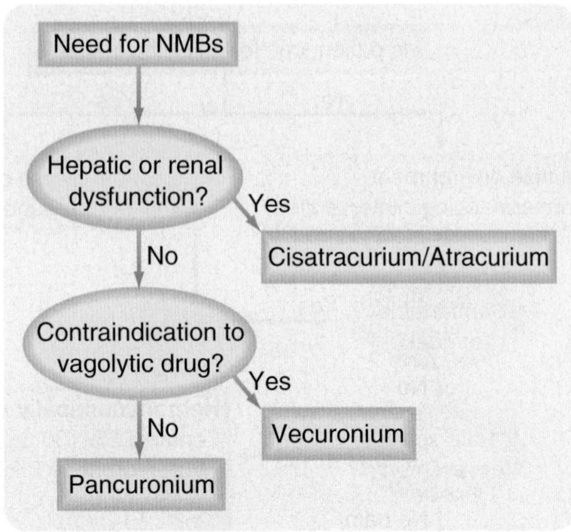


**FIGURE 23-2** Algorithm for NMB in the ICU. (Adapted from Murray MJ, Cowen J, DeBlock H, et al: Clinical practice guidelines for sustained neuromuscular blockade in the adult critically ill patient. Crit Care Med 30:141–156, 2002.)

that the level of sedation can be optimized. Prolonged recovery from paralysis is associated with the steroidal NMBs, and critical -illness myopathy syndromes have been reported in patients receiving NMBs and corticosteroids. Although not seemingly related to specific NMB agents, prolonged exposure to NMBs appears to be the key risk factor. Consequently, similar to continuous sedation regimens, patients on continuous NMBs should have daily medication withdrawal to allow some muscle activity and reassess the need for NMBs, unless otherwise contraindicated.

## CARDIOVASCULAR SYSTEM

## Hemodynamic Monitoring

### Arterial Catheters

Arterial catheter placement is indicated if vasoactive drugs are being administered, continuous monitoring of systemic arterial pressure is required, or frequent arterial blood gas monitoring is needed. The primary complications associated with arterial catheters are infections, arterial thrombosis, and ischemic injuries. A widespread misconception is that the infectious risk associated with arterial catheters is much lower than that of a central venous catheter, but recent reviews of a number of ICUs has found no significant difference in the colonization and infection rates of arterial lines and central venous catheters.[7] Arterial catheters must be placed under sterile conditions. Thrombosis with distal ischemia can be minimized by placing catheters in arteries with good collateral circulation. Thus, the radial or dorsalis pedis arteries are preferred to the brachial or femoral arteries. Allen's test should be performed prior to placement of a radial artery catheter to document adequate collateral flow from the ulnar artery. Ulnar arterial lines are never acceptable because most hands are dominantly perfused by this artery. It appears that placement of difficult arterial lines may be facilitated by the use of ultrasound, likely resulting in fewer attempts. Best medical practice dictates that the need for indwelling medical devices, including arterial lines, in an ICU patient be evaluated daily and that all devices be removed from the patient as soon as possible to minimize nosocomial infections.[8]

Stiffness and resistance of a catheter and measuring system, catheter whip, and distance from the heart all contribute to variance between the actual and measured systolic (SBP) and diastolic (DBP) blood pressures. Thus, MAP is the most accurate measurement obtained and can be determined using the following formula:

$$MAP = DBP + \frac{1}{3}(SBP - DBP)$$

### Central Venous Catheters

Central venous catheter placement may be indicated for long-term venous access to provide parenteral nutrition or chemotherapeutic agents or to measure central venous pressure (CVP). The most common complications associated with central venous catheter insertion include dysrhythmias, pneumothorax (up to 5% following subclavian vein placement), arterial puncture with resultant intimal flap, pseudoaneurysm formation, hemorrhage or arteriovenous fistulization, air or catheter embolism, and even death. These complications represent technical errors, which emphasizes the importance of knowledge of anatomy and proper insertion techniques. Additionally, catheter-related bloodstream infections are a major cause of preventable morbidity and mortality in ICU patients that can be diminished by adherence to full barrier precautions, a chlorhexidine-alcohol skin preparation at the time of insertion, and removal of catheters as soon as possible.[8]

Measurement of CVP can be helpful in assessing right heart function, but it must be remembered that right-sided heart function is an unreliable predictor of left-sided heart function in critically ill patients. Although CVP is widely assumed to be a good indicator of a patient's volume status, it has been shown to be relatively inaccurate in a diverse group of patients. In mechanically ventilated patients, intracardiac pressures are increased during the inspiratory phase, whereas the end-expiratory pressure is usually the lowest pressure recorded. Conversely, during spontaneous respiration, intracardiac pressures decrease as negative intrathoracic pressure is generated; thus, the end-expiratory pressure is typically the highest pressure recorded. Measurement should be made at end expiration because it is relatively independent of the ventilatory status. If more information is desired, or if the patient's clinical status or response to therapy seems incongruous, a pulmonary arterial catheter (PAC) or one of the newer modalities for noninvasive hemodynamic monitoring may be useful (see later).

### Pulmonary Arterial Catheters

PACs allow the direct measurement of CVP, right atrial pressure, pulmonary arterial pressure, right ventricular end-diastolic pressure, pulmonary artery wedge pressure (PAWP), and mixed venous oxygen saturation ($Svo_2$) and indirect calculations of left heart filling pressures and cardiac output. Insertion of a PAC is warranted in any patient with severe cardiopulmonary derangement and is most useful in guiding therapy by repeated monitoring of hemodynamic parameters rather than making a primary diagnosis. It provides information about volume status, and cardiac performance and helps determine the need for volume, inotropic support, and vasoactive drugs. Complications associated with PAC placement include those associated with central venous catheter placement, plus arrhythmias, conduction defects, pulmonary infarction, pulmonary artery rupture, valvular damage, and knotting or catheter entrapment. Pulmonary artery rupture is probably the most feared complication and has been reported to be caused by distal catheter positioning or rapid balloon inflation, or occurring in the setting of noncompliant pulmonary vessels (i.e., pulmonary hypertension). Prophylactic lidocaine may help prevent dysrhythmias in patients with irritable myocardium. Floating a PAC in a patient with left heart block can be particularly hazardous, because the catheter may interfere with conduction in the right bundle, resulting in complete heart block. This is particularly problematic in patients with a new-onset left heart block, which is widely considered to be a contraindication to a PAC.

Placement of a PAC relies on the correct interpretation of pressure tracings from the distal catheter transducer. The catheter should be inserted from 15 to 20 cm and the balloon inflated. Passage into the right ventricle is usually obvious because it is accompanied by wide excursions in the pressure tracing. As the catheter is continuously advanced, exit into the pulmonary artery is heralded by much higher diastolic pressures, with gradually decreasing pressure waves during diastole and an obvious dicrotic notch. A dampened waveform usually signals the wedge position. The balloon should be deflated and the catheter should be incrementally moved back to achieve a minimum insertion to acquire a proper wedge tracing with reinflation. There is significant variability in how much length of catheter is inserted to reach the wedge position, typically ranging from 50 to 75 cm. A chest x-ray should confirm the position of the catheter in the pulmonary arterial trunk; one should look for complications of central venous access if the PAC was inserted through a freshly inserted introducer sheath.

There are also newer noninvasive approaches to hemodynamic monitoring, including pulse contour cardiac output analysis, lithium dilution, and peripheral catheter transpulmonary thermodilution, although no studies to date have demonstrated superior outcomes with these new technologies compared with the PAC. Despite early studies that showed promise in using the transpulmonary thermodilution technique to estimate intrathoracic blood volume, cardiac filling pressures, and preload, a more recent larger, prospective, multicenter multinational study did not show any clinical benefit compared with a PAC.[9] Even though there is a paucity of data supporting the use of these newer technologies in the critically ill, it is still worth pursuing randomized prospective data because it is hoped that these technologies will afford the ICU clinician additional noninvasive options for hemodynamic monitoring and patient care.

Esophageal Doppler, a technique introduced over 30 years ago, can measure blood flow velocity in the descending aorta continuously to determine cardiac output and stroke volume. Although the pulmonary artery catheter relies on pressure measurements that can be affected by a number of neural and hormonal influences and thermodilution principles, the esophageal Doppler system directly measures flow velocity, so it is a potentially more direct indicator of cardiac performance.[10] Esophageal Doppler measurement of left ventricular outflow stroke volume is similar to the technique of transesophageal echocardiography; studies have shown that placement of the catheter and probe is relatively easy and can rapidly produce data that can instantaneously and continuously yield cardiac output. When measured against the standard of thermodilution, measurements were found to be in good correlation with those of the PAC and that the variations in hemodynamics of individual patients yielded similar changes in cardiac output between the two monitoring methods.[10] Significant disadvantages and drawbacks of esophageal Doppler monitoring include its invasiveness, its almost universal requirement for deep sedation and mechanical ventilation, and frequent need for repositioning. Also, the angle between the probe and flow of blood remain fairly constant and relies on many assumptions—for example, that the esophagus is exactly parallel to the descending aorta, blood flow remains fairly constant in distribution between the brachiocephalic, descending aortic, and coronary circulations, and the flow velocity is fairly uniform between blood flowing in the center of the descending aorta and the peripheral aspects of the vessel.

Bioimpedance plethysmography is another technique that is evolving with regard to clinical practicality and use. This technique relies on the significant changes in impedance of the thoracic cavity that occur throughout the cardiac cycle and on changes of lung conductivity with differing degrees of blood volume or edema present. Surface potentials between two electrodes across the chest are measured frequently to estimate stroke volume, cardiac output, and amount of lung water. Its accuracy and clinical usefulness in the management of hemodynamically abnormal patients are still under investigation. The technique is entirely noninvasive and may even be used in an outpatient setting.

## Cardiovascular Dysfunction

### Shock

Shock is simply defined as perfusion that is inadequate to meet the body's metabolic needs. Management of the patient in shock is focused on the following: (1) identifying the presence of shock; (2) searching for and treating immediately life-threatening conditions; and (3) treating shock based on the underlying pathophysiology (see Chapter 5).

Shock commonly presents with hypotension, but it is important to recognize that it can exist in the presence of normal blood pressure. Other signs of shock may include tachycardia, bradycardia, tachypnea, mental status changes, cutaneous hypoperfusion (cool skin, sluggish capillary refill), oliguria, myocardial ischemia, hypoxemia, and metabolic acidosis. Once shock is identified, the first step is to identify and correct immediately life-threatening abnormalities. These could include loss of airway or inadequate ventilation, compression of the heart or great vessels, dysrhythmias, hemorrhage, or anaphylaxis. A rapid assessment of the ABCs can help direct lifesaving interventions, such as endotracheal intubation or mechanical ventilation, tube thoracostomy, pericardiocentesis, fluid resuscitation or transfusion, and administration of antidysrhythmic or vasoactive medications.

After addressing immediate threats to life, it is important to identify and treat the underlying cause of shock. Shock may be broadly classified into five categories: hypovolemic, cardiac compressive, neurogenic, septic, and cardiogenic. Hypovolemic shock may be caused by third spacing of fluid, gastrointestinal or insensible losses, or hemorrhage. Hypovolemic shock secondary to acute blood loss is more accurately termed *hemorrhagic shock*. A crystalloid (isotonic saline) bolus (20 mL/kg) should be administered immediately, and repeated if necessary. In addition to its therapeutic benefit, the response to fluid may help confirm the assessment of hypovolemia. Glucose-containing fluids should be avoided because they may stimulate an osmotic diuresis. If hemorrhage is suspected and the hemodynamic response to crystalloid is not satisfactory, a blood transfusion should be initiated without delay and a search for the source of hemorrhage aggressively undertaken. The rapidity of resuscitation is predicated on the patient's condition; restoration of normal blood pressure, heart rate (HR), skin color, mentation, and urine output signify a reversal of hypoperfusion. The need for continued resuscitation may be estimated by additional measurements (see later, "End Points of Resuscitation"). In the setting of hemorrhagic shock or ongoing bleeding, it is prudent to restore hemoglobin (Hb) to near-normal levels in the acute phase.

Cardiac or great vessel compressive shock may be caused by tension pneumothorax or massive hemothorax, which can impede venous return by shifting the mediastinum and kinking of the vena cava, or pericardial tamponade, which prohibits cardiac diastolic filling. Tube thoracostomy relieves mediastinal shift associated with tension pneumothorax or hemothorax, and may provide definitive management of the problem. Pericardial tamponade may be caused by blood, transudative fluid, or air in the pericardium. A hemodynamically unstable patient with pericardial tamponade should undergo immediate decompression, either via thoracotomy or sternotomy or pericardiocentesis. The latter may be performed under ultrasound guidance and a catheter left in with a stopcock to allow intermittent drainage while transporting the patient for definitive management, thoracotomy or pericardial window. The appearance of hemodynamic stability must be interpreted with caution, however, because ongoing subendocardial ischemia may compromise long-term recovery from the insult. Thus, the confirmation of pericardial tamponade calls for action—fluid resuscitation and plans for decompression—without delay. Neurogenic shock is typically seen in the setting of a spinal cord injury resulting in loss of vasomotor tone. The treatment is judicious fluid administration with α-adrenergic vasopressors, as needed. Other causes of shock such as hemorrhage must be aggressively sought because, in the acute trauma setting, neurogenic shock should be considered a diagnosis of exclusion.

Septic shock represents cardiovascular collapse associated with an infectious process and represents the final stage on the continuum from systemic inflammatory response syndrome (SIRS) to sepsis and septic shock. Management of septic shock involves treating the underlying infectious process (source control), administering appropriate antibiotics (see later, "Sepsis"), and volume resuscitation. Cardiogenic shock refers to primary pump failure and is associated with high cardiac filling pressure and diminished cardiac output. Although fluid administration is a key component in treating shock, no matter what the cause, each type of shock requires additional interventions; thus, the prompt identification of shock's cause is critical to a good outcome.

### Support of Circulation

To reverse shock, one must ensure adequate perfusion of tissues. The factors that determine perfusion are the $O_2$ content of the blood ($CaO_2$), pumping function of the heart, and tone of the vasculature. Thus, $O_2$ delivery ($DO_2$) is the product of $CaO_2$ (mL $O_2$/100 mL blood), and the cardiac output (CO; liters/min). The $DO_2$ is usually indexed to body surface area, so the cardiac index (CI) is used in the calculation and the result is reported in mL $O_2$/min/m$^2$:

$$Do_2 = Cao_2 \times CI \times 10$$

The $Cao_2$ consists of the $O_2$ that is carried by Hb and that which is dissolved into the blood itself:

$$CaO_2 = [Hb \times Sao_2 \times 1.39] + [0.003 \times Pao_2]$$

Where Hb is the concentration (in g/dL), $Sao_2$ is the arterial $O_2$ saturation (%) and $Pao_2$ is the partial pressure of $O_2$ (mm Hg) in arterial blood. Usually, the fraction of $O_2$ that is dissolved in blood is inconsequential; an exceptional situation is a patient with a critically low Hb (e.g., a Jehovah's Witness who is profoundly anemic) or a patient treated in a hyperbaric chamber, in which the $Pao_2$ may be several-fold higher than normal. To optimize $Do_2$ to tissues, one should try to maximize the $Sao_2$ and provide a normal concentration of Hb. The usual guidelines for transfusion (see later) do not apply to the patient in shock, especially hemorrhagic shock. Once the $Cao_2$ is maximized, CO must be addressed. The CO is equal to stroke volume multiplied by HR, and is influenced by cardiac rhythm and contractility as well as vascular tone. The approach to augmenting CO begins with ensuring a perfusing HR and rhythm and good contractility of the heart.

### Dysrhythmias

Dysrhythmias are common in the ICU and correct interpretation of the rhythm is the key to proper treatment. In a patient with cardiopulmonary arrest, it is helpful to diagnose the rhythm with quick-look paddles. The most recent algorithm from the American Heart Association stresses the need for almost continuous cardiopulmonary resuscitation (CPR) and presents guidelines for CPR, including advanced cardiac life support; it is updated approximately every 5 years (Box 23-1). For ventricular fibrillation or pulseless ventricular tachycardia, defibrillation with 360 J (monophasic) or 120 to 200 J (biphasic) should be delivered but should not be repeated or stacked without resuming another cycle of CPR because this interrupts chest compressions and decreases coronary perfusion pressure . If the phase type of the defibrillator is unknown, 200 J should be selected; automatic external defibrillators will administer their preprogrammed electrical dose. If electrical defibrillation is not successful, CPR should continue and the following steps should be taken:

1. Infuse epinephrine (1 mg IV) or vasopressin 40 U (IV).
2. Epinephrine may be redosed every 3 to 5 minutes but should not be administered for 10 minutes following a vasopressin bolus, which is typically given as a one-time dose.
3. CPR should be continued throughout this process and additional shocks should be delivered after every five cycles of CPR if a rhythm potentially amenable to defibrillation is present.

It cannot be overstated that maintaining adequate chest compressions, with minimal interruption and early defibrillation, are the most important components of CPR.

Asystole should be verified by rotating leads and high-quality CPR should be initiated. Epinephrine (1 mg IV) or a one-time dose of vasopressin (40 U IV) should be given.

**BOX 23-1 Guidelines for Management of Cardiopulmonary Arrest**

**Ventricular Fibrillation and Pulseless Ventricular Tachycardia**

Give one shock (monophasic, 360 J; biphasic, 100-200 J).
CPR; additional countershocks if shockable rhythm obtained
Epinephrine, 1 mg IV, repeat every 3-5 min; *or* vasopressin, 40U IV (may be given to replace first or second dose of epinephrine)
Consider amiodarone (300 mg IV), lidocaine (1-1.5 mg/kg), magnesium (1-2 g IV).
If no shockable rhythm, revert to asystole or pulseless electrical activity (PEA) algorithm.

**Asystole or Pulseless Electrical Activity**

Verify with lead rotation.
Epinephrine, 1 mg IV, repeat every 3-5 min; *or* vasopressin, 40 U IV (may be given to replace first or second dose of epinephrine)
Consider atropine (1 mg IV every 3-5 min, up to three doses).
If shockable rhythm, revert to ventricular fibrillation–ventricular tachycardia algorithm.

Adapted from ECC Committee, Subcommittees and Task Forces of the American Heart Association: American Heart Association Guidelines for Cardiopulmonary Resuscitation and Emergency Care, Part 7.2: Management of Cardiac Arrest. Circulation 112(Suppl):IV1–IV59, 2005.

Atropine (1 mg IV) should also be given and repeated every 5 minutes, for a total of three doses. Countershock should only be given if fine ventricular fibrillation is suspected. There is no role for antiarrhythmics or defibrillation in asystolic cardiac arrest (see Box 23-1).

Patients without cardiac arrest are approached differently. Unstable patients with bradycardia (HR $< 60$ beats/min) should be treated promptly with transcutaneous pacing. Atropine (1 mg) and epinephrine (2 to 10 μg/min) can be adjuncts if pacing is not readily available. When approaching any patient with a cardiac dysrhythmia, a 12-lead electrocardiogram (ECG) and rhythm strip should be obtained. If the QRS complex is found to be wide and rapid, cardioversion and amiodarone are indicated because this is most likely ventricular in origin. If the QRS is narrow and the patient is hemodynamically unstable, synchronized cardioversion is warranted. The differential diagnosis includes supraventricular tachycardias, atrial fibrillation, atrial flutter, multifocal atrial tachycardia, and uncertain tachycardias, all of which require different treatments. A detailed discussion of the management of these rhythm abnormalities is beyond the scope of this chapter and expert consultation may be necessary.

Sinus tachycardia is the most common tachycardia in the ICU and is not a dysrhythmia per se, but can be an appropriate response to fever, pain, sympathetic stimulation, hypotension, sepsis, or inflammation. Therapy should be directed at the underlying cause. If the QRS width is unclear, adenosine (6 mg, repeated once) may be administered and typically will facilitate the identification of the underlying rhythm. If the rate does not slow, treat it as a wide complex tachycardia; if it slows, treat it as a narrow complex tachycardia.

The most common sustained dysrhythmia is atrial fibrillation, with a prevalence of 5% in patients older than 65 years.

Numerous stresses in the perioperative period may trigger new-onset atrial fibrillation or loss of rate control in the patient with chronic atrial fibrillation. Cardioversion should be performed for hemodynamic instability; otherwise, rate control is attempted while the underlying cause (e.g., myocardial ischemia, fluid overload, electrolyte imbalances, hypoxemia, acidosis, pulmonary embolism [PE]) is identified and treated. IV amiodarone, calcium channel blockers, or beta blockers are usually effective in rapid conversion; digoxin takes several hours for maximal effect. There are also a number of new medications that can be used for conversion of atrial fibrillation to sinus rhythm, notably the class III antiarrhythmic agent dofetilide. However, potential drug-related complications such as torsades de pointes and the need for renal dosing limit their usefulness and make rate control and use of beta blockers and calcium channel blockers the preferred medical management for atrial fibrillation.[11] In patients who have had atrial fibrillation for less than 48 hours, or who are already on warfarin, no anticoagulation is necessary. If the precise time of onset is not known, however, it is probably safest to anticoagulate prior to cardioversion or perform cardioversion under guidance by transesophageal echocardiography. A number of randomized trials have addressed rate control and rhythm conversion in patients with atrial fibrillation. Conversion may be detrimental in some patient populations because of toxicities of antiarrythmic medications but may provide some benefit in terms of improved quality of life and left ventricular function in patients with heart failure.

### Pump Dysfunction

In patients with inflammatory or cardiogenic shock, cardiac pump function may be disturbed because of circulating myocardial depressants or ischemia. The clinical manifestations of the failing heart may include pulmonary edema (left heart failure), peripheral edema and distended neck veins (right heart failure), or both. Once $CaO_2$ has been maximized and a perfusing rhythm has been ensured, the next step is to optimize CO. The principal determinants of CO are preload, afterload, and contractility. At a minimum, CVP monitoring should be instituted; if CVP and MAP are both low, volume replacement is warranted. If CVP is high and MAP is low, however, a PAC should be inserted for monitoring of PAWP and CO. If PAWP and CO are both high, the patient may have been overresuscitated; fluids should be slowed or stopped and diuretic therapy considered in severe cases. Low PAWP and CO may be associated with inflammatory shock, anaphylaxis, and hepatic or autonomic dysfunction. If the PAWP and CO are both low, administer fluid boluses of crystalloid to increase PAWP by 3 to 5 mm Hg and remeasure the CO; if it improves, repeat until the patient stabilizes. If PAWP is high and CO is low, then an inotropic agent or afterload-reducing agent may be warranted. If the patient is normotensive, an afterload reducer may be helpful. Sodium nitroprusside and nitroglycerin are most frequently used, but angiotensin-converting enzyme inhibitors or hydralazine may also be considered. Nitroprusside (0.5 μg/kg/min) is advantageous because of its rapid onset and reversibility and rare intolerance or tachyphylaxis. A byproduct is cyanide, which is converted to thiocyanate and excreted by the kidneys. Cyanide toxicity may be heralded by increasing mixed $SvO_2$; it is treated by administering 3% sodium nitrite (10 mL) followed by methylene blue (1 mg/kg). Thiocyanate levels higher than 10 mg/dL may necessitate hemodialysis. Nitroglycerin (5 μg/min, titrated up to 300 μg/min) is a good choice for patients with elevated preload and afterload, and especially those with pulmonary edema.

Hypotensive patients may require medication to augment cardiac contractility, increase systemic arterial vasoconstriction, or both. There are several agents that may be used, each having a unique profile of activity on adrenergic receptors (Table 23-2). $\alpha_1$-Adrenergic receptors have a primary effect on systemic arterial vasoconstriction, and lesser effects on systemic veins and pulmonary arteries. $\beta_1$-Adrenergic receptors act primarily on the heart, increasing HR, contractility, and atrioventricular conduction. $\beta_2$-Adrenergic receptors increase HR and contractility, but are also vasodilatory to the systemic and pulmonary vasculature. Dopaminergic receptors modulate arterial vasodilatation and, to a lesser degree, cardiac contractility, but the effects of dopamine are unpredictable and the side effects may be substantial; therefore, enthusiasm for its use in the ICU has been waning.

Three of the most commonly used medications for hypotensive patients are epinephrine, norepinephrine, and phenylephrine. In the past, dopamine was widely used but, as noted,

**Table 23-2 Effects of Selected Vasoactive Agents**

| | | Receptor Activity | | | Hemodynamic Response | | | |
|---|---|---|---|---|---|---|---|---|
| **DRUG** | **DOSAGE (μG/KG/MIN)** | **α** | **$\beta_1$** | **$\beta_2$** | **HR** | **MAP** | **CO** | **SVR** |
| Dopamine | 3-5 | – | ++ | – | ↑ | ↑ | ↑ | → |
| | 5-20 | ++ | ++ | – | ↑↑ | ↑↑ | ↑ | ↑↑ |
| Dobutamine | 2-20 | – | ++ | + | ↑↑ | ↑ | ↑ | ↓ |
| Norepinephrine | 1-20 μg/min | ++ | + | – | ↑ | ↑↑ | ↑ | ↑↑ |
| Phenylephrine | 10-100 μg/min | ++ | – | – | → | ↑↑ | ↓ | ↑↑ |
| Epinephrine | 0.005-0.02 | – | ++ | ++ | ↑↑ | ↑ | ↑ | ↓ |
| | 0.01-0.1 | ++ | ++ | + | ↑↑ | ↑↑ | ↑ | ↑↑ |
| Isoproterenol | 0.03-0.15 | – | ++ | + | ↑↑ | → | ↑ | ↓ |
| Amiodarone | 5-10 | | | | → | → | ↑↑ | ↓ |
| Milrinone | 0.3-1.5 | | | | → | → | ↑↑ | ↓ |

*SVR*, Systemic vascular resistance.

interest in its use has faded in the ICU. Epinephrine is a potent α- and β-adrenergic agonist; it increases myocardial contractility as well as vasoconstriction. It increases myocardial $O_2$ consumption and is arrhythmogenic, so its usefulness in the ICU is limited to patients with profound hypotension, especially those with concomitant bradycardia. Norepinephrine's primary value is to increase MAP by increasing systemic vascular resistance via the α-adrenergic receptor. It may have deleterious effects on CO in high afterload states such as cardiogenic shock; however, it does increase heart rate and myocardial contractility via β-adrenergic stimulation so it is particularly useful for patients with myocardial dysfunction and peripheral vasodilation. Phenylephrine is a pure α-adrenergic agonist and, as such, can be helpful in increasing SBP through its action on the vasculature while not affecting the heart at all. It is commonly used by anesthesiologists and may be particularly useful in reversing the vasodilation caused by epidural anesthetics or spinal cord injury, but it is associated with tachyphylaxis, which limits its effectiveness.

Vasopressin is commonly used by critical care physicians; it is not an adrenergic drug but instead functions through an independent G protein–coupled receptor and thus may be useful for patients who are refractory to catecholamines. Its main function in the body appears to be regulation of water balance but, in shock, it is a potent vasopressor, irrespective of the level of circulating endogenous vasopressin. In septic shock, it is typically administered in doses up to 0.04 U/min, which mimic physiologic levels and avoids some of the adverse effects associated with higher doses, such as myocardial or splanchnic ischemia. One of the primary advantages of vasopressin in septic shock is that it continues to have an effect in the setting of profound metabolic acidosis, whereas adrenergic agents typically have decreased efficacy in acidemic states. Despite this, vasopressin was found to be no more beneficial than norepinephrine in terms of 28-day mortality in a fairly large multicenter randomized trial of patients in septic or severe septic shock.[12] Also, vasopressin is a potent peripheral vasoconstrictor; in shock states, these effects can worsen splanchnic and renal ischemia more than adrenergic agents such as norepinephrine that provide some inotropic and chronotropic effects.

In patients who have an adequate MAP but need augmented myocardial contractility, inotropic drugs are indicated. Generally, these drugs have vasodilatory effects, so it is important to ensure adequate preload prior to infusion. Dobutamine (5 to 15 μg/kg/min) can be effective, but it does increase myocardial oxygen demand and may be arrhythmogenic. Isoproterenol is a powerful synthetic β-adrenergic agonist that is no longer used in clinical practice because of its associated arrhythmogenicity. The phosphodiesterase inhibitors amrinone and milrinone are thought to act by inhibiting the breakdown of cyclic adenosine monophosphate (cAMP). They increase CO and reduce preload and afterload; amrinone may cause profound vasodilation and its long-term administration is associated with thrombocytopenia and gastrointestinal side effects. Milrinone is a more potent inotrope with fewer side effects but it is also associated with vasodilation and arrhythmias. It causes pulmonary vascular vasodilation and may be helpful in treating myocardial dysfunction in the setting of pulmonary hypertension. The phosphodiesterase inhibitors appear to be able to increase myocardial contractility without affecting myocardial oxygen demand by reducing wall stress, which counteracts the increased oxygen requirement to support enhanced contractility (Table 23-2).

## Resuscitation

### Fluids

Fluid resuscitation is the initial maneuver whenever a shock state is recognized. Crystalloid is typically administered to expand the intravascular volume, but only about one third of the fluid will remain in the intravascular space. Additionally, in many shock states, there may be cellular dysfunction, resulting in loss of capillary integrity and massive fluid extravasation and causing widespread tissue edema. For many decades, a debate about the advantages and disadvantages of crystalloid versus colloid fluid resuscitation has persisted. Although colloids provide more effective volume expansion than crystalloid solutions because of their ability to remain in the vascular space, prospective, randomized, clinical trials (PRCTs) have demonstrated that survival is no better and possibly worse when albumin is given instead of crystalloid.[13] This argument has been countered by meta-analyses showing that the administration of albumin reduces morbidity in acutely ill hospitalized patients[14] and may have beneficial effects in a wide range of clinical settings. Whatever the outcome of this debate, it is apparent that many more studies will be required before a definitive conclusion is reached. However, in the case of severe hemorrhagic shock, it is certain that the usual transfusion triggers and colloid-crystalloid debate do not apply, and Hb should be restored to near-normal levels.

There has also been some recent enthusiasm for the use of synthetic colloid analogues—namely, hydroxyethyl starch solutions—for septic, hypovolemic, or hemorrhagic shock states; it is thought that a much larger percentage of the synthetic solutions would remain in the intravascular space compared with that of crystalloid. No clinical studies have shown any benefit in using these solutions in surgical or critically ill patients; investigations of fluid resuscitation end points have found that the volume of these starch solutions required to reach these end points far exceeds the expected amount in relation to the amount of crystalloids given.[17] Actually, almost equal volumes of the synthetic starch solutions and crystalloid were given to reach the resuscitation end points. There are also serious potential deleterious effects of synthetic starch solutions, including coagulopathy, with decreased levels of circulating factor VIII and von Willebrand factor, platelet dysfunction, nephrotoxicity, and pruritus. Other studies have also shown an increased need for renal replacement therapy (RRT) in patients with sepsis who have been given synthetic starch solutions. Newer hydroxyethyl starch (HES) solutions of different compositions (e.g., HES 130/0.4) are still unproven in terms of their potential to cause less hemostatic compromise or renal failure. Recent reports of these synthetic solutions have questioned their overall safety in critically ill surgical patients; thus, it is probably prudent to avoid using these agents at this time.[15]

### End Points of Resuscitation

Although fluid resuscitation may normalize many clinical parameters such as HR, blood pressure, skin color, mentation, and urine output, it does not ensure that the $O_2$ debt has been repaid. Thus, there should be an objective measure of the success of resuscitation in meeting tissue metabolic needs. In the early 1990s, Bishop and colleagues[16] have identified values for CI

(4.5 liter/min/$m^2$), $DO_2$ (600 mL $O_2$/min/$m^2$) and $O_2$ consumption ($\dot{V}O_2$; 170 mL $O_2$/min/$m^2$) above which survival could be predicted in critically ill patients. Subsequent PRCTs testing these resuscitation goals offered mixed results. Kern and Shoemaker[17] have reviewed published data and suggested that if hemodynamic optimization is applied to subgroups with an expected mortality of 20% or higher, prior to the development of organ failure, and the goal of increased $DO_2$ is achieved, then survival will be improved. It is difficult to prove definitively that early aggressive resuscitation benefits critically ill patients, but it is important to augment $DO_2$ whenever possible, because this is the basis of goal-directed resuscitation.[18] It must be recognized, however, that not all patients respond in the same way. For example, Moore and associates[19] have reported that 38% of severely injured patients are unable to attain a $\dot{V}O_2$ of 150 mL $O_2$/min/$m^2$, despite supranormal $DO_2$. This group appeared to have defective aerobic metabolism, leading to a higher incidence of multiple organ failure (MOF). Thus, routine resuscitation to supranormal targets may be unnecessary and inappropriate when shock is readily reversed, fruitless when the patient does not respond, and even detrimental when it results in the abdominal compartment syndrome (ACS).

Recently, there have been inquiries into the potential detriments and benefits of supranormal fluid resuscitation or conservative fluid administration strategies. These inquiries are mainly based on the theorized mechanism of overzealous fluid resuscitation causing increased cardiac filling pressures and resultant pulmonary edema and impaired gas exchange. Post hoc analysis of the Fluid and Catheter Treatment Trial (FACTT) from 2006 has shown that surgical patients managed with a conservative fluid strategy that aimed for lower CVPs, PCWPs, and urine output than those managed with a liberal strategy have significantly fewer days on a ventilator, without any increase in mortality or renal failure.[20] Further study is warranted to continue to assess the potential benefits of such conservative fluid strategies in a wider range of surgical patients.

Alternative parameters that may serve as resuscitation end points include mixed venous oxygen saturation ($SvO_2$), end-tidal carbon dioxide ($ETCO_2$), gastric intramucosal pH (pHi), base deficit, and arterial lactate levels. $SvO_2$ is an indicator of $O_2$ extraction and is used to calculate $\dot{V}O_2$. Continuous monitoring of $SvO_2$ can provide early clues about inadequate perfusion (e.g., hemorrhage, myocardial ischemia, shock) before it becomes fully manifested, but intermittent measurements are not as helpful. Fortunately, continuous $SvO_2$ monitoring PACs are readily available and offer valuable insight into the status of a patient's hemodynamics, provided that the clinician understands the limitations of this parameter. Furthermore, although a low value may be helpful in prompting clinical action, a normal or high $SvO_2$ may be misleading. For example, in severe sepsis or preterminal shock, there can be significant shunting, with little $O_2$ being delivered to tissue beds or mitochondrial dysfunction preventing oxygen uptake, resulting in a high $SvO_2$. Assessing serum lactate levels or base deficit in conjunction with the $SvO_2$ measurement can be particularly helpful in this setting and provides more information than either parameter alone. In general, overreliance on any one parameter is unwise and can result in inappropriate and harmful therapeutic interventions. A classic example is vigorous fluid administration to correct type B lactic acidosis, in which tissue perfusion is maintained and the acidosis is caused by factors such as metformin, antiviral agents, or even acute alcohol intoxication, and the patient needlessly develops pulmonary edema or congestive failure.

The $ETCO_2$ reflects alveolar $CO_2$. Decreased CO or increased pulmonary dead space may decrease $ETCO_2$ and increase the arterial-$ETCO_2$ difference, which has been associated with nonsurvival. Splanchnic circulation is the first to be compromised in shock and the last to be restored. Gastric tonometry measures the pHi in the stomach, which strongly reflects mesenteric tissue ischemia. A pHi value threshold of 7.3 or higher has compared favorably with supranormal $DO_2$ and $\dot{V}O_2$ (600 and 150 mL/min/$m^2$, respectively) as an end point.

The major drawbacks to the widespread use of gastric tonometry are technologic limitations, cost, and inconvenience. A number of investigators have measured transcutaneous $O_2$ and $CO_2$ levels, as well as skeletal muscle oxyhemoglobin. Early results have been encouraging in a military setting with tissue oxygen monitors placed in the thenar muscle bed guiding trauma resuscitations and have correlated well with clinical findings of hemorrhagic shock in small series of patients. This technology promises a useful device for guiding and monitoring massive resuscitations; however, its usefulness for other forms of shock resuscitation remains unknown.[2] Arterial lactate levels and base deficit are measures of global tissue perfusion and can be particularly helpful in predicting which patient will experience an adverse outcome, because the time to normalization strongly correlates with mortality and morbidity.[21] In addition to their prognostic significance, these parameters allow the degree of physiologic derangement to be quantified, and they serve as targets for ongoing resuscitation, but it appears that lactate levels may offer an improved predictive ability compared with base deficit.

The Surviving Sepsis Campaign, an international multiorganization effort to reduce the mortality associated with sepsis, is noteworthy for assembling a concise set of resuscitation principles that stresses early targeted physiologic goals.[22] This evidence-based campaign began in 2002 and was updated in 2004 and 2008, with the goal of improving the management of severely septic and septic shock patients. Elements of the guidelines were "bundled" into two sets of targets: (1) the resuscitation bundle, which sets goals of care, data to be gathered, and tasks to be accomplished within 6 hours of a septic patient's presentation; and (2) a second management bundle, less geared toward data gathering and more dedicated to actual management of the physiologic derangements of sepsis. The resuscitation bundle guides early fluid resuscitation and vasopressor support based on the presence of hypotension and/or elevated lactate levels, and targets a MAP higher than 65 mm Hg. If this goal is unmet, CVP is targeted to 8 mm Hg or higher or a central venous oxygen saturation of 70% or higher. In the next phase, the administration of corticosteroids for septic shock, consideration of activated protein C, glucose control, and maintenance of lower ventilatory plateau pressure are addressed.[22] For all septic patients, it must be emphasized that identification of the cause of sepsis is crucial so that eradication or source control can be carried out; without it, the elements of this bundle stand little chance of reducing septic mortality.

With the establishment of these management principles, the campaign recruited over 250 hospital sites and has recently reported a steady decrease in in-hospital mortality of over 15,000 septic patients. This is the largest prospective evaluation of patients with severe sepsis that has ever been conducted.[22] Interestingly, the longer a hospital used these guidelines, the better the survival benefit, and bundle compliance correlated with reductions in septic deaths. Although the campaign has been successful in reducing sepsis-related mortality, this success may be dependent more on an organized approach to caring for septic patients rather than on the actual components of the bundles themselves because the bundles sometimes contained elements that were or remain controversial or were subsequently shown to be ineffective in treating sepsis. With few exceptions, every prospective, goal-directed clinical trial that has shown a survival advantage has espoused the principles of the supranormal $Do_2$ strategy—volume loading with or without transfusion plus inotropic support as needed to meet a predetermined goal. The optimal algorithm for fluids and inotropes remains to be determined, but it is clear that a defined end point is desirable. Rather than selecting a goal that simply confirms the act of resuscitation, it is more appropriate to select an end point that confirms a response to resuscitation.

## Perioperative Cardiac Support

### Cardiac Risk Assessment

Cardiovascular complications are frequent following noncardiac surgery. It has been estimated that 50,000 patients will have a perioperative myocardial infarction and another 1 million patients will have a cardiac complication annually.[23] As our population ages, cardiac complications will continue to increase, requiring increased vigilance in assessing and minimizing cardiac risk. In the setting of an acute surgical emergency, the preoperative risk assessment is limited to vital signs, volume status, and electrocardiography. There is no opportunity for further risk assessment or risk reduction; however, in less urgent circumstances, evaluation proceeds based on the presence of risk factors (Table 23-3). If the patient has no risk factors, no further testing or treatment is necessary. One or two risk factors do not by themselves warrant additional testing, but in the presence of a past medical history consistent with coronary artery disease, noninvasive testing is prudent. Three or more risk factors mandate noninvasive testing[23]; however, the optimal noninvasive test is debatable. Exercise (stress) electrocardiography is generally advocated as the initial test, but it is not suitable for patients who have noninterpretable ECGs or who are unable to exercise. In these cases, an imaging test that simulates exercise, such as dipyridamole thallium scanning, is necessary. Also, imaging is indicated for patients with poor myocardial function or previous revascularization to assess myocardial viability. The choice of imaging, radionuclide perfusion imaging versus echocardiography, depends primarily on local expertise. An abnormal noninvasive test results mandates cardiac catheterization with coronary arteriography. Recent investigations have shown that patients with left main or multivessel coronary artery disease have lower mortality and less frequent need for repeat revascularization with coronary artery bypass surgery than with percutaneous angioplasty or stenting, whereas single-vessel disease may be treated by coronary angioplasty.[24] Ultimately, revascularization should be limited to those patients with a clear need, independent of the need for noncardiac surgery.

**Table 23-3 Risk Factors for Perioperative Cardiac Complications in Patients Undergoing Noncardiac Surgery**

| RISK FACTOR | ODDS RATIO |
|---|---|
| Diabetes mellitus | 3.0 (1.3-7.1) |
| Renal insufficiency | 3.0 (1.4-6.8) |
| High-risk surgery | 2.8 (1.6-4.9) |
| Ischemic heart disease | 2.4 (1.3-4.2) |
| Congestive heart failure | 1.9 (1.1-3.5) |
| Poor functional status | 1.8 (0.9-3.5) |

Patients who will not be referred for revascularization, but who have cardiac risk factors, should receive medical therapy aimed at minimizing perioperative cardiac risk. A number of clinical trials have not proven a benefit of perioperative monitoring with a PAC but beta blockers should be administered to all patients at risk for cardiac events who are scheduled to undergo surgery.[25] If possible, beta blocker therapy should be instituted well in advance of the operation, with studies supporting better outcomes (e.g., cardiac death, nonfatal myocardial infarction) when shorter acting agents such as bisoprolol or metoprolol are started as early as 1 month preoperatively, targeting a resting HR of 50 to 70 beats/min. HMG-CoA (3-hydroxy-3-methylglutaryl-coenzyme A) reductase inhibitors (statins), with their known ability to stabilize coronary plaque, have also shown potential for improving perioperative outcomes in patients with cardiac risk factors. The amount of prospective data to support their perioperative use is limited but it seems that the benefits of plaque stabilization likely significantly outweigh the risks of statin-induced myopathy or rhabdomyolysis.

### Heart Failure

Heart failure may be encountered in the perioperative period, particularly in emergent surgery in patients with significant medical comorbidities. Shock should be managed as noted. Less severe episodes may be manifest by tachycardia, low CO, and pulmonary (if left-sided failure) or peripheral (if right-sided failure) edema. The most common cause of heart failure in the surgical ICU is myocardial ischemia, but it may also represent decompensation of chronic heart failure. Thus, the history and physical examination should be supplemented with electrocardiography and cardiac enzyme analysis. Chest radiographs may be helpful to identify pulmonary pathology; invasive monitoring with a PAC facilitates determination of filling pressures, CO, and pulmonary and systemic resistance and helps distinguish cardiogenic from noncardiogenic pulmonary edema. The PAC is less helpful for differentiating systolic from diastolic dysfunction; thus, echocardiography may be a more useful tool for patients with acute heart failure. Echocardiography provides information on chamber size, ventricular and valvular function, and indirect measurements of pressures, as well as identifying extracardiac problems such as pericardial effusion. Diuretics and vasodilators are the mainstays of treatment for heart failure. Diuretics improve pulmonary congestion and reduce ventricular end-diastolic volume, improving myocardial $\dot{V}o_2$. Loop diuretics are the class of choice in the acute setting because of their reliable efficacy, short onset, and potency.

Vasodilators, including angiotensin-converting enzyme inhibitors (ACEIs), hydralazine, and nitrates, are also used. ACEIs prevent the formation of angiotensin II, a potent vasoconstrictor and stimulus for aldosterone secretion. In addition to decreasing afterload, they augment stroke volume and are therefore generally preferred, particularly in patients with a depressed (<40%) left ventricular ejection fraction. They provide symptomatic improvement, as well as a long-term survival advantage. Hydralazine and nitroglycerin are second-line agents for patients who cannot tolerate ACEI therapy. The cardiac glycoside digoxin has a limited role in the treatment of acute heart failure. In patients with diastolic failure, inotropes may exacerbate failure, and treatment with agents capable of reducing myocardial wall tension may be needed. Beta blockers help attenuate the sympathetic overactivity associated with heart failure and decrease myocardial $\dot{V}O_2$; however, careful monitoring is required when even small doses of beta blockers are administered because of their negative inotropic and chronotropic effects.

Mechanical support, including intra-aortic balloon pumps or left ventricular assist devices (LVADs), may be required as a bridge to heart transplantation or for cardiogenic shock patients after bypass. Although there are marked limitations on the number of heart donors, the number of patients who will become candidates for cardiac transplantation caused by heart failure is inevitably going to increase because there are more than 5 million people in the United States with clinically significant congestive heart failure. Over the last 2 decades, the number of patients undergoing orthotopic cardiac transplantation annually has quadrupled. VADs and their role as a bridge to transplantation have become increasingly important and have been shown to be a successful up to 70% of the time in patients younger than 60 years. The devices most commonly used are the LVAD and BiVAD (biventricular assist device); these are not only useful as a bridge to transplantation, but also for older patients to manage advanced heart failure while they recover from critical illness related to failure of other organ systems.

Intra-aortic balloon pump counterpulsation is now the most commonly used method of mechanical assistance for patients with cardiogenic shock after acute myocardial infarction and is a class I recommendation of the American Heart Association/American College of Cardiology in this setting.[26] The initial goal is to manage a patient's cardiogenic shock medically but if this is unsuccessful, the decision to place and use an intra-aortic balloon pump should be done in a timely fashion because delays its placement are associated with worse outcomes. Unfortunately, there are little data at this time to show that intra-aortic balloon pump therapy provides significant clinical benefit in patients after acute myocardial infarction (AMI) or in AMI patients after percutaneous angioplasty or stent placement. Further study in this group is warranted.

## RESPIRATORY SYSTEM

### Respiratory Failure

Acute respiratory failure, common in the surgical ICU, can be caused by decreased oxygenation without hypercapnia (hypoxemic or type I respiratory failure) or hypoxia with $CO_2$ retention (hypercapnic or type II respiratory failure). The causes of respiratory failure are numerous and may include preexisting cardiopulmonary or neuromuscular disease that compromises respiratory mechanics, gas exchange, or ventilatory drive. A number of factors also affect postsurgical or critically ill patients—respiratory mechanics may be compromised by the acute disease process, the surgical intervention, or pain, gas exchange may be adversely affected by fluid shifts, direct lung injury, or systemic inflammation, with resultant acute lung injury (ALI), and ventilatory drive or airway protection may be depressed because of analgesics or sedatives. To minimize the morbidity and mortality associated with respiratory failure, it is critically important to recognize it, ascertain the cause, and initiate treatment.

Signs and symptoms of acute respiratory failure include shortness of breath, anxiety, altered mental status, cyanosis, use of accessory muscles of respiration, stridor, tachypnea, tachycardia, and hypoxia. The initial evaluation includes a rapid assessment to ensure airway patency and air movement. Stridor implies impending airway obstruction and is an airway emergency. Vital signs, including pulse oximetry, should be obtained and supplemental $O_2$ should be provided immediately as other causes of the respiratory failure are sought. A chest x-ray and ABG analysis are mandatory; other studies such as electrocardiography, bronchoscopy, ventilation-perfusion ($\dot{V}/\dot{Q}$), and/or chest CT scanning should be considered based on the clinical scenario. There are several options for the delivery of supplemental $O_2$, including nasal cannula, face tent, face mask, noninvasive positive-pressure systems, and endotracheal intubation with mechanical ventilation. The choice is dictated by the patient's condition and ventilatory needs. Indications for intubation and mechanical ventilation can be given by the SOAP mnemonic: excessive ***s***ecretions requiring pulmonary toilet; impaired ***o***xygenation requiring positive pressure ventilation; ***a***irway obstruction or inability to protect the airway; and compromised ***p***ulmonary function (i.e., inability to generate adequate respiratory effort or to meet minute ventilatory needs).

The amount of $O_2$ that must be supplied is the lowest amount that provides adequate $CaO_2$ in the blood. As previously discussed, this is directly related to the Hb concentration and $SaO_2$. Therefore, as in the setting of shock, consideration should be given to restoring near-normal Hb levels in patients with acute respiratory failure. Pulse oximetry and ABG analysis will yield information on $SaO_2$ and $PaO_2$ respectively. Although related, $PaO_2$ and $SaO_2$ have a complex relationship, as indicated by the Hb-$O_2$ dissociation curve (Fig. 23-3). At low levels of $O_2$ tension (point A to point B), increases in $PaO_2$ translate into only small increases in the percentage of $O_2$ bound to Hb but, during midrange $O_2$ tension (point B to point C), the relationship of $PaO_2$ to $O_2$-Hb binding is almost linear, with significant increases in $SaO_2$ resulting from increases in $PaO_2$. This relationship is not

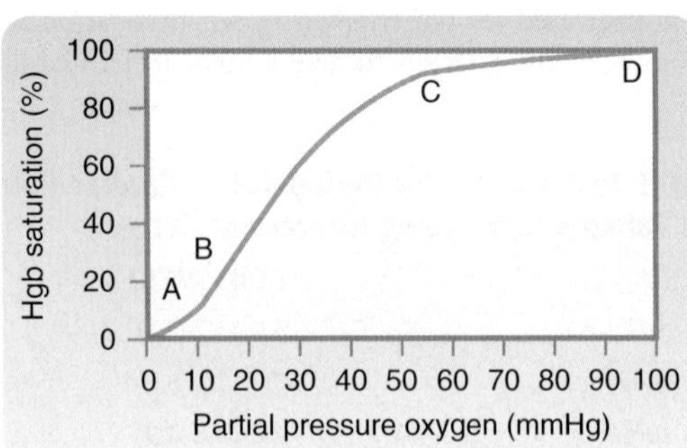


**FIGURE 23-3** Oxygen-hemoglobin (Hgb) dissociation curve. A sigmoid-shaped curve shows maximal oxygen loading in the lung and unloading of $O_2$ in the periphery occurring over a very narrow range of $PAO_2$.

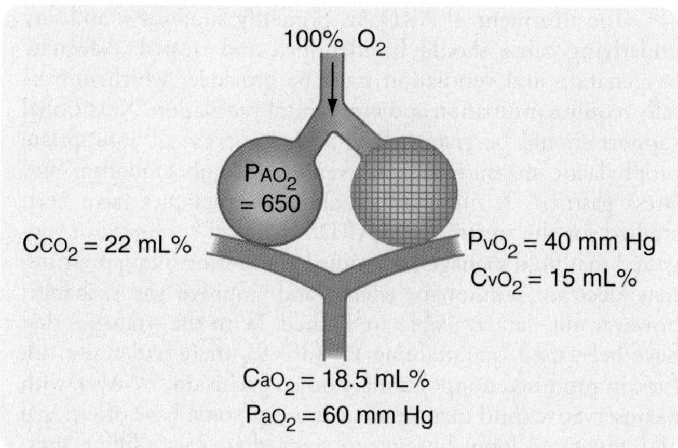


**FIGURE 23-4** Model of the two-alveolus theory of lung function. In the presence of alveolar collapse or alveolar flooding *(hatched area)*, nonoxygenated venous blood on the right is allowed to shunt past the alveolus with no oxygen transfer, for a $Pao_2$ of 40 mm Hg and oxygen content of 15 mL%. Despite a normal alveolus on the left and normal oxygen content after passing by the alveolus ($O_2$ content, 22 mL%), the mixing of right and left blood flow gives the systemic blood a $Po_2$ of 60 mm Hg and a low $O_2$ content of 18.5 mL%. (From Hall JB, Wood LD: Acute hypoxemic respiratory failure. In Hall JB, Schmidt GA, Wood LDH [eds]: Principles of critical care, New York, 1992, McGraw-Hill.)

linear at higher $O_2$ tension (point C to point D), so that continued increases in $Pao_2$ result in very little increase in $Sao_2$. The goal in acute respiratory failure is to achieve a $Pao_2$ that lies on the upper plateau of the curve.

Hypoxemia is affected by inspired $O_2$, ventilation, shunting, and ($\dot{V}/\dot{Q}$ matching. ($\dot{V}/\dot{Q}$ matching is the balance between ventilation and perfusion at the alveolar level. It is a continuum, ranging from complete shunt (perfused but nonventilated space) to dead space (ventilated but nonperfused space). Alveolar collapse (e.g., atelectasis, alveolar flooding with fluid and/or proteinaceous debris) results in a shunt. Blood that perfuses such an alveolus returns to the left atrium with low $CaO_2$, essentially the same as that of mixed venous blood. Dead space ventilation occurs in the conducting airways, where perfusion is limited and essentially no gas exchange occurs. Ultimately, $Pao_2$ represents the sum total of gas exchange (Fig. 23-4). Defects can be quantified as the alveolar-arterial $O_2$ gradient ($AaDo_2$):

$$AaDo_2 = PAO_2 - Pao_2$$

where

$$PAO_2 = [FIO_2 \times (PATM - PH_2O)] - PACO_2$$

PATM is the atmospheric pressure (760 mm Hg at sea level, 627 mm Hg at 5280 feet), $PH_2O$ is the vapor pressure of water (40 mm Hg), and $PACO_2$ is the alveolar pressure of $CO_2$, which can be calculated from $Paco_2$ divided by the respiratory quotient (normally = 0.8). Thus, as an example, for an individual breathing room air at sea level and having $Paco_2$ = 40 mm Hg:

$$PAO_2 = [0.21 \times (760 - 47)] - (40/0.8) = (0.21 \times 713) - 50 = 150 - 50 = 100 \text{ mm Hg}$$

At 5280 feet, $PAO_2$ = 72 mm Hg and, at sea level breathing 100% $O_2$, $PAO_2$ = 663 mm Hg. Subtracting the $Pao_2$ from $PAO_2$ quantifies the $AaDo_2$. In healthy individuals, ventilation and perfusion are well matched and the $AaDo_2$ is low (10 to 25 mm Hg), reflecting only dead space ventilation in the conducting airways and shunting of small amounts of blood via bronchial vessels and thebesian veins. An elevated $AaDo_2$ suggests impaired gas exchange. Nonpulmonary causes of right-to-left shunting include atrial septal defect, pulmonary arteriovenous malformations, severe sepsis, and cirrhosis. There are numerous pulmonary causes of pulmonary dysfunction, including aspiration, atelectasis, pneumonia, pulmonary contusion, PE, pulmonary edema, and ALI–acute respiratory distress syndrome (ARDS).

Aspiration is a common problem in the ICU and may lead to chemical pneumonitis, ventilator-associated pneumonias, and even ARDS. Aspiration occurs because of impairment in laryngeal competence and glottic closure or from gastric reflux caused by ileus or gastric outlet obstruction. It is facilitated by indwelling tubes that breach normal protective mechanisms. If the aspiration event is significant, initial manifestations result from the mechanical effects of airway obstruction. Patients with a diminished sensorium are at particular risk and will not cough to expel the aspirate, resulting in more severe effects. Soon after, the chemical injury becomes evident, with bronchoconstriction and fluid sequestration in the alveoli. An inflammatory response follows, with the release of leukocyte- and platelet-derived inflammatory mediators and leak of protein-rich fluid into the alveoli. Pulmonary function progressively worsens throughout these phases and the resultant hypoxemia may be severe. Because of immunosuppression and compromised airway defenses, bacterial pneumonia is a major risk during the clinical course. Treatment of aspiration is to clear the airways of debris mechanically, decompress the stomach to prevent further events, and provide supportive respiratory care (e.g., bronchodilators, bronchoscopy, mechanical ventilation) as needed. There is no role for corticosteroids or prophylactic antibiotics because these will serve only to select for bacterial resistance; however, the physician should remain vigilant for true pneumonia.

Atelectasis is most often seen in postsurgical or immobilized patients. Alveolar collapse leads to shunting, with ensuing hypoxemia. Additional findings are related to the degree of atelectasis and include diminished breath sounds and reduced lung volumes, elevated hemidiaphragms, and consolidation on chest x-ray. Associated fever may be significant but usually abates with reinflation; however, collapsed alveoli are prone to bacterial colonization, leading to the development of pneumonia. Treatment is aimed at reexpansion of collapsed alveoli, so the maintenance of airway patency and pulmonary toilet is of prime importance. Pain management is pivotal to balance pain-induced splinting with sedation and hypoventilation.

Pneumonia is common in the ICU, particularly among ventilated patients and those with direct lung injury. The clinical presentation involves fever, leukocytosis, hypoxia, distinct radiographic infiltrate, and purulent sputum, with high numbers of bacterial organisms and neutrophils. Respiratory support, pulmonary toilet, and antibiotics are the fundamentals of treatment; however, preventive measures such as back rest elevation, good oral hygiene, daily interruption of sedation, and avoidance of aspiration are paramount. The diagnosis and management of pneumonia are discussed in Chapter 12. Pulmonary contusion is associated with chest wall injury, so pulmonary dysfunction stems not only from disruption of respiratory mechanics with hypoventilation secondary to pain, but to disruption of lung tissue, with alveolar hemorrhage and fluid sequestration overwhelming the innate alveolar protective mechanisms. Chest wall trauma greatly impairs actions such as deep breathing and coughing, so pulmonary toilet is compromised, further predisposing the patient to atelectasis and pneumonia. The initial presentation of pulmonary contusion varies widely and it typically worsens during the ensuing 24 to 48 hours with evolution of the inflammatory response and fluid shifts resulting in blossoming. Management is supportive, with respiratory support and pulmonary toilet, but the contusion remains fertile ground for the development of pneumonia (see Chapter 58).

Pulmonary edema is a potentially catastrophic event, initially manifested by hypoxemia. Clinical signs include dyspnea, tachypnea, hypoxemia, bilateral rhonchi or rales, and frothy sputum. Patients may have signs of hypervolemia, with congestive heart failure, distended neck veins, and peripheral edema. Radiographic findings include redistribution of blood flow (cephalization), perivascular cuffing, enlarged cardiac silhouette, and pleural effusions. The underlying cause may be volume overload or left-sided heart failure. In patients with cardiopulmonary or renal dysfunction, invasive hemodynamic monitoring may be warranted to clarify the diagnosis and optimize therapy. Hypoxemia and hypercapnia are treated supportively, and inotropic support is provided as needed. Diuretic and nitrates may be administered to decrease preload; hydralazine, ACEIs, or nitroprusside can be used to promote afterload reduction. Noninvasive ventilation may buy time for diuretics and other therapies to become effective but the threshold to intubate should remain low.

### Acute Lung Injury and Acute Respiratory Distress Syndrome

ALI and ARDS are clinical syndromes of pulmonary dysfunction that may result from any number of infectious, inflammatory, tissue injury, or cellular shock conditions. Criteria for the diagnosis of ARDS include an acute onset, bilateral pulmonary infiltrates on chest x-ray, absence of cardiogenic pulmonary edema (i.e., PAWP <18 mm Hg), and hypoxemia ($PaO_2/FIO_2$ ≤200).[27] On the same continuum, ALI is a milder form, with $PaO_2/FIO_2$ ranging from 201 to 300.

The mortality of ARDS approaches 50%, with most deaths attributed to MOF. The pathogenesis of ARDS progresses through three stages. The first stage, coinciding with the acute onset of respiratory failure, is known as the exudative phase. Disruption of the alveolar epithelium results in the influx of protein-rich edema fluid and leukocytes into the alveolus. Destruction of type II pneumocytes disrupts normal alveolar fluid transport and surfactant production, contributing to alveolar flooding and collapse. Alveolar macrophages release proinflammatory cytokines that attract and activate neutrophils, provoking tissue injury. Some patients have an uncomplicated course with resolution of the process, whereas others progress to the fibroproliferative phase. Mesenchymal cells fill the alveolar space and initiate fibrosis, with collagen and fibronectin accumulating in the lung. In the final stage, the resolution phase, alveolar edema is resolved as type II pneumocytes repopulate the epithelium, protein is cleared, and there is gradual remodeling of granulation tissue and fibrosis.

The treatment of ARDS is primarily supportive and any underlying cause should be identified and treated. Adequate oxygenation and ventilation must be provided, which universally requires intubation and mechanical ventilation. Nutritional support should be given, along with initiation of appropriate prophylactic measures against venous thromboembolism and stress gastritis. A number of adjunctive therapies have been studied for the treatment of ARDS. Clinical studies have suggested that fluid management aimed at lowering filling pressures may decrease pulmonary edema and improve gas exchange; however, the data available are limited. With the strategies that have been used (maintaining PAWP <8), there is definite risk for compromised nonpulmonary organ perfusion.[20,28] Also, with a conservative fluid management strategy, some have often used and advocated loop diuretics to reach these lower filling pressures but patients with ALI and ARDS often have concurrent pneumonia and other infectious states with tenuous hemodynamics, which preclude the use of diuretics. Surfactant replacement therapy has been successful in neonates, but has not been proven beneficial in adults with ARDS, nor have nitric oxide and other vasodilators, despite earlier studies showing encouraging results. Corticosteroids were never found to be beneficial when administered early in the course of ARDS; however, as the pathophysiology became better understood, this therapy was applied to the later fibroproliferative phase of ARDS. Early results were encouraging, but later trials have shown that this may result in increased mortality. Accordingly, the role of corticosteroids in the management of ARDS remains unclear and they must be used with caution because they predispose patients to an increased risk of infection. There is also recent published evidence that enteral feedings rich in fish oil, specifically omega-3 polyunsaturated fatty acids and arginine, provide clinical benefit. Omega-3 polyunsaturated fatty acids have been shown to improve oxygenation and decrease mortality, overall complications, and ICU length of stay.[29]

A number of methods have been used to ventilate patients with ARDS, including more conventional means such as pressure control ventilation, volume control ventilation, inverse ratio ventilation, and some of the so-called salvage or rescue modes, such as high-frequency jet, percussive, or oscillatory ventilation, extracorporeal membrane oxygenation (ECMO), and extracorporeal carbon dioxide removal. It is now apparent that a strategy of lung protective ventilation using a tidal volume ($V_T$) of 6 mL/kg is associated with mortality reduction, as evidenced by the National Institutes of Health's ARDS Network study.[30] In this multicenter PRCT, patients were randomized to a $V_T$ of 12 mL/kg versus 6 mL/kg, plateau pressures were maintained at less than 50 and less than 30 cm $H_2O$, respectively, in the traditional and lung protective groups, and respiratory acidosis was treated by increasing minute ventilation or adding a bicarbonate infusion. The trial was stopped after enrolling 861 patients because interim analysis showed that in-hospital mortality was reduced from 40% to 31%[30] in the lower $V_T$ group. The results of this study differed from earlier studies (smaller trials) but obtained results that were substantiated in follow-up studies; thus, this approach has gained widespread acceptance as the ventilatory strategy of choice for treating ARDS.

High-frequency percussive ventilation (HFPV) and high-frequency oscillatory ventilation (HFOV) are more commonly used and have been referred to as rescue or salvage modes for ARDS.[31] Their use has largely been limited to patients who have remained hypoxemic on the more conventional modes, such as pressure or volume control ventilation. The exudative and fibroproliferative phases of ARDS cause a marked decrease in lung compliance and the high peak airway pressures generated by the conventional modes can result in significant barotrauma. Both HFPV and HFOV create far lower peak pressures but maintain or slightly increase mean airway pressures compared with the conventional modes, which is one mechanism whereby they improve oxygenation. The other hypothesized mechanisms of improvement of oxygenation by HFPV include changes in flow patterns (bulk, convective flow) and molecular diffusion; however, it is beyond the scope of this chapter to provide further details. There is a significant amount of literature showing improved outcomes with HFPV for inhalation injury, but the investigation into its benefits for non–thermally injured trauma or surgical patients with ARDS is evolving. Some retrospective data show that HFPV improves oxygenation in ARDS while not changing mean airway pressures significantly,[31] so additional research is needed. However, HFPV and HFOV are now considered as salvage methods for difficult to oxygenate ARDS patients. Airway pressure release ventilation (APRV) is another potentially useful mode of ventilation for patients with ALI and ARDS. APRV maintains a higher mean airway pressure while avoiding the higher peak pressures of conventional modes of ventilation; it can improve oxygenation and possibly reduce barotrauma.[32] The more consistent alveolar recruitment may also improve ventilation-perfusion matching and improve overall gas exchange. Also, patients can have spontaneous respirations with APRV, which this may lead to greater patient comfort and decreased use of sedation. Presently, however, there is no evidence showing improved clinical outcomes with APRV, only that it is a ventilation method that can be used safely for these patients.

Prone positioning has been proposed as a means to improve oxygenation by increasing end-expiratory lung volume, improving ($\dot{V}/\dot{Q}$ matching, and changing chest wall mechanics. In a multicenter PRCT conducted more than 10 years ago, prone positioning improved oxygenation but not survival in a subset of patients with severe hypoxemia; however, this was before ARDS trials introduced lung protective strategies, such as lower $V_T$ ventilation. Since then, randomized investigations have still not found a survival benefit in the prone positioning strategy, which has continued to show increased drawbacks and complication rates, most notably in the need for increased sedation, use of neuromuscular blockade, hemodynamic instability, and patient device displacement. Care of the patient in the prone position is labor-intensive and meticulous attention must be paid to minimize complications, such as pressure ulceration and accidental extubation.

Positive end-expiratory pressure (PEEP) can improve oxygenation by recruiting collapsed alveoli and increasing functional residual capacity. Conventional ventilation generally calls for the minimal PEEP necessary to provide acceptable oxygenation. However, in the setting of ARDS, there may be benefit to increasing PEEP to improve oxygenation and protect the lung by preventing the repetitive shearing forces of recruitment or derecruitment of alveoli, reducing cyclic reopening and stretch during mechanical breaths. The optimal level of PEEP may be determined by incrementally increasing PEEP to maximize the $PaO_2/FIO_2$ ratio; however, some have argued that this ignores lung mechanics. A lung pressure-volume curve may be generated for a given patient and the lower inflection point (PFLEX), the point at which the slope increases in steepness, representing a pressure at which most alveolar units are open, may be identified. Alternatively, the PEEP may be titrated to maximal compliance, which may be easier to measure at the bedside. Available evidence seems to support the concept that higher levels of PEEP in ARDS may limit stretch trauma to the lung and may have beneficial effects on outcomes.[27]

## Ventilatory Support

### Noninvasive Ventilatory Support

Many patients require more support than a passive $O_2$ delivery device. Several noninvasive ventilatory interventions can support oxygenation and ventilation, and possibly obviate the need for endotracheal intubation and mechanical ventilation. Intermittent positive pressure breathing aids in clearance of secretions but is labor intensive and, because it is not continuously applied, does not permanently recruit alveoli. Continuous positive airway pressure (CPAP) applied by a tight-fitting mask can maintain and restore functional residual capacity and, therefore, provides a temporary salutary effect on oxygenation as the underlying cause of hypoxia is treated. This intervention has little if any effect on ventilation and requires a nasogastric tube because of associated aerophagia. Also, a decreased level of consciousness is a relative contraindication to the tight-fitting mask because the patient may vomit and may not be able to remove the mask from his or her face, resulting in aspiration. Bilevel positive airway pressure (BiPAP) also uses a tight-fitting mask, but requires a ventilator to deliver a high airway pressure during spontaneous patient-initiated breaths and a lower baseline pressure during exhalation (like PEEP). It may provide enough assistance to prevent fatigue and stave off endotracheal intubation. Similar to CPAP, BiPAP should be considered a short-term therapy that allows for the identification and treatment of the underlying derangement. Continued close monitoring is necessary for patients on CPAP and BiPAP because their condition may deteriorate precipitously. A cautionary note must be sounded regarding the use of noninvasive ventilation to treat postextubation respiratory failure because this may be associated with a higher mortality than standard therapy.[33]

### Mechanical Ventilation

As noted, there are four primary indications for endotracheal intubation and mechanical ventilation, as given earlier by the mnemonic SOAP. The first variable to set is the trigger—that is, the variable that will initiate inspiration. The trigger may be a time interval or a threshold rate of air flow. The second variable to set is an inspiratory limit, which may be a volume, pressure, or maximum air flow rate. The third variable to set is the cycle, which may be a volume, pressure, or time. Based on these variables, the ventilator will deliver one of three types of breaths, mandatory, assisted, or spontaneous. A mandatory breath is triggered, limited, and cycled by the machine. An assisted breath is triggered by the patient, but is limited and cycled by the ventilator. A spontaneous breath is triggered, limited, and cycled by the patient.

### Volume-Cycled Ventilation

This type of ventilation delivers a preset $V_T$ with each breath. Advantages include delivery of a reliable minute volume and ease of use. The major disadvantage is potential for high airway pressures and resulting lung injury. The different modes of volume-cycled ventilation include controlled mandatory ventilation (CMV), assist control ventilation (AC), and intermittent mandatory ventilation (IMV). With CMV, the patient receives a set number of fixed-volume breaths, but is unable to increase minute ventilation by triggering additional breaths. CMV is typically only used in patients in the operating room under general anesthesia. AC differs from CMV in that the patient can trigger additional breaths. Every triggered breath will be a full machine-cycled breath. AC is used when full ventilatory support is required but is not suitable for the agitated patient who is tachypneic because it may lead to severe respiratory alkalosis. IMV allows spontaneous breathing. It delivers intermittent fixed-volume breaths and allows the patient to breathe spontaneously between mechanical breaths. Synchronized IMV (SIMV) allows the mechanical breaths to be triggered by the patient's own respiratory effort and avoids stacking of breaths. Varying degrees of pressure support may be added to the spontaneous breaths to assist the patient. SIMV is a useful mode of ventilation when attempting to wean the patient or when there is patient-ventilator asynchrony. In general, volume-cycled ventilation is the most uncomfortable for the patient and may result in significant patient-ventilator dyssynchrony, requiring significant amounts of sedatives.

### Pressure-Cycled Ventilation

Pressure-controlled ventilation is designed to protect the lung from alveolar overdistention and epithelial injury. A set pressure is applied to the ventilatory circuit during each breath, allowing the lungs to expand based on thoracic compliance. The major advantages are lower mean and peak airway pressures and an exponential decelerating flow pattern, which tends to be more comfortable for the patient. The major disadvantage is fluctuating minute ventilation in the presence of changing lung compliance. Pressure-cycled breaths can be delivered in an analogous fashion to volume-cycled breaths in an AC or SIMV mode. Pressure-support ventilation (PSV) is a spontaneous ventilatory mode. A negative inspiratory force created by the patient will trigger the ventilator to apply a certain pressure to the ventilator circuit. PSV is the most comfortable mode of ventilation because the patient can control all the elements of inspiration and expiration; accordingly, PSV has become the mode of choice for weaning patients off mechanical ventilation. The major disadvantage of PSV is that minute ventilation cannot be ensured and hypoventilation and apnea can occur; thus, patients must have an intact respiratory drive and be carefully monitored.

### Difficult to Ventilate Patients

Patients with severe lung disease can be a challenge to oxygenate and ventilate. On volume-cycled ventilator modes, airway pressures may climb; on pressure-cycled modes, the delivered $V_T$ may decrease. The goals include maintaining airway pressures less than 35 to 40 cm $H_2O$, and an $Sa_{O_2}$ of 90% or higher. Definitive recommendations for optimal ventilator strategies are not available, but there are a number of maneuvers that may be attempted. Prone positioning, inhaled nitric oxide, and permissive hypercapnia have been discussed earlier. Inverse ratio ventilation involves lengthening inspiratory time to more than 50% of the respiratory cycle, which increases the mean airway pressure and recruits air spaces by auto-PEEP in a manner similar to that of applied PEEP. Inverse ratio ventilation should be used with caution in patients with diminished dynamic compliance, such as chronic obstructive pulmonary disease (COPD), asthma, and ARDS, given their propensity for air trapping. Air trapping should be suspected in a patient whenever an increased minute volume results in an increased $P_{CO_2}$. In severe cases, pharmacologic paralysis, which relaxes the chest wall musculature and allows for synchronization of ventilator and patient while decreasing $V_{O_2}$ and $CO_2$ production, may be required. Tracheal gas insufflation provides 2 to 10 liters/min of 100% $O_2$ delivered 1 cm above the carina. It decreases $Pa_{CO_2}$ by washing out the proximal anatomic dead space and can be useful when permissive hypercapnia is being used to attenuate respiratory acidosis.

A tracheostomy may be necessary to facilitate weaning and discontinuation of mechanical ventilation in some patients because it can decrease dead space ventilation and the work of breathing and improve patient comfort, thus decreasing sedation requirements and improving pulmonary toileting and clearance of secretions. The timing of tracheostomy for respiratory failure is a controversial topic. Older studies suggested that the procedure be performed on patients who have remained on mechanical ventilation longer than 14 to 20 days; however, more recent data have shown decreases in ICU length of stay and duration of mechanical ventilation without increased complication rates when tracheostomy is performed within 7 days of the occurrence of respiratory failure.[34] This has been further supported by studies showing the same benefits in a mixed population of medical, surgical, and trauma patients who underwent tracheostomy within 3 days of the initiation of mechanical ventilation. Percutaneous tracheostomy is an attractive modality because it is more convenient than traditional tracheostomy done in the operating room and may be associated with reduced costs, transport complications, delays, and postoperative hemorrhage and infection than open techniques.

ECMO or $CO_2$ removal may offer enough lung protection to salvage critically ill patients, but expertise and availability are often limited. Their use is best restricted to rescue patients with severe respiratory failure unresponsive to other modalities of advanced ventilatory support in the hope that the patients' lungs will recover while avoiding further exposure to the potentially injurious aspects of mechanical ventilation.[35] The influenza A (H1N1) pandemic led to the investigation of ECMO as a means to treat the many patients who suffered from H1N1-associated ARDS.[35] Although the initial results in terms of survival and recovery of pulmonary function are promising, only observational data exist at this time and it must be remembered that prior investigations into ECMO for ARDS have uniformly failed to show any survival benefit. The exception to this is a recent randomized trial (CESAR 2009) in the UK of 180 patients with severe, acute respiratory failure; some survival benefit without significant disability was noted in patients treated with ECMO when compared with conventional ventilation.[36,37]

### Weaning from Mechanical Ventilation

Patients who are intubated for pulmonary failure usually require a period of weaning to regain strength and to prove their ability to ventilate and oxygenate themselves. When considering removing a patient from the ventilator, it is important first to ensure that the underlying problem leading to intubation has been rectified and the patient is otherwise stable. Then, one may make the same SOAP assessment as when determining the need for intubation:

1. Are the ***s***ecretions too much for the patient to handle?
2. Is the patient ***o***xygenating adequately (i.e., $Pa{O_2}/F{IO_2}$ >200, which requires that $F{IO_2}$ ≤0.40 to 0.50 and PEEP <5 to 8 cm $H_2O$)?
3. Can the patient protect his or her ***a***irway?
4. Is ***p***ulmonary function adequate?

Ideally, the patient is assessed while breathing spontaneously and a number of parameters may be obtained to assess pulmonary function. Negative inspiratory force (>−20 to −30 cm $H_2O$), minute ventilation (<10 to 15 liters/min), VT (>5 mL/kg), and respiratory rate (<30 breaths/min) are all useful indicators. Perhaps the most reliable single test is the frequency (f)/VT ratio, the Tobin or Rapid Shallow Breathing Index.[37] A value higher than 105 predicts failure of extubation with a 95% likelihood, whereas a value lower than 80 predicts success in 95% of patients. There are four primary methods of weaning. Multiple daily T piece trials may be performed with extubation once the patient can tolerate several hours. This is labor-intensive and may cause the patient undue stress, particularly if she or he is intubated with a small-diameter endotracheal tube. A single T piece trial may be performed daily with extubation if it is successful. If this trial is unsuccessful, the patient is rested for 24 hours and the test is repeated the following day. IMV and PSV weaning are popular, without a clear-cut advantage of one over the other. It is clear, however, that trials of spontaneous breathing shorten weaning time, so daily sedation holidays and spontaneous breathing trials are mandatory.

Prior to extubating a patient, the bedside clinician should systematically review the patient's overall condition in addition to the previously mentioned SOAP assessment, focusing on factors other than respiratory mechanics. Upper airway edema and obstruction should be ruled out by checking for an endotracheal tube cuff leak. An unambiguous and objective method of doing this requires the patient to cough around the endotracheal tube with the cuff down and a finger occluding the tube's lumen; however, care must be taken to prevent aspiration of secretions pooled above the balloon prior to its deflation. The chart and anesthesia record should be reviewed to ensure that the initial intubation was straightforward in case the patient needs to be reintubated. Patients intubated after multiple attempts, bronchoscopic assistance, or via a retrograde intubation are best extubated under controlled circumstances rather than in the middle of the night. Finally, factors necessitating increased ventilatory demand should be corrected, if possible, such as acid-base disturbances, hepatic or renal failure, high fever, sepsis, pronounced anxiety, and agitation. Patients who are difficult to sedate and alternate between agitation and oversedation may benefit from the $\alpha_2$-adrenergic agonist dexmedetomidine which exerts only minimal effects on hemodynamic stability or respiratory drive.[6]

## GASTROINTESTINAL SYSTEM

### Stress Gastritis

Stress-related mucosal lesions are the result of gastric acid acting on compromised (i.e., poorly perfused and/or immunologically incompetent) gastric mucosa. These lesions have been reported to develop in 25% to100% of ICU patients within 24 to 48 hours of admission, with clinically significant bleeding manifesting in only 5% to10% of patients. Based on these data, routine stress ulcer prophylaxis is provided in most ICUs; however, it is probably not necessary for every ICU patient. The evolution of care in ICUs has provided earlier and better resuscitation and nutritional support, resulting in improved mucosal perfusion and preserved integrity. Risk factors for stress gastritis include mechanical ventilation longer than 48 hours, coagulopathy, significant burns, and head injury. Patients with risk factors should receive prophylaxis until they are taking a gastric enteral diet at more than 50% of caloric intake goals because gastric feeding represents one of the most effective means of preventing stress gastritis. Prophylactic agents include antacids, sucralfate, histamine $H_2$ receptor antagonists, and proton pump inhibitors, with the latter becoming the mainstay of therapy because of their long duration of action and efficacy. Antacids have not been proven effective for at-risk ICU patients and should not be considered a first-line agent. Sucralfate is a sucrose-based polymer that is activated in an acidic environment and binds to exposed gastric mucosa and ulcer craters, forming a protective barrier. It also stimulates local prostaglandin synthesis and can be given as an elixir by mouth or via nasogastric tube. Early trials suggested a lower risk of nosocomial pneumonia compared with $H_2$ receptor antagonists, which was attributed to the preservation of an acidic gastric environment and reduced bacterial proliferation. The major disadvantage of sucralfate is its interference with absorption of other medications, such as antibiotics, warfarin, and phenytoin. The $H_2$ receptor antagonists have potent acid reducing properties. Concerns regarding $H_2$ receptor antagonists include the development of tachyphylaxis and increased gastric bacterial colonization leading to the development of pneumonia. A large multicenter PRCT comparing the use of sucralfate to ranitidine in ICU patients with risk factors has determined that $H_2$ receptor antagonists are superior to sucralfate in preventing clinically important bleeding whereas the rate of ventilator associated pneumonia was similar between the groups. Although proton pump inhibitors have been shown to be superior to $H_2$ receptor antagonists in the treatment of peptic ulcer disease, clinical trials demonstrating their superiority in preventing stress gastritis are lacking.[38] Additionally, an association has been made between PPI usage and community-acquired *Clostridium difficile* colitis.

### Selective Digestive Decontamination

Selective digestive decontamination (SDD) is a strategy aimed at reducing the bacterial load in the intestine based on the theory that gut bacteria translocate to the systemic circulation, inciting an inflammatory response that leads to MOF (see later).[39] Although the phenomenon of microbial translocation has been documented in animals and suggested in some human studies, there is no convincing evidence that translocation of bacteria is responsible for adverse clinical outcomes. Conversely, there is evidence that inflammatory mediators may traverse the gut in times of stress, aided by gut hypoperfusion and the loss of mucosal integrity, immunoglobulins, and enterocytes. SDD is designed to reduce the load of gram-negative aerobic and anaerobic pathogens in the gut. A typical formulation includes a paste of polymyxin, tobramycin, and amphotericin or colistin applied to the oral mucosa, a slurry administered into the stomach, and a third-generation cephalosporin administered IV. Another strategy is selective oral decontamination (SOD), in which a similarly constituted paste or slurry is created and applied to the oral mucosa but no IV agents are given. Studies in a varied population of critically ill patients have shown a subtle mortality benefit from SDD and SOD compared with a regimen of standard care. Howver, SDD and SOD strategies are controversial and other studies have yielded mixed results, with some showing markedly increased complications rates of hospital-acquired and surgical site infections. Despite this, ongoing research suggests that SDD may be beneficial, particularly in surgical ICU patients.

### Abdominal Compartment Syndrome

The abdomen is a closed space, bound by the relatively nonexpansile fascia of the abdominal musculature and, as such, is susceptible to a compartment syndrome analogous to that seen in the lower extremities. ACS is fundamentally defined as increased intra-abdominal pressure (IAP) associated with adverse physiologic consequences.[40] ACS has usually been described in patients with massive abdominal or pelvic hemorrhage, often following damage control laparotomy, but it may be encountered in various clinical scenarios. Circumferential torso burn eschar, reduction of a large ventral hernia, or military antishock trousers may significantly increase IAP. Bowel distention caused by obstruction or ileus, ascites, or pneumoperitoneum may also lead to ACS. Pancreatitis or surgical dissection may result in profound retroperitoneal edema. Edema of the bowel may result from prolonged evisceration during surgery, which elongates and narrows mesenteric veins and lymphatics; it may also be related to ischemia or reperfusion of the bowel aggravated by resuscitation with large volumes of crystalloid solutions. Secondary ACS refers to ACS in the absence of abdominal or pelvic pathology and is entirely caused by edema and ascites following shock and aggressive resuscitation. In this setting, particularly in nontrauma patients, it may represent a state of irreversible shock, with loss of capillary integrity.

The organ systems that appear most affected by ACS are the cardiovascular, pulmonary, and renal systems. Cardiovascular effects of increased IAP include decreased CO because of diminished venous return and a markedly increased systemic vascular resistance. Ensuring adequate volume status is a key feature of ACS management and can be used to temporize the situation while arrangements are made for urgent decompression. Increased IAP diminishes diaphragmatic excursion, decreases pulmonary compliance, and creates high airway pressures, with diminishing VT and resultant respiratory acidosis. Renal dysfunction, oliguria progressing to anuria because of ACS, appears to be caused by direct parenchymal compression and shunting of renal plasma flow. Visceral blood flow is similarly affected, leading to intestinal necrosis, hepatic dysfunction, and gut anastomotic breakdown. Intracranial hypertension is also aggravated by ACS. Decompressive celiotomy can reverse these changes immediately, but untreated ACS leads to lethal organ failure, with collective mortality rates exceeding 50%.[40]

The recognition of ACS is not difficult once the diagnosis is considered. Those at highest risk include severely injured patients who require abdominal packing for abbreviated or staged laparotomy, particularly those with a coagulopathy caused by core hypothermia or cirrhosis. It is prudent to screen patients at high risk for developing ACS, particularly those acutely resuscitated from shock, those who require vasopressors, and those who are receiving large volumes of crystalloid fluids or blood products. The findings of a tensely distended abdomen, progressive oliguria in spite of adequate CO, or hypoxia with increasing airway pressures are sufficient to justify abdominal decompression. Physical findings alone may be inaccurate in the critically ill patient; thus, bladder pressures can be measured to determine an elevated IAP and correlate it with physiologic parameters; therefore, bladder pressure has become the objective measure for confirming ACS. The level of IAP at which ACS occurs is patient-specific, so the diagnosis and treatment are based on the patient's physiologic responses to increased IAP. Rough correlations can be made between the level of IAP elevation and the need for decompression (Table 23-4). Although significant alterations in physiology can be demonstrated with an IAP between 10 and 15 mm Hg (grade I), it is doubtful that abdominal decompression is warranted at this level. With an IAP between 15 and 25 mm Hg (grade II), the need for treatment should be based on the patient's clinical condition; however, in the absence of oliguria, hypoxia, or significantly elevated airway pressure, abdominal decompression is difficult to justify.

**Table 23-4 Grading System for Abdominal Compartment Syndrome**

| GRADE | INTRA-ABDOMINAL PRESSURE (MM HG) | TREATMENT |
|---|---|---|
| I | 10-14 | Normovolemic resuscitation |
| II | 15-24 | Hypovolemic resuscitation |
| III | 25-35 | Decompression |
| IV | >35 | Emergency reexploration |

Continued monitoring is clearly indicated because signs and symptoms of intra-abdominal hypertension progress insidiously. Most patients with an IAP between 25 and 35 mm Hg (grade III) ultimately require decompression. All patients with an IAP higher than 35 mm Hg (grade IV) require immediate decompression because they may deteriorate to cardiac arrest at any time. Percutaneous drainage of ascitic fluid may be a temporizing maneuver, but operative decompression is usually necessary. At the time of decompression, an abdominal closure that affords additional intra-abdominal domain is indicated. Of the various dressings described, the most effective appears to be based on some type of vacuum, either commercially available or home-made, so that bowel edema and lateral retraction of the fascia are minimized and peritoneal fluid is controlled.[41]

Every reasonable effort should be made to achieve definitive abdominal closure within several days, because the lateral retractive forces of the broad flat muscles of the abdominal wall can make primary closure difficult. If the abdomen cannot be closed, absorbable or biologic meshes and skin grafts should be used to minimize the risk of intestinal fistulas. Interestingly, vacuum-assisted wound dressings may facilitate early definitive abdominal closure, as well as late closure many weeks after the initial operation.[42] Care of the patient with an open abdomen is an evolving area of surgery but efforts should generally focus on protecting the bowel from fistula formation, optimizing nutrition, treating infections and organ failure, and closing the fascia as soon as possible.

### Nutritional Support

The neuroendocrine response to critical illness and injury includes the release of stress hormones (e.g., epinephrine, glucagon, cortisol) and inflammatory mediators that culminate in a hypercatabolic state (see Chapter 4). Endogenous nutrient substrates are mobilized, depleting glucose and fat stores and breaking down lean muscle mass. Subsequently, visceral protein stores are eroded, resulting in organ system and immune dysfunction. Presently, we have little ability to modulate the systemic inflammatory response in critical illness but the preferred therapeutic strategy of administering exogenous substrate in the form of nutritional therapy (the preferred term of the American Society for Parenteral and Enteral Nutrition) is now the norm.[43] Nutritional therapy should be considered if the following are seen: (1) the patient has been without nutrition for 5 to 7 days; (2) the duration of illness is expected to exceed 10 days; or (3) the patient was premorbidly malnourished. A recent unintended weight loss of 15% to 20% suggests moderate malnutrition; loss of over 20% implies severe caloric malnutrition. Serum protein levels, such as albumin, prealbumin, transferrin, and retinol-binding protein, may be measured but they are usually negatively affected by severe illness and inflammatory states and are considered highly unreliable markers of nutritional status. Once the decision is made to provide support, the next step is to determine the nutritional needs of the patient. A practical rule of thumb is based on weight, so that for most patients, 25 to 30 kcal/kg/day should be adequate. A more precise number for the basal energy expenditure (BEE, in kcal/day) may be estimated by the Harris-Benedict equations.

For males:

$$\text{BEE} = 66 + (13.7 \times \text{weight}) + (5 \times \text{height}) - (6.8 \times \text{age})$$

For females:

$$\text{BEE} = 665 + (9.6 \times \text{weight}) + (1.8 \times \text{height}) - (4.7 \times \text{age})$$

where weight is measured in kilograms, height in centimeters, and age in years. The BEE estimate is then multiplied by a stress factor ranging from 1.25 to 1.75, depending on the severity of illness or injury. In stable mechanically ventilated patients in whom overfeeding or underfeeding would be particularly detrimental, whose energy expenditure is significantly altered from expected values, or who are not responding as expected to calculated regimens, indirect calorimetry can be used to calculate the measured energy expenditure (MEE, also in kcal/day):

$$\text{MEE} = [(3.9 \times \text{V}_{\text{O}_2}) + 1.1 + \text{V}_{\text{CO}_2}] \times 1.44 - (2.8 \times \text{U}_{\text{UN}})$$

where $V_{O_2}$ and $CO_2$ production ($V_{CO_2}$) reflect that during a 30-minute period. The preferred ratio of nonprotein calories to nitrogen varies with stress level. In minimally stressed patients, 200 to 300 : 1 is appropriate, but should be decreased to 150 : 1 in moderately stressed and 100 : 1 or less in severely stressed patients. In patients with hepatic or renal failure, protein restriction may be warranted. An alternative method of determining protein needs is weight- and stress-based: 1.5 for mild, 2.0 for moderate, and 2.5 g protein/kg for severe stress.

Finally, measurement of urine urea nitrogen ($U_{UN}$) can help determine protein needs because as stress-related catabolism increases, nitrogen excretion (and $U_{UN}$) increases. The $U_{UN}$ represents 90% of excreted nitrogen. Protein losses (g/day) may be calculated based on 24-hour $U_{UN}$:

$$\text{Protein loss} = [\text{U}_{\text{UN}} + (4\text{ g insensible} + \text{nonurea nitrogen loss})]$$

The goal of nutritional support is to provide a positive nitrogen balance of 3 to 5 g/day, so additional protein must be added beyond the calculated requirements. To calculate the protein requirements, multiply nitrogen requirements by 6.25. Patients should be assessed serially to ensure that they are receiving adequate amounts of protein because most standard enteral formulas tend to have higher ratios of nonprotein to protein calories for energy provision than are optimal for a postoperative or injured patient.[43]

The optimal route and method for delivery of nutritional support remain controversial. In general, a patient with a functioning gastrointestinal tract should be fed enterally; the goal should be to initiate these feedings as soon as a patient is hemodynamically normal because the immunomodulating and promoting effects of the feeding are most likely to occur within the first 24 to 72 hours after surgery or injury. Enteral feeding preserves gut mucosal integrity, barrier function, secretory IgA production, and normal flora, which may be one explanation for the reduction in septic complications and improved survival seen in enterally fed patients with severe injuries, acute pancreatitis, inflammatory bowel disease, and liver transplantation. Furthermore, the safety and feasibility of early postoperative enteral feeding have been proven and avoiding parenteral nutrition and the central venous access required results in significantly lower rates of bacteremia and central catheter–associated sepsis. Also, enteral nutrition is associated with lower rates of pneumonia, has significantly lower cost, likely results in a more stable glycemic profile, and is associated with improved return of cognition in traumatic brain injury patients when compared with parenteral nutrition. Conversely, there are some conflicting data and no evidence of clear overall superiority of enteral nutrition over parenteral nutrition. Parenteral delivery of nutrition can ensure adequate provision of nutrients and should be used when enteral feeding is not tolerated, when frequent stoppages occur to limit caloric delivery because of the need for procedures or reoperation, or in the presence of short gut or high-output or proximal gastrointestinal fistulae. In critically ill patients, postpyloric feeding was thought to be safer; however, no significant differences have been shown in rates of aspiration or ventilator-associated pneumonia between gastric and postpyloric feeding techniques. Postpyloric feeding can be used as a backup method for patients intolerant of gastric feeding who have repeated high gastric residual volumes or those who clinicians believe are at unacceptably high risk for aspiration. Regardless of the route of enteral nutrition used, tube feeding protocols (e.g., starting and advancing feed rates, residual volume tolerance) executed and managed by ICU nurses result in higher rates of intended caloric delivery.

Immune-enhancing diets provide specific nutrients (e.g., glutamine, arginine, nucleotides, omega-3 fatty acids) that exert favorable immunomodulatory effects. Glutamine is an oxidative fuel for enterocytes and other rapidly replicating cells and is said to be conditionally essential. Arginine promotes normal T cell function, aids in wound healing, and is necessary for the metabolism of ammonia. Nucleotides enhance the replication of rapidly dividing cells as well as promote immune responsiveness. The omega-3 fatty acids compete with omega-6 fatty acids (specifically arachidonic acid) in cyclooxygenase metabolism, resulting in the production of prostaglandins in series

3 (eicosapentaenoic acid) and leukotrienes in series 5. These eicosanoids are less inflammatory and immunosuppressive than the prostaglandins in series 2 and the leukotrienes in series 4 produced by arachidonic acid. The addition of glutamine to enteral formulas should be considered in burn and trauma patients because there are some limited data showing decreased hospital and ICU length of stay; however, further study is needed and the costs of adding glutamine to tube feeds are not inconsequential. Although several clinical trials have suggested significant benefits with these diets, study results are mixed and a mortality benefit is lacking[44]; thus, patients not meeting the criteria for immune-modulating formulations should receive standard enteral formulations.

## ACUTE KIDNEY INJURY

Acute kidney injury (AKI, formerly known as acute renal failure [ARF]) is a deadly problem, with mortality rates exceeding 30%, which more than doubles if dialysis is required. AKI, a term coined by the Acute Dialysis Quality Initiative, is now the preferred term to describe a newfound decrease in renal function and use of the RIFLE criteria (***r***isk, ***i***njury, failure, ***l***oss, ***e***nd-stage renal disease [ESRD] has been shown to be the most sensitive method for detecting AKI early after its occurrence (Box 23-2).[45] Its onset is heralded by oliguria (<0.5 mL/kg/hr, or <400 mL/24 hr) or a rising serum creatinine level, which should prompt a search for its cause (prerenal, renal parenchymal, or postrenal). The first step is a physical examination to look for signs of hypovolemia, heart failure, shock, obstruction, ACS, or rash. The most common cause of oliguria in surgical patients is prerenal hypovolemia. A Foley catheter should be inserted to exclude bladder outlet obstruction and monitor the urine output closely. Next, a fluid bolus (500 to 1000 mL, or 10% of the circulating blood volume) should be administered, except in patients in whom severe heart failure is suspected; in that case, measurement of PAWP is more helpful in directing therapy. If the patient does not respond to fluid administration, a more extensive evaluation must be undertaken and invasive hemodynamic monitoring is warranted to measure filling pressures and assess cardiac function. A spot urine sodium ($U_{Na}$) level may be helpful in distinguishing prerenal from renal parenchymal causes of AKI because $U_{Na}$ less than 20 mEq/liter is consistent with a prerenal cause and $U_{Na}$ higher than 40 mEq/liter with a renal parenchymal cause. By measuring sodium and creatinine levels in the urine and plasma, the fractional excretion of sodium ($FE_{Na}$) may be calculated as a percentage:

$$FE_{Na} = [(U_{Na} \times P_{Cr})/(P_{Na} \times U_{Cr})] \times 100$$

**BOX 23-2 RIFLE Criteria**

***R***isk: ↑ creatinine level × 1.5 *or* ↓ GFR > 25% *or* UO < 0.5 mL/kg/hr q6h
***I***njury: ↑ creatinine level × 2 *or* ↓ GFR > 50% *or* UO < 0.5 mL/kg/hr q12h
***F***ailure: ↑ creatinine level × 3 *or* ↓ GFR > 75% *or* UO < 0.3 mL/kg/hr q24h *or* anuria q12h
***L***oss: Persistent AKI: complete loss of kidney function > 4 wk
***E***SRD: End-stage renal disease > 3 mo

*GFR*, Glomerular filtration rate; *UO*, urine output.

$FE_{Na}$ less than 1% indicates a prerenal cause of AKI, whereas $FE_{Na}$ higher than 3% suggests a renal parenchymal or postrenal problem. The patient's medications should be reviewed for nephrotoxic agents and postrenal pathology may be identified by renal ultrasonography. Urinalysis can also provide clues to the underlying cause: high urine specific gravity and low pH are consistent with prerenal AKI; tubular casts are indicative of renal parenchymal dysfunction; hemoglobinuria is consistent with a transfusion reaction, vasculitis, or rhabdomyolysis; myoglobinuria is suggestive of rhabdomyolysis; and eosinophilia is associated with interstitial nephritis. These laboratory investigations are less helpful in older patients, those with chronic renal dysfunction, or patients who have received diuretics or osmotic agents in the previous 24 hours.

The management of prerenal AKI is to augment renal perfusion through volume loading and inotropic support as needed. Unfortunately, renal vasoconstriction may be an unwanted side effect of such inotropic agents. Formerly, low-dose (0.3 to 3 μg/kg/min) dopamine was advocated for the treatment of AKI to dilate the renal vasculature and stimulate diuresis; however, evidence to support this is lacking. Nephrotoxic drugs, including contrast agents, should be avoided, and renally excreted drugs should be dose-adjusted. The creatinine clearance ($C_{Cr}$, in mL/min) can be used for medication dose adjustment:

$$C_{Cr} = (U_{Cr} \times V)/P_{Cr}$$

where UCr is urine creatinine concentration (mg/dL), V is urine volume (mL/min) and $P_{Cr}$ is plasma creatinine concentration (mg/dL). A 24-hour collection is most accurate, but a 4-hour sample may be used. An immediate calculation may be made using the Cockcroft-Gault approximation:

$$C_{Cr} = [(140 - \text{age}) \times \text{weight}]/(P_{Cr} \times 72)$$

where weight is measured in kilograms. In women, the value is multiplied by 0.85. A normal $C_{Cr}$ value is 95 mL/min in women and 120 mL/min in men. In cases of rhabdomyolysis and transfusion reactions, clearance of circulating myoglobin or Hb may be achieved by forcing diuresis (>100 mL/hr) with crystalloids and osmotic diuretics; however, success with this technique is variable. Obstructing lesions should be treated, comorbid conditions addressed, and nutritional support provided. Although the conversion of oliguric to nonoliguric AKI with diuretics may facilitate volume management, it is often unsuccessful and there is insufficient evidence that it improves outcomes. Diuretic usage in AKI remains controversial, with some studies suggesting an increased risk of nonrecovery of renal function and mortality and others not suggesting this.

RRT may be indicated for symptomatic fluid overload, severe electrolyte or acid-base disorders, sepsis, or uremic complications such as encephalopathy or pericarditis. There are, however, no specific criteria to guide the timing or institution of replacement therapies and the decision to do so is based on clinical assessment. Several options for RRT exist, including intermittent techniques such as peritoneal dialysis or hemodialysis. Peritoneal dialysis is appropriate in chronic renal failure patients who do not have peritonitis or have not undergone recent abdominal surgery but has limited applications in the ICU. Hemodialysis provides efficient removal of fluid, solutes, and some toxins, but may be associated with hemodynamic instability because of the high flow rates required and is relatively resource-intensive. Continuous RRT techniques offer the advantage of improved hemodynamic stability and relatively less resource use, but require some type of anticoagulation and have not been proven superior to hemodialysis in improving outcomes except in some limited clinical trials. Interestingly, RRT has been shown to remove cytokines and inflammatory mediators from the blood of septic patients without having a significant impact on survival. Continuous hemofiltration may be used to remove fluid and solutes in patients who only suffer from fluid overload, but continuous venovenous hemodialysis (CVVHD) is the most commonly used method in the ICU. It uses a double-lumen central venous catheter and pumps blood through a filter against the counterflow of dialysate before returning it to the patient. Initially, there was significant enthusiasm for increased flow rates in continuous renal replacement therapies, leading to better clinical outcomes, but more recent randomized trials have shown no reduction in mortality, ICU length of stay, or duration on a ventilator with these higher intensity therapy and flow rates.[46] Continuous arteriovenous hemodiafiltration (CAVHD) is similar but requires a large-bore arterial cannula and adequate patient arterial pressure to drive the process and, as such, has fallen out of favor.

Given the significant morbidity and mortality associated with AKI, prevention is the ideal strategy. This involves careful attention to fluid balance and perfusion, proper dosing and monitoring of medications, and avoidance of nephrotoxic drugs. Radiographic contrast material causes 10% to 15% of hospital-acquired AKI. Hydration and the use of nonionic contrast agents may help reduce this incidence. Hydration with sodium bicarbonate before a contrast load has been shown to be an effective means of preventing AKI in patients with preexisting renal insufficiency.

## HEPATIC DYSFUNCTION

Liver disease should be suspected in patients with a history of alcohol or IV drug abuse, blood transfusions, or presence of tattoos. Physical stigmata of liver disease include jaundice, malnutrition, muscle wasting, encephalopathy, gynecomastia, testicular atrophy, spider angiomas, palmar erythema, ascites, fetor hepaticus, and caput medusae. Laboratory findings reveal an elevated bilirubin level, prolonged prothrombin time, hypoalbuminemia, and increased or normal transaminase levels, depending on the stage of the liver failure. Critically ill patients may develop secondary liver failure, manifested by cholestatic jaundice, impaired synthetic activity, and altered mental status. Treatment is directed at the underlying condition, but failure to correct this problem often results in MOF and death. Primary liver failure may represent an exacerbation of chronic liver disease or may be an acute problem caused by viral illness, drugs, or other toxins. In cases of acute liver failure, the cause and extrahepatic complications (e.g., fluid, electrolyte, and coagulation abnormalities; renal, pulmonary, and immune dysfunction) are treated medically. Cerebral edema is present in 80% of patients dying of fulminant hepatic failure, so aggressive management, including early ICP monitoring, is critical. Orthotopic liver transplantation may prove lifesaving, but must be considered before irreversible brain damage or MOF develops.

Patients with an exacerbation of chronic liver disease usually present with a complication that must be treated. Variceal hemorrhage is the most dramatic presentation and carries a high mortality (see Chapter 54). Patients with ascites and acute physiologic decompensation should undergo diagnostic paracentesis and cell count to exclude bacterial peritonitis. A white blood cell count higher than 500/mm$^3$ suggests bacterial peritonitis. Primary bacterial peritonitis occurs in over 20% of cirrhotic patients with ascites. It is typically monomicrobial (*Pneumococcus*) and is treated by antibiotic therapy alone, but its associated 1-year mortality is 50%. Polymicrobial peritonitis is indicative of an intra-abdominal abscess or perforated viscus. Patients showing signs of intra-abdominal hypertension secondary to tense ascites may require large-volume paracentesis to alleviate symptoms. Medical management of ascites includes sodium (1 to 2 g/day) and water restriction and diuresis. Spironolactone is preferred because it inhibits sodium reabsorption, but furosemide may be required in advanced cases. Large-volume paracentesis is generally well tolerated, but albumin replacement (7 to 9 g/liter) should be considered beforehand and may decrease renal insufficiency and encephalopathy. Management of hepatic encephalopathy begins with reversal of precipitating factors, such as removing drugs with CNS effects, treating infections, and correcting fluid and electrolyte abnormalities. Ammonia formation and elimination are addressed by administering neomycin and lactulose, respectively.

The hepatorenal syndrome is a functional renal problem seen in patients with end-stage liver disease that is caused by a combination of systemic vasodilation, relative hypovolemia, and increased activity of the renin-angiotensin-aldosterone system. It is marked by azotemia, oliguria, extremely low urinary sodium level (<10 mEq/liter), and high urinary osmolality. The prognosis is dismal, but systemic vasoconstriction using vasopressin, terlipressin, or ornipressin has shown promising results, whereas octreotide has proven largely ineffective.[47] Care is largely supportive and orthotopic liver transplantation may be curative. Nutritional support should limit protein to 1 to 1.2 g/kg/day and provide 25 to 35 kcal/kg/day, with 30% to 40% of nonprotein calories in the form of fat.

## ENDOCRINE SYSTEM

### Adrenal Insufficiency

The hypothalamic-pituitary-adrenal axis (HPAA) is activated by physiologic stress, resulting in proportional increases in corticotropin-releasing hormone, adrenocorticotropic hormone, and cortisol levels (see Chapter 41). Stress may unmask adrenal insufficiency, with potentially devastating consequences. Patients with potential adrenal insufficiency may be identified based on a history of chronic or recent steroid administration or clinical findings consistent with hypercortisolism or Cushing's syndrome (e.g., hypertension, diabetes, truncal obesity, hirsutism, buffalo hump) or primary adrenal insufficiency or Addison's disease (e.g., thin build, hyperpigmented, constitutional complaints). In this setting, steroids should be administered based on the patient's history and degree of expected surgical stress. Patients on long-term therapeutic doses of corticosteroids should be maintained on them perioperatively and postoperatively on doses equivalent to their daily exogenous total dosage. Usually, they do not require true stress-dose steroid administration, but in cases of volume-refractory hypotension there should be a low threshold for giving these doses. Patients who present for surgery or who have been injured who were maintained on physiologic replacement doses for adrenal insufficiency or with dysfunction of the HPAA are likely unable to mount an adequate cortisol response; they need the equivalent of 50 mg of hydrocortisone on the day of surgery for a minor operation and then their daily maintenance dose should be continued. For major surgery, these patients should receive from 75 to 150 mg of hydrocortisone intraoperatively; the doses should be continued three times daily for 48 to 72 hours.[48] The risks and complications of using stress-dose corticosteroids mainly involve hyperglycemia and an uncertain degree of immunosuppression; it is thought that the benefits of treating patients with such a regimen outweigh the risks in most cases.

An acute adrenal (addisonian) crisis may be difficult to diagnose in the ICU and presents with unexplained hypotension, fever, abdominal pain, or weakness. If adrenal crisis is suspected in a patient with fluid-unresponsive hypotension that begins to require vasopressor support, hydrocortisone or dexamethasone should be administered empirically while awaiting confirmatory laboratory values and investigation (e.g., for hyponatremia, hyperkalemia, hypoglycemia, azotemia, cortisol level <20 μg/dL). Dexamethasone does not interfere with the serum assay of cortisol but hydrocortisone does. If adrenal insufficiency is present, hydrocortisone should be continued at 200 to 300 mg/day in divided doses. Relative adrenal insufficiency has become an emerging problem in the ICUs and manifests as hypotension refractory to fluid and/or vasopressor therapy. If there is a concern about adrenal insufficiency, a random (baseline) serum cortisol level should be measured because there is a loss of diurnal variation of cortisol secretion in critical illness. Previously, a cosyntropin (250-μg) stimulation test was performed but this is now controversial and may be omitted. A baseline random cortisol level higher than 34 μg/dL suggests normal adrenal function and no further testing is required, but a cortisol level lower than 15 μg/dL is consistent with hypoadrenalism and corticosteroids should be administered. For cortisol levels between 15 and 34 μg/dL, the response to cosyntropin stimulation may define adrenal insufficiency; failure to increase the cortisol level by at least 9 μg/dL over baseline is consistent with hypoadrenalism. This should prompt corticosteroid therapy but, as noted, this practice is no longer recommended. In patients with septic shock, hydrocortisone replacement therapy has been shown in a randomized controlled trial to facilitate vasopressor weaning and lower mortality in patients with relative adrenal insufficiency.[49]

The sedative and hypnotic agent etomidate is often used to facilitate intubation and can cause marked adrenal insufficiency for up to 48 to 72 hours after its administration. Etomidate inhibits the conversion of 11β-deoxycortisol into cortisol and limits overall steroid synthesis. Patients' medications should always be reviewed to determine whether this agent was given and stress-dose corticosteroids should be ordered promptly if etomidate-induced adrenal insufficiency is suspected.

### Glucose Disorders

Diabetic ketoacidosis (DKA) is typically seen in patients with type 1 diabetes mellitus, caused by noncompliance with insulin therapy or acute illness or injury. Patients typically present with symptoms of nausea, abdominal pain, excessive thirst, or fatigue; however, hemodynamically instability and an altered level of consciousness are possible. A classic finding is Kussmaul breathing (rapid, deep respirations) and an acetone or fruity breath odor. Laboratory findings include hyperglycemia, a high anion gap metabolic acidosis, and ketosis. Hyperkalemia is common despite total body potassium deficit. Mortality from DKA can approach 10% to 15%, so aggressive treatment is critical. Normal saline is infused to replace intravascular volume, along with regular insulin (0.1 to 0.2-U/kg bolus followed by 0.1 U/kg/hr), and frequent glucose monitoring. Glucose should be added to the fluid resuscitation once the serum glucose level falls below 250 mg/dL. The insulin infusion should be titrated but continued until the ketoacidosis resolves. Hypokalemia and hypophosphatemia commonly develop during therapy and should be aggressively corrected.

Hyperosmolar nonketotic dehydration syndrome (HONK) is more common in patients who have sufficient insulin to prevent ketoacidosis, but not hyperglycemia. Its precipitating factors and clinical presentation are similar to those of DKA, but mental status changes are more common and pronounced. The hyperglycemia of HONK is more extreme, generally exceeding 800 mg/dL; however, ketoacidosis is absent. Osmotic diuresis leads to dehydration and hypernatremia, but the sodium level can be misleading because of hyperglycemic pseudohyponatremia. The free water deficit may be calculated based on the corrected serum sodium level (add 1.6 mmol/liter for every 100-mg/dL elevation in the glucose level):

$$\text{Free water deficit} = 0.6 \times \text{weight}\,[1 - (140/\text{serum Na})]$$

where weight is in kilograms and free water deficit in liters. Treatment of HONK is similar to that for DKA except that fluid resuscitation needs to be more aggressive.

Hyperglycemia in the absence of a diagnosis of diabetes mellitus is common in critically ill patients. The phenomenon of stress-related hyperglycemia appears to be related to insulin resistance resulting from the release of counterregulatory hormones (e.g., glucagon, epinephrine, norepinephrine, glucocorticoids, growth hormone) and cytokines (e.g., tumor necrosis factor, interleukin [IL]-1 and IL-6). It may be present on ICU admission and typically resolves as the catabolic illness subsides; however, ongoing metabolic dysregulation and protracted hyperglycemia may persist in some patients, particularly those with untreated infection or ongoing inflammation. Consequences of protracted hyperglycemia center around infectious complications in critically ill surgical and injured patients. However, one PRCT has demonstrated improved survival associated with intensive insulin therapy (maintenance of glucose level between 80 and 110 mg/dL, compared with 180 to 200 mg/dL).[41] However, these findings have been challenged by several PRCTs that could not reproduce that result. Recently, a meta-analysis comparing outcomes in patients managed with goal blood glucose levels of 81 to 108 mg/dL (intensive regimen) versus those with blood glucose levels lower than180 mg/dL (conventional regimen) has shown a mortality increase and significantly more episodes of severe hypoglycemia (glucose level <40 mg/dL) in the intensive glucose treatment group.[50] Episodes of severe hypoglycemia have been shown to be associated with mortality from cardiovascular causes and may be particularly detrimental in patients with traumatic brain injury. Thus, at present, the target for blood glucose control centers on a level of 150 mg/dL, a value that was shown over 20 years ago to be associated with less infectious complications in surgical patients.

## HEMATOLOGIC SYSTEM

### Venous Thromboembolism

#### Deep Venous Thrombosis

ICU patients typically manifest all three components of Virchow's triad that contribute to risk for venous thrombosis—stasis, endothelial injury, and hypercoagulability. Surveillance ultrasonography and venography studies in trauma and medical ICUs have determined the incidence of deep venous thrombosis (DVT) in 30% to 40% of patients; in these patients, DVTs that extend to the thigh in approximately 40% to 50% will result in a PE. The mortality rate of an untreated PE is 25%; thus, it is prudent for every institution to have a formal prevention strategy for venous thromboembolism (VTE) and PE. High-risk factors that justify prophylaxis include the following: major general surgery (thoracic or abdominal operations under general anesthesia, lasting ≥30 minutes), neurosurgical procedures, coronary artery bypass surgery, surgery for gynecologic malignancies, major urologic surgery, multiple trauma, hip fracture, spinal cord injury, surgery or chemotherapy for malignancy, congestive heart failure, and respiratory failure.

There are additional risk factors that are not sufficient to justify prophylaxis, but which may in combination warrant or alter prophylaxis: prior VTE, age older than 40 years, obesity, recent presence of a central venous catheter, prolonged immobility, hormone replacement therapy, antiphospholipid antibody syndrome, and hereditary risk factors. Because ICU patients generally have at least one risk factor, DVT prophylaxis should be considered routine; however, these patients also often have increased risk factors for bleeding complications because of coagulopathy, thrombocytopenia, or platelet dysfunction, so the decision should be reviewed carefully. All patients should have intermittent pneumatic compression devices applied. If there is no contraindication, low-molecular-weight heparin (LMWH), low-dose unfractionated heparin (LDUH), adjusted-dose heparin, or oral anticoagulants should be administered. LMWH has been proven to be superior to LDUH for trauma and joint replacement patients, but evidence is increasing that standard dosing of LMWH may result in inadequate levels of anti–factor X (Xa) in ICU patients.[51] Fondaparinux sodium, a synthetic pentasaccharide that inhibits Xa, appears promising in major orthopedic surgery and possibly as a therapy for heparin-induced thrombocytopenia (see later). The use of prophylactic inferior vena caval filters is controversial. In general, their use should be limited to high-risk patients who have contraindications to anticoagulation or to those with recurrent PE; however, the advent of removable filters has probably lowered the threshold for their placement. This modality remains relatively new so the available evidence to guide their use is still being developed.

The clinical signs and symptoms of DVT (e.g., leg pain, swelling, rubor, fever) are unreliable in the ICU and most patients with ultrasound-proven DVT will have no subjective complaints or physical findings. Venography had been considered the gold standard for diagnosis, but it is invasive, requires a contrast load, and is rapidly becoming a test of the past as familiarity and experience with it wanes. Imaging with CT or MRI is expensive and requires moving the patient but may have a role in detecting pelvic vein thrombus not readily seen on ultrasonography. On the other hand, duplex ultrasonography is noninvasive, portable, and has sensitivity and specificity of more than 95%, making it an excellent screening tool; however, its usefulness for detecting proximal clot is limited. Literature has supported use of the D-dimer assay, noting its high negative predictive value, but D-dimer is insufficient to exclude DVT in patients who have a moderate to high clinical probability based on pretest assessment. However, the combination of a normal D-dimer concentration and low pretest probability is likely adequate to rule out VTE.

Treatment of DVT has typically been with IV unfractionated heparin (UFH) but because of its more consistent and predictable response, favorable dosing, and equivalent efficacy, with fewer bleeding complications, LMWH is now preferred. Previous enthusiasm for using UFH, which was based on the decreased need for monitoring anti-Xa levels, may be decreasing because recent studies have shown that patients are frequently underdosed, even when it is used as prophylactic anticoagulation.[51] Attention should be paid to the potential for bioaccumulation because of its exclusive renal clearance, especially in patients with $C_{Cr}$ lower than 30 mL/min. Also, as noted, monitoring of activated Xa levels is probably warranted in critically ill and morbidly obese patients. LMWH also affords the option of long-term treatment, obviating the need for warfarin, but this requires injection therapy rather than oral administration. Treatment for VTE is generally for 3 to 12 months, with the duration depending largely on a patient's likelihood of recurrence compared with the risk of a bleeding event, with the highest risk of recurrence occurring in the first 3 months and in those patients with malignancy or cardiovascular disease. Thrombolytic therapy should be considered for limb-threatening thrombosis of the iliofemoral system, but otherwise it offers little additional benefit to offset its bleeding risk. Upper extremity DVT should be treated as aggressively as lower extremity DVT, because the rate of PE exceeds 10%.

#### Pulmonary Embolism

PE is a common and likely underdiagnosed problem in the ICU setting because its clinical manifestations are nonspecific (e.g., tachypnea, hypoxemia, tachyarrhythmias) and associated with many other conditions in ICU patients. Fortunately, most PEs are clinically insignificant, but hypotension may be seen with moderate-sized PEs. If PE is clinically suspected and the clinical situation allows, UFH should be administered empirically while a diagnosis is pursued. Systemic lytic therapy should be considered for moderate to severe cases when hemodynamic instability or signs of marked right heart strain are present. If the clinical suspicion for PE is low, a noninvasive study such as a D-dimer assay or duplex ultrasonography may be used, but a normal D-dimer level in this setting can obviate the need for further testing. If the PE is moderate to severe, a more definitive test is needed. Pulmonary angiography is considered the gold standard, but it is invasive and requires interventional radiologic capability. Ventilation-perfusion scanning, the former first-line test, is only valuable if it is negative or there is a high probability. Spiral CT pulmonary angiography is fairly accurate in diagnosing PE and may demonstrate additional or alternative pathology. Catastrophic PE, such as seen with a large saddle embolus, may cause sudden death. Immediate cardiopulmonary resuscitation is required, with large doses of heparin or thrombolytics. The Trendelenburg procedure, a surgical thrombectomy of the pulmonary artery, is an option but is rarely indicated and infrequently successful.

## Heparin-Induced Thrombocytopenia

Up to 15% of patients who receive heparin experience acute thrombocytopenia, which resolves spontaneously and has limited clinical sequelae. It is caused by platelet clumping or transient sequestration of platelets and is termed *HIT type I*. HIT type II is caused by heparin-associated antiplatelet antibodies (platelet factor 4 [PF4), which develop in 1% to 3% of patients on UFH and 0.1% of patients on LMWH. HIT type II leads to platelet activation and aggregation, resulting in a severe VTE phenomenon, which typically occurs 8 days (average) after the beginning of heparin administration, less if a patient was previously sensitized. The diagnosis of HIT should be suspected if a patient develops resistance to anticoagulation, thromboembolic events, a fall in the platelet count of more than 50% or an absolute platelet count less than 100,000/mm$^3$. If HIT is suspected, all forms of heparin should be stopped and the patient tested for PF4. If there are no antibodies, heparin can be resumed; however, if anti-PF4 antibodies are found, heparin needs to be discontinued and alternative anticoagulants are required. Patients with PF4 antibodies requiring ongoing VTE prophylaxis are usually treated with direct thrombin inhibitors such as lepirudin, argatroban, bivalirudin, or danaparoid, which bind thrombin and block its activity, or factor Xa inhibitors such as fondaparinux, idraparinux, and razaxaban. Of these agents, lepirudin, argatroban, and danaparoid are currently U.S. Food and Drug Administration (FDA)–approved for use for this indication. Anti-PF4 antibodies tend to fade over weeks to months, so patients may receive heparin if future retesting is negative. The role for long-term anticoagulation with warfarin remains unclear but it is generally used.

## Blood Transfusions

Anemia is a widespread problem in critically ill patients because of injury, surgery, diagnostic tests, and decreased erythropoiesis resulting in frequent blood transfusions. A large, recent, retrospective cohort study has reported that 67% of patients were transfused during their stay, with higher rates of transfusion associated with increased ICU length of stay and prolonged mechanical ventilation.[52] Clinical trials have indicated that Hb tends to reach a steady-state level of approximately 8.5 g/dL in ICU patients and that moderate anemia (Hb, 7 to 10 g/dL) is well tolerated in healthy individuals, but some ICU patients with excessive metabolic demands may not tolerate the associated decrease in $Do_2$.[44] Transfusion therapy is not without risk because blood is altered during storage; transfusion may incite electrolyte and acid-base disturbances, coagulopathy, and diminished oxygen-delivering capacity. Despite improved safety of the current blood supply, there is still the potential of viral infections, incompatibility resulting in hemolytic reactions, anaphylaxis, and febrile reactions. Blood transfusions have significant immunosuppressive properties and can improve the survival of renal allografts, but are also associated with an increased recurrence of cancers and postoperative infections. There is also growing evidence in a number of prospective cohort studies that blood transfusion is associated with an increased risk of ALI and ARDS. ALI was prospectively observed in 8% of patients who underwent transfusion of any blood product. These investigations have also reported a dose-response relationship between the number of transfusions and incidence of ARDS.[53] There is also an association between increased length of storage of blood products and a recipient's neutrophil activation, another possible mechanism for transfusion-related lung injury. Finally, blood transfusion has also been identified as a robust independent predictor of postinjury MOF and has been shown to be associated with markedly increased mortality rates, length of hospital stay, and higher expense. Thus, the transfusion trigger is being constantly revised as our understanding of the risk-benefit ratio of blood transfusion continues to evolve.

A multicenter PRCT has examined the effects of a restrictive transfusion strategy, transfusing for an Hb level less than 7 g/dL and maintaining an Hb level of 7 to 9 g/dL, compared with a liberal strategy (maintaining an Hb level of 10 to 12 g/dL).[44] The in-hospital mortality was lower among the restrictive strategy group. In this same group, 30-day mortality was lower in the subset of patients who were less acutely ill (Acute Physiology and Chronic Health Evaluation [APACHE] score ≤20) and younger (<55 years), but not those with clinically significant cardiac disease. Based on the current literature, a rational set of transfusion guidelines may be constructed (Box 23-3).

Recognizing the detrimental effects of low $Do_2$ and blood transfusion, alternatives to transfusion are being investigated. In the operating room, practical alternatives include preoperative autologous blood donation, normovolemic hemodilution, induced hypotension to reduce blood loss, and red blood cell (RBC) salvage systems; however, these are not feasible in the ICU. Autotransfusion involves the recovery and readministration of shed blood from body cavities, wounds, and drains. The blood is collected in a reservoir containing an anticoagulant, and reinfused after washing and/or filtering. There is almost no risk of transmission of infectious disease and transfusion reactions are essentially eliminated. Conversely, shed blood recovered from body cavities is defibrinated and essentially depleted of clotting factors, so dilutional coagulopathy may result from

**BOX 23-3 Transfusion Guidelines**

**Packed Red Blood Cells**

- Hemoglobin <7 g/dL
- Acute blood volume loss >15%
- >20% decrease in blood pressure or blood pressure <100 mm Hg because of blood loss
- Hemoglobin <10 g/dL accompanied by symptoms (e.g., chest pain, dyspnea, fatigability, light-headedness, orthostatic hypotension) or in the presence of significant cardiac disease
- Hemoglobin <11 g/dL for patients at risk for MOF

**Fresh-Frozen Plasma**

- Prothrombin time >17 sec
- Clotting factor deficiency (<25% of normal value)
- Massive transfusion (1 U/5 U red blood cells) or if clinically bleeding
- Severe traumatic brain injury

**Platelets**

- Platelet count <10,000/μL
- Platelet count <10,000 to 20,000/μL with bleeding
- Platelet count <50,000 acutely after severe trauma
- Bleeding time >15 min

**Cryoprecipitate**

- Fibrinogen <100 mg/dL
- Hemophilia A, von Willebrand disease
- Severe traumatic brain injury

major autotransfusion. Because the blood has been partially clotted, with subsequent lysis, transfusion of these products of fibrinolysis can activate the patient's coagulation system and result in disseminated intravascular coagulation. There is also a risk of contamination of the shed blood, particularly during gastrointestinal surgery or trauma. Inability to predict who will benefit and its labor intensity limits its cost-effectiveness and practicality.

The anemia of critical illness is associated with a blunted increase in circulating erythropoietin concentrations in response to physiologic stimuli and stress. Although there was some optimism from prospective randomized data in the 1990s showing that the scheduled administration of recombinant human erythropoietin reduces blood transfusion requirements, this was recently contradicted in a large multicenter prospective trial.[54] The same group that had initially shown reduced transfusion requirements with scheduled erythropoietin was now unable to repeat this finding in a multicenter investigation, and attributed this to more restrictive and lower hemoglobin triggers for transfusion. An association was shown between scheduled erythropoietin administration and decreased mortality in trauma patients admitted for more than 48 hours, a finding that was also present in their earlier studies; postulated beneficial mechanisms of erythropoietin other than hematopoiesis and include its potential antiapoptotic activity and cytokine properties.[54]

### Blood Substitutes

Blood products require typing and cross matching, have a limited shelf life, and are not immediately available in all health care facilities or clinical settings. Consequently, Hb substitutes that will provide physiologic $O_2$-carrying capacity and volume expansion without adverse effects or risks have been the subject of active investigation (Box 23-4). In the last 3 decades, two strategies of blood substitutes have been developed and tested clinically, perfluorocarbon (PFC) emulsions and Hb solutions. PFCs have a solubility for $O_2$ that is 10 to 20 times higher than that of blood, but have no special affinity for $O_2$, and thus their efficacy relies on maintaining a high $PaO_2$. They offer no discrete benefit compared with crystalloid solutions and have been associated with unacceptable toxicities.

The Hb tetramer is the active ingredient of the RBC and is durable and functions independently to transport $O_2$ outside its cell membrane. Unfortunately, unmodified tetrameric Hb is unsuitable for clinical use because it dissociates into heterodimers and extravasates, scavenging nitric oxide and resulting in unwanted vasoconstriction, hypertension, and significant toxicities. Unmodified tetrameric Hb is further hindered by its low $O_2$ half-saturation pressure (P50) and relatively high osmolality. Modification of Hb, therefore, has at least four major objectives: (1) minimize toxicity; (2) prolong intravascular retention; (3) decrease $O_2$ affinity; and (4) reduce colloid osmotic pressure. There are at least four Hb-based RBC substitutes that have been investigated in clinical trials. The primary differences in the Hb solutions lie in the source and technical aspects of polymerization. Diaspirin cross-linked Hb, derived from outdated human blood, has been one of the most widely studied solutions but clinical experience has been disappointing. A multicenter randomized trial in patients with hemorrhagic shock found that mortality was higher in the study group (46%) compared with a saline resuscitation group (17%). The cause of the excessive death rate was not known but is theorized to be caused by its negative effect on nitric oxide. Another product, *o*-raffinose polymerized Hb, was shown in phase II clinical trials that it may be effective in reducing the need for transfusions in patients undergoing coronary artery bypass grafting; however, this compound was similarly hindered by its pressor effect. A glutaraldehyde polymerized bovine Hb product has a reduced $O_2$ affinity that promotes $O_2$ unloading in the tissues. In clinical trials, it was able to reduce the need for transfusions, but at the cost of increased systemic vascular resistance and methemoglobinemia. Finally, human Hb-based glutaraldehyde polymerized pyridoxylated stroma-free Hb (Poly SFH-P) solution (PolyHeme, Northfield Laboratories, Chicago) has a near-normal P50, and essentially all unreacted tetramer is removed in a purification process. Clinical trials have demonstrated the safety and physiologic function of PolyHeme, as well as its ability to decrease transfusions of allogeneic blood. It has been most valuable in situations in which allogeneic packed red blood cells or whole blood are unavailable, notably injured patients in a shock state who were not in the immediate vicinity of a trauma center. Unlike the other solutions described, there is no evidence that it increases systemic or pulmonary vascular resistance because the transfusion-related hyperinflammatory response appears to be blunted by PolyHeme.

The principles of hemostatic resuscitation have also been investigated recently, especially in injured patients who have suffered significant degrees of blood loss.[55] With the now extensive experience in civilian and military injuries, there has been an increasing appreciation for the significant coagulopathy associated with massive blood loss, consumption of clotting factors, and dilution of these factors from high-volume crystalloid and packed red cell transfusions. The principles of hemostatic resuscitation involve administering more equal ratios of fresh-frozen plasma (FFP) to packed red cells than had been previously to replace lost and diluted clotting factors in patients who suffered significant blood loss from injuries or subsequent surgery. Recent retrospective data have shown a significantly decreased mortality and trauma ICU length of stay when a 1 : 1 packed red cell-to-FFP ratio was administered to patients with trauma-induced coagulopathy when compared with a 1 : 4 packed red cell-to-FFP ratio.[55] Accordingly, the early aggressive use of FFP and platelets appears warranted in all hemorrhaging patients requiring blood component therapy.

**BOX 23-4 Ideal Blood Substitute**

- Physiologic loading and unloading of $O_2$
- Volume expansion capability
- Immediate availability
- Universal compatibility
- No adverse physiologic effects
- Freedom from disease transmission
- Long-term storage capability

## SEPSIS AND MULTIPLE ORGAN FAILURE

### Sepsis

The earliest reports of the MOF syndrome, in the 1970s, linked the syndrome to sepsis. In the ensuing decade, it became clearer that the systemic manifestations of gram-negative sepsis could result from noninfectious stimuli. To clarify terminology in this area, the American College of Chest Physicians and the Society of Critical Care Medicine published a consensus description and definition of SIRS (Box 23-5). These definitions are important so that clinicians can communicate effectively, conveying a true sense of a patient's illness as well as identifying those who might be candidates for adjunctive therapies.

An epidemiologic study based on hospital discharge databases from seven states, representing 25% of the United States population at that time, determined that severe sepsis affects 751,000 patients annually (2.3/100 hospital discharges), with 29% mortality.[18] As the U.S. population ages, it is anticipated that the incidence of sepsis will increase roughly 1.5%/year. Not every infection, however, causes sepsis. Its occurrence depends on a combination of bacterial virulence factors (e.g., adherence properties, resistance to phagocytosis or antibiotics, endotoxin from gram-negative bacteria, exotoxin from gram-positive bacteria) and host factors (e.g., immune status and immune response, epithelial barrier function, gender, genetic factors).

The fundamental strategy in managing septic patients involves fluid resuscitation and treatment of the underlying infection, or source control, plus the administration of appropriate antibiotics. Suitable empirical antibiotic therapy for severe sepsis includes carbapenems, third- or fourth-generation cephalosporin with additional anaerobic coverage, or antipseudomonal penicillins. Agents with activity against methicillin-resistant *Staphylococcus aureus* should be used if there is a reasonable concern that this organism is present (e.g., nosocomial infection, chronic health facility resident). Source control refers to the drainage of abscesses, débridement of devitalized tissue, removal of infected foreign bodies, and definitive management of the source (e.g., appendectomy, cholecystectomy). Resuscitation of patients should follow the principles outlined earlier. The benefits of early goal-directed therapy, targeting CVP at 8 to 12 mm Hg, MAP, 65 to 90 mm Hg, and central venous $So_2$, 70% or higher, have been demonstrated in a prospective clinical trials.[56] In this study, in-hospital mortality was reduced in all patients, including the subgroup with severe sepsis and septic shock.

**BOX 23-5 Systemic Inflammatory Response Syndrome and Sepsis: Definitions**

**SIRS**

Two or more of the following:

- Temperature >38° C *or* <35° C
- Heart rate >90 beats/min
- Respiratory rate >20 breaths/min *or* $Paco_2$ <32 mm Hg
- WBC count >12,000 or <4000/mm$^3$

**Sepsis**

SIRS + documented infection

**Severe Sepsis**

Sepsis + organ dysfunction or hypoperfusion (e.g., lacticacidosis, oliguria, altered mental status)

**Septic Shock**

Sepsis + organ dysfunction + hypotension (SBP <90 mm Hg *or* SBP >90 mm Hg with vasopressors)

Septic shock is an abnormal vasodilatory distribution of cardiac output, in which CO may be normal or increased. Septic shock is often refractory to catecholamines, which may be a manifestation of vasopressin deficiency. Thus, there is a role for vasopressin administration in patients with septic shock, especially those patients with catecholamine-refractory septic shock in whom vasopressin infusion may result in an immediate and sustained increase in MAP. The increased recognition of adrenal insufficiency in critically ill patients has prompted a resurgence in glucocorticoid therapy for sepsis and critical care in general, as noted. In the seminal study of steroids in septic shock, steroids were shown to reverse shock, reduce vasopressor requirements, moderate organ dysfunction scores, and improve survival.[49]

There are a number of adjunctive therapies that have shown promise in preclinical studies or small clinical trials, but large multicenter PRCTs have not demonstrated survival benefits. These include ibuprofen, prostaglandin E1, pentoxifylline, *N*-acetylcysteine, selenium, antithrombin-3, IV immunoglobulins, hemofiltration, recombinant tissue factor pathway inhibitor, p55 tumor necrosis factor (TNF), receptor fusion protein, and antibodies to TNF-$\alpha$ and endotoxin. Only recombinant human activated protein C (APC) has been shown to improve survival in patients with severe sepsis. APC is an endogenous protein that promotes fibrinolysis and inhibits thrombosis and inflammation; it is an important modulator of the coagulation and inflammation associated with severe sepsis. In a multicenter PRCT of 1690 randomized severe sepsis patients, APC reduced mortality from 31% to 25%.[57] The only significant adverse effect was an increase in bleeding complications in the APC group (3.5% versus 2.0%; $P = .06$).

Although new potentially beneficial therapies for sepsis have begun to emerge, there have also been more studies seeking more sensitive and specific biomarkers for sepsis. Finding such a biomarker, which might be manifest earlier in the course of developing sepsis to guide therapies, prognosis, and even antibiotic duration has been another aspect of these investigations. Unfortunately, it is often difficult in the ICU to distinguish inflammatory states from infectious states because relying on traditional means such as leukocyte counts, C-reactive protein (CRP), erythrocyte sedimentation rate (ESR), and presence of fever can be unreliable, especially in patients with prolonged ICU stays. Procalcitonin has been evaluated as a means to delineate sepsis from other noninfectious causes of SIRS; there have been some initially promising data from small, single-center studies showing a greater sensitivity compared with white blood cell (WBC) count and CRP in detecting infection when daily procalcitonin levels were followed, even in situations in which the change in procalcitonin levels were subtle. There is also emerging support for using procalcitonin as a marker in long-term, critically ill patients because WBC and CRP tend to become even less accurate markers for these patients. All this enthusiasm is tempered by the cost and clinical impracticality of drawing and determining daily procalcitonin levels, so further study will likely focus on the benefit of following them on less frequently.

## Multiple Organ Failure

MOF has been called a syndrome of surgical progress, because its emergence was the result of advances in treating circulatory shock, renal failure, and pulmonary insufficiency. MOF as a distinct entity was first described in the 1970s, when a number

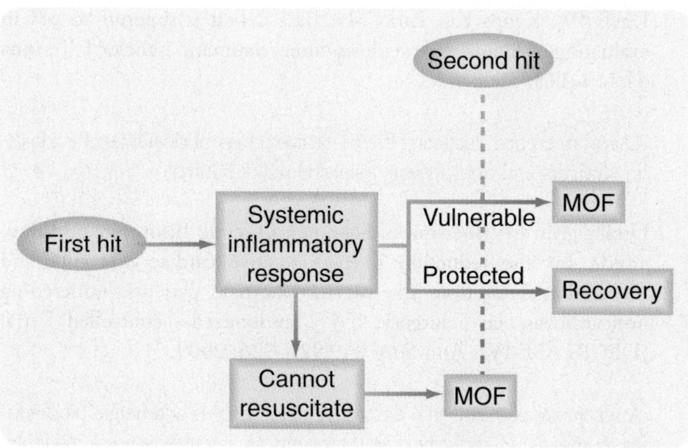


**FIGURE 23-5** The two-event model of MOF. An initial insult results in systemic hyperinflammation. If the insult or inflammatory response is exaggerated or perpetuated, overt MOF may develop. More commonly, the host endures multiple sequential insults. A second insult during a vulnerable period amplifies the systemic inflammatory response to produce MOF.

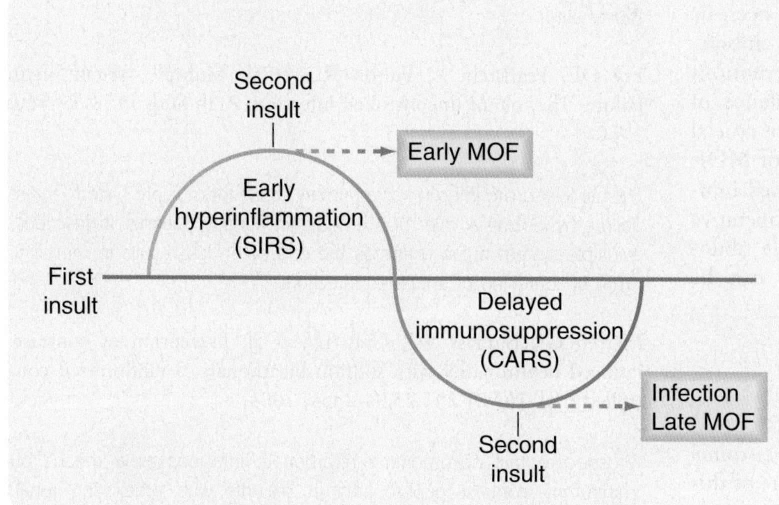


**FIGURE 23-6** A dysfunctional inflammatory or immune response leads to MOF. The amplitude of the early SIRS is related to the initial insult. A CARS may result in delayed immunosuppression. Sequential insults superimposed on the hyperinflammatory or immunosuppressed state may result in MOF.

of groups described the progressive failure of organ systems with a sequential pattern. Mortality associated with MOF ranges from 40% to 100% and is directly related to the number and duration of organ systems that fail. However, neither the incidence nor the mortality of the syndrome has improved significantly, and it remains a leading cause of death in the ICU.

Early reports of MOF implicated infection as the primary causative factor, but subsequent studies have emphasized that overt clinical infections are not a requisite to MOF. Approximately one third of patients dying of MOF will have positive blood cultures, with no identifiable source. It is now believed that MOF represents the culmination of generalized and excessive neuroendocrine, immune, and inflammatory responses. The cascade may be precipitated by a wide variety of insults, broadly classified as tissue injury, cellular shock, inflammation, and infection. Evidence has supported the concept that multiple insults are likely responsible for MOF.

In the two-event model of MOF (Fig. 23-5), the host experiences sequential insults so that the subsequent systemic inflammatory response exceeds the typical response elicited by either insult alone. The initial insult primes the inflammatory response and patients enter a state of systemic hyperinflammation (i.e., SIRS). If the insult or inflammatory response is exaggerated or perpetuated, patients enter a state of malignant systemic hyperinflammation (severe SIRS) that can evolve into overt MOF, independent of other factors. The more common scenario involves multiple sequential insults. A second insult during a vulnerable period amplifies SIRS to produce MOF. The progression appears to be dependent on the type of insult, with a bimodal pattern to the development of MOF. Early MOF, occurring within 72 hours of the initial insult, seems to be precipitated by cellular shock. In contrast, late MOF (typically, 6 to 8 days postevent) is usually related to an infection. Although the initial insult determines the patient's susceptibility, there is little direct evidence that any one insult is more likely than another to lead to MOF. It seems that the pivotal risk factor is a dysfunctional inflammatory or immune response (Fig. 23-6). The amplitude of the early systemic inflammatory response is related to the initial insult. Negative feedback mechanisms downregulate this response in an attempt to limit self-destructive inflammation. This compensatory anti-inflammatory response syndrome (CARS) may result in delayed immunosuppression and increased susceptibility to infection. In this paradigm, a second insult during early hyperinflammation or delayed immunosuppression will have the same net effect, deterioration into MOF.

Despite 30 years of clinical and basic science research and studies of many failed antimediators, the mortality rates for patients in MOF remain largely unchanged. This fact, along with our inability to modify the syndrome significantly, indicates the overriding importance of adopting strategies to prevent the development of MOF. Avoiding so-called second insults can be accomplished in three distinct areas—resuscitation, operative interventions, and critical care. Resuscitation end points such as clearance of lactate and base deficit represents repayment of the oxygen debt and may minimize the cellular injury resulting from shock. Even the choice of resuscitation fluid is important. Hypertonic saline appears to have favorable immunomodulatory properties, whereas transfusion of banked blood serves as a second insult.

In one of the seminal articles describing MOF,[58] more than 50% of MOF cases were caused by an intraoperative error or perioperative blunder. Meticulous surgical technique, minimizing tissue trauma, avoidance of hematomas and blood loss requiring transfusions, adequate débridement of necrotic tissue, timely and appropriate antibiotic therapy, and embracing the concept of damage control surgery are all interventions whereby operative management can lessen the incidence of MOF. Avoidance and timely treatment of the ACS are crucial because it represents one of the only reversible forms of MOF. Finally, maintaining a high index of suspicion for missed injuries and intra-abdominal catastrophes in the postoperative period, and remaining amenable to exploring hostile abdomens, are additional ways that the risk of MOF can be lessened.

## CONCLUSION

The purpose of this chapter was to provide a brief but focused overview of surgical critical care so that health care personnel can continue to take effective care of their patients. Part of this efficacy is using management strategies that have been shown to have a real impact on morbidity and mortality, such as lung protective ventilation, early and adequate nutrition, restrictive blood transfusion practices, DVT and stress gastritis prophylaxis, and source control in septic patients. This list is by no means all-inclusive but is part of the strategy to minimize the development of complications and reduce the potential of developing MOF.

## SELECTED REFERENCES

Annane D, Sebille V, Charpentier C, et al: Effect of treatment with low doses of hydrocortisone and fluodrocortisone on mortality in patients with septic shock. JAMA 288:862–871, 2002.

Key article showing a reduction in mortality by physiologic corticosteroid replacement therapy in patients in septic shock with relative adrenal insufficiency.

Bernard GR, Vincent JL, Laterre PF, et al: Efficacy and safety of recombinant human activated protein C for severe sepsis. N Engl J Med 344:699–709, 2001.

First article dealing with the benefits of recombinant activate protein C in patients with severe sepsis.

Davis JW, Kaups KL, Parks SN: Base deficit is superior to pH in evaluating clearance of acidosis after traumatic shock. J Trauma 44:114–118, 1998.

Classic reference illustrating the predictive power of clearance of acidosis in survivors and nonsurvivors following major trauma.

Dunkelgrun M, Boersma E, Schouten O, et al: Bisoprolol and fluvastatin for the reduction of perioperative cardiac mortality and myocardial infarction in intermediate-risk patients undergoing noncardiovascular surgery: A randomized controlled trial (DECREASE-IV). Ann Surg 249:921–926, 2009.

A recent randomized trial describing the role of α-adrenergic blockade as a means of reducing cardiac events in intermediate-risk patients undergoing noncardiac surgical procedures by decreasing myocardial demand. This study also showed trends to improved outcomes in these same patients with use of the HMG CoA reductase inhibitor fluvastatin.

Fry DE, Pearlstein L, Fulton RL, et al: Multiple system organ failure: The role of uncontrolled infection. Arch Surg 115:136–140, 1980.

First article to cite infection as a primary cause for multiple system organ failure by looking at over 500 emergency surgical patients. It describes multiple system organ failure as the end point that results in mortality from uncontrolled or untreated infection.

Merten GJ, Burgess WP, Gray LV, et al: Prevention of contrast-induced nephropathy with sodium bicarbonate: a randomized controlled trial. JAMA 291:2328–2334, 2004.

Prospective trial documenting bicarbonate infusions as a means of minimizing contrast nephropathy in patients with preexisting renal insufficiency.

Tobin MJ: Advances in mechanical ventilation. N Engl J Med 344:1986–1996, 2001.

Classic review of ventilator strategies and weaning from mechanical ventilation.

Van den Berghe G, Wouters P, Weekers F, et al: Intensive insulin therapy in critically ill patients. N Engl J Med 345:1359–1367, 2001.

Seminal article listing the beneficial effects of keeping a patient's blood glucose level less than 110 mg/dLin the ICU. Several subsequent PRCTs failed to reproduce the results of this trial; thus, this article serves as a cautionary reminder of the dangers of embracing a single study to establish clinical practice.

Ventilation with lower tidal volumes as compared with traditional tidal volumes for acute lung injury and the acute respiratory distress syndrome. The Acute Respiratory Distress Syndrome Network. N Engl J Med 342:1301–1308 2000.

Seminal article establishing the benefit of lung protective ventilation in patients with ARDS.

Vincent JL: Vasopressin in hypotensive and shock states. Crit Care Clin 22: 187–197, 2006.

A review of clinical and basic science data examining the effect of vasopressin therapy in hemorrhagic and septic shock states, emphasizing that vasopressin has shown positive effects on blood pressure and urine output, but a mortality benefit remains to be proven.

## REFERENCES


1. Stevens RD, Bhardwaj A: Approach to the comatose patient. Crit Care Med 34:31–41, 2006.
2. Guenther U, Popp J, Koecher L, et al: Validity and reliability of the CAM-ICU flowsheet to diagnose delirium in surgical ICU patients. J Crit Care 25:144–151, 2010.
3. Arias-Rivera S, Sanchez-Sanchez Mdel M, Santos-Diaz R, et al: Effect of a nursing-implemented sedation protocol on weaning outcome. Crit Care Med 36:2054–2060, 2008.
4. Popping DM, Elia N, Marret E, et al: Protective effects of epidural analgesia on pulmonary complications after abdominal and thoracic surgery: A meta-analysis. Arch Surg 143:990–999, 2008.
5. Tonnelier JM, Prat G, Le Gal G, et al: Impact of a nurses' protocol-directed weaning procedure on outcomes in patients undergoing mechanical ventilation for longer than 48 hours: A prospective cohort study with a matched historical control group. Crit Care 9:R83–R89, 2005.
6. MacLaren R, Forrest LK, Kiser TH: Adjunctive dexmedetomidine therapy in the intensive care unit: A retrospective assessment of impact on sedative and analgesic requirements, levels of sedation and analgesia, and ventilatory and hemodynamic parameters. Pharmacotherapy 27:351–359, 2007.
7. Lucet JC, Bouadma L, Zahar JR, et al: Infectious risk associated with arterial catheters compared with central venous catheters. Crit Care Med 38:1030–1035, 2010.
8. Pronovost P, Needham D, Berenholtz S, et al: An intervention to decrease catheter-related bloodstream infections in the ICU. N Engl J Med 355:2725–2732, 2006.
9. Uchino S, Bellomo R, Morimatsu H, et al: Pulmonary artery catheter versus pulse contour analysis: A prospective epidemiological study. Crit Care 10:R174, 2006.
10. Cholley BP, Singer M: Esophageal Doppler: Noninvasive cardiac output monitor. Echocardiography 20:763–769, 2003.
11. Roukoz H, Saliba W: Dofetilide: A new class III antiarrhythmic agent. Expert Rev Cardiovasc Ther 5:9–19, 2007.
12. Russell JA, Walley KR, Singer J, et al: Vasopressin versus norepinephrine infusion in patients with septic shock. N Engl J Med 358:877–887, 2008.
13. Roberts I, Alderson P, Bunn F, et al: Colloids versus crystalloids for fluid resuscitation in critically ill patients. Cochrane Database Syst Rev (4):CD000567, 2004.
14. Vincent JL, Navickis RJ, Wilkes MM: Morbidity in hospitalized patients receiving human albumin: A meta-analysis of randomized, controlled trials. Crit Care Med 32:2029–2038, 2004.
15. Hartog C, Reinhart K: CONTRA: Hydroxyethyl starch solutions are unsafe in critically ill patients. Intensive Care Med 35:1337–1342, 2009.
16. Bishop MH, Shoemaker WC, Appel PL, et al: Relationship between supranormal circulatory values, time delays, and outcome in severely traumatized patients. Crit Care Med 21:56–63, 1993.
17. Kern JW, Shoemaker WC: Meta-analysis of hemodynamic optimization in high-risk patients. Crit Care Med 30:1686–1692, 2002.
18. Angus DC, Linde-Zwirble WT, Lidicker J, et al: Epidemiology of severe sepsis in the United States: Analysis of incidence, outcome, and associated costs of care. Crit Care Med 29:1303–1310, 2001.
19. Moore FA, Haenel JB, Moore EE, et al: Incommensurate oxygen consumption in response to maximal oxygen availability predicts postinjury multiple organ failure. J Trauma 33:58–65, 1992.
20. Wiedemann HP: A perspective on the fluids and catheters treatment trial (FACTT). Fluid restriction is superior in acute lung injury and ARDS. Cleve Clin J Med 75:42–48, 2008.
21. Davis JW, Kaups KL, Parks SN: Base deficit is superior to pH in evaluating clearance of acidosis after traumatic shock. J Trauma 44:114–118, 1998.
22. Levy MM, Dellinger RP, Townsend SR, et al: The Surviving Sepsis Campaign: Results of an international guideline-based performance improvement program targeting severe sepsis. Crit Care Med 38:367–374, 2010.
23. Fleisher LA, Eagle KA: Clinical practice. Lowering cardiac risk in noncardiac surgery. N Engl J Med 345:1677–1682, 2001.
24. Hannan EL, Wu C, Walford G, et al: Drug-eluting stents vs. coronary-artery bypass grafting in multivessel coronary disease. N Engl J Med 358:331–341, 2008.
25. Dunkelgrun M, Boersma E, Schouten O, et al: Bisoprolol and fluvastatin for the reduction of perioperative cardiac mortality and myocardial infarction in intermediate-risk patients undergoing noncardiovascular surgery: A randomized controlled trial (DECREASE-IV). Ann Surg 249:921–926, 2009.
26. Prondzinsky R, Lemm H, Swyter M, et al: Intra-aortic balloon counterpulsation in patients with acute myocardial infarction complicated by cardiogenic shock: The prospective, randomized IABP SHOCK Trial for attenuation of multiorgan dysfunction syndrome. Crit Care Med 38:152–160, 2010.
27. Villar J, Kacmarek RM, Perez-Mendez L, et al: A high positive end-expiratory pressure, low tidal volume ventilatory strategy improves outcome in persistent acute respiratory distress syndrome: A randomized, controlled trial. Crit Care Med 34:1311–1318, 2006.
28. Wiedemann HP, Wheeler AP, Bernard GR, et al: Comparison of two fluid-management strategies in acute lung injury. N Engl J Med 354:2564–2575, 2006.
29. Singer P, Shapiro H: Enteral omega-3 in acute respiratory distress syndrome. Curr Opin Clin Nutr Metab Care 12:123–128, 2009.
30. Ventilation with lower tidal volumes as compared with traditional tidal volumes for acute lung injury and the acute respiratory distress syndrome. The Acute Respiratory Distress Syndrome Network. N Engl J Med 342:1301–1308, 2000.
31. Eastman A, Holland D, Higgins J, et al: High-frequency percussive ventilation improves oxygenation in trauma patients with acute respiratory distress syndrome: A retrospective review. Am J Surg 192:191–195, 2006.
32. Myers TR, MacIntyre NR: Respiratory controversies in the critical care setting. Does airway pressure release ventilation offer important new advantages in mechanical ventilator support? Respir Care 52:452–458; discussion 458–460, 2007.
33. Esteban A, Frutos-Vivar F, Ferguson ND, et al: Noninvasive positive-pressure ventilation for respiratory failure after extubation. N Engl J Med 350:2452–2460, 2004.

**34.** Zagli G, Linden M, Spina R, et al: Early tracheostomy in intensive care unit: A retrospective study of 506 cases of video-guided Ciaglia Blue Rhino tracheostomies. J Trauma 68:367–372, 2010.

**35.** Davies A, Jones D, Bailey M, et al: Extracorporeal membrane oxygenation for 2009 influenza A(H1N1) acute respiratory distress syndrome. JAMA 302:1888–1895, 2009.

**36.** Peek GJ, Mugford M, Tiruvoipati R, et al: Efficacy and economic assessment of conventional ventilatory support versus extracorporeal membrane oxygenation for severe adult respiratory failure (CESAR): A multicentre randomised controlled trial. Lancet 374:1351–1363, 2009.

**37.** Tobin MJ: Advances in mechanical ventilation. N Engl J Med 344:1986–1996, 2001.

**38.** Leontiadis GI, Sharma VK, Howden CW: Proton pump inhibitor treatment for acute peptic ulcer bleeding. Cochrane Database Syst Rev (1):CD002094, 2006.

**39.** Deitch EA, Xu D, Kaise VL: Role of the gut in the development of injury- and shock-induced SIRS and MODS: The gut-lymph hypothesis; a review. Front Biosci 11:520–528, 2006.

**40.** Burch JM, Moore EE, Moore FA, et al: The abdominal compartment syndrome. Surg Clin North Am 76:833–842, 1996.

**41.** van den Berghe G, Wouters P, Weekers F, et al: Intensive insulin therapy in the critically ill patients. N Engl J Med 345:1359–1367, 2001.

**42.** Miller RS, Morris JA, Jr, Diaz JJ, Jr, et al: Complications after 344 damage-control open celiotomies. J Trauma 59:1365–1371, 2005.

**43.** McClave SA, Martindale RG, Vanek VW, et al: A.S.P.E.N. Board of Directors; American College of Critical Care Medicine; Society of Critical Care Medicine: Guidelines for the Provision and Assessment of Nutrition Support Therapy in the Adult Critically Ill Patient: Society of Critical Care Medicine (SCCM) and American Society for Parenteral and Enteral Nutrition (A.S.P.E.N.). JPEN J Parenter Enteral Nutr 33:277–316, 2009.

**44.** Hebert PC, Wells G, Blajchman MA, et al: A multicenter, randomized, controlled clinical trial of transfusion requirements in critical care. Transfusion Requirements in Critical Care Investigators, Canadian Critical Care Trials Group. N Engl J Med 340:409–417, 1999.

**45.** Joannidis M, Metnitz B, Bauer P, et al: Acute kidney injury in critically ill patients classified by AKIN versus RIFLE using the SAPS 3 database. Intensive Care Med 35:1692–1702, 2009.

**46.** Bellomo R, Cass A, Cole L, et al: Intensity of continuous renal-replacement therapy in critically ill patients. N Engl J Med 361:1627–1638, 2009.

**47.** Pomier-Layrargues G, Paquin SC, Hassoun Z, et al: Octreotide in hepatorenal syndrome: A randomized, double-blind, placebo-controlled, crossover study. Hepatology 38:238–243, 2003.

**48.** Marik PE, Varon J: Requirement of perioperative stress doses of corticosteroids: A systematic review of the literature. Arch Surg 143:1222–1226, 2008.

**49.** Annane D, Sebille V, Charpentier C, et al: Effect of treatment with low doses of hydrocortisone and fludrocortisone on mortality in patients with septic shock. JAMA 288:862–871, 2002.

**50.** Finfer S, Chittock DR, Su SY, et al: Intensive versus conventional glucose control in critically ill patients. N Engl J Med 360:1283–1297, 2009.

**51.** Malinoski D, Jafari F, Ewing T, et al: Standard prophylactic enoxaparin dosing leads to inadequate anti-Xa levels and increased deep venous thrombosis rates in critically ill trauma and surgical patients. J Trauma 68:874–880, 2010.

**52.** Zilberberg MD, Stern LS, Wiederkehr DP, et al: Anemia, transfusions and hospital outcomes among critically ill patients on prolonged acute mechanical ventilation: A retrospective cohort study. Crit Care 12:R60, 2008.

**53.** Gajic O, Rana R, Winters JL, et al: Transfusion-related acute lung injury in the critically ill: Prospective nested case-control study. Am J Respir Crit Care Med 176:886–891, 2007.

**54.** Corwin HL, Gettinger A, Fabian TC, et al: Efficacy and safety of epoetin alfa in critically ill patients. N Engl J Med 357:965–976, 2007.

**55.** Duchesne JC, Islam TM, Stuke L, et al: Hemostatic resuscitation during surgery improves survival in patients with traumatic-induced coagulopathy. J Trauma 67:33–37, 2009.

**56.** Rivers E, Nguyen B, Havstad S, et al: Early goal-directed therapy in the treatment of severe sepsis and septic shock. N Engl J Med 345:1368–1377, 2001.

**57.** Bernard GR, Vincent JL, Laterre PF, et al: Efficacy and safety of recombinant human activated protein C for severe sepsis. N Engl J Med 344:699–709, 2001.

**58.** Eiseman B, Beart R, Norton L: Multiple organ failure. Surg Gynecol Obstet 144:323–326, 1977.

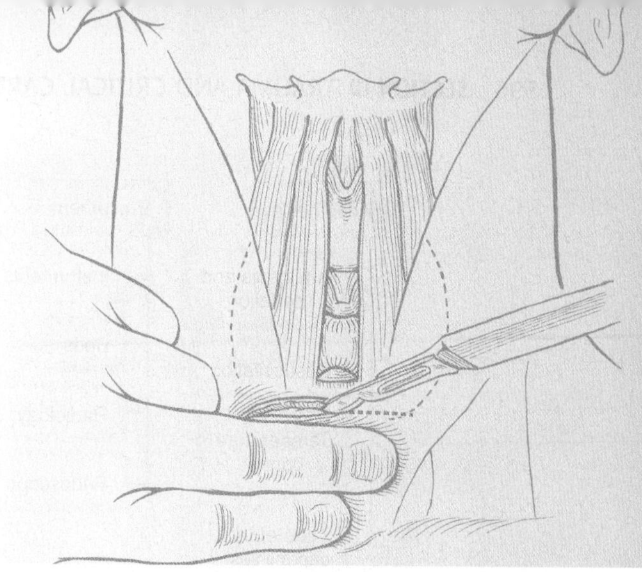

CHAPTER 24

# BEDSIDE SURGICAL PROCEDURES

Oliver L. Gunter, Jose J. Diaz, and Addison K. May



A number of factors have combined to increase the frequency and appropriateness of operative procedures performed at the bedside in the intensive care unit (ICU) for critically ill surgical patients. These include the following: increasing severity of illness in critically ill surgical patients; acceptance of staged and damage control management strategies for severe abdominal, soft tissue, and orthopedic pathology; advances in endoscopic and percutaneous techniques; increasing competition for operating room (OR) space; difficulty of transporting severely critically ill patients; and resource cost of repetitive operative procedures. For abdominal procedures, in particular, the introduction of the open abdominal approach for the management of abdominal catastrophes and abdominal compartment syndrome has created the need for frequent and repetitive abdominal procedures that can safely and efficiently be done at the bedside. Also, acceptance by many surgeons of the usefulness of early tracheostomy with the introduction of percutaneous tracheostomy and endoscopically guided feeding access has resulted in a number of procedures being performed at the ICU bedside that formerly had been performed in the OR. As an example, over the 9-year period between July 2001 and December 2009, our Division of Trauma and Surgical Critical Care performed more than 13,000 bedside surgical procedures, including more than 2800 tracheostomies, 1240 gastrostomy or gastrojejunostomy tubes, 4000 bronchoscopies, and 900 laparotomies. Our monthly bedside laparotomy rate has increased from 1.9/month during 1996 to 2000 to 8.7/month during 2001 to 2009. During these two time periods, the indications for laparotomy shifted significantly from emergency indications toward the elective and semielective indications of washout or closure—27% of laparotomies were performed for elective and semielective indications during the earlier time period, which increased to 75% in the later time period.[1,2]

Documenting the safety and cost-effectiveness of bedside surgical procedures is made difficult by the breadth of procedures, diverse populations, and variable indications for these procedures. For the most common procedures, sufficient data support safety and cost-effectiveness. Early reports of combined analyses of common bedside procedures, including percutaneous dilational tracheostomy (PDT), percutaneous endoscopic gastrostomy (PEG) placement, inferior vena cava (IVC) filter placement, and laparotomies have demonstrated results with similar complication rates as those performed in the OR, with a significant cost reduction.[3-5] Also, other reports examining PDT, PEG, and bedside laparotomy individually have also shown these procedures to be safer and more cost-effective than those performed in the OR.[1,2,6-9] Bedside procedures avoid the risk and difficulties introduced by the required transport of the patient for procedures performed in the OR. Although progress has been made in regard to the safe transport of critically ill, high-risk patients, serious adverse events and death can occur.[10] A small group of patients are simply not transportable because of the severity of pulmonary dysfunction or the rapidity with which the underlying process must be addressed. In this population, rapidly performed bedside procedures can be lifesaving.

Although bedside operative procedures can be performed safely, with complication rates equal to those in the OR suite, doing so mandates that cases be appropriately selected and that appropriate safety practices be consistently implemented. The ICU represents a complex environment in which to perform complex processes and procedures. Recognition of the potential for error and adverse events in these settings is important. Based on the experience of industrial safety practices and those of other organizations, prevention of error and adverse events requires standardization of processes and elimination of variability.[11] Protocols and safety practices specifically for bedside operative procedures should be in place to ensure that these procedures are safely performed, with low infection rates and the assurance of comfort and anesthesia. In this chapter, we will discuss the rationale for bedside surgical procedures and the process of bringing the OR to the ICU:

- Systematic safety methodologies and practices to ensure safe performance of bedside procedures
- Selection of patients for bedside surgical procedures
- Specific considerations for common bedside procedures
    - Bedside laparotomy
    - Percutaneous tracheostomy
    - Percutaneous endoscopic feeding tubes
    - Bronchoscopy

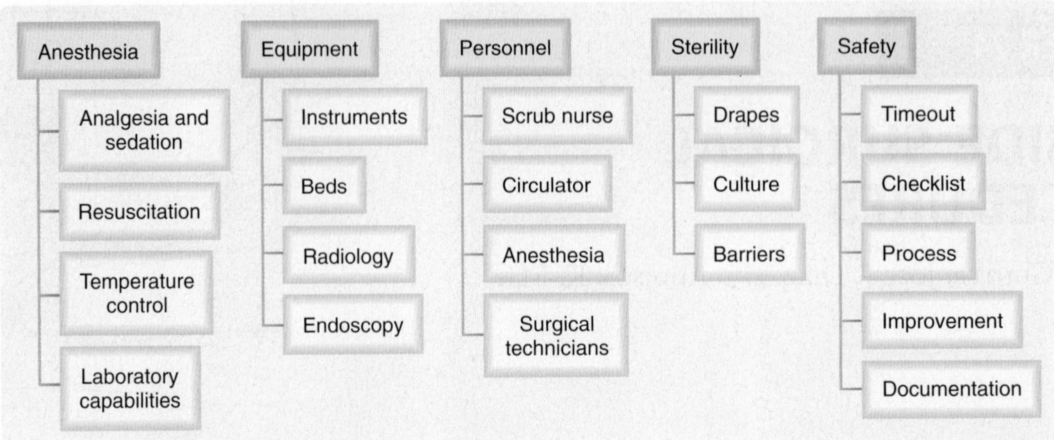


**FIGURE 24-1** Resources available in the operating room.

## RATIONALE FOR BEDSIDE SURGICAL PROCEDURES

For good reasons, most surgical procedures are performed in the OR. The centralization of resources including anesthesia personnel and equipment, surgical equipment, radiology, specialized nursing and procedural support staff, and safety policies and principles make the modern surgical suite an ideal venue for most operations (Fig. 24-1). The supply of ORs, although not fixed, frequently cannot meet the demands of surgery and require significant resources to expand.

The transport of a critically ill patient from an ICU to the OR and back ties up many personnel, including nursing, transport, respiratory care, and anesthesia staff. Furthermore, the change of venue and personnel caring for the patient necessitates detailed communication for a handoff, and represents a potential source of medical error. Thus, the transport of a patient from the ICU to the OR is a potential drain on resources and should be evaluated in the same manner as other treatments by assessing risk versus benefit. This, combined with long turnover times frequently observed in this patient population, can grind the usual efficiency of the OR to a halt. As the complexity and severity of illness of the average critical care patient have increased, so too has their immobility.

## TAKING THE OPERATING ROOM TO THE INTENSIVE CARE UNIT

By creating and applying a well-constructed system, the major benefits of the OR can be reproduced at the bedside (Fig. 24-2). As seen in this figure, there are a number of factors required to create and maintain a successful system for performing bedside procedures. Management guidelines may include standard operating procedures, preprocedure checklists, including timeout procedures, and sedation protocols. Dedicated procedure support personnel not only decrease the variability in how an individual procedure is performed, they also play important roles in guideline compliance, both of which are significant factors in reducing error. Appropriate access to supplies may require temporary storage of core equipment in an individual ICU with standardized restocking mechanisms, thus streamlining the supply chain. Finally, a facilitative mindset among staff is vital to the success of such a system.

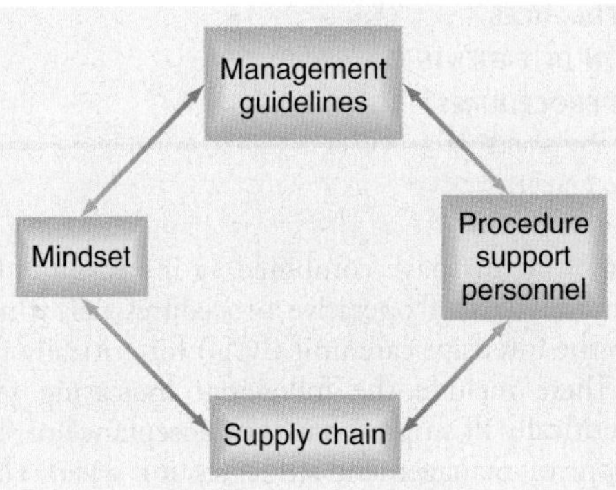


**FIGURE 24-2** Fundamentals vital to the success of bedside surgical procedures.

## SAFETY PRACTICES

To ensure the safety of operative procedures performed at the bedside, systematic measures should be undertaken to ensure the appropriate selection of patients and adequate expertise of support personnel, reduce procedural variability, and prevent communication errors. Implementation of the World Health Organization (WHO) "Safe Surgery Saves Lives" program has been associated with a significant global reduction in perioperative morbidity and mortality.[12] Objectives outlined for procedures performed in the OR also apply to those done at the bedside. These are the 10 safety objectives outlined in the WHO guidelines[13]:

1. The team will operate on the correct patient at the correct site.
2. The team will use methods known to prevent harm from administration of anesthetics, while protecting the patient from pain.
3. The team will recognize and effectively prepare for life-threatening loss of airway or respiratory function.
4. The team will recognize and effectively prepare for risk of high blood loss.
5. The team will avoid inducing an allergic or adverse drug reaction for which the patient is known to be at significant risk.

6. The team will consistently use methods known to minimize the risk for surgical site infection.
7. The team will prevent inadvertent retention of instruments and sponges in surgical wounds.
8. The team will secure and accurately identify all surgical specimens.
9. The team will effectively communicate and exchange critical information for the safe conduct of the operation.
10. Hospitals and public health systems will establish routine surveillance of surgical capacity, volume, and results.

The use of specifically trained personnel to support bedside operative procedures in the ICU greatly facilitates reduction in variability, compliance with standard operative procedures, reduction of communication errors, and maintenance of appropriate skill sets. Depending on the volume of procedures to be supported, these personnel can be unit- or service-specific or can be used to support bedside procedures on numerous services in a number of ICUs. Limiting this procedure support role to a small number of individuals allows a greater degree of expertise to be developed and has, in our experience, been extremely valuable in maintaining procedural safety. This is particularly true with handling of the airway and endotracheal tube during percutaneous tracheostomies. Also, these personnel are charged with the development and monitoring of safety practices and ensures their application during all procedures.

Management guidelines, protocols, and standard operating procedures should be in place before the routine performance of bedside operative procedures. They should be in line with those developed for the OR and be easily accessible and compliance monitored. Because of variations in specific personnel and practice patterns in various ICUs, our documents are customized to each location to ensure their appropriate application during bedside operative procedures. These documents should address issues such as the selection of appropriate cases, mandatory personnel, equipment, medications, and monitoring. An example of our bedside operative guideline is provided in Box 24-1.[2] All patients should have blood pressure, electrocardiogram (ECG), pulse oximetry, and ventilation routinely monitored throughout the procedures. Adequate personnel must be present to allow performance of the procedure, monitoring of sedation and anesthesia, medication administration, manipulation of ventilation if required, and documentation. The actual number of individuals required varies, depending on procedure and that person's expertise. Both analgesia and sedation must be ensured with appropriate medications under the direction of the critical care staff. In addition, guidelines and protocols should include standards for adequate preparation, equipment, and instrument accounting.

The use of preprocedure time-out and procedural checklists aids in the implementation of appropriate safety practices. Use of these tools helps limit communication errors and facilitates compliance with standard operating procedures, and can be used to assist in documentation and compliance monitoring. Again, these tools should be consistent with practices used in the OR to reduce variability, where appropriate. Figure 24-3 provides an example of a procedural checklist. Ideally, these tools can be combined with forms required for documentation and information can be captured for quality and performance analysis.

Ensuring a high degree of safety of bedside operative procedures and providing documentation of them, when required, mandates that mechanisms for tracking procedure performance, compliance monitoring, and adverse event review and reporting be developed and be in place. These must be applicable locally to facilitate consistent, nonvariable performance and interface with global hospital safety mechanisms and initiatives. Development of processes to map flow charts and diagrams facilitates the integration of unit-specific, departmental, and hospital-wide processes and helps delineate lines of communication and authority.

**BOX 24-1 Bedside Surgery Protocol**

**Indications**

Decompressive celiotomy for abdominal compartment syndrome

Exploratory celiotomy for intra-abdominal hemorrhage after damage control and packing

Reexploration of a previously open abdomen for washout or closure

Exploratory celiotomy to rule out intra-abdominal sepsis in a patient with ventilatory requirements that prohibit safe transport to the OR

**Protocol**

ICU attending and operating surgeon will be present for the entire surgical procedure.

Informed consent obtained (if possible)

Preprocedure checklist to be reviewed by the bedside nurse

Bedside nurse and a respiratory therapist will monitor patient and record procedure (conscious sedation sheet)

Indications to proceed to the OR (level 1):

- Surgical bleeding
- Dead bowel
- Need to open another body cavity
- Surgeon preference

For laparotomies:

- A sterile perimeter will be set up in the patient's room. All individuals must wear a surgical head covering and mask.
- The ICU attending will oversee anesthetic management of the patient.
- General anesthesia–narcotics, benzodiazepines, propofol, paralytics, ventilator management
- A sterile hand wash is performed by the operating team.
- Preoperative antibiotics are indicated only if a new surgical wound is to be made (e.g., cefazolin [Ancef], 1-2 g IV).
- A povidone-iodine (Betadine)–chlorhexidine abdominal preparation will be used.
- A standard Bovie will be set up (when indicated).
- Wall suction canisters set up
- 4-liter warm irrigation with normal saline
- A standard bedside celiotomy tray will be set up with suture on a sterile field.

Adapted from Vanderbilt University Medical Center, Division of Trauma & Surgical Critical Care: Emergency general surgery protocols: Bedside surgery protocol, 2005 (http://www.mc.vanderbilt.edu/surgery/trauma/Protocols/EGS BedsideSurgery.pdf).

| SICU Procedure "TIME-OUT" Check List | | |
|---|---|---|
| Complete this form (a) just prior to beginning the procedure and (b) at the location where the procedure is to be performed | | |
| Patient's Name: ______________________ Medical record number: __________ | | |
| Procedure Type: ☐ Planned non-emergent ☐ Not planned non-emergent ☐ Emergent | | |
| **VERIFICATION** | | |
| 1. Invasive procedure to be performed: | Circle one | |
| 2. H&P completed if patient admitted within past 24 hours | Yes | No |
| 3. Informed consent obtained? (Verified by Bedside RN and Procedure RN) | Yes | No |
| 4. Correct patient identity? ☐ Arm Band ☐ MRN ☐ Consent If procedure is emergent, Bedside RN, Procedure RN, and Physician performing procedure need to verify patient ID and initial this form. | Yes | No |
| 5. Agreement on procedure (Agreement b/w Physician performing procedure and Procedure RN) | Yes | No |
| 6. Correct side/site verified and marked? ☐ NA ☐ Right ☐ Left ☐ Site: (Verified and marked by Physician performing procedure and Procedure RN) | Yes | No |
| 7. Correct equipment available? (Verified by Physician performing procedure and Procedure RN) | Yes | No |
| 8. Required resources available? (Verified by Physician performing procedure and Procedure RN) | Yes | No |
| 9. Ready to setup procedure? (Verified by Procedure RN) | Yes | No |
| 9. Ready to proceed with procedure? (Verified by Procedure RN) | Yes | No |
| TIME-OUT: All individuals performing and assisting with the procedure are to review the checklist and sign below. | | |
| Physician performing procedure: | | |
| Procedure RN name: | | |
| Bedside RN name: | | |
| Other: | Other: | Other: |
| Staff calling "TIME-OUT": (Title and signature) | | |

**FIGURE 24-3** Surgical ICU procedure time-out checklist.

## SELECTION OF PATIENTS

As noted, bedside operative procedures can be performed with similar risk of complications as when performed in the OR, at lower cost, and without transport risks, if selected appropriately.[1-3,5,8-10] However, there are no randomized studies and few retrospective reviews that have evaluated the safety of bedside operative procedures or helped delineate appropriate patient populations and operative procedures. Both the safety and efficacy of bedside procedures will vary, depending on the local experience and application of safety practices. As experience is gained, indications may broaden and the frequency of bedside procedures will increase.

The decision to perform an operative procedure at the bedside should consider the balance between the difficulty and risk of transport, complexity of operation, ability to achieve timely OR space, and safety, ease, and cost savings of performing the procedure at bedside. The vast majority of major operative procedures should be performed in the OR and, in general, the indications for bedside operative procedures fall into two categories: (1) the patient is too unstable for transport to the operating room and the procedure is a required, lifesaving intervention; or (2) the procedure is modest enough that the difficulties of transport, scheduling, and cost of OR seem unjustified.[14] Factors that generally favor performance of procedures in the OR include complex procedures, bleeding risk from major vascular structures, need for insertion of prosthetic materials, significant lighting requirements, and lengthy procedures. Commonly performed bedside procedures include percutaneous and open tracheostomy, percutaneous endoscopic gastrostomy or gastrojejunostomy tube placement, bronchoscopy, soft tissue débridement, decompressive laparotomy for abdominal hypertension, washout and packing removal following a damage control laparotomy, placement of IVC filters, and damage control orthopedic procedures. Occasionally, very critically ill patients can be temporized at the bedside by the performance of a bedside operative procedure, with subsequent implementation of the definitive operation in the OR.

## BEDSIDE PROCEDURES

### Laparotomy

Bedside laparotomy was initially a procedure of last resort in patients too sick to proceed to the OR, such as a heroic attempt to identify reversible intra-abdominal pathology as the patient was near death.[2] However, the recognition of the abdominal compartment syndrome (ACS) as a frequent complication of the resuscitation of acutely ill patients and acceptance of the damage control approach to the management of acutely ill patients with intra-abdominal pathology has resulted in a dramatic increase in the application of bedside laparotomy in more controlled settings.[1,14-16] Both damage control and the management of ACS use an open abdomen approach, in which the fascia remains open and necessitates the use of various temporary abdominal closure techniques. Indications for bedside laparotomy can be classified as emergent or semielective. Common emergent indications include the following: (1) decompressive laparotomy for abdominal compartment syndrome; (2) control and packing for recurrent bleeding following a previous damage control laparotomy; and (3) suspicion of intra-abdominal infection in patients too critically ill to be transported to the operating room. The common semielective indications include the following: (1) pack removal following damage control laparotomy; (2) irrigation and débridement of the open abdomen; (3) source control for sepsis caused by intra-abdominal pathology; and (4) management of traumatic abdominal defects.

The most common emergent indication for a bedside laparotomy is for decompression of abdominal hypertension. Recognition and understanding of the pathophysiology of increased intra-abdominal pressure leading to organ system dysfunction, termed *abdominal compartment syndrome,* has increased significantly since Kron and colleagues first described the measurement of intra-abdominal pressure as an indication for abdominal reexploration.[15,17-19] ACS can be classified as primary, caused by intra-abdominal processes, or secondary, caused by bowel edema and intra-abdominal fluid secondary to the treatment and resuscitation of extra-abdominal pathology. Increasing intra-abdominal pressure leads to alterations in abdominal perfusion pressure, restricted venous return, and reduction of pulmonary compliance. These alterations can, in turn, lead to cardiac failure, pulmonary decompensation, and oliguria. Severe elevations in abdominal pressure can lead to organ hypoperfusion and ischemia, although the pressure at which this occurs may vary, depending on mean arterial pressure. Grading systems for the degree of abdominal hypertension have been proposed with grades III (21 to 25 mm Hg) and IV (>25 mm Hg) considered to be significantly elevated, defining ACS.[20] Management of ACS may involve only measures to ensure adequate abdominal perfusion pressures at lower pressures; however, as intra-abdominal pressure increases, abdominal decompression by laparotomy is indicated. Appropriate treatment requires recognition of the development of this syndrome. Thus, routine monitoring of bladder pressures is essential in those requiring significant resuscitation after abdominal procedures and patients being resuscitated from a significant shock (base deficit >10 mmol/liter) who receive 6 liters or more of crystalloid or 6 U or more of packed red blood cells (PRBCs) in a 6-hour period.[15]

The acceptance of damage control, an abbreviated laparotomy to salvage trauma patients with exsanguination, has led to an increased application of bedside laparotomy for control of recurrent bleeding within the abdomen before correction of the patient's systemic physiology and for removal of abdominal packs, irrigation, and débridement.[21] Bedside laparotomy is common in most level I trauma centers in which damage control and temporary abdominal closure for the patient in extremis are frequently used. Numerous methods of temporary abdominal closure have been described and continue to evolve. We prefer the use of negative-pressure systems and experience with the application of these systems is required for patient management.

The open abdominal approach is also applied to the general surgery population, usually for the management of necrotizing pancreatitis, necrotizing soft tissue infection of the abdominal wall, diffuse peritonitis in patients at high risk of failure of source control, and mesenteric ischemia.[2,14] Damage control techniques with staged gastrointestinal reconstruction, serial abdominal washouts for source control, and delayed abdominal wall closure can be used in the management of these complex patients. Controlled trials of these techniques are limited and the indications and settings in which the open abdominal approach is most appropriate have not been fully determined.

## Tracheostomy

Open tracheostomy and PDT can be performed safely at the bedside in the ICU.[8,9,22,23] The ease and convenience of bedside tracheostomy and the acceptance of early tracheostomy in critically ill surgical patients likely has led to a dramatic increase in their performance at the bedside. Indications for tracheostomy in surgical patients include the following:

- Presence of pathologic conditions predicting prolonged mechanical intubation, inability to protect the airway, or both
- Airway edema and high-risk airway following maxillofacial surgery and trauma
- High-risk airway because of cervical immobilization for fracture fixation
- Need for a surgical airway because of the inability to intubate the patient.

Not all of these indications are straightforward in their identification and clinical decision making remains difficult. However, perioperative mortality related to PDT in randomized studies appears to be less than 0.2%.[6,8,9,22,24] In this context, tracheostomy should be considered for patients who are at high risk of airway loss. Timing of tracheostomy remains controversial in patients with predicted prolonged mechanical ventilation. Some studies have supported early tracheostomy (up to 7 days) versus delayed tracheostomy (after 7 days), with shorter ICU stays and less mechanical ventilation, but with no difference in mortality in both trauma and nontrauma populations.[25] However, a randomized study of medical ICU patients has demonstrated a significant reduction in mortality (32% versus 62%), pneumonia (5% versus 25%), and accidental extubation (0% versus 6%) when early tracheostomy (48 hours) was compared with delayed tracheostomy (14 to 16 days) for patients predicted to require 14 days of mechanical ventilation.[26] The early group also had significantly decreased ICU length of stay and ventilator days.

PDT has become the procedure of choice for the elective tracheostomy in the critically ill adult patient. Ciaglia and associates[27] first described elective PDT in 1985 and, since that time, a number of modifications to the technique have been made. When comparing PDT with standard surgical tracheostomy performed in the OR, PDT demonstrates decreased wound infection, clinically relevant bleeding, and mortality.[8,22] Percutaneous tracheostomy has also been demonstrated to be more cost-effective in the critically ill ICU patient.[6,9,23] Long-term complications have not been adequately studied in randomized trials to draw conclusions.

Our most commonly used commercial percutaneous tracheostomy kit is the Ciaglia Blue Rhino (Cook Critical Care, Bloomington, Ind). which is practical, easy to use, and safe.[28] Reported perioperative complications of percutaneous tracheostomy include the following:

- Peristomal bleeding from injury to the anterior jugular veins or thyroid isthmus
- Injury of the trachea and/or the esophagus by laceration through the back wall of the trachea
- Extraluminal placement by creating a false tract during placement of the tracheostomy tube
- Loss of airway

Major perioperative complications can be minimized by using the safety measures outlined earlier. We have found that specifically trained support personnel managing the airway are particularly helpful in limiting airway mishaps. Also, one of two techniques should be used to ensure proper positioning of the tracheostomy tube and minimize risk of loss of airway by inadvertent extubation[29] during the procedure with bronchoscopic guidance or a semiopen technique with blunt dissection to the anterior trachea.[30,31] However, bronchoscopic guidance does not eliminate severe tracheal injuries and involvement of experienced personnel is important to prevent these complications. PDT tracheostomies can be performed safely in morbidly obese patients; however, care must be taken when selecting the size and length of the tracheostomy tube.[32] Because no studies have appropriately described methods of selecting the appropriate length of tracheostomy tube, we routinely place proximally extended tracheostomy tubes rather than standard-length tubes in patients with a body mass index (BMI) greater than 35 or in patients with severe anasarca.

The long-term incidence of serious tracheal stenosis after percutaneous tracheostomy is low, with reports as low as 6%,[33,34] and this usually occurs early in the subglottic position. Subclinical tracheal stenosis is found in 40% of patients.[35]

## Percutaneous Endoscopic Gastrostomy

Gauderer and coworkers first described the PEG in 1980 for access into the stomach for enteral feedings using a pull technique.[36] There have been various other techniques described since then. The principle of a sutureless approximation of the stomach to the anterior abdominal wall has allowed the pull technique to become the most popular method used. The other two most commonly used techniques are the push and introducer techniques, both of which require the use of stay sutures to approximate the stomach to the anterior abdominal wall. Newer percutaneous gastrojejunostomy (PEGJ) tubes combine both gastric and jejunal ports to allow distal feeding and proximal decompression.

Accepted primary indications for a PEG or PEGJ include the inability to swallow, high risk of aspiration, severe facial trauma, and indications for mechanical ventilation for longer than 4 weeks.[7,37] Other indications include nutritional access for debilitated and demented patients suffering from severe malnutrition. PEG tubes have been associated with reducing overall hospital cost.[38]

A number of gastrostomy and gastrojejunostomy tubes are commercially available. Most allow simple gastrostomy assess, with or without a valve. Some are flush with the skin and only require a tube to be attached during feeding. For critically ill patients, with increased risk of aspiration, multilumen percutaneous endoscopic transgastric jejunostomy tubes are available. These tubes allow drainage of the stomach while feeding the proximal jejunum. A third lumen connects to a balloon that maintains apposition of the gastric and abdominal walls.[39] Although feeding can be started on the same day as the PEG is placed, most critically ill patients are not started on feedings for 24 hours.[40] There are a number of contraindications for PEG placement, including the following:

- No endoscopic access
- Severe coagulopathy
- Gastric outlet obstruction
- Survival <4 weeks
- Inability to bring the gastric wall in approximation to the abdominal wall

There are a few relative contraindications, such as the inability to transilluminate through the anterior abdominal wall, gastric varices, and diffuse gastric cancer. Anterior wall inflammation or infection should be treated prior to the procedure. Ascites can be drained before the procedure and is not an absolute contraindication.[41] PEG tubes may be placed in the presence of a ventriculoperitoneal shunt or a dialysis catheter; however, placement should be separated by 1 to 2 weeks or more.[42,43] History of a previous or recent laparotomy is not a contraindication for PEG; however, a discrete indentation of the stomach when palpating the anterior abdominal wall and adequate transillumination should be ensured.[44]

PEG is thought to be a safe procedure whether it is performed in the gastrointestinal (GI) laboratory, OR, or at bedside in the ICU. However, because PEG tube placement is frequently performed in debilitated or critically ill patients, complications are associated with a higher mortality than would be expected for most elective procedures.[29] Free intraperitoneal air after PEG is common and can persist for as long as 4 weeks.[45] Abdominal wall infection can occur as an early complication of PEG placement; an ample skin incision that prevents creation of a closed space around the feeding tube and preprocedure antibiotics have both been demonstrated to decrease the incidence of PEG site infections.[46,47] Dislodgment of the PEG tube from the stomach can occur and may be life-threatening. This may occur acutely through the application of traction on the gastrostomy tube, thus pulling it partially or completely through the abdominal wall. Alternatively, the tube may necrose through the stomach wall if the PEG flange or balloon applies too much pressure on the gastric wall. If this complication occurs prior to development of a fibrous tract during the initial 10 to 14 days, it should be considered a surgical emergency, because gastric contents would spill into the abdominal cavity. Operative closure of the gastrostomy is required. To minimize the risk of this complication, methods that prevent inadvertent movement of the gastrostomy tube should be used and meticulously followed. These include ensuring adequate fixation of the tube to the external abdominal wall, recording and routine verification of the immediate post-procedure gastrostomy tube position at the skin surface, and application of binders or other devices that limit the inadvertent application of traction of the tube.

## Bronchoscopy

Fiberoptic bronchoscopy of the surgical patient is indicated for diagnostic and therapeutic indications. Under the therapeutic indication, bronchoscopy can be used to insert an endotracheal tube, remove foreign bodies inadvertently aspirated and mucous plugs, reversing atelectasis in mechanically ventilated patients, suctioning of thick tenacious secretions, and diagnosis of obstructive pneumonia.[48]

Diagnostic bronchoscopy is most commonly used for obtaining pulmonary specimens for the diagnosis and management of pneumonia.[49] Quantitative cultures obtained via fiberoptic bronchoscopy have been demonstrated to eliminate the diagnosis of pneumonia in almost 50% of patients with clinical signs of pneumonia, decrease inappropriate antibiotic use, and improve mortality when compared with nonquantitative techniques. Standardization of culture techniques should be undertaken.[50]

The risks associated with bronchoscopy are related more to the need for conscious sedation and to the medications required if performed in a nonintubated patient. This could result in depressed mental status progressing to hypoventilation, airway vulnerability, and the risk of aspiration. The risks of the procedure itself are pneumothorax, hypoxia, airway hyperreactivity, pulmonary hemorrhage, and systemic hypotension or hypertension.

## SELECTED REFERENCES

Byhahn C, Wilke HJ, Halbig S, et al: Percutaneous tracheostomy: Ciaglia blue rhino versus the basic Ciaglia technique of percutaneous dilational tracheostomy. Anesth Analg 91:882–886, 2000.

Primary article describing the most common technique currently used for percutaneous dilational tracheostomy.

Delaney A, Bagshaw SM, Nalos M: Percutaneous dilatational tracheostomy versus surgical tracheostomy in critically ill patients: A systematic review and meta-analysis. Crit Care 10:R55, 2006.

This most current meta-analysis of PDT versus standard open surgical tracheostomy supports the benefits of PDT.

Diaz JJ, Jr, Mejia V, Subhawong AP, et al: Protocol for bedside laparotomy in trauma and emergency general surgery: A low return to the operating room. Am Surg 71:986–991, 2005.

Primary article examining outcomes of bedside laparotomy with a protocol for indications and support.

Fagon JY: Diagnosis and treatment of ventilator-associated pneumonia: Fiberoptic bronchoscopy with bronchoalveolar lavage is essential. Semin Respir Crit Care Med 27:34–44, 2006.

Review of the indications, benefits, and performance of bronchoscopy for the diagnosis of pneumonia.

Griffiths J, Barber VS, Morgan L, Young JD: Systematic review and meta-analysis of studies of the timing of tracheostomy in adult patients undergoing artificial ventilation. BMJ 330:1243, 2005.

Meta-analysis of studies evaluating the timing of tracheostomy. Early tracheostomy was defined as less than 7 days.

Meduri GU, Chastre J: The standardization of bronchoscopic techniques for ventilator-associated pneumonia. Chest 102:557S–564S, 1992.

Extensive review of the techniques and limitations of quantitative culture in diagnosing pneumonia.

Moore AF, Hargest R, Martin M, Delicata RJ: Intra-abdominal hypertension and the abdominal compartment syndrome. Br J Surg 91:1102–1110, 2004.

Review of the pathophysiology and treatment of abdominal compartment syndrome.

Rumbak MJ, Newton M, Truncale T, et al: A prospective, randomized, study comparing early percutaneous dilational tracheotomy to prolonged translaryngeal intubation (delayed tracheotomy) in critically ill medical patients. Crit Care Med 32:1689–1694, 2004.

Primary article examining the benefit of tracheostomy at 48 hours versus 14 days. This study demonstrated a significant reduction in complications and mortality when performed early.

Shapiro MB, Jenkins DH, Schwab CW, Rotondo MF: Damage control: Collective review. J Trauma 49:969–978, 2000.

Collective review of the history, indications, and performance of damage control laparotomy.

Van Natta TL, Morris JA, Jr, Eddy VA, et al: Elective bedside surgery in critically injured patients is safe and cost-effective. Ann Surg 227:618–624, 1998.

First report of the safety and effectiveness of bedside surgical procedures.

## REFERENCES

1. Diaz JJ, Jr, Mauer A, May AK, et al: Bedside laparotomy for trauma: Are there risks? Surg Infect (Larchmt) 5:15–20, 2004.
2. Diaz JJ, Jr, Mejia V, Subhawong AP, et al: Protocol for bedside laparotomy in trauma and emergency general surgery: A low return to the operating room. Am Surg 71:986–991, 2005.
3. Porter JM, Ivatury RR, Kavarana M, et al: The surgical intensive care unit as a cost-efficient substitute for an operating room at a Level I trauma center. Am Surg 65:328–330, 1999.
4. Porter JM, Ivatury RR: Preferred route of tracheostomy—percutaneous versus open at the bedside: A randomized, prospective study in the surgical intensive care unit. Am Surg 65:142–146, 1999.
5. Van Natta TL, Morris JA, Jr, Eddy VA, et al: Elective bedside surgery in critically injured patients is safe and cost-effective. Ann Surg 227:618–624, 1998.
6. Bowen CP, Whitney LR, Truwit JD, et al: Comparison of safety and cost of percutaneous versus surgical tracheostomy. Am Surg 67:54–60, 2001.
7. Carrillo EH, Heniford BT, Osborne DL, et al: Bedside percutaneous endoscopic gastrostomy. A safe alternative for early nutritional support in critically ill trauma patients. Surg Endosc 11:1068–1071, 1997.
8. Freeman BD, Isabella K, Lin N, et al: A meta-analysis of prospective trials comparing percutaneous and surgical tracheostomy in critically ill patients. Chest 118:1412–1418, 2000.
9. Freeman BD, Isabella K, Cobb JP, et al: A prospective, randomized study comparing percutaneous with surgical tracheostomy in critically ill patients. Crit Care Med 29:926–930, 2001.
10. Beckmann U, Gillies DM, Berenholtz SM, et al: Incidents relating to the intra-hospital transfer of critically ill patients. An analysis of the reports submitted to the Australian Incident Monitoring Study in Intensive Care. Intensive Care Med 30:1579–1585, 2004.
11. Pronovost PJ, Thompson DA: Reducing defects in the use of interventions. Intensive Care Med 30:1505–1507, 2004.
12. Haynes AB, Weiser TG, Berry WR, et al: A surgical safety checklist to reduce morbidity and mortality in a global population. N Engl J Med 360:491–499, 2009.
13. World Health Organization: Safe surgery saves lives: The Second Global Patient Safety Challenge, 2009 (http://www.who.int/patientsafety/safesurgery/en).
14. Mayberry JC: Bedside open abdominal surgery. Utility and wound management. Crit Care Clin 16:151–172, 2000.
15. Biffl WL, Moore EE, Burch JM, et al: Secondary abdominal compartment syndrome is a highly lethal event. Am J Surg 182:645–648, 2001.
16. Miller RS, Morris JA, Jr, Diaz JJ, Jr, et al: Complications after 344 damage-control open celiotomies. J Trauma 59:1365–1371, 2005.
17. Kirkpatrick AW, Balogh Z, Ball CG, et al: The secondary abdominal compartment syndrome: Iatrogenic or unavoidable? J Am Coll Surg 202:668–679, 2006.
18. Leppaniemi A, Kemppainen E: Recent advances in the surgical management of necrotizing pancreatitis. Curr Opin Crit Care 11:349–352, 2005.
19. Moore AF, Hargest R, Martin M, et al: Intra-abdominal hypertension and the abdominal compartment syndrome. Br J Surg 91:1102–1110, 2004.
20. Sugrue M: Abdominal compartment syndrome. Curr Opin Crit Care 11:333–338, 2005.
21. Shapiro MB, Jenkins DH, Schwab CW, et al: Damage control: Collective review. J Trauma 49:969–978, 2000.
22. Delaney A, Bagshaw SM, Nalos M: Percutaneous dilatational tracheostomy versus surgical tracheostomy in critically ill patients: A systematic review and meta-analysis. Crit Care 10:R55, 2006.
23. Heikkinen M, Aarnio P, Hannukainen J: Percutaneous dilational tracheostomy or conventional surgical tracheostomy? Crit Care Med 28:1399–1402, 2000.
24. Griffiths J, Barber VS, Morgan L, et al: Systematic review and meta-analysis of studies of the timing of tracheostomy in adult patients undergoing artificial ventilation. BMJ 330:1–5, 2005.
25. Arabi Y, Haddad S, Shirawi N, et al: Early tracheostomy in intensive care trauma patients improves resource utilization: A cohort study and literature review. Crit Care 8:R347–R352, 2004.
26. Rumbak MJ, Newton M, Truncale T, et al: A prospective, randomized, study comparing early percutaneous dilational tracheotomy to prolonged translaryngeal intubation (delayed tracheotomy) in critically ill medical patients. Crit Care Med 32:1689–1694, 2004.
27. Ciaglia P, Firsching R, Syniec C: Elective percutaneous dilatational tracheostomy. A new simple bedside procedure; preliminary report. Chest 87:715–719, 1985.
28. Byhahn C, Wilke HJ, Halbig S, et al: Percutaneous tracheostomy: Ciaglia blue rhino versus the basic ciaglia technique of percutaneous dilational tracheostomy. Anesth Analg 91:882–886, 2000.
29. Lockett MA, Templeton ML, Byrne TK, et al: Percutaneous endoscopic gastrostomy complications in a tertiary-care center. Am Surg 68:117–120, 2002.
30. Paran H, Butnaru G, Hass I, et al: Evaluation of a modified percutaneous tracheostomy technique without bronchoscopic guidance. Chest 126:868–871, 2004.
31. Polderman KH, Spijkstra JJ, de Bree R, et al: Percutaneous dilatational tracheostomy in the ICU: Optimal organization, low complication rates, and description of a new complication. Chest 123:1595–1602, 2003.
32. Heyrosa MG, Melniczek DM, Rovito P, et al: Percutaneous tracheostomy: A safe procedure in the morbidly obese. J Am Coll Surg 202:618–622, 2006.
33. Fikkers BG, Briede IS, Verwiel JM, et al: Percutaneous tracheostomy with the Blue Rhino trademark technique: Presentation of 100 consecutive patients. Anaesthesia 57:1094–1097, 2002.

**34.** Norwood S, Vallina VL, Short K, et al: Incidence of tracheal stenosis and other late complications after percutaneous tracheostomy. Ann Surg 232:233–241, 2000.

**35.** Walz MK, Peitgen K, Thurauf N, et al: Percutaneous dilatational tracheostomy—early results and long-term outcome of 326 critically ill patients. Intensive Care Med 24:685–690, 1998.

**36.** Gauderer MW, Ponsky JL, Izant RJ, Jr: Gastrostomy without laparotomy: A percutaneous endoscopic technique. J Pediatr Surg 15:872–875, 1980.

**37.** Adams GF, Guest DP, Ciraulo DL, et al: Maximizing tolerance of enteral nutrition in severely injured trauma patients: A comparison of enteral feedings by means of percutaneous endoscopic gastrostomy versus percutaneous endoscopic gastrojejunostomy. J Trauma 48:459–464, 2000.

**38.** Harbrecht BG, Moraca RJ, Saul M, et al: Percutaneous endoscopic gastrostomy reduces total hospital costs in head-injured patients. Am J Surg 176:311–314, 1998.

**39.** Shang E, Kahler G, Meier-Hellmann A, et al: Advantages of endoscopic therapy of gastrojejunal dissociation in critical care patients. Intensive Care Med 25:162–165, 1999.

**40.** Stein J, Schulte-Bockholt A, Sabin M, et al: A randomized prospective trial of immediate vs. next-day feeding after percutaneous endoscopic gastrostomy in intensive care patients. Intensive Care Med 28:1656–1660, 2002.

**41.** Wejda BU, Deppe H, Huchzermeyer H, et al: PEG placement in patients with ascites: A new approach. Gastrointest Endosc 61:178–180, 2005.

**42.** Schulman AS, Sawyer RG: The safety of percutaneous endoscopic gastrostomy tube placement in patients with existing ventriculoperitoneal shunts. JPEN J Parenter Enteral Nutr 29:442–444, 2005.

**43.** Taylor AL, Carroll TA, Jakubowski J, et al: Percutaneous endoscopic gastrostomy in patients with ventriculoperitoneal shunts. Br J Surg 88:724–727, 2001.

**44.** Eleftheriadis E, Kotzampassi K: Percutaneous endoscopic gastrostomy after abdominal surgery. Surg Endosc 15:213–216, 2001.

**45.** Dulabon GR, Abrams JE, Rutherford EJ: The incidence and significance of free air after percutaneous endoscopic gastrostomy. Am Surg 68:590–593, 2002.

**46.** Ahmad I, Mouncher A, Abdoolah A, et al: Antibiotic prophylaxis for percutaneous endoscopic gastrostomy—a prospective, randomised, double-blind trial. Aliment Pharmacol Ther 18:209–215, 2003.

**47.** Sharma VK, Howden CW: Meta-analysis of randomized, controlled trials of antibiotic prophylaxis before percutaneous endoscopic gastrostomy. Am J Gastroenterol 95:3133–3136, 2000.

**48.** Labbe A, Meyer F, Albertini M: Bronchoscopy in intensive care units. Paediatr Respir Rev 5 Suppl A:S15–19, 2004.

**49.** Fagon JY: Diagnosis and treatment of ventilator-associated pneumonia: Fiberoptic bronchoscopy with bronchoalveolar lavage is essential. Semin Respir Crit Care Med 27:34–44, 2006.

**50.** Meduri GU, Chastre J: The standardization of bronchoscopic techniques for ventilator-associated pneumonia. Chest 102:557S–564S, 1992.

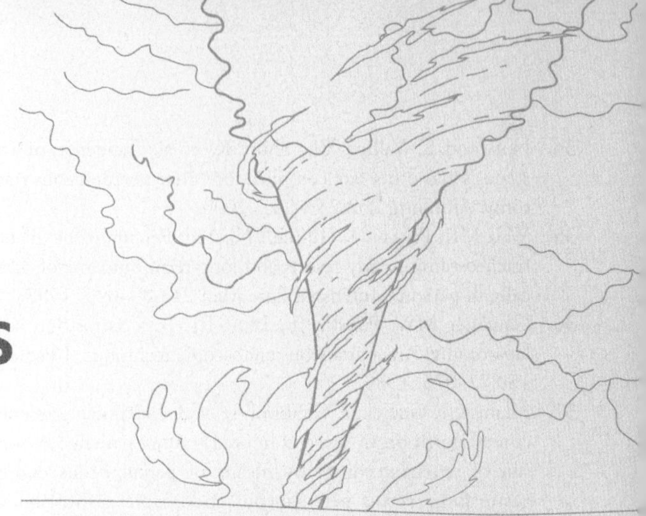

CHAPTER 25

# THE SURGEON'S ROLE IN MASS CASUALTY INCIDENTS

Asher Hirshberg and Michael Stein



In the past decade, there has been a surge of interest among surgeons in the medical consequences of mass casualty incidents and civilian disasters. The megaterrorist acts of 9/11 focused attention on the wave of urban terrorism that is sweeping across the globe, causing tens of thousands of casualties each year and challenging trauma and emergency systems from New York to Bali and from Madrid to Mumbai. At the same time, a series of large-scale natural disasters, such as the 2004 tsunami in Southeast Asia, which claimed almost 250,000 lives in 10 countries, and Hurricane Katrina, which devastated New Orleans in August 2005, helped focus public attention on the medical consequences of natural catastrophes. As this chapter is being written, the horrible consequences of the Haiti earthquake in January 2010 are becoming clear and the unique challenges facing medical teams and other relief workers are the center of much media attention.

Until recently, the medical response to mass casualty incidents and disasters has not been part of the traditional body of knowledge of general surgery. However, as growing numbers of surgeons are involved in their institutions' disaster planning, and treating casualties of urban bombings, school shootings, train accidents, or natural disasters, interest in this topic has grown.

Despite this increased interest, many surgeons remain unsure about their role in mass casualty incidents because they think of disasters primarily as logistic rather than medical challenges. The prevailing view has always been that trauma care in disasters is similar to that in normal daily practice, only more of the same. This is a dangerous misconception. A mass casualty incident is a unique challenge to surgeons and trauma systems because the large number of casualties affects how individual patients are treated inside and outside the hospital. Furthermore, urban terrorism and natural disasters confront surgeons with unusual injury patterns and unique clinical problems not seen in their daily practice. Preparing for these challenges requires, therefore, not only special planning and training but, most importantly, a different way of thinking about trauma care. The aim of this chapter is to provide a concise overview of the medical response to civilian mass casualty incidents and disasters from the perspective of the clinical surgeon practicing in a hospital that is part of a modern trauma system.

## KEY CONCEPTS

### Classification of Disasters and Implications for Trauma Care

In a mass casualty incident (MCI), a medical system is suddenly confronted by a large number of casualties needing care within a short period of time. This unexpected surge creates a discrepancy between the number of patients and the resources available to treat them. An MCI can be classified by cause (natural versus man-made), duration, location, and many other characteristics, but there is no single universally accepted classification of disasters. From the clinical perspective of medical care, it is important to distinguish among three classes of disaster scenarios and understand the implications for trauma care (Table 25-1).[1,2]

#### Multiple Casualty Incidents

These involve dozens of casualties and can be effectively managed using local hospital resources. In other words, the arriving casualties strain the hospital resources beyond normal daily operations, but do not overwhelm them.

#### Mass Casualty Incidents

These involve hundreds of casualties arriving at a single institution. Despite an effective disaster response, this number exceeds the capacity of the emergency department (ED) and the hospital. As a result, some severely wounded patients will not receive the level of care they require, and others will experience significant delays. Therefore, the term *mass casualty* implies some degree of failure to provide optimal trauma care to all severe casualties.

#### Major Medical Disasters

These typically result in many thousands of casualties and destruction of organized community support systems. In this scenario, the resources to treat critically injured casualties have been largely destroyed. External medical teams supported by appropriate logistic envelopes can make a difference in the management of severely injured survivors, although help usually arrives late and deals primarily with delayed complications.

In this chapter, MCI is used as a generic term describing a large-scale event. When referring to a specific disaster class or scenario (e.g., multiple casualty incident), it is fully spelled out.

**Table 25-1 Classification of Disasters and Implications for Trauma Care**

| DISASTER CLASS | TOTAL NUMBER OF CASUALTIES | IMPLICATIONS FOR TRAUMA CARE |
|---|---|---|
| Multiple casualty | Less than ED capacity | Standards of care are maintained for all severe casualties. |
| Mass casualty | More than ED capacity | Care of some severe casualties is delayed or suboptimal. |
| Major disaster | ED and hospital overwhelmed | Most severely injured patients die or survive without any medical care. |

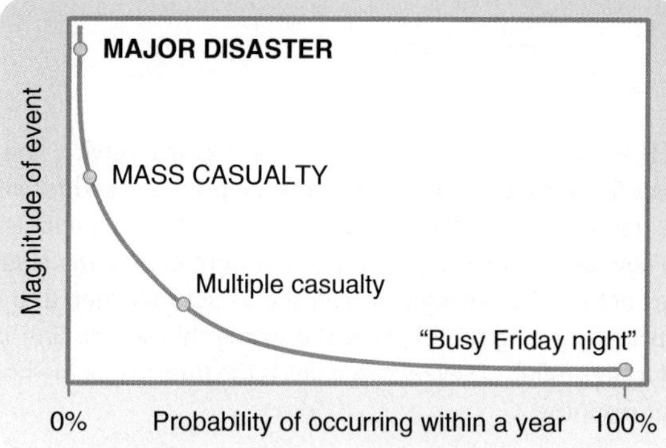


**FIGURE 25-1** Graphic depiction of the inverse relationship between the magnitude of disaster scenarios and their frequency. Although most surgeons will not encounter a major natural disaster during their careers, busy Friday nights are a regular feature in most urban trauma centers.

The magnitude of a MCI is inversely related to its frequency (Fig. 25-1). The overwhelming majority of practicing surgeons will not encounter a major medical disaster in their communities, whereas most hospitals occasionally face limited multiple casualty incidents. In fact, busy Friday nights, a single trauma team on call coping with a cluster of severely injured patients arriving together is situation that occurs frequently in every urban trauma center. It represents the lowermost end of a spectrum of magnitudes, with a major earthquake or a devastating Tsunami at the other extreme. The sad paradox of disaster preparedness is that the most time and effort is spent on preparing and training for the largest and least likely doomsday scenarios instead of improving the response to limited but more realistic threats.

### Injury Severity Distribution

A key feature of every MCI is the injury severity distribution of the casualties. Regardless of the cause or magnitude of the MCI, only about 10% to 15% of survivors presenting to a hospital will be severely wounded, of whom roughly one third will have immediate life-threatening injuries (Fig. 25-2). Most others sustain minor trauma or nonurgent injuries.[3] For example, during the London subway bombings in July 2005, the Royal London Hospital received 194 casualties within 3 hours, but only 27 (14%) were severely injured. Of these, only 8 casualties (4% of the total) were critically wounded.[4] Although the death toll at the scene depends on the cause of the MCI, and is very high when structural collapse is involved, the injury severity distribution is a constant feature of MCIs. This means that even though the total number of casualties may be high, the overwhelming majority will not require a high level of trauma care and are not urgent. These considerations form the rationale for planning an effective medical response.

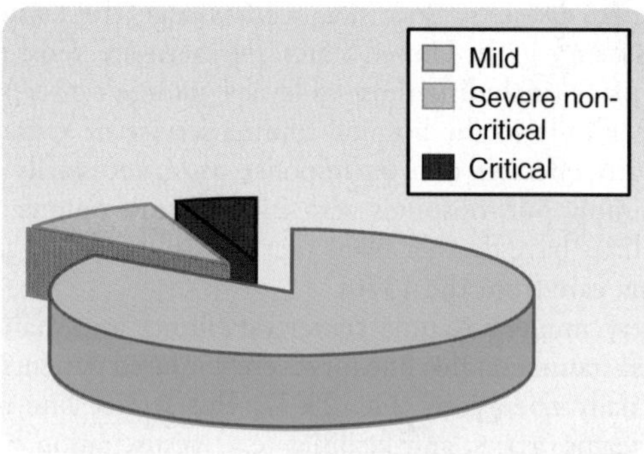


**FIGURE 25-2** Generic injury severity distribution for disaster scenarios. Of all survivors arriving in the hospital, the overwhelming majority (85%) will have only minor injuries. Of the severely injured (ISS > 9), only one third, or 1 in 20 arrivals, will be critically injured with life-threatening injuries. This injury severity distribution forms the basis for planning the hospital disaster response.

## MASS CASUALTY AND MODERN TRAUMA SYSTEMS

### Goal of the Hospital Disaster Responses

A well-known underlying principle of medical disaster response is to do the greatest good for the greatest number of casualties, but it is crucial to understand the precise clinical implications of this principle for trauma care.

Bearing in mind the injury severity distribution, a MCI is "a needle in a haystack" situation in which a small group of severely injured patients who require immediate high-level trauma care is immersed within a much larger group of casualties with minor injuries, who can tolerate delays and even suboptimal care without adversely affecting their outcome.[1] The ultimate goal of the entire hospital disaster response is, therefore, to provide this small group of critically injured patients with a level of care that approximates the care provided to similarly injured patients on a normal working day. This goal has never been formally declared by the American College of Surgeons[2] or any other professional organization, but it has always been implicitly understood by surgeons and trauma care providers and is certainly an expectation of the public. In a multiple casualty incident, this goal can be achieved by effective triage and priority-driven trauma care. In a mass casualty incident, it can still be achieved by diverting trauma assets and resources from the less severely injured to the critically wounded—but at a cost. Contrary to popular belief, the casualties whose management is delayed and compromised in a mass casualty scenario are not the mild ones but the severely injured patients with non–life-threatening injuries.

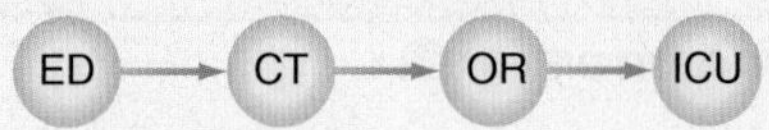


**FIGURE 25-3** Schematic depiction of the trauma service line of a hospital. The service line consists of resource, assets, and facilities in which trauma care providers treat severely injured patients. The typical flow of a severely injured patient is from the trauma resuscitation bay of the ED to imaging, usually the CT scanner, then to the OR, and finally to a surgical ICU bed. Preserving this service line in the face of a large influx of severe casualties is the true goal of the hospital disaster response.

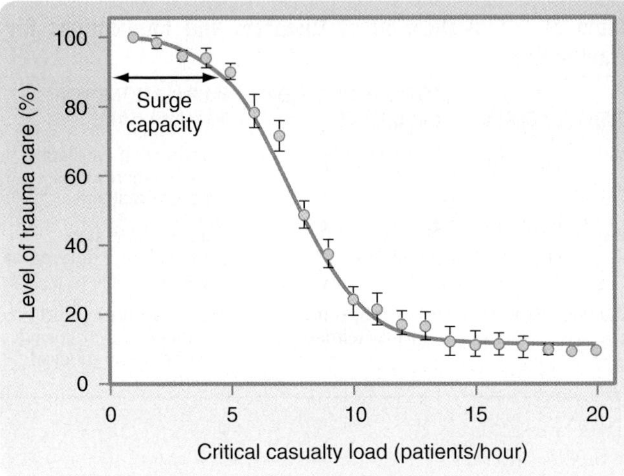


**FIGURE 25-4** Graphic depiction of the results of a computer simulation of the flow of casualties of urban bombing through the trauma service line of the Ben Taub General Hospital, a level 1 trauma center in Houston. The model predicts a sigmoid-shaped relationship between the casualty load and global level of trauma care. The level of care for a single patient on a normal working day is defined as 100%. The *upper flat portion* of the curve corresponds to a multiple casualty incident, the *steep portion* represents a mass casualty situation, and the *lower flat portion* represents a major medical disaster. The surge capacity of the hospital trauma service line is the maximal critical casualty load that can be managed without a precipitous drop in the level of care. This simulation is based on clinical profiles of casualties treated at the Rabin Medical Center in Petach Tikva, Israel. (From Hirshberg A, Scott BG, Granchi T, et al: How does casualty load affect trauma care in urban bombing incidents? A quantitative analysis. J Trauma 58:686–693, 2005.)

## The Trauma Service Line in Disasters

There is a strange dissociation between the dramatic advances in trauma systems in the past 30 years and current disaster planning. The U.S. National Response Framework (NRF), which lays out the guiding principles for all levels of a unified national response to disasters, does not acknowledge the existence of trauma systems in the United States. Furthermore, most hospital disaster plans (including those of level 1 trauma centers) do not refer specifically to the hospital trauma service or system, even though any effective disaster response must necessarily rely on them. Simply put, hospitals with 21st century trauma services and facilities have disaster plans that are still based on concepts of trauma care from the 1970s.

Every modern trauma center establishes and maintains a dedicated trauma service line for severely injured patients during normal daily operations (Fig. 25-3). This service line includes trauma teams, assets, and facilities (e.g., resuscitation bays and operating rooms), all readily available to treat seriously injured patients. The trauma service line of a hospital provides the resources for optimal care of individual patients, but has limited capabilities to treat multiple badly injured patients simultaneously. The goal of an effective disaster response is therefore to preserve the hospital trauma service line in the face of an unusually large number of casualties. From the trauma care perspective, success in dealing with an MCI is not streamlining the flow of 40 or 60 casualties through the ED, but rather preserving the capability to provide optimal trauma care to the three or four critically injured (but salvageable) casualties among them.[5]

## Casualty Load and Surge Capacity

Many hospital administrators have an exaggerated view of the capacity of their institutions because hospital disaster planning is typically based on counting ED gurneys and hospital beds, rather than on the rate at which casualties are treated (or processed) by the hospital trauma system. In reality, as the MCI unfolds and progressively more casualties arrive, finding an available resuscitation bay and staffing it with experienced trauma teams becomes increasingly difficult.[1]

From the trauma care perspective, the arrival rate of severe casualties is a more meaningful metric of the burden on a trauma system than the absolute number of casualties. The casualty load is the arrival rate of severe casualties per hour, and an increasing casualty load eventually leads to degradation of trauma care as severely injured patients compete for the limited assets and resources. An intact trauma service line provides each severe casualty with a trauma team, resuscitation bay, and other resources, such as an available computed tomography (CT) scanner, operating room, and intensive care bed. The point beyond which this level of care cannot be maintained for new arrivals represents the surge capacity of the trauma service line of the hospital.[6] Surge capacity is, therefore, a dynamic measure of the processing capacity of the trauma service line, and cannot be derived from static calculations of ED gurneys and staff. Using a similar definition, a surge capacity can also be defined separately for each trauma-related facility in the hospital.

An increasing casualty load adversely affects the quality of trauma care for the severely injured because many casualties compete for the same limited trauma assets and resources. Analysis using a computer model[6] describes this relationship as a sigmoid-shaped curve (Fig. 25-4). The upper flat portion of the curve represents an intact trauma service line, where the level of care for severe casualties approximates the care given to a single patient on a normal working day. This is a multiple casualty incident. The steep portion represents a gradually failing trauma service line, corresponding to a mass casualty scenario. The lower flat portion represents a failed (or nonexistent) service line overwhelmed by a major medical disaster.

The surge capacity of the trauma service line is the point beyond which the level of care begins to drop. An effective disaster response shifts the curve to the right, increasing the surge capacity and resulting in a more gradual degradation of the level of care. An empirical estimate[7] puts the surge capacity at one severely injured patient per hour for every 100 hospital beds, providing a practical yardstick that can be used in disaster planning.

## Mass Casualty and Modern Trauma Systems

The overwhelming majority of urban terrorist bombings are multiple casualty incidents that do not exceed the surge capacity of individual hospitals. However, in the past decade, terrorist groups have made repeated attempts to increase the magnitude of these MCIs by coordinated multiple simultaneous bombings. The two best documented examples were the Madrid trains bombing (March 2004)[8] and the London subway bombing (July 2005).[4] However, these incidents clearly demonstrated that modern emergency medical services (EMS) and trauma systems in large metropolitan areas serve as effective buffers that mitigate the medical impact of a large-scale event by distributing casualties among hospitals. With 2253 casualties in Madrid and more than 700 in London, rapid dispersion of the casualties among several hospitals resulted in each participating hospital facing only a multiple casualty incident with a handful of critical patients. This strong buffering mechanism was, however, conspicuously absent in the U.S. Embassy bombing in Nairobi, Kenya, in 1998, where more than 4000 casualties flooded the Kenyatta National Hospital.[9] This inadequately documented MCI is the only truly overwhelming urban mass casualty incident in recent history. This is a key point that is worth reemphasizing: no hospital in a metropolitan area that has a functioning EMS system has ever been overwhelmed by a MCI.

A major difficulty in trying to learn useful lessons from past incidents is the paucity of clinical data. Most published reports provide only global statistics, such as the total number of casualties and the mortality among the critically injured (critical mortality), with few clinical details about the trauma care of individual patients. Difficulties and problems in trauma care must be inferred between the lines, such as an alarmingly high number of negative laparotomies, which are hidden in the data of the main reports from the Madrid and London bombings. Interestingly, in the entire body of literature on disaster medicine, no hospital has ever reported having preventable morbidity and mortality. In view of the high public profile and emotional impact of such incidents, factual detailed clinical reports about trauma care in MCIs are unlikely to be published.

The keys to an effective medical response to any MCI are robust trauma systems and well-functioning trauma centers. Unfortunately, trauma centers in the United States are currently in the midst of a major crisis. The public and its elected representatives simply do not associate the well-being of trauma centers with the medical response to disasters. Thus, while the national grid of functioning trauma centers is being eroded by lack of public support, huge resources are allocated to preparing hospitals for so-called all-hazard scenarios, which have become a top priority despite their extremely small likelihood. The public clearly does not realize this dangerous paradox. Without a strong national grid of trauma centers, no effective disaster response will be possible for doomsday scenarios or just plain civilian MCIs.

## Medical Care at the Scene

Most MCIs in an urban environment follow a typical timeline that can be divided into four distinct phases (Table 25-2).[10] The initial chaotic phase begins immediately after the inciting event.

**Table 25-2 Typical Timeline of Urban Mass Casualty Incident**

| SCENE PHASE | CHARACTERISTICS | IMPLICATIONS FOR THE ED |
|---|---|---|
| Chaotic | No organized medical care; mild casualties go to nearest hospital | First wave: A few walking wounded |
| Organized effort | Key is effective triage; priority-driven transport of casualties | Second wave: Main body of casualties |
| Site clearing | Remaining casualties transported | |
| Late | Sporadic mild casualties | Third wave: Slow trickle of mild casualties |

Without any organized medical effort, many minor casualties and those with acute stress reaction run from the scene and find their way to the nearest hospitals. The organized effort phase begins when a prehospital responder takes charge at the scene and initiates a systematic medical effort while also ensuring the safety and security of the medical teams. The most important aspect of this phase is effective field triage, which allows priority-driven transport of casualties to hospitals. This is followed by the site-clearing phase, the duration of which depends on the specific circumstances of the incident (i.e., magnitude, structural collapse, or need for prolonged extrication). It ends when the last live casualty is transported from the scene. The late phase is a poorly defined period when minor casualties who initially ran from the scene decide to seek medical attention, often after being persuaded by family and friends.

From the hospital perspective, this timeline translates into a characteristic casualty arrival pattern consisting of three waves (see Table 25-2). The first wave consists of a small cluster of casualties with minor injuries who arrive in hospital on their own. After a variable interval, the main body of casualties begins to pour in, presenting a wide variety of injury severities. Finally, a slow trickle of late arrivals with minor injuries or acute stress reaction continues over many hours.[10]

Because the time from injury to definitive care is a key determinant of mortality, the dominant approach of prehospital teams in an urban setting is to "scoop and run." The emphasis is on triage and rapid transport; interventions are largely restricted to airway management and control of external hemorrhage. However, in a rural or remote MCI, transport can be a bottleneck because of limited means or long distances and may mandate some form of trauma care at the scene.

Field triage schemes are based on a rapid assessment of clinical and physiologic parameters. Until recently, the dominant algorithm in the United States was START (*s*imple *t*riage *a*nd *r*apid *t*reatment), which sorts casualties into four categories—immediate, delayed, minor, and deceased.[11] Criticism of START, which results in excessive overtriage, has led to the recent introduction of the SALT triage scheme (*s*ort, *a*ssess, *l*ife-saving interventions, *t*reatment and/or transport), which combines global assessment of the casualties (e.g., walking versus laying still) with a more detailed yet brief assessment of vital signs.[12] SALT has been endorsed by the American College of Surgeons and other professional organizations dealing with mass casualty triage. Although it is promoted as a universal triage scheme for MCIs, its main usefulness is at the scene rather than for hospital triage at the ED door.

## CLINICAL ASPECTS OF HOSPITAL DISASTER PLANS

### Hospital Disaster Response

The ultimate goal of the hospital disaster plan is to rapidly augment the surge capacity of the trauma service line with its support elements, such as the blood bank and emergency laboratory. An emergency operations center (EOC) coordinates the institutional effort.

Each service or facility in the hospital response envelope activates a facility-specific disaster protocol designed to increase the processing capacity (or surge capacity) of the facility quickly to accommodate a sudden large influx of casualties. The underlying principle of these protocols is suspension of normal daily activities while rapidly mobilizing staff reinforcements.

Full activation of the entire disaster plan of a large hospital takes time, disrupts normal daily activities, is expensive, and is also usually unnecessary, because the overwhelming majority of MCIs that any hospital is likely to face are limited events. It makes sense, therefore, to base the hospital disaster plan on a tiered response.[13] The plan for a limited MCI centers primarily on the ED and relies on in-house staff and resources. A plan for large-scale MCIs recruits reinforcement staff and additional facilities outside the ED. Although this tiered approach is not yet a formal part of the hospital disaster planning in the United States, it makes clinical and administrative sense and is implicitly adopted by a growing number of institutions.

From the perspective of trauma care, the hospital response consists of two distinct phases.[10] During the initial phase, the incident is still evolving, casualties are arriving, and their ultimate number is unknown. Therefore, the key consideration is to preserve the trauma service line for the next critical arrival. The definitive phase begins when casualties are no longer arriving, the overall casualty number is known, and the hospital response envelope has been fully deployed. The clinical focus shifts to providing definitive care to all casualties in a graded, priority-oriented fashion.

### Preparing to Receive Casualties

The person authorized to initiate the hospital disaster response can be either a hospital administrator or a local decision maker in the ED (e.g., the charge nurse or the attending emergency physician). The former approach reflects a top-down command mentality and comes at a price of expediency, especially outside normal working hours. The latter is in line with a flexible approach of empowering local managers to make decisions, facilitating a rapid response.

The characteristic time lag between the notification to expect incoming casualties and the actual arrival of the first wave is a window of opportunity to initiate the opening steps of the institutional response. Actions taken during this brief window have a profound effect on the subsequent response. Nowhere is this window more crucial than in the ED, where a rapid evacuation plan is activated to create empty gurneys and physical space for a large number of incoming casualties.[14] Based on their medical condition, ED patients can be discharged, admitted to the floors, or transferred to a predesignated location within the hospital. Other priorities are to position a triage officer outside (not inside) the ED and improvise additional trauma bays close to the trauma resuscitation area. The command chain in the ED must be clear to all, and the entire staff must be briefed and given specific roles. For example, in the trauma resuscitation area, staff members are assigned to specific teams and told explicitly who will take the first, second, and subsequent critical arrivals. Emergency carts containing additional medical supplies are deployed in predesignated areas.

### Incident Command and Clinical Decision Making

Hospital disaster plans are traditionally based on a top-down organizational hierarchy stemming from the incident command structure developed in the 1970s to streamline the field management of large-scale incidents.[3] However, the implementation of these top-down organizational structures during a real incident is problematic because most MCIs are brief and limited in scope. The rapid dynamics of an urban MCI far outpace the deployment of the top-down hospital command structure, so that by the time the hospital has an incident command center up and running, the incident is long over. More importantly, the top-down hierarchical tree means that when a problem arises, it is communicated upward in anticipation of a solution, which will inevitably be delayed. In a real incident, local managers frequently solve problems by communicating horizontally among themselves.

The shortcomings of the rigid top-down command structure were glaringly obvious during the response to Hurricane Katrina in 2005[15] and stood in sharp contrast to many small-scale successes led by resourceful local managers who collaborated with peers in their professional or organizational networks. It is becoming increasingly clear that an effective disaster response at any level must be based on such collaborative networks rather than on rigid top-down chains of command.[16]

Few hospital administrators realize that the major driving forces that propel the hospital disaster response are clinical decisions made at the bedside. The movement of severe casualties among facilities is essentially flow between decision points, because no casualty enters (or leaves) a facility unless a clinical decision has been made by a trauma care provider. In a traditional top-down command structure, executive decisions are made at the top and implemented by the lower echelons. In a hospital coping with an MCI, the situation is reversed, because the crucial decisions are made at the bedside and the role of the higher organizational echelons is to support and facilitate the implementation of these clinical decisions.[14]

The effective response of every facility in the trauma service line to a sudden large casualty load always hinges on a small group of local managers whose clinical decisions drive the entire effort. In the ED, these are the surgeon in charge, attending emergency physician, charge nurse, and triage officer. These decision makers understand the overarching goals of the hospital plan and should be empowered to solve problems independently instead of merely reporting them. They should be trained to improvise and communicate horizontally with other local managers. Such collaborative network architectures provide flexibility, adaptability, and speed and are resilient when parts of the system fail unexpectedly.

Surgeons must also be aware of a fundamental change in the medical decision making process during an MCI. In everyday clinical practice, trauma team leaders enjoy full autonomy in their clinical decisions regarding treatment priorities and the use of resources and facilities. In an MCI, a large number of severely injured patients compete for these same resources and facilities. Key clinical decisions must therefore be made by the surgeon in charge, who can visualize the "big picture" of the institutional situation, and the autonomy of the individual team leader no longer exists.[17] For example, the decision to take a patient with a penetrating abdominal injury and intra-abdominal bleeding to the operating room is not automatic nor can it be made by the trauma team leader alone, because it depends on other casualties and on the situation in the operating rooms. The surgeon in charge is not merely a coordinator or supervisor but actually makes key clinical decisions about individual patients.

## Hospital Triage

Triage is the central element of the hospital disaster response with implications far beyond the ED door.[18] There is a wide discrepancy between the theory of triage and the harsh reality of sorting arriving casualties on the ambulance dock. Most hospital plans call for an experienced trauma surgeon to stand at the ED entrance and sort arriving casualties based on a brief assessment of physiologic parameters (e.g., palpable peripheral pulse or respiratory distress). Popular schemes divide casualties into five categories—immediate (life-threatening injuries), delayed (severe injuries that can wait for definitive care), minimal (walking wounded), dead, and expectant (hopeless; Table 25-3).

Experience from real MCIs has shown that triage on the ambulance dock cannot be based on physiologic parameters simply because the triage officer has time for only a rapid cursory glance at each arrival. The triage decision must therefore rely on a global impression of the patient's clinical condition.[19] Furthermore, it is often impossible to distinguish immediate from delayed casualties based on this rapid cursory glance, and pronouncing death on the ambulance dock without a thorough examination and cardiac monitor is also an unrealistic expectation. Most problematic is the hopeless (or expectant) category, because such determinations often depend on the available resources; the same critical casualty may be deemed salvageable if the casualty load is light (or if the patient is an early arrival) or hopeless when the ED is overwhelmed.[1] For all these reasons, realistic triage on the ambulance dock should be viewed as a screening test for severe casualties who require immediate access to the hospital trauma service line.

The quality of triage has traditionally been expressed in terms of overtriage and undertriage rates.[19] The former is the erroneous assignment of nonsevere casualties to the trauma resuscitation area, whereas the latter is the erroneous assignment of severe casualties to a regular ED gurney. Overtriage is a system problem because these patients compete with severe casualties for trauma teams and facilities. Undertriage, on the other hand, is a medical error that may affect preventable morbidity and mortality. It has been suggested recently that hospital triage should be viewed as any other diagnostic screening test, using specificity and sensitivity rates, which do not directly correspond with overtriage and undertriage, as measures of triage accuracy.[20]

The major goal of effective triage is to facilitate better use of limited trauma resources. The key resource most needed by a severely injured patient is the specific attention of a trauma team. The price of inaccurate triage can therefore be quantified in terms of trauma team workload. A recently published computer model has shown that increasing triage accuracy reduces this workload.[20]

It is important to underscore that triage does not end on the ambulance dock. It is, in fact, a reiterative process whereby each casualty is sequentially and repeatedly assessed as he or she progresses along the trauma service line. Each reevaluation increases the accuracy of the overall process and increases the likelihood that the patient will be triaged correctly and allocated the appropriate resources for the best possible clinical outcome.

**Table 25-3 Traditional and Realistic Hospital Triage Categories**

| | Triage Mode | |
|---|---|---|
| **TRADITIONAL CATEGORIES** | **SINGLE-STEP** | **SEQUENTIAL** |
| Immediate<br>Expectant<br>Dead | Severe (to shock room) | Critical (to shock room) |
| Delayed<br>Minimal | All others (to ED holding) | Delayed (to ED holding)<br>Minimal (treated outside ED) |

## Clinical Implications of Triage Modes

From the perspective of the trauma service line of the hospital, there are two realistic modes for triage on the ambulance dock (see Table 25-3). Single-step triage is the simple binary decision mode whereby casualties are sorted into severe (roughly corresponding to an Injury Severity Score [ISS] of more than 9, or 15% of the casualties) and all others. The former are assigned a trauma team in the trauma resuscitation area; the rest are treated in the ED holding area. Sequential (two-step) triage further sorts severe casualties into critical (or immediate; ISS > 15) or urgent (or delayed; ISS = 9 to15) categories. The former (approximately 5% of the casualties) are assigned a full trauma team in a resuscitation bay to address immediate life-threatening injuries, whereas the latter are treated by one team per several casualties in the holding area. In this mode, mild casualties (walking wounded) are directed to a designated area outside the ED.

Sequential triage can be performed by two triage officers working in sequence (one on the ambulance dock, the other inside the ED) or by a single officer making two triage decisions in rapid sequence. The first decision separates mild casualties, who go to a designated area outside the ED, from the severely injuries, who enter the ED. The second decision determines which casualties will receive a full dedicated trauma team.

Single-step triage works well in limited multiple casualty incidents, in which the total number of expected casualties is below the bed capacity of the ED. Sequential triage is needed only in large-scale incidents that exceed this capacity. It is important to emphasize that sequential triage is not merely a refined triage scheme with an additional category, but rather a dramatic qualitative change in trauma care. In this mode, roughly two of every three severely injured patients will receive a lower level of trauma care than they would get on a normal working day. The decision to use sequential triage is therefore the most important medical leadership decision during the early stages of a MCI.

Any disaster response entails a necessary compromise to do the most good to the greatest number of casualties. However, as sequential triage shows, it is in the treatment of urgent casualties with severe (but not immediately life-threatening) injuries that this compromise is the most evident. Although it is intuitively assumed that this lower level of care will not directly affect outcome, this crucial point has never been addressed in published reports of past MCIs.

## Trauma Care in the Initial Phase

During the initial phase of a MCI (Box 25-1), the hospital operates two parallel (but separate) service lines for incoming casualties.[14] The first is a high-priority line with neither queues nor delays. It is reserved for severe casualties and includes the staff and resources that treat severely wounded patients during normal daily operations, from the trauma resuscitation bay in the ED to the surgical intensive care unit (SICU; see Fig. 25-3). This service line is staffed by the experienced trauma care providers who deal with severely injured patients daily.

The second service line is designated for the mildly injured, who require mostly treatment of trivial injuries and ruling out occult significant trauma. Here, the role of trauma care providers is to supervise and guide hospital staff who are not trauma care providers but are called up to help in the ED.

It is interesting to note that the roles of the trauma surgeon and trauma-trained nurse in MCIs have never been formally defined in published guidelines, and are conspicuously absent from templates for hospital disaster plans. Depending on the structure and size of the trauma service at a specific institution, surgeons and nurses with trauma experience may be assigned to perform triage, be in charge of the trauma resuscitation area, or have medical control of other parts of the hospital response envelope. The underlying principle is that trauma surgeons and nurses should be positioned where they can have the most impact on the overall clinical result. Their roles should be defined well in advance and incorporated into the institutional disaster plan.

Critical casualties who enter the trauma service line are treated in a fashion similar to that of everyday care, with an emphasis on expediency, rapid turnover times, and using smaller trauma teams. The crucial difference is that all major clinical decisions are referred to the surgeon in charge who roams in the trauma resuscitation area and acts as coordinator and ultimate clinical decision maker.[17] Clinical and administrative control are maintained through frequent rounding on all casualties in the ED by the surgeon in charge, charge nurse, and ED attending physician. The product of these rounds is a list of casualties, their diagnoses, and their disposition (or plan). Knowing the total number of casualties and their injuries and dispositions, as well as the situation at each trauma service point, allows the surgeon in charge to consider clinical priorities against available resources and determine a feasible solution for each critical casualty.

**BOX 25-1 Goals and Principles of Trauma Care in the Initial Phase**

**Goals**

Optimal trauma care for critical casualties
Minimal acceptable care for all others

**Principles**

Two parallel but separate service lines
Conservation of trauma assets and resources
Centralized clinical decision making
Loss of continuity of care

The guiding principle for the care of noncritical casualties during the initial phase is minimal acceptable care, which means empirical trauma care along the line of first aid in the field.[21] The aim is to buy time, conserve trauma resources, and delay definitive care while offloading the trauma service line. This concept of minimal acceptable care is based on experience with civilian casualties of war, in which some two thirds of casualties survive for 1 week after injury without any medical care, and nonoperative management buys time and improves survival.[22] Thus, the clinical suspicion of a long bone fracture is treated by empirical splinting and analgesia and the patient is rapidly admitted to a floor bed without imaging. Penetrating abdominal trauma with peritoneal signs but no hemodynamic compromise is treated with IV fluids, antibiotics, nasogastric suction, analgesia, and admission to a floor bed until the definitive care phase. One of the hallmarks of this temporizing philosophy is to limit access to the CT scanner only to patients for whom the scan is absolutely essential or potentially lifesaving (e.g., a head injury with lateralizing signs or a deteriorating level of consciousness).

Another distinguishing feature of trauma care in disasters is discontinuity of care, because in most real-life events, teams are assigned to service points rather than to individual critical patients. Thus, a critical casualty may be resuscitated in the shock room by one team, the imaging studies reviewed by a second team, and the operation performed by a third. Few hospital disaster plans currently address this crucial issue and incorporate solutions (e.g., case managers) to mitigate the potential adverse effects of this loss of continuity of care.[23]

Although the CT scanner is a classic bottleneck in the flow of casualties along the trauma service line, operating room availability is not a major concern because only very few casualties require emergency surgery during the initial phase.[21,24] Even in large-scale MCIs, such as the simultaneous terrorist bombings in Madrid (2004) and London (2005), there was a time window of more than 1 hour between activation of the disaster response and the first operative procedure.

Contrary to the situation in the operating room (OR), the availability of ICU beds is a source of grave concern. This is especially true in urban bombing incidents, in which approximately one of every four admitted casualties will need an intensive care bed. This high demand comes in the face of a severe SICU bed shortage in most trauma centers. The hospital disaster response must therefore include protocols for rapidly generating a substantial number of vacant intensive care beds available for incoming casualties.[25] This is typically accomplished by transferring nonventilated patients to floor beds or by using nonsurgical intensive care facilities within the hospital. The postanesthesia care unit is often the first to be used to accommodate an overflow of ventilated patients. Critically injured nonoperated patients from an urban bombing will need an SICU bed approximately 4 to 5 hours after arrival in the hospital, and operated casualties take even longer.[4] These long intervals allow the hospital to prepare beds, transfer patients, and mobilize staff reinforcements to achieve a substantial surge in intensive care capacity.

## Definitive Care Phase

During this phase, casualties are no longer arriving, their ultimate number is known, and the disaster response envelope of the hospital is fully deployed. It is now possible to take stock and proceed with definitive care for all admitted casualties.[10,21,25]

The central tool in this phase is a series of detailed rounds by members of the trauma service on all admitted casualties, making a detailed and priority-driven treatment plan for each one. The deliverables of these rounds are prioritized lists of patients in need of imaging, consults, operative procedures, and transfer to other institutions. In other words, the minimal acceptable care of the initial phase now transforms into priority-driven definitive care in which the more urgent clinical problems are addressed first.

The definitive care phase consumes considerable time and resources,[26] so even limited multiple casualty incidents may disrupt the normal daily activities of the trauma service line and related facilities for 24 to 48 hours after the last casualties have arrived. Return to normal daily activities is therefore gradual and the timeline differs among facilities. The ED can return to normal relatively quickly, but the intensive care unit (ICU) often requires additional staffing and support for several days. The Israeli experience with urban bombings contains useful descriptions of the a general ICU coping with multiple casualty incidents, the importance of planning to relieve staff at regular intervals, and the use of staff reinforcements, nursing students, and volunteers.[25,27]

During the definitive care phase, consideration should be given to the need for secondary distribution of casualties by transferring some of them to other institutions. Interhospital transfer of burn patients to burn centers is a self-evident example. Such transfers are more problematic when the indication is mostly logistic, such as the desire to shorten waiting times for nonurgent operations (e.g., internal fixation of long bone fractures). Financial and administrative issues, as well as considerations of institutional prestige, often create barriers to interhospital transfer—to the detriment of patients.

An urban bombing is an example of a short MCI, in which the main body of casualties arrives within approximately 2 hours of the explosion. When structural collapse is involved, prolonged extrication and site-clearing activities extend the initial phase, but there is still a clear distinction between the initial and definitive care phases. However, in some types of MCIs, such as natural disasters or civilian trauma care in areas of conflict, an ongoing stream of casualties blurs the distinction between the phases and poses an ongoing challenge to the hospital trauma service line and its logistic supply chains. The hospital disaster response must therefore include plans for such a rolling MCI, in which maintenance of capabilities and preservation of resources over time become a central issue. Strict rationing of staff working hours, maintaining a supply chain for critical items such as blood products, and preparing for the need to have hospital personnel reside in-house for many days are all elements of such a plan for a rolling MCI.

A crucial final step before return to normal daily operations is a formal debriefing. This activity takes place as soon as possible after the incident. Ideally, all staff (hospital and prehospital) who took part in the effort should participate. The debriefing should be carefully structured to cover all key areas of clinical and administrative activity while allowing free input from any participant who wishes to make a point. The aim is to learn lessons and identify barriers to the hospital response that can later be incorporated into the hospital disaster plan.

## SURGEON'S ROLE IN NATURAL DISASTERS

The medical aid stampede during the first few weeks after the Haiti earthquake in January 2010 demonstrated how little surgeons know about their role in natural disasters, as many volunteers with good intentions rushed to the stricken country in improvised teams, only to discover how little good intentions and surgical skills alone can achieve.

There are fundamental differences between the medical response to an urban MCI and organizing medical aid to a major natural disaster. In the former, a functioning trauma system is coping with an unusually large casualty load over a brief period (from hours to several days). In the latter, the catastrophic event compromises or destroys infrastructure and community support systems (including trauma and health care systems) in the disaster area. External medical assets and resources must therefore be imported into the disaster area to reinforce, support, or replace compromised local assets over a period of many weeks, months, and sometimes years.[28]

The vulnerability of the population affected by a major natural disaster is determined primarily by its poverty level because poor countries have a weaker infrastructure, and hence suffer more devastation, but have fewer resources with which to cope. Thus, the 2010 Haiti earthquake, with some 230,000 dead, stands in dramatic contrast to the 1989 earthquake near San Francisco, which was of a similar magnitude yet resulted in only 63 deaths.

### Injury Patterns in Natural Disasters

It is important to know the typical injury patterns seen in various types of natural disasters.[29] In a major earthquake, the most important wounding mechanisms are falling debris and entrapment underneath collapsed buildings. Immediate search and rescue efforts by survivors in their immediate vicinity save more lives than the organized (but delayed) rescue efforts of external agencies. During the first few hours after an earthquake, survivors present with a wide variety of extremity and visceral injuries, but later the prevailing patterns are extremity injuries and a high incidence of crush injuries. Only a small fraction of the overall number of casualties is extricated alive after 48 hours underneath the rubble, approximately 300 patients in the Haiti earthquake of January 2010 that killed 250,000. Delayed extrication translates into a high incidence of crush syndrome and acute renal failure, as seen after the Marmara earthquake in Turkey in 1999.[30,31]

The 2004 tsunami in Southeast Asia caused twice as many dead than injured survivors, in whom the dominant injury patterns were extremity fractures and soft tissue wounds.[32] In a volcanic eruption, injuries are caused by falling rocks, exposure to ash (a strong respiratory irritant), and inhalation injury from volcanic gases. The leading cause of death is suffocation. Knowing the characteristic injury patterns for each type of natural disaster is an obvious prerequisite for planning a medical relief effort.

### Initiating the Medical Relief Effort

Contrary to the popular notion of the heroic medical volunteer racing to the rescue, there is a formal methodology for initiating a medical response to a natural disaster. The crucial first step is a rapid needs assessment, a formal mission that is carried out as soon as possible after the catastrophe.[28,33] A United Nations Disaster Assessment and Coordination (UNDAC) team, typically composed of two to six experts, travels quickly to the disaster area to assess the immediate needs and report them to the international community. The rapid needs assessment, conducted in close collaboration with local authorities and facilities, defines not only the extent of the damage to local infrastructure and medical resources, but also estimates the numbers of casualties, types of injuries, and key priorities for disaster relief. Medical needs are often assigned a lower priority than essentials such as water, food, and shelter. Without an expert needs assessment and subsequent careful planning of the mission tailored to the specific profile of the disaster, the effort will not be effective. Improvised initiatives of enthusiastic individuals are likely to end up as part of the problem rather than part of the solution.

### Trauma Care in the Disaster Area

The medical response to a major natural disaster consists of two distinct phases.[28] During the immediate phase, the first days and weeks following the catastrophe, the main goal is to provide trauma care to the injured. In the late phase, in the subsequent months or even years, the focus is on supporting the reconstruction of local medical services and facilities in the disaster area.

During the immediate phase, by the time outside medical help with surgical capabilities arrives, casualties with severe visceral injuries have either been treated already or have not survived. Therefore, the clinical focus shifts to the management of extremity and soft tissue injuries that may be neglected or infected and to specific complications, such as renal failure from crush syndrome. Another important component of the work of outside medical teams is to provide solutions to ongoing surgical emergencies in the afflicted population. In the absence of surgical facilities in the disaster area, even simple, straightforward, nontrauma emergencies such as an incarcerated hernia or an obstetric condition requiring an urgent cesarean section may lead to preventable mortality.

In the immediate phase, the surgical management of extremity injuries follows the well-established principles of the management of war wounds. The focus is on simple and traightforward procedures rather than on complex reconstructions, which are not a feasible option. Muscle compartments should be decompressed liberally and early nonviable or heavily contaminated tissue must be excised while carefully preserving intact skin and viable soft tissue. Wounds are left open for delayed primary closure or reexcision if needed. Nonsalvageable or mangled extremities should undergo early amputation, with the stump left open for delayed primary closure.[28]

The composition and surgical capabilities of a team deployed to a disaster area must be carefully considered in view of the clinical needs in the field. A typical team consists of torso and extremity surgeons with trauma experience. More important than specific surgical skills is the ability to work in an austere environment in a spirit of collaboration with local and other external medical teams. Here, again, the trained professional team with disaster relief experience, supported by a robust logistic, security, and communications envelope has a much better chance of rendering effective medical care than an ad hoc team of enthusiastic volunteers. Such an effort relies on data-driven planning based on a competent rapid needs assessment, is limited in scope and duration, and has well-defined realistic goals.

**Table 25-4 Classification of Blast Trauma**

| CLASS OF BLAST INJURY | MECHANISM |
|---|---|
| Primary | Wounding of air-filled viscera as direct result of the blast wave |
| Secondary | Penetrating trauma from bomb fragments and other projectiles of varying mass and velocity |
| Tertiary | Casualties propelled by the blast wind, resulting in standard patterns of blunt trauma |
| Quaternary | Burns, crush, and all other trauma mechanisms that are not included above |

## BLAST TRAUMA: CLINICAL PATTERNS AND SYSTEM IMPLICATIONS

Urban bombing incidents result in unusually severe and challenging patterns of injury, where up to one third of casualties admitted to hospital have an ISS higher than 15, a rate three times higher than that seen in a typical civilian trauma practice. The overall number of casualties and rate of immediate on-scene mortality are determined by the size of the explosive charge, structural failure of the building, and indoor detonation, which results in a greatly amplified blast wave. Suicide bombers are particularly devastating weapons of urban terror because they specifically target crowded indoors locations or large open space gatherings to maximize the effect of the explosion.[21]

Blast trauma is viewed by trauma surgeons as a multidimensional injury because it often combines blast, penetrating, blunt, and burn mechanisms in the same casualty. The results are injury patterns of higher severity and complexity and a greater burden on the trauma service line of the hospital. The classification of blast injuries is given in Table 25-4.

### Primary Blast Injury

The most common clinical sign of blast injury is eardrum perforation. These perforations usually heal spontaneously but may result in various degrees of hearing loss in up 25% of patients. Eardrum perforation is a useful marker of the proximity of the patient to the detonation but is not a reliable predictor of lung injury.[34] All arriving casualties should therefore be screened for tympanic membrane rupture in the ED; those with a perforation should undergo an audiometric assessment for hearing loss within 24 hours, regardless of symptoms. Although it is customary to admit otherwise asymptomatic patients with eardrum perforation for overnight observation because of their proximity to the detonation and concerns over the insidious onset of a blast lung injury, this practice is not evidence-based.

The blast wave from the detonation disrupts the alveolar-capillary interface of the lung, resulting in a spectrum of blast lung injury ranging in severity from mild pulmonary contusion with intra-alveolar hemorrhage to severe and rapidly evolving acute respiratory distress syndrome (ARDS).[35] Blast lung injury is uncommon, occurring in only 5% to 8% of live casualties in urban bombings, but its severity is the key determinant of mortality among early survivors. Blast may also cause barotrauma (pneumothorax and bronchoalveolar fistula), air embolism, and upper airway mucosal damage.

Mild blast lung injury presents with localized infiltrates on chest x-ray. It is managed similarly to a mild lung contusion and has a good outcome. Patients with severe lung injury typically present with rapidly worsening hypoxia, develop bilateral diffuse infiltrates, and require early aggressive respiratory support along the lines of managing ARDS. Pneumothorax should be actively sought and immediately decompressed in these patients. Mortality is in excess of 60% in these severe cases.[36]

Blast lung injury in the setting of an urban bombing poses an exceptional burden on the surgical ICU.[25,27] The trauma service line encounters several patients with severe and rapidly worsening hypoxia who arrive within a short time of each other. Each of these patients requires emergency endotracheal intubation in the trauma resuscitation area and subsequent advanced ventilatory support, and sometimes invasive hemodynamic monitoring in an ICU. This logistic nightmare scenario is almost unique to urban bombing incidents and translates into a huge medical, organizational, and staffing challenge.[14] The presence of associated injuries (e.g., burns or penetrating visceral trauma) adds to the complexity of an already difficult situation. These patients require not only an intensive care bed but, more importantly, the personal and undivided attention of a team of experienced critical care providers.

Intestinal blast trauma varies in severity from subserosal hemorrhage to full-thickness perforation.[37] Clinically important bowel blast injury is rare in urban bombings, occurring in less than 2% of live casualties, but is the most common form of trauma in an immersion blast from an underwater explosion. The clinical pitfall with these injuries is a delayed presentation, with some casualties developing peritoneal signs 48 hours or more after the explosion. The injury may affect any portion of the bowel but a propensity for the terminal ileum has been described.[38] Intraoperatively, a common dilemma is how much contused but nonperforated bowel to resect. The concern is that traumatized bowel may eventually progress to a delayed perforation. This decision is an operative judgment call.

### Secondary Blast Injury

Penetrating trauma from fragments of the bomb casing or from metal projectiles added to an improvised explosive device (IED) can cause a wide array of injuries, ranging from superficial skin lacerations to lethal visceral wounds. From the perspective of the hospital trauma service line, the key consideration is the need for extensive imaging to locate penetrating fragments and define their trajectories because a physical examination is a poor predictor of the depth of penetration. The most expedient method is to use a helical CT scan to locate multiple projectiles rapidly and delineate their trajectories.[39] However, this makes the CT scanner a bottleneck to patient flow[24] and requires setting priorities and rationing access to the scanner during the initial phase of the hospital response.

Penetrating trauma by multiple projectiles may result in deep soft tissue wounds that bleed profusely. Because these wounds are typically located on the posterior aspect of the torso and extremities, the associated blood loss is often underestimated. In patients who are taken to the OR for emergency surgery (e.g., for celiotomy) it is therefore advisable to log-roll the patient and rapidly pack the wounds with gauze before the main surgical procedure.[40]

Whereas classic management principles for traumatic wounds have called for débridement of each wound and removal of embedded foreign bodies, this is often not a realistic option in casualties with multiple (sometimes dozens) of asymptomatic penetrating wounds. These multiple débridements consume OR time and resources and end up causing more tissue damage than the original injury. A common sense approach is to address only symptomatic or infected projectiles and those in problematic locations (e.g., intra-articular).

### Tertiary and Quaternary Blast Injuries

When casualties are propelled against stationary objects by the explosion, the results are standard patterns of blunt trauma. However, these tertiary blast injuries are typically combined with other types of trauma caused by the blast. This complicates the clinical picture and presents unusual dilemmas in terms of treatment priorities and resource allocation.[21]

Quaternary blast trauma refers mostly to burns and crush injuries.[35] Superficial flash burns, typically involving large body areas, are caused by the explosion itself, and are markers of proximity to the blast. They are common among casualties found dead at the scene and have also been shown to be predictors of blast lung injury.[41] The ignition of flammable materials and clothes causes deep burns of variable extent, sometimes in conjunction with inhalation injury. A large number of burn casualties, many of them brought initially to hospitals that do not have a dedicated burn service, pose an extraordinary burden on regional burn systems that generally have a limited surge capacity, even during normal daily operations. Secondary distribution of these patients to other, often geographically remote, burn centers outside the immediate vicinity of the bombing site is a key feature of MCIs involving a large number of burned casualties, such as the Bali nightclub bombing in Indonesia in 2002.[42]

## CONCLUSION

The central message of this chapter is that amidst the wailing sirens of approaching ambulances, the terrible sights on television, the hectic activity of medical teams, and the emotional outrage of the public, surgeons must not forget their core mission in disasters. This core mission is to preserve the trauma service line of the hospital and remain focused on providing optimal trauma care to the next critical casualty. Contrary to the tendency among disaster planners and hospital administrators to prepare for nightmare megascenarios that surgeons are unlikely ever to encounter in their professional careers, the emphasis should be to on preparing for realistic MCIs that affect every institution from time to time.

Surgeons must remember that the ultimate goal of the entire hospital disaster plan is to provide a small group of critically injured casualties with a level of trauma care comparable to the care given to similarly injured patients on a normal working day. The many mildly injured patients are the noise, the casualties that are seen and heard on the evening news. The surgeon's role is to focus on the few casualties who are silent, those whose battle for survival unfolds away from the cameras, in the shock room, operating room, and ICU. Strange as it may seem, it is these very few critically injured patients who are the crux of the entire effort.

## SELECTED REFERENCES

Aylwin CJ, Konig TC, Brennan NW, et al: Reduction in critical mortality in urban mass casualty incidents: Analysis of triage, surge, and resource use after the London bombings on July 7, 2005. Lancet 368:2219–2225, 2006.

This report paints a detailed picture of the hospital response to the London subway bombings, including individual timelines for severe casualties. although it shows how a modern trauma centers copes with a large-scale event, it does not provide details on preventable morbidity and mortality.

Cushman JG, Pachter HL, Beaton HL: Two New York City hospitals' surgical response to the September 11, 2001, terrorist attack in New York City. J Trauma 54:147–154, 2003.

A classic report of the main hospital response to the World Trade Center destruction on 9/11 with a discussion of the tiered hospital response plan.

Frykberg ER: Medical management of disasters and mass casualties from terrorist bombings: how can we cope? J Trauma 53:201–212, 2002.

This is the first overview of the medical response to urban terrorism that emphasizes the role of effective triage and looks at the medical response in quantitative terms.

Hirshberg A, Scott BG, Granchi T, et al: How does casualty load affect trauma care in urban bombing incidents? A quantitative analysis. J Trauma 58:686–693, 2005.

A computer model was used to simulate the response of a major U.S. trauma center to an urban bombing using casualty profiles from an Israeli hospital. The model predicts the now classic sigmoid-shaped relationship between the level of trauma care and increasing casualty load and defines surge capacity of the hospital trauma service line.

Welling DR, Ryan JM, Burris DG, et al: Seven sins of humanitarian medicine. World J Surg. 2010;34:466–470.

A must-read for any surgeon contemplating participation in a humanitarian disaster relief effort, this editorial explains how good intentions can end up causing more damage than good.

## REFERENCES


1. Hirshberg A, Holcomb JB, Mattox KL: Hospital trauma care in multiple-casualty incidents: A critical view. Ann Emerg Med 37:647–652, 2001.
2. Committee on Trauma, American College of Surgeons: Disaster planning and management. In Committee on Trauma, American College of Surgeons: Resources for optimal care of the injured patient, Chicago, 2006, American College of Surgeons, pp 125–131.
3. O'Neill PA: The ABC's of disaster response. Scand J Surg 94:259–266, 2005.
4. Aylwin CJ, Konig TC, Brennan NW, et al: Reduction in critical mortality in urban mass casualty incidents: Analysis of triage, surge, and resource use after the London bombings on July 7, 2005. Lancet 368:2219–2225, 2006.
5. Hirshberg A: Multiple casualty incidents: Lessons from the front line. Ann Surg 239:322–324, 2004.
6. Hirshberg A, Scott BG, Granchi T, et al: How does casualty load affect trauma care in urban bombing incidents? A quantitative analysis. J Trauma 58:686–693, 2005.
7. De Boer J: Order in chaos: modelling medical management in disasters. Eur J Emerg Med 6:141–148, 1999.
8. Gutierrez de Ceballos JP, Turegano Fuentes F, Perez Diaz D, et al: Casualties treated at the closest hospital in the Madrid, March 11, terrorist bombings. Crit Care Med 33:S107–S112, 2005.
9. Macintyre AG, Weir S, Barbera JA: The international search and rescue response to the U.S. Embassy bombing in Kenya: The medical team experience. Prehosp Disaster Med 14:215–221, 1999.
10. Stein M, Hirshberg A: Medical consequences of terrorism. The conventional weapon threat. Surg Clin North Am 79:1537–1552, 1999.
11. Kahn CA, Schultz CH, Miller KT, et al: Does START triage work? An outcomes assessment after a disaster. Ann Emerg Med 54:424–430, 430 e421, 2009.
12. SALT mass casualty triage: Concept endorsed by the American College of Emergency Physicians, American College of Surgeons Committee on Trauma, American Trauma Society, National Association of EMS Physicians, National Disaster Life Support Education Consortium, and State and Territorial Injury Prevention Directors Association. Disaster Med Public Health Prep 2:245–246, 2008.
13. Cushman JG, Pachter HL, Beaton HL: Two New York City hospitals' surgical response to the September 11, 2001, terrorist attack in New York City. J Trauma 54:147–154, 2003.
14. Hirshberg A, Stein M: Trauma care in mass casualty incidents. In Feliciano DV, Mattox KL, Moore EE, editors: Trauma, ed 6, New York, 2008, McGraw Hill.
15. McSwain N, Jr: Disaster preparedness perspective from 90.05.32w, 29.57.18n. Crit Care 10:108, 2006.
16. Mattox KL: Hurricanes Katrina and Rita: Role of individuals and collaborative networks in mobilizing/coordinating societal and professional resources for major disasters. Crit Care 10:205, 2006.
17. Almogy G, Belzberg H, Mintz Y, et al: Suicide bombing attacks: Update and modifications to the protocol. Ann Surg 239:295–303, 2004.
18. Frykberg ER: Medical management of disasters and mass casualties from terrorist bombings: How can we cope? J Trauma 53:201–212, 2002.
19. Frykberg ER: Triage: Principles and practice. Scand J Surg 94:272–278, 2005.
20. Hirshberg A, Frykberg EF, Mattox KL, Stein M: Triage and trauma workload in mass casualty: A computer model. J Trauma 69:1074–1081, 2010.
21. Stein M: Urban bombing: A trauma surgeon's perspective. Scand J Surg 94:286–292, 2005.
22. Coupland RM: Epidemiological approach to surgical management of the casualties of war. BMJ 308:1693–1697, 1994.
23. Einav S, Schecter WP, Matot I, et al: Case managers in mass casualty incidents. Ann Surg 249:496–501, 2009.
24. Hirshberg A, Stein M, Walden R: Surgical resource utilization in urban terrorist bombing: A computer simulation. J Trauma 47: 545–550, 1999.
25. Shamir MY, Rivkind A, Weissman C, et al: Conventional terrorist bomb incidents and the intensive care unit. Curr Opin Crit Care 11:580–584, 2005.
26. Einav S, Aharonson-Daniel L, Weissman C, et al: In-hospital resource utilization during multiple casualty incidents. Ann Surg 243:533–540, 2006.

27. Aschkenasy-Steuer G, Shamir M, Rivkind A, et al: Clinical review: The Israeli experience: Conventional terrorism and critical care. Crit Care 9:490–499, 2005.
28. Ryan JM: Natural disasters: the surgeon's role. Scand J Surg 94:311–318, 2005.
29. Redmond AD: Natural disasters. BMJ 330:1259–1261, 2005.
30. Erek E, Sever MS, Serdengecti K, et al: An overview of morbidity and mortality in patients with acute renal failure due to crush syndrome: The Marmara earthquake experience. Nephrol Dial Transplant 17:33–40, 2002.
31. Sever MS, Erek E, Vanholder R, et al: Lessons learned from the catastrophic Marmara earthquake: Factors influencing the final outcome of renal victims. Clin Nephrol 61:413–421, 2004.
32. Dries D, Perry JF, Jr: Tsunami disaster: A report from the front. Crit Care Med 33:1178–1179, 2005.
33. Redmond AD: Needs assessment of humanitarian crises. BMJ 330:1320–1322, 2005.
34. Leibovici D, Gofrit ON, Shapira SC: Eardrum perforation in explosion survivors: Is it a marker of pulmonary blast injury? Ann Emerg Med 34:168–172, 1999.
35. Born CT: Blast trauma: The fourth weapon of mass destruction. Scand J Surg 94:279–285, 2005.
36. Pizov R, Oppenheim-Eden A, Matot I, et al: Blast lung injury from an explosion on a civilian bus. Chest 115:165–172, 1999.
37. Cripps NP, Cooper GJ: Risk of late perforation in intestinal contusions caused by explosive blast. Br J Surg 84:1298–1303, 1997.
38. Paran H, Neufeld D, Shwartz I, et al: Perforation of the terminal ileum induced by blast injury: Delayed diagnosis or delayed perforation? J Trauma 40:472–475, 1996.
39. Sosna J, Sella T, Shaham D, et al: Facing the new threats of terrorism: radiologists' perspectives based on experience in Israel. Radiology 237:28–36, 2005.
40. Bala M, Rivkind AI, Zamir G, et al: Abdominal trauma after terrorist bombing attacks exhibits a unique pattern of injury. Ann Surg 248:303–309, 2008.
41. Almogy G, Luria T, Richter E, et al: Can external signs of trauma guide management? Lessons learned from suicide bombing attacks in Israel. Arch Surg 140:390–393, 2005.
42. Fisher D, Burrow J: The Bali bombings of 12 October, 2002: Lessons in disaster management for physicians. Intern Med J 33:125–126, 2003.

# SECTION IV

# TRANSPLANTATION AND IMMUNOLOGY

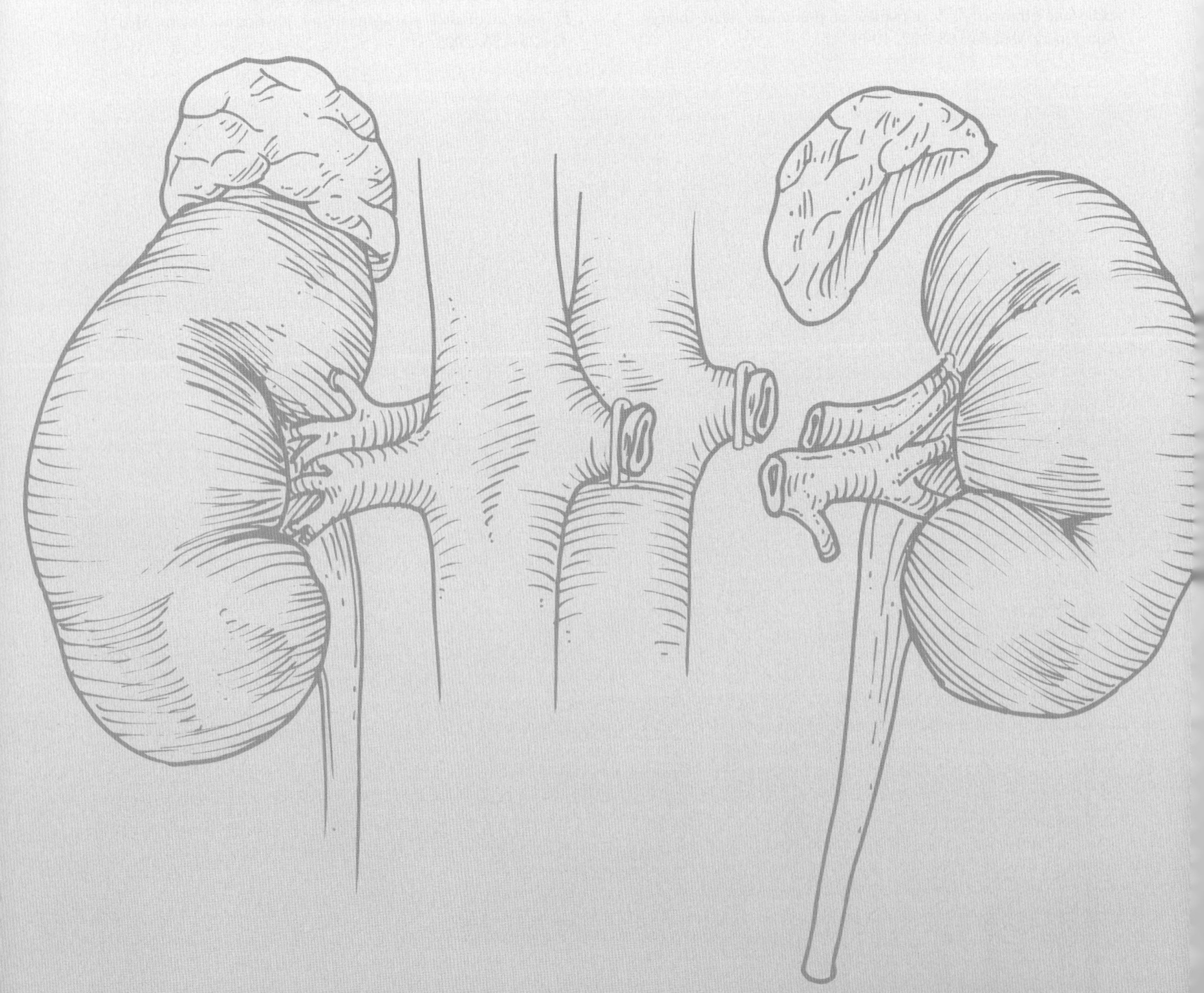

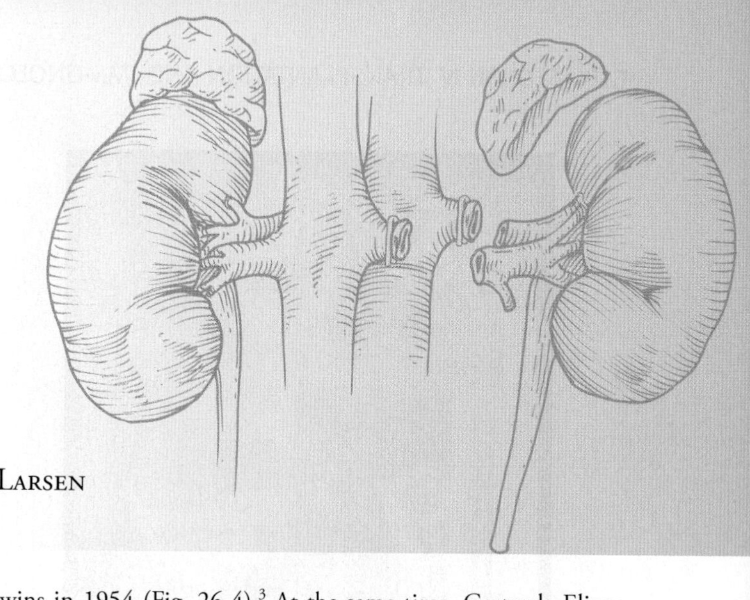

CHAPTER 26

# TRANSPLANTATION IMMUNOBIOLOGY AND IMMUNOSUPPRESSION

Andrew B. Adams, Allan D. Kirk, and Christian P. Larsen



Transplantation has revolutionized the treatment of end-stage organ failure. Today, there are over 25,000 transplantations performed annually and more than 100,000 patients are currently listed and awaiting an organ. The concept of tissue transplantation is certainly not new. As early as 800 BC, skin grafts were performed in India to conceal amputation of the nose, a punishment for adultery. History also is replete with legends and myths recounting the replacement of limbs and organs. One of the first references specifically to solid organ replacement as a therapeutic solution occurred when Tua-Ho, of China, reportedly replaced diseased organs with healthy ones approximately 200 AD. A more well-known myth of early transplantation derived from the miracle of Saints Cosmas and Damian (brothers and subsequently patron saints of physicians and surgeons), in which they successfully replaced the gangrenous leg of the Roman deacon Justinian with a leg from a recently deceased Ethiopian (Fig. 26-1). However, it was not until the French surgeon Alexis Carrel developed a method for joining blood vessels in the late 19th century that the transplantation of organs became technically feasible and verifiable accounts of transplantation began (Fig. 26-2). He was awarded the Nobel Prize in Medicine in 1912 "in recognition of his work on vascular suture and the transplantation of blood vessels and organs." Having established the technical component, Carrel himself noted that there were two issues to be resolved "regarding the transplantation of tissues and organs . . . the surgical and the biological." He had solved one aspect, the surgical, but he also understood that "it will only be through a more fundamental study of the biological relationships existing between living tissues"[1] that the more difficult problem of the biology would come to be solved. Forty years would pass before another set of eventual Nobel Prize winners, including Peter Medawar, would begin to define the process whereby one individual rejects another's tissue (Fig. 26-3).[2] Shortly thereafter, Joseph Murray, Nobel Laureate 1990, performed the first successful renal transplant between identical twins in 1954 (Fig. 26-4).[3] At the same time, Gertrude Elion, who worked as an assistant to George Hitchings at Wellcome Research Laboratories, developed several new immunosuppressive compounds, including 6-MP and Aza. Murray and Roy Calne subsequently introduced these agents into clinical practice, permitting nonidentical transplantation to be successful. Elion and Hitchings later shared the Nobel Prize in 1988 for their work on "the important principles of drug development." The subsequent discovery of increasingly potent agents to suppress the rejection response has led to the success in allograft survival that we enjoy today. It is this collaboration between scientists and surgeons that has driven our understanding of the immune system as it relates to transplantation. In this chapter, we will provide a primer on rejection in the context of the broader immune response, review the specific agents that are used to suppress the rejection response, and provide a glimpse into the future of the field of immunology and the immune response.

## THE IMMUNE RESPONSE

The process of rejection did not evolve as a response to prevent the relatively recent developments in transplantation, but is part of a system that has developed over thousands of years to protect against invasion by pathogens and prevent subsequent disease. To understand the rejection process and, in particular, to appreciate the consequences of pharmacologic suppression of rejection, a general understanding of the immune response as it functions in a physiologic setting is required.

The immune system has evolved to include two complementary divisions to respond to disease, the innate and acquired immune systems. Broadly speaking, the innate immune system recognizes general characteristics that have through selective pressure come to represent universal pathologic challenges to our species (e.g., ischemia, necrosis, trauma, certain nonhuman cell surfaces).[4] Conversely, the acquired arm recognizes specific structural aspects of foreign substances, usually peptide or carbohydrate moieties, recognized by receptors generated randomly and selected to avoid self-recognition. Although the two systems differ in their specific responsibilities, they act in concert to influence each other to achieve an optimal overall response.

### Acquired Immunity

The distinguishing feature of the acquired immune system is specific recognition and disposition of foreign elements, as well as the ability to recall prior challenges and respond appropriately. Highly specific receptors (see later) have evolved to distinguish

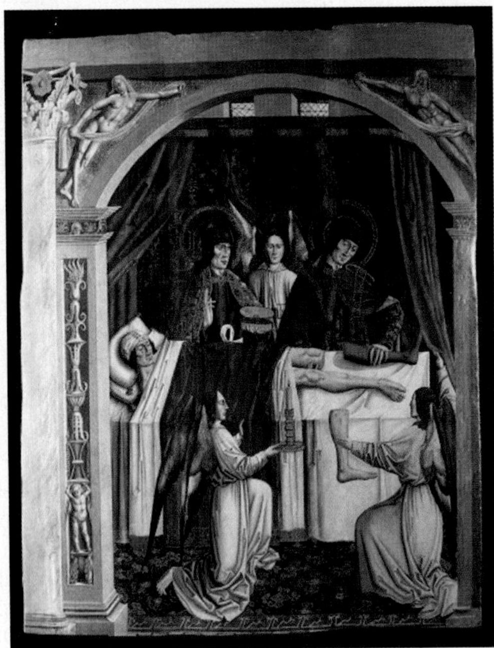

**FIGURE 26-1** Painting of Cosmas and Damian (15th C.), patron saints of physicians and surgeons. The legend of the Miracle of the Black Leg depicts the removal of the diseased leg of the Roman, Justinian, and replacement with the leg of a recently deceased Ethiopian man. (Courtesy Wellcome Library, London.)

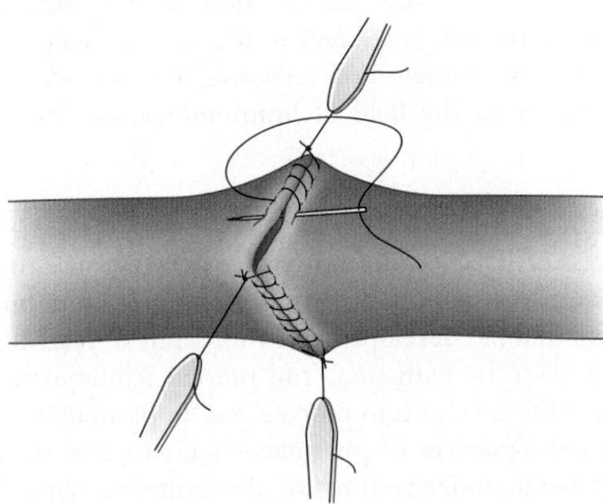

**FIGURE 26-2** Triangulation technique of vascular anastomosis by Alexis Carrel. (From Edwards WS, Edwards PD: Alexis Carrel: Visionary surgeon, Springfield, Ill, 1974, Charles C Thomas, pp 64–83.)

foreign from normal tissue through antigen binding. The term *antigen* is used to describe a molecule that can be recognized by the acquired immune system. An epitope is the portion of the antigen, generally a carbohydrate or peptide moiety, that actually serves as the binding site for the immune system receptor and is the base unit of antigen recognition. Thus, there may be one or many epitopes on any given antigen. The acquired response is divided into two distinct arms, cellular and humoral. The predominant effector cell in each arm is the T cell and B cell, respectively. Accordingly, the two main types of receptors that the immune system uses to recognize any given epitope are the T cell receptor (TCR) and B cell receptor, or antibody. In general, individual T or B lymphocytes express identical receptors, each of which only binds to a single epitope. This mechanism establishes the specificity of the acquired immune response. The antigenic encounter alters the immune system so that future challenges with the same antigen provoke a more rapid and vigorous response, a phenomenon known as immunologic memory. There are vast differences in the way each division of the acquired immune response identifies an antigen. The B cell receptor or antibody can identify its epitope directly without preparation of the antigen, either on an invading pathogen itself or as a free-floating molecule in the extracellular fluid. T cells, however, only recognize their specific epitope after it has been processed and bound to a set of proteins, unique to the individual, which are responsible for presentation of the antigen. This set of proteins, crucial to antigen presentation, is termed *histocompatibility proteins* and, as their name suggests, were defined through studies examining tissue transplantation. The case of the immune response in tissue transplantation is unique and will be discussed in its own section.

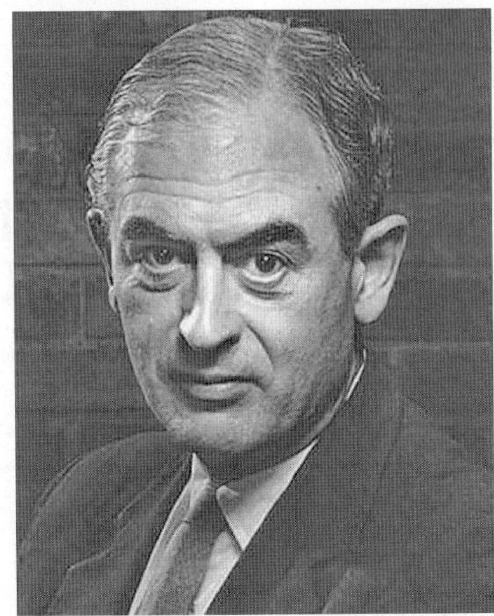

**FIGURE 26-3** Sir Peter Medawar. (Courtesy Bern Schwartz Collection, National Portrait Gallery, London.)

## Major Histocompatibility Locus: Transplantation Antigens

The major histocompatibility complex (MHC) refers to a cluster of highly conserved polymorphic genes on the sixth human chromosome. Much of what we know about the details of the immune response grew from initial studies defining the immunogenetics of the MHC. Studies began in mice, in which the MHC gene complex, termed *H-2,* was described by Gorer and Snell as a genetic locus that segregated with transplanted tumor survival. Subsequent serologic studies identified a similar genetic locus in humans called the HLA (human leukocyte antigen) locus. The products of these genes are expressed on a wide variety of cell types and play a pivotal role in the immune response. They are also the antigens primarily responsible for human transplant rejection and their clinical implications will be discussed later.

MHC molecules play a role in the innate and acquired immune systems. Their predominant role, however, lies in antigen presentation within the acquired response. As noted, the TCR does not recognize its specific antigen directly; rather, it

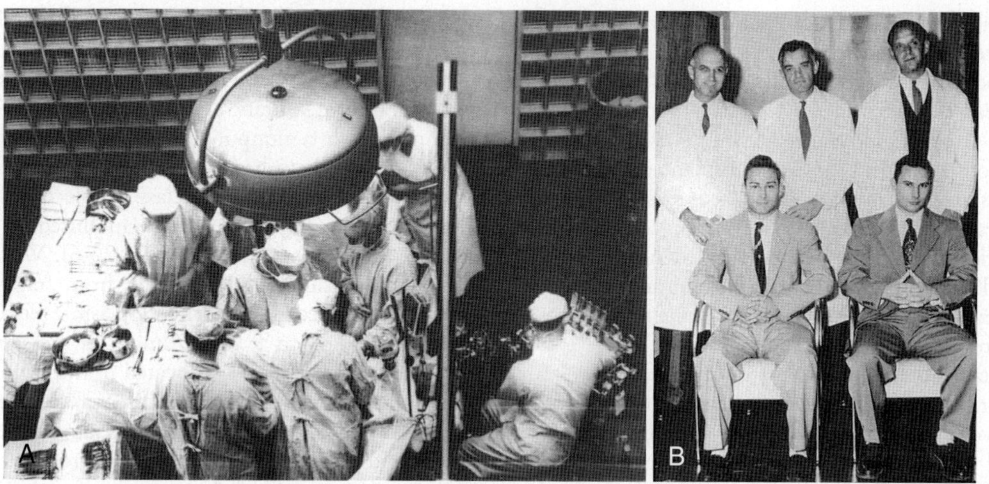


**FIGURE 26-4 A,** The first identical twin kidney transplantation, performed on December 23, 1954. **B,** Herrick twins (seated) with transplantation team. (Courtesy Harvard Medical Library, Francis A. Countway Library of Medicine, Center for the History of Medicine, Boston.)

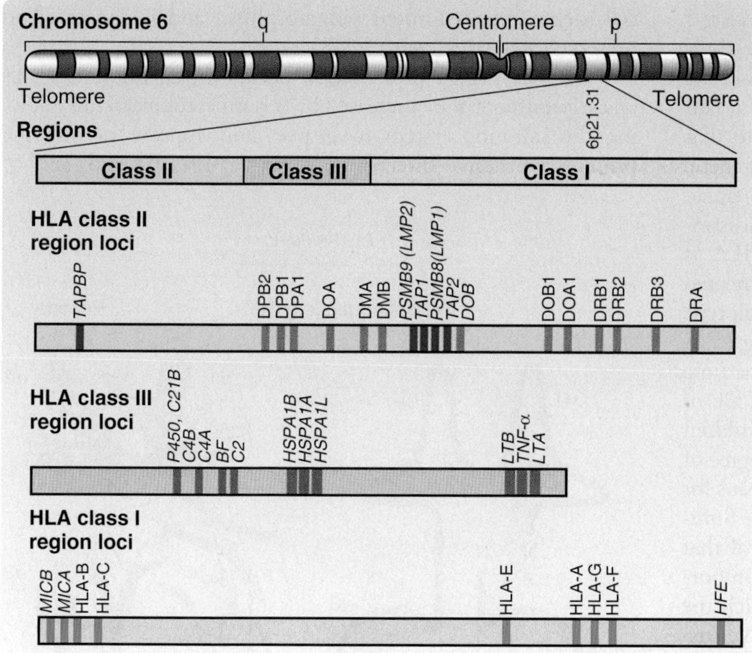


**FIGURE 26-5** Location and organization of the HLA complex on human chromosome 6. The complex is conventionally divided into three regions, I, II, and III. Class III genes are not related to class I and class II genes, structurally or functionally. (Adapted from Klein J, Sato A: The HLA system—first of two parts. N Engl J Med 343:702–709, 2000.)

binds to the processed antigen that is bound to cell surface proteins. It is the MHC molecule that binds the peptide antigen and interacts with the TCR, a process called antigen presentation. Thus, all T cells are restricted to an MHC for their response. There are two classes of MHC molecules, class I and class II. In general, $CD8^+$ T cells bind to antigen in class I MHC and $CD4^+$ T cells bind to antigen in class II MHC.

### Human Histocompatibility Complex

The antigens primarily responsible for human allograft rejection are those encoded by the HLA region of chromosome 6 (Fig. 26-5). The polymorphic proteins encoded by this locus include class I molecules (HLA-A, -B, and -C) and class II molecules (HLA-DR, -DP, and -DQ). There are additional class I genes with limited polymorphism (E, F, G, H, and J) but they are not currently used in tissue typing for transplantation and are not considered here. There are class III genes as well, but they are not cell surface proteins involved in antigen presentation directly but include molecules pertinent to the immune response by various mechanisms—tumor necrosis factors-α (TNF-α) and TNF-β, components of the complement cascade, nuclear transcription factor β, and HSP 70. Other conserved genes in HLA include genes necessary for class I and class II presentation of peptides, such as the peptide transporter proteins TAP-1 and TAP-2 and proteosome proteases LMP-2 and LMP-7.[5] Although other polymorphic genes, referred to as minor histocompatibility antigens, exist in the genome outside of the HLA locus, they play a more limited role in transplant rejection and will not be covered here. It is, however, important to point out that even HLA-identical individuals are subject to rejection on the basis of these minor differences. The blood group antigens of the ABO system must also be considered transplantation antigens and their biology is critical to humoral rejection.

Although initially identified as transplantation antigens, class I and class II MHC molecules actually play vital roles in all immune responses, not just those to transplanted tissue. HLA class I molecules are present on all nucleated cells. In contrast, class II molecules are found almost exclusively on cells associated with the immune system (e.g., macrophages, dendritic cells, B cells, activated T cells) but can be upregulated and appear on other parenchymal cells in the setting of cytokine release caused by an immune response or injury.

The importance of MHC gene products to transplantation stems from their polymorphism. Unlike most genes, which are identical in a given species, polymorphic gene products differ in detail while still conforming to the same basic structure. Thus, polymorphic MHC proteins from one individual are foreign alloantigens to another individual. Recombination within the HLA locus is uncommon, occurring in approximately 1% of molecules. Consequently, the HLA type of the offspring is predictable. The unit of inheritance is the haplotype, which consists of one chromosome 6, and therefore one copy of each class I and class II locus (HLA-A, -B, -C, -DR, -DP, and -DQ). Thus, donor-recipient pairings that are matched at all HLA loci are referred to as HLA-identical allografts and those matched at half of the HLA loci are referred to as haploidentical. Note that HLA-identical allografts still differ genetically at other genetic loci and are distinct from isografts. Isografts are organs transplanted between identical twins, are immunologically indistinguishable, and thus do not reject. The genetics of HLA is particularly important in understanding clinical living-related donor (LRD) transplantation. Each child inherits one haplotype from each parent; therefore, the chance of siblings being HLA identical is 25%. Haploidentical siblings occur 50% of the time and completely nonidentical or HLA-distinct siblings 25% of the time. Biologic parents are haploidentical with their children unless there has been a rare recombination event. The degree of HLA match can also improve if the parents are homozygous for a given allele, thus giving the same allele to all children. Similarly, if the parents share the same allele, the likelihood of that allele being inherited improves to 50%. This is even more important in the field of bone marrow transplantation, in which the risks of donor-mediated cytotoxicity and resultant graft-versus-host disease become a more relevant issue.

Each class I molecule is encoded by a single polymorphic gene that is combined with the nonpolymorphic protein $\beta_2$-microglobulin ($\beta_2$M; chromosome 15) for expression. The polymorphism of each class I molecule is extreme, with 30 to 50 alleles/locus. Class II molecules are made up of two chains, $\alpha$ and $\beta$, and individuals differ not only in the alleles represented at each locus, but also in the number of loci present in the HLA class II region. The polymorphism of class II is thus increased by combinations of $\alpha$ and $\beta$ chains, as well as of hybrid assembly of chains from one class II locus to another. As the HLA sequence varies, the ability of various peptides to bind to the molecule and be presented for T cell recognition changes. Teleologically, this extreme diversity is thought to improve the likelihood that a given pathogenic peptide will fit into the binding site of these antigen-presenting molecules, thus preventing a single viral agent from evading detection by T cells of an entire population.[6]

**Class I Major Histocompatibility Complex** The three-dimensional structure of class I molecules (HLA-A, -B, and -C) was first elucidated in 1987.[7] The class I molecule is composed of a 44-kDa transmembrane glycoprotein ($\alpha$ chain) in a noncovalent complex with a nonpolymorphic 12-kDa polypeptide called $\beta_2$-M. The $\alpha$ chain has three domains, $\alpha$-1, $\alpha$-2, and $\alpha$-3. The critical structural feature of class I molecules is the presence of a groove formed by two $\alpha$ helices mounted on a $\beta$-pleated sheet in the $\alpha$-1 and $\alpha$-2 domains (Fig. 26-6). Within this groove, a nine-amino-acid peptide, formed from fragments of proteins being synthesized in the cell's endoplasmic reticulum, is mounted for presentation to T cells. Almost all the significant sequence polymorphism of class I is located in the region of the peptide-binding groove and in areas of direct T cell contact. The assembly of class I is dependent on association of the $\alpha$ chain with $\beta_2$-M and native peptide within the groove. Incomplete molecules are not expressed. In general, all peptides made by a cell are candidates for presentation, although sequence alterations in this region favor certain sequences over others. The $\alpha$-3 immunoglobulin-like domain, which is the domain closest to the membrane and interacts with the CD8 molecule on the T cell, demonstrates limited polymorphism and is conserved to preserve interactions with $CD8^+$ T cells.

Human class I presentation occurs on all nucleated cells and expression can be increased by certain cytokines, thus allowing the immune system to inspect and approve of ongoing protein synthesis. Interferons (IFN-$\alpha$, IFN-$\beta$, and IFN-$\gamma$)

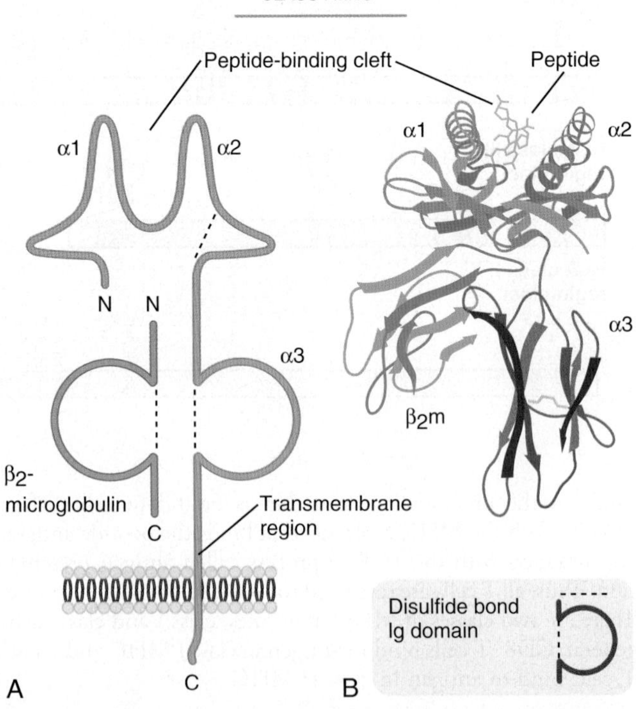


**FIGURE 26-6** Structure of the MHC class I molecule. Class I molecules are composed of a polymorphic $\alpha$ chain noncovalently attached to the nonpolymorphic $\beta_2$-microglobulin ($\beta_2$M). **A,** Schematic diagram. **B,** Ribbon diagram shows the extracellular structure of a class I molecule with a bound peptide. (Adapted from Abbas AK, Lichtman AH, Pillai S: Cellular and molecular immunology, ed 6, Philadelphia, 2010, Saunders-Elsevier.)

induce an increase in the expression of class I molecules on a given cell by increasing levels of gene expression. T cell activation occurs when a given T cell encounters a class I MHC molecule carrying a peptide from a nonself protein presented in the proper context (e.g., viral protein is processed in an infected cell and the peptide fragments are presented on class I molecules for T cell recognition). So-called cross-presentation may also occur, in which certain antigen-presenting cells (APCs)—namely, a subset of dendritic cells— have the ability to take up and process exogenous antigen and present it on class I molecules to $CD8^+$ T cells.[8] In the case of transplantation, this activation is not only possible when foreign peptide is identified after the donor MHC has been processed and presented on recipient APCs, but more commonly occurs when a T cell interacts directly with the nonself class I MHC, the so-called direct alloresponse.

**Class II MHC** The class II molecules are products of the HLA-DR, HLA-DQ, and HLA-DP genes. The structural features of class II molecules are strikingly similar to those of class I molecules.

The three-dimensional structure of class II molecules was inferred by sequence homology to class I in 1988 and eventually proven by x-ray crystallography in 1993 (Fig. 26-7).[9] The class II molecules contain two polymorphic chains, one approximately 32 kDa and the other approximately 30 kDa. The peptide-binding region is composed of the α-1 and β-1 domains.

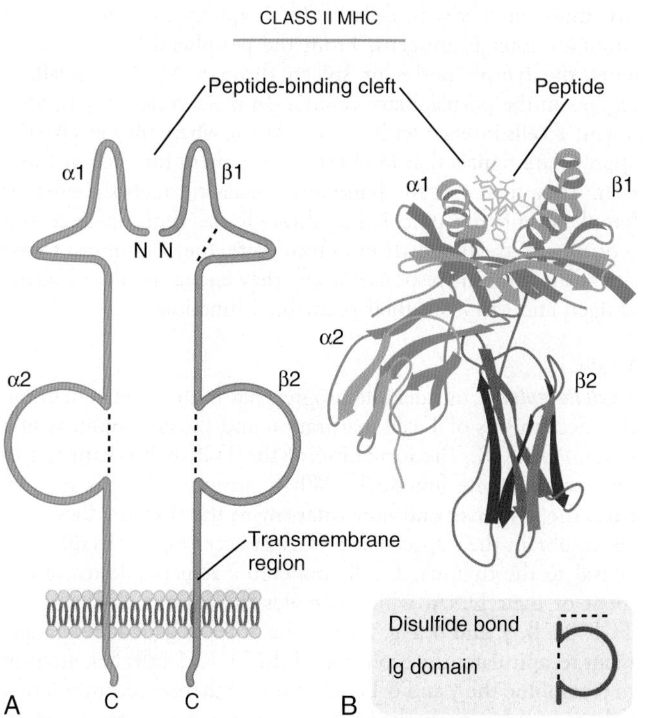


**FIGURE 26-7** Structure of the MHC class II molecule. Class II molecules are composed of a polymorphic α chain noncovalently attached to a polymorphic β chain. **A,** Schematic diagram. **B,** Ribbon diagram shows the extracellular structure of a class II molecule with a bound peptide. (Adapted from Abbas AK, Lichtman AH, Pillai S: Cellular and molecular immunology, ed 6, Philadelphia, 2010, Saunders-Elsevier.)

The immunoglobulin-like domain is composed of the α-2 and β-2 segments. Similar to the class I immunoglobulin-like α-3 domain, there is limited polymorphism in these segments and the β-2 domain, in particular, is involved in the binding of the CD4 molecule, helping to restrict class II interactions to $CD4^+$ T cells. Class II molecule assembly requires association of both the α chain and β chains in combination with a temporary protein called the invariant chain.[10] This third protein covers the peptide-binding groove until the class II molecule is out of the endoplasmic reticulum and is sequestered in an endosome. Proteins that are engulfed by a phagocytic cell are degraded at the same time as the invariant chain is removed, allowing peptides of external sources to be associated with and presented by class II. In this way, the acquired immune system can inspect and approve of proteins that are present in circulation or that have been liberated from foreign cells or pathogens through the phagocytic process. Accordingly, class II molecules, in contrast to class I molecules, are confined to cells related to the immune response, particularly APCs (e.g., macrophages, dendritic cells, B cells, and monocytes). Class II expression can also be induced on other cells, including endothelial cells under the appropriate conditions. After binding class II molecules, $CD4^+$ T cells participate in APC-mediated activation of $CD8^+$ T cells and antibody-producing B cells. In the case of transplanted organs, ischemic injury at the time of transplantation accentuates the potential for T cell activation by the upregulation of class I and class II molecules locally on the recipient. The trauma of surgery and ischemia also upregulate class II molecules on all cells of an allograft, making nonself-MHC more abundant. Host $CD4^+$ T cells may then recognize donor MHC directly (direct alloresponse) or after antigen processing (indirect alloresponse) and then proceed to participate in rejection.

### HLA Typing: Implications for Transplantation

For the reasons already discussed, closely matched transplants are less likely to be recognized and rejected than are similar grafts differing by multiple alleles at the MHC. HLA matching has a clear influence on the prolongation of graft survival. Humans have two different HLA-A, -B, and -DR alleles—one from each parent, six in total. Although clearly important, the HLA-C, -DP, and -DQ loci are administratively dismissed in general organ allocation. Although current immunosuppressive regimens negate much of the impact of matching, there have been several studies that have demonstrated improvements in renal allograft survival when the six primary alleles are matched between donor and recipient, a so-called six-antigen match (Fig. 26-8). Historically, MHC match has been defined using two cellular assays, the lymphocytotoxicity assay and the mixed lymphocyte reaction (MLC). Both assays define MHC epitopes but do not comprehensively define the entire antigen or the exact genetic disparity involved. Techniques now exist for precise genotyping via molecular techniques that distinguish the nucleotide sequence of an individual's MHC.

The MLC is performed by incubating recipient T cells with irradiated donor cells in the presence of $^3$H-thymidine; the irradiation treatment ensures that the assay only measures the proliferation of recipient T cells. If the cells differ at the class II MHC locus, recipient $CD4^+$ T cells produce interleukin-2 (IL-2), which stimulates proliferation. Proliferating cells incorporate the labeled nucleotide into their newly manufactured DNA, which can be detected and quantified. Class II

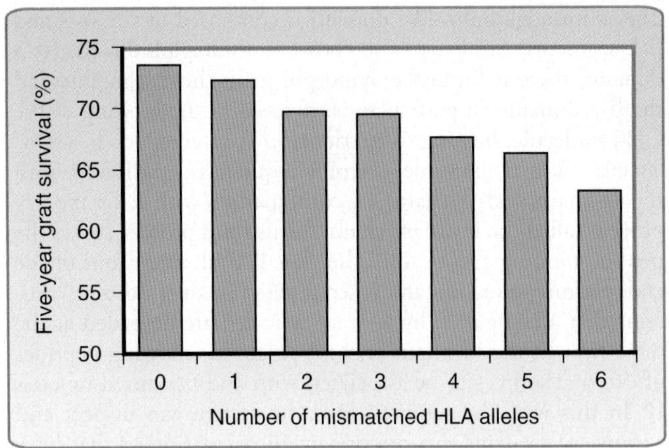


**FIGURE 26-8** Influence of HLA matching on renal allograft survival. Matching HLA alleles between donor and recipient significantly improves renal allograft survival. The data shown are for deceased donor renal allografts stratified by number of matched HLA alleles. (Data from U.S. Organ Procurement and Transplant Network and the Scientific Registry of Transplant Patients: 2008 OPTN/SRTP annual report: Transplant data 1998–2007 [http://optn. transplant.hrsa.gov/ar2008].)

polymorphism can be detected by this assay, but it takes several days to complete one assay. Thus, the use of MLC as a prospective typing assay is limited to LRDs. The specific MHC alleles are not identified with this assay per se; instead, they are inferred from a series of reactions. Although this assay has been extremely valuable historically, it has now been largely supplanted by more modern molecular techniques. The lymphocytotoxicity assay involves taking serum from individuals with anti-MHC antibodies of known specificity and mixing it with lymphocytes from the individual in question. Exogenous complement is added, as well as a vital dye that is not taken up by intact cells. If the antibody binds to MHC, it activates the complement and leads to cell membrane disruption, and the cell takes up the vital stain. Microscopic examination of the cells can then determine whether the MHC antigen was present on the cells. This, too, has been supplanted by more modern methods of MHC-specific antibody detection.

The sequencing of the class I and class II HLA loci has allowed several genetic-based techniques to be used for histocompatibility testing. These methods include restriction fragment length polymorphism (RFLP), oligonucleotide hybridization, and polymorphism-specific amplification using the polymerase chain reaction and sequence-specific primers (PCR-SSP). Of these methods, the PCR-SSP technique is most commonly used for class II typing. Serologic techniques are still the predominant method for class I typing because of the complexity of class I sequence polymorphism. It is important to note that sequence polymorphisms that do not alter the TCR-MHC interface are unlikely to affect allograft survival; thus, the enhanced precision of molecular typing may provide more information than is actually clinically relevant.

### Cellular Components of the Acquired Immune System

The key cellular components of the immune system, T cells, B cells, and antigen-presenting cells, are hematopoietically derived and arise from a common progenitor stem cell. The development of the lymphoid system begins with pluripotent stem cells in the liver and bone marrow of the fetus. As the fetus matures, the bone marrow becomes the primary site of lymphopoiesis. B cells were named after the primary lymphoid organ that produces B cells in birds, the bursa of Fabricius. In humans and most other mammals, precursor B cells remain within the bone marrow as they mature and fully develop. Although precursor T cells also originate in the bone marrow, they soon migrate to the thymus, the primary site of T cell maturation, where they become "educated" to self and acquire their specific cell surface receptors and the ability to generate effector function. Mature lymphocytes are then released from the primary lymphoid organs, the bone marrow and thymus, to populate the secondary lymphoid organs, including lymph nodes, spleen, and gut, as well as peripheral tissues. Each of these cells has a unique role in establishing the immune response. The highly coordinated network is regulated in part through the use of cytokines (Table 26-1).

Both B and T cells are integral components of a highly specific response that must be prepared to recognize a seemingly endless array of pathogens. This is accomplished through a unique method that allows for random generation of almost unlimited receptor specificity, yet controls the ultimate product by eliminating or suppressing those that might ultimately react against self and enable an autoimmune response. There are fundamental differences in the manner in which T and B cells recognize antigen. B cells are structured to respond to whole antigen and, in response, synthesize and secrete antibody that can interact with antigen at distant sites. T cells, on the other hand, are responsible for cell-mediated immunity and, of necessity, must interact with cells in the periphery to neutralize and eliminate foreign antigens. From the peripheral blood, T cells enter the lymph nodes or spleen through highly specialized regions in the postcapillary venules. In the secondary lymphoid organ, T cells interact with specific APCs, where they receive the appropriate signals that in effect, license them for effector function. They then exit the lymphoid tissues through the efferent lymph, eventually percolating through the thoracic duct and returning to the bloodstream. From there, they can return to the site of the immune response, where they encounter their specific antigen and carry out their predefined functions.

#### T Cells

***T Cell Receptor*** Considerable progress has been made in defining the mechanisms of T cell maturation and the development of a functional TCR. The formation of the TCR is fundamental to understanding its function.[11] When precursor T cells migrate from the fetal liver and bone marrow to the thymus, they have yet to obtain their specialized TCR or accessory molecules. On arrival to the thymus, T cells undergo a remarkable rearrangement of their DNA, which encodes the various chains of the TCR ($\alpha$, $\beta$, $\gamma$, and $\delta$; Fig. 26-9). The order of genetic rearrangement recapitulates the evolution of the TCR. T cells first attempt to recombine the $\gamma$ and $\delta$ TCR genes and then, if recombination fails to yield a properly formed receptor, resort to the more diverse $\alpha$ and $\beta$ TCR genes. The $\gamma\delta$ configuration is typically not successful and thus most T cells are $\alpha\beta$ T cells. T cells expressing the $\gamma\delta$ TCR have more primitive functions, including recognition of heat shock proteins and activity similar to natural killer (NK) cells, as well as MHC recognition, whereas $\alpha\beta$ T cells are more typically limited to recognition of MHC complexed with processed peptide.

**Table 26-1 Summary of Cytokines**

| CYTOKINE | SOURCE | PRINCIPAL CELLULAR TARGETS AND BIOLOGIC EFFECTS |
|---|---|---|
| IL-1 | Macrophages, endothelial cells, some epithelial cells | Endothelial cell: Activation (inflammation, coagulation)<br>Hypothalamus; Fever<br>Liver: Synthesis of acute-phase proteins |
| IL-2 | T cells | T cells: Proliferation, ↑ cytokine synthesis, survival, potentiate Fas-mediated apoptosis, promote regulatory T cell development<br>NK cells: Proliferation, activation<br>B cells: Proliferation, antibody synthesis (in vitro) |
| IL-3 | T cells | Immature hematopoietic progenitor cells: Stimulate differentiation into myeloid lineage, proliferation of myeloid lineage cells |
| IL-4 | CD4$^+$ T cells (Th2), mast cells | B cells: Isotype switching to IgE<br>T cells: Th2 differentiation, proliferation<br>Macrophages: Inhibit IFN-γ mediated activation<br>Mast cells: Stimulate proliferation |
| IL-5 | CD4$^+$ T cells (Th2) | Eosinophils: Activation, ↑ production<br>B cells: Proliferation, IgA production |
| IL-6 | Macrophages, endothelial cells, T cells | Liver: ↑ synthesis of acute-phase proteins<br>B cells: Proliferation of antibody-producing cells |
| IL-7 | Fibroblasts, bone marrow stromal cells | Immature hematopoietic progenitor cells: Stimulate differentiation into lymphoid lineage<br>T and B cells: Important for survival during development as well as for T cell memory |
| TNF | Macrophages, T cells | Endothelial cells: Activation (inflammation, coagulation)<br>Neutrophils: Activation<br>Hypothalamus: Fever<br>Liver: ↑ synthesis of acute-phase proteins<br>Muscle, fat: Catabolism (cachexia)<br>Many cell types: apoptosis |
| IFN-γ | T cells (Th1, CD8$^+$ T cells), NK cells | Macrophages: Activation (increased microbicidal functions)<br>B cells: Isotype switching to IgG subclasses, which facilitate complement fixation and opsonization<br>T cells: Th1 differentiation<br>Various cells: ↑ expression of class I and class II MHC, ↑ antigen processing and presentation to T cells |
| Type I IFNs (IFN-α, IFN-β) | Macrophages, IFN-α; fibroblasts, IFN-β | All cells: Stimulate antiviral activity, including ↑ class I MHC expression<br>NK cells: Activation |
| TGF-β | T cells, macrophages, other cell types | T cells: Inhibit proliferation and effector functions<br>B cells: Inhibit proliferation, ↑ IgA production<br>Macrophages: Inhibit activation, stimulates angiogenic factors<br>Fibroblasts: Increased collagen synthesis |
| Lymphotoxin (LT) | T cells | Lymphoid organogenesis<br>Neutrophils: Increased recruitment and activation |
| IL-8 | Lymphocytes, monocytes | Stimulate granulocyte activity, chemotactic activity |
| IL-9 | Activated Th2 cells, lymphocytes | Enhance proliferation of T cells, mast cells |
| IL-10 | Macrophages, T cells (mainly regulatory T cells) | Macrophages, dendritic cells: Inhibit IL-12 production, stimulate expression of costimulatory molecules and class II MHC |
| IL-11 | Bone marrow stromal cells | Megakaryocytes: Thrombopoiesis<br>Liver: Induces acute-phase proteins<br>B cells: Stimulate T-dependent antibody production<br>T cells: May skew toward Th2 phenotype |
| IL-12 | Macrophages, dendritic cells | T cells: Th1 differentiation<br>NK and T cells: IFN-γ synthesis, increased cytotoxic activity |
| IL-13 | CD4$^+$ T cells (Th2), NKT cells, mast cells | B cells: Isotype switching to IgE<br>Epithelial cells: Increased mucus production<br>Fibroblasts and macrophages: Increased collagen synthesis |
| IL-14 | T cells, some B cell tumors | B cells: Enhance proliferation of activated B cells, stimulate immunoglobulin production |
| IL-15 | Macrophages, others | NK cells: Proliferation<br>T cells: Proliferation (memory CD8$^+$ T cells) |
| IL-17 | T cells | Endothelial cells: Increased chemokine production<br>Macrophages: Increased chemokine, cytokine production<br>Epithelial cells: GM-CSF and G-CSF production |
| IL-18 | Macrophages | NK and T cells: IFN-γ synthesis |
| IL-23 | Macrophages, dendritic cells | T cells: Maintenance of IL-17 producing T cells |
| IL-27 | Macrophages, dendritic cells | T cells: Inhibit production of IL-17/Th17 cells, promote Th1 differentiation<br>NK cells: IFN-γ synthesis |

Adapted from Abbas AK, Lichtman AH, Pillai S: Cellular and molecular immunology, ed 6, Philadelphia, 2010, Saunders-Elsevier.

*G-CSF,* Granulocyte-colony stimulating factor; *GM-CSF,* granulocyte-macrophage colony-stimulating factor.

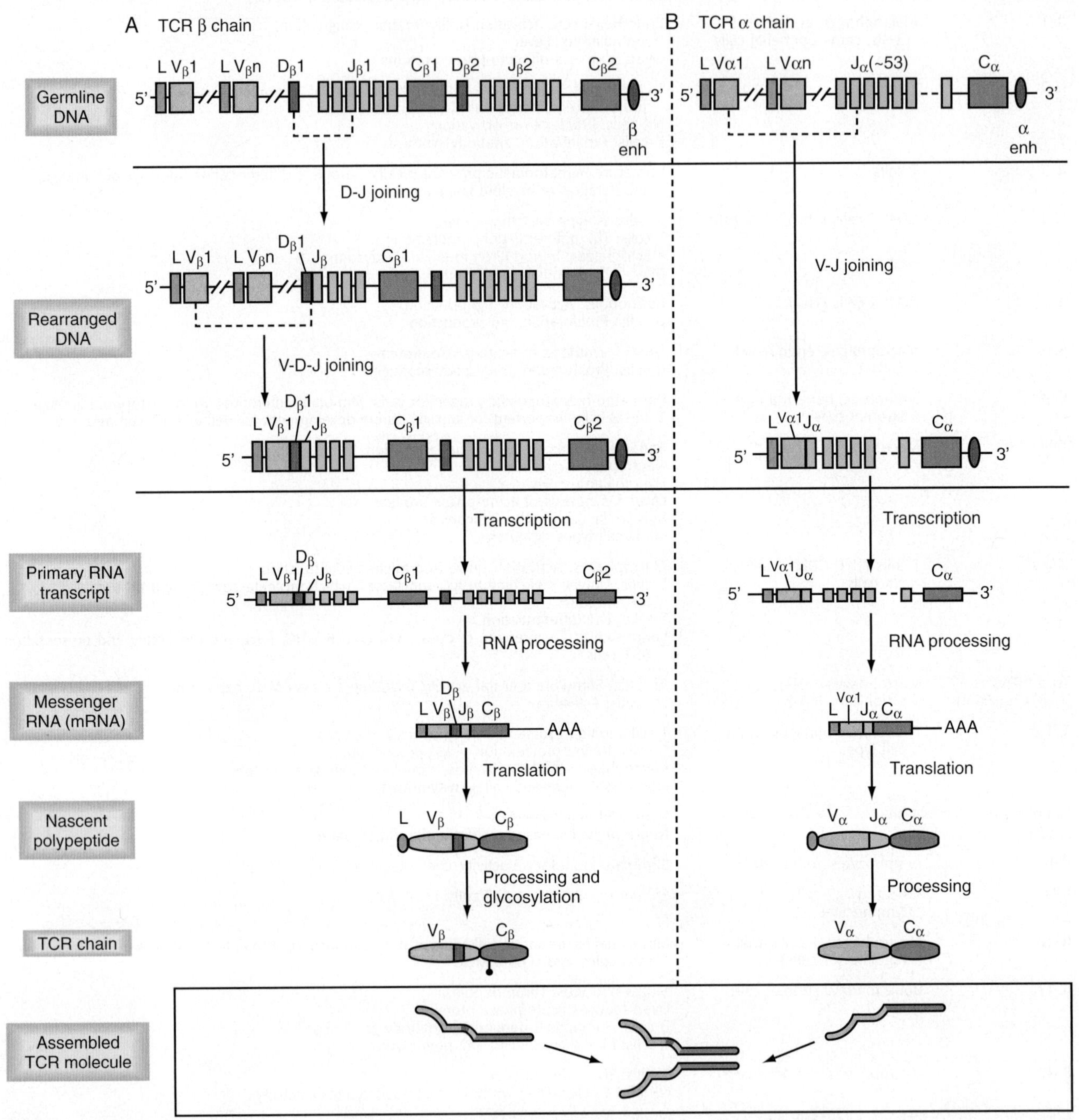


**FIGURE 26-9** TCR recombination and expression (α and β loci shown here). There is an elaborate genetic rearrangement that leads to the formation of a diverse repertoire of T cell receptors. Genomic DNA is spliced under the direction of specific enzymes active during T cell development in the thymus. Random segments from regions known as variable (V), joining (J), diversity (D), and constant (C) are brought together to form a unique gene responsible for a unique TCR chain. The γ and δ loci recombine first and, if successful, a γδ TCR is formed. If unsuccessful, then α and β regions recombine to form an αβ TCR. Approximately 95% of T cells progress to express an αβ TCR. (Adapted from Abbas AK, Lichtman AH, Pillai S: Cellular and molecular immunology, ed 6, Philadelphia, 2010, Saunders-Elsevier.)

Regardless of the genes used, individual cells recombine to express a TCR with only a single specificity. The rearrangements occur randomly, resulting in a population of T cells capable of binding $10^9$ different specificities, essentially all combinations of MHC and peptide. As a result, the frequency of naïve T cells available to respond to any given pathogen is relatively small, between 1 in 200,000 to 500,000. These developing T cells also express both CD4 and CD8, accessory molecules, which strengthen the TCR binding to MHC. These accessory molecules further increase the binding repertoire of the population to include class I or class II MHC molecules. If the process of T cell maturation ended at this stage, there would be a host of T cells that could recognize self-MHC–peptide complexes, resulting in an uncontrolled global

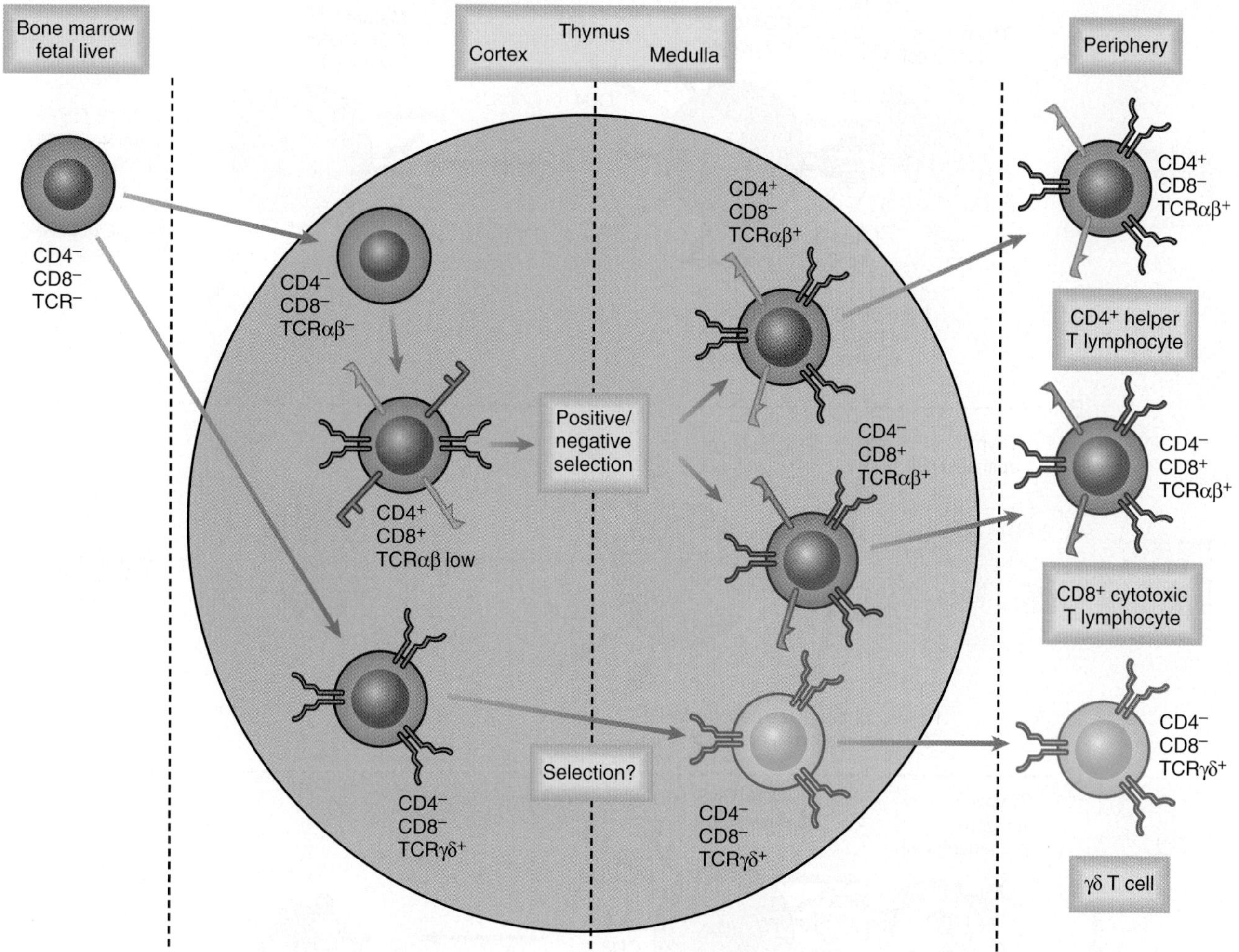


**FIGURE 26-10** T cell maturation. Initially, T cell precursors arrive in the thymic cortex lacking CD4, CD8, or a TCR and are referred to as double-negative. The genes responsible for the expression of the TCR chains subsequently undergo a series recombination events, resulting in expression of a γδ TCR or, more commonly (>90%), an αβ TCR on the cell surface. γδ T cells proceed through a distinct selection process that is independent of MHC restriction. αβ T cells acquire expression of both CD4 and CD8 and are then referred to as double-positive. They then proceed to undergo the process of positive and negative selection and ultimately express only CD4 or CD8, depending on which class of MHC they restrict to. (Adapted from Abbas AK, Lichtman AH, Pillai S: Cellular and molecular immunology, ed 6, Philadelphia, 2010, Saunders-Elsevier.)

autoimmune response. To avoid the release of autoreactive T cells, developing cells undergo a process following recombination known as thymic selection (Fig. 26-10).[12] Cells initially interact with the MHC-expressing cortical thymic epithelium, which produces hormones (thymopoietin and thymosin) as well as cytokines (e.g., IL-7), which are critical to T cell development. If binding does not occur to self-MHC, those cells are useless to the individual—because they cannot bind self cells to assess for viral infection—and they undergo programmed self-destruction via apoptosis, a process called positive selection (Fig. 26-11). Cells surviving positive selection then move to the thymic medulla and, normally, eventually lose CD4 or CD8. If binding to self-MHC in the medulla occurs with an unacceptably high affinity, programmed death again results; this process is called negative selection. The precise nature of this affinity threshold remains a matter of intense investigation and involves interaction with hematopoietic cells that reside in the thymus. The only cells released into the periphery are those that can bind self-MHC and avoid activation. Whereas T cells are restricted to bind self-MHC–peptide complexes without activation, the selection process does not consider foreign MHC. Thus, by random chance, some cells with appropriate affinity for self-MHC survive and have an inappropriately high affinity for the MHC molecules of other individuals. In the setting of transplantation, these recipient T cells are able to recognize donor MHC-peptide complexes because there are sufficient conserved motifs shared between donor and self-MHC molecules. However, because donor MHC was not present during the thymic education process, the binding of donor MHC by an alloreactive T cell leads to activation, and rejection ensues. The precursor frequency or the number of alloreactive T cells is much higher than the 1 in 200,000 or 500,000 T cells available to react toward any given antigen. Because T cells are selected to bind self-MHC, the frequency specific for a similar, nonself-MHC (i.e., alloreactive) is between 1% and 10% of all T cells.

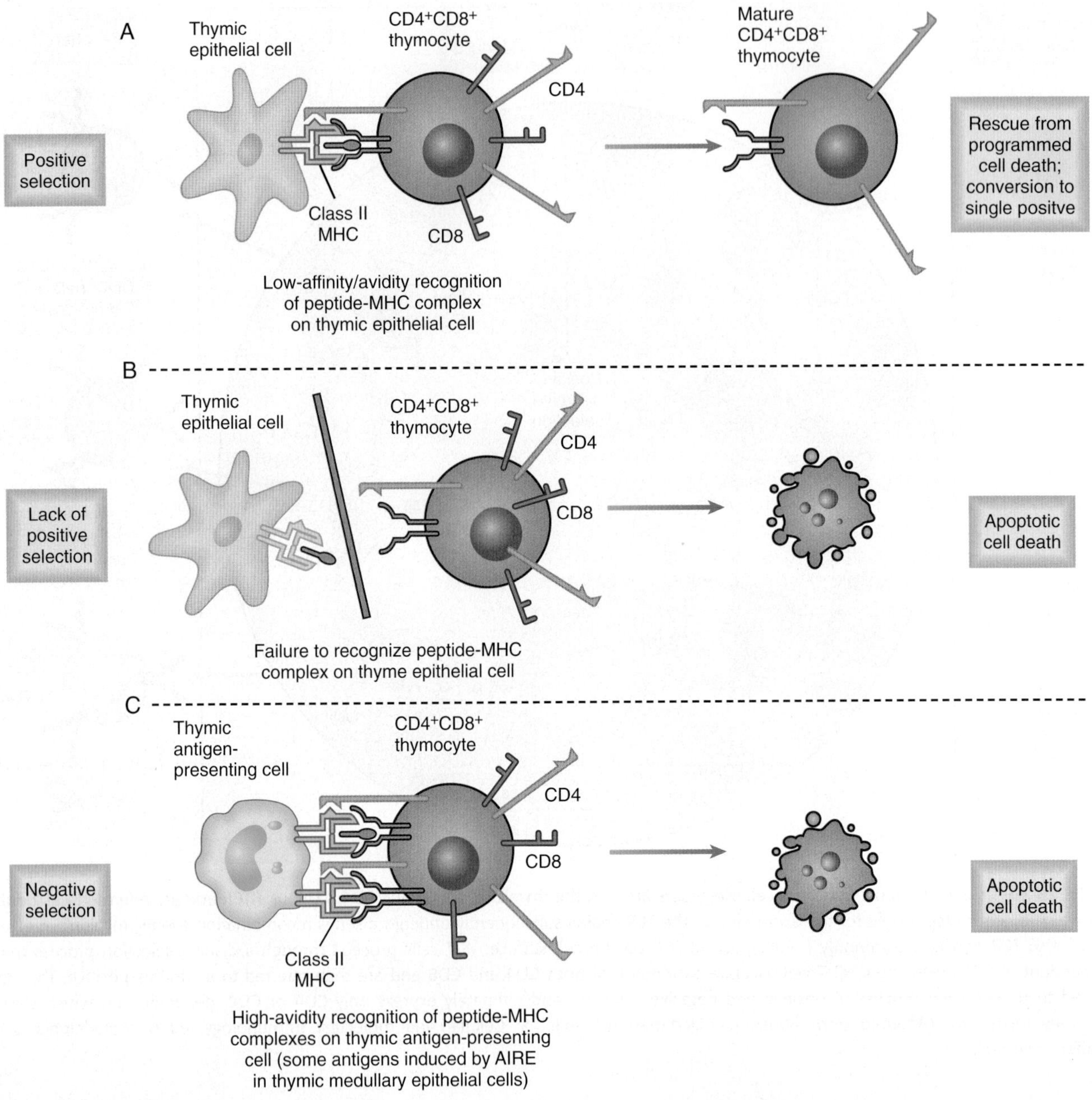

**FIGURE 26-11** Thymic selection. αβ T cells must go through positive and negative selection within the thymus to become a functional T cell. **A, B,** Positive selection. **A,** Double-positive thymocytes are required to interact with self MHC–endogenous peptide complexes expressed on mainly thymic epithelial cells to receive survival signals. **B,** Thymocytes whose TCR does not recognize self-MHC fail to receive the essential survival signals and go on to be deleted from the repertoire via programmed cell death. This process ensures that all mature T cells are restricted to self-MHC. **C,** Negative selection. T cells that are positively selected migrate through the thymic medulla to undergo negative selection. Negative selection is the process whereby self-reactive T cells are eliminated. If thymocytes bind with high avidity (i.e., strongly) to self-MHC–peptide complexes on bone marrow–derived thymic dendritic cells, they receive signals that promote apoptosis. (Adapted from Abbas AK, Lichtman AH, Pillai S: Cellular and molecular immunology, ed 6, Philadelphia, 2010, Saunders-Elsevier.)

In addition to thymic selection, it is now clear that mechanisms exist for peripheral modification of the T cell repertoire. Many of these mechanisms are in place for the removal of T cells following an immune response and downregulation of activated clones. CD95, a molecule known as Fas, is a member of the TNF receptor superfamily and is expressed on activated T cells. Under appropriate conditions, binding of this molecule to its ligand, CD178, promotes programmed cell death of a cohort of activated T cells. This method is dependent on TCR binding and the activation state of the T cell. Complementing this deletional method to TCR repertoire control are nondeletional mechanisms that selectively anergize (make unreactive) specific T cell clones. In addition to signaling through the TCR complex, T cells require additional costimulatory signals (see later). TCR binding only leads to T cell activation if the costimulatory signals are present, generally delivered via APCs. In the absence of costimulation, the cell remains unable to proceed toward activation and, in some cases, becomes refractory to activation, even with the appropriate signals. Thus, TCR binding that occurs to self in the absence of appropriate antigen presentation or active inflammation results in an aborted activation and prevents self-reactivity.

***T Cell Activation*** T cell activation is a sophisticated series of events that has only recently been more fully described. As noted, the TCR, unlike antibody, only recognizes its ligand in the context of MHC. By requiring that T cells only respond to antigen encountered when it is physically embedded on self-cells, the system avoids constant activation by soluble molecules.

T cells can then specifically recognize and destroy cells that make peptide products of mutation or viral infection. Because the number of potential antigens is high, and the likelihood is that self-antigens vary minimally from foreign antigens, the nature of the TCR-binding event has evolved so that a single interaction with an MHC molecule is not sufficient to cause activation. In fact, a T cell must register a signal from approximately 8000 TCR–ligand interactions with the same antigen before a threshold of activation is reached.[13] Each event results in the internalization of the TCR. Because resting T cells have low TCR density, sequential binding and internalization over several hours is required. Transient encounters are not sufficient. This threshold is reduced considerably by appropriate costimulation signals (see later).

As discussed in the previous section, most TCRs are heterodimers composed of two transmembrane polypeptide chains, α and β. The αβ-TCR is noncovalently associated with several other transmembrane signaling proteins, including CD3 (composed of three separate chains, γ, δ, and ε), and ζ chain molecules, as well as the appropriate accessory molecule from the T cell. This is either CD4 or CD8, which associates with its respective MHC molecule. Together, these proteins are known as the TCR complex. When the TCR is bound to an MHC molecule and the proper configuration of accessory molecules stabilize its binding, a signal is initiated by intracytoplasmic protein tyrosine kinases (PTKs). These PTKs include p56lck (on CD4 or CD8), p59Fyn, and ZAP70; the latter two are associated with CD3. Repetitive binding signals combined with the appropriate costimulation eventually activate phosphokinase C-gamma (PLC-γ1), which in turn hydrolyzes the membrane lipid phosphatidyl inositol biphosphate (PIP2), thereby releasing inositol triphosphate (IP3) and diacyl glycerol (DAG). IP3 binds to the endoplasmic reticulum, causing a release of calcium that induces calmodulin to bind to and activate calcineurin. Calcineurin dephosphorylates the critical cytokine transcription factor nuclear factor of activated T cells (NFAT), prompting it, with the transcription factor nuclear factor κB (NF-κB), to initiate the transcription of cytokines, including IL-2 and its receptor (Fig. 26-12). Resting T cells express only low levels of the IL-2 receptor (IL-2R; CD25) but, with activation, IL-2R expression is increased. As the activated T cell begins to produce IL-2 secondary to events initiated by TCR activation, the cytokine begins to work in autocrine and paracrine fashions, potentiating DAG activation of protein kinase C (PKC). PKC is important in activating many gene regulatory steps critical for cell division. This effect, however, is restricted only to T cells that have undergone activation after encountering their specific antigen, leading to IL-2R expression. Thus, the process limits proliferation and expansion to only those clones specific for the offending antigen. As the antigenic stimulus is removed, IL-2R density decreases and the TCR complex is reexpressed on the cell surface. There is a negative feedback system between the TCR and the IL-2R, resulting in a highly regulated and efficient system that is only reactive in the presence of antigen and ceases to function once antigen is removed. Many of these steps in T cell activation have been targeted in the development of immunosuppressive agents. These will be discussed in detail later in this chapter.

***Costimulation*** As noted, recognition of the antigenic peptide–MHC complex via TCR binding is usually not sufficient alone to generate a response in a naïve T cell. Additional signals, through so-called costimulatory pathways, are required for optimal T cell activation.[14,15] In fact, receipt of TCR complex signaling, often referred to as signal 1, in the absence of costimulation, or signal 2, not only fails to achieve activation but can lead to a state of inaction, or anergy (Fig. 26-13). An anergic T cell is now unable to respond, even if given both appropriate stimuli.[16] This characteristic of the immune system is thought to be one of the major mechanisms in tolerance to self-antigens in the periphery, crucial in the prevention of autoimmunity. Researchers have exploited this discovery using antibodies or receptor fusion proteins designed to block interactions between key costimulatory molecules at the time of antigen exposure. Most research to date has focused on the interactions of two costimulatory pathways, the CD28-B7 pathway (immunoglobulin-like superfamily members) and CD40-CD154 pathway (tumor necrosis factor [TNF]–TNFR superfamily members). There have been, however, many additional pairings in these same families and others that have been found to have distinct roles in costimulatory function (Table 26-2).

CD28, present on T cells, and the B7 molecules CD80 and CD86 on APCs, were among the first costimulatory molecules to be described. Ligation of CD28 is necessary for optimal IL-2 production and can lead to the production of additional cytokines, such as IL-4 and IL-8, and chemokines such as RANTES, and protect T cells from activation-induced apoptosis through the upregulation of antiapoptotic factors such as Bcl-x. CD28 is expressed constitutively on most T cells, whereas the expression of CD80 and CD86 is largely restricted to professional APCs (e.g., dendritic cells, monocytes, macrophages. The kinetics of CD80-CD86 expression is complex but is typically increased with the induction of the immune response. Another ligand for CD80 and CD86 is CTLA-4 (CD152). This molecule is upregulated and expressed on the surface of T cells following activation, and it binds the B7 receptors with 10 to 20 times greater affinity than CD28. CTLA-4 has been shown to have a negative regulatory effect on T cell activation and proliferation, an observation supported by the fact that CTLA-4 deficient mice develop a lymphoproliferative disorder. The therapeutic potential of costimulation blockade was first made apparent through the use of an engineered fusion protein composed of the extracellular portion of the CTLA-4 molecule and a portion of the human immunoglobulin (Ig) molecule. This compound binds CD80 and CD86 and prevents costimulation via CD28. Several clinical trials in autoimmunity have demonstrated the efficacy of CTLA4-Ig (abatacept). More recently, a higher affinity, second-generation version, LEA29Y (belatacept),

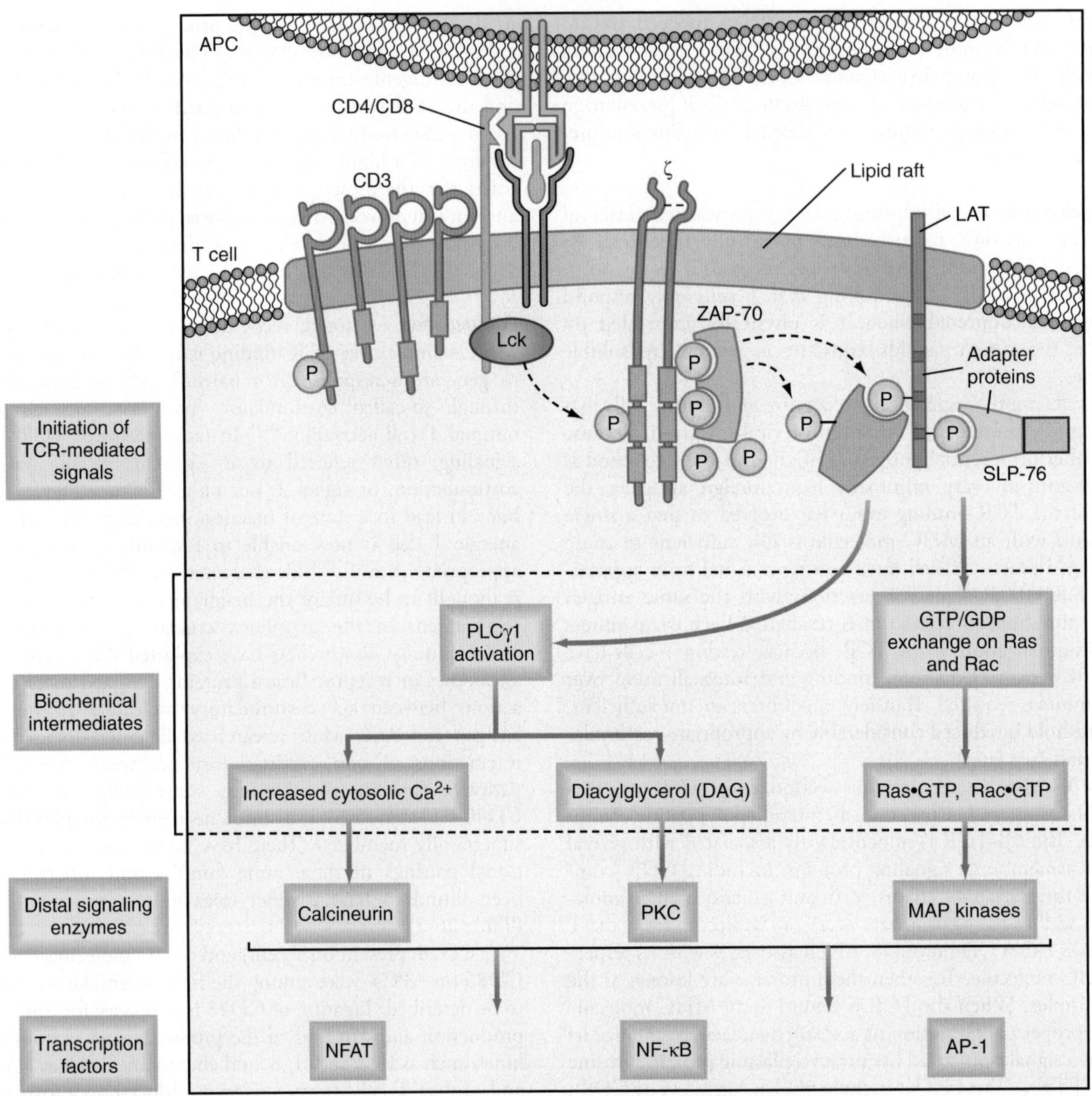


**FIGURE 26-12** T cell activation. On antigen recognition, there is a clustering of TCR complexes and coreceptors, which initiates a cascade of signaling events within the T cell. Tyrosine kinases associated with the coreceptors (e.g., Lck) phosphorylate CD3 and the ζ chain. ζ-chain association protein kinase (Zap-70) subsequently associates with these regions and becomes activated. Zap-70 phosphorylates various adaptor and coreceptor proteins, ultimately activating numerous cellular enzymes, including calcineurin, PKC, and several MAP kinases. These enzymes then activate transcription factors that promote the expression of various genes involved in proliferation and T cell responses. (Adapted from Abbas AK, Lichtman AH, Pillai S: Cellular and molecular immunology, ed 6, Philadelphia, 2010, Saunders-Elsevier.)

has been tested in renal transplantation trials, with success as a replacement for calcineurin inhibitors.

Closely related to the CD28-B7 pathway is the CD40-CD154 (CD40L) pathway. Evidence for the crucial role of the CD40-CD154 pathway in the immune response was seen following the observation that hyper-IgM syndrome results from a mutational defect in the gene encoding for CD154. In addition to defects in the generation of T cell–dependent antibody responses, patients with hyper-IgM syndrome also have defects in T cell–mediated immune responses. CD40 is a cell surface molecule expressed on endothelium, B cells, dendritic cells, and other APCs. Its ligand, CD154, is primarily found on activated T cells. Upregulation of CD154 following TCR signaling allows for signals to be sent to the APC via CD40; in particular, it is a critical signal for B cell activation and proliferation. CD40 binding is required for APCs to stimulate a cytotoxic T cell response. It leads to the release of activating cytokines, particularly IL-12, and the upregulation of B7 molecules. It also initiates innate functions of APCs, including nitric oxide synthesis and phagocytosis. Interestingly, CD154 is also released in soluble form by activated platelets. Thus, sites of trauma that attract activated platelets simultaneously recruit the ligand required to activate tissue-based APCs, providing a link between innate and acquired immunity. Antibody preparations to CD154 have

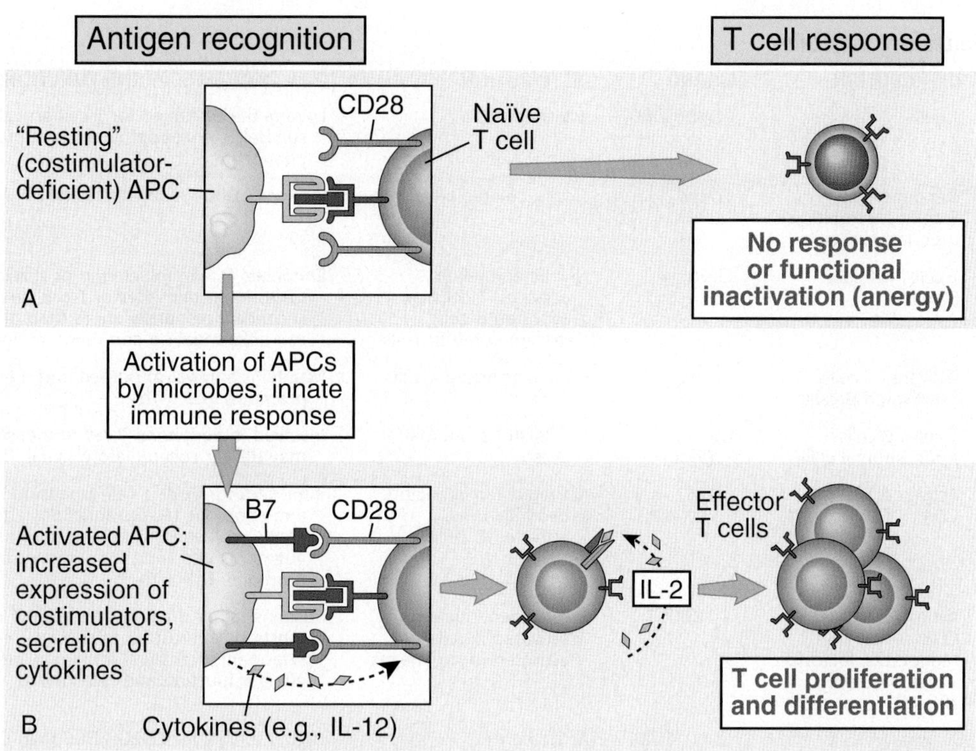


**FIGURE 26-13** T cell costimulation. Naïve T cells require multiple signals for efficient activation. **A,** Signal 1 occurs when the TCR recognizes its putative MHC-peptide combination. In the absence of any additional signals, there is an aborted response, or anergy, a state in which the cell is no longer available for stimulation. **B,** TCR signaling in conjunction with signals received through costimulatory molecules, signal 2, promote effective T cell activation and function. (Adapted from Abbas AK, Lichtman AH, Pillai S: Cellular and molecular immunology, ed 6, Philadelphia, 2010, Saunders-Elsevier.)

shown great promise in experimental models but clinical trials were halted over concern for unexpected thrombotic complications. There continues to be hope that anti-CD154 antibodies that bind distinct epitopes or antibodies directed toward CD40 may circumvent this issue.

Since earlier investigations, other pairings of molecules have been characterized and shown to demonstrate costimulatory activity. CD278 (inducible costimulator, or ICOS) is a CD28 superfamily expressed on activated T cells and its ligand, CD275 (ICOSL, or B7-H2), is expressed on APCs. Unlike CD28, ICOS is not present on naïve T cells but, instead, expression is upregulated after T cell activation and persists on memory T cells. Several studies have demonstrated a unique role for ICOS in the generation of helper T type 2 cell (Th2) responses. A CTLA-4 homologue has also been identified, PD-1 (CD279), and its ligands, PD-L1 (CD274) and PD-L2 (CD273; both B7 family members), have been shown to be involved in negative regulation of the immune response. Several members of the TNF-TNFR superfamily have been shown to play important roles in T cell costimulation, including CD134-CD252 (OX40-OX40L), CD137-CD137L (41BB-41BBL), CD27-CD70, CD95-CD178 (Fas-FasL), CD30-CD153, and RANK-TRANCE. Also, many other adhesion molecules (e.g., intercellular adhesion molecule [ICAM], selectins, integrins) control the movement of immune cells through the body, monitor their trafficking to specific areas of inflammation, and strengthen the TCR-MHC binding interaction nonspecifically. They differ from costimulation molecules in that they enhance the interaction of the T cell with its antigen without influencing the quality of the TCR response. Almost all are upregulated by cytokines released during T cell and endothelial activation.

***T Cell Effector Functions*** As noted, during thymic education, most T cells initially express both CD4 and CD8 molecules, but T cells subsequently become $CD4^+$ or $CD8^+$, depending on which MHC class they restrict to. Thus, these accessory molecules govern which type of MHC and, by extension, which types of cells a given T cell can interact with and evaluate. Because there is almost ubiquitous expression of class I MHC, all cell types are surveyed. These class I molecules display peptides that are generated within the cell (e.g., peptides from normal cellular processes or from internal viral replication). T cells responsible for inspecting all cells express the accessory molecule CD8, which in turn binds to class I, and specifically stabilizes a TCR interaction with a class I–presented antigen. Thus, $CD8^+$ T cells evaluate most cell types and mediate the destruction of altered cells. Appropriately, they have been termed *cytotoxic T cells.*

APCs are the predominant cell type that expresses class II in addition to class I MHC molecules. Class II molecules display peptides that have been sampled from surrounding extracellular spaces via phagocytosis and thus usually represent the presentation of newly acquired antigen. Cells initiating an immune response need to have access to this newly processed antigen. CD4 binds class II MHC and stabilizes the interaction of the TCR with the class II–peptide complex. Thus, under physiologic conditions, $CD4^+$ T cells are first alerted to an invasion of the

**Table 26-2 Costimulatory Molecules**

| RECEPTOR | DISTRIBUTION | LIGAND | DISTRIBUTION | PRINCIPAL EFFECTS AND FUNCTIONS |
|---|---|---|---|---|
| CD28 | T cells | CD80/CD86 | Activated APCs | Lowers the threshold for T cell activation, promotes survival, ↑ antiapoptotic factors, promotes Th1 phenotype |
| CD40 | Dendritic cells, B cells, macrophages, endothelial cells | CD154 | T cells, soluble platelets | Induces CD80-CD86 expression on APCs |
| CD27 | T cells, NK cells B cells | CD70 | Thymic epithelium, activated T cells, activated B cells, mature dendritic cells | Enhances T cell proliferation or survival, acts after CD28 to sustain effector T cell survival, influences secondary responses more than primary, promotes B cell differentiation and memory formation |
| CD30 | Activated T cells, activated B cells | CD153 | B cells, activated T cells | Maintains survival of primed and memory T cells, promotes Th2 > Th1 |
| CD95 (Fas) | T cells, B cells APCs, stromal cells | CD178 (FasL) | T cells, APCs, stromal cells | Involved in peripheral T cell homeostasis via fratricide, may deliver costimulatory signal |
| CD134 (OX-40) | Activated T cells $CD4^+$ > $CD8^+$ | CD252 (OX-40L) | Activated T cells mature dendritic cells, activated B cells | Important for $CD4^+$ T cell expansion, survival, ↑ anti-apoptotic factors, functions after CD28 to sustain $CD4^+$ T cell survival, enhances cytokine production, augments effector and memory $CD4^+$ T cell function, promotes Th2 > Th1 |
| CD137 (4-1BB) | Activated T cells $CD8^+$ > $CD4^+$, Monocytes, follicular dendritic cells, NK cells | 4-1BBL | Mature dendritic cells, activated B cells, activated macrophages | Sustains rather than initiates $CD8^+$ T cells responses, functions after CD28 to sustain T cell survival, important in antiviral immunity, promotes $CD8^+$ effector function and cell survival |
| CD152 (CTLA-4) | Activated T cells | CD80/CD86 | Activated APCs | Higher affinity for CD80-CD86 than CD28, inhibits T cell response |
| HVEM | T cells, monocytes, immature dendritic cells | CD258 (LIGHT) | Activated lymphocytes, immature dendritic cells, NK cells | Augments T cell responses, $CD8^+$ > $CD4^+$, promotes dendritic cells maturation |
| | | CD272 (BTLA) | Activated T cells, B cells, dendritic cells | Negative costimulator, inhibits IL-2 production, BTLA remains expressed on Th1 but not Th2 |
| | | CD160 | NK cells, cytolytic $CD8^+$ T cells, $\gamma\delta$ T cells | Negative regulator of $CD4^+$ T cell activation, inhibits proliferation and cytokine production |
| CD265 (RANK) | Dendritic cells | CD254 (TRANCE) | Activated T cells $CD4^+$ > $CD8^+$ | Enhances dendritic cell survival, upregulates Bcl-xl, (?) enhances IFN-γ production |
| CD279 (PD-1) | T cells | CD274 (PD-L1) | T cells, B cells, APCs, some parenchymal cells | Inhibits activation, proliferation and acquisition of effector cell function Th1 > Th2 |
| | | CD273 (PD-L2) | Dendritic cells, macrophages | Inhibits activation, proliferation, and acquisition of effector cell function, Th2 > Th1 |
| CD278 (ICOS) | Activated T cells, memory T cells | CD275 (ICOSL) | Dendritic cells B cells, macrophages | Promotes survival *and* expansion of effector T cells, (?) promotes Th2 responses |
| GITR | Treg, $CD8^+$ T cells, B cells, macrophages | GITR L | B cells, dendritic cells, macrophages endothelial cells | Marker for Treg, allows proliferation of Tregs Promotes T cell proliferation and cytokine production, negative regulator for NK function |

body by hematopoietically derived APCs that present their newly acquired antigen in the form of processed peptide in a class II molecule. As a consequence of their MHC restriction, these subpopulations of T cells have several different functions. $CD4^+$ T cells typically contribute to the response in a helper or regulatory role, whereas $CD8^+$ T cells are much more likely to play a part in cell elimination via cytotoxic functions.

Following activation, $CD4^+$ T cells initially play a critical role in the expansion of the immune response. After encountering an APC that expresses the specific antigenic peptide–MHC II pairing, the $CD4^+$ T cell can then signal back to the APC to elicit factors that allow for $CD8^+$ T cell activation. This process is accomplished via expression of specific costimulatory molecules and the release of certain cytokines. This so-called licensing of $CD8^+$ T cells for cytotoxic function is a key step within the immune response. This partly describes how $CD4^+$ T cells become helper cells. More recently, there has been further elucidation of their cellular differentiation into well-defined specific Th subsets. Two distinct Th populations have been described, based on their pattern of cytokine synthesis—Th1 cells induce a cell-mediated response whereas Th2 cells promote a humoral response (Fig. 26-14). These two distinct populations differ in their pattern of cytokine synthesis.

The main cytokines driving the Th1 response are interferon-γ (IFN-γ) and tumor necrosis factor (TNF). The predominant role of IFN-γ is to enhance macrophage function and activity and promote cell-mediated immunity. Activated macrophages then proceed to ingest and kill invading microbes and,

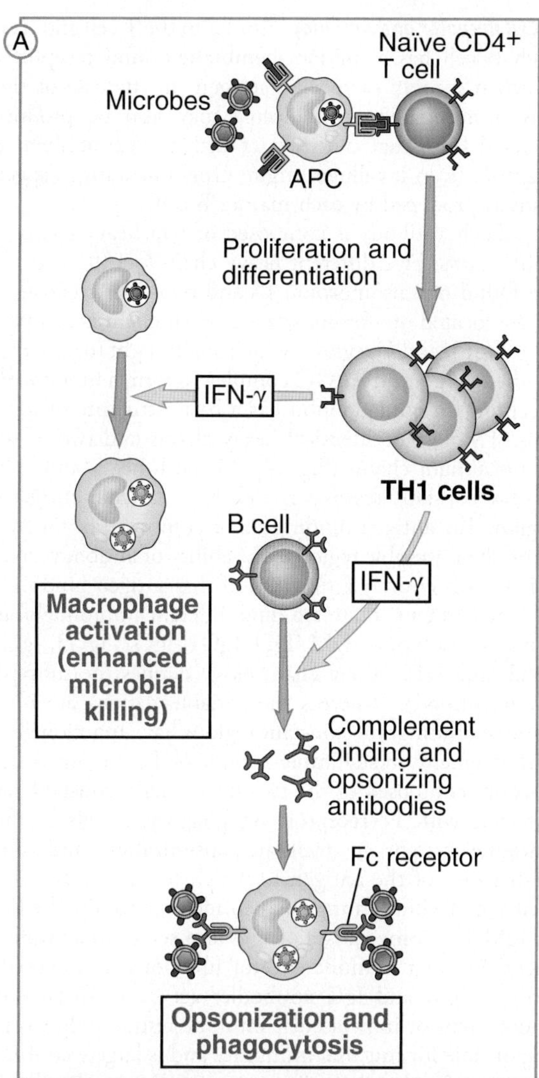


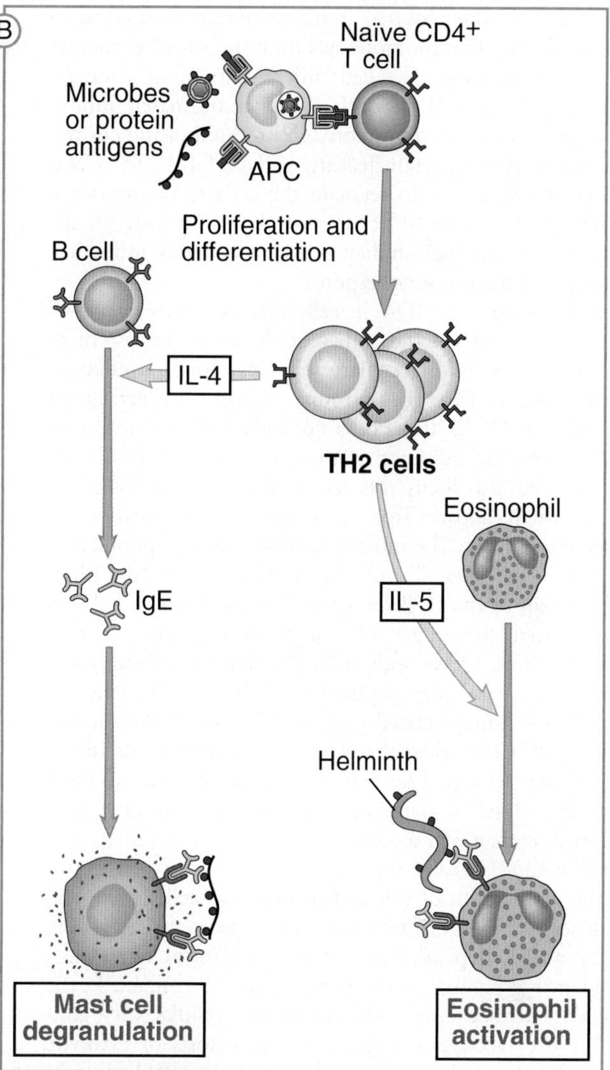


| Ⓒ Property | TH1 subset | TH2 subset |
|---|---|---|
| Cytokines produced | | |
| IFN-γ, IL-2, TNF | +++ | - |
| IL-4, IL-5, IL-13 | - | +++ |
| IL-10 | +/- | ++ |
| IL-3, GM-CSF | ++ | ++ |
| Cytokine receptor expression | | |
| IL-12R β chain | ++ | - |
| IL-18R | ++ | - |
| Chemokine receptor expression | | |
| CCR3, CCR4 | +/- | ++ |
| CXCR3, CCR5 | ++ | +/- |
| Ligands for E- and P-selectin | ++ | +/- |
| Antibody isotypes stimulated | IgG2a (mouse) | IgE; IgG1 (mouse)/ IgG4 (humans) |
| Macrophage activation | +++ | - |

**FIGURE 26-14** Helper T cell subsets. Naïve CD4+ T cells may differentiate into distinct lineages, such as Th1 and Th2 cells. **A,** Th1 cells produce IFN-γ, which activates macrophages to kill intracellular microbes. **B,** Th2 cells produce cytokines (e.g., IL-4, IL-5), which stimulate IgE production and activate eosinophils in response to parasitic infection. (Adapted from Abbas AK, Lichtman AH, Pillai S: Cellular and molecular immunology, ed 6, Philadelphia, 2010, Saunders-Elsevier.)

at the same time, the acquired immune system is directed to produce antibodies that promote opsonization, thereby enhancing the overall process. Th2 cell differentiation, in contrast, results in the release of IL-4 and IL-5, which ultimately inhibit macrophage activation and promote IgE production and eosinophil activation. An important feature of these $CD4^+$ Th cells is the ability of one subset to regulate the activity of the other. Thus, the initial steps in differentiation depend greatly on the surrounding immunologic milieu, which ultimately influences the character of the immune response.

Another subset of $CD4^+$ T cells that has been described to play a critical role in the ability of the immune system to temper its response is the regulatory T cell (Treg) population. They can downregulate the immune response by acting on effector cells or APCs. These cells not only have the ability to suppress cytokines, adhesion molecules, and costimulatory signals, but can also focus this response by the expression of integrins, which allows Treg to home to the location of immune engagement. The most extensively studied population of Treg are those $CD4^+$ T cells that express CD25 (the high-affinity α chain of the IL-2 receptor).[17] These $CD4^+$ $CD25^+$ T cells have been the target of numerous attempts to alter immune function. Other molecules that have been suggested to be unique to regulatory populations include glucocorticoid-induced TNFR family-related gene (GITR) and forkhead box P3 (FoxP3). It is now clear that Treg plays a crucial role in the control of day to day immune activation; absence of these cells has led to lethal lymphoproliferative autoimmune syndromes in several animal models.

Unlike $CD4^+$ T cells, the function of $CD8^+$ T cells is primarily the elimination of infected or defective cells. As noted, licensing occurs via APC interactions and subsequent cell killing occurs by a $Ca^{2+}$-dependent secretory mechanism or a $Ca^{2+}$-independent mechanism that requires direct cell contact. In the $Ca^{2+}$-dependent mechanism, the rise in intracellular $Ca^{2+}$ concentration after activation triggers the exocytosis of cytolytic granules. These granules contain a lytic protein called perforin and serine proteases called granzymes. Perforin polymerization forms defects in the target cell's membrane, allowing granzyme activity to lyse the cell. In the absence of $Ca^{2+}$, T cells can induce apoptosis of a target cell via a Fas-dependent mechanism. It occurs when surface CD95 (Fas) is bound by its ligand, CD178 (FasL). Cytotoxic T cells upregulate CD178 on activation, which in turn binds CD95 on target cells and causes programmed cell death.

**B Cells** The primary lymphoid organ responsible for B cell differentiation is the bone marrow. Similar to all other cells in the immune system, B cells are derived from pluripotent bone marrow stem cells. IL-7, produced by bone marrow stromal cells, is a growth factor for pre–B cells. IL-4, IL-5, and IL-6 are cytokines that stimulate the maturation and proliferation of mature primed B cells. The principal function of B cells is to produce antibodies against foreign antigens—that is, the humoral immune response—and be involved in antigen presentation. B cell development occurs through several stages, with each stage representing a change in the genomic content at the antibody loci. During the differentiation process, there is an elegant series of nucleotide rearrangements that results in an almost unlimited array of specificities, allowing for a diverse recognition repertoire.

***B Cell Receptor and Antibody*** Similar to the T cell and its receptor, each B cell has a unique membrane-bound receptor through which it recognizes specific antigen. In the case of the B cell, this immunoglobulin molecule may also be produced in a secreted form that can interact with the extracellular environment far from it cellular origin. Only one antigen-specific antibody is produced by each mature B cell.

Each antibody is composed of two heavy chains and two light chains. Five different heavy chain loci (μ, γ, α, ε, and δ) are found on chromosome 14 and two light chain loci (κ and λ) are located on chromosome 2. Each chain is composed of V, D and/or J, and C regions, which are brought together randomly by the RAG-1 and RAG-2 complex to form a functional antigen receptor. Immunoglobulin has a basic structure of four chains, two of which are identical heavy chains and two of which are identical light chains (Fig. 26-15). Both heavy and light chains have a constant region, as well as a variable antigen-binding region. The antigen-binding site is composed of the heavy- and light-chain variable regions. The ability of antibody to neutralize microbes is entirely a function of this antigen-binding region.

In humans, there are nine different immunoglobulin subclasses or isotypes—IgM, IgD, IgG1, IgG2, IgG3, IgG4, IgA1, IgA2, and IgE. Heavy chain usage defines the subtype of any given antibody. Whereas the variable regions are involved in antigen binding, the constant regions have functionality as well. The fragment crystallizable region, or Fc region, is in the tail portion, composed of the two heavy chain constant regions. It interacts with Fc receptors on phagocytic cells of the innate immune system to facilitate opsonization and subsequent destruction of the antigen to which the antibody is bound, as well as to facilitate antigenic peptide processing. The Fc portion of IgM and some classes of IgG also serves to activate complement. Distinct immune effector functions are assigned to each isotype. IgM and IgG antibodies act in a pivotal role in the endogenous or intravascular immune response. IgA is primarily responsible for mucosal immunity and is largely confined to the gastrointestinal and respiratory tracts. Resting B cells that have not yet been exposed to antigen express IgD and IgM on their cell surfaces. Following interaction with antigen, the first isotype produced is IgM, which is quite efficient at binding complement to facilitate phagocytosis or cell lysis. Further activation or differentiation of the B cell occurs after interactions with $CD4^+$ T cells. B cells undergo isotype switching, which results in a decrease in IgM titer, with a concomitant rise in IgG titer. Unlike the TCR, the Ig loci undergo continued alteration after B cell stimulation to improve the affinity and functionality of the secreted antibody. A primed B cell may undergo further mutation within the variable regions that leads to increased affinity of antibody, termed *somatic hypermutation.* Such B cells are retained to provide the ability to generate a more vigorous response if the antigen happens to be reencountered (Fig. 26-16).

***B Cell Activation*** When antigen is bound by two surface antibodies (or a multimeric form of antibody), the antibodies are brought together on the cell surface in a process known as cross linking. This is the event that stimulates B cell activation, proliferation, and differentiation into a plasma cell (antibody-producing cell). Like the T cell, the threshold for B cell activation is high. This can be lowered 100-fold by costimulation signals received by the transmembrane complex CD19-CD21. B cells can also internalize antigens bound to surface antibodies and

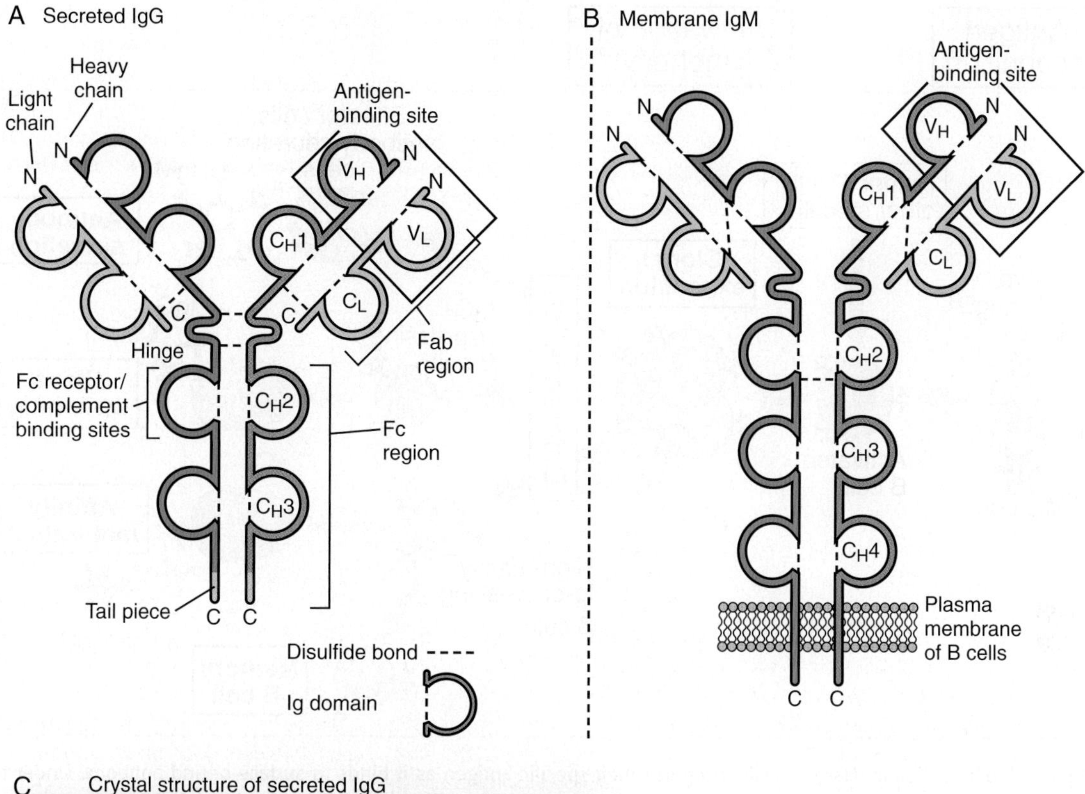


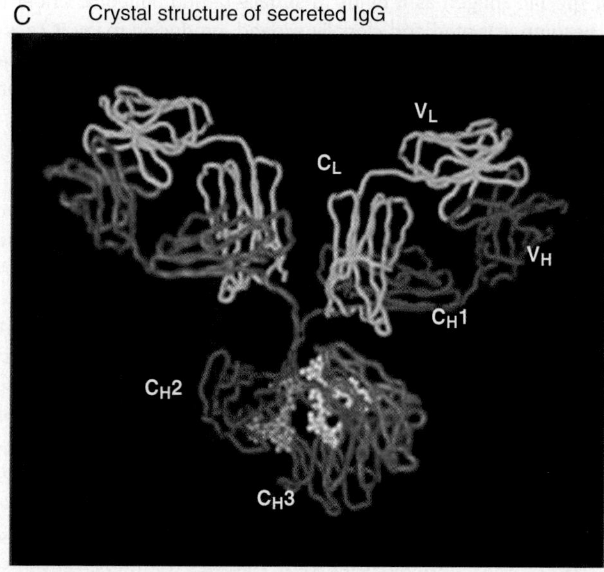


**FIGURE 26-15** Structure of immunoglobulin. **A,** Representation of secreted IgG molecule. The antigen binding regions are formed by the variable regions of light ($V_L$) and heavy ($V_H$) chains. The constant region of the heavy chain ($C_H$) is responsible for the Fc receptor and complement binding sites. **B,** Schematic diagram of membrane-bound IgM. The membrane form of the antibody has C-terminal transmembrane and cytoplasmic portions that anchor the molecule in the plasma membrane. **C,** X-ray crystallography representation of IgG molecule. Heavy chains are colored blue and red, light chains are colored green, and carbohydrates are shown in gray. (Adapted from Abbas AK, Lichtman AH, Pillai S: Cellular and molecular immunology, ed 6, Philadelphia, 2010, Saunders-Elsevier.)

process them for presentation to T cells, thus participating in antigen presentation. As noted, B cells may provide and receive certain costimulatory signals. For example, B cells express CD40 and, when bound by CD154 expressed on activated T cells, the result is upregulation of B7 molecules on the B cell and delivery of important costimulatory signals to T cells.

Plasma cells (activated B cells) are distinguished histologically by their hypertrophied Golgi apparatus. They secrete large amounts of monoclonal (single-specificity) antibody. In addition to being secreted following exposure to an antigen, antibody can be present as part of a natural repertoire in circulation for initial response to common pathogens. Antigen exposure generally

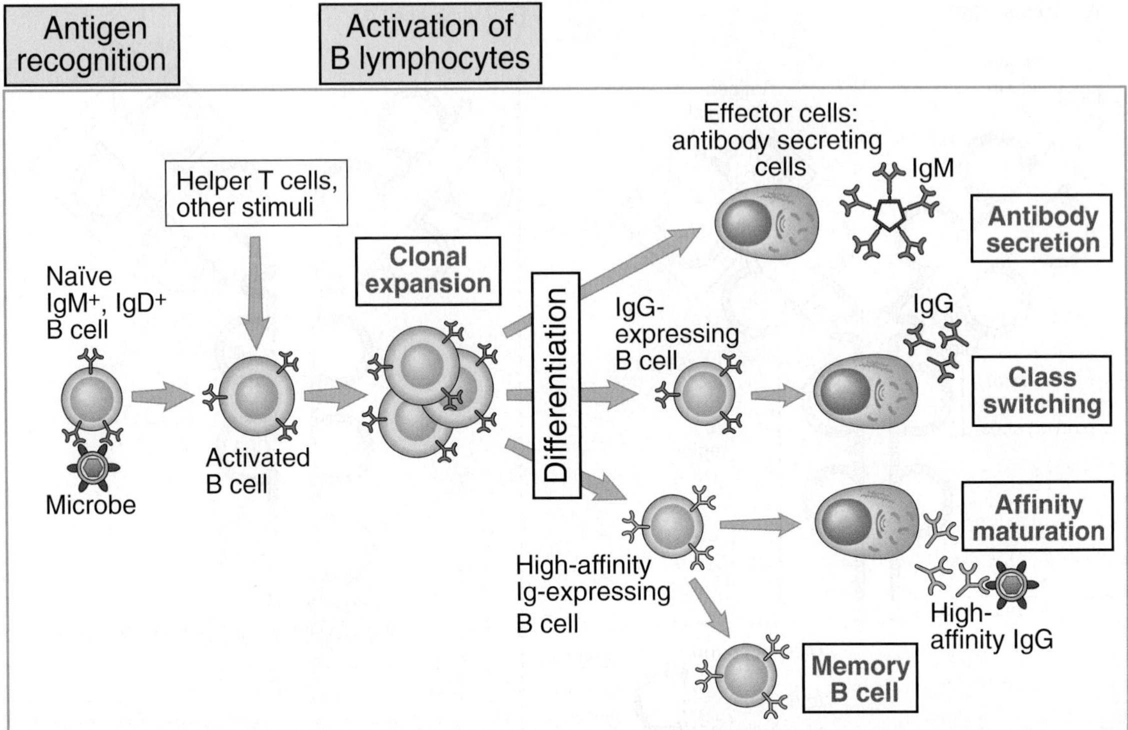


**FIGURE 26-16** B cell differentiation. Naïve B cells recognize their specific antigen as it binds to surface-bound antibody. Under the influence of helper T cells, costimulatory signals, and other stimuli, B cells become activated and clonally expand, producing many B cells of the same specificity. They also differentiate into antibody-secreting cells, plasma cells. Some of the activated B cells undergo heavy chain class switching and affinity maturation. Ultimately, a small subset becomes long-lived memory cells, primed for future responses. (Adapted from Abbas AK, Lichtman AH, Pillai S: Cellular and molecular immunology, ed 6, Philadelphia, 2010, Saunders-Elsevier.)

leads to B cell affinity maturation and isotype switching, and produces high-affinity IgG antibodies. Naturally occurring antibodies, however, are generally IgM antibodies, with low affinity, and are generally thought to respond to a broad array of carbohydrate epitopes found on many common bacterial pathogens. Natural antibody is responsible for ABO blood group antigen responses and discordant xenograft rejection (see later, "Xenotransplantation").

## Innate Immunity

The innate immune system is thought to be a holdover from an evolutionarily distant response to foreign pathogens. In contrast to the acquired immune system, which uses an innumerable host of specificities to identify any possible antigen, the innate system uses a select number of protein receptors to identify specific motifs consistent with foreign, altered, or damaged tissues. These receptors can exist on cells, such as macrophages, neutrophils, and NK cells, or free in the circulation, as is the case for complement. Although they fail to exhibit the specificity of the TCR or antibody, they are broadly reactive against common components of pathogenic organisms—for example, lipopolysaccharides on gram-negative organisms or other glycoconjugates. Thus, the receptors of innate immunity are the same from one individual to another within a species and, in general, do not play a role in the direct recognition of a transplanted organ. They do, however, exert their effects indirectly through the identification of injured tissue (e.g., as is the case when an ischemic damaged organ is moved from one individual to another).

Once activated, the innate system performs two vital functions. It initiates cytolytic pathways for the destruction of the offending organism, primarily through the complement cascade (Fig. 26-17). In addition, the innate system can convey the encounter to the acquired immune system for a more specific response through byproducts of complement activation via activation of APCs. Macrophages and dendritic cells engulf not only foreign organisms that have been bound by complement, but can also distinguish pathogens, because they can be identified through receptors for foreign carbohydrates (e.g., mannose receptors). Recently, a highly evolutionarily conserved family of proteins known as Toll-like receptors (TLRs) has been described as playing an important role as activation molecules for innate APCs. They bind to pathogen-associated molecular patterns (PAMPs) motifs common to pathogenic organisms. Some examples of TLR ligands include lipopolysaccharide (LPS), flagellin (from bacterial flagella), double-stranded viral RNA, unmethylated CpG islands of bacterial and viral DNA, zymosan (β-glucan found in fungi), and numerous heat shock proteins (HSPs).

### Monocytes

Mononuclear phagocytes are also bone marrow-derived and initially emerge as monocytes within peripheral blood. In the setting of certain inflammatory signals, they home to sites of injury or inflammation, where they mature and become macrophages. Their function is to acquire, process, and present antigen as well as serve as effector cells in certain situations. Once activated, they elaborate various cytokines that regulate the local

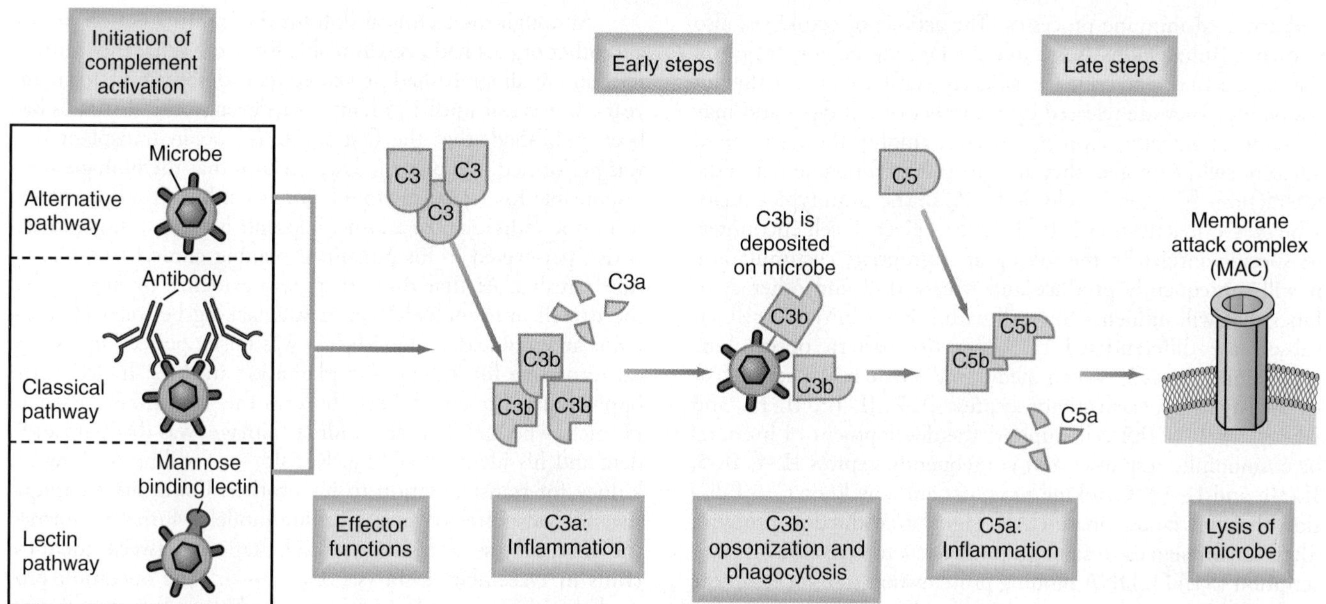


**FIGURE 26-17** Complement activation. There are three distinct pathways that lead to complement activation. All three pathways lead to production of C3b, which initiates the late steps of complement activation. C3b binds to the microbe and promotes opsonization and phagocytosis. C5a stimulates the local inflammatory response and catalyzes formation of the membrane attack complex (MAC), which results in microbial cell membrane disruption and death by lysis. (Adapted from Abbas AK, Lichtman AH, Pillai S: Cellular and molecular immunology, ed 6, Philadelphia, 2010, Saunders-Elsevier.)

immune response. They play a significant role in facilitating the acquired T cell response through antigen presentation and their cytokines induce substantial tissue dysfunction in sites of inflammation. Thus, their recruitment to sites of T cell activation, such as in transplant rejection, exacerbates the dysfunction evoked by direct T cell cytotoxic mechanisms.

### Dendritic Cells

Dendritic cells are specialized macrophages that are regarded as professional APCs. They are the most potent cells that present antigen and are distributed throughout the lymphoid and nonlymphoid tissues of the body. Immature dendritic cells can be found along the gut mucosa, within the skin, and at other sites of antigen entry. Once they have encountered antigen in sites of injury, they undergo a process of maturation, including the upregulation of MHC class I and class II molecules as well as various costimulatory molecules. They also begin to migrate toward peripheral lymphoid tissue (i.e., lymph nodes) where they can interact with antigen-specific T cells and potentiate their activation. The dendritic cell is involved in the licensing of $CD8^+$ T cells for cytotoxic function, stimulates T cell clonal expansion, and provides signals for Th differentiation to a Th1 or Th2 response. There are also subsets of dendritic cells, which serve distinct functions in inducing and regulating the cellular response. For example, myeloid dendritic cells (DC1) are more immunogenic, whereas plasmacytoid dendritic cells (pDCs) are more tolerogenic and may work to suppress the immune response.

### Natural Killer Cells

NK cells are large granular lymphocytes with potent cytolytic function that constitute a critical component of innate immunity. They were initially discovered during studies focused on tumor immunology. There was a small subset of lymphocytes that exhibited the ability to lyse tumor cells in the absence of prior sensitization, described as naturally reactive. These so-called natural killer cells exhibited rapid cytolytic activity and existed in a relatively mature state (i.e., morphology characteristic of activated cytotoxic lymphocytes—large size, high protein synthesis activity, with abundant endoplasmic reticulum, and rapid killing activity). Further studies have indicated that NK cells lyse cell targets that lack expression of self MHC class I, termed the *missing self hypothesis,* a situation that could arise because of viral infection with suppression of self class I molecules, or in tumors under strong selection pressure of killer T cells. Since those initial studies, NK cells have been found to express cell surface inhibitory receptors, which include killer inhibitory receptors (KIRs). These molecules function to deliver inhibitory signals when they bind class I MHC molecules, thus preventing NK-mediated cytolysis on otherwise healthy host cells. NK cells produce various cytokines, including IFN-γ; these may function to activate macrophages, which can in turn eliminate host cells infected by intracellular microbes. Similarly to macrophages, NK cells express cell surface Fc receptors that bind antibody and participate in antibody-dependent cellular cytotoxicity (ADCC). NK cells also play an important role in the immune response after bone marrow transplantation and xenotransplantation. Their role in solid organ transplantation is less well defined.

### Cytokines

Cell surface receptors provide an interface through which adjacent cells can transfer signals vital to the immune response. Although this cell to cell contact is a critical component of cellular communication, soluble mediators are also used extensively to accomplish similar tasks. These polypeptides, termed *cytokines,* are critical to the development and function of the innate and acquired immune processes. The actions of cytokines, also known as interleukins (see Table 26-1), may be autocrine (on the same cell) or paracrine (on adjacent cells) but are usually not endocrine. They are released by a number of cell types and may function to activate, suppress, or even amplify the response of adjacent cells. As noted, they are particularly fundamental to the interactions between T cells and APCs. The prototypical cytokine of T cell activation is IL-2. Once a given T cell encounters its specific antigen in the setting of appropriate costimulation, it will subsequently produce and release IL-2 and other cytokines that will influence any cell within its vicinity. Th cellular subsets are differentiated based on the pattern of cytokine expression. Th1 cells, which mediate cytotoxic responses such as delayed-type hypersensitivity, express IL-2, IL-12, IL-15, and IFN-γ, whereas Th2 cells support the development of humoral or eosinophilic responses and consequently express IL-4, IL-5, IL-10, and IL-13. Cytokine receptors are now known to function through Janus kinase (JAK) signal transduction proteins. They convey signals to signal transducers and activators of transcription (STAT), DNA binding proteins that translocate to the nucleus to influence gene transcription. As is the case with most of the immune response this pathway is tightly regulated. For example, suppressors of cytokine signaling (SOCS) proteins act in a negative feedback loop to inhibit STAT phosphorylation by binding and inhibiting JAKs or competing with STATs for phosphotyrosine binding sites on cytokine receptors. There is evidence emerging for the involvement of SOCS proteins in human disease, which raises the possibility that therapeutic strategies based on the manipulation of SOCS activity might be of clinical benefit. In addition to cytokines, there are a host of other soluble, small-molecule mediators that are released during an immune response or with other types of inflammation. These function to increase blood flow to the area and improve the exposure of the area to lymphocytes and the innate immune system.

## Transplantation Immunity

The study of modern transplantation immunology is traditionally attributed to the experiments of Sir Peter Medawar, fueled by attempts to use skin transplantation as a treatment for burned aviators during World War II. While monitoring the victims with autologous (syngeneic) and homologous (allogeneic) skin grafts, he noted that not only did all allogeneic grafts universally fail promptly, but also secondary grafts from the same donor were rejected even more vigorously, suggesting immune involvement. He pursued this hypothesis with extensive experiments in rabbits, wherein he confirmed his previous observation and noted the presence of a heavy lymphocyte infiltrate in the rejecting graft. It was Mitchison, working in the early 1950s, who definitively identified a role for lymphocytes in the rejection of foreign tissue. Subsequent studies in tumor immunology, as well as work by Snell using strains of genetically identical mice, identified the genetic basis for graft rejection as the MHC, known in humans as HLA and in mice as the H-2 locus. These series of experiments, over a short period of several years, demonstrated that rejection of transplanted tissue was an immunologic process, implicated lymphocytes as the principal effector cells, and identified the MHC as the source of the primary source of antigen in the rejection response. These pivotal studies laid the groundwork for the transition of transplantation from the experimental to the clinical realm.

Although the technical skill for the transplantation of skin and other organs had been available for some time, the vigorous rejection of allografts had prevented its widespread use for many years. It was not until 1954, after Medawar's critical studies had been published, that the first successful organ transplantation was performed. Despite Medawar's claim that the biologic force responsible for rejection would "forever inhibit transplantation from one individual to another," Joseph Murray, a surgeon scientist, persevered in his pursuit of making clinical transplantation a reality. At that time, there was evidence to suggest that the overall immunologic barrier was lacking between identical twins and, coincidentally, Murray was busily perfecting a surgical technique for kidney transplantation in dogs. In 1954, the opportunity presented itself to test the hypothesis. Richard Herrick, who had incurable kidney damage, was the first candidate and his identical sibling, Ronald, was willing to donate a kidney for transplantation to his brother. Using the technique that he had perfected in the canine model, Murray performed the first successful kidney transplantation between identical twins in December 1954 (see Fig. 26-4).[3] The operation proceeded without complications and the kidney functioned well, without the need for immunosuppressive therapy. Despite this landmark advance in transplantation, the vast majority of individuals in need of a transplant were not identical twins and the focus of the field was appropriately directed toward the development of methods to control the rejection response.

During the 1950s and 1960s, several discoveries were made that were of the utmost importance for future successes in transplantation. Following Gorer and Snell's description of the murine MHC system, Jean Dausset described the equivalent in humans using antibodies developed against HLA. This led to the first serologically based typing system for human transplantation antigens. Snell and Dausset shared the Nobel Prize in Medicine in 1980 for their observations.

In the late 1960s, Terasaki reported on the significance of preformed antibody directed against donor MHC molecules and its impact on kidney graft survival. He developed the microlymphocyte cytotoxicity test, allowing for pretransplantation detection of recipient-derived antidonor antibody. This formed the basis for the crossmatch assay that is used today to screen potential donor-recipient pairings. These techniques, along with the development of new immunosuppressive compounds, including 6-mercaptopurine (6-MP) and azathioprine, led to the first successful kidney transplantation between relatives who were not identical twins, and also to the first successful transplantation using a kidney from a deceased donor.

Although early attempts at immunosuppression permitted extended allograft survival in select patients, both the reproducibility and durability of results were far from adequate. In the 1970s, investigators sought novel treatments to improve the success rate for transplantation; these modalities included thoracic duct drainage and the use of antilymphocyte serum. Despite these efforts, the results for kidney transplantation remained poor, with the best centers achieving 1-year survival rates of 70% for living-related kidney grafts and 50% for deceased donor kidney transplants. Then, a chance discovery of a promising agent from a fungal isolate dramatically changed the outlook for kidney and other types of transplantation. Borel identified an active metabolite, cyclosporin A (cyclosporine), which showed selective in vitro inhibition of lymphocyte cultures but no significant myelotoxic effects (see later for more details). Promising results in dogs eventually led to clinical trials in humans, and the modern era of transplantation had begun.

The introduction of cyclosporine ushered in the most dramatic improvement in the field of transplantation. Liver and heart transplantation survival rates doubled, and the improved immunosuppression encouraged transplantation teams around the world to begin broader investigational use, transplanting lung, small bowel, and pancreas. Now, with the use of cyclosporine and newer agents, 1-year graft survival has exceeded 90% for almost all organs except the small intestine. Despite the discovery and clinical introduction of ever-increasingly potent immunosuppressants, the field of transplantation has many areas in need of improvement. Drug-related side effects and the intractable problem of chronic rejection still plague physicians. The focus of the current research is the development of a clinically applicable strategy to promote transplantation tolerance, thereby eliminating the pitfalls and shortcomings of current immunosuppressive therapy.

## REJECTION

There are three classic definitions of rejection that are based not only on the predominant mediator, but also the timing of the process (Fig. 26-18).

1. Hyperacute rejection occurs within minutes to days after transplantation and is primarily mediated by preformed antibody.
2. Acute rejection is a process mediated by T cells, although it is often accompanied by an acquired antibody response, and generally occurs within the first few weeks to months of transplantation but can occur at any time.
3. Chronic rejection is the most common cause of long-term allograft loss and is an indolent fibrotic process that occurs over months to years. It is thought to be secondary to T and B cell processes but is difficult to separate completely from nonimmune mechanisms of chronic organ damage (e.g., drug toxicity, cardiovascular comorbid diseases).

### Hyperacute Rejection

Although essentially untreatable, hyperacute rejection is almost universally preventable with the proper use of the lymphocytotoxic crossmatch assay or other means of detecting donor-specific antibodies before transplantation. This form of rejection occurs when donor-specific antibodies are present in the recipient's system prior to transplantation. These antibodies may be the result of natural processes, such as the formation of antibody to blood group antigens or the product of prior exposure to antigens with similar enough specificities as those expressed by the donor that cross-reactivity can occur. In the latter case, prior sensitization is usually the result of prior transplantation, transfusion, or pregnancy, but may also be the result of prior environmental antigen exposure. As expected, a hyperacute rejection can occur within the first minutes to hours following graft reperfusion. Antibodies bind to the donor tissue, initiate complement-mediated lysis, endothelial cell activation, resulting in a procoagulant state, and immediate graft thrombosis (Fig. 26-19).

Similar to the lymphocytotoxicity assay described earlier, which is used for MHC class I typing, the crossmatch assay is performed by mixing cells from the donor with serum from the recipient and adding complement, if needed. Lysis of the donor cells indicates that antibodies directed against the donor are present in the recipient serum; this is called a positive crossmatch. Thus, a negative crossmatch assay coupled with proper ABO matching will effectively prevent hyperacute rejection in 99.5% of transplantations. Newer crossmatch techniques have become increasingly sophisticated, including those directed at class I and class II antibodies, flow cytometric techniques, and bead-based screening assays to exclude non-HLA antibodies. Because a given patient's sensitivity status may change over time, a more common technique for screening a patient's sensitization status is to screen a potential recipient's serum against a panel of random donor cells representing the likely regional donor pool. Known as the panel-reactive antibody (PRA) assay, the results are expressed as a percentage of the panel in the randomly selected cell set that lyses when recipient serum is added. Thus, a nonsensitized patient would be given a score of 0% and a highly sensitized patient might have a PRA up to 100%. These screening tests can now be performed without the need for cells by using polystyrene beads coated with HLA antigens. In this situation, the laboratory detects all anti-HLA antibodies and calculates a PRA based on the expected frequency of the HLA types in the donor pool. There are now clinical protocols to attempt desensitization that use plasmapheresis and/or intravenous immune globulin (IVIg) to reduce circulating antibody.[18] A more promising method is to avoid crossmatch-positive donor-recipient pairs with paired donor exchange.

### Acute Rejection

Of the three types of rejection, only acute rejection can be successfully reversed once it is established. T cells constitute the core element responsible for acute rejection, often termed *T cell–mediated rejection* (TCMR). There is also a form of acute rejection that is particularly aggressive and involves vascular invasion by T cells, termed *acute vascular rejection.* Finally, a more recently recognized form of acute rejection mediated by the humoral immune system, termed *antibody-mediated rejection* (ABMR), will be discussed briefly. With the advent of more effective immunosuppression, allograft loss from acute cellular rejection has become increasingly rare. Acute rejection can occur at any time after the first few postoperative days, the time needed to mount an acquired immune response, and most commonly occurs within the first 6 months after transplantation. Without adequate immunosuppression, the cellular response will progress over the course of days to a few weeks, ultimately destroying the allograft. As noted, there are two main pathways through which rejection can proceed, the direct and indirect alloresponses (Fig. 26-20). In either case, allospecific T cells encounter their appropriate antigen, processed donor MHC peptides presented on self-MHC or via direct recognition of donor MHC, undergo activation, and promote similar responses. The precursor frequency of T cells specific for direct or indirect allorecognition differs. Indirect allorecognition is similar to any given pathogen. Donor MHC protein is processed into peptides and presented on self-MHC. The number of T cells specific for this antigen is approximately 1 in 200,000 to 500,000. Direct allorecognition, however, has a much higher precursor frequency. These T cells recognize donor MHC directly without processing (Fig. 26-21). Given that the T cells are selected to recognize self-MHC molecules and that there are similarities between donor and recipient MHC, it is no surprise that a substantial number of T cells are alloreactive. Some estimates have suggested that approximately 1% to 10% of all T cells are directly alloreactive. This high

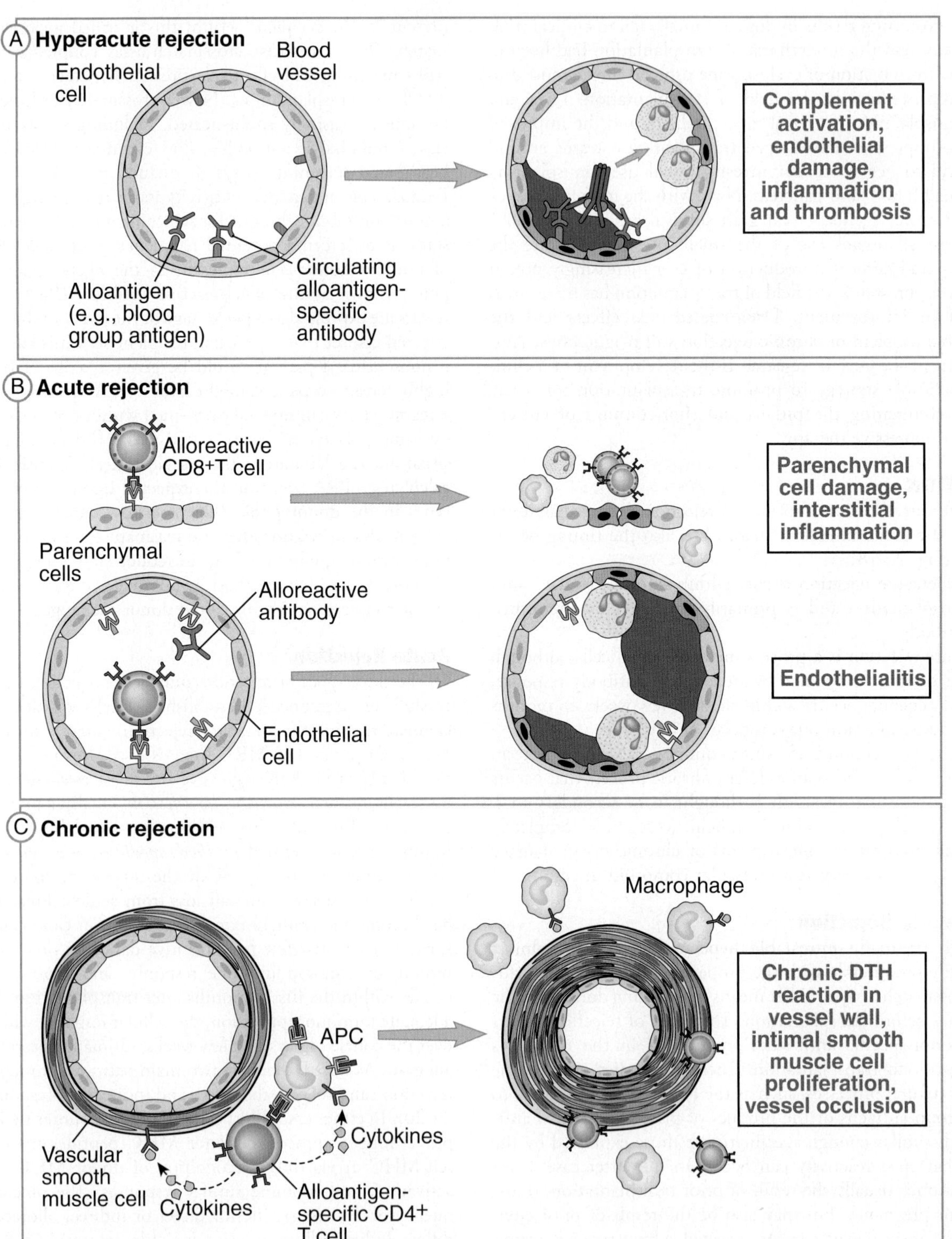


**FIGURE 26-18** Mechanisms of rejection. **A,** Hyperacute rejection occurs when preformed antibodies react with donor antigens on the vascular endothelium of the graft. Subsequent complement activation triggers rapid intravascular thrombosis and graft necrosis. **B,** Acute rejection is predominantly mediated by a cellular infiltrate of alloreactive T cells, which attack donor cells in the organ parenchyma and occasionally donor vessels/endothelium, termed acute vascular rejections. Alloreactive antibodies also develop and contribute to acute humoral or antibody-mediated rejection. **C,** Chronic rejection is characterized by graft arteriosclerosis and fibrosis. Immune- and nonimmune-mediated mechanisms are responsible for abnormal proliferation of cells within the intima and media of the vessels of the graft, eventually leading to luminal occlusion. (Adapted from Abbas AK, Lichtman AH, Pillai S: Cellular and molecular immunology, ed 6, Philadelphia, 2010, Saunders-Elsevier.)

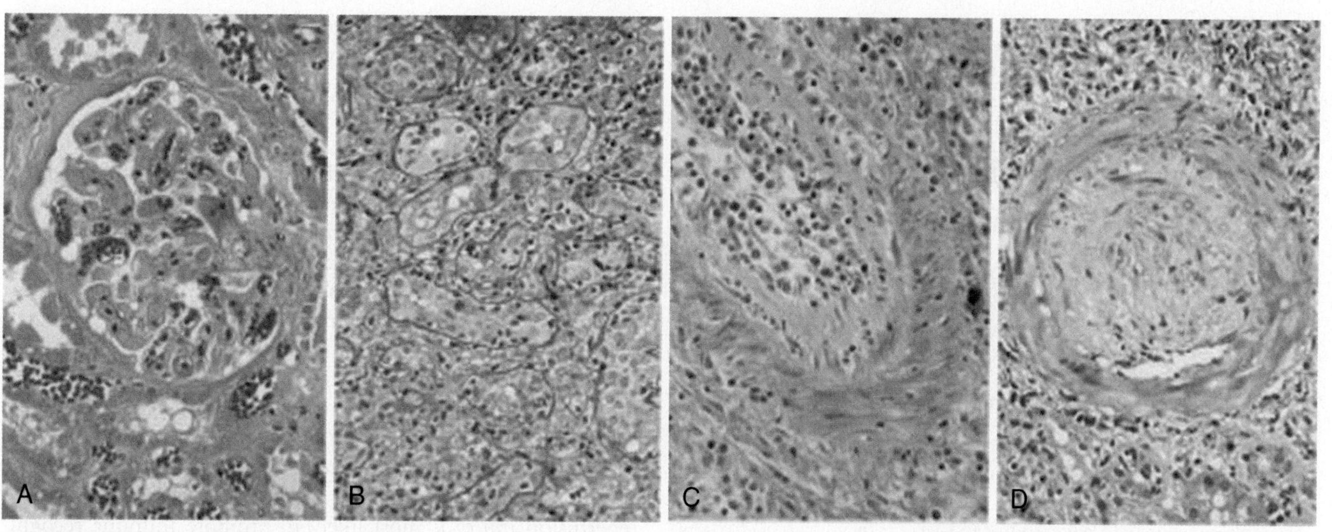


**FIGURE 26-19** Histology of rejection. **A,** Hyperacute rejection of a kidney allograft, with characteristic endothelial damage, thrombus, and early neutrophil infiltrates. **B,** Acute rejection of kidney, with inflammatory cells within the connective tissue around the tubules and between tubular epithelial cells. **C,** Acute rejection of a kidney allograft, with an inflammatory reaction within a graft vessel, resulting in endothelial disruption. **D,** Chronic rejection in a transplanted kidney with graft arteriosclerosis. The vascular lumen has been replaced with smooth muscle cells and a fibrotic response. (Adapted from Abbas AK, Lichtman AH, Pillai S: Cellular and molecular immunology, ed 6, Philadelphia, 2010, Saunders-Elsevier.)

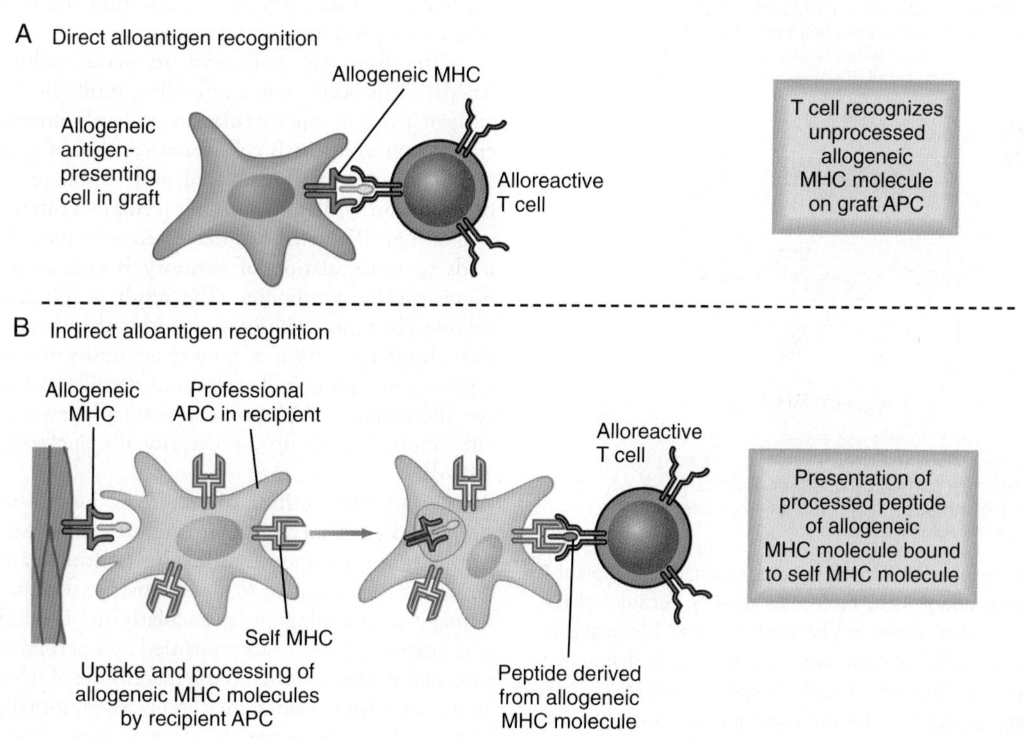


**FIGURE 26-20** Direct versus indirect allorecognition. **A,** Direct allorecognition occurs when recipient T cells bind directly to donor MHC molecules on graft cells. **B,** Indirect allorecognition results when recipient antigen-presenting cells take up donor MHC and process the alloantigen. Allopeptides are then presented on recipient (self) MHC molecules in standard fashion to alloreactive T cells. (Adapted from Abbas AK, Lichtman AH, Pillai S: Cellular and molecular immunology, ed 6, Philadelphia, 2010, Saunders-Elsevier.)

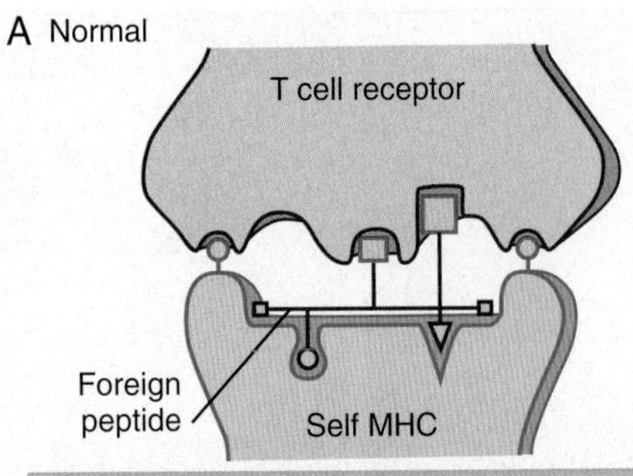
A Normal
T cell receptor
Foreign peptide
Self MHC
Self MHC molecule presents foreign peptide to T cell selected to recognize self MHC weakly, but may recognize self MHC-foreign peptide complexes well

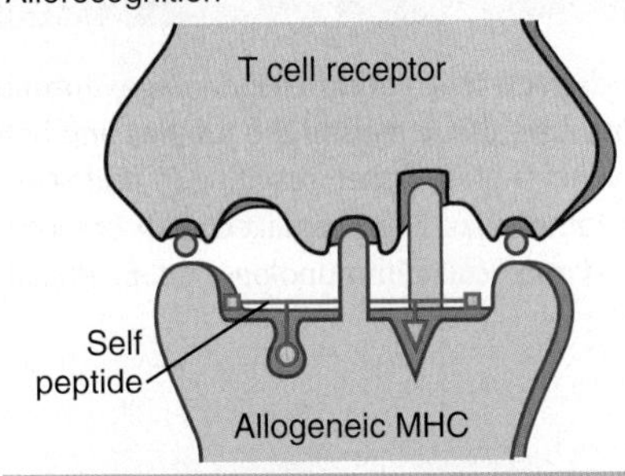
B Allorecognition
T cell receptor
Self peptide
Allogeneic MHC
The self MHC-restricted T cell recognizes the allogeneic MHC molecule whose structure resembles a self MHC-foreign peptide complex

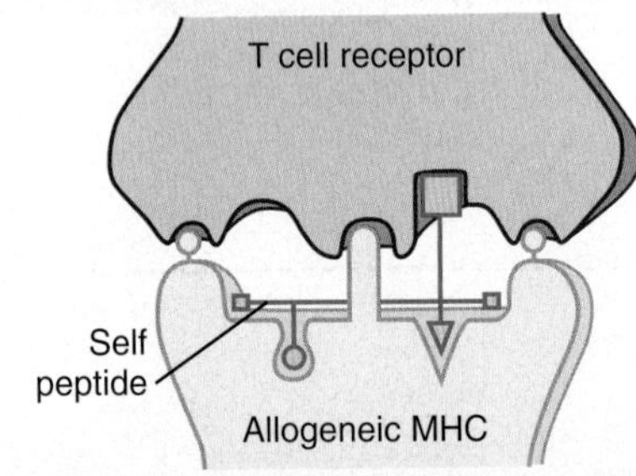
C Allorecognition
T cell receptor
Self peptide
Allogeneic MHC
The self MHC-restricted T cell recognizes a structure formed by both the allogeneic MHC molecule and the bound peptide

**FIGURE 26-21** Molecular basis for direct allorecognition. Recipient T cells may recognize donor MHC molecules directly because of the similarities between MHC alleles but become activated because only T cells strongly reactive to self-MHC were deleted in the thymus via negative selection. **A,** Normally, T cells encounter self-MHC complexed with foreign peptide and become activated in the appropriate situation. **B,** T cells may encounter allogeneic MHC complexed with endogenous peptide and mistakenly react because the structure of the foreign MHC molecule itself resembles self-MHC bound with foreign peptide. **C,** Alternatively, the combination of self-peptide and allogeneic MHC may promote activation. (Adapted from Abbas AK, Lichtman AH, Pillai S: Cellular and molecular immunology, ed 6, Philadelphia, 2010, Saunders-Elsevier.)

precursor frequency likely overwhelms many of the regulatory processes in place to control the much lower cell frequencies involved in physiologic immune responses. Once activated, these alloreactive T cells move to destroy the graft. Subsequently, there is massive infiltration of T cells and monocytes into the allograft, resulting in destruction of the organ through direct cytolysis and a general inflammatory milieu that leads to generalized parenchymal dysfunction and endothelial injury, resulting in thrombosis (see Fig. 26-19).

The bulk of current immunosuppressive agents are directed toward T cells themselves or interruption of pathways essential to their activation or effector functions. In an effort to prevent acute cellular rejection, induction therapy may be used during the initial post-transplantation stages. These agents will be discussed in the next section, but often will be antibody therapies that serve to deplete or inactivate T cells globally during the immediate postoperative period of engraftment, when reperfusion injury is most likely to promote immune recognition. Immunosuppressive regimens are frequently scheduled initially to favor an intense regimen in the immediate postoperative period and then tapered to lower, less toxic levels over time.

T cell–specific treatments lead to the prevention of acute rejection in approximately 70% of transplantations and, when it does occur, it can usually be reversed. Similar to hyperacute rejection resulting from preformed antibody responses, T cell presensitization will result in an accelerated form of cellular rejection mediated by memory T cells. It generally occurs within the first 2 to 3 days after transplantation and is often accompanied by a significant humoral response.

The humoral equivalent to acute cellular rejection is ABMR. This occurs when offending antibodies specific for alloantigen exist in the circulation at levels undetectable by the crossmatch assay, or B cell clones capable of producing donor-specific antibody are activated and stimulated to produce de novo allo antibodies. The former scenario is often seen in patients with a high PRA that has decreased over time. Transplantation leads to restimulation of memory B cells responsible for the donor-specific antibodies. The result is initial graft function, followed by rapid deterioration within the first few postoperative days. Implementation of a more aggressive immunosuppressive regimen, including higher doses of steroids combined with nonspecific antibody depletion via plasmapheresis or IVIg (nonspecific immunoglobulin) is occasionally successful in reversing ABMR.

Prompt recognition of acute rejection is essential to ensure prolonged graft survival. Untreated rejection leads to expansion of the immune response to involve multiple pathways, some of which are less sensitive to T cell–specific therapies. In addition, damage to the allograft, particularly for the kidney, pancreas, and heart, is generally accompanied by a permanent loss of function that is proportional to the magnitude of involvement. Most acute rejection episodes are initially asymptomatic until the secondary effects of organ dysfunction occur. By this time, the rejection process has proceeded to a point that is often more difficult to reverse. Accordingly, monitoring for acute rejection is usually initially intense, particularly during the first year following transplantation. In general, any unexplained graft dysfunction should prompt biopsy and evaluation for the lymphocytic infiltration, antibody deposition, and/or parenchymal necrosis characteristic of acute rejection.

### Chronic Rejection

Although the mechanisms of acute and hyperacute rejection have been well described, chronic rejection remains poorly understood. True chronic rejection is an immune-based process derived from repeated or indolent TCMR or ABMR, but the clinical phenotype of chronic graft fibrosis and deterioration is often secondary to a combination of immune and nonimmune effects. Appropriately, the term *chronic rejection* has been replaced by more descriptive terms: *interstitial fibrosis and tubular atrophy* (IF-TA) or *chronic allograft nephropathy* for the kidney, *chronic coronary vasculopathy* for the heart, *vanishing bile duct syndrome* for the liver, and *bronchiolitis obliterans* for the lungs.[19] The process is insidious, usually occurring over a period of years, but can be accelerated and occur within the first year. Regardless of the organ involved, it is characterized by parenchymal replacement by fibrous tissue with a relatively sparse lymphocytic infiltrate, but may contain macrophages or dendritic cells (see Fig. 26-19). Organs with epithelium show a disappearance of epithelial cells as well as endothelial destruction. The events that ultimately trigger this response are certainly related to the transplantation itself, including but not limited to the response to alloantigen and to the ischemia-reperfusion injury associated with the actual transfer of the organ itself. These events set the stage for expression of various soluble factors, including transforming growth factor-β (TGF-β), leading to a remodeling of the parenchyma and ensuing fibrous replacement. Chronic inflammatory insults can also evoke a process of epithelial to mesenchymal dedifferentiation, leading to epithelial cells that regress into fibrocytes. To date, these processes remain essentially untreatable once identified, but there are several factors that have been identified that predispose toward the development of chronic rejection. The most important of these is prior acute rejection episodes. Thus, the more effective immune control is exerted to limit acute rejection episodes in the early post-transplantation stages, the less likely chronic rejection is to occur.

## IMMUNOSUPPRESSION

Current immunosuppressive therapies in transplantation achieve excellent results, especially in terms of relatively short-term patient and allograft survival rates. Despite tremendous progress over the past 50 years, all agents designed to prevent rejection remain nonspecific to the alloimmune response. Given the redundancy of the immune system, recipients almost always need a number of agents to control the normal immune response adequately. In addition, none of these therapies specifically inhibit the response to the allograft; instead, most immunosuppressants target the immune response globally. In other words, all drugs that prevent rejection do so at the cost of preventing the normal host response to bacterial and viral infections, as well as tumor surveillance. Although some of the newer therapies are more precise in their mechanisms, many target not only the mediators of the immune response but also any cells undergoing maturation or division. Consequently, there are many nonimmune side effects associated with immunosuppressive therapy that can directly or indirectly contribute to graft dysfunction. Also, the social costs are not trivial, considering that transplant recipients may have to take dozens of pills daily at an annual cost of approximately $10,000 to $15,000.

As noted, the most critical time period for immunoprotection is the first few days to months post- transplantation. The graft is fresh and there is a heightened state of inflammation secondary to inevitable graft injury from ischemia or reperfusion, as well as the physical transfer of the organ itself. In addition, this is the time of initial antigen exposure, which will play a large role in establishing a lasting state of immune unresponsiveness. For this reason, immunosuppression is extremely intense in the early postoperative period and normally tapered thereafter. This initial conditioning of the recipient's immune system is known as induction immunosuppression. It usually involves complete deletion, or at least aggressive diminution of the T cell response, and consequently is only tolerated for a short period of time without lethal consequences. After this initial period, the agents used to prevent acute rejection for the remainder of the patient's life are called maintenance immunosuppressants. As noted, these medications still carry with them many immune and nonimmune side effects that may also ultimately contribute to long-term graft failure. Immunosuppressants used to reverse an acute rejection episode are called rescue agents. They are generally the same as those used for induction therapy. The mechanisms of action of the various immunosuppressants are described here and detailed in Table 26-3.

### Corticosteroids

Steroids, in particular glucocorticoids, remain one of the most commonly used medications to prevent rejection. They are almost exclusively used in combination with other agents, with which they seem to act synergistically to improve graft survival. They may also be used in higher doses as rescue therapy for acute rejection episodes. Although steroids possess potent immunosuppressive properties, they can contribute significantly to the morbidity of transplantation because of their effects on wound healing and propensity to cause diabetes, hypertension, and osteoporosis. More recently, because of these side effects, there has been an emphasis on developing steroid-minimizing or steroid-sparing protocols.

Although the Nobel prize was awarded over 50 years ago for work on the hormones of the adrenal cortex, the mechanism of the immunosuppressive effect of glucocorticoids was only elucidated.[20] Similar to other steroid hormones, glucocorticoids bind to an intracellular receptor after passing into the cytoplasm through nonspecific mechanisms. The receptor-steroid complex then enters the nucleus, where it acts as a transcription factor. One of the most important genes upregulated is IκB gene. This protein binds to and inhibits the function of NF-κB, a key activator of proinflammatory cytokines and an important transcription factor involved in T cell activation. Through this mechanism, steroids also act to diminish the transcription of IL-1 and TNF-α by APCs and to prevent the upregulation of MHC expression. Phospholipase A2, and consequently the entire arachidonic acid cascade, is also inhibited. They decrease the leukocyte response to various chemokines and chemotactins; by inhibiting vasodilators such as histamine and prostacyclin, they consequently dampen the inflammatory response globally. This broad anti-inflammatory response quickly mollifies the intragraft environment and thus substantially improves graft function, long before the offending cells have actually left the graft. The most commonly used oral glucocorticoid formulation is prednisone; its IV equivalent is methylprednisolone.

**Table 26-3 Summary of Immunosuppressive Drugs**

| DRUG | DESCRIPTION | MECHANISM OF ACTION | NONIMMUNE TOXICITY AND COMMENTS |
|---|---|---|---|
| Prednisone | Corticosteroid | Binds nuclear receptor and enhances transcription of IκB, which inhibits NF-κB and T cell activation | Diabetes, weight gain, psychological disturbances, osteoporosis, ulcers, wound healing, adrenal suppression |
| Cyclosporine | 11-amino-acid cyclic peptide from *Tolypocladium inflatum* | Binds to cyclophilin; complex inhibits calcineurin phosphatase and T cell activation | Nephrotoxicity, hemolytic-uremic syndrome, hypertension, neurotoxicity, gingival hyperplasia, skin changes, hirsutism, post-transplantation diabetes, hyperlipidemia |
| Tacrolimus (Prograf) | Macrolide antibiotic from *Streptomyces tsukubaensis* | Binds to FKBP12; complex inhibits calcineurin phosphatase and T cell activation | Effects similar to cyclosporine but with lower incidence of hypertension, hyperlipidemia, skin changes, hirsutism, and gingival hyperplasia but higher incidence of post-transplantation diabetes and neurotoxicity |
| Sirolimus (rapamycin) | Triene macrolide antibiotic from *Streptomyces hygroscopicus* from Easter Island (Rapa Nui) | Binds to FKBP12; complex inhibits target of rapamycin and IL-2–dependent T cell proliferation | Hyperlipidemia, increased toxicity of calcineurin inhibitors, thrombocytopenia, delayed wound healing, delayed graft function, mouth ulcers, pneumonitis, interstitial lung disease |
| Everolimus | Derivative of sirolimus, similar mechanism and toxicities | | |
| Mycophenolate mofetil (Cellcept) | Mycophenolic acid from *Penicillium stoloniferum* | Inhibits synthesis of guanosine monophosphate nucleotides; blocks purine synthesis preventing proliferation of T and B cells | Gastrointestinal symptoms (mainly diarrhea), neutropenia, mild anemia |
| Azathioprine (Imuran) | Prodrug that undergoes hepatic metabolism to form 6-mercaptopurine | Converts 6-mercaptopurine to 6-thioinosine-5′-monophosphate, which is converted to thioguanine nucleotides that interfere with DNA and purine synthesis | Leukopenia, bone marrow depression, liver toxicity (uncommon) |
| Antithymocyte globulin | Polyclonal IgG from rabbits or horses immunized with human thymocytes | Blocks T cell membrane proteins (e.g., CD2, CD3, CD45), causing altered function, lysis, and prolonged T cell depletion | Cytokine release syndrome, thrombocytopenia, leukopenia, serum sickness |
| Muromonab-CD3 (OKT3) | Anti-CD3 murine monoclonal antibody | Binds CD3 associated with the TCR, leading to initial activation and cytokine release, followed by blockade of function, lysis, T cell depletion | Severe cytokine release syndrome, pulmonary edema, acute renal failure, CNS changes |
| Basiliximab | Anti-CD25 chimeric monoclonal antibody | Binds to high-affinity chain of IL-2R (CD25) on activated T cells, causing depletion and preventing IL-2–mediated activation | Hypersensitivity reaction, uncommon |
| Dacluzimab | Anti-CD25 humanized monoclonal antibody | Similar to that of basiliximab | Hypersensitivity reaction, uncommon |
| Rituximab | Anti-CD20 chimeric monoclonal antibody | Binds to CD20 on B cells and causes depletion | Infusion or hypersensitivity reactions, uncommon |
| Alemtuzumab | Anti-CD52 humanized monoclonal antibody | Binds to CD52 expressed on most T and B cells, monocytes, macrophages, NK cells, causing lysis and prolonged depletion | Mild cytokine release syndrome, neutropenia, anemia, autoimmune thrombocytopenia, thyroid disease |
| FTY720 | Sphingosine-like derivative of myriocin from the fungus *Isaria sinclairii* | Functions as antagonist for sphingosine-1-phosphate receptors on lymphocytes, enhancing homing to lymphoid tissues and preventing egress, causing lymphopenia | Reversible first-dose bradycardia, potentiated by general anesthetics and beta blockers, nausea, vomiting, diarrhea, increased liver enzyme levels |
| Belatacept (LEA29Y) | High-affinity homologue of CTLA-4 Ig | Binds to CD80-CD86 and prevents costimulation via CD28 | Clinical trials—preliminary results suggest equal efficacy to CsA but improved glomerular filtration rate |

Adapted from Abbas AK, Lichtman AH, Pillai S: Cellular and molecular immunology, ed 6, Philadelphia, 2010, Saunders-Elsevier.

## Antiproliferative Agents

### Azathioprine

The purine analogue azathioprine was first described in the 1960s and remained a mainstay of immunosuppression for the next 30 years.[21] It is still used today in organ transplantation and for the treatment of some autoimmune diseases. Similar to other antiproliferative agents, it is a nucleotide analogue that targets cells undergoing rapid division; in the case of an immune response, its goal is to limit the clonal expansion of T and B cells. Azathioprine undergoes hepatic conversion to several active metabolites, including 6-MP and 6-thioinosine-5′-monophosphate. These derivatives inhibit DNA synthesis by alkylating DNA precursors and interfering with DNA repair mechanisms. In addition, they inhibit the enzymatic conversion of inosine monophosphate (IMP) to adenosine monophosphate (AMP) and guanosine monophosphate (GMP), effectively depleting the cell of adenosine. The effects of azathioprine are relatively nonspecific and, like other antiproliferative agents, it acts on all rapidly dividing cells that require nucleotide synthesis. Consequently, its predominant toxicities are seen in the bone marrow, gut mucosa, and liver. It is primarily used as a maintenance agent in combination with other medications, such as a corticosteroid and calcineurin inhibitor.

### Mycophenolate Mofetil

Mycophenolate mofetil (MMF) is an immunosuppressive agent with a similar mechanism of action as azathioprine It is derived from the fungus *Penicillium stoloniferum.* Once ingested, it is metabolized in the liver to the active moiety, mycophenolic acid. The active compound inhibits IMP dehydrogenase, the enzyme that controls the rate of synthesis of GMP in the de novo pathway of purine synthesis, a critical step in RNA and DNA synthesis. Importantly, however, is the presence of a salvage pathway for GMP production in most cells except lymphocytes (hypoxanthine-guanine phosphoribosyl transferase–catalyzed GMP production directly from guanosine). Thus, MMF exploits a critical difference between lymphocytes and other body tissues, resulting in relatively lymphocyte-specific immunosuppressive effects. MMF blocks the proliferative response of both T and B cells, inhibits antibody formation, and prevents the clonal expansion of cytotoxic T cells.

There have been numerous clinical trials to evaluate MMF. Specifically, MMF has been shown to decrease the rate of biopsy-proven rejection and the need for rescue therapy compared with azathioprine.[22] Appropriately, MMF has replaced azathioprine in most immunosuppressive protocols as the third agent in the standard three-drug regimen, although recent evidence has suggested that its therapeutic difference is less pronounced when used with more modern immunosuppressive regimens. It has also been used in combination with a calcineurin inhibitor or sirolimus by many centers in steroid-sparing protocols. However, MMF is not effective enough to use without steroids or calcineurin inhibitors. The major clinical side effects include leukopenia and diarrhea.

## Calcineurin Inhibitors

### Cyclosporine

Jean-Francois Borel is credited with the discovery of cyclosporin A (CsA; cyclosporine) in 1972 while working as a microbiologist for Sandoz Laboratories (now Novartis). He apparently was vacationing in Norway and collected soil samples for analysis in search of new antibiotics. Although the samples failed to show any significant antimicrobial activity, they did show potent immunosuppressive characteristics. Further studies demonstrated that the active component is a cyclic, nonribosomal, peptide of 11 amino acids produced by the fungus *Tolypocladium inflatum.*[23] The mechanism of action of CsA is mediated primarily through its ability to bind the cytoplasmic protein cyclophilin. The CsA-cyclophilin complex binds to the calcineurin-calmodulin complex within the cytoplasm and blocks calcium-dependent phosphorylation and activation of nuclear factor of activated T cells (NFAT), a critical transcription factor involved in T cell activation, including upregulation of the IL-2 transcript (Fig. 26-22). The result is blockade of IL-2 production. Thus, CsA is used as a maintenance agent, blocking the initiation of an immune response, but is ineffective as a rescue agent once IL-2 has already been produced. In addition, CsA acts to increase the transcription of TGF-β, a cytokine involved in the normal processes that limit the immune response by inhibiting T cell activation, reducing regional blood flow and stimulating tissue remodeling and wound repair. As will be discussed later, the toxicity and side effects of CsA may in large part be related to the effects of TGF-β.

CsA has poor water solubility and consequently must be given as a suspension or emulsion. This becomes a particular concern in liver transplantation because the oral absorption of CsA is dependent on bile flow; fortunately, this has been addressed by the development of a microemulsion form that is less bile-dependent. CsA is metabolized by the hepatic cytochrome P-450 enzymes and blood levels are therefore influenced by agents that affect the P-450 system. P-450 inhibitors, which include ketoconazole, erythromycin, calcium channel blockers, and grapefruit juice, result in higher CsA levels, whereas inducers of P-450, including rifampin, phenobarbital, and phenytoin, result in lower CsA levels.

The discovery of CsA and its subsequent development as an immunosuppressant contributed enormously to the advancement of organ transplantation. It was first approved for clinical use in 1983, then led to a substantial improvement in the outcome of deceased donor renal transplantation, and permitted the widespread practice of heart and liver transplantation. Although its potent immunosuppressive activity was welcomed, its attendant toxicities were less than ideal. As noted, CsA induces the expression of TGF-β and much of the toxicity of CsA can be linked to increased TGF-β activity. One of the most important side effects of CsA is renal toxicity. CsA has a significant vasoconstrictor effect on proximal renal arterioles, causing a 30% decrease in renal blood flow. This action is most likely mediated through increased TGF- β levels, which act to increase the transcription of endothelin, a potent vasoconstrictor, activating the renin-angiotensin pathway and resulting in hypertension.[24] The remodeling effects of TGF- β also induce fibrin deposition, which is thought to play a role in the fibrosis typically seen during chronic allograft nephropathy. Also, CsA frequently causes neurologic side effects, consisting of tremors, paresthesias, headache, depression, confusion, somnolence and, rarely, seizures. Hypertrichosis (increased hair growth) is another frequent side effect, mainly occurring on the face, arms, and back in up to 50% of patients. Gingival hyperplasia may also occur, and CsA may promote malignant transformation of some cell types. The use of CsA in combination with corticosteroids has permitted a lowering of the CsA dose, resulting in decreased toxicity, particularly nephrotoxicity.

### Tacrolimus

Tacrolimus was isolated from Japanese soil samples in 1984 as part of an effort to discover novel immunosuppressants. A macrolide, produced by the fungus *Streptomyces tsukubaensis*, tacrolimus was found to possess potent immunosuppressive properties.[25] Similar to CsA, it blocks the effects of NFAT, prevents cytokine transcription, and arrests T cell activation.[26] The intracellular target is an immunophilin protein distinct from cyclophilin, known as FK-binding protein (FK-BP). In vitro tacrolimus was found to be 100 times more potent in blocking IL-2 and IFN-γ production than CsA. Tacrolimus, like CsA, also increases TGF-β transcription, leading to the beneficial and toxic effects of this cytokine. The side effect profile for tacrolimus is similar to that of CsA with regard to renal toxicity but

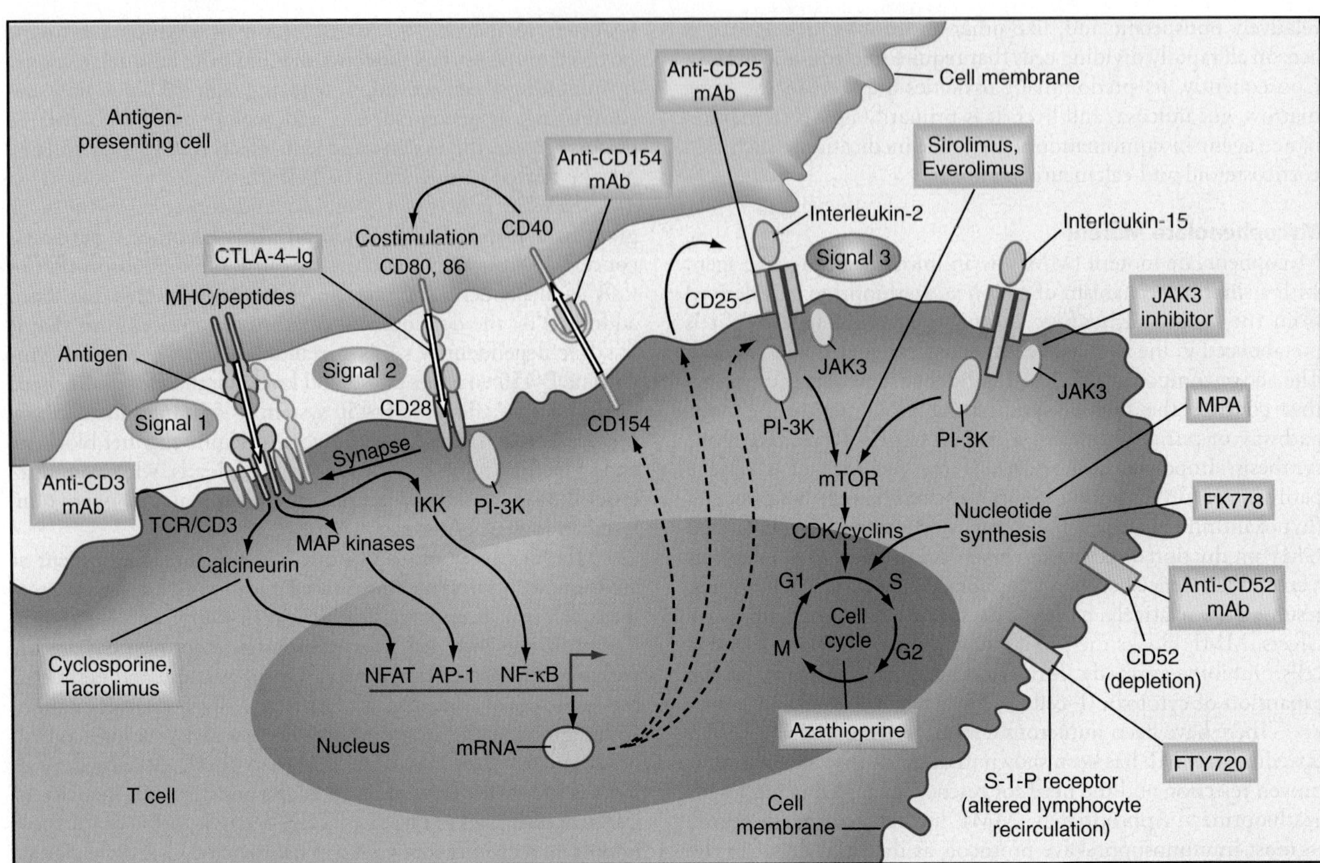


**FIGURE 26-22** Molecular mechanisms of immunosuppression. Immunosuppressants may be small molecules, antibodies, or fusion proteins that block various pathways critical for T cell activation. TCR binding facilitates kinase activity by CD3 and the coreceptors (CD4 or CD8). The costimulatory molecules CD28, CD154, and others determine the relative potency of these signals. TCR signal transduction proceeds via a calcineurin-dependent pathway, resulting in dephosphorylation of NFAT, which subsequently enters the nucleus and acts in concert with NF-κB to facilitate cytokine gene expression. IL-2 functions in an autocrine fashion, binding to the IL-2R once the high-affinity chain (CD25) is expressed, to promote cell division. Cyclosporine and tacrolimus block TCR signal transduction by inhibiting calcineurin. Sirolimus and everolimus target mTOR to block IL-2R signaling effectively. Azathioprine and MMF-MPA interrupt the cell cycle by interfering with nucleic acid metabolism. Monoclonal antibodies (e.g., OKT3, anti–IL-2R, alemtuzumab [Campath], anti-CD154) or fusion proteins (e.g., CTLA4-Ig, belatacept) function to deplete T cells or interrupt key surface interactions required for T cell function. (From Halloran PF: Immunosuppressive drugs for kidney transplantation. N Engl J Med 351:2715–2729, 2004.)

the cosmetic side effects, such as abnormal hair growth and gingival hyperplasia, are substantially reduced when compared with CsA. Neurotoxicity, including tremors and mental status changes, is more pronounced with tacrolimus as is its diabetogenic effect. Tacrolimus has been shown to be extremely effective for liver transplantation and has become the drug of choice for most centers.

## Lymphocyte Depletion Preparations

Most of the current induction regimens involve the use of some antilymphocyte antibody preparation. Their mechanism of action is probably not fully understood but involves some combination of selective or nonselective depletion and/or inactivation. They cause profound immunosuppression, placing the recipient at increased risk for opportunistic infections or lymphoma, and are consequently generally limited to short-term use, days to weeks.

### Antilymphocyte Globulin

Antilymphocyte globulin preparations are produced by immunizing another species with an inoculum of human lymphocytes, followed by collection of the sera and purification of the gamma globulin fraction. The result is a polyclonal antibody preparation that contains antibodies directed at a multitude of antigens on lymphocytes. More recently, preparations have used human thymocytes as the immunogen. The two most commonly used preparations are rabbit antithymocyte globulin (RATG) and horse antithymocyte globulin (ATGAM). RATG seems to be more effective than ATGAM at reducing the incidence of acute rejection episodes and consequently is the preferred preparation at most U.S. transplantation centers.[27] The polyclonal preparation consists of hundreds of antibodies that coat dozens of epitopes over the surface of the T cell. The result is T cell clearance through complement-mediated lysis and opsonization. In addition to simple depletion mechanisms, the antiserum also interferes with effective TCR signaling and can promote inappropriate cross linking of key cell surface molecules, including adhesion and costimulatory receptors, resulting in unresponsiveness or anergy.[28]

These preparations are used as induction agents and as rescue treatment for acute rejection episodes. Most commonly, RATG is used as part of a multidrug induction protocol that includes a calcineurin inhibitor, an antiproliferative such as MMF, and prednisone. A frequent strategy in renal transplantation is the sequential use of RATG followed by a calcineurin inhibitor to avoid the nephrotoxic effects of the calcineurin inhibitor in the early post-transplantation period, and to maximize the effects of RATG by depleting or inactivating most T cells at the critical time of graft introduction. More recently, RATG has been used as a key component of newer steroid-minimizing or calcineurin inhibitor–free regimens.[29,30]

Many of the side effects associated with RATG administration are related to its polyclonal composition. Surprisingly, only a small fraction of the known specificities are actually directed at defined T cell epitopes. One major side effect is profound thrombocytopenia secondary to platelet-specific antibodies within the polyclonal preparation. In addition to T cell depletion, leukopenia and anemia may result. Overimmunosuppression is also a concern; given that these preparations are extremely effective at T cell depletion, there is an increase in viral reactivation and primary viral infections, including cytomegalovirus (CMV), Epstein-Barr virus (EBV), herpes simplex virus (HSV), and varicella-zoster virus (VZV). The effect on EBV-specific T cells also predisposes treated patients to a higher incidence of EBV-associated lymphoid malignancies. Overall, however, the drug is well tolerated by most transplant recipients. The most common symptoms are the result of transient cytokine release following antibody binding. Chills and fevers occur in up to 20% of patients, but this cytokine release syndrome is usually treatable with antipyretics and antihistamines. In addition, this response is often tempered in patients receiving corticosteroids as part of the induction regimen.

### Muromonab-CD3

Muromonab-CD3 (OKT3), a murine monoclonal antibody directed against the human CD3 ε chain (a component of the TCR signaling complex; see Fig. 26-12), was approved by the U.S. Food and Drug Administration (FDA) in 1986. It was the first commercially available monoclonal antibody preparation for use in organ transplantation. Similar to the polyclonal preparations, there are several proposed mechanisms of action for OKT3. On binding to CD3, OKT3 triggers internalization of the TCR complex, preventing antigen recognition and subsequent signal transduction. It also labels cells for elimination via opsonization and phagocytosis. Adequate dosing is usually monitored by flow cytometry and staining for $CD3^+$ T cells in recipients' blood samples; depletion to less than 10% of baseline is considered an adequate response. Interestingly, several days after OKT3 administration, T cells reappear, as detected by $CD4^+$ or $CD8^+$ cells in the peripheral blood; however, these cells lack TCR expression and are unable to generate an antigen-specific response. OKT3 not only functions to impair naïve T cell activation, but it is also effective during acute rejection episodes by interfering with the function of primed antigen-specific T cells. OKT3 has been shown to be superior to conventional steroid therapy in reversing rejection and consequently improves allograft survival.[31]

Unfortunately, because OKT3 is a mouse antibody, it can elicit an immune response itself and the recipient will generate antimurine antibodies directed against the structural regions of the antibody or the actual binding site. The presence of antimurine antibodies limits the desired effect and eventually precludes further use of OKT3. In addition, the cytokine release syndrome associated with OKT3 administration can be vigorous; resulting in hypotension, pulmonary edema, and myocardial depression. A high dose of a steroid is often given IV as premedication prior to the first few administrations of OKT3 in an attempt to minimize adverse reactions. Subsequent dosing is less likely to result in symptoms because most target cells available for degranulation have been removed from the periphery. Because of this vigorous response and its immunogenicity, OKT3 has recently (2009) been withdrawn from production and is generally unavailable. There are newer monoclonal antibodies, chimeric or humanized, with a similar mechanism of action and specificity as OKT3; these include otelixizumab, teplizumab, and visilizumab. They are currently being investigated for the treatment of autoimmune conditions such as Crohn's disease, ulcerative colitis, and type 1 diabetes.

### Anti–Interleukin-2 Receptor Antibodies

As discussed earlier, the cytokine IL-2 plays a critical role in T cell activation and function. After antigen recognition and signal transduction via the TCR complex, expression of IL-2 and its receptor are markedly upregulated. The receptor consists of three chains, α (CD25), β (CD122), and the common cytokine receptor γ chain (CD132). These chains associate in a noncovalent manner to form the IL-2 receptor complex. The α chain, CD25, is a type I transmembrane protein responsible for the high-affinity binding of IL-2 on activated T cells; it is critical for T cell clonal expansion (see Fig. 26-22). Given its importance in the cellular response two monoclonal antibodies have been developed and are now approved for use in transplantation, daclizumab and basiliximab.[32,33] The two antibodies differ in their composition in that daclizumab is humanized and basiliximab is a mouse-human chimeric antibody. Both are directed against CD25 and function to block IL-2 binding. Because CD25 is preferentially expressed on recently activated T cells, the antibodies are semiselective in their effects, presumably only affecting T cells specific for the allograft that have been activated at the time of graft implantation. Once the T cell response is well under way, effector T cells are much less dependent on CD25 expression and these antibodies are much less effective. Therefore, both anti-CD25 antibodies are used during the induction phase only. Much like antithymocyte globulin (ATG), they have been shown to prevent or reduce the frequency of acute rejection when used in combination with the standard three-drug regimen. More recently, they have been used as part of regimens to reduce or eliminate calcineurin inhibitors or within steroid minimization protocols. Both antibodies are well tolerated clinically because they do not cause the same side effects as those seen with OKT3 or even ATG, such as the cytokine release syndrome. Unlike OKT3, both daclizumab and basiliximab are the products of genetic engineering, with the structural components of the mouse antibody having been replaced with human IgG; thus, they are less likely to invoke a neutralizing antibody response themselves.

## Other Immunoglobulin Therapies

### Rituximab

Rituximab is a murine antihuman CD20 chimeric antibody that was initially developed for the treatment of B cell lymphoma and has since been used in the treatment of post-transplantation lymphoproliferative disorder (PTLD). CD20 is a cell surface protein expressed on all mature B cells but not on plasma cells. Rituximab binds to CD20 and facilitates ADCC and complement-dependent cytotoxicity of B cells, as well as promoting programmed cell death. More recently, rituximab has been used in a wide variety of autoimmune disorders. It has also been used as a component in some investigational strategies designed as induction therapy in highly sensitized transplant recipients undergoing kidney transplantation, and even in ABO-incompatible pairings. CD20 is not expressed on antibody-producing plasma cells. As such, its role in limiting aggressive forms of rejection may relate to the role of B cells in antigen presentation.

### Alemtuzumab

Similar to rituximab, alemtuzumab was originally developed in the oncology field for the treatment of lymphoma. It is a humanized antibody against human CD52, a cell surface protein expressed on most mature lymphocytes and monocytes, but not their stem cell precursors. It has been used not only in patients with lymphoma but also for autoimmune processes, such as multiple sclerosis and rheumatoid arthritis. Administration of alemtuzumab is extremely effective at reducing the number of T cells, both in the peripheral blood and in secondary lymphoid organs. In addition, it depletes, to a lesser extent, B cells and monocytes. Unlike other strategies, this depletion may last for weeks to months after dosing. Investigational studies in transplantation using alemtuzumab as an induction agent have allowed for the minimization of immunosuppression, particularly when combined with a calcineurin inhibitor.[34,35] Its optimal use in transplantation remains to be established.

### Intravenous Immunoglobulin

IVIg is composed of pooled plasma fractions from thousands of donors and essentially contains a representative sample of all antibodies found in that population. It is used frequently in the treatment of several autoimmune diseases, such as idiopathic thrombocytopenic purpura (ITP), Guillain-Barré syndrome, and myasthenia gravis, as well as in patients with severe immunodeficiencies featuring low or absent antibody levels. IVIg is also used in organ transplantation, specifically for the treatment of humoral rejection or prior to transplantation in a highly sensitized recipient in an attempt to reduce the PRA and potential positive cross-match. More recently, it has also been used as part of ABO-incompatible protocols. IVIg likely works through several mechanisms to alter the immune response, including neutralization of circulating auto antibodies and alloantibodies via anti-idiotypic antibodies and selective downregulation of antibody production through Fc-mediated mechanisms.[36]

## Newer Immunosuppressive Agents

### Mammalian Target of Rapamycin Inhibitors

Rapamycin (sirolimus) was isolated from a soil sample taken from Easter Island, a Polynesian island also known as Rapa Nui—hence, the name Rapamycin. It is a macrolide derived from the bacterium *Streptomyces hygroscopicus,* with potent immunosuppressive properties. Everolimus is a derivative of rapamycin that possesses similar properties. Both are similar in structure to tacrolimus and bind to the same intracellular target, FK-BP, but neither agent affects calcineurin activity and consequently does not inhibit expression of NFAT or IL-2. Instead, the sirolimus–FK-BP complex inhibits the mammalian target of rapamycin (mTOR), specifically the mTOR complex 1 (see Fig. 26-22). mTOR is also called FRAP (FK-BP–rapamycin-associated protein) or RAFT (rapamycin and FK-BP target). RAFT-1 is a critical kinase involved in the IL-2 receptor signaling pathway. The result is inhibition of p70 S6 kinase activity, an enzyme essential for ribosomal phosphorylation and arrest of cell cycle progression.[37] Other receptors are also affected, including those for IL-4, IL-6, and platelet-derived growth factor (PDGF).

Both sirolimus and everolimus are potent inhibitors of rejection in experimental models. Sirolimus and tacrolimus can act synergistically to impair rejection but the combination results in intolerable toxicity, specifically calcineurin inhibitor–mediated nephrotoxicity. More often, sirolimus is used as an alternative to calcineurin inhibitors in a multidrug regimen or combined with other agents, allowing a reduction in the dose and minimizing side effects, including calcineurin inhibitor–related nephrotoxicity and steroid-specific side effects. In addition to their immunosuppressive properties, mTOR inhibitors also have been shown to have promising antitumor effects. For example, sirolimus has been shown to promote programmed cell death in B cell lymphomas and everolimus has demonstrated activity against EBV. Thus, both agents may play an important role in the prevention of PTLD. Sirolimus and everolimus have also been used in the development of drug-eluting coronary stents and to limit the rate of in-stent restenosis because of their antiproliferative properties. There is an increased incidence of hypercholesterolemia and hypertriglyceridemia with both agents that often require treatment with cholesterol-lowering agents or discontinuation of the drug. Oral ulcers, wound-healing complications (in particular, an increased incidence of lymphoceles), and elevated levels of proteinuria and thrombocytopenia remain frequent problems and limit universal application.

### Beletacept

Costimulation is a critical component of naïve T cell activation and has been extensively studied as a potential target for manipulation in organ transplantation. One of the most important pathways is the interaction between CD28 and CD80-CD86. As described earlier, signaling through CD28 allows for effective IL-2 production and promotes cell survival through the upregulation of antiapoptotic molecules. CD152 (CTLA-4) is another cell surface molecule expressed on activated T cells that is more effective in binding CD80 and CD86 than CD28. Once activated, T cells begin to express CD152, which interacts with CD80 and CD86 with a higher affinity and effectively blocks CD28 binding. CD152 then delivers an inhibitory signal to the T cell as part of a downregulatory mechanism for the immune response. A fusion protein consisting of the extracellular component of CTLA-4 and the heavy chain of human IgG1 was developed to block CD28–CD80-CD86 interactions, and consequently impairs costimulation and T cell activation (see Fig. 26-22). CTLA4-Ig (abatacept) is used clinically for several autoimmune indications, including rheumatoid arthritis and psoriasis.[38,39] Further efforts to improve the efficacy of CTLA4-Ig have resulted in a novel mutant form, LEA29Y (belatacept). LEA29Y is a second-generation CTLA4-Ig molecule that differs by two amino acid residues within the binding domain, resulting in increased affinity for CD80 and CD86. The resultant improvement in binding affinity has led to more potent immunosuppressive properties in vitro and in vivo.[40] Belatacept has since been used in preclinical nonhuman primate studies and phase III clinical trials in human renal transplantation. It has demonstrated efficacy equivalent to that of cyclosporine in renal transplant recipients receiving MMF and steroids and appears to promote superior renal function as a calcineurin inhibitor–free regimen.[41] One potential drawback is that it must be administered parenterally. Instead of a few pills every day, the patient must come into the clinic or an infusion center every few weeks for his or her maintenance therapy. This requirement to receive the drug in a health care environment may improve drug adherence.

### Fingolimod

Fingolimod (FTY720) has a unique mechanism of action that results in the sequestration of lymphocytes in lymph nodes, thereby preventing them from participating in allograft rejection or autoimmunity. It is derived from the fungus *Isaria sinclairii* and is an analogue of sphingosine. FTY720 requires phosphorylation by sphingosine kinase 2 to become active, after which it binds to a sphingosine-1-phosphate receptor, specifically S1PR1 (see Fig. 26-22). Binding of S1PR1 by FTY70-P results in aberrant internalization of the receptor. Lack of the receptor on the cell surface deprives lymphocytes of the signals necessary for egress from secondary lymphoid organs and functionally traps them within lymph nodes. Unfortunately, despite promising experimental data, FTY720 has failed to show an improvement in efficacy for the prevention of renal allograft rejection in two large phase III studies. A common side effect was self-limited bradycardia, which had been documented in earlier safety trials. The phase III trials, however, revealed a surprising decrease in renal function in the FTY720 treatment arm. Also, there were a worrisome number of patients who developed macular edema. Given that there was no documented benefit in efficacy and new, unexpected side effects had appeared, clinical trials were halted for renal transplantation. Trials have continued in autoimmune conditions, such as multiple sclerosis. A recent phase III clinical trial has suggested that FTY720 is superior to IFN-$\alpha$1a in the treatment of multiple sclerosis.[42]

### Deoxyspergualin

Deoxyspergualin (DSG; Gusperimus) is a derivative of the antitumor antibiotic spergualin, which was isolated from *Bacillus laterosporus* in 1981. DSG was found to have both antiproliferative and immunosuppressive properties. Although the mechanism of action for DSG is not completely understood, there is evidence that it mediates its effect predominantly via modulation of the APC. It prevents the nuclear translocation of NF-κB, reportedly through its interaction with the intracellular chaperones Hsp70 and Hsp90.[43] As noted earlier, NF-κB is a critical transcription factor required by a number of cell types for an optimal immune response, in particular T cell activation and survival. Similar to the effect of glucocorticoids, there is decreased transcription of IL-1 and TNF-$\alpha$ by APCs, reduction in MHC expression, and diminished costimulation. DSG has effectively prolonged allograft survival in various experimental models. Disappointingly, early clinical studies have not been as promising; for now, DSG will likely have a minor role in the field of transplantation.[35]

## Complications of Immunosuppression

The development of immunosuppressive agents was the key step in the advancement of the field of transplantation, but these same agents are also responsible for much of the morbidity associated with organ transplantation. All current immunosuppressants function to a greater or lesser degree in a nonspecific fashion—that is, global immunosuppression instead of donor-specific or allospecific immunosuppression. The consequence is occasional overzealous suppression of the immune system, resulting in infectious complications, primarily viral infections, and an increased risk of malignancy. Also, many of these agents modify the function of proteins and pathways required for normal cell function and their inhibition consequently results in undesired, nonimmune side effects, including direct organ injury.

### Risk of Infection

There is a fine balance between sufficient immunosuppression to prevent rejection and preservation of the host response to nontransplantation antigens and pathogens. Introduction of tissue from one individual to another always allows for the potential transfer of a new organism. Currently, an extensive battery of testing is performed on the donor and recipient prior to transplantation. These examinations have greatly decreased the potential exposure to the recipient but no test is perfect, and testing can be limited by available technology and the time interval between explant and implant. Some infections may still be transferred unknowingly for various reasons, including early infection and lack of seropositivity. Infections may be donor-derived, such as a CMV-positive organ placed into a CMV-negative recipient, or may arise from less commonly transferred viruses, resulting in primary infections of human immunodeficiency virus (HIV), hepatitis C or B virus (HCV or HBV), tuberculosis, *Trypanosoma cruzi,* West Nile virus, lymphocytic choriomeningitis virus, or rabies.[44]

The threat comes not only from exposure to new pathogens but, more importantly, from those to which the recipient has likely already been exposed and harbors in a dormant state. Normally, these pathogens are controlled after the initial infection and remain quiescent. After the immune system is rendered impotent by pharmacologic suppression, these pathogens can be reactivated and quickly become uncontrollable. Recipient-derived infections are more common after transplantation than donor-derived infections. One common example is CMV reactivation. Most people have been exposed to CMV at some point in their lives. On transplantation and induction immunosuppressive therapy, CMV reactivation can occur, resulting in pneumonitis, hepatitis, pancreatitis, or colitis. CMV has also been implicated in the lesions of heart transplant recipients with chronic rejection, highlighting the interplay between the immune response and chronic viral infections or the inflammation they may induce. Other recipient-derived infections include tuberculosis, certain parasites (e.g., *Strongyloides stercoralis, T. cruzi*), viruses (e.g., CMV, EBV, HSV, VZV, HBV, HCV, and HIV), and endemic fungi (e.g., *Pneumocystis jiroveci,*

*Histoplasma capsulatam, Coccidioides immitis,* and *Paracoccidioides brasiliensis*).

Fortunately, patterns of opportunistic infections after transplantation have been altered by the use of routine antimicrobial prophylaxis. The risk for reactivation is highest approximately 6 to 12 weeks after transplantation and again after periods of increased immunosuppression for acute rejection episodes. Transplantation programs use various prophylactic regimens, depending on the organs transplanted. Many regimens include pneumococcal vaccine, hepatitis B vaccine, trimethoprim-sulfamethoxazole for *Pneumocystis* pneumonia and urinary tract infections, ganciclovir or valganciclovir for CMV, and clotrimazole troche or nystatin for oral and esophageal fungal infections. As immunosuppressive strategies have evolved, causing increases in allograft and patient survival, the specific pathogens and pattern of infection have also evolved. For example, the polyomaviruses BK and JC have recently been recognized to play a more important role in transplantation than previously understood. Infection with BK has been found in association with a progressive nephropathy and ureteral obstruction, and the JC virus has been associated with progressive multifocal leukoencephalopathy. Detection of BK viral DNA in blood and urine has been useful for monitoring response to therapy, which includes minimizing immunosuppression and treatment with antiviral therapies.

### Risk for Malignancy

The immune system not only plays a critical role in defending the host against attack from pathogens, it also plays an important role in the surveillance and detection of cancer, particularly those driven by viral infection. The consequence is an almost 10-fold increase in malignancy rates. Skin cancers, particularly squamous cell cancers, are the most common malignant conditions in transplant recipients and account for substantial morbidity and mortality.[45] As expected, virally mediated tumors tend to occur more frequently in transplant recipients. For example, human papillomavirus is associated with cancer of the cervix, HBV and HCV with hepatocellular carcinoma, and human herpesvirus 8 with Kaposi's sarcoma. EBV, in particular, can be associated with the development of PTLD, a broad term used to describe EBV-associated lymphomas that occur in transplant recipients. PTLD varies from asymptomatic to life- threatening; accordingly, treatment varies from simple reduction or withdrawal of immunosuppression to vigorous chemotherapeutic regimens. More recently, patients have been treated with antiviral agents targeting EBV or even chemotherapy, including antibody therapy against the tumor cells, such as rituximab.

### Nonimmune Side Effects

Although current immunosuppressants have become increasingly more specific, they are generally still directed at pathways that play an important role in systems other than immunity. Thus, inhibition of a pathway for the sake of immunosuppression can also lead to unintended consequences if the target is critical to other processes. For example, calcineurin inhibitors are potent suppressors of T cell activation but their activity not only decreases IL-2 transcription, but also increases TGF-β expression. Elevated levels of TGF-β result in an increase in endothelin expression and eventually lead to hypertension. In addition, TGF-β may play a critical role in the development of chronic allograft nephropathy, previously thought to be immune-mediated but now likely to be at least partly secondary to nonimmune side effects secondary to calcineurin inhibitor use.

Histologic evidence of calcineurin inhibitor–associated nephrotoxicity is essentially universal in renal transplants by 10 years. Furthermore, these deleterious effects are not limited only to renal transplant recipients. The incidence of chronic renal failure in nonrenal transplant recipients is an astonishing 16.5%.[46] New-onset diabetes post-transplantation is also an important problem, particularly in those receiving tacrolimus or steroids. The incidence of new-onset immunosuppressive-related diabetes mellitus approaches 30% in the first 2 years following renal transplantation, conferring a significantly higher risk of death. In addition to renal failure, hypertension, and diabetes, immunosuppressive therapy can also lead to hyperlipidemia, anemia, and accelerated cardiovascular disease, which is a leading cause of death in long-term transplantation survivors. Thus, it appears that the very reagents that ushered in a new era of success in organ transplantation have proven to be major contributors in the demise of the transplanted organ and/or recipient. Clearly, there is a pressing clinical need to develop novel immunosuppressive agents that are more specific yet less toxic, or to devise strategies to induce immune tolerance so that long-term immunosuppression may eventually be eliminated altogether.

## TOLERANCE

Immunologic tolerance has been thought of as the holy grail of transplantation biology. Self-tolerance (see earlier) involves regulation of the immune response to prevent undesired effects toward host tissues or proteins. This is established and maintained through central (i.e., thymic selection and deletion) and peripheral mechanisms. The ability to inactive the host response selectively toward only the transplanted donor antigens while maintaining immunocompetence would be highly desirable. This would avoid the need for lifelong immunosuppression, with its associated toxicities, and would eliminate chronic rejection, the major cause of late graft failure.

It has been more than 50 years since the first reports of acquired tolerance. The discovery of neonatal transplant tolerance has been credited to Ray Owen, a geneticist who studied the inheritance of red blood cell antigens in cattle. In 1945, he reported that dizygotic twins had mixtures of their own cells and their twin partner cells. Earlier observations had demonstrated that bovine dizygotic twins develop a fusion of their placentas during embryonic life. This results in a common intrauterine circulation and the unabated passage of sex hormones, explaining the phenomenon of freemartin cattle. Owen also recognized that this common circulation allows for the exchange of hematopoietic cells during embryonic life and the establishment of a chimeric state. Interestingly, these calves do not develop isoantibodies to their twin, suggesting a state of immunologic tolerance.

Peter Medawar acknowledged the importance of Owen's observation and predicted that an exchange of skin grafts between dizygotic calves could verify the tolerance hypothesis. Together with his postdoctoral fellow, Rupert Billingham, he performed a series of grafting experiments that provided direct support for the concept of neonatally acquired transplant tolerance. Subsequent experiments by Billingham, Leslie Brent, and Medawar demonstrated that neonatally acquired transplant tolerance could be achieved in mice by the inoculation of embryos or IV injection of newborn mice with allogeneic cells. Medawar shared the Nobel Prize in Medicine in 1960 for the discovery of acquired immunologic tolerance.

Just as there are a number of methods to provide for self-tolerance in any given individual, there have been many strategies proposed to induce transplantation tolerance exploiting these pathways. These include clonal deletion or elimination of donor-reactive cells, clonal anergy–functional inactivation of donor-reactive cells, and regulation or suppression of donor-reactive cells. There are rare reports in which patients have discontinued immunosuppression for various reasons and have not experienced rejection. Ongoing studies in this small patient population have sought to determine which mechanisms are responsible for graft maintenance in the absence of immunosuppression. There are numerous reports of tolerance in experimental models but most of these have not been substantiated when translated to higher animal models, such as nonhuman primates. Although there are several exciting avenues of research and even clinical trials in humans, there is currently no proven regimen to induce transplantation tolerance that would be widely applicable. Discussed here are some strategies of particular interest that are now under investigation.[47]

## T Cell Ablation

Most currently used immunosuppressive regimens involve the use of induction therapy. Many rely on some form of antilymphocyte preparation, usually RATG, to eliminate or inactivate recipient cells at the time of transplantation. They are used in the very early post- transplantation period, which corresponds to when ischemia and reperfusion of the graft, accompanied by the surgical trauma, significantly increase immune recognition. These preparations successfully remove T cells from the circulation for several days and those that are present remain anergic for some time. Use of these agents has significantly reduced the rate of acute rejection and allowed for minimization of immunosuppression in several different protocols. Even more effective depleting agents have been tested in nonhuman primate models in attempts to reset the T cell repertoire and induce tolerance to the allograft. A T cell–specific immunotoxin was developed that results in almost complete depletion of all recipient T cells. Reconstitution does not occur for approximately 1 month. In this model, approximately 50% of the animals developed tolerance following pretransplantation T cell depletion. There was no rejection and the emerging T cell repertoire displayed donor-specific hyporesponsiveness, with preserved responses to third parties.

Based on these studies, a number of groups have undertaken clinical trials using early recipient T cell depletion. Several studies have used alemtuzumab to induce profound T cell depletion. Despite achieving depletion equivalent to that obtained using anti–CD3 immunotoxin with respect to kinetics, magnitude, and effectiveness in the secondary lymphoid tissues, treatment with alemtuzumab alone or in combination with deoxyspergualin is not sufficient to induce tolerance in adult humans.[35] The failure of these T cell–centric approaches suggests that other components of the immune system, such as B cells, NK cells, or monocytes, may need to be specifically targeted to achieve tolerance. Although depletion alone has not been able to establish tolerance, it has allowed for minimization of immunosuppression to single-agent monotherapy in some cases and likely facilitates other protolerant approaches.

## Costimulation Blockade

As noted earlier, T cell activation requires not only interaction between the TCR complex and MHC-bound peptide but also sufficient costimulatory signals to promote a successful response. TCR ligation in the absence of appropriate costimulation results in T cell inactivation or anergy. This mechanism is used presumably as a mechanism of peripheral tolerance to control any aberrant, self-reactive T cells that may have escaped the thymic selection process. Researchers have tried to exploit this through the development of antibodies or fusion proteins designed to block these costimulatory interactions. Interruption of costimulatory pathways at the time of transplantation should thus selectively inactivate or anergize only those cells specific for donor antigen, leaving nonreactive cells unaffected. Preexisting immunity and innate responses should be unaffected by this approach. There are a number of animal models of transplantation in which this has proven to be the case, particularly with the simultaneous blockade of the CD28 and CD40 pathways. This approach in rodents and primates has resulted in prolonged survival of cardiac and renal allografts, without the need for any subsequent immunosuppression and with no infectious or malignant side effects. The extrapolation of these results to clinical practice has so far been disappointing. In the only human tolerance trial of costimulation blockade, hu5C8, a humanized anti-CD154 monoclonal antibody demonstrated limited efficacy and was associated with potential thromboembolic toxicity. As noted, newly developed agents that block the CD28 pathway are now being tested as maintenance agents, which may pave the way for their use in future tolerance trials.

## Mixed Chimerism

Mixed hematopoietic chimerism is associated with a particularly robust form of donor-specific tolerance. This approach involves central and peripheral mechanisms for induction and maintenance of tolerance. Mixed chimerism refers to a recipient who possesses self- and donor-derived hematopoietic cells after bone marrow transplantation. Similar to the normal physiologic process, donor marrow elements migrate to the thymus and participate in thymic selection, resulting in the central deletion of potentially donor-reactive T cells. Presumably, similar events occur within the bone marrow for B cell selection. The peripheral compartment can be pharmacologically deleted in a nonspecific fashion at the time of transplantation or, alternatively, donor antigen delivered at the time of bone marrow infusion engages donor-reactive cells in the absence of appropriate costimulation. This results in peripheral deletion, anergy, or regulation, resulting in donor-specific nonresponsiveness.

In humans, successful bone marrow transplantation allows for the acceptance of subsequent organ allografts from the same donor in the absence of immunosuppression. Conventional bone marrow transplantation regimens, however, are typically myeloablative in nature and the associated toxicities are too great to use as part of a solid organ tolerance trial. Newer advances in nonmyeloablative techniques with less toxicity have since led to the clinical application and testing of mixed chimerism-based strategies. An initial trial to test the efficacy of a mixed chimerism strategy to induce tolerance was performed in highly selected patients suffering from end-stage renal failure and multiple myeloma. These patients simultaneously received bone marrow and a kidney from an HLA-identical sibling. The regimen led to chimerism in all six patients; four had transient chimerism and the remaining two progressed into full chimeras. Three patients remain operationally tolerant without any immunosuppression after a reported follow-up of up to 7 years. Recently, the same group of investigators reported on a similar protocol in haploidentical living-related donor-recipient pairs, which resulted in the successful induction of transient chimerism and tolerance. None of these patients possessed concomitant indications for bone marrow transplantation, such as multiple myeloma, as was the case in the first trial. One allograft was lost to irreversible humoral rejection but, remarkably, the other four recipients have sustained stable renal allograft function for up to 5 years after complete withdrawal of immunosuppressive drugs. The conditioning regimen required resulted in profound T, B, and NK cell depletion and substantial myelosuppression, leading to severe leukopenia and capillary leak syndrome. Interestingly, the biologic phenomenon that inspired the protocol, mixed chimerism, was not achieved in any patient, suggesting that the predominant effect is one of intensive induction. Although there is still a significant need to develop regimens to induce transplantation tolerance, this effort will have to be balanced with the exceptional patient and allograft outcomes presently available with current immunosuppressive therapies.

## XENOTRANSPLANTATION

The most pressing problem in clinical transplantation is the shortage of organs available. More than 100,000 individuals are currently listed and are awaiting organ transplantation. Many more individuals could benefit from transplantation but, given the shortage of organs, are not currently considered. Those that are placed on the transplantation list must often wait a long time before an organ becomes available, during which their clinical status can deteriorate, diminishing their ability to withstand surgery. An alternative source of organs could be from another species, a process known as xenotransplantation. In addition to increasing the supply of available organs, xenotransplantation also offers some of the same benefits realized with living donors, such as decreased ischemic time and injury and optimization of the recipient's health status. There are potential novel disadvantages with xenotransplantation, such as zoonotic viral transmission. Xenografts may be concordant and discordant, depending on the proximity of the particular species in evolution to humans. This proximity markedly influences the immune response and the implications are discussed here.

### Concordant Xenografts

Concordant xenografts refer to transplants between closely related species; for humans, these include Old World monkeys and apes. The critical element defining an animal as concordant is the assembly of carbohydrate antigens on the cell surface. Similar to humans, concordant species lack galactosyl transferase and, as a result, their carbohydrates are the typical blood group antigens that lack the N-linked disaccharide galactose-α-1,3-galactose (α-Gal). Thus, the natural antibodies present in the circulation of potential human recipients can be predicted by straightforward blood group typing, thereby avoiding the problem of hyperacute rejection. Even though hyperacute rejection is not a threat, the typical mechanisms of graft rejection remain, including acute cellular rejection, acute vascular rejection and, presumably, chronic rejection. Surprisingly, most of the critical molecular elements responsible for antigen presentation and T cell–mediated rejection are evolutionarily conserved in mammals. That is, MHC molecules, adhesion proteins, and costimulatory molecules are similar across species and are adequate for immune function. Consequently, concordant xenografts undergo cellular and humoral rejection in a similar fashion as would a totally MHC mismatched allograft in the absence of immunosuppression.

Several experimental models of concordant xenograft transplantation, as well as occasional ventures into the clinical arena, have clearly demonstrated that concordant xenotransplantation is feasible. The most famous case occurred almost 25 years ago, when clinicians transplanted a baboon heart into an infant born with hypoplastic heart syndrome. The child survived for 20 days after transplantation before eventually succumbing to primarily humoral-mediated rejection.[48] This foray into the realm of clinical xenotransplantation highlighted the ethical issues associated with primate to human transplantation. Widespread application of concordant xenografts would quickly deplete the supply of nonhuman primates, particularly when a loss rate extrapolated from poorly matched allografts is taken into consideration. In addition, there is significant concern that zoonotic transfer of disease—in particular, retroviral transmission—will put the patient and public at undue risk. Given these factors, it is unlikely that concordant xenotransplantation will ever gain widespread application.

### Discordant Xenografts

As noted, transplant concordance among species is predominantly determined based on the expression of the enzyme galactosyl transferase. This enzyme is responsible for differential expression of carbohydrate moieties on the cell surface on discordant species, primarily α-Gal expression. When considering human recipients, discordant xenograft donors would include New World monkeys and other mammals but, for physiologic concerns (e.g., organ size, availability), pigs would be the preferred animal donor. When organs from discordant species are transplanted into humans, they rapidly undergo hyperacute rejection. The primary mechanism relies on the presence of preformed IgM antibodies against cell surface carbohydrate moieties, particularly α-Gal. These so-called natural antibodies are similar to those antibodies that define the blood group antigens. On transplantation, they bind to the endothelial cells on the donor organ and, in concert with complement, precipitate an irreversible reaction of cell damage, thrombosis, and immediate graft failure. As with concordant xenografts, the remainder of the acquired and innate immune responses may also play an important role in the rejection process.

Despite the aggressive immune response elicited by discordant xenograft transplantation, enthusiasm and research continues toward establishing a xenogeneic source of donor organs. Several groups have now developed transgenic pigs that express human complement regulator proteins such as CD59, CD55 (DAF, decay-accelerating factor), and membrane cofactor protein. Other groups have developed α-1,3-galactosyltransferase knockout animals, which would eliminate the expression of α-Gal, removing the major target of complement activation. Baboons transplanted with hearts from DAF transgenic pigs enjoy prolonged survival when compared with control pig donors. With additional treatments, including conventional immunosuppression, anti-C5 monoclonal antibody, cobra venom factor, and soluble complement receptor type 1, hyperacute rejection can be prevented and survival can be extended from minutes to weeks. Although there are significant barriers before clinical application, genetic engineering may conceivably allow for an endless supply of made to order organs.

## NEW AREAS OF TRANSPLANTATION

### Islet Cell Transplantation

The concept of islet cell transplantation to treat diabetes is not new, but reliable reversal of diabetes after islet transplantation is a relatively recent accomplishment. Techniques for islet isolation underwent refinement for most of the latter half of the 20th century. Clinical application of this technique, however, was largely hampered by the lack of efficient isolation techniques and immunosuppressive regimens that included diabetogenic drugs such as steroids, which promoted diabetes themselves and resulted in poor outcomes (≈10% of recipients became insulin-independent after transplantation). In 2000, a group from Edmonton, Alberta, demonstrated successful, consistent insulin independence after islet transplantation. The principal change was the development of a steroid-free immunosuppressive protocol, which included low-dose tacrolimus, sirolimus, and daclizumab.

The initial report ignited incredible enthusiasm within the diabetes community, but this early optimism has since been tempered by less promising long-term results. In a subsequent multicenter trial, less than half of 36 patients achieved insulin independence 1 year after transplantation and those who initially did achieve independence lost it over time. In addition to the questions of long-term efficacy, islet transplantation is associated with substantial costs and there are questions about its safety and ultimate usefulness. Despite these setbacks, there is tremendous promise for the field of islet transplantation, including research focusing on ex vivo islet expansion, including the use of stem cells, newer and more effective but less toxic immunosuppressive protocols, tolerance regimens, and xenotransplantation.

### Composite Tissue Transplantation

Composite tissue transplantation involves the transfer of a number of tissue types within one graft, including skin, fat, muscle, nerves, blood vessels, tendon, and bone. Annually, there are millions of patients with lost limbs or extensive soft tissue injuries who could benefit from reconstruction with composite tissue transfer. Several of these cases have been highlighted in the media over the last few years and the ethical debate over non–lifesaving transplantation has generated extensive discussion. The first successful hand transplantation was performed in Lyon, France, in 1998 and since then a total of 40 hands have been transplanted on 32 patients worldwide. Many have recovered remarkable levels of function, including being able to tie shoes, dial a cell phone, turn a door knob, and throw a ball, as well as sensitivity to hot and cold. Unfortunately, some patients have required amputation of the transplanted hand(s) after uncontrolled rejection, most of which has been attributed to noncompliance. Shortly after the early reports of hand transplantation, there have been numerous descriptions of other successful composite tissue allografts, including larynx, trachea,[49] and, more recently, face.[50]

The first successful face composite allograft was reported by a group of surgeons from France in 2005. Not long after, in 2008, the first near-total human face transplantation in the United States was performed on a patient with severe midface trauma after a gunshot wound. In contrast to her condition prior to transplantation, after the surgery she was able to breathe through her nose, smell, taste, speak intelligibly, eat solid foods, and drink from a cup (Fig. 26-23).[50] Unlike traditional solid organ transplantation, many cases of composite tissue transplantation provoke ethical, economic, and clinical dilemmas. Some have argued that subjecting recipients to the risks of surgery and lifelong immunosuppression for a non–life-sustaining transplant may not be appropriate. Nevertheless, these transplants can totally transform the life of a severely disabled or disfigured patient, improving form and function. With the advent of increasingly less toxic immunosuppressants and possible tolerance strategies, composite tissue transplantation will be become an ever-increasing part of standard clinical treatment.

## CONCLUSION

More than 50 years have passed since the first successful solid organ transplant. Today, thousands of patients with end-stage diseases undergo lifesaving transplantation each year. The concept of replacing a diseased organ with a healthy one is simple in concept, yet the details of managing the rejection response can become complex. The immune system typically generates a highly organized but regulated response when challenged. Many of the principal details of the normal immune response were described by researchers who were examining the mechanisms of allograft rejection. In fact, many surgeons earned a Nobel Prize in Medicine for their significant contributions to the field.

Although short-term allograft survival rates have steadily improved, there are still many issues that could be improved. The availability of adequate donor organs remains the most pressing issue, restricting most potential recipients from receiving a life-sustaining transplant. There continues to be progress in xenotransplantation and tissue engineering; this may provide for an unlimited supply of safe transplantable organs. As noted, there are significant drawbacks to nonselective immunosuppressive therapy, including increased risk of infections and malignancy, economic constraints, and long-term effects (e.g., renal insufficiency, diabetes, hyperlipidemia, cardiovascular disease). Targeted immunosuppressive agents continue to be developed and tested. Ultimately, the goal would be risk-free, donor-specific immunosuppression. The development of a safe, widely applicable regimen that produces transplant tolerance reliably would eliminate many problems currently associated with organ transplantation. The infancy and growth of organ transplantation are one of the medical miracles of the last century. Challenges remain, but transplantation surgeons and scientists will undoubtedly be at the forefront of discovery and innovation as we move forward.

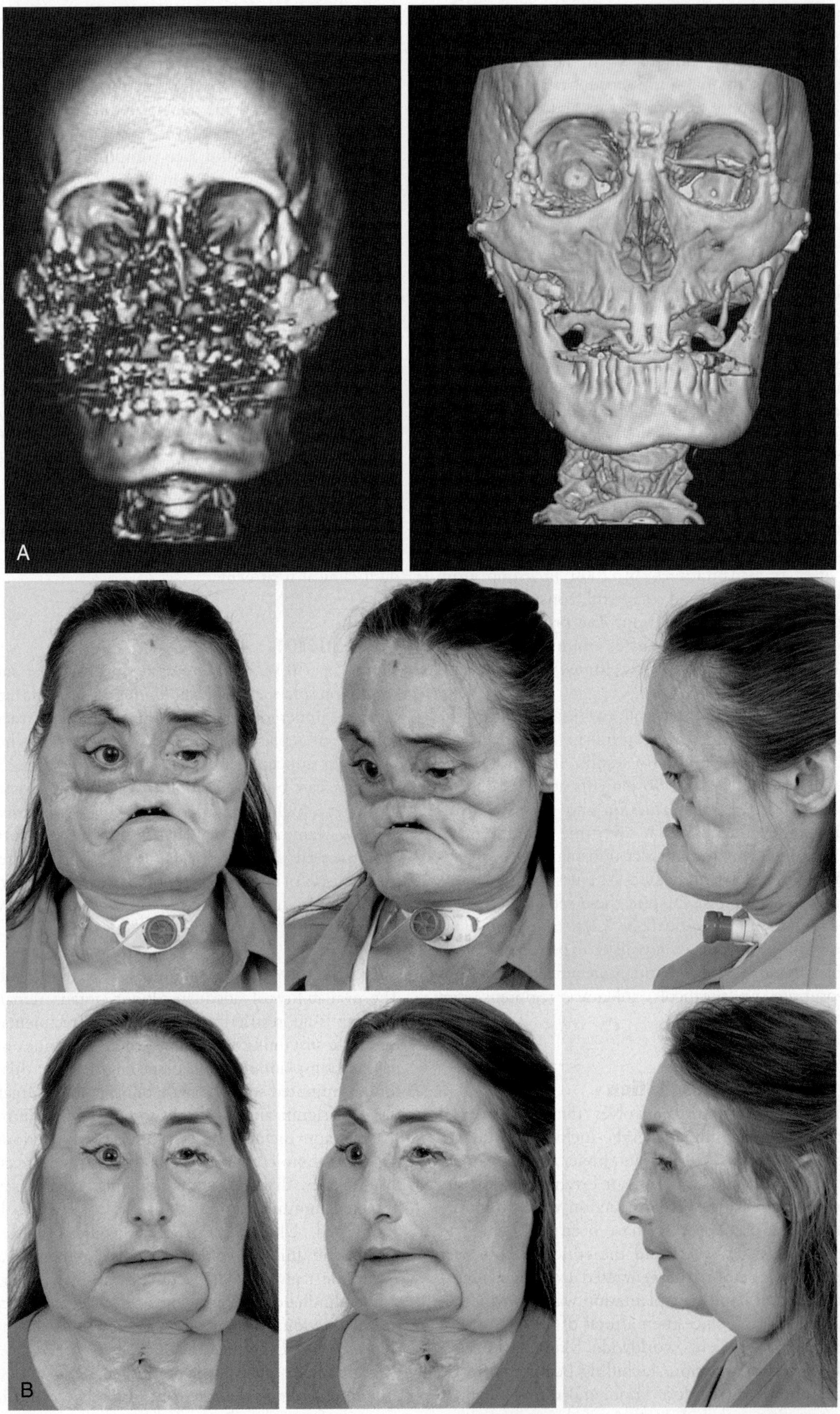

**FIGURE 26-23** Human face transplantation. **A,** CT scan of recipient before and 3 months after near-total face transplantation. **B,** Profiles of recipient before and 6 months after reconstruction. (From Siemionow M, Papay F, Alam D, et al: Near-total human face transplantation for a severely disfigured patient in the USA. Lancet 374:203–209, 2009.)

## SELECTED REFERENCES

Abbas AK, Lichtman AH, Pillai S: Cellular and molecular immunology, ed 6, Philadelphia, 2010, Saunders/Elsevier.

Concise, well developed textbook of immunology.

Brent L: A history of transplantation immunology, San Diego, 1997, Academic Press.

An interesting historical prospective on the development of transplantation immunology.

Fishman JA: Infection in solid-organ transplant recipients. N Engl J Med 357:2601–2614, 2007.

Insightful review of infection in transplantation.

Halloran PF: Immunosuppressive drugs for kidney transplantation. N Engl J Med 351:2715–2729, 2004.

Excellent overview of clinical transplantation and immunosuppression.

Kirk AD: Induction immunosuppression. Transplantation 82:593–602, 2006.

Review of induction immunosuppression, including an analysis of important clinical trials.

Newell KA, Larsen CP, Kirk AD: Transplant tolerance: Converging on a moving target. Transplantation 81:1–6, 2006.

Review of the current concepts of transplantation tolerance.

## REFERENCES

1. Carrel A: Landmark article, Nov 14, 1908: Results of the transplantation of blood vessels, organs and limbs. JAMA 250: 944–953, 1983.
2. Billingham RE, Brent L, Medawar PB: Actively acquired tolerance of foreign cells. Nature 172:603–606, 1953.
3. Murray JE, Lang S, Miller BF: Observations on the natural history of renal homotransplants in dogs. Surg Forum 5:241–244, 1955.
4. Dempsey PW, Allison ME, Akkaraju S, et al: C3d of complement as a molecular adjuvant: Bridging innate and acquired immunity. Science 271:348–350, 1996.
5. Campbell RD, Trowsdale J: Map of the human MHC. Immunol Today 14:349–352, 1993.
6. Parham P, Ohta T: Population biology of antigen presentation by MHC class I molecules. Science 272:67–74, 1996.
7. Bjorkman PJ, Saper MA, Samraoui B, et al: Structure of the human class I histocompatibility antigen, HLA-A2. Nature 329: 506–512, 1987.
8. Bevan MJ: Cross-priming. Nat Immunol 7:363–365, 2006.
9. Brown JH, Jardetzky TS, Gorga JC, et al: Three-dimensional structure of the human class II histocompatibility antigen HLA-DR1. Nature 364:33–39, 1993.
10. Teyton L, O'Sullivan D, Dickson PW, et al: Invariant chain distinguishes between the exogenous and endogenous antigen presentation pathways. Nature 348:39–44, 1990.
11. Davis MM, Bjorkman PJ: T-cell antigen receptor genes and T-cell recognition. Nature 334:395–402, 1988.
12. Kappler JW, Roehm N, Marrack P: T cell tolerance by clonal elimination in the thymus. Cell 49:273–280, 1987.
13. Viola A, Lanzavecchia A: T cell activation determined by T cell receptor number and tunable thresholds. Science 273:104–106, 1996.
14. Chambers CA, Allison JP: Co-stimulation in T cell responses. Curr Opin Immunol 9:396–404, 1997.
15. Larsen CP, Pearson TC: The CD40 pathway in allograft rejection, acceptance, and tolerance. Curr Opin Immunol 9:641–647, 1997.
16. Schwartz RH: A cell culture model for T lymphocyte clonal anergy. Science 248:1349–1356, 1990.
17. Wood KJ, Sakaguchi S: Regulatory T cells in transplantation tolerance. Nat Rev Immunol 3:199–210, 2003.
18. Gloor JM, DeGoey SR, Pineda AA, et al: Overcoming a positive crossmatch in living-donor kidney transplantation. Am J Transplant 3:1017–1023, 2003.
19. Gourishankar S, Halloran PF: Late deterioration of organ transplants: A problem in injury and homeostasis. Curr Opin Immunol 14:576–583, 2002.
20. Rhen T, Cidlowski JA: Antiinflammatory action of glucocorticoids—new mechanisms for old drugs. N Engl J Med 353:1711–1723, 2005.
21. Calne RY, Murray JE: Inhibition of the rejection of renal homografts in dogs by Burroughs Wellcome 57-322. Surg Forum 12:118–120, 1961.
22. Sollinger HW: Mycophenolate mofetil for the prevention of acute rejection in primary cadaveric renal allograft recipients. U.S. Renal Transplant Mycophenolate Mofetil Study Group. Transplantation 60:225–232, 1995.
23. Borel JF, Feurer C, Gubler HU, et al: Biological effects of cyclosporin A: A new antilymphocytic agent. Agents Actions 6:468–475, 1976.
24. Kirk AD, Jacobson LM, Heisey DM, et al: Posttransplant diastolic hypertension: associations with intragraft transforming growth factor-beta, endothelin, and renin transcription. Transplantation 64:1716–1720, 1997.
25. Kino T, Hatanaka H, Miyata S, et al: FK-506, a novel immunosuppressant isolated from a Streptomyces. II. Immunosuppressive effect of FK-506 in vitro. J Antibiot (Tokyo) 40:1256–1265, 1987.
26. Fruman DA, Klee CB, Bierer BE, et al: Calcineurin phosphatase activity in T lymphocytes is inhibited by FK 506 and cyclosporin A. Proc Natl Acad Sci U S A 89:3686–3690, 1992.
27. Hardinger KL, Rhee S, Buchanan P, et al: A prospective, randomized, double-blinded comparison of thymoglobulin versus Atgam for induction immunosuppressive therapy: 10-year results. Transplantation 86:947–952, 2008.
28. Merion RM, Howell T, Bromberg JS: Partial T-cell activation and anergy induction by polyclonal antithymocyte globulin. Transplantation 65:1481–1489, 1998.
29. Swanson SJ, Hale DA, Mannon RB, et al: Kidney transplantation with rabbit antithymocyte globulin induction and sirolimus monotherapy. Lancet 360:1662–1664, 2002.
30. Matas AJ, Kandaswamy R, Gillingham KJ, et al: Prednisone-free maintenance immunosuppression—a 5-year experience. Am J Transplant 5:2473–2478, 2005.
31. Ortho Multicenter Transplant Study Group: A randomized clinical trial of OKT3 monoclonal antibody for acute rejection

of cadaveric renal transplants. N Engl J Med 313:337–342, 1985.

**32.** Vincenti F, Kirkman R, Light S, et al: Interleukin-2-receptor blockade with daclizumab to prevent acute rejection in renal transplantation. Daclizumab Triple Therapy Study Group. N Engl J Med 338:161–165, 1998.

**33.** Nashan B, Moore R, Amlot P, et al: Randomised trial of basiliximab versus placebo for control of acute cellular rejection in renal allograft recipients. CHIB 201 International Study Group. Lancet 350:1193–1198, 1997.

**34.** Calne R, Friend P, Moffatt S, et al: Prope tolerance, perioperative campath 1H, and low-dose cyclosporin monotherapy in renal allograft recipients. Lancet 351:1701–1702, 1998.

**35.** Kirk AD, Hale DA, Mannon RB, et al: Results from a human renal allograft tolerance trial evaluating the humanized CD52-specific monoclonal antibody alemtuzumab (CAMPATH-1H). Transplantation 76:120–129, 2003.

**36.** Samuelsson A, Towers TL, Ravetch JV: Anti-inflammatory activity of IVIg mediated through the inhibitory Fc receptor. Science 291:484–486, 2001.

**37.** Kuo CJ, Chung J, Fiorentino DF, et al: Rapamycin selectively inhibits interleukin-2 activation of p70 S6 kinase. Nature 358:70–73, 1992.

**38.** Kremer JM, Westhovens R, Leon M, et al: Treatment of rheumatoid arthritis by selective inhibition of T-cell activation with fusion protein CTLA4Ig. N Engl J Med 349:1907–1915, 2003.

**39.** Abrams JR, Lebwohl MG, Guzzo CA, et al: CTLA4Ig-mediated blockade of T-cell costimulation in patients with psoriasis vulgaris. J Clin Invest 103:1243–1252, 1999.

**40.** Larsen CP, Pearson TC, Adams AB, et al: Rational development of LEA29Y (belatacept), a high-affinity variant of CTLA4-Ig with potent immunosuppressive properties. Am J Transplant 5:443–453, 2005.

**41.** Vincenti F, Larsen C, Durrbach A, et al: Costimulation blockade with belatacept in renal transplantation. N Engl J Med 353:770–781, 2005.

**42.** Cohen JA, Barkhof F, Comi G, et al: Oral fingolimod or intramuscular interferon for relapsing multiple sclerosis. N Engl J Med 362:402–415, 2010.

**43.** Nadler SG, Tepper MA, Schacter B, et al: Interaction of the immunosuppressant deoxyspergualin with a member of the Hsp70 family of heat shock proteins. Science 258:484–486, 1992.

**44.** Fishman JA: Infection in solid-organ transplant recipients. N Engl J Med 357:2601–2614, 2007.

**45.** Euvrard S, Kanitakis J, Claudy A: Skin cancers after organ transplantation. N Engl J Med 348:1681–1691, 2003.

**46.** Ojo AO, Held PJ, Port FK, et al: Chronic renal failure after transplantation of a nonrenal organ. N Engl J Med 349:931–940, 2003.

**47.** Newell KA, Larsen CP, Kirk AD: Transplant tolerance: Converging on a moving target. Transplantation 81:1–6, 2006.

**48.** Bailey LL, Nehlsen-Cannarella SL, Concepcion W, et al: Baboon-to-human cardiac xenotransplantation in a neonate. JAMA 254: 3321–3329, 1985.

**49.** Delaere P, Vranckx J, Verleden G, et al: Tracheal allotransplantation after withdrawal of immunosuppressive therapy. N Engl J Med 362:138–145, 2010.

**50.** Siemionow M, Papay F, Alam D, et al: Near-total human face transplantation for a severely disfigured patient in the USA. Lancet 374:203–209, 2009.

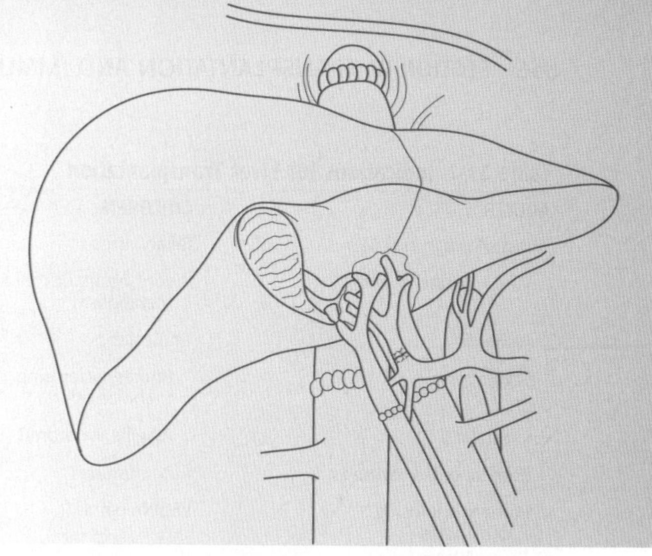

CHAPTER 27

# LIVER TRANSPLANTATION

Nancy L. Ascher



## HISTORY

The ability to replace the human liver successfully reflects the rich history of transplantation. Transplantation moved beyond the exchange of skin and tissue with the development of vascular techniques. Sewing blood vessels together, as described by Alexis Carrel at the outset of the 20th century, made it possible for researchers to implant whole organs for the first time. This development set the stage for the implantation of organs into humans.

The kidney was the first organ in which transplantation was attempted. Lack of dialysis provided the need and the production of urine was an immediate visible marker of transplantation success. Work was undertaken for the other solid organs, but the technical aspects were more challenging than for kidney transplantation. Early progress in kidney transplantation was related to the technical ease of the kidney transplantation surgery compared with that of others; the immunologic problems hampered progress until the development of the immunosuppressive agent azathioprine. The first successful human kidney transplantation was in 1954.[1] It avoided the need for immunosuppression because it was a live donor kidney transplant exchanged between identical twins; this case was proof of concept that solid organ transplantation could successfully be achieved. The field of kidney transplantation was further fueled by the U.S. government underwriting the support of patients with end-stage renal disease, which fostered advances in kidney transplantation and hemodialysis. The parallel development of the concept of brain death[2] resulted in a potential source of donor organs for the nascent field of transplantation.

The first human liver transplantation was performed in 1963 by Dr. Thomas Starzl. The patient suffered from biliary atresia, had coagulopathy, and did not survive the surgery.[3] Additional attempts in Berlin, Boston, and Paris were also unsuccessful. Subsequent initial successes in orthotopic liver transplantation were in patients with liver cancer. These patients had less portal hypertension and relatively straightforward surgery but were not long-term survivors secondary to recurrent disease, technical problems, and lack of adequate immunosuppression.

In the early 1980s, liver transplantation in the United States was limited to a handful of programs; initial results were poor, with less than 30% 1-year survival. A major advance came with the clinical introduction of cyclosporine for immunosuppression in solid organ transplantation.[4] Its use in liver transplant recipients allowed for further developments in this field.

As success in liver transplantation increased, more centers initiated programs and increasing numbers of patients availed themselves of this therapy. In attempts to provide timely transplantation to patients with the greatest need, local regional and national distribution schemes were developed and allocation to patients on the waiting list became based on need rather than on time on the list (see later, "Organ Shortage, Model for End-Stage Liver Disease, and Liver Distribution").

The increasing disparity between available brain dead deceased donor livers and potential recipients has led to a number of advances that serve to increase the donor pool. These include split liver transplantation, live donor liver transplantation, and the use of donors after cardiac death. These topics will be covered in detail.

## INDICATIONS AND CONTRAINDICATIONS

### Indications

As the outcome of liver transplantation has improved, the indications have expanded to include any patient with compromise of life from chronic liver insufficiency, chronic liver disease with acute decompensation, acute liver failure, and enzyme deficiencies (Table 27-1). Liver transplantation is also indicated to a limited degree for patients with primary liver tumors.

The first issue regarding candidacy for transplantation is whether a given patient would benefit from liver replacement. The second issue that must be addressed is whether the patient can withstand the challenge of a liver transplantation surgery. Compromise in cardiac or pulmonary function may prohibit the patient as a candidate. In some cases, failure of an additional

**Table 27-1 Indications for Liver Transplantation**

| ADULTS | | CHILDREN | |
|---|---|---|---|
| Noncholestatic cirrhosis | 65 | Biliary atresia | 58 |
| Viral hepatitis B and C | | Inborn errors of metabolism | 11 |
| Alcoholic* | | Cholestatic | 9 |
| Cryptogenic | | Primary sclerosing cholangitis | |
| Cholestatic | 14 | Alagille syndrome | |
| Primary biliary cirrhosis | | Autoimmune | 4 |
| Primary sclerosing cholangitis | | Viral hepatitis | 2 |
| Autoimmune | 5 | Miscellaneous | 16 |
| Malignant neoplasm | 2 | | |
| Miscellaneous | 14 | | |

*Most alcoholic patients are coinfected with the hepatitis C virus.

organ system may dictate combination transplantations. Although kidney-liver transplantations are relatively common, heart-liver and lung-liver transplantations are rarely performed.[5]

Regardless of the specific cause of liver disease, patients with chronic liver disease who have deteriorated tend to present with common signs and symptoms. These include coagulopathy, thrombocytopenia, muscle wasting, gynecomastia, ascites, varices, encephalopathy, and renal insufficiency. These physiologic perturbations may lead to life-threatening complications; patients with ascites are susceptible to spontaneous bacterial peritonitis or the development of a peritoneal-pleural fistula. Gastrointestinal bleeding is the potential complication of varices.

An acute exacerbation of chronic liver disease can be triggered by sepsis, gastrointestinal bleeding, or progressive renal insufficiency. Some diseases, such as Wilson's disease or autoimmune hepatitis, may present with an acute decompensation without a prior diagnosis of liver disease.

The production of many essential proteins originates in the liver. The inborn errors of metabolism reflect failure of production of crucial enzymes in the liver. Liver transplantation cures the disease by replacing the liver cells with competent metabolic pathways; it is recommended for those diseases in which there is no central nervous system compromise.

## Fulminant Hepatic Failure

Fulminant hepatic failure refers to the acute onset of liver failure with the absence of previous liver disease. The entity is defined as the presence of encephalopathy within 8 weeks of jaundice.

In addition to encephalopathy, the disease is characterized by jaundice, coagulopathy, metabolic acidosis, and renal insufficiency. Encephalopathy may progress to coma. Once a patient reaches stage 4 encephalopathy, the rate of successful treatment without transplantation ranges from 5% to 20%, depending on the cause.[6] Its most common cause in the United States and England is acetaminophen overdose,[7] either accidental or intentional. In Asia, acute hepatitis from hepatitis B viral infection is the most common cause.[8] In a significant number of cases the specific cause is unknown. Acetaminophen overdose carries a relatively good prognosis without transplantation if the metabolic functions related to the liver are maintained.

The key to successful liver transplantation for fulminant hepatic failure is early recognition and listing for transplantation, avoidance of cerebral edema, prevention of infection, and timely transplantation. Brain death from cerebral edema is a common cause of death in these patients. Depending on the cause and potential for liver regeneration, the liver assist device or hepatocyte transplantation may be an alternative to liver transplantation, but these modalities are experimental at this time.

## Hepatitis C and Liver Transplantation

Chronic hepatitis C infection is the most common indication for transplantation in the West. In the United States, it is estimated that 5 million individuals are infected with hepatitis C. In approximately 20% of these patients, a chronic injury state develops in the liver, with progression to cirrhosis and liver insufficiency. Hepatitis C can be subdivided into five groups or serotypes. The most common U.S. serotype is genotype 1. Type 1 is less responsive to antiviral medication than genotype 2 or 3.

Hepatitis C infection recurs after transplantation because the virus resides in tissues other than the liver. The aggressiveness of the recurrent hepatitis C after liver transplantation cannot be predicted; risk factors include donor age, treatment for acute rejection, and level of hepatitis C viremia at the time of transplantation.[9] Another factor that predicts hepatitis C reinfection severity after transplantation is the treatment for rejection after transplantation (with additional steroids or antilymphocyte preparations).[10] Transplantation of a liver from a donor older than 40 years is associated with a greater risk of recurrent cirrhosis than from a younger donor. Hepatitis C treatment with interferon and ribavirin is effective in approximately 50% of patients prior to transplantation and in 30% to 40% of patients post-transplantation.[11] It has been suggested that pretransplantation treatment of patients for whom a live donor has been identified can be followed by planned transplantation as a rescue therapy. The success of pretransplantation treatment of hepatitis C depends on the level of viremia in the recipient. The limitations to treatment with interferon and ribavirin are bone marrow suppression and the systemic inflammatory response associated with their administration. In cirrhotic patients, splenic sequestration of platelets and neutrophils limit preoperative therapy with interferon and ribavirin.

Chronic hepatitis C infection is also an important risk factor for the development of hepatocellular carcinoma (HCC). It has been estimated that the current rise in the incidence of HCC reflects the United States hepatitis C epidemic of the 1960s through 1970s.[12]

## Hepatitis B

Chronic hepatitis B infection is the most common cause of chronic liver disease in endemic regions of Asia and Africa, and the most common cause of death from hepatitis worldwide.[13]

The hepatitis B vaccine is effective in inducing the formation of antibodies that will protect against hepatitis B exposure. As the use of hepatitis B vaccine spreads worldwide, one can look forward to an overall decrease in the incidence of hepatitis B infection over time.

In the past, hepatitis B was a major problem after transplantation, with rapid reinfection of the graft. Effective therapy with antiviral agents and hyperimmune globulin has largely eradicated disease recurrence after transplantation.

### Primary Biliary Cirrhosis

Primary biliary cirrhosis is a form of autoimmune cholestatic liver disease, with inflammatory injury to the bile ducts. It is a chronic cause of hepatic insufficiency and is characterized by autoimmune markers and some response to immunosuppressants.[14] This disease is more common in females. The disease may recur years after transplantation but its recurrence is unlikely to progress to the need for retransplantation.

### Primary Sclerosing Cholangitis

This is an autoimmune disease that is more frequent in males. It progresses over the years to a cholestatic picture associated with scarring of the intrahepatic and extrahepatic bile ducts. The disease is associated with ulcerative colitis in approximately 90% of patients. In a small number of patients (<10%), the process is associated with cholangiocarcinoma.[15] The bile duct involvement in primary sclerosing cholangitis dictates the use of choledochojejunostomy in patients undergoing liver transplantation. Primary sclerosing cholangitis may also recur after transplantation, although its recurrence is rare.

### Alcoholic Liver Disease

Chronic alcohol abuse may cause scarring in the liver, leading to cirrhosis with decompensation. Patients who stop the use of alcohol can prevent progression of the disease. Alcoholic liver disease may be seen in association with other chronic insults to the liver, such as chronic hepatitis C and, in this setting, is more likely to progress to decompensation. Most transplantation centers require abstinence from alcohol after transplantation and a period of abstinence (usually 6 months) prior to transplantation to demonstrate the patient's understanding of the contribution of alcohol to the disease and a commitment to abstinence.

### Nonalcoholic Steatohepatitis

Nonalcoholic steatohepatitis[16] reflects a pending epidemic of liver disease associated with the epidemic of obesity and metabolic syndrome in the United States. Fatty infiltration of the liver, with inflammation and subsequent injury and fibrosis, are the histologic features. The associated metabolic syndrome and diabetes dictate evaluation of the coronary arteries of these potential recipients. Nonalcoholic steatohepatitis may recur after transplantation.

### Biliary Atresia

Biliary atresia is the most common indication for liver transplantation in the pediatric patient. The incidence is 1 in 40,000 live births and is a major concern in the infant with persistent jaundice after birth. Its diagnosis is made with liver biopsy and the finding of an absent extrahepatic bile duct at the time of laparotomy. Its cause is unclear.

Affected infants are treated with hepaticojejunostomy (Kasai procedure). The success of this procedure is dictated by surgery soon after birth and the size of the bile ducts in the bile duct plate. Post–Kasai cholangitis may hasten the need for transplantation. An early indication for transplantation in children is a failure to grow. Intervention with transplantation at this stage may allow catch-up growth. At transplantation, the Roux-en-Y procedure is required for biliary drainage.

### Contraindications

Patients with liver disease are extensively evaluated to determine their candidacy for transplantation. Cardiac, pulmonary, and renal functions are assessed. Patients are also seen by a social worker or other mental health professional for psychosocial evaluation. Each patient is individually evaluated to determine the risk-benefit ratio. There are generally accepted absolute and relative contraindications to transplantation. In general, contraindications reflect the expectation of a poor outcome.

Systemic infections are considered contraindications to transplantation and uncontrolled bacterial and fungal infections are absolute contraindications to transplantation. Infections in the liver, such as cholangitis, may be an exception to this rule. HIV infection is considered by some groups to be a contraindication but several studies have shown outcomes comparable to those of matched control patients if the virus is controlled.[17]

Failure of another organ may be a contraindication to transplantation if that organ cannot be replaced or expected to recover. Kidney transplantation accompanies liver transplantation in 5% of cases. On occasion, liver-heart transplantation is performed for diseases such as amyloidosis; combined liver-lung transplantation for diseases such as cystic fibrosis has been performed in rare circumstances.[5]

Patients with chronic liver disease can develop pulmonary manifestations of their liver disease. Portopulmonary hypertension is considered a contraindication with persistent pulmonary artery pressures higher than 50 mm Hg in the presence of elevated pulmonary vascular resistance.[18] Hepatopulmonary syndrome becomes a contraindication to transplantation when the $PaO_2$ does not demonstrate marked improvement with the administration of 100% oxygen.[19]

Inability to care for the transplanted organ adequately because of continued drug or alcohol abuse or lack of commitment to immunosuppressive drugs is considered a contraindication to transplant. Continued commitment to immunosuppressive drugs is difficult to assess pretransplantation; in some series, noncompliance has been reported to be up to 35%.[20]

Anatomic considerations may be relative contraindications to liver transplantation. The presence of portal vein thrombosis may be overcome by removal of the thrombose or jump graft to the superior mesenteric vein. With complete thrombosis of the portal system, portal inflow from the infrahepatic vena cava has been used, although use of this procedure is rare and morbidity is high.

Metastatic HCC is considered an absolute contraindication to transplantation, related to poor outcome from metastatic disease. The risk of metastatic disease after liver transplantation is dependent on the size and number of HCC(s) in the liver. The Milan criteria for liver transplantation for HCC (single nodule <5 cm, or less than three nodules, the largest of which is <3 cm) are used to predict the risk of recurrent disease after transplantation. Patients who meet these criteria have a risk of recurrence that is less than 20% whereas patients outside the criteria have a recurrence rate of approximately 60%.[21] The Milan criteria are currently used to define acceptable candidates for transplantation in the United States; patients who meet Milan criteria are given extra priority for transplantation. There is a controversy regarding transplantation for patients outside the Milan criteria and there is an interest in finding other methods of identifying those patients who have a low recurrence risk after transplantation. In the future, molecular biomarkers may prove reliable for selecting patients who will benefit from transplantation.

## Organ Shortage, Model for End-Stage Liver Disease, and Liver Distribution

The decision of whether a patient is a candidate for transplantation and what priority a given patient should have is dictated in part by the relative shortage of deceased donor donors. Despite substantial governmental and community efforts, the needs of the 15,000 patients awaiting transplantation are not met by the approximately 5000 or so donors.[22]

With recognition of the improved outcomes of liver transplantation in the 1980s, transplantation programs proliferated. Livers were allocated to programs and teams rather than patients, with the transplantation center selecting the most appropriate recipient for a given donor. Because of the concept that the organs should be allocated to patients rather than centers, lists of patients were created and ordered according to the patient's time waiting on the list and the organs offered to the patients.

The current system of liver distribution in the United States depends first on the level of the local organ procurement organization, then to the 11 United Network for Organ Sharing (UNOS) regions, and then shared on a national basis. A patient's priority on the waiting list is based on his or her medical status as determined by the model for end-stage liver disease (MELD) score, which reflects the likelihood of death within 3 months. The MELD score assigns points that reflect the severity of liver disease. The score is based on a formula that considers bilirubin and creatinine levels and the international normalized ratio (INR).[23]

## Model for End-Stage Liver Disease Formula

$$\begin{aligned}\text{MELD score} = {} & (0.957 \times \log_e \text{ creatinine [mg/dL]}) + \\ & (0.378 \times \log_e \text{ bilirubin [mg/dL]}) + \\ & (1.120 \times \log_e \text{ INR}) + 0.643\end{aligned}$$

The components of the MELD score were chosen because they represent objective criteria that can be reviewed and verified as compared with ascites and encephalopathy, which were used previously (as part of the Childs-Pugh score) but are subjective and cannot be readily verified. The use of the MELD score to determine liver distribution has led to a significant decrease in the rate of death of potential recipients on the waiting list because it allows livers to be directed to the sickest patients. Patients with a high MELD score at the time of transplantation have slightly poorer survival following transplantation (Table 27-2).

For patients with low MELD scores, less than 15, the risk of death while waiting for transplantation is less than the risk of death after transplantation.[24] The current allocation system therefore discourages transplantation of patients with MELD scores less than 15 by allocating a liver to all the higher MELD score patients in the region before allowing local use in patients with scores less than 15. These last two concepts, that sicker patients have a greater risk of poor outcome after liver transplantation and that relatively healthy patients, whose outcomes are worse with transplantation than if they remained on the waiting list, suggest that both pretransplantation and posttransplantation outcomes should be considered in the allocation of livers. Currently, the use of the MELD score only weighs the pretransplantation outcomes, and death on the waiting list has been reduced since the initiation of MELD. It has been proposed that the MELD score be replaced as a means to distribute organs with a system that determines potential survival benefit after transplantation, or a combination of survival benefit prior to and after transplantation for patients with chronic liver disease.[25]

For some patients, the risk of death or dropout from the list may not be reflected in the laboratory values in the MELD score. For example, patients with HCC benefit from transplantation, even when their laboratory test results are normal. To allow transplantation, an exception is made and additional MELD points are assigned to these patients.[26] This approach is used to transplant these patients prior to their tumors becoming so extensive that patients fall outside the limits of criteria for liver transplantation. It is also used for diseases such as amyloidosis.

Pediatric donors are distributed to pediatric patients preferentially. The scoring used in pediatric patients is referred to as the pediatric end-stage liver disease (PELD) score.[27]

Patients with acute liver failure such as fulminant hepatic failure are given the highest priority (status 1) for donor organs to avoid the development of cerebral edema and other fatal outcomes. Status 1 supersedes the MELD score in the organ allocation process.

**Table 27-2 Concordance With 3-Month Mortality**

| SCORE | CONCORDANCE (%) | 95% CONFIDENCE INTERVAL (%) |
|---|---|---|
| MELD | 0.88 | 0.85, 0.90 |
| Childs-Turcote-Pugh (CTP) | 0.79 | 0.75, 0.83 |

# LIVE DONOR LIVER TRANSPLANTATION

Regardless of the distribution scheme used for deceased donor transplants, the need for potential liver transplant recipients far exceeds the supply. As a consequence of this disparity, a number of alternatives have been used to increase the supply, including live donor liver transplantation. The basis for this approach includes the work of Otte and colleagues,[28] who pared down adult-sized livers for use in pediatric patients, as well as the observation that the liver can regenerate after major liver resection for cancer.

Subsequently, Millis and associates[29] at the University of Chicago thoughtfully raised the medical and ethical issues of pediatric patients dying while awaiting liver transplantation as the foundation for the development of a live donor transplant program. This program yielded outstanding patient survival, greatly reduced death on the waiting list for the pediatric patients, and led the way for the development of adult to adult live donor liver transplantation. The development was further fueled in Asia by the absence of brain death legislation and the cultural and religious reluctance to embrace the brain death concept.

The long history of live donor kidney transplantation has provided the cultural, ethical, and medical framework on which to build live donor liver transplantation, but the issues regarding live donor liver transplantation have been more complex. Long-term studies of kidney transplant donors showed low operative mortality and the same long-term morbidity as age-matched controls, with no higher incidence of the need for dialysis over time.[30] To date, there are no long-term evaluations of live donors but concern exists regarding their long-term course in terms of hepatic reserve and bile duct problems.

It rapidly became clear that operative mortality for live donor liver transplantation was significant, with early death from pulmonary emboli in those who donated the lateral segment of their liver and the highly publicized death of a right lobe donor in the United States in 2002. Subsequent deaths throughout the world have underscored the concern for the risks of the procedure. Current estimates are that the risk of death from liver donation is 1 in 500 to 1000 and the risk of death from kidney donation is 1 in 3000.[31]

The balance between adequate liver mass for the recipient and risk to the donor underscores the challenges for progress in this field. The other major factor is that the perceived need for live donor liver transplantation varies across the United States because there are regional inequities in the availability of organs.[22] In the United States, live donor liver transplantation for adult patients decreased significantly after the institution of the MELD system and has stayed low, constituting less than 5% of liver transplantations carried out.[22] In Asia, without the alternative of deceased donor transplantation, an increasing number of live donor transplantations are performed, with expanding recipient indications, and centers have experience with large numbers of live donor liver transplantations.[32]

A number of groups have been rethinking the use of left lobe grafts, largely because of concern over donor safety. The physiologic strains on the donor of the left lobe appear to be less; there have been no reports of a left lobe donor requiring liver transplantation after donation as compared with right lobe donation, for which the need for emergent donor transplantation has been reported.[31] The reservation about using the smaller piece of liver from left lobe donation is that the high portal flow generated by the enlarged spleen, and other vascular manifestations of portal hypertension, results in injury to the graft from hyperperfusion and endothelial damage. It has been estimated that the weight of the graft should be more than 0.8% of the recipient's body weight to prevent injury from hyperperfusion. The small left lobe grafts (generally, 30% to 40% of the total liver mass) may be protected from harm by decreasing portal vein blood flow by performing porta caval shunts, ligating the splenic artery, or performing splenectomy. Another strategy has been to use two left lobe donors for a single recipient, a strategy that attempts to minimize risk to the donor by using the left lobe from two donors while maximizing liver mass in the recipient.[33] The potential risk to two donors is the major concern to this approach. However, excellent outcomes have been reported with low live donor morbidity.

Of live liver donors, 30% to 40% suffer one or more postoperative complications[34]; the most include pulmonary emboli, portal vein thrombosis, bile duct injury, and liver insufficiency secondary to a resection that is too extensive.

The result of the potential for death among live liver donors has led to a more clearly delineated informed consent process in the transplant community, the use of a donor advocate to ensure that the concern for donor safety is paramount, and the clear separation of donor and recipient teams to ensure that the donor is treated without ulterior motives, which might occur if the same team cared for both the donor and recipient. Long-term follow-up will be necessary to determine whether the long-term sequelae of liver donors is as benign as for living kidney donors.

The recent application of hand-assisted laparoscopic techniques for living donor right hepatic lobectomy may have a similar impact as laparoscopic donor nephrectomy in increasing live liver donation. This technique, using a midline incision for the hand port, needs wider application to realize its potential impact.[35]

There appears to be a learning curve with live donor liver transplantation. Centers with extensive experience note decreased rates of complications compared with inexperienced centers. Additionally, groups in Asia with extensive experience have outstanding records of low complications in their live donor experience.

The recipient outcomes from live liver donors are superior to those for patients waiting and those receiving deceased donor transplants.[36] These differences are primarily explained by the opportunity to perform live donor liver transplantation when the recipient is in relatively good health, rather than relying on the MELD system, which distributes deceased donor livers to the most gravely ill hosts. Controlling for recipient condition and comparing recipients of live donor versus deceased donor transplants also favors outcomes in the recipients of live donor grafts; this may reflect the same factors that are operative in live donor kidney transplantation—the use of an organ that is free of preservation insult, avoidance of the negative effects of brain death on organ viability, and the immunologic advantage of a live donor graft (most often immunologically related). In the early days of adult to adult live liver donation, high MELD score recipients were found to have poor outcomes and many centers limited transplantation with partial grafts to recipients with a MELD score less than 25. More recently, excellent outcomes have been reported in high MELD score recipients of live liver donors.[37] This is likely to result in increased live liver donor transplantation in this group of patients.

Living donor transplantation, however, does suffer from the increased complications in the recipient related to the bile duct anastomosis. Because the branch rather than the trunk of the bile duct is used in living donor transplantation, as in deceased donor transplantation, the rate of biliary complications is roughly twice as high in living donor transplantation.

## TECHNICAL ASPECTS OF LIVER TRANSPLANTATION

Unlike the kidney transplant (placed in a heterotrophic position in the iliac fossa), the liver is placed orthotopically—in its native position within the abdomen. The procedure involves removal of the host liver and replacement with a whole or partial graft. Figure 27-1 demonstrates a completed orthotopic liver transplantation.

Removal of the host liver is often challenging because of the portal hypertension and coagulopathy that frequently accompany chronic liver disease. After mobilization of the liver, the bile duct is divided and vascular clamps are placed on the suprahepatic vena cava, infrahepatic vena cava, portal vein, and hepatic artery. The anhepatic phase of the surgery relates to the period during which the new liver is sewn in and the patient is without a liver. An alternative to the conventional implantation technique in which the suprahepatic vena cava, infrahepatic vena cava, portal vein, and hepatic artery are sewn in sequence is the piggyback technique. This technique leaves the vena cava intact and involves an anastomosis between the donor suprahepatic

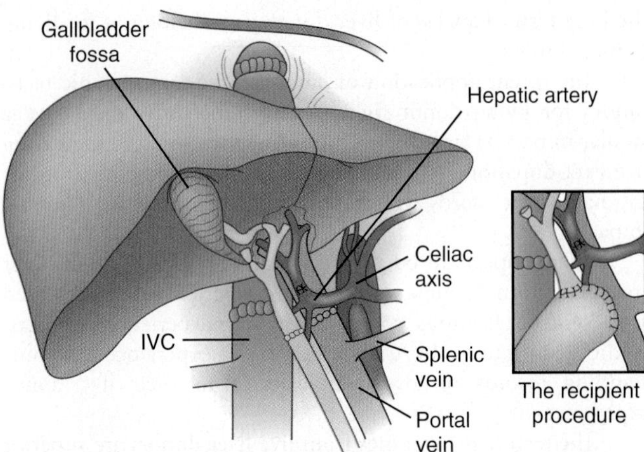


**FIGURE 27-1** Orthotopic liver transplant. *Left,* A choledochocholedochostomy (duct to duct) anastomosis. *Inset,* A choledochojejunostomy.

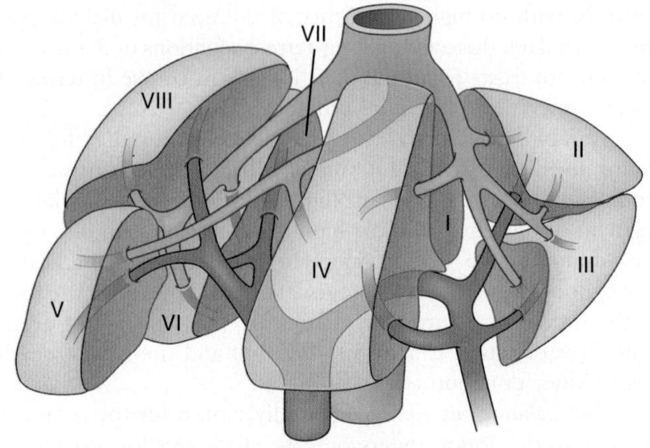


**FIGURE 27-2** Anatomic segments of the liver.

cava and the confluence of two or three hepatic veins, depending on the specific anatomy. In this technique, the donor infrahepatic cava is oversewn. The piggyback method may shorten the anhepatic phase and has the potential for improved cardiovascular stability because it leaves the vena caval flow intact during the anhepatic phase.

Some centers use venovenous bypass, in which shunt tubing is placed in the host portal vein and infrahepatic cava and returned to the central venous circulation to maintain vascular stability during the anhepatic phase. Centers that do not use the bypass technique rely more on anesthesia support of the blood pressure through volume administration and pressers.

The piggyback technique is necessary for patients undergoing live donor liver or split liver transplantation when a donor vena cava is not available. In the case of a right lobe graft (segments 5 to 8), the venous drainage is the right hepatic vein; the inflow is the right hepatic artery and right portal vein.

The anhepatic phase ends with reperfusion of the graft, with inflow from the portal vein and outflow through the vena cava. Subsequently, arterial inflow is reestablished and biliary drainage is accomplished through a choledochocholedochostomy or choledochojejunostomy (usually in the case of biliary atresia or sclerosing cholangitis, in which the host duct is unsuitable), when appropriate.

## Split Liver Transplant

The identification of separate units within the liver with unique blood supply, venous drainage and biliary drainage makes possible the use of a single deceased donor liver applicable for two recipients. Figure 27-2 demonstrates the segments of liver (1 to 8) that can be defined by their separate venous and arterial inflow, venous outflow, and biliary drainage.

Usually, the split is done between a child (receiving segments 2 and 3 or segments 2, 3, and 4) and an adult (receiving segments 1, 4, 5, 6, 7, and 8 or segments 1, 5, 6, 7, and 8). The right lobe graft most commonly includes the donor vena cava and right hepatic artery; the pediatric graft is based on the celiac trunk providing the left hepatic artery, left portal vein, and left hepatic vein.

The splitting of a deceased donor liver for use in two adult patients has been infrequent. Inadequate left lobe mass may be a problem.

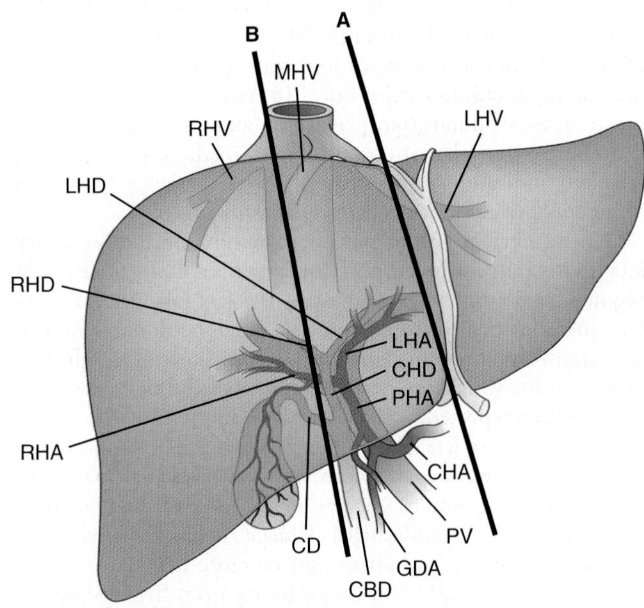


**FIGURE 27-3** Planes of dissection for the 2-3 hepatectomy *(line A)* and for a right-left lobe split *(line B).*

## Live Donor Operation

### Segment 2-3 Hepatectomy

Figure 27-3 depicts the line of resection for a segment 2-3 hepatectomy (line A) in the setting of an adult to child live donor liver operation or for a cadaveric split for an adult and child (line A).

The use of segments 2 and 3 is most appropriate for infants and small children (up to 5 years of age). The operation can be performed through a midline incision. The round ligament is divided, retracted, and mobilized. The left triangular ligament is taken down. The left hepatic artery and left portal vein are mobilized. Numerous branches from the left port vein to segments 1 and 4 are ligated and divided. The left hepatic vein is mobilized. A resection line is drawn from the right edge of the left hepatic vein, coursing approximately 1 cm to the right of the falciform ligament to the bile duct plate, which sits

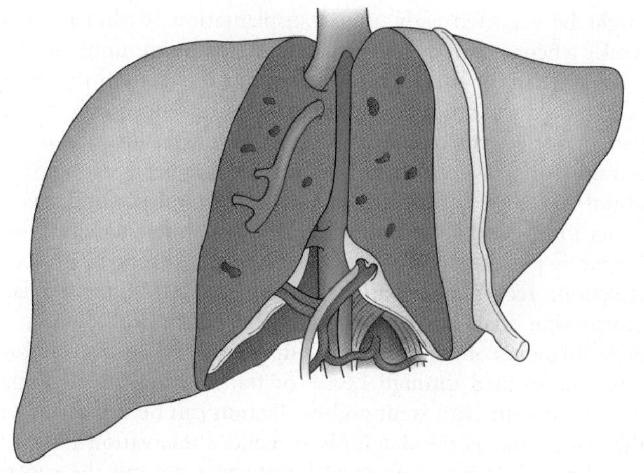

**FIGURE 27-4** Plane of donor dissection for right and/or left live donor liver transplantation and for split liver ttransplantation.

superiorly above the left portal vein as it enters segment 2-3. The liver parenchyma is carefully divided with clipping or ligature of large vessels and ducts. The plane just to the right of the falciform is usually used because it usually yields a single 2-3 bile duct for reimplantation. After the parenchymal dissection medially, the segment 2-3 is lifted superiorly and dissected free from segment 1. This results in an isolated segment 2-3 with left hepatic artery, left portal vein, and left hepatic vein, along with the segment 2-3 duct. The segment 2-3 is flushed through the left portal vein and left hepatic artery.

### Right Lobe Dissection for Live Donor Liver Transplantation

The right lobe (segments 5 to 8) is most commonly used for adult to adult live donor liver transplantation. The right lobe represents 60% to 80% of the liver mass. A bilateral subcostal incision is made, or midline incision is done if laparoscopic division of the coronary ligaments is used. A cholecystectomy is performed. The right hepatic artery and right portal vein are isolated and temporarily occluded to establish the line of demarcation, which is used to plan the plane of resection (Fig. 27-4; also see Fig. 27-3, resection line B). This line typically runs at the left edge of the gallbladder fossa to the medial aspect of the right hepatic vein. The right lobe is mobilized by division of the right triangular ligaments and suture ligation of the perforating veins between the right lobe and infrahepatic vena cava. The right hepatic vein and accessory right hepatic veins (>5 mm) are isolated. The right hepatic duct is mobilized; it may be divided prior to or after the parenchymal dissection.

Various techniques may be used to divide the parenchyma; preferred is the dissection with the Cavitron ultrasonic surgical aspirator (CUSA; Cooper Medical, Santa Clara, Calif), which allows for the identification of vessels and ducts for ligation. Venous branches from segments 5 and 8 may be preserved for reimplantation; there is controversy as to whether this is necessary to prevent venous outflow obstruction and congestion of the graft. Once the parenchymal dissection is complete and the right duct divided, vascular clamps are placed on the right hepatic artery, right portal vein and right hepatic vein for resection of the right lobe.

### Left Lobe Dissection for Live Donor Liver Transplantation

The left lobe graft is based on segments 2, 3, 4, and 5, with inflow from the left hepatic artery and left portal vein and outflow from the middle and left hepatic veins, which frequently have a confluent trunk at the vena cava (see Fig. 27-3, resection line B). The operation includes the parenchymal dissection along Cantlie's line, the same line as for the right hepatic lobectomy. The middle and left hepatic veins may need to be taken separately or as a single trunk, depending on the level of confluence of these vessels. The parenchymal dissection is done in the same manner as for right hepatic lobectomy, with care to clip or suture-ligate large vessels and bile ducts.

### Implantation of Partial Liver Graft

The piggyback technique is the basis for implantation of a split liver graft or a graft from a live donor. If the split liver comes intact with a vena cava, a conventional transplantation procedure may be done.

The piggyback technique involves ligation and division of the perforating veins from the right lobe of the host liver to the vena cava. Accessory right hepatic veins are also sacrificed. The venous anastomosis is usually created between the graft hepatic vein and a wide cavotomy, typically using one of the recipient hepatic vein orifices. Depending on whether the donor graft is the right or left lobe, either the right or left hepatic artery branches from the recipient may be used for inflow. Similarly, inflow may be from the right or left portal vein branch. If a left lobe graft is used and a portal caval shunt is planned to decompress the portal system to prevent portal hyperperfusion, the right portal vein branch may be used to create the shunt to the vena cava and the left portal vein branch used for inflow into the donor portal vein branch. Biliary drainage is achieved through a duct to duct anastomosis or a Roux-en-Y anastomosis to the donor duct, depending on the duct sizes. Care must be used to avoid tension on this anastomosis.

## EARLY COMPLICATIONS OF LIVER TRANSPLANTATION

Early signs that a newly implanted liver is functioning are acid clearance, normalization of clotting parameters, and bile production; these signs may be apparent within a few minutes after reperfusion. Primary nonfunction refers to a condition in which the transplanted liver does not work. It is rare (<2%), and is fatal without retransplantation. Ultrasonography with Doppler may be useful to eliminate vascular thromboses as a cause. Hepatic artery thrombosis occurs in 2% to 4% of adult transplantation procedures[38] but have a threefold to fourfold higher incidence in children. Although early thrombectomy of the hepatic artery may prevent retransplantation in some patients, most patients require retransplantation. Portal venous thrombosis may be unnoticed but may present with gastrointestinal bleeding or coagulopathy, and require therapy for new or persistent portal hypertension. Other complications include bleeding, inadequate production of clotting factors (poor initial function), and inadequate replacement of factors at the time of transplantation (e.g. platelet or fresh-frozen plasma replacement). The need to reoperate on a given patient is dictated by cardiovascular stability, liver function, presence of abdominal compartment syndrome (which may be manifest by acute or progressive renal failure), and total blood products used. Bile duct stricture or leak is a complication that may be seen early after transplantation, or later; its cause likely reflects compromised blood supply of the donor and/or recipient duct. The first line of therapy for an anastomotic stricture is dilation and stent placement performed through endoscopic retrograde cholangiopancreatography (ERCP) or via a transhepatic route. Strictures that persist or recur after dilation or stenting are treated surgically, with conversion to a choledochojejunostomy.

### Outcome

Progress in the technical and immunologic aspects of liver transplant has led to excellent graft and patient survival, with 1- and 5-year patient survival rates of 88% and 75%, respectively.[22] Results depend on the specific disease for which the transplantation is performed.

## EXTENDED CRITERIA DONORS

Although liver transplantation is successful using both live and deceased donors, it is increasingly difficult to find a perfect deceased donor. The ideal liver donor (young and otherwise completely healthy) is increasingly rare, because the cause of death for most donors has shifted from trauma to cerebrovascular accidents. Using UNOS data, Feng and coworkers[39] have defined the factors increasing the risk of failure after live transplantation into a formula called the donor risk index. Factors contributing to risk using livers from donation after brain death include advanced donor age, fatty infiltration, and the use of split livers from these donors. The donor risk issues must be taken in context of the recipient for whom it is used. The use of an older donor is particularly hazardous in the hepatitis C virus (HCV)–positive recipient. The risk to the recipient is more rapid development of cirrhosis after transplantation. This risk is apparent with a donor age older than 40 years and becomes more pronounced with a donor age older than 60 years. Many transplantation programs balance the recipient's risk of death based on the MELD score to the risk of recurrent cirrhosis in HCV-positive patients.

Another donor source, the use of which has increased significantly over the past 5 years, is the donor after cardiac death. These are donors who do not meet brain death criteria and become donors after they are removed from life support and experience cessation of cardiac function. Most centers use a 30-minute cutoff from the time of withdrawal of life support to the perfusion of the organ as a criterion for accepting such donors. Even with these criteria, the recipients of livers from cardiac death donors have increased mortality and significant morbidity, largely from bile duct complications.[40] However, the increased risk from the use of any donor must be examined in the context of potential benefit to a given recipient. Recipients with high MELD scores and high likelihood of dying without transplantation show survival benefit from the use of high-risk donors after brain death, as well as from livers from donors after cardiac death.

## EVALUATION OF ABNORMAL LIVER FUNCTION TEST RESULTS

Abnormal liver function test results do not differentiate the specific problem that may be present in the liver; vascular occlusion, bile duct stricture, preservation injury, recurrent hepatitis, and rejection may all present with nonspecific abnormalities. The time after transplantation can be an important clue about the cause of the laboratory abnormalities. Preservation injury might be expected early after transplantation (within the first week) when recurrent hepatitis and rejection are unlikely. The nonspecificity of liver function tests and the overlap in timing of these complications dictate an organized approach to the patient with perturbations in laboratory test results. The use of ultrasonography is recommended to evaluate hepatic artery and portal vein flow and bile duct caliber. If the ultrasound reveals intact inflow and absent bile duct dilation, a percutaneous liver biopsy is performed and used to make the diagnosis of acute rejection, recurrent hepatitis, or preservation injury. Biliary obstruction may be manifested by bile duct proliferation or pericholangitis on biopsy, but the diagnosis rests on cholangiography performed through ERCP or transhepatic cholangiography. Treatment with stent and/or dilation can be carried out at the same time as the diagnosis is made. Preservation injury is manifested by vacuolization of hepatocytes around the central vein; no treatment is necessary because the process is self-limited and reversible. An ischemic pattern on biopsy with hepatocyte dropout or necrosis, combined with an abnormal ultrasound, may prompt hepatic angiography to evaluate the possibility of hepatic artery stenosis or median arcuate ligament syndrome. Hepatic artery stenosis may be treated with balloon dilation or stenting, with or without anticoagulation.

Liver rejection is diagnosed by the presence of a portal inflammatory infiltrate, bile duct injury, and endothelial injury, known as endotheliitis. The portal infiltrate is usually a mixture of lymphocytes, neutrophils, and eosinophils. Rejection is generally first treated with increased steroids or change in immunosuppressive therapy. In patients with underlying hepatitis C, increased steroids are avoided in favor of increasing immunosuppression to avoid enhanced viral replication induced by steroids. Typically, the increased immunosuppression would be an increase in the tacrolimus or mycophenolate dose.

Recurrent hepatitis C generally occurs later than the complications noted, but may be seen within a few weeks of transplantation. Distinguishing recurrent hepatitis C from rejection using liver biopsy can be difficult. The time after transplantation can be an important clue to deciding whether it is rejection or recurrent hepatitis C, with recurrent hepatitis C usually occurring more than 6 weeks after transplantation and rejection usually occurring within 6 weeks of transplantation. Recurrent hepatitis C may be treated with a combination of interferon and ribavirin.

Hepatic artery occlusion is an indication for retransplantation if it occurs in the early postoperative period. It is associated with progressive saccular dilation of the biliary tree secondary to occlusion and the development of liver abscesses. If the hepatic artery occludes slowly over time, adequate collaterals may develop and obviate the need for retransplantation.

## IMMUNOSUPPRESSION AFTER LIVER TRANSPLANTATION

The liver has been referred to as a privileged organ because, in general, the need for immunosuppression decreases over time and, unlike the situation in kidney and heart transplantation, chronic rejection is uncommon.

The mainstay of immunosuppression after liver transplantation is the use of a combination of a calcineurin inhibitor (tacrolimus or cyclosporine), steroids (methylprednisolone), and antiproliferative agent (e.g., mycophenolate mofetil). The calcineurin inhibitors are used in 95% of transplantation centers, despite their known nephrotoxicity. These agents are also associated with hypertension, diabetes, and neurologic effects, including seizures.[41] The major advantages of the mycophenolate derivatives are their lack of renal toxicity, although their toxicities include gastrointestinal irritation[42] and bone marrow suppression. Steroid-free protocols may be useful in terms of a de novo diabetes mellitus, cytomegalovirus (CMV), cholesterol levels and, in HCV patients, the recurrence of HCV hepatitis.[43]

Sirolimus (rapamycin) is a mammalian target of rapamycin (mTOR) inhibitor that effectively decreases interleukin-2 (IL-2) production by a mechanism distinct from that of the calcineurin inhibitors. Its antineoplastic effect makes it attractive for use in patients with HCC as an indication for transplantation.[44] Because sirolimus inhibits wound healing, some groups avoid its use in the immediate postoperative period. The U.S. Food and Drug Administration (FDA) has a black box warning about the early use of sirolimus because it has been associated with hepatic artery thrombosis.

## RETRANSPLANTATION AND RECURRENT DISEASE

Rejection, although frequent early after transplantation, is rarely the cause of graft failure. This is in contradistinction to other types of solid organ transplantations in which chronic rejection is a common cause of the need for retransplantation. Recurrent disease is most frequently the cause of graft failure in patients with chronic hepatitis C infection. Recurrent disease may, rarely, be the cause of graft failure in patients with chronic hepatitis B infection, primary biliary cirrhosis, sclerosing cholangitis, nonalcoholic steatohepatitis, and autoimmune liver disease. Alcoholic liver disease may recur if the patient returns to alcohol. HCC may also recur, but its recurrence rarely causes graft failure and is not always limited solely to the graft.

## ROLE OF LIVER TRANSPLANTATION FOR HEPATOCELLULAR CARCINOMA

There is considerable controversy as to whether patients with HCC are better served with liver transplantation versus liver resection. In the early days of liver transplantation, a number of first transplantations were done in patients with cancer. The immediate postoperative success likely reflected less severe liver disease and absent portal hypertension. Although the operation and early post-transplantation course could be judged as a success in these patients, they succumbed with recurrent cancer. As a consequence, liver transplantation for HCC was not pursued on a large scale for many years. Mazzaferro and colleagues[21] have clearly defined those patients with HCC who were likely to have survival that matched other indications for transplantation. This group defined the Milan criteria, which selected candidates with good short- and long-term outcomes and a low rate of tumor recurrence. The Milan criteria dictate that transplantation be limited to patients with a single tumor smaller than 5 cm or no more than three tumors, the largest of which must be less than 3 cm. These criteria have been applied throughout the world and adapted by the central agency distributing livers in the United States (UNOS) to provide the basis for additional points to modify the MELD score. The Milan criteria, based on the pathology of the explanted organ, has been challenged because preoperative imaging may be inaccurate in as many as 30% of patients, both in overestimating and underestimating the number and size of cancers. Additionally, the criteria have been challenged as being too restrictive by a number of groups who have demonstrated excellent short- and long-term survival; they expanded the criteria to include bigger solitary tumors and/or an increase in the number of tumors.[45,46]

HCC most commonly develops on the background of chronic scarring of the liver—cirrhosis. In the setting of cirrhosis, the issue of hepatic reserve and potential for decompensation limits the suitability of resection as a first-line approach to patients with cirrhosis and HCC. The other limitation of resection as definitive treatment for HCC is the potential for recurrence in the remaining liver. Because HCC occurs in the background of chronic liver disease, its occurrence reflects a field effect and therefore the potential evolution to HCC in other portions of the liver.

Data from patients followed after resection or radiofrequency ablation have demonstrated that 40% to 50% of patients will have recurrence by 3 years.[47] Although outcomes from resection have improved significantly over the past 20 years, with 1-year patient survival that matches the outcomes of liver transplantation, the 5-year disease-free survival for resection is far lower than the outcomes for transplantation when treating tumors of the same size.[48]

The major limitation in the use of transplantation as treatment for HCC is the limited number of donors. The disparity between the number of potential deceased donors and patients listed for transplantation is significant; HCC is increasingly the indication for transplantation, accounting for 25% of transplantations done in 2008.[22] The use of live donors or extended-criteria deceased donors has not yet met the continued need. Use of transplantation in a patient with HCC removes from the donor pool a lifesaving organ from a patient who may not have an alternative therapy, such as resection. It is hoped that better patient selection using biologic markers of the tumor or of the remnant liver may predict those patients at highest risk of recurrence after resection and funnel those patients toward transplantation and the remaining patients, at low risk for recurrence, would undergo resection.

It has been suggested that liver resection be used as first-line therapy for HCC, with salvage transplantation if and when the cancer recurs.[49] One could consider this a "poor man's" biologic marker using the remnant liver's biology over time to delineate those patients at risk for recurrence. This approach would avoid unnecessary transplantation and unwarranted immunosuppression in patients in whom the tumor does not recur. However, this is hampered by the fact that many patients recur outside the criteria for transplantation, with multiple intrahepatic tumors, and that transplantation after resection may be more difficult.

The recurrence after resection may be more aggressive and likely to be outside of transplantation criteria, because of extensive tumor within the liver or as the result of metastatic disease. There are conflicting data in the literature in this regard.[50,51]

## ROLE OF CELLULAR TRANSPLANTATION IN LIVER REPLACEMENT

The replacement of the liver involves a major surgical procedure, with complex technical and immunologic aspects. The notion, therefore, of using cells instead of the entire organ is an attractive alternative.

The use of hepatocyte transplantation makes the most logical sense for replacing missing enzymes in which only a small number of cells would be needed to correct deficiencies.

Examples of such defects include urea cycle defects such as ornithine transcarbamylase deficiency and the defect in bilirubin conjugation, Crigler-Najjar syndrome. Animal models have demonstrated the possibility of at least temporary correction of enzyme deficits using hepatocyte transplantation.[52]

Hepatocytes could also be used in fulminant hepatic failure in which the hepatic scaffolding is left intact, and a few case reports have suggested its usefulness.[52] Hepatocyte transplantation has also been used in chronic liver disease but the results have not been convincing.[52] When advanced liver disease is associated with portal hypertension, it is unlikely to be of benefit.

The potential role for the use of hepatocytes or stem cells from the host has expanded with the reintroduction of these cells and is the hope for the future. This approach may avoid the need for liver replacement and may also obviate the need for immunosuppression.[53]

## SELECTED REFERENCES

Baker TB, Jay CL, Ladner DP, et al: Laparoscopy-assisted and open living donor right hepatectomy: A comparative study of outcomes. Surgery 146:817–823, 2009.

> The use of minimally invasive surgery (MIS) for live donor kidney transplantation markedly increased the donor pool. This article reports results of the application of MIS for live donor liver transplantation.

Feng S, Goodrich NP, Bragg-Gresham JL, et al: Characteristics associated with liver graft failure: The concept of a donor risk index. Am J Transplant 6:783–790, 2006.

> It is recognized that the outcome after liver transplantation must take into account comorbid conditions in the recipient. This article articulates the donor factors that also influence post-transplantation survival.

Kamath PS, Wiesner RH, Malinchoc M, et al: A model to predict survival in patients with end-stage liver disease. Hepatology 33:464–470, 2001.

> This article describes the scoring system currently used to distribute livers in the United States. It also predicts for chance of death without liver replacement.

Mazzaferro V, Regalia E, Doci R, et al: Liver transplantation for the treatment of small hepatocellular carcinomas in patients with cirrhosis. N Engl J Med 334:693–699, 1996.

> This landmark article demonstrates for the first time that patients with small HCC undergoing liver transplantation have comparable results to patients with other diagnoses.

Pillai AA, Levitsky J: Overview of immunosuppression in liver transplantation. World J Gastroenterol 15:4225–4233, 2009.

> This article provides a broad overview of the drugs used for immunosuppression in liver transplantation.

Schaubel DE, Guidinger MK, Biggins SW, et al: Survival benefit-based deceased-donor liver allocation. Am J Transplant 9:970–981, 2009.

> Avoidance of death before transplantation and survival benefit after transplantation are blended together to dictate a new potential distribution of livers for transplantation.

Yao FY: Liver transplantation for hepatocellular carcinoma: Beyond the Milan criteria. Am J Transplant 8:1982–1989, 2008.

> The outcomes after liver transplantation using the Milan criteria represent excellent results but exclude a large number of patients. Expanding the criteria serves more patients without sacrificing outcome.

## REFERENCES


1. Murray G, Holden R: Transplantation of kidneys, experimentally and in human cases. Am J Surg 87:508–515, 1954.
2. A definition of irreversible coma. Report of the Ad Hoc Committee of the Harvard Medical School to Examine the Definition of Brain Death. JAMA 205:337–340, 1968.
3. Starzl TE, Groth CG, Brettschneider L, et al: Orthotopic homotransplantation of the human liver. Ann Surg 168:392–415, 1968.
4. Borel JF, Feurer C, Gubler HU, et al: Biological effects of cyclosporin A: A new antilymphocytic agent. Agents Actions 6:468–475, 1976.
5. Kotru A, Sheperd R, Nadler M, et al: Combined lung and liver transplantation: The United States experience. Transplantation 82:144–145; author reply 145, 2006.
6. Ostapowicz G, Fontana RJ, Schiodt FV, et al: Results of a prospective study of acute liver failure at 17 tertiary care centers in the United States. Ann Intern Med 137:947–954, 2002.
7. Marudanayagam R, Shanmugam V, Gunson B, et al: Aetiology and outcome of acute liver failure. HPB (Oxford) 11:429–434, 2009.
8. Lee WM: Etiologies of acute liver failure. Semin Liver Dis 28:142–152, 2008.
9. Roche B, Samuel D: Risk factors for hepatitis C recurrence after liver transplantation. J Viral Hepat 14(Suppl 1):89–96, 2007.
10. Everson GT: Impact of immunosuppressive therapy on recurrence of hepatitis C. Liver Transpl 8:S19–S27, 2002.
11. Berenguer M: Systematic review of the treatment of established recurrent hepatitis C with pegylated interferon in combination with ribavirin. J Hepatol 49:274–287, 2008.
12. El-Serag HB, Mason AC: Rising incidence of hepatocellular carcinoma in the United States. N Engl J Med 340:745–750, 1999.
13. Beasley RP: Hepatitis B virus. The major etiology of hepatocellular carcinoma. Cancer 61:1942–1956, 1988.
14. Liermann Garcia RF, Evangelista Garcia C, McMaster P, et al: Transplantation for primary biliary cirrhosis: Retrospective analysis of 400 patients in a single center. Hepatology 33:22–27, 2001.
15. Gow PJ, Chapman RW: Liver transplantation for primary sclerosing cholangitis. Liver 20:97–103, 2000.
16. Younossi ZM: Review article: Current management of non-alcoholic fatty liver disease and non-alcoholic steatohepatitis. Aliment Pharmacol Ther 28:2–12, 2008.
17. Tan-Tam CC, Frassetto LA, Stock PG: Liver and kidney transplantation in HIV-infected patients. AIDS Rev 11:190–204, 2009.
18. Saner FH, Nadalin S, Pavlakovic G, et al: Portopulmonary hypertension in the early phase following liver transplantation. Transplantation 82:887–891, 2006.

**19.** Martinez-Palli G, Taura P, Balust J, et al: Liver transplantation in high-risk patients: Hepatopulmonary syndrome and portopulmonary hypertension. Transplant Proc 37:3861–3864, 2005.

**20.** Dew MA, DiMartini AF, De Vito Dabbs A, et al: Rates and risk factors for nonadherence to the medical regimen after adult solid organ transplantation. Transplantation 83:858–873, 2007.

**21.** Mazzaferro V, Regalia E, Doci R, et al: Liver transplantation for the treatment of small hepatocellular carcinomas in patients with cirrhosis. N Engl J Med 334:693–699, 1996.

**22.** Health Resources, Services Administration, U.S. Department of Health & Human Services: Organ Procurement and Transplantation Network, 2011 (http://optn.transplant.hrsa.gov).

**23.** Kamath PS, Wiesner RH, Malinchoc M, et al: A model to predict survival in patients with end-stage liver disease. Hepatology 33:464–470, 2001.

**24.** Martin AP, Bartels M, Hauss J, et al: Overview of the MELD score and the UNOS adult liver allocation system. Transplant Proc 39:3169–3174, 2007.

**25.** Schaubel DE, Guidinger MK, Biggins SW, et al: Survival benefit-based deceased-donor liver allocation. Am J Transplant 9:970–981, 2009.

**26.** Ioannou GN, Perkins JD, Carithers RL, Jr: Liver transplantation for hepatocellular carcinoma: impact of the MELD allocation system and predictors of survival. Gastroenterology 134:1342–1351, 2008.

**27.** Barshes NR, Lee TC, Udell IW, et al: The pediatric end-stage liver disease (PELD) model as a predictor of survival benefit and post-transplant survival in pediatric liver transplant recipients. Liver Transpl 12:475–480, 2006.

**28.** Otte JB, de Ville de Goyet J, Alberti D, et al: The concept and technique of the split liver in clinical transplantation. Surgery 107:605–612, 1990.

**29.** Millis JM, Cronin DC, Brady LM, et al: Primary living-donor liver transplantation at the University of Chicago: Technical aspects of the first 104 recipients. Ann Surg 232:104–111, 2000.

**30.** Segev DL, Muzaale AD, Caffo BS, et al: Perioperative mortality and long-term survival following live kidney donation. JAMA 303:959–966, 2010.

**31.** Trotter JF, Adam R, Lo CM, et al: Documented deaths of hepatic lobe donors for living donor liver transplantation. Liver Transpl 12:1485–1488, 2006.

**32.** Hwang S, Lee SG, Lee YJ, et al: Lessons learned from 1,000 living donor liver transplantations in a single center: How to make living donations safe. Liver Transpl 12:920–927, 2006.

**33.** Song GW, Lee SG, Hwang S, et al: Dual living donor liver transplantation with ABO-incompatible and ABO-compatible grafts to overcome small-for-size graft and ABO blood group barrier. Liver Transpl 16:491–498, 2010.

**34.** Ghobrial RM, Freise CE, Trotter JF, et al: Donor morbidity after living donation for liver transplantation. Gastroenterology 135:468–476, 2008.

**35.** Baker TB, Jay CL, Ladner DP, et al: Laparoscopy-assisted and open living donor right hepatectomy: a comparative study of outcomes. Surgery 146:817–823, 2009.

**36.** Berg CL, Gillespie BW, Merion RM, et al: Improvement in survival associated with adult-to-adult living donor liver transplantation. Gastroenterology 133:1806–1813, 2007.

**37.** Selzner M, Kashfi A, Cattral MS, et al: Live donor liver transplantation in high MELD score recipients. Ann Surg 251:153–157, 2010.

**38.** Stewart ZA, Locke JE, Segev DL, et al: Increased risk of graft loss from hepatic artery thrombosis after liver transplantation with older donors. Liver Transpl 15:1688–1695, 2009.

**39.** Feng S, Goodrich NP, Bragg-Gresham JL, et al: Characteristics associated with liver graft failure: The concept of a donor risk index. Am J Transplant 6:783–790, 2006.

**40.** Skaro AI, Jay CL, Baker TB, et al: The impact of ischemic cholangiopathy in liver transplantation using donors after cardiac death: The untold story. Surgery 146:543–552; discussion 552–543, 2009.

**41.** Pillai AA, Levitsky J: Overview of immunosuppression in liver transplantation. World J Gastroenterol 15:4225–4233, 2009.

**42.** Sollinger HW: Mycophenolates in transplantation. Clin Transplant 18:485–492, 2004.

**43.** Sgourakis G, Radtke A, Fouzas I, et al: Corticosteroid-free immunosuppression in liver transplantation: A meta-analysis and meta-regression of outcomes. Transpl Int 22:892–905, 2009.

**44.** Watson CJ, Friend PJ, Jamieson NV, et al: Sirolimus: A potent new immunosuppressant for liver transplantation. Transplantation 67:505–509, 1999.

**45.** Yao FY: Liver transplantation for hepatocellular carcinoma: Beyond the Milan criteria. Am J Transplant 8:1982–1989, 2008.

**46.** Marsh JW, Schmidt C: The Milan criteria: No room on the metro for the king? Liver Transpl 16:252–255, 2010.

**47.** Ng KK, Poon RT, Lo CM, et al: Analysis of recurrence pattern and its influence on survival outcome after radiofrequency ablation of hepatocellular carcinoma. J Gastrointest Surg 12:183–191, 2008.

**48.** Morris-Stiff G, Gomez D, de Liguori Carino N, et al: Surgical management of hepatocellular carcinoma: Is the jury still out? Surg Oncol 18:298–321, 2009.

**49.** Poon RT, Fan ST, Lo CM, et al: Long-term survival and pattern of recurrence after resection of small hepatocellular carcinoma in patients with preserved liver function: Implications for a strategy of salvage transplantation. Ann Surg 235:373–382, 2002.

**50.** Hu RH, Ho MC, Wu YM, et al: Feasibility of salvage liver transplantation for patients with recurrent hepatocellular carcinoma. Clin Transplant 19:175–180, 2005.

**51.** Cucchetti A, Vitale A, Gaudio MD, et al: Harm and benefits of primary liver resection and salvage transplantation for hepatocellular carcinoma. Am J Transplant 10:619–627, 2010.

**52.** Fitzpatrick E, Mitry RR, Dhawan A: Human hepatocyte transplantation: State of the art. J Intern Med 266:339–357, 2009.

**53.** Locke JE, Shamblott MJ, Cameron AM: Stem cells and the liver: Clinical applications in transplantation. Adv Surg 43:35–51, 2009.

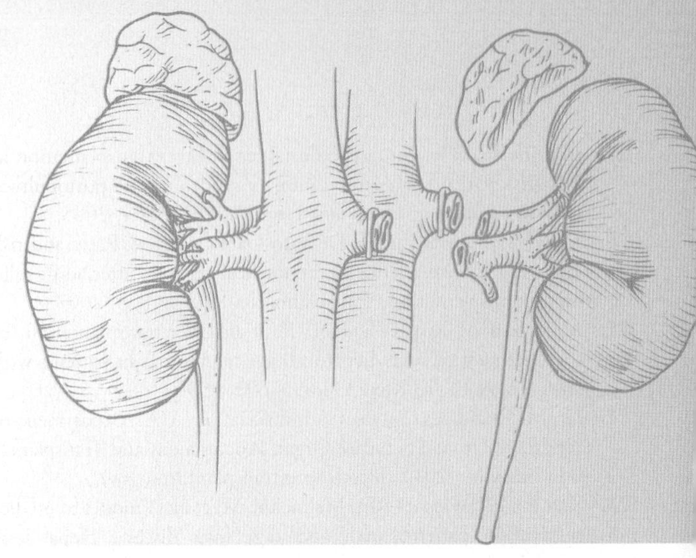

# CHAPTER 28

# KIDNEY AND PANCREAS TRANSPLANTATION

Yolanda Becker



## HISTORICAL PERSPECTIVE

Interest in transplanting organs into humans dates back to the early 1900s. Floresco described anastomosis of the renal graft to the iliac fossa in 1905. In 1906, Jaboulay attempted to use a pig kidney to cure a patient with acute nephritis. He anastomosed the renal xenograft to the brachial arteries of the patient and urine was noted for 1 hour postreperfusion. Alexis Carrel was developing techniques of triangulation of vascular anastomoses by performing various organ transplants in animals and received the Nobel Prize in 1912. However, organ function was minimal and further attempts at organ transplantation were abandoned. However, in the early 1950s, Medawar and colleagues described the prevention of rejection in mice and human organ transplantation was again attempted. The first successful renal transplantation was performed by Murray in 1954 between identical twins. Other major milestones in transplantation have included the discovery of cyclosporine and other effective immunosuppressive medications, description of the histocompatibility antigens, and perfecting of preservation solutions (Table 28-1).

The history of the discovery of diabetes and insulin is fascinating and well-documented. Pancreas transplantation has also developed as a durable way to provide constant insulin to the type 1 diabetic. The first pancreas transplantation in an animal was performed by Hedon in 1913, who attempted placement of a pancreas allograft in the neck of pancreatectomized dogs. The first successful human pancreas transplantation was performed by William Kelly and Richard Lillehei at the University of Minnesota. They transplanted a duct-ligated segmental pancreas graft simultaneously with a kidney graft from the same deceased donor. The pancreas was placed into the left iliac fossa but, unfortunately, had to be removed on the seventh postoperative day. Management of the exocrine pancreas secretions remained problematic, with many revisions over the years from using a donor duodenal button technique, bladder drainage, duct ablation via injection, and finally enteric drainage. This chapter describes aspects of kidney and pancreas transplantation. Patient selection for transplantation with a kidney or pancreas is considered first. Organ procurement, preservation, transplant technique, and outcomes of kidney and pancreas transplantation are discussed independently.

## KIDNEY TRANSPLANTATION

### Indications

Kidney transplantation offers patients better long-term outcomes than dialysis. The quality of life is improved and survival is projected to be 10 years longer than if the patient remains on dialysis.[1] During the past decade, the kidney waiting list has grown and the death of candidates who die while waiting has doubled. This reflects a change in demographics in the recipient waiting list, with patients listed at older ages and an increasing number of patients being inactive on the waiting list.[2]

The most common causes of renal disease have evolved over the last 10 years. Overall, the percentage of patients with diabetes and hypertension as the cause of failure has increased from 24% to 28% and the percentage of glomerular disease has declined from 42% to 21%.[2] In addition, the incidence of chronic kidney disease has also rapidly increased, from 209,000 patients in 1991 to 472,000 in 2004. Coresh and associates[3] have noted that the higher prevalence of diabetes, hypertension, and higher body mass index (BMI) explains this trend. Similarly, the waiting list for kidney transplantation continues to grow every year. Potential recipients are also older than in past decades, with the group aged 50 to 64 years seeing the greatest increase (Fig. 28-1) This change in demographics has certainly presented challenges in preparation of these patients for transplantation and immunosuppression. It is also estimated that by 2015, the annual incidence of end-stage renal disease will be 136,000 patients/year and the prevalence will be 712,000 patients/year.

### Patient Selection

The evaluation of patients as appropriate candidates for transplantation can be an arduous process. Patients with end-stage kidney disease have significant comorbidities and these must be taken into account when evaluating for transplantation. Guidelines for evaluation of these patients have been established.[4] Emphasis should be placed on determining the original cause of renal disease so that the patient can be given reasonable expectations for graft survival. A graded association has been reported between reduced glomerular filtration rate (GFR) and risk of death and cardiovascular events.[5] Mortality rates are more than 20%/year with dialysis. Long-term follow-up of kidney transplant recipients has shown a clear survival advantage over

**Table 28-1 Major Milestones in the History of Transplantation**

| YEAR | MILESTONE |
|---|---|
| 1954 | Dr. Joseph Murray performs the first successful kidney transplantation between identical twins. |
| 1966 | Kelly and Lillihei perform the first pancreas transplantation. |
| 1967 | First simultaneous kidney and pancreas transplantation. |
| 1970s | Borel, Stahelin, Calne, and White initiate trials of use of cyclosporine in transplantation. |
| 1980s | Belzer and Southard develop University of Wisconsin Solution (Viaspan). |
| 1990 | Dr. Murray receives the Nobel Prize in Medicine. |
| 1990 | Scharp and Lacy report the first successful human clinical islet transplantation. |

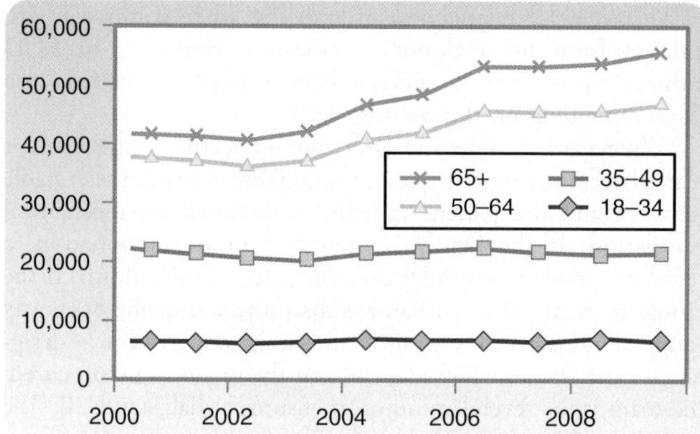


**FIGURE 28-1** Additions to the UNOS-OPTN (Organ Procurement and Transplantation Network) waiting list by age. (OPTN/UNOS Ethics Committee Report: Waiting list patient characteristics at end of year; kidney waiting list; active waitlist patients, 1999 to 2008 [http://www.ustransplant.org/annual_reports/current/501a_age_ki.htm]).

**BOX 28-1 Contraindications for Renal Transplantation**

**Absolute**
- Active malignancy
- Active infection
- Unreconstructable peripheral vascular disease
- Severe cardiac or pulmonary disease
- Active IV drug abuse

**Relative**
- Life expectancy
- History of nonadherence to medication regimen
- History of noncompliance with dialysis
- Financial barriers
- Psychiatric issues
- Renal disease with high recurrence rate

**Table 28-2 Primary Renal Diseases and Recurrence Rates**

| DISEASE | RECURRENCE RATE (%) | GRAFT LOSS (%) |
|---|---|---|
| Diabetes | 100 | Low until 10 yrs post-transplant |
| Focal segmental glomerulosclerosis | 20–30, first transplant; 80, second transplant | 40–50 |
| Membranoproliferative glomerulonephritis (MPGN) type 1 | 20–30 | 20–60 |
| MPGN type 2 | 50–100 | 10 |
| IgA nephropathy | 40–50 | 30 |
| Membranous nephropathy | 40 | Up to 50 |
| Hemolytic uremic syndrome | 30 | 20–30 |
| Systemic lupus | 30 | Rare |
| Polycystic kidney disease | 0 | 0 |

remaining on dialysis.[6] Studies have also shown significant improvements in quality of life measures.[7]

The first step in the evaluation process is referral to a transplantation center. Many factors may affect the ability of the patient to be seen for evaluation. Furth and coworkers[8] have shown that lower socioeconomic status, female gender, and lower level of education results in fewer referrals. There has been concern that geographic distance to a transplantation center might negatively influence access to care. However, a study of rural populations has shown that remote or rural residence is not associated with a longer waiting list time.

Recipients must be carefully evaluated for surgical risk as well as their ability to tolerate long-term immunosuppression. With improvements in perioperative management, the indications for kidney transplantation have increased. The absolute and relative contraindications for transplantation are shown in Box 28-1. HIV infection was once a contraindication to transplantation, but select patients have good results with transplantation as a treatment modality for HIV-associated nephropathy.[9] According to the National Kidney Foundation Kidney Disease Outcomes Quality Initiative (NKF KDOQI) guidelines, patients with a GFR of 30 mL/min/1.72 m$^2$ or less, and/or chronic kidney disease (CKD), stage 3 or 4, should be referred to a nephrologist (http://www.kidney.org/professionals/kdoqi/index.cfm). Patients whose GFR falls below 20 should be evaluated as possible kidney transplant recipients if they do not have an absolute contraindication.

Common causes of renal failure leading to the need for replacement therapy include diabetes, hypertension, glomerular disease, interstitial disease, cystic disease, and chronic allograft nephropathy, with subsequent failure of a transplanted kidney. Kidney disease can recur in the allograft with varying frequency. Some diseases may lead to transplant failure with an inability to retransplant, such as aggressive focal sclerosing glomerulonephritis. Common primary renal diseases and their probability of recurrence are listed in Table 28-2.[10–15]

Screening of potential recipients should begin with a detailed history, paying particular attention to the original cause of disease. The length of time on dialysis has been noted to be an independent risk factor for poorer outcomes.[16] The past medical history should include exposures to infectious diseases (especially tuberculosis, cytomegalovirus, Epstein-Barr virus, and hepatitis) as well as malignancy. Cardiac risk factors should be evaluated. A family history of renal disease or other systemic illnesses should be documented. Routine screening examinations such as Pap smear, mammography, colonoscopy, dental prophylaxis, and bone density scanning should be carried out as recommended by clinical practice guidelines. Prostate-specific antigen levels should be checked in men older than 50 years. In addition, the patient should be questioned about thrombotic events such as miscarriages, multiple dialysis access events, deep venous thrombosis, or pulmonary embolus so that a hypercoagulable profile can be obtained. The ability of the patient to tolerate immunosuppression should be evaluated. This not only involves consideration of the medical conditions, but also the ability to comply with a complex medical regimen and the financial ability to obtain the medications.

As noted, end-stage kidney disease patients are at increased risk for cardiovascular disease.[5] Hence, a careful preoperative cardiac screening must be completed. However, there is little consensus about the optimal screening algorithm. Patients should have a baseline electrocardiogam (ECG) obtained, recognizing that almost 75% will have evidence of left ventricular hypertrophy. The patient's risk profile should be assessed to see whether any risk factors can be modified (e.g., diet, weight management). Low-risk patients include those who have good functional capacity and no previously identified cardiac disease. These are typically patients with isolated renal disease such as immunoglobulin A (IgA) nephropathy or polycystic kidney disease, and with little comorbidity. Moderate-risk patients should undergo stress testing. It is important to ensure that the stress is diagnostic and a reasonable heart rate is achieved. Moderate-risk patients include those without cardiac symptoms but who have diabetes, prior history of heart disease, or two or more other risk factors for coronary disease (e.g., smoking, strong family history, hyperlipidemia, hypercholesterolemia). High-risk patients include those with a positive noninvasive test result, long-standing diabetes, or a history of severe congestive heart failure. These patients require cardiac catheterization prior to being accepted for the transplant list. Cardiac revascularization should occur prior to transplantation. If the patient requires lifelong clopidogrel (Plavix), there will be an increased risk of bleeding.[17] Patients are required by federal guidelines to be reevaluated on a yearly basis. At any reevaluation, the patient's cardiac status should be routinely reviewed and updated.

A full physical examination should be completed. Renal patients are at increased risk for cerebrovascular events[18]; therefore, if carotid bruits are discovered, patients should be screened for significant carotid stenosis. Atrial fibrillation can also be discovered on physical examination. The femoral, dorsalis pedis, and posterior tibial arteries should be palpated and any bruits documented. If the pulses are abnormal, or the patient has undergone previous amputation for vascular disease, noncontrast abdominal and pelvic CT scans should be obtained to assess the level of peripheral vascular disease. Iliac inflow might be significantly compromised, which would prevent the patient from having a successful outcome. If inflow is compromised, then one can consider whether a revascularization is warranted prior to or at the time of transplantation.[19]

Kidney organs can be obtained from living or deceased donors. The demand for kidney transplant and appropriate organs has continually increased given the increase in the burden of ESRD. Although living related donor (LRD) and living unrelated donor (LURD) numbers have increased in recent years, expanding the deceased donor pool is crucial. In 2003, the National Organ Breakthrough Collaborative was launched. The intent of this national effort was to increase the conversion rate (number of families consenting to donation in appropriate potential donors) to 75%. An update in 2005 sought to increase donors organs further by increasing the average organs transplanted/donor to 3.75.[20] Deceased donor kidneys are placed in three broad categories: extended-criteria donor (ECD), standard criteria donor (SCD), and donor after cardiac death (DCD). As part of the effort to increase the pool of potential kidney organs, an emphasis was placed on ECD and DCD kidneys. In the past, these donor organs had a high rate of discard and there were no uniform DCD policies across the country. ECD kidneys are obtained from donors older than 60 years or from donors aged 50 to 59 years with at least two of the following criteria: cerebrovascular accident as cause of death, terminal creatinine higher than 1.5 mg/dL, or a history of hypertension. Kidneys from donors meeting the criteria for ECD have a 1.7 relative risk of graft loss when compared with kidneys from other donors.[21] However, recipients of ECD kidneys clearly have a survival benefit when compared with those remaining on the waiting list.[22]

In regard to donation after cardiac death, the health care team determines that the patient is unlikely to make a reasonable recovery and the patient is being maintained on mechanical ventilation. If the family is interested in organ donation, a request is made to consider donation after cardiac death. If the family consents, the ventilator is disconnected in the operating room or intensive care unit. If the heart stops within a designated time frame, which depends on the organ to be procured, the team waits several minutes to ensure cardiac standstill. The patient is then declared dead by the health care team (not a member of the organ recovery team) and the organs are procured en bloc.

### Living Donor Selection

The first successful living kidney donation was performed in 1954. Since that time, data continue to show that living kidney donation provides the best graft and patient survival results.[23] Donors may or may not be genetically related to their intended recipient. In some cases, living donors are anonymous. There are now reports of extended altruistic donor chains. In these cases, an initial donor-recipient pair cannot go forward with transplantation usually because of ABO incompatibility or sensitization of the recipient. A reciprocal exchange with another incompatible pair allows for a domino transplantation, with multiple exchanges with as many as 10 kidney transplant chains reported.[24] The 5-year survival of an unrelated kidney transplant is the same as that from a related donor. Interestingly, the outcome from a completely mismatched donor and one who is haploidentical is also similar. The underlying premise of living donation is that the donor will not suffer any medical consequences from the donation and has minimal surgical risk.

Currently accepted eligibility criteria include the following: age, 18 to 70 years, BMI less than 35, no cancer or active infection, and adequate renal function. ABO compatibility is also a consideration. However, recipients can undergo desensitization protocols and transplantation can be performed across ABO barriers. The donor should be informed in these circumstances of an increased risk of rejection of the kidney by the recipient.

**BOX 28-2 Contraindications to Living Kidney Donation**

BMI > 40
Diabetes
Active malignancy
HIV-positive
GFR < 70
Significant albuminuria
Hypertension requiring multiple medications
Pelvic or horseshoe kidney
Significant psychiatric impairment
Nephrolithiasis with a high chance of recurrence (cystine, struvite)

There is some individual variation among transplantation centers concerning acceptable GFR or BMI values. Relative contraindications include renal stones, impaired glucose tolerance, with a family history of type 2 diabetes, GFR of 70 to 80, hypertension, and BMI higher than 35. Absolute contraindications are listed in Box 28-2. For screening, all donors should have a thorough history and physical examination completed. Potential donors should be asked about nonsteroidal anti-inflammatory drug (NSAID) use in addition to questions about any medical illnesses. Potential donors should be made aware of the need to be away from work for a period of time and their willingness to donate free of coercion should be ascertained. An ECG and chest x-ray should be obtained. Routine laboratory work should include urinalysis, complete blood count (CBC), liver function tests, determination of creatinine (Cr) level, with estimated GFR (eGFR), lipid profile, microalbumin level, and oral glucose toleranc test. Prostate-specific antigen (PSA) levels should be obtained in men. Mammograms and Pap smears should be obtained in women of appropriate age. Radiographic evaluation of the anatomy of the renal arteries, veins, and collecting system should be performed and can be done via computed tomography (CT) angiography, magnetic resonance imaging (MRI), or arteriography, based on local expertise. In addition, all donors must be evaluated by an independent donor advocate (IDA). The IDA is not influenced by a relationship with the intended recipient or the transplantation center. The donor and recipient pair must also adhere to the National Organ Transplant Act of 1984, which states that "It is unlawful for any person to knowingly acquire, receive, or otherwise transfer any human organ for valuable consideration for use in human transplantation." Many transplantation centers ask potential donors to undergo a psychological or psychiatric evaluation.

Potential donors should be informed that the risk of perioperative mortality, regardless of surgical technique, is approximately 0.03%.[23] Matas and colleagues[25] have surveyed 234 United Network for Organ Sharing (UNOS)-listed kidney transplantation programs and found that reoperation is required in 0.4% of patients undergoing open nephrectomy, 1.0% in hand-assisted laparoscopic nephrectomy, and 0.9% in total laparoscopic nephrectomy.

Donor nephrectomy may be performed via open or laparoscopic techniques. The open technique is performed through a flank incision. Currently, over 50% of the donor nephrectomy procedures in the United States are performed laparoscopically. There are variations in the technique of laparoscopic donor nephrectomy. Some centers use a hand-assisted approach whereas others perform the procedure entirely laparoscopically and make a Pfannenstiel incision to retrieve the kidney. Some centers perform a single-incision donor nephrectomy and dissect the renal hilum using instruments placed through a GelPort, which is ultimately the site of kidney retrieval. If unexpected anatomy or bleeding is encountered, it is important to convert to open techniques promptly to prevent any donor complications or prolonged surgery.

## Laparoscopic Surgical Technique

The right or left kidney can be procured laparoscopically. The left renal anatomy is generally preferred because the renal vein is longer. Many studies have shown that the right kidney can be procured safely.[23] A left kidney dissection is described here because it is more commonly done. A 5-mm entry site is placed in the left lower quadrant and a Veress needle is used to insufflate the abdomen to a pressure of 10 to 15 mm Hg. A 12-mm port is placed at the umbilicus. Two additional 5-mm ports are placed, one at the left costal margin and the last in the midaxillary line to retract the kidney.

The left colon and splenic flexure are taken down at the line of Toldt with the harmonic scalpel. The ureter and gonadal vein complex are identified at the pelvic brim and isolated from surrounding tissue. The renal vein is identified by following the gonadal vein to its entry point. The artery is identified and lymphatic tissue overlying the artery and vein is divided using the harmonic scalpel.

The adrenal gland is visualized at the upper pole of the kidney and divided from that site. The adrenal vein is dissected free from surrounding tissue and transected. The kidney is retracted medially and the posterior and lateral attachments outside of Gerota's fascia are divided with the harmonic scalpel. A Pfannenstiel incision is made approximately three fingerbreadths above the pubis. The rectus abdominis muscles are split at the midline and a purse-string 0 Vicryl suture is sewn in the peritoneum. Electrocautery is used to enter the peritoneum and an Endo Catch bag is introduced for retrieval of the kidney. The ureter and gonadal vein are transected with the linear endo GIA white load stapler at the pelvic brim. The artery is isolated and divided with an endo GIA white load linear cutting stapler. The vein is also divided using the endo GIA stapler. The kidney is placed in the Endo Catch bag, brought out through the Pfannenstiel incision, and given to the recipient surgeon for flushing.

## Open Surgical Technique

The patient is placed in the lateral decubitus position. A subcostal incision is made from the tip of the 12th rib anteriorly, extending approximately 10 to 12 cm. The latissimus dorsi and posterior serratus are divided. The external and internal oblique muscles are divided, starting at the posterior border. The retroperitoneal space is exposed and Gerota's fascia is identified. The 12th rib may need to be resected to allow for better exposure. However, this will increase the risk of a postoperative pneumothorax (0.09%).[25] Gerota's fascia is then incised. The ureter is identified and dissected down to the iliac vessels, at which point it is clipped and divided, preserving an appropriate length for subsequent transplantation. Tissue overlying the renal artery and vein is identified and divided. At this point, the kidney is isolated on its vascular pedicle. When the recipient team is ready, a right angle clamp is placed on the renal artery and the artery is divided. A Satinsky clamp is placed around the inferior vena cava for a right nephrectomy or on the renal vein for a left nephrectomy. The renal vein is divided and the kidney is given to the recipient team. The renal artery stump is then suture-ligated. The renal vein stump is oversewn with 5-0 Prolene sutures in a running fashion.

## Postoperative Care and Follow-Up

Postoperatively, the patient should be kept well-hydrated and careful attention paid to urine output. The diet can be advanced quickly in open or laparoscopic cases. The most common complications include urinary retention and ileus. Other less common complications include bleeding, deep venous thrombosis or pulmonary embolus, rhabdomyolysis, and injury to the bowel, bladder, or spleen. Patients who undergo laparoscopic donor nephrectomy tend to have shorter hospital stays (2 to 4 days) compared with patients who have undergone open nephrectomy (3 to 7 days).[23]

The long-term consequences of kidney donation have been carefully reviewed. However, a long-term donor registry has still not been created. Survival and the development of end-stage kidney disease do not appear to be affected by living donation. In a study of 3698 kidney donors from 1963 to 2007 at a single center, it was shown that end-stage renal disease (ESRD) developed in 180 cases/million persons/year in donors compared with 268 cases/million persons/year in the general population.[26] Scores of physical and mental health in this population were significantly better than those of the general U.S. population. In summary, living donation is a safe procedure that does not adversely affect the future health of carefully screened people. Previous living kidney donors enjoy an excellent quality of life and the rate of change in GFR has not been found to exceed that of the general population.

## Deceased Donors

As noted earlier, organs are procured from standard criteria or extended-criteria donors. Procurement occurs after declaration of death, either brain death (Box 28-3) or cardiac death. The University of Wisconsin has created a tool to determine the likelihood of progression to cardiac death to allow centers to inform families better (Fig. 28-2).[27] A complete neurologic examination must first be completed when the patient has a core temperature above 32° C and there is no evidence of drug intoxication, poisoning, or neuromuscular blocking agents. There can be no other medical conditions that could confound the clinical assessment, such as severe electrolyte, acid-base, or endocrine disturbances or hypotension. A complete clinical neurologic examination includes documentation of coma, the absence of brainstem reflexes, and apnea. Confirmatory testing is also completed, as outlined in Box 28-3.

A careful medical and social history is obtained from the medical record and family. Potential donors are excluded if there is active infection or malignancy. Renal function and urine output are assessed. If a donor has high-risk behavior, as defined by the Centers for Disease Control and Prevention (CDC) for transmission of HIV, the donor may need to be excluded from consideration (Box 28-4). When managing a donor, it is important to monitor urine output carefully. Vasopressin may need to be given if diabetes insipidus develops. Many organ procurement specialists administer hormonal therapy to stabilize the donor after the catecholamine release that is common in acute brain death.[28] This catecholamine release can result in significant decrease in thyroid hormone, cortisol, and insulin levels.

**BOX 28-3 Confirmatory Testing Criteria for Determination of Brain Death**

**Cerebral Angiography**

The contrast medium should be injected under high pressure in anterior and posterior circulation.

No intracerebral filling should be detected at the level of entry of the carotid or vertebral artery to the skull.

The external carotid circulation should be patent.

The filling of the superior longitudinal sinus may be delayed.

**Electroencephalography**

A minimum of eight scalp electrodes should be used.

Interelectrode impedance should be between 100 and 10,000 Ω.

The integrity of the entire recording system should be tested.

The distance between electrodes should be at least 10 cm.

The sensitivity should be increased to at least 2 μV for 30 min with the inclusion of appropriate calibrations.

The high-frequency filter setting should not be set below 30 Hz and the low-frequency setting should not be above 1 Hz.

Electroencephalography should demonstrate a lack of reactivity to intense somatosensory or audiovisual stimuli.

**Transcranial Doppler Ultrasonography**

There should be bilateral insonation. The probe should be placed at the temporal bone above the zygomatic arch or the vertebrobasilar arteries through the suboccipital transcranial window.

The abnormalities should include a lack of diastolic or reverberating flow and documentation of small systolic peaks in early systole. A finding of a complete absence of flow may not be reliable because of inadequate transtemporal windows for insonation.

**Cerebral Scintigraphy (Tc-99m Hexametazime)**

The isotope should be injected within 30 min after its reconstitution.

A static image of 500,000 counts should be obtained at several time points—immediately, between 30 and 60 min later, and at 2 hr.

A correct IV injection may be confirmed with additional images of the liver demonstrating uptake (optional).

From Wijdicks EF: The diagnosis of brain death. N Engl J Med 344:1215–1221, 2001.

### Kidney Procurement and Preparation

The retroperitoneum is fully exposed. The ureters are identified and divided as close to the bladder as possible. When procuring the right kidney, it is important to preserve the vena cava cuff so that the renal vein can be lengthened, if needed, to facilitate the recipient operation.

On the back table, Gerota's fascia is removed. The renal artery and vein are identified. The ureter is identified and the periureteric tissue is preserved, as well as the tissue along the lower pole of the kidney, to prevent ureter ischemia. If any lower pole renal arteries are identified, these must be reconstructed to ensure adequate blood supply to the ureter.

DCD TOOL SCORE

| Points | Expiration in <60 minutes | Expiration in <120 minutes |
|---|---|---|
| 7–11 | 4–24% | 10–40% |
| 12–17 | 34–87% | 51–91% |
| 18–23 | 92–98% | 94–98% |

UW DCD EVALUATION TOOL

| Criteria | Assigned Points | Pt. Score |
|---|---|---|
| ***Spontaneous Respirations After 10 min.*** | – | |
| Rate >12 | 1 | |
| Rate <12 | 3 | |
| TV >200 cc | 1 | |
| TV <200 cc | 3 | |
| NIF >20 | 1 | |
| NIF <20 | 3 | |
| ***No Spontaneous Respirations*** | 9 | |
| ***BMI*** | | |
| <25 | 1 | |
| 25–29 | 2 | |
| >30 | 3 | |
| ***Vasopressors*** | | |
| No Vasopressors | 1 | |
| Single Vasopressor | 2 | |
| Multiple Vasopressors | 3 | |
| ***Patient Age*** | | |
| 0–30 | 1 | |
| 31–50 | 2 | |
| 51+ | 3 | |
| ***Intubation*** | | |
| Endotracheal tube | 3 | |
| Tracheostomy | 1 | |
| ***Oxygenation After 10 minutes*** | | |
| O2 Sat >90% | 1 | |
| O2 Sat 80–89% | 2 | |
| O2 Sat <79% | 3 | |
| **Final Score** | | |
| Date of Extubation Time of Extubation | | |
| Date of Expiration Time of Expiration | | |
| **Total Time** | | |

**FIGURE 28-2** Tool for predicting progression to cardiac death (Adapted from Lewis J, Peltier J, Nelson H, et al: Development of the University of Wisconsin Donation After Cardiac Death Evaluation Tool. Prog Transplant 13:265–273, 2003.)

**BOX 28-4 High-Risk Donor*: Behavior and History Exclusionary Criteria**

- Men who have had sex with another man in the preceding 5 yr
- Persons who report nonmedical IV, IM, or subsequence injection of drugs in the preceding 5 yr
- Persons with hemophilia or related clotting disorders who have received human-derived clotting factor concentrates
- Men and women who have engaged in sex in exchange for money or drugs in the preceding 5 yr
- Persons who have had sex in the preceding 12 mo with any person described in items 1 to 4 above or with a person known or suspected to have HIV infection
- Persons who have been exposed in the last 12 mo to known or suspected HIV-infected blood
- Inmates of correctional systems

*For transmission of HIV, according to the Centers for Disease Control and Prevention.

**Table 28-3 Composition of Viaspan Preservation Solution**

| UNIVERSITY OF WISCONSIN (UW) SOLUTION (VIASPAN) | CONCENTRATION |
|---|---|
| Lactobionic acid | 100 mmol/liter |
| KOH (5 M) | 20 mL |
| NaOH (5 M) | 5 mL |
| Adenosine | 5 mmol/liter |
| Allopurinol | 3 mmol/liter |
| $KH_2PO_4$ | 25 mmol/liter |
| HES | 5 g% |
| Glutathione | 3 mmol/liter |
| Raffinose | 30 mmol/liter |
| $MgSO_4$ | 5 mmol/liter |
| Insulin | 40 U/liter |
| Dexamethasone | 8 mg/liter |
| Bactrim | 2 mL/liter |

### Preservation and Storage

Once the kidneys are procured, they must be transported to the respective transplantation centers by the organ procurement organization (OPO). During this time, the kidneys experience changes because of cold ischemia. The goal of preservation is to extend the period of organ viability. Delayed graft function (DGF) significantly increases at 24 hours. Various preservation solutions have been developed over the years. The predominant storage solution used in the United State is Viaspan (DuPont Pharma, Dublin). The composition of Viaspan is shown in Table 28-3.

Kidneys may be stored in a static cold solution. However, there is increasing evidence supporting the use of pulsatile machine perfusion in the preservation of kidneys. Using this technology, flow is maintained throughout the kidney and vasoconstriction can be minimized. A recent study by Moers and associates[29] has shown that machine perfusion significantly decreases the risk of DGF and the recipient's Cr level is significantly lower for the first 2 weeks following transplantation. Interestingly, there was no difference seen when a subgroup analysis of DCD, ECD and SCD kidneys was completed. However, if DGF did develop, the duration was 3 days shorter in machine-perfused kidneys (10 versus 13 days; $P = .04$).

### Recipient Operation

The kidney is usually placed in a retroperitoneal position in the recipient. The donor renal vein is anastomosed to the common iliac vein and the donor artery is anastomosed to the recipient common or external iliac artery. It should be noted that if the recipient has significant upstream iliac atherosclerotic disease, this may affect transplantation outcomes. The ureter is then spatulated and an end-to-side anastomosis is completed to the bladder mucosa. A ureteral stent is placed, which is then removed 4 to 6 weeks postoperatively.

## Postoperative Surgical Complications

The overall rate of technical complications in kidney transplantation is low (5% to 10%). Most complications present as a sudden decrease in urine output. However, some recipients experience DGF, so urine output is not a reliable marker of a surgical complication. Daily monitoring of serum Cr and hemoglobin levels is crucial in the first days following kidney transplantation. Other parameters such as $\beta_2$-microglobulin ($\beta_2$M) can also be helpful to differentiate early rejection from a surgical complication. The most common surgical complications are outlined here.

### Hemorrhage

If the kidney transplant was placed in the retroperitoneal space and no window was created to the peritoneal cavity, bleeding will be limited. Patients will commonly present with the acute onset of flank pain and there may be a palpable mass at the incision site. An acute decrease in hematocrit or hemoglobin level may also be seen. Because of compression of the kidney parenchyma, patients will sometimes present with hypertension rather than expected hypotension. Many patients are on beta blockers, so tachycardia is also not a reliable sign. The patient must be examined and a high clinical suspicion should be maintained. Risk factors include obesity, antiplatelet agents, and anticoagulation.[30] An ultrasound can be helpful if time permits. Often, the bleeding site cannot be identified and evacuation of a large hematoma is completed. The kidney should be biopsied because hyperacute rejection can lead to kidney swelling and disruption of the parenchyma as the cause of the bleed (Fig. 28-3).

### Venous Thrombosis

Venous thrombosis occurs in 0.5% to 4% of cases and usually presents within the first week postoperatively.[31] The patient may develop sudden hematuria or decrease in urine output. Ultrasound confirms the diagnosis. The transplanted renal vein might be kinked at the time of the original procedure because of compression in the retroperitoneal position or possibly external compression for a lymphocele or hematoma. Dialysis patients also have a high incidence of hypercoagulable states. A preoperative hypercoagulable workup should be completed if the patient reports multiple dialysis access thromboses, especially of native fistulas, a history of deep venous thrombosis or pulmonary embolus, or a high incidence of miscarriages. The graft is usually

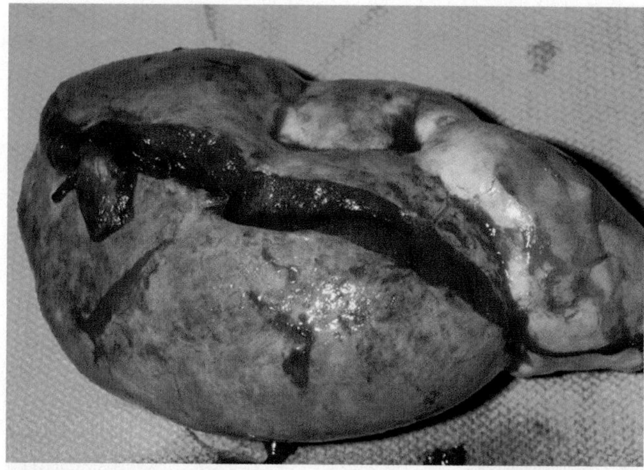

**FIGURE 28-3** Acute rejection causing kidney parenchymal disruption and hemorrhage.

unable to be salvaged. There are case reports of salvage if the patient is able to be taken to the operaating room (OR) within the hour after the diagnosis.[32] However, this is rare, and usually a transplant nephrectomy is required.

### Arterial Thrombosis

This is a rare complication, occurring in less than 1% of cases. The patient may have sudden cessation of urine output, or the failure of the $\beta_2$M levels to decrease post-transplantation may herald the problem. Ultrasound is diagnostic. If there is normal anatomy and a single renal artery, the chance of salvage is minimal. The kidney will not tolerate warm ischemia and a transplant nephrectomy is warranted. In rare cases, if a segmental artery or upper pole branch is affected, the remaining renal mass may be able to sustain the patient for a period of time. However, if a lower pole artery is thrombosed, the ureter becomes ischemic and a urine leak may develop from ureteral necrosis.

### Arterial Stenosis

Stenosis of the renal artery is a late complication. The incidence varies from 1% to 23%. Patients usually present with an asymptomatic rise in the creatinine level. Some may have bilateral lower extremity edema and worsening hypertension. MRI or CT angiography (CTA) can be performed to confirm the diagnosis. Patients may have upstream iliac disease, which will mimic transplantation renal artery stenosis because the transplant is still ischemic. Many modalities can be used to treat the stenosis. If the native iliac artery is diseased, balloon angioplasty can be successful. Figure 28-4 demonstrates native iliac artery atherosclerotic disease. In this case, the renal artery was anastomosed to the recipient's hypogastric artery at the initial operation because of native atherosclerotic disease. Balloon angioplasty of transplantation renal artery stenosis has success rates ranging from 20% to 80%. Another alternative is using an ABO-compatible deceased donor iliac artery as a bypass graft from the native iliac artery to a point beyond the renal artery stenosis.[33]

### Urologic Complications

The blood supply to the ureter comes from a number of sources, including the gonadal artery, superior and inferior vesicular arteries, and common iliac and hypogastric arteries. During procurement of the donor kidney, it is important to avoid injuring the periureteric tissue in the golden triangle—an anatomic area defined by the renal artery, lower pole of the kidney, and ureter. Approximately 15% to 20% of donors have a lower pole renal artery that is a major source of arterial inflow to the ureter. Complications of the ureter include leak, obstruction, and/or stenosis. Stenosis may occur early or late and occurs in 2% to 15% of recipients.[34] Early in the course of transplantation, stenosis may be caused by extrinsic compression from a lymphocele or acute ischemia. Polyoma BK virus is a cause of late multiple strictures. Patients usually present with an asymptomatic rise in creatinine levels. If a leak is present, patients may report significant pelvic pain. If the diagnosis is obstruction or stenosis, an ultrasound will demonstrate hydronephrosis (Fig. 28-5) and may also reveal a lymphocele obstructing the ureter. The acute obstruction can be relieved by placing a percutaneous nephrostomy tube. A more definitive study can then be performed to

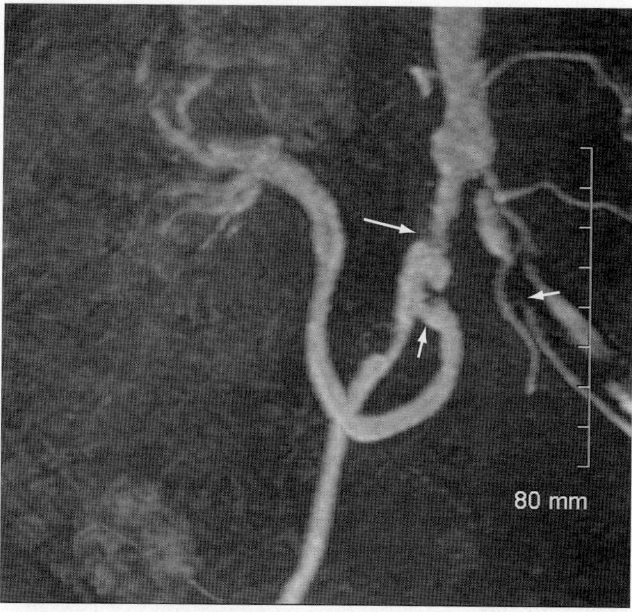


**FIGURE 28-4** Angiogram demonstrating native iliac disease limiting arterial inflow to the transplanted kidney.

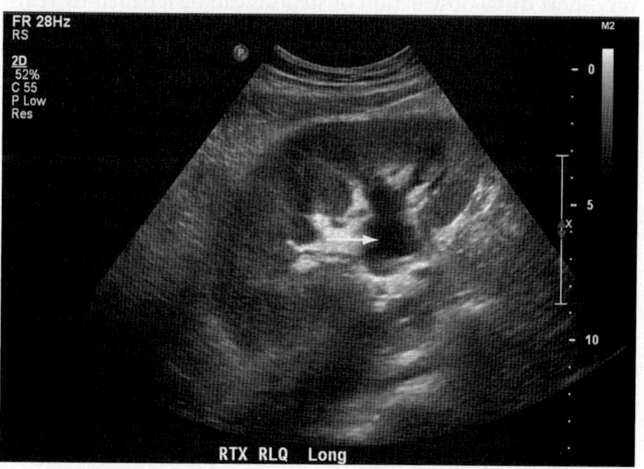


**FIGURE 28-5** Ultrasound demonstrating hydronephrosis.

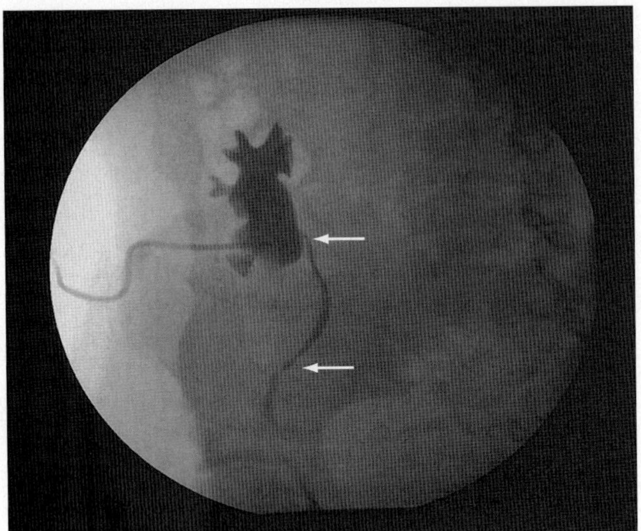

**FIGURE 28-6** Percutaneous nephrostogram demonstrating obstruction.

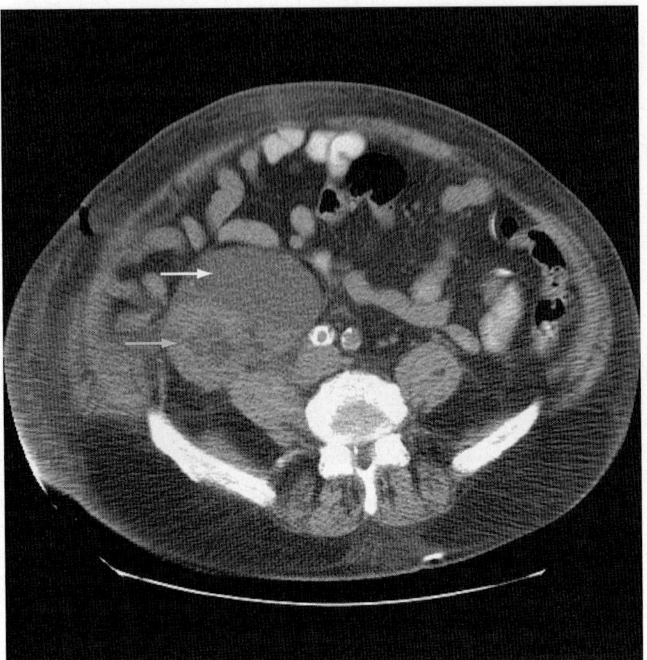

**FIGURE 28-7** CT scan demonstrating a lymphocele. *Yellow arrow,* kidney transplant; *white arrow,* lymphocele.

demonstrate the exact location of the obstruction (Fig. 28-6). A very short distal obstruction or stenosis can be repaired by reimplanting the ureter. A long stricture or very proximal stricture will need to be repaired by performing an ureteropyelostomy and using the native ureter. It is very important to determine that the patient has a normal native ureter prior to this reconstruction.

Urine leak can also develop. This occurs in 1% of cases overall, but accounts for 25% of all urologic complications.[34] Patients present with pain and swelling at the transplant site, usually within the first week after transplantation. The creatinine level is also elevated. The diagnosis can be made by aspirating the perinephric fluid and checking the creatinine level. A nuclear medicine scan can also be performed. Delayed images will reveal the urine leak when the contrast is seen outside the bladder. Placement of a double J stent at the time of transplantation may decrease the risk of this complication. Graft loss is rare with urologic complications.

### Lymphocele

During the routine recipient operation, the lymphatics overlying the iliac vessels are divided. Approximately 1% to 18% of recipients can develop a lymphocele when these lymphatics leak.[30] Careful ligation at the time of transplantation can help decrease the incidence of this complication, but it does not completely eliminate the risk. Many lymphoceles are asymptomatic. However, some patients may present with a swollen leg and increased creatinine levels because of compression on the iliac vein or transplanted ureter. CT is diagnostic (Fig. 28-7). The treatment of symptomatic lymphoceles is surgical, with a peritoneal communication being established by an open technique or laparoscopically. Percutaneous aspiration has poor results with a high rate of recurrence and also carries the risk of infecting the fluid collection. A large single-center study at the University of California San Francisco has compared the two techniques.[35] The recurrence rate after surgical repair was 6.7% overall, regardless of technique. With the open technique, a large peritoneal window can be created. However, laparoscopic techniques have been successful, with less postoperative pain and a slight decrease in length of hospital stay. Care must be taken not to injure the transplanted ureter when creating a window using either technique. There has been an increased risk of this injury with laparoscopic methods. The lymphocele fluid should be sent for creatinine level determination at the time of surgery to ensure that there is no occult urine leak.

### Infections

Infectious complications are common following transplantation, mainly because of the use of immunosuppressive therapy. Up to 80% of recipients experience a urinary tract infection. There is a 1% to 10% chance of wound infections immediately following surgery. As expected, diabetes, obesity, and the use of steroids increases the risk. Viral infections are also common in the first 3 months following transplantation because this is when the patient is on the highest levels of maintenance immunosuppression and the effects of induction therapy are the most pronounced. Common viral infections include cytomegalovirus (CMV), Epstein-Barr Virus (EBV), and polyomavirus BK. For this reason, many transplantation centers will treat patients in the early post- transplantation phase with antivirals, including ganciclovir, acyclovir, and valganciclovir. Another common opportunistic infection is *Pneumocystis jiroveci,* and trimethoprim-sulfamethoxazole (Bactrim) or pentamidine is used as prophylaxis.

## Outcomes

Transplantation offers patients a better quality of life when compared with dialysis. It is also a cost-effective form of kidney replacement therapy associated with improved survival, especially if the patient can be transplanted prior to the initiation of dialysis.[16] As noted by Womer and Kaplan,[20] the number of deceased donor kidneys has increased over the last decade.

**Table 28-4 Kidney Graft Survival (years)**

| | Survival (%) | | |
|---|---|---|---|
| **DONOR** | **1** | **5** | **10** |
| Deceased donor, non-ECD | 91.7 | 70.4 | 43.7 |
| ECD | 84.8 | 54.8 | 26.3 |
| Living donor | 95.7 | 80.8 | 57.9 |

From U.S. Department of health and Human Services: OPTN/SRTR annual report, 2009 (http://www.ustransplant.org/annual_reports/current/default.htm).

Living donation has remained relatively stable. Patient survival is excellent at 1 year, with LRD recipients having a survival rate of 98% and recipients of deceased donor kidneys having a survival rate of 95%. At 5 years, recipients of LRD or LURD kidneys have a survival rate of 90%, which exceeds that of non-ECD recipients, whose survival rate is 83%. Recipients of ECD kidneys have a 5-year survival rate of 69%. These figures can be affected by recipient selection. Graft survival is shown in Table 28-4. The most common cause of graft loss is progressive interstitial fibrosis that ultimately leads to kidney failure.

## PANCREAS TRANSPLANTATION

Diabetes is a major health concern in the United States and is the single leading cause of ESRD. Diabetic retinopathy is a leading cause of blindness. In 1999, the American Diabetes Association clinical guidelines advocated whole-organ pancreas transplantation as a viable treatment option for type 1 diabetes. The guidelines state that "pancreas transplantation should be considered an acceptable therapeutic alternative to continued insulin therapy in diabetic patients with imminent or established ESRD who have had or plan to undergo kidney transplantation, because the successful addition of a pancreas does not jeopardize patient survival, may improve kidney survival, and will restore normal glycemia" (www.guideline.gov). In the 2004 International Pancreas Transplant Registry, over 23,000 pancreas transplants were performed worldwide. Successful pancreas transplantation can improve the quality of life of patients with type 1 diabetes by eliminating the need for frequent glucose monitoring and decreasing the need for strict dietary monitoring. In addition, patients and their families no longer need to monitor for life-threatening hypoglycemic events.

The history of pancreas transplantation has been marked by the limitations of surgical complications and rejection. In the early era of pancreas transplantation, 25% of grafts were lost because of technical issues. With improvements in technique and immunosuppression, 1-year patient survival for pancreas alone and simultaneous kidney and pancreas (SPK) transplantation is over 95% in the current Scientific Registry of Transplant Recipients (SRTR) report and 1-year pancreas graft survival is 86% for kidney-pancreas transplantation nationally.[36] Patients who undergo SPK transplantation have better renal graft function when compared with patients receiving a kidney alone, without an increase in surgical complications.[37]

### Patient Selection

Patients requiring pancreas transplantation are usually type 1 diabetics with a clear C-peptide deficiency. Given that insulin therapy can mitigate the complications of hyperglycemia, patients who are accepted as transplant recipients must balance the effects of lifelong immunosuppression and potential surgical risk with the opportunity to improve their quality of life and perhaps decrease the progression of microvascular complications. Patients may undergo SPK transplantation, pancreas transplantation alone (PTA), or pancreas transplantation following kidney transplantation from a different donor (pancreas after kidney [PAK]). For patients choosing PTA, there should be clear documentation of significant hypoglycemic events as well as stable renal function. Because patients will require calcineurin inhibitor therapy after PTA, a GFR higher than 70 to 80 and less than 1 g of proteinuria is required in our program. In addition, these patients should be informed that PTA has been shown to be an independent risk factor for renal failure.[38] In PAK candidates, a GFR higher than 50 is required to maintain renal function, with a temporary increase in immunosuppression. Patients with minimal secondary complications are the best candidates for pancreas transplantation. However, it has been shown that many of the secondary complications of diabetes are ameliorated by a constant euglycemic state.[39]

Diabetes is a major risk factor for atherosclerosis, so careful screening for cardiac disease and peripheral vascular disease is necessary. Cardiovascular disease is the leading cause of death among type 1 diabetics. The evaluation of the cardiac reserve of a pancreas transplantation candidate is controversial. Bates and coworkers[40] have shown that noninvasive studies in this patient population are notoriously unreliable. Although concerns about preserving renal function are important, correcting cardiac lesions pretransplantation is paramount to a successful outcome. Given the burden of disease in this population, cardiac catheterization is recommended for evaluation. A careful physical examination, paying particular attention to the peripheral dorsalis pedis and posterior tibial pulses, and the presence of carotid bruits, can help determine whether further screening studies are required.

There have been case reports of patients with type 2 diabetes who have undergone pancreas transplantation with successful outcomes. In a study at the University of Minnesota, 17 patients underwent SPK, PAK, or PTA transplantation for type 2 diabetes. The average age at onset of diabetes was 35.7 and the BMI at time of transplant was 27. In this cohort, there was one early death. Four patients died, with a mean of 2.2 years from the time of transplantation to death. Three of these patients were insulin-independent at the time of death and 11 of the 12 remaining patients have remained insulin-free.[41] In select patients, pancreas transplantation may be a reasonable treatment for insulin-resistant diabetes.

### Pancreas Donor

There are no clear-cut chemical criteria for the evaluation of a pancreas donor. A clinical judgment must be made at the time of procurement to determine the quality of the pancreas. The ideal pancreas is neither fatty nor edematous (Fig. 28-8). Pancreas transplantation can be safely procured from donors after cardiac death, with outcomes similar to donation after brain death. In DCD, I recommend warm ischemia times of less than 45 minutes.[39] The ideal age range is 10 to 45 minutes. Because of the increased risk of graft thrombosis, leaks, and decreased survival, caution should be used when using organs from older donors.[40] Pediatric donors can be safely used. In a study at the University of Wisconsin, there were 142 pancreas donors younger than 18 years. The average donor weight was 24.5 ±

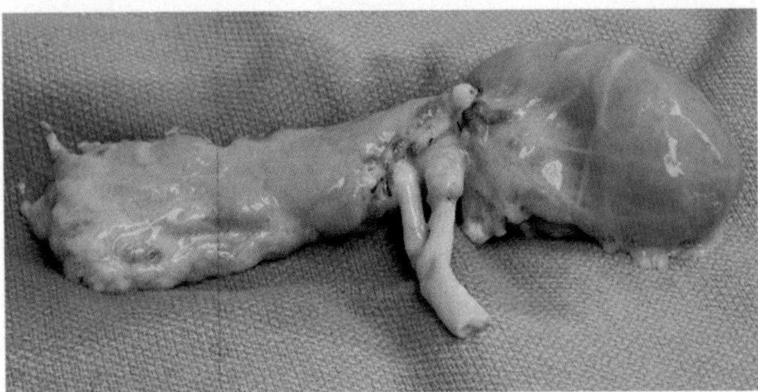

**FIGURE 28-8** Photograph of the ideal pancreas for transplantation.

5 kg. The aggregate outcome in the pediatric donors is compared with that of adult donors in Table 28-5. The lower limit of age in this study was 3 years old and the lower weight limit was 25 kg.[42]

## Pancreas Procurement, Preparation, and Transplantation

During procurement, minimal handling of the pancreas is optimal. A generous midline incision is made and a median sternotomy is accomplished. It is most common to procure the liver and pancreas en bloc and then separate the organs in ice to minimize warm ischemia time. The right and left colon are mobilized and a Kocher maneuver is carried out to free the duodenum and head of the pancreas. The gastrohepatic ligament is carefully inspected to identify a replaced left hepatic artery. The gastrohepatic ligament is divided, as well as the omentum, along the greater curvature of the stomach. The pancreas is visualized and inspected for fibrosis or masses. The splenic attachments are freed and the tail of the pancreas is mobilized from its attachments, taking care to stay away from the pancreatic parenchyma. The left gastric artery is ligated and divided. The pancreas is mobilized to the level of the vena cava. The bowel mesentery is ligated and divided. Our center prefers silk ligatures rather than stapled ligatures to ensure that small mesenteric vessels do not retract and cause a significant hematoma at the head of the pancreas transplant on reperfusion. The stomach is divided at the level of the pylorus using a TA stapler and the small bowel is divided using a GIA 55 or 75 stapler just distal to the ligament of Treitz. The superior mesenteric artery (SMA) root is identified. The aorta is cross-clamped and 2 liters of University of Wisconsin (UW) solution (Viaspan) is flushed through the organs. The pancreas and liver block are removed.

At the back table, the SMA is identified and care is taken to preserve a replaced right hepatic artery, if present. The splenic artery is identified and a small 6-0 Prolene suture is used to mark the splenic artery as it enters the pancreatic body. The splenic artery is then divided. Division of the portal vein must be done carefully to ensure adequate length for liver and pancreas transplant recipients. At least 1 cm of portal vein should be preserved for the pancreas anastomosis. Extension of the portal vein for pancreas transplantation results in an unacceptable risk of transplant thrombosis.

Once the pancreas and liver are separated, the pancreas is bathed in UW solution and further back table preparation is done. The spleen is removed from the tail of the pancreas. A probe is placed in the splenic artery and SMA to check patency. The duodenal segment is prepared. The segment is stapled with a GIA

**Table 28-5 Pancreas Graft Outcomes**

| | Age (yr) | |
|---|---|---|
| **OUTCOME** | **<18 (*N* = 63)** | **>18 (*N* = 237)** |
| GFR | 65.6 ± 16 | 58.3 ± 17* |
| 5-yr Glc | 85.3 ± 13 | 95.2 ± 29* |
| 5-yr HbA1C | 5.47 ± 0.98 | 5.86 ± 3.5† |
| 5-yr kidney | 85.0% | 83.2% |
| 5-yr pancreas | 85.3% | 79.8% |

*GFR*, Glomerular filtration rate; *Glc*, glucose; *HbA1C*, hemoglobin A1C.

*$P \leq .002$.

†$P = .013$.

55 stapler just distal to the pylorus, taking care to preserve the pancreatic duct drainage. The excess distal small bowel is also shortened using a GIA stapler. Both staple lines are oversewn using 3-0 silk in a Lembert fashion. The portal vein is dissected. There is usually one small peripancreatic venous branch that can be safely ligated and divided, thereby lengthening the portal vein. The splenic artery and SMA are clearly identified. The excess celiac plexus tissue between the arteries is carefully ligated and divided. Extreme care must be taken to prevent injury to the pancreas at this point. Several figure-of-eight silk sutures are placed in this area to prevent bleeding after reperfusion. The vascular reconstruction is then completed. The iliac artery is used as a y-graft and an end-to-end anastomosis of the external and internal iliac arteries to the pancreas splenic artery and SMA respectively is completed using 6-0 Prolene sutures in a running fashion.

The recipient is then prepared. A midline incision is made and the iliac arteries are exposed for systemic drainage. The pancreas transplant is usually placed on the right side to prevent undue stretching of the venous anastomosis. For systemic venous drainage, the portal vein is anastomosed to the distal vena cava in an end-to-side fashion. The iliac artery graft is sutured to the common iliac artery of the recipient. For portal drainage, the donor portal vein is anastomosed to the recipient, proximal superior mesenteric vein. A path is created in the small bowel mesentery so that the arterial y-graft can be anastomosed to the iliac artery, usually the right. The vascular clamps are then removed. Slow sequential removal of the clamps is essential to prevent hematoma formation. The venous clamp is slowly removed and venous bleeding is controlled. The distal arterial clamp is removed and hemorrhage controlled. The proximal arterial clamp is removed. For enteric drainage of exocrine secretions, the bowel anastomosis is then completed from the duodenal transplant stump side to side to the recipient midjejunum. If necessary, a Roux-en-Y drainage may also be performed, if needed, to prevent tension on the transplant duodenal stump. I prefer a hand-sewn double layer anastomosis because stapled anastomoses are associated with an increased risk of bleeding. The exocrine secretions may also be drained to the bladder. A 4- to 5-cm cystostomy is made on the anterior dome of the bladder. A two-layer anastomosis is completed, with an outer layer of nonabsorbable 3-0 or 4-0 sutures and the inner layer created using absorbable 4-0 to 5-0 sutures.

After completion of the exocrine drainage anastomosis, another careful inspection of the graft should be accomplished to identify any delayed bleeding that might have developed after warming of the transplant.

## Drainage Techniques: Endocrine and Exocrine Secretions

### Bladder Drainage or Enteric Drainage

Managing the exocrine secretions of the pancreas transplant remains a challenge. Many techniques have been used over the years, including duct exclusion via injection, duct ligation, and even open drainage to the peritoneal cavity. In the past, the duodenal stump was thought to be a cause for rejection and the size was minimized via a button technique, or the stump was eliminated altogether and a direct duct anastomosis was completed. However, all these techniques were complicated by significant leak rates. The duodenal stump is now left intact and anastomosed to the bladder or bowel (see earlier).

Bladder drainage offers the advantages of decreasing the risk of enteric content contamination from the native enterotomy and allowing monitoring of urinary amylase as an early diagnostic tool for determining transplant dysfunction or rejection. However, significant metabolic acidosis may develop, as well as urinary tract complications. There is a high incidence of urinary tract infections, dysuria, urethritis, and urethral disruption.[39] Leaks can occur in the early postoperative course and patients may present with abdominal discomfort, or there may be an asymptomatic rise in the amylase or lipase level. Urinary anastomotic leaks are can be diagnosed with a bladder contrast CT with delayed images. If the CT scan does not show a significant amount of intra-abdominal fluid, a Foley catheter can be placed for 7 to 10 days. In my experience, a normal amylase level with normoglycemia represents clinical resolution of the leak and no further images studies are required. However, if a large amount of fluid is seen, the patient will require prompt laparotomy with consideration of transplantation pancreatectomy if there is significant compromise of the duodenal stump.

Evidence of better outcomes has emerged after conversion of bladder drainage to enteric drainage in a subset of patients.[43] Given the good outcomes in patients who have undergone conversion of bladder to enteric drainage, and the fact that enteric drainage is more physiologic, interest was renewed in enteric drainage beginning in early 2000. Follow-up studies have shown that the enteric drainage is not associated with significant increases in infection and, by using this technique, the complications of bladder drainage can be avoided. Currently, the vast majority of pancreas transplantations are performed with enteric drainage of the exocrine secretions, with only 20% of programs reporting the use of bladder drainage to the International Pancreas and Islet Transplant Association (IPITA) database.

### Systemic Drainage Versus Portal Drainage

Hyperinsulinemia has been noted in pancreas transplant recipients who have systemic drainage, likely because of the loss of the first-pass effect of hepatic degradation. Stratta and colleagues[44] began to champion portal drainage, which was proposed to be more physiologic and would not result in a proatherosclerotic state caused by hyperinsulinemia. In long-term studies comparing systemic drainage and portal drainage, there has been no clear advantage seen in portal drainage. Although theoretical concern exists about atherosclerosis, no definitive metabolic advantages of portal drainage have been proven. In a comprehensive review, Young noted that currently, there is no incontrovertible evidence that systemic hyperinsulinemia is proatherosclerotic, whereas recent metabolic studies on systemic drainage and portal drainage have shown that there is no benefit to portal drainage.[44a] At this point, the choice of systemic drainage or portal drainage lies with the surgeon.

## Surgical Complications

### Leak

Leak from the enteric anastomosis was the Achilles heel of early attempts at pancreas transplantation. The incidence varies from 2% to 10%.[45] Enteric leak presents with signs and symptoms similar to those of intestinal perforation, including abdominal pain, nausea and vomiting, fever, and tachycardia. Patients may have an elevated white blood cell (WBC) count, but this is often nonspecific because patients are receiving steroids. The amylase levels are not always affected. However, serum creatinine levels are often elevated and can signal ongoing infection. It is important to note that as a consequence of immunosuppression, transplant recipients may not display overt signs of infection or leak, and a high index of suspicion is critical for timely diagnosis and treatment. Clinical suspicion may be sufficient to mandate reoperation, but radiographic imaging can often provide confirmatory evidence in equivocal cases. The most useful imaging test in this setting is CT with oral contrast. Findings include free or loculated intraperitoneal fluid, extraluminal air, and contrast extravasation.[46]

Enteric leak almost always requires reoperation. Early leaks are most often anastomotic and treatment depends on the size of the leak and condition of the donor duodenum. Simple oversewing may be sufficient for small leaks. If part of the duodenum is compromised, that portion may be resected and the remaining duodenum shortened. If the original anastomosis was performed in a side-to-side fashion, a Roux-en-Y limb may be created to divert the intestinal stream away from the graft. In the case of significant leak with sepsis or advanced peritonitis, or in the setting of devitalized tissue, graft pancreatectomy is the procedure of choice.

Most leaks occur in the first several weeks post-transplantation. However, there is a subset of patients who experience leaks late in their transplantation course. Predisposing factors include biopsy-proven rejection, CMV infection, blunt abdominal trauma, and obstructive uropathy. In a series of patients with bladder drainage, 9 of 25 cases of leaks resolved with Foley catheter treatment only. In the remainder, direct suture repair or conversion to enteric drainage was successful.[47] In my experience, when leaks from the bladder anastomosis occur after 10 years, the duodenal stump can be thin-walled and conversion is associated with a higher rate of anastomotic leak from the newly created enteric anastomosis.[39] Thus, I recommend that enteric conversion in transplantation over 10 years be created with a Roux-en-Y anastomosis to divert the intestinal stream. I also place perianastomotic drains at the time of the conversion.

### Vascular Complications

**Thrombosis** Graft thrombosis represents the most common nonimmunologic cause of pancreas transplantation failure.[49] An analysis of UNOS data through June 2004 has demonstrated graft loss rates caused by thrombosis ranging from 2.7% in bladder-drained SPK transplantation to 8% in enteric-drained

PTA transplantation. The choice of exocrine drainage affected graft thrombosis rates only in SPK transplantation (2.7% for bladder drained versus 5.4% for enteric drained). Although thrombosis rates have improved considerably when compared with previous eras of analysis, it remains the most common cause of early technical graft loss.

A number of risk factors have been identified for graft thrombosis. In the donor, advanced age, cerebrovascular cause of death, hemodynamic instability, and massive resuscitation confer a high risk. Using a venous interposition graft to extend the portal vein may also increase the risk for thrombosis.[39] Recipient factors likely also play a part in graft thrombosis. Coagulopathy related to uremia may confer protection from thrombosis in recipients of SPKs, while the diabetic state is known to be associated with hypercoagulability. At the University of Wisconsin, I routinely use intraoperative IV heparin for PAK and PTA, but not for SPK transplantation.

Most graft thromboses occur early after transplantation and are suspected in the setting of graft tenderness, hyperglycemia, elevation in serum amylase and lipase levels, or decrease in urinary amylase levels for bladder-drained pancreas transplants. Patients with arterial thrombosis may have an acute rise in glucose levels without pain because the graft is not swollen after arterial thrombosis. Graft thrombosis leads to a rapid decline in the patient's clinical status, with hypotension and tachycardia developing soon after the rise in glucose level. Emergent exploratory laparotomy with transplantation pancreatectomy is often necessary. In the case of partial arterial thrombosis, the graft may occasionally be rescued with a combination of mechanical or pharmacologic thrombolysis and/or resection. The appearance of the graft on re exploration is critical. It is usually obvious whether there is sufficient viable pancreas to save.

Pancreas transplantation ultrasound is the initial diagnostic test of choice. Doppler flow imaging can provide an overall view of parenchymal vascularity and flow signals should be identified in the arterial and venous systems. Limitations of ultrasonography include operator dependence and interference from surrounding structures and overlying bowel.

Percutaneous thrombolysis or thrombectomy may be of benefit in selected patients, especially those with partial venous thrombosis.[45]

**Bleeding** Immediate post-transplantation bleeding can occur from the pancreatic parenchyma, particularly near the SMA or splenic arteries. The patient presents with hypotension, tachycardia, and abdominal distention. It is my practice to place several figure-of- eight superficial silk sutures in the peripancreatic tissue lying between the SMA and splenic arteries to prevent bleeding in this difficult to approach area.

Delayed gastrointestinal (GI) bleeding can also occur from the enteric anastomosis. This usually presents from postoperative days 6 to 10 and is self-limited. Patients present with a sudden drop in hemoglobin level and are usually hemodynamically stable. It is important to correct any coagulopathy that might be preexisting. Single doses of vasopressin, 0.3 μg/kg, as well as initiation of an octreotide infusion, 25 μg/hr, are also helpful in limiting blood loss. Endoscopy or radiographic studies are usually not diagnostic in this case. However, if the patient becomes hemodynamically unstable, another diagnosis, such as duodenal ulcer, should be considered.

Late GI bleeding can ensue as a result of CMV infection, duodenal ulcers of the duodenal stump from ischemia, or rejection. Arterioenteric fistulas may develop and cause massive GI bleeding.[48]

### Other Considerations

Infections, bowel obstruction, and pancreatitis can also occur following transplantation. Usually, these do not require open surgical therapy but must be considered in the differential diagnosis of transplant dysfunction.

**Infection** Following pancreas transplantation, infection may develop in the superficial or deep wound spaces. The appropriate use of perioperative antibiotics can limit this complication. Pancreas transplant recipients should be treated with 48 hours of gram-positive, gram-negative, and fungal coverage.

Surgical site infection, most commonly from gram-positive organisms, may occur in up to 50% of patients.[45] Superficial wound infections are generally treated with local wound care and additional antibiotics. Deep space, or intra-abdominal, infections are less common, but carry a significantly greater morbidity. Signs and symptoms of intra-abdominal infection are similar to those for enteric leak. Ultrasound and CT are the mainstays of diagnosis.

The stable patient with a localized abscess can generally be treated with percutaneous abscess drainage. Patients with widespread infection or hemodynamic instability should be reexplored. Cultures should be obtained to focus antimicrobial therapy. Intra-abdominal infection, especially when in close proximity to the vascular anastomosis, may predispose to pseudoaneurysm formation. Unexplained intra-abdominal bleeding in a patient with a history of abdominal abscess should raise the possibility of an anastomotic pseudoaneurysm.

**Pancreatitis** Graft pancreatitis is common following transplantation, occurring in as many as 35% of patients.[45] Early pancreatitis is likely related to reperfusion injury to the graft. The diagnosis is made in the setting of abdominal pain and hyperamylasemia. It is important to rule out the possibility of acute rejection, although abdominal pain is less likely with rejection. CT imaging of the graft reveals a swollen hypervascular organ, often with a significant amount of surrounding fluid. My treatment of graft pancreatitis includes aggressive fluid resuscitation, withholding of enteral nutrition, with institution of total parenteral nutrition (TPN), as required, treatment of superimposed or concurrent infection, and supportive management. Most cases of pancreatitis are self-limited.

**Bowel Obstruction** Significant intra-abdominal dissection is required in pancreas transplantation. In contrast to the retroperitoneal kidney transplantation alone, the intraperitoneal nature of the pancreas operation increases the risk of bowel complications. Small bowel obstruction may be caused by postsurgical adhesions or internal hernia formation.

Patients typically present with nausea, vomiting, obstipation, and abdominal pain. Plain x-rays demonstrate air fluid levels and CT confirms the diagnosis. In the stable patient, resuscitation and nasogastric tube decompression may be sufficient. Unstable patients or those with peritonitis should be explored in the operating room.

### Outcomes

The total number of pancreas transplantations performed in the United States from 1966 to 2008 reported to the International Pancreas Transplant Registry (IPTR)–UNOS registry was 22,618.[36,45] Pancreas transplantationis a safe and reliable treatment for type 1 diabetes. Normoglycemia is restored and patients demonstrate normal hemoglobin (Hg) A1C levels. Importantly, patients do not suffer from hypoglycemic unawareness. Early efforts at pancreas transplantation were hindered by surgical complications and difficulty with the diagnosis and treatment of rejection. However, with improvements in surgical technique, immunosuppressive therapy, and tissue typing, outcomes significantly improved from 2000 to 2010. Graft survival is comparable to that for other transplants with a 1-year patient survival rate of more than 95% and survival at 3 years of more than 90%.[49] I have found that patient survival at 1, 10, and 20 years is 97%, 80% and 58%, respectively, with pancreas graft survival of 88%, 63%, and 36% over the same time frame. Acute rejection rates have fallen to below 10% in the current era of immunosuppression with prednisone, mycophenolate mofetil, and tacrolimus.[39] A major consideration for pancreas transplantation is the potential for prevention of the secondary complications of diabetes. However, there are no randomized clinical trials comparing the efficacy of pancreas transplantation to tight glycemic control with insulin therapy. It has become increasingly apparent that benefits might not be seen until 5 to 10 years after transplantation.[50] Peripheral neuropathy improves after 1 year, as shown by increased nerve conduction velocity. In addition, in a comparison of neuropathy in patients 10 years post-transplantation, those with functioning pancreas grafts had stable nerve action amplitudes whereas those patients with failed grafts showed a steady decline.[51] There has been debate about the effect of consistent normoglycemia on diabetic retinopathy. The grade of disease pretransplantation may affect the response. Those with severe disease pretransplantation may still progress to blindness. However, in long-term follow-up studies, retinopathy was found to stabilize and conjunctival microcirculation improve in patients undergoing successful transplantation.[52]

The major cause of death in pancreas transplant recipients is cardiovascular disease. A careful preoperative screening is necessary in these patients to treat any silent cardiac disease prior to transplantation. Sollinger and and associates[39] have found that 72% of pretransplantation patients were screened with coronary angiography from 2005 to 2007. In addition to normalization of HgA1C levels and near-normal fasting glucose levels, patients enjoy freedom from hypoglycemic events, which significantly improves the quality of life for the patients and their families.

## ISLET TRANSPLANTATION

There has been renewed interest in islet transplantation since the report by Shapiro and coworkers[53] of seven patients who were insulin-free 1 year after islet transplantation on a steroid-free protocol of immunosuppression. The advantage of using islets is the avoidance of a complex intra-abdominal surgical procedure. In patients with severe peripheral vascular disease, islet injection may offer their only hope of becoming insulin-free. Transplanting only the islets also obviates the need to manage the complications secondary to the exocrine secretions of the pancreas. The patient and physician must consider the balance between the secondary complications of diabetes and the side effects of immunosuppression. Initial attempts at islet transplantation in the early 1970s failed, primarily because of difficulties in obtaining sufficient yields.

### Isolation Techniques

Pancreas organs that are not to be used for whole-organ transplantation are allocated for use in experimental islet isolation. These organs tend to be from fattier donors or those with complex vascular anatomy, and occasionally from trauma victims who have undergone splenectomy when the tail of the pancreas was compromised. The organ is procured in standard fashion. Collagenase is infused to separate the islets and the preparation is purified using density gradient centrifugation. Special techniques for transport are used, including two-layer technique in which the pancreas is sandwiched between a layer of Viaspan (UW solution) and perfluorodecalin infused with oxygen.[51] Many different sites for implantation were tested in experimental models. Infusion into the portal vein has been found to be the most reliable in human clinical trials. Portal pressure is carefully monitored during the infusion and many centers use concurrent heparin infusions to prevent portal vein thrombosis.

### Outcomes

The initial excitement over the Edmonton protocol has faded somewhat over the subsequent years. In recent studies, patients who received islet cell transplants had an acceleration of nephropathy, likely because of side effect from immunosuppression.[50] Unfortunately, all the commonly used immunosuppressants also have negative effect on the islets, including decreased insulin gene transcription, decreased synthesis of insulin in vivo and in vitro, and decreased stability of insulin messenger RNA. There is no assay to predict islet quality reliably. There is also no reliable way to diagnose rejection until hyperglycemia occurs and, at that point, the islet allograft is usually lost. Since the original successful transplantation in 1990, approximately 1500 transplants have been reported to the Collaborative Islet Transplant Registry (CITR). A total of 325 recipients have been transplanted, with 649 preparations from 712 donors.[51] It is clear that multiple injections are required to obtain at least 6000 islet cell equivalents/kg body weight. CITR data have shown that 70% of patients are insulin-independent after 1 year, but this is not durable, because only 35% were euglycemic at 3 years. However, many patients retain some allograft function, despite the need for insulin. These patients had a decrease in frequency of hypoglycemic events.

There is guarded optimism about the future of islet transplantation. It is clear that restoring euglycemia, even for short periods, and prevention of hypoglycemic events are important. With improvements in procurement and isolation techniques, as well as refinements in immunosuppressive combinations, there may yet be a place for clinical islet transplantation.

## SELECTED REFERENCES

Ibrahim HN, Foley R, Tan L, et al: Long-term consequences of kidney donation. N Engl J Med 360:459–469, 2009.

This is the most comprehensive review of outcomes following kidney donation. It is crucial to review the data in this paper with potential recipients to complete informed consent.

Kidney Disease: Improving Global Outcomes (KDIGO) Transplant Work Group: KDIGO clinical practice guideline for the care of kidney transplant recipients. Am J Transplant 9(Suppl 3):S1–S155, 2009.

This article should be reviewed for most current recommendations for the care of transplant recipients.

Leichtman AB, Cohen D, Keith D, et al: Kidney and pancreas transplantation in the United States, 1997–2006: The HRSA Breakthrough Collaboratives and the 58 DSA Challenge. Am J Transplant 8:946–957, 2008.

This article succinctly outlines the challenges of organ supply and reviews proposals to increase organ donation. The demographics of the recipient waiting list is also analyzed.

Lipshutz GS, Wilkinson AH: Pancreas-kidney and pancreas transplantation for the treatment of diabetes mellitus. Endocrinol Metab Clin North Am 36:1015–1038, 2007.

A detailed review of the basic tenets of pancreas transplantation as well as surgical and medical complications.

Moers C, Smits JM, Maathuis MH, et al: Machine perfusion or cold storage in deceased-donor kidney transplantation. N Engl J Med 360:7–19, 2009.

A landmark article discussing the various methods or organ preservation and a large retrospective review with important clinical ramifications.

Shapiro AM, Lakey JR, Ryan EA, et al: Islet transplantation in seven patients with type 1 diabetes mellitus using a glucocorticoid-free immunosuppressive regimen. N Engl J Med 343:230–238, 2000.

A classic article that launched a reinvigoration of the field of pancreas islet transplantation.

## REFERENCES


1. Wolfe RA, Ashby VB, Milford EL, et al: Comparison of mortality in all patients on dialysis, patients on dialysis awaiting transplantation, and recipients of a first cadaveric transplant. N Engl J Med 341:1725–1730, 1999.
2. Leichtman AB, Cohen D, Keith D, et al: Kidney and pancreas transplantation in the United States, 1997–2006: The HRSA Breakthrough Collaboratives and the 58 DSA Challenge. Am J Transplant 8:946–957, 2008.
3. Coresh J, Selvin E, Stevens LA, et al: Prevalence of chronic kidney disease in the United States. JAMA 298:2038–2047, 2007.
4. Kidney Disease: Improving Global Outcomes (KDIGO) Transplant Work Group: KDIGO clinical practice guideline for the care of kidney transplant recipients. Am J Transplant 9(Suppl 3):S1–S155, 2009.
5. Go AS, Chertow GM, Fan D, et al: Chronic kidney disease and the risks of death, cardiovascular events, and hospitalization. N Engl J Med 351:1296–1305, 2004.
6. Meier-Kriesche HU, Ojo AO, Port FK, et al: Survival improvement among patients with end-stage renal disease: Trends over time for transplant recipients and wait-listed patients. J Am Soc Nephrol 12:1293–1296, 2001.
7. Muehrer RJ, Becker BN: Life after transplantation: New transitions in quality of life and psychological distress. Semin Dial 18:124–131, 2005.
8. Furth SL, Hwang W, Neu AM, et al: Effects of patient compliance, parental education and race on nephrologists' recommendations for kidney transplantation in children. Am J Transplant 3:28–34, 2003.
9. Frassetto LA, Tan-Tam C, Stock PG: Renal transplantation in patients with HIV. Nat Rev Nephrol 5:582–589, 2009.
10. Artero M, Biava C, Amend W, et al: Recurrent focal glomerulosclerosis: Natural history and response to therapy. Am J Med 92:375–383, 1992.
11. Cochat P, Fargue S, Mestrallet G, et al: Disease recurrence in paediatric renal transplantation. Pediatr Nephrol 24:2097–2108, 2009.
12. Chadban S: Glomerulonephritis recurrence in the renal graft. J Am Soc Nephrol 12:394–402, 2001.
13. Dabade TS, Grande JP, Norby SM, et al: Recurrent idiopathic membranous nephropathy after kidney transplantation: N surveillance biopsy study. Am J Transplant 8:1318–1322, 2008.
14. Loirat C, Fremeaux-Bacchi V: Hemolytic uremic syndrome recurrence after renal transplantation. Pediatr Transplant 12:619–629, 2008.
15. Goral S, Ynares C, Shappell SB, et al: Recurrent lupus nephritis in renal transplant recipients revisited: It is not rare. Transplantation 75:651–656, 2003.
16. Abecassis M, Bartlett ST, Collins AJ, et al: Kidney transplantation as primary therapy for end-stage renal disease: A National Kidney Foundation/Kidney Disease Outcomes Quality Initiative (NKF/KDOQITM) conference. Clin J Am Soc Nephrol 3:471–480, 2008.
17. Chan KE, Lazarus JM, Thadhani R, et al: Anticoagulant and antiplatelet usage associates with mortality among hemodialysis patients. J Am Soc Nephrol 20:872–881, 2009.
18. Seliger SL, Gillen DL, Longstreth WT, Jr, et al: Elevated risk of stroke among patients with end-stage renal disease. Kidney Int 64:603–609, 2003.
19. Brekke IB, Lien B, Sodal G, et al: Aortoiliac reconstruction in preparation for renal transplantation. Transpl Int 6:161–163, 1993.
20. Womer KL, Kaplan B: Recent developments in kidney transplantation—a critical assessment. Am J Transplant 9:1265–1271, 2009.
21. Sung RS, Christensen LL, Leichtman AB, et al: Determinants of discard of expanded criteria donor kidneys: Impact of biopsy and machine perfusion. Am J Transplant 8:783–792, 2008.
22. Ojo AO, Hanson JA, Meier-Kriesche H, et al: Survival in recipients of marginal cadaveric donor kidneys compared with other recipients and wait-listed transplant candidates. J Am Soc Nephrol 12:589–597, 2001.
23. Davis CL, Delmonico FL: Living-donor kidney transplantation: A review of the current practices for the live donor. J Am Soc Nephrol 16:2098–2110, 2005.
24. Rees MA, Kopke JE, Pelletier RP, et al: A nonsimultaneous, extended, altruistic-donor chain. N Engl J Med 360:1096–1101, 2009.
25. Matas AJ, Bartlett ST, Leichtman AB, et al: Morbidity and mortality after living kidney donation, 1999–2001: Survey of United States transplant centers. Am J Transplant 3:830–834, 2003.
26. Ibrahim HN, Foley R, Tan L, et al: Long-term consequences of kidney donation. N Engl J Med 360:459–469, 2009.

27. Lewis J, Peltier J, Nelson H, et al: Development of the University of Wisconsin donation After Cardiac Death Evaluation Tool. Prog Transplant 13:265–273, 2003.
28. Wijdicks EF: The diagnosis of brain death. N Engl J Med 344:1215–1221, 2001.
29. Moers C, Smits JM, Maathuis MH, et al: Machine perfusion or cold storage in deceased-donor kidney transplantation. N Engl J Med 360:7–19, 2009.
30. Humar A, Matas AJ: Surgical complications after kidney transplantation. Semin Dial 18:505–510, 2005.
31. Sadej P, Feld RI, Frank A: Transplant renal vein thrombosis: Role of preoperative and intraoperative Doppler sonography. Am J Kidney Dis 54:1167–1170, 2009.
32. Fathi T, Samhan M, Gawish A, et al: Renal allograft venous thrombosis is salvageable. Transplant Proc 39:1120–1121, 2007.
33. Shames BD, Odorico JS, D'Alessandro AM, et al: Surgical repair of transplant renal artery stenosis with preserved cadaveric iliac artery grafts. Ann Surg 237:116–122, 2003.
34. Dinckan A, Tekin A, Turkyilmaz S, et al: Early and late urological complications corrected surgically following renal transplantation. Transpl Int 20:702–707, 2007.
35. Fuller TF, Kang SM, Hirose R, et al: Management of lymphoceles after renal transplantation: Laparoscopic versus open drainage. J Urol 169:2022–2025, 2003.
36. Chronic Disease Research Group of the Minneapolis Medical Research Foundation: Scientific registry of transplant recipients, 2011 (http://www.srtr.org).
37. Gutierrez P, Marrero D, Hernandez D, et al: Surgical complications and renal function after kidney alone or simultaneous pancreas-kidney transplantation: A matched comparative study. Nephrol Dial Transplant 22:1451–1455, 2007.
38. Scalea JR, Butler CC, Munivenkatappa RB, et al: Pancreas transplant alone as an independent risk factor for the development of renal failure: A retrospective study. Transplantation 86:1789–1794, 2008.
39. Sollinger HW, Odorico JS, Becker YT, et al: One thousand simultaneous pancreas-kidney transplants at a single center with 22-year follow-up. Ann Surg 250:618–630, 2009.
40. Bates JR, Sawada SG, Segar DS, et al: Evaluation using dobutamine stress echocardiography in patients with insulin-dependent diabetes mellitus before kidney and/or pancreas transplantation. Am J Cardiol 77:175–179, 1996.
41. Nath DS, Gruessner AC, Kandaswamy R, et al: Outcomes of pancreas transplants for patients with type 2 diabetes mellitus. Clin Transplant 19:792–797, 2005.
42. Fernandez LA, Turgeon NA, Odorico JS, et al: Superior long-term results of simultaneous pancreas-kidney transplantation from pediatric donors. Am J Transplant 4:2093–2101, 2004.
43. van de Linde P, van der Boog PJ, Baranski AG, et al: Pancreas transplantation: Advantages of both enteric and bladder drainage combined in a two-step approach. Clin Transplant 20:253–257, 2006.
44. Stratta RJ, Gaber AO, Shokouh-Amiri MH, et al: A prospective comparison of systemic-bladder versus portal-enteric drainage in vascularized pancreas transplantation. Surgery 127:217–226, 2000.
44a. Young CJ: Are there still roles for exocrine bladder drainage and portal venous drainage for pancreatic allografts? Curr Opin in Org Trans 14(1):90–94, 2009.
45. Goodman J, Becker YT: Pancreas surgical complications. Curr Opin Organ Transplant 14:85–89, 2009.
46. Lall CG, Sandrasegaran K, Maglinte DT, et al: Bowel complications seen on CT after pancreas transplantation with enteric drainage. AJR Am J Roentgenol 187:1288–1295, 2006.
47. Nath DS, Gruessner A, Kandaswamy R, et al: Late anastomotic leaks in pancreas transplant recipients—clinical characteristics and predisposing factors. Clin Transplant 19:220–224, 2005.
48. Troppmann C: Complications after pancreas transplantation. Curr Opin Organ Transplant 15:112–118, 2010.
49. Gruessner AC, Sutherland DE, Gruessner RW: Pancreas transplantation in the United States: A review. Curr Opin Organ Transplant 15:93–101, 2010.
50. Morath C, Schmied B, Mehrabi A, et al: Simultaneous pancreas-kidney transplantation in type 1 diabetes. Clin Transplant 23(Suppl 21):115–120, 2009.
51. Sutherland DE, Gruessner RW, Dunn DL, et al: Lessons learned from more than 1,000 pancreas transplants at a single institution. Ann Surg 233:463–501, 2001.
52. Shipman KE, Patel CK: The effect of combined renal and pancreatic transplantation on diabetic retinopathy. Clin Ophthalmol 3:531–535, 2009.
53. Shapiro AM, Lakey JR, Ryan EA, et al: Islet transplantation in seven patients with type 1 diabetes mellitus using a glucocorticoid-free immunosuppressive regimen. N Engl J Med 343:230–238, 2000.

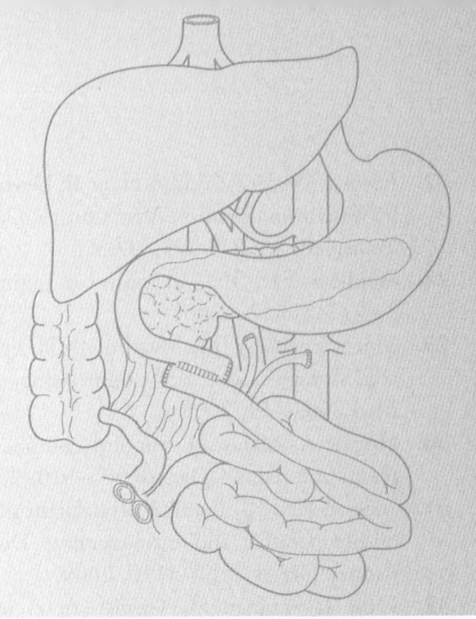

CHAPTER 29

# SMALL BOWEL TRANSPLANTATION

Abigail E. Martin and Debra L. Sudan



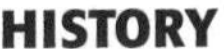

## HISTORY

Disease processes that lead to an inability to sustain oneself via normal enteral nutrition remain a therapeutic challenge to patients and physicians alike. The terms *short gut syndrome* and *short bowel syndrome* are often used to describe patients who are dependent on total parenteral nutrition (TPN) because of significant loss of bowel length from a variety of causes, ranging from congenital malformations to traumatic injury to ischemic loss. Prior to the availability of TPN, short bowel syndrome was almost always fatal and, even with current therapies, extremely short remnant bowel length, less than 50 cm of jejunoileum in adults, is associated with a 43% 5-year mortality.[1] However, the term *short bowel syndrome* excludes a subset of patients who may have a normal or near-normal intestinal length. Inflammatory illnesses such as Crohn's disease, motility disorders such as intestinal pseudo-obstruction, and diseases of the enterocytes such as intestinal epithelial dysplasia share the same devastating consequence of being unable to sustain oneself via enteral means. For this reason, the term *intestinal failure* represents a more accurate and fully inclusive term when describing patients who are unable to tolerate enteral feedings.

Dudrick and associates' seminal work[2] in the laboratory showing that puppies could achieve near-normal growth patterns while exclusively sustained via hyperalimentation was one of the most significant medical breakthroughs of the century. Long-term TPN support increased patient survival, but also introduced a new set of problems, including potentially life-threatening infections and technical difficulties for maintaining access. As more patients were sustained for longer periods with TPN, cholestasis leading to liver failure was increasingly recognized as a potentially fatal complication.[3] Until recently, transplantation or death appeared to be inevitable once a patient developed parenteral nutrition–associated liver disease (PNALD). However, a new investigational fish oil–based lipid formulation has been reported to prevent or even reverse TPN-induced cholestasis,[4] and may be the next major breakthrough in this field.

Early investigational models of intestinal transplantation were being developed long before the advent of TPN, but were doomed to failure because of a lack of understanding of immunology. The first investigation of intestinal transplantation as novel therapy for intestinal failure is attributed to Alexis Carrel in 1905.[5] Approximately 50 years later, in 1959, after the earliest successful kidney transplantation in Boston, Lillehei and colleagues[6] at the University of Minnesota published their successful work transplanting intestines using a canine model. Starzl and associates[7] in Pittsburgh reported transplanting a cluster of organs, including the intestine, in dogs in 1960. The first published human intestinal transplantation was performed by Lillehei and coworkers[8] in 1967, but the patient unfortunately did not survive because of thromboembolic complications. Over the next few years, there were several other unsuccessful attempts in humans,[9] primarily because of the inability to control rejection, resulting in overwhelming infections. Given the apparent success of parenteral nutritional support, there was diminished enthusiasm for further clinical trials of intestinal transplantation.

The advent of cyclosporine immunosuppression in the early 1980s coincided with descriptions of life-threatening complications associated with long-term TPN and led to renewed interest in the field of intestinal transplantation. Cohen and coworkers[10] in Toronto reported the first isolated intestinal transplantation using cyclosporine in 1985 but, unfortunately, the 26-year-old recipient died on postoperative day 9. Over the next 5 years, several successful intestinal transplants procedures were performed by Deltz,[11] Starzl,[12] and colleagues, resulting in patient survival ranging from 6 months to longer than 20 years.[13] In the early 1990s, substantial improvements in control of rejection accompanied the introduction of tacrolimus immunosuppression, and individual centers were able to demonstrate consistent successes.[14,15] In the United States, over 1800 intestinal transplantation were performed through the end of 2009, based on Organ Procurement and Transplantation Network (OPTN) data (http://optn.transplant.hrsa.gov).

## NONTRANSPLANTATION THERAPIES FOR SHORT BOWEL SYNDROME

Although nontransplantation surgery is not the focus of this chapter, several novel surgical approaches were developed with the goal of maximizing function of the remaining intestine in short bowel syndrome. These surgical therapies play an important role in the history of the treatment of intestinal failure and are therefore mentioned briefly here. As early as the 1950s, the surgical creation of segments of antiperistaltic loops of bowel was proposed in an attempt to slow transit time in patients with limited intestinal length.[16] Subsequently, it was recognized that the normal adaptive response to short bowel syndrome is to develop gradual dilation of the remnant segment, but this can lead to substantial dysmotility and bacterial overgrowth. Over time, this practice has been abandoned because of resulting dysmotility and bacterial overgrowth in these antiperistaltic loops. Tapering of these dilated bowel segments by excision of a portion of the bowel along the antimesenteric border to produce a more normal diameter can then improve forward motion of chyme, thus avoiding the need for resection of the dysmotile segment and further loss of length.[17] In 1980, Bianchi[18] described a novel alternative to resection and simple tapering consisting of separating distended bowel loops longitudinally so that two smaller diameter loops of bowel are created and reanastomosed in an isoperistaltic fashion. The resulting bowel is twice the length, but with only half of the original diameter (Fig. 29-1). Given the technical challenges involved, when more potent immunosuppression became available, attention was largely refocused on intestinal transplantation.

Kim and coworkers[19] in Boston developed a technically simpler nontransplantation alternative to the longitudinal tapering and lengthening called serial transverse enteroplasty (STEP). This technique is performed by alternate staple firings from opposite directions across the distended loops of bowel in a zigzag pattern, resulting in a decreased final bowel diameter that allows for more normal motility and absorption (see Fig. 29-1). An International STEP Data Registry has been created to allow for the assessment of long-term follow-up of the efficacy and safety of the STEP procedure; the most recent publication has described the results in the first 38 patients undergoing the procedure at 19 centers.[20] Another large single-center series has described 21 additional patients, which along with the registry demonstrate that application of STEP in carefully selected intestinal failure patients can avoid the need for transplantation in 50% to 60% of cases.[21] Furthermore, in contrast to the Bianchi lengthening, STEP can be applied as a secondary lengthening procedure after primary Bianchi or STEP, with success rates similar to those after the initial lengthening.[22] Clearly, a multidisciplinary approach with expertise in TPN management, nontransplantation surgical procedures, and intestinal transplantation is necessary to optimize care of the individual patient with intestinal failure.

## INDICATIONS FOR INTESTINAL TRANSPLANTATION

The underlying causes of intestinal failure in pediatric patients referred for intestinal transplantation are more likely to result from loss of length caused by congenital diseases when compared with adult patients (Table 29-1). The Intestinal Transplant Registry (ITR) has reported the three most common underlying disease states leading to transplantation in children as gastroschisis (21%), volvulus (17%), and necrotizing enterocolitis (12%).[23] In contrast, the most common indications for intestinal transplantation in adults are ischemia (23%), Crohn's disease (14%), and trauma (10%). Although the most common indications fall under the category of short bowel syndrome, children and adults may suffer from diseases that result in dysmotility or

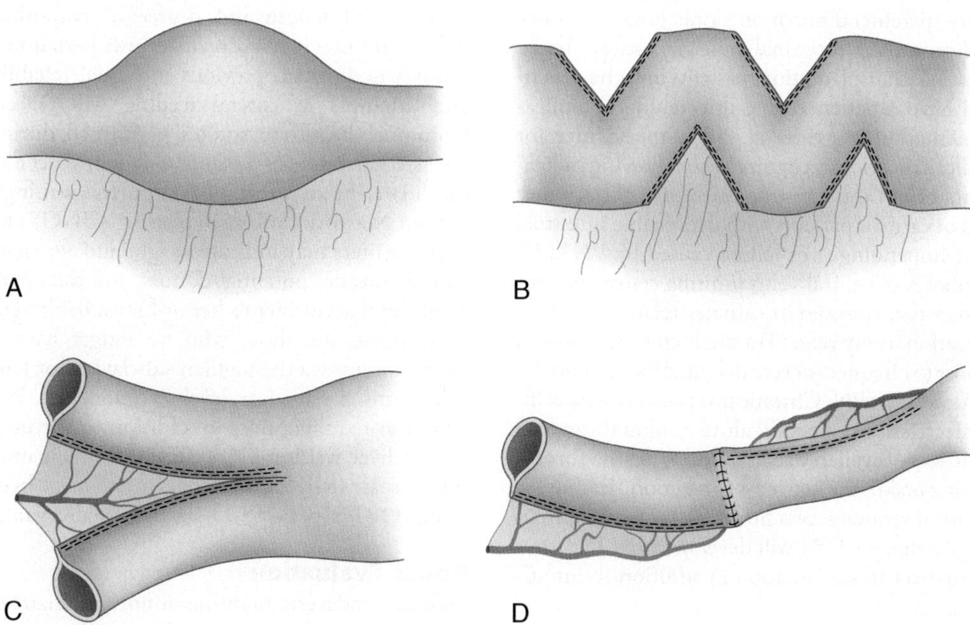


**FIGURE 29-1** **A,** Distended bowel. **B,** Stepwise transverse enteroplasty, showing alternating staple lines, thus reducing the diameter while increasing length. **C,** Bianchi enteroplasty, part 1. This is a longitudinal division of a loop of distended bowel so that the two leaves of the mesentery each supply one of the divided segments. **D,** Bianchi enteroplasty, part 2. The divided segments are anastomosed to create a loop of bowel that is twice the length of the original loop, but with only half the original diameter.

**Table 29-1 Underlying Indications for Intestinal Transplantation**

| PEDIATRIC | INCIDENCE (%) | ADULT | INCIDENCE (%) |
|---|---|---|---|
| Gastroschisis | 21 | Ischemia | 23 |
| Volvulus | 17 | Crohn's disease | 14 |
| Necrotizing enterocolitis | 12 | Trauma | 10 |
| Pseudo-obstruction | 9 | Desmoid tumors | 9 |
| Intestinal atresia | 8 | Motility disorders | 8 |
| Retransplant | 8 | Volvulus | 7 |
| Hirschsprung's disease | 7 | Short gut, other | 7 |
| Microvillous inclusion disease | 6 | Retransplant | 6 |
| Malabsorption, other | 4 | Miscellaneous | 5 |
| Short gut, other | 4 | Other tumors | 4 |
| Other | 4 | Gardner's syndrome | 3 |
| Motility | 2 | | |
| Tumor | 1 | | |

From Intestinal Transplant Association (ITA): Intestine transplant registry: 25 years of follow-up results (http://intestinaltransplantassociation.com).

**Table 29-2 Some Diagnostic Studies for Pretransplantation Evaluation**

| DIAGNOSTIC STUDIES | EXAMPLES |
|---|---|
| Laboratory evaluation | Serum chemistries, liver function tests, complete blood count, prothrombin time–international normalized ratio (PT-INR), partial thromboplastin time (PTT), platelet count, albumin, prealbumin |
| Serologies for infectious diseases | CMV, EBV, hepatitis panel, HIV |
| Endoscopy | Upper gastrointestinal (UGI) series, colonoscopy with biopsies |
| Pathology | Percutaneous liver biopsy |
| Radiographic evaluation | UGI with small bowel follow-through, CT of abdomen and pelvis, Doppler ultrasonography or magnetic resonance venography |

malabsorption, resulting in poor enteral function. For patients with short bowel syndrome, the remnant intestinal length and presence or absence of an ileocecal valve have been identified as predictive factors as to whether rehabilitation will be successful.[24]

Dependence on parenteral nutrition alone, however, is not considered an indication for intestinal transplantation. To be considered for intestinal transplantation, patients must be dependent on TPN and have experienced life-threatening complications of hyperalimentation. As early as 2000, the Center for Medicare and Medicaid Services recognized the following indications for transplantation of the intestine, with or without other organs, as standard of care for patients with irreversible intestinal failure: (1) overt or impending liver failure caused by PNALD; (2) multiple thromboses of central veins limiting central venous access; (3) more than two episodes of catheter-related infection requiring hospitalization in any year; (4) a single episode of fungal line infection; and/or (5) frequent severe dehydration, despite IV fluid supplementation and TPN. Chronic line infections, specifically fungal line infections, can be difficult to clear and can lead to venous occlusion, loss of available access sites, or death. Thrombosis can also occur outside the setting of infection, leading to loss of potential central venous access sites. In addition, approximately 50% of all patients on TPN will develop PNALD,[25] thus potentially requiring liver transplantation in addition to intestinal transplantation.

In 2001, the American Society of Transplantation issued a position paper concerning indications for pediatric intestinal transplantation. In addition to the criteria noted, they also proposed that intestinal transplantation be considered for patients with intestinal failure that almost always results in early death, despite optimal nutrition, and for patients with high morbidity, poor quality of life, or fluid or electrolyte abnormalities who cannot be successfully managed on an outpatient basis.[26] Despite establishment of these criteria a decade ago, many referrals for intestinal transplantation continue to occur late in the patient's clinical course. Currently, 75% of patients on the waiting list for intestinal transplantation also require a liver, thus placing more strain on an already limited organ supply.[27]

## EVALUATION

### Recipient Evaluation

After referral to an intestinal transplantation center, the patient undergoes evaluation to determine the extent of complications of intestinal failure and degree of comorbidities. Historical details and previous hospital records pertaining to surgical procedures performed, previous intestinal rehabilitation attempts, and attempts at enteral feeding will be closely examined. Common diagnostic studies performed during the evaluation are listed in Table 29-2. Once a patient is deemed an appropriate candidate, he or she is placed on the waiting list within their United Network for Organ Sharing (UNOS) region. Transplantation centers may indicate weight and age spans for which they would consider potential donors, and each patient is assigned a status level according to her or his available venous access. Level 1 recipients are those who no longer have adequate central venous access via the jugular, subclavian, or femoral vein and all others are classified as level 2 candidates. Potential recipients who also require a liver in addition to the intestine, are placed on the liver waiting list according to their model for end-stage liver disease (MELD) or pediatric end-stage liver disease (PELD) score (OPTN policy 3.11 on intestinal organ allocation).

### Donor Evaluation

Potential cadaveric intestine donors are matched to appropriate size- and blood type–compatible recipients according to UNOS policies—first locally, then regionally, and finally nationally. When centers are evaluating a potential donor, consideration is given to existing intestinal pathology or past surgical history, such as extensive resection or Roux-en-Y reconstruction.

Donors may be deemed inappropriate based on Epstein–Barr virus (EBV) and cytomegalovirus (CMV) serologies, which could lead to post-transplantation lymphoproliferative disorder and severe enteritis in the recipients, respectively. Another consideration is the size of the donor compared with the recipient, because significant loss of abdominal domain after extensive resection may not allow accommodation of organs from larger or even size-matched donors. In these cases, an ideal donor should have a weight 50% to 75% that of the recipient. Furthermore, long cold ischemia times of the intestinal allograft may lead to loss of mucosal integrity and bacterial translocation or intestinal perforation in the donor organ. Therefore, consideration is given to any factor that could potentially increase the cold ischemia time, such as prior abdominal surgery in the donor and travel time between the recipient and donor medical centers. Close communication must occur between the donor and recipient teams to optimize timing. As with all cadaveric organs, the final evaluation occurs during the procurement operation, during which the intestine is closely inspected for anatomic or perfusion defects that might preclude its use. Overall, intestine is recovered from potential donors less frequently than any other solid organ, but rates of recovery have been increasing over time.[28]

## ANATOMIC CONSIDERATIONS

Isolated intestinal transplants include the entire jejunum and ileum and their associated mesentery. Use of isolated intestine is limited to patients who lack or have reversible PNALD despite intestinal failure and TPN dependence. Unfortunately, because of the frequency of end-stage liver disease in potential recipients, most require a combined transplant of the intestine with the liver. The nomenclature of grafts that include other organs with the intestine has been complicated by the inconsistent use of terms among various centers. For example, a liver-intestine graft may refer to individual liver and intestine grafts from the same donor, but with each implanted separately. This requires reconstruction of the biliary drainage and complex vascular anastomoses. More commonly a liver-intestine, or multivisceral graft, includes the head or entire pancreas, whether or not the recipient retains his or her native pancreas, because of the shared blood supply of the duodenum and pancreas with the liver and intestine grafts. Others use the term *multivisceral* or *modified mutivisceral transplants* only when the stomach, colon, and/or spleen are included as part of the graft. A more reliable and perhaps simpler approach would be simply to name the organs included in the graft.

Decisions as to which organs should be included are made based on the recipient's underlying disease process and vary slightly based on individual center experience. Some centers have included stomach in the allograft for recipients suffering from gastroparesis preoperatively, with good functional results, whereas other centers have reported that the transplanted stomach may also suffer from gastroparesis.[29] Historically, the right and transverse colon, which receive their arterial supply based on the superior mesenteric artery, were included as part of the intestinal transplant. The colon was placed orthotopically and anastomosed to the recipient colon or brought out as an end colostomy. An early series from Pittsburgh has described increased risk of graft loss[14] and the practice was largely abandoned. Recent reports dispute this finding and a few centers now include the colon routinely.[30]

### Surgical Technique

#### Isolated Intestinal Transplantation

In adult and older pediatric donors without significant aberrations in anatomy, isolated intestine can be safely procured while still allowing for use of the liver and pancreas from the same donor.[31] During the donor operation for an isolated intestinal graft, the jejunum is divided at the ligament of Treitz and the ileum at its terminus. After a careful dissection of the mesentery from the retroperitoneal organs and colon and systemic flushing with preservation solution, the superior mesenteric artery (SMA) and superior mesenteric vein (SMV) are divided at the mesenteric root just distal to the middle colic vessels. In the neonatal donor, or other situations in which the isolated pancreas is not placed separately for transplantation, the SMA is divided at the level of the aorta and the portal vein is divided at the superior border of the pancreas to provide longer vessels to the intestinal allograft. Carotid or iliac arteries and iliac or jugular veins are also procured from the cadaveric donor to allow for vascular reconstruction. During the recipient operation, arterial inflow is established by direct anastomosis of the donor SMA to the recipient infrarenal aorta or by interposition of a donor arterial conduit. Venous outflow from the allograft is provided by anastomosis of the donor SMV to the recipient portal vein or inferior vena cava, with or without an interposition of donor venous conduit. The continuity of the bowel is established proximally and distally using standard techniques for enteric anastomoses. Finally, a distal ileostomy is created to allow for routine monitoring of the graft (Fig. 29-2).

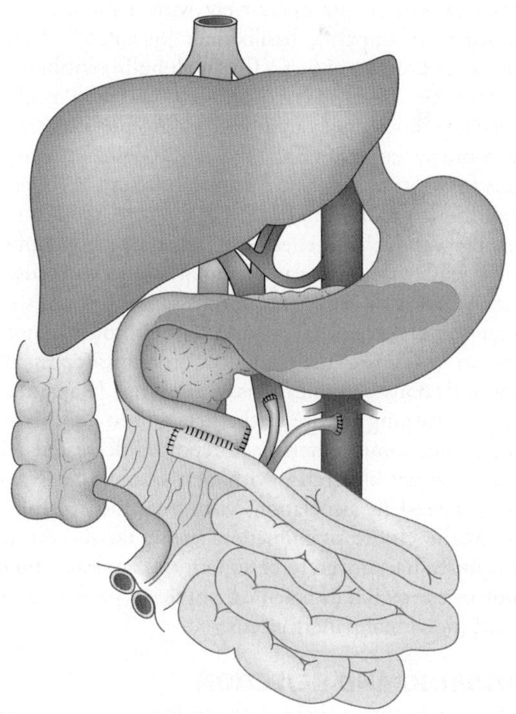

**FIGURE 29-2** Isolated intestinal transplant. Arterial inflow is established through anastomosis with the infrarenal aorta. The donor superior mesenteric vein is anastomosed to the native portal vein. The proximal graft jejunum is anastomosed to the recipient duodenum and the distal ileum is brought out as an ileostomy.

### Liver-Intestine-Pancreas Transplantation

During procurement of a combined liver-intestine transplant, the liver, duodenum, pancreas, spleen, and small bowel are generally procured en bloc, thus avoiding any hilar dissection. The celiac and SMA arteries are left on an aortic cuff or a conduit of donor aorta. The spleen is removed during back table preparation in most programs. During the recipient operation, the liver is excised, along with most of the remnant small bowel, to make room for the intestinal allograft. At times, the recipient duodenum, pancreas, spleen, and a portion of the stomach may also be excised because of prior fistula or injury during liver explantation, or to provide space for the donor organs in the recipient abdominal cavity. Using the donor thoracic aorta as a conduit, the donor celiac trunk and SMA are anastomosed to the recipient supraceliac or infrarenal aorta.[32] The suprahepatic inferior vena cava anastomosis, either caval replacement or piggyback fashion, allows for venous drainage of all transplanted organs because the donor portal system remains intact. When the recipient foregut is retained, a portocaval or splenorenal shunt procedure must be performed to allow for venous drainage of the native stomach, pancreas, spleen, and duodenum to prevent formation of esophagogastric varices from venous outflow obstruction. As in isolated intestinal transplantation, bowel continuity is reestablished through standard proximal and distal bowel anastomoses and an ileostomy is fashioned to allow for monitoring of the graft (Fig. 29-3).

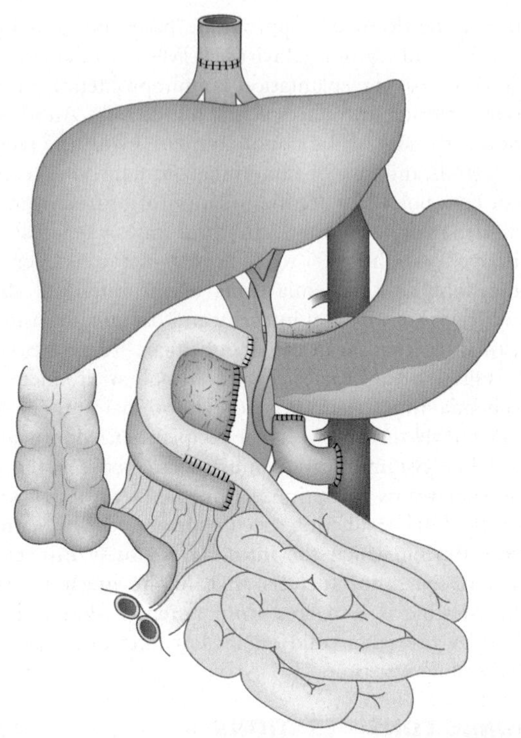

**FIGURE 29-3** Liver-intestine-pancreas transplant. The donor celiac and superior mesenteric arteries are left on an aortic conduit, which is anastomosed to the recipient aorta. Venous outflow is via the anastomosis between the donor hepatic veins and the recipient suprahepatic inferior vena cava (IVC). The donor duodenum and head of the pancreas (shown) or the entire donor pancreas are left intact to preserve the donor common bile duct. The donor jejunum is anastomosed to the native stomach, duodenum (shown), or proximal jejunum, depending on the native remnant anatomy.

## IMMUNOSUPPRESSION

The increased immunogenicity of the intestine often requires more potent immunosuppression regimens than are typically used with other solid organs. Most centers use induction immunosuppression intraoperatively with a monoclonal (e.g., alemtuzumab [Campath], basiliximab [Simulect], daclizumab [Zenapax]) or polyclonal (e.g., Thymoglobulin) antibody preparation. Induction therapy has been associated with a substantial decrease in the incidence of early rejection, but no single agent has been proven superior. Tacrolimus (FK-506, Prograf) forms the basis for most maintenance immunotherapy regimens, with cyclosporine (Sandimmune) use limited to patients unable to tolerate the various side effects of tacrolimus. Mycophenolate mofetil (CellCept) usage varies among centers because of its gastrointestinal side effects. Steroids are also widely used, although some centers have avoided their routine use in an attempt to minimize maintenance immunosuppression and decrease infectious complications.[33] Sirolimus (Rapamune) has a black box warning for use in the first month after liver transplantation, but some centers have reported decreased rejection rates in intestinal allografts, with or without the liver, when sirolimus is used in association with a calcineurin inhibitor.[34] Similar to the choice of induction agent, no specific maintenance regimen has proven to be superior to another, and centers continue to use regimens based on physician preference, experience, and individual patient needs.

## MONITORING AND REJECTION

Historically, rejection was seen frequently in intestinal transplant recipients, with some series reporting a 100% incidence.[35] More recently, some centers have reported a decrease in the incidence of rejection associated with improved patient survival.[33,36] Acute cellular rejection usually occurs within the first year post-transplantation but can occur at any time. The most frequent clinical signs and symptoms of rejection may mimic those of viral gastroenteritis, including unexplained fever, abdominal pain and/or cramping, and increased stoma or stool output. Rejection remains closely associated with rates of graft failure and mortality.[33] Unlike hepatic or renal transplantation, no convenient serochemical marker exists to monitor intestinal function. Stool calprotectin and serum citrulline levels have been proposed as potential markers of intestinal function, but none are widely used at this time.[37] Ileoscopies provide a method of visualizing the mucosa and obtaining tissue for pathologic examination. Routine ileoscopy and biopsy typically begins between postoperative days 5 and 7. Most centers will repeat the ileoscopy once or twice weekly for the first month, with the frequency decreasing the further from transplantation and in the absence of significant problems.[38]

Histopathologically, acute cellular rejection is characterized by an inflammatory response that is localized to the lamina propria and crypts. In mild forms, the mucosa remains intact but there are increased numbers of apoptotic bodies seen in the crypts. Moderate acute cellular rejection shows markedly increased inflammation within the lamina and an increase in apoptotic bodies within the crypts. The damage to crypts is so marked in severe acute cellular rejection that the intestinal architecture is lost and mucosal ulcerations are present. Although the mechanism is presently unclear, the liver appears to have a protective effect for rejection of the intestine, with some centers reporting a higher incidence or severity of acute cellular rejection in isolated intestinal transplants when compared with intestinal transplants in combination with the liver.[39]

Once rejection has been established, treatment usually consists of large steroid doses and ensuring that maintenance immunosuppressive medications are at target levels. Repeat ileoscopy and biopsy will evaluate for resolution of rejection. Resistant cases may be treated with more intense immunosuppression, including infliximab (a murine monoclonal antibody to tumor necrosis factor-α [TNF-α]; Remicade) or thymoglobulin (rabbit antithymocyte globulin), with or without additional maintenance immunosuppressants (e.g., sirolimus, mycophenolate mofetil). During treatment for rejection, the combination of increased immunosuppression and potential compromise of the gut mucosal barrier can lead to secondary infections, so a high index of suspicion for infections must be maintained.[39]

Chronic rejection in intestinal allografts leading to graft loss can lead to retransplantation in up to 13% of recipients.[38,40] Most patients experience multiple episodes of acute cellular rejection prior to a diagnosis of chronic rejection. Clinically, these patients may have chronic diarrhea despite adequate treatment of their acute rejection or may develop obstructive symptoms from graft scarring. On ileoscopy, the bowel can have a variable appearance; the mucosa may appear normal, be replaced by granulation tissue, or may show evidence of ulcerations and fibrosis. Similar to other solid organs, an obliterative arteriopathy is a major feature, although this may not be seen in the mucosal biopsies from ileoscopy and full-thickness biopsy may be required for a definitive diagnosis. Comparable to acute cellular rejection, chronic rejection rates appear to be higher for isolated intestinal transplants than for intestines transplanted with other organs.[27] In severe cases, an allograft enterectomy may be performed to reduce symptoms prior to retransplantation. However, in patients receiving a liver and intestine, this is not always feasible, because removing the intestine could adversely affect portal inflow to the liver.

## COMPLICATIONS

Despite the advances in intestinal transplantation, it remains an operation with high morbidity, and reported complication rates approach 50%.[38] Postoperative hemorrhage may caused by recipient coagulopathy, amplified by the extensive dissection usually required as a result of multiple adhesions from previous surgeries. Biliary complications can be largely avoided in liver-intestine transplants by including the duodenum and pancreas, thus avoiding any hilar dissection, but may still be a factor in procedures in which a bile duct anastomosis is required or from preservation injury caused by prolonged cold ischemia. Vascular complications are rare, but thrombosis of arterial inflow or venous outflow conduits can lead to a sudden deterioration in the patient and graft loss. Other technical complications, such as bowel anastomotic leaks and wound complications, can be catastrophic, but are addressed in the intestinal allograft recipient using standard surgical principles.

Infection is a serious risk in the short and long term and can lead to significant morbidity and mortality. Bacterial infections are prevalent, with one retrospective series reporting a 94% incidence of bacterial infection after intestinal transplantation.[41] A number of preoperative and intraoperative factors contribute to a high rate of bacterial infection, including prolonged operative time, preexisting liver disease, preexisting infections, uniform need for chronic central venous access, and multiple blood transfusions. Ischemia reperfusion injury may also lead to loss of the gut mucosal barrier and bacterial translocation in the immediate postoperative period. Rejection leads to a similar impairment of the gut mucosal barrier, but later in the postoperative course. Bacterial infections can manifest as intra-abdominal infection, catheter-related infections, pneumonia, or wound infections, with central line infections being the most common.[42] Organisms include typical gut flora such as *Escherichia coli, Klebsiella, Enterobacter,* and enterococci and, commonly, polymicrobial infections. Special consideration should also be given to fungal infections; most centers use antifungals as part of their routine perioperative antibiotics.

Viral infections are also common in patients receiving intestinal transplants, with approximately two thirds of patients developing such infections.[41] CMV is a common pathogen post–intestinal transplantation, which often affects the allograft. The reported incidence ranges from 25% in isolated intestine recipients to 40% in recipients who receive multiple organs.[41] The presentation of CMV infection ranges from fever, increased stoma or stool output, cramping, and abdominal pain to intestinal ulceration, bleeding, perforation, or frank ischemia. Because these symptoms may mimic those of rejection, biopsy of the allograft may be needed to differentiate the two. The presence of CMV inclusion bodies on slides (with hematoxylin and eosin [H&E] stain) confirms the diagnosis of CMV enteritis, and questionable findings can be confirmed with immunohistochemistry stains specific for CMV virus. Fortunately, with appropriate antimicrobial treatment, typically ganciclovir (Cytovene) and/or CMV immunoglobulin (CytoGam), and reduction in immunosuppression, graft loss can be avoided in most cases. Because of the potential for severe sepsis or death from primary CMV infections, some centers avoid transplantation of a CMV-positive donor intestine into a CMV-negative recipient.

EBV also presents a unique challenge to intestinal transplant recipients because of the higher rates of post-transplantation lymphoproliferative disorder (PTLD) when compared with other solid organ transplant recipients. In intestinal transplant recipients, the reported incidence of PTLD is 10% to 20%[43] compared with kidney recipients (1% to 2%), liver recipients (2% to 3%), and heart recipients (3% to 5%). PTLD has a variable presentation, ranging from lymphadenopathy to solid masses at extranodal sites, such as the transplanted intestine or within the lung, liver, or central nervous system. EBV-associated PTLD usually presents within the first year after intestinal transplantation and, therefore, some centers use a routine screening program using a serum quantitative EBV polymerase chain reaction (PCR) assay for the first 6 to 12 months. Risk factors for the development of PTLD include an EBV-positive donor to EBV-negative recipient and the use of muromonab-CD3 (Orthoclone OKT3) as a rescue agent.[43] No specific maintenance agent or protocol has been specifically implicated as a risk factor. Pediatric patients are also more likely to develop PTLD, with 15.3% of pediatric recipients developing PTLD compared with only 5% of adult recipients.[23] Although computed tomography (CT) scanning is often used in evaluating for PTLD when there is clinical suspicion, diagnosis requires confirmation by biopsy of affected tissue. Reduction of immunotherapy is the first line of treatment, but more resistant cases may require antivirals, chemotherapy, and/or anti-CD20 monoclonal antibodies (e.g., Rituximab) that target the EBV-infected B cells. Despite these treatments, EBV-associated PTLD has a mortality rate of 25% to 60%.[44]

Graft-versus-host disease (GVHD) occurs when donor lymphoid cells begin to target recipient tissues, most notably the epithelial cells in the skin and intestine. Because of the large amount of lymphoid tissue present in the intestine, it was predicted that an intestine recipient might be at higher risk for GVHD but surprisingly, it has been relatively uncommon.[35,45] The reported incidence ranges from 0% to 14% and is most frequently associated with patients with concomitant severe combined immunodeficiency.[35,46] Increasing immunosuppression, mainly through the increase or addition of steroids or antithymocyte globulin, has been the mainstay of treatment, but the outcome varies according to severity; in many cases, this proves fatal.

## OUTCOMES

### Patient and Graft Survival

Since the earliest cases, survival rates for grafts and patients have steadily improved. In 1997, the 1-year adjusted graft survival for all intestinal transplant patients was only 55.6% but improved to 69.6% in 2006.[47] Over the same period, 1-year adjusted patient survival improved from 60.4% in 1997 to 78.4% in 2006.[47] There were early differences noted in terms of patient and graft survival between recipients of isolated intestinal transplants and intestinal transplants that included a liver (Table 29-3). Comparison data for deceased donor liver transplants are included in the table. The most common reason for death after intestinal transplantation is infection. Sepsis accounted for 46% of patient deaths in the ITR, followed by rejection (11%), respiratory failure (6.6%), PTLD (6.1%), and technical complications (6.1%).[23]

In general, graft function after transplantation is good in survivors. According to the 2003 report from the ITR, of the 406 patients who survived longer than 6 months after transplantation, 81% were completely weaned from TPN. Another 3.9% required only IV fluid supplementation and 6.4% required partial TPN supplementation to enteral feeds.[40] According to the same database, graft loss occurred in 160 of 989 patients (16.2%).[40] The most common reason for graft loss was rejection, occurring in 56.3% of patients, followed by vascular complications (20.6%), other reasons (13.1%), sepsis (8.8%), and lymphoma (1.2%). When divided into the pediatric versus adult patient population, children younger than 18 years were more likely to lose their grafts as a result of rejection (62.4% versus 47.8%) and lymphoma (2.2% versus 0%) than adults.[23]

### Costs and Quality of Life

Estimates of the annual cost for home TPN range from $75,000 to $150,000, excluding the cost of hospitalizations for complications from TPN, such as line sepsis or dysfunction.[48] Despite the high initial cost of the intestinal transplantation procedure and hospitalization, when average costs of immunosuppressive medications and subsequent hospitalizations are considered, transplantation becomes cost-effective when compared with home TPN, usually between 1 and 3 years after transplantation.[48] In addition to the assessment of cost-effectiveness, studies have attempted to evaluate potential improvements in quality of life after intestinal transplantation, but these are limited. The ITR has reported that of patients who survive longer than 6 months post-transplantation, 85% reported a Karnofsky score higher than 90%, implying a good to excellent quality of life, with minimal symptoms.[23] DiMartini and colleagues[49] have reported that patients perceive an equal or better quality of life measures after transplantation, compared with remaining on home TPN. Studies in pediatric intestinal recipients are more difficult to perform because of the young age of most recipients with intestinal failure and the lack of appropriate and reliable tools for assessing this age group. Sudan and associates[50] have reported that parents of intestine recipients perceive a slightly worse quality of life measure than the patients themselves, but the children rate their quality of life similar to that of normal age-matched children. Long-term studies of cognitive development and motor skills in pediatric intestinal recipients do not exist to date.

## CONCLUSIONS

The field of intestinal transplantation has expanded greatly over the last several decades. The widespread use of home TPN has allowed for longer lives for many patients, but has also led to the development of PNALD and catheter-related complications in a subset of patients for whom intestinal transplantation may hold the best hope of survival. Since 2000, intestinal transplantation is no longer considered experimental; improvements in

**Table 29-3 Graft and Patient Survival (%)***

| TRANSPLANT | SURVIVAL | 1 YEAR (2005-2006)† | 3 YEARS (2003-2006)† | 5 YEARS (2001-2006)† | 10 YEARS (1996-2006)† |
|---|---|---|---|---|---|
| Intestine | Graft survival | 68.3 | 57.4 | 36.3 | 25.2 |
| | Patient survival | 81.4 | 70.6 | 56.2 | 46.4 |
| Liver-intestine | Intestine graft survival | 73.1 | 59.7 | 50.6 | 35.8 |
| | Liver graft survival | 73.1 | 60.0 | 51.1 | 36.3 |
| | Patient survival | 73.4 | 60.6 | 54.8 | 38.1 |
| Liver (deceased donor) | Graft survival | 82.4 | 73.4 | 67.6 | 53.4 |
| | Patient survival | 87.1 | 78.7 | 73.3 | 59.5 |

Data from U.S. Organ Procurement and Transplantation Network and the Scientific Registry of Transplant Recipients: 2008 OPTN/SRTR annual report: Transplant data 1999-2007 (http://optn.transplant.hrsa.gov/ar2008).

*For intestine, intestine-liver, and liver transplants at 1, 3, 5, and 10 years post-transplantation.

†Years in parentheses represent years of treatment.

morbidity and mortality have led to acceptance of intestinal transplantation as a standard treatment for intestinal failure. The current challenges in the field include the following:

1. The need for multi-institutional studies to identify
   - Patients at the earliest possible time in their disease process who will inevitably require transplantation
   - Factors associated with the most efficacious timing of performing intestinal transplantation
   - The most effective induction and maintenance immunosuppression strategies
   - Biomarkers that can replace ileoscopy and biopsy for routine monitoring of the intestinal allograft
2. The lack of consistent nomenclature for the technical aspects of the various procedures
3. The lack of clear indications and risks of inclusion or exclusion of other organs (e.g., stomach, colon, spleen)

In addition, only a limited number of centers have established expertise in intestinal transplantation worldwide, leading to differential access to multidisciplinary management of intestinal failure based on location and extensive regulatory requirements, which make it difficult for new programs to develop. These challenges are balanced by continued efforts at widespread education about the availability and outcomes of intestinal transplantation and the hard-working efforts of pioneers to expand clinical and scientific discoveries in the field.

## SELECTED REFERENCES


Bianchi A: Intestinal loop lengthening—a technique for increasing small intestinal length. J Pediatr Surg 15:145–151, 1980.

Dr. Bianchi's first description of his novel bowel-lengthening procedure.

Deltz E, Schroeder P, Gebhardt H, et al: Successful clinical small bowel transplantation—report of a case. Clinical Transplantation 3:89–91, 1988.

A case report of what is considered the first successful small intestine transplant.

Dudrick SJ, Rhoads JE, Vars HM: Growth of puppies receiving all nutritional requirements by vein. Fortschr Parenteral Ernahrung 2:16–18, 1967.

This is Dr. Dudrick's landmark paper in which he demonstrated survival in puppies using only hyperalimentation.

Fryer J: Intestinal transplantation: Current status. Gastroenterol Clin N Am 36:145–159, 2007.

A review of intestinal transplantation and its current practices.

Grant D, Abu-Elmagd K, Reyes J, et al: 2003 report of the intestine transplant registry: A new era has dawned. Ann Surg 241:607–613, 2005.

This is a summary of data from the Intestinal Transplant Registry database that includes statistics compiled from intestinal transplant recipients at transplant centers from 21 countries.

Kaufman S, Atkinson J, Bianchi A, et al: Indications for pediatric intestinal transplantation: A position paper of the American Society of Transplantation. Pediatr Transplant 5:80–87, 2001.

A thorough review of commonly accepted indications for intestinal transplantation.

Kim H, Fauza D, Garza J, et al: Serial transverse enteroplasty (STEP): A novel bowel lengthening procedure. J Pediatr Surg 38:425–429, 2003.

A description of the STEP procedure, which is an alternative bowel lengthening procedure to the Bianchi operation.

Starzl TE, Rowe MI, Todo S, et al: Transplantation of multiple abdominal viscera. JAMA 261:1449–1457, 1989.

This paper describes two children who received multivisceral transplants, one of whom is considered the first successful case of liver-intestine transplantation.


## REFERENCES


1. Howard L, Heaphey L, Fleming CR, et al: Four years of North American registry home parenteral nutrition outcome data and their implications for patient management. JPEN J Parenter Enteral Nutr 15:384–393, 1991.
2. Dudrick SJ, Rhoads JE, Vars HM: Growth of puppies receiving all nutritional requirements by vein. Fortschr Parenteral Ernahrung 2:16–18, 1967.
3. Touloukian RJ, Downing SE: Cholestasis associated with long-term parenteral hyperalimentation. Arch Surg 106:58–62, 1973.
4. Gura K, Duggan C, Collier S, et al: Reversal of parenteral nutrition-associated liver disease in two infants with short bowel syndrome using parenteral fish oil: Implications for future management. Pediatrics 118:e197–201, 2006.
5. Carrell A: Landmark article, Nov 14, 1908: Results of the transplantation of blood vessels, organs and limbs. JAMA 250:944–953, 1905.
6. Lillehei R, Goott B, Miller F: The physiological reponse of the small bowel of the dog to ischemia, including prolonged in vitro preservation of the bowel with successful replacement of survival. Ann Surg 150:543–560, 1959.
7. Starzl T, Kaupp HJ: Mass homotransplantation of abdominal organs in dogs. Surg Forum 11:28–30, 1960.
8. Lillehei R, Idezuke Y, Feemster J, et al: Transplantation of stomach, intestine, and pancreas: Experimental and clinical observations. Surgery 62:721–741, 1967.
9. Alican F, Hardy J, Cayirli M, et al: Intestinal transplantation: Laboratory experience and report of a clinical case. Am J Surg 121:150–159, 1971.
10. Cohen Z, Silverman R, Wassef R, et al: Small intestinal transplantation using cyclosporine. Report of a case. Transplantation 42: 613–621, 1986.
11. Deltz E, Schroeder P, Gebhardt H, et al: Successful clinical small bowel transplantation—report of a case. Clinical Transplantation 3:89–91, 1988.
12. Starzl T, Rowe M, Todo S, et al: Transplantation of multiple abdominal viscera. JAMA 261:1449–1457, 1989.
13. Margreiter R: The history of intestinal transplantation. Transplant Rev 11:9–21, 1997.

14. Todo S, Reyes J, Furukawa H, et al: Outcome analysis of 71 clinical intestinal transplantations. Ann Surg 222:270–280, 1995.
15. Langnas A, Shaw BJ, Antonson D, et al: Preliminary experience with intestinal transplantation in infants and children. Pediatrics 97:443–448, 1996.
16. Hammer J, Seay P, Johnston R, et al: The effect of antiperistaltic bowel segments on intestinal emptying time. Arch Surg 79:537–541, 1959.
17. Thompson J: Surgical rehabilitation of intestine in short bowel syndrome. Surgery 135:465–470, 2004.
18. Bianchi A: Intestinal loop lengthening—a technique for increasing small intestinal length. J Pediatr Surg 15:145–151, 1980.
19. Kim H, Fauza D, Garza J, et al: Serial transverse enteroplasty (STEP): A novel bowel lengthening procedure. J Pediatr Surg 38:425–429, 2003.
20. Modi B, Javid P, Jaksic T, et al: First report of the international serial transverse enteroplasty data registry: indications, efficacy, and complications. J Am Coll Surg 204:365–371, 2007.
21. Sudan D, Thompson J, Botha J, et al: Comparison of lengthening procedures for patients with short bowel syndrome. Ann Surg 246:593–601, 2007.
22. Andres A, Thompson J, Grant W, et al: Repeat surgical bowel lengthening with the STEP procedure. Transplantation 85:1294–1299, 2008.
23. Intestinal Transplant Association (ITA): Intestine transplant registry: 25 years of follow-up results (http://intestinaltransplantassociation.com).
24. Carbonnel F, Cosnes J, Chrvret S, et al: The role of anatomic factors in nutritional autonomy after extensive samll bowel resection. J Parenter Enteral Nutr 20:275–280, 1996.
25. Fishbein T, Matsumoto C: Intestinal replacement therapy: timing and indications for referral of patients to an intestinal rehabilitation and transplant program. Gastroenterology 130:S147–S151, 2006.
26. Kaufman S, Atkinson J, Bianchi A, et al: Indications for pediatric intestinal transplantation: A position paper of the American Society of Transplantation. Pediatr Transplant 5:80–87, 2001.
27. Fryer J: The current status of intestinal transplantation. Curr Opin Organ Transplant 13:266–272, 2008.
28. Tuttle-Newhall J, Krishnan S, Levy M, et al: Organ donation and utilization in the United States: 1998-2007. Am J Transplant 9:879–893, 2009.
29. Loinaz C, Mittal N, Kato T, et al: Multivisceral transplantation for pediatric intestinal pseudo-obstruction: Single center's experience of 16 cases. Transplant Proc 36:312–313, 2004.
30. Kato T, Selvaggi G, Gaynor J, et al: Inclusion of donor colon and ileocecal valve in intestinal transplantation. Transplantation 86:293–297, 2008.
31. Abu-Elmagd K, Fung J, Bueno J, et al: Logistics and technique for procurement of intestinal, pancreatic, and hepatic grafts from the same donor. Ann Surg 232:680–687, 2000.
32. Sudan D, Iyer K, Deroover A, et al: A new technique for combined liver/small intestinal transplantation. Transplantation 72:1846–1848, 2002.
33. Abu-Elmagd K, Costa G, Bond G, et al: Evolution of the immunosuppressive strategies for the intestinal and multivisceral recipients with special reference to allograft immunity and achievement of partial tolerance. Transplant Int 22:96–109, 2009.
34. Lauro A, Dazzi A, Ercolani G, et al: Rejection episodes and 3-year graft survival under sirolimus and tacrolimus treatment after adult intestinal transplantation. Transplant Proc 39:1629–1631, 2007.
35. Sudan D, Kaufman S, Shaw B, et al: Isolated intestinal transplantation for intestinal failure. Am J Gastroenterol 95:1506–1515, 2000.
36. Sudan D, Shinnakotla S, Horslen S, et al: Basiliximab decreases the incidence of acute rejection after intestinal transplantation. Transplant Proc 34:940–941, 2002.
37. Avitzur Y, Grant D: Intestine transplantation in children: Update 2010. Pediatr Clin North Am 57:415–431, 2010.
38. DeLegge M, Alsolaiman M, Barbour E, et al: Short bowel syndrome: Parenteral nutrition versus intestinal transplantation. Where are we today? Dig Dis Sci 52:876–892, 2006.
39. Fryer J: Intestinal transplantation: Current status. Gastroenterol Clin N Am 36:145–159, 2007.
40. Grant D, Abu-Elmagd K, Reyes J, et al: 2003 report of the intestine transplant registry: A new era has dawned. Ann Surg 241:607–613, 2005.
41. Guaraldi G, Cocchi S, Codeluppi M, et al: Outcome, incidence, and timing of infectious complications in small bowel and multivisceral organ transplantation patients. Transplantation 80:1742–1748, 2005.
42. Oltean M, Herlenius G, Gabel M, et al: Infectious complications after multivisceral transplantation in adults. Transplant Proc 38:2683–2685, 2006.
43. Quintini C, Kato T, Gaynor J, et al: Analysis of risk factors for the devlopment of post-transplant lymphoproliferative disorder among 119 children who received primary intestinal transplants at a single center. Transplant Proc 38:1755–1758, 2006.
44. Abu-Elmagd K, Mazariegos G, Costa G, et al: Lymphoproliferative disorders and de novo malignancies in intestinal and multivisceral recipients: improved outcomes with new outlooks. Transplantation 88:926–934, 2009.
45. Mazariegos G, Abu-Elmagd K, Jaffe R, et al: Graft versus host disease in intestinal transplantation. Am J Transplant 4:1459–1465, 2004.
46. Gilroy R, Coccia P, Talmadge J, et al: Donor immune reconstitution after liver-small bowel transplantation for multiple intestinal atresia with immunodeficiency. Blood 103:1171–1174, 2004.
47. U.S. Organ Procurement and Transplantation Network and the Scientific Registry of Transplant Recipients: 2008 OPTN/SRTR annual report: Transplant data 1999-2007 (http://optn.transplant.hrsa.gov/ar2008).
48. Sudan D: Cost and quality of life after intestinal transplantation. Gastroenterology 130:S168–S162, 2006.
49. DiMartini A, Rovera G, Graham T, et al: Quality of life after small intestinal transplantation and among home parenteral nutrition patients. J Parenter Enteral Nutr 22:357–362, 1998.
50. Sudan D, Horslen S, Botha J, et al: Quality of life after pediatric intestinal transplantation: The perception of pediatric recipients and their parents. Am J Transplant 4:407–413, 2004.

# SECTION V

# SURGICAL ONCOLOGY

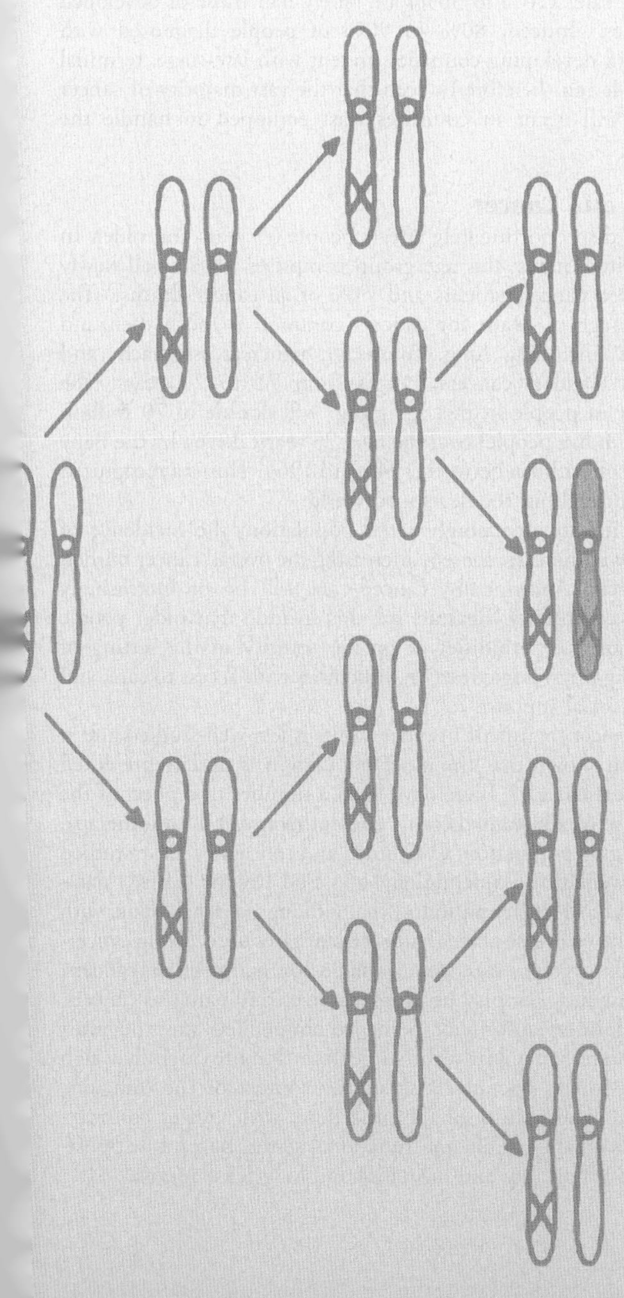

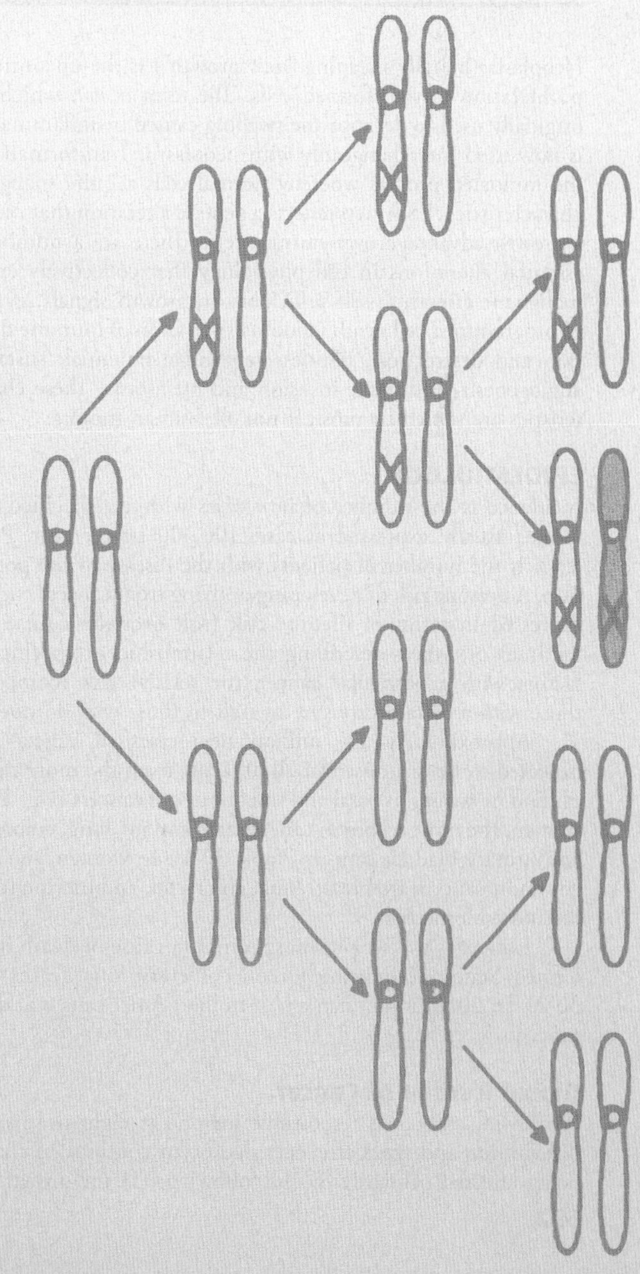

CHAPTER 30

# TUMOR BIOLOGY AND TUMOR MARKERS

Marcus C.B. Tan, S. Peter Goedegebuure, and Timothy J. Eberlein

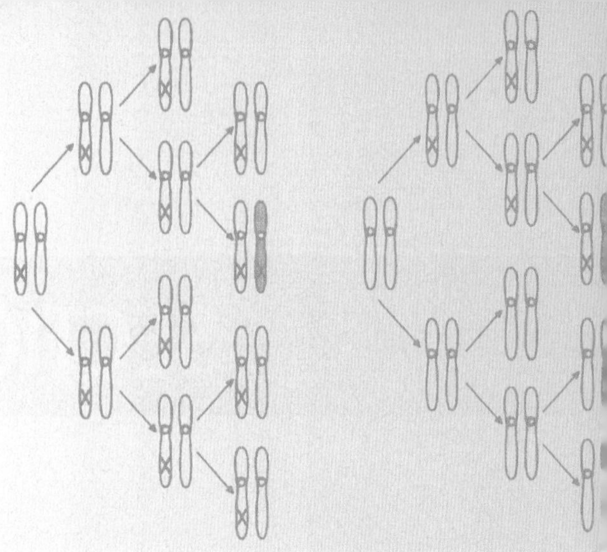

EPIDEMIOLOGY
TUMOR BIOLOGY
CARCINOGENESIS
TUMOR MARKERS

Neoplasia (literally meaning "new growth") is the uncontrolled proliferation of transformed cells. The term *tumor,* which was originally used to describe the swelling caused by inflammation, is now used interchangeably with neoplasm. Transformation is the multistep process whereby normal cells acquire malignant characteristics. Each step reflects a genetic alteration that confers a growth advantage over normal cells. There are a number of essential alterations in cell physiology that collectively enable malignant growth[1,2]; self-sufficiency in growth signals, evasion of programmed cell death (apoptosis), evasion of immune detection and destruction, limitless replicative potential, sustained angiogenesis, and tissue invasion and metastasis. These characteristics are shared by most, if not all, human tumors.

## EPIDEMIOLOGY

Incidence is the number of new cases within a specified time frame, usually expressed as cases/100,000 people/year. Prevalence is the number of patients with the disease in the population. A person's risk of developing or dying from cancer is usually expressed in terms of lifetime risk (risk over the course of a lifetime) or, when describing the relationship of specific risk factors with a particular cancer, the relative risk (comparing those with a certain exposure or trait to those who do not).

Approximately 1.5 million new cases of cancer were expected to be diagnosed in 2010, apart from the more than 1 million new cases of basal and squamous cell cancers (Fig. 30-1). In men, the most common cancers are prostate, lung, colorectal, and urinary bladder cancers (Table 30-1). In women, the most common cancers are breast, lung, colorectal, and uterine (cervical and endometrial).

Cancer is the second most common cause of death in the United States, accounting for one of every four deaths (Fig. 30-2). In 2010, more than a half-million Americans will die of cancer.

### Global Burden of Cancer

Worldwide, cancer is responsible for one in eight deaths. The distribution and types of cancer that occur continue to change, being affected primarily by the following: (1) the growth and aging of populations; (2) the increasing encroachment of modifiable risk factors (e.g., cigarette smoking, Western diet, physical inactivity) in developing countries; and (3) the relatively slower decrease in infection-related cancers.[3] By 2020, 70% of all cancer-related deaths will be in developing countries, in which survival rates (20% to 30%) are barely half those of developed countries.[4] Indeed, 80% to 90% of people diagnosed with cancer in developing countries present with late-stage, terminal cancer. It can therefore be seen that the vast majority of cancer deaths will occur in countries least equipped to handle the burden.

### Aging and Cancer

Cancer disproportionately affects people 65 years and older. In the United States, this age group comprises 56% of all newly diagnosed cancer patients and 71% of all cancer deaths.[5] The median age of death for cancers common to both men and women (including lung, colorectal, pancreas, stomach, and urinary bladder) cancers, ranges from 71 to 77 years. The number of people in this age group will double to 70 million (or one in five people) over the next 25 years, driven by the Baby Boom cohort born between 1946 and 1964. This is a recognized trend throughout the developed world.

With an increasingly older population, the incidence of cancer will increase, thereby increasing the overall cancer burden on society. Additionally, cancer care will be of increasingly greater complexity. Reasons for this include that older people have more comorbidities of greater severity in the setting of declining physiologic reserve, difficulties with access to care, and lack of social support.

Cancer treatment in older adults is less well-studied and it has been shown that the older population is underrepresented in clinical trials.[6–8] There have been a number of reports of the underuse of adjuvant therapy, chemotherapy and radiotherapy, in the aging population. O'Connell and colleagues[9] have studied the Surveillance, Epidemiology, and End Results (SEER) database (1988–1997), and found that although older patients with colorectal or breast cancer had excellent rates of receiving cancer-directed surgery, rates were variable for many other cancers, including lung, esophagus, stomach, liver, and pancreas cancers. Surgical intervention not being recommended was the most common reason. Clearly, the surgeon must more carefully weigh an individual's operative risk in the context of the difficulty, length and morbidity of the procedure, with greater consideration for quality of life and functional status, beyond just post-operative mortality and mortality and long-term survival.

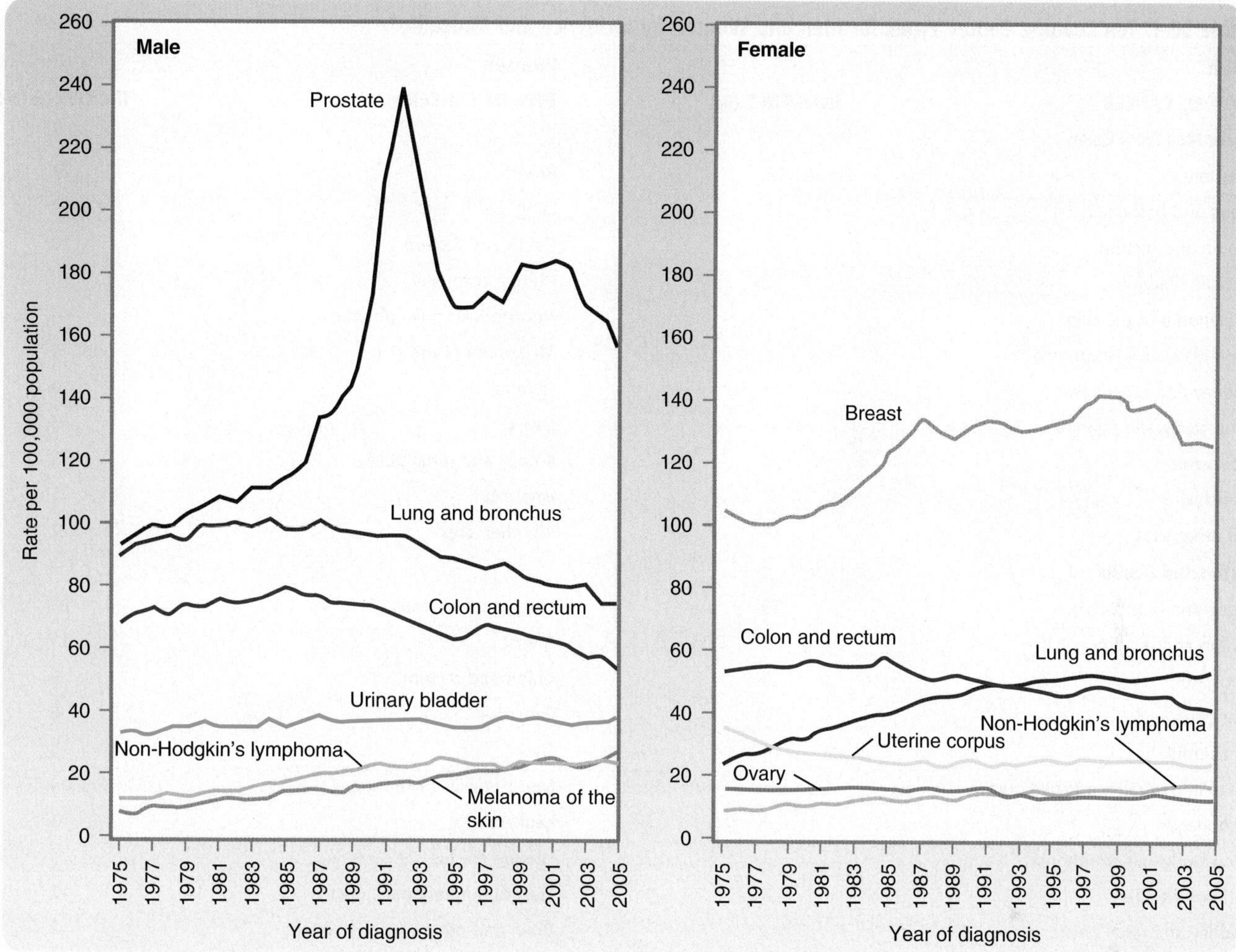


**FIGURE 30-1** Annual age-adjusted cancer incidence rates for males and females for selected cancers in the United States, 1975-2005. (From Jemal A, Siegel R, Ward E, et al: Cancer statistics, 2009. CA Cancer J Clin 59:225–249, 2009.)

## Obesity and Cancer

Prevalence of overweight (body mass index [BMI], 25 to 30) and obesity (BMI ≥ 30) in most developed countries, and in urban areas of many less developed countries, has been increasing markedly over the past 25 years. In the United States, approximately one third of the population is now classified as obese. Although obesity has long been recognized as an important cause of diabetes and cardiovascular disease, the relationship between obesity and cancer has received less attention. Epidemiologic studies indicate that adiposity contributes to the increased incidence and/or death from cancers of the colon, breast (in postmenopausal women), endometrium, kidney (renal cell), esophagus (adenocarcinoma), gastric cardia, pancreas, gallbladder, and liver (hepatocellular carcinoma). It has been estimated that 15% to 20% of all cancer deaths in the United States can be attributed to overweight and obesity.[10]

The mechanisms whereby obesity increases cancer risk appear to involve the metabolic and endocrine effects of obesity via their alterations in peptide and steroid hormone levels. For example, greater amounts of adipose tissue lead to increased circulating levels of free fatty acids. This, in turn, causes liver, muscle and other tissues to increase their usage of fats for energy production, thereby reducing their need for uptake and metabolism of glucose and eventually leading to hyperglycemia. This functional insulin resistance forces an increase in pancreatic insulin secretion. Epidemiologic and experimental evidence suggests that chronic hyperinsulinemia increases the risk of cancers of the colon and endometrium, and probably other tumors (e.g., those of the pancreas and kidney).

Circulating levels of estrogens are strongly related to adiposity. For cancers of the breast (in postmenopausal women) and endometrium, the effects of overweight and obesity on cancer risk are largely mediated by increased estrogen levels. For patients with breast cancer, adiposity has been associated with poorer survival and increased likelihood of recurrence, an effect that persisted after adjustment for tumor stage and grade, hormone receptor status, and adjuvant therapy.

# TUMOR BIOLOGY

Much has been learned about the multistep process of tumorigenesis. A well-documented example of tumor development is presented in Table 30-2. The transformation of melanocytes into malignant melanoma can be divided histopathologically and clinically into five major identifiable steps. Successive genetic changes each confer a growth advantage, leading to the progressive conversion of normal cells into cancer cells. This process is

**Table 30-1 Ten Leading Cancer Types for Men and Women by Incidence and Mortality***

| **Men** | | **Women** | |
|---|---|---|---|
| **TYPE OF CANCER** | **INCIDENCE (%)** | **TYPE OF CANCER** | **INCIDENCE (%)** |
| **Estimated New Cases** | | | |
| Prostate | 25 | Breast | 27 |
| Lung and bronchus | 15 | Lung and bronchus | 14 |
| Colon and rectum | 10 | Colon and rectum | 10 |
| Urinary bladder | 7 | Uterine corpus | 6 |
| Melanoma of the skin | 5 | Non-Hodgkin's lymphoma | 4 |
| Non-Hodgkin's lymphoma | 5 | Melanoma of the skin | 4 |
| Kidney and renal pelvis | 5 | Thyroid | 4 |
| Oral cavity and pharynx | 3 | Ovary | 3 |
| Leukemia | 3 | Kidney and renal pelvis | 3 |
| Pancreas | 3 | Pancreas | 3 |
| All other sites | 19 | All other sites | 22 |
| **Estimated Deaths** | | | |
| Lung and bronchus | 30 | Lung and bronchus | 26 |
| Colon and rectum | 9 | Breast | 15 |
| Prostate | 9 | Colon and rectum | 9 |
| Pancreas | 6 | Pancreas | 6 |
| Leukemia | 4 | Ovary | 5 |
| Liver and intrahepatic bile duct | 4 | Non-Hodgkin's lymphoma | 4 |
| Esophagus | 4 | Leukemia | 3 |
| Non-Hodgkin's lymphoma | 3 | Uterine corpus | 3 |
| Urinary bladder | 3 | Liver and intrahepatic duct | 2 |
| Kidney and renal pelvis | 3 | Brain and other nervous system | 2 |
| All other sites | 25 | All other sites | 25 |

Adapted from Jemal A, Siegel R, Ward E, et al: Cancer statistics, 2009. CA Cancer J Clin 59:225–249, 2009.
*Excluding basal and squamous cell skin cancers, and in situ carcinomas except urinary bladder.

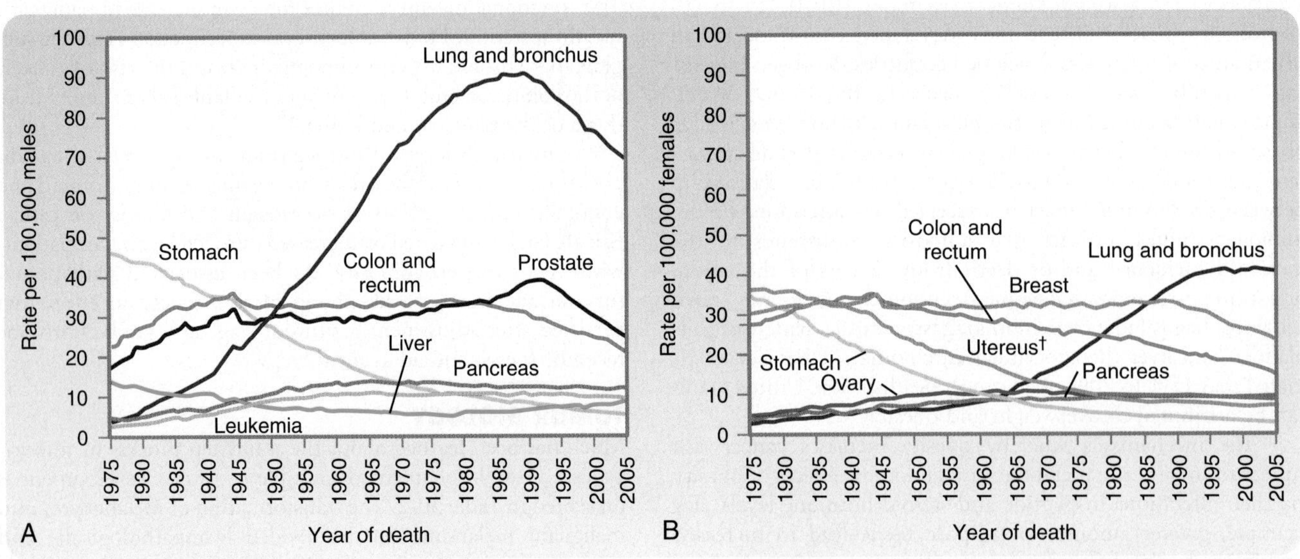


**FIGURE 30-2** Annual age-adjusted cancer mortality rates for males and females with selected cancers in the United States, 1930-2005. (From Jemal A, Siegel R, Ward E, et al: Cancer statistics, 2009. CA Cancer J Clin 59:225–249, 2009.)

**Table 30-2 Stepwise Progression from Melanocyte to Metastatic Melanoma**

| STEP* | CHARACTERISTICS |
|---|---|
| 1 | Common melanocytic nevus |
| 2 | Dysplastic nevus |
| 3 | Radial growth phase of melanoma |
| 4 | Vertical growth phase of melanoma |
| 5 | Metastatic melanoma |

Adapted from Clark WH Jr, Elder DE, Guerry Dt, et al: A study of tumor progression: the precursor lesions of superficial spreading and nodular melanoma. Hum Pathol 15:1147–1165, 1984.

*Common acquired and congenital nevi without cytologic atypia (step 1) may progress into dysplastic nevi with clear atypical histologic and cytologic features (step 2). Most of these lesions are stable, but a few may progress to a malignant melanoma that tends to grow outward along the radius of the plaque (step 3). Within the plaque, a nodule develops of fast-growing cells that expand in a vertical direction, invading the dermis and elevating the epidermis (step 4). Finally, the tumor metastasizes (step 5).

associated with a number of distinct changes in cell physiology (Fig. 30-3),[1,2] each of which is discussed in detail here.

## Self-Sufficiency in Growth Signals

Cells within normal tissues are largely instructed to grow by neighboring cells (paracrine signals) or via systemic (endocrine) signals. Similarly, cell to cell growth signaling also occurs in the vast majority of tumors. The immediate tumor cell environment (the stroma) contains resident nonmalignant cells such as parenchymal cells, epithelial cells, fibroblasts, and endothelial cells. In addition, most tumors are characterized by infiltrating immune cells such as lymphocytes, polymorphonuclear cells, mast cells, and macrophages. In some tumors, these cooperating cells may eventually transform themselves, coevolving with the tumor cells to sustain the growth of the latter. Finally, basement membranes form the extracellular matrix (ECM), which provides a scaffold for proliferation of fibroblast and endothelial cells. Together, tumor cells and stroma produce factors (autocrine and paracrine factors) that in cell-bound, matrix-bound, or soluble form directly or indirectly influence tumor development. Autocrine factors secreted by tumor cells promote growth of tumor cells but may also stimulate neighboring cells. In addition, tumor cells secrete paracrine factors that act on host cells or ECMs, generating a supportive microenvironment. For example,

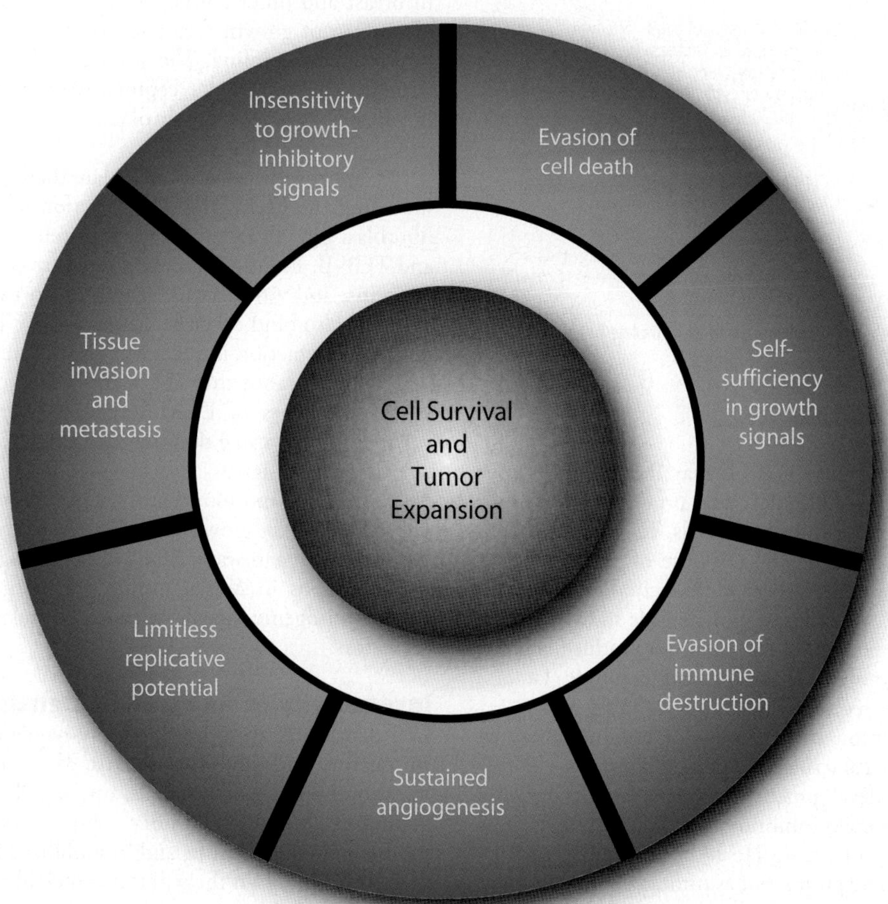


**FIGURE 30-3** Changes in cell physiology associated with progressive conversion of normal cells into tumor cells. The indicated traits are common to the vast majority of human cancers, together conferring cell survival and/or tumor expansion. (Adapted from Hanahan D, Weinberg RA: The hallmarks of cancer. Cell 100:57–70, 2000.)

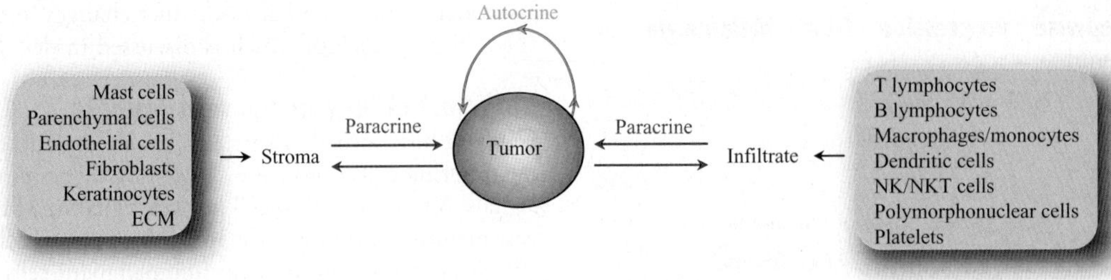

**FIGURE 30-4** Paracrine and autocrine growth mechanisms. Both stromal cells and infiltrate secrete paracrine factors that affect tumor development. Additionally, tumor cells secrete autocrine as well as paracrine factors that, in turn, act on stromal cells and infiltrating cells.

**Table 30-3 Cells and Soluble Factors Affecting Tumor Development***

| CELLS | SOLUBLE FACTORS |
|---|---|
| **Stroma** | |
| Parenchymal cells<br>Endothelial cells<br>Fibroblasts<br>Mast cells<br>Extracellular matrix<br>Keratinocytes | Growth factors, growth inhibitors, nutritional factors, hormones, degradative enzymes, cytokines, angiogenesis factors |
| **Infiltrate** | |
| T lymphocytes<br>B lymphocytes<br>Natural killer cells<br>Natural killer T cells<br>Macrophages, monocytes<br>Dendritic cells<br>Polymorphonuclear cells<br>Platelets | Cytokines, chemokines, cytolytic factors, angiogenesis factors, growth (inhibitory) factors, degradative enzymes, cytostatic factors, antibodies |
| **Tumor** | |
| | Chemokines, cytokines, angiogenesis factors, degradative enzymes, growth (inhibitory) factors |

*The list of cells and soluble factors is not meant to be complete but to illustrate the complexity of factors affecting tumor development.

transforming growth factor-β (TGF)-β may induce angiogenesis, production of ECM molecules, and production of other cytokines by fibroblasts and endothelial cells. To state it simply,, tumor growth is dependent on the response of tumor cells to paracrine and autocrine factors (Fig. 30-4, such as angiogenesis factors, growth factors, chemokines (polypeptide signaling molecules originally characterized by their ability to induce chemotaxis), cytokines, hormones, enzymes, and cytolytic factors, which may promote or reduce tumor growth (Table 30-3).

During the evolution of a tumor, its responsiveness to growth signals changes. Paracrine growth mechanisms are dominant during the early development of tumor. Tumors become resistant to paracrine growth inhibitors and gain responsiveness to paracrine growth promoters. However, autocrine growth mechanisms become more prominent as tumors develop further. The observation that in late-stage tumors, metastatic tumor cells tend to spread more randomly throughout the body suggests that autocrine growth mechanisms may be more dominant than paracrine growth mechanisms. Advanced breast cancers, for example, lose hormone responsiveness. It is even possible for a tumor to grow completely autonomously (acrine state) and be independent of growth factors and inhibitors (Fig. 30-5).

To achieve growth self-sufficiency, growth signaling pathways are altered. This involves the alteration of extracellular growth signals, transmembrane transducers of those signals, or intracellular signaling pathways that translate those signals into action. Growth factor receptors are overexpressed in many cancers. Receptor overexpression may enable the cancer cell to respond to low levels of growth factor that normally would not trigger proliferation. For example, the epidermal growth factor receptor (EGFR) and the Her2/neu receptor are overexpressed in breast and other epithelial cancers. Additionally, gross overexpression of growth factor receptors can elicit growth factor–independent signaling. The latter can also be achieved through structural alteration of receptors, such as truncated versions of the EGFR that lack much of its cytoplasmic domain and are constitutively activated.

Cancer cells can also modulate their stromal environment, including the ECM, through secretion of factors such as basic fibroblast growth factor (bFGF), platelet-derived growth factor, and TGF-β. ECM components, such as collagens, fibronectins, laminins, and vitronectins, may bind to two or more receptors and may also bind other ECM molecules. The matrix molecule-receptor interaction induces signals that influence cell behavior, including entrance into the active cell cycle. Cancer cells can switch the types of ECM receptors (e.g., integrins, heparan sulfate proteoglycans) that they express, favoring ones that transmit progrowth signals.

The third and most complex mechanism for acquisition of self-sufficiency in growth signals stem from changes in intracellular signaling pathways. Many of the oncogenes, such as activating mutations in *KRAS*, mimic normal growth signaling and induce mitogenic signals without stimulation from upstream regulators.

## Insensitivity to Antigrowth Signals

Cell division is an ordered, tightly regulated process involving stimulatory and inhibitory signals. Thus, in addition to acquiring stimulatory growth signals, tumor cells need to overcome or neutralize growth inhibitory signals. These signals include soluble growth inhibitors and immobilized inhibitors embedded in the ECM and on the surfaces of neighboring cells. Similar to many of the stimulatory signals, the growth inhibitory signals are transduced by transmembrane receptors coupled to intracellular signaling pathways that target genes regulating the cell cycle. The cell cycle can be divided into an interphase and a mitotic (M) phase (Fig. 30-6).[11] The interphase is further

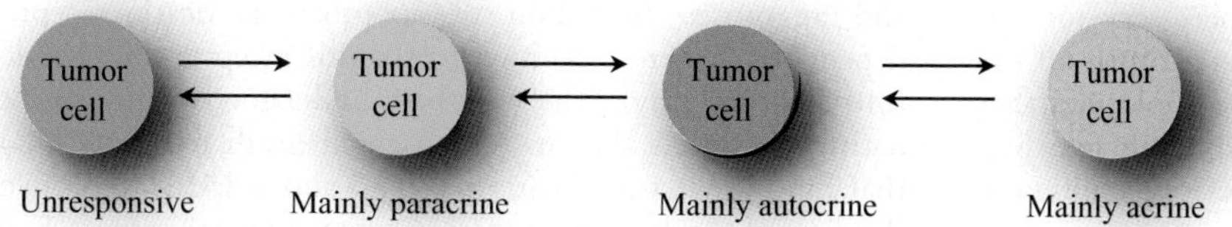


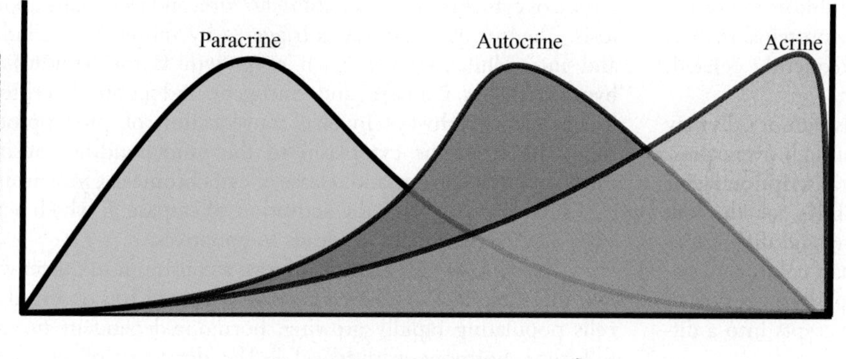


**FIGURE 30-5** Changes in contribution of growth mechanisms to tumor development. During tumor progression, the contribution of paracrine growth mechanisms decreases and the tumor becomes more dependent on autocrine growth mechanisms. At later stages, the tumor may even become independent of growth mechanisms (acrine state).

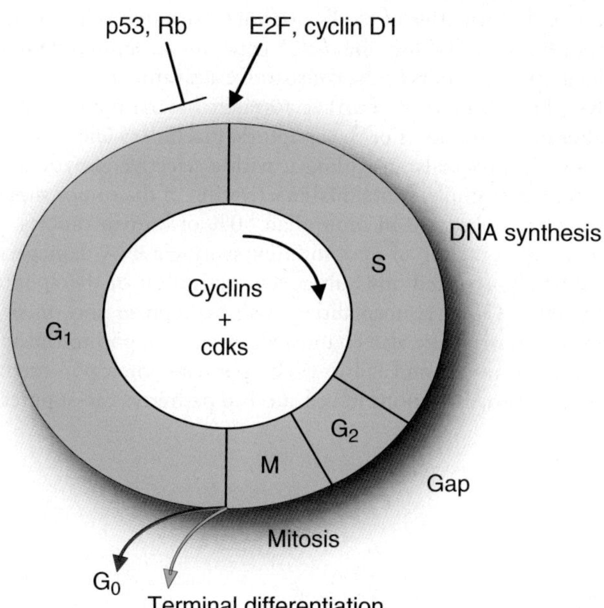


**FIGURE 30-6** Schematic overview of the cell cycle. Cell division is governed by cyclin proteins and CDKs. After mitosis, a cell can terminally differentiate, enter a quiescent state, or reenter the cell cycle. A critical point in the cell cycle control is the transition from $G_1$ to S. After passing this checkpoint, the cell is committed to division. Tumor suppressor genes such as the retinoblastoma *(Rb)* and *p53* gene block $G_1$ to S transition, whereas oncogenes such as *cyclin D1* and *E2F* promote transition.

subdivided into two gap phases ($G_1$ and $G_2$), separated by a phase of DNA synthesis (S phase). The two gap phases involve crucial regulatory events that prepare the cell for DNA replication and mitosis.

Central to cell cycle progression are the cyclin-dependent kinases (CDKs) that bind to the cyclin proteins. These proteins are regulated by numerous other proteins, including tumor suppressors and oncogenes that induce stimulatory or inhibitory signals. Antigrowth signals can block cell division by two distinct mechanisms. Cells may be forced to exit the cell cycle into a quiescent ($G_0$) state (Fig. 30-6).

Alternatively, cells may be induced to enter a postmitotic state, usually associated with terminal differentiation. Much of the signaling pathways that enable normal cells to respond to antigrowth signals are associated with the cell cycle block, specifically with the components governing the restriction point in the $G_1$ phase of the cell cycle. The restriction point marks the point between early and late $G_1$ phase passage that represents an irreversible commitment to undergo one cell division. Cells monitor their external environment during this period and, on the basis of sensed signals, decide whether to proliferate, be quiescent, or enter into a postmitotic state. At the molecular level, many and perhaps all antiproliferative signals involve the retinoblastoma protein (pRb) and its two family members, p107 and p130.[11] pRb is a key negative regulator at the restriction point. In quiescent cells, pRb is hypophosphorylated and blocks cell division by binding E2F transcription factors that control the expression of many genes essential for progression from the $G_1$ into the S phase (see Fig. 30-6). In contrast, growth stimulatory signals induce phosphorylation of pRb that does not bind E2F factors and is considered functionally inactive. Similarly, disruption of the pRb pathway liberates E2Fs and thus allows cell proliferation, rendering cells insensitive to antigrowth factors that normally operate along this pathway to block advance through the $G_1$ phase of the cell cycle. For example, TGF-β prevents the phosphorylation of pRb that inactivates pRb and thereby blocks advance through $G_1$. In some tumors, such as breast, colon, liver, and pancreatic cancers, TGF-β responsiveness is lost through downregulation of TGF-β receptors or through the expression of mutant, dysfunctional receptors. In others, such as colon, lung, and liver cancers, the cytoplasmic Smad4 protein, which transduces signals from ligand-activated TGF-β receptors to downstream targets, may be eliminated through mutation of its encoding gene. Alternatively, in cervical carcinomas induced by human papillomavirus (HPV), the viral oncoprotein E7 binds pRb and thereby induces dissociation of E2F and subsequent transcription of genes necessary for cell cycle progression. In addition, cancer cells can also turn off the expression of integrins and other cell adhesion molecules that send antigrowth signals. In summary, the antigrowth signaling pathways converging onto Rb and the cell cycle are disrupted in most human cancers.

Cyclin-CDK complexes, essential for cell cycle progression, are regulated by two families of cyclin-CDK inhibitors in normal cells. However, in tumor cells, these regulatory proteins, such as the p16 member of the INK4 family, are frequently deleted, allowing tumor cells to bypass cell cycle arrest.

In addition to avoiding antigrowth signals, tumor cells may also avoid terminal differentiation, such as through overexpression of the oncogene c-*myc,* which encodes a transcription factor regulating the expression of cyclins and CDKs, or through upregulation of ID (***i***nhibitor of ***D***NA-binding and differentiation) family members. Similarly, during human colon carcinogenesis, inactivation of the APC/β-catenin pathway serves to block the egress of enterocytes in the colonic crypts into a differentiated postmitotic state.

## Evasion of Cell Death

The growth of tumors is determined by the ability of tumor cells to proliferate, offset by cell death. Most, if not all, types of tumors are characterized by defects in cell death–signaling pathways and are resistant to cell death. Cell death in tumors is caused primarily by programmed cell death, or apoptosis, which is the most common and well-defined form of cell death.[12] Apoptosis is a physiologic cell suicide program essential for embryonic development, functioning of the immune system, and maintenance of tissue homeostasis. Apoptosis is characterized by disruption of membranes and chromosomal degradation in a matter of hours. The general apoptosis signaling pathway involves the release of cytochrome c from mitochondria that activates various caspases (a family of at least 10 proteases) in sequence (Fig. 30-7).

Activation of caspase cascades leads to DNA fragmentation and apoptosis. Induction of apoptosis is death receptor–dependent (extrinsic pathway) or death receptor–independent (intrinsic pathway). The two best understood death receptor pathways include the Fas receptor and death receptor (DR)-5 that bind the extracellular Fas ligand and TRAIL, respectively. Binding of the ligands triggers the activation of caspase 8 and promotes the cascade of procaspase activation, leading to the release of cytochrome c from mitochondria and eventually apoptosis. The intrinsic pathway is triggered by various extracellular and intracellular stresses, such as growth factor withdrawal, hypoxia, DNA damage, and oncogene induction. Receptor-independent pathways involve translocation of proapoptotic molecules from the cytoplasm to the mitochondria, causing mitochondrial damage and release of cytochrome c. Cytochrome c is directly involved in the activation of caspase 9, which activates caspase 3, which then leads to apoptosis.

The concept that apoptosis forms a constraint to cancer was first put forth in 1972, when massive apoptosis was observed in cells populating rapidly growing, hormone-dependent tumors following hormone withdrawal.[13] The discovery of the *bcl-2* oncogene as having antiapoptotic activity led to the investigation of apoptosis in cancer at the molecular level.[14] Bcl-2 promotes the formation of B cell lymphomas through a chromosomal translocation linking the *bcl-2* gene to an immunoglobulin locus, which results in the constitutive activation of *bcl2,* driving lymphocyte survival. Further research has demonstrated that altering components of the apoptotic machinery allows a cell to resist death signals, providing it with a selective growth advantage. For example, functional inactivation of the tumor suppressor p53 is observed in more than 50% of human cancers. p53 is a key regulator of apoptosis by sensing DNA damage that cannot be repaired and subsequent activation of the apoptotic pathway. Other abnormalities, such as hypoxia and oncogene overexpression, are also channeled, in part via p53 to the apoptotic machinery, and fail to elicit apoptosis when p53 function is lost. Also, alterations in cell survival pathways can suppress or

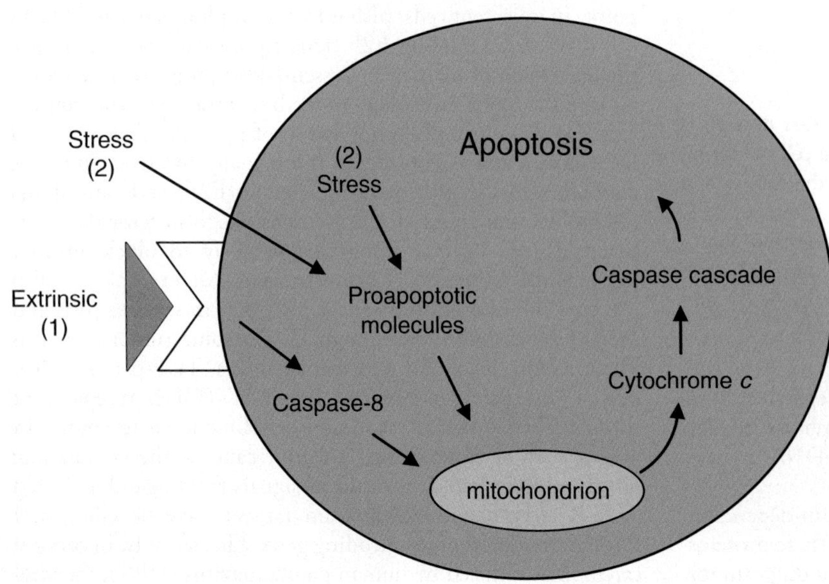


**FIGURE 30-7** Apoptotic pathways. Extracellular and intracellular stresses can induce apoptosis in tumor cells. Extracellular triggering can occur through a receptor-dependent (1) or receptor-independent (2) pathway. Both pathways induce the release of cytochrome c from mitochondria, which triggers the activation of various caspases in sequence, ultimately leading to apoptosis.

alter apoptosis. For example, the PI3 kinase-AKT pathway, which transmits antiapoptotic survival signals, is likely involved in inhibiting apoptosis in many human tumors. This signaling pathway can be activated by extracellular factors such as insulin-like growth factor 1 (IGF-1), IGF-2, or interleukin-3 (IL-3), intracellular signals from Ras, or loss of the pTEN tumor suppressor that negatively regulates the PI3 kinase–AKT pathway. A final example is the discovery of a nonsignaling decoy receptor for Fas ligand in a high fraction of lung and colon carcinoma cell lines. Expression of this decoy receptor dilutes the death signal mediated through Fas.

Nonapoptotic types of cell death include necrosis, autophagy, and mitotic catastrophe. Necrosis is normally induced by pathophysiologic conditions such as infection, inflammation, or ischemia. Necrosis is characterized by unregulated cell destruction. Autophagy, on the other hand, is characterized by the proteolysis of long-lived proteins and organelle components in lysosomes.[15] Cells that undergo excessive autophagy undergo apoptosis. Autophagy is triggered by growth factor withdrawal, hypoxia, DNA damage, and differentiation and developmental triggers.[12] Finally, aberrant mitosis caused by failure of the $G_2$ checkpoint to block mitosis when DNA is damaged, can lead to cell death, known as mitotic catastrophe. The signaling pathways involved in these types of nonapoptotic cell death are less well defined compared with those that regulate apoptosis, but it is clear that defects in nonapoptotic cell death pathways have been linked to cancer. For example, amplification of the MDM2 oncogene, which negatively regulates expression of p53, results in inadequate expression of p53 and thereby loss of tumor suppressor function. Another example is the deletion of the autophagy-regulating gene *becklin-1* in high percentages of ovarian, breast, and prostate cancers. In addition to cell death, cells can undergo permanent growth arrest, known as senescence, when repair of damaged DNA fails. Senescent cells lose their clonogenicity, but defects in the senescent program contribute to tumor development.

## Limitless Replication Potential

Acquired disruption of cell to cell signaling by itself does not ensure expansive tumor growth on its own. This is caused by the intrinsic programmed decline in replication potential that limits the multiplication of normal somatic cells. This program must be disrupted in order for a clone of cells to develop into a macroscopic tumor. Normal cells have a finite replicative potential. Once a cell population has progressed through a certain number of doublings, they stop growing, a process termed *senescence.*

With the exception of stem cells, activated lymphocytes, and germline cells, normal cells have a limited replicative potential. Stem cells give rise to progenitor cells that can progress through a certain number of doublings, with an increasing degree of differentiation. Fully differentiated cells do not have replicative potential. The number of doublings is controlled by telomeres, the ends of chromosomes that are composed of several thousand repeats of a short 6-bp sequence element.[16] Telomeres prevent end to end chromosomal fusion. However, each DNA replication is associated with a loss of 50 to 100 base pairs of telomeric DNA from the ends of every chromosome. The progressive shortening of telomeres through successive cycles of replication eventually causes them to lose their ability to protect the ends of chromosomal DNA. When the critical length is bridged, the unprotected chromosomal ends participate in end to end chromosomal fusions, yielding a karyotype disarray that almost inevitably results in the death of the affected cell. Telomeric attrition is negated by the enzyme telomerase, which elongates telomeric DNA. Telomerase activity is high during embryonic development and in certain cell populations, such as adult stem cells. However, many tumors are characterized by elevated telomerase activity. Alternatively, telomeres are maintained through recombination-based interchromosomal exchanges of sequence information. Thus, by maintaining a telomere length above a critical threshold, the tumor cells have unlimited proliferative potential and are considered immortal.

Recently, evidence has been obtained for the existence of cancer stem cells or cancer-initiating cells that give rise to tissue-specific progenitor cells and phenotypically diverse cancer cells with limited replicative potential.[17] Unlike mature, terminally differentiated tissue cells, cells with the capacity for self-renewal would live long enough for the stepwise accumulation of genetic mutations over time. Small populations of putative cancer stem cells have now been identified in many of the common cancers based on their ability to replicate, whereas most cancer cells have no or limited ability to proliferate. The most likely origin of cancer stem cells is normal adult stem cells that replace short-lived mature cells in tissues such as skin, gut, and blood. When normal stem cells divide, one of the daughter cells inherits stem cell capabilities, whereas the other cell is launched along the differentiation pathway. In cancer stem cells, the genes regulating self-renewal, such as *Bmi-1*, are overexpressed, thereby suppressing the default pathway of differentiation.

## Sustained Angiogenesis

Based on the observation that many individuals who died of non–cancer-related causes had in situ tumors at the time of autopsy, physicians and scientists have concluded these microscopic tumors are in a dormant state. Tumor dormancy occurs because the body blocks the tumor from recruiting its own blood supply to provide tumor cells with the required oxygen and nutrients. The growth of new blood vessels, angiogenesis, is a highly regulated process to ensure supply to all cells in an organ. Surprisingly, the microscopic tumors lack the ability to induce angiogenesis, and only an estimated 1 in 600 acquire angiogenic activity. Research pioneered by Judah Folkman has demonstrated that naturally occurring endogenous angiogenesis inhibitors prevent tumors from expanding.[18] The angiogenesis inhibitors keep the tumors in check by counterbalancing the angiogenic signals. These signals are mediated by soluble factors and their receptors on endothelial cells, as well as integrins and adhesion molecules mediating cell-matrix and cell-cell interactions. Angiogenic activity is induced by growth factors such as vascular endothelial growth factor (VEGF), basic and acidic fibroblast growth factor (FGF), and platelet-derived growth factor. Each binds to transmembrane tyrosine kinase receptors displayed primarily by endothelial cells connected to intracellular signaling pathways. Angiogenesis inhibitors are associated with specific tissues or circulate in the blood. The first inhibitor, interferon-$\alpha$ (IFN-$\alpha$), was reported in 1980, and an additional 26 endogenous inhibitors have been identified since then. These include thrombospondin, tumstatin, canstatin, endostatin, and angiostatin.

Evidence for the importance of inducing and sustaining angiogenesis in tumors is overwhelming. For example, the switch of dormant human tumors into fast-growing tumors in immunocompromised mice is associated with an angiogenesis gene signature. Most telling are the results of clinical studies with the anti-VEGF antibody, bevacizumab (Avastin), the first angiogenesis inhibitor approved by the U.S. Food and Drug Administration (FDA) for the treatment of colon cancer. Bevacizumab significantly prolongs the survival of patients with advanced cancer. Similarly, a dominant-interfering version of the VEGF receptor 2 has been shown to impair neovascularization and growth of subcutaneous tumors in mice.

The ability to induce and sustain angiogenesis seems to be acquired in a discrete step (or steps) during tumor development via a switch to the angiogenic phenotype.[18,19] Tumors appear to activate the angiogenic switch by changing the balance between total angiogenic stimulation and total angiogenic inhibition.[20] This usually occurs when the angiogenesis stimulators overwhelm the angiogenesis inhibitors. In some tumors, these changes may be linked. It is likely that such disruption in the angiogenic balance is under control of the genetic makeup of the individual tumor cell and its microenvironment. Angiogenesis inducers and inhibitors may be genetically controlled by tumor suppressor genes such as *p53,* whereas oncogenes such as *ras* may downregulate transcription of endogenous inhibitors or activate inducers. For example, bcl2 activation leads to significantly increased expression of VEGF and angiogenesis. Another dimension of regulation is through proteases, which can control the bioavailability of angiogenic activators and inhibitors. Thus, a variety of proteases can release bFGF stored in the ECM, whereas plasmin, a proangiogenic component of the clotting system, can cleave itself into an angiogenesis inhibitor form called angiostatin. Another angiogenesis inhibitor, endostatin, is an internal fragment of the basement membrane collagen XVIII. Finally, hypoxia and other metabolic stressors, mechanical stress from proliferating cells, or inflammatory immune responses can trigger angiogenesis. The coordinated expression of proangiogenic and antiangiogenic signaling molecules and their modulation by proteolysis appear to reflect the complex homeostatic regulation of normal tissue angiogenesis and vascular integrity. Different types of tumors use distinct molecular strategies to activate the angiogenic switch.

Key in the formation of new blood vessels are endothelial cells via the production or expression of angiogenesis-promoting factors. These factors include proinflammatory cytokines such as IL-6, VEGF, and hematopoietic growth factors such as colony-stimulating factors that recruit and activate bone marrow–derived progenitor cells. Among the progenitor cells are myeloid precursors that further promote the proinflammatory responses at the tumor and actively contribute to angiogenesis by producing matrix metalloprotease-9 (MMP-9), a critical regulator of tumor angiogenesis through the induced release of VEGF. Bone marrow–derived endothelial precursors foster tumor blood vessel assembly.

### Tissue Invasion and Metastasis

Progressing tumors give rise to distant metastases that are the cause of 90% of human cancer deaths. The formation of tumor metastases is characterized by the detachment of some tumor cells from the primary tumor and infiltration into the bloodstream or lymphatics (intravasation). The reciprocal process occurs at other locations in the body (extravasation). Both intravasation and extravasation are characterized by changes in ECMs and their interactions with tumor cells. The cell-cell and cell-matrix interactions are mediated through cell adhesion molecules (CAMs), primarily by members of the immunoglobulin and calcium-dependent cadherin families,[21] hyaluronan receptor CD44, selectins, and integrins,[22] which link cells to ECM substrates. Studies have shown that the molecules mediating adhesion are also capable of signal transduction. As such, changes in expression of adhesion molecules will alter signaling pathways and, conversely, signaling molecules can directly affect the function of adhesion molecules in tumor cells.

Epithelial (E)-cadherin is the prototype cadherin responsible for cell polarity and organization of epithelium. E-cadherin function is lost in most epithelial tumors during progression to tumor malignancy, and may in fact be a prerequisite for tumor cell invasion and metastasis formation. In normal cells, extracellular domains of E-cadherin on opposing cells couple and form cell-cell junctions (Fig. 30-8). The cytoplasmic cell-adhesion complex is linked to the actin cytoskeleton through catenins ($\alpha$, $\beta$, $\gamma$). Mechanisms that include mutational inactivation of the E-cadherin or $\beta$-catenin genes, transcriptional repression, or proteases of the extracellular cadherin domain induce loss of E-cadherin function.[21] This prevents catenins from binding and leads to their accumulation in the cytoplasm. Inactivation of nonsequestered $\beta$- and $\gamma$-catenin is dependent on the presence of the tumor suppressor gene *APC* and an inactive Wnt signaling pathway (Fig. 30-8). However, when *APC* function is lost, as is the case in many colon cancers or in case of Wnt activation, $\beta$-catenin is not degraded but instead translocates to the nucleus; here transcription is activated of genes involved in cell proliferation and tumor progression, such as *c-myc, cyclin D1, CD44,* and others.

Changes in expression of CAMs in the immunoglobulin superfamily also appear to play critical roles in the processes of invasion and metastasis.[2,21] Neuronal (N)-CAM, for example, undergoes a switch in expression from a highly adhesive isoform to poorly adhesive (or even repulsive) forms in Wilms' tumor, neuroblastoma, and small cell lung cancer. In invasive pancreatic cancer and colorectal cancers, the overall expression of N-CAM is reduced.

Selectins are a family of transmembrane molecules consisting of E-, L- (leukocyte), and P (platelet)-selectin, that normally mediate blood cell–endothelial cell interactions. However, alterations in the expression level of selectins and/or their ligands, such as the E- and L-selectin ligand, CD44, have been associated with increased invasiveness and poor survival in several malignancies (e.g., breast cancer, colorectal cancer).

Changes in integrin expression are also evident in invasive and metastatic cells. For invading and metastasizing cells to be successful, they need to adapt to changing tissue microenvironments. This is accomplished through shifts in the spectrum of integrin $\alpha$ and $\beta$ subunits displayed on the cell surface by the migrating cells. The large extracellular domain of integrins can bind to ECM molecules such as collagens, laminin, and fibronectin, ligands associated with vascular and coagulation physiology, such as thrombospondin and factor X, or with other CAMs. Each integrin molecule consists of an $\alpha$ subunit and $\beta$ subunit, but a particular $\beta$ subunit can dimerize with several different $\alpha$ subunits. These novel permutations result in different integrin subtypes—24 combinations have now been described—having distinct substrate preferences. Also, integrins may exhibit different specificities when expressed on different cell types. Thus

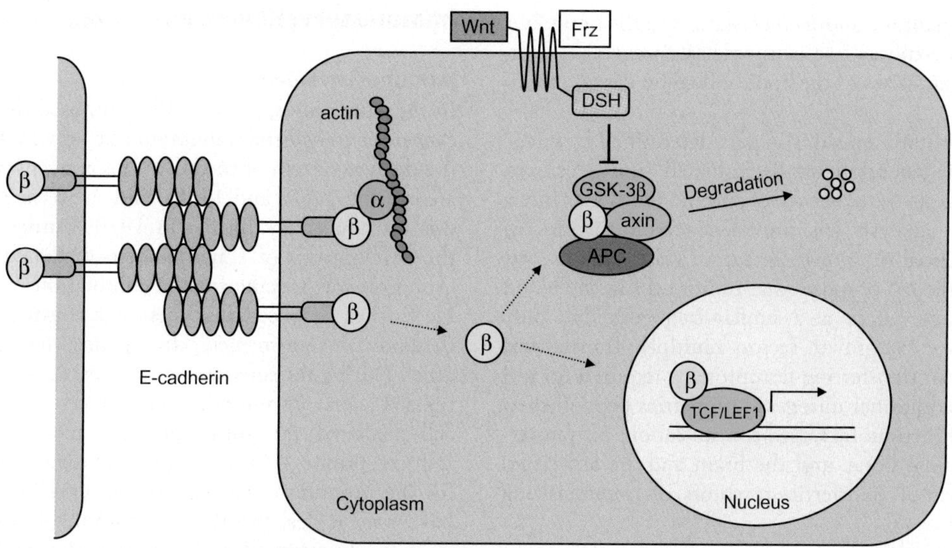


**FIGURE 30-8** Loss of E-cadherin permits tumor progression. Functional loss of E-cadherin to sequester β-catenin leads to the accumulation of β-catenin in the cytoplasm. Similarly, Wnt signaling inactivates GSK-3β, which leads to the stabilization of β-catenin instead of its degradation. Also, loss of APC function may result in the accumulation of β-catenin in the cytoplasm. This leads to the translocation of β-catenin to the nucleus, where it binds the T cell–specific transcription factor/lymphoid enhancer factor-1 (TCF/LEF-1), inducing a genetic program that leads to tumor progression. *α,* α-Catenin; *APC,* adenomatous polyposis coli; *β,* β-catenin; *Frz,* frizzled (transmembrane receptor for Wnt growth factors); *DSH,* disheveled; *GSK-3β,* glycogen synthase kinase 3β.

carcinoma cells facilitate invasion by shifting their expression of integrins from those that favor ECM present in normal epithelium to other integrins that preferentially bind the degraded stromal components produced by extracellular proteases.[2] For example, expression of $\alpha_4\beta_1$, which binds fibronectin, correlates with the progression of melanoma. The changes are incompletely understood because of the large number of distinct integrin genes, by the even larger number of heterodimeric receptors resulting from combinatorial expression of various α and β receptor subunits, and by increasing evidence of complex signals emitted by the cytoplasmic domains of these receptors. Changes in integrin expression may also be essential for the expansion of the tumor stem cell compartment by inhibiting differentiation or apoptosis.[23]

The second general parameter of the invasive and metastatic capability involves extracellular proteases that regulate ECM turnover. It has become clear that tumor progression may involve an increased expression of proteases, decreased expression of protease inhibitors, and inactive zymogen forms of proteases that are converted into active enzymes. Expression of the protease tenascin, which neutralizes adhesion to fibronectin, is increased 10-fold in invasive breast carcinoma compared with normal breast tissue. MMPs are overexpressed in melanoma, invasive breast carcinoma, and invasive squamous cell carcinoma. Matrix-degrading proteases are characteristically associated with the cell surface by synthesis with a transmembrane domain, binding to specific protease receptors, or association with integrins. It is possible that docking of active proteases on the cell surface can facilitate invasion by cancer cells into nearby stroma, across blood vessel walls, and through normal epithelium cell layers. Nevertheless, it is difficult to ascribe unambiguously the functions of particular proteases solely to this capability, given their evident roles in other hallmark capabilities, including angiogenesis and growth signaling, which in turn contribute directly or indirectly to their invasive or metastatic capability. A further complexity derives from the many cell types involved in protease expression and display, including stromal and inflammatory cells.

The activation of extracellular proteases and altered binding specificities of cadherins, CAMs, selectins, and integrins are clearly central to the acquisition of invasiveness and metastatic potential. The clonal and genetic diversity of tumors permits adhesion and detachment from the same matrix. Some tumor cells in a primary tumor may have the correct genotype and phenotype to permit detachment from the surrounding tissue and entry into blood vessels or lymphatic vessels. Similarly, extravasation may be mediated by a few tumor cells that express the required receptors for certain ECM molecules. In general, those mutations that confer escape from homeostatic control mechanisms in the host or that give the tumor cell a growth advantage over others are favorably selected. Thus, tumor clones that best complement the environment with the expression of particular ECM receptors may thrive because this provides an advantage over other clones. However, the regulatory pathways and molecular mechanisms that govern these changes are incompletely understood, and appear to differ from one tissue environment to another.

## Outgrowth at Preferred Sites

Invasion and metastatic spread of tumor cells do not appear to be random processes. In 1889, Paget observed that breast carcinoma often metastasized to the liver, lungs, bone, adrenals, or brain. He hypothesized that tumor cells (the seed) would grow only in selective environments (the soil), in which conditions supported tumor growth—hence, the so-called seed-and-soil hypothesis. Since then, additional studies have confirmed this.

For example, malignant melanoma metastasizes to the brain, but ocular malignant melanoma frequently metastasizes to the liver. Prostate cancer metastasizes to the bone and colon carcinoma to the liver.

Although metastatic spread is in part determined by circulation patterns, the retention of disseminated tumor cells in distant organs suggests the existence of specific molecular interactions. Molecular analysis has provided several theories to explain the preferential outgrowth of tumor cells. One theory, the growth factor theory, proposes that tumor cells in the blood or lymphatics invade organs at a similar frequency, but only those that find favorable growth factors multiply. Transferrins, for example, are iron-transferring ferroproteins required for cell growth that have additional mitogenic properties beyond their iron-transporting function. Increased concentrations of transferrin are found in lung, bone, and the brain and are associated with elevated levels of transferrin receptors on metastasizing tumor cells.

Another theory, the adhesion theory, proposes that endothelial cells lining the blood vessels in certain organs express adhesion molecules that bind tumor cells and permit extravasation. A third theory is that chemokines secreted by the target organ can enter the circulation and selectively attract tumor cells that express receptors for the chemokines. Evidence for the importance of chemokines in tumor progression has been obtained for breast cancer cells preferentially metastasizing in bone marrow, liver, lymph nodes, and lung.[24] These organs were found to secrete CXCL12, which is the ligand for the chemokine receptor, CXCR4, enriched on breast cancer cells compared with normal breast epithelial cells. A similar phenomenon was observed for melanoma cells that were found to express elevated levels of the receptors CXCR4, CCR7, and CCR10 compared with normal melanocytes. Lymph nodes, lung, liver, bone marrow, and skin express the highest levels of the ligands for these receptors and are the preferred sites for metastatic spread of melanomas. Because chemokines are now known to affect angiogenesis and expression of cytokines, adhesion molecules, and proteases, in addition to inducing migration, it appears that chemokines and their receptors play an essential role in the successful outgrowth of tumors at preferential sites.

Detailed analyses of primary tumors have indicated that gene functions mediating metastatic activities are present early in the disease. These functions result from genetic or epigenetic alterations. The genes can be grouped into classes such as metastasis-initiating genes, which control invasion, angiogenesis, circulation, and bone marrow mobilization. Similarly, metastasis progression genes control extravasation, survival, and reinitiation, whereas metastasis virulence genes regulate organ-specific colonization. These intrinsic properties of the tumor, together with its cellular origin, determine the organ specificity and temporal course of metastasis formation.

Central to the mechanisms dictating metastatic predisposition are bone marrow–derived progenitor cells expressing the VEGF receptor 1 (VEGFR1) and VLA-4, which are prompted by the primary tumor to establish premetastatic niches before arrival of metastatic tumor cells.[25] Tumor-secreted humoral factors induce fibronectin (a VLA-4 ligand) expression on fibroblasts and fibroblast-like cells in specific distant organs. Simultaneously, the VEGFR1$^+$, VLA-4$^+$ cells leave the bone marrow and migrate to the premetastatic niche, where they form cellular clusters that permit the development of metastases.

## Immunosurveillance and Immunoediting

### Immunosurveillance

In the early 1900s, Paul Ehrlich proposed that the frequency of cancerous transformations would be very high if it were not for the defense system of the host. This concept was later substantiated in the 1950s and 1960s, and the term *immunosurveillance* was introduced by Burnet in 1970. Burnet hypothesized that the development of T lymphocyte–mediated immunity during evolution was specific for the elimination of transformed cells. He further proposed that there is a continuous surveillance of the body for transformed cells—hence, the term *immunosurveillance*. During the subsequent years, experiments in immunosuppressed and immunodeficient mice demonstrated that T cell–mediated immunity provides protection against virally induced tumors. However, no conclusive evidence was obtained for the immunosurveillance of cancer. More recent discoveries have made it clear that the earlier studies were performed in mice erroneously assumed to be immunodeficient. When tested in truly immunoincompetent mice, evidence for immune surveillance of cancer was obtained; immunodeficient mice were significantly more susceptible to the formation of chemically induced tumors and spontaneous tumors than immunocompetent mice.[1] This suggests that the unmanipulated immune system is capable of recognizing and eliminating primary tumors.

Does immunosurveillance of cancer exist in humans? Evaluation of long-term studies in transplant patients who were immunosuppressed and patients with immunodeficiencies has shown an increased incidence of virally induced tumors, such as non-Hodgkin's lymphoma, Kaposi's sarcoma, and carcinomas of the genitourinary and anogenital regions. However, they also showed a higher incidence of tumors with no apparent viral cause, such as malignant melanoma, lung cancer, pancreatic cancer, colon cancer, and kidney cancer. More conclusive were observations from patients with paraneoplastic neurologic degenerations (PNDs).[26] These patients develop autoimmune neurologic disease in discrete regions of the nervous system, mediated through antibodies and cytotoxic T cells against neuronal antigens. Clinical examination reveals systemic malignancies, usually breast or ovarian adenocarcinoma or small cell lung cancer that are generally small, show limited spread, and are sensitive to treatment. Importantly, the presence of antineuronal T cells and antibodies in all PND patients studied is associated with clinical and pathologic evidence of suppression of tumor growth. Some cancer patients mount a PND immune response but do not develop neurologic disease. These patients have smaller tumors and longer survival than those without such immune responses. Finally, extensive studies on immune infiltrate in primary human cancers have established that the presence of memory T cells, particularly of the T helper 1 subtype, and cytotoxic T cells are prognostic factors for disease-free and overall survival at all stages of clinical disease.[27] The data from mouse and human studies combined suggest that immunosurveillance of cancer does exist, mediated through immune cells and soluble factors. Although the immune system may eliminate most transformed cells, some cells manage to escape and may develop into tumors.

### Immunoediting

The continuous pressure of the immune system in an immunocompetent host determines to a great degree if and how tumors

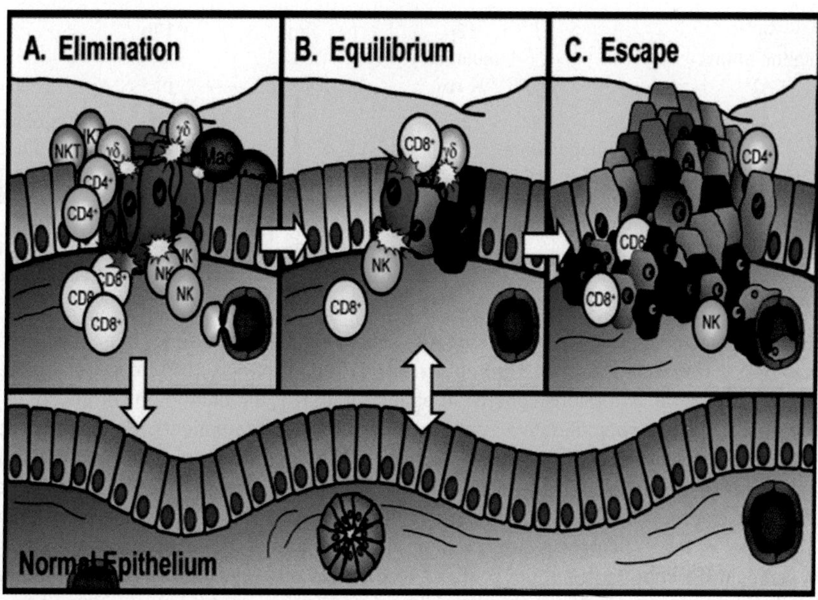


**FIGURE 30-9** Schematic overview of immunoediting. When developing tumors disrupt local tissue structures, proinflammatory cytokines are released and, together with secreted chemokines, attract innate immune cells, such as macrophages, NK cells, NKT cells, and γδ cells. Innate immune cells can recognize and lyse tumor cells directly, but can also induce an adaptive immune response mediated by T and B lymphocytes. Although most tumor cells are eliminated (elimination phase, A), tumor cell variants may survive and expand. However, the activated immune system keeps the tumor in check by eliminating those tumor cells that are sufficiently immunogenic (equilibrium phase, B). The immunologic pressure may cause selection toward tumor cell variants with reduced immunogenicity that are capable of escaping from immune recognition (escape phase, C). These variants can expand in an immunologically intact environment. (From Dunn GP, Old LJ, Schreiber RD: The three Es of cancer immunoediting. Annu Rev Immunol 22:329–360, 2004.)

evolve, a process termed *immunoediting* (Fig. 30-9).[1] In this process, the immune system plays a dual role in the interactions between the tumor and host. On one hand, the immune system effectively eliminates highly immunogenic tumor cells. At the same time, however, the immune system fails to eliminate tumor cells with reduced immunogenicity, thereby selecting for tumor variants that have acquired immune evasion mechanisms. Over time, this selection leads to the outgrowth of tumor cells that fail to induce an effective immune response. As such, the interactions between an intact immune system and tumor cells evolve through three phases—the elimination phase, equilibrium phase, and escape phase. The recognition and elimination of transformed cells is a concerted effort between innate and adaptive immunity, representing the two arms of the immune system. Local disruption of tissue that occurs as a result of expansion of transformed cells is associated with the release of chemokines and proinflammatory cytokines such as IFNs, IL-1, IL-6, and tumor necrosis factor-α (TNF-α) that trigger innate immunity.

The innate immune system represents the first line of defense against transformed cells (and microorganisms). The most important outcome of these initial events is the production of IFN-γ by activated innate immune cells. IFN-γ has direct antitumor effects and further boosts tumor cell lysis by innate immune cells. The resulting availability of tumor antigen triggers an adaptive immune response. Key in this process is the uptake of tumor antigen by antigen-presenting cells, primarily dendritic cells. The dendritic cells migrate to tumor-draining lymph nodes and stimulate T and B lymphocytes. The development of adaptive immunity represents the second line of defense against tumors and, together with innate immunity, could completely eliminate the tumor. However, this does not always occur, and may lead to what is referred to as the equilibrium phase. This phase is characterized by a balance between tumor growth and tumor elimination, as the name suggests. Antitumor immunity leads to destruction of immunogenic tumor cells, whereas tumor cells with reduced immunity go unnoticed.

Over time, genetic instability and heterogeneity of the tumor cells may give rise to tumor variants better able to withstand the immunologic pressure. Contributing to the failure of the immune system are tumor-induced immune suppressor mechanisms. Once this point has been reached, referred to as the escape phase, the immune system can no longer contain the tumor, and the tumor grows progressively. In the last 15 years, a number of mechanisms have been identified through which tumors escape from elimination by the immune system. These mechanisms include host-related factors, tumor-related factors, and a combination of both. Among host-related factors are treatment-related immunosuppression, acquired or inherited immunodeficiency, and aging. The list of tumor-related escape mechanisms includes loss of major histocompatibility complex (MHC) alleles, reduced antigen processing and/or presentation, decreased expression of costimulatory molecules required for T cell recognition, secretion of immunosuppressive factors (TGF-β, IL-10), stimulation of suppressor cells, and mechanisms that actively induce tolerance or apoptosis in activated immune cells.

## CARCINOGENESIS

### Cancer Genetics

As stated at the beginning of this chapter, malignant transformation is the process whereby a clonal population of cells acquires

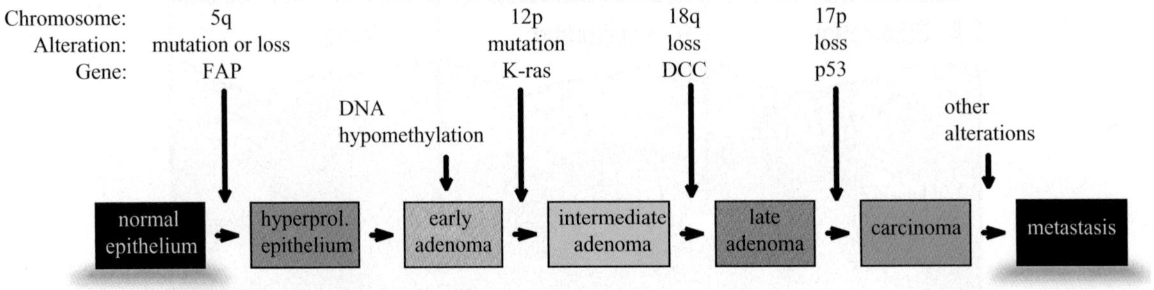

Chromosome: 5q | 12p | 18q | 17p
Alteration: mutation or loss | mutation | loss | loss
Gene: FAP | K-ras | DCC | p53
DNA hypomethylation
other alterations
normal epithelium → hyperprol. epithelium → early adenoma → intermediate adenoma → late adenoma → carcinoma → metastasis

**FIGURE 30-10** Genetic model for colorectal tumorigenesis. Tumorigenesis proceeds through a series of genetic alterations involving oncogenes *(ras)* and tumor suppressor genes (particularly those on chromosomes 5q, 12p, 17p, and 18q). In general, the three stages of adenomas represent tumors of increasing size, dysplasia, and villous content. In patients with FAP, a mutation on chromosome 5q (*APC* gene) is inherited. This alteration may be responsible for the hypoproliferative epithelium present in these patients. Hypomethylation is present in very small adenomas in patients with or without polyposis, and this alteration may lead to aneuploidy, resulting in the loss of suppressor gene alleles. The *ras* gene mutation appears to occur in one cell of a preexisting small adenoma and, through clonal expansion, produces a larger and more dysplastic tumor. Allelic deletions of chromosome 17p and 18q usually occur at a later stage of tumorigenesis than deletions of chromosome 5q or *ras* gene mutations. The order of these changes is not invariant, however, and accumulation of these changes, rather than their order with respect to one another, seems most important. Tumors continue to progress once carcinomas have formed and the accumulated loss of suppressor genes on additional chromosomes correlates with the ability of the carcinomas to metastasize and cause death. (From Fearon ER: A genetic model for colorectal tumorigenesis. Cell 61:759–767, 1990.)

alterations that confer a growth advantage over normal cells. Many of these alterations occur at the genetic level, involving the gain of function by oncogenes or the loss of function by tumor suppressor genes. A multistep model for colorectal tumorigenesis has been described (Fig. 30-10). Designation as an oncogene or tumor suppressor gene relates to the directionality of effect, without implications about molecular detail. The original name for what came to be known as tumor suppressor genes was, in fact, antioncogenes.

Genetic mutations inherited from one's parents and present in all cells of the body are called germline (or constitutional) mutations; in contrast, somatic mutations are acquired during an individual's lifetime and cannot be passed on to one's children. Somatic mutations, which account for most mutations in cancer, may be caused by exposure to carcinogens in the form of radiation, chemicals, or chronic inflammation (see later).

A tumor that arises in an individual may be classified as hereditary or sporadic. In hereditary cases, a germline mutation is responsible for the predisposition to neoplasia. The index case, or proband, is the individual who is first diagnosed as having the syndrome, even if earlier generations are later recognized as also having the syndrome. If the patient with a tumor does not have an inherited predisposition, and the tumor's genetic mutations are all somatic, the tumor is classified as sporadic. In some hereditary cancer syndromes, the germline mutation causes a tendency for the cell to accumulate somatic mutations.

Although hereditary cancer syndromes are rare, their study has provided powerful insights into more common forms of cancer (Table 30-4). Key germline mutations in hereditary cancers are often the same as somatic mutations present in sporadic cancers. *p53* is the most commonly mutated gene in human cancer and, if inherited in a mutant form, causes Li-Fraumeni syndrome. Familial adenomatous polyposis (FAP) is caused by a germline mutation in the adenomatous polyposis gene *(APC)* gene. More than 80% of sporadic colorectal cancers also have a somatic mutation of this same gene. Similarly, a mutation in the RET proto-oncogene is responsible for the predisposition to develop the familial form of medullary thyroid cancer (MTC). Somatic mutations of *RET* are found in approximately 50% of sporadic MTCs.

Predisposition in familial cancer syndromes is generally inherited in an autosomal dominant fashion. Exceptions include ataxia-telangiectasia and xeroderma pigmentosa, which are transmitted in an autosomal recessive manner. Not all inherited genetic mutations have complete penetrance. There is almost complete penetrance of colorectal cancer in FAP and of medullary thyroid cancer in multiple endocrine neoplasia type 2 (MEN2). In contrast, penetrance is less than 50% for pheochromocytoma in neurofibromatosis. Penetrance can also vary considerably for different characteristics of the same syndrome. However, the factors determining penetrance remain largely unknown.

There are a number of features of hereditary cancers that distinguish them phenotypically from their sporadic counterparts. The former tend to cause the development of multifocal bilateral cancer at an early age, whereas in the latter, cancer occurs later and is usually unilateral. Hereditary cancers will display clustering of the same cancer type in relatives and may be associated with other conditions, such as mental retardation and pathognomonic skin lesions.

## Familial Cancer Syndromes

### Retinoblastoma

Retinoblastoma is a pediatric retinal tumor that holds an important place in the history of cancer genetics because the causative gene, *RB1*, was the first tumor suppressor gene to be cloned. Most cases are detected by age 7 years, but bilateral disease presents earlier, usually within the first year of life. It is associated with extraocular malignancies, including sarcomas, melanomas, and central nervous system tumors. Distinct sporadic and hereditary forms of retinoblastoma have long been recognized, with predisposition conferred by a germline mutation in approximately 40% of cases. Knudson reasoned that the germline

**Table 30-4 Familial Cancer Syndromes**

| SYNDROME | GENES | LOCATIONS | CANCER SITES AND ASSOCIATED TRAITS |
|---|---|---|---|
| Breast, ovarian syndrome | *BRCA1*<br>*BRCA2* | 17q21<br>13q12.3 | Cancers of the breast, ovary, colon, prostate<br>Cancers of the breast, ovary, colon, prostate, gallbladder and biliary tree, pancreas, stomach; melanoma |
| Cowden disease | *PTEN* | 10q23.3 | Cancer of the breast, endometrium, and thyroid |
| Familial adenomatous polyposis (FAP) | *APC* | 17q21 | Colorectal carcinoma, duodenal and gastric neoplasms, medulloblastomas, osteomas |
| Familial melanoma | *p16; CDK4* | 9p21; 12q14 | Melanoma, pancreatic cancer, dysplastic nevi, atypical moles |
| Hereditary diffuse gastric cancer | *CDH1* | 16q22 | Gastric cancer |
| Hereditary nonpolyposis colorectal cancer | *hMLH1; hMSH2; hMSH6; hPMS1; hPMS2* | 3p21; 2p22-21; 2p16; 2q31.1; 7p22.2 | Colorectal cancer, endometrial cancer, transitional cell carcinoma of the ureter and renal pelvis, carcinomas of the stomach, small bowel, pancreas, and ovary |
| Hereditary papillary renal cell carcinoma | *MET* | 7q31 | Renal cell cancer |
| Hereditary paraganglioma and pheochromocytoma | *SDHB; SDHC; SDHD* | 1p36.1-p35; 1q21; 11q23 | Paraganglioma, pheochromocytoma |
| Juvenile polyposis coli | *BMPRIA*<br>*SMAD4/DPC4* | 10q21-q22<br>18q21.1 | Juvenile polyps of the gastrointestinal tract, gastrointestinal malignancies |
| Li-Fraumeni syndrome | *p53*<br>*hCHK2* | 17p13<br>22q12.1 | Breast cancer, soft tissue sarcoma, osteosarcoma, brain tumors, adrenocortical carcinoma, Wilms' tumor, phyllodes tumor (breast), pancreatic cancer, leukemia, neuroblastoma |
| Multiple endocrine neoplasia type 1 (MEN1) | *MEN1* | 11q13 | Pancreatic islet cell tumors, parathyroid hyperplasia, pituitary adenomas |
| Multiple endocrine neoplasia type 2 (MEN2) | *RET* | 10q11.2 | Medullary thyroid cancer, pheochromocytoma, parathyroid hyperplasia |
| MYH-associated adenomatous polyposis | *MYH* | 1p34.3-p32.1 | Cancer of the colon, rectum, breast, stomach |
| Neurofibromatosis type 1 | *NF1* | 17q11 | Neurofibromas, neurofibrosarcoma, acute myelogenous leukemia, brain tumors |
| Neurofibromatosis type 2 | *NF2* | 22q12 | Acoustic neuromas, meningiomas, gliomas, ependymomas |
| Nevoid basal cell carcinoma | *PTC* | 9q22.3 | Basal cell carcinoma |
| Peutz-Jeghers syndrome | *STK11* | 19p13.3 | Gastrointestinal carcinomas, breast cancer, testicular cancer, pancreatic cancer, benign pigmentation of the skin and mucosa |
| Retinoblastoma | *RB* | 13q14 | Retinoblastoma, sarcomas, melanoma, malignant neoplasms of the brain and meninges |
| Tuberous sclerosis | *TSC1; TSC2* | 9q34; 16p13 | Multiple hamartomas, renal cell carcinoma, astrocytoma |
| von Hippel-Lindau syndrome | *VHL* | 3p25 | Renal cell carcinoma, hemangioblastomas of the retina and central nervous system, pheochromocytoma |
| Wilms' tumor | *WT* | 11p13 | Wilms' tumor, aniridia, genitourinary abnormalities, mental retardation |

From Marsh D, Zori R: Genetic insights into familial cancers—update and recent discoveries. Cancer Lett 181:125–164, 2002.

mutation is necessary but not by itself sufficient for tumorigenesis, because some children with an affected parent do not develop a tumor, but later produce an affected child, indicating that they are carriers of the germline mutation. Most affected children with an affected parent develop tumors bilaterally. It was further hypothesized that hereditary retinoblastoma requires two mutations, one of which is germline and the other somatic. In children with unilateral disease and no family history, both mutations are somatic. The hereditary and nonhereditary forms of the tumor require the same number of events, the two-hit hypothesis (Fig. 30-11). The RB1 protein product is a key regulator of the cell cycle and its loss results in failure of retinoblasts to differentiate properly.

### Li-Fraumeni Syndrome

In 1969, Li and Fraumeni reported a new familial syndrome involving sarcomas of soft tissue and bone, breast cancers (the most common malignancy in this syndrome), brain tumors, leukemias, adrenocortical carcinomas, and other cancers. The syndrome that now bears their name has been defined as (1) a proband diagnosed with sarcoma before the age of 45 years, with (2) a first-degree relative with any cancer diagnosed before the age of 45 years, plus (3) an additional first- or second-degree relative with a sarcoma at any age or with any cancer in someone younger than 45 years. Half of Li-Fraumeni kindreds have mutations in the *TP53* gene, which produces the protein p53. Inheritance is in an autosomal dominant fashion. Penetrance is 50%

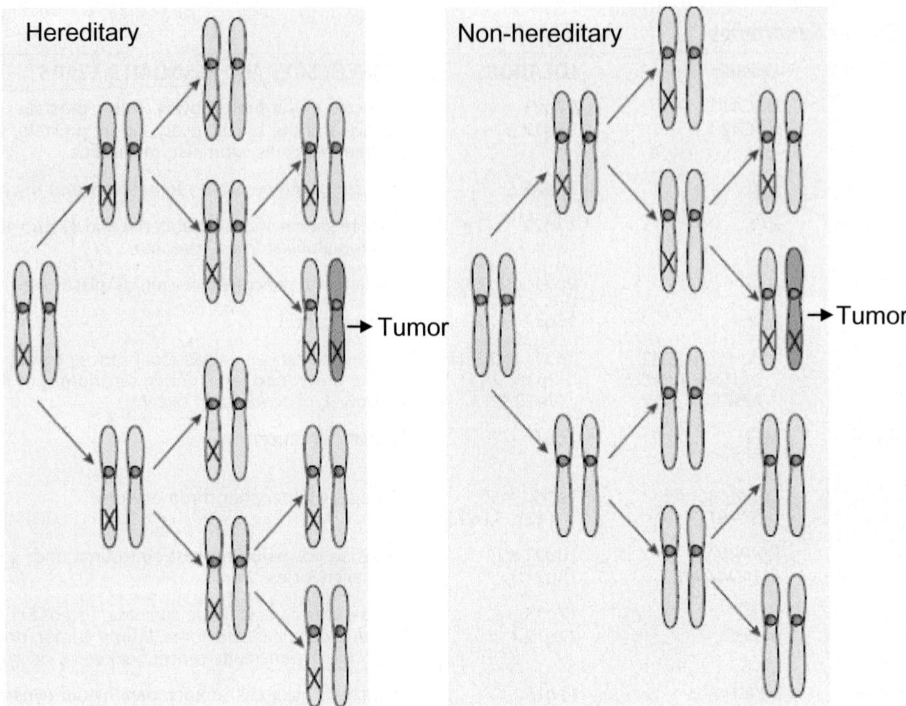


**FIGURE 30-11** Two genetic hits to cancer. In hereditary retinoblastoma, all retinoblasts are heterozygous for the mutant allele (X); they all have already sustained one hit. In contrast, the preneoplastic clone in nonhereditary retinoblastoma must acquire this mutation before sustaining the second hit to complete malignant transformation. (Adapted from Knudson AG: Two genetic hits [more or less] to cancer. Nat Rev Cancer 1:157–162, 2001.)

by age 40 and 90% by age 60. Patients exhibit increased sensitivity to radiation; the irradiated field is susceptible to the development of new malignancies. For kindreds that lack germline *TP53* mutations, a number of candidate genes have been proposed, including the cell cycle checkpoint kinases *CHK1* and *CHK2,* which phosphorylate p53 directly. It is likely that other such causative genes serve similar tumor suppressive functions to p53 or are involved in the regulation of p53.

### Familial Adenomatous Polyposis

FAP accounts for 1% of the total colorectal cancer burden. It is an autosomal dominant condition caused by mutation in the *APC* gene, located on chromosome 5q21. Penetrance is extremely high, with more than 90% of affected individuals developing colorectal cancer. It is characterized clinically by the development of 300 or 400 to more than 1000 adenomatous polyps that carpet the colon. The first clear FAP kindreds were described in 1925 by the surgeon Lockhart-Mummery. The phenotype usually emerges during the second and third decades of life. The polyps are macroscopically and microscopically indistinguishable from sporadic adenomatous polyps; each individual polyp does not have a greater propensity to undergo malignant degeneration than a sporadic polyp. Rather, it is the sheer number of polyps that makes the collective risk of malignancy so high. Untreated individuals typically present with colorectal cancer at 35 to 40 years of age, approximately 30 years earlier than the median age for sporadic colorectal cancer. Extracolonic manifestations of FAP include upper gastrointestinal polyps, desmoid tumors (15%), and thyroid cancer (1% to 2%; usually papillary). Polyps of the stomach and duodenum are present in more than 90% of patients by age 70, with two thirds of duodenal polyps located in the periampullary region. Duodenal adenocarcinoma is the third leading cause of death in FAP, after metastatic colorectal carcinoma and desmoid tumors. Desmoid tumors are locally invasive fibromatoses that occur within the abdomen or abdominal wall. Patients with FAP have a relative risk of developing desmoid disease 850 times greater than that of the general population.

The *APC* gene was first localized in 1987 and cloned in 1991, after mutation analyses of FAP kindreds. It encodes a 300-kDa protein, expressed in various cell types, whose major function is as a scaffolding protein, affecting cell adhesion and migration. It is part of a protein complex, modulated by the Wnt signaling pathway, which regulates the phosphorylation and degradation of β-catenin. When *APC* is mutated, β-catenin is not phosphorylated and accumulates in the cytoplasm, where it binds to the Tcf family of transcription factors, altering the expression of various genes involved in cell proliferation, migration, differentiation, and apoptosis. More than 700 disease-causing mutations in the *APC* gene have been reported. The most common of these involve a frameshift mutation (68%), nonsense mutation (30%) or large deletion (2%). Most of these mutations are located in what is referred to as the *mutation cluster region*, at the 5′ end of exon 15.

The location of the mutation plays a role in determining the phenotype. Mutations between 976 and 1067 are associated with a threefold to fourfold increased risk of developing duodenal adenomas. Congenital hypertrophy of the retinal pigment epithelium is associated with mutations between codons 463 and 1387. Gardner's syndrome is associated with mutations between codons 1403 and 1578[28] and, in addition to colorectal cancer (CRC), manifests osteomas of the mandible or skull, epidermal cysts, and multiple skin and soft tissue tumors, especially desmoids and thyroid tumors. Attenuated FAP is a phenotypically distinct variant of FAP in which (1) affected individuals have fewer than 100 adenomas, (2) the polyps are more proximally distributed in the colon, and (3) the onset of CRC is about 15 years later than in patients with FAP. Mutations responsible for this variant occur in the extreme upstream or downstream portions of the *APC* gene.

*MYH*-associated polyposis (MAP) is a syndrome caused by mutations in the human MutY homologue (*MYH*) gene. It accounts for about one third of patients who have attenuated polyposis but who test negative for *APC* mutations. Unlike FAP, MAP is inherited in an autosomal recessive manner. Phenotypically, MAP-associated colorectal cancer is indistinguishable from attenuated FAP although it presents later, at about the age of 50 years. The polyps are distributed throughout the colon, although there are conflicting data about right- and left-sided tumor predominance. Extracolonic manifestations include breast cancer (18%) and upper gastrointestinal polyps (one third).[29] The *MYH* gene encodes a DNA glycosylase involved in the base excision repair pathway, important in preventing mutations caused by oxidative damage. *Y165C* and *G382D* mutations account for more than 80% of all mutations discovered thus far. Penetrance is estimated at 50%. Homozygotes or compound heterozygotes for germline mutations of the *MYH* gene have a 93-fold increased risk of colorectal cancer.[30] Mutation leads to chromosomal instability, in which there is an accelerated rate of chromosomal misaggregation during cell division. This leads to aneuploidy, which has been recognized as an early genetic change in the stepwise carcinogenesis of FAP and MAP tumors. Polyps-bearing *MYH* mutations have twice the overall incidence of aneuploidy compared with those in patients with FAP. Evidence suggests that carriers of single mutated alleles are unlikely to have more than a 50% increased risk of colorectal cancer.

### Hereditary Nonpolyposis Colorectal Cancer

Also known as Lynch syndrome, hereditary nonpolyposis colorectal cancer (HNPCC) accounts for 2% of all colorectal cancers. It is an autosomal dominant condition, caused by mutations in DNA mismatch repair genes. When originally described by Lynch, kindreds were subclassified into types I and II based on whether they only developed colorectal cancer (type I) or whether extracolonic cancers were present (type II). Penetrance is high. The broad phenotype of HNPCC is of right-sided predominance of colonic cancers (70% proximal to the splenic flexure) that appear at an earlier age (median age of diagnosis, 45 years), with increased likelihood of synchronous and metachronous cancers. Extracolonic malignancies occur, especially of the endometrium and ovary. Although the actual incidence of adenomatous polyps is the same as for those who develop sporadic colorectal cancer, once a tumor develops, there is an increased rate of tumor progression (accelerated carcinogenesis). This is because the rate of genetic mutation in HNPCC tumors is two to three times higher than in normal cells. A colonic adenoma may progress to carcinoma within 2 to 3 years, in contrast to the 8 to 10 years typical of sporadic cases.

Mutations in DNA mismatch repair genes cause microsatellite instability. Microsatellites are genomic regions in which short DNA sequences are repeated. During replication of these sequences, slippage of the DNA polymerase complex can occur, resulting in the formation of daughter strands that contain too many or too few copies of these sequences. Mutations may occur when these microsatellites are misaligned. The mutations then persist when the DNA mismatch repair proteins fail to correct the errors. This causes inactivation of tumor suppressor genes, such as *TGF-β RII, IGFRII,* and *BAX.* Mutations in a number of DNA mismatch repair genes have been identified in patients with HNPCC. Mutations in *MSH2* and *MLH1* account for about two thirds of cases. *MSH6* mutations account for a further 10% of cases. Other mismatch repair genes in which mutations lead to HNPCC include *PMS1* and *PMS2.* It should be noted that 15% of sporadic colorectal cancers have microsatellite instability, but this occurs through methylation silencing of the *hMLH1* gene, rather than through mutation, as in HNPCC.

### *BRCA1* and *BRCA2*

About 5% to 10% of all breast cancers are hereditary and attributable to mutations in high-penetrance susceptibility genes. However, only two of these have been identified, *BRCA1* and *BRCA2.* In high-risk kindreds, 25% have mutations in either of these genes. Although the estimated risk of breast cancer is 80% for a 70-year-old woman with a germline mutation in *BRCA1* or *BRCA2,* different mutations vary in their risk of malignancy.

Carriers are at risk for other cancers, especially of the ovary. The risk of ovarian cancer in a patient who is a carrier for *BRCA1* or *BRCA2* is 60% and 27%, respectively. Approximately 5% of all ovarian cancers are attributed to *BRCA1* germline mutations. The risk of ovarian cancer for patients with *BRCA2* mutations is lower, approximately 15% to 20%. Male carriers are at greater risk for prostate cancer. *BRCA2* mutation is also associated with an increased risk of melanoma and cancers of the pancreas, stomach, gallbladder, and biliary system.

The *BRCA1* gene is located on the long arm of chromosome 17. It is a large gene of approximately 100,000 nucleic acids and more than 250 different mutations have been reported. The sheer number of mutations makes the task of identifying the specific mutation in a new kindred very difficult. The *BRCA2* gene is an even larger gene then *BRCA1* and about 100 mutations have been reported. As for *BRCA1,* the vast majority of alterations are frameshift or nonsense mutations, which produce a truncated protein. Both *BRCA1* and *BRCA2* are tumor suppressor genes; they are nonfunctional in malignant cells as a result of combined germline mutation followed by inactivation of the second allele in the tumor (the Knudson two-hit hypothesis). These genes have key roles in DNA damage repair, regulation of gene expression, and cell cycle control.

### Multiple Endocrine Neoplasia

**Type 1** MEN1 is an autosomal dominant condition characterized phenotypically by tumors of the parathyroid gland (leading to hyperparathyroidism), pancreatic islet cells, and pituitary gland. Affected individuals can also develop lipomas, adenomas of the adrenal and thyroid glands, cutaneous angiofibromas, and carcinoid tumors.

Mutations in the tumor suppressor gene, called *MEN1,* located on chromosome 11q13, are responsible for this syndrome; 80% of mutations identified result in the loss of function of the gene product, called menin. Menin is a 67-kDa protein predominantly found in the nucleus. It binds with a variety of proteins active in the regulation of transcription, DNA repair, and organization of the cytoskeleton. None of these menin pathways has been found to be critical in *MEN1* tumorigenesis, although a number of candidates, such as JunD, have been proposed.

**Type 2** All affected individuals with MEN 2 develop MTC, subclassified into types A and B. MEN2A is characterized by pheochromocytoma (50%) and hyperparathyroidism (25%). In addition to MTC and pheochromocytoma, MEN2B is characterized by mucosal neuromas on the tongue, lips, and subconjunctival areas, intestinal ganglioneuromatosis and a Marfanoid body habitus. Most cases of MEN 2B are the result of spontaneous, new *RET* mutations.

Both types are caused by germline mutations in the *RET* (***re***arranged during ***t***ransfection) proto-oncogene, located on chromosome 10q11. It encodes a transmembrane tyrosine kinase receptor, which is expressed on a wide variety of neuroendocrine and neural cells, including thyroid C, adrenal medullary, and autonomic ganglion cells. Once mutated, the receptor constitutively activates various signaling pathways, including p38-MAPK and JNK pathways.

### Von Hippel-Lindau Syndrome

Von Hippel-Lindau syndrome is a rare autosomal dominant syndrome characterized by the development of highly vascularized tumors in a number of organs. These include hemangioblastomas of the retina and central nervous system, renal cysts that develop into clear cell renal cell cancer, and pheochromocytomas. It is caused by mutations in the *VHL* gene. Penetrance is 90% by the age of 65 years; the mean age of diagnosis 26 years. Since the discovery of the role of the *VHL* gene in this syndrome, mutations of this same gene have been found in most sporadic clear cell renal cell carcinomas. The loss of *VHL* function is a critical event during renal cell carcinogenesis, as supported by experiments in which the introduction of wild-type *VHL* into *VHL*-deficient renal cancer cell lines resulted in suppression of tumor growth.

The protein product of the *VHL* gene, pVHL, functions as a tumor suppressor and is part of the cell's response mechanism to hypoxia. Under conditions of low cellular oxygen tension, hypoxia inducible factor (HIF)-1 and HIF-2 regulate genes involved in metabolism, angiogenesis, erythropoiesis, and cell proliferation. pVHL targets the $\alpha$ subunit of HIF for oxygen-dependent proteolysis. Therefore, lack of pVHL results in persistence of the HIF complex, with increased HIF transcriptional activity and upregulation of HIF target genes, including *VEGF, GLUT-1,* and the erythropoietin gene *(Epo),* independent of cellular oxygen levels. pVHL also has roles in regulating extracellular matrix turnover and microtubule stability.

## Cancer Epigenetics

Epigenetic inheritance is defined as cellular information, other than the nucleotide sequence, that is heritable during cell division. There are three main interrelated forms—DNA methylation, genomic imprinting, and histone modification. These epigenetic templates control gene expression and can be transmitted to daughter cells independently of the DNA sequence.

One of the best studied types of epigenetic changes is the cytosine methylation at CpG dinucleotides. CpG islands (CGIs) are approximately 1-kb stretches of DNA containing clusters of CpG dinucleotides that are usually unmethylated in normal cells and are often located near the 5′ ends of genes. Methylation of promoter CGIs is associated with a closed chromatin structure and transcriptional silencing of the associated gene. This has been shown to be a common event in carcinogenesis. Tumor-suppressor genes such as *CDKN2A, RB, VHL,* and *BRCA1* are inactivated by hypermethylation of their promoter CGIs.

Conversely, genes that are hypomethylated, leading to increased transcription, have been identified. For example, promoter CpG demethylation has been shown to lead to overexpression of cyclin D2 and maspin in gastric cancer.[31] DNA hypomethylation has also been associated with genomic instability. Loss of methylation is particularly severe in pericentromeric satellite sequences, and cancers of the ovary and breast frequently contain unbalanced chromosomal translocations, with breakpoints in the pericentromeric regions of chromosomes 1 and 16. The demethylation of these satellite sequences may predispose to their breakage and recombination.

Genomic imprinting refers to the conditioning of maternal and paternal genomes during gametogenesis, so that a specific parental allele is more abundantly (or exclusively) expressed in the offspring. In Wilms' tumors, loss of imprinting has been demonstrated to lead to pathologic biallelic expression of *IGF2.* This appears to occur in combination with hypermethylation of regions of the reciprocally imprinted *H19* gene. These two phenomena are the earliest detectable genetic changes in this cancer, strongly suggesting a gatekeeper role for epigenetic alterations in cancer.

CGI methylation is associated with a condensed chromatin structure, which blocks the access of transcription factors to DNA promoter sites, leading to transcriptional silencing. The modification of histones, such as by acetylation, methylation, or phosphorylation, is important in the compaction of chromatin structure. Studies of colorectal cancer have suggested that the combination of DNA hypermethylation, together with histone modifications, play a critical role in the maintenance of gene silencing.[32] This is a new area of research.

## Carcinogens

Any agent that can contribute to tumor formation is referred to as a carcinogen; it can be chemical, physical, or biologic. The International Agency for Research on Cancer (IARC) maintains a registry of human carcinogens available on the Internet (www.iarc.fr). The compounds are categorized into five groups based on epidemiologic studies, animal models, and short-term mutagenesis tests. Group 1 contains what are considered to be proven human carcinogens. Group 2A agents are probable human carcinogens; there is limited evidence of carcinogenicity in humans but sufficient evidence to prove carcinogenicity in experimental animals. The group 2B category includes agents that are possibly carcinogenic to humans, in which there is limited evidence of carcinogenicity in humans and less than sufficient evidence of carcinogenicity in experimental animals. There is inadequate evidence for carcinogenicity in humans or experimental animals for agents included in group 3. Group 4 agents are probably not carcinogenic to humans.

### Chemical Agents

Chemicals that initiate carcinogenesis are extremely diverse in structure and function, and include natural and synthetic products (Tables 30-5 and 30-6). They fall into one of two categories:

**Table 30-5 International Agency for Research on Cancer: Selected Group 1 Chemical Carcinogens**

| CHEMICAL CARCINOGEN | MEANS OF EXPOSURE | PREDOMINANT TUMOR TYPE |
|---|---|---|
| Aflatoxins | Ingestion of contaminated maize and peanuts grown in hot, humid climates | Hepatocellular carcinoma |
| Arsenic | Ingestion; also inhalation by smelter workers | Skin cancer |
| Asbestos | Inhalation | Mesothelioma, lung cancer |
| Benzene | Inhalation, especially in gasoline-related industries or in the production of other chemicals from benzene | Leukemia |
| Benzidine | Inhalation by workers in the dye industry | Cancer of the urinary bladder |
| Beryllium | Inhalation by workers in the refining of the metal and production of beryllium-containing products; also those in the aircraft, aerospace, electronics, and nuclear industries | Lung cancer |
| Cadmium | Inhalation by workers in cadmium production and refining, nickel-cadmium battery manufacturing, other cadmium-related industries | Lung cancer |
| Chromium compounds | Inhalation during chromium plating, chromate production, welding | Lung cancer |
| Ethylene oxide | Inhalation during production of various industrial chemicals (e.g., ethylene glycol) | Leukemia, lymphoma |
| Nickel | Inhalation, ingestion or skin contact in nickel or nickel alloy production plants, welding, or electroplating operations | Lung cancer, nasal cancer |
| Radon | Inhalation in underground mines | Lung cancer |
| Vinyl chloride | Inhalation during production of polyvinyl chloride (PVC) | Hepatic angiosarcoma, HCC, brain tumors, lung cancer, hematopoietic malignancies |
| Coal tars | Inhalation, transcutaneous absorption in a variety of industrial settings | Skin cancer, scrotal cancer |
| Tobacco smoke | Inhalation | Lung cancer, oral cancer, pharyngeal cancer, laryngeal cancer, esophageal cancer |

Adapted from International Agency for Research on Cancer: IARC monographs on the evaluation of carcinogenic risks to humans, 2011 (http://monographs.iarc.fr/ENG/Monographs/PDFs/index.php).

**Table 30-6 International Agency for Research on Cancer: Selected Group 1 Pharmaceutical Carcinogens**

| PHARMACEUTICAL CARCINOGENS | PREDOMINANT TUMOR TYPE |
|---|---|
| Azathioprine | Non-Hodgkin's lymphoma, squamous cell skin cancer, HCC, cholangiocarcinoma |
| Cyclophosphamide | Cancer of the urinary bladder, leukemia |
| Chlorambucil | Leukemia |
| Tamoxifen | Endometrial cancer |
| Estrogens (OCP, HRT) | Cancer of the breast and endometrium |

*HRT,* Hormone replacement therapy; *OCP,* oral contraceptive pill.

Adapted from International Agency for Research on Cancer: IARC monographs on the evaluation of carcinogenic risks to humans, 2011 (http://monographs.iarc.fr/ENG/Monographs/PDFs/index.php).

(1) direct-acting compounds, which do not require chemical transformation for their carcinogenicity; and (2) indirect-acting compounds, or procarcinogens, which require metabolic conversion in vivo for their carcinogenic effects. All these compounds, or their active metabolites in the latter category, share the essential property of being highly reactive electrophiles (have electron-deficient atoms) that can react with nucleophilic (electron-rich) sites in the cell. These reactions are nonenzymatic and result in the formation of covalent adducts between the chemical carcinogens and, almost always, DNA.

The vast majority of chemical carcinogens require metabolic activation for their carcinogenic effects. The metabolic pathway that produces the active metabolite may be only one of a number of metabolic pathways required for the degradation of the parent compound. Thus, the carcinogenic potency of the carcinogen is determined not just by the reactivity of the electrophilic derivative(s), but also by the balance between the metabolic activation and inactivation reactions. Most of the known carcinogens are metabolized by cytochrome P-450–dependent monooxygenases. Because these enzymes are essential for the activation of procarcinogens, individual susceptibility to carcinogenesis is regulated in part by polymorphisms in the genes that encode these enzymes. For example, the product of the P-450 gene *CYP1A1* metabolizes polycyclic aromatic hydrocarbons such as benzo(a)pyrene. Approximately 10% of whites have a highly inducible form of this enzyme that is associated with an increased risk of lung cancer in smokers. Light smokers with the susceptible genotype of *CYP1Q1* have a sevenfold higher risk of developing lung cancer as compared with smokers without the permissive genotype. Age, gender, and nutritional status also have an effect on the metabolism of carcinogens and thus their probability of inducing malignancy.

DNA is the primary target of chemical carcinogens. The ability of these compounds to induce mutations is termed *mutagenic potential.* The Ames test is the most common method for evaluating mutagenic potential and measures the ability of a chemical to induce mutations in the bacterium *Salmonella typhimurium.* Most known chemical carcinogens score positive on the Ames test, so it is a useful screening test. However, not all compounds with mutagenic potential in vitro also have in vivo effects. Although there is no one mutation unique to all chemical carcinogens, individual compounds have been found to induce characteristic changes in DNA. For example, aflatoxin B1 induces a G:C → T:A transconversion in codon 249 of the *TP53* gene (249ser *p53* mutation). Individuals from areas in which there is a high level of exposure to aflatoxin B1 develop hepatocellular carcinoma (HCC) with this characteristic mutation. This mutation is an otherwise uncommon occurrence in HCC caused by other agents, such as the hepatitis B virus.

The carcinogenicity of some chemicals is augmented by the subsequent administration of other agents, called promoters, which are by themselves nontumorigenic. These include phorbol esters, hormones, and phenols. Their fundamental characteristic is their ability to induce cell proliferation. Promotion may involve a number of compounds acting as promoters, which act on different regulatory pathways. The end result is the clonal expansion of initiated cells.

### Radiation Carcinogens

The two most important forms of radiation causing malignant change in humans are ultraviolet (UV) and ionizing radiation (IR). Although IR has been found to cause a variety of cancers, UV radiation is principally implicated as a cause of skin cancers. There is typically a long latency period between radiation exposure and the clinical development of cancer.

UV radiation is a known risk factor for squamous cell carcinoma, basal cell carcinoma, and possibly malignant melanoma. The degree of risk depends on the type of UV rays, intensity of exposure, and quantity of melanin present in the skin. The UV portion of the electromagnetic spectrum can be divided into three wavelength ranges—UVA (320 to 400 nm), UVB (280 to 320 nm), and UVC (200 to 280 nm). Of these, UVB is the most important. UVC, also a potent mutagen, is filtered out by the planetary ozone layer. The carcinogenicity of UVB is caused by its formation of pyrimidine dimers in DNA. This damage may be repaired by the nucleotide excision repair pathway. This is a multistep process involving recognition of the damaged DNA strands, their incision and removal, and synthesis of a patch containing the correct nucleotide sequence, which is then annealed to the DNA structure. With excessive sun exposure, it is postulated that the capacity of this pathway is overwhelmed, and some DNA that is damaged remains unrepaired. Xeroderma pigmentosa, a family of autosomal recessive disorders characterized by extreme photosensitivity and a 2000-fold increased risk of skin cancer, is caused by mutations in the genes involved in nucleotide excision repair. Mutations in the *ras* and *p53* genes occur early in skin cancers, mainly at dipyrimidine sequences.

IR includes electromagnetic (x-rays, gamma rays) and particulate (alpha particles, beta particles, protons, neutrons) forms. Ionizing radiation is a carcinogen and therapeutic agent—low-dose exposure can increase an individual's risk of developing cancer but, when given at high doses, it can slow or stop tumor growth. IR has many effects on tissues, affecting cells and their microenvironment. IR leads to a rapid, global, and persistent activation of the microenvironment. Inflammation leads to the production of reactive oxygen species (ROS) and/or reactive nitrogen species (RNS) by tissue macrophages or neutrophils. Long-term sublethal exposure to these inflammatory products may cause genomic instability in parenchymal cells, eventually leading to chromosomal abnormalities and/or gene mutations. In addition, has become apparent that irradiated stroma has a persistent activated phenotype. Irradiated stroma has been shown to contribute to the selection and proliferation of malignant clones in animal models.

Survivors of the atomic bombs dropped on Hiroshima and Nagasaki in 1945 developed leukemias after an average latency period of 7 years, but have also suffered an increased incidence of solid organ tumors (e.g., breast, colon, thyroid, lung). Irradiation of the head and neck in childhood is associated with a high incidence of thyroid cancer in adulthood.

There is a defined vulnerability of different tissues to radiation-induced carcinogenesis. Most vulnerable are the hematopoietic cell line, causing leukemias (except chronic lymphocytic leukemia), followed by the thyroid gland. In the intermediate category are breast, lung, and salivary glands. The skin, bone, and gastrointestinal tract are relatively radioresistant.

### Infectious Carcinogens

One of the first observations that cancer may be caused by transmissible agents was by Peyton Rous in 1911, when he demonstrated that cell-free extracts from sarcomas in chickens could transmit sarcomas to other animals injected with these extracts. This was subsequently discovered to represent the viral transmission of cancer by the Rous sarcoma virus.

Infectious agents (Table 30-7) may cause or increase the risk of malignancy via a number of mechanisms, including direct transformation, expression of oncogenes that interfere with cell cycle checkpoints or DNA repair, expression of cytokines or other growth factors, and alteration of the immune system.

**Viral Carcinogenesis** Approximately 15% of all human tumors worldwide are caused by viruses. This number reflects predominantly two malignancies, cervical cancer caused by HPV, and

**Table 30-7 International Agency for Research on Cancer: Selected Group 1 Infectious Carcinogens**

| INFECTIOUS CARCINOGENS | PREDOMINANT TUMOR TYPE |
|---|---|
| Epstein-Barr virus | Burkitt's lymphoma, Hodgkin's disease, immunosuppression-related lymphoma, nasopharyngeal carcinoma |
| Hepatitis B | Hepatocellular carcinoma |
| Hepatitis C | Hepatocellular carcinoma |
| Human immunodeficiency virus type 1 | Kaposi's sarcoma |
| Human papillomavirus types 16 and 18 | Cervical cancer, anal cancer |
| Human T cell lymphotropic virus type I (HTLV-1) | Adult T-cell leukemia |
| *Helicobacter pylori* | Gastric adenocarcinoma |
| *Opisthorchis viverrini* | Cholangiocarcinoma, HCC |
| *Schistosoma haematobium* | Cancer of the urinary bladder |

Adapted from International Agency for Research on Cancer: IARC monographs on the evaluation of carcinogenic risks to humans, 2011 (http://monographs.iarc.fr/ENG/Monographs/PDFs/index.php).

HCC, caused by hepatitis B virus (HBV, a DNA virus) and HCV.

***Principles of Viral Carcinogenesis*** Human tumor viruses display different mechanisms of cell transformation and fall into direct- and indirect-acting categories (Box 30-1). Direct-acting viruses carry one or more oncogenes, whereas indirect-acting agents appear not to possess an oncogene. Both types establish long-term persistent infections in their target cell types.

***Small DNA Tumor Viruses*** Because of their limited genetic content, small DNA tumor viruses (e.g., HPV) are dependent on the host cell machinery to replicate the viral genome. Virus-encoded nonstructural proteins stimulate resting cells to enter the S phase to provide the enzymes and environment conducive to viral DNA replication. Because of this ability to usurp cell cycle control, these proteins are also responsible for cell transformation. The binding of viral oncoproteins to cellular tumor suppressor proteins p53 and pRb is fundamental to the effects of the small DNA tumor viruses on host cells. For example, the E6 oncoprotein of HPV forms a complex with p53, targeting it for ubiquitin-mediated degradation.

***Hepatitis B Virus*** The development of HCC after HBV infection probably involves a combination of indirect and direct mechanisms (Fig. 30-12). Chronic liver injury secondary to persistent viral infection leads to necrosis, inflammation, and hepatocyte regeneration. The constitutive induction of liver cell progression into the cell cycle overwhelms DNA repair mechanisms in the presence of mutational events. This may induce fixed DNA mutations and chromosomal rearrangements, which are major determinants of cell transformation; concurrently, fibrosis disrupts the normal lobular structure and modifies cell-cell and cell-extracellular matrix interactions, with further loss of control over cell growth. Integration of HBV DNA into the host genome occurs in 90% of HBV-related HCC cases and has been postulated as an early event in chronic viral infection. Thus far, no specific genes have been identified to be the preferential target for HBV insertion. However, the insertion itself may induce general genomic instability. Dysregulation of cellular genes controlling immortalization *(hTERT)*, proliferation (*MAPK1*, cyclin A), and viability (TNF receptor–associated protein 1) has been

**BOX 30-1 Principles of Viral Carcinogenesis**

- Viruses can cause neoplasia in animals and humans.
- Tumor viruses frequently establish persistent infections in natural hosts.
- Viral infections are more common than virus-related tumor formation.
- Long latent periods usually elapse between initial viral infection and tumor appearance.
- Host factors are important determinants of virus-induced tumorigenesis.
- Viruses may be direct- or indirect-acting carcinogenic agents.
- Viruses are seldom complete carcinogens.
- Viral strains may differ in oncogenic potential.
- Oncogenic viruses modulate growth control pathways in cells.
- In tumors affected by viral carcinogenesis, viral markers are usually present in neoplastic cells.
- One virus may be associated with more than one type of neoplasia.

Adapted from Butel JS: Viral carcinogenesis: Revelation of molecular mechanisms and etiology of human disease. Carcinogenesis 21:405–426, 2000.

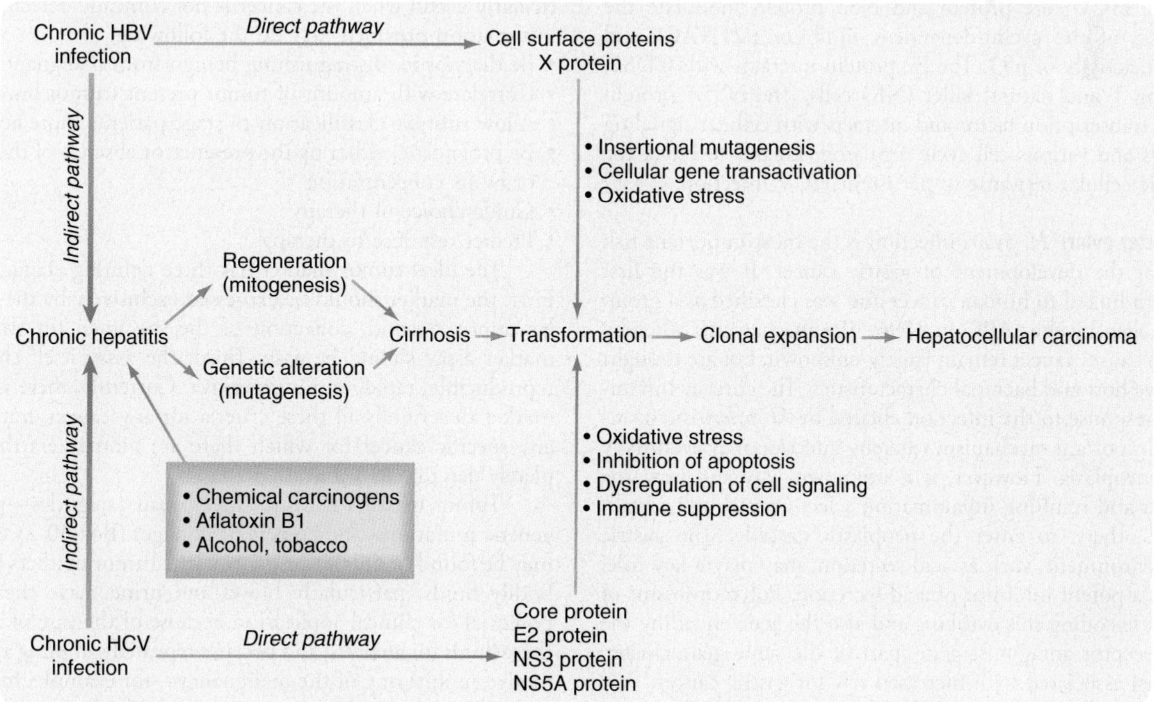


**FIGURE 30-12** Mechanisms of viral-induced hepatic carcinogenesis. (Adapted from Fung J, Lai CL, Yuen MF: Hepatitis B and C virus–related carcinogenesis. Clin Microbiol Infect 15:964–970, 2009.)

observed.[33] HBV cell surface proteins have been shown to increase hepatocyte proliferation and may contribute to carcinogenesis by accumulating in the endoplasmic reticulum (ER), thereby inducing ER stress. The HBV X protein (HBx) may also act as a potential viral oncoprotein. It is a potent transcriptional activator, acting on a number of viral and cellular promoters. It influences signal transduction pathways in the cytoplasm and mitochondrion. HBx also binds p53 and inhibits several critical p53-mediated processes, including DNA sequence–specific binding, transcriptional transactivation and apoptosis.

***RNA Viruses: Human T Cell Lymphotropic Virus Type 1 and Hepatitis C Virus*** After viral infection, the single-stranded RNA viral genome is transcribed into a double-stranded DNA copy, which is then integrated into the chromosomal DNA of the cell. Retroviral infection is permanent. Oncogenic retroviruses carry oncogenes derived from cellular genes, which for the most part are involved in mitogenic signaling and growth control. Examples of such proto-oncogenes are protein kinases, G proteins, growth factors and transcription factors. Alternatively, retroviruses that do not possess oncogenes may cause tumors during integration into the cellular genome. If this occurs near normal cellular proto-oncogenes, the strong promoter and enhancer sequences of the provirus, which allow viral replication, will also affect the expression of proto-oncogenes. This mechanism is termed *proviral insertional mutagenesis.*

***Hepatitis C Virus*** Unlike retroviruses, HCV (an RNA flavivirus) does not appear to cause integration of its DNA into the cellular genome.[34] The predominant mechanism of HCV in the development of HCC appears to be indirect—that is, by the induction of chronic hepatocellular injury, combined with inflammation and liver cell regeneration. However, a number of HCV proteins have been implicated in its carcinogenic activity.[35] Both the HCV core protein and NS3 protein modulate the expression of the cyclin-dependent inhibitor p21WAF1 and affect the activity of p53. The E2 protein interacts with CD82, inhibiting T and natural killer (NK) cells. The NS5A protein acts as a transcription factor and interacts with cellular signaling pathways and various cell cycle regulatory kinases to block the apoptotic cellular response to persistent HCV infection.

**Helicobacter pylori** *H. pylori* infection is the most important risk factor for the development of gastric cancer. It was the first bacterium linked to human cancer and was classified as a group 1 carcinogen by the IARC in 1996. The mechanisms whereby *H. pylori* causes cancer remain largely unknown, but are thought to involve host and bacterial characteristics. The chronic inflammatory response to the infection elicited by *H. pylori* is considered an important mechanism whereby infection may eventually lead to neoplasia. However, it is unknown why and how the infection and resulting inflammation select certain individuals, but not others, to enter the neoplastic cascade. The gastric microenvironment, such as acid secretion, may play a key role. IL-1β is a potent inhibitor of acid secretion. Polymorphisms of the gene encoding this cytokine and also the gene encoding the IL-1β receptor antagonist gene, part of the same gene cluster, have been associated with increased risk for gastric cancer.

Infection with strains of *H. pylori* that carry the cytotoxin-associated antigen A gene *(cagA)* is associated with gastric carcinoma. The *cagA* gene product, CagA, is delivered into gastric epithelial cells by the bacterial type IV secretion system—in essence, a molecular syringe. Once intracellular, CagA is tyrosine-phosphorylated by SRC family kinases and then can specifically bind and activate the cellular oncoprotein SHP2. Thus, it can be seen that CagA deregulation of SHP2 mimics a situation in which SHP2 acquires a gain-of-function mutation. CagA is thought to be important during the early phases of gastric carcinogenesis—in particular, the progression from superficial gastritis to atrophic gastritis to intestinal metaplasia. However, the presence of CagA alone is not sufficient for the transformation of gastric epithelial cells into a malignant phenotype.

### Chronic Inflammation

Chronic inflammation in the absence of infection has long been linked with the development of cancer. Examples include the development of squamous cell carcinoma of the skin in areas of chronic ulceration (Marjolin's ulcer) and the high risk for colorectal cancer in patients with ulcerative colitis. However, the exact mechanistic changes that occur during chronic inflammation that lead to malignant transformation have begun to be elucidated. For example, in ulcerative colitis–associated colorectal cancer, a dual mechanism has been proposed. Ulceration of the epithelium exposes underlying cell layers to the contents of the bowel lumen. The intestinal flora triggers the nuclear factor κB (NF-κB) pathway in macrophages, causing them to release proinflammatory agents such as prostaglandins, chemokines, and interleukins that indirectly promote survival of transformed epithelial cells.

## TUMOR MARKERS

Tumor markers are indicators of cellular, biochemical, molecular, or genetic alterations whereby neoplasia can be recognized. They are surrogate measures of the biology of the cancer, providing insight into the clinical behavior of the tumor. This is particularly useful when the cancer is not clinically detectable. The information provided may do the following:

- Be diagnostic, distinguishing benign from malignant disease
- Correlate with amount of tumor present (tumor burden)
- Allow subtype classification to stage patients more accurately
- Be prognostic, either by the presence or absence of the marker or by its concentration
- Guide choice of therapy
- Predict response to therapy

The ideal tumor marker has three defining characteristics. First, the marker should be expressed exclusively by the particular tumor. Second, collection of the specimen for the tumor marker assay should be easy. Third, the assay itself should be reproducible, rapid, and inexpensive. Currently, there is no one marker that fulfills all these criteria for any cancer, nor is there any specific cancer for which there are biomarkers that completely describe its behavior.

Tumor markers fall into three broad categories—proteins, genetic mutations, and epigenetic changes (Box 30-2). All three may be found in the tumor tissue itself. Tumor markers found in bodily fluids, particularly blood and urine, have the greatest potential for clinical application because of the ease of access to these fluids for analysis, and because repeated sampling allows for in vivo monitoring of the malignancy—for example, for disease progression or recurrence, metastasis, and response to therapy.

Rather than provide an exhaustive review of all tumor markers, this section will outline the major categories of tumor

**BOX 30-2 Potential Nonprotein Tumor Markers**

**RNA-based markers**
Overexpressed or underexpressed transcripts
Regulatory RNAs (e.g., micro-RNAs)

**DNA-based markers**
Single-nucleotide polymorphisms (SNPs)
Chromosomal translocations–*bcr-abl* (Philadelphia)
Changes in DNA copy number
Microsatellite instability
Epigenetic changes (e.g., differential promoter-region methylation)

From Ludwig JA, Weinstein JN: Biomarkers in cancer staging, prognosis and treatment selection. Nat Rev Cancer 5:845–856, 2005.

markers and focus on the evidence for the tumor markers in clinical use.

## Protein Tumor Markers

Proteins were the first type of tumor marker identified and hence are considered the classic tumor markers. However, despite decades of research, few are in clinical use. Those routinely used are often limited by poor sensitivity and specificity. Their serum or plasma levels generally correlate with tumor burden because they are shed from the expanding neoplasm.

### Carcinoembryonic Antigen

Carcinoembryonic antigen (CEA) is probably the most studied cancer tumor marker and its main clinical use is for patients with cancer of the colon and rectum. It is an oncofetal protein that is normally present during fetal life but can be present in low concentrations in healthy adults. Structurally, it is a glycoprotein with a molecular weight of 200 kDa; it is a component of the glycocalyx, located on the luminal side of the cell membrane of normal epithelial intestinal cells. CEA is a member of a large family of proteins related to the immunoglobulin gene superfamily. The molecule itself is secreted into the circulation and is also found in the mucous secretions of the stomach, small intestine, and biliary tree. Although its exact function is unknown, CEA has been shown to be involved in cell adhesion and can inhibit apoptosis induced by loss of anchorage to the ECM.

**Testing** Immunoassay kits allow determination of serum CEA levels accurately, reproducibly, and relatively inexpensively. Normal serum levels are lower than 2.5 ng/mL, borderline if 2.5 to 5.0 ng/mL, and elevated if higher than 5.0 ng/mL. Borderline levels occur with benign disorders such as inflammatory bowel disease (IBD), pancreatitis, cirrhosis, chronic obstructive pulmonary disease (COPD), and smoking can also increase CEA; the upper limit of normal in smokers should be considered as being 5 ng/mL.

**Screening** CEA is not useful as a screening test because of its low sensitivity in early-stage disease. Elevated CEA levels occur in only 5% to 40% of patients with localized disease.

**Prognosis** Elevated CEA levels reflect the burden of tumor present. The degree of CEA elevation correlates with increasing stage of disease; therefore, CEA levels have prognostic value. Preoperative serum CEA is an independent predictor of survival—the higher the preoperative serum level, the poorer the prognosis. This effect persists even after patients are stratified for resectability and extent of local tumor invasion. The 5-year survival is significantly worse in patients with elevated preoperative CEA levels compared with those with a normal preoperative CEA level. Furthermore, 5-year survival is higher in those patients whose elevated preoperative CEA level normalized postoperatively. Finally, patients with elevated preoperative CEA levels have higher recurrence rates compared with those with normal CEA levels.

**Monitoring** The most common application of CEA is monitoring patients for recurrent disease. CEA is most sensitive for hepatic or retroperitoneal metastasis and relatively insensitive for local, pulmonary, or peritoneal involvement. Approximately 75% of patients with recurrent CRC have an elevated serum CEA level before developing symptoms. However, the pattern or magnitude of the rise in the CEA level is of no value in distinguishing localized recurrence from distant disease. However, because elevations of CEA levels may be transient, repeat measurement should be performed as confirmation of the trend. A confirmed rising trend in CEA level should prompt evaluation for recurrent disease.

Because CEA reflects tumor burden, it is useful for monitoring response to chemotherapy in patients with metastatic cancer. An elevated CEA level is an independent factor associated with poor survival and progression on 5-fluorouracil chemotherapy in patients with metastatic colorectal cancer. Patients with advanced cancer whose CEA levels fall during chemotherapy survive significantly longer than those whose CEA levels do not change or increase.

### α-Fetoprotein

α-Fetoprotein (AFP) is used in the detection and management of HCC. It is an oncofetal antigen, consisting of a single-chain polypeptide with a molecular weight of 700 kDa. Levels are elevated in the fetus, fall to low levels after birth, and are elevated during pregnancy. It is synthesized by hepatocytes and endodermally derived gastrointestinal tissues.

**Testing** AFP is measured using immunoassay kits, an enzyme-linked immunoassay (ELISA) or radioimmunoassay (RIA). The upper limit of normal for a healthy nonpregnant adult is less than 25 ng/mL. There are no detectable levels of AFP in 10% to 20% of HCCs. Levels are also raised in nonseminomatous testicular cancer, for which it is valuable tumor marker (see later). significant elevations (>5 ng/mL) of serum AFP levels are seen in 20% of patients with gastric or pancreatic cancer and 5% of patients with colorectal or lung cancer. Elevated levels are also seen in hepatitis, IBD, and cirrhosis.

**Screening** AFP has an estimated sensitivity of 25% to 75%, specificity of 76% to 94%, and positive predictive value (PPV) of 9% to 50%. However, it should be noted that the sensitivity and specificity vary with the cutoff value chosen. If set at 20 ng/mL, the sensitivity and specificity are 30% and 87%, respectively, but if raised to 100 and 400 ng/mL, sensitivity and specificity vary from 72% to 56% and 70% to 94%, respectively.

The combination of AFP and ultrasound improves screening efficacy. One surveillance study of 1125 patients with HCV has reported a sensitivity of 100% with a combination AFP and ultrasound compared with a sensitivity of 75% for AFP alone and 87% for ultrasound alone.[36] Cost-effectiveness analysis calculates the costs of each additional life year gained, in terms of quality-adjusted life-years (QALYs). A QALY less than $50,000 is considered cost-effective. In the United States, studies have suggested that surveillance of patients with HCV-related cirrhosis with a combination of AFP and an imaging modality (ultrasound or CT) would gain QALYs at an acceptable cost.[37–39]

**Prognosis** AFP concentration reflects tumor size, with levels higher than 400 ng/mL associated with larger tumors. As a result, it has been shown that AFP level correlates with stage and prognosis. The rate of increase, expressed as AFP doubling time, has also been associated with a poorer prognosis.

**Monitoring** The AFP level has been shown to decline after resection or ablation. Following complete resection, AFP levels should decrease and remain lower than 10 ng/mL. Shirabe and colleagues[40] have found that in patients with HCC whose preoperative AFP level was higher than 100 ng/mL and in whom the postoperative AFP did not fall below 20 ng/mL, early recurrence in the first postoperative year should be strongly suspected. For those patients whose AFP levels normalize postoperatively, a subsequent rise in AFP level over the course of serial serum measurements has been found to be the best indicator of recurrent disease. It was the first measured abnormality in 34% of these patients. However, in some patients who had elevated serum levels of AFP with their original HCC, postoperative levels of AFP were unreliable in detecting recurrence. Five patients (12%) did not have elevated serum levels despite the presence of recurrent disease.

Tumor regrowth after treatment with chemoembolization does not correlate with the rate of AFP level increase or tumor burden. AFP levels usually decline in response to effective chemotherapy. Monitoring of the AFP level, therefore, avoids prolonged use of ineffective and potentially toxic chemotherapy.

### Carbohydrate Antigen 19-9

Carbohydrate antigen 19-9 (CA 19-9) is widely used as a serum marker of pancreatic cancer, but its use is limited to monitoring responses to therapy, not as a diagnostic marker. It is a mucin-type glycoprotein expressed on the surface of pancreatic cancer cells and was initially detected by monoclonal antibodies raised against colon cancer cell lines in a mouse model. The CA 19-9 epitope is normally present within the biliary tree. Biliary tract disease, acute and chronic, can elevate serum CA 19-9 levels.

**Testing** CA 19-9 is detected using an immunoassay, with the upper limit of normal for a healthy adult being 37 U/mL. Sensitivities of CA 19-9 in the diagnosis of pancreatic cancer range from 67% to 92%, with specificities ranging from 68% to 92%. The usefulness of CA 19-9 as a diagnostic marker is limited in a number of ways. First, patients with a negative Lewis a ($Le^a$) blood group antigen cannot synthesize CA 19-9, and therefore it should not be used as a serologic marker in these individuals, who make up approximately 10% of the population. Second, patients with benign biliary tract disease can have levels of up to 400 U/mL, with 87% having concentrations higher than 70 U/mL. Significant numbers of patients with pancreatitis, acute or chronic, also have elevated levels. Third, in addition to pancreas cancer, CA 19-9 levels are also elevated in patients with other cancers, including those of the biliary tree (95%), stomach (5%), colon (15%), liver (HCC, 7%) and (lung 13%). For the latter, CA 19-9 levels add little clinically useful information to the determination of CEA levels.

**Screening** CA 19-9 is not useful as a screening modality because of its low sensitivity in early-stage disease. With increasing levels of CA 19-9, the diagnosis of pancreatic cancer becomes more accurate. When a cutoff level of 100 U/mL is used, a number of studies have demonstrated that although sensitivity ranges from 60% to 84%, specificity for pancreas cancer is 95% or higher. Levels higher than 1000 U/mL are almost diagnostic of pancreatic cancer. Because of its frequent elevation in benign biliary tract disease, CA 19-9 is not useful for distinguishing benign from malignant distal CBD strictures.

**Prognosis** In patients with pancreatic cancer who have CA 19-9 detectable in their serum, the level has been shown to correlate with tumor burden. For example, higher CA 19-9 levels typically correlate with higher tumor stage and more than 95% of patients with unresectable disease have levels higher than 1000 U/mL. Of patients who undergo curative resection, those whose CA 19-9 levels returned to normal survived longer than those whose levels fell but never normalized.

**Monitoring** Serial measurement of CA 19-9 is used to monitor response to therapy. A rise in CA 19-9 level after curative resection has been shown to precede clinical or CT evidence of recurrence by 2 to 9 months. In patients with unresectable or metastatic disease, failure of CA 19-9 levels to fall with chemotherapy reflects poor tumor response. However, in both settings, the lack of alternative effective therapies limits the usefulness of serial monitoring of CA 19-9.

### Prostate-Specific Antigen

Prostate-specific antigen (PSA) is a serine protease formed in the prostatic epithelium and secreted into the prostatic ducts. Its function is to digest the gel that is formed in seminal fluid after ejaculation. Under normal circumstances, only small amounts of PSA leak into the circulation. With enlargement of the gland (e.g., in patients with benign prostatic hyperplasia [BPH]) or distortion of its architecture, serum PSA levels increase. Thus, PSA is considered a tissue-specific rather than a prostate cancer-specific marker; patients who have undergone curative radical prostatectomy, and women, have no detectable PSA.

**Testing** PSA level is detected with an immunoassay. In addition to BPH, other situations in which serum PSA levels may be elevated include prostatitis, prostatic massage, prostatic biopsy, and digital rectal examination. Initial studies set the upper limit of normal for PSA at 4 ng/mL, with levels higher than 10 ng/mL suspicious for malignancy and levels of 4 to 10 ng/mL being indeterminate. Since then, it has been found that the upper limit of the normal range of PSA increases with age. The limit is 2.5 ng/mL for those aged 40 to 49 years, 3.5 ng/mL for those 50 to 59, 4.5 ng/mL for those 60 to 69, and 6.5 ng/mL for those 70 and older. The rate of increase of PSA in a normal 60-year-old man is 0.04 ng/mL/year.

Expressing PSA relative to prostatic volume and time have also helped discriminate cancer from benign conditions when the PSA level is lower than 1 0 ng/mL but higher than the upper limit of normal for the patient's age. PSA density is defined as the ratio of PSA to prostatic volume, as measured by transrectal ultrasound or magnetic resonance imaging (MRI). Higher PSA densities are more suggestive of malignancy compared with BPH because the amount of PSA released per gram of prostate cancer is significantly higher than that released from normal prostatic tissue.

The ratio of free to total PSA has also been found to improve the specificity of prostate cancer diagnosis in the PSA range of 4 to 10 ng/mL. PSA slope (also known as PSA velocity) is the rate of change of the concentration of PSA over time. For individuals with initial levels lower than 4.0 ng/mL, a PSA slope greater than 0.75 ng/mL/year is considered significant; for patients whose baseline level is higher than 4.0 ng/mL, a slope of higher than 0.4 ng/mL is considered significant.

**Screening** PSA is widely used as a screening tool for prostate cancer, enabling early detection and diagnosis of this disease. However, its use has been called into question by the results of two recent trials.[41] The European Randomized Study of Screening for Prostate Cancer (ERSPC) randomized 162,387 men to screening with PSA or no screening. With a median follow-up of 9 years, there were 214 prostate cancer deaths in the screening group and 326 in the control group, resulting in an adjusted rate ratio for death of 0.8 for the screening group. In other words, to prevent one death from prostate cancer, more than 1400 men need to be screened and 48 men treated. In the Prostate, Lung, Colorectal, and Ovary Cancer (PLCO) trial, 76,693 U.S. men were randomized; with an average of 7 years of follow-up, mortality between the screened and control groups did not differ (rate ratio for death, 1.1). These data have added to concerns regarding overdiagnosis and overtreatment of this disease, with the associated effects on the patient's quality of life. Autopsy studies have found that prostate cancer can be found in 55% of men in their fifth decade of life and 64% in their seventh decade, indicating that a significant proportion of these cancers are not lethal. Only one in eight screen-detected cancers is likely to kill its host if left untreated.

**Monitoring Response to Therapy** After operative resection, the PSA level is expected to normalize after 2 to 3 weeks. Patients whose PSA level remained elevated 6 months after radical prostatectomy eventually developed recurrent disease. In contrast, it takes 3 to 5 months for the PSA level to normalize after radiotherapy. However, failure of the PSA level to normalize after radiotherapy also predicts relapse. An increase in the serum PSA level is usually the first sign of local recurrence or metastatic progression. In patients with advanced disease, PSA levels are also used to monitor response to systemic therapy.

### Carbohydrate Antigen 125

Carbohydrate antigen 125 (CA 125) is a carbohydrate epitope on a glycoprotein carcinoma antigen. It is present in the fetus and in derivatives of the coelomic epithelium, including the peritoneum, pleura, pericardium, and amnion. In healthy adults, CA 125 has been detected by immunohistochemistry in the epithelium of the fallopian tubes, endometrium, and endocervix. However, neither adult nor fetal ovarian epithelium expresses CA 125.

**Testing** CA 125 levels are measured using an immunoassay, with the upper limit of normal set at 35 U/mL. Elevated levels are detected in 80% of patients with ovarian cancer. In patients with ovarian masses, an elevated CA 125 level has a sensitivity of 75% and a specificity of approximately 90% for malignancy. It is also detectable in a high percentage of patients with cancer of the fallopian tube, endometrium, and cervix, as well as in nongynecologic malignancies of the pancreas, colon, lung, and liver. Benign conditions in which the CA 125 level is elevated include endometriosis, adenomyosis, uterine fibroids, pelvic inflammatory disease, cirrhosis, and ascites. As for CA 19-9 in patients with pancreas cancer, CA 125 is an adjunct to diagnosis, rather than being diagnostic itself.

**Screening** By itself, CA 125 is not useful as a screening tool for ovarian cancer because of its poor specificity. However, the United Kingdom Collaborative Trial of Ovarian Cancer Screening has evaluated the effectiveness of CA 125 in postmenopausal women. In this study, women classified as high risk according to their CA 125 level have been further screened with transvaginal ultrasound. Final results from this trial are expected in 2014.

**Prognosis** Patients with elevated CA 125 levels at the time of diagnosis have a worse prognosis compared with patients with normal levels. Absolute levels of CA 125 do not correlate clearly with tumor stage, although with increasing stage, a greater percentages of patients has elevated CA 125 levels—50% of stage I patients, 70% of stage II patients, 90% of stage III patients, and 98% of stage IV patients.

**Monitoring Response to Therapy** CA 125 is of value in monitoring disease course. Partial or complete response to therapy is associated with a decrease in the CA 125 level in more than 95% of patients. Increasing levels of CA 125 correlate with disease recurrence and precede clinical or imaging evidence of recurrence by a median of 3 months. When rising CA 125 levels are used as an indication for second-look laparotomies, recurrent disease is found in approximately 90% of patients.

CA 125 levels in peritoneal fluid may be more sensitive than serum levels. Thus, in patients whose serum CA 125 level normalizes during therapy, peritoneal fluid CA 125 levels may be better able to distinguish patients with residual disease from those without. The upper limit of normal for peritoneal fluid CA 125 is 200 U/mL.

### α-Fetoprotein and Human Chorionic Gonadotropin in Testicular Germ Cell Tumors

Nonseminomatous testicular cancers comprise several different histologic types, including embryonal carcinoma, syncytiotrophoblasts (choriocarcinoma), yolk sac tumors, and teratomas. Marker expression can be predicted on the basis of the predominant histologic type. Human chorionic gonadotropin (hCG) is detected in more than 90% of choriocarcinomas, whereas AFP is expressed by 90% to 95% of yolk sac tumors, 20% of teratomas, and 10% of embryonal carcinomas.

**Diagnosis** Of patients with proven nonseminomatous testicular germ cell tumors, approximately 50% will have elevated serum levels of hCG and 60% of AFP, whereas either marker is elevated in 90% of cases. The determination of both marker levels is important, because almost 50% of these tumors secrete only one of these substances. In addition to the high rate of marker positivity, there have been few cases of spuriously elevated serum levels of hCG or AFP in patients without testicular cancer. The presence of a testicular tumor in combination with an elevated level of AFP or hCG is suspicious for testicular cancer, without being diagnostic. Elevated levels of these markers in a man younger than 40 years without signs of a testicular tumor may indicate extratesticular germ cell cancer.

**Prognosis** An absolute AFP concentration higher than 500 ng/mL or hCG level higher than 1000 ng/mL predicts a poor prognosis. These tumor markers are useful in identifying biologically distinct categories of morphologically similar tumors. In one study that studied pretreatment levels of AFP and hCG, 92% of patients with normal levels of both markers achieved complete remission, compared with 26% of those with elevated AFP levels only, 46% of those with elevated hCG levels only, and 35% of those with elevations of both. Similarly, when comparing groups of patients with similar disease burdens, those with elevated marker levels have a worse prognosis compared with those with normal marker levels.[42]

**Monitoring** In most patients with nonseminomatous germ cell tumors, tumor marker levels correlate with response to chemotherapy. The rate of marker decline (half-life), calculated from weekly determinations after the initiation of chemotherapy, can be used to identify early those patients who respond poorly to chemotherapy. Half-lives longer than 3.5 days for hCG or longer than 7 days for AFP suggest that patients require aggressive therapy, such as high-dose chemotherapy in combination with stem cell transplantation. However, there is a significant percentage of patients whose levels of tumor markers fall despite failure of their tumors to regress with therapy.

After completion of primary therapy, increasing marker concentrations, even in the absence of other features of recurrence, may lead to salvage chemotherapy. Therefore, it is important to exclude false-positive results. The level of hCG should be measured in the urine, in which the concentration should be similar to that of serum. In contrast, interfering substances are not excreted into the urine. Intensive chemotherapy may induce hypogonadism, with associated hCG levels of up to 5 to 10 IU/liter. It can be differentiated from relapse by the measurement of luteinizing hormone (LH) and follicle-stimulating hormone (FSH) levels; like the postmenopausal state in women, levels higher than 30 to 50 IU/liter indicate that the hCG is derived from the pituitary.

## DNA-Based Markers

Specific mutations in oncogenes, tumor suppressor genes, and mismatch repair genes can serve as biomarkers. These mutations may be germline mutations, such as the *RET* proto-oncogene of MEN2 and the *APC* gene of FAP, or somatic mutations, such as the occurrence of *p53* mutations in a wide variety of tumors. Chromosomal abnormalities, such as the 9:22 translocation that creates the *bcr-abl* oncogene, are also useful biomarkers. Specific single-nucleotide polymorphisms have been identified that are associated with increased risk for specific cancers, and haplotype assessment has been shown to predict susceptibility to several cancers, including prostate, breast, lung, and colon.

DNA-based markers are beginning to have a profound influence on clinical practice. For example, HER-2/neu amplification status is now being routinely used to guide treatment with trastuzumab in patients with breast cancer. In April 2009, the American Society of Clinical Oncology released a provisional clinical opinion (PCO)[43] addressing the usefulness of *KRAS* gene mutation testing in patients with metastatic colorectal carcinoma to predict response to anti-EGFR monoclonal antibody (MoAb) therapy with cetuximab or panitumumab. In summarizing the results of five randomized trials and another five single-arm studies, they recommended that all patients with metastatic colorectal carcinoma who are candidates for anti-EGFR antibody therapy should have their tumor tested for the *KRAS* mutation. If the *KRAS* mutation in codon 12 or 13 is detected, these patients should not receive anti-EGFR antibody therapy as part of their treatment. This represents the first major step toward individualized treatment for patients with metastatic colorectal cancer.

In a similar fashion, somatic *EGFR* mutations have been found to represent an important mechanism of resistance to tyrosine kinase inhibitors (TKIs) in non–small cell lung cancer (NSCLC). Deletions in exon 19 and L858R are associated with the response of NSCLC to gefitinib or erlotinib monotherapy, whereas mutations in exon 20 (particularly the T790M point mutation) confer resistance to erlotinib and gefitinib.[44] As a result, *EGFR* mutation analysis is being used to identify patients who are likely to respond to monotherapy with TKIs.

### Epigenetic Changes

Testing for epigenetic changes is still at an early stage and has not yet reached the clinic. However, it has great potential for a number of reasons. First, DNA assays for aberrant methylation are easier and more sensitive than those for point mutations. Second, cancer-specific DNA methylation patterns can be detected in tumor-derived free DNA in the bloodstream and in epithelial tumor cells shed into the lumen. This ease of access to the sample medium may facilitate efforts at detection and monitoring of cancer. Third, DNA methylation profiles are more chemically and biologically stable than RNA or most proteins. Thus, they may be more reliably detected in diverse biologic fluids. Methylation biomarker studies have been performed in a variety of cancers, including breast, esophageal, gastric, colorectal, and prostate. The sources of the DNA have included plasma, serum, urine, sputum, and saliva. A number of general observations have been made. Targeted biologic fluid sources of DNA, such as urine for bladder cancer, tend to have higher clinical sensitivities than serum or plasma analysis. In contrast, the specificity of plasma or serum detection of tumor-specific markers has been found to be extremely high, approximately 100%. Combining DNA methylation assays may complement existing screening methods of high sensitivity but low specificity, such as PSA for prostate cancer. Use of methylation target panels in these studies improved the clinical sensitivity of the assay.

### Potential Applications

**Early Detection** Although abnormal epigenetic silencing of genes can occur at any time during carcinogenesis, it appears to occur most frequently early in the transformation process. Aberrant crypt foci, which contain preneoplastic hyperplastic colonic epithelial cells, have been found to contain abnormal methylation in promoter regions of genes involved in the abnormal activation of the Wnt signaling pathway.[45] Detection of abnormal methylation patterns in histologically normal cells may emerge as useful markers for cancer risk assessment.

**Predict Response to Therapy** Methylation of specific genes can be linked to the biologic behavior of the tumor. A number of studies have reported an association between DNA methylation markers and response to chemotherapy. The most extensive work has been done on CpG hypermethylation of the O-6-methylguanine DNA methyltransferase (MGMT) gene, which appears to confer sensitivity to various alkylating chemotherapeutic agents. MGMT methylation was associated with prolonged survival in glioma patients treated with carmustine and in patients with large, diffuse B cell lymphoma who were treated with cyclophosphamide as part of multidrug regimens.[46] Widschwendter and colleagues[47] have studied the correlation between methylation profiles and hormone receptor status in breast cancer. In particular, they found that methylation of the *ESR1* gene and the *PGR* gene were the best predictors of progesterone and estrogen receptor status, respectively. Furthermore, *ESR1* methylation outperformed hormone receptor status as a predictor of clinical response in patients treated with tamoxifen. Individual methylation markers, such as of the E-cadherin promoter, have also been linked to breast cancer metastasis.

**Prognostication** Abnormal methylation of combinations of genes has been associated with a poor outcome.

Conversely, it should be noted that loss of methylation is being increasingly recognized as an important event in carcinogenesis.[31] Hypomethylated CpG islands have been associated with the activation of nearby genes. For example, hypomethylation of the promoter for the cancer–testis antigen CAGE correlates with the gene's increased expression; it is found in premalignant lesions of the stomach.[48] Similar examples of demethylated promoters activating their downstream genes have been found in a number of other cancers, including those of the colon, pancreas, liver, uterus, lung, and cervix. In a study of ovarian carcinogenesis,[49] the hypomethylation of centromeric and juxtacentromeric satellite DNA was found to be increased in tumors of advanced stage or high grade, and this strong hypomethylation was an independent marker of poor prognosis. Furthermore, genome-wide hypomethylation has also been detected in cancer cells, and may contribute to genomic instability.[45]

DNA methylation profiles, examining hypermethylation and hypomethylation, may provide greater insights into tumor behavior than either profile alone.

## RNA-Based Markers

RNA-based markers have been identified in the context of global mRNA expression using high-throughput technologies. These microarrays (gene chips) allow the expression of 30,000 to 40,000 human genes to be measured in a single experiment. Statistical modeling then allows the selection of groups of genes, fingerprints, that best distinguish disease states.

Sparano and Paik[50] have described an algorithm to predict the likelihood of distant recurrence in patients with node-negative, tamoxifen-treated breast cancer, based on the expression of 21 genes in tumor tissue. This multigene assay, known as Oncotype DX, includes 16 tumor-associated genes and 5 reference genes, with the result expressed as a recurrence score (RS). Higher expression levels of favorable genes result in a lower RS, whereas higher expression levels of unfavorable genes result in a higher RS. Validation studies have demonstrated that this assay is more accurate in predicting clinical outcome in ER-positive, lymph node–negative breast cancer patients treated with tamoxifen than traditional clinicopathologic characteristics. Several studies have found that use of this test has altered the treatment choice in approximately 25% of patients. In an effort to integrate genetic testing into clinical testing further, the Trial Assigning Individualized Options for Treatment (Rx), or TAILORx, will use this 21-gene assay to assign treatment based on whether patients have a low RS (hormonal therapy alone) or high RS (chemohormonal therapy), with those having a mid-range RS being randomly assigned to chemohormonal therapy (standard treatment arm) or hormonal therapy alone (experimental arm). Patient accrual is expected to be completed by the end of 2009.

The MammaPrint assay is another multigene assay, using 70 genes, designed to individualize treatment for patients with estrogen receptor–positive or estrogen receptor–negative, lymph node–negative breast cancer. Its accuracy to select early-stage breast cancer patients who are highly likely to develop distant metastases and therefore may benefit most from adjuvant chemotherapy is being tested prospectively in the MINDACT (Microarray In Node-Negative Disease May Avoid ChemoTherapy) clinical trial.[51]

## Proteomic Profiling

Proteomics is the study of all the proteins expressed by the genome. Ultimately, genetic mutations are manifested at the protein level, involving derangements of protein function and communication within diseased cells and with their microenvironment. Execution of the disease process occurs through altered protein function. Protein tumor biomarkers are thought to be low-abundance proteins (of concentrations in the nanomolar range), shed from tumor cells or from the tumor-host interface into the circulation. Detection and measurement of these proteins provide information about the clinical behavior of the cancer. Proteomic profiling using mass spectrometry technologies generate complex fingerprints of ion peaks corresponding to protein concentrations, which can be correlated with disease states. A number of studies, using samples from blood (plasma or serum), urine, and pancreatic juice, have demonstrated the feasibility of this technology for biomarker discovery and for the early detection of ovarian, breast, prostate, and pancreatic cancers. Identification of reproducible protein signatures of specific diseases has the potential to achieve much higher diagnostic sensitivity and specificity than currently available biomarkers. Proteomic profiling lacks a standardized methodology and remains time- and labor-intensive. However, these technologies are still not ready for routine clinical use. Their principal role is in protein biomarker discovery. Candidate biomarkers discovered through this process can be validated using standard immunometric techniques after the development of specific antibodies.

Clearly, the future holds great promise for the greater use of biomarkers in the clinical management of patients with cancer (Table 30-8). It is expected that combinations of tumor markers,

**Table 30-8 Biomarkers and Biologically Targeted Therapies**

| CANCER | BIOMARKER | THERAPY |
|---|---|---|
| Breast | Estrogen receptor, progesterone receptor | Tamoxifen, aromatase inhibitors |
| Lymphoma | CD20 | Rituximab |
| Chronic myelogenous leukemia (CML) | *Bcr-abl* | Imatinib |
| Gastrointestinal stromal tumor (GIST) | *c-kit* | Imatinib |
| Non–small cell lung cancer | *EGFR* mutation | Geftinib |
| Breast | *HER2/neu* | Trastuzumab |

From Ludwig JA, Weinstein JN: Biomarkers in cancer staging, prognosis and treatment selection. Nat Rev Cancer 5:845–856, 2005.

Biomarker expression is being increasingly used, independently of formal staging criteria, to decide which patients receive biologically targeted therapies.

and of different types of tumor markers, will be developed and then incorporated into formal staging criteria. There will also be further delineation of the role of tumor markers in predicting the response to biologic and other types of therapies.

## SELECTED REFERENCES


Allegra CJ, Jessup JM, Somerfield MR, et al: American Society of Clinical Oncology provisional clinical opinion: Testing for KRAS gene mutations in patients with metastatic colorectal carcinoma to predict response to anti-epidermal growth factor receptor monoclonal antibody therapy. J Clin Oncol 27:2091–2096, 2009.

This paper summarizes the role and rationale for KRAS mutation testing to determine treatment in patients with metastatic colorectal cancer.

Almog N: Molecular mechanisms underlying tumor dormancy. Cancer Letters 294:139–146, 2010.

A review of the scientific evidence that tumors acquire the ability to induce angiogenesis.

Clark WH, Jr, Elder DE, Guerry DT, et al: A study of tumor progression: The precursor lesions of superficial spreading and nodular melanoma. Hum Pathol 15:1147–1165, 1984.

This paper summarizes observations of tumor progression and defines the series of proliferative lesions that constitute the progression from melanocytic neoplasia to malignant melanoma. Based on their observations, the authors provide a paradigm for the development of neoplasia in general and provide a list of six lesional steps.

Dunn GP, Old LJ, Schreiber RD: The immunobiology of cancer immunosurveillance and immunoediting. Immunity 21:137–148, 2004.

This paper reviews the evidence for immune surveillance of cancer.

Fearon ER, Vogelstein B: A genetic model for colorectal tumorigenesis. Cell 61:759–767, 1990.

The first genetic model for tumorigenesis involving a series of genetic mutations, including mutational activation of oncogenes and inactivation of tumor suppressor genes.

Feinberg AP, Tycko B: The history of cancer epigenetics. Nat Rev Cancer 4:143–153, 2004.

Excellent overview of the development and progress of the emerging field of cancer epigenetics, with a discussion of hypomethylation, hypermethylation, loss of imprinting, and chromatin modification.

Hanahan D, Weinberg RA: The hallmarks of cancer. Cell 100:57–70, 2000.

The authors provide a comprehensive overview of the common physiologic and molecular characteristics of cancer.

Knudson AG: Two genetic hits (more or less) to cancer. Nat Rev Cancer 1:157–162, 2001.

This paper provides a perspective on the number of genetic mutations that lead to cancer by using retinoblastoma as a model.

Korsmeyer SJ: Chromosomal translocations in lymphoid malignancies reveal novel proto-oncogenes. Annu Rev Immunol 10:785–807, 1992.

Review of chromosomal translocations in lymphoid tumors that led to the discovery of novel proto-oncogenes, including the family of oncogenes regulating programmed cell death and the first discovered family member, bcl-2.

Sparano JA, Paik S: Development of the 21-gene assay and its application in clinical practice and clinical trials. J Clin Oncol 26:721–728, 2008.

This paper reviews the use of the Oncotype DX assay in the clinical decision making for patients with node-negative, tamoxifen-treated breast cancer.


## REFERENCES


1. Dunn GP, Old LJ, Schreiber RD: The immunobiology of cancer immunosurveillance and immunoediting. Immunity 21:137–148, 2004.
2. Hanahan D, Weinberg RA: The hallmarks of cancer. Cell 100:57–70, 2000.
3. Thun MJ, DeLancey JO, Center MM, et al: The global burden of cancer: Priorities for prevention. Carcinogenesis 31:100–110, 2010.
4. Sener SF, Grey N: The global burden of cancer. J Surg Oncol 92:1–3, 2005.
5. Yancik R: Population aging and cancer: A cross-national concern. Cancer J 11:437–441, 2005.
6. Hutchins LF, Unger JM, Crowley JJ, et al: Underrepresentation of patients 65 years of age or older in cancer treatment trials. N Engl J Med 341:2061–2067, 1999.
7. Lewis JH, Kilgore ML, Goldman DP, et al: Participation of patients 65 years of age or older in cancer clinical trials. J Clin Oncol 21:1383–1389, 2003.

8. Trimble EL, Carter CL, Cain D, et al: Representation of older patients in cancer treatment trials. Cancer 74:2208–2214, 1994.
9. O'Connell JB, Maggard MA, Ko CY: Cancer-directed surgery for localized disease: Decreased use in the elderly. Ann Surg Oncol 11:962–969, 2004.
10. Calle EE, Rodriguez C, Walker-Thurmond K, et al: Overweight, obesity, and mortality from cancer in a prospectively studied cohort of U.S. adults. N Engl J Med 348:1625–1638, 2003.
11. Burkhart DL, Sage J: Cellular mechanisms of tumour suppression by the retinoblastoma gene. Nat Rev Cancer 8:671–682, 2008.
12. Okada H, Mak TW: Pathways of apoptotic and non-apoptotic death in tumour cells. Nat Rev Cancer 4:592–603, 2004.
13. Kerr JF, Wyllie AH, Currie AR: Apoptosis: A basic biological phenomenon with wide-ranging implications in tissue kinetics. Br J Cancer 26:239–257, 1972.
14. Korsmeyer SJ: Chromosomal translocations in lymphoid malignancies reveal novel proto-oncogenes. Annu Rev Immunol 10:785–807, 1992.
15. Kelekar A: Autophagy. Ann N Y Acad Sci 1066:259–271, 2005.
16. Shin JS, Hong A, Solomon MJ, et al: The role of telomeres and telomerase in the pathology of human cancer and aging. Pathology 38:103–113, 2006.
17. Zhou BB, Zhang H, Damelin M, et al: Tumour-initiating cells: Challenges and opportunities for anticancer drug discovery. Nat Rev Drug Discov 8:806–823, 2009.
18. Folkman J: Angiogenesis. Annu Rev Med 57:1–18, 2006.
19. Naumov GN, Folkman J, Straume O: Tumor dormancy due to failure of angiogenesis: Role of the microenvironment. Clin Exp Metastasis 26:51–60, 2009.
20. Hanahan D, Folkman J: Patterns and emerging mechanisms of the angiogenic switch during tumorigenesis. Cell 86:353–364, 1996.
21. Cavallaro U, Christofori G: Cell adhesion and signalling by cadherins and Ig-CAMs in cancer. Nat Rev Cancer 4:118–132, 2004.
22. Makrilia N, Kollias A, Manolopoulos L, et al: Cell adhesion molecules: role and clinical significance in cancer. Cancer Invest 27:1023–1037, 2009.
23. Janes SM, Watt FM: New roles for integrins in squamous-cell carcinoma. Nat Rev Cancer 6:175–183, 2006.
24. Zlotnik A: Chemokines and cancer. Int J Cancer 119:2026–2029, 2006.
25. Kaplan RN, Riba RD, Zacharoulis S, et al: VEGFR1-positive haematopoietic bone marrow progenitors initiate the premetastatic niche. Nature 438:820–827, 2005.
26. Roberts WK, Deluca IJ, Thomas A, et al: Patients with lung cancer and paraneoplastic Hu syndrome harbor HuD-specific type 2 CD8+ T cells. J Clin Invest 119:2042–2051, 2009.
27. Pages F, Galon J, Dieu-Nosjean MC, et al: Immune infiltration in human tumors: A prognostic factor that should not be ignored. Oncogene 29:1093–1102, 2010.
28. Fearon ER: Human cancer syndromes: Clues to the origin and nature of cancer. Science 278:1043–1050, 1997.
29. Nielsen M, Franken PF, Reinards TH, et al: Multiplicity in polyp count and extracolonic manifestations in 40 Dutch patients with MYH-associated polyposis coli (MAP). J Med Genet 42:e54, 2005.
30. Galiatsatos P, Foulkes WD: Familial adenomatous polyposis. Am J Gastroenterol 101:385–398, 2006.
31. Feinberg AP, Tycko B: The history of cancer epigenetics. Nat Rev Cancer 4:143–153, 2004.
32. Kondo Y, Shen L, Issa JP: Critical role of histone methylation in tumor suppressor gene silencing in colorectal cancer. Mol Cell Biol 23:206–215, 2003.
33. Chemin I, Zoulim F: Hepatitis B virus–induced hepatocellular carcinoma. Cancer Lett 286:52–59, 2009.
34. Butel JS: Viral carcinogenesis: Revelation of molecular mechanisms and etiology of human disease. Carcinogenesis 21:405–426, 2000.
35. Anzola M: Hepatocellular carcinoma: role of hepatitis B and hepatitis C viruses proteins in hepatocarcinogenesis. J Viral Hepat 11:383–393, 2004.
36. Izzo F, Cremona F, Ruffolo F, et al: Outcome of 67 patients with hepatocellular cancer detected during screening of 1125 patients with chronic hepatitis. Ann Surg 227:513–518, 1998.
37. Arguedas MR, Chen VK, Eloubeidi MA, et al: Screening for hepatocellular carcinoma in patients with hepatitis C cirrhosis: A cost-utility analysis. Am J Gastroenterol 98:679–690, 2003.
38. Lin OS, Keeffe EB, Sanders GD, et al: Cost-effectiveness of screening for hepatocellular carcinoma in patients with cirrhosis due to chronic hepatitis C. Aliment Pharmacol Ther 19:1159–1172, 2004.
39. Saab S, Ly D, Nieto J, et al: Hepatocellular carcinoma screening in patients waiting for liver transplantation: A decision analytic model. Liver Transpl 9:672–681, 2003.
40. Shirabe K, Takenaka K, Gion T, et al: Significance of alpha-fetoprotein levels for detection of early recurrence of hepatocellular carcinoma after hepatic resection. J Surg Oncol 64:143–146, 1997.
41. Eckersberger E, Finkelstein J, Sadri H, et al: Screening for prostate cancer: A review of the ERSPC and PLCO trials. Rev Urol 11:127–133, 2009.
42. Birch R, Williams S, Cone A, et al: Prognostic factors for favorable outcome in disseminated germ cell tumors. J Clin Oncol 4:400–407, 1986.
43. Allegra CJ, Jessup JM, Somerfield MR, et al: American Society of Clinical Oncology provisional clinical opinion: Testing for KRAS gene mutations in patients with metastatic colorectal carcinoma to predict response to anti-epidermal growth factor receptor monoclonal antibody therapy. J Clin Oncol 27:2091–2096, 2009.
44. Linardou H, Dahabreh IJ, Bafaloukos D, et al: Somatic EGFR mutations and efficacy of tyrosine kinase inhibitors in NSCLC. Nat Rev Clin Oncol 6:352–366, 2009.
45. Baylin SB, Ohm JE: Epigenetic gene silencing in cancer—a mechanism for early oncogenic pathway addiction? Nat Rev Cancer 6:107–116, 2006.
46. Laird PW: The power and the promise of DNA methylation markers. Nat Rev Cancer 3:253–266, 2003.
47. Widschwendter M, Siegmund KD, Muller HM, et al: Association of breast cancer DNA methylation profiles with hormone receptor status and response to tamoxifen. Cancer Res 64:3807–3813, 2004.
48. Cho B, Lee H, Jeong S, et al: Promoter hypomethylation of a novel cancer/testis antigen gene CAGE is correlated with its aberrant expression and is seen in premalignant stage of gastric carcinoma. Biochem Biophys Res Commun 307:52–63, 2003.
49. Widschwendter M, Jiang G, Woods C, et al: DNA hypomethylation and ovarian cancer biology. Cancer Res 64:4472–4480, 2004.
50. Sparano JA, Paik S: Development of the 21-gene assay and its application in clinical practice and clinical trials. J Clin Oncol 26:721–728, 2008.
51. Mook S, Van't Veer LJ, Rutgers EJ, et al: Individualization of therapy using Mammaprint: From development to the MINDACT Trial. Cancer Genomics Proteomics 4:147–155, 2007.

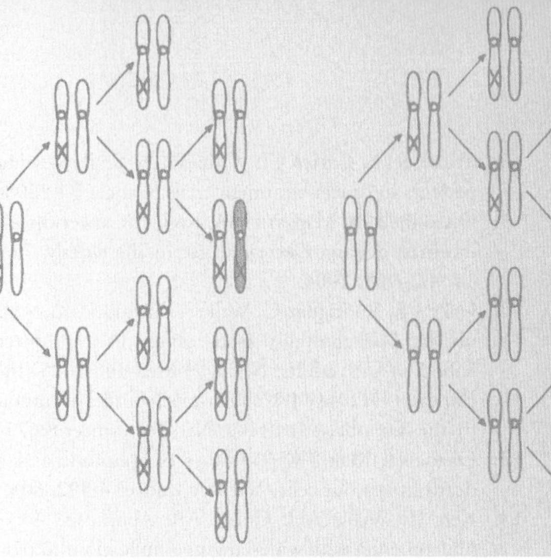

CHAPTER 31

# TUMOR IMMUNOLOGY AND IMMUNOTHERAPY

James S. Economou, James C. Yang, and James S. Tomlinson



The immune system is our most powerful defense against infectious disease[1] and the mediator of rejection in transplantation. In a small subset of patients, modern immune-based therapies can also effect dramatic and durable rejection of bulky metastatic melanoma and renal cell cancer. This attests to the capacity of the adaptive, and perhaps innate, immune system to recognize and destroy malignancies. These complete responses, however few, are durable, and patients rarely relapse, which is even more remarkable. Perhaps the most important observation, which has been confirmed repeatedly over the last 2 decades, is that the human immune system recognizes self-antigens expressed in the context of major histocompatibility complex (MHCs) on the cell surface. Almost half of the human T cell repertoire recognizes self—these generally low-affinity self-reactive T cells having escaped thymic deletion—which underscores the reality that antitumor immune responses are frequently autoimmune in nature. The immune system has evolved mechanisms of immunologic tolerance which allow for discrimination between self and nonself. Therefore, there is a wealth of potential immune targets for solid and hematopoietic malignancies, which include normal self-proteins and tumor-specific mutations, against which human T cells can be activated, expanded, and become specifically cytotoxic. Genome-based scientific advances have provided promising recombinant immunomodulatory molecules as well.[2] Thus, there is broad potential in human cancer immunotherapy, if we could only understand all the biologic rules.

## OVERVIEW OF TUMOR IMMUNOLOGY

### T Lymphocytes and Natural Killer Cells

Bone marrow–derived progenitor cells enter the thymus, from which T cells eventually emerge. In the thymus, an enormous repertoire of T cell receptors is randomly generated by recombinations and mutations in α and β chains of the T cell receptor (TCR). Progenitors with TCRs of high affinity for self-antigens undergo deletion (negative selection). Some of those with low affinity for self-antigens survive and are positively selected, so that a significant percentage of self-reactive T cells emerge from the thymus. Only a very small percentage of the cells entering and proliferating within the thymus survive this education process. Several types of T cells emerge into the periphery. $CD8^+$ T cells recognize antigen in the context of MHC class I molecules, express αβ TCR, have cytotoxic activity, and produce cytokines. $CD4^+$ T cells recognize antigen in the context of MHC class II molecules. There are several subsets of $CD4^+$ T cells (Fig. 31-1). Among the better recognized are Th1 cells (helper type 1 T cells) that secrete interleukin-2 (IL-2), tumor necrosis factor α (TNF-α), and interferon-γ (IFN-γ) and Th2 cells, which produce IL-4, IL-5, IL-6, IL-10, and IL-13. Th1 cells promote cytotoxicity and inflammation whereas Th2 cells assist in the stimulation of B cells to produce antibody. T helper cells will favor a Th1 (cell-mediated) or Th2 (humoral) immune response, but a subset of regulatory cells (Treg cells) plays a critical role in dampening autoimmunity. These Treg constitute 5% to 10% of $CD4^+$ cells and express the transcription factor Foxp3. Mutation of the Foxp3 gene in humans and mice leads to multiorgan autoimmune disease. A fourth type of T cell subtype is the so-called Th17 cell, which preferentially produces IL-17, IL-21, and IL-22 and is important in the pathogenesis of autoimmune diseases.

$CD4^+$ T cells also play an important role in the initiation and maintenance of $CD8^+$ T cell responses.[3] They may do this through a variety of mechanisms. Activated $CD4^+$ T cells can interact with dendritic cells (DCs), professional antigen-presenting cells, through an interaction between the CD40 receptor and its ligand, CD40L. This activation, or licensing, of DCs allows these antigen-presenting cells to promote the differentiation of $CD8^+$ T cells and establish a durable memory T cell response. $CD4^+$ T cells also produce IL-2 and IFN-γ, which could potentially support CD8 function. Thus, the importance of $CD4^+$ T cells in shaping a productive antitumor response has been incorporated into many tumor immunotherapy strategies.

Another T cell subset (γδ) represents a minor population (1% to 10%) of $CD3^+$ T cells that is even more enriched in mucosal epithelium, which expresses TCRs that recognize bacterial and viral antigens. Natural killer T (NKT) cells express phenotypic markers of T and NK cells and express a specific family of TCRs that recognize glycolipid antigens presented by CD1d molecules. These NKT cells are thought to help initiate T cell responses through the production of large amounts of the cytokines IFN-γ and IL-4.

Mature T cells have a broad repertoire of αβ TCR, with diverse antigen specificity. This diverse TCR repertoire is generated during T cell differentiation by a process of gene

**Glossary of Terms**

1MT—1-methyltryptophan
ADCC—antibody-dependent cellular cytotoxicity
BCG—Bacille Calmette-Guérin
CAR—chimeric antigen receptor
CCL—cc chemokine
CCR—cc chemokine receptor
CDC—complement-dependent cytotoxicity
CDR—complementarity-determining region
CEA—carcinoembryonic antigen
cGy—centigray
COX-2—cyclooxygenase-2
CpG—unmethylated CG dinudeotides
CTL—cytotoxic T lymphocytes
CTLA-4 cytotoxic T lymphocyte-associated antigen-4
DC—dendritic cell
EGFR—epidermal growth factor receptor
FDA—U.S. Food and Drug Administration
Foxp3—forkhead box P3
GM-CSF granulocyte macrophage-colony stimulating factor
HAMA—human antimouse antibody
HIV—human immunodeficiency virus
HLA—human leukocyte antigen
hTERT—human telomerase reverse transcriptase
IDO—indoleamine 2,3-dioxygenase
IFN—interferon
Ig—immunoglobulin
IL—interleukin
LAK—lymphokine-activated killer cell
mAb—monoclonal antibody
MDSC—myeloid-derived suppressor cell
MHC—major histocompatibility complex
NHL—non-Hodgkin's lymphoma
NK—natural killer
PARP—poly (ADP-ribose) polymerase
PD-1—programmed death-1
PD-L1—programmed death receptor ligand-1
PGE2—prostaglandin E2
PRR—pattern recognition receptor
PSA—prostate-specific antigen
PSMA—prostate-specific membrane antigen
RAIT—radioimmunotherapy
RCC—renal cell cancer
SEREX—serologic expressive cloning
SOCS—suppressor of cytokine signaling
TCR—T cell receptor
TGF-β—transforming growth factor β
Th—T helper cell
TLR—Toll-like receptor
TNF—tumor necrosis factor
TRAIL—TNF-related apoptosis-inducing ligand
Treg cell—T regulatory cell
VEGF—vascular endothelial growth factor
VEGFR—vascular endothelial growth factor receptor

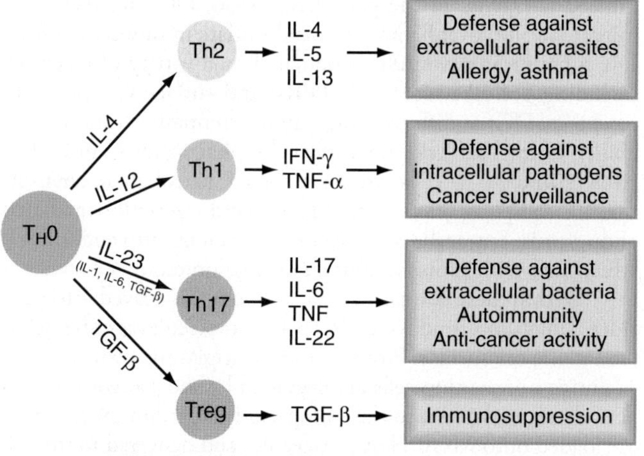


**FIGURE 31-1** $CD4^+$ T cell subsets and their properties.

rearrangement of variable (V), joining (J), and diversity (D) gene segments. TCRs are composed of α and β chains; it is estimated that recombination events could potentially yield a repertoire exceeding $10^{12}$ unique TCRs. These TCRs recognize antigen in the context of MHC proteins found on the surface of cells. Proteins within the cell are digested in the proteasome complex into short peptide fragments (8- to 12-amino-acid residues), which are transported to the cell surface bound in the groove of MHC class molecules; the specific peptide sequence presented is determined by the MHC (in humans, also called HLA [human leukocyte antigen]) allele. These class I–restricted peptides are recognized by $CD8^+$ T cells. This provides the immune system with a continuous surveillance system for intracellular pathogens, such as viruses, so that infected cells can be quickly recognized and killed. The activation of resting T cells requires engagement of the correct MHC-peptide complex by the TCR (so-called signal 1) and additional costimulatory signals (signal 2). Professional antigen-presenting cells (DCs) provide the molecule B7 (either CD80 or CD86), which engages the CD28 receptor on the T cell, a requirement for T cell activation. T cells then upregulate another receptor, cytotoxic T lymphocyte–associated antigen 4 (CTLA-4), which also binds B7 but with a higher affinity than CD28. Engagement of CTLA-4 induces an inhibitory signal that downregulates T cell activation. This is a natural immunomodulatory mechanism for dampening immune responses. Monoclonal antibodies that bind to CTLA-4 can block this interaction and inhibit the negative regulatory signaling. Studies in human subjects have demonstrated that CTLA-4 blockade can break peripheral tolerance to self-antigens and induce antitumor and antiself autoimmune responses. Other examples of potential signaling interactions between DCs and T cells are shown in Figure 31-2 (see later).

Although much emphasis in antitumor immunity has been focused on adaptive responses (T lymphocytes and antibodies), effector cells of the innate immune system, specifically NK cells, can act alone or in concert with adaptive immunity.[2,4] NK cells are innate immune cells because they can recognize and kill target cells without prior sensitization. These cells contain activating and inhibitory cell surface receptors and, when their

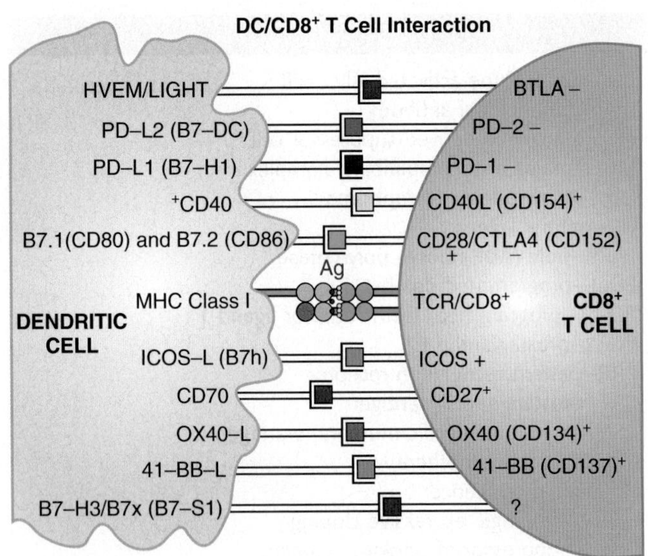


FIGURE 31-2 Potential receptor-ligand interactions between dendritic cells and CD8+ T cells.

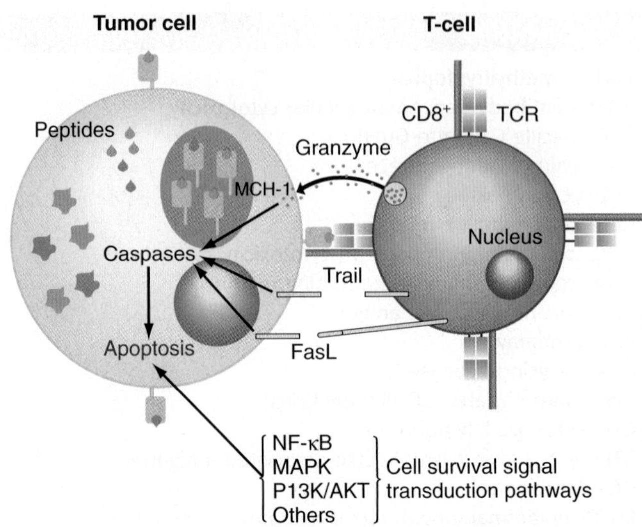


FIGURE 31-3 Mechanisms of target cell killing by cytotoxic lymphocytes.

activating receptors are engaged without concomitant ligation of their inhibitory receptors, can kill targets directly. NK cells have been traditionally viewed as providing a first line of defense, attacking virally infected cells. NK cells can also interact with the adaptive immune system. They can modulate the function of professional antigen-presenting cells (e.g., DCs), promote the generation of Th1 responses, and potentially dampen autoimmune immunopathology. Because their inhibitory receptors engage MHC molecules, NK cells specifically recognize cells that have lost MHC class I molecules; this can occur during viral infections or malignant transformation. NK cells are strongly activated by exogenous cytokines such as interleukin 2 (IL-2) and are then termed *lymphokine-activated killer cells* (LAK cells). LAK cells have greatly enhanced cytotoxicity for a much broader range of target cells.

The cytotoxic pathways initiated by the activation of CTLs (cytotoxic T lymphocytes) and NK cells are the granule-exocytosis pathway, releasing membrane-destructive perforin and granzymes, and the death receptor pathways mediated by TNF-α, TRAIL, and FasL on binding their cognate receptors on the target cell surface (Fig. 31-3).[5] These receptors activate the caspase cascade involving caspase-8 autoprocessing, activation of caspase-3, and cleavage of death substrates (e.g., poly[ADP-ribose] polymerase, PARP), with subsequent induction of apoptosis. Another mechanism inducing apoptosis, which is more typical for some chemotherapeutic drugs, uses a mitochondrial pathway involving permeabilization of the mitochondrial membrane and mitochondrial collapse. Mitochondrial integrity is preserved by a balance between antiapoptotic (e.g., Bcl-2, Bcl-xL, Bfl-1/A1, Mcl-1) and proapoptotic Bcl-2 family members (e.g., Bax, Bid, Bad, Bik, Bcl-xS). Mitochondrial destabilization will facilitate the cytosolic release of apoptogenic molecules, which expedites caspase-9 activation and in turn activates caspase-3, leading to apoptosis. The expression of these gene products is tightly regulated by the activity of survival signaling pathways (nuclear factor κB [NF-κB], AKT/PI3K, ERK1/2, p38, and JNK).

## Antigen-Presenting Cells

DCs are professional antigen-presenting cells; their role is to take up, process, and present antigen to the immune system,[6] and they are essential during the initial activation of resting T cells. There are different subtypes of DCs, with specialized functions that depend on their anatomic location. DCs are found in lymphoid tissues, in the skin, and on the mucosal surfaces of many organs. DCs in the gastrointestinal tract can sample bacteria in the intestinal lumen and initiate secretory immunoglobulin A (IgA) responses. In the lung, DCs help maintain tolerance to inhaled allergens. In the peripheral blood, DC precursors can migrate to sites of inflammation and initiate immune responses. DC function is powerfully modulated by a variety of receptors including Toll-like receptors (TLRs) and surface C-type lectin receptors. DCs at different stages in differentiation vary in their ability to migrate, take up antigen by phagocytosis, and effectively stimulate T cells. Immature DCs patrol their environment, sampling by pinocytosis and receptor-mediated endocytosis. Extracellular antigens are taken up into endosomes, which fuse with protease-containing lysosomes.

Within these compartments, antigens are cleaved into peptides, which can bind to MHC class II molecules and be delivered to the cell surface. Proteins in the cytoplasmic compartment of antigen-presenting cells are degraded by the proteosome and actively transported into the endoplasmic reticulum, where they are loaded onto MHC class I molecules and delivered to the cell surface. Some exogenous or environmental antigens can also find their way into the MHC class I antigen presentation pathway; this is termed *cross-presentation* and is an important mechanism for generating CD8+ class I–restricted T cell responses (Fig. 31-4). DCs can acquire antigen in the periphery and travel to lymph nodes, where they interact with T cells and present antigen. DCs originate from pluripotent stem cells from bone marrow, enter the blood, and localize to almost all tissues and lymphoid organs. There are a number of different subsets of DCs, including myeloid DCs (these include DCs found in deep epithelial tissues and Langerhans cells present in the epidermis) and plasmacytoid DCs, which are a major source of type I IFN.

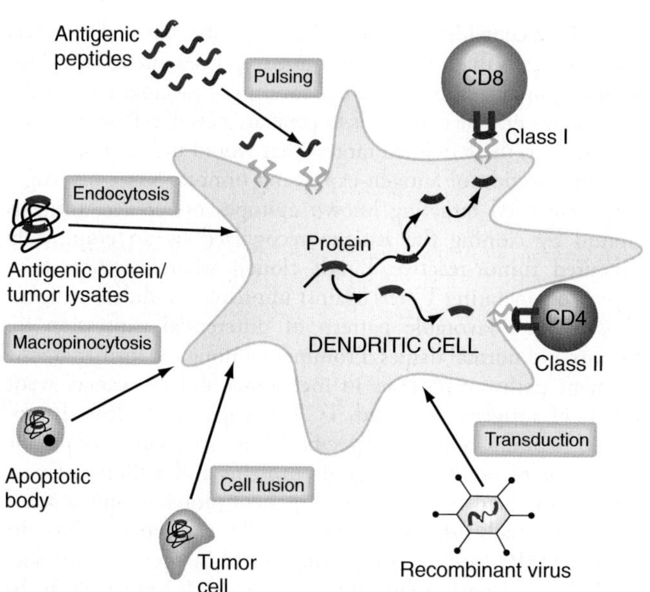


**FIGURE 31-4** Tumor antigen acquisition and processing by dendritic cells.

DCs have cell surface receptors termed *pattern recognition receptors* (PRRs) that screen the environment for pathogens. The TLR family is the best characterized; these can recognize bacterial products (e.g., lipopolysaccharide [LPS], flagellin), viral products such as double-stranded RNA, and specific CpG-rich DNA motifs, more common in microbial genomes. These signals, along with various proinflammatory cytokines, can deliver a danger signal to DCs that establishes the context within which they see and present antigens. TLR signaling drives immature DCs into a more mature phenotype, with much higher expression of MHC, costimulatory molecules, and DC-derived cytokines, such as IL-12. Immature DCs are migratory and highly efficient in antigen capture, whereas mature DCs are less mobile but more efficient in processing and presenting antigen in an immunostimulatory context.

Distinct sets of molecules govern migration of DCs to and from the periphery and to lymph nodes. Prominent among these signals include a variety of chemokines and their receptors (e.g., CCR7, CCL19, CCL21). Signals that induce maturation of immature DCs include CD40 ligand delivered by T cells, as well as signals by NK cells, a variety of proinflammatory cytokines (e.g., IL-1, TNF, IL-6), and engagement of TLR and C type lectins. The context of antigen presentation and the maturational phenotype of DCs will determine and shape the type of T cell response. Immature DCs have the potential to be tolerogenic, perhaps because they present antigen without an appropriate costimulatory second signal. Activated mature DCs have greater potency in activating and expanding antigen-reactive T cells. This is an oversimplified overview of the complex central role of various DC subset in regard to orchestrating adaptive and innate antitumor responses.

## Antibody

Cell surface and circulating antigens can be recognized by Igs (antibody molecules). Igs serve as membrane-associated receptors on the surface of B cells, which can then be secreted as soluble molecules as these cells differentiate into plasma cells. There are five distinct classes of immunoglobulin molecules: IgG, IgA, IgM, IgD, and IgE. There are several isotypes of IgG and IgA. The basic structure of antibody molecules include two identical light and two identical heavy polypeptide chains linked by interchain disulfide bridges. Variable regions within the heavy and light chains create a so-called hypervariable region responsible for antigen binding. Antibody binding to antigen is reversible and of variable avidity. The C terminal portion of certain antibody classes can bind to Fc receptors, which are expressed among a range of mononuclear cells. Antibody binding to antigen and engagement of one of these cells can trigger phagocytosis or antibody-dependent cell-mediated cytotoxicity (ADCC).

The complement system is composed of a series of plasma proteins, many of which exist as proenzymes that require cleavage for activation. Surface-bound IgG and IgM antibodies can activate complement through the so-called classical pathway, a byproduct of which is the assembly of complement proteins that effect transmembrane pore formation in target cells. Complement byproducts can also promote chemotaxis of mononuclear cells that release cytokines. Thus, complement activation can only not kill targets, but can label them as pathogens for elimination. The alternative pathway allows complement activation without antibody.

## Tumor Antigens

A molecular understanding of tumor recognition has been achieved only recently. The first molecularly defined antigen recognized by a tumor-reactive T cell was only discovered in 1991.[7] This advance first required elucidation of the biology of antigen processing and presentation and its interaction with MHC molecules, which occurred in the late 1980s. These discoveries showed that when antigens were presented by MHC class I molecules, they were largely derived from intrinsic cytoplasmic proteins. These were degraded (predominantly in the proteosome) to specific 8- to 12-amino-acid peptides, which were actively transported into the endoplasmic reticulum, where they were loaded onto nascent MHC class I molecules, specifically binding to the antigen groove of a particular presenting MHC allele. These MHC-peptide complexes are then exported to the cell surface and are the actual entities that engage a specific TCR. Antigens presented by class II MHC molecules are often environmental proteins taken up by professional antigen-presenting cells (DCs) by endocytosis; these endosomes fuse with lysosomes, which mediate degradation of those exogenous proteins into short amino acid fragments that are loaded onto class II molecules and again displayed on the cell surface as peptide-MHC complexes. One cannot discern from its sequence or structure whether a particular TCR recognizes a class I– or class II– restricted antigen. Mature T cells also express the CD8 or CD4 coreceptor and these bind to invariant portions on all class I or class II MHC molecules, respectively. This additional ligation increases the affinity of the T cell interaction with the antigen-presenting cell. Therefore, T cells expressing CD4 typically recognize antigens presented by MHC class II molecules and $CD8^+$ T cells usually recognize class I–presented antigens.

Cancer cells can overexpress or abnormally express a variety of self-antigens, including some with sequence mutations. Because of the ability of the human T cell repertoire to recognize self, most of these could potentially serve as targets for cancer vaccines. The characteristics of an ideal cancer antigen include immunogenicity, with elicitation of T cell and/or antibody responses. A gene product associated with the neoplastic process (e.g., an oncogene) and with a high degree of specificity and level of expression could also serve as a good antigen candidate. It is generally believed that optimally designed cancer vaccines using and incorporating such tumor antigens would carry the highest likelihood of therapeutic efficacy.

A comprehensive analysis of human cancer antigens has identified 46 that are immunogenic in clinical trials, with 20 having suggestive therapeutic efficacy.[8] Examples of general classes of tumor antigens include the following: (1) MAGE-1, -2, and -3, BAGE, and RAGE, which are nonmutated antigens expressed in a variety of tumor cells; (2) lineage-specific tumor antigens, such as the melanocyte-melanoma lineage antigens MART-1/Melan-A (MART-1), gp100 protein, mda 7 protein, tyrosinase, and tyrosinase-related-protein (TRP-1 and -2), and the prostate antigens—prostate-specific membrane antigen (PSMA) and prostate-specific antigen (PSA); (3) epitopes derived from genes mutated in tumor cells and/or genes expressed at different levels in tumor compared with normal cells, such as mutated *ras*, *bcr/abl* rearrangement, and *p53*; (4) epitopes derived from oncoviral processes, such as human papillomavirus (HPV), and proteins E6 and E7; and (5) nonmutated proteins with a tumor-selective expression, including carcinoembryonic antigen (CEA), PSA, Her2/neu, and α-fetoprotein, among a rapidly growing list. Although the immune system has been widely exposed to some of these in fetal life or later, responses can still be generated to these proteins when adequately presented to the immune system (Box 31-1).

**BOX 31-1 Tumor Antigens Recognized by T Cells**

- Tissue differentiation antigens: Specialized proteins with a functional role in the tumor's tissue of origin.
  - Melanoma and melanocytes–proteins involved in pigment production (e.g., tyrosinase, gp100, and MART-1)
- Tumor-testis antigens: Family of proteins expressed by tumors and germline tissues, but not other normal tissues
  - Some identified by cloning antigens using native T-cells with tumor reactivity
  - Others found by serologic expression cloning (SEREX) using high-affinity IgGs in serum of some cancer patients (leading to discovery of T cell epitopes in these proteins)
  - Examples are the MAGE family of proteins and NY-ESO-1
- Proteins overexpressed after transformation: Often contribute to malignant transformation or growth but are also normal proteins with conventional functions
  - Examples–normal p53 molecule (overexpressed when a mutant allele is present), erbB-2, and hTERT (from telomerase)
- Tumor-specific mutations
  - Mutation occurs in normal protein within a peptide naturally processed and presented from that protein
  - Mutations contributing to transformation or tumor growth most significant (immune evasion by mutation loss less likely)
  - Examples are CDK4, β-catenin, HLA-A*1101 (all in melanoma)

The recent identification of the specific molecular targets on tumor cells that provoke immune responses opened the door to new approaches to the age-old concept of vaccinating patients against cancer. The concept is to generate new T cell or antibody responses to these defined targets that would induce the regression or rejection of antigen-expressing tumors. Some investigators have tried targeting known epitopes on proven antigens (found by cloning the antigen recognized by an empirically procured tumor-reactive T cell clone), whereas others have explored generating T cells against unproven candidate antigens chosen by a favorable pattern of differential expression on tumors and normal tissues. Prominent among the former are the pigment pathway proteins in melanoma and the cancer testis family of antigens. As noted, TCRs engage small, cleaved, processed peptides bound to specific MHC molecules. From the thousands of potential antigenic proteins and millions of possible amino acid fragments within these proteins, only a select few are actually liberated enzymatically, transported into the correct MHC-loading compartment within the cell, and successfully bind with good affinity to an MHC molecule to be exported and displayed on the cell surface. Beginning antigen discovery and selection with a tumor-reactive T cell ensures that there is a successfully processed and presented peptide epitope involved, but cannot ensure that the antigen from which it is derived will be well expressed on tumors but not on normal tissues. On the other hand, selecting an attractive candidate tumor antigen based on known expression data does not guarantee that protein will contain a peptide epitope that will be processed and presented and be immunogenic.

### Immunosuppressive Tumor Microenvironment

There is abundant evidence that cancer cells have acquired an array of defense mechanisms to thwart destruction by the immune system.[9] These are summarized in Box 31-2. Most human cancers present peptide epitopes in the context of MHC molecules that can be recognized by antigen-reactive T cells, but tumor cells themselves do not present antigen in an immunostimulatory context. The human T cell repertoire that recognizes tumor self-antigens generally have TCRs of low affinity and require additional signaling through costimulatory molecules, such as B7-1/B7-2 (CD80-CD86) for optimal T cell activation and expansion. Without these other signals, T cells can become anergic. Tumor cells can also downregulate antigen expression by a variety of mechanisms, such as epigenetic silencing, loss of MHC expression, and loss of function of the intracellular machinery that processes and transports peptides to the cell surface. These antigen loss variants and lack of costimulatory signaling impose limitations on tumor cells, autonomously initiating antitumor immune responses.

The immune system also has complex and generally fine-tuned downregulatory signaling so that immune responses can be appropriately modulated.[10] Shutting down an acute immune response after 1 to 2 weeks may be appropriate for a viral infection, but can be an impediment to rejecting a large mass of malignant tissue. Many autoimmune processes and transplant rejection, which can serve to model tumor rejection, are chronic ongoing events and tumor immunotherapy will require the circumvention of the normal protective mechanisms that prevent these occurrences.

In addition to CTLA-4 signaling (see earlier), negative signaling can also be transduced through programmed death

**BOX 31-2 Cancer Cell Defense Mechanisms**

- T regulatory (Treg) cells: $CD4^+$-$CD25^+$ T cell population, which inhibits T cell function and proliferation
  - In mice, deletion of these cells can induce autoimmunity
  - Shown to affect tumor rejection by T cells in mice adversely
  - Circumstantial evidence for a role in humans
- CTLA-4 (CD152): Inhibitory receptor induced by T cell activation that binds to CD80 and CD86 ligands
  - Blockade can induce tumor regression in some patients
- PD-1 (CD279; programmed death-1): Another inhibitory receptor on T cells, prevalent on lymphocytes in the tumor microenvironment
  - Binds to ligand PD-L1 (CD274); also present on some human tumors
- SOCS (suppressors of cytokine signaling): Family of proteins that binds and inhibits kinases in the JAK/STAT pathway through which a number of cytokines signal
- Myeloid suppressor cells: Cells of myeloid lineage that inhibit T cells
  - Inhibit by a variety of putative mechanisms, including effects on DCs and modulation of arginine and nitric oxide metabolism
  - Accumulate in tumor-bearing state
- TGF-β: Multifunctional and complex cytokine with many effects on the immune response, some of which are inhibitory

receptor 1 (PD-1). DCs express the programmed death receptor ligand (PD-L1 or B7-H1); its expression by DCs can skew T cells toward an unresponsive phenotype. DCs found within the tumor microenvironment have been shown to express high levels of PD-L1, which contribute to decreased T cell function in the tumor microenvironment. Some tumor cells themselves can present this inhibitory ligand and expression of PD-L1 by renal cancer is associated with a poorer clinical outcome. Blockade of this PD-L1–PD-1 interaction using decoy receptors or antibodies is effective in improving immune therapies in animal models and is currently undergoing clinical testing.

A small subpopulation of $CD4^+$ T cells (5% to 10%) constitutively express the α chain of the IL-2 receptor, CD25; most of these cells also express a transcription factor Foxp3 (a forkhead–winged helix family member), GITR (glucocorticoid-induced tumor necrosis factor receptor), as well as CTLA-4. These cells, Treg, produce immunosuppressive cytokines such as IL-10 and TGF-β and can also inhibit through cell contact–dependent mechanisms. Mice or patients with a genetic mutation in Foxp3 lack these Treg cells and develop a fulminant and lethal autoimmune disorder. Murine data have clearly shown that Treg cells are responsible for suppressing the self-reactive T cell repertoire and the clinical manifestations from genetic loss of Foxp3 suggest this may also be true in humans. Human Treg are enriched in tumor specimens and in draining lymph nodes of many solid tumors and there is emerging evidence supporting a dominant role in suppressing self-reactive antitumor immune responses. Moderating Treg cell function could potentially favor antitumor immune responses. The use of lymphodepleting strategies prior to adoptive cell therapy, which clearly enhances the antitumor biology of adoptively transferred T cells, may be caused in part by the depletion of host resident Treg cells.

Myeloid-derived suppressor cells (MDSCs) and tumor-associated macrophages are found in increased numbers in the bone marrow, blood, and lymphoid organs of tumor-bearing mice. These MDSCs include granulocytes and immature myelomonocytic precursors. They clearly suppress T cell function through a variety of mechanisms. Although not as well studied in human solid tumors, MDSCs have been isolated and have an immunosuppressive phenotype.

Tumors themselves, and at times tumor stroma, can produce immunosuppressive substances; a prominent factor is transforming growth factor-β (TGF-β). TGF-β directly inhibits cytotoxic T cell activation, cytokine production, helper T cell responses, and activation of DCs and can promote the differentiation of Treg cells. Inhibition of TGF-β can have a salutary effect on antitumor immunity. T cells rendered insensitive to TGF-β signaling using a dominant-negative receptor have enhanced function in vivo. Neutralizing antibodies, small molecules inhibitors, and engineered T cells are currently under study in clinical trials. Vascular endothelial growth factor (VEGF) is important in angiogenesis but can also inhibit the function of DC. Thus, anti-VEGF therapy could also function through an immune mechanism. An isoform of the enzyme cyclooxygenase-2 (COX-2) is overexpressed in many tumors and catalyzes the synthesis of prostaglandin E2 (PGE2). PGE2 has a generally adverse impact on the immune system, particularly on DC and T cell function. Clinical trials combining selective COX-2 inhibitors with antitumor vaccines are supported by preclinical studies and are undergoing clinical testing.

Amino acid metabolism can profoundly affect immune cell function; two key amino acids in this respect are arginine and tryptophan. Indoleamine 2, 3-dioxygenase (IDO) metabolizes the essential amino acid L-tryptophan and arginase metabolizes arginine. High levels of either enzyme are associated with functional inhibition of T cells and other cell populations, such as DCs. IDO overexpression has been observed in a variety of human cancers and can be an independent adverse prognostic factor. IDO can also be induced in DCs and macrophages in the tumor microenvironment by Treg cells. A specific small molecule inhibitor of IDO, 1-methyl-tryptophan (1MT) and a similar inhibitor for arginase, N-methylarginine, are being studied preclinically and clinically.

## Animal Models of Tumor Immunotherapy

Realistic murine models of tumor immunology require the establishment of syngeneic mouse strains in which over 20 generations of sibling or parent-offspring matings result in a stable genome, in which every locus is homozygous. Fully autologous tumors from these strains had to be established to ensure that tumor rejection was not caused by allorejection. Even now, slow mutational drift in murine strains or extensively passaged tumor lines can corrupt the biology of immune tumor rejection; diligent efforts are needed to ensure the integrity and provenance of the mice and the tumors used. In the 1950s, these strains of mice allowed Prehn and Main[11] to use carcinogen-induced syngeneic sarcomas; they have shown that unique and shared tumor-specific transplantation antigens exist in immunization challenge experiments.

Accurate modeling of immune tumor rejection is critical. The vast majority of early tumor rejection data were generated using tumor prevention models or treating very early micrometastases within a few days of tumor inoculation, when there is not yet invasion, stroma, or angiogenesis. In some cases, essentially an in vivo tumor lysis assay was done, with tumor cells and tumor-reactive immune cells mixed and coinjected, evaluating subsequent tumor outgrowth. It is now apparent that many immune mechanisms that can kill circulating tumor cells or prevent implantation and invasion will not induce regression of an established vascularized tumor. A striking example is the use of lymphokine-activated killer cells (LAK cells; NK cells activated in vitro with high levels of interleukin-2), which have shown active lysis of human and murine tumors in vitro. By adoptive transfer in mice, they are highly effective 1 to 3 days after IV tumor inoculation but completely ineffective 4 days after tumor injection. Subsequent clinical trials with high numbers of LAK cells generated in vitro have confirmed that they do not contribute to tumor rejection in patients. However, in contradistinction, murine models transferring activated tumor reactive T cells can cause regression of tumors as large as 1 cm in diameter, and the same approach has been highly effective in early clinical trials.

## STRATEGIES FOR CLINICAL TUMOR IMMUNOTHERAPY

Evaluation of tumor immune therapies currently lack response criteria and accurate biomarkers that adequately describe the antitumor biologic events taking place.[12] The clinical trial endpoints that have been well established for cytotoxic chemotherapies are viewed as being inadequate. For example, some patients with apparently progressive disease undergoing CTLA-4 blockade still experience long-term survival. Also, some patients achieving a complete or partial response by the usual criteria may require many months to evolve. Moreover, commonly used surrogate immunologic endpoints of immunotherapy, which generally involve serial sampling and assays of immunologic reactivity of peripheral blood T cell function or measurement of antibody responses, are generally considered inadequate for reflecting the events taking place in the tumor microenvironment. Investigators studying cancer immunotherapies are continually refining biomarkers to predict immune responsiveness, define underlying mechanisms, and predict clinical benefit.

Autoimmune responses are characterized by a phenomenon known as epitope or determinant spreading. Self-reactive driver T cell clones attack normal tissues, which release their intracellular contents and are then taken up and presented by professional antigen-presenting cells (DCs). In a proinflammatory environment, this promotes the progressive accumulation of effector cells recognizing antigenic epitopes on different portions of the original inciting protein antigen and to other proteins expressed by that cell. This phenomenon of intramolecular and intermolecular determinant spreading has been observed in a number of clinical immunotherapy trials in patients who have achieved a complete clinical response. It is still not clear whether epitope spreading is causally important to tumor rejection or is a simple reflection of a particularly immunocompetent patient or innately immunogenic tumor. However, these observations suggest that a broad oligoclonal T cell response may be advantageous for a number of reasons, including mitigating the risk of antigen loss variants in a heterogenous tumor population.

### Cytokine Therapy

The cellular immune system often communicates among its component cells or exerts its effector functions using secreted proteins that bind to specific receptors, which then activate or inhibit other cell populations. These secreted proteins are referred to as cytokines and, most often, they act in a paracrine fashion, exerting their action on cells in their local environment. Thus, the family of interleukins, which currently includes 35 members, was originally thought to be used for communication among leukocytes and the interferons were first thought to be targeting virally infected cells and disrupting replication. It is now clear that these initial concepts were simplistic and excessively constrained, and the true scope of interactions for the cytokines is protean. In the clinical arena, several cytokines have been demonstrated to be of use but are often administered in pharmacologic doses as systemic agents.

The first agent to be used as a therapeutic agent was IFN-α. Currently, there are more than 12 species of interferons, grouped into IFN-α, IFN-β, and IFN-γ; and these differ in regard to which cells produce them and to which receptors they bind. On the other hand, all the IFN-α agents have similar activities and are also somewhat similar to IFN-β, so that these are collectively referred to as type I interferons. There is only one species of IFN-γ, which is made only by T cells, type II interferon, and is thought to have a central in vivo role in tumor immunotherapy and rejection. The first source of IFN-α for clinical use was from stimulated blood bank–derived leukocytes from which a mixed preparation of IFN-α was purified. This was initially used in attempts to treat viral diseases, but was soon applied to patients with cancer. The first evidence for anticancer activity was seen in patients with renal cancer and chronic myelogenous leukemia (CML). Subsequently, activity was seen against hairy cell leukemia and HIV-associated Kaposi's sarcoma. The objective response rates seen with advanced renal cancer were approximately 10% and complete responses were rare. These findings served primarily to show that cytokine therapy could be active against cancer, but IFN for all these diseases has largely been superseded by other, more effective approaches.

IL-2 was the first cytokine to demonstrate curative outcomes consistently from immunotherapy in patients with widely metastatic cancer. The advent of protein production from recombinant DNA technology has provided the means to test large amounts of this cytokine given systemically. Multiorgan toxicity is observed with high-dose administration, including hypotension, capillary leak, transient hepatic and renal insufficiency, and mental status changes, which are in many ways reminiscent of events in sepsis. Toxicity is managed by judicious limitations on IL-2 dosing, fluid management, and supportive care, because these toxicities are almost always self-limiting and fully reversible. In experienced hands, the treatment-related mortality of high-dose IL-2 should be no more than 1%, with some investigators describing more than 800 consecutive courses given, with no deaths.[13] Initial studies of IL-2 included tumors of many histologic types, but it soon became apparent that the two most consistently responsive cancers were melanoma and renal cell cancer (RCC). For patients with metastatic disease, the objective response rates (partial and complete) for melanoma and RCC were approximately 15% and 20%, respectively.[14,15] The frequency of response was not remarkable, but it became clear that some of these patients (4% to 7%) would achieve complete regression of widespread disease that have proven to

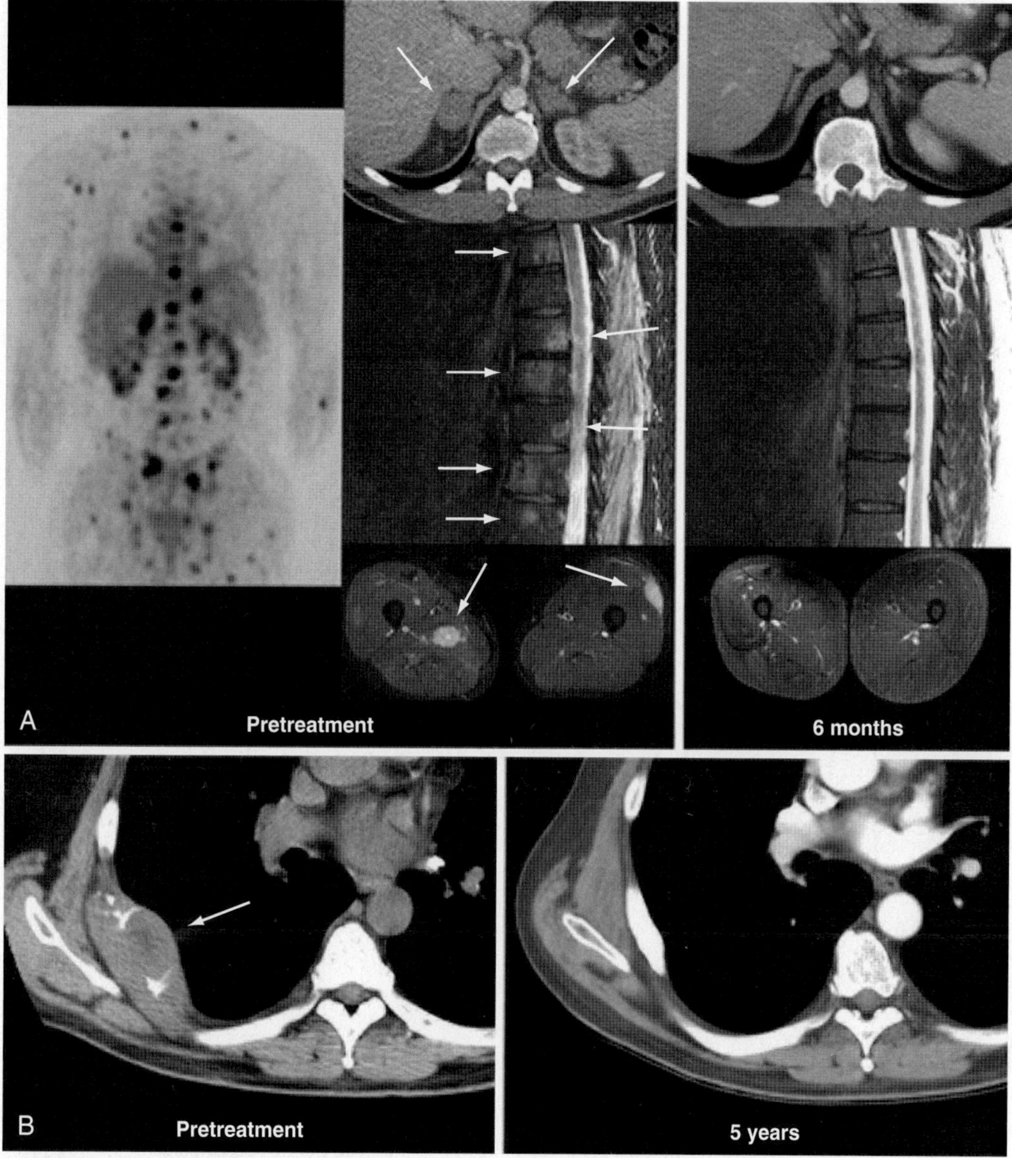


**FIGURE 31-5** Complete responses to high-dose interleukin-2. **A,** Patient with diffuse metastatic melanoma by computed tomography (CT) *(left)* and PET scanning who received high-dose IL-2 therapy and had complete regression of all measurable disease, which is still ongoing 2 years later. **B,** Patient with multiple bone metastases from RCC, with a complete response sustained 5 years later.

be durable more than 20 years later (Fig. 31-5).[16,17] The ability to cure widely metastatic solid tumors with any systemic treatment is rare, with a few exceptions. However, for patients with RCC and melanoma, those achieving a complete response rarely relapsed (Fig. 31-6). Despite much investigation, there are few predictors of patients who will respond to IL-2. For patients with metastatic clear cell renal cancer, two randomized studies have suggested that high dose IL-2 regimens produce higher response rates (21% to 23% partial and complete responses with high-dose treatments versus 10% to 13% with lower dose regimens) and more durable responses than low-dose regimens, but were underpowered to evaluate differences in overall survival.[18]

There have been numerous attempts to combine cytokines with other biologic or chemotherapeutic agents to improve efficacy. One in common use is melanoma-specific chemotherapy followed by IL-2, often termed *biochemotherapy.* Using combinations of cisplatin, vinblastine, and dacarbazine (DTIC) with IL-2 and IFN-α, investigators reported early phase II data suggesting an augmented response rate over IL-2 or chemotherapy alone in patients with metastatic melanoma. Subsequent randomized trials against IL-2 alone or chemotherapy alone have varied on whether response rates are augmented with biochemotherapy but, in general, have failed to show any survival benefit and demonstrated increased toxicity from the combination. Combinations of IL-2 and IFN had a similar history, with increased toxicity and possibly augmented responses in phase II trials, but without confirmation of synergy with these two agents in subsequent randomized studies.

Use of biologic therapies in the adjuvant setting after complete resection of high-risk local regional melanoma remains controversial. The U.S. Food and Drug Administration (FDA) has approved the use of high-dose IFN-α (1 month of maximal

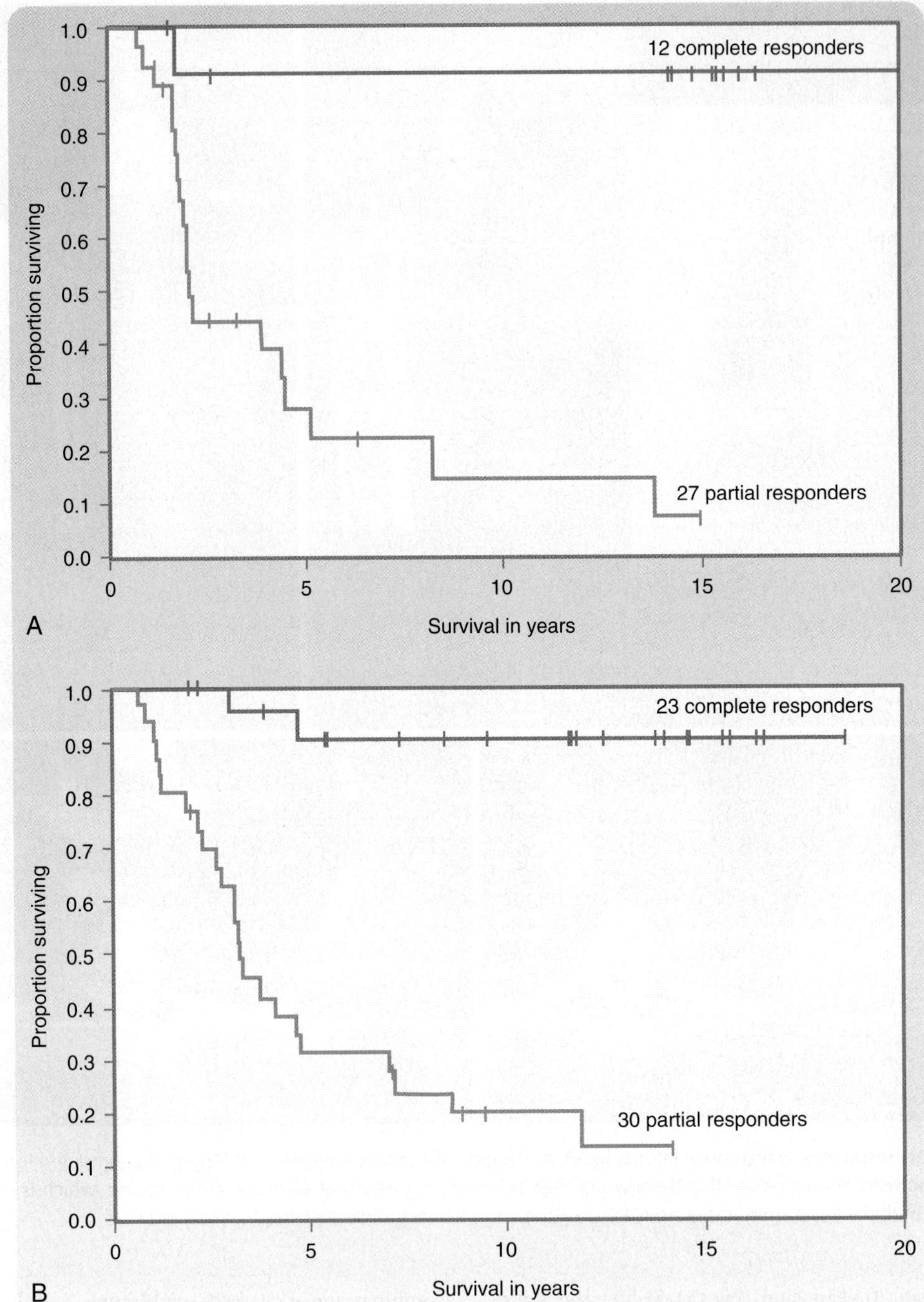


**FIGURE 31-6** Overall survival with long-term follow-up of patients with metastatic melanoma **(A)** and renal cancer **(B)** responding to IL-2. Complete responses to high-dose interleukin-2 in these two malignancies are very durable, whereas partially responding patients typically relapse, although many experience substantial benefit.

dose IV therapy followed by 11 months of lower dose SC treatment) after resection of node-positive melanoma, based on a randomized prospective study showing a delay in time to progression and borderline improved overall survival. In subsequent follow-up, the survival benefit in the original study was no longer significant and a larger randomized study showed delayed time to progression, with no survival benefit.[19] Underpowered attempts to demonstrate a benefit of adjuvant IL-2 administration for high-risk melanoma have never suggested a benefit. This may not be surprising, because a drug that achieves dramatic regressions in a small minority of patients in the metastatic setting may require enormous studies to evaluate it properly in the adjuvant setting.

Several other cytokines are highly promising. IL-15 is a T cell growth factor, but it also inhibits antigen-induced cell death of T cells, in contrast to IL-2. It is made by DCs and macrophages and is necessary for the maintenance of $CD8^+$ memory cells and NK cell development. IL-15 could potentially be used as an adjuvant for vaccines and to support adoptive T cell therapy. IL-7 is another T cell growth factor; T cells expanding in a lymphopenic environment require IL-7 for homeostatic expansion. IL-7 is required for T cell development and causes dramatic increases in total body $CD4^+$ and $CD8^+$ T cells when administered to human subjects. IL-7 could potentially be used as a vaccine adjuvant and in support of adoptive cell therapy. Flt 3 ligand (Flt3L) is a hematopoietic growth factor that induces the expansion and differentiation of DC progenitors. Administration of Flt3L to human subjects increases DC numbers in peripheral blood, lymph nodes, and even tumors. Flt3L could potentially be used in combination with vaccines, adoptive cell therapy, and DC mobilization. IL-12 promotes cytokine release, particularly IFN-γ, from T cells and NK cells and induces TH1 polarization. As a stand-alone drug, IL-12 has significant toxicity and only modest antitumor activity, but may prove to be an effective vaccine adjuvant or enhancer of T cell transfer.

## Vaccines

Successful presentation of a peptide epitope on an MHC molecule does not automatically result in a brisk T cell response. To initiate a good T cell response, an antigen must be presented to the immune system along with appropriate costimulatory molecules (signal 2, where the peptide MHC complex is signal 1) or they may be rendered anergic instead of reactive. The CD28 receptor usually serves this coreceptor function, although other mechanisms exist. Another important principle is that even well-presented unmutated self-proteins are weak immunogens because of the presence of central tolerance. This is a protective mechanism wherein immune responses to these proteins are attenuated by deletion of the most avid self-reactive T cell clones in the thymus during T cell development, presumably to avoid autoimmunity. Thus, the proteins of greatest usefulness in general vaccine approaches (shared, unmutated, tumor-associated antigens) may be the weakest immunogens because high-avidity T cells against these normal cellular proteins have been deleted on the thymus.

Early cancer vaccine strategies used autologous or allogeneic cell-based vaccines. These efforts were based on science generated in the early 1950s using carcinogen-induced murine tumor models. Whole-cell vaccines contain multiple antigens, which could be cross-presented by host antigen-presenting cells (DCs) whose function could be further enhanced with an adjuvant. Vaccine formulations generally incorporated nonspecific immune-activating adjuvant agents. Older adjuvants include alum and the tuberculosis vaccine BCG (Bacille Calmette-Guérin). Other adjuvants such as imiquimod or unmethylated CG dinucleotides (CpG ODN) activate pattern recognition receptors such as TLRs, found on professional antigen-presenting cells (DCs). Another effect of these adjuvants was the prolonged release of antigen from a tissue depot to provide a chronic source of immune stimulation. The results of these whole tumor cell vaccines trials have been disappointing. The largest study to date involved an allogeneic cancer vaccine using three melanoma cell lines (Canvaxin) in patients with stage III or resected stage IV melanoma. More than 1000 patients were randomized to receive allogeneic melanoma cells incorporated in BCG or BCG alone after surgery. The study was closed prematurely; not only was there no improvement in survival, but there appeared to be a borderline survival disadvantage in the experimental melanoma vaccine arm.

A modification of whole cell tumor vaccines is the use of tumor cells genetically engineered to produce cytokines with the goal of dramatically improving immunogenicity. The use of viral vectors to introduce granulocyte macrophage-colony stimulating factor (GM-CSF; or perhaps other cytokines such as IL-7 or IL-12) into tumor cells provides a tumor cell vaccine that attracts professional antigen-presenting cells to the vaccine injection site. These recruited DCs have enhanced antigen uptake with cross-presentation to both T and B cells. Autologous and allogeneic GM-CSF modified tumor vaccines have been studied and have been found to be safe and effective in eliciting T cell and antibody responses to define tumor antigens. However, an improvement in survival in metastatic disease when compared with or added to standard therapy was not observed in recently conducted randomized trials.

The identification of tumor rejection antigens has allowed epitope mapping to determine specific peptide sequences presented by MHC class I and class II molecules to antigen-reactive $CD8^+$ and $CD4^+$ T cells, respectively. Presenting these individual peptides to the immune system incorporated with adjuvants or pulsed onto ex vivo prepared DCs represents the next refinement in vaccine strategies. The former strategy, using adjuvants, requires that these peptides find their way to antigen-presenting cells in vivo, where they can be presented in an immunostimulatory context. A number of clinical trials, primarily in patients with melanoma, but also with breast, colon, lung, or hepatocellular cancer, have shown that these peptide-based vaccines can expand tumor antigen peptide epitope-reactive T cells and produce occasional clinical responses.

Because the proximal event in the induction of an adaptive antitumor immune response is antigen presentation through DCs, there has been considerable clinical trial activity using ex vivo generated DC populations loaded with tumor antigen and then administered as a cell-based vaccine. The most common strategy has been to load tumor peptide antigens onto the surface of DCs by using high peptide concentrations to displace endogenous peptide on DC surface MHC molecules. These DCs are generated from human subjects by retrieving peripheral blood mononuclear cells and differentiating them in cell culture using GM-CSF and IL-4. After 1 week of culture, these monocyte precursors differentiate into immature DCs, which have a high capacity to take up antigen. These DCs can be further differentiated using additional maturation signals, such as endotoxin, CD40L or TNF-α, where they have much higher immunostimulatory properties. Many clinical trials have been conducted with peptide-loaded DCs, both immature and mature, and have consistently demonstrated expansion of antigen-reactive T cells with a low but reproducible clinical response rate.

Other strategies for delivering tumor antigen to DC populations have been studied experimentally and in clinical trial settings.[20] These include providing DCs with whole protein, apoptotic tumor cells or DNA or RNA-based vectors encoding tumor-associated antigens (see Fig. 31-4). Although all these approaches have the potential to allow DCs to process and present a number of antigenic epitopes to the immune system in the context of class I and class II with enhanced immunogenicity, improvement in the low baseline clinical response rate (5% to 7%) has not been observed.

Prostate cancer has historically not been viewed as an immunologically responsive tumor. Several phase III immunotherapy trials have been conducted in patients with metastatic castrate-resistant prostate cancer using an autologous monocyte-based vaccine loaded with a prostatic acid phosphatase–GM-CSF fusion protein. This cell-based vaccine appeared to improve median survival to a level of statistical significance and will undoubtedly renew interest in DC-based clinical vaccine approaches.

DNA-based vaccines represent another way to stimulate immune responses in patients.[21] The simplest method is the direct injection of plasmid DNA with a promoter-enhancer sequence driving expression of the tumor antigen. IM injection of plasmid DNA results in its being taken up by myocytes. In animals, plasmid DNA has been shown to reside episomally for extended periods and to express low levels of tumor antigen protein. The local tissue damage creates danger signals, which attract professional antigen-presenting cells. These take up the tumor antigen being expressed, which is then processed and cross-presented to the immune system. Weak immunity to self-antigens can be significantly enhanced with the incorporation of certain cytokines or chemokine genes whose paracrine production attracts larger numbers of antigen-presenting cells and provides for their further maturation.

However, the most effective DNA vaccines that have been studied clinically involve the incorporation of genes encoding tumor-associated antigens into recombinant viral vectors. Use of recombinant poxviruses such as vaccinia and adenoviral vectors generate significantly higher levels of transgene expression, creating a more robust proinflammatory environment and resulting in higher levels of activation of antigen-reactive T cells. These two viruses can be hampered by preexisting immunity to the viral vector because of remote exposure, so other studies have been using avian poxviruses not typically seen before and not replication-competent in humans. Still, any immunogenic vector cannot be used repeatedly, so prime boost vaccination strategies, incorporating plasmid or DC priming to generate starting populations of specific T cells and then switching to a recombinant viral boost, may prove more effective.

Ideally, antigen should be delivered to DC cells in a specific manner, which can be accomplished with antibodies (that target specific DC receptors) or recombinant viral vectors (that have altered tropism achieved by pseudotyping their envelopes). These DC-specific in vivo DNA vaccines could include more than one tumor antigen and potentially proinflammatory or costimulatory genes in their payload. DNA cancer vaccines that can be directly administered to human subjects have the obvious advantage of being off the shelf reagents, which obviates the labor-intensive step of ex vivo cell manipulation.

The vigorous application of vaccination against cancer-associated antigens has led to modest success in causing cancer regression. Dozens of vaccine approaches against dozens of target antigens in hundreds of clinical trials have largely been unsuccessful against measurable metastatic disease. Many trials have reported infrequent anecdotal responses, primarily in patients with melanoma confined to the skin and nodal sites, which appear to be somewhat more amenable to immunotherapy in general. A review of over 1200 patients vaccinated for cancer reported an overall objective response rate of 3.6%.[22] In many cases, analyses of these trials have shown that there is little evidence for the generation of significant numbers of new tumor-reactive T cells. Even in cases in which large populations of antigen-reactive T cells were generated by vigorous vaccination schedules in patients with no documented recurrence, patients still relapsed with tumors that continued to express antigen and the appropriate MHC molecule. This broad clinical experience reinforces the view that a better understanding of basic immune biology is needed to overcome these limitations of cancer vaccine therapies.

### Immunomodulatory Strategies

Recent clinical experience has validated that some tumors survive immunologic rejection because of cell immunosuppressive factors. Murine data have demonstrated that a wealth of mechanisms exist to suppress or curtail immune responses appropriately to avoid toxicity (e.g., autoimmunity) or conserve immunologic resources. These include a requirement for two signals to initiate most immune responses successfully, the existence of Treg cells, and a host of inhibitory receptors on T cells that are induced by chronic or maximal stimuli. Mice with genetic knockouts for many of these pathways show fatal or debilitating autoimmunity or lymphoproliferation. It has also been recently shown that within the tumor microenvironment, with its chronic antigenic stimuli, many of these mechanisms are active.

However, the first compelling data that such factors have clinical significance was only obtained in 2003, when a blocking antibody to the inhibitory receptor CTLA-4 was first given to patients with metastatic melanoma. This receptor binds to the same ligands (B7) as a positive T cell costimulatory receptor, CD28, yet its function is to inhibit T cell responses (Fig. 31-7). CTLA-4 expression is induced in response to successful T cell stimulation and mice congenitally lacking CTLA-4 die of overwhelming lymphocytosis. In a proportion of patients with melanoma, CTLA-4 blocking antibody induced objective tumor regression, with some patients achieving complete responses, now maintained beyond 5 years (Figs. 31-8 and 31-9). A subset

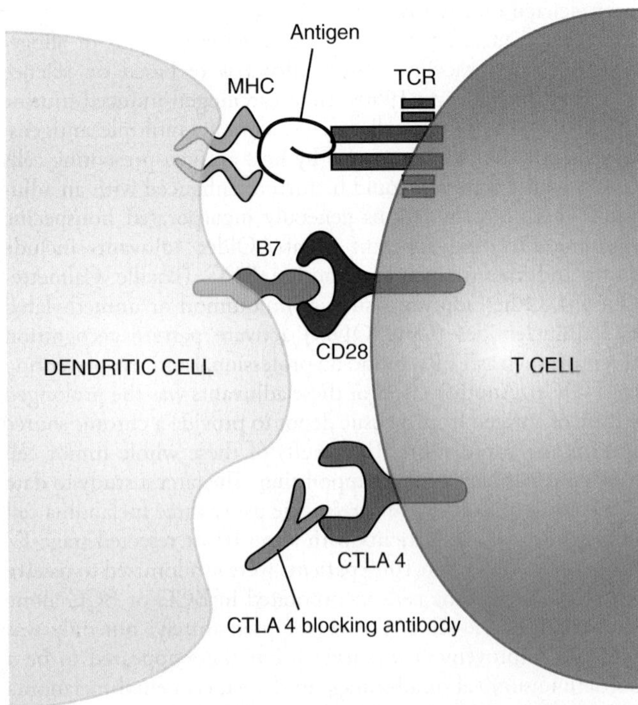


**FIGURE 31-7** Interruption of CTLA-4 downregulatory signaling by CTLA-4 blocking antibody.

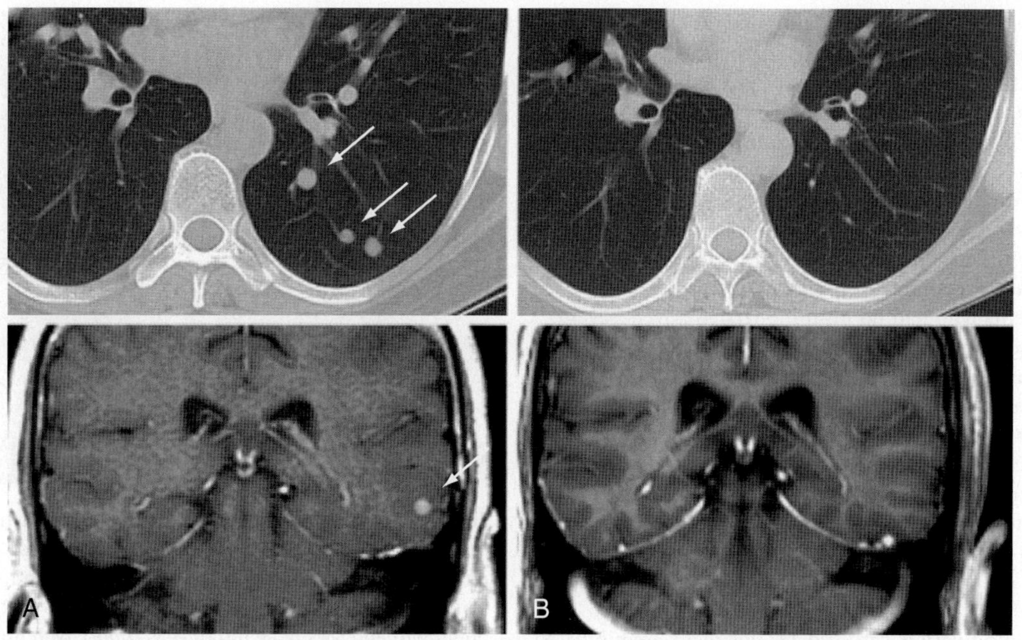


**FIGURE 31-8** Regression of lung and brain metastases from melanoma in a patient treated with ipilimumab (anti–CTLA-4 antibody). **A,** Patient with lung, subcutaneous, and brain metastases received ipilimumab and showed tumor progression at 6 weeks. **B,** He then developed immune-mediated hypopituitarism and had a complete regression of all disease, which is ongoing 7 years later.

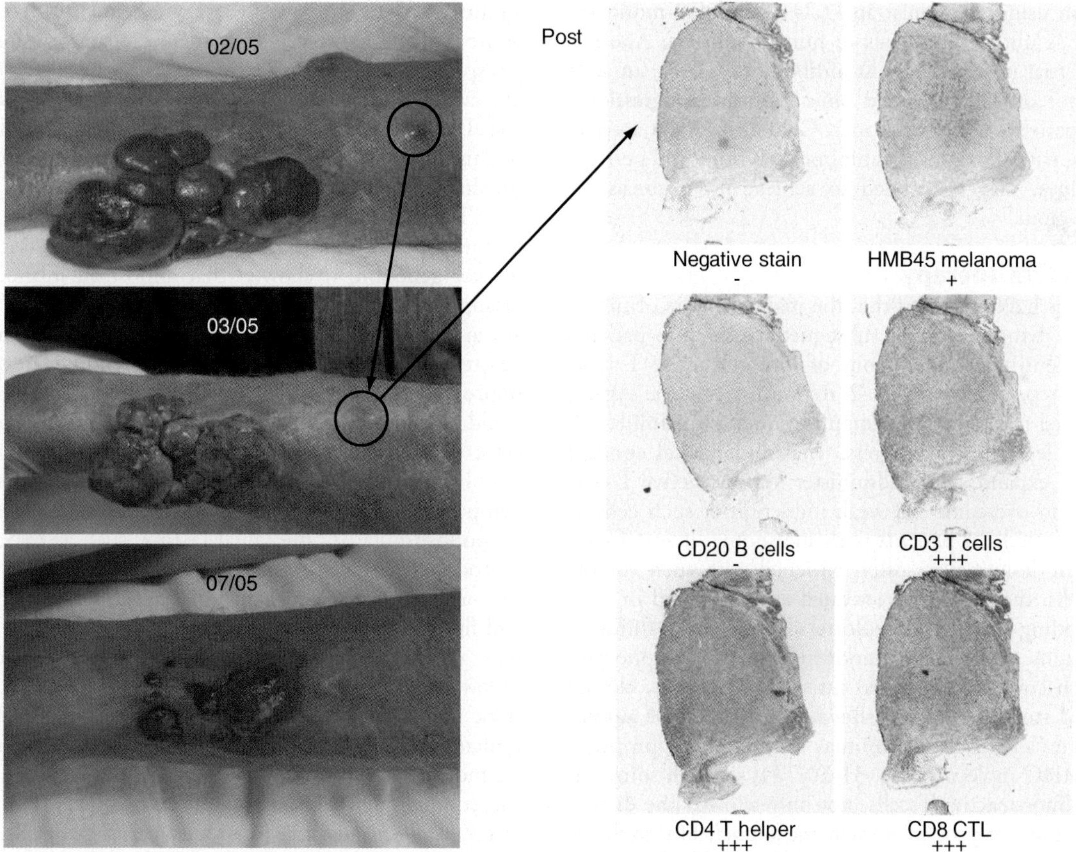


**FIGURE 31-9** Partial regression of metastatic melanoma induced by CTLA-4 blockade accompanied by dense infiltration of immune effector cells. (Adapted from Ribas A, Comin-Anduix B, Economou JS, et al: Intratumoral immune cell infiltrates, FoxP3, and indoleamine 2,3-dioxygenase in patients with melanoma undergoing CTLA4 blockade. Clin Cancer Res 15:390–399, 2009.)

of patients given CTLA-4 blocking antibody developed autoimmune adverse events, including colitis, dermatitis, and endocrinopathies, and there was an association between the development of these adverse events and the likelihood of an objective tumor response. In 139 patients with melanoma given CTLA-4 antibody, most in combination with a peptide vaccination, the overall response rate (partial responses and complete responses [PR + CR]) was 17%; there was a 28% response rate among those 50 patients experiencing a severe grade 3 or 4 adverse event, including all complete responders, versus a 2% response rate in 53 patients who had no immune-related adverse event.[23] In a small phase II trial, responses were also seen in patients with renal cancer, but consistent objective tumor regressions have yet to be documented for other tumor types. Therefore, in cancers with proven immunogenicity, immunologic inhibition mediated by CTLA-4 seems to be one mechanism preventing tumor rejection in some patients. With the wealth of new inhibitory mechanisms purported to be capable of constraining antitumor immunity, this field seems poised for progress, particularly using combinations of agents to overcome redundant tolerogenic pathways.

Immune modulation can also be positively manipulated by stimulation of coreceptors, which enhances immunity. 4-1BB (CD137) is a receptor-like protein expressed on $CD4^+$ and $CD8^+$ T cells after activation; cross linking 4-1BB with a ligand or antibody delivers a costimulatory signal to the T cell. Preclinical animal studies have demonstrated enhanced tumor rejection in established tumor models. This strategy for immunomodulation using an agonist anti-CD137 human monoclonal antibody is undergoing trials in human subjects. Another early clinical trial using an agonist antibody to CD40, an activating receptor on DCs, showed objective tumor regressions, again all in patients with melanoma. Combining such activating strategies, with blocking of inhibitory receptors and perhaps adding vaccines, may be needed to achieve more consistent clinical regressions.

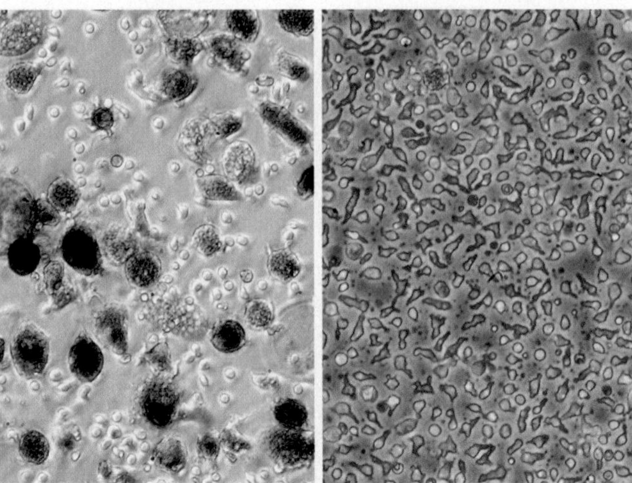

**FIGURE 31-10** Outgrowth of TILs from resected metastatic melanoma in culture with IL-2. Photomicrograph of fresh melanoma after enzymatic dispersal *(left)* showing tumor cells and small infiltrating lymphocytes. After several weeks of culture in IL-2, there is T cell outgrowth and lysis of all tumor cells *(right)*, with most cultures then demonstrating immunologic recognition of HLA-appropriate tumor cells on in vitro assay.

## T Cell Adoptive Therapy

Murine models have indicated that the main effectors of tumor rejection are T lymphocytes, so subsequent research in patients focused on identifying populations of tumor reactive T lymphocytes from patients with IL-2 responsive cancers. Again, the unexplained tendency for human melanoma to stimulate T cell responses led to early progress. The fundamental concept was to isolate, expand, and readminister tumor-reactive T cells as the means to overcome the weak induction of such cells in vivo by vaccination. In patients with melanoma, it was found that metastatic lesions were often enriched with such tumor-reactive T cells; they could be activated and expanded in vitro simply by adding IL-2 to the culture medium. Two thirds of resected lesions contained tumor-infiltrating lymphocytes (TILs), which could be expanded into T cell cultures, cleared all cocultured tumor cells, and showed recognition of autologous tumor or allogeneic melanomas sharing the appropriate presenting MHC molecule (Fig. 31-10). TILs, a rich source of polyclonal tumor-reactive T cells, not only allowed the discovery of numerous antigens in human melanoma, but could be used directly for adoptive transfer of autologous T cell populations for therapy. The initial attempt at such an approach used huge numbers of cells grown in vitro (a median of $2 \times 10^{11}$ cells was given) and concomitant high-dose systemic IL-2 was administered to support TIL survival and in vivo function.[24] Some patients also received a single preparatory dose of cyclophosphamide based on empirical murine data. An overall objective response rate of 33% was seen, and was not influenced by prior IL-2 failure. However, the major shortcoming of this study was that most responses were of short duration (median, 7 months).

The first protocol administering genetically modified cells to patients was used to track TILs after administration using a marker gene and it showed that almost all infused TILs had disappeared from the circulation within days.[25,26] The next advance was the finding that lymphodepleting the recipient before adoptive transfer could enhance lymphocyte survival and improve T cell persistence. Murine models suggest that this could be caused by the following: (1) removal of suppressive Treg cells; (2) stimulation of T cell growth factors in response to lymphodepletion (homeostatic proliferation); (3) reduction in competition for these homeostatic cytokines; and (4) increased immunostimulatory microbial factors, such as LPS. In clinical protocols, a reduced intensity, nonmyeloablative allotransplant regimen was used, consisting of high-dose cyclophosphamide and fludarabine. When peripheral leukocyte counts were essentially zero, a median of $5 \times 10^{10}$ cultured TILs were given, again followed by systemic IL-2 support. In 43 patients with metastatic melanoma, an overall response rate of 49% was seen, and updated results have shown a median duration of response of 13 months; 14% of responses were sustained at 4 years.[27] Two subsequent cohorts of 25 patients each added 200 or 1200 cGy of total body irradiation (with autologous stem cell support) to the preparative regimen prior to TIL infusion and objective response rates of 52% and 72% were seen[28] (Figs. 31-11 and 31-12). In these 93 total patients, of whom 86% had metastatic visceral tumor involvement and 84% had prior IL-2, the

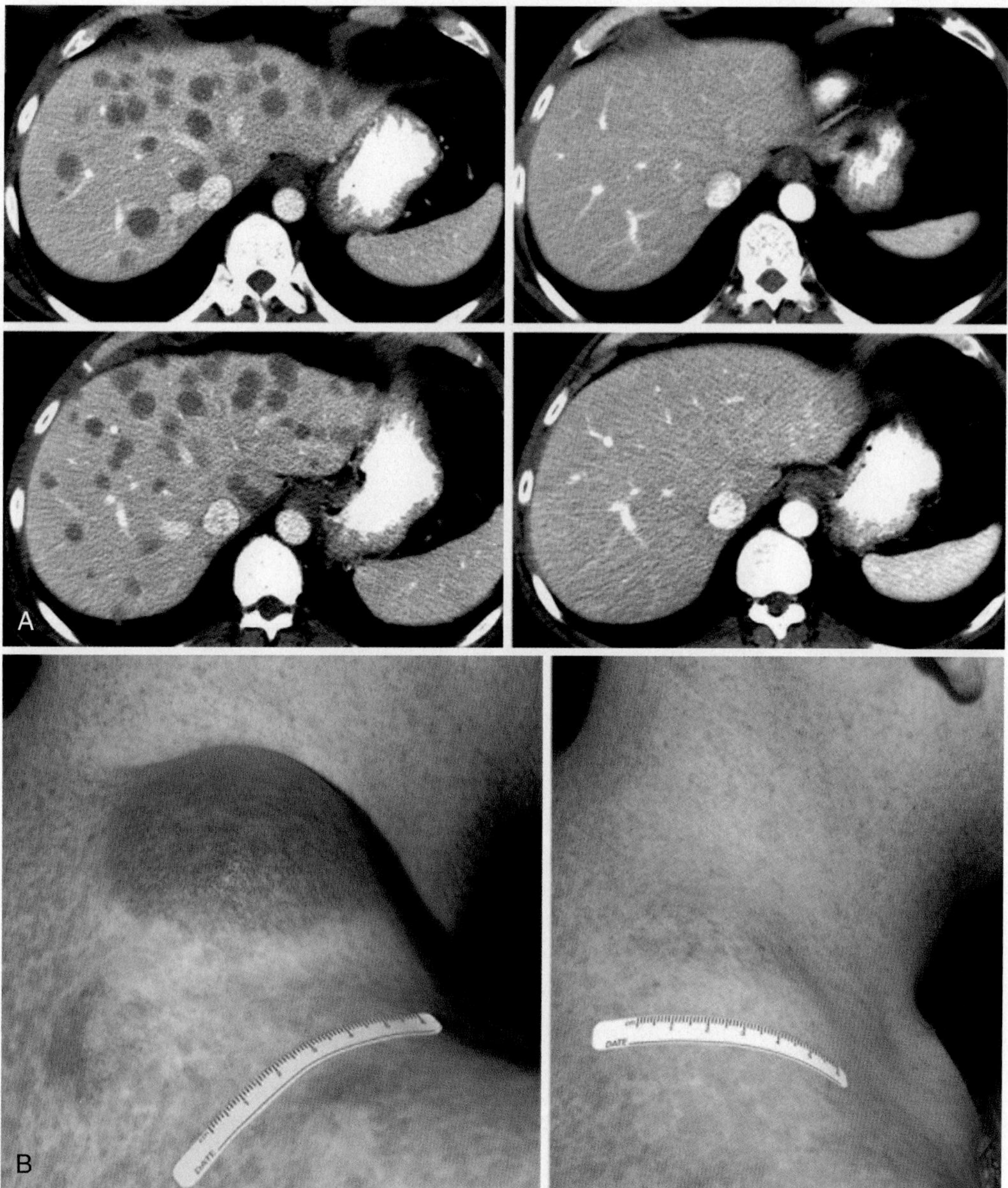

**FIGURE 31-11** Clinical responses in patients with metastatic melanoma to adoptive transfer of in vitro expanded TILs with systemic IL-2, following preparative lymphodepletion. Responses can be durable and rapid. **A,** Patient with extensive liver disease remains free of disease over 5 years after one T cell transfer. **B,** Another patient showed rapid regression of bulky subcutaneous disease only 12 days after cell transfer, sustaining a complete response, currently at 4 years.

estimated 3-year actuarial survival was 34%, with 22% of all patients achieving complete regressions (Fig. 31-13). Another report of the transfer of a $CD4^+$ T cell clone, generated in vitro from peripheral blood and reactive with the tumor testis antigen NY-ESO-1, to a patient with melanoma described a complete response of over 2 years' duration, documenting that other T cell populations may also have efficacy in adoptive transfer.

Ongoing efforts in T cell adoptive transfer include the genetic engineering of T cells to express high-affinity TCRs specific for defined tumor antigens.[29] This can be accomplished using retroviral vectors encoding the α and β TCR chains, or single chimeric receptors (CARs). Preliminary clinical trials (Fig. 31-14) have demonstrated that objective tumor regressions can be achieved with these genetically engineered T cells.[30,31]

## Monoclonal Antibody Therapy

The concept of the immune system providing targeted therapy in the treatment of disease has its origins in experiments performed in 1890 by von Behring and Kitasato. They determined that immunity to infectious diseases could be transferred from one rat to the next through a serum transfusion; they coined the term *passive serotherapy.* The first application of passive serotherapy in the treatment of cancer was performed in 1895 by Hericourt and Richet when they immunized dogs with human sarcoma and transferred the serum to patients in an attempt to provide cancer immunity. After almost 100 years since the first cancer immunotherapy trial, the FDA approved the first monoclonal antibody (mAb) to be used in the treatment of cancer. Today, therapeutic mAbs are considered to be the fastest growing

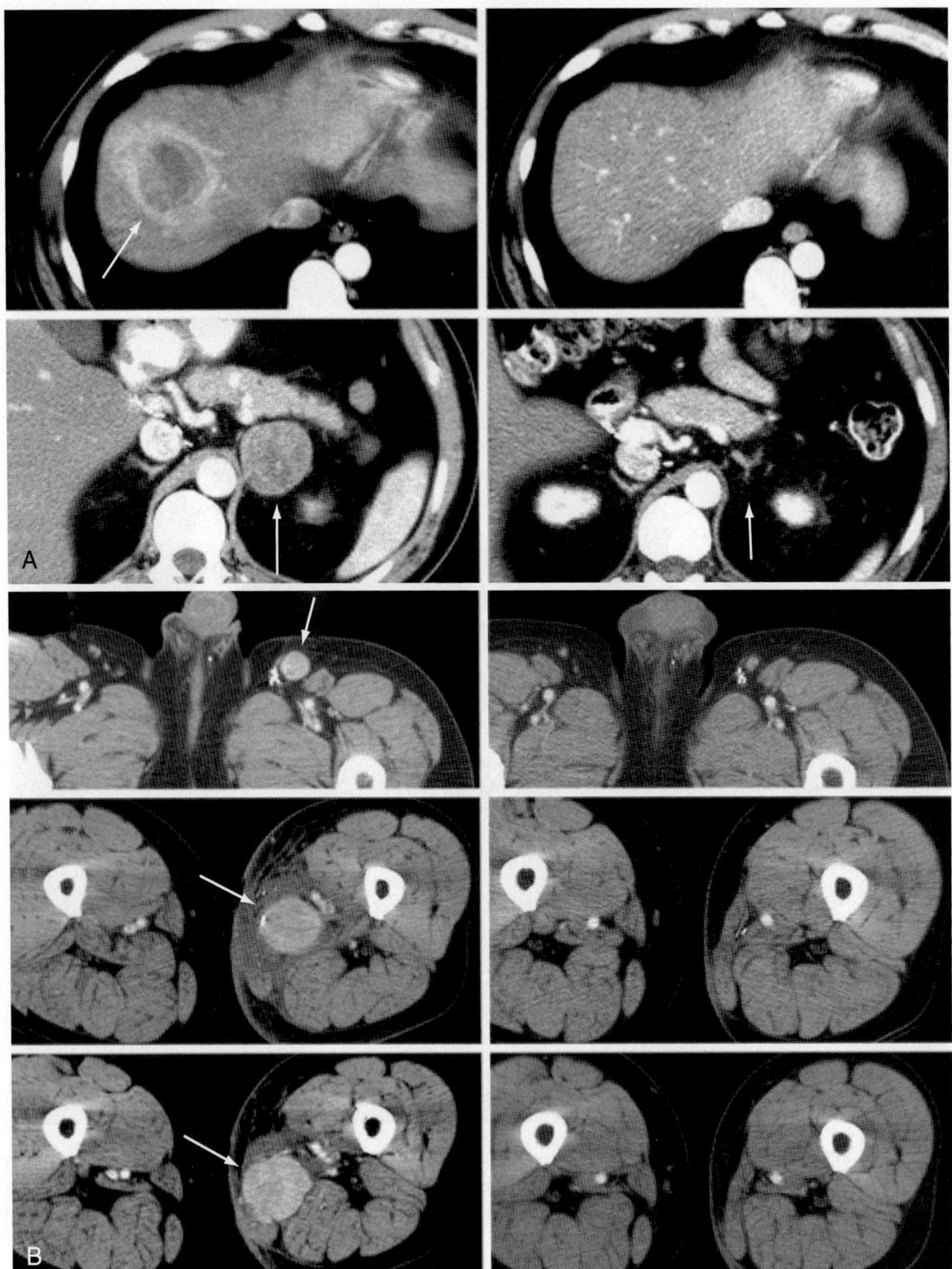


**FIGURE 31-12** Almost all sites of metastatic melanoma can respond to adoptive cell transfer. Single adoptive transfers into two patients with liver and adrenal metastases **(A)** and nodal and intramuscular metastases **(B)** have resulted in ongoing complete regressions at 38 and 33 months, respectively.

class of new therapeutic agents. Although many had predicted the therapeutic potential of mAbs over the past century, it wasn't until mouse hybridoma technology was developed by Kohler and Milstein in 1975 that the ability to produce mAbs directed against a specific target antigen became a reality.[32,33]

Unfortunately, mAbs created from mouse hybridoma technology were specific but limited in their therapeutic potential secondary to xenogeneic reasons. First, they are recognized by the immune system as foreign and stimulate the production of ***h***uman ***a***nti-***m***ouse ***a***ntibodies, commonly referred to as the HAMA response. This immunogenic response usually limits murine mAbs to a single dose. Secondly, murine mAbs are unable to activate other effector functions (e.g., complement, NK cells, phagocytes) of the human immune system. Finally, murine mAbs suffer from a much reduced serum half-life when compared with human antibodies, resulting in decreased time of exposure to the target antigen. To overcome many of these limitations, molecular engineering techniques were developed to generate antibodies in

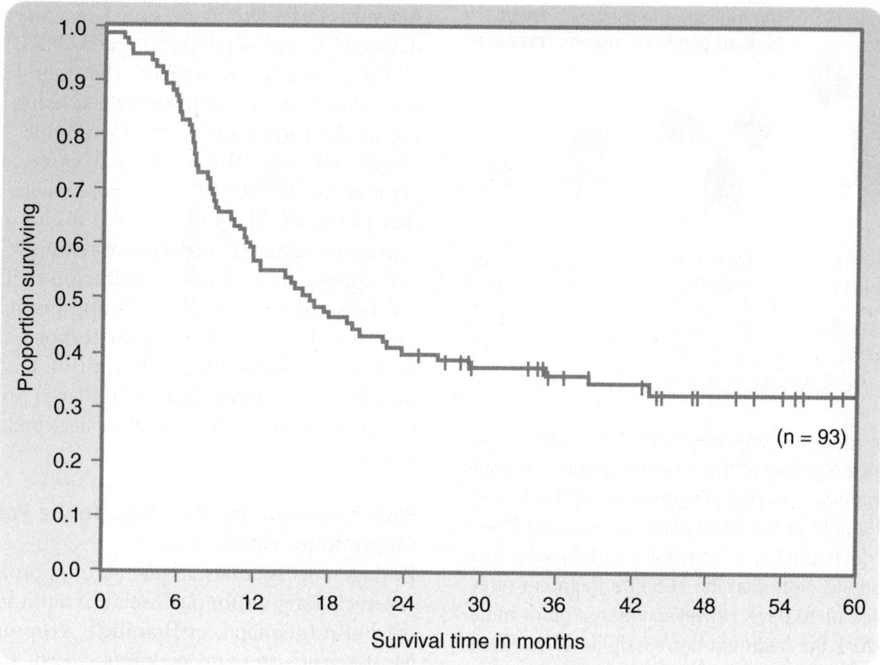


**FIGURE 31-13** Overall survival of 93 patients with metastatic melanoma (86% with visceral metastases) given TILs and IL-2 after preparative lymphodepletion. Estimated actuarial survival at 3 and 5 years are 36% and 32%, respectively.

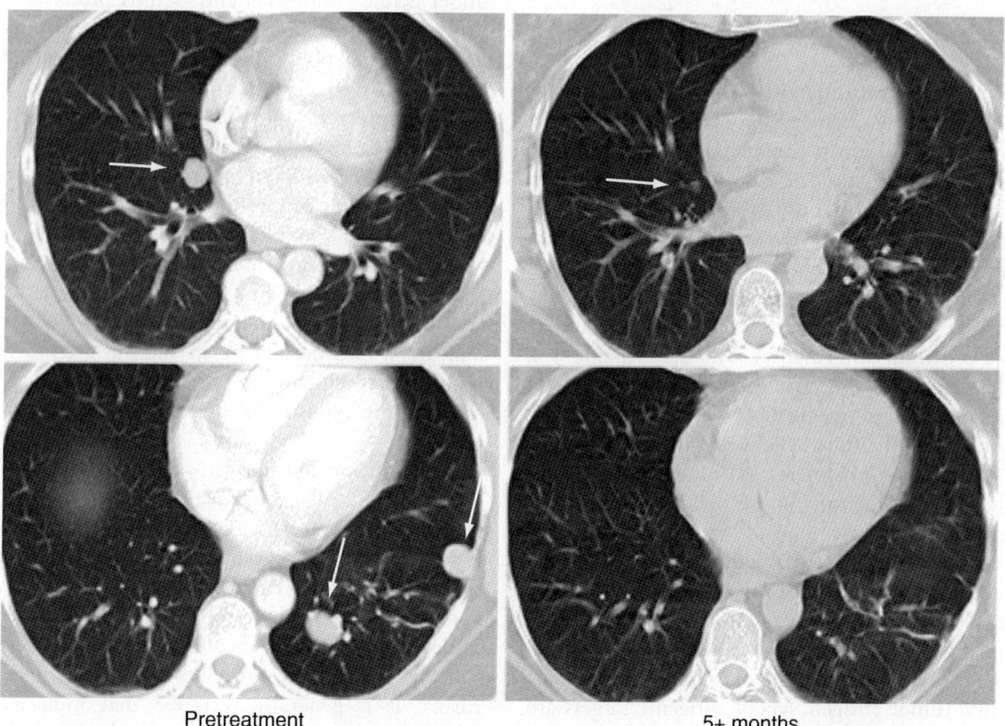


**FIGURE 31-14** Patient with metastatic melanoma responding to MART melanoma antigen TCR-engineered T cell adoptive immunotherapy.

which the murine sequences were partially or fully replaced by human protein sequences. A chimeric mAb refers to a murine antibody in which the variable regions responsible for the antigen specificity remain murine and the constant region (Fc) is replaced by human sequences. A humanized mAb refers to an mAb created by engrafting murine complementarity-determining regions (CDRs) onto a human mAb variable region. Most recently, fully human antibodies have been produced via human hybridomas and transgenic mice expressing human immunoglobulin genes.[34] Also, engineered mAb fragments have been developed and characterized that have unique pharmacokinetic and therapeutic properties (Fig. 31-15).[35,36]

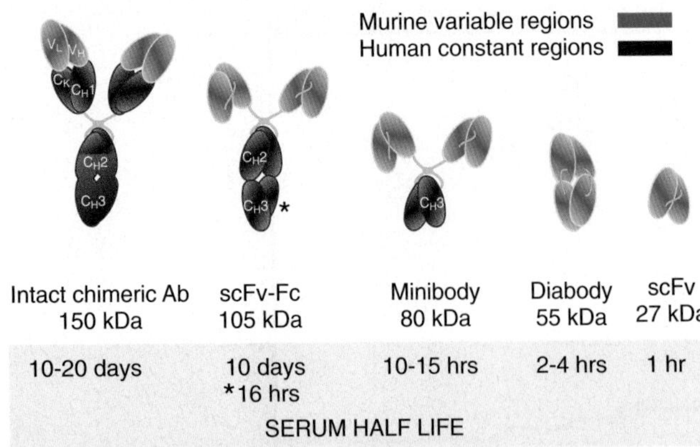


**FIGURE 31-15** Chimeric mAb and engineered Ab fragments. A chimeric intact mAb is depicted, showing the retained murine domains *(green)* and human domains *(purple).* Engineered antibody fragments are depicted to the right of the intact chimeric antibody. These fragments are listed in decreasing size from right to left, with their corresponding serum half-life. Note that the 105-kDa fragment (scFv-Fc) normally has a half-life of 10 days. However, when a point mutation is introduced *(red star),* the fragment has a half-life of 16 hours, comparable to the much smaller 80-kDa minibody fragment. This is the result of a point mutation introduced into the FcRn binding region in the $C_{H3}$ domain, which decreases the fragments affinity for the FcRn, resulting in a much decreased serum half-life.

mAbs account for approximately 25% of new biotech (genetically-engineered) drugs in development. To date, the FDA has approved over 21 mAb fragments to treat various diseases, such as cancer, autoimmune diseases, and transplant rejection, with many more currently in clinical trials (Table 31-1). The U.S. Adopted Name Council, in collaboration with the World Health Organization (WHO) International Nonproprietary Names Committee, has established guidelines for the naming of new mABs. Each name is comprised of four syllables, with each syllable providing information. The first syllable is a unique prefix; the second syllable describes the indication. For example, all mAbs intended to treat tumors will have the second syllable of -tu- for *tu*mor. The third syllable identifies the source of the antibody (murine, -o-; chimeric, -xi-; human, -u-). The last syllable is always -mab identifying the therapeutic agent as a monoclonal antibody.

To highlight the clinical potential and challenges to mAb therapeutics, the remaining portion of this section will describe mAb therapy as it pertains to cancer.[37,38] The mechanism of action used by mAbs in the fight against cancer can be divided into two types. The first results from the physical binding of the mAb to the specific tumor antigen. Many antigenic targets are cell surface receptors connected to signaling pathways, which are important in cancer progression. The best example of this is trastuzumab (Herceptin), which blocks signaling through an overexpressed growth factor receptor (Her2/neu) in a subset of breast cancers. Second, and perhaps more important, a mAb directed against a tumor antigen can activate the patient's own immune system to attack the tumor tissue. This mechanism is mediated through interactions of the Fc region of the antibody and effector cells of the immune system bearing the Fcγ receptor, such as natural killer cells, phagocytes, and neutrophils. Activation of these professional phagocytes leads to tumor cell destruction and is referred to as ADCC.[39] Also, the Fc domain of the antibody can activate the complement system through interactions with complement-activating protein (C1q), resulting in the formation of the membrane attack complex, which causes cell lysis. This is referred to as complement-dependent cytotoxicity (CDC). Furthermore, there is mounting evidence that mAbs are likely to enhance tumor antigen (TA) presentation by professional antigen-presenting cells such as DCs, which may ultimately lead to the induction of TA-specific cytotoxic T cell responses and result in lasting immunity. Amplification of the immune response to other tumor antigens may also occur because it is likely after ADCC or CDC that many tumor peptides have the opportunity to undergo professional antigen presentation, with the potential of also inciting a cytotoxic T cell response.[40,41]

### Factors Governing the Therapeutic Potential of Monoclonal Antibodies

Endogenous IgG has a half-life of approximately 3 weeks. This relatively long serum persistence is a result of its interaction with the FcRn (neonatal, or Brambell, receptor) on endothelial cells. Most serum proteins are pinocytosed, followed by progressive acidification of the endosome, which eventually fuses with a lysosome and results in the destruction of entrapped proteins. IgG, however, binds the FcRn of the endosomal membrane under acidic conditions and is thus protected from lysosomal degradation; it is shuttled back to the serum and released from FcRn under a physiologic pH (7.4). Site-specific mutagenesis has identified the specific amino acid residues responsible for the Fc-FcRn interaction that leads to the long serum half-life of IgG antibodies. Thus, by introducing specific amino acid changes into the Fc region of an engineered antibody, one can tailor the pharmacokinetic properties to fit the clinical or therapeutic indication.[42] For example, by substitution of one amino acid (H310A), the serum half-life of an engineered chimeric mAb fragment was reduced by 90%, from 10 days to 16 hours. One can imagine therapeutic applications in which a shorter serum half-life would be beneficia,l such as a conjugated mAb with toxin or radionuclide in which rapid clearance would serve to decrease the exposure of the normal tissues of the body to the toxin.

Monoclonal antibodies of the IgG subtype are large (150-kDa) proteins. Their relatively large size may limit their ability to penetrate tissues to bind the targeted tumor antigen. It is estimated that the average intervessel distance in tumors is approximately 40 to 100 μM. Obviously, in hypoxic areas of a tumor, this distance is probably increased. Therefore, a smaller molecule will be able to diffuse or penetrate further and more quickly. Also, small molecules have different clearance mechanisms. It is generally accepted that molecules smaller than 80 kDa are below the renal threshold and are able to clear solely through the kidney. To this end, protein engineers have been able to create very small antibody fragments that retain the antigen-binding specificity but no longer retain the ability to bind the FcRn. The smallest of these entities is the single-chain Fv, with a molecular weight of 27 kDa. Many of these fragments, with ultrashort half-lives, are being tested in mouse models for the ability to target tumors for imaging, diagnostics, and potential transport of larger toxic molecules and chemotherapeutic agents to the tumor.

**Table 31-1 FDA-Approved Monoclonal Antibody-Based Therapeutics**

| GENERIC NAME | TRADE NAME | DESCRIPTION | FDA APPROVAL YEAR |
|---|---|---|---|
| Muromonab-CD3 | Orthoclone OKT3 | Murine mAb used to deplete T cells to treat transplant rejection | 1986 |
| Abciximab | ReoPRo | Chimeric mAb targeting ant-GPIIb/IIa to inhibit platelet aggregation | 1994 |
| Imciromab pentetate | Myoscint | Murine Fab fragment against myosin; this mAb fragment is conjugated to diethylenetriamine pentaacetic acid and a radionuclide, indium-111, which is used in nuclear imaging of damaged cardiac muscle. | 1996 |
| Arcitumomab | CEA-Scan | Murine mAb fragment (Fab) targeting CEA expressed on tumor cells and conjugated to radionuclide (technetium-99) used fornuclear imaging of colorectal cancer cells | 1996 |
| Rituximab | Rituxan | Chimer mAb against CD20 expressed on non-Hodgkin's lymphoma cells | 1997 |
| Daclizumab | Zenapax | Humanized mAb targeting anti-CD25 | 1997 |
| Basiliximab | Sumlect | Chimeric mAb targeting anti-CD25 | 1998 |
| Palivizumab | Synagis | Humanized mAb targeting RSV | 1998 |
| Infliximab | Remicade | Chimeric mAb targeting TNF-α | 1998 |
| Trastuzumab | Herceptin | Humanized mAb targeting HER2/neu | 1998 |
| Gemtuzumab-ozgamicin | Mylotarg | Humanized mAb targeting CD33 on tumor cells with conjugated immunotoxin targeting | 2000 |
| Alemtuzumab | Campath-1H | Humanized mAb targeting CD52 of tumor cells | 2001 |
| Ibritumomab-tiuxetan | Zevalin | Murine mAb targeting CD20 with conjugated radionuclide (Yttrium-90) | 2002 |
| Adalimumab | Humira | Human mAb targeting TNF-α in the treatment of autoimmune diseases | 2002 |
| Omalizumab | Xolair | Humanized mAb targeting IgE in the treatment of allergic asthma | 2003 |
| Tositumomab–iodine-131 | Bexxar | Anti-CD20 murine mAb targeting IgG2a antibodies conjugated with radionuclide (iodine-131) used to treat non-Hodgkin's lymphoma | 2003 |
| Efalizumab | Raptiva | Humanized mAb targeting CD11a in the treatment of moderate to severe psoriasis (Immunosuppressant) | 2003 |
| Cetuximab | Erbitux | Chimeric mAb targeting the EGFR expressed on tumor cells | 2004 |
| Bevacizumab | Avastin | Humanized mAb targeting VEGF to decrease angiogenic signaling in tumors | 2004 |
| Natalizumab | Tysabri | Humanized mAb targeting the α4 integrin subunit in the treatment of multiple sclerosis and Crohn's disease | 2004 |
| Ranibizumab | Lucentis | Humanized mAb targeting VEGF-α in the treatment of age-related macular degeneration | 2006 |
| Panitumumab | Vectibix | Human mAb targeting EGFR expressed on tumor cells | 2006 |
| Eculizumab | Soliris | Humanized mAb targeting complement protein C5 in the treatment of paroxysmal nocturnal hemoglobinuria | 2007 |
| Ustekinumab | Slellara | Human mAb targeting cytokines IL-12 and IL-23 in the treatment of plaque psoriasis | 2009 |
| Ofatumumab | Arzerra | Human mAb targeting CD20 and used in the treatment of chronic lymphocytic leukemia and follicular lymphomas | 2009 |
| Tocilizumab | Actemra | Humanized mAb targeting the IL-6 receptor used in the treatment of rheumatoid arthritis (RA) | 2010 |

Compared with traditional chemotherapy, the side effect profile of nonconjugated mAb immunotherapy is rather mild. Most of the toxicity is related to hypersensitivity reactions caused by the protein sequences of mouse origin. Although fatal infusion reactions are rare, they have been reported. These reactions usually occur during or just after the first dose of the mAb. Other side effects may occur as a result of the binding of the mAb to its cognate Ag. For example, cetuximab, a chimeric mAb that binds the epidermal growth factor receptor, is associated with skin eruptions secondary to the blockade of epidermal growth factor receptor signaling. Also, bevacizumab (Avastin), an mAb which binds the VEGF, is associated with hemorrhagic and thrombotic events associated with the decreased signaling through the VEGF receptor (VEGFR).

## Unconjugated Antibodies

As noted, the treatment of disease with unconjugated mAbs became popular in the 1980s, after murine mAbs became available secondary to hybridoma technology. These early therapeutic mAbs suffered from poor clinical efficacy and immunogenicity secondary to HAMA, leading to the termination of most clinical mAb studies. It wasn't until the development of chimeric, humanized, and fully human therapeutic mAbs that clinical efficacy was routinely witnessed in mAb studies. Although many therapeutic mAbs start as murine mAbs, much of the murine antibody is replaced by human IgG protein sequences. For example, a chimeric IgG molecule is approximately 75% human and 25% murine. A humanized murine mAb is approximately 95% human, with only the CDRs of the variable region remaining murine.

Rituximab is an excellent example of the development of an mAb clinically effective against a cancer after transitioning to the chimeric form of the antibody from the parent murine mAb. Rituximab, but not its parent murine mAb, has demonstrated cytotoxicity in experimental systems. Rutiximab is a chimeric mAb directed against a cell surface antigen found on mature B cells of non-Hodgkin's lymphoma (NHL) and was the first mAb to be approved by the FDA, in 1997, for use in the treatment of a human malignancy. Initially, rituximab was used as a single-agent therapy for recurrent or refractory low-grade B cell lymphomas and demonstrated an overall response rate of 48% and a complete response rate of 10%.[43] The cytotoxic activity of rituximab is thought to be a combination of CDC and ADCC; this clarifies the inactivity of the parent murine mAb, which lacks the human Fc region to interact with the serum complement protein (C1q) and the Fcγ receptor of the professional phagocytes to elicit ADCC. Evidence in support of ADCC as the mechanism of action was the finding that Fcγ receptor polymorphisms predict response rates in patients with follicular lymphoma treated with rituximab. With high response rates and limited toxicity in the setting of recurrent or refractory NHL, studies were undertaken to investigate rituximab as a first-line therapy. Initially, rituximab was shown to increase the sensitivity of chemotherapy-resistant cell lines, which spawned a trial of rituximab added to first-line chemotherapy regimen of cyclophosphamide, doxorubicin, vincristine, and prednisolone (CHOP). The addition of rituximab to CHOP, commonly referred to as R-CHOP, resulted in a 95% overall response rate, including a 55% complete response rate. Long-term follow-up revealed a statistically improved survival without significant differences in toxicity.

Trastuzumab is a humanized antibody derived from a murine mAb directed against HER-2/neu. This receptor tyrosine kinase is a member of the epidermal growth factor receptor (EGFR) family, which was noted to be overexpressed because of gene amplification in approximately 25% of breast cancers. Therefore, the strategy was undertaken to target this overexpressed cell surface receptor that was associated with a more aggressive biology in an attempt to disrupt the cancer-promoting mitogenic signaling through antibody blockade of this receptor. Initial phase II trials, conducted in the setting of metastatic HER-2/neu–positive breast cancers, demonstrated modest objective response rates of 12% to 16%. Given the evidence for single-agent activity, further trials were conducted with trastuzumab in combination with standard chemotherapy regimens, which demonstrated a doubling of the response rates (25% to 57%) compared with chemotherapy alone. Additionally, in the adjuvant setting, trastuzumab has been associated with a 50% reduction in 1-year recurrence rates in phase III trials.[44,45] The mechanism of action responsible for the response rates of trastuzumab in the treatment of breast cancer has not been fully elucidated. Although some studies have provided evidence that the interruption of intracellular signaling by HER2/neu plays a major role in its antitumor activity; others consider ADCC to be a major component of the antitumor activity of trastuzumab. Cardiomyopathy is the major side effect of trastuzumab therapy, especially when combined with taxanes and anthracyclines.

Cetuximab (Erbitux) also targets a receptor tyrosine kinase, EGFR. This chimeric mAb binds to the receptor in a nonactivating manner with a much higher affinity than the natural ligands. This causes receptor blockade and eventual internalization of the receptor, leading to an overall decrease in receptor signaling. Cetuximab was approved for use in the treatment of colorectal cancer in 2004 based on a trial that compared cetuximab with cetuximab plus irinotecan in patients with metastatic disease. The addition of cetuximab to irinotecan demonstrated superior activity. Interestingly, cetuximab demonstrated moderate response rates in previously chemoresistant patients and appeared to be synergistic when combined with chemotherapy.[46] Recently, cetuximab has been approved for use in squamous cell head and neck cancers in combination with radiotherapy.[47] The addition of cetuximab to radiotherapy has decreased local regional recurrence by 32% and significantly improved overall survival. Toxicity associated with cetuximab therapy is an acneform skin rash. There is some evidence that the severity of the skin rash is associated with improved antitumor activity. Moreover, some medical oncologists are proposing that dosing should be escalated until a rash forms.

Bevacizumab (Avastin) is a humanized mAb that targets VEGF, the soluble ligand of the VEGFR expressed on endothelial cells. Signaling through VEGFR is thought to play a major role in the development of new vessels or angiogenesis. Many tumors are known to be associated with increased production of VEGF, leading to increased tumor angiogenesis, which is thought to play an important role in cancer progression and metastases. Bevacizumab has been approved for use in the treatment of metastatic colorectal cancer.[48] Currently, it is combined with fluorouracil and oxaliplatin or irinotecan as first-line therapy for metastatic colorectal cancer. A proposed mechanism of action is actually to normalize tumor vasculature, which helps in the delivery of cytotoxic chemotherapy. Also, bevacizumab has received FDA approval for use in some patients with other cancers, such as RCC (combined with IFN-α), non–small cell lung cancer, breast cancer, and glioblastoma. Associated toxicities reported are delayed wound healing and hemorrhagic events. It is customary to delay elective surgical procedures until 6 weeks after the last dose of bevacizumab.

### Immunoconjugates

Antibodies conjugated to radionuclides were among the first immunoconjugates. External beam radiation delivers focused high-dose radiation delivered over several weeks to treat local areas of disease. Targeted ***ra***dio***i***mmuno***t***herapy (RAIT) such as that provided by an immunoconjugate could be delivered IV as a systemic therapy to treat tumors throughout the body. Another important difference between external beam radiation is that the radiation energy source is delivered to the site of the tumor; thus, the tumor is continually exposed to the radiation. Radionuclides can be categorized with respect to the characteristics of the energy emitted on nuclear decay. Some radionuclides are considered high-energy beta emitters (yttrium-90 and rhenium-188) and the path length of cytotoxic radiation can penetrate a tumor up to a distance of 1 cm. This relatively long path length of cytotoxic radiation could overcome some of the limitations of radioimmunoconjugates, such as poor tumor penetration or heterogenous antigen expression by achieving a large bystander effect. Radionuclides such as lutetium-177 and iodine-131 are considered medium-energy beta emitters whose energy can traverse approximately 1 mm. If one considers the diameter of a cell to be approximately 10 μm, then the bystander effect should encompass approximately 100 cells in all directions. One could imagine that radioimmunoconjugates transporting medium energy beta emitters could be used in the treatment of micrometastatic disease. Using these radionuclides may limit the radiation dose to the normal tissue surrounding the small tumor deposits.

Two anti CD-20 IgG radioimmunoconjugates are currently FDA-approved for the treatment of NHL. Ibritumomab (Zevalin) is conjugated to yttrium-90 and tositumomab (Bexxar) is conjugated to iodine-131. Interestingly, both are murine mAbs, yet the feared HAMA response rarely occurs. The lack of this immunogenic response is thought to be related to the destruction of the CD20-positive B cell population, which would elicit the HAMA response. Both of these radioimmunoconjugates are associated with high response rates. Patients treated with tositumomab had an overall response rate of 67 and patients with bulky disease also demonstrated a significant clinical response. Also, in a head to head comparison of tositumomab conjugated to I-131 versus the unconjugated antibody, the addition of the radionuclide improved overall response rates and complete response rates were tripled.[49] Moreover, these complete responses proved to be durable when compared with responses achieved by rituximab, an unconjugated anti-CD20 mAb. The primary toxicity associated with RAIT is the exposure of the highly sensitive bone marrow to radioactivity, resulting in dose limiting myelosuppression.

## CONCLUSION

Future work in human tumor immunotherapy will need to define and then address the underlying mechanisms that limit a productive antitumor response (Fig. 31-16). These include strategies to optimize the delivery of defined tumor antigens to professional antigen-presenting cells, such as DCs, and in an immunostimulatory context to initiate a robust $CD8^+$ and $CD4^+$ T cell response. Provision of adequate precursors, through genetic engineering of T cells or hematopoietic stem cells, may also be needed. T cell activation and expansion can be promoted in vivo through a variety of strategies that include blocking of negative regulatory signaling and provision of cytokines. As antigen-reactive effector T cells enter a tumor, they encounter a hostile immunosuppressive microenvironment. Tumor cell targets have also frequently acquired constitutively active survival pathways. However, there are promising strategies being developed to address each of these limiting steps, as evidenced by the progressive improvement in clinical tumor immunotherapy occasioned by our better understanding of the underlying basic science.

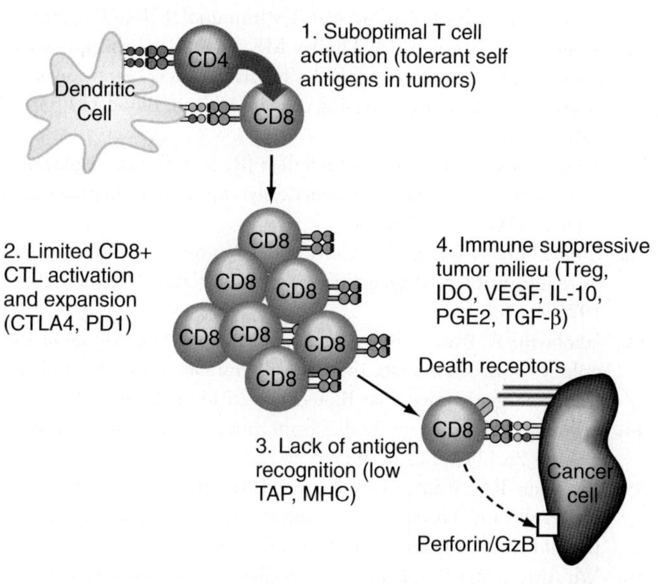


**FIGURE 31-16** Steps required to achieve a productive antitumor immune response.

## SELECTED REFERENCES

Cheever MA: Twelve immunotherapy drugs that could cure cancers. Immunol Rev 222:357–368, 2008.

An overview of the most promising strategies to enhance antitumor immunity.

Dudley ME, Wunderlich JR, Yang JC, et al: Adoptive cell transfer therapy following non-myeloablative but lymphodepleting chemotherapy for the treatment of patients with refractory metastatic melanoma. J Clin Oncol 23:2346–2357, 2005.

A phase II study showing the effectiveness of adoptively transferring cultured melanoma-reactive T cells to a patient after preparative lymphodepletion. The response rate of 51% and the achievement of durable complete responses in some patients illustrate the potential of this approach to immunotherapy

Jakobovits A, Amado RG, Yang X, et al: From XenoMouse technology to panitumumab, the first fully human antibody product from transgenic mice. Nat Biotechnol 25:1134–1143, 2007.

One of the major drawbacks to therapeutic monoclonal antibody development and efficacy is because of the immunogenicity of murine protein sequences. This review summarizes the powerful development of a transgenic mouse (XenoMouse), in which, the mouse antibody production genes were replaced by human immunoglobulin heavy and light-chain loci. Panitumumab was the first fully human mAb developed by immunizing the XenoMouse against a cancer cell line that overexpresses EGFR.

Rosenberg SA, Lotze MT, Yang JC, et al: Experience with the use of high-dose interleukin-2 in the treatment of 652 cancer patients. Ann Surg 210:474–484, 1989.

A broad experience in the use of IL-2 to treat melanoma and renal cancer, documenting its ability to cause regressions and some apparent cures of metastatic disease.

van der Bruggen P, Traversari C, Chomez P, et al: A gene encoding an antigen recognized by cytolytic T lymphocytes on a human melanoma. Science 254:1643–1647, 1991.

A groundbreaking description of the first molecular characterization of a tumor-associated antigen recognized by a T cell. This was an impressive accomplishment, following so quickly after the first understanding of how antigens are processed, presented by MHC, and recognized by T cells. It proved to be the MAGE-1 antigen on a melanoma, presented by HLA-A1.

## REFERENCES

1. Loose D, Van de Wiele C: The immune system and cancer. Cancer Biother Radiopharm 24:369–376, 2009.
2. Cheever MA: Twelve immunotherapy drugs that could cure cancers. Immunol Rev 222:357–368, 2008.
3. Zhang S, Zhang H, Zhao J: The role of CD4 T cell help for CD8 CTL activation. Biochem Biophys Res Commun 384:405–408, 2009.
4. Topham NJ, Hewitt EW: Natural killer cell cytotoxicity: How do they pull the trigger? Immunology 128:7–15, 2009.
5. Chavez-Galan L, Arenas-Del Angel MC, Zenteno E, et al: Cell death mechanisms induced by cytotoxic lymphocytes. Cell Mol Immunol 6:15–25, 2009.
6. Ferrantini M, Capone I, Belardelli F: Dendritic cells and cytokines in immune rejection of cancer. Cytokine Growth Factor Rev 19:93–107, 2008.
7. van der Bruggen P, Traversari C, Chomez P, et al: A gene encoding an antigen recognized by cytolytic T lymphocytes on a human melanoma. Science 254:1643–1647, 1991.
8. Cheever MA, Allison JP, Ferris AS, et al: The prioritization of cancer antigens: A National Cancer Institute pilot project for the acceleration of translational research. Clin Cancer Res 15:5323–5337, 2009.
9. Pittet MJ: Behavior of immune players in the tumor microenvironment. Curr Opin Oncol 21:53–59, 2009.
10. Peggs KS, Quezada SA, Allison JP: Cancer immunotherapy: Co-stimulatory agonists and co-inhibitory antagonists. Clin Exp Immunol 157:9–19, 2009.
11. Prehn RT, Main JM: Immunity to methylcholanthrene-induced sarcomas. J Natl Cancer Inst 18:769–778, 1957.
12. Wolchok JD, Hoos A, O'Day S, et al: Guidelines for the evaluation of immune therapy activity in solid tumors: Immune-related response criteria. Clin Cancer Res 15:7412–7420, 2009.
13. Kammula US, White DE, Rosenberg SA: Trends in the safety of high-dose bolus interleukin-2 administration in patients with metastatic cancer. Cancer 83:797–805, 1998.
14. Smith FO, Downey SG, Klapper JA, et al: Treatment of metastatic melanoma using interleukin-2 alone or in conjunction with vaccines. Clin Cancer Res 14:5610–5618, 2008.
15. Klapper JA, Downey SG, Smith FO, et al: High-dose interleukin-2 for the treatment of metastatic renal cell carcinoma: A retrospective analysis of response and survival in patients treated in the surgery branch at the National Cancer Institute between 1986 and 2006. Cancer 113:293–301, 2008.
16. Rosenberg SA, Yang JC, White DE, et al: Durability of complete responses in patients with metastatic cancer treated with high-dose interleukin-2: Identification of the antigens mediating response. Ann Surg 228:307–319, 1998.
17. Rosenberg SA, Lotze MT, Yang JC, et al: Experience with the use of high-dose interleukin-2 in the treatment of 652 cancer patients. Ann Surg 210:474–484; discussion 484–475, 1989.
18. Yang JC, Sherry RM, Steinberg SM, et al: Randomized study of high-dose and low-dose interleukin-2 in patients with metastatic renal cancer. J Clin Oncol 21:3127–3132, 2003.
19. Kirkwood JM, Ibrahim JG, Sondak VK, et al: High- and low-dose interferon alfa-2b in high-risk melanoma: First analysis of intergroup trial E1690/S9111/C9190. J Clin Oncol 18:2444–2458, 2000.
20. Smits EL, Anguille S, Cools N, et al: Dendritic cell-based cancer gene therapy. Hum Gene Ther 20:1106–1118, 2009.
21. Draper SJ, Heeney JL: Viruses as vaccine vectors for infectious diseases and cancer. Nat Rev Microbiol 8:62–73, 2010.
22. Rosenberg SA, Yang JC, Restifo NP: Cancer immunotherapy: Moving beyond current vaccines. Nat Med 10:909–915, 2004.
23. Downey SG, Klapper JA, Smith FO, et al: Prognostic factors related to clinical response in patients with metastatic melanoma treated by CTL-associated antigen-4 blockade. Clin Cancer Res 13:6681–6688, 2007.
24. Rosenberg SA, Yannelli JR, Yang JC, et al: Treatment of patients with metastatic melanoma with autologous tumor-infiltrating lymphocytes and interleukin 2. J Natl Cancer Inst 86:1159–1166, 1994.
25. Rosenberg SA, Aebersold P, Cornetta K, et al: Gene transfer into humans—immunotherapy of patients with advanced melanoma, using tumor-infiltrating lymphocytes modified by retroviral gene transduction. N Engl J Med 323:570–578, 1990.
26. Dubinett SM, Patrone L, Huang M, et al: Interleukin-2-responsive wound-infiltrating lymphocytes in surgical adjuvant cancer immunotherapy. Immunol Invest 22:13–23, 1993.
27. Dudley ME, Wunderlich JR, Yang JC, et al: Adoptive cell transfer therapy following non-myeloablative but lymphodepleting chemotherapy for the treatment of patients with refractory metastatic melanoma. J Clin Oncol 23:2346–2357, 2005.
28. Dudley ME, Yang JC, Sherry R, et al: Adoptive cell therapy for patients with metastatic melanoma: Evaluation of intensive myeloablative chemoradiation preparative regimens. J Clin Oncol 26:5233–5239, 2008.
29. June CH, Blazar BR, Riley JL: Engineering lymphocyte subsets: Tools, trials and tribulations. Nat Rev Immunol 9:704–716, 2009.
30. Johnson LA, Morgan RA, Dudley ME, et al: Gene therapy with human and mouse T-cell receptors mediates cancer regression and targets normal tissues expressing cognate antigen. Blood 114:535–546, 2009.
31. Morgan RA, Dudley ME, Wunderlich JR, et al: Cancer regression in patients after transfer of genetically engineered lymphocytes. Science 314:126–129, 2006.
32. Kohler G, Milstein C: Continuous cultures of fused cells secreting antibody of predefined specificity. Nature 256:495–497, 1975.
33. Jakobovits A, Amado RG, Yang X, et al: From XenoMouse technology to panitumumab, the first fully human antibody product from transgenic mice. Nat Biotechnol 25:1134–1143, 2007.
34. Lonberg N: Human antibodies from transgenic animals. Nat Biotechnol 23:1117–1125, 2005.
35. Beckman RA, Weiner LM, Davis HM: Antibody constructs in cancer therapy: Protein engineering strategies to improve exposure in solid tumors. Cancer 109:170–179, 2007.
36. Wu AM, Senter PD: Arming antibodies: Prospects and challenges for immunoconjugates. Nat Biotechnol 23:1137–1146, 2005.
37. Griggs J, Zinkewich-Peotti K: The state of the art: Immune-mediated mechanisms of monoclonal antibodies in cancer therapy. Br J Cancer 101:1807–1812, 2009.

**38.** Campoli M, Ferris R, Ferrone S, et al: Immunotherapy of malignant disease with tumor antigen-specific monoclonal antibodies. Clin Cancer Res 16:11–20, 2010.

**39.** Steplewski Z, Lubeck MD, Koprowski H: Human macrophages armed with murine immunoglobulin G2a antibodies to tumors destroy human cancer cells. Science 221:865–867, 1983.

**40.** Weiner LM, Dhodapkar MV, Ferrone S: Monoclonal antibodies for cancer immunotherapy. Lancet 373:1033–1040, 2009.

**41.** Selenko N, Majdic O, Jager U, et al: Cross-priming of cytotoxic T cells promoted by apoptosis-inducing tumor cell reactive antibodies? J Clin Immunol 22:124–130, 2002.

**42.** Olafsen T, Kenanova VE, Wu AM: Tunable pharmacokinetics: modifying the in vivo half-life of antibodies by directed mutagenesis of the Fc fragment. Nat Protoc 1:2048–2060, 2006.

**43.** McLaughlin P, Grillo-Lopez AJ, Link BK, et al: Rituximab chimeric anti-CD20 monoclonal antibody therapy for relapsed indolent lymphoma: Half of patients respond to a four-dose treatment program. J Clin Oncol 16:2825–2833, 1998.

**44.** Piccart-Gebhart MJ, Procter M, Leyland-Jones B, et al: Trastuzumab after adjuvant chemotherapy in HER2-positive breast cancer. N Engl J Med 353:1659–1672, 2005.

**45.** Romond EH, Perez EA, Bryant J, et al: Trastuzumab plus adjuvant chemotherapy for operable HER2-positive breast cancer. N Engl J Med 353:1673–1684, 2005.

**46.** Jonker DJ, O'Callaghan CJ, Karapetis CS, et al: Cetuximab for the treatment of colorectal cancer. N Engl J Med 357:2040–2048, 2007.

**47.** Bonner JA, Harari PM, Giralt J, et al: Radiotherapy plus cetuximab for squamous-cell carcinoma of the head and neck. N Engl J Med 354:567–578, 2006.

**48.** Hurwitz H, Fehrenbacher L, Novotny W, et al: Bevacizumab plus irinotecan, fluorouracil, and leucovorin for metastatic colorectal cancer. N Engl J Med 350:2335–2342, 2004.

**49.** Davis TA, Kaminski MS, Leonard JP, et al: The radioisotope contributes significantly to the activity of radioimmunotherapy. Clin Cancer Res 10:7792–7798, 2004.

CHAPTER 32

# MELANOMA AND CUTANEOUS MALIGNANCIES

Kelly M. McMasters and Marshall M. Urist

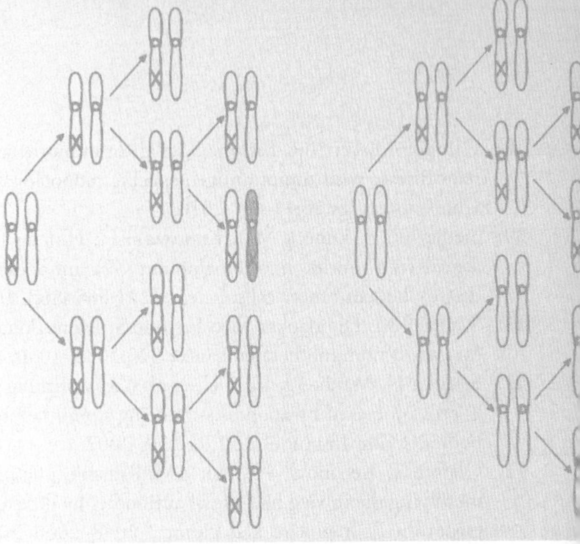

CUTANEOUS MELANOMA
CUTANEOUS MALIGNANCIES: NONMELANOMA SKIN CANCER

## CUTANEOUS MELANOMA

In 1787, Hunter published one of the first accounts of a patient with melanoma. Laennec, who found metastatic melanoma deposits in distant viscera, described melanoma as cancer noire, or the black cancer, in 1806. He subsequently named the disease melanosis in 1812.[1]

### Epidemiology and Causes

Skin cancer is the most common form of cancer, accounting for at least half of all malignancies. Melanoma is a cancer of melanocytes, cells of neural crest origin that migrate during fetal development to several organs and tissues, but predominantly to the skin. Melanocytes in the skin are positioned along the basement membrane at the dermal-epidermal junction.

Melanoma is now the fifth most common cancer in men and the sixth most common cancer in women in the United States. Although melanoma accounts for less than 5% of skin cancer cases, it causes the vast majority of skin cancer deaths.[2] The incidence is greatest in Australia and lowest in Japan among developed countries (Fig. 32-1).[3] The American Cancer Society has estimated that approximately 70,230 new melanomas were diagnosed in the United States in 2010. The incidence of melanoma has risen sharply in the past few decades (Fig. 32-2).[4] During the 1970s, its incidence rose at a rate of about 6%/year. Fortunately, the increase slowed to less than 3%/year during the 1980s and 1990s and, since 2000, it has been relatively stable. It is estimated that there were 8790 deaths from melanoma in 2010 in the United States. The death rate has been stable since 1990, although it continues to rise gradually for men aged 65 years or older (Fig. 32-3).

Cutaneous melanoma is predominantly a disease of whites. The degree of pigmentation in the skin is a relative protective factor against cutaneous melanoma. Risk factors for melanoma include high-risk skin type (e.g., those with blue eyes, blond or red hair, fair complexion), reaction to sun exposure (e.g., freckling, inability to tan, propensity for sunburn), a history of severe blistering sunburns, intense intermittent sun exposure, upper socioeconomic status, family history of melanoma, large number of nevi, giant congenital nevi, presence of dysplastic nevi, immunosuppression, history of prior melanoma or other skin cancers, and xeroderma pigmentosum. The average annual age-adjusted melanoma incidence/100,000 persons is 18.4 for whites compared with 2.3 for Hispanics, 1.6 for Asians, 1.0 for Native Americans, and 0.8 for African Americans. Melanoma is slightly more common in males than in females.[5,6]

Melanoma affects patients at all stages of life. Although the median age of melanoma patients is about 50 years, it occurs in a wide age distribution. The incidence is greatest in older patients, but it is one of the most common cancers in young adults and adolescents. Because of the relatively young median age of melanoma patients, melanoma ranks among the worst cancers in terms of years of life lost per malignancy.

The causes of melanoma are not completely defined, but it is clear that exposure to ultraviolet (UV) radiation is a key causative factor. UV wavelengths are classified as UVA or UVB; UVA has the longer wavelength, 320 to 400 n, and UVB ranges from 290 to 320 nm. UVA, the predominant UV wavelength in tanning beds and lights, penetrates more deeply into the skin than UVB. Although UVA radiation has long been known to play a major role in skin aging and wrinkling, growing evidence has implicated UVA radiation in the cause of nonmelanoma skin cancers as well as melanomas. In melanoma centers around the country, teenagers and young adults are often found with melanoma, predominantly young women who almost universally have been tanning bed users. UV radiation exposure from the sun is a major risk factor, especially among those with fair skin who are more susceptible to sunburns. As compared with nonmelanoma skin cancers, which appear to be related more to chronic repeated sun exposure, melanoma might be related more to intermittent sun or UV radiation exposure. UVB damages the skin's more superficial epidermal layers and is the chief cause of sunburn; it has long been implicated in the development of melanoma.[7]

### Precursor Lesions

Although melanomas frequently arise de novo, they can develop within precursor lesions, such as dysplastic nevi and congenital nevi. In general, a dysplastic nevus is a 6- to 15-mm macular (flat) pigmented skin lesion with indistinct margins and variable color, although the clinical distinction between a nevus with or without dysplasia is often difficult. Dysplastic nevi are typically described as having mild, moderate, or severe dysplasia. Those with moderate or severe dysplasia should be excised with negative margins; wide local excision (WLE) is unnecessary. Those with mild dysplasia usually do not require excision with negative margins and can be observed.

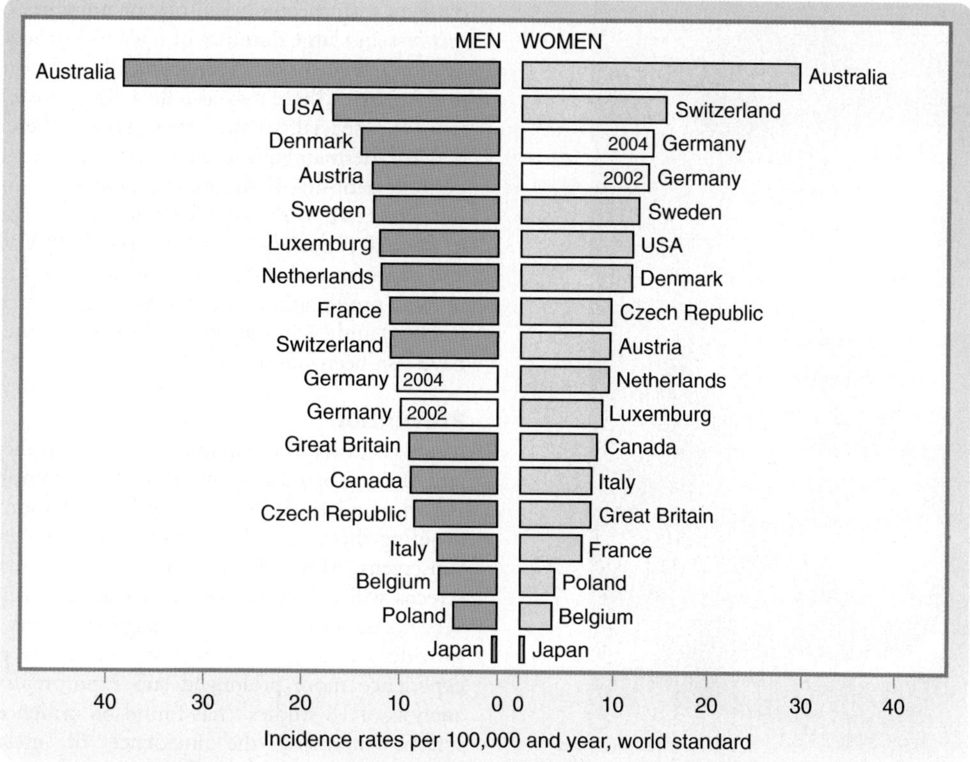


**FIGURE 32-1** Age-standardized (world standard population) incidence rates from 17 countries worldwide for the year 2002. (From Garbe C, Ulrike L: Melanoma epidemiology and trends. Clin Dermatol 27:3–9, 2009.)

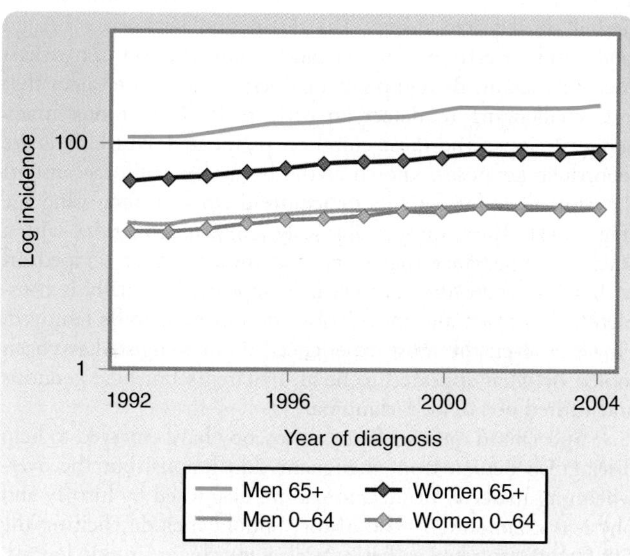


**FIGURE 32-2** Age-adjusted incidence of malignant melanoma/100,000 according to age and gender, 1992-2004. The y axis is a logarithmic scale. (From Linos E, Swetter SM, Cockburn MG, et al: Increasing burden of melanoma in the United States. J Invest Dermatol 129: 1666–1674, 2009.)

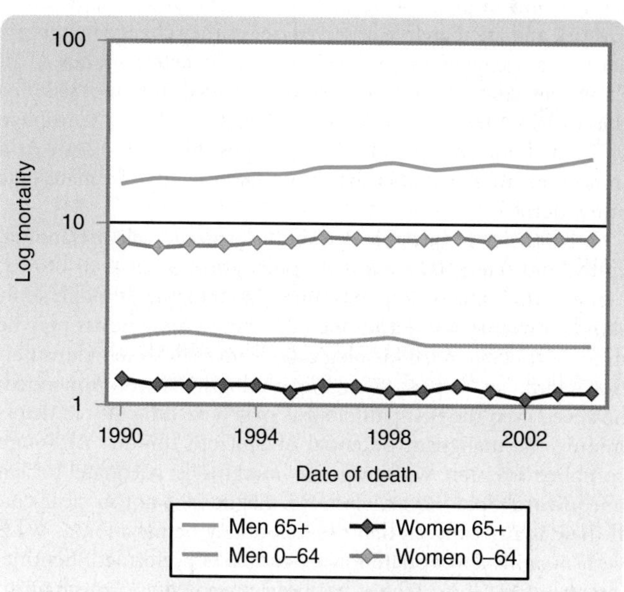


**FIGURE 32-3** Age-adjusted mortality rates from melanoma/100,000 according to age and gender, 1990-2004. (From Linos E, Swetter SM, Cockburn MG, et al: Increasing burden of melanoma in the United States. J Invest Dermatol 129:1666–1674, 2009.)

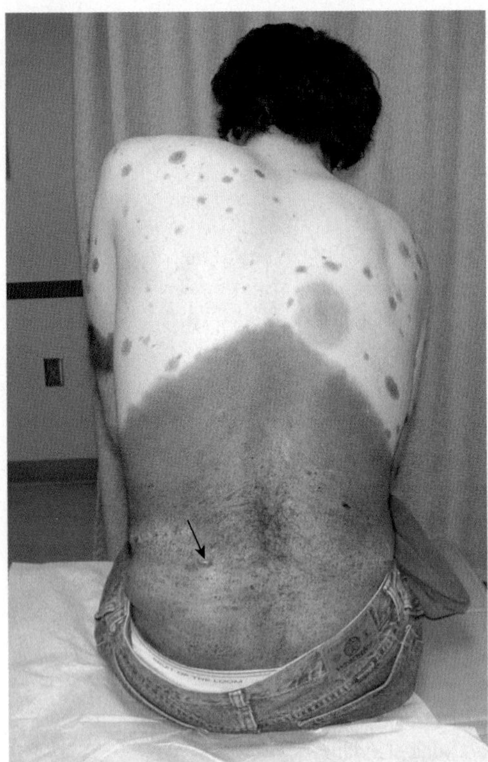

**FIGURE 32-4** Giant congenital nevus of the trunk with a melanoma *(arrow)* on the lower back.

The risk of those with congenital nevi is proportional to the size and number of nevi. Small congenital nevi represent a low risk and are therefore observed unless they change in appearance. Giant congenital nevi (>20 cm in diameter) are rare (1 in 20,000 newborns), but carry an increased lifetime risk for the development of melanoma of up to 10%. Complete excision should be considered, when possible (Fig. 32-4). At a minimum, these patients should undergo regular dermatologic evaluation.[8]

Spitz nevus (juvenile melanoma, spindle cell melanoma, epithelioid cell melanoma) is a rapidly growing, pink or brown, benign skin lesion arising most often in children, although adult skin lesions may also have spitzoid features. Spitz nevus may be difficult to distinguish histologically from melanoma. Consultation with an expert dermatopathologist is recommended; however, even the best pathologists may have difficulty in determining the malignant potential of Spitzoid tumors. Although complete excision with negative margins is adequate for an unequivocal Spitz nevus, often the diagnosis is not so clear-cut. If there is any concern that the lesion may be melanoma, WLE with margins appropriate for melanoma is performed. Sentinel lymph node (SLN) biopsy has been proposed as a mechanism to clarify the malignant potential in indeterminate cases, although this is controversial.[9]

### Familial Melanoma

A hereditary basis has been established for a minority of patients with melanoma. Variously termed *dysplastic nevus syndrome, familial atypical multiple mole-melanoma* (FAMMM) *syndrome,* and *B-K mole syndrome,* among others, these syndromes include patients with melanoma in one or more first- or second-degree relatives and large numbers of melanocytic nevi (often 50 to 100 or more), some of which are clinically and histologically atypical or dysplastic. There may also be a family history of other malignancies, especially pancreatic cancer. These patients require detailed dermatologic evaluation several times annually, with periodic biopsies of the most suspicious lesions. Mutations in the gene *CDKN2A* in the 9p21 region have been demonstrated in familial melanoma kindreds. The *CDKN2A* gene is complex and codes for *p16* and *p14ARF,* which both function to suppress cellular proliferation. Mutations in cyclin-dependent kinase 4 (CDK4) and cyclin-dependent kinase inhibitor 2A (CDKN2A) have also been implicated.[5,10]

## Prevention

Much excessive UV radiation exposure, in the form sunbathing and tanning bed use, is intentional and completely preventable. Recommendations for reducing UV radiation exposure include avoiding these activities, use of protective clothing, and use of sunscreens. Although most experts believe that the use of sunscreens will reduce the risk of melanoma, this topic is controversial, because some have suggested that sunscreens may provide a false sense of security and allow persons at risk to experience more prolonged sun exposure. However, a meta-analysis of 18 studies[11] has found no evidence that use of sunscreens increased the incidence of melanoma.[5] Regular dermatologic evaluation of patients with suspicious pigmented skin lesions is prudent.

## Diagnosis

Melanoma presents most commonly as an irregular pigmented skin lesion that has grown or changed over time. Melanomas most commonly arise de novo, but may also arise within a congenital or acquired nevus. The distinction between a benign nevus and an early melanoma can be difficult, even for experienced clinicians. Benign pigmented lesions are so prevalent that it is challenging to detect an early melanoma among many benign lesions. The most common pigmented skin lesions are seborrheic keratoses, known as the barnacles of life because of the propensity for patients to acquire them with increasing age (Fig. 32-5). These are typically scaly, waxy, raised lesions with a stuck-on appearance that seem as if they could be scraped off with a fingernail; the characteristic appearance usually is completely diagnostic and these lesions do not need to be removed. However, even the most experienced dermatologists have been fooled by what appeared to be an irritated seborrheic keratosis and turned out to be melanoma.

Specialized tools such as dermoscopy have emerged to help distinguish benign from malignant skin lesions, but the overwhelming majority of melanomas are diagnosed by history and physical examination. The history should include eliciting the risk factors described earlier, as well as any change in skin lesions, including itching and bleeding. The physical examination requires only the simplest of preparations; the patient must undress. Although it is widely recognized that skin examination should be part of the routine physical examination by primary care physicians and others, it is rarely performed. It may take only 1 minute to perform a complete skin survey, which admittedly is not the same as a detailed dermatologic examination, but many lives have been saved by early detection of melanomas by physicians who took the time to evaluate the skin.

The ABCDEs of melanoma are used to guide the decision about performing a biopsy—***a***symmetrical irregular ***b***orders, variable shades of ***c***olor, ***d***iameter greater than 6 mm, and ***e***volution, or change over time. However, many melanomas do not follow these rules. Amelanotic melanomas are not pigmented and may present as a raised pink or flesh-colored skin lesion. A high index of clinical suspicion is needed, and particular attention should be paid to any history of change in a lesion. If a patient presents with a skin lesion that has changed in size, color, or shape, and/or is itching or bleeding, a biopsy should be performed. To tell a patient that it will just be observed means that it will be ignored. There should be a low threshold for performance of biopsy. Fortunately, locally advanced melanomas are now infrequently encountered, given the increased awareness of this disease (Fig. 32-6).

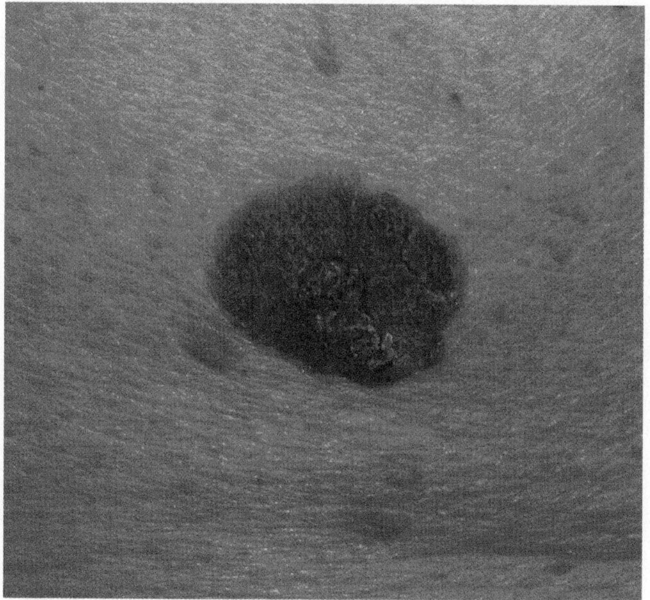

**FIGURE 32-5** Seborrheic keratosis.

## Biopsy

Primary care physicians, as well as dermatologists and surgeons, should be trained to perform a skin biopsy. There are three basic types of skin biopsy—excisional, incisional (including punch biopsy), and shave biopsy. An excisional biopsy is the most appropriate and prudent method of diagnosing and completely removing a pigmented skin lesion in most cases. Most patients who have a pigmented lesion that is of concern want it completely removed in any case, even if it is benign. Using local anesthesia, a narrow margin excision is performed, which includes subcutaneous fat to get a full-thickness biopsy, and the defect is closed with sutures. Attention should be paid to the orientation of the excision, because a fusiform excision should be oriented in such a way as to prepare for the possibility that the lesion is a melanoma and may require WLE. Specifically, a longitudinal orientation on the extremities is best and, in other areas, consideration should be given to the orientation that would allow closure with the least tension and best cosmetic outcome in case wide excision is needed. Therefore, excisional biopsy is best for most small pigmented lesions.

For larger lesions, it may be appropriate first to get a tissue diagnosis prior to performing complete excision; this is accomplished by a full-thickness incisional biopsy. The simplest way to perform an incisional biopsy is by use of a punch biopsy. A punch biopsy is performed using a disposable instrument that removes a cylinder of skin and subcutaneous tissue (2 to 8 mm in diameter) by simply twisting the instrument into the anesthetized skin, followed by closure with one or two simple sutures (Fig. 32-7). Punch biopsies of at least 4 mm should be performed, because a 2-mm punch often does not provide adequate tissue for pathologic evaluation. The punch biopsy should be

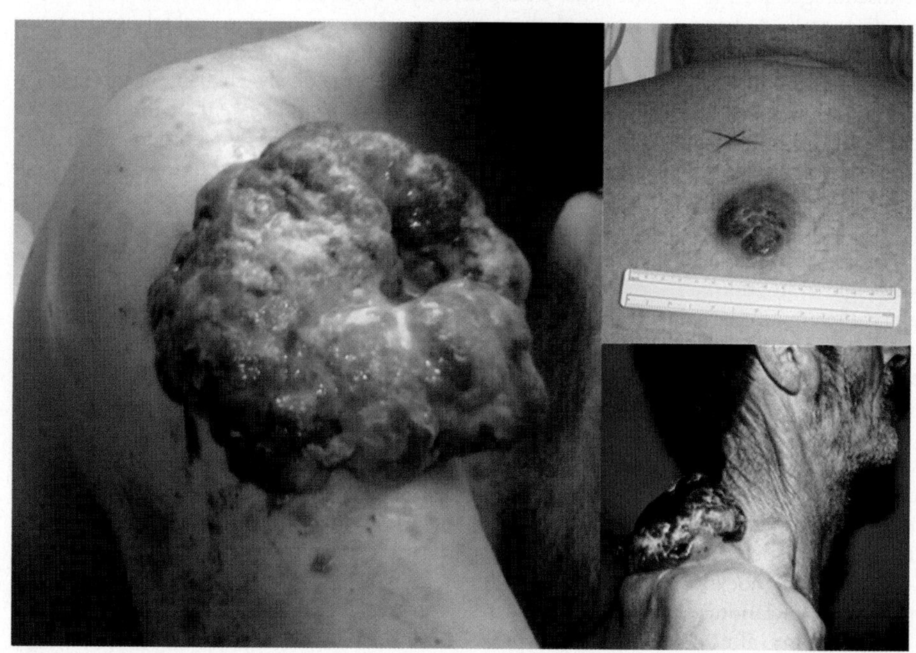

**FIGURE 32-6** Locally advanced melanomas.

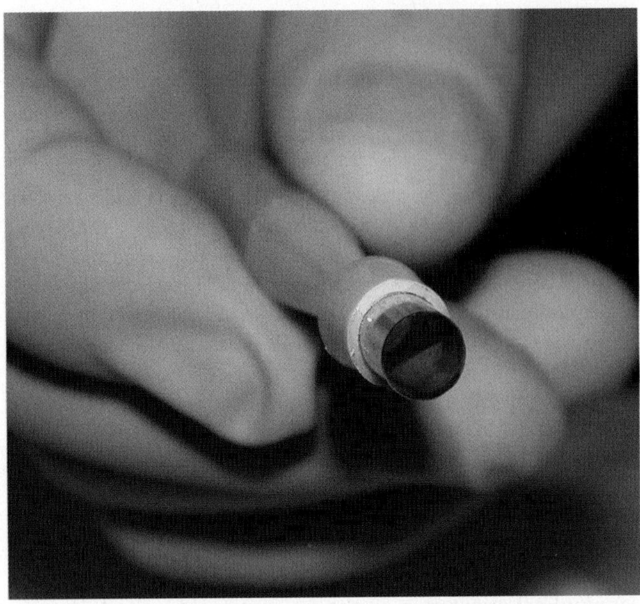

**FIGURE 32-7** Disposable instrument used for punch biopsy.

performed through the thickest area(s) of the lesion, and multiple punch biopsies can be performed to sample larger lesions. Shave biopsies are frequently performed by dermatologists and are appropriate for many nonpigmented skin lesions. This is a good way to diagnose squamous cell and basal cell carcinoma. A shave biopsy is performed by elevating the skin lesion with forceps or inserting a small needle beneath the lesion, followed by shaving the lesion with a razor blade or scalpel. Hemostasis is achieved using topical agents such as ammonium chloride or by electrocautery. The patient then treats the area with topical antibiotic ointment and it is allowed to heal by secondary intention. Because a shave biopsy is quick and simple to perform and does not require sutures, it is a popular method of biopsy. However, shave biopsy should generally be discouraged for pigmented lesions, because if a melanoma is diagnosed, a shave biopsy may transect directly through the melanoma and not allow an accurate assessment of tumor thickness as the base of the lesion is cauterized. Therefore, shave biopsy should not be used when melanoma is suspected. To circumvent this problem, dermatologists often perform deep shave or saucerization biopsies, which completely remove the lesion down to subcutaneous fat if there is any concern for melanoma. In the hands of experienced clinicians, this can be an effective biopsy technique. All pigmented lesions should be sent for pathologic evaluation.[12] Ablation of pigmented skin lesions using cryotherapy, cautery, or lasers should be specifically discouraged; there are many examples of disastrous delays in diagnosis as a result of such practices.

## Pathology

Over the past several years, there has been a dramatic increase in the diagnosis of equivocal lesions whose biologic behavior cannot be predicted with absolute certainty. There is a spectrum that ranges from mild to severe dysplasia to atypical melanocytic proliferation to melanoma in situ to early invasive melanoma. Part of the increase in the incidence of melanoma almost certainly results from a lower threshold on the part of pathologists to diagnose such equivocal lesions as melanoma because of the potential consequences of a missed diagnosis of melanoma. It is now common for a pathology report to contain a long description that essentially states that the lesion may be anything from a severely dysplastic nevus to early invasive melanoma. In such cases, the prudent decision is to treat such lesions as an early invasive melanoma with a 1-cm margin WLE. Melanoma in situ is considered a premalignant precursor lesion that has a significant likelihood of progression to invasive melanoma. Because it does not invade beyond the basement membrane, it does not have access to blood vessels and lymphatics and does not generally have metastatic potential.

Histologically, invasive cutaneous melanoma is divided into four major types based on growth pattern and location. These forms are lentigo maligna melanoma, superficial spreading melanoma, acral lentiginous melanoma, and nodular melanoma. Melanomas arise as proliferations of melanocytes in the basal layer of the skin. As they multiply, these cells expand radially in the epidermis and superficial dermal layer, termed the *radial growth phase.* With time, the growth begins in a vertical direction as the skin lesion may become palpable, the so-called vertical growth phase. Nodular melanomas are an exception to this pattern, wherein the vertical growth phase is present early in tumor development. The vertical growth phase allows invasion into the deeper layers of the skin, where the tumor may achieve metastatic potential by invasion of blood and lymphatic vessels.[13]

The histologic subtype of melanoma is not, in general, a major factor in prognosis; tumor thickness, ulceration, and other factors determine the prognosis. However, some histologic subtypes are more likely to be detected at a more advanced stage. Lentigo maligna melanoma occurs most commonly on the face of older individuals with sun-damaged skin and presents as a flat, dark, variably pigmented lesion, with irregular borders and a history of slow development (Fig. 32-8). Lentigo maligna melanomas may become large prior to diagnosis, because the slow progression may escape the patient's notice. Overall, the prognosis of lentigo maligna melanomas is better than for the other histopathologic types because of the often superficial nature of these tumors. However, lentigo maligna melanomas can pose challenging management problems because of their propensity to develop in cosmetically challenging areas (e.g., face), and the fact that the histologic extent of the lesion may extend well beyond the clinically apparent borders of the pigmented lesion. Thus, achieving negative margins may be challenging. Before embarking on complex tissue flaps for closure, it is prudent to ensure negative margins. This may necessitate delaying the closure until the final pathology report indicates negative margins of excision.

The most common histologic type is superficial spreading melanoma (Fig. 32-9). It is not necessarily associated with sun-exposed skin. As the name suggests, superficial spreading melanoma initially appears as a flat pigmented lesion growing in the radial dimension. If allowed to progress, these melanomas develop a vertical growth phase and invade more deeply into the skin.

Acral lentiginous melanoma (ALM) is classified by its anatomic site of origin. These tumors develop in the subungual areas, beneath the fingernails and toenails, and on the palms of the hand and soles of the feet (Fig. 32-10). This is the most common type of melanoma in black patients. The histologic

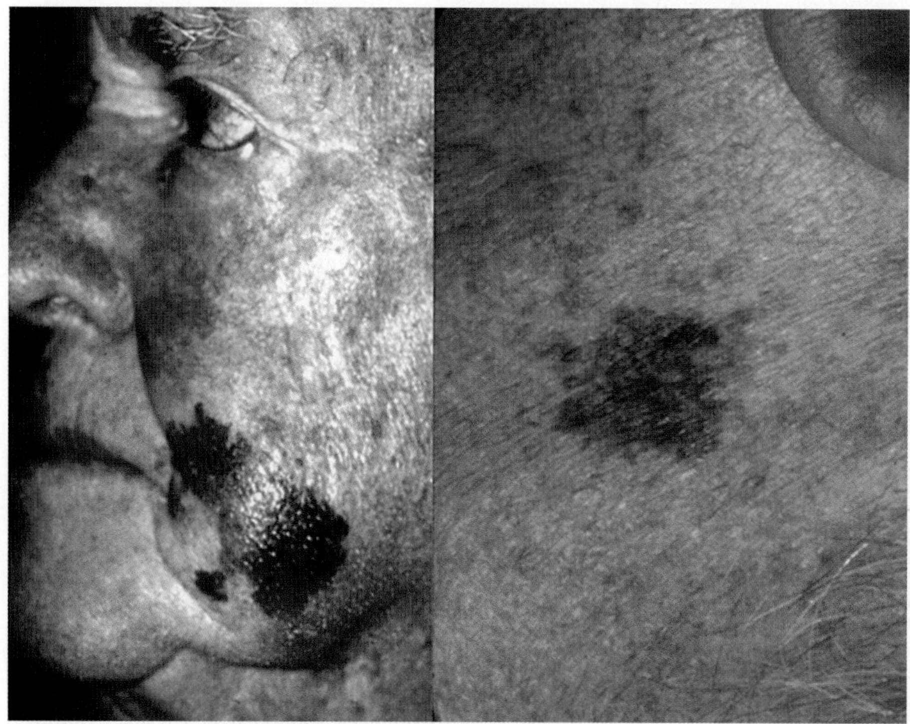

**FIGURE 32-8** Lentigo maligna melanomas.

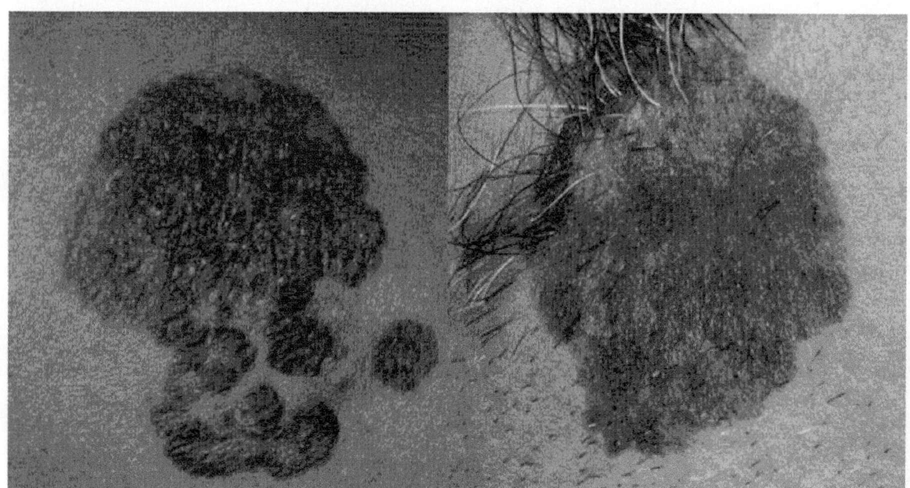

**FIGURE 32-9** Superficial spreading melanomas.

appearance of ALMs is similar to melanomas arising on the mucous membranes. The diagnosis is often made at an advanced stage, which accounts for the poor prognosis of these tumors in general. Subungual acral lentiginous melanomas are often mistaken for a subungual hematomas, leading to a delay in diagnosis. A key feature distinguishing a subungual melanoma from a subungual hematoma is that for subungual hematoma, the pigment should migrate distally with growth of the nail. Biopsy of subungual melanomas can be accomplished by performing a digital block with local anesthesia and removing the nail or performing a punch biopsy through the nail itself.

Nodular melanomas are raised papular lesions that develop a vertical growth pattern early in their course (Fig. 32-11). These melanomas often have a poor prognosis because of greater average tumor thickness and frequent ulceration.

Desmoplastic melanoma is a specific type of amelanotic melanoma, which commonly arises on the head and neck. Desmoplastic melanomas often exhibit neurotropism and have a greater propensity for local recurrence, with a decreased risk of nodal metastasis.

## Prognostic Factors

Most patients with newly-diagnosed melanoma are anxious and concerned that they may die of this disease. However, it must be recognized that approximately 87% of melanoma patients are cured of their cancer, largely because of early detection. It is

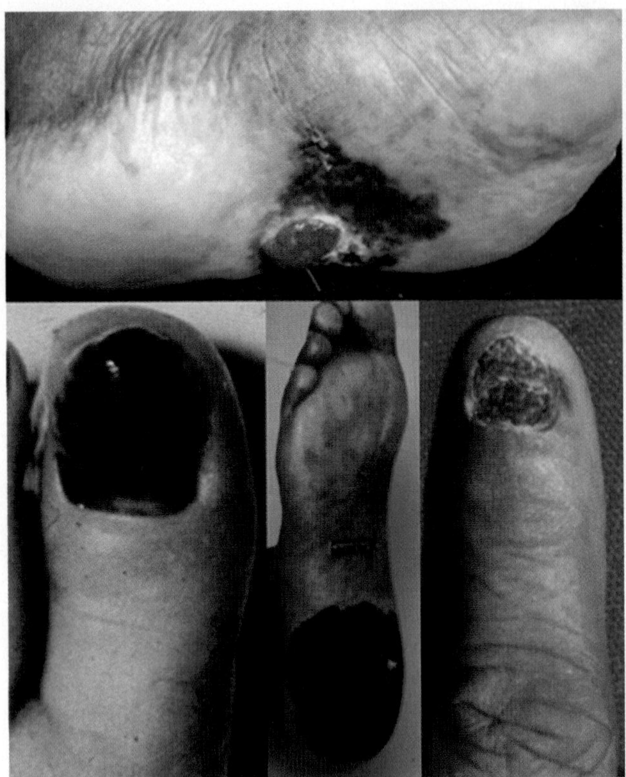

FIGURE 32-10 Acral lentiginous melanoma.

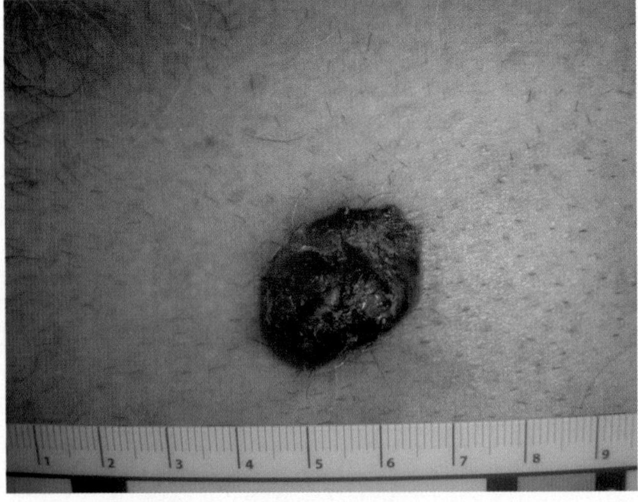

FIGURE 32-11 Nodular melanoma.

therefore of substantial importance to stratify risk and predict prognosis to guide appropriate management decisions.

In 1969, Dr. Wallace Clark described a classification of melanoma based on the level of invasion into the anatomic layers of the skin. Henceforth known as Clark's level of invasion, this classification scheme correlated with survival (Fig. 32-12).[14] Clark level I tumors represent melanoma in situ and are limited to the epidermis; therefore, these lesions do not have metastatic potential. Clark level II melanomas extend into the papillary dermis, level III fill the papillary dermis, level IV to the reticular dermis, and level V extend to the subcutaneous fat. In 1970, Dr. Alexander Breslow described a simpler system based on measurement of the vertical thickness of the melanoma in millimeters, now known as Breslow's thickness.[15] As the thickness of the melanoma increases, the prognosis worsens.

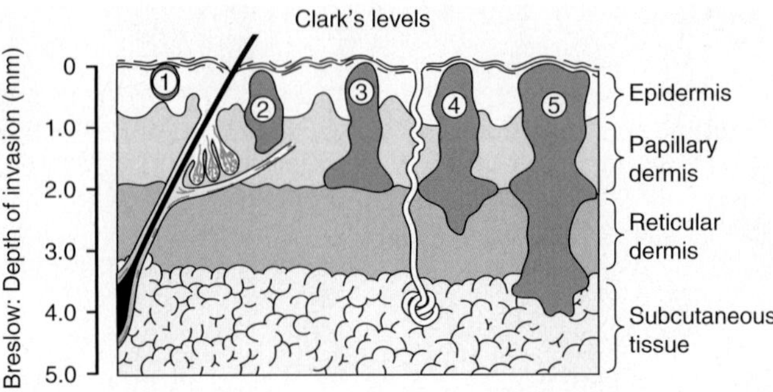


FIGURE 32-12 Clark's level of invasion.

Melanomas are commonly considered to be thin (<1-mm Breslow thickness), intermediate thickness (>1 to 4 mm), and thick (>4 mm). Over time, Breslow thickness has largely supplanted Clark level, because it has been shown to be a more accurate method of predicting prognosis. Clark level continues to be reported routinely, even though it is a weak prognostic factor. It is not uncommon that confusion arises among patients and referring physicians regarding the significance of Clark level and melanoma stage; there is obviously a large difference between a Clark level IV melanoma, which may have a very good prognosis, and stage IV melanoma, indicating distant metastatic disease.

The status of the regional lymph nodes is the single most important prognostic factor predicting survival. Metastasis to the regional lymph nodes increases the chances of mortality from melanoma substantially. The other major prognostic factors, in order of importance, are Breslow thickness, ulceration, age, anatomic location of the primary tumor, and gender. Mitotic rate is a more recently validated prognostic factor that may also be important to consider, especially among patients with thin melanomas. Ulceration has emerged as a robust predictor of prognosis. Ulceration is defined pathologically as the absence of an intact epithelium overlying the melanoma. Patients with ulcerated melanomas have a worse prognosis than those with nonulcerated melanomas, even among patients with regional nodal metastasis. Why patients with ulcerated melanomas have a worse prognosis is unclear, but ulceration appears to be a phenotypic marker for worse tumor biology and greater propensity for invasion and metastasis. Older patients have a greater risk of melanoma mortality than younger patients, despite the fact that younger patients are more likely to have nodal metastasis. Patients with axial (trunk, head, and neck) melanomas have a worse prognosis than those with extremity tumors. Regression has not been shown to be an important factor predicting nodal metastasis or survival. Women have a better prognosis than men, for reasons that are unclear.[16]

In an ongoing effort, the American Joint Committee on Cancer (AJCC) Melanoma Staging Committee, led by Dr. Charles Balch, has analyzed multi-institutional data from North America, Europe, and Australia, which an evidence-based staging system to be developed that predicts prognosis with exquisite accuracy.

## Staging

Staging for cutaneous melanoma uses the tumor-node-metastasis (TNM) system of classification as defined by the AJCC (Tables 32-1 and 32-2). The 2009 version (seventh) of the staging system is based on analysis of a database of over 30,000 patients.[17] The important prognostic factors in the staging system include Breslow thickness, ulceration, nodal status, and presence of other manifestations of lymphatic spread (e.g., satellite lesions, in-transit disease), as well as the presence of distant metastatic disease. The principal change from the previous (sixth) version is that a mitotic rate of one mitosis/mm$^2$ or more is now used, instead of Clark level, to discriminate T1a from T1b tumors based on the finding that the mitotic rate is a more powerful predictor of prognosis (Table 32-3). This system provides excellent discrimination of survival among various stages of disease (Fig. 32-13). Based on the work of Balch, collaborators from the AJCC staging committee developed an online tool for the assessment of prognosis based on individual patient characteristics (www.melanomaprognosis.org).

## Initial Evaluation

Most melanoma patients who seek surgical consultation will have already been diagnosed with melanoma. The first and most important evaluation of a patient diagnosed with melanoma is a thorough history and physical examination. The history should elicit factors related to the primary melanoma (e.g., duration, change over time, symptoms such as itching and bleeding) and other factors, such as sun exposure, tanning bed use, immunosuppression, prior history of cancer, and family history. Melanoma may be localized or may metastasize to regional or distant sites. Regional metastasis refers to the lymphatic spread of tumor to the regional lymph nodes, those in the immediate lymphatic drainage pathway from the site of the primary tumor. In-transit melanoma is a form of regional lymphatic metastasis in which the tumor spreads within the draining lymphatic channels and becomes evident as cutaneous or subcutaneous nodules between the site of the primary tumor and regional lymph nodes (Fig. 32-14). Distant metastasis refers to the hematogenous spread of melanoma to distant organs. Although uncommon at the time of initial diagnosis, it is also important to elicit symptoms of metastatic disease, such as any masses, neurologic symptoms or headaches, anorexia, weight loss, bone pain, or respiratory symptoms. A detailed physical examination should specifically include a complete skin examination, with inspection and palpation of the skin to detect any other suspicious skin lesions, including detection of in-transit disease. Palpation of the cervical, axillary, and inguinal lymph nodes should be performed, and palpation of the epitrochlear or popliteal nodes, as appropriate for distal upper or lower extremity melanomas, respectively. When present, all symptoms and signs of metastasis require further radiologic evaluation.

The National Comprehensive Cancer Network (NCCN), a consortium of oncologists from National Cancer Institute–designated cancer centers, provides consensus-based guidelines for cancer treatment. These guidelines for the management of primary melanoma are available online (www.nccn.org).

**Table 32-1 TNM Staging Categories for Cutaneous Melanoma**

| T CLASSIFICATION | THICKNESS | ULCERATION STATUS AND MITOSES |
|---|---|---|
| T1 | ≤1.0 mm | a: Without ulceration and mitosis <1/mm$^2$<br>b: With ulceration or mitoses ≥1/mm$^2$ |
| T2 | 1.01-2.0 mm | a: Without ulceration<br>b: With ulceration |
| T3 | 2.01-4.0 mm | a: Without ulceration<br>b: With ulceration |
| T4 | >4.0 mm | a: Without ulceration<br>b: With ulceration |
| **N CLASSIFICATION** | **NO. OF METASTATIC NODES** | **NODAL METASTATIC MASS** |
| N1 | One node | a: Micrometastasis*<br>b: Macrometastasis† |
| N2 | Two or three nodes | a: Micrometastasis*<br>b: Macrometastasis†<br>c: In-transit met(s)/satellite(s) without metastatic nodes |
| N3 | Four or more metastatic nodes, or matted nodes, or in-transit metastases-satellite(s) with metastatic node(s) | |
| **M CLASSIFICATION** | **SITE** | **SERUM LDH LEVEL** |
| M1a | Distant skin, subcutaneous, or nodal mets | Normal |
| M1b | Lung metastases | Normal |
| M1c | All other visceral metastases<br>Any distant metastasis | Normal<br>Elevated |

From Balch CM, Gershenwald JE, Soong SJ, et al: Final version of 2009 AJCC melanoma staging and classification. J Clin Oncol 27:6199–6206, 2009.

*Micrometastases are diagnosed after sentinel lymph node biopsy and completion lymphadenectomy (if performed).

†Macrometastases are defined as clinically detectable nodal metastases confirmed by therapeutic lymphadenectomy or when nodal metastasis exhibits gross extracapsular extension.

**Table 32-2 Stage Groupings for Cutaneous Melanoma**

| Clinical Staging* | | | | Pathologic Staging† | | | |
|---|---|---|---|---|---|---|---|
| | T | N | M | | T | N | M |
| 0 | Tis | N0 | M0 | 0 | Tis | N0 | M0 |
| IA | T1a | N0 | M0 | IA | T1a | N0 | M0 |
| IB | T1b<br>T2a | N0<br>N0 | M0<br>M0 | IB | T1b<br>T2a | N0<br>N0 | M0<br>M0 |
| IIA | T2b<br>T3a | N0<br>N0 | M0<br>M0 | IIA | T2b<br>T3a | N0<br>N0 | M0<br>M0 |
| IIB | T3b<br>T4a | N0<br>N0 | M0<br>M0 | IIB | T3b<br>T4a | N0<br>N0 | M0<br>M0 |
| IIC | T4b | N0 | M0 | IIC | T4b | N0 | M0 |
| III | Any T | Any N | M0 | IIIA | T1–4a<br>T1–4a | N1a<br>N2a | M0<br>M0 |
| | | | | IIIB | T1–4b<br>T1–4b<br>T1–4a<br>T1–4a<br>T1–4a | N1a<br>N2a<br>N1b<br>N2b<br>N2c | M0<br>M0<br>M0<br>M0<br>M0 |
| | | | | IIIC | T1–4b<br>T1–4b<br>T1–4b<br>Any T | N1b<br>N2b<br>N2c<br>N3 | M0<br>M0<br>M0<br>M0 |
| IV | Any T | Any N | Any M | IV | Any T | Any N | Any M |

From Balch CM, Gershenwald JE, Soong SJ, et al: Final version of 2009 AJCC melanoma staging and classification. J Clin Oncol 27:6199–6206, 2009.

*Clinical staging includes microstaging of the primary melanoma and clinical and/or radiologic evaluation for metastases. By convention, it should be used after complete excision of the primary melanoma, with clinical assessment for regional and distant metastases.

†Pathologic staging includes microstaging of the primary melanoma and pathologic information about the regional lymph nodes after partial or complete lymphadenectomy. Pathologic stage 0 or stage IA patients are the exception; they do not require pathologic evaluation of their lymph nodes.

**Table 32-3 Multivariate Cox Regression Analysis of Pathologic Factors by T Category for Stages I and II Melanoma***

| T CATEGORY | BRESLOW THICKNESS | ULCERATION | MITOTIC RATE | CLARK LEVEL |
|---|---|---|---|---|
| T1 | 12.8 ($P$ = .0003) | 3.8 ($P$ = .05) | 20.8 ($P$ < .0001) | 1.9 ($P$ = .17) |
| T2 | 4.9 ($P$ = .03) | 16.2 ($P$ < .0001) | 15.9 ($P$ < .0001) | 0.2 ($P$ = .65) |
| T3 | 4.1 ($P$ = .04) | 15.4 ($P$ < .0001) | 12.2 ($P$ = .0005) | 1.4 ($P$ = .24) |
| T4 | 0.2 ($P$ = .69) | 14.2 ($P$ = .0002) | 9.1 ($P$ = .003) | 2.7 ($P$ = .10) |

From Balch CM, Gershenwald JE, Soong SJ, et al: Final version of 2009 AJCC melanoma staging and classification. J Clin Oncol 27:6199–6206, 2009.

*With mitotic rate data available. When mitotic rate is considered in the multivariate model, the Clark level is no longer a significant factor predicting overall survival. Data are chi-square values and *P* values.

### Extent of Disease Evaluation

Clinical stages 0 and I patients do not require any further tests. Stage II patients may undergo chest x-ray, although it is considered optional. Formerly, liver function tests such as lactate dehydrogenase (LDH) levels were commonly performed; however, there is no evidence that blood tests are helpful for detecting metastatic disease and need not be performed for patients with clinically localized melanoma.

There is controversy regarding the extent of imaging evaluation appropriate for patients with melanoma. For most stages I and II patients, additional imaging studies are unnecessary, although imaging evaluation may be appropriate in patients with thick primary tumors (stage IIC). The role of imaging tests for stage III patients with disease detected by sentinel node biopsy is controversial. Because the probability of detecting true-positive findings on studies such as positron emission tomography (PET) and computed tomography (CT) scanning is extraordinarily low in patients with microscopic nodal metastasis; there is a real danger of false-positive results, but these imaging tests should be ordered and interpreted with caution. Patients with clinically detectable nodal metastasis should undergo imaging studies to evaluate for the presence of distant metastatic disease, because the distinction between stages III and IV disease is important in determining the appropriate treatment options. Furthermore, for patients with stage IV melanoma, imaging evaluation is necessary to determine the extent of disease and whether resection is appropriate. In such cases, PET, CT, and magnetic resonance imaging (MRI) of the brain are generally recommended.[18]

## Treatment

### Surgical Management

**Wide Local Excision** The operation to resect the primary melanoma is known as WLE. The appropriate margins for excision have long been a topic of controversy. In 1857, Norris suggested WLE for a primary melanoma to prevent local recurrence and advocated a 5-cm margin, a recommendation that would be followed for over a century.[19] Until the 1960s, all melanomas were considered to be aggressive tumors and were often treated with very wide margin excision. Current guidelines for WLE are given in Table 32-4.

Melanoma in situ is generally adequately treated by a 0.5-cm margin excision; this is not based on any randomized data, but on clinical experience with this disease entity. However, given that there is significant interobserver variability among pathologists in its diagnosis,[20] and that early invasive melanoma may be diagnosed after WLE if the entire lesion was not removed during the initial biopsy, it is often prudent to perform a 1-cm WLE for melanoma in situ that occurs in anatomic areas that easily allow a 1-cm margin with primary closure (e.g., the trunk).

Several randomized studies have been performed to assess the margin width for intermediate-thickness melanomas.[21,22] The first trial, conducted by the World Health Organization, randomized 612 patients with melanomas 2-mm thick or less to WLE using a 1- or 3-cm margin. Local recurrence as a site of first recurrence was observed in four patients, all with melanomas larger than 1 to 2 mm thick who were in the 1-cm margin group; however, this did not significantly affect overall survival. The Intergroup Melanoma Trial randomized 462 patients with melanomas of the trunk or proximal extremities between 1-mm and 4-mm Breslow thickness to receive WLE with a 2-cm or 4-cm margin. After a median follow-up of 10 years, the incidence of local recurrence was the same for patients undergoing 2-cm or 4-cm margin excision (2.1% versus 2.6%,

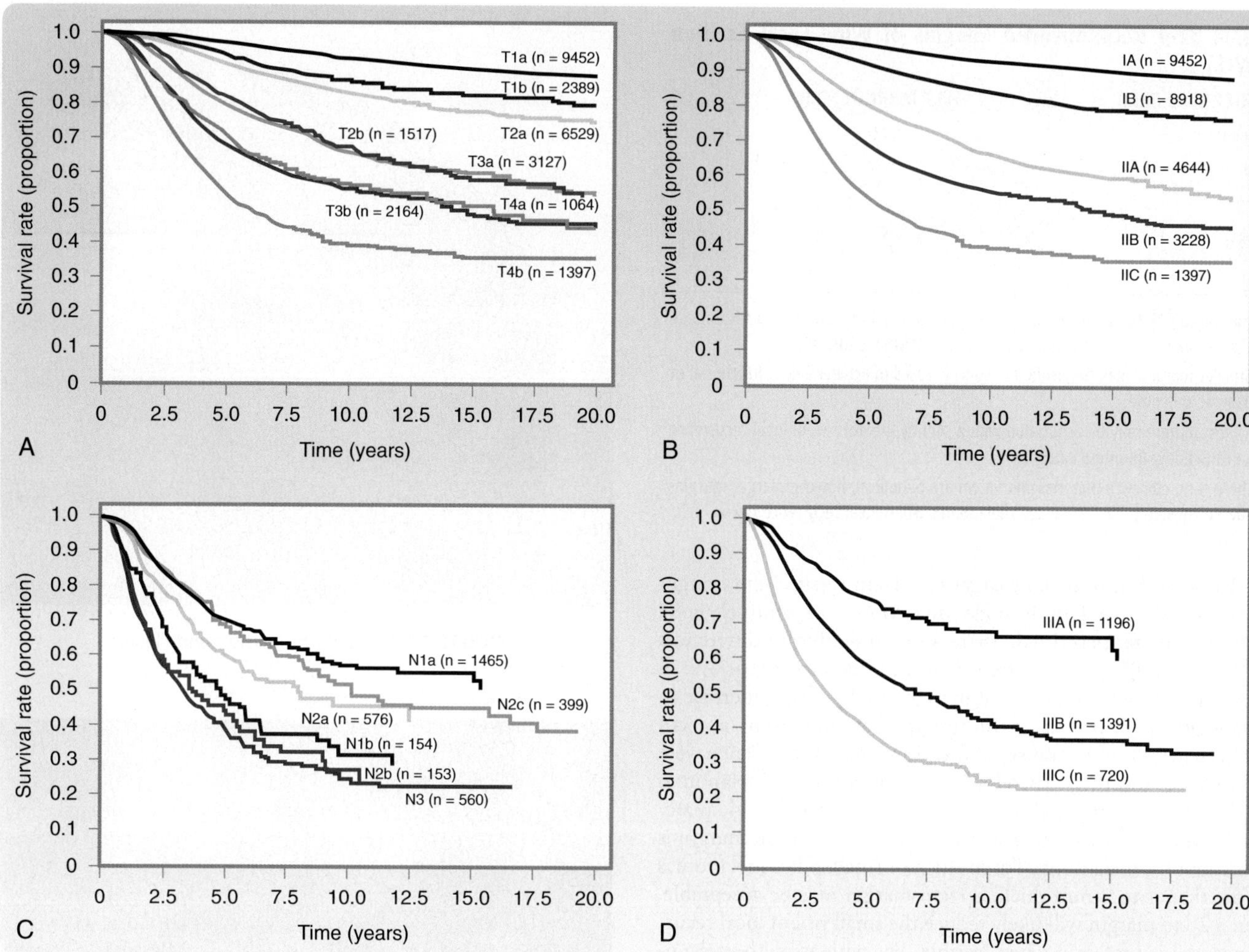

**FIGURE 32-13** Survival curves from the AJCC Melanoma Staging Database comparing the different T categories **(A)** and stage groupings for stages I and II **(B)** melanoma. For patients with stage III disease, survival curves are shown comparing the different N categories **(C)** and stage groupings **(D)**. (From Balch CM, Gershenwald JE, Soong SJ, et al: Final version of 2009 AJCC melanoma staging and classification. J Clin Oncol 27:6199-6206, 2009.)

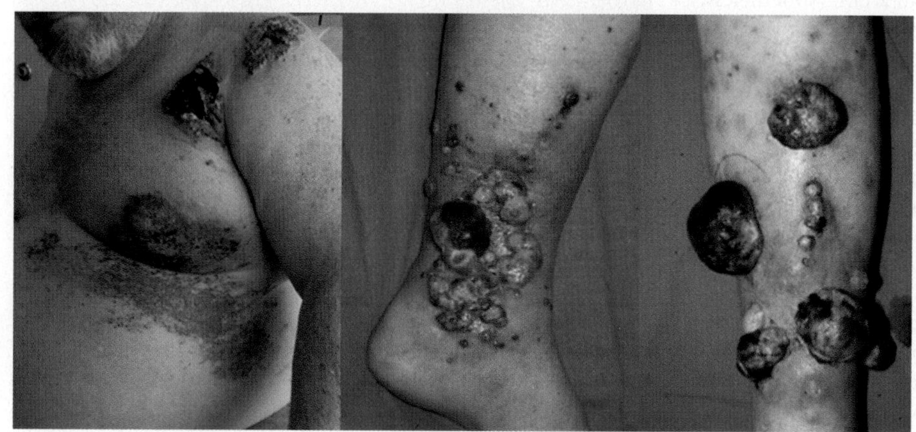

**FIGURE 32-14** In-transit melanoma.

respectively); there was no significant difference in overall survival. Factors significantly associated with local recurrence were ulceration, thickness, and anatomic location of the primary melanoma; head and neck melanomas had a much greater risk of local recurrence. The Swedish Melanoma Trial and the French Melanoma Trial compared 2-cm versus 5-cm WLE in patients with melanomas less than 2-mm Breslow thickness. Neither trial showed an advantage for a 5-cm margin excision in terms of local recurrence, disease-free survival, or overall survival. The British Collaborative Trial randomized 900 patients with

**Table 32-4 Recommended Margins of Wide Local Excision (WLE)**

| THICKNESS (MM) | WLE MARGIN (CM)* |
|---|---|
| In situ | 0.5 |
| <1 | 1 |
| 1-2 | 1-2† |
| >2-4 | 2 |
| >4 | 2‡ |

From Balch CM, Gershenwald JE, Soong SJ, et al: Final version of 2009 AJCC melanoma staging and classification. J Clin Oncol 27:6199–6206, 2009.

*Smaller margins may be justified in specific cases to achieve better functional or cosmetic outcome.

†A 1-cm margin may be associated with a slightly greater risk of local recurrence in this Breslow thickness category.

‡There is no evidence that margins >2 cm are beneficial; however, larger margins may be considered for advanced melanomas when local recurrence risk is high.

melanomas 2 mm thick or larger to a 1-cm versus 3-cm margin excision; elective lymph node dissection and sentinel node biopsy were not permitted. There were no significant differences in local and in-transit recurrence, disease-free survival, or overall survival. However, there was a marginally significant increase in locoregional recurrence in the group that underwent a 1-cm WLE when local, in-transit, and regional nodal recurrence were considered together. Therefore, for patients with melanomas 2 mm thick or larger, a 1-cm margin is considered inadequate.

Taken together, these studies suggest that a 1-cm margin is sufficient for melanomas 1 mm thick or smaller. For melanomas more than 1 to 2 mm thick, a 1-cm margin may be acceptable, but a 2-cm margin will likely reduce the small risk of local recurrence and is preferred when feasible. For patients with melanomas more than 2 mm thick, a 2-cm margin is appropriate. There are no data to conclude that a 3-cm margin is better than a 2-cm margin. Appropriate margins of excision for thick melanomas (>4 mm thick) have not been studied in the context of randomized trials; however, retrospective analysis has suggested that there is no advantage for margins more than 2 cm. Nonetheless, it may be appropriate to perform wider margin excision for locally advanced melanomas when the risk of recurrence is high.[21,22]

WLE can be performed under local anesthesia in most cases, although general anesthesia is preferred for patients who undergo concomitant sentinel node biopsy or lymphadenectomy. The appropriate margins of excision are measured from the edge of the lesion or previous biopsy scar. Usually, this represents a fusiform incision that encompasses the margins of excision to allow primary closure (Fig. 32-15). WLE is performed to remove the skin and subcutaneous tissue down to the muscular fascia. Excision of the fascia is not necessary in most cases, but may be performed for patients with thick primary tumors. The specimen is submitted for permanent section pathology; frozen section analysis of margins is not performed. In most cases, the incision is closed by mobilizing the skin without the need for complex tissue rearrangement or skin grafting. Complex tissue flaps or skin grafts are rarely necessary, except for melanomas of the head and neck and distal extremities (Fig. 32-16). Tumors arising in proximity to structures such as the nose, eye, and ear may require a compromise of the conventional margins to avoid deformities or disabilities. Subungual melanomas are treated with amputation of the distal digit to provide a 1-cm margin from the tumor. For fingers, ray amputations are unnecessary because the melanoma commonly involves only the distal phalanx; usually, amputation at the distal interphalangeal joint is sufficient. In all cases, resection should achieve histologically negative margins. It should be noted that the recommended margins of excision are the clinically measured margins; it is unnecessary to re-excise the melanoma if the final pathology report indicates that the measured distance from the

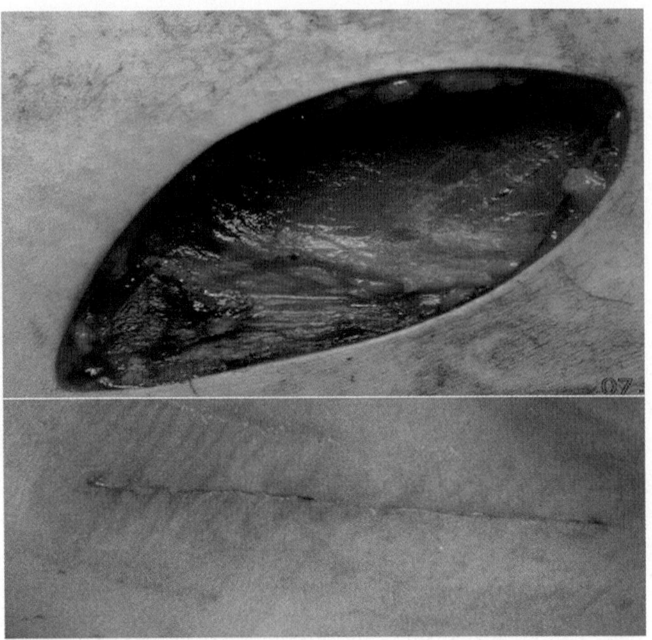

**FIGURE 32-15** Fusiform incision and closure.

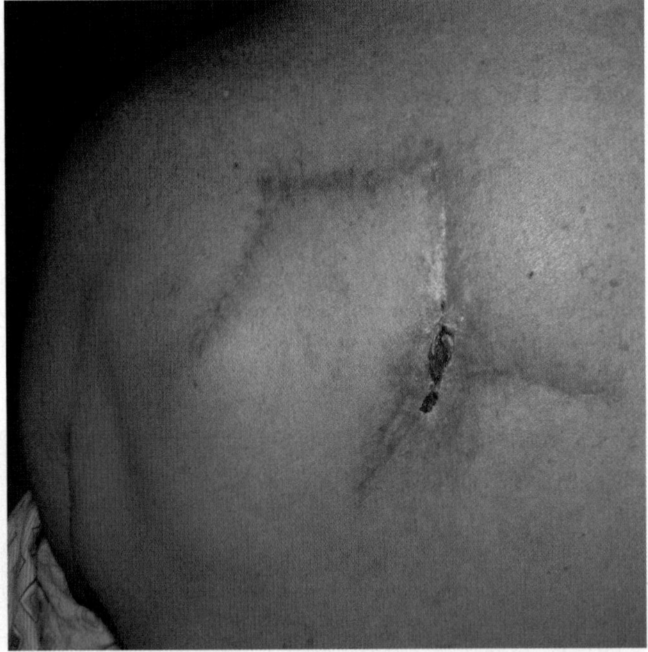

**FIGURE 32-16** Unnecessarily complex closure.

melanoma to the edge of the excised skin is less than the recommended margin, unless the margin is involved or almost involved by tumor.

Mohs micrographic surgery involves the sequential tangential excision of skin cancers with immediate pathologic margin assessment. It is used most often for skin cancers such as squamous cell and basal cell carcinomas, with good results. Mohs surgery is used in some centers for melanoma in situ, especially on the face, to minimize the cosmetic defect while still achieving negative margins of excision. Although there have been several single-institution reports indicating that Mohs surgery results in low local recurrence rates for melanoma in situ, it remains controversial. Mohs surgery for invasive melanoma should be discouraged, because there are no randomized prospective trials to compare it to conventional WLE.[22]

### Management of the Regional Lymph Nodes

It is important to understand the proper terminology regarding the operations performed for regional lymph nodes. Lymph node dissection is described as elective if performed for patients without clinical evidence of nodal metastasis—that is, those without palpable nodes or imaging studies to suggest regional nodal disease. Therapeutic lymph node dissection refers to lymphadenectomy performed for palpable or clinically evident disease. Completion lymph node dissection is the operation performed after finding nodal metastasis by SLN biopsy.

**Elective Lymph Node Dissection** In 1892, Herbert Snow reported the propensity for melanoma to metastasize to the regional lymph nodes and advocated that treatment of melanoma with curative intent should include elective lymph node dissection.[1] Snow's manuscript sparked controversy over elective lymph node dissection that lasted for an entire century. As described by Snow, melanoma commonly metastasizes initially to the regional lymph nodes. In fact, patients rarely develop distant metastases without ever developing nodal metastasis. Most patients with melanoma present without clinical evidence of nodal metastasis, although approximately 20% of patients with melanomas 1 mm thick or larger will develop palpable nodal disease if left untreated. The rationale for elective lymph node dissection stemmed from the concept that regional nodal metastases might metastasize in turn to distant sites, and that the greater the tumor burden in the regional nodes, the greater the chance for distant metastasis. Early removal of microscopic nodal metastases was therefore thought to improve survival. This argument was bolstered by the fact that remains true today: some patients with nodal metastasis are cured by regional lymph node dissection, and the likelihood of cure is proportional to the disease burden in the nodes. Retrospective studies have provided support for this concept.

This controversy led to several randomized prospective trials, none of which has demonstrated an overall survival benefit for elective lymph node dissection.[22,23] In the Intergroup Melanoma Trial, 740 patients with melanoma 1 to 4 mm thick were randomized to elective lymph node dissection or nodal observation. Although there was no survival difference between the groups overall, subgroup analysis has suggested that some patients may benefit from elective lymph node dissection, specifically, patients younger than 60 years, those without ulcerated melanomas, those with melanomas 1- to 2-mm Breslow thickness, and those with extremity melanomas. In 1998, a World Health Organization (WHO) study evaluated 240 patients with truncal melanomas 1.5 mm thick or larger randomized to elective lymph node dissection or nodal observation and found no survival advantage for elective lymph node dissection. However, subgroup analysis revealed a significant improvement in 5-year survival when the patients with occult nodal metastasis detected at elective lymph node dissection were compared with those in the observation arm. These patients developed nodal metastasis and underwent therapeutic lymph node dissection (48% versus 27%, respectively; $P = .04$). This provided some support for the notion that early removal of nodal metastasis is more efficacious than waiting for the patients to develop large palpable nodes. Two other studies have failed to demonstrate a survival benefit for elective lymph node dissection.

The problem with elective lymph node dissection is that only approximately 20% of patients with melanomas 1 mm thick or larger have nodal metastases at the time of presentation. Therefore, 80% of patients (those without nodal metastases) cannot possibly benefit from lymphadenectomy. Because the morbidity of lymph node dissection can be substantial, including wound complications, chronic pain, and lymphedema, there was little enthusiasm for elective lymph node dissection in the absence of a demonstrable survival benefit. The entire controversy regarding elective lymph node biopsy, however, evaporated with the advent of SLN biopsy.

**Sentinel Lymph Node Biopsy** In 1977, Robinson and colleagues[24] published a study on the use of cutaneous lymphoscintigraphy to identify the lymph nodes draining truncal melanomas with ambiguous drainage patterns. Because truncal melanomas can potentially drain to cervical, axillary, or inguinal lymph nodes, the decision regarding which nodal basin(s) should undergo elective lymph node dissection was based on Sappey's classic anatomic studies (performed in the 19th century). Lymphoscintigraphy involves the use of a radioactive agent that is injected into the skin around the melanoma. The radioactive tracer particles are taken up by the lymphatic channels and captured in the draining lymph nodes. Although it now seems obvious that the first node(s) in the nodal basin to receive the radioactive tracer should also be the first nodes to receive metastatic tumor cells, the concept of a sentinel node was not actually established until the pioneering work of Dr. Donald Morton. An SLN is the first lymph node(s) to receive lymphatic drainage from the site of the primary tumor. In 1992, Morton and coworkers[25] published the first report of SLN biopsy for melanoma and found that the sentinel node accurately determines the presence or absence of microscopic nodal metastasis.

Since that time, thousands of articles have been published to validate the SLN hypothesis in a variety of malignancies, and SLN biopsy has become a standard method of staging the regional nodes in melanoma and breast cancer.[26] A landmark study by Gershenwald and associates[27] at M.D. Anderson Cancer Center has demonstrated that SLN biopsy is the single most important factor predicting prognosis in melanoma patients without clinical evidence of nodal metastasis. Because sentinel node biopsy is a minimally invasive procedure that usually involves removal of one or two lymph nodes, it has been shown to be associated with fewer complications than a complete lymph node dissection.[28]

***Indications*** SLN biopsy is a staging procedure to determine the nodal status of patients with melanoma. Although SLN biopsy is a minimally invasive procedure, it is not without morbidity and certainly not without cost. Like other staging tests (e.g., PET, CT), it should not be overused in low-risk patients. Because of the significant risk of nodal metastasis, there is general agreement that SLN biopsy is appropriate for patients with intermediate thickness melanomas (1- to 4-mm Breslow thickness). Patients with thin melanomas (<1-mm thick) have a low risk of nodal metastasis overall (<5%), but this subgroup represents about 65% of all melanoma patients; therefore, a substantial number of node-positive patients may be missed if SLN biopsy is never performed. A thorough analysis of the literature has identified ulceration and mitotic rate as important factors to consider in the decision to perform SLN biopsy for patients with thin melanomas.[29] Although ulceration is infrequently identified in patients with thin melanomas (4% to 9%) and limited data are available to determine the impact of ulceration on the risk of nodal metastasis in this population, the powerful prognostic significance of ulceration overall suggests that SLN biopsy should be considered for all ulcerated melanomas, regardless of thickness. A mitotic rate of $1/mm^2$ or higher has been shown to be an important predictor of nodal metastasis in thin melanoma patients. Conveniently, ulceration and mitotic rate are now used in the most recent edition of the AJCC melanoma staging system to discriminate T1a from T1b melanomas.[17] Therefore, SLN biopsy for T1b melanomas is recommended. Breslow thickness should also be considered in the thin melanoma category. The incidence of SLN metastasis among patients with melanomas 0.75 mm thick or smaller was 2.7% and 6.2% for those with melanomas 0.75 to 1 mm thick. Whether all patients with melanomas 0.75 to 1.0 mm thick should undergo SLN biopsy is controversial; the high-risk group might be better discriminated by considering ulceration and mitotic rate. Factors that have not been universally demonstrated to increase the risk of nodal metastasis include age, gender, regression, Clark level, vertical growth phase, and tumor-infiltrating lymphocytes. Kesmodel and coworkers[30] have used tumor mitotic rate to develop a risk classification tree for patients with thin vertical growth phase melanomas (Fig. 32-17). This model provides a useful framework for considering the risk of nodal metastasis as well.

The role of SLN biopsy for patients with thick melanomas (>4 mm) has also been questioned. Patients with thick melanomas are at high risk for systemic metastases. This has led to the dogma that no patients with thick melanoma could ever benefit from SLN biopsy or lymph node dissection. However, a number of studies have shown that thick melanoma patients with tumor-negative SLN have a better prognosis than those with tumor-positive SLN. Because there is a continuum of risk that does not abruptly end at 4-mm Breslow thickness and because some thick melanoma patients with nodal metastases can be cured by resection of nodal metastases, SLN biopsy should be performed in this population.[31]

Although the benefit remains unproven, there are also intriguing reports of SLN biopsy for patients with locally recurrent or in-transit melanoma.

***Technical Details*** The technical details of proper SLN biopsy are worthy of attention. First, all patients should undergo preoperative lymphoscintigraphy, typically performed on the same day as the operation to perform SLN biopsy and WLE. Technetium-99 sulfur colloid (0.5 mCi) should be injected into the dermis, raising a wheal, in four aliquots around the melanoma or biopsy site. It is important to inject the tracer into the normal skin approximately 0.5 cm away from the melanoma or scar from the biopsy, not into the melanoma or biopsy scar. A common mistake is to inject the radioactive tracer too deeply, into the subcutaneous tissue, which will result in failure to detect a sentinel node. If no sentinel nodes are identified after the initial injection, repeat injection should be performed with the proper technique by an experienced clinician. In almost all cases, this will result in identification of sentinel nodes. Imaging is performed with a gamma camera, with dynamic and static images that allow identification of lymphatic channels and sentinel nodes (Fig. 32-18). Although patterns of lymphatic drainage may be generally predicted by the anatomic studies of Sappey, lymphoscintigraphy often identifies lymph nodes in locations that might not be anticipated. This is especially true for melanomas in ambiguous lymphatic drainage areas, such as the trunk, head, or neck, where anatomic predictions of nodal spread are unreliable. In such cases, it is possible to identify sentinel nodes in more than one nodal basin. Furthermore, it is not uncommon to identify sentinel nodes outside the traditional cervical, axillary, and inguinal nodal basins. So-called interval, intercalated, or in-transit nodes may be found in subcutaneous locations or between muscle groups. For distal upper or lower extremity melanomas, it is important to assess the presence of epitrochlear or popliteal sentinel nodes, respectively (Fig. 32-19). These interval nodes have the same risk of harboring melanoma cells as sentinel nodes in traditional nodal basins; therefore, it is recommended that they be removed at the time of sentinel node biopsy.[32] In addition, 85% of the time the interval lymph node is the only positive node, even for those patients with other SLN

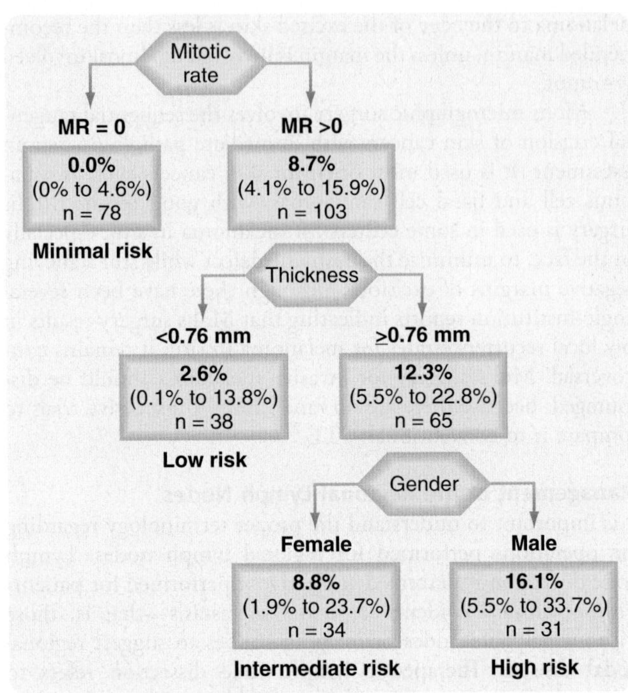


**FIGURE 32-17** Risk classification tree for patients with thin vertical growth phase melanomas. (From Kesmodel SB, Karakousis GC, Botbyl JD, et al: Mitotic rate as a predictor of sentinel lymph node positivity in patients with thin melanomas. Ann Surg Oncol 12:449–458, 2005.)

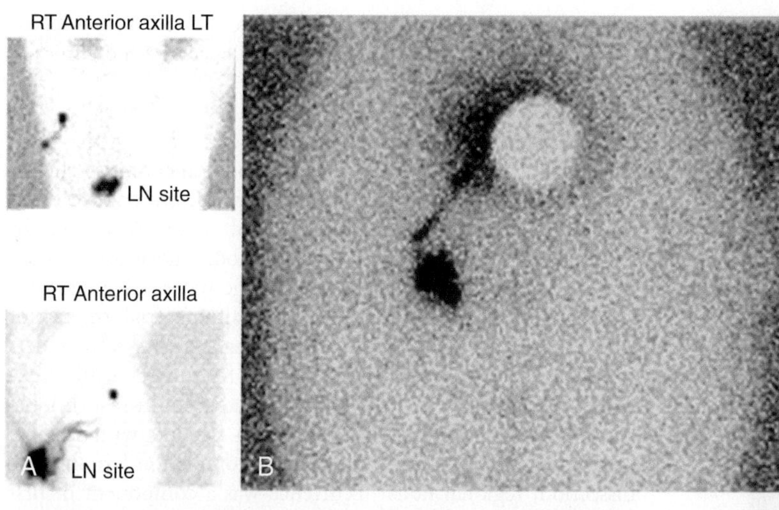


**FIGURE 32-18** Lymphoscintigraphy is used to determine the location of the sentinel nodes. **A,** Melanoma of the back with lymphatic channels leading to the axilla. **B,** Periumbilical melanoma with lymphatic drainage to the left groin.

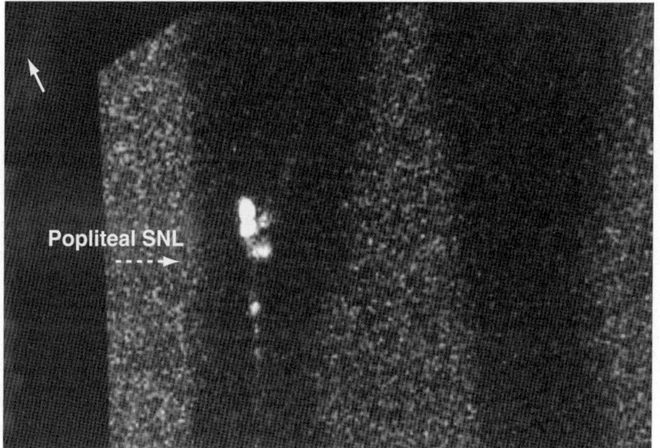


**FIGURE 32-19** Popliteal SLN lymphoscintigram.

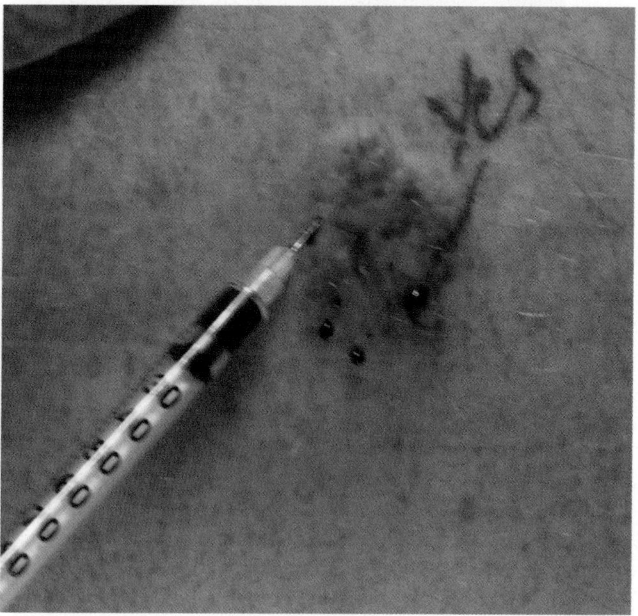


**FIGURE 32-20** Vital blue dye (e.g., isosulfan blue) injected into the dermis around the melanoma.

identified in traditional basins. Therefore, all sentinel nodes identified by preoperative lymphoscintigraphy should be removed.

At operation, which is generally performed under general anesthesia, a vital blue dye (e.g., isosulfan blue) is injected into the dermis around the melanoma site in a manner similar to that for injection of the radioactive tracer (Fig. 32-20). This combined lymphatic mapping technique allows for the identification of the sentinel nodes in 99% of patients.[33] Because the blue dye will not persist in the sentinel nodes for prolonged periods, it is injected just before the operation. One to 5 mL of blue dye is used, depending on the size of the melanoma site. Because the blue dye will persist in the skin for many months after injection, it is best to inject it within the margins of the planned WLE. A hand-held gamma probe is used to identify the location of the sentinel node(s), and dissection is performed to identify blue lymphatic channels entering into a blue, radioactive lymph node, which is removed (Fig. 32-21). A sentinel node, in practical terms, is defined as any lymph node that is the most radioactive node in the nodal basin, any node that is blue, which indicates a direct lymphatic drainage pathway from the primary tumor, any node that has a radioactive count of 10% or higher of the most radioactive node in that basin, or any node that is palpably suspicious for tumor. Following these guidelines will minimize the false-negative rate of sentinel node biopsy.[34] The average number of sentinel nodes identified is two per nodal basin. Although multiple radioactive lymph nodes may be evident within a nodal basin on lymphoscintigraphy, many of these represent second-echelon nodes that are more likely to be imaged; there is often a poor correlation between the number of nodes visualized on the lymphoscintigram and the number of SLNs identified. SLN(s) should be sent for permanent section histopathology with immunohistochemical stains for melanoma markers (e.g., S-100, HMB-45); immediate frozen section histology should be avoided because even expert pathologists have difficulty diagnosing micrometastatic melanoma in the SLN on frozen sections.

SLN biopsy is more challenging in the head and neck than for other regions, likely because of the rich lymphatic drainage network in this location. Correspondingly, the false-negative rate for SLN biopsy is generally higher for melanomas in these

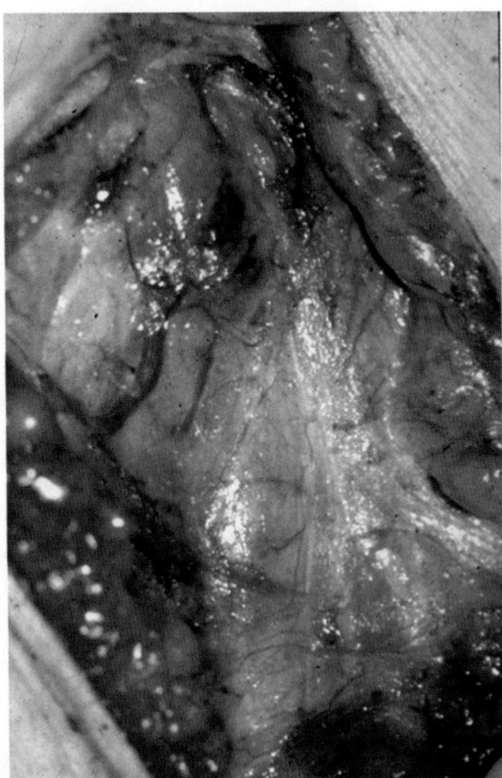

**FIGURE 32-21** Dissection showing blue lymphatic channels entering into a blue radioactive lymph node.

locations.[35] Precise knowledge of the anatomy in this region is essential to avoid inadvertent neurologic injury. Parotid SLN can be identified and removed, usually without the need for superficial parotidectomy. However, if there is any concern for facial nerve injury, superficial parotidectomy may be a safer option. A common site for cervical SLN is directly adjacent to the spinal accessory nerve, which should be visualized and preserved.

### Multicenter Selective Lymphadenectomy Trial

In 1994, the first Multicenter Selective Lymphadenectomy Trial (MSLT-I) was initiated by Dr. Morton. In this study, 1347 patients with melanomas 1.2 to 3.5 mm wide were randomized to receive WLE alone or WLE with sentinel node biopsy to determine whether sentinel node biopsy, with completion lymph node dissection for those that had metastatic disease in the sentinel nodes, improved disease-free and overall survival compared with nodal observation.[36] The 5-year disease-free survival rate for the sentinel node group was significantly improved (78.3%) compared with the nodal observation group (78.3% versus 73.1%, respectively; $P$ = .009); however, the 5-year melanoma-specific survival rates were similar (87.1 versus 86.6, respectively). In a subgroup analysis considering only patients with nodal metastasis, there was a significant difference in 5-year survival, 72.3% versus 52.4% ($P$ = .004) comparing those with sentinel node metastases to those who developed palpable nodal disease in the observation group, respectively. Some have suggested that sentinel node biopsy may detect tiny nodal micrometastases that have no clinical significance, but the fact that the same number of patients in each group (16%) were found to have nodal metastasis suggests that microscopic tumor deposits found at sentinel node biopsy will likely become clinically evident if not resected.

### Lymph Node Dissection

**Completion** Patients with sentinel node metastasis should undergo completion lymph node dissection. Some have questioned the need for completion lymph node dissection for patients with SLN metastases because nodal metastasis is often not found beyond the SLN. In two large prospective randomized trials, MSLT-I and the Sunbelt Melanoma Trial, the rate of tumor-positive nonsentinel nodes among patients who underwent completion lymph node dissection for tumor-positive sentinel nodes was 16%.[36,37] In a retrospective multi-institutional study by Wong and colleagues[38] of 134 patients with sentinel node metastases who did not undergo completion lymph node dissection, regional nodal recurrence was a component of first recurrence in 15% of patients. Therefore, the risk of nodal recurrence if completion lymph node dissection is not performed may be estimated as at least 15%. Several studies have tried to identify subgroups of sentinel node-positive patients who may be at low risk of nonsentinel node metastasis. Although tumor burden within the SLN appears to affect the risk of nonsentinel node metastasis, there is currently no consensus regarding which patients may safely avoid completion lymphadenectomy.[39] If a patient has SLN identified in more than one nodal basin (e.g., axilla and groin) and is found to have a tumor-positive SLN in only one of those nodal basins, completion lymph node dissection should only be performed for the basin in which metastatic disease is identified.

The goals of completion lymph node dissection are two—cure and regional disease control. Regional disease control is an important goal of therapy, because some patients may develop unresectable nodal metastases that cause pain and suffering. In MSLT-I, the rate of regional nodal recurrence after completion lymph node dissection was 4.2%[36]; in the Sunbelt Melanoma Trial, it was 4.9%. Therefore, although it remains uncertain whether completion lymph node dissection cures more patients or improves overall survival, it does appear to provide excellent regional disease control. Until the results of MSLT-II are available, it recommended that patients with metastatic disease in the SLN undergo completion lymphadenectomy.

**Therapeutic Lymph Node Dissection** Patients with nodal metastasis suspected by palpation or imaging studies should undergo confirmation with fine-needle aspiration (FNA) biopsy in most cases. In some cases, palpable nodes may be benign; lymph node dissection for patients who have benign lymphadenopathy should be avoided. If necessary, excisional biopsy may confirm the diagnosis. After imaging evaluation to assess for the presence of distant metastatic disease (brain MRI and/or PET-CT scanning are appropriate), therapeutic lymph node dissection will result in long-term survival and potential cure of a significant fraction of patients. Prognosis depends on the extent of the nodal disease. The number of involved lymph nodes appears to have greater prognostic significance than the size of the nodes, but there is a clear range of prognoses, depending on whether the nodes have microscopic versus macroscopic evidence of melanoma as well. The survival of stage III melanoma patients who undergo lymph node dissection ranges from approximately 25% to 75%, depending on the nodal tumor burden.[16,36]

**Extent** Because of the lack of effective adjuvant therapy agents, lymphadenectomy should be as complete as possible. There is a marked difference, for example, in the axillary lymph node dissection performed for breast cancer as compared with melanoma. In breast cancer, a level I or II lymph node dissection is performed to gain important staging information, but effective hormonal therapy, chemotherapy, and radiation therapy make regional recurrence uncommon. For melanoma patients, a thorough level I, II, or III axillary dissection should be performed, which will reduce the likelihood of nodal recurrence. Level II nodes exist in a fat pad that extends cephalad to the axillary vein. The conventional wisdom in breast cancer is not to extend the lymph node dissection cephalad to the axillary vein, and not to remove level III nodes, because of the supposed increased risk of lymphedema. However, failure to clear these level II and III nodes completely is not an infrequent cause of nodal recurrence in melanoma patients after axillary lymphadenectomy. Therefore, complete removal of all fibrofatty tissue around the axillary vein, thoracodorsal and medial pectoral neurovascular bundles, and long thoracic nerve should be performed. If necessary to clear bulky level II and III nodes, the pectoralis minor muscle may be divided near its insertion on the coracoid process; rarely, the pectoralis major muscle may need to be divided. If a tumor involves the axillary vein, it may be ligated and divided, often with less consequence in terms of edema than one might anticipate.

Inguinal lymph node dissection includes the superficial inguinal (femoral) lymph nodes and deep or pelvic (internal iliac, external iliac, and obturator) nodes. In most cases of lower extremity melanoma metastatic to inguinal sentinel nodes, a superficial inguinal lymph node dissection is sufficient. Some surgeons prefer to include a deep dissection for patients with buttock or truncal primary tumors that metastasize to superficial inguinal SLN. For patients with palpable nodal disease, the deep nodes should be dissected in most cases. Metastasis to Cloquet's node, the most proximal femoral lymph node that lies beneath the inguinal ligament medial to the common femoral vein, has been used by some to determine the need for pelvic lymph node dissection. Surveillance with imaging studies after finding involved inguinal nodes is recommended, because pelvic nodal recurrence is difficult to detect by palpation until it is bulky and extensive. Once this has occurred, regional disease control is lost and patients may suffer the consequences.

A functional neck dissection, sparing the internal jugular vein and spinal accessory nerve, is usually sufficient. The need for superficial parotidectomy may be guided by the lymphoscintigraphy and SLN results. Epitrochlear or popliteal lymphadenectomy is infrequently necessary, but requires careful attention to the particular anatomy in these regions (Fig. 32-22).[40,41]

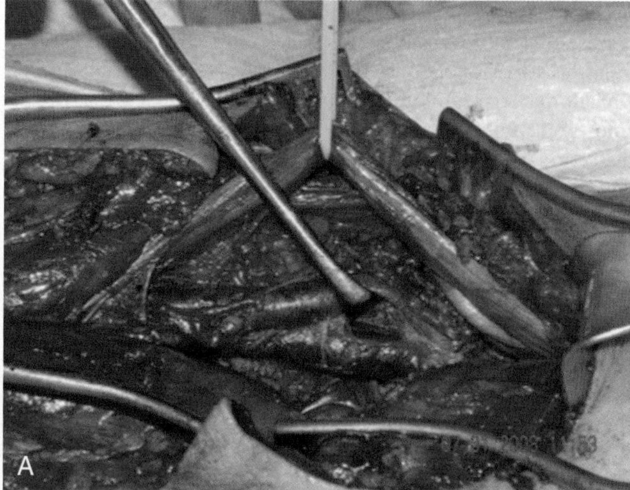


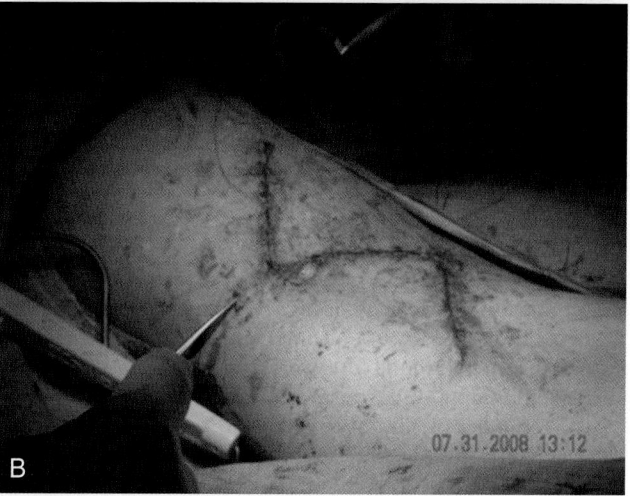


**FIGURE 32-22 A,** Popliteal lymphadenectomy. **B,** Popliteal lymphadenectomy closure.

## Adjuvant Therapy

**Systemic Therapy** The only adjuvant therapy approved by the U.S. Food and Drug Administration (FDA) is high-dose interferon alfa-2b. Interferon alfa-2b is administered at a dose near the maximally tolerated dose, with 1 month of IV therapy followed by 11 months of subcutaneous injections three times weekly. High-dose interferon has substantial adverse effects, including flu-like symptoms, fatigue, malaise, anorexia, neuropsychiatric side effects, and potential hepatic toxicity. The benefit of high-dose interferon alfa-2b has been evaluated in four prospective randomized trials.[42] The first trial, conducted by the Eastern Cooperative Oncology Group (ECOG) in conjunction with other cooperative groups, was E-1684, started in 1984, which demonstrated a disease-free and overall survival benefit for treatment with interferon. Most of the high-risk melanoma patients enrolled in this study had palpable nodal disease (stage III). However, a second larger trial, E1690, demonstrated a marginal improvement in disease-free survival but no difference in overall survival. A third study, E1694, randomized patients to high-dose interferon versus a ganglioside vaccine (GM2). This study was stopped early because of the clear superiority of interferon compared with the vaccine in terms of disease-free and overall survival, which was initially interpreted as evidence of a beneficial effect of interferon rather than a detrimental effect of the vaccine. However, a prospective randomized trial with this GM2 vaccine conducted by the European Organization for Research and Treatment of Cancer (EORTC) has demonstrated a significant detrimental effect of this vaccine compared with a placebo group. This casts significant doubt regarding the interpretation of the results of the study of E1694. The EORTC trial 18991 randomized patients to 5 years of pegylated IFN-a2b (PEG-IFN) versus observation. In this trial, the PEG-IFN dosing schedule was comparable to that of the high-dose interferon regimen. This study demonstrated improvement in disease-free survival, but no benefit in terms of a distant metastasis-free interval or overall survival. Finally, the Sunbelt Melanoma Trial randomized patients with a single positive sentinel node (all of whom underwent completion lymph node dissection) to observation versus high-dose interferon alfa-2b. Although somewhat underpowered to detect small differences in disease-free or overall survival, this study showed neither trends nor significant differences to suggest a benefit from high-dose interferon in this population. The 5-year survival rate for sentinel node–positive patients (without interferon) in the Sunbelt Melanoma Trial and MSLT-I were 67% and 72%, respectively, indicating that such patients with clinically occult nodal metastasis have an intermediate, rather than high, risk of mortality.

Intermediate doses of interferon were evaluated in patients with stage IIB or III disease in EORTC trial 18952, demonstrating improvement in disease-free survival, but no improvement in distant metastasis-free interval or overall survival for patients who received interferon. Seven clinical trials have evaluated low-dose interferon; four demonstrated an improvement in disease-free survival but only one demonstrated improvement in overall survival.[42]

Taken together, the results of these studies suggest that adjuvant interferon therapy may prolong the time to recurrence, but is unlikely to cure more patients. Lower doses may provide the same disease-free survival advantage as high-dose interferon. Given the cost and toxicity of high-dose interferon alfa-2b, use of this adjuvant therapy has become controversial and is not used in many centers around the world. However, it is the only current FDA-approved treatment option outside of clinical trials. A number of clinical trials have investigated other adjuvant therapies, including melanoma vaccines. The results to date have not identified any additional beneficial adjuvant therapy agents, and some appear to be frankly harmful. Participation in clinical trials of novel agents is encouraged to identify more effective, less toxic therapies. Observation for patients with tumor-positive SLN after completion lymphadenectomy is also a reasonable option.

### Radiation Therapy

Adjuvant radiation therapy for melanoma is not used routinely, because melanoma is generally considered to be relatively resistant to irradiation. However, radiation therapy is used in many centers in an attempt to improve locoregional disease control, especially for high-risk head and neck melanomas, in which the risk of local recurrence and in-transit disease is greater than for other sites. Retrospective data have also suggested there may be a benefit of radiation therapy for regional disease control in patients with multiple tumor-involved lymph nodes or extracapsular extension after lymph node dissection. A recent Australian prospective trial[43] randomized 217 patients with a significant risk of regional recurrence after lymphadenectomy to adjuvant radiotherapy versus observation. The risk factors included the number of positive nodes (at least one for parotid, two for neck and axilla, and three for groin), lymph node size (30 mm or larger for parotid, neck, and axilla; 40 mm or larger for groin), or extracapsular extension of tumor. With a median follow-up of 27 months, there was a significant improvement in regional recurrence in the radiation therapy versus observation group (19% versus 31%, respectively), although there was no difference in overall survival. This is the first prospective randomized trial to demonstrate a benefit for adjuvant radiation therapy for patients with nodal metastasis. Further studies are necessary to define the subgroups of patients who may benefit from radiotherapy.

### Follow-Up After Treatment of Melanoma

There is no consensus on the best way to monitor patients for recurrence after treatment of melanoma. However, some general principles should be considered. All patients who have been diagnosed with melanoma have a lifetime risk of developing a second primary melanoma that is approximately 8%, as well as an increased risk of other skin cancers. Therefore, all melanoma patients should undergo at least an annual complete dermatologic examination for life. In general, most recurrences are detected by the patient, fewer by routine history and physical examination, and fewer still by routine laboratory or imaging tests. Most recurrences (75%) will be detected in the first 3 years after treatment of the primary melanoma, although it is possible to detect metastatic disease decades afterward. There is little evidence that early detection of distant metastatic disease will alter the patient's outcome. Therefore, the follow-up strategy should be tailored to the individual patient's risk of metastasis. Stage 0, I, and IIA patients are at low risk of recurrence and should be followed by history and physical examination at least every 6 months for the first 3 years and at least annually there after. Although laboratory tests such as hematocrit and lactate dehydrogenase (LDH) levels, and routine chest x-ray have been used in some centers, there is no evidence that these tests are useful for the early detection of metastatic disease; these tests are not required. A careful history to elicit symptoms such as new cutaneous or subcutaneous lesions, nodal masses, pain, headaches, neurologic changes, weight loss, and gastrointestinal and pulmonary symptoms, is essential. Patients should be informed about the common symptoms and signs of recurrence so that they can report important changes arising between scheduled examinations. Physical examination should include a complete skin inspection and palpation to detect regional nodal or in-transit recurrence. For stage IIB, IIC, and III melanoma patients, a reasonable follow-up schedule would be a history and physical examination every 3 or 4 months for the first 3 years, every 6 months for the next 2 years, and annually thereafter. The use of laboratory tests and imaging tests such as CT, MRI, or PET-CT is controversial but, for patients with stage IIB, IIC, or III melanoma, is not unreasonable. Patients with stage IV melanoma will have regular clinical, laboratory, and radiologic evaluations to monitor the response to treatment.[18]

### Treatment of Recurrent or Metastatic Disease

**Local Recurrence** Local recurrence is defined as a tumor appearing in the skin or subcutaneous tissues within 2 cm of the scar or skin graft of the WLE site. Local recurrence risk increases with tumor thickness and has been reported to be 0.2%, 2%, 6%, and 13% for melanomas 0.75 mm or smaller, larger than 0.75 to 1.5 mm, larger than1.5 to 4 mm, and larger than 4 mm, respectively. Local recurrence reflects aggressive biologic behavior of the melanoma and portends a poor prognosis; long-term survival is less than 20% for patients who experience local recurrence. The treatment of local recurrence is surgical resection, with histologically negative margins. Although WLE guidelines for primary tumors do not apply to local recurrences, it is prudent to attempt at least a 1-cm margin of excision around the recurrence and even to resect the entire prior wide excision scar. SLN biopsy for local recurrence may detect regional nodal metastasis, but its value in this situation is unclear.

**In-Transit Disease** In-transit recurrence represents endolymphatic disease manifested by cutaneous or subcutaneous tumor nodules between the primary tumor site and regional nodal basin(s). In-transit lesions may be palpable but not visible, and are frequently not pigmented; they may be pink or flesh-colored. Such patients should have an imaging evaluation to detect distant metastatic disease, although many patients with in-transit disease may live for many years without developing metastasis beyond locoregional sites. Limited in-transit disease is adequately treated by resection. As with local recurrence, SLN biopsy is of unclear value but may be considered. Although recurrence of in-transit disease after resection is the rule rather than the exception, many patients with limited in-transit disease may be managed for years with sequential excision of in-transit lesions, and with good quality of life. Radiation therapy for in-transit disease is generally futile and may be harmful. Local injection of refractory in-transit disease with agents such as Bacille Calmette-Guérin (BCG), interferon, and interleukin-2 may, in some cases, result in complete response. Laser and other ablative therapies may be considered. However, the evidence to support such treatments is largely anecdotal.

More extensive or recurrent in-transit disease, when confined to the upper or lower extremity, may be treated by hyperthermic isolated limb perfusion (HILP) with L-phenylalanine mustard (melphalan). Creech and colleagues first performed HILP at Tulane University in the 1950s. The concept is that higher chemotherapeutic drug concentrations may be achieved regionally while limiting systemic toxicity. HILP is performed by cannulation of the major extremity artery and vein, with hyperthermic (40° to 42° C) perfusion using a pump oxygenator after tourniquet isolation of the proximal extremity. Several single-institution studies have demonstrated overall response rates of approximately 80%, with 40% to 60% complete responses.[44] Unfortunately, complete responses may be short-lived, because many patients will experience recurrence within approximately1 year. However, complete response appears to predict a better prognosis. In a study by Kroon and Thompson[45] in the Sydney Melanoma Unit, the 5-year survival rate for nonresponders and partial responders was 7%, whereas the 10-year survival rate for complete responders was 49%. HILP achieved long-term control of in-transit disease in 57% of complete responders.

Repeat perfusion can be performed in patients who recur, but should only be attempted in patients who responded well to the initial perfusion. The toxicity of HILP can be substantial, including compartment syndrome, neuropathy, skin reaction, blistering, and lymphedema; toxicity resulting in amputation may occur in 1% to 3% of patients. Thompson and coworkers[46] have also pioneered the use of isolated limb infusion (ILI), which is a less invasive method of delivering regional chemotherapy, in which percutaneous catheters are placed instead of open operative insertion of cannulas into the major artery and vein supplying the extremity, followed by pneumatic tourniquet isolation (Fig. 32-23). Perfusion with ILI is accomplished by manual circulation using a syringe. ILI is therefore less resource-intensive than HILP, because it does not require use of a pump oxygenator

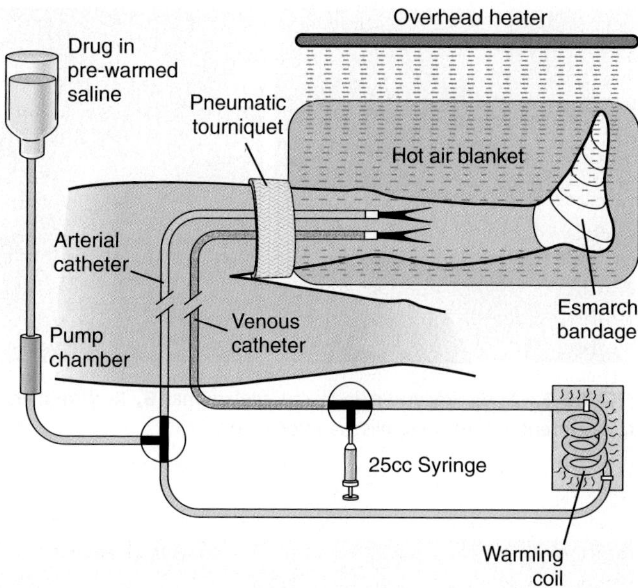


**FIGURE 32-23** Schematic illustration of the circuit used for isolated infusion of a lower limb. (From Kroon HM, Thompson JF: Isolated limb infusion: A review. J Surg Oncol 100:169–177, 2009.)

and perfusion team; it appears to be associated with response rates that are almost comparable to that of HILP. However, limb toxicity is no less than with HILP (Fig. 32-24). ILI is especially appealing for treatment of patients with in-transit disease who do not require regional lymphadenectomy or who have undergone prior HILP.

Based on encouraging results using therapeutic HILP, a randomized trial was designed to test the value of perfusion in patients with high-risk melanoma (>1.5 mm thickness).[46] Over 800 patients participated in this trial comparing WLE to WLE with HILP. After more than a 6-year median follow-up, there was no improvement in overall survival, although the number of in-transit metastases was reduced from 6.6% to 3.3%. Therefore, HILP is recommended only for patients with established in-transit metastases.

Some nonrandomized studies have suggested that the addition of tumor necrosis factor-α (TNF-α) to melphalan may improve the response to HILP. A study conducted by the American College of Surgeons Oncology Group (ACOSOG) randomized 124 patients with extremity in-transit melanoma to receive melphalan alone or melphalan plus TNF-α. The study revealed no benefit to the addition of TNF-α to melphalan in HILP. At 3 months after treatment, overall response rates were 64% versus 69%; complete response rates were 25% versus 26% in the groups treated with melphalan versus melphalan plus TNF-α, respectively. Limb toxicity was greater in the TNF-α–treated group. Therefore, this study found no benefit for the inclusion of TNF-α.[46]

Amputation for extensive regional recurrence is seldom indicated. These patients carry a high risk of having other distant metastases; therefore, long-term disease-free survival is not achieved by resection.

**Regional Nodal Recurrence** Regional nodal recurrence is treated by lymphadenectomy (see earlier, "Therapeutic Lymph Node

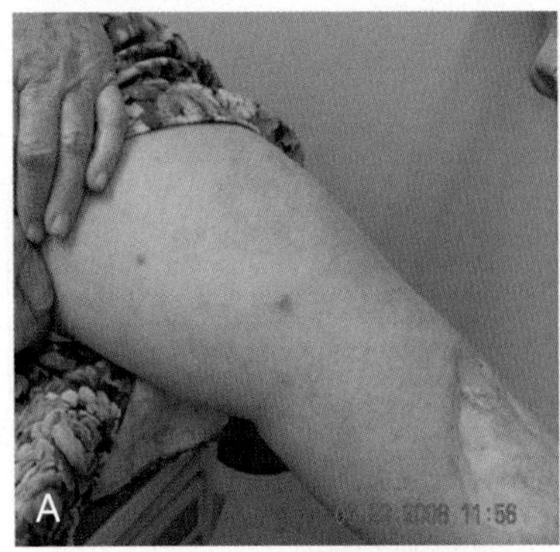


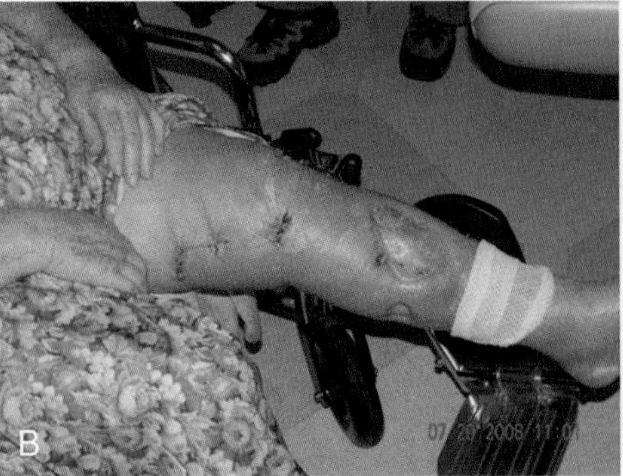


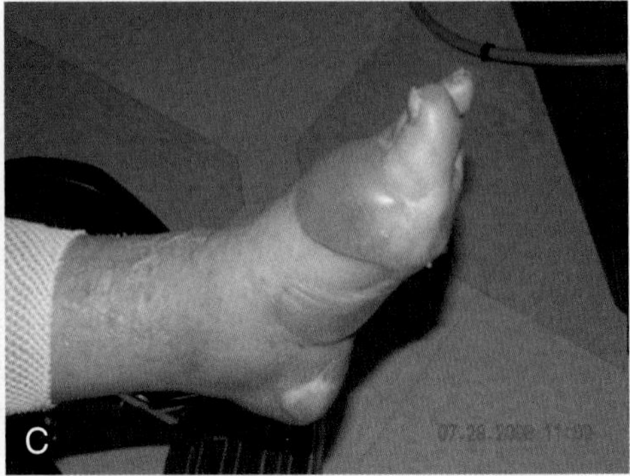


**FIGURE 32-24** **A,** Recurrent in-transit melanoma. **B,** Recurrent in-transit leg erythema after hyperthermic isolated limb perfusion (HILP). **C,** Recurrent in-transit leg blisters after HILP.

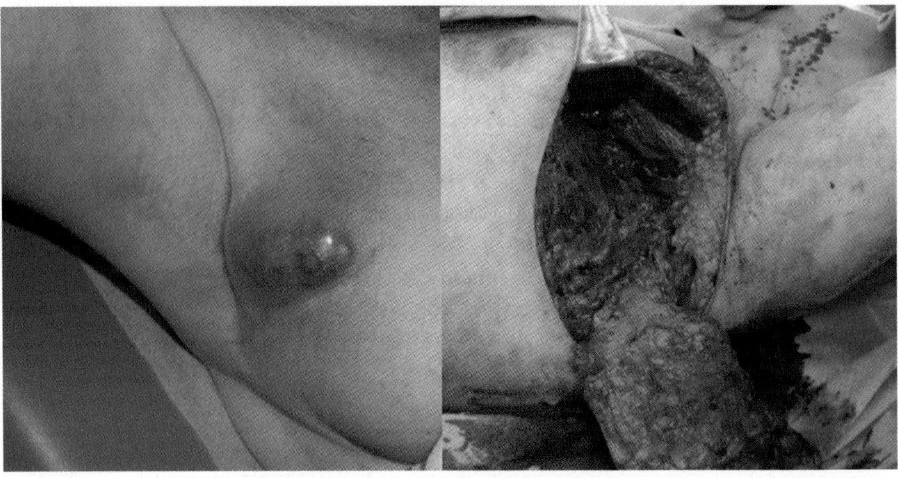

**FIGURE 32-25** Advanced nodal disease.

Dissection"); consideration should be given to adjuvant systemic and radiation therapy based on the extent of disease. Advanced regional nodal disease can pose a serious threat to loss of regional disease control (Fig. 32-25). Such nodal metastases may invade and encase neurovascular structures and may ulcerate through the skin, causing pain, bleeding, infection, and decreased quality of life.

**Distant Metastases** The most common sites of initial distant metastases are in the brain, lung, liver and, less commonly, the skin, distant lymph nodes, bone, and gastrointestinal tract. The median survival of patients with stage IV melanoma is approximately 7 months. Most patients will develop multiple sites of distant metastasis not amenable to resection. However, resection should be considered, when possible, for patients with stage IV melanoma, including brain metastases. Several studies have documented 5-year survival rates of 20% to 40% after resection of selected patients with distant metastases. Because these survival rates are similar to those of patients who undergo therapeutic lymph node dissection for palpable nodal disease, resection should be considered as first-line therapy whenever complete extirpation of all disease can be reasonably accomplished. In fact, the best treatment for melanoma at any stage is complete resection of all sites of disease. One should never overlook the opportunity to render a melanoma patient surgically free of cancer; some patients at every stage will enjoy long-term survival.[47]

Patients with unresectable metastatic disease should be considered for systemic therapy or palliative care. Melanoma is generally resistant to conventional chemotherapeutic agents. Two agents are approved by the FDA for stage IV melanoma, dacarbazine (DTIC) and high-dose interleukin-2 (IL-2). DTIC results in response rates of approximately 15 but no studies have demonstrated that DTIC prolongs survival. Combination cytotoxic chemotherapy has not been shown to be superior to single agent therapy. High-dose IL-2 is associated with substantial toxicity, is administered in an intensive care unit setting, and results in complete response rates of approximately 6%. However, complete response rates may be durable and some patients are presumably cured. Combination biochemotherapy, which typically combines three chemotherapeutic agents (cisplatin, vinblastine, dacarbazine) with interferon and IL-2, is associated with substantial toxicity but may result in overall response rates of up to 50% and complete response rates of up to 15%. However, biochemotherapy has not been shown to improve overall survival in randomized trials.[48]

Radiation therapy may provide useful palliation of bone and central nervous system metastases. Stereotactic radiation therapy benefits some patients with brain metastases. In general, however, radiation therapy provides little benefit for metastatic melanoma in other sites.

## Special Situations and Noncutaneous Melanoma

### Unknown Primary Melanoma

In some cases, melanoma is detected in lymph nodes or other organs without evidence of a primary melanoma; unknown primary melanoma is most common in lymph nodes. This occurs in less than 2% of all melanoma cases and less than 5% of all patients who present with metastatic melanoma. In such cases, investigation should be carried out to search for a primary melanoma. Some believe that melanoma may sometimes arise primarily in benign nevus cells that are found in lymph nodes; this would account for some cases of nodal melanoma when no primary melanoma is ever found. However, cutaneous melanoma is known to undergo spontaneous regression in rare cases, presumably as a result of an immune response to the primary tumor. Therefore, a history of a prior pigmented skin lesion that has disappeared or clinical evidence of vitiligo should be sought. Not infrequently, patients will provide a history of prior skin lesions that have been excised, cauterized, or treated with lasers. Pathology review of any prior skin lesions excised should be performed. A complete skin examination should be performed, including the scalp, external auditory canal, nail beds, external genitalia, and perianal area. Mucosal melanomas may be sought by examination and endoscopic evaluation of the oral cavity and nasopharynx, as well as the anus and rectum. Women should undergo a thorough pelvic examination. An ophthalmology examination should be performed to evaluate for ocular melanomas.

In the case of a lymph node metastasis, therapeutic lymph node dissection is performed with the assumption that it represents stage III, rather than stage IV, disease. The prognosis of patients with unknown primary melanomas who present with lymph node involvement is no worse than, and perhaps better than, those with known primary melanomas of similar stage.

### Melanoma During Pregnancy

Melanoma that presents during pregnancy poses difficult clinical issues. It is possible that the growth rate of the tumor is affected by hormonal changes during pregnancy. The prognosis for patients treated during pregnancy is no different from nonpregnant patients of a similar stage. SLN biopsy can be considered with caution. Although there is obvious concern for radiation exposure, data from patients with breast cancer have indicated that there is little risk to the fetus from lymphoscintigraphy. Because of the unknown risk to the fetus from isosulfan blue dye injection, as well as an approximately 1 in 10,000 risk of anaphylactic reaction, vital blue dye probably should not be used during pregnancy. General anesthesia is best avoided during the first trimester of pregnancy. One cautious approach for intermediate or thick melanomas during pregnancy is to perform WLE with a 1-cm margin under local anesthesia, await delivery, and then perform an additional 1-cm margin excision with SLN biopsy. There is no therapeutic benefit for the early termination of pregnancy.

### Noncutaneous Melanomas

In embryogenesis, melanocytes arise in the neural crest area and migrate to many sites other than the skin. Less than 10% of melanomas arise in these areas, which include the eye, mucosal surfaces, and unknown primary sites.

Ocular melanoma is the most common malignancy arising in the eye. In the eye, melanocytes are found in the retina and uveal tract (iris, ciliary body, and choroids). The options for treatment are photocoagulation, partial resection, radiation, or enucleation. Although ocular and cutaneous melanomas have several common histologic features, their clinical course is different. Ocular melanoma rarely metastasizes to lymph nodes because the uveal tract has no lymphatic vessels. Ocular melanomas have a peculiar pattern of metastasis—almost always, and often exclusively, to the liver. Surgical resection of liver metastases from ocular melanoma is rarely possible. Although a CT scan may sometimes suggest a single liver metastasis from ocular melanoma, this imaging modality may vastly underestimate the burden of disease. MRI of the liver is a more sensitive test, which will often demonstrate hundreds of small metastases. There are no accepted effective treatments for ocular melanoma metastatic to the liver.

The most common sites of origin for melanomas arising on the mucous membranes are the head and neck (oral cavity, oropharynx, nasopharynx, and paranasal sinuses), anal canal, rectum, and female genitalia. Compared with melanomas arising on the skin, mucosal melanomas are more advanced and have a uniformly poor prognosis. These tumors should be excised to negative margins. Extensive local resections do not affect survival, although locoregional control may be improved. For anorectal melanomas, abdominoperineal resection may reduce the incidence of locoregional recurrence but does not improve survival. In general, lymph node dissection is not indicated unless patients have clinically evident lymphadenopathy. SLN biopsy is being investigated for patients with vulvar and anal melanoma, although the benefit is unclear. The overall prognosis for patients with mucosal melanomas is uniformly poor, with less than a 10% 5-year survival.

# CUTANEOUS MALIGNANCIES: NONMELANOMA SKIN CANCER

## Squamous Cell Carcinoma and Basal Cell Carcinoma

Squamous cell carcinoma (SCC) and basal cell carcinoma (BCC) are the most common types of malignant neoplasms in the world. Just as with melanoma, the incidence of these cancers is rising each year. Current predictions are that this disease will develop in one in five Americans during their lifetime. Fortunately, mortality rates for nonmelanoma skin cancer (NMSC) are declining, and this decrease is attributed to early detection and effective treatment. Patients in whom any type of skin cancer develops undergo long-term periodic surveillance. After the initial diagnosis of BCC or SCC, the risk for development of an additional skin cancer is estimated to be 35% in 3 years and 50% in 5 years. In addition, there is a risk for other common malignancies such as lung cancer.

### Squamous Cell Carcinoma

By some estimates, NMSC develops in more than 1 million people annually; however, accurate statistics are problematic for a disease that is often treated without a histologic diagnosis. Although BCC is the most common type of NMSC, SCC has a higher mortality rate. As is true with other types of skin cancer, the incidence of SCC is increasing. There is a disproportionate increasing risk for women as opposed to men.[49]

Causes of SCC include the following: sunlight, susceptible phenotype, and compromised immunity, in addition to environmental conditions and diseases. Sunlight is thought to be the major causative factor because most SCCs occur on sun-exposed surfaces of the head and neck. In susceptible individuals (those with fair skin, blonde hair, and blue eyes), increasing sun exposure carries a growing risk for the development of SCC. Individuals with dark complexions have a lower risk, even with prolonged sun exposure. Specifically, UVB is thought to be the form of UV radiation that causes this disease. Most of the evidence for UV radiation comes from population-based studies in Australia, where individuals of Celtic origin moved to a geographic area in which they were subjected to higher sun exposure. The pattern of skin cancer appearing in this population indicated that exposure to UV radiation earlier in life was a major risk factor because individuals who moved to Australia after adolescence had a lower incidence of skin cancer than those who moved during their childhood. The risk for skin cancer increases with occupational or recreational sun exposure, advancing age, and proximity to the equator. The amount of sun exposure is also proportional to the incidence of precursor skin changes for SCC—namely, nevi, atrophy, and actinic keratosis.

It is postulated that UV radiation affects the skin in two ways that result in an increased incidence of SCC. First, there is a direct carcinogenic effect on frequently dividing keratinocytes in the basilar layer of the epidermis. Unrepaired mutations result in tumor promotion and growth. The second mechanism relates to depression of the cutaneous immune surveillance response, which in turn inhibits tumor rejection. The *p53* tumor suppressor gene is mutated in more than 90% of SCCs.[50]

Occupational and environmental exposures to arsenic, organic hydrocarbon, ionizing radiation, and cigarette smoke have been associated with increasing risk for SCCs. Genetic disorders, including xeroderma pigmentosum and albinism, are associated with increased risk for many types of skin cancer. Chronic conditions of the skin, such as burn scars (Marjolin's ulcer), draining sinuses, infections, and ulcers, can predate the development of SCCs. Previously healed wounds that break down or chronic wounds that will not heal undergo biopsy for the presence of SCC.

Impaired immunity, especially cell-mediated immunity, is a well-established cause of SCCs of the skin. It was found that the largest population of chronically immunosuppressed patients had undergone organ transplantation (Fig. 32-26).[51] Immunosuppressive drugs such as azathioprine, cyclosporine, and prednisone have been linked to a more than 50% increase in the risk for SCC. The intensity of immunosuppression and duration of therapy are associated with the risk for development of malignancies. After 10 years of immunosuppression, malignancies develop in 10% of patients and this figure increases to 40% after 20 years. Conditions associated with acquired impaired cell-mediated immunity, including lymphomas, leukemias, and autoimmune diseases, all increase the risk for SCCs. Human papillomavirus, an infection associated with immunosuppression, is proposed as a causative factor for the development of SCCs.

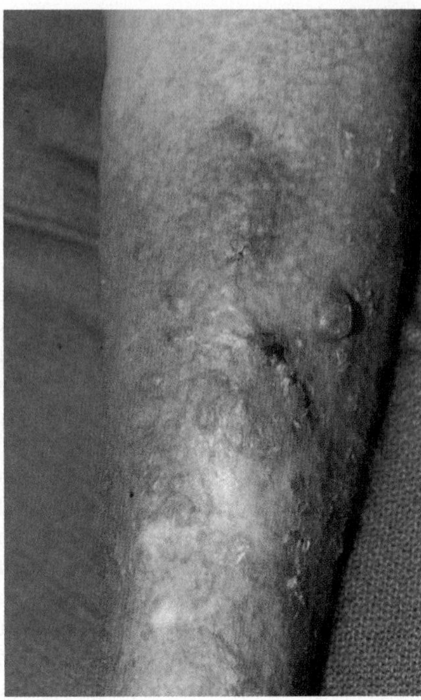

**FIGURE 32-26** Multiple squamous cell carcinomas on the upper extremity of a patient 11 years after kidney transplantation.

Most SCCs begin with a proliferation of keratin cells in the basal layer of the epidermis that appear as red or pink areas, clinically termed *actinic keratoses* (solar keratoses).[52] Local symptoms may wax and wane over a period of many months. Lesions are scaling, with an uneven surface and an erythematous base. Individual lesions are usually smaller than 1 cm in diameter and appear in chronically sun-damaged skin. The diagnosis is clinical and histologic because actinic keratoses have many features in common with SCC in situ microscopically. The overall risk for malignant conversion to invasive SCC is low and estimated to be in the range of 1 in 1000 lesions/year. When the reddened area begins to develop a plaquelike thickening, it is termed *Bowen's disease,* which appears histologically as SCC in situ and may vary from small lesions (<1 cm) to large areas, especially in the anogluteal region.

Invasive SCCs are palpable scaling lesions that become ulcerated centrally and have elevated edges (Fig. 32-27). They may be confused with keratoacanthoma, a benign lesion that can also thicken and ulcerate. Biopsy may be required to differentiate between these two conditions.

Most SCCs can be treated locally with excellent results (see later, "Treatment Options for Squamous and Basal Cell Carcinoma"). Recurrence is associated with tumor size, degree of differentiation, depth of invasion, perineural involvement, immune status of the patient, and anatomic site. Local recurrence is associated with an increased risk for regional and distant metastases. The first site of metastasis is usually the regional lymph nodes.

### Basal Cell Carcinoma

In contrast to SCCs and actinic keratoses, there is no precursor skin lesion for BCCs. These lesions may have an appearance that varies from nodules in the skin to a large nonhealing sore, with

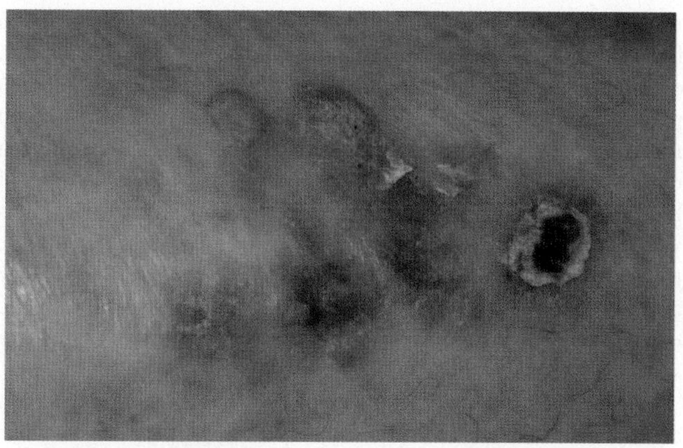

**FIGURE 32-27** Squamous cell carcinoma appearing as areas of thickened, red, scaling skin.

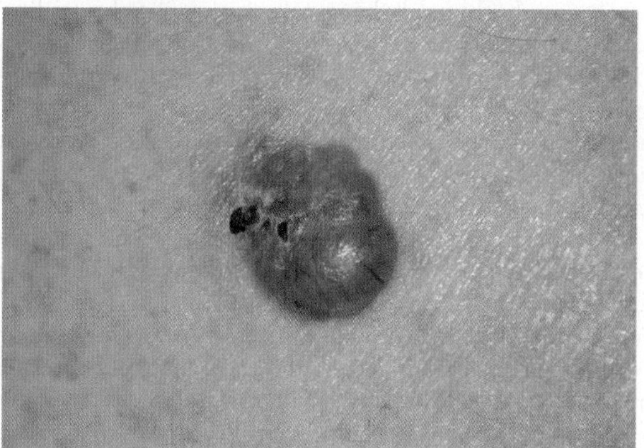

**FIGURE 32-28** Nodular basal cell carcinoma.

drainage and crusting. In comparison to SCCs, they have a slow growth rate, which can lead to a delay in diagnosis.[53]

BCCs grow in distinct patterns, described as nodular, pigmented, cystic, and superficial. The nodular growth pattern is characterized by a well-defined elevated lesion with a waxy appearance (Fig. 32-28). As the lesion grows, pearly opalescent nodules develop along the margins. A central depression with umbilication is a classic sign. Distinct blood vessels (telangiectasia) may be seen across the surface of the tumor mass. Although most BCCs are pink or skin-colored, they may also have shades of brown or black pigmentation, thereby mimicking a benign mole or melanoma. Cystic BCCs are less common but have a distinctive appearance. Their surface is translucent, and they may appear blue or gray and be confused with a blue nevus. Superficial BCCs (20%) are more macular than other growth patterns and may extend over the surface of the skin in a multicentric pattern. The center can ulcerate and the margins can become ill defined. These lesions may appear very similar to those of psoriasis, tinea, or eczema. They may also be multiple, pink or red, small, slightly elevated lesions that pepper the skin. This more aggressive growth pattern is associated with extension well beyond visible changes in the skin surface, and lesions can penetrate deep into the underlying subdermis. The white scarring varieties of this growth pattern are termed *morpheaform BCC* (Fig. 32-29).

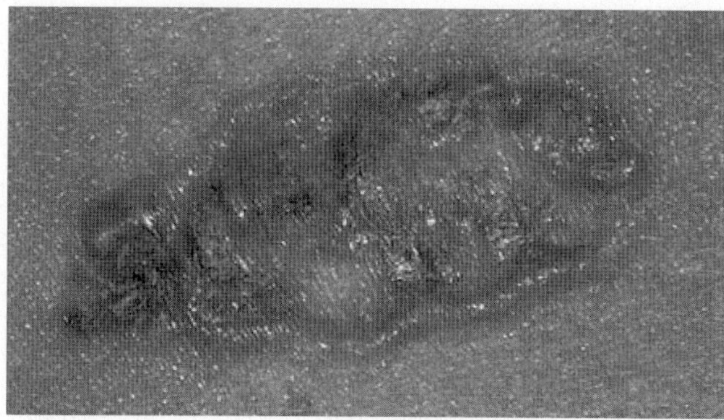

**FIGURE 32-29** Basal cell carcinoma growing in a morpheaform pattern.

BCCs commonly infiltrate locally but rarely metastasize. Metastases are associated with advanced patient age and neglected large lesions. The primary site has often been resected on multiple occasions before metastases appear. The median survival time for the rare patients with metastatic disease is less than 1 year.

### Treatment Options for Squamous and Basal Cell Carcinoma

NMSC is staged by different criteria than melanoma. The T stage is determined by the largest diameter of the lesion on the skin surface and by invasion of extradermal structures.[54] The overall favorable prognosis and the fact that a number of primary skin cancers develop in many patients make this staging system less useful in planning treatment compared with the melanoma staging system.

Actinic keratoses and the precursor lesions of SCC are usually treated with cryotherapy; however, alternative treatments include topical 5-fluorouracil, electrodessication and curettage, $CO_2$ laser, dermabrasion, and chemical peel. Tissue biopsy is indicated when the actinic keratosis is raised or recurrent after topical therapy.

Because a number of techniques are available, the strategy for surgical treatment of SCCs and BCCs begins with an assessment for high-risk factors (Table 32-5). Considerations include size, location, primary versus recurrent, histology, and individual patient factors. All appropriate options are reviewed with the patient, in addition to making a specific recommendation. Surgical resection techniques include histopathologic analysis to define the margins of resection. In contrast, field therapies treat a generalized area but do not define the status of margins. Such approaches include radiation therapy, cryosurgery, curettage, and electrodessication.

Standard surgical excision is the preferred treatment for most SCCs and BCCs. This procedure is usually performed under local anesthesia. The width of the margin for resection is not as well defined as in the treatment of melanoma. A minimum acceptable margin is one that is found to be free of carcinoma histologically, commonly a 3- to 4-mm area of normal-appearing skin. The risk for local recurrence is less when wider margins are obtained, especially in the presence of micronodular, infiltrative, and morpheaform histologic patterns. With these methods, the local cure rate is greater than 90%. An alternative surgical approach is the use of Mohs' micrographic excision (MME),

**Table 32-5 Nonmelanoma Skin Cancer: Risk Factors for Local Recurrence Based on Characteristics of the Primary Tumor**

| | Risk | |
|---|---|---|
| **FACTOR** | **LOW** | **HIGH** |
| Location | | |
| Trunk and extremities | <20 mm | $^{3}$20 mm |
| Forehead and neck | <10 mm | $^{3}$10 mm |
| Central part of the face | <6 mm | $^{3}$6 mm |
| Borders | Well defined | Poorly defined |
| Incidence | Primary | Recurrent |
| Immunosuppression | Negative | Positive |
| Previous radiation therapy, chronic inflammation | Negative | Positive |
| Rapid growth rate | Negative | Positive |
| Neurologic symptoms | Negative | Positive |
| Differentiation | Well | Moderate or poorly |
| Perineural/vascular invasion | Negative | Positive |

Adapted with permission from the NCCN Clinical Practice Guidelines in Oncology (NCCN Guidelines®) for Basal and Squamous Cell Skin Cancers v.1.2012. © 2011 National Comprehensive Cancer Network, Inc. All rights reserved. The NCCN Guidelines™ and illustrations herein may not be reproduced in any form for any purpose without the express written permission of the NCCN. To view the most recent and complete version of the NCCN Guidelines, go online to NCCN.org. NATIONAL COMPREHENSIVE CANCER NETWORK®, NCCN®, NCCN GUIDELINES®, and all other NCCN Content are trademarks owned by the National Comprehensive Cancer Network, Inc.

which has a high rate of local tumor control with the use of horizontal frozen sections. The high success rate of MME is attributed to examination of a greater proportion of the margin of excision, in addition to mapping the precise location of any margins found to be positive. Excisions in positive areas continue until clear margins are obtained. MME is ideal under high-risk conditions and for anatomic areas in which it is important to preserve as much tissue as possible, such as around the eye, nose, mouth, and ear.[55]

Although field therapy techniques (e.g., cryotherapy, topical fluorouracil, electrodessication) do not define the margins of treatment histologically, they may still be effective for local tumor control. Cryotherapy is best suited for small superficial lesions and can be expected to achieve local control rates of greater than 90%. Treated areas may heal slowly by secondary intention and leave pale scars.

Radiation therapy is highly effective for the treatment of BCC and SCC, especially for preserving wide areas of skin in the head and neck region. Radiation is also useful in treating areas at high risk for recurrence after extensive surgical excision.

## Uncommon Cutaneous Malignancies

Among the hundreds of specific types of skin conditions and tumors, four uncommon skin malignancies are important for the general surgeon to understand and be prepared to manage. Cutaneous angiosarcoma is a rare, aggressive, soft tissue sarcoma derived from blood or lymphatic vessel endothelium. It is most often seen on the face and scalp of older white men. In addition, angiosarcoma has been observed as a consequence of chronic lymphedema after axillary dissection for breast cancer (Stewart-Treves syndrome). Angiosarcoma may also arise in irradiated tissues after intervals of 10 to 20 years. The typical finding is a flat, painless, often pruritic macule or plaque with a red, blue, or purple color that develops into a mass and ulcerates if left in place. Histologically, angiosarcomas are high grade and often multifocal, with skip areas of normal-appearing skin. When compared with other sarcomas, there is a high incidence of lymph node metastasis (~15%). Treatment consists of resection with histologically negative margins and irradiation of the involved field. Lymph node dissection is indicated if adenopathy appears before distant metastases are identified. There is no consensus about the role of adjuvant chemotherapy. The 5-year survival rate is less than 40%.

Dermatofibrosarcoma protuberans is a low-grade sarcoma arising from dermal fibroblasts. Lesions appear as smooth nodules in or immediately beneath the skin (trunk, 40%; head-neck, 40%) in midadult life. Because of their slow growth, lesions are commonly 1 to 2 cm at diagnosis. Their external appearance belies their true character because tumor cells frequently invade the underlying soft tissues, thereby leading to incomplete excision and local recurrence. Treatment consists of WLE, with a 3-cm margin. Specimen orientation and pathologic analysis of margins are required. Distant metastases are uncommon and are preceded by two or more local recurrences. Radiation therapy has been used effectively after resection of recurrences.

Extramammary Paget's disease (EMPD) is a rare form of adenocarcinoma that arises from apocrine glands of the skin, most commonly in the perianal area, vulva, and scrotum. The clinical appearance is that of an erythematous plaque, but white or depigmented areas with crusts and scaling may also be present. The size is variable, from smaller than 1 cm to an entire area in the anogenital region. Because EMPD can have many clinical characteristics in common with eczema, bacterial and fungal infections, and nonspecific dermatitis, the diagnosis is often made by biopsy of lesions not responding to standard therapies. In most cases, EMPD is confined to the epidermis and is well controlled with excision. When invasion of the deeper structures occurs, the disease becomes increasingly difficult to control and the mortality rate increases to about 50%. Because EMPD is also associated with an increased risk for simultaneous internal malignancies in the genitourinary and gastrointestinal tracts (~40%), a complete workup includes a survey of these locations. Standard treatment is surgical resection extending to histologically clear margins, which may require a number of procedures because the histologic changes are best seen on permanent section. Patients require close clinical follow-up because local recurrences are common.[47] Radiation therapy has been reported to reduce the incidence of local recurrence after excision.

Kaposi's sarcoma, a low-grade soft tissue malignancy, arises from lymphatic vascular endothelial cells in the skin. The incidence is increasing because it is most often seen in patients with acquired immunodeficiency syndrome (AIDS) and other immunosuppressed states, such as organ transplantation. In patients infected with human immunodeficiency virus (HIV), human herpesvirus-8 has been identified as the causative agent of Kaposi's sarcoma. There is also a classic variant seen on the lower extremities of older men of Eastern European and Mediterranean descent. The clinical picture is variable; asymptomatic purple to brown bruises develop and progress to spots, plaques, or nodules on both lower extremities. Local symptoms appear late as the tumors become advanced. In AIDS patients, skin changes respond best to aggressive antiretroviral therapy. Symptomatic skin lesions can be treated with radiation therapy, intralesional injection of chemotherapeutic agents, cryotherapy, or excision.

Merkel cell carcinoma, derived from neuroendocrine cells, is indistinguishable histologically from small cell carcinoma arising in the lung or any other site. The initial workup includes a chest radiograph to rule out a pulmonary primary. From any site of origin, small cell carcinoma is a highly malignant tumor with a propensity to spread locally and regionally to nodes and distant sites. In the skin, it appears as a rapidly growing, red-blue nodule, most frequently in the head and neck area of older individuals. The diagnosis is confirmed by biopsy, and the primary treatment is WLE (2 to 3 cm), with histologically confirmed negative margins. SLN biopsy has been used successfully to identify patients with occult regional lymphatic metastases (10% to 30%), but there is no evidence that patients benefit other than by improved regional tumor control. SLN biopsy–negative patients have significantly better survival than biopsy-positive patients.[48] Involved-field irradiation has been shown to reduce the local recurrence rate and some reports have suggested a survival benefit; however, all studies have been too small and uncontrolled to draw definitive conclusions.[56] Although metastases may be responsive to chemotherapy, there is little evidence to support adjuvant systemic therapy. Overall, the prognosis is poor, with variable mortality rates of 55% to 79%.[57]

Many other cutaneous lesions and conditions are associated with malignancy but are beyond the scope of this chapter. However, the important principles in the management of these entities are the same as those reviewed earlier:

1. Clinicians must have a low threshold for biopsy of new or changing skin lesions.
2. The diagnosis is made by biopsy and histologic analysis.
3. If appropriate, surgical excision is performed, with histologically defined negative margins.
4. Further treatment and follow-up schedules will be determined by the specific diagnosis.

## SELECTED REFERENCES


Andtbacka RH, Gershenwald JE: Role of sentinel lymph node biopsy in patients with thin melanoma. J Natl Compr Canc Netw 7:308–317, 2009.

This paper provides an excellent summary and analysis of the data regarding the use of SLN biopsy for patients with thin melanomas.

Balch CM, Gershenwald JE, Soong SJ, et al: Final version of 2009 AJCC melanoma staging and classification. J Clin Oncol 27:6199–6206, 2009.

The latest proposed melanoma staging system is described in detail based on extensive data analysis from the AJCC staging committee.

Balch CM, Soong SJ, Gerschenwald JE, et al: Prognostic factors analysis of 17,600 melanoma patients: Validation of the American Joint Committee on Cancer melanoma staging system. J Clin Oncol 19:3622–3634, 2001.

This article provides an extensive analysis of prognostic factors in melanoma, which formed the basis for revision of the staging system.

Breslow A: Thickness, cross-sectional areas and depth of invasion in the prognosis of cutaneous melanoma. Ann Surg 172:902–908, 1970.

The original description of the Breslow thickness classification for melanoma.

Clark WH, Jr, From L, Bernadino EA, et al: The histogenesis and biologic behavior of primary human malignant melanomas of the skin. Cancer Res 29:705–727, 1969.

Clark's original description of this classification system of melanoma.

Coit DG, Andtbacka R, Bichakjian CK, et al: Melanoma. J Natl Compr Canc Netw 7:250–275, 2009.

Current NCCN guidelines for melanoma evaluation and treatment are provided.

Eggermont AM, Testori A, Marsden J, et al: Utility of adjuvant systemic therapy in melanoma. Ann Oncol 20:vi30–4, 2009.

The utility, or futility, of systemic therapy is reviewed and discussed.

Garbe C, Leiter U: Melanoma epidemiology and trends. Clinics Dermatol 27:3–9, 2009.

This paper provides an excellent updated summary of melanoma epidemiology worldwide.

Kroon HM, Thompson JF: Isolated limb infusion: A review. J Surg Oncol 100:169–177, 2009.

The use of hyperthermic isolated limb perfusion is analyzed and discussed in detail.

Landry CS, McMasters KM, Scoggins CR: The evolution of the management of regional lymph nodes in melanoma. J Surg Oncol 96:316–621, 2007.

The history and evolution of management of regional lymph nodes for patients with melanoma are reviewed.

McMasters KM, Reintgen DS, Ross MI, et al: Sentinel lymph node biopsy for melanoma: Controversy despite widespread agreement. J Clin Oncol 19:2851–2855, 2001.

A thorough discussion of the rationale for sentinel node biopsy in melanoma is provided.

Morton DL, Wen DR, Wong JH, et al: Technical details of intraoperative lymphatic mapping for early stage melanoma. Arch Surg 127:392–399, 1992.

Thisis an original description of SLN biopsy for melanoma.

Morton DL, Thompson JF, Cochran AJ, et al: Sentinel-node biopsy or nodal observation in melanoma. N Engl J Med 355:1307–1317, 2006.

Results of the landmark MSLT-I study are presented to analyze the benefits of SLN biopsy.

Ollila DW: Complete metastasectomy in patients with stage IV metastatic melanoma. Lancet Oncol 7:919–924, 2006.

The role of surgical resection of distant metastases has been controversial. This paper presents the evidence to support surgical resection in patients with stage IV melanoma.

Santillan AA, Cherpelis BS, Glass LF, et al: Management of familial melanoma and nonmelanoma skin cancer syndromes. Surg Oncol Clin N Am 18:73–98, 2009.

The molecular genetics and progress in understanding familial melanoma and skin cancer syndromes is reviewed in detail.

Wargo JA, Tanabe K: Surgical management of melanoma. Hematol Oncol Clin North Am 23:565–581, 2009.

This is an excellent review of the surgical principles and appropriate management for melanoma patients.

## REFERENCES


1. Neuhaus SJ, Clark MA, Thomas JM: Dr. Herbert Lumley Snow, MD, MRCS (1847–1930): The original champion of elective lymph node dissection in melanoma. Ann Surg Oncol 11:875–878, 2004.
2. Jemal A, Siegel R, Ward E: Cancer statistics, 2009. CA Cancer J Clin 59:225–249, 2009.
3. Garbe C, Leiter U: Melanoma epidemiology and trends. Clinics Dermatol 27:3–9, 2009.
4. Linos E, Swetter SM, Cockburn MG, et al: Increasing burden of melanoma in the United States. J Invest Dermatol 129:1666–1674, 2009.
5. Thompson JF, Scolyer RA, Kefford RF: Cutaneous melanoma in the era of molecular profiling. Lancet 374:362–365, 2009.
6. Cormier JN, Xing Y, Ding M, et al: Ethnic differences among patients with cutaneous melanoma. Arch Intern Med 166:1907–1914, 2006.
7. von Thaler AK, Kamenisch Y, Berneburg M: The role of ultraviolet radiation in melanomagenesis. Exp Dermatol 19:81–88, 2010.
8. Arneja JS, Gosain AK: Giant congenital melanocytic nevi. Plast Reconstr Surg 120:26e-40e, 2007.
9. Kamino H: Spitzoid melanoma. Clin Dermatol 27:545–555, 2009.
10. Santillan AA, Cherpelis BS, Glass LF, et al: Management of familial melanoma and nonmelanoma skin cancer syndromes. Surg Oncol Clin N Am 18:73–98, 2009.
11. Dennis LK, Beane Freeman LE, VanBeek MJ: Sunscreen use and the risk for melanoma: A quantitative review. Ann Intern Med 139:966–978, 2003.
12. Tran KT, Wright NA, Cockerell CJ: Biopsy of the pigmented lesion—when and how. J Am Acad Dermatol 59:852–871, 2008.
13. Piris A, Mihm MC, Jr: Progress in melanoma histopathology and diagnosis. Hematol Oncol Clin North Am 23:467–480, 2009.
14. Clark WH, Jr, From L, Bernadino EA, et al: The histogenesis and biologic behavior of primary human malignant melanomas of the skin. Cancer Res 29:705–727, 1969.
15. Breslow A: Thickness, cross-sectional areas and depth of invasion in the prognosis of cutaneous melanoma. Ann Surg 172:902–908, 1970.
16. Balch CM, Soong S-J, Gerschenwald JE, et al: Prognostic factors analysis of 17,600 melanoma patients: Validation of the American Joint Committee on Cancer melanoma staging system. J Clin Oncol 19:3622–3634, 2001.
17. Balch CM, Gershenwald JE, Soong SJ, et al: Final version of 2009 AJCC melanoma staging and classification. J Clin Oncol 27:6199–6206, 2009.
18. Coit DG, Andtbacka R, Bichakjian CK, et al: Melanoma. J Natl Compr Canc Netw 7:250–275, 2009.
19. Norris W: Eight cases of melanosis with pathological and therapeutic remarks on that disease, London, 1857, Longman, Brown, Green, Longman, and Roberts.
20. Santillan AA, Messina JL, Marzban SS, et al: Pathology review of thin melanoma and melanoma in situ in a multidisciplinary melanoma clinic: Impact on treatment decisions. J Clin Oncol 28:481–486, 2010.
21. Sladden MJ, Balch C, Barzilai DA, et al: Surgical excision margins for primary cutaneous melanoma.Cochrane Database Syst Rev 7:CD004835, 2009.
22. Wargo JA, Tanabe K: Surgical management of melanoma. Hematol Oncol Clin North Am 23:565–581, 2009.
23. Landry CS, McMasters KM, Scoggins CR: The evolution of the management of regional lymph nodes in melanoma. J Surg Oncol 96:316–321, 2007.
24. Robinson DS, Sample WF, Fee HJ, et al: Regional lymphatic drainage in primary malignant melanoma of the trunk determined by colloidal gold scanning. Surg Forum 28:147–148, 1977.
25. Morton DL, Wen DR, Wong JH, et al: Technical details of intraoperative lymphatic mapping for early stage melanoma. Arch Surg 127:392–399, 1992.
26. McMasters KM, Reintgen DS, Ross MI, et al: Sentinel lymph node biopsy for melanoma: Controversy despite widespread agreement. J Clin Oncol 19:2851–2855, 2001.
27. Gershenwald JE, Thompson W, Mansfield PF, et al: Multi-institutional melanoma lymphatic mapping experience: The prognostic value of sentinel lymph node status in 612 stage I or II melanoma patients. J Clin Oncol 17:976–983, 1999.
28. Wrightson WR, Wong SL, Edwards MJ, et al: Complications associated with sentinel lymph node biopsy for melanoma. Ann Surg Oncol 10:676–680, 2003.
29. Andtbacka RH, Gershenwald JE: Role of sentinel lymph node biopsy in patients with thin melanoma. J Natl Compr Canc Netw 7:308–317, 2009.
30. Kesmodel SB, Karakousis GC, Botbyl JD, et al: Mitotic rate as a predictor of sentinel lymph node positivity in patients with thin melanomas. Ann Surg Oncol 12:449–458, 2005.
31. Gajdos C, Griffith KA, Wong SL, et al: Is there a benefit to sentinel lymph node biopsy in patients with T4 melanoma? Cancer 115:5752–5760, 2009.
32. McMasters KM, Chao C, Wong SL, et al: Interval sentinel lymph nodes in melanoma. Arch Surg 137:543–547, 2002.
33. Gershenwald JE, Tseng CH, Thompson W, et al: Improved sentinel lymph node localization in patients with primary melanoma with the use of radiolabeled colloid. Surgery 124:203–210, 1998.
34. McMasters KM, Reintgen DS, Ross MI, et al: Sentinel lymph node biopsy for melanoma: How many radioactive nodes should be removed? Ann Surg Oncol 8:192–197, 2001.
35. Chao C,Wong SL, Edwards MJ, et al: Sentinel lymph node biopsy for head and neck melanomas. Ann Surg Oncol 10: 21–26, 2003.

**36.** Morton DL, Thompson JF, Cochran AJ, et al: Sentinel-node biopsy or nodal observation in melanoma. N Engl J Med 355: 1307–1317, 2006.

**37.** McMasters KM, Ross MI, Reintgen DS, et al: Final results of the Sunbelt Melanoma Trial. J Clin Oncol 26(Suppl):abstr 9003, 2008.

**38.** Wong SL, Morton DL, Thompson JF, et al: Melanoma patients with positive sentinel nodes who did not undergo completion lymphadenectomy: A multi-institutional study. Ann Surg Oncol 13:809–816, 2006.

**39.** Cadili A, McKinnon G, Wright F, et al: Validation of a scoring system to predict non-sentinel lymph node metastasis in melanoma. J Surg Oncol 101:191–194, 2010

**40.** Sholar A, Martin RC, 2nd, McMasters KM: Popliteal lymph node dissection. Ann Surg Oncol 12:189–193, 2005.

**41.** Tanabe KK: Lymphatic mapping and epitrochlear lymph node dissection for melanoma. Surgery 121:102–104, 1997.

**42.** Eggermont AM, Testori A, Marsden J, et al: Utility of adjuvant systemic therapy in melanoma. Ann Oncol 20(Suppl 6):vi30–vi34, 2009.

**43.** Burmeister B, Henderson M, Thompson J, et al: Adjuvant radiotherapy improves regional (lymph node field) control in melanoma patients after lymphadenectomy: Results of an intergroup randomized trial (TROG 02.01/ANZMTG 01.02). Int J Radiat Oncol Biol Phys 75:S2, 2009.

**44.** Kroon BB, Noorda EM, Vrouenraets BC, et al: Isolated limb perfusion for melanoma. Surg Oncol Clin N Am 17:785–794, 2008.

**45.** Sanki A, Kam PC, Thompson JF: Long-term results of hyperthermic, isolated limb perfusion for melanoma: A reflection of tumor biology. Ann Surg 245:591–596, 2007.

**46.** Kroon HM, Thompson JF: Isolated limb infusion: A review. J Surg Oncol 100:169–177, 2009.

**47.** Ollila DW: Complete metastasectomy in patients with stage IV metastatic melanoma. Lancet Oncol 7:919–924, 2006.

**48.** Atkins MB, Hsu J, Lee S, et al: Phase III trial comparing concurrent biochemotherapy with cisplatin, vinblastine, dacarbazine, interleukin-2, and interferon alfa-2b with cisplatin, vinblastine, and dacarbazine alone in patients with metastatic malignant melanoma (E3695): A trial coordinated by the Eastern Cooperative Oncology Group. J Clin Oncol 26:5748–5754, 2008.

**49.** Hussain SK, Sundquist J, Hemminki K: Incidence trends of squamous cell and rare skin cancers in the Swedish national cancer registry point to calendar year and age-dependent increases. J Invest Dermatol 130:1323–1328, 2010.

**50.** Brash DE: Roles of the transcription factor p53 in keratinocyte carcinomas. Br J Dermatol 154(Suppl 1):8–10, 2006.

**51.** Ulrich C, Kanitakis J, Stockfleth E, et al: Skin cancer in organ transplantation recipients—where do we stand? Am J Transpl 8:2192–2198, 2008.

**52.** Fu W, Cockerell CJ: The actinic (solar) keratosis. Arch Dermatol 139:66–70, 2003.

**53.** Rubin AI, Chen EH, Ratner D: Current concepts: Basal cell carcinoma. N Engl J Med 353:2262–2269, 2005.

**54.** Greene FL, Page DL, Fleming ID, et al, editors: AJCC cancer staging manual, ed 6, New York, 2002, Springer-Verlag.

**55.** Kuijpers DI, Thissen MR, Neumann MH: Basal cell carcinoma: Treatment options and prognosis, a scientific approach to a common malignancy. Am J Clin Dermatol 3:247–259, 2002.

**56.** Eng TY, Boersma MG, Fuller CD, et al: A comprehensive review of the treatment of Merkel cell carcinoma. Am J Clin Oncol 30:624–636, 2007.

**57.** Zhan FQ, Packianathan VS, Zeitouni NC: Merkel cell carcinoma: A review of current advances. J Natl Compr Canc Netw 7:333–339, 2009.

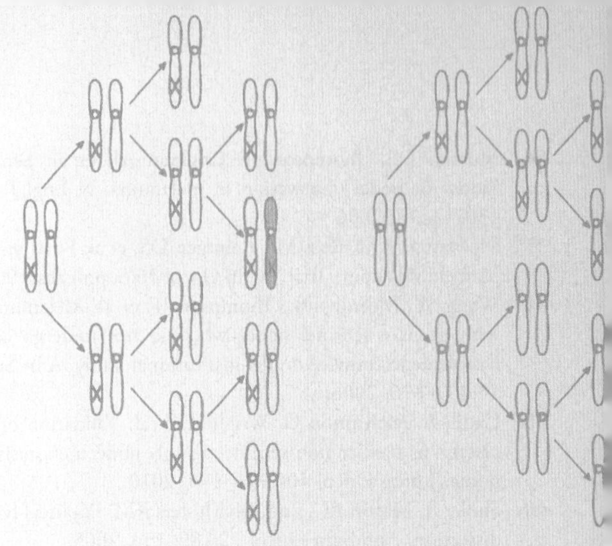

CHAPTER 33

# SOFT TISSUE SARCOMAS

Samuel Singer



Soft tissue sarcomas are rare and unusual neoplasms, accounting for approximately 1% of adult human cancers and 15% of pediatric malignancies. Sarcomas affect more than 10,600 patients/year in the United States and approximately 4000 patients will die each year from inoperable forms of soft tissue sarcoma.[1] Sarcomas continue to carry biologic and clinical interest and significance disproportionate to their clinical frequency because of their often clearly defined molecular genetics and the vast expansion of cytogenetic and molecular genetic information that has been discovered over the past 10 years. Soft tissue sarcomas may develop in any anatomic site and this feature, together with the more than 50 histologic types and subtypes, continues to pose a challenge in diagnosis and management. Our understanding of the histology-specific natural history and of the most important clinicopathologic factors that predict outcome and response to therapy has improved our ability to select an optimal treatment plan for the patient diagnosed with soft tissue sarcoma. Most sarcoma types remain resistant to conventional chemotherapy, which means that approximately 40% of newly diagnosed patients will eventually die of disease. Therefore, there exists an urgent unmet need for new therapies targeting the underlying genetic aberrations driving sarcomagenesis. This chapter focuses on the biology, epidemiology, molecular genetics, histopathology, clinical features, and management of soft tissue sarcomas among adults (older than 16 years).

## DISTRIBUTION, AGE, AND CAUSES

Although soft tissue sarcomas may occur in any anatomic site, 45% occur in the extremity, most commonly in the thigh, followed in order of frequency by visceral (20%), retroperitoneal (15%), truncal or thoracic (10%), and other locations (10%). Soft tissue sarcomas become more common with increasing age, with the translocation-associated sarcomas having a median age of onset in the 1930s and the complex sarcoma types having a median age of onset in the 1950s or 1960s.

Most cases of soft tissue sarcoma are thought to be sporadic and their cause is unknown. In rare cases, genetic factors, environmental factors, prior radiation therapy, viral infections, and immunodeficiency have been associated with the development of sarcoma. In addition, sarcomas have been reported to arise in scar tissue, fracture sites, or anatomic regions associated with prior soft tissue trauma. Genetic syndromes such as neurofibromatosis, familial adenomatous polyposis, and the Li-Fraumeni syndrome have all been shown to be associated with the development of soft tissue sarcoma. Desmoid tumors occur in patients with familial adenomatous polyposis, a disorder caused by the germline adenomatous polyposis coli (APC) gene mutation. Malignant peripheral nerve sheath tumors develop in a benign nerve sheath in approximately 2% of patients with neurofibromatosis. The Li-Fraumeni syndrome is a rare, highly penetrant, familial cancer phenotype usually associated with germline mutations in the *p53* tumor suppressor gene.[2] Of patients with this syndrome, 80% develop cancer by age 45 and soft tissue or bone sarcomas of diverse histology arise as the index tumor in 36% of patients. Heritable retinoblastoma gene *(RB1)* mutations are associated with an increased risk of bone and soft tissue sarcoma. For example, patients with *RB1* mutations have a 36% cumulative incidence over 50 years of developing sarcoma in previously irradiated tissue.[3] Most of the excess cancer risks in hereditary retinoblastoma survivors can be prevented by limiting exposures to DNA damaging agents such as radiotherapy, tobacco, and ultraviolet (UV) light,[4] emphasizing the importance of avoiding the use of radiation in sarcoma patients with a known germline mutation in *RB1.*

A soft tissue sarcoma (STS) is one of the most common types of radiation-associated tumors in the general population.[5] Although a clear dose-response relationship for radiation-associated malignancies is not established, it is generally accepted that carcinomas arise in tissues exposed to lower doses, whereas sarcomas are induced in heavily radiated tissues (most patients have received 50 Gy or more) in or close to the radiation fields. The median interval between radiation exposure and the development of sarcoma is 10 years (range, 1.3 to 74 years) and this varies by histologic type, with the shortest latency observed in liposarcoma (median, 4.3 years; range, 3 to 17 years), and the longest in leiomyosarcoma (median, 23.5 years; range, 7.0 to 74.0 years).[6] Radiation-associated sarcomas are associated with inferior survival compared with sporadic soft tissue sarcoma, even if one adjusts for known prognostic factors such as histologic type, size, age, margin status, and site.[6]

Several studies have reported an increased incidence of soft tissue sarcoma after relatively high level occupational exposure to phenoxyacetic herbicides, chlorophenols, and dioxins. However, more recent case-control studies have not confirmed this association and have shown no positive correlation between dioxin concentrations and soft tissue sarcoma risk. In fact, sarcoma risk was highest among those having the lowest dioxin level.[7,8]

## MOLECULAR GENETICS

Knowledge of the genomic alterations in soft tissue sarcoma is limited to only the most recurrent alterations. These alterations segregate sarcoma into two major groups. The first group consists of sarcoma types with near-diploid, simple karyotypes that bear few chromosomal rearrangements but have pathognomonic alterations, such as the translocations in myxoid round cell liposarcoma (MRC) [t(12;16)(q13;p11), t(12;22)(q13;q12)] and synovial sarcomas (SSs) [t(X;18)(p11;q11)], *APC/β-catenin* mutations in desmoid tumors, and activating mutations in *KIT* or *PDGFRA* in gastrointestinal stromal tumors (GISTs).[9-11] Discovery of these last mutations has led to the clinical deployment of imatinib for the treatment of GIST,[12] providing a model for genotype-directed therapies in molecularly defined sarcoma subtypes. Conversely, the second group consists of sarcomas with complex karyotypes, including dedifferentiated and pleomorphic liposarcomas, leiomyosarcomas, pleomorphic malignant fibrous histiocytoma, and myxofibrosarcomas. Sarcomas in this group have no known characteristic mutations or fusion genes, although abnormalities are frequently observed in the Rb, p53, and specific growth factor signaling pathways. Thus, a significant subset of soft tissue sarcoma is characterized by recurrent and specific chromosomal aberrations that can be diagnostically and, occasionally, prognostically useful (Table 33-1). The fusion gene translocations include 13 different gene fusions involving the *EWS* gene or *EWS* family members *(TLS, TAF2N)* found in five different sarcomas and 11 other types of fusions in eight other sarcoma types.

If conventional cytogenetics is not available, molecular genetic techniques (e.g., reverse transcription polymerase chain reaction and fluorescence in situ hybridization) are useful as diagnostic adjuncts. In addition, investigation of molecular changes of genes at the sites of chromosomal alterations has led to the identification of novel genes and the characterization of their mechanisms of deregulation. The tumor suppressor genes best studied in sarcoma are p53, *RB1,* and *NF1.* Inactivation of these genes is involved in the tumorigenesis of several sarcomas. The major mechanisms of *p53* pathway inactivation in sarcomas include *p53* point mutations, homozygous deletion of *CDKN2A,* which encodes both p14ARF and p16, and *MDM2* amplification. In sarcomas with specific reciprocal translocations, p53 pathway alteration is a rare event but, when present, is a strong prognostic factor, associated with significantly decreased survival in synovial sarcoma,[13] myxoid liposarcoma,[14] and Ewing's sarcoma–peripheral neuroectodermal tumor (PNET).[15] Decreased survival and poor response to chemotherapy in Ewing's sarcoma–PNET was associated with deletion of *CDKN2A,* representing a type of p53 pathway alteration through loss of the *CDKN2A* alternative product p14ARF.[15] In contrast, in sarcomas with nonspecific genetic alterations and complex karyotypes, *p53* pathway alteration is more common and has weaker prognostic value, often requiring large numbers of patients to achieve statistical significance, as demonstrated in several studies of mixed adult soft tissue sarcoma. Its high prevalence in this class of sarcomas may account for its limited ability to define distinct clinical prognostic subsets in these tumors.

In addition to serving as specific and powerful diagnostic markers, fusion genes resulting from translocations encode chimeric proteins that are important determinants of tumor biology, acting as abnormal transcription factors that alter the transcription of a number of downstream genes and pathways. The structures of these chimeric proteins play a prominent role in the pathogenesis of sarcoma; this has been shown by the impact of relatively minor cytogenetic variability, as a result of variant molecular breakpoints, on tumor phenotype and clinical behavior.[16,17] Although the diagnostic significance of sarcoma genomic aberrations has been known for more than 20 years, these same aberrations have only recently become useful as potential therapeutic targets. For example, the identification of the *COL1A1-PDGFB1* gene fusion leading to constitutive expression of the platelet-derived growth factor (and its receptor, presumably through an autocrine or paracrine loop) in dermatofibrosarcoma protuberans (DFSP) has paved the way for targeted therapy with imatinib in patients with advanced disease.[18,19] The recent discovery that angiosarcomas show distinct upregulation of vascular-specific receptor tyrosine kinases, including TIE1, KDR, SNRK, TEK, and FLT1, by expression profiling and that 10% of patients harbor *KDR* mutations with evidence for ligand-dependent kinase activation provides a basis for treating angiosarcoma patients with vascular endothelial growth factor receptor (VEGFR) tyrosine kinase inhibitors.[20] In a multicenter phase II trial of sorafenib, a small-molecule B-raf and VEGFR inhibitor, in a cohort of patients with metastatic or recurrent sarcoma, only patients with angiosarcoma showed a significant response to therapy, with 5 of 37 patients (14%) having a partial response.[21]

## EVALUATION

### Clinical Evaluation and Diagnosis

Benign soft tissue tumors outnumber sarcomas by at least 100 to 1, with most benign lesions located superficially to the fascia. The most frequent benign lesion is a lipoma, which frequently goes untreated. Because excisional biopsy may often cause difficulties with further patient management, it is generally recommended to obtain a diagnostic biopsy prior to definitive treatment for all soft tissue masses larger than 5 cm, unless an obvious subcutaneous lipoma, and for all subfascial or deep-seated masses, almost irrespective of size.

Patients with extremity sarcoma usually present with a painless mass, often with no functional impact, although pain is noted at presentation in up to 33% of patients. Delay in diagnosis is common, with the most common differential diagnosis for extremity and trunk lesions being a hematoma or a pulled muscle. Physical examination should include assessment of the size of the mass, its depth in relation to superficial fascia, and its relationship to neurovascular and bony structures. Generally, in an adult, any soft tissue mass that is symptomatic or enlarging, any superficial mass that is larger than 5 cm, and all deep-seated masses irrespective of size should be sampled. Biopsy technique is important. For most soft tissue masses, an open incisional biopsy or core needle biopsy is usually preferred. Ideally, the initial diagnostic procedure should be performed at

**Table 33-1 Cytogenetic and Molecular Abnormalities in Sarcomas**

| HISTOLOGIC TYPE | CYTOGENETIC EVENT | GENE REARRANGEMENT OR MOLECULAR ABNORMALITY | FREQUENCY (%) | DIAGNOSTIC |
|---|---|---|---|---|
| Synovial sarcoma | t(X;18)(p11;q11) | | >90 | Yes |
| | | *SYT-SSX1* fusion | 66 | Yes |
| | | *SYT-SSX2* fusion | 33 | Yes |
| | | *SYT-SSX4* fusion | <1 | Yes |
| Myxoid, round cell liposarcoma | t(12;16)(q13;p11) | *TLS-CHOP* fusion | >90 | Yes |
| | t(12;22)(q13;q12) | *EWS-CHOP* fusion | <5 | Yes |
| Ewing's sarcoma | t(11;22)(q24;q12) | *EWS-FLI1* fusion | >80 | Yes |
| | t(21;22)(q22;q12) | *EWS-ERG* fusion | 10-15 | Yes |
| | t(7;22)(p22;q12) | *EWS-ETV1* fusion | <2 | Yes |
| | t(17;22)(q12;q12) | *EWS-E1AF* fusion | <2 | Yes |
| | t(2;22)(q33;q12) | *EWS-FEV* fusion | <2 | Yes |
| | inv(22)(q12q12) | *EWS-ZSG fusion* | <2 | Yes |
| Alveolar rhabdomyosarcoma | t(2;13)(q35;q14) | *PAX3-FKHR* fusion | >75 | Yes |
| | t(1;13)(p36;q14) | *PAX7-FKHR* fusion | 10-20 | Yes |
| Embryonal rhabdomyosarcoma | Trisomies 2q, 8, and 20 | | >75 | Yes |
| | | LOH at 11p15 | >75 | Yes |
| Extraskeletal myxoid chondrosarcoma | t(9;22)(q22;q12) | EWS-NR4A3 fusion | >75 | Yes |
| | t(9;17)(q22;q11) | TAF2N-NR4A3 fusion | <10 | Yes |
| | t(9;15)(q22;q21) | TCF12-NR4A3 fusion | <10 | Yes |
| Endometrial stromal tumor | t(7;17)(p15;q21) | JAZF1-JJAZ1 | 30 | Yes |
| Dermatofibrosarcoma protuberans | Rings derived from t(17;22) | COL1A1-PDGFB1 fusion | >75 | Yes |
| | t(17;22)(q22;q13.1) | *COL1A1-PDGFB1* fusion | 10 | Yes |
| Desmoplastic small round cell tumor | t(11;22)(p13;q12) | *EWS-WT1* fusion | >75 | Yes |
| Clear cell sarcoma | t(12;22)(q13;q12) | *EWS-ATF1* fusion | >75 | Yes |
| Infantile fibrosarcoma | t(12;15)(p13;q25) | ETV6-NTRK3 fusion | >75 | Yes |
| Alveolar soft part sarcoma | t(X;17)(p11;q25) | ASPL-TFE3 fusion | >90 | Yes |
| Inflammatory myofibroblastic tumor | 2p23 rearrangement | *ALK* fusion genes | 50 | Yes |
| Gastrointestinal stromal tumor | Monosomies 14 and 22 | | >75 | Yes |
| | Deletion of 1p | | >25 | No |
| | | *KIT* or *PDGFRA* mutation | >90 | Yes |
| Desmoid fibromatosis | Trisomies 8 and 20 | | 30 | Yes |
| | Deletion of 5q | *APC* inactivation by mutation/ deletion | 10 | Yes |
| | | *β-Catenin* mutations | 85 | Yes |
| Well-differentiated or dedifferentiated liposarcoma | 12q rings and giant markers | *MDM2* and *CDK4* amplification | >85 | Yes |
| Leiomyosarcoma | Complex* | | >90 | No |
| | Deletions of 1p | | >50 | No |
| | | *RB1* point mutations, deletions | ? | No |
| Pleomorphic liposarcoma | Complex* | | >90 | No |
| Pleomorphic malignant fibrous histiocytoma and myxofibrosarcoma | Complex* | | >90 | No |
| Malignant peripheral nerve sheath tumor | Complex* | | 90 | No |
| | | *NF-1* mutation, loss, or deletion | >50 | No |

*Complex karyotypes containing multiple numeric and structural chromosomal aberrations.

the center at which the patient will be treated. This facilitates proper placement of the biopsy site (or incision) and also avoids the complications and diagnostic difficulties that can arise if such biopsy samples are handled infrequently. Limb masses are generally best sampled through a longitudinal incision so that the entire biopsy tract can be excised at the time of definitive resection. The incision should be centered over the mass in its most superficial location. No tissue flap should be raised, and meticulous hemostasis should be ensured to prevent cellular dissemination by hematoma. Excisional biopsy is recommended only for small cutaneous or subcutaneous tumors, usually smaller than 5 cm, in which a wide reexcision (if required) is usually straightforward. Fine-needle aspiration biopsy has a limited role in diagnosing extremity soft tissue tumors but may be of value in the documentation of recurrence. An analysis of 164 soft tissue masses for the value of core needle biopsy has suggested that 83% of specimens obtained at initial biopsy are adequate for diagnosis. Of the adequate biopsy specimens, 95% correlated with the final resection diagnosis for malignancy, 88% for histologic grade, and 75% for histologic subtype. Core needle biopsy can be then advocated as the first step in the diagnostic armamentarium. The high diagnostic accuracy, ease of performance, low cost, and low complication rate make this technique attractive. If tissue is inadequate or there is any indecision, repeat core biopsy under image guidance or an open, linearly placed incisional biopsy is then indicated. Tumor histologic type and grade are correctly identified in most patients and can be used to define the optimal treatment plan and extent of surgery required for definitive therapy.

Patients with intra-abdominal or retroperitoneal sarcomas often experience nonspecific abdominal discomfort and gastrointestinal symptoms before diagnosis. The diagnosis is usually suspected on finding a soft tissue mass on abdominal computed tomography (CT) or magnetic resonance imaging (MRI). Fine-needle aspiration biopsy or CT-guided core biopsy has a limited role in the routine diagnostic evaluation of these patients. CT-guided core biopsy is indicated if abdominal lymphoma, germ cell tumor, or carcinoma is strongly suspected as part of the differential diagnosis. Preoperative percutaneous biopsy is also indicated for patients who present with distant metastasis or advanced local disease that on abdominal or pelvic imaging appears to be surgically difficult to remove completely without substantial morbidity. In most patients, exploratory laparotomy should be performed and the diagnosis made at operation, unless the patient's tumor is clearly unresectable or the patient will be undergoing preoperative investigational treatment.

## Evaluation of Extent of Disease

All patients require a thorough history and physical examination. MRI examination is usually the preferred procedure for imaging extremity soft tissue masses. MRI enhances the contrast between tumor and adjacent structures and provides excellent three-dimensional definition of fascial planes. Also, it aids in guiding biopsies, planning surgery, evaluating response to therapy, and restaging and in the long-term follow-up for local recurrence. MRI accurately defines tumor size, multiplicity, and location but only infrequently can predict histologic diagnosis and biologic behavior reliably. CT is a predominantly anatomic imaging modality. It is limited in the differentiation of subtle soft tissue differences. Therefore, CT plays mainly a complementary role to MRI in evaluation of the extent of tumor. MRI, with its superior soft tissue contrast resolution, is the dominant imaging modality for the evaluation of extremity sarcomas. CT is useful for evaluation of the tumor matrix, especially for small calcifications and the evaluation of subtle cortical involvement. MRI is limited in the detection of small calcifications within a mass because calcium distorts the magnetic field. CT may also be useful in patients for whom MRI is contraindicated or cannot be tolerated.

Once the diagnosis and grade are known, evaluation for sites of potential metastasis can be performed. Lymph node metastases occur in less than 3% of adult soft tissue sarcomas. For extremity lesions, the lung is the principal site for metastasis; for visceral lesions and some histologic types of retroperitoneal sarcoma, the liver is the principal site. Thus, patients with low-grade extremity lesions require a chest radiograph and most of those with high-grade lesions require a chest CT scan. CT is the most commonly used modality to evaluate pulmonary metastases. However, it is more expensive than radiographs, delivers a higher radiation dose, and may give false-positive results because of small, indeterminate pulmonary nodules. One study has correlated thoracotomy with CT and found that only 60% of nodules smaller than 6 mm were malignant.[22] It is unclear whether there is a better imaging modality to evaluate metastases smaller than 1 cm. Patients with visceral and retroperitoneal lesions should have their liver imaged as part of the initial abdominal CT or MRI. Newer techniques, such as $^{18}$F-fluorodeoxyglucose positron emission tomography (FDG-PET), are being used to evaluate distant metastases and, when combined with CT and conventional imaging, may improve the diagnostic accuracy of preoperative staging. However, overstaging remains a problem in 12% of patients and PET-CT remains limited for evaluating pulmonary metastases smaller than 1 cm.[23] FDG-PET lacks specificity in its ability to help distinguish between low-grade malignancies and benign entities. An additional concern is that several high-grade sarcoma types, such as round cell liposarcoma and many low-grade sarcomas, do not reliably show uptake for FDG, further limiting its routine use for staging sarcoma patients.

## Pathologic Evaluation

There are more than 50 histologic types of soft tissue sarcoma, many of which are associated with distinctive clinical, therapeutic, or prognostic features. Detailed descriptions of the histopathologic classification and guidelines for the histologic reporting of soft tissue sarcoma have been published elsewhere.[24] To summarize, the most commonly found are liposarcoma, leiomyosarcoma, pleomorphic malignant fibrous histiocytoma (pMFH), GIST, desmoids, myxofibrosarcoma, and synovial sarcoma (Fig. 33-1). Histopathology is anatomic site–dependent. The common subtypes in the extremities are liposarcoma, pMFH, myxofibrosarcoma, and synovial sarcoma; in retroperitoneal and intra-abdominal sites, liposarcoma and leiomyosarcoma are the most common histiotypes, whereas in the visceral location, gastrointestinal stromal tumors, leiomyosarcoma, and desmoids are found almost exclusively (Fig. 33-2). Liposarcoma is further classified into three biologic groups encompassing five histologic subtypes, based on strict morphologic features and cytogenetic aberrations—well-differentiated, dedifferentiated, myxoid, round cell, and pleomorphic.[24] The well-differentiated and dedifferentiated subtypes account for 42% and 21% of liposarcomas, respectively, and are more commonly found in the retroperitoneal location; the myxoid, round cell, and pleomorphic subtypes account for 25% and 8% of liposarcomas, respectively, and are usually located in the extremity (Fig. 33-3).

Age is also a factor in histopathology, with the translocation-associated sarcomas often presenting at an age approximately 2 decades earlier than the more complex sarcoma types. In childhood, embryonal rhabdomyosarcoma is most common, synovial sarcoma has a peak incidence among individuals in their 20s and 30s, myxoid and round cell liposarcomas have a peak incidence among those in their 30s, and well-differentiated or dedifferentiated liposarcoma, leiomyosarcoma, pMFH, and myxofibrosarcoma are the predominant types in the older population, with a peak incidence among those in their 50s to 60s (Fig. 33-4). The designation MFH is currently being reevaluated, with many of these tumors being reclassified as myofibrosarcoma, pleomorphic sarcoma, or dedifferentiated liposarcoma.

Because none of the existing grading systems are ideal and applicable to all tumor types, sarcoma histologic type and liposarcoma subtype are generally important determinants of prognosis and predictors of distinctive patterns of behavior. Biologic behavior is currently best predicted based on histologic type, histologic grade, tumor size, and depth. Although many

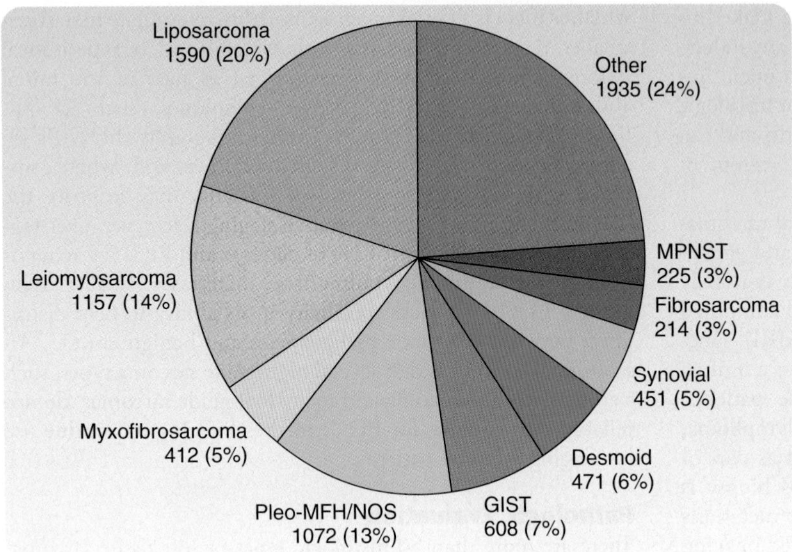


**FIGURE 33-1** Histology distribution of 8135 patients with soft tissue sarcoma treated at Memorial Sloan-Kettering Cancer Center from July 1, 1982, through June 30, 2009. These data include extremity, trunk, visceral, and retroperitoneal tumors. *GIST,* Gastrointestinal stromal tumor; *MFH,* malignant fibrous histiocytoma; *MPNST,* malignant peripheral nerve sheath tumor.

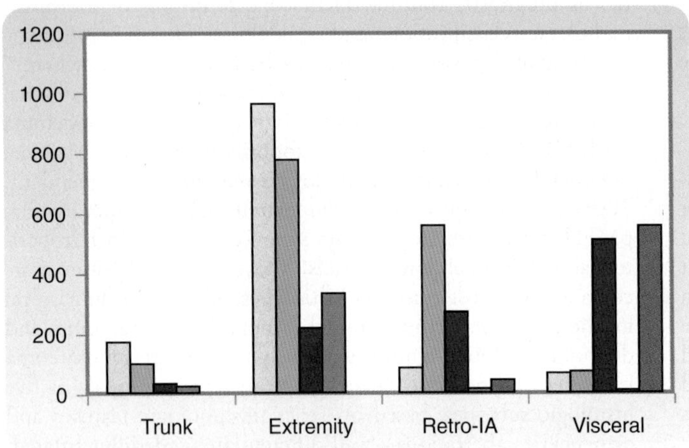


**FIGURE 33-2** Site-specific histology distribution for 4841 patients with soft tissue sarcoma treated at Memorial Sloan-Kettering Cancer Center from July 1, 1982, through June 30, 2009. *Yellow,* pleomorphic MFH/sarcoma NOS; *green,* liposarcoma; *red,* leiomyosarcoma; *blue,* synovial sarcoma; *brown,* GIST.

published series have combined all the histologic types of sarcoma, the significance of such subtyping is exemplified by liposarcoma, in which the five subsets (well-differentiated, dedifferentiated, myxoid, round cell, and pleomorphic) have totally different biology, patterns of behavior, and response to chemotherapy.[24-27] A further clear demonstration is the importance of myogenic differentiation in pleomorphic sarcomas, which is associated with a substantially increased risk of metastasis.[28] In a postoperative nomogram based on a database of 2136 adult patients from Memorial Sloan-Kettering Cancer Center (MSKCC), histologic type was found to be one of the most important predictors of sarcoma-specific death, with malignant peripheral nerve sheath tumors having the highest risk of mortality.[29] A more recent liposarcoma-based nomogram has further highlighted the importance of histologic subtype in enhancing assessment of disease-specific survival for the individual patient.[30]

## HISTOLOGIC GRADING AND PROGNOSTIC FACTORS FOR OUTCOME

The histologic type of sarcoma does not always provide sufficient information for predicting the clinical outcome and, therefore, may be inadequate to inform therapeutic decisions completely. Grading, based on histologic parameters only, evaluates the degree of malignancy and probability of distant metastasis. Several grading systems based on various histologic parameters have been published and proved to correlate with prognosis. The two most important parameters appear to be mitotic index and the extent of tumor necrosis. In general, the two most widely used grading systems are the National Cancer Institute (NCI) system developed by Costa and colleagues and the FNCLCC system developed by the French Federation of Cancer Centers Sarcoma Group. Both are three-tier systems (high, intermediate, and low). A comparative study of these three-tier systems has shown a slightly increased ability of the FNCLCC system to predict distant metastasis development and tumor mortality compared with the NCI system.[31] However, studies evaluating the interobserver reproducibility of the FNCLCC system have shown a 60% to 75% agreement for tumor grade and a 61% to 75% agreement for histologic type.[32] This high level of disagreement (25% to 40%), even among expert sarcoma pathologists, emphasizes the importance of histologic peer review and the need for developing more objective systems for sarcoma grading and classification. In fact, neither the FNCLCC system nor the NCI system has been formally endorsed by the World Health Organization[24] or Association of Directors of Anatomic and Surgical Pathology.

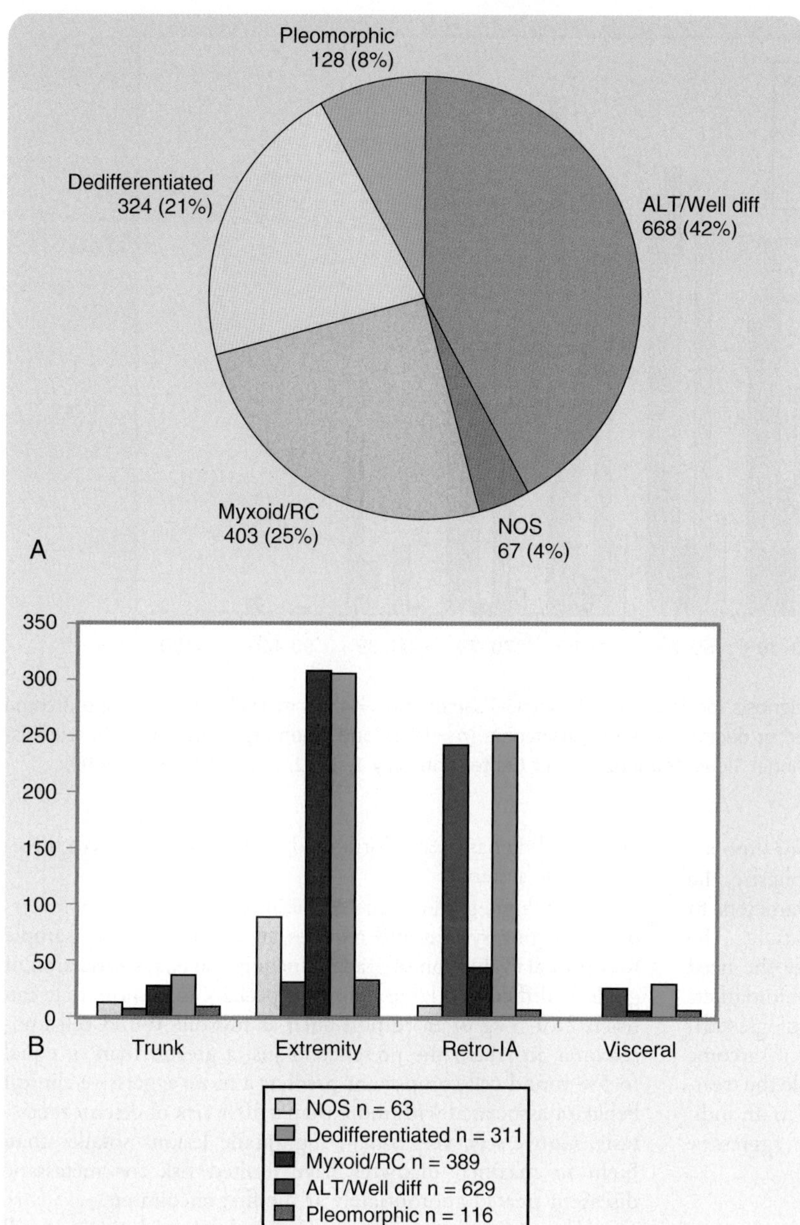


**FIGURE 33-3** Patients with liposarcoma treated at Memorial Sloan-Kettering Cancer Center from July 1, 1982, through June 30, 2009. **A,** Histologic subtype distribution of 1508 patients with liposarcoma. These data include extremity, trunk, visceral, and retroperitoneal tumors. **B,** Site-specific histologic subtype distribution for 1508 patients with liposarcoma.

MSKCC has had a long-standing interest and expertise in the staging and prognosis of soft tissue sarcoma and has developed a staging system that is highly predictive of systemic relapse based on size, grade, and tumor depth. In the MSKCC system, grade is classified as high or low based on degree of tumor differentiation, cellularity, necrosis, and mitotic activity. The use of these rigorous criteria has resulted in an excellent correlation with clinical outcome in many histologic types (e.g., liposarcoma, myxofibrosarcoma, malignant peripheral nerve sheath tumor [MPNST]) among patients in our prospective sarcoma database. In addition, this system avoids the management dilemma of an intermediate grade, which in most institutions would be lumped with and treated as a high-grade sarcoma. I recognize that in certain situations (approximately 5% to 10% of cases), the distinction between low- and high-grade tumors can be difficult, and therefore an intermediate grade would seem the most suitable. These difficult cases can be graded most appropriately by using systematic sampling and thorough examination. With a three-tier system, a larger subgroup of tumors will fall into the intermediate category, which could result in potential overtreatment of patients whose grade 2 tumors might be treated as high-grade tumors.

MSKCC researchers have developed a nomogram that adds to the prognostic value of size, grade (low versus high), and tumor depth, with the addition of age, site, and histopathology to refine predictions further of probability of sarcoma-specific survival.[29] Although there is widespread use of some form of grading system in the diagnosis and management of sarcomas, there is also agreement that currently no grading system performs well for every type of sarcoma. For a number of reasons, certain histologic types of sarcoma do not lend themselves well to grading. To address some of these issues, my group has

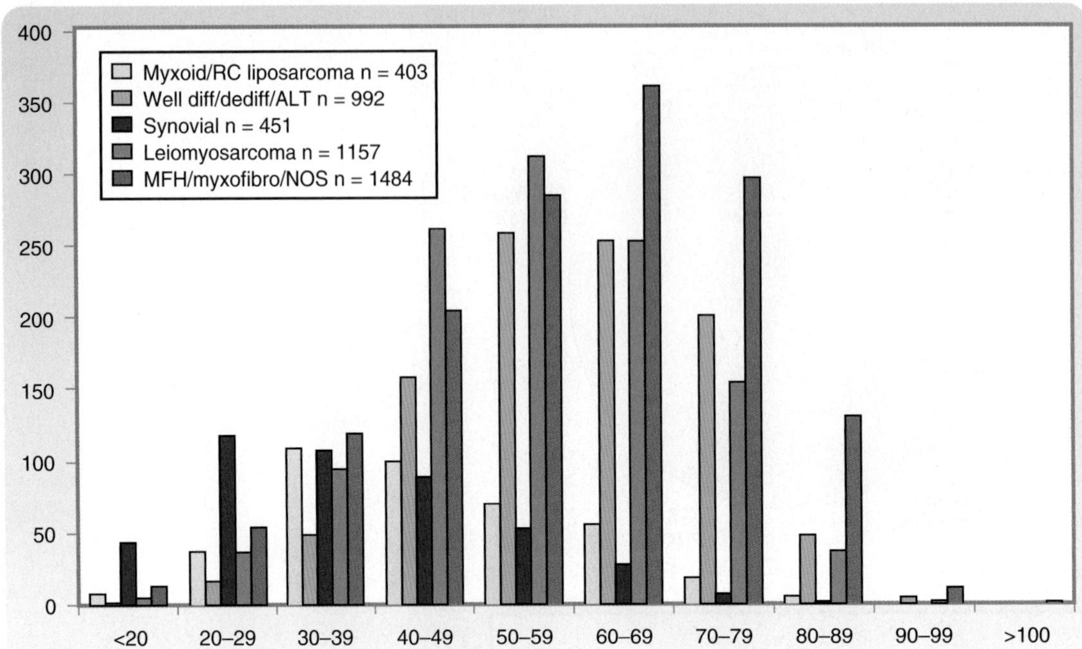


**FIGURE 33-4** Distribution by age at presentation and diagnosis for patients with synovial sarcoma ($n$ = 451), myxoid–round cell liposarcoma ($n$ = 403), leiomyosarcoma ($n$ = 1157), well-differentiated or dedifferentiated liposarcoma ($n$ = 992), and pleomorphic malignant fibrous histiocytoma or myxofibrosarcoma ($n$ = 1484) seen at Memorial Sloan-Kettering Cancer Center from July 1, 1982, through June 30, 2009.

recently developed histology-specific nomograms for liposarcoma,[30] synovial sarcoma,[33] and GIST[34] that emphasize the importance of assessing clinical and histologic parameters to improve prognostic accuracy for the individual patient. The limitations of the present grading systems emphasize the need to develop histology-specific molecular or genetic biomarkers that can be combined with conventional clinicopathologic variables to improve objective and accurate assessment of sarcoma prognosis for the individual patient. This would enable the treating physician to design a treatment strategy tailored to an individual patient's risk of relapse and potential for an aggressive clinical course.

## STAGING

Current staging systems are based on histologic and clinical information. The major staging system used for soft tissue sarcoma was developed by the American Joint Committee on Cancer (AJCC) and appears to be clinically useful and of prognostic value. This TNM system incorporates histologic type, histologic grade, tumor size, depth, regional lymph node involvement, and distant metastasis. It accommodates two-, three-, and four-tiered grading systems. The present 2010 AJCC soft tissue sarcoma grading system (Table 33-2) incorporates four major changes compared with the previous 2002 AJCC grading system[35]:

1. It now excludes the following histologic types: GIST, fibromatosis (desmoid tumor), Kaposi's sarcoma and infantile fibrosarcoma.
2. Angiosarcoma, extraskeletal Ewing's sarcoma, and dermatofibrosarcoma protuberans have been added to the list of histologic types.
3. N1 disease has been reclassified as stage III rather than stage IV disease.
4. Grading has been reformatted from a four-grade to a three-grade system.

Histologic grade is one of the most important parameters of the staging system and requires an adequate biopsy sample for optimal evaluation of grade. Unequivocal characterization of grade is difficult in large lesions, especially in tumors that can reach 2 or 3 kg or in tumors such as myxoid–round cell liposarcoma, in which the presence of just a greater than or equal to 5% round cell componant predicts a more aggressive clinical behavior associated with more than a 50% risk of distant metastasis. Conversely, very small, high-grade lesions smaller than 5 cm in maximal diameter have limited risk for metastatic disease if treated appropriately at the first encounter.

The staging system continues to undergo evolution and still fails to account adequately for sarcomas located in the retroperitoneum. Analysis of the primary extremity soft tissue sarcomas seen at Memorial Sloan-Kettering Cancer Center from July 1, 1982 to June 30, 2009 suggests that the probability of metastasis by stage is best discriminated in the new AJCC 2010 staging system (Table 33-3). Figure 33-5 shows the excellent discrimination by stage for distant recurrence-free survival using the AJCC 2010 system. It is important to emphasize that staging systems (1) apply to risk of metastasis or disease-specific survival or overall survival and (2) are almost exclusively confined to extremity lesions. There is as yet no adequate staging system for retroperitoneal or intra-abdominal lesions.

## MANAGEMENT

### Extremity and Superficial Trunk Sarcoma

Although surgery remains the principal therapeutic modality for soft tissue sarcoma, the extent of surgery required, along with the optimum combination of radiotherapy and chemotherapy,

**Table 33-2 American Joint Committee on Cancer 2010 Staging System for Soft Tissue Sarcoma**

| HISTOLOGIC GRADE (G) | FEATURES |
|---|---|
| GX | Grade cannot be assessed |
| G1 | Grade 1 |
| G2 | Grade 2 |
| G3 | Grade 3 |
| G4 (???) | |
| **PRIMARY TUMOR (T)** | **FEATURES** |
| TX | Primary tumor cannot be assessed |
| T0 | No evidence of primary tumor |
| T1 | Tumor ≤5 cm in greatest dimension* |
| T1a | Superficial tumor |
| T1b | Deep tumor |
| T2 | Tumor >5 cm in greatest dimension* |
| T2a | Superficial tumor |
| T2b | Deep tumor |
| **REGIONAL LYMPH NODES (N)** | **FEATURES** |
| NX | Regional lymph nodes cannot be assessed |
| N0 | No regional lymph node metastasis |
| N1† | Regional lymph node metastasis |
| **Distant Metastasis (M)** | |
| M0 | No distant metastasis |
| M1 | Distant metastasis present |

**Anatomic Stage and Prognostic Groups**

| STAGE | T | N | M | G |
|---|---|---|---|---|
| | **Prognostic Group** | | | |
| IA | T1a | N0 | M0 | G1, GX |
| | T1b | N0 | M0 | G1, GX |
| IB | T2a | N0 | M0 | G1, GX |
| | T2b | N0 | M0 | G1, GX |
| IIA | T1a | N0 | M0 | G2, G3 |
| | T1b | N0 | M0 | G2, G3 |
| IIB | T2a | N0 | M0 | G2 |
| | T2b | N0 | M0 | G2 |
| III | T2a, T2b | N0 | M0 | G3 |
| | Any T | N1 | M0 | Any G |
| IV | Any T | Any N | M1 | Any G |

From Edge S, Byrd D, Compton C, et al (eds): AJCC Cancer Staging Manual, ed 7, New York, 2010, Springer.

*Superficial tumor is located exclusively above the superficial fascia without invasion of the fascia; deep tumor is located exclusively beneath the superficial fascia, superficial to the fascia with invasion of or through the fascia, or both superficial yet beneath the fascia.

†Presence of positive nodes (N1) in M0 tumors is considered stage III.

**Table 33-3 Primary Extremity Soft Tissue Sarcoma: Distant Metastases by American Joint Committee on Cancer Stage***

| STAGE | TOTAL NO. OF PATIENTS | DISTANT METASTASES (%) |
|---|---|---|
| **Staging System (1997)** | | |
| 1A | 136 | 2 (1%) |
| 1B | 28 | 3 (11%) |
| 2A | 224 | 28 (13%) |
| 2B | 362 | 72 (20%) |
| 2C | 33 | 13 (40%) |
| 3A | 302 | 105 (35%) |
| 3B | 325 | 156 (48%) |
| **Staging System (2002)** | | |
| 1 | 388 | 33 (9%) |
| 2 | 395 | 85 (22%) |
| 3 | 627 | 261 (42%) |
| **Staging System (2010)*** | | |
| 1 | 739 | 49 (7%) |
| 2 | 507 | 99 (20%) |
| 3 | 1022 | 467 (46%) |

From Memorial Sloan-Kettering Cancer Center, July 1, 1982 to June 30, 2009.

*Excludes desmoid and dermatofibrosarcoma protuberans.

remains controversial. The important clinical and pathologic prognostic variables should be used by the surgeon to design the most effective treatment plan for the individual patient based on the predicted patterns of spread for certain sarcoma histologic types, with the aim of minimizing local recurrence, maximizing function, and improving overall survival. An algorithm for the management of soft tissue sarcoma of the extremity and trunk is shown in Figure 33-6. Surgical excision remains the dominant modality of curative therapy. Whenever possible, function- and limb-sparing procedures should be performed. As long as the entire tumor is removed, less radical procedures have not been demonstrated to affect local recurrence or outcome adversely.[36] The surgical objective should be complete removal of the tumor, with negative margins and maximal preservation of function. Also, when possible, tumors should be excised with 1 to 2 cm of normal tissue because of the propensity for local, unappreciated spread. Conversely, deliberate sacrifice of major neurovascular structures can generally be avoided, provided the surgeon pays meticulous attention to dissection and the preservation of intact fascial barriers.

Resection of bone is rarely required given the low incidence of direct bone invasion for soft tissue sarcoma. For sarcoma that closely approximates bone, the periosteum, if removed intact, can serve as a sufficient intact fascial margin. The extent of resection is often determined by the histologic type. For example, histologic types such as myxofibrosarcoma (formally myxoid MFH), a tumor that predominates in the extremities of older patients, are often multifocal and may spread considerable distances along fascial planes. Thus, the surgical plan should be designed to encompass all suspicious regions of enhancement on MRI and these areas should be excised with extensive lateral (2- to 3-cm) margins and 1- to 2-cm deep soft tissue margins if this can be accomplished with minimal functional loss. The most extensive resection is clearly amputation. This is rarely indicated in soft tissue sarcoma because, at present, limb-sparing operations are possible in

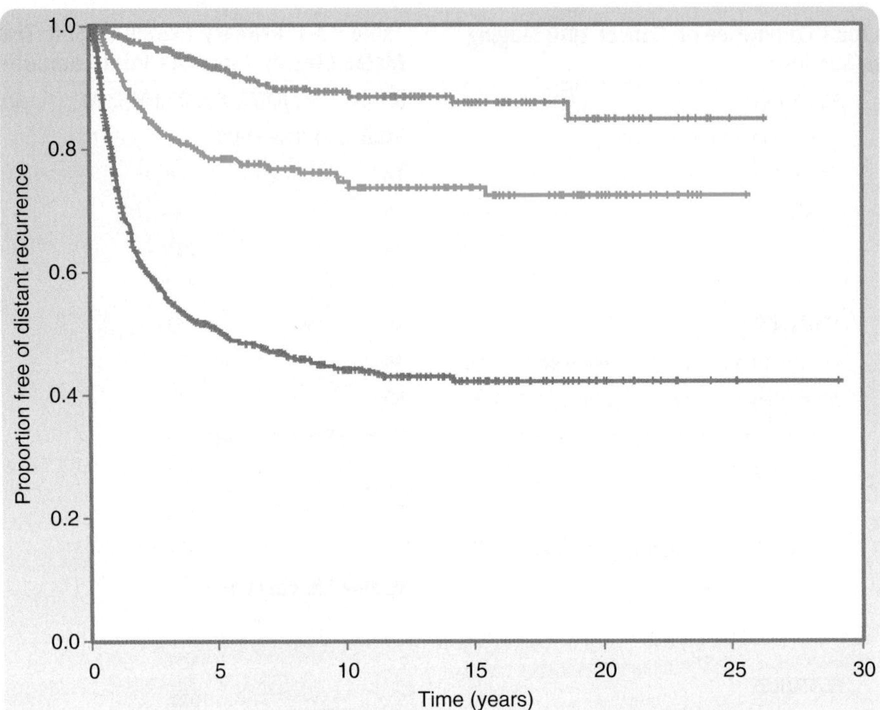


**FIGURE 33-5** Distant recurrence-free survival for patients with primary extremity soft tissue sarcoma (*N* = 2263) by AJCC 2010 stage seen at Memorial Sloan-Kettering Cancer Center from July 1, 1982, through June 30, 2009 (excludes desmoid and dermatofibrosarcoma protuberans).

95% of patients. Experience over the last 27 years at MSKCC has indicated that the 50% amputation rate in the late 1960s is now less than 5%. Amputation should mainly be reserved for patients with tumors that cannot be completely resected by any other means, who are without evidence of metastatic disease, and who have the propensity for good long-term functional rehabilitation. Often, these are patients with large, low-grade tumors causing considerable cosmetic and functional deformity that can be rendered symptom- and disease-free by a major amputation.

The effectiveness of adjuvant radiation for improving local control has been clearly shown, not only through retrospective data,[37] but also by two prospective randomized trials that have compared surgery alone with surgery and radiation.[38,39] This includes using brachytherapy for high-grade lesions or external beam radiation therapy for large (>5 cm) high- or low-grade lesions. For subcutaneous or intramuscular high-grade sarcomas smaller than 5 cm, or any size low-grade sarcoma, surgery alone should be considered if adequate wide excision with a good 1-cm cuff of surrounding fat and muscle can be achieved. For certain low-grade histologic types, 1-cm margins are not required for excellent local control. In the case of atypical lipomas or well-differentiated liposarcoma of the extremities, only complete excision, with a minimal surrounding margin is required, because most of these patients will not recur following a limited or microscopic positive margin excision as long as the excision is complete. Thus, radiation therapy is rarely indicated for this histologic type unless there is a significant sclerosing component combined with a microscopic positive margin.[26] For most deep, high-grade sarcoma types, larger than 5 cm, if the excision margin is close, particularly with extramuscular involvement, or if a local recurrence would result in the sacrifice of a major neurovascular bundle or amputation, then adjuvant radiation therapy should be added to the surgical resection to reduce the probability of local failure.[39] Irrespective of grade, postoperative irradiation is probably used more than is strictly necessary. Several studies have shown that a significant subset of subcutaneous and intramuscular sarcomas can be treated by wide excision alone, with a local recurrence rate of only 8% to 20%.[40-42]

The value of chemotherapy depends on the histologic type of sarcoma. Neoadjuvant chemotherapy is almost always indicated for the treatment of Ewing's sarcoma–PNET and rhabdomyosarcoma, because of the high risk of microscopic metastasis at diagnosis and high response rate with this therapy. The potential for cure in these chemotherapy-sensitive, small, blue round cell tumor types is inversely proportional to the volume and spread of disease at initial diagnosis. For patients with other histologic types of high-grade sarcoma, the role of chemotherapy remains controversial. This is because, given the rarity of these tumors, the randomized trials have enrolled relatively small patient populations with heterogeneous groups of histologic types or subtypes. Fourteen randomized phase III trials have examined the effectiveness of postoperative adjuvant chemotherapy versus no treatment to increase survival in high-risk soft tissue sarcoma patients presenting with localized disease. Most of these trials were performed between 1977 and 2000, and all used combinations of anthracyclines with dacarbazine or ifosfamide or used doxorubicin as a single agent.[43,44] In most trials, a lower risk for local recurrence was observed in patients

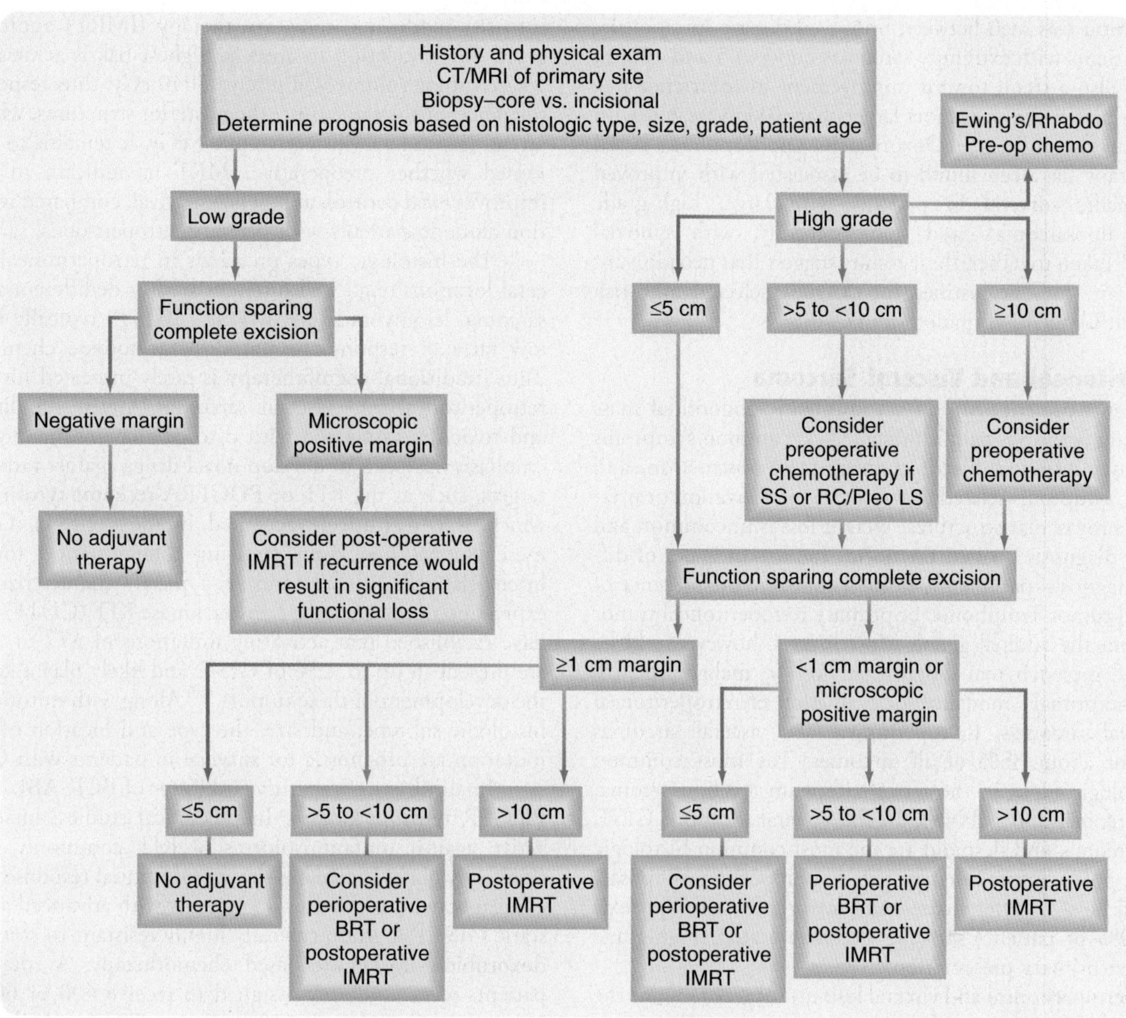


**FIGURE 33-6** Algorithm for the management of primary (with no metastases) extremity or trunk soft tissue sarcoma, using a biologic rationale (i.e., size and grade of tumor). *BRT,* Brachytherapy; *EBRT,* external beam radiation therapy; *RC/Pleo LS,* round cell–pleomorphic liposarcoma.

receiving adjuvant chemotherapy. Some trials showed a lower risk for metastatic progression, but only a few reported longer survival times.

A meta-analysis of all published studies has confirmed a significantly lower risk for relapse, local or metastatic, but with only a 4% (nonsignificant) lower risk for death.[43] A more recent trial from the Italian Sarcoma Group has shown a significantly longer overall survival duration for patients with high-risk sarcoma of the extremities receiving adjuvant chemotherapy with ifosfamide,[44] but the overall survival benefit was not sustained with additional follow-up. Thus, in an unselected population of patients with high-grade soft tissue sarcoma, adjuvant chemotherapy has not reproducibly demonstrated its capacity to improve overall survival or relapse-free survival and is rarely indicated, except in a clinical trial. Presently, there is an urgent need to select patients with sarcoma types most likely to benefit from chemotherapy and then test this subgroup of patients prospectively with a control arm. The preoperative use of neoadjuvant combination chemotherapy (usually with doxorubicin [Adriamycin] and ifosfamide) for adult soft tissue sarcoma has several potential advantages, particularly for the treatment of locally advanced tumors:

1. It can make subsequent surgery easier.
2. It may treat micrometastatic disease early before the acquisition of resistance.
3. It leaves the vasculature intact for improved drug delivery.
4. It enables assessment of therapeutic response or resistance to therapy.

A retrospective analysis of patients with high-grade extremity sarcoma from prospectively acquired databases of patients from MSKCC and Dana Farber Cancer Institute (DFCI) was used to determine the impact of neoadjuvant chemotherapy on outcome.[45] A stratified Cox proportional hazards model was used to compare the disease-specific survival of 74 patients treated with neoadjuvant chemotherapy and surgery with 282 patients treated with surgery alone and to account for differences in known prognostic factors (e.g., size, histology, age). Neoadjuvant chemotherapy was associated with an overall improvement in disease-specific survival for the complete cohort of patients; this improvement appeared to be driven by the benefit of neoadjuvant chemotherapy in patients with extremity sarcomas larger than 10 cm. In this high-risk group, there was a 21% improvement in disease-specific survival at 3 years. Conversely, no association was seen between improved disease-specific survival in patients with extremity sarcomas between 5 and 10 cm. There was also a trend toward improvement in recurrence-free survival in patients with tumors larger than 10 cm treated with neoadjuvant chemotherapy. Doxorubicin- and ifosfamide-based chemotherapy has been found to be associated with improved disease-specific survival in patients with large, high-grade extremity liposarcoma[25] and, more recently, with synovial sarcoma.[46] Taken together, these results suggest that neoadjuvant chemotherapy may be justified for carefully selected high-risk patients with large high-grade tumors.

## Retroperitoneal and Visceral Sarcoma

Most patients present with an asymptomatic abdominal mass although, on occasion, pain is present. Less common symptoms include gastrointestinal bleeding, incomplete obstruction, and neurologic symptoms related to retroperitoneal invasion or pressure on neurovascular structures. Weight loss is uncommon and incidental diagnosis is often the norm. Important issues of differential diagnosis, particularly in the young, are the presence of a germ cell tumor, lymphoma, or primary retroperitoneal tumor arising from the adrenal gland. Most lesions, however, will be tumors of mesenchymal origin, benign or malignant. CT remains the primary modality for evaluation of retroperitoneal and visceral sarcomas. Retroperitoneal and visceral sarcomas account for about 35% of all sarcomas. The most common histopathologic types in the retroperitoneum are liposarcoma, leiomyosarcoma, and MPNST. In the visceral location, GIST, leiomyosarcoma, and desmoid are the most common histologic types (Fig. 33-2). Approximately 55% of retroperitoneal liposarcomas will be well-differentiated and low grade, with approximately 40% of patients showing dedifferentiated, high-grade histology at primary presentation.

For retroperitoneal and visceral lesions, surgery remains the dominant therapeutic modality,[27,47] with the most important prognostic factors for survival in retroperitoneal sarcoma being completeness of resection, histologic subtype, and grade. Although resection of adjacent organs is common,[27] proof that a more extensive resection of adjacent organs has an impact on long-term survival seems limited. Despite an aggressive surgical approach, local control is still a major problem, and multifocal unresectable tumors recur in many patients, particularly those with liposarcoma. The role of radiation therapy for retroperitoneal sarcoma is not well defined and is in need of further investigation. In theory, preoperative or postoperative irradiation to this site is desirable but, in reality, it is often not possible to deliver full-dose radiation therapy (60 to 66 Gy) to areas at risk because the dose is limited by the large treatment volume required and sensitivities of adjacent normal tissues, such as bowel, kidney, liver, and spinal cord.

Brachytherapy or intraoperative radiation therapy at the time of surgical resection may be used to treat a localized area at high risk of microscopic or gross residual disease when further surgical excision is not possible. However, care must be taken to avoid excessive morbidity and mortality that could result from aggressive brachytherapy, particularly when combined with external beam radiation therapy. Therefore, the ideal radiation approach is the one that could dose-escalate preoperative radiation. With conventional radiation, it is impossible to escalate preoperative radiation beyond 5040 cGy without incurring excessive toxicity. However, with a dose-painting, preoperative, intensity-modulated radiation therapy (IMRT) approach, targeted dose escalation to areas at highest risk is achievable. The whole tumor volume will receive 5040 cGy, thus respecting the tolerance; at the same time, the posterior structures, where there are no intestines, will receive 6000 cGy. It remains to be determined whether preoperative IMRT in addition to resection improves local control, and hence survival, compared with resection alone in patients with primary retroperitoneal sarcoma.

The histologic types prevalent in retroperitoneal and visceral locations (e.g., well-differentiated or dedifferentiated liposarcoma, leiomyosarcoma, MPNST, GIST) typically have very low rates of response to traditional cytotoxic chemotherapy. Thus, traditional chemotherapy is rarely indicated for operable retroperitoneal and visceral sarcomas. Given the limitations and toxicities associated with cytotoxic chemotherapy, current emphasis has been to develop novel drugs against rational drug targets, such as the KIT or PDGFRA receptor tyrosine kinase, which is constitutively activated in most GISTs. GISTs are mesenchymal neoplasms showing differentiation toward the interstitial cells of Cajal and are typically characterized by the expression of the receptor tyrosine kinase KIT (CD117). Studies have established that activating mutations of *KIT* or *PDGFRA* are present in up to 92% of GISTs and likely play a key role in the development of these tumors.[9,10] Along with mitotic activity, histologic subtype, and size, the type and location of the *KIT* mutation are prognostic for survival in patients with GIST.[48]

Imatinib is a competitive inhibitor of BCR-ABL, KIT, and PDGFR tyrosine kinases. In preclinical studies, imatinib was active against mutant isoforms of KIT commonly found in GIST.[11] A phase II trial has shown substantial response rates and clinical benefit of imatinib in patients with advanced and metastatic GIST,[12] a group typically highly resistant to conventional doxorubicin-ifosfamide–based chemotherapy. A total of 147 patients were randomly assigned to receive 400 or 600 mg of imatinib daily. Overall, 79 patients (53.7%) had a partial response and 41 patients (27.9%) had stable disease. No patient had a complete response to the treatment. Early resistance to imatinib was noted in 20 patients (13.6%). Therapy was well tolerated, although mild to moderate edema, diarrhea, and fatigue were common. Gastrointestinal or intra-abdominal hemorrhage occurred in approximately 5% of patients. There were no significant differences in toxic effects or response between the two doses. Thus, inhibition of the KIT signal transduction pathway with tyrosine kinase inhibitors benefits over 80% of patients with advanced GIST. Studies have consistently shown that patients with GISTs harboring KIT exon 11 mutations achieve the best responses to imatinib therapy and longer median overall and progression-free survival compared with other GIST mutations. For example, the presence of KIT exon 9-activating mutations is an adverse prognostic factor for response to imatinib, increasing the relative risk of progression by 171% and the relative risk of death by 190%, compared with exon 11 mutations in an analysis of 377 GISTs from patients in a phase III trial.[49] In patients with KIT exon 9 mutations, treatment with higher dose imatinib (800 mg/day) resulted in a significantly superior median progression-free survival relative to treatment with imatinib 400 mg/day, with a 61% reduction in the relative risk of progression.[49] These results support the notion that patients with KIT exon 9 mutations may gain particular benefit from high-dose imatinib compared with patients with other mutations, and highlight the importance of mutational testing for patients with GIST before the initiation of tyrosine kinase inhibitor therapy.

The role of imatinib therapy in the adjuvant setting for the treatment of GIST has been evaluated in a randomized phase III, double-blind, placebo-controlled multicenter trial.[50] Eligible patients had complete gross resection of a primary GIST, which was at least 3 cm in size and positive for the KIT protein by immunohistochemistry. Patients were randomly assigned to imatinib 400 mg ($n$ = 359) or to placebo ($n$ = 354) daily for 1 year after surgical resection. With a median follow-up for surviving patients of 19.7 months, the estimated 1-year recurrence-free survival was 98% (95% confidence index [CI], 96 to 100) in the imatinib group versus 83% (95% CI, 78 to 88) in the placebo group. At this time, there is no difference in overall survival. Longer patient follow-up is necessary to establish whether adjuvant imatinib increases the cure rate of surgery alone for localized primary GIST. Acquired resistance is a frequent event in patients with metastatic GIST who initially respond to imatinib. GIST progression occurs at a median of 18 to 24 months,[51] usually from the development of a secondary mutation in the KIT gene.[52] Once clinical progression develops, increased doses of imatinib or sunitinib (a multitarget tyrosine kinase inhibitor) can restore GIST response in some patients, at least temporarily.[53]

Given the problems with the development of acquired resistance in the setting of advanced disease, it remains to be determined if early treatment with imatinib therapy in the adjuvant setting will also lead to the development of resistant clones or to complete eradication of subclinical microscopic disease. Thus, the role of adjuvant imatinib for the treatment of localized primary GIST and optimal duration of treatment remains a subject of debate. Until additional follow-up data are available it is prudent to suggest that adjuvant imatinib therapy should only be administered within clinical trials.

## Treatment of Recurrent Disease

Despite optimum multimodality limb-sparing treatment for extremity soft tissue sarcoma, a significant number of patients will develop distant metastasis. For extremity lesions, the most common site of metastasis is the lung. It is the only site of recurrence in approximately 50% of all patients. Extrapulmonary metastasis is relatively uncommon and usually occurs as a late manifestation of widely disseminated disease. Patients whose primary tumors are controlled or controllable, who have no extrathoracic disease, who are medically fit for thoracotomy, and for whom complete resection of all lung disease appears possible should undergo thoracotomy with the intent of resecting all disease. Patients with unresectable pulmonary metastases or extrapulmonary metastatic sarcoma in more than a single site have a uniformly poor prognosis and are best treated with systemic chemotherapy. The role of chemotherapy in advanced sarcoma is controversial and, at present, the treatment of metastatic sarcoma represents palliative, not curative, therapy.

Current active drugs that have significant response rates include doxorubicin, ifosfamide, and dacarbazine, but none has had a major impact on long-term survival. The combination of mesna, ifosfamide, doxorubicin, and dacarbazine (MAID) has been shown to have a 47% response rate and a 10% complete response rate. Randomized prospective clinical trials on combination chemotherapy regimens such as MAID and other ifosfamide-doxorubicin combinations with cytokine support have shown statistically improved rates of antitumor response. However, these do not translate into improvements in survival and come at the cost of increased toxicity and a decrease in quality of life. In an analysis of 1897 patients with primary extremity soft tissue sarcomas, isolated distant metastasis to lung developed in 508 patients (27%) and 138 (7%) underwent pulmonary metastasectomy.[54] Five-year postmetastasis disease-specific survival for patients undergoing pulmonary resection for metastatic soft tissue sarcoma of the extremity was 29% compared with 6% for the patients with clinically unresectable disease who were treated with chemotherapy alone. In the group undergoing pulmonary metastasectomy, preoperative chemotherapy was found to have no impact on the disease-specific survival or progression-free survival of patients undergoing pulmonary resection for metastatic extremity soft tissue sarcoma compared with patients treated with metastasectomy alone. The independent factors found on multivariate analysis to be statistically associated with prolonged, postmetastasis, disease-specific survival were complete pulmonary metastasectomy ($P$ = .026; hazard ratio [HR] = 0.52) and disease-free interval longer than 1 year ($P$ = .014; HR = 0.53). Therefore, pulmonary resection alone, without conventional chemotherapy, should be considered a valid and evidence-based approach for patients with metastatic extremity sarcoma.

Despite improvements in imaging and surgical techniques and the use of multimodality therapy, local recurrence remains a significant problem for patients with extremity soft tissue sarcoma. The local recurrence rate after treatment of primary extremity sarcoma ranges from 6% to 20% in published series.[37,40] Local recurrence in an extremity often presents as a nodular mass or series of nodules arising in the surgical scar. Treatment of these local recurrences may be particularly challenging, because it may be difficult to design a surgical plan that encompasses the entire previously resected tumor bed and maintains sufficient function. In general, approximately 80% of patients presenting with a local recurrence can be effectively treated with limb-sparing surgery. In an analysis of 1421 patients who underwent surgical treatment for primary extremity sarcoma at MSKCC between 1982 and 2002, a total of 179 (13%) subsequently developed an isolated local recurrence and underwent complete surgical resection.[55] The median interval to initial local recurrence was 16 months; 65% developed a local recurrence by 2 years and 90% by 4 years. Independent prognostic factors for disease-specific survival after local recurrence were a high histologic grade, large local recurrence tumor size, and short local recurrence-free interval. Patients who developed a local recurrence larger than 5 cm in less than 16 months had a 4-year disease-specific survival of 18%, compared with 81% for patients who developed a local recurrence smaller than 5 cm in more than 16 months. A patient who presents with a large local recurrence that develops in a short interval should be considered to have a biologically aggressive tumor, with a high tumor-specific mortality. These high-risk patients, depending on their histologic type, may be excellent candidates for systemic neoadjuvant therapy trials.

Local recurrence following complete resection of primary retroperitoneal liposarcoma is common, with 50% of well-differentiated and 80% of dedifferentiated tumors recurring within 5 years.[27] Retroperitoneal recurrences are often detected on routine screening with imaging or patients may present with pain or nonspecific symptoms. After a workup to determine the extent of disease, patients with isolated local recurrence should be carefully evaluated for reresection.

Current chemotherapy is ineffective for most patients and toxicity limits adequate dosing by radiation therapy, so complete surgical resection remains the most effective treatment modality. The most difficult decision in retroperitoneal liposarcoma is selecting those patients most likely to benefit from reoperation and the timing of the reoperation; a period of watchful monitoring is often appropriate. A recent analysis of 105 patients who had at least one local recurrence following complete resection of a primary retroperitoneal liposarcoma at MSKCC was performed to determine factors that determine survival and would assist with selecting patients most likely to benefit from surgery.[56] Of these 105 patients, 61 underwent complete resection of their first local recurrence. Local recurrence size, primary histologic variant and grade, and local recurrence growth rate were found to be independent predictors of disease-specific survival. Despite aggressive operative management, patients with a local recurrence growth rate more than 1 cm/month were associated with poor outcomes, similar to those of patients who were not treated with resection. Only patients with local recurrence growth rates less than 0.9 cm/month were associated with improved survival following aggressive resection of the local recurrence.

Based on these results, for patients presenting with asymptomatic local recurrence and growth rates exceeding or equal to 1 cm/month, I now recommend treatment with systemic chemotherapy or novel targeted therapy trials. Surgery is only considered for this subgroup if patients develop symptoms unresponsive to medical management, such as obstruction or bleeding. For patients with local recurrence growth rates less than 1 cm/month, immediate surgery is recommended for all symptomatic patients and for asymptomatic patients whose local recurrence is impinging on critical structures, particularly if further growth may result in the need to sacrifice critical organs or the tumor has a solid appearance on CT scan (suspicious for dedifferentiation). Many asymptomatic patients with a well-differentiated–appearing local recurrence that is well away from critical structures may be safely followed off any therapy and monitored to determine whether they develop other sites of disease before complete surgical resection is recommended. Such an approach can extend the interval between surgical resections and enables the surgeon to be more confident that all known disease sites are being encompassed with the planned procedure.

## SUMMARY

Soft tissue sarcomas are relatively rare, with an annual incidence of about 10,600 cases in the United States. Primary therapy is predicated on surgical resection with an adequate margin of normal tissue. For high-risk patients, local control is improved with postoperative adjuvant radiation therapy. Local recurrence rates vary, depending on anatomic site. In extremity lesions, 15% of patients will develop locally recurrent disease, with a median disease-free interval of 18 months. Treatment results for localized extremity recurrence may approach those for primary disease. Isolated pulmonary metastases may be resected, with 30% 5-year survival rates after complete resection. Adjuvant or neoadjuvant chemotherapy has not been proven to result in longer overall survival times after optimal resection of the primary sarcoma. In patients with retroperitoneal and visceral sarcoma, complete resection remains the dominant factor for the outcome. As opposed to extremity sites, local recurrence in this site is a common cause of death. Patients with unresectable pulmonary metastases or extrapulmonary metastatic sarcoma have a uniformly poor prognosis and are best treated with systemic chemotherapy, reserving surgical resection for meaningful palliation. There is an urgent need to develop novel targeted therapies that are histologically and molecular type–specific for the more than 4000 patients who will die each year from inoperable forms of soft tissue sarcoma.

## SELECTED REFERENCES

Baldini EH, Goldberg J, Jenner C, et al: Long-term outcomes after function-sparing surgery without radiotherapy for soft tissue sarcoma of the extremities and trunk. J Clin Oncol 17:3252–3259, 1999.

Pisters PW, Pollock RE, Lewis VO, et al: Long-term results of prospective trial of surgery alone with selective use of radiation for patients with T1 extremity and trunk soft tissue sarcomas. Ann Surg 246:675–681, 2007.

These studies suggest that there may be a select subset of patients with soft tissue sarcoma in whom carefully performed function-sparing surgery may serve as definitive therapy and in whom adjuvant radiotherapy may not be necessary.

Brennan MF, Lewis JJ: Diagnosis and management of soft tissue sarcoma, London, 2002, Martin Dunitz.

Brennan MF, Singer S, Maki RG, O'Sullivan B: Sarcomas of the soft tissues and bone. In DeVita VT, Hellman S, Rosenberg SA, editors: Cancer principles and practice of oncology, Philadelphia, 2005, Lippincott Williams & Wilkins, p 1584.

Singer S, Demetri GD, Baldini EH, Fletcher CDM: Management of soft-tissue sarcomas: An overview and update. Lancet Oncol 1:75–85, 2000.

These reviews summarize the subject in a single monograph or text.

Antonescu CR, Besmer P, Guo T, et al: Acquired resistance to imatinib in gastrointestinal stromal tumor occurs through secondary gene mutation. Clin Cancer Res 11:4182–4190, 2005.

Dematteo RP, Ballman KV, Antonescu CR, et al: Adjuvant imatinib mesylate after resection of localised, primary gastrointestinal stromal tumour: A randomised, double-blind, placebo-controlled trial. Lancet 373:1097–1104, 2009.

Demetri GD, von Mehren M, Blanke CD, et al: Efficacy and safety of imatinib mesylate in advanced gastrointestinal stromal tumors. N Engl J Med 347:472–480, 2002.

Heinrich MC, Corless, CL, Demetri, GD, et al: Kinase mutations and imatinib response in patients with metastatic gastrointestinal stromal tumor. J Clin Oncol 21:4342–4349, 2003.

Singer S, Rubin BP, Lux ML, et al: Prognostic value of *KIT* mutation type, mitotic activity, and histologic subtype in gastrointestinal stromal tumors. J Clin Oncol 20:3898–3905, 2002.

These studies demonstrate the importance of *KIT* and PDGFRA activation and mutations in GIST pathogenesis, and the rationale for and application of KIT tyrosine kinase inhibitors for targeted therapy of GIST. The importance of *KIT* mutation type for predicting response to imatinib and the development of secondary mutations as a mechanism for acquired resistance to imatinib is described in the Antonescu and Heinrich references. Early results from a randomized phase III trial of adjuvant imatinib following resection of primary localized GIST are presented in the Dematteo reference.

Park JO, Qin LX, Prete FP, et al: Predicting outcome by growth rate of locally recurrent retroperitoneal liposarcoma: The one centimeter per month rule. Ann Surg 250:977–982, 2009.
Singer S, Antonescu CR, Riedel E, et al: Histologic subtype and margin of resection predict pattern of recurrence and survival for retroperitoneal liposarcoma. Ann Surg 238:358–370, 2003.

These studies provide an extensive description of outcome and prognostic factors for patients with primary and locally recurrent retroperitoneal liposarcomas.

Pisters P, Leung D, Woodruff J, et al: Analysis of prognostic factors in 1041 patients with localized soft tissue sarcomas of the extremity. J Clin Oncol 14:1679–1689, 1996.

This report provides data on prognostic factors for extremity soft tissue sarcoma from a large single-institution series.

Pisters PW, Harrison LB, Leung DH, et al: Long-term results of a prospective randomized trial of adjuvant brachytherapy in soft tissue sarcoma. J Clin Oncol 14:859–868, 1996.
Yang JC, Chang AE, Baker AR, et al: Randomized prospective study of the benefit of adjuvant radiation therapy in the treatment of soft tissue sarcomas of the extremity. J Clin Oncol 16:197–203, 1998.

These studies confirm the benefit of adjuvant radiation therapy in patients with completely resected localized extremity sarcoma.

## REFERENCES


1. Jemal A, Siegel R, Ward E, et al: Cancer statistics, 2009. CA Cancer J Clin 59:225–249, 2009.
2. Malkin D, Li FP, Strong LC, et al: Germline p53 mutations in a familial syndrome of breast cancer, sarcomas, and other neoplasms. Science 250:1233–1238, 1990.
3. Kleinerman RA, Tucker MA, Tarone RE, et al: Risk of new cancers after radiotherapy in long-term survivors of retinoblastoma: An extended follow-up. J Clin Oncol 23:2272–2279, 2005.
4. Fletcher O, Easton D, Anderson K, et al: Lifetime risks of common cancers among retinoblastoma survivors. J Natl Cancer Inst 96:357–363, 2004.
5. Kirova YM, Gambotti L, De Rycke Y, et al: Risk of second malignancies after adjuvant radiotherapy for breast cancer: A large-scale, single-institution review. Int J Radiat Oncol Biol Phys 68:359–363, 2007.
6. Gladdy RA, Qin L, Moraco N, et al: Do radiation associated soft tissue sarcomas have the same prognosis as sporadic soft tissue sarcomas? J Clin Oncol. In Press.
7. Tuomisto J, Pekkanen J, Kiviranta H, et al: Dioxin cancer risk—example of hormesis? Dose Response 3:332–341, 2006.
8. Tuomisto JT, Pekkanen J, Kiviranta H, et al: Soft-tissue sarcoma and dioxin: A case-control study. Int J Cancer 108:893–900, 2004.
9. Heinrich MC, Corless CL, Duensing A, et al: PDGFRA activating mutations in gastrointestinal stromal tumors. Science 299:708–710, 2003.
10. Hirota S, Isozaki K, Moriyama Y, et al: Gain-of-function mutations of c-kit in human gastrointestinal stromal tumors. Science 279:577–580, 1998.
11. Tuveson DA, Willis NA, Jacks T, et al: STI571 inactivation of the gastrointestinal stromal tumor c-KIT oncoprotein: Biological and clinical implications. Oncogene 20:5054–5058, 2001.
12. Demetri GD, von Mehren M, Blanke CD, et al: Efficacy and safety of imatinib mesylate in advanced gastrointestinal stromal tumors. N Engl J Med 347:472–480, 2002.
13. Antonescu CR, Leung DH, Dudas M, et al: Alterations of cell cycle regulators in localized synovial sarcoma: A multifactorial study with prognostic implications. Am J Pathol 156:977–983, 2000.
14. Perrone F, Tamborini E, Suardi S, et al: Re: Oda et al. Frequent alteration of p16INK4a/p14ARF and p53 pathways in the round cell component of myxoid/round cell liposarcoma: p53 gene alterations and reduced p14ARF expression both correlate with poor prognosis. J Pathol 207:410–421, 2005.
15. Huang HY, Illei PB, Zhao Z, et al: Ewing sarcomas with p53 mutation or p16/p14ARF homozygous deletion: A highly lethal subset associated with poor chemoresponse. J Clin Oncol 23:548–558, 2005.
16. Ladanyi M, Antonescu CR, Leung DH, et al: Impact of SYT-SSX fusion type on the clinical behavior of synovial sarcoma: A multi-institutional retrospective study of 243 patients. Cancer Res 62: 135–140, 2002.
17. Sorensen PH, Lynch JC, Qualman SJ, et al: PAX3-FKHR and PAX7-FKHR gene fusions are prognostic indicators in alveolar rhabdomyosarcoma: A report from the children's oncology group. J Clin Oncol 20:2672–2679, 2002.
18. Maki RG, Awan RA, Dixon RH, et al: Differential sensitivity to imatinib of 2 patients with metastatic sarcoma arising from dermatofibrosarcoma protuberans. Int J Cancer 100:623–626, 2002.
19. McArthur GA, Demetri GD, van Oosterom A, et al: Molecular and clinical analysis of locally advanced dermatofibrosarcoma protuberans treated with imatinib: Imatinib Target Exploration Consortium Study B2225. J Clin Oncol 23:866–873, 2005.
20. Antonescu CR, Yoshida A, Guo T, et al: KDR activating mutations in human angiosarcomas are sensitive to specific kinase inhibitors. Cancer Res 69:7175–7179, 2009.
21. Maki RG, D'Adamo DR, Keohan ML, et al: Phase II study of sorafenib in patients with metastatic or recurrent sarcomas. J Clin Oncol 27:3133–3140, 2009.
22. Margaritora S, Porziella V, D'Andrilli A, et al: Pulmonary metastases: Can accurate radiological evaluation avoid thoracotomic approach? Eur J Cardiothorac Surg 21:1111–1114, 2002.
23. Tateishi U, Yamaguchi U, Seki K, et al: Bone and soft-tissue sarcoma: Preoperative staging with fluorine 18 fluorodeoxyglucose PET/CT and conventional imaging. Radiology 245:839–847, 2007.
24. Fletcher C, Unni K, Mertens F, editors: Pathology and genetics of tumors of soft tissue and bone. World Health Organization Classification of Tumors, Lyon, France, 2002, International Agency for Research on Cancer Press, p 427.
25. Eilber FC, Eilber FR, Eckardt J, et al: The impact of chemotherapy on the survival of patients with high-grade primary extremity liposarcoma. Ann Surg 240:686–695, 2004.
26. Kooby DA, Antonescu CR, Brennan MF, et al: Atypical lipomatous tumor/well-differentiated liposarcoma of the extremity and trunk wall: Importance of histological subtype with treatment recommendations. Ann Surg Oncol 11:78–84, 2004.

27. Singer S, Antonescu CR, Riedel E, et al: Histologic subtype and margin of resection predict pattern of recurrence and survival for retroperitoneal liposarcoma. Ann Surg 238:358–370, 2003.
28. Massi D, Beltrami G, Capanna R, et al: Histopathological re-classification of extremity pleomorphic soft tissue sarcoma has clinical relevance. Eur J Surg Oncol 30:1131–1136, 2004.
29. Kattan M, Leung D, Brennan M: Postoperative nomogram for 12-year sarcoma-specific death. J Clin Oncology 20:791–796, 2002.
30. Dalal KM, Kattan MW, Antonescu CR, et al: Subtype specific prognostic nomogram for patients with primary liposarcoma of the retroperitoneum, extremity, or trunk. Ann Surg 244:381–391, 2006.
31. Guillou L, Coindre J, Bonichon F, et al: Comparative Study of the National Cancer Institute and French Federation of Cancer Centers Sarcoma Group grading systems in a population of 410 adult patients with soft tissue sarcoma. J Clin Oncol 15:350–362, 1997.
32. Alvegard TA, Berg NO: Histopathology peer review of high-grade soft tissue sarcoma: The Scandinavian Sarcoma Group experience. J Clin Oncol 7:1845–1851, 1989.
33. Canter RJ, Qin LX, Maki RG, et al: A synovial sarcoma-specific preoperative nomogram supports a survival benefit to ifosfamide-based chemotherapy and improves risk stratification for patients. Clin Cancer Res 14:8191–8197, 2008.
34. Gold JS, Gonen M, Gutierrez A, et al: Development and validation of a prognostic nomogram for recurrence-free survival after complete surgical resection of localised primary gastrointestinal stromal tumour: a retrospective analysis. Lancet Oncol 10:1045–1052, 2009.
35. Edge SB, Byrd DR, Compton CC, et al, editors: AJCC cancer staging manual, ed 7, New York, 2009, Springer.
36. Rosenberg SA, Tepper J, Glatstein E, et al: The treatment of soft-tissue sarcomas of the extremities: Prospective randomized evaluations of (1) limb-sparing surgery plus radiation therapy compared with amputation and (2) the role of adjuvant chemotherapy. Ann Surg 196:305–315, 1982.
37. Alektiar KM, Brennan MF, Healey JH, et al: Impact of intensity-modulated radiation therapy on local control in primary soft-tissue sarcoma of the extremity. J Clin Oncol 26:3440–3444, 2008.
38. Pisters PW, Harrison LB, Leung DH, et al: Long-term results of a prospective randomized trial of adjuvant brachytherapy in soft tissue sarcoma. J Clin Oncol 14:859–868, 1996.
39. Yang JC, Chang AE, Baker AR, et al: Randomized prospective study of the benefit of adjuvant radiation therapy in the treatment of soft tissue sarcomas of the extremity. J Clin Oncol 16:197–203, 1998.
40. Alektiar KM, Leung D, Zelefsky MJ, et al: Adjuvant radiation for stage II-B soft tissue sarcoma of the extremity. J Clin Oncol 20:1643–1650, 2002.
41. Baldini EH, Goldberg J, Jenner C, et al: Long-term outcomes after function-sparing surgery without radiotherapy for soft tissue sarcoma of the extremities and trunk. J Clin Oncol 17:3252–3259, 1999.
42. Pisters PW, Pollock RE, Lewis VO, et al: Long-term results of prospective trial of surgery alone with selective use of radiation for patients with T1 extremity and trunk soft tissue sarcomas. Ann Surg 246:675–681, 2007.
43. Sarcoma Meta-analysis Collaboration: Adjuvant chemotherapy for localised resectable soft-tissue sarcoma of adults: Meta-analysis of individual data. Lancet 350:1647–1654, 1997.
44. Frustaci S, Gherlinzoni F, De Paoli A, et al: Adjuvant chemotherapy for adult soft tissue sarcomas of the extremities and girdles: Results of the Italian randomized cooperative trial. J Clin Oncol 19:1238–1247, 2001.
45. Grobmyer SR, Maki RG, Demetri GD, et al: Neo-adjuvant chemotherapy for primary high-grade extremity soft tissue sarcoma. Ann Oncol 15:1667–1672, 2004.
46. Eilber FC, Brennan MF, Eilber FR, et al: Chemotherapy is associated with improved survival in adult patients with primary extremity synovial sarcoma. Ann Surg 246:105–113, 2007.
47. Dematteo RP, Gold JS, Saran L, et al: Tumor mitotic rate, size, and location independently predict recurrence after resection of primary gastrointestinal stromal tumor (GIST). Cancer 112:608–615, 2008.
48. Singer S, Rubin BP, Lux ML, et al: Prognostic value of KIT mutation type, mitotic activity, and histologic subtype in gastrointestinal stromal tumors. J Clin Oncol 20:3898–3905, 2002.
49. Debiec Rychter M, Sciot R, Le Cesne A, et al: KIT mutations and dose selection for imatinib in patients with advanced gastrointestinal stromal tumours. Eur J Cancer 42:1093–1103, 2006.
50. Dematteo RP, Ballman KV, Antonescu CR, et al: Adjuvant imatinib mesylate after resection of localised, primary gastrointestinal stromal tumour: A randomised, double-blind, placebo-controlled trial. Lancet 373:1097–1104, 2009.
51. Blanke CD, Rankin C, Demetri GD, et al: Phase III randomized, intergroup trial assessing imatinib mesylate at two dose levels in patients with unresectable or metastatic gastrointestinal stromal tumors expressing the kit receptor tyrosine kinase: S0033. J Clin Oncol 26:626–632, 2008.
52. Antonescu CR, Besmer P, Guo T, et al: Acquired resistance to imatinib in gastrointestinal stromal tumor occurs through secondary gene mutation. Clin Cancer Res 11:4182–4190, 2005.
53. Demetri GD, van Oosterom AT, Garrett CR, et al: Efficacy and safety of sunitinib in patients with advanced gastrointestinal stromal tumour after failure of imatinib: A randomised controlled trial. Lancet 368:1329–1338, 2006.
54. Canter RJ, Qin LX, Downey RJ, et al: Perioperative chemotherapy in patients undergoing pulmonary resection for metastatic soft-tissue sarcoma of the extremity: A retrospective analysis. Cancer 110:2050–2060, 2007.
55. Eilber FC, Brennan MF, Riedel E, et al: Prognostic factors for survival in patients with locally recurrent extremity soft tissue sarcomas. Ann Surg Oncol 12:228–236, 2005.
56. Park JO, Qin LX, Prete FP, et al: Predicting outcome by growth rate of locally recurrent retroperitoneal liposarcoma: The one centimeter per month rule. Ann Surg 250:977–982, 2009.

CHAPTER 34

# BONE TUMORS

HERBERT S. SCHWARTZ AND GINGER E. HOLT

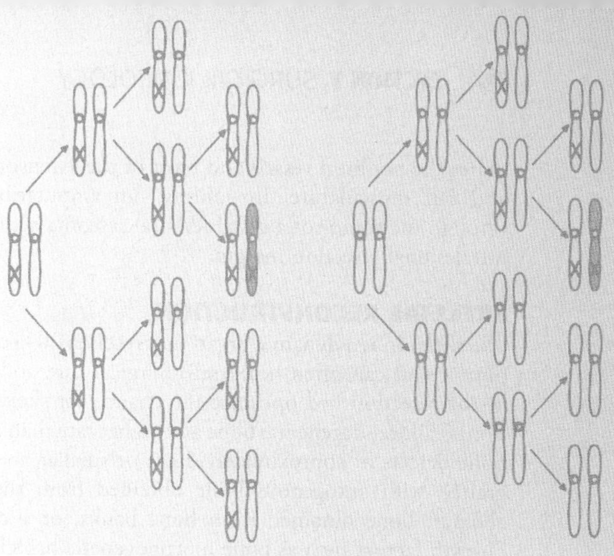



Orthopedic oncology is a complex surgical discipline that involves the care and management of individuals with primary and secondary neoplasms of the musculoskeletal system. The neoplasms may be benign or malignant. This chapter deals with bone tumors only.

Management of bone tumors is more difficult than treatment of neoplasms in other organ sites because of the need for skeletal stability. Adequate oncologic resection must be followed by skeletal reconstruction and restoration of function. With benign lesions, the process of reconstruction may be facilitated by bone's unique property of regenerating, even in adults. For malignant lesions, bone cannot be relied on to heal and aggressive unconventional reconstruction is required. Care must be taken, from biopsy to definitive treatment. An inappropriately placed skeletal biopsy may result in a fracture. Bone biopsy may be extensive and require cement along with internal fixation to prevent an iatrogenic fracture.

Biopsy is a complex cognitive skill in the skeleton. Fine-needle, core, or surgical biopsy tracts harbor malignant cells. Therefore, definitive surgical resection of cancer requires removing the biopsy tract, all iatrogenic contamination, and the bone tumor in an en bloc resection. This requires extensive exposure with wide flaps and mobilization of neurovascular structures. Inappropriately placed biopsy or needle puncture sites can complicate placement of the definitive surgical incision or require multiple incisions, thereby jeopardizing limb salvage. Key structures may be contaminated by the biopsy tract. It has been conclusively shown in several studies that surgeons inexperienced in musculoskeletal oncology principles have a three to four times increased rate of complications from a poorly placed biopsy site.[1-3] Unfortunately, this results in unnecessarily complex revision surgery and, in some cases, amputation instead of limb salvage.

Staging of skeletal sarcomas is straightforward and has remained relatively unchanged since its original description by Enneking and colleagues.[4] Roman numeral I refers to a low-grade skeletal sarcoma as interpreted by the pathologist. Roman numeral II is high grade. Roman numeral III signifies metastasis, whether regional or distant. The letter A refers to intracompartmental tumor localization, whereas the letter B refers to extracompartmental growth of the primary skeletal sarcoma. A bone tumor that begins in the femur and grows into the quadriceps musculature is extracompartmental because it has grown out of its original compartment into another. Pathologic fractures can be thought of as extracompartmental tumors. The Enneking system has five stages, IA, IB, IIA, IIB, and III. Stage IIB tumors are high risk. Stage III represents metastases of any type. The staging system of the American Joint Committee on Cancer has not been universally adopted for skeletal sarcomas.

Bone tumor management can best be summarized by three factors. The first is the adequacy of oncologic resection. The second is the type and extent of skeletal reconstruction. The third is the functional outcome anticipated by the specific type of skeletal reconstruction. All three factors must be weighed and discussed with the patient and caregivers to decide on the optimal management for a particular individual. Adequacy of the surgical oncologic margin is not always the prime consideration; surgical resection for palliation is often important.

## ONCOLOGIC RESECTION

There are four types of surgical resection, each of which is defined by their margin. The margin represents the surgical dissection plane relative to the pseudocapsule and the neoplasm itself. Intralesional resections are exemplified by curettage. The surgical dissection plane goes through the tumor itself and potentially leaves gross tumor behind. Marginal resections generate a dissection plane at the periphery of the tumor through its pseudocapsule (e.g., subperiosteal long bone dissection). Theoretically, microscopic tumor may be left behind. Wide surgical margins have a dissection plane through a cuff of normal tissue. The cuff of normal tissue may be 1 cm or 1 m distant to the tumor. Theoretically, only satellite malignant cells may be left behind. With radical resection margins, the entire compartment in which the tumor resides is resected. For example, a tumor that originates in the distal end of the femur would undergo radical resection if the entire femur were removed, from the hip joint to the knee joint. Local recurrence rates are inversely proportional to how radical the surgical procedure is. It is common for a limb salvage procedure to achieve a more radical margin than amputation. For example, limb salvage resection of a distal femoral sarcoma can achieve a wide surgical margin that spares the popliteal vessels and most of the extensor mechanism and calf musculature. In contrast, an amputation that goes through the tumor of a distal femoral sarcoma achieves only an intralesional resection margin.

## SKELETAL RECONSTRUCTION

The skeleton is a dynamic organ that receives 20% of the cardiac output and can often heal itself. Surgical care and preparation of the resection bed optimize the chance for skeletal regeneration. Children regenerate bone at a higher rate than adults. Small bone defects of approximately 5 cm or smaller are often bone-grafted with autogenous bone obtained from the iliac crest, allograft bone obtained from bone banks, or a combination. Growth factors such as bone morphogenetic protein 2 (BMP2) and BMP7 are being used to potentiate osteoinduction. Demineralized bone matrix is a commercially derived allograft product that retains the noncellular protein constituents of normal bone and may facilitate osteogenesis.

Larger skeletal defects require more complex reconstruction strategies. If a joint is close by, reconstruction often involves the use of an arthroplasty or arthrodesis. These two options frequently require the application of a metal or structural bone allograft spacer. Occasionally, a vascularized autograft such as a fibula may be used by itself or in conjunction with skeletal reconstruction. An intercalary segmental defect involves the shaft of a long bone and does not require joint reconstruction. In these cases, structural bone allografts and metal spacers are used along with internal fixation, such as intramedullary rods or plates and screws.

### Function

The long-term functional outcome after skeletal reconstruction is directly related to the durability of the implant. Metallic implants offer good immediate function, but suffer from metal fatigue after millions of repetitive loading cycles, and long-term failure eventually occurs. In contrast, bone autografts or allografts provide short-term partial stability (protected weight bearing) but have the potential long-term advantage of permanent osteogenic ingrowth along with revascularization, leading to intact viable bone. The weight-bearing needs of the lower extremities are different from those of the high-demand, non–weight-bearing functions of the upper extremities. The axial skeleton has a mixture of high-demand and load-bearing requirements. Skeletal reconstruction in children requires calculation for limb growth. The more complicated the reconstruction, the higher the infection rate. Infections of metallic endoprostheses or large structural allografts can often be devastating and result in amputation. Terminal cancer patients who require skeletal reconstruction have different functional needs, immediate functional use with inconsequential long-term demands.

## GENETICS

Alterations in DNA by inheritance, carcinogen exposure, sporadic replication or housekeeping error, mutation, chromosomal rearrangement, amplification, deletion, or change in expression can be oncogenic. Neoplastic cells that acquire such a genetic change may begin a multistep process that confers a potential growth advantage. Further genetic change leads to more mutations and the creation of clones of cells that acquire malignant characteristics.

Benign and malignant skeletal neoplasms have a host of DNA alterations catalogued by the absence or presence of suppressor genes, oncogenes, translocations, and chromosome gains or losses. Table 34-1 lists these genetic alterations for some selected bone tumors[5]; this table is meant to be a summary rather than an exhaustive list.

In contrast, skeletal metastases (e.g., carcinomas) manipulate the normal bone microenvironment to create osteolytic bone destruction while promoting the growth and spread of cancer cells.[6,7] Cell adhesion molecules are used for both cell to

**Table 34-1 Genetic Alterations for Some Bone Tumors**

| | Neoplasia | | | DNA Alterations | | |
|---|---|---|---|---|---|---|
| **SKELETAL TUMOR** | **SUPPRESSOR GENE** | **ONCOGENE** | **TRANSLOCATIONS** | **CHROMOSOME LOSS** | **CHROMOSOME GAIN** | **PROTEIN CHANGE** |
| Osteosarcoma | *RB, p53, INK4A, INK2A* | *CDK4, FOS, cMYC, MDM2, MET* | | 6q, 13q, 15q, 17p, 18q | 1q, 5p, 6p, 7q, 8q, 12q, 17p, 19q, 7p, 12q, 21q | |
| Ewing's sarcoma | *KCMF1* | CD99 | t(11;22)(q24;q12) *EWS-FLI1* t(21;22)(q22;q12) *EWS-ERG* | | | |
| Chondrosarcoma | | | | 1p, 5q, 6p, 9p, 14q, 22q | 7p, 12q, 21q | |
| Osteochondroma | *EXT1, EXT2* | | | | | |
| Endochondroma | | | | | 12q | IHH-PTHrP (Indian hedgehog–parathyroid hormone-related protein) |
| Aneurysmal bone cyst | | | t(16;17)(q22;p13) *CHD11-USP6* | | | |
| Fibrous dysplasia | | *GNAS1* | | 20q | | GS |
| Giant cell tumor | | *TPX2* | Telomeric fusions | | 20q | RANKL |

cell and cell to matrix binding. Deregulation of matrix metalloproteinases disrupts the delicate balance of matrix homeostasis by increasing proteolytic activity. Degradation of the extracellular matrix results in cancer cell invasion. Angiogenesis stimulators such as vascular endothelial growth factor, fibroblast growth factor, and transforming growth factor-β are triggered by cancer cells to promote their own growth. Parathyroid hormone–related protein is released by certain tumor cells acting on the same receptors for parathyroid hormones to promote osteoclast-mediated bone resorption. Osteoclastogenesis is also promoted by interleukin-6, interleukin-8, and RANKL (receptor activator of nuclear factor κB ligand). There is a complex interaction among many cell receptors, cytokines, growth factors, and proteases in the metastatic bone microenvironment.

## BENIGN BONE TUMORS

### Incidence

The incidence of benign bone tumors far exceeds that of skeletal sarcomas. In our clinical experience, there are at least five benign bone tumors for every primary malignant bone neoplasm. Unni and Inwards[8] have found that approximately 54% of benign bone tumors are chondrogenic. Osteochondroma and enchondroma are the most common benign tumors. Both can be polyostotic. Osteochondromas are surface neoplasms of bone, whereas enchondromas are located intraosseously. The true prevalence of these tumors is unknown because many go undetected and unreported.

### Overview

The significance of benign bone tumors is that they occur more frequently in the pediatric population than in adults. Fractures are often the initial mode of expression. A pathologic fracture may occur during running or other activities, with pain being the initial symptom. Frequently, benign bone tumors are detected in the pediatric or adult population as an incidental radiographic discovery. A patient with rotator cuff tendinitis may complain of shoulder pain and a plain radiograph identifies an incidental abnormality in the proximal humeral metaphysis, which by itself is asymptomatic. Benign bone tumors grow with the child and generally stop growing when the child reaches skeletal maturity. In children and adults, surgical indications include deformity (angular or limb length inequality), pain, pathologic fracture, and malignant transformation.

### Surgical Oncology

Most benign bone tumors can be resected safely with an intralesional resection margin. These procedures typically consist of intralesional curettage. The goal is a local recurrence rate between 10% and 20%. In the skeletally immature patient, physeal injury must be avoided.

Reconstruction of benign bone tumors after curettage is often accomplished with a combination of bone grafting and stabilization of impending or completed fractures. Bone grafting can be performed with autogenous bone or allograft. Many allograft preparations are commercially available, including demineralized bone matrix from an American Association of Tissue Banks–approved bone bank.[9] Adequate curettage demands a large bone portal to access the intraosseous cavity, which, however, severely compromises the biomechanical integrity of the bone and requires operative stabilization. Stabilization can be done extracorporeally, such as with a cast or splint. Internal bone stabilization can be accomplished with a combination of rods, plates, pins, or screws. The goal is to achieve osteogenesis, preserve skeletal growth, and gain strength within weeks.

### Function

The functional outcome after intralesional resection, fixation, and bone grafting, especially in a child, is excellent. Limb length inequalities, especially overgrowth, may occur when the procedure is performed in a young child. The younger the child, the more conservative are the internal fixation techniques. Casting is preferred because joint stiffness is seldom a problem in this patient population.

### Examples

#### Enchondroma

Enchondroma (Fig. 34-1) is a benign proliferation of hyaline cartilage typically found in long bones, but it may also occur in the axial skeleton. Cartilage anlage or islands retain chondroid features and continue to grow until skeletal maturity, when they begin to undergo calcification. Their long-term physiologic activity is why they remain scintigraphically active decades later on a bone scan. An enchondroma typically begins in the metaphysis and extends into the diaphysis. It seldom occurs in the epiphysis of long bones. Polyostotic syndromes may occur, often with unilateral predominance. Ollier's disease is the eponym associated with multiple skeletal enchondromas. Maffucci's syndrome is Ollier's disease associated with multiple subcutaneous hemangiomas. In the pediatric population, management involves maintaining a strong, straight, and

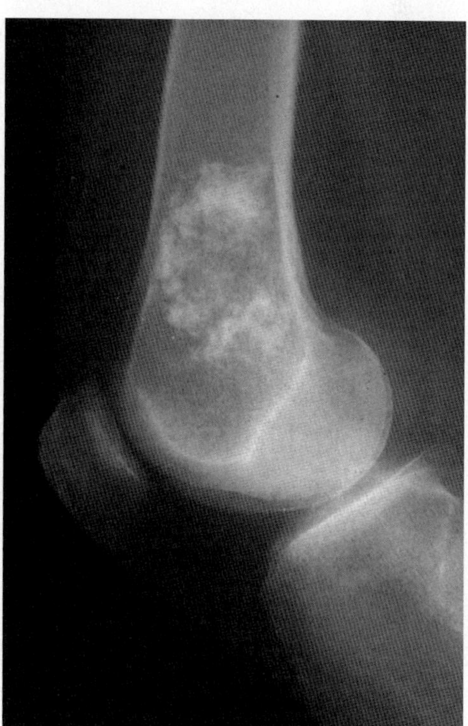

**FIGURE 34-1** Plain radiograph of an enchondroma of the distal end of the femur, lateral projection. Note the heavy calcification of the benign chondroid matrix.

symmetrical bone of appropriate length. After skeletal maturity, malignant transformation is rare. However, the greater the tumor burden, the greater the late malignant transformation rate. Therefore, patients with Ollier's disease often have a higher incidence of chondrosarcoma formation than those with solitary disease. The more axially located tumors of the pelvis, spine, and scapula have the worst prognosis. Interestingly, individuals with Maffucci's syndrome have the same elevated incidence of chondrosarcoma formation; however, this unique patient population frequently succumbs to the development of occult carcinomas.[10]

Treatment of enchondromas is conservative and serial radiographic evaluation remains the mainstay of treatment. When necessary, albeit rare, intralesional curettage and bone grafting result in excellent outcomes. Enchondromas are particularly common in the small bones of the hands and feet. Histopathologic interpretation of benign cartilage tumors is difficult because it is extremely dependent on the clinical findings and plain radiographic appearance of the tumor. Rarely, cytogenetic abnormalities are identified in enchondromas. It appears that abnormalities in 12q13-15 appear to be common in benign and malignant cartilaginous neoplasms.[5]

### Fibrous Dysplasia

Fibrous dysplasia (Fig. 34-2) is not a true neoplasm but represents dysplasia in the fibro-osseous proliferation of bone. It may be monostotic or polyostotic. The cause appears to be a postfertilization mutation in the gene encoding the α-activating subunit of the G (guanine nucleotide binding) protein that participates in guanosine triphosphatase activity. The mutation occurs on chromosome 20 at location 20q13.2. It appears to be a missense point mutation at the arginine 201 amino acid that leads to constitutive activation of the formation of cyclic adenosine monophosphate.[11,12] Fibrous dysplasia may be monostotic, polyostotic, or associated with an endocrinopathy syndrome known as McCune-Albright syndrome. This disorder occurs more often in females and is characterized by the triad of polyostotic fibrous dysplasia predominating on one side, precocious puberty (may be manifested as vaginal bleeding within the first few months of life), and large macules, often overlying the involved bone. Treatment is similar to that for other benign bone tumors but it is important to realize that complete extirpation of the tumor is unnecessary. The bone is biomechanically weak, and therefore treatment is aimed at structural stabilization. Rarely, late sarcomatous transformation occurs. The incidence of fibrous dysplasia parallels that of giant cell tumor.

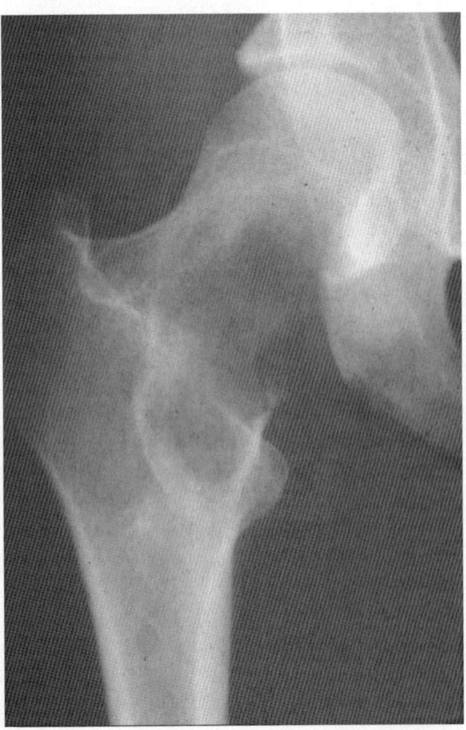

**FIGURE 34-2** Fibrous dysplasia shown on a plain anteroposterior (AP) radiograph of the right hip. Note the partially ossified matrix of the tumor with loss of normal bone trabeculae.

### Giant Cell Tumor

Giant cell tumor (Fig. 34-3) represents approximately 20% of benign bone tumors. It is the most aggressive benign tumor and threatens the true definition of a benign cancer because benign pulmonary metastases develop in approximately 1% to 2% of giant cell tumors.[13] In these cases, the metastatic focus in the lung does not meet the histopathologic criteria for malignancy and is identical in appearance to the benign bone tumor in the skeleton. Survival rates are approximately 80% with aggressive treatment. Local recurrence rates after treatment of giant cell tumor in a bone can be as high as 40% but can be halved through aggressive surgical treatment, often with the use of local adjuvants,[14] including high-speed turbine burring, polymethylmethacrylate bone cement, liquid nitrogen, phenol, and argon beam laser. This tumor typically develops in the epiphysis of long bones, although it may occur in the flat bones of the pelvis, often between the ages of 20 and 40 years, and is manifested as an intra-articular displaced pathologic fracture. Management involves radiographic pulmonary examination, aggressive local treatment with a large surgical approach and exposure of the bone cavity, and aggressive local intralesional resection, with or without adjuvant therapy. Reconstruction demands stability and bone grafting alone is frequently inadequate. Cement provides

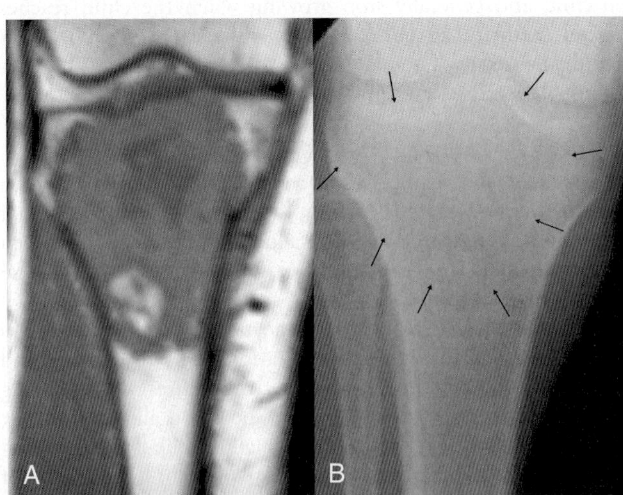


**FIGURE 34-3** Giant cell tumor of bone involving the proximal tibia, seen on magnetic resonance imaging (MRI) scan **(A)** and indicated by *arrows* on a plain radiograph **(B)**.

immediate stability but is associated with the potential for late arthritic development in the adjacent joint.

The tumor often extends to subchondral bone under the articular cartilage. The spectrum of biologic behavior of this capricious tumor is not well understood. The cytogenetics of giant cell tumor is fascinating but does not belie its true biologic potential. The presence of telomere to telomere chromosomal translocations (telomeric associations) in giant cell tumor is a rarely reported cytogenetic phenomenon in human neoplasia.[15] Giant cell tumor also has the unique ability to grow in a variety of microenvironments and therefore represents a challenge to the surgeon, inasmuch as iatrogenic implantation and metastases are distinctly common occurrences.

Patients require long-term follow-up because recurrences may develop several years postoperatively. Giant cell tumors in the spine, sacrum, and pelvis present greater surgical challenges. Preoperative embolization is often required because intraoperative tumor hemorrhage is significant. Radiation treatment may have a role in primary giant cell tumors of the axial skeleton or in recurrent refractory giant cell tumors in a long bone. There is strong evidence, however, that irradiation of giant cell tumors increases the chance for malignant transformation to a frank giant cell sarcoma decades later.[16] New systemic treatment options include a fully human monoclonal antibody to RANKL which has shown significant positive response rates when treating unresectable disease.[17]

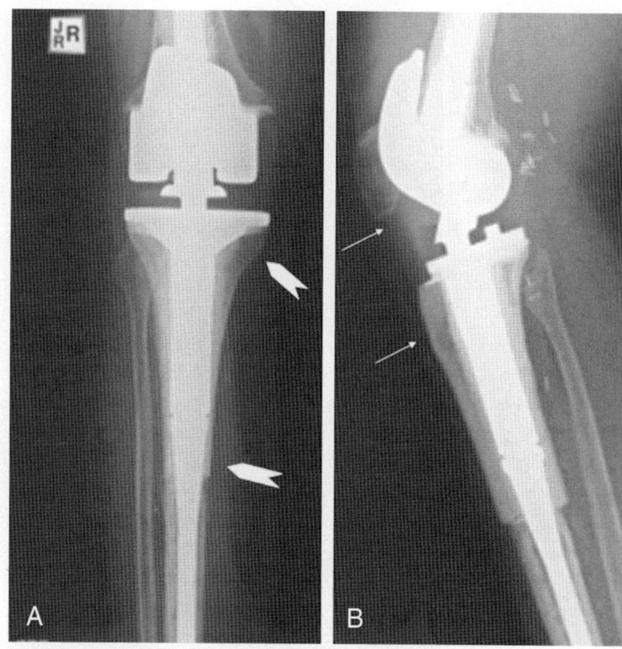

**FIGURE 34-4** Limb salvage resection and reconstruction with allograft tibia and prosthetic knee arthroplasty. **A,** Anterior-posterior projection. **B,** Lateral projection. The arrows point to the sutured patellar tendons of the host and allograft.

## SKELETAL SARCOMAS

### Incidence

Approximately 2300 skeletal sarcomas are diagnosed each year in the United States.[18] This incidence translates into approximately one new case/100,000 population/year. Osteosarcoma is the most common primary malignant neoplasm of bone; it represents one third of cases and often occurs in teenagers. Chondrosarcoma accounts for 25% of skeletal sarcomas, followed by Ewing's sarcoma at 16%. The incidence of skeletal sarcomas is approximately equal in the pediatric and adult populations.

### Overview

The need for complex skeletal reconstruction, often using large metallic endoprosthetic implants, structural allografts, or both, ushered in the era of neoadjuvant chemotherapy and limb salvage (Fig. 34-4). Many skeletal sarcomas are sensitive to chemotherapy. In the 1970s, intensive chemotherapy was administered to many teenagers with nonmetastatic osteosarcoma of the extremities after biopsy.[19] While a custom endoprosthesis was being fabricated, treatment continued with systemic cytotoxic chemotherapy. After several months, the tumor was surgically removed and the implant inserted to preserve the limb. The resected bone tumor was then examined histopathologically for the necrotic effect of preoperative or neoadjuvant chemotherapy.

### Surgical Oncology

Wide surgical margins are preferred for the treatment of skeletal sarcomas. For many skeletal sarcomas, resection follows neoadjuvant chemotherapy. Chemotherapy facilitates limb salvage by allowing easier dissection and mobilization of critical neurovascular structures. The surgical goal is a local recurrence rate of less than 7%. Early studies by Simon,[20] Link,[21] and their associates documented equivalent local recurrence and survival rates with limb salvage and amputation for distal femoral osteosarcoma. Cure rates are approximately 67% for extremity sarcomas, whereas axial tumors in the pelvis or spine have a worse prognosis (33%) for a similar tissue type.[22,23]

Reconstruction of large skeletal defects requires the use of metallic endoprostheses, structural allografts, or combinations called allograft-prosthesis composites. Reconstruction strategies are more complicated in the pediatric population because future growth must be predicted and accounted for.

### Function

It has been demonstrated that limb salvage is more cost-effective over a period of decades than immediate amputation in the teenage population.[24] Implant survival is complicated in the short term by infection (allografts) and in the long term by aseptic loosening (metal).[25] Ten-year implant survival rates for metallic prostheses range from 50% to 80% in the proximal tibia, distal femur, and proximal femur.[26] Wound healing, especially while administering chemotherapy, is enhanced with healthy local flaps. This is especially true around the knee, where gastrocnemius flaps are necessary to cover the prosthesis and restore function to the extensor mechanism.

### Examples

#### Osteosarcoma (Osteogenic Sarcoma)

Osteosarcoma, or osteogenic sarcoma (Fig. 34-5), is defined as a malignant tumor that produces neoplastic osteoid. Neoplastic cartilage or fibrous tissue may be present. There are many types of osteosarcoma; they vary by location (intraosseous, surface, or extraskeletal), grade, or cause. Spontaneous osteosarcomas are most common, but some osteosarcomas occur in the genetic syndromes of Li-Fraumeni, hereditary retinoblastoma, and in

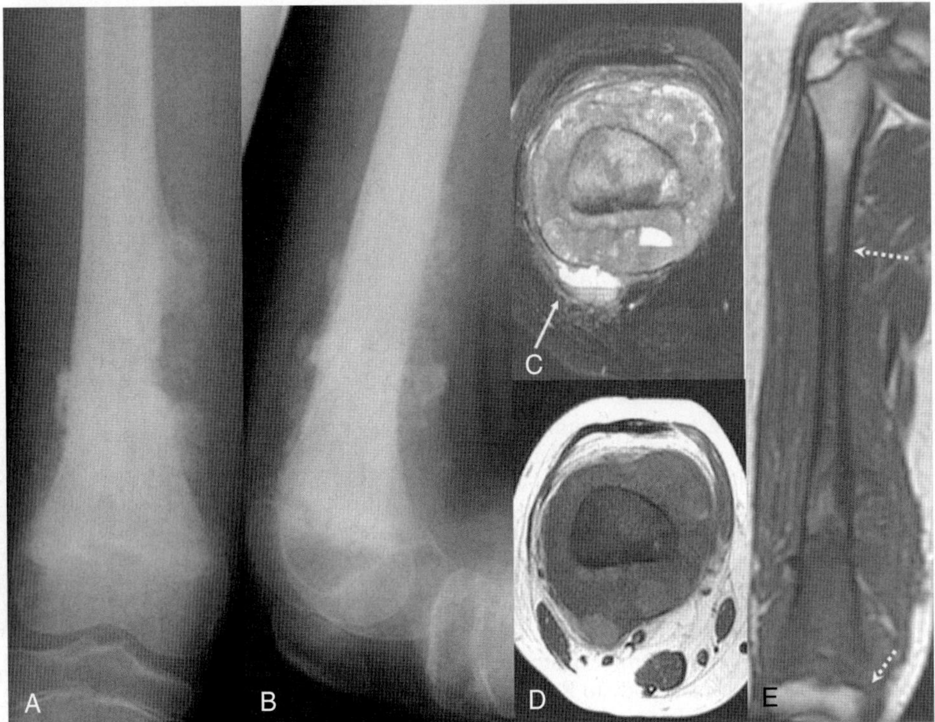


FIGURE 34-5 Osteosarcoma. AP **(A)** and lateral **(B)** radiographs show malignant intramedullary and extramedullary bone formation. T2-weighted **(C)** and T1-weighted **(D)** MRI scans demonstrate a large circumferential soft tissue mass, with extension into the posterior compartment (**C,** *arrow*). **E,** Coronal MRI scan shows tumor extending from the diaphysial femur to the distal physis *(arrow).*

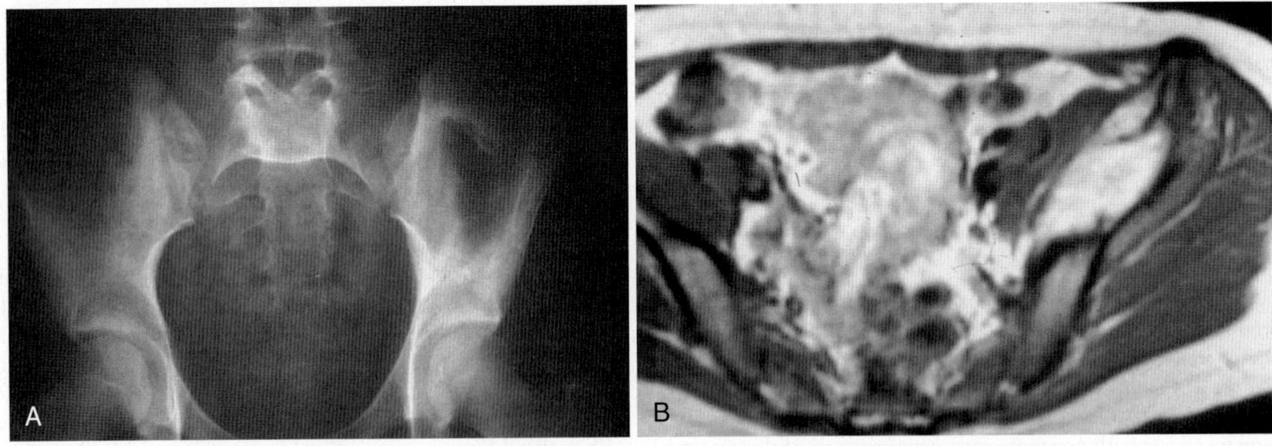


FIGURE 34-6 Ewing's sarcoma. **A,** AP plain radiograph of the pelvis. Note the destructive and permeative changes in the left pelvis (ilium). **B,** Axial T2-weighted MRI scan demonstrating the white tumor infiltrating the left ilium and breaking out into the musculature as an extraosseous soft tissue mass.

postradiation scenarios.[27-29] There is a bimodal age of tumor occurrence. Conventional osteosarcomas occur in the first 2 decades of life, whereas post-treatment or secondary (malignant transformation) osteosarcomas occur much later. Postradiation skeletal sarcomas of the chest wall have become more common with the gaining popularity of lumpectomy and radiation treatment for mammary carcinoma.[30]

Survival is best predicted by the degree of chemotherapy-induced necrosis.[31] Nonmetastatic extremity osteosarcoma with more than 90% chemotherapy-induced necrosis has a survival rate of 80% at 5 years; pelvic osteosarcoma with less than 90% chemotherapy-induced necrosis has a survival rate of approximately 30%.[22,23]

## Ewing's Sarcoma

Ewing's sarcoma (Fig. 34-6) and primitive neuroectodermal tumors are small, blue cell (microscopic appearance) malignancies of bone that cytogenetically represent the same entity. They share a common translocation, t(11;22)(q24;q12), in 85% of cases. Molecular cloning of the translocation reveals fusion between the 5′ end of the *EWS* gene from the 22q12 chromosome and the 3′ end of the 11q24 *FLI1* gene.[32-34] This tumor is exquisitely sensitive to chemotherapy and radiation treatment. Neither modality alone or in combination is sufficient to maximize the cure rate, however. Surgical extirpation in conjunction with chemotherapy is the preferred treatment. Reconstruction options follow those for other skeletal sarcomas.

### Chondrosarcoma

Chondrosarcoma (Fig. 34-7) is a malignant skeletal neoplasm that produces hyaline cartilage. Several pathologic subtypes exist in which the neoplastic cells produce unusual matrices. Histopathology alone does not predict biologic behavior. Rather, a combination of histopathology, age, location, and radiographic appearance yields the best predictor of tumor aggressiveness. A low-grade cartilage tumor of the phalanx may have the same microscopic appearance as a pelvic chondrosarcoma. It would be exceedingly rare to die of a phalanx cartilage tumor; however, local control is notoriously difficult to achieve in pelvic chondrosarcomas, and long-term cure rates require massive resection. Secondary chondrosarcomas occur after malignant transformation of a benign cartilage tumor, such as enchondroma or osteochondroma.[35] There is increasing molecular evidence that growth plate chondrocyte signaling pathways are recapitulated in cartilage neoplasia (Indian hedgehog–parathyroid hormone–related protein axis).

## SKELETAL METASTASES

### Incidence

Skeletal metastases are approximately 500 times more common than skeletal sarcomas.[18] Approximately 1.2 million new cases of carcinoma are diagnosed each year in the United States. Osteophytes include prostate, thyroid, breast, lung, and kidney cancer.

### Overview

Adults are more commonly afflicted with skeletal metastases than children. The prevalence of individuals with skeletal metastases continues to rise as cancer therapies improve with time. Pathologic fractures and impending pathologic fractures represent common problems for the orthopedic oncologist. The workup for a metastatic skeletal carcinoma of unknown primary origin consists only of a computed tomography CT scan of the chest, abdomen, and pelvis, a bone scan, serum protein electrophoresis, and assay for prostate-specific antigen.[36] Physical examination of the breast and prostate is mandatory. Bisphosphonate therapy diminishes osteoclast resorption of bone and preserves the biomechanical integrity of the skeleton.

### Surgical Oncology

Intralesional resection after tissue confirmation of the diagnosis minimizes the chance of local recurrence. Treatment goals include whole-bone prophylaxis with intramedullary locked nails, plates, and cement or a combination of these. Postoperative radiation therapy must include delivery to the entire bone from joint to joint. A surgical goal of a local recurrence rate less than 15% is preferred. Isolated metastases, such as from renal cell carcinoma or melanoma, can be treated aggressively if they are indeed isolated and occur after a long hiatus (several years) after the primary. Cures, in such cases, are not rare.

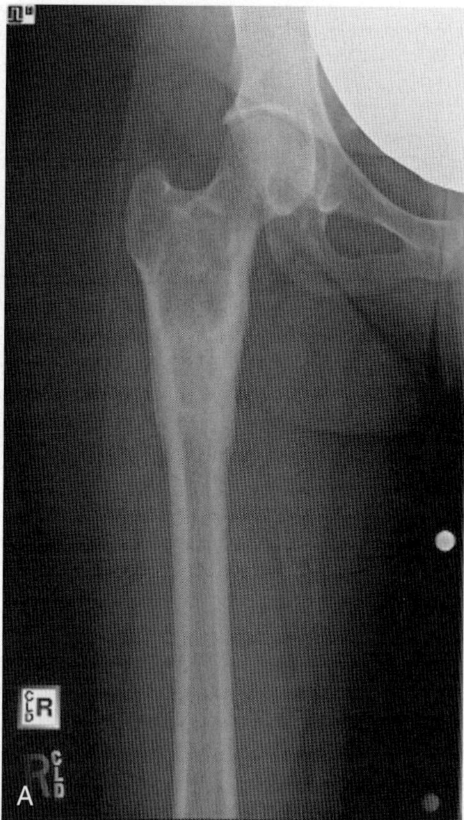


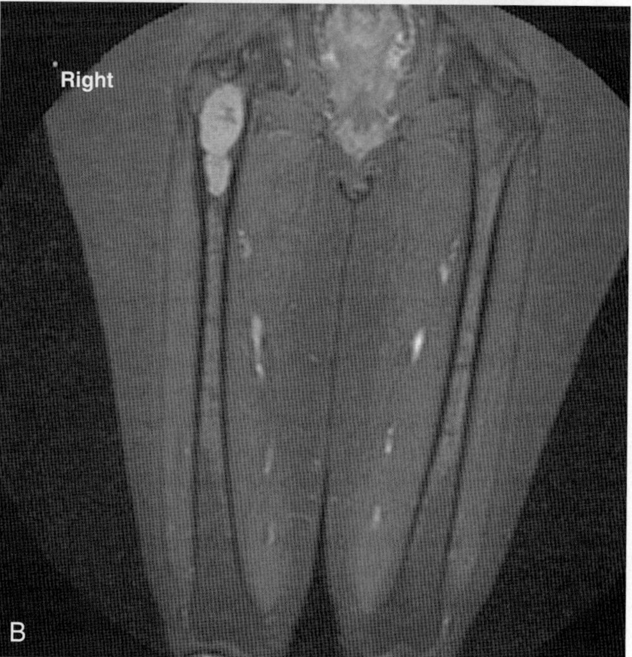


**FIGURE 34-7** Chondrosarcoma. **A,** AP plain radiograph of the right proximal femur showing expansion of the bone from the poorly mineralized malignant chondroid matrix. **B,** Coronal MRI scan demonstrating the extent of the tumor into the intramedullary space.

Reconstructive goals consist of choosing an implant durable enough to outlive the patient. The bone cannot be expected to heal after tumor resection and chemoradiation therapy. Therefore, cement and metal must be used to preserve biomechanical integrity, especially in weight-bearing joints (Fig. 34-8) and the spine.

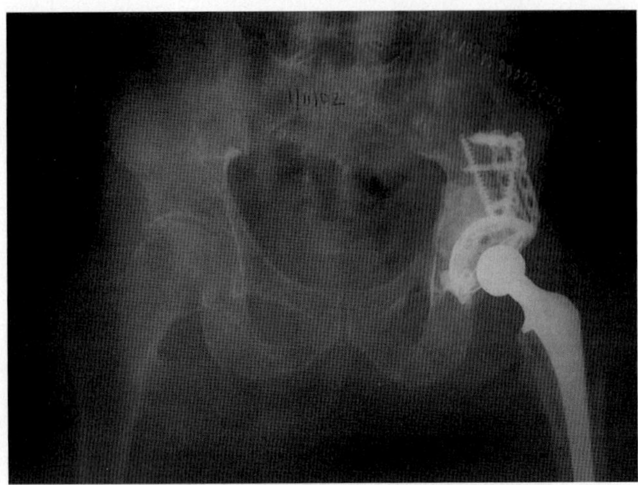

**FIGURE 34-8** Carcinoma metastatic to the left acetabulum. After resection, reconstruction was accomplished with cement, screws, and total hip arthroplasty.

A variety of surgical techniques are used to reconstruct a skeleton that is symptomatic and has metastatic carcinoma. Examples requiring different techniques include a weight-bearing long bone such as the femur, a non–weight-bearing long bone such as the humerus, and a flat bone such as the pelvis. Aggressive surgical management of premyelopathic isolated spinal metastases in conjunction with radiotherapy is preferred over radiation therapy alone.[37]

### Function

Palliative relief of pain and maximization of function are the goals of surgery. The goal is to keep the patient pain-free, mobile, and independent. Bisphosphonates significantly diminish osteoclast function and therefore bone resorption. They have become an important tool in preventing pathologic fractures in patients with metastatic disease while preserving function.

## FUTURE CONSIDERATIONS

Advances in the treatment of skeletal malignancies will require better understanding of the molecular causes of the disease. Implants will improve, but material and biomechanical principles are still at a plateau in development. In contrast, knowledge of the genetic causes of sarcomas and the microenvironment surrounding them has been growing rapidly. Identifying skeletal sarcoma biomarkers of high-risk biologic behavior may at some point stratify patients by metastatic potential early in the cancer treatment course. Examining the microenvironment of bone may identify molecular triggers of matrix lysis and endothelial invasion. Targeted therapies that downgrade the growth and invasive potential of cancers offer the hope of prolonged survival through new treatment paradigms.

## SELECTED REFERENCES

Aurias A, Rimbaut C, Buffe D, et al: Chromosomal translocations in Ewing's sarcoma. N Engl J Med 309:496–497, 1983.

This study included cytogenetic investigations of Ewing's sarcoma, identifying the 11;22 chromosomal translocation.

Enneking WF, Spanier SS, Goodman MA: A system for the staging of musculoskeletal sarcoma. Clin Orthop Relat Res 153:106–120, 1980.

This surgical staging system for musculoskeletal sarcomas stratifies bone and soft tissue tumors by the grade of biologic aggressiveness, anatomic setting, and presence of metastasis. It consists of three stages: I, low grade; II, high grade; and III, presence of metastases. These stages are subdivided by whether the lesion is anatomically confined within a compartment, or beyond a compartment in ill-defined fascial planes and spaces. It has proven to be the most correlative system for predicting sarcoma outcomes.

Link MP, Goorin AM, Miser AW, et al: The effect of adjuvant chemotherapy on relapse-free survival in patients with osteosarcoma of the extremity. N Engl J Med 314:1600–1606, 1986.

This study concluded that the natural history of osteosarcoma of the extremity has remained stable over 20 years and that adjuvant chemotherapy increases the chances of relapse-free survival of patients with high-grade osteosarcoma.

Mankin HJ, Mankin CJ, Simon MA: The methods of biopsy revisited. J Bone Joint Surg Am 78:656–663, 1996.

This investigation showed significant rates in error of diagnosis and technique, which resulted in complications and also adversely, affected the care of patients with musculoskeletal tumors. These data differed when the biopsy was carried out in a treatment center rather than in a referring institution. On the basis of these observations, whenever possible, it was concluded that the procedure should be done in a treatment center rather than in a referring institution.

Rosen G, Marcove RC, Caparros B, et al: Primary osteogenic sarcoma: The rationale for preoperative chemotherapy and delayed surgery. Cancer 42:2163–2177, 1979.

This was the first reported use of neoadjuvant chemotherapy in the treatment of malignant tumors. Patients with primary osteogenic sarcomas (31 patients) were treated with preoperative chemotherapy followed by tumor resection. Histologic examination of primary tumor removed at surgery revealed varying degrees of tumor destruction, from very little effect to no evidence of viable tumor, attributable to the effect of chemotherapy.

Rougraff BT, Kneisl JS, Simon MA: Skeletal metastasis of unknown origin: A prospective study of a diagnosis strategy. J Bone Joint Surg Am 75:1276–1281, 1993.

In 85% of patients, the primary site of metastatic origin was identified by CT scans of the chest, abdomen, and pelvis. This diagnostic strategy was simple and highly successful for the identification of the site of an occult malignant tumor before biopsy in patients who had skeletal metastases of unknown origin. In a patient presenting with a skeletal lesion suspicious for a metastatic lesion with an unknown primary, CT is the recommended diagnostic modality to identify the primary lesion.

Simon MA, Aschliman MA, Thomas N, et al: Limb-salvage treatment versus amputation for osteosarcoma of the distal end of the femur. J Bone Joint Surg Am 68:1331–1337, 1986.

This study compared three groups of patients who had had a limb-sparing procedure, above-knee amputation, or disarticulation of the hip for osteosarcoma of the distal femur. The use of a limb salvage procedure for osteosarcoma of the distal end of the femur did not shorten the disease-free interval or compromise long-term survival.

## REFERENCES


1. Mankin HJ, Mankin CJ, Simon MA: The methods of biopsy revisited. J Bone Joint Surg Am 78:656–663, 1996.
2. Randall RL, Bruckner JD, Papenhausen MD, et al: Errors in diagnosis and margin determination of soft tissue sarcoma initially treated at non-tertiary centers. Orthopedics 27:209–212, 2004.
3. Trovik CK: Scandinavian Sarcoma Group Project. Acta Orthop Scand Suppl 300:1–31, 2001.
4. Enneking WF, Spanier SS, Goodman MA: A system for the staging of musculoskeletal sarcoma. Clin Orthop Relat Res 153:106–120, 1980.
5. Sandberg AA, Bridge JA: Updates on the cytogenetics and molecular genetics of bone and soft tissue tumors: Osteosarcomas and related tumors. Cancer Genet Cytogenet 145:1–30, 2003.
6. Roodman GD: Mechanisms of bone metastasis. N Engl J Med 350:1655–1664, 2004.
7. Kang Y, Siegel PM, Shu W, et al: A multigenic program mediating breast cancer metastasis to bone. Cancer Cell 3:537–549, 2003.
8. Unni KK, Inwards CY: Dahlin's bone tumors: General aspects and data on 11,087 cases, ed 6, Philadelphia, 2009, Lippincott Williams & Wilkins.
9. Joyce MJ: Safety and FDA regulations for musculoskeletal allografts. Clin Orthop Relat Res 435:22–30, 2005.
10. Altay M, Bayrakci K, Yildiz Y, et al: Secondary chondrosarcoma in cartilage bone tumors: Report of 32 patients. J Orthop Sci 12:415–423, 2007.
11. Ding C, Deng Z, Levine MA: A highly sensitive PCR method detects activating mutations of the GNAS1 gene in peripheral blood cells of patients with McCune-Albright syndrome or isolated fibrous dysplasia. J Bone Miner Res 16(Suppl 1):S417–S422, 2001.
12. Weinstein LS, Shenker A, Gejman PV, et al: Activating mutations of the stimulating G protein in the McCune-Albright syndrome. N Engl J Med 325:1688–1695, 1991.
13. Dominkus M, Ruggieri P, Bertoni F, et al: Histologically verified lung metastases in benign giant cell tumours—14 cases from a single institution. Int Orthop 30:499–504, 2006.
14. Turcotte RE, Wunder JS, Isler MH, et al: Giant cell tumor of long bone: A Canadian Sarcoma Group study. Clin Orthop Relat Res 397:248–258, 2002.
15. Schwartz HS, Jenkins RB, Dahl RJ, et al: Cytogenetic analyses on giant cell tumor of bone. Clin Orthop Relat Res 240:250–260, 1989.
16. Rock MG, Sim FH, Unni KK: Secondary malignant giant cell tumor of bone. J Bone Joint Surg Am 68:1073–1079, 1986.
17. Thomas DM, Skubitz KM: Giant cell tumour of bone. Curr Opin Oncol 21:338–344, 2009.
18. Jemal A, Siegel R, Ward E, et al: Cancer statistics, 2009. CA Cancer J Clin 59:225–249, 2009.
19. Rosen G, Marcove RC, Caparros B, et al: Primary osteogenic sarcoma: The rationale for preoperative chemotherapy and delayed surgery. Cancer 42:2163–2177, 1979.
20. Simon MA, Aschliman MA, Thomas N, et al: Limb salvage treatment versus amputation for osteosarcoma of the distal end of the femur. J Bone Joint Surg Am 68:1331–1337, 1986.
21. Link MP, Goorin AM, Miser AW, et al: The effect of adjuvant chemotherapy on relapse-free survival in patients with osteosarcoma of the extremity. N Engl J Med 314:1600–1606, 1986.
22. Pakos EE, Nearchou AD, Grimer RJ, et al: Prognostic factors and outcomes for osteosarcoma: An international collaboration. Eur J Cancer 45:2367–2375, 2009.
23. Goorin AM, Schwartzentruber DJ, Devidas M, et al: Presurgical chemotherapy combined with immediate surgery and adjuvant chemotherapy for nonmetastatic osteosarcoma: Pediatric Oncology Group POG 8651. J Clin Oncol 21:1574–1580, 2003.
24. Grimer RJ, Carter SR, Pynsent PB: The cost-effectiveness of limb salvage for bone tumors. J Bone Joint Surg Br 79:558–561, 1997.
25. Mankin HJ, Hornicek FJ, Raskin KA: Infection in massive bone allografts. Clin Orthop Relat Res 432:210–216, 2005.
26. Jeys LM, Kulkarni A, Grimer RJ, et al: Endoprosthetic reconstruction for the treatment of musculoskeletal tumors of the appendicular skeleton and pelvis. J Bone Joint Surg Am 90:1265–1271, 2008.
27. Li FP, Fraumeni JF, Mulvihill JJ, et al: A cancer family syndrome in 24 kindreds. Cancer Res 48:5358–5362, 1988.
28. Draper GJ, Sanders BM, Kingston JE: Second primary neoplasms in patients with retinoblastoma. Br J Cancer 53:661–671, 1986.
29. Yap J, Chuba PJ, Thomas R, et al: Sarcoma as a second malignancy after treatment for breast cancer. Int J Radiat Oncol Biol Phys 52:1231–1237, 2002.
30. Holt, GE, Thomson AB, Griffin AM, et al: Multifocality and post-radiation sarcomas. Clin Orthop Relat Res 450:67–75, 2006.
31. Picci P, Bacci G, Campanacci M, et al: Histologic evaluation of necrosis in osteosarcoma induced by chemotherapy. Regional mapping of viable and nonviable tumor. Cancer 56:1515–1521, 1985.
32. Aurias A, Rimbaut C, Buffe D, et al: Chromosomal translocations in Ewing's sarcoma. N Engl J Med 309:496–497, 1983.
33. deAlava E, Gerald WL: Molecular biology of the Ewing's sarcoma/primitive neuroectodermal tumor family. J Clin Oncol 18:204–213, 2000.
34. Hu-Lieskovan S, Zhang J, Wu L, et al: EWS-FLI1 fusion protein up-regulates critical genes in neural crest development and is responsible for the observed phenotype of Ewing's family of tumors. Cancer Res 65:4633–4644, 2005.
35. Bovee JVMG, Cleton-Jansen A, Taminiau AHM, et al: Emerging pathways in the development of chondrosarcoma of bone and implications for targeted treatment. Lancet 6:599–607, 2005.
36. Rougraff BT, Kneisl JS, Simon MA: Skeletal metastasis of unknown origin: A prospective study of a diagnosis strategy. J Bone Joint Surg Am 75:1276–1281, 1993.
37. Patchell RA, Tibbs PA, Regine WF, et al: Direct decompressive surgical resection in the treatment of spinal cord compression caused by metastatic cancer: A randomized trial. Lancet 366: 643–648, 2005.

# SECTION VI

# HEAD AND NECK

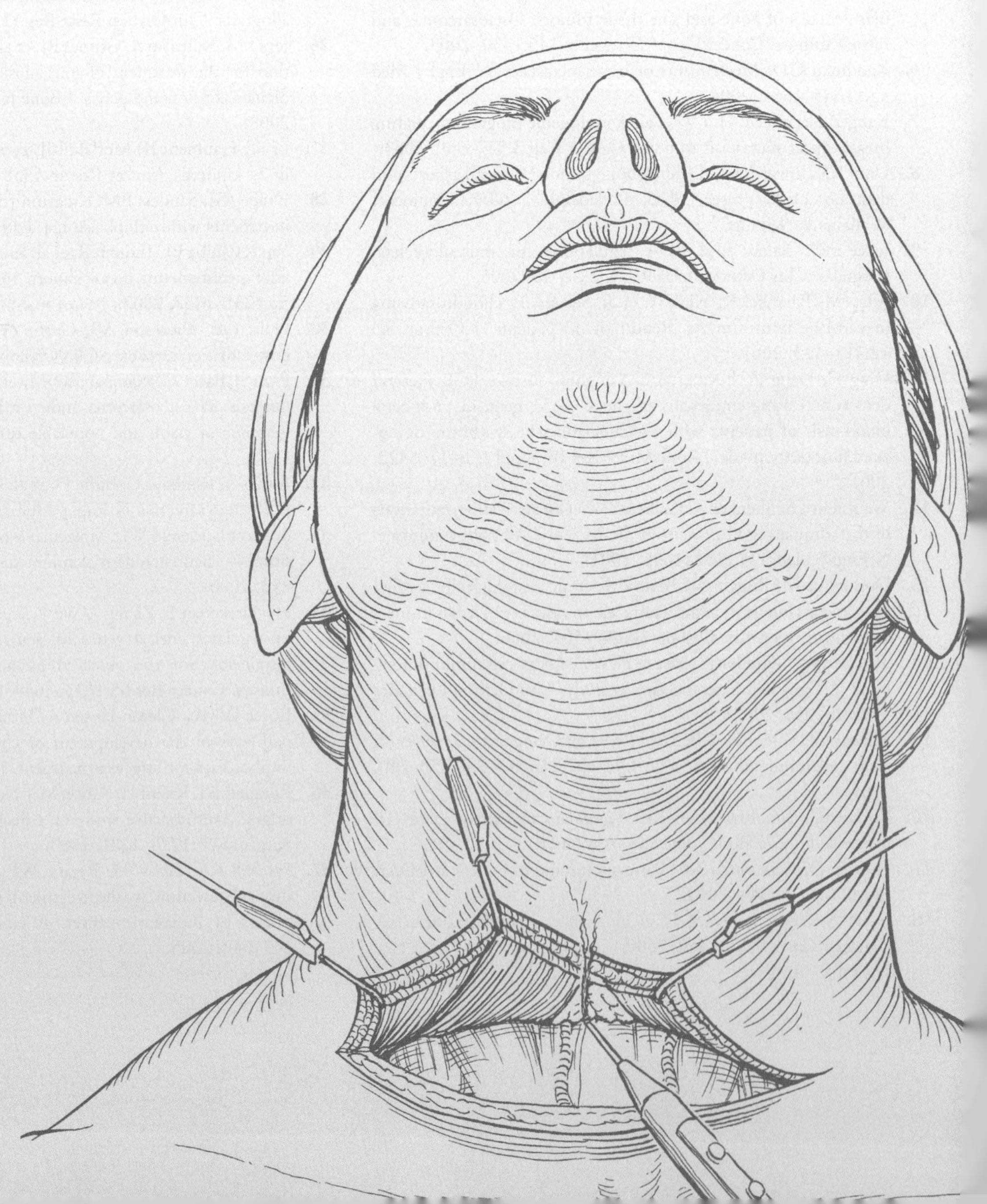

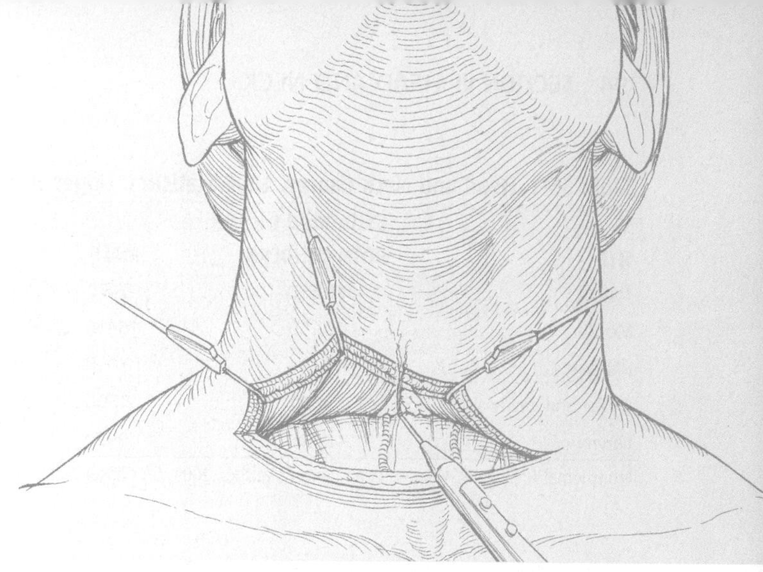

# CHAPTER 35

# HEAD AND NECK

Robert R. Lorenz, Marion E. Couch, and Brian B. Burkey



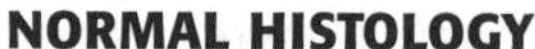

## NORMAL HISTOLOGY

The normal histology of the upper aerodigestive tract varies in each site. A complete review of the thyroid and parathyroid glands is beyond the scope of this chapter. The nasal vestibule is considered a cutaneous structure and is lined by keratinizing squamous epithelium. The limen nasi, or mucocutaneous junction, is where the epithelium changes to a ciliated pseudostratified columnar (respiratory) epithelium to line the nasal cavities. The exception is the olfactory epithelium at the roof of the nasal cavity, which is composed of bipolar, spindle-shaped olfactory neural cells with surrounding supporting cells. The paranasal sinuses are also lined by respiratory epithelium, but it tends to be thinner and less vascular than that of the nasal cavity. The nasopharyngeal lining varies from squamous to respiratory epithelium in an inconsistent manner. The adenoidal pad is composed of lymphoid tissue containing germinal centers without capsules or sinusoids. The oral cavity is lined by nonkeratinized stratified squamous epithelium with minor salivary glands throughout the submucosa and within the muscular tissue of the tongue. Although the oropharynx is lined by squamous epithelium, Waldeyer's ring is formed by lymphoid tissues of the palatine tonsils, adenoids, lingual tonsils, and adjacent submucosal lymphatics. The tonsils contain germinal centers without capsules or sinusoids but, unlike the adenoids, the tonsils have crypts lined by stratified squamous epithelium.

The hypopharynx is lined by nonkeratinizing, stratified squamous epithelium. Seromucous glands are found throughout the submucosa of the hypopharynx, in the lower two thirds of the epiglottis, and in the potential space between the true and false vocal folds known as the ventricle. Nonkeratinizing stratified squamous epithelium lines the epiglottis and true vocal fold. Pseudostratified, ciliated respiratory epithelium lines the false vocal fold, ventricle, and subglottis. The thyroid, cricoid, and arytenoid cartilages are composed of hyaline cartilage, whereas the epiglottis, cuneiform, and corniculate cartilages are composed of elastic-type cartilage. The external ear is a cutaneous structure lined with keratinizing squamous epithelium and associated adnexal structures. The external third of the external auditory canal is unique in that it contains modified apocrine glands that produce cerumen. The middle ear is lined with respiratory epithelium.

Numerous noncancerous changes in squamous epithelium can be seen in the upper aerodigestive tract. Leukoplakia, which describes any white mucosal lesion, and erythroplasia, which describes any red mucosal lesion, are both clinical descriptions and should not be used as diagnostic terms (Fig. 35-1). Erythroplakia is more often indicative of an underlying malignant lesion. Hyperplasia refers to thickening of the epithelium secondary to an increase in the total number of cells. Parakeratosis is an abnormal presence of nuclei in the keratin layers, whereas dyskeratosis refers to any abnormal keratinization of epithelial cells and is found in dysplastic lesions. Koilocytosis is a descriptive term for the vacuolization of squamous cells and is suggestive of viral infection, especially human papillomavirus (HPV).

## EPIDEMIOLOGY

The American Joint Committee on Cancer (AJCC) staging system divides sites of malignancy originating in the head and neck into six major groups: lip and oral cavity, pharynx, larynx, nasal cavity and paranasal sinuses, major salivary glands, and thyroid.[1] Of the sites arising from the aerodigestive tract, laryngeal cancer remains the most common cause of death (Table 35-1), whereas pharyngeal cancer has emerged as exhibiting the highest incidence over the past several years. Although there clearly remains a male preponderance in aerodigestive tract malignancies, the male-to-female ratio has been steadily decreasing because of the direct association between tobacco as a causative agent and the increased incidence of female smokers. Tobacco abuse increases the odds ratio for the development of laryngeal cancer by 15 : 1, whereas alcohol abuse carries an odds ratio of 2 : 1. Combined abuse of alcohol and tobacco is not additive in terms of the odds ratio but multiplicative. More recent studies have suggested that the epidemiology of head and neck cancer is shifting to mirror a change in the cause.[2] In the United States, during the period from 1973 to 2003, the incidence rate for cancer sites causally related to HPV infection significantly increased (tongue base and tonsil subsites of the oropharynx), whereas significant declines in incidence were observed for oral cancers not causally related to HPV. In

**Table 35-1 Head and Neck Cancer, 2009 Statistics: Upper Aerodigestive Tract**

| | Estimated Incidence | | | Estimated Deaths | | |
|---|---|---|---|---|---|---|
| **SITE** | **BOTH GENDERS** | **MALE** | **FEMALE** | **BOTH GENDERS** | **MALE** | **FEMALE** |
| Tongue | 10,530 | 7470 | 3060 | 1910 | 1240 | 670 |
| Mouth | 10,750 | 6450 | 4300 | 1810 | 1110 | 700 |
| Pharynx | 12,610 | 10,020 | 2590 | 2230 | 1640 | 590 |
| Other oral cavity | 1830 | 1300 | 530 | 1650 | 1250 | 400 |
| Larynx | 12,290 | 9920 | 2370 | 3660 | 2900 | 760 |

From Jemal A, Siegel R, Ward E, et al: Cancer statistics, 2009. CA Cancer J Clin 59:225–249, 2009.

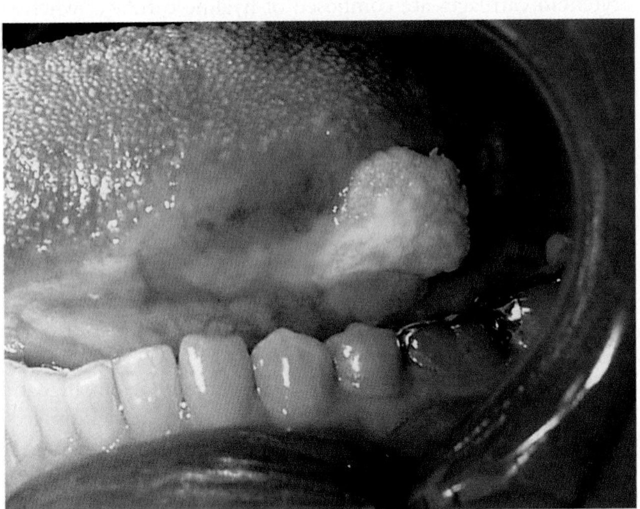

**FIGURE 35-1** Leukoplakic lesion on the left mobile tongue. On biopsy, this lesion was determined to be hyperkeratosis without invasive cancer.

addition, HPV-associated cancers tended to be younger in age by 3 to 5 years and were less likely to be associated with alcohol or tobacco use. Worldwide, the highest incidence rates in males exceeded 30/100,000 in areas of France, Hong Kong, India, Spain, Italy, and Brazil, as well as in U.S. blacks, with dramatic increases in oral cancer being seen in Central and Eastern Europe, most notably Hungary, Poland, Slovakia, and Romania.[3] The highest female rates are higher than 10/100,000 and are found in India, where chewing of betel quid and tobacco is common. Although aggregate rates are slowly declining in certain areas, such as India, Hong Kong, and Brazil, as well as in U.S. whites, rates are increasing in most other regions of the world. In addition to alcohol and tobacco consumption as causative factors, other risk factors include HPV and Epstein-Barr virus infection, Plummer-Vinson syndrome, metabolic polymorphisms, malnutrition, and occupational exposure to mutagenic agents. According to the National Cancer Database, squamous cell carcinoma (SCC) is the most common head and neck tumor of the major head and neck sites (88.9%), adenocarcinoma is the most common of the major salivary glands (56.4%), SCC is the most common of the sinonasal tract (43.6%), and lymphoma is the most common of the sites classified as other (82.5%).[4]

## CARCINOGENESIS

HPV infection is now recognized as a causative agent for oropharyngeal carcinoma. Based on the molecular cause, HPV-positive and HPV-negative head and neck SCCs (HNSCCs) may be considered as two distinct cancers.[5] High-risk HPV strains (subtypes 16 and 18) suppress apoptosis and activate cell growth when the HPV E6 and E7 proteins disrupt regulatory cell cycle and DNA repair pathways. Malignant transformation begins with inactivation of the p53 tumor suppressor gene by E6, whereas E7 inactivates the retinoblastoma tumor suppressor protein (Rb). E6 targets the cellular ubiquitin-protein ligase E6-AP, which then targets p53 for ubiquitination and degradation; this results in unregulated cell growth. E7 associates with Rb and p21 by blocking the interaction of Rb with E2F, which initiates uncontrolled cell proliferation.[5] Viruses such as HPV can usurp cellular processes, but often the development of carcinoma is the result of a stepwise accumulation of genetic alterations.[6] Tobacco, a well-known risk factor, was one of the first carcinogens to be linked with p53 mutations. One tobacco carcinogen, benzo[α]pyrene diol epoxide, induces genetic damage by forming covalently bound DNA adducts throughout the genome, including p53. Damage induced by benzo[α]pyrene diol epoxide and other carcinogens is repaired with the nucleotide excision repair system. Several studies have demonstrated that sequence variations in nucleotide excision repair genes contribute to HNSCC susceptibility.[7]

Many years after Slaughter proposed field cancerization, Califano and colleagues described the molecular basis for histopathologic changes in HNSCC.[8] Samples of dysplastic mucosa and benign hyperplastic lesions displayed loss of heterozygosity at specific loci (9p21, 3p21, 17p13). In particular, loss of heterozygosity at 9p21 or 3p21 is one of the earliest detectable events leading to dysplasia in this tumor progression model. From dysplasia, further genetic alteration in 11q, 13q, and 14q results in carcinoma in situ. The high rate of recurrence of HNSCC is believed to result from histopathologically benign squamous cell epithelium harboring a clonal population with genetic alterations.[8] Studies using microsatellite analysis and X chromosome inactivation have verified that metachronous and synchronous lesions from distinct anatomic sites in HNSCC often originate from a common clone. This evidence confirms that genetically altered mucosa is difficult to cure in the HNSCC patient because it is on the path to tumorigenesis, as predicted by this model. Indeed, HNSCC patients have a 3% to 7% annual incidence of secondary lesions in the upper aerodigestive tract, esophagus, or lung. A synchronous second primary lesion is defined as a tumor detected within 6 months of the index tumor. The occurrence of a second primary lesion more than 6 months after the initial lesion is referred to as metachronous. A second primary will develop in the aerodigestive tract of 14% of patients with HNSCC over the course of their lifetime, with more than half of these lesions occurring within the first 2 years of the index tumor.

There is also evidence to suggest that changes in the programming of cells, including stem cells, may also be involved in tumorigenesis in HNSCC because of the epithelial to mesenchymal transition.[9] Abnormalities in cadherins, tight junctions, and desmosomes lead to a decrease in cell-cell adherence and loss of polarity, increasing the mobility of these cells. As epithelial cells disassemble their junctional structures, undergo extracellular matrix remodeling, and begin expressing proteins of mesenchymal origin, they become migratory. When the process of epithelial to mesenchymal transition becomes pathologic, regulatory checkpoints are deficient. Thus, in the carcinogenic process, epithelial to mesenchymal transition may cause changes that contribute to tumor invasion and metastasis, enabling cancer cell dissemination.[9]

Epidermal growth factor receptor (EGFR) signaling has been strongly implicated in tumor progression in HNSCC. The ErbB family is comprised of four structurally related receptor tyrosine kinases. EGFR mRNA and protein are preferentially expressed in HNSCC compared with surrounding normal tissues, suggesting a significant role in carcinogenesis. EGFR is overexpressed in up to 80% to 100% of HNSCC tumors, with advanced-stage and poorly differentiated carcinomas more frequently demonstrating overexpression.[10] The most common mutation, *EGFRvIII,* occurs in up to 40% of HNSCCs. This mutant receptor is only found in cancer cells and has an in-frame deletion of exons 2 to 7, which results in a constitutively active receptor. The fact that *EGFRvIII* is not found in normal tissues makes this an attractive target for therapy. The two classes of therapies are monoclonal antibodies to EGFR receptor subunits and small-molecule EGFR tyrosine kinase inhibitors (TKIs). When ligands bind to one of the ErbB receptors, a dimer forms and the receptor's intracellular tyrosine residues then undergoes ATP-dependent autophosphorylation. Once phosphorylated, the receptor has the potential to trigger many different intracellular downstream pathways. The Janus kinase–signal transducers and activators of transcription (JAK–STAT), along with the phospholipase-Cγ–protein kinase C (PLCγ–PKC) pathways are activated in association with EGFR phosphorylation.

An emerging potential target for molecular-based cancer therapy is the insulin-like growth factor-1 receptor (IGF-1R) and its ligands, insulin growth factor-1 (IGF-1) and insulin growth factor-2 (IGF-2).[11] With activation of the receptor, downstream signaling events include phosphorylation of insulin receptor substrate-1 (IRS-1), activation of mitogen-activated protein kinases (MAPKs), and stimulation of the phosphatidylinositol-3 kinase (PI3K) pathway. This activation of both the Ras-MAPK-ERK and PI3K-Akt pathways is similar to the downstream signaling seen with EGFR autophosphorylation.

With the advent of increasingly sophisticated molecular detection techniques, such as DNA microarrays, large numbers of genetic markers can now be tested with greater ease. As single molecular markers, most studied to date have failed to demonstrate sufficient predictive potential in terms of incidence or prognosis. However, although single markers may not prove to have enough clinical applicability, panels of different molecular markers may offer more promising diagnostic and prognostic value.

## STAGING

Staging of head and neck cancer follows the TNM classification established by the AJCC.[1] The T classification refers to the extent of the primary tumor and is specific to each of the six sites of origin, with subclassifications within each site. The N classification refers to the pattern of lymphatic spread within the neck nodes and is the same for most head and neck sites, except thyroid, nasopharynx, mucosal melanoma, and skin (Table 35-2). In the new seventh edition of the AJCC Cancer Staging Manual,[1] a descriptor has been added as ECS+ or ECS–, depending on the presence or absence of nodal extracapsular spread (ECS). Clinical staging of the neck is based primarily on palpation, although radiographic studies, including computed tomography (CT) and magnetic resonance imaging (MRI), have been shown to be accurate in detecting positive nodes. If the CT criteria of nodes with central necrosis or size larger than 1.0 cm are used to determine positivity, only 7% of pathologically positive lymph nodes would be missed, and these smaller nodes are most often found in necks with more extensive disease. Metastatic disease is reported simply as Mx (cannot be assessed), M0 (no distant metastases are present), or M1 (metastases present). The most common sites of distant spread are the lungs and bones, whereas hepatic and brain metastases occur less frequently. The risk for distant metastases is more dependent on nodal staging than on primary tumor size.

After complete resection of the primary and nodal disease, pathologic staging may be reported. This is designated by a preceding "p," as in pTNM. It must be remembered when

**Table 35-2 Metastatic Staging of Regional Lymph Nodes (N)**

| STAGE | DESCRIPTION |
|---|---|
| NX | Regional lymph nodes cannot be assessed |
| N0 | No regional lymph node metastasis |
| N1* | Metastasis in a single ipsilateral lymph node, ≤3 cm in greatest dimension |
| N2* | Metastasis in a single ipsilateral lymph node, >3 cm but not >6 cm in greatest dimension, or in multiple ipsilateral lymph nodes, none >6 cm in greatest dimension, or in bilateral or contralateral lymph nodes, none >6 cm in greatest dimension |
| N2a* | Metastasis in single ipsilateral lymph node >3 cm but not >6 cm in greatest dimension |
| N2b* | Metastasis in multiple ipsilateral lymph nodes, none >6 cm in greatest dimension |
| N2c* | Metastasis in bilateral or contralateral lymph nodes, none >6 cm in greatest dimension |
| N3* | Metastasis in a lymph node >6 cm in greatest dimension |

From Edge SB, Byrd DR, Compton CC, et al [eds]: AJCC cancer staging manual, ed 7, New York, 2010, Springer-Verlag.

*A designation of U or L may be used for any N stage to indicate metastasis above the lower border of the cricoid (U) or below the lower border of the cricoid (L). Similarly, clinical or radiologic extracapsular spread (ECS) should be recorded as E– or E+, and histopathologic ECS should be designated as En (none), Em (microscopic), or Eg (gross).

measuring a pathologic mucosal specimen that tumor size may decrease up to 30% after resection. Although clinical T staging is of primary concern, pathologic N staging allows detection of occult microscopic disease and is useful in determining prognosis. Site-specific staging systems are discussed according to the primary site. The major change in the 2010 edition of the AJCC staging system for HNSCC sites, in addition to the ECS + or – descriptor, is the addition of a separate classification for mucosal melanoma of the head and neck, a very rare tumor.[1]

## CLINICAL OVERVIEW

### Evaluation

Proper treatment of HNSCC requires careful evaluation and accurate staging, both clinically and radiographically. Patients with HNSCC are initially evaluated in a similar manner, regardless of the site of tumor. Patient histories focus on symptomatology of the tumor, including the duration of symptoms, detection of masses, location of pain, and presence of referred pain. Special attention is paid to numbness, cranial nerve weakness, dysphagia, odynophagia, hoarseness, disarticulation, airway compromise, trismus, nasal obstruction, epistaxis, and hemoptysis. Alcohol and tobacco use histories are elicited. Office examination includes nasopharyngeal and laryngeal visualization with a mirror or fiberoptic endoscope. The examiner should be especially vigilant for second primary tumors and not be preoccupied by the obvious primary lesion. Contrast-enhanced CT and MRI of the head and neck may be performed for evaluation of the tumor and detection of occult lymphadenopathy. CT scanning is best at evaluating bony destruction, whereas MRI can determine soft tissue involvement and is excellent at evaluating parotid and parapharyngeal space tumors. Chest radiography or chest CT is performed to rule out synchronous lung lesions. Levels of serum tumor markers such as alkaline phosphatase and calcium may be determined, but such tests are not standard.

Direct laryngoscopy and examination under anesthesia are commonly performed as part of the evaluation of HNSCC. These procedures allow the physician to evaluate tumors without patient discomfort and with muscle paralysis, as well as evaluate the oropharynx, hypopharynx, and larynx and obtain biopsy samples. Pathologic confirmation of cancer is mandatory before initiating treatment. Concurrent bronchoscopy and esophagoscopy have historically been recommended for the detection of synchronous second primaries of the aerodigestive tract, which occur in 4% to 8% of patients who have one head and neck malignancy. With a normal chest radiograph or CT scan, bronchoscopy has a low yield for discovering bronchial tree second primaries. A barium esophagogram may substitute for esophagoscopy in patients at low risk for the development of esophageal tumors.

#### Positron Emission Tomography

$^{18}$F-fluorodeoxyglucose is a glucose analogue that is preferentially absorbed by neoplastic cells and can be detected by positron emission tomography (PET). The role of PET has been investigated in the initial evaluation of patients with HNSCC.[12] PET is more sensitive than CT in identifying the primary lesion, but cannot detect unknown primary tumors with more than 50% sensitivity. More than one third of patients have a change in their TNM score based on PET findings, and 14% of patients are assigned a different stage when it is added to the diagnostic workup. PET evaluates neck metastases with sensitivity equal to that of CT but with fewer false-positive results. PET can detect a higher percentage of lung metastases than chest radiography, bronchoscopy, or CT, but the specificity ranges from 50% to 80%, and how to treat a patient with a positive PET and an otherwise negative lung workup is still in question. In approximately 10% of patients, a synchronous second primary cancer is detected in various sites, including the stomach, pancreas, colon, and thyroid. Patients with tumors that demonstrate high uptake on PET have a worse prognosis than patients with less avid tumors and also have less response to radiation therapy. The exact role of PET in the initial evaluation of HNSCC is still under investigation and its use is becoming more routine, but is not within the current standard of care.

### Lymphatic Spread

The cervical lymphatic nodal basins contain between 50 and 70 lymph nodes per side and are divided into seven levels (Figs. 35-2 and 35-3).

1. Level I is subdivided:
   - Level IA is bounded by the anterior belly of the digastric muscle, hyoid bone, and midline.
   - Level IB is bounded by the anterior and posterior bellies of the digastric muscle and the inferior border of the mandible. Level IB contains the submandibular gland.
2. Level II is bounded superiorly by the skull base, anteriorly by the stylohyoid muscle, inferiorly by a horizontal plane extending posteriorly from the hyoid bone, and posteriorly by the posterior edge of the sternocleidomastoid muscle. Level II is further subdivided:
   - Level IIA is anterior to the spinal accessory nerve.
   - Level IIB, or the so-called submuscular triangle, is posterior to the nerve.
3. Level III begins at the inferior edge of level II and is bounded by the laryngeal strap muscles anteriorly, by

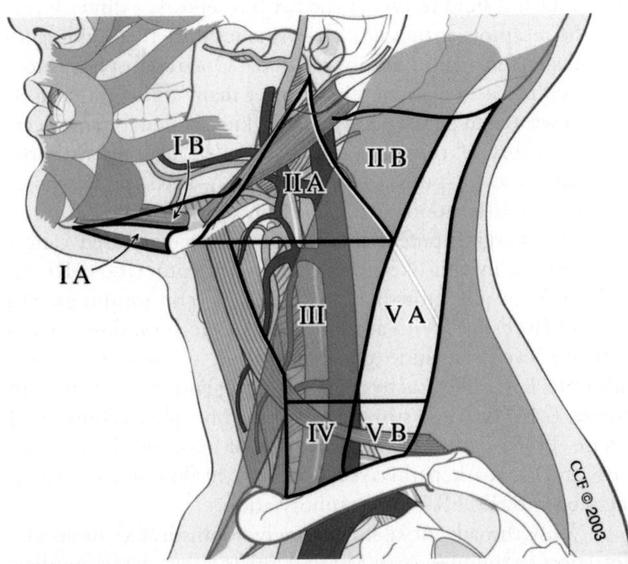


**FIGURE 35-2** Diagram of cervical lymph node levels I through V. Level II is divided into regions A and B by the spinal accessory nerve. (Courtesy Cleveland Clinic Foundation, 2003.)

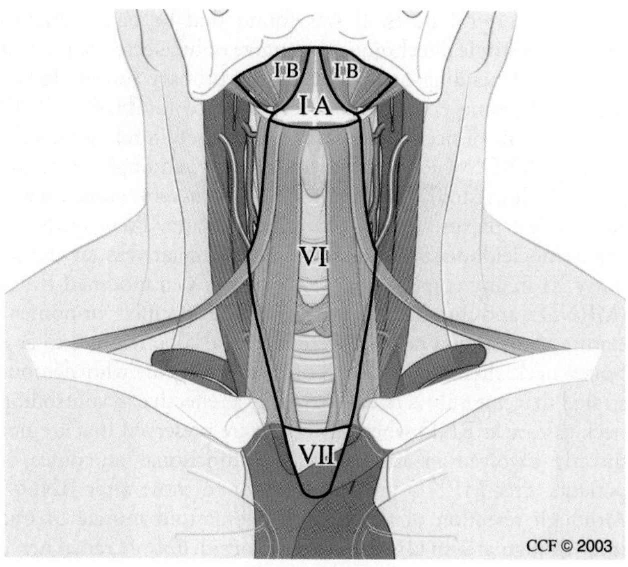


**FIGURE 35-3** Diagram of anterior lymph node levels I, VI, and VII. Although large in area, most level VI lymph nodes are confined to the paratracheal region. (Courtesy Cleveland Clinic Foundation, 2003.)

the posterior border of the sternocleidomastoid muscle posteriorly, and by a horizontal plane extending posteriorly from the inferior border of the cricoid cartilage.

4. Level IV begins at the inferior border of level III and is bounded anteriorly by the strap muscles, posteriorly by the posterior edge of the sternocleidomastoid muscle, and inferiorly by the clavicle.
5. Level V is posterior to the posterior edge of the sternocleidomastoid muscle, anterior to the trapezius muscle, superior to the clavicle, and inferior to the base of skull.
6. Level VI is bounded by the hyoid bone superiorly, the common carotid arteries laterally, and the sternum inferiorly. Although level VI is large in area, the few lymph nodes that it contains are mostly in the paratracheal regions near the thyroid gland.
7. Level VII (superior mediastinum) lies between the common carotid arteries and is superior to the aortic arch and inferior to the upper border of the sternum.

Lymphatic drainage usually occurs in a superior to inferior direction and follows predictable patterns based on the primary site. Primary tumors of the lip and oral cavity generally metastasize to nodes in levels I, II, and III, although skip metastases may occur in lower levels. The upper lip primarily metastasizes ipsilaterally, whereas the lower lip has ipsilateral and contralateral drainage. Tumors in the oropharynx, hypopharynx, and larynx usually metastasize to levels II, III, and IV. Tumors of the nasopharynx spread to the retropharyngeal and parapharyngeal lymph nodes, as well as to levels II through V. Other sites that metastasize to the retropharyngeal lymph nodes are the soft palate, posterior and lateral oropharynx, and hypopharynx. Tumors of the subglottis, thyroid, hypopharynx, and cervical esophagus spread to levels VI and VII. In addition to the lower lip, the supraglottis, base of the tongue, and soft palate have a high incidence of bilateral metastases.

## Therapeutic Options

Therapeutic options for patients with HNSCC include surgery, radiation therapy, chemotherapy, and combination regimens. In general, early-stage disease (stage I or II) is treated by surgery or radiation therapy. Late-stage disease (stage III or IV) is best treated by a combination of surgery and radiation therapy or chemotherapy and radiation therapy, or all three modalities, depending on the site of the primary. Because surgery was the first therapeutic option available to physicians, it has the longest track record of the three and established the head and neck surgeon as the leader of the treatment team for HNSCC. Photon irradiation is superior to surgery for eradicating microscopic disease and is an excellent alternative to surgery for early lesions. Tonsil, tongue base, and nasopharyngeal primary tumors are especially responsive to photon irradiation. Neutron and proton irradiation are used much less often in the head and neck, although experience has grown with their role in salivary gland malignancies and skull base cancers, respectively. Electrons are not commonly used in the head and neck for noncutaneous tumors. With the advent of intensity-modulated radiation therapy, which can reduce the photon dosage to surrounding normal tissue through computer three-dimensional planning, the dogma that patients may not receive more than 7200 cGy to tissue of the head and neck has been called into question. Hyperfractionation is the practice of administering radiation more than once daily, and results of the European Organization for Research and Treatment of Cancer have determined that hyperfractionation for HNSCC produces greater locoregional control than conventional once-daily regimens.[13] Radiation therapy is not as effective in treating large-volume, low-grade neoplasms or tumors in close proximity to the mandible because of the risk for osteoradionecrosis. The loss of salivary function with irradiation of the oral and oropharyngeal cavity can be disabling to patients, and its impact should not be minimized in the decision making process.

A landmark chemotherapy trial for HNSCC was the Veterans Affairs larynx trial, published in 1991.[14] Although chemotherapy alone is not curative in HNSCC, its role as a radiation sensitizer was established in this study. Two thirds of patients treated with radiation therapy and chemotherapy were able to keep their larynx, and survival was equal to that of patients treated with laryngectomy and radiation therapy. Recurrences after radiation therapy have been shown to be multifocal in the bed of the original tumor and the salvage surgeon should be familiar with the original tumor location and volume. Chemotherapy is commonly used in the treatment of incurable HNSCC, such as unresectable and metastatic disease, and can provide excellent symptom control in these patients.

Data from two large-scale, independent trials have examined the benefit of adding chemotherapy to postoperative irradiation for HNSCC.[15,16] Both the European Organization for Research and Treatment of Cancer Trial and the Radiation Therapy Oncology Group 9501/Intergroup treated advanced-stage, high-risk patients with cisplatin concurrently with postoperative radiation therapy and compared the outcomes with those of patients undergoing postoperative irradiation alone. In the Radiation Therapy Oncology Group, the 2-year locoregional control rate was 82% for the group receiving chemoradiation therapy versus 72% for the radiation therapy–alone group. Disease-free survival was significantly longer in the chemoradiation therapy patients, although overall survival was not significantly different between the groups. Not unexpectedly, significantly more toxicity and treatment morbidity were seen in the combined-treatment group, and further prognostic indicators about which patients are at high risk for failure are needed to predict which groups warrant this more intensive adjuvant therapy.

The neck should be treated when there are clinically positive nodes or the risk for occult disease is more than 20%, based on the location and stage of the primary lesion. The decision to perform neck dissection or irradiate the neck is related to treatment of the primary lesion. If the index tumor is being treated with radiation and the neck is N0 (no clinically detectable disease) or N1, the nodes are usually treated with irradiation. For surgically treated primary lesions, N0 or N1 neck disease may also be treated surgically. Negative prognostic factors such as extracapsular spread of tumor, perineural invasion, vascular invasion, fixation to surrounding structures, and multiple positive nodes are indicators for postoperative adjuvant radiation therapy. For N2 or N3 neck disease, neck dissection with planned postoperative radiation therapy is performed. When chemoradiation therapy protocols are used in treating the primary lesion and there is a complete response in the primary tumor and an N2 or N3 neck, planned neck dissection 8 weeks after chemoradiation therapy will contain cancer in up to one third of specimens.[17] If the neck mass persists, the percentage of residual disease increases to two thirds. When patients have advanced neck disease that involves the carotid artery or deep neck musculature, radiation or chemoradiation therapy is given preoperatively in the hope that the tumor will reduce in size and become resectable. CT scans notoriously carry a high false-positive rate for determining carotid encasement. When carotid resection is necessary, the associated morbidity is high (major neurologic injury in 17%), with a 22% 2-year survival rate, and the decision to resect should be weighed carefully.

Radical neck dissection (RND) was attributed to Crile in 1906 and was considered the gold standard for the removal of nodal metastases (Fig. 35-4). Through a subsequent close reading of Crile's surgical notes, it was found that he had begun to modify his surgical technique to remove only selected regions of the neck, depending on the site of the primary tumor. Today, this has become common surgical practice for HNSCC. All modifications of neck dissection are described in relation to the standard RND, which removes nodal levels I through V and the sternocleidomastoid muscle, internal jugular vein, cranial nerve XI, cervical plexus, and submandibular gland. Preservation of the sternocleidomastoid muscle, internal jugular vein, or cranial nerve XI in any combination is referred to as a modified RND (MRND), and the structures preserved are specified for nomenclature. A modified neck dissection may also be referred to as a Bocca neck dissection, named after the surgeon who demonstrated that not only is MRND equally as effective in controlling neck disease as RND when structures are preserved that are not directly involved in tumor, but the functional outcomes of patients after MRND are also superior to those after RND.[18] Although resection of the sternocleidomastoid muscle or one internal jugular vein is relatively nonmorbid, loss of cranial nerve XI leaves a denervated trapezius muscle, which can cause a painful chronic frozen shoulder.

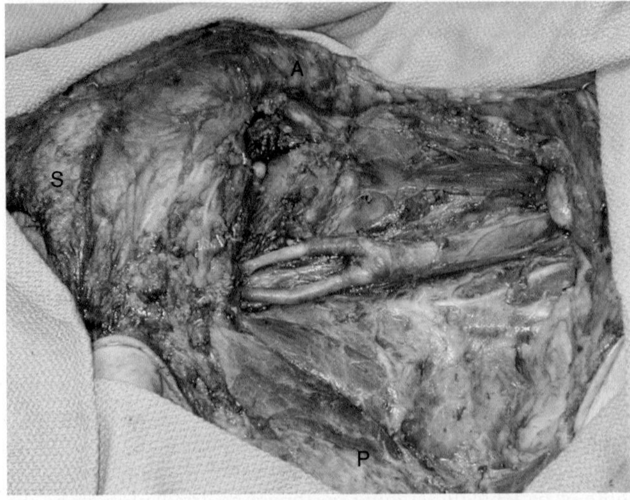


**FIGURE 35-4** Proper appearance of the right neck after a radical neck dissection. In addition to all lymphatic tissue, the three structures of the internal jugular vein, sternocleidomastoid muscle, and spinal accessory nerve have been resected. *A,* Anterior; *P,* posterior; *S,* superior.

RND or MRND can be performed for removal of detectable nodal disease. Preservation of any of levels I through V during neck dissection is referred to as selective neck dissection and is based on knowledge of the patterns of spread to neck regions. Selective neck dissection is performed on a clinically negative (N0) neck, with preservation of nodal groups carrying less than a 20% chance of being involved with metastatic disease. Regional control has been shown to be as effective after selective neck dissection as after MRND in patients with a clinically negative neck. Recent studies evaluating treatment of an N0 neck have investigated the use of sentinel lymph node biopsy, which attempts to predict the disease status of the neck based on the first echelon of nodes that drain the tumor.[19] Although sentinel lymph node biopsy has been used extensively with melanoma, its use in HNSCC has come about more gradually. Early results using isosulfan blue dye alone have suggested that this technique cannot consistently identify the sentinel node in HNSCC. More recent results using a gamma probe have been more encouraging, although the isolated node should be serial step–sectioned at a thickness of 150 nm and be examined through permanent processing. The current recommendations are that the technique should be restricted to early-stage (T1 or T2) oral and oropharyngeal cancers, with clinically N0 necks; this continues to be an investigational tool pending validation by large randomized clinical trials.

## ANATOMIC SITES

### Lip

Anatomically, the lip is considered a subsite of the oral cavity. The lip begins at the junction of the vermilion border and skin and is composed of the vermilion surface, which refers to the mucosa that contacts the opposing lip. It is divided into the upper lip, lower lip, and oral commissures. Most lip cancers occur on the lower lip (90% to 95%) and less often on the upper lip (2% to 7%) and commissures (1%). White men 50 to 80 years of age are the most common group in which lip cancer develops. Sun exposure and pipe smoking are associated with lip cancer. Although SCC is the most common lip cancer (90%), the most common cancer of the upper lip is basal cell carcinoma.

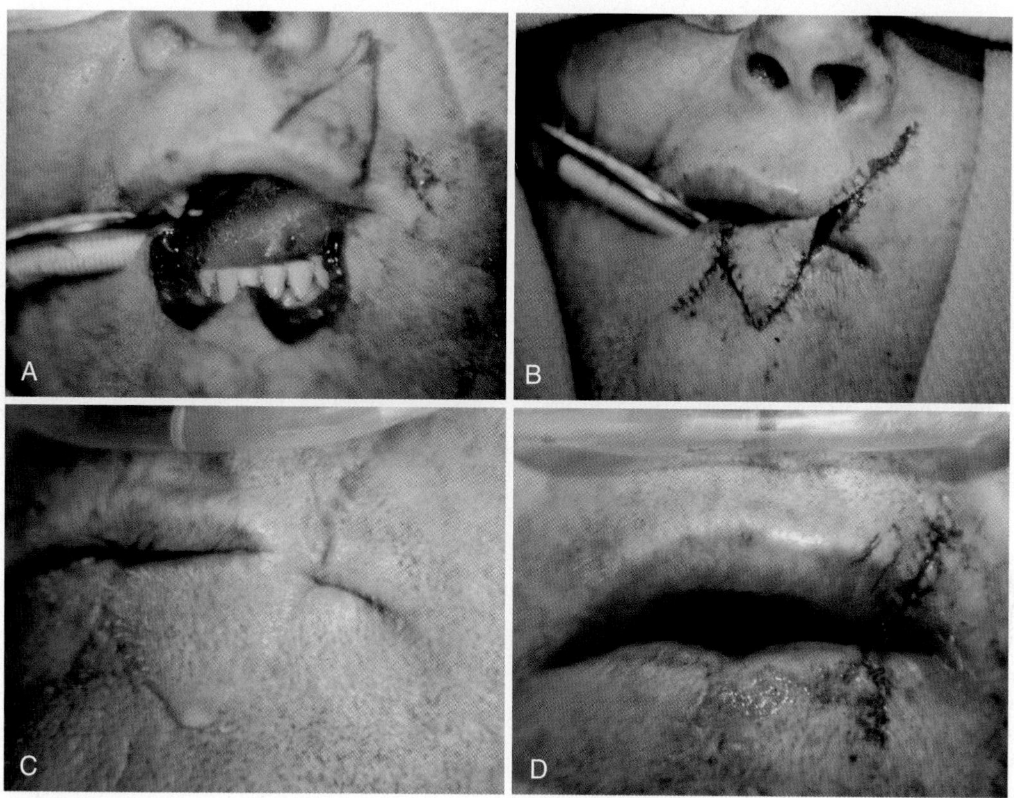

**FIGURE 35-5** **A,** Squamous cell carcinoma resected from the lower lip, leaving approximately 25% of normal tissue. **B,** Abbé flap uses upper lip tissue pedicled on the labial artery. **C,** Prior to division of the flap after 6 weeks of healing. **D,** Appearance after pedicle division.

Other lip cancers include variants of SCC (e.g., spindle cell and adenoid squamous carcinoma), as well as mucosal melanoma and minor salivary gland cancers.

The most common clinical manifestation of lip cancer is an ulcerative lesion on the vermilion or skin surface. Palpation is necessary to determine the submucosal extent of the lesion and possible fixation to underlying bone. Sensation of the chin should be tested to determine involvement of the mental nerve. Poor prognostic indicators include nerve involvement, fixation to the maxilla or mandible, cancer arising on the upper lip or commissure, positive nodal disease, and age younger than 40 years at diagnosis. The most frequently involved nodal basins are the submental and submandibular levels. A depth of tumor invasion of 4 mm has been shown to be a cutoff above which the incidence of cervical nodal disease is significantly increased.[20]

Similar to the rest of the oral cavity, lip cancer staging is based on size at initial evaluation. Early-stage disease may be treated by surgery or radiation therapy with equal success. Local surgery (wide local excision) with negative margin control of at least 3 mm is the preferred treatment, with supraomohyoid neck dissection performed for tumors with clinically negative necks but deeper primary invasion or size larger than 3 cm. Neck dissection with postoperative radiation therapy for patients with clinically evident neck disease has an acceptable 91% regional control rate in the neck.[21] The overall 5-year cure rate of 90% drops to 50% in the presence of neck metastases. Postoperative irradiation is also indicated for advanced-stage primary disease, tumors with perineural involvement, or close or positive margins at the time of resection.

The goals of lip reconstruction include reinstitution of oral competence, cosmesis, and maintenance of dynamic function while allowing adequate access for oral hygiene. Fortunately, the surgeon can remove up to half of the lip and still close the defect primarily, particularly defects in the lower lip, which contains more excess tissue than the upper lip. A lower lip wedge excision should not be carried below the mental crease unless the tumor dictates its excision. Care is taken to achieve close approximation of the white line on either side of the defect at the vermilion border because the eye is drawn to any mismatch that exists at this critical aesthetic location.

Defects encompassing between half and two thirds of the lip require augmentation. The Estlander and Abbé flaps are lip switch flaps based on the sublabial or superior labial artery. The Estlander flap is used when the defect involves the commissure, whereas the Abbé flap is used for more midline defects and requires second-stage division of the pedicle (Fig. 35-5). The Karapandzic flap consists of circumoral incisions with circular rotation of the skin flaps while maintaining innervation of the orbicularis oris musculature. This one-stage procedure is used for defects involving more than two thirds of the lip. Microstomia is a potential complication from these types of flap reconstructions, and denture use may not be possible. For defects larger than two thirds, the Webster, Gillies, or Bernard types of repairs may also be used.

## Oral Cavity

Because the oral cavity begins at the skin-vermilion junction, the lips are considered part of the oral cavity for staging purposes. Other subsites in the oral cavity include the buccal mucosa, upper and lower alveolar ridges, retromolar trigone, floor of mouth, hard palate, and oral tongue. The tongue is divided into the oral tongue (two thirds of the tongue volume), anterior to the circumvallate papillae, and the base of tongue, which is not considered part of the oral cavity but rather the oropharynx. Staging of the oral cavity is based on size: T1, 0 to 2 cm; T2, 2 to 4 cm; T3, 4 to 6 cm; and T4, tumors larger than 6 cm or invading adjacent structures, including bone (cortical bone of the mandible or maxilla, not superficial erosion or tooth sockets), deep tongue musculature, or facial skin. SCC accounts for 90% of tumors located in these subsites, with a male preponderance in the fifth and sixth decades of life. There is a close association with alcohol and tobacco abuse.

### Oral Tongue

The oral tongue begins at the junction between the tongue and floor of mouth and extends posteriorly to the circumvallate papillae. Tumors appear as exophytic, ulcerative, or submucosal masses that may be associated with tenderness or irritation with mastication. Benign tumors tend to be submucosal and include leiomyomas, neurofibromas, and granular cell tumors. Although granular cell tumors can arise in the larynx, they occur more frequently in the tongue and can be confused with SCC because of overlying pseudoepitheliomatous hyperplasia. Complete excision is curative, but histologic borders are notorious for extending beyond gross disease, and negative intraoperative margins are mandatory.

SCC is the most common type of malignancy, but leiomyosarcomas and rhabdomyosarcomas are also encountered (rarely). Neurotropic malignancies may involve the lingual or hypoglossal nerves, so tongue deviation or loss of sensation should be examined closely. Treatment of oral tongue cancer is primarily surgical, with wide local excision and negative margin control. The development of cervical metastases is related to the depth of invasion, perineural spread, advanced T stage, and tumor differentiation. Infiltration of more than 4 to 5 mm into the tongue musculature increases the incidence of occult cervical metastases. Metastases from the anterior of the tongue most frequently spread to the submental and submandibular regions. Tumors located more posteriorly often metastasize to levels II and III. Indications for postoperative radiation therapy include evidence of perineural or angiolymphatic spread and/or positive nodal disease.

Small tumors may be removed by wide local excision and primary closure or closure by secondary intention. Excision of larger tumors requires partial glossectomy or hemiglossectomy. Extirpation may result in significant dysfunction in terms of disarticulation and dysphagia from an inability to contact the palate, sense oral contents, or manipulate the tongue against the alveolus or lips. Reconstructive efforts should focus on maintaining tongue mobility without excess bulk. Split-thickness skin grafts, primary closure, or healing by secondary intention of larger tongue defects often results in tongue tethering. Thin, pliable fasciocutaneous flaps (e.g., the radial forearm free flap) are the preferred reconstructive technique for such defects. A palatal augmentation prosthesis may assist in maintaining palatal contact, important for speech and posterior propulsion of food boluses.

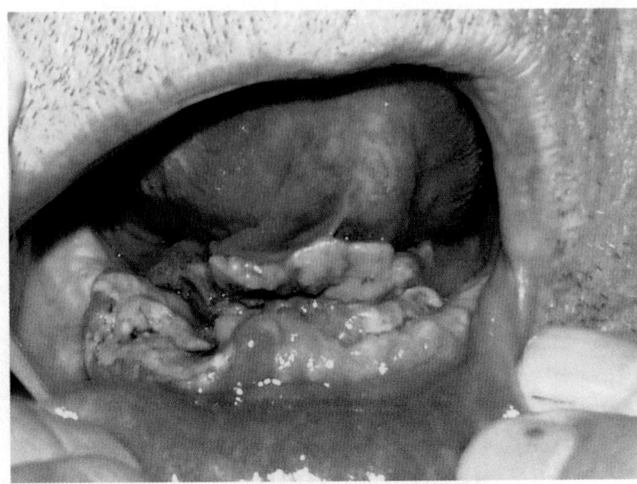

**FIGURE 35-6** 62-year-old man with squamous cell carcinoma of the anterior floor of mouth invading the mandible.

### Floor of the Mouth

The floor of the mouth extends from the inner surface of the mandible medially to the ventral surface of the tongue and from the anteriormost frenulum posteriorly to the anterior tonsillar pillars. The mucosa of the floor of the mouth contains the openings of the sublingual gland and submandibular gland (via Wharton's ducts). The muscular floor is composed of the genioglossus, mylohyoid, and hyoglossus muscles, with the lingual nerve located immediately submucosally.

Bimanual palpation can often determine fixation of tumors of the floor of the mouth to the mandible. CT demonstrates the depth of mandibular bony invasion, and widening of the cranial neural foramen, such as the foramen ovale, suggests neurotropic intracranial spread in advanced tumors. Determining mandibular invasion is of utmost importance for preoperative planning (Fig. 35-6). Invasion into the tongue musculature necessitates partial glossectomy concurrently with removal of the lesion on the floor of the mouth.

Treatment of lesions on the floor of the mouth is primarily surgical, with excision of the involved tongue or mandible as necessary to obtain negative margins. Removal of bone with soft tissue in continuity is commonly referred to as a commando or composite resection. Involvement of the neck may occur by direct extension of tumor through the floor of the mouth musculature or by lymphatic spread. The primary lesion and neck specimen should be taken in continuity so that accompanying lymphatic channels are resected. Adjuvant radiation therapy has similar indications as in oral tongue cancers. The primary goal of reconstruction is separation of the oral cavity from the neck by creating a watertight oral closure. This prevents orocutaneous salivary fistula formation. Secondary goals are maintaining tongue mobility, creating a lingual-alveolar sulcus, and preserving mandibular continuity. Local flaps for soft tissue reconstruction include the platysmal and submental myocutaneous pedicled flaps. Larger defects, including mandibular resection, require complex reconstruction, which is most often performed with free flaps.

### Alveolus

The alveolus and its accompanying gingiva constitute the dental surfaces of the maxilla and mandible and extend from the gingivobuccal sulcus laterally to the floor of the mouth and hard palate medially. Posteriorly, the alveolus extends to the pterygopalatine arch and ascending ramus of the mandible, also referred to as the retromolar trigone. Because of the tight attachment between the mucosa and underlying bone, treatment of alveolar SCC often involves treatment of the maxilla or mandible. Of gingival carcinomas, 70% occur on the lower gum. The periosteum of the mandible is a strong tumor barrier, and tumors that abut the bone may often be resected along with the adjacent periosteum only. Tumors adherent to the periosteum should undergo excision with marginal mandibulectomy, which involves resection of the superior or inner cortical portions of the mandible, with preservation of a continuous rim. Even superficial tumors that invade the outermost part of the mandible may be resected with a marginal mandibulectomy, although this is not oncologically sound if the tumor is a recurrence after radiation therapy. Segmental mandibulectomy entails excision of the full thickness of the mandible, thus interrupting mandibular continuity, and is indicated for patients with gross bone invasion by tumor. Primary radiation therapy for mandibular tumors is not a viable treatment option because of the high likelihood of osteoradionecrosis and poor response of involved bone to radiation therapy.

### Buccal Mucosa

The buccal mucosa extends from the inner surface of the opposing surfaces of the lips to the alveolar ridges and pterygomandibular raphe. Buccal cancer is uncommon and represents 5% of all oral cavity carcinomas. Smoking, alcohol abuse, lichen planus, dental trauma, snuff dipping, and tobacco chewing are causative factors associated with buccal cancer. Approximately 65% of patients with buccal cancer are initially found to have extension beyond the cheek mucosa. Lymphatic drainage is to the submandibular lymph nodes; however, tumors in the posterior aspect of the cheek may spread to level II initially. Stage I cancers have historically been treated by surgery and did not involve elective neck dissection because of the low rate of occult metastases. More recent studies, however, have suggested high rates of local recurrence for lesions treated by surgery alone, and adjuvant radiation therapy has been suggested, even for early-stage lesions.[22] Deep invasion may require through and through excision of cheek skin, thus necessitating internal and external linings, usually with a fasciocutaneous free flap.

### Palate

The hard palate is defined as the area medial to the maxillary alveolar ridges and extending posterior to the edge of the palatine bone. Chronic inflammatory lesions such as viral lesions, zoster, and pemphigoid can mimic neoplasms, and biopsy is indicated for persistent lesions. Necrotizing sialometaplasia is a benign, self-limited process of the minor salivary glands that has a predilection for the palate and can clinically mimic malignancy. The most common intraoral site for Kaposi's sarcoma is the palate in immunosuppressed patients. Torus palatinus is a benign exostosis of the midline hard palate and may require surgery if it interferes with denture wearing.

Minor salivary gland tumors, along with SCC, make up most hard palate tumors. Adenoid cystic carcinoma, mucoepidermoid carcinoma, adenocarcinoma, and polymorphous low-grade adenocarcinoma are common malignancies of salivary gland origin that tend to arise at the junction of the hard and soft palate. Malignancies of the hard palate are treated by local excision, if found early, but most commonly require resection of bone because of close adherence of the mucosa to the palate. Inferior maxillectomy, subtotal maxillectomy, or total maxillectomy is indicated for progressively destructive tumors extending into the maxillary antrum. Adjuvant radiation therapy is given for advanced lesions. Reconstruction may be accomplished with soft tissue flaps for small defects, obturation with a dental prosthesis for defects with some remaining hard palate, or bony free tissue transfer for extensive palatal resections.

### Oropharynx

The borders of the oropharynx include the circumvallate papillae anteriorly, plane of the superior surface of the soft palate superiorly, plane of the hyoid bone inferiorly, pharyngeal constrictors laterally and posteriorly, and medial aspect of the mandible laterally. The oropharynx includes the base of the tongue, inferior surface of the soft palate and uvula, anterior and posterior tonsillar pillars, glossotonsillar sulci, pharyngeal tonsils, and lateral and posterior pharyngeal walls. Similar to the oral cavity, T staging in the oropharynx is dependent on size. T4 tumors may extend out of the oropharynx posteriorly into the parapharyngeal space, inferiorly into the larynx, or laterally into the mandible.

Of tumors of the oropharynx, 90% are SCCs. Other tumors include lymphoma of the tonsils or tongue base or salivary gland neoplasms arising from minor salivary glands in the soft palate or tongue base. Initial symptoms include sore throat, bleeding, dysphagia and odynophagia, referred otalgia, and voice changes, including a muffled quality or hot potato voice. Trismus suggests involvement of the pterygoid musculature. Imaging studies should focus on invasion through the pharyngeal constrictors, bony involvement of the pterygoid plates or mandible, invasion of the parapharyngeal space or carotid artery, involvement of the prevertebral fascia, and extension into the larynx. Lymph node metastases generally occur in the upper jugular chain (levels II to IV), although lesions may skip to lower levels and spread to level V; such lesions are more common with oropharyngeal tumors than with tumors of the oral cavity. Bilateral metastases are more common with tongue base and soft palate lesions, especially those with midline lesions.

Treatment of oropharyngeal SCC has focused increasingly on conservation therapy with chemotherapy and radiation therapy. Many tumors of the oropharynx are poorly differentiated and respond well to radiation. Chemotherapy has been used as a radiation sensitizer in a number of studies and the local control rate achieved has been 90%, even in stage IV disease, although overall survival has not improved over more traditional surgery and radiation therapy.[23] A recent study of the cause of tonsil and tongue base cancers has suggested that when the disease is associated with HPV infection, the prognosis is significantly improved over non-HPV tumors. In a phase II trial of investigational therapy in patients with oropharyngeal and laryngeal cancers (ECOG 2399), patients with HPV positive tumors had a 73% reduction in risk of progression and a 64% reduction in risk of death when compared with HPV-negative patients.[24] This landmark study was the first to demonstrate that tumor HPV status is a strong and favorable prognostic marker in uniform patient populations with similar treatment protocols. Many physicians are advising that tumor HPV status should be incorporated as a stratification factor in patients with oropharyngeal cancer, although basing treatment protocols on HPV status has yet to be definitively investigated.

Surgery is necessary for primary disease that involves the mandible, for resectable recurrent disease, and it has a role in very early superficial tumors that do not justify a full course of radiation therapy. Extensive surgery of the tongue base significantly alters a patient's ability to swallow. Reconstruction of the tongue with preservation of the larynx requires surgical techniques that maintain tongue mobility and suspend the larynx and neotongue to prevent aspiration.

Resection or contracture after irradiation of the soft palate may result in velopharyngeal insufficiency, which is manifested clinically as nasal regurgitation of liquids and solids and hypernasal speech. Augmentation of the soft palate may be performed surgically or via palatal obturation. Although a palatal obturator requires cleaning and is not permanent, patients can remove it for sleep. With surgical augmentation of the palate, a balance between reducing velopharyngeal insufficiency and causing obstructive sleep apnea is difficult to achieve. After tongue base resection, an inferiorly directed palatal obturator assists in achieving the contact at the tongue base that is necessary for the projection of food posteriorly during the oral and pharyngeal phases of swallowing.

## Hypopharynx

The hypopharynx is the portion of the pharynx that extends inferiorly from the horizontal plane of the top of the hyoid bone to a horizontal plane extending posteriorly from the inferior border of the cricoid cartilage. The hypopharynx includes both piriform sinuses, lateral and posterior hypopharyngeal walls, and postcricoid region. The postcricoid area extends inferiorly from the two arytenoid cartilages to the inferior border of the cricoid cartilage, thereby connecting the piriform sinuses and forming the anterior hypopharyngeal wall. The piriform sinuses are inverted, pyramid-shaped potential spaces medial to the thyroid lamina; they begin at the pharyngoepiglottic folds and extend to the cervical esophagus at the inferior border of the cricoid cartilage.

Hypopharyngeal cancer is more common in men 55 to 70 years of age with a history of alcohol abuse and smoking. The exception is in the postcricoid area, in which cancers are more common worldwide in women. This is directly related to Plummer-Vinson syndrome, a combination of dysphagia, hypopharyngeal and esophageal webs, weight loss, and iron deficiency anemia, usually occurring in middle-aged women. In patients who fail to undergo treatment consisting of dilation, iron replacement, and vitamin therapy, postcricoid carcinoma may develop just proximal to the web.

Hypopharyngeal tumors are manifested as a chronic sore throat, dysphagia, referred otalgia, and a foreign body sensation in the throat. A high index of suspicion should be maintained because similar symptoms may be seen with the more common gastroesophageal reflux disease. In advanced disease, hoarseness may develop from direct involvement of the arytenoid, recurrent laryngeal nerve, or paraglottic space. The rich lymphatics that drain the hypopharyngeal region contribute to the fact that 70% of patients with hypopharyngeal cancer are initially seen with palpable lymphadenopathy. Patients with hypopharyngeal cancer have the highest rate of synchronous malignancies and the highest rate of development of second HNSCC primaries of any of the head and neck sites. Staging for hypopharyngeal cancer is based on the number of involved subsites or size of the tumor.

Physical examination for hypopharyngeal lesions includes fiberoptic endoscopy. Having the patient blow against closed lips and pinching the nose closed will inflate the potential spaces of the piriformis and assist in visualization of the tumor. Palpation of the larynx may demonstrate a loss of laryngeal crepitus. A fixed larynx suggests posterior extension into the prevertebral fascia and unresectability. Barium swallow may demonstrate mucosal abnormalities associated with an exophytic tumor and is useful for determining the extent of involvement of the cervical esophagus. It also assists in determining the presence and amount of aspiration present. CT can be used to determine the presence of thyroid cartilage invasion, direct extension into the neck, and pathologic lymphadenopathy. Biopsy of the hypopharynx usually requires direct laryngoscopy under general anesthesia.

The most common area for lymphatic spread is the upper jugular nodes, even with inferior tumors. Other regions include the paratracheal and retropharyngeal nodes. The presence of contralateral cervical metastases or level V involvement is a grave prognostic indicator. Treatment of hypopharyngeal cancer yields poor results in comparison to other sites in the head and neck, presumably because of the late stage of the disease at diagnosis. For early lesions confined to the medial wall of the piriform or posterior pharyngeal wall, radiation or chemoradiation therapy is effective as a primary treatment modality. Seldom is laryngeal-sparing partial pharyngectomy possible. Small tumors of the medial piriform wall or pharyngoepiglottic fold may be amenable to conservation surgery, but they must not involve the piriform apex and the patient must have mobile vocal cords and adequate pulmonary reserve.

The most common treatment of hypopharyngeal cancer is laryngopharyngectomy and bilateral neck dissection, including the paratracheal compartments, along with adjuvant radiation therapy. Trials of neoadjuvant chemotherapy followed by concomitant chemotherapy and radiation therapy have shown promise in organ preservation in hypopharyngeal cancer.[25] The estimated 5-year laryngeal preservation rate is 35%, and induction chemotherapy appears to decrease the rate of death from distant metastases.

After total laryngectomy and partial pharyngectomy, primary closure may be possible if at least 4 cm of viable pharyngeal mucosa remains. Primary closure using less than 4 cm of mucosa generally leads to stricture and an inability to swallow effectively. A pedicled cutaneous flap such as a pectoralis myocutaneous flap can be used to augment any remaining mucosa in these cases. When total laryngopharyngectomy with esophagectomy has been performed, a gastric pull-up may be used for reconstruction. More recently, free flap reconstruction with enteric flaps or tubed cutaneous flaps, such as radial forearm or anterolateral thigh flaps, has been used to reconstruct the total pharyngectomy defect.

## Larynx

The three-dimensional boundaries of the larynx are complex, and exacting definitions are necessary before understanding the pathologic conditions affecting this organ system. The anterior border of the larynx is composed of the lingual surface of the epiglottis, thyrohyoid membrane, anterior commissure, and anterior wall of the subglottis, which consists of the thyroid cartilage, cricothyroid membrane, and anterior arch of the cricoid cartilage. The posterior and lateral limits of the larynx are the arytenoids and interarytenoid region, aryepiglottic folds, and posterior wall of the subglottis, which is composed of the mucosa covering the cricoid cartilage. The superior limits are the tip and lateral borders of the epiglottis. The inferior limit is made up of the plane passing through the inferior edge of the cricoid cartilage.

For staging purposes, the larynx is divided into three regions—supraglottis, glottis, and subglottis. The supraglottis is composed of the epiglottis, laryngeal surfaces of the aryepiglottic folds, arytenoids, and false vocal folds. In addition to these supraglottic subsites, the epiglottis is divided into the suprahyoid and infrahyoid epiglottis, for a total of five supraglottic subsites. The inferior limit of the supraglottis is a horizontal plane through the ventricles, which is the lateral recess between the true and false vocal folds. This plane is also the superior border of the glottis; this is composed of the superior and inferior surfaces of the true vocal folds, extends inferiorly from the true vocal folds, and is 1 cm thick. Also included in the glottis are the anterior and posterior commissures. The subglottis extends from the lower border of the glottis to the lower margin of the cricoid cartilage.

Innervation of the larynx includes the superior laryngeal nerve, which supplies the cricothyroid and inferior constrictor muscles and contains afferent sensory fibers from the mucosa of the false vocal folds and piriform sinuses. The recurrent laryngeal nerve supplies motor innervation to all the intrinsic muscles of the larynx and sensation to the mucosa of the true vocal folds, subglottic region, and adjacent esophageal mucosa. The normal functions of the larynx are to provide airway patency, protect the tracheobronchial tree from aspiration, provide resistance for Valsalva maneuvers and coughing, and facilitate phonation. Tumors that involve the larynx impair these functions to a variable degree, depending on location, size, and depth of invasion.

Glottic tumors are often manifested early as hoarseness because the vibratory edge of the true vocal fold is normally responsible for the quality of the voice and is sensitive to even small lesions. Signs of airway compromise occur later in disease progression, when tumor bulk obstructs the glottic opening. Impaired movement of the vocal fold may cause hoarseness, aspiration, impaired cough, or obstructive symptoms. Impaired movement is caused by tumor bulk, direct invasion of the thyroarytenoid muscle, invasion of the cricoarytenoid joint, or invasion of the recurrent nerve. Hemoptysis occurs with hemorrhagic lesions.

When compared with glottic tumors, supraglottic lesions are relatively indolent and are initially seen at a later stage of disease (Fig. 35-7). Patients often complain of a sore throat or odynophagia. Referred otalgia is caused by Arnold's nerve, the vagal branch that supplies part of the ear sensation. Bulky tumors of the epiglottis are often associated with a hot potato or muffled voice quality because of airway compromise. Dysphagia may cause weight loss and malnutrition. Subglottic tumors are rare and most often manifest as airway obstruction, vocal fold immobility, or pain.

The respiratory and squamous epithelia of the larynx are most often the cause of laryngeal neoplasms, benign and malignant. Laryngeal papillomatosis is a benign exophytic growth of squamous epithelium with a tendency to recur, despite surgical excision. It has a bimodal distribution, referred to as the juvenile type and adult type. Granular cell tumors are also benign but may be confused with SCC because of a characteristic pseudoepitheliomatous hyperplasia that overlies this subepithelial lesion. Less frequent benign lesions include chondromas and rhabdomyomas. Non-neoplastic lesions of the larynx include vocal fold nodules and polyps, contact ulcers, subglottic stenosis, amyloidosis, and sarcoidosis. Finally, with exposure to carcinogens (e.g., tobacco), the epithelium of the larynx may undergo a series of precancerous changes, clinically referred to as leukoplakia (any white lesion of the mucosa) or erythroplakia (a red lesion), that consist of hyperplasia, metaplasia, or variable degrees of dysplasia.

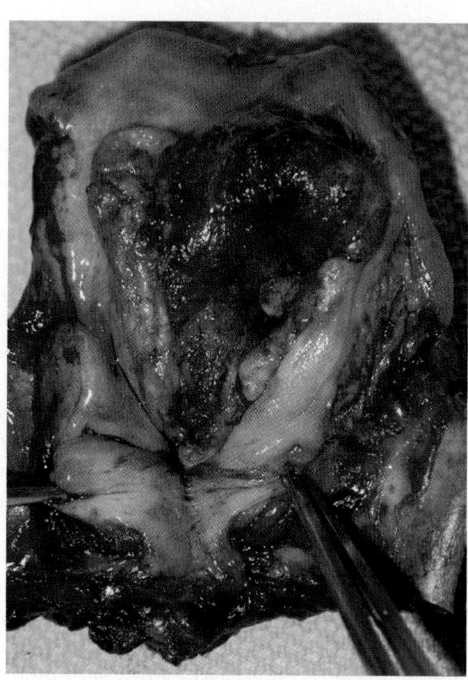

**FIGURE 35-7** Pathologic specimen from a supracricoid laryngectomy for squamous cell carcinoma. The tumor involves almost the entire laryngeal surface of the epiglottis, as well as the anterior commissure of the true vocal folds. Both vocal folds have been resected back to the vocal processes of the arytenoids, which are preserved to continue phonation and protect the airway from aspiration.

The most common malignant lesion of the larynx is SCC, which is often classified as SCC in situ, microinvasive SCC, or invasive SCC. Spindle cell carcinoma and basaloid SCC are rare and represent more aggressive variants of SCC. Verrucous carcinoma is a highly differentiated variant of SCC that is locally destructive but does not metastasize and should respond to complete surgical excision. The nonepithelial components of the larynx may also undergo malignant transformation, leading to tumors of salivary origin such as adenocarcinoma, adenoid cystic carcinoma, and mucoepidermoid carcinoma. Other tumors include neuroendocrine carcinoma, adenosquamous carcinoma, chondrosarcoma, synovial sarcoma, and distant metastases from other organ systems.

The staging system for laryngeal cancers is based on subsite involvement and vocal fold mobility. Office examination includes flexible laryngoscopy to assess the location and functional impairment. Stroboscopic laryngoscopy can detect subtle impairment of true fold mucosal waves that suggest significant tumor penetration. Direct laryngoscopy under anesthesia allows examination of all laryngeal subsites, along with the ability to perform biopsy. Specific sites that are important to examine in supraglottic tumors include the ventricle, anterior commissure, vallecula, base of the tongue, piriform sinus, and preepiglottic space. Key areas of glottic involvement include the false vocal fold, ventricle, anterior commissure, arytenoids, subglottis, and posterior commissure or postcricoid mucosa. Under general anesthesia, paralysis of the vocal fold is differentiated from arytenoid fixation by palpation of the vocal process portion of the arytenoid.

CT is routinely performed for laryngeal lesions and images the preepiglottic and paraglottic regions and extent of cartilage involvement, as well as determining direct extension into the deep neck structures. For the natural barriers and pathways of direct tumor spread, see the landmark histopathologic work of Kirchner.[26] CT examination should be performed with contrast agents and thin (1.5-mm) cuts through the larynx. Lymph node metastases are also identified by CT. The lymphatic drainage of the larynx differs in the supraglottic and glottic regions. Supraglottic epidermoid cancers metastasize early, with up to 50% of lesions having positive nodes. Contralateral and bilateral nodal metastases are common with supraglottic lesions because of the embryologic development of the supraglottis as a midline structure. Lymphatic drainage exits along the course of the superior laryngeal neurovascular pedicle and pierces the thyrohyoid membrane to drain to the subdigastric and superior jugular groups of nodes (levels II and III). Lymphatic drainage of tumors in the glottic and subglottic areas exits via the cricothyroid ligament and drains to the prelaryngeal (delphian) node, paratracheal nodes, and deep cervical nodes in the region of the inferior thyroid artery. Tumors confined to the glottis are only rarely associated with regional disease (4%), and positive nodes, when present, are most often ipsilateral.

Decision making in the treatment of laryngeal cancer is governed by tumor location and characteristics of tumor aggressiveness, as well as the patient's overall constitution and lifestyle. Poor prognostic factors include size, nodal metastasis, perineural invasion, and extracapsular spread. Low-grade epidermoid lesions of the larynx, such as dysplasia and carcinoma in situ, can be managed with local excision, such as microscopic excision of the mucosa. Concurrent denuding of the mucosa of both vocal folds near the anterior commissure can lead to the formation of an anterior web, which reduces voice quality and is a difficult complication to correct. Successful treatment of low-grade lesions includes close follow-up, with repeat office or operative laryngoscopy, as well as strict smoking cessation. For invasive disease, multiple treatment options are available, including conservation surgery and aggressive surgery, radiation therapy, and chemoradiation therapy. In general, conservation of the larynx in early-stage disease is key and can be accomplished with laryngeal preservation surgery or radiation therapy. Later stage disease that is still confined to the larynx is generally treated by chemoradiation therapy, with total laryngectomy used for salvage.

Laryngeal preservation surgery includes endoscopic surgery with cold steel, endoscopic laser resection, and open surgery, with preservation of some portion of the larynx to maintain the ability to talk. Transoral laser microsurgery, promoted by Ambrosch and colleagues[27] in Germany, has been used to treat not only all stages of laryngeal cancer but also oropharyngeal and hypopharyngeal tumors. Challenging the dogma that non–en bloc resection of tumors promotes locoregional recurrence, they have demonstrated comparable cancer survival while decreasing perioperative morbidity. In supraglottic cancers, this group reported 100% 5-year control rates for T1 and 89% for T2, with excellent functional outcomes, including minimal aspiration and short recovery periods.[27]

In recurrent glottic tumors after failure of radiation therapy, transoral laser microsurgery has demonstrated an overall 3-year survival rate of 74%, comparable to that of total laryngectomy.[28] Although laser microsurgery requires significant technical expertise, acceptance of this oncologic technique has been increasing, changing the approach to upper aerodigestive tract malignancies.

Open conservation laryngeal surgery entails maintaining a conduit for air flow through the remnant of the larynx to permit the ability to talk without aspiration. When deciding whether a patient is a candidate for laryngeal preservation surgery, factors such as pulmonary function and cardiovascular status must be examined, because these patients will often have to tolerate some amount of aspiration or airway compromise.

Pulmonary function testing, such as spirometry and arterial blood gas analysis, is performed preoperatively. An excellent functional test is to have the patient climb two flights of stairs successively without becoming short of breath. The least invasive of the open procedures is open cordectomy, which is indicated for small midfold lesions and for which 100% and 97% 5-year control rates for T1 and T2 lesions, respectively, have been reported.[29] Reconstruction is performed with a false vocal fold flap. For lesions involving the anterior commissure with less than 10 mm of inferior extension, an anterior frontal partial laryngectomy may be performed.

Conservation surgery options for more extensive tumors include vertical partial laryngectomy, supracricoid laryngectomy, and supraglottic laryngectomy. For T1 or T2 glottic lesions, vertical partial laryngectomy plus reconstruction with a false vocal cord pull-down or local muscle flap is indicated, as long as the cartilage is not involved. For T3 lesions not involving the preepiglottic space or arytenoid cartilage, supracricoid laryngectomy with cricohyoidopexy or cricohyoidoepiglottopexy is possible (Fig. 35-8). Excellent disease control has been achieved with this technique, largely because of removal of the paraglottic space and thyroid cartilage. Naudo and coworkers have shown that removal of feeding tubes and respiration without a tracheotomy can be achieved in 98% of patients.[30] The standard supraglottic laryngectomy preserves both true vocal folds, both arytenoids, the tongue base, and the hyoid bone (Fig. 35-9). Because there are numerous extensions of this operation, in which more than the standard structures are resected, cure rates are difficult to compare but, in general, T1 and T2 local control rates range from 85% to 100%, with decreased control for higher stage lesions.

If a decision has been made to undergo nonsurgical therapy, the patient must be able to complete the full course of radiation therapy, which usually includes 5 to 7 weeks of continuous daily therapy visits. Previous irradiation is a contraindication to further radiation therapy. Finally, the patient must be reliable in adhering to follow-up for years after treatment because recurrences may be indolent and difficult to detect.

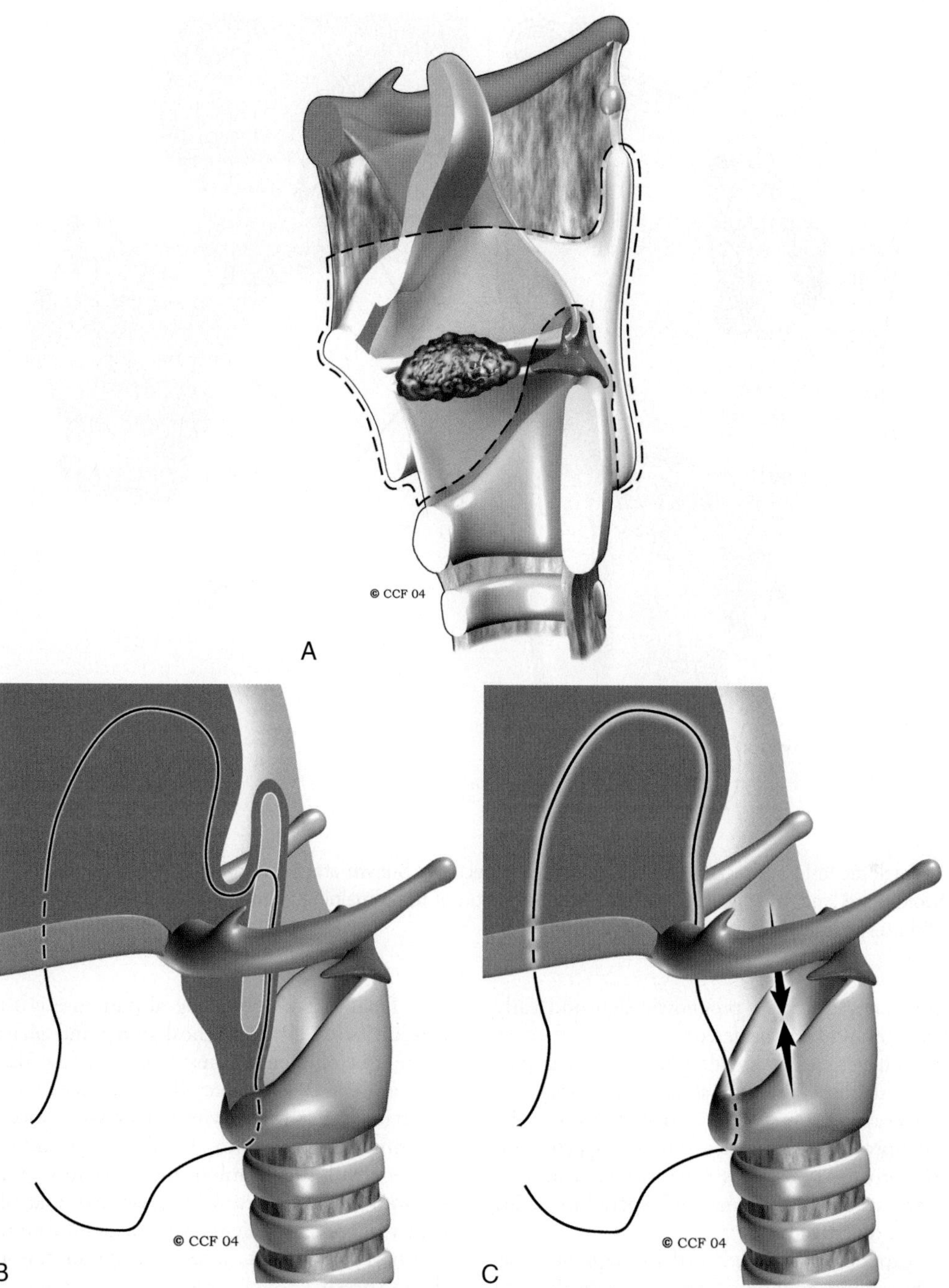


**FIGURE 35-8 A,** Lesion of the glottis deemed removable by supracricoid laryngectomy. The *dotted line* demonstrates resection of the true vocal fold to the arytenoid cartilages, including the entire laryngeal cartilage and paraglottic spaces laterally. **B,** Reconstruction by cricohyoidoepiglottopexy, with the cricoid cartilage sutured directly to the epiglottic remnant and hyoid bone, or cricohyoidopexy **(C),** with the cricoid sutured to the hyoid bone and tongue base directly. (Courtesy Cleveland Clinic Foundation, 2004.)

For neoadjuvant or concurrent chemotherapy, the patient must have sufficient constitutional health to withstand the chemotherapeutic agents. For early laryngeal cancer (T1 or T2), irradiation provides excellent disease control, with good to excellent post-therapy voice quality. For professional voice users with early lesions, irradiation is usually the choice of therapy.

The combination of chemotherapy and radiation therapy for advanced-stage disease (stages III and IV) was first brought into the mainstream with the Veterans Affairs larynx trial in 1991.[14] Induction chemotherapy followed by radiation therapy was found to provide 2-year survival equal to that after total laryngectomy with postoperative radiation therapy, in addition to being able to preserve the larynx in 64% of patients. More recently, trials with concurrent chemotherapy and radiation therapy have demonstrated even better local control of advanced laryngeal cancers. Pretreatment vocal cord fixation does not preclude conservative nonsurgical therapy, but persistent

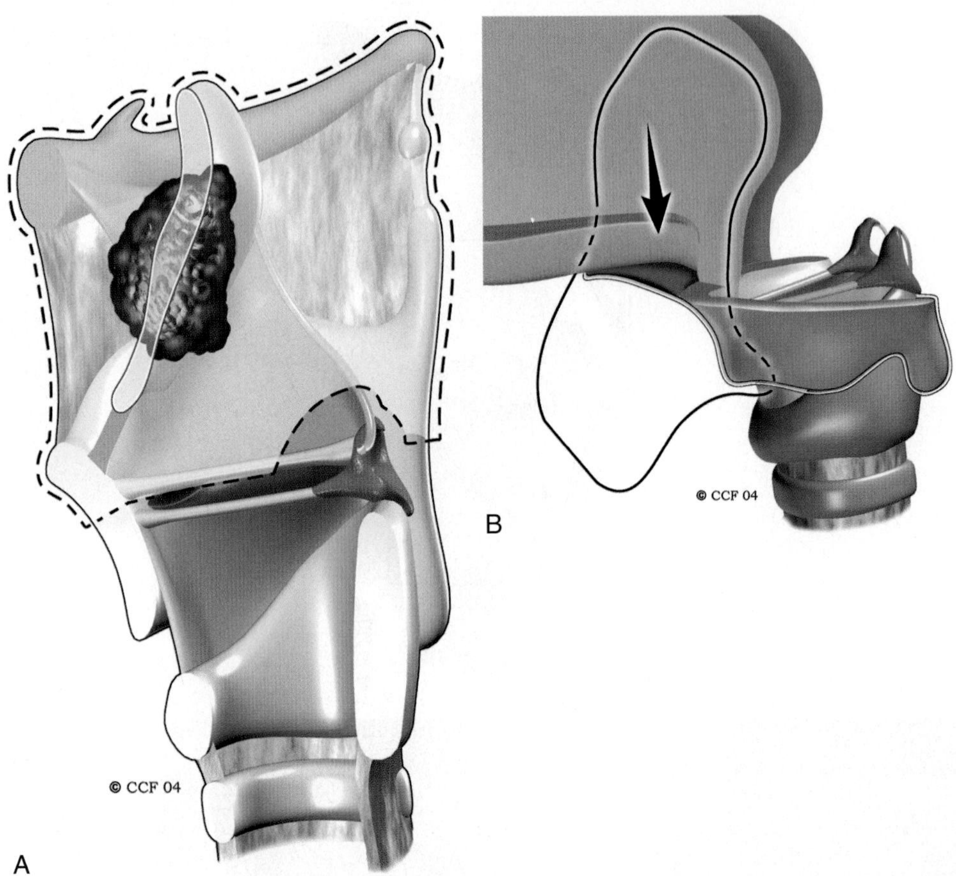


**FIGURE 35-9 A,** Supraglottic lesion, resectable by supraglottic laryngectomy. Shown are the borders of resection *(dotted line),* including the false vocal folds, hyoid bone, and preepiglottic space. **B,** Reconstruction of the remaining inferior segment of the thyroid cartilage sutured to the tongue base. (Courtesy Cleveland Clinic Foundation, 2004.)

immobility posttreatment is a poor prognostic sign and early surgical intervention should be considered.[31]

In patients who have disease extending outside the larynx, who fail conservative therapy (although some failures may still be amenable to conservation surgery), or who are not otherwise candidates for organ-preserving strategies, total laryngectomy is still commonly performed. It involves a permanent tracheostoma and loss of the voice, with permanent separation of the upper respiratory and digestive tracts.

Patients may experience a period of depression or social withdrawal after becoming aphonic. Speech and swallowing rehabilitation have become an integral part of laryngeal cancer treatment and should begin preoperatively. Speech rehabilitation options include speech with an electrolarynx, esophageal speech, and tracheoesophageal puncture. The electrolarynx is considered the easiest of the three methods to use and consists of a vibratory sound wave generator that is usually placed directly on the submandibular area or cheek. The patient mouths words to produce a monotone, electronic-sounding speech. Becoming understandable can take considerable time and patience.

Esophageal speech is produced by swallowing air into the esophagus and expulsing the air back through the pharynx, which vibrates as the air passes. The ability to master esophageal speech takes a motivated patient to be able to control the release of air through the upper esophageal sphincter, which occurs in only 20% of laryngectomized patients.

Finally, tracheoesophageal puncture is a surgically created conduit between the tracheal stoma and pharynx that is made at the time of laryngectomy or secondarily. This conduit is fitted with a one-way valve that allows passage of air posteriorly from the trachea to the pharynx but prevents food and liquid from entering anteriorly into the airway. By occluding the stomal opening with the thumb during exhalation, the patient can pass air into the pharynx, which vibrates and allows remarkable clarity of speech. Patients who are good candidates for tracheoesophageal puncture have an 80% success rate of achieving fluent speech.

Swallowing rehabilitation is a second role of the speech therapist when rehabilitating a laryngeal cancer patient, whether treated surgically or nonsurgically. Partial laryngectomy patients may have impaired pharyngeal movement and sensation, impaired vocal fold movement, decreased laryngeal elevation, and decreased subglottic pressure with poor cough, all contributing to possible aspiration.

Specially designed swallowing maneuvers and training in regard to food consistency are offered by the speech therapist to maintain an oral diet, although some patients may require gastric feeding or conversion to total laryngectomy if aspiration persists. Even laryngectomized patients have difficulty relearning the act of swallowing. Radiation therapy and chemotherapy, although organ-preserving, cause fibrosis, decreased sensation and movement, and decreased lubrication, which have a negative impact on swallowing. Furthermore, because of the exposed circumferential ulcerated mucosa of the pharynx that occurs with chemoradiation therapy, pharyngeal stenosis may develop during the recovery phase and necessitate dilation and even pharyngeal augmentation surgery with healthy nonirradiated tissue. Thus, the speech therapist and surgeon must work as a team to rehabilitate a larynx cancer patient.

## Nasal Cavity and Paranasal Sinuses

The nasal cavity consists of the nares, vestibule, septum, lateral nasal wall, and roof. The paranasal sinuses include the frontal, maxillary, ethmoid, and sphenoid sinuses. The lateral nasal wall includes the highly vascular inferior, middle, superior and, occasionally, supreme turbinates, as well as the ostiomeatal complex and nasolacrimal duct and orifice. The frontal sinuses are two asymmetrical air cavities within the frontal bone that drain into the nasal cavity via the frontal recesses. The ethmoid sinuses are a complex bony labyrinth directly beneath the anterior cranial fossa. The lamina papyracea is the paper-thin lateral wall of the ethmoid sinus that constitutes the medial wall of the orbit. The anterior ethmoids drain into the middle meatus (inferior to the middle turbinate), whereas the posterior ethmoids drain via the sphenoethmoidal recess. The sphenoid sinus lies in the middle of the sphenoid bone and also drains via the sphenoethmoidal recess. The vital structures of the optic nerves, carotid arteries, and cavernous sinuses are contained within the lateral walls of the sphenoid sinus, whereas the sella turcica and optic chiasm lie superiorly within the roof. The maxillary sinuses drain into the middle meatus and are bound posteriorly by the pterygopalatine and infratemporal fossae.

Tumors of the nasal cavity and paranasal sinuses tend to be seen initially at a late stage because their symptoms are often attributed to more mundane causes. Symptoms include epistaxis, nasal congestion, headache, and facial pain. Orbital involvement produces proptosis, orbital pain, diplopia, epiphora, and even vision loss. Nerve involvement is heralded by numbness in the distribution of the infraorbital nerve. A variety of benign tumors occur in the nasal region. Sinonasal papilloma (or schneiderian papilloma) is classified into three groups:

1. Septal papillomas (50%) arise on the septum. They are exophytic and not associated with malignant degeneration.
2. Inverted papilloma (47%).
3. Cylindrical cell papillomas (3%) arise on the lateral nasal wall or from the paranasal sinuses and are associated with malignant degeneration (10% to 15%), usually into SCC.

Previously believed to require radical extirpation, sinonasal papillomas require only local surgical excision with negative margins.

Other benign nasal lesions include hemangioma, benign fibrous histiocytoma, fibromatosis, leiomyoma, ameloblastoma, myxoma, hemangiopericytoma (a benign, aggressive lesion with a tendency to metastasize), fibromyxoma, and fibro-osseous and osseous lesions, such as fibrous dysplasia, ossifying fibroma, and osteoma. Intracranial tissues may extend into the nasal area and give rise to encephaloceles, meningoceles, and pituitary tumors. CT and MRI demonstrate the intracranial connection, and biopsy without previous imaging is unwarranted because of the risk for cerebrospinal fluid (CSF) leakage or uncontrollable bleeding from vascular tumors.

Malignancies of the sinonasal tract represent only 1% of all cancers or 3% of upper respiratory tract malignancies and have a 2 : 1 male-to-female ratio. Because respiratory epithelium can differentiate into squamous or glandular histology, SCC and adenocarcinoma represent two of the most common sinonasal cancers.[4] Sinonasal carcinoma is related to exposure to nickel, Thorotrast (used as a radiographic contrast agent in the United States from about 1930 to the mid-1950s), and softwood dust. Chronic exposure to hardwood dust or leatherworking has been associated with adenocarcinoma of the sinonasal tract. Other malignancies include olfactory neuroblastoma, malignant fibrous histiocytoma, midline malignant reticulosis (also known as lethal midline granuloma or polymorphic reticulosis), osteosarcoma, chondrosarcoma, mucosal melanoma, lymphoma, fibrosarcoma, leiomyosarcoma, angiosarcoma, teratocarcinoma, and metastases from other organ systems, especially renal cell carcinoma.

Since the publication of the 2002 AJCC staging manual, the nasal cavity and ethmoid sinuses have been considered as separate primary sites, in addition to the maxillary sinus.[1] The staging system is only for carcinomatous malignancies and does not include the frontal or sphenoid sinuses as separate sites because of the rarity of tumors arising in these sites. Staging is partly dependent on local spread of the tumor. Ohngren's line extends from the medial canthus to the mandibular angle. Maxillary tumors superior to Ohngren's line have a poorer prognosis than those inferior to the line because of the proximity to the orbit and cranial cavity. Local spread of tumors may occur along nerves or vessels or directly through bone. Advanced tumors of the maxillary sinuses commonly involve the pterygopalatine and infratemporal fossae. Widening of the foramen rotundum (V2) or foramen ovale (V3) on imaging suggests neural spread with intracranial involvement (Fig. 35-10). Because olfactory neuroblastomas are believed to arise from the olfactory neuroepithelium, these tumors commonly involve the cribriform plate and spread intracranially toward the frontal lobes. Sphenoidal tumors may include extension to the cavernous sinuses, carotid arteries, optic nerves, or the ophthalmic or maxillary branches of the trigeminal nerves. Lymph node metastases are in general uncommon (15%), and elective neck dissection or irradiation of a

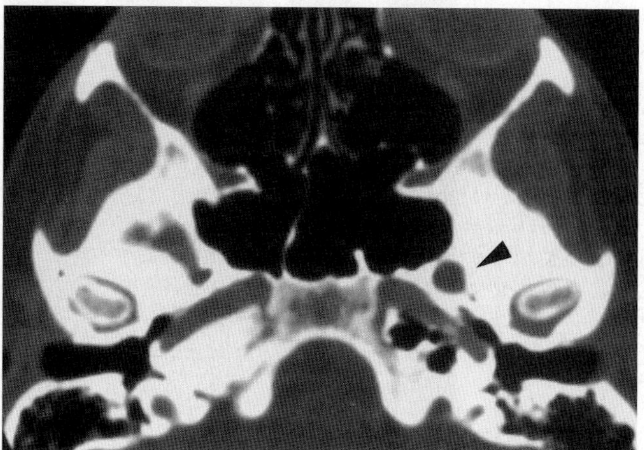

**FIGURE 35-10** CT scan of 38-year-old woman with adenoid cystic carcinoma demonstrating perineural spread along V3 and widening of the foramen ovale *(arrowhead).* (Courtesy Dr. J. Netterville.)

clinically negative neck is most often unwarranted. Involved nodal groups include the retropharyngeal, parapharyngeal, submental, and upper jugulodigastric nodes.

The standard treatment of sinonasal malignancies is surgical resection, with postoperative radiation or chemoradiation therapy used for high-grade histology or advanced local disease. Because these cancers can involve the dentition, orbits, or brain, treatment requires a multidisciplinary team, including a head and neck surgeon, neurosurgeon, ophthalmologist, prosthodontist, oral surgeon, and reconstructive surgeon. After a preoperative workup consisting of imaging, endoscopy, and biopsy, a tumor map and operative plan are formulated. Vascular tumors are embolized by an interventional radiologist, preferably within 24 hours of surgery. Patients with tumors requiring skull base exploration may need a lumbar drain to decompress the dura from the cranium and reduce the risk for postoperative CSF leakage. Routine prophylactic use of a tracheotomy for craniofacial surgery to reduce the risk for postoperative pneumocephalus is controversial.

Low-grade tumors limited to the lateral nasal wall, ethmoid sinuses, or septum have increasingly been removed with endoscopic techniques. A lateral rhinotomy incision is the classic open approach for a medial maxillectomy and entails removal of the lateral nasal wall. If the tumor involves the inferior maxilla, an inferior maxillectomy, including removal of the hard palate and the medial, lateral, and posterior maxillary sinus walls, is performed. For tumors more superior in the maxillary sinus, a total maxillectomy, including excision of the roof, is performed. If the bone of the floor of the orbit is involved, removal with postoperative reconstruction is indicated. If the orbital periosteum is involved with tumor, it may be resected with preservation of the orbit, although more extensive involvement of fat or muscle necessitates orbital exenteration (Fig. 35-11).[32]

If the anterior cranial floor is involved with tumor, as it often is in olfactory neuroblastomas, craniofacial resection is indicated. This procedure combines a craniotomy approach with a transfacial approach. Surgical disruption of the cribriform region causes postoperative anosmia. Reconstruction of the anterior cranial fossa requires separation of the cranial vault from the nasal cavity with a pericranial flap, temporoparietal fascial flap, fascia lata free graft or, when extensive resection has been performed, a microvascular free flap. Unresectable lesions include those with brain involvement, carotid artery encasement, or bilateral optic nerve involvement.

Radiation therapy and chemotherapy for sinonasal malignancies are being used with increasing frequency. Sinonasal undifferentiated carcinoma, rhabdomyosarcoma, and midline reticulocytosis are examples of aggressive cancers in which neoadjuvant chemotherapy and radiation therapy play an integral role. Combining chemotherapy with radiation therapy and surgery for treatment of advanced sinonasal SCC has met with variable success.

### Nasopharynx

The nasopharynx begins at the posterior nasal choana and ends at the horizontal plane between the posterior edge of the hard palate and posterior pharyngeal wall. The nasopharynx includes the vault, lateral walls, which contain the eustachian tube orifices and the fossae of Rosenmüller, roof, which is made up of the sphenoid rostrum, and posterior wall, which consists of the basiocciput or clivus. Both malignant and benign tumors of the nasopharynx are usually related to the normal histology, which includes squamous and respiratory epithelium, the lymphoid tissues of the adenoids, and deeper tissues, including fascia, cartilage, bone, and muscle. Benign tumors of the nasopharynx are rare and include fibromyxomatous polyps, papillomas, teratomas, and pedunculated fibromas. Angiofibroma, a benign tumor that affects young males, is the most common benign tumor of the nasopharynx. Rathke's pouch cysts arise high in the nasopharynx at the sphenovomerian junction. The cyst develops from a remnant of ectoderm that normally invaginates to form the anterior pituitary and may become infected later in life. Thornwaldt's bursa is located more inferiorly and arises from a remnant of the caudal notochord; it can contain a jelly-like material. It may also become infected in later life, and marsupialization is most often all that is required to treat it and

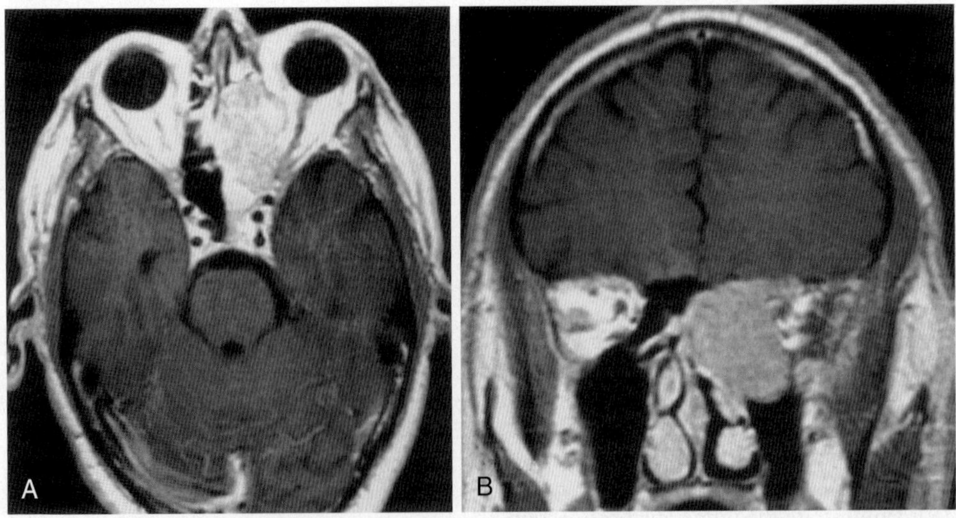


**FIGURE 35-11** **A,** Axial MRI scan of patient with adenosquamous carcinoma of the ethmoids involving the orbital fat. Orbital exenteration was necessary. **B,** Coronal MRI scan of the same patient demonstrating tumor extension to the floor of the anterior cranial fossa. (Courtesy Dr. J. Netterville.)

Rathke's pouch cysts. Craniopharyngiomas, extracranial meningiomas, encephaloceles, hemangiomas, paragangliomas, chordomas (which can cause extensive destruction), and antral-choanal polyps can also be seen in the nasopharynx.

The clinical findings in patients with nasopharyngeal tumors include symptoms of nasal obstruction, serous otitis with effusion and associated conductive hearing loss, epistaxis, and nasal drainage. Findings such as a cervical mass, headache, otalgia, trismus, and cranial nerve involvement suggest malignancy. Examination of the nasopharynx was historically performed with a mirror and has greatly been improved with the use of a rigid or flexible nasopharyngoscope in the office. CT is excellent for determining bony destruction and widening of foramina. MRI is used to assess soft tissue involvement and intracranial extension, as well as nerve, cavernous sinus, and carotid involvement.

Angiofibromas are vascular lesions found exclusively in males, usually develop during puberty, and are commonly referred to as juvenile nasopharyngeal angiofibromas. Although they are benign tumors, angiofibromas often erode bone and cause significant structural and functional dysfunction, as well as bleeding. CT findings of a nasopharyngeal mass, anterior bowing of the posterior wall of the antrum, erosion of the sphenoid bone, erosion of the hard palate, erosion of the medial wall of the maxillary sinus, and displacement of the nasal septum in an adolescent male are highly suggestive of angiofibroma (Fig. 35-12). Surgery after embolization is the primary treatment modality and understanding the location of origin is critical for complete tumor extirpation. Tumors originate at the posterolateral wall of the roof of the nasal cavity, at the sphenopalatine foramen. Whether performed endoscopically or via an open approach, such as lateral rhinotomy or the Caldwell-Luc operation, complete removal of all tumor and bone in the sphenopalatine region is crucial to decrease the possibility of recurrence. Radiation has been successfully used as treatment for these tumors but, given the young age at diagnosis and the lifelong risks associated with radiation exposure, is usually reserved for unresectable angiofibromas and recurrences.

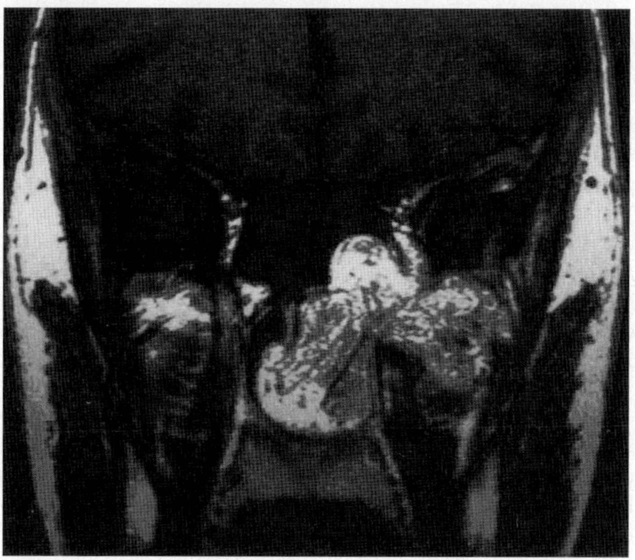

**FIGURE 35-12** MRI scan of a 16-year-old boy with a left-sided juvenile angiofibroma. The tumor arose in the pterygomaxillary region and has extended into the nasopharynx and infratemporal fossa. (Courtesy Dr. J. Netterville.)

Possible malignancies include nasopharyngeal carcinoma, low-grade nasopharyngeal papillary adenocarcinoma, lymphoma, rhabdomyosarcoma, malignant schwannoma, liposarcoma, and aggressive chordoma. The staging system of malignant tumors of the nasopharynx is for epithelial tumors only and is based on confinement to the nasopharynx or spread to surrounding structures. Although nasopharyngeal carcinoma accounts for only 0.25% of all cancers in North America, it represents approximately 18% of all malignancies in China.[33] There is a strong correlation with Epstein-Barr virus, which has been demonstrated in all histologic subtypes of nasopharyngeal carcinoma. The World Health Organization has divided nasopharyngeal carcinoma into three histologic variants—keratinizing (25%), nonkeratinizing (15%), and undifferentiated (60%)—although more recent classifications combine nonkeratinizing and undifferentiated tumors.[33] The most common initial sign is neck node metastases, especially to the posterior cervical triangle, and inferiorly positioned positive nodes predict poor outcomes. Treatment is based on radiation therapy to the primary site and bilaterally in the neck. With the addition of cisplatin and 5-fluorouracil, the rate of distant metastases decreases and disease-free and overall survival increase.[34] Intracavitary irradiation is used to provide a boost at the primary site for advanced tumors and is used in cases of reirradiation. Surgery is reserved for persistent neck disease or for selected cases of local recurrence. It is unique that the risk for recurrence with nonkeratinizing and undifferentiated carcinoma appears to be chronic and does not level off at 5 years, as it does with most other cancers. Rhabdomyosarcoma is the most frequent soft tissue sarcoma in the pediatric population and is the most common sarcoma occurring in the head and neck. Excluding the orbit, the most common site in the head and neck is the nasopharynx. Treatment is based on multimodality therapy consisting of nonradical surgery and radiotherapy, plus multiagent chemotherapy.

Although surgery of the nasopharynx is used primarily for benign pathologies, a number of approaches have been described, both endoscopic and open, for the surrounding skull base region. The recent development of endoscopic skull base tumor resection has gained significantly in popularity, although the limits of the technique have yet to be clearly defined.[35] Endoscopic techniques not only avoid facial incisions but also allow shorter hospital stays. The most commonly described tumor removed via transnasal techniques is an inverting papilloma, which is excised in piecemeal fashion. Success has also been reported with the endoscopic removal of mucoceles. Numerous open surgical approaches have been described to obtain access to the central skull base. For tumors of the nasopharynx, the transpalatal approach offers excellent visualization. The transfacial approach of lateral rhinotomy with unilateral or bilateral medial maxillectomy creates a facial incision but offers greater lateral exposure. The midfacial degloving procedure allows excellent bilateral exposure of the maxillae, paranasal sinuses, and nasopharynx without facial incisions. The posterior wall of the maxillary sinus may be removed to allow access to the pterygomaxillary fossa and deeper infratemporal fossa. For disease located more laterally, the transmastoid, transcochlear, and translabyrinthine approaches described by Fisch are used alone or in combination with more anterior approaches.

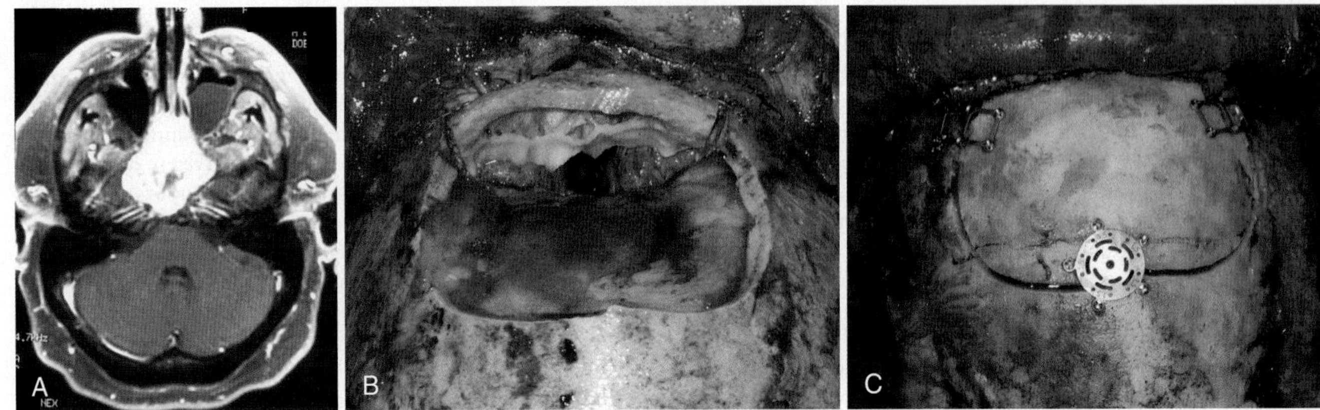

**FIGURE 35-13** **A,** MRI scan of a 42-year-old man with a midline fibromyxoid sarcoma. **B,** Bicoronal incision with a combined subfrontal bar and craniotomy, allowing full access to the central anterior skull base. **C,** Replacement of the cranial bone along with a pericranial flap harvested from deep surface of bicoronal flap for reconstructing of skull base.

More extensive approaches include the lateral facial split and mandibular swing, frontal-orbital or frontal-orbital-zygomatic approach, and maxillary swing and, for disease of the high nasopharynx, the subfrontal approach affords excellent medial exposure (Fig. 35-13).

## Pituitary Surgery

Although neurosurgery maintains the discipline responsible for the comprehensive management of hypophyseal disease, a collaboration between otolaryngologists with endoscopic sinus surgery skills and neurosurgeons has resulted in the development of minimally invasive pituitary surgery.[35] The endoscopic transnasal transsphenoidal approach provides excellent visualization of the operative field and avoids intraoral or anterior nasal incisions, nasal packing, and postoperative complications, such as septal deviation and lip anesthesia. Length of hospital stay, use of lumbar drains, and the need for nasal packing have been demonstrated to be significantly reduced with minimally invasive pituitary surgery as compared with open traditional approaches. Reconstruction of the sella by minimally invasive endoscopic repair has demonstrated that normal sphenoidal function can be maintained while obtaining excellent results in terms of a low incidence of CSF leakage and harvest site morbidity (Fig. 35-14).[36]

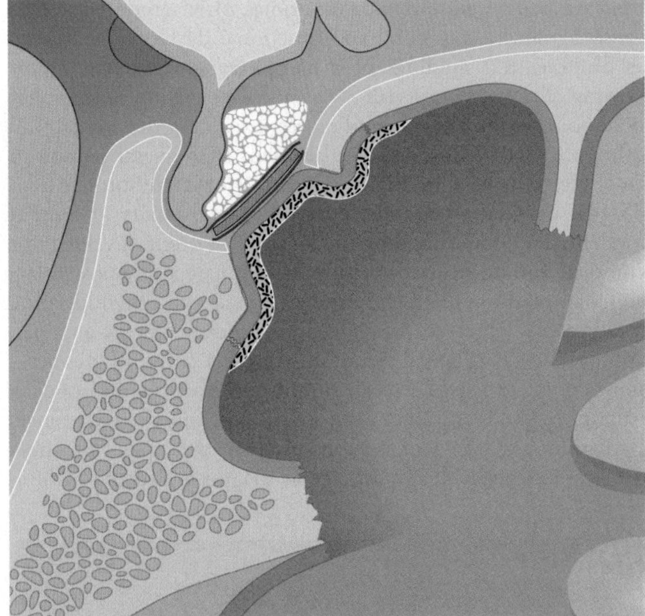

**FIGURE 35-14** After endoscopically opening the sphenoid sinus in the minimally invasive hypophysectomy technique and resecting the pituitary tumor, sellar reconstruction is performed in a layered fashion. The sellar defect is partially filled with Gelfoam or fat, followed by layers of acellular human dermis, cartilage, acellular human dermis, mucosa, and fibrin glue. (From Lorenz RR, Dean RL, Chuang J, Citardi MJ: Endoscopic reconstruction of anterior and middle cranial fossa defects using acellular dermal allograft. Laryngoscope 113:496–501, 2003.)

## Ear and Temporal Bone

When referring to tumors of the ear, the structures commonly involved include the external ear, middle ear, and inner ear. The external ear consists of the auricle or pinna and the external auditory canal to the tympanic membrane. The middle ear contains the tympanic cavity proper, ossicles, eustachian tube, epitympanic recess, and mastoid cavity. The borders of the middle ear include the tympanic membrane and squamous portion of the temporal bone laterally, petrous temporal bone medially, tegmen tympani or roof superiorly, carotid canal anteriorly, mastoid posteriorly, and floor of the tympanic bone inferiorly. The inner ear is contained within the petrous portion of the temporal bone and consists of the membranous and osseous labyrinth and internal auditory canal.

Evaluation of ear and temporal bone neoplasms requires appropriate physical examination and audiologic and vestibular testing, as well as radiologic assessment. Findings of hearing loss, vertigo, eustachian tube dysfunction with serous otitis media, cranial nerve deficits, pulsatile tinnitus, drainage, and deep boring pain are often associated with tumors and must be thoroughly evaluated. CT plays a crucial role in evaluating the temporal bone because of the complex anatomy contained within bony confines. MRI with gadolinium contrast is complementary and is used to define soft tissue anatomy (Fig. 35-15).

Neoplasms of the pinna are most often related to sun exposure and include basal cell carcinoma and SCC.

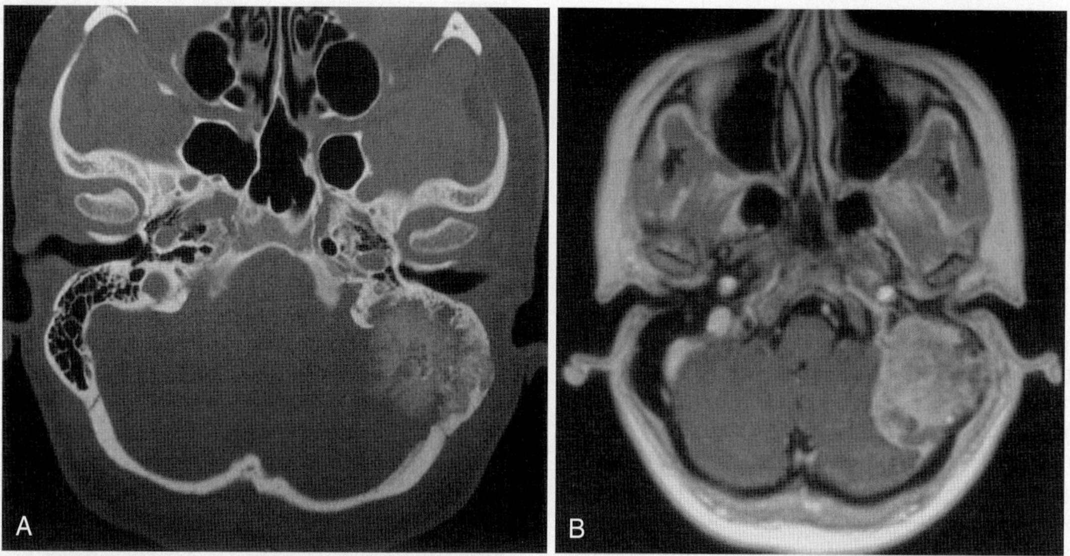


**FIGURE 35-15 A,** CT scan of a 19-year-old woman with osteosarcoma of the left temporal bone and bony destruction of the mastoid. **B,** MRI is useful for determining the extent of the tumor and the lack of brain invasion. (Courtesy Dr. J. Netterville.)

Keratoacanthoma is a benign tumor characterized by rapid growth and spontaneous involution and may be confused with SCC. In the external auditory canal, ceruminal gland adenocarcinomas, adenoid cystic carcinoma, and atypical fibroxanthomas may arise. Within the temporal bone, benign neoplasms include adenoma, paraganglioma (at the tympanic membrane and at the jugular bulb), acoustic neuroma, and meningioma. SCC is the most common cancer of the temporal bone; others include adenocarcinoma of middle ear or endolymphatic sac origin. In the pediatric population, soft tissue sarcomas such as rhabdomyosarcoma predominate. Metastases are an underrecognized cause of petrous bone tumors.

Malignancies of the pinna are treated similarly to skin cancers elsewhere on the face. Mohs microsurgery with frozen section control of margins minimizes the amount of normal tissue resected with the cutaneous malignancy. Involvement of underlying cartilage leads to more disseminated growth, necessitating partial or total auriculectomy. If the extent of disease is great, lateral temporal bone resection may be indicated, with attempted preservation of the facial nerve and inner ear. When the facial nerve or parotid gland is involved, lateral temporal bone resection with parotidectomy is performed. Radiation therapy may be used uncommonly for primary treatment or, more commonly, for adjuvant treatment in the case of perineural spread or poorly differentiated tumors.

Treatment of tumors involving the middle ear and bony canal consists of en bloc resection of structures at risk for involvement. Rarely, when the tumor involves only the external canal without bony destruction, sleeve resection of the canal can be performed. Lateral temporal bone resection removes the bony and cartilaginous canal, tympanic membrane, and ossicles. Subtotal temporal bone resection involves removal of the ear canal, middle ear, petrous bone, temporomandibular joint, and facial nerve. Involvement of the petrous apex necessitates total temporal bone resection, with removal of the carotid artery. SCC within the petrous apex is considered incurable, although adenoid cystic carcinoma and select low-grade sarcomas may be excised with total temporal bone resection. The goals of reconstruction of temporal bone defects are protection from CSF leaks and coverage of vital structures and remaining bone to prepare for postoperative radiation therapy. Techniques for facial nerve rehabilitation are covered below in the section on salivary gland malignancies. A prosthetic ear provides acceptable rehabilitation when a total auriculectomy has been performed.

## Salivary Gland Neoplasms

The major salivary glands include the parotid glands, submandibular glands, and sublingual glands. There are also approximately 750 minor salivary glands scattered throughout the submucosa of the oral cavity, oropharynx, hypopharynx, larynx, parapharyngeal space, and nasopharynx. Salivary gland neoplasms are rare and constitute 3% to 4% of head and neck neoplasms. Most neoplasms arise in the parotid gland (70%), whereas tumors of the submandibular gland (22%) and sublingual and minor salivary glands (8%) are less common. The ratio of malignant to benign tumors varies by site as well—parotid gland, 80% benign and 20% malignant; submandibular gland and sublingual gland, 50% benign and 50% malignant; and minor salivary glands, 25% benign and 75% malignant.

The parotid gland is the largest salivary gland and is divided into the superficial lobe and deep lobe by the facial nerve. On imaging, the lobes can be differentiated by the retromandibular vein, which is commonly found at the division of the lobes. Deep lobe tumors lie within the parapharyngeal space. Stensen's duct is approximately 5 cm long; it pierces the buccal fat pad and opens in the oral cavity, opposite the second maxillary molar. The submandibular glands are closely associated with the lingual nerve in the submandibular triangle and empty via Wharton's duct into the papilla, just lateral to the frenulum. The sublingual gland lies on the inner table of the mandible and secretes via tiny openings (ducts of Rivinus) directly into the floor of the mouth or via several ducts that unite to form the common sublingual duct (Bartholin), which then merges with Wharton's duct.

Numerous non-neoplastic diseases commonly affect the salivary glands. Sialadenitis is an acute, subacute, or chronic inflammation of a salivary gland. Acute sialadenitis commonly affects the parotid and submandibular glands and can be caused by bacterial (usually *Staphylococcus aureus*) or viral (mumps) infection. Chronic sialadenitis results from granulomatous inflammation of the glands and is commonly associated with sarcoidosis, actinomycosis, tuberculosis, and cat scratch disease. Sialolithiasis is the accumulation of obstructive calcifications within the glandular ductal system, more common in the submandibular gland (90%) than in the parotid (10%). When the calculi become obstructive, stasis of saliva may cause infection and create a painful, acutely swollen gland. Benign lymphoepithelial lesions of the salivary glands are non-neoplastic glandular enlargements associated with autoimmune diseases, such as Sjögren's syndrome.

Salivary gland neoplasms are most often manifested as slow-growing, well-circumscribed masses. Symptoms such as pain, rapid growth, nerve weakness, and paresthesias and signs of cervical lymphadenopathy and fixation to skin or underlying muscles suggest malignancy. When the initial symptom is complete unilateral facial paralysis, Bell's palsy may be misdiagnosed as the cause, and it is important to remember that all patients with Bell's palsy will show some improvement in facial movement within 6 months of the onset of weakness. Trismus is associated with involvement of the pterygoid musculature by deep parotid lobe malignancies. Bimanual palpation of submandibular masses assists in determining fixation to surrounding structures. CT and MRI tend to show irregular tumor borders and obliteration of fat planes in the parapharyngeal space with deep parotid lobe cancers. The accuracy of fine-needle aspiration cytology of the salivary glands has been well established. The sensitivity, specificity, and accuracy of parotid gland aspirates in one series were 92%, 100%, and 98%, respectively.[37] Excision of the gland is used to confirm the final diagnosis.

Benign tumors of the salivary glands include pleomorphic adenomas, various monomorphic adenomas (e.g., Warthin's tumor, oncocytomas, basal cell adenomas, canalicular adenomas, and myoepitheliomas), various ductal papillomas, and capillary hemangiomas. Pleomorphic adenomas account for 40% to 70% of all tumors of the salivary glands and usually occur in the tail of the parotid. Like all benign parotid tumors, the treatment of choice is surgical excision with a margin of normal tissue (e.g., superficial parotidectomy). In the parotid gland, if excision is possible without complete removal of the affected lobe, the postoperative cosmetic appearance will be superior to that in patients in whom a complete lobe is removed. Shelling out of pleomorphic adenomas is to be avoided because it has been shown to correlate with increased rates of recurrence.[38] The facial nerve should not be sacrificed when removing a benign lesion (Fig. 35-16). Warthin's tumor, or papillary cystadenoma lymphomatosum, is the second most common benign parotid tumor and occurs most often in older white men. Because of the high mitochondrial content within oncocytes, the oncocyte-rich Warthin tumor and oncocytomas will incorporate technetium-99m and appear as hot spots on radionuclide scans. If fine-needle aspiration suggests a slow-growing Warthin tumor with confirmatory technetium scanning in a patient with contraindications to surgery, the tumor may be closely monitored because it has no malignant potential.

Malignant salivary tumors are staged according to size; T1 is smaller than 2 cm, T2 is 2 to 4 cm, T3 is larger than 4 cm (or any tumor with macroscopic extraparenchymal extension), and T4 involves invasion of surrounding tissues. Malignant salivary tumors are listed in Box 35-1. Mucoepidermoid carcinoma is the most common malignant tumor of the parotid gland and can be divided into low-grade and high-grade tumors. High-grade lesions have a propensity for both regional and distant metastases and corresponding shorter survival rates than low-grade mucoepidermoid carcinomas. Adenoid cystic carcinoma constitutes 10% of all salivary neoplasms, with two thirds occurring in the minor salivary glands. The histologic types of adenoid cystic carcinoma are tubular, cribriform, and solid, listed in order from best to worst prognosis. An indolent growth pattern and a relentless propensity for perineural invasion characterize adenoid cystic carcinoma. Regional lymphatic spread is uncommon, although distant metastases occur within the first 5 years after diagnosis and may remain asymptomatic for decades. Malignant mixed tumors include cancers originating from pleomorphic adenomas, termed *carcinoma ex pleomorphic adenoma,* and de novo malignant mixed tumors. The risk for malignant transformation of benign pleomorphic adenomas is 1.5% within

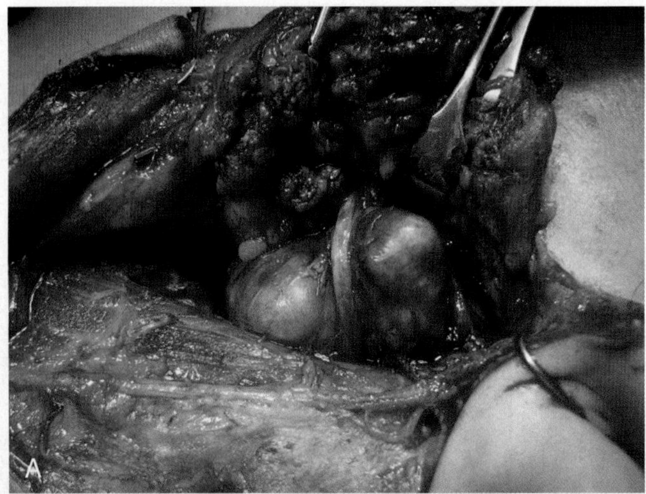

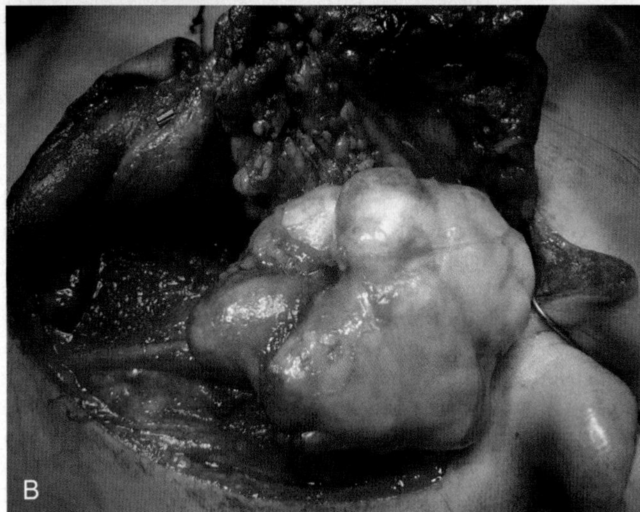

**FIGURE 35-16 A,** 32-year-old woman with a deep parotid lobe pleomorphic adenoma. The facial nerve is displaced laterally. **B,** Once the mass is separated from the prestyloid space, it is delivered around the facial nerve, emptying the compressed parapharyngeal space and avoiding facial nerve injury.

**BOX 35-1 Tumors of the Major and Minor Salivary Glands**

**Benign**
Pleomorphic adenoma
Warthin's tumor
Capillary hemangioma
Oncocytoma
Basal cell adenoma
Canalicular adenoma
Myoepithelioma
Sialadenoma papilliferum
Intraductal papilloma
Inverted ductal papilloma

**Malignant**
Acinic cell carcinoma
Mucoepidermoid carcinoma
Adenoid cystic carcinoma
Polymorphous low-grade adenocarcinoma
Epithelial-myoepithelial carcinoma
Basal cell adenocarcinoma
Sebaceous carcinoma
Papillary cystadenocarcinoma
Mucinous adenocarcinoma
Oncocytic carcinoma
Salivary duct carcinoma
Adenocarcinoma
Myoepithelial carcinoma
Malignant mixed tumor
Squamous cell carcinoma
Small cell carcinoma
Lymphoma
Metastatic carcinoma
Carcinoma ex pleomorphic adenoma

the first 5 years but increases to 9.5% once the benign tumor has been present for more than 15 years.[39] Most salivary gland lymphomas are of the non-Hodgkin's variety (85%). The risk for malignant lymphoma in patients with Sjögren's syndrome is 44-fold higher than in the normal population. Metastatic tumors are most often derived from cutaneous carcinomas and melanomas from the scalp, temporal area, and ear. Distant metastatic tumors are rare but may arise from the lung, kidneys, and breasts.

Treatment of salivary gland malignancies is en bloc surgical excision. Radiation therapy is administered postoperatively for high-grade malignancies demonstrating extraglandular disease, perineural invasion, direct invasion of surrounding tissue, or regional metastases. For tumors confined to the superficial lobe of the parotid gland, lateral lobectomy with preservation of the facial nerve may be performed. Gross tumor should not be left in situ but, if the facial nerve can be preserved by peeling tumor off the nerve, the nerve should be preserved and radiation therapy used for microscopic residual disease. For cancers of the deep lobe, total parotidectomy is performed. Elective neck dissections are performed for high-grade malignancies, such as high-grade mucoepidermoid carcinoma. In patients with gross facial nerve involvement, temporal bone resection is performed and the nerve is sacrificed proximally to obtain a negative margin. When the facial nerve is removed, rehabilitation with a simultaneous nerve graft may be performed in the hope of producing facial muscular tone. Although the primary goal of facial nerve rehabilitation is protection of the cornea from chronic exposure, other concerns include oral competency, nasal valve maintenance, and cosmesis. Upper lid gold weights, lateral tarsorrhaphies, static fascial slings, dynamic muscular slings, and delayed reinnervation procedures are also used for facial rehabilitation. Submandibular gland and minor salivary gland malignancies are treated similarly to parotid gland cancers, by en bloc resection. Submandibular gland malignancies are removed with level I contents and accompanying MRND. Gross involvement of the hypoglossal or lingual nerves requires sacrificing them and obtaining a negative margin by following the nerves toward the skull base. Adenoid cystic cancers are highly neurotropic; treatment consists of removal of gross tumor with radiation therapy for the microscopic disease that is assumed to exist at the periphery of the tumor.

## Neck and Unknown Primary

The workup of a neck mass is different in children than in adults because of differing causes. Cervical masses are common in children and most often represent inflammatory processes or congenital abnormalities. Of pediatric neck masses that are persistent, 2% to 15% that are removed will be malignant. Pediatric evaluation requires thorough head and neck examination, including endoscopy of the nasopharynx and larynx. The most common cause of cervical adenopathy is viral upper respiratory tract infections. The associated lymphadenopathy generally subsides within 2 weeks, although mononucleosis-related lymphadenopathy may persist for 4 to 6 weeks. The location of the mass, as well as its character, most often leads to the diagnosis. Lymphadenopathy not attributable to viral infections may represent a less common infectious process. Bacterial cervical adenitis is most often caused by group A beta-hemolytic streptococci or *S. aureus.* Scrofula is cervical adenitis secondary to tuberculosis and is relatively uncommon in industrialized countries, although atypical mycobacteria may also cause cervical adenitis. Cat scratch disease should be suspected if there is a history of cat contact, and indirect fluorescence antibody testing for *Bartonella henselae* should be performed. Midline masses include thyroglossal duct cysts, enlarged lymph nodes, dermoid cysts, hemangiomas, and pyramidal lobes of the thyroid. Nonlymphoid masses anterior to the sternocleidomastoid muscle are usually branchial cleft cysts. A soft compressible mass of the posterior triangle may represent a lymphangioma (or cystic hygroma), which usually develops before the age of 2 years. Cervical teratomas are present at birth and may involve compression of the airway or esophagus. Malignancies most commonly encountered in pediatric neck masses include sarcomas, lymphomas, and metastatic thyroid carcinoma.

In adults, neck masses represent malignancies more often than in children. It should be emphasized that persistent masses larger than 2 cm represent cancer in 80% of cases. In addition to head and neck examination, CT assists in evaluating not only the masses but also potential primary sites. Fine-needle aspiration (<22-gauge needle) is performed as one of the initial steps in the workup of neck masses; it has an overall accuracy of 95% for benign neck masses and 87% for malignant masses (Fig. 35-17).[40] As in children, the location of the mass has a bearing on the likelihood of diagnosis: midline masses may represent thyroglossal duct cysts, dermoid tumors, delphian nodes, thyroid

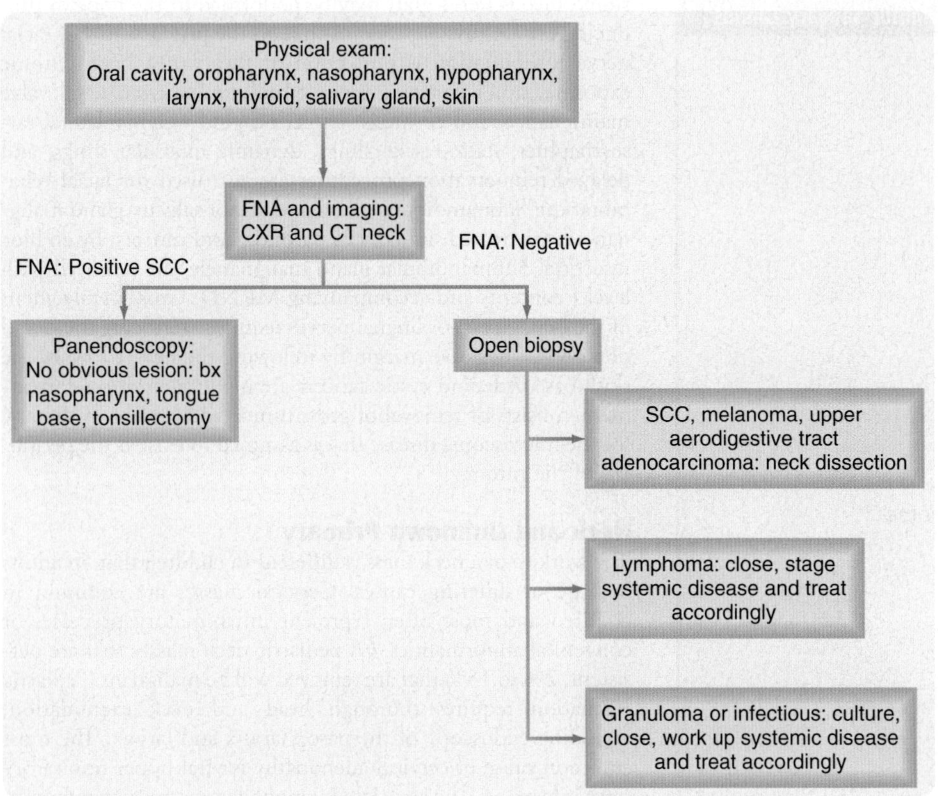


**FIGURE 35-17** Workup of an asymptomatic unilateral neck mass in adults. *CXR,* Chest x-ray; *FNA,* fine-needle aspiration.

masses, lipomas, or sebaceous cysts. Thyroglossal duct cysts represent the vestigial tract of descent that the thyroid followed from the foramen cecum to its normal location below the cricoid. The cyst may become enlarged later in life concurrent with an upper respiratory tract infection. Surgical excision should include the central portion of the hyoid bone (Sistrunk procedure), or recurrence is more likely.

Persistent lateral neck masses in adults may represent enlarged benign or malignant lymph nodes, neuromas or neurofibromas, carotid body tumors, branchial cleft cysts, lipomas, sebaceous cysts, parathyroid cysts, or a primary soft tissue tumor. Enlarged lymph nodes may be have an infectious cause, similar to those in the pediatric population, lymphoma, regional metastases from SCC, melanoma, thyroid carcinoma, or salivary gland tumors, or distant metastases. Usually, lymphadenopathy in an adult is indicative of metastatic HNSCC, with lymphoma being less likely. Metastatic SCC is most frequently from the nasopharynx, oropharynx, or hypopharynx and its presence is a negative prognostic indicator. In all cases of metastases to the neck, lymphadenectomy as treatment is valuable only in cases of SCC, salivary gland tumors, melanoma, and thyroid carcinoma. Otherwise, removal of metastatic lymph nodes is indicated for diagnosis only, and systemic treatment must be initiated. In cases of multiple lymph node enlargement, a diagnosis of HIV infection, toxoplasmosis, or fungal infection should be investigated.

Less frequently, benign neck masses can develop in adults. The branchial cleft apparatus that persists after birth may give rise to a number of neck masses. First branchial cleft cysts develop in the preauricular or submandibular area, are intimately associated with the external auditory canal and parotid gland, and may require dissection of the facial nerve during excision. Second and third branchial cleft cysts and tracts develop anterior to the sternocleidomastoid muscle and often become symptomatic after upper respiratory tract infections. Although the second branchial cleft communicates with the ipsilateral tonsillar fossa, the third communicates with the piriform sinus. Removal of the cyst and tract necessitates dissection along the course of embryologic descent. Second branchial cleft tracts course between the internal and external carotid arteries. Third branchial cleft tracts course posterior to both branches of the carotid artery. Occasionally, a carcinoma may be found within the cyst. Debate continues about whether the carcinoma represents a cystic metastasis from the tongue base or tonsil or whether cancer may occur de novo within a branchial cleft cyst.[41]

Carotid body tumors or chemodectomas are more properly referred to as paragangliomas and arise from the branchiomeric paraganglia at the carotid body. These tumors are usually benign, unifocal, and nonhereditary; they are manifested as a nonpainful mass at the carotid bifurcation and have a characteristic lyre sign on carotid arteriography (Fig. 35-18). Because of their highly vascular nature, biopsy is contraindicated. Preoperative embolization is performed for tumors larger than 3 cm. The most frequent sequela from resection is cranial nerve injury, most commonly of the superior laryngeal nerve, but also the vagal nerve or hypoglossal nerve with large tumors.[42] Tumors larger than 5 cm are associated with a need for concurrent carotid artery replacement. The term *first-bite syndrome* was coined to describe the phenomenon of pain with the initiation of mastication; it is believed to be caused by removal of the sympathetic nerves surrounding the carotid bifurcation and reinnervation of the parotid secretory glands by parasympathetic fibers. Excision

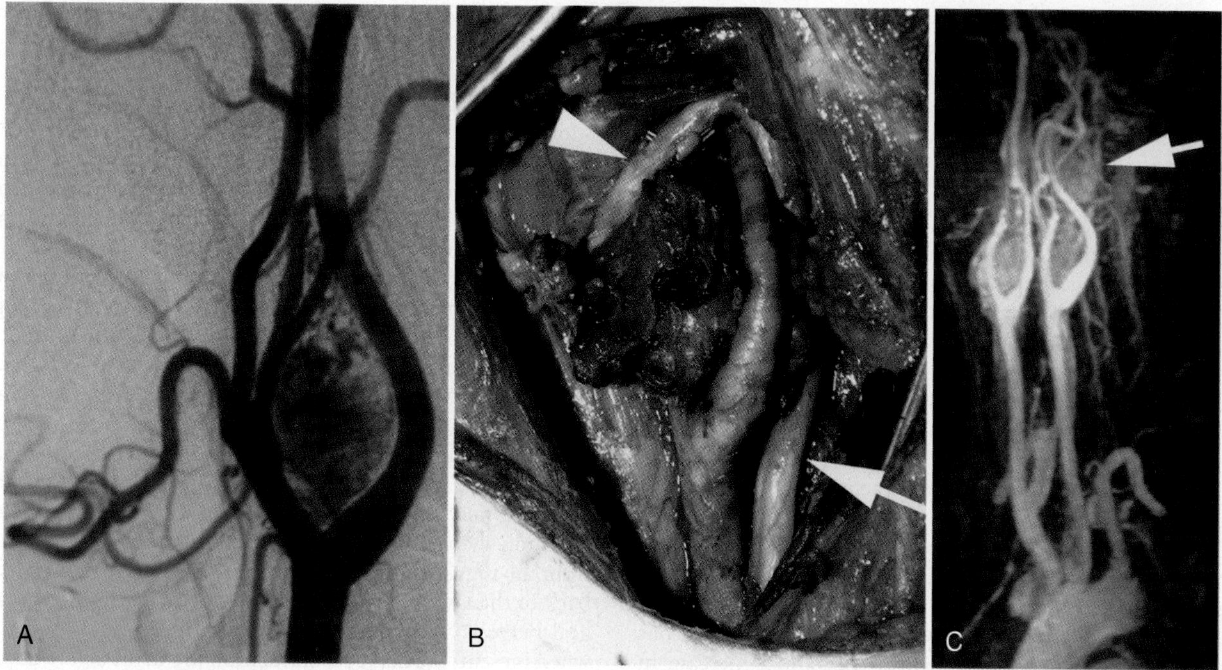


**FIGURE 35-18 A,** Characteristic lyre sign on an arteriogram of a carotid body paraganglioma demonstrating splaying of the internal and external carotid arteries. **B,** The tumor lies between the arteries, superficial to the vagus nerve *(arrow)* and deep to the hypoglossal nerve *(arrowhead)*. **C,** MR angiography scan of a different patient demonstrating bilateral carotid body tumors in addition to a separate, more superior, left vagal paraganglioma *(arrow)*. (Courtesy Dr. J. Netterville.)

of bilateral carotid body tumors may lead to baroreceptor failure, with wide fluctuations in blood pressure.

Tumors of the parapharyngeal space are distinguished by their location; they are prestyloid, usually of salivary gland origin, or poststyloid, usually vascular or neurogenic in origin. Initial symptoms may consist of a superior neck mass, fullness of the parotid gland or tonsillar fossa, trismus, dysphagia, Horner's syndrome, or cranial nerve impairment. Tumors include paraganglioma, salivary gland neoplasms, schwannoma or neurilemoma, lipoma, sarcoma, and lymphadenopathy. Access to these tumors is usually performed transcervically and care must be taken to preserve uninvolved structures, such as the carotid artery and major cranial nerves (Fig. 35-19). A mandibulotomy approach is rarely required.

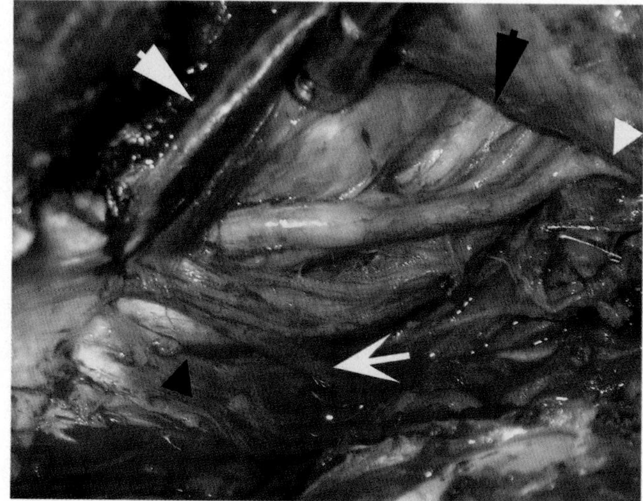

**FIGURE 35-19** Left poststyloid space after removal of a parapharyngeal space tumor and lateral temporal bone resection. The carotid is seen anteriorly *(black arrowhead)* where it enters the skull base, whereas the internal jugular vein *(large white arrowhead)* is retracted posteriorly. The vagus nerve *(large black arrowhead)* is intimately associated with the hypoglossal nerve *(small white arrowhead)*, and separation of the two nerves at this level often leads to vocal cord paralysis. The glossopharyngeal nerve is seen anteriorly *(large white arrow)*.

## TRACHEOTOMY

Tracheotomy is generally used for patients requiring prolonged mechanical ventilation to reduce the risk of damage to the larynx, assist ventilation and pulmonary hygiene, and improve patient comfort and oral care. There is no hard rule about how long a translaryngeal endotracheal tube can be left in place. Some laryngologists recommend conversion to a tracheotomy after 3 days of intubation, although most use 2 to 3 weeks as a limit. Other common reasons for tracheotomy include chronic aspiration, acute airway obstruction secondary to facial or laryngeal trauma or oral or deep neck space infections, or perioperatively during radical cancer ablation.

The term *tracheotomy* implies formation of an opening that will close spontaneously once the tracheotomy tube has been decannulated. Closure via secondary intention generally occurs over a period of 5 to 7 days and the healing process should not be hastened by suturing the overlying skin closed, or an abscess may form in this highly contaminated wound. The term *tracheostomy* implies the formation of a permanent opening that remains open after removal of the tube. The surgeon can form a tracheostomy by suturing an inferiorly based tracheal ring flap to the skin at the time of surgery. Although this flap allows safer replacement of the tracheal tube should it become accidentally decannulated, once the mucocutaneous junction forms, a surgical procedure with rotational skin flaps is required to close the tracheostomy. A permanent tracheostomy should be considered for patients with extended mechanical ventilation, chronic aspiration, obstructive sleep apnea, and/or uncorrectable upper airway obstruction.

Preoperative assessment should include a history of previous tracheotomy or neck surgery, laryngeal pathology, bleeding difficulties, or cervical spine injuries. Perioperative complications of tracheotomy include bleeding, aspiration, pneumothorax and pneumomediastinum, recurrent laryngeal nerve injury, and hypoxia. Long-term problems include the formation of granulation tissue at the skin and within the trachea, collapse of tracheal cartilage and airway obstruction, and tracheoinnominate artery and tracheoesophageal fistulas.

Although the traditional open tracheotomy technique is still primarily used and preferred, percutaneous tracheotomy is being done more often. There have been reports of increased and decreased complication rates with the percutaneous technique versus the open technique.[43,44] Although one might suspect that the trauma from dilating the tracheal rings in the percutaneous technique might be associated with a substantial increase in long-term tracheal stenosis, this does not always seem to be the case; percutaneous tracheotomies have become common in many intensive care units in patients with favorable anatomy and supportive clinical settings.

## VOCAL CORD PARALYSIS

More appropriately termed *vocal fold immobility,* loss of vocal cord function remains a common occurrence. The recurrent laryngeal nerve supplies all the laryngeal musculature except for the cricothyroid muscle, which is supplied by the superior laryngeal nerve. Paralysis of the laryngeal muscles may occur from a lesion in the central nervous system or, usually, with peripheral nerve involvement (90%). Once the vagus nerve exits the jugular foramen, the superior laryngeal nerve divides superiorly in the parapharyngeal space and passes deep to the carotid artery. On the left side, the recurrent laryngeal nerve separates from the vagus nerve in the thorax, passes around the aortic arch at the ductus arteriosus, and travels superiorly in the tracheoesophageal groove to the cricothyroid joint. Probably as a result of the left recurrent nerve's longer course, left vocal cord paralysis is more common than on the right. The right recurrent nerve separates from the vagus and passes around the right subclavian artery and back to the larynx (Fig. 35-20). A nonrecurrent recurrent laryngeal nerve is a rare finding (0.5% to 1.0%) on the right side; when present, the nerve separates from the vagus before descending into the chest, passes directly to the larynx, and is associated with a retroesophageal right subclavian artery. Approaches to the

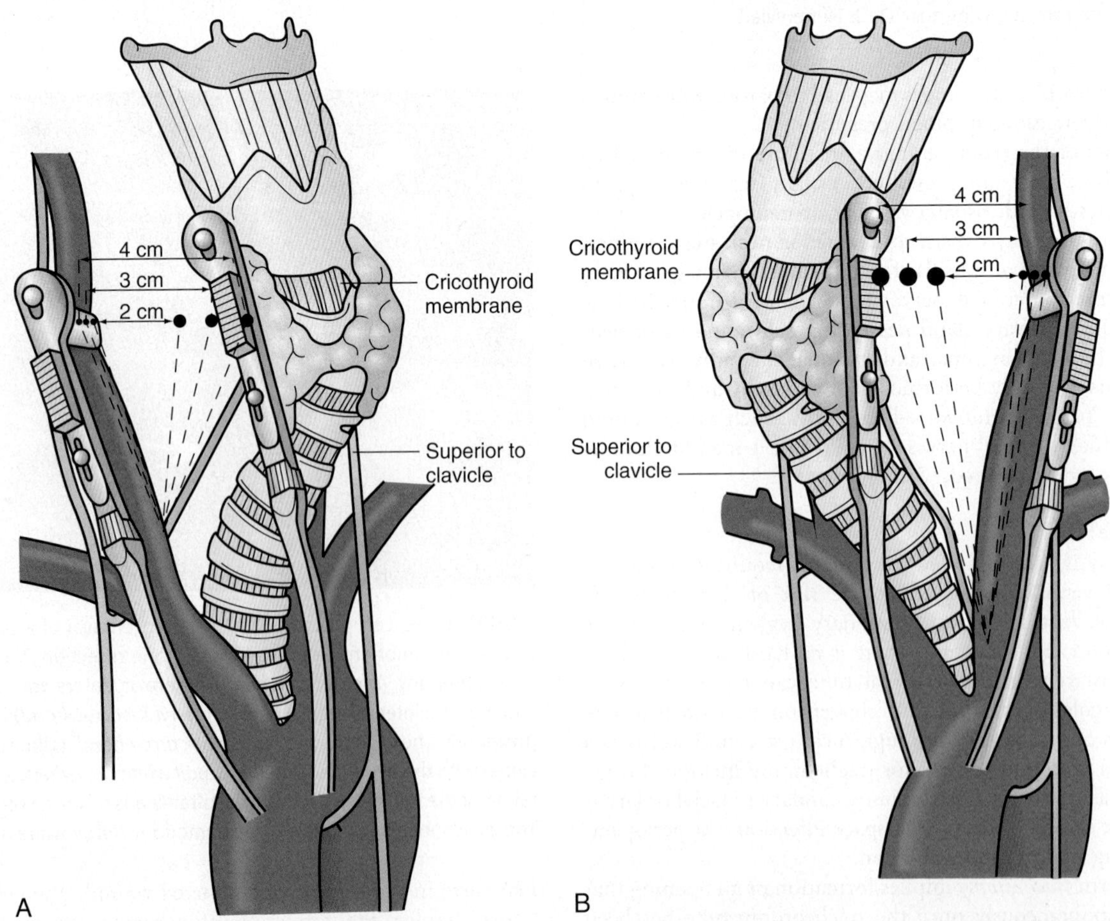


**FIGURE 35-20** Anatomy of the right **(A)** and left **(B)** recurrent laryngeal nerves. The more diagonal course on the right side predisposes patients to traction injury during anterior cervical neck surgery. (From Netterville JL, Koriwchak MJ, Winkle M, et al: Vocal fold paralysis following the anterior approach to the cervical spine. Ann Otol Rhinol Laryngol 105:85–91, 1996.)

cervical spine should generally be performed from the left to reduce traction injury on the recurrent nerve because right-sided approaches have been associated with a higher rate of laryngeal nerve injury.[45]

Dysfunction of the superior laryngeal nerve usually occurs after thyroidectomy because the nerve is in close proximity to the superior thyroid vascular pedicle and affected patients may have difficulty achieving precision in pitch, noticeable usually in professional voice users. Injury to the recurrent laryngeal nerve results in vocal fold paresis or paralysis. Patients with unilateral vocal cord immobility may have hoarseness, ineffective cough, dysphagia, aspiration, or airway compromise or may be completely asymptomatic because of their ability to compensate. Definitive diagnosis is made via laryngoscopy and subtle weakness may require stroboscopic examination. Causes of paralysis include surgical trauma (usually thyroidectomy), malignancies of the thyroid, mediastinum, esophagus, or larynx, mediastinal compression, viral neuropathy, collagen vascular disease, sarcoidosis, diabetic neuropathy, and other reported factors. The cause remains unknown in 20% of patients. Because re-creating volitional abduction and adduction of the vocal cord is not currently feasible, the goal of treatment entails creating sufficient medialization of the involved vocal cord to allow efficient voicing and cough, as well as reduce hoarseness and aspiration. Medialization may be accomplished with intracordal injection of various substances, including fat, Gelfoam, and human cadaveric collagen preparations. Because of the risk for granuloma formation, Teflon injection is rarely used today. Medialization thyroplasty, with or without concurrent arytenoid adduction, consists of a surgically created window in the thyroid cartilage with the insertion of Silastic, hydroxyapatite, or Gore-Tex and has shown excellent results. Laryngeal reinnervation via an ansa cervicalis–recurrent laryngeal nerve anastomosis provides medialization with tone to the paralyzed cord but takes several months to become effective.[46] Bilateral vocal fold paralysis is an uncommon scenario manifested by both vocal folds remaining near the midline position. Patients maintain a strong voice because the vocal folds continue to vibrate, but they might suffer life-threatening airway obstruction and stridor and require immediate reintubation or tracheotomy.

## RECONSTRUCTION

Perhaps the area of head and neck surgery that has undergone the most advancement in the past 25 years is reconstruction, fueled largely by the advent of microvascular free flaps. Today, there is almost no defect that cannot be repaired, which this has afforded the ablative surgeon more leeway in obtaining tumor-free margins. The head and neck region is unique in the intricacy of its form and function, and careful reconstruction is needed to return patients back to their premorbid condition. Focus is usually on speech, swallowing, and cosmesis when considering rehabilitative goals. Swallowing may be impaired by resection of local tissues of the oral cavity, oropharynx, hypopharynx, larynx, and cervical esophagus. Loss of innervation, sensory or motor, locally or at the skull base, can severely impair swallowing. Irradiation leads to fibrosis of local tissues, as well as loss of saliva and taste, and may cause stenosis years after treatment is finished. Speech rehabilitation of speech has been discussed earlier (see "Larynx"). Because of the proximity and complexity of the airway and digestive tracts at the oral cavity, oropharynx, larynx, and hypopharynx, the ability to maintain the two functions is closely related. Frequently, aspiration occurs when the swallowing process is impeded. Although a tracheotomy tube helps protect the airway somewhat from aspiration and allows increased pulmonary suctioning, it also tethers the larynx to the skin and often exacerbates dysphagia. Once dysfunction has occurred, the physician is hampered by trying to maintain balance among airway, speech, and swallowing, and one function may have to be further impaired to improve another. In a severely dysfunctional upper airway, total sacrifice of one function may have to be accepted, and laryngectomy or a permanent gastric tube may be required.

Cosmetic deformities are most obvious in the head and neck area. Functional deficits not only occur in speech and swallowing but also affect eyelid function, oral competence, and maintenance of a nasal and oral airway. General principles of facial restoration include reconstructing the underlying bony framework, replacing skin with skin of matching quality, minimizing scar visibility and contracture, and reconstructing in zones of facial units. Skin should be matched by color, thickness, and hair-bearing units, when possible. The aesthetic facial units include the forehead, eyes and periorbital area, midface, nose (which itself contains several subunits), and lips and mentum. A spectrum of reconstructive options exists, with healing by secondary intention and primary closure at one end and extensive reconstruction such as microvascular free flaps at the other. The option that is selected depends on the location and severity of the defect, overall health of the patient, available donor sites for flaps, status of the tissue adjacent to the defect (irradiated, infected, previously operated), and functionality of the area to be reconstructed. Not only must the reconstructive surgeon choose which option is best for a given defect, but secondary and tertiary options should be also planned in case of flap failure or recurrent disease.

Healing by secondary intention is an excellent option in several clinical scenarios. Mucosal defects with an underlying layer of vascularized muscle or bone that will not contract to the point of impeding function may be left to close by secondary intention. Examples include small tonsillectomy defects, tongue resections, and some laryngeal mucosal defects. Primary closure is likely to be the most commonly used option for closure of cutaneous defects. Attempts should be made to keep incisions within the lines of relaxed skin tension. These lines are caused by muscular insertion into the skin and form when there is mimetic motion. Incisions that parallel the lines of relaxed skin tension not only respect the aesthetic units of the face but also have the least amount of tension along them, which decreases scarring. A Z-plasty may be used to reorient an unfavorable line of closure into a relaxed skin tension line.

Skin grafts are generally used for oral cavity, ear, or maxillectomy defects, and for coverage of donor sites, such as the radial forearm and fibular free flaps and deltopectoral flap. Skin grafts are completely dependent for nutrition on the tissue over which they are placed and can heal well over muscle, perichondrium, and periosteum. They do not take well over bone or cartilage, nor on tissue that has been irradiated or infected or is hypovascular. Split-thickness skin grafts contain the epidermis and a portion of the dermis and are harvested with a dermatome at approximately 0.012- to 0.018-inch thickness. Thinner grafts require less nutrients to remain viable but will also contract more when healing. Grafts may be meshed to allow greater surface coverage, but these types of grafts are generally restricted to the scalp or over muscle because of a less cosmetic result. A nonadherent antibiotic-impregnated bolster is commonly used to maintain stability between the split-thickness skin graft and recipient bed for 5 days to allow transmission of nutrients and capillary ingrowth while healing. Harvest sites include the anterior and lateral aspects of the thighs and buttocks.

Full-thickness skin grafts are characterized by a better color match, texture, and contour and less contracture but success rates lower than with split-thickness skin grafts. Commonly used donor sites include the postauricular, upper eyelid, and supraclavicular fossa skin. Composite grafts are occasionally needed for cartilage and skin reconstruction of the nasal ala and may be harvested from the conchal bowl without significantly affecting the appearance of the pinna. Acellular cadaveric human dermis that has been prepared by removing immunogenic cells while leaving the collagen matrix intact has grown in popularity as a skin graft substitute and avoids the need for a donor site.

Local skin flaps have an excellent tissue match because of their proximity to the defect. Commonly used designs include advancement, rotation, transposition, rhomboid, and bilobed flaps. Similar to primary closure, local flaps should be designed to be incorporated into the lines of relaxed skin tension. Although local flaps depend on the subdermal plexus of capillaries, regional flaps have an axial blood supply. This latter vascular pedicle is necessary for flap viability because greater distances are spanned by the flap and it is contained within the subcutaneous fascia, as in a fasciocutaneous flap, or within an underlying muscle, as in a myocutaneous flap. The deltopectoral, or Bakamjian, flap was one of the early regional flaps and was used extensively in head and neck reconstruction. Based on the intercostal perforating branches from the internal mammary artery, the flap is based medially and is designed over the upper pectoralis and deltoid regions. Because of the pliability of the transferred skin, it can be swung upward for skin defects or pharyngeal reconstruction.

Perhaps the development with the most significant impact on head and neck reconstruction was introduction of the pectoralis myocutaneous flap in 1978. Based on the pectoral branch of the thoracoacromial artery, the artery pierces the pectoralis muscle from the deep surface. A skin paddle designed over the muscle, or simply the muscle itself, may be transferred to reconstruct defects up to the nasopharynx. Historically, the pectoralis muscle was tunneled under the intervening skin to preserve the ipsilateral deltopectoral flap in case it was needed for future coverage. Division of the pectoral nerve branches ensures atrophy of the muscle and reduces the bulge over the clavicle. In addition to reconstruction of mucosal defects with the vascularized skin, coverage of an exposed carotid artery is an excellent use of the myogenous flap. The trapezius muscle offers multiple soft tissue flaps that may be rotated into head and neck defects. The lower trapezius myocutaneous flap, based on the dorsal scapular artery, has already been referred to as an excellent choice for lateral temporal bone defects. Finally, the submental and platysmal flaps are based on the facial artery and provide excellent local flap coverage for oral and oropharyngeal defects.

A free flap entails removal of composite tissue from a distant site, along with its blood supply, and reimplantation of the vasculature in the reconstructive field. Although the first successful human microvasculature transfer was a jejunal interposition flap in 1959, the modern era of microvasculature reconstruction did not arise until the 1970s, with improvements in instrumentation and technique. The current selection of donor sites allows the benefit of choosing among sites with large-caliber, long vascular pedicles that are anatomically consistent. In addition to favorable vascularity, optimal donor sites allow a simultaneous two-team approach of ablation and harvesting, possibility of a sensate flap, composite transfer of bone stock capable of accepting osseointegrated implants, transfer of secretory mucosa, or any combinations of these options. Patient selection for free flap reconstruction is of critical importance. Advanced age is not a contraindication to microvascular reconstruction, although previous recipient bed irradiation, contraction of tissues after secondary reconstruction, or previous free flap failure should raise concern in the reconstructive surgeon. Complete loss of a free tissue transfer should occur in less than 5% of cases.

The radial aspect of the forearm has emerged as the workhorse of soft tissue free flaps in head and neck reconstruction. A fasciocutaneous flap with sensate capabilities, the radial forearm flap is based on the radial artery and its venae comitantes, cephalic vein, or both for drainage. Variations of the flap include harvest of partial radius bone or palmaris longus tendon for bony or suspensory reconstruction, respectively. The main advantage of the radial forearm flap is the thinness and pliability of the harvested skin, which makes it ideal not only for external cutaneous defects but also for reconstruction of the floor of the mouth or tongue (Fig. 35-21), soft palate and oropharyngeal wall, and pharynx, and for skull base reconstruction. Although the donor site is more cosmetically obvious than other donor sites, long-term morbidity of the harvest is minimal. Other soft tissue flaps include the lateral arm flap, anterolateral thigh and lateral thigh flaps, latissimus dorsi flap, and rectus abdominis flap. The lateral arm flap is an excellent alternative to the radial forearm flap when the patient exhibits a dominant radial artery supply to the hand, which is a contraindication to use of the forearm site. The lateral arm flap is based on the posterior branches of the radial collateral vessels. It offers slightly more bulk than the radial forearm flap does but is compromised to some extent by vessels that are smaller in caliber. Experience with thigh flaps has shown excellent results in tubed reconstruction of the pharynx. Both the latissimus dorsi and rectus abdominis flaps can be transferred as myogenous or myocutaneous flaps. Although skin match is not ideal, these flaps are best suited to large defects, including skull base repair or maxillectomy defects with orbital exenteration (Fig. 35-22). Harvest of the rectus abdominis may lead to the complication of postoperative hernia formation.

Enteric flaps include the gastro-omental flap and the jejunal flap. Disadvantages of these donor sites include the need for a laparotomy, which may preclude a two-team approach. In addition, the acceptable ischemia time is shortest with the enteric flaps because of their high tissue oxygen and nutrient demand. Unlike other donor sites, the pedicle of these flaps cannot be divided even years postoperatively because the flap tissues do not incorporate blood supply from the surrounding tissue bed. The main advantages of enteric flaps are their pliability and ability to continue secreting mucus. In an irradiated patient who suffers from xerostomia, enteric reconstruction of recurrent oral or oropharyngeal tumors affords the opportunity to improve his or her quality of life significantly. The omentum of the gastro-omental flap may be draped into the neck to provide contour and bulk to a neck that has previously been dissected.

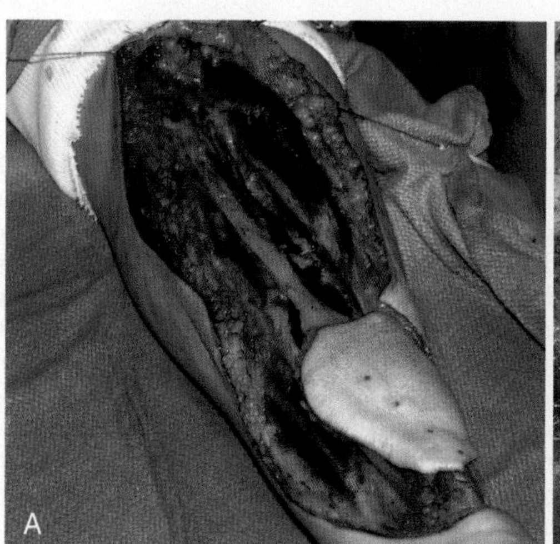


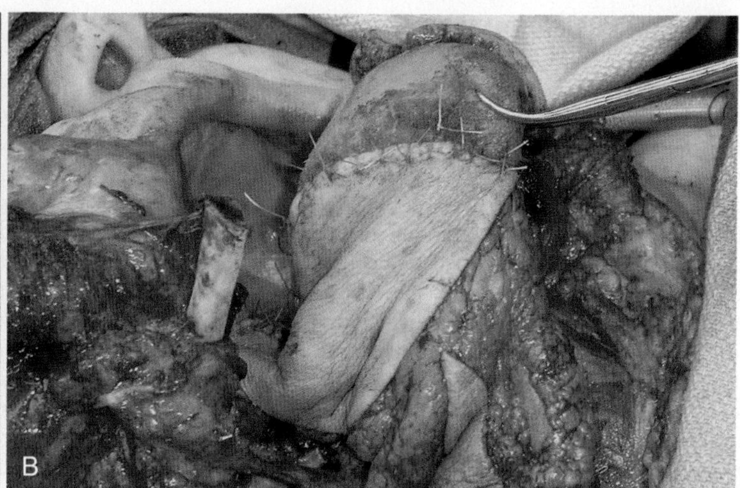


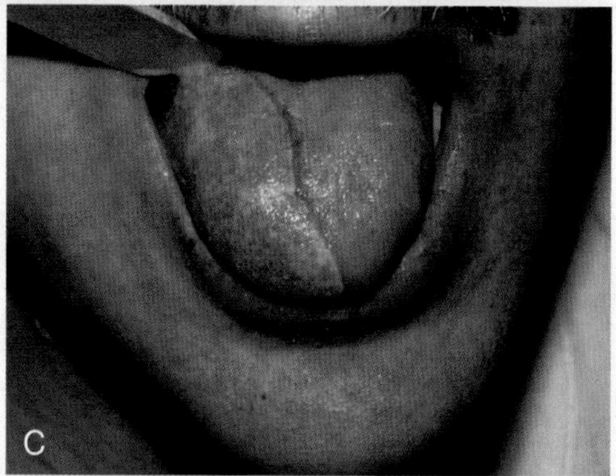


**FIGURE 35-21 A,** Harvest of a radial forearm fasciocutaneous free flap based on the radial artery. **B,** Right hemiglossectomy for squamous cell carcinoma of the right mobile tongue reconstructed with a radial forearm flap. **C,** Postoperative result 1 year later demonstrating excellent contour and tongue mobility.

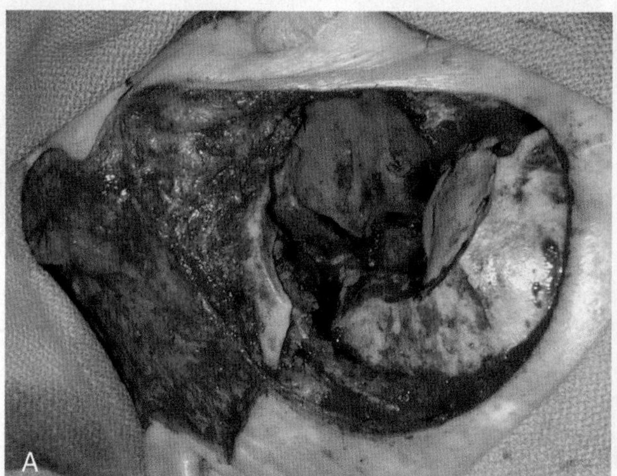


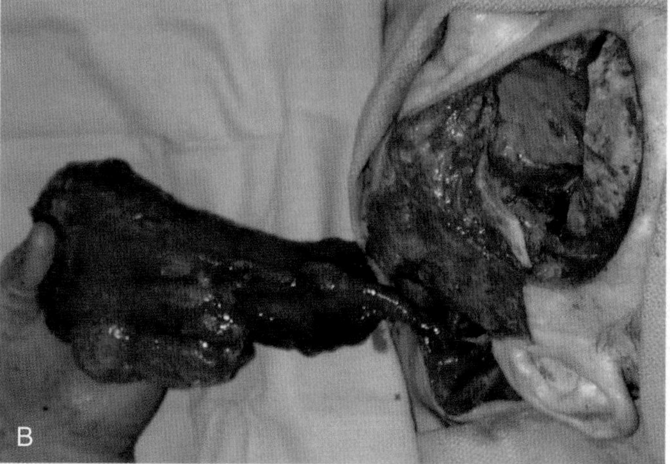


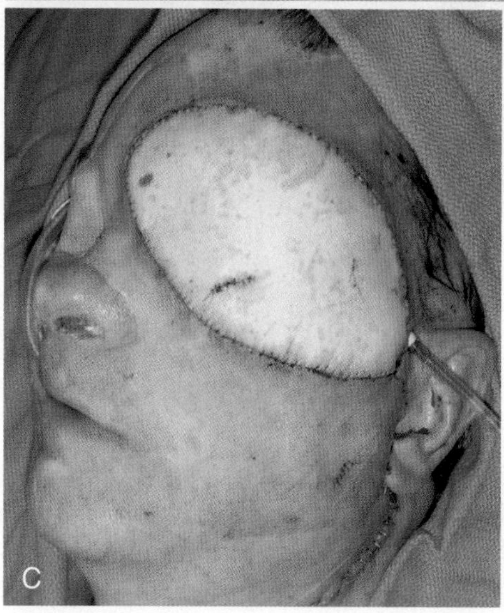


**FIGURE 35-22 A,** Resection of a recurrent skin squamous cell carcinoma invading the left orbit, paranasal sinuses, and frontal lobe dura. **B,** A rectus abdominis myocutaneous free flap has been revascularized with microvascular techniques into the recipient vessels of the neck, with the flap inset into place **(C)** for cutaneous and skull base reconstruction.

The most commonly used osseous free flaps include the fibula, scapula, and iliac crest. The fibular free flap is based on the peroneal artery and vein, and the blood supply to the foot should be investigated before harvesting this flap.[47] Up to 25 cm of fibula may be harvested for mandibular or maxillary reconstruction with an osseous or osteocutaneous graft, and donor site morbidity is minimal (Fig. 35-23). The bone stock of the fibula is sufficient to allow osseointegrated implantation for dentition or prosthetic anchors. The iliac crest osteocutaneous free flap allows even greater bone stock and is already naturally shaped in the form of a mandibular angle. Like the rectus abdominis flap, the iliac crest is hampered by the potential for postoperative hernias and has a relatively short vascular pedicle. Although the scapular free flap has the least bone stock of the three osseous flaps, it offers the advantage of simultaneous muscular, cutaneous, and bony reconstruction based on separate pedicles, thus allowing tremendous versatility in flap orientation. The megaflap includes the lateral border of the scapula based on the angular artery or the periosteal branch of the circumflex scapular artery, scapular or parascapular skin paddle based on cutaneous branches of the circumflex scapular artery, and latissimus dorsi and serratus anterior muscles supplied by the thoracodorsal artery. All arterial branches lead to the subscapular artery where it branches from the axillary artery, and revascularization of all segments may be accomplished with a single arterial anastomosis.

Perhaps the ultimate in head and neck reconstruction lies in the possibility of replacing ablated tissue with identical cadaveric donor tissue. In 1998, the first successful human laryngeal transplantation was performed with microvascular reconstruction (Fig. 35-24).[48] Not only the larynx but also the pharynx, thyroid, parathyroids, and trachea were transplanted. Since the initial laryngeal transplant, further transplants of both the larynx and trachea have been performed successfully, but until nontoxic

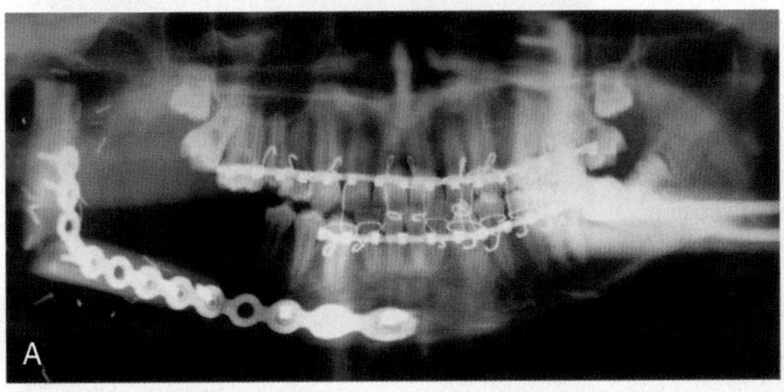


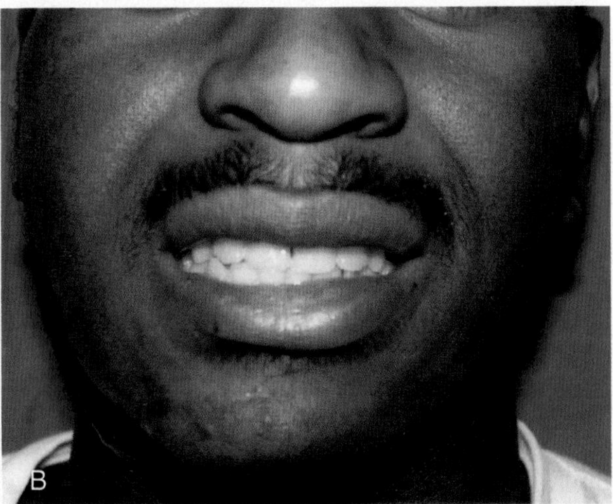


**FIGURE 35-23 A,** Immediate postoperative radiograph of a 35-year-old man after resection of an osteosarcoma of the mandibular ramus and reconstruction with a fibular osseocutaneous free flap. **B,** At 6 months postoperatively, the patient's dental occlusion has been preserved, along with excellent facial contour.

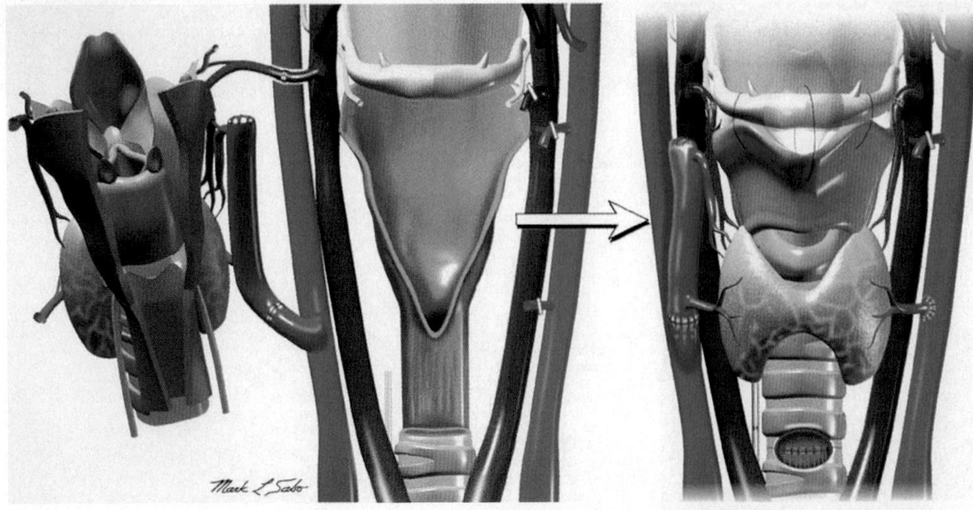

**FIGURE 35-24** Schematic of the first successful laryngeal transplantation, performed in 1998. Not only was the larynx transplanted, but the thyroid, parathyroids, pharynx, and five rings of trachea accompanied the vascularized and innervated organ. (From Strome M, Stein J, Esclamado R, et al: Laryngeal transplantation and 48-month follow-up. N Engl J Med 344:1676–1679, 2001.)

immunosuppressive drugs and protection against fostering tumor recurrence have been developed, nonvital organ transplantation are unlikely to become commonplace.

## SELECTED REFERENCES

Bocca E, Pignataro: A conservation technique in radical neck dissection. Ann Otol Rhinol Laryngol 76:975–987, 1967.

A landmark paper demonstrating equal control of metastatic neck disease with radical neck dissection and modified radical neck dissection while avoiding the morbidity of unnecessary removal of neck structures.

Fakhry C, Westra WH, Li S, et al: Improved survival of patients with human papillomavirus-positive head and neck squamous cell carcinoma in a prospective clinical trial. J Natl Cancer Inst 100:261–269, 2008.

A recent phase II trial that suggests that when HNSCC is associated with HPV infection, the prognosis is significantly improved over non-HPV tumors. This landmark study was the first to demonstrate that tumor HPV status is a favorable prognostic marker in uniform patient populations with similar treatment protocols. Many physicians advise that tumor HPV status should be incorporated as a stratification factor in patients with oropharyngeal cancer, although basing treatment protocols on HPV status has yet to be definitively investigated.

Naudo P, Laccourreye O, Weinstein G, et al: Complications and functional outcome after supracricoid partial laryngectomy with cricohyoidoepiglottopexy. Otolaryngol Head Neck Surg 118:124–129, 1998.

This paper describes the outstanding functional results of supracricoid laryngectomy in terms of speech and swallowing while obtaining excellent local control of disease.

The Department of Veterans Affairs Laryngeal Cancer Study Group: Induction chemotherapy plus radiation compared with surgery plus radiation in patients with advanced laryngeal cancer. N Engl J Med 324:1685–1690, 1991.

This multi-institutional randomized trial demonstrated equal success between chemoradiation therapy and surgery with irradiation for laryngeal carcinoma while allowing patients who responded to the conservation treatment to keep their larynx.

## REFERENCES

1. Edge SB, Byrd DR, Compton CC, et al, editors: AJCC cancer staging manual, ed 7, New York, 2010, Springer-Verlag.
2. Chaturvedi AK, Engels EA, Anderson WF, et al: Incidence trends for human papillomavirus–related and unrelated oral squamous cell carcinomas in the United States. J Clin Oncol 26:612–619, 2008.
3. Johnson N: Tobacco use and oral cancer: a global perspective. J Dent Educ 65:328–339, 2001.
4. Cooper JS, Porter K, Mallin K, et al: The National Cancer Database report on cancer of the head and neck: 10-year update. Head Neck 31:748–758, 2009.
5. Gillison ML: Current topics in the epidemiology of oral cavity and oropharyngeal cancers. Head Neck 29:779–792, 2007.
6. Stadler M, Patel M, Couch M, et al: Molecular biology of head and neck cancer. Hemat Oncol Clin N Am 22:1099–1124, 2008.
7. Li C, Hu Z, Lu J, et al: Genetic polymorphisms in DNA base-excision repair genes ADPRT, XRCC1, and APE1 and the risk of squamous cell carcinoma of the head and neck. Cancer 110:867–875, 2007.
8. Califano J, van der Riet P, Westra W, et al: Genetic progression model for head and neck cancer: Implications for field cancerization. Cancer Res 56:2488–2492, 1996.
9. Hugo H, Ackland ML, Blick T, et al: Epithelial-mesenchymal and mesenchymal-epithelial transitions in carcinoma progression. J Cell Physiol 213:374–383, 2007.
10. Kalyankrishna S, Grandis JR: Epidermal growth factor receptor biology in head and neck cancer. J Clin Oncol 24:2666–2672, 2006.
11. Pollak MN, Schernhammer ES, Hankinson SE: Insulin-like growth factors and neoplasia. Nat Rev Cancer 4:505–518, 2004.
12. Kutler DI, Wong RJ, Kraus DH: Functional imaging in head and neck cancer. Curr Oncol Rep 7:137–144, 2005.
13. Bourhis J, Wibault P, Lusinchi A, et al: Status of accelerated fractionation radiotherapy in head and neck squamous cell carcinomas. Curr Opin Oncol 9:262–266, 1997.
14. The Department of Veterans Affairs Laryngeal Cancer Study Group: Induction chemotherapy plus radiation compared with surgery plus radiation in patients with advanced laryngeal cancer. N Engl J Med 324:1685–1690, 1991.
15. Bernier J, Domenge C, Ozashin M, et al: Postoperative irradiation with or without concurrent chemotherapy for locally advanced head and neck cancer. N Engl J Med 350:1945–1952, 2004.
16. Cooper JS, Pajak TF, Forastiere AA, et al: Postoperative concurrent radiotherapy and chemotherapy for high-risk squamous cell carcinoma of the head and neck. N Engl J Med 350:1937–1944, 2004.
17. Roy S, Tibesar RJ, Daly K, et al: Role of planned neck dissection for advanced metastatic disease in tongue base or tonsil squamous cell carcinoma treated with radiotherapy. Head Neck 24:474–481, 2002.
18. Bocca E, Pignataro O: A conservation technique in radical neck dissection. Ann Otol Rhinol Laryngol 76:975–987, 1967.
19. Kuriakose MA, Trivedi NP: Sentinel node biopsy in head and neck squamous cell carcinoma. Curr Opin Otolaryngol Head Neck Surg 17:100–110, 2009.
20. O'Brien CJ, Lauer CS, Fredricks S, et al: Tumor thickness influences prognosis of T1 and T2 oral cavity cancer—but what thickness? Head Neck 25:937–945, 2003.
21. Gooris PJ, Vermey A, de Visscher JG, et al: Supraomohyoid neck dissection in the management of cervical lymph node metastases of squamous cell carcinoma of the lower lip. Head Neck 24:678–683, 2002.
22. Strome SE, To W, Strawderman M, et al: Squamous cell carcinoma of the buccal mucosa. Otolaryngol Head Neck Surg 120:375–379, 1999.
23. Adelstein DJ, Saxton JP, Rybicki LA, et al: Multiagent concurrent chemoradiotherapy for locoregionally advanced squamous cell head and neck cancer: Mature results from a single institution. J Clin Oncol 24:1064–1071, 2006.
24. Fakhry C, Westra WH, Li S, et al: Improved survival of patients with human papillomavirus–positive head and neck squamous cell carcinoma in a prospective clinical trial. J Natl Cancer Inst 100:261–269, 2008.

25. Lefebvre JL, Chevalier D, Luboinski B, et al: Larynx preservation in piriform sinus cancer: Preliminary results of a European Organization for Research and Treatment of Cancer phase III trial. EORTC Head and Neck Cancer Cooperative Group. J Natl Cancer Inst 88:890–899, 1996.
26. Kirchner JA: Vocal fold histopathology: A symposium, San Diego, Calif, 1986, College-Hill Press.
27. Ambrosch P, Kron M, Steiner W: Carbon dioxide laser microsurgery for early supraglottic carcinoma. Ann Otol Rhinol Laryngol 107:680–688, 1998.
28. Steiner W, Vogt P, Ambrosch P, Kron M: Transoral carbon dioxide laser microsurgery for recurrent glottic carcinoma after radiotherapy. Head Neck 26:477–484, 2004.
29. Muscatello L, Laccourreye O, Biacabe B, et al: Laryngofissure and cordectomy for glottic carcinoma limited to the mid third of the mobile true vocal cord. Laryngoscope 107:1507–1510, 1997.
30. Naudo P, Laccourreye O, Weinstein G, et al: Complications and functional outcome after supracricoid partial laryngectomy with cricohyoidoepiglottopexy. Otolaryngol Head Neck Surg 118:124–129, 1998.
31. Solares CA, Wood B, Rodriguez CP, et al: Does vocal cord fixation preclude nonsurgical management of laryngeal cancer? Laryngoscope 119:1130–1134, 2009.
32. Imola MJ, Schramm VL: Orbital preservation in surgical management of sinonasal malignancy. Laryngoscope 112:1357–1365, 2002.
33. Vasef MA, Ferlito A, Weiss LM: Clinicopathological consultation: Nasopharyngeal carcinoma, with emphasis on its relationship to Epstein-Barr virus. Ann Otol Rhinol Laryngol 106:348–356, 1997.
34. Al-Sarraf M, LeBlanc M, Giri PB, et al: Chemoradiotherapy versus radiotherapy in patients with advanced nasopharyngeal cancer: Phase III randomized Intergroup Study 0099. J Clin Oncol 16:1310–1317, 1998.
35. Jia WH, Huang QH, Liao J, et al: Trends in incidence and mortality of nasopharyngeal carcinoma over a 20–25 year period (1978/1983–2002) in Sihui and Cangwu counties in southern China. BMC Cancer 6:178, 2006.
36. Lorenz RR, Dean RL, Chuang J, Citardi MJ: Endoscopic reconstruction of anterior and middle cranial fossa defects using acellular dermal allograft. Laryngoscope 113:496–501, 2003.
37. Stewart CJ, MacKenzie K, McGarry GW, et al: Fine-needle aspiration cytology of salivary gland: A review of 341 cases. Diagn Cytopathol 22:139–146, 2000.
38. Witt RL: The significance of the margin in parotid surgery for pleomorphic adenoma. Laryngoscope 112:2141–2154, 2002.
39. Seifert G: Histopathology of malignant salivary gland tumours. Eur J Cancer B Oral Oncol 28B:49–52, 1992.
40. Amedee RG, Dhurandhar NR: Fine-needle aspiration biopsy. Laryngoscope 111:1551–1557, 2001.
41. Zimmermann CE, von Domarus H, Moubayed P: Carcinoma in situ in a lateral cervical cyst. Head Neck 24:965–969, 2002.
42. Cohen SM, Burkey BB, Netterville JL: Surgical management of parapharyngeal space masses. Head Neck 27:669–675, 2005.
43. van Heurn LW, Goei R, de Ploeg I, et al: Late complications of percutaneous dilatational tracheotomy. Chest 110:1572–1576, 1996.
44. Kost KM: Endoscopic percutaneous dilatational tracheotomy: A prospective evaluation of 500 consecutive cases. Laryngoscope 115:1–30, 2005.
45. Netterville JL, Koriwchak MJ, Winkle M, et al: Vocal fold paralysis following the anterior approach to the cervical spine. Ann Otol Rhinol Laryngol 105:85–91, 1996.
46 Lorenz RR, Teker AM, Strome M, et al: Ansa cervicalis-to-recurrent laryngeal nerve anastomosis for unilateral vocal fold paralysis: A single institutional experience. Ann Otol Rhinol Laryngol 117:40–45, 2008.
47. Lorenz RR, Esclamado R: Preoperative magnetic resonance angiography in fibular free flap reconstruction of head and neck defects. Head Neck 23:844–850, 2001.
48. Strome M, Stein J, Esclamado R, et al: Laryngeal transplantation and 40-month follow-up. N Engl J Med 344:1676–1679, 2001.

# SECTION VII

# BREAST

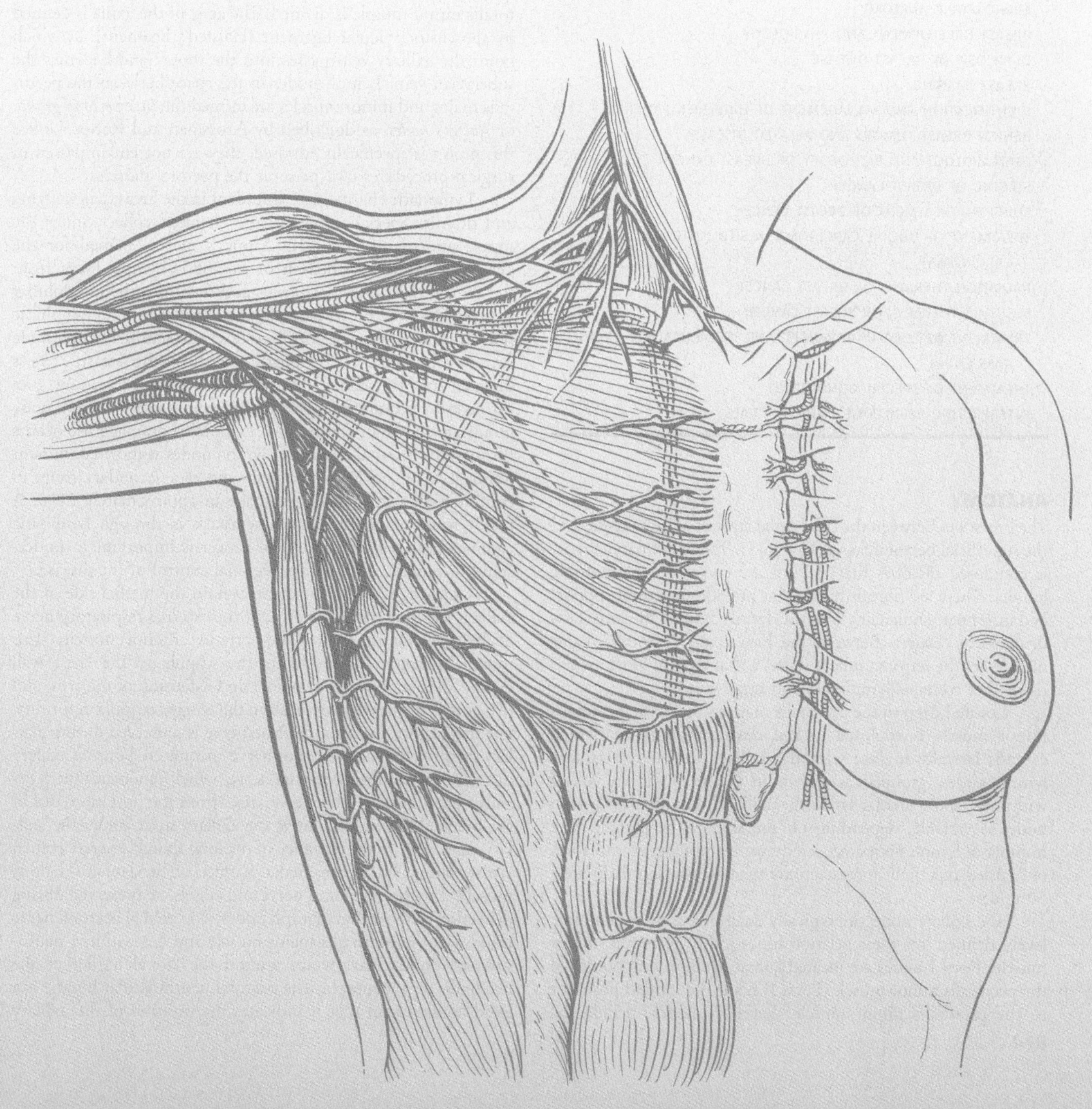

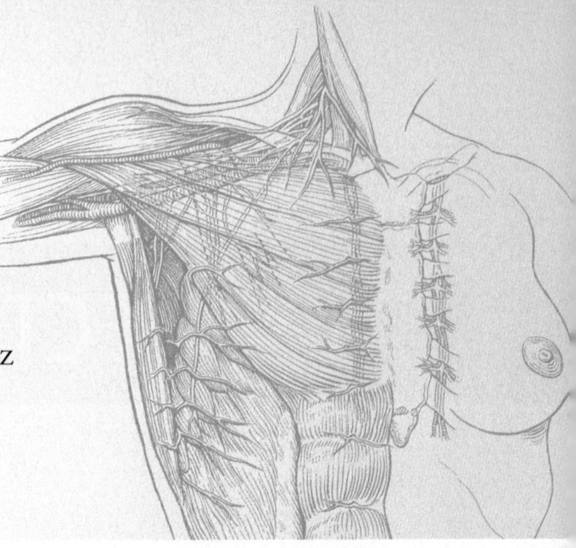

CHAPTER 36

# DISEASES OF THE BREAST

Kelly K. Hunt, Marjorie C. Green, and Thomas A. Buchholz



## ANATOMY

The breast lies between the subdermal layer of adipose tissue and the superficial pectoral fascia (Fig. 36-1). The breast parenchyma is composed of lobes that in turn are comprised of multiple lobules. There are fibrous bands that provide structural support and insert perpendicularly into the dermis, termed the *suspensory ligaments of Cooper.* Between the breast and pectoralis major muscle lies the retromammary space, a thin layer of loose areolar tissue that contains lymphatics and small vessels.

Located deep to the pectoralis major muscle, the pectoralis minor muscle is enclosed in the clavipectoral fascia, which extends laterally to fuse with the axillary fascia. The axillary lymph nodes, grouped as shown in Figure 36-2, are found within the loose areolar fat of the axilla; the number of lymph nodes is variable, depending on the size of the patient. The number of lymph nodes recovered from pathologic examination of Halsted-type radical mastectomy specimens is approximately 50 nodes.

The axillary nodes are typically described as three anatomic levels defined by their relationship to the pectoralis minor muscle. Level I nodes are located lateral to the lateral border of the pectoralis minor muscle. Level II nodes are located posterior to the pectoralis minor muscle. Level III nodes include the subclavicular nodes medial to the pectoralis minor muscle. The level III nodes are easier to visualize and remove when the pectoralis minor muscle is divided. The apex of the axilla is defined by the costoclavicular ligament (Halsted's ligament), at which point the axillary vein passes into the thorax and becomes the subclavian vein. Lymph nodes in the space between the pectoralis major and minor muscles are termed the *interpectoral group,* or *Rotter's nodes,* as described by Grossman and Rotter. Unless this group is specifically exposed, they are not encompassed in surgical procedures that preserve the pectoral muscles.

Lymphatic channels are abundant in the breast parenchyma and dermis. Specialized lymphatic channels collect under the nipple and areola and form Sappey's plexus, named for the anatomist who described them in 1885. Lymph flows from the skin to the subareolar plexus and then into the interlobular lymphatics of the breast parenchyma. Appreciation of lymphatic flow is important for performing successful sentinel lymph node surgery (see later). Of lymphatic flow from the breast, 75% is directed into the axillary lymph nodes. A minor amount goes through the pectoralis muscle and into more medial lymph node groups, as shown in Figure 36-2. Lymphatic drainage also occurs through the internal mammary lymph nodes as the predominant drainage in up to 5% of patients and as a secondary route in combination with axillary drainage in approximately 20%. A major route of breast cancer metastasis is through lymphatic channels; the regional spread of cancer is important to understand to provide optimal locoregional control of the disease.

Coursing close to the chest wall on the medial side of the axilla is the long thoracic nerve, or the external respiratory nerve of Bell, which innervates the serratus anterior muscle. This muscle is important for fixing the scapula to the chest wall during adduction of the shoulder and extension of the arm, and division of the nerve may result in the winged scapula deformity. For this reason, the long thoracic nerve is preserved during axillary surgery. The second major nerve encountered during axillary dissection is the thoracodorsal nerve, which innervates the latissimus dorsi muscle. This nerve arises from the posterior cord of the brachial plexus and enters the axillary space under the axillary vein, close to the entrance of the long thoracic nerve. It then crosses the axilla to the medial surface of the latissimus dorsi muscle. The thoracodorsal nerve and vessels are preserved during dissection of the axillary lymph nodes. The medial pectoral nerve innervates the pectoralis major muscle and lies within a neurovascular bundle that wraps around the lateral border of the pectoralis minor muscle. The pectoral neurovascular bundle is a good landmark in that it indicates the position of the axillary

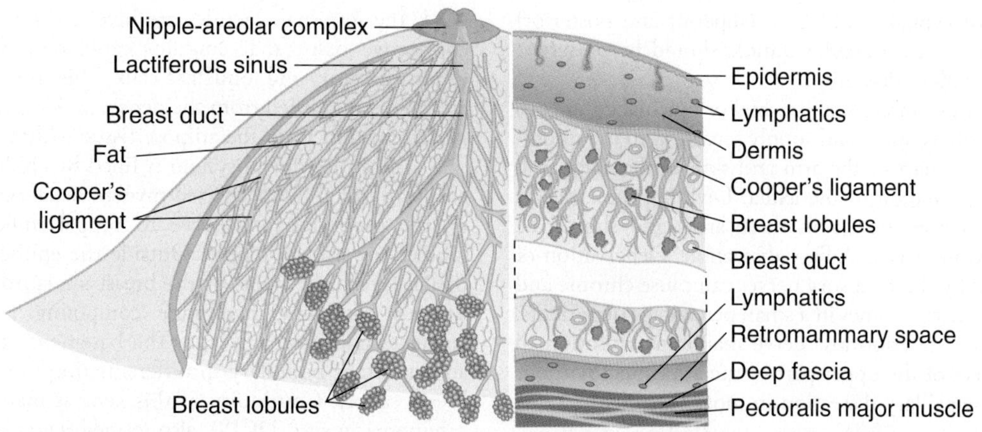


**FIGURE 36-1** Cut-away diagram of a mature resting breast. The breast lies cushioned in fat between the overlying skin and pectoralis major muscle. Both the skin and retromammary space under the breast are rich with lymphatic channels. Cooper's ligaments, the suspensory ligaments of the breast, fuse with the overlying superficial fascia just under the dermis, coalesce as the interlobular fascia in the breast parenchyma, and then join with the deep fascia of breast over the pectoralis muscle. The system of ducts in the breast is configured like an inverted tree, with the largest ducts just under the nipple and successively smaller ducts in the periphery. After several branching generations, small ducts at the periphery enter the breast lobule, which is the milk-forming glandular unit of the breast.

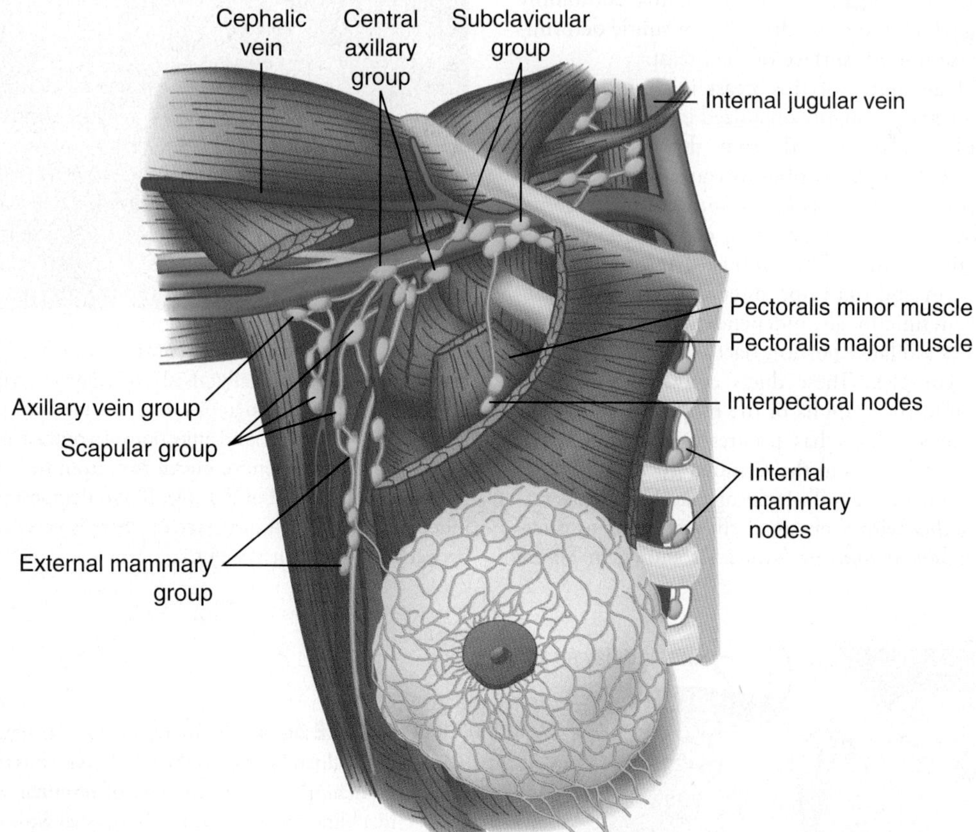


**FIGURE 36-2** Contents of the axilla. In this diagram, there are five named and contiguous groupings of lymph nodes in the full axilla. Complete axillary dissection, as done in the historical radical mastectomy, removes all these nodes. However, note that the subclavicular nodes in the axilla are continuous with the supraclavicular nodes in the neck and nodes between the pectoralis major and minor muscles, called the *interpectoral nodes* in this diagram (also known as *Rotter's lymph nodes*). The sentinel lymph node is functionally the first node in the axillary chain and, anatomically, is usually found in the external mammary group. (From Donegan WL, Spratt JS: Cancer of the breast, ed 3, Philadelphia, 1988, WB Saunders, p 19.)

vein, which is just cephalad and deep (superior and posterior) to the bundle. This neurovascular bundle should be preserved during standard axillary dissection.

The large sensory intercostal brachial or brachial cutaneous nerves span the axillary space and supply sensation to the undersurface of the upper part of the arm and skin of the chest wall along the posterior margin of the axilla. Dividing these nerves results in cutaneous anesthesia in these areas and should be explained to patients before axillary dissection. Denervation of the areas supplied by these sensory nerves can cause chronic and uncomfortable pain syndromes in a small percentage of patients. Preservation of the superiormost nerve maintains sensation to the posterior aspect of the upper part of the arm intact without compromising the axillary dissection in most patients.

## MICROSCOPIC ANATOMY

The mature breast is composed of three principal tissue types: (1) glandular epithelium; (2) fibrous stroma and supporting structures; and (3) adipose tissue. Lymphocytes and macrophages are also found within the breast. In adolescents, the predominant tissues are epithelium and stroma. In postmenopausal women, the glandular structures involute and are largely replaced by adipose tissue. Cooper's ligaments provide shape and structure to the breast as they course from the overlying skin to the underlying deep fascia. Because they are anchored into the skin, infiltration of these ligaments by carcinoma commonly produces tethering which can cause dimpling or subtle deformities on the otherwise smooth surface of the breast.

The glandular apparatus of the breast is composed of a branching system of ducts, roughly organized in a radial pattern spreading outward and downward from the nipple-areolar complex (see Fig. 36-1). It is possible to cannulate individual ducts and visualize the lactiferous ducts with contrast agents. Figure 36-3 demonstrates the arborization of branching ducts, which end in terminal lobules. The contrast dye opacifies only a single ductal system and does not enter adjacent and intertwined branches from functionally independent ductal branches. Each major duct has a dilated portion (lactiferous sinus) below the nipple-areolar complex. These ducts converge through a constricted orifice into the ampulla of the nipple.

Each of the major ducts has progressive generations of branching and ultimately ends in the terminal ductules or acini (Fig. 36-4). These acini are the milk-forming glands of the lactating breast and, together with their small efferent ducts or ductules, are known as *lobular units* or *lobules*. As shown in Figure 36-4, the terminal ductules are invested in a specialized loose connective tissue that contains capillaries, lymphocytes, and other migratory mononuclear cells. This intralobular stroma is clearly distinguished from the denser and less cellular interlobular stroma and from the adipose tissue within the breast.

The entire ductal system is lined by epithelial cells, which are surrounded by specialized myoepithelial cells that have contractile properties and serve to propel milk formed in the lobules toward the nipple. Outside the epithelial and myoepithelial layers, the ducts of the breast are surrounded by a continuous basement membrane containing laminin, type IV collagen, and proteoglycans. The basement membrane layer is an important boundary in differentiating in situ from invasive breast cancer. Continuity of this layer is maintained in ductal carcinoma in situ (DCIS), also termed *noninvasive breast cancer* (see later, "Pathology"). Invasive breast cancer is defined by penetration of the basement membrane by malignant cells invading the stroma.

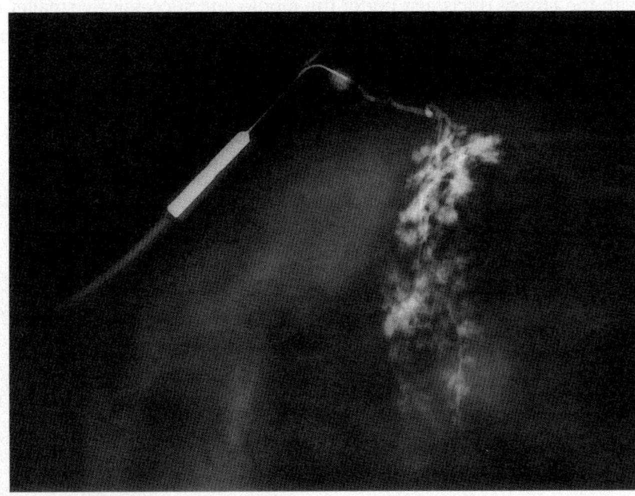

**FIGURE 36-3** Injection of contrast into a single ductal system (ductogram). Occasionally used to evaluate surgically significant nipple discharge, ductography is performed by cannulation of an individual duct orifice and injection of contrast material. This ductogram opacifies the entire ductal tree, from the retroareolar duct to the lobules at the end of the tree. It also demonstrates the functional independence of each duct system; there is no cross-communication between independent systems.

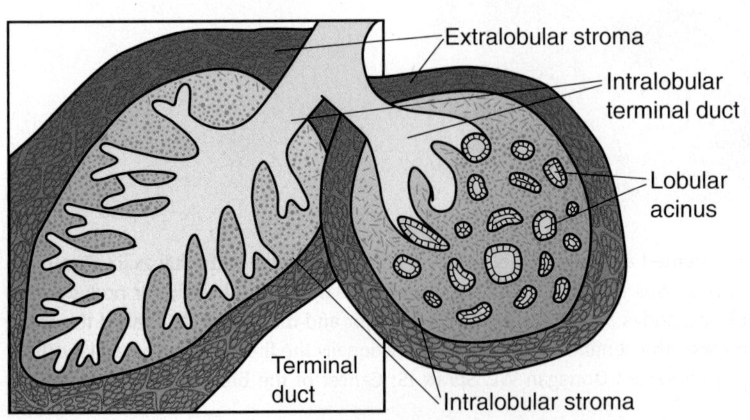


**FIGURE 36-4** Mature resting lobular unit. At the distal end of the ductal system is the lobule, which is formed by multiple branching events at the end of terminal ducts, each ending in a blind sac or acini, and is invested with specialized stroma. The lobule is a three-dimensional structure but is seen in two dimensions in a histologic thin section, shown in the *lower right*. The intralobular terminal ductule and acini are invested in loose connective tissue containing a modest number of infiltrating lymphocytes and plasma cells. The lobule is distinct from the denser interlobular stroma, which contains larger breast ducts, blood vessels, and fat.

## BREAST DEVELOPMENT AND PHYSIOLOGY

### Normal Development and Physiology

Prior to puberty, the breast is composed primarily of dense fibrous stroma and scattered ducts lined with epithelium. In the United States, puberty, as measured by breast development and the growth of pubic hair, begins between the ages of 9 and 12 years, and menarche (onset of menstrual cycles) begins at approximately 12 to 13 years of age. These events are initiated by low-amplitude pulses of pituitary gonadotropins, which raise serum estradiol concentrations. In the breast, this hormone-dependent maturation (thelarche) entails increased deposition of fat, the formation of new ducts by branching and elongation, and the first appearance of lobular units. This process of growth and cell division is under the control of estrogen, progesterone, adrenal hormones, pituitary hormones, and the trophic effects of insulin and thyroid hormone. There is evidence that local growth factor networks are also important. The exact timing of these events and the coordinated development of both breast buds may vary from the average in individual patients. The term *prepubertal gynecomastia* refers to symmetrical enlargement and projection of the breast bud in a young girl before the average age of 12 years, unaccompanied by the other changes of puberty. This process, which may be unilateral, should not be confused with neoplastic growth and is not an indication for biopsy.[1]

The postpubertal mature or resting breast contains fat, stroma, lactiferous ducts, and lobular units. During phases of the menstrual cycle or in response to exogenous hormones, the breast epithelium and lobular stroma undergo cyclic stimulation. It appears that the dominant process is hypertrophy and alteration of morphology rather than hyperplasia. In the late luteal (premenstrual) phase, there is an accumulation of fluid and intralobular edema. This accumulation of edema can produce pain and breast engorgement.

These physiologic changes can lead to increased nodularity and may be mistaken for a malignant tumor. Ill-defined masses in premenopausal women are generally observed through the course of the menstrual cycle prior to intervention. With pregnancy, there is diminution of the fibrous stroma and the formation of new acini or lobules, termed the *adenosis of pregnancy.* After birth, there is a sudden loss of placental hormones, which, combined with continued high levels of prolactin, is the principal trigger for lactation. The actual expulsion of milk is under hormonal control and is caused by contraction of the myoepithelial cells that surround the breast ducts and terminal ductules. There is no evidence for innervation of these myoepithelial cells; their contraction appears to occur in response to the pituitary-derived peptide oxytocin. Stimulation of the nipple appears to be the physiologic signal for continued pituitary secretion of prolactin and acute release of oxytocin. When breastfeeding ceases, there is a fall in the prolactin level and no stimulus for release of oxytocin. The breast then returns to a resting state and to the cyclic changes induced when menstruation resumes.

Menopause is defined by cessation in menstrual flow for at least 1 year; in the United States, it usually occurs between the ages of 40 and 55 years, with a median age of 51 years. Menopause may be accompanied by symptoms such as vasomotor disturbances (hot flashes), vaginal dryness, urinary tract infections, and cognitive impairment (possibly secondary to interruption of sleep by hot flashes). Menopause results in involution and a general decrease in the epithelial elements of the resting breast. These changes include increased fat deposition, diminished connective tissue, and the disappearance of lobular units. The persistence of lobules, hyperplasia of the ductal epithelium, and even cyst formation can all occur under the influence of exogenous ovarian hormones, usually in the form of postmenopausal hormone replacement therapy (HRT). Physicians should inquire about the menstrual history, onset of menses, and cessation of menses in postmenopausal women and record the use of HRT. HRT can lead to increased breast density, which may lower the sensitivity of mammography.

### Fibrocystic Changes and Breast Pain

The condition previously referred to as *fibrocystic disease* represents a spectrum of clinical, mammographic, and histologic findings and is common during the fourth and fifth decades of life, generally lasting until menopause. An exaggerated response of breast stroma and epithelium to a variety of circulating and locally produced hormones and growth factors is frequently characterized by the constellation of breast pain, tenderness, and nodularity. Symptomatically, the condition is manifested as premenstrual cyclic mastalgia, with pain and tenderness to touch. This can be worrisome to many women; however, breast pain is not usually a symptom of breast cancer. Haagensen[1] has recorded the symptoms of women with breast carcinoma and found pain as an unprompted symptom in 5.4% of patients. In women with breast pain and an associated palpable mass, the presence of the mass is the focus of evaluation and treatment. Normal ovarian hormonal influences on breast glandular elements frequently produce cyclic mastalgia, generally pain in phase with the menstrual cycle. Noncyclic mastalgia is more likely idiopathic and difficult to treat. Women 30 years and older with noncyclic mastalgia should undergo breast imaging with mammography in addition to a physical examination. If examination reveals a mass, this should become the focus of subsequent evaluation. Occasionally, a simple cyst may cause noncyclic breast pain, and aspiration of the cyst will usually resolve the pain. Most patients with simple cysts do not require any further evaluation unless it is a complex cyst with solid intracystic components.

Patients with fibrocystic changes have clinical breast findings that range from mild alterations in texture to dense, firm breast tissue with palpable masses. The appearance of large palpable cysts completes the picture. Mammographically, fibrocystic changes are usually seen as diffuse or focal radiologically dense tissue. By ultrasound, cysts exist in up to one third of all women 35 to 50 years of age, with most of them being nonpalpable. However, palpable cysts or multiple small cysts are typical of fibrocystic disease. Cysts, with or without fibrocystic disease, are uncommon in women older than 60 and younger than 30 years.

Histologically, in addition to macrocysts and microcysts, identified solid elements include adenosis, sclerosis, apocrine metaplasia, stromal fibrosis, and epithelial metaplasia and hyperplasia. Depending on the presence of epithelial hyperplasia, fibrocystic change is classified as nonproliferative, proliferative without atypia, or proliferative with atypia. All three alterations can occur alone or in combination and to a variable degree and, in the absence of epithelial atypia, represent the histologic spectrum of normal breast tissue. However, atypical epithelial hyperplasia (atypical ductal hyperplasia [ADH]) is a risk factor for the development of breast cancer. Atypical proliferations of ductal epithelial cells confer increased risk for breast cancer; however, fibrocystic change is not itself a risk factor for the development of breast malignancy.

## Abnormal Development and Physiology

### Absent or Accessory Breast Tissue

Absence of breast tissue (amastia) and absence of the nipple (athelia) are rare anomalies. Unilateral rudimentary breast development is more common, as is adolescent hypertrophy of one breast with lesser development of the other. In contrast, accessory breast tissue (polymastia) and accessory nipples (supernumerary nipples) are both common. Supernumerary nipples are usually rudimentary and occur along the milk line from the axilla to the pubis in males and females. They may be mistaken for a small mole; however, accessory nipples are usually only removed for cosmetic reasons. True polythelia refers to more than one nipple serving a single breast, which is rare. Accessory breast tissue is commonly located above the breast in the axilla. Rudimentary nipple development may be present, and lactation is possible with more complete development. Accessory breast tissue may be seen as an enlarging mass in the axilla during pregnancy and persists as excess tissue in the axilla after lactation is complete. The accessory mammary tissue may be removed surgically if it is large or cosmetically deforming or to prevent enlargement during future pregnancy.

### Gynecomastia

Hypertrophy of breast tissue in men is a clinical entity for which there is frequently no identifiable cause. Pubertal hypertrophy occurs in boys between the ages of 13 years and early adulthood and senescent hypertrophy is diagnosed in men older than 50 years. Gynecomastia in teenage boys is common and may be bilateral or unilateral. Unless it is unilateral or painful, it may pass unnoticed and regress with adulthood. Pubertal hypertrophy is generally treated by observation without surgery. Surgical excision may be discussed if the enlargement is unilateral, fails to regress, or is cosmetically unacceptable. Hypertrophy in older men is also relatively common. The enlargement is frequently unilateral, although the contralateral breast may enlarge with time. A number of commonly used medications, such as digoxin, thiazides, estrogens, phenothiazines, and theophylline, may exacerbate senescent gynecomastia. In addition, gynecomastia may be a systemic manifestation of hepatic cirrhosis, renal failure, and malnutrition. In both age groups, the mass is smooth, firm, and symmetrically distributed beneath the areola. It is frequently tender, which is often the reason for seeking medical attention. Both pubertal and senescent gynecomastia may be managed nonoperatively and can be fully characterized with ultrasonography. There is little confusion with carcinoma occurring in the male breast. Carcinoma is not usually tender, is asymmetrically located beneath or beside the areola, and may be fixed to the overlying dermis or to the deep fascia. A dominant mass suspected of being carcinoma should be examined with core needle biopsy. Mammography and ultrasound can also be useful tools to discriminate between gynecomastia and a suspected malignancy of the breast in older men.

### Nipple Discharge

The appearance of discharge from the nipple of a nonlactating woman is a relatively common condition and is rarely associated with an underlying carcinoma. In one review of 270 subareolar biopsies for discharge coming from one identifiable duct and without an associated breast mass, carcinoma was found in only 16 patients (5.9%). In these cases, the fluid was bloody or tested strongly positive for occult hemoglobin. In another series of 249 patients, breast carcinoma was found in 10 (4%). In 8 of these patients, a mass lesion was identified in addition to the discharge. In the absence of a palpable mass or a suspicious mammogram, discharge is rarely associated with cancer.

It is important to establish whether the discharge comes from one breast or from both breasts, whether it comes from multiple duct orifices or from just one, and whether the discharge is grossly bloody or contains blood. A milky discharge from both breasts is termed *galactorrhea.* In the absence of lactation or a history of recent lactation, galactorrhea may be associated with increased production of prolactin. Radioimmunoassay for serum prolactin is diagnostic. However, true galactorrhea is rare and is diagnosed only when the discharge is milky (contains lactose, fat, and milk-specific proteins). Unilateral discharge coming from one duct orifice is often treated surgically when there is a significant amount of discharge (Fig. 36-5). However, the underlying cause is rarely a breast malignancy.

The most common cause of spontaneous nipple discharge from a single duct is a solitary intraductal papilloma in one of the large subareolar ducts under the nipple. Subareolar duct ectasia producing inflammation and dilation of large collecting ducts under the nipple is common and usually involves discharge from multiple ducts. Cancer is a very unusual cause of discharge in the absence of other signs. In summary, nipple discharge that is bilateral and comes from multiple ducts is not usually a surgical problem. Bloody discharge from a single duct often requires surgical excision to establish a diagnosis and control the discharge. A diagnosis of intraductal papilloma is found in most of these cases.

### Galactocele

A galactocele is a milk-filled cyst that is round, well circumscribed, and easily movable within the breast. It generally occurs after the cessation of lactation or when feeding frequency has curtailed significantly. Haagensen[1] has reported that galactoceles may occur up to 6 to 10 months after breastfeeding has ceased. The pathogenesis of galactocele is unknown, but it is thought that inspissated milk within ducts is responsible. The tumor is usually located in the central portion of the breast or under the nipple. Needle aspiration produces thick creamy material that may be tinged dark green or brown. Although it appears purulent, the fluid is sterile. Treatment is needle aspiration, and withdrawal of thick milky secretion confirms the diagnosis; surgery is reserved for cysts that cannot be aspirated or those that become infected.

## DIAGNOSIS OF BREAST DISEASE

### Patient History

It is important for the examiner to determine the patient's age and obtain a reproductive history, including age at menarche, age at menopause, and history of pregnancies, including age at first full-term pregnancy. A previous history of breast biopsies should be obtained, including the pathologic findings, especially proliferative breast disease. If the patient has had a hysterectomy, it is important to determine whether the ovaries were removed. In premenopausal women, a recent history of pregnancy and

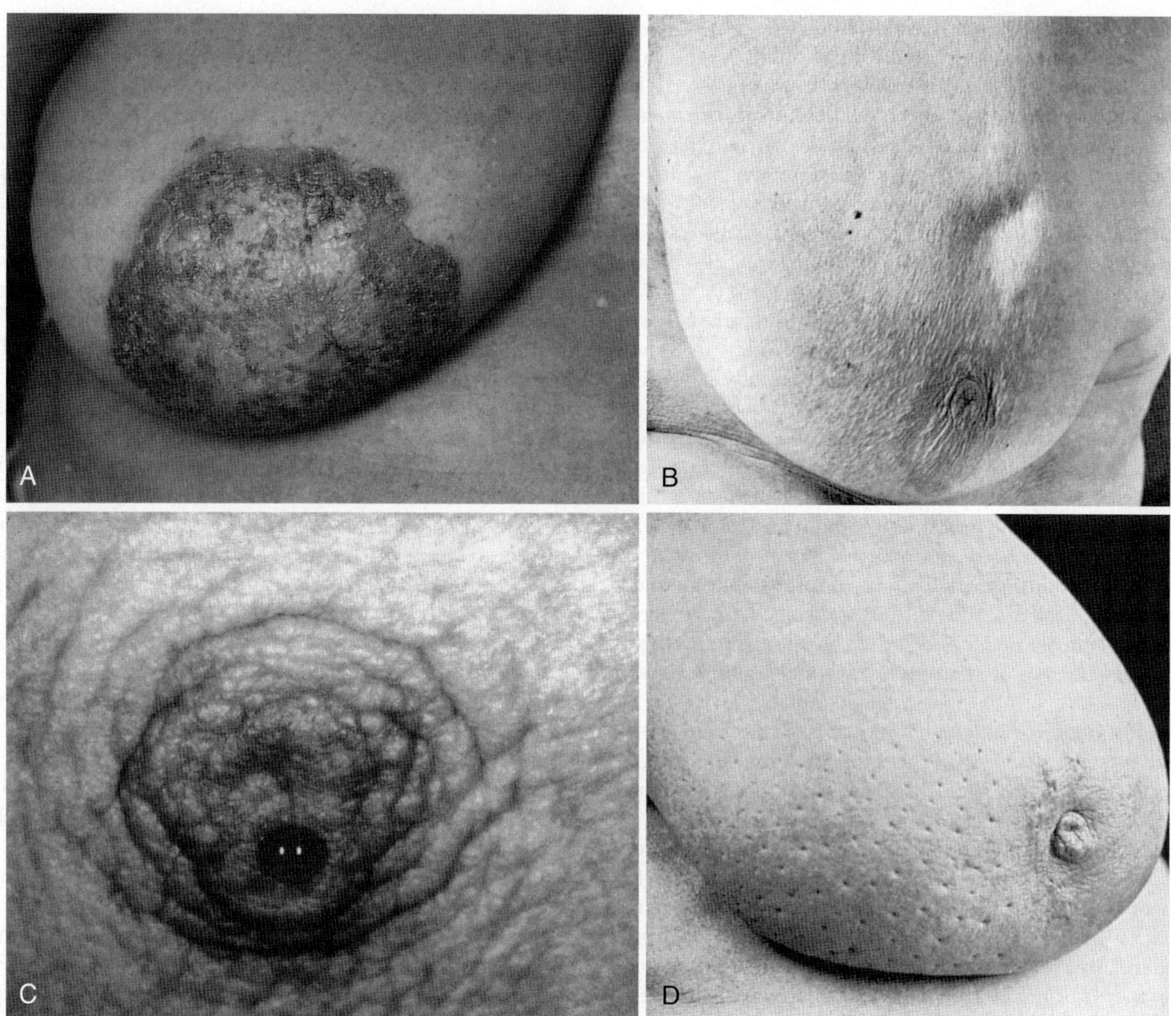


**FIGURE 36-5** Common physical findings during breast examination. **A,** Paget's disease of the nipple. Malignant ductal cells invade the epidermis without traversing the basement membrane of the subareolar duct or epidermis. The disease appears as a psoriatic rash that begins on the nipple and spreads off onto the areola and into the skin of the breast. **B,** Skin dimpling. Traction on Cooper's ligaments by a scirrhous tumor is distorting the surface of the breast and producing a dimple best seen with angled indirect lighting during abduction of the arms upward. **C,** Nipple discharge. Discharge from multiple ducts or bilateral discharge is a common finding in healthy breasts. In this case, the discharge is from a single duct orifice and may signify underlying disease in the discharging duct. In this patient, a papilloma was the source of her symptoms. **D,** Peau d'orange (skin of the orange) or edema of the skin of the breast. This finding may be caused by dependency of the breast, lymphatic blockage (from surgery or radiation), or mastitis. The most feared cause is inflammatory carcinoma, in which malignant cells plug the dermal lymphatics—the pathologic hallmark of the disease.

lactation should be noted. The history should include any use of HRT or hormones used for contraception. The family history should detail any cancer of the breast and ovaries and the menopausal status of any affected relatives.

With respect to the specific breast complaint, questioning should include history of a mass, breast pain, nipple discharge, and any skin changes. If a mass is present, one should inquire as to how long it has been present and whether it changes with the menstrual cycle. If a cancer diagnosis is suspected, inquiry about constitutional symptoms, bone pain, weight loss, respiratory changes, and similar clinical indications can direct investigations that could reveal evidence of metastatic disease.

## Physical Examination

The examination begins with the patient in the upright sitting position with careful visual inspection for obvious masses, asymmetries, and skin changes. The nipples are inspected and compared for the presence of retraction, nipple inversion, or excoriation of the superficial epidermis such as that seen with Paget's disease (see Fig. 36-5*A*). The use of indirect lighting can unmask subtle dimpling of the skin or nipple caused by a carcinoma that places Cooper's ligaments under tension (see Fig. 36-5*B*). Simple maneuvers such as stretching the arms high above the head or tensing the pectoralis muscles may accentuate asymmetries and dimpling. If carefully sought, dimpling of the skin or nipple retraction is a sensitive and specific sign of underlying cancer.

Edema of the skin produces a clinical sign known as *peau d'orange* (see Fig. 36-5*D*). When combined with tenderness, warmth and swelling of the breast, these signs and symptoms are the hallmark of inflammatory carcinoma and may be mistaken for acute mastitis. The inflammatory changes and edema are caused by obstruction of dermal lymphatic channels with emboli of carcinoma cells. Occasionally, a bulky tumor may produce obstruction of lymph channels that results in overlying skin edema. This is not typically the case with inflammatory carcinoma, where there is usually no discrete palpable mass but diffuse changes throughout the breast parenchyma. In 40 patients with inflammatory carcinoma described by Haagensen,[1] erythema and edema of the skin were present in all cases, a palpable mass or localized induration was noted in 19 patients, and no localized tumor was present in 21 patients.

Involvement of the nipple and areola can occur with carcinoma of the breast, especially when the primary tumor is located in the subareolar position. Direct involvement may result in retraction of the nipple. Flattening or inversion of the nipple can be caused by fibrosis in certain benign conditions, especially subareolar duct ectasia. In these cases, the finding is frequently bilateral and the history confirms that the condition has been present for many years. Unilateral retraction or retraction that develops over a period of weeks or months is more suggestive of carcinoma. Centrally located tumors that go undetected for a long period of time may directly invade and ulcerate the skin of the areola or nipple. Peripheral tumors may distort the normal symmetry of the nipples by traction on Cooper's ligaments.

A condition of the nipple that is commonly associated with an underlying breast cancer is Paget's disease. First described by Sir James Paget in 1874, Paget's disease has histologically distinct changes within the dermis of the nipple. There is often an underlying intraductal carcinoma in the large sinuses just under the nipple (see Fig. 36-5*A*). Carcinoma cells invade across the junction of epidermal and ductal epithelial cells and enter the epidermal layer of the skin of the nipple. Clinically, this produces a dermatitis that may appear eczematoid and moist or dry and psoriatic. It begins in the nipple, although it can spread to the skin of the areola. Many benign skin conditions such as eczema frequently begin on the areola, whereas Paget's disease originates on the nipple and secondarily involves the areola.

Palpation of the breast tissue and regional lymph nodes follows visual inspection. While the patient is still in the sitting position, the examiner supports the patient's arm and palpates each axilla to detect the presence of enlarged axillary lymph nodes. The supraclavicular and infraclavicular spaces are similarly palpated for enlarged nodes. Palpation of the breast is always done with the patient lying supine on a solid examining surface, with the arm stretched above the head. Palpation of the breast while the patient is sitting is often inaccurate because the overlapping breast tissue may feel like a mass or a mass may go undetected within the breast tissue. The breast is best examined with compression of the tissue toward the chest wall, with palpation of each quadrant and the tissue under the nipple-areolar complex. Palpable masses are characterized according to their size, shape, consistency, and location and whether they are fixed to the skin or underlying musculature. Benign tumors, such as fibroadenomas and cysts, can be as firm as carcinoma; usually, these benign entities are distinct, well circumscribed, and movable. Carcinoma is typically firm but less circumscribed, and moving it produces a drag of adjacent tissue. Cysts and fibrocystic changes can be tender with palpation of the breast; however, tenderness is rarely a helpful diagnostic sign. Most palpable masses are self-discovered by patients during casual or intentional self-examination.

## Biopsy

### Fine-Needle Aspiration Biopsy

Fine-needle aspiration (FNA) biopsy is a common tool used in the diagnosis of breast masses. It can be done with a 22-gauge needle, an appropriate-sized syringe, and an alcohol preparation pad. The aspirate must be properly prepared on a slide for cytologic examination to be clinically useful. The main usefulness of FNA biopsy is differentiation of solid from cystic masses, but it may be performed whenever a new, dominant, unexplained mass is found in the breast. The routine performance of FNA to distinguish solid from cystic breast masses has largely been replaced by ultrasonography. With a mammographically identified mass or a palpable mass, ultrasonography can quickly discriminate solid from cystic masses, which this may often obviate the need for aspiration. Cyst fluid is usually turbid and dark green or amber and can be discarded if the mass totally disappears and the fluid is not bloody. If the FNA of a suspected cyst does not reveal cyst fluid, the next step to consider is a core needle biopsy, usually with mammographic or ultrasonographic guidance. If the cyst aspiration reveals blood-tinged fluid or fluid is produced but the mass fails to resolve completely, consideration should be given to pneumocystography or image-guided core needle biopsy. It is not uncommon for cysts to reaccumulate fluid after initial aspiration. If the cyst is demonstrated to be a simple cyst on breast imaging, no further intervention is required. If the cyst is classified as a complex cyst, further imaging and evaluation should be considered to rule out an underlying carcinoma.

If the mass is solid and the clinical situation is consistent with carcinoma, cytologic examination of the aspirated material is performed. The needle is repeatedly inserted into the mass while constant negative pressure is applied to the syringe. Suction is released and the needle is withdrawn. The scanty fluid and cellular material within the needle are submitted in physiologically buffered saline (Normosol) or fixed immediately on slides in 95% ethyl alcohol. Because the cytologic evaluation will not discriminate between noninvasive and invasive breast cancers, most clinicians recommend core needle biopsy for definitive histologic diagnosis prior to surgical intervention. A positive result on FNA biopsy allows the surgeon to begin informed discussions with the patient; however, definite plans for treatment should be based on the histologic diagnosis from a core needle biopsy.

### Core Needle Biopsy

Core needle biopsy is the method of choice to sample nonpalpable, image-detected breast abnormalities. This technique is also preferred for the diagnosis of palpable lesions. Core needle biopsy can be performed under mammographic (stereotactic), ultrasonographic, or magnetic resonance imaging (MRI) guidance. Mass lesions that are visualized on ultrasonography can be sampled under ultrasonographic guidance; calcifications and densities that are best seen on mammography are sampled under stereotactic guidance. During stereotactic core needle biopsy, the breast is compressed, most often with the patient lying prone on the stereotactic core biopsy table. A robotic arm and biopsy device are positioned by computed analysis of triangulated mammographic images. After local anesthetic is injected, a small skin incision is made and an 11-gauge core biopsy needle is inserted into the lesion to obtain the tissue sample with vacuum assistance. There are standards for the appropriate number of core samples to be obtained based on the type of abnormality being sampled and a clip should be placed to mark the site of the lesion, particularly for small lesions that may be difficult to find after extensive sampling. The specimens should be placed in a Petri dish and imaged to confirm that the targeted lesion has been adequately sampled. A similar approach is used for ultrasonographic and MRI-guided biopsy of lesions.

Specimen radiography of excised cores is performed to confirm that the targeted lesion has been sampled and to direct pathologic assessment of the tissue. A postbiopsy mammogram confirms that a defect has been created within the target lesion and that the marking clip is in the correct position. Wire localization and surgical excision are required if the lesion cannot be adequately sampled by core biopsy approaches, or if there is discordance between the imaging abnormality and pathologic findings.

**Interpretation of Core Needle Biopsy Results** The limited sample size obtained by core biopsy techniques requires proper interpretation of the pathology results. Most patients undergoing core biopsy will have benign findings and may return to routine screening, with no other intervention required. If a malignancy is detected, histologic subtype, grade, and receptor status should be determined from the core biopsy sample. The patient may proceed to definitive treatment of the cancer if it is an early-stage breast cancer. Patients with locally advanced or inflammatory breast cancer should be treated with systemic chemotherapy prior to surgical intervention. Depending on the size of the imaging abnormality, approximately 10% to 20% of patients with a diagnosis of DCIS on core biopsy will be found to have some invasive carcinoma at definitive surgery.

The diagnosis of breast lesions using a minimally invasive procedure, such as core needle biopsy, is the preferred approach. The use of excisional breast biopsy as a diagnostic procedure increases costs and results in delays to definitive surgery for patients with cancer.[2] Fewer than 10% of patients who undergo core biopsy will have inconclusive results and require wire-localized surgical biopsy for definitive diagnosis. Biopsy results that are not concordant with the targeted lesion (e.g., a spiculated mass on imaging and normal breast tissue on core biopsy) also require surgical excision. When ADH is found on core biopsy, surgical excision will reveal DCIS or invasive carcinoma in up to 20% of cases because of difficulty distinguishing ADH and DCIS in a limited tissue sample. A finding of a cellular fibroadenoma on core biopsy requires excision to rule out a phyllodes tumor.

## BREAST IMAGING

Breast imaging techniques are used to detect small, nonpalpable breast abnormalities, evaluate clinical findings, and guide diagnostic procedures. Mammography is the primary imaging modality for screening asymptomatic women. During mammography, the breast is compressed between Plexiglas plates to reduce the thickness of the tissue through which the radiation must pass, separate adjacent structures, and improve resolution. Two views of each breast are obtained on a screening mammogram, mediolateral oblique and craniocaudal. A diagnostic mammogram is indicated for further evaluation of abnormalities identified on a screening mammogram or of clinical findings or symptoms. Magnification views are obtained to evaluate calcifications and compression views are used to provide additional detail when a mass lesion is suspected. Mammographic sensitivity is limited by breast density, with as many as 10% to 15% of clinically evident breast cancers having no associated mammographic abnormality. Digital mammography acquires digital images and stores them electronically, thereby allowing manipulation and enhancement of images to facilitate interpretation. Digital mammography appears to be superior to traditional film-screen mammography for detecting cancer in younger women and those with dense breasts. Mammography in women younger than 30 years, whose breast tissue is dense with stroma and epithelium, may produce an image without much definition. As women age, the breast tissue involutes and is replaced by fatty tissue. On mammography, fat absorbs relatively little radiation and provides a contrasting background that favors detection of small lesions. Computer-assisted diagnosis (CAD) has been shown to increase the sensitivity and specificity of mammography and ultrasound over review by the radiologist alone.

### Screening Mammography

Screening mammography is performed in asymptomatic women with the goal of detecting breast cancer that is not yet clinically evident. This approach assumes that breast cancers identified through screening will be smaller, have a better prognosis, and require less aggressive treatment than cancers identified by palpation. The potential benefits of screening are weighed against the cost of screening and the number of false-positive studies that prompt additional workup, biopsies, and patient anxiety.

Eight prospective randomized trials of screening mammography have been performed, with almost 500,000 women participating. The impact of mammographic screening on breast cancer mortality has been assessed by age group at specific intervals by the U.S. Preventive Services Task Force and the most recent report resulted in a change in recommendations for breast cancer screening. Based on the review of eight trials in women aged 39 to 49 years, screening mammography reduced the risk for breast cancer death by 15% (relative risk [RR], 0.85; credible interval [CrI], 0.75 to 0.96). In the six trials that included women aged 50 to 59, there was a reduction in risk of 14% (RR, 0.86; CrI, 0.75 to 0.99). There were two trials that included women aged 60 to 69 and, in this age group, there was a reduction in risk of 32% (RR, 0.68; CrI, 0.54 to 0.87). There was only one trial that included women older than 70 years, and it was concluded that there were insufficient data to recommend routine screening in this age group. Based on these results, the most recent U.S. Preventive Services Task Force report recommended biennial screening mammography for women aged 50 to 74 years and recommended against screening for those aged 40 to 49 and women older than 75 years of age.[2] The recommendations were based on the risk reduction, number of women needed to invite for screening to prevent one breast cancer death, and potential for harm from additional testing and biopsies (Table 36-1).

At present, the American Cancer Society continues to recommend annual screening mammography for women older than 40 years and suggests that this practice should continue as long as the woman is in good health. Younger women with a significant family history, histologic risk factors, or history of previous breast cancer may also benefit from screening with MRI. Although the randomized trials did not enroll women

**Table 36-1 Effect on Breast Cancer Mortality and False-Positive Mammograms by Age Group in Breast Cancer Screening Trials**

| AGE GROUP (YR) | NO. OF TRIALS | BREAST CANCER MORTALITY, RR (95% CRI) | NO. NEEDED TO INVITE FOR SCREENING TO PREVENT ONE BREAST CANCER DEATH (95% CRI) | FALSE-POSITIVE MAMMOGRAMS/ SCREENING ROUND* |
|---|---|---|---|---|
| 39-49 | 8 | 0.85 (0.75-0.96) | 1904 (929-6378) | 97.8 |
| 50-59 | 6 | 0.86 (0.75-0.99) | 1339 (322-7455) | 86.6 |
| 60-69 | 2 | 0.68 (0.54-0.87) | 377 (230-1050) | 79.0 |
| 70-74 | 1 | 1.12 (0.73-1.72) | Not available | 68.8 |

Adapted from Nelson HD, Tyne K, Naik A, et al; U.S. Preventive Services Task Force: Screening for breast cancer: Systematic evidence review update for the U.S. Preventive Services Task Force. Ann Intern Med 151:727, 2009.

*Per 1000 screened.

older than 74 years, breast cancer risk increases with advancing age, and the sensitivity and specificity of mammography are highest in older women, whose breast tissue has usually been replaced by fat. It is reasonable to continue mammographic screening in older women who are in good general health who would otherwise be considered appropriate surgical candidates.

## Ultrasonography

Ultrasonography is useful in determining whether a lesion detected by mammography is solid or cystic. Ultrasonography can be useful for discriminating lesions in the patient with dense breasts. However, it has not been found to be a useful screening tool because it is highly dependent on the operator performing the freehand screening and there is a lack of standardized screening protocols. The American College of Radiology Imaging Network (ACRIN) has performed a trial (ACRIN 6666) in high-risk women in whom mammography and ultrasonography were performed in randomized order to compare the sensitivity, specificity, and diagnostic yield of ultrasonography plus mammography compared with mammography alone.[3] The investigators found that the combination of ultrasonography and mammography allowed for an increased diagnostic yield of 4.2 cancers/1000 women. However, the use of ultrasonography resulted in more false-positive events and required more callbacks and biopsies. There are no data available showing that the use of screening ultrasonography can reduce mortality caused by breast cancer.

## Magnetic Resonance Imaging

MRI is increasingly being used for the evaluation of breast abnormalities. It is useful for identifying the primary tumor in the breast in patients who present with axillary lymph node metastases without mammographic evidence of a primary breast tumor (unknown primary). MRI may also be useful for assessing the extent of the primary tumor, particularly in young women with dense breast tissue, and for evaluating invasive lobular cancers. Some surgeons will use MRI preoperatively to determine eligibility for breast conservation; however, there is no level 1 evidence to support its routine use for this purpose. MRI has shown usefulness as a screening tool in patients with known *BRCA* gene mutations and for detecting contralateral breast cancers in women diagnosed with a unilateral cancer on mammography. The sensitivity of MRI for invasive cancer is higher than 90%, but is only 60% or less for DCIS. The specificity of MRI is only moderate, with significant overlap in the appearance of benign and malignant lesions. A meta-analysis of 22 studies reporting the detection of contralateral breast cancer by MRI has revealed a mean incremental cancer detection rate of 4.1% and a positive predictive value (PPV) of 47.9%. This high rate of detection may be partially the result of selection bias; however, it is of significant concern that more than 50% of the abnormalities detected on MRI are false- positives, resulting in the need for additional imaging studies and biopsies. The comparative effectiveness of MRI in breast cancer (COMICE) trial was a multicenter trial that recruited 1623 women aged 18 years or older with newly diagnosed breast cancer to assess the clinical efficacy of contrast-enhanced MRI.[4] Patients had standard clinical and radiological examination and then were randomized to undergo MRI or no further imaging. The primary end point was reexcision rates or need for mastectomy within 6 months. There was no statistically significant difference in reoperative rates between patients who did or did not undergo MRI. Of note, the contralateral breast cancer detection rate in the COMICE trial was 1.6%, significantly lower than that reported in other trials. This trial has been criticized because MRI-guided biopsy was not available at all centers to assess suspicious findings identified on MRI. This led to a number of mastectomies without pathologic verification of additional disease, which would have precluded breast-conserving therapy.

## Nonpalpable Mammographic Abnormalities

Mammographic abnormalities that cannot be detected by physical examination include clustered microcalcifications and areas of abnormal density (e.g., masses, architectural distortions, asymmetries) that have not produced a palpable finding (Fig. 36-6). The Breast Imaging Reporting and Data System (BI-RADS) is used to categorize the degree of suspicion of malignancy for a mammographic abnormality (Table 36-2). To avoid unnecessary biopsies for low-suspicion mammographic findings, probably benign lesions are designated BI-RADS 3 and are monitored with a schedule of short-interval mammograms over a 2-year period. Biopsy is performed only for lesions that progress during follow-up.

Diagnostic biopsy of a nonpalpable mammographic lesion should be performed by image-guided core needle biopsy. Because 75% to 80% of patients for whom biopsy is recommended will have benign findings, the less invasive and less

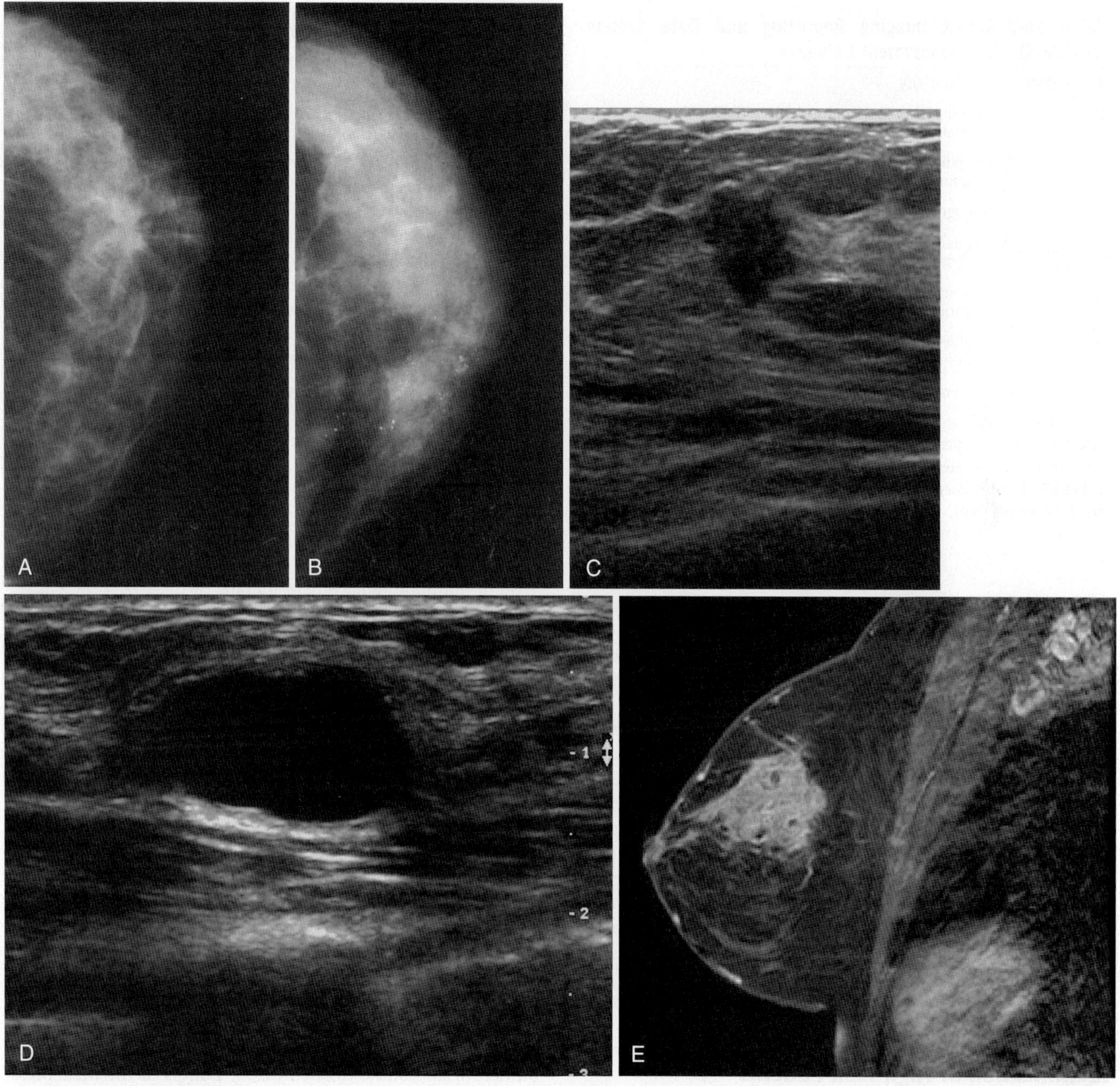


**FIGURE 36-6** Mammographic, ultrasonographic, and MRI findings in breast disease. **A,** Stellate mass in the breast. The combination of a density with spiculated borders and distortion of surrounding breast architecture suggests a malignancy. **B,** Clustered microcalcifications. Fine, pleomorphic, and linear calcifications that cluster together suggest the diagnosis of ductal carcinoma in situ. **C,** Ultrasound image of breast cancer. The mass is solid, contains internal echoes, and displays an irregular border. Most malignant lesions are taller than they are wide. **D,** Ultrasound image of a simple cyst. By ultrasound, the cyst is round with smooth borders, there is a paucity of internal sound echoes, and there is increased through-transmission of sound, with enhanced posterior echoes. **E,** Breast MRI showing gadolinium enhancement of a breast cancer. Rapid and intense gadolinium enhancement reflects increased tumor vascularity. Lesion contour and size may also be assessed by MRI.

costly image-guided core needle biopsy approach is preferred whenever feasible.

### Wire-Localized Surgical Excision

Nonpalpable breast lesions should be assessed with image-guided core biopsy, as appropriate, based on the type of abnormality. If the diagnosis is not concordant with imaging findings or there is ADH in a field of microcalcifications that may represent DCIS, most patients should proceed to excisional biopsy for definitive diagnosis. To ensure that the abnormality is completely excised, a localizing wire is placed adjacent to the lesion under mammographic or ultrasonographic guidance. The wire is placed though an introducer needle and has a hook that engages within the breast parenchyma at or near the abnormality to hold it in position after the introducer is withdrawn. Images with the wire in place are made available in the operating room

**Table 36-2 Breast Imaging Reporting and Data System (BI-RADS): Final Assessment Category**

| CATEGORY | DEFINITION |
|---|---|
| 0 | Incomplete assessment–need additional imaging evaluation or prior mammograms for comparison |
| 1 | Negative–nothing to comment on; usually recommend annual screening |
| 2 | Benign finding–usually recommend annual screening |
| 3 | Probably benign finding (<2% malignant)–initial short-interval follow-up suggested |
| 4 | Suspicious abnormality (2%-95% malignant)–biopsy should be considered |
| 5 | Highly suggestive of malignancy (>95% malignant)–appropriate action should be taken |
| 6 | Known biopsy–proven malignancy |

Adapted from Liberman L, Abramson AF, Squires FB, et al: The breast imaging reporting and data system: Positive predictive values of mammographic feature and final assessment categories. AJR Am J Roentgenol 171:35, 1998; and Liberman L, Menell JH: Breast imaging reporting and data systems (BI-RADS). Radiol Clin North Am 40:409, 2002.

to guide the surgeon. It is generally recommended that the surgical incision be placed directly over the lesion that is marked by the hook of the localizing wire, and not where the wire enters the skin. Depending on the size of the breast and length of the localization wire, the hook may be a long distance from the skin entry site. Placing the surgical incision over the site of the hook wire will minimize the amount of normal breast tissue excised during the biopsy procedure. Depending on the size of the lesion and the suspicion of malignancy, it is generally wise to excise a border of normal tissue around the lesion to ensure complete removal, with a negative margin. After excision, the specimen is sent for specimen radiography to confirm that the targeted lesion has been excised. Patients who have a diagnosis of benign findings on excision should undergo a new baseline mammography 4 to 6 months following the surgical procedure.

## IDENTIFICATION AND MANAGEMENT OF HIGH-RISK PATIENTS

### Identification of High-Risk Patients

#### Risk Factors for Breast Cancer

Identification of factors associated with an increased incidence of breast cancer development is important in general health screening for women (Box 36-1). Risk factors for breast cancer can be divided into seven broad categories—age, family history of breast cancer, hormonal factors, proliferative breast disease, irradiation of the breast or chest wall at an early age, personal history of malignancy, and lifestyle factors.

**BOX 36-1 Risk Factors for Breast Cancer**

**Risk Factors That Cannot be Modified**

Increasing age
Female gender
Menstrual factors
Early age at menarche (onset of menses prior to age 12 yr)
Older age at menopause (onset beyond age 55 yr)
Nulliparity
Family history of breast cancer
Genetic predisposition (*BRCA1* and *BRCA2* mutation carriers)
Personal history of breast cancer
Race, ethnicity (white women have increased risk compared with others)
History of radiation exposure

**Risk Factors That Could be Modified**

Reproductive factors
Age at first live birth (full-term pregnancy after age 30 yr)
Parity
Lack of breast-feeding
Obesity
Alcohol consumption
Tobacco smoking
Use of hormone replacement therapy
Decreased physical activity
Shift work (night shifts)

**Histologic Risk Factors**

Proliferative breast disease
ADH
ALH
LCIS

**Age and Gender** Age is probably the most important risk factor for breast cancer development. The age-adjusted incidence of breast cancer continues to increase with advancing age of the female population. Breast cancer is rare in persons younger than 20 years, and cases in these women constitute less than 2% of the total cases. Thereafter, the incidence increases to 1 in 233 from ages 30 to 39 years, 1 in 69 from ages 40 to 49, 1 in 42 from ages 50 to 59, 1 in 29 from ages 60 to 69, and 1 in 8 by age 80 years. Alternatively stated, women now have an average risk of 12.2% of being diagnosed with breast cancer at some time during their lives. Gender is also an important risk factor because the vast majority of breast cancers occur in women. Breast cancer does occur in men, however, although it is less than 1% of the incidence in females, with 1970 cases of invasive breast cancer having been anticipated in 2010 (out of a total burden of 209,060 estimated cases). Lumps in the male breast are more likely to be benign and the result of gynecomastia (see earlier) or other noncancerous tumors.

**Personal History of Breast Cancer** A history of mammary cancer in one breast increases the likelihood of a second primary cancer in the contralateral breast. The magnitude of risk depends on the age at diagnosis of the first primary cancer, estrogen receptor status of the initial breast cancer, and use of adjuvant systemic chemotherapy and hormonal therapy. In absolute terms, the actual risk varies from 0.5% to 1%/year in younger patients to 0.2% in older patients.[1,5]

**Histologic Risk Factors** Histologic abnormalities diagnosed by breast biopsy represent an important category of breast cancer risk factors. Lobular carcinoma in situ (LCIS) is a relatively uncommon condition that is observed predominantly in younger premenopausal women. It is typically an incidental finding at biopsy for another condition and does not present as a palpable mass or suspicious microcalcifications on mammography. Haagensen[1] reported that LCIS was found in 3.6% of more than 5000 biopsies performed for benign disease. In a review of 297 patients with LCIS treated by biopsy and careful observation, it was determined that the actuarial probability of carcinoma developing at the end of 35 years was 21.4%. When compared with the Connecticut Tumor Registry data, a risk ratio (ratio of observed to expected cases) of 7 : 1 was calculated. Significantly, 40% of the carcinomas that subsequently developed were purely in situ lesions, the invasive cancers that developed were predominantly ductal and not lobular in histology, and 50% of the carcinomas occurred in the contralateral breast. Thus, LCIS is not considered a breast cancer but rather a histologic marker for increased breast cancer susceptibility, which is estimated at slightly less than 1%/year longitudinally.

A conservative approach is favored for most patients with a diagnosis of LCIS. The three options that can be discussed with the patient are close observation, chemoprevention with tamoxifen or raloxifene, and bilateral mastectomy. LCIS predisposes to subsequent carcinoma and the risk is lifelong and equal for both breasts. A 5-year course of tamoxifen provides a 56% reduction in breast cancer risk.[6] For those who elect surgery in preference to observation, bilateral total mastectomy remains the procedure of choice.

Benign breast disease produces a spectrum of histologic changes and is broadly divided into histologic lesions that display proliferative epithelial alterations and those that display nonproliferative epithelial alterations. Nonproliferative changes include mild to moderate hyperplasia of luminal cells within breast ducts; these changes do not significantly increase a woman's lifetime risk for development of breast cancer. Proliferative changes within the breast ductal system are associated with an increased risk of developing breast cancer. Dupont and Page have divided proliferative lesions into those with epithelial hyperplasia with atypia and those without atypia; proliferative lesions without atypia sometimes are termed *severe hyperplasia.*

Subsequent studies have adhered to this classification scheme—nonproliferative lesions, proliferative breast epithelium without atypia (severe hyperplasia), and proliferative changes with atypia. ADH and atypical lobular hyperplasia (ALH) are both categorized as proliferative changes with atypia. The risk ratio for breast cancer in women with ADH or ALH is approximately four to five times the risk for development of breast cancer in the general population. A family history of breast cancer and atypical hyperplasia increases the risk to almost nine times that of the general population. Thus, the annual risk for development of breast cancer in a woman with LCIS is slightly less than 1%/year and, with ADH or ALH, it is between 0.5% and 1%/year. These estimates are influenced by age at diagnosis, menopausal status, and family history. An overview of histologic risk factors is presented in Table 36-3.[7]

**Table 36-3 Histologic Risk Factors for Development of Breast Cancer**

| HISTOLOGIC DIAGNOSIS | ESTIMATES, RR* |
|---|---|
| Nonproliferative disease† | 1.0 |
| Proliferative disease without atypia‡ | 1.3-1.9 |
| Proliferative disease with atypia§ | 3.7-4.2 |
| and a strong family history | 4-9 |
| Lobular carcinoma in situ | >7 |

Data from Hartmann LC, Sellers TA, Frost MH, et al: Benign breast disease and the risk of breast cancer. N Engl J Med 353:229, 2005; London SJ, Connolly JL, Schnitt SJ, Colditz GA: A prospective study of benign breast disease and the risk of breast cancer. JAMA 267:1780, 1992; and Dupont WD, Parl FF, Hartmann WH, et al: Breast cancer risk associated with proliferative breast disease and atypical hyperplasia. Cancer 71:1258, 1993.

*Ratio of observed incidence over the incidence in women without proliferative disease.

†Fibrocystic change with no, usual, or mild hyperplasia.

‡Fibrocystic change with hyperplasia greater than mild or usual, papilloma, papillomatosis, sclerosing adenosis, radial scar, and other findings.

§Any diagnosis of atypical ductal or lobular hyperplasia, or both.

**Family History and Genetic Risk Factors** Many studies have examined the relationship of family history and the risk for breast cancer. First-degree relatives (mothers, sisters, and daughters) of patients with breast cancer have a twofold to threefold excess risk for development of the disease. Risk is much higher if affected first-degree relatives had premenopausal onset and bilateral breast cancer. Risk is not significantly increased in women with distant relatives affected with breast cancer (cousins, aunts, grandmothers), although breast cancer in paternal aunts may be associated with a genetic predisposition. In families with multiple affected members, particularly with bilateral and early-onset cancer, the absolute risk in first-degree relatives approaches 50%, consistent with an autosomal dominant mode of inheritance in these families.

Genetic factors are estimated to be responsible for 5% to 10% of all breast cancer cases, but they may account for 25% of cases in women younger than 30 years. In 1990, King and colleagues identified a region on the long arm of chromosome 17 (17q21) that contained a cancer susceptibility gene. The *BRCA1* gene was discovered in 1994; it is now known that mutations in *BRCA1* account for up to 40% of familial breast cancers. One year later, a second susceptibility gene, *BRCA2,* was discovered. In addition to increased breast cancer risk, women with mutations in *BRCA1* or *BRCA2* are at increased risk for ovarian cancer (45% lifetime risk for *BRCA1* carriers).

Deleterious mutations in *BRCA1* or *BRCA2* are rare in the general population. The frequency of mutations is approximately 1 in 1000 (0.1%) in the American population. Certain relatively closed populations may have higher prevalence rates and show preference for certain mutations, termed *founder mutations,* including the 185delAG and 5382insC mutations in *BRCA1,* which are found in up to 1.0% of the Ashkenazi Jewish population (Jews of Eastern European descent), and the C4446T mutation in French Canadian families. *BRCA1* is a large gene with 22 coding exons and more than 500 mutations; many of these are unique and limited to a given family, which makes genetic testing technically difficult. *BRCA1* is a tumor suppressor gene with disease susceptibility inherited in an autosomal dominant fashion. Germline mutations inactivate a single inherited allele of *BRCA1* in every cell and this precedes a somatic event in breast epithelial cells, which eliminates the remaining allele and causes the cancer. The gene product may provide negative regulation of cell growth and is also involved in recognition and repair of genetic damage.

The *BRCA2* gene is located on chromosome 13 and accounts for up to 30% of familial breast cancers; unlike *BRCA1*, it is associated with increased breast cancer risk in males. Women with a mutation in *BRCA2* also have a 20% to 30% lifelong risk for ovarian cancer. Founder mutations of *BRCA2* include the 617delT mutation present in 1.4% of the Ashkenazi population, 8765delAG mutation in the French Canadian population, and 999del15 mutation in the Icelandic population. In Iceland, 7% of unselected female breast cancer patients and 0.6% of the general population carry the 999del15 mutation.

The penetrance of *BRCA1* and *BRCA2* refers to the chance that carriers of mutations in these genes will actually develop breast cancer. The initial estimates of this chance were high, but a more recent estimate has placed the penetrance of *BRCA1* and *BRCA2* mutations at 56% (95% confidence interval [CI], 40% to 73%). It is reasonable to quote lifelong rates of breast cancer between 50% and 70% for carriers of *BRCA1* or *BRCA2* mutations.

The histopathology of *BRCA1*-associated breast cancer is unfavorable when compared with *BRCA2*-associated cancer and includes tumors that are high grade, hormone receptor–negative, and aneuploid, with an increased S phase fraction. There is a strong association between the basal-like breast cancer subtype and *BRCA1* mutations. Women who carry a *BRCA1* mutation and contract breast cancer are highly likely to have a basal-like breast cancer; up to 10% of basal-like tumors arise in women found to have a mutation. The same is not true for *BRCA2*-associated cancers, which are more commonly hormone receptor–positive. Overall mortality rates in patients with *BRCA1*- or *BRCA2*-associated breast cancer are similar to those in women with sporadic breast cancer. Because the risk for development of breast cancer is high in carriers of a *BRCA* gene mutation, the use of prophylactic surgery is considered to be the most rational approach. The use of MRI is encouraged for women who prefer to undergo an intensive screening program. The efficacy of chemoprevention in *BRCA* mutation carriers is unclear, especially in those with *BRCA1* mutations who tend to develop estrogen receptor–negative breast cancers.

**Reproductive Risk Factors** Reproductive milestones that increase a woman's lifetime estrogen exposure are thought to increase her breast cancer risk. These include onset of menarche before 12 years of age, first live childbirth after age 30, nulliparity, and menopause after age 55 years. There is a 10% reduction in breast cancer risk for each 2-year delay in menarche; the risk doubles with menopause after age 55. Those having a full-term first pregnancy before age 18 have half the risk for development of breast cancer than women whose first pregnancy is after age 30. There is no increased risk associated with induced abortion. Breastfeeding has been reported to reduce breast cancer risk and this may be secondary to a decrease in the number of lifetime menstrual cycles. When compared with gender, age, histologic risk factors, and genetics, reproductive risk factors are relatively mild in terms of their contribution to risk (RR, 0.5 to 2.0). However, these factors, unlike family history or histologic factors, have a large influence on breast cancer prevalence in populations.[7]

**Exogenous Hormone Use** Therapeutic or supplemental estrogen and progesterone are taken for a variety of conditions, with the two most common scenarios being contraception in premenopausal women and HRT in postmenopausal women. Other indications for use include menstrual irregularities, polycystic ovaries, fertility treatment, and hormone insufficiency states. Studies have suggested that breast cancer risk is increased in current or past users of oral contraceptives, a risk that decreases as the interval after cessation of use increases.[8,9]

The use of HRT was studied by the Women's Health Initiative,[8] a prospective, randomized controlled trial in which healthy postmenopausal women 50 to 79 years of age received various dietary and vitamin supplements and postmenopausal HRT. The study assessed the benefits and risks associated with HRT, a low-fat diet, and calcium and vitamin D supplementation and their effects on rates of cancer, cardiovascular disease, and osteoporosis-related fractures. A total of 16,608 women were randomized to receive combined conjugated equine estrogens (e.g., Premarin, 0.625 mg/day) plus medroxyprogesterone acetate (2.5 mg/day) or placebo from 1993 to 1998 at 40 centers in the United States. Screening mammography and clinical breast examinations were performed at baseline and yearly thereafter. The study reached a stopping rule at 5.2 years of follow-up, at which time there were 245 cases of breast cancer (invasive and noninvasive) in the combined HRT group versus 185 cases in the placebo group. When compared with placebo, the combination of estrogen and progesterone, specifically PremPro, increased the risk of developing breast cancer in postmenopausal women with an intact uterus. Of greater concern was that women on estrogen plus progesterone were more likely to be diagnosed with a breast cancer at a more advanced stage, and there was a substantial increase in the number of women with abnormal mammograms. Women who had a hysterectomy were randomized to estrogen only versus placebo and, after 7 years of follow-up, 10,739 women receiving conjugated equine estrogens (e.g., Premarin) at a dose of 0.625 mg daily or a placebo had equivalent rates of breast cancer (RR, 0.80; 95% CI, 0.62 to 1.04).[9] There was a statistically significant difference between the treatment and control groups in the need for short-interval mammographic follow-up examinations, which was higher in the group that received Premarin (36.2% versus 28.1%). These data show that women receiving combination HRT with estrogen and progesterone for 5 years have approximately a 20% increased risk for the development of breast cancer. Women who take estrogen-only formulations (because of previous hysterectomy) do not appear to suffer an increased incidence of breast cancer.

### Risk Assessment Tools

A model for assessing breast cancer risk was developed from case-control data in the Breast Cancer Detection Demonstration Project (available for clinical use at http://cancer.gov/bc risktool; also known as the *Gail model*). It was determined that age, race, age at menarche, age at first live birth, number of previous breast biopsies, presence of proliferative disease with atypia, and number of first-degree female relatives with breast cancer influenced the risk for breast cancer. The model does not include detailed information about genetic factors and may underestimate the risk for a *BRCA1* or *BRCA2* mutation carrier and overestimate the risk in a noncarrier. It should not be used in women with a diagnosis of LCIS or DCIS. The Gail model for breast cancer risk was used in the design of the Breast Cancer Prevention Trial, which randomly assigned women at high risk (>1.67%) to receive tamoxifen or a placebo, and in the Study of Tamoxifen and Raloxifene (STAR),[10] which randomly assigned women at high risk to receive tamoxifen or raloxifene. The Gail model assesses population risk using nongenetic factors, whereas the hereditary and familial models assess genetic and familial risk of breast cancer. The Claus model is another risk assessment model, which is based on assumptions about the prevalence of high-penetrance breast cancer susceptibility genes. The Claus model incorporates more information about family history and provides individual estimates of breast cancer risk according to decade of life based on knowledge of first- and second-degree relatives with breast cancer and their age at diagnosis.

There have been several models designed to assess the risk for an individual harboring a mutation in *BRCA1* or *BRCA2*. This can be useful in determining the need for genetic testing. The Couch model predicts risk for a mutation in the *BRCA1* gene. The BRCAPro model was developed by Myriad Genetics Laboratories and provides estimates for the risk of *BRCA1* and *BRCA2* mutations. The Tyrer model incorporates personal risk factors and genetic analysis to give a more comprehensive and individual risk assessment. Such models have estimated that the incidence of clinically significant *BRCA1* or *BRCA2* mutations in the general population is approximately 1 in 300 to 500. Indications for consideration of genetic testing include a personal history of young age at diagnosis (<50 years), bilateral breast cancer, breast and ovarian cancer in the same individual, and male breast cancer. Other factors that may be an indication for testing are a family history (maternal or paternal) of two or more individuals with breast and ovarian cancer, close male relative with breast cancer, close relative with early-onset breast or ovarian cancer (<50 years), and known *BRCA1* or *BRCA2* mutation.

## Management of High-Risk Patients

In practice, clinicians assess risk factors and consider those that are important to individual patients in making recommendations about screening and intervention. Increased risk for breast cancer is defined as a 5-year calculated risk of 1.7% or higher using the National Cancer Institute (NCI) risk calculator. This is the average risk for a woman who is 60 years old; it has been used in the design of the U.S. prevention trials. This risk calculator is not applicable to women with a history of invasive breast cancer, DCIS, or LCIS. The model does not make adjustments for a first-degree relative with premenopausal or bilateral breast cancer and genetic mutations are not considered in the calculation. The clinician must understand that risk may be significantly underestimated if these factors are present and, therefore, the risk calculation should be made within the context of the patient's overall personal and family history. However, even with these limitations, the Gail model provides a valuable starting point for the evaluation of breast cancer risk assessment. This risk assessment can provide a context for recommendations for primary prevention strategies and screening appropriate to the individual's risk level. For women found to be at high risk for the development of breast cancer, options include close surveillance with clinical breast examination, mammography, and breast MRI (depending on the lifetime risk), or interventions to reduce risk, such as chemoprevention with tamoxifen or raloxifene or a bilateral prophylactic mastectomy or oophorectomy.

### Close Surveillance

Surveillance guidelines for individuals at high risk for breast cancer were established in 2002 by the National Comprehensive Cancer Network and the Cancer Genetics Studies Consortium. These guidelines are based primarily on expert opinion; screening guidelines for high-risk individuals are not established by prospective trials.

Recommendations for women in a family with a breast and ovarian cancer syndrome include monthly breast self-examination beginning at 18 to 20 years of age, semiannual clinical breast examination beginning at age 25, and annual mammography beginning at age 25, or 10 years before the earliest age at onset of breast cancer in a family member. Nonetheless, studies of women with known *BRCA1* or *BRCA2* mutations have found that 50% of the detected breast cancers were diagnosed as interval cancers; that is, they occurred between screening episodes and not during the course of routine screening. This observation has prompted many groups to add annual screening MRI to mammography, with some doing both simultaneously and others staggering the two examinations. If not done previously, genetic counseling is offered to those with a strong family history of early-onset breast and ovarian cancer, including a discussion of genetic testing for *BRCA1* and *BRCA2* mutations.

### Chemoprevention for Breast Cancer

The drugs currently approved for reducing breast cancer risk are tamoxifen and raloxifene. Tamoxifen is an estrogen antagonist with proven benefit for the treatment of estrogen receptor (ER)–positive breast cancer. Raloxifene is a selective ER modulator (SERM). Tamoxifen has been used in the adjuvant setting for breast cancer for several decades and is known to reduce the incidence of a second primary breast cancer in the contralateral breast of women who received the drug as adjuvant therapy for a first breast cancer. Findings from the overview analysis of the Early Breast Cancer Trialists' Collaborative Group (EBCTCG) have demonstrated that adjuvant tamoxifen reduces the risk for a second breast cancer in the unaffected breast by 47%. Four prospective randomized trials have been completed evaluating tamoxifen as chemoprevention in healthy women known to be at increased risk for breast cancer. The National Surgical Adjuvant Breast and Bowel Project (NSABP) recently reported findings of the STAR trial, which compared tamoxifen versus raloxifene.[10] Trials are ongoing assessing the role of aromatase inhibitors (AIs) as chemoprevention in postmenopausal women.

The NSABP P-1 trial randomized 13,388 women aged 35 to 59 years with a diagnosis of LCIS, women whose risk for breast cancer was moderately increased (RR, 1.66 over a 5-year period), and women 60 years or older to tamoxifen or placebo. The risk estimates were based on the Gail model of risk (see earlier). In this study, tamoxifen reduced the risk for invasive breast cancer by 49% through 69 months of follow-up, with a risk reduction of 59% in the subgroup with LCIS and 86% in those with ADH or ALH. The reduction in risk was noted only for ER-positive cancers. Tamoxifen treatment for 5 years was not without side effects and complications. In the tamoxifen treatment arm, endometrial cancers resulting from estrogen-like effects of the drug on the endometrium were increased by a factor of approximately 2.5. Pulmonary embolism (RR, 3) and deep venous thrombosis (RR, 1.7) were also more common in women who received tamoxifen. Data on the efficacy of tamoxifen for reduction of breast cancer risk in *BRCA1* and *BRCA2* mutation carriers are limited because mutation testing was not routinely performed on P-1 study participants. Tamoxifen is most effective at reducing the incidence of ER-positive breast cancers, so its role in *BRCA1* mutation carriers (who more often develop ER-negative breast cancers) is questionable. Several other tamoxifen prevention trials were conducted at around the same time as the NSABP P-1 trial, including the Italian Tamoxifen Prevention Study, Royal Marsden Hospital Tamoxifen Prevention Pilot Trial, and International Breast Cancer Intervention Study (IBIS-1). The Italian and Royal Marsden studies did not show any benefit of tamoxifen over placebo in terms of reduced incidence of breast cancer. There were some differences in the study population and trial designs, which may explain the negative results as compared with the P-1 trial. The IBIS-1 trial showed a 33% reduction in the incidence of breast cancer, slightly lower than that in P-1 but confirming the risk reduction benefit of tamoxifen. Subsequently, a meta-analysis of all the tamoxifen prevention trials found that tamoxifen reduced the risk of breast cancer by 38%. This analysis also confirmed the increased risks of endometrial cancer and venous thromboembolic events seen with tamoxifen use.

The NSABP P-2 trial (STAR trial)[10] compared tamoxifen with raloxifene in postmenopausal women. This comparison was based on the findings from the MORE trial, which included more than 10,000 women who received placebo versus raloxifene for the prevention and treatment of osteoporosis. At an average 3 years of follow-up, there was a 54% reduction in the incidence of breast cancer and no increase in uterine cancer. The STAR trial enrolled 19,747 women at increased risk for breast cancer and demonstrated that tamoxifen and raloxifene reduced the risk for invasive breast cancer by approximately 50%. Raloxifene had a more favorable toxicity profile, the number of uterine cancers was reduced by 36% compared with tamoxifen, and women taking raloxifene had 29% fewer episodes of venous thrombosis and a reduced incidence of pulmonary embolism.

### Prophylactic Mastectomy

Prophylactic mastectomy has been shown to reduce the chance of developing breast cancer in high-risk women by 90%. Hartmann and coworkers[11] have reported on a retrospective review of 639 women with a family history of breast cancer who underwent prophylactic mastectomy. The women were divided into high-risk ($n = 214$) and moderate-risk ($n = 425$) groups, with high-risk patients defined as those with a family history suggestive of an autosomal dominant predisposition to breast cancer. For women of moderate risk, the number of expected breast cancers was calculated according to the Gail model. Based on this model, 37.4 breast cancers were expected to have developed and 4 cancers actually did, for an incidence risk reduction of 89%. For women in the high-risk cohort, the Gail model would underestimate the risk for the development of breast cancer. Thus, the expected number of breast cancers was calculated by using three different statistical models from a control study of the high-risk probands (sisters). Three breast cancers developed after prophylactic mastectomy, for an incident risk reduction of at least 90%.

Several groups have reported on prospective studies in *BRCA1* and *BRCA2* mutation carriers treated with prophylactic mastectomy versus surveillance and have shown that mastectomy is highly effective in preventing breast cancers compared with a significant number of events in women not choosing preventive mastectomy. More recently, results of risk-reducing mastectomy (RRM) and risk-reducing salpingo-oophorectomy (RRSO) were reported in *BRCA1* and *BRCA2* mutation carriers followed in 22 centers as part of the PROSE consortium.[12] None of the participants who underwent RRM developed a subsequent breast cancer compared with 7% of the women who did not undergo RRM. The use of RRSO reduced the incidence of ovarian cancers from 5.8% to 1.1% and the incidence of breast cancers from 19.2% to 11.4%. RRSO was associated with a significant reduction in breast cancer–specific mortality, ovarian cancer– specific mortality, and all-cause mortality. The available data suggest that *BRCA* mutation carriers should be counseled to consider risk-reducing surgeries as a strategy to reduce cancer incidence and improve survival.

Women who undergo annual mammographic screening have an overall 80% chance of surviving the breast cancer once it has been detected. Coupled with penetrance figures in the range of 50% to 60% for mutation carriers, the chance of *BRCA1* or *BRCA2* mutation carriers dying from breast cancer is approximately 10% if they choose not to undergo risk-reducing surgery.[11]

The use of risk-reducing surgery in women who are not known to have deleterious mutations in *BRCA1* or *BRCA2* remains controversial. Recent trends have suggested that more women with newly diagnosed breast cancer are choosing to undergo contralateral prophylactic mastectomy as a risk reduction strategy for contralateral breast cancer. Determining which patients may benefit from this approach has been challenging. Bedrosian and colleagues[13] used the Surveillance, Epidemiology, and End Results (SEER) database to study this and found that there was an improvement in breast cancer–specific mortality of 4.8% at 5 years in women with stage I or II breast cancer with ER-negative disease who underwent contralateral prophylactic mastectomy. There was a lower incidence of contralateral breast cancers in women with ER-positive disease who did not undergo prophylactic mastectomy compared with their ER-negative counterparts.

### Summary: Risk Assessment and Management

Understanding risk factors for the development of disease provide clues to pathogenesis and identifies patients likely to benefit from risk-reducing strategies. Although breast cancer can develop in both genders, women are at greatly increased risk and breast cancer in men is uncommon. Age is a strong determinant of risk and is part of the NCI risk assessment tool. Family history is most significant when breast cancer affects young first-degree relatives (mothers, sisters, and daughters) and when cases of ovarian cancer are found in the same side of the family, and may preclude the use of the NCI tool for accurate risk assessment. The most significant histologic risk factors for the development of breast cancer are ADH, ALH, and LCIS. A personal history of breast cancer predisposes to contralateral breast cancer.

## BENIGN BREAST TUMORS AND RELATED DISEASES

### Breast Cysts

Cysts within the breast parenchyma are fluid-filled, epithelial-lined cavities that may vary in size from microscopic to large palpable masses containing as much as 20 to 30 mL of fluid. A palpable cyst develops in at least 1 in every 14 women, and 50%

of cysts are multiple or recurrent. The pathogenesis of cyst formation is not well understood; however, cysts appear to arise from destruction and dilation of lobules and terminal ductules. Microscopic studies have shown that fibrosis at or near the lobule, combined with continued secretion, results in unfolding of the lobule and expansion of an epithelial-lined cavity containing fluid.[1,5]

Cysts are influenced by ovarian hormones, a fact that explains their variation with the menstrual cycle. Most cysts occur in women older than 35 years; the incidence steadily increases until menopause and sharply declines thereafter. New cyst formation in older women is generally associated with exogenous hormone replacement.

Intracystic carcinoma is exceedingly rare. Rosemond has reported that only three cancers were identified in more than 3000 cyst aspirations (0.1%). Other investigators have confirmed this low incidence. There is no evidence of increased risk for breast cancer associated with cyst formation.

A palpable mass can be confirmed to be a cyst by direct aspiration or ultrasonography. Cyst fluid can be straw-colored, opaque, or dark green and may contain debris. Given the low risk for malignancy within a cyst, if the mass resolves following aspiration and the cyst contents are not grossly bloody, the fluid does not need to be sent for cytologic analysis. If the cyst recurs multiple times (more than twice is a reasonable rule), pneumocystography should be performed to evaluate for a sold component and core or FNA biopsy should be performed to evaluate the solid elements. Surgical removal of a cyst is usually not indicated but may be required if the cyst recurs multiple times, or based on the needle biopsy results.

## Fibroadenoma and Other Benign Tumors

Fibroadenomas are benign solid tumors composed of stromal and epithelial elements. Fibroadenoma is the second most common tumor in the breast (after carcinoma) and is the most common tumor in women younger than 30 years. In contrast to cysts, fibroadenomas most often arise in the late teens and in women during their early reproductive years. Fibroadenomas are rarely seen as new masses in women after the age of 40 or 45 years. Clinically, they present as firm masses that are easily movable and may increase in size over a period of several months. They slide easily under the examining fingers and may be lobulated or smooth. On excision, fibroadenomas are well-encapsulated masses that may detach easily from surrounding breast tissue. Mammography is of little help in discriminating between cysts and fibroadenomas; however, ultrasonography can readily distinguish between them because each has specific characteristics. FNA biopsy can also be used to confirm the imaging findings.

Fibroadenomas are benign tumors, although neoplasia may develop in the epithelial elements within them. Cancer in a newly discovered fibroadenoma is exceedingly rare; 50% of neoplasias that involve fibroadenomas are LCIS, 35% are infiltrating carcinomas, and 15% are intraductal carcinoma.

Once a tissue diagnosis confirms that the breast mass is a fibroadenoma, the patient can be reassured without the need for surgical excision. If the patient is bothered by the mass or it continues to increase in size, the mass can be excised or treated with cryoablation under ultrasonographic guidance. The mass may remain palpable following cryoablation or, in other cases, the mass may calcify, causing it to feel more firm on palpation.

Two subtypes of fibroadenoma are recognized. *Giant fibroadenoma* is a descriptive term applied to a fibroadenoma that attains an unusually large size, typically greater than 5 cm. The term *juvenile fibroadenoma* refers to the occasional large fibroadenoma that occurs in adolescents and young adults and histologically is more cellular than the usual fibroadenoma. Although these lesions may display remarkably rapid growth, surgical removal is curative.

## Hamartoma and Adenoma

These lesions are benign proliferations of variable amounts of epithelium and stromal supporting tissue. A hamartoma is a discrete nodule that contains closely packed lobules and prominent, ectatic extralobular ducts. On physical examination, mammography, and gross inspection, a hamartoma is indistinguishable from fibroadenoma. Page and Anderson have described an adenoma or tubular adenoma as a benign cellular neoplasm of ductules packed closely together so that they form a sheet of tiny glands without supporting stroma. During pregnancy and lactation, these tumors may increase in size, and histologic examination shows secretory differentiation. Biopsy is required to establish the diagnosis.

## Breast Abscess and Infections

Infections of the breast fall into two general categories, lactational infections and chronic subareolar infections associated with duct ectasia. Lactational infections are thought to arise from entry of bacteria through the nipple into the duct system and are characterized by fever, leukocytosis, erythema, and tenderness. Infections are most often caused by *Staphylococcus aureus* and may be manifested as cellulitis with breast parenchymal inflammation and swelling, termed *mastitis,* or as abscesses. Treatment requires antibiotics and frequent emptying of the breast. True abscesses require surgical drainage because they are generally multiloculated.

In women who are not lactating, a chronic relapsing form of infection may develop in the subareolar ducts of the breast that is variously known as *periductal mastitis* or *duct ectasia*. This condition appears to be associated with smoking and diabetes. The infections that arise are most often mixed infections that include aerobic and anaerobic skin flora. A series of infections with resulting inflammatory changes and scarring may lead to retraction or inversion of the nipple, masses in the subareolar area and, occasionally, a chronic fistula from the subareolar ducts to the periareolar skin. Palpable masses and mammographic changes may result from the infection and scarring; these can make surveillance for breast cancer more challenging.

Subareolar infections may initially be manifested as subareolar pain and mild erythema. If treated at this stage, warm soaks and oral antibiotics may be effective. Antibiotic treatment generally requires coverage for aerobic and anaerobic organisms. If an abscess has developed, incision and drainage are required, in addition to antibiotics. Repeated infections are treated by excision of the entire subareolar duct complex after the acute infection has resolved completely, together with IV antibiotic coverage. Rarely, patients will have recurrent infections requiring excision of the nipple and areola.

A presumed infection of the breast generally clears promptly and completely with antibiotic therapy. If erythema or edema persists, a diagnosis of inflammatory carcinoma should be considered.

### Papillomas and Papillomatosis

Solitary intraductal papillomas are true polyps of epithelial-lined breast ducts. Solitary papillomas are most often located close to the areola but may be present in peripheral locations. Most papillomas are smaller than 1 cm but can grow to as large as 4 or 5 cm in size. Larger papillomas may appear to arise within a cystic structure, probably representing a greatly expanded duct. Papillomas are not associated with an increased risk for breast cancer.

Papillomas located close to the nipple are often accompanied by bloody nipple discharge. Less frequently, they are discovered as a palpable mass under the areola or as a density seen on a mammogram. Treatment is excision through a circumareolar incision. For peripheral papillomas, the differential diagnosis is between papilloma and invasive papillary carcinoma.

It is important to distinguish papillomatosis from solitary or multiple papillomas. Papillomatosis refers to epithelial hyperplasia, which commonly occurs in younger women or is associated with fibrocystic change. Papillomatosis is not composed of true papillomas but has hyperplastic epithelium that may fill individual ducts like a true polyp but has no stalk of fibrovascular tissue.

### Sclerosing Adenosis

Adenosis refers to an increased number of small terminal ductules or acini. It is frequently associated with a proliferation of stromal tissue producing a histologic lesion, sclerosing adenosis, which can be confused with carcinoma both grossly and histologically. These lesions can be associated with deposition of calcium, which can be seen on a mammogram in a pattern indistinguishable from the microcalcifications of intraductal carcinoma. Sclerosing adenosis is the most common pathologic diagnosis in patients undergoing needle-directed biopsy of microcalcifications in many series. Sclerosing adenosis is frequently listed as one of the component lesions of fibrocystic disease; it is common and has no significant malignant potential.

### Radial Scar

Radial scars belong to a group of abnormalities known as *complex sclerosing lesions*. They can appear similar to carcinomas mammographically because they create irregular spiculations in the surrounding stroma. These lesions contain microcysts, epithelial hyperplasia, adenosis, and a prominent display of central sclerosis. The gross abnormality is rarely more than 1 cm in diameter. Larger lesions may form palpable tumors and appear as a spiculated mass with prominent architectural distortion on a mammogram. These tumors can even result in skin dimpling by producing traction on surrounding tissues. They generally require excision to rule out an underlying carcinoma. Radial scars are associated with a modestly increased risk for breast cancer.

### Fat Necrosis

Fat necrosis can mimic cancer by producing a palpable mass or density on a mammogram that may contain calcifications. Fat necrosis may follow an episode of trauma to the breast or be related to a prior surgical procedure or radiation treatment. The calcifications are characteristic of fat necrosis and can often be imaged on ultrasonography as well. Histologically, the lesion is composed of lipid-laden macrophages, scar tissue, and chronic inflammatory cells. This lesion has no malignant potential.

## EPIDEMIOLOGY AND PATHOLOGY OF BREAST CANCER

### Epidemiology

In 2010, a total of 209,060 cases of invasive breast cancer and almost 54,010 cases of in situ breast cancer were diagnosed in the United States. Breast cancer continues to be the second leading cause of cancer-related deaths. second to lung cancer, with approximately 40,000 deaths caused by breast cancer annually. Breast cancer is also a global health problem, with more than 1 million cases of breast cancer diagnosed worldwide each year. The overall incidence of breast cancer was rising until approximately 1999 because of increases in the average life span, lifestyle changes that increase the risk for breast cancer, and improved survival from other diseases. The rates began to decrease from 1999 to 2006 by approximately 2%/year. This decrease has been attributed to a reduction in the use of HRT after the initial results of the Women's Health Initiative were published but may also be the result of a reduction in the use of screening mammography (70.1% of women 40 years and older were screened in 2000 versus 66.4% in 2005). Survival rates in women with breast cancer have steadily improved over the last several decades, with 5-year survival rates of 63% in the early 1960s, 75% from 1975 to 1977, 79% from 1984 to 1986 and 90% from 1995 to 2005. The largest decrease in death rates caused by breast cancer have been in women younger than 50 years (3.2%/year), although they have also decreased in women older than 50 (2%/year). The decreased mortality from breast cancer is thought to be the result of earlier detection via mammographic screening, improvements in therapy, and a decreased incidence of breast cancer. The current treatment of breast cancer is guided by pathology, staging, and recent insights into breast cancer biology. There is an increased emphasis on defining disease biology and status in individual patients, with the subsequent tailoring of therapies toward that individual.

### Pathology

#### Noninvasive Breast Cancer

Noninvasive neoplasms are broadly divided into two major types, LCIS and DCIS (Box 36-2). LCIS was initially believed to be a malignant lesion, but is now regarded more as a risk factor for the development of breast cancer. LCIS is recognized by its conformity to the outline of the normal lobule, with expanded and filled acini (Fig. 36-7). DCIS is a more heterogeneous lesion morphologically, and pathologists recognize four broad categories—papillary, cribriform, solid, and comedo types; the latter three types are shown in Figure 36-7. DCIS is recognized as discrete spaces filled with malignant cells, usually with a recognizable basal cell layer made up of presumably normal myoepithelial cells. The four morphologic categories of DCIS are rarely seen as pure lesions, but in reality are often mixed. The papillary and cribriform types of DCIS are generally of lower grade and may take a longer period of time to transform to invasive cancer. The solid and comedo types of DCIS are generally higher grade lesions.

**BOX 36-2 Classification of Primary Breast Cancer**

**Noninvasive Epithelial Cancers**
LCIS
DCIS or intraductal carcinoma
- Papillary, cribriform, solid, and comedo types

**Invasive Epithelial Cancers (percentage of total)**
Invasive lobular carcinoma (10%)
Invasive ductal carcinoma
- Invasive ductal carcinoma, NOS (50%-70%)
- Tubular carcinoma (2%-3%)
- Mucinous or colloid carcinoma (2%-3%)
- Medullary carcinoma (5%)
- Invasive cribriform carcinoma (1%-3%)
- Invasive papillary carcinoma (1%-2%)
- Adenoid cystic carcinoma (1%)
- Metaplastic carcinoma (1%)

**Mixed Connective and Epithelial Tumors**
Phyllodes tumors, benign and malignant
Carcinosarcoma
Angiosarcoma
Adenocarcinoma

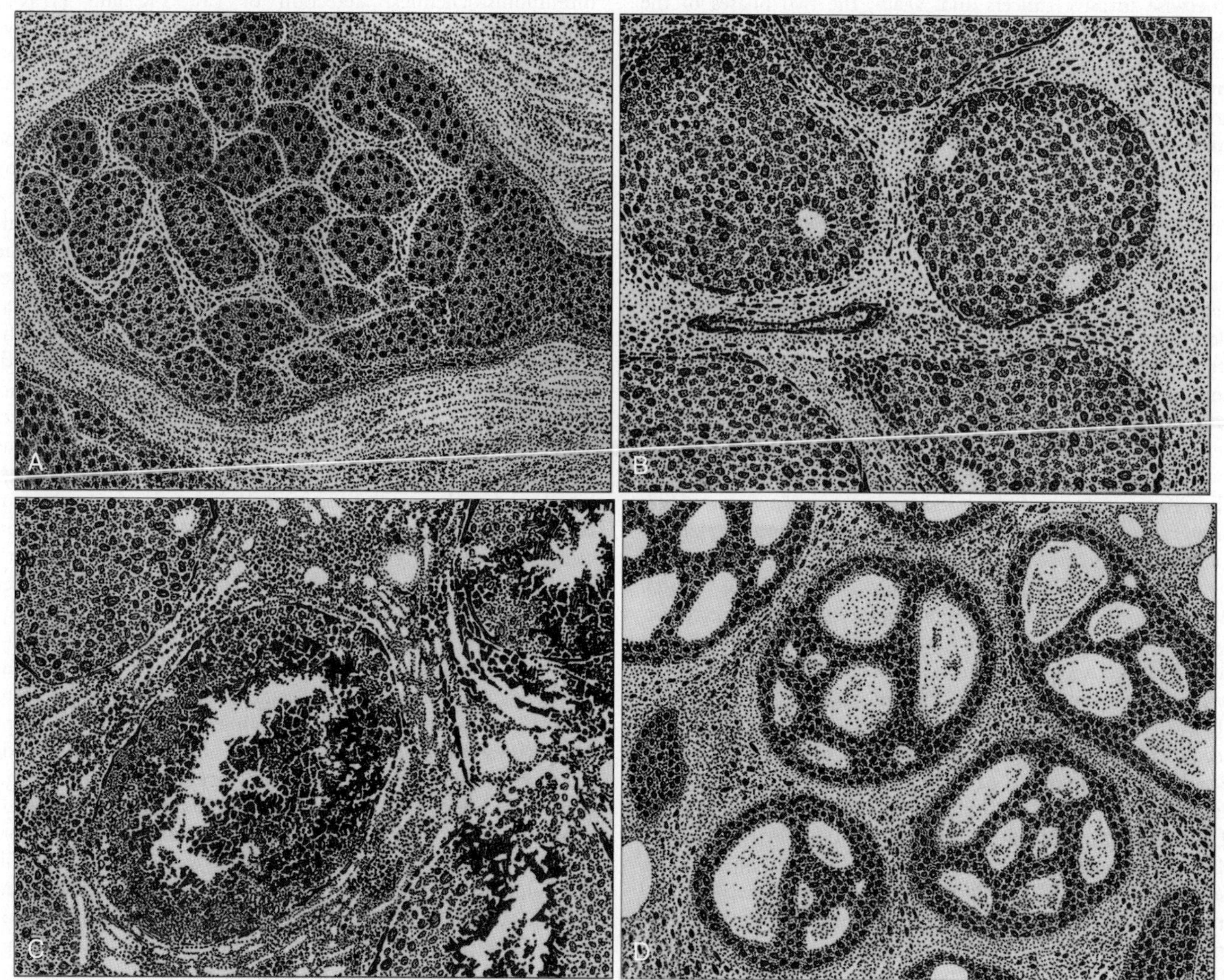


**FIGURE 36-7** Noninvasive breast cancer. **A,** LCIS. The neoplastic cells are small with compact, bland nuclei and are distending the acini but preserving the cross-sectional architecture of the lobular unit. **B,** DCIS, solid type. The cells are larger than in LCIS and are filling the ductal rather than the lobular spaces. However, the cells are contained within the basement membrane of the duct and do not invade the breast stroma. **C,** DCIS, comedo type. In comedo DCIS, the malignant cells in the center undergo necrosis, coagulation, and calcification. **D,** DCIS, cribriform type. In this type, bridges of tumor cells span the ductal space and leave round, punched-out spaces.

As the cells inside the ductal membrane grow, they have a tendency to undergo central necrosis, perhaps because the blood supply to these cells is located outside the basement membrane. The necrotic debris in the center of the duct undergoes coagulation and finally calcifies, thereby leading to the tiny, pleomorphic, and frequently linear forms of microcalcifications seen on mammograms. In some patients, an entire ductal tree may be involved in the malignancy, and the mammogram shows typical calcifications from the nipple extending posteriorly into the interior of the breast (termed *segmental calcifications*). For reasons that are not completely understood, DCIS transforms into an invasive cancer, usually recapitulating the morphology of the cells inside the duct. In other words, low-grade cribriform DCIS tends to be associated with a low-grade invasive lesion that retains some cribriform features. There is no tendency for the grade to advance with invasion. DCIS frequently coexists with otherwise invasive cancers and, again, the two phases of the malignancy are in step with each other morphologically.

### Invasive Breast Cancer

Invasive cancers are recognized by their lack of overall architecture, infiltration of cells haphazardly into a variable amount of stroma, or formation of sheets of continuous and monotonous cells without respect for form and function of a glandular organ. Pathologists broadly divide invasive breast cancer into lobular and ductal histologic types, which probably does not reflect histogenesis and only imperfectly predicts clinical behavior. Invasive lobular cancer tends to permeate the breast in a single-file nature, which explains why it remains clinically occult and often escapes detection on mammography or physical examination until the extent of the disease is large. Ductal cancers tend to grow as a more cohesive mass; they form discrete abnormalities on mammograms and are often palpable as a discrete lump in the breast at a smaller size compared with lobular cancers. The growth pattern of these lesions is shown in Figure 36-8, invasive ductal cancer in Figure 36-8*A* and invasive lobular cancer in Figure 36-8*B*.

Invasive ductal cancer, also known as *infiltrating ductal carcinoma*, is the most common form of breast cancer; it accounts for 50% to 70% of invasive breast cancers. When this cancer does not take on special features, it is called *infiltrating ductal carcinoma*. Invasive lobular carcinoma accounts for up to 10% of breast cancers, and mixed ductal and lobular cancers have been increasingly recognized and described in pathology reports. When infiltrating ductal carcinomas take on differentiated features, they are named according to the features that they display. If the infiltrating cells form small glands lined by a single row of bland epithelium, they are called *infiltrating tubular carcinoma* (see Fig. 36-8*D*). The infiltrating cells may secrete copious amounts of mucin and appear to float in this material. These lesions are called *mucinous* or *colloid tumors* (see Fig. 36-8*C*). Both tubular and mucinous tumors are usually low grade (grade I) lesions and represent about 2% or 3% each of invasive breast carcinomas.

In contrast, bizarre invasive cells with high-grade nuclear features, many mitoses, and lack of an in situ component characterize medullary cancer. The malignancy forms sheets of cells in an almost syncytial fashion, surrounded by an infiltrate of small mononuclear lymphocytes. The borders of the tumor push into the surrounding breast rather than infiltrate or permeate the stroma. This tumor is shown in Figure 36-8*E*, which demonstrates the bizarre and pleomorphic nuclear features of the cells. In its pure form, it accounts for only approximately 5% of breast cancers; however, some pathologists have described a so-called *medullary variant* that has some features of the pure form of the cancer. These tumors are uniformly high grade, ER- and progesterone receptor (PR)–negative, and negative for the human epidermal growth factor receptor 2 (HER-2/neu; HER-2) cell surface receptor. Tumors that lack expression of ER, PR and HER-2 are often called *triple-negative breast cancers*. Gene expression profiling and microarray analysis of breast cancers have revealed that triple-negative breast cancers are distinctly different from other ductal breast cancers and may also express molecular markers found in basal or myoepithelial cells. The term *basal-like breast cancer* describes a specific subtype of breast cancer as defined by microarray analysis, whereas triple-negative breast cancer is a definition determined by the lack of immunohistochemical detection of ER, PR and HER-2. Although there may be some overlap between triple-negative and basal-like breast cancers, the categories were developed using differing technologies and they are not always the same entity.

The different histologic subtypes of breast cancer have some relationship with prognosis, although this is influenced by tumor size, histologic grade, hormone receptor status, HER-2 status, lymph node status, and other prognostic variables. Infiltrating ductal carcinoma, not otherwise specified (NOS), is the most common form of breast cancer. Its prognosis is variable, modified by histologic grade and expression of molecular markers. Basal-like cancer, or medullary cancer in older classifications, is commonly an aggressive form of breast cancer and, because it is triple receptor–negative, there are no targeted treatments for this form of cancer. Infiltrating lobular breast cancers carry an intermediate prognosis, whereas tubular and mucinous cancers have the best overall prognosis. These generalizations, based on histologic subtype, are useful only in the context of tumor size, grade, and receptor status. Modern classification schemes are replacing these older morphologic descriptions with the determination of molecular markers and breast cancer subtype by microarray analysis.

**Molecular Markers and Breast Cancer Subtypes** There are numerous pathways and molecular markers that have been reported to affect breast cancer outcomes, including steroid hormone receptor pathway (ER and PR), human epidermal growth factor receptor pathway (HER family), angiogenesis, cell cycle (e.g., cyclin-dependent kinases [CDKs]), apoptosis modulators, proteasome, cyclooxygenase-2 (COX-2), peroxisome proliferator-activated receptor-γ (PPAR-γ), insulin-like growth factors (IGF family), transforming growth factor-γ (TGF- γ), platelet-derived growth factor (PDGF), and p53. Most these markers are not routinely tested on breast cancer specimens at the time of diagnosis nor would it be feasible to do so.

Incorporating predictive markers into the routine testing of breast cancers could help predict which patients would be most likely to benefit from therapies directed at that marker. The best example of this is the ER. Before the discovery of the ER, all breast cancers were considered potentially sensitive to endocrine therapy. Now, pathologic assessment of ER is performed on all primary tumors and predicts which patients should receive therapy directed at ER with endocrine therapy. Patients whose tumors are ER negative can be spared 5 years of endocrine

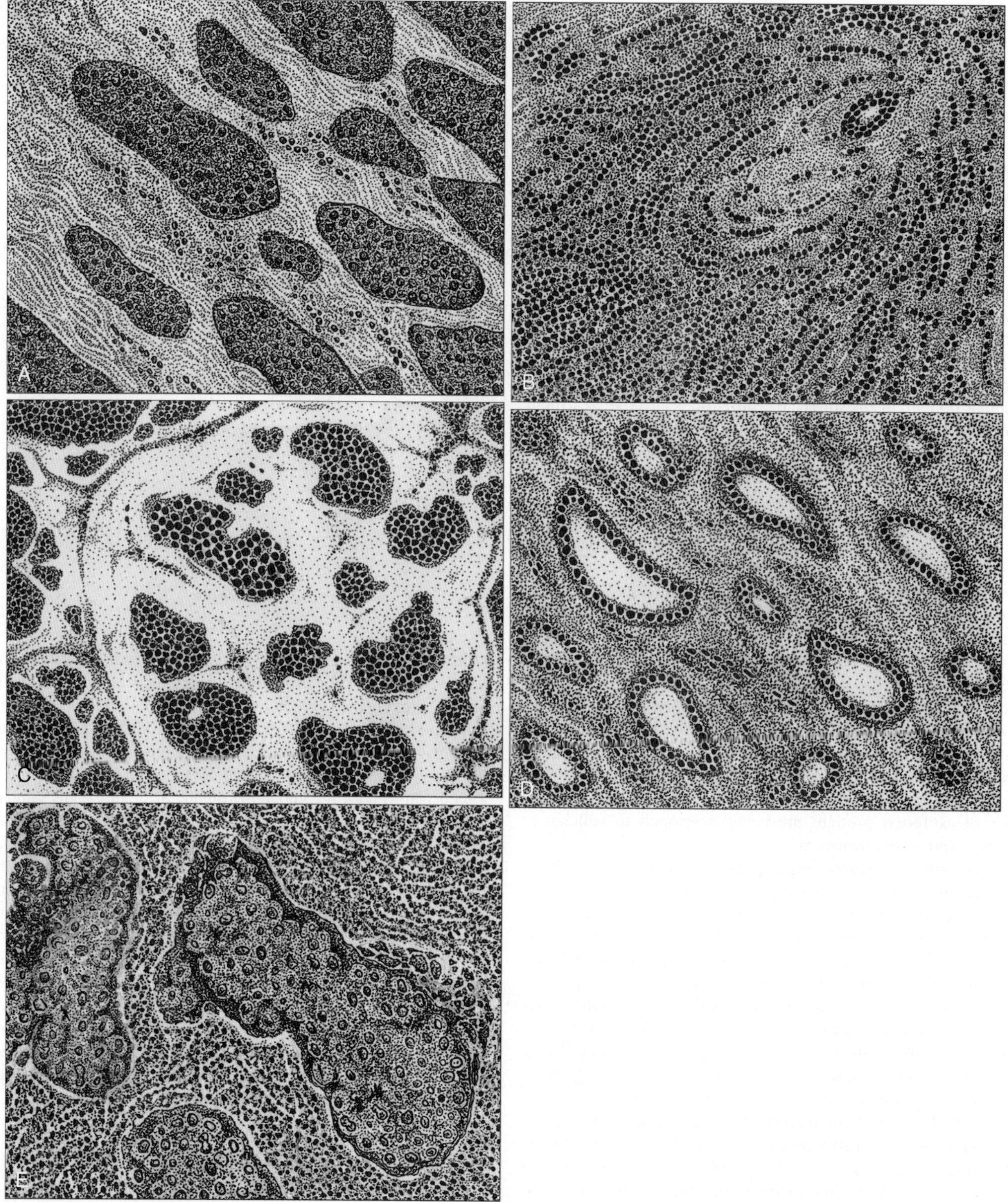


**FIGURE 36-8** Invasive breast cancer. **A,** Invasive ductal carcinoma, NOS. The malignant cells invade in haphazard groups and singly into the stroma. **B,** Invasive lobular carcinoma. The malignant cells invade the stroma in a characteristic single-file pattern and may form concentric circles of single-file cells around normal ducts (targetoid pattern). **C,** Mucinous or colloid carcinoma. The bland tumor cells float like islands in lakes of mucin. **D,** Invasive tubular carcinoma. The cancer invades as small tubules, lined by a single layer of well-differentiated cells. **E,** Medullary carcinoma. The tumor cells are large and very undifferentiated, with pleomorphic nuclei. The distinctive features of this tumor are the infiltrate of lymphocytes and the syncytium-appearing sheets of tumor cells.

therapy. A second important predictive factor in breast cancer, discovered in 1985, is HER-2 or erb-B2/neu protein. This protein is the product of the *erb-B2* gene and is amplified in approximately 20% of human breast cancers. The extracellular domain of the receptor is present on the surface of breast cancer cells and an intracellular tyrosine kinase enzyme links the receptor to the internal machinery of the cell. The tyrosine kinase of HER-2 is activated by growth factors binding to partners and cross-stimulating the HER-2 kinase. Amplification leads to protein overexpression, generally measured clinically by immunohistochemistry and scored on a scale from 0 to 3+. Alternatively, fluorescent in situ hybridization (FISH) directly detects the quantity of HER-2 gene copies; there are normally two copy numbers. Research has shown that inhibition of the function of the HER-2 receptor–like protein slows the growth of HER-2–amplified tumors in laboratory models and in clinical trials. Trastuzumab is a humanized antibody directed against the extracellular domain of the surface receptor and is effective treatment for HER-2–positive breast cancer (see later). HER-2 testing is now a standard part of pathologic reporting on the primary tumor and is a predictive marker for HER-2–directed therapies.

A logical classification scheme for invasive breast cancer is based on the expression of ER status and HER-2 proteins. It has the advantage of directing treatment choices. ER-positive tumors receive endocrine therapies and HER-2–positive cancers are treated with HER-2 inhibitors. However, breast cancer is a heterogeneous disease, and different breast cancers behave in different ways. For example, some ER-positive tumors are indolent and not life-threatening, whereas other ER-positive tumors are very aggressive. In an attempt to subclassify the disease further, investigators are turning to global assessment of gene expression by using microarrays; these are composed of oligonucleotide probes to almost every known expressed sequence of DNA in the human genome. Similar technologies based on single-nucleotide polymorphisms (SNPs) in the cancer DNA and profiles of expressed proteins are being developed to subclassify cancers and direct treatment.

A typical microarray experiment is shown in Figure 36-9, commonly known as a *heat map*; the colors indicate levels of gene expression. Such a portrayal of the disease shows how different ER-positive tumors are from ER-negative tumors and underscores the modern concept that subclassification needs not only to define different groups of breast cancer but also to guide treatment.[14] In Figure 36-9, HER-2–positive tumors form two clusters (in green at the top), although these clusters are fused together in many depictions. HER-2–positive tumors cluster similarly and are responsive to inhibitors of the HER-2 tyrosine kinase–linked surface receptor (e.g., trastuzumab). An unexpected finding, emphasized recently, is the uniqueness of tumors that are both ER-negative and HER-2–negative. These cancers, also negative for PR, are called *triple-negative cancers.* They express proteins in common with myoepithelial cells at the base of mammary ducts and are also called *basal-like cancers* (see earlier). Because they do not express ER or HER-2, new treatments are required. Women who carry a deleterious mutation in *BRCA1* (but not *BRCA2*) are much more likely to contract a basal-like cancer than another subtype. In summary, categorizing breast cancer according to the expression of molecular targets of treatments is practical and appears to agree with nonbiased classifications based on gene expression. Classification schemes reflect biology and predict treatment efficacy.

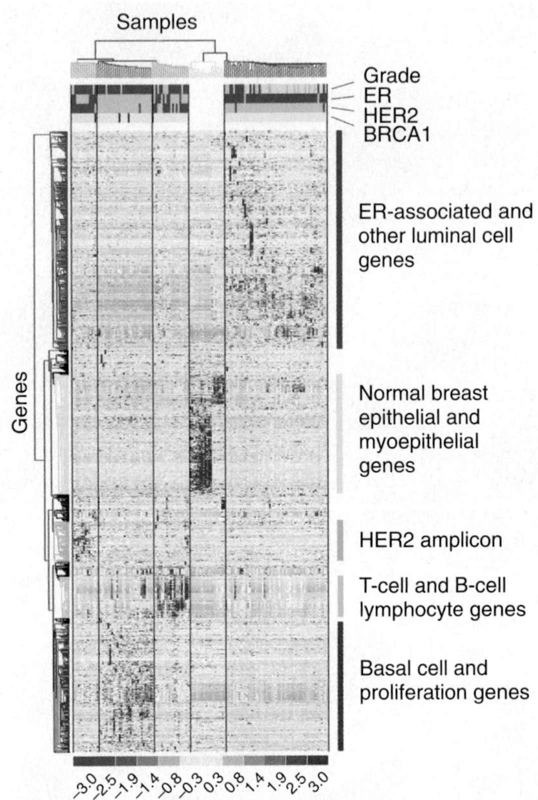


**FIGURE 36-9** Microarray representation of human breast cancer. This portrayal of global gene expression is called a *heat map*, with shades of red indicating high gene expression and shades of blue indicating low gene expression relative to a mean across tissue samples. Tissue samples are present across the top in columns and individual genes are in rows down the side; the intersection is an individual gene in a particular sample. A computer-clustering algorithm aligns samples with similar gene expression and genes with similar expression patterns in the samples (two-way clustering). This illustration provides an unbiased look at breast cancer according to gene expression. The dendrogram at the top depicts the degree of similarity of the tissue samples: yellow, normal breast epithelium; blue, predominantly ER-positive cancers; red, basal-like or triple-negative cancers; and green, HER-2–positive cancers (in two clusters defined by the degree of lymphocytic infiltrate). The *stripes* at the top indicate grade (shades of darker purple are higher grades), ER expression (purple is positive; green is negative), and HER-2 (purple is positive; green is negative). *BRCA1* mutation was determined for other reasons in this experiment. (Courtesy Dr. Andrea Richardson, Department of Pathology, Brigham and Women's Hospital, Boston.)

In addition to classification, molecular markers are used to select patients for systemic treatment (e.g., chemotherapy, endocrine therapy) and to predict the response of patients to these pharmacologic treatments. The simplest example is the use of ER or HER-2 status to predict the response to endocrine treatment or trastuzumab. Multiple gene products may be used in combination for these determinations. Microarray experiments use thousands of gene transcripts (mRNAs) to provide a snapshot of an individual cancer's molecular phenotype. To adapt this technology for clinical application, investigators have selected critical assemblies of gene products that provide the same predictive ability as a nonbiased, genome-wide analysis. The most advanced is a 21-gene test that can be used on paraffin-embedded tumor material from breast surgical specimens (Oncotype DX assay, a 21-gene recurrence score assay).[15] Originally designed to predict the recurrence of ER-positive, node-negative breast cancer treated with adjuvant endocrine therapy, the 21-gene recurrence score assay provides a recurrence score for ER-positive breast cancer that is used clinically to determine whether women with high-risk ER-positive breast cancer should receive adjuvant chemotherapy in addition to tamoxifen (an endocrine therapy; see later). Another multigene assay for determining prognosis is the MammaPrint assay. The MammaPrint assay uses fresh tissue prior to formalin fixation and analyzes data from 70 genes to develop a risk profile. The test provides a simple readout of low-risk or high-risk disease. This tool can be used for risk assessment in patients with ER-positive and ER-negative tumors. It is likely that tests based on critical combinations of genes will increasingly be used to assist clinical decision making when treating breast cancer.

### Other Tumors of the Breast

**Phyllodes Tumors** Tumors of mixed connective tissue and epithelium constitute an important group of unusual primary breast tumors. On one end of the spectrum is the benign fibroadenoma, which is characterized by a proliferation of connective tissue and a variable component of ductal elements that may appear compressed by the swirls of fibroblastic growth. Clinically more challenging are the phyllodes tumors, which contain a biphasic proliferation of stroma and mammary epithelium. First called *cystosarcoma phyllodes*, the name has been changed to phyllodes tumor in recognition of its usually benign course. However, with increasing cellularity, an invasive margin, and sarcomatous appearance, these tumors may be classified as malignant phyllodes tumors. Benign phyllodes tumors are recognized as firm lobulated masses that can range in size, with an average size of approximately 5 cm (larger than average fibroadenomas). Histologically, these tumors are similar to fibroadenomas, but the whorled stroma forms larger clefts lined by epithelium that resemble clusters of leaflike structures. The stroma is more cellular than a fibroadenoma, but the fibroblastic cells are bland and mitoses are infrequent.

Mammographically, these lesions are seen as round densities with smooth borders and are indistinguishable from fibroadenomas. Ultrasonography may reveal a discrete structure with cystic spaces. The diagnosis is suggested by the larger size, history of rapid growth, and occurrence in older patients. Cytologic analysis is unreliable in differentiating a low-grade phyllodes tumor from a fibroadenoma. Core needle biopsy is preferred, although it is difficult to classify phyllodes tumors with benign or intermediate malignant potential based on a limited sampling. Thus, the final diagnosis is best made by excisional biopsy, followed by careful pathologic review.

Local excision of a benign phyllodes tumor is curative, similar to that for a fibroadenoma. The intermediate tumors, also called *borderline phyllodes tumors*, are those in which it is difficult to assign a benign label. These tumors are treated by excision, with margins of at least 1 cm to prevent local recurrence. Affected patients are at some risk for local recurrence, most often within the first 2 years after excision, and close follow-up with examination and imaging allows early detection of recurrence. Finally, frankly malignant stromal sarcomas are at the other end of the spectrum. Malignant phyllodes tumors are treated similar to soft tissue sarcomas that occur on the trunk or extremities. Complete surgical excision of the entire tumor with a margin of normal tissue is advised. When the tumor is large with respect to the size of the breast, this may require total mastectomy. Similar to other soft tissue sarcomas, regional lymph node dissection is not required for staging or locoregional control.

Metastases from malignant phyllodes tumors occur via hematogenous spread; common sites include lung, bone, abdominal viscera, and mediastinum. The optimal palliative treatment of patients with metastatic phyllodes tumors has not been determined. The systemic therapeutic agents used for sarcomas have resulted in minimal success.

**Angiosarcoma** This vascular tumor may occur de novo in the breast or within the dermis of the breast after irradiation for breast cancer. Angiosarcoma has also been seen to develop in the upper extremity of patients with lymphedema, historically after radical mastectomy. Angiosarcoma arising in the absence of previous radiation therapy or surgery generally forms an ill-defined mass within the parenchyma of the breast. In contrast, angiosarcomas caused by prior radiation therapy arise in the irradiated skin as purplish vascular proliferations that may go unrecognized for a period of time. The differential diagnosis is frequently between malignant angiosarcoma and atypical vascular proliferations in irradiated skin. Histologically, the tumor is composed of an anastomosing tangle of blood vessels in the dermis and superficial subcutaneous fat. The atypical and crowded vessels invade through the dermis and into subcutaneous fat. These tumors are graded by the appearance and behavior of the associated endothelial cells. Pleomorphic nuclei, frequent mitoses, and stacking of the endothelial cells lining neoplastic vessels are features seen in higher grade lesions. Rarely seen in hemangiomas, necrosis is common in high-grade angiosarcomas. Clinically, radiation-induced angiosarcoma is identified as a reddish brown to purple raised rash within the radiation portals and on the skin of the breast. As the disease progresses, tumors protruding from the surface of the skin may predominate.

Mammography is unrevealing in most cases of angiosarcoma. In the absence of metastatic disease at initial evaluation, surgery is performed to secure negative skin margins and usually involves a total mastectomy. A split-thickness skin graft or myocutaneous flap may be needed to replace a large skin defect created by the resection. Metastasis to regional nodes is extraordinarily rare and axillary dissection is not required.

Patients remain at high risk for local recurrence after resection of angiosarcoma. For patients who present with primary angiosarcoma of the breast, radiation therapy is of benefit in the locoregional treatment. Patients with radiation-related angiosarcoma are not candidates for further radiotherapy. Metastatic spread occurs hematogenously, most commonly to the lungs and bone and less frequently to abdominal viscera, brain, and even the contralateral breast. Chemotherapy is generally recommended in the adjuvant setting and may improve outcomes of patients with angiosarcoma. For those free of metastatic disease at initial evaluation, the median time to recurrence after mastectomy is 8 months and the median survival is 2 years.

## STAGING OF BREAST CANCER

Breast cancer stage is determined prior to any treatment with physical examination and imaging studies (clinical staging) and on definitive surgical treatment by pathologic examination of the primary tumor and regional lymph nodes (pathologic staging). Staging is performed to group patients into risk categories that define prognosis and guide treatment recommendations for patients with a similar prognosis. Breast cancer is classified with the TNM classification system, which groups patients into four stage groupings based on the size of the primary tumor (T), status of the regional lymph nodes (N), and presence or absence of distant metastasis (M). The most widely used system is that of the American Joint Committee on Cancer (AJCC). This system is updated every 6 to 8 years to reflect current understanding of tumor behavior. Some of the most significant changes in the most recent update (seventh edition) include a more stringent classification of isolated tumor cells based on the number of cells and whether the cells are almost confluent or nonconfluent; stage I breast cancers have been subdivided to IA and IB, with IB classifying T1 tumors associated with micrometastasis (N1mi) in the lymph nodes, and a new category of M0(i+) for patients with circulating tumor cells, disseminated tumor cells (bone marrow micrometastases), or cells found incidentally in other tissues that do not exceed 0.2 mm. Table 36-4 presents the TNM working guide; stage groupings are shown in Table 36-5.

Metastasis to ipsilateral axillary nodes predicts outcome after surgical treatment more powerfully than tumor size. Prior to the incorporation of systemic therapies in the management of breast cancer patients, treatment with surgery alone revealed an almost linear decrement in survival rate with increasing nodal involvement. Although staging is an important part of the initial assessment of breast cancer patients, it is largely based on anatomic variables and does not incorporate other important prognostic factors. The new staging form has a place to record other variables, including tumor grade, ER status, PR status, HER-2/neu status, circulating tumor cells, disseminated tumor cells (bone marrow), multigene recurrence score, and response to chemotherapy. These variables are not currently part of the staging system but it is hoped that future versions will incorporate the most important biologic variables in order for the stage groupings to reflect expected outcomes more accurately. Some prefixes and suffixes are used with the cTNM (clinical) and pTNM (pathologic) staging systems to designate special cases. These do not affect the stage group but indicate that they must be analyzed separately. They include the "m" suffix, which signifies multiple primary tumors, pT(m) NM, the "y" prefix, which denotes patients who have received systemic therapy, ypTNM, and the "r" prefix, which indicates a recurrent tumor, rTNM. In clinical practice, physicians use the anatomic stage grouping in addition to important biologic factors to determine risk and guide treatment recommendations.

## SURGICAL TREATMENT OF BREAST CANCER

### Historical Perspective

Through the mid-20th century, breast cancer was thought to arise in the breast and progress to other sites largely via centrifugal spread. In this model, more extensive surgical procedures were expected to reduce mortality by resecting locoregional disease before it could spread to distant sites. This model was supported, in part, by the results of the Halsted radical mastectomy, which was the first procedure that demonstrated improvements in breast cancer survival relative to the local excision of tumors. Introduced in the 1890s, the radical mastectomy included removal of the breast, overlying skin, and underlying pectoralis muscles in continuity with the regional lymph nodes along the axillary vein to the costoclavicular ligament. The procedure often required a skin graft to cover the large skin defect that was created. This approach was well suited to breast cancer biology of the time, when most tumors were locally advanced, frequently with chest wall or skin involvement and extensive axillary nodal disease. Radical mastectomy provided improved local control and led to an increasing population of long-term survivors. Radical mastectomy continued as the mainstay of surgical therapy into the 1970s.

A large number of women continued to die of metastatic breast cancer after radical mastectomy and even more extensive surgical procedures, including en bloc resection of the internal mammary and supraclavicular nodes, were used but failed to improve survival. This eventually led to a shift in the theory of primary centrifugal spread to the more modern theory that breast cancer spreads both centrifugally to adjacent structures and embolically via lymphatics and blood vessels to distant sites.

In the modern era, breast cancer treatment includes local and regional approaches (surgery and radiation therapy) in addition to medical therapies designed to treat systemic disease. Multimodality treatment approaches were the first to show significant improvements in both locoregional control and survival. As breast cancer was being recognized at earlier stages, the radical mastectomy was abandoned for more conservative approaches in combination with radiation therapy. This has allowed for dramatic reductions in the extent of surgery required for local control of breast cancer, with decreases in treatment-related morbidity. It is recognized that breast cancer is a heterogeneous disease and current treatment strategies take into account properties of the individual patient's tumor, as well as the size and location of tumor, to guide treatment.

### Initial Surgical Trials of Local Therapy for Operable Breast Cancer

For further information about clinical trials and their significance, see later section, "Interpreting Results of Clinical Trials."

#### Radical Mastectomy Versus Total Mastectomy, With or Without Radiation Therapy

The NSABP B-04 trial randomized patients with clinically negative nodes to radical mastectomy, total mastectomy with irradiation of the chest wall and regional nodes, or total mastectomy alone with delayed axillary dissection if nodes became clinically enlarged. Patients with clinically positive nodes were randomized to radical mastectomy or total mastectomy with irradiation of the chest wall and regional lymphatics. At 25 years of follow-up, overall survival and disease-free survival were equivalent in all treatment arms between the node-positive and node-negative groups.[16] In the clinically node-negative patients who underwent radical mastectomy, 38% were found to have nodal metastases at surgery, yet only 18% of patients undergoing total mastectomy without dissection or radiation therapy developed axillary recurrence requiring delayed dissection. Despite the differences in the timing of their treatment, these patients had

**Table 36-4 TNM Classification for Breast Cancer (Pathologic Staging)**

| **Primary Tumor (T)** | |
|---|---|
| TX | Primary tumor cannot be assessed |
| T0 | No evidence of primary tumor |
| Tis | Carcinoma in situ |
| Tis (DCIS) | Ductal carcinoma in situ |
| Tis (LCIS) | Lobular carcinoma in situ |
| Tis (Paget's) | Paget's disease of the nipple not associated with invasive carcinoma or carcinoma in situ (DCIS and/or LCIS) in the underlying breast parenchyma. |
| T1 | Tumor ≤20 mm in greatest dimension |
| T1mi | Tumor ≤1 mm in greatest dimension |
| T1a | Tumor >1 mm but ≤5 mm in greatest dimension |
| T1b | Tumor >5 mm but ≤10 mm in greatest dimension |
| T1c | Tumor >10 mm but ≤20 mm in greatest dimension |
| T2 | Tumor >20 mm but ≤50 mm in greatest dimension |
| T3 | Tumor >50 mm in greatest dimension |
| T4 | Tumor of any size with direct extension to the chest wall and/or to the skin |
| T4a | Extension to the chest wall, not including only pectoralis muscle adherence or invasion |
| T4b | Ulceration and/or ipsilateral satellite nodules and/or edema of the skin |
| T4c | Both T4a and T4b |
| T4d | Inflammatory carcinoma |
| **Regional Lymph Nodes (N)** | |
| pNX | Regional lymph nodes cannot be assessed |
| pN0 | No regional lymph node metastasis |
| pN0(i–) | No regional lymph node metastasis histologically, negative IHC |
| pN0(i+) | Malignant cells in regional lymph node(s) no greater than 0.2 mm |
| pN0(mol–) | No regional lymph node metastasis histologically, negative molecular findings (IHC) |
| pN0(mol+) | Positive molecular findings (RT-PCR), but no metastasis detected by histology or IHC |
| pN1 | Micrometastases; or metastases in one to three axillary nodes; and/or in internal mammary nodes with metastases detected by sentinel lymph node biopsy but not clinically detected |
| pN1mi | Micrometastases (>0.2 mm and/or >200 cells but none >2.0 mm) |
| pN1a | Metastases in one to three axillary nodes; at least one metastasis >2.0 mm |
| pN1b | Metastases in internal mammary nodes with micrometastasis or macrometastases detected by sentinel lymph node biopsy (not clinically detected) |
| pN1c | Metastases in one to three axillary nodes and in internal mammary nodes with micrometastases or macrometastases detected by sentinel lymph node biopsy but not clinically detected |
| pN2 | Metastases in four to nine axillary nodes; or in clinically detected internal mammary lymph nodes in the absence of axillary lymph node metastases |
| pN2a | Metastases in four to nine axillary nodes (at least one tumor deposit >2.0 mm) |
| pN2b | Metastases in clinically detected internal mammary lymph nodes in the absence of axillary lymph node metastases |
| pN3 | Metastases in ten or more axillary nodes; or in infraclavicular (level III axillary nodes); or in clinically detected ipsilateral internal mammary lymph nodes in the presence of one or more positive level I, II axillary nodes; or in more than three axillary lymph nodes and internal mammary lymph nodes, with micrometastases or macrometastases detected by sentinel lymph node biopsy but not clinically detected; or in ipsilateral supraclavicular lymph nodes |
| **Distant Metastases (M)** | |
| M0 | No clinical or radiographic evidence of distant metastases |
| cM0(i+) | No clinical or radiographic evidence of distant metastases, but deposits of molecularly or microscopically detected tumor cells in circulating blood, bone marrow, or other nonregional nodal tissue that are no larger than 0.2 mm in a patient without symptoms or signs of metastases |
| M1 | Distant detectable metastases as determined by classic clinical and radiographic means and/or histologically proven larger than 0.2 mm |

From Edge SB, Byrd DR, Compton CC, et al (eds): AJCC cancer staging manual, ed 7, New York, 2010, Springer-Verlag.

equivalent survival with delayed axillary dissection. The results of this trial led to the conclusion that the mode and time of treatment of axillary nodes does not alter disease-free survival or overall survival. Immediate removal, delayed removal, or irradiation produced equivalent clinical results.

**Table 36-5 Stage Groupings for Breast Cancer**

| ANATOMIC STAGE | PROGNOSTIC GROUP | | |
|---|---|---|---|
| 0 | Tis | N0 | M0 |
| IA | T1 | N0 | M0 |
| IB | T0<br>T1 | N1mi<br>N1mi | M0<br>M0 |
| IIA | T0<br>T1<br>T2 | N1<br>N1<br>N0 | M0<br>M0<br>M0 |
| IIB | T2<br>T3 | N1<br>N0 | M0<br>M0 |
| IIIA | T0<br>T1<br>T2<br>T3<br>T3 | N2<br>N2<br>N2<br>N1<br>N2 | M0<br>M0<br>M0<br>M0<br>M0 |
| IIIB | T4<br>T4<br>T4 | N0<br>N1<br>N2 | M0<br>M0<br>M0 |
| IIIC | Any T | N3 | M0 |
| IV | Any T | Any N | M1 |

### Clinical Trials Comparing Breast-Conserving Therapy With Mastectomy

Six prospective clinical trials have randomized more than 4500 patients to mastectomy versus breast-conserving therapy (Table 36-6). In all these trials, there was no survival advantage for the use of mastectomy over breast preservation. Ipsilateral breast recurrence rates were higher in patients undergoing breast-conserving surgery, but local recurrences could be salvaged by mastectomy at the time of recurrence, with no significant detriment in survival rates. Data from these trials have served to define predictors of local recurrence after lumpectomy and have led to modifications in surgical and radiation techniques to reduce local recurrence.

**NSABP B-06: Mastectomy Versus Lumpectomy With Irradiation Versus Lumpectomy Alone** A total of 1851 patients with tumors up to 4 cm in diameter and clinically negative lymph nodes were randomized in B-06 to receive modified radical mastectomy, lumpectomy alone, or lumpectomy with postoperative irradiation of the breast without an extra boost to the lumpectomy site.[17] All patients with histologically positive axillary nodes received chemotherapy. At 20 years of follow-up, overall survival and disease-free survival were the same in all three treatment arms (Fig. 36-10).

NSABP B-06 provided valuable information about rates of ipsilateral breast cancer recurrence after lumpectomy, with or without breast irradiation. At 20 years of follow-up, local recurrence rates were 14.3% in women treated with lumpectomy and radiation therapy and 39.2% in women treated with

**Table 36-6 Randomized Trials Comparing Breast Conservation vs Mastectomy**

| TRIAL | NO. OF PATIENTS | MAX TUMOR SIZE (CM) | SYSTEMIC THERAPY | FOLLOW-UP (YR) | % SURVIVAL LUMPECTOMY + XRT | % SURVIVAL MASTECTOMY | LOCAL RECURRENCE (BCT) (%) |
|---|---|---|---|---|---|---|---|
| NSABP B-06[a] | 1851 | 4 | Yes | 20 | 47 | 46 | 14* |
| Milan Cancer Institute[b] | 701 | 2 | Yes | 20 | 44 | 43 | 8.8* |
| Institute Gustave-Roussy[c] | 179 | 2 | No | | 73 | 65 | 13 |
| National Cancer Institute[d] | 237 | 5 | Yes | 10 | 77 | 75 | 16 |
| EORTC[e] | 868 | 5 | Yes | 10 | 65 | 66 | 17.6 |
| Danish Breast Cancer Group[f] | 905 | None | Yes | 6 | 79 | 82 | 3 |

*BCT,* Breast-conserving therapy; *EORTC,* European Organization for Research and Treatment of Cancer; *NSABP,* National Surgical Adjuvant Breast and Bowel Project; *XRT,* radiation therapy.

*Includes only women whose excision margins were negative.

Data from the following sources:

[a]Fisher B, Anderson S, Bryant J, et al: Twenty-year follow-up of a randomized trial comparing total mastectomy, lumpectomy, and lumpectomy plus irradiation for the treatment of invasive breast cancer. N Engl J Med 347:1233, 2002.

[b]Veronesi U, Cascinelli N, Mariani L, et al: Twenty-year follow-up of a randomized study comparing breast-conserving surgery with radical mastectomy for early breast cancer. N Engl J Med 347:1227, 2002.

[c]Arriagada R, Le M, Rochard F, et al: Conservative treatment versus mastectomy in early breast cancer: Patterns of failure with 15 years of follow-up data. J Clin Oncol 14:1558, 1996.

[d]Jacobson J, Danforth D, Cowan K, et al: Ten-year results of a comparison of conservation with mastectomy in the treatment of stage I and II breast cancer. N Engl J Med 332:907, 1995.

[e]van Dongen J, Voogd A, Fentiman I, et al: Long-term results of a randomized trial comparing breast-conserving therapy with mastectomy: European Organization for Research and Treatment of Cancer 10801 Trial. J Natl Cancer Inst 92:1143, 2000.

[f]Blichert-Toft M, Rose C, Andersen J, et al: Danish randomized trial comparing breast conservation therapy with mastectomy: Six years of life-table analysis. Danish Breast Cancer Cooperative Group. J Natl Cancer Inst Monogr 11:19, 1992.

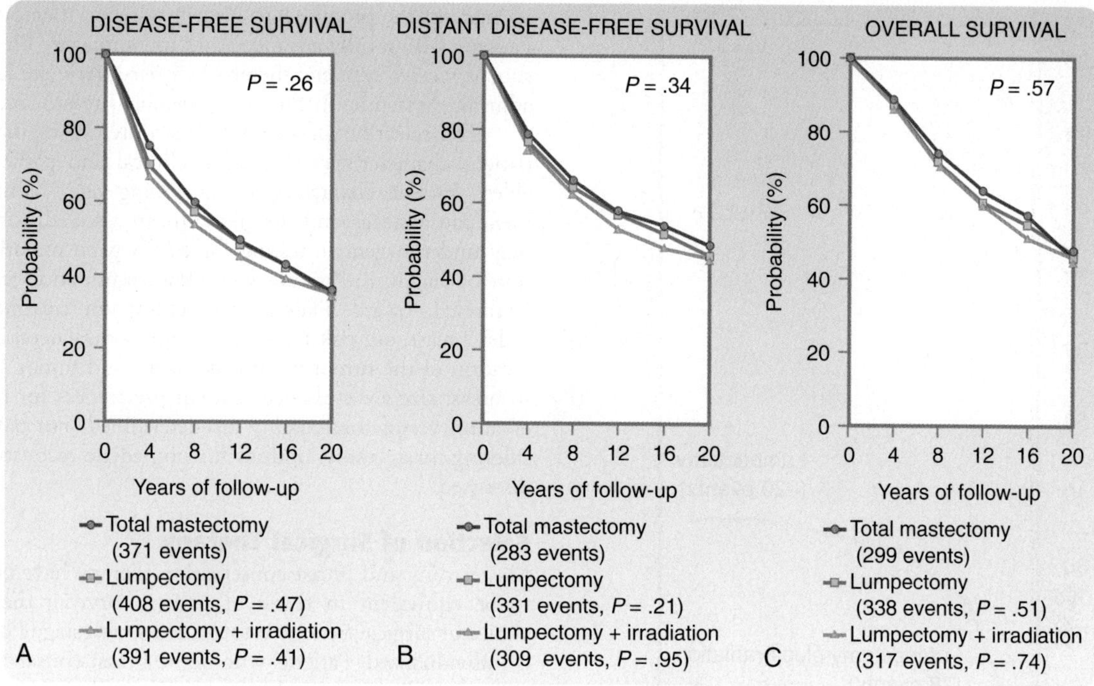


**FIGURE 36-10** Disease-free survival **(A)**, distant disease-free survival **(B)**, and overall survival **(C)** after 20 years of follow-up in the NSABP protocol B-06. There were no significant differences in the three randomized arms of this trial. (From Fisher B, Anderson S, Bryant J, et al: Twenty-year follow-up of a randomized trial comparing total mastectomy, lumpectomy, and lumpectomy plus irradiation for the treatment of invasive breast cancer. N Engl J Med 347:1233–1241, 2002.)

lumpectomy alone ($P < .001$; Fig. 36-11). For patients with positive nodes who received chemotherapy, the local recurrence rate was 44.2% for lumpectomy alone as opposed to 8.8% for lumpectomy plus radiation therapy.

**Milan I Trial** The Milan I trial enrolled patients with smaller tumors and used more extensive surgery and radiation therapy than the NSABP B-06 trial. The Milan trial randomized 701 women with tumors up to 2 cm in size and clinically negative nodes to receive radical mastectomy versus quadrantectomy with axillary dissection and postoperative irradiation. Patients with pathologically positive nodes received chemotherapy. Overall survival at 20 years was not different in the two groups. Locoregional failures were different between groups with chest wall recurrence after radical mastectomy in 2.3% of women and ipsilateral breast tumor recurrence after quadrantectomy and radiation therapy in 8.8% of women (20-year follow-up). Contralateral breast cancer rates were identical, approximately 0.66%/year for all women, refuting the hypothesis that irradiation increases the incidence of contralateral breast cancers. Local failure rates were higher in younger women after quadrantectomy, with rates of 1%/year in women younger than 45 years and only 0.5%/year in older women.

**Other Trials of Breast Conservation** Three other randomized trials in patients with operable breast cancer found no survival benefit of mastectomy over breast-conserving therapy. The European Organization for Research and Treatment of Cancer (EORTC) Trial 10801 randomized 868 women to modified radical mastectomy or lumpectomy and irradiation and found no difference in survival at 10 years. Importantly, this trial included tumors up to 5 cm, and 80% of women enrolled had tumors larger than 2.0 cm. Positive margins were allowed, and the results showed lower rates of local recurrence with clear versus involved margins.

The Institut Gustave-Roussy trial randomized 179 women with tumors smaller than 2 cm to modified radical mastectomy versus lumpectomy with a 2-cm margin of normal tissue around the cancer. No differences were observed between the two surgical groups in risk for death, metastases, contralateral breast cancer, or locoregional recurrence at 15 years of follow-up.

The NCI (United States) trial randomized 237 women with tumors 5 cm or smaller to compare lumpectomy with axillary dissection and radiation therapy versus modified radical mastectomy. There were no differences seen in overall survival or disease-free survival rates at 10 years.

## Planning Surgical Treatments

It is critical to establish the diagnosis of breast cancer firmly prior to initiating definitive surgical treatment. Biopsy of a palpable or image-detected lesion with core needle biopsy is the approach of choice for diagnosis. Open surgical biopsy is reserved for lesions not amenable to core biopsy or when core biopsy has proved nondiagnostic. FNA biopsy can be useful for diagnosing breast lesions, although its high false-negative rate means that a negative result requires additional workup. FNA biopsy is also unable to distinguish invasive from in situ lesions reliably. Examination of biopsy material should provide information about tumor histologic type and grade, ER and PR status, HER-2 status, and presence of lymphovascular invasion.

A history and physical examination, in addition to appropriate imaging studies, are important to establish the extent of disease and assign a clinical stage. The most common sites of

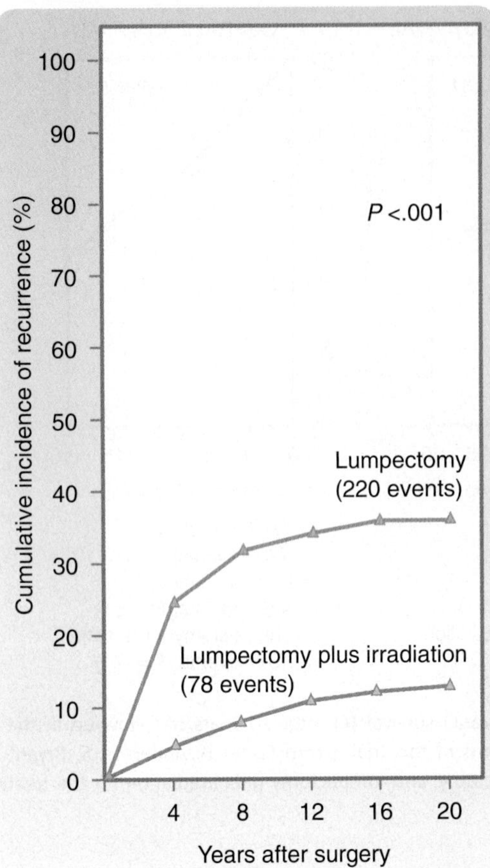


**FIGURE 36-11** Cumulative incidence of a first recurrence of cancer in the treated conserved breast during 20 years of follow-up in the NSABP protocol B-06. The data presented here are for patients achieving a pathologically tumor-free margin after lumpectomy. There were 570 women treated by lumpectomy alone and 567 treated by lumpectomy and ipsilateral breast irradiation. (From Fisher B, Anderson S, Bryant J, et al: Twenty-year follow-up of a randomized trial comparing total mastectomy, lumpectomy, and lumpectomy plus irradiation for the treatment of invasive breast cancer. N Engl J Med 347:1233–1241, 2002.)

distant metastases from breast cancer are the liver, lungs, and bones. The National Comprehensive Cancer Network provides guidelines for the use of laboratory and radiologic testing in patients at initial diagnosis based on clinical stage. Computed tomography (CT) scans, bone scans, and other imaging studies are generally reserved for patients with abnormalities on blood chemistry tests or chest radiographs and for patients with locally advanced or inflammatory breast cancer. Thorough imaging of the ipsilateral and contralateral breast is performed to look for additional areas of concern other than the index lesion. Breast MRI may be used in select cases to define the extent of tumor and look for additional breast lesions.

In the absence of metastatic disease, the first intervention for patients with early-stage breast cancer is surgery to excise the tumor and surgically stage the regional lymph nodes, when appropriate. Assessment of the primary tumor size and regional lymph nodes defines the pathologic stage and provides an estimate of the prognosis to inform systemic therapy decisions. Patients with locally advanced and inflammatory breast cancers should receive systemic therapy before surgery (see later, "Neoadjuvant Systemic Therapy for Operable Breast Cancer").

The selection of surgical procedures takes into account patient characteristics and other clinical and pathologic variables. Patient characteristics, including age, family history, menopausal status, and overall health, are assessed. Some patients may undergo genetic testing for *BRCA* gene mutations at the time of diagnosis. Patients with a known mutation are generally counseled toward bilateral mastectomy for treatment of the index breast and risk reduction of the contralateral breast. The location of the tumor within the breast and tumor size relative to breast size are evaluated. Patient preferences for breast preservation versus mastectomy are determined. For patients considering mastectomy, options for immediate reconstruction are discussed.

## Selection of Surgical Therapy

Mastectomy and breast conservation therapy have been shown to be equivalent in terms of patient survival; therefore, the choice of surgical treatment for patients with stage I or II disease is individualized. Patients who desire breast-conserving surgery must be willing to attend postoperative radiation treatment sessions and to undergo postoperative surveillance of the treated breast. Consideration should be made for consultation with a radiation oncologist before the planned surgery. Patients are advised about the risks and long-term sequelae of radiation therapy. A mastectomy is generally recommended for patients who have contraindications to radiation therapy.

A significant factor in determining whether breast conservation therapy is feasible is the relationship between tumor size and breast size. In general, the tumor must be small enough in relation to the breast size so that the tumor can be resected with adequate margins and acceptable cosmesis. In patients with large tumors for whom systemic chemotherapy will likely be recommended in the postoperative (adjuvant) setting, the use of preoperative chemotherapy may be considered because it can significantly reduce the size of the tumor, allowing more patients to undergo breast-conserving surgery. If chemotherapy is administered prior to surgery, it may decrease the tumor size sufficiently to permit breast-conserving surgery in patients who would not otherwise appear to be good candidates. Another strategy is to consider local tissue rearrangement or pedicled myocutaneous flaps (latissimus dorsi) to fill the defect resulting from breast-conserving surgery. Patients with multicentric tumors are usually served best by mastectomy because it is difficult to perform more than one breast-conserving surgery in the same breast with acceptable cosmesis. Although high nuclear grade, presence of lymphovascular invasion, and negative steroid hormone receptor status have all been linked to increased local recurrence rates, none of these factors are considered absolute contraindications to breast conservation.

### Eligibility for Breast Conservation

Randomized trials have demonstrated the efficacy of breast-conserving surgery for a wide variety of breast cancers and have defined eligibility for breast conservation. With these criteria and current surgical and radiation approaches, local recurrence rates after lumpectomy and radiation therapy are now less than 5% at 10 years in many large centers.

**Tumor Size** Tumors up to 5 cm in size, tumors with clinically positive nodes, and tumors with both lobular and ductal histology were included in the randomized trials. In current practice, lumpectomy is considered in cases in which the tumor can be excised to clear margins and leave an acceptable cosmetic result.

**Margins** Local recurrence rates are reduced when 2- to 3-mm microscopically clear margins are obtained on all aspects of the lumpectomy specimen. Margins should be clear for invasive cancer and DCIS.

**Histology** Invasive lobular cancers and cancers with an extensive intraductal component are eligible for lumpectomy if clear margins are achieved. Atypical hyperplasia and LCIS at resection margins do not increase local recurrence rates.

**Patient Age** Local recurrence rates are somewhat higher for younger versus older women. Local recurrence rates are reduced in patients of all ages with the use of radiation therapy. A radiation boost to the tumor bed has been shown to reduce local failures after lumpectomy, particularly in younger women.

## Surgical Procedures for Breast Cancer

### Breast-Conserving Surgery

**Technical Aspects** Excision of the primary tumor with preservation of the breast has been referred to by many terms, including *lumpectomy, partial mastectomy, segmental mastectomy, segmentectomy, tylectomy,* and *wide local excision.* Breast-conserving surgery removes the malignancy with a surrounding rim of grossly normal breast parenchyma. This procedure is depicted in Figure 36-12, which shows the completed lumpectomy and skin incision for the axillary component of the procedure. A more extensive local procedure, quadrantectomy, used in some European trials of breast conservation, removes 2 to 3 cm of adjacent breast and skin over the tumor. These more extensive margins and skin excision have not been shown to improve survival and are not used in current approaches to breast conservation.

The breast conservation specimen that is removed is oriented and its edges inked prior to sectioning. Specimen radiography should be performed for all nonpalpable lesions or if there are microcalcifications associated with the palpable tumor. If a margin appears to be close or is positive histologically on intraoperative assessment, reexcision to remove more tissue will frequently achieve a clear margin and allow conservation of the breast. Orientation of the surgical specimen allows focal reexcision of involved margins rather than global reexcision and improves the cosmetic result by reducing the amount of normal breast parenchyma that is excised.

The surgical defect created after lumpectomy is closed in cosmetic fashion. There is increasing interest in the use of advancement flap closure and other oncoplastic surgical techniques to maximize the cosmetic result.

Surgical staging of the axilla is usually performed through a separate incision in most patients undergoing breast conservation. Sentinel lymph node dissection (see Fig. 36-12*B*) has largely replaced anatomic axillary node dissection in patients with clinically negative axillary nodes. For patients who require axillary dissection, the extent of the dissection is identical to the

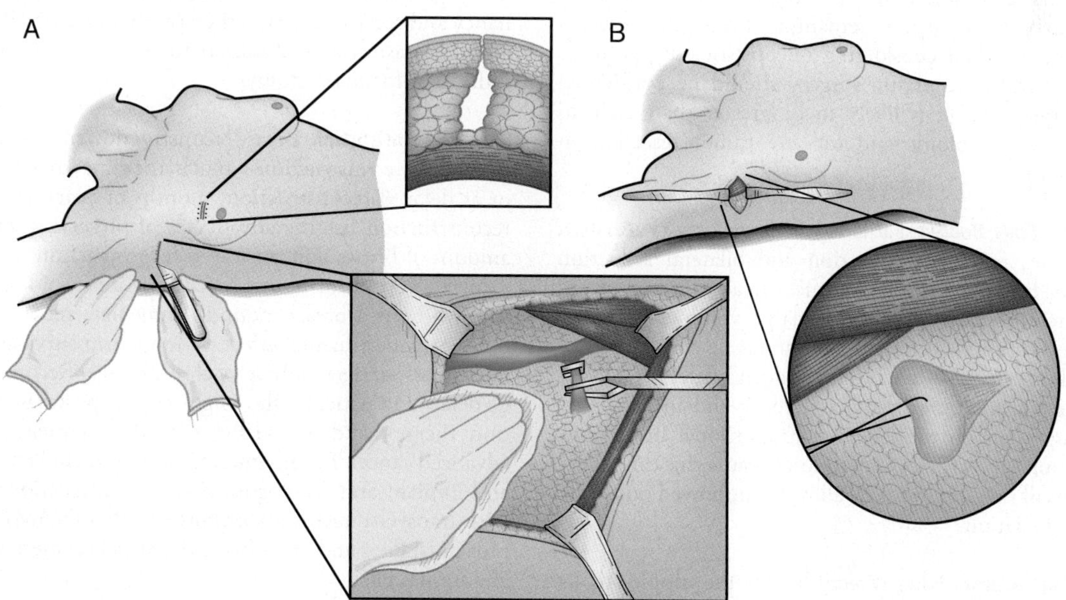


**FIGURE 36-12** Breast-conserving surgery. **A,** Incisions to remove malignant tumors are placed directly over the tumor, without tunneling. A transverse incision in the low axillary region is used for sentinel node biopsy or axillary dissection. The axillary dissection is identical to the procedure for a modified radical mastectomy. The boundaries of the operation are the axillary vein superiorly, the latissimus dorsi muscle laterally, and the chest wall medially. The inferior dissection enters the tail of Spence (the axillary tail of the breast). *Inset,* Excision cavity of the lumpectomy. **B,** In sentinel node biopsy, a similar transverse incision is made, which may be located by percutaneous mapping with the gamma probe if radiolabeled colloid is used. It is extended through the clavipectoral fascia and the true axilla is entered. The sentinel node is located by its staining with dye, radioactivity, or both, and dissected free as a single specimen.

axillary component of the modified radical mastectomy (see Fig. 36-12*A*).

**Cosmetic Challenges** The term *oncoplastic surgery* has been popularized in recent years to stress the importance of achieving the best possible aesthetic result in the context of resecting the tumor with adequate oncologic margins. The goal is to retain as much of the natural breast size and contour as possible to provide optimal cosmesis and symmetry with the opposite breast. When the primary tumor is resected using an incision directly over the tumor and then closing the skin without reapproximating any breast tissue, several deformities can occur. These include volumetric deformity from a large parenchymal resection, retraction deformity when the seroma resorbs at the operative site, skin–pectoral muscle adherence deformity, in which the skin adheres to the underlying pectoral muscle, and lower pole deformity with downward turning of the nipple caused by excision of a tumor in the lower hemisphere of the breast. These deformities can make it difficult for patients to wear athletic clothing or bathing suits because significant asymmetry may be evident. It is important to correct these deformities prior to radiation therapy because the irradiation may further accentuate any asymmetry and make it more challenging to correct the defect in the future.

The surgeon should consider oncoplastic techniques when the following situations occur: (1) a significant area of skin will be resected with the tumor; (2) a large-volume resection is expected; (3) the tumor is in an area associated with poor cosmetic outcomes (e.g., lower hemisphere below the nipple); or (4) resection may lead to nipple malposition.

***Extent of Breast Resection*** It is not the absolute breast volume that will be resected but rather the ratio of the anticipated defect to the volume of the remaining breast parenchyma that is important when considering oncoplastic surgery techniques. In general, oncoplastic surgery should be considered when the surgical defect is likely to be greater than 20% to 30% of the breast volume and for any tumor resection in the lower breast.

***Breast Size and Body Habitus*** Patients with large breasts are often good candidates for tumor resection and bilateral reduction mammaplasty. Breast reduction strategies can allow for improved aesthetic outcomes after resection of large volumes of breast tissue at any location. Obese patients should be considered for this approach because they are often poor candidates for autologous tissue reconstruction after mastectomy and implants are often not large enough to recreate a proportional breast size. Breast reduction surgery is a good option because this can relieve the symptoms of macromastia and allow for improved outcomes after breast irradiation.

***Tumor Location*** Tumors lying directly under the nipple-areolar complex and those located between the nipple-areolar complex and inframammary fold require special attention to avoid nipple-areolar complex distortion and contour deformity. In general, there must be an adjustment of skin and well-vascularized breast parenchyma to correct for the removal of breast tissue in these areas. As noted, deformities in the contour will be exacerbated by radiation and may be more challenging to correct at a later date.

**Timing of Oncoplastic Surgery** Immediate reconstruction of the partial mastectomy defect is almost always preferred to a delayed approach. Oncoplastic techniques such as tissue advancement and local tissue rearrangement at the initial surgical procedure tend to provide the optimal solution. This approach has not been associated with delay in delivery of adjuvant systemic therapy or radiation delivery. In general, local tissue transfer and breast reduction surgery cannot be performed on the irradiated breast; thus, it is preferable to perform the procedure prior to radiation. Tissue expanders and implants are not recommended to fill partial mastectomy defects because radiation may lead to capsular contracture, distortion, and infection.

If a cosmetic defect occurs following breast-conserving surgery and radiation, reconstruction of the treated breast is generally not recommended for up to 1 to 2 years after radiation therapy has been completed. In irradiated tissue, there is a higher rate of tissue necrosis, seroma formation, and infection. The use of vascularized tissue from outside the radiation field is the favored approach. If the main deformity is caused by asymmetry with the contralateral breast, a mastopexy of the contralateral breast can be considered. In general, surgical procedures on the irradiated breast should be minimized because healing and recovery are impaired, even when the skin appears healthy.

### Mastectomy

**Indications** Certain tumors still require mastectomy, including those that are large relative to breast size, those with extensive calcifications on mammography, tumors for which clear margins cannot be obtained on wide local excision, and patients with contraindications to breast irradiation. Contraindications to the use of radiation therapy include previous breast or chest wall irradiation, active lupus or scleroderma, and pregnancy, although many patients pregnant at diagnosis can complete their pregnancy and receive radiation therapy after delivery. Patient preference for mastectomy or a desire to avoid radiation is also a valid indication for mastectomy.

**Breast Reconstruction** Breast reconstruction may be performed as immediate reconstruction—that is, the same day as mastectomy—or as delayed reconstruction, months or years later. Immediate reconstruction has the advantages of preserving the maximum amount of breast skin for use in reconstruction, combining the recovery period for both procedures, and avoiding a period of time without a breast mound. Immediate reconstruction does not have a detrimental effect on long-term survival, local recurrence rates, or detection of local recurrence. Reconstruction may be delayed in patients who might require postmastectomy radiation therapy and is usually delayed in patients with locally advanced cancer. Reconstruction options include tissue expander and implant and autologous tissue reconstructions, most often with transverse rectus abdominis muscle (TRAM) flaps, latissimus dorsi flaps and, more recently, muscle-preserving perforator abdominal flaps.

**Technical Details**

***Simple and Modified Radical Mastectomy*** Simple or total mastectomy refers to complete removal of the mammary gland, including the nipple and areola. Sentinel lymph node surgery for axillary staging may be performed through the mastectomy incision or through a separate axillary incision. Modified radical mastectomy refers to removal of the mammary gland, nipple,

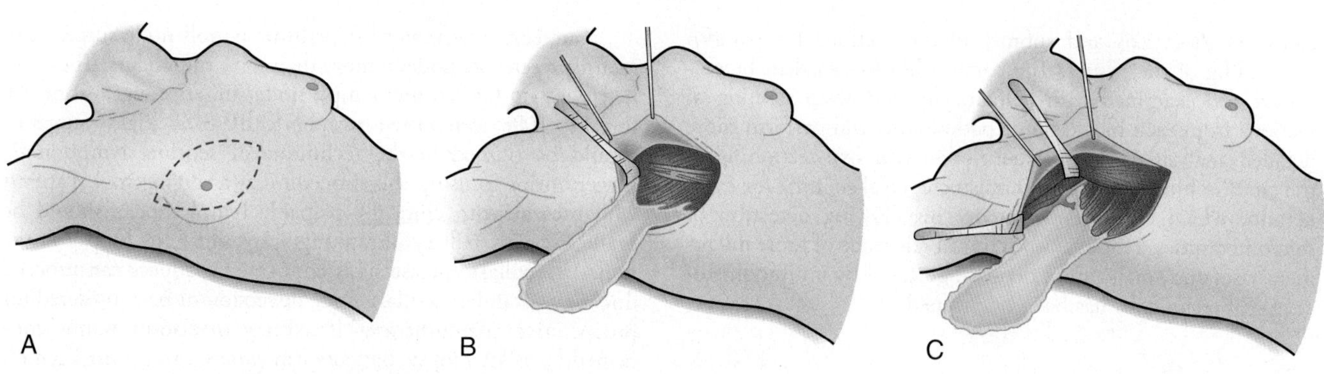


**FIGURE 36-13** Total mastectomy with and without axillary dissection. **A,** Skin incisions are generally transverse and surround the central breast and nipple-areolar complex. **B,** Skin flaps are raised sharply to separate the gland from the overlying skin and then the gland from the underlying muscle. Simple mastectomy divides the breast from the axillary contents and stops at the clavipectoral fascia. **C,** In modified radical mastectomy, dissection continues into the axilla and generally extends up to the axillary vein, with removal of level I and II nodes. Division of a branch of the axillary vein is shown, with separation of the node-bearing axillary fat from the axillary vein at the superior aspect of the dissection.

and areola, with the addition of a complete axillary lymph node dissection (Fig. 36-13).

An elliptical skin incision is planned to include the nipple and areola and usually any previous excisional biopsy scars (see Fig. 36-13A). Skin flaps are raised to separate the underlying gland from the overlying skin along the subdermal plexus (see Figs. 36-13*B* and *C*). If immediate reconstruction is not planned, sufficient skin is taken to allow smooth closure of skin flaps without redundant skin folds. This will facilitate comfortable use of a breast prosthesis in the future. If immediate reconstruction is planned, a skin-sparing mastectomy may be performed in which only the nipple-areola complex is removed and the maximum amount of skin is left for use in the reconstruction. Nipple-areola–sparing mastectomy has been used with increasing frequency for patients undergoing prophylactic mastectomy for risk reduction. There are also some early reports suggesting that it may be appropriate for some select patients with a diagnosis of breast cancer.

Breast tissue is separated from the underlying pectoralis muscle and the pectoral fascia is generally taken with the breast specimen. In a total mastectomy (see Fig. 36-13*B*), breast tissue is separated from the axillary contents and all breast tissue superficial to the fascia of the axilla is removed. In a modified radical mastectomy, the levels I and II axillary lymph nodes are taken with the axillary breast tissue (see Fig. 36-13*C*). Level I nodes are those inferior to the axillary vein and lateral to the pectoralis minor muscle and level II nodes are those posterior to the pectoralis minor.

## Lymph Node Staging

The pathologic status of the axillary lymph nodes is one of the most important prognostic factors in patients with breast cancer. Identification of metastatic tumor deposits in the axillary nodes indicates a poorer prognosis and often prompts a recommendation for more aggressive systemic and locoregional therapies.

Axillary lymph node dissection has long been a routine component of the surgical management of breast cancer patients. It provides prognostic information about axillary nodal status and also plays a therapeutic role in removing axillary disease in patients with positive nodes. The surgical procedure includes clearance of node-bearing tissue between the pectoralis major and latissimus dorsi muscles from the edge of the breast tissue in the low axillary region to the axillary vein and removal of the nodes posterior to the pectoralis minor muscle. Unfortunately, axillary dissection is often the main source of morbidity in patients with early-stage breast cancer. The immediate problems include acute pain and paresthesias, need for hospitalization, reduced range of motion at the shoulder joint, and need for a drain in the surgical bed for a period of 2 weeks or more. Long-term problems resulting from axillary dissection include lymphedema of the ipsilateral arm, numbness, chronic pain, and reduced range of motion at the shoulder joint.

The technique of sentinel lymph node dissection was developed to reduce the morbidity associated with axillary surgery while still providing accurate staging information. Because many patients now present with clinically node-negative disease, sentinel lymph node dissection can identify those with proven node-positive disease who may benefit from completion axillary dissection. Those patients with a negative sentinel lymph node can avoid the morbidity of axillary dissection. Identification of the first, or sentinel, node(s) draining the area of the primary tumor in the breast allows for this more selective approach to the axilla. The sentinel node(s) is the most likely node to contain metastatic disease, if present, and therefore the pathologist can focus the examination on the sentinel node(s) without the added cost and time required to examine the full axillary contents. In sentinel lymph node surgery, radiolabeled colloid and/or blue dye is injected into breast tissue at the site of the primary tumor; this then passes through the lymphatics to the first draining node, where the material accumulates. The procedure can also be performed with injection of the mapping agents at the subareolar position or in a subdermal location overlying the site of the primary tumor. The sentinel node is identified as a blue node, radioactive node or both. If the pathologic analysis of the sentinel node is negative for evidence of metastasis, the likelihood that other nodes are involved is sufficiently low that axillary lymph node dissection is not required. Published studies have confirmed the proof of concept and numerous subsequent studies have shown that the technique is accurate.

Identification of the sentinel node(s) allows for a more detailed analysis of the lymph node most likely to have a positive yield. In general, pathologists will section the sentinel node along its short axis and submit all the sections for paraffin embedding of the tissues. The paraffin blocks can then be sectioned and examined with hematoxylin and eosin staining of sections from each block. Some pathologists will perform more detailed analysis of the sentinel nodes with step-sectioning of the paraffin blocks and immunohistochemical staining for cytokeratin, which enhances sensitivity by allowing detection of micrometastases. However, the clinical relevance of these micrometastases and small tumor deposits detected by immunohistochemical techniques has been questioned.[18]

## Sentinel Node Technique

Lymphatic mapping can be performed with a combination of technetium-labeled sulfur colloid and a vital blue dye (isosulfan blue [Lymphazurin]) or with a single agent for localization of the sentinel lymph node. A number of studies have shown that using the combination technique results in the lowest possible false-negative rate. Preoperative lymphoscintigraphy can provide information on the specific nodal basins draining the primary tumor and can also demonstrate the number of sentinel nodes in each nodal basin. Using a peritumoral injection technique, approximately 70% of patients will have drainage to the axilla, 20% will have drainage to both the axilla and internal mammary nodal basin, 2% to 3% will have drainage to the internal mammary nodal basin alone, and approximately 8% will not show any drainage to the regional nodal basins. If a subareolar or subdermal injection technique is used, drainage is seen only to the axillary nodal basins. If preoperative lymphoscintigraphy demonstrates drainage to the internal mammary lymph nodes, an internal mammary sentinel node biopsy can be considered. The inability to demonstrate a sentinel lymph node on preoperative lymphoscintigraphy does not preclude the success of identifying a sentinel node intraoperatively but may indicate a higher chance of identifying positive lymph nodes. A dose of 2.5 mCi of technetium-labeled sulfur colloid can be injected on the day prior to surgery for the preoperative lymphoscintigraphy. This allows for adequate activity to remain in the sentinel nodes for the intraoperative lymphatic mapping procedure the following day, without the need for reinjection.

In the operating suite, 3 to 5 mL of blue dye is injected peritumorally and the injection site is massaged to facilitate passage of the dye through the lymphatics. A handheld gamma probe is used to transcutaneously localize the area of increased radioactivity and this helps to guide placement of the incision for the sentinel node procedure. After the incision is made, localization of an area of increased radioactivity is made with the hand-held gamma probe and the surgeon visualizes blue lymphatic channels leading to the sentinel node. Dissection is performed to avoid prematurely disrupting the afferent lymphatics. If a blue-stained lymphatic channel or a specific area of radioactivity ("hot spot") cannot be identified, resection of the primary tumor can be performed to remove the site of injection, decreasing the background shine-through radioactivity. The sentinel node may then be identified and removed and the nodal basin is checked again to confirm that the level of radioactivity has decreased. If the level of radioactivity remains high, additional sentinel nodes may remain in the nodal basin and additional dissection should be completed to remove all sentinel nodes. Published studies have demonstrated an average of two or three sentinel nodes per patient.

Surgeons experienced in sentinel lymph node surgery can identify a sentinel node in more than 95% of patients. The false-negative rate for sentinel lymph node surgery ranges from 0% to up to 10%, as reported in the NSABP B-32 trial.[19] Surgeons should be trained in the technique of sentinel lymph node surgery prior to using this procedure as a staging tool. Patients who present with clinically palpable lymph nodes should be evaluated with axillary ultrasonography and FNA biopsy of the nodes. If axillary metastasis is confirmed, patients can proceed directly to standard axillary node dissection or be considered for preoperative chemotherapy. If axillary metastasis is not confirmed by FNA biopsy, patients can proceed to sentinel lymph node surgery for staging.

Some studies have shown that patients who have undergone previous excisional biopsy of the primary tumor are more likely to have a false-negative sentinel lymph node.[19] The lymphatics may be disrupted by the biopsy, which can affect drainage patterns of the area surrounding the excisional biopsy site. To avoid this scenario, core needle biopsy is the preferred diagnostic approach in patients suspected of having breast cancer.

Sentinel lymph node surgery was reported in older studies to be less accurate in patients treated with preoperative chemotherapy. A meta-analysis of the published studies on sentinel node surgery after chemotherapy has suggested that this technique is accurate; a recent comparison has shown that false-negative rates after chemotherapy compare favorably with those observed in patients who undergo surgery first.[20] Patients with documented metastasis prior to the initiation of chemotherapy should undergo standard axillary node dissection on completion of chemotherapy.

Morbidity rates are substantially lower with sentinel node dissection compared with axillary dissection. Another advantage is that sentinel lymph node dissection can be performed as an outpatient procedure and does not require a drain. Patients have more rapid return to full mobility and are able to return to work and other activities weeks sooner than after axillary dissection. Long-term morbidity, including lymphedema, numbness, and chronic pain, is greatly reduced.

Sentinel node dissection has been shown to provide reliable pathologic staging of the axilla, with false-negative rates generally lower than 5% in experienced hands. Axillary recurrence rates have been shown to be extremely low after a negative sentinel node biopsy without axillary dissection. A negative sentinel node biopsy is now widely accepted as sufficient to establish a patient as node-negative, with no further axillary treatment required.[19]

When the sentinel node contains metastatic disease, the likelihood of additional involved nodes is directly proportional to the size of the breast primary, presence of lymphatic vascular invasion, and size of the lymph node metastasis. In approximately 50% of patients with positive sentinel nodes, the sentinel node is the only positive node. In the presence of a positive sentinel node, treatment guidelines have dictated completion axillary lymph node dissection (ALND) as the standard. This is most commonly achieved with a completion level I and II axillary dissection. Although ALND has been standard practice for patients with positive SLNs, the need for ALND in all patients with a positive SLN has come into question because many patients have small-volume metastases and the sentinel node is often the only positive node. A meta-analysis of studies evaluating patients with positive sentinel nodes has shown that 53% of patients have additional positive nodes at ALND.[21] In the case of micrometastatic disease in the sentinel nodes, the rate of nonsentinel node involvement is as low as 20% and, for patients with isolated tumor cells, it is below 12%. This has led to a trend of omitting ALND in selected patients with positive sentinel nodes. An analysis of the SEER data from 1998 to 2004 revealed that up to 16% of sentinel node–positive patients did not undergo ALND. This was seen more commonly in older patients with low-grade, ER-positive tumors. During this time frame, the number of patients with micrometastasis in the sentinel node who did not undergo ALND increased from 21% to 38%. A review of the National Cancer Data Base (NCDB) data from 1998 to 2005 revealed similar findings, with 20.8% of sentinel–node positive patients avoiding ALND. There were no differences seen in axillary recurrence rates or survival for patients who had sentinel node surgery only versus those who underwent ALND.

One factor that may have contributed to the decrease in ALND for patients with positive sentinel nodes is the emergence of the use of nomograms, which can predict the probability of disease burden in the undissected nonsentinel nodes. For patients with micrometastasis in one of several sentinel nodes, or those with disease detected by immunohistochemistry only, the estimated risk of additional positive nodes remaining in the axilla is low. The first nomogram developed was published by researchers from the Memorial Sloan Kettering Cancer Center (MSKCC) and is available to clinicians on the Internet (http://nomograms.mskcc.org/Breast/index.aspx). A more recent tool, developed at the M.D. Anderson Cancer Center, includes the important variable of sentinel node metastasis size. This nomogram is also available on the Internet (http://www3.mdanderson.org/app/medcalc/bc_nomogram2/index.cfm?pagename=nsln). Both these nomograms have been validated to estimate the degree of additional nodal involvement based on characteristics of the patient, primary tumor, number of sentinel nodes, and other factors. These and other nomograms can be used by the surgeon, in combination with clinical judgment and other available information, to estimate the risk of additional positive nonsentinel nodes in an individual patient.

The American College of Surgeons Oncology Group (ACOSOG) initiated a prospective randomized trial in 1999 designed specifically to evaluate the impact of ALND on locoregional recurrence and survival in patients with early-stage breast cancer.[22] The ACOSOG Z0011 trial enrolled patients with clinical T1 or T2 breast cancer with one or two positive sentinel nodes who were planned for breast-conserving surgery and whole-breast irradiation and then randomized them to undergo completion ALND or no further surgery (sentinel node surgery alone). The primary end point of Z0011 was overall survival with locoregional recurrence as a secondary end point. Patients who participated in Z0011 had relatively favorable disease characteristics; median age was 55 years, 70% had T1 tumors, 82% had ER-positive tumors, 71% had only one positive sentinel node, and 44% had micrometastases. At a median follow-up of 6.3 years, local recurrence was seen in 3.6% ($n$ = 29) of the ALND group versus 1.8% ($n$ = 8) of the sentinel node only group. Axillary recurrences were reported in 0.5% ($n$ = 2) of patients in the ALND group versus 0.9% ($n$ = 4) in the sentinel node only group. There were no differences in overall survival (91.9% after ALND versus 92.5% after sentinel node only; $P$ = .24) or disease-free survival at 5 years (82.2% after ALND versus 83.8% after sentinel node only). The Z0011 study investigators concluded that the routine use of ALND was not justified in all patients with early-stage breast cancer found to have a positive sentinel node. The results of this study are practice-changing. It is now widely believed that ALND may be safely omitted in select patients with clinically node-negative disease who have a positive sentinel node and are similar to the participants in the Z0011 trial—women with T1 or T2, clinically node-negative breast cancer who undergo breast-conserving surgery and whole-breast irradiation who have one or two positive sentinel nodes and are planned for adjuvant systemic therapy. Patients with a positive sentinel node undergoing mastectomy and those undergoing breast-conserving surgery who are planned for accelerated partial-breast irradiation (APBI) should continue to undergo ALND as standard practice.

Axillary lymph node dissection remains the standard of care for patients with locally advanced breast cancer or inflammatory breast cancer, for those with a positive sentinel node who are planned for mastectomy, and for those with a positive sentinel node after neoadjuvant chemotherapy.

## TREATMENT OF DUCTAL CARCINOMA IN SITU (INTRADUCTAL CARCINOMA)

DCIS, or intraductal cancer, currently accounts for approximately 25% of all newly diagnosed breast cancers, with more than 54,000 new cases diagnosed in 2010. Most DCIS is characterized by an area of clustered calcifications on a screening mammogram, without an associated palpable abnormality. Rarely, DCIS will be manifested as a palpable mass or as unilateral, single-duct nipple discharge.

Mammographic findings in patients with DCIS include clustered calcifications without an associated density in 75% of patients, calcifications coexisting with an associated density in 15%, and a density alone in 10%. The calcifications seen on a mammogram generally correspond to areas within the central involved duct in which there is often necrosis and debris. DCIS calcifications tend to cluster closely together, are pleomorphic, and may be linear or branching, thus suggesting their ductal origin.

DCIS is viewed as a precursor of invasive ductal cancer and treatment aims to remove the DCIS to prevent progression to invasive disease. Because the risk for metastatic disease in patients with DCIS without demonstrable invasion is rare (<1%), systemic chemotherapy is not required. Hormonal therapy may be used for prevention of new primary tumors and to improve local control after breast-conserving therapy but is generally only recommended when the DCIS is positive for ER on immunohistochemistry.

Treatment recommendations for an individual patient with DCIS are based on the extent of disease within the breast, histologic grade, ER status, and presence of microinvasion, as well as patient age and preference. Treatment options for DCIS include mastectomy, breast-conserving surgery with irradiation, and breast-conserving surgery alone. When the patient is treated with breast conservation or unilateral mastectomy, there is also the option of adjuvant hormonal therapy with tamoxifen as risk reduction for future breast cancers.[23]

### Mastectomy

Breast cancer mortality after treatment of DCIS by total mastectomy is 1%, which is the standard against which breast-conserving approaches are compared (Table 36-7). Local

**Table 36-7 Recurrence and Mortality Rates After Mastectomy for Ductal Carcinoma in Situ**

| STUDY (YEAR) | DATES OF STUDY | NO. OF PATIENTS | FOLLOW-UP (YR) | NONCLINICAL (%) | NO. OF RECURRENCES | NO. DEAD OF DISEASE |
|---|---|---|---|---|---|---|
| Farrow (1970)[a] | 1949-1967 | 181 | 5-20 | 0 | 6 | 4 |
| Brown et al (1976)[b] | 1952-1975 | 39 | 1-15 | 10 | 0 | 0 |
| Carter and Smith (1977)[c] | 1960-1975 | 28 | 1-14 | | 1 | 1 |
| Sunshine et al (1985)[d] | 1960-1980 | 73 | 10-year minimum | 0 | 4 | 3 |
| Von Rueden and Wilson (1984)[e] | 1960-1981 | 45 | Not reported | 8 | 1 | 0 |
| Ashikari et al (1971)[f] | 1960-1969 | 92 | 11 year maximum | 40 | 0 | 0 |
| Schuh et al (1986)[g] | 1965-1984 | 49 | 5.5 mean | 33 | 1 | 1 |
| Kinne et al (1989)[h] | 1970-1976 | 101 | 11.5 median | 58 | 1 | 1 |
| Lagios et al (1982)[i] | 1975-1980 | 42 | Not reported | | 0 | 0 |
| Fisher et al (1986)[j] | 1976-1984 | 27 | 5 | | 1 | 1 |
| Arnesson et al (1989)[k] | 1978-1984 | 28 | 6.4 median | 100 | 0 | 0 |
| Ward et al (1992)[l] | 1979-1983 | 123 | 10 | 11 | 1 | ? |
| Silverstein (1997)[m] | 1979-1990 | 98 | 4.9 median | 62 | 1 | 0 |
| Total | | 926 | | | 17 (2%) | 11(1%) |

Data from the following sources:

[a]Farrow JH: Current concepts in the detection and treatment of the earliest of the early breast cancers. Cancer 25:468, 1970.

[b]Brown PW, Silverman J, Owens E, et al: Intraductal "noninfiltrating" carcinoma of the breast. Arch Surg 111:1063, 1976.

[c]Carter D, Smith RL: Carcinoma in situ of the breast. Cancer 40:1189, 1977.

[d]Sunshine JA, Moseley MS, Fletcher WS, et al: Breast carcinoma in situ: A retrospective review of 112 cases with a minimum 10-year follow-up. Am J Surg 150:44, 1985.

[e]Von Rueden DG, Wilson RE: Intraductal carcinoma of the breast. Surg Gynecol Obstet 158:105, 1984.

[f]Ashikari R, Hajdu SI, Robbins GF: Intraductal carcinoma of the breast (1960-1969). Cancer 28:1182, 1971.

[g]Schuh ME, Nemoto T, Penetrante R, et al: Intraductal carcinoma: Analysis of presentation, pathologic findings, and outcome of disease. Arch Surg 121:1303, 1986.

[h]Kinne DW, Petrek JA, Osborne MP, et al: Breast carcinoma in situ. Arch Surg 124:33, 1989.

[i]Lagios MD, Westdahl PR, Margolin FR, et al: Duct carcinoma in situ: Relationship of extent of noninvasive disease to the frequency of occult invasion, multicentricity, lymph node metastases, and short-term treatment failures. Cancer 50:1309, 1982.

[j]Fisher ER, Sass R, Fisher B, et al: Pathologic findings from the National Surgical Adjuvant Breast Project (Protocol 6). I: Intraductal carcinoma (DCIS). Cancer 57:197, 1986.

[k]Arnesson LG, Smeds S, Fagerberg G, et al: Follow-up of two treatment modalities for ductal cancer in situ of the breast. Br J Surg 76:672, 1989.

[l]Ward BA, McKhann CF, Ravikumar TS: Ten-year follow-up of breast carcinoma in situ in Connecticut. Arch Surg 127:1392, 1992.

[m]Silverstein MJ (ed): Ductal carcinoma in situ of the breast. Baltimore, 1997, Williams & Wilkins, p 443.

recurrences are rare and suggest malignant transformation of residual glandular tissue. Metastatic disease in patients with pure DCIS is suggestive of a histologically unrecognized invasive carcinoma in the mastectomy specimen or the development of a contralateral primary.

Reasons to select total mastectomy for treatment of DCIS include the following:

1. Diffuse suspicious mammographic calcifications suggestive of extensive disease
2. Inability to obtain clear margins with breast-conserving surgery
3. Likelihood of a poor cosmetic result after breast-conserving surgery
4. Patient not motivated to preserve her breast
5. Contraindications to radiation therapy

Contraindications to breast irradiation include the following:

1. Previous irradiation of the breast or chest wall
2. Collagen vascular disease (scleroderma or active lupus)
3. First- or second-trimester pregnancy

## Breast Conservation Therapy

As in the case of invasive breast cancer, breast conservation for DCIS requires resection to microscopically clear margins. The use of adjuvant whole-breast radiation therapy has been demonstrated in prospective randomized trials to decrease the risk for local recurrence. The use of hormonal therapy in ER-positive DCIS can further decrease the risk for local recurrence and also reduces the risk for development of new contralateral and ipsilateral breast cancers.

The use of radiation after lumpectomy has been investigated in four prospective randomized trials and the results of these studies have been remarkably consistent. The NSABP B-17 trial randomized 818 women with DCIS to lumpectomy alone versus lumpectomy plus 50 Gy of postoperative whole-breast irradiation, and 12-year actuarial recurrence data showed that the addition of radiation decreased the ipsilateral recurrence rate from 30.8% in patients undergoing excision alone to 14.9% in patients undergoing excision with irradiation ($P < .000005$).[24] The use of radiation therapy resulted in a decrease in the incidence of invasive breast cancer (16.4% versus 7.1%; $P < .00001$), with a smaller decrease in the incidence of in situ recurrence

**Table 36-8 Randomized Trials of Lumpectomy for Ductal Carcinoma in Situ: Impact of Radiation Therapy and Tamoxifen**

| | | | Local Recurrence Rates (%) | | | |
|---|---|---|---|---|---|---|
| TRIAL | NO. OF PATIENTS | FOLLOW-UP (YR) | LUMPECTOMY | LUMPECTOMY + XRT | LUMPECTOMY + XRT + TAMOXIFEN | *P* VALUE |
| NSABP B-17[a] | 818 | 12 | 30.8 | 14.9 | | <.000005 |
| EORTC 10853[b] | 1010 | 4.25 | 16 | 9 | | <.005 |
| UK ANZ | 1701 | 5 | 20 | 8 | 6 | <.0001 |
| SweDCIS | 1067 | 5 | 7 | 22 | | <.0001 |
| NSABP B-24[c] | 1804 | 7 | | 9 | 6 | 0.04 |

*EORTC,* European Organization for Research and Treatment of Cancer; *NSABP,* National Surgical Adjuvant Breast and Bowel Project; *SweDCIS,* Swedish ductal carcinoma in situ trial; *UK ANZ,* United Kingdom, Australia and New Zealand; *XRT,* Radiation therapy.

Data from the following sources:

[a]Fisher B, Dignam J, Wolmark N, et al: Lumpectomy and radiation therapy for the treatment of intraductal breast cancer: Findings from National Surgical Adjuvant Breast and Bowel Project B-17. J Clin Oncol 16:441, 1998.

[b]Julien JP, Bijker N, Fentiman IS, et al: Radiotherapy in breast-conserving treatment for ductal carcinoma in situ: First results of the EORTC randomised phase III trial 10853. EORTC Breast Cancer Cooperative Group and EORTC Radiotherapy Group. Lancet 355:528, 2000.

[c]Fisher B, Land S, Mamounas E, et al: Prevention of invasive breast cancer in women with ductal carcinoma in situ: An update of the National Surgical Adjuvant Breast and Bowel Project experience. Semin Oncol 28:400, 2001.

(14.1% versus 7.8%; $P < .001$; Table 36-8). The EORTC 10853 trial randomized 1010 women with DCIS to lumpectomy alone versus lumpectomy plus 50 Gy of radiation therapy.[25] Radiation use improved the 10-year rates of breast recurrence from 26% to 15% ($P < .0001$) and the rates of invasive recurrences from 13% to 8% ($P = .0011$). The UK ANZ (United Kingdom, Australia, and New Zealand) trial was a third large randomized trial that simultaneously evaluated the benefit of radiation therapy and tamoxifen after breast conservation surgery for patients with DCIS.[26] This trial, which enrolled 1701 patients, also demonstrated that radiation therapy reduced the risk of overall breast cancer recurrence (hazard ratio [HR], 0.38; $P <$ .0001) and invasive breast cancer recurrence (HR, 0.45; $P =$ .01). Finally, the SweDICS trial enrolled 1067 patients with DCIS; after a median follow-up of 5 years, a cumulative incidence of breast recurrence of 22% in the group that underwent surgery only versus 7% in the group that received surgery plus radiation ($P < .0001$) was reported.

Attempts have been made to identify subsets of DCIS for which wide excision without irradiation would provide sufficient local control. Silverstein[27] derived the Van Nuys criteria from a series of DCIS patients treated by wide excision, with and without radiation therapy. They proposed a system to identify patients who do not need radiation therapy based on low DCIS nuclear grade, small size of the lesion, age of the patient, and width of the surgical margin. They have reported low breast recurrence rates with surgery alone for patients with favorable Van Nuys scores. However, in a prospective trial testing this approach, investigators from Harvard enrolled 158 patients from the most favorable Van Nuys subset (low- or intermediate-grade DCIS <2.5 cm, with a minimum 1-cm margin on excision) and were not able to reproduce their results; they stopped the trial early because the rates of recurrence exceeded the predefined stopping rules. Most recently, the first result of a relatively large prospective single-arm study investigating surgery that achieved a 3 mm or greater negative margin without radiation for favorable subsets of patients with DCIS has been reported by Eastern Cooperative Oncology Group (ECOG) investigators.[28] Patients with low- or intermediate-grade DCIS measuring 2.5 cm or smaller had a 5-year rate of ipsilateral breast recurrence of only 6.1%. In contrast, patients with high-grade disease had a much higher 5-year rate of recurrence, 15.3%. In summary, these data suggest that most patients with DCIS should be recommended to receive whole-breast irradiation following lumpectomy. The one subgroup who appears to have favorable outcome are those patients with small-, low-, or intermediate-grade lesions.

## Role of Tamoxifen

The use of tamoxifen has been shown to reduce the risk for development of new breast cancers in high-risk women, including those with previous breast cancer (see earlier, "Chemoprevention for Breast Cancer"). To evaluate the benefit of tamoxifen for DCIS, the NSABP B-24 protocol randomized 1804 women who underwent lumpectomy and radiation therapy for DCIS to 5 years of tamoxifen versus placebo.[23] Study criteria allowed enrollment of patients with positive margins, and ER measurements were not performed. At 7 years of follow-up, the addition of tamoxifen to lumpectomy and radiation therapy decreased the incidence of recurrent ipsilateral breast cancers from 9% to 6% and the risk for a new contralateral breast cancer was reduced by 47% (an absolute reduction of 2%; see Table 36-8).

Combining the results of NSABP B-17 and NSABP B-24 at 7 years of follow-up, the total ipsilateral and contralateral breast cancer recurrence rate was 30% for excision alone, 17% for excision with radiation therapy, and 10% for excision, irradiation, and tamoxifen. Subsequent analyses have demonstrated that the benefit from tamoxifen is seen only in women whose DCIS is ER-positive. Patients at highest risk for local recurrence, and therefore those most likely to benefit from tamoxifen, were patients with positive margins, comedo necrosis, a mass on physical examination, and age younger than 50 years. For individual patients, the benefits of tamoxifen are weighed against its side effects, including risk for endometrial carcinoma, thromboembolic events, hot flashes, and cataracts.

### Sentinel Node Biopsy

DCIS, by definition, represents breast cancer contained within an intact basement membrane and without access to lymphatic or vascular channels. However, when axillary dissection is performed during mastectomy for intraductal disease, positive nodes can be seen in up to 3.6% of cases, as identified in a review of more than 10,000 patients in the National Cancer Database. These positive nodes probably result from the presence of microinvasion in the primary tumor that was not detected on routine pathologic analysis.

Patients with small, mammographically detected areas of DCIS have very low rates of occult invasion, so surgical staging of the axilla is not necessary. However, in women undergoing breast-conserving surgery for larger areas of DCIS, particularly those with high-grade histology or when the suspicion for microinvasion is high, sentinel node surgery to evaluate the lymph nodes may be considered.

Sentinel node surgery is currently recommended when mastectomy is performed for DCIS because up to 20% of patients with DCIS on a diagnostic core needle biopsy will be found to have invasive cancer on detailed evaluation of the mastectomy specimen. The addition of sentinel node surgery to mastectomy adds minimal morbidity and, because sentinel node mapping is no longer possible after mastectomy, avoids the need for axillary dissection if invasive cancer is identified.

## RADIATION THERAPY FOR BREAST CANCER

### After Breast-Conserving Surgery

For patients with invasive breast cancer treated with breast-conserving surgery, adjuvant radiation to the breast has been conclusively demonstrated to reduce the probability of a breast recurrence and improve outcome. The EBCTCG has published a meta-analysis of the data from 7300 women who participated in randomized trials of breast-conserving surgery, with or without radiation therapy.[29] In this analysis, radiation was found to reduce the 10-year rate of in-breast recurrence from 29% to 10% for patients with negative lymph nodes and from 47% to 13% for patients with positive lymph nodes. Importantly, this improvement in local control led to a reduction in the 15-year breast cancer mortality and overall death rate. On the basis of these data, radiation treatments should be considered as a standard. Most trials attempting to define subgroups who could potentially avoid radiation after lumpectomy have been unsuccessful, with the one potential exception of patients older than 70 years who undergo lumpectomy and adjuvant hormonal therapy for a stage I ER-positive breast cancer.[30]

Historically, radiation treatments after lumpectomy have consisted of a 6- to 8-week treatment course, which can be a hardship for patients. An important Canadian trial was successful in comparing a more abbreviated whole-breast irradiation treatment schedule. Based on long-term outcome results from this study, it is reasonable to treat a postmenopausal patient with a non– high-grade, estrogen receptor–positive, stage I breast cancer with a 16-fraction course of treatment, shortening the overall treatment time to approximately 3 weeks. In addition to this approach, there has been significant interest in shortening the treatment course to 1 week or less but focusing the radiation treatment exclusively to the area around the tumor bed. This approach, called *partial-breast irradiation*, may be performed with brachytherapy catheters, balloon catheters, or external beam radiation. Results from large phase III clinical trials comparing this approach with conventional whole breast treatment have yet to mature. Nonetheless, the approach has proven to be popular with physicians and patients. Recently, the American Society for Radiation Oncology (ASTRO) published a consensus statement highlighting appropriate selection criteria that should be considered if patients are to be treated with this approach outside the context of a clinical trial.[31]

### Postmastectomy Radiation Therapy

For patients with T1N0 or T2N0 breast cancer, mastectomy and sentinel lymph node dissection provide effective local control and radiation therapy is not required.[32] In contrast, it is clear that patients with stage III breast cancer have high rates of locoregional recurrence after treatment with a modified radical mastectomy and adjuvant or neoadjuvant chemotherapy. Clinical trial data indicate that postmastectomy radiation can significantly improve the outcome of patients who have a 20% to 40% risk of locoregional recurrence.

Three prospective randomized trials have addressed the role of postmastectomy irradiation. In the Danish Trials, premenopausal women with stage II or III breast cancer were randomized to chemotherapy alone or chemotherapy plus chest wall and nodal irradiation (protocol 82b); postmenopausal women were randomized to tamoxifen alone or tamoxifen plus radiation therapy (protocol 82c).[33] In the British Columbia study, premenopausal women with node-positive breast cancer were randomized to chemotherapy alone or chemotherapy plus chest wall and nodal irradiation.[34] In addition to the expected benefit in reducing locoregional recurrences, postmastectomy irradiation also resulted in a significant improvement in overall survival in all three trials (Table 36-9). In 2005, the EBCTCG published the results of their meta-analysis of postmastectomy radiation trials, which included data from 9933 patients treated with mastectomy or axillary clearance, with or without postmastectomy radiation.[32] Postmastectomy radiation therapy decreased the 15-year isolated locoregional recurrence rate for patients with lymph node–positive disease from 29% to 8% and reduced the 15-year breast cancer mortality rate from 60% (no radiation) to 55% (radiation). The most recent analysis from this group has suggested that similar benefits are noted for patients with one to three positive lymph nodes as those with four or more positive lymph nodes.

There is consensus that patients with four or more positive lymph nodes, or other features that lead to stage III disease, should be recommended to receive radiation. However, the use of postmastectomy radiation for patients with stage II disease is controversial. This is because a number of U.S. series have indicated that locoregional recurrence rates after a standard modified radical mastectomy and adjuvant chemotherapy are only 12% to 15%, much lower than that reported in the clinical trials and the EBCTCG meta-analysis. Based on this disparity, it is reasonable to consider postmastectomy radiation only for selected patients with stage II disease, such as those with extracapsular extension, lymphovascular space invasion, age 40 years or younger, close surgical margins, a nodal positivity ratio of 20% or greater, and those patients who have undergone less than a standard axillary level I or II dissection.

**Table 36-9 Trials of Systemic Therapy With or Without Irradiation After Mastectomy**

| | No. of Patients | | | Local Recurrence Rate (%) | | | Overall Survival (%) | | |
|---|---|---|---|---|---|---|---|---|---|
| TRIAL | SYSTEMIC THERAPY + XRT | SYSTEMIC THERAPY ALONE | TOTAL | SYSTEMIC THERAPY + XRT | SYSTEMIC THERAPY ALONE | *P* VALUE | SYSTEMIC THERAPY + XRT | SYSTEMIC THERAPY ALONE | *P* VALUE |
| DBCG 82b (10 yr; chemo)[a] | 852 | 856 | 1708 | 9 | 32 | <0.001 | 54 | 45 | <0.001 |
| DBCG 82c (10 yr; tamoxifen)[b] | 686 | 689 | 1375 | 8 | 35 | <0.001 | 45 | 38 | 0.03 |
| DBCG 82c (combined 18 yr) | 1538 | 1545 | 3083 | 14 | 49 | <0.001 | 37 | 27 | |
| British Columbia Trial (20 yr)[c] | 164 | 154 | 318 | 13 | 25 | 0.003* | 64 | 54 | 0.003* |

*chemo,* Chemotherapy; *DBCG,* Danish Breast Cancer Group; *XRT,* radiation therapy.

*Aggregate *P* value for comparisons at various follow-up intervals; this is the 10-year result.

Data from the following sources:

[a]Overgaard M, Hansen Per S, Overgaard J, et al: Postoperative radiotherapy in high-risk premenopausal women with breast cancer who receive adjuvant chemotherapy. N Engl J Med 337:949, 1997.

[b]Overgaard M, Jensen M-B, Overgaard J, et al: Postoperative radiotherapy in high-risk postmenopausal breast cancer patients given adjuvant tamoxifen: Danish Breast Cancer Cooperative Group DBCG 82c randomized trial. Lancet 353:1641, 1999.

[c]Ragaz J, Jackson S, Le N, et al: Adjuvant radiotherapy and chemotherapy in node-positive premenopausal women with breast cancer. N Engl J Med 337:956, 1997.

## SYSTEMIC THERAPY FOR BREAST CANCER

Despite advances in locoregional therapy, a significant proportion of women with breast cancer will develop metastatic disease within 5 to 10 years after diagnosis. For most patients who develop metastatic breast cancer, this is a fatal condition. A systemic approach of treatment with medications is used to treat and prevent recurrence of possible microscopic metastatic disease. For women with advanced stage IV breast cancer, systemic therapy is given in efforts to palliate symptoms from cancer and potentially to prolong survival. Current thinking places the metastatic event early in the progression of breast cancer, probably before initial clinical evaluation in most patients. This concept argues for a systemic approach to breast cancer, administered in concert with local treatment. The missing link is the ability to detect occult metastatic disease accurately and select appropriate patients to receive systemic treatment.

### Goals of Therapy and Determination of Risk of Harm

For stages I to III invasive breast cancer, the goals of treatment for patients are curative. Treatment is considered in the context of the potential benefits of therapy based on reduction of risk of recurrence, as well as the potential harm of treatment. In addition, patient preferences are strongly considered when determining adjuvant therapy use. For some patients, their personal belief is that the reduction in risk of recurrence with therapy is not worth the adverse effects of the treatment, in particular for chemotherapy. Often, several long discussions regarding therapy are essential when determining the treatment that best suits an individual patient.

With increasing stage of disease is an associated increased risk in the development of systemic recurrence. Not only does the volume (extent) of disease present at diagnosis affect the risk of cancer recurrence, the biologic characteristics of an individual tumor also influence the risk of recurrence. The most commonly used biomarkers—ER, PR, and HER-2—affect prognosis and are also predictive of response to different therapies. In very general terms, tumors that have low levels of expression of estrogen and PR, as well as tumors with high levels of HER-2, are associated with worse cancer outcomes when compared with tumors that are strongly estrogen- and PR-positive and HER-2–negative or normal. For most patients, risk of recurrence is estimated based on population-based statistics. Current federal and international guidelines use stage and biologic characteristics in the development of treatment recommendations (Table 36-10).

Recently, multigene assays (e.g., 21-gene recurrence score assay and MammaPrint assay) have been developed in an attempt to identify a specific molecular phenotype of an individual patient's tumor and then to use this phenotype in predicting the response to therapy or provide information regarding prognosis.[35] For example, the Oncotype DX assay was developed from a candidate pool of 250 genes and narrowed to a specific 21-gene panel based on three independent studies of the candidate genes.[15] This assay was validated first in a patient population with ER-positive, lymph node–negative breast cancer (NSABP B-14). It was found to be prognostic in terms of estimating overall survival and predictive for benefits from differing therapies, with higher recurrence scores estimating increased benefit from chemotherapy and lower scores estimating lesser benefit from chemotherapy and increased benefit from endocrine therapy. This assay was also validated in subsequent studies. The Oncotype DX (21-gene recurrence score) assay is a tool available to assist clinicians in estimating the benefits of therapy for patients with lymph node–negative, ER-positive breast cancer.

**Table 36-10 Decision Making for Medical Therapy**

| STAGE | MEDICAL THERAPY | COMMENTS |
|---|---|---|
| **I (<1cm)** | | |
| Hormone receptor–positive | Endocrine therapy ± chemotherapy | Consider genomic testing |
| Hormone receptor–negative | Consider chemotherapy | |
| HER-2–positive | Strongly consider trastuzumab based chemotherapy | |
| **I (>1cm)** | | |
| Hormone receptor–positive | Endocrine therapy ± chemotherapy | Consider genomic testing |
| Hormone receptor–negative | Chemotherapy | |
| HER-2–positive | Trastuzumab based chemotherapy | |
| **II (LN negative)** | | |
| Hormone receptor–positive | Endocrine therapy ± chemotherapy | Consider genomic testing |
| Hormone receptor–negative | Chemotherapy | |
| HER-2–positive | Trastuzumab-based chemotherapy | |
| **II (LN positive), III** | | |
| Hormone receptor–positive | Chemotherapy* + endocrine therapy | *Consider tumor grade; extent of disease; % HR positive; markers of proliferation (Ki67); patient health |
| Hormone receptor–negative | Chemotherapy | |
| HER-2–positive | Trastuzumab based chemotherapy | |

*LN,* Lymph node.

*The decision to use chemotherapy in patients with hormone receptor-positive disease is multifactorial. Consideration should be given to grade, percent of cells that are hormone receptor positive, proliferative rate and overall patient health and co-morbidities.

There are areas of uncertainty regarding its use that are still under investigation. For patients with low-risk recurrence scores, chemotherapy appears to add marginal benefit on reducing the risk of distant recurrence, whereas high-risk recurrence scores are associated with marked benefit from chemotherapy. The magnitude of benefit from chemotherapy is uncertain, however, for the group with intermediate- risk scores and was the subject of a recently completed cooperative group trial (TAILORx). These assays are used in the context of patient characteristics (e.g., general health, age) and extent of disease (e.g., tumor size) and are not the sole determinants of the type of medical therapy prescribed. It is expected that as assays (currently available or under development) are evaluated further in clinical studies, their ability to tailor medical therapy to an individual will improve.

Adjuvant! Online (www.adjuvantonline.com) is an online tool that has been designed to help physicians determine the 10-year risk of recurrence and death caused by breast cancer for an individual patient. This validated tool also informs the clinician about how specific interventions, such as chemotherapy, hormone therapy, or a combination of the two, are expected to affect survival.[36] These estimates of prognosis are based largely on the SEER registry estimates. The primary factors incorporated in this model include age, comorbidity, estrogen receptor status, grade, tumor size, and nodal status. HER-2 status is not currently in the model but is expected to be added in future updated versions. Once the clinician inputs patient and tumor-related information, this online tool provides graphics to depict 10-year recurrence-free and overall survival estimates for an individual patient, as well as estimates adjusted for the use of chemotherapy and/or endocrine therapy.

The Adjuvant! Online program does have limitations because it is based on registry information and relapse data, and cause of death may be inaccurate from these registries. Also, it does not incorporate information about HER-2 positivity or risk-stratify for breast cancer in women younger than 35 years. In some cases, estimating recurrence and breast cancer–related death information with estimates of survival may be distressing to patients. However, the design does allow the physician and patient to have an interactive discussion regarding the risks and benefits of therapies, and how these therapies may affect risk of recurrence and death caused by breast cancer. Some newer additions to the website include diagrams and patient education tools that may enhance this dialogue.

## Chemotherapy

Metastatic disease is the principal cause of death from breast cancer. Patients who benefit from chemotherapy or hormonal therapy do so because metastasis is prevented, cured, or delayed. The first prospective trials of systemic treatment combined oophorectomy, to deprive patients of estrogens, with radical mastectomy. Since these early trials, hundreds of prospective studies have involved thousands of women.

Medications used to treat early breast cancer have their foundation as treatment of advanced disease. In general, treatments that are used effectively to improve outcome for patients with incurable breast cancer are estimated to have increased impact on outcomes for patients with earlier stages of breast cancer, in whom smaller volumes of disease, and potentially less resistance to therapy, will be present. When medications are identified that improve outcomes for patients with incurable stage IV breast cancer, they are often brought forward into clinical studies for earlier stages of disease. Chemotherapy is generally used with combinations of medications in an effort to take advantage of nonoverlapping toxicities and maximize different mechanisms of action in targeting tumor cells. The concept of using non–cross-resistant therapies (i.e., drugs with different mechanisms of action to overcome cancer cell resistance to therapy) has dominated the development of adjuvant (after surgery) and neoadjuvant (before surgery) chemotherapy regimens. The duration of therapy is usually somewhere between four and eight cycles of treatment, depending on which regimen is used. Longer durations of chemotherapy with the same agents (>6 months) have not improved survival and are no longer used.

The largest comprehensive analysis of the benefits of chemotherapy is from the EBCTCG. This group meets every 5 years to review outcome data from breast cancer trials conducted worldwide. The most recently available data regarding adjuvant chemotherapy was published in 2005[37] and summarizes data from randomized trials that were initiated by 1995. The authors presented data from trials evaluating adjuvant chemotherapy versus no chemotherapy (60 trials) as well as cyclophosphamide, methotrexate, and 5-fluorouracil (CMF)–type chemotherapy versus anthracycline-based chemotherapy (17 trials). For younger women (<50 years), polychemotherapy reduces the risk of death by 30% and the risk of relapse by 37% compared with the use of no chemotherapy. For women older than 50 years, a reduction in the risk of death (12%) and relapse (19%) was also seen, even though the magnitude of benefit was less.

The main classes of chemotherapeutics used to treat early-stage breast include anthracyclines (e.g., doxorubicin, epirubicin) and taxanes (e.g., paclitaxel, docetaxel). The anthracyclines, whose activity is via action as both a topoisomerase II inhibitor and antimetabolite, have high levels of activity in the treatment of breast cancer. When used for the treatment of metastatic breast cancer as a single agent, responses to therapy are generally seen in from 45% to 80% of patients. The EBCTCG analysis[37] noted that anthracyclines add additional benefit when compared with nonanthracycline, CMF-type therapies, with a 16% reduction of death and 11% reduction in the risk of recurrence. Anthracyclines are associated with the potential long-term toxicity of cardiomyopathy, which may lead to congestive heart failure, often many years after treatment. The risk of cardiac dysfunction from anthracyclines is dose-dependent and current anthracycline-containing chemotherapy regimens have a risk of cardiac dysfunction from 1.5% to 3%. An additional dangerous risk from anthracycline-based chemotherapy is the risk of the development of leukemia (<1%).

Taxanes (microtubule inhibitors) have significant activity in the treatment of metastatic breast cancer and are active not only in tumors previously unexposed to chemotherapy, but also active in anthracycline-resistant tumors. A number of clinical trials have evaluated the use of taxanes as treatment of early-stage breast cancer. A meta-analysis regarding the use of taxanes in 13 different studies has described improvement in both DFS (hazard ratio [HR], 0.83; 95% confidence interval [CI], 0.79 to 0.87; $P < .0001$) and OS (HR 0.85; 95% CI 0.79-0.91; $P < .0001$).[38] The antitumor activity of paclitaxel is dependent on the timing of delivery of therapy—that is, more frequent administration of paclitaxel improves outcomes.[39] The activity of docetaxel is less dependent on timing of treatment and is generally used on an every 3-week schedule of administration. Both taxanes, when given at their optimal dose and schedule, have shown equivalence in outcome, as noted in the ECOG 1199 trial. This study randomized patients with lymph node–positive breast cancer to receive paclitaxel or docetaxel weekly or every 3 weeks after completion of an anthracycline based regimen. Weekly paclitaxel and every 3-week docetaxel were associated with the most favorable outcomes in terms of disease control and adverse effects when compared with every 3-week administration of paclitaxel. The taxanes are associated with the potential permanent toxicity of peripheral neuropathy but do not cause long-term increased risk of second cancers and/or cardiac dysfunction.

**BOX 36-3 Commonly Used Chemotherapy Regimens**

**Non–Trastuzumab-Based Regimens**

AC (doxorubicin, cyclophosphamide)
TC (docetaxel, cyclophosphamide)
TAC (docetaxel, doxorubicin, cyclophosphamide)
Dose-dense chemotherapy: AC followed by paclitaxel, administration every 2 wk
AC followed by paclitaxel administered weekly
AC followed by docetaxel
FAC (5-fluorouracil, doxorubicin, cyclophosphamide)
FEC (5-fluorouracil, epirubicin, cyclophosphamide)
CMF (cyclophosphamide, methotrexate, 5-fluorouracil)
FAC or FEC followed by paclitaxel weekly or docetaxel

**Trastuzumab-Based Regimens**

AC followed by paclitaxel weekly + trastuzumab → trastuzumab maintenance
AC followed by docetaxel + trastuzumab → trastuzumab maintenance
TCH (docetaxel, carboplatin, trastuzumab) → trastuzumab maintenance
Chemotherapy followed by trastuzumab maintenance ERA

**Neoadjuvant Therapy**

Paclitaxel weekly + trastuzumab followed by FEC + trastuzumab

Adapted from Carlson RW, Allred DC, Anderson BO, et al: Breast cancer. Clinical practice guidelines in oncology. J Natl Compr Canc Netw 7:122, 2009.

A variety of chemotherapy regimens are used in the United States in the systemic treatment of breast cancer patients (Box 36-3). Selection of a specific chemotherapy regimen is based on the potential risks of the regimen in context of the benefits of therapy. For example, the third-generation anthracycline- or taxane-containing chemotherapy regimens are associated with an approximately 50% to 60% reduction in the risk of relapse. Each of these regimens has variable toxicities and clinicians tailor the regimen prescribed in an attempt to maximize benefit and minimize harm. Most chemotherapy regimens used in routine practice were investigated for patients with lymph node–positive disease; however, the proportional reduction in risk of recurrence is thought to be similar for patients with high-risk, lymph node–negative breast cancer. Several studies have specifically targeted this population and found benefit from chemotherapy. Retrospective analyses of clinical studies have suggested that anthracyclines may have limited benefit when used as treatment in hormone-receptor positive, HER-2 normal breast cancers. A recent clinical trial evaluated a taxane-only–based chemotherapy regimen (docetaxel, cyclophosphamide) in comparison to an anthracycline-based regimen (doxorubicin, cyclophosphamide) in efforts to lower long-term toxicity risks to patients while maintaining anticancer activity.[40] The taxane-based regimen, TC, improved DFS and OS when compared with an anthracycline-based regimen, AC (DFS 86% TC versus 80% AC; HR, 0.67; 95% CI, 0.50 to 0.94; $P = .015$). In an ongoing clinical trial, the NSABP (B-46-I/07132) is comparing taxane-only based regimens against an anthracycline-taxane regimen and may further clarify the role of anthracyclines in more modern systemic therapy for breast cancer.

Chemotherapy is most commonly administered in the adjuvant setting following completion of surgery. There are theoretical advantages regarding delivery of chemotherapy prior to surgery (neoadjuvant setting), including the potential for encountering lower volume of microscopic metastatic disease, potential decrease in drug resistance by treating tumors before resistance has developed, intact vascular system, improved rates of breast conservation, and ability to evaluate the in vivo response to treatment. In theory, the ability to evaluate response to therapy may help avoid administration of ineffective therapy and allow the clinician to tailor individual therapy. Neoadjuvant chemotherapy does have potential disadvantages in terms of loss of prechemotherapy prognostic information (e.g., axillary lymph node status, actual invasive tumor size) as well as potential impact for decision making with respect to postmastectomy radiation therapy. Overall, however, a number of clinical trials have shown equivalence in survival for administration of therapy in the neoadjuvant setting versus the adjuvant setting. A meta-analysis of nine randomized studies ($N$ = 3946) has shown equivalence in survival as well as locoregional recurrence for neoadjuvant versus adjuvant therapy.[41] In routine practice, neoadjuvant chemotherapy is used outside of clinical trials for patients with locally advanced or inoperable breast cancer, patients with inflammatory breast cancer, or those who might benefit from reduction of tumor size in an effort to enhance the ability to perform breast conservation. In general, chemotherapy regimens that are routinely used in the adjuvant setting may also be used in the neoadjuvant setting.

### Trastuzumab-Based Chemotherapy Regimens

Trastuzumab is a humanized monoclonal antibody developed to target the extracellular domain of the HER-2 receptor. HER-2 gene amplification or protein overexpression occurs in approximately 25% to 30% of breast cancers. Amplification leads to protein overexpression, measured clinically by immunohistochemistry and scored on a scale from 0 to 3+. Alternatively, FISH directly detects the quantity of HER-2 gene copies, with a normal copy number of two. Research has shown that inhibition of the function of the HER-2 receptor–like protein slows the growth of HER-2–amplified tumors in laboratory models and in clinical trials. When used as a single agent for treatment of metastatic breast cancer, response is seen in approximately 30% of patients.

Combined with chemotherapy, trastuzumab is even more powerful in the preclinical setting, with biologic synergy seen with multiple agents. Trastuzumab-based chemotherapy regimens improve disease-free and overall survival for patients with metastatic disease. Given the promising activity seen for metastatic disease, a number of adjuvant studies and neoadjuvant studies were conducted and have demonstrated improved outcomes for patients with stages I to III breast cancer. The HERceptin Adjuvant (HERA) trial ($N = 5090$) enrolled patients with HER-2–positive breast cancers and randomized patients to trastuzumab (for 1 or 2 years) versus observation after completion of chemotherapy.[42] Data regarding 2 years of therapy is not yet available; however, when comparing 1 year of trastuzumab versus observation, trastuzumab reduced the risk of a breast cancer–related event by 46% (HR, 0.54; 95% CI, 0.43 to 0.67; $P < .001$) and improved overall survival by 34% (HR, 0.66; 95% CI, 0.47 to 0.91; $P < .0115$).

The NSABP B-31 and NCCTG-N9831 adjuvant trials were similar in study design; the results from both studies were combined for initial analysis.[43] Patients in the control arm of these studies received AC followed by paclitaxel. Trastuzumab was added in the experimental groups, either concurrently with paclitaxel or sequentially after the paclitaxel. The patients who received trastuzumab had a reduction in breast cancer–related events by 52% (DFS HR, 0.48; 95% CI, 0.39 to 0.61; $P < .001$). There was toxicity noted with the addition of trastuzumab and patients receiving trastuzumab-based therapy in NSABP B-31(AC followed by paclitaxel-trastuzumab) had an increased risk of cardiac dysfunction, with a 3-year event rate of 4.1% versus a control arm rate of 0.8%. Patients who initiated therapy with lower ejection fractions, who were older and/or had hypertension, were at highest risk of cardiac dysfunction. The BCIRG 006 trial used a nonanthracycline-containing regimen as one of its treatment groups and showed equivalence in outcome between AC followed by docetaxel-trastuzumab (AC→TH) versus docetaxel combined with carboplatin and trastuzumab (TCH).[44] Both treatment groups were superior in terms of DFS to the control group treatment of AC followed by docetaxel, with a HR of 0.61 (95% CI, 0.48 to 0.76; $P < .001$) for the AC→TH arm and a HR of 0.67 for the TCH group (95% CI, 0.54 to 0.83). Patients receiving TCH had markedly reduced cardiac toxicity (0.37%) versus the AC→TH arm (1.87%). Current and ongoing studies for patients with HER-2– positive disease are evaluating the tyrosine kinase inhibitor lapatinib as well as the trastuzumab-drug conjugate TDM1. Trastuzumab-based therapy has significantly changed outcomes for patients with what is considered an aggressive biologic subtype of breast cancer, and ongoing efforts to identify other targets to enhance therapy are underway.

## Endocrine Therapy

One of the original targeted therapy approaches was the use of oophorectomy to reduce systemic estrogen production as a treatment for breast cancer. Most breast cancers (>60%) have the presence of the ER and/or PR; interruption of the production of estrogen or the ability of estrogen to interact with the ER has been associated with improved disease-free and overall survival for women with metastatic breast cancer. This therapeutic approach is associated with a generally favorable side effect profile with each class of agents when contrasted with the adverse effects from chemotherapy.

### Tamoxifen

Tamoxifen is a selective estrogen receptor modulator that has antagonistic and weak agonistic effects. Clinical trials using tamoxifen as treatment for early-stage breast cancer began in the 1970s. In 2005, the EBCTCG meta-analysis reported data of more than 80,000 women treated in clinical studies.[37] Tamoxifen administered for 5 years was found to improve outcomes by reducing the risk of recurrence of breast cancer for patients with hormone receptor–positive disease by 41% (recurrence rate ratio, 0.59; standard error [SE], 0.03). The risk of death from breast cancer was reduced by approximately one third (death rate ratio, 0.66; SE, 0.04). Tamoxifen was shown to be of benefit for premenopausal and postmenopausal women and has a similar magnitude of benefit for patients with lymph node–positive versus lymph node–negative disease. The duration of therapy with tamoxifen was also evaluated; 5 years of therapy were found to be superior to only 1 to 2 years of therapy in terms of breast cancer recurrence (15.2% proportionate reduction; $P < .001$) and death from breast cancer (7.9% proportionate reduction; $P = .01$). There is uncertain benefit of longer durations of tamoxifen beyond 5 years because the agonistic effects of tamoxifen become more profound and there is an increasing risk of adverse events. Results from NSABP B-14 have shown no improvement in disease-free or overall survival for 10 years of therapy with tamoxifen versus 5 years of tamoxifen treatment.

Tamoxifen causes reduction of cell proliferation and has direct antagonistic effects when combined with chemotherapy. SWOG 8814 has found that patients who receive concurrent tamoxifen with anthracycline-based chemotherapy have numeric but nonsignificant reductions in disease-free and overall survival.[45] Tamoxifen is generally a well-tolerated medication, with the most common side effect being hot flashes or vasomotor symptoms, occurring in less than 50% of patients treated. In postmenopausal women, the estrogen-like agonist effect of tamoxifen will improve bone density, whereas in premenopausal women the agent is antagonistic to bone health. Potentially serious but rare effects include increased risk of thromboembolic disease and uterine cancer.

#### Ovarian Ablation

The EBCTCG meta-analysis evaluated premenopausal women who were treated with ovarian ablation or suppression and found that this treatment approach reduces the risk of relapse and death from breast cancer.[37] When compared with the use of CMF chemotherapy, the use of ovarian ablation with goserelin as treatment for lymph node–positive, premenopausal stage II breast cancer resulted in equivalent outcome in terms of DFS (HR, 1.01; $P = .94$) and OS (HR, 0.99; $P = .94$). Even with this high level of activity, the optimal role for the use of the addition of ovarian ablation in addition to modern chemotherapy and/or other antihormone therapies is controversial and is the subject of ongoing clinical trials.

#### Aromatase Inhibitors

AIs block the conversion of the hormone androstenedione into estrone by inhibition of the aromatase enzyme. This enzyme is present in adipose tissue, breast tissue, breast tumor cells, and other sites. Multiple generations of medications that block the aromatase enzyme have been evaluated; however, less specific agents such as aminoglutethimide also suppress production of other hormones, and this is associated with unacceptable side effects. Selective or third-generation AIs purely block the final step conversion of hormones into estrogen and are not associated with the broad hormone suppression seen with earlier AIs. These agents, which include anastrozole, exemestane, and letrozole, are not able to suppress ovarian function completely in a premenopausal or perimenopausal woman and are restricted for use in postmenopausal women.

Several different trial designs have been used to evaluate AIs in the adjuvant setting. Direct comparisons of 5 years of a selective AI versus 5 years of tamoxifen have demonstrated improvement in cancer outcomes for anastrozole and letrozole.[46] The ATAC (***a***rimidex, ***t***amoxifen, ***a***lone or in ***c***ombination) trial has demonstrated that 5 years of anastrozole significantly improve DFS by 17% when compared with 5 years of tamoxifen (HR, 0.83; 95% CI, 0.73 to 94; $P = .05$). In addition to reducing the risk of distant recurrence (distant DFS HR, 0.86; 95% CI, 0.74 to 0.99; $P = 0.04$), anastrozole reduced the risk of the development of contralateral breast cancers by 42%.[46]

The selective AIs have also been evaluated when given sequentially for 2 to 3 years after the use of tamoxifen for 2 to 3 years compared with 5 years of tamoxifen treatment.[47] The use of all three modern AIs after 2 to 3 years of tamoxifen has shown improved cancer outcomes when compared with the use of tamoxifen alone. In addition, extended adjuvant therapy with 5 years of the AI letrozole after 5 years of tamoxifen was shown to improve outcome when compared with placebo. The use of letrozole versus placebo reduced the risk of breast cancer events by 43% ($P < .008$).

The ideal use of AIs in the treatment of postmenopausal breast cancer patients with ER-positive disease is not known. The risk of recurrence of ER-positive breast cancer persists beyond 5 years after diagnosis and there is significant interest in evaluating the extended use of antiestrogen therapy to lower the risk of recurrence. Ongoing studies are evaluating the extended use of AIs beyond 5 years, and even beyond 10 years. In addition, it is not clear whether tamoxifen is an essential component in the adjuvant treatment for the postmenopausal patient population. Given the multiple studies demonstrating consistently improved outcomes with the selective AIs, the American Society of Clinical Oncology (ASCO) released a clinical practice guideline in 2010, which stated that postmenopausal women should receive a selective AI at some point during their cancer therapy.[48] Selective AIs as a group have similar adverse effects, including hot flashes, vasomotor symptoms, joint symptoms, myalgias, bone loss, and vaginal dryness.

#### Summary of Medical Therapy for Early-Stage Breast Cancer

Most patients diagnosed with early stage (I to III) invasive breast cancer will be offered medical therapy in an effort to improve disease-free and overall survival. In addition, the use of antiestrogen therapy as treatment of hormone receptor–positive breast cancer will also act to help lower the risk of new breast cancers. The use of medical therapy is guided by tumor characteristics (e.g., stage, molecular markers), patient characteristics (e.g., age, general health, personal preferences), and a careful balance of benefits of therapy versus potential risks of treatment. As advances in molecular analysis of tumors progress, it is likely that treatment recommendations and options will be refined toward a patient's tumor profile and more general guidelines, as are currently used, will not be implemented as often.

### Neoadjuvant Systemic Therapy for Operable Breast Cancer

Administration of systemic chemotherapy or hormonal therapy before surgery can result in a significant reduction in tumor size in 50% to 80% of patients with locally advanced breast cancer. This preoperative, or neoadjuvant, therapy can convert inoperable tumors to operable ones, convert tumors that would require mastectomy to eligibility for lumpectomy, and shrink larger tumors to allow an improved cosmetic outcome with breast-conserving surgery. This approach also allows for the study of tumor biology via serial analysis of tumor tissue before, during, and after treatment and has been used to study the efficacy and mechanism of action of systemic therapy agents.

Several prospective randomized trials have evaluated the efficacy of chemotherapy and hormonal therapy administered before (neoadjuvant) versus after (adjuvant) definitive surgery. These studies all demonstrated increased rates of breast conservation with the use of systemic therapy before surgery. The NSABP B-18 trial included 1523 patients and found no survival advantage (or detriment) in patients who received preoperative doxorubicin and cyclophosphamide chemotherapy versus the same regimen delivered postoperatively. The breast conservation rate was higher in women completing preoperative chemotherapy, and in-breast recurrence after preoperative therapy was not significantly different from that in women who underwent lumpectomy before adjuvant chemotherapy. Response to preoperative therapy was found to correlate with prognosis. At 9 years of follow-up, the disease-free survival rate in patients achieving a complete pathologic response in the preoperative arm (no evidence of tumor at surgery) was 75%, as opposed to 58% in patients who had any residual invasive disease left after chemotherapy.

The neoadjuvant approach is now commonly used for operable patients who would require mastectomy but could become candidates for breast conservation if their primary tumor size could be reduced before surgery. By the end of systemic therapy, 10% to 15% of such patients will have complete resolution of their tumors by clinical examination and imaging but might have microscopic residual disease. Consequently, a metallic clip is placed at the primary tumor site under image guidance before initiating chemotherapy to allow identification of the original tumor site for excision.

Management of the axilla in patients undergoing neoadjuvant therapy has evolved. Some centers perform sentinel node surgery before neoadjuvant therapy in patients with clinically negative nodes to inform systemic and radiation therapy decisions. Advocates of sentinel node surgery before neoadjuvant chemotherapy cite concerns about lower rates of successful mapping and higher false-negative rates after neoadjuvant therapy. Other centers now favor sentinel node surgery after neoadjuvant therapy for any patient whose axilla is clinically negative after therapy to obtain more information about the status of the nodes after neoadjuvant therapy. Studies have now shown the status of the axillary nodes after chemotherapy to be the strongest predictor of outcome. In addition, the chemotherapy can eradicate microscopic disease in the regional nodes in up to 40% of patients, reducing the need for complete axillary lymph node dissection at the time of surgical intervention. Complete axillary dissection remains the standard for all patients receiving neoadjuvant therapy who have biopsy-proven, node-positive disease at initial presentation.

In practice, the neoadjuvant approach is used routinely for patients with inoperable locally advanced breast cancer, including those with inflammatory breast cancer, those with large, fixed, or erosive lesions not amenable to mastectomy, and those with advanced nodal disease that is fixed, bulky, or causing arm edema. Most of these patients will then undergo mastectomy, radiation therapy, and possibly additional systemic therapy. In this setting, neoadjuvant chemotherapy serves as a remarkable research platform, in which it is possible to learn more about tumor biology and drug responses in an expedited time frame as compared with the adjuvant approach, in which long-term survival is the end point. More recently, there has been much interest in treating operable patients in the neoadjuvant setting because the response to systemic therapy can result in improvements in the clinical management of these patients. Patient selection is based on tumor characteristics beyond tumor size alone and therapies are targeted to specific subtypes with the greatest potential for affecting locoregional and systemic outcomes. Patients are monitored carefully during treatment and the pathologic assessment of the regional nodes can guide clinicians in determining how much additional therapy is warranted after a complete response or residual disease.

There are some key concepts that have been gleaned from the results of neoadjuvant therapy trials completed over the last few years. First, the use of neoadjuvant chemotherapy as a research platform has led to the identification of patient and tumor characteristics that can predict response to therapy. This allows clinicians to define better the population of patients who are most likely to benefit from the use of neoadjuvant chemotherapy. The use of targeted therapies, such as trastuzumab, in combination with chemotherapy can be safely administered in the neoadjuvant setting in HER-2–positive breast cancer patients, resulting in markedly increased rates of pathologic complete response. In the context of targeted therapy, patients with ER-positive disease can be treated with endocrine therapy in the neoadjuvant setting with significant response rates and increased rates of breast-conserving surgery. This approach is optimal in postmenopausal women with ER-positive tumors for whom endocrine therapy provides more protection against risk of recurrence and of death caused by breast cancer over standard chemotherapy. Finally, as new and more targeted regimens have led to an increasing population of patients with a clinical complete response to neoadjuvant therapy, accurately assessing the residual tumor burden in the breast and regional nodes will become increasingly important in terms of defining prognosis and determining further therapy that is needed.

## TREATMENT OF LOCALLY ADVANCED AND INFLAMMATORY BREAST CANCER

Patients with locally advanced breast cancer include those with large primary tumors (>5 cm), tumors involving the chest wall, skin involvement, ulceration or satellite skin nodules, inflammatory carcinoma, bulky or fixed axillary nodes, and clinically apparent internal mammary or supraclavicular nodal involvement (stages IIB, IIIA, and IIIB disease). Central to treatment is the concept that the disease is advanced on the chest wall, in regional lymph nodes, or both, with no evidence of metastasis to distant sites. These patients are recognized to be at significant risk for the development of subsequent metastases, and treatment must address the risk for local and systemic relapse. Experience before the 1970s demonstrated that surgery alone provided poor local control, with local relapse rates in the range of 30% to 50% and mortality rates of 70%. Similar results were reported when radiation therapy was the sole modality of treatment. Current management includes surgery, radiation therapy, and systemic therapy, with the sequence and extent of treatment determined by specifics of the patient's circumstance.

Inflammatory breast cancer remains the most aggressive subtype of breast cancer but fortunately is rare, constituting approximately 5% of all breast tumors. The hallmark of inflammatory breast cancer is diffuse tumor involvement of the dermal lymphatic channels within the breast and overlying skin, often without an underlying tumor mass. Inflammatory breast cancer is clinically manifested as erythema, edema, and warmth of the breast as a result of lymphatic obstruction. There may be no mammographic abnormality beyond skin thickening, and a palpable mass is not required for the diagnosis. The term *peau d'orange* is used to describe the orange peel appearance of the skin resulting from edema and dimpling at sites of hair follicles (see Fig. 36-5*D*). The history should describe a rapid onset of the disease, with progression over a period of weeks to 3 months. Neglected breast cancer primaries that lead to secondary inflammatory changes within the breast should not be categorized as inflammatory breast cancer. Inflammatory cancer is a clinical diagnosis and can occur with tumors of ductal or lobular histology. The pathologic hallmark of inflammatory cancer is the presence of tumor cells within dermal lymphatics, but this can be often missed because of sampling error and therefore is not a prerequisite to diagnosis. Axillary nodal metastases are common, and there is a significant risk for distant metastases.

Current treatment approaches emphasize aggressive use of combined-modality treatment, including neoadjuvant chemotherapy, mastectomy, and radiation therapy, with hormonal therapy in ER-positive tumors and trastuzumab for HER-2–positive tumors. The results of this multimodality treatment now show relapse-free survival rates of 50% or higher at 5 years as compared with a single-institution historical series showing a 7% 5-year survival rate in patients receiving less aggressive treatment.[49]

## TREATMENT OF SPECIAL CONDITIONS

### Breast Cancer in Older Adults

Several studies have explored options that reduce the extent of surgery and radiation therapy for older women with breast cancer. Two recent trials randomized older women to lumpectomy with or without irradiation. In the Cancer and Leukemia Group B (CALGB) 9343 trial,[30] 647 women 70 years or older with ER-positive tumors 2 cm or smaller and clinically negative nodes received lumpectomy and tamoxifen and were randomized to irradiation or no irradiation. At 5 years' follow-up, survival was identical, and the in-breast recurrence rate was only 4% in the no-radiation arm versus 1% in the radiation arm. The death rate from breast cancer was 1% at 5 years in this population, with a 17% death rate from other causes.

Fyles and associates have reported the results of a Canadian trial with more inclusive eligibility criteria in which 769 women aged 50 years or older with tumors up to 5 cm and positive or negative ER status were enrolled. All patients underwent wide excision, received tamoxifen, and were randomized to irradiation or no irradiation. Recurrence rates were significantly higher overall in patients who did not receive radiation therapy. However, in an unplanned analysis of a subset of 193 women older than 60, the local recurrence rate was only 1.2% without radiation versus no recurrences with radiation therapy.

These low rates of local recurrence and the significant rates of death from other comorbid conditions have led to the acceptance of wide excision and hormonal therapy without irradiation for selected older patients with small ER-positive tumors and clinically negative axillary nodes. Axillary surgery has been omitted in such patients in the past; however, sentinel node surgery can easily be incorporated, with minimal morbidity.

### Paget's Disease

Paget's disease accounts for 1% or less of breast malignancies. It is characterized clinically by nipple erythema and irritation with associated pruritus and may progress to crusting and ulceration. The condition may spread outward from the nipple and onto the areola and surrounding skin of the breast (see Fig. 36-5). The differential diagnosis of scaling skin and erythema of the nipple-areola complex includes eczema, contact dermatitis, postradiation dermatitis, and Paget's disease. A biopsy of the skin of the nipple should be performed; a specimen containing Paget cells secures the diagnosis.

Pathologically, a Paget cell is a large, pale-staining cell with round or oval nuclei and large nucleoli located between the normal keratinocytes of the nipple epidermis. Paget cells spread into the lactiferous sinuses under the nipple and upward to invade the overlying epidermis of the nipple. Paget cells do not invade through the dermal basement membrane and therefore are categorized as carcinoma in situ.

More than 95% of patients with Paget's disease have an underlying breast carcinoma. Paget's disease may be accompanied by a palpable mass in just over 50% of patients. Invasive breast cancer will be identified in patients with a palpable mass and Paget's disease in over 90% of patients.

Treatment of Paget's disease includes mastectomy with axillary staging or wide local excision of the nipple and areola to achieve clear margins, axillary staging, and radiation therapy. For many patients, lumpectomy and irradiation will provide an acceptable cosmetic appearance and avoid the more extensive surgery of mastectomy and reconstruction. Nipple-areolar reconstruction can be performed 4 to 6 months following radiation therapy. For patients considering lumpectomy, thorough preoperative evaluation is required to rule out occult multicentric disease.

### Male Breast Cancer

Breast cancer occurring in the mammary gland of men is infrequent; it accounts for 0.8% of all breast cancers, less than 1% of all newly diagnosed male cancers, and 0.2% of male cancer deaths. Annually, in the United States, 1500 new cases and 400 deaths are reported. The median age at diagnosis is 68 years, 5 years older than in women.

Risk factors include increasing age, radiation exposure, and factors related to abnormalities in estrogen and androgen balance, including testicular disease, infertility, obesity, and cirrhosis. Risk factors related to a genetic predisposition include Klinefelter's syndrome (47,XXY karyotype), family history, and *BRCA* gene mutations, particularly *BRCA2* mutations. Gynecomastia is not a risk factor.

Histologically, 90% of male breast cancers are invasive ductal carcinomas. Approximately 80% are ER-positive, 75% are PR-positive, and 35% overexpress HER-2. The remaining 10% are DCIS. Given the absence of terminal lobules in the normal male breast, lobular carcinoma, both invasive and in situ, is rarely seen.

Most men with breast cancer have a breast mass. The differential diagnosis includes gynecomastia, primary breast

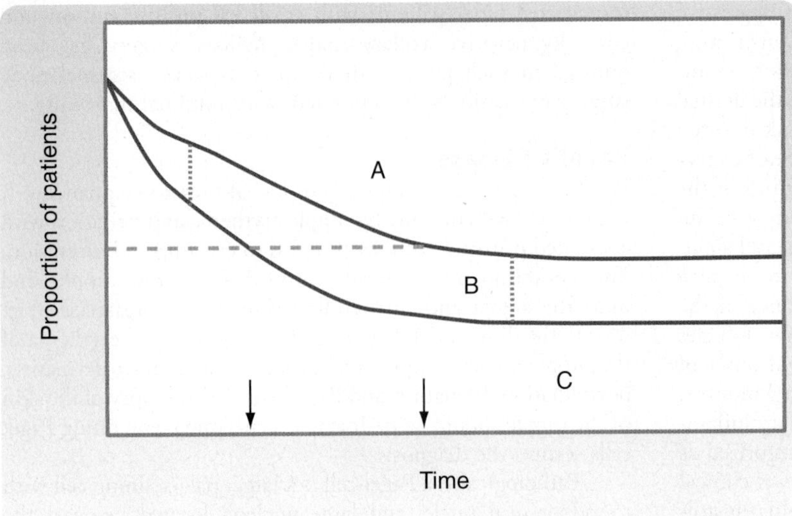


**FIGURE 36-14** Interpretation of actuarial curves used in clinical trials comparing two groups of patients. See text for details.

carcinoma, metastatic carcinoma to the breast, sarcoma, and breast abscess. In addition to local pain and axillary adenopathy, other initial symptoms may include nipple retraction, ulceration, bleeding, and discharge. Evaluation includes breast imaging studies and diagnostic needle core biopsy.

Prognostic factors in male breast cancer are the same as in female breast cancer and include nodal involvement, tumor size, histologic grade, and hormone receptor status. When matched for age and stage, survival is similar to that in women.

Treatment of carcinoma in the male breast depends on the stage and local extent of the tumor, with treatment choices similar to those for women. Small tumors may be treated by local excision and irradiation or by mastectomy. Sentinel node biopsy has been shown to be effective for staging male breast cancer. Breast tumors in men more commonly involve the pectoralis major muscle, probably because breast tissue in men is scant. If the underlying pectoral muscle is involved, modified radical mastectomy with excision of the involved portion of muscle is adequate treatment and may be combined with postoperative radiation therapy.

Adjuvant systemic therapy for male breast cancer is used as for female breast cancer. Most male breast cancers are hormone receptor–positive. Adjuvant hormonal therapy with tamoxifen or AIs is indicated for node-positive and high-risk, node-negative patients. Adjuvant chemotherapy is used in men at substantial risk for metastatic disease.

## INTERPRETING RESULTS OF CLINICAL TRIALS

Survival curves are the most familiar method of comparing groups of patients in randomized trials involving different therapies. To estimate the survival curve for any group of individuals, investigators use the life table method, also called the *actuarial method.* Kaplan and Meier proposed a popular modification of these general methods that suits clinical trials, and the resulting curves are often called *Kaplan-Meier curves.* This method tabulates the number of patients surviving as a proportion of the total number of patients reaching the interval of time in question after entering the trial. Survival or death is only one outcome that can be expressed in actuarial terms. Others include disease-free survival, event-free survival, and freedom from local failure, which can all be expressed in actuarial terms.

Comparisons between groups (e.g., treated versus control) can be described in several ways, each of which has limitations and ambiguities. As shown in Figure 36-14, the simplest way is to measure the absolute difference between the curves at any specified interval of time during follow-up, as demonstrated by the vertical dashed lines between the Kaplan-Meier curves. Alternatively, for any specific proportion of patients, there is a different time until relapse or death between the two curves, as shown by the horizontal dashed line in the figure. For example, the median survival time is the length of survival free of relapse or death for 50% of patients. Differences in median survival times between treated and control patients may be significant, even though absolute differences are small. For most treatment comparisons, there are three groups to consider. Some patients will remain free of recurrence or death with the control treatment, shown as the area under the lower curve (C). Other patients are destined to fail both the experimental and control treatments, shown as the area above the experimental curve (upper curve, A). It is only the patients falling between the two curves (B) who benefit (or are harmed) by the experimental treatment. The concept of proportional benefit is important when evaluating adjuvant chemotherapy or hormonal therapy for breast cancer; only a small proportion of treated patients benefit from receiving postoperative adjuvant treatments.

A popular way to express the difference between control and experimental groups is to cite the proportional reduction in treatment failures. For example, the proportional reduction in mortality is the difference in survival between the two groups at an interval divided by the percentage of patients who have died in the control group in the same interval. For the same proportional reduction in mortality, the absolute difference in survival varies greatly; it is generally larger for groups of patients with a higher risk of dying (e.g., node-positive versus node-negative patients). To calculate the proportional increase in survival, the absolute difference between the control and experimental curves in a specified interval is divided by the total surviving in the experimental group (assuming that it is larger). For groups with poor survival, small absolute differences lead to larger estimates of the percent increase in survival.

## SELECTED REFERENCES

Clarke M, Collins R, Darby S, et al; Early Breast Cancer Trialists' Collaborative Group (EBCTCG): Effects of radiotherapy and of differences in the extent of surgery for early breast cancer on local recurrence and 15-year survival: An overview of the randomised trials. Lancet 366:2087–2106, 2005.

Overview analysis by the Early Breast Cancer Trialists' Collaborative Group showing the benefit of radiotherapy on survival in breast cancer patients.

Domchek S, Friebel TM, Singer CF, et al: Association of risk-reducing surgery in BRCA1 or BRCA2 mutation carriers with cancer risk and mortality. JAMA 304:967–975, 2010.

First trial to demonstrate survival benefit of risk-reducing surgery in *BRCA1* and *BRCA2* mutation carriers.

Early Breast Cancer Trialists' Collaborative Group (EBCTCG): Effects of chemotherapy and hormonal therapy for early breast cancer on recurrence and 15-year survival: An overview of the randomised trials. Lancet 365:1687–1717, 2005.

Overview analysis by the Early Breast Cancer Trialists' Collaborative Group showing the benefit of chemotherapy and hormonal therapy on survival based on stage of disease and hormone receptor status.

Fisher B, Costantino JP, Wickerham DL, et al: Tamoxifen for prevention of breast cancer: Report of the National Surgical Adjuvant Breast and Bowel Project P-1 Study. J Natl Cancer Inst 90:1371–1388, 1998.

The first report of a randomized trial for breast cancer prevention in a high risk population. Patients were assessed for risk based on the Gail model and randomly assigned to receive five years of tamoxifen or placebo. The use of tamoxifen reduced breast cancer incidence by approximately 50%.

Fisher B, Jeong JH, Anderson S, et al: Twenty-five-year follow-up of a randomized trial comparing radical mastectomy, total mastectomy, and total mastectomy followed by irradiation. N Engl J Med 347:567–575, 2002.

Report showing no difference in survival between radical mastectomy and total mastectomy with or without radiation.

Fisher B, Anderson S, Bryant J, et al: Twenty-year follow-up of a randomized trial comparing total mastectomy, lumpectomy, and lumpectomy plus irradiation for the treatment of invasive breast cancer. N Engl J Med 347:1233–1241, 2002.

Randomized trial showing no difference in survival between total mastectomy and breast conserving surgery with or without radiation.

Giuliano AE, Hunt KK, Ballman KV, et al: Axillary dissection vs no axillary dissection in women with invasive breast cancer and sentinel node metastasis. JAMA 305:569–575, 2011.

Randomized trial showing no benefit to completion axillary lymph node dissection in selected early stage patients with positive sentinel lymph nodes.

Hartmann LC, Sellers TA, Frost MH, et al: Benign breast disease and the risk of breast cancer. N Engl J Med 353:229–237, 2005.

Identified risk factors for breast cancer development after a diagnosis of benign breast disease based on histologic classification and family history.

Krag DN, Anderson SJ, Julian TB, et al: Sentinel-lymph-node resection compared with conventional axillary-lymph-node dissection in clinically node negative patients with breast cancer: Overall survival findings from the NSABP B-32 randomised phase 3 trial. Lancet Oncology 11:927–933, 2010.

Randomized trial of sentinel lymph node dissection versus axillary dissection in early stage breast cancer. There was no difference in overall survival or locoregional recurrence amongst the patients having sentinel node surgery versus standard axillary surgery.

Perou CM, Sorlie T, Eisen MB, et al: Molecular portraits of human breast tumours. Nature 406:747–752, 2000.

First description of molecular subtypes of breast cancer using microarray analysis.

Rossouw JE, Anderson GL, Prentice RL, et al: Risks and benefits of estrogen plus progestin in healthy postmenopausal women: principal results from the Women's Health Initiative randomized controlled trial. JAMA 288:321–333, 2002.

Demonstrated risks and benefits of hormone replacement therapy in postmenopausal women. Long-term follow-up of participants in the Women's Health Initiative.

Weaver DL, Ashikaga T, Krag DN, et al: Effect of occult metastases on survival in node-negative breast cancer. N Engl J Med 364:412–421, 2011.

Demonstrated that occult metastases identified in sentinel lymph nodes of early-stage breast cancer patients do not have clinical relevance.

## REFERENCES

1. Haagensen C: Diseases of the breast, ed 3, Philadelphia, 1986, WB Saunders.
2. Nelson H, Tyne K, Naik A, et al: U.S. Preventive Services Task Force: Screening for breast cancer: Systematic evidence review update for the U.S. Preventive Services Task Force. Ann Intern Med 151:727–737, 2009.
3. Berg WA, Blume JD, Cormack JB, et al: Combined screening with ultrasound and mammography compared with mammography alone in women at elevated risk of breast cancer: Results of the first-year screen in ACRIN 6666. JAMA 299:2151–2163, 2008.
4. Turnbull L, Brown S, Harvey I, et al: Comparative effectiveness of MRI in breast cancer (COMICE) trial: A randomised controlled trial Lancet 375:563–571, 2010.
5. Rosen PR: Rosen's breast pathology, ed 2, Philadelphia, 2001, Lippincott Williams & Wilkins.
6. Fisher B, Costantino JP, Wickerham DL, et al: Tamoxifen for prevention of breast cancer: Report of the National Surgical Adjuvant Breast and Bowel Project P-1 Study. J Natl Cancer Inst 90:1371–1388, 1998.

7. Hartmann LC, Sellers TA, Frost MH, et al: Benign breast disease and the risk of breast cancer. N Engl J Med 353:229–237, 2005.
8. Rossouw JE, Anderson GL, Prentice RL, et al: Risks and benefits of estrogen plus progestin in healthy postmenopausal women: Principal results from the Women's Health Initiative randomized controlled trial. JAMA 288:321–333, 2002.
9. Stefanick ML, Anderson GL, Margolis KL, et al: Effects of conjugated equine estrogens on breast cancer and mammography screening in postmenopausal women with hysterectomy. JAMA 295:1647–1657, 2006.
10. Vogel VG, Costantino JP, Wickerham DL, et al: Effects of tamoxifen vs raloxifene on the risk of developing invasive breast cancer and other disease outcomes: The NSABP Study of Tamoxifen and Raloxifene (STAR) P-2 trial. JAMA 295:2727–2741, 2006.
11. Hartmann LC, Schaid DJ, Woods JE, et al: Efficacy of bilateral prophylactic mastectomy in women with a family history of breast cancer. N Engl J Med 340:77–84, 1999.
12. Domchek SM, Friebel TM, Singer CF, et al: Association of risk-reducing surgery in BRCA1 or BRCA2 mutation carriers with cancer risk and mortality. JAMA 304:967–975, 2010.
13. Bedrosian I, Hu CY, Chang GJ: Population-based study of contralateral prophylactic mastectomy and survival outcomes of breast cancer patients. J Natl Cancer Inst 102:401–409, 2010.
14. Perou CM, Sorlie T, Eisen MB, et al: Molecular portraits of human breast tumours. Nature 406:747–752, 2000.
15. Paik S, Shak S, Tang G, et al: A multigene assay to predict recurrence of tamoxifen-treated, node-negative breast cancer. N Engl J Med 351:2817–2826, 2004.
16. Fisher B, Jeong JH, Anderson S, et al: Twenty-five-year follow-up of a randomized trial comparing radical mastectomy, total mastectomy, and total mastectomy followed by irradiation. N Engl J Med 347:567–575, 2002.
17. Fisher B, Anderson S, Bryant J, et al: Twenty-year follow-up of a randomized trial comparing total mastectomy, lumpectomy, and lumpectomy plus irradiation for the treatment of invasive breast cancer. N Engl J Med 347:1233–1241, 2002.
18. Weaver DL, Ashikaga T, Krag DN, et al: Effect of occult metastases on survival in node-negative breast cancer. N Engl J Med 364:412–421, 2011.
19. Krag DN, Anderson SJ, Julian TB, et al: Sentinel-lymph-node resection compared with conventional axillary-lymph-node dissection in clinically node negative patients with breast cancer: Overall survival findings from the NSABP B-32 randomised phase 3 trial. Lancet Oncology 11:927–933, 2010.
20. Hunt KK, Yi M, Mittendorf EA, et al: sentinel lymph node surgery after neoadjuvant chemotherapy is accurate and reduces the need for axillary dissection in breast cancer patients. Ann Surg 250:558–566, 2009.
21. Kim T, Giuliano AE, Lyman GH: Lymphatic mapping and sentinel lymph node biopsy in early-stage breast carcinoma: A meta-analysis. Cancer 106:4–16, 2006.
22. Giuliano AE, Hunt KK, Ballman KV, et al: Axillary dissection vs no axillary dissection in women with invasive breast cancer and sentinel node metastasis. JAMA 305:569–575, 2011.
23. Fisher B, Dignam J, Wolmark N, et al: Tamoxifen in treatment of intraductal breast cancer: National Surgical Adjuvant Breast and Bowel Project B-24 randomised controlled trial. Lancet 353:1993–2000, 1999.
24. Fisher B, Dignam J, Wolmark N, et al: Lumpectomy and radiation therapy for the treatment of intraductal breast cancer: Findings from National Surgical Adjuvant Breast and Bowel Project B-17. J Clin Oncol 16:441–452, 1998.
25. Julien JP, Bijker N, Fentiman IS, et al: Radiotherapy in breast-conserving treatment for ductal carcinoma in situ: First results of the EORTC randomised phase III trial 10853. EORTC Breast Cancer Cooperative Group and EORTC Radiotherapy Group. Lancet 355:528–533, 2000.
26. Houghton J, George WD, Cuzick J, et al: Radiotherapy and tamoxifen in women with completely excised ductal carcinoma in situ of the breast in the UK, Australia, and New Zealand: Randomised controlled trial. Lancet 362:95–102, 2003.
27. Silverstein MJ: The University of Southern California/Van Nuys prognostic index for ductal carcinoma in situ of the breast. Am J Surg 186:337–343, 2003.
28. Hughes LL, Wang M, Page DL, et al: Local excision alone without irradiation for ductal carcinoma in situ of the breast: A trial of the Eastern Cooperative Oncology Group. J Clin Oncol 27:5319–5324, 2009.
29. Clarke M, Collins R, Darby S, et al: Effects of radiotherapy and of differences in the extent of surgery for early breast cancer on local recurrence and 15-year survival: An overview of the randomised trials. Lancet 366:2087–2106, 2005.
30. Hughes KS, Schnaper LA, Berry D, et al: Lumpectomy plus tamoxifen with or without irradiation in women 70 years of age or older with early breast cancer. N Engl J Med 351:971–977, 2004.
31. Smith BD, Arthur DW, Buchholz TA, et al: Accelerated partial breast irradiation consensus statement from the American Society for Radiation Oncology (ASTRO). Int J Radiat Oncol Biol Phys 74:987–1001, 2009.
32. Clarke M, Collins R, Darby S, et al; Early Breast Cancer Trialists' Collaborative Group (EBCTCG): Effects of radiotherapy and of differences in the extent of surgery for early breast cancer on local recurrence and 15-year survival: An overview of the randomised trials. Lancet 366:2087–2106, 2005.
33. Nielsen HM, Overgaard M, Grau C, et al: Study of failure pattern among high-risk breast cancer patients with or without postmastectomy radiotherapy in addition to adjuvant systemic therapy: Long-term results from the Danish Breast Cancer Cooperative Group DBCG 82 b and c randomized studies. J Clin Oncol 24:2268–2275, 2006.
34. Ragaz J, Olivotto IA, Spinelli JJ, et al: Locoregional radiation therapy in patients with high-risk breast cancer receiving adjuvant chemotherapy: 20-year results of the British Columbia randomized trial. J Natl Cancer Inst 97:116–126, 2005.
35. van de Vijver MJ, He YD, van't Veer LJ, et al: A gene-expression signature as a predictor of survival in breast cancer. N Engl J Med 347:1999–2009, 2002.
36. Ravdin PM, Siminoff LA, Davis GJ, et al: Computer program to assist in making decisions about adjuvant therapy for women with early breast cancer. J Clin Oncol 19:980–991, 2001.
37. Early Breast Cancer Trialists' Collaborative Group (EBCTCG): Effects of chemotherapy and hormonal therapy for early breast cancer on recurrence and 15-year survival: An overview of the randomised trials. Lancet 365:1687–1717, 2005.
38. De Laurentiis M, Cancello G, D'Agostino D, et al: Taxane-based combinations as adjuvant chemotherapy of early breast cancer: A meta-analysis of randomized trials. J Clin Oncol 26:44–53, 2008.
39. Citron ML, Berry DA, Cirrincione C, et al: Randomized trial of dose-dense versus conventionally scheduled and sequential versus concurrent combination chemotherapy as postoperative adjuvant

treatment of node-positive primary breast cancer: First report of Intergroup Trial C9741/Cancer and Leukemia Group B Trial 9741. J Clin Oncol 21:1431–1439, 2003.

**40.** Jones S, Holmes FA, O'Shaughnessy J, et al: Docetaxel with cyclophosphamide is associated with an overall survival benefit compared with doxorubicin and cyclophosphamide: 7-Year follow-up of US Oncology Research Trial 9735. J Clin Oncol 27:1177–1183, 2009.

**41.** Mauri D, Pavlidis N, Ioannidis JP: Neoadjuvant versus adjuvant systemic treatment in breast cancer: A meta-analysis. J Natl Cancer Inst 97:188–194, 2005.

**42.** Piccart-Gebhart MJ, Procter M, Leyland-Jones B, et al: Trastuzumab after adjuvant chemotherapy in HER2-positive breast cancer. N Engl J Med 353:1659–1672, 2005.

**43.** Romond EH, Perez EA, Bryant J, et al: Trastuzumab plus adjuvant chemotherapy for operable HER2-positive breast cancer. N Engl J Med 353:1673–1684, 2005.

**44.** Slamon D, Eiermann W, Robert N, et al: BCIRG 006: 2nd interim analysis phase III randomized trial comparing doxorubicin and cyclophosphamide followed by docetaxel (AC→T) with doxorubicin and cyclophosphamide followed by docetaxel and trastuzumab (AC→TH) with docetaxel, carboplatin and trastuzumab (TCH) in Her2neu positive early breast cancer patients, 2006 (http://www.bcirg.org/NR/rdonlyres/euynx4wi7wx6yq4qenuxw5ok6bbclmm5ckfz5vyo7kdkrbg5iq4ketb23g4epbwzpld5vhqbsiolga72y2itf7plpqb/BCIRG+006+-+Final+Abstract+SABCS.pdf).

**45.** Albain KS, Barlow WE, Ravdin PM, et al: Adjuvant chemotherapy and timing of tamoxifen in postmenopausal patients with endocrine-responsive, node-positive breast cancer: A phase 3, open-label, randomised controlled trial. Lancet 374:2055–2063, 2009.

**46.** Howell A, Cuzick J, Baum M, et al: Results of the ATAC (Arimidex, Tamoxifen, Alone or in Combination) trial after completion of 5 years' adjuvant treatment for breast cancer. Lancet 365:60–62, 2005.

**47.** Boccardo F, Rubagotti A, Aldrighetti D, et al: Switching to an aromatase inhibitor provides mortality benefit in early breast carcinoma: Pooled analysis of 2 consecutive trials. Cancer 109:1060–1067, 2007.

**48.** Burstein HJ, Prestrud AA, Seidenfeld J, et al: American Society of Clinical Oncology clinical practice guideline: Update on adjuvant endocrine therapy for women with hormone receptor-positive breast cancer. J Clin Oncol 28:3784–3796, 2010.

**49.** Cristofanilli M, Gonzalez-Angulo AM, Buzdar AU, et al: Paclitaxel improves the prognosis in estrogen receptor negative inflammatory breast cancer: The M.D. Anderson Cancer Center experience. Clin Breast Cancer 4:415–419, 2004.

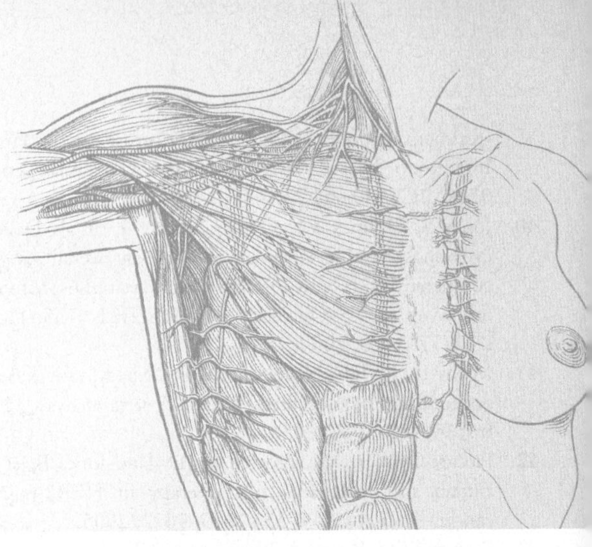

CHAPTER 37

# BREAST RECONSTRUCTION

Kendall R. Roehl, Bradon J. Wilhelmi, and Linda G. Phillips



## ROLE OF THE GENERAL SURGEON IN BREAST RECONSTRUCTION

Breast cancer is an extremely emotional topic because of its anatomic location and the importance of the female breast in today's society. Therefore, it is imperative for surgeons performing breast surgery to have a basic understanding of which patients are candidates for breast reconstruction and of the reconstructive options. Most patients start their inquiry about breast reconstruction with the surgeon who will be performing the mastectomy. They might ask, "What will it look like when you are done?" or "Will I have to live without a breast?" It is at this point that a general surgeon greatly influences a woman's decision to pursue breast reconstruction.

Although the reconstructive surgeon goes into detail about the surgical options, risks, and expected outcomes, ablative surgeons must be prepared for at least a basic discussion with patients. Whether breast implants versus autogenous tissue will be used, where the scars will be, and how long the recovery will take are all questions that most patients want answered. The decision about whether they undergo breast reconstruction can be influenced by the bias of ablative surgeons. Oncologic surgeons are trained to place priority on ablation of the tumor; however, care standards now dictate that we also be sensitive to the resulting deformity. Only through a close alliance between the surgical oncologist and reconstructive surgeon can the patient's emotional, physical, and oncologic needs be addressed.

## HISTORY

In the late 1800s, the prognosis of patients with breast cancer was poor. Notable surgeons such as Volkmann, Czerny, and Billroth reported local recurrence rates ranging from 52% to 85%. Within 2 decades of these reports, William Halsted presented his successful treatment of breast cancer, with only a 6% recurrence rate. The halstedian theory of breast cancer treatment would remain the mainstay of breast cancer surgery for the next 60 years. He believed that "the slightest inattention to detail and or attempts to hasten convalescence by such plastic operations as are feasible only when a restricted amount of skin is removed may sacrifice his patient to the disease." So, concerned with the possibility of inadequate skin excision, Halsted went on to say that "To attempt to close the breast wound more or less regularly by any plastic method is hazardous, and in my opinion, to be vigorously discounted." Therefore, true attempts at breast reconstruction would have to wait for almost 50 years.

Despite Halsted's condemnation of reconstructive procedures, it was recognized that the sizable defects left after this radical surgery did need to be closed. Although primary closure was often used, skin grafting of larger wounds was acceptable. Even though plastic procedures had been reported by Legueu and Graeve of France and Warren of the United States, these were merely chest wall closure techniques and not true breast mound reconstructions.

The first attempt at true breast reconstruction occurred in 1895, when Vincent Czerny transplanted a large lipoma from his patient's flank to the mastectomy site. In recounting this case, Dr. Robert Goldwyn noted that 1 year after surgery, the patient was doing well and had good breast symmetry. In this particular case, the mastectomy was performed for fibrocystic disease and not cancer. Tansini described the first use of the latissimus dorsi myocutaneous flap in 1906. Unfortunately, this remarkable operation would not gain acceptance for another 70 years.

In 1942, Sir Harold Gillies of England started using a tubed pedicle technique of breast reconstruction. In this operation, he would "waltz" a flap from the abdomen to the chest to reconstruct the breast. Although this technique was successful, the multiple procedures and prolonged treatment course precluded its widespread application.

Since approximately 1970, many advances in reconstructive surgery have occurred and been applied to breast reconstruction. The development of breast implants was the first of these revolutions. In 1963, the silicone breast implant was introduced for breast augmentation and was quickly adopted for breast reconstruction. In 1963, Cronin and Gerow[1] presented a series of patients who received implants for reconstruction of mastectomy defects. For the first time, the plastic surgeon had a procedure that could simulate the missing breast without the need for multiple procedures and a prolonged treatment course. In many ways, it was the simplicity and safety of breast implants that ignited interest in breast reconstruction. By the later 1970s, reconstruction was being performed immediately after breast ablation.[2-4]

The development of muscle, musculocutaneous, and fasciocutaneous flaps and microsurgical transplantation has had a tremendous impact on breast reconstruction. The ideal material to reconstruct any defect is similar to tissue. Until the early 1970s, such tissue was available only in limited quantities for breast reconstruction. The landmark work by Manchot[5] on vascular territories of the body was rediscovered, and surgeons were then able to exploit this basic knowledge to design flaps based on the axial patterns of named blood vessels. These technical developments allowed surgeons to rearrange tissues reliably and more precisely reconstruct all types of defects, including those of the breast.[6]

## PATIENT SELECTION

Women have a number of reasons for choosing to undergo breast reconstruction, including no need for an external prosthesis, fewer limitations with regard to clothing, regaining femininity, and feeling whole again. Others choose not to undergo reconstruction because they feel too old for the procedure or are afraid of complications.[7,8] Given the myriad of options in breast reconstruction, the surgery should be tailored to the patient's wishes as well as her underlying health. There are a small number of relative contraindications to breast reconstruction. Extreme age, severe cardiovascular disease or other comorbidities, extreme obesity, and advanced breast disease are possible reasons why breast reconstruction may not be reasonable.

Often, women are faced with the choice, in early disease, of breast conservation therapy (BCT) versus mastectomy. Studies have shown equivalent survival outcomes when comparing the modalities of BCT with radiation and mastectomy. These decisions are often made in conjunction with the ablative surgeon. Patient satisfaction with these two modalities is varied. Pusic and colleagues[9] have surveyed women who underwent lumpectomy/XRT, mastectomy, and mastectomy with reconstruction. Similar to Reaby's report,[7] women who chose reconstruction were younger, white, and more educated. Interestingly, comfort with nudity was much lower in the mastectomy-alone group and quality of life varied with age. Younger women (<55 years) were least happy with mastectomy alone, whereas those older than 55 years were least satisfied with lumpectomy. Ultimately, the choice is that of the breast cancer patient and must be individualized.

After the advent of BCT, many women chose this option to preserve as much of their native breast as possible. The current paradigm has shifted, and more women are choosing to undergo mastectomy. This shift is multifactorial and includes dissatisfaction with the cosmesis of BCT–external radiation therapy (XRT) breasts, skin preservation mastectomies (nipple-sparing and areolar-sparing), improved reconstructive options (silicone gel prostheses and perforator flap reconstructions), genetic testing for *BRCA-1* and *BRCA -2* genes, necessitating bilateral mastectomies, increase in contralateral prophylactic mastectomy, and bilateral reconstruction in younger women. In addition, women who are now often diagnosed at younger ages, with higher lifetime risks, may have more aggressive disease or multifocal tumors.

Similarly, BCT is also evolving. It is now possible to minimize the effects of radiation on the breast after lumpectomy via oncoplastic techniques. These include breast reduction strategies to obliterate the dead space of lumpectomy–segmental mastectomy and to counteract the contractile forces seen after radiation therapy. These techniques are used by a breast surgeon or plastic surgeon. All these techniques will be discussed further.[10,11]

## TIMING

The timing of breast reconstruction after mastectomy has progressed from delayed to immediate because of advances and refinements in breast reconstructive techniques and recognition of beneficial psychological effects.[7,9,10,12] Because studies have shown a psychological benefit, cost-effectiveness, cosmetic advantage, and no increased risk for complications or oncologic risk with immediate breast reconstruction, it has become the preferred timing of reconstruction. In 1990, the American Society of Plastic and Reconstructive Surgeons reported that members performed 38% immediate versus 62% delayed reconstructions. In a more recent study, 75% of reconstructions were performed immediately.[13]

Because most local tumor recurrences are in the skin and/or subcutaneous adipose tissue or in the axilla, there are few reasons to delay reconstruction. Therefore, immediate reconstruction has become commonplace in America.[14] It affords psychological benefits to women and is the opportune time to preserve the normal footplate of the breast—most importantly, the inframammary fold. This can be more difficult in a delayed reconstruction setting. Skin flaps are also more pliable in the immediate setting. Currently, most women with stage I or II cancer are candidates for immediate reconstruction. There are caveats to this with certain chemotherapeutic agents and the need for adjuvant radiotherapy, in which immediate reconstruction is not possible. These can interfere with postoperative healing and aesthetic outcome, respectively.

One must also consider, however, the possibility of complications with immediate reconstruction. In patients in whom reconstructions have complications such as delayed wound healing, infection, mastectomy flap loss, and flap necrosis, the initiation of chemotherapy and radiation therapy may require delay, and thus compromise, in cancer treatment. All these must be considered by the ablative and reconstructive surgeons, as well as the patient, to determine the appropriate timing of reconstruction.

## PROCEDURE SELECTION AND SURGICAL PLANNING

The options for surgical breast reconstruction are varied and include partial and total reconstruction. Total breast reconstruction involves two common modalities, the use of an expander or implant, autologous tissue, and some combination of the two. Any of these procedures must not delay adjuvant cancer therapies. The most common procedures performed are the following (Box 37-1):

- Tissue expander placement, with later exchange for an implant
- Immediate permanent implant placement
- Latissimus dorsi with implant
- Autologous tissue (pedicled)
- Autologous tissue (free)

The choice among these therapies must take into account the need for skin resection, adjuvant radiation therapy, patient size and aesthetic desires, and activity level. Consideration of the opposite breast, and of available donor tissue, must be determined. Ideally, reconstructive surgeons would merely be filling

**BOX 37-1 Options for Breast Reconstruction**

Autogenous
- Abdominal-based flaps
  - TRAM
  - Single pedicle
  - Double pedicle
  - Free flap*
  - Deep inferior epigastric perforator flap*
- Upper abdominal horizontal flap
- Vertical abdominal flap
- Tubed abdominal flap

Latissimus dorsi musculocutaneous flap
Gluteal flap*
- Superiorly based
- Inferiorly based

Rubens flap*
Thoracoepigastric flap
Lateral thigh flap*
Breast-splitting procedure†
Alloplastic
- Silicone gel implant
- Silicone implant with saline fill
  - Smooth wall
  - Textured wall
  - Round
  - Anatomic shaped
- Silicone injection†

Combination procedures
- Latissimus dorsi flap with implant
- TRAM flap with implant

*Requires microsurgical procedure.
†Historical note only.

**BOX 37-2 Implant Reconstruction**

**Indications**
Bilateral reconstruction
Patient requesting augmentation in addition to reconstruction
Patient not suited for long surgery
Lack of adequate abdominal tissue
Patient unwilling to have additional scars on her back or abdomen
Small breast mound, with minimal ptosis

**Relative Contraindications**
Young age (may need an implant replaced multiple times)
Patient unwilling to adhere to follow-up
Very large breast
Very ptotic breast
Silicon allergy
Implant fear
Previous failed implants
Need for adjuvant radiation therapy

the empty space left after removal of the gland, with preservation of the normal footplate of the breast. This is not always the case. Usually, except for advanced and inflammatory disease, some version of skin-sparing mastectomy can be performed. Breast surgeons also offer nipple- and areolar-sparing mastectomies. These allow for more aesthetically pleasing reconstructions because they confine the scar to the area around the skin paddle of a flap, if used. There is no increased cancer risk or recurrence with skin-sparing mastectomy, as long as the skin flaps are not too thick. Conversely, the thickness of the skin determines flap survival, and very thin flaps often become necrotic. In large-breasted women, the skin incisions for mastectomy may be modified to allow easy access for the general surgeon and the ability to have scar symmetry for the reconstructive surgeon. Breast reduction patterns can be used for the mastectomy, as well as the contralateral symmetry procedure.

Breast reconstruction is more than just providing a mound on the chest wall. Of utmost importance is the ability to create symmetry. Nice reconstructions can be a great disappointment if they do not match the contralateral native breast. For the most part, autologous reconstruction provides better symmetry. This is less of an issue in the case of bilateral reconstruction. In planning reconstructions, one must consider not only the size and shape of the opposite breast, but also the position on the chest wall, location of the inframammary fold, height, size, and color of the nipple-areolar complex, and amount of breast ptosis.

## Implant-Based Reconstructions

Implant reconstructions are performed in those women who have a reasonable amount of good-quality skin after mastectomy, enough to cover an implant completely and provide a natural shape. They are advantageous in that they are relatively quick procedures, with minimal morbidity to the patient. Implant reconstruction is best used for a bilateral reconstruction because it is the best opportunity for symmetry. With implant-only reconstructions, it is difficult to mimic the natural ptosis and contour of the contralateral breast, except in the cases of young women with relatively small, youthful-appearing breasts (Box 37-2).

Initially, these reconstructive procedures were performed with placement of the implant in the subcutaneous pocket. This fell out of favor because of visible rippling of the implant beneath a thin layer of skin and a greater complication risk of capsular contracture. Currently, these implants are placed in a submuscular pocket beneath the pectoralis major. Some surgeons provide for full muscle coverage, with the assistance of the serratus anterior and rectus abdominis fascia inferiorly. Others provide coverage of the inferior pole of the implant with bioprosthetic material (e.g., human, porcine, bovine dermal allografts) to help create a natural inframammary fold and contoured reconstruction and provide an additional layer between the implant and inferior mastectomy skin flap. This material is sutured to the pectoralis major muscle superiorly and then inferiorly to the previously marked or designated inframammary fold (Figs. 37-1 and 37-2).[13,15,16] Either method helps fix the pectoralis major and keeps it from migrating superiorly, exposing more of the implant.

Often, these forms of reconstruction are begun with placement of a tissue expander at the time of mastectomy. This is to allow for little stress on the tenuous mastectomy flaps initially

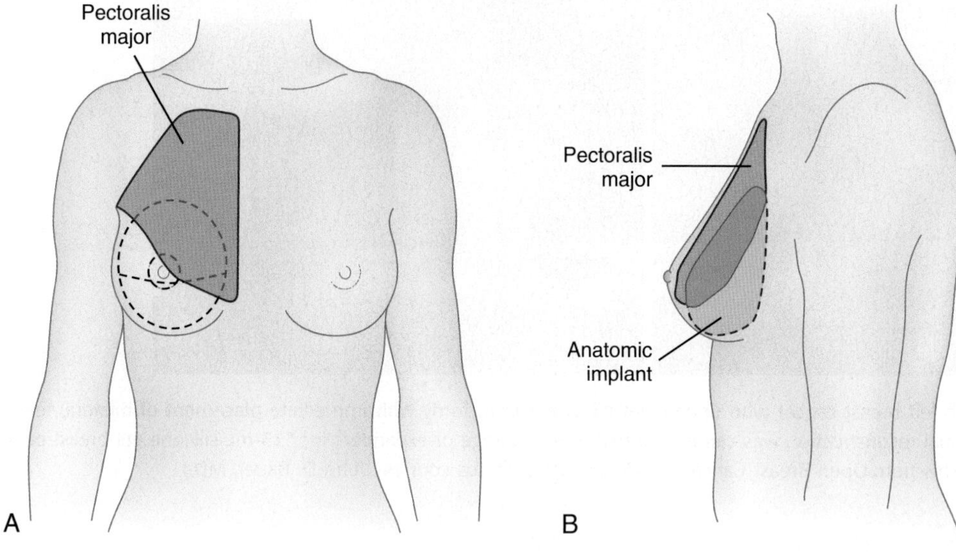


**FIGURE 37-1** Schematic representation of implant position, pectoralis position, and chest wall. The pectoralis muscle cannot cover the inferior pole of the breast; thus, bioprosthetic material is needed in the area of greatest expansion. (Breuing KH, Warren SM: Immediate bilateral breast reconstruction with implants and inferolateral AlloDerm slings. Ann Plast Surg 55:232–239, 2005.)

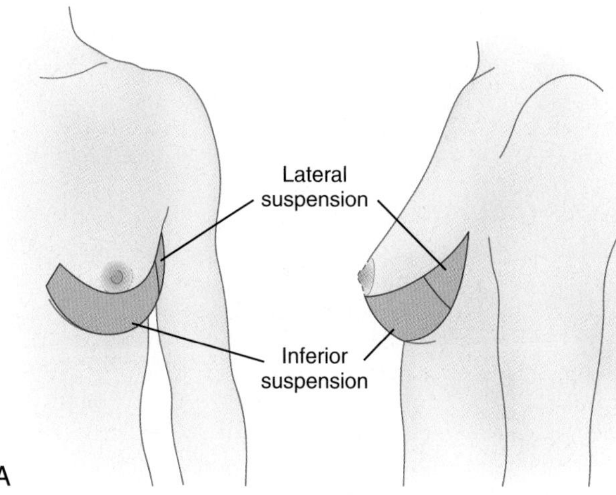


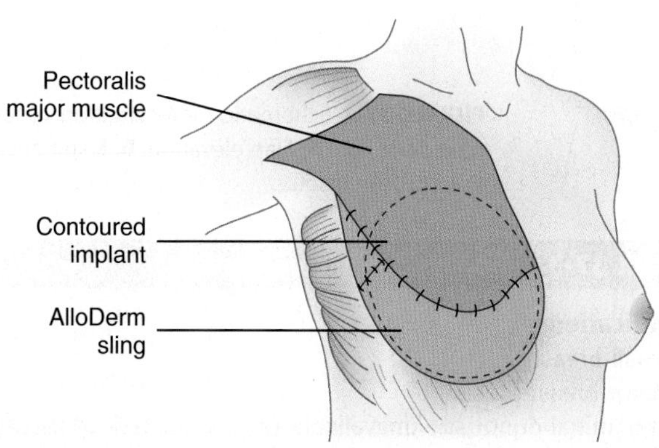


**FIGURE 37-2** Schematic representation of chest wall, breast, pectoralis muscle, bioprosthetic sling, and implant. Bioprosthetic material is sutured to the inferior border of the pectoralis muscle superiorly, the inframammary fold inferiorly, and curved laterally along the chest wall to re-create the footprint of the breast for expansion. (Breuing KH, Warren SM: Immediate bilateral breast reconstruction with implants and inferolateral AlloDerm slings. Ann Plast Surg 55:232–239, 2005.)

or for progressive stretching of the skin to place a larger implant than would have been safe at the time of mastectomy. Expanders are silicone shell prostheses that have an integrated or remote port for the injection of saline in the clinical setting. Most surgeons expand the skin to a slightly larger size to provide for a large pocket with some ptosis. There is a period of 4 to 8 weeks prior to exchange of the expanders for implants to allow for maturation of the capsule and limit the rapid shrinkage of expanded skin.

In general, implant-based reconstructions provide for a round-shaped, youthful breast mound without ptosis (Fig. 37-3). Some would refer to this as less natural. It requires multiple clinic visits to provide for expansion and then a subsequent procedure to place the permanent implants, which requires a time commitment from the patient. Over time, implant reconstructions tend to change because of the effects of gravity, the body's response to foreign objects (capsule formation), and aging of the implants themselves. This occurs linearly with time, so that 86% of women are pleased with their results at 2 years versus 54% at 5 years.[17]

## Combination Reconstruction

Use of autologous tissue in conjunction with an implant was first done in the 1970s. There is often a need for additional tissue after mastectomy to create a sizable breast and a natural breast drape to prevent the development of ptosis. This form of reconstruction generally uses myocutaneous latissimus dorsi muscle based on the thoracodorsal artery pedicle, as described by Schneider and associates.[18] It is a broad flat muscle that spans the back from the tip of the scapula superiorly to the spine medially and the iliac crest inferiorly. Usually, the muscle is taken with an overlying skin paddle to replace the removed nipple-areolar complex or larger deficits in the case of traditional mastectomy, as popularized by Bostwick and coworkers.[19] The skin paddle is centered over the muscle and attempts are made to hide the donor site scar within the bra line. In smaller breasted women, entire reconstructions can be made of the latissimus dorsi, its overlying fat, and the subscapular fat pad (known as the extended latissimus flap); otherwise, an implant is added. The latissimus dorsi serves as a sling inferiorly, attached to the superior

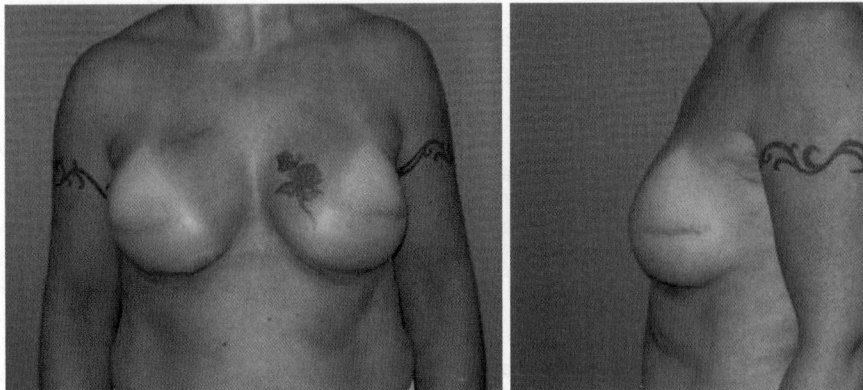

**FIGURE 37-3** 41-year-old woman with left breast cancer who underwent bilateral mastectomy with immediate placement of bilateral tissue expanders with bioprosthetic slings. Final reconstruction was carried out with the exchange of expanders for 533-mL silicone gel breast prostheses. (From Roehl KR: Breast reconstruction. Open Breast Cancer J 2:25–37, 2010. Photos courtesy John D. Bauer, MD.)

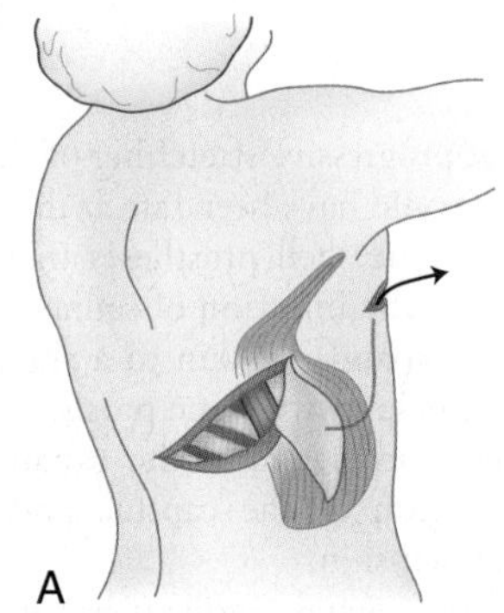


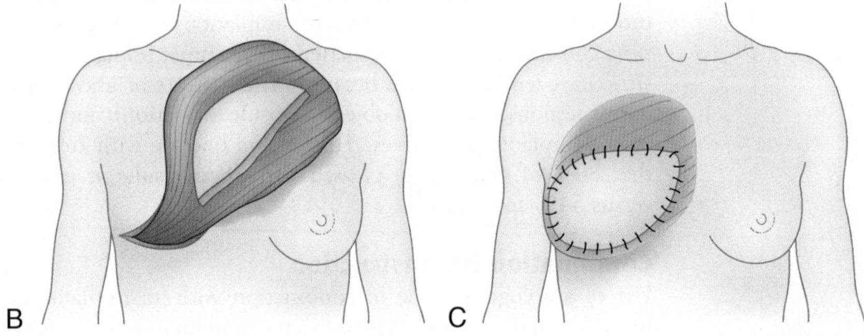


**FIGURE 37-4** Schematic representation of latissimus dorsi flap. **A,** Flap elevation. **B,** Flap transposition. **C,** Flap inset.

pectoralis to provide full muscle coverage of the implant (Fig. 37-4).

This flap, performed in a single-stage fashion, is ideal for relatively small-breasted women with some ptosis, but can be used to create larger reconstructed breasts in a staged fashion. It is also used for the reconstruction of lateral partial mastectomy defects. The latissimus flap is advantageous because of its proximity to the breast and reliable circulation. It is the workhorse for reconstruction of unilateral defects in thin women with minimal donor sites and in smaller breasted women, and as salvage for any failed breast reconstruction. Its disadvantages, however, are a large scar on the back and the likelihood of donor site complications (see later; Box 37-3).

**BOX 37-3 Latissimus Dorsi Reconstruction**

**Indications**

Small breast
Minor breast ptosis
Abdominal donor site unavailable (e.g., scars, lack of tissue)
Salvage of previous breast reconstruction

**Relative contraindications**

Planned postoperative radiation therapy
Bilateral reconstruction
Significant breast ptosis

**Contraindications**

Previous lateral thoracotomy
Very large breast in a patient who does not desire reduction

## Autologous Reconstruction

### Pedicled Flap

Today, the gold standard in breast reconstruction with autogenous tissue is the transverse rectus abdominis myocutaneous (TRAM) flap because of the lower abdominal tissue's similarities in consistency with breast tissue. The first description of the RAM flap used in breast reconstruction, by Robbins in 1979, was with a vertical skin island. The TRAM flap as we know it, with a horizontal lower abdominal skin paddle, was first described by Hartrampf in 1982.[20] This orients the donor scar into a more acceptable abdominoplasty location. Although this location of the skin paddle provides for a better arc of rotation, the ensuing blood supply to this large volume of tissue is more distal and therefore tenuous. This donor area of skin and adipose tissue has a dual blood supply for the superior and inferior epigastric systems. Pedicled flaps are thus supplied by the proximal superior epigastric vessels and the inferior system must be divided for transfer. The small vessels connecting the superior and inferior systems, known as choke vessels, are then dilated to increase perfusion once the deep system is ligated. Studies by Moon and Taylor[21] have further elucidated the perfusion zones of the lower abdomen skin territory. They found rich perforating blood vessels that arise out of the rectus to supply the overlying skin and fat. Perfusion is best overlying the rectus muscle (zone I) on the side (pedicle) used, followed by the region overlying the contralateral rectus muscle (zone II). Next is the ipsilateral outer region of tissue (zone III), and the region perfused the least is the farthest from the rectus pedicle (zone IV; Fig. 37-5).

This type of reconstruction is advantageous in that it replaces like with like tissue and provides an acceptable donor scar and improvement of abdominal contour. The limitations include the following:

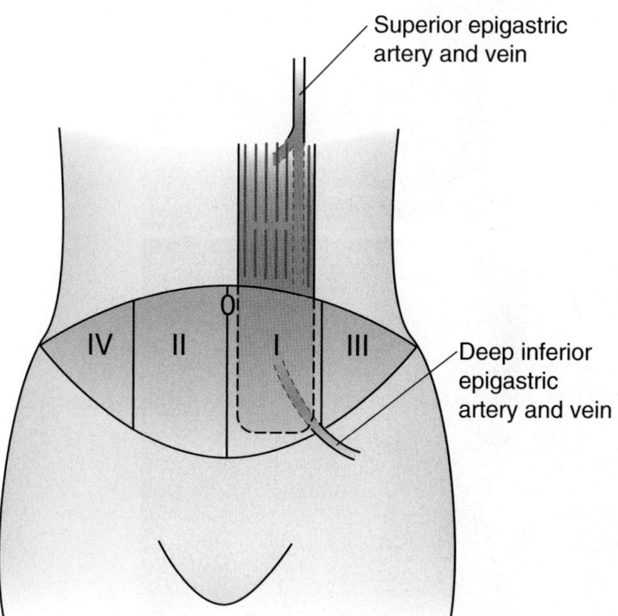


FIGURE 37-5 Vascular territories of the abdominal wall provided by a unilateral TRAM flap (as determined by Moon and Taylor[21]). Blood flow is best in zone I, followed by zones II, III, and IV, respectively.

1. This tissue has high metabolic demands that are sometimes not met, so that portions of the flap go on to form fat necrosis or die.
2. There is a longer recovery period after this surgery, with increased abdominal discomfort and the risk for abdominal weakness and/or hernia formation.

Its use can also be limited by previous abdominal operations and scars. Women who are obese, smokers, or have medical comorbidities (especially diabetes) are at greater risk for these complications (Box 37-4).

### Abdominal-Based, Gluteal-Based, and Inner Thigh–Based Flaps

**Abdominal-Based Flaps** As noted, the dominant blood supply to the lower abdomen is the deep inferior epigastric system. Perfusion of the skin and fat based on this system is thus more reliable. It became evident that performing this flap as a free tissue transfer would be beneficial. Free abdominal-based flaps have less partial flap and fat necrosis than pedicled flaps and avoid the epigastric bulge of the muscle that occurs in pedicled flaps. In free TRAM flaps, the skin and fat of the lower abdomen are connected via the deep inferior epigastric artery and vein to the blood supply in the axilla (thoracodorsal vessels, originally) or, more recently, with the internal mammary artery and vein. This procedure is often done in conjunction with the mastectomy, except in advanced disease, for which adjuvant radiation may be required (Figs. 37-6 to 37-8).

Holmstrom,[22] in 1979, was the first to perform this type of reconstruction. Since then, this and its further refined flaps have become the gold standard for microvascular autologous breast reconstruction. Original reports from this procedure revealed a partial flap loss rate of 7.1%, total flap loss rate of 1.4%, and fat necrosis in 12% of smokers, but only 3% in nonsmokers. Abdominal bulge occurred in about 5% initially but became less as smaller amounts of rectus muscle were harvested, transitioning to the muscle-sparing (ms) TRAM.[23] Further refinements of this operation have been made to preserve abdominal wall strength.

The quest to minimize abdominal wall morbidity led to the development of the msTRAM flap, in which only the muscle surrounding the perforating vessels is taken, the DIEP (deep

**BOX 37-4 Transverse Rectus Abdominis Muscle Flap Reconstruction**

**Indications**
Breasts of all sizes
Breast ptosis

**Relative Contraindications**
Smoking
Abdominal liposuction
Previous abdominal surgery
Pulmonary disease
Obesity

**Contraindications**
Previous abdominoplasty
Patient unable to tolerate a 4- to 6-week recovery period
Patient unable to tolerate a longer procedure

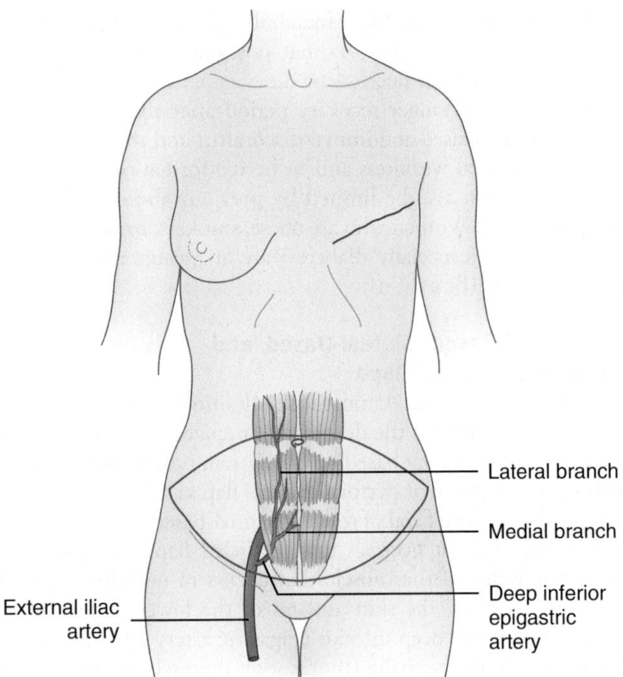


FIGURE 37-6 Schematic of lower abdomen markings for autologous reconstruction based on the medial and lateral row of perforators, which are based on the deep inferior epigastric artery system.

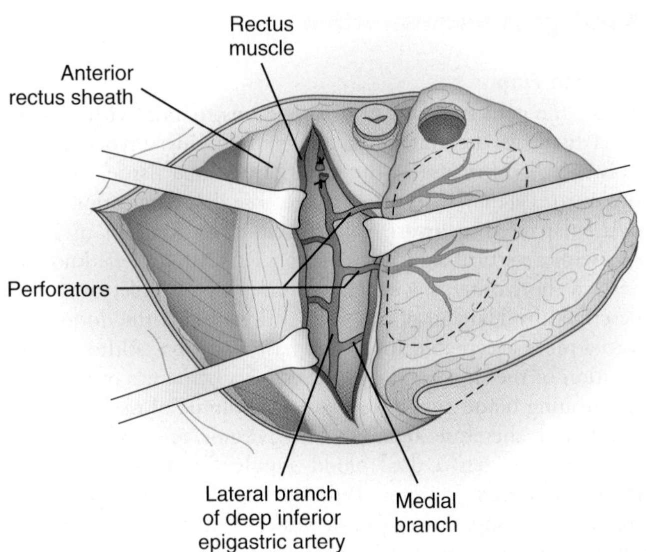


**FIGURE 37-7** Anatomy of the deep inferior epigastric artery flap. Shown are perforating vessels of the lateral row, after splitting the rectus abdominis muscle, as they enter the skin and subcutaneous tissue.

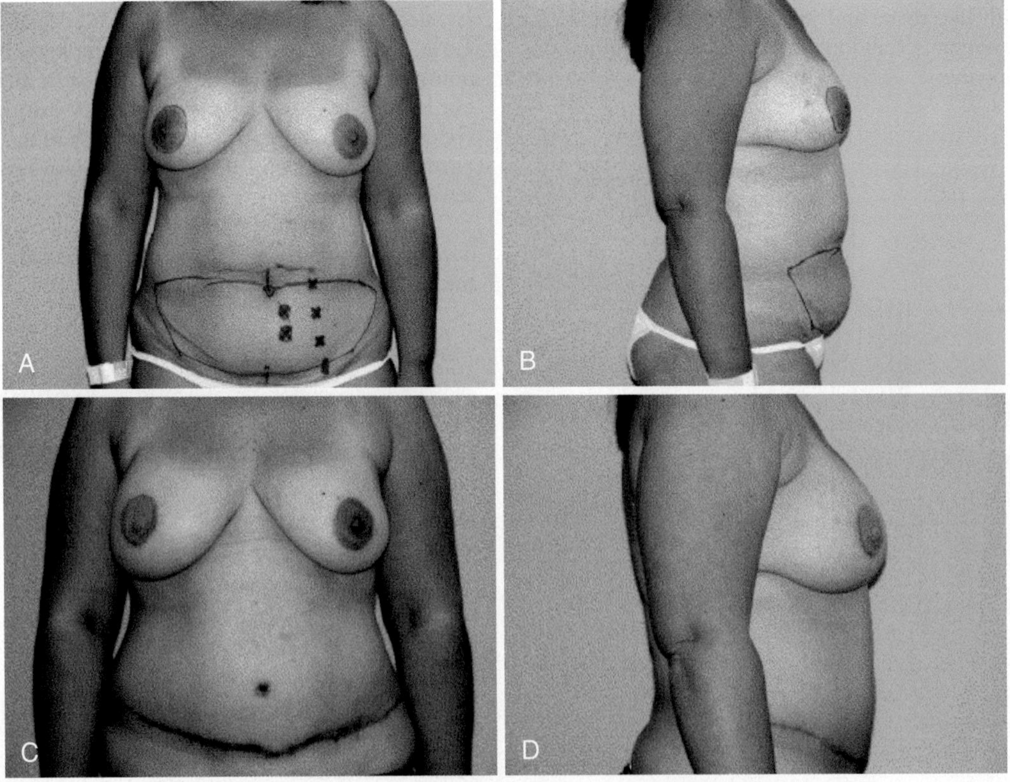


**FIGURE 37-8** **A, B,** Preoperative views of patient with right breast cancer for mastectomy and DIEP reconstruction. **C, D,** Patient approximately 3 months after breast revision, nipple creation, and tattooing. (Granzow JW, Levine JL, Chiu ES, et al: Breast reconstruction with the deep inferior epigastric perforator flap: history and an update on current technique. J Plast Reconstr Aesthet Surg 59:571–579, 2006.)

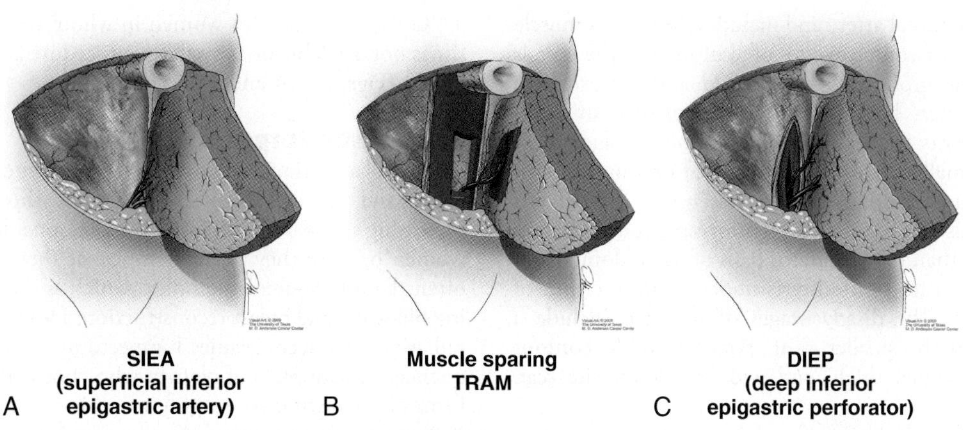


**FIGURE 37-9** Schematic representation of the SIEA flap in which abdominal wall fascia is undisturbed **(A)**, DIEP flap, in which all muscle is spared **(B)**, and msTRAM flap, in which a small window of muscle is taken around the supplying perforators **(C)**. (© 2009 The University of Texas M.D. Anderson Cancer Center.)

inferior epigastric artery perforator) flap, in which no muscle is taken and the perforating vessels are dissected out in a chain, and the SIEA (superficial inferior epigastric artery) flap, when a suitable SIEA is available (about 30%) provides a pedicle that does not penetrate the rectus muscle at all (and thus there is no abdominal wall morbidity and shorter recovery time; Fig. 37-9).[24-26]

The choice of flap is often determined by the patient's anatomy. When the SIEA flap is available and of reasonable caliber, often more than 1.5 mm, it is often chosen because it results in the least amount of abdominal morbidity. Difficulties with this flap can occur because the artery is small and there may be some discrepancy between the SIEA and internal mammary artery. In addition, the SIEA will only support half of the abdominal skin and fat so it is favorable for small breast reconstructions and for bilateral cases. The choice between DIEP and msTRAM is by the surgeon. When the anatomy is favorable and reasonable caliber perforators are available in a formation that allows for minimal disruption of rectus muscle, a DIEP flap is chosen. When the vessels are smaller or their orientation is not favorable for muscular dissection, an msTRAM flap is used. Flap perfusion is often better with an msTRAM. DIEP rates of partial flap loss and fat necrosis are often higher, and thus abdominal wall preservation is sometimes at the expense of flap perfusion and overall breast outcome.[27] Often, preoperative imaging studies are used to evaluate the vascular system of the anterior abdominal wall. Computed tomography (CT) angiography, conventional angiography, and even staging CT scans performed during cancer workup have been used to visualize the perforators supplying the anterior abdominal skin and subcutaneous tissue. These can provide some guidance for perforator selection and often decrease dissection times.

**Gluteal-Based Flaps** Breast reconstruction can also be performed using tissue from the gluteal region based on the superior or the inferior gluteal arteries and their overlying skin and subcutaneous tissue. This is commonly performed in women who desire autologous breast reconstruction but have little adiposity in the lower abdomen. The buttock provides a reasonable amount of fat that is firm and provides sufficient volume and projection in breast reconstruction. Originally described as a musculocutaneous flap, gluteal artery perforator (GAP) flaps (superior GAP [SGAP] and inferior GAP [IGAP] flaps) had a number of donor site complications, including significant seroma, contour deformity, and sciatica from nerve compression. They have evolved into a perforator flap design, similar to the evolution of the TRAM flap to the DIEP. Perforator design limits the deformity at the donor site and lessens the incidence of sciatica. The disadvantages of these flaps include difficulty of dissection, short pedicle length, and size discrepancy of the gluteal vein when anastomosing it with the internal mammary vein. These flaps are technically challenging but provide a good amount of autologous tissue for reconstruction of one or even both breasts (Figs. 37-10 to 37-13).[28-31]

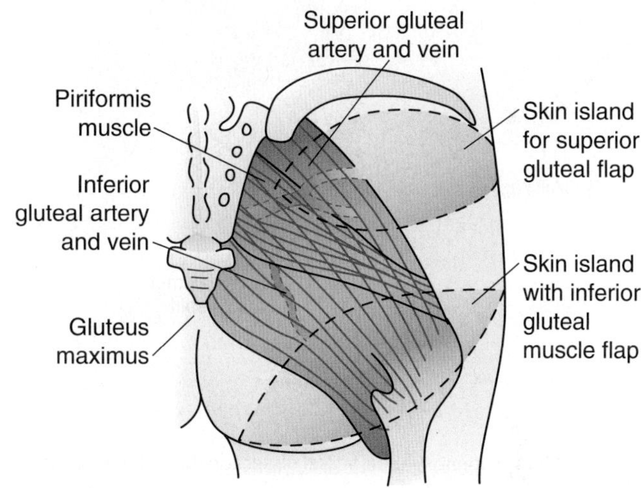


**FIGURE 37-10** Skin island location of the SGAP and IGAP flaps. The skin paddle can be oriented over the superior or inferior gluteal artery.

**Inner Thigh–Based Flaps** Additionally, breast reconstruction can be performed using the upper inner thigh tissue. This is ideal for women without abdominal or gluteal tissue to use as a donor site. Similarly, some women are opposed to the donor scar on the buttock or abdomen and would prefer reduction in the excess fat or skin in the inner thigh region. The transverse upper gracilis (TUG) flap is based on the ascending branch of the medial circumflex femoral artery and includes the gracilis muscle and the overlying horizontal paddle of skin or fat. The scar is camouflaged in the groin and gluteal fold and a reasonable amount of tissue can be obtained to reconstruct small to moderate-sized breasts in the immediate setting. Because these flaps are slightly smaller than their abdominal or gluteal counterparts with regard to skin, they are less useful for delayed reconstruction. This flap is rather straightforward and dissection is somewhat easier than the perforator flaps of the abdomen and buttock. Minimal to no morbidity is noticed with sacrifice of the gracilis muscle. The disadvantages of this flap include a shorter pedicle length, smaller skin island, possible contour deformity of the medial thigh, and widened donor site scar.

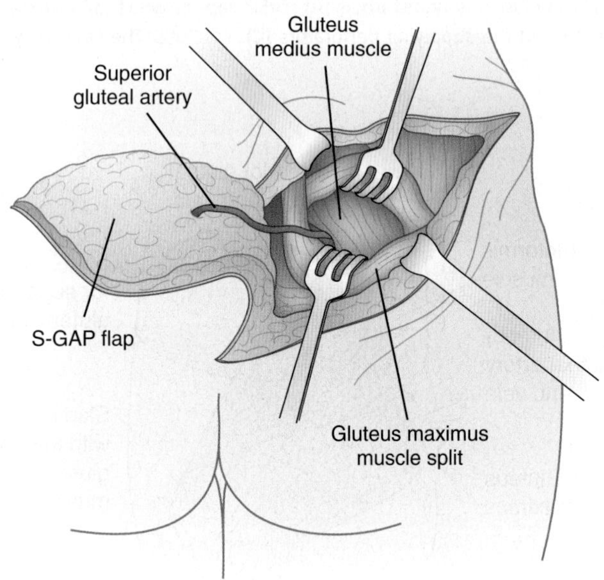


**FIGURE 37-11** Superior gluteal vessel dissection through the retracted gluteus maximus muscle.

TUG flaps are ideal for women in whom the abdominal donor site is not available or as a salvage procedure after reconstruction failure (Figs. 37-14 and 37-15).[32-34]

## Oncoplastic Surgery

Breast conservation has comparable outcomes in cancer treatment, and up to 40% of women chose this option in 1991, increasing to 60% by 2002. BCT is a reasonable choice for many women because they preserve much of their native breast and often the nipple-areola complex, which is the most disappointing phase of total breast reconstruction. However, the adjunctive radiation that accompanies lumpectomy is not without consequence. At least 30% of women who choose BCT require some form of reconstructive surgery to achieve better symmetry and 86% observe asymmetry.[35] Breast revision can be difficult after radiation therapy, with complication rates of 50% in the radiated breast. Thus, women were formerly offered reduction of the normal breast for symmetry in clothing and minimal to no surgery on the radiated side. In an attempt to improve cosmetic outcomes, we now can provide preemptive treatment at the time of lumpectomy to improve contour and aesthetic deformity after the effects of radiation. This is done in the form of breast rearrangement after the cancerous tissue is removed. These types of procedures are ideal for the large-breasted woman, when resection is 20% of breast volume, when tumor location is central, medial, or inferior, when she desires smaller breasts, or when she has significant breast ptosis and/or asymmetry (Fig. 37-16).

Oncoplastic procedures are performed immediately or 1 to 2 weeks after lumpectomy, once final pathology is available. They include rearrangement of the remaining breast tissue through a variety of techniques, often adhering to breast reduction principles. In addition, more tissue can be brought into the breast to correct the volume deficit, often in the form of a latissimus dorsi flap. Indications for these procedures depend on the patient's preoperative breast size, available remaining breast tissue, and overall goals for ultimate breast size and shape. All these procedures are done prior to radiation to prevent the

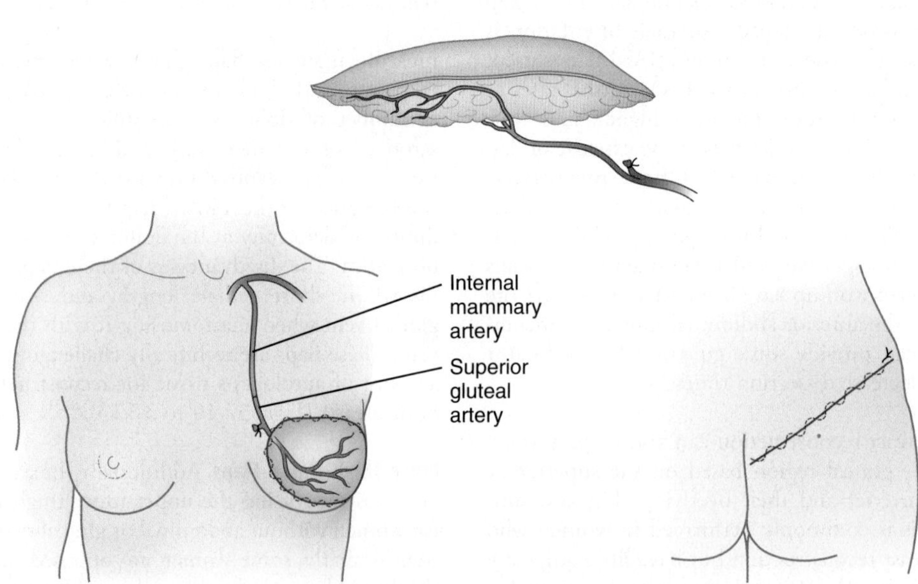


**FIGURE 37-12** Schematic of the gluteal perforator flap, inset into the defect via the internal mammary vessels, and donor site closure. (Granzow JW, Levine JL, Chiu ES, et al: Breast reconstruction with gluteal artery perforator flaps. J Plast Reconstr Aesthet Surg 59:614–621, 2006.)

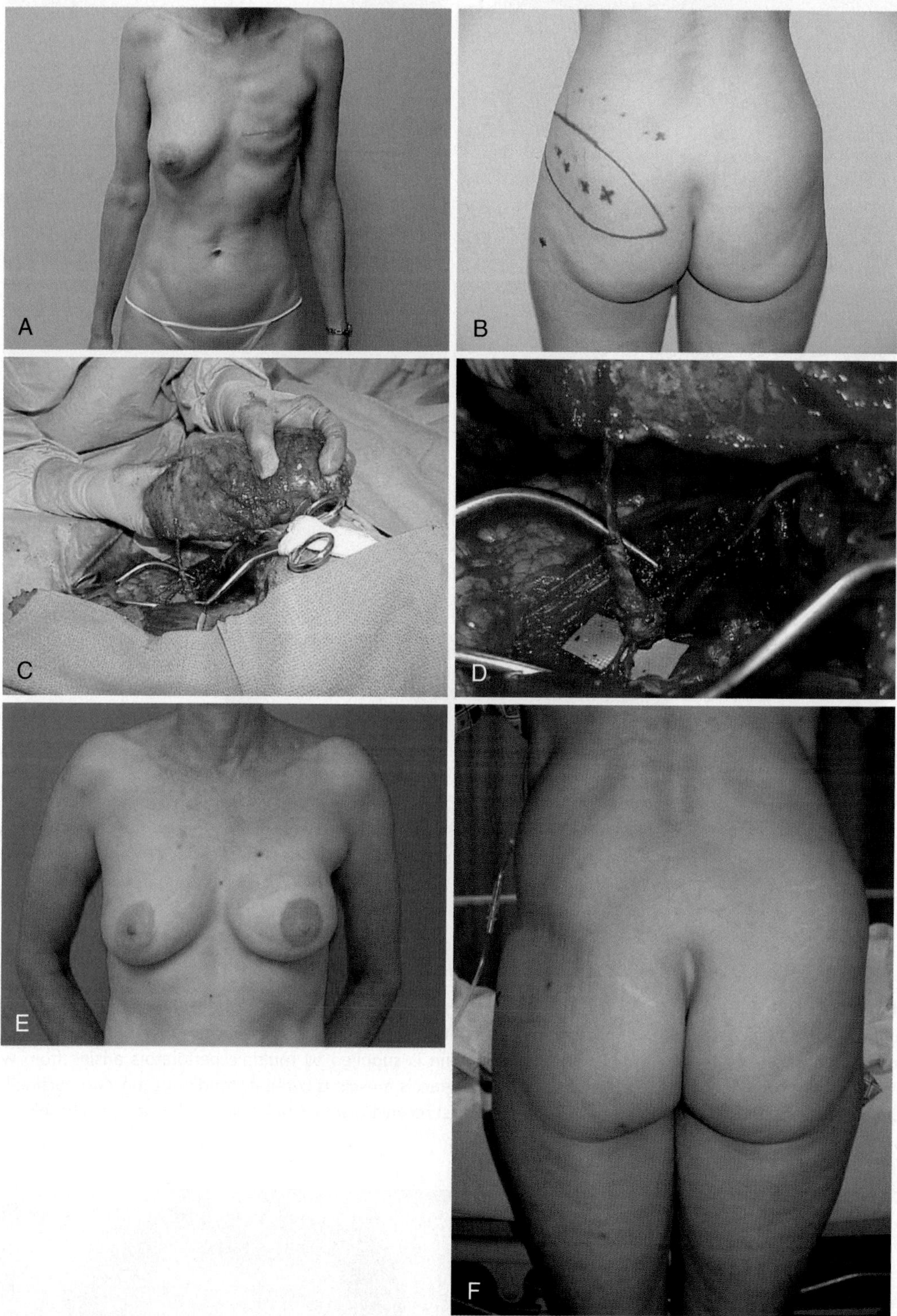


**FIGURE 37-13** **A, B,** Preoperative view and markings. **C, D,** Intraoperative views of flap and superior gluteal artery perforator vessels. **E, F,** Postoperative views (anterior and posterior) 21 months after surgery. (Granzow JW, Levine JL, Chiu ES, et al: Breast reconstruction with gluteal artery perforator flaps. J Plast Reconstr Aesthet Surg 59:614–621, 2006.)

contracture of the lumpectomy defect and distortion of the nipple-areolar complex. Although this technique is rather new, recent outcomes are judged to be good. In many cases, these women still require contralateral balancing procedures after the completion of radiation.[36-38]

## COMPLICATIONS

Complications can be encountered with any form of breast reconstruction and may cause delay in adjuvant chemotherapy. They include partial or total flap loss, mastectomy flap loss, wound breakdown, and infection. Complications are known to

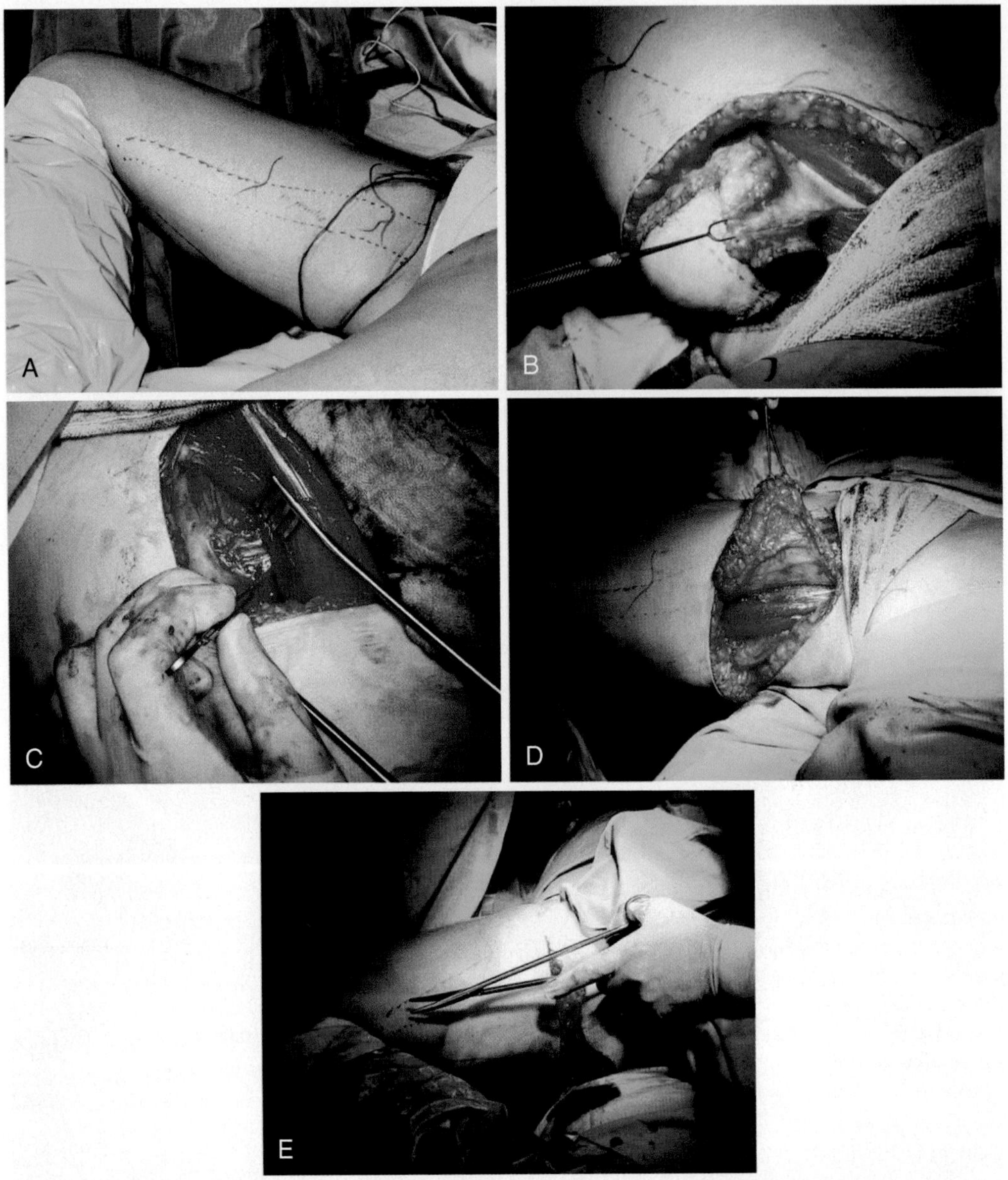

**FIGURE 37-14** **A,** *Top left,* Typical marking of the TUG flap. **B,** *Top, right,* The anterior portion of the flap is dissected first of the underlying adductor longus. The pedicle, medial circumflex femoral artery, is identified at the dorsal border of this muscle. **C,** *Center, left,* Posterior portion of the skin island is lifted off the underlying muscle. The overlying skin is supplied by multiple perforators arising from within the gracilis. **D** and **E,** *Center, right and bottom,* After complete skin dissection, the gracilis muscle is cut at its tendinous junction. (Schoeller T, Huemer GM, Wechselberger G: The transverse musculocutaneous gracilis flap for breast reconstruction: Guidelines for flap and patient selection. Plast Reconstr Surg 122:29–38, 2008.)

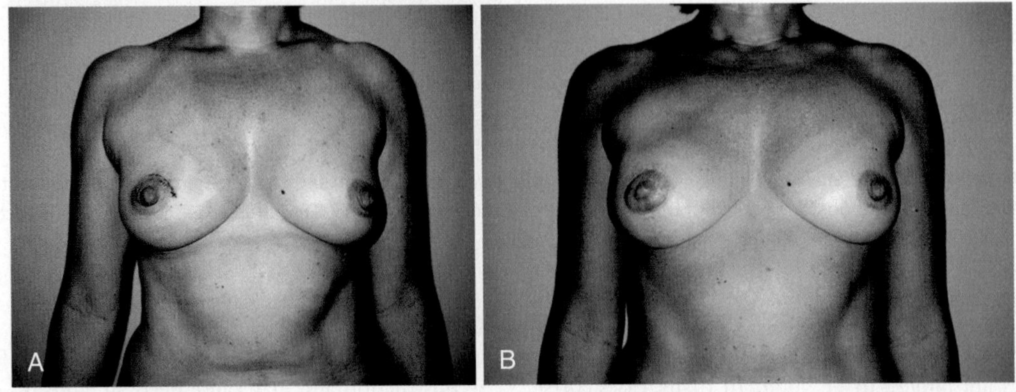

**FIGURE 37-15** **A,** Patient with right breast cancer before *(left)* and after *(right)* unilateral right breast reconstruction using TUG flap. **B,** 33 months after reconstruction. (Schoeller T, Huemer GM, Wechselberger G: The transverse musculocutaneous gracilis flap for breast reconstruction: Guidelines for flap and patient selection. Plast Reconstr Surg 122:29–38, 2008.)

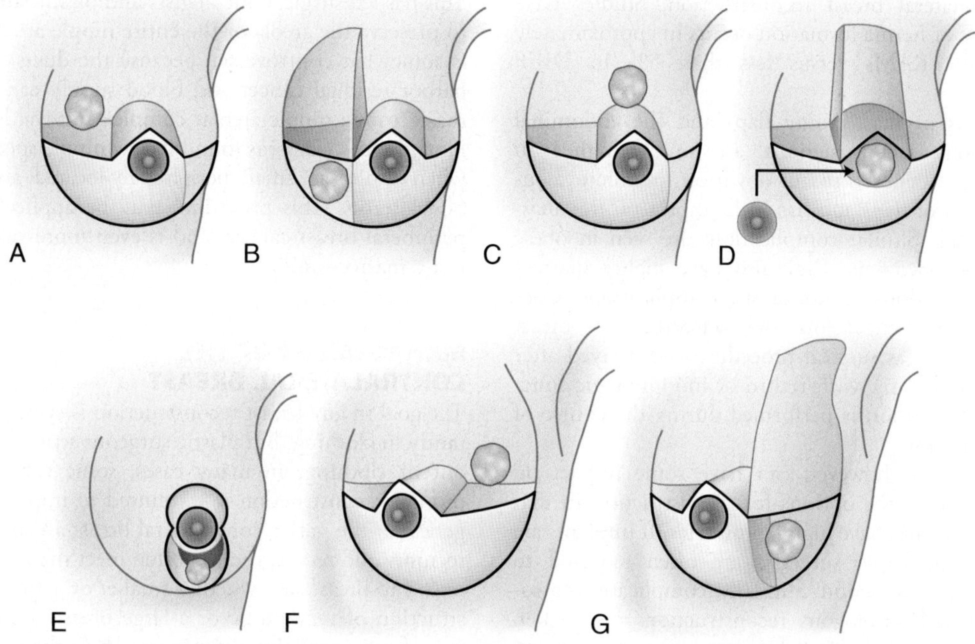


**FIGURE 37-16** Guidelines for design of the nipple pedicle to repair a partial mastectomy defect using the breast reduction technique by tumor location *(pink)*. **A,** (Above, left) Upper inner quadrant, showing the inferomedial pedicle *(white)*. The retained medial component *(yellow)* fills the defect on closure of the Wise skin pattern and maintains the cleavage of the breast. **B,** (Above, second from left) Lower inner quadrant, showing the inferolateral pedicle. The retained lateral component provides additional blood supply to the nipple-areola complex. A thick layer of subcutaneous tissue is maintained on the medial aspect of the Wise skin pattern flap to fill the defect on closure of the Wise skin pattern and maintain cleavage of the breast. **C,** (Above, second from right) Upper central quadrant, showing the inferomedial pedicle. The retained medial component provides a cosmetic advantage and additional blood supply to the nipple-areola complex in patients with very large ptotic breasts. **D,** (Above, right) Middle central quadrant, showing the amputative design with a free nipple graft and maintenance of a thick layer of subcutaneous tissue on the central aspect of the Wise skin pattern flap *(yellow)*. **E,** (Below, left) Lower central quadrant, showing the vertical scar reduction mammaplasty. **F,** (Below, center) Upper outer quadrant, showing the inferomediolateral pedicle. The retained lateral component fills the defect on closure of the Wise skin pattern. **G,** (Below, right) Lower outer quadrant, showing the inferomedial pedicle. The retained medial component provides a cosmetic advantage and additional blood supply to the nipple-areola complex. A thick layer of subcutaneous tissue is maintained on the lateral aspect of the Wise skin pattern flap to fill the defect *(yellow)*. (Kronowitz SJ, Kuerer HM, Buchholz TA, et al: A management algorithm and practical oncoplastic surgical techniques for repairing partial mastectomy defects. Plast Reconstr Surg 122:1631–1647, 2008.)

be higher in women who require adjuvant radiation therapy and, more commonly, with implant-based reconstructions (15% without radiation and up to 42% with radiation).[17,39,40] Symmetry is also affected by radiation therapy; thus, implant-based reconstructions are not the best option for women requiring radiation therapy.

The most common complication with implant-based reconstructions is capsular contracture, which can occur regardless of implant type or placement position. Treatment may require capsulectomy, capsulotomy, change in implant position or type, and/or implant removal, with some other form of reconstruction. Additional complications include infection, seroma, skin slough, necrosis, deflation, and unacceptable appearance.

Satisfaction with this modality of reconstruction tends to decline over time regardless of type, volume, patient age, or type of mastectomy.[17] Thus, implant-based reconstruction is best suited for thin patients with inadequate autologous donor sites or for women who opt not to undergo more lengthy procedures. Implants can also be used to enhance autologous reconstructions to improve symmetry and women's aesthetic wishes.

Complications associated with flap reconstruction include mastectomy flap issues, partial or total flap loss, and problems related to the flap donor site. For the latissimus dorsi flap, back seroma is the most common complication. In addition, many women require the addition of an implant to achieve adequate volume and thus accrue all the possible implant-related complications. Abdomen-based reconstructions have possible partial flap loss, total flap loss, and fat necrosis, which can present later as a firm suspicious nodule. Fat necrosis occurs in approximately 50% of pedicled TRAMs versus 17% in those procedures performed in a free fashion.[41] Complications associated with the abdominal donor site include flap necrosis, abdominal weakness, bulge, and hernia. Partial flap loss is more common with pedicled reconstructions and total flap loss is more common with free transfer of the abdominal tissue. Partial flap loss rates for free tissue transfers are approximately 2% for msTRAM, 7% for DIEP, 3% for SIEA, and 4% for GAP flaps. Fat necrosis also occurs in about 3% of msTRAM and 7% and 9% for SIEA and DIEP flaps, respectively. Abdominal weakness and bulge have been reported to occur less in the DIEP setting, especially with bilateral breast reconstruction. Studies have revealed that bulge or hernia formation occurs in approximately 15% of pedicled TRAMs versus less than 5% in DIEP flaps.[41-44]

Complications of mastectomy flaps and the abdominal wall in autologous reconstructions are much higher in smokers. Smoking is believed to cut down on the microvascular distal circulation of flaps and has little impact on the anastomosis of free flaps. Similar complications are seen in obese and morbidly obese women. They also have higher mastectomy flap loss and abdominal donor site complications. Chemotherapy has little effect on the outcomes of breast reconstruction, as long as surgical procedures are delayed after neoadjuvant chemotherapy, with return of immunologic function, and little intervention is performed during the course of adjuvant chemotherapy.

Radiation therapy, however, can have some impact on reconstruction. It limits the options for reconstruction in that implant-based procedures have high failure rates. If implants are used, additional and larger surgeries are often required to salvage the breast reconstruction. Similarly, complications associated with irradiated autologous reconstructions are higher. Early complications are similar in delayed and immediate reconstruction with adjuvant radiation therapy. Immediate reconstruction followed by radiation has complication rates of 87% versus 8.6% in those that have delayed reconstruction after radiation therapy. In those who have immediate reconstruction, 28% require additional flap surgery to correct contour deformities.[45]

## NIPPLE-AREOLAR RECONSTRUCTION

The focus of all the procedures described is creation of a breast mound. This provides the woman with symmetry in clothing and a bra. For many women, this is satisfactory and they want no further operative intervention. Other women would like completion of their reconstruction to mirror the normal contralateral breast, which requires the creation of a nipple and areolar complex. Often, these procedures are done some months after the initial mound reconstruction to allow for settling of the reconstruction. This allows for symmetrical positioning of the created nipple. In addition, a period of time after radiation should be allotted because the breast reconstruction will undergo some amount of contraction. This is usually 2 to 3 months after creation of the breast mound or completion of adjuvant therapy.

The nipple itself can be created via a myriad of local flap techniques using the skin of the reconstructed breast mound. A number of local flap designs have been proposed and all have relatively similar results. Over the first year, they undergo some amount of contraction, up to 50%, so all are initially made rather large, accordingly. The areolar reconstruction can be performed in one of two ways. Some surgeons opt to use a full-thickness skin graft, usually from the groin for the native darker pigmentation. Others choose to use medical tattoo pigments that are chosen from a color wheel to match the contralateral native areola. Creation of the areola usually occurs 4 to 6 weeks after creation of the nipple. Nipple tattoo tends to fade over time and requires occasional touchup.

In general, nipple areolar reconstruction is the least satisfying portion of the overall breast reconstruction experience. The reconstructed nipple and areola have little projection compared with normal and is insensate and less than the aesthetic normal. This has led surgical oncologists and plastic surgeons to attempt to preserve the areola or the entire nipple areolar complex. This is somewhat controversial because the ducts in the nipple can harbor residual cancer and blood supply can be tenuous after mastectomy; nipple-areolar complex survival is not guaranteed. Nonetheless, cancer is found in few nipple specimens, especially when tumors are small, peripherally located, and have a negative nodal status. This procedure may be applicable to early-stage peripheral breast cancers and is even more valuable in prophylactic mastectomies.

## MANAGEMENT OF THE CONTRALATERAL BREAST

The goal in any breast reconstruction is symmetry, most importantly in clothing, but plastic surgeons strive for symmetry, even out of clothing. In many cases, some revision of the breast mound reconstruction is warranted to improve shape and surgeries on the native contralateral breast are also necessary. Mastectomy and reconstruction often meet the patient's desires with regard to breast size, whether smaller or larger. Complete reconstruction of very ptotic or a large breast is often difficult with any of reconstructive techniques. Thus, the techniques used are augmentation mammaplasty, mastopexy (lifting), and reduction mammaplasty.

The incidence of contralateral cancer is rather low, but is approximately 1%/year. Therefore, young women often choose a prophylactic mastectomy. Also, *BRCA*-positive women are encouraged to undergo bilateral mastectomies because their incidence of breast cancer is 80% or higher in their lifetime. In the case of bilateral mastectomies, reconstruction is best when the same procedure is performed on both sides.

## SURVEILLANCE

Reconstructed breasts are easy to monitor for local recurrence because it is most often within the skin. Any firm or suspicious mass should be biopsied without delay. The result is often fat necrosis in autologous tissue reconstructions. Routine mammography of breast reconstructions is not necessary. Ultrasound and magnetic resonance imaging (MRI) are the most commonly used radiographic modalities. Recurrence is usually managed with surgical excision, adjuvant chemotherapy, and/or radiation therapy. The reconstruction infrequently has to be removed in its entirety—only in the case of multifocal recurrence or involvement of the flap pedicle itself.

## CONCLUSIONS

Breast reconstruction is a vital component in the treatment of breast cancer for many women. It is often the optimistic portion of a devastating diagnosis. Reconstruction lessens the psychological and physical burden of the diagnosis for many women. When possible, immediate reconstruction is preferred because it has not been shown to increase oncologic risk or delay adjuvant therapy, provides for better aesthetic outcomes, and results in less depression. It is also more cost-effective. Planning and decision making for reconstruction must be individualized to each patient to achieve her desires in the safest and most reasonable fashion. There are advantages and disadvantages of each procedure; decision making should be individualized for the patient and her reconstructive surgeon to determine the most rational radiotherapy.

## SELECTED REFERENCES

Granzow JW, Levine JL, Chiu ES, et al: Breast reconstruction using perforator flaps. J Surg Oncol 94:441–454, 2006.

The authors described the use of SIEA, DIEP, and GAP flaps for breast reconstruction with preservation of muscle at donor sites. The procedures and donor sites are well described and illustrated.

Grotting JC, Urist MM, Maddox WA, et al: Conventional TRAM flap versus free microsurgical TRAM flap for immediate breast reconstruction. Plast Reconstr Surg 83:828–841, 1989.

The authors described use of the lower abdomen skin paddle and rectus abdominis muscle as a free flap for microvascular tissue transfer in breast reconstruction, with several advantages over the pedicled TRAM flap.

Guerra AB, Metzinger SE, Bidros RS, et al: Breast reconstruction with gluteal artery perforator (GAP) flaps: A critical analysis of 142 cases. Ann Plast Surg 52:118–125, 2004.

The authors described their experience in reconstructing mastectomy defects with the free gluteal artery perforator flaps from the superior and inferior systems in 142 patients. Results and surgical refinements, advantages, disadvantages, and lessons learned are presented.

Hartrampf CR, Scheflan M, Black PW: Breast reconstruction with a transverse abdominal island flap. Plast Reconstr Surg 69:216–225, 1982.

The authors described reconstruction of mastectomy defects with a transversely oriented skin paddle based on perforators from the rectus abdominis muscle.

Khoo A, Kroll SS, Reece GP, et al: A comparison of resource costs of immediate and delayed breast reconstruction. Plast Reconstr Surg 101:964–968, 1998.

This report evaluated the cost of delayed versus immediate breast reconstruction in 276 patients and concludes that mastectomy with immediate breast reconstruction is significantly less expensive than mastectomy followed by delayed reconstruction.

Singletary SE: Skin-sparing mastectomy with immediate breast reconstruction: The M. D. Anderson Cancer Center experience. Ann Surg Oncol 3:411–416, 1996.

This report on 545 patients undergoing skin-sparing mastectomies and immediate breast reconstruction indicated a low regional recurrence rate of 2.6%. This recurrence was found to be a function of tumor biology and disease stage, not use of immediate breast reconstruction or skin-sparing mastectomy.

Stevens LA, McGrath MH, Druss RG, et al: The psychological impact of immediate breast reconstruction for women with early breast cancer. Plast Reconstr Surg 73:619–628, 1984.

This prospective study evaluated the psychological effects of immediate versus delayed breast reconstruction. The patient's mood, body image, sexuality, femininity, and social and occupational functioning were found to be superior in the group who underwent immediate breast reconstruction.

Warren AG, Morris DJ, Houlihan MJ, et al: Breast reconstruction in a changing breast cancer treatment paradigm. Plast Reconstr Surg 121:1116–1126, 2008.

The authors provide an overview of the current trends in breast cancer treatment, including breast conservation, oncoplastic surgery, sentinel lymph node biopsy, and skin-sparing mastectomy. With regard to reconstruction, new silicone implants, perforator flap reconstructions, and the use of acellular dermal matrix in implant reconstructions are discussed.

## REFERENCES

1. Cronin TD, Gerow FJ: Augmentation mammaplasty: A new natural feel prosthesis. In Broadbent TR, editors: Transactions of the Third International Congress of Plastic Surgery, Amsterdam, 1963, Excerpta Medica.
2. Mandel MA: Subcutaneous mastectomy with immediate reconstruction of the large breast. Surg Gynecol Obstet 146:90–92, 1978.
3. Pontes R: Single-stage reconstruction of the missing breast. Br J Plast Surg 26:377–380, 1973.
4. Snyderman RK, Guthrie RH: Reconstruction of the female breast following radical mastectomy. Plast Reconstr Surg 47:565–567, 1971.
5. Manchot C: Die Hautarterien des Menschlichen Korpers, Leipzig, 1889, Vogel.
6. Ryan JJ: A lower thoracic advancement flap in breast reconstruction after mastectomy. Plast Reconstr Surg 70:153–160, 1982.
7. Reaby LL: Reasons why women who have mastectomy decide to have or not to have breast reconstruction. Plast Reconstr Surg 101:1810–1818, 1998.
8. Stevens LA, McGrath MH, Druss RG, et al: The psychological impact of immediate breast reconstruction for women with early breast cancer. Plast Reconstr Surg 73:619–628, 1984.
9. Pusic A, Thompson TA, Kerrigan CL, et al: Surgical options for the early-stage breast cancer: Factors associated with patient choice and postoperative quality of life. Plast Reconstr Surg 104:1325–1333, 1999.
10. McGuire KP, Santillan AA, Kaur P, et al: Are mastectomies on the rise? A 13-year trend analysis of the selection of mastectomy versus breast conservation therapy in 5865 patients. Ann Surg Oncol 16:2682–2690, 2009.
11. Warren AG, Morris DJ, Houlihan MJ, et al: Breast reconstruction in a changing breast cancer treatment paradigm. Plast Reconstr Surg 121:1116–1126, 2008.
12. Khoo A, Kroll SS, Reece GP, et al: A comparison of resource costs of immediate and delayed breast reconstruction. Plast Reconstr Surg 101:964–968, 1998.
13. Gamboa-Bobadilla GM: Implant breast reconstruction using acellular dermal matrix. Ann Plast Surg 56:22–25, 2006.
14. Singletary SE: Skin-sparing mastectomy with immediate breast reconstruction: The M. D. Anderson Cancer Center experience. Ann Surg Oncol 3:411–416, 1996.
15. Breuing KH, Warren SM: Immediate bilateral breast reconstruction with implants and inferolateral AlloDerm slings. Ann Plast Surg 55:232–239, 2005.
16. Spear SL, Parikh PM, Reisin E, et al: Acellular dermis-assisted breast reconstruction. Aesthetic Plast Surg 32:418–425, 2008.
17. Clough KB, O'Donoghue JM, Fitoussi AD, et al: Prospective evaluation of late cosmetic results following breast reconstruction:

I. Implant reconstruction. Plast Reconstr Surg 107:1702–1709, 2001.

18. Schneider WJ, Hill HL, Jr., Brown RG: Latissimus dorsi myocutaneous flap for breast reconstruction. Br J Plast Surg 30:277–281, 1977.
19. Bostwick J, 3rd, Scheflan M: The latissimus dorsi musculocutaneous flap: A one-stage breast reconstruction. Clin Plast Surg 7:71–78, 1980.
20. Hartrampf CR, Scheflan M, Black PW: Breast reconstruction with a transverse abdominal island flap. Plast Reconstr Surg 69:216–225, 1982.
21. Moon HK, Taylor GI: The vascular anatomy of rectus abdominis musculocutaneous flaps based on the deep superior epigastric system. Plast Reconstr Surg 82:815–832, 1988.
22. Holmstrom H: The free abdominoplasty flap and its use in breast reconstruction. An experimental study and clinical case report. Scand J Plast Reconstr Surg 13:423–427, 1979.
23. Garvey PB, Buchel EW, Pockaj BA, et al: DIEP and pedicled TRAM flaps: A comparison of outcomes. Plast Reconstr Surg 117:1711–1719, 2006.
24. Chevray PM: Breast reconstruction with superficial inferior epigastric artery flaps: A prospective comparison with TRAM and DIEP flaps. Plast Reconstr Surg 114:1077–1083, 2004.
25. Man LX, Selber JC, Serletti JM: Abdominal wall following free TRAM or DIEP flap reconstruction: A meta-analysis and critical review. Plast Reconstr Surg 124:752–764, 2009.
26. Grotting JC, Urist MM, Maddox WA, et al: Conventional TRAM flap versus free microsurgical TRAM flap for immediate breast reconstruction. Plast Reconstr Surg 83:828–841, 1989.
27. Granzow JW, Levine JL, Chiu ES, et al: Breast reconstruction using perforator flaps. J Surg Oncol 94:441–454, 2006.
28. Guerra AB, Metzinger SE, Bidros RS, et al: Breast reconstruction with gluteal artery perforator (GAP) flaps: A critical analysis of 142 cases. Ann Plast Surg 52:118–125, 2004.
29. Allen RJ, Levine JL, Granzow JW: The in-the-crease inferior gluteal artery perforator flap for breast reconstruction. Plast Reconstr Surg 118:333–339, 2006.
30. Granzow JW, Levine JL, Chiu ES, et al: Breast reconstruction with gluteal artery perforator flaps. J Plast Reconstr Aesthet Surg 59:614–621, 2006.
31. Guerra AB, Soueid N, Metzinger SE, et al: Simultaneous bilateral breast reconstruction with superior gluteal artery perforator (SGAP) flaps. Ann Plast Surg 53:305–310, 2004.
32. Arnez ZM, Pogorelec D, Planinsek F, et al: Breast reconstruction by the free transverse gracilis (TUG) flap. Br J Plast Surg 57:20–26, 2004.
33. Fattah A, Figus A, Mathur B, et al: The transverse myocutaneous gracilis flap: Technical refinements. J Plast Reconstr Aesthet Surg 63:305–313, 2010.
34. Schoeller T, Huemer GM, Wechselberger G: The transverse musculocutaneous gracilis flap for breast reconstruction: guidelines for flap and patient selection. Plast Reconstr Surg 122:29–38, 2008.
35. Bajaj AK, Kon PS, Oberg KC, et al: Aesthetic outcomes in patients undergoing breast conservation therapy for the treatment of localized breast cancer. Plast Reconstr Surg 114:1442–1449, 2004.
36. Losken A, Hamdi M: Partial breast reconstruction: Current perspectives. Plast Reconstr Surg 124:722–736, 2009.
37. Kronowitz SJ, Kuerer HM, Buchholz TA, et al: A management algorithm and practical oncoplastic surgical techniques for repairing partial mastectomy defects. Plast Reconstr Surg 122:1631–1647, 2008.
38. Berry M, Fitoussi AD, Curnier A, et al: Oncoplastic breast surgery: A review and systematic approach. J Plast Reconstr Aesthet Surg 63:1233–1243, 2010.
39. Chawla AK, Kachnic LA, Taghian AG, et al: Radiotherapy and breast reconstruction: complications and cosmesis with TRAM versus tissue expander/implant. Int J Radiat Oncol Biol Phys 54:520–526, 2002.
40. Benediktsson K, Perbeck L: Capsular contracture around saline-filled and textured subcutaneously-placed implants in irradiated and non-irradiated breast cancer patients: Five years of monitoring of a prospective trial. J Plast Reconstr Aesthet Surg 59:27–34, 2006.
41. Schusterman MA, Kroll SS, Miller MJ, et al: The free transverse rectus abdominis musculocutaneous flap for breast reconstruction: One center's experience with 211 consecutive cases. Ann Plast Surg 32:234–241, 1994.
42. Blondeel N, Vanderstraeten GG, Monstrey SJ, et al: The donor site morbidity of free DIEP flaps and free TRAM flaps for breast reconstruction. Br J Plast Surg 50:322–330, 1997.
43. Nahabedian MY, Dooley W, Singh N, et al: Contour abnormalities of the abdomen after breast reconstruction with abdominal flaps: The role of muscle preservation. Plast Reconstr Surg 109:91–101, 2002.
44. Bottero L, Lefaucheur JP, Fadhul S, et al: Electromyographic assessment of rectus abdominis muscle function after deep inferior epigastric perforator flap surgery. Plast Reconstr Surg 113:156–161, 2004.
45. Tran NV, Chang DW, Gupta A, et al: Comparison of immediate and delayed free TRAM flap breast reconstruction in patients receiving postmastectomy radiation therapy. Plast Reconstr Surg 108:78–82, 2001.

# SECTION VIII

## ENDOCRINE

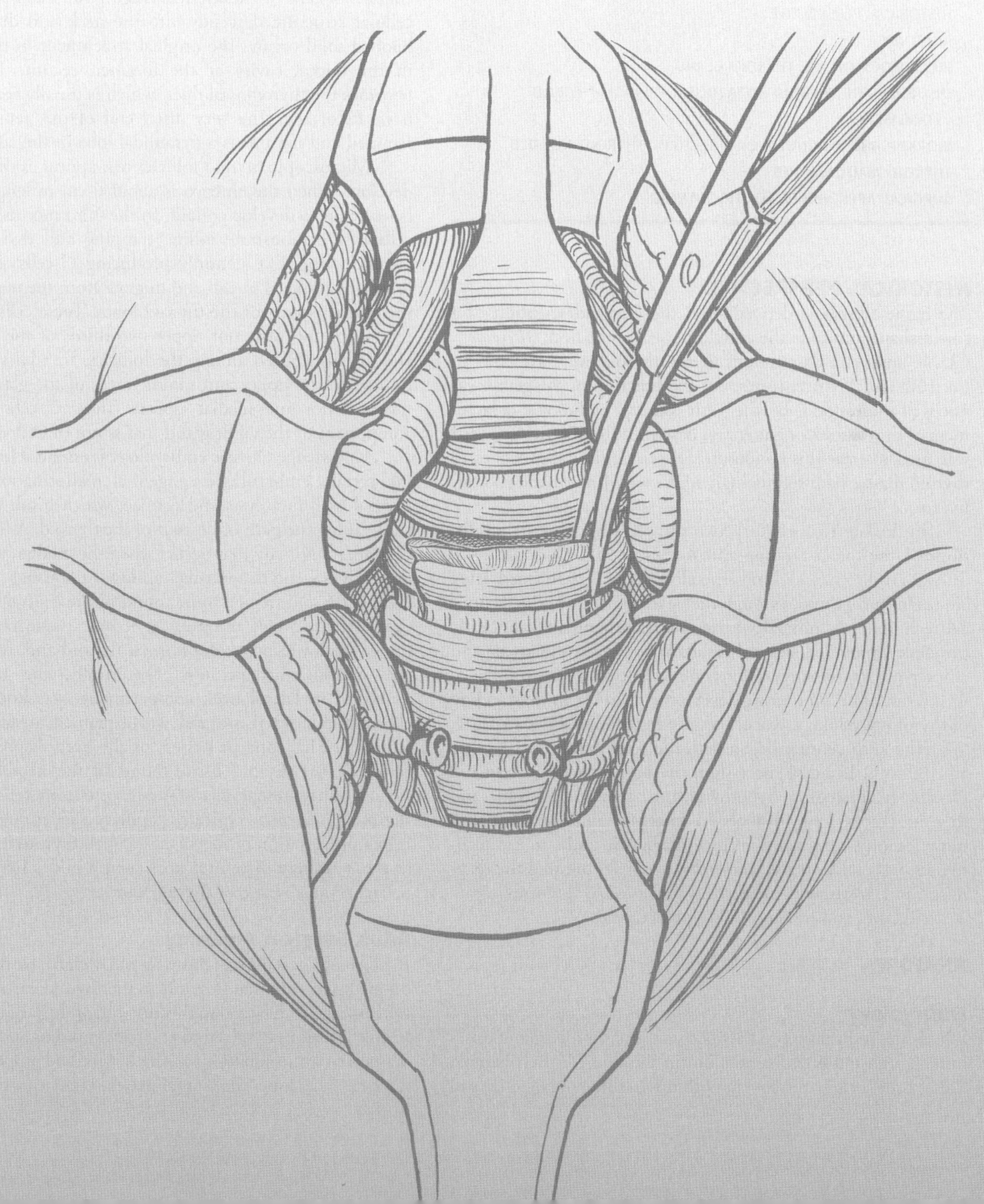

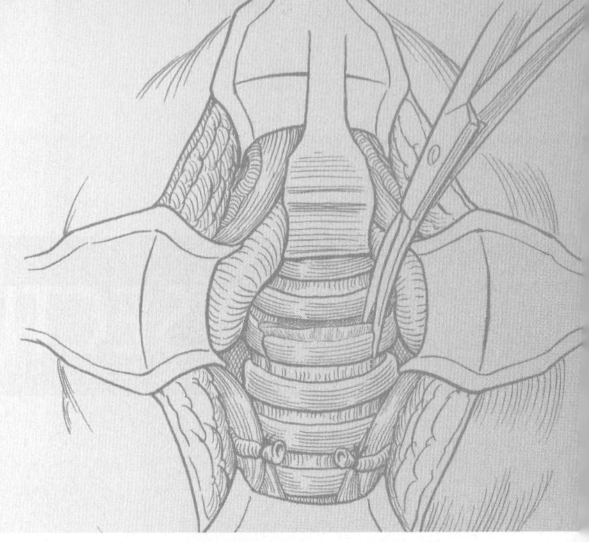

CHAPTER 38

# THYROID

Philip W. Smith, Leslie J. Salomone, and John B. Hanks



## HISTORICAL PERSPECTIVE

The name *thyroid* is derived from the Greek description of a shield-shaped gland in the anterior aspect of the neck (*thyroides*). Classic anatomic descriptions of the thyroid were available in the 16th and 17th centuries, but the function of the gland was not well understood. By the 19th century, pathologic enlargement of the thyroid, or goiter, was described. Iodine-rich seaweed was used to treat this condition. Direct surgical approaches to thyroid masses had frighteningly high complication and mortality rates.

In the late 19th century, two surgeon-physiologists revolutionized the understanding and treatment of thyroid diseases. Theodor Billroth and Emil Theodor Kocher established large clinics in Europe and, through the development of skilled surgical techniques combined with newer anesthetic and antiseptic principles, provided surgical results that proved the safety and efficacy of thyroid surgery for benign and malignant problems. As a result of his pioneering developments in the understanding of thyroid physiology, Kocher received the Nobel Prize in 1909.

The 20th century began with the contributions of Kocher and Billroth. In rapid succession, the understanding of altered physiology, including hypothyroidism, hyperthyroidism, and thyroid cancer, and advances in imaging, epidemiology and, most recently, minimally invasive diagnostic and surgical techniques, have taken place. These advances have allowed the diagnosis and treatment of thyroid diseases to become rapid, cost-effective, and low-morbidity procedures.

## ANATOMY

### Embryology

The tissue bud that ultimately becomes the thyroid gland arises initially as a midline diverticulum in the floor of the pharynx. This tissue originates in the primitive alimentary tract and consists of cells of endodermal origin. The main portion of this cellular structure descends into the neck and develops into a bilobed solid organ. The original attachment in the pharynx is in the buccal cavity at the foramen cecum. This structure becomes the thyroglossal duct, which is usually reabsorbed after 6 weeks of age. The very distal end of this remnant may be retained and mature as a pyramidal lobe in the adult thyroid.

Microscopic thyroid follicles first appear as the lateral lobes develop. When the embryo is about 6 cm in length, these follicles begin to develop colloid. In the third month, the follicular cells first demonstrate iodine trapping and thyroid hormone secretion begins. Calcitonin-producing C cells arise from the fourth pharyngeal pouch and migrate from the neural crest into the lateral aspects of the thyroid lobes. These cells migrate into the lateral and posterior upper two thirds of the thyroid lobes and are distributed among the follicles. In adults, they remain limited to the upper and middle areas of the gland, usually in the posterior and medial aspects. These C cells are the only component of the adult gland that is not of endodermal origin.

Knowledge of basic embryology is essential for understanding certain embryologic congenital malformations, including thyroglossal duct cysts and fistulae, which result from retained tissue along the path of descent of the thyroid. A lingual thyroid is another anomaly that occurs when the median thyroid anlage does not descend in a normal fashion. In unusual circumstances, ectopic thyroid tissue can be found in the central compartment of the neck. Small amounts of ectopic tissue may be located under the lower poles of a normal thyroid and, occasionally, in the anterior mediastinum. Historically, the thyroid tissue described in lateral neck compartments was known as lateral aberrant thyroid tissue and was explained as an embryologic variation. This concept has essentially been disproved, and it is believed that thyroid tissue found in the neck lateral to the jugular vein represents metastatic deposits from well-differentiated thyroid carcinoma, typically papillary cancer, and may be the initial presentation of this disease. Small thyroid follicles located at the periphery of central neck lymph nodes may occasionally occur in the absence of thyroid cancer.

### Adult Surgical Anatomy

A normally developed adult thyroid weighs 10 to 20 g; it is a bilobed structure that lies next to the thyroid cartilage in a position anterior and lateral to the junction of the larynx and trachea. In this position, the thyroid encircles approximately 75% of the diameter of the junction of the larynx and upper part of the trachea. The lobes lie lateral to the trachea and esophagus, anteromedial to the carotid sheath and posteromedial to the sternocleidomastoid, sternohyoid, and sternothyroid muscles. The two lateral lobes are joined at the midline by an isthmus, whose superior edge is situated at or just below the cricoid cartilage. A pyramidal lobe is present in about 30% of patients and represents the most distal portion of the thyroglossal duct. In an adult, it may be a prominent structure that can extend from the midline of the isthmus as far cephalad as the hyoid bone.

A thin layer of connective tissue surrounds the thyroid. This tissue is part of the fascial layer that invests the trachea. This fascia is different from the thyroid capsule and, during surgery, can easily be separated from the capsule, whereas the true capsule of the thyroid cannot. This fascia coalesces with the thyroid capsule posteriorly and laterally to form a suspensory ligament known as the ligament of Berry, which is the primary point of fixation of the thyroid to surrounding structures. The ligament of Berry is closely attached to the cricoid cartilage and has important surgical implications because of its relationship to the recurrent laryngeal nerve.

## Laryngeal Nerves

### Recurrent Laryngeal Nerve

The recurrent laryngeal nerves (Fig. 38-1) ascend on either side of the trachea and each lies just lateral to the ligament of Berry as it enters the larynx. There are a number of important variations. In about 25% of patients, the recurrent laryngeal nerve is contained within the ligament as it enters the larynx. On the right side, the recurrent laryngeal nerve originates from the vagus nerve as it crosses the subclavian artery; it then passes posterior to the subclavian artery and ascends in a position lateral to the trachea along the tracheoesophageal groove. During neck dissection, the right recurrent laryngeal nerve can usually be found no further than 1 cm lateral to or within the tracheoesophageal groove, at the level of the lower border of the thyroid. As it ascends to the midportion of the thyroid, however, the nerve assumes its position within the tracheoesophageal groove. At this location, the nerve might divide into one, two, or more branches as it enters the first or second ring of the trachea, with the most important branch disappearing beneath the inferior border of the cricothyroid muscle. The nerve can usually be found immediately anterior or posterior to a main arterial trunk of the inferior thyroid artery at this level. Unusually, a nonrecurrent right laryngeal nerve can arise directly from the vagus and course medially into the larynx. This nonrecurrent anatomy is found in 0.5% to 1.5% of patients and occurs in the setting of arterial anomalies, most commonly an aberrant right subclavian artery (arteria lusoria), which could potentially be predicted from vascular findings on preoperative neck ultrasound prior to cervical exploration.[1] There have also been reports of patients who have both a recurrent and nonrecurrent laryngeal nerve on the right. These two nerves usually would join in a position beneath the lower border of the thyroid.[2]

On the left side, the recurrent laryngeal nerve separates from the vagus as that nerve traverses the arch of the aorta. The left recurrent laryngeal nerve then passes inferiorly and medially to the aorta at the ligamentum arteriosum and begins to ascend toward the larynx, where it enters the tracheoesophageal groove as it ascends to the level of the lower lobe of the thyroid. A nonrecurrent left laryngeal nerve is associated with more extensive and less common arch and great vessel anomalies than those associated with nonrecurrent right laryngeal nerves and is therefore rare.[1]

Both recurrent laryngeal nerves are consistently found within the tracheoesophageal groove when they are within 2.5 cm of their entrance into the larynx. These nerves pass inferior or posterior to an arterial branch of the inferior thyroid artery and eventually enter the larynx at the level of the cricothyroid articulation, on the caudal border of the cricothyroid muscle. At this level, the nerve courses immediately adjacent to the superior parathyroid gland, inferior thyroid artery, and posteriormost aspect of the thyroid. Great care is needed during surgical dissection in this area because the nerve is essentially tethered as it dives beneath the cricothyroid muscle and can be

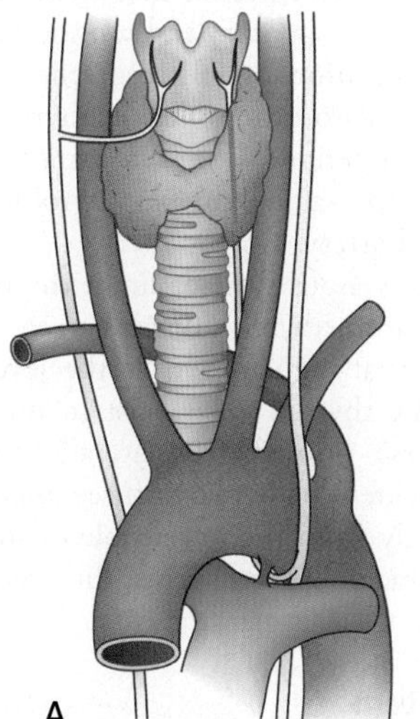


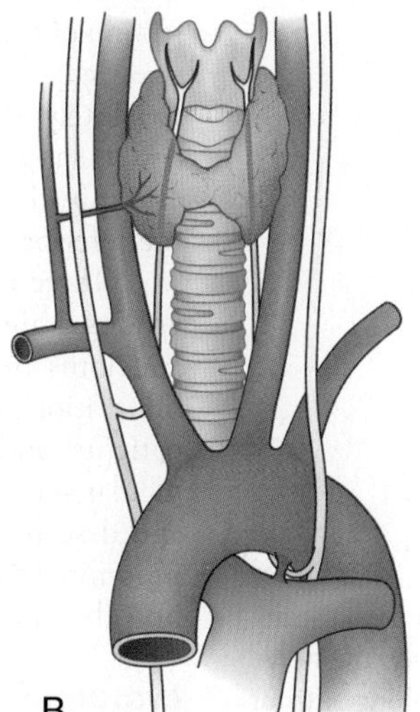


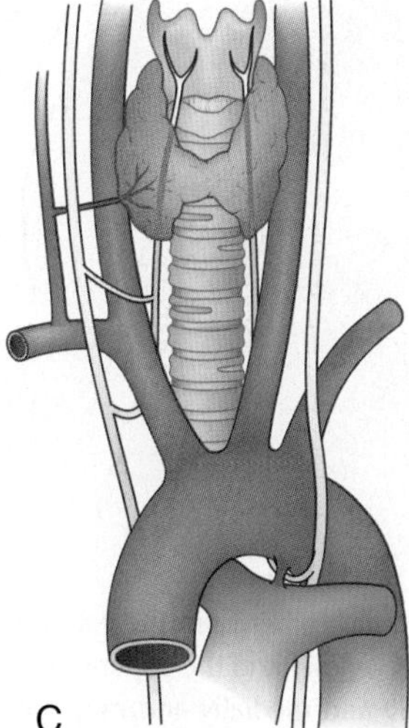


**FIGURE 38-1** Anomalous variations in the course of the right recurrent laryngeal nerve. **A,** A nonrecurrent laryngeal nerve arises from the vagus and courses medially into the larynx in the setting of an aberrant origin of the right subclavian artery. **B,** The normal course of the recurrent laryngeal nerve arises from the vagus after it passes beneath the subclavian artery. **C,** The unusual coexistence of the nonrecurrent and the recurrent laryngeal nerve join to form a common distal nerve.

stretched by overly vigorous dissection. A small branch of the inferior laryngeal artery crosses the nerve at the level of the ligament of Berry, so bleeding in this area should be addressed with great caution to avoid nerve injury.

The recurrent laryngeal nerve has mixed motor, sensory, and autonomic functions and innervates the intrinsic laryngeal muscles. Damage to a recurrent laryngeal nerve results in mixed pathology, the most important of which is paralysis of the vocal cord on the side affected. Such damage might result in a cord that remains in a medial position or just lateral to the midline. A normal voice, albeit weakened, can still be present if the remaining functioning contralateral cord is able to approximate the paralyzed cord. If the vocal cord remains paralyzed in an abducted position and closure cannot occur, a severely impaired voice and ineffective cough can result. If the recurrent laryngeal nerves are damaged bilaterally, complete loss of voice or airway obstruction may occur and possibly require emergency intubation and tracheostomy. Occasionally, bilateral damage can result in cords taking an abducted position, which, although allowing airway movement, may result in upper respiratory infection because of ineffective cough and aspiration.[2]

### Superior Laryngeal Nerve

The superior laryngeal nerve (Fig. 38-2) separates from the vagus nerve at the base of the skull and descends toward the superior pole of the thyroid along the internal carotid artery. At the level of the hyoid cornu, it divides into two branches. The larger internal branch has sensory function and enters the thyrohyoid membrane, where it innervates the larynx. The smaller external branch continues to travel along the lateral surface of the inferior pharyngeal constrictor muscle and usually descends anteriorly and medially, along with the superior thyroid artery. Within 1 cm of the entrance of the superior thyroid artery into the thyroid capsule, the nerve generally takes a medial course and enters the cricothyroid muscle, which it innervates. This relationship is important because during thyroid lobectomy, the external branch is not usually visualized because it has already entered the inferior pharyngeal muscle fascia. This nerve is at risk of being severed or entrapped, however, if the superior pole vessels are ligated at too great a distance above the superior pole of the thyroid. Damage to the external branch can result in severe loss of voice quality or strength. Although such loss may not be as clinically devastating as recurrent laryngeal nerve damage, it is extremely bothersome to patients whose occupation demands good voice quality.[2]

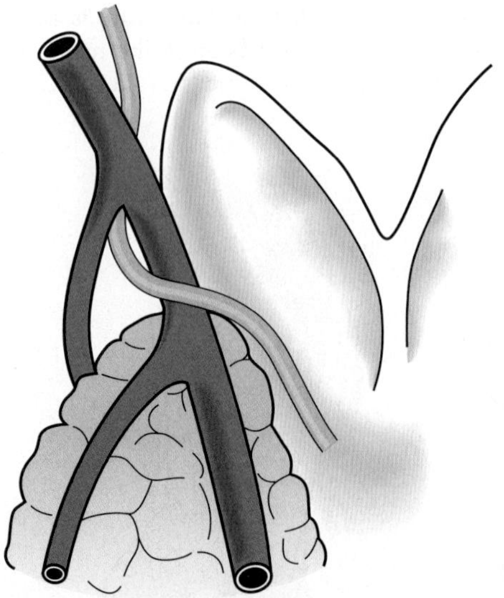

**FIGURE 38-2** Relationship between the external branch of the superior laryngeal nerve *(yellow)* and the superior thyroid artery. The nerve can course inferiorly and medially and may run partly along with or around the artery or branches of the artery as they enter the superior lobe of the thyroid. (From Duh QY: Surgical anatomy and embryology of the thyroid and parathyroid glands and recurrent and external laryngeal nerves. In Clark OH, Duh QY [eds]: Textbook of endocrine surgery, Philadelphia, 1997, WB Saunders, p 11.)

## Blood Supply

The arterial supply to the thyroid gland consists of four main arteries, two superior and two inferior. The superior thyroid artery is the first branch of the external carotid artery and arises immediately above the bifurcation of the common carotid artery. The superior thyroid artery gives off the superior laryngeal artery, courses medially onto the surface of the inferior pharyngeal constrictor muscle, and enters the apex of the superior pole. As the superior thyroid artery proceeds medially, it is adjacent to the external branch of the superior laryngeal nerve, and thus care must be taken to not damage it when controlling the artery (see Fig. 38-2).

The inferior thyroid artery takes its origin from the thyrocervical trunk. This artery originates from the subclavian artery and ascends into the neck on either side behind the carotid sheath, arches medially, and enters the thyroid gland posteriorly, usually near the ligament of Berry. There is generally no direct arterial supply that enters the thyroid inferiorly. However, a thyroidea ima artery may be present in less than 5% of patients and usually arises directly from the innominate artery or from the aorta.

The inferior thyroid artery has important anatomic relationships. The recurrent laryngeal nerve is usually directly adjacent (in an anterior or posterior position) to the inferior thyroid artery, within 1 cm of its entrance into the larynx. Careful dissection of the artery is mandatory and cannot be completed until knowledge of the position of the recurrent laryngeal nerve is absolutely defined. Also, the inferior thyroid artery almost always supplies the superior and inferior parathyroid glands, and care must be taken to evaluate the parathyroids after division of the inferior thyroid artery.

Three pairs of venous systems drain the thyroid. Superior venous drainage is immediately adjacent to the superior arteries and joins the internal jugular vein at the level of the carotid bifurcation. Middle thyroid veins exist in more than 50% of patients and course immediately laterally into the internal jugular vein. There are usually two or three inferior thyroid veins and descend directly from the lower pole of the gland into the innominate and brachiocephalic veins; they veins often descend into the tail of the thymus gland.

## Lymphatic System

The relationship of the thyroid gland to its lymphatic drainage is most important when considering surgical treatment of thyroid carcinoma. The thyroid gland and its neighboring structures have rich lymphatics that drain the thyroid in almost every direction. Within the gland, lymphatic channels are present immediately beneath the capsule and communicate between lobes through the isthmus. This drainage connects to structures directly adjacent to the thyroid, with numerous lymphatic channels into the regional lymph nodes. Clinically, it is useful to divide the lymph nodes between the central and lateral neck; the boundary between them is marked by the carotid sheath. The lateral neck zones are further subdivided (Fig. 38-3). Most thyroid cancers drain directly to central nodal basins (level VI), except those in the superior third of the gland, which may drain directly to the lateral compartment. These regional lymph nodes occupy a pretracheal position immediately superior to the isthmus, paratracheal nodes, tracheoesophageal groove lymph nodes, mediastinal nodes in the anterior and superior position, jugular lymph nodes in the upper, middle, and lower distribution, and retropharyngeal and esophageal lymph nodes. Laterally, cervical lymph nodes within the posterior triangle may be involved in patients with widespread thyroid cancer (levels II, III, IV). Also, lymph nodes within the submaxillary triangle may be involved. Papillary carcinoma of the thyroid is commonly associated with adjacent nodal metastasis and medullary carcinoma has a strong predilection for metastatic lymphatic involvement, generally within the central compartment (level VI).

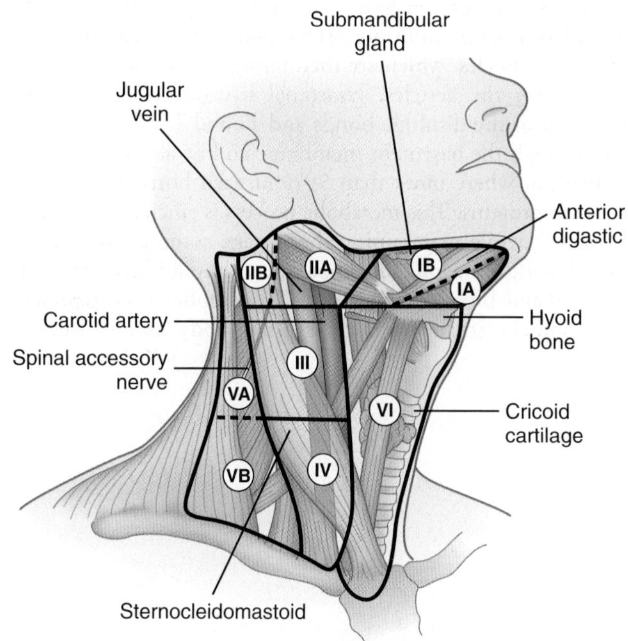


**FIGURE 38-3** Lymph node compartments separated into levels and sublevels. Level VI contains the thyroid gland and the adjacent nodes bordered superiorly by the hyoid bone, inferiorly by the innominate (brachiocephalic) artery, and laterally on each side by the carotid sheaths. The level II, III, and IV nodes are arrayed along the jugular veins on each side, bordered anteromedially by level VI and laterally by the posterior border of the sternocleidomastoid muscle. The level III nodes are bounded superiorly by the level of the hyoid bone, and inferiorly by the cricoid cartilage; levels II and IV are above and below level III, respectively. The level I node compartment includes the submental and submandibular nodes, above the hyoid bone, and anterior to the posterior edge of the submandibular gland. Finally, the level V nodes are in the posterior triangle, lateral to the lateral edge of the sternocleidomastoid muscle. Levels I, II, and V can be further subdivided as noted in the figure. The inferior extent of level VI is defined as the suprasternal notch. Many authors also include the pretracheal and paratracheal superior mediastinal lymph nodes above the level of the innominate artery (sometimes referred to as level VII) in central neck dissection.

### Parathyroid Glands

The thyroid sheath encases the lateral and posterior portion of each thyroid lobe and, as such, frequently provides a covering for the superior parathyroid gland. When the superior portion of the thyroid lobe is dissected and rolled medially, an area containing fat beneath this fascia is apparent. The superior parathyroid gland almost always lies within this fatty area, beneath the thyroid sheath in a posterior position relative to the superior part of the thyroid lobe. The inferior parathyroid gland may also be located within the thyroid sheath on the posterior aspect of the lower portion of the lobe and, like the superior gland, is usually encased in a small amount of fat. The position of the inferior parathyroid is more variable, however, and can be located along the branches of the inferior thyroid vein lateral or inferior to the lowermost portion of the thyroid lobe. Because of the similar consistency and color of the parathyroids and the fat that surrounds them, parathyroids in both positions are most easily found by following the smaller branches of the inferior thyroid artery into the parathyroid substance.

The superior and inferior parathyroid glands have a single end artery that supplies them medially from the inferior thyroid artery. If the main trunk of the inferior thyroid artery is sacrificed for dissection, both parathyroids on that side become devascularized because there is usually no collateral blood supply to maintain viability. Careful dissection should attempt to divide only the branches of the inferior thyroid entering the thyroid capsule during excision. With careful technique, good vascular supply to the superior and inferior parathyroid can be maintained, even when total thyroidectomy is performed. In some cases, there may be arterial supply to the superior parathyroid from the superior thyroid artery, although this generally does not occur.

## PHYSIOLOGY OF THE THYROID GLAND

The thyroid gland weighs 10 to 20 g in normal adults and is responsible for the production of two families of metabolic hormones, the thyroid hormones, thyroxine ($T_4$) and triiodothyronine ($T_3$), and the calcium-regulating hormone, calcitonin. The spherical thyroid follicular unit is the important site of thyroid hormone production. The follicular unit is made up of a single layer of cuboidal follicular cells that encompass a central depository of colloid filled mostly with thyroglobulin (Tg), the protein in which $T_4$ and $T_3$ are synthesized and stored.

### Iodine Metabolism

Iodine is essential for the production of thyroid hormones. It can be efficiently absorbed from the gastrointestinal (GI) tract in the form of inorganic iodide and rapidly enters the extracellular iodide pool. The thyroid gland is responsible for storing 90% of total body iodide at any given time, with less than 10% existing in the extracellular pool. Iodide is stored in the thyroid as preformed thyroid hormone or as an iodinated amino acid.

Iodide is transported from the extracellular space into the follicular cells against a chemical and electrical gradient via an intrinsic transmembrane protein located in the basolateral membrane of the thyroid follicular cells.[3] Once inside the cells, iodide rapidly diffuses to the apical surface, where it is quickly moved to exocytic vesicles. Here, it is rapidly oxidized and bound to Tg. Transport of iodide into follicular cells is regulated by thyroid-stimulating hormone (TSH) from the pituitary gland, as well as by the follicular content of iodide.

The relationship between iodine ingestion and thyroid disease has been known for more than 100 years. At the turn of the 20th century, the practice of iodine supplementation of food and water came about as a result of careful study in areas in which iodine insufficiency was found and linked to endemic goiter. Significant iodine deficiency still occurs in various undeveloped parts of the world. Surprisingly, an evaluation of urinary iodine excretion in the U.S. population in 1998 indicated that a substantial number of people were currently iodine-deficient here as well.[4] Iodine deficiency can result in nodular goiter, hypothyroidism, and cretinism, and possibly the development of follicular thyroid carcinoma (FTC). The World Health Organization has been involved in providing dietary iodine supplementation to treat entire populations in certain areas of the world. In situations in which iodine excess occurs, disorders such as Graves' disease and Hashimoto's thyroiditis can occur.

## Thyroid Hormone Synthesis

Once organic iodide is efficiently oxidized and bound, it couples to Tg with tyrosine moieties to form iodotyrosines in a single conformation (monoiodotyrosine [MIT]) or a coupled conformation (diiodotyrosine [DIT]; Fig. 38-4). The formation of DIT and MIT is dependent on an important intracellular catalytic agent, thyroid peroxidase, which has been well characterized and is an integral part of the initial process of organification and storage of inorganic iodide. This enzyme, along with Tg, is remarkably specific to the thyroid follicular cells, making both important in the diagnosis and management of autoimmune thyroid disease and well-differentiated thyroid cancer.

MIT and DIT are biologically inert. Coupling of these two residues gives rise to the two biologically active thyroid hormones, $T_4$ and $T_3$. $T_4$ is formed by the coupling of two molecules of DIT, whereas $T_3$ is formed by the coupling of one molecule of MIT with one molecule of DIT. In normal circumstances, formation of $T_4$ predominates. Both $T_3$ and $T_4$ are bound to Tg and stored in the colloid in the center of the follicular unit, which allows quicker secretion of the hormones than if they had to be synthesized de novo. This rapid and metabolically active process normally results in the storage of about 2 weeks' worth of thyroid hormone in the organism under normal circumstances.[5] Most thyroid hormone released from the thyroid gland is $T_4$, which is deiodinated in peripheral extrathyroidal tissues and converted to $T_3$.

Release of $T_4$ and $T_3$ is regulated by the apical membrane of the follicular cell via lysosomal hydrolysis of the colloid that contains the Tg-bound hormones. The apical membrane of the thyroid cell forms multiple pseudopodia and incorporates Tg into small vesicles, which are then brought into the cell apparatus. Within the vesicles, lysosomal hydrolysis results in the reduction of the disulfide bonds and $T_3$ and $T_4$ are then free to pass through the basement membrane and be absorbed into the circulation, where more than 99% of each hormone is bound to serum proteins. This metabolic process is efficient in releasing $T_3$ and $T_4$ while maintaining the storage components, Tg and colloid, within the follicular apparatus. Although sensitive assays of peripheral blood can measure Tg, peripheral Tg represents an extremely small fraction of total body stores. Residual

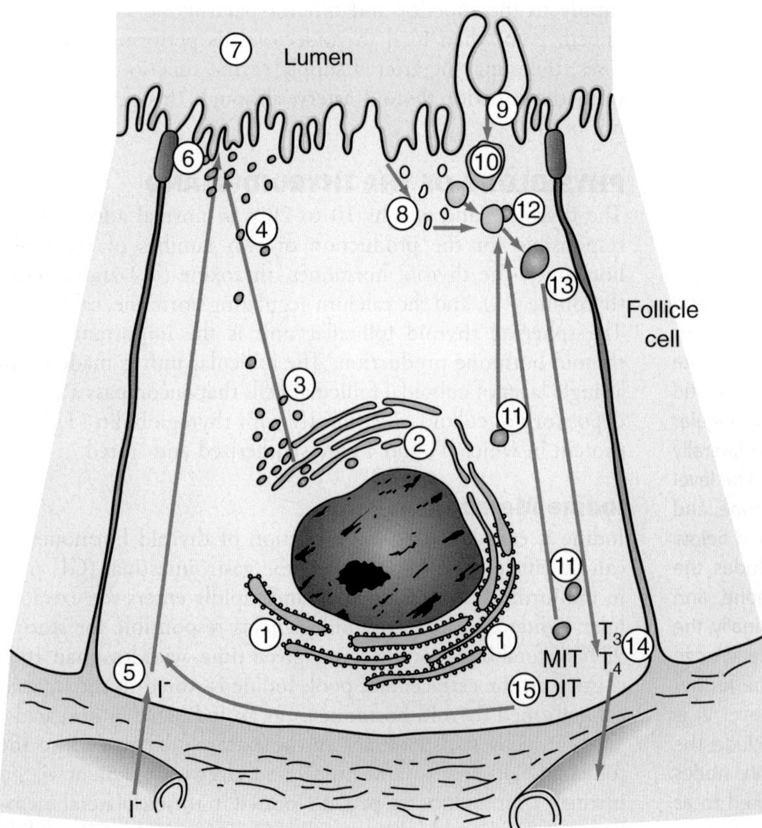


**FIGURE 38-4** Diagrammatic scheme of thyroid hormone formation and secretion. 1, Tg and protein synthesis in the rough endoplasmic reticulum. 2, Coupling of the Tg carbohydrate units in the smooth endoplasmic reticulum and Golgi apparatus. 3, Formation of exocytotic vesicles. 4, Transport of exocytotic vesicles with noniodinated Tg to the apical surface of the follicle cell and into the follicular lumen. 5, Iodide transport at the basal cell membrane. 6, Iodide oxidation, Tg iodination, and coupling of iodotyrosyl to iodothyronyl residues. 7, Storage of iodinated Tg in the follicular lumen. 8, Endocytosis by micropinocytosis. 9, Endocytosis by macropinocytosis (pseudopods). 10, Colloid droplets. 11, Lysosome migrating to the apical pole. 12, Fusion of lysosomes with colloid droplets. 13, Phagolysosomes with Tg hydrolysis. 14, $T_3$ and $T_4$ secretion. 15, MIT and DIT deiodination.

iodotyrosines undergo peripheral breakdown, deiodination, and recycling and can then be added to the recently absorbed iodide stores and become available for the synthesis of new thyroid hormone (Fig. 38-5).[5]

### Thyroglobulin

Tg is a 660-kDa glycoprotein specific to the follicular cell that is the primary component of the colloid matrix necessary for iodination and hormonogenesis. Tg facilitates the conversion of MIT and DIT into $T_3$ and $T_4$. This process is accompanied by the escape of small amounts of Tg into the peripheral bloodstream, where it can be assayed. TSH enhances the whole process of endocytosis, proteolysis, and release through an adenylate cyclase system. Excess peripheral levels of iodine inhibit further release by enhancing Tg resistance to proteolysis.

Peripheral Tg can be measured to evaluate benign or malignant thyroid neoplasms. Measurement of peripheral Tg has predictive value for the recurrence of well-differentiated thyroid carcinoma, locally or in metastatic deposits after initial total thyroidectomy.[6] However, the usefulness of measuring serum Tg levels prior to the initial resection of a known or suspected well-differentiated thyroid cancer is unknown and its routine measurement is not recommended.[7]

### Calcitonin

Calcitonin is a 32–amino acid polypeptide secreted by the parafollicular cells, or C cells, located superolaterally in each thyroid lobe. Calcitonin acts principally to inhibit calcium absorption by osteoclasts and thereby to lower peripheral serum calcium levels. Increased peripheral levels of serum calcium stimulate calcitonin secretion. Calcitonin secretion can be stimulated clinically by the infusion of calcium, pentagastrin, and alcohol.

The specific action of calcitonin takes place on the surface receptors of osteoclasts but its effect does not result in a clinically apparent marked decrease in calcium levels. In fact, patients with clinical calcitonin excess syndromes, such as medullary carcinoma of the thyroid (MTC), usually have little alteration in peripheral calcium metabolism. Basal or stimulated calcitonin levels are sensitive markers for primary or recurrent MTC.

## Regulation of Thyroid Hormone Secretion

The hypothalamic-pituitary-thyroid axis regulates thyroid hormone production and release in a classic endocrine feedback system. The major regulator of thyroid gland activity is the glycoprotein TSH, which is a major growth factor for the thyroid. TSH stimulates thyroid cell growth and differentiation, as well as iodine uptake and organification and release of $T_3$ and $T_4$ from Tg. Also, TSH has been shown to stimulate the growth and invasive characteristics of some well-differentiated thyroid cancer cell lines in vitro.

TSH is a 28-kDa glycoprotein secreted in a pulsatile fashion by the anterior pituitary gland. It has two components; the α subunit is common to other anterior pituitary hormones but the β subunit is unique to TSH and determines the hormone's biologic specificity. Once TSH activates the receptor (TSH-R), it interacts with a guanine nucleotide–binding protein (G protein), stimulating the production of cyclic adenosine monophosphate (cAMP). This cAMP pathway is an important hormone-synthesizing event. Receptors coupled with G proteins have seven transmembrane-spanning domains, with cytoplasmic and extracellular loops. The first three of these cytoplasmic loops have important relationships in mediating the TSH-dependent increase in cAMP production and therefore in stimulating

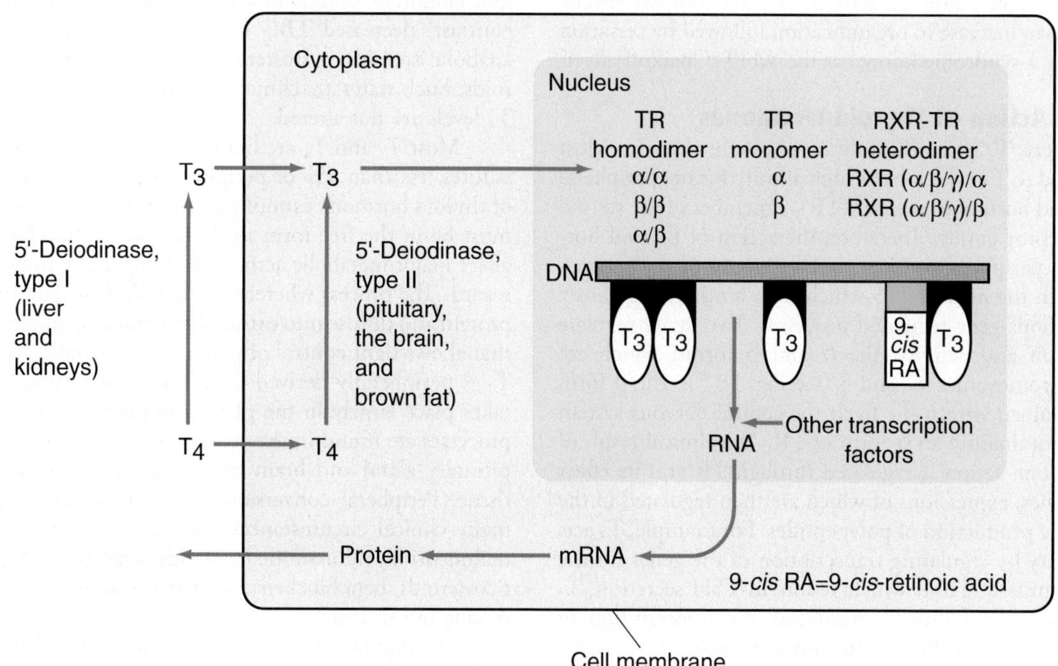


**FIGURE 38-5** Cellular and molecular events involved in thyroid hormone function. $T_4$ is converted in the periphery and in the cytoplasm of the cell into $T_3$. $T_3$ travels to the nucleus, where it binds to the thyroid hormone receptor (TR; homodimer, monomer, or heterodimer). TR binding leads to RNA transcription in association with other transcription factors; messenger RNA is subsequently expressed and then translated into protein.

thyroid hormone production. The receptors that respond to TSH have been identified and cloned. Specific mutations in the genetics of this system have been identified and are associated with follicular thyroid neoplasms.[8]

The feedback loop is an important regulator of TSH secretion. Increased thyrotropin-releasing hormone (TRH) from the paraventricular nucleus of the hypothalamus and reduced levels of $T_3$ stimulate release of TSH from the anterior pituitary. TRH is a three–amino acid peptide that passes through the hypothalamic portal system into the median eminence and through the pituitary stalk to the anterior pituitary. Peripheral thyroid hormone levels may, in addition to stimulating release of TSH from the anterior pituitary, enhance TRH secretion.

Many pathologic states result in increased peripheral levels of $T_3$ and $T_4$, which decrease TSH secretion by a negative feedback loop. Peripheral $T_4$ is locally deiodinated in the pituitary and converted to $T_3$, which then directly inhibits the release and synthesis of TSH. The condition that usually decreases TSH secretion is classified as primary hyperthyroidism. It has many causes, including many types of thyroiditis, Graves' disease, autonomously functioning thyroid nodules, and conditions that increase human chorionic gonadotrophin (hCG) levels, such as gynecologic malignancies and overuse of exogenous thyroid hormone. Decreased levels of TSH can also be caused by abnormalities at the level of the pituitary and/or hypothalamus, which are collectively termed *central hypothyroidism.* These conditions are much rarer than primary hyperthyroidism.

Although TSH is the primary regulator of thyroid hormone synthesis, intrinsic autoregulatory mechanisms are alternative routes whereby the thyroid can control intraglandular stores of thyroid hormones. In areas in which dietary iodide is excessive, the thyroid gland has an autoregulated process that inhibits the uptake of iodide into follicular cells. The reverse is true in iodide deficiency. Excessively large doses of iodide have complex effects. These include an increase in organification followed by cessation of production, a syndrome known as the Wolff- Chaikoff effect.

## Peripheral Action of Thyroid Hormones

In the periphery, $T_3$ is significantly more potent than $T_4$. Most $T_4$ is converted to $T_3$, which has a high affinity for the peripheral nuclear thyroid hormone receptor (TR), a member of the steroid hormone receptor family. Therefore, the action of thyroid hormones in the periphery consists predominantly of the interaction of $T_3$ with the nuclear TR, which then binds to regulatory regions in various gene-regulated processes. Two genes regulate TR production and activity, the $\alpha$ and $\beta$ forms, which are located on chromosomes 17 and 3 (see Fig. 38-5). The $\beta$ form of TR is contained within the liver; the central nervous system contains predominantly an $\alpha$ form of TR. The clinical result of thyroid hormone action is regulated through TR and its effect on various genes, expressions of which are then regulated in the nucleus via the production of polypeptides. For example, $T_3$ acts on the pituitary by regulating transcription of the genes for the $\alpha$ and $\beta$ subunits of TSH, which results in TSH secretion. $T_3$ affects cardiac contractility by regulating the transcription of myosin heavy chain production in cardiac muscle.

Of circulating $T_3$ and $T_4$, 80% is bound to thyroxine-binding globulin (TBG) in the periphery. A number of medications and clinical scenarios alter serum levels of TBG or the affinity of TBG for circulating thyroid hormone (Box 38-1). Also, $T_4$ is bound to prealbumin and albumin. In pregnancy and

**BOX 38-1 Drugs Affecting Thyroid Hormone Serum Transport Proteins**

**Increased TBG Concentration**
Estrogen
Heroin, methadone
Clofibrate
5-Fluorouracil
Tamoxifen

**Decreased TBG Concentration**
Androgens and anabolic steroids
Glucocorticoids
Nicotinic acid

**Interfere with Binding to TBG**
Salicylates
Carbamazepine
Diazepam
Furosemide
Sulfonylureas
NSAIDs
Heparin (IV)
Enoxaparin

Adapted from Degroot LJ, Jameson JL: Endocrinology, ed 5, Philadelphia, 2005, Elsevier Saunders.

other clinical situations with elevated estrogen levels, such as oral contraceptives, menopausal estrogen replacement therapy, and tamoxifen or raloxifene use (selective estrogen receptor modulators), TBG levels are significantly increased, thereby resulting in higher levels of bound $T_4$ (total) in the periphery. Other causes of increased TBG concentrations include heroine or methadone use, clofibrate, and 5-flurouracil (chemotherapeutic agent). In contrast, decreased TBG levels are caused by agents such as anabolic steroids (testosterone), nicotinic acid, and corticosteroids. Such states are clinically euthyroid, however, because free $T_4$ levels are not altered.

Most $T_3$ and $T_4$ are bound to the extent that free $T_4$ constitutes less than 1% of peripheral hormone. The bound form of thyroid hormone cannot pass from the extracellular space and must be in the free form to diffuse into extracellular tissues to affect major metabolic activity. $T_3$ is especially important in this regard. The process whereby $T_3$ and $T_4$ dissociate from binding protein and diffuse into extracellular tissues is an efficient process that allows tight control of peripheral metabolic activities. Most $T_3$ is peripherally derived from the deiodination of $T_4$, which takes place largely in the plasma and liver. Other deiodination processes are found in the central nervous system, especially the pituitary gland and brain tissues, as well as in brown adipose tissue. Peripheral conversion of $T_4$ to $T_3$ can be impaired in many clinical circumstances, such as overwhelming sepsis and malnutrition, thionamide (propylthiouracil) use, high-dose corticosteroids, beta blockers, iodinated contrast agents, and amiodarone use (Box 38-2).

The half-life of $T_3$ is approximately 8 to 12 hours and free levels disappear rapidly from the peripheral circulation. In adults, the half-life of $T_4$ is approximately 7 days because of the efficient and significant degree of binding to carrier proteins. Therefore, thyroid hormones generally have a slow turnover time in the peripheral circulation and the body is ensured of at least

**BOX 38-2 Agents Affecting Extrathyroidal Metabolism of the Thyroid Hormone**

**Inhibit Conversion of $T_4$ to $T_3$**
Propylthiouracil (PTU)
Glucocorticoids
Propranolol
Interleukin-6
Iodinated contrast agents
Amiodarone
Clomipramine

**Stimulate Thyroid Hormone Degradation**
Diphenylhydantoin
Carbamazepine
Phenobarbital
Rifampin
Ritonavir
Sertraline

**Decrease GI Absorption of Thyroid Hormone**
Cholestyramine
Calcium carbonate
Ferrous dulfate
Sucralfate
Aluminum hydroxide

Adapted from Degroot LJ, Jameson JL: Endocrinology, ed 5, Philadelphia, 2005, Elsevier Saunders.

a 7- to 10-day supply of $T_4$ available for peripheral metabolism. A number of medications are known to stimulate the degradation of thyroid hormone (see Box 38-2).

### Inhibition of Thyroid Synthesis

**Drugs** Antithyroid medications are an option for the treatment of thyroid excess states. The thionamide class of antithyroid drugs includes propylthiouracil (PTU) and methimazole (Tapazole). This class of drugs acts by inhibiting the organification and oxidation of inorganic iodine, as well as by inhibiting linkage of the initial iodotyrosine molecules MIT and DIT. In addition to these effects, PTU inhibits the peripheral conversion of $T_4$ to $T_3$. Because of this added capability, PTU is a popular choice for the rapid treatment of hyperthyroid conditions. Methimazole has longer activity and requires a single daily dose; it is the preferred agent in nonpregnant individuals. Both drugs can cause agranulocytosis but this occurs in less than 1% of cases. Other side effects include rash, arthralgias, neuritis, and liver dysfunction (potentially worse with PTU).

Exogenous glucocorticoids can effectively suppress the pituitary-thyroid axis. Also, they can act in the periphery to inhibit the peripheral conversion of $T_4$ to $T_3$. This effectively lowers serum $T_3$ levels, thus allowing steroids to be used as a rapid inhibitory agent for hyperthyroid conditions. Steroids can also lower serum TSH concentration. The rapid action of steroids makes them a potentially important primary treatment of severe, previously untreated, or resistant hyperthyroidism; however, they are not without potential side effects.

Patients with thyrotoxicosis have increased adrenergic stimulation. Although beta blockers do not directly inhibit thyroid hormone synthesis per se, they are valuable in controlling peripheral sensitivity to catecholamines by blocking their effects. Therefore, cardiovascular symptoms such as an increased pulse rate, tremor, and anxiety can be improved, but the hypermetabolic state can remain or progress with this treatment alone.

**Iodine** Iodine, given in large doses after the administration of an antithyroid medication, can inhibit thyroid hormone release by altering the organic binding process (Wolff-Chaikoff effect). This stunning effect is transient, but iodine supplementation can be used to treat hyperactivity of the gland in preparation for surgery.

## Tests of Thyroid Function

### Evaluation of the Pituitary-Thyroid Feedback Loop

Measurement of serum TSH by an ultrasensitive radioimmunoassay (RIA) is an important screening test for the diagnosis of thyroid dysfunction. This assay is especially important for the delineation of hypothyroidism and hyperthyroidism from euthyroid states. Because of its sensitivity, TSH values can detect thyroid dysfunction before clinical manifestations are noted (e.g., subclinical hypothyroidism or hyperthyroidism). The sensitivity of the TSH assay is less affected by nonthyroidal disease processes and remains unaffected by changes in thyroid hormone–binding proteins.

### Serum Triiodothyronine and Thyroxine Levels

Thyroid production is initially screened by measuring serum free $T_4$ and $T_3$ levels directly by RIA. Assays for total $T_4$ and $T_3$, which measure free and protein-bound hormone, can be affected by changes in hormone production or hormone binding to serum proteins; therefore, accurate evaluation of thyroid function requires measurement of free $T_4$ and $T_3$ levels.

### Calcitonin

In patients with thyroid masses and in whom multiple endocrine neoplasia type 2 (MEN2) syndrome or isolated medullary carcinoma is suspected, a baseline calcitonin level can be obtained. If there is doubt about the diagnosis, pentagastrin- or calcium-stimulated calcitonin evaluation, a 4- to 5-hour test, can be performed. Also, calcitonin can be used as a screening test in families with MEN2 syndrome to document clinically inapparent disease. The routine use of calcitonin determination in the workup of thyroid nodules in otherwise nonsuspicious clinical scenarios is not cost-effective and is not recommended.

### Radioactive Iodine Uptake

Radioactive iodine uptake directly evaluates thyroid gland function; however, it has become less widely used because of more precise biochemical measurements of $T_3$, $T_4$, and TSH and improved thyroid ultrasonography. This test has involved the oral administration of iodine-123 ($^{123}I$) and calculated uptake with radioscintigraphy. A normal result is 15% to 30% uptake of the radionuclide after about 24 hours. A number of clinical situations alter the 24-hour uptake of radioiodine, leading to an abnormal result (Box 38-3). Use of $^{123}I$ is preferable because of its shorter half-life and lesser radiation exposure than with the use of $^{131}I$, which is used to radioablate thyroid neoplasms. Indications for the use of radioscintigraphy include the evaluation of a solitary thyroid nodule, thyroid remnant survey after surgery, detection of functioning thyroid cancer metastases, and evaluation of focal functional thyroid abnormalities.

**BOX 38-3 Factors Affecting 24-Hour Radioiodine Uptake**

**Increased Uptake**
Hyperthyroidism, including Graves' disease, toxic nodule, thyroid hormone resistance
Nontoxic goiter—Hashimoto's thyroiditis
Decreased renal clearance of iodine (renal insufficiency, severe heart failure)
Iodine deficiency (endemic or sporadic dietary, pregnancy)
TSH administration

**Decreased Uptake**
Hypothyroidism (primary or secondary)
TSH resistance
Thyroid hormone replacement, suppression
Iodine excess (dietary, drugs)

Adapted from Degroot LJ, Jameson JL: Endocrinology, ed 5, Philadelphia, 2005, Elsevier Saunders.

### Thyroid Autoantibody Levels

Thyroid antigens are produced in autoimmune thyroid disorders (thyroid-stimulating immunoglobulin [TSI], antimicrosomal and antithyroid peroxidase antibodies), including Graves' disease and Hashimoto's thyroiditis. Detection of autoantibodies can be extremely important if either of these autoimmune conditions is suspected. About 95% of patients with Hashimoto's thyroiditis and 80% with Graves' disease have detectable antimicrosomal antibodies. In Graves' disease, circulating antibodies have a high affinity for TSH-R on thyroid follicular cells. Assays now have greater sensitivity and may allow earlier detection of Graves' disease and more accurate monitoring of the effects of thyroid medication.

## DISORDERS OF THYROID METABOLISM—BENIGN THYROID DISEASE

## Hypothyroidism

A delicate balance between central production and peripheral action of $T_3$ and $T_4$ is required for a euthyroid state in the periphery. Clinical hypothyroidism is usually a result of failure of the thyroid to produce sufficient hormone (i.e., primary hypothyroidism), although states of limited activity or resistance to thyroid hormone in the periphery can also occur, although these are extremely rare. In many underdeveloped countries, lack of sufficient iodine intake results in a large proportion of hypothyroid conditions. In more developed countries, most cases of adult hypothyroidism are caused by Hashimoto's thyroiditis, radioactive iodine therapy, or surgical removal. An increasing number of commonly used pharmacologic agents also cause primary hypothyroidism.

### Metabolic Consequences of Iodine Deficiency

The chronic physiologic changes that result from a lifetime of iodine deficiency involve anatomic and metabolic alterations of varying significance. As a result of chronic deficient iodine intake, production of $T_4$ and $T_3$ is decreased, thereby resulting in gradually increasing thyroid clearance of iodine and decreased renal excretion. Chronic preferential production of $T_3$ rather than $T_4$ occurs, as well as enhanced peripheral conversion of $T_4$ to $T_3$. By making the production of $T_3$ and clearance of the metabolically active hormone as efficient as possible, clinical hypothyroidism is largely avoided by a biochemical pattern of low serum $T_4$ levels with elevated TSH levels and normal or above-normal levels of $T_3$. In the most severe cases, serum $T_3$ and $T_4$ concentrations are low and the serum TSH level is elevated. Iodine deficiency can lead to a preventable disease referred to as endemic goiter, which in its most severe form results in endemic cretinism. This clinical scenario includes neurologic impairment, stunted growth, mental deficiency, and overt hypothyroidism caused by profound iodine deficiency in utero.

Although countries in Southeast Asia, including India, Indonesia, and China, account for most of the total population of the world at risk for iodine deficiency (approximately 12 million), mild to moderate iodine deficiency can still be seen in a number of European countries, including Italy, Spain, Hungary, Poland, and Yugoslavia. In areas with the most severe iodine deficiency, clinical signs and symptoms of goiter appear at an earlier age.

The prevalence increases dramatically in the later childhood years, with a peak at puberty. The incidence of goiter decreases during adulthood but remains slightly higher in women. Diffuse enlargement of the thyroid gland often occurs, accompanying the physiologic changes in response to iodine deficiency. Thyroid follicles demonstrate a hypertrophic response, with a reduction in follicular spaces. As the iodine deficiency becomes more severe, follicles can become inactive and distended with colloid. Focal areas of nodular hyperplasia may develop and form nodules, some of which may become hot nodules and have an autonomous function. Others become inactive and inert. Necrosis, scarring, and hemorrhage can occur and result in fibrous ingrowth; all these disorders are accompanied by marked enlargement of the gland, often in an asymmetric pattern.

### Postradiation Hypothyroidism

Planned clinical hypothyroidism can be the result of treatment of certain disorders by $^{131}I$. This treatment has become increasingly popular for patients with hyperthyroid conditions, especially Graves' disease and toxic multinodular goiter. Between 50% and 70% of patients who receive more than 10 mCi are at risk of becoming clinically hypothyroid. For patients undergoing this type of treatment, continued thyroid monitoring is necessary, at least on an annual basis.

External beam mediastinal radiation for lymphoma or for head and neck cancer is associated with subclinical hypothyroidism. This becomes particularly important for patients who have previously undergone thyroid resection for a benign or malignant disease process.

### Postsurgical Hypothyroidism

If $^{131}I$ therapy is not available for patients with hyperthyroidism or Graves' disease, subtotal or total thyroidectomy effectively produces hypothyroidism. The incidence of permanent postoperative hypothyroidism varies with the skill of the operating surgeon and amount of thyroid that is ablated. The rate of complications, however, such as recurrent laryngeal nerve damage and hypocalcemia, is increased with more aggressive surgical ablation. Other factors affecting the postoperative development of hypothyroidism include antithyroid drug administration, dietary iodine availability, and lymphocytic infiltration of the remaining tissue.

### Pharmacologic Hypothyroidism

**Antithyroid Drugs** If administered in excess, methimazole and PTU can cause hypothyroidism. Careful monitoring of patients taking these drugs and understanding the disease process for which they are given are mandatory when managing these patients.

**Amiodarone, Lithium, Cytokines** Most drugs cause hypothyroidism by interfering with thyroid hormone release from the gland and/or direct toxicity to the thyroid itself. The commonly used antiarrythmic, amiodarone, is iodine-rich, containing 37% iodine by weight. Patients on amiodarone receive a 50- to 100-fold excess of iodine daily. In 14% to 18% of patients treated with amiodarone, there is clinically apparent thyroid dysfunction, which can be a hyperthyroid or hypothyroid state. Amiodarone induced thyrotoxicosis occurs more frequently in populations that are iodine-depletes at baseline, whereas in the United States, an area of higher iodine intake, hypothyroidism predominates.[9]

Amiodarone effects hypothyroidism via several mechanisms. It inhibits 5′-deiodinase activity, which results in a decreased conversion of $T_4$ to $T_3$, inhibits the entry of thyroid hormone into peripheral tissues, and has a direct cytotoxic effect on follicular cells. Patients with preexisting Hashimoto's thyroiditis are at particular risk for amiodarone-induced hypothyroidism and the large iodine load may cause an acute Wolff-Chaikoff effect. The presentation is that of clinical hypothyroidism; treatment consists of exogenous thyroid hormone administration.[9]

Although amiodarone-induced thyrotoxicosis is rare in the United States, it represents a clinical challenge when it occurs. The presentation often is not of typical hyperthyroidism, but rather may present as an exacerbation of the cardiac disease that is being treated with amiodarone. Depending on the specific presentation, treatment of amiodarone-induced thyrotoxicosis may include discontinuation of amiodarone, administration of methimazole or glucocorticoids, and potassium perchlorate. In patients for whom amiodarone withdrawal is not feasible and medical therapy is not successful, total thyroidectomy may be indicated.[9]

Lithium, still used to treat bipolar disorder, inhibits the cAMP-dependent pathway of hormone formation and may thereby inhibit the formation of thyroid hormone. Hypothyroidism in patients taking lithium is seen more frequently in those with underlying Hashimoto's thyroiditis, although it can occur in patients with normal thyroid function.

The effects of cytokines on the development of hypothyroidism may be the aggravation of an underlying thyroiditis. The exact nature of the effects of cytokines on the development of Hashimoto's thyroiditis is unclear. It is known that hypothyroidism can develop in patients undergoing treatment with interferon-alfa or interleukin-2 for hepatitis or certain malignant diseases; in such cases, the hypothyroidism is reversible with discontinuation of these drugs. This is particularly important for patients with underlying Hashimoto's thyroiditis, and taking a careful history is essential.

### Diagnosis

If primary hypothyroidism is suspected based on the clinical scenario, serum TSH and free $T_4$ levels should be assessed. These laboratory tests will demonstrate low free $T_4$ and elevated TSH levels.

### Treatment

Levothyroxine is a safe and effective treatment for hypothyroidism once the diagnosis has been made. It is available in oral, intramuscular, and IV preparations. The vast majority of patients can be treated with oral medication once daily. The initial dose is calculated according to the patient's weight. Patients with severe clinical hypothyroidism are monitored closely and gradually started on increasing doses because of sensitivity to the hormone as a result of chronic depletion of catecholamines in the myocardium, especially in older patients and those with a cardiac history.

## Thyroiditis

### Hashimoto's Thyroiditis

The major cause of hypothyroidism in the adult population is Hashimoto's thyroiditis, autoimmune-mediated destruction of thyrocytes. The disorder predominates in women (4 to 10 : 1 female preponderance). A complex immunologic phenomenon results in the formation of immune complexes and complement in the basement membrane of follicular cells. This leads to alterations in thyroid cell function that impair $T_3$ and $T_4$ production. These cellular reactions ultimately result in the infiltration of lymphocytes and resultant fibrosis, which decreases the number and efficiency of individual follicles. As this immune phenomenon continues, the presence of TSH-blocking antibodies can be detected. Thyroid peroxidase antibodies (anti-TPO Abs) are produced that are probably key mediators in the initial complement fixation process. As the immune process continues, changes in thyroid function can be altered by levels of these antibodies. Ultimately, a clinical hypothyroid state can occur in patients with persistent TSH-blocking antibodies.

### Acute Suppurative Thyroiditis

Acute suppurative thyroiditis is extremely rare and is usually the result of a severe pyogenic infection of the upper airway. The process results in severe localized pain and is generally unilateral. Abscess drainage followed by the administration of antibiotics is effective, and long-term deleterious effects on thyroid function are rare.

### Subacute Thyroiditis

Subacute thyroiditis occurs predominantly in women (2 : 1) in the United States, England, and Japan. The mean age of patients is in the 40s in most series. The exact cause is not known, although it is believed to have a viral or autoimmune origin. In the vast majority of patients, a history of an upper respiratory infection before the onset of thyroiditis can be elicited. Patients have diffuse swelling in the cervical area and a sudden increase in pain. Approximately two thirds of patients demonstrate fever, weight loss, and severe fatigue. Fine-needle aspiration (FNA) can be diagnostic if it demonstrates giant cells of an epithelioid foreign body type, which characterize the lesion. Microscopic pathology shows large follicles infiltrated by mononuclear cells, neutrophils, and lymphocytes. Treatment with corticosteroids or nonsteroidal anti-inflammatory drugs (NSAIDs) is effective in relieving symptoms. However, the disease process generally continues, unaffected by these medications.

### Riedel's Struma

Riedel's thyroiditis (struma) is a rare entity characterized by a firm thyroid secondary to a chronic inflammatory process involving the entire gland. Symptoms of severe discomfort can occur because of extension into the trachea, esophagus, and laryngeal nerve. As a result, patients may have impending airway obstruction or dysphagia. Unilateral involvement of symptoms may suggest a malignancy and lead to surgical intervention. The findings at surgery can also be impressive because the process can extend into the trachea and esophagus, with the obliteration of anatomic planes and landmarks. Surgical pathology reveals dense fibrous tissue and almost total obliteration of normal follicular architecture. Grossly, direct involvement of the process can result in severe tracheal and esophageal obstruction.

Treatment with thyroid hormone replacement, corticosteroids, or tamoxifen may be effective. Immediate tracheal or esophageal obstruction may require a surgical approach to relieve symptoms. Such surgery should be performed by an experienced thyroid surgeon. No consensus exists on the surgical management of this rare disease but, in general, only the constricting portion of the thyroid is removed.[10]

## Hyperthyroidism

Disease processes associated with increased thyroid secretion result in a predictable hypermetabolic state. Increased thyroid secretion can be caused by primary alterations within the gland (e.g., Graves' disease, toxic nodular goiter, toxic thyroid adenoma) or central nervous system disorders and increased TSH-produced stimulation of the thyroid. Most hyperthyroid states occur because of primary malfunction. Even more unusual hyperthyroid states can result from mismanaged exogenous thyroid ingestion, molar pregnancy with increased release of human chorionic gonadotropin and, very unusually, thyroid malignancy with overproduction of thyroid hormone. Classic symptoms of hyperthyroidism or thyrotoxicosis include sweating, unintentional weight loss despite increased appetite, heat intolerance, increased thirst, menstrual disturbance, anxiety, diarrhea, palpitations, hair loss, and sleep disturbance. More severe signs of thyrotoxicosis are high-output cardiac failure, congestive heart failure with peripheral edema, and arrhythmias such as ventricular tachycardia and atrial fibrillation.

### Hyperthyroid Disorders

**Graves' Disease** Grave's disease is the most common cause of hyperthyroidism (diffuse toxic goiter). This disease entity was originally described by an Irish physician, Dr. Robert Graves, in 1835. Women between the ages of 20 and 40 years are most commonly affected. The hyperthyroidism in Graves' disease is caused by stimulatory autoantibodies to TSH-R. Although several theories about the stimulus that initiates production of these antibodies have been proposed, there is no universal agreement about the cause of the process. Genetic susceptibility to this disease is possible, as evidenced by the increased probability of Graves' disease in monozygotic twins.[11] Graves' disease generally presents with the classic triad of complaints: (1) signs and symptoms of thyrotoxicosis; (2) a visibly enlarged neck mass consistent with a goiter that may demonstrate an audible bruit secondary to increased vascular flow; (and 3) exophthalmos. Tracheal compression can result in symptoms of airway obstruction, although acute compression with respiratory distress is exceedingly rare.

The ocular consequences of prolonged and untreated thyrotoxicosis, such as proptosis, supraorbital and infraorbital swelling, and conjunctival swelling and edema, can be severe. The ophthalmopathy is believed to be caused by stimulation of the overexpressed TSH-R in the retro-orbital tissues of Graves' patients. In its most severe form, spasm of the upper eyelid, resulting in retraction and visualization of a larger amount of sclera than normal, can lead to lid lag and exacerbation of the already swollen conjunctiva. All these pressure-related phenomena can progress to decreased oculomuscular movements, ophthalmoplegia, and diplopia. Optic nerve damage and blindness can be a long-term consequence if the underlying condition is not corrected. Currently, however, this is rarely seen with improved screening assays that detect Graves' disease at early stages. Sustained hyperthyroidism is treated aggressively to remove the stimulus to the retro-orbital tissues.

**Toxic Nodular Goiter and Toxic Adenoma** Toxic nodular goiter, also known as Plummer's disease, refers to a nodule contained in an otherwise goitrous thyroid gland that has autonomous function. Increased thyroid hormone production occurs independently of TSH control. Such patients generally have a milder course and are older than those with Graves' disease. The thyroid in these patients may be diffusely enlarged or associated with retrosternal goiters. Initial symptoms are mild, peripheral thyroid hormone levels are elevated, and TSH levels are suppressed. Antithyroid antibody levels are usually not detected. The diagnosis is generally confirmed after clinical suspicion, and an $^{131}$I radionuclide scan is performed to localize one or two autonomous areas of function while the rest of the gland is suppressed (Fig. 38-6). Toxic nodular goiter can be treated with thionamides, radioiodine therapy, or surgery; however, the latter two are preferred because these nodules rarely resolve with prolonged thionamide

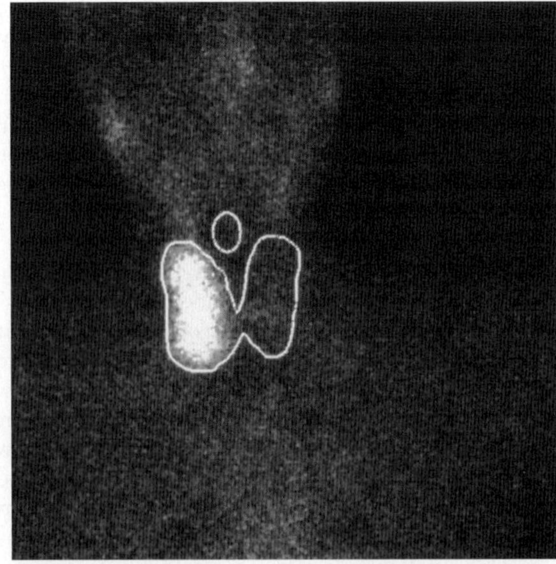

**FIGURE 38-6** 131I scan demonstrating an area of increased uptake in the right lobe of a 32-year-old woman with increased thyroid function test values and a palpable nodule. This scan is consistent with a toxic or hyperfunctioning nodule.

therapy. Radioiodine is widely used for patients with toxic adenomas, although it is not as effective as for those with Graves' disease.[12] Most patients are euthyroid after radioiodine therapy because the radioiodine preferentially accumulates in hyperfunctioning nodules. The surgical approach is lobectomy or near-total thyroidectomy, particularly when clinical symptoms are pronounced. In the case of a single hyperfunctioning adenoma, lobectomy is generally curative.

## Diagnosis

An enlarged smooth thyroid mass and signs and symptoms of thyrotoxicosis suggest the diagnosis of hyperthyroidism. A cost-effective workup can include an extensive history, physical examination, and thyroid function tests. In addition to elevated levels of $T_3$ and $T_4$, a decreased or undetectable level of TSH is demonstrated. Thyroid antibodies are usually elevated. In most cases, an $^{123}$I radionuclide scan demonstrates elevated uptake throughout an enlarged gland. Ultrasound or computed tomography (CT) of the neck can be used to evaluate clinical landmarks (Fig. 38-7). However, the absolute requirement of CT and ultrasound for preoperative assessment is not universally accepted.

## Treatment

When a diagnosis of hyperthyroidism has been made, therapy is initiated rapidly to ameliorate symptoms and decrease thyroid hormone synthesis. This is particularly crucial for patients with vision-threatening exophthalmos usually seen only with Graves' disease. Beta blocker therapy can lessen the adrenergic (excitatory) symptoms of thyrotoxicosis. PTU or methimazole effectively block synthesis of thyroid hormone. Radioactive iodine ablation therapy and surgical ablation are also effective for normalizing serum thyroid hormone levels. Proper patient education about the risks and benefits of each treatment option is advisable.

PTU and methimazole inhibit the organification of intrathyroid iodine, as well as the coupling of iodotyrosine molecules to form $T_3$ and $T_4$. PTU has the additive effect of blocking peripheral conversion of $T_4$ to $T_3$. This is important because peripheral access to $T_3$ and $T_4$ has a number of hyperdynamic and hypermetabolic effects. Also, the peripheral adrenergic effects of thyrotoxicosis can be modulated by the use of beta blocking agents such as propranolol. Corticosteroids in combination with beta blockers can help gain rapid control of the

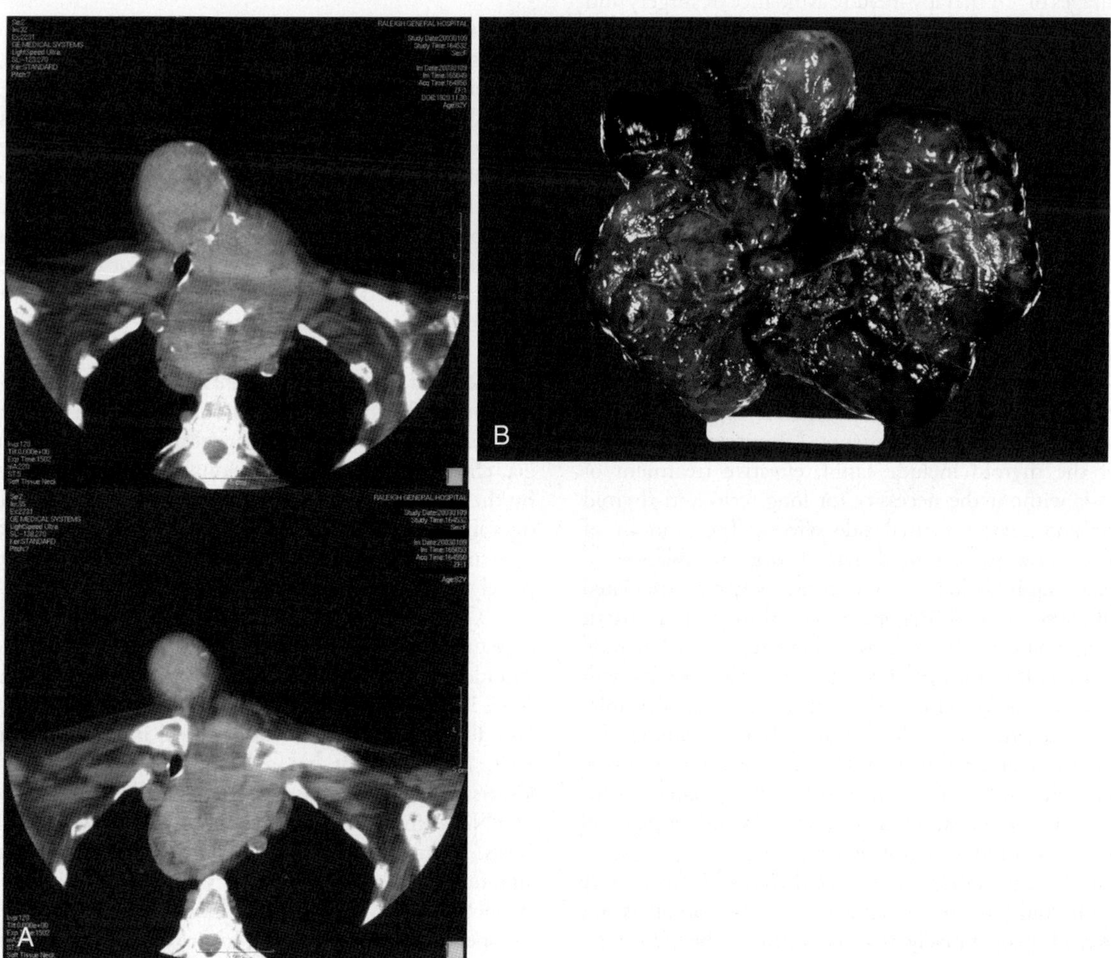


**FIGURE 38-7 A,** CT scan at the level of the thoracic inlet demonstrating a heterogeneous, large thyroid mass that has involved both lobes of the thyroid and displaced the trachea. It has extended into the anterior mediastinum. This patient ultimately proved to have a large multinodular goiter. **B,** Gross picture of the resected multinodular goiter.

hypermetabolic effects of increased peripheral $T_4$ and $T_3$. Patients may choose a trial of antithyroid medication over radioactive iodine therapy. The goal of this therapy is to attain euthyroidism; however, hypothyroidism may result and necessitate thyroid hormone replacement. Antithyroid medication is effective for gaining rapid control of thyrotoxicosis, but the relapse rate after discontinuation of medication approaches 50% within 12 to 18 months after cessation. Also, patients need to be monitored for side effects of the drugs, which may include granulocytopenia and, in rare cases, aplastic anemia. Other side effects include fever, polyarteritis, and rash.

Radioiodide ablation with $^{131}I$ is the therapy of choice in the United States for Graves' disease. It is also a good option for the treatment of toxic adenoma and toxic multinodular goiter. It ablates the thyroid within 6 to 18 weeks.[12] Patients with mild, well-tolerated hyperthyroidism can safely proceed to radioactive iodine ablation immediately. However, those who are older or severely thyrotoxic may require pretreatment with a thionamide. The overall cure rate with radioactive iodine is 90%. Hypothyroidism will develop in cured individuals—hence the need for careful measurement of thyroid hormone and TSH levels at regular intervals after therapy. Most patients are candidates for radioactive iodine; exceptions include women who are pregnant or lactating or those with a suspicious nodule.

Advantages of $^{131}I$ therapy include avoidance of surgery and the associated risks of recurrent laryngeal nerve damage, hypoparathyroidism, or postsurgical recurrence. The use of $^{131}I$ therapy might be more cost-effective over time, but the financial advantage is not as clear if repeated $^{131}I$ therapy is needed. Additional disadvantages include exacerbation of cardiac arrhythmias, particularly in older patients, possible fetal damage in pregnant women, worsening ophthalmic problems, and rare but possibly life-threatening thyroid storm.

Over the last 20 years, surgical ablation for Graves' disease has been advocated less frequently in the United States. It is primarily indicated for patients who have an obstructive goiter with compressive symptoms, have a fear of radioactivity, are noncompliant, have had an adverse effect with thionamide drugs, or there is concern for concomitant malignancy. Additional candidates are pregnant patients. Advantages of surgical ablation of the thyroid include rapid, effective treatment of thyrotoxicosis without the necessity for long-term anti-thyroid medications and their potential side effects. The amount of residual tissue is a subject of debate. Complete ablation of thyroid tissue requires total thyroidectomy, which is associated with the highest rates of hypoparathyroidism and recurrent laryngeal nerve damage. Some groups have reported that total thyroidectomy is the most effective way to treat patients with severe Graves' disease because it offers the lowest rate of relapse. It may be that patients, particularly those with ophthalmopathy, are stabilized most successfully by total thyroidectomy. Removal of the entire antigenic focus is the most likely explanation for this observation. Other subtotal resections include near-total thyroidectomy or subtotal thyroidectomy.

Careful documentation of euthyroid status before surgery in all hyperthyroid patients is mandatory. If the patient is not properly treated preoperatively, thyroid storm can be life threatening. Fortunately, this complication is rarely encountered if appropriately anticipated. Thyroid storm is manifested by severe tachycardia, fever, confusion, vomiting to the point of dehydration, and adrenergic overstimulation to the point of mania and coma after thyroid resection in an uncontrolled hyperthyroid patient. Treatment of a patient with overt thyroid storm includes rapid fluid replacement and institution of antithyroid drugs, beta blockers, iodine solutions, and steroids. In life-threatening circumstances, peritoneal dialysis or hemodialysis may be effective in lowering $T_4$ and $T_3$ levels.

## Nonfunctioning Goiter

### Multinodular Goiter

The term *multinodular goiter* describes an enlarged, diffusely heterogeneous thyroid gland. Initial findings may include diffuse enlargement, but asymmetrical nodularity of the mass often develops. The cause of this mass is usually iodine deficiency. Initially, the mass is euthyroid, but with increasing size, elevations in $T_3$ and $T_4$ levels can occur and gradually progress to clinical hyperthyroidism. Workup and diagnosis involve evaluation of thyroid function test results. Ultrasound and radioisotopic scanning demonstrate heterogeneous thyroid substance. Nodules with poor uptake can appear as lesions suggestive of malignancy. The incidence of carcinoma in multinodular goiter has been reported to be 5% to 10%. Therefore, FNA for diagnosis and resection for suspicious lesions should be strongly considered.

### Substernal Goiter

A substernal goiter is an unusual manifestation of intrathoracic extension of an enlarged thyroid that generally occurs as a result of multinodular goiter. Most intrathoracic or substernal goiters are termed *secondary* because they are enlargements or extensions of multinodular goiters based on the inferior thyroid vasculature. They expand downward into the anterior mediastinum. The extremely rare (~1%) *primary* substernal goiter arises as aberrant thyroid tissue within the anterior or posterior mediastinum; it is based on the intrathoracic vasculature and not supplied by the inferior thyroid artery.

### Special Considerations for Patients With Goiter

Patients with an enlarged thyroid mass (>5 cm) can have a spectrum of symptoms ranging from minimal to severe dysphagia, choking, and pain. Occasionally, the diagnosis is suggested by the presence of an anterior mediastinal mass on chest radiography. In 10% to 20% of cases, an asymptomatic patient may have no palpable abnormality in the cervical area and a completely intrathoracic lesion.

CT is the preferred imaging study and full neck and chest CT scans should be obtained (see Fig. 38-7). Benign goiters have rounded smooth borders. Thyroid malignancies generally have more ill-defined borders and may have evidence of invasion. CT also allows the evaluation of regional lymph nodes and metastasis. If the patient has a history of cervical pain and night sweats, a diagnosis of lymphoma should be considered. The use of FNA with CT guidance is important to secure a tissue diagnosis. Magnetic resonance imaging (MRI) does not usually add significant information to a well-performed CT scan. For patients with an intrathoracic lesion and a history of coughing, preoperative bronchoscopy can provide important information about vocal cord status and possible luminal invasion by a malignancy.

Almost all goiters and other thyroid masses are initially approached surgically through a cervical incision. Goiters are usually mobilized easily, even when they are substernal. The blood supply is generally based on the inferior thyroid artery, which is in its normal position and allows even large substernal masses to be mobilized into the neck. Careful attention must be directed to the location of the esophagus, trachea, and recurrent laryngeal nerves. The esophagus can be injured by overaggressive manipulation of the thyroid mass. The recurrent laryngeal nerve is usually displaced posteriorly and inferiorly; however, it can be draped anteriorly over the mass and damaged in that position. Great care must be exercised in mobilization of the mass until the nerve is identified. The cervical incision is extended to a median sternotomy if there is significant bleeding from the anterior mediastinum, if the anatomy and location of the recurrent laryngeal nerve are in doubt, or if the mass cannot be mobilized through the surgical field.

## WORKUP AND DIAGNOSIS OF A SOLITARY THYROID NODULE

The ultimate decision to proceed to surgical intervention after detection of a solitary nodule depends on the findings of a structured and cost-effective workup and predicted prognosis (Fig. 38-8). Ultimately, this evaluation focuses on determining the presence or absence of a disorder of function or malignancy. Most patients with a solitary thyroid nodule will have a nonfunctioning benign lesion; however, thyroid cancer must be considered in all patients. Deciding between conservative management and surgical therapy relies on careful analysis of the clinical findings, risk assessment, imaging, and diagnostic testing.[7,13]

### Incidence

Increasing numbers of thyroid nodules are being found incidentally, possibly because of the increasing availability and sophistication of imaging techniques. Palpable thyroid nodules are present in 1% of men and 5% of women, and ultrasound-detectable thyroid nodules are present in 19% to 67% of unselected patients. The frequency of both palpable and nonpalpable thyroid nodules rises with age. Most of these nodules are benign but, overall, 5% to 15% are thyroid cancers (Fig. 38-9).[7]

### Initial Evaluation

The workup of a patient with a solitary nodule begins with a careful history and physical examination. Clinical evidence of hyperthyroidism should be evaluated. An important part of the evaluation focuses on risk factors for malignancy. The highest risk for malignancy in a thyroid nodule exists in children, males, adults younger than 30 or older than 60 years, and those exposed to radiation. The examiner should seek a thorough history of exposure to radiation, from occupational sources or from therapeutic radiation of the head or neck, especially during childhood. A personal and family history should be assessed for specific endocrine disorders, including familial medullary carcinoma, MEN2, or papillary thyroid cancer, a history of polyposis, including Gardner's syndrome, or Cowden's syndrome.

On physical examination, it is important to include thorough palpation of the thyroid, as well as the anterior and posterior cervical triangles, with attention to associated lymphadenopathy. The size and consistency of the nodule should be determined. Multiple nodules or diffuse nodularity are more

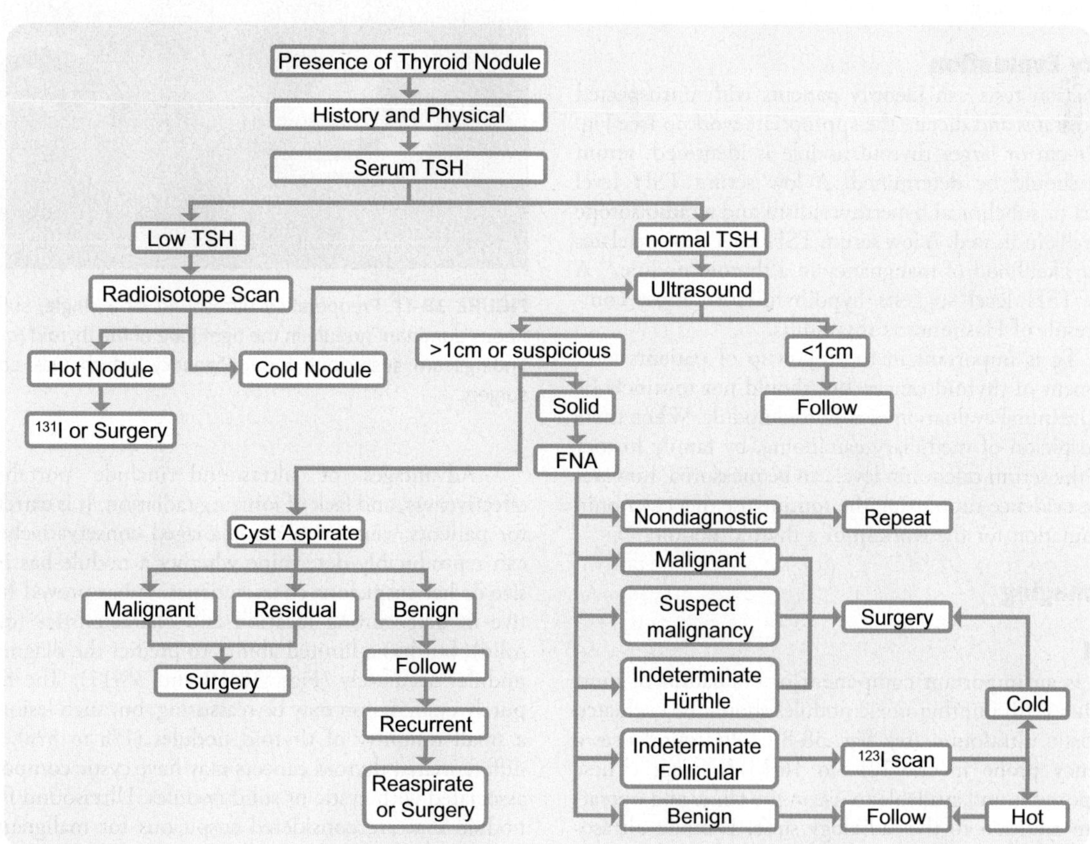


**FIGURE 38-8** Workup of a solitary thyroid nodule.

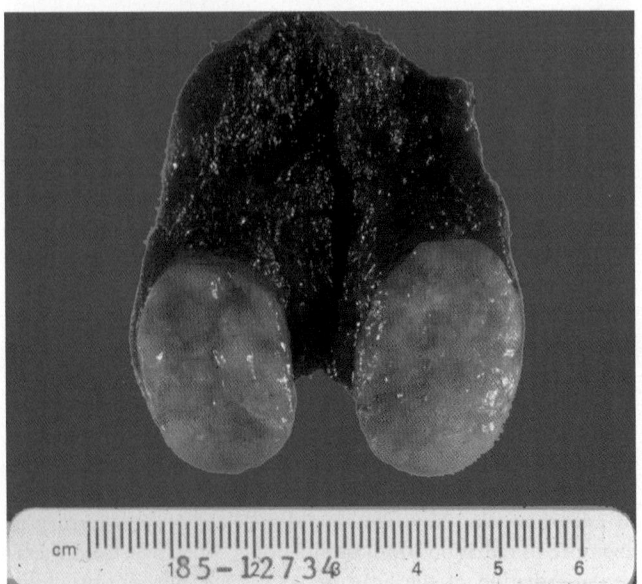


**FIGURE 38-9** This solid 2- × 2.5-cm solid nodule was confirmed as a benign follicular adenoma on permanent section pathology.

associated with a benign diagnosis, whereas a firm solitary nodule, particularly in older men, is more suggestive of malignancy. Nodules that are present on ultrasound, but not palpable on physical examination have the same size-adjusted risk of malignancy as those that are palpable. Rapid growth and clinical indicators of potential invasion, such as pain or hoarseness, are suggestive, but not diagnostic of malignancy.

## Laboratory Evaluation

Thyroid function tests can identify patients with unsuspected hyperthyroid states and dictate the appropriate workup (see Fig. 38-8). If a 1-cm or larger thyroid nodule is identified, serum TSH levels should be determined. A low serum TSH level denotes overt or subclinical hyperthyroidism and a radioisotope scan is generally indicated. A low serum TSH level also correlates with a lower likelihood of malignancy in a thyroid nodule.[14] A high serum TSH level suggests hypothyroidism, most commonly the result of Hashimoto's thyroiditis.

Serum Tg is important in the followup of patients after initial treatment of thyroid cancer, but should not routinely be checked in the initial evaluation of a thyroid nodule. When there is clinical suspicion of medullary carcinoma, by family history or by FNA, the serum calcitonin level can be measured; however there is little evidence supporting the routine use of a calcitonin level determination for the workup of a thyroid nodule.[7,13]

## Thyroid Imaging

### Ultrasound

Ultrasound is an important component of evaluation of most thyroid nodules. All nonthyrotoxic nodules should be evaluated with diagnostic ultrasound (see Fig. 38-8). Ultrasound uses a high-frequency probe in the 7.5- to 16-MHz range. These devices are portable and available to use in the clinic and operating room, in addition to the radiology suite. B-mode ultrasonography can be used preoperatively or intraoperatively. Ultrasound is increasingly being used to assist in FNA.

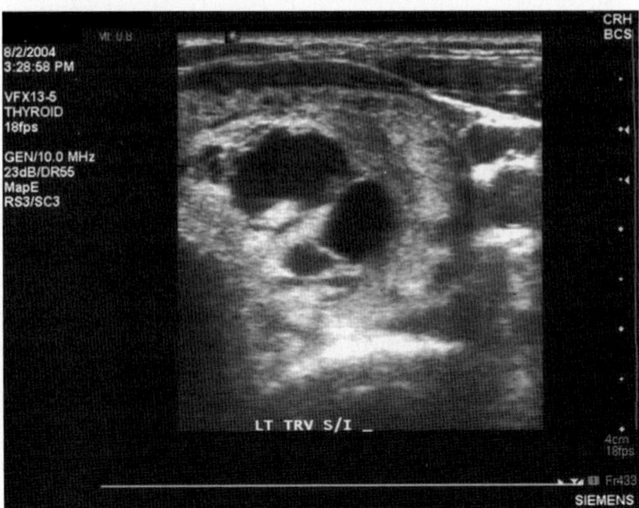


**FIGURE 38-10** Preoperative ultrasound demonstrating a large left thyroid nodule that has solid and cystic components. This lesion was a colloid nodule and was treated by lobectomy.

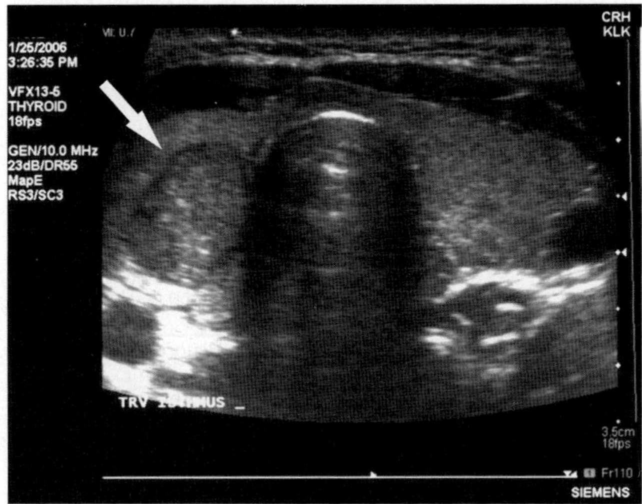


**FIGURE 38-11** Preoperative ultrasound of a single, solid homogeneous dominant nodule in the right lobe of the thyroid *(arrow)*. These findings are suspicious for malignancy, which was confirmed by surgery.

Advantages of ultrasound include portability, cost-effectiveness, and lack of ionizing radiation. It is extremely useful for patients who are being managed conservatively because it can reproducibly determine whether a nodule has increased in size or has suspicious characteristics. It has proved highly effective in determining location and characteristics (cystic versus solid), but has a limited ability to predict the diagnosis of solid nodules accurately (Figs. 38-10 and 38-11). The finding of a purely cystic lesion may be reassuring, but such lesions represent a small minority of thyroid nodules (1% to 5%). Also, well-differentiated thyroid cancers may have cystic components or be associated with cystic or solid nodules. Ultrasound findings in a nodule that are considered suspicious for malignancy include microcalcifications, hypervascularity, infiltrative margins, being hypoechoic compared with surrounding parenchyma, and

**Table 38-1 Ultrasonographic Features of Thyroid Cancer**

| | | | Predictive Value (%) | |
|---|---|---|---|---|
| IMAGING FEATURE | SENSITIVITY (%) | SPECIFICITY (%) | POSITIVE | NEGATIVE |
| Microcalcifications | 26-59 | 86-95 | 24-71 | 42-94 |
| Hypoechogenicity | 27-87 | 43-94 | 11-68 | 74-94 |
| Irregular margins or no halo | 17-78 | 39-85 | 9-60 | 39-98 |
| Solid | 69-75 | 53-56 | 16-27 | 88-92 |
| Intranodular vascularity | 54-74 | 79-81 | 24-42 | 86-97 |
| More tall than wide | 33 | 93 | 67 | 75 |

Data from Frates MC, Benson CB, Charboneau JW, et al: Management of thyroid nodules detected at US: Society of Radiologists in Ultrasound consensus conference statement. Radiology 237:794–800, 2005.

having a shape that is taller than its width on transverse view (Table 38-1).[15]

The size of a nodule on ultrasound is important in determining the need for further evaluation, such as needle biopsy. In general nodules that are smaller than 1 cm in greatest dimension are not further evaluated (see Fig. 38-8). Further workup of nodules smaller than 1 cm may be indicated for nodules such as those with suspicious characteristics on ultrasound and those associated with suspicious lymphadenopathy by ultrasound or clinical examination, patients with a family history of papillary thyroid cancer, history of radiation exposure, prior personal history of thyroid cancer, and $^{18}$F-fluorodeoxyglucose (FDG)/ positron emission tomography (PET)–positive lesions.

### Radioisotope Scanning

Whereas ultrasound allows anatomic evaluation, radionuclide scans allow assessment of thyroid function. If a dominant thyroid nodule larger than 1 cm is found to be associated with a suppressed serum TSH level, a radionuclide scan using technetium-99m pertechnetate ($^{99m}$Tc) or $^{123}$I should be obtained to determine whether the nodule is hyperfunctioning (see Figs. 38-6 and 38-8).[7] In euthyroid or hypothyroid patients with thyroid nodules, radioisotope scanning is not routinely indicated.

$^{99m}$Tc is taken up rapidly by the normal activity of follicular cells. It is trapped by follicular cells, but not organified. $^{99m}$Tc has a short half-life and low radiation dose. Its rapid absorption allows quick evaluation of increased uptake (hot) or hypofunctioning (cold) areas of the thyroid. Because screening with $^{99m}$Tc shows uptake in the salivary glands and major vascular structures, interpretation of thyroid pathology requires expertise.

$^{123}$I and $^{131}$I iodine scintigraphy is also used to evaluate the functional status of the gland (see Fig. 38-6). Both are trapped by active follicular cells and organified. Advantages of scanning with $^{123}$I include a low dose of radiation (100 μCi) and short half-life (12 to 13 hours). $^{123}$I is a good choice for evaluating suspected lingual thyroids or substernal goiters. $^{131}$I has a longer half-life (8 days) and emits higher levels of β-radiation. $^{131}$I is optimal for imaging thyroid carcinoma and is the screening modality of choice for the evaluation of distant metastasis. Malignancy has been shown to occur in 15% to 20% of cold nodules and in 5% to 9% of warm or hot nodules. Therefore, although suggestive, malignancy of a nodule can neither be confirmed nor excluded based on radionuclide uptake.

PET with $^{18}$F-fluorodeoxyglucose can be used to provide three-dimensional reconstruction images. There has been increasing enthusiasm for its use in detecting primary and metastatic thyroid cancer. Interestingly, 1% to 2% of PET scans identify so-called thyroid incidentalomas when evaluating other solid malignancies. Although most PET-avid incidentalomas in the thyroid are benign, the incidence of malignancy in those that have progressed to resection has been reported to be as high as 33%.[16] The appropriateness of PET in the workup or follow-up of thyroid nodules remains debatable.

### Computed Tomography and Magnetic Resonance Imaging

It is fairly well agreed that CT and MRI do not add significantly to the workup of uncomplicated thyroid nodules that are otherwise well characterized by ultrasound. Either modality, however, may be helpful for evaluating for local extension in more advanced stages of thyroid cancer. CT or MRI is particularly appropriate for a suspicious mass (or biopsy-proven cancer) with palpable cervical lymph nodes. Also, either can be used for postoperative follow-up, particularly for suspicion of recurrent disease. CT or MRI is advisable in preoperative planning for larger thyroid masses that show significant tracheal deviation suggestive of a substernal goiter on chest radiographs.

CT and MRI are both equally sensitive and specific for the evaluation of thyroid masses. Consideration must be given to the use of IV contrast for CT evaluation of a possible cancer. Although the use of IV contrast improves anatomic definition, the large iodine load may interfere with subsequent plans for radioactive iodine imaging or therapy.[7]

## Fine-Needle Aspiration Biopsy

FNA with a small-gauge needle (23 to 27 gauge) is a cost-effective and valuable tool and is now an accepted key modality for the evaluation of patients with thyroid nodules. Essentially all dominant nonfunctioning thyroid nodules that are 1 cm or larger should be evaluated by FNA biopsy if a decision for operative intervention has not already been made (see Fig. 38-8). Lesions that are smaller than 1 cm but that may still warrant FNA have been described earlier. Use of small gauge needles has allowed a marked drop in the complication rate associated with the use of large-bore or core needle biopsies while maintaining diagnostic accuracy. Also, experience in performing the biopsy and interpreting the results are important to the success of this technique. In a series of 561 patients, FNA was found to have a sensitivity of 86% and a specificity of 91%.[17] Another series

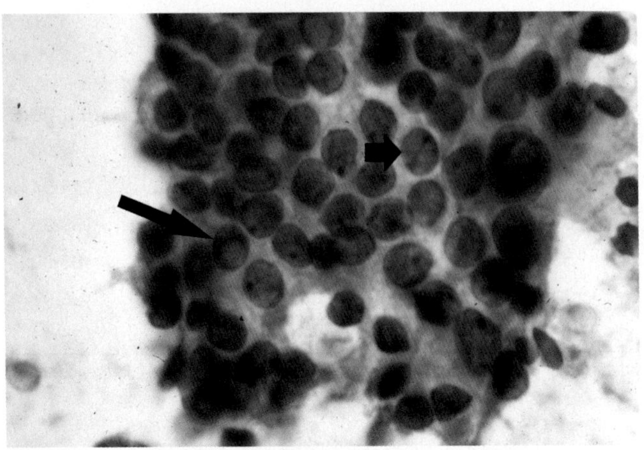

**FIGURE 38-12** FNA of a thyroid mass allows determination of individual cellular morphology. Cells in this aspirate demonstrate intranuclear grooving *(fat arrow),* as well as ground-glass cytoplasmic inclusions *(thin arrow)* (so-called Orphan Annie eyes). These cellular features confirm the diagnosis of papillary carcinoma of the thyroid.

of 240 patients found a 4% rate of false-positive and false-negative FNA results.[18] Accurate diagnosis of benign lesions has significantly decreased rates of surgery in patients with thyroid nodules. Currently, preoperative FNA is replacing the use of intraoperative, frozen section pathologic analysis.

For palpable nodules, FNA biopsy may be performed without image guidance. However, ultrasound guidance may be used for FNA biopsy of palpable lesions, especially heterogenous lesions. Ultrasound guidance is recommended for nonpalpable, posteriorly located, or cystic nodules and results in a lower rate of nondiagnostic cytology and sampling errors.

Results of FNA biopsy may be broadly grouped in several ways, including the following: (1) malignant, (2) indeterminate or suspicious, (3) benign, and (4) nondiagnostic. In cases of nondiagnostic cytology, repeat FNA using ultrasound guidance is indicated and yields diagnostic cytology in 50% to 75% of cases.[19] Lesions in which FNA is persistently nondiagnostic are known to have a significant rate of malignancy and therefore must continue to be followed closely or excised. The finding of a malignant diagnosis on FNA is associated with a high rate of accuracy, approaching 100%, and this finding should prompt resection. Certain discrete cytologic characteristics of papillary carcinoma allow the use of FNA to be extremely accurate in securing this particular diagnosis (Fig. 38-12). If FNA biopsy demonstrates suspicion of papillary carcinoma or Hürthle cell neoplasm, no radionuclide scan is needed and resection should be planned, particularly for higher risk patients or those with a prior history of radiation exposure. The secure FNA diagnosis of medullary or anaplastic carcinoma may require interpretation by an experienced cytopathologist.

Diagnosis of follicular cancer is based on the demonstration of capsular or vascular invasion by follicular cells, not on cellular cytology alone. When FNA reveals follicular cells, although most of these cases are benign (follicular adenoma), the diagnosis or exclusion of follicular carcinoma ultimately depends on complete histologic examination of the resected specimen. Large series have shown malignancy in 6% to 20% of thyroid lesions when follicular cells are demonstrated on FNA.[20] When FNA demonstrates follicular neoplasm, lobectomy or total thyroidectomy should be considered unless a concordant autonomously functioning nodule is demonstrated on $^{123}I$ uptake scan (see Fig. 38-6 and 38-8).[7] When FNA results are suspicious but not confirmatory of malignancy, it appears that more than 50% of such FNA results are associated with malignancy. If the FNA findings are indeterminate, repeat aspiration, resection, or close conservative follow-up of the nodule is suggested.[18] The use of molecular markers such as BRAF, galectin, and others to predict malignancy in the setting of indeterminate FNA will likely play a significant role in decision making for these patients in the future.[21]

The presence of colloid and macrophages in the aspirate strongly suggests a benign lesion. The patient must understand, however, that this diagnosis depends only on the aspirated material. Tissue immediately adjacent to or contained within another part of the nodule may harbor malignant cells. The false-negative rate of FNA has been reported to be between 1% and 6%.[13] Therefore, benign nodules diagnosed by FNA are monitored sequentially with ultrasound to ensure that their characteristics do not change. A repeat ultrasound should be performed 6 to 18 months after the initial FNA. If this shows stable ultrasound findings, further ultrasound examinations should be performed every 3 to 5 years. However, if ultrasound shows more than a 50% change in volume, or a 20% increase in two dimensions, FNA should be repeated under ultrasound guidance.[7]

FNA can also be used for lesions that are determined to be cystic by ultrasound. A larger bore needle can be used to aspirate the cystic fluid. Examination of most cystic fluid results in benign cytologic findings; however, an occasional papillary carcinoma can be manifested as a cyst and diagnosed by cytologic examination of cystic fluid. Cysts that have a residual palpable mass after aspiration and those aspirated with benign cytology but then recur should be considered for resection.[7]

Patients with multiple thyroid nodules have an equivalent risk of harboring malignancy as those with a solitary nodule, but each individual nodule has a lower risk than a solitary nodule. A reasonable approach for those patients with multiple thyroid nodules larger than 1 cm is preferential FNA biopsy of those nodules with suspicious ultrasonographic features. Furthermore, if radionuclide scanning demonstrates a hypofunctioning nodule in a patient with multiple nodules, FNA should be considered for the cold nodules.[7]

## Decision Making and Treatment

Decision making about thyroid nodules depends on the structured use of the modalities described and consideration of the clinical setting (Table 38-2; also see Fig. 38-8). All patients with a thyroid nodule undergo thyroid function tests (at least for serum TSH). If the patient is hyperthyroid, a radiouptake scan is used to confirm a hot nodule. If this is the case, the patient is carefully monitored with thyroid suppression and seen again after 6 months for confirmation of successful suppression and reevaluation. If suppressive therapy fails, surgery (usually lobectomy) is highly effective, but not generally required (see earlier, "Toxic Nodular Goiter and Toxic Adenoma").

In a patient with a thyroid nodule and normal thyroid function test results, ultrasound is performed. Cystic lesions on ultrasound are usually benign; however, cystic papillary carcinomas, although rare, do occur. Cystic lesions are aspirated; bloody or suspicious aspirates can be sent for cytologic examination. After aspiration, these patients are seen again in 6 months.

**Table 38-2 Thyroid Nodules**

| DIAGNOSIS | FACTORS ASSOCIATED WITH DIAGNOSIS | FACTORS THAT CONFIRM THE DIAGNOSIS | FACTORS ASSOCIATED WITH WORSE PROGNOSIS |
|---|---|---|---|
| **Benign** | | | |
| Colloid | Multinodular goiter; FNA shows colloid and macrophages | Surgery | – |
| Hyperfunctioning nodule | Hyperthyroidism | $^{131}$I scan | – |
| **Malignant** | | | |
| Papillary carcinoma | Radiation exposure; previous surgery for papillary carcinoma | FNA or surgery | Male gender; age > 40 yr; size > 3 cm; tall cell variant |
| Follicular carcinoma | Follicular cells by FNA | Permanent section pathology | Male gender; age > 40 yr; size > 3 cm; poorly differentiated cell type |
| Medullary carcinoma | MEN2A and MEN2B; elevated calcitonin level | Surgery; FNA; calcitonin levels; *ret* oncogene | MEN2B and sporadic |
| Anaplastic carcinoma | Rapid progression of tumor mass; pain, hoarseness | FNA; surgery | Diagnosis |

Patients with recurrent cysts are considered surgical candidates.

For patients whose nodules on ultrasound are solid or have mixed solid-cystic components, decision making depends on additional information. Depending on the history, examination, and imaging risk factors for malignancy, some patients will choose excision, regardless of further workup. In most patients, FNA is indicated if a decision for surgery has not already been made. FNA can be used to diagnose papillary cancer and is strongly suggestive of medullary cancer or anaplastic cancer. It cannot confirm follicular cancer, nor can it confirm a completely benign diagnosis. Therefore, risk assessment is crucial when advising patients with a solid nodule for whom the diagnosis is not secure with FNA. Colloid nodules are usually suggested by a mixed solid-cystic appearance on ultrasound, and FNA shows colloid and macrophages. If not otherwise suspicious, these lesions can be monitored closely with serial ultrasonography every 6 months to establish stability. Alterations in the appearance of the suspicious lesion indicate a need for surgery (Figs. 38-13 and 38-14).[7,13]

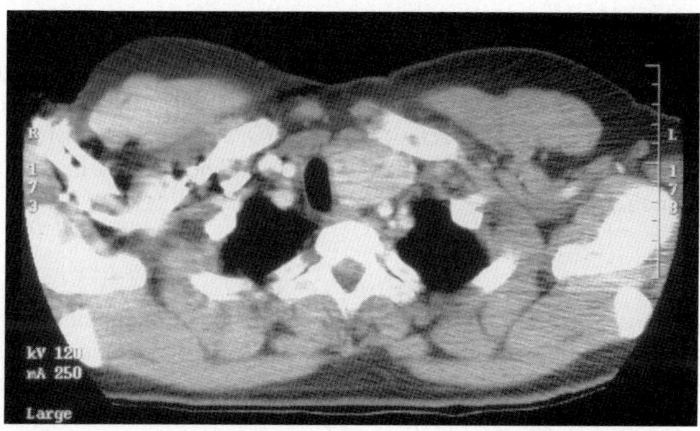


**FIGURE 38-13** CT findings of a 4-cm mass in the left lobe of a 40-year-old man suggesting an infraclavicular or substernal location. The mass ultimately proved to be papillary carcinoma.

The increased availability of ultrasound appears to have affected the incidence of small thyroid cancers in the United States. Most seem to be asymptomatic papillary carcinomas smaller than 1 cm. The fact that these lesions are highly curable and associated with almost nonexistent mortality needs to be taken into account when deciding whether to perform FNA and proceed to surgery.[22]

The practice of using exogenous thyroid replacement to suppress endogenous TSH to suppress a thyroid nodule is losing favor. It previously was believed that nodules that grew on suppressive therapy were likely malignant, whereas those that shrank were likely benign. This is neither sensitive nor specific, because only 20% to 30% of nodules were found to shrink on suppressive therapy and up to 13% of proven papillary cancers in one series decreased in size on suppressive therapy.[23]

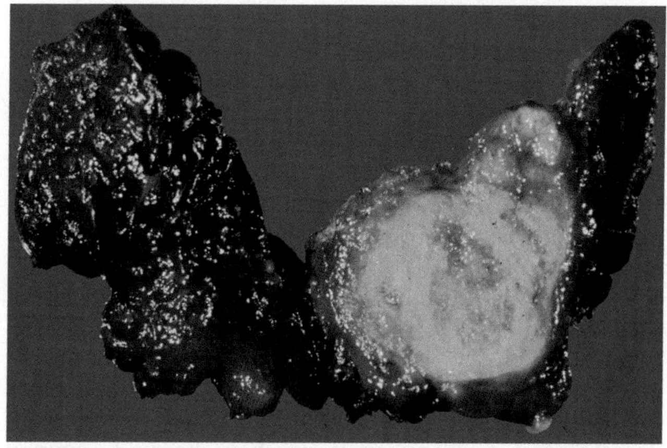

**FIGURE 38-14** This 4- to 5-cm right lobe mass was removed as part of total thyroidectomy. Permanent section pathology revealed papillary carcinoma.

The finding of a thyroid nodule in a child or pregnant patient can be of particular concern to the patient, family, and referring clinicians. Although the frequency of malignancy may be higher in children than in adults, the evaluation should generally proceed in the same fashion as for an adult.[7] In pregnant

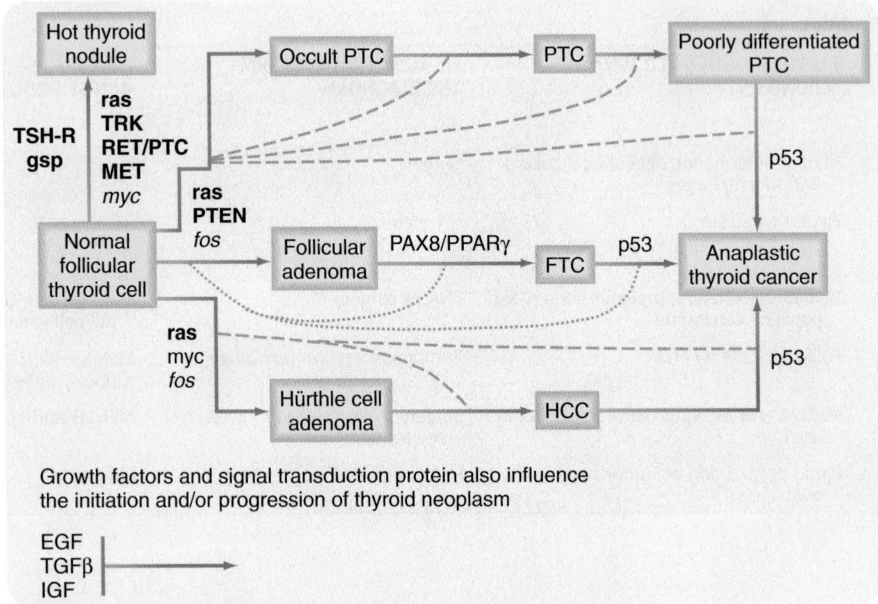


**FIGURE 38-15** Genetic events that occur in thyroid oncogenesis (the main genetic events are in boldface). The *dashed lines* for each histologic type of thyroid cancer indicate that an adenoma to carcinoma progression is not necessarily always the sequence of progression in carcinogenesis. *EGF,* Epidermal growth factor; *FTC,* follicular thyroid carcinoma; *HCC,* Hürthle cell carcinoma; *IGF,* insulin-like growth factor; *PPARγ,* peroxisome proliferator–activated receptor-γ; *PTC,* papillary thyroid carcinoma; *TGFβ,* transforming growth factor-β; *TSH-R,* thyroid-simulating hormone receptor. (From Kebebew E: Thyroid oncogenesis. In Clark OH [ed]: Textbook of endocrine surgery, ed 2, Philadelphia, 2005, Elsevier Saunders, p 289.)

patients, it is not clear whether the incidence of malignancy for a given nodule is different than that in nonpregnant patients. The evaluation of a thyroid nodule discovered in pregnancy is the same as in the nonpregnant patient except that radionuclide scans are contraindicated. If a nodule is found to represent papillary cancer during pregnancy and remains stable by midgestation or is diagnosed in the second half of pregnancy, surgery may be deferred until the patient is postpartum. This practice is believed not to affect the oncologic outcome.[7]

## THYROID MALIGNANCIES

Thyroid cancer represents approximately 3% of all malignancies in the United States, with about 48,020 cases in the United States annually. These cases were predicted to result in 1740 deaths in the United States in 2011.[24] Almost 75% of cases occur in women, making this the sixth most common malignancy in women. The incidence of papillary thyroid cancer has been increasing rapidly in men and women, increasing 189% in the United States between 1973 and 2003.[25]

Of thyroid cancers, 90% to 95% are categorized as well-differentiated tumors arising from the follicular cells. Papillary, follicular, and Hürthle cell carcinomas are included in this category. Medullary thyroid cancer accounts for about 6% of thyroid cancers (20% to 30% of which occur on a familial basis, including MEN2A and MEN2B). Anaplastic carcinoma is an aggressive malignancy responsible for less than 1% of thyroid carcinomas in the United States. Prognosis mirrors incidence in that papillary cancer, which is the most common thyroid malignancy, also generally carries a good prognosis, whereas anaplastic cancer is far less common and bears a grim prognosis.

### Thyroid Oncogenesis

#### Genetic Alterations

Genetic processes that lead to thyroid neoplasia include two important categories, mutated proto-oncogenes, which result in altered protein production and in accelerated growth, and loss of function in growth suppression genes, allowing unregulated cell growth. Most of these genetic abnormalities are acquired, but between 5% and 10% of papillary thyroid cancers are believed to be familial.[21] Several known oncogenes have been associated with thyroid tumors but few are limited to specific thyroid malignancies. The working model for oncogenes causing papillary and follicular cancer is not as well understood; it appears that at least three gene categories of locations or actions are important (Fig. 38-15; Table 38-3).

Genetic alterations that lead to constitutive activation of the mitogen-activated protein kinase (MAPK) pathway are common in papillary carcinoma. This is a downstream effect of a pathway that includes the RET and NTRK1 transmembrane proteins. Mutations in the RET and NTRK1 tyrosine kinases result in chimeric products known as RET-PTC and TRK, respectively. These rearrangements occur in up to 40% of sporadic papillary carcinomas and may be associated with a less favorable prognosis.[26]

The *PTC-RET* proto-oncogene has received perhaps the most attention in thyroid tumorigenesis studies and has been well characterized.[27] The *PTC-RET* proto-oncogene encodes for a membrane receptor tyrosine kinase and is the most frequent genetic alteration in papillary thyroid cancer (PTC), despite the absence of the RET protein product in normal thyroid follicular cells. This proto-oncogene may well be involved in the normal

**Table 38-3 Main Genes Involved in Thyroid Oncogenesis: Classification, Tumor Types, and Prevalence**

| GENES | HISTOLOGIC TYPE | PREVALENCE (%) | COMMENT |
|---|---|---|---|
| **Receptor** | | | |
| *TSH* | Autonomous follicular adenoma | 3-82 | TSH activation mutations not oncogenic |
| *TRK* | PTC | 6-20 | Tyrosine kinase receptor, somatic mutation absent in benign thyroid neoplasms |
| *RET-PTC* | PTC | 2.5-85, higher with radiation exposure | Tyrosine kinase receptor, somatic mutation; higher prevalence with radiation exposure; possibly associated with more aggressive tumors; five chimeric subtypes have been identified |
| *Met* | PTC, FTC | ~75 PTC | Tyrosine kinase receptor, somatic mutation |
| | | ~25 FTC | Possibly associated with aggressive tumors |
| | | | Overexpressed mostly in PTC and poorly differentiated DTC |
| *c-erb-2* | PTC | ~50 PTC | Tyrosine kinase activity, similar to epidermal growth factor receptor |
| | | | Overexpressed in PTC, but oncogene is not overamplified |
| **Signal Transduction Proteins** | | | |
| *ras* | PTC, FTC, HCC, autonomous follicular adenoma | 7-92 (~30 overall) | Early event in carcinogenesis; may be associated with aggressive PTC |
| *gsp* | Autonomous follicular adenoma | 7-28 | Early event in carcinogenesis; similar frequency in benign and malignant thyroid neoplasms; coexisting *ras* and *gsp* mutations in same tumor may be associated with aggressive DTC |
| **Tumor Suppressor Genes and Nuclear Oncogenes** | | | |
| *PAX8-PPAR*$\gamma$ | FTC | 75 | Presence of this fusion oncoprotein may be used to differentiate follicular adenoma from carcinoma |
| *p53* | Poorly DTC, ATC | ~75 | p53 immunohistochemistry may be predictive of tumor aggressiveness; believed to occur as a late genetic event in thyroid carcinogenesis |
| *PTEN* | Benign follicular adenoma, infrequently in DTC | 26 of benign,6 of malignant | Higher rate in benign than malignant tumor questions presence of a strict adenomatocarcinoma sequence |

From Kebebew E: Thyroid oncogenesis. In Clark OH (ed): Textbook of endocrine surgery, ed 2, Philadelphia, 2005, Elsevier Saunders, p 289.

differentiation of neuronal cells. Cells of neural crest origin appear to have increased expression of this gene because it has been found in neuroblastoma, pheochromocytoma, and MTC tissue. Alterations in this system have been shown to result in developmental abnormalities in a number of other neuronal tissues, as well as in patients with Hirschsprung's disease. Expression of the *RET* oncogene is predominantly found in malignant tissue. It has not been detected to any substantial degree in nonmalignant thyroid disease processes. Thyroid malignancies expressing this oncogene may have a predilection for distant metastasis. In addition, the *RET* proto-oncogene is associated with a high frequency of missense mutations in patients with MEN2A and genetic analysis for this mutation allows a secure diagnosis in children before the clinical appearance of MTC.

The downstream pathway of the *RET* and *NTRK1* mutations includes RAS, BRAF, MEK, and ultimately activation of MAPK. Of all the isoforms of RAF kinase, the B type (BRAF) is the most potent stimulator of MAPK signaling. BRAF is implicated in PTC, and has been seen in anaplastic thyroid cancer, but not FTC. The prevalence of *BRAF* mutations is highest in tall cell variant PTC. Activating mutations of *BRAF* induce the MAPK pathway and initiate malignant transformation. Several groups have reported that *BRAF* mutations are found in as many as 70% of PTC operative specimens. Cohen and colleagues[28] have found a 94% concordance in evaluating preoperative FNA specimens with the postoperative result in documented papillary cancer cases. Xing and associates[29] have found that the *BRAF* gene is associated with an increased likelihood of postoperative tumor recurrence, extrathyroidal invasion, and lymph node metastases. Interestingly, *BRAF* mutations appear to be less common in childhood PTC, which also generally have a more favorable prognosis.[30] Recently, an experience of testing preoperative FNA specimens for *BRAF* mutations in patients with PTC has demonstrated a significant association of *BRAF* mutation with poorer clinicopathologic outcomes of PTC.[31] This may prove useful in tailoring the extent of surgery based on preoperative risk stratification.

The *ras* gene family encodes signal transduction G proteins that play an important role in the regulation of cell growth and differentiation. Mutational activation of this oncogene results in the production of an inactive form of an enzyme (guanosine triphosphatase) that is ineffective in inactivating protein degradation. As many as 40% of thyroid tumors may have one of three *ras* gene point mutations (H-*ras*, K-*ras*, or N-*ras*) and *ras* mutations may occur in benign and malignant thyroid neoplasms, including follicular adenomas, follicular cancers, and follicular variant papillary cancers.[32] Patients who live in iodine-deficient areas may have an incidence of *ras* mutations that is slightly decreased in comparison to those in iodine-sufficient areas. K-*ras* mutations appear more frequently in radiation-induced papillary cancers. Follicular cancers with *ras* mutations are more aggressive than those without *ras* mutations, and *ras* mutations may also be found in undifferentiated and anaplastic thyroid cancers.[33] It appears that tumor oncogenesis may be related not only to the prevalence of certain mutations, but also to other genetic factors, as well as environmental factors, such as iodine availability.

Tumor suppressor genes also play a role in thyroid malignancy. Loss of function of the *p53* tumor suppressor gene is one of the most common genetic alterations seen across all human cancers and is associated with radiation exposure. The *p53* gene product plays an important role in cell cycle progression. Inactivating mutations of *p53* appear to be associated with more aggressive PTC and FTC and are a late event in thyroid cancer progression; they have been associated with the development of anaplastic thyroid cancer.[34]

### Ionizing Radiation

Ionizing radiation can cause genetic mutations leading to malignant transformation. This association is much stronger for thyroid cancer than for other malignancies, and radiation is the only well-established environmental risk factor for thyroid malignancy. The risk of developing thyroid cancer after exposure to radiation is greater in those exposed during childhood and increases with higher doses of radiation delivered to the thyroid. This is true for exposure to ionizing radiation given for medical purposes and for environmental exposures. The association with radiation is much stronger for papillary than for follicular cancer.

The use of external beam radiation in children and young adults in the 1950s and 1960s for acne and tonsillitis has been shown to result in an increased incidence of well-differentiated carcinoma (usually papillary) at any time, generally 5 years after exposure. Also, patients who receive external radiation for a soft tissue malignancy, such as Hodgkin's lymphoma, have an increased incidence of thyroid nodules and cancer (as many as 30% to 35% of those exposed). Acute environmental exposures, such as those seen following the Chernobyl nuclear event, also have significant impact. The incidence of thyroid cancer in children in some areas affected by Chernobyl peaked at 100 times that seen prior to the accident.[35]

## Papillary Carcinoma

Papillary carcinoma is the most common of the thyroid neoplasms and is usually associated with an excellent prognosis, particularly in young female patients. Of thyroid carcinomas, 70% to 80% are diagnosed are papillary carcinoma. The incidence of well-differentiated thyroid carcinoma, particularly PTC, increased 189% in the United States between 1973 and 2003; this is the most rapid increase in incidence of any malignancy in the United States.[25] This increased incidence is believed to be at least partly the result of enhanced detection of previously unknown small papillary cancers, although other factors such as environmental exposure cannot be excluded. Papillary cancer may actually occur much more commonly than it is diagnosed, with autopsy series finding small (<1 cm) papillary cancers in as many of 30% of people who have died of other causes. This suggests that small papillary cancers may be of minimal clinical significance.

The most important risk factor for papillary cancer is childhood radiation exposure from medical or environmental sources. Other important risk factors for papillary thyroid cancer include a history of thyroid cancer in a first-degree relative and the presence of a familial syndrome that includes thyroid cancer, such as Werner syndrome, Carney complex, and familial polyposis. Papillary cancer occurs in a 2.5:1 female-to-male ratio and the peak incidence occurs between the ages of 30 and 50 years.

### Pathologic Classification

The pathologic diagnosis of papillary carcinoma depends on the findings of well-recognized papillary cytomorphology. Individual cellular morphology may be used to make the diagnosis of papillary carcinoma and, for this reason, the diagnosis of papillary cancer may be made definitively based on FNA cytology. Findings of papillary cancer on FNA include intranuclear inclusion bodies and cellular grooving (see Fig. 38-12). Also, the finding of calcified clumps of cells, known as psammoma bodies and most likely caused by sloughed papillary projections, is diagnostic of papillary cancer. Alternately, the neoplasm may form well-defined follicles, with only minimal papillary architecture. The latter group is classified as the follicular variant of papillary carcinoma and constitutes about 10% of papillary cancers. Classic papillary carcinoma and the follicular variant of papillary carcinoma have similar prognostic implications.

Other subtypes of papillary carcinoma include insular, columnar, and tall cell carcinomas which are more unpredictably aggressive in their biologic behavior. Although these subtypes are rare, they tend to occur in older patients, and the prognosis is less favorable. These latter groups represent perhaps less than 1% of all papillary carcinomas (Fig. 38-16).

### Clinical Features

Papillary cancer most typically presents as a thyroid nodule; its evaluation has been described earlier. However, an increasing number of thyroid nodules are now being discovered incidentally on imaging. Clinical features suspicious for malignancy include painless and firm masses, fixation to surrounding structures, associated hoarseness, presence of ipsilateral adenopathy, and presence of the risk factors described. Papillary cancers may be partially cystic on ultrasound. Occasionally, a metastatic papillary cancer will present as a painless lateral neck mass that is confirmed to be nodal metastatic thyroid cancer, even with a normal thyroid examination. Thorough head and neck examination, often aided by office-based ultrasound, allows characterization of the mass, and FNA is generally indicated.

Most patients with papillary carcinoma can expect an excellent prognosis, with the 10-year survival rate above 95% for the most favorable stages. Various factors in the clinical findings and pathologic staging, however, may alter the excellent prognosis (Table 38-4). In 1979, Cady and coworkers[36] first evaluated a clinical scoring system and reported a 30-year study of a group of patients in which the investigators attempted to place the patients into risk stratification groups. These studies described the AMES clinical scoring system, which is based on ***a***ge, distant ***m***etastasis, ***e***xtent of the primary tumor, and ***s***ize of the primary tumor. Hay and associates[37] reported the Mayo Clinic experience and developed their own scoring scale, the AGES clinical scoring system, based on ***a***ge, pathologic ***g***rade of tumor, and ***e***xtent and ***s***ize of the primary tumor. Both the AMES and AGES clinical scoring systems have proved beneficial in predicting the prognosis of papillary and follicular cancer (see Table 38-4).

Age at diagnosis is the most important prognostic factor in well-differentiated thyroid cancer. Diagnosis at an age younger than 40 years is associated with excellent survival. In women, this age benefit is extended to 50 years. Also, absence of distant

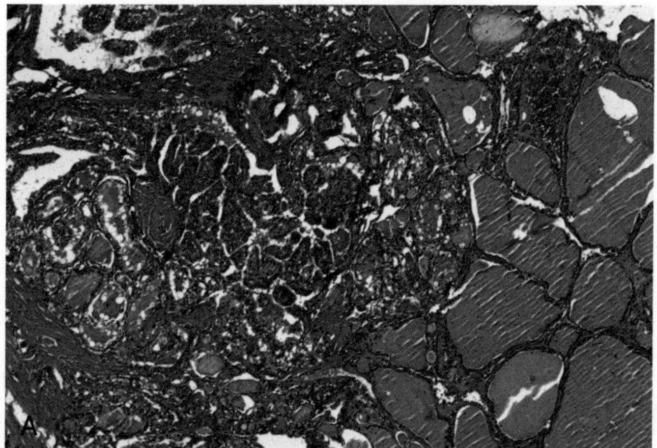

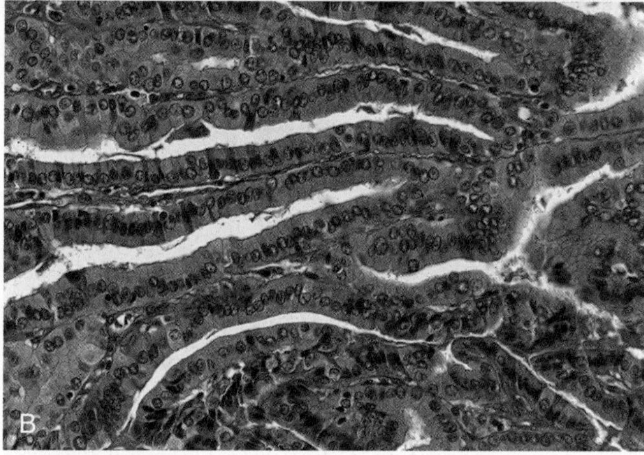

**FIGURE 38-16 A,** Thyroid mass showing papillary projections consistent with papillary carcinoma (H&E stain, ×100). **B,** Papillary carcinoma with cells with an increased height-to-width ratio in a single row. This is the so-called tall cell variant of papillary carcinoma, which is associated with a poorer prognosis than well-differentiated papillary cancer (H&E stain, ×400).

**Table 38-4 Prognostic Risk Classification for Patients With Well-Differentiated Thyroid Cancer (AMES or AGES)**

| | Risk | |
|---|---|---|
| **PARAMETER** | **LOW** | **HIGH** |
| Age (yr) | <40 | >40 |
| Gender | Female | Male |
| Extent | No local extension, intrathyroidal, no capsular invasion | Capsular invasion, extrathyroidal extension |
| Metastasis | None | Regional or distant |
| Size | <2 cm | >4 cm |
| Grade | Well differentiated | Poorly differentiated |

*AGES,* ***A****ge,* ***p****athologic grade of tumor,* ***e****xtent and* ***s****ize of the primary tumor; AMES,* ***a****ge, distant* ***m****etastasis,* ***e****xtent of primary tumor,* ***s****ize of primary tumor.*

metastasis at the time of initial treatment and size smaller than 4 cm are important positive predictors. Even those patients with distant spread to the lungs still have significant survival of up to 50% at 10 years; however, those with brain metastases have a median 1-year survival. Tumor size larger than 4 cm and extension of the primary tumor through the capsule of the lesion and into surrounding soft tissue increase the risk for mortality. Small tumors generally have excellent prognoses, but may still present with clinically evident recurrence. The impact of lymphatic metastases on prognosis depends on patient age. In a large series in younger patients (<45 years), the presence of lymph node metastases had no effect on the excellent overall survival, but in those patients older than 45 years, the presence of lymph node metastases increased the risk of death by 46%.[38]

Multicentricity can be anticipated in as many as 70% of patients with papillary cancer and may represent intraglandular metastasis or multiple primary tumors. Also, cervical lymph node metastases are common, particularly in children, who have up to a 50% incidence of clinically detectable nodal disease and up to a 90% rate of microscopically detectable nodal disease at the time of initial presentation; however, this does not appreciably affect mortality. The presence of lymph node metastasis in patients with contained intrathyroidal primary papillary carcinoma also does not affect long-term survival. If there is gross or microscopic extension of a primary papillary carcinoma through the thyroid capsule, a poor prognosis and possibly a higher rate of lymph node metastasis may be anticipated.[39,40] Because multicentricity and lymph node metastases are common, complete ultrasound of the thyroid and central and lateral neck nodal basins should be performed prior to thyroidectomy for known or suspected malignancy.[7] Although papillary cancer typically disseminates via lymphatic spread, distant metastases do occur and are present in 3% to 5% of patients at the time of diagnosis. The two most common sites of spread are to the lungs and bones.

Study of DNA ploidy has been used to evaluate clinical prognosis. Increased nuclear DNA (aneuploidy) was believed to increase the risk for mortality. Universal agreement about this concept does not exist, however. Information on DNA ploidy may have some implications for prognosis but has had no definite impact on therapeutics.

### Treatment

The primary treatment of differentiated thyroid cancer, including papillary and follicular thyroid cancer, is surgical ablation. Several factors enter into surgical decision making. As noted, although well-differentiated cancers generally have a good prognosis, there are high rates of multicentricity within the thyroid and high rates of lymph node metastases, and recurrence is not infrequent. Furthermore, although more aggressive resections of the thyroid and lymphatic beds expose the patient to more potential morbidity, they facilitate radioiodine therapy, thyroxine suppression, and surveillance. With these considerations in mind, the objectives of initial therapy include the following: (1) remove the primary tumor and involved cervical lymph nodes; (2) minimize treatment related morbidity; (3) stage the disease accurately; (4) facilitate postoperative radioiodine therapy, if appropriate; (5) permit accurate long term surveillance; and (6) minimize risk of recurrence or metastasis.[7]

Appropriate surgical options and terminology for known or suspected thyroid malignancy include the following: (1) hemithyroidectomy or thyroid lobectomy, with or without isthmusectomy; (2) near-total thyroidectomy, defined by leaving less than 1 g of tissue adjacent to the recurrent laryngeal nerve at the ligament of Berry on one side; and (3) total thyroidectomy, defined by removal of all visible thyroid tissue. Nodulectomy or leaving more than 1 g of thyroid tissue in a subtotal thyroidectomy is not considered an appropriate surgical option for thyroid malignancy (Table 38-5).[7] The advantages of total or near-total thyroidectomy include the efficient use of radioiodine postoperative treatment. Radioablation is much less effective and requires a larger dosage if residual thyroid exists. Advantages of a procedure less than total or near-total thyroidectomy are decreased rates of bilateral recurrent laryngeal nerve damage and hypoparathyroidism.

For patients who do not have a biopsy-proven thyroid malignancy, the surgical option selected should balance the likelihood of cancer with potential morbidity. Because of the higher likelihood of malignancy, the following patients with undiagnosed nodules should undergo a total or near-total thyroidectomy as their initial resection: patients with larger than 4-cm tumors, those with marked atypia on biopsy, those with FNA results suspicious for papillary cancer, those with a family history of thyroid cancer, patients with a history of radiation exposure, and men older than 50 years. In patients without these high-risk findings and without a diagnosis of malignancy, thyroid lobectomy is an appropriate initial resection and serves as a diagnostic biopsy.[7]

Papillary cancers smaller than 1 cm in diameter are defined as microcarcinoma. In patients who have cytologic and imaging diagnosis of a solitary intrathyroidal papillary microcarcinoma, no clinically involved cervical lymph nodes, and no history of head and neck radiation, a unilateral thyroid lobectomy and isthmusectomy is an appropriate resection. Patients with a diagnosed thyroid cancer larger than 1 cm or a smaller than 1 cm papillary cancer with clinically positive nodal disease, multicentricity, or a history of head and neck radiation, the initial thyroid resection should be a total or near-total thyroidectomy, which will most likely be followed with radioablation.[7]

The management of central and lateral neck lymph nodal basins has been a topic of active debate in the multidisciplinary literature. The anatomically defined nodal regions of the central and lateral neck are shown in Figure 38-3. Although some patient groups, particularly those younger than 45 years, appear not to have significant prognostic impact of lymphatic spread, large registry studies have shown that in all patients with papillary thyroid cancer, there is a small but statistically significant decrease in long-term survival in those with lymphatic metastases compared with those without.[41] Therefore, it is currently recommended that all patients with known or suspected papillary cancer undergo a thorough physical examination and complete ultrasound of the central and lateral neck prior to resection of the thyroid lesion. If clinically positive adenopathy is detected in the central neck, a therapeutic level VI or central neck lymph node dissection should be performed at the time of total or near-total thyroidectomy. There is an emerging hypothesis that prophylactic level VI dissection should be routinely performed, even in those patients with clinically uninvolved nodes, but this remains a topic of debate. Those who support this practice have noted that there is a high frequency of pathologically positive but clinically negative nodal spread, and that some studies report lower rates of recurrent disease following routine central neck dissection.[42] Conversely, others studies find a higher rate of transient hypocalcemia, permanent hypoparathyroidism and nerve injury, and no evidence of benefit following prophylactic central neck dissection.[7, 43]

**Table 38-5 Indications for Interventional Procedures**

| PROCEDURE | ADVANTAGE | DISADVANTAGES AND COMPLICATIONS | INDICATION |
|---|---|---|---|
| FNA | Accurate diagnosis of malignancy | Cannot confirm benign diagnosis; capsular hemorrhage | Tissue diagnosis of ultrasound-determined solid nodule; prior nondiagnostic result |
| Open biopsy | Direct visualization | Requires an operating room, possibly general anesthesia | Complex case in which FNA has failed to give a diagnosis |
| Nodulectomy (less than a lobectomy) | None | Difficult second operation to complete lobectomy if cancer is diagnosed | None |
| Lobectomy (with isthmectomy) | Lower rates of hypocalcemia and nerve damage | May require completion thyroidectomy if cancer is diagnosed | Strong suspicion of benign disease; well-differentiated, low-risk PTC, <1 cm |
| Near-total thyroidectomy | Lower rates of hypocalcemia and nerve damage | Possible recurrence in residual thyroid tissue | Benign multinodular disease; small nodule on side of complete lobectomy; hyperthyroidism |
| Total thyroidectomy | Use of postoperative $^{131}I$ most efficacious; use of post–thyroglobulin levels for recurrence | Higher rate of hypocalcemia and nerve damage | Extensive multinodular disease; hyperthyroidism; >1 cm thyroid cancer (nonpalpable lymph nodes) |
| Modified radical lymph node dissection | Decreased rate of recurrence | Cranial nerve XII injury; loss of sensation over the ear and lateral cervical area; (left) thoracic duct leak and lymphocele; Horner's syndrome | Palpable or ultrasound-positive adenopathy with diagnosis of PTC, FTC, or medullary cancer |
| Median sternotomy | Exposure of mediastinal contents | Bleeding; nonunion of sternum (if complete sternotomy); increased hospital stay | Extension of malignancy into anterior mediastinum; inability to mobilize a large substernal goiter |
| Central neck (level VI) lymph node dissection | Decreased risk for recurrence | Increased risk for hypocalcemia and nerve damage | Medullary carcinoma; palpable or ultrasound-positive adenopathy with diagnosis of PTC or FTC |

The management of lateral neck lymph node basins has similarly been a topic of debate. Currently, consensus supports a practice of ipsilateral therapeutic lateral neck dissection for patients who have biopsy-proven metastatic lateral cervical disease. This should be undertaken as a formal clearance of a defined lymph node level, rather than isolated resection of the involved node, or berry picking.[7] Studies have shown that despite an almost 30% rate of micrometastases in lateral lymph nodes, there is little benefit of prophylactic lateral neck dissection for clinically negative nodes.[43]

It is not infrequent to diagnose well-differentiated thyroid cancer or multicentricity after completing a diagnostic thyroid lobectomy or total thyroidectomy performed for what was believed to be benign disease, such as symptomatic multinodular goiter. This presents the clinical question of whether completion thyroidectomy and/or lymphadenectomy should be carried out. Completion thyroidectomy offers the benefit of complete clearance of multifocal disease, facilitating radioiodine therapy, and enabling surveillance with determination of a serum Tg level. The downside involves a reoperative intervention, which carries a risk of technical complications. Current recommendations are that completion thyroidectomy should be performed if the original recommendation would have been total or near-total thyroidectomy if the pathology were known preoperatively. In other words, completion thyroidectomy should be performed, except in those patients with small (<1 cm), unifocal, intrathyroidal, node-negative and otherwise low-risk papillary cancers. In patients that meet these low-risk criteria, thyroid lobectomy may be considered an adequate resection and no further surgical intervention is required.[7]

For patients with lower stage disease, surgical resection generally results in excellent 5- to 10-year survival rates, exceeding 90%. With larger lesions, survival may decrease, especially in older men, and postoperative $^{131}$I therapy has been advocated for those with known metastases, extrathyroidal extension, and tumors larger than 4 cm.[7,35] Recurrence in local or regional lymph nodes after initial surgery is treated by completion thyroidectomy, if residual tissue exists, plus regional lymph node dissection. Radioiodine therapy is used as adjunctive therapy. Distant metastases are rare but have a poor prognosis (Fig. 38-17). Patients who have undergone thyroidectomy will require exogenous thyroid hormone replacement, which also provides the benefit of suppressing TSH and therefore suppressing a stimulus to further growth of differentiated thyroid cancers.[7]

The Mayo Clinic has published a follow-up series of patients with papillary cancer dating back to 1940.[37] In the first 10 years of the study (1940-1949), lobectomy was the primary procedure and was performed in almost 70% of cases. Since 1950, near-total or total thyroidectomy has essentially been the standard procedure and resulted in significantly improved survival in comparison to the earlier group. Cause-specific mortality and local recurrence rates have remained stable since then and over the last 50 years of the study, despite the more frequent use of postoperative radiation. Other studies have shown a benefit to postoperative $^{131}$I therapy.

The presence of distant metastatic disease may be evaluated with chest radiography, radionuclide scanning, CT, and other modalities, as guided by clinical suspicion. In patients after total thyroidectomy, postoperative Tg levels may be followed to monitor for recurrence, although preoperative Tg levels are not needed.[6,7,35]

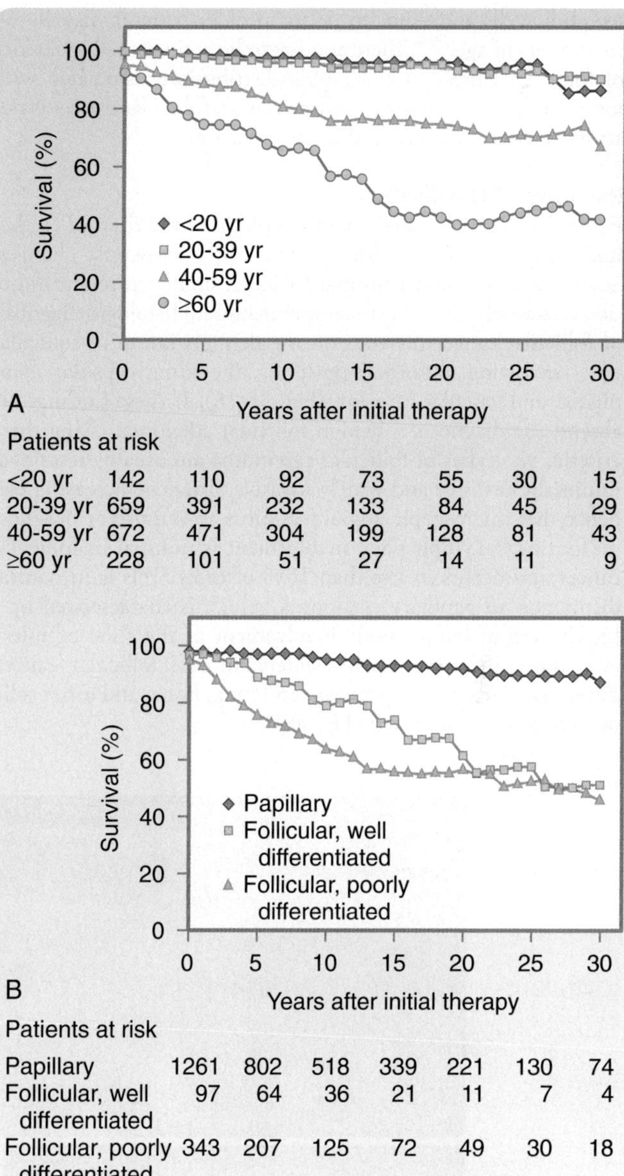


**FIGURE 38-17** Survival rates of 1701 patients with papillary or follicular carcinoma (no distant metastasis at time of diagnosis). Overall survival rates were 82% at 10 years, 72% at 20 years, and 60% at 30 years. Patients were followed at the Institut Gustav-Roussy in France. **A,** Effect of age at diagnosis on mortality for combined groups. **B,** Survival rate according to histologic subtype. (From Schlumberger ML: Medical progress: Papillary and follicular thyroid carcinoma. N Engl J Med 338:297–306, 1998.)

## Follicular Carcinoma

Follicular thyroid cancer is the second category of well-differentiated thyroid cancer and constitutes about 10% of all thyroid malignancies. Follicular cancer is a disease of an older population compared with papillary cancer, with a peak incidence between ages 40 and 60 years. It occurs more commonly in women, with a ratio of approximately 3 : 1. A subtype of follicular cancer, known as Hürthle cell carcinoma, consists of oxyphilic cells and tends to occur in older patients, usually 60 to 75 years of age.[35,40] There appears to be an increased incidence of follicular cancer in geographic distributions associated with iodine deficiency. Unlike papillary cancer, follicular cancer is not strongly associated with radiation exposure.

## Pathologic Classification

Follicular cancer is a malignant neoplasm of the thyroid epithelium that can have a wide spectrum of microscopic changes, anywhere from almost normal follicular architecture and function to severely altered cellular architecture. Histologic diagnosis of follicular cancer depends on the demonstration of follicular cells occupying abnormal positions, including capsular, lymphatic, and vascular invasion (Fig. 38-18). If these findings are absent, the diagnosis is benign follicular adenoma. Using these criteria, two types of follicular carcinoma are usually described, minimally invasive and widely invasive. There is increasing evidence that microscopic angioinvasion is an important prognostic finding.[44] Lymph node involvement is unusual in follicular cancer and occurs in less than 10% of cases. This is in contradistinction to papillary carcinoma, which is characterized by a higher rate of lymph node involvement at the time of initial evaluation. In patients with widely invasive follicular cancer, distant spread is more common, and lung, bone, and other solid organs are often involved (Fig. 38-19).[44]

## Clinical Features

Follicular cancer, like papillary cancer, typically manifests as a painless thyroid mass, which is evaluated as described earlier. Follicular cancer and multinodular goiter can coexist in as many as 10% of cases. Although the findings of hoarseness and firm

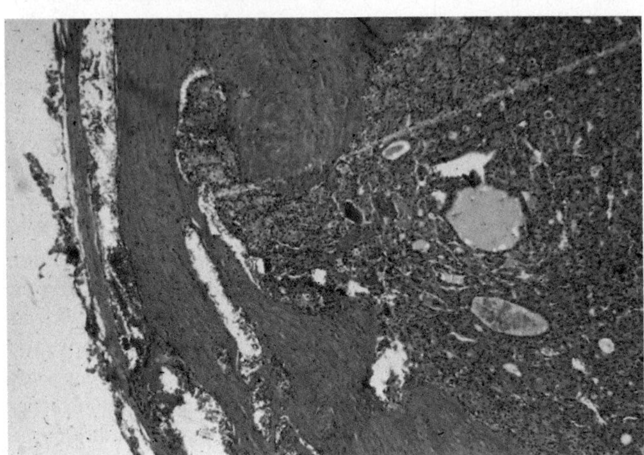

**FIGURE 38-18** Follicular lesion. This high-power examination reveals capsular invasion by follicular cells and allows the diagnosis of follicular cancer (H&E stain, ×100).

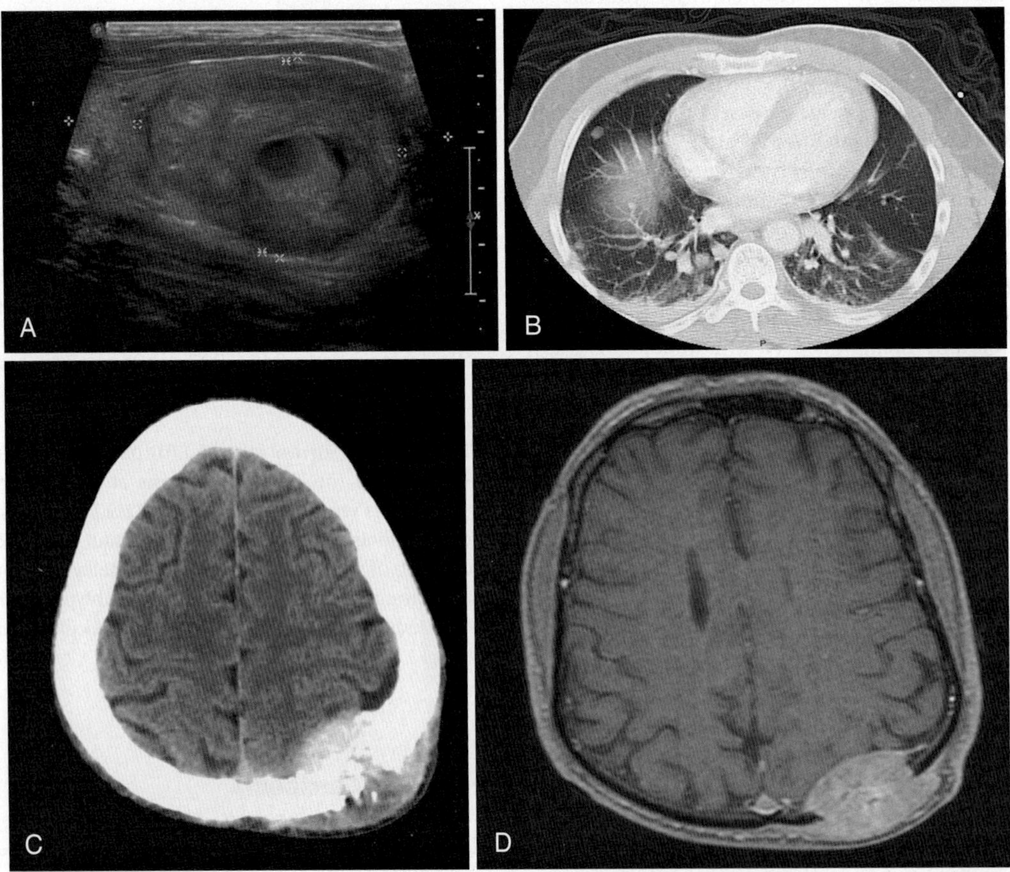


**FIGURE 38-19** Metastatic follicular cancer. All images are of the same patient. **A,** Preoperative ultrasound demonstrates a 6.7-cm mass in the left lobe of the thyroid; pathology demonstrates follicular cancer. **B,** CT scan of the chest demonstrates multiple pulmonary metastases. **C,** CT scan of the head demonstrates left parietal bone metastasis. **D,** MRI scan of the head demonstrates left parietal bone metastasis with an epidural component and mass effect on the brain.

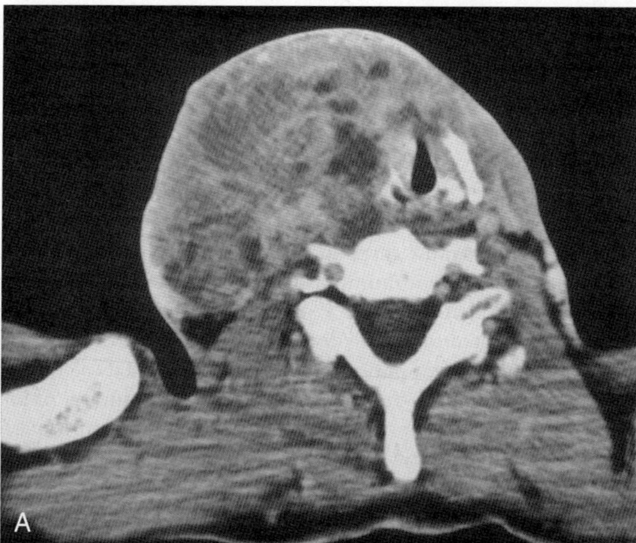


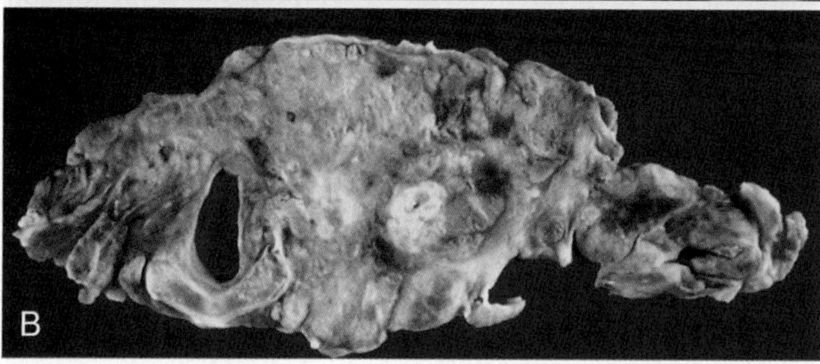


**FIGURE 38-20 A, B,** Rapidly enlarging thyroid mass in a 70-year-old man. The CT scan **(A)** demonstrates displacement of the larynx and lateral involvement of both jugular veins. This patient died within 6 months of rapidly progressing follicular cancer.

fixation of the mass on clinical evaluation suggest advanced disease and a poor prognosis, these circumstances are again found in a minority of cases. In such cases, a diligent search for aggressive extension into the trachea and for distant metastasis, particularly in older patients, is carried out with CT or MRI of the neck and chest (Fig. 38-20).[39]

Laboratory workup usually reveals a euthyroid state. The incidence of thyrotoxicosis in association with a thyroid malignancy, including follicular cancer, is approximately 2%. Preoperative imaging may be of some assistance in assessing the extent of a palpable mass. Ultrasound can determine the size and multicentricity of the malignancy; however, follicular cancer is usually manifested as a solitary mass. Radionuclide scanning can determine whether a mass is functioning or is cold, although a minority of cold nodules actually prove to be malignant.

Although FNA cytology is important in the workup of thyroid nodules, it is of limited value in the preoperative diagnosis of follicular cancer. Diagnosis of follicular cancer requires demonstration of cellular invasion of the capsule or vascular or lymphatic channels. These ultrastructural characteristics cannot be determined on FNA. Also, intraoperative frozen section has been notoriously ineffective in making a definitive diagnosis of follicular cancer.[17,20]

Unlike papillary cancer, follicular thyroid cancer typically spreads via hematogenous routes, which occurs in 10% to 15% of cases. The most common sites for metastatic deposits are lytic bone lesions and lung (see Fig. 38-19).

Prognosis is less favorable for follicular than for papillary cancer and is best in young patients with limited capsular or vascular invasion. As with papillary cancer, age is the most important predictor of survival, with a 95% 10-year survival in those younger than 40 years and an 80% 10-year survival between 40 and 60 years. Follicular cancers in older patients also are less likely to respond to radioiodine therapy. Size of the primary tumor is an important prognostic indicator although, unlike papillary cancer, even small follicular cancers should be considered clinically significant.

#### Treatment

Treatment of follicular carcinoma is primarily surgical. The diagnosis of the carcinoma cannot be determined by preoperative FNA or intraoperative frozen section diagnosis of a follicular lesion. The surgeon is left to select the most efficacious treatment of a follicular lesion, which, lacking the obvious gross characteristics of malignancy and widely invasive follicular cancer, is most likely a benign lesion. If the lesion is 2 cm or smaller and well contained within one thyroid lobe, an argument may be made for thyroid lobectomy and isthmusectomy. If the lesion is larger than 2 cm, the surgeon may well proceed with total thyroidectomy. If the follicular lesion is larger than 4 cm, the risk for cancer is higher than 50%, and total thyroidectomy is an obvious choice. In general, the recommendations for surgical management of follicular cancer mirror those of papillary cancer (see earlier). Also, as noted, follicular neoplasms excised by thyroid lobectomy may turn out to be follicular cancers on final pathology. Current recommendations support performing completion thyroidectomy if total thyroidectomy would have been offered if the diagnosis had been secured preoperatively.[7]

The prognosis after treatment of follicular cancer depends on age. Patients younger than 40 years have the best prognosis, with survival rates approaching 95% at 5 and 10 years. Series comparing follicular cancer with PTC have shown a poorer prognosis for follicular cancer, although this disparity is more prominent after 10 to 15 years. Poorly differentiated follicular cancer and well-differentiated follicular cancer have 60% and 80% 10-year survival rates, respectively (see Fig. 38-17).[39]

#### Postoperative Treatment

Accepted postsurgical management of well-differentiated papillary and follicular thyroid cancers involves the use of radioiodine ablation and long-term monitoring of Tg. $^{131}$I contains high-energy (gamma rays) and medium-energy (beta particles), which enhances the therapeutic effect. Patients are usually withheld from thyroid replacement therapy so that TSH levels may become elevated, rendering the thyroid iodine avid and thus maximizing the effect of $^{131}$I. Several studies have suggested that $^{131}$I ablation reduces disease-specific mortality in patients with primary tumors measuring at least 1 cm.[35]

If a patient has undergone complete thyroid ablation, Tg levels should be undetectable. The recent development of human recombinant TSH has redefined the efficacy of monitoring stimulated Tg levels as evidence of recurrence. It is possible that the use of human recombinant TSH can detect tumor recurrence at earlier and allow earlier treatment. Despite these advances, the use of Tg to monitor tumor recurrence remains imperfect.[6] As many as 15% to 30% of patients with thyroid carcinoma have anti-Tg antibodies, which seriously compromises the use of Tg as a tumor marker.[45]

## Hürthle Cell Carcinoma

Hürthle cell carcinoma is a subtype of FTC that closely resembles FTC, both grossly and on microscopic examination. The tumor contains an abundance of oxyphilic cells, or oncocytes. These cells are derived from follicular cells and have abundant granular acidophilic cytoplasm. Some studies have suggested that Hürthle cell carcinoma may have a worse clinical prognosis than standard FTC; however, there is no uniform agreement on these findings. Hürthle cell carcinoma appears in an older age group and is very unusual in children.

### Prognosis and Treatment

Hürthle cell carcinoma is manifested in much the same fashion as follicular cell neoplasms. The use of preoperative FNA raises many of the same issues; the finding of Hürthle cells leaves open the question of invasiveness and the diagnosis of malignancy. Treatment is surgical, following the same general principles as for the workup of a follicular neoplasm. There is debate as to whether patients with a predominance of Hürthle cells on FNA of a dominant thyroid nodule should undergo total thyroidectomy, or if lobectomy may be appropriate.[46,47]

Unlike papillary and follicular cancer, spread to local lymph nodes in Hürthle cell carcinoma is a poor prognostic event, associated with almost 70% mortality. Hürthle cell carcinoma is associated with a worse prognosis than FTC, which may be in part be caused by its poor uptake of iodine, thus rendering radioiodine ablation less effective. There is a significantly higher rate of recurrence than that seen in FTC.

## Medullary Carcinoma

Medullary carcinoma of the thyroid accounts for 4% to 10% of thyroid cancers. The malignancy originates in the parafollicular or C cells, which reside in the upper poles of the thyroid lobes and are of neural crest origin. MTC occurs most commonly in a sporadic form (80%) and the remainder as an autosomal dominant inherited disorder, such as MEN2A, MEN2B, and familial medullary thyroid cancer (FMTC). FMTC is a variant of MEN 2A, which includes MTC, but not the other features of MEN2A. MTCs arising in MEN2A usually has a more favorable long-term outcome than those arising in MEN2B or sporadic MTC.[35,48]

### Clinical Features

A patient with a sporadic medullary carcinoma typically has either of two manifestations: (1) a palpable mass in the thyroid that is present in most cases and for which a diagnosis can be made with FNA with immunohistochemistry; or (2) the finding of an elevated calcitonin level. Excess secretion of calcitonin has been demonstrated to be an effective marker for the presence of MTC and the presence of both a mass and an elevated calcitonin level is almost diagnostic of MTC. However, the finding of an elevated basal calcitonin level in the absence of a thyroid mass might require further workup, including repeat basal calcitonin measurement and a calcium-stimulated or gastrin-stimulated test. This calcitonin excess is not clinically associated with hypocalcemia, but may, rarely, result in symptoms of diarrhea and flushing in patients with advanced disease. Carcinoembryonic antigen (CEA) may also be elevated in some MTCs.

The MEN2 and FMTC syndromes involve different germline-activating mutations in the *RET* protooncogene. Also, 40% to 50% of sporadic MTC specimens have acquired *RET* mutations. Patients with inherited MTC syndromes initially develop C cell hyperplasia, which is a preneoplastic lesion in these patients, although C cell hyperplasia has little to no malignant potential in patients without *RET* mutations. Because of the high penetrance of MTC and the early development of C cell hyperplasia and MTC, family members of patients with MEN2 should be screened at an early age for the *RET* protooncogene. In MEN2B kindreds, *RET* testing should be performed shortly after birth and before age 5 years in FMTC and MEN2A kindreds.[48] The workup of these patients includes a detailed and in-depth family history to inquire about the characteristics of MEN2 in the patient and family members (Fig. 38-21). If MTC is suspected, the presence of other components of MEN2 syndrome must be considered; serum calcium and urinary catecholamine levels must be measured to evaluate for hyperparathyroidism and pheochromocytoma.

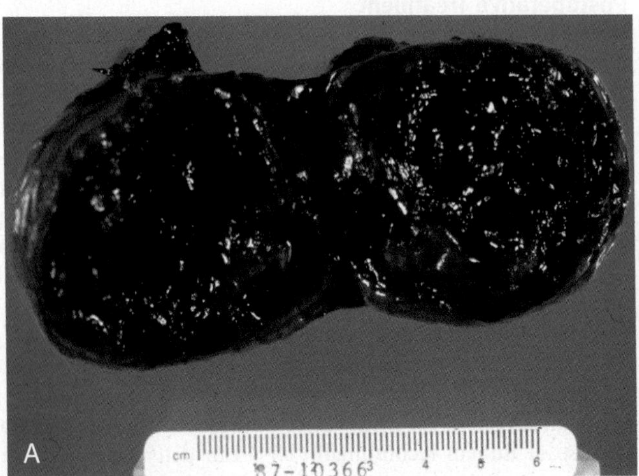


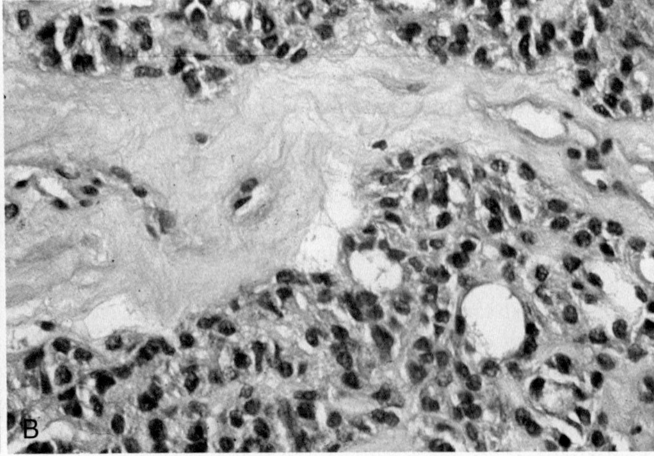


**FIGURE 38-21 A,** This 4-cm solitary mass in a thyroid lobe was removed by total thyroidectomy. **B,** Cells consistent with medullary carcinoma with amyloid infiltrate (H&E stain, ×400).

Pheochromocytoma, in particular, must be excluded prior to considering interventions in patients with MTC.

### Treatment

Most patients with MTC or a syndromic predisposition to MTC should undergo at least a total thyroidectomy. Total thyroidectomy allows complete removal of the gland and a search for multicentricity. Whereas in sporadic MTC the lesion is generally contained within one lobe, in MEN2 the malignancy involves the upper halves of both lobes. Patients with the MEN2B *RET* mutation are recommended to undergo prophylactic total thyroidectomy within the first year of life. Other patients with germline *RET* mutations should undergo prophylactic total thyroidectomy before age 5 years, although it may be appropriate to wait beyond 5 years with particular *RET* mutations. Level VI nodal dissection may be omitted in MEN2B patients younger than 1 year and MEN2A and FMTC patients younger than 5 years who are undergoing prophylactic thyroidectomy unless there are thyroid nodules larger than 5 mm, elevated calcitonin levels, or evidence of lymph node metastasis.[48]

Even in the absence of germline *RET* mutations, patients with known or suspected MTC without evidence of advanced disease should undergo total thyroidectomy with prophylactic level VI nodal dissection. The presence of nodal metastasis in the central neck mandates bilateral level VI nodal dissection; opinion varies regarding the addition of a lateral neck dissection on the side ipsilateral to the level VI disease. The presence of clinically or ultrasound-detectable disease in the lateral neck warrants total thyroidectomy and level VI and lateral compartment nodal dissection. If preoperative evaluation reveals distant metastatic disease, less aggressive surgery in the neck may be warranted to decrease the risk of morbidity caused by potential laryngeal nerve injury and hypoparathyroidism. However, palliative surgery may be indicated for patients with neck pain or airway compromise.[48]

If MTC is diagnosed postoperatively in a patient undergoing less than total thyroidectomy, further operative intervention is indicated to complete therapy as though the diagnosis were known preoperatively, including completion thyroidectomy and nodal dissection, as indicated. An exception to this are patients with an incidental finding of MTC in a thyroid lobectomy in which the MTC is sporadic and unifocal, there is no C cell hyperplasia, and an otherwise normal ultrasound of the neck, negative surgical margin, and normal serum calcitonin level are all confirmed.[48]

All prophylactic thyroidectomies for patients with *RET* mutations should be performed in experienced centers and attention should be given to preserving recurrent laryngeal nerve and parathyroid function. Dissection of the central lymph node compartment allows appropriate staging of this process. A successful operation with a good prognosis is predicted for patients with smaller masses and in whom calcitonin levels are undetectable after surgery. The literature has described the use of basal and stimulated calcitonin tests to monitor for recurrence because stimulated calcitonin values may rise before basal calcitonin levels. Unfortunately, documentation of recurrent MTC by biochemical means is often associated with unresectable recurrence in distant metastatic locations, including the lung and liver.[35] Recent reports have suggested that radioactive iodine scanning and therapy have little role in MTC, unless there is a concomitant PTC or FTC.[48]

## Anaplastic Thyroid Cancer

Anaplastic thyroid carcinoma represents approximately 1% of all thyroid malignancies. In contrast to a frequently positive prognosis in well-differentiated thyroid cancers, it is the most aggressive form of thyroid cancer, with a disease-specific mortality approaching 100%. A typical manifestation is an older patient with dysphagia, cervical tenderness, and a painful, rapidly enlarging neck mass. Patients frequently have a history of prior or coexistent differentiated thyroid cancer, and up to 50% have a history of goiter. Superior vena cava syndrome can also be part of the findings. The clinical situation deteriorates rapidly into tracheal obstruction and rapid local invasion of surrounding structures.

### Pathology

Grossly, the tumor is locally invasive, with a firm whitish appearance. On microscopic evaluation, giant cells with intranuclear cytoplasmic invaginations can be seen. There is a wide variety of cell types, ranging from moderately differentiated to extremely poorly differentiated cells (Fig. 38-22). Occasionally, squamous cell elements or islands of more recognizable differentiated thyroid carcinoma, such as papillary carcinoma, can be identified within the locus of the tumor. This has led to speculation that anaplastic carcinoma might arise from more well-differentiated carcinoma; however, there has been no solid proof of this theory.[35]

### Treatment

The results of any surgical treatment of anaplastic thyroid carcinoma are tempered by its rapidly progressive clinical course. Distant spread is present in 90% of patients at the time of diagnosis, usually to the lungs, and most reports of resection are not optimistic. FNA is accurate in 90% of cases, thus making open biopsy an uncommon surgical indication. Three types of cell populations have been classified—small spindle cell, giant cell, and squamous. All have a poor prognosis. *p53* mutations are found in 15% of tumors, a much higher rate than noted with well-differentiated cancers. Postoperative external beam radiation or adjunctive chemotherapy adds little to the overall prognosis, but should be considered.[49]

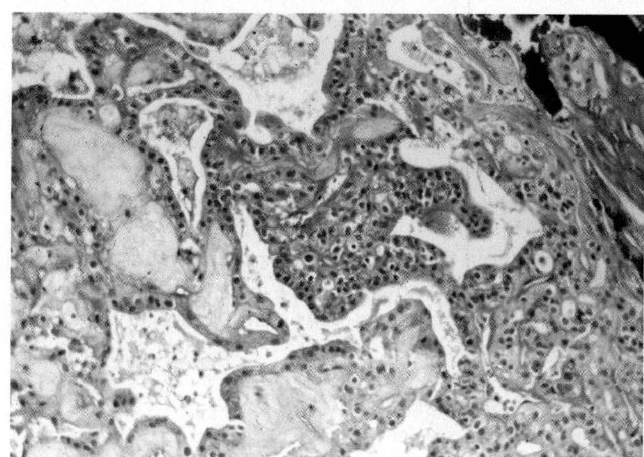

**FIGURE 38-22** Thyroid mass with a population of poorly differentiated cells, many of which are multinucleated. This is consistent with anaplastic carcinoma of the thyroid (H&E stain, ×200).

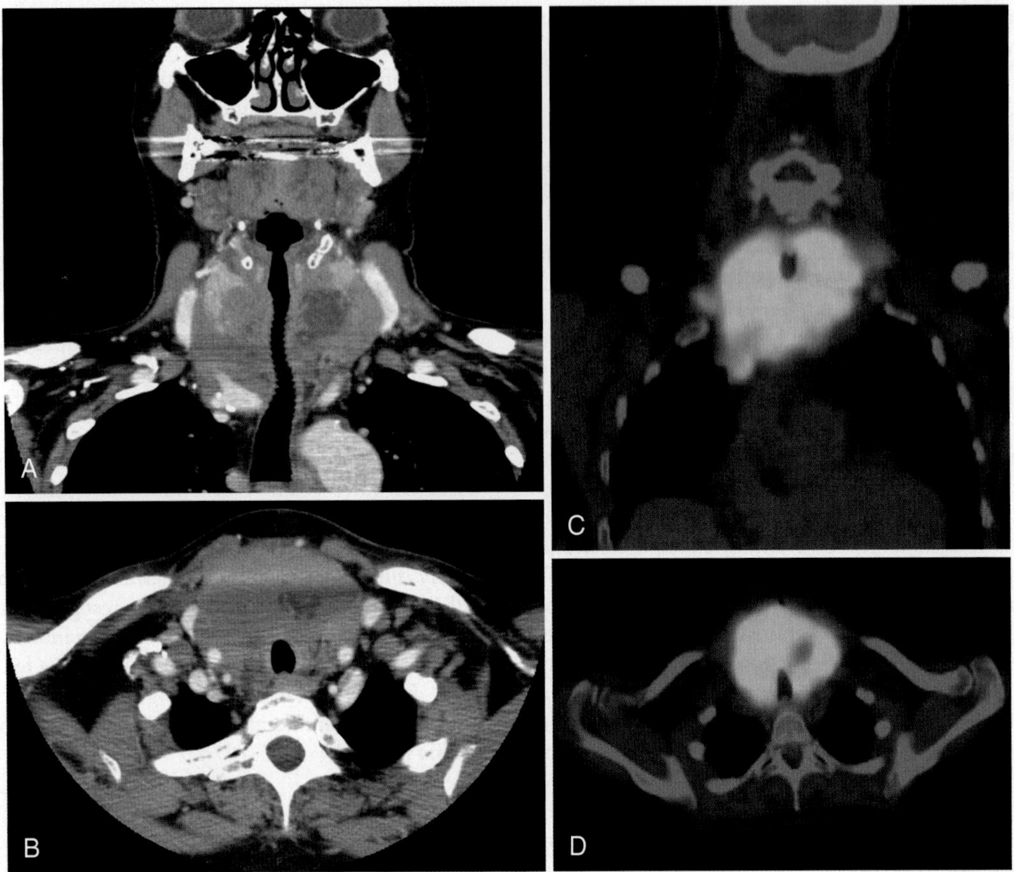


**FIGURE 38-23** B cell lymphoma of the thyroid. All images are of the same patient. Coronal **(A)** and axial **(B)** CT projections demonstrate a diffuse thyroid mass encasing the trachea, with necrotic components. Abnormal FDG-PET activity is demonstrated within this mass by PET-CT fusion imaging in coronal **(C)** and axial projections **(D)**.

It appears that if anaplastic carcinoma is initially confirmed to be resectable, some small improvement in survival may be seen following resection. The finding of distant metastasis or invasion into locally unresectable structures, such as the trachea or vasculature of the anterior mediastinum, leads to a more conservative surgical approach, such as tracheostomy. Because the prognosis is so grim in this disease, end-of-life planning and consideration of palliation must be part of the very early management and counseling of these patients.

### Lymphoma

Primary thyroid lymphoma, although rare, has been recognized more frequently. The diagnosis is considered in patients with a goiter, especially one that has apparently grown significantly in a short period. Other initial symptoms include hoarseness, dysphagia, and fever. Thyroid lymphoma occurs four times more frequently in women than in men. Approximately 50% of primary thyroid lymphomas occur in the setting of preexisting Hashimoto's thyroiditis.

#### Workup and Diagnosis

Patients with lymphoma undergo the standard workup for a thyroid mass or goiter. Suspicious signs are rapid enlargement and diffuse pain. The physical examination demonstrates a firm, slightly tender, fixed mass, frequently with substernal extension. There may be local symptoms, including vocal cord paralysis. A minority of patients have symptoms of lymphoma. Ultrasound may demonstrate a classic pseudocystic pattern. FNA can be diagnostic in this situation using flow cytometry for monoclonality to confirm the diagnosis. Thyroid lymphomas are almost all non-Hodgkin's lymphomas and most are B cell in origin. A subgroup of mucosa-associated lymphoid tissue (MALT) lymphomas occur in 6% to 27% of patients in some series.[50] If FNA is nondiagnostic, core needle biopsy or open biopsy can be considered. If the diagnosis is confirmed or highly suspicious, additional evaluation includes neck, chest, and abdominal CT or MRI to assess for extrathyroidal disease and may demonstrate disease completely encircling the trachea. The addition of PET imaging may be considered (Fig. 38-23). Approximately 50% of patients will have disease confined to the thyroid, 5% will have disease on both sides of the diaphragm or diffuse organ involvement, and the remainder will have locoregional nodal disease.

#### Treatment

Patients with impending airway compromise will frequently have rapid relief with the initiation of chemotherapy, particularly the glucocorticoid component, potentially avoiding the need for a surgical airway. Treatment philosophies differ with regard to chemotherapy or surgical ablation. Use of the CHOP regimen (***c***yclophosphamide, ***h***ydroxydaunomycin [doxorubicin], ***v***incristine, and ***p***rednisolone) has been associated with excellent survival. Surgical resection, including near-total or total thyroidectomy, is believed to enhance these results, particularly for MALT lymphomas, but likely has little role in patients with extrathyroidal disease. There can be a significant amount of pericapsular edema and swelling, with loss of normal tissue planes. There is likely no role for aggressive resections that might increase operative morbidity in the neck.

MALT lymphomas are usually diagnosed at an earlier stage and have an indolent course. Diffuse and mixed large cell lymphomas behave more aggressively and are often initially found to have widespread involvement. Five-year survival rates for MALT lymphomas approach 100%, whereas rates for large cell and mixed large cell lymphoma are 71% and 78%, respectively.

## SURGICAL APPROACHES TO THE THYROID

### Cervical Approach

Before any cervical exploration, the patient must be appropriately positioned, with the neck extended. We favor full muscle relaxation, which allows optimal positioning and facilitates exposure through limited incisions. After positioning, and before skin preparation, an excellent opportunity to perform neck ultrasound is available. A transverse incision is made about two fingerbreadths above the clavicular heads. The incision is placed so that it provides a direct approach to the thyroid gland and its adjacent structures while allowing optimal postoperative cosmetic results. If possible, the incision incorporates normal skin lines to aid in optimal cosmetic healing. The lateral borders of the incision can approach the medial borders of the sternocleidomastoid muscle but can be lengthened if the lateral aspect of the neck is to be investigated. The skin incision is carried through subcutaneous fat and the platysmal muscle, and superior and inferior flaps are dissected in a bloodless plane beneath the platysmal layer. The anterior jugular veins are identified, and any that are crossing or running along the midline can be divided (Fig. 38-24).

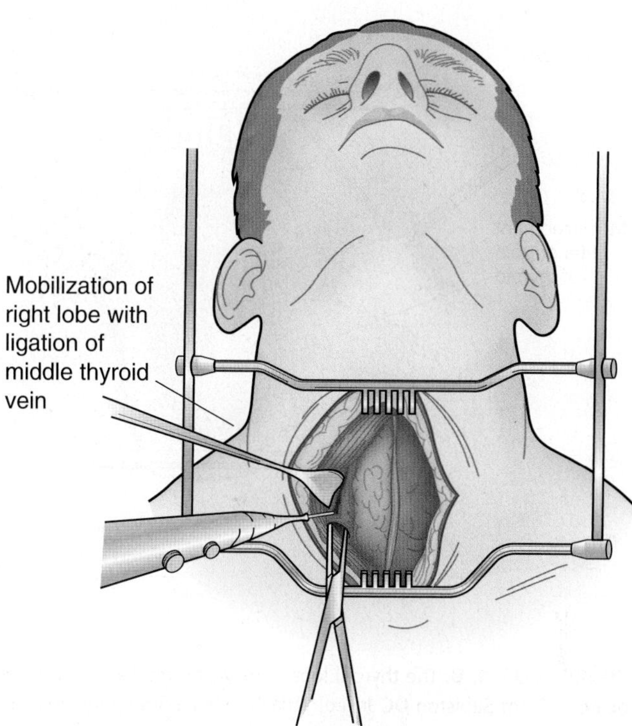


**FIGURE 38-24** A Mahorner retractor is inserted, and towels (not shown) are placed so that only the incision is exposed. The strap muscles (sternohyoid and sternothyroid) are then separated by dividing the tissues in the avascular midline plane from the thyroid cartilage to the suprasternal notch. The thyroid lobe is exposed by mobilizing the strap muscles away from the lobe by means of lateral retraction on the muscles. The middle vein is exposed, divided, and ligated. (From Sabiston DC Jr [ed]: Atlas of general surgery, Philadelphia, 1995, WB Saunders.)

The midline raphe can be identified between the sternohyoid muscles; this raphe is divided in a bloodless plane from the thyroid cartilage superiorly to the sternal notch inferiorly. As the plane immediately beneath the sternohyoid muscles is entered, one encounters the isthmus of the thyroid in the midline and each of the lobes laterally. Above and below the isthmus are the cartilaginous rings of the trachea. Blunt finger dissection can separate the sternohyoid muscle from the thyroid capsule medially and identify the sternothyroid muscles in a deep and lateral position. The sternothyroid muscles do not meet in the midline and must be separated off the thyroid capsule to gain lateral exposure to the thyroid. In patients who have previously undergone FNA, it may be that the planes under the sternothyroid muscle are obliterated by recent hemorrhage or scarring. If the patient has previously had thyroid surgery, these muscle groups will be densely adherent to the trachea and perhaps the tracheoesophageal groove. Great care must be used in this case to identify the parathyroids and recurrent laryngeal nerve.

When the recurrent laryngeal nerve has been identified on either side, it is mandatory to track it through any scar tissue or thyroid carcinoma. Every effort must be made to avoid sacrificing the nerve. In rare situations, such as anaplastic thyroid carcinoma, aggressive well-differentiated carcinoma, or obvious involvement with other head and neck tumors, the nerve may be sacrificed. If a recurrent laryngeal nerve is found to have been injured during the course of an otherwise uncomplicated operation, every attempt is made to repair it initially with microscope-aided visualization and a microvascular technique (8-0 or 9-0 monofilament sutures).

Dissection between the sternohyoid and sternothyroid muscles gains exposure to the lateral and deeper structures. Exposure of these lateral structures is enhanced by placing medial traction on the thyroid lobe on the side being dissected. Care must be taken to divide the middle thyroid vein before it is placed under excessive traction by this maneuver. With lateral retraction of the muscles and medial retraction of the thyroid lobe, the common carotid is quickly defined. On the left side, the esophagus is more prominent because of its more lateral position at this level in the neck. Definition of this area can be enhanced by placement of an esophageal stethoscope, which allows easier palpation of the esophagus.

In the case of complicated lateral thyroid masses, lymphadenopathy, or previous surgery, it may be necessary to gain exposure laterally by dividing the sternohyoid and sternothyroid muscles. It is rarely necessary to divide these two muscles, however, because lateral traction generally provides good exposure. If transection of the sternohyoid or sternothyroid muscle is necessary, it is done superiorly to minimize denervation because both these muscle groups are innervated from a caudal direction through the ansa hypoglossi nerves.

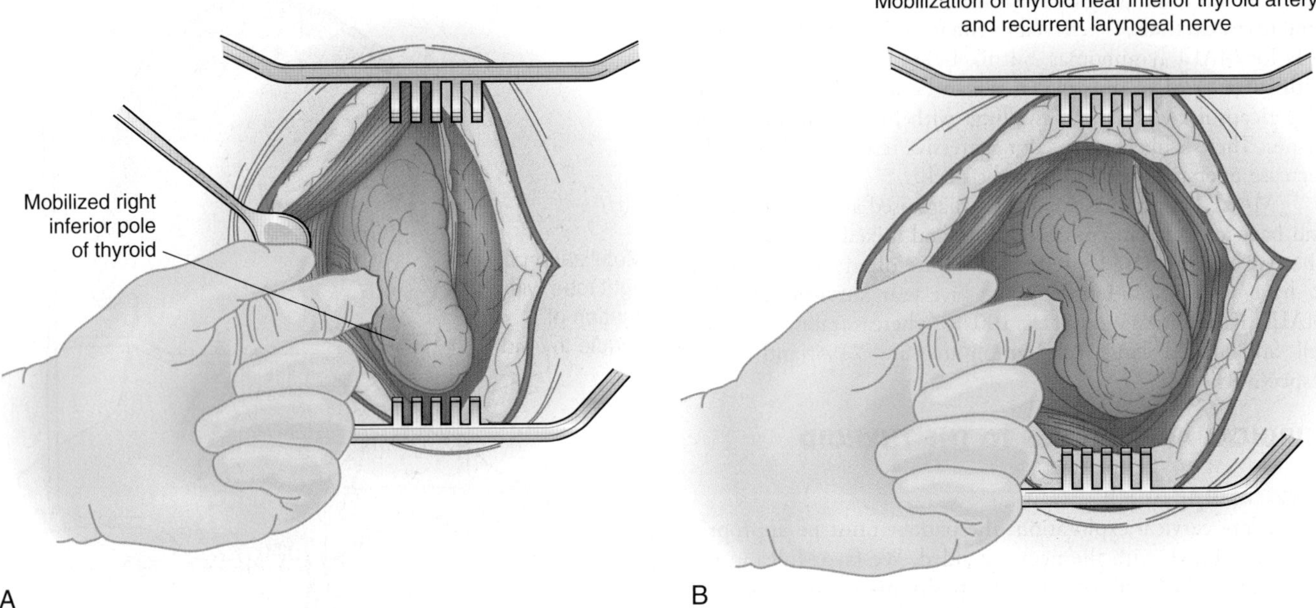


**FIGURE 38-25 A, B,** The thyroid lobe is retracted medially to expose the area where the parathyroid glands and recurrent laryngeal nerve are located. (From Sabiston DC Jr [ed]: Atlas of General Surgery. Philadelphia, WB Saunders, 1995.)

By gaining access to the plane immediately above the thyroid sheath and placing lateral traction on the strap muscles of the neck, the operating surgeon should be able to visualize the entirety of the anterior surface of the thyroid, even in reoperative cases. Traction on the thyroid lobes in a medial direction helps identify a dissection plane for gaining access to the superior pole vessels (Figs. 38-25 and 38-26). To skeletonize the superior pole vessels, one needs to have good exposure laterally between the common carotid artery and superior aspect of the ipsilateral thyroid lobe. One can then enter behind or posterior to the superior thyroid pole, adjacent to the cricothyroid muscle. Careful dissection in this area avoids injury to the external laryngeal nerve. Most patients (75% to 80%) have external laryngeal nerves that run on the cricothyroid muscle and are separate from the superior vessels; however, this leaves a significant number of patients in whom the nerve runs in close proximity to the superior pole vessels and could be divided if care is not exercised. After the superior pole vessels are carefully dissected and identified, they can be double-ligated adjacent to their entrance into the thyroid lobe. After the superior thyroid vessels and middle thyroid veins have been divided, continued medial retraction of the thyroid lobe allows the posterior aspect of the thyroid lobe to be visualized. The superior parathyroids are usually found lying in small deposits of fat in this area, within the thyroid sheath (Figs. 38-27 and 38-28).

Further mobilization of the thyroid lobe allows exposure of the tracheoesophageal groove and recurrent laryngeal nerve (Figs. 38-29 to 38-33). Minimal dissection of the lower vessels entering the thyroid is undertaken and no division is carried out until the recurrent laryngeal nerve is seen and positively identified. On the right side, care is taken when dissecting in the posterolateral aspects of the trachea because the esophagus is not well palpated in this area. In patients undergoing thyroid reoperations, this area is extremely treacherous because of scar tissue. It is generally advisable, if the recurrent laryngeal nerve is not immediately visible at the level of the thyroid lobe, to proceed

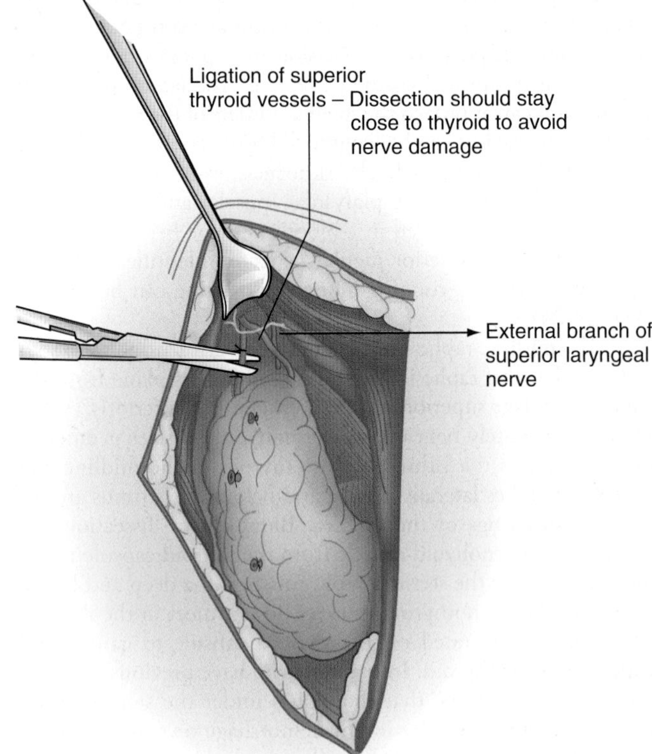


**FIGURE 38-26** Downward traction exposes the superior pole vessels, including branches of the superior thyroid artery. The external laryngeal nerve courses along the cricothyroid muscle, just medial to the superior pole vessels. To avoid injury to this nerve, which controls tension of the vocal cords, the superior pole vessels are divided individually as close as possible to the point at which they enter the thyroid gland. (From Sabiston DC Jr [ed]: Atlas of general surgery, Philadelphia, 1995, WB Saunders.)

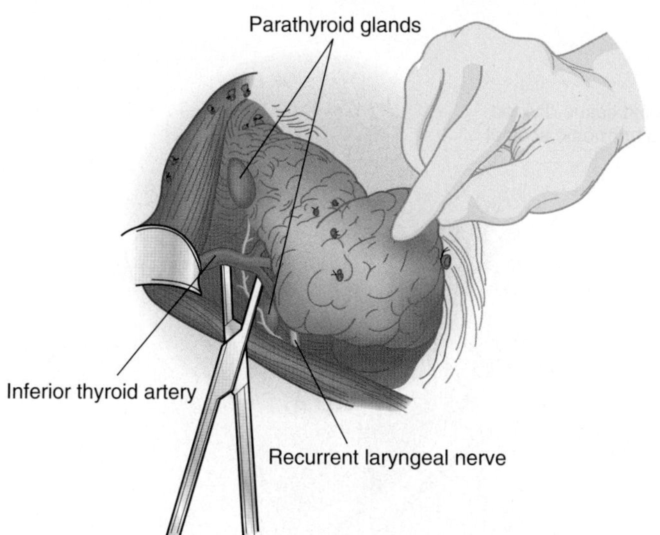


**FIGURE 38-27** As the thyroid is retracted medially, gentle dissection is used to expose the parathyroid glands, inferior thyroid artery, and recurrent laryngeal nerve. The recurrent nerve usually passes behind the inferior thyroid but occasionally lies anterior to it. It is best found by careful dissection just inferior to the artery. The nerve can then be traced upward, and its position in relation to the thyroid can be determined. Parathyroid glands that lie on the thyroid surface can be mobilized with their vascular supply and thus preserved. (From Sabiston DC Jr [ed]: Atlas of general surgery, Philadelphia, 1995, WB Saunders.)

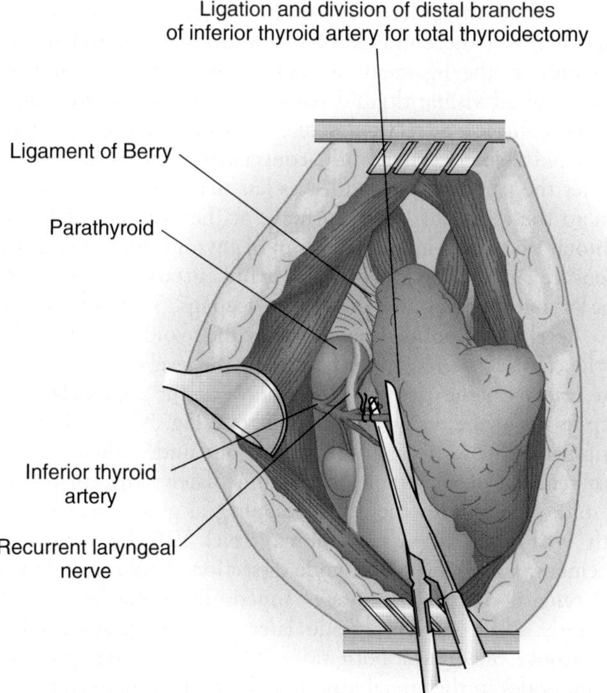


**FIGURE 38-28** To perform a total lobectomy, branches of the inferior thyroid artery are divided at the surface of the thyroid gland. The inferior thyroid veins can now be ligated and divided. Superiorly, the connective tissue (ligament of Berry), which binds the thyroid to the tracheal rings, is carefully divided. Several small accompanying vessels are usually present; the recurrent nerve is closest to the thyroid and most vulnerable at this point. Division of the ligament allows the thyroid to be mobilized medially. (From Sabiston DC Jr [ed]: Atlas of general surgery, Philadelphia, 1995, WB Saunders.)

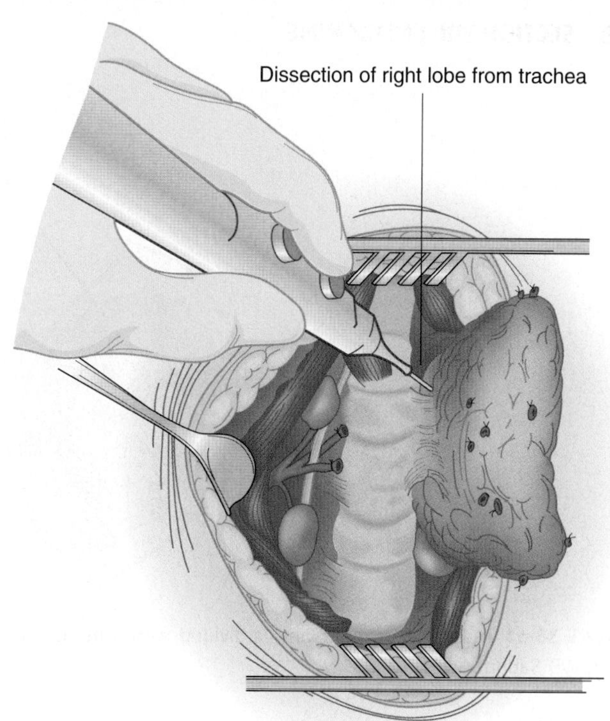


**FIGURE 38-29** Dissection of the thyroid from the trachea can be performed with the cautery by division of the loose connective tissue between these structures. Dissection is extended under the isthmus and the specimen is divided so that the isthmus is included with the resected lobe. The pyramidal lobe is also included, if present. (From Sabiston DC Jr [ed]: Atlas of general surgery, Philadelphia, 1995, WB Saunders.)

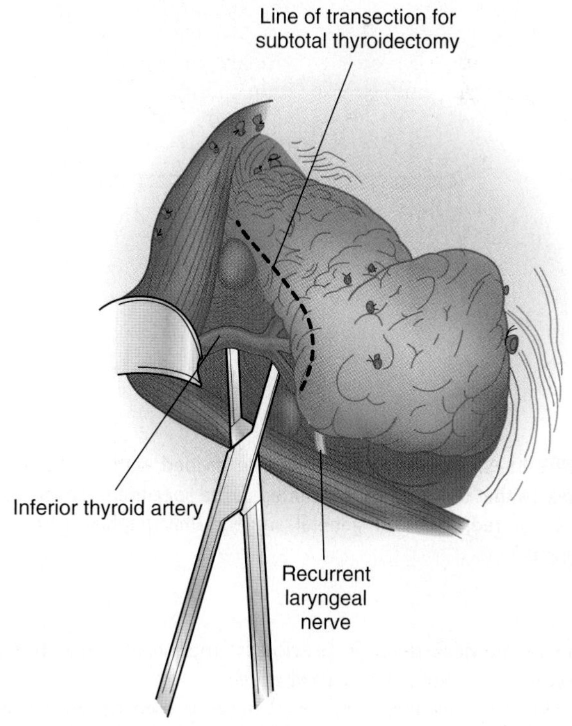


**FIGURE 38-30** Subtotal lobectomy necessitates identification of the parathyroid glands, inferior thyroid artery, and recurrent laryngeal nerve, as described earlier. The line of resection is selected to preserve the parathyroid glands and their blood supply and to protect the recurrent laryngeal nerve. This is based on the inferior thyroid artery or its major branches. (From Sabiston DC Jr [ed]: Atlas of general surgery, Philadelphia, 1995, WB Saunders.)

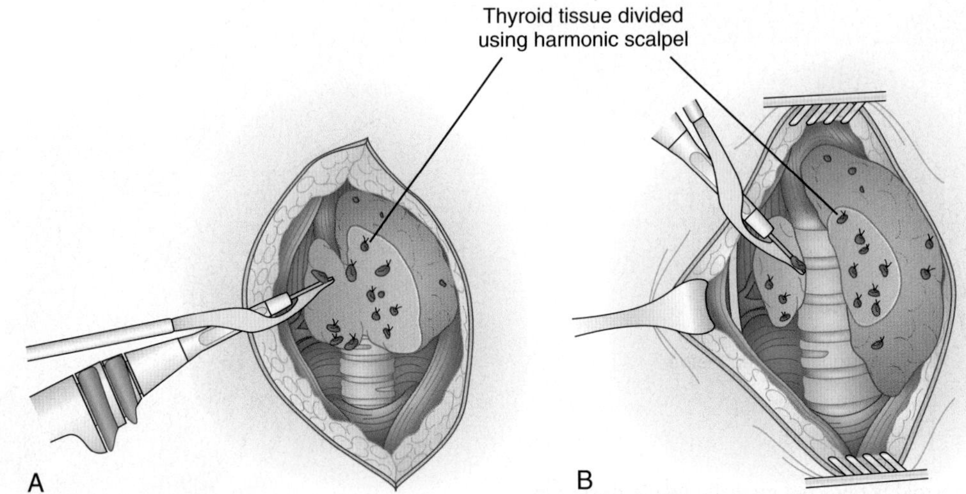


**FIGURE 38-31 A, B,** The thyroid gland is divided with a harmonic scalpel. (From Sabiston DC Jr [ed]: Atlas of general surgery, Philadelphia, 1995, WB Saunders.)

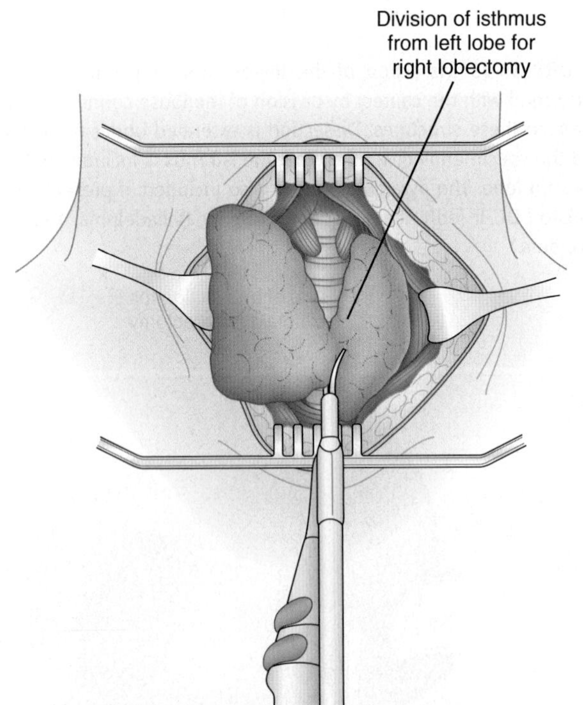


**FIGURE 38-32** The thyroid can now be divided with the harmonic scalpel so that the isthmus is included in the specimen. (From Sabiston DC Jr [ed]: Atlas of general surgery, Philadelphia, 1995, WB Saunders.)

lower in the neck tissue in previously undissected areas to gain access to the recurrent laryngeal nerve.

After the recurrent laryngeal nerve is seen on either side, the pace of the operation may be increased; the inferior vessels may be divided while the course of the recurrent laryngeal nerve is visualized directly. Continued medial traction on the lobe then identifies the cephalad course of the nerve to the point at which it disappears under the ligament of Berry or into its final destination, the caudal border of the cricothyroid muscle. The ligament of Berry is in a position just anterior and slightly medial to the nerve's entrance underneath the cricothyroid muscle; this structure, with a small rim of thyroid tissue, can be ligated with silk suture or a harmonic scalpel. After division of the ligament of Berry, the attachment of the thyroid medially on the trachea can be divided with low-energy Bovie dissection or a harmonic scalpel (see Fig. 38-29).

Terminology for thyroid surgery is inconsistent in the literature. Total thyroidectomy involves division of all thyroid tissue between the entrance of the recurrent laryngeal nerves bilaterally at the ligament of Berry, and results in complete removal of all visible thyroid tissue. Near-total thyroidectomy involves complete dissection on one side while leaving a remnant of thyroid tissue laterally on the contralateral side, which incorporates the parathyroids and leaves less than 1 g of tissue adjacent to the recurrent laryngeal nerve at the ligament of Berry. Subtotal thyroidectomy leaves a rim of thyroid tissue bilaterally to ensure parathyroid viability and avoid entrance of the recurrent laryngeal nerves into the larynx (see Figs. 38-28 to 38-32).

Level VI is bounded superiorly by the hyoid bone, laterally by the carotid arteries, and inferiorly by the level of the innominate artery on the right, and lies between the superficial and deep layers of the deep cervical fascia (see Fig. 38-3).[51] Central lymph node dissection can be carried out under direct vision, with removal of all lymph nodes immediately adjacent to the thyroid, especially in the tracheoesophageal groove in patients with well-differentiated carcinoma (level VI). By consensus statement, a level VI lymph node dissection should include the prelaryngeal or delphian nodes superiorly, pretracheal nodes inferiorly, and paratracheal nodes laterally in the tracheoesophageal groove on one or both sides.[51] If a patient has palpable lymph nodes in the lateral aspect of the neck, a more complete modified radical neck dissection is performed.

Postoperative monitoring of thyroid and parathyroid function is extremely important. The surgeon is obligated to evaluate and inform the patient and referring physician of the details of the resection and its expected impact on postoperative function. A calcium assay is performed within 24 hours of surgery. If no signs of hypocalcemia are present, particularly if the surgeon has visualized the glands during surgery, no calcium

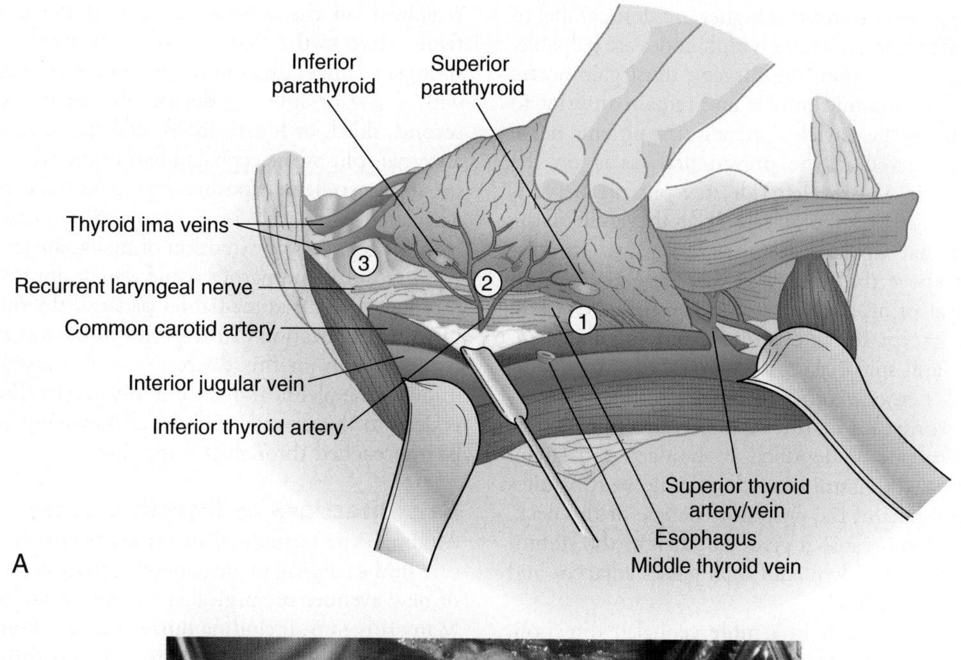


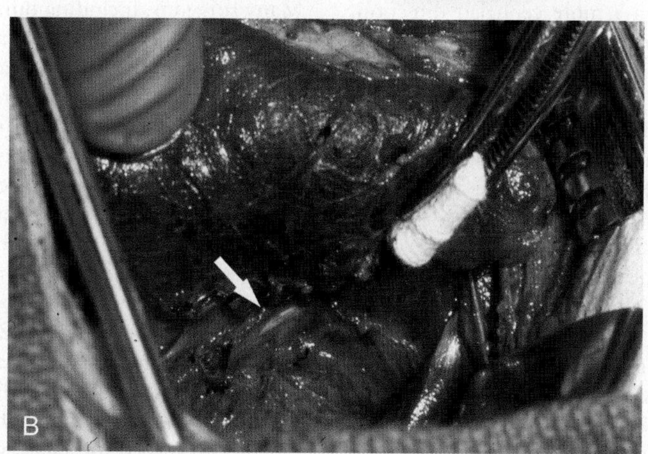


**FIGURE 38-33 A,** During thyroidectomy, the recurrent laryngeal nerve is at greatest risk for injury at the ligament of Berry (1), during ligation of branches of the inferior thyroid artery (2), and at the thoracic inlet (3). **B,** Intraoperative photograph of the recurrent laryngeal nerve in the tracheoesophageal groove *(white arrow).* (A from Kahky MP, Weber RS: Intraoperative problems: Complications of surgery of the thyroid and parathyroid glands. Surg Clin North Am 73:307-321, 1993.)

supplementation may be necessary. If symptoms occur or if the surgeon is concerned about the patient's parathyroid status, daily supplements of 1500 to 3000 mg of elemental calcium may be started.

If the patient was euthyroid before surgery, it is reasonable to expect that replacement may not be needed for at least 10 days, even after total thyroidectomy. This allows time for complete evaluation of the specimen by pathology. Thyroid replacement generally requires a daily dose of 1.6 μg/kg of levothyroxine (Synthroid). Most endocrinologists believe that the levothyroxine dose needs to be adjusted to keep TSH levels at low-normal values after resection for cancer or suppressive therapy.

## Modified Radical Neck Dissection

There is some controversy about when to perform a modified radical neck dissection for thyroid carcinoma. However, it is safe to say that this operation is most widely performed in patients with documented disease in whom obvious and palpable lymphadenopathy lateral to the carotid sheath exists at the time of the original diagnosis or occurs after preceding thyroid surgery. Current consensus recommendations have been reviewed (see earlier) and the use of selected removal of palpable nodes in the lateral compartment (so-called berry picking) has largely been abandoned. In our practice, modified radical neck dissection is primarily reserved for patients with thyroid carcinoma and clinically palpable cervical lymph node metastases. This can be accomplished with an en bloc dissection that removes all the lymphatic and adipose tissue in the lateral neck compartment while avoiding the cosmetic or functional abnormality associated with the removal of muscle groups that is used in the classic radical neck dissection. The sternocleidomastoid muscle and spinal accessory nerve are spared.[52]

A cervical skin incision is used for the operation, which is standard for most thyroid surgeries. It is extended laterally and superiorly along the border of the sternocleidomastoid muscle.

Occasionally, it is necessary to make a higher incision parallel to the previous surgical incision if higher lymph nodes are palpable. In initiating the neck dissection, the surgeon must gain access deep to the sternocleidomastoid muscle and remain anterior to the carotid sheath above the clavicle. Laterally, the phrenic nerve is identified and preserved in the prevertebral fascia on the anterior scalene muscle. On the left side, the phrenic nerve is immediately adjacent to the thoracic duct at the level of the junction of the internal jugular and subclavian veins. The dissection begins just above the clavicle in this area. The goal of dissection is removal of all tissue between the superficial and prevertebral fascia, except for the carotid artery, jugular vein, vagus, and phrenic and spinal accessory nerves. Also, the sympathetic chain and sternocleidomastoid muscle must be preserved. Dissection continues in the cephalad direction, where the spinal accessory nerve is identified at the deep and lateral surface of the sternocleidomastoid muscle. The nerve runs inferiorly in the lateral aspect of the posterior triangle of the neck. The nerve can be traced because it gives a branch to the sternocleidomastoid muscle at this level and then passes adjacent and posterior to the digastric muscle.

As the dissection proceeds in a more cephalad direction, the hypoglossal nerve is encountered; it crosses anteriorly to the internal carotid artery and internal jugular vein but deep to the anterior facial vein. It follows the stylohyoid muscle into the submandibular triangle and innervates the muscles of the tongue. If one chooses to ligate the internal jugular vein, care must be taken not to injure the hypoglossal nerve as it crosses in this area.

Medially, the surgeon must take care not to injure the cervical sympathetic chain, which lies deep to the carotid sheath, just anterior to the prevertebral fascia. The retropharyngeal lymphatics connect with the cervical and jugular lymphatics across the chain in this area and may have metastatic deposits of thyroid cancer. Injury to the sympathetic chain in this area results in Horner's syndrome, which includes ptosis, miosis, anhidrosis, and increased skin temperature on the involved side.

On completion of a modified radical dissection, a triangle of fibrofatty tissue, which may or may not include the internal jugular vein, is dissected free and oriented for pathology. It is not usually necessary to extend dissection into the suprahyoid area unless there is extensive lymph node involvement, which occurs only in a few patients with well-differentiated thyroid carcinoma (~1%). Great care is taken when dissecting structures in the lateral aspect of the neck, including the sympathetic chain and recurrent laryngeal and spinal accessory nerves, unless they are obviously and grossly involved with tumor.

## Median Sternotomy

Exploration of the anterior mediastinal space is within the armamentarium of an experienced thyroid surgeon. Almost every benign and malignant thyroid tumor can be removed through cervical exploration. Occasionally, a median sternotomy may be necessary for patients who need a reoperation, have large invasive tumors, have low-lying thyroid glands and a large tumor, or have previously undergone radioiodine ablation or external beam radiation.

Initial exploration usually involves a cervical incision. If a median sternotomy is then required, a midline incision is made from the middle of the cervical wound and extended inferiorly and onto the manubrium. Before dividing the sternum, access is gained on the superior border of the manubrium and all tissues deep to the sternum are swept away bluntly with cotton sponges or finger dissection. The midline sternal incision is made with a saw or splitting device and carried to the level of the second, third, or fourth intercostal space, as needed. We prefer a sternal split of the cephalad half of the sternum, which usually provides excellent exposure and avoids the possible instability associated with full sternotomy. Substernal thyroid masses, including goiters or extension of malignancies, as well as ectopic parathyroid adenomatous tissue, can be approached through this incision. The anteromedial fat pad and thymus can be dissected to gain visualization of the pericardium superiorly. As one proceeds laterally in this dissection, care must be taken to avoid injuring the pleura and the phrenic nerves. The innominate vein is deep to the thymus. Almost all low-lying thyroid masses can be approached through this incision.

## New Directions in Thyroid Surgery

Although the techniques described here remain the standard of care in the surgical management of thyroid pathology, a number of new avenues of surgical intervention are being investigated. Many surgeons, including ourselves, have found that traditional surgical technique may be accomplished through more limited skin incisions. This requires careful positioning and appropriate use of self-retaining retractors, and is facilitated by paralysis. Other techniques allow even more limited cervical incisions or relocation of the incision away from the neck and, in one case, the skin incision was entirely eliminated. The appropriate application and safety profile of all these techniques is still being defined and must be measured against traditional thyroidectomy, which is well tolerated and has a low rate of morbidity.

Minimally invasive video-assisted thyroidectomy (MIVAT) involves the use of a 1.5- to 2-cm anterior cervical incision, an endoscopic camera placed into the wound for visualization, self-retaining retractors, and dedicated surgical instruments. This technique is generally applied to lobectomy for benign disease, but has been used for small, well-differentiated thyroid cancers and even to total thyroidectomy for malignancy, although total thyroidectomy requires a bilateral approach. This approach does result in longer operative times, which improve after a learning curve, and is believed to have the same rate of technical complication as traditional thyroidectomy. Prior neck surgery, large-volume thyroid (>25 mL), large lesion, and lymphatic metastasis are considered contraindications to this technique.[53,54]

Kang and colleagues,[55] in South Korea, have championed the use of a transaxillary, gasless, robotically assisted approach to thyroidectomy. A 5- to 6-cm incision is made in the axilla and a subcutaneous plane is created anterior to the pectoralis, between the heads of the sternocleidomastoid muscle, and deep to the strap muscles. A second incision (<1 cm) is also required on the anterior chest. Using these incisions, a self-retaining retractor, and robotic surgical system, total thyroidectomy may be performed. This approach has been applied to benign disease and small malignancies. The authors include an ipsilateral level VI nodal dissection in all cases. They reported a 1% rate of permanent recurrent laryngeal nerve injury and a 3-day mean hospital stay.

There is a single reported case of thyroid lobectomy performed with no skin incision. This technique involved several incisions in the floor of the mouth, through which instruments were tunneled to a subplatysmal plane, the neck insufflated, and endoscopic thyroidectomy undertaken. With the exception of a small hematoma, the patient reported to have undergone this procedure had a good recovery, but no series is yet available to establish efficacy and safety.[56]

## Complications of Surgery

The advantage of complete removal of disease-bearing tissue and efficient subsequent application of postprocedure radioiodine ablation after total thyroidectomy must be weighed against lesser procedures, such as lobectomy, in terms of surgical complications. The most significant complications are postprocedure hypocalcemia secondary to devascularization of the parathyroid and significant hoarseness caused by recurrent laryngeal nerve injury, induced by traction or division (see Fig. 38-33).

### Hypocalcemia

Rates of postprocedure hypocalcemia are approximately 5%; it resolves in 80% of cases in approximately 12 months.[57] Therefore, every effort is made to evaluate the parathyroid tissue intraoperatively. For glands that appear to be devascularized, the use of immediate parathyroid autotransplantation of 1-mm fragments of saline-chilled tissue into pockets made in the sternocleidomastoid or brachioradialis muscle is extremely effective for avoiding hypocalcemia.

### Nerve Injury

**Superior Laryngeal Nerve** The superior laryngeal nerve has two branches, an internal branch that supplies sensory fibers to the larynx and an external branch that supplies motor fibers to the cricothyroid muscles and tenses the vocal cords. The external branch can run closely adherent to the superior thyroid artery, and care must be exercised during dissection in this area. Injury to the branch causes voice changes, huskiness, poor volume voice fatigue, and an inability to sing at higher ranges.[2,58]

**Recurrent Laryngeal Nerve** As noted, the recurrent laryngeal nerve arises from the vagus and is a mixed motor, sensory, and autonomous nerve that innervates the adductor and abductor muscles (see Fig. 38-33). Unilateral injury is classically described as a paralyzed vocal cord, with loss of movement from the midline. A wide spectrum of injuries to the voice, swallowing mechanisms, or both can occur because of the mixed fibers contained within the nerve.[2] A temporary or permanent voice change can result, which is extremely distressing to the patient.

### Bleeding

Other complications such as bleeding and wound hematomas may require immediate reexploration, which is done in the operating room unless airway compromise dictates otherwise. These complications can be avoided by meticulous hemostasis at closing, which results in less than a 1% rate of occurrence.[58]

Complication rates appear to be affected by surgeon experience. A study in Maryland of 5860 patients reported the lowest complication rates in patients of surgeons who performed more than 100 neck explorations annually.[59]

## SELECTED REFERENCES

Cady B, Sedgwick CE, Meissner WA, et al: Risk factor analysis in differentiated thyroid cancer. Cancer 43:810–820, 1979.

A classic paper exploring the important prognostic factors in well-differentiated thyroid cancers, particularly highlighting the importance of age and gender.

Cooper DS, Doherty GM, Haugen BR, et al: Revised American Thyroid Association management guidelines for patients with thyroid nodules and differentiated thyroid cancer. Thyroid 19:1167–1214, 2009.

A thorough update of the original 2006 consensus statement of the American Thyroid Association on the management of thyroid nodules and differentiated thyroid cancer; must be read by anyone managing thyroid pathologies.

Hartl DM, Travagli JP, Leboulleux S, et al: Clinical review: Current concepts in the management of unilateral recurrent laryngeal nerve paralysis after thyroid surgery. J Clin Endocrinol Metab 90:3084–3088, 2005.

An excellent discussion of the pathophysiology of surgically induced damage to the external branch of the superior laryngeal and recurrent laryngeal nerves; must be read by all thyroid surgeons.

Hay ID, Thompson GB, Grant CS, et al: Papillary thyroid carcinoma managed at the Mayo Clinic during six decades (1940-1999): Temporal trends in initial therapy and long-term outcome in 2444 consecutively treated patients. World J Surg 26:879–885, 2002.

Another excellent Mayo Clinic contribution in the area of thyroid cancer that possibly represents the longest study of this cancer. It confirms the use of more extensive resection and postoperative radioablation and substantiates the data with 50 years of follow-up.

Schlumberger MJ: Papillary and follicular thyroid cancer. N Engl J Med 338:297–306, 1998.

An excellent update on the topic, with 93 references. Modern controversies and classic observations are well discussed and presented. The author's experience with 1700 patients is included in the discussion.

Sherman SI: Thyroid carcinoma. Lancet 361:501–511, 2003.

An excellent seminar on the diagnosis, treatment, and follow-up monitoring of all four cancer groups. This review includes 168 references and an excellent discussion.

## REFERENCES

1. Huang SM, Wu TJ: Neck ultrasound for prediction of right nonrecurrent laryngeal nerve. Head Neck 32:844–849, 2010.
2. Hartl DM, Travagli JP, Leboulleux S, et al: Clinical review: Current concepts in the management of unilateral recurrent laryngeal nerve paralysis after thyroid surgery. J Clin Endocrinol Metab 90:3084–3088, 2005.
3. Spitzweg C, Heufelder AE, Morris JC: Thyroid iodine transport. Thyroid 10:321–330, 2000.
4. Hollowell JG, Staehling NW, Hannon WH, et al: Iodine nutrition in the United States. Trends and public health implications: Iodine excretion data from National Health and Nutrition Examination Surveys I and III (1971-1974 and 1988-1994). J Clin Endocrinol Metab 83:3401–3408, 1998.

5. Chopra I: Nature, source, and relative significance of circulating thyroid hormones. In Braverman LE, Utiger RE, editors: Werner and Ingbar's the thyroid, ed 7, Philadelphia, 1996, Lippincott-Raven, pp 111–124.
6. Mazzaferri EL, Robbins RJ, Spencer CA, et al: A consensus report of the role of serum thyroglobulin as a monitoring method for low-risk patients with papillary thyroid carcinoma. J Clin Endocrinol Metab 88:1433–1441, 2003.
7. Cooper DS, Doherty GM, Haugen BR, et al: Revised American Thyroid Association management guidelines for patients with thyroid nodules and differentiated thyroid cancer. Thyroid 19:1167–1214, 2009.
8. Duh QY, Grossman RF: Thyroid growth factors, signal transduction pathways, and oncogenes. Surg Clin North Am 75:421–437, 1995.
9. Martino E, Bartalena L, Bogazzi F, et al: The effects of amiodarone on the thyroid. Endocr Rev 22:240–254, 2001.
10. Lorenz K, Gimm O, Holzhausen HJ, et al: Riedel's thyroiditis: Impact and strategy of a challenging surgery. Langenbecks Arch Surg 392:405–412, 2007.
11. Tomer Y, Barbesino G, Greenberg DA, et al: Mapping the major susceptibility loci for familial Graves' and Hashimoto's diseases: evidence for genetic heterogeneity and gene interactions. J Clin Endocrinol Metab 84:4656–4664, 1999.
12. Franklyn JA: The management of hyperthyroidism. N Engl J Med 330:1731–1738, 1994.
13. Castro MR, Gharib H: Continuing controversies in the management of thyroid nodules. Ann Intern Med 142:926–931, 2005.
14. Boelaert K, Horacek J, Holder RL, et al: Serum thyrotropin concentration as a novel predictor of malignancy in thyroid nodules investigated by fine-needle aspiration. J Clin Endocrinol Metab 91:4295–4301, 2006.
15. Frates MC, Benson CB, Charboneau JW, et al: Management of thyroid nodules detected at US: Society of Radiologists in Ultrasound consensus conference statement. Radiology 237:794–800, 2005.
16. Are C, Hsu JF, Ghossein RA, et al: Histological aggressiveness of fluorodeoxyglucose positron-emission tomogram (FDG-PET)–detected incidental thyroid carcinomas. Ann Surg Oncol 14:3210–3215, 2007.
17. Sabel MS, Staren ED, Gianakakis LM, et al: User of fine-needle aspiration biopsy and frozen section in the management of the solitary thyroid nodule. Surgery 122:1021–1026, 1997.
18. Sclabas GM, Staerkel GA, Shapiro SE, et al: Fine-needle aspiration of the thyroid and correlation with histopathology in a contemporary series of 240 patients. Am J Surg 186:702–709; discussion 709–710, 2003.
19. Braga M, Cavalcanti TC, Collaco LM, et al: Efficacy of ultrasound-guided fine-needle aspiration biopsy in the diagnosis of complex thyroid nodules. J Clin Endocrinol Metab 86:4089–4091, 2001.
20. Boyd LA, Earnhardt RC, Dunn JT, et al: Preoperative evaluation and predictive value of fine-needle aspiration and frozen section of thyroid nodules. J Am Coll Surg 187:494–502, 1998.
21. Kouniavsky G, Zeiger MA: Thyroid tumorigenesis and molecular markers in thyroid cancer. Curr Opin Oncol 22:23–29, 2010.
22. Davies L, Welch HG: Increasing incidence of thyroid cancer in the United States, 1973-2002. Jama 295:2164–2167, 2006.
23. Mazzaferri EL, Young RL: Papillary thyroid carcinoma: A 10-year follow-up report of the impact of therapy in 576 patients. Am J Med 70:511–518, 1981.
24. Siegel R, Ward E, Brawley O, et al: Cancer statistics, 2011. CA Cancer J Clin 61:212–236, 2011.
25. Albores-Saavedra J, Henson DE, Glazer E, et al: Changing patterns in the incidence and survival of thyroid cancer with follicular phenotype—papillary, follicular, and anaplastic: A morphological and epidemiological study. Endocr Pathol 18:1–7, 2007.
26. Bongarzone I, Vigneri P, Mariani L, et al: RET/NTRK1 rearrangements in thyroid gland tumors of the papillary carcinoma family: Correlation with clinicopathological features. Clin Cancer Res 4:223–228, 1998.
27. Kim DS, McCabe CJ, Buchanan MA, et al: Oncogenes in thyroid cancer. Clin Otolaryngol Allied Sci 28:386–395, 2003.
28. Cohen Y, Rosenbaum E, Clark DP, et al: Mutational analysis of BRAF in fine needle aspiration biopsies of the thyroid: A potential application for the preoperative assessment of thyroid nodules. Clin Cancer Res 10:2761–2765, 2004.
29. Xing M, Westra WH, Tufano RP, et al: BRAF mutation predicts a poorer clinical prognosis for papillary thyroid cancer. J Clin Endocrinol Metab 90:6373–6379, 2005.
30. Kumagai A, Namba H, Saenko VA, et al: Low frequency of BRAFT1796A mutations in childhood thyroid carcinomas. J Clin Endocrinol Metab 89:4280–4284, 2004.
31. Xing M, Clark D, Guan H, et al: BRAF mutation testing of thyroid fine-needle aspiration biopsy specimens for preoperative risk stratification in papillary thyroid cancer. J Clin Oncol 27:2977–2982, 2009.
32. Zhu Z, Gandhi M, Nikiforova MN, et al: Molecular profile and clinical-pathologic features of the follicular variant of papillary thyroid carcinoma. An unusually high prevalence of ras mutations. Am J Clin Pathol 120:71–77, 2003.
33. Garcia-Rostan G, Zhao H, Camp RL, et al: Ras mutations are associated with aggressive tumor phenotypes and poor prognosis in thyroid cancer. J Clin Oncol 21:3226–3235, 2003.
34. Parameswaran R, Brooks S, Sadler G: Molecular pathogenesis of follicular cell derived thyroid cancers. Int J Surg 8:186–193, 2010.
35. Sherman SI: Thyroid carcinoma. Lancet 361:501–511, 2003.
36. Cady B, Sedgwick CE, Meissner WA, et al: Risk factor analysis in differentiated thyroid cancer. Cancer 43:810–820, 1979.
37. Hay ID, Thompson GB, Grant CS, et al: Papillary thyroid carcinoma managed at the Mayo Clinic during six decades (1940-1999): Temporal trends in initial therapy and long-term outcome in 2444 consecutively treated patients. World J Surg 26:879–885, 2002.
38. Zaydfudim V, Feurer ID, Griffin MR, et al: The impact of lymph node involvement on survival in patients with papillary and follicular thyroid carcinoma. Surgery 144:1070–1077, 2008.
39. Schlumberger MJ: Papillary and follicular thyroid carcinoma. N Engl J Med 338:297–306, 1998.
40. Hundahl SA, Cady B, Cunningham MP, et al: Initial results from a prospective cohort study of 5583 cases of thyroid carcinoma treated in the united states during 1996. U.S. and German Thyroid Cancer Study Group. An American College of Surgeons Commission on Cancer Patient Care Evaluation study. Cancer 89:202–217, 2000.
41. Podnos YD, Smith D, Wagman LD, et al: The implication of lymph node metastasis on survival in patients with well-differentiated thyroid cancer. Am Surg 71:731–734, 2005.
42. Sywak M, Cornford L, Roach P, et al: Routine ipsilateral level VI lymphadenectomy reduces postoperative thyroglobulin levels in papillary thyroid cancer. Surgery 140:1000–1005, 2006.

**43.** Wada N, Duh QY, Sugino K, et al: Lymph node metastasis from 259 papillary thyroid microcarcinomas: Frequency, pattern of occurrence and recurrence, and optimal strategy for neck dissection. Ann Surg 237:399–407, 2003.

**44.** D'Avanzo A, Treseler P, Ituarte PH, et al: Follicular thyroid carcinoma: Histology and prognosis. Cancer 100:1123–1129, 2004.

**45.** Kinder BK: Well-differentiated thyroid cancer. Curr Opin Oncol 15:71–77, 2003.

**46.** Alaedeen DI, Khiyami A, McHenry CR: Fine-needle aspiration biopsy specimen with a predominance of Hurthle cells: A dilemma in the management of nodular thyroid disease. Surgery 138:650–656, 2005.

**47.** Melck A, Bugis S, Baliski C, et al: Hemithyroidectomy: The preferred initial surgical approach for management of Hurthle cell neoplasm. Am J Surg 191:593–597, 2006.

**48.** Kloos RT, Eng C, Evans DB, et al: Medullary thyroid cancer: Management guidelines of the American Thyroid Association. Thyroid 19:565–612, 2009.

**49.** Pasieka JL: Anaplastic thyroid cancer. Curr Opin Oncol 15:78–83, 2003.

**50.** Bojunga J, Zeuzem S: Molecular detection of thyroid cancer: an update. Clin Endocrinol (Oxf) 61:523–530, 2004.

**51.** Carty SE, Cooper DS, Doherty GM, et al: Consensus statement on the terminology and classification of central neck dissection for thyroid cancer. Thyroid 19:1153–1158, 2009.

**52.** Attie JN: Modified neck dissection in treatment of thyroid cancer: A safe procedure. Eur J Cancer Clin Oncol 24:315–324, 1988.

**53.** Miccoli P, Minuto MN, Ugolini C, et al: Minimally invasive video-assisted thyroidectomy for benign thyroid disease: An evidence-based review. World J Surg 32:1333–1340, 2008.

**54.** Del Rio P, Sommaruga L, Pisani P, et al: Minimally invasive video-assisted thyroidectomy in differentiated thyroid cancer: A 1-year follow-up. Surg Laparosc Endosc Percutan Tech 19:290–292, 2009.

**55.** Kang SW, Lee SC, Lee SH, et al: Robotic thyroid surgery using a gasless, transaxillary approach and the da Vinci S system: The operative outcomes of 338 consecutive patients. Surgery 146:1048–1055, 2009.

**56.** Wilhelm T, Metzig A: Endoscopic minimally invasive thyroidectomy: First clinical experience. Surg Endosc 24:1757–1758, 2010.

**57.** Mazzaferri EL, Kloos RT: Clinical review 128: Current approaches to primary therapy for papillary and follicular thyroid cancer. J Clin Endocrinol Metab 86:1447–1463, 2001.

**58.** Zarnegar R, Brunaud L, Clark OH: Prevention, evaluation, and management of complications following thyroidectomy for thyroid carcinoma. Endocrinol Metab Clin North Am 32:483–502, 2003.

**59.** Sosa JA, Bowman HM, Tielsch JM, et al: The importance of surgeon experience for clinical and economic outcomes from thyroidectomy. Ann Surg 228:320–330, 1998.

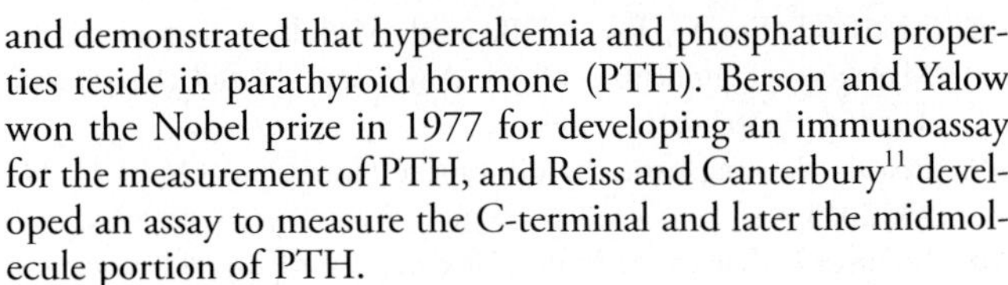

CHAPTER 39

# THE PARATHYROID GLANDS

Julie Ann Sosa and Robert Udelsman

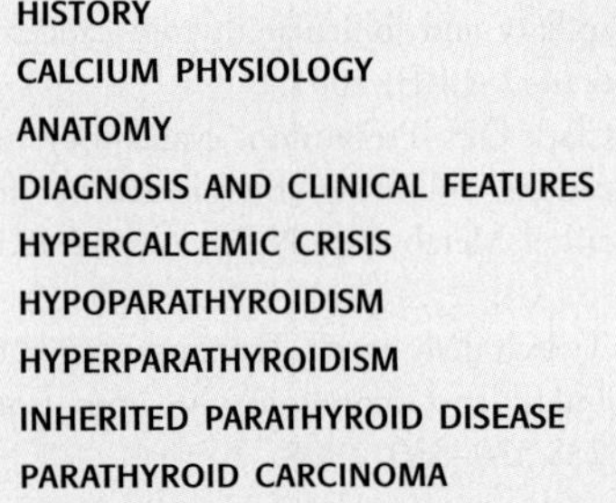



The clinical features, diagnosis, and treatment of parathyroid disease have changed radically over the past 25 years as a result of technologic advances in the fields of laboratory medicine, radiology, medicine, and surgery. In particular, there have been many technical advances in the surgical management of primary hyperparathyroidism (HPT).

## HISTORY

Advances in parathyroid surgery have been colorful and international. Although the Swedish medical student Ivar Sandstrom is credited with first describing the "glandularae parathyrtreoidae" in 1880,[1] Sir Richard Owen made the original description in 1850.[2] Understanding of parathyroid function predated appreciation of the glands themselves; tetany was described in 1879 in a patient who underwent thyroidectomy (and incidental parathyroidectomy), and the connection between the parathyroids and tetany was identified in 1891.[3] Famous patients with HPT include Albert Gahne, a Viennese tram car conductor who underwent two separate parathyroid resections in the 1920s by Felix Mandl for what was most likely parathyroid carcinoma,[4] and Captain Charles Martell, a Merchant Marine captain who underwent seven operations and was eventually found to have a mediastinal parathyroid adenoma.[5] Both men succumbed to their disease and the consequences of its treatment.

The relationship between chronic renal disease and HPT was first suggested by Albright and colleagues in 1934.[6] Castleman and Mallory[7] described the pathologic finding of parathyroid hyperplasia of chief cells with marked gland enlargement. Stanbury and associates[8] described renal rickets, azotemic osteomalacia, and azotemic HPT and also performed the first subtotal parathyroidectomy as definitive therapy for renal osteitis fibrosa. Rasmussen and Craig[9] and, independently, Berson and coworkers,[10] extracted a stable homogeneous parathyroid polypeptide and demonstrated that hypercalcemia and phosphaturic properties reside in parathyroid hormone (PTH). Berson and Yalow won the Nobel prize in 1977 for developing an immunoassay for the measurement of PTH, and Reiss and Canterbury[11] developed an assay to measure the C-terminal and later the midmolecule portion of PTH.

Introduction of the serum channel autoanalyzer in the mid-1960s ushered in a new era of parathyroid surgery in that it facilitated earlier diagnosis of primary HPT. There was an increase in incidence of the disease and asymptomatic patients became commonplace. Additional technical advances have included improved preoperative localization with sestamibi scans, often using single-photon emission computed tomography (SPECT), the rapid intraoperative PTH assay, and the use of minimally invasive parathyroidectomy (MIP) with unilateral neck exploration through a small incision and regional anesthesia in the ambulatory setting.

## CALCIUM PHYSIOLOGY

Calcium exists in extracellular plasma in a free ionized state, as well as bound to other molecules. So-called normal plasma levels of total calcium vary among laboratories, but the range of (bound and unbound) calcium is usually between 8.5 and 10.2 mg/dL (2.2 and 2.5 mmol/liter). The biologically inert bound fraction (55% of the total) binds to proteins. Changes in albumin alter total calcium levels significantly because most protein-bound calcium associates with albumin (80%). A small percentage of calcium is associated with other proteins, such as β-globulins, or with nonprotein molecules, such as phosphate and citrate. Mathematical formulas correcting for disparate albumin levels (e.g., corrected calcium = 0.8-mg/dL decrease for every 1.0-mg/dL decrease in albumin; [total calcium + 0.025] × [40 − albumin]) are notoriously inaccurate. Consequently, ionized calcium levels are measured when required. Forty-five percent of the total calcium is biologically active and exists in the ionized form, with a normal level of 4.5 to 5.0 mg/dL. Ionized calcium levels are inversely affected by the pH of blood; a 1-unit rise in pH will decrease the ionized calcium level by 0.36 mmol/liter.[12] Accordingly, patients who are hypocalcemic and hyperventilate can enhance their hypocalcemic symptoms, including perioral paresthesia, tingling in the fingers and toes, muscle cramping, and seizures.

Levels of calcium are highly modulated through a delicate interplay among PTH, calcitonin, and vitamin D acting on target organs such as bone, kidney, and the gastrointestinal (GI) tract (Table 39-1; Fig. 39-1). Chief cells in the parathyroid

**Table 39-1 Actions of Major Calcium-Regulating Hormones**

| HORMONE | BONE | KIDNEY | INTESTINE |
|---|---|---|---|
| Parathyroid hormone | Stimulates resorption of calcium and phosphate | Stimulates resorption of calcium and conversion of 25(OH)$D_3$; inhibits resorption of phosphate and bicarbonate | No direct effects |
| Vitamin D | Stimulates transport of calcium | Inhibits resorption of calcium | Stimulates calcium and phosphate absorption |
| Calcitonin | Inhibits resorption of calcium and phosphate | Inhibits resorption of calcium and phosphate | No direct effects |

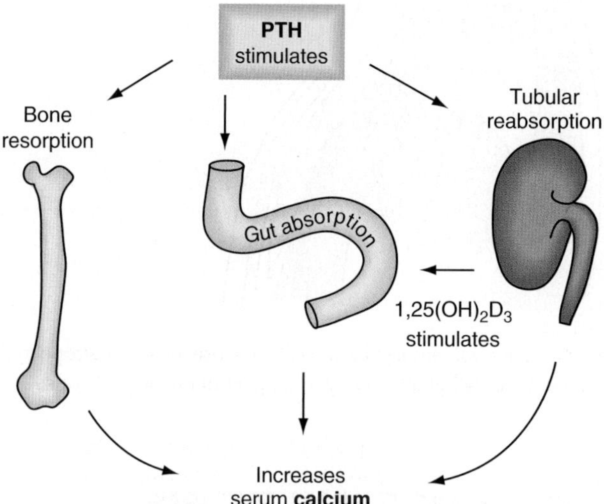


**FIGURE 39-1** Calcium homeostasis and PTH.

glands secrete PTH, an 84–amino acid protein, whenever serum calcium levels fall. PTH binds to its peripheral receptors and stimulates osteoclasts to increase bone resorption, to the kidney to increase calcium resorption and renal production of 1,25-dihydroxyvitamin $D_3$ (1,25[OH]$_2D_3$), and to the intestine to increase absorption of calcium and phosphate. Together, these processes raise the serum calcium level. The recently cloned calcium-sensing receptors (CaSRs) in the parathyroid glands detect changes in calcium levels, which results in a negative feedback loop that decreases PTH production.

Calcitonin is a 32–amino acid protein secreted by the parafollicular cells of the thyroid gland in response to high calcium levels. Its actions oppose those of PTH. Calcitonin rapidly inhibits bone resorption, thereby leading to a transient decrease in serum calcium levels. Although calcitonin plays a significant homeostatic function in other species, its effects on calcium metabolism in humans is not significant when a person is exposed to chronically elevated calcitonin levels. Accordingly, patients with extensive medullary carcinoma of the thyroid who have extraordinarily high serum calcitonin levels are usually eucalcemic.

Vitamin D is ingested or synthesized in precursor form, which then undergoes two hydroxylation steps before becoming biologically active. The first hydroxylation at carbon 25 occurs in the liver and the second hydroxylation at carbon 1 occurs in the kidney in response to increased PTH levels. 1,25(OH)$_2D_3$ increases calcium and phosphate resorption from the GI tract and stimulates bone resorption, which raises calcium levels. As a result, patients who are deficient in 1,25(OH)$_2D_3$ have an impaired ability to absorb calcium from their GI tract.

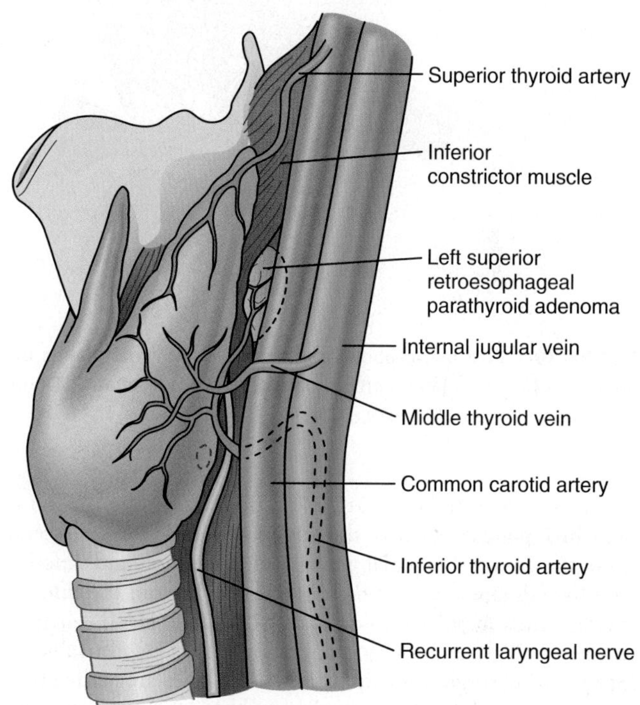


**FIGURE 39-2** Anatomic relationship of a left superior parathyroid adenoma to nearby structures, including the recurrent laryngeal nerve, carotid sheath, and its blood supply from the inferior thyroid artery. Aberrantly located parathyroid glands can be found behind the esophagus and in the carotid sheath, thymus, and mediastinum.

## ANATOMY

There are usually four parathyroid glands, which lie on the posterior surface of the thyroid. The superior glands are normally located on the posteromedial aspect of the thyroid near the tracheoesophageal groove, whereas the inferior parathyroids are more widely distributed in the region below the inferior thyroid artery (Fig. 39-2). Common sites for ectopic parathyroids are the thyrothymic ligament, superior thyroid poles, tracheoesophageal groove, retroesophageal space, and carotid sheath (Fig. 39-3).[13] The percentage of individuals with supernumerary glands varies in published series from 2.5% to 22%.[14] The average weight of a normal parathyroid gland is 35 to 40 mg; in adults, its color turns to yellow as the fat content

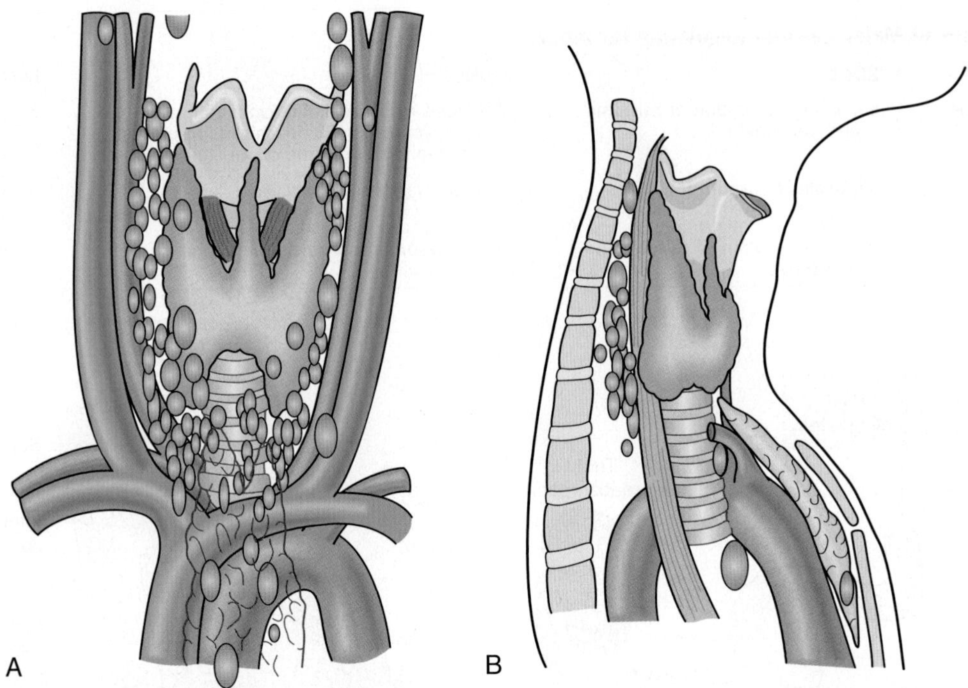


**FIGURE 39-3** Possible locations of enlarged parathyroid glands in the neck and superior mediastinum with the use of an anteroposterior projection **(A)** and a lateral projection **(B).** (From Udelsman R, Donovan PI: Remedial parathyroid surgery: Changing trends in 130 consecutive cases. Ann Surg 244:471–479, 2006.)

increases. The inferior parathyroids originate from the third branchial pouch, whereas the superior parathyroids descend from the fourth branchial pouch. The superior and inferior parathyroid glands receive their blood supply from the inferior thyroid artery in 80% of cases. Each parathyroid gland generally receives a single end-artery blood supply that is vulnerable to injury during surgical manipulation. The glands are made up of chief and oxyphil cells, as well as fibrovascular stroma and adipose tissue.

Primary HPT can be produced by three different pathologic lesions. A parathyroid adenoma is a benign encapsulated neoplasm responsible for 80% to 90% of cases. It usually affects a single gland, but 2% to 5% of patients with primary HPT have adenomas in two glands (double adenomas). Hyperplasia is a proliferation of parenchymal cells that affects all the parathyroid glands; it accounts for 10% to 15% of cases of primary HPT and all cases of secondary HPT. Most patients with primary HPT caused by multigland hyperplasia have sporadic disease. It is also associated with multiple endocrine neoplasia (MEN) type 1 (primary HPT combined with lesions of the pancreas and pituitary) and type 2A (primary HPT, medullary thyroid cancer, and pheochromocytoma) syndromes. Parathyroid carcinoma is a slow-growing, invasive neoplasm of parenchymal cells responsible for less than 1% of cases of primary HPT. Although fibrosis and mitotic activity are common, they are not specific for malignancy. The diagnosis of carcinoma is restricted to tumors that show invasion of blood vessels, perineural spaces, soft tissues, thyroid gland, or other adjacent structures, or to tumors with documented metastases. It is often difficult for the pathologist to make this diagnosis, especially if there is only a frozen section analysis of a resected parathyroid gland.

## DIAGNOSIS AND CLINICAL FEATURES

Primary HPT is the third most common endocrine disorder, after diabetes mellitus and thyroid disease. Middle-aged and older women are most commonly affected by the disease. It is characterized by hypersecretion of PTH, leading to hypercalcemia. Box 39-1 lists the differential diagnosis for hypercalcemia. The diagnosis is made by demonstrating elevated serum calcium and intact PTH (iPTH) levels and normal or increased urinary calcium levels in the setting of normal renal function. In up to 15% of patients, serum PTH levels fall within the upper normal range, but these levels are inappropriate relative to the elevated serum calcium levels. A 24-hour urine collection can help exclude the diagnosis of benign familial hypocalciuric hypercalcemia (BFHH), which results in mild increases in blood calcium and iPTH levels but low urinary calcium. Whereas the calcium-to-creatinine (Ca/Cr) clearance ratio is typically less than 0.01 in patients with BFHH, the ratio is usually more than 0.02 in primary HPT. BFHH is a generally benign condition transmitted in an autosomal dominant fashion that cannot be corrected by parathyroidectomy.

The clinical entity termed *normocalcemic primary hyperparathyroidism* has recently been described.[15] It appears to be an early form of primary HPT in which patients have serum calcium levels in the high-normal range associated with an elevated serum PTH level. When these patients are symptomatic, surgical intervention is appropriate.

When HPT is seen in the setting of chronic renal failure, it is termed *secondary HPT.* This is a discrete clinical entity from primary HPT. Other less common causes of secondary HPT include malabsorptive and other metabolic disorders. Renal failure leads to hyperphosphatemia and decreased renal conversion of 25-hydroxycholecalciferol to

**BOX 39-1 Differential Diagnosis of Hypercalcemia***

**Parathyroid**
Primary hyperparathyroidism: Sporadic, Familial

**Nonparathyroid Endocrine**
Thyrotoxicosis
Pheochromocytoma
Acute adrenal insufficiency
Vasointestinal polypeptide hormone–producing tumor (VIPoma)

**Malignancy**
Solid tumors
Lytic bone metastases
Lymphoma and leukemia
Parathyroid hormone–related peptide
Excess production of 1,25$(OH)_2D_3$
Other factors (cytokines, growth factors)

**Granulomatous Diseases**
Sarcoidosis
Tuberculosis
Histoplasmosis
Coccidiomycosis
Leprosy

**Medications**
Calcium supplementation
Thiazide diuretics
Lithium
Estrogens, antiestrogens, testosterone in breast cancer
Vitamin A or D intoxication

**Other**
Benign familial hypocalciuric hypercalcemia
Milk-alkali syndrome
Immobilization
Paget's disease
Acute and chronic renal insufficiency
Aluminum excess
Parenteral nutrition

Adapted from Mulder JE, Bilezikian JP: Acute management of hypercalcemia. In Bilezikian JP, Marcus R, Levine MA (eds): The parathyroids, ed 2, San Diego, Calif, 2001, Academic Press, p 730.
*Malignancy is the most common cause of hypercalcemia in the inpatient setting; primary hyperparathyroidism is the most common cause in the outpatient setting.

1,25-dihydroxycholecalciferol, thereby resulting in diminished intestinal calcium absorption. Both these effects lead to chronic hypocalcemia, which stimulates PTH secretion and parathyroid hyperplasia. As many as 90% of patients with chronic renal failure have evidence of secondary HPT. With prolonged stimulation of the parathyroids, a disorder termed *tertiary HPT* can develop in patients with chronic renal failure or those with long-standing secondary HPT who undergo kidney transplantation. Autonomous hyperfunction develops and the parathyroids no longer respond to calcium feedback inhibition, which results in hypercalcemia.

Before advent of the serum channel autoanalyzer, patients with primary HPT were typically seen with the clinical manifestations of hypercalcemia, including painful bones, kidney stones, abdominal groans, "psychic moans," and fatigue overtones. Until the 1970s, 75% of patients presented with nephrolithiasis. Today, however, a biochemical diagnosis is usually made before the appearance of symptoms, and many patients are asymptomatic or minimally symptomatic. Less than 20% of primary HPT patients have renal symptoms and less than 5% have evidence of osteitis fibrosis cystica. Bone turnover is increased in up to 80% of patients with primary HPT, and serial measurements demonstrate a rapid fall in bone resorption within 2 weeks of parathyroidectomy.

Most contemporary series, however, demonstrate that at least 50% of patients today have a nonrenal nonosseous manifestation, and several series have demonstrated that 30% to 40% of patients are asymptomatic. Nonspecific complaints such as fatigue, lethargy, and depression are most commonly cited. Hypertension has been noted in approximately one third of patients with HPT, and a significant inverse relationship between mean arterial pressure and the glomerular filtration rate has been noted in these patients.

## HYPERCALCEMIC CRISIS

Occasionally, patients with primary HPT are initially seen after symptoms and extremely high serum calcium levels have developed. Management of a so-called hypercalcemic crisis involves urgent medical and surgical strategies. Pharmacologic agents associated with or adversely affected by hypercalcemia need to be discontinued; specifically, digoxin potentiates arrhythmias in the setting of hypercalcemia. These patients are almost always severely dehydrated, and initial management requires hydration with normal saline. Medical management promotes the renal excretion of calcium. Once a patient with primary HPT is stabilized and serum calcium levels have been reduced to levels acceptable for induction of anesthesia (general or locoregional, if a minimally invasive surgical technique is anticipated), expedient efforts are made to localize the parathyroid disease in anticipation of urgent parathyroidectomy.

IV fluids, preferably normal saline, are administered at a rapid rate (200 to 300 mL/hr) to reverse the intravascular volume contraction and promote the renal excretion of calcium. Bedside vigilance to prevent fluid overload is essential. Loop diuretics are added to the regimen to reduce the risk for volume overload and inhibit calcium resorption in the loop of Henle. Patients with renal failure often cannot tolerate such large-volume resuscitation; instead, they undergo dialysis with a low-calcium dialysate.

Glucocorticoids lower calcium by inhibiting the effects of vitamin D. They also have been shown to decrease intestinal absorption of calcium, increase renal calcium excretion, and inhibit osteoclast-activating factor. Glucocorticoids are particularly effective in the setting of hypercalcemia secondary to granulomatous disease, in which the hypercalcemia stems from vitamin D toxicity. The initial dose of hydrocortisone is 200 to 400 mg/day IV for 3 to 5 days. Glucocorticoids are ineffective in most cases of hypercalcemia associated with malignancy.

Hypercalcemia of malignancy occurs by two mechanisms: (1) as a direct result of extensive osseous metastases; and (2) indirectly by release of parathyroid hormone–related peptide (PTHrP) by some tumors. Treatment of hypercalcemia of malignancy includes surgery, chemotherapy, or radiation therapy, or any combination of these, to treat the underlying cancer, as well as the administration of pharmacologic agents. Gallium nitrate, a compound that inhibits osteoclast resorption and lowers calcium levels, can be used at 200 $mg/m^2$ daily IV for 5 days.

In this setting, gallium nitrate and pamidronate, a bisphosphonate (see later), have been equivalent in controlling hypercalcemia in small studies.

Calcitonin acts quickly (within 24 to 48 hours) to lower serum calcium levels and is more effective when used in combination with glucocorticoids. In a small, double-blind randomized trial of 50 cancer patients, however, calcitonin (up to 8 IU/kg SC or IM for 5 days) was less effective than gallium nitrate. Because preparations of calcitonin are extracted from salmon, patients with preformed antibodies or those with previous exposure to calcitonin can demonstrate an allergic reaction consisting of respiratory distress, flushing, nausea, vomiting, and tingling in the extremities.

Bisphosphonates are pyrophosphate analogues that have a high affinity for hydroxyapatite in bone. They potently inhibit osteoclast activity for up to 1 month. In hypercalcemia of malignancy, pamidronate (90 mg IV) or zoledronic acid (4 mg IV as initial treatment, 8 mg on retreatment) normalizes calcium levels in most patients. Although a single dose of pamidronate lowers calcium levels, evidence has suggested that zoledronic acid might become the bisphosphonate of choice because of its rapid onset of action and ability to lengthen the time to relapse by twofold. However, zoledronic acid also has been associated with compromised renal function.

## HYPOPARATHYROIDISM

Hypoparathyroidism is an endocrine disorder in which hypocalcemia and hyperphosphatemia are the result of a deficiency in PTH secretion or action. The most common cause of hypoparathyroidism is damage to the parathyroid glands during thyroidectomy, but it can also occur after parathyroid exploration (see later, "Postoperative Complications"). The signs and symptoms of hypocalcemia are caused by neuromuscular excitability from reduced plasma ionized calcium. Early manifestations include perioral numbness and tingling in the fingers. Anxiety or confusion can follow, and it is important for the surgical team to reassure patients early to reduce psychiatric and neurocognitive symptoms. Anxiety often results in hyperventilation, which can then lead to respiratory alkalosis and a further reduction in the serum calcium level. Tetany, marked by carpopedal spasm, convulsions, or laryngospasm (or any combination of the three), may follow and can be fatal. Physical examination includes testing for a Chvostek sign, which is contraction of the facial muscles after tapping on the facial nerve anterior to the ear. Approximately 15% of normal individuals have a positive Chvostek sign, however.

There are also inherited forms of hypoparathyroidism. It can occur as part of a multiglandular endocrine deficiency syndrome (type 1), usually characterized by hypoparathyroidism, adrenal insufficiency, and mucocutaneous candidiasis. This syndrome generally develops in childhood, and not all patients express the classic triad. Idiopathic hypoparathyroidism also occurs sporadically in adults and is associated with antiparathyroid antibodies. Some cases might be related to incomplete penetrance of familial multiglandular syndrome type 1.

Disorders in which there is abnormal or absent formation of the parathyroid glands are associated with hypocalcemia. For example, DiGeorge's syndrome occurs when the third and fourth branchial pouches develop abnormally. Transient neonatal hypocalcemia, a self-limited disorder, is more common than the genetic disorders that lead to permanent hypoparathyroidism. Parathyroid gland function can be impaired by infiltrative involvement of the glands in diseases such as hemochromatosis, Wilson's disease, sarcoidosis, tuberculosis, or amyloidosis. Exposure to external radiation or very large doses of $^{131}I$ for Graves' disease or well-differentiated thyroid cancer has rarely been associated with hypocalcemia. Finally, abnormalities in magnesium levels are associated with a reversible abnormality of PTH secretion.

Pseudohypoparathyroidism is an uncommon metabolic disorder characterized by biochemical hypoparathyroidism, increased PTH secretion, and target tissue unresponsiveness to the biologic action of PTH. In addition to functional hypoparathyroidism, many of these patients exhibit a distinctive constellation of developmental and skeletal defects, collectively termed *Albright's hereditary osteodystrophy,* including a round face, short stature, obesity, brachydactyly, heterotopic ossification, and mental retardation. Several forms of pseudohypoparathyroidism have been described and a diagnostic classification system has been developed (types 1a to 1c and 2).

## HYPERPARATHYROIDISM

### Primary Hyperparathyroidism

#### Effects of Surgery

Even though a National Institutes of Health (NIH) consensus conference was conducted in 1990, another workshop was held in 2002, and an international workshop was held in 2008 on the management of asymptomatic primary HPT, there is still no consensus among endocrinologists and endocrine surgeons about whether to administer nonoperative medical therapy and monitor patients or to refer them for early parathyroidectomy. Criteria for surgery have been established according to the best evidence to date (Box 39-2).[16] To some extent, the role of parathyroidectomy in asymptomatic patients with mild to moderate hypercalcemia is debated because the natural history of the disease is still not well understood. Overall, rapid increases in the serum calcium level, progression of symptoms of complications, or both are uncommon in patients with borderline hypercalcemia. However, because of the long-term deleterious effects on bone mineralization, the pendulum has shifted to surgical intervention.[17]

Neuromuscular symptoms of primary HPT vary in expression and response to parathyroidectomy among series. However, proximal muscle weakness detected by examination of the isokinetic strength of knee extension and flexion appears to have a

**BOX 39-2 Criteria for Surgical Referral**

- Serum calcium concentration >1 mg/dL (>0.25 mM/liter) above the upper limits of normal
- Bone density at the lumbar spine, hip, or distal end of the radius that is >2 SD below peak bone mass (T-score <–2.5)
- All individuals with primary hyperparathyroidism and <50 yr
- Patients for whom medical surveillance is undesirable or impossible

Adapted from Bilezikian JP, Khan AA, Potts JT Jr: Third International Workshop on the Management of Asymptomatic Primary Hyperthyroidism: Guidelines for the management of asymptomatic primary hyperparathyroidism: summary statement from the third international workshop. J Clin Endocrinol Metab 94:335–339, 2009.

**Table 39-2 Preoperative Imaging in Patients With Primary Hyperparathyroidism**

| IMAGING MODALITY | SENSITIVITY | SPECIFICITY | COST | SAFETY |
|---|---|---|---|---|
| **Noninvasive** | | | | |
| Sestamibi | Moderate | Moderate | Moderate | Safe |
| Sestamibi SPECT | High | High | Moderate | Safe |
| Ultrasound | Moderate | Moderate | Low | Safe |
| 4D-CT | High | High | High | Radiation |
| MRI | Low | Moderate | Moderate | Safe |
| PET-CT | ? | ? | High | Radiation |
| **Invasive** | | | | |
| Angiography | Moderate | Moderate | Very high | Hematoma, CVA, nephropathy* |
| Venous localization | High | High | Very high | Hematoma, nephropathy* |
| Ultrasound, biopsy | High | High | Moderate | Hematoma, infection |

*4D-CT,* Four-dimensional CT; *CVA,* cerebrovascular accident (stroke); *PET,* positron emission tomography; *SPECT,* single-photon emission CT.
*IV contrast nephropathy.

higher prevalence and good response to parathyroidectomy, as does respiratory muscle capacity. Psychiatric symptoms such as mental dullness, confusion, and depression are a focus of ongoing investigations. In a study by Roman and coworkers,[18] 55 patients with primary HPT and benign euthyroid thyroid disease referred for surgery were evaluated preoperatively and postoperatively with validated psychometric and neurocognitive instruments. Patients with primary HPT reported more symptoms of depression preoperatively that improved postoperatively. Preoperatively, patients with primary HPT also showed greater delays in spatial learning. All subjects learned across the neurocognitive trials, but primary HPT patients were more delayed. After surgery, primary HPT patients improved and functioned at a level equivalent to that of patients with thyroid disease. The authors concluded that primary HPT may be associated with a deficit in spatial learning and processing that improves after parathyroidectomy. Several other studies have supported the possibility that patients with primary HPT may exhibit neurocognitive changes, and that these traits may show some improvement after parathyroidectomy.

Significant increases in bone mineral density in the lumbar spine and hip occur after parathyroidectomy, and these improvements are durable. Changes in bone remodeling and density are apparent within 6 months of surgery. Cohort studies have shown that fracture risk declines after parathyroidectomy. No effect of successful surgery has been noted on hypertension or renal impairment. Urinary calcium excretion and the incidence of nephrolithiasis are reduced by surgery. Currently, there are still no convincing data proving that surgical cure increases life expectancy. A Swedish case-control study conducted retrospectively demonstrated that 23 patients who underwent parathyroidectomy had a hazard ratio for death of 0.89 in comparison to matched controls in the normal population, but the numbers were too small to achieve statistical significance.[19]

### Noninvasive Preoperative Localization

A major advance has been improvements in imaging techniques. This has led to the development of more localized surgery, with the opportunity for short operation times, the use of local or regional anesthesia, and limited or no hospital stay. There is now consensus—as marked by the recommendation of the 2002 NIH workshop and the 2008 international workshop—that preoperative localization is imperative before primary exploration if unilateral exploration is desired. Localization continues to be essential before all remedial parathyroidectomies (Table 39-2).

Several noninvasive preoperative localization modalities are available, including technetium-99m ($^{99m}$Tc) sestamibi scintigraphy, ultrasonography, computed tomography (CT), magnetic resonance imaging (MRI), and thallous chloride-201($^{201}$Tl) – $^{99m}$Tc-pertechnetate subtraction scanning. Most recently, four-dimensional CT and positron emission tomography (PET)-CT fusion studies have also been used with success for parathyroid localization. There is general consensus that the single best study is sestamibi, especially when combined with SPECT, and it is now the most common nuclear medicine study performed. In 1989, $^{99m}$Tc, used for cardiac imaging, also was noted to be avidly taken up by parathyroid tissue. The study works by mitochondrial uptake of $^{99m}$Tc-sestamibi, and parathyroid cells typically have a large number of mitochondria. Sestamibi, a monovalent lipophilic cation, diffuses passively across cell membranes and concentrates in mitochondria. Hence, it is preferentially concentrated in adenomatous and hyperplastic parathyroid tissue because of increased blood supply, higher metabolic activity, and absence of P-glycoprotein on the cell membrane (Fig. 39-4). Sestamibi imaging can be performed preoperatively for MIP planning or on the morning of surgery in the operating room in conjunction with the use of a gamma probe to guide the surgeon during surgery.[20]

A meta-analysis of the sensitivity and specificity of sestamibi scanning in 6331 cases has demonstrated values of 91% and 99%, respectively, and suggested that 87% of patients with sporadic primary HPT would be candidates for unilateral exploration. Routine preoperative screening becomes cost-effective when more than 51% of patients are suitable for a unilateral operation. The sensitivity of sestamibi is limited in multiglandular disease. In one large study, scintigraphy localized at least one gland in all patients, but only 62% of the total number of hyperplastic glands. SPECT, which allows localization of structures in the anteroposterior plane, is particularly helpful in

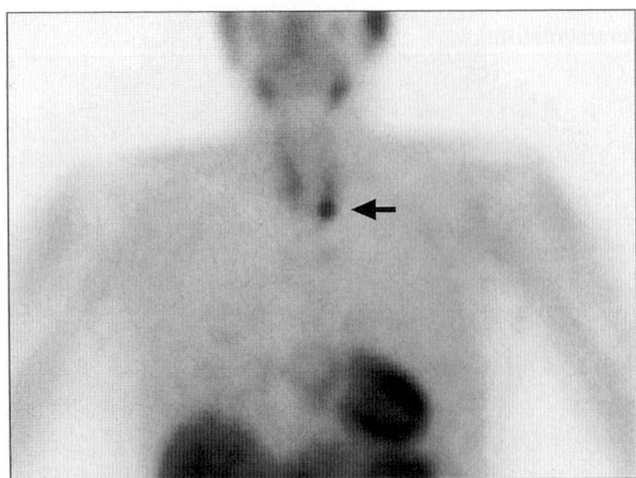

**FIGURE 39-4** Sestamibi scan demonstrating a left inferior parathyroid adenoma *(arrow)*. Physiologic areas of increased tracer uptake include the thyroid, salivary glands, heart, and liver.

detecting smaller lesions and adenomas located behind the thyroid. The overall sensitivity for localizing adenomas smaller than 500 mg ranges considerably, from 53% to 92%.

A significant limitation of sestamibi scans is related to the coexistence of thyroid pathology or other metabolically active tissue (e.g., lymph nodes or thyroid cancer) that can mimic parathyroid adenomas by causing false-positive results on sestamibi scans. This limitation can be overcome in part by using the double-tracer subtraction technique of sestamibi, in which both thyroid and parathyroid nodular abnormalities can be diagnosed simultaneously, or in combination with neck ultrasonography to distinguish thyroid lesions and parathyroid adenomas preoperatively. Sestamibi scans are now being performed with simultaneous CT imaging to yield correlative functional and anatomic localization.

Ultrasound is effective, noninvasive, and inexpensive, but its limitations include operator dependency and restriction to application in the neck because it cannot image mediastinal parathyroid lesions (Fig. 39-5).[21] It has a 48% to 74% true-positive rate. Ultrasound often is used in combination with sestamibi, in which case the combined true-positive rate rises to 90%. CT and MRI provide cross-sectional imaging and are useful for visualizing mediastinal tumors and glands within the tracheoesophageal groove. MRI does not involve the use of radiation, and parathyroid adenomas often appear intense on T2-weighted images. CT is less expensive and has a sensitivity of 70% and a specificity of nearly 100%. In a study of 42 surgical patients with primary HPT in which alternative preoperative localization strategies were compared, sensitivity was highest for sestamibi using the $^{99m}$Tc subtraction technique (95%), followed by $^{201}$Tl-$^{99m}$Tc subtraction (86%), CT (83%), and ultrasound (81%).[22]

Four-dimensional CT (4D-CT), a novel imaging modality similar to CT angiography, is derived from three-dimensional (3D)-CT scanning with an added dimension from the changes in perfusion of contrast over time. It generates detailed multiplanar images of the neck and allows the visualization of differences in the perfusion characteristics of hyperfunctioning parathyroid glands (i.e., rapid uptake and washout). Therefore,

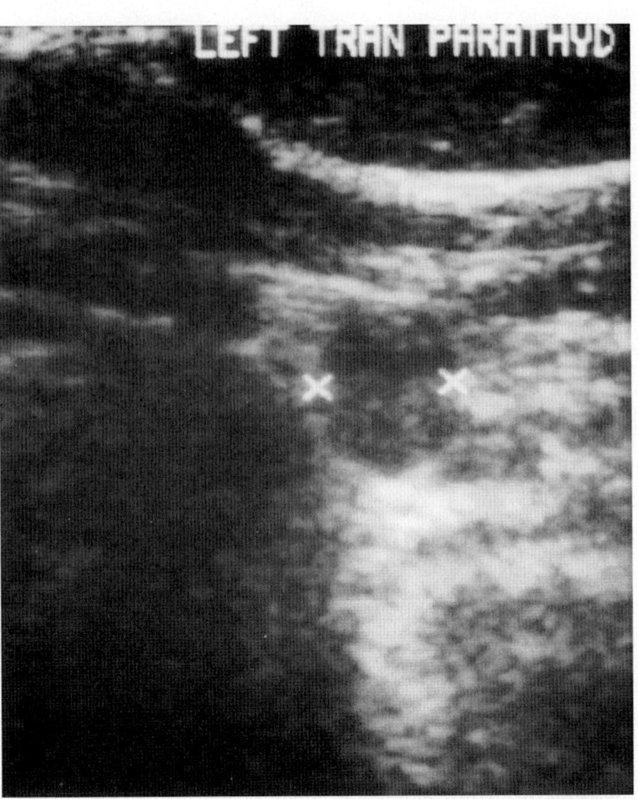


**FIGURE 39-5** Ultrasound image of a hypoechoic parathyroid adenoma (with tumor perimeter marked).

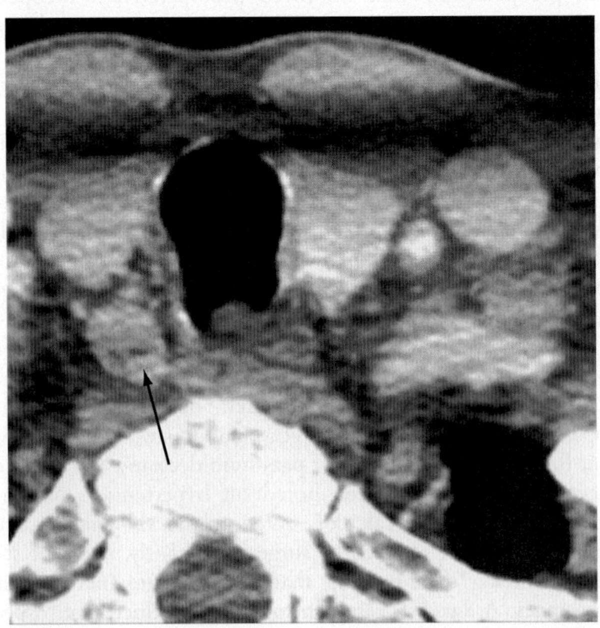

**FIGURE 39-6** 4D-CT showing increased uptake on delayed phase imaging of a parathyroid adenoma *(arrow)*.

4D-CT images provide anatomic and functional information (Fig. 39-6). In a study of 75 patients with primary HPT, 4D-CT demonstrated improved sensitivity (88%) over sestamibi (65%) and ultrasonography (57%) when the imaging studies were used to lateralize hyperfunctioning parathyroid glands to one side of the neck.[23]

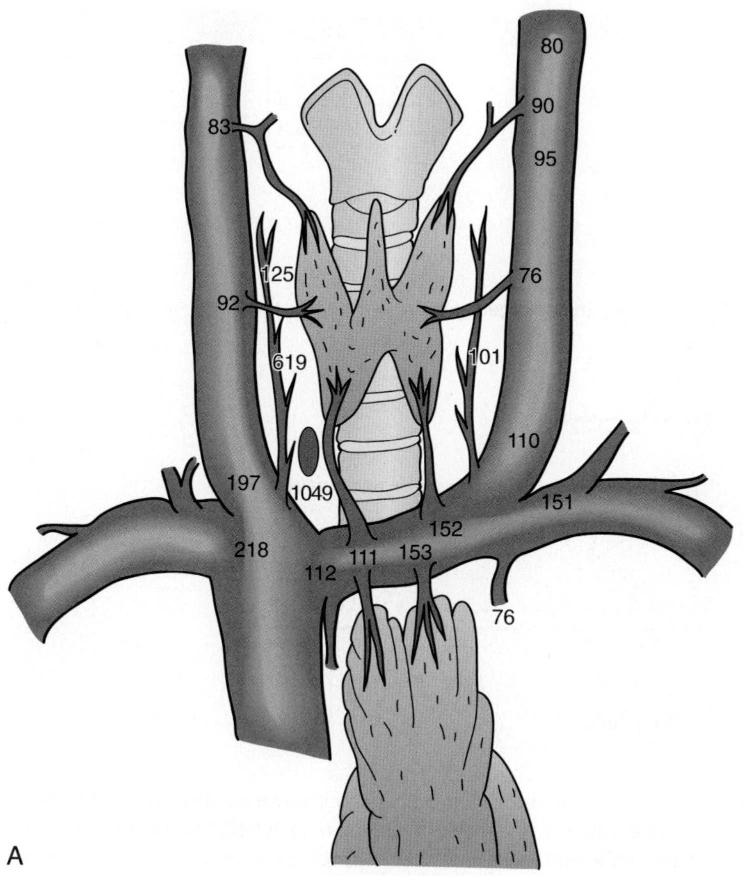


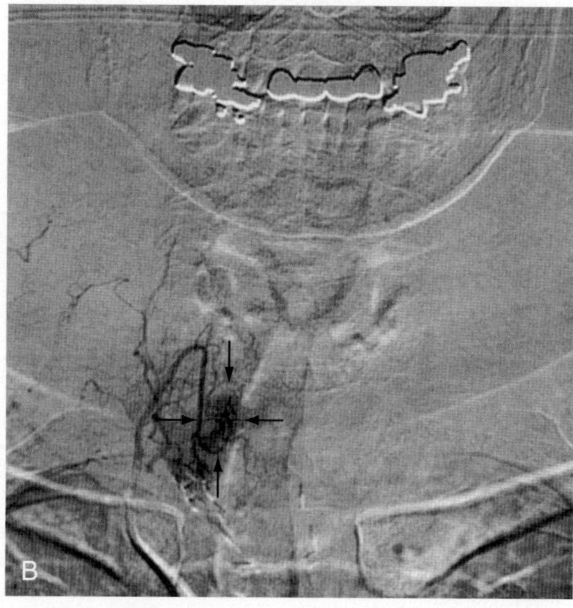


**FIGURE 39-7 A,** Venous localization mapping PTH levels at different cervical sampling sites. The 1049 level is consistent with a right posterior parathyroid adenoma. **B,** Corresponding angiogram showing the adenoma as a classic blush in the right posterior position (*arrows*). (From Udelsman R, Aruny JE, Donovan PI, et al: Rapid parathyroid hormone analysis during venous localization. Ann Surg 237:714–719, 2003.)

## Localization

**Invasive Preoperative Localization** A subset of patients who require reexploration will have negative, discordant, or nonconvincing noninvasive localization studies. Current guidelines recommend that these patients undergo invasive localization in the form of selective arteriography in conjunction with venous sampling for PTH (Fig. 39-7). This technique requires catheterization of multiple veins in the neck and mediastinum, from which blood samples are obtained. In the past, samples were collected, stored on ice, and sent to the laboratory, and the serum was later analyzed by immunoradiometric assay (IRMA) for iPTH. Rapid PTH measurement is now being performed in the angiography suite. Results are available quickly, so interventional radiologists can obtain additional samples from a region in which a subtle, but potentially significant, PTH gradient is detected. Because parathyroid adenomas have increased vascularity, they have a characteristic blush on arteriography. Although these studies have a sensitivity of only 60%, they yield few false-positive results. This use of interventional radiology rarely causes serious complications such as visual field defects or other cerebrovascular events, but such studies are time-consuming and expensive and must be performed only at centers with expertise.

In the remedial setting, ultrasound localization can be used to guide fine-needle aspiration of a lesion suspicious for a parathyroid adenoma.[24] This technique can be used with rapid PTH measurement of the parathyroid aspirate in the ultrasound suite to give ultrasonographers immediate feedback so that they can continue searching for an abnormal parathyroid gland if the aspirate of the suspicious lesion is negative.

**Intraoperative Localization** The rapid intraoperative PTH assay can be used to confirm adequate removal of hypersecreting parathyroids and predict a curative procedure. Its use is associated with reduced operating time. The first reported application of the assay was in 1988, but it has been refined since then, largely because of the work of Boggs and associates.[25] The rapid PTH assay is an IRMA that uses chemiluminescent acridinium esters as a label. In the presence of hydrogen peroxide and sodium hydroxide triggers, the acridinium esters are oxidized to an excited state, and subsequent return to the ground state causes an emission of light that can be quantified. The amount of bound labeled antibody is directly proportional to the concentration of PTH in the sample. A certified clinical laboratory technician ideally performs the assay inside the operating room or in its proximity; results of the assay are available in as little as 9 minutes.

A peripheral blood specimen is obtained immediately before surgery. Repeat blood samples are then drawn intraoperatively immediately after resection of the enlarged gland(s) to capture a potential hormone spike caused by manipulation of the gland during extirpation, and then 5 and 10 minutes after excision (Fig. 39-8). These protocols have been designed

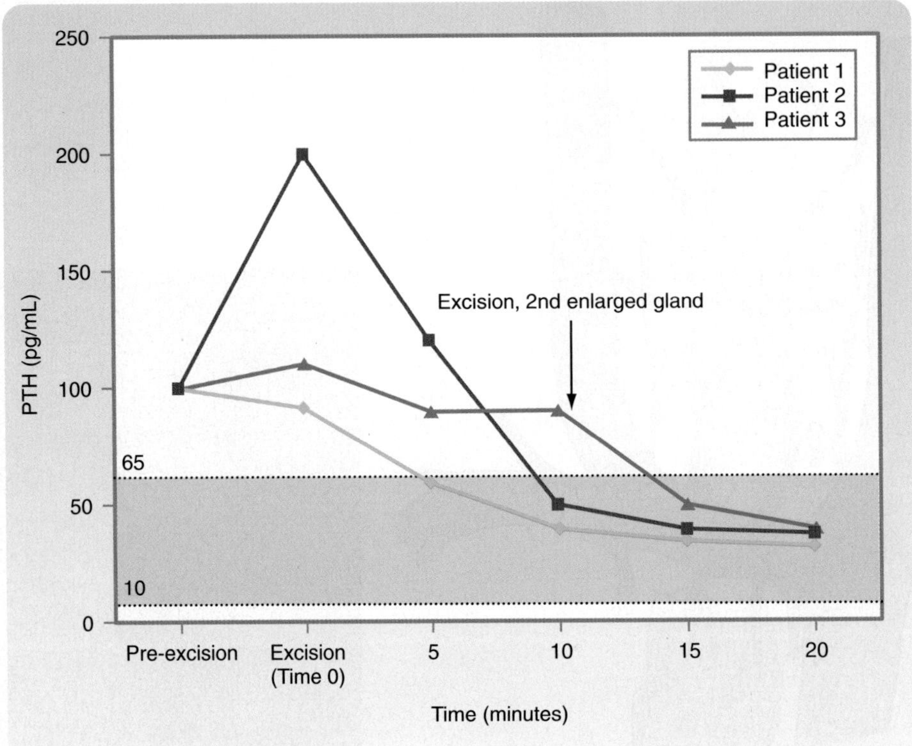


**FIGURE 39-8** Intraoperative PTH values of patients with primary hyperparathyroidism undergoing minimally invasive parathyroidectomy. Patient 1 demonstrates classic PTH degradation, patient 2 shows a spike in PTH at excision as a result of surgical manipulation of the adenoma, and patient 3 shows failure of PTH to decline after excision of the first gland and adequate decline after excision of the second adenoma (double adenoma). The *lavender* region represents the normal range of the rapid PTH assay (10-65 pg/mL).

to account for the half-life of PTH, which is approximately 3.5 to 4 minutes. A 50% reduction in the PTH level from baseline is used as an indication that the exploration has been successful, and this has proved to be predictive of cure in 96% of cases.[26]

The rapid PTH assay is especially helpful when the surgeon has difficulty distinguishing between thyroid tissue, lymph nodes, or a parathyroid adenoma. Aspiration of parathyroid tissue yields substantially higher hormone values than the upper limit of the standard curve; levels higher than 1500 pg/mL confirm the tissue diagnosis. Intraoperative ex vivo PTH aspiration has become a useful alternative to frozen section for identification of the parathyroid gland. It is also much faster and less expensive.

Operative failure rates for initial and remedial parathyroidectomy appear to have decreased significantly in centers that use this intraoperative adjunct. Irvin[27] has demonstrated that operative failure rates from initial parathyroidectomy have decreased significantly with the use of the rapid PTH assay, from 6% to 1.5%; long-term recurrence is 4.8%. Although experience seems to vary, even in the more difficult field of reoperation, the use of intraoperative PTH testing has been reported to increase success rates to 89%.[28] Critics have emphasized that false-negative predictions from the test lead to unnecessary exploration and that surgeons who depend on hormone measurement for intraoperative decisions cease to be cost-effective. Overall, although there continues to be some controversy, the largest endocrine surgery centers use the assay as an important adjunct to MIP. In patients with multigland disease in particular, intraoperative PTH testing has been shown to be essential; in a recent review of 519 patients, the assay changed operative management in 17% of all patients and in 82% of patients who had incorrect or negative preoperative imaging.[29]

In radioguided parathyroidectomy, developed in 1996, 10 to 20 mCi of $^{99m}$Tc-sestamibi is injected IV 2 to 4 hours before surgery, and the adenoma is localized intraoperatively with a hand-held quantitative gamma counter with a 9- to 14-mm probe.[30] Gamma counts are obtained at the start of the operation in all four quadrants of the neck, through the skin, and after the incision, under the strap muscles. Care is taken not to interpret radioactivity emitted by the heart. Exploration in which counts are highest focuses surgery and reduces operative time. The activity of the removed parathyroid is checked with the gamma probe to confirm cure. The excised adenoma emits radioactivity at least 20% and often 50% in excess of the postexcision background. Finally, the postexcision radioactivity in all four quadrants of the neck should equalize.

Theoretically, use of the gamma probe can expedite some of the intraoperative decision making associated with routine parathyroidectomy by providing functional feedback to the surgeon. This has been shown to be particularly helpful in the setting of false-positive sestamibi scans, ectopic parathyroid adenomas, and remedial parathyroidectomy in which attempts at localization have been suboptimal. Still, intraoperative use of the gamma probe has not been embraced by most experienced endocrine surgeons because it yields little additional information over that obtained by adequate preoperative localization and the intraoperative PTH assay.

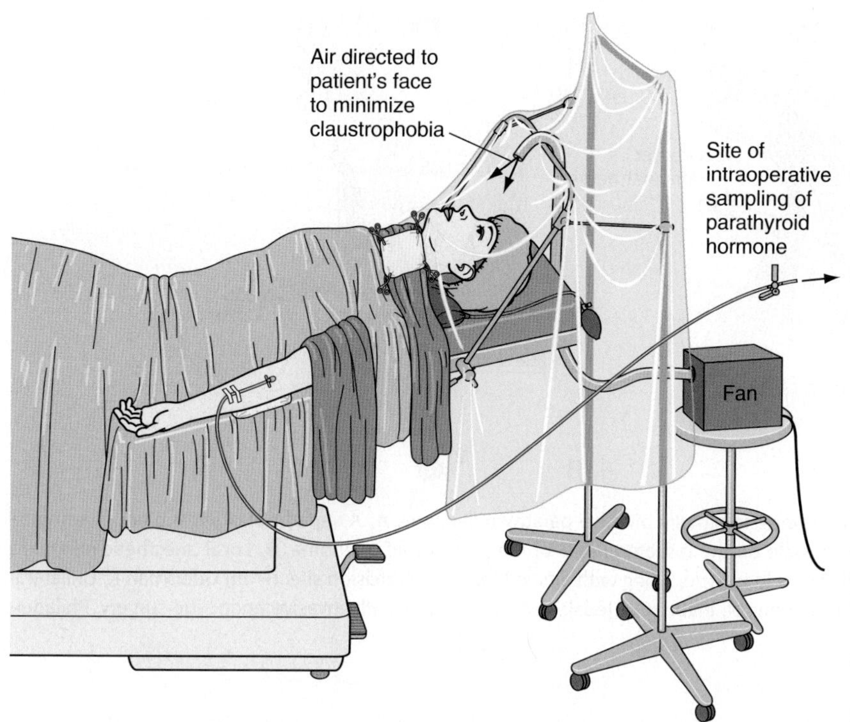


**FIGURE 39-9** Organization of an ambulatory operating room used for minimally invasive parathyroidectomy. A large-bore IV line facilitates sedation and performance of the rapid parathyroid hormone assay. At the head of the bed, cool air blows over the patient to minimize claustrophobia. (From Udelsman R: Unilateral neck exploration under local or regional anesthesia. In Gagner M, Inabnet W [eds]: Textbook of minimally invasive endocrine surgery, Philadelphia, 2002, JB Lippincott.)

**Bilateral Neck Exploration** The classic approach to the surgical management of primary HPT traditionally has been bilateral neck exploration under general anesthesia, with intraoperative, histopathologic frozen section examination of excised parathyroid tissue. Ideally, all the parathyroid glands are identified, and the surgeon removes the pathologically enlarged gland or glands. Historically, patients were admitted to the hospital for 1 or 2 days and failure rates in the best series were consistently less than 3% to 5%. Standard bilateral neck exploration is still considered an excellent operation, with a complication rate in the 1% to 2% range and a cure rate (defined as normocalcemia 6 months postoperatively) higher than 95%.

### Parathyroidectomy

**Minimally Invasive Parathyroidectomy** Because 85% of primary HPT results from a single adenoma and is cured by excision of the culprit gland, directed surgery after accurate preoperative localization has been used with increased frequency. MIP involves the use of unilateral neck exploration under regional or local anesthesia in the ambulatory setting.

The initial approach to unilateral surgery for primary HPT was advocated by Roth and colleagues[31] in 1975, with selection of the side to be explored based on palpation or imaging, including esophagography, venography, or angiography. If an enlarged and normal gland were found on the initial side, contralateral exploration was deferred. Intraoperative staining with Sudan black was performed. Wang[32] advocated a similar approach and argued that bilateral exploration increased the risk, cost, and morbidity associated with parathyroidectomy for primary HPT. Tibblin and associates,[33] in 1982, advocated unilateral parathyroidectomy, which they defined as removal of both the adenoma and normal gland from one side. Excised tissue stained with oil red O, which stains fat droplets, was studied under the microscope during surgery, and the decision to stop the operation was based on demonstration of a reduction in intracytoplasmic fat droplets in the excised adenomatous parathyroid tissue. Both techniques would fail, however, in the setting of double adenomas on the contralateral side if the random choice of which side to explore was in error.

Bergenfelz and coworkers[34] have reported the results of a prospective, randomized controlled trial comparing unilateral with bilateral neck exploration. In this study of 91 patients, comparisons were made among patients assigned to preoperative sestamibi localization, unilateral neck exploration, and use of the rapid PTH assay (cases) and patients assigned to bilateral neck exploration (controls). Patients who underwent unilateral neck exploration had a lower incidence of early postoperative hypocalcemia requiring the administration of supplemental calcium. There were no statistical differences among complication rates, cost, and operative time between the two treatment groups. The study was not blinded and was flawed by a high crossover rate; only 62% of patients assigned to unilateral neck exploration actually underwent the assigned operation. The rest underwent bilateral neck exploration, probably because sestamibi had a sensitivity of only 71% in the study.

Today, MIP requires preoperative localization (typically with sestamibi, combined with SPECT) followed by limited exploration, often using cervical block anesthesia and the intraoperative PTH assay to confirm the adequacy of resection (Fig. 39-9). Patients with known multigland hyperplasia are not generally offered MIP. However, if such a patient is encountered during MIP, bilateral neck exploration can often be accomplished with the technique or the procedure can be converted to general anesthesia, if necessary. The vast majority of patients undergoing MIP are discharged on the day of surgery. They are monitored carefully as outpatients, and serum calcium and iPTH levels are measured within the first week of follow-up.

The skin incision is small, typically 2 to 4 cm. A superficial cervical block is administered posterior and deep to the sternocleidomastoid muscle on the ipsilateral side of the

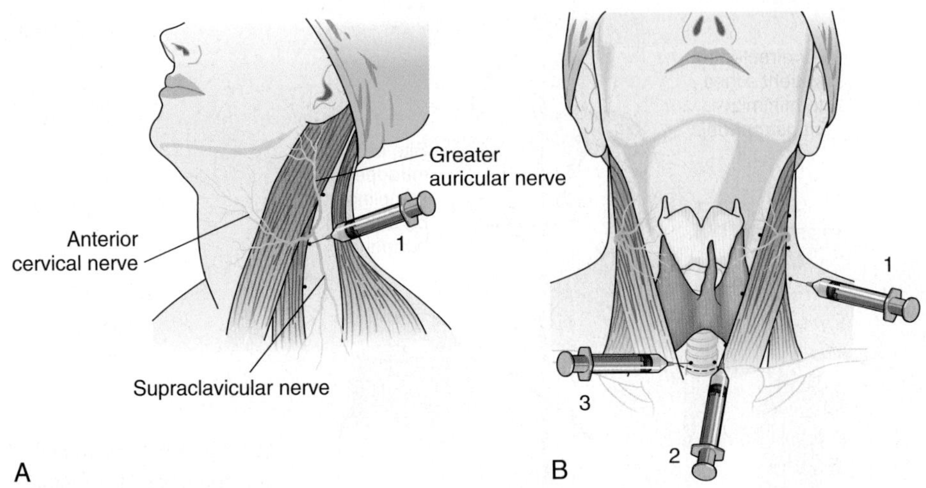


**FIGURE 39-10** Cervical block performed by a surgeon during minimally invasive parathyroidectomy. **A,** A superficial cervical block is administered posterior and deep to the sternocleidomastoid muscle on the ipsilateral side of the parathyroid adenoma. **B,** Local anesthetic infiltrated along the anterior border of the ipsilateral sternocleidomastoid muscle, along with a field block at the incision site. (From Udelsman R: Unilateral neck exploration under local or regional anesthesia. In Gagner M, Inabnet W [eds]: Textbook of minimally invasive endocrine surgery, Philadelphia, 2002, JB Lippincott.)

sestamibi-localized adenoma (Fig. 39-10*A* and *B*). In most patients, 1% lidocaine with or without 1 : 100,000 epinephrine is used; it can be supplemented during the operation, if required. Care is always taken to aspirate before delivering the anesthetic to avoid intravascular administration. We have found that by also infiltrating along the anterior border of the sternocleidomastoid muscle, as well as performing a local field block, excellent analgesia is obtained in almost all cases. The total volume of lidocaine required is typically 18 to 25 mL.

The regional block is performed in the operating room and IV supplementation is administered by the anesthesia staff. Propofol is discontinued at least 5 minutes before PTH sampling because it may interfere with the PTH assay. Sedation with fentanyl, midazolam, or both is used to minimize patient anxiety while maintaining an awake conscious patient who can phonate. Bilateral neck exploration under regional anesthesia, first shown by LoGerfo, can be performed safely and effectively.[35] In a series of 236 patients undergoing MIP, 62% had a nonlocalizing sestamibi scan preoperatively or no scan at all, but only 4 required conversion to general anesthesia. A simultaneous procedure was performed in 23% and 85% underwent bilateral neck exploration. The average operating time in the series was 43 minutes for parathyroid procedures and 66 minutes for combined parathyroid/thyroid procedures.

A focused exploration is performed according to the results of the preoperative imaging study, and the intraoperative PTH assay is used to confirm the adequacy of resection in the operating room (Fig. 39-11). The success of MIP has been confirmed by evidence of cure and complication rates that are at least as good as those achieved with conventional bilateral exploration. Specifically, in a series of 656 consecutive parathyroidectomies (401 of which were performed in standard fashion and 255 with MIP) between 1990 and 2001, there were no significant differences in complication rates (3% and 1.2%, respectively) or cure rates (97% and 99%, respectively).[36] MIP was associated with a 50% reduction in operating time (1.3 hours for MIP versus 2.4 hours for the standard operation), a sevenfold reduction in length of hospital stay (0.24 versus 1.64 days, respectively), and a mean savings of $2693/procedure, which represents a reduction in total hospital charges by almost 50%.

**Video-Assisted Parathyroidectomy** The technique of video-assisted parathyroidectomy was introduced and pioneered by Miccoli and colleagues.[37] It does not require steady gas flow, but rather a brief insufflation of carbon dioxide to establish the operative space, which is then maintained by external retraction. Preoperative localization is essential and general anesthesia is typically used, although local anesthesia might be feasible.

A 15-mm skin incision is created 1 cm above the sternal notch to accommodate tactile assessment, suction irrigation, and dissection and retraction equipment. The incision can be moved, depending on the location of the adenoma. Another 10-mm trocar site is made vertically in the midline below the strap muscles and above the thyroid gland on the ipsilateral side of the suspected adenoma to accommodate the insufflator at the start of the case; a 30-degree, 5-mm endoscope is then inserted with two retractors for moving the thyroid medially and the strap muscles laterally. Suction irrigation is feasible because continuous insufflation is not required.

A multi-institution series from Italy, Germany, the United States, and Turkey included 123 patients enrolled between 1997 and 1999 who were successfully evaluated with preoperative localization studies and had no evidence of multiglandular disease, thyroid malignancy, large thyroid mass, or previous neck surgery or irradiation.[38] The rapid PTH assay was used as an adjunct. All patients were cured by the video-assisted technique. Conversion to open parathyroidectomy occurred in 11% of patients, and 2 patients experienced recurrent laryngeal nerve palsy. The operating time was 55 minutes (average), with a median hospital stay of 1.5 days.

**Endoscopic Parathyroidectomy** Advances in laparoscopy and endoscopy have been applied to parathyroidectomy. Patients with mediastinal parathyroid adenomas can undergo

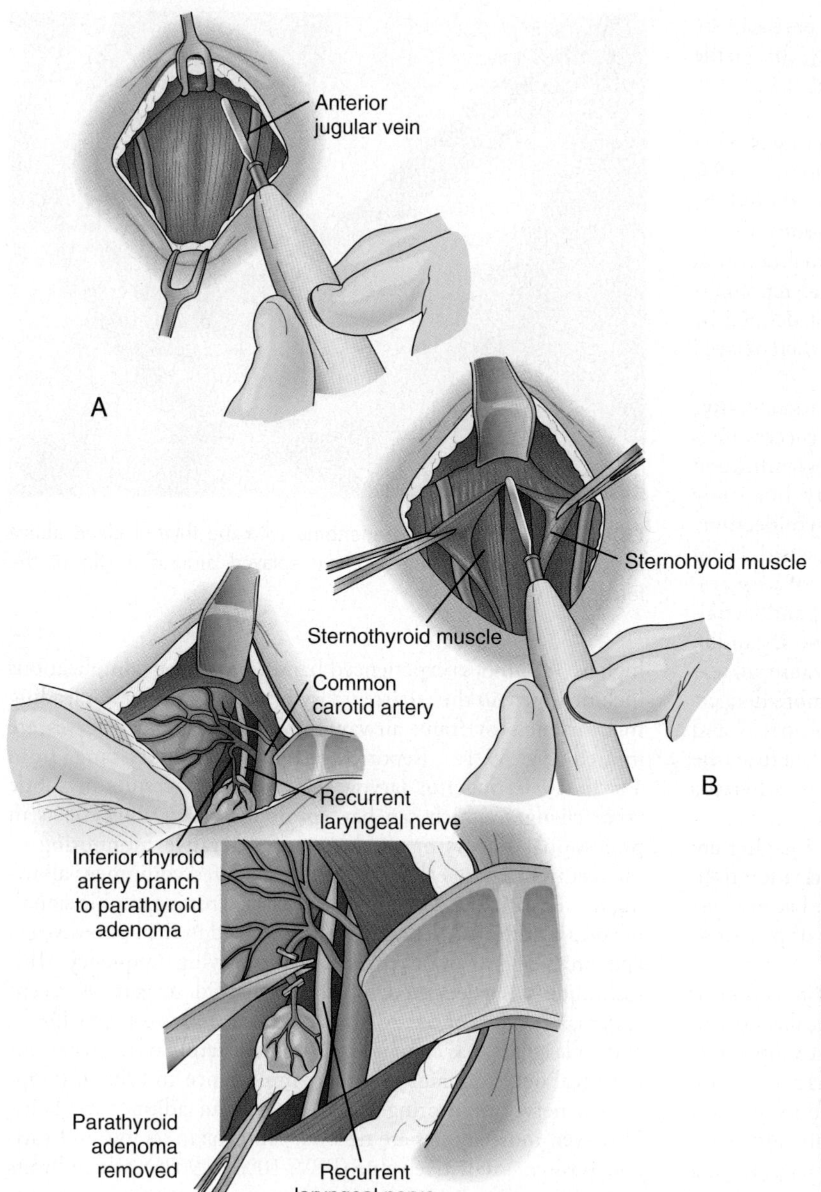


**FIGURE 39-11** Technique of minimally invasive parathyroidectomy. **A,** A small transverse cervical skin incision is made, the platysma is divided, and the anterior jugular veins are preserved. **B,** The raphe between the strap muscles is divided in the midline. **C,** The parathyroid adenoma is excised, with care taken to preserve the recurrent laryngeal nerve and minimize manipulation of the tumor during ligation of the end artery. (From Udelsman R: Unilateral neck exploration under local or regional anesthesia. In Gagner M, Inabnet W [eds]: Textbook of minimally invasive endocrine surgery, Philadelphia, 2002, JB Lippincott.)

thoracoscopic removal. In one study,[39] after preoperative imaging localized the disease to the mediastinum, the patients were placed in the right lateral decubitus position, and parathyroidectomies were performed through three thoracoscopic ports in less than 3.5 hours, with no morbidity. One patient's tumor recurred, however.

The first endoscopic removal of a parathyroid in the neck was reported by Gagner in 1996. In a patient with familial hypercalcemia, the neck was explored with the use of four 5-mm ports and carbon dioxide insufflation; 3.5 glands were excised, and the patient was cured. However, the operation took 5 hours and was complicated by intraoperative hypercapnea and postoperative subcutaneous emphysema.

Endoscopic parathyroidectomy has since been modified. It is generally reserved for patients with single-gland disease and requires preoperative imaging to localize the culprit parathyroid adenoma and guide the operation. Generally, access for the endoscope is obtained at the manubrium and two additional ports are inserted laterally in the neck, anterior to the sternocleidomastoid muscle and ipsilateral to the parathyroid tumor. In this way, it is similar to the lateral approach used for conventional remedial neck exploration. The operative space is created between the platysma and strap muscles by using insufflation at low pressure (5 to 8 mm Hg), and the strap muscles and thyroid are mobilized to expose the parathyroid.

Variations on this technique exist. Henry suggested that all three trocars can be inserted along the anterior border of the sternocleidomastoid muscle on the ipsilateral side of the adenoma, thus reducing the need for constant insufflation. Dulucq described excellent results with insertion of the endoscope at the manubrium and the other two trocars on opposite sides of the neck. Regardless of technique, there is a significant learning curve associated with endoscopic parathyroidectomy. Even with low insufflation pressure, there can still be problems with small amounts of blood obscuring the field of view, metabolic disturbances from carbon dioxide absorption, and subcutaneous emphysema. Finally, the operative space can be lost during suction, and there is no opportunity for tactile assessment.

**Remedial Parathyroidectomy** Remedial parathyroidectomy is often required for symptomatic persistent and recurrent HPT. However, the threshold for surgical intervention should be higher, given the complex nature of these reexplorations. Persistent HPT is defined by an inability to achieve normalization of the serum calcium level after initial exploration and represents an immediate technical failure. Recurrent disease is defined by initial normalization of the serum calcium level but then delayed hypercalcemia after 6 months of eucalcemia.

Preoperative localization and use of the rapid intraoperative PTH assay are important adjuncts for enhancing success rates during remedial parathyroid surgery. Perhaps the best indication for 4D-CT is in the setting of remedial neck surgery. In a study of 45 patients who underwent reoperative parathyroidectomy after preoperative localization using 4D-CT, the sensitivity of 4D-CT for localization was 88% compared with 54% for sestamibi; it more often correctly localized ($P < .0003$) and lateralized ($P < .005$) hyperfunctional parathyroid tissue than sestamibi. Reoperative neck exploration is more difficult because of scar tissue and distortion of normal tissue planes. It is more dangerous because of a greater chance of injury to the recurrent and superior laryngeal nerves. Therefore, reviewing the data from the initial exploration (noting the location of the parathyroids encountered, biopsied, or excised from the operative and pathology reports) and obtaining adequate preoperative imaging are essential for guided surgical exploration. In cases of reexploration, it can be useful to have cryopreservation available because the only remaining parathyroid tissue might be the site of persistent or recurrent disease.

Many surgeons have shown that radioguided resection of parathyroid glands can facilitate intraoperative localization in selected patients with primary HPT, especially in the reoperative setting. In a recent study of 769 patients who had sestamibi scanning and then surgery, radioguided parathyroidectomy was equally effective in patients with negative (nonlocalizing) sestamibi scans undergoing surgery, and use of the gamma probe led to the detection of all parathyroid glands, including ectopically located ones.[40]

Experience with parathyroid surgery is still the most important predictor of success in reoperative parathyroidectomy. The lateral approach to parathyroidectomy, first described by Feind—specifically, dissection between the anterior border of the sternocleidomastoid muscle and the posterior border of the strap muscles—can be invaluable. This approach provides a dissection plane more likely to be free of scar tissue from the previous exploration than the traditional anterior approach. It is sometimes necessary to perform a partial or (rarely) complete median sternotomy at the time of reexploration for parathyroids located in the mediastinum. Success rates of 85% to 95% can be achieved by experienced endocrine surgeons in the remedial setting.

## Postoperative Complications

There is good evidence that clinical outcomes are related to the experience of the surgeon performing the parathyroidectomy; high-volume endocrine surgeons have higher cure rates and lower complication rates. The rate of persistent HPT can be as high as 30% in less experienced hands. Operative complications include injury to the recurrent laryngeal nerve or nerves, leading to hoarseness or frank airway compromise if both nerves are injured (Fig. 39-12). Reported rates of nerve injury range from 1% to 10%. Superior laryngeal nerve injury results in subtle voice changes, which can have profound deleterious effects in professional singers or speakers. Intraoperative monitoring of the recurrent laryngeal nerve using specialized equipment allowing for recording and documenting of electromyographic signals of vocal cord function have been introduced in the last few years, and are being used in practice with varying frequency. This technique has been used mostly in thyroid surgery. A recent systematic review of the existing literature on this topic by Dralle and colleagues[41] has concluded that visualization of the recurrent laryngeal nerve remains of utmost importance and that intraoperative nerve monitoring could provide an adjunct modality. However, more studies are necessary to explain its low and variable positive predictive value (PPV; 10% to 90%), which limits its usefulness for intraoperative nerve management.

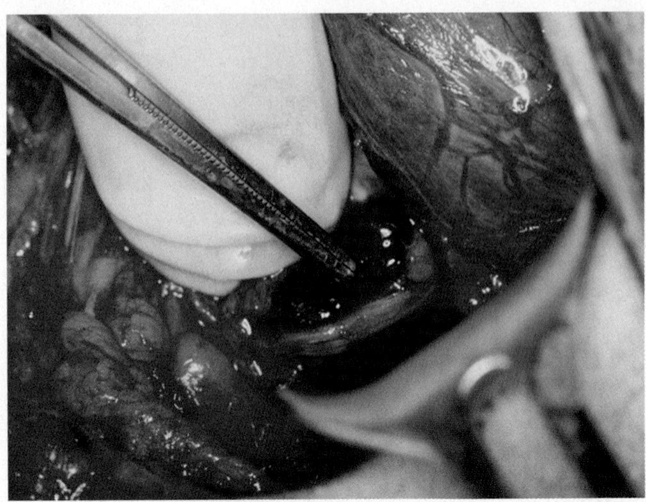

**FIGURE 39-12** Parathyroid adenoma with the thyroid gland above and the recurrent laryngeal nerve splayed around it (tip of the forceps).

Hematomas and wound infections are uncommon. The risk for these complications is theoretically less when exploration is confined to one side of the neck.

Hypoparathyroidism from injury to or removal or devascularization of the remaining parathyroids can occur and result in hypocalcemia (see earlier, "Hypoparathyroidism"). Transient postoperative hypocalcemia is not uncommon. Risk factors for the development of hypocalcemia after parathyroidectomy include subtotal or 3.5-gland parathyroidectomy, bilateral neck exploration, removal of the parathyroids together with the thyroid gland, or history of previous neck dissection. For such patients, a calcium gluconate infusion needs to be available to facilitate rapid administration. The drip is prepared by diluting 10 ampules of calcium gluconate in 1 liter of normal saline. The initial rate of infusion is 30 mL/hr, which needs to be titrated according to symptoms and serial serum calcium levels. Coincident electrolyte abnormalities, such as hypomagnesemia, need to be corrected to facilitate correction of the hypocalcemia. Oral calcium and vitamin D analogues are used for long-term management.

### Treatment Controversies

The optimal clinical treatment of patients with asymptomatic primary HPT has not yet been established. The principal debate is whether patients should be treated with early surgery or whether surveillance or medical therapy can be used safely until symptoms develop. Although consensus-based recommendations have existed for more than 15 years regarding optimal management of the disease, there continues to be substantial variation in the practice patterns of endocrine surgeons and endocrinologists. A cross-sectional survey of North American members of the American Association of Endocrine Surgeons has demonstrated that even among a group of highly experienced surgeons, criteria for parathyroidectomy vary widely and appear to be associated with surgeon experience. High-volume surgeons (>50 cases/year) had significantly lower thresholds for surgery with respect to abnormalities in preoperative creatinine clearance, bone densitometry changes, and levels of iPTH and urinary calcium than their low-volume colleagues (1 to 15 cases/year). In addition, their criteria for surgery diverged from NIH guidelines. It is interesting to note that there was a statistically significant association between several self-reported surgical outcomes and surgeon volume, a finding that has been shown with administrative data for several complex procedures.

A national survey of endocrinologists in the United States was conducted to examine the treatment of patients with primary HPT and awareness of NIH recommendations.[42] Data regarding practice demographics and annual primary HPT case volume were also collected. High-volume physicians were more aware of the NIH guidelines than low-volume physicians. Marked variations in treatment were noted, with 7% of all physicians referring more than 90% of their asymptomatic patients for surgery and 31% referring less than 10%. Adherence to monitoring recommendations for nonoperatively treated patients ranged widely, depending on the indication. Surgical referral practices varied as well, with 25% of endocrinologists referring patients because of mild hypercalcemia, 39% because of moderate hypercalcemia, 31% because of severe hypercalcemia, and 4% reporting that hypercalcemia by itself was not a sufficient reason to refer for parathyroidectomy. These results challenged the endocrine community to examine the evidential basis for decisions made in the treatment of primary HPT.

As awareness of the importance of skeletal health has increased, some community physicians and bone specialists have begun to measure PTH levels in the context of an evaluation for low bone density. There has been some difficulty in clarifying a diagnosis of primary HPT in patients with normal serum calcium levels but variable PTH levels. Mild elevation of PTH concentrations has been observed in several scenarios, such as in older individuals, blacks relative to whites, those with low calcium intake, obese individuals, and those with vitamin D deficiency or insufficiency. Serum levels of 25-hydroxyvitamin D should also be measured in patients with elevated serum PTH levels and, if vitamin D insufficiency is present, it should be treated. Serum calcium and iPTH levels should be reevaluated after vitamin D repletion.[43]

Patients with elevated PTH levels and consistently normal serum calcium levels, in whom secondary causes of hyperparathyroidism have been excluded, may represent the earliest presentation of primary HPT. It is believed that during this early phase, termed *normocalcemic hyperparathyroidism,* elevated serum PTH levels cause a reduction in cortical bone density. Data on this early entity are sparse but, in a longitudinal cohort study of 37 patients with normocalcemic HPT followed with annual physical examinations, biochemical indices, and bone mineral density studies, Lowe and associates[15] have found that many of these patients had a history of kidney stones (14%), fragility fractures (11%), and osteoporosis (57%) over the course of up to 8 years. During follow-up, 40% developed further signs of primary HPT, such as hypercalcemia, renal stones, fractures, or bone loss. The authors concluded that normocalcemic HPT can have substantial skeletal involvement and may represent an early form of symptomatic, rather than asymptomatic, primary HPT.

### Medical Alternatives

There are no long-term medical therapies for which data are convincing regarding their efficacy or safety in the treatment of primary HPT. Three classes of agents—bisphosphonates, selective estrogen receptor modulators, and calcimimetics—have shown preliminary efficacy on surrogate markers of severity of disease, including serum calcium and bone density, but these effects have not been verified based on clinical outcomes.

Bisphosphonates such as etidronate, alendronate, and pamidronate have been used in the treatment of Paget's disease, osteoporosis, and hypercalcemia of malignancy (see earlier). IV pamidronate appears to be the most effective for the acute treatment of hypercalcemia associated with primary HPT. Limitations of long-term treatment include poor GI drug absorption, a rise in PTH levels with increased renal tubular resorption and GI absorption of calcium, and their expense.

Bone mineral density has been a primary end point in studies of hormonal therapy in patients with primary HPT. The risk-benefit equation for determining the usefulness of hormone replacement therapy is complex, however, because estrogen replacement therapy does not reduce PTH concentrations in patients with primary HPT. In addition, unopposed estrogen increases the risk for endometrial hyperplasia and carcinoma, as well as the risk for venous thromboembolism, and it may cause vaginal bleeding or increase the risk for breast cancer. As a result, selective estrogen receptor inhibitors such as raloxifene and tamoxifen have been used in a preliminary fashion. In one report of 11 postmenopausal women with mild primary HPT, the mean serum calcium level declined 0.7 mg/dL over a 7-month follow-up.

Discovery of the CaSR and its molecular role in mineral metabolism represented a major scientific advance. The CaSR is a low-affinity, G protein–coupled receptor found in high concentrations on the surface of parathyroid cells, as well as on thyroid C cells secreting calcitonin, and in the nephron, brain, bone, and other tissues. Activation of the CaSR by small changes in extracellular ionized calcium accounts for the steep inverse relationship between PTH and small changes in the blood calcium level, as well as the sharp comcomitant rise in the urinary calcium level. Alterations of the receptor are responsible for BFHH, severe infantile HPT, and hereditary forms of hypoparathyroidism. Acquired alterations in CaSR might play a role in the pathophysiologic features of primary and secondary HPT. Parathyroids obtained from uremic patients with secondary HPT have been shown to exhibit reduced expression of CaSR on the surface of parathyroid cells; data from patients with parathyroid adenomas or carcinomas are more inconsistent.

The CaSR became the target for the development of compounds that enhance the affinity of the CaSR for calcium and reduce PTH secretion. Experience with the compound R-568 in patients with primary or secondary HPT demonstrated a dose-dependent reduction in PTH and blood calcium levels, with larger doses causing more sustained effects. The long-term role of calcimimetic agents such as cinacalcet has yet to be determined for the treatment of primary HPT, but it has become established as a mainstay in the management of secondary HPT (see later).

A cost-effectiveness analysis has shown that parathyroidectomy is more cost-effective than observation for managing asymptomatic primary HPT patients who do not meet NIH criteria for parathyroidectomy.[44] Treatment outcomes, their probabilities, and costs (in 2005 dollars) were identified based on literature and cost database review, and outcomes were weighted using quality of life usefulness factors. The incremental cost-effectiveness ratio for parathyroidectomy was $4778/quality-adjusted life-year (QALY) gained. Operation remained cost-effective until the average cost of parathyroidectomy increased from the estimated value of $4778 to $14,650. Pharmacologic therapy was not cost-effective unless the annual cost of therapy decreased from an estimated $7406 (for cinacalcet) to $221. Although the NIH guidelines recommended surgery for patients younger than 50 years, an additional cost-effectiveness analysis with Markov modeling has demonstrated that parathyroidectomy is the optimal strategy for many patients with asymptomatic primary HPT who are older than 50 years. Cost-effectiveness was optimal when life expectancy reached 5 years for outpatient parathyroidectomy and 6.5 years for inpatient surgery. Observation was the optimal strategy at all shorter life expectancies. Pharmacologic management was not optimal at any life expectancy.

## Secondary Hyperparathyroidism in Renal Failure

### Pathogenesis

Although renal osteodystrophy was recognized for many years, Slatopolsky and Bricker first postulated in 1973 that uremic hyperphosphatemia leads to hypocalcemia, which in turn leads to HPT. This then becomes a compensatory mechanism serving to maintain phosphate balance in uremia. The trade-off was normalization of calcium and phosphate levels at the cost of sustained high PTH levels. It is now believed that the pathogenesis of secondary HPT has multiple contributing factors, including possible genetic mutations, altered vitamin D metabolism and resistance, impaired calcemic response to PTH, retention of phosphorus, and altered metabolism of PTH. In all cases of secondary HPT, the failing kidney is unable to hydroxylate vitamin $D_2$ to active vitamin $D_3$ (calcitriol).

The pathways leading to secondary HPT seem to have different predominating factors, depending on the severity of the renal failure. In early renal failure, possible mutations in CaSR and a generalized defect in calcitriol receptors could lead to incipient secondary HPT. Subtle changes in calcitriol and serum phosphate levels and the direct action of phosphate on the parathyroids may further potentiate HPT. Altered calcitriol levels and receptor binding seem to begin to alter PTH secretion. In progressing renal failure, calcitriol deficiency becomes more important and phosphate retention plays a major role in worsening secondary HPT. Changes in calcium set points, increasing skeletal resistance to PTH, and decreased metabolic clearance of PTH contribute to the clinical syndrome of secondary HPT.

### Indications for Surgery

Although secondary HPT is typically managed initially with nonoperative strategies, there are pathophysiologic sequelae of chronic renal failure that serve as indications for parathyroidectomy. *Renal osteodystrophy* is a term used to describe the multiple skeletal complications of ESRD, including osteitis fibrosa cystica, osteomalacia, and adynamic bone disease. It is a disorder of bone remodeling and is affected by HPT. Osteitis fibrosa cystica is marked by marrow fibrosis with increased bone remodeling as a result of the increased number and activity of osteoclasts, as well as higher rates of bone formation. It is associated with osteopenia, bone cysts, brown tumors, and decreased bone strength, resulting in long bone fractures because of dystrophic bone formation. High levels of PTH coupled with increased cytokine production and low calcitriol levels cause this condition. Osteomalacia is characterized by lower bone turnover, mineralization deficiency, and accumulation of unmineralized osteoid. Deposition of aluminum and other heavy metals associated with ESRD leads to defective mineralization. The incidence has declined, although the disease has not disappeared completely. Osteomalacia is marked by skeletal deformity, fractures, and pain. It is refractory to vitamin D administration. Adynamic bone disease is characterized by hypocellular bone surfaces with little or no evidence of remodeling; it is common in patients with normal or low PTH levels or severe diabetes and aluminum intoxication. It has been associated with long-term peritoneal dialysis. It can cause fractures and microfractures leading to bone pain.

The diagnosis of bone complications from secondary HPT can be established by bone biopsy, along with measurement of serum alkaline phosphatase, PTH, and serum aluminum concentrations, as well as bone scintigraphy. Radiographic examination of the hands, skull, and long bones will show osteopenia, periosteal bone resorption and, occasionally, cysts. Medical control of osteodystrophy includes a low-phosphate diet, addition of calcium-based phosphate binders, and limitation of magnesium intake because magnesium inhibits mineralization. Maintaining positive calcium balance and aiming for a serum concentration on the high end of normal to suppress overactivity of the parathyroids are also beneficial.

Administration of vitamin D analogues has been used to treat secondary HPT and correct the endogenous deficiency of chronic renal failure. The calcimimetic agents (e.g., cinacalcet) have revolutionized the medical management of secondary HPT in chronic renal failure patients undergoing dialysis. These drugs directly lower PTH levels by increasing the sensitivity of the CaSR to extracellular calcium.[45] The starting dose of the drug is 30 mg/day; it is titrated every 2 to 4 weeks to a maximum of 180 mg/day in divided doses to achieve a target PTH level.

Uremic pruritus, or severe itching with end-stage renal failure, has been postulated to occur as a result of increased calcium salt deposition in the dermis without visible skin lesions. Parathyroidectomy appears to relieve these symptoms within a few days. General weakness is common in uremic patients, particularly in those with secondary HPT. Chou and coworkers[46] have described a series of 56 patients with ESRD and secondary HPT who were evaluated by muscle strength flexion and extension, as well as overall activity. Patients then underwent parathyroidectomy, with resolution of the secondary HPT. At 3 months, all patients showed an increase in muscle force measurements and improvement in physical activity. Finally, anemia is common in uremic patients. It is believed that PTH may directly inhibit renal and extrarenal production of erythropoietin. Excess PTH secretion in secondary HPT can lead to marrow fibrosis, thereby potentiating anemia. There are more complex effects mediated by PTH that affect hemoglobin levels, including intracellular and extracellular calcium and phosphate levels, osteoclast resorption, and erythropoietic progenitor cell response to exogenous erythropoietin. Improvements in anemia have been reported after parathyroidectomy.

Calciphylaxis is a rare, severe, and life-threatening complication of secondary HPT characterized by calcification of the media of small to medium-sized arteries; it results in ischemic damage in dermal and epidermal structures. Calcification can lead to nonhealing ulcers, gangrene, sepsis, and death. Women maintained on hemodialysis are almost three times as likely to develop the disease as men. The diagnosis of calciphylaxis is usually based on clinical findings of characteristic skin lesions and can be supported by microscopic examination of skin biopsy samples. Lesions are mottled and painful and advance to hard tender plaques that develop central ulceration and then eschar. Serum calcium and PTH levels can be normal or slightly elevated. Parathyroidectomy is effective for some patients in slowing progression of the disease and allowing eventual healing of the wounds, with intensive local therapy. Overall, calciphylaxis involving the trunk, shoulder, buttock, or thigh has a poorer prognosis than in patients with distal extremity disease.

### Surgical Strategies

Generally, preoperative imaging before initial parathyroidectomy for secondary HPT is not indicated because bilateral neck exploration is required for identification of all glands, given that the underlying pathology is parathyroid hyperplasia. Imaging techniques are indicated for reoperative parathyroidectomy when heterotopic or supernumerary glands cannot be identified, despite adequate first-time surgical exploration. The sensitivity and specificity of imaging are limited in patients with ESRD, perhaps because of variations in size and function among the different glands, despite increased metabolic activity overall.

After the first successful surgical intervention by Stanbury in 1960, subtotal parathyroidectomy became the standard operative strategy. In 1975, with the demonstration by PTH assay of parathyroid autograft function after forearm autotransplantation, total parathyroidectomy with heterotopic autotransplantation became popular.[47] Total parathyroidectomy without autotransplantation has been described but is not widely used because it appears to have long-term detrimental effects on bone. The debate over which procedure is better has been longstanding. Both approaches require thorough neck exploration through a cervical incision. When performing subtotal parathyroidectomy, it is well advised to choose the most easily accessible gland for the vascularized remnant. Usually, this will be an inferior gland because of its more anterior location. If the remnant appears ischemic, a second gland is chosen. Surgery consists of removal of three (or more, if supernumerary glands are identified) glands in toto and 50% to 75% removal of one gland with preservation of a viable, histologically confirmed remnant. Marking the remnant with a titanium clip enables later identification if recurrence develops in the remnant. Use of intraoperative PTH level measurements can help ensure that adequate tissue has been resected. Cervical thymectomy should be performed in all patients undergoing surgery for secondary HPT because supernumerary, intrathymic parathyroid glands are a common cause of persistent or recurrent disease.

Subtotal parathyroidectomy has several advantages. A well-vascularized eutopic gland will maintain function, in contrast to an autotransplanted gland, which would need to undergo neovascularization. This might be particularly important in a noncompliant patient who is less likely to take calcium and vitamin D supplementation faithfully postoperatively. Choosing an accessible gland and marking it with a clip for potential identification make reexploration easier. Finally, avoiding an arm incision allows easier hemodialysis access. Its disadvantages are that a second neck surgery is necessary if HPT recurs, and hypoparathyroidism with significant hypocalcemia may develop if the remnant is not well vascularized. However, because it is advantageous to avoid remedial cervical exploration, heterotopic parathyroid transplantation is attractive.

Total parathyroidectomy with autotransplantation removes all identified glands and uses an easily accessible area, most commonly the forearm or the sternocleidomastoid muscle, as the site for implantation. The gland to be transplanted is minced into 1-mm pieces and 12 to 18 pieces are embedded in well-vascularized muscle and marked with a stitch or clip. Some groups use a technique of injection into subcutaneous tissue. Neovascularization occurs over a period of several weeks. The principal advantage of this technique is that residual parathyroid function is easily monitored and recurrences can be treated by partial resection under local anesthesia without the need for cervical reexploration. There are several disadvantages. More aggressive medical treatment is necessary postoperatively to maintain adequate serum calcium levels and avoid serious hypocalcemic complications. Autograft failure can lead to hypoparathyroidism, which can be profound. Retrieval of all small grafts may be difficult at reoperation. Implantation into muscle may interfere with hemodialysis access in the future; invasive growth of autografts into muscle and adjacent tissue requiring radical resection has been described. Finally, supernumerary glands may still be present in the neck, thereby resulting in two potential sites of recurrence.

Subtotal parathyroidectomy seems to be the preferred surgical approach in most but not all patients. The recurrence rate of secondary HPT varies from 5% to 17%, and the incidence is directly related to the length of patient survival. The residual parathyroid tissue in the neck or forearm will grow and cause recurrent disease if survival is prolonged and patients do not receive a renal transplant. Nodular proliferation in glands seems to predispose to recurrence more often than homogeneous gland hyperplasia. Cryopreservation of excised tissue (if available) is a good strategy when total parathyroidectomy with autotransplantation is planned in case the autograft is nonfunctional.

## Tertiary Hyperparathyroidism

Tertiary HPT occurs in two settings. The first is in a subset of patients with secondary HPT in whom the parathyroid glands become autonomous and hypercalcemia develops. The second was first recognized by St. Goar, who described how secondary HPT can persist, even after patients underwent renal transplantation and postulated that the parathyroids became autonomous. Theoretically, reversal of parathyroid hyperplasia should be expected after successful renal transplantation. Nevertheless, studies have shown that hypercalcemia can persist in 8.5% to 53% of transplant recipients. Of these, less than 1% requires parathyroidectomy for tertiary HPT. Transplant patients may have additional factors that can contribute to persistent tertiary HPT; glucocorticoids, cyclosporine, thiazide diuretics, and alterations in the glomerular filtration rate as a result of tubular injury or rejection episodes can influence parathyroid function and bone response. Accordingly, patients with severe secondary HPT should not undergo renal transplantation until their secondary HPT has been treated.

It is known that hypercalcemia may adversely affect renal graft function. Therefore, calcium levels higher than 11 mg/dL may need to be addressed more aggressively. Patients with symptomatic bone disease or other serious sequelae of uremic HPT may benefit from surgery. Otherwise, given the finding that HPT will resolve after transplantation in most cases, medical treatment may be indicated. Surgical treatment of tertiary HPT after renal transplantation is not common and is reserved for patients without resolution of symptoms, for those with hormonal and chemical abnormalities such as elevated or increasing iPTH levels and an increase in serum calcium levels to higher than 12.0 mg/dL that persists more than 1 year after transplantation, and for those with acute hypercalcemia (calcium level > 12.5 mg/dL) in the immediate post-transplantation period.

## INHERITED PARATHYROID DISEASE

Surgical management of HPT in the setting of inherited parathyroid disease differs depending on the specific syndromes, and the complexity is magnified by the patient's predisposition to persistent or recurrent HPT. The basic principles of surgery are to achieve and maintain normocalcemia for as long as possible, avoid iatrogenic hypocalcemia and other perioperative complications, and facilitate future surgery, should it be indicated.[48]

### Multiple Endocrine Neoplasia

#### Type 1

MEN1 syndrome consists of primary HPT resulting from parathyroid hyperplasia associated with lesions of the pancreas and pituitary. HPT is the most common and usually the first glandular manifestation; it typically occurs in the third to fifth decades of life. The parathyroid glands are asymmetrically enlarged and there is a high incidence of supernumerary glands (up to 20%). Parathyroid surgery in patients with MEN1 is thought of as a debulking or palliative procedure because recurrence is inevitable if survival is unlimited; it is indicated to treat and prevent the complications of HPT. Controversy exists regarding the timing of the procedure. Although early parathyroidectomy may reduce the exposure to long-term HPT and the associated osteopenia, it also might predispose to an earlier recurrence of HPT and the possibility of difficult reoperations.

The initial surgical procedure of choice in a patient with MEN1 and HPT is subtotal parathyroidectomy or total parathyroidectomy with heterotopic autotransplantation of resected parathyroid tissue; transcervical thymectomy is also performed at the initial operation. Subtotal parathyroidectomy requires identification of all parathyroids, and a remnant the size of a normal parathyroid is left in situ and marked with a surgical clip to facilitate remedial surgery. Total parathyroidectomy is accompanied by immediate heterotopic transplantation of 12 to 18 1-mm pieces of fresh parathyroid into individual pockets typically created in the brachioradialis muscle of the nondominant forearm. Reoperative debulking surgery of the forearm graft can then be performed, when necessary, under local anesthesia. Because parathyroid remnants can become ischemic or necrose and result in permanent hypoparathyroidism, cryopreservation of parathyroid tissue is performed at the time of total parathyroidectomy whenever possible.

#### Type 2A

MEN2A is marked by the findings of medullary thyroid cancer, pheochromocytoma, and primary HPT. HPT in MEN2A is the least common manifestation and occurs in 20% to 30% of patients. HPT in MEN2A differs from MEN1 in several important features, and the indications for parathyroidectomy and diagnostic criteria are more similar to those of sporadic primary HPT. When compared with HPT in MEN1, HPT in MEN2A tends to be milder and more often asymptomatic because of a single adenoma, although multiglandular hyperplasia does occur. Therefore, curative resection can be less aggressive. Enlarged parathyroids encountered during thyroidectomy for medullary thyroid cancer in a normocalcemic patient are resected. Most but not all endocrine surgeons leave normal-appearing parathyroids in situ, although total parathyroidectomy with autotransplantation to the forearm has been advocated by some.

### Familial Hyperparathyroidism

Other less common forms of familial HPT include the HPT–jaw tumor syndrome (HPT-JT), familial isolated hyperparathyroidism (FIHPT), and a number of syndromes marked by mutations in CaSR, including autosomal dominant mild HPT (ADMH), familial hypercalcemia with hypercalciuria, and neonatal severe HPT (NSHPT). Recommendations for parathyroid surgery in these settings are still evolving, although some general principles exist. HPT is the most common feature of HPT-JT and is associated with a high incidence of severe hypercalcemia and a risk for parathyroid carcinoma. In general, HPT may be treated similarly to MEN2A, with resection of grossly enlarged parathyroids unless parathyroid cancer is suspected. An alternative but rarely used strategy is total parathyroidectomy to achieve a theoretically lower risk for carcinoma.

In FIHPT, if uniglandular disease is encountered, adenoma resection can be performed, whereas multiglandular hyperplasia is treated by subtotal parathyroidectomy. In this setting, the rapid intraoperative PTH assay can be helpful to ensure that an adequate resection is performed. Parathyroid surgery for syndromes associated with CaSR abnormalities has variable results. NSHPT is manifested in neonates as severe hypercalcemia and is typically lethal unless total parathyroidectomy is performed in the first months of life. For patients with ADMH, radical subtotal parathyroid resection or total parathyroidectomy with autotransplantation can be performed. Diffuse to nodular neoplasia was found on pathologic examination and, in one study, persistent hypercalcemia was noted in 60% of patients undergoing the less radical procedure.

## PARATHYROID CARCINOMA

Parathyroid carcinoma is rare. It tends to occur a decade earlier than adenomas, and the gender ratio is approximately equal, in contrast to the female preponderance with adenomas.[49] A history of previous neck radiation is a risk factor for the development of parathyroid adenomas, but the role of radiation in the development of parathyroid carcinoma is less clear. Parathyroid carcinoma has also been reported rarely in patients with secondary HPT.

Most patients with carcinomas have marked hypercalcemia (>14 mg/dL) and are more likely to have associated bone and renal disease than those with adenomas. Hypercalcemia is usually manifested as muscle weakness, fatigue, depression, nausea, and polyuria. Suspicion also is raised by an extremely high iPTH level, a palpable neck mass on physical examination, significant uptake on sestamibi scan, or ultrasound evidence of invasion with loss of planes between the parathyroid and thyroid, occasionally with lymphadenopathy.

If a large, gray-white, locally invasive parathyroid carcinoma is suspected on exploration, an initial aggressive surgical approach involving en bloc tumor resection, ipsilateral thyroid lobectomy, and resection of adjacent soft tissues is performed because this is the only potentially curative treatment. If the procedure is being performed with a minimally invasive technique, the surgery is converted to general anesthesia if necessary to facilitate a thorough oncologic operation. A frozen section biopsy is not performed before resection because it could lead to capsular rupture and potentially spread tumor cells within the neck.

En bloc resection is associated with a 40% local recurrence rate and an overall survival rate of 89% (mean follow-up, 119 months).[50] Parathyroid carcinomas tend to recur locally after incomplete excision. Distant metastases generally develop in the lungs, liver, and bone; they can occasionally be treated by resection of individual tumor deposits. Generally, control of hypercalcemia by surgical resection of metastases or local recurrence is more effective than medical treatment. Overall, adverse prognostic factors for survival are simple parathyroidectomy alone, the presence of nodal or distant metastases at initial evaluation, nonfunctional status of the tumor, and a high index of the cancer antigen Ki-67 (>10%). There are no effective chemotherapeutic agents, although cinacalcet (the calcimimetic agent described earlier) has been approved by the U.S. Food and Drug Administration for symptomatic control of hypercalcemia. In select patients, adjuvant external beam radiation appears to decrease the rate of local recurrence and may improve disease-free survival, particularly in high-risk patients. Most patients with metastatic or locally unresectable disease die of the metabolic effects of uncontrolled hypercalcemia. There are still no generally accepted staging systems for parathyroid carcinoma.

## SELECTED REFERENCES

Akerström G, Malmaeus J, Bergström R: Surgical anatomy of human parathyroid glands. Surgery 95:14–21, 1984.

This large autopsy study increased understanding of the most common eutopic and ectopic locations of parathyroid glands.

Bilezikian JP, Khan AA, Potts JT, et al: Guidelines for the management of asymptomatic primary hyperparathyroidism: Summary statement from the third international workshop. J Clin Endocrinol Metab 94:335–339, 2009.

This recent revision of the management principles for patients with asymptomatic primary HPT represents the combined opinions of many medical and surgical leaders in the treatment of primary HPT, as well as a synthesis of published medical evidence.

Boggs JE, Irvin GL, Molinari AS, et al: Intraoperative parathyroid hormone monitoring as an adjunct to parathyroidectomy. Surgery 120:954–958, 1996.

In this landmark article, 89 patients with hyperparathyroidism had plasma samples measured for iPTH levels during parathyroidectomy. Prediction of postoperative calcium levels by means of the rapid PTH assay had a sensitivity of 97%, specificity of 100%, and overall accuracy of 97%, which led the authors to conclude that the assay should be considered as a routine intraoperative adjunct.

Roman SA, Sosa JA, Mayes L, et al: Parathyroidectomy improves neurocognitive deficits in patients with primary hyperparathyroidism. Surgery 138:1121–1129, 2005.

This prospective study compares patients with primary hyperparathyroidism undergoing parathyroidectomy and patients with benign euthyroid disease undergoing thyroidectomy. It shows that primary hyperparathyroidism appears to be associated with a spatial learning and processing deficit that improves after surgery and raises the question of whether neurocognitive symptoms should be considered as criteria for parathyroidectomy.

Udelsman R, Donovan P: Remedial parathyroid surgery: Changing trends in 130 consecutive cases. Ann Surg 244:471–479, 2006.

This large clinical series demonstrates that remedial parathyroidectomy can be performed safely with a cure rate higher than than 94% when done by an experienced endocrine surgeon. Novel preoperative imaging techniques are useful, and minimally invasive parathyroidectomy can be used in a subset of these patients.

Udelsman R, Pasieka JL, Sturgeon C, et al: Surgery for asymptomatic primary hyperparathyroidism: Proceedings of the third international workshop. J Clin Endocrinol Metab 94:366–372, 2009.

This is the most recent review of the indications for surgical treatment in primary HPT.

## REFERENCES


1. Sandstrom IV: On a new gland in man and several mammals. Bull Inst Hist Med 6:192–222, 1938.
2. Owen R: On the anatomy of the Indian rhinoceros (Rh. unicornis, L). Tran Zool Soc Lond 4:31–58, 1862.
3. Gley ME: Sur les functions du corps thyroide. CR Soc Biol 43:841–843, 1891.
4. Mandl F: Attempt to treat generalized fibrous osteitis by extirpation of parathyroid tumor. Zentralbl Chir 53:260–264, 1926.
5. Bauer W, Albright F, Aub JC: A case of osteitis fibrosa cystica (osteomalacia?) with evidence of hyperactivity of the parathyroid bodies: A metabolic study. J Clin Invest 8:228–248 1930.
6. Albright F, Baird PC, Cope O, et al: Studies on the physiology of parathyroid glands—renal complications of hyperparathyroidism. Am J Med Sci 187:49–65, 1934.

7. Castleman B, Mallory TB: Parathyroid hyperplasia in chronic renal insufficiency. Am J Pathol 13:553–558, 1937.
8. Stanbury SW, Lumb GA, Nicholson WF: Elective subtotal parathyroidectomy for renal hyperparathyroidism. Lancet 1:793–799, 1960.
9. Rasmussen H, Craig LC: Purification of parathyroid hormone by use of countercurrent distribution. J Am Chem Soc 81:5003, 1959.
10. Berson SA, Yalow RS, Aurbach GD, et al: Immunoassay of bovine and human parathyroid hormone. Proc Natl Acad Sci U S A 49:613–617, 1963.
11. Reiss E, Canterbury JM: A radioimmunoassay for parathyroid hormone in man. Proc Soc Exp Biol Med 128:501–504, 1968.
12. Wang S, McDonnell EH, Sedor FA, et al: pH effects on measurements of ionized calcium and ionized magnesium in blood. Arch Pathol Lab Med 126:947–950, 2002.
13. Udelsman R, Donovan PI: Remedial parathyroid surgery: Changing trends in 130 consecutive cases. Ann Surg 244:471–479, 2006.
14. Akerström G, Malmaeus J, Bergström R: Surgical anatomy of human parathyroid glands. Surgery 95:14–21, 1984.
15. Lowe H, McMahon DJ, Rubin MR, et al: Normocalcemic primary hyperparathyroidism: Further characterization of a new clinical phenotype. J Clin Endocrinol Metab 92:3001–3005, 2007.
16. Bilezikian JP, Khan AA, Potts Jr, JT: Third International Workshop on the Management of Asymptomatic Primary Hyperthyroidism: Guidelines for the management of asymptomatic primary hyperparathyroidism: summary statement from the third international workshop. J Clin Endocrinol Metab 94:335–339, 2009.
17. Udelsman R, Pasieka JL, Sturgeon C, et al: Surgery for asymptomatic primary hyperparathyroidism: Proceedings of the Third International Workshop. J Clin Endocrinol Metab 94:366–372, 2009.
18. Roman SA, Sosa JA, Mayes L, et al: Parathyroidectomy improves neurocognitive deficits in patients with primary hyperparathyroidism. Surgery 138:1121–1128, 2005.
19. Lundgren E, Lind L, Palmer M, et al: Increased cardiovascular mortality and normalized serum calcium in patients with mild hypercalcemia followed up for 25 years. Surgery 130:978–985, 2001.
20. Lindqvist V, Jacobsson H, Chandanos E, et al: Preoperative $^{99m}$Tc-sestamibi scintigraphy with SPECT localizes most pathologic parathyroid glands. Langenbecks Arch Surg 394:811–815, 2009.
21. Jabiev AA, Lew JI, Solorzano CC: Surgeon-performed ultrasound: A single-institution experience in parathyroid localization. Surgery 146:569–575, 2009.
22. Geatti O, Shapiro B, Orsolon PG, et al: Localization of parathyroid enlargement: Experience with technetium-99m methoxyisobutylisonitrile and thallium-201 scintigraphy, ultrasonography and computed tomography. Eur J Nucl Med 21:17–22, 1994.
23. Rodgers SE, Hunter GJ, Hamberg LM, et al: Improved preoperative planning for directed parathyroidectomy with 4-dimensional computed tomography. Surgery 140:932–940, 2006.
24. Maser C, Donovan P, Santos F, et al: Sonographically guided fine needle aspiration with rapid parathyroid hormone assay. Ann Surg Oncol 13:1690–1695, 2006.
25. Boggs JE, Irvin GL, 3rd, Molinari AS, et al: Intraoperative parathyroid hormone monitoring as an adjunct to parathyroidectomy. Surgery 120:954–958, 1996.
26. Lew JI, Irvin GL, III: Focused parathyroidectomy guided by intraoperative parathormone monitoring does not miss multiglandular disease in patients with sporadic primary hyperparathyroidism: A 10-year outcome. Surgery 146:1021–1027, 2009.
27. Solorzano CC, Mendez W, Lew JI, et al: Long-term outcome of patients with elevated parathyroid hormone levels after successful parathyroidectomy for sporadic primary hyperparathyroidism. Arch Surg 143:659–663, 2008.
28. Richards ML, Thompson GB, Farley DR, et al: Reoperative parathyroidectomy in 228 patients during the era of minimal-access surgery and intraoperative parathyroid hormone monitoring. Am J Surg 196:937–942, 2008.
29. Carneiro-Pla DM, Solorzano CC, Irvin GL, III: Consequences of targeted parathyroidectomy guided by localization studies without intraoperative parathyroid hormone monitoring. J Am Coll Surg 202:715–722, 2006.
30. Adil E, Adil T, Fedok F, et al: Minimally invasive radioguided parathyroidectomy performed for primary hyperparathyroidism. Otolaryngol Head Neck Surg 141:34–38, 2009.
31. Roth SI, Wang CA, Potts JT, Jr: The team approach to primary hyperparathyroidism. Hum Pathol 6:645–648, 1975.
32. Wang CA: Surgical management of primary hyperparathyroidism. Curr Probl Surg 22:1–50, 1985.
33. Tibblin S, Bondeson AG, Ljungberg O: Unilateral parathyroidectomy in hyperparathyroidism due to single adenoma. Ann Surg 195:245–252, 1982.
34. Bergenfelz A, Lindblom P, Tibblin S, et al: Unilateral versus bilateral neck exploration for primary hyperparathyroidism: A prospective randomized controlled trial. Ann Surg 236:543–551, 2002.
35. Bergenfelz A, Kanngiesser V, Zielke A, et al: Conventional bilateral cervical exploration versus open minimally invasive parathyroidectomy under local anaesthesia for primary hyperparathyroidism. Br J Surg 92:190–197, 2005.
36. Udelsman R: Six hundred fifty-six consecutive explorations for primary hyperparathyroidism. Ann Surg 235:665–670, 2002.
37. Miccoli P, Berti P, Ambrosini CE: Perspectives and lessons learned after a decade of minimally invasive video-assisted thyroidectomy. ORL J Otorhinolaryngol Relat Spec 70:282–286, 2008.
38. Lorenz K, Miccoli P, Monchik JM, et al: Minimally invasive video-assisted parathyroidectomy: Multi-institutional study. World J Surg 25:704–707, 2001.
39. Alesina PF, Moka D, Mahlstedt J, et al: Thoracoscopic removal of mediastinal hyperfunctioning parathyroid glands: Personal experience and review of the literature. World J Surg 32:224–231, 2008.
40. Chen H, Sippel RS, Schaefer S: The effectiveness of radioguided parathyroidectomy in patients with negative technetium Tc 99m-sestamibi scans. Arch Surg 144:643–648, 2009.
41. Dralle H, Sekulla C, Lorenz K, et al: Intraoperative monitoring of the recurrent laryngeal nerve in thyroid surgery. World J Surg 32:1358–1366, 2008.
42. Mahadevia PJ, Sosa JA, Levine MA, et al: Clinical management of primary hyperparathyroidism and thresholds for surgical referral: A national study examining concordance between practice patterns and consensus panel recommendations. Endocr Pract 9:494–503, 2003.
43. Eastell R, Arnold A, Brandi ML, et al: Diagnosis of asymptomatic primary hyperparathyroidism: Proceedings of the Third International Workshop. J Clin Endocrinol Metab 94:340–350, 2009.
44. Zanocco K, Angelos P, Sturgeon C: Cost-effectiveness analysis of parathyroidectomy for asymptomatic primary hyperparathyroidism. Surgery 140:874–881, 2006.

45. Riccardi D, Brown EM: Physiology and pathophysiology of the calcium-sensing receptor in the kidney. Am J Physiol Renal Physiol 298:F485–499, 2010.
46. Chou FF, Lee CH, Chen JB: General weakness as an indication for parathyroid surgery in patients with secondary hyperparathyroidism. Arch Surg 134:1108–1111, 1999.
47. Wells SA, Jr, Gunnells JC, Shelburne JD, et al: Transplantation of the parathyroid glands in man: Clinical indications and results. Surgery 78:34–44, 1975.
48. Carling T, Udelsman R: Parathyroid surgery in familial hyperparathyroid disorders. J Intern Med 257:27–37, 2005.
49. DeLellis RA: Parathyroid carcinoma: An overview. Adv Anat Pathol 12:53–61, 2005.
50. Iihara M, Okamoto T, Suzuki R, et al: Functional parathyroid carcinoma: Long-term treatment outcome and risk factor analysis. Surgery 142:936–943, 2007.

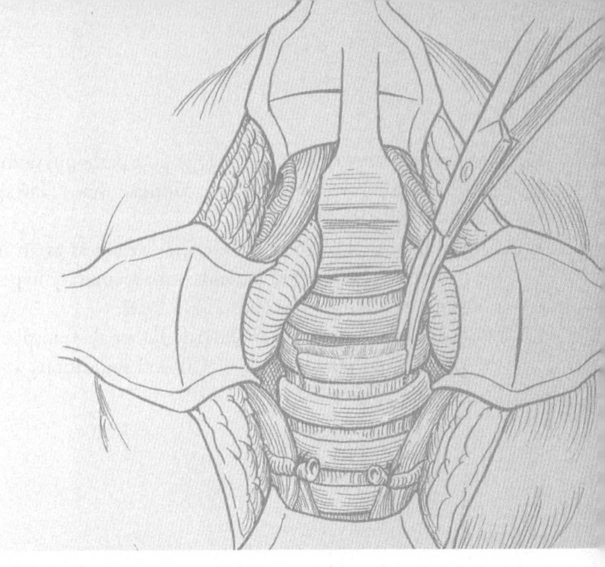

CHAPTER 40

# ENDOCRINE PANCREAS

Taylor S. Riall and Courtney M. Townsend, Jr.



The pancreas is a digestive organ located in the retroperitoneum (Fig. 40-1) that has endocrine and exocrine function. The endocrine cells are organized in discrete clumps throughout the pancreas, called islets of Langerhans. The primary physiologic function of the endocrine pancreas can be summarized as regulation of body energy, largely through hormonal control of carbohydrate metabolism. The islets secrete hormones directly into the bloodstream in endocrine fashion. Insulin is the hormone of energy storage, while glucagon is the hormone of energy release. Additional pancreatic endocrine hormones, such as somatostatin, play a role in the complex regulation of pancreatic exocrine secretion and digestion.

The pancreas was first identified by a Greek anatomist and surgeon, Herophilus (335-280 BC). In medieval Persia, in 1025, Avicenna provided the first detailed account of diabetes mellitus in the *Canon of Medicine.* He described a patient with an abnormal appetite, collapse of sexual function, and the sweet taste of diabetic urine. In 1889, Minkowski and von Mering, who were studying fat absorption in dogs after pancreatectomy, noted that the urine attracted flies. On analysis of the urine, they documented glucosuria and ketonuria. They also noted that surgical removal of the pancreas led to eventual coma and death. In 1869, while a medical student, Paul Langerhans described collections of pale staining cells within the pancreas, the islets that now bear his name (see Fig. 40-1). Eugene Opie was the first to associate diabetes with microscopic hyaline changes in the islets of Langerhans. Frederick Banting and Charles Best in Toronto discovered insulin in 1922. Banting and Best surgically ligated the pancreas of one set of dogs, leading to atrophy of the exocrine pancreas. They then removed and homogenized the pancreas and injected the homogenized extract into a diabetic dog, temporarily reversing this condition; a few injections each day could keep it healthy and free of symptoms. Banting and Best were awarded a Nobel Prize for this work.

Adult human pancreatic islets contain multiple cell types (Table 40-1). Alpha (A) cells secrete glucagon, beta (B) cells secrete insulin, delta (D) cells secrete somatostatin and vasoactive intestinal peptide (VIP), and F cells secrete pancreatic polypeptide (PP). Gastrin-producing cells are normally present in the fetal pancreas only. Islet cell tumors may secrete one or more of these hormones. The resulting syndromes are named for the peptide whose clinical symptoms predominate.

In this chapter, we will cover the histomorphology, embryology, and physiology of the endocrine pancreas. We will briefly highlight new technologies, including autologous islet cell transplantation for chronic pancreatitis and allogeneic islet cell transplantation for type 1 diabetes. Our focus will be on the diagnosis and management of endocrine tumors of the pancreas.

## HISTOMORPHOLOGY OF ISLETS

In the human fetus, pancreatic islets comprise approximately one third of the pancreatic mass. In the adult pancreas, there are approximately $10^6$ islets in the adult pancreas, accounting for less than 2% of the overall pancreatic mass. The average islet contains approximately 3000 cells and ranges in diameter from 40 to 900 μm. Each pancreatic islet should be considered a microorganism with a complex and definite organization, with only intact islet architecture enabling normal endocrine function.

The islet cell types are not distributed evenly within the islets. B cells constitute approximately 70% of the islet cell mass and are located centrally within the islet.[1] Insulin is the main secretory product of B cells, but they have also been shown to secrete amylin and cholecystokinin (CCK; see Table 40-1).[2] The A cells, located in the periphery, secrete glucagon and constitute approximately 10% of the islet cell mass. The D cells are evenly distributed throughout the islet and constitute approximately 5% of the islet cell mass. D cells secrete somatostatin and $D_2$ cells secrete VIP. Also located peripherally, F cells secrete PP. B and D cells are concentrated in the body and tail of the pancreas and F cells are concentrated in the head and uncinate process. This distribution is important clinically, because resection of different parts of the pancreas will have varying endocrine effects.

Pancreatic islets have a rich portal microcirculation that has significance in endocrine to endocrine cell signaling. Afferent arterioles enter the islet in an area of discontinuity in the peripheral, non-B cell mantle of cells. The order of islet cellular perfusion and interaction is from the B cell core outward to the mantle, and the mantle is further subordered with most D cells downstream or distal to most A cells. This allows B cells to inhibit A cell secretion and A cells to stimulate D cell secretion.[3]

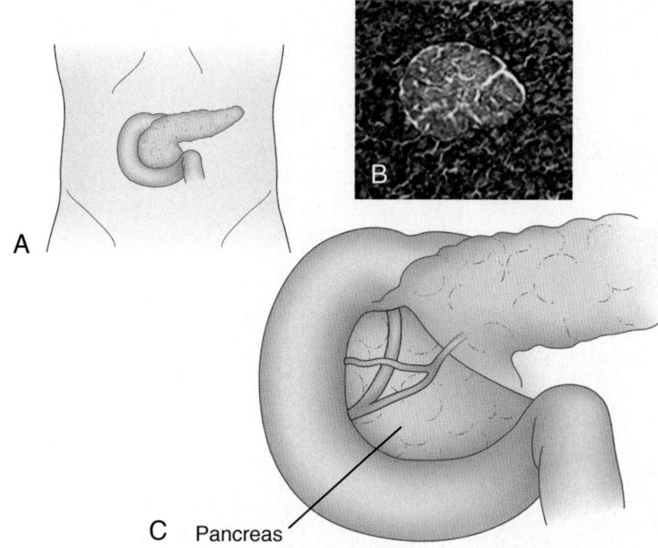


**FIGURE 40-1** **A,** The pancreas is noted in its retroperitoneal position at the level of the second lumbar vertebra. **B,** Relationship of the head of the pancreas in the C loop of the duodenum, with the pancreatic duct and common bile duct emptying into the ampulla of Vater. **C,** On microscopic view, the endocrine cells are located in nests, called islets of Langerhans, which are distributed throughout the pancreas (Trichrome stain, ×10).

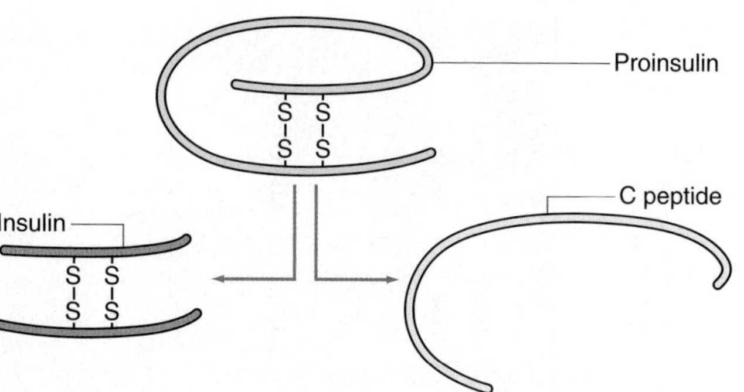


**FIGURE 40-2** Diagram of insulin synthesis. Proinsulin, synthesized by the endoplasmic reticulum, is packaged within secretory granules of the beta cell, where it is cleaved to insulin and C-peptide. Equimolar amounts of insulin and C-peptide are secreted into the bloodstream. (From Andersen DK, Brunicardi FC: Pancreatic anatomy and physiology. In Greenfield LJ, Mulholland MW, Oldham KT, et al [eds]: Surgery: Scientific principles and practice, ed 2, Philadelphia, 1997, Lippincott-Raven, p 869.)

Pancreatic endocrine secretion also regulates pancreatic exocrine secretion through the islet-acinar axis of the pancreas. Insulin stimulates pancreatic exocrine secretion, amino acid transport, and synthesis of protein and enzymes, whereas glucagon acts in a counterregulatory fashion, inhibiting the same processes. The role of somatostatin is controversial. Somatostatin may have a direct inhibitory effect on pancreatic acinar cells, which possess somatostatin receptors. It may also act through an inhibitory effect on islet B cells.

## EMBRYOLOGY OF THE ENDOCRINE PANCREAS

During the fifth week of gestation, the pancreas begins forming at the junction of the foregut and midgut. It begins as two endodermal pancreatic buds, the dorsal bud and ventral bud, which eventually fuse to form the pancreas. The acinar cells and islet cells differentiate from the endodermal cells found in the embryonic buds. In humans, the first glucagon-producing cells are seen in 3-week-old embryos and the first islets of endocrine tissue appear at approximately 10 weeks. During this early developmental period, predominantly glucagon-positive islet cells initially appear in the tail of the pancreas. Subsequently, there is a major amplification of endocrine cell numbers, particularly B cells. The mature pancreas consists of the endocrine islets of Langerhans, digestive enzyme-secreting acinar cells contained in clusters of acini, and acinar-draining ducts, with accompanying blood vessels and lymphatics.

Islet cells were initially believed to arise from neural crest cells. Gittes and Rutter[4] have studied the patterns of expression of hormonal messenger RNA and concluded that both endocrine and exocrine cells of the pancreas arise from the foregut endoderm, a view that is now generally accepted. Early glucagon-positive endocrine cells convert to nonepithelial cells and lose connection with the lumen and tight junctions. This conversion to a nonepithelial location of endocrine cells has been postulated to entail a change in cell division polarity, from perpendicular to the basement membrane to parallel to the basement membrane. There also appears to be downregulation of *pdx1,* a key marker of early pancreatic progenitor cells, in these endocrine progenitor cells as they become nonepithelial. This conversion process has been postulated to parallel mesenchymal to mesenchyme transformation.

## ENDOCRINE PHYSIOLOGY

The primary function of the endocrine pancreas is regulation of body energy. This is achieved primarily through control of carbohydrate metabolism. Insulin secreted by the endocrine pancreas functions to story energy by decreasing blood glucose levels and increasing glucose transport into cells, except beta cells, hepatocytes, and cells of the central nervous system. Insulin also stimulates protein synthesis and inhibits the breakdown of glycogen and fat stores. Glucagon functions antagonistically to insulin, increasing blood glucose levels through stimulation of glycogenolysis, lipolysis, and gluconeogenesis.

### Insulin

Insulin is a 56–amino acid polypeptide with a molecular weight of 6 kDa. It consists of two polypeptide chains (A and B) joined by two disulfide bridges. Although the amino acid sequence varies among species, the locations of the disulfide bridges are highly conserved and are critical for its biologic activity. Insulin is synthesized as a precursor peptide, called proinsulin; the two polypeptide chains are joined by means of connecting peptide (C peptide). In response to pancreatic B cell stimulation by glucose, proinsulin is synthesized in the endoplasmic reticulum and transported to the Golgi complex, where it is cleaved into insulin and the residual C peptide (Fig. 40-2). Insulin is then moved via microtubules into secretory granules, where it is released directly into the bloodstream via exocytosis. C peptide and insulin are secreted in equimolar amounts.

There is significant secretory reserve of insulin within the pancreas. Destruction or removal of 80% of the pancreatic islet cell mass is necessary before endocrine dysfunction becomes

**Table 40-1 Endocrine Cells of the Pancreas and Tumor Syndromes**

| CELL | CONTENT | ISLET CELLS (%) | SECRETORY GRANULE SIZE | TUMOR SYNDROMES | CLINICAL FEATURES | DIAGNOSTIC HORMONE LEVELS | MALIGNANT (%) | MULTIPLE (%) | MEN1 | AT SURGERY: % IDENTIFIED/ % RESECTABLE |
|---|---|---|---|---|---|---|---|---|---|---|
| A | Glucagon, glicentin (TRH, CCK, endorphin, PYY, pancreastatin) | 15 | 225 | Glucagonoma | Necrolytic migratory erythema, diabetes, anemia | Normal = <150 pg/mL Tumor = 200-2000 pg/mL | Nearly all | Rare | Few | 98/35 |
| B | Insulin (TRH, CGRP, amylin, pancreastatin, prolactin) | 65 | 300 | Insulinoma | Hypoglycemic symptoms (catecholamine release) plus mental confusion | >5 μU/mL in the face of hypoglycemia | 10 | 10 | 10% | 80-100/>90 |
| D | Somatostatin (met-encephalon) | 5 | 200-235 | Somatostatinoma | Diabetes, gallstones, steatorrhea | Normal = 10-25 pg/mL Tumor = 100-400 pg/mL | Nearly all | 0 | — | 100/60 |
| $D_2$ | VIP | <1 | 120 | VIPoma (watery diarrhea, hypokalemia, achlorhydria [WDHA] [Verner-Morrison]) | High-volume secretory diarrhea, hypokalemia, metabolic acidosis, hypochlorhydria | Normal = <200 pg/mL Tumor = 225-2000 pg/mL | 50 | Rare | Few | 100/70 |
| EC | Substance P and serotonin | <1 | 325 | ? | — | — | — | — | — | — |
| G* | Gastrin (ACTH-related peptides) | — | 300 | Gastrinoma (Zollinger-Ellison syndrome) | Abdominal pain with ulcer disease, massive gastric hypersecretion, secretory diarrhea that can be halted by nasogastric asporation | Normal = <100 pg/mL Suspicous = >1000 pg/mL With secretin text, ↑ >200 pg/mL diagnostic | 70 | — | 25% | 50-85/79 Of the 70% pancreatic, <20 duodenal, all ectopic, 80 |
| PP (F) | Pancreatic polypeptide (met-enkephalin, PHI) | 15 | 140 | Tumors (PPomas) are without endocrine symptoms | — | — | — | — | Frequent | — |
| Prob B | Ghrelin† | ? | ? | None Known | N/A | | | | | |

Adapted from Bonner-Weir S: Anatomy of the islet of Langerhans. In Samols E (ed): The endocrine pancreas, New York, 1991, Raven Press, p 16; and Marx M, Newman JB, Guice KS, et al: Clinical significance of gastrointestinal hormones. In Thompson JC, Greeley GH Jr, Rayford PL, Townsend CM Jr (eds): Gastrointestinal endocrinology, New York, 1987, McGraw-Hill, p 416.

*CGRP,* calcitonin gene–related peptide; *PHI,* peptide histidine isoleucine; *TRH,* thyrotropin-releasing hormone.

*Gastrin is present in fetal but not in normal adult pancreatic islets.

†Broglio F, Gottero C, Benso A, et al: Ghrelin and the endocrine pancreas. Endocrine 22:19–24:2003.

clinically apparent in the form of type 1 (insulin-dependent) diabetes. Defects in the synthesis and cleavage of insulin can lead to rare forms of diabetes mellitus, such as Wakayama syndrome and proinsulin syndrome.[5]

The B cell is sensitive to even small changes in glucose concentration and is maximally stimulated at concentrations of 400 to 500 mg/dL. In response to glucose, the endocrine pancreas immediately reacts with a short burst of stored insulin (4 to 6 minutes), followed by a sustained secretion of insulin, which requires active synthesis of the hormone within the islet cell. Insulin has a 7- to 10-minute half-life and is primarily metabolized by the liver. Excess insulin is then slowly metabolized by the liver, kidneys, and skeletal muscles. Brain cells and red blood cells do not take up insulin.

Insulin binds to a specific 300-kDa glycoprotein cell surface receptor, which has been isolated and well characterized. After receptor stimulation, glucose is actively transported across cell membranes throughout the body by 55-kDa membrane-bound glucose transporters. There are several classes of glucose transporters, with varying affinities for glucose. Stimulation of the insulin receptor is dependent on insulin concentration. Insulin resistance, present in type 2 diabetes, can be the result of decreased numbers of receptors or a decreased affinity of receptors for insulin. Sulfonylurea compounds, which act independently of glucose concentration, also stimulate insulin secretion and are used in the treatment of type 2 diabetes, in which the primary defect is peripheral insulin resistance.

Orally administered glucose has a greater effect on insulin secretion than an equivalent amount of glucose administered IV, even though blood glucose levels might be the same. This effect is called the enteroinsular axis and is related to the release of enteric peptide hormones from the proximal gastrointestinal tract, which augment nutrient-induced insulin secretion. These insulinotropic factors, called incretins, act directly on the B cells and include gastric inhibitory polypeptide (GIP), glucagon, glucagon-like peptide-1, CCK, amino acids (arginine, lysine, and leucine), and free fatty acids. Humoral inhibitors of insulin secretion include somatostatin, amylin, leptin, and pancreastatin.

Insulin secretion is also under neuronal control. Vagal (cholinergic) stimulation leads to the release of insulin. Alpha-sympathetic stimulation strongly inhibits insulin release, whereas beta-sympathetic fibers stimulate it. Insulin release is stimulated by the peptidergic nerve release of gastrin-releasing peptide (GRP), CCK, gastrin, enkephalin, and VIP, whereas insulin release is inhibited by neurotensin, substance P, and somatostatin. A loss of pancreatic innervation in the setting of pancreatic transplantation or islet cell transplantation can result in changes in the pattern and quality of insulin secretion.

## Glucagon

Glucagon is a 29–amino acid, straight chain polypeptide with a molecular weight of 3.5 kDa. Secreted by the A cells, the primary function of glucagon is to elevate blood glucose levels through stimulation of glycogenolysis and gluconeogenesis in the hepatocytes. Glucagon secretion is tightly controlled by neural, hormonal, and nutrient factors. A and B cells respond primarily to serum glucose concentration, but in a reciprocal fashion. Insulin and glucagon are counterregulatory hormones and function together to maintain glucose homeostasis. Dysfunctional secretion of glucagon may play a role in the elevation of blood glucose levels in diabetes. The diabetes resulting from total pancreatectomy is very brittle and difficult to control because of the lack of endogenous glucagon to balance exogenously administered insulin. Like epinephrine, cortisol, and growth hormone, glucagon is considered a stress hormone because it increases metabolic fuel in the form of glucose during stress. Glucagon secretion is stimulated by sympathetic neural transmitters, epinephrine, and the amino acids arginine and alanine. Insulin and somatostatin have a suppressive effect on glucagon secretion.

## Somatostatin

Somatostatin, secreted by islet D cells, is a 14–amino acid polypeptide weighing 1.6 kDa. Although it is logical to think that somatostatin modulates the secretion of other islet hormones, its actual function within the pancreas remains unknown. Although exogenous administration of somatostatin has been shown to inhibit the release of insulin, glucagon, and PP, and to inhibit gastric, pancreatic, and biliary secretion, endogenous somatostatin has not been proven to influence the secretion of other islet hormones directly.

A synthetic octapeptide, octreotide, has been developed, which mimics the pharmacologic action of somatostatin. It has a longer half-life in the serum than endogenous somatostatin and is a more potent inhibitor of growth hormone, glucagon, and insulin secretion than the natural hormone. The potent inhibitory effect of octreotide has been used to treat exocrine and endocrine disorders of the pancreas, including secretory diarrhea, bowel fistulas, pancreatic fistulas, and endocrine hypersecretory syndromes.

## Pancreatic Polypeptide

PP is a 36–amino acid, 4.2-kDa polypeptide secreted by the F cells of the pancreatic islet. The physiologic role of PP remains unclear; its clinical usefulness is limited to its role as a marker for other endocrine tumors of the pancreas. Cholinergic innervation predominantly regulates PP secretion. As a result, surgical vagotomy ablates the increased PP response normally observed after meals. In diabetes and normal aging, PP secretion is increased, resulting in increased circulating PP levels. Absence of PP may play a role in the diabetes observed after total pancreatectomy or after chronic atrophic pancreatitis.

## Other Peptide Hormones

Other peptides are secreted by the pancreatic islets. These include neuropeptides such as VIP, amylin, galanin, and serotonin. VIP is a 28–amino acid, 3.3-kDa polypeptide that stimulates insulin release and inhibits gastric secretion. It is found not only throughout the gastrointestinal tract, but in the respiratory tract, where it causes vasodilation and bronchodilation. Amylin, a 36–amino acid polypeptide, is secreted by B cells and inhibits the secretion and uptake of insulin. Amylin deposits in the pancreas of patients with type 2 diabetes have been implicated in the pathogenesis of the disease. Pancreastatin is part of a larger ubiquitous molecule, chromogranin A, which inhibits insulin secretion. Gastrin-producing cells are present in the fetal pancreas, but not in the normal adult pancreas. Many additional peptides, including thyrotropin-releasing hormone, glicentin, CCK, peptide YY, GRF, calcitonin gene–related peptide, prolactin, adrenocorticotropic hormone (ACTH), parathyroid hormone–related protein, and ghrelin have been reported in normal islets and in islet cell tumors.

## SURGICAL TREATMENT OF DIABETES

### Autologous Islet Cell Transplantation

Autologous islet cell transplantation has a role in patients with severe chronic pancreatitis. Surgical resection of all or part of the pancreas for this disease can significantly improve quality of life by eradicating or reducing intractable pain, allowing the return of a normal appetite with subsequent needed weight gain, and reducing the number of hospital admissions. A major disadvantage of a total pancreatectomy, however, is that it renders the patient a brittle diabetic. Partial resections can also greatly reduce the insulin-secreting capacity of the already compromised pancreas, sometimes necessitating exogenous insulin after surgery. Regardless, even without pancreatic resection a significant number of patients with chronic pancreatitis will progress to develop diabetes or impaired glucose tolerance. Because of the loss of insulin, glucagon, and PP, the type of diabetes that develops in patients with chronic pancreatitis is similar to that following pancreatic resection.

Total or partial pancreatectomy with islet autotransplantation is being offered in several centers in the United States. This option has the potential to treat the symptoms of chronic pancreatitis definitively while preventing the onset of diabetes in certain patients. Other patients remain or become insulin-dependent but retain significant insulin and glucagon secretion and the benefits of endogenous C peptide production, thus making the resulting diabetes easier to control. Our dedicated islet isolation facility and a diagrammatic representation of the process are shown in Figure 40-3. Patients undergo pancreatectomy; the pancreatic tissue is immediately digested with the use of enzyme solutions containing collagenase and neutral proteases and the islet cells are purified. The islet cells are then returned to the patient via infusion into the portal vein. The islet cells engraft in the liver and produce insulin and C peptide and glucose levels are measured to evaluate the function of the transplanted islets.

Depending on center expertise and experience, variable results following pancreatic islet autotransplantation have been reported. Insulin independence is as high as 40% to 50% initially in some patients,[6-8] but there is a notable decline in islet function over time, with increased insulin requirements in the 10 years following transplantation, with only about 10% of patients remaining insulin-independent. Although insulin-independence is not always achieved, most patients are C peptide positive and have diabetes that is more manageable. In addition, all studies have demonstrated improvement in pain and other symptoms of chronic pancreatitis.[9,10] Success rates depend on the number of isolated and transplanted islets and transplanted islets as well as the cause of the pancreatic disease. Patients who are not diabetic before autotransplantation and younger patients (especially preadolescents) achieve the best results. The most feared procedure-related complication is thrombosis of the portal vein, occurring in less than 1% of cases.

### Immune Therapy, Pancreatic Transplantation, and Islet Allotransplantation

Type 1 diabetes results from autoimmune destruction of pancreatic islets. Immune treatment for type 1 diabetes is currently being investigated. There is a growing body of evidence to suggest that the autoimmunity observed in patients with type 1 diabetes is the result of an imbalance between autoaggressive and

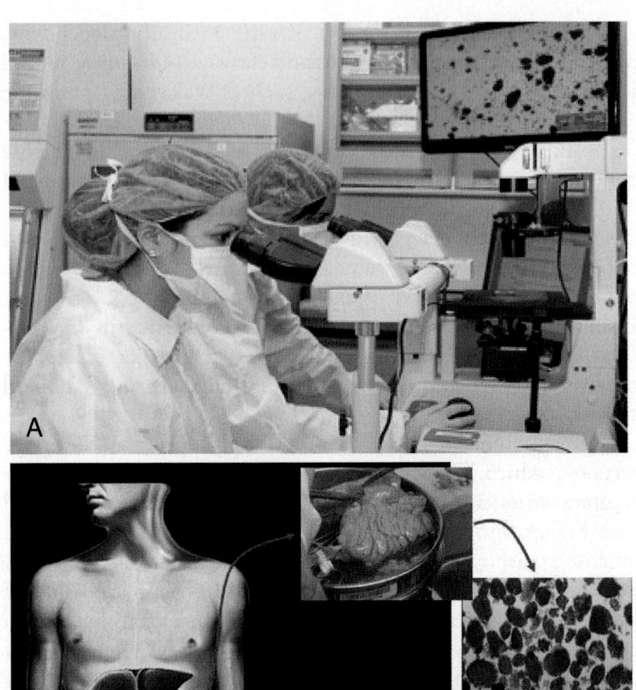


**FIGURE 40-3 A,** Dedicated islet isolation facility at our center (University of Texas Medical Branch). **B,** The screen in the upper right hand corner shows isolated islets stained red from a patient undergoing total pancreatectomy and islet autotransplantation. **C,** Pancreatic islet autotransplantation. The patient undergoes partial or total pancreatectomy. The pancreatic tissue is immediately digested with using enzyme solutions containing collagenase and neutral proteases and the islet cells are purified. The islet cells are then returned to the patient via infusion into the portal vein.

regulatory T cell subsets.[11,12] Vaccination with selected T cell receptor autoantigens has been shown to generate autoantibodies and the autoaggressive T cell clones, which are reacting to beta cells. The induction of a lasting, robust immune response generating autoantigen-specific regulatory T cells provides strong justification for further testing of this therapy for type 1 diabetes.

The current surgical treatment for type 1 diabetes is transplantation of allogeneic islet cell tissue by means of whole organ transplantation or transplantation of isolated islets, usually infused into the portal vein. Pancreatic transplantation was first performed in 1966 by Kelly and colleagues. From 1966 through 2008, over 30,000 pancreas transplantations have been reported to the International Pancreas Transplant Registry, including more than 22,000 from the United States.[13] Whole organ pancreas transplants restore euglycemia almost immediately following transplantation, and 1-year graft survival rates in the United States have improved to 85% for simultaneous pancreas-kidney transplants, 78% for pancreas after kidney transplants, and 76% for pancreas-only transplants. Recipients experience immediate normal fasting and postprandial glucose levels, and hemoglobin

A1c levels return to normal. With the observed decrease in morbidity and mortality, recipients who become insulin-independent report a better quality of life, despite the need for immunosuppression. They also experience stabilization or improvements in retinopathy, nephropathy, neuropathy, and microvascular and macrovascular diseases normally associated with poor glucose control. Therefore, for the select group of patients with labile diabetes who do not respond well to conventional approaches or insulin pumps, whole pancreas transplantation remains the gold standard for treatment.

Allogeneic islet cell transplantation is the other option. Currently, long-term insulin independence remains elusive for patients undergoing allogeneic islet transplantation. The data show that even with patients who receive multiple infusions, few remain normoglycemic over time. Data from the Collaborative Islet Transplant Registry (CITR) have demonstrated that 70% of patients achieve insulin independence within the first year (including patients with multiple infusions) but, by the third year, the percentage of patients who remain euglycemic is closer to 35%.[13a] The partial pancreatic endocrine function confers some benefit, with decreased occurrence of severe hypoglycemic events, abatement of hypoglycemic unawareness, persistent C peptide levels, improvement in glycemic control, and stabilization of diabetic complications.

Whole pancreas transplantation procedures currently outnumber islet transplantation procedures. Pancreas transplantation is associated with a higher surgical morbidity, whereas islet transplantation is a less invasive method of achieving insulin independence. However, pancreas transplantation is associated with a higher success rate. In addition, islet cell transplantation requires two donors per recipient to maintain graft function.[14] Stem cell therapy offers the potential of producing an unlimited source of cells, and a growing number of studies have demonstrated successful in vitro differentiation and expansion of embryonic cells of murine and human origin from pancreatic ducts that express insulin and respond to glucose stimulation.

## ISLET CELL TUMORS

### Overview and History

Endocrine tumors of the pancreas in the United States are rare, with an estimated incidence of 5 to 10 cases/1 million population annually. These tumors are 1000 to 2000 times more common in autopsy statistics, indicating that most are benign and nonfunctional. Endocrine tumors of the pancreas vary greatly in the mode of onset, severity of symptoms, location, functionality, and malignant potential.[15] The incidence of malignancy in these tumors varies from approximately 10% in insulinomas to almost 100% in glucagonomas and somatostatinomas (see Table 40-1). On hematoxylin and eosin–stained sections, all pancreatic endocrine tumors look similar. Malignancy is determined by the presence or absence of metastases and immunostaining allows for the identification of the endocrine content of the cells (Fig. 40-4). Over time, they may vary significantly in secretion of hormone products and biologic aggressiveness. Although the tumor syndromes are classically attributed to pancreatic islet tumors, tumors are often found in extrapancreatic locations, such as the duodenum and peripancreatic soft tissue. Almost all insulinomas, glucagonomas, and VIPomas arise from the pancreas, whereas most gastrinomas occur in the duodenum.

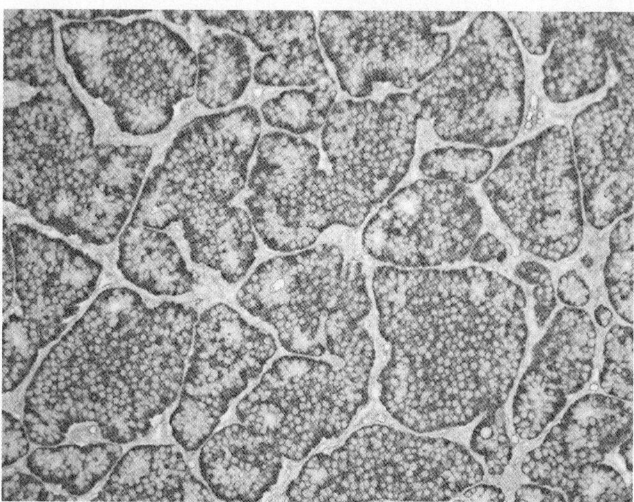

**FIGURE 40-4** Pathology of a pancreatic endocrine tumor stained positive for chromogranin, a neuroendocrine tumor marker. The chromogranin is cystoplasmic and stains brown. (Courtesy Dr. Christine Iacobuzio-Donahue, Johns Hopkins University School of Medicine, Baltimore.)

Stomatostatinomas are equally divided between the pancreas and proximal small bowel.

The morbidity from pancreatic endocrine tumors is a result of both secretion of active gastrointestinal hormones and the malignant potential. Secretion of hormones by functional tumors leads to the characteristic syndromes and physiologic derangements associated with these rare neoplasms. Although multiple hormones may be produced by a single tumor, the syndrome is recognized and named for the clinical signs and symptoms associated with the predominant endocrine agent.

In 1908, Nichols described a pancreatic adenoma consisting of islet cell tissue. In 1935, Whipple and Frantz were the first to report an association between a clinical syndrome and an islet cell tumor. They described hyperinsulinism and the associated symptoms that became known as Whipple's triad—the appearance during fasting of neuroglycopenic symptoms of hypoglycemia, low blood glucose (<45 mg/dL), and relief of symptoms by the administration of glucose. Over the next 25 years, additional syndromes associated with islet cell tumors were described. In 1942, Becker described a patient with severe dermatitis, anemia, and diabetes who also had an islet cell tumor; McGarvan later identified the cause of the syndrome as glucagon-secreting islet cell carcinoma of the pancreas. In 1955, Zollinger and Ellison described two patients with a fulminant peptic ulcer diathesis, acid hypersecretion, and non–beta islet cell tumors of the pancreas.[16] It was later determined that the secretagogue was gastrin. The first description of watery diarrhea and hypokalemia related to an islet cell tumor was by Priest and Alexander in 1957. In 1958, Verner and Morrison described two patients who died from refractory watery diarrhea and hypokalemia and an associated islet cell tumor. Later, this syndrome was clearly defined when patients with this constellation of symptoms and islet cell tumors were found to have high circulating levels of VIP. The development and refinement of sensitive radioimmunoassay techniques in 1956 allowed for the detection of micromolar concentrations of circulating peptides and greatly contributed to our understanding of these syndromes.

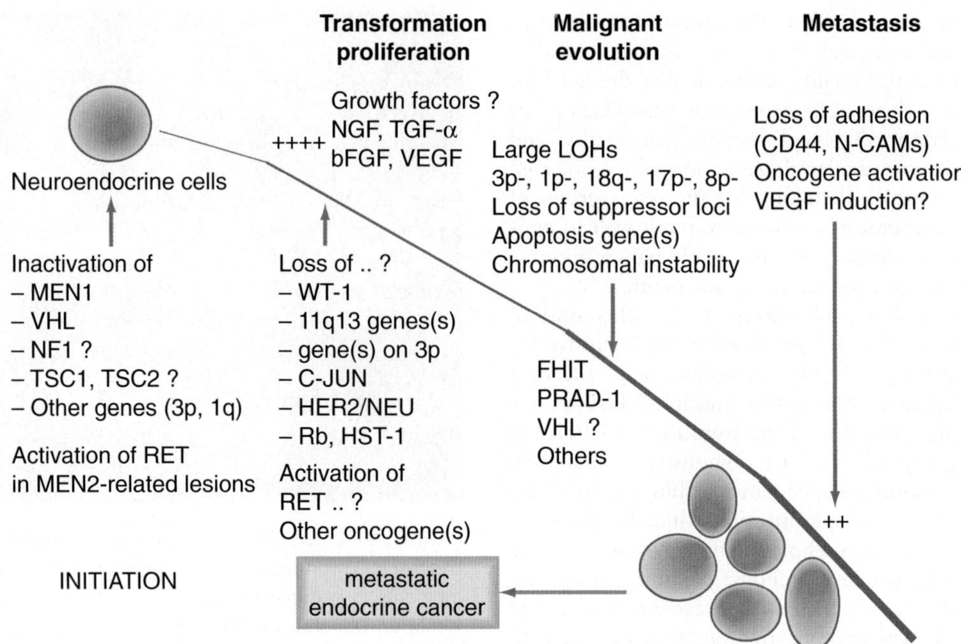


**FIGURE 40-5** Summary of the major events involved in tumor initiation, progression, and pathogenic mechanisms involved in metastasis. bFGF, Basic fibroblast growth factor; FHIT, fragile histidine triad; MEN1, multiple endocrine neoplasia type 1; NF1, neurofibromatosis type 1 (neurofibromin); NGF, nerve growth factor; PRAD-1, parathyroid adenoma–related protein; TGFα, transforming growth factor-α; TSC1, TSC2, tuberous sclerosis genes; VEGF, vasculoendothelial growth factor; VHL, von Hippel-Lindau genes. (From Calender A: Molecular genetics of neuroendocrine tumors. Digestion 62[Suppl 1]:3–18, 2000.)

## Molecular Genetics of Islet Cell Tumors

Similar to the adenoma-carcinoma sequence in colorectal cancer, tumorigenesis of islet cells and other neuroendocrine cells involves an accumulation of a number of genetic events, including activation of oncogenes and inactivation of tumor suppressor genes (Fig. 40-5). This progression is distinct from that of pancreatic adenocarcinoma. Mutations in the *k-ras, p53, dpc4, myc, fos, jun, src,* and retinoblastoma (mainly *RB1*) genes are not seen. Transcriptional silencing is believed to play a role in islet cell tumorigenesis. More than 90% of gastrinomas and nonfunctioning neuroendocrine tumors had homozygous deletions or epigenetic silencing by 5′ CpG island methylation.[17] Loss of heterozygosity (LOH) at chromosome 11q is common in functional pancreatic endocrine tumors, whereas LOH at chromosome 6q is associated with the development of nonfunctional tumors.[18] One third of patients with sporadic pancreatic endocrine tumors have allelic loss on chromosome loci *3p35, 3p27,* and *11p13,* suggesting that these loci encode tumor suppressor genes critical for the development of endocrine tumors. This allelic loss is associated with malignant clinical disease.[19] More than 90% of these tumors demonstrate silencing of the tumor suppressor gene *p16/MTS.* Evers and colleagues[20] have shown amplification of the proto-oncogene *HER-2/neu,* but not *p53* or *ras* in gastrinomas. Others have reported an increase only in aggressive tumors.[21] Studies of insulinomas have shown that the G protein $G_s$ has threefold greater expression in insulinoma when compared with normal islet cells, suggesting that it may be involved in unregulated insulin secretion or tumorigenesis. Activation of the *myc* oncogene, *TGF-α,* and *ras* genes may be early genetic events in insulinoma tumorigenesis. Loss of the sex chromosome (X in women and Y in men) has been identified in pancreatic endocrine tumors and appears to be associated with an aggressive phenotype.

Although most pancreatic endocrine tumors occur sporadically, others can be associated with genetic syndromes. The most common genetic syndrome associated with pancreatic endocrine tumors is multiple endocrine neoplasia type 1 (MEN1). The syndrome is also characterized by pancreatic endocrine tumors, parathyroid hyperplasia, and pituitary adenomas. Pancreatic endocrine tumors occur in 30% to 80% of patients with MEN1 and are the most common cause of tumor-related death in MEN1 patients. MEN1 is caused by mutations or allelic deletions in the tumor suppressor gene, *MENIN,* on chromosome 11q13 and is inherited in an autosomal dominant fashion. Mutation or allelic deletion causes loss of tumor suppressor function and predisposes patients to neoplastic growth in the parathyroid, pituitary, and pancreatic endocrine tissue. Patients with MEN1-associated pancreatic endocrine tumors tend to be younger (30 to 40 years old), more likely to have malignant disease, and more likely to have multicentric disease than patients with sporadic tumors. Approximately 50% of patients with MEN1-associated neuroendocrine tumors will present with metastatic disease.[22] Gastrinomas are the most common functional pancreatic endocrine tumors occurring in MEN1 patients (54% of functional MEN1-associated tumors). PPomas, which are not associated with a functional syndrome, occur most commonly in more than 80% of MEN1 cases.

Management of patients with MEN1 and pancreatic endocrine tumors requires recognition and staged treatment of associated tumors. Patients suspected of having MEN1 should undergo biochemical screening for gastrin, insulin and proinsulin, PP, glucagon, and chromogranin A (a tumor marker elaborated by most pancreatic endocrine tumors). Hyperparathyroidism, if present, should be treated first because correction of hypercalcemia will improve the outcome of treatment for the pancreatic endocrine tumor.

## Diagnosis

### Functional Pancreatic Endocrine Tumors

**Insulinoma** Insulinoma is the most common functioning tumor of the endocrine pancreas, with an incidence of 1/1 million population annually in the United States. The average age at diagnosis is 45 years. Despite the predominance of beta cells in the body and tail of the pancreas, 97% of insulinomas are located in the pancreas, with equal distribution in the head, body, and tail. The remaining 3% are located in the duodenum, splenic hilum, or gastrocolic ligament. Insulinomas are typically small, with an average size of 1.0 to 1.5 cm. Because of their rich vascular supply, they are hyperattenuating when compared with surrounding pancreatic tissue on contrast-enhanced computed tomography (CT) or magnetic resonance imaging (MRI; Fig. 40-6).

The diagnostic hallmark of the syndrome is the so-called Whipple's triad, namely fasting-induced neuroglyopenic symptoms of hypoglycemia (diaphoresis, shaking, mental confusion, obtundation, and seizures), low blood glucose levels (40 to 50 mg/dL), and relief of symptoms after the administration of glucose. Many patients have had symptoms for years before diagnosis. The symptom complex may vary among patients. Some have symptoms related to sympathetic nervous system overactivity in response to hypoglycemia, including fatigue, weakness, fearfulness, hunger, tremor, diaphoresis, and tachycardia. In others, a central nervous system disturbance predominates, with apathy, irritability, anxiety, confusion, excitement, loss of orientation, blurred vision, delirium, stupor, coma, and/ or seizures. Patients with insulinomas often report a significant weight gain associated with the onset of symptoms as they compensate by eating frequently to prevent hypoglycemia.

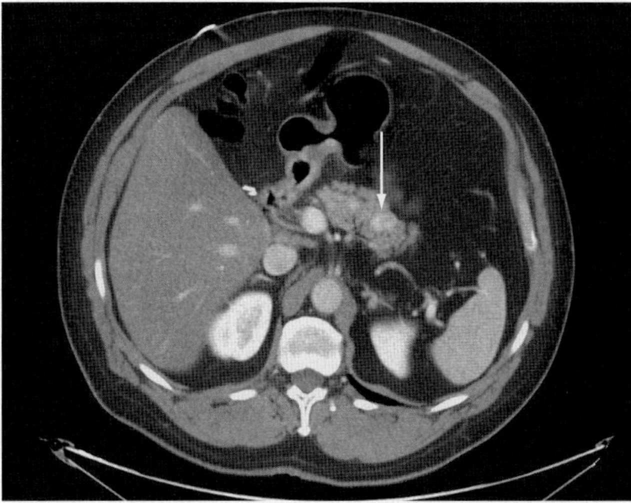

**FIGURE 40-6** Three-dimensional spiral, pancreas protocol CT scan demonstrating a hyperattenuating 1.5-cm lesion in the tail of the pancreas *(arrow)* in a patient with a 4-year history of episodic symptomatic hypoglycemia. On 72-hour monitored fast, patients demonstrated symptomatic hypoglycemia and associated high insulin and C peptide levels in 22 hours.

Whipple's triad can be emulated by other entities, including surreptitious administration of insulin or sulfonylurea compounds, rare soft tissue tumors and, occasionally, reactive hypoglycemia. The diagnosis of insulinoma is usually made with a monitored 72-hour fast. The fast is monitored for two reasons; the first is to prevent life-threatening hypoglycemia and the second is to rule out the possibility of factitious hypoglycemia as a result of exogenous insulin administration. Insulin, glucose, proinsulin, and C peptide levels are measured every 6 hours until the glucose level is lower than 60 mg/dL and then every 1 to 2 hours, or until the patient becomes symptomatic. Proinsulin, the precursor peptide to insulin is secreted by insulinomas. Similar to their normal beta cell counterparts, proinsulin is cleaved into C peptide in the Golgi complex and released into the bloodstream as functional insulin and the associated C peptide cleavage product. Exogenous insulin is already cleaved, so C peptide levels would be low in the setting of high insulin levels with surreptitious insulin administration. C peptide levels should be measured to confirm an endogenous source of insulin if there is any suspicion of hypoglycemia from surreptitious insulin injections. Urine should be checked for elevated sulfonylurea levels, suggesting surreptitious administration of oral hypoglycemia agents.

During the fast, approximately two thirds to three quarters of patients with insulinomas will experience hypoglycemic symptoms in the first 24 hours, and 95% will experience symptoms by 72 hours. An inappropriately high level of serum insulin (>5 μU/mL) in the setting of hypoglycemia is highly suggestive, but not diagnostic of insulinoma, because this may occur in hyperinsulinism from other causes. Therefore, evaluating the insulin-to-glucose ratio is also useful. A ratio higher than 0.3 occurs with insulinoma (μU/mL of insulin/[mg/dL of glucose]). Less commonly, a ratio of 0.3 can occur in the obese patient as a result of insulin resistance, but such patients should not be hypoglycemic. C peptide levels higher than 1.2 μg/mL with a glucose level lower than 40 mg/dL are also highly suggestive of an insulinoma. Provocative testing is rarely indicated to confirm the diagnosis of insulinoma and may cause dangerously profound hypoglycemia. When necessary, testing is performed in a carefully monitored setting with stimulation of insulin release using glucagon or tolbutamide and serial measurements of insulin and glucose levels.

**Gastrinoma** Gastrinomas are the second most common functional pancreatic endocrine tumor, with an incidence of 1/2.5 million population. The mean age of patients at diagnosis is 50 years and they are slightly more common in men (60%). Gastrinomas produce Zollinger-Ellison syndrome (ZES) because of islet cell tumor overproduction of gastrin, which is normally synthesized by G cells located in the antral mucosa of the stomach. The syndrome consists of hypergastrinemia, subsequent severe peptic ulceration and, often, severe diarrhea. The cell of origin is not clear, because the normal adult pancreas has no gastrin-producing cells. The gastrin produced by islet cell tumors is not subject to the normal stimulation by amino acids and peptides in the stomach or gastric distention. In addition, these tumors are not suppressed by a high luminal pH and can be stimulated (instead of inhibited) by secretin. All gastrinomas

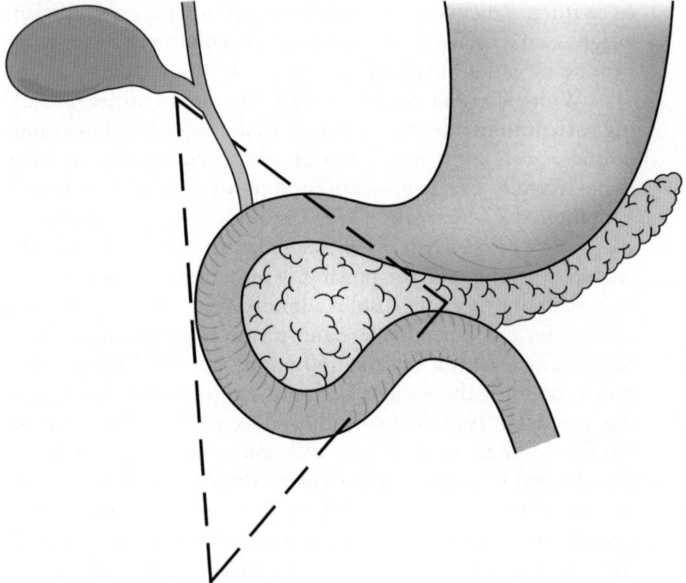

**FIGURE 40-7** Anatomic triangle in which approximately 90% of gastrinomas are found. (From Stabile BE, Morrow DJ, Passaro E Jr: The gastrinoma triangle: Operative implications. Am J Surg 147: 25–31, 1984.)

also produce chromogranin A, leading to elevated serum levels and positive immunostaining (see Fig. 40-4).

The main symptoms are those caused by peptic acid hypersecretion, with abdominal pain being the chief complaint in about 75% of patients. Almost two thirds of patients have diarrhea, and in 10% to 20% diarrhea is the only symptom. A unique characteristic of this acid-induced diarrhea is that it is halted by nasogastric aspiration of gastric secretions, a feature that separates it from all other secretory diarrheas. Most patients have peptic ulcers; duodenal ulcers are the most common, but jejunal ulceration may be found (both patients in the original report by Zollinger and Ellison had jejunal ulcers). Approximately one third of patients have signs and symptoms of gastroesophageal reflux disease, and this number appears to be increasing. Ninety percent of gastrinomas are located within the gastrinoma triangle, bounded by the lines connecting the cystic duct, the junction between the second and third portions of the duodenum, and the junction between the neck and body of the pancreas (Fig. 40-7). Gastrinomas are located in the duodenum in over 60% of patients. There is a pronounced proximal to distal gradient within the duodenum, with most arising in the first portion and none in the fourth portion.

ZES must be excluded in all patients with intractable peptic ulcers, severe esophagitis, or persistent secretory diarrhea. The diagnosis depends on the presence of hypergastrinemia in the presence of increased secretion of gastric acid. Most laboratories have an upper limit of normal of 100 pg/mL for fasting levels of gastrin. Levels of 100 to 1000 pg/mL are occasionally seen in non-ZES patients, and levels higher than 1000 pg/mL are highly suggestive of gastrinoma, provided that the patient makes gastric acid. Patients with pernicious anemia and patients on PPIs can have very high gastrin levels but make no gastric acid. All PPIs should be stopped 2 weeks prior to testing gastrin levels to diagnose ZES. An elevated serum gastrin level coupled with a pH lower than 2 in the gastric aspirate is almost diagnostic of ZES. A gastric pH higher than 3 without acid-suppressing medications or prior acid-reducing operations almost excludes ZES as the potential cause of hypergastrinemia. Other causes of hypergastrinemia, which fall into two categories—

**Table 40-2 Causes of Hypergastrinemia**

| HIGH GASTRIC ACID OUTPUT | NORMAL, LOW, OR NO GASTRIC ACID OUTPUT |
|---|---|
| ZES (gastrinoma) | $H_2$ receptor antagonist therapy |
| Gastric outlet obstruction | PPI therapy |
| G cell hyperplasia | Prior acid-reducing procedure |
| Retained gastric antrum | Atrophic gastritis, pernicious anemia, gastric cancer, vitiligo, achlorhydria, vagotomy, renal failure |

hypergastrinemia associated with high and low gastric acid output—must be excluded (Table 40-2). If the diagnosis is in doubt, the secretin provocation test is highly useful. In this test, the fasting gastrin level is measured before secretin (2 IU/kg) is administered IV, and further samples for determination of gastrin are obtained 2, 5, 10, and 20 minutes after the administration of secretin. An increase of more than 200 pg/mL in the gastrin value after administration of secretin is found in 87% of patients, with no false-positive results. False-negative results may be caused by the presence of *Helicobacter pylori.*

Once the diagnosis is established, acid secretion needs to be controlled to prevent complications and relieve symptoms. The best results are achieved with PPIs, but these often require dosing higher than that used for simple peptic ulcer or gastroesophageal reflux disease. PPIs have been shown to be safe and effective at high doses and should be given at the dosage required to decrease gastric acid output to less than 5 mEq/hr.

Gastrinomas are sporadic in 75% of patients and are associated with MEN1 in 25%. It is important to consider the diagnosis of MEN1 in patients with ZES, because 20% of patients with ZES have MEN-associated disease.[22] These patients should be tested for hyperparathyroidism which, if present, should be treated first because it can complicate the management of their gastrinoma. The average age at onset is usually 5 to 10 years earlier with MEN-associated gastrinomas. Gastrinomas in

**Table 40-3 Comparison of Clinical and Laboratory Characteristics of Patients With Gastrinoma (Benign or Malignant)**

| | Clinical Course (All Patients, %) | |
|---|---|---|
| **CHARACTERISTICS*** | **BENIGN†** | **MALIGNANT†** |
| Percentage of patients | 76 | 24 |
| Initially with liver metastases | 0 | 19 |
| Liver metastases developing later | 0 | 5 |
| Gender | Predominantly male (68) | Predominantly female (67) |
| MEM I at initial evaluation | 21 | Uncommon (6) |
| Time from onset to diagnosis | Long (mean, 5.9 yr) | Short (mean, 2.7 yr) |
| Serum gastrin level‡ | Moderately elevated (mean, 1711 pg/mL) | Very elevated (mean, 5157 pg/mL) |
| Size of primary tumor | Small (≤1 cm) | Large (>3 cm) |
| Location of primary tumor | Primarily duodenum (66) | Primarily pancreatic (92) |
| Survival at 10 yr | Excellent (96) | Poor (30) |
| Flow cytometry of tumor | Low S phase (mean, 3.3)<br>High percentage of nontetraploid aneuploid (32)<br>Multiple stem line aneuploid rare | High S phase (mean, 5.1)<br>Low percentage of nontetraploid aneuploid<br>Multiple stem line aneuploid frequent |

From Jensen RT: Gastrin-producing tumors. Cancer Treat Res 89:304, 1997.

*All characteristics were significantly different ($P < .0001$) between the two groups.

†The benign or nonaggressive course was not associated with the development of liver metastases ($n = 140$), whereas patients in whom the gastrinoma pursued a malignant or aggressive course had liver metastases at the initial evaluation ($n = 36$) or later, during follow-up ($n = 9$).

‡Normal serum gastrin level <100 pg/mL.

MEN1 patients are more likely to occur in the duodenum and are more likely to be multiple, complicating their management.[23-25] The most common pancreatic endocrine syndrome seen in MEN1 patients is gastrinoma (54%), followed by insulinoma (21%), glucagonoma (3%), and VIPoma (1%). Nonfunctioning PPomas are seen in 80% of patients with MEN1. Of MEN1 patients, 60% to 80% have duodenal gastrinomas, which are metastatic to the lymph nodes in 85% at presentation. They tend not to metastasize to the liver, whereas sporadic tumors larger than 3 cm tend to do so.

It is believed that gastrinoma may take an aggressive or relatively benign clinical course (Table 40-3). The aggressive form, seen in about 25% of all patients, is more frequent in women and those with MEN1 syndrome. The aggressive form is associated with larger pancreatic tumors, liver metastases, and worse long-term survival; 90% of aggressive tumors are located in the pancreas. Their 10-year survival rate of 30% is in stark contrast to the 96% survival observed in patients with the nonaggressive form. The salient factors influencing prognosis in these aggressive tumors include liver metastases, incomplete resection, and DNA flow cytometry showing a high index of aneuploidy.[26]

**VIPomas** VIP is a small peptide normally found in the brain, G cells of the antrum, adrenal medulla, gut mucosa, pancreatic neurons, and $D_2$ cells of the pancreas. VIPomas usually arise from pancreatic islet $D_2$ cells and release high levels of VIP, producing the Verner-Morrison syndrome. This syndrome is also known as WDHA syndrome (***w***atery ***d***iarrhea, ***h***ypokalemia, ***a***chlorhydria) or pancreatic cholera. Overall, these tumors are exceedingly rare, with an incidence of 1/10 million population. Most patients are diagnosed with VIPomas at middle age but approximately 10% of patients are diagnosed before the age of 10 years. Elevated VIP levels in these young patients are most commonly caused by ganglioneuromas, ganglioblastomas, or neuroblastomas, instead of pancreatic tumors. More than two thirds are malignant (see Table 40-1) and at the time of presentation more than 70% of patients have metastatic disease. Ninety percent of lesions are found in the pancreas and 10% have been described in the colon, bronchus, liver, adrenal gland, and sympathetic ganglia. Tumors are generally solitary and are usually diagnosed when larger than 3 cm. VIPomas are found in the pancreatic body and tail in 75% of patients. Approximately 10% of patients with VIPomas have MEN1.

Superphysiologic levels of VIP cause the symptoms associated with Verner-Morrison syndrome. The diagnostic triad in Verner-Morrison syndrome is a secretory diarrhea, high levels of circulating VIP, and a pancreatic tumor. Profuse, watery, iso-osmotic secretory diarrhea is the most common presenting symptom and may exceed a volume of 3 to 5 liters/day. The diagnosis of VIPoma is unlikely if the stool volume is less than 700 mL/day. VIP acts directly on intestinal epithelial cells to activate adenylate cyclase, thus increasing cyclic adenosine monophosphate (cAMP) levels within colonocytes, which stimulates the hypersecretion of fluid into the lumen, resulting in watery diarrhea. The diarrhea is further exacerbated because cAMP inhibits sodium reabsorption and stimulates chloride secretion, causing increased fluid and electrolyte shifts into the intestinal lumen. The diarrhea persists despite fasting, which qualifies it as a secretory diarrhea and, despite nasogastric aspiration, which differentiates it from the diarrhea of ZES. Conditions to be considered in the differential diagnosis are laxative abuse, bacterial and parasitic diarrhea, carcinoid syndrome, which has an elevated level of 5-hydroxyindoleacetic acid in urine, and ZES, which has an elevated serum gastrin level. Of these, VIPomas alone show elevated levels of VIP; normal levels are lower than 200 pg/mL and VIPoma patients have levels ranging from 225 to

2000 pg/mL. Levels of VIP should be measured after an overnight fast.

Weight loss, crampy abdominal pain, dehydration, electrolyte abnormalities, and metabolic acidosis (from fluid and bicarbonate loss) are common with Verner-Morrison syndrome. Hypokalemia may be profound because patients can lose more than 400 mEq of potassium/day, which may lead to disturbances of cardiac rhythm and even sudden death in extreme cases. Almost 75% of patients have hypochlorhydria or achlorhydria and decreased levels of magnesium and phosphorus are often present. The profound electrolyte abnormalities and dehydration need to be corrected prior to definitive surgical management.

**Glucagonomas** Glucagonomas are exceedingly rare, with an estimated incidence of 1/20 million population.[27] They are two- to threefold more common in women. Compared with other pancreatic endocrine tumors, they tend to be larger, averaging 5 to 10 cm in size at the time of diagnosis. These tumors almost always arise in the pancreas and 65% to 75% are found in the body or tail, corresponding to the normal distribution of alpha cells in the pancreas. Glucagonomas are malignant in 50% of cases; 80% of patients with malignant glucagonomas have liver metastases at the time of diagnosis. Most glucagonomas are sporadic; however, 5% to 17% are associated with MEN1. As with other pancreatic endocrine tumors, patients with MEN1-associated glucagonomas tend to be younger and have more advanced disease at the time of diagnosis.

The glucagonoma syndrome is a rare syndrome, with a classic presentation of the 4Ds: diabetes, dermatitis, deep vein thrombosis, and depression. It is also characterized by a severe catabolic state with weight loss, depletion of fat and protein stores, and associated vitamin deficiencies. The syndrome was first described in 1942 by dermatologists who noted the relationship between pancreatic tumor and severe unrelenting dermatitis. The characteristic skin lesion, a necrolytic migrating erythema (Fig. 40-8), is noted in approximately two thirds of patients and often appears before other symptoms of the syndrome. The cause is believed to be severe amino acid deficiency, although trace element deficiency and general malnutrition probably contribute. Parenteral administration of amino acids was found to result in the disappearance of the skin lesions.[28] The catabolic state induced by unregulated, hypersecretion of glucagon causes hyperglycemia, depletion of the circulating pool of amino acids, and depletion of fat stores. Diabetes develops in 76% to 94% of patients with glucagonoma at some point during their illness, but is usually mild. The diagnosis of glucagonoma is established by measuring glucagon levels; a fasting glucagon level higher than 50 pmol/L is considered diagnostic.

**Somatostatinomas** Somatostatinomas are exceedingly rare, with fewer than 100 cases reported in the literature. The tumor was first described in 1977 in two separate reports. The full syndrome of steatorrhea, diabetes mellitus, hypochlorhydria, and gallstones was characterized in 1979.[29] Inhibition of pancreatic enzyme and hormone secretion by unregulated hypersecretion of somatostatin causes steatorrhea, diabetes, malabsorption, and cholelithiasis caused by reduced gallbladder emptying.[29] Because the symptoms are nonspecific, the diagnosis of somatostatinoma is rarely made preoperatively. When suspected, the diagnosis can be confirmed by documenting an elevated fasting somatostatin level higher than 14 mol/liter.

Somatostatinomas are usually solitary and 85% are larger than 2 cm. More than 60% are found in the pancreas, usually the head, with the remainder in the duodenum or elsewhere in the small intestine. Patients are typically 50 to 60 years old at the time of diagnosis. Ninety percent are malignant, with metastases to the liver or lymph nodes commonly noted at the time of diagnosis.[30] Somatostatinomas are rarely associated with MEN1 but are associated with von Recklinghausen's disease and pheochromocytomas.

**Other Functional Pancreatic Endocrine Tumors** Pancreatic endocrine tumors that produce other hormones have been described, but are extremely rare. There have been case reports of pancreatic endocrine tumors that secrete gastrin-releasing factor (GRF), parathyroid hormone–related peptide (PTHrP), PP, ACTH, calcitonin, enteroglucagon, CCK, gastric inhibitory peptide,

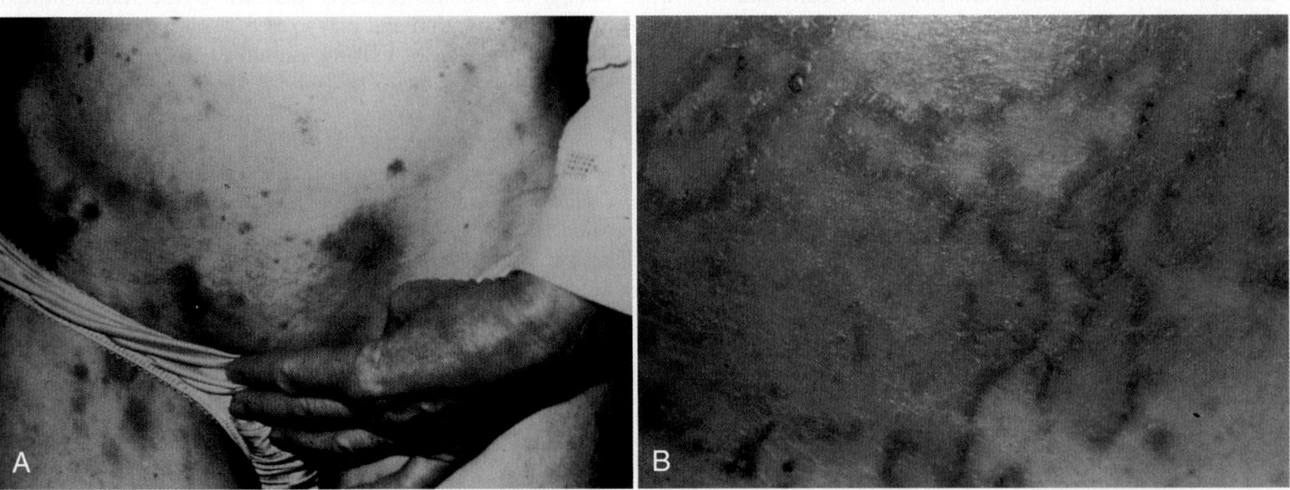


**FIGURE 40-8** Characteristic necrolytic migrating erythematous dermatitis of the glucagonoma syndrome. **A,** Confluent patches with superficial necrosis. **B,** Close-up showing serpiginous margins. (Courtesy Dr. Hugo V. Villar.)

luteinizing hormone, neurotensin, or ghrelin have also been described. GRFomas are invariably associated with MEN1 and only 30% arise in the pancreas. Patients with ACTH-secreting tumors have Cushing's syndrome and usually have other endocrine syndromes, most commonly ZES. Usually malignant, neurotensinomas cause hypokalemia, weight loss, hypotension, cyanosis, flushing, and diabetes. PPomas are associated with high circulating levels of PP, but no associated clinical syndrome. Unless associated with MEN1, they are large and solitary. In addition, elevated PP levels are often seen in other endocrine tumor syndromes. PP, neurotensin, and calcitonin-secreting tumors are sometimes classified as nonfunctional because the hormone products have little biologic consequence and rarely cause symptoms.

### Nonfunctional Neuroendocrine Tumors

Of pancreatic endocrine tumors, 20% are nonfunctional, defined as a pancreatic tumor of endocrine origin, with no definable hormonal syndrome. Patients with nonfunctioning islet tumors are late in seeking help and finally do so because of symptoms of tumor progression. At presentation, most tumors are malignant and have metastasized by the time of diagnosis. On microscopic examination, nonfunctional tumors do not appear different than their functional counterparts; the endocrine origin of these tumors is usually identified by positive immunostaining for chromogranin A or synaptophysin.

Two thirds of nonfunctional pancreatic endocrine tumors are malignant and 60% to 80% of malignant tumors have metastasized to distant sites at the time of diagnosis. These tumors are typically larger than their functional counterparts (4 to 5 cm versus 1 to 2 cm, respectively) when initially discovered. Patients may present with abdominal pain and jaundice secondary to compression of adjacent structures. This is particularly common with PPomas that occur predominantly within the head of the pancreas.

## Imaging and Localization

### Imaging Modalities

Once the diagnosis of a functional pancreatic endocrine tumor is made, cross-sectional imaging with CT or MRI is the first step in localization. The sensitivity of dual-phase CT in the localization of functioning islet cell tumors is 71% to 82%[31] and is directly related to the size of the tumor. The vast majority of noninsulinoma or nongastrinoma pancreatic endocrine tumors will be identified on cross-sectional imaging. Insulinomas and gastrinomas, which are smaller at presentation, are more difficult to localize. As a result, CT technique, including thinner collimation (1.25-mm cuts) and multiple-phase imaging, is critical to improving sensitivity of CT for these small lesions. Capturing the vascular blush in the arterial phase is critical for identification and differentiation from other types of pancreatic tumors (see Fig. 40-6), which is less pronounced in the venous phase. In addition, the use of water instead of oral contrast may assist in identifying small duodenal gastrinomas.[32]

The ability of MRI to demonstrate contrast between normal pancreatic parenchyma and small pancreatic endocrine tumors make this modality a useful primary technique for localization. As with CT, size is directly related to sensitivity. Pancreatic endocrine tumors demonstrate low-signal intensity on T1-weighted images and high-signal intensity on T2-weighted images. In one large series of insulinomas, contrast-enhanced MRI identified all lesions larger than 3 cm, 50% of lesions 1 to 2 cm, and no lesions smaller than 1 cm.[33] The overall sensitivity of MRI for detecting pancreatic endocrine tumors is 85%.[34]

If unable to localize a pancreatic endocrine tumor on CT or MRI, endoscopic ultrasound (EUS) should be performed. EUS has an overall sensitivity of 93% for tumors of all sizes.[35,36] This modality has a greater sensitivity when compared with CT and MRI for detecting tumors smaller than 3 cm. Similar to CT and MRI, however, EUS has a limited ability to detect small duodenal tumors, with a sensitivity of only 50% in this setting. EUS also allows for fine-needle aspiration (FNA) of tumors for a pathologic diagnosis. This is especially useful for nonfunctional tumors without a classic CT appearance of pancreatic endocrine tumors. An FNA confirming a diagnosis of pancreatic endocrine tumor will dictate an aggressive approach, given the good prognosis of advanced pancreatic endocrine tumors relative to pancreatic adenocarcinoma.

Another useful modality is somatostatin receptor scintigraphy (SRS). In this technique, 6 mCi of $^{111}$In-labeled octreotide is given IV. Body images are obtained with a gamma camera at 4 and 24 hours. The abundance of somatostatin receptors on certain types (but not all) of pancreatic endocrine tumors makes SRS a useful adjunct in localization, if tumors are not evident on CT or MRI. Somatostatin receptors are present in more than 90% of gastrinomas; in contrast, pancreatic adenocarcinomas do not possess somatostatin receptors. They are also present in a significant portion of glucagonomas and nonfunctioning endocrine tumors. The sensitivity for SRS is over 80% for all pancreatic endocrine tumors excluding insulinomas; it has an overall sensitivity of 80% to 100% and specificity higher than 90% for gastrinomas. This technique is also useful for detecting hepatic metastases from noninsulinoma endocrine tumors (Fig. 40-9). Although sensitive, SRS may not show the exact location of a tumor but only indicates its general vicinity within a few centimeters.

For small insulinomas and gastrinomas that have not been identified with CT, MRI, SRS (gastrinomas only), or EUS, angiographic techniques may be useful. Angiography will detect approximately 70% of insulinomas larger than 5 mm, showing a characteristic vascular blush that corresponds to the highly vascular nature of insulinomas (Fig. 40-10). If standard radiographic techniques are unsuccessful, portal venous sampling for insulin or gastrin levels, with or without arterial stimulation with calcium or secretin injection, may allow localization to a region of the pancreas (head, body, or tail) to aid in operative planning (Fig. 40-11). This technique does not absolutely localize the tumor, but provides accurate information on the region of the pancreas from which the high levels of hormones are released. Arterial stimulation by injecting calcium or secretin into the celiac and superior mesenteric arteries can further increase the likelihood of localization with simultaneous portal venous sampling for appropriate hormone levels. Calcium stimulates insulin release from insulinomas, whereas secretin stimulates gastrin release from gastrinomas. Arterial stimulation venous sampling has a sensitivity higher than 90%.[37,38]

In the unlikely event that preoperative studies cannot localize the tumor, blind exploration with intraoperative ultrasound, combined with careful palpation and exploration of the entire pancreas and duodenum, will identify most tumors. Carrying

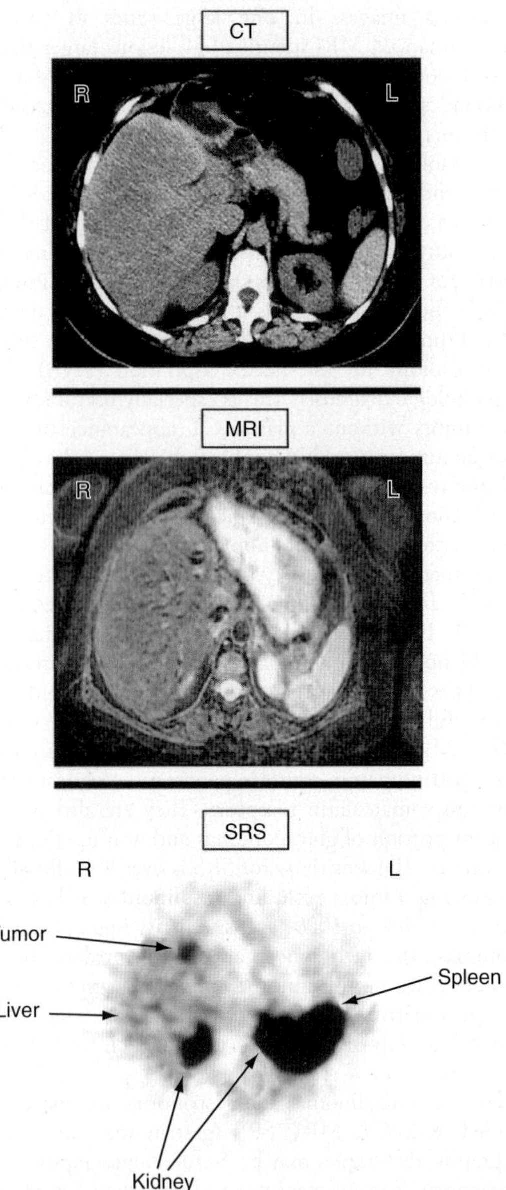


**FIGURE 40-9** Comparison of CT, MRI, and SRS in a patient with Zollinger-Ellison syndrome. Neither the CT scan *(top)* nor MRI *(middle)* localized a gastrinoma. SRS, however, showed a focus in the left lobe of the liver. At surgery, the patient had two 1-cm left lobe liver metastases and a small duodenal tumor (0.3-cm gastrinoma plus an adjacent lymph node). This result demonstrates the enhanced sensitivity of SRS but also shows that it frequently misses small tumors. (From Norton JA, Jensen RT: Resolved and unresolved controversies in the surgical management of patients with Zollinger-Ellison syndrome. Ann Surg 240;757–773, 2004.)

out effective intraoperative pancreatic ultrasound requires complete mobilization of the pancreas. Duodenal gastrinomas are usually difficult to localize preoperatively by any technique because of their small size. Small duodenal tumors may be seen in the operating room using intraoperative esophagogastroduodenoscopy. This transilluminates the duodenal wall and allow for the visualization of small submucosal tumors.

### Localization

**Insulinoma** After the biochemical diagnosis of insulinoma (Fig. 40-12) is made, CT or MRI should be performed. If the tumor is localized, the surgeon proceeds to resection. If not, EUS should be performed. If the tumor remains unlocalized, angiography with or without stimulation should be performed. Only in the event of all of the above being negative should blind exploration and intraoperative ultrasound be performed. SRS is not useful for insulinomas.

**Gastrinoma** For patients with biochemically confirmed ZES, the first step of the algorithm for localizing a gastrinoma (see Fig. 40-12) should include CT. If CT fails to localize the tumor, SRS should be performed because almost all gastrinomas express somatostatin receptors. If not localized, EUS and/or MRI should be used to evaluate for small pancreatic lesions. If localization has still not been accomplished, angiography with or without stimulation should be performed next. If not found by other techniques, it may be reasonable to proceed with operative exploration to localize definitively and treat the tumor at the same operation.

**Other Endocrine Tumors** VIPomas, glucagonomas, and somatostatinomas are usually larger and easily localized by CT. SRS can be performed if CT is not informative. Most nonfunctional neuroendocrine tumors are diagnosed initially by CT based on symptoms of abdominal pain or jaundice.

## Treatment

The treatment of endocrine tumors is surgical, performed by open or laparoscopic approaches. In most cases, a partial pancreatic resection is performed, such as pancreatic head resection, distal pancreatic resection, or enucleation. In open procedures, the incision is dictated by operator preference, either a midline incision from the xiphoid to below the umbilicus or a bilateral subcostal incision. The entire abdomen must be explored, with particular attention paid to possible liver metastases. If the tumor is not localized preoperatively, the entire pancreas needs to be mobilized. This is done by dividing the gastrocolic ligament from left to right, incising the posterior lining of the lesser sac along the inferior and superior margins of the pancreas, and mobilizing the C loop of the duodenum medially with an extensive Kocher maneuver. The head of the pancreas is palpated carefully and examined anteriorly and posteriorly; the body and tail of the pancreas are palpated, any ligamentous attachments to the spleen are divided, the spleen is delivered into the wound, and the tail is rotated anteriorly to allow palpation and visualization.

Several groups of surgeons have shown the applicability of laparoscopy to endocrine pancreatic tumors, especially insulinomas and nonfunctioning adenomas. The technique is particularly applicable to small solitary benign islet tumors in the body and tail. As with open resection, the most common complication is pancreatic fistula, most often seen after enucleation. The use of laparoscopic ultrasound is vital and allows for the selection of the most efficient resection technique.

Intraoperative ultrasonography is essential for islet cell tumors, especially insulinomas and gastrinomas, that cannot be localized preoperatively. Higher resolution (7.5- to 10-MHz) transducers are used for the pancreas; because of its greater depth of penetration, a 5-MHz transducer is better for the liver. Islet

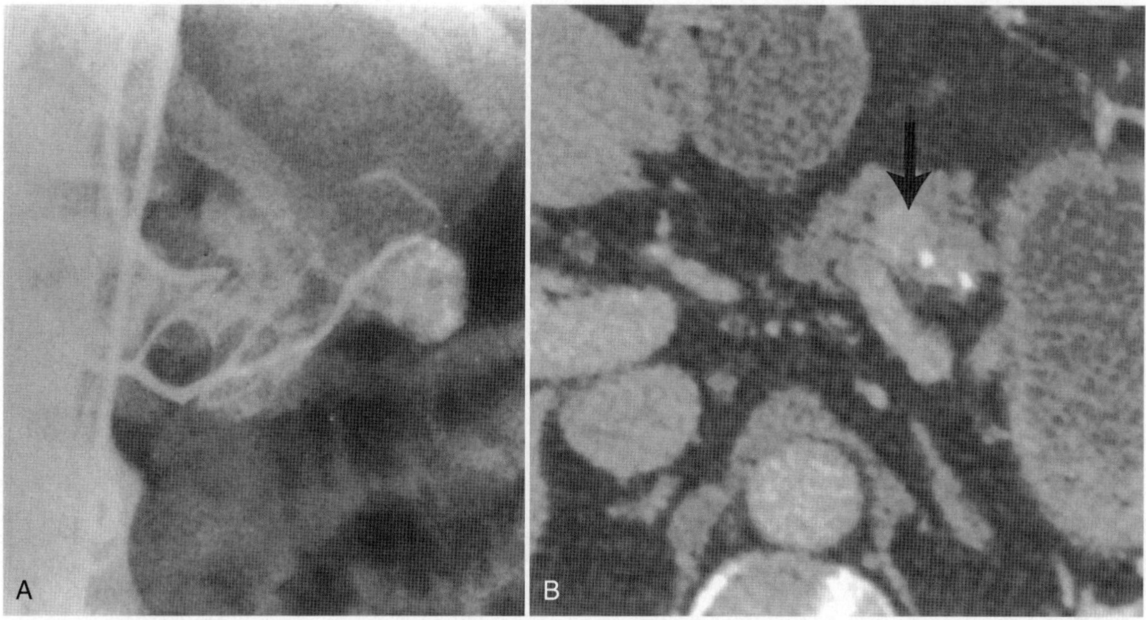


**FIGURE 40-10** Arteriographic demonstration of an insulinoma. **A,** Selective injection into the specific dorsal pancreatic artery demonstrates the tumor precisely. **B,** Insulinoma with triphasic enhancement on CT. The mass in the pancreatic body (*arrow*) demonstrates early and prolonged enhancement with washout during the portal venous phase; note that the maximal difference in enhancement between the tumor and normal pancreas occurs during the pancreatic phase (shown). (**A** from Edis AJ, McIlrath DC, Ven Heerden JA, et al: Insulinoma: Current diagnosis and surgical management. Curr Prob Surg 13:1–45, 1976; **B** from Ros PR, Mortelé KJ: Imaging features of pancreatic neoplasms. JBR-BTR 84:239–249, 2001.)

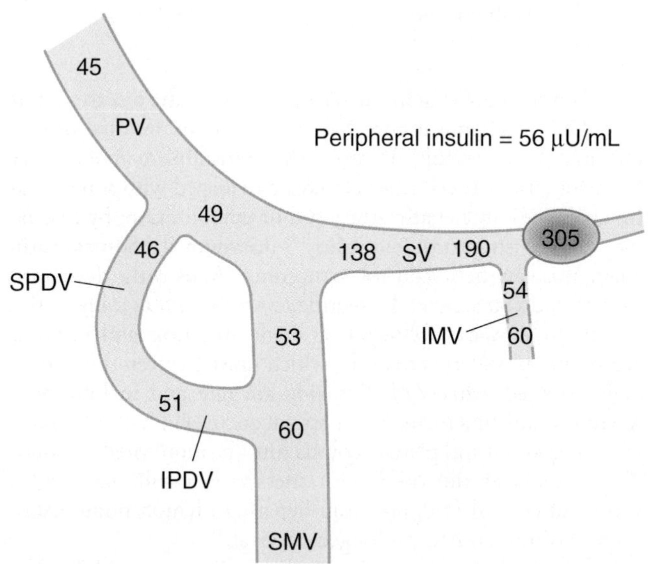


**FIGURE 40-11** Transhepatic selective venous sampling of the portal vein and its tributaries for insulin. Venous insulin levels are greatly elevated in the distal splenic vein *(shaded circle).* Intraoperative ultrasound and palpation of the pancreas failed to reveal an insulinoma. Distal pancreatectomy was performed on the basis of the portovenous sampling gradient shown here, and the pathologists confirmed the presence of a 1-cm insulinoma. IMV, Inferior mesenteric vein; IPDV, inferior pancreaticoduodenal vein; PV, portal vein; SMV, superior mesenteric vein; SPDV, superior pancreaticoduodenal vein; SV, splenic vein. Insulin concentrations are given in μU/mL. (From Norton JA, Shawker TH, Doppman JL, et al: Localization and surgical treatment of occult insulinomas. Ann Surg 212:615–620, 1990.)

tumors are detected as sonolucent masses, generally of uniform consistency. Several reports have attested to the high degree of accuracy of intraoperative ultrasound. The color Doppler attachment allows the detection of adjacent vessels and aids in identification of the pancreatic ductal system, which shows up as a lucent tube without flow. Identification of the ductal system is useful to prevent pancreatic fistula formation.

### Insulinoma

Surgical resection is the mainstay of treatment and is the only curative option for insulinoma. After localization, surgical resection of insulinoma is usually curative because most tumors tend to be small, benign, and solitary. Preoperatively, it is important to prevent severe hypoglycemic attacks. Glucose infusions must be used in the perioperative period, especially when patients are taking nothing by mouth. Administration of diazoxide decreases beta cell release of insulin (usually 3 mg/kg/day, divided into two or three daily doses) and should be used to prevent or attenuate symptoms of hypoglycemia prior to surgical intervention once the diagnosis is made.

Once a tumor has been identified intraoperatively, the location should correlate with preoperative localization studies. If not, multiple lesions need to be considered. Because more than 90% of insulinomas are benign, enucleation is usually preferred, when possible, to preserve functional pancreatic mass. Enucleation should not be performed if the tumor is within 2 mm of the main pancreatic duct, which can be identified on intraoperative ultrasound. In all enucleations, careful dissection is necessary to avoid entry into the main pancreatic duct. Resection via distal pancreatectomy, central pancreatectomy, or pancreaticoduodenectomy may be necessary for tumors abutting the main pancreatic duct or for large tumors. Many surgeons advocate

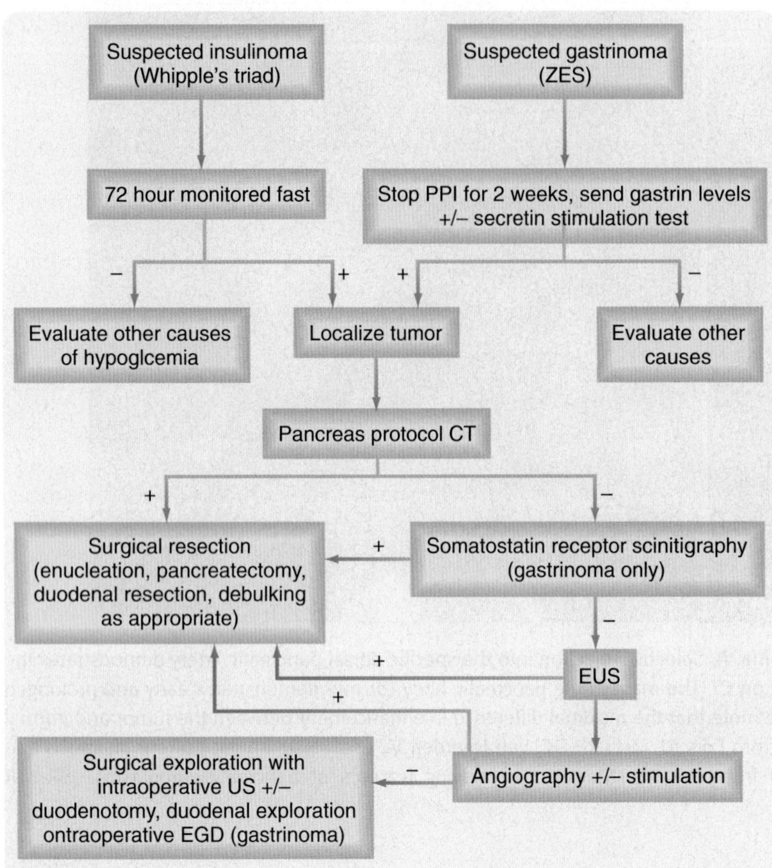


**FIGURE 40-12** Algorithm for biochemical evaluation, localization, and management of insulinomas and gastrinomas.

placement of a Silastic drain adjacent to the enucleation site to control any leak of pancreatic secretions postoperatively. Insulinomas are well suited for laparoscopic resection or enucleations. More extensive pancreatic resections for malignant tumors are best resected through an open approach. In the rare case in which the tumor cannot be localized with preoperative or intraoperative techniques, blind resection of any part of the pancreas is not recommended.

When no tumor can be identified, biopsies should be taken from the pancreatic tail to evaluate for nesidioblastosis. A revival of interest in adult nesidioblastosis has suggested a noninsulinoma pancreatogenous hypoglycemia syndrome.[39] These rare cases appear to resemble nesidioblastosis in neonates. The number of confirmed cases is low but, rarely, surgeons may need to consider empirical distal pancreatectomy.

Life expectancy should be normal after the complete excision of a benign insulinoma. More extensive resections are required for complete excision of malignant insulinomas and for patients with MEN1 or multifocal disease. The 10% of patients with hyperinsulinism who have MEN1 syndrome have multiple islet tumors, one of which is usually dominant and responsible for the excessive insulin output. These are probably best managed by resecting the area of the pancreas that shows the highest insulin output on selective portovenous sampling or selective intra-arterial calcium challenge. However, MEN1 patients may require a combination of partial pancreatic resection—distal pancreatectomy or pancreaticoduodenectomy—and enucleation for multiple lesions in the pancreas. In general, total pancreatectomy is not indicated for insulinoma.

Tumor debulking in the setting of metastatic disease results in a 95% biochemical cure rate because some residual disease may not be functional.[40] Persistent hyperinsulinism after surgery for metastatic islet cell tumors may be managed with somatostatin analogues, by hepatic artery tumor embolization, by diazoxide, or by streptozotocin plus 5-fluorouracil. Somatostatin analogues can help control symptoms. A recently developed somatostatin analogue, lanreotide, remains biologically active for up to 2 weeks following a single injection and controls symptoms as well as octreotide, which must be given three times daily. The side effects of diazoxide are rare and include fluid retention and hirsutism. With streptozocin and 5-fluorouracil, white blood cell and platelet counts must be monitored carefully. Ten patients at the NIH with metastatic insulinoma had a variety of clinical findings, from hepatic to lymph node metastases; 9 of the 10 had prolonged survival.[41]

Even with metastatic disease, the median survival following resection is approximately 5 years. Streptozotocin, with or without 5-fluorouracil, is associated with improved survival in metastatic pancreatic endocrine tumors.

### Gastrinoma

Although gastrinomas have a high rate of malignancy, they are more likely to be cured than cancer of any other abdominal viscera. Operative treatment of gastrinomas is indicated when curative resection appears possible based on preoperative imaging or for palliative cytoreduction for symptom control. The presence or absence of malignant disease is the most important prognostic indicator. The goals of surgery are twofold, potentially curative resection of the primary tumor and prevention of malignant progression.

Every attempt is made to localize the tumor before surgery (see earlier). Gastric secretion is controlled during the perioperative period with oral or parenteral PPIs. If not localized preoperatively, finding tumors in the pancreas may be difficult, but finding duodenal tumors is more difficult. Exploration includes the entire abdomen, from the undersurface of the diaphragm to the pelvic floor, with particular attention paid to the liver, right subhepatic and paraduodenal area, and pelvic cul-de-sac and ovaries. The entire small bowel and colon are examined carefully, with the surgeon looking for lymph nodes in the mesentery or attached to the wall of the bowel. The entire pancreas should be mobilized to allow for thorough palpation and intraoperative ultrasound. The surgeon should carefully inspect the gastrinoma triangle (see Fig. 40-7) to confirm the location of the tumor. Intraoperative ultrasound should be routinely performed to identify small pancreatic lesions or liver metastases. Transillumination of the duodenum with intraoperative endoscopy may help identify small submucosal lesions. After transillumination of the duodenum with intraoperative endoscopy, the duodenal wall can be gently palpated between the surgeon's fingers through a 3-cm duodenotomy on the anterolateral surface of the second portion of the duodenum, allowing for the detection of gastrinomas smaller than 1 cm. Duodenotomy will detect 25% to 30% of tumors not seen on preoperative imaging.

We have found small primary gastrinomas free in the small bowel mesentery, adjacent to the duodenum, in the wall of the stomach, above the confluence of the right and left hepatic ducts, and as a cystic tumor attached to the lesser curvature of the stomach. Gastrinomas have been reported in the ovary and colon. Any suspicious nodules are excised and sent for frozen section biopsy.

Enucleation of gastrinomas should be reserved for small well-encapsulated tumors in the pancreas. Large unencapsulated lesions deep within the gland may require segmental resection, including distal pancreatectomy or pancreaticoduodenectomy. Pancreaticoduodenectomy may increase disease-free survival in patients with MEN1 because, following local excision, recurrent tumors are most commonly found in the duodenum.[22,42,43] In 5% to 8% of cases, the surgeon is unable to localize a gastrinoma intraoperatively.[44] In this case, blind pancreatic resection is not indicated. Detailed inspection of peripancreatic, periduodenal, and portohepatic lymph nodes should be performed because resection of grossly positive lymphatic spread may increase disease-free survival. Unfortunately, with long follow-up, almost 50% of patients initially free of disease show symptomatic or biochemical (i.e., a positive secretin test result) recurrence by 5 years.

More than 50% of patients with gastrinomas have metastatic disease at the time of diagnosis. Treatment of metastatic disease has undergone serial changes but is still unsatisfactory. Radiation therapy and chemotherapy are largely ineffective. The combination of doxorubicin, streptozotocin, and 5-fluorouracil has a low, temporary response rate, but is highly toxic and has no impact on survival. Chemoembolization or radiofrequency ablation of hepatic metastases may be effective in reducing tumor burden within the liver. Similarly, octreotide and interferon-$\alpha$ are associated with few temporary and partial responses. Surgical treatment of distant metastases by debulking appears to be useful, and some patients with solitary localized metastatic disease have prolonged postoperative disease-free survival.

For patients with unresectable, symptomatic metastatic disease, treatment should focus on symptom control (i.e., reduction of acid production). Pharmacologic control of acid secretion with PPIs has rendered total gastrectomy and other surgical acid-reducing procedures unnecessary. Symptoms are controlled in more than 90% of patients, starting with dosages of 60 to 80 mg pantoprazole daily, although higher dosages may be required. Efficacy can be demonstrated by measuring basal acid output (BAO); PPI dosage should be titrated to keep BAO lower than 10 mEq/hr (or <5 mEq/hr if the patient had a prior acid-reducing procedure). One of the few remaining indications for total gastrectomy in patients with ZES is the presence of gastric carcinoid tumors, which may arise from prolonged hypergastrinemia. However, gastric carcinoids occur in fewer than 10% of patients with MEN1 and ZES; thus, gastrectomy is rarely required. Gastrectomy may also be indicated for patients who are unable to tolerate PPIs and cannot achieve acid secretion control through other means. Total gastrectomy cures all symptoms produced by excessive acid but has no effect on survival for metastatic disease. Octreotide, used to decrease gastrin release and subsequent acid secretion, is rarely effective without concurrent PPI use.

The role of routine surgical exploration for resection or cure in patients with ZES has been controversial since the original description of this disease in 1955, especially because medical therapy of acid hypersecretion is so effective. In a report of 151 patients operated on between 1981 and 1998, 123 of whom had sporadic gastrinomas and 28 had ZES-MEN1, the overall 10-year survival rate was 94%; 34% of patients with sporadic gastrinomas were free of disease at 10 years, whereas none of the ZES-MEN1 patients were free of disease.[45] A later study by the same group compared outcomes in 35 nonsurgical patients and 160 patients who underwent resection. The two groups did not differ in clinical, laboratory, or tumor imaging results. At surgery, 94% had a tumor removed, 51% were cured immediately, and 41% were cured at last follow-up. Significantly more nonsurgical patients developed liver metastases (29% versus 5%), died of any cause (54 versus 21%), or died a disease-related death (23% versus 1%). Disease-specific survival at 15 years was 98% for operated and 74% for unoperated patients. The conclusion from these and other studies is that all patients with the sporadic form of ZES, without metastatic disease, need to be offered surgical exploration. The role of surgery in patients with MEN-associated ZES remains less clear.

The best predictor of survival for patients with gastrinoma is the presence of liver metastases, whereas lymph node metastases are not predictive.[46] Patients with bulky metastatic disease have a 5-year survival lower than 50%, whereas 90% of patients without metastases are alive after 5 years. Resection of all gross disease and metastases may provide palliation of symptoms and may prolong survival. Norton and colleagues[15] have reported 5-year survival rates of almost 100% for patient without liver metastases. Patients who had no synchronous liver lesions but developed them metachronously had a 5-year survival of almost 100% and a 10-year survival rate of 80%. Finally, patients presenting with synchronous liver metastases had a 5-year survival rate of approximately 45%. Aggressive surgical therapy is indicated, because patients have been known to live more than 20 years with residual disease.

### Other Functional and Nonfunctional Endocrine Tumors

The treatment of VIPomas begins with aggressive preoperative hydration and correction of electrolyte abnormalities and acid-base disturbances. Octreotide is commonly used preperatively to reduce diarrhea volume and facilitate fluid and electrolyte replacement. If diarrhea persists despite octreotide therapy, addition of a glucocorticoid may be helpful.

Patients with glucagonomas have typically lost a significant amount of weight and lean body mass. Treatment begins with medical therapy to improve their nutritional condition, with supplemental enteral nutrition in excess of basic caloric needs. Octreotide is often required in conjunction with enteral nutrition to reverse the catabolic state. IV infusions of amino acids may be required to reverse symptoms and improve dermatitis. Prophylaxis against thromboembolism should be instituted early during hospitalization to prevent perioperative deep vein thrombosis and pulmonary embolism, which occur commonly and are significant causes of morbidity and mortality in these patients. There is little necessary in the way of specific preoperative preparation for somatostatinomas and nonfunctional endocrine tumors.

Resection is the treatment of choice for VIPomas, glucagonomas, somatostatinomas, and nonfunctional pancreatic endocrine tumors and remains the only curative option. Because these tumors tend to be invasive, simple enucleation is often inadequate and partial pancreatic resection is usually recommended. Unfortunately, the frequent presence of synchronous metastases may make complete excision impossible. Palliative resection of recurrences and metastatic foci may be helpful to control symptoms, but improvement in overall survival is unlikely. In a review of the literature, 86% of VIPomas were resected and 23% of patients died of disease from 12 to 52 months after diagnosis or surgery.[47] Other forms of therapy for metastatic disease have been used anecdotally, including hepatic artery embolization, radiofrequency ablation, liver transplantation, radioactive octreotide, chemotherapy, and cryotherapy. Adjuvant chemotherapy has not been shown to be beneficial.

Following resection, 5-year survival for patients with glucagonoma is almost 85% if no metastases are present. Five-year survival is approximately 60% in patients with metastatic disease.[48] Dacarbazine is uniquely effective against glucagonoma as compared with other pancreatic endocrine tumors, and complete remission has been reported in several cases.[49] The overall 5-year survival for nonfunctional pancreatic endocrine tumors is approximately 50%.[50]

## SUMMARY

The endocrine cells of the pancreas are located within the islets of Langerhans, which are dispersed throughout the pancreas. The role of hormones produced by the islet cells can be summarized as the regulation of total body energy, largely achieved by hormonal control of carbohydrate metabolism. Insulin is the hormone of energy storage and glucagon is the hormone of energy release. Insulin stores energy by decreasing blood glucose levels, increasing protein synthesis, decreasing glycogenolysis, decreasing lipolysis, and increasing glucose transport into cells Glucagon acts in a counterregulatory fashion, releasing energy by increasing blood glucose levels via stimulation of glycogenolysis, gluconeogenesis, and lipolysis.

Tumors of any of these cells may secrete a number of hormones, serially or simultaneously. The syndromes produced are named for the peptide whose symptoms predominate. Thus, the endocrine pancreas may produce insulinomas, glucagonomas, somatostatinomas, VIPomas, PPomas, or gastrinomas. Islet cell tumors can also be nonfunctional. All pancreatic endocrine tumors are rare (estimated at ~5 cases/1 million population/year), so time is required to develop logical strategies for treatment. Management of these tumors has undergone evaluation, but surgical management remains the mainstay of treatment and the only curative option for all pancreatic endocrine tumors. The presence or absence of metastatic disease is the primary determinant of long-term survival. Long-term survival is almost more than 90% for resected benign endocrine tumors. Although long-term survival is lower with metastatic endocrine tumors of the pancreas when compared with benign lesions, metastatic endocrine tumors have a better prognosis than pancreatic adenocarcinoma. An aggressive surgical approach to these tumors, often with debulking, is indicated.

## SELECTED REFERENCES

Ellison EC, Sparks J, Verducci JS, et al: 50-year appraisal of gastrinoma: Recommendations for staging and treatment. J Am Coll Surg 202:897–905, 2006.

This review of 106 patients with gastrinoma seen over a 50-year period at Ohio State University Hospital (where ZES was first described) reiterates the conclusion that survival is influenced by tumor size and distant metastases (chiefly hepatic), but not by lymph node spread.

Norton JA: Neuroendocrine tumors of the pancreas and duodenum. Curr Probl Surg 31:77–156, 1994.

This review of the immense National Institutes of Health experience in the surgical management of endocrine tumors of the pancreas and duodenum provides a useful method for students of these syndromes. Especially helpful are discussions of localization methods for insulinomas and gastrinomas and the variabilities brought about by MEN1 syndrome. Norton concludes that almost all these tumors can be located and that aggressive surgical management is highly beneficial. Localizing plus removing duodenal gastrinomas is of paramount importance in achieving improved ZES cure rates.

Norton JA, Jensen RT: Resolved and unresolved controversies in the surgical management of patients with Zollinger-Ellison syndrome. Ann Surg 240:757–773, 2004.

In this extensive review, two of the leading authorities on ZES evaluate the signal controversies in surgical management. They report that the cure rate in patients with ZES and MEN1 is low without pancreaticoduodenectomy, but that the final role for this resection is not yet clear. In patients with the sporadic form of ZES, cure rates of 34% at 10 years for local resection favor an aggressive approach. They confirm division of ZES into benign and malignant (24%) forms, with long-term survival rates of 30% in the malignant form (usually associated with hepatic spread) to 96% for the nonaggressive group. They note that total gastrectomy should be reserved only for some patients with aggressive gastric carcinoid tumors.

Orci L: Macro- and micro-domains in the endocrine pancreas. Diabetes 31:538–565, 1982.

In this 1981 Banting Lecture, Orci summarizes 2 decades of his work on the histomorphology and cytomorphology of islets; the subcellular organization of the beta cell in the biosynthesis and release of insulin, cellular environment of beta cells, and cross-talk between beta and neighboring islet cells are discussed. The illustrations alone invite the reader into a new world with, for example, electron micrographs showing freeze fracture replicas across the Golgi apparatus of a B cell.

Phan GQ, Yeo CJ, Hruban RH, et al: Surgical experience with pancreatic and peripancreatic neuroendocrine tumors: Review of 125 patients. J Gastrointest Surg 2:473–482, 1998.

This article reviews the outcomes of 125 patients undergoing resection for pancreatic endocrine tumors; 48% had nonfunctional tumors and 52% had functional tumors, of which 55% were insulinomas, 36% were gastrinomas, 5% were VIPomas, 3% were glucagonomas, and 1% were ACTHomas. Tumors were benign in 48% of patients and malignant in 52%. The overall 2-, 5-, and 10-year actuarial survival rates were 82%, 65%, and 47%, repectively. The 5-year survival for patients with functional tumors was 77% compared with 52% for those with nonfunctional tumors and 91% and 49% for benign versus malignant tumors.

Vardanyan M, Parkin E, Gruessner C, et al: Pancreas vs. islet transplantation: A call on the future. Curr Opin Organ Transplant 15:124–130, 2010.

This review compares whole pancreas transplantation to allogeneic islet cell transplantation for type 1 diabetes. The authors conclude that the major benefit of pancreas transplantation is the reversal of diabetes improvement of diabetes complications. Although the procedure requires major surgery and lifelong immunosuppression, it remains the gold standard for patients with type 1 diabetes who do not respond to conventional therapy. Allogeneic islet transplantation is a promising alternative, but patient outcomes remain less than optimal and significant progress is required for this procedure to be considered a reliable therapy.

## REFERENCES


1. Orci L: Macro- and micro-domains in the endocrine pancreas. Diabetes 31:538–565, 1982.
2. Cooper GJ, Day AJ, Willis AC, et al: Amylin and the amylin gene: structure, function and relationship to islet amyloid and to diabetes mellitus. Biochim Biophys Acta 1014:247–258, 1989.
3. Samols E, Stagner JI, Ewart RB, et al: The order of islet microvascular cellular perfusion is B–A-D in the perfused rat pancreas. J Clin Invest 82:350–353, 1988.
4. Gittes GK, Rutter WJ: Onset of cell-specific gene expression in the developing mouse pancreas. Proc Natl Acad Sci U S A 89:1128–1132, 1992.
5. Nanjo K, Sanke T, Miyano M, et al: Diabetes due to secretion of a structurally abnormal insulin (insulin Wakayama). Clinical and functional characteristics of [LeuA3] insulin. J Clin Invest 77:514–519, 1986.
6. Bellin MD, Carlson AM, Kobayashi T, et al: Outcome after pancreatectomy and islet autotransplantation in a pediatric population. J Pediatr Gastroenterol Nutr 47:37–44, 2008.
7. Ris F, Morel P, Bosco D, et al: [Islet autotransplantation to prevent diabetes after pancreatectomy for benign disease of the pancreas.] Rev Med Suisse 3:1627–1628, 1630–1631, 2007.
8. Webb MA, Illouz SC, Pollard CA, et al: Islet auto transplantation following total pancreatectomy: A long-term assessment of graft function. Pancreas 37:282–287, 2008.
9. Argo JL, Contreras JL, Wesley MM, et al: Pancreatic resection with islet cell autotransplant for the treatment of severe chronic pancreatitis. Am Surg 74:530–536, 2008.
10. Dixon J, DeLegge M, Morgan KA, et al: Impact of total pancreatectomy with islet cell transplant on chronic pancreatitis management at a disease-based center. Am Surg 74:735–738, 2008.
11. Eisenbarth GS: Type 1 diabetes mellitus. A chronic autoimmune disease. N Engl J Med 314:1360–1368, 1986.
12. Orban T, Farkas K, Jalahej H, et al: Autoantigen-specific regulatory T cells induced in patients with type 1 diabetes mellitus by insulin B-chain immunotherapy. J Autoimmun 34:408–415, 2010.
13. Gruessner AC, Sutherland DE, Gruessner RW: Pancreas transplantation in the United States: A review. Curr Opin Organ Transplant 15:93–101, 2010.

13a. Alejandro R, Barton FB, Hering BJ, et al: Update from the collaborative islet transplant registry. Transplantation 86:1783–1788, 2008.

14. Vardanyan M, Parkin E, Gruessner C, et al: Pancreas versus islet transplantation: A call on the future. Curr Opin Organ Transplant 15:124–130, 2010.
15. Norton JA: Neuroendocrine tumors of the pancreas and duodenum. Curr Probl Surg 31:77–156, 1994.
16. Zollinger RM, Ellison EH: Primary peptic ulcerations of the jejunum associated with islet cell tumors of the pancreas. Ann Surg 142:709–723, 1955.
17. Muscarella P, Melvin WS, Fisher WE, et al: Genetic alterations in gastrinomas and nonfunctioning pancreatic neuroendocrine tumors: An analysis of p16/MTS1 tumor suppressor gene inactivation. Cancer Res 58:237–240, 1998.
18. Rigaud G, Missiaglia E, Moore PS, et al: High-resolution allelotype of nonfunctional pancreatic endocrine tumors: Identification of two molecular subgroups with clinical implications. Cancer Res 61:285–292, 2001.
19. Chung DC, Smith AP, Louis DN, et al: A novel pancreatic endocrine tumor suppressor gene locus on chromosome 3p with clinical prognostic implications. J Clin Invest 100:404–410, 1997.
20. Evers BM, Rady PL, Sandoval K, et al: Gastrinomas demonstrate amplification of the HER-2/neu proto-oncogene. Ann Surg 219:596–601, 1994.
21. Goebel SU, Iwamoto M, Raffeld M, et al: Her-2/neu expression and gene amplification in gastrinomas: Correlations with tumor biology, growth, and aggressiveness. Cancer Res 62:3702–3710, 2002.
22. Gibril F, Schumann M, Pace A, et al: Multiple endocrine neoplasia type 1 and Zollinger-Ellison syndrome: A prospective study of 107 cases and comparison with 1009 cases from the literature. Medicine (Baltimore) 83:43–83, 2004.
23. Thompson JC, Hirose FM, Lemmi CA, et al: Zollinger-Ellison syndrome in a patient with multiple carcinoid-islet cell tumors of the duodenum. Am J Surg 115:177–184, 1968.
24. Doherty GM: Multiple endocrine neoplasia type 1: Duodenopancreatic tumors. Surg Oncol 12:135–143, 2003.
25. Tonelli F, Fratini G, Falchetti A, et al: Surgery for gastroenteropancreatic tumours in mùltiple endocrine neoplasia type 1: Review and personal experience. J Intern Med 257:38–49, 2005.
26. Norton JA, Jensen RT: Resolved and unresolved controversies in the surgical management of patients with Zollinger-Ellison syndrome. Ann Surg 240:757–773, 2004.

27. Boden G: Glucagonomas and insulinomas. Gastroenterol Clin North Am 18:831–845, 1989.
28. Norton JA, Kahn CR, Schiebinger R, et al: Amino acid deficiency and the skin rash associated with glucagonoma. Ann Intern Med 91:213–215, 1979.
29. Krejs GJ, Orci L, Conlon JM, et al: Somatostatinoma syndrome. Biochemical, morphologic and clinical features. N Engl J Med 301:285–292, 1979.
30. Harris GJ, Tio F, Cruz AB, Jr: Somatostatinoma: A case report and review of the literature. J Surg Oncol 36:8–16, 1987.
31. Van Hoe L, Gryspeerdt S, Marchal G, et al: Helical CT for the preoperative localization of islet cell tumors of the pancreas: Value of arterial and parenchymal phase images. AJR Am J Roentgenol 165:1437–1439, 1995.
32. Sheth S, Hruban RK, Fishman EK: Helical CT of islet cell tumors of the pancreas: Typical and atypical manifestations. AJR Am J Roentgenol 179:725–730, 2002.
33. Boukhman MP, Karam JM, Shaver J, et al: Localization of insulinomas. Arch Surg 134:818–822; discussion 822–813, 1999.
34. Thoeni RF, Mueller-Lisse UG, Chan R, et al: Detection of small, functional islet cell tumors in the pancreas: Selection of MR imaging sequences for optimal sensitivity. Radiology 214:483–490, 2000.
35. Muller MF, Meyenberger C, Bertschinger P, et al: Pancreatic tumors: evaluation with endoscopic US, CT, and MR imaging. Radiology 190:745–751, 1994.
36. Proye C, Malvaux P, Pattou F, et al: Noninvasive imaging of insulinomas and gastrinomas with endoscopic ultrasonography and somatostatin receptor scintigraphy. Surgery 124:1134–1143; discussion 1143–1134, 1998.
37. Jackson JE: Angiography and arterial stimulation venous sampling in the localization of pancreatic neuroendocrine tumours. Best Pract Res Clin Endocrinol Metab 19:229–239, 2005.
38. Frucht H, Howard JM, Slaff JI, et al: Secretin and calcium provocative tests in the Zollinger-Ellison syndrome. A prospective study. Ann Intern Med 111:713–722, 1989.
39. Anlauf M, Wieben D, Perren A, et al: Persistent hyperinsulinemic hypoglycemia in 15 adults with diffuse nesidioblastosis: Diagnostic criteria, incidence, and characterization of beta-cell changes. Am J Surg Pathol 29:524–533, 2005.
40. Doherty GM, Doppman JL, Shawker TH, et al: Results of a prospective strategy to diagnose, localize, and resect insulinomas. Surgery 110:989–996, 1991.
41. Hirshberg B, Cochran C, Skarulis MC, et al: Malignant insulinoma: Spectrum of unusual clinical features. Cancer 104:264–272, 2005.
42. Simonenko VB, Dulin PA, Makanin MA: [Somatostatin analogues in treatment of gastrointestinal and pancreatic neuroendocrine tumors.] Klin Med (Mosk) 84:4–8, 2006.
43. Norton JA, Jensen RT: Current surgical management of Zollinger-Ellison syndrome (ZES) in patients without multiple endocrine neoplasia-type 1 (MEN1). Surg Oncol 12:145–151, 2003.
44. Norton JA, Doppman JL, Jensen RT: Curative resection in Zollinger-Ellison syndrome. Results of a 10-year prospective study. Ann Surg 215:8–18, 1992.
45. Norton JA, Fraker DL, Alexander HR, et al: Surgery to cure the Zollinger-Ellison syndrome. N Engl J Med 341:635–644, 1999.
46. Ellison EC, Sparks J, Verducci JS, et al: 50-year appraisal of gastrinoma: Recommendations for staging and treatment. J Am Coll Surg 202:897–905, 2006.
47. Ghaferi AA, Chojnacki KA, Long WD, et al: Pancreatic VIPomas: Subject review and one institutional experience. J Gastrointest Surg 12:382–393, 2008.
48. Stacpoole PW: The glucagonoma syndrome: Clinical features, diagnosis, and treatment. Endocr Rev 2:347–361, 1981.
49. Marynick SP, Fagadau WR, Duncan LA: Malignant glucagonoma syndrome: Response to chemotherapy. Ann Intern Med 93:453–454, 1980.
50. Phan GQ, Yeo CJ, Hruban RH, et al: Surgical experience with pancreatic and peripancreatic neuroendocrine tumors: Review of 125 patients. J Gastrointest Surg 2:473–482, 1998.

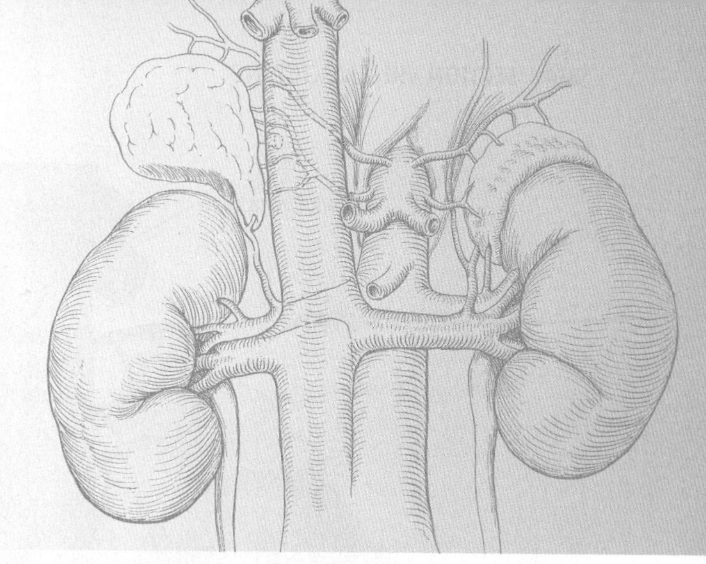

CHAPTER 41

# THE ADRENAL GLANDS

Michael W. Yeh and Quan-Yang Duh

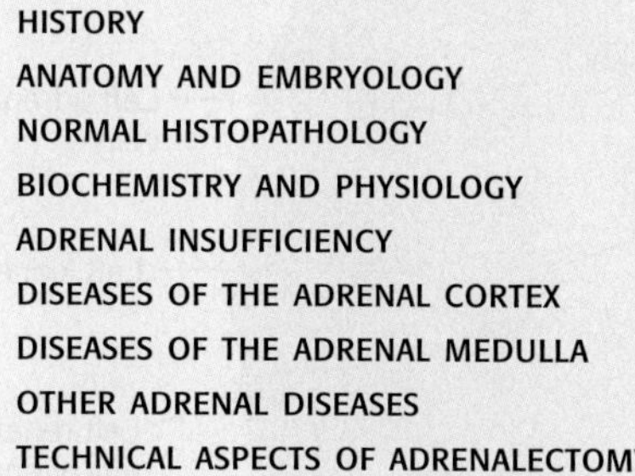

HISTORY
ANATOMY AND EMBRYOLOGY
NORMAL HISTOPATHOLOGY
BIOCHEMISTRY AND PHYSIOLOGY
ADRENAL INSUFFICIENCY
DISEASES OF THE ADRENAL CORTEX
DISEASES OF THE ADRENAL MEDULLA
OTHER ADRENAL DISEASES
TECHNICAL ASPECTS OF ADRENALECTOMY

## HISTORY

The adrenal glands were first described by the Italian anatomist Bartolomeo Eustachi in 1563. The German comparative anatomist Albert von Kölliker (1817-1905), who noted the presence of the adrenals in a number of vertebrate species, is credited with first identifying two distinct portions of the adrenal gland, the cortex and the medulla. Although Thomas Addison described the clinical features of primary adrenal failure in 1855, it was not until almost a century later that the adrenal hormones were fully isolated and characterized. Adrenaline (or epinephrine) was first isolated from adrenal extract at the turn of the century. Steroid hormones were crystallized from cortical extract *(cortin)* by Swiss and American investigators in the 1930s, but their highly similar chemical structures made isolation of the individual compounds challenging. Edward Kendall, Tadeus Reichstein, and Philip Hench jointly received the 1950 Nobel Prize in Physiology or Medicine for their groundbreaking work on the adrenocortical hormones. The Austrian-born endocrinologist Hans Selye first described the stress response in mammals in 1936 and made major contributions to the understanding of the hypothalamic-pituitary-adrenal (HPA) axis. Roger Guillemin, Andrew Schally, and Rosalyn Yalow were awarded the Nobel Prize in Physiology or Medicine in 1977 for characterizing the peptide hormones of the brain that underlie the HPA axis as we now understand it.[1,2]

## ANATOMY AND EMBRYOLOGY

### General and Developmental Aspects

The adrenal glands are paired, mustard-colored structures positioned superior and slightly medial to the kidneys in the retroperitoneal space (Fig. 41-1). They are flattened and roughly pyramidal (right) or crescent-shaped (left), weighing approximately 4 g each. The adrenals are among the most highly perfused organs in the body, receiving 2000 mL/kg/min of blood, after only the kidney and thyroid. In most respects, the cortex and medulla can be considered as two completely distinct organs that happen to colocalize during development. The two portions have disparate embryologic origins. The primordial cortex arises from the coelomic mesodermal tissue near the cephalic end of the mesonephros during the fourth to fifth week of gestation. Biosynthetic activity can be detected as early as the seventh week. Cortical cell mass dominates the fetal adrenal at 4 months of development and steroidogenesis reaches is maximum during the third trimester. The adrenal medulla arises from the ectodermal tissues of the embryonic neural crest. It develops in parallel with the sympathetic nervous system, beginning in the fifth to sixth week of gestation. From their original position adjacent to the neural tube, neural crest cells migrate ventrally to assume a para-aortic position near the developing adrenal cortex. There, they differentiate into chromaffin cells that make up the adrenal medulla.

This course of embryologic development yields certain surgically relevant sequelae. Both cortical and medullary tissue can be found at extra-adrenal sites (Fig. 41-2). The range of potential sites is wider for chromaffin tissue than for cortical tissue. Pheochromocytomas may arise in extra-adrenal sites more commonly than previously believed (see later). When extra-adrenal, pheochromocytomas are also termed *paragangliomas.*

### Relationships

The right adrenal gland abuts the posterolateral surface of the retrohepatic vena cava. The right adrenal fossa is bounded by the right kidney inferolaterally, diaphragm posteriorly, and bare area of the liver anterosuperiorly. The left adrenal gland lies between the left kidney and aorta, with its inferior limb extending farther caudad toward the renal hilum than the right adrenal. The other relationships of the left adrenal gland are the diaphragm posteriorly and the tail of the pancreas and splenic hilum anteriorly. Each adrenal gland is enveloped by its proper capsule, in addition to sharing Gerota's fascia with the kidneys. The adrenal capsules are immediately associated with the perirenal fat.

### Vasculature

Knowledge of the macroscopic vascular anatomy of the adrenal glands is essential to proper surgical management. It is important to conceptualize that although the arterial supply is diffuse,

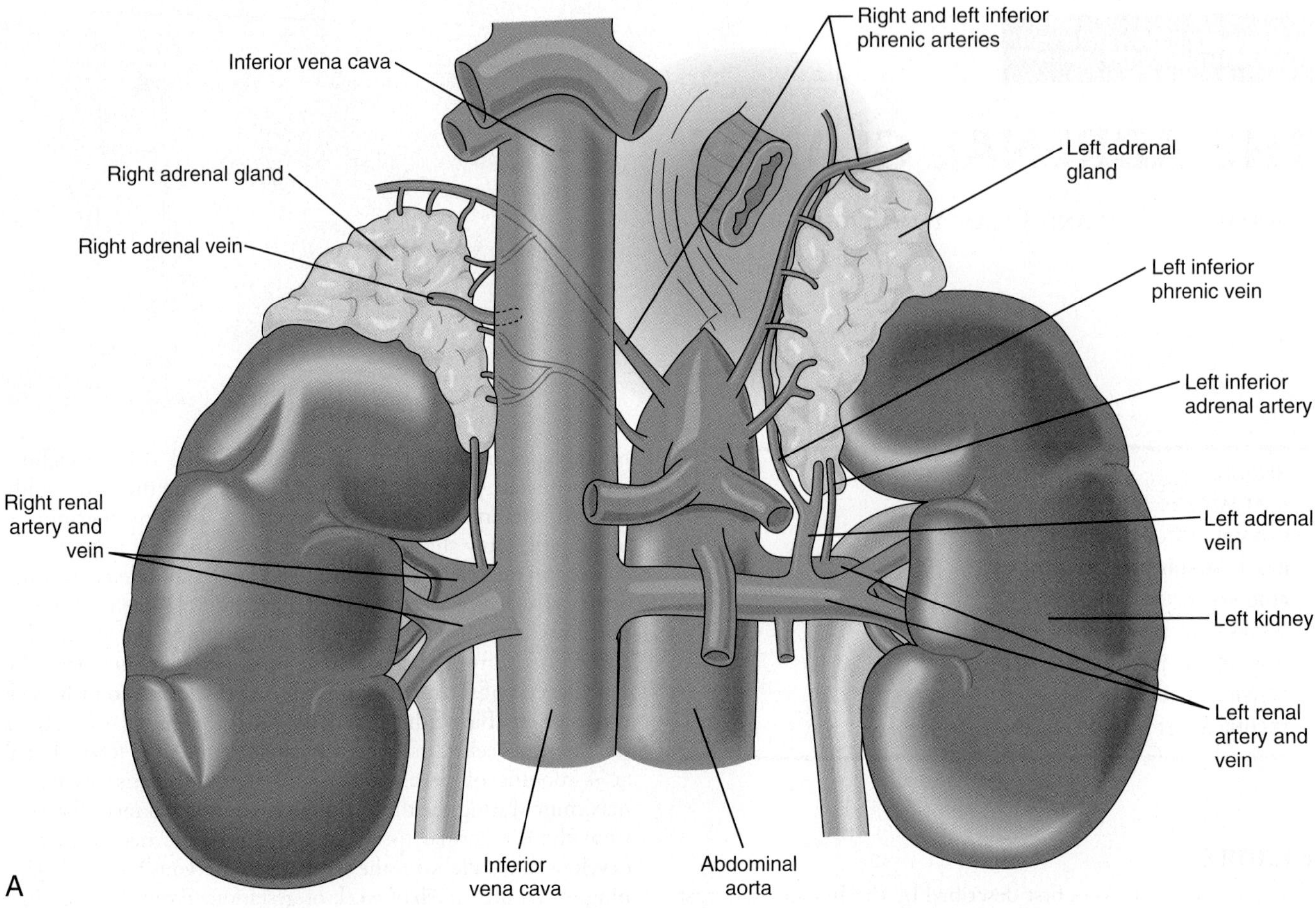


**FIGURE 41-1** Anatomy of the adrenal glands. ***A,*** Left and right adrenal glands in situ.

the venous drainage of each gland is usually solitary. The arterial supply arises from three distinct vessels—the superior adrenal arteries from the inferior phrenic arteries, small middle adrenal arteries from the juxtaceliac aorta, and inferior adrenal arteries from the renal arteries. Of these, the inferior is the most prominent and is commonly a single identifiable vessel. The left adrenal vein is approximately 2 cm long and drains into the left renal vein after joining the inferior phrenic vein. The right adrenal vein is typically as short as it is wide (0.5 cm) and drains directly into the vena cava. This configuration presents a surgical challenge that will be discussed in more detail later in this chapter. In up to 20% of individuals, the right adrenal vein may drain into an accessory right hepatic vein or into the vena cava, at or near the confluence of the vein. Vigilance about this variant and others (Fig. 41-3) may reduce the likelihood of intraoperative venous hemorrhage during a right adrenalectomy.

## NORMAL HISTOPATHOLOGY

The cortex is approximately 2 mm thick and comprises more than 80% of the mass of the gland. It is made up of three layers (Fig. 41-4). The outer zona glomerulosa is a thin layer of relatively small cells with moderately eosinophilic, lipid-poor cytoplasm. It has an undulating inner border and normally does not form a complete circumferential layer. Most of the adrenal cortex is formed by the zona fasciculata, a middle layer composed of long radial columns of large, clear, lipid-laden cells. The inner zona reticularis is made up of small nests of compact eosinophilic cells. The adrenal medulla consists of clusters and short cords of chromaffin cells, which are large, polyhedral, and packed with basophilic secretory granules. Catecholamines within these granules yield a brown-colored reaction when treated with chromium salts, giving the cells their name. In contrast to the cortex, the adrenal medulla is richly endowed with autonomic nerve fibers and ganglion cells. Sympathetic fibers synapse directly with the chromaffin cells, constituting an interface between the nervous and endocrine systems.

The microvasculature of the adrenal gland functionally unifies the cortex and medulla. The adrenal arteries arborize extensively before entering the capsule to form a subcapsular plexus. Blood flows centripetally through capillaries in the zona glomerulosa and zona fasciculata before forming a deep plexus within the zona reticularis. From there, steroid-enriched postcapillary blood enters the medulla, where cortisol drives expression of phenylethanolamine N-methyl transferase (PNMT). PNMT is responsible for the conversion of norepinephrine to epinephrine. This microvascular arrangement is essentially a portal system between the cortex and medulla.

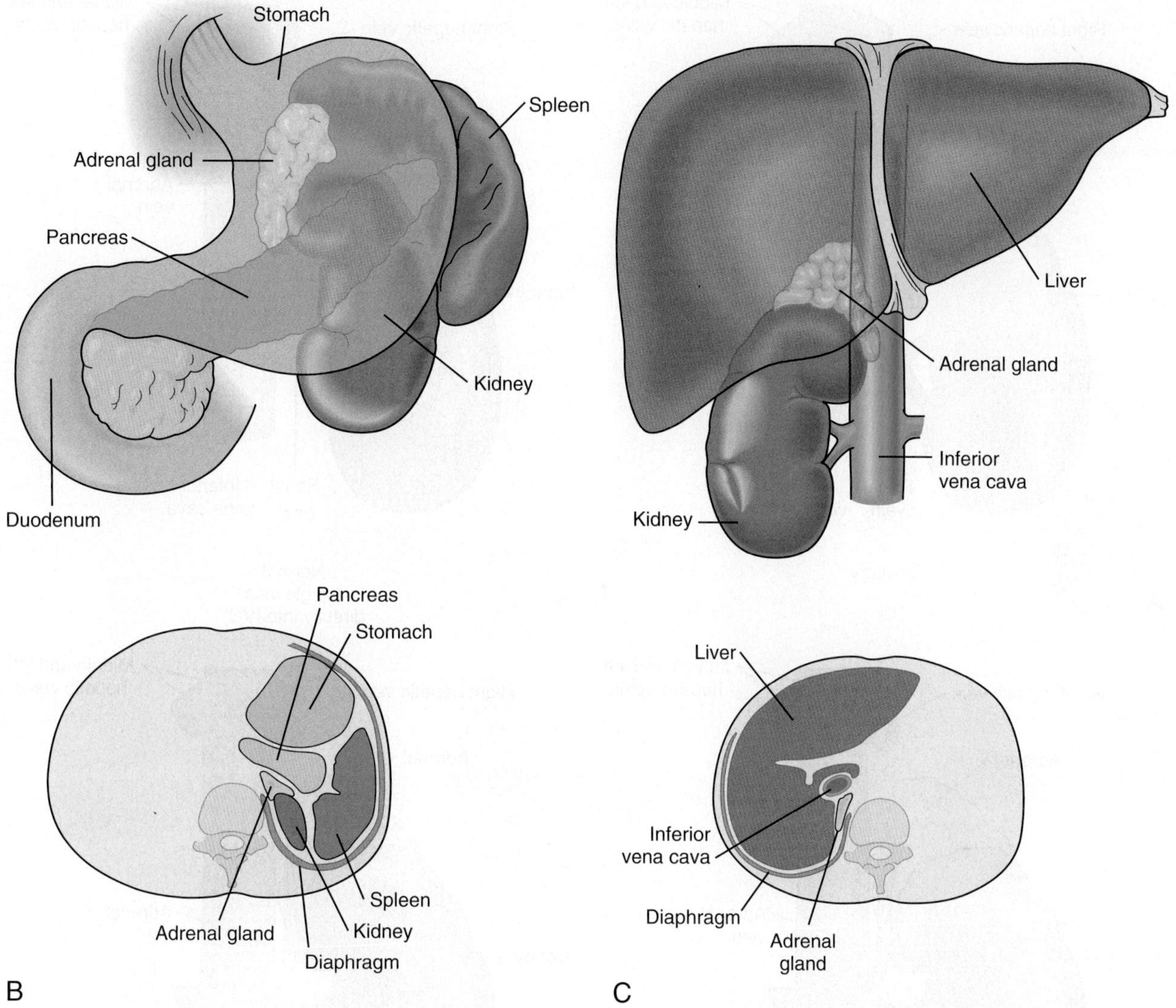

**FIGURE 41-1, cont'd B,** Relationships of the left adrenal gland. **C,** Relationships of the right adrenal gland.

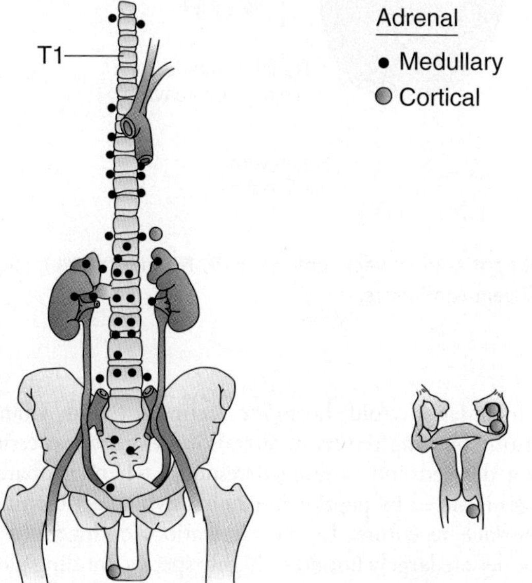


**FIGURE 41-2** Sites of extra-adrenal cortical and medullary tissue.

## BIOCHEMISTRY AND PHYSIOLOGY

### Adrenal Steroid Biosynthesis

Adrenal steroid biosynthesis begins with the transport of cholesterol to the inner mitochondrial membrane by the steroidogenic acute regulatory protein (StAR; Fig. 41-5). Cholesterol then undergoes a series of oxidative reactions catalyzed predominantly by membrane-associated enzymes belonging to the cytochrome P450 (CYP) family. Cleavage of the cholesterol side chain yields the hormonally inactive compound pregnenolone, the immediate precursor to the adrenal steroid hormones. Serial oxidation by CYP17 converts pregnenolone and progesterone into the major adrenal sex steroids, dehydroepiandrosterone (DHEA) and androstenedione. Additional enzymatic steps confined to the gonads generate testosterone, estrone, and estradiol from androstenedione. Oxidation of 17-hydroxypregnenolone by 3β-hydroxysteroid dehydrogenase (3β-HSD), followed by action of CYP21A2 and CYP11B1 yields cortisol, the active glucocorticoid hormone in humans. Aldosterone is generated by the oxidation of corticosterone by CYP11B2 within the zona glomerulosa. CYP17

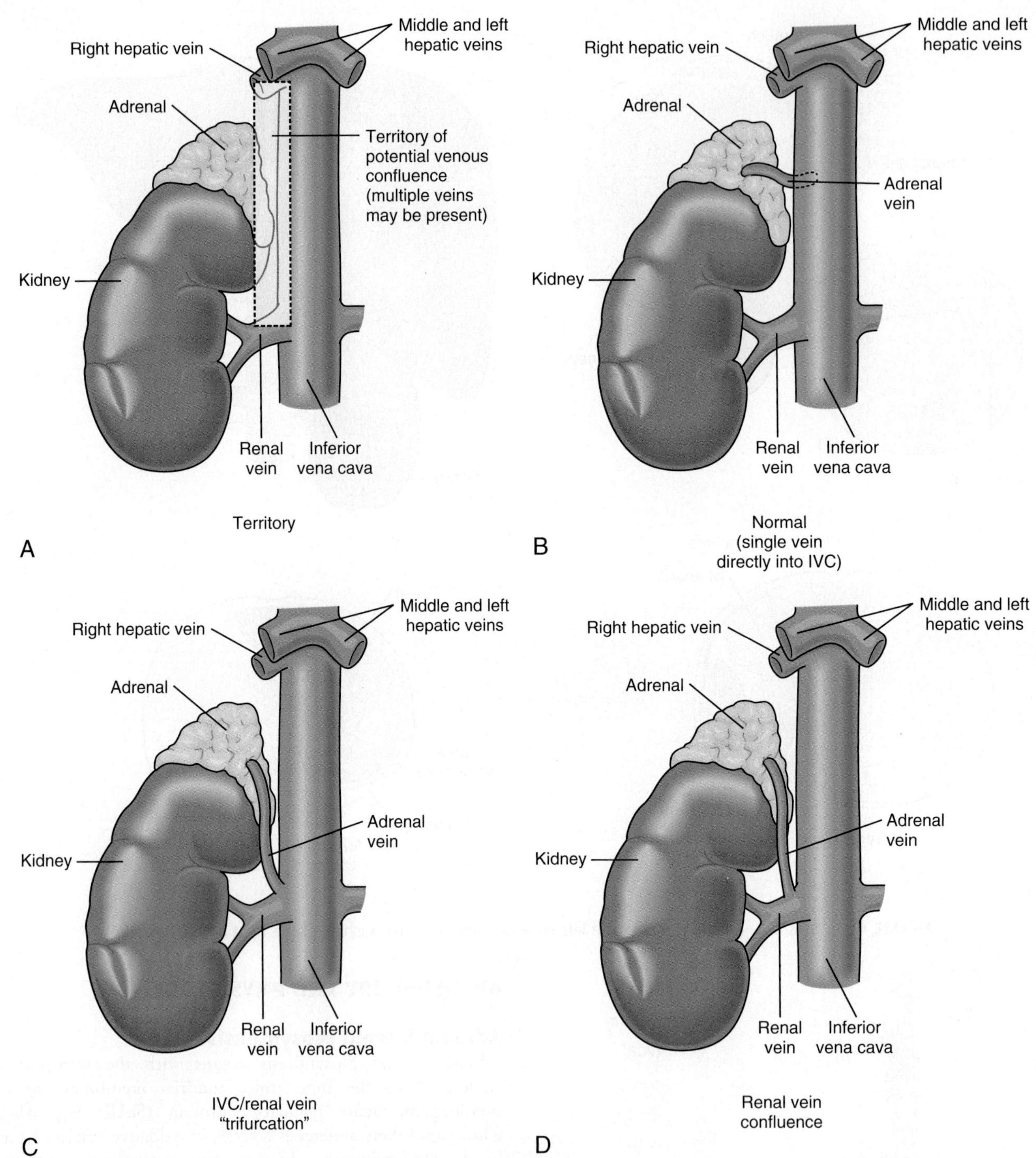


**FIGURE 41-3** Variations in right adrenal vein anatomy. **A,** Territory of potential right adrenal vein confluence. **B,** Normal (>80%); single vein directly into the inferior vena cava (IVC). **C,** IVC–renal vein trifurcation. **D,** Renal vein confluence.

expression is confined to the zona fasciculata and zona reticularis, accounting for the synthesis of glucocorticoids and adrenal sex steroids in these regions.

## Steroid Hormone Physiology and Metabolism

Steroid hormones belong to a general class of low-molecular-weight, lipophilic signaling molecules that act by entering cells and binding to intracellular receptors. This group of hormones also includes thyroid hormone, retinoids, and vitamin D. Hormone binding results in alterations in gene expression that show a delayed and prolonged response when compared with changes induced by peptide hormones, which act by binding to cell surface receptors. In the circulation, endogenous steroid hormones are largely bound to highly specific binding globulins. Serum levels of these proteins—and hence free hormone levels—can be altered by certain physiologic and disease states such as

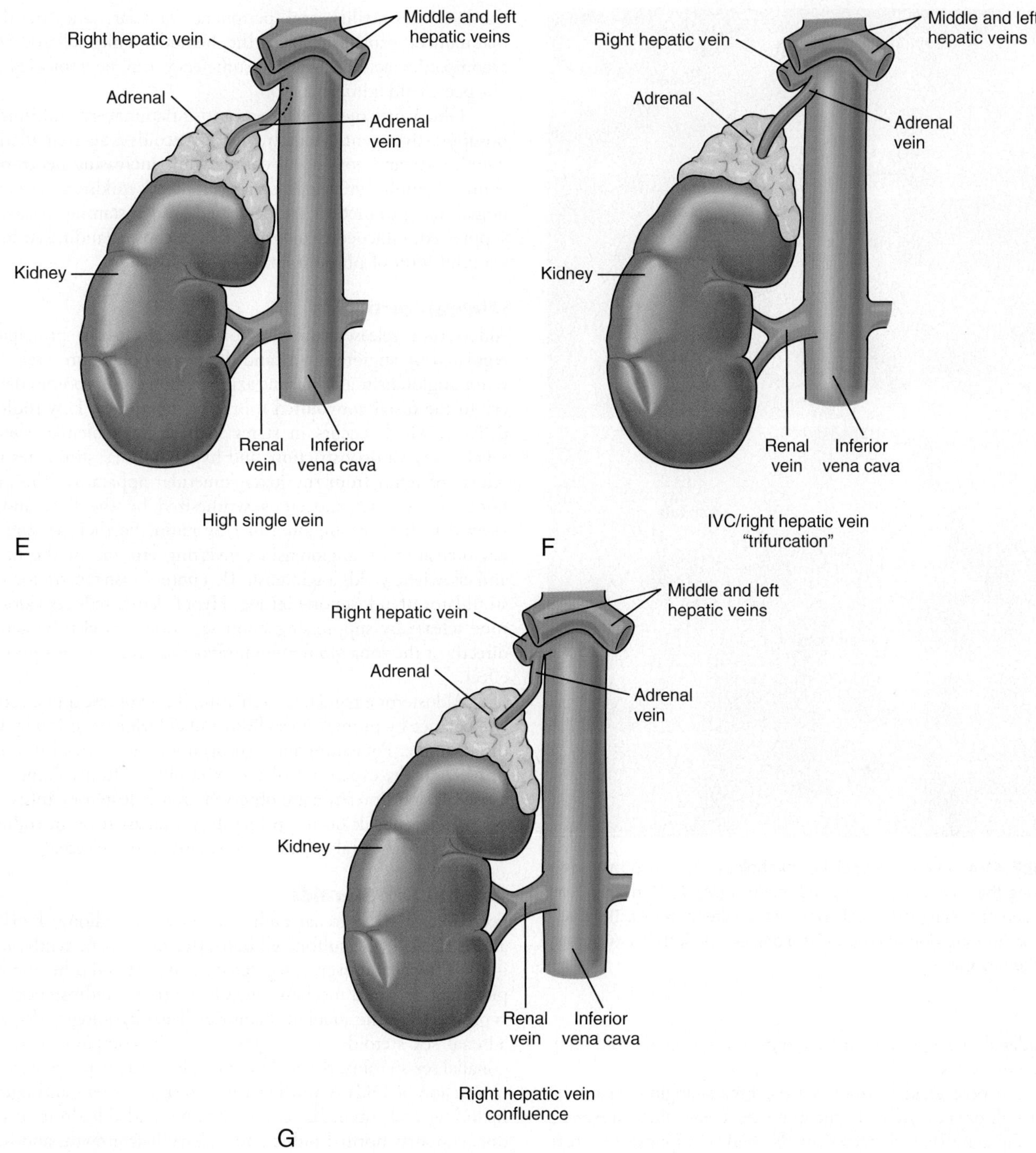


**FIGURE 41-3, cont'd E,** High single vein into the IVC. **F,** IVC–right hepatic vein trifurcation. **G,** Right hepatic vein confluence.

pregnancy, nephrotic syndrome, and cirrhosis. Metabolism of endogenous and pharmacologic steroids generally proceeds via hydroxylation, sulfonation, and/or conjugation to glucuronic acid in the liver, followed by urinary excretion. The regulation and physiologic actions of individual steroid hormones are discussed here.

## Glucocorticoids

The release of corticotropin-releasing factor (CRF) into the hypothalamic-pituitary portal system by hypothalamic neurons results in adrenocorticotropic hormone (ACTH) secretion by the anterior pituitary. ACTH binds to a G protein–coupled receptor on the adrenocortical cell surface and stimulates glucocorticoid secretion. Steroidogenesis is acutely upregulated via increased StAR-mediated cholesterol transport and pregnenolone synthesis by CYP11A1. ACTH is released in a pulsatile fashion that normally displays a circadian rhythm. The highest levels of ACTH, and thus cortisol, are generally detected on waking, with levels gradually declining throughout the day to reach a nadir in the early evening. This pattern must be

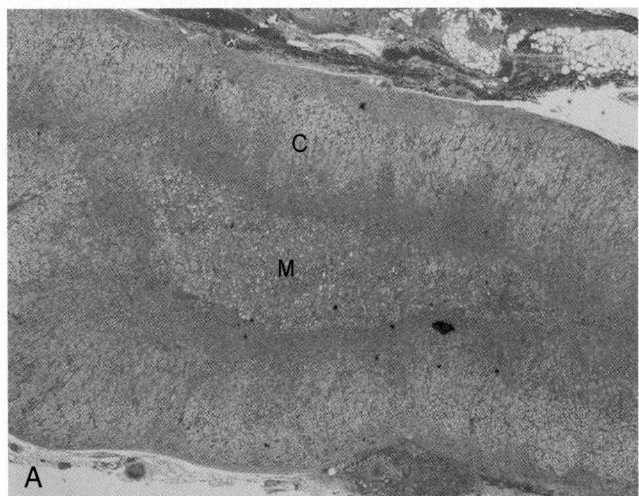


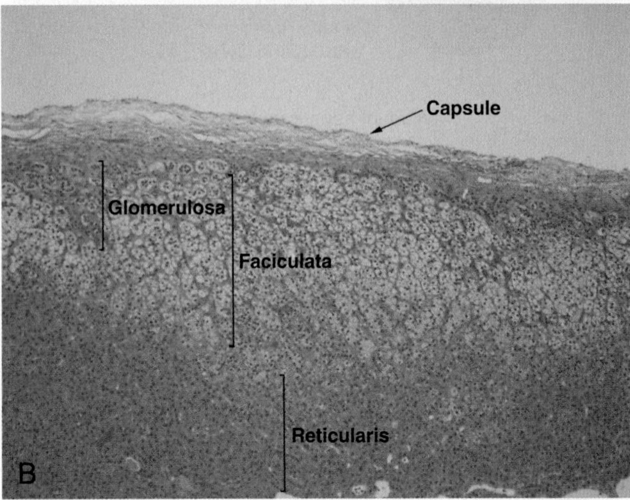


**FIGURE 41-4** Normal adrenal histopathology. **A,** Low-power view showing the adrenal cortex (C) and medulla (M). **B,** Medium-power view demonstrating individual layers of the adrenal cortex. The thickness of the zona glomerulosa varies along its length (H&E). (Courtesy Dr. Anthony Gill.)

considered when evaluating patients for glucocorticoid deficiency or excess.

Glucocorticoid hormones have broad-ranging effects on almost all organ systems in the body. As a rule, they generate a catabolic state that characterizes the body's response to stress. The hormones are so named because they cause alterations in carbohydrate, protein, and lipid metabolism that have the net effect of increasing blood glucose concentrations. Hepatic glucose output is elevated by the upregulation of gluconeogenesis and net glycogen deposition occurs. Glucose uptake by peripheral tissues is directly inhibited. Glucocorticoids stimulate lipolysis with release of free fatty acids into the circulation and a general state of insulin resistance is induced, resulting in protein catabolism. Fatty acids and amino acids serve as energy sources and substrates for gluconeogenesis. In the cardiovascular system, glucocorticoids exert a permissive and enhancing effect on catecholamine signaling by sensitizing arterial smooth muscle cells to β-adrenergic stimulation and increasing catecholamine concentrations in neuromuscular junctions. Cardiac contractility and peripheral vascular tone are thus maintained, explaining why the hemodynamic collapse that accompanies acute adrenal insufficiency can be remedied by glucocorticoid administration.

Glucocorticoids are potent anti-inflammatory and immunosuppressive agents. Acutely, glucocorticoids reduce circulating lymphocyte and eosinophil counts while increasing neutrophil counts. Lymphocyte apoptosis is promoted, cytokine and immunoglobulin production are decreased, and histamine release is suppressed. Glucocorticoids also reduce prostaglandin synthesis via inhibition of phospholipase A2.

## Mineralocorticoids

Aldosterone release from the zona glomerulosa is principally regulated by angiotensin II and the blood potassium level. The renin-angiotensin-aldosterone axis is responsive to sodium delivery to the distal convoluted tubule of the kidney. Low sodium delivery, which occurs in states such as hypovolemia, shock, renal artery vasoconstriction, and hyponatremia, stimulates the release of renin from the juxtaglomerular apparatus. The prohormone angiotensinogen is synthesized by the liver and is cleaved to inactive angiotensin I by renin. Further cleavage of angiotensin I by angiotensin-converting enzyme in the lungs and elsewhere yields angiotensin II, a potent vasoconstrictor and stimulator of aldosterone release. Hypokalemia reduces aldosterone release by suppressing renin secretion and also by acting directly at the zona glomerulosa. Hyperkalemia has the opposite effect.

Aldosterone regulates circulating fluid volume and electrolyte balance by promoting sodium and chloride retention by the distal tubule. Potassium and hydrogen ion are secreted into the urine. Acutely, expansion of the extracellular fluid volume and a rise in blood pressure are observed after aldosterone infusion. Negative feedback occurs primarily via an increase in sodium delivery to the distal tubule, suppressing renin release.

## Adrenal Sex Steroids

Secretion of the adrenal androgens androstenedione, DHEA, and DHEA-S (the sulfonated derivative of DHEA, synthesized in the adrenal and liver) is regulated by ACTH and other incompletely understood mechanisms. Of the three, androstenedione is produced in the smallest quantities. The physiologic effects of adrenal sex steroids are generally weak in comparison to the gonadal sex steroids, particularly in males. In females, peripheral conversion of DHEA and DHEA-S to more potent androgens, including androstenedione, testosterone, and dihydrotestosterone, supports normal pubic and axillary hair growth, and may play a role in maintaining libido and a sense of well-being.

## Catecholamine Biosynthesis and Physiology

Synthesis of catecholamines in the adrenal medulla begins with the hydroxylation of tyrosine, a rate-limiting step that generates dihydroxyphenylalanine (L-dopa) in the cytosol (Fig. 41-6). Decarboxylation of L-dopa generates dopamine, which is then β-hydroxylated to form norepinephrine. Epinephrine is created by the action of PNMT, which, unlike the other enzymes involved in catecholamine synthesis, is localized to the chromaffin cells of the adrenal medulla and organ of Zuckerkandl. Sympathetic stimulation of the adrenal medulla results in the release of stored catecholamines into the circulation. Basal levels of adrenal catecholamine secretion are normally low, although

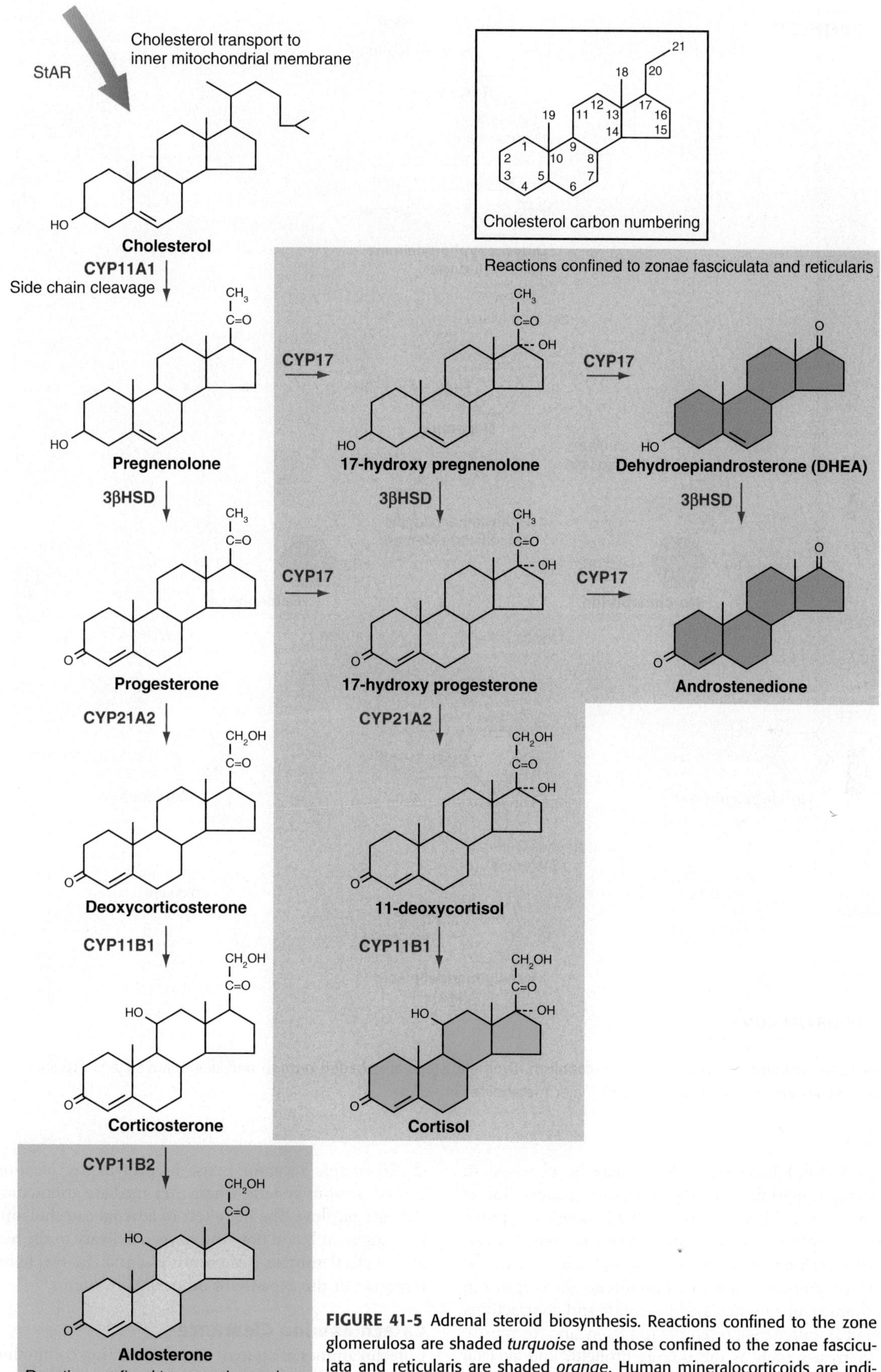


**FIGURE 41-5** Adrenal steroid biosynthesis. Reactions confined to the zone glomerulosa are shaded *turquoise* and those confined to the zonae fasciculata and reticularis are shaded *orange*. Human mineralocorticoids are indicated in *yellow*, glucocorticoids in *green*, and sex steroids in *blue*.

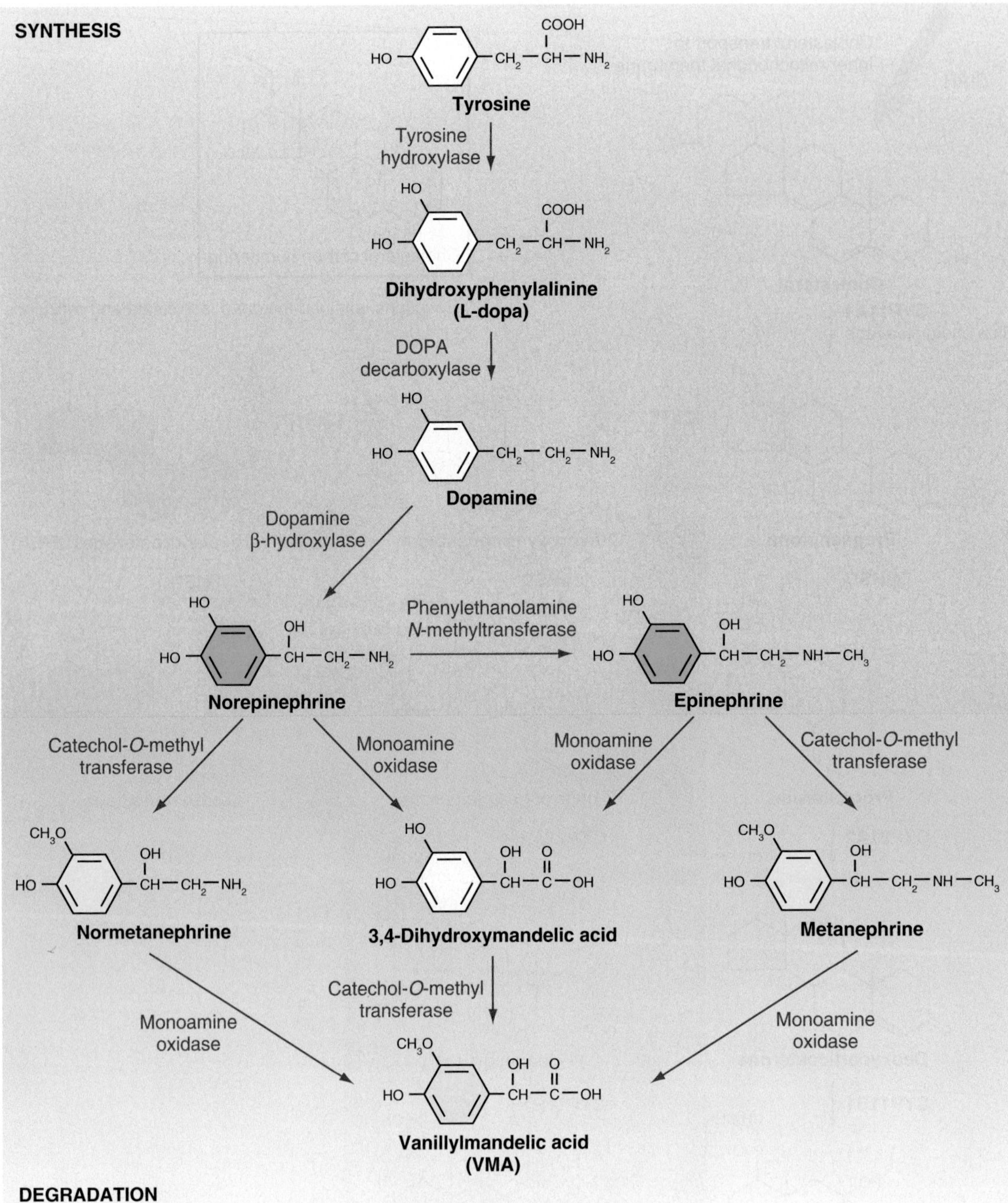


**FIGURE 41-6** Catecholamine biosynthesis and metabolism. Synthetic steps are shaded *orange* and degradative steps are shaded *turquoise*. Major catecholamines are indicated in *green* and major metabolites in *yellow*.

large (up to 50-fold) increases in levels may be observed in response to major physiologic or psychological stressors. Target tissue responses are mediated by α- and β-adrenergic receptors. α-Adrenergic receptors display greater affinity for norepinephrine compared with epinephrine, and the opposite is true for β-adrenergic receptors. Stimulation of $\beta_1$-adrenergic receptors in the myocardium results in increased heart rate and contractility. Stimulation of $\beta_2$-adrenergic receptors results in smooth muscle relaxation in tissues such as the uterus, bronchi, and skeletal muscle arterioles. $\alpha_1$-Adrenergic receptors mediate vasoconstriction in tissues such as the skin and gastrointestinal tract. $\alpha_2$-Adrenergic receptors exist in presynaptic locations in the central nervous system, where they mediate attenuation of sympathetic outflow. The net effect of adrenal catecholamine release is to augment blood flow and oxygen delivery to the brain, heart, and skeletal muscle, which are essential to the fight-or-flight response, at the expense of other organ systems.

## Catecholamine Clearance

Catecholamines are potent and short-acting compounds, with a plasma half-life of approximately 1 minute. Their presence in synapses and the circulation exhibits tight negative regulation

**Table 41-1 Properties of Endogenous and Commonly Used Pharmacologic Glucocorticoids***

| COMPOUND | IV/PO[*] | COMMON TRADE NAME | RELATIVE POTENCY | DAILY PHYSIOLOGIC DOSE (MG) | DOSING INTERVAL |
|---|---|---|---|---|---|
| Cortisol = hydrocortisone | Both | Cortef (PO)<br>Solu-Cortef (IV) | 1× | 20 | q8-12h |
| Cortisone | PO | – | 0.8× | 25 | q8-12h |
| Prednisone | PO | – | 4× | 5 | q24h |
| Prednisolone | PO | – | 4× | 5 | q24h |
| Methylprednisolone | Both | Medrol (PO)<br>Solu-Medrol (IV) | 5× | 4 | q24h |
| Dexamethasone[†] | Both | Decadron | 25× | 1 | q24h |

*Oral and intravenous dosages are similar.
†Does not cross-react with the cortisol assay.

by reuptake and degradation. Degradation pathways merit some discussion because they generate the metabolites commonly measured in the biochemical evaluation of pheochromocytoma (see later). Epinephrine and norepinephrine are inactivated by one or both of the enzymes monoamine oxidase (MAO) and catechol-*O*-methyl transferase (COMT; see Fig. 41-6). Initial methylation by COMT yields metanephrine and normetanephrine, which can be detected in plasma and urine. Their relatively stable plasma levels, which contrast with the high-amplitude fluctuations seen in plasma epinephrine and norepinephrine levels, make them attractive diagnostic markers.[3] The sequential action of MAO and COMT generates the major final product, vanillylmandelic acid (VMA). Catecholamine metabolites are excreted in the urine, sometimes after sulfonation or conjugation to glucuronic acid in the liver.

## ADRENAL INSUFFICIENCY

### Types of Adrenal Insufficiency

#### Primary Adrenal Insufficiency (Addison's Disease)

Originally described in patients with tuberculous destruction of the adrenal glands, this rare disease presents with weakness and fatigue, anorexia, nausea or vomiting, weight loss, hyperpigmentation, hypotension, and electrolyte disturbances (hyponatremia and hyperkalemia). Hyperpigmentation, previously believed to be caused by elevated levels of POMC and its cleavage product alpha–melanocyte-stimulating hormone (α-MSH) is now believed to result from ACTH-induced melanogenesis.[4] Hormonal insufficiency caused by intrinsic adrenal disease arises from three general mechanisms—congenital adrenal dysgenesis/hypoplasia, defective steroidogenesis, and adrenal destruction. Of these, adrenal destruction from autoimmune causes is the most common, followed by infectious adrenalitis (e.g., tuberculous, fungal, viral), adrenal replacement by metastatic tumor, and adrenal hemorrhage (Waterhouse-Friderichsen syndrome [WFS]). The latter occurs in the setting of septicemia caused by meningococcal or other organisms and is more common in pediatric and asplenic patients.

#### Secondary Adrenal Insufficiency

Secondary adrenal insufficiency is a relatively common disorder resulting from ACTH deficiency, often occurring in the setting of pharmacologic steroid withdrawal. Patients receiving high supraphysiologic doses of glucocorticoids (more than the equivalent of 20 mg prednisone daily; see Table 41-1) for more than 5 days and those receiving low supraphysiologic doses for more than 3 weeks are at risk for HPA axis suppression. Surgical cure of Cushing's syndrome (see later) similarly results in glucocorticoid withdrawal. The rate of recovery from HPA axis suppression varies in accordance with the duration and severity of previous glucocorticoid excess, and the need for glucocorticoid supplementation may last several years.[5] Other less common causes of secondary adrenal insufficiency include panhypopituitarism caused by neoplastic or infiltrative replacement, granulomatous disease, and pituitary hemorrhage or infarction. Pituitary infarction may occur in the setting of severe postpartum hemorrhage (Sheehan's syndrome).

#### Adrenal Insufficiency in the Critically Ill

Studies have suggested that critically ill patients with sepsis or systemic inflammatory response syndrome (SIRS) may be affected by acute reversible dysfunction of the HPA axis. The incidence of the disorder is approximately 30% in critically ill patients, although this figure may be higher in those with septic shock. Whether these patients incur increased mortality because of adrenal insufficiency remains to be defined. Proposed mechanisms of reversible HPA axis dysfunction include adrenal ACTH resistance and decreased responsiveness of target tissues to glucocorticoids. Glucocorticoid supplementation in septic patients has been the topic of at least 14 randomized controlled trials. Among these studies, there appears to be an inverse relationship between survival benefit and glucocorticoid dose, with physiologic (i.e., replacement) doses yielding a median relative survival benefit of 1.33 and high supraphysiologic doses demonstrating significant harm. Although the data remains controversial, evidence has suggested that patients with vasopressor-dependent septic shock may benefit from 5- to 7-day courses of glucocorticoids in the dosage range of 400 mg/day or less of hydrocortisone or equivalent.[6]

#### Adrenal Crisis

Acute adrenal insufficiency, or adrenal crisis, is a life-threatening condition that typically occurs in individuals with already marginal adrenocortical function who are subjected to a significant acute physiologic stressor, such as infection or trauma. Sudden and complete loss of adrenal function, as occurs with WFS and certain hypercoagulable states, can also manifest with adrenal crisis. Clinical findings include shock, abdominal pain, fever, nausea and vomiting, electrolyte disturbances and, occasionally, hypoglycemia. Mineralocorticoid deficiency, resulting in an inability to maintain sodium and intravascular volume, is the primary pathogenetic mechanism, although diminished cardiovascular responsiveness to catecholamines caused by glucocorticoid deficiency also plays a role. The treatment of adrenal crisis centers around large-volume (>2 liters) IV resuscitation with isotonic saline and glucocorticoid administration in the form of hydrocortisone (100 mg IV every 6 to 8 hours) or dexamethasone (4 mg IV every 24 hours). Dexamethasone is long-acting and carries the advantage of not interfering with biochemical assays of endogenous glucocorticoid production. Ironically, mineralocorticoid replacement is not an early priority, because the sodium- and fluid-retaining effects of mineralocorticoids do not manifest until several days after administration. Fluid and electrolyte balance can be rapidly achieved by saline infusion.

## Diagnosis and Treatment

### Diagnosis

As is true for most endocrine disorders, the diagnosis of adrenal insufficiency depends on maintaining sufficient clinical suspicion for the disease. The clinical manifestations have been discussed earlier. Surgeons are most likely to encounter patients with adrenal insufficiency in the intensive care unit, trauma suite, or operating room when treating patients with steroid-dependent chronic illnesses. Routine and provocative biochemical testing is necessary to confirm the diagnosis (Fig. 41-7). The first step is to document inadequate cortisol production, which can be done by measuring morning levels of cortisol in the serum or saliva. In most patients, morning serum cortisol concentration higher than 15 μg/dL or morning salivary cortisol concentration higher than 5.8 ng/mL effectively excludes adrenal insufficiency. Patients whose levels fall below these thresholds should undergo provocative testing. A high-dose cosyntropin stimulation test is performed by administering 250 μg cosyntropin and measuring serum cortisol levels 30 to 60 minutes later. A positive test (i.e., a stimulated cortisol level lower than 18 μg/dL) is strongly suggestive of adrenal insufficiency. After the diagnosis of adrenal insufficiency has been made, a morning ACTH level is determined to differentiate between primary and secondary adrenal insufficiency.

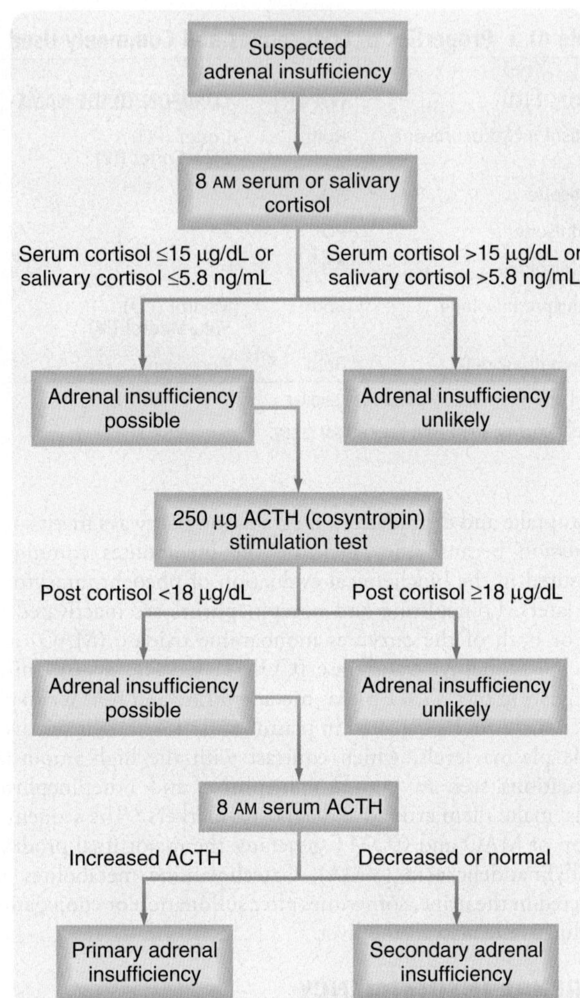


**FIGURE 41-7** Algorithm for the diagnosis of adrenal insufficiency. The adequacy of cortisol production is initially assessed with morning cortisol level measurement. Patients with low or borderline values undergo provocative ACTH stimulation testing, with serum cortisol levels measured before and 30 to 60 minutes after the administration of ACTH. Failure to mount an adequate response to ACTH usually establishes the diagnosis of adrenal insufficiency. The cause of adrenal insufficiency is then investigated with a morning ACTH level measurement.

### Treatment

The treatment of adrenal crisis has been discussed. The goal of maintenance therapy for chronic adrenal insufficiency is to replace physiologic glucocorticoid and mineralocorticoid levels. Daily adult cortisol production is in the range of 10 to 20 mg, which can be replaced by the long-acting, orally bioavailable agent prednisone at a dosage of 5 mg/day. Typical mineralocorticoid replacement consists of fludrocortisone, 0.1 mg/day. Commensurate increased dosages of glucocorticoids are needed during periods of minor and major physiologic stress, such as mild infections (minor) and trauma, significant infections, burns, or elective surgery (major).

## Perioperative Steroid Administration

Recommendations concerning glucocorticoid administration during elective surgery have been based primarily on uncontrolled retrospective studies. The need for supraphysiologic doses of glucocorticoids in this setting has generally been overstated. Patients with secondary adrenal insufficiency caused by chronic glucocorticoid treatment for autoimmune or inflammatory conditions have a 1% to 2% risk of hypotensive crisis without perioperative glucocorticoid coverage. To prevent this rare but hazardous complication, chronic glucocorticoid users should, at the least, be maintained on their usual glucocorticoid dosage throughout the perioperative period. Supplementation above this level should be given in short courses according to the guidelines listed in Table 41-2.[7] Patients undergoing unilateral adrenalectomy should only be given supplemental glucocorticoids if the underlying diagnosis is Cushing's syndrome.

**Table 41-2 Perioperative Glucocorticoid Regimens for Patients With Secondary Adrenal Insufficiency***

| DEGEREE OF SURGICAL STRESS | EXAMPLES | DAILY GLUCOCORTICOID DOSE |
|---|---|---|
| Minor | Procedures under local anesthesia, most outpatient procedures, inguinal hernia repair | Hydrocortisone, 25 mg or equivalent |
| Moderate | Routine abdominal, peripheral, vascular, or orthopedic surgery | Hydrocortisone, 50-75 mg or equivalent |
| Major | Resection of gastrointestinal cancer, cardiopulmonary bypass | Hydrocortisone, 100-150 mg or equivalent |

Adapted from Salem M, Tainsh RE Jr, Bromberg J, et al: Perioperative glucocorticoid coverage. A reassessment 42 years after emergence of a problem. Ann Surg 219:416–425, 1994.

*Caused by chronic pharmacologic steroid use.

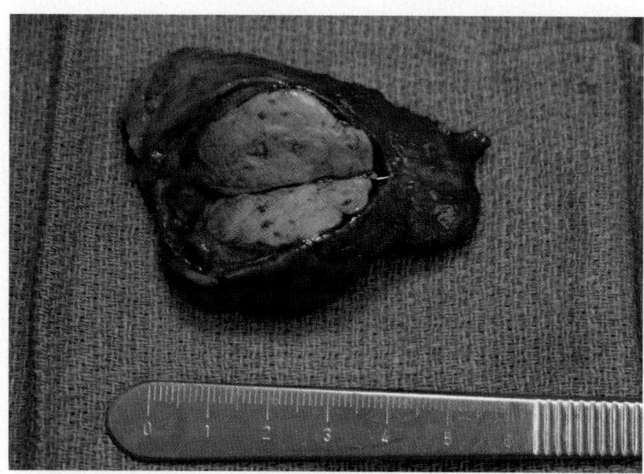

**FIGURE 41-8** Classic canary yellow aldosteronoma.

**Table 41-3 Causes of Primary Hyperaldosteronism (%)***

| CAUSE | Screening SELECTIVE | NONSELECTIVE |
|---|---|---|
| Aldosterone-producing adenoma | 60 | 30 |
| Bilateral adrenal hyperplasia (idiopathic hyperaldosteronism) | 35 | 65 |
| Aldosterone-producing adrenocortical carcinoma | <1 | <1 |
| Familial hyperaldosteronism | | |
| Type 1 (glucocorticoid-remediable aldosteronism) | <1 | <1 |
| Type 2 (non-glucocorticoid-remediable aldosteronism) | <1 | <1 |

*Rates of specific pathologies are highly dependent on the pattern of screening (selective versus nonselective).

## DISEASES OF THE ADRENAL CORTEX

## Primary Hyperaldosteronism

### Epidemiology and Clinical Features

Primary hyperaldosteronism, the unregulated release of excess aldosterone from one or both adrenal glands, was first described by Jerome Conn in 1954. Primary hyperaldosteronism classically presents with resistant hypertension and hypokalemia, although studies have revealed that most patients may be normokalemic, depending on the population screened. Hypokalemia is likely a manifestation of severe or late-stage disease. The prevalence of primary hyperaldosteronism has been the topic of considerable debate. It was generally believed to affect approximately 1% of hypertensives. Widespread application of the aldosterone-to-renin ratio (see later) as a screening test in certain centers has led to reports of a 10% to 40% prevalence of primary hyperaldosteronism among hypertensive patients.[8] There is some consensus that these higher figures reflect strong referral bias, and that the actual prevalence in unselected hypertensive patients is likely to be 7% or less. Nonselective use of the aldosterone-to-renin ratio to identify patients with primary hyperaldosteronism is known to decrease the fraction of patients with surgically correctible disease (unilateral aldosteronoma) significantly, although the absolute number of surgically treatable cases has increased.[9]

The mean age at diagnosis for primary hyperaldosteronism is approximately 50 years and the disease has a slight male predilection. Most patients are asymptomatic, although patients with significant hypokalemia may complain of muscle cramps, weakness, or paresthesias. Patients typically have moderate to severe hypertension that is refractory to medical therapy. It is common for them to require two to four antihypertensive medications. Responsiveness to spironolactone may be seen, a feature that is predictive of a good response to surgical treatment.

Primary hyperaldosteronism is a potentially curable cause of significant cardiovascular disease. A study comparing 124 subjects with biochemically confirmed primary hyperaldosteronism with hypertensive controls matched for age and systolic blood pressure has revealed that primary hyperaldosteronism is associated with a significantly increased risk of stroke, myocardial infarction, atrial fibrillation, and left ventricular hypertrophy.[10] These results add to existing evidence indicating that the adverse cardiovascular sequelae of primary hyperaldosteronism are more pronounced than those caused by blood pressure elevation alone. Successful removal of an aldosteronoma leads to regression of many of these adverse physiologic changes.

The most common causes of primary hyperaldosteronism are unilateral aldosterone-producing adenomas (aldosteronomas; Fig. 41-8) and bilateral adrenal hyperplasia (also termed *idiopathic hyperaldosteronism;* Table 41-3). In the past, aldosteronoma was present in more than 60% of cases, but this number has decreased substantially as nonselective screening with the aldosterone-to-renin ratio has been applied. This phenomenon may reflect increased detection of hyperplasia, which is characterized by milder biochemical abnormalities than aldosteronoma.

### Diagnosis and Localization

**Biochemical Diagnosis** The goal of diagnostic testing is to identify and lateralize aldosteronomas. There is some consensus that biochemical screening should be performed in all patients with hypertension and unexplained hypokalemia, as well as those with hypertension sufficiently resistant to medical therapy to warrant investigation for secondary hypertension. Establishing the diagnosis of primary hyperaldosteronism begins with determining the ratio of plasma aldosterone concentration to plasma renin activity (expressed here as ng/dL divided by ng/[mL • hr]; Fig. 41-9). This test should be performed after discontinuation of interfering medications, such as spironolactone, angiotensin-converting enzyme (ACE) inhibitors, diuretics, and β-adrenergic blockers. Variable cutoff values have been used in the literature, but a value of 30 yields a sensitivity of approximately 90%.[11] A subset of patients with essential hypertension will have suppressed renin levels, which may result in false elevations of the aldosterone-to-renin ratio. Thus, the inclusion of an absolute aldosterone concentration higher than 15 mg/dL increases the specificity of initial screening. Patients who test positive and are younger than 30 years should be genetically screened for glucocorticoid-remediable aldosteronism (familial hyperaldosteronism type I), especially if they have a family history of early-onset hypertension. This rare autosomal dominant condition results in abnormal regulation of aldosterone synthesis by ACTH and can be medically treated.

Confirmatory biochemical testing is aimed at demonstrating inappropriately high (nonsuppressible) aldosterone levels by creating a state of hypervolemia–sodium excess. This is done with IV saline loading (2 to 3 liters of isotonic saline given over 4 to 6 hours, followed by measurement of plasma aldosterone) or oral salt loading (200 mEq = 5000 mg sodium daily over 3 days, followed by measurement of 24-hour urine aldosterone excretion). Some centers administer high-dose fludrocortisone (0.1 mg every 6 hours) during oral salt loading to increase the specificity of suppression testing, but this method has not been widely adopted.

**Localization** After the diagnosis has been confirmed, localization is performed with anatomic imaging, selective venous sampling, and sometimes functional scanning. The fact that most aldosteronomas are smaller than 15 mm in maximum dimension poses some challenges to localization. Thin-cut (3-mm) adrenal computed tomography (CT) scanning is the preferred initial localization test (Fig. 41-10).

The next step in the localization algorithm is selective adrenal venous sampling (AVS). This test relies on the simultaneous measurement of cortisol and aldosterone levels in the peripheral circulation and left and right adrenal veins (Fig. 41-11). More than a fivefold elevation of the cortisol concentration in a sample relative to peripheral blood indicates successful cannulation of an adrenal vein (positive control). Lateralization is indicated by an unbalanced ratio of aldosterone to cortisol in the left and right adrenal veins, with the ratio on one side being fourfold higher than the other to identify the culprit gland.

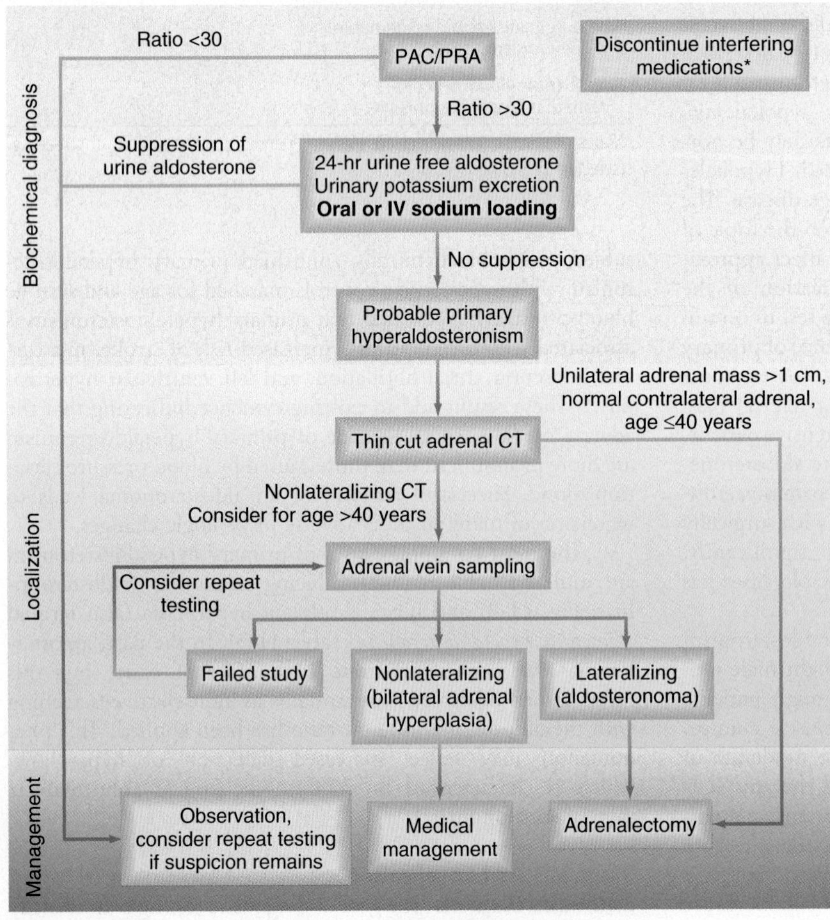


**FIGURE 41-9** Algorithm for diagnosis, localization, and management of primary hyperaldosteronism. Initial screening is done with the PRA/PAC ratio being determined, followed by confirmatory testing with sodium loading. After the biochemical diagnosis has been established, noninvasive localization is attempted with CT. Patients with clear CT evidence of a unilateral abnormality can proceed to adrenalectomy with a >90% cure rate. AVS is done in patients with equivocal CT findings and older patients, especially those older than 60 years, because nonfunctional cortical adenomas are found in 4% or more of this population and can cause false-positive CT localization. PAC, Plasma aldosterone concentration, in ng/dL; PRA, plasma renin activity, in ng/(mL • hr).

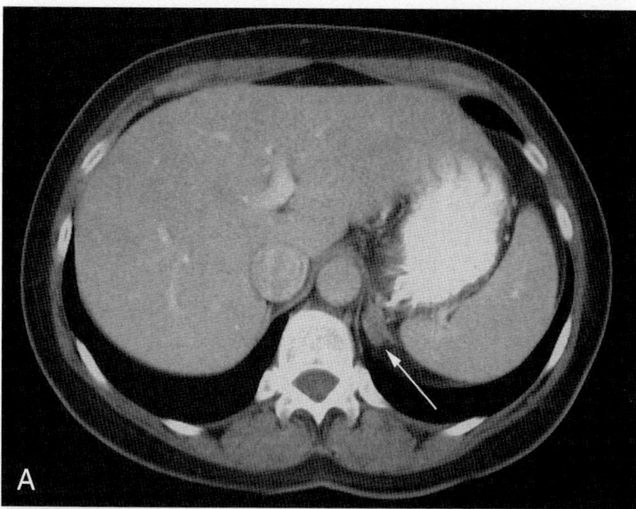


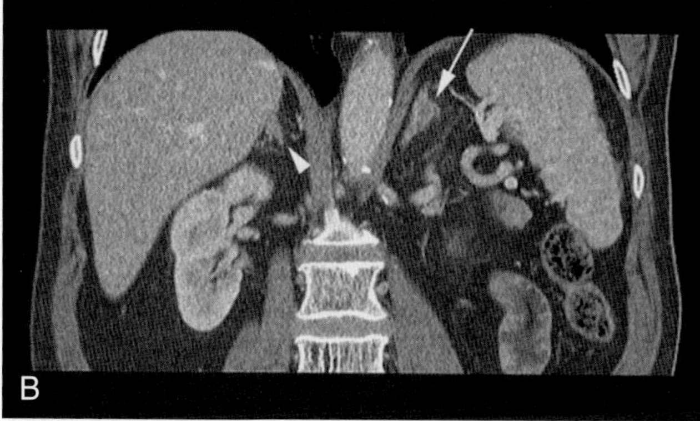


**FIGURE 41-10** Appearance of aldosteronoma on anatomic imaging. **A,** Venous phase, contrast-enhanced CT demonstrating a 2-cm left aldosteronoma *(arrow)*. **B,** Late arterial phase, coronal CT demonstrating a 1.7-cm left aldosteronoma *(arrow)* and a normal right adrenal gland *(arrowhead)*.

Considerable controversy exists over which patients should undergo AVS, an invasive procedure with a 90% technical success rate in experienced hands. There is consensus that AVS should be applied in all cases in which the biochemical diagnosis of primary hyperaldosteronism has been confirmed and thin-cut adrenal CT reveals no abnormalities or bilateral abnormalities. Of the remaining patients who have a unilateral mass on CT scan, a small but not insignificant fraction (2% to 10%) will represent false-positive localization and have persistent hyperaldosteronism after unilateral adrenalectomy. In these patients, the adrenal mass represents a nonfunctioning cortical adenoma and the true underlying diagnosis is a contralateral microaldosteronoma or bilateral adrenal hyperplasia, the latter of which is not surgically remediable.

Because patients 40 years and older are more likely to possess nonfunctioning adrenal cortical adenomas, some have advocated AVS in all older patients[12] and others have recommended universal application of this test in the workup of primary hyperaldosteronism.[13] It has been our practice to perform AVS selectively. Patients found to have a unilateral cortical adrenal mass larger than 1 cm in diameter and a normal contralateral adrenal gland on CT can proceed to directly to adrenalectomy, whereas those without definitive CT localization undergo AVS. This strategy has yielded cure rates in excess of 95%.[14]

Practically speaking, approximately 20% to 30% of patients being evaluated for primary hyperaldosteronism undergo AVS when it is applied to select patients. The usefulness of the test is limited by its low success rate in most reports (40% to 80%), with the most common reason for incomplete AVS being failure to cannulate the right adrenal vein. Frequently, however, sufficient lateralizing information is provided during AVS to guide surgical treatment, even when the study is not bilaterally selective.[15]

### Surgical Management and Outcomes

Laparoscopic adrenalectomy is the preferred procedure for the management of aldosteronoma and most other adrenal tumors.[16] Cure of primary hyperaldosteronism is defined by clinical and biochemical end points. Reductions in blood pressure, antihypertensive medication requirements, plasma and urine aldosterone levels, and resolution of hypokalemia (if previously present) are observed as soon as 24 hours after successful surgery. Overall cure rates range from 75% to 95% at subspecialty centers, depending on the specific criteria for cure that are used. In general, more than 80% of patients can expect normalization of blood pressure or a significant reduction in antihypertensive medication requirements (typically, from three or four medications down to one). In some patients, depending on the degree of preoperative sodium overload, blood pressure may take several weeks to improve. Our practice is to stop all antihypertensive medications immediately after surgery, with the exception of beta blockers and clonidine, which must be tapered to avoid a rebound phenomenon. For those patients who continue to be hypertensive in the short term, medications may be added back temporarily, as needed, until the blood pressure gradually reaches a new equilibrium over time.

A subset of patients with the following preoperative features display reduced benefit from surgical treatment and continue to require antihypertensive medications after operation: men older than 45 years, family history of hypertension, longstanding hypertension, and nonresponse to spironolactone. These indicate a component of essential hypertension and, in some cases, irreversible cardiovascular alterations caused by chronic disease. Based on these features, patients should be appropriately counseled as to what they should expect to gain from surgery.

## Cushing's Syndrome

### Epidemiology and Clinical Features

The clinical features of glucocorticoid excess were first documented by Harvey Cushing in 1912. He described a young woman of "extraordinary appearance" who developed obesity, hirsutism, amenorrhea, easy bruising, and extreme muscle weakness. The principal differential diagnosis to be considered when evaluating patients for Cushing's syndrome is obesity, an increasingly common condition. A subset of signs and symptoms, including easy bruising, muscle weakness, hypertension, plethora (a red facial appearance caused by thinning of the skin), and hirsutism, may allow discrimination between Cushing's syndrome and obesity based on clinical features (Fig. 41-12). The most common cause of Cushing's syndrome is pharmacologic glucocorticoid use for the treatment of

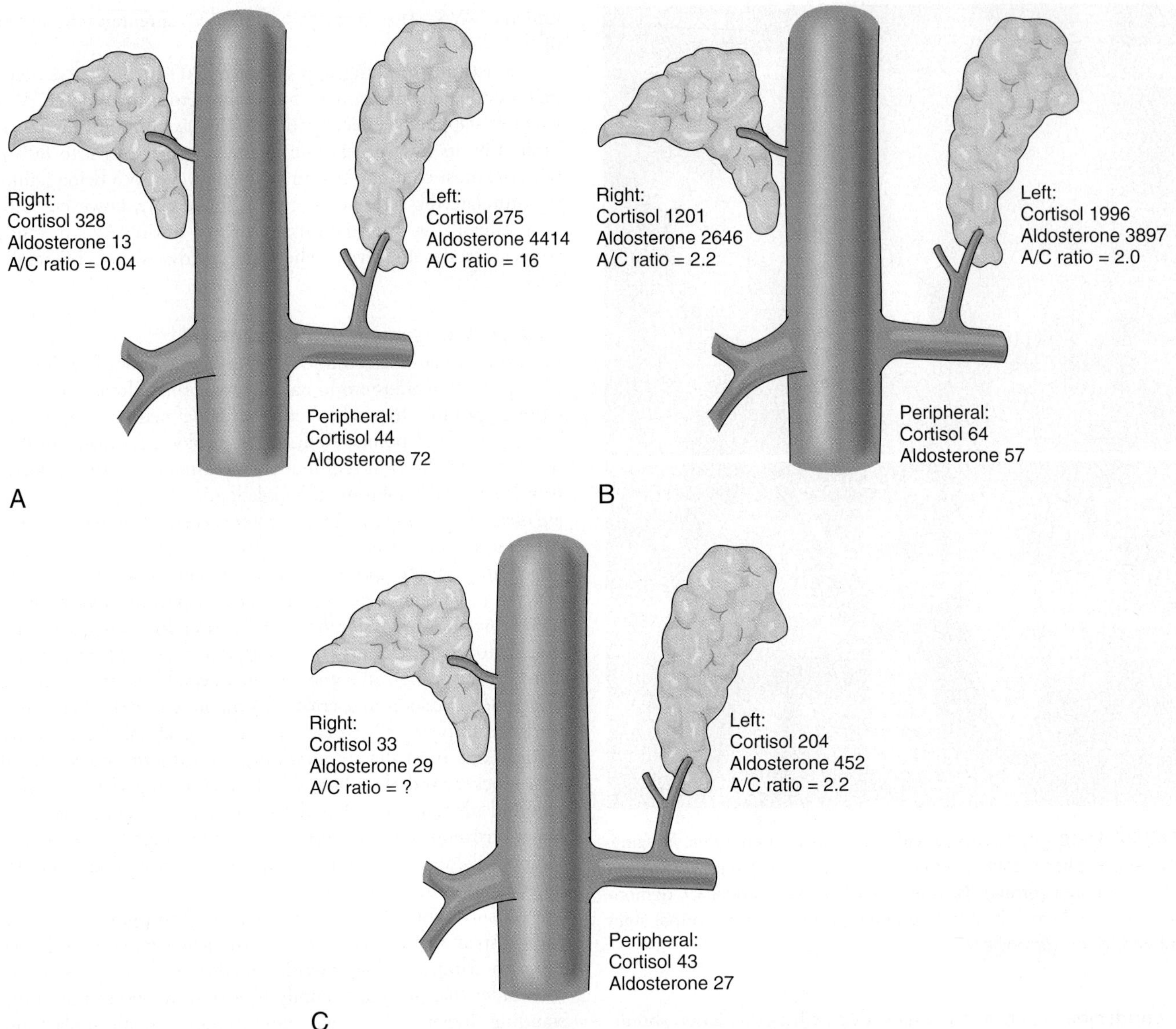


**FIGURE 41-11** Possible outcomes of AVS for primary hyperaldosteronism. Aldosterone is expressed in ng/dL, cortisol in µg/dL. **A,** Successful study lateralizing strongly to the left adrenal. **B,** Successful study, nonlateralizing. Stimulation with ACTH yielded high adrenal vein cortisol levels. **C,** Failed study. The right adrenal vein was not cannulated.

inflammatory disorders. Endogenous Cushing's syndrome is rare, affecting 5 to 10 individuals/million. Of these, most affected individuals (75%) will have Cushing's disease—that is, glucocorticoid excess caused by an ACTH-hypersecreting pituitary adenoma. The remainder will be split between primary adrenal Cushing's syndrome (15%) and ectopic ACTH syndrome (<10%), the latter of which usually is caused by from neuroendocrine tumors or bronchogenic malignancies arising in the thorax.

Cushing's syndrome is a lethal disease. The physiologic derangements resulting from glucocorticoid excess, including hypertension (present in >70% of cases), hyperglycemia, and truncal obesity, ultimately yield a fivefold excess mortality, primarily because of cardiovascular complications.[17] Thus, all efforts should be made to identify and appropriately treat patients with Cushing's syndrome.

### Biochemical Diagnosis and Localization

The diagnosis of Cushing's syndrome is reliant on demonstration of inappropriate cortisol secretion or the loss of physiologic negative feedback. Normally, cortisol release follows a predictable circadian rhythm, peaking approximately 1 hour after waking and reaching a nadir around midnight. Thus, inappropriate cortisol secretion can be detected as elevated cortisol release over a 24-hour period or as a higher than expected level in the late evening. Traditionally, lack of negative feedback has been assessed using dexamethasone suppression testing and other types of provocative tests, many of which are cumbersome and require inpatient hospitalization. The development of late evening salivary cortisol testing has provided an attractive and feasible alternative to suppression testing.

More than 90% of circulating cortisol is bound to plasma proteins. Unbound cortisol can be detected in the urine and

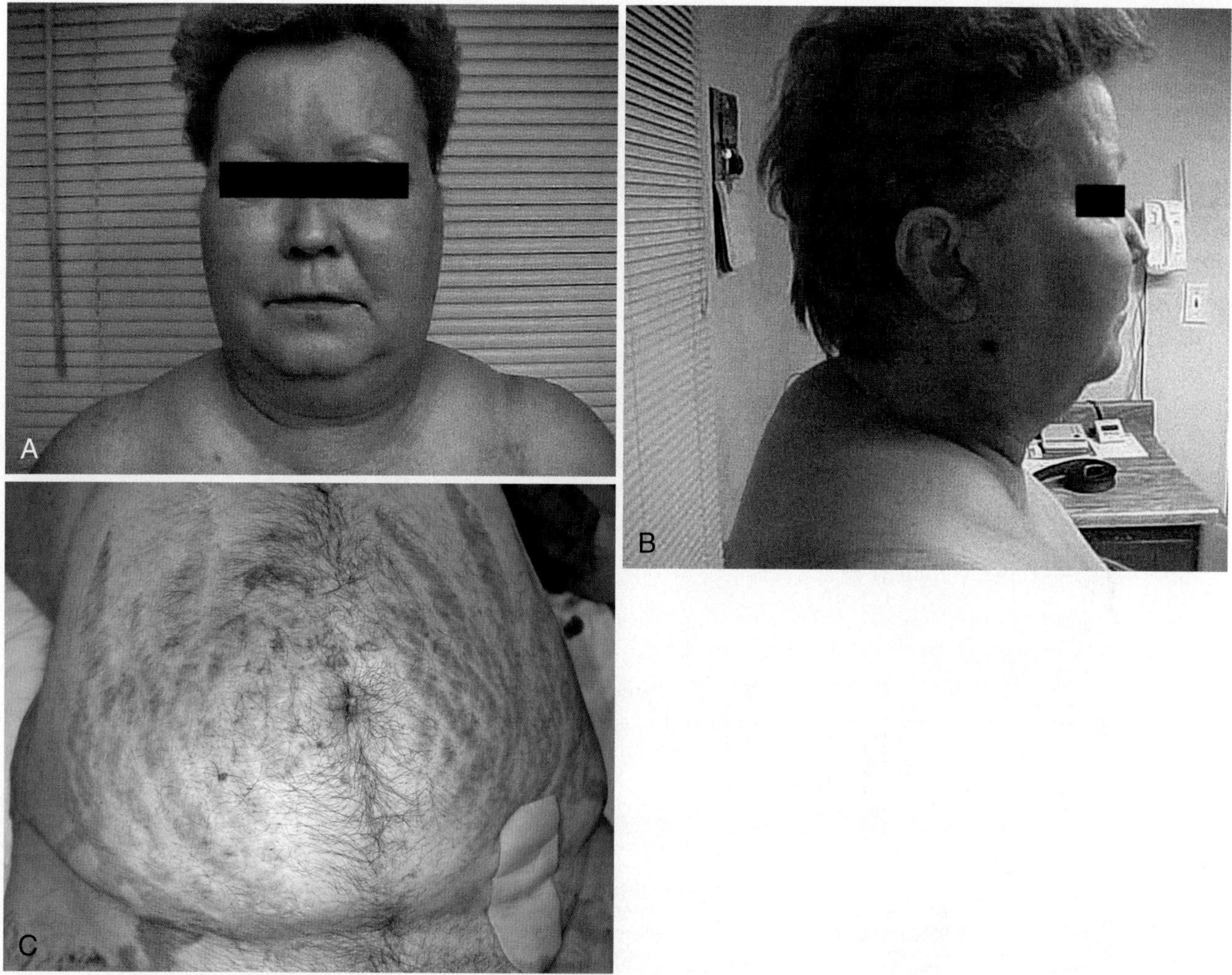

**FIGURE 41-12** Clinical manifestations of Cushing's syndrome. **A,** Moon facies, plethora, and excess supraclavicular fat in a woman with Cushing's syndrome. **B,** Buffalo hump in a woman with Cushing's syndrome. **C,** Purple abdominal striae in a man with Cushing's syndrome.

saliva, and assessment of these body fluids forms the basis of biochemical screening for Cushing's syndrome (Fig. 41-13); 24-hour urine collection for urine free cortisol should be performed at least twice for initial screening. Unequivocally elevated levels should prompt immediate further testing to determine the cause and subtype of Cushing's syndrome (i.e., primary adrenal cause versus pituitary cause versus ectopic ACTH syndrome). Patients with moderately elevated 24-hour urine cortisol levels should undergo confirmatory testing with two late evening (bedtime) cortisol measurements. A high cutoff value of 550 ng/mL has a sensitivity of 93% and specificity of 100%.[18]

Primary adrenal Cushing's syndrome, also termed *ACTH-independent Cushing's syndrome,* is caused by autonomous adrenal cortisol production and therefore is generally associated with an undetectable ACTH level (<5 pg/mL) because of feedback inhibition. The underlying pathology is variable, with solitary adrenal adenoma found in approximately 90% of cases, adrenocortical carcinoma in less than 10%, and bilateral micronodular or macronodular hyperplasia in less than 1%. Almost all these lesions, except micronodular hyperplasia, are readily apparent on CT scans.

Hypercortisolemia associated with normal or elevated ACTH levels is indicative of ACTH-dependent Cushing's syndrome, most commonly caused by a pituitary corticotroph microadenoma (Cushing's disease). Suspicion for ACTH-dependent Cushing's syndrome should prompt pituitary imaging and high-dose dexamethasone suppression testing—that is, serum or urine cortisol measurement after administration of 2 mg dexamethasone every 6 hours over 48 hours. Dexamethasone is chosen because it does not cross-react with biochemical assays for cortisol. Corticotroph adenomas are commonly suppressed in response to high-dose dexamethasone administration, whereas ectopic ACTH sources are completely lacking in feedback inhibition. Slightly more than 50% of corticotroph microadenomas are visible on pituitary magnetic resonance imaging (MRI). Detection of a pituitary mass larger than 6 mm in diameter in a patient with ACTH-dependent Cushing's syndrome that is suppressed with high-dose dexamethasone justifies proceeding to pituitary surgery.[19] In the absence of a demonstrable mass, bilateral inferior petrosal sinus ACTH sampling (IPSS) with CRF stimulation should be pursued. Demonstration of a central to peripheral ACTH gradient in a study performed by a skilled physician is sufficient to diagnose Cushing's disease.

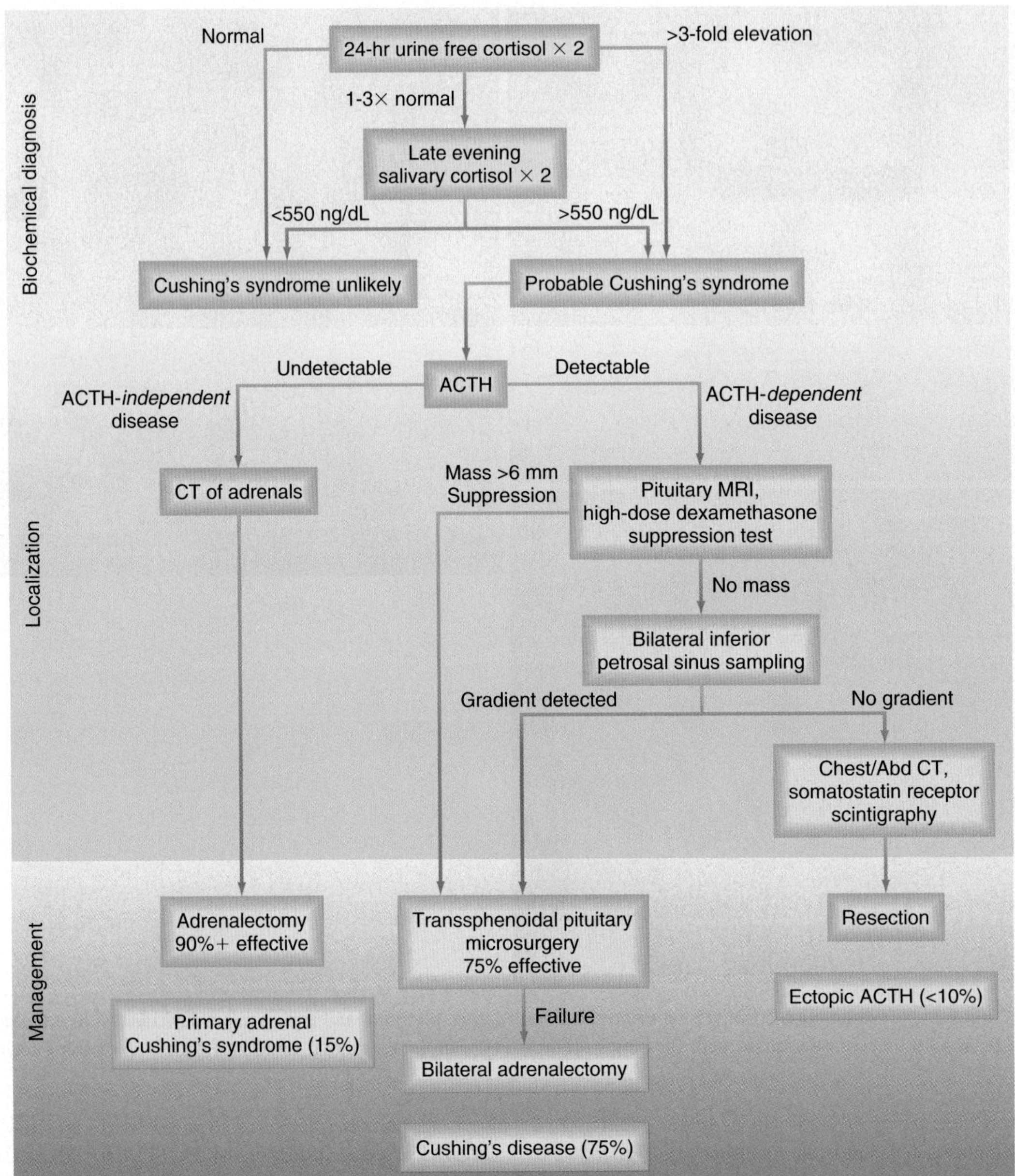


**FIGURE 41-13** Algorithm for the diagnosis, localization, and management of endogenous Cushing's syndrome. A biochemical diagnosis can be established with an unequivocally elevated 24-hour urine free cortisol level (greater than a threefold elevation) or an elevated late evening salivary cortisol. Most cases of Cushing's syndrome are caused by Cushing's disease (pituitary corticotroph microadenoma), in which the plasma ACTH level is elevated. An undetectable ACTH level establishes the diagnosis of ACTH-independent Cushing's syndrome and prompts adrenal imaging. Bilateral adrenalectomy is considered for patients with Cushing's disease not cured by trans-sphenoidal surgery.

The absence of a clear gradient should prompt CT imaging of the chest and abdomen and, occasionally, somatostatin receptor scintigraphy to identify an ectopic ACTH source.

## Surgical Management and Outcomes

Perioperative and postoperative glucocorticoid administration is obviously essential in the care of patients with Cushing's syndrome. For patients undergoing adrenalectomy for Cushing's syndrome, perioperative stress dose steroids (e.g., hydrocortisone, 100 mg IV, every 8 hours for 24 hours) are recommended. In the most common scenario of resection of a solitary adrenal Cushing's adenoma, steroids can usually be tapered to physiologic replacement levels over the course of several weeks. However, a subset of patients with Cushing's syndrome of longer duration and severity will demonstrate lasting HPA axis suppression, requiring glucocorticoid supplementation for longer periods, sometimes longer than 1 year.

The management of patients who undergo pituitary surgery for Cushing's disease is variable. In some centers, glucocorticoids are withheld during the immediate postoperative period to provide a window during which early remission may be assessed.[20] A subnormal morning cortisol level on postoperative day 1 or 2 is indicative of cure. Glucocorticoid supplementation is then resumed until the HPA axis recovers, usually for at least 6 months. Because of the significant risk of postoperative adrenal crisis in patients with Cushing's syndrome of all subtypes, glucocorticoid management is ideally done in conjunction with an experienced endocrinologist.

Adrenalectomy is more than 90% effective in the treatment of primary adrenal Cushing's syndrome. Resolution of symptoms typically takes months to years,[21] and certain deleterious physiologic effects regarding bone density, body composition, and inflammation are extremely persistent.[22,23] Failures may result from local and occasionally distant tumor recurrence in the case of malignant disease. Pituitary microsurgery for Cushing's disease, typically performed via a transnasal transsphenoidal approach, is approximately 90% successful in expert hands. Remission rates may be improved by reoperation or pituitary irradiation for patients whose basal cortisol levels do not fall appropriately after initial surgery. Laparoscopic bilateral adrenalectomy should be considered for patients in whom pituitary surgery has failed.[24]

### Special Case: Subclinical Cushing's Syndrome

The term *subclinical Cushing's syndrome* has been used to describe patients with incidentally discovered adrenal masses (see later, "Incidentally Discovered Adrenal Mass") who display biochemical evidence of cortisol hypersecretion without overt signs or symptoms of Cushing's syndrome. This disease entity has been incompletely characterized with respect to its physiologic consequences and natural history. Clear-cut definitions for the diagnosis of subclinical Cushing's syndrome, such as cutoff values for biochemical tests and objective assessment guidelines for the presence or absence of clinical features, are lacking.

Hypertension, dyslipidemia, and impaired glucose tolerance appear to be more prevalent among individuals with subclinical Cushing's syndrome compared with normal individuals. However, adrenalectomy for this entity has not been consistently demonstrated to yield health benefits, and progression to overt Cushing's syndrome occurs in less than 10% of cases. A recent randomized controlled trial comparing surgery with observation in 45 patients with subclinical Cushing's syndrome noted more frequent resolution of hypertension in the surgically treated group.[25] At present, patients found to have subclinical hypercortisolism should be monitored for the development of adverse cardiovascular and metabolic features, with most experts agreeing that surgery should be performed selectively in patients exhibiting progressive disease. However, lower biochemical thresholds for surgical treatment should be considered in patients with larger (3- to 4-cm) tumors and those whose tumors enlarge on serial imaging studies.

## Sex Steroid Excess

Adrenal tumors causing clinical features of sex steroid excess are rare. Most of these tumors are virilizing (as opposed to feminizing), and may present at a late stage in association with an advanced adrenal malignancy. Almost all feminizing tumors are malignant, whereas approximately one third of virilizing tumors are malignant. Of adrenocortical carcinomas, 20% cause virilization, with most these cases occurring in children. An additional 24% of adrenocortical carcinomas will display mixed features of Cushing's syndrome and virilization.[26] Virilizing tumors may be biochemically detected using measurements of 24-hour urine testosterone, DHEA, and DHEA-S. Although laparoscopic adrenalectomy remains the preferred procedure for most sex steroid–secreting tumors, the high probability of malignancy merits close radiographic and intraoperative monitoring for evidence of invasion and/or metastasis. Open adrenalectomy should be performed for malignant tumors.

## Adrenocortical Carcinoma

Adrenocortical carcinoma is a rare tumor, with an annual incidence of approximately 1/million. Almost all cases occur in patients aged 40 to 50 years, although there is a minor peak in occurrence among children younger than 5 years. They demonstrate no significant gender predilection. At the time of presentation, adrenocortical carcinomas tend to be very large (mean tumor size, 9 to 13 cm) and have usually spread beyond the confines of the adrenal gland.[27] Historically, overall 5-year survival rates have been in the 15% to 20% range. Among patients who undergo surgical resection, 5-year survival is approximately 40%, a figure that has essentially remained unchanged over the past 2 decades.[28] A higher risk of death is associated with increasing patient age, poorly differentiated or high-grade tumors, positive surgical margins, and the presence of distant metastases. More than 50% of adrenocortical carcinomas are functional. Cushing's syndrome is most commonly seen, followed by virilization. Radiographic evaluation is primarily performed with CT, which typically reveals a heterogenous mass with irregular or indistinct borders, central necrosis, and invasion of adjacent structures (Fig. 41-14). Metastases to lymph nodes, liver, and lungs may be found.

Treatment of adrenocortical carcinoma centers around radical open surgery. Complete resection can be achieved in up to 70% of patients in experienced hands. This frequently involves en bloc resection of adjacent organs and/or regional lymphadenectomy. Particular care must be taken when dealing with right-sided adrenocortical carcinomas larger than 9 cm, because direct tumor extension into the inferior vena cava and sometimes the right heart may be observed. Tumors demonstrating intravascular extension may need to be resected while the patient is on cardiopulmonary bypass to reduce the likelihood of lethal intraoperative tumor embolization.[29]

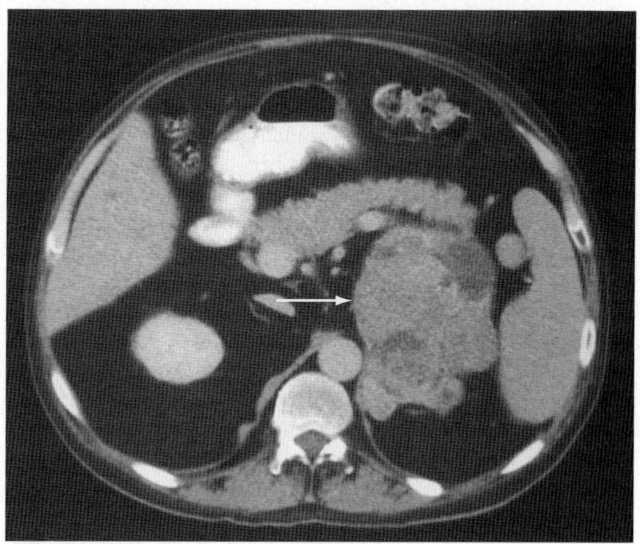

**FIGURE 41-14** CT scan demonstrating a 10-cm left adrenocortical carcinoma. Note the areas of central necrosis *(arrow)*.

Patients who undergo incomplete resection of adrenocortical carcinomas have extremely limited life expectancy (median survival < 1 year). Even those who undergo successful surgery are prone to developing local recurrence and metastases, which typically occur within 2 years. The principle chemotherapeutic agent for the treatment of adrenocortical carcinoma is mitotane (*o,p′*-DDD [1,1-dichloro-2-{*o*-chlorophenyl}-2-{*p*-chlorophenyl} ethane]), a derivative of the insecticide DDT that is a direct adrenocortical toxin. Mitotane has been used clinically as an adjuvant to surgery and as primary therapy in individuals with unresectable or metastatic disease. A multinational retrospective study examining the efficacy of adjuvant mitotane following radical surgery has demonstrated a significant improvement in recurrence-free survival.[30] The use of mitotane is limited by significant, dose-dependent gastrointestinal and neurologic toxicity. The ongoing multinational FIRM-ACT trial compares etoposide, doxorubicin, cisplatin, and mitotane versus streptozotocin and mitotane in patients with locally advanced or metastatic adrenocortical carcinoma, with the intent of defining standard initial combination chemotherapy for this disease. A number of other trials are examining targeted agents such as epidermal growth factor (EGF) inhibitors, insulin-like growth factor 1 (IGF-1) inhibitors, antiangiogenic agents, and broad-spectrum tyrosine kinase inhibitors. There is also an emerging interest in individualized therapy based on genomic and expression profiling of tumors.[31]

## DISEASES OF THE ADRENAL MEDULLA

### Pheochromocytoma

#### Epidemiology and Clinical Features

The first account of pheochromocytoma was published in 1886 by Felix Frankel, who described a young woman suffering from intermittent attacks of palpitations, anxiety, vertigo, and headache. Autopsy revealed bilateral adrenal tumors that stained brown when treated with chromium salts. Because of the characteristic positive chromaffin reaction, these adrenomedullary tumors are termed *pheochromocytoma* (dusky-colored tumor, from the Greek *phaios,* dusky). Successful surgical management of pheochromocytoma was initially described in 1926 by César Roux and Charles Mayo.[32]

Pheochromocytoma affects approximately 0.2% of hypertensive individuals. Men and women are affected equally. The peak incidence in sporadic cases is between the ages of 40 and 50 years, whereas familial cases tend to manifest earlier. A subset of patients present with the classic triad of headache, diaphoresis, and palpitations, although almost all patients will display at least one of these symptoms. Hypertension is present in 90% of cases and may be episodic or sustained. The principle challenge in making the diagnosis of pheochromocytoma arises from the fact that essential hypertension is common and the clinical features suggestive of pheochromocytoma are nonspecific. In fact, only 0.5% of patients with hypertension and suggestive features will ultimately prove to have the disease. The differential diagnosis of pheochromocytoma is wide, encompassing diverse processes such as hyperthyroidism, hypoglycemia, coronary artery disease, heart failure, stroke, drug-related effects, and panic disorder. Pheochromocytoma has been described as a biologic time bomb because of the potentially lethal cardiovascular effects of the bioactive compounds secreted by these tumors. Thus, despite the challenges in diagnosis, clinicians should screen for this disease aggressively and seek appropriate treatment for affected patients.

Previously, pheochromocytoma was termed the *10% tumor,* suggesting that 10% are bilateral, 10% malignant, 10% extra-adrenal, and 10% familial. Discoveries regarding the genetic underpinnings of pheochromocytoma have challenged these old axioms.

#### Biochemical Diagnosis and Localization

Establishing the biochemical diagnosis of pheochromocytoma is based on the detection of elevated levels of catecholamines and their metabolites in bodily fluids. Measurements of 24-hour urine levels of these compounds have long been the cornerstone of biochemical testing, and are still the most reliable tests available. In 2002, measurement of free (unconjugated) metanephrines in plasma was introduced as an alternative screening tool for pheochromocytoma. Plasma-free metanephrine testing carries an extremely high sensitivity, approaching 99%, and, being a one-time blood test, is more convenient than 24-hour urine testing. However, the specificity of plasma-free metanephrine testing is 89% at best, with specificities at most laboratories likely to be in the 85% range or below. Given that pheochromocytoma is a rare diagnosis that is sought within a large pool of hypertensive individuals, false-positive test results are a major problem. It has been estimated that false-positive test results outnumber true-positive test results as much as 30 : 1 when plasma-free metanephrine testing is used as a principal screening tool.[33]

Therefore, the primary usefulness of plasma-free metanephrine testing is to exclude pheochromocytoma when the test is negative (Fig. 41-15). When positive, confirmatory testing with 24-hour urine levels of catecholamines and their metabolites is required. Many drugs and conditions are capable of confounding catecholamine-based testing, contributing further to the problem of false-positive results. These include sympathomimetics (present in many cold remedies), phenoxybenzamine (frequently initiated when suspicion for pheochromocytoma is raised), acetaminophen (which interferes with the plasma-free metanephrine assay), many psychotropic drugs (notably tricyclic antidepressants), and major physical or psychological stressors. Tests performed during episodes of acute pain, critical illness, or urgent hospitalization may be misleading. The presence of confounding factors is extremely common in the population being screened, because they represent manifestations or treatments of competing diagnoses. Clearly, biochemical testing should be ideally performed when the patient is as free as practically possible of all confounding factors.

The operating characteristics of catecholamine-based plasma and urine tests are listed, along with corresponding cutoff values, in Table 41-4. Cutoff values for 24-hour urine tests are deliberately set high to maximize specificity; these values are approximately double the upper 95% reference range in most laboratories. A urine collection may be considered positive if total metanephrines or any single catecholamine fraction (e.g., epinephrine, norepinephrine, dopamine) is elevated above its cutoff value. This approach maintains high specificity and yields an acceptable sensitivity of 88%.[34] Importantly, it takes into account the fact that pheochromocytomas synthesize and metabolize catecholamines, and that tumors may possess

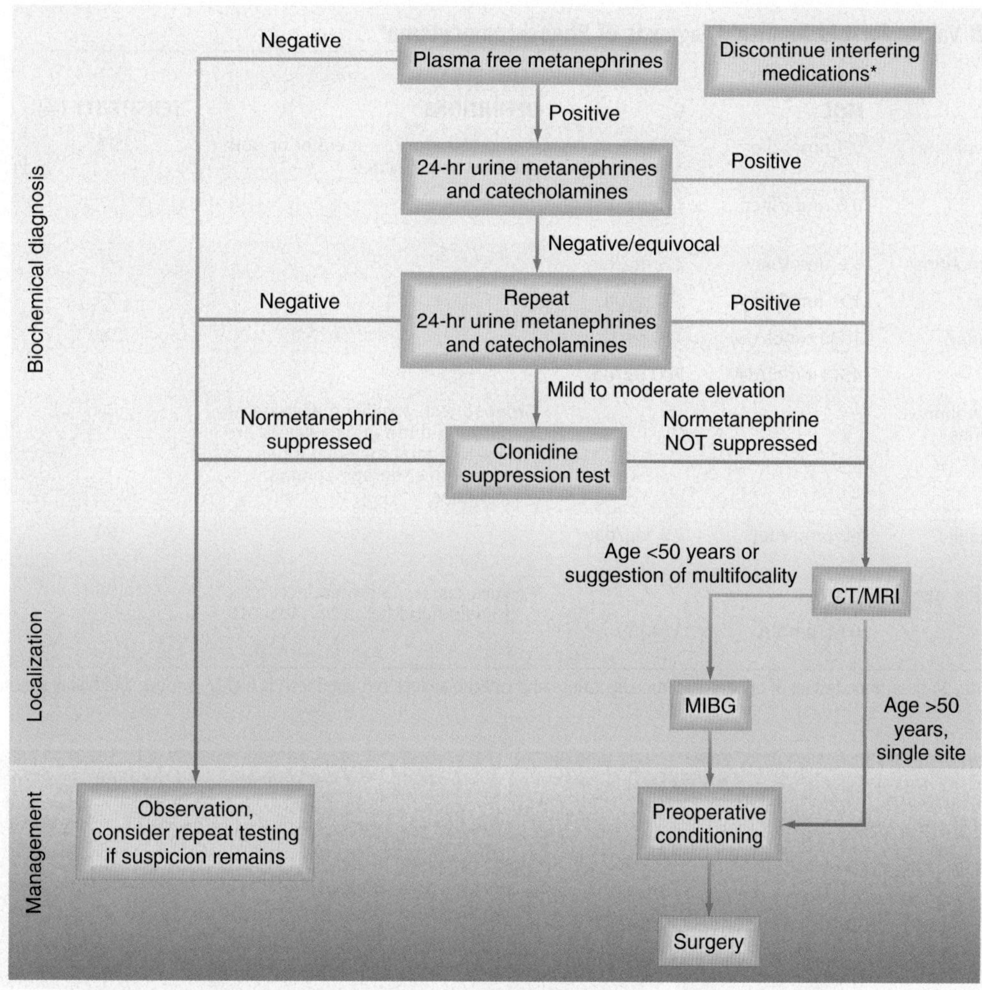


**FIGURE 41-15** Algorithm for the diagnosis, localization, and management of pheochromocytoma. Initial plasma free metanephrine testing can effectively exclude the diagnosis if negative. Twenty-four-hour urine collection for catecholamines and their metabolites is generally performed twice, with cutoffs approximately twice the upper limit of normal being criteria for positivity (see Table 41-4). Clonidine suppression testing can be used for the small fraction of patients in whom the diagnosis remains uncertain after urine testing. Localization with CT or MRI follows biochemical confirmation of the diagnosis, with MIBG scanning performed for younger patients and those otherwise at risk for multifocal disease. Phenoxybenzamine is given in escalating doses for at least 2 weeks before surgery.

heterogenous secretory profiles, depending on their relative expression of synthetic and degradative enzymes (see Fig. 41-6).

Two 24-hour urine collections for catecholamines and their metabolites are sufficient to make (or exclude) the diagnosis of pheochromocytoma in almost all cases. Clonidine suppression testing, the measurement of plasma-free normetanephrine levels after the oral administration of 0.3 mg clonidine, may help clarify equivocal test results. Anatomic localization may be performed with MRI or CT. MRI is slightly more sensitive, but CT often yields better anatomic definition for operative planning (Fig. 41-16). Scintigraphy with $^{131}$I- or $^{123}$I-labelled metaiodobenzylguanidine (MIBG; see Fig. 41-17) should be performed in select patients in whom multifocal disease is suspected. MIBG scanning is highly specific for pheochromocytoma, but carries a sensitivity of only 77% to 90%. Positron emission tomography (PET) and PET-CT using novel radionuclides such as $^{18}$F-L-dihydroxyphenylalanine ($^{18}$F-DOPA; see Fig. 41-16D) and $^{18}$F-dopamine are highly sensitive and superior to MIBG scanning in the imaging of pheochromocytoma.[35,36] However, the availability of these techniques remains confined to a small number of academic centers worldwide.

## Perioperative Care

Throughout the first half of the 20th century, perioperative mortality rates in the treatment of pheochromocytoma ranged from 26% to 50%. Currently, the mortality rate in most specialized centers is approximately 1%. This dramatic improvement can largely be ascribed to advances in pharmacology, physiology, anesthesia, and perioperative medical care. The adverse perioperative hemodynamic changes most commonly observed with pheochromocytoma are intraoperative hypertension and postoperative hypotension. Intraoperative hypertension may be caused by stimulation of catecholamine release by anesthetic induction agents as well as by direct manipulation of the tumor. Postoperative hypotension may be profound. It results from a state of hypovolemia created by the presence of excess circulating

**Table 41-4 Cutoff Values for Biochemical Diagnosis of Pheochromocytoma***

| | Cutoff Value | | | | |
|---|---|---|---|---|---|
| **TEST*** | **MOL** | **G** | **DEFINITIONS** | **SENSITIVITY (%)** | **SPECIFICITY (%)** |
| Plasma-free metanephrine | 0.3 nmol/liter | 59 μg/L | Paired test, positive if either or both values are elevated | 99 | 85-89 |
| Plasma-free normetanephrine | 0.6 nmol/liter | 110 μg/L | | | |
| Urinary total metanephrines | 6.6 μmol/day | 1.3 mg/day | | 71 | 99.6 |
| Urinary epinephrine | 191 nmol/day | 35 μg/day | | 29 | 99.6 |
| Urinary norepinephrine | 1005 nmol/day | 170 μg/day | | 50 | 99.6 |
| Urinary dopamine | 4571 nmol/day | 700 μg/day | | 8 | 100 |
| Urinary total metanephrines **and** catecholamines | — | | Grouped test, positive if any one of following three urinary values are elevated: total metanephrines, epinephrine, norepinephrine, dopamine | 88 | 99 |
| Urinary vanillylmandelic acid | 40 μmol/day | 7.9 mg/day | | 64 | 95 |
| Clonidine suppression test | | | Positive result = elevated level after clonidine and fall of less than 40 | 96 | 100 |
| Plasma-free normetanephrine | 0.61 nmol/L | 112 μg/L | | | |

*When performed twice, 24-hour urine testing of urinary total metanephrines and catecholamines (grouped test) is highly sensitive and highly specific.

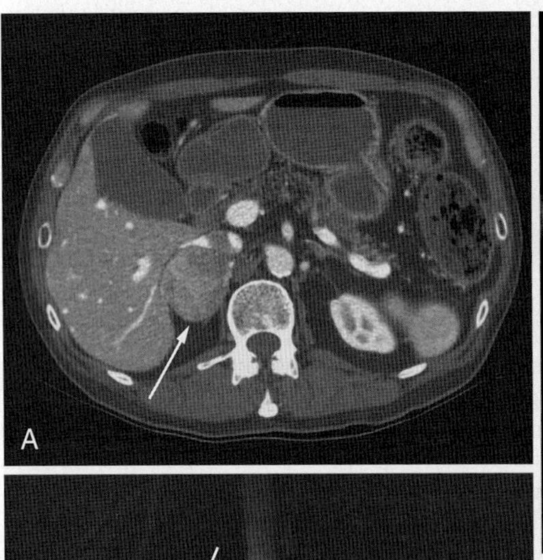


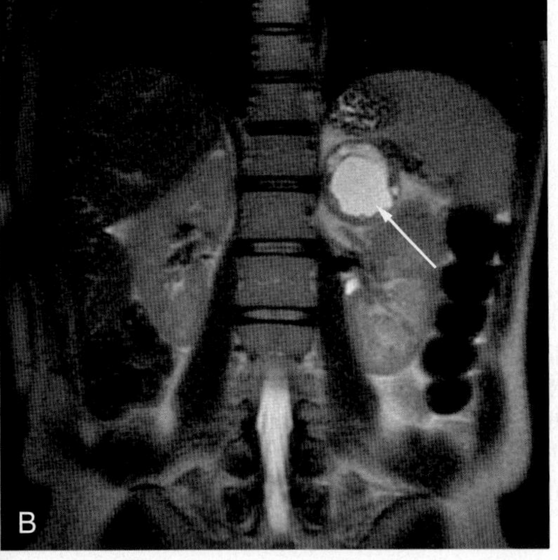


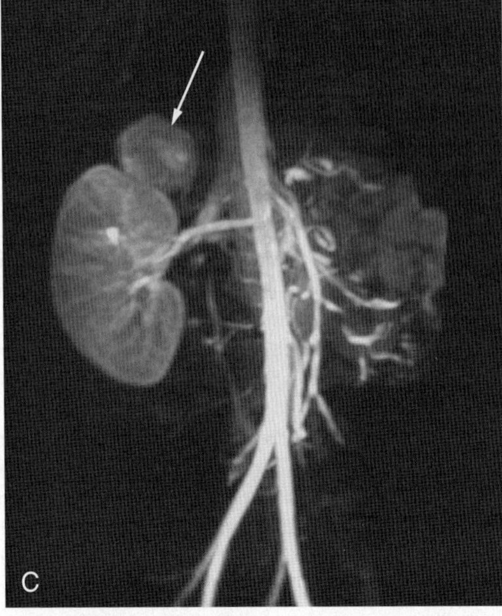


**FIGURE 41-16** Appearance of pheochromocytoma on anatomic imaging. **A,** Venous phase, contrast-enhanced CT scan demonstrating a right adrenal pheochromocytoma *(arrow).* The heterogeneity in the inferior vena cava represents swirling of contrast, not tumor thrombus or invasion. **B,** Coronal T2-weighted MRI scan demonstrating a left adrenal pheochromocytoma with central cystic change *(arrow).* **C,** Left anterior oblique MR angiographic reconstruction demonstrating a right adrenal pheochromocytoma *(arrow).*

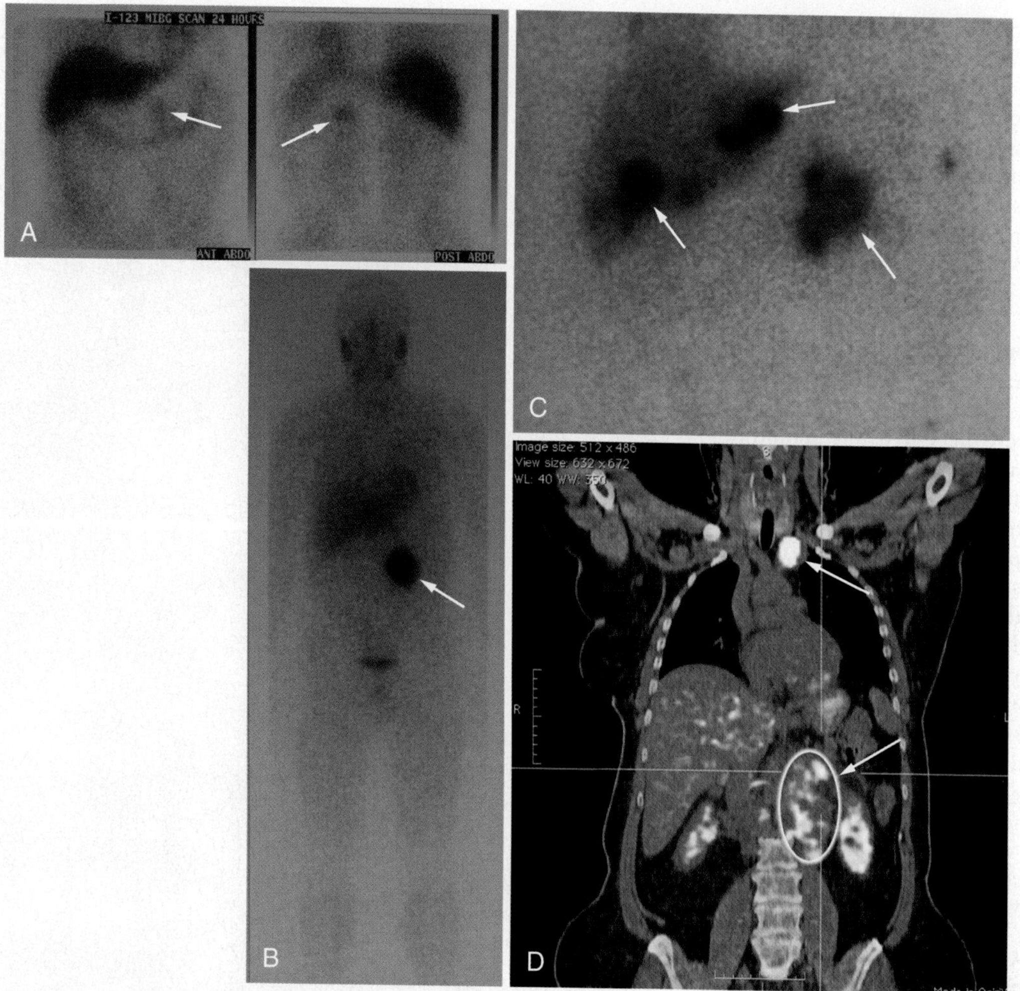


**FIGURE 41-17** Appearance of pheochromocytoma on functional imaging (MIBG scanning). **A,** $^{123}$I-MIBG scan of the abdomen demonstrating an isolated left adrenal pheochromocytoma *(arrows).* Physiologic radiotracer uptake is noted in the liver, right colon, and transverse colon. **B,** Whole-body $^{131}$I-MIBG scan demonstrating a large, left, para-aortic extra-adrenal pheochromocytoma *(arrow).* Physiologic radiotracer uptake is noted in the liver, salivary glands, and bladder. **C,** $^{131}$I-MIBG scan of the abdomen demonstrating malignant pheochromocytoma, with local recurrence in the left adrenal bed and liver metastases *(arrows).* **D,** $^{18}$F-DOPA PET-CT scan in a patient with malignant multifocal pheochromocytoma. Diffuse uptake above background is seen in the region of the left adrenal gland and left periaortic region, where a locally invasive tumor was found at surgery *(arrow).* A second area of intense tracer uptake is seen in the left paratracheal region, where a carotid sheath paraganglioma was found *(arrow).* The patient is an *SDHB* mutation carrier.

catecholamines. Sudden withdrawal of this stimulus after tumor removal leads to peripheral arteriolar vasodilation and a dramatic increase in venous capacitance, which together may precipitate cardiovascular collapse. In their early report of a large successful case series, investigators at the Mayo clinic described the use of intraoperative α-adrenergic blockade followed by aggressive volume repletion and the administration of α-adrenergic agonists in the immediate postoperative period.[37]

The principles of perioperative care remain much the same. As soon as the biochemical diagnosis of pheochromocytoma has been confirmed, α-adrenergic blockade should be initiated to protect against hemodynamic lability. Our practice is to start with phenoxybenzamine 10 mg twice daily. The dosage can be titrated upward every 2 to 3 days to a maximum of 40 mg three times daily to achieve normalization of heart rate and blood pressure. The period of preoperative conditioning should last at least 2 weeks to allow for adequate reversal of α-adrenergic receptor downregulation. This restores sensitivity to vasopressor agents, which can then be used to treat the patient postoperatively. Phenoxybenzamine is a nonspecific, noncompetitive (irreversible), long-acting (half-life of 24 hours) α-adrenergic antagonist. Although its use is associated with the side effects of postural hypotension and significant nasal congestion, it is generally favored over $\alpha_1$-adrenergic selective agents, such as prazosin and doxazosin. Nasal congestion can actually serve as a useful indicator of adequate blockade. Furthermore, phenoxybenzamine provides the most complete alpha blockade among available agents, and its pharmacokinetics permit serum drug levels to decay in parallel with catecholamine levels postoperatively.

Beta blockers may be administered after adequate alpha blockade has been achieved for the subset of patients with persistent tachycardia. Beta blockers should never be the first agent administered, because a decrease in peripheral vasodilatory beta receptor stimulation results in unopposed α-adrenergic tone, which may exacerbate hypertension. Preoperative volume expansion with isotonic fluids has been advocated in the past. However, in our experience, the need for this is significantly reduced when aggressive preoperative alpha blockade has been achieved, because the resultant increase in venous capacitance restores euvolemia. Clinical suspicion for hypovolemia should remain high in the postoperative period and patients should be aggressively resuscitated if they become hypotensive or oliguric. Some patients may require vasopressors after tumor removal, especially if preoperative alpha blockade is incomplete.

### Surgical Management and Outcomes

Successful operative treatment of pheochromocytoma is dependent on close communication between the surgeon and anesthesiologist. Invasive hemodynamic monitoring is required and fluid management must be meticulous. Manipulation of the tumor should be minimized and the anesthetic team should be prepared to administer supplemental IV alpha and beta blockers, as well as vasopressors, when necessary.

Surgery is curative in more than 90% of pheochromocytoma cases. Although these tumors are highly vascular and tend to adhere to adjacent structures (Fig. 41-18), most of them can be removed successfully using a laparoscopic approach. Laparoscopic resection is contraindicated when preoperative imaging demonstrates local invasion. Advances in surgical technique have resulted in reduced operative complication rates. Specifically, functional image-guided focused exploration has replaced bilateral adrenal and retroperitoneal exploration, leading to diminished rates of solid organ injury. The largest North American series on pheochromocytoma, published in 2010, described 108 operations, 90% of them laparoscopic.[38] The perioperative morbidity rate was 13% and there were no deaths.

### Molecular Genetics of Pheochromocytoma

A number of reports describing novel germline mutations have demonstrated that familial pheochromocytomas are much more common than previously believed. Before 2000, pheochromocytoma was known to be associated with multiple endocrine neoplasia type 2 syndromes (40% to 50% penetrant), von Hippel-Lindau syndrome (10% to 20% penetrant), and neurofibromatosis type 1 (1% to 5% penetrant). The discovery that neuroendocrine cells of the carotid body proliferate in response to hypoxic stimuli has led to the identification of mutations in the succinate dehydrogenase gene family in kindreds affected with pheochromocytoma or paraganglioma. Succinate dehydrogenase, which is made up of four subunits, is localized to the mitochondria and catalyzes essential steps in oxidative phosphorylation. Germline mutations in the B and D subunits, inherited in an autosomal dominant fashion, have been identified in approximately 10% of apparently sporadic pheochromocytoma cases. Thus, there is a consensus that 21% to 30% of pheochromocytomas are familial.[39]

Familial cases manifest at an earlier age and are more likely to be multifocal. Succinate dehydrogenase B mutation carriers have high rates of extra-adrenal (abdominal or thoracic) pheochromocytomas and malignant disease, whereas succinate dehydrogenase D carriers tend to manifest with multiple tumors and hormonally inactive paragangliomas of the head and neck. The lifetime penetrance of succinate dehydrogenase mutations is estimated at more than 75%.[40] Several clinical features are known to be predictive of mutation carrier status and should prompt genetic testing. These include age younger than 45 years, multiple tumors, extra-adrenal location, and previous head and neck paraganglioma.[41]

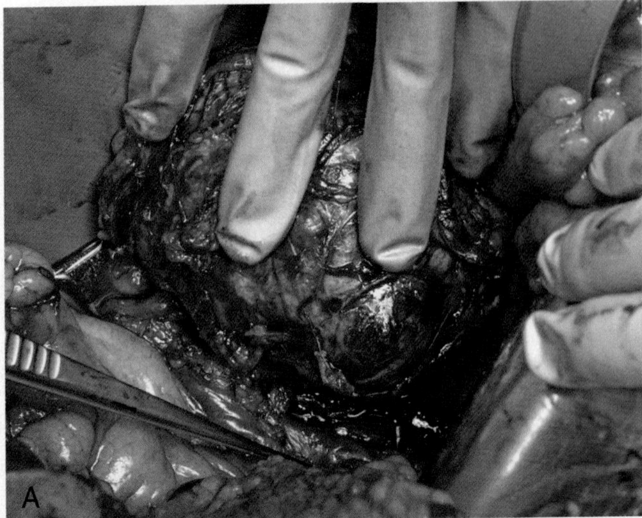


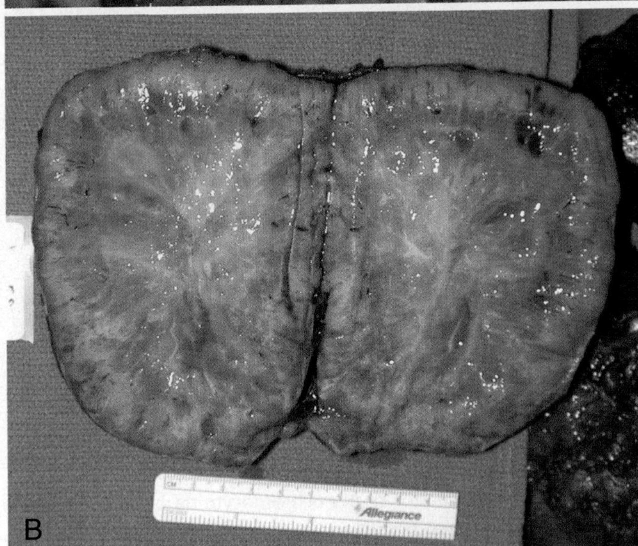


**FIGURE 41-18** Gross appearance of pheochromocytoma. **A,** Open resection of a left para-aortic extra-adrenal pheochromocytoma (depicted in Fig. 41-17B) via an infracolic approach. The patient's head is to the right. The tumor is being rotated medially by the surgeon's hand to reveal the left ureter, indicated by forceps. **B,** Left adrenal pheochromocytoma. (**A,** Courtesy Dr. Stan Sidhu.)

### Malignant Pheochromocytoma

Depending on the underlying genotype, 2.5% to 40% of pheochromocytomas are malignant. Survival at 5 years ranges from 20% to 45%. No histopathologic criteria for determining malignancy have demonstrated the ability to predict the clinical course accurately. Thus, malignancy is defined by the development of metastases (i.e., tumor implants distant from the primary mass in locations in which neuroectodermal tissues are not normally found). The latter criterion distinguishes metastatic disease from possible multifocal primary disease. The most common sites of metastasis are the axial skeleton, lymph nodes, liver, lung, and kidney. Treatment of primary and recurrent disease centers on surgical resection, which, even in the absence of cure, may have significant palliative benefits in terms of managing mass effect in critical anatomic locations and reducing the systemic impact of catecholamine excess.[42]

Malignant pheochromocytomas are minimally responsive to radiotherapy and chemotherapy. In a recent phase II study, high-dose $^{131}$I-MIBG radionuclide therapy was shown to achieve a complete or partial response rate of 22% in select patients with metastatic pheochromocytoma.[43] Significant hematologic toxicities were observed and long-term benefit remains uncommon. Chronic medical management of catecholamine excess should be performed with $\alpha_1$-adrenergic selective blockers because of their favorable side effect profile.

## OTHER ADRENAL DISEASES

### Incidentally Discovered Adrenal Mass (Incidentaloma)

#### Epidemiology and Differential Diagnosis

Incidentally discovered adrenal masses, also termed *clinically inapparent adrenal masses* or *incidentalomas,* are discovered through imaging performed for unrelated nonadrenal disease. Their existence as a clinical entity is a byproduct of advanced medical imaging. Incidentalomas were first described in the early 1980s, when CT scanners became more prevalent in developed nations, and they have become a common clinical problem as the use of CT and MRI has become widespread. Incidentalomas have been found in 2.1% of autopsies and 1% to 4% of abdominal imaging studies.[44] The prevalence has increased to more than 4% in patients older than 60 years.

The differential diagnosis of adrenal incidentaloma is wide and includes secreting and non-ecreting neoplasms (Fig. 41-19). In patients with a history of malignancy, metastatic disease is the most likely cause of adrenal masses, particularly when bilateral (see later, "Metastases to the Adrenal Gland"). In those without a clear history of malignancy, at least 80% of incidentalomas will turn out to be nonfunctioning cortical adenomas or other benign lesions, which do not require surgical management. Thus, in most patients, the most important aspect of management is to distinguish the subset of adrenal masses that are likely to have a clinical impact from the large proportion that are not.

#### Clinical Evaluation and Surgical Management

The workup of the adrenal incidentaloma integrates hormonal evaluation with size criteria. The principles and methods of hormonal evaluation have been discussed in the tumor-specific sections (see earlier) and are generally applicable to incidentalomas. However, one conceptual difference is that the biochemical thresholds that prompt operative treatment are somewhat lower in patients with an initial radiographic presentation (incidentalomas) as compared with those with an initial clinical presentation. This is because tumor size, which correlates strongly with risk of malignancy, contributes an additive effect in favor of surgical management.

Evaluation begins with history taking, with a focus on prior malignancy, hypertension, and symptoms of glucocorticoid or sex steroid excess. Biochemical investigations for hormonally active tumors are followed by consideration of size criteria (Fig. 41-20). In a general sense, surgery is recommended for hormonally active tumors and those that carry a significant risk of malignancy. Adrenocortical carcinomas comprise less than 2% of adrenal tumors measuring 4 cm or smaller and roughly 6% of those measuring 4 to 6 cm. Tumors larger than 6 cm carry a more than 25% risk of malignancy. Because studies have consistently found that CT and MRI underestimate adrenal tumor size by approximately 20%, an effect that is exaggerated in smaller tumors, our practice is to remove all incidentalomas measuring 5 cm or larger and to consider strongly removal of those measuring 3 to 5 cm.[45] Factors that should be considered in surgical decision making for this latter group include suspicious imaging characteristics (e.g., heterogeneity, high attenuation, irregular margins), patient age and surgical risk, growth on interval imaging, and patient preference. If observation is chosen, patients should undergo repeat imaging in 6 to 12 months, given the fact that 5% to 25% of adrenal masses may increase in size.

It must be emphasized that CT-guided fine-needle aspiration (FNA) is rarely helpful in the evaluation of adrenal masses and may be hazardous. The diagnosis of primary adrenal malignancy cannot reliably be made based on cytologic criteria alone. Therefore, the use of FNA is generally confined to patients with a history of extra-adrenal malignancy in whom the clinician seeks to establish the diagnosis of metastatic disease. In all cases, pheochromocytoma must be excluded prior to attempting such a procedure to avoid precipitating a potentially fatal hypertensive crisis.

As with the other disease processes that have been discussed, most adrenal incidentalomas can be removed laparoscopically, except for those displaying obvious malignant features on imaging. No upper size limit to this approach has been established, and tumors measuring 15 cm have been successfully removed laparoscopically by experienced surgeons.

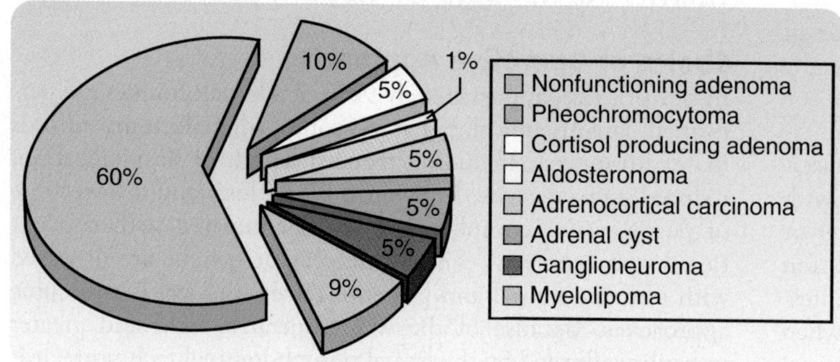


**FIGURE 41-19** Differential diagnosis of adrenal incidentaloma in patients without a history of malignancy. Approximate proportions of the various pathologies are shown.

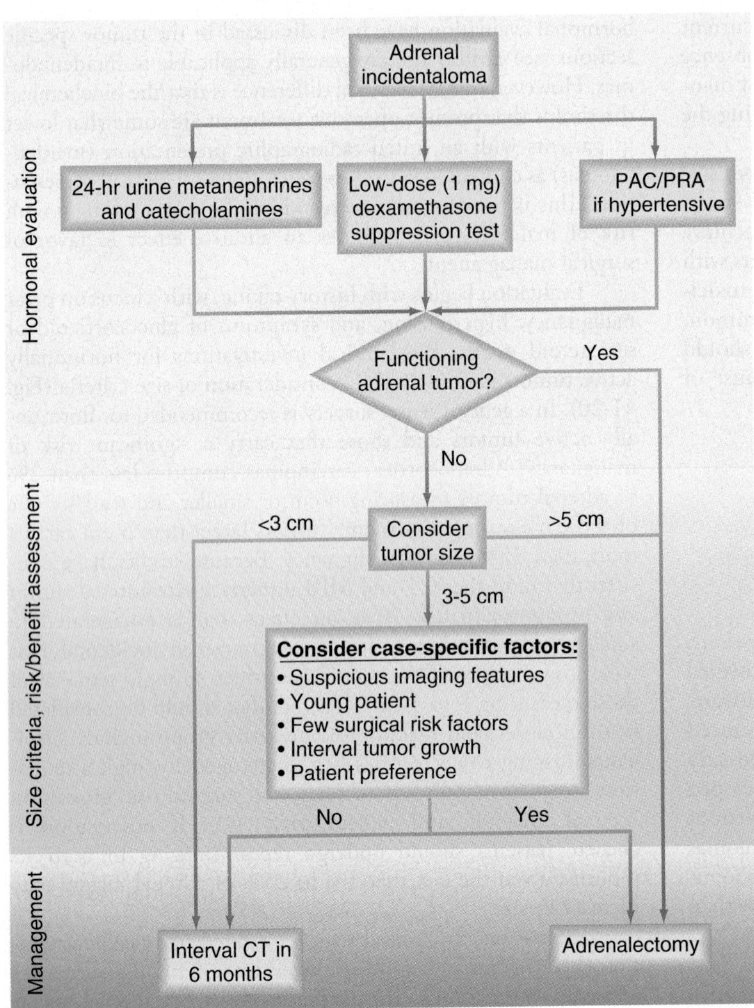


**FIGURE 41-20** Algorithm for the management of an adrenal incidentaloma. Adrenalectomy is recommended for all patients with functional tumors. For nonfunctioning tumors, the risk for malignancy is assessed according to size. Tumors larger than 5 cm on CT carry a >25% risk for malignancy and need to be removed. Those <3 cm can be safely observed. Case-specific factors must be considered for intermediate-sized tumors. PAC, Plasma aldosterone concentration, in ng/dL; PRA, plasma renin activity, in ng/(mL • hr).

## Metastases to the Adrenal Gland

### Epidemiology and Clinical Features

The adrenal glands are common sites of metastasis because of their rich vascular supply. Autopsy studies have revealed that approximately 25% of patients with carcinomas eventually develop adrenal involvement. In 50% of these cases, metastatic disease is bilateral. The primary cancers that most often spread to the adrenals are those of the lung, gastrointestinal tract, breast, kidney, pancreas, and skin (melanoma). Patients with isolated adrenal metastases represent a very small subset of the total. However, these individuals are of particular interest to the surgeon and oncologist because evidence has indicated that resection of isolated adrenal metastases may improve survival. Depending on the underlying pathology, 5-year survival rates of approximately 25% can be achieved after adrenalectomy.

### Clinical Evaluation and Surgical Management

Evaluation of patients presenting with isolated adrenal metastases must involve careful exclusion of extra-adrenal disease with CT or MRI—including the head in cases of breast cancer or melanoma, and triphasic contrast-enhanced CT evaluation of the liver plus 3-mm slices through the lungs for gastrointestinal malignancies—as well as bone and PET scanning, when appropriate. Patients presenting with isolated bilateral adrenal metastases (Fig. 41-21) must be evaluated for adrenal insufficiency because of replacement of all normal adrenal tissue with tumor, which may occur in up to 30% of these patients. This is best performed with measurement of morning cortisol and ACTH levels. Cortical insufficiency should be adequately treated prior to operation to avoid perioperative adrenal crisis.

Most adrenal metastases are well-encapsulated and are thus amenable to laparoscopic resection. Complete adrenal metastasectomy has yielded mean survival rates of 20 to 30 months in most series[46] as compared with 12 months for patients with incomplete resection and 6 months for patients not undergoing surgical therapy.

## TECHNICAL ASPECTS OF ADRENALECTOMY

### Choice of Operative Approach

In our practice, approximately 90% of adrenalectomies are performed laparoscopically. Laparoscopic adrenalectomy affords many advantages, including reduced length of hospitalization, reduced pain, decreased operative blood loss, and a lower rate of postoperative complications when compared with conventional open surgery.[47] Similar degrees of benefit are observed with transabdominal and posterior retroperitoneal laparoscopic approaches. Because of the wider operative field and greater versatility afforded by the lateral transabdominal technique, it is

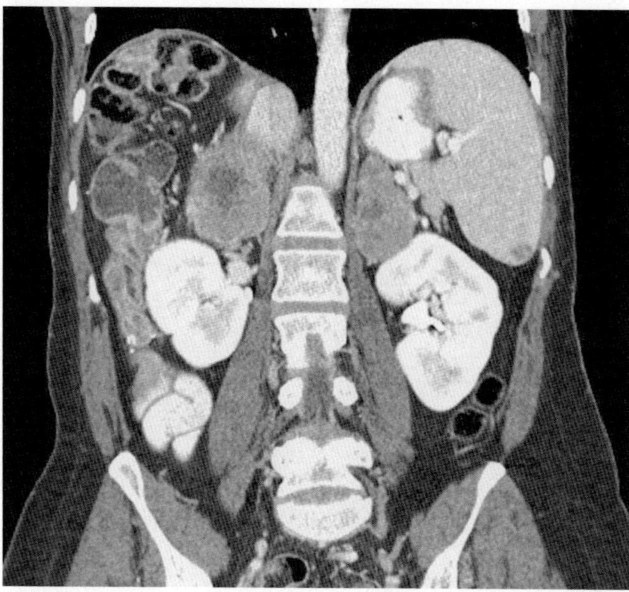

**FIGURE 41-21** Isolated bilateral 7-cm adrenal metastases from colorectal cancer causing adrenal insufficiency. The patient had undergone previous right colectomy and right hepatectomy. Bilateral adrenal metastasectomy was performed laparoscopically.

our favored approach and will be discussed in greater detail. The lateral transabdominal approach can be used to handle very large tumors and previous abdominal surgery does not alter the success rate significantly when the procedure is performed by an experienced surgeon.[48] The overall conversion rate to open adrenalectomy is less than 5% in large series.

As noted, open adrenalectomy should be performed for primary adrenal tumors demonstrating features suspicious for malignancy, such as large size (>8 cm), clinical feminization, hypersecretion of multiple steroid hormones, or any of the following imaging attributes: local or vascular invasion, regional adenopathy, and metastases. For open adrenalectomy, we also prefer a transabdominal approach, which is performed via a subcostal incision (see later).

## Laparoscopic Lateral Transabdominal Adrenalectomy

### Patient Preparation and Positioning

Drawsheets and a full-length beanbag are placed on the operating table in advance. It is important that the table be capable of flexion and have a kidney rest that can be elevated. The patient is initially positioned supine for the induction of anesthesia and placement of a urinary catheter. Intermittent pneumatic compression devices are applied to the legs. The placement of an orogastric or nasogastric tube for gastric decompression is frequently helpful, particularly when treating left-sided lesions. The patient is then turned on his or her side (80-degree lateral decubitus position), with the side of the lesion facing upward (Fig. 41-22). At this point, the patient is carefully positioned cephalocaudally so that the 10th rib is directly over the break point in the table. The table is flexed and the beanbag rigidified in a position that supports the buttocks and back while leaving the umbilicus, an important surface landmark, exposed. Flexing the table and raising the kidney rest serve to widen the space between

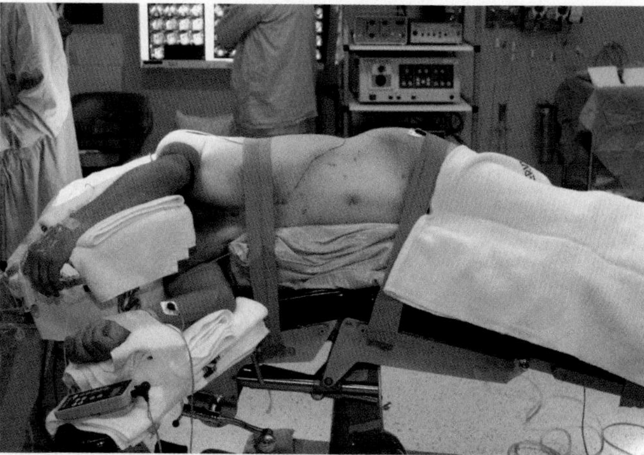

**FIGURE 41-22** Patient positioning for left lateral transabdominal laparoscopic adrenalectomy.

the costal margin and iliac crest and to drop the iliac crest away from the plane of the laparoscopic instruments. Wide cloth tape is used to secure the patient to the table at the chest, hips, and lower extremities. Great care must be taken to protect bony prominences and points of potential peripheral nerve compression in the extremities. The surgical preparation is carried from the nipple line to the pubis and from the umbilicus to the midline of the back.

Careful positioning is essential for technical success in laparoscopic adrenalectomy. As will be discussed, the surgeon is reliant on gravity to serve as a retractor for providing the necessary exposure. Having the patient securely fixed to the table permits the often extreme positioning with respect to pitch (Trendelenburg, reverse Trendelenburg) and roll (tilting left, right), that are necessary during the operation.

### Technique

**Left Adrenal** Initial peritoneal access is achieved 2 cm inferior to the costal margin in the midclavicular line (Palmer's point). This can be performed with the Veress technique in most cases. We generally use three radially dilating trocars and a fourth may be added in cases in which the spleen and pancreatic tail require additional retraction. The ports are equally distributed along the costal margin, with the posterior port placed as far lateral-posterior as permitted by the position of the colon (Fig. 41-23). It is advisable to leave at least 5 cm (4 fingerbreadths) between each port to minimize external interference of the laparoscopic instruments. For tissue dissection, we use the hook monopolar cautery and an energy-based tissue sealing or dividing device.

The lateral attachments of the spleen are taken down first, with the goal of rotating the left upper quadrant viscera anteromedially. Care must be taken to avoid a capsular tear of the spleen, which may arise from undue tension on a congenital or acquired adhesive band. Splenic mobilization is continued until the greater curvature of stomach becomes visible at its apex, at which point the spleen and tail of the pancreas are allowed to fall anteriorly with rightward tilting of the table and gentle use of the fan retractor, if necessary. It is critical to achieve the correct plane of dissection precisely during this part of the procedure because the tail of the pancreas and splenic vessels are potentially vulnerable to injury. In patients with large or inferiorly positioned tumors, the splenic flexure of the colon must be

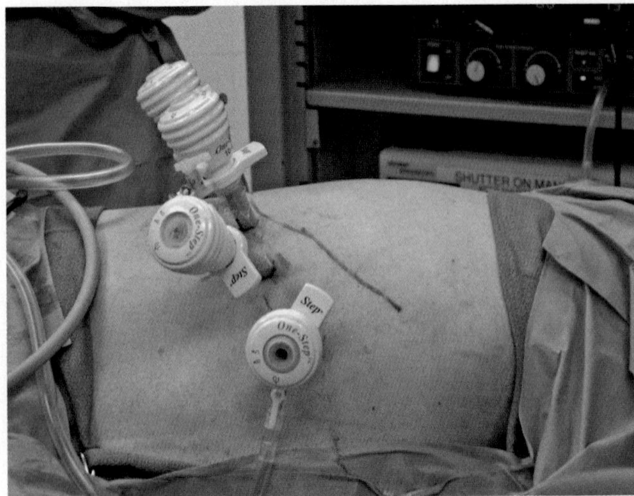

**FIGURE 41-23** Port placement for right laparoscopic adrenalectomy. The patient is lying right-side up, with the head toward the right. The marked line denotes the costal margin. Ports are placed approximately 2 cm inferior to the costal margin, spaced about 4 fingerbreadths apart.

mobilized caudally by dividing the splenocolic ligament. We use an open book technique, which involves developing the cleftlike plane just medial to the adrenal gland and lateral to the aorta (Fig. 41-24). The left-hand page of the book is comprised of the spleen, tail of the pancreas, and greater curvature of the stomach. The right-hand page of the book is made up by the kidney and adrenal tumor. The left crus of the diaphragm is a useful landmark that leads the surgeon to the left inferior phrenic vein.

As mentioned in the anatomy section of this chapter, the left inferior phrenic vein courses along the medial aspect of the left adrenal gland before joining with the left adrenal vein. By developing the cleft of the open book, moving from superior to inferior, the adrenal vein is encountered at the inferomedial aspect of the adrenal gland. The small adrenal arteries that lie within this plane can be handled with energy-based coagulation. The left adrenal vein is carefully dissected out, aggressively coagulated or clipped, and divided. The inferior tip of the left adrenal gland may extend low, approaching the renal hilum within millimeters. However, because the left adrenal vein is rather long (2 cm), it is generally not necessary to expose the renal vasculature during left adrenalectomy. Many patients have a superior pole renal artery branch that approaches the inferior aspect of the left adrenal gland. Injury to this structure must be carefully avoided by keeping dissection close to the adrenal capsule while the specimen is elevated away from the medial aspect of the superior pole of the left kidney.

The adrenal gland is liberated by completing dissection circumferentially and posteriorly, taking the specimen off the superior pole of the kidney and posterior abdominal wall. These attachments are deliberately divided last because they aid in suspending the adrenal gland on the lateral-superior wall of the operative field, providing exposure of the medial vascular plane during the critical initial portion of the procedure. The tumor is placed into a resilient catchment device, morcellated, and extracted. If noncutting trocars are used, only the skin will need to be closed.

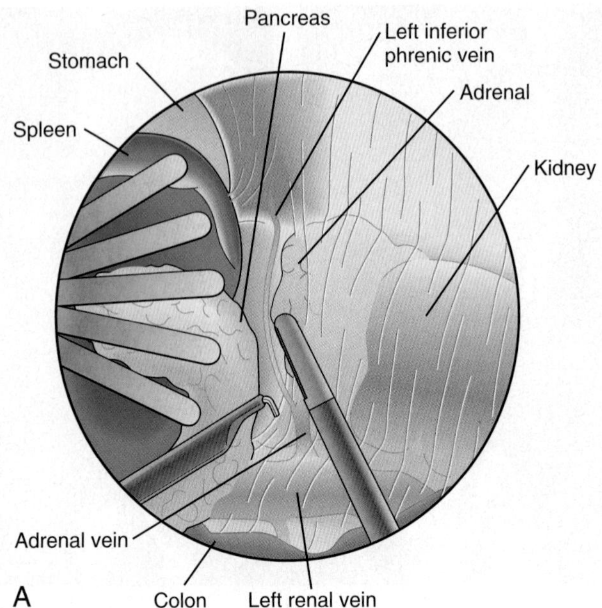


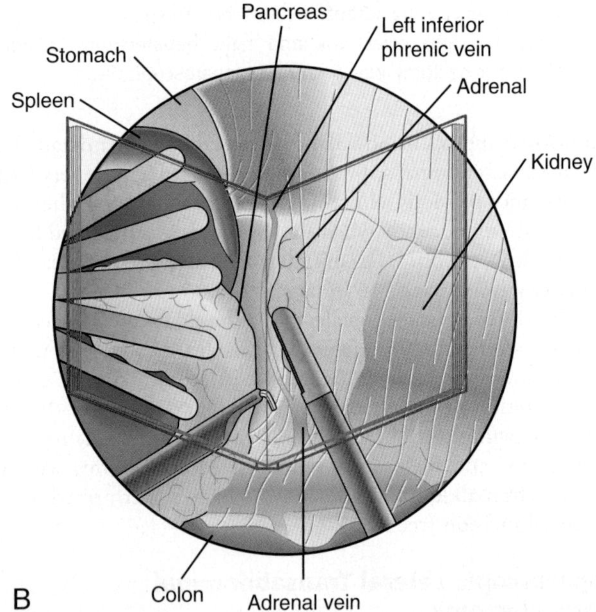


**FIGURE 41-24** Technique of left laparoscopic adrenalectomy. The spleen and pancreatic tail have been mobilized and retracted anteromedially to expose the adrenal gland. The cleft of the open book is developed in a superior to inferior direction to identify the inferior phrenic vein and adrenal vein.

**Right Adrenal** Laparoscopic right adrenalectomy is, in some respects, a mirror image of the procedure just described. During right adrenalectomy, the left-hand page of the open book is made up by the kidney and adrenal tumor and the right-hand page is comprised of the bare area of the liver (Fig. 41-25). To gain access to the appropriate plane, the right triangular ligament of the liver must first be completely mobilized and the liver allowed to rotate anteromedially. On the right side, the colon usually lies well inferior to the operative field. When developing the space between the adrenal gland and inferior vena cava from superior to inferior, the surgeon must be mindful

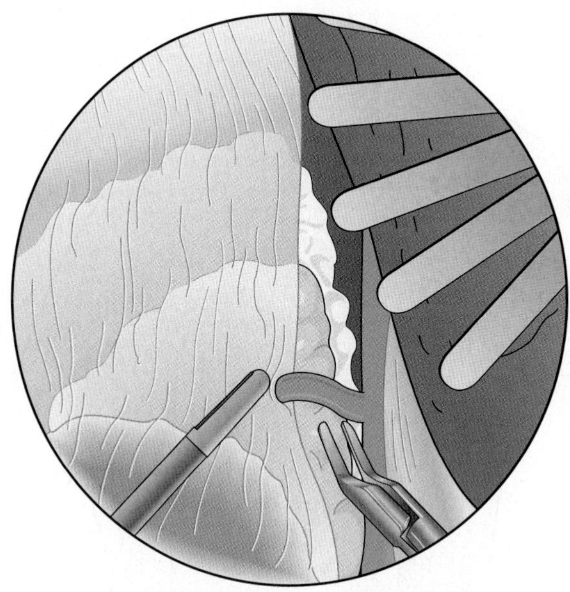

FIGURE 41-25 Technique of right laparoscopic adrenalectomy. The liver has been mobilized and retracted medially to expose the adrenal gland and IVC. The space just medial to the adrenal gland is developed to identify the adrenal vasculature.

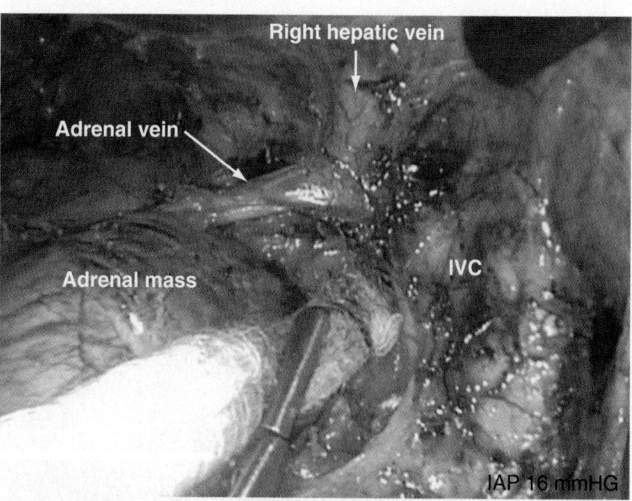


FIGURE 41-26 Right adrenal vein variant. This solitary adrenal vein arises from the superior apex of the gland and drains into the confluence of the IVC and right hepatic vein, as shown in Figure 41-3*F*.

of adrenal vein variants, as illustrated in the anatomy section of this chapter (see Fig. 41-3). The right adrenal vein is a potentially perilous structure to manage, because it is short, wide, variable, and confluent with thin-walled, large capacitance vessels (the inferior vena cava in more than 80% of cases, followed by the renal vein and, uncommonly, the right hepatic vein) that can bleed briskly if directly injured (e.g., by the cautery), lacerated from undue traction on adjacent structures, or sheared by clips. A significant second adrenal vein may be found in up to 10% of patients. By methodically dissecting one layer at a time and moving from superior to inferior, all potential adrenal vein variants can be encountered in a controlled fashion (Fig. 41-26). The adrenal vein must be dissected out delicately, definitively ligated (usually with two clips on the patient side), and then divided. Loss of control of the adrenal vein stump should be avoided; should this occur, conversion to an open procedure may be necessary. A conceptual contrast between left and right adrenalectomy is that left adrenalectomy centers on identification of the correct plane of dissection and right adrenalectomy centers on the avoidance of venous bleeding.

Of note, the junction of the inferior vena cava and right renal vein is frequently difficult to identify. In vivo, the transition is a gradual curve, rather than the 90-degree takeoff depicted in anatomy texts. Therefore, it cannot be used as a reliable anatomic landmark for identification of the adrenal vein. After control of the vein, the remaining mobilization of the right adrenal gland is straightforward because the inferomedial limb generally does not reach as far down toward the renal hilum as on the left side.

## Posterior Retroperitoneoscopic Adrenalectomy

Posterior retroperitoneoscopic adrenalectomy was popularized in 1994 by Walz and associates.[49] The technique has undergone a series of refinements so that now a subset of lean patients with tumors smaller than 4 cm in diameter can be managed using a novel single access technique.[50] The retroperitoneal approach has several advantages, including avoidance of mobilization of the solid organs that is necessary with transabdominal approaches, eliminating the need for repositioning during bilateral adrenalectomy, and avoidance of anterior adhesions in patients with extensive prior abdominal surgery. One disadvantage is the relatively small working space, which makes the retroperitoneal technique best suited for tumors less than 7 cm in diameter.

A prone position is used, with supports placed under the lower chest and pelvic girdle so that the abdomen is allowed to hang anteriorly (Fig. 41-27*A*). Three ports are placed inferior to the 12th rib (see Fig. 41-27*B*) using a direct cut-down technique for initial access. Relatively high insufflation pressures of 20 to 28 mm Hg are used and have caused no complications in regard to air emboli, hypercapnea, or clinically significant soft tissue emphysema. The working space is initially created by bluntly dissecting the retroperitoneal contents anteriorly away from the ports. The upper pole of the kidney is mobilized and reflected inferiorly to expose the adrenal gland. Mobilization of the adrenal gland begins near the paraspinous muscles, at the inferomedial aspect of the gland. This is where the left adrenal vein is almost always encountered early in the procedure (see Fig. 41-27*C*). On the right side, the vein is encountered slightly later as dissection proceeds superiorly. The small adrenal arteries that run within the medial vascular space are coagulated. After the superior apex of the adrenal gland is mobilized, dissection proceeds circumferentially to include the periadrenal fat.

### Complications and Postoperative Care

Potential technical complications include venous hemorrhage and bleeding from solid organ capsular injuries. Small amounts of bleeding can often be managed with coagulation or direct pressure using a rolled Kittner gauze. Hollow viscous injuries are uncommon but may be associated with procedures performed in patients with prior major abdominal surgery. Pancreatic injuries and fistulas have been reported with left-sided procedures; these are rare complications, as are port site hernias and port site metastases in cases of malignancy. Patients undergoing laparoscopic adrenalectomy for Cushing's syndrome are at

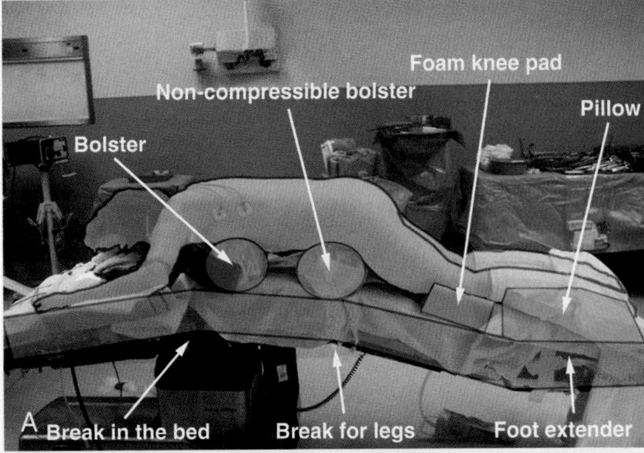


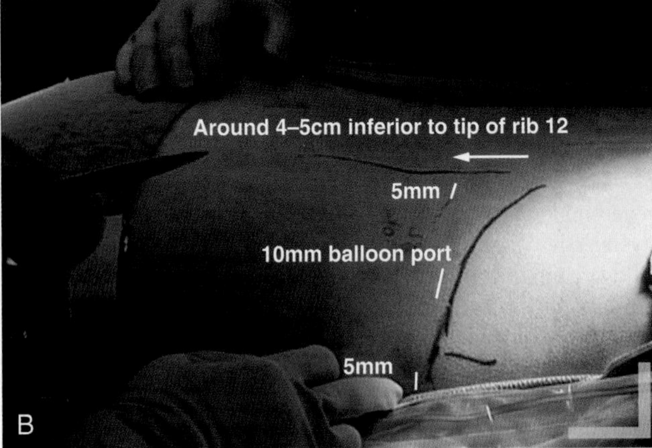


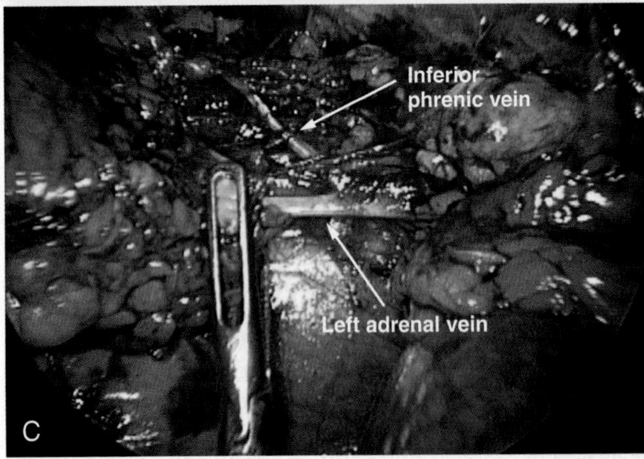


**FIGURE 41-27** **A,** Patient positioning for posterior retroperitoneoscopic adrenalectomy. **B,** Port placement for posterior retroperitoneoscopic adrenalectomy. **C,** Posterior view of the left adrenal vein. The left inferior phrenic vein can be seen superiorly. Adrenal tissue is being retracted to the left-hand side of the photograph. (Courtesy Dr. James Lee.)

risk for surgical site infections because of their catabolic and immunosuppressed state. These include port site infections in 5% of patients and, rarely, subphrenic abscesses requiring catheter drainage. One complication specific to the retroperitoneal approach is injury of the subcostal nerve, which occurs in 8% of patients and is usually temporary.

Patients who undergo laparoscopic adrenalectomy recover rapidly. Most patients, including approximately 50% of those treated for pheochromocytoma, can leave the hospital on the first postoperative day. In the treatment of adrenal tumors, successful outcomes hinge on excellent perioperative medical management as much as technical skill, particularly in cases of pheochromocytoma and Cushing's syndrome. These considerations have been discussed earlier.

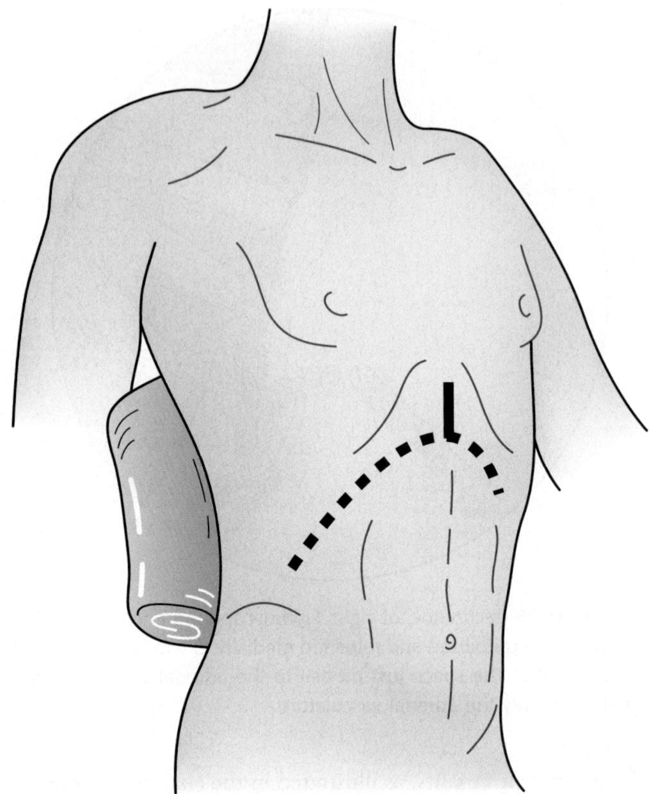

**FIGURE 41-28** Patient positioning for open right adrenalectomy.

## Open Anterior Transabdominal Adrenalectomy

### Patient Preparation and Positioning

Neuraxial blockade (use of an epidural catheter) is routinely used for intraoperative and postoperative anesthetic or analgesic management. The patient is positioned supine, with the ipsilateral side slightly elevated on a bolster (Fig. 41-28). A urinary catheter, orogastric or nasogastric tube, and intermittent pneumatic compression devices are placed. The surgical preparation is carried from the nipple line to the pubis and down to the table on either side.

### Technique

**Left Adrenal** We prefer to use a subcostal incision, which may be extended across the midline (chevron), with or without a vertical upper midline extension, to achieve wide exposure. The left adrenal can be exposed by entering the lesser sac through the gastrocolic ligament and incising the retroperitoneum inferior to the tail of the pancreas or by rotating the spleen, pancreatic tail, and stomach anteromedially, as described earlier in the section on laparoscopic adrenalectomy. We use the latter approach in our practice. The splenic flexure of the colon is mobilized inferiorly and the plane medial to the adrenal gland is developed. The adrenal vein is isolated, tied in continuity, and

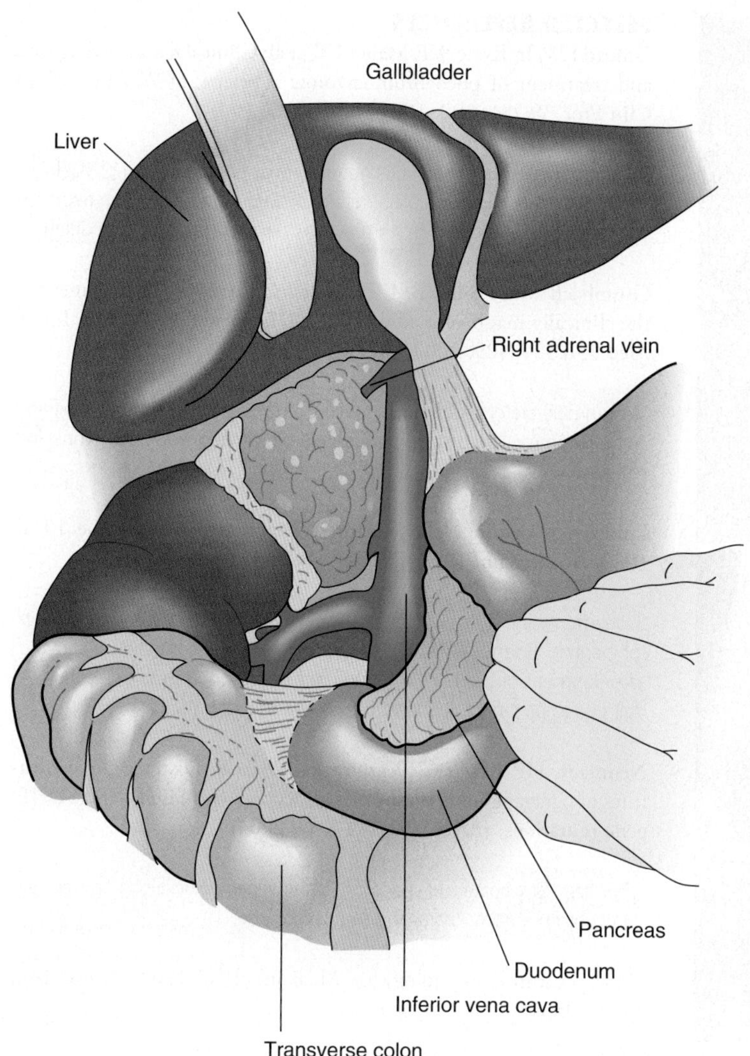


**FIGURE 41-29** Open right adrenalectomy. The right lobe of the liver and the hepatic flexure of the colon have been completely mobilized. The retroperitoneum is entered and the duodenum and head of the pancreas reflected medially (Kocher maneuver) to expose the adrenal gland and IVC.

divided. The small adrenal arteries can be ligated or electrocoagulated and the specimen removed after circumferential dissection is completed.

**Right Adrenal** Open right adrenalectomy begins with complete mobilization of the right lobe of the liver, including the lateral attachments and the falciform ligament. The adrenal can be exposed by rotating the liver medially or, more commonly, retracting the inferoposterior segments cephalad using long padded retractors (liver, renal vein, Deaver, or Harrington types). The retroperitoneum is entered by performing a Kocher maneuver (Fig. 41-29) and the inferior vena cava is exposed by medial reflection of the duodenum. The plane between the adrenal gland and inferior vena cava is developed first. Vascular structures, which may be numerous in highly angiogenic tumors, are ligated sequentially. The adrenal vein is isolated, securely tied, and divided. Loss of control of the adrenal vein stump may be managed with the application of a side-biting (Satinsky) vascular clamp. As noted, open adrenalectomy is generally performed in cases of suspected or known malignancy. Locally invasive right-sided adrenal tumors can be challenging to manage, given their frequent invasion of adjacent venous structures (Fig. 41-30). It

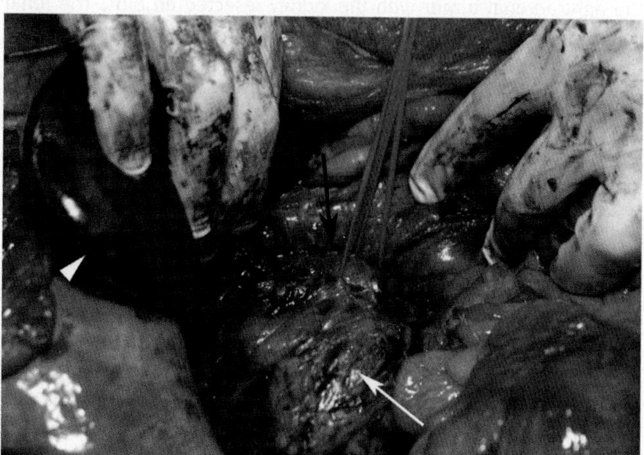

**FIGURE 41-30** Open resection of a right adrenocortical carcinoma invading the IVC. The patient's head is to the left. The liver *(white arrowhead)* is retracted cephalad. The *white arrow* indicates the tumor and the *black arrow* indicates the IVC, which is encircled with vessel loops.

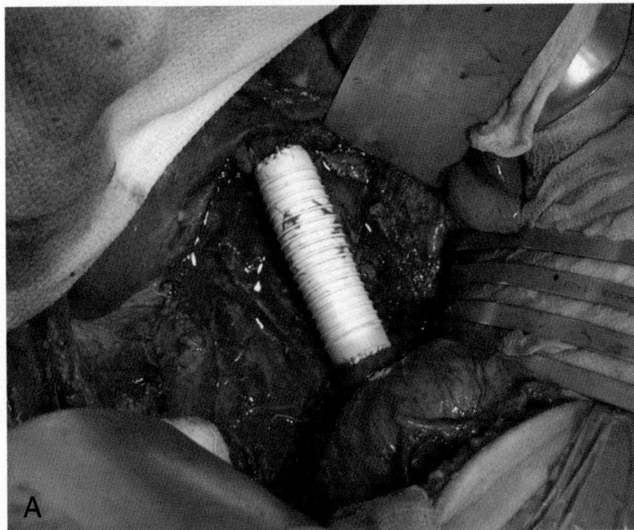


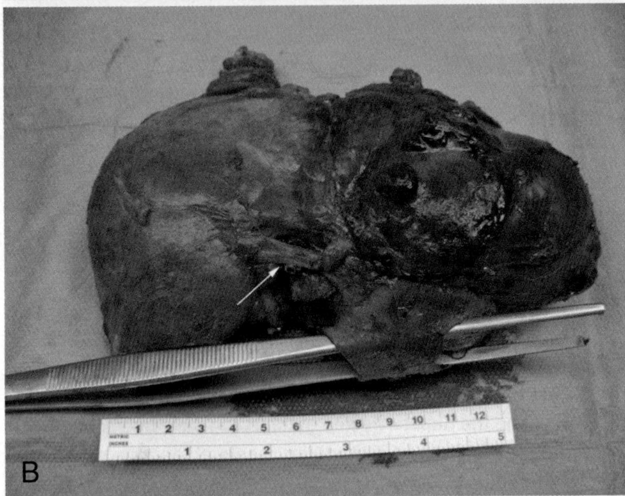


**FIGURE 41-31** Open resection of a right adrenocortical carcinoma requiring vascular reconstruction. **A,** The infrahepatic IVC has been replaced with a polytetrafluoroethylene graft. The liver can be seen superiorly and the colon inferiorly. **B,** Ex vivo specimen consisting of the right adrenal tumor with the kidney resected en bloc. The renal vein is indicated by the *arrow*. Forceps have been placed through the resected segment of the IVC.

is our practice to involve an experienced vascular or liver surgeon in the management of tumors with extensive venous invasion. Locally invaded organs, most commonly the kidney, should be resected en bloc with the primary mass. Complete radical resection is a critical determinant of survival in patients with malignant adrenal tumors; in some cases, this can only be achieved if immediate venous reconstruction is performed (Fig. 41-31).

### Complications and Postoperative Care

Technical complications of open adrenalectomy include venous hemorrhage, tumor embolization in cases with intravascular tumor extension, and solid organ injury. Postoperative complications are similar to those associated with other major abdominal procedures. Most patients experience return of bowel function within 3 to 4 days and are able to leave the hospital on postoperative days 5 to 7.

## SELECTED REFERENCES

Gifford RW, Jr, Kvale WF, Maher FT, et al: Clinical features, diagnosis and treatment of pheochromocytoma: A review of 76 cases. Mayo Clin Proc 39:281–302, 1964.

A landmark account of the biochemical, pharmacologic, and physiologic advances that allowed collaborators at the Mayo Clinic to treat 76 patients with pheochromocytoma while experiencing only one death.

Grumbach MM, Biller BM, Braunstein GD, et al: Management of the clinically inapparent adrenal mass ("incidentaloma"). Ann Intern Med 138:424–429, 2003.

A summary statement from the NIH Consensus Development Program with recommendations on incidentaloma workup and indications for surgery.

Lindsten J, editor: Nobel Lectures, Physiology or Medicine 1971-1980, Amsterdam, 1992, Elsevier.

Documents the formidable challenges surmounted in the identification of peptide hormones, found in such minute concentrations, and the development of the radioimmunoassay necessary for their detection. A full transcript can be found at http://www.nobelprize.org.

Neumann HP, Pawlu C, Peczkowska M, et al: Distinct clinical features of paraganglioma syndromes associated with SDHB and SDHD gene mutations. JAMA 292:943–951, 2004.

The first description of genotype-phenotype associations in familial pheochromocytoma/paraganglioma syndrome.

Nobel Lectures, Physiology or Medicine 1942-1962, Amsterdam, 1964, Elsevier.

An account of the clinical discoveries and advances in organic chemistry that led to the identification, isolation, and artificial synthesis of adrenal cortical hormones. A full transcript can be found at http://www.nobelprize.org.

Sukor N, Kogovsek C, Gordon RD, et al: Improved quality of life, blood pressure, and biochemical status following laparoscopic adrenalectomy for unilateral primary aldosteronism. J Clin Endocrinol Metab 95:1360–1364, 2010.

This prospective pilot study examines an array of short-term outcomes after surgical treatment of hyperaldosteronism.

Terzolo M, Angeli A, Fassnacht M, et al: Adjuvant mitotane treatment for adrenocortical carcinoma. N Engl J Med 356:2372–2380, 2007.

The extreme rarity of adrenocortical carcinoma has been a major obstacle in the systematic study of this disease. This landmark multinational report, which involved 177 patients from 55 European centers, was the first to demonstrate the beneficial effect of adjuvant mitotane.

Walz MK, Alesina PF, Wenger FA, et al: Posterior retroperitoneoscopic adrenalectomy—results of 560 procedures in 520 patients. Surgery 140:943–948, 2006.

The largest single institution series on this procedure, written by the developers of the technique.

Welbourn RB: Early surgical history of phaeochromocytoma. Br J Surg 74:594–596, 1987.

Describes the initial achievements of American and European surgeons in regard to the successful treatment of pheochromocytoma.

## REFERENCES


1. Nobel Lectures, Physiology or Medicine 1942-1962, Amsterdam, 1964, Elsevier.
2. Lindsten J, editor: Nobel Lectures, Physiology or Medicine 1971-1980, Amsterdam, 1992, Elsevier.
3. Lenders JW, Pacak K, Walther MM, et al: Biochemical diagnosis of pheochromocytoma: Which test is best? JAMA 287:1427–1434, 2002.
4. Nieman LK, Chanco Turner ML: Addison's disease. Clin Dermatol 24:276–280, 2006.
5. Shen WT, Lee J, Kebebew E, et al: Selective use of steroid replacement after adrenalectomy: Lessons from 331 consecutive cases. Arch Surg 141:771–774, 2006.
6. Minneci PC, Deans KJ, Banks SM, et al: Meta-analysis: The effect of steroids on survival and shock during sepsis depends on the dose. Ann Intern Med 141:47–56, 2004.
7. Axelrod L: Perioperative management of patients treated with glucocorticoids. Endocrinol Metab Clin North Am 32:367–383, 2003.
8. Kaplan NM: The current epidemic of primary aldosteronism: Causes and consequences. J Hypertens 22:863–869, 2004.
9. Mulatero P, Stowasser M, Loh KC, et al: Increased diagnosis of primary aldosteronism, including surgically correctable forms, in centers from five continents. J Clin Endocrinol Metab 89:1045–1050, 2004.
10. Milliez P, Girerd X, Plouin PF, et al: Evidence for an increased rate of cardiovascular events in patients with primary aldosteronism. J Am Coll Cardiol 45:1243–1248, 2005.
11. Doi SA, Abalkhail S, Al-Qudhaiby MM, et al: Optimal use and interpretation of the aldosterone-renin ratio to detect aldosterone excess in hypertension. J Hum Hypertens 20:482–489, 2006.
12. Young WF, Stanson AW, Thompson GB, et al: Role for adrenal venous sampling in primary aldosteronism. Surgery 136:1227–1235, 2004.
13. White ML, Gauger PG, Doherty GM, et al: The role of radiologic studies in the evaluation and management of primary hyperaldosteronism. Surgery 144:926–933, 2008.
14. Tan YY, Ogilvie JB, Triponez F, et al: Selective use of adrenal venous sampling in the lateralization of aldosterone-producing adenomas. World J Surg 30:879–885, 2006.
15. Harvey A, Kline G, Pasieka JL: Adrenal venous sampling in primary hyperaldosteronism: comparison of radiographic with biochemical success and the clinical decision-making with "less than ideal" testing. Surgery 140:847–853, 2006.
16. Sukor N, Kogovsek C, Gordon RD, et al: Improved quality of life, blood pressure, and biochemical status following laparoscopic adrenalectomy for unilateral primary aldosteronism. J Clin Endocrinol Metab 95:1360–1364, 2010.
17. Lindholm J, Juul S, Jorgensen JO, et al: Incidence and late prognosis of Cushing's syndrome: A population-based study. J Clin Endocrinol Metab 86:117–123, 2001.
18. Papanicolaou DA, Mullen N, Kyrou I, et al: Nighttime salivary cortisol: A useful test for the diagnosis of Cushing's syndrome. J Clin Endocrinol Metab 87:4515–4521, 2002.
19. Newell-Price J, Bertagna X, Grossman AB, et al: Cushing's syndrome. Lancet 367:1605–1617, 2006.
20. Esposito F, Dusick JR, Cohan P, et al: Clinical review: Early morning cortisol levels as a predictor of remission after transsphenoidal surgery for Cushing's disease. J Clin Endocrinol Metab 91:7–13, 2006.
21. Sippel RS, Elaraj DM, Kebebew E, et al: Waiting for change: Symptom resolution after adrenalectomy for Cushing's syndrome. Surgery 144:1054–1060, 2008.
22. Barahona MJ, Sucunza N, Resmini E, et al: Persistent body fat mass and inflammatory marker increases after long-term cure of Cushing's syndrome. J Clin Endocrinol Metab 94:3365–3371, 2009.
23. Barahona MJ, Sucunza N, Resmini E, et al: Deleterious effects of glucocorticoid replacement on bone in women after long-term remission of Cushing's syndrome. J Bone Miner Res 24:1841–1846, 2009.
24. Findling JW, Raff H: Cushing's syndrome: Important issues in diagnosis and management. J Clin Endocrinol Metab 91:3746–3753, 2006.
25. Toniato A, Merante-Boschin I, Opocher G, et al: Surgical versus conservative management for subclinical Cushing syndrome in adrenal incidentalomas: A prospective randomized study. Ann Surg 249:388–391, 2009.
26. Ng L, Libertino JM: Adrenocortical carcinoma: Diagnosis, evaluation and treatment. J Urol 169:5–11, 2003.
27. Soon PS, Sidhu SB: Adrenocortical carcinoma. Cancer Treat Res 153:187–210, 2010.
28. Bilimoria KY, Shen WT, Elaraj D, et al: Adrenocortical carcinoma in the United States: Treatment utilization and prognostic factors. Cancer 113:3130–3136, 2008.
29. Yeh MW, Lisewski D, Campbell P: Virilizing adrenocortical carcinoma with cavoatrial extension. Am J Surg 192:209–210, 2006.
30. Terzolo M, Angeli A, Fassnacht M, et al: Adjuvant mitotane treatment for adrenocortical carcinoma. N Engl J Med 356:2372–2380, 2007.
31. Bussey KJ, Demeure MJ: Genomic and expression profiling of adrenocortical carcinoma: Application to diagnosis, prognosis and treatment. Future Oncol 5:641–655, 2009.
32. Welbourn RB: Early surgical history of phaeochromocytoma. Br J Surg 74:594–596, 1987.
33. Sawka AM, Prebtani AP, Thabane L, et al: A systematic review of the literature examining the diagnostic efficacy of measurement of fractionated plasma free metanephrines in the biochemical diagnosis of pheochromocytoma. BMC Endocr Disord 4:2, 2004.
34. Kudva YC, Sawka AM, Young WF, Jr: Clinical review 164: The laboratory diagnosis of adrenal pheochromocytoma: The Mayo Clinic experience. J Clin Endocrinol Metab 88:4533–4539, 2003.
35. Timmers HJ, Chen CC, Carrasquillo JA, et al: Comparison of 18F-fluoro-L-DOPA, 18F-fluoro-deoxyglucose, and 18F-fluorodopamine PET and 123I-MIBG scintigraphy in the localization of pheochromocytoma and paraganglioma. J Clin Endocrinol Metab 94:4757–4767, 2009.
36. Imani F, Agopian VG, Auerbach MS, et al: 18F-FDOPA PET and PET/CT accurately localize pheochromocytomas. J Nucl Med 50:513–519, 2009.

**37.** Gifford RW, Jr, Kvale WF, Maher FT, et al: Clinical features, diagnosis and treatment of pheochromocytoma: A review of 76 cases. Mayo Clin Proc 39:281–302, 1964.

**38.** Shen WT, Grogan R, Vriens M, et al: One hundred two patients with pheochromocytoma treated at a single institution since the introduction of laparoscopic adrenalectomy. Arch Surg 145:893–897, 2010.

**39.** Benn DE, Robinson BG: Genetic basis of phaeochromocytoma and paraganglioma. Best Pract Res Clin Endocrinol Metab 20:435–450, 2006.

**40.** Neumann HP, Pawlu C, Peczkowska M, et al: Distinct clinical features of paraganglioma syndromes associated with SDHB and SDHD gene mutations. Jama 292:943–951, 2004.

**41.** Erlic Z, Rybicki L, Peczkowska M, et al: Clinical predictors and algorithm for the genetic diagnosis of pheochromocytoma patients. Clin Cancer Res 15:6378–6385, 2009.

**42.** Adjalle R, Plouin PF, Pacak K, et al: Treatment of malignant pheochromocytoma. Horm Metab Res 41:687–696, 2009.

**43.** Gonias S, Goldsby R, Matthay KK, et al: Phase II study of high-dose [131I]metaiodobenzylguanidine therapy for patients with metastatic pheochromocytoma and paraganglioma. J Clin Oncol 27:4162–4168, 2009.

**44.** Grumbach MM, Biller BM, Braunstein GD, et al: Management of the clinically inapparent adrenal mass ("incidentaloma"). Ann Intern Med 138:424–429, 2003.

**45.** Sturgeon C, Kebebew E: Laparoscopic adrenalectomy for malignancy. Surg Clin North Am 84:755–774, 2004.

**46.** Sebag F, Calzolari F, Harding J, et al: Isolated adrenal metastasis: The role of laparoscopic surgery. World J Surg 30:888–892, 2006.

**47.** Shen WT, Kebebew E, Clark OH, et al: Reasons for conversion from laparoscopic to open or hand-assisted adrenalectomy: Review of 261 laparoscopic adrenalectomies from 1993 to 2003. World J Surg 28:1176–1179, 2004.

**48.** Morris L, Ituarte P, Zarnegar R, et al: Laparoscopic adrenalectomy after prior abdominal surgery. World J Surg 32:897–903, 2008.

**49.** Walz MK, Alesina PF, Wenger FA, et al: Posterior retroperitoneoscopic adrenalectomy—results of 560 procedures in 520 patients. Surgery 140:943–948, 2006.

**50.** Walz MK, Alesina PF: Single access retroperitoneoscopic adrenalectomy (SARA)—one step beyond in endocrine surgery. Langenbecks Arch Surg 394:447–450, 2009.

CHAPTER 42

# MULTIPLE ENDOCRINE NEOPLASIA SYNDROMES

Terry C. Lairmore and Jeffrey F. Moley



Genetic changes in a tumor suppressor gene and a proto-oncogene result in the multiple endocrine neoplasia (MEN) types 1 and 2 syndromes, respectively. These hereditary cancer syndromes are characterized by neoplastic transformation in multiple target endocrine tissues, as well as pathologic involvement of nonendocrine tissues. The associated endocrine tumors may be benign or malignant and may develop synchronously or metachronously. Within an affected endocrine target tissue, a diffuse preneoplastic hyperplasia typically precedes the development of microscopic invasion or grossly evident multifocal carcinoma. In the MEN syndromes, the genetic predisposition to multiple endocrine neoplasms with malignant potential is conferred on otherwise healthy, young individuals. Importantly, the discovery of the specific genetic basis for the MEN1 and 2 syndromes has allowed the development of strategies for direct genetic testing and early surgical intervention. Early thyroidectomy is indicated for patients with a genetic diagnosis of MEN2, with the aim of preventing the subsequent development of regional or distant medullary thyroid carcinoma metastases. The optimal early surgical intervention to prevent metastatic spread of the potentially malignant neuroendocrine tumors (NETs) in patients with a genetic diagnosis of MEN1 remains clinically controversial.

The MEN syndromes are characterized by differing patterns of involvement. MEN1 is characterized by the development of multiglandular parathyroid disease, NETs of the gastroenteropancreatic system, adenomas of the anterior pituitary gland, foregut and thymic carcinoids, and other associated nonendocrine neoplasms, such as facial angiofibromas, lipomas, and collagenomas. The MEN2A syndrome is characterized by the development of medullary thyroid carcinoma (MTC), pheochromocytomas, and parathyroid tumors, whereas MEN2B consists of MTC, pheochromocytomas, mucosal neuromas, skeletal abnormalities, ganglioneuromatosis of the gastrointestinal tract, and what has been termed a distinctive *marfanoid habitus.*

## MULTIPLE ENDOCRINE NEOPLASIA TYPE 1

### Genetic Studies and Pathogenesis

The *MEN1* tumor suppressor gene, whose mutations are responsible for the MEN1 syndrome, was originally mapped to human chromosome 11q13 by genetic linkage studies and tumor DNA deletion mapping, and was identified by positional cloning in 1997.[1] *MEN1* is a putative tumor suppressor gene, whose protein product likely has diverse actions that confer a negative influence or brake on cellular growth and proliferation, so that loss of its function results in unregulated cell growth or neoplastic transformation. As a tumor suppressor gene, development of MEN1 requires two genetic hits involving both allelic copies of the gene to result in loss of function. The first mutation is inherited in the germline and is present in every cell; the second somatic mutation occurs in an individual cell of an involved target tissue and results in tumor formation. According to the two-hit model of tumorigenesis, the first event is a mutation inherited in the germline that confers susceptibility to neoplastic change in the involved tissues. Elimination of the remaining functional copy of the gene in a single cell through a chance somatic mutational event, or second hit (such as a gene deletion), results in clonal expansion and cancer development. The occurrence of individual second hits in several target organ cells explains the multifocal involvement characteristically observed in affected endocrine tissues. Somatic mutations in the *MEN1* gene occur frequently in sporadic parathyroid adenomas, insulinomas and gastrinoma, pituitary tumors, and bronchial carcinoids, indicating that loss of the *MEN1* gene contributes to the development of a subset of nonhereditary endocrine tumors.

The *MEN1* gene consists of 10 exons (9 coding and 1 untranslated) and encodes a 610–amino acid protein termed *menin.*[1] Menin is ubiquitously expressed in endocrine and nonendocrine tissues. The menin protein sequence is highly conserved evolutionarily, with the murine *Men1* gene demonstrating 98% homology. Knockout of both *Men1* alleles in mice results in embryonic lethality, demonstrating that menin is essential for early development and has a broader role in the regulation of cell growth that is not limited to the endocrine tissues affected in MEN1. An excellent mouse animal model for the study of MEN1 tumorigenesis exists. Heterozygous *Men1*± mice demonstrate somatic loss of the wild-type *Men1* allele in tumors[2] and develop a constellation of endocrine tumors remarkably similar to the human MEN1 syndrome.

Menin is now known to have diverse influences in the regulation of gene transcription, cell cycle progression, apoptotic pathways, DNA processing and repair, cytoskeletal integrity, and genome stability. Menin is predominantly a nuclear protein that binds to Jun, a member of the AP-1 transcription factor family, and represses JunD-mediated transcription.[3] In addition, menin has been shown to interact physically with a diverse variety of

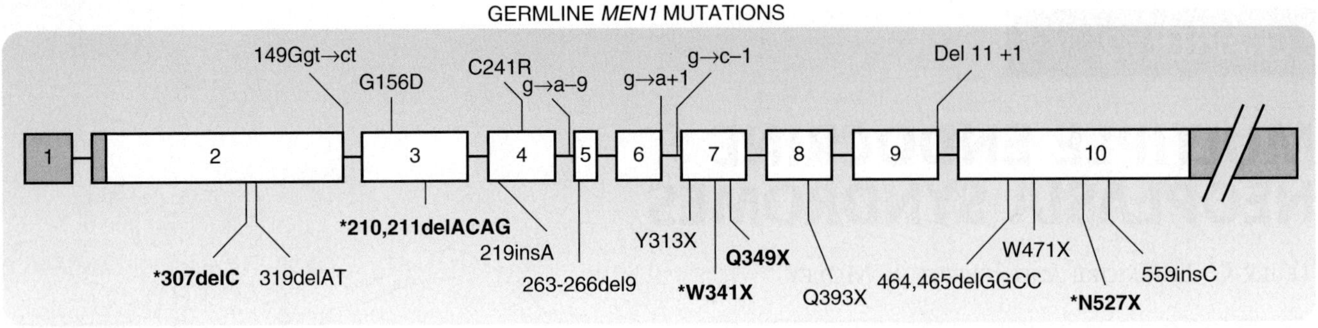

**FIGURE 42-1** Germline mutations in the *MEN1* gene in a set of 25 independent kindreds. The mutations are distributed throughout the nine coding exons of the gene. The genetic alterations may include missense, nonsense, frameshift, and RNA-splicing defects that may occur anywhere throughout the coding exons and immediately flanking intron sequences. Five splicing defects and two missense mutations are depicted above the *MEN1* gene, and seven nonsense and six frameshift mutations are depicted below the *MEN1* gene. (From Mutch MG, Dilley WG, Sanjurjo F, et al: Germline mutations in the multiple endocrine neoplasia type 1 gene: Evidence for frequent splicing defects. Hum Mutat 13:175–185, 1999.)

other proteins that comprise transcription factors, DNA-processing factors, DNA repair proteins, and cytoskeletal proteins (e.g., Smad3, NF-κB, nm23, Pem, FANCD2, RPA2, ASK). Overexpression of menin has been shown to diminish the tumorigenic phenotype of Ras-transformed NIH-3T3 cells, consistent with its putative tumor suppressor function. In addition, studies have suggested a possible role for menin in repressing telomerase activity in somatic cells, perhaps explaining in part its tumor suppressor properties. Although there is now rapidly expanding evidence regarding diverse menin interactions and influences on a variety of cellular functions and pathways, the full complexity of the tumor suppressor role of menin in MEN1 and sporadic endocrine tumorigenesis has not yet provided a comprehensive understanding of the mechanisms involved.

Menin upregulates certain cyclin-dependent kinase (CDK) inhibitors by increasing histone H3 lysine 4 (H3K4) methylation and inhibits $G_0$ or $G_1$ to S phase transition. These findings suggest that by promoting histone modifications within specific gene promoters, menin promotes the maintenance of transcription of critical cell cycle regulators essential for normal endocrine cell growth control.

To date, more than 1330 independent mutations have been identified in the *MEN1* gene.[4] *MEN1* mutations may be nonsense, missense, frameshift, deletions, and RNA splicing defects. These diverse mutations may occur throughout the coding sequence and intron-exon junctions of the gene, as demonstrated in a representative study of *MEN1* germline mutations (Fig. 42-1).[5] Approximately two thirds of the reported mutations in the *MEN1* gene result in premature termination of translation and truncation of the C-terminal portion of the menin protein. No clear genotype-phenotype correlation has been established for MEN1, although phenotypic variants (isolated hyperparathyroidism, frequent prolactinomas) have been described.[6]

Direct genetic testing can detect disease-associated germline mutations in the *MEN1* gene and identify affected individuals. The clinical application of genetic testing has associated limitations. The detection of a disease-associated mutation in a family with a previously defined specific genetic change is straightforward. However, in a newly identified MEN1 family for whom the specific mutation is not known in advance, a comprehensive search of the coding sequence and intron-exon junctions is necessary to search for all possible mutations; only approximately 85% to 90% of these novel families will have the specific mutation identified by standard genetic screening. For this reason, a negative comprehensive screen for mutations in the *MEN1* gene does not exclude involvement with MEN1. Formal genetic counseling and informed consent, including disclosures relevant to the privacy of medical information and the potential impact of the genetic information on treatment, are essential to a comprehensive program of genetic testing.

Because no clear correlation has been found between specific mutations in the *MEN1* gene and phenotype of the affected patients, the use of genetic testing for the prediction of malignant potential and prognosis is not possible at present.[7] When an index-suspected MEN1 patient is diagnosed clinically, genetic evaluation of that patient and first-degree relatives should be performed. Presymptomatic individuals who test positive for an *MEN1* mutation should then undergo more frequent and intensive biochemical testing, with special emphasis on the potentially malignant pancreaticoduodenal and intrathoracic tumors. Close observation and frequent surveillance of patients with *MEN1* mutations allows for much earlier detection of biochemical abnormalities associated with neoplasia.[8] Conversely, a negative genetic test result in a patient from a family whose specific mutation is known would obviate further lifelong screening or testing, with the associated costs and psychological impact.

## Clinical Features and Management

The principal feature that develops in almost all individuals inheriting an *MEN1* mutation is hypercalcemia caused by multiglandular parathyroid tumors. Patients may also develop NET of the pancreas and duodenum, bronchial and thymic carcinoids, and adenomas of the anterior pituitary. In addition, bronchial and thymic carcinoids, thyroid nodules, adrenocortical nodular hyperplasia, lipomas, ependymomas, and cutaneous angiofibromas occur with increased frequency in patients with MEN1. Clinically, MEN1 is defined as the occurrence of neoplasms in at least two target endocrine tissues (parathyroid, endocrine pancreas, pituitary) in an individual; familial MEN1 is defined as the additional occurrence of at least one tumor type in a first-degree relative.

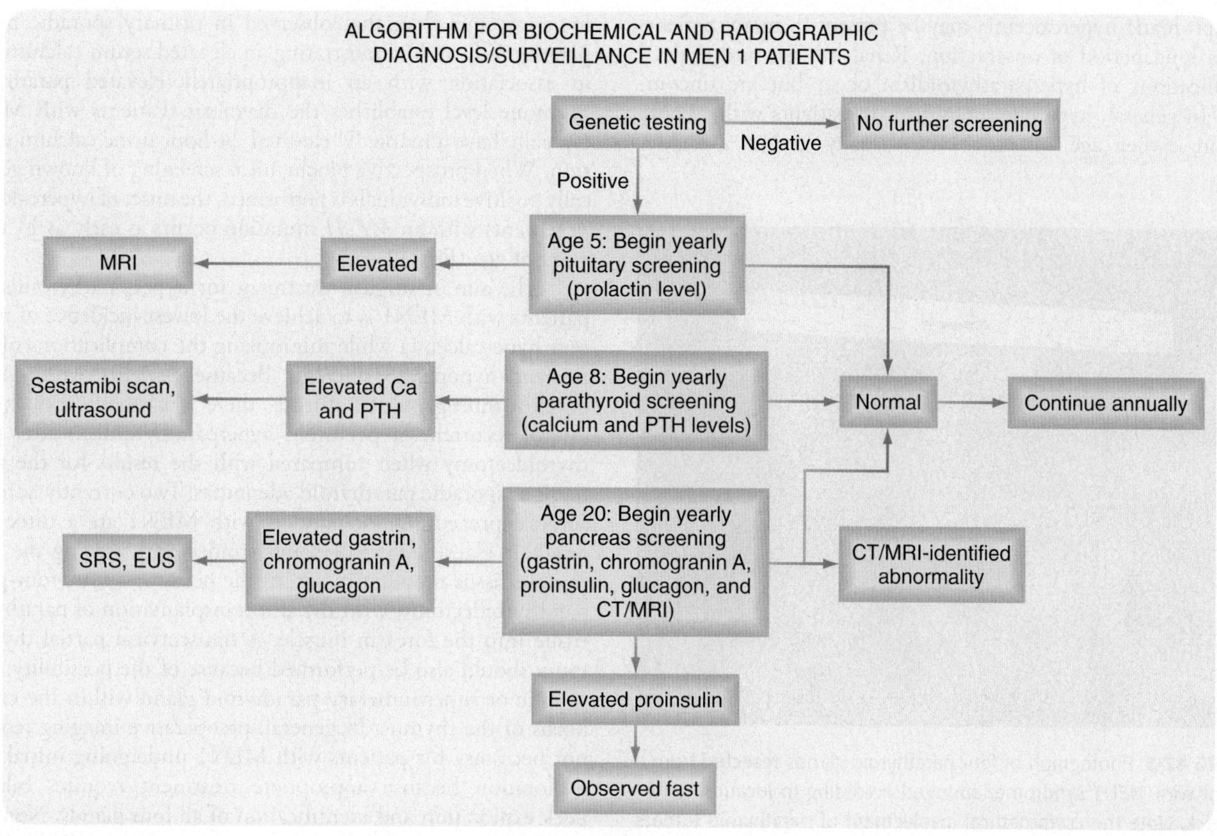


**FIGURE 42-2** Clinical and biochemical surveillance in patients with MEN1. (From Whaley JG, Lairmore TC: Multiple endocrine neoplasia type 1: Current diagnosis and management. In Morita SY, Dackiw APB, Zeiger MA [eds]: McGraw-Hill's manual of endocrine surgery, New York, 2009, McGraw-Hill, pp 334–347.)

Males and females are affected equally with MEN1, as predicted by the autosomal dominant inheritance pattern. MEN1 has been described in many geographic regions and ethnic groups, and no racial predilection has been demonstrated. The MEN1 trait is transmitted with almost 100% penetrance, but with variable expressivity, so that each affected person may exhibit some but not necessarily all components of the syndrome. The most common abnormality in MEN1 is multiple parathyroid tumors, which eventually develop in 98% to 100% of affected individuals. Duodenopancreatic NET, which carries a malignant potential, occurs in approximately 30% to 80% of patients, whereas pituitary tumors become clinically evident in approximately 15% to 50% of affected patients. At autopsy, pathologic involvement in all three endocrine tissues has been described in almost all patients. When compared with sporadic endocrine tumors, the endocrine tumors arising in association with the familial MEN1 syndrome are characterized by an earlier age of onset, multifocal involvement within a target endocrine tissue, and development of concurrent neoplasms in multiple endocrine tissues.

The clinical manifestations of patients with MEN1 depend on the endocrine tissue involved, specific hormone overproduced, or local mass effect and malignant progression of the neoplasm. Previously, complications related to hormone excess, such as severe ulcer disease or hypoglycemia, were the most frequent presenting complaints. At present, the principal cause of mortality in patients with MEN1 is malignant progression of duodenopancreatic neuroendocrine cancers or intrathoracic malignant carcinoids. Current recommendations indicate that annual biochemical testing, including determination of pancreatic polypeptide, gastrin, glucagon, and chromogranin A levels, should begin at approximately age 15 to 20 years in presymptomatic affected individuals.[9] It is now recommended to begin biochemical screening for pituitary adenomas in carriers of MEN1 mutations at 5 years of age. Some have recommended screening for hyperparathyroidism as early as the age of 8 years in MEN1 mutation carriers, but the peak incidence of clinically apparent HPT is in the late second or early third decade. A summary of our recommendations for the clinical and biochemical surveillance of patients with MEN1 is shown in Figure 42-2.

## Parathyroid Glands

The most common endocrine abnormality (>98% affected individuals) in MEN1 is multiglandular parathyroid tumors. The parathyroid tumors in MEN1 are clonal, resulting from inactivation of both alleles of the *MEN1* tumor suppressor gene by two separate events, and are therefore multiple adenomas from a strict genetic standpoint.[10] In contrast, fewer than 15% of patients with sporadic primary hyperparathyroidism have multiglandular involvement. The typical enlargement of parathyroid glands in MEN1 patients is asymmetrical at any point in the intervention (Fig. 42-3).

Hypercalcemia is usually the first biochemical abnormality detected in patients with MEN1, and may precede the clinical onset of a pancreatic NET or pituitary neoplasm by several years.

Asymptomatic hypercalcemia may be present in many patients over a long period of observation. Renal lithiasis and skeletal complications of hyperparathyroidism occur but are uncommon. In general, hyperparathyroidism in patients with MEN1 has an earlier age of onset and usually causes a milder hypercalcemia than that observed in primary sporadic hyperparathyroidism. Demonstrating an elevated serum calcium level in association with an inappropriately elevated parathyroid hormone level establishes the diagnosis. Patients with MEN1 typically have a markedly elevated 24-hour urine calcium excretion. When prospective biochemical screening of known genetically positive individuals is performed, the onset of hypercalcemia in patients with an *MEN1* mutation occurs as early as 11 to 14 years of age (Fig. 42-4).

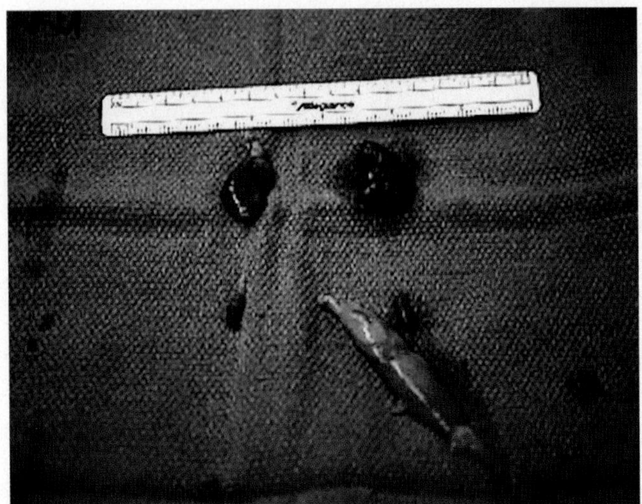

**FIGURE 42-3** Photograph of four parathyroid glands resected from a patient with MEN1 syndrome, arranged according to location within the neck. Note the asymmetrical involvement of parathyroid tumors with two markedly enlarged upper glands and more modestly enlarged lower glands. The left inferior parathyroid was located within the cranial horn of the thymus.

The aim of surgical treatment for hyperparathyroidism in patients with MEN1 is to achieve the lowest incidence of recurrent hypercalcemia while minimizing the complications of permanent hypoparathyroidism. Because patients with MEN1 develop multiglandular disease, there is a significantly higher rate of recurrent or persistent hyperparathyroidism after parathyroidectomy when compared with the results for the treatment of sporadic parathyroid adenomas. Two currently accepted surgical procedures for patients with MEN1 are a three-and-one-half–gland (subtotal) parathyroidectomy, leaving the parathyroid tissue remnant in situ in the neck, or a total four-gland parathyroidectomy, with IM autotransplantation of parathyroid tissue into the forearm muscle. A transcervical partial thymectomy should also be performed because of the possibility of an ectopic or supernumerary parathyroid gland within the cranial horns of the thymus. In general, preoperative imaging tests are not necessary for patients with MEN1 undergoing initial neck exploration because appropriate treatment requires bilateral neck exploration and identification of all four glands. Noninvasive imaging tests, such as parathyroid nuclear medicine (sestamibi) scanning and ultrasound may be useful for parathyroid localization prior to reoperative surgery.

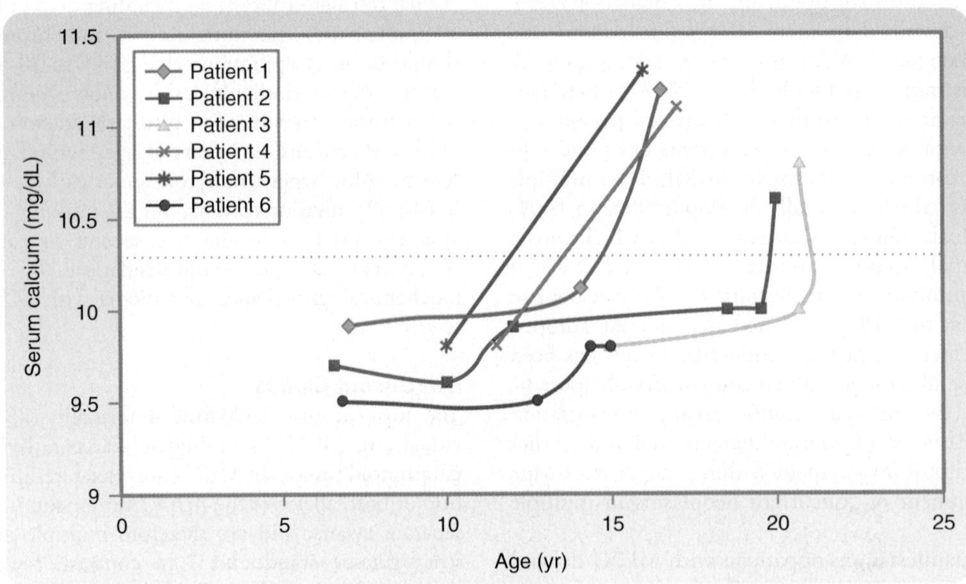


**FIGURE 42-4** Serum calcium levels versus age in six patients genetically positive for MEN1. The data were obtained prospectively based on genetic diagnosis. Each patient's curve is represented by a different color and data point symbol according to the legend in the upper left corner. The serum calcium level (mg/dL) is plotted as a function of age (years). The upper limit of normal for calcium is indicated by the *dotted line*. In this selected subset of genetically positive patients followed prospectively, a rapid rise in calcium levels is evident between the ages of 10 and 15 years. (From Lairmore TC, Piersall LD, DeBenedetti MK, et al: Clinical genetic testing and early surgical intervention in patients with multiple endocrine neoplasia type 1 [MEN1]. Ann Surg 239:637–645, 2004.)

Debate continues regarding the optimal surgical procedure for hyperparathyroidism in patients with MEN1. The incidence of recurrent hyperparathyroidism following any surgical treatment for the multiglandular disease in MEN1 is approximately 30% to 40% 5 years postsurgery, reflecting the genetic first-hit predisposition in every parathyroid cell. Recurrences are related to how long the patient is followed and the performance of thymectomy.[11] A potential advantage of total parathyroidectomy and heterotopic autotransplantation to the forearm is the ability to manage recurrent hyperparathyroidism, if it develops, by excision of a portion of the grafted parathyroid tissue under local anesthesia, obviating the morbidity of repeat neck exploration. Subtotal resection is believed by many to achieve equivalent results without a purported higher risk of permanent hypocalcemia from autograft failure.[12] Currently, both treatments appear to provide essentially equivalent results, and the answer to this question awaits a randomized, prospective clinical trial. Delayed transplantation of cryopreserved autologous parathyroid tissue can salvage a proportion of patients with permanent postoperative hypocalcemia following either procedure. In one study,[13] approximately 60% of delayed, cryopreserved parathyroid autografts showed evidence of graft function based on venous parathyroid hormone (PTH) gradients between the grafted and nongrafted arms; 40% of autografts achieved full competency without supplements.

### Pancreas and Duodenum

The second most frequent component of MEN1 is the development of NETs of the duodenum or pancreas. Depending on the method of study, 30% to 80% of patients with MEN1 develop clinically evident tumors. These tumors, along with the intrathoracic carcinoids, carry a significant malignant potential and result in most of the MEN1 disease-related morbidity and mortality. The pathologic change is typically multifocal, and diffuse islet cell hyperplasia and microadenoma formation may be present in areas of the pancreas distant from grossly evident tumor. Gastrinomas frequently occur within the wall of the duodenum or in extrapancreatic sites. The pancreaticoduodenal tumors in patients with MEN1 produce symptoms caused by hormone oversecretion or mass effect from the tumor growth itself; these are characterized by a high malignant potential.

Several radiographic imaging methods are available for the preoperative detection of the gastroenteropancreatic NETs. A cross-sectional imaging test (computed tomography [CT] or magnetic resonance imaging [MRI]) should be performed as an initial test in almost all patients to exclude a very large primary neoplasm or metastases. Biphasic thin slice CT has been reported to have a sensitivity of 94.4% for pancreatic NETs. However, the sensitivity decreases with smaller tumors (<2 cm), multiple tumors (as is often the case with MEN1), tumors located in extrapancreatic locations (e.g., duodenal wall), or tumors located in the distal tail of the pancreas. MRI is advocated by some and can detect smaller tumors; however, no clear advantage of MRI over CT has been shown.

Endoscopic ultrasonography (EUS) is an excellent imaging modality for NETs of the pancreas and duodenum but is dependent on availability and operator skill in selected centers. In 1992, Rosch and colleagues[14] have reported a sensitivity of 82% and specificity of 95% of EUS in detecting pancreatic NETs that had not been localized by transabdominal ultrasound or CT. However, the detection rate decreases with distal progression along the pancreatic tail, likely because of increased distance from the gastric or duodenal lumen. EUS is an effective and relatively noninvasive localizing test (after initial CT), but is dependent on the skill and experience of the operator and availability.

Somatostatin receptor scintigraphy (SRS) may also be used to localize these tumors. In the subpopulation of MEN1 patients, one study found that the specificity and positive predictive value of SRS for pancreatic tumors are 25% and 100%, respectively, whereas specificity and positive predictive value of SRS for duodenal gastrinomas are 72% and 100%, respectively.[15] In this study, all pancreatic NETs were detected by EUS or SRS.

Finally, selective pancreatic arteriography with provocative stimulation by selected secretagogues and measurement of increment hormone secretion in the hepatic vein is an invasive test, but may be the most accurate single localizing study.[16] This test provides regional localization of functional tumors (e.g., insulinoma, gastrinoma) within the pancreas and is especially useful for patients with MEN1 who characteristically have multiple tumors.

Pancreatic NETs that are nonfunctioning or that secrete pancreatic polypeptide are probably the most frequent NETs that occur in patients with MEN1. The most common functional NET in patients with MEN1 is gastrinoma. The presenting signs and symptoms in patients with hypergastrinemia (Zollinger-Ellison syndrome [ZES]) include epigastric pain, reflux esophagitis, secretory diarrhea, and weight loss. Currently, with highly effective proton pump inhibitors (PPIs) for medical therapy, active peptic ulcer disease is present in less than 20% of patients at the time of diagnosis. Patients may infrequently present with a severe ulcer diathesis as well as stricture or perforation of the esophagus caused by severe reflux esophagitis. Gastrinoma is diagnosed by the documentation of gastric acid hypersecretion (>15 mEq/liter in patients without surgery or >5 mEq/liter in patients with prior ulcer surgery), associated with elevated fasting levels of serum gastrin (>100 pg/mL). The diagnosis can be confirmed by an abnormal secretin test result.

Gastrinomas that develop in patients with MEN1 are usually malignant (≈80%), as indicated by the presence of regional lymph node or distant metastases. Gastrinomas were previously believed to be located predominantly in the head of the pancreas within the gastrinoma triangle. More recent data have suggested that gastrinomas in patients with MEN1 occur most frequently within the wall of the duodenum (Fig. 42-5). Because of the small size of these neoplasms, the primary gastrinoma may not be localized preoperatively by CT scanning or angiography. Endoscopic ultrasound has been used successfully to localize gastrinomas within the wall of the duodenum or head of the pancreas. There is controversy about the development of primary gastrinoma within lymph nodes. Although occasional patients have been biochemically cured after resection of gastrinoma within lymph nodes, it is unclear whether an occult gastrinoma primary was missed within the pancreas or wall of the duodenum.

The value of surgical resection for intended cure of gastrinoma in patients with MEN1 is controversial. Although most evidence indicates that patients with ZES and MEN1 rarely demonstrate long-term biochemical cure following operation,[17] localized resection of a potentially malignant NET is indicated in an attempt to control the tumoral process and prevent subsequent malignant dissemination. The recognition that primary

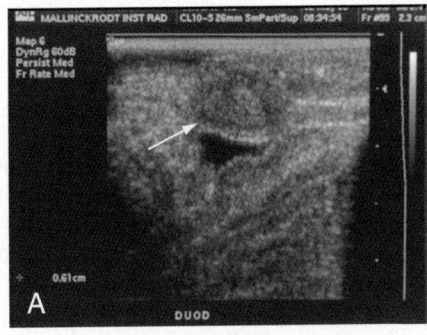

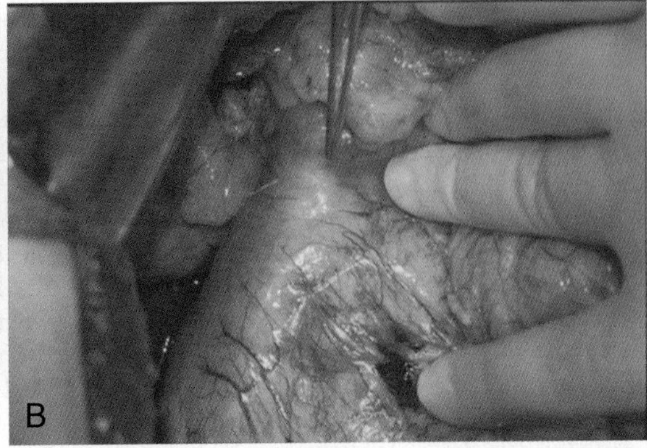


**FIGURE 42-5** Gastrinoma in the duodenal wall from patient with MEN1. **A,** Intraoperative ultrasound demonstrating a circumscribed hypoechoic tumor in the submucosa of the duodenal wall, demonstrated just superior to the duodenal lumen. **B,** Gross appearance of the duodenal wall tumor from the serosal surface.

gastrinomas occur frequently in the duodenal wall, combined with efforts to perform an extensive regional lymphadenectomy or even pancreaticoduodenectomy, may improve the success rate of surgery for ZES in the setting of MEN1.[18] Newer strategies, including rapid intraoperative gastrin determinations, are also being used in the surgical management of gastrinoma. Total gastrectomy is rarely indicated for patients with gastrinoma because medical therapy effectively prevents most of the symptoms or complications resulting from the acid hypersecretion. The availability of PPIs allows effective medical therapy for patients with unresectable gastrinoma or extensive metastatic disease. However, careful observation of the stomach by repeated endoscopy is necessary because long-term administration of PPIs to patients with MEN1 and ZES has been associated with the development of gastric carcinoid tumors. Patients with primary hyperparathyroidism should undergo parathyroidectomy because normalization of the serum calcium level improves the ZES.[19]

The second most common clinically evident pancreatic NETs in patients with MEN1 are insulinomas. These are usually small (<2 cm) and occur with even distribution throughout the pancreas. Patients typically present with recurrent symptoms of neuroglycopenia—sweating, dizziness, confusion, or syncope. Documenting symptomatic hypoglycemia in association with inappropriately elevated plasma levels of insulin and C-peptide during a supervised 72-hour fast confirms the diagnosis of insulinoma. Insulinomas may be occult and are infrequently localized by conventional preoperative imaging studies such as CT, ultrasound, MRI, or angiography.

There is no ideal medical therapy for insulinoma; therefore, the preferred treatment is accurate localization and surgical resection of the functioning tumor to correct life-threatening hyperinsulinemia. Patients with MEN1 characteristically develop multiple NETs, which may complicate identification of the specific functional tumor responsible for the hyperinsulinism. Preoperative regional localization of the functioning tumor within the pancreas may be provided by selective catheterization of the arteries supplying the pancreas, followed by injection of an insulin secretagogue (calcium gluconate) and measurement of insulin gradients in the hepatic veins. The operative approach includes complete mobilization of the pancreas and careful examination of the gland by inspection and palpation.

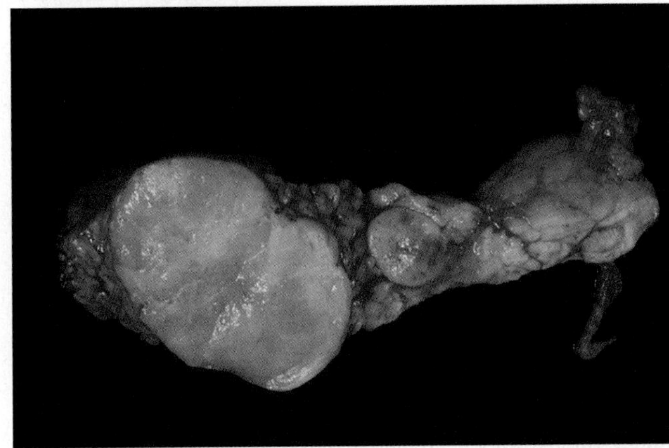

**FIGURE 42-6** Multiple neuroendocrine tumors of the pancreas in a distal pancreatectomy specimen from a patient with MEN1.

Intraoperative ultrasound is essential for the identification of small tumors, especially within the pancreatic head or uncinate process.[20] Small benign insulinomas are amenable to enucleation. Partial pancreatectomy may be required for multiple or potentially malignant tumors.[16] If the insulinoma is not identified, despite an exhaustive intraoperative search, blind subtotal pancreatectomy is not recommended. Approximately 10% of insulinomas occurring in patients with MEN1 are malignant. Patients with malignant insulinoma and disseminated metastases may respond to treatment with streptozotocin and some control of hypoglycemia may be achieved by the administration of diazoxide or octreotide.

Other functional NETs of the pancreas, such as glucagonoma, somatostatinoma, and tumors secreting vasoactive intestinal peptide or pancreatic polypeptide, occur rarely in association with MEN1.

The involvement of NETs within the pancreas of patients with MEN1 is characteristically multifocal (Fig. 42-6). Controversy exists regarding the optimal timing and most appropriate operation to perform for NETs of the pancreas and duodenum in patients with MEN1. The controversy reflects uncertainty about the natural history of small, potentially benign or nonfunctional tumors, which must be weighed against the risks of early and/or repeat major pancreatic interventions carrying a significant risk of morbidity. Some are reluctant to advocate routine or early pancreatic exploration in young, otherwise healthy patients for small nonfunctional tumors, which might be clinically insignificant. On the other hand, these tumors have a malignant potential, and delay in diagnosis and effective treatment carry the risk of the development of local or distant metastasis. It is obviously desirable to intervene early to prevent malignant dissemination while minimizing morbidity and mortality (from cancer or surgery). Complicating factors include the lack of genotype-phenotype correlation in MEN1, which might otherwise allow genetic stratification of those at higher risk of malignant progression, and failure of recent studies to identify a clear relationship between the size of the tumor and risk of regional lymph node or distant metastases.[21]

The spectrum of clinical strategies proposed ranges from the most aggressive approach, consisting of early surgical exploration and resection of tumors when the patient's peptide tumor markers become elevated (even without radiographically detectable tumors), to the most conservative approach, advocating operation only for tumors exceeding approximately 1.0 cm in size on radiographic imaging or demonstrating hormone hyperfunction.[16,22,23] The malignant potential of these neoplasms is clear, with up to 50% of patients eventually developing regional lymph node or distant metastases. Many groups now recommend early operation and excision of these tumors to prevent malignant progression.[24] One recent large retrospective study has suggested improved overall survival in patients undergoing surgery, especially younger patients with localized tumors and those with hormonally functional tumors.[21] The operative strategy for NET in patients with MEN1 must be aimed at extirpation of all grossly evident tumors, with preservation of pancreatic exocrine and endocrine function and avoidance of excessive operative morbidity. These factors are complex and must be individualized to the patient.

### Pituitary Gland

Adenomas of the anterior pituitary gland occur in a variable proportion of patients with MEN1. The most frequent pituitary tumor in patients with MEN1 is a prolactinoma. Pituitary tumors cause symptoms by hypersecretion of hormones or compression of adjacent structures. Large adenomas may cause visual field defects by pressure on the optic chiasm or manifestations of hypopituitarism through compression of the adjacent normal gland. Prolactin-secreting tumors result in amenorrhea and galactorrhea in women or hypogonadism in men. MEN1 patients with pituitary tumors may exhibit acromegaly resulting from growth hormone overproduction or Cushing's disease caused by an adrenocorticotropic hormone (ACTH)–producing pituitary tumor.

Medical treatment with a dopamine agonist such as bromocriptine or cabergoline is effective in controlling the hyperprolactinemia in most patients with prolactinomas. Growth hormone–producing tumors causing acromegaly or ACTH-producing tumors are usually treated by surgical resection; medical therapy for growth hormone–secreting tumors includes somatostatin analogues such as octreotide and lanreotide. Trans-sphenoidal pituitary microsurgery or radiation therapy are indicated infrequently for rapidly enlarging, nonfunctional macroadenomas that are unresponsive to medical therapy or result in local compressive symptoms because of their mass effect.

### Other Tumors

Bronchial and thymic carcinoids, benign thyroid tumors, benign and malignant adrenocortical tumors, lipomas, ependymomas of the central nervous system (CNS), and facial cutaneous angiofibromas and collagenomas occur with increased frequency in patients with MEN1. Approximately 30% of patients with MEN1 develop adrenal masses or bilateral nodular adrenal hyperplasia. Surgical removal of adrenocortical tumors larger than 3.0 cm may prevent development of adrenal malignancy. Thymectomy to prevent development of malignant thymic carcinoid may be considered in male patients, especially smokers.

## MULTIPLE ENDOCRINE NEOPLASIA TYPE 2 SYNDROMES

The MEN2 syndromes include MEN2A, MEN2B, and familial, non-MEN medullary thyroid carcinoma (FMTC). The hallmark of the MEN2 syndromes is MTC, which occurs with almost complete penetrance. Additional manifestations are of variable penetrance and include pheochromocytoma in MEN2A and MEN2B and hyperparathyroidism in MEN2A (Table 42-1; Fig. 42-7). The MEN2 syndromes have an autosomal dominant pattern of inheritance and are caused by activating mutations in the *RET* proto-oncogene on chromosome 10 (Fig. 42-8).[25] The clinical features and tumor behavior seen in the MEN2 syndromes are closely correlated with the specific germline mutation present in the *RET* gene. Management of patients

**Table 42-1 Clinical Features of Multiple Endocrine Neoplasia Syndromes**

| CLINICAL SETTING | FEATURES OF MTC | INHERITANCE PATTERN | ASSOCIATED ABNORMALITIES | GENETIC DEFECT |
|---|---|---|---|---|
| Sporadic MTC | Unifocal | None | None | Somatic *RET* mutations in >20% of tumors |
| MEN2A | Multifocal, bilateral | Autosomal dominant | Pheochromocytomas, hyperparathyroidism | Germ-line missense mutations in extracellular cysteine codons of *RET* |
| MEN2B | Multifocal, bilateral | Autosomal dominant | Pheochromocytomas, mucosal neuromas, megacolon, skeletal abnormalities | Germline missense mutation in tyrosine kinase domain of *RET* |
| FMTC | Multifocal, bilateral | Autosomal dominant | None | Germline missense mutations in extracellular or intracellular cysteine codons of *RET* |

Adapted from Moley JF, Lairmore TC, Phay JE: Hereditary endocrinopathies. Curr Probl Surg 36:653–764, 1999.

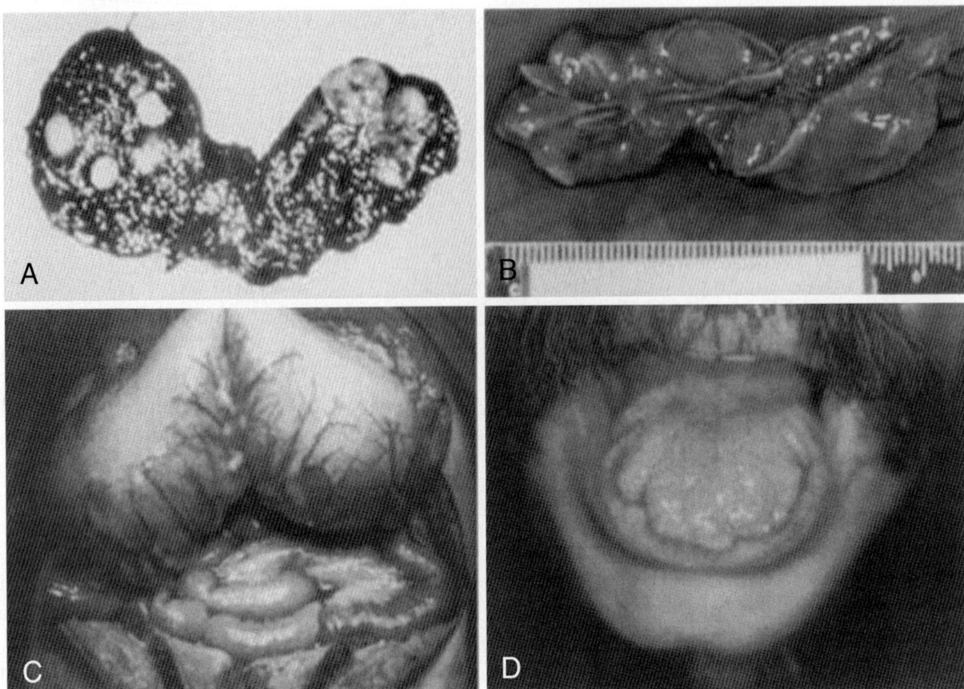


**FIGURE 42-7** Features of MEN2A and 2B syndromes. **A,** Bisected thyroidectomy specimen showing multifocal, bilateral MTC tumors. **B,** Adrenalectomy specimen from patient with MEN2B showing pheochromocytoma. **C,** Megacolon in patient with MEN2B. **D,** Tongue nodules in patient with MEN2B. (**A,** Courtesy Dr. S. A. Wells; **B-D,** courtesy Dr. R. Thompson; From Moley JF: Medullary thyroid cancer. In Clark OH, Duh QY [eds]: Textbook of endocrine surgery, Philadelphia, 1997, WB Saunders.)

and families affected by these syndromes should be informed by an understanding of the genotype-phenotype correlation associated with the specific *RET* mutation present in family members.

Understanding the genetic basis of the MEN2 syndromes has led to a paradigm shift in the screening and treatment of affected patients and their families. Treatment now focuses on early identification of *RET* mutation carriers and early thyroidectomy to prevent MTC, when possible. This section will describe the genetics, clinical features, diagnosis, and management of patients with the MEN2 syndromes.

## Genetics and Clinical Features

### *RET* Proto-Oncogene

The *RET* (***re***arranged during ***t***ransfection) proto-oncogene encodes a receptor tyrosine kinase protein involved in growth, differentiation, and migration of developing tissues. The full-length protein includes an extracellular, cysteine-rich, ligand-binding domain, transmembrane domain, intracellular juxtamembrane domain, and intracellular tyrosine kinase domain (see Fig. 42-8). The mutations responsible for MTC are missense mutations that result in single amino acid changes that cause gain of function alterations in the protein. There are consistent associations between the specific *RET* mutation (genotype) and clinical phenotype of patients with familial forms of MTC.[26] This includes age of onset, aggressiveness of MTC, and presence or absence of other endocrine neoplasms. MEN2B patients expressing the M918T mutation have the most aggressive forms of MTC, with evidence of disease often present in early infancy. MEN2A patients have a variable course of MTC disease presentation and progression, whereas FMTC patients demonstrate an indolent form that more often presents in the later decades of life. *RET* mutations in MEN2 are inherited in an autosomal dominant fashion. Thus, MEN2 carriers confer a 50% risk of genetic transmission to their offspring.

*RET* is expressed in multiple tissues descended from the neural crest, including the thyroid parafollicular cells (C cells), parathyroid glands, adrenal chromaffin cells, enteric ganglia, and other peripheral and central neurons. Based on studies in animal models, *RET* signaling is necessary for the normal development of the kidney, parasympathetic nervous system, gut-associated lymphoid tissue, and enteric nervous system. *RET* knockout mice demonstrate features that include renal agenesis and aberrant gut neurophysiology. In humans, inactivating (loss of function) mutations in *RET* are associated with Hirschsprung's disease, a defect in migration and development of enteric neurons, which causes megacolon in infancy. Activating (gain of function) germline mutations in *RET* are associated with the MEN2 syndromes, and activating somatic mutations are associated with sporadic thyroid carcinomas. This mechanism differs from MEN1 and most other hereditary cancer syndromes (including hereditary breast cancer and colon cancer), which are caused by loss of function mutations in the predisposition gene (tumor suppressor genes).

The RET protein has four known ligands that induce its activation—glial cell line–derived neurotrophic factor (GDNF), artemin, persephin, and neurturin, known collectively as the GDNF family ligands (GFLs). RET activation by each of these GFLs is mediated through one of four ligand-specific coreceptors, belonging to the GDNF family receptors

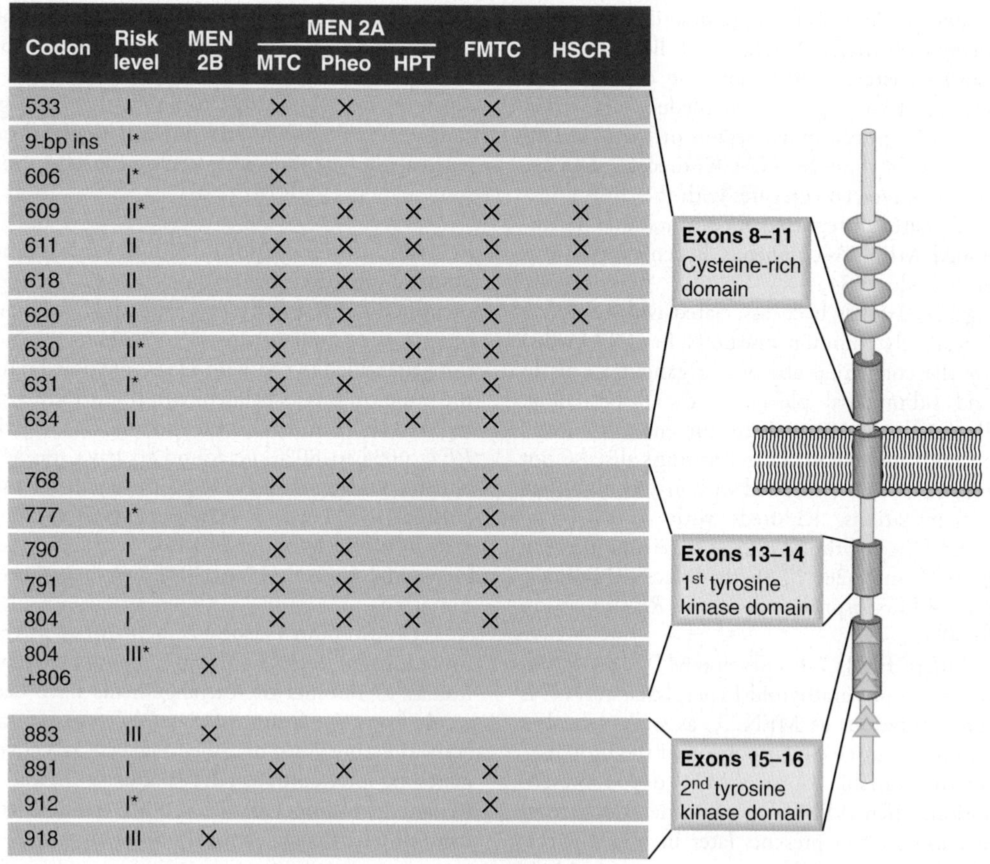

| Codon | Risk level | MEN 2B | MEN 2A MTC | MEN 2A Pheo | MEN 2A HPT | FMTC | HSCR |
|---|---|---|---|---|---|---|---|
| 533 | I | | × | × | | × | |
| 9-bp ins | I* | | | | | × | |
| 606 | I* | | × | | | | |
| 609 | II* | | × | × | × | × | × |
| 611 | II | | × | × | × | × | × |
| 618 | II | | × | × | × | × | × |
| 620 | II | | × | × | | × | × |
| 630 | II* | | × | | × | × | |
| 631 | I* | | × | × | | × | |
| 634 | II | | × | × | × | × | |
| 768 | I | | × | × | | × | |
| 777 | I* | | | | | × | |
| 790 | I | | × | × | | × | |
| 791 | I | | × | × | × | × | |
| 804 | I | | × | × | × | × | |
| 804 +806 | III* | × | | | | | |
| 883 | III | × | | | | | |
| 891 | I | | × | × | | × | |
| 912 | I* | | | | | × | |
| 918 | III | × | | | | | |



**FIGURE 42-8** *RET* mutation sites associated with MEN2 syndromes. Codons previously reported in association with MEN2 syndromes are listed by structural domain within the RET protein. Risk level is based on consensus guidelines or more recent clinical reports. Previously reported phenotypes for each codon are shown. *FMTC,* Familial medullary thyroid carcinoma; *HSCR,* Hirschsprung's disease; *HPT,* hyperparathyroidism; *MTC,* medullary thyroid carcinoma; *Pheo,* pheochromocytoma; ***, risk level based on recent clinical reports (not available at publication of the consensus guidelines). (From Traugott AL, Moley JF: The RET protooncogene. Cancer Treat Res 153:303–319, 2010.)

α (GFRα). These GFRα coreceptors are anchored to the plasma membrane by a glycosylphosphatidylinositol residue, likely facilitating their interaction with the membrane-bound RET protein. Normal RET activation occurs with the assembly of a dimeric complex including two RET proteins, two ligand molecules, and two GFRα coreceptors. Current evidence indicates that this entire complex is necessary for RET signaling and that ligand binding and downstream activation require the coreceptor.

The dimerized RET receptor complex activates a number of intracellular signaling pathways implicated in cell survival and differentiation. These include the Ras/ERK and PI3K/Akt pathways, which are important in cell proliferation, differentiation, and survival. Additional pathways activated by RET include p38MAPK, phospholipase C-γ (PLCγ), JNK, and ERK5, suggesting additional roles for RET in cell differentiation, migration, and cytokine production. Activated RET also has a phosphorylated serine residue (S696) in the juxtamembrane domain. This site has been implicated in Rac-mediated migration of enteric neural crest cells during normal development. An inactivating mutation at this site in mice has resulted in a lack of enteric neurons in the distal colon, similar to the phenotype of Hirschsprung's disease in humans.

### Multiple Endocrine Neoplasia Type 2A and Familial, Non–Multiple Endocrine Neoplasia Medullary Thyroid Carcinoma

In the 1960s, Sipple and Steiner described the association of thyroid cancer with pheochromocytoma and hyperparathyroidism, respectively.[27] MEN2A is characterized by a hereditary predisposition to MTC. Penetrance of this feature is almost complete—that is, almost all patients who inherit a germline MEN2A-associated mutation in the *RET* proto-oncogene develop MTC. MEN2A patients will all develop MTC during their lifetime, although the age of onset varies from early childhood to adulthood, depending on the specific mutation and kindred. Of MEN2A patients, 40% to 50% will develop pheochromocytoma, which may or may not be synchronous with MTC in its presentation. Pheochromocytoma occurs in 42% to 46% of MEN2A patients overall, although the prevalence varies from 5% to 100% in different kindreds. The degree of penetrance for pheochromocytoma in MEN2A correlates with specific *RET* mutations, with the highest expression in carriers of mutations at codon 634.[28] Parathyroid hyperplasia, in one or multiple glands, results in primary hyperparathyroidism in 20% to 35% of MEN2A patients overall and this also varies by kindred.

Cutaneous lichen amyloidosis has been described in several kindreds and patients with MEN2A. Cutaneous lichen amyloidosis is a rare disorder characterized by amyloid deposition in the papillary dermis, resulting in pruritic cutaneous plaques that are often localized to the interscapular region or extensor surfaces of the extremities. In these MEN2A kindreds, cutaneous lichen amyloidosis phenotype cosegregates with the clinical features of MEN2A. To date, all reported *RET* mutations in kindreds with combined MEN2A–cutaneous lichen amyloidosis features have been in codon 634.

Hirschsprung's disease has been associated with MEN2A and FMTC. This relatively common disease (1 in 5000 births) is characterized by the congenital absence of ganglion cells in the myenteric and submucosal plexus of the distal colon. Newborn Hirschsprung's disease patients present with distal bowel obstruction and megacolon. Hirschsprung's disease not associated with MEN2 is often associated with inactivating (loss of function) *RET* mutations. Kindreds with cosegregating MEN2A-FMTC and Hirschsprung's disease have mutations in *RET* codons 609, 618, and 624.[26,29] In the affected kindreds, reported penetrance of Hirschsprung's disease in *RET* mutation carriers is 16% to 50%.

Patients who inherit FMTC also develop MTC but do not have pheochromocytoma or parathyroid hyperplasia. FMTC is caused by the same mutations as MEN2A, as well as by less common mutations in the intracellular portion of the protein.[30] MEN2A patients have a variable course of MTC disease presentation and progression, whereas FMTC patients demonstrate an indolent form that more often presents later in life. There is considerable overlap between the RET codons affected in FMTC and those in MEN2A, which supports the theory that FMTC is a variant of MEN2A and not a distinct clinical entity. Occasional patients with FMTC will never manifest clinical evidence of MTC (symptoms or a palpable neck mass), although biochemical testing and histologic evaluation of the thyroid demonstrates MTC.

The most common mutations associated with MEN2A/FMTC occur in exons 10 and 11, within the extracellular cysteine-rich domain of the RET protein. Cysteine residues at codons 609, 611, 618, 620, 630, and 634 fall within this region. The amino acid changes caused by these mutations de-stabilize the normal tertiary structure of the RET protein, which results in ligand-independent dimerization and persistent intracellular signaling by RET.

### Multiple Endocrine Neoplasia Type 2B

In MEN2B, as in MEN2A, all patients develop MTC. All MEN2B individuals have mucosal neuromas, and 40% to 50% of patients develop pheochromocytomas. MEN2B patients do not develop hyperparathyroidism. MTC in MEN2B presents at a very young age, in infancy, and appears to be the most aggressive form of hereditary MTC. These patients often have a distinct physical appearance with a prominent mid–upper lip, everted eyebrows, multiple tongue nodules, and marfanoid body habitus (see Fig. 42-7). The mucosal neuromas are unencapsulated thickened proliferations of nerves that occur principally on the lips and tongue, but can also be found on the gingiva, buccal mucosa, nasal mucosa, vocal cords, and conjunctiva. MEN2B patients also develop ganglioneuromas of the intestine in the submucosal and myenteric plexus. All MEN2B patients have a megacolon and usually have chronic bowel problems. Intestinal dysfunction may manifest early in life with poor feeding, failure to thrive, constipation, or pseudo-obstruction. Adults with this disorder may have dysphagia from esophageal dysmotility. Rarely, a patient can present with toxic megacolon. MEN2B patients, however, do not develop Hirschsprung's disease, as do some patients with MEN2A.

### *RET* Mutations in Sporadic Thyroid Carcinomas

Somatic mutations or rearrangements involving *RET* have been identified in 40% to 50% of sporadic MTCs and in up to 70% of sporadic papillary thyroid carcinomas.[31] Most of the mutations identified in sporadic MTCs are point mutations involving the same codons associated with the MEN2 syndromes, including 918, 634, and 883. Of sporadic MTCs with alterations of *RET*, 60% to 80% are found to have the M918T mutation. Patients with sporadic MTCs bearing a *RET* mutation (particularly M918T) have a more advanced stage at diagnosis, increased rates of recurrent or persistent disease after resection, and poorer long-term survival (10 to 20 years) than those without a *RET* mutation.

Chromosomal rearrangements of *RET*, rather than point mutations, are associated with sporadic papillary thyroid carcinomas. A number of rearrangements have been reported that result from the fusion of the *RET* tyrosine kinase domain to activating portions of other genes. Collectively, these fusion genes are referred to as RET–papillary thyroid carcinomas and, to date, 13 distinct variants, resulting from rearrangement events from different genes, have been described.[32]

## Screening and Genetic Testing

Before the genetic basis of MEN2 was well characterized, pentagastrin-stimulated calcitonin testing was used to screen for MEN2 and MTC in patients at risk for inheriting an MEN2 syndrome. Occasional false-positive and false-negative tests, however, resulted in unnecessary surgery or a missed opportunity to intervene early. Sequencing of the *RET* gene to detect germline mutations is now the standard screening test for MEN2 syndromes. *RET* mutation testing can identify young carriers at an earlier stage of disease, often before they develop cancer, and it has lower false-positive and false-negative rates than calcitonin testing. It is recommended that patients or their parents meet with a genetic counselor prior to testing. Genetic counseling is an important component of informed consent and education for these patients, who are facing a major event that will affect their own and their family's lives.

*RET* mutation testing should be performed routinely for at-risk members of MEN2 and FMTC families. If possible, testing should occur at birth, because carrier status determines the need for clinical screening and preventive surgery. In families in which the inherited *RET* mutation is already known, *RET* sequencing can be limited to the site of the known mutation. Those family members who are negative for their kindred's known mutation have the same risk for MEN2 as the general population, and they need no other screening. When an MTC patient with no known family history of MTC or MEN2 is found to have a *RET* mutation (index case), all first-degree family members should be offered genetic counseling and testing.

*RET* mutation testing is also indicated for adult or pediatric patients who present with MTC or pheochromocytoma, regardless of any family history of endocrine tumors. Approximately 5% to 7% of patients believed to have sporadic MTC are found to have a germline *RET* mutation. Up to 24% of pheochromocytomas are hereditary, with 5% resulting from *RET* mutations.[33] Infants presenting with Hirschsprung's disease should undergo *RET* mutation testing. All reported cases of MEN2A associated with Hirschsprung's disease have occurred in patients with mutations in exon 10 of *RET* at codons 609, 618, and 620.

## Medullary Thyroid Carcinoma

MTC comprises 3% to 9% of all thyroid cancers and arises from thyroid C cells. MTC may be sporadic (75% of cases) or hereditary, occurring in all patients with the MEN2 syndromes (25% of cases). Hereditary MTCs are often multifocal and bilateral. Multicentric C cell hyperplasia has been shown to precede the development of hereditary MTC.[34] MTC is a relatively indolent malignancy, with reported 10-year survival rates ranging from 69% to 89%.[35] Unlike differentiated thyroid cancer, MTC cells do not concentrate radioactive iodine and are not sensitive to manipulation of thyroid-stimulating hormone (TSH). These features must be considered when planning therapy for a patient with MTC.[36]

Patients with established MTC may present with a palpable thyroid mass or nodule. Symptoms of dysphagia, shortness of breath, or hoarseness are present in approximately 15% of cases. Metastases to regional cervical lymph nodes are present in up to 75% of patients who present with palpable disease.[37] The most frequent sites of lymphatic spread are to the central compartment of the neck (level VI), followed by the ipsilateral jugular nodes (levels II to V) and then the contralateral cervical nodes. Other frequent metastatic sites include the mediastinum, lungs, liver, and bone.[30]

Calcitonin is made by thyroid C cells and MTC cells. It is a sensitive and specific tumor marker that may be measured in blood in the basal state or after the administration of the secretagogues calcium and pentagastrin (no longer available in the United States). Calcitonin levels are almost always elevated in patients with MTC. Measurement of calcitonin levels is helpful for screening patients at risk for MTC and for post-treatment follow-up. Following primary surgery for MTC, persistent or recurrent elevations of calcitonin levels indicate persistent regional nodal metastasis or distant metastasis. Some MTCs also secrete carcinoembryonic antigen, but its long half-life and lower specificity make it a less useful marker.

On CT scanning, MTCs appear as nodules with calcifications and may demonstrate extrathyroidal disease. Fine-needle aspiration of the palpable thyroid nodule or cervical lymph node metastasis is a sensitive means for establishing the diagnosis of MTC. Ultrasound examination of the neck is a useful technique for identifying cervical lymph node metastases.[38]

## Treatment

### Surgery for Established Medullary Thyroid Carcinoma

Recently published guidelines for clinicians contain recommendations for the management of MTC in a number of relevant clinical settings that will be useful to clinicians treating these patients.[30] Patients with established MTC (palpable or present on imaging studies, with elevated calcitonin levels) should undergo total thyroidectomy, central neck dissection, and unilateral or bilateral dissection of levels II through V nodes (Figs. 42-9 and 42-10). The decision to resect lateral nodes depends on the extent of central neck node involvement and on the results of preoperative imaging; ultrasound examination of the cervical nodes, with preoperative marking of abnormal or suspicious nodes, is helpful for planning the extent of surgery.[37-39] In patients with central lymph node metastases and negative imaging of the lateral neck, however, consideration should be given to doing at least an ipsilateral level II to IV compartment lymph node dissection because of the high likelihood of microscopic nodal involvement.

Central node dissection often compromises the blood supply of parathyroid glands. Preservation of parathyroid function may be achieved by a combination of careful preservation of glands on a vascular pedicle, where possible, and autotransplantation of devascularized glands. At our institution, the

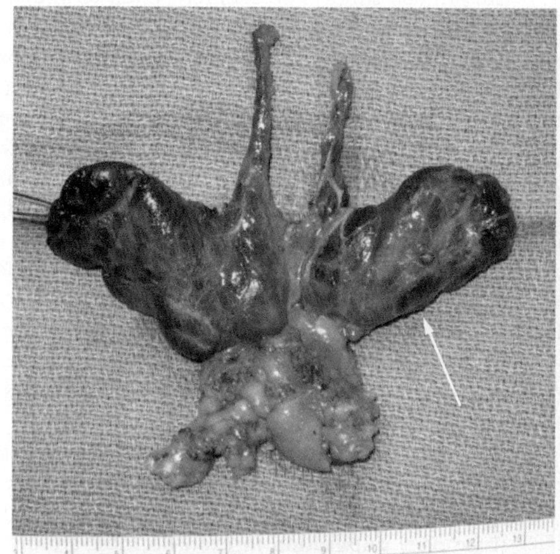

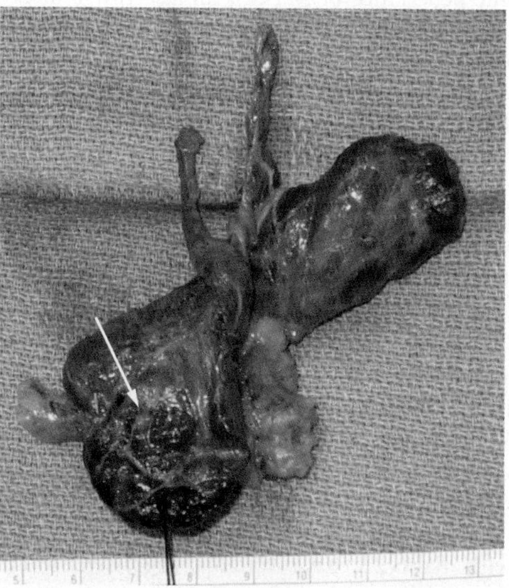

**FIGURE 42-9** Total thyroidectomy and central neck dissection in a MEN2A patient with multifocal MTC. *Arrows* indicate visible MTC tumors.

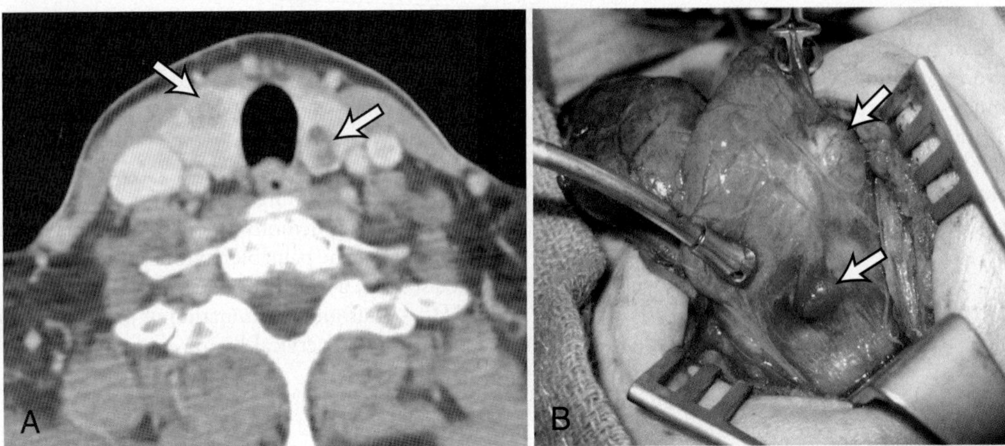


**FIGURE 42-10** **A,** CT scan showing multiple bilateral foci of medullary thyroid carcinoma in an older patient with MEN2A. **B,** Operative photograph of the same patient showing focus of MTC in thyroid *(top arrow)* and enlarged parathyroid *(bottom arrow).*

approach has been to resect and autotransplant the two parathyroids on the side of the primary tumor, as well as the contralateral lower parathyroid, leaving the contralateral upper parathyroid in situ on a vascular pedicle, if possible. All removed parathyroids should be carefully minced into 1- × 3-mm fragments; these fragments are transplanted into individual muscle pockets (two to three fragments per pocket) that are then closed with a suture.[40] Transplantation of whole minced glands into a single pocket is discouraged. Parathyroid fragments may be transplanted into individual muscle pockets in the sternocleidomastoid muscle in cases of sporadic disease, FMTC, or MEN2B. They may be transplanted into the nondominant forearm in cases of MEN2A when there is a significant risk of future hyperparathyroidism (e.g., codon 634 *RET* mutation carriers). The reason for this difference is the risk of subsequent graft-dependent hyperparathyroidism in some MEN2A patients, which is more easily localized and treated if the grafts are in the forearm.

### Preventive Surgery

Although the age of onset and rate of disease progression may differ, the lifetime penetrance of MTC is almost 100% in carriers of *RET* mutations associated with MEN2 syndromes. Therefore, all patients diagnosed with MEN2 should undergo a total thyroidectomy. A number of studies have demonstrated improved biochemical cure rates and/or decreased recurrence rates from early thyroidectomy, performed after positive screening by calcitonin testing or *RET* mutation testing.[41]

Patients with MEN2B have the most aggressive form of MTC, with invasive disease reported in patients younger than 1 year of age.[30] MEN2B mutations are the highest risk level, designated as level III.[9] These patients should have preventative surgery early in the first year of life, if possible. Identification and preservation of parathyroid glands can be extremely difficult in these infants because of their small size, translucent appearance, and presence of exuberant thymic and perithyroidal nodal tissue. These procedures should be performed by surgeons experienced in parathyroid operations and pediatric thyroidectomy.

Patients with MEN2A have variably aggressive MTC. Mutations in codons 634, 620, 618, and 611 are considered high risk (level II). Patients with level II mutations should undergo a total thyroidectomy at 5 to 6 years of age. There is evidence that the risk of lymph node metastasis is very low in MEN2A patients younger than 8 years, with normal calcitonin levels.[40,42] Central lymph node dissection is associated with a higher risk of hypoparathyroidism and recurrent laryngeal nerve injury and should be reserved for patients with elevated calcitonin levels (see Fig. 42-9).[34,43]

A larger subset of *RET* mutations, associated with MEN2A and/or FMTC, are considered lowest risk (level I). These include mutations at codons 768, 790, 791, 804, and 891.[30] For patients with low-risk level I mutations, total thyroidectomy is recommended, and surgery before age 5 to 10 years is appropriate. As with the level II mutations, the need for central lymph node dissection should be guided by calcitonin levels and clinical features of the patient and kindred.

Our group at Washington University has reported long-term follow-up on a series of 50 young patients with MEN2A following total thyroidectomy, central node dissection, and total parathyroidectomy, with autotransplantation of all the parathyroid tissue into the muscle of the nondominant forearm during the primary surgical procedure.[40] Long-term disease control was excellent. Long-term parathyroid function was normal (no supplementation) in 47 of 50 patients. Other groups have reported good results with selective removal lymph nodes and parathyroids in young at-risk patients.[44] Follow-up studies have indicated that the likelihood of nodal metastases in MEN2A and FMTC patients is extremely low in patients younger than 8 years and in patients with a basal calcitonin level lower that 40 pg/mL.[40,42] Thus, it is now our practice to perform a total thyroidectomy, leaving the parathyroids in situ, if possible, in children with a low calcitonin level (<40 pg/mL). In patients with an elevated calcitonin level, we a perform total thyroidectomy, central node dissection, and parathyroid autotransplantation. In either case, these operations should only be performed by surgeons experienced in thyroid and parathyroid surgery in children.

Since publication of the consensus guidelines, a number of new mutations have been described in association with MEN2 syndromes at codons 912, 630, 631, 606, and 533 and a 9-bp (base pair) duplication in exon 8. These are uncommon mutations and, because of lack of clinical experience, their penetrance and aggressiveness are not well characterized.

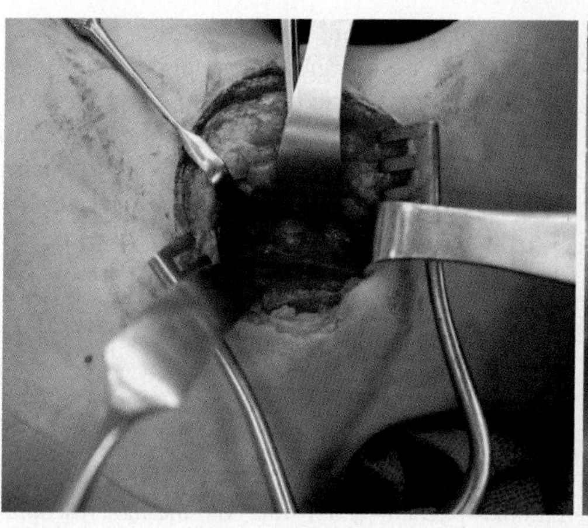

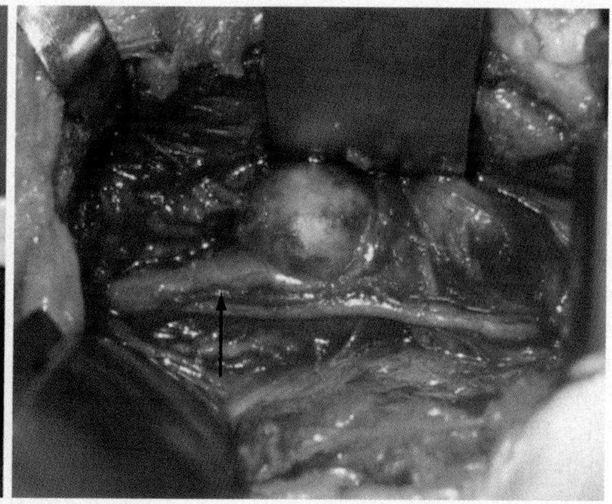

**FIGURE 42-11** Reoperation—left central neck dissection in a young patient with MEN2B. Note the large size of the recurrent laryngeal nerve *(arrow)* and the nodule of recurrent medullary thyroid carcinoma adjacent to the cricoid. (From Moley JF: Medullary thyroid carcinoma: Management of lymph node metastases. J Natl Compr Canc Netw 8:549–556, 2010.)

## Follow-Up

Following thyroidectomy, thyroid hormone replacement is required for life. Patients may need several weeks of oral calcium and vitamin D until parathyroid function recovers. Intermittent calcitonin testing may be done to monitor for persistent or recurrent MTC.

The term *biochemical cure* is used to refer to patients with normal calcitonin levels after surgery for MTC. Complete postoperative normalization of calcitonin levels has been associated with decreased long-term risk of MTC recurrence, although the evidence is less clear for a survival benefit. A persistent or recurrent elevation in the calcitonin level indicates residual or recurrent MTC and warrants additional investigation by imaging, at a minimum. However, because most MTCs have a fairly indolent course, patients with biochemical evidence of recurrent disease may not have corollary imaging findings for some time.

## Management of Recurrent and Metastatic Disease

Patients with findings of recurrent disease localized to the neck should undergo reoperation when possible, with the goal of removing all remaining disease. These procedures may result in long-term survival benefit and prevent complications of recurrence in the neck (Fig. 42-11).[37] External beam radiation therapy is effective in palliation of bone metastases, but consistent benefit has not been shown for recurrent disease in the neck.[45] Previous clinical response rates for chemotherapy in patients with locally advanced or metastatic MTC have been disappointing. The understanding of MTC molecular oncogenesis, however, has resulted in the identification of novel molecular targets for treatment. Most current targeted molecular therapies fall under the classification of tyrosine kinase inhibitors. Vandetanib (ZD6474, Zactima) is a recently developed anilinoquinazoline compound engineered to inhibit vascular endothelial growth factor receptor (VEGFR), endothelial growth factor receptor (EGFR), and RET tyrosine kinases selectively. In a study of 30 patients with advanced hereditary MTC, Wells and colleagues[46] have reported a 20% partial response rate and a more than 50% reduction of calcitonin level in 24 of 30 patients. At present, there are several other ongoing and completed institutional and multi-institutional phase II trials for MTC patients with unresectable, measurable, and locally advanced MTC.

## Pheochromocytoma

Pheochromocytomas are neoplasms arising from chromaffin cells in the adrenal medulla, which synthesize and secrete catecholamines. Patients with pheochromocytoma may present with symptoms of catecholamine excess, including headache, hypertension, palpitations, tremors, and anxiety. This unregulated catecholamine secretion can have devastating consequences, including stroke, myocardial infarction, and sudden death.

Approximately 40% to 50% of all patients with MEN2A or MEN2B develop pheochromocytomas, with a mean age of diagnosis from 30 to 40 years. In rare cases, the age of onset may be as young as 5 to 10 years, although this is usually in the setting of MEN2B.[9,30] Two studies have indicated that the penetrance and age at diagnosis differ between kindreds and correlate somewhat with specific *RET* mutations, with the highest penetrance associated with mutations at codons 918 or 634.[28,47] Pheochromocytomas are rarely seen in patients with mutations of exon 10 (codon 609, 611, 620). The specific amino acid change in the codon may also affect expression of features in MEN2. In MEN2A patients with amino acid substitutions at codon 618, the penetrance of pheochromocytoma is variable—C618R shows a 41% penetrance, C618G shows a 24% penetrance, and C618Y shows a 0% penetrance.

Unlike sporadic presentations of pheochromocytoma, which may be malignant or in an extra-adrenal location (paraganglioma), cases associated with MEN2 are almost always benign and confined to the adrenal medulla. These tumors are usually multifocal in MEN2 patients and are bilateral in more than 50% of cases.

Screening for pheochromocytomas should be done in all patients diagnosed with MEN2A or MEN2B. Numerous studies have shown that measurement of plasma and/or 24-hour urine metanephrine levels is more sensitive and specific than measurement of catecholamine levels or other metabolites for detecting pheochromocytoma.[48] Pheochromocytoma screening should begin at the age when thyroidectomy would be considered, based on the risk level of the patient's *RET* mutation and family history.[30] If negative, testing should be done annually thereafter. Positive or borderline results mandate additional investigation by imaging, usually adrenal CT or MRI.

MEN2 patients with pheochromocytoma should undergo partial or total adrenalectomy. The surgical management of unilateral disease has been the subject of some controversy, because many patients will eventually develop pheochromocytoma on the contralateral side. Some authors have recommended bilateral adrenalectomies for all MEN2 patients with pheochromocytoma. Patients who have had both adrenals removed, however, have a significant risk of adrenal insufficiency and addisonian crisis. Pheochromocytomas are not malignant in MEN2 patients, and the interval between the development of a pheochromocytoma on one side and the other side is more than 10 years.[49] For these reasons, most surgeons now recommend removing only the affected adrenal in the setting of unilateral pheochromocytoma in MEN2 patients, with annual screening thereafter.

Laparoscopic adrenalectomy has gained favor as a preferred surgical approach for many MEN2 patients. The conversion rate to an open procedure is less than 10%.[49] It is considered appropriate for lesions confined to the adrenal and smaller than 9 to 10 cm, depending on the capability of the surgeon. Laparoscopic adrenalectomy has been associated with shorter hospital stay, decreased postoperative pain, and faster recovery as compared with open adrenalectomy.[50]

### Primary Hyperparathyroidism

The overall reported prevalence of primary hyperparathyroidism in MEN2A patients is between 10% and 35%, although this is highly variable between kindreds. This is not a clinical feature of FMTC or MEN2B. The age of onset tends to be later than that of MTC, so hyperparathyroidism is rarely the initial presenting complaint that leads to a diagnosis of MEN2A. In more than 80% of cases, parathyroid hyperplasia will be identified in multiple glands (see Fig. 42-10). Inappropriate secretion of PTH leads to hypercalcemia and can result in osteoporosis, kidney stones, musculoskeletal pain, depression, and other nonspecific symptoms. Hyperparathyroidism in MEN2A is most commonly associated with the C634R mutation.

Patients known to have MEN2A should be screened with a serum calcium level determination annually. If the calcium level is elevated, the PTH level should be measured. Inappropriate elevation of the PTH level is diagnostic in a patient with MEN2A.

The treatment for hyperparathyroidism in MEN2A is four-gland parathyroidectomy with autotransplantation to the nondominant forearm muscle. This is done even if one or more glands appear grossly normal because of the likelihood that parathyroid hyperplasia will also develop in the normal-appearing glands in the future. Patients with a new diagnosis of MEN2A should be screened before undergoing thyroidectomy, because a positive finding will preclude preservation of the parathyroids in situ. Many MEN2A patients who underwent preventive thyroidectomy in childhood will have had their parathyroids removed and autotransplanted at the time of the previous surgery. If hyperparathyroidism manifests in a patient with a forearm graft, the graft can be explored and partly excised. Patients who previously underwent thyroidectomy without removal of the parathyroids will need a reexploration of the neck.

### Conclusions

The management of MEN2 syndromes has changed significantly since they were first characterized in the mid-20th century. The advent of mutation testing in the RET and menin proto-oncogenes, and our growing understanding of the relationships between genotype and phenotype, has refined the diagnostic and prognostic capabilities for the MEN syndromes. Preventive surgery based on mutation analysis may prove to be a cure for MTC in young MEN2 patients. More accurate identification of those at risk has reduced the need for screening in many members of MEN kindreds. As more is learned about the pathogenesis of this disease, treatment can be further tailored to improve outcomes for individual patients.

## SELECTED REFERENCES

Brunt LM, Lairmore TC, Doherty GM, et al: Adrenalectomy for familial pheochromocytoma in the laparoscopic era. Ann Surg 235:713–720, 2002.

Summary of a large institutional experience with laparoscopic removal of pheochromocytomas from patients with the MEN2 syndromes.

Chandrasekharappa SC, Guru SC, Manickam P, et al: Positional cloning of the gene for multiple endocrine neoplasia-type 1. Science 276:404–407, 1997.

Original article reporting the cloning of the *MEN1* gene.

Kloos RT, Eng C, Evans DB, et al: Medullary thyroid cancer: Management guidelines of the American Thyroid Association. Thyroid 19:565–612, 2009.

Recently published guidelines for management of patients with MEN2 written by a panel of experts.

Skinner MA, Moley JA, Dilley WG, et al: Prophylactic thyroidectomy in multiple endocrine neoplasia type 2A. N Engl J Med 353:1105–1113, 2005.

This article reports 50 consecutive preventative thyroidectomies with parathyroid autotransplantation and central neck dissection in patients with MEN2A with more than a 5-year follow-up.

Thompson NW: Management of pancreatic endocrine tumors in patients with multiple endocrine neoplasia type 1. Surg Oncol Clin N Am 7:881–891, 1998.

This article describes a large personal experience with pancreatic tumors in patients with the MEN1 syndrome.

## REFERENCES

1. Chandrasekharappa SC, Guru SC, Manickam P, et al: Positional cloning of the gene for multiple endocrine neoplasia-type 1. Science 276:404–407, 1997.
2. Crabtree JS, Scacheri PC, Ward JM, et al: A mouse model of multiple endocrine neoplasia, type 1, develops multiple endocrine tumors. Proc Natl Acad of Sci U S A 98:1118–1123, 2001.
3. Agarwal SK, Guru SC, Heppner C, et al: Menin interacts with the AP1 transcription factor JunD and represses JunD-activated transcription. Cell 96:143–152, 1999.
4. Lemos MC, Thakker RV: Multiple endocrine neoplasia type 1 (MEN1): Analysis of 1336 mutations reported in the first decade

following identification of the gene. Hum Mutat 29:22–32, 2008.

5. Mutch MG, Dilley WG, Sanjurjo F, et al: Germline mutations in the multiple endocrine neoplasia type 1 gene: Evidence for frequent splicing defects. Hum Mutat 13:175–185, 1999.
6. Kassem M, Kruse TA, Wong FK, et al: Familial isolated hyperparathyroidism as a variant of multiple endocrine neoplasia type 1 in a large Danish pedigree. J Clin Endocrinol Metab 85: 165–167, 2000.
7. Piecha G, Chudek J, Wiecek A: Multiple endocrine neoplasia type 1. Eur J Intern Med 19:99–103, 2008.
8. Lairmore TC, Piersall LD, DeBenedetti MK, et al: Clinical genetic testing and early surgical intervention in patients with multiple endocrine neoplasia type 1 (MEN1). Ann Surg 239:637–645, 2004.
9. Brandi ML, Gagel RF, Angeli A, et al: Guidelines for diagnosis and therapy of MEN type 1 and type 2. J Clin Endocrinol Metab 86:5658–5671, 2001.
10. Doherty GM, Lairmore TC, DeBenedetti MK: Multiple endocrine neoplasia type 1 parathyroid adenoma development over time. World J Surg 28:1139–1142, 2004.
11. Balsalobre Salmeron MD, Rodriguez Gonzalez JM, et al: Causes and treatment of recurrent hyperparathyroidism after subtotal parathyroidectomy in the presence of multiple endocrine neoplasia 1. World J Surg 34:1325–1331, 2010.
12. Elaraj DM, Skarulis MC, Libutti SK, et al: Results of initial operation for hyperparathyroidism in patients with multiple endocrine neoplasia type 1. Surgery 134:858–864, 2003.
13. Cohen MS, Dilley WG, Wells SA, Jr, et al: Long-term functionality of cryopreserved parathyroid autografts: A 13-year prospective analysis. Surgery 138:1033–1040, 2005.
14. Rosch T, Lightdale CJ, Botet JF, et al: Localization of pancreatic endocrine tumors by endoscopic ultrasonography. N Engl J Med 326:1721–1726, 1992.
15. Proye C, Malvaux P, Pattou F, et al: Noninvasive imaging of insulinomas and gastrinomas with endoscopic ultrasonography and somatostatin receptor scintigraphy. Surgery 124:1134–1143, 1998.
16. Lairmore TC, Chen VY, DeBenedetti MK, et al: Duodenopancreatic resections in patients with multiple endocrine neoplasia type 1. Ann Surg 231:909–918, 2000.
17. Norton JA, Fraker DL, Alexander R, et al: Surgery to cure the Zollinger-Ellison syndrome. N Engl J Med 341:635–644, 1999.
18. Thompson NW: Management of pancreatic endocrine tumors in patients with multiple endocrine neoplasia type 1. Surg Oncol Clin N Am 7:881–891, 1998.
19. Norton JA, Cornelius MJ, Doppman JL: Effect of parathyroidectomy in patients with hyperparathyroidism and multiple endocrine neoplasia type I. Surgery 102:958–966, 1987.
20. Doherty GM, Doppman JL, Shawker TH, et al: Results of a prospective strategy to diagnose, localize, and resect insulinomas. Surgery 110:989–996, 1991.
21. Kouvaraki MA, Shapiro SE, Cote GJ, et al: Management of pancreatic endocrine tumors in multiple endocrine neoplasia type 1. World J Surg 30:643–653, 2006.
22. Bartsch DK, Fendrich V, Langer P, et al: Outcome of duodenopancreatic resections in patients with multiple endocrine neoplasia type 1. Ann Surg 242:757–764, 2005.
23. Thompson NW: Current concepts in the surgical management of multiple endocrine neoplasia type 1 pancreatic-duodenal disease. Results in the treatment of 40 patients with Zollinger-Ellison syndrome, hypoglycaemia or both. J Intern Med 243:495–500, 1998.
24. Tonelli F, Fratini G, Nesi G, et al: Pancreatectomy in multiple endocrine neoplasia type 1-related gastrinomas and pancreatic endocrine neoplasias. Ann Surg 244:61–70, 2006.
25. Mulligan LM, Kwok JB, Healey CS, et al: Germ-line mutations of the RET proto-oncogene in multiple endocrine neoplasia type 2A. Nature 363:458–460, 1993.
26. Eng C, Clayton D, Schuffenecker I, et al: The relationship between specific RET proto-oncogene mutations and disease phenotype in multiple endocrine neoplasia type 2. International RET mutation consortium analysis. JAMA 276:1575–1579, 1996.
27. Sipple J: The association of pheochromocytoma with carcinomas of the thyroid gland. Am J Med 31:163–166, 1961.
28. Quayle FJ, Fialkowski EA, Benveniste R, et al: Pheochromocytoma penetrance varies by RET mutation in MEN2A. Surgery 142:800–805, 2007.
29. Moore SW, Zaahl MG: Multiple endocrine neoplasia syndromes, children, Hirschsprung's disease and RET. Pediatr Surg Int 24:521–530, 2008.
30. Kloos RT, Eng C, Evans DB, et al: Medullary thyroid cancer: Management guidelines of the American Thyroid Association. Thyroid 19:565–612, 2009.
31. Elisei R, Cosci B, Romei C, et al: Prognostic significance of somatic RET oncogene mutations in sporadic medullary thyroid cancer: A 10-year follow-up study. J Clin Endocrinol Metab 93:682–687, 2008.
32. Arighi E, Borrello MG, Sariola H: RET tyrosine kinase signaling in development and cancer. Cytokine Growth Factor Rev 16: 441–467, 2005.
33. Neumann HP, Bausch B, McWhinney SR, et al: Germ-line mutations in nonsyndromic pheochromocytoma. N Engl J Med 346:1459–1466, 2002.
34. Dralle H, Gimm O, Simon D, et al: Prophylactic thyroidectomy in 75 children and adolescents with hereditary medullary thyroid carcinoma: German and Austrian experience. World J Surg 22:744–750, 1998.
35. Hundahl SA, Fleming ID, Fremgen AM, et al: A National Cancer Data Base report on 53,856 cases of thyroid carcinoma treated in the U.S., 1985-1995 [see comments]. Cancer 83:2638–2648, 1998.
36. Moley JF, Fialkowski EA: Evidence-based approach to the management of sporadic medullary thyroid carcinoma. World J Surg 31:946–956, 2007.
37. Moley JF: Medullary thyroid carcinoma: Management of lymph node metastases. J Natl Compr Canc Netw 8:549–556, 2010.
38. Kouvaraki MA, Shapiro SE, Fornage BD, et al: Role of preoperative ultrasonography in the surgical management of patients with thyroid cancer. Surgery. 134:946–954, 2003.
39. Dralle H: Lymph node dissection and medullary thyroid carcinoma. Br J Surg 89:1073–1075, 2002.
40. Skinner MA, Moley JA, Dilley WG, et al: Prophylactic thyroidectomy in multiple endocrine neoplasia type 2A. N Engl J Med 353:1105–1113, 2005.
41. Gagel RF, Tashjian AH, Jr., Cummings T, et al: The clinical outcome of prospective screening for multiple endocrine neoplasia type 2A. An 18-year experience. N Engl J Med 318:478–484, 1988.

42. Machens A, Niccoli-Sire P, Hoegel J, et al: Early malignant progression of hereditary medullary thyroid cancer. N Engl J Med 349:1517–1525, 2003.
43. Sosa JA, Tuggle CT, Wang TS, et al: Clinical and economic outcomes of thyroid and parathyroid surgery in children. J Clin Endocrinol Metab 93:3058–3065, 2008.
44. Lips CJ, Landsvater RM, Hoppener JW, et al: Clinical screening as compared with DNA analysis in families with multiple endocrine neoplasia type 2A. N Engl J Med. 331:870–871, 1994.
45. Brierley J, Tsang R, Simpson WJ, et al: Medullary thyroid cancer: Analyses of survival and prognostic factors and the role of radiation therapy in local control. Thyroid 6:305–310, 1996.
46. Wells SA, Gosnell JE, Gagel RF, et al: Vandetanib for the treatment of patients with locally advanced or metastatic hereditary medullary thyroid carcinoma. J Clin Oncol 28:767–772, 2010.
47. Machens A, Brauckhoff M, Holzhausen HJ, et al: Codon-specific development of pheochromocytoma in multiple endocrine neoplasia type 2. J Clin Endocrinol Metab 90:3999–4003, 2005.
48. Eisenhofer G, Lenders JW, Linehan WM, et al: Plasma normetanephrine and metanephrine for detecting pheochromocytoma in von Hippel-Lindau disease and multiple endocrine neoplasia type 2. N Engl J Med 340:1872–1879, 1999.
49. Rodriguez JM, Balsalobre M, Ponce JL, et al: Pheochromocytoma in MEN2A syndrome. Study of 54 patients. World J Surg 32:2520–2526, 2008.
50. Brunt LM, Lairmore TC, Doherty GM, et al: Adrenalectomy for familial pheochromocytoma in the laparoscopic era. Ann Surg 235:713–720, 2002.

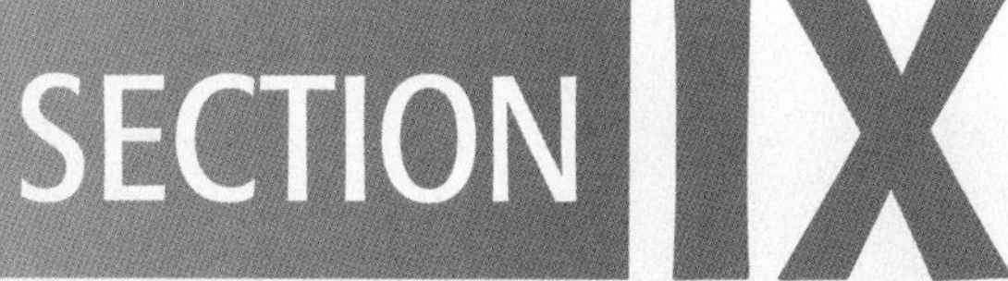

# SECTION IX

# ESOPHAGUS

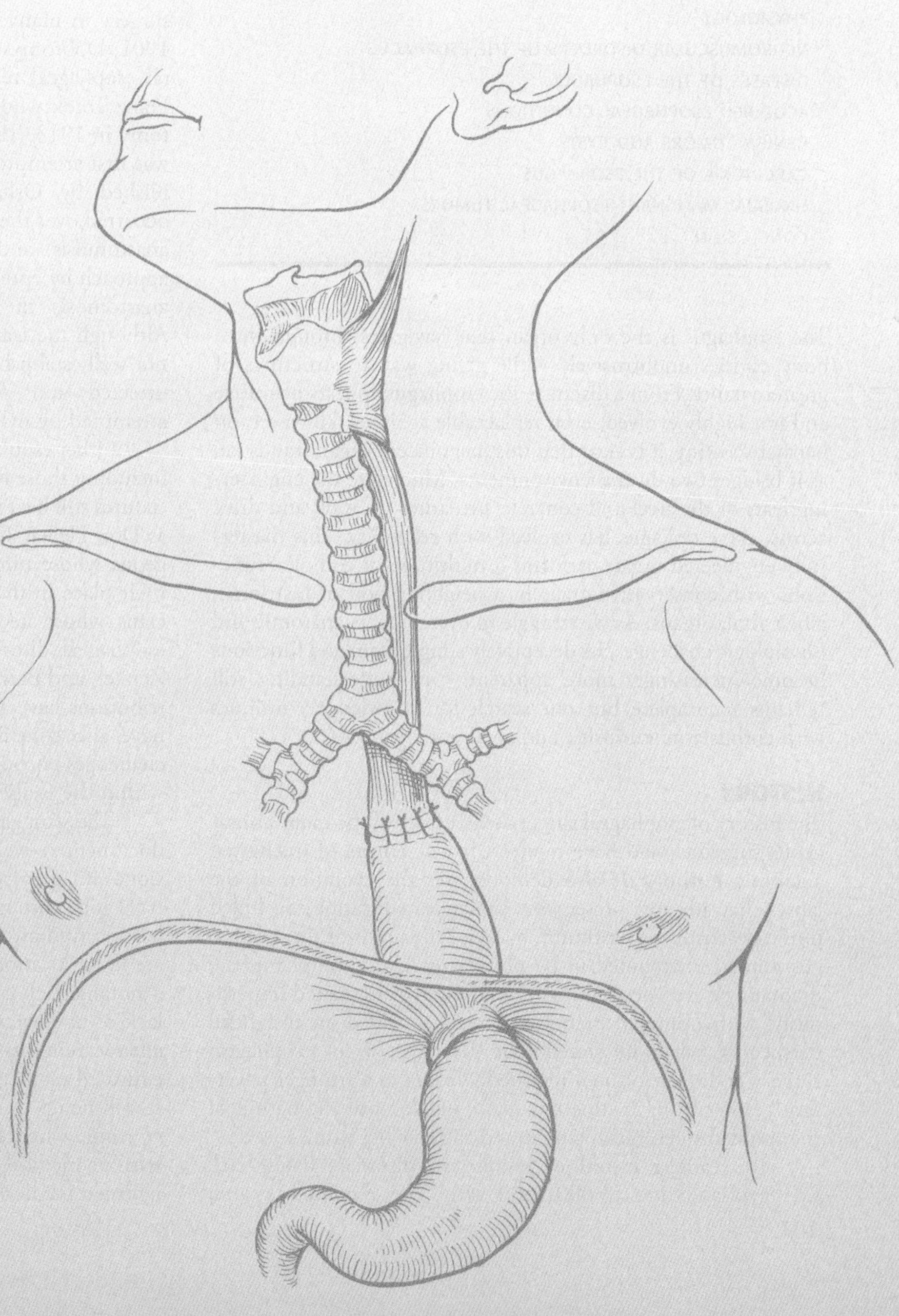

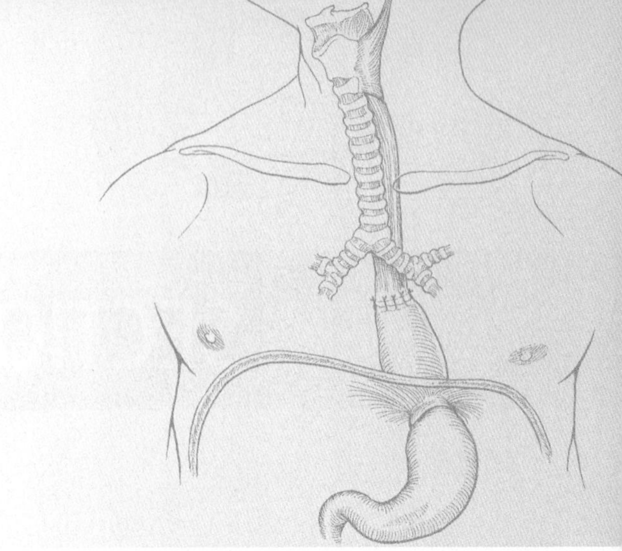

CHAPTER 43

# ESOPHAGUS

Mary S. Maish



The esophagus is the only organ that navigates through three body cavities unobtrusively while giving way to structures of greater vitality. From a distance, the esophagus appears primitive and not highly evolved, even replaceable at times. However, on harsher scrutiny, it is clear that this magnificent organ stands tall as it bridges two diverse environments. Much like the engineering feats of the steel and concrete structures we walk and drive across, the esophagus has evolved with reliability. This masterfully engineered organ performs a multitude of complex functions with conservative grace in a neighborhood of histrionic, albeit vital, organs. As we struggle to overcome its anatomic and physiologic challenges, its deceptively simple form and functions become increasingly more apparent. Our understanding still remains incomplete but our search for knowledge continues with enthusiasm, curiosity, and great anticipation.

## HISTORY

The history of esophageal surgery tells a story of the many courageous surgeons who have pioneered their efforts in uncharted anatomic territory. It also demonstrates the evolution of the lapses that are now present in esophageal education. Secluded in the posterior mediastinum, many of the needs of the esophagus remain unattended to by physicians. Until complaints are dramatic or even devastating, the symptoms are treated impetuously, with nominal attention. Emslie provided an insightful perspective when he stated that "The history of esophageal surgery is the tale of men repeatedly losing to a stronger adversary yet persisting in this unequal struggle until the nature of the problems became apparent and the war [is] won."

The earliest record of esophageal disorders dates back to Egyptian times (3000-2500 BC). The *Surgical Papyrus,* discovered in 1862 by Edwin Smith, described the successful treatment of "a gaping wound of the throat penetrating the gullet." At the turn of the century, there were significant improvements in anesthesia that allowed for the growth of surgery in many areas, including surgery of the esophagus. In 1901, Dobromysslow performed the first intrathoracic segmental esophageal resection and primary anastomosis, but it was Franz Torek who pioneered the first subtotal esophagogastrectomy in 1913. The use of the stomach to replace the esophagus was first attempted by Leipzin in 1920 and successfully accomplished by Oshava in 1933. A number of modifications occurred over the next 40 years, including changes in approach, anastomosis, and conduits. Ivor Lewis (1946) modified the approach by entering the right chest, and McKewon placed the anastomosis in the neck to eliminate intrathoracic leaks. Although the transhiatal approach had been attempted, it was not well established until 1978, when Orringer and Sloan[1] resurrected and perfected this operation, which had been attempted by many before them.

Other esophageal surgeries evolved in a similar time frame, including those for achalasia, reflux, and diverticula. These procedures still bear the names of historically famous surgeons, such as Dor, Heller, Toupet, Belsey, and Nissen. Along with the surgeons whose nimble fingers and brave hearts have established their place in the archives of esophageal surgery are the physicians whose keen observations and critical minds identified esophageal disorders that now bear their names. Boerhaave, Zenker, and Barrett are among the many physicians whose contributions have also been historically noteworthy. Many others have also contributed significantly toward understanding the challenges encountered by those whose professional passions lie within the walls of the esophagus.

The struggles with surgery of the esophagus that have been documented over the years are reflected in the social and professional image of the esophagus. Unlike some other organs that have gone through a seemingly glamorous phase, the esophagus has received attention only for dysfunction and disorder. There are few educational tools to help understand the esophagus and a notable lack of esophageal education has resulted in a gross lack of understanding by many physicians. As the incidence of adenocarcinoma of the esophagus continues to increase, well-educated esophagologists and surgeons will be in great demand. It will be up to the academic physicians of the 21st century to continue where history has left off and establish the esophagus, with its medical and surgical challenges, on the forefront of the national medical agenda.

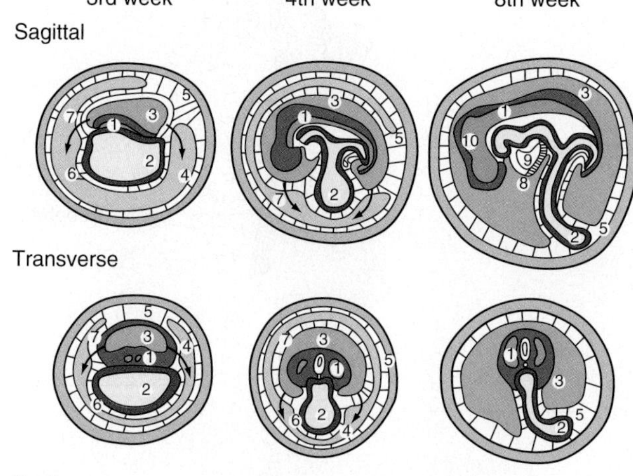


**FIGURE 43-1** Early embryologic development. (Adapted from Pearson FG, Cooper JD, Deslauriers J, et al: Esophageal surgery, ed 2, New York, 2002, Churchill Livingstone, p 20.)

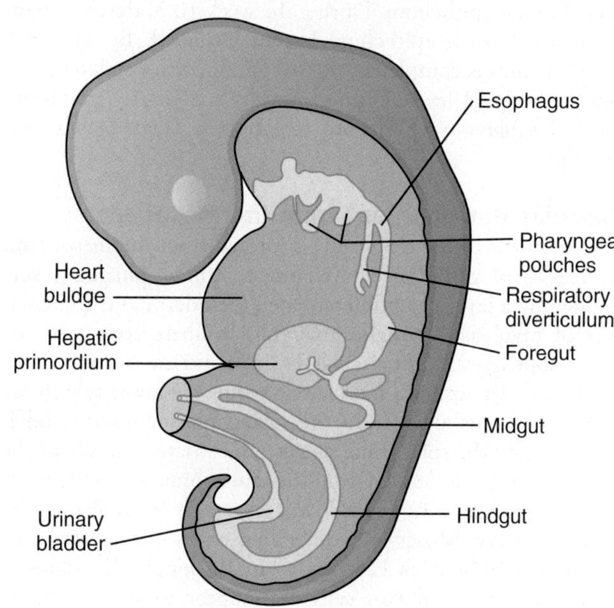


**FIGURE 43-2** The developing gut.

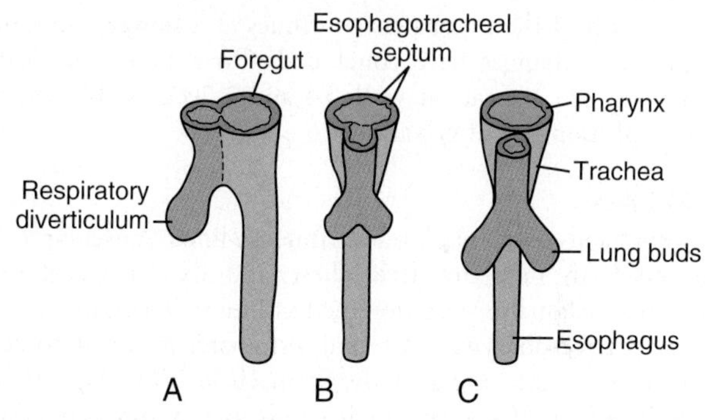


**FIGURE 43-3** Partitioning of the foregut. **A,** Week 4; **B,** week 8; **C,** week 14. (Adapted from Sadler TW [ed]: Medical embryology, Philadelphia, 2003, Lippincott Williams & Wilkins, p 290.)

## EMBRYOLOGY

Evolutionary biologists, creationists, and proponents of the theory of intelligent design alike would probably all agree that the process of human development is amazingly intricate and well executed. The development of the esophagus is among those remarkable feats, and a few moments to appreciate the product of years of precise development will establish a sound basis on which normal and abnormal esophageal form and function can be understood. The development of the esophagus begins in week 3 of gestation and, by the 14th week, the fetus takes its first swallow. To give life to the esophagus, there are several aspects of esophageal development that must be described carefully—initial formation of the gut tube, molecular regulation of the gut tube, differentiation of the endoderm (the lining of the esophagus), and derivation of the muscular layers from the mesoderm.

### Formation of the Gut Tube

During the embryonic period of development, cephalocaudal (Fig. 43-1) and lateral folding of the embryo occurs. As a result, a portion of the endoderm-lined yolk sac cavity is incorporated into the embryo to form the primitive gut. The primitive gut forms a blind-ending tube consisting of the foregut, midgut, and hindgut (Fig. 43-2). The foregut gives rise to the esophagus. It extends from the pharyngeal tube as far caudally as the liver outgrowth. By the end of week 3 of development, the primitive foregut develops a ventral diverticulum from which the tracheobronchial tree develops. The tracheoesophageal septum gradually partitions this diverticulum from the dorsal portion of the foregut, resulting in a ventral respiratory primordium and dorsal esophagus (Fig. 43-3). During weeks 4 and 5 of development, the rapid growth of the heart and liver allows the esophagus to stretch. As it elongates, the esophageal lumen is almost completely obliterated at the level of the carina. The dorsal esophageal embrace of the trachea results in close approximation of the tracheal bifurcation to the front wall of the esophagus, further narrowing the esophageal lumen.

### Molecular Regulation of the Gut Tube

Differentiation of various regions of the gut and its derivatives is dependent on a reciprocal interaction between the endoderm (epithelium) of the gut tube and surrounding splanchnic mesoderm. The mesoderm dictates the type of structure that will form, such as the esophagus forming from the foregut, through an HOX code. The induction of the HOX code is a result of sonic hedgehog (SHH) that is expressed throughout the gut endoderm. In the foregut, expression of SHH in the endoderm promotes the expression of the HOX code in the mesoderm. Once specified by this code, the mesoderm instructs the endoderm to form the various components of the foregut.[2]

### Differentiation of the Endoderm

Early in gestation the mesoderm is HOX-coded to instruct the endoderm to form the epithelial lining of the digestive tract. At the end of the embryonic period, from weeks 6 to 8 of gestation, the epithelium becomes two to five cells thick and remains stratified columnar epithelium. During the week 10 of development, stratified columnar epithelium becomes ciliated. By week 12, the epithelium is completely ciliated and growth is taking place only at the basal level. During months 4 and 5 of gestation, stratified squamous epithelium replaces the ciliated columnar epithelium.

### Muscular Development from the Mesoderm

The remainder of the esophagus is formed from the mesoderm. By week 6 of gestational development, the esophagus is surrounded by a layer of undifferentiated mesoderm and a circular layer of myoblasts. Longitudinal muscle fibers appear in the lower esophagus as the circular layer of muscle becomes well established. The smooth muscle that forms the lower two thirds of the esophagus arises from the splanchnic mesoderm and is innervated by the splanchnic plexus. The striated muscle of the upper esophagus is derived from the caudal branchial arches and appears from weeks 12 to 15. It will eventually be innervated by the vagus nerve. Muscular proliferation peaks during weeks 11 and 12, so that by week 12 of gestation, the longitudinal muscle is well defined. Ganglion cells also appear in the myenteric plexus, whereas the longitudinal muscle becomes well defined between weeks 10 and 12 of gestation. Furthermore, the muscularis mucosa becomes well defined, and typical mucosal folds formed by longitudinal mesenchymal ridges can be appreciated.

Growth of the esophagus continues at a slower pace after morphologic changes have concluded. On a functional level, swallowing first appears at week 14 and is well established by the end of month 4 of gestation.

## ANATOMY

The esophagus is a two-layered, mucosa-lined muscular tube that travels through the neck, chest, and abdomen and rests unobtrusively in the posterior mediastinum. It commences at the base of the pharynx at C6 and terminates in the abdomen, where it joins the cardia of the stomach at T11 (Fig. 43-4). Along its 25- to 30-cm course, it winds its way through a path yielding to structures of more vital efforts. The cervical esophagus begins as a midline structure that deviates slightly to the left of the trachea as it passes through the neck into the thoracic inlet. At the level of the carina, it deviates to the right to accommodate the arch of the aorta. It then winds its way back under the left mainstem bronchus and remains slightly deviated to the left as it enters the diaphragm through the esophageal hiatus at the level of the 11th thoracic vertebra. In the neck and upper thorax, the esophagus is secured between the vertebral column posteriorly and the trachea anteriorly. At the level of the carina, the heart and pericardium lie directly anterior to the thoracic esophagus. Immediately before entering the abdomen, the esophagus is pushed anteriorly by the descending thoracic aorta that accompanies the esophagus through the diaphragm into the abdomen separated by the median arcuate ligament.

The journey through the muscular esophagus begins and ends with two distinct high-pressure zones, the upper (UES) and lower esophageal sphincter (LES). After passing through the UES, four esophageal segments are encountered—the pharyngeal, cervical, thoracic, and abdominal esophagus. The LES is the outlet through which passage into the stomach is then facilitated.

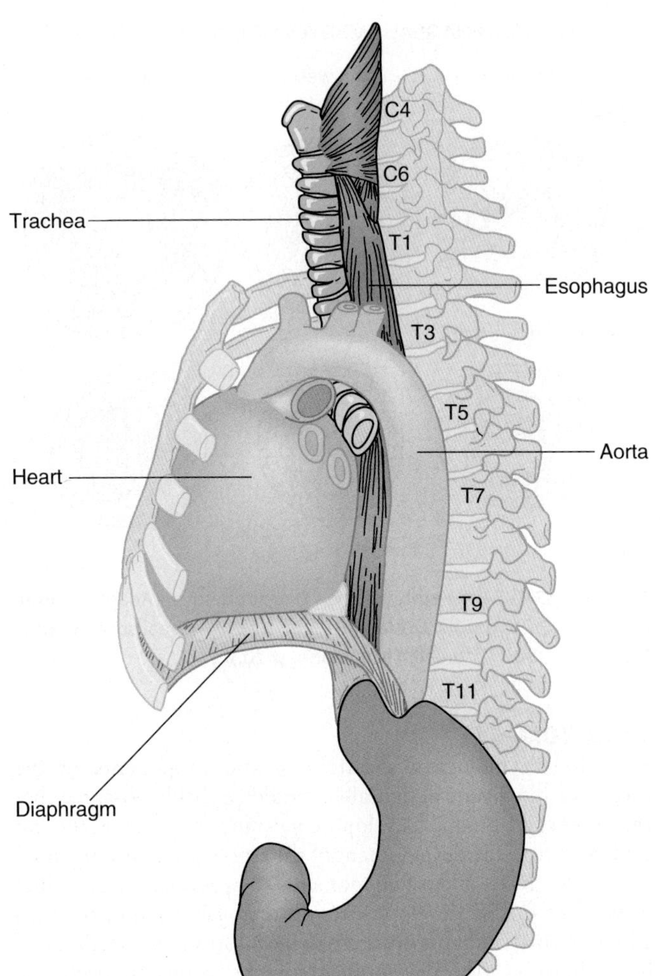


**FIGURE 43-4** Course of the esophagus.

### Esophageal Inlet

The high-pressure zone at the inlet of the esophagus is the UES, which anatomically marks the end of a complex configuration of muscles that begins in the larynx and posterior pharynx and ends in the neck. The pharyngeal constrictor muscles are three consecutive muscles that begin at the base of the palate and end at the crest of the esophagus. The superior and middle pharyngeal constrictor muscles, as well as the oblique, transverse, and posterior cricoarytenoid muscles, are immediately proximal to the UES and serve to anchor the pharynx and larynx to structures in the mouth and palate. These muscles also aid in deglutition and speech, but are not responsible for the high pressures noted in the UES. The inferior pharyngeal constrictor muscle is the final bridge between the pharyngeal and esophageal musculature.

Inserting into the median pharyngeal raphe, the inferior pharyngeal constrictor muscle is composed of two consecutive muscle beds—the thyropharyngeus and cricopharyngeus muscles—that originate bilaterally from the lateral portions of the thyroid and cricoid cartilages, respectively. The transition between the oblique fibers of the thyropharyngeus muscle and the horizontal fibers of the cricopharyngeus muscle creates a point of potential weakness, known as Killian's triangle (site of a Zenker's diverticulum). The cricopharyngeus muscle is responsible for generating a high-pressure zone that marks the position

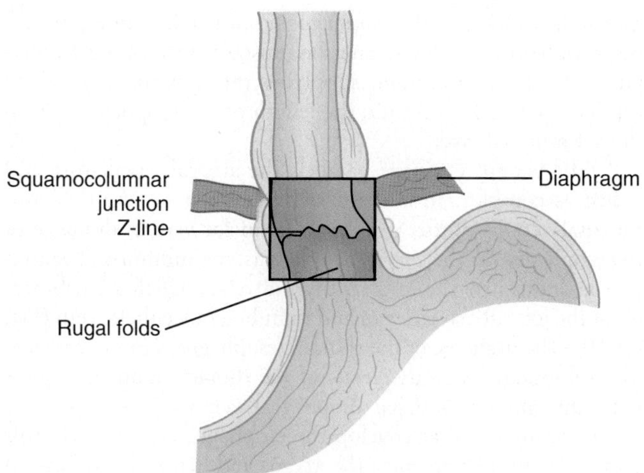


FIGURE 43-5 Z-line.

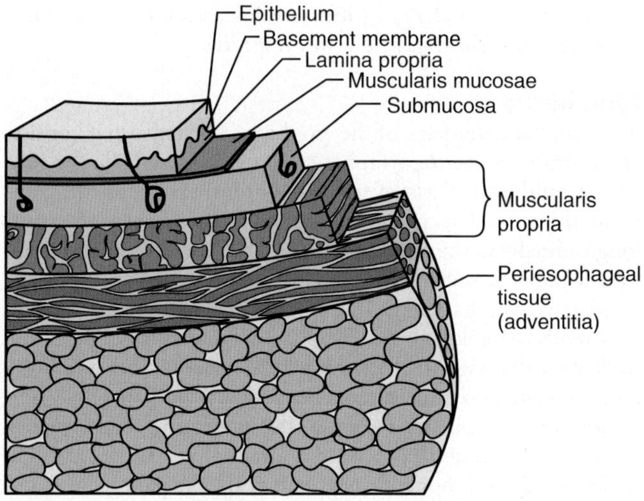


FIGURE 43-6 Layers of the esophagus. (Adapted from Pearson FG, Cooper JD, Deslauriers J, et al: Esophageal surgery, ed 2, New York, 2002, Churchill Livingstone, p 124.)

of the UES and esophageal introitus. Its distinctive bowing array of muscle fibers is unique and serves to transition into the circular esophageal musculature. This point of transition is flanked by the longitudinal esophageal muscles that extend superiorly to attach to the midportion of the posterior surface of the cricoid cartilage and form the V-shaped area of Laimer.

## Esophageal Layers

The esophagus is comprised of two proper layers, the mucosa and muscularis propria. It is distinguished from the other layers of the alimentary tract by its lack of a serosa. The mucosa is the innermost layer and consists of squamous epithelium for most of its course. The distal 1 to 2 cm of esophageal mucosa transitions to cardiac mucosa or junctional columnar epithelium at a point known as the Z-line (Fig. 43-5). Within the mucosa, there are four distinct layers—the epithelium, basement membrane, lamina propria, and muscularis mucosae. Deep to the muscularis mucosae lays the submucosa (Fig. 43-6). Within it is a plush network of lymphatic and vascular structures, as well as mucous glands and Meissner's neural plexus.

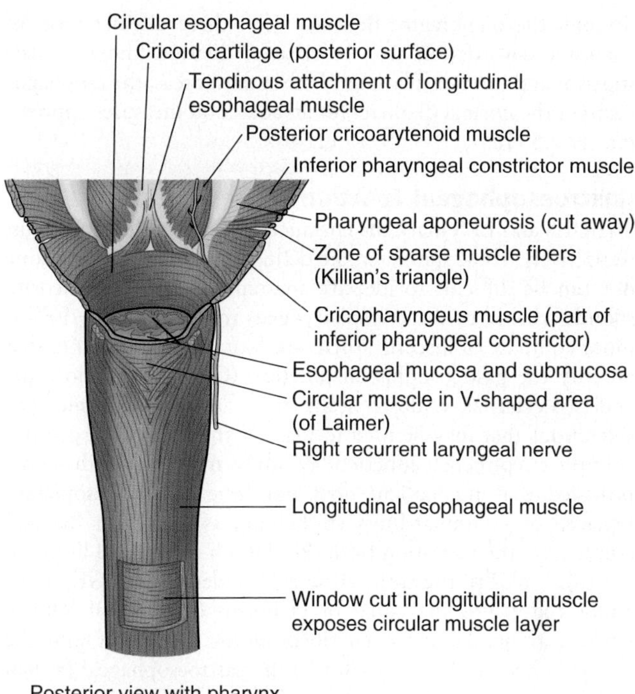


FIGURE 43-7 Muscles of the esophagus.

Enveloping the mucosa, directly abutting the submucosa, is the muscularis propria. Below the cricopharyngeus muscle, the esophagus is composed of two concentric muscle bundles, an inner circular and outer longitudinal (Fig. 43-7). Both layers of the upper third of the esophagus are striated, whereas the layers of the lower two thirds are smooth muscle. The circular muscles are an extension of the cricopharyngeus muscle and traverse through the thoracic cavity into the abdomen, where they become the middle circular muscles of the lesser curvature of the stomach. The collar of Helvetius marks the transition of the circular muscles of the esophagus to oblique muscles of the stomach at the incisura (cardiac notch). Between the layers of esophageal muscle is a thin septum comprised of connective tissue, blood vessels, and an interconnected network of ganglia known as Auerbach's plexus. Enshrouding the inner circular layer, the longitudinal muscles of the esophagus begin at the cricoid cartilage and extend into the abdomen, where they join the longitudinal musculature of the cardia of the stomach. The esophagus is then wrapped by a layer of fibroalveolar adventitia.

## Anatomic Narrowing

The esophageal silhouette resembles an hourglass. There are three distinct areas of narrowing that contribute to its shape. Measuring 14 mm in diameter, the cricopharyngeus muscle is the narrowest point of the gastrointestinal tract and marks the superiormost portion of the hourglass-shaped esophagus. Located just below the carina, where the left mainstem bronchus and aorta abut the esophagus, the bronchoaortic constriction at the level of the fourth thoracic vertebra creates the center narrowing and measures 15 to 17 mm. Finally, the diaphragmatic constriction, measuring 16 to 19 mm, marks the inferior portion of the hourglass and is located where the esophagus passes through the diaphragm. Between these three distinct areas of anatomic constriction are two areas of dilation known as the superior and inferior dilations. Within these areas, the esophagus resumes the normal diameter for an adult and measures approximately 2.5 cm.

### Gastroesophageal Junction

The UES and LES mark the entrance and exit to the esophagus, respectively. These sphincters are defined by a high-pressure zone but can be difficult to identify anatomically. The UES corresponds reliably to the cricopharyngeus muscle, but the LES is more complex to discern. There are four anatomic points that identify the gastroesophageal junction (GEJ), two endoscopic and two external. Endoscopically, there are two anatomic considerations that may be used to identify the GEJ. The squamocolumnar epithelial junction (Z-line) may mark the GEJ provided that the patient does not have a distal esophagus replaced by columnar-lined epithelium, as seen with Barrett's esophagus. The transition from the smooth esophageal lining to the rugal folds of the stomach may also identify the GEJ accurately. Externally, the collar of Helvetius (or loop of Willis), where the circular muscular fibers of the esophagus join the oblique fibers of the stomach, and the gastroesophageal fat pad are consistent identifiers of the GEJ (Fig. 43-8).

### Vasculature

The rich vascular and lymphatic structures that nourish and drain the esophagus serve as a surgical safety net and a highway for metastases. The vasculature is divided into three segments, cervical, thoracic, and abdominal. The cervical esophagus receives most of its blood supply from the inferior thyroid arteries, which branch off of the thyrocervical trunk on the left and the subclavian artery on the right (Fig. 43-9). The cricopharyngeus muscle, which marks the inlet of the esophagus, is supplied by the superior thyroid artery. The thoracic esophagus receives its blood supply directly from four to six esophageal arteries coming off the aorta, as well as esophageal branches off the right and left bronchial arteries. It is supplemented by descending branches off the inferior thyroid arteries, intercostal arteries, and ascending branches of the paired inferior phrenic arteries. The abdominal esophagus receives its blood supply from the left gastric artery and paired inferior phrenic arteries. All the arteries that supply blood to the esophagus terminate in a fine capillary network before they penetrate the muscular wall of the esophagus. After penetrating and supplying the muscular layers, the capillary network continues the length of the esophagus within the submucosal layer.

The venous drainage parallels the arterial vasculature and is just as complex. In all parts of the esophagus, the rich submucosal venous plexus is the first basin for venous drainage of the esophagus. In the cervical esophagus, the submucosal venous plexus drains into the inferior thyroid veins, which are tributaries of the left subclavian vein and right brachiocephalic vein (Fig. 43-10). The drainage of the thoracic esophagus is more intricate. The submucosal venous plexus of the thoracic esophagus joins with the more superficial esophageal venous plexus and the venae comitantes that envelop the esophagus at this level. This plexus, in turn, drains into the azygos and hemiazygos veins on the right and left sides of the chest, respectively. The intercostal veins also drain into the azygos venous system. The abdominal esophagus drains into the systemic and portal venous systems through the left and right phrenic veins and left gastric (coronary) vein and short gastric veins, respectively.

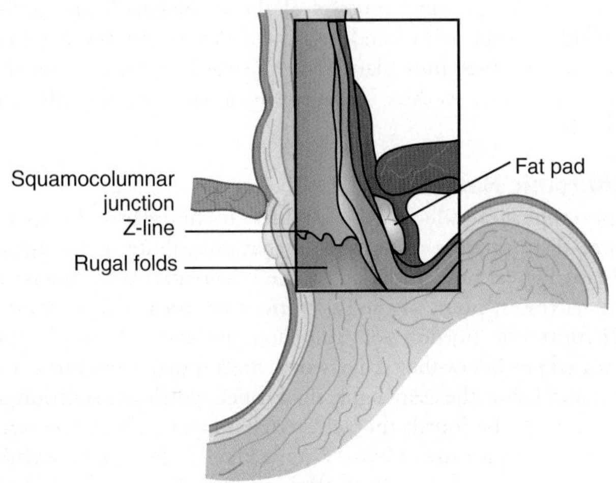


**FIGURE 43-8** Identifiers of the gastroesophageal junction.

### Lymphatics

The lymphatic drainage of the esophagus is extensive; it consists of two interconnecting lymphatic plexuses arising from the submucosa and muscularis layers. The submucosal lymphatics penetrate the muscularis propria and drain into the plexus that runs longitudinally in the esophageal wall. They then egress and drain into regional lymph node beds. In the upper two thirds of the esophagus, lymphatic flow is upward, whereas in the distal third, flow tends to be downward. Esophageal lymphatics begin in the neck with drainage to the paratracheal lymph nodes anteriorly and deep lateral cervical and internal jugular nodes laterally and posteriorly. Once inside the chest, the lymphatics form a matrix of interconnecting channels that drain into the mediastinal lymph nodes and thoracic duct. Anteriorly, the paratracheal and subcarinal lymph nodes, and the paraesophageal, retrocardiac, and infracardiac nodes, all drain the esophagus.

Other mediastinal stations, such as the para-aortic and inferior pulmonary ligament nodes, can also receive drainage from the thoracic esophagus. Posteriorly, nodes along the esophagus and azygos veins are the primary sites of drainage (Fig. 43-11). The intricate lymphatic network of the esophagus allows for rapid spread of infection and tumor into three body cavities. It stands to reason that the rich arterial supply to the esophagus makes it one of the more durable organs in the body with respect to surgical manipulation, whereas its comprehensive venous and lymphatic drainage create an oncologic challenge to controlling cellular migration. These anatomic complexities lead to surgical challenges when treating esophageal cancer and other esophageal diseases.

### Innervation

The innervation to the esophagus is sympathetic and parasympathetic (Fig. 43-12). The cervical sympathetic trunk arises from the superior ganglion in the neck. It extends next to the esophagus into the thoracic cavity, where it terminates in the cervicothoracic (stellate) ganglion. Along the way, it gives off branches to the cervical esophagus. The thoracic sympathetic trunk continues on from the stellate ganglion, giving off branches to the esophageal plexus, which envelops the thoracic esophagus

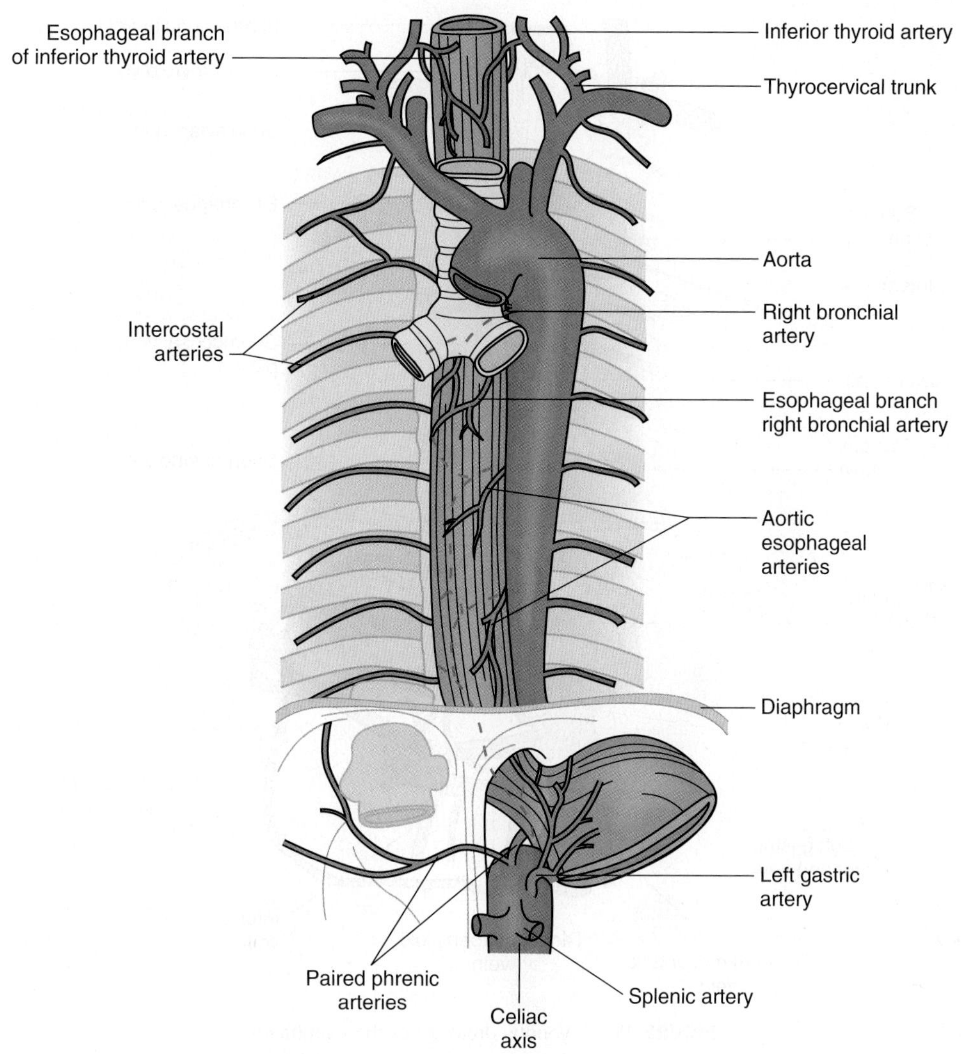


**FIGURE 43-9** Arterial supply to the esophagus.

anteriorly and posteriorly. Inferiorly, the greater and lesser splanchnic nerves innervate the distal thoracic esophagus. In the abdomen, the sympathetic fibers lay posteriorly alongside the left gastric artery.

The parasympathetic fibers arise from the vagus nerve, which gives rise to the superior and recurrent laryngeal nerves. The superior laryngeal nerve branches into the external and internal laryngeal nerves that supply motor innervation to the inferior pharyngeal constrictor muscle and cricothyroid muscle and sensory innervation to the larynx, respectively (Fig. 43-13). The right and left recurrent laryngeal nerves come off the vagus nerve and loop underneath the right subclavian artery and aortic arch, respectively. They then travel upward in the tracheoesophageal groove to enter the larynx laterally underneath the inferior pharyngeal constrictor muscle. Along the way, they innervate the cervical esophagus, including the cricopharyngeus muscle. Unilateral injury to the superior or recurrent laryngeal nerve results in hoarseness and aspiration from laryngeal and UES dysfunction. In the thorax, the vagus nerve sends fibers to the striated muscle and parasympathetic preganglionic fibers to the smooth muscle of the esophagus. A weblike nervous plexus envelops the esophagus throughout its thoracic extent. These sympathetic and parasympathetic fibers penetrate through the muscular wall, forming networks between the muscle layers to become Auerbach's plexus and within the submucosal layer to become Meissner's plexus (Fig. 43-14). They provide an intrinsic autonomic nervous system within the esophageal wall that is responsible for peristalsis. The parasympathetic fibers coalesce 2 cm above the diaphragm into the left (anterior) and right (posterior) vagus nerves, which descend anteriorly onto the fundus and lesser curvature and posteriorly onto the celiac plexus, respectively.

## PHYSIOLOGY

Chicago architect Louis Sullivan is well known for his progressive philosophy that form should follow function. In anatomy this is demonstrated often, and there is no better illustration of this principle in the human body than the esophagus. The primary function of the esophagus is to transport material from the pharynx to the stomach. Secondarily, the esophagus needs to constrain the amount of air that is swallowed and the amount of material that is refluxed. Its form has evolved nicely to enable it to function seamlessly. The esophagus usually measures 30 cm, extending from the pharynx down onto the cardia of the

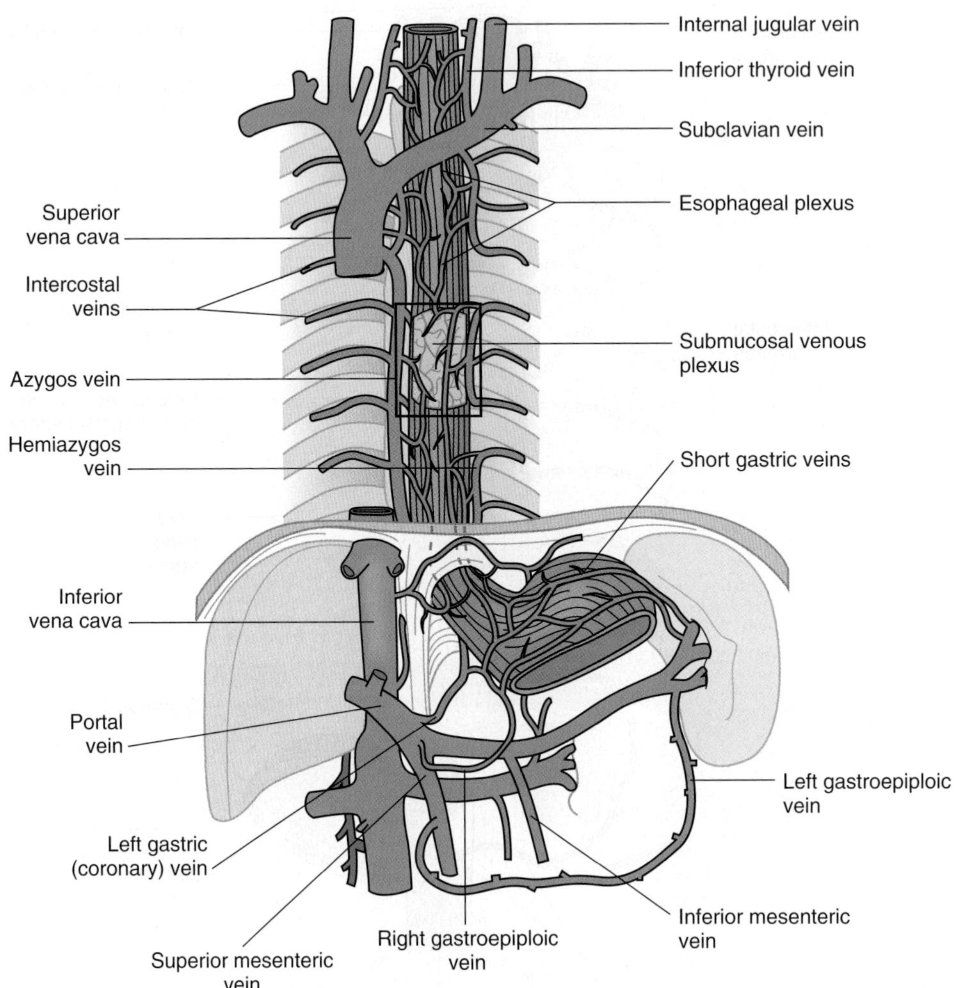


**FIGURE 43-10** Venous drainage of the esophagus.

stomach. Under ideal physiologic conditions, the concentric muscular configuration permits effortless unidirectional flow of material from the top to the bottom of the esophagus. The UES, 4 to 5 cm in length, remains in a constant state of tone (mean, 60 mm Hg), preventing a steady flow of air into the esophagus, whereas the tone in the LES (mean, 24 mm Hg) remains elevated just enough to prevent excessive material from refluxing back up into the esophagus (Table 43-1). Transport of a food bolus from the mouth through the esophagus into the stomach begins with swallowing and ends with postrelaxation contraction of the LES, requiring coordinated peristaltic contractions in transit. The material in transit can move easily because the esophageal neuromuscular form provides all functions necessary to power the food bolus through three body cavities.

## Swallowing

There are three phases to swallowing, oral, pharyngeal, and esophageal. Six events occur during the oropharyngeal phase of swallowing (Fig. 43-15). These rapid series of events last about 1.5 seconds and, once initiated, are completely reflexive.

1. Elevation of the tongue. Food is taken into the mouth and mixed with saliva to prepare a soft bolus for transport. The tongue pushes the bolus into the posterior oropharynx.
2. Posterior movement of the tongue. The tongue moves posteriorly and thrusts the food bolus into the hypopharynx.
3. Elevation of the soft palate. Simultaneously, as the tongue moves the food bolus into the hypopharynx, the soft palate is elevated to close off the passage into the nasopharynx.
4. Elevation of the hyoid. To help bring the epiglottis under the tongue, the hyoid bone moves anteriorly and upward.
5. Elevation of the larynx. The change in position of the hyoid elevates the larynx and opens up the retrolaryngeal space, further facilitating the movement of the epiglottis under the tongue.
6. Tilting of the epiglottis. Finally, the epiglottis tilts back, covering the opening of the larynx to prevent aspiration.

### Esophageal Phase

**Upper Esophageal Sphincter** The esophageal phase of swallowing is initiated by the actions during the pharyngeal phase. To allow passage of the food bolus, the UES relaxes and the peristaltic contractions of the posterior pharyngeal constrictors propel the bolus into the esophagus. The pressure differential generated between the positive pressure in the cervical esophagus and the negative intrathoracic pressure sucks the bolus into the thoracic esophagus. Within 0.5 second of the initiation of swallowing,

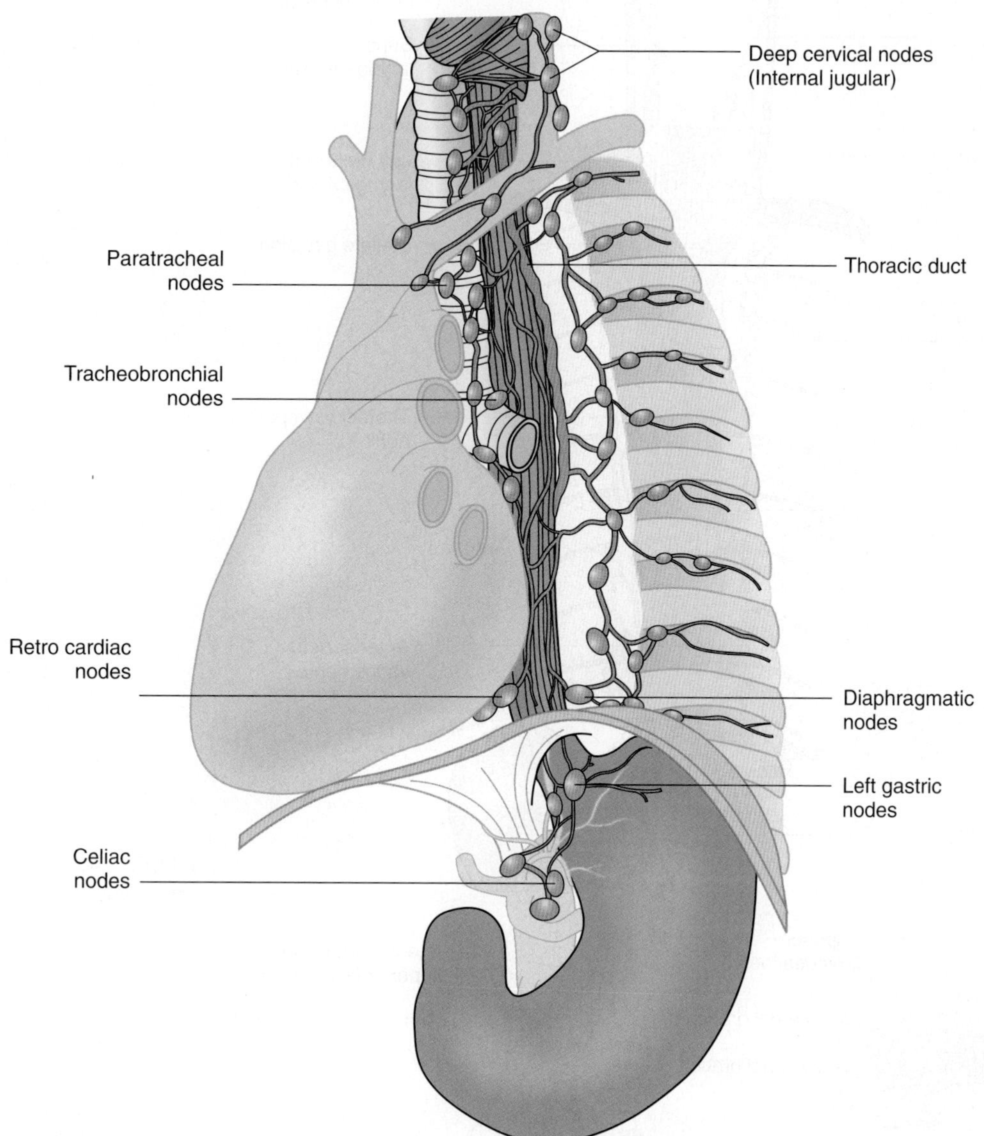


**FIGURE 43-11** Lymphatic drainage of the esophagus.

the UES closes, reaching close to 90 mm Hg. This postrelaxation contraction lasts 2 to 5 milliseconds, initiates peristalsis, and prevents reflux of the bolus back into the pharynx. The UES pressure returns to resting pressure (60 mm Hg) as the wave travels into the midesophagus (Fig. 43-16).

**Peristalsis** There are three types of esophageal contractions, primary, secondary, and tertiary. Primary peristaltic contractions are progressive and move down the esophagus at a rate of 2 to 4 cm/sec and reach the LES about 9 seconds after the initiation of swallowing (Fig. 43-17). They generate an intraluminal pressure from 40 to 80 mm Hg. Successive swallows will follow with a similar peristaltic wave unless swallowing is repeated rapidly, at which time the esophagus will remain relaxed until the last swallow occurs, and peristalsis will follow. Secondary peristaltic contractions are also progressive but are generated from distention or irritation of the esophagus, rather than voluntary swallowing. They can occur as an independent local reflex to clear the esophagus of material that was left behind after the progression of the primary peristaltic wave. Tertiary contractions are nonprogressive, nonperistaltic, monophasic or multiphasic, simultaneous waves that can occur after voluntary swallowing or spontaneously between swallows throughout the esophagus. They represent uncoordinated contractions of the smooth muscle that are responsible for esophageal spasm.

**Lower Esophageal Sphincter** The final phase of esophageal bolus transit occurs through the LES. Although this is not a true sphincter, there is a distinct high-pressure zone that measures 2 to 5 cm in length and generates a resting pressure of 6 to 26 mm Hg. The LES is located in the chest and abdomen. A minimum total length of 2 cm, with at least 1 cm of intra-abdominal length, is required for normal LES function. The transition from the intrathoracic to the intra-abdominal sphincter is noted on a manometric tracing and is known as the respiratory inversion point (RIP; Fig. 43-18). At this point, the pressure of the esophagus changes from negative to positive with inspiration and positive to negative with expiration.

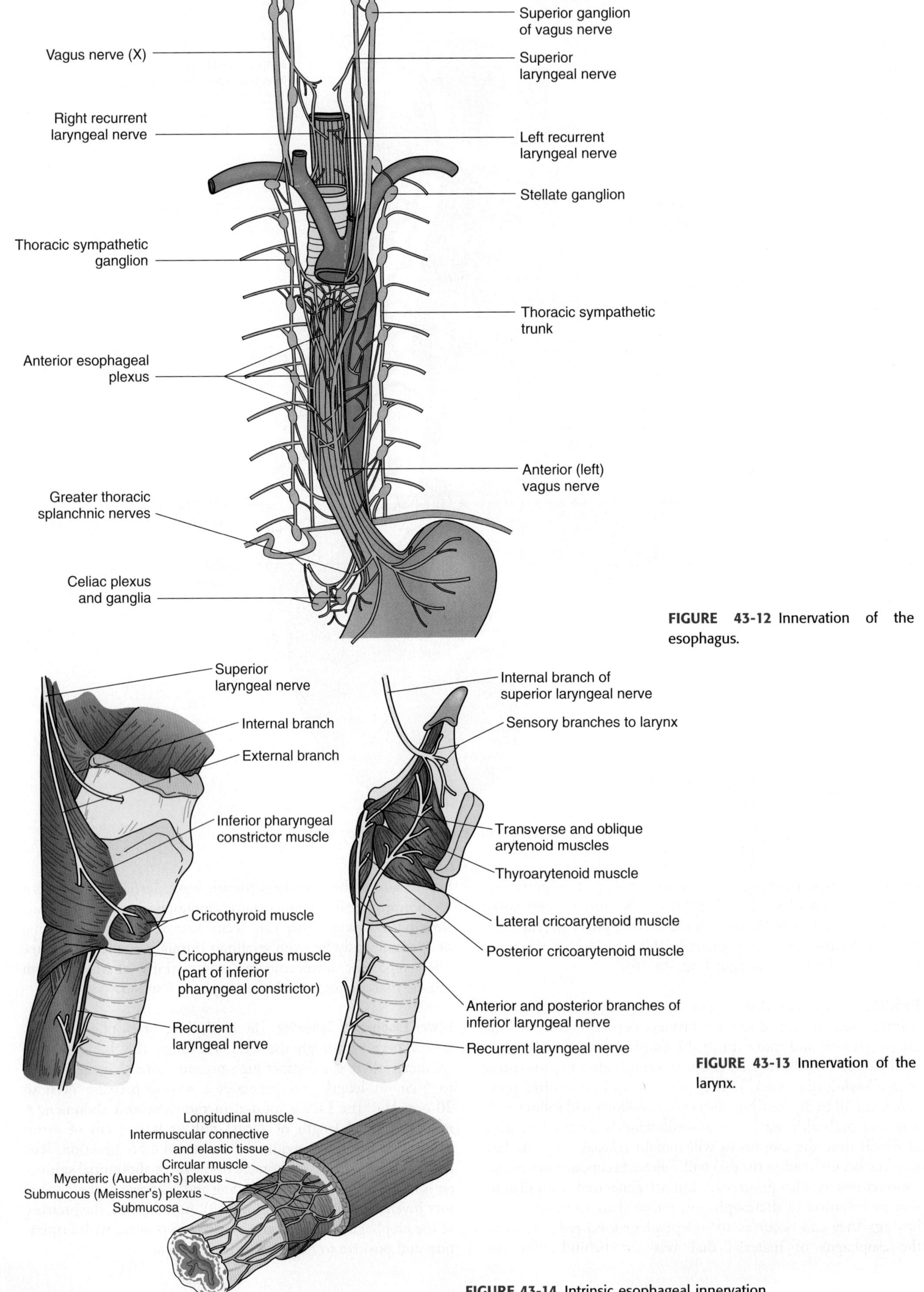


**FIGURE 43-12** Innervation of the esophagus.

**FIGURE 43-13** Innervation of the larynx.

**FIGURE 43-14** Intrinsic esophageal innervation.

**Table 43-1 Normal Manometric Values**

| PARAMETER | VALUE |
|---|---|
| **Upper Esophageal Sphincter** | |
| Total length | 4.0-5.0 cm |
| Resting pressure | 60.0 mm Hg |
| Relaxation time | 0.58 sec |
| Residual pressure | 0.7-3.7 mm Hg |
| **Lower Esophageal Sphincter** | |
| Total length | 3-5 cm |
| Abdominal length | 2-4 cm |
| Resting pressure | 6-26 mm Hg |
| Relaxation time | 8.4 sec |
| Residual pressure | 3 mm Hg |
| **Esophageal Body Contractions** | |
| Amplitude | 40-80 mm Hg |
| Duration | 2.3-3.6 sec |

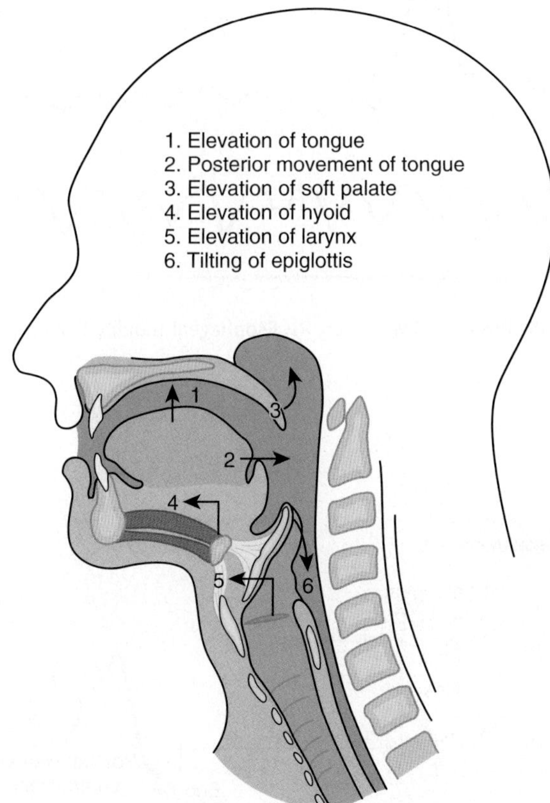


**FIGURE 43-15** Phases of oropharyngeal swallowing. (Adapted from Zuidema GD, Orringer MB: Shackelford's surgery of the alimentary tract, ed 3, Philadelphia, 1991, WB Saunders, p 95.)

Peristaltic contractions alone do not generate enough force to open up the LES. Vagal-mediated relaxation of the LES occurs 1.5 to 2.5 seconds after pharyngeal swallowing and lasts 4 to 6 seconds. This flawlessly timed relaxation is needed to allow efficient transport of a food bolus out of the esophagus and into the stomach. A postrelaxation contraction of the LES occurs after the peristaltic wave has passed through the esophagus, allowing the LES to return to its baseline pressure (Fig. 43-19), reestablishing a barrier to reflux.

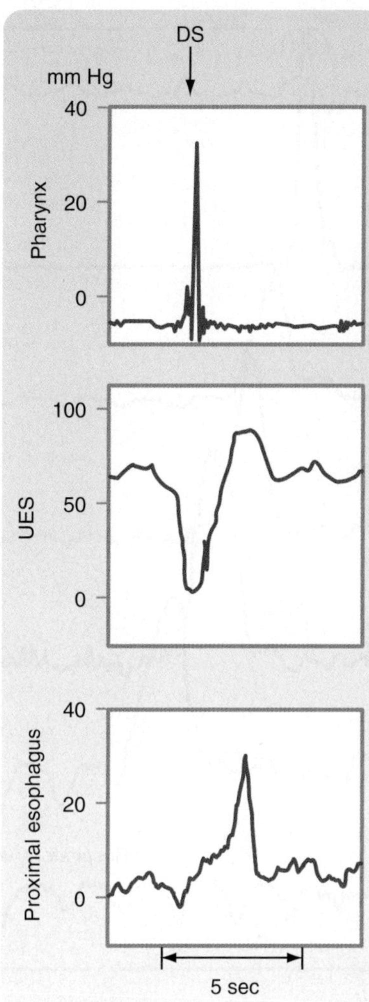


**FIGURE 43-16** Manometry of the upper esophageal sphincter. (Adapted from Pearson FG, Cooper JD, Deslauriers J, et al: Esophageal surgery, ed 2, New York, 2002, Churchill Livingstone, p 480.)

## Reflux Mechanism

Not all reflux is abnormal. Healthy individuals have occasional episodes of gastroesophageal reflux that is a result of spontaneous opening of the LES. The competence of the LES and its ability to establish a barrier to reflux depends on several factors—adequate pressure and length, radial symmetry, and motility of the esophagus and stomach. A competent sphincter is at least 2 cm and carries a pressure between 6 and 26 mm Hg. Radial asymmetry and abnormal peristalsis prevent proper closure and allow free refluxing of gastric material into the distal esophagus. Abnormal esophageal motility and poor gastric emptying result in inadequate esophageal clearance that also encourages reflux. Finally, neurotransmitters, hormones, and peptides that regulate the LES can increase or decrease tone. All these anatomic and physiologic disruptions can result in reflux through the LES and are implicated in the development of gastroesophageal reflux disease (GERD).

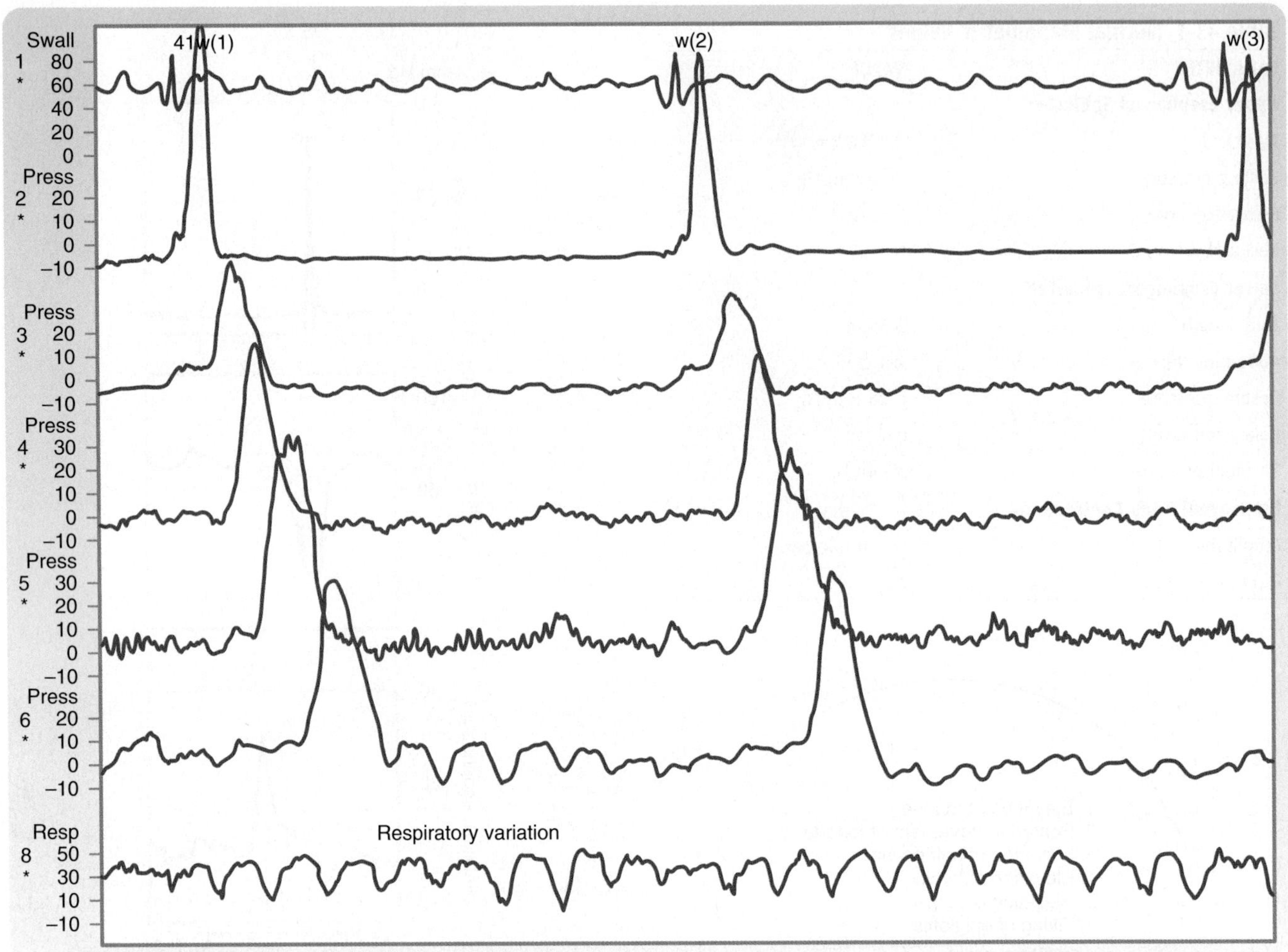

**FIGURE 43-17** Normal esophageal peristalsis. (From Bremner CG, DeMeester TR, Bremner RM, Mason RJ: Esophageal motility testing made easy, St Louis, 2001, Quality Medical Publishing, p 35.)

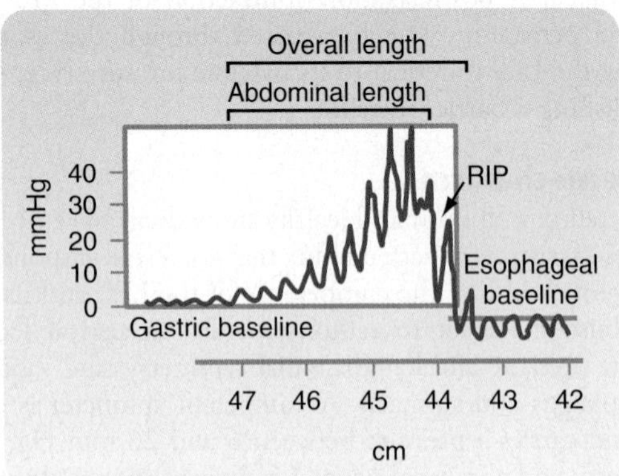


**FIGURE 43-18** Normal lower esophageal sphincter. (From Bremner CG, DeMeester TR, Bremner RM, Mason RJ: Esophageal motility testing made easy, St Louis, 2001, Quality Medical Publishing, p 15.)

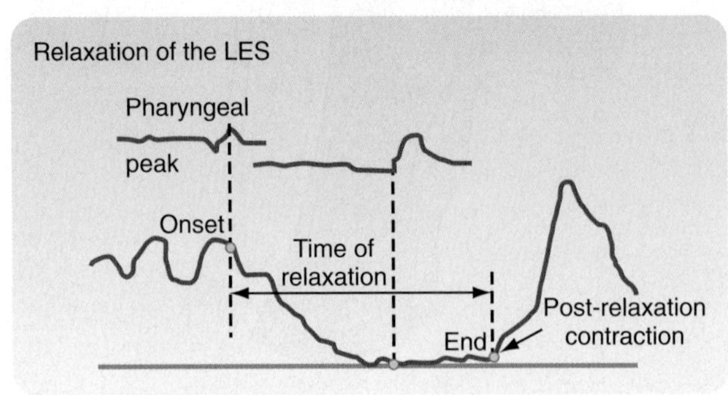


**FIGURE 43-19** Relaxation of the lower esophageal sphincter. (From Bremner CG, DeMeester TR, Bremner RM, Mason RJ: Esophageal motility testing made easy, St Louis, 2001, Quality Medical Publishing, p 24.)

## NEUROMUSCULAR DISORDERS OF THE ESOPHAGUS

### Diverticula

Historically, esophageal diverticula were thought to be a primary disorder that resulted in motility abnormalities. It is now well established that most diverticula are a result of a primary motor disturbance or an abnormality of the UES or LES. Diverticula were originally classified according to their location and, as a convention, they are classifications to which we still adhere. Esophageal diverticula can occur in several places along the esophagus. The three most common sites of occurrence are pharyngoesophageal (Zenker's), parabronchial (midesophageal), and epiphrenic (supradiaphragmatic). True diverticula involve all layers of the esophageal wall, including mucosa, submucosa, and muscularis. A false diverticulum consists of mucosa and submucosa only. Pulsion diverticula are false diverticula that occur because of elevated intraluminal pressures generated from abnormal motility disorders. These forces cause the mucosa and submucosa to herniate through the esophageal musculature. Both a Zenker's diverticulum and an epiphrenic diverticulum fall under the category of false pulsion diverticula. Traction, or true, diverticula result from external inflammatory mediastinal lymph nodes adhering to the esophagus as they heal and contract, pulling the esophagus during the process. Over time, the esophageal wall herniates, forming an outpouching, and a diverticulum ensues.

### Pharyngoesophageal (Zenker's) Diverticulum

Originally described by Zenker and Von Ziemssen, the pharyngoesophageal diverticulum (Zenker's diverticulum) is the most common esophageal diverticulum found today. It usually presents in older patients in the seventh decade of life and has been postulated to be a result of loss of tissue elasticity and muscle tone with age. It is specifically found herniating into Killian's triangle, between the oblique fibers of the thyropharyngeus muscle and the horizontal fibers of the cricopharyngeus muscle (Fig. 43-20). As the diverticulum enlarges, the mucosal and submucosal layers dissect down the left side of the esophagus into the superior mediastinum, posteriorly along the prevertebral space. Zenker's diverticulum is often referred to as *cricopharyngeal achalasia* and is managed accordingly.

**Symptoms and Diagnosis** Until the Zenker's diverticulum begins to enlarge, patients are often initially asymptomatic. Commonly, patients complain of a sticking in the throat. A nagging cough, excessive salivation, and intermittent dysphagia often are signs of progressive disease. As the sac increases in size, regurgitation of foul-smelling, undigested material is common. Halitosis, voice changes, retrosternal pain, and respiratory infections are especially common in older adults. Patients learn to compensate for the difficulties by avoiding social situations. The most serious complication from an untreated Zenker's diverticulum is aspiration pneumonia or lung abscess. In an older patient, this can be morbid and sometimes fatal.

Diagnosis is made by barium esophagraphy (Fig. 43-21). At the level of the cricothyroid cartilage, the diverticulum can be seen filled with barium resting posteriorly alongside the esophagus. Lateral views are critical to obtain because this is usually a posterior structure. Neither esophageal manometry nor endoscopy is needed to diagnose Zenker's diverticulum.

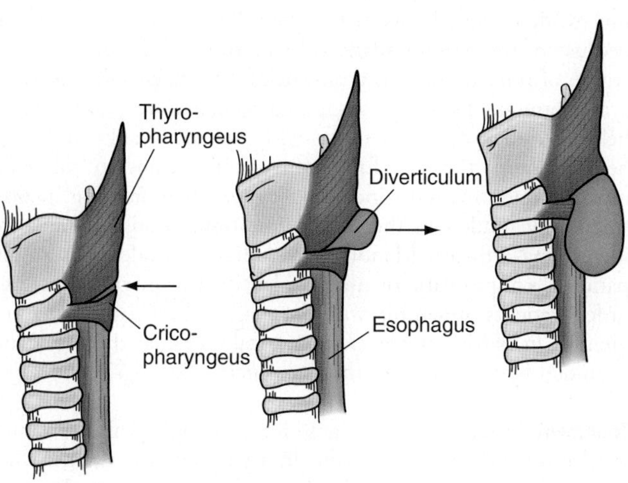


**FIGURE 43-20** Zenker's diverticulum.

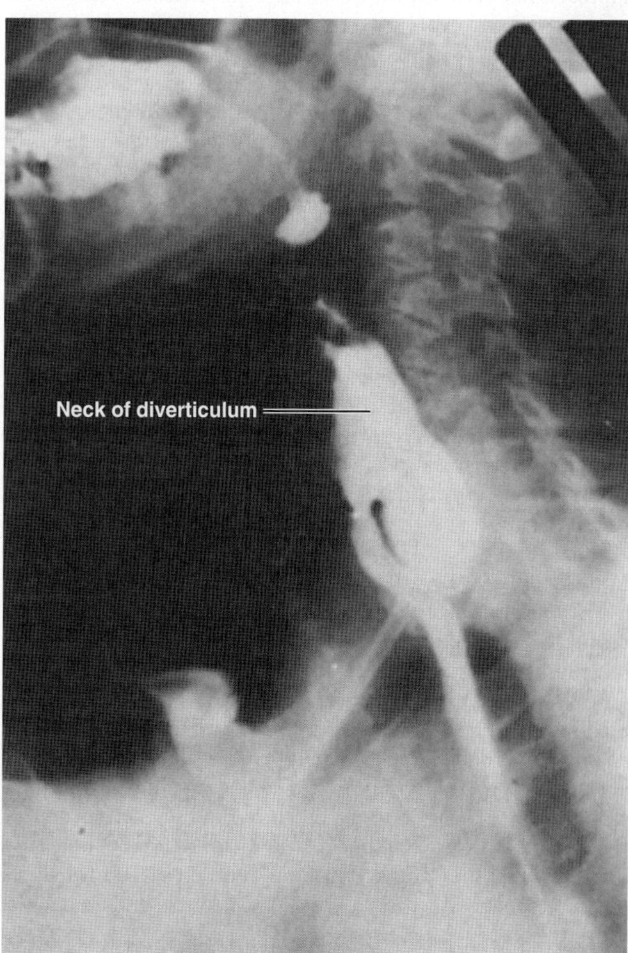


**FIGURE 43-21** Barium swallow showing Zenker's diverticulum. (Adapted from Trastek VF, Deschamps C: Esophageal diverticula. In Shields TW, Locicero J III, Ponn RB [eds]: General thoracic surgery, ed 5, Philadelphia, 1999, Lippincott Williams & Wilkins, p 1841.)

**Treatment** Surgical or endoscopic repair of a Zenker's diverticulum is the gold standard of treatment. Traditionally, an open repair through the left neck was advocated. However, endoscopic exclusion has gained popularity in many centers throughout the United States. Two types of open repair are performed, resection and surgical fixation of the diverticulum. The diverticulectomy and diverticulopexy are performed through an incision in the left neck. Under general anesthesia, they both require about 1 hour to complete. In all cases, a myotomy of the proximal and distal thyropharyngeus and cricopharyngeus muscles is performed. In cases of a small diverticulum (<2 cm), a myotomy alone is often sufficient. In frail patients who may be subject to a higher rate of cervical esophageal leak, a diverticulopexy, without resection, may be performed and will prevent symptoms from recurring.[3] In most patients with good tissue or a large sac (>5 cm), excision of the sac is indicated. The postoperative stay is approximately 2 to 3 days, during which the patient remains unable to eat or drink.

An alternative to open surgical repair is the endoscopic Dohlman procedure, which has become more popular. Endoscopic division of the common wall between the esophagus and diverticulum using a laser or stapler has also been successful. Because of the configuration of the inline stapling device, this approach has been advocated for larger diverticula. The risk for an incomplete myotomy increases with smaller diverticula, smaller than 3 cm. This method divides the distal cricopharyngeus muscle while obliterating the sac. The esophagus and diverticulum form a common channel. The technique requires maximal extension of the neck and can be difficult to perform in older patients with cervical stenosis. It is done transorally under general anesthesia in approximately 1 hour. The postoperative course is slightly shorter, with patients taking liquids the following day and requiring only a single overnight hospital stay. Thus, this technique has gained favor and is advocated for patients with diverticula between 2 and 5 cm.

The results of open repair versus endoscopic repair have been well studied. For diverticula 3 cm or less in size, surgical repair is superior to endoscopic repair in eliminating symptoms. For any diverticulum larger than 3 cm, the results are the same.[4] Both the hospital stay and length of inanition are shorter with an endoscopic procedure. Regardless of the method of repair, patients do well and the results are excellent.

### Midesophageal Diverticula

Midesophageal diverticula were first described in the 19th century. Historically, inflamed mediastinal lymph nodes from an infection with tuberculosis accounted for most cases (Fig. 43-22). Infections with histoplasmosis and resultant fibrosing mediastinitis have now become more common. Inflammation of the lymph nodes exerts traction on the wall of the esophagus and leads to the formation of a true diverticulum in the midesophagus. This continues to be an important mechanism for these traction diverticula but it is now believed that some may also be caused by a primary motility disorder, such as achalasia, diffuse esophageal spasm (DES), or nonspecific esophageal motility (NEM) disorder.

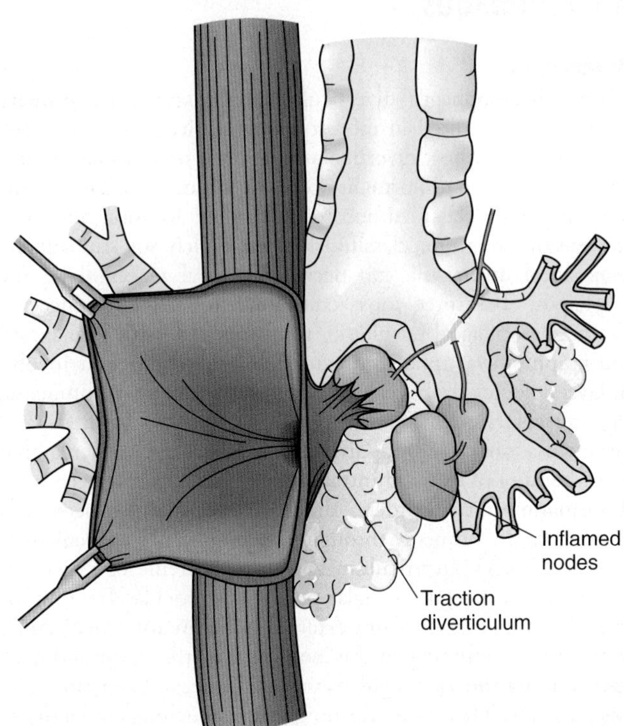


**FIGURE 43-22** Midesophageal diverticulum. (Adapted from Peters JH, DeMeester TR: Esophagus and diaphragmatic hernia. In Schwartz SI, J Fischer JE, Spencer FC, et al [eds]: Principles of surgery, ed 7, New York, 1998, McGraw-Hill, p 1130.)

**Symptoms and Diagnosis** Most patients with a midesophageal diverticulum are asymptomatic. They are often incidentally found during a workup for some other complaint. Dysphagia, chest pain, and regurgitation can be present and are usually indicative of an underlying primary motility disorder. Patients presenting with a chronic cough are under suspicion for development of a bronchoesophageal fistula. Rarely, hemoptysis can be a presenting symptom, indicating infectious erosion of lymph nodes into major vasculature and the bronchial tree. In this case, the diverticulum is an incidental finding of lesser importance.

The diagnosis of the anatomic structure, as well as the size and location of an esophageal diverticulum, is made through barium esophagraphy. Lateral views are needed to determine from which side of the esophagus the diverticulum is protruding. Midesophageal diverticula typically present on the right because of the overabundance of structures in the midthoracic region of the left chest. It is also helpful to make a diagnosis of a concomitant fistula. A computed tomography (CT) scan is helpful to identify any mediastinal lymphadenopathy and may help lateralize the sac. Endoscopy is important to rule out mucosal abnormalities, including cancer, that may be inconspicuously hidden in the sac. In addition, endoscopy aids in identifying a fistula. Manometric studies are undertaken in all patients, symptomatic or not, to identify a primary motor disorder. Patients presenting with dysphagia, chest pain, or regurgitation in particular are manometrically evaluated. Treatment is guided by the results of the manometric findings.

**Treatment** Determining the cause for midesophageal diverticula is critical for guiding treatment. In asymptomatic patients who have inflamed mediastinal lymph nodes from tuberculosis or histoplasmosis, medical treatment with antituberculin or antifungal agents is indicated. If the diverticulum is smaller than 2 cm, it can be observed. If patients progress to become symptomatic or if the diverticulum is 2 cm or larger, surgical intervention is indicated. Usually, midesophageal diverticula have a wide mouth and rest close to the spine. Therefore, a diverticulopexy can be performed where the diverticulum is suspended from the thoracic vertebral fascia. In patients with severe chest pain or dysphagia and a documented motor abnormality, a long esophagomyotomy is also indicated.

### Epiphrenic Diverticula

Epiphrenic diverticula are found adjacent to the diaphragm in the distal third of the esophagus, within 10 cm of the GEJ. They are most often related to thickened distal esophageal musculature or increased intraluminal pressure. They are pulsion, or false, diverticula that are often associated with DES, achalasia and, most commonly, NEM disorders. In patients in whom a motility abnormality cannot be identified, a congenital (Ehlers-Danlos syndrome) or traumatic cause is considered. As with midesophageal diverticula, epiphrenic diverticula are more common on the right side and tend to be wide-mouthed.

**Symptoms and Diagnosis** Most patients with epiphrenic diverticula present asymptomatically. They may present with dysphagia or chest pain, which is indicative of a motility disturbance. The diagnosis is often made during the workup for a motility disorder and the diverticulum is found incidentally. Other symptoms, such as regurgitation, epigastric pain, anorexia, weight loss, chronic cough, and halitosis, are indicative of an advanced motility abnormality resulting in a sizable epiphrenic diverticulum.

A barium esophagram is the best diagnostic tool to detect the presence of an epiphrenic diverticulum (Fig. 43-23). The size, position, and proximity of the diverticulum to the diaphragm can all be clearly delineated. The underlying motility disorder is often identified as well; however, manometric studies need to be undertaken to evaluate the overall motility of the esophageal body and LES. An endoscopy is performed to evaluate for mucosal lesions, including esophagitis, Barrett's esophagus, and cancer.

**Treatment** The treatment of an epiphrenic diverticulum is similar to that of a midesophageal diverticulum. These types of diverticula also have a wide mouth and rest close to the spine. Small (<2 cm) diverticula can be suspended from the vertebral fascia and need not be excised. In patients with severe chest pain, dysphagia, or a documented motor abnormality, a long esophagomyotomy is indicated. If a diverticulopexy is performed, the myotomy is begun at the neck of the diverticulum and extended onto the LES. If a diverticulectomy is pursued, a vertical stapling device is placed across the neck and the diverticulum is excised. The muscle is closed over the excision site and a long myotomy is performed on the opposite esophageal wall, extending from the level of the diverticulum onto the LES. If a large hiatal hernia is also present, the diverticulum is excised, a myotomy performed, and the hiatal hernia repaired. Failure to repair the hernia results in a high incidence of postoperative reflux.

### Motor Disorders

Motility disorders of the esophagus run on a continuum from hypomotile to hypermotile dysfunction, with intermediate types

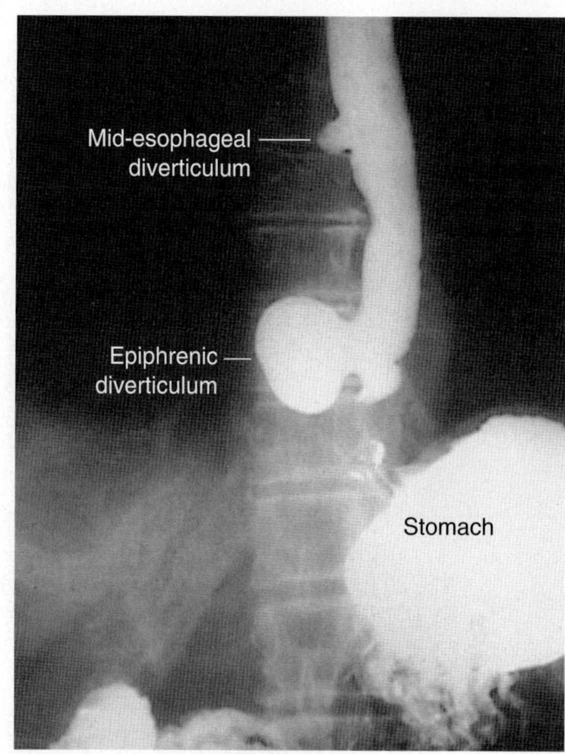


**FIGURE 43-23** Barium swallow showing mid and distal esophageal diverticula. (Adapted from Pearson FG, Cooper JD, Deslauriers J, et al: Esophageal surgery, ed 2, New York, 2002, Churchill Livingstone, p 508.)

in between. There are primary and secondary motor disorders of the esophagus. Most esophageal motility disorders fall into one of five primary motor disorders: achalasia, DES, nutcracker esophagus, hypertensive LES, and ineffective esophageal motility (IEM; Table 43-2). The use of esophageal manometry has demonstrated a number of nonspecific abnormalities reflecting a spectrum of various stages of destruction of esophageal motor function that do not fit into a specific classification. Secondary motor disorders of the esophagus result from progression of other diseases, such as collagen vascular and neuromuscular diseases, and result in NEM disorders. Although the underlying pathologies are different, the presenting symptoms of primary and secondary motility disorders may be similar. A careful assessment must be done to ensure an accurate diagnosis and appropriate treatment plan.

**Achalasia** The literal meaning of the term *achalasia* is "failure to relax," which is said of any sphincter that remains in a constant state of tone with periods of relaxation. It is the best understood of all esophageal motility disorders. The incidence is 6/100,000 persons/year and is seen in young women and middle-aged men and women alike. Its pathogenesis is presumed to be idiopathic or infectious neurogenic degeneration.[5] Severe emotional stress, trauma, drastic weight reduction, and Chagas' disease (parasitic infection with *Trypanosoma cruzi*) have also been implicated. Regardless of the cause, the muscle of the esophagus and LES are affected. Prevailing theories support the model that the destruction of the nerves to the LES is the primary pathology and that degeneration of the neuromuscular function of the

**Table 43-2 Manometric Features of Primary and Nonspecific Esophageal Motility Disorders**

| FEATURE | NORMAL | ACHALASIA | VIGOROUS ACHALASIA | HYPERTENSIVE LES | DIFFUSE ESOPHAGEAL SPASM | NUTCRACKER ESOPHAGUS | INEFFECTIVE ESOPHAGEAL MOTILITY | NONSPECIFIC ESOPHAGEAL MOTILITY DISORDER |
|---|---|---|---|---|---|---|---|---|
| Symptoms | None | Dysphagia<br>Chest pressure<br>Regurgitation | Dysphagia<br>Chest pain | Dysphagia | Chest pain<br>Dysphagia | Dysphagia<br>Chest pain | Dysphagia<br>Heartburn<br>Chest pain | Dysphagia<br>Chest pain |
| Esophagram | Normal | Bird's beak<br>Dilated esophagus | Abnormal | Distal obstruction | Corkscrew esophagus | Normal progressive contractions | Slow transit<br>Incomplete emptying | Slow transit<br>Incomplete emptying |
| Endoscopy | Normal | Patulous esophagus | Normal | Normal | Hyperperistalsis | Hyperperistalsis | Nonspecific | Nonspecific |
| LES pressure | 15-25 mm Hg | Hypertensive (>26 mm Hg) | Normal or hypertensive | Hypertensive (>26 mm Hg) | Normal or slightly elevated | Normal | Normal or low | Normal |
| LES relaxation | Follows swallowing | Incomplete<br>Residual pressure (>5 mm Hg) | Partial or absent | Normal | Normal | Normal | Normal | Incomplete (>90%)<br>Residual pressure (>5 mm Hg) |
| Amplitude pressure | 50-120 mm Hg | Decreased (<40 mm Hg) | Normal | Normal | Normal | Hypertensive (>180 mm Hg) (>400 mm Hg) | Decreased (<30 mm Hg) | Decreased (<35 mm Hg) |
| Contraction waves | Progressive | Simultaneous<br>Mirrored<br>Pressurized | Simultaneous<br>Repetitive | Normal | Simultaneous<br>Repetitive | Long duration (>6 sec) | Nontransmitted (>30%) | Nontransmitted (>20%)<br>Triple-peaked, retrograde<br>Prolonged (>6 sec) |
| Peristalsis | Normal | None | None | Normal | None | Hypertensive peristalsis | Abnormal | Abnormal |

body of the esophagus is secondary. This degeneration results in hypertension of the LES and failure of the LES to relax on pharyngeal swallowing, as well as pressurization of the esophagus, esophageal dilation, and resultant loss of progressive peristalsis.

Vigorous achalasia is seen in a subset of patients presenting with dysphagia. In these patients, the LES is hypertensive and fails to relax, as seen in achalasia. Furthermore, the contractions of the esophageal body continue to be simultaneous and nonperistaltic. However, the amplitude of the contractions in response to swallowing is normal or high, which is inconsistent with classic achalasia. It is postulated that patients in the early development of achalasia may not have abnormalities in the esophageal body that are seen in later stages of the disease. Patients presenting with vigorous achalasia may be in this early phase and will go on to develop abnormal esophageal body contractions.

Achalasia is also known to be a premalignant condition of the esophagus. Over a 20-year period, a patient will have up to an 8% chance of developing carcinoma. Squamous cell carcinoma is the most common type identified and is thought to be the result of long-standing air-fluid levels in the body of the esophagus, causing mucosal irritation and inducing metaplasia. Adenocarcinoma tends to appear in the middle third of the esophagus, below the air-fluid level where the mucosal irritation is the greatest. No specific surveillance program has yet to be initiated in patients with treated achalasia.

***Symptoms and Diagnosis*** The classic triad of presenting symptoms consists of dysphagia, regurgitation, and weight loss. However, heartburn, postprandial choking, and nocturnal coughing are commonly seen. The dysphagia that patients experience begins with liquids and progresses to solids. Most patients describe eating as a laborious process during which they must pay special attention to the process. They eat slowly and use large volumes of water to help wash the food down into the stomach. As the water builds up pressure, retrosternal chest pain is experienced and can be severe until the LES opens, which provides quick relief. Regurgitation of undigested, foul-smelling foods is common and, with progressive disease, aspiration can become life-threatening. Pneumonia, lung abscess, and bronchiectasis often result from long-standing achalasia. The dysphagia progresses slowly over years and patients adapt their lifestyle to accommodate the inconveniences that accompany this disease. Patients often do not seek medical attention until their symptoms are advanced and will present with marked distention of the esophagus.

The diagnosis of achalasia is usually made from an esophagram and a motility study. The findings may vary, depending on the advanced nature of the disease. The esophagram will show a dilated esophagus with a distal narrowing referred to as the classic bird's beak appearance of the barium-filled esophagus (Fig. 43-24). Sphincter spasm and delayed emptying through the LES, as well as dilation of the esophageal body, are observed. A lack of peristaltic waves in the body and failure of relaxation of the LES are noted. Lack of a gastric air bubble is a common finding on the upright portion of the esophagram and is a result of the tight LES not allowing air to pass easily into the stomach. In the more advanced stage of disease, massive esophageal dilation, tortuosity, and a sigmoidal esophagus (megaesophagus) are seen (Fig. 43-25).

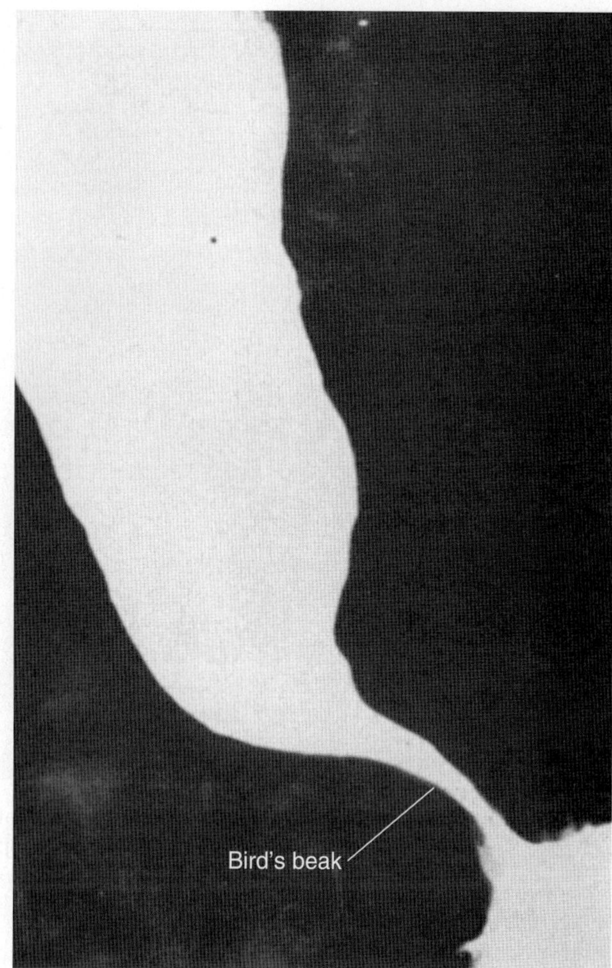


**FIGURE 43-24** Barium swallow showing achalasia. (Adapted from Dalton CB: Esophageal motility disorders. In Pearson FG, Cooper JD, Deslauriers J, et al [eds]: Esophageal surgery, ed 2 New York, 2002, Churchill Livingstone, p 519.)

Manometry is the gold standard test for diagnosis and will help eliminate other potential esophageal motility disorders. In typical achalasia, the manometry tracings show five classic findings, two abnormalities of the LES and three of the esophageal body. The LES will be hypertensive, with pressures usually higher than 35 mm Hg but, more importantly, will fail to relax with deglutition (Fig. 43-26). The body of the esophagus will have a pressure above baseline (pressurization of the esophagus) from incomplete air evacuation, simultaneous mirrored contractions with no evidence of progressive peristalsis, and low-amplitude waveforms indicating a lack of muscular tone (Fig. 43-27). These five findings provide a diagnosis of achalasia. An endoscopy is performed to evaluate the mucosa for evidence of esophagitis or cancer. It otherwise contributes little to the diagnosis of achalasia.

***Treatment*** There are surgical and nonsurgical treatment options for patients with achalasia; all are directed toward relieving the obstruction caused by the LES. Because none of them addresses the issue of decreased motility in the esophageal body, they are all palliative treatments. Nonsurgical treatment options include

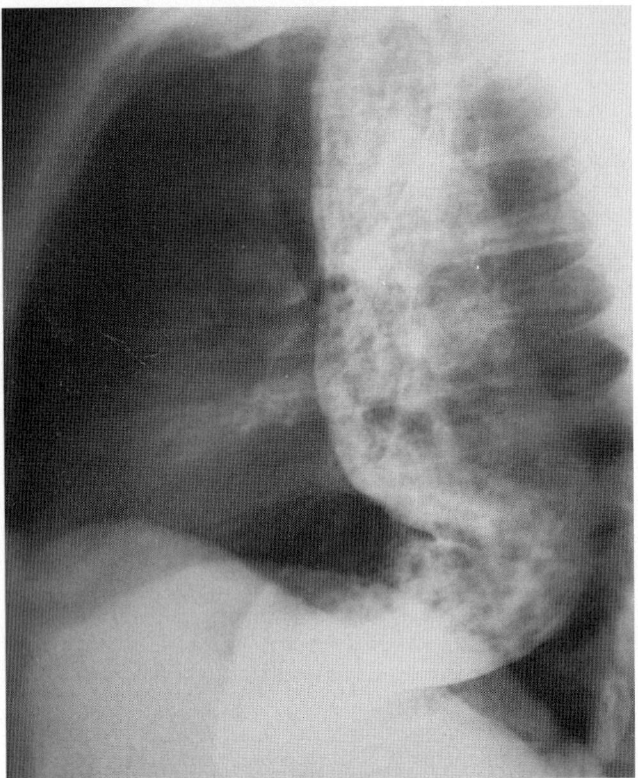

**FIGURE 43-25** Barium swallow showing megaesophagus. (From Orringer MB: Disorders of esophageal motility. In Sabiston DC [ed]: Textbook of Surgery, ed 15, Philadelphia, 1997, WB Saunders, p 719.)

medications and endoscopic interventions but usually are only a short-term solution to a lifelong problem. In the early stage of the disease, medical treatment with sublingual nitroglycerin, nitrates, or calcium channel blockers may offer hours of relief of chest pressure before or after a meal.[6] Bougie dilation up to 54 Fr may offer several months of relief but requires repeated dilations to be sustainable. Injections of botulinum toxin (Botox) directly into the LES blocks acetylcholine release, preventing smooth muscle contraction, and effectively relaxes the LES. With repeated treatments, Botox may offer symptomatic relief for years, but symptoms recur more than 50% of the time within 6 months. Dilation with a Gruntzig-type (volume-limited, pressure control) balloon is effective in 60% of patients and has a risk for perforation less than 4%; however, perforation is life-threatening and must be weighed carefully in otherwise unhealthy patients.

Surgical esophagomyotomy offers superior results and is less traumatic than balloon dilation.[7] The current technique is a modification of the Heller myotomy that was described originally by a laparotomy in 1913.[8] Various changes have been made to the originally described procedure but the modified laparoscopic Heller myotomy is now the operation of choice. It is done open or with video or robotic assistance. The decision to perform an antireflux procedure remains controversial. Most patients who have undergone a myotomy will experience some symptoms of reflux. The addition of a partial antireflux procedure, such as a Toupet or Dor fundoplication, will restore a barrier to reflux and decrease postoperative symptoms. This is especially true in patients whose esophageal clearance is greatly impaired.[9]

Esophagectomy is considered in any symptomatic patient with tortuous esophagus (megaesophagus), sigmoid esophagus, failure of more than one myotomy, or an undilatable reflux stricture. Fewer than 60% of patients undergoing repeat myotomy benefit from surgery, and fundoplication for treatment of reflux strictures has even more dismal results. In addition to definitively treating the end-stage achalasia, esophageal resection also eliminates the risk for carcinoma. A transhiatal esophagectomy with[10] or without preservation of the vagus nerve offers a good long-term result.

***Results*** Results of medical, interventional, and surgical procedures all point to surgery as the safest and most effective treatment of achalasia. When comparing balloon dilation to Botox injections, remission of symptoms occurred in 89% versus 38% of patients at 1 year, respectively. Studies done to compare balloon dilation versus surgery have shown perforation rates of 4% and 1% and mortality rates of 0.5% and 0.2%, respectively. Results were considered excellent in 60% of patients undergoing balloon dilation and in 85% of those undergoing surgery. Studies of laparoscopic versus open myotomy have all demonstrated superior results with a minimally invasive technique. Shorter length of stay, less pain, and excellent relief of dysphagia with an improved heartburn score have all been documented with a laparoscopic approach. Furthermore, laparoscopic myotomy appears to be safe and effective, even after treatment with Botox or balloon dilation or with a massively dilated esophagus. Although most patients present fairly early in their disease process, end-stage achalasia is still found in a small percentage of patients. In these late presentations, a surgical myotomy is not likely to be effective.

**Diffuse Esophageal Spasm** DES is a poorly understood hypermotility disorder of the esophagus. Although it presents in a similar fashion to achalasia, it is five times less common. It is seen most often in women and is often found in patients with multiple complaints. The cause of the neuromuscular physiology is unclear. The basic pathology is related to a motor abnormality of the esophageal body that is most notable in the lower two thirds of the esophagus. Muscular hypertrophy and degeneration of the branches of the vagus nerve in the esophagus have been observed. As a result, the esophageal contractions are repetitive, simultaneous, and of high amplitude.

***Symptoms and Diagnosis*** The clinical presentation of DES is typically that of chest pain and dysphagia. These symptoms may be related to eating or exertion and may mimic those of angina. Patients will complain of a squeezing pressure in the chest that may radiate to the jaw, arms, and upper back. The symptoms are often pronounced during times of heightened emotional stress. Regurgitation of esophageal contents and saliva is common, but acid reflux is not. However, acid reflux can aggravate the symptoms, as can cold liquids. Other functional gastrointestinal complaints, such as irritable bowel syndrome and pyloric spasm, may accompany DES, whereas other gastrointestinal problems, such as gallstones, peptic ulcer disease, and pancreatitis, all trigger DES.

The diagnosis of DES is made by esophagraphy and manometric studies. The classic picture of the corkscrew esophagus or pseudodiverticulosis on an esophagram is caused by the presence of tertiary contractions and indicates advanced disease

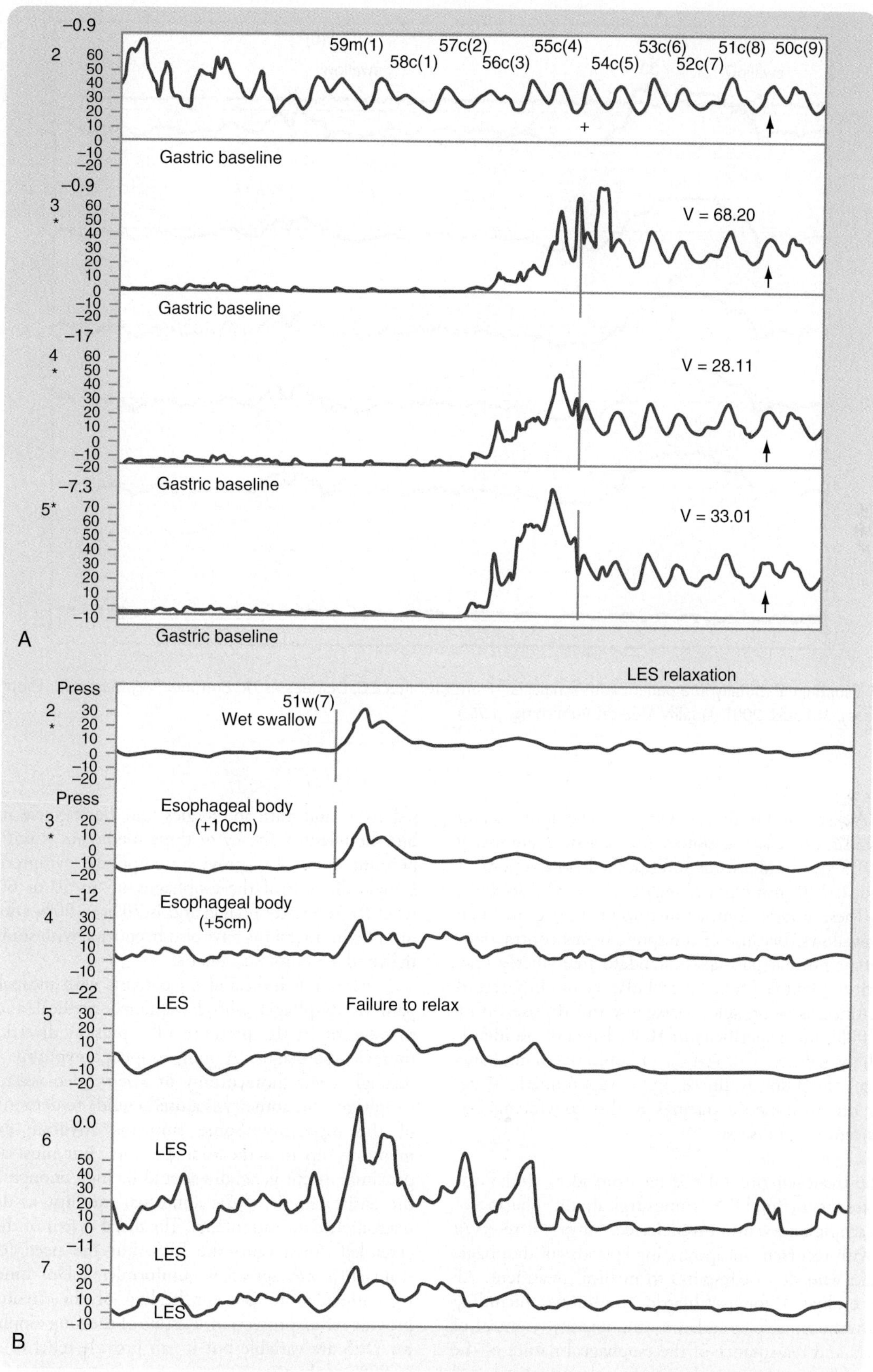


**FIGURE 43-26** Motility of the lower esophageal sphincter in a patient with achalasia. (Adapted from Pearson FG, Cooper JD, Deslauriers J, et al: Esophageal surgery, ed 2, New York, 2002, Churchill Livingstone, p 520.)

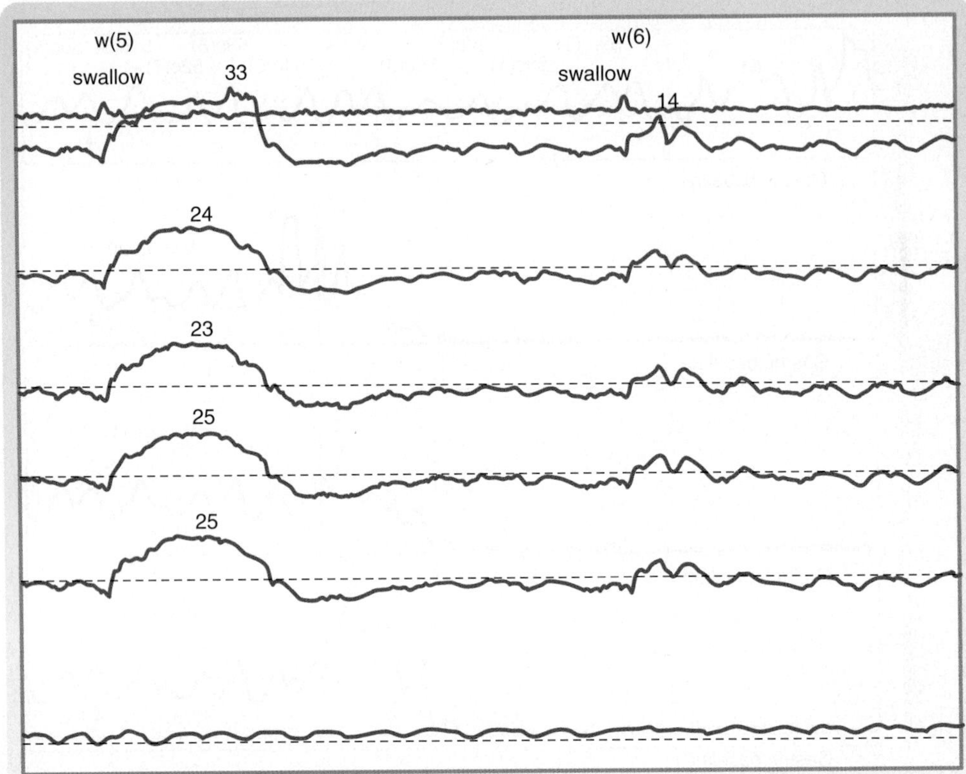


**FIGURE 43-27** Esophageal motility in a patient with achalasia. (From Bremner CG, DeMeester TR, Bremner RM, Mason RJ: Esophageal motility testing made easy, St Louis, 2001, Quality Medical Publishing, p 75.)

(Fig. 43-28). A distal bird beak narrowing of the esophagus and normal peristalsis can also be noted. The classic manometry findings in DES are simultaneous multipeaked contractions of high amplitude (>120 mm Hg) or long duration (>2.5 seconds; Fig. 43-29). These erratic contractions occur after more than 10% of wet swallows. Because of the spontaneous contractions and intermittent normal peristalsis, standard manometry may not be enough to identify DES. An ambulatory motility record has been identified as being able to diagnose this disease with a sensitivity of 90% and a specificity of 100% based on an identified set of abnormalities. Correlation of subjective complaints with evidence of spasm (induced by a vagomimetic drug, bethanechol) on manometric tracings is also convincing evidence of this capricious disease.

***Treatment*** The treatment for DES is far from ideal. Today the mainstay of treatment for DES is nonsurgical, and pharmacologic or endoscopic intervention is preferred. Surgery is reserved for patients with recurrent incapacitating episodes of dysphagia and chest pain who do not respond to medical treatment. All patients are evaluated for psychiatric conditions, including depression, psychosomatic complaints, and anxiety. Control of these disorders and reassurance of the esophageal nature of the chest pain that they are experiencing is often therapeutic in and of itself. If dysphagia is a component of a patient's symptoms, steps must be taken to eliminate trigger foods or drinks from the diet. Similarly, if reflux is a component, acid suppression medications are helpful. Nitrates, calcium channel blockers, sedatives, and anticholinergics may be effective in some cases, but the relative efficacy of these medicines is not known. Peppermint may also provide temporary symptomatic relief.[11] Bougie dilation of the esophagus up to 50 or 60 Fr provides relief for severe dysphagia and is 70% to 80% effective. Botulinum toxin injections have also been tried with some success, but the results are not sustainable.

Surgery is indicated for patients with incapacitating chest pain or dysphagia who have failed medical and endoscopic therapy, or in the presence of a pulsion diverticulum of the thoracic esophagus. A long esophagomyotomy is performed through a left thoracotomy or a left video-assisted technique. Esophageal manometry is a useful guide to determine the extent of the myotomy. Some surgeons advocate extending the myotomy up into the thoracic inlet, but most agree that the proximal extent generally should be high enough to encompass the entire length of the abnormal motility, as determined by manometric measurements. The distal extent of the myotomy is extended down onto the LES, but the need to include the stomach is not agreed on uniformly. A Dor fundoplication is recommended to prevent healing of the myotomy site and provide reflux protection. Results of the long esophagomyotomy for DES are variable but it can provide relief of symptoms up to 80% of the time.

**Nutcracker Esophagus** Recognized in the late 1970s as a distinct entity, nutcracker esophagus is a hypermotility disorder also known as supersqueeze esophagus. It is described as

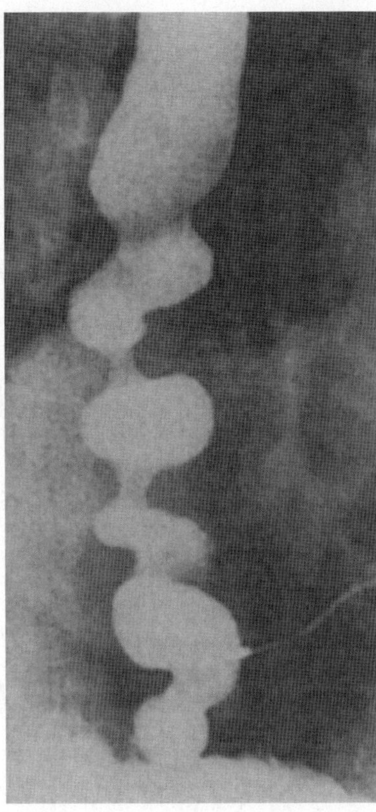

**FIGURE 43-28** Barium esophagram of diffuse esophageal spasm. (Adapted from Peters JH, DeMeester TR: Esophagus and diaphragmatic hernia. In Schwartz SI, J Fischer JE, Spencer FC, et al [eds]: Principles of surgery, ed 7, New York, 1998, McGraw-Hill, p 1129.)

an esophagus with hypertensive peristalsis or high-amplitude peristaltic contractions. It is seen in patients of all ages, with equal gender predilection, and is the most common of all esophageal hypermotility disorders. Like DES, the pathophysiology is not well understood. It is associated with hypertrophic musculature that results in high-amplitude contractions of the esophagus and is the most painful of all esophageal motility disorders.

***Symptoms and Diagnosis*** Patients present in a similar fashion to patients with DES with chest pain and dysphagia. Odynophagia is also noted, but regurgitation and reflux are uncommon. An esophagram may or may not reveal any abnormalities. The gold standard of diagnosis is the subjective complaint of chest pain with simultaneous objective evidence of peristaltic esophageal contractions 2 standard deviations (SDs) above the normal values on manometric tracings. Amplitudes higher than 400 mm Hg are common (Fig. 43-30). The LES pressure is normal and relaxation occurs with each wet swallow. Ambulatory monitoring can help distinguish this disorder from DES. This is of critical importance because a subset of DES patients with dysphagia can be helped with esophagomyotomy, but surgery is of questionable value in patients with a nutcracker esophagus.

***Treatment*** The treatment of nutcracker esophagus is medical. Calcium channel blockers, nitrates, and antispasmodics may offer temporary relief during acute spasms. Bougie dilation may offer some temporary relief of severe discomfort but has no long-term benefits. Patients with nutcracker esophagus may have triggers and are counseled to avoid caffeine, cold, and hot foods.

**Hypertensive LES** The condition known as hypertensive LES was first described as a separate entity by Code and colleagues.[12] It was observed in patients presenting with dysphagia, chest pain, and manometric findings of an elevated LES. However, the manometric findings are not consistent with achalasia. The LES pressure is above normal and relaxation will be incomplete but may not be consistently abnormal. The motility of the esophageal body may be hyperperistaltic or normal. The pathogenesis is not well understood, but it has been theorized that it may be a similar process to that of achalasia in evolution.

***Symptoms and Diagnosis*** Patients with hypertensive LES present with chest pain or dysphagia. Acid reflux and regurgitation are experienced less commonly. Diagnosis is made by manometry. An esophagram may show narrowing at the GEJ with delayed flow and abnormalities of esophageal contraction; however, these are nonspecific findings. Manometry tracings demonstrate elevated LES pressure (>26 mm Hg) and normal relaxation of the LES. About 50% of the time, peristalsis in the esophageal body is normal. In the remainder, abnormal contractions are noted to be hypertensive peristaltic or simultaneous waveforms.

***Treatment*** The treatment of hypertensive LES is with endoscopic and surgical intervention. Botox injections alleviate symptoms temporarily and hydrostatic balloon dilation may provide long-term symptomatic relief. Surgery is indicated for patients who fail interventional treatments and those with significant symptoms. A laparoscopic modified Heller esophagomyotomy is the operation of choice. In patients with normal esophageal motility, a partial antireflux procedure (e.g., Dor or Toupet fundoplication) is added.

**Ineffective Esophageal Motility** IEM was first recognized as a separate disturbance by Castell in 2000.[13] It is defined as a contraction abnormality of the distal esophagus and is usually associated with GERD. It may be secondary to inflammatory injury of the esophageal body because of increased exposure to gastric contents. Dampened motility of the esophageal body leads to poor acid clearance in the lower esophagus. Once altered motility is present, the condition appears to be irreversible.

***Symptoms*** The symptoms of IEM are mixed but patients usually present with symptoms of reflux and dysphagia. Heartburn, chest pain, and regurgitation are noted. Diagnosis is made by manometry. IEM is defined as a contraction abnormality of the distal esophagus in which the total of the number of low-amplitude contractions (<30 mm Hg) plus nontransmitted contractions exceeds 30% of wet swallows. A barium esophagram demonstrates nonspecific abnormalities of esophageal contraction but will not further distinguish IEM from other motor disorders.

***Treatment*** The best treatment of IEM is prevention, which is associated with effective treatment of GERD. Once altered motility occurs, it appears to be irreversible.

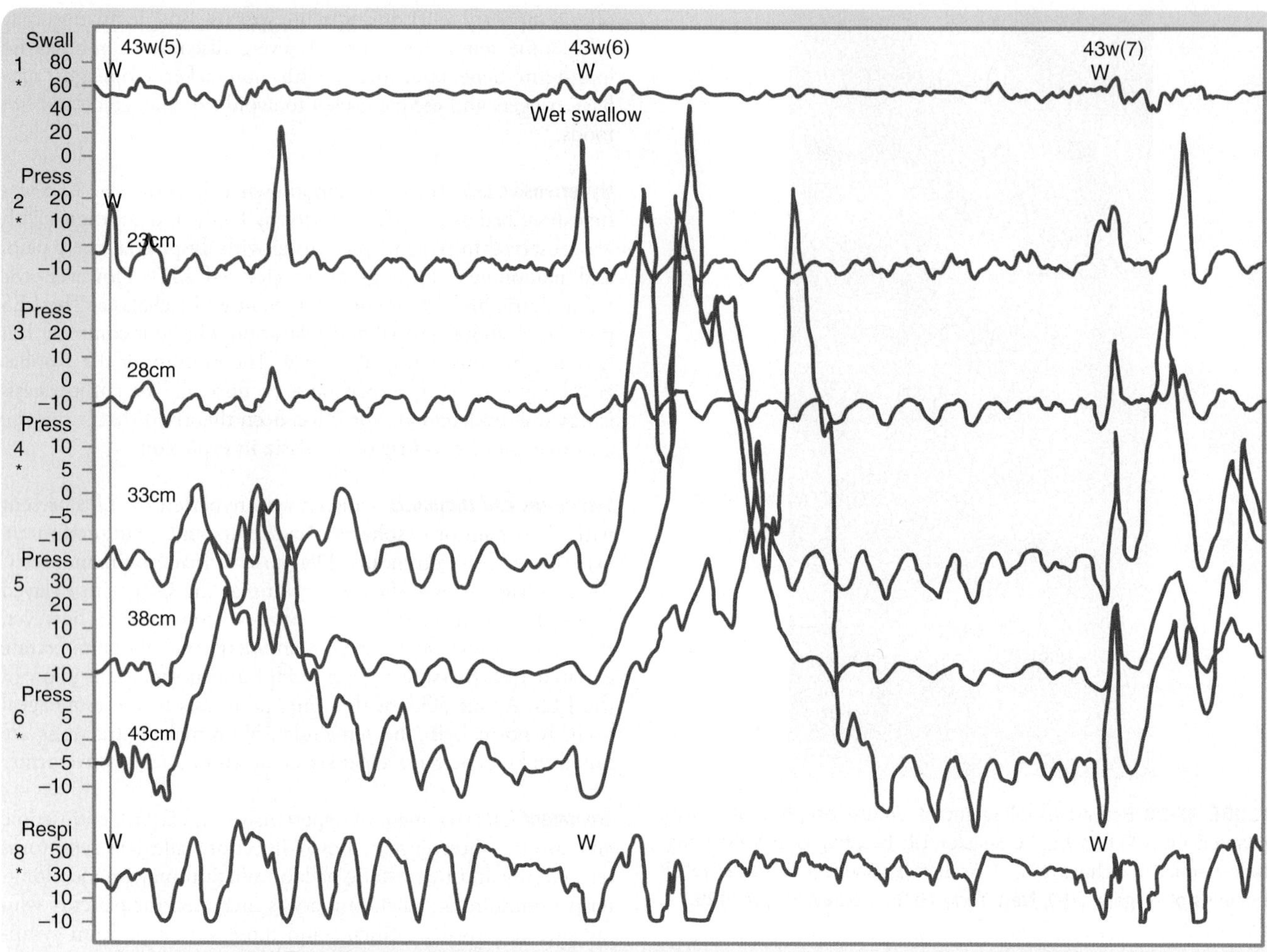


**FIGURE 43-29** Manometry findings in diffuse esophageal spasm. (From Bremner CG, DeMeester TR, Bremner RM, Mason RJ: Esophageal motility testing made easy, St Louis, 2001, Quality Medical Publishing, p 83.)

**Nonspecific Esophageal Motor Disorders** Patients with manometric findings that do not fit into one of the five classic patterns are placed in the category of nonspecific esophageal motor disorders. These nonspecific abnormalities support the understanding that esophageal motility disorders are a spectrum of abnormalities that reflect various stages of destruction of esophageal motor function. The pathogenesis of NEM is multifaceted and has no any single isolated cause. Several collagen vascular disorders are known to cause abnormalities of esophageal motility, including scleroderma, dermatomyositis, polymyositis, and lupus erythematosus. All affect the neuromuscular esophageal architecture, resulting in poor esophageal motility.

***Symptoms and Diagnosis*** Patients with NEM present with chest pain and dysphagia and tend to experience more reflux symptoms and regurgitation than patients with other defined disorders. Diagnostic tests include barium esophagraphy and manometric studies. Esophagraphy is helpful to rule out disorders with defined abnormalities and identifies abnormal esophageal body contractions as well as abnormalities of the LES. Manometry is critical to determine the nature of the motor abnormalities that the patient is experiencing. The LES can be normal or hypertensive, but incomplete relaxation (residual >5 mm Hg) is noted. Contractions of the esophageal body will follow one or more of the following patterns: nontransmitted, triple-peaked, retrograde, low-amplitude (<35 mm Hg), or prolonged duration (>6 seconds). Interruption of normal peristalsis at various esophageal levels is also common. Some patients will have characteristic waveforms that can be ascribed to an underlying collagen vascular disorder. Patients with scleroderma will have low-amplitude simultaneous contractions of the esophageal body, similar to those seen with achalasia, but the LES is noted to have normal or low pressure.

***Treatment*** Treatment of NEM is difficult because a primary diagnosis is evasive. Those with collagen vascular or neuromuscular disorders are treated for their primary medical condition, which often results in improved esophageal motility. For those whose underlying condition remains undiagnosed, combination therapy, including medications and therapeutic interventions, can be applied, as guided by the prevailing manometric findings.

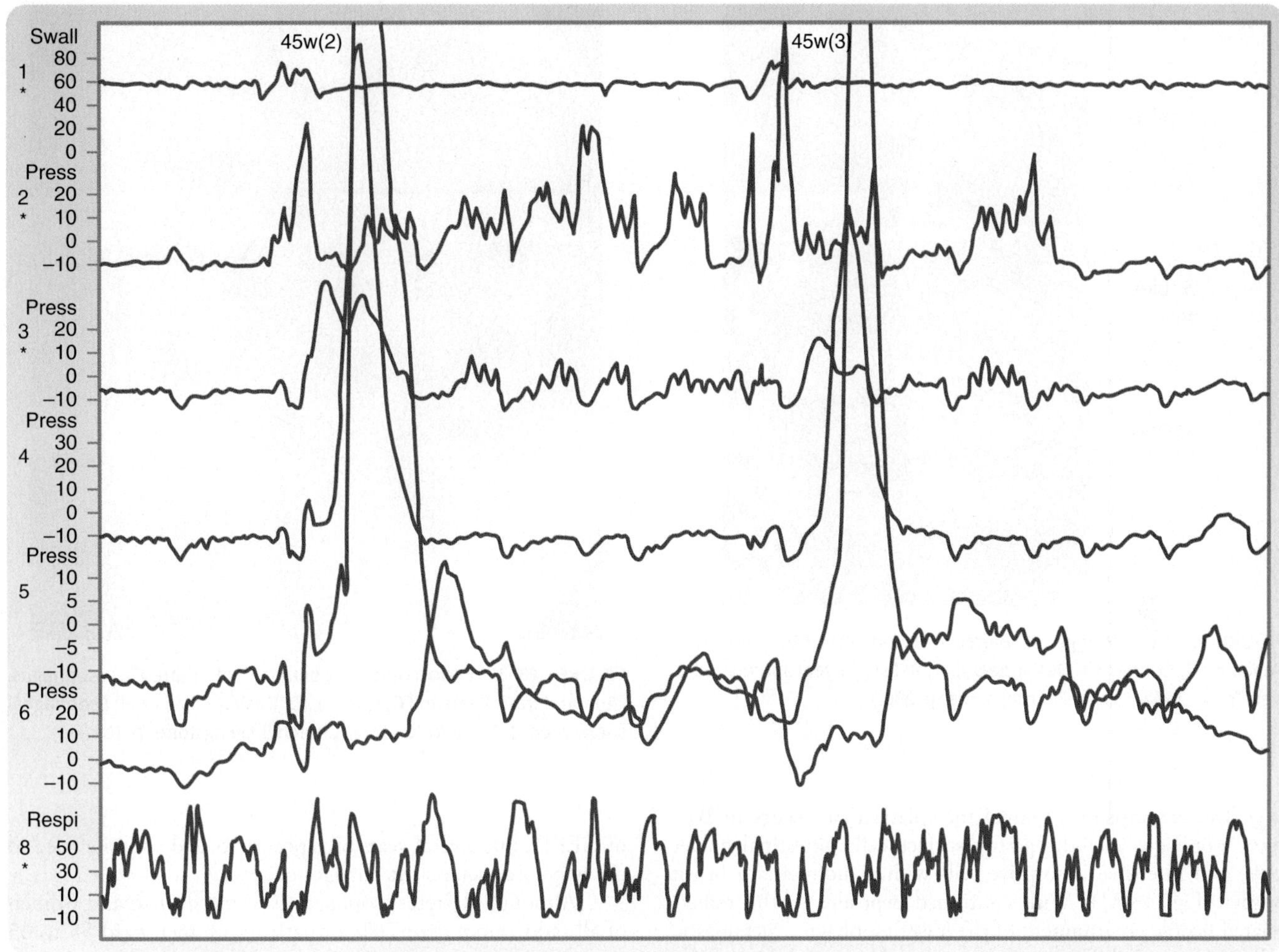


**FIGURE 43-30** Manometry findings in nutcracker esophagus. (From Bremner CG, DeMeester TR, Bremner RM, Mason RJ: Esophageal motility testing made easy, St Louis, 2001, Quality Medical Publishing, p 85.)

## DISEASES OF THE ESOPHAGUS

### Barrett's Esophagus

#### Historical Perspective

In the 1950s, a British surgeon, Dr. Norman Barrett, proposed that sections of the gastrointestinal tract are defined by their mucosa. He went on to say that the esophagus ended at the squamocolumnar junction and that ulcers within columnar mucosa distal to the squamous esophageal mucosa were within "a pouch of stomach . . . drawn up by scar tissue into the mediastinum." In 1953, Allison and Johnstone demonstrated that this distal pouch of stomach had no peritoneal covering, normal esophageal musculature, and typical esophageal mucous glands. They concluded that this segment represents a columnar-lined distal esophagus, not stomach. Agreeing with their findings, Barrett retracted his opinion. Despite his initial misinterpretation, this condition bears his name.

#### Background

To adapt to the ever-changing environments that it encounters, the human body has built-in mechanisms that facilitate the necessary adjustments. Metaplasia is one of those mechanisms and has been viewed teleologically as an attempt to protect vulnerable tissues from a hostile environment. The process of metaplasia, in which one type of fully differentiated (adult) cell replaces another type of adult cell, occurs in a number of organs. In most organs that exhibit epithelial metaplasia, stratified squamous epithelium replaces an inflamed columnar mucosa. In contrast, Barrett's esophagus is a condition whereby an intestinal columnar epithelium replaces the stratified squamous epithelium that normally lines the distal esophagus. Chronic gastroesophageal reflux is the factor that injures the squamous epithelium and promotes repair through columnar metaplasia. Although these metaplastic cells may be more resistant to injury from reflux, they also are more prone to malignancy. Of patients with GERD, 10% develop Barrett's esophagus. Even more unsettling is the 40-fold increase in risk for developing esophageal carcinoma in patients with Barrett's esophagus. Prospectively following 100 patients with Barrett's esophagus for 1 year will result in one patient developing adenocarcinoma, an incidence of 1%/year.[14] This is a similar risk to that of patients with a 20-pack-year smoking history developing lung cancer.

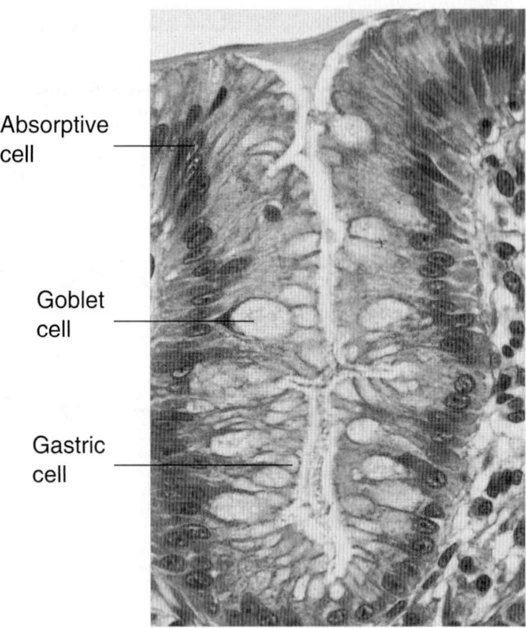


**FIGURE 43-31** Histology of Barrett's esophagus. (Adapted from Pearson FG, Cooper JD, Deslauriers J, et al: Esophageal surgery, ed 2, New York, 2002, Churchill Livingstone, p 286.)

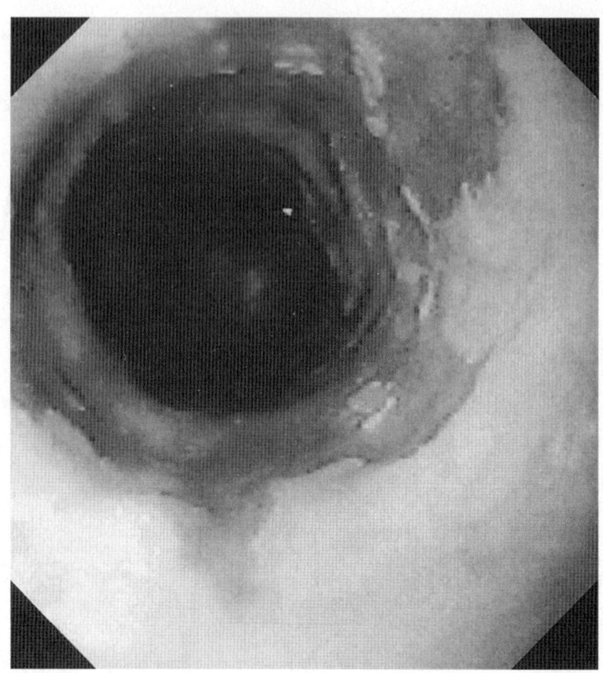

**FIGURE 43-32** Endoscopic appearance of Barrett's esophagus. (Adapted from Pearson FG, Cooper JD, Deslauriers J, et al: Esophageal surgery, ed 2, New York, 2002, Churchill Livingstone, p 151.)

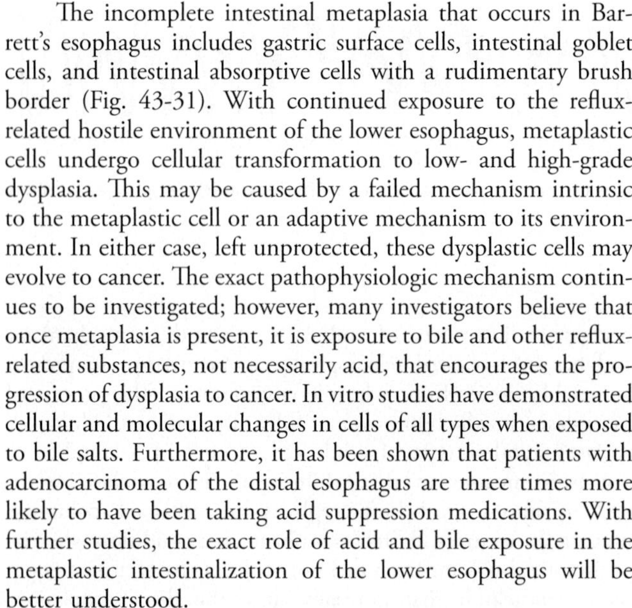

The incomplete intestinal metaplasia that occurs in Barrett's esophagus includes gastric surface cells, intestinal goblet cells, and intestinal absorptive cells with a rudimentary brush border (Fig. 43-31). With continued exposure to the reflux-related hostile environment of the lower esophagus, metaplastic cells undergo cellular transformation to low- and high-grade dysplasia. This may be caused by a failed mechanism intrinsic to the metaplastic cell or an adaptive mechanism to its environment. In either case, left unprotected, these dysplastic cells may evolve to cancer. The exact pathophysiologic mechanism continues to be investigated; however, many investigators believe that once metaplasia is present, it is exposure to bile and other reflux-related substances, not necessarily acid, that encourages the progression of dysplasia to cancer. In vitro studies have demonstrated cellular and molecular changes in cells of all types when exposed to bile salts. Furthermore, it has been shown that patients with adenocarcinoma of the distal esophagus are three times more likely to have been taking acid suppression medications. With further studies, the exact role of acid and bile exposure in the metaplastic intestinalization of the lower esophagus will be better understood.

A number of other causes have been investigated in the development of Barrett's esophagus. Infectious causes, such as *Helicobacter pylori,* have been investigated, although it has not been shown to be associated with an increase in esophageal metaplasia of the esophagus. Genetic abnormalities play a role that is not well defined. An incompetent LES, with or without a hiatal hernia, plays an important role in the development of GERD and Barrett's esophagus. Factors that have been implicated in the pathophysiology of the LES are age, obesity, stress, caffeinated products, alcohol, tobacco, and a number of foods, including spicy, fatty, and acidic foods. Once the LES is rendered incompetent, esophagitis may appear within 1 year of symptoms of GERD, but several years of exposure to acid and bile need to occur before metaplastic changes occur.

Although Barrett's esophagus is found in men and women of all races, more than 70% of patients are men aged 55 to 63 years. White men predominate (up to 20 : 1) over African American men.[15] Men have a 15-fold increased incidence over women with adenocarcinoma of the esophagus, but women with Barrett's esophagus are increasing in number as the differences in the Western lifestyle between men and women diminish. Many Asian cultures have a high rate of squamous cell carcinoma of the esophagus, not related to Barrett's esophagus, and a low rate of adenocarcinoma in which Barrett's esophagus has been implicated. This strongly suggests that cultural lifestyles play an important role in the evolution of Barrett's esophagus.

### Symptoms and Diagnosis

Many patients harboring intestinal metaplasia in their distal esophagus are asymptomatic. Most patients present with symptoms of GERD. Heartburn, regurgitation, acid or bitter taste in the mouth, excessive belching, and indigestion are some of the common symptoms associated with GERD. Recurrent respiratory infections, adult asthma, and infections in the head and neck also are common complaints. The diagnosis of Barrett's esophagus is made by endoscopy and pathology. The presence of any endoscopically visible segment of columnar mucosa within the esophagus (Fig. 43-32) that identifies intestinal metaplasia on pathology defines Barrett's esophagus. Most patients are found to have intestinal metaplasia on a routine endoscopy done for GERD. Other diagnostic tests, such as manometry and barium esophagraphy, are useful for determining adjunctive esophageal pathology but offer little to obtaining a diagnosis of intestinal metaplasia.

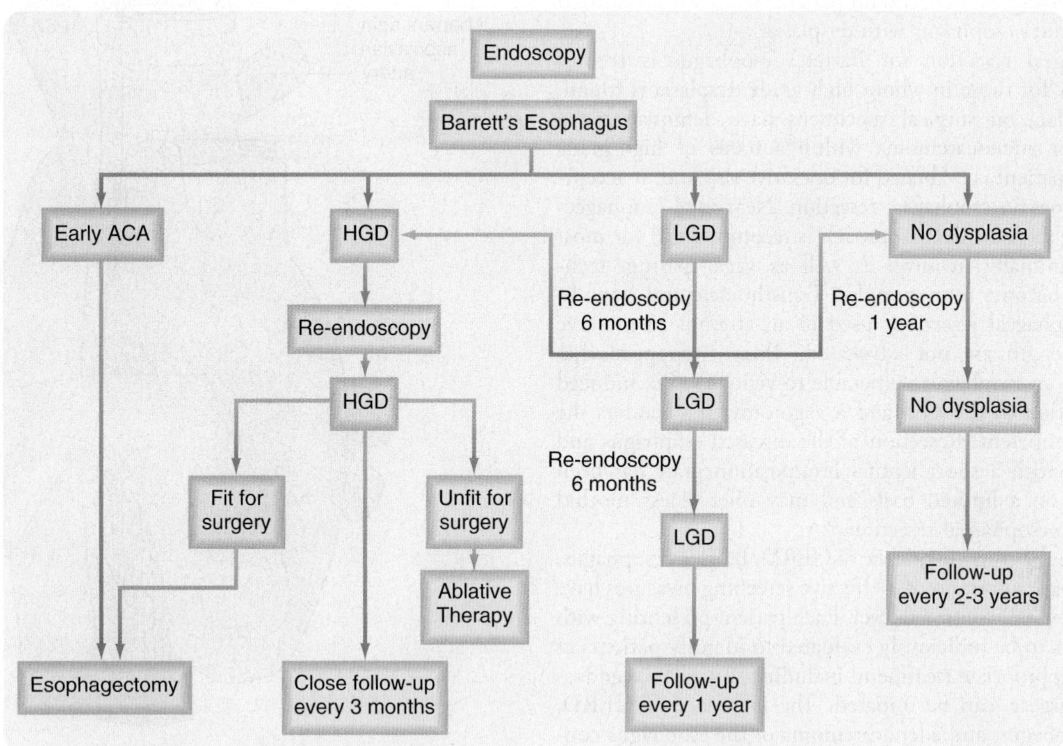


**FIGURE 43-33** Grade of dysplasia and proposed follow-up algorithm for the treatment of Barrett's esophagus. ACA, Adenocarcinoma; HGD, high-grade dysplasia; LGD, low-grade dysplasia. (Adapted from Pearson FG, Cooper JD, Deslauriers J, et al: Esophageal surgery, ed 2, New York, 2002, Churchill Livingstone, p 742.)

### Treatment

Until the pathophysiologic mechanisms of Barrett's esophagus are well understood, the treatment of this disease will remain controversial. Current treatment is hindered by the interest and educational bias of the diagnosing physician and is greatly lacking in continuity and sound scientific data. There are several accepted treatment options—surveillance endoscopy, antireflux surgery with or without continued surveillance endoscopy, ablative therapy, endoscopic mucosal resection, and esophageal resection. In general, gastroenterologists advocate aggressive surveillance programs with high-dose acid suppression and surgeons advocate antireflux surgery to correct the dysfunctional LES. It is likely that there is role for each and that a cohesive treatment plan will be established.

Annual surveillance endoscopy is recommended for all patients with a diagnosis of Barrett's esophagus, regardless of the length of the segment. Practice guidelines put out by the American College of Gastroenterology suggest that surveillance be extended to every 2 to 3 years for individuals with no evidence of dysplasia on two consecutive annual endoscopic examinations (Fig. 43-33). For patients with low-grade dysplasia, surveillance endoscopy is performed at 6-month intervals for the first year and then annually thereafter if there has been no change. Patients undergoing surveillance are placed on acid suppression medication and monitored for changes in their reflux symptoms.

Controversy surrounds the benefits of antireflux surgery in patients with Barrett's esophagus. Those in favor of surgery argue that medical therapy and endoscopic surveillance may treat the symptoms but fail to address the problem. The problem is the functional impairment of the LES, which leads to chronic reflux and metaplastic transformation of the lower esophageal mucosa. Surgery renders the LES competent and restores the barrier to reflux. Studies have demonstrated regression of metaplasia to normal mucosa up to 57% of the time[16] in patients who have undergone antireflux surgery. Furthermore, antireflux surgery encourages regression of low-grade dysplasia to intestinal metaplasia, or Barrett's esophagus. Those who oppose surgery argue that adequate surveillance is impossible after a fundoplication, placing patients at risk for developing cancer in a hidden segment of Barrett's esophagus.

Ablative therapy for Barrett's esophagus is an additional treatment option that has become more popular, mainly proposed for patients with high-grade dysplasia. Photodynamic therapy (PDT) is the most common ablative method used. Complications include persistent metaplasia in more than 50% of patients,[17] as well as esophageal strictures in up to 34% of patients. Combined ablative therapies with PDT and laser therapy have also been tried but have limited acceptance. Endoscopic mucosal resection (EMR) has gained favor for the treatment of Barrett's esophagus with low-grade dysplasia. Also, it has been used as a diagnostic tool to rule out cancer in a focus of Barrett's esophagus with high-grade dysplasia. Because of an increase in stricture rate with larger resections, it is not advocated for long-segment Barrett's esophagus. It is acceptable for patients with high-grade dysplasia who are not acceptable candidates for esophageal resection and useful for patients who have an isolated focus of Barrett's esophagus with dysplasia.

Esophageal resection for Barrett's esophagus is recommended only for those in whom high-grade dysplasia is found. Pathologic data on surgical specimens have demonstrated a 40% risk for adenocarcinoma within a focus of high-grade dysplasia. A patient is evaluated for operative risk and, if acceptable, undergoes an esophageal resection. Near-total esophagectomy through a transhiatal approach is recommended for most patients. Minimally invasive, as well as vagal-sparing, techniques have become more popular. Transthoracic and transabdominal esophageal resections used in an attempt to preserve esophageal length are not advocated. These two approaches leave behind an esophagus vulnerable to vicious reflux induced by the resection of the LES and a vagotomy that renders the pylorus incompetent. Resection of the diseased esophagus and replacement with a short jejunal interposition graft has been investigated on a limited basis and may offer a less morbid alternative to esophageal resection.[18]

Despite the rising incidence of GERD, Barrett's esophagus, and esophageal cancer, no cost-effective screening measures have been instituted on a national level. Each patient presenting with GERD needs to be judiciously evaluated to identify patients at risk so that appropriate treatment, including surveillance endoscopy and surgery, can be initiated. The incidence of GERD, Barrett's esophagus, and adenocarcinoma of the esophagus continue to rise and, without serious consideration, these diseases will result in an epidemic in the years ahead.

## Rings, Slings, and Webs

Many diseases that affect the esophagus are morbid and lead to devastating consequences. Vascular and esophageal rings, pulmonary artery slings, and esophageal webs are challenging but rewarding conditions for the surgeon to treat. All these abnormalities cause compression of the esophagus by extrinsic compression, as with vascular rings and pulmonary artery slings, or intrinsic compression, as with esophageal webs and Schatzki's rings.

### Vascular Rings and Pulmonary Artery Slings

Vascular rings and pulmonary slings occur as a result of developmental abnormalities of the great vessels that cause compression of the esophagus. The most common aortic arch anomaly that creates an incomplete vascular ring is when the right subclavian artery arises from the descending aorta and travels behind the esophagus to complete its course to the right upper extremity (Fig. 43-34). Although it does not form a complete vascular ring, it may cause significant posterior compression of the esophagus. Anomalous formation of a right aortic arch with a left ligamentum arteriosum and a resultant retroesophageal left subclavian artery will form a complete ring that will also cause posterior esophageal compression. A pulmonary artery sling is an anomaly of the pulmonary arterial trunk whereby the left pulmonary artery arises from the right pulmonary artery, instead of from the main pulmonary artery trunk (Fig. 43-35). To complete its course to the left lung, it traverses between the trachea and esophagus and causes significant anterior compression of the esophagus. Pulmonary artery slings are commonly associated with intracardiac defects and other developmental abnormalities of the foregut.

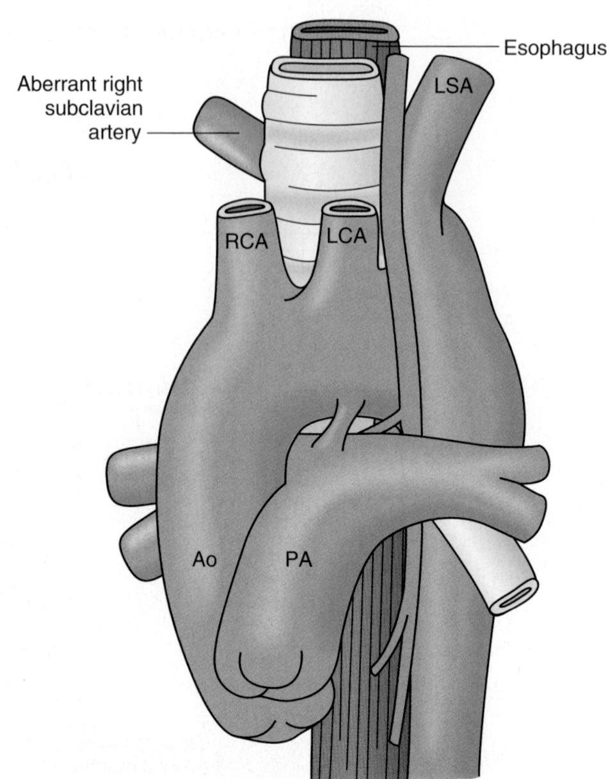


**FIGURE 43-34** Left aortic arch with right subclavian artery. *Ao,* Aorta; *LCA,* left coronary artery; *LSA,* left subclavian artery; *PA,* pulmonary artery; *RCA,* right coronary artery. (Adapted from Lamberti JL, Mainwaring RD: Tracheoesophageal compressive syndromes of vascular origins: Rings and slings. In Baue A, Geha AS, Hammond GL, et al [eds]: Glenn's thoracic and cardiovascular surgery, ed 6, vol 2, Stamford, Conn, 1996, Appleton & Lange, p 1096.)

**Symptoms and Diagnosis** Vascular rings and pulmonary artery slings cause dysphagia. Recurrent respiratory infections and difficulty breathing are also common symptoms. The tightness of the ring or sling will determine the age of clinical presentation and severity of symptoms. Aberrant right subclavian anomalies cause mild dysphagia to solids but not liquids. The term *dysphagia lusoria* (Latin for a "sport of nature") describes the error of ascribing dysphagia to the radiologic finding of this anomaly. Nevertheless, it can be found in children and adults of all ages and needs to be considered in the differential diagnosis of dysphagia. Pulmonary artery slings may also cause dysphagia and are more often accompanied by significant respiratory problems.

Any patient presenting with dysphagia should undergo barium esophagraphy. This radiographic study will reveal extrinsic anterior (Fig. 43-36) or posterior compression of the esophagus. It can be followed with angiography or high-resolution contrast CT (HRCT) to identify the anomalous anatomy.

**Treatment** In symptomatic patients, vascular rings and pulmonary artery slings are repaired. Patients with aberrant right subclavian artery anomalies may be asymptomatic and need no repair. Pulmonary artery slings all require repair to avoid narrowing of the left pulmonary artery and tracheal stenosis that develop with time. Open sternotomy with cardiopulmonary

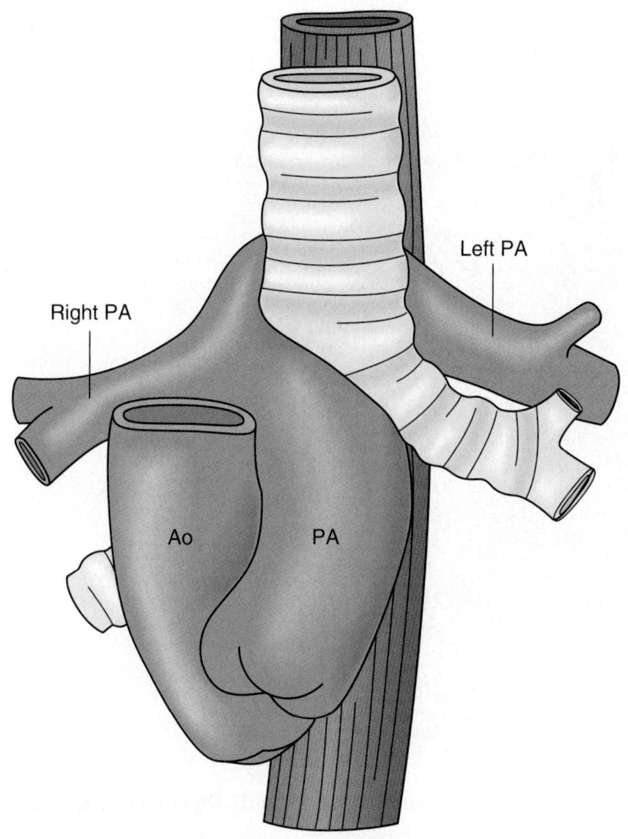


**FIGURE 43-35** Pulmonary artery sling. (Adapted from Lamberti JL, Mainwaring RD: Tracheoesophageal compressive syndromes of vascular origins: Rings and slings. In Baue A, Geha AS, Hammond GL, et al [eds]: Glenn's thoracic and cardiovascular surgery, ed 6, vol 2, Stamford, Conn, 1996, Appleton & Lange, p 1098.)

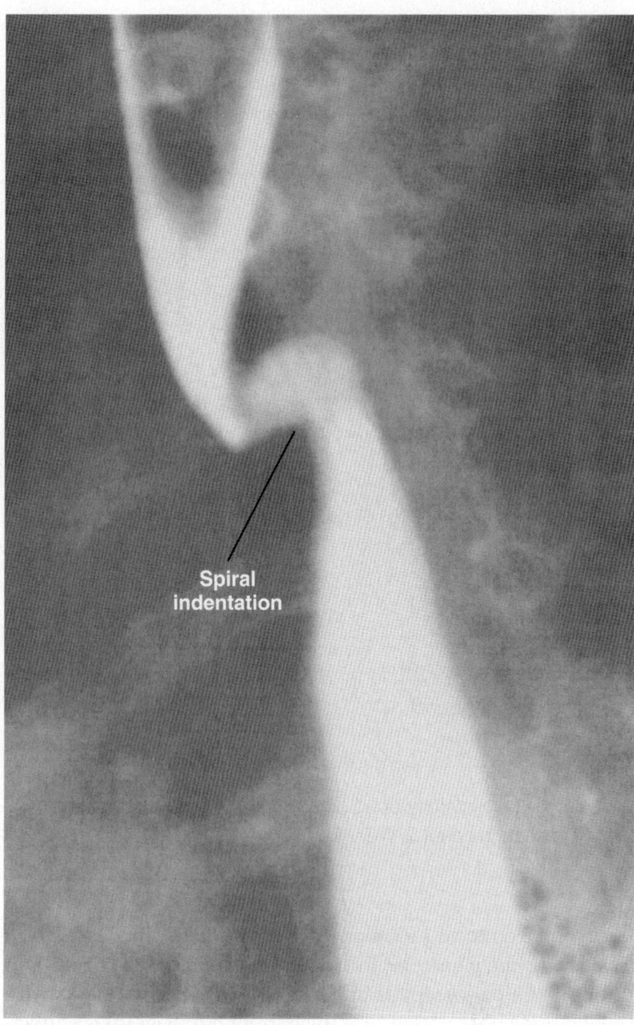


**FIGURE 43-36** Barium esophagram in a patient with an aberrant right subclavian artery showing anterior compression of the esophagus. (Adapted from Lamberti JL, Mainwaring RD: Tracheoesophageal compressive syndromes of vascular origins: Rings and slings. In Baue A, Geha AS, Hammond GL, et al [eds]: Glenn's thoracic and cardiovascular surgery, ed 6, vol 2, Stamford, Conn, 1996, Appleton & Lange, p 1099.)

bypass is required and anatomic repositioning of the great vessels is performed. The results are usually good and the dysphagia resolves almost 100% of the time.

## Esophageal Rings

Esophageal rings were first described by Schatzki and Gary in 1945. Despite the lack of recognition he may have suffered, Gary, along with his colleague Schatzki, made a significant contribution to medical science by describing this acquired anomaly. Lying precisely at the squamocolumnar mucosal GEJ, this ring consists of a concentric symmetrical narrowing representing an area of restricted distensibility of the lower esophagus. It consists of esophageal mucosa above and gastric mucosa below, with variable amounts of muscularis mucosae, connective tissue, and submucosal fibrosis in between (Fig. 43-37). It does not have a component of true esophageal muscle nor is it associated with esophagitis.

The cause of Schatzki's ring is not well understood. It is often accompanied by a small hiatal hernia and some have advocated that it is a result of reflux esophagitis. Another theory is that overcontractility of circular esophageal musculature at the level of the inferior esophageal sphincter, combined with the sliding gastric mucosa of the hiatal hernia, results in persistent apposition of the two mucosal layers and fibrosis of the submucosal layer below.

**Symptoms and Diagnosis** Most patients with Schatzki's rings present with dysphagia. The dysphagia is usually to solid foods only and comes on abruptly, with almost complete obstruction. The term *episodic aphagia* is often ascribed to patients with Schatzki's ring, describing the intermittent obstruction of the nondistensible ring by large pieces of meat. Lower retrosternal pressure and pain accompany an acute obstruction and are followed by salivation and the secretion of copious thick mucus from the esophagus. Patients are unable to eat or drink anything and there is little a patient can do to relieve the obstruction. Forced vomiting may cause esophageal rupture, and spontaneous passage of the food bolus into the stomach usually occurs within a few minutes.

Diagnosis of a Schatzki's ring is made with barium esophagraphy (Fig. 43-38). The patient is placed into the prone position, turned slightly onto the right side, and asked to take in a large breath just as the bolus of barium is reaching

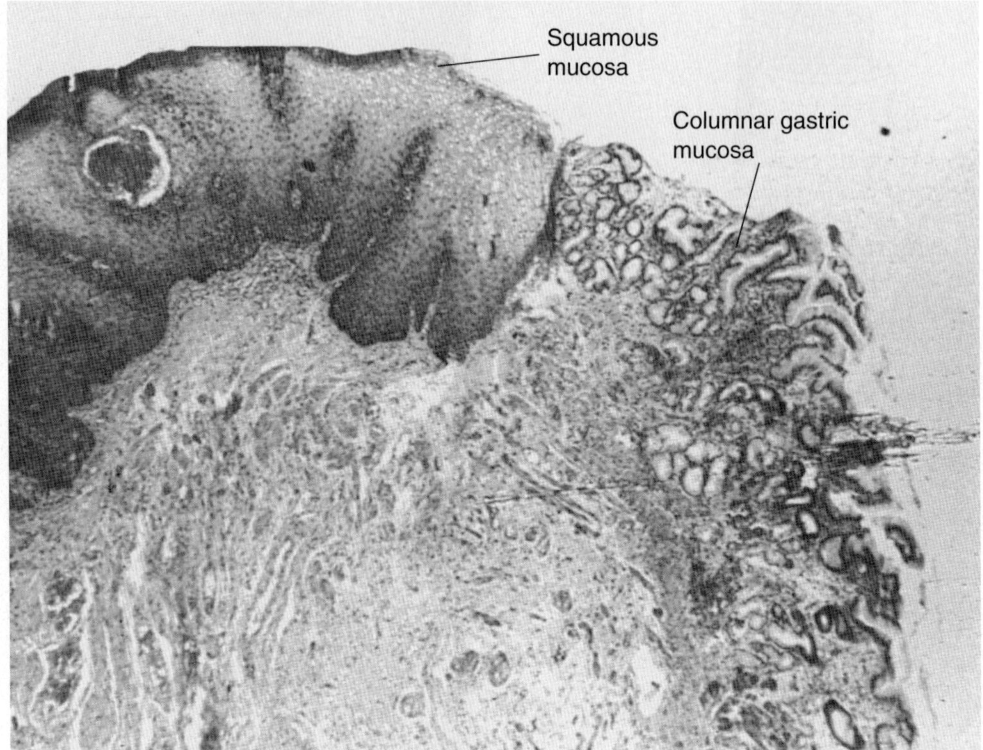


**FIGURE 43-37** Histology of a Schatzki's ring. (Adapted from Wilkins EW Jr: Rings and webs. In Pearson FG, Cooper JD, Deslauriers J, et al [eds]: Esophageal surgery, ed 2, New York, 2002, Churchill Livingstone, p 300.)

the esophagogastric junction. In this position, the ring is well visualized, but it may be missed if the patient is in an upright position. An endoscopy is indicated if the patient presents with foreign body obstruction or if the barium esophagram is equivocal. Upper endoscopy is performed with placement of an overtube to facilitate complete evacuation of the esophagus.

**Treatment** Asymptomatic patients incidentally found to have a Schatzki's ring require no treatment. Patients presenting with acute obstruction require immediate attention. The administration of oral papain in a 2.5% solution is useful for proteolytic digestion of impacted protein food. It is administered in 5-mL aliquots every 30 minutes, for a total of four doses. IV meperidine (25 to 50 mg) may also be used in small doses to encourage spontaneous dislodgment of the impacted food bolus. Esophagoscopy, rigid or flexible, with the use of an overtube facilitates safe extraction. General anesthesia may be desirable to protect the airway adequately. Various instruments are used to extract the food. Pushing the food into the stomach can result in perforation and is only done if the distal lumen is noted at the time of endoscopy. After the food is dislodged, a complete evaluation of the esophageal mucosa is carried out. If there is any question of the integrity of the mucosa, an esophagram is obtained.

In a patient presenting with symptoms of dysphagia in which Schatzki's ring is found, treatment is disruption of the ring by oral dilation. A 50-Fr tapered Maloney bougie is used. Symptoms are relieved for up to 18 months. Sequential bougienage dilation is carried out as symptoms recur. Surgery is not indicated for the treatment of Schatzki's ring and can cause devastating esophageal strictures that are much more difficult to manage. Surgical intervention is reserved for patients who fail bougienage or have intractable reflux. In these few scenarios, intraoperative bougienage followed by a Nissen fundoplication is recommended, but excision of the ring is not indicated.

### Esophageal Webs

Esophageal webs are thin membranous structures that partially or completely compromise the esophageal lumen. They usually only involve the mucosa and part of the submucosa and are composed of squamous cell epithelium above and below the web (Fig. 43-39). This distinguishes the web from a Schatzki's ring, which is composed of esophageal epithelium above and gastric epithelium below the ring. Esophageal webs are not involved in any motility disorder, although a similar radiographic appearance may be noted to accompany some motility abnormalities with no corresponding mucosal abnormality.

Webs may be congenital or acquired and are present throughout the esophagus in men and women of all ages. Congenital webs are rare and are found in young children. They may occur at any level but more commonly are found in the lower two thirds of the esophagus. They are thought to be the result of a failure of coalescence of esophageal vacuoles, which normally leads to complete luminal patency between 25 and 31 days of embryologic development. The congenital web is more likely to be circumferential or eccentric and may be thick and rough rather than thin and diaphanous. Any esophageal web found later in life needs to have been accompanied by a significant history of dysphagia throughout childhood and is considered to be congenital; otherwise, it is considered an acquired condition.

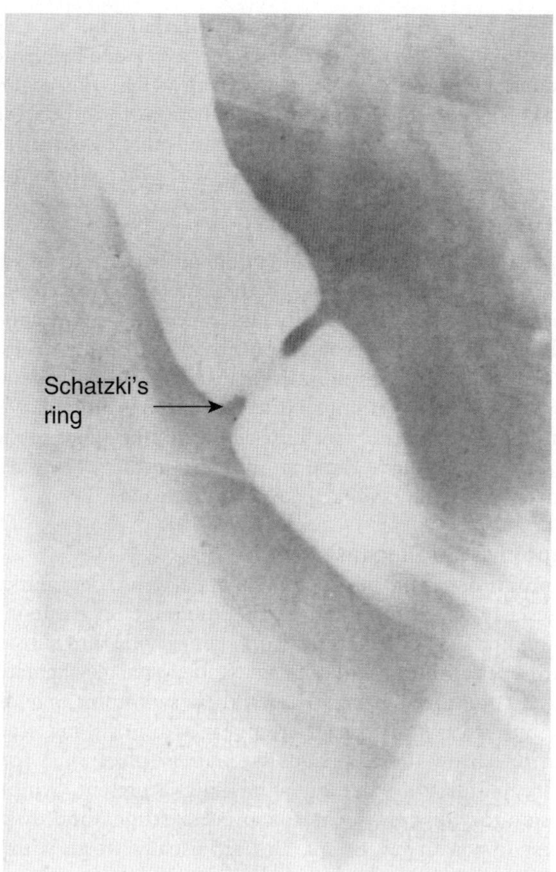


**FIGURE 43-38** Barium esophagram of a Schatzki's ring. (Adapted from Wilkins EW Jr: Rings and webs. In Pearson FG, Cooper JD, Deslauriers J, et al [eds]: Esophageal surgery, ed 2, New York, 2002, Churchill Livingstone, p 298.)

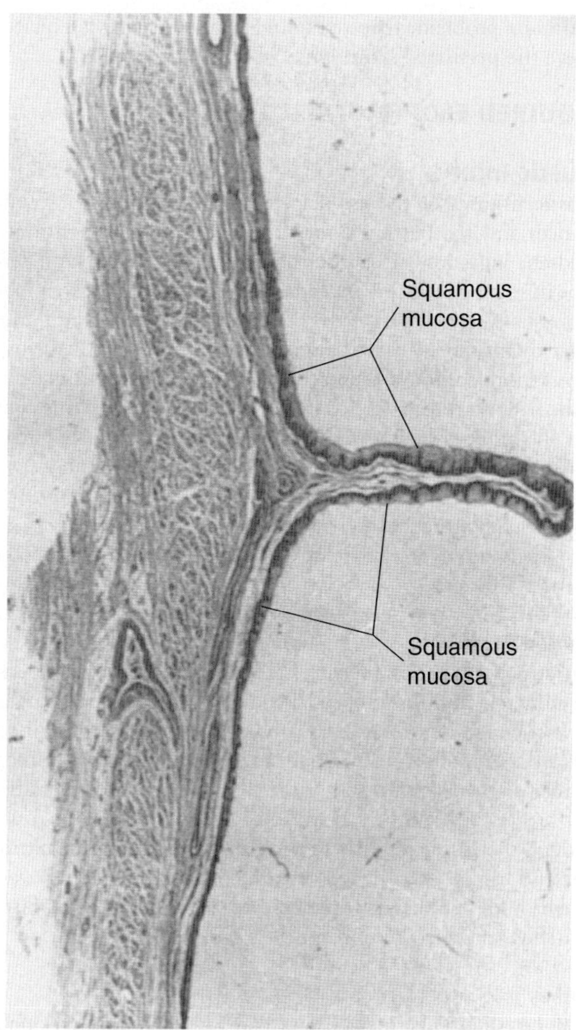


**FIGURE 43-39** Histology of an esophageal web. (Adapted from Wilkins EW Jr: Rings and webs. In Pearson FG, Cooper JD, Deslauriers J, et al [eds]: Esophageal surgery, ed 2, New York, 2002, Churchill Livingstone, p 302.)

Acquired esophageal webs are more common than congenital webs and are usually found in the anterior cervical esophagus, causing focal narrowing in the postcricoid area. They are covered on both sides with squamous epithelium and are usually a thin mucosal fold that protrudes into the lumen. These webs are seen in patients with Plummer-Vinson syndrome (edentulous, middle-aged, malnourished women with atrophic oral mucosa, glossitis, spoon-shaped fingernails, and iron deficiency anemia), pemphigoid, and ulcerative colitis. They are also associated with a slight increase in squamous cell cancer of the esophagus.

**Symptoms and Diagnosis** In children, symptoms of poor feeding may not begin until the child is taking in solid foods. Congenital webs often are imperforate, allowing liquids to pass through easily. Almost complete luminal obstruction results in regurgitation of nonbilious feeds in early infancy. Most adults with acquired esophageal webs are asymptomatic. Symptoms of solid food dysphagia, especially with meat or bread, are otherwise common. The swallowing difficulty may come and go and can be aggravated by specific foods. An evaluation for dysphagia always begins with a barium esophagraphy. This dynamic study will identify an esophageal web accurately and is useful to rule out other obstructing lesions. Endoscopy may be performed; however, the blind passage of the endoscope may take the instrument past the web without ever seeing it.

**Treatment** The management of an esophageal web depends on the nature of the web. Thin webs are treated with membranous disruption through an endoscope or bougie. Piecemeal excision with a biopsy forceps or laser lysis is also an option, but is not routinely performed. Balloon dilation is advocated by some and has good results. Similar to angioplasty, this technique involves the use of fluoroscopically guided balloon dilators inflated with water-soluble contrast material under carefully monitored pressure. The membrane is disrupted under controlled circumstances so that perforation is avoided. Results are favorable, but the technique has not been widely supported. Laser lysis has gained popularity and may prove to be the treatment of choice in the future. Surgical mucosal resection is reserved for patients with thick rings refractory to bougienage. A transcervical or transthoracic approach to the esophagus is used. A longitudinal myotomy and circumferential excision of the web are performed. Circumferential reapproximation of the mucosa is done with interrupted absorbable sutures, followed by longitudinal closure of the muscle. Treatment of all types results in good long-term results, with few recurrences of dysphagia. If recurrent dysphagia becomes a problem, repeated bougienage is usually adequate to relieve the persistent symptoms.

## ACQUIRED ESOPHAGEAL CONDITIONS

### Caustic Injury

Caustic injuries of the esophagus can have devastating consequences and the best cure for this condition is prevention. In children, ingestion of caustic materials is accidental and tends to be in small quantities. In teenagers and adults, however, ingestion usually is deliberate during suicide attempts, and much larger quantities of caustic liquids are consumed. Alkali ingestion is more common than acid ingestion because of its lack of immediate symptoms. Acids cause an immediate burning sensation in the mouth, whereas alkali does not. The consequences of alkali ingestion are much more devastating and almost always lead to significant destruction of the esophagus, resulting in long-term dysfunction.

There are acute and chronic phases in caustic esophageal injuries. The acute phase is dependent on the severity and location of the injury, type of substance ingested (acid versus alkali), form of the substance (liquid versus solid), quantity and concentration of the substance ingested, amount of residual food in the stomach, and duration of tissue contact. The chronic phase of caustic ingestion focuses on subsequent strictures and disruption of the swallowing mechanism, which become significant problems several months after the injury. There are several sites that are prone to injury because of a relative delay in transit through the esophagus. These correlate to the anatomic narrowings and can be seen in the proximal esophagus at the level of the UES, midesophagus where the aorta abuts the left mainstem bronchus, and distal esophagus just proximal to the LES.

#### Causes

**Alkali Ingestion** Alkaline substances dissolve tissues by liquefactive necrosis, deeply penetrating the tissues they touch. There are three phases of tissue injury from alkali ingestion (Table 43-3):

Phase 1. The acute necrotic phase lasts 1 to 4 days after injury, during which coagulation of intracellular proteins results in cell necrosis. The surrounding tissues develop an intense inflammatory reaction.

Phase 2. The ulceration and granulation phase is next. It begins 3 to 5 days after injury and lasts approximately 3 to 12 days. During this phase, the tissues slough and granulation tissue begins to fill in the ulcerated base left behind. The esophagus is at its weakest point during this second phase.

Phase 3. In the third phase, cicatrization and scarring begin and the newly formed connective tissue begins to contract, resulting in esophageal narrowing. This occurs 3 weeks after the initial injury. Adhesions form between areas of granulation, resulting in bands that constrict the esophagus significantly. During this time, efforts are aimed at reducing stricture formation.

**Acid Ingestion** Ingestion of acid is difficult because its ingestion causes an immediate burning in the mouth. When compared with lye ingestion, the quantity and concentration are modest. Acid substances cause coagulative necrosis, forming an eschar that limits tissue penetration. In some cases, acid burns result in full-thickness injury, although in most cases, it is limited. Within 48 hours, the extent to which the acid will injure the esophagus is already determined. These injuries tend to be less severe and relatively spare the esophagus over the stomach.

#### Symptoms and Diagnosis

Symptoms of caustic burns to the esophagus are determined by the severity of the burn and parallel the stages of tissue injury. During phase 1, patients may complain of oral and substernal pain, hypersalivation, odynophagia and dysphagia, hematemesis, and vomiting. During phase 2, these symptoms may disappear, only to have dysphagia reappear as fibrosis and scarring begin to narrow the esophagus throughout phase 3. A fever is usually an indicator that esophageal injury is present. Symptoms of respiratory distress, such as hoarseness, stridor, and dyspnea, suggest upper airway edema and are usually worse with acid ingestion. Pain in the back and chest may indicate a perforation of the mediastinal esophagus, whereas abdominal pain may indicate abdominal visceral perforation. Studies have demonstrated that asymptomatic patients tend to have minimal injury to the esophagus, whereas in symptomatic patients, especially with three or more symptoms, hematemesis or respiratory distress are likely to represent severe injury.[19]

Diagnosis is initiated with a physical examination specifically evaluating the mouth, airway, chest, and abdomen. Careful inspection of the lips, palate, pharynx, and larynx is done. Auscultation of the lungs is critical to determine the degree of upper airway involvement. The abdomen is examined for signs of perforation. Early endoscopy is recommended 12 to 24 hours after ingestion to identify the grade of the burn (Table 43-4). Radiographic examination in adults is not a useful tool at initial presentation but is helpful in later stages to assess stricture formation. Serial chest and abdominal radiographs are indicated to follow patients with questionable chest and abdominal examinations. A CT scan is indicated for a patient with an equivocal

**Table 43-3 Three Phases of Tissue Injury from Alkali Ingestion**

| PHASE | TISSUE INJURY | ONSET | DURATION | INFLAMMATORY RESPONSE |
|---|---|---|---|---|
| 1 | Acute necrosis | 1-4 days | 1-4 days | Coagulation of intracellular proteins<br>Inflammation |
| 2 | Ulceration and granulation | 3-5 days | 3-12 days | Tissue sloughing<br>Granulation of ulcerated tissue bed |
| 3 | Cicatrization and scarring | 3 wk | 1-6 mo | Adhesion formation<br>Scarring |

**Table 43-4 Endoscopic Grading and Treatment of Corrosive Esophageal and Gastric Burns**

| DEGREE OF BURN | ENDOSCOPIC EVALUATION | TREATMENT |
|---|---|---|
| First degree | Mucosal hyperemia<br>Edema | 48-hr observation<br>Acid suppression |
| Second degree | Limited hemorrhage<br>Exudates<br>Ulceration<br>Pseudomembrane formation | Aggressive IV resuscitation<br>IV antibiotics<br>Acid suppression |
| Third degree | Mucosal sloughing<br>Deep ulcerations<br>Massive hemorrhage<br>Complete luminal obstruction<br>Charring<br>Perforation | Inhaled steroids<br>Fiberoptic intubation (if needed) |

endoscopic examination in whom there is a strong index of suspicion for a perforation.

### Treatment

The treatment of caustic lesions of the esophagus is determined by the extent of the injury and addresses the injuries that occur in the acute and chronic phases.

**Acute Phase** Management of the acute phase is aimed at limiting and identifying the extent of the injury. It begins with neutralization of the ingested substance. If a patient presents within the first hour of ingestion, neutralization is attempted. Alkalis (including lye) are neutralized with half-strength vinegar or citrus juice. Acids are neutralized with milk, egg whites, or antacids. Emetics and sodium bicarbonate need to be avoided because they can increase the chance of perforation. Further treatment is guided by the extent of injury identified endoscopically and the patient's underlying condition.

***No Evidence of Burn*** Early observation is safe for those asymptomatic patients whose physical examination and initial endoscopy are negative. Oral nutrition may be resumed when a patient can swallow saliva painlessly.

***First-Degree Burn*** In patients with endoscopically identified first-degree burns, 48 hours of observation is indicated. Oral nutrition can be resumed when a patient can swallow saliva painlessly. A repeat endoscopy and barium esophagram are done in follow-up at intervals of 1, 2, and 8 months, at which time 60%, 80%, and almost 100% of strictures will have developed, respectively.

***Second- and Third-Degree Burns*** Patients with second- and third-degree burns to the esophagus are triaged similar to burn patients. Massive fluid shifts, renal failure, and sepsis can occur rapidly, and underestimation of the extent of injury can lead to fatal outcomes. Resuscitation is aggressively pursued. The patient is monitored in the intensive care unit (ICU) and kept NPO with IV fluids. IV antibiotics and a proton pump inhibitor are started. In patients with evidence of acute airway involvement, aerosolized steroids may be used to relieve airway obstruction. Fiberoptic intubation may be needed and must be available. The use of steroids to prevent stricture formation is controversial. It has been suggested that although steroids will decrease the rate of stricture formation, they will also mask symptoms of peritonitis.

The management of second- and third-degree burns of the esophagus is multifaceted and has several acceptable options. Aggressive resuscitation and placement of an esophageal stent are one option. Oral nutrition is resumed when a patient can swallow saliva painlessly. Alternatively, a feeding tube or central venous catheter is placed and the patient is kept NPO until oral pain subsides. If the diagnosis is not secured with endoscopy, an exploratory laparoscopy (in stable patients) or laparotomy (in unstable patients) is performed. A viable stomach and esophagus are left in situ, a feeding jejunostomy tube is placed, and an esophageal stent is placed in the operating room endoscopically. A questionable esophagus and stomach are left in situ and a second-look operation is planned for 36 hours. Management at 36 hours is dictated by the findings at that time. If full-thickness necrosis or perforation of the esophagus or stomach is found at any time, an emergent exploratory laparotomy is indicated. The esophagus and stomach and all affected surrounding organs and tissues are resected, an end-cervical esophagostomy is performed, and a feeding jejunostomy is placed (Fig. 43-40). Postoperatively, the patient is monitored in the ICU and managed aggressively.

**Chronic Phase** Treatment in the chronic phase of caustic esophageal injuries is aimed at managing the problems and challenges that occur as a result of the burn injury, including strictures, esophageal reconstruction, and fistulas.

***Strictures*** There are a variety of ways to deal with strictures caused by caustic burns of the esophagus. The best treatment is prevention. Early stent placement is advocated by most. There is some evidence that early bougienage is also effective. However, before reepithelialization, bougie dilation may add insult to injury. If a stent is placed during the acute phase, it is left in place for 21 days, at which time it is removed. At 3 weeks, 3 months, and 6 months, a barium esophagram is performed to evaluate for stricture formation, gastric outlet obstruction, and linitis plastica appearance. An endoscopy is performed to determine the extent of reepithelialization. After reepithelialization, patients with strictures are aggressively treated with bougie dilations. Patients with esophageal strictures undergo bougie dilation regardless of their symptoms. Waiting until symptoms arise results in long-term strictures that often fail bougie dilation and ultimately require esophageal resection. Dilations are performed daily for 2 to 3 weeks, every other day for 2 to 3 weeks, and then weekly for months. An adequate lumen needs to be reestablished within 6 to 12 months, lengthening the intervals between dilations as time passes. Retrograde dilation may also be successful in case antegrade dilation is not. If endoscopic dilation fails to reestablish an adequate lumen (40 Fr), surgical intervention is necessary (Fig. 43-41).

***Reconstruction*** Restoration of the alimentary tract is delayed until 6 to 12 months. By this time, the patient has recovered from the acute insult, scar formation is mostly complete, and failed endoscopic treatment of strictures is terminated. In patients whose esophagus and stomach remain in situ, resection of the damaged organs is recommended. The incidence of

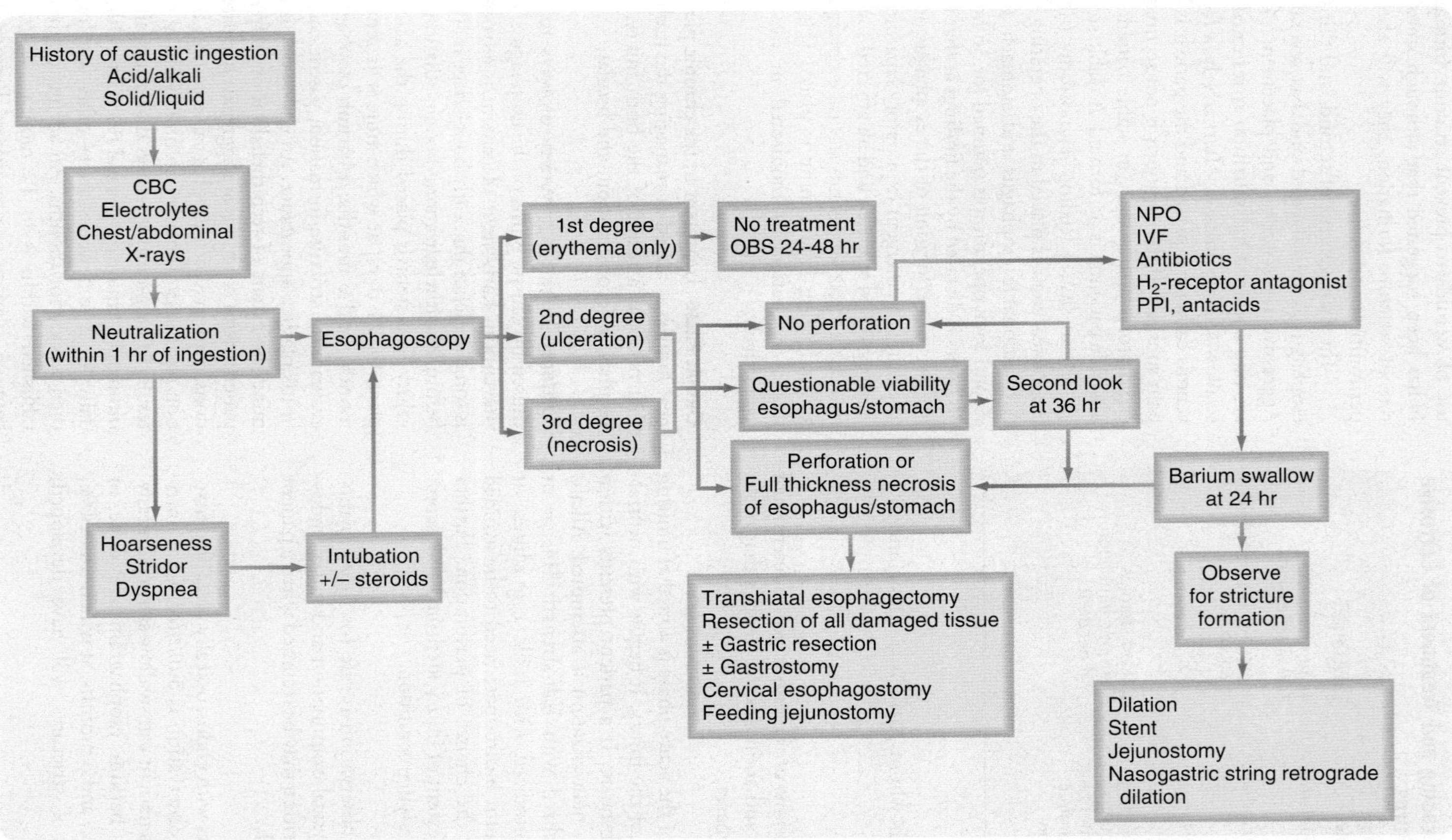


**FIGURE 43-40** Management of caustic injury of the esophagus: acute phase. *CBC,* Complete blood count; *IVF,* IV fluids; *OBS,* observe; *PPI,* proton pump inhibitor. (Adapted from Zwischenberger JB, Savage C, Bidani A: Surgical aspects of esophageal disease. Am J Respir Crit Care Med 164:1037–1040, 2001.)

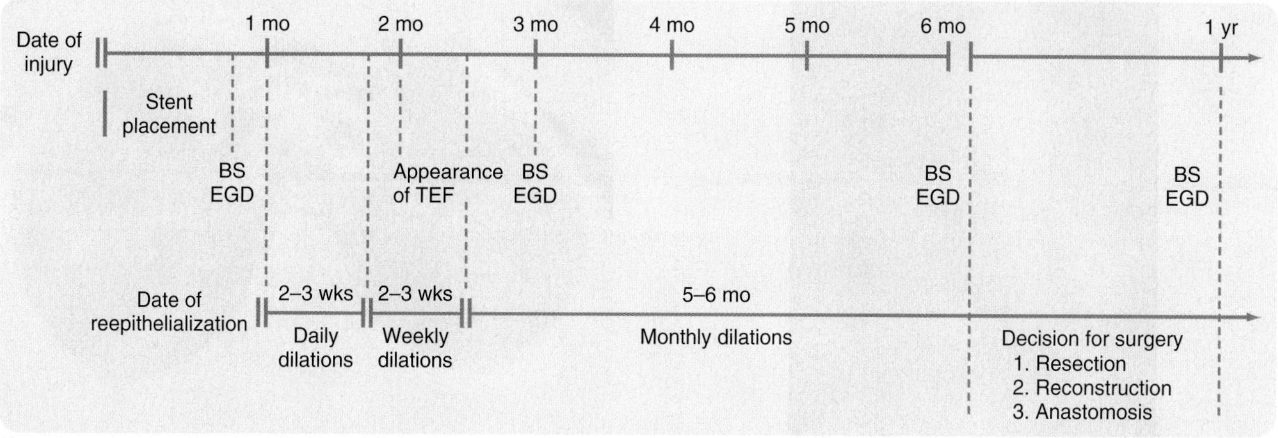


**FIGURE 43-41** Management of caustic injury of the esophagus, chronic phase. *BS,* Barium swallow; *EGD,* esophagogastroduodenoscopy; *TEF,* transesophageal fistula.

esophageal cancer in patients with caustic injury is 1000-fold greater than in the general population. Unless there is prohibitive risk, the esophagus and excessively scarred portions of the stomach must be resected. Transhiatal resection of the scarred esophagus can be fraught with danger, and transthoracic mobilization is recommended. Operative management needs to be preplanned. The type and route of the conduit, as well as the site of proximal anastomosis, is carefully considered. A gastric pull-up is preferred but, if only a portion of the stomach is viable, the distal portion of the stomach can be combined with a jejunal interposition. For a long-segment interposition graft, the colon is preferred. The esophageal replacement graft is placed in the posterior mediastinal space, if possible, and in the retrosternal position when the posterior mediastinum is excessively scarred. The site of the proximal anastomosis is determined by the extent of injury to the hypopharynx and proximal esophagus.

## Esophageal Perforation

Perforation of the esophagus is a surgical emergency. Early detection and surgical repair within the first 24 hours results in 80% to 90% survival; after 24 hours, survival decreases to less than 50%. On presentation, patients suspected of having a perforation based on initial history and physical examination are evaluated quickly so that surgical intervention may be initiated promptly. Perforation from forceful vomiting (Boerhaave's syndrome), foreign body ingestion, or trauma accounts for 15%, 14%, and 10% of cases, respectively. Most esophageal perforations occur after endoscopic instrumentation for a diagnostic or therapeutic procedure, including dilation, stent placement, and laser fulguration. Other iatrogenic causes that have been noted include difficult endotracheal intubation, blind insertion of a minitracheostomy, and inadvertent injury during dissections in the neck, chest, and abdomen.

### Boerhaave's Syndrome

Hermann Boerhaave first described this syndrome after performing an autopsy on Baron Jan van Wassenaer. After relieving postprandial discomfort by self-induced vomiting, the baron died from a distal esophageal perforation that was later noted at autopsy. It has since been elucidated that recurrent emesis disrupts the normal vomiting reflex that enables sphincter relaxation, resulting in an increase in intrathoracic esophageal pressure and perforation. Postemetic rupture of the esophagus, now termed *Boerhaave's syndrome,* is only one of many causes of esophageal rupture. Similar findings are noted with blunt thoracic trauma, epileptic seizures, defecation, and childbirth, all of which are associated with increased intra-abdominal pressure. A tear in the esophageal mucosa, known as a Mallory-Weiss tear, also occurs after persistent retching, but is not associated with perforation.

**Symptoms and Diagnosis** Symptoms of neck, substernal, or epigastric pain are consistently associated with esophageal perforation and generate a high index of suspicion. Vomiting, hematemesis, or dysphagia may also occur. In addition, a history of trauma, advanced esophageal cancer, violent retching, as seen in Boerhaave's syndrome, swallowing of a foreign body, or recent instrumentation must raise the question of esophageal perforation. Cervical perforations may present with neck ache and stiffness caused by contamination of the prevertebral space. Thoracic perforations present with shortness of breath and retrosternal chest pain lateralizing to the side of perforation. Abdominal perforations present with epigastric pain that radiates to the back if the perforation is posterior. Signs of perforation change over time. A patient may present early with tachypnea, tachycardia, and low-grade fever but have no other overt signs of perforation. With increased mediastinal and pleural contamination, patients progress toward hemodynamic instability and shock. On examination, subcutaneous air in the neck or chest, shallow decreased breath sounds, and/or a tender abdomen are all suggestive of perforation. Laboratory values of significance are an elevated white blood cell count and an elevated salivary amylase level in the blood or pleural fluid.

Diagnosis of an esophageal perforation may be made radiographically. A chest roentgenogram may demonstrate a hydropneumothorax. Contrast esophagraphy is performed using barium for a suspected thoracic perforation and Gastrografin for an abdominal perforation. Barium is inert in the chest but causes peritonitis in the abdomen, whereas aspirated Gastrografin can cause life-threatening pneumonitis. Most perforations are found above the GEJ on the left lateral wall of the esophagus (Fig.

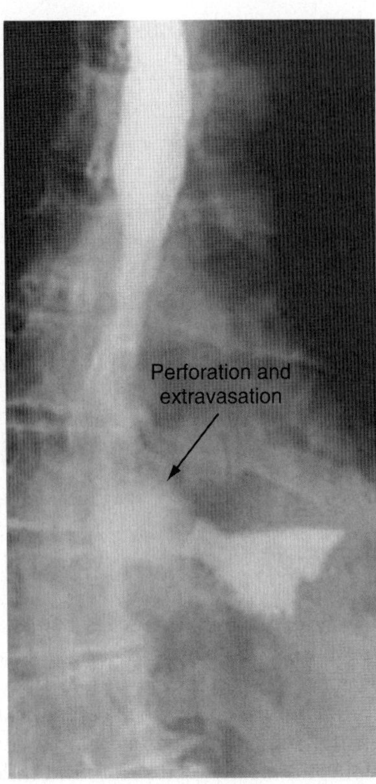


**FIGURE 43-42** Barium esophagram of a perforated esophagus. Note the extravasation of contrast into the left chest. (Adapted from Duranceau A: Perforation of the esophagus. In Sabiston DC [ed]: Textbook of Surgery, ed 15, Philadelphia, 1997, WB Saunders, p 761.)

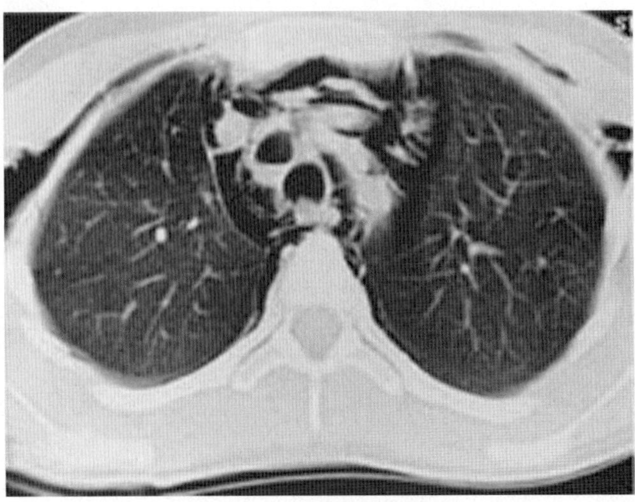

**FIGURE 43-43** CT scan of a perforated esophagus. Note the air and fluid in the mediastinum. (Adapted from Duranceau A: Perforation of the esophagus. In Sabiston DC [ed]: Textbook of Surgery, ed 15, Philadelphia, 1997, WB Saunders, p 761.)

43-42), which results in a 10% false-negative result in the contrast esophagram if the patient is not placed in the lateral decubitus position. The chest CT scan shows mediastinal air and fluid at the site of perforation (Fig. 43-43). A surgical endoscopy needs to be performed if the esophagram is negative or if operative intervention is planned. Mucosal injury is suggested if blood, mucosal hematoma, or a flap is seen or if the esophagus is difficult to insufflate.

**Treatment** The management of patients with esophageal perforation takes place in the ICU and operating room. Patients with an esophageal perforation can progress rapidly to hemodynamic instability and shock. If perforation is suspected, appropriate resuscitation measures with the placement of large-bore peripheral IV catheters, urinary catheter, and secured airway are undertaken before the patient is sent for diagnostic testing. IV fluids and broad-spectrum antibiotics are started immediately, and the patient is monitored in an ICU. The patient is kept NPO and nutritional access needs are assessed. A nasogastric tube is placed only after management decisions are made. These conservative measures are often lifesaving and, in patients who do not undergo surgery, are life-sustaining.

Surgery is not indicated for every patient with a perforation of the esophagus and management is dependent on several variables—stability of the patient, extent of contamination, degree of inflammation, underlying esophageal disease, and location of perforation (Fig. 43-44*A*). A stable patient will have a number of treatment options based on other variables. An unstable patient will need rapid assessment and expeditious treatment, depending on the degree of contamination. In patients who remain clinically stable, with no signs of progressive sepsis, a contained perforation may be treated conservatively. The patient is kept NPO and nutrition is maintained by enteral access. A temporary endoluminal stent may be placed endoscopically and removed after 6 to 12 weeks. Interval esophagraphy or esophagoscopy is done to determine when the perforation is healed. Partial resolution of the perforation is treated with continuation of conservative therapy. Persistence or progression of the perforation without evidence of healing is treated by surgical intervention in the stable patient. During the course of conservative management, if a patient's clinical condition deteriorates or the perforation is no longer contained, surgical intervention is advised. In an unstable patient with a contained perforation, a temporary stent may be placed and conservative measures initiated. In an unstable patient with a free perforation, surgical intervention with débridement of devitalized tissue, esophageal diversion or resection, creation of an esophagostomy, wide drainage, placement of a gastrostomy, and feeding jejunostomy is indicated.

The most critical variable that determines the surgical management of an esophageal perforation is the degree of inflammation surrounding the perforation. When patients present within 24 hours of perforation, inflammation is generally minimal and primary surgical repair is recommended. With time, inflammation progresses and tissues become friable and may not be amenable to primary repair. The so-called golden period for primary closure of an esophageal perforation is within the first 24 hours. Although primary repair is usually possible within this time period, it is by no means a magical cutoff time. If a healthy bed of tissue is encountered during surgical exploration, primary repair of the perforation is acceptable at any time. If a severe inflammatory reaction or mediastinitis is present and the tissues are not amenable to primary repair, a muscle flap procedure is

MANAGEMENT OF THORACIC AND ABDOMINAL ESOPHAGEAL PERFORATIONS

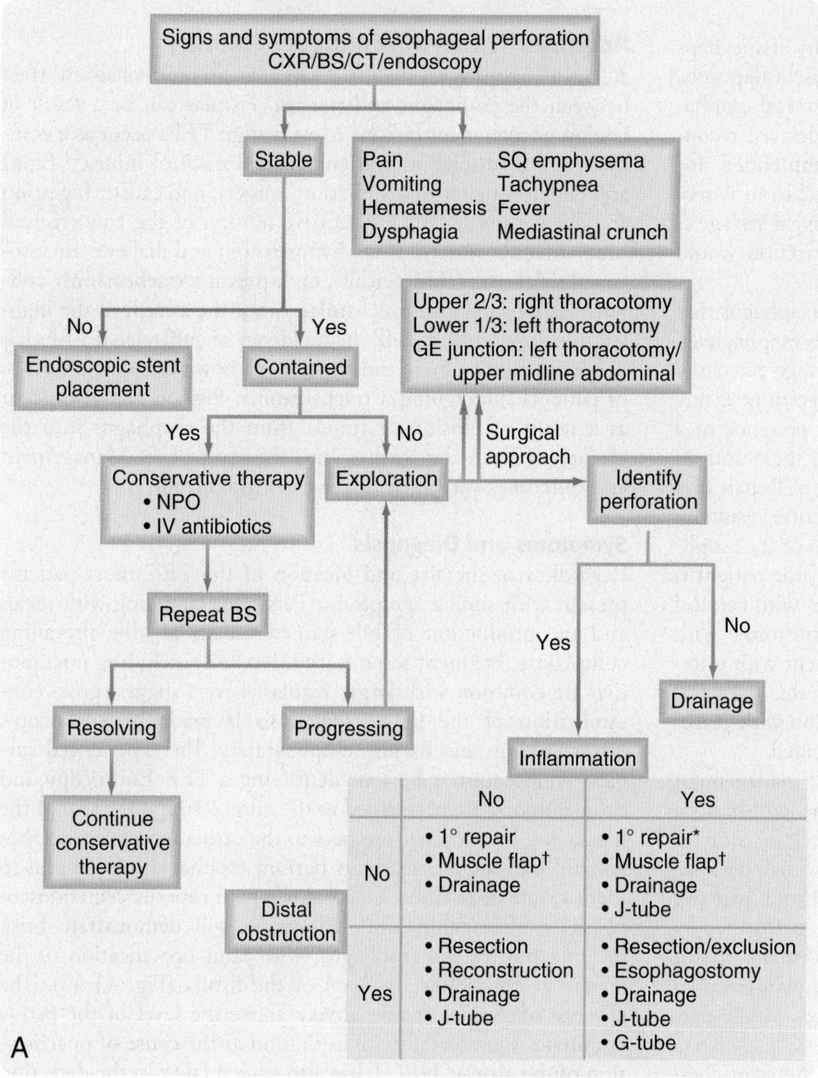


MANAGEMENT OF CERVICAL ESOPHAGEAL PERFORATIONS

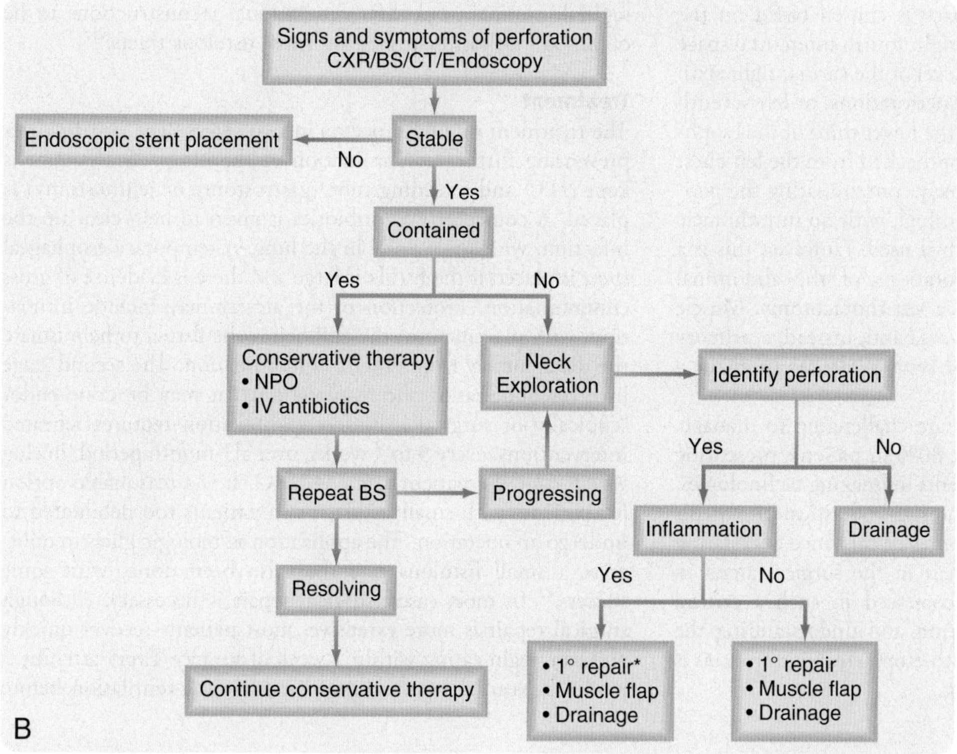


**FIGURE 43-44 A,** Management of thoracic and abdominal perforations of the esophagus. **B,** Management of cervical perforations of the esophagus. *BS,* Barium swallow. *Assess ability to do a primary repair. †Gastric fundoplication used in the abdomen in place of a flap.

performed. All repairs are buttressed with healthy tissue flaps and widely drained. If primary repair or the muscle flap fails, resection or exclusion of the esophagus with a cervical esophagostomy, gastrostomy, feeding jejunostomy, and delayed reconstruction is recommended. Resection is recommended for patients with mid- to high-level perforations. Exclusion is recommended for low perforations in which esophageal salvage is possible or in any unstable patient for whom resection would not be tolerated.

There are four underlying conditions of the esophagus that affect the treatment of a free perforation of the esophagus—resectable carcinoma, megaesophagus from end-stage achalasia, severe peptic strictures, or a history of caustic ingestion. If any of these is a factor, primary repair, even in the presence of a healthy tissue bed, is not recommended. Each of these entities is associated with distal narrowing and obstruction. Repair of a perforation without resolution of a distal obstruction results in fistula formation. In these circumstances, resection of the esophagus with immediate reconstruction is preferred if the patient is stable. In an unstable patient, esophageal resection with cervical esophagostomy, gastrostomy, and feeding jejunostomy with delayed reconstruction is recommended. In a patient with unresectable cancer, an esophageal stent is placed. If this does not contain the leak, esophageal exclusion and diversion with placement of a gastrostomy and jejunostomy are indicated.

The final variable to consider in the surgical management of esophageal perforations is the location of the perforation. Cervical perforations are approached through a neck incision on the same side of the perforation (see Fig. 43-44*B*). Small perforations may be difficult to find and drainage without primary closure often is adequate. If primary repair is performed, a muscle flap is usually not required, but the placement of soft drains is necessary. In case of a large perforation that is attempted to be closed primarily, a flap from a rotated strap muscle may be used to buttress the repair.

Thoracic perforations are approached from the right chest for the upper two thirds of the esophagus and the left chest for the lower third. The intercostal space is chosen based on the location of the perforation; it is the right fourth intercostal space if the perforation is at or above the level of the carina, right sixth intercostal space for midesophageal perforations, or left seventh intercostal space for perforations of the lower third of the esophagus. Abdominal perforations are approached from the left chest or abdomen. If the perforation is freely contaminating the peritoneal space and is truly intra-abdominal, with no intrathoracic component, an abdominal approach is used. However, this is a rare circumstance and most perforations of the abdominal esophagus are approached through a left thoracotomy. Muscle flaps are not easily accessible in this area and, instead, a primary repair in this location is buttressed with a pleural patch or a fundoplication.

Perforations of the esophagus are challenging to manage. The mortality rate had been almost 80% in patients presenting with free perforation but advancements in imaging technologies, improved surgical techniques, and progress of critical care medicine have vastly improved the outcomes of this once devastating acquired disease. There are few areas in the surgical arena in which knowledge and skill have coalesced in such a critical manner. Recognizing the presentation and understanding the detailed management of patients with esophageal perforations is essential and will often be lifesaving.

## Acquired Tracheoesophageal Fistulas

A tracheoesophageal fistula (TEF) is an epithelialized tract between the esophagus and trachea. Fistulas can be a result of benign or malignant factors. Most benign TEFs occur as a complication of intubation and cuff-related tracheal injury.[20] Blunt and penetrating trauma, radiation, surgery, and caustic ingestion are also common causes. Excessive motion of the endotracheal tube, infections, steroid use, hypotension, and diabetes are associated risk factors. Historically, high-pressure tracheostomy cuffs were responsible for most fistulas. Since the advent of the high-volume, low-pressure cuff, the incidence of cuff-related TEFs has decreased significantly and fistulas are now seen in only 0.5% of patients undergoing a tracheostomy. Fistulas can also occur as a result of erosion of tumor from the esophagus into the trachea or from the trachea into the esophagus. Management and outcomes vary with the cause of the fistula.

### Symptoms and Diagnosis

Regardless of the size and location of the TEF, most patients present with similar symptoms. Persistent coughing with meals and the production of bile-stained mucus are the prevailing complaints. Frequent respiratory infections, including pneumonia, are common with larger fistulas. Fevers suggest gross contamination of the lungs. Diagnosis is made by endoscopy, bronchoscopy, and barium esophagraphy. The experienced surgical endoscopist is best at identifying a TEF. Endoscopy and bronchoscopy are performed at the same setting. The size of the fistula and location with respect to the carina, vocal cords, UES, and LES are noted clearly. A barium esophagram is helpful to identify laterality and is essential when an experienced endoscopist is not available. The radiograph will demonstrate brisk opacification of the esophagus, with faint opacification of the airway at and below the level of the fistula (Fig. 43-45). The absence of barium in the airway above the level of the fistula eliminates the possibility of aspiration as the cause of opacification of the airway. HRCT has also gained favor in the detection of tracheoesophageal fistulas. Technologic advances have allowed sagittal, coronal, and three-dimensional reconstructions to be obtained that can help identify small fistulous tracts.[21]

### Treatment

The treatment of a TEF occurs in two stages. The first involves preventing further contamination of the lungs. The patient is kept NPO and a feeding tube (gastrostomy or jejunostomy) is placed. A course of IV antibiotics is given to help clear up the infection, which is usually in the lung. A temporary esophageal stent is placed if the fistula is large and there is evidence of gross contamination. Protection of the airway may include intubation, with placement of the cuff below the fistula to help isolate the distal airway from enteric contamination. The second stage involves obliterating the fistulous tract; it may be done endoscopically or surgically. Endoscopic ablation requires repeated interventions, every 3 to 4 weeks, over a 3-month period, during which time the patient remains NPO. It is a reasonable option for patients with small fistulas or in patients too debilitated to undergo an operation. The application of biologic glues to obliterate a small fistulous tract has also been done, with some success.[22] In most cases, surgical repair is necessary. Although surgical repair is more extensive, most patients recover quickly and can begin eating within 1 week of surgery. Every attempt is made to wean the patient from mechanical ventilation before

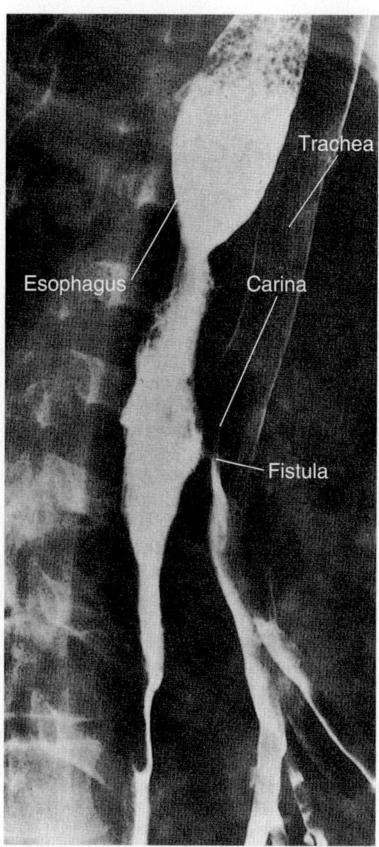


**FIGURE 43-45** Barium esophagram of a tracheoesophageal fistula. (Adapted from Little AG: Esophageal bypass. In Pearson FG, Cooper JD, Deslauriers J, et al [eds]: Esophageal surgery, ed 2, New York, 2002, Churchill Livingstone, p 896.)

definitive intervention because postoperative positive-pressure ventilation increases the rate of dehiscence of the repair.

Surgical repair of a TEF takes place in three stages. The first is exposure of the fistulous tract through a cervical or thoracotomy incision. Stage 2 is segmental resection of the trachea and primary repair of the esophagus. Stage 3 is harvesting an appropriate muscle flap and placing it between the trachea and esophagus to encourage healing, contain leaks, and prevent future fistulization. Although it may not be necessary to resect a segment of the trachea associated with the fistulous tract, it has been noted that in the case of repair of a postintubation TEF, tracheal resection and primary anastomosis decrease the rate of tracheal stenosis, even in the absence of obvious tracheal damage.[23]

### Other Esophageal Fistulas

Other types of fistulas involving the esophagus can occur after surgical manipulation. Fistulas from the esophagus or replacement grafts, such as the stomach or colon, can form in any part of the airway, pleural space, or mediastinum. Breakdown of anastomotic sites or gastric staple lines can cause localized infections that erode into the airway or mediastinum. Although most esophageal fistulas to the airway occur at the level of the trachea, fistulas to the bronchi and distal airways can also occur. Traction diverticula, localized mediastinal infections, and ischemic perforations of esophageal replacement conduits can lead to the formation of fistulas to the distal airways. Patients present with symptoms of a TEF and treatment is similar to that of patients presenting with esophageal perforations.

## BENIGN TUMORS AND CYSTS

Benign tumors of the esophagus are unusual and constitute less than 1% of all esophageal neoplasms. They can be found in the muscular wall or in the lumen of the esophagus and are identified as solid tumors, cysts, or fibrovascular polyps (Table 43-5). Approximately 60% of benign esophageal lesions are leiomyomas, 20% are cysts, 5% are polyps, and the remaining 5% are other neoplasms. Intramural lesions are solid tumors or cysts and are made up of smooth muscle and fibrous tissue in variable proportions. Leiomyomas are the most common, whereas the others (e.g., papillomas, fibromas, myomas, lipomas, neurofibromas, hemangiomas, adenomas, and glomus tumors) are rare.

### Leiomyoma

Leiomyomas constitute 60% of all benign esophageal tumors. They are found in men slightly more often than women and tend to present in the fourth and fifth decades. They originate from the mesenchymal layer of embryologic development and are found in the distal two thirds of the esophagus more than 80% of the time. They are usually solitary and remain intramural, causing symptoms as they enlarge. They have been classified as a gastrointestinal stromal tumor (GIST). GIST tumors are the most common mesenchymal tumors of the gastrointestinal tract and can be benign or malignant. Almost all GIST tumors occur from mutations of the c-*KIT* oncogene, which codes for the expression of *c-KIT* (CD117). Identification of this molecular marker is considered the most specific criterion for this diagnosis.[24] A true leiomyoma, or a non-GIST (c-*KIT*–negative) tumor, is rare. All leiomyomas are benign; malignant transformation occurs rarely.

#### Symptoms and Diagnosis

Many leiomyomas are asymptomatic and it is believed that most go undetected over a lifetime. Dysphagia and pain are the most common symptoms and can result from even the smallest tumors. Location and size tend not to correlate with symptoms consistently; however, tumors nestled between the spine and airway often will cause dysphagia, even when the tumor is only 1 cm in size. A chest radiograph is not usually helpful to diagnose a leiomyoma but, on a barium esophagram, a leiomyoma has a characteristic appearance. A smooth, well-defined, noncircumferential mass with distinct borders is seen (Fig. 43-46). During endoscopy, extrinsic compression is seen and the overlying mucosa is noted to be intact. Despite this compression, the endoscope is easily passed distally as the esophagus accommodates. Diagnosis also can be made by an endoscopic ultrasound (EUS), which will demonstrate a hypoechoic mass in the submucosa or muscularis propria. Endoscopic biopsy is avoided because subsequent mucosal adherence to the mass increases the chance of a mucosal perforation during surgical resection.

#### Treatment

Leiomyomas are slow-growing tumors with rare malignant potential that continue to grow and become progressively symptomatic over time. Although observation is acceptable in patients with small (<2 cm) asymptomatic tumors or other significant comorbid conditions, surgical resection is advocated for most

**Table 43-5 Histogenetic Classification of Benign Esophageal Tumors**

| ESOPHAGEAL WALL TISSUE OF ORIGIN | TUMOR TYPE | TISSUE TYPE |
|---|---|---|
| **Mucosa** | | |
| Epithelial lining | | |
| Normal stratified squamous epithelium | Squamous cell papilloma | Epithelial |
| Acquired metaplastic columnar epithelium | True adenoma (rare) or adenomatous hyperplasia | Epithelial |
| Lamina propria | | |
| Simple esophageal cardiac mucous gland | Mucus retention cyst | Epithelial |
| | True adenoma (rare) | Epithelial |
| Epithelial lining plus lamina propria | Inflammatory pseudotumor | Mesenchymal |
| | Fibrovascular polyp | Mesenchymal |
| Muscularis mucosae | Leiomyoma | Nonepithelial |
| Inflamed gastric mucosal fold at gastroesophageal junction | Inflammatory reflux polyp | Reflux polyp–fold complex |
| **Submucosa** | | |
| Esophageal mucous gland proper | Mucus retention cyst | Epithelial |
| | Adenoma | Epithelial |
| Vascular connective tissue | Fibrovascular polyp (fibrolipoma, fibromyxoma) | Mesenchymal |
| Blood vessel | Hemangioma | Mesenchymal |
| Schwann cell | Granular cell tumor | Mesenchymal |
| | Neurilemoma | Mesenchymal |
| **Muscularis Propria** | | |
| Striated muscle (upper one third) | Rhabdomyoma | Mesenchymal |
| Smooth muscle (lower two thirds) | Leiomyoma | Mesenchymal |
| Nerve fiber | Neurofibroma | Mesenchymal |
| Schwann cell | Granular cell tumor | Mesenchymal |
| | Neurilemoma | Mesenchymal |
| **Tunica Adventitia** | | |
| Connective tissue | Fibroma | Mesenchymal |
| Nerve plexus | Schwannoma (neurilemoma) | Mesenchymal |
| **Ectopic Tissues** | | |
| Sebaceous gland | Adenoma | Epithelial |
| Tracheobronchial rests | Choristoma | Mixed tissues |

From Shamji F, Todd TRJ: Benign tumors. In Pearson FG, Cooper JF, Deslauriers J, et al (eds): Esophageal surgery, ed 2, Philadelphia, 2002, Churchill Livingstone, p 639.

patients. There are no known medical treatments for esophageal leiomyomas; however, imatinib (a tyrosine kinase inhibitor), as targeted therapy used on other GIST tumors, may have some benefit for esophageal leiomyomas. Surgical enucleation of the tumor remains the standard of care and is performed through a thoracotomy or with video or robotic assistance. Lesions of the proximal and midesophagus are removed through the right chest; those of distal origin are removed through the left chest. Morbidity is low, less than 5%, and includes inadvertent mucosal injury and pneumonia. The mortality rate is lower than 2% and success in relieving dysphagia approaches 100%.[25]

## Esophageal Cysts

Esophageal cysts are the second most common benign lesion of the esophagus. They can be congenital or acquired. Congenital cysts arise from persistent vacuoles in the wall of the foregut during embryologic development. They are lined with simple columnar, pseudostratified ciliated columnar, or stratified squamous epithelium. They are found within or in close proximity to the esophageal wall. Over time, they fill with mucus and increase in size, causing symptoms of obstruction. Most congenital cysts will present within the first year of life and are found in the upper third of the esophagus. Cysts of the lower two thirds present in childhood. Acquired cysts are probably a result of obstruction of the excretory ducts of esophageal glands. They are found in the lower esophagus and tend to present later in life.

### Symptoms and Diagnosis

Most cysts, congenital or acquired, remain asymptomatic until they are large enough to obstruct the esophageal lumen. Symptoms of dysphagia or recurrent respiratory infections from aspiration of cystic fluid or a fistulous tract to the airway are common. Large cysts may impinge on the airway, causing symptoms of shortness of breath and dyspnea on exertion. Diagnosis is made with a barium esophagram or CT scan (Fig. 43-47). A smooth oval mass will appear to be obstructing the lumen of the esophagus similar to that seen with a leiomyoma. EUS is helpful to distinguish a cyst from a solid mass and aids in cyst aspiration for diagnosis.

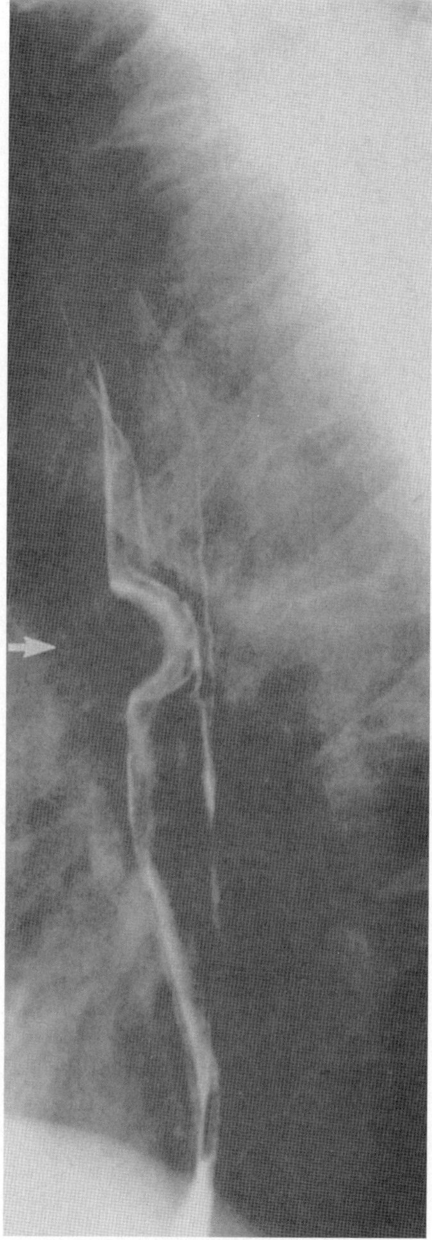

**FIGURE 43-46** Barium esophagram showing a leiomyoma. Note the characteristic smooth, distinct borders of the mass. (From Shamji F, Todd TR: Benign tumors. In Pearson FG, Cooper JD, Deslauriers J, et al [eds]: Esophageal surgery, ed 2, New York, 2002, Churchill Livingstone, p 640.)

### Treatment

Left untreated, an esophageal cyst will increase in size, resulting in obstruction, infection, or rupture. Cyst aspiration alone is not adequate because fluid will reaccumulate. Surgical resection of the cyst needs to be considered for all patients, whenever possible. Extramucosal resection or enucleation is preferred and is done through a neck incision or thoracotomy. A fistulous tract to the airway may be present and must be sought. If one is found, it is ligated and divided.

### Fibrovascular Polyps

Fibrovascular polyps are uncommon tumors of the esophagus and are found in men aged 60 to 70 years. Most (85%) are located in the cervical esophagus below the cricopharyngeus muscle. They are composed of edematous connective tissue containing blood vessels and fatty tissue. They begin as small mucosal tumors and elongate over time; some can grow to a substantial size and have extremely long pedicles. The pedicle can be thin or thick and extremely vascular. The overlying mucosa may be ulcerated from trauma and infection. Although they are benign lesions, some polyps may harbor carcinoma and need to be evaluated thoroughly.

### Symptoms and Diagnosis

Pedunculated polyps are usually asymptomatic until they grow large enough to cause dysphagia caused by obstruction of the esophageal lumen. Bleeding from mucosal ulcerations may occur and result in a slow gastrointestinal bleed. Diagnosis is made by endoscopy or barium esophagraphy. Endoscopic evaluation may miss small lesions because the polyp surface appears similar to that of normal esophageal mucosa. The thickness of the pedicle and size of the tumor mass is noted. Biopsies of the overlying mucosa are undertaken to rule out cancer. A barium esophagram demonstrates an irregular filling defect of the esophagus, with distal narrowing (Fig. 43-48A) and CT identifies the intraluminal mass within the esophagus (see Fig. 43-48*B*).

### Treatment

All fibrovascular polyps are removed. Left untreated, they will continue to grow and obstruct the esophageal lumen. Endoscopic removal by electrocautery ligation is indicated if the mass is small (<2 cm) or if the pedicle is not richly vascular. Larger polyps can be removed endoscopically but they are difficult to pull through the esophagus past the cricopharyngeus muscle. There is a risk for airway obstruction with endoscopic removal of large polyps that do not pass through the pharynx easily. Surgical resection is recommended for all masses that are longer than 8 cm or have a richly vascularized pedicle (see Fig. 43-48*C*). Depending on the location of the mass, resection is approached through a cervical incision or thoracotomy.

## CARCINOMA OF THE ESOPHAGUS

Esophageal cancer is the fastest growing cancer in the United States. It remains the sixth most common malignancy, with an incidence of 20/100,000, and represents 4% of newly diagnosed cancers in North America. Worldwide, esophageal cancer is even more prevalent, reaching an incidence of 160/100,000 in parts of South Africa and China and 540/100,000 in Kazakhstan. Squamous cell carcinoma still accounts for most esophageal cancers diagnosed. However, in the United States, esophageal adenocarcinoma is noted in up to 70% of patients presenting with esophageal cancer. The distribution of esophageal cancer across gender, age, and race is affected by the cell type. The male-to-female ratio for squamous cell cancer is 3 : 1; in contrast, this ratio for adenocarcinoma is 15 : 1 in the fifth decade of life. Squamous cell cancer is rarely seen before the age of 30 years, with the highest mortality rates seen in men between 60 and 70 years of age. Adenocarcinoma is seen infrequently before the age of 40 years and increases in incidence with age. Racial discrepancies are observed. Adenocarcinoma is a disease affecting white

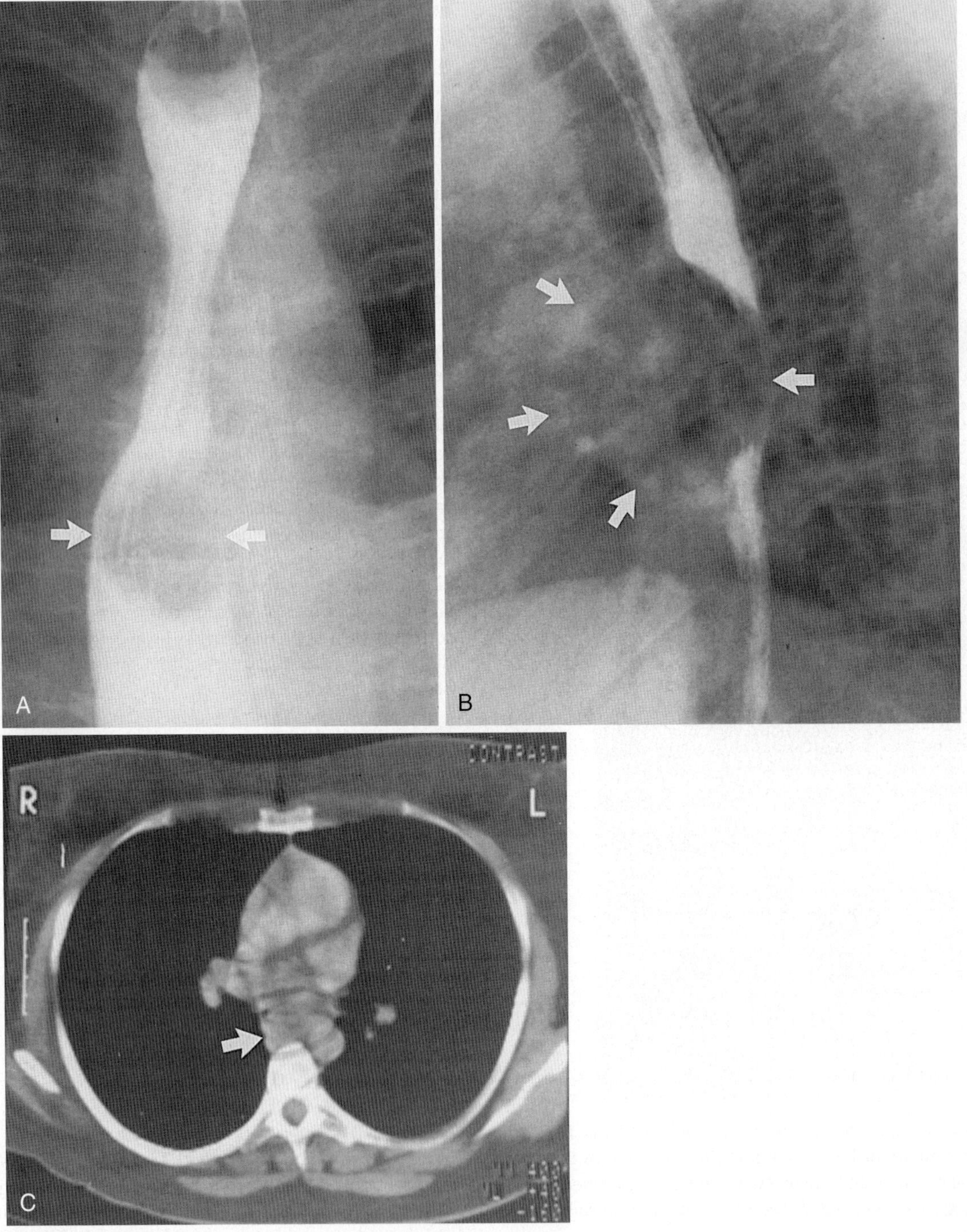


**FIGURE 43-47** Barium esophagram and CT scan of an esophageal cyst *(arrows)*. **A,** AP chest radiograph. **B,** Lateral chest radiograph. **C,** CT scan of the chest. (Adapted from Orringer MB: Tumors of the esophagus. In In Sabiston DC [ed]: Textbook of Surgery, ed 15, Philadelphia, 1997, WB Saunders, p 746.)

men, whereas squamous cell carcinoma predominantly affects African American men.

Squamous cell carcinomas arise from the squamous mucosa that is native to the esophagus and is found in the upper and middle thirds of the esophagus 70% of the time. This type of cancer is caused by exposure to environmental factors. Smoking and alcohol both increase the risk for foregut cancers by fivefold. Combined, the risk increases from 25- to 100-fold. Food additives, including nitrosamines found in pickled and smoked foods, long-term ingestion of hot liquids, and vitamin (vitamin A) and mineral deficiencies (zinc, molybdenum) have been implicated. Other disorders that expose the esophagus to mucosal trauma, including caustic ingestion, achalasia, bulimia, tylosis (an inherited autosomal dominant trait), Plummer-Vinson syndrome, external beam radiation, and esophageal diverticula have known associations with squamous cell cancer.

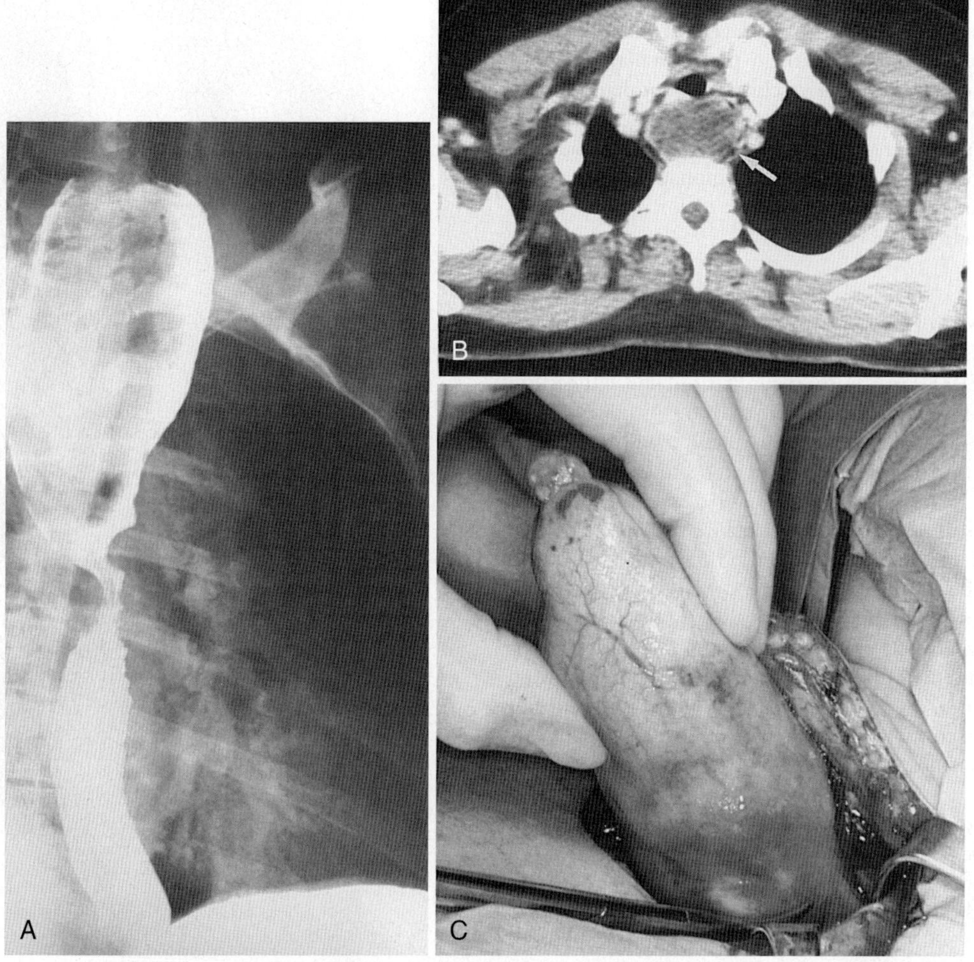


**FIGURE 43-48** Barium esophagram **(A)** and CT scan **(B)** of an esophageal polyp. **C,** Resection of a large esophageal polyp. (Adapted from Orringer MB: Tumors of the esophagus. In Sabiston DC [ed]: Textbook of Surgery, ed 15, Philadelphia, 1997, WB Saunders, p 747.)

The 5-year survival rate varies but can be as high as 70% with polypoid lesions and as low as 15% with advanced tumors.

Once a relatively unusual disease, esophageal adenocarcinoma now accounts for almost 70% of all esophageal carcinomas diagnosed in the United States and Western countries. There are a number of factors responsible for this shift in cell type:

1. Increasing incidence of GERD
2. Western diet
3. Increased use of acid-suppression medications

Intake of caffeine, fats, and acidic and spicy foods all lead to decreased tone in the LES and an increase in reflux. As an adaptive measure, the squamous-lined distal esophagus changes to become lined with metaplastic columnar epithelium (Barrett's esophagus). Progressive changes from metaplastic (Barrett's esophagus) to dysplastic cells may lead to the development of esophageal adenocarcinoma. Histologically, esophageal adenocarcinoma arises from one of three sites:

1. Submucosal glands of the esophagus
2. Heterotopic islands of columnar epithelium
3. Malignant degeneration of metaplastic columnar epithelium (Barrett's esophagus)

There are several intrinsic diseases of the esophagus that are considered premalignant. Patients with Plummer-Vinson syndrome, a disease of iron and vitamin deficiency that results in atrophy of the oropharyngeal and esophageal mucosa, have an increased risk for developing squamous cell cancers of the cervical esophagus. Tylosis, an uncommon familial syndrome characterized by thickening of the skin of the soles and palms, has an estimated 40% increased risk for developing squamous cell carcinoma that appears to be genetically linked. Achalasia, a disorder of esophageal motility, is associated with a 16-fold increased risk for squamous cell cancer in late-stage disease. Both esophageal strictures and diverticula have been reported to be associated with a small but increased risk for esophageal cancer. Patients with aerodigestive tract cancers are also at increased risk for developing esophageal squamous tumors. Barrett's esophagus, or metaplastic columnar epithelium in the esophagus, is associated with a 40-fold increased risk for adenocarcinoma of the esophagus. No specific infectious agents have been identified as a cause of esophageal cancer, but many remain under investigation. Genetic alterations accounting for cellular and molecular changes (as in the *p53* gene) have been associated with an increased risk for esophageal cancer.

Regardless of the cell type, esophageal cancer asserts aggressive biologic behavior. With only two layers to the esophageal wall, tumors rapidly infiltrate through the muscular wall into surrounding structures. The rich vascular and lymphatic supply facilitates spread to regional lymph nodes. Advanced disease is common at the time of presentation and contributes to the high mortality rate. Spread of disease follows lymphatic drainage patterns so that drainage tends to be to local, regional, and then to distant lymph node beds.

### Symptoms

The symptoms of esophageal cancer vary with the stage of the disease. Early-stage cancers may be asymptomatic or mimic symptoms of GERD. Heartburn, regurgitation, and indigestion are symptoms of reflux, but cancer may be lurking within. Most patients with esophageal cancer present with dysphagia and weight loss, symptoms that usually indicate advanced disease. Because of the distensibility of the esophagus, a mass can obstruct two thirds of the lumen before symptoms of dysphagia are noted. Furthermore, the symptoms of dysphagia and weight loss may be slowly progressive and well compensated for over a period of months. It is not until the esophageal lumen is narrowed from an average of 24 to 12 mm that dysphagia is noted. Many patients will be symptomatic before narrowing occurs to this degree, but medical treatment is often not sought until the symptoms are disabling. Effortless weight loss is welcomed by most, although its true significance goes unappreciated.

Choking, coughing, and aspiration from a tracheoesophageal fistula, as well as hoarseness and vocal cord paralysis from direct invasion into the recurrent laryngeal nerve, are ominous signs of advanced disease. Systemic metastases to liver, bone, and lung can present with jaundice, excessive pain, and respiratory symptoms.

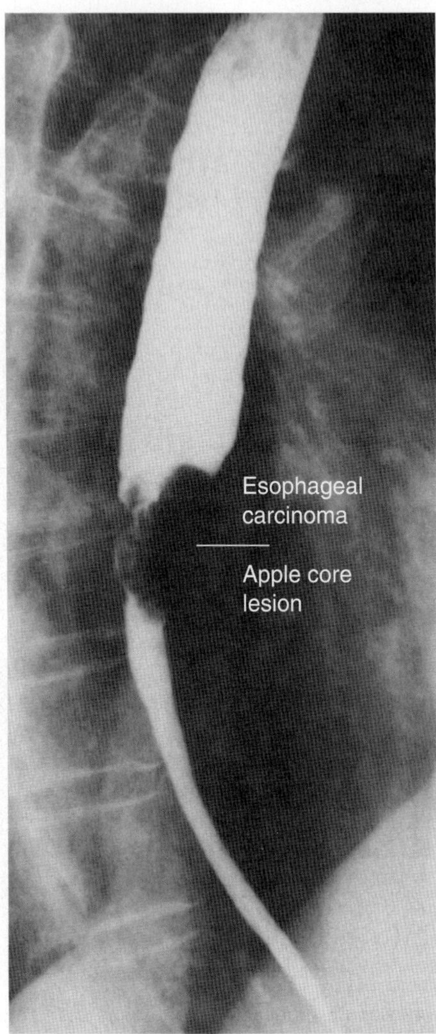


**FIGURE 43-49** Carcinoma of the esophagus. Note the appearance of an apple core lesion. (From Jaffer NM, Chia SH: Radiology, computed tomography and magnetic resonance imaging. In Pearson FG, Cooper JD, Deslauriers J, et al [eds]: Esophageal Surgery, ed 2, New York, Churchill Livingstone, 2002, p 88.)

### Diagnosis

A number of modalities are available to diagnose and stage esophageal cancer. Radiologic tests, endoscopic procedures, and minimally invasive surgical techniques all add value to a solid staging workup in a patient with esophageal cancer.

#### Esophagraphy

A barium esophagram is recommended for any patient presenting with dysphagia. The esophagram provides an overview of anatomy and function. It can differentiate intraluminal from intramural lesions and discriminate between intrinsic (from a mass protruding into the lumen) and extrinsic (from compression of a structures outside the esophagus) compression. The classic finding of an apple core lesion in patients with esophageal cancer is recognized easily (Fig. 43-49). Although the esophagram will not be specific for cancer, it is a good first test to perform in patients presenting with dysphagia and a suspicion of esophageal cancer.

#### Endoscopy

The diagnosis of esophageal cancer is best made from an endoscopic biopsy. During endoscopy, it is critical to document the following:

1. Location of the lesion (with respect to distance from the incisors)
2. Nature of the lesion (e.g., friable, firm, polypoid)
3. Proximal and distal extent of the lesion
4. Relationship of the lesion to the cricopharyngeus muscle, GEJ, and gastric cardia
5. Distensibility of the stomach

Each of these points is important for the management of esophageal cancer and helps guide surgical therapy. Incontrovertibly, any patient undergoing surgery for esophageal cancer must have an endoscopy performed by the operating surgeon before entering the operating room for a definitive resection.

#### Computed Tomography

There are additional diagnostic modalities used for accurate staging. A CT scan of the chest and abdomen is important to assess the length of the tumor, thickness of the esophagus and stomach, regional lymph node status (including cervical, mediastinal, and celiac lymph nodes), and distant disease to the liver

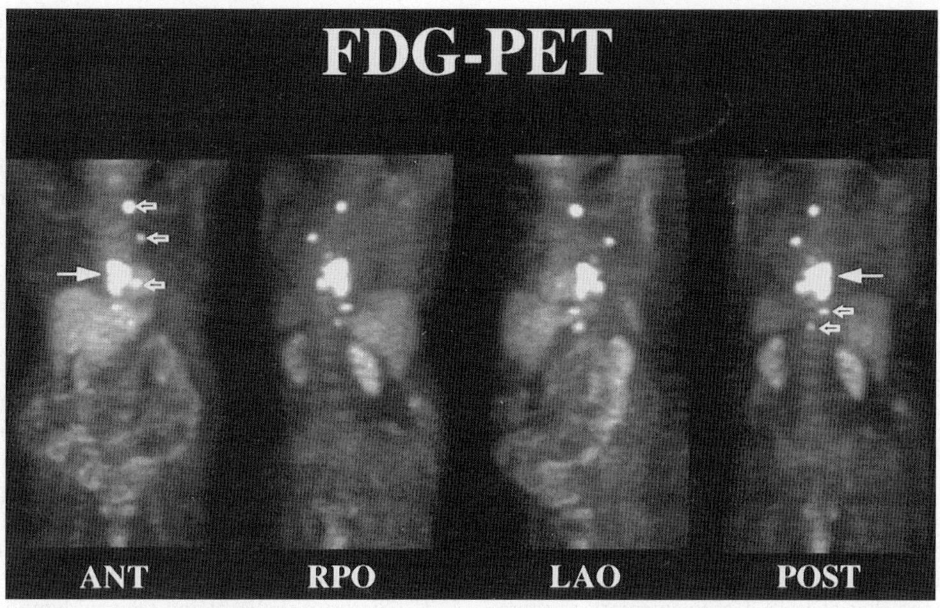


**FIGURE 43-50** FDG-PET scan of an esophageal cancer. *ANT,* Anterior; *LAO,* left anterior oblique; *POST,* posterior; RPO, right posterior oblique. (From Dehdashti F, Siegel BA: Positron emission tomography. In Pearson FG, Cooper JD, Deslauriers J, et al [eds]: Esophageal surgery, ed 2, New York, 2002, Churchill Livingstone, p 117.)

and lungs. It is also helpful for determining T4 lesions, in which the lesion is invading surrounding structures. It may identify a fistula or other anatomic variations, such as a deviated trachea. Although a CT scan is helpful, its accuracy is only 57% for T staging, 74% for N staging, and 83% for M staging.[26] Many unresectable tumors by CT scan are deemed resectable at the time of surgery. It is an important piece of the diagnostic workup but its findings must be interpreted judiciously, and only as a part of the total picture.

### Positron Emission Tomography

An $^{18}$F-fluorodeoxyglucose (FDG)–positron emission tomography (PET) scan evaluates the primary mass, regional lymph nodes, and distant disease (Fig. 43-50). Its sensitivity and specificity slightly exceed those of a CT scan; however, they remain low for definitive staging. The sensitivity and specificity of PET for evaluating metastatic disease are as high as 88% and 93%, respectively. For evaluation of lymph node disease, PET has a sensitivity (72%), specificity (86%), and accuracy (76%) equivalent to CT.[27] As with CT, the ability of PET to evaluate local and regional lymph node disease is dependent on the location of the tumor, size of the lymph node, and technique of the scanner. Although its role is evolving, PET appears to be an important piece of the diagnostic workup but is not reliable enough as a single diagnostic modality.

### Magnetic Resonance Imaging

Magnetic resonance imaging (MRI) is not performed routinely and adds to the staging of esophageal cancer in few circumstances. To identify involvement of vascular and neural tissues, MRI is helpful. It can accurately detect T4 lesions and metastatic lesions in the liver but overstages T and N status, with only a 74% accuracy.

### Endoscopic Ultrasound

EUS is the most critical component of esophageal cancer staging. The information obtained from EUS will help guide medical and surgical therapy. The experienced endoscopic ultrasonographer can identify the depth and length of the tumor, degree of luminal compromise, status of regional lymph nodes, and involvement of adjacent structures. In addition, biopsy samples can be obtained of the mass and lymph nodes in the paratracheal, subcarinal, paraesophageal, celiac, lesser curvature, and gastrohepatic regions. EUS tends to overstage T status and understage N status. The accuracy of EUS for T staging correlates directly with increasing T stage. For T1 lesions, EUS is 84% accurate, and it approaches 95% accuracy in estimating T4 lesions. Size and location of the lymph node influence the accuracy, so that lymph nodes smaller than 1 cm tend to be evaluated less accurately. The overall sensitivity (78%) and specificity (60%) of EUS for evaluating lymph nodes are poor but improve dramatically for evaluating celiac lymph nodes, for which the sensitivity and specificity are 72% and 97%, respectively.

### Endoscopic Mucosal Resection

EMR is performed with a double-channel endoscope with a soft plastic cap at its tip. The cap is placed over the top of the lesion, suction is applied, and a snare is brought down over the top of the lesion. A biopsy specimen of 1 to 1.5 cm will contain mucosa and submucosa. In skilled hands, EMR provides essential staging information that guides treatment. It may also be used as a therapeutic modality for premalignant and early malignant conditions. An additional diagnostic and therapeutic tool has been explored by Japanese and German researchers. Endoscopic submucosal dissection (ESD) is a technique that uses hook cautery and scissors to resect a lesion down to the level of the muscularis propria. This is technique that has not yet gained enough experience worldwide; however, the future is promising.

### Minimally Invasive Surgical Modalities

Bronchoscopy, mediastinoscopy, thoracoscopy, and laparoscopy are all useful staging tools. Bronchoscopy is performed in any patient presenting with a cough or evidence of a cervical esophageal cancer. It is helpful to rule out a tracheoesophageal fistula or growth of tumors into the trachea. Mediastinoscopy is used in the workup for esophageal cancer. It is used to biopsy suspicious lymph nodes that may indicate advanced disease and that are not amenable to endoultrasonographic biopsy. Using video-assisted thoracoscopic surgery technology, lymph nodes in the thoracic inlet, mediastinum (including paratracheal, subcarinal, and paraesophageal lymph nodes), and along the thoracic duct and into the diaphragmatic hiatus can be evaluated. Metastatic lesions in the lung or extension of tumor into the pericardium, aorta, azygos vein, trachea, or diaphragm are noted with an accuracy of 93%.[28] Laparoscopy also has some usefulness for staging esophageal cancer. The extent of tumor can be determined and biopsies of the celiac axis, perihepatic, and GEJ lymph nodes can be performed. The addition of a laparoscopic ultrasound probe allows visualization of nodes as small as 3 mm in diameter, similar to that of EUS. Complementary to thoracoscopy, laparoscopy is an additional method for providing accurate staging information, with low risk to the patient.

## Staging

The most critical aspect of treating a patient with esophageal cancer is determining an accurate clinical stage. The data obtained in the process of staging the patient are more important than the stage within which the patient falls. Precise staging at the time of presentation allows for the most appropriate treatment and results in the best chance for long-term survival.

The staging of esophageal cancer has been transformed through a variety of systems and still remains controversial. The American Joint Committee on Cancer (AJCC) staging criteria were instituted in 1988 and are currently the most widely adopted staging system (Table 43-6). However, recognizing the flaws in the AJCC system, in 1997 Ellis proposed a staging system based on the criteria defined by Skinner that restructures the T status (Table 43-7). The AJCC classification uses the TNM (tumor, lymph node, metastasis) system to stratify patients and estimate prognosis, whereas the Ellis classification uses the WNM (wall penetration, lymph node, metastasis) system. In the AJCC system, the T represents the depth of the tumor (T1, submucosal; T2, muscularis propria; T3, adventitia; T4, surrounding structures), the N represents involvement of lymph nodes (N0, none; N1, any), and the M represents metastatic disease to nonregional lymph nodes or distant sites (M0, none; M1a, regional lymph nodes; M1b, distant lymph nodes). In the Ellis classification, the W represents the depth of wall penetration (W0, muscularis mucosae; W1, submucosa and muscularis propria; W2, adventitia), N represents the number of positive lymph nodes (N0, none; N1, one to four; N2, >4), and M represents distant disease (M0, none; M1, any; Fig. 43-51). In both systems, the depth of invasion and extent of local and regional lymph node involvement affect prognosis. However, the Ellis classification emphasizes not only that the depth of invasion is important, but also that the number of lymph nodes affects survival. A comparison between the two systems is presented in Table 43-8 and Figure 43-52.

The T1 status has been classified further.[29] In this staging system, the mucosa and submucosal layers are subdivided to identify tumors with extension into the epithelium, lamina propria, muscularis mucosae, and superficial, middle, and deep submucosal layers. This study has shown that the depth of tumor directly relates to lymph node involvement. Tumors confined to the epithelial layer have no associated lymph node involvement. Lesions penetrating the lamina propria and muscularis mucosae are associated with lymph node involvement 5% and 18% of the time, respectively. Superficial and deep submucosal lesions have an associated 50% and 55% lymph node involvement, respectively.

## Treatment

Traditionally, staging systems were used to guide therapy and assess long-term outcomes (Fig. 43-53). As technology, medical therapy, and knowledge of the biology of tumors continue to advance, staging systems are changing and becoming less functional. When a patient presents with esophageal cancer, the following variables are considered (Table 43-9):

1. Histology, location, and local extent (depth of invasion) of the primary tumor
2. Status of the local and regional lymph nodes
3. Presence of distant lymph nodes or systemic disease
4. Overall condition of the patient (including nutritional status and ability to swallow)
5. Intended goal of treatment, curative or palliative

These variables guide management and help develop appropriate treatment plans that may include chemotherapy, radiotherapy, endoscopic procedures, and surgical resection. Although treatment is controversial at all stages and varies among oncologists, radiation oncologists, gastroenterologists, and surgeons, and among surgeons themselves, multimodality therapy with chemotherapy, radiation therapy, endoscopic procedures, and surgical resection is appropriate for most patients presenting with esophageal cancer (Fig. 43-54).

### Histology, Location, and Local Extent of Primary Tumor

There are two predominant cells types of esophageal cancer, adenocarcinoma and squamous cell carcinoma. Adenocarcinoma represents more than 70% of esophageal cancers in the United States but, worldwide, squamous cell cancers are predominant. The histology of the tumor is important because it guides treatment in two ways: (1) squamous cell tumors are more sensitive to chemoradiotherapy and are treated aggressively with nonsurgical therapy; (2) adenocarcinomas are not as sensitive to chemoradiotherapy and are often imbedded in long segments of Barrett's esophagus, necessitating a more aggressive surgical approach. Patients with squamous cell tumors may achieve a complete response to chemoradiotherapy, making the need for surgical intervention uncertain and not very compelling. However, most studies have supported multimodality therapy for the treatment of squamous cell tumors. Surgery is strongly advocated for most patients with adenocarcinoma because a complete response to chemotherapy is seen only 25% of the time in this cell type. Little is known about the biology of esophageal tumors, but as more studies are carried out and published, future medical therapies will be targeted at the biology, not the histology, of the tumor. This is already well established in other malignancies, such as breast cancer.

The location of the tumor also directs the management of esophageal cancer. Of all esophageal tumors present in the cervical esophagus, 8% are almost always squamous cell cancers.

**Table 43-6 Tumor-Node-Metastasis (TNM) Staging of Esophageal Carcinoma**

| **Primary Tumor (T)*** | |
|---|---|
| TX | Primary tumor cannot be assessed |
| T0 | No evidence of primary tumor |
| Tis | High-grade dysplasia† |
| T1 | Tumor invades lamina propria, muscularis mucosae, or submucosa |
| T1a | Tumor invades lamina propria or muscularis mucosae |
| T1b | Tumor invades submucosa |
| T2 | Tumor invades muscularis propria |
| T3 | Tumor invades adventitia |
| T4 | Tumor invades adjacent structures |
| T4a | Resectable tumor invading pleura, pericardium, or diaphgragm |
| T4b | Unresectable tumor invading other adjacent structures, such as aorta, vertebral body, trachea, etc. |
| **Regional Lymph Nodes (N)‡** | |
| NX | Regional lymph nodes cannot be assessed |
| N0 | No regional lymph node metastasis |
| N1 | Metastasis in 1-2 regional lymph nodes |
| N2 | Metastasis in 3-6 regional lymph nodes |
| N3 | Metastasis in seven or more regional lymph nodes |
| **Distant Metastasis (M)** | |
| M0 | No distant metastasis |
| M1 | Distant metastasis |

**Stage Grouping**

| STAGE | T | N | M | GRADE | TUMOR LOCATION¶ |
|---|---|---|---|---|---|
| **Squamous Cell Carcinoma§** | | | | | |
| 0 | Tis (HGD) | N0 | M0 | 1, X | Any |
| IA | T1 | N0 | M0 | 1, X | Any |
| IB | T1<br>T2-3 | N0<br>N0 | M0<br>M0 | 2-3<br>1, X | Any<br>Lower, X |
| IIA | T2-3<br>T2-3 | N0<br>N0 | M0<br>M0 | 1, X<br>2-3 | Upper, middle<br>Lower, X |
| IIB | T2-3<br>T1-2 | N0<br>N1 | M0<br>M0 | 2-3<br>Any | Upper, middle<br>Any |
| IIIA | T1-2<br>T3<br>T4a | N2<br>N1<br>N0 | M0<br>M0<br>M0 | Any<br>Any<br>Any | Any<br>Any<br>Any |
| IIIB | T3 | N2 | M0 | Any | Any |
| IIIC | T4a<br>T4b<br>Any | N1-2<br>Any<br>N3 | M0<br>M0<br>M0 | Any<br>Any<br>Any | Any<br>Any<br>Any |
| IV | Any | Any | M1 | Any | Any |
| **Adenocarcinoma** | | | | | |
| 0 | Tis (HGD) | N0 | M0 | 1, X | |
| IA | T1 | N0 | M0 | 1-2, X | |
| IB | T1<br>T2 | N0<br>N0 | M0<br>M0 | 3<br>1-2, X | |
| IIA | T2 | N0 | M0 | 3 | |
| IIB | T3<br>T1-2 | N0<br>N1 | M0<br>M0 | Any<br>Any | |
| IIIA | T1-2<br>T3<br>T4a | N2<br>N1<br>N0 | M0<br>M0<br>M0 | Any<br>Any<br>Any | |
| IIIB | T3 | N2 | M0 | Any | |
| IIIC | T4a<br>T4b<br>Any | N1-2<br>Any<br>N3 | M0<br>M0<br>M0 | Any<br>Any<br>Any | |
| IV | Any | Any | M1 | Any | |

From Edge S, Byrd D, Compton C, et al (eds): AJCC cancer staging manual, ed 7, New York, 2010, Springer.

*1. At least maximal dimension of the tumor must be recorded. 2. Multiple tumors require the T(m) suffix.

†High-grade dysplasia includes all noninvasive neoplastic epithelia that was formerly called carcinoma in situ, a diagnosis that is no longer used for columnar mucosae anywhere in the gastrointestinal tract.

‡Number must be recorded for total number of regional nodes sampled and total number of reported nodes with metastasis.

§Or mixed histology, including a squamous component or not otherwise specified (NOS).

¶Location of the primary cancer site is defined by the position of the upper (proximal) edge of the tumor in the esophagus.

**Table 43-7 Wall Penetration-Node-Metastasis (WNM) Staging of Esophageal Carcinoma**

| STAGE | FEATURES |
|---|---|
| **W: Wall Penetration** | |
| W0 | Intramucosal mucosa penetration |
| W1 | Intramural mucosa penetration |
| W2 | Transmural mucosa penetration |
| **N: Regional Lymph Nodes** | |
| Nx | Regional lymph nodes cannot be assessed |
| N0 | No regional lymph node metastases |
| N1 | Four lymph nodes metastases or fewer |
| N2 | More than four lymph node metastases |
| **M: Distant Metastases** | |
| Mx | Distant metastases cannot be assessed |
| M0 | No distant metastases |
| M1 | Distant metastases present |

**Stage Grouping**

| STAGE | W | N | M |
|---|---|---|---|
| 0 | W0 | N0 | M0 |
| I | W0<br>W1 | N1<br>N0 | M0<br>M0 |
| II | W1<br>W2 | N1<br>N0 | M0<br>M0 |
| III | W2<br>W1<br>W0 | N1<br>N2<br>N2 | M0<br>M0<br>M0 |
| IV | Any W | Any N | M1a |

From Ellis FH Jr, Heatley GJ, Krasna MJ, et al: Esophagogastrectomy for carcinoma of the esophagus and cardia: a comparison of findings and results after standard resection in three consecutive eight-year intervals with improved staging criteria. J Thorac Cardiovasc Surg 113:836–846; discussion 846-838, 1997.

These tumors may be locally aggressive and are managed with chemoradiotherapy, followed by segmental resection of the cervical esophagus. Upper thoracic and midthoracic tumors account for 3% and 32% of esophageal tumors, respectively, and may be squamous cell cancers or adenocarcinomas. Near-total esophagectomy through a thoracotomy is usually required to remove all the disease in this part of the esophagus. The remaining tumors are found in the lower esophagus (25%) and cardia of the stomach (32%) and tend to be adenocarcinomas. Distal esophagectomy, through a transabdominal or transthoracic approach, in patients with no known Barrett's esophagus or total gastrectomy in those with Barrett's esophagus is appropriate for early disease. Near-total esophagectomy, through a transhiatal or transthoracic approach, is recommended for patients who have tumors in segments of Barrett's esophagus or tumors of considerable length.

The depth of invasion of a tumor, the T status, is another important variable in determining stage and treatment of esophageal cancer. T1 lesions are divided into intramucosal and submucosal lesions that are associated with lymph node metastasis 18% and 50% of the time, respectively. Conservative esophageal resections, such as vagal-sparing, transhiatal, or minimally invasive esophagectomy, are recommended for any T1 lesion. For localized intramucosal tumors of limited extent, EMR[30] and ESD are acceptable alternatives to esophagectomy. There is almost no role for chemoradiotherapy in the treatment of T1 lesions. Surgical or endoscopic resection alone carries a good long-term survival, as high as 88% in some series.

Treatment of lesions that extend into the muscularis propria, T2 lesions, remains controversial. The rate of lymph node metastasis is up to 60%; the need for chemoradiotherapy or a radical lymphadenectomy has been debated. Aggressive surgical resection can stand alone, but outcomes may improve if chemoradiotherapy is added. Neither approach is supported in the literature. Advocates of en bloc esophagectomy have argued that a wide envelope of tissue surrounding the lesion improves long-term outcomes. Advocates of a less invasive resection for T2 lesions have argued that the transhiatal resection obtains an adequate radial margin, with less morbidity. A

**Table 43-8 Comparison Between WNM and TNM Classification Systems**

| WNM 5-YR SURVIVAL (%) | WNM STAGE | WNM CLASS | TNM CLASS | TNM STAGE | TNM 5-YR SURVIVAL (%) |
|---|---|---|---|---|---|
| 88 | 0 | W0 N0 M0 | Tis N0 M0<br>T1 N0 M0 | 0<br>1 | 100<br>79 |
| 50 | 1 | W0 N1 M0 | NE | NE | NE |
| 50 | 1 | W1 N0 M0 | T1 N0 M0<br>T2 N0 M0 | 1<br>2A | 79<br>38 |
| 23 | 2 | W1 N1 M0 | T1 N1 M0<br>T2 N1 M0 | 2B | 27 |
| 23 | 2 | W2 N0 M0 | T3 N0 M0<br>T4 N0 M0 | 2A | 38 |
| 11 | 3 | W2 N1 M0 | T3 N1 M0<br>T4 N1 M0 | 3 | 14 |
| 11 | 3 | W1 N2 M0 | T1 N1 M0<br>T2 N1 M0 | 2B | 27 |
| 11 | 3 | W0 N2 M0 | NE | NE | NE |
| 0 | 4 | Wx Nx M1 | Tx Nx M1 | 4 | 0 |

*NE,* No equivalent.

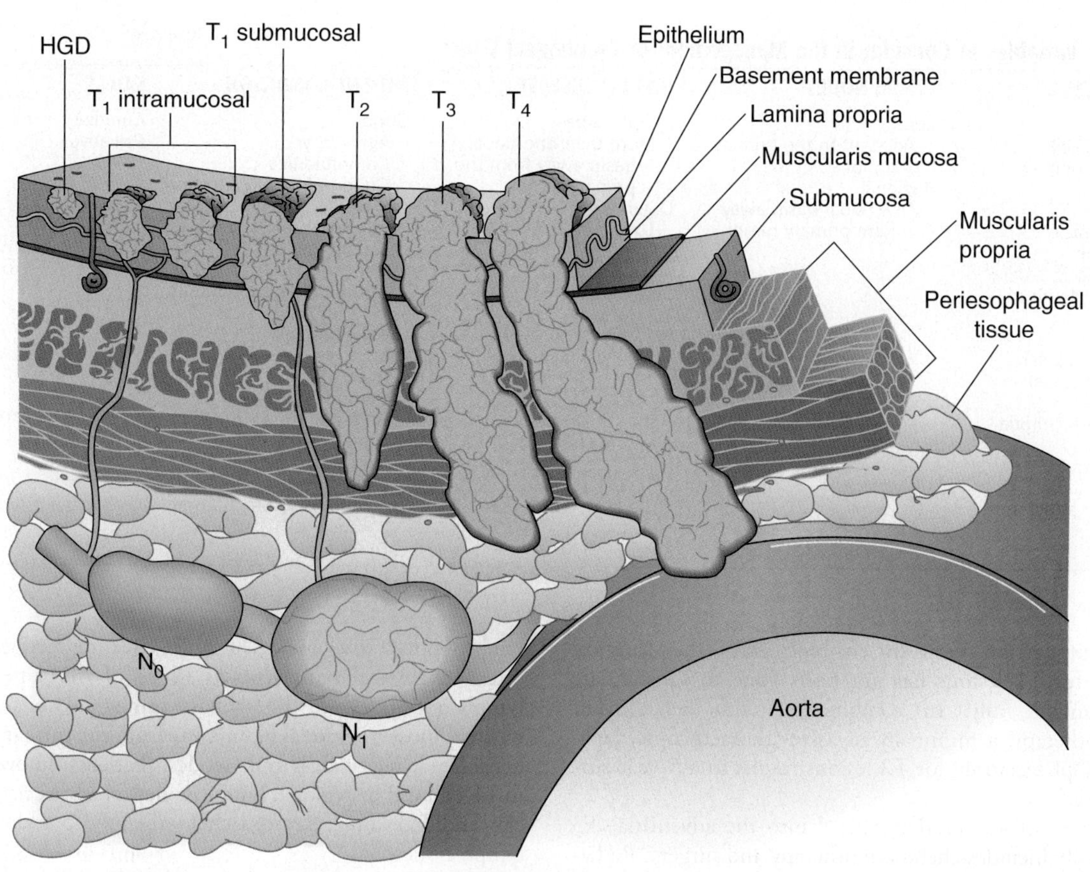


**FIGURE 43-51** Primary tumor status (T) is defined by depth of invasion. Regional lymph node (N) is defined by the absence (N0) or presence (N1) of regional nodal metastases. HGD, High-grade dysplasia. (From Rice WR: Diagnosis and staging of esophageal carcinoma. In Pearson FG, Cooper JD, Deslauriers J, et al [eds]: Esophageal surgery, ed 2, New York, 2002, Churchill Livingstone, p 687.)

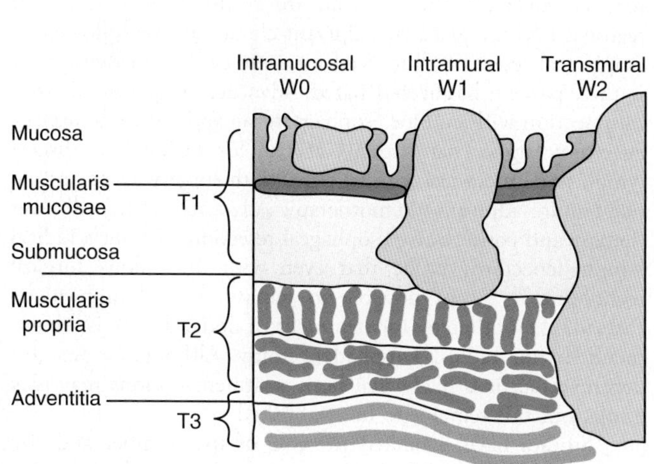


**FIGURE 43-52** Comparison between the TNM and WNM staging systems. (Adapted from DeMeester TR, Attwood SEA, Smyrk TC, et al: Surgical therapy in Barrett's esophagus. Ann Surg 212:530, 1990.)

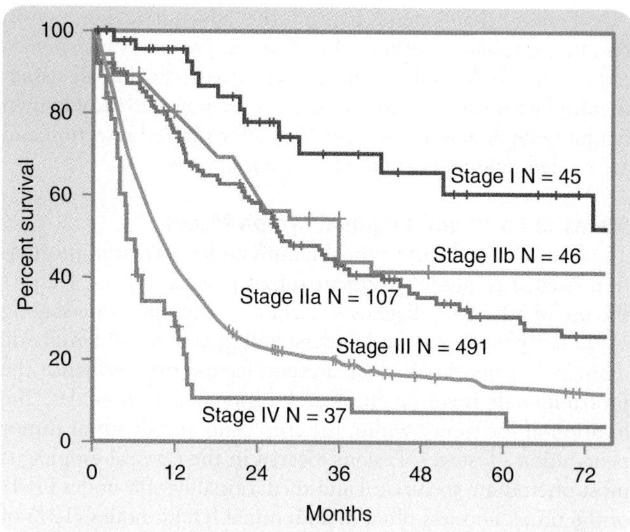


**FIGURE 43-53** Cumulative survival curves. (From Law SYW, Wong J: Management of squamous cell carcinoma of the esophagus. In Pearson FG, Cooper JD, Deslauriers J, et al [eds]: Esophageal surgery, ed 2, New York, 2002, Churchill Livingstone, p 719.)

**Table 43-9 Variables to Consider in the Management of Esophageal Cancer**

| PRIMARY TUMOR | LYMPH NODES | DISTANT DISEASE | PATIENT CONDITION | GOALS |
|---|---|---|---|---|
| Histology<br>Squamous cell<br>Adenocarcinoma<br>Location<br>Cervical<br>Upper thoracic<br>Midthoracic<br>Distal thoracic, cardia<br>Local extent, depth of invasion<br>T1<br>A: Intramucosal<br>B: Submucosal<br>T2<br>Muscularis propria<br>T3<br>Adventitia<br>T4<br>Adjacent structures | Local<br>Adjacent to the primary tumor<br>Regional<br>One nodal basin away from primary tumor | Lymph nodes<br>More than one nodal basin away from the primary tumor<br>Organ<br>Lung<br>Liver<br>Other<br>Systemic | Good<br>Age <75 yr<br>Comorbidities <3<br>Good pulmonary function tests<br>Cardiac reserve<br>Weight loss <10%<br>Nutrition: Serum albumin >3.4 g/dL<br>No dysphagia<br>Fair<br>Age >75 yr<br>Comorbidities ≥3<br>Poor pulmonary function tests<br>No cardiac reserve<br>Weight loss >10%<br>Nutrition: Serum albumin <3.4 g/dL<br>Dysphagia | Curative<br>Palliative |

scientific comparison between en bloc and other surgical approaches for T2 lesions has not been done to substantiate either argument fully. In combination with neoadjuvant chemoradiotherapy, a minimally invasive (thoracoscopic, laparoscopic) esophagectomy for T2 lesions results in a 5-year survival of 70%.[31]

Treatment of lesions that extend into the adventitia, T3 lesions, usually includes chemoradiotherapy and surgery. Radiation therapy controls the primary tumor and may reduce the extent of surgical resection margins. Chemotherapy controls tumor spread to local and regional lymph nodes that occurs up to 80% of the time with T3 lesions. Neoadjuvant chemoradiotherapy followed by surgery may improve survival for T3 lesions with known lymph node involvement but adversely affects surgical morbidity and mortality. The need for neoadjuvant therapy or aggressive surgical resection and radical lymphadenectomy for T3 lesions remains debated.

Lesions that extend beyond the adventitia, T4 lesions, require aggressive multimodality therapy. Neoadjuvant chemoradiotherapy followed by surgical resection removing all tissues involved with tumor is recommended. Lesions with any known lymph node disease are not considered for surgical resection and are treated definitively with chemoradiotherapy.

### Status of Local and Regional Lymph Nodes

The status of local and regional lymph nodes is critical information needed to guide treatment for esophageal cancer. Despite the use of advanced diagnostic techniques, lymph node staging is still fairly inaccurate and understanding patterns of lymphatic drainage is important. There are two factors that influence the probability of involved local and regional lymph nodes, the location of the tumor within the esophagus and depth of tumor penetration (T stage). Lesions located in the cervical esophagus most often drain to cervical and mediastinal lymph nodes (46% of the time), and less often to abdominal lymph nodes (12% of the time). In contrast, midesophageal tumors drain most often to mediastinal lymph nodes (53% of the time) and abdominal lymph nodes (40% of the time), and less often to cervical lymph nodes (29% of the time). Not surprisingly, lower esophageal and cardia tumors most often drain into abdominal and mediastinal lymph nodes (74% and 58% of the time, respectively) and less often to cervical lymph nodes (27% of the time). Involved lymph nodes next to the primary tumor are considered local, whereas those one nodal basin away from the primary tumor are considered regional lymph nodes. Patients known to have involved local or regional lymph nodes remain acceptable surgical candidates but also need chemotherapy to address involved lymph nodes.

The depth of tumor penetration (T stage) affects lymph node involvement (LNI) in the following manner: intramucosal T1 lesions (18% LNI), submucosal T1 lesions (55% LNI), T2 lesions (60% LNI), and T3 lesions (80% LNI). Patients who are at low risk (<50% LNI) for regional lymph node involvement are not given chemotherapy and are not likely to benefit from a radical lymphadenectomy. Conservative esophageal resections, such as the vagal-sparing, transhiatal, or minimally invasive esophagectomy, with a limited lymph node dissection, are adequate for these patients. If the surgical specimen reveals involvement of lymph nodes, adjuvant chemotherapy is given in an attempt to treat regional and possibly distant lymph nodes that may be involved. Patients who are at risk (>50% LNI) for regional LNI are given neoadjuvant chemotherapy followed by esophageal resection. The need for a radical lymphadenectomy in these patients has been debated. Advocates of aggressive surgical resection with en bloc esophagectomy and radical lymphadenectomy argue that patients at risk for regional or distant lymph node metastasis can be cured with surgery alone and do not require adjuvant chemotherapy. Advocates of neoadjuvant therapy and conservative esophageal resection without a radical lymphadenectomy argue that even with meticulous surgical technique, it is not possible to remove every lymph node. Instead, chemotherapy for treatment of nodal disease is recommended, not radical lymphadenectomy. Although it remains controversial, it is likely that both treatment options may play a role, but this remains to be established.

Studies have evaluated the role of the number and size of involved lymph nodes in determining the need for adjuvant chemotherapy. The WNM staging system suggests a significant difference in 5-year survival between patients with negative nodes and those with five or more involved lymph nodes (22.5%

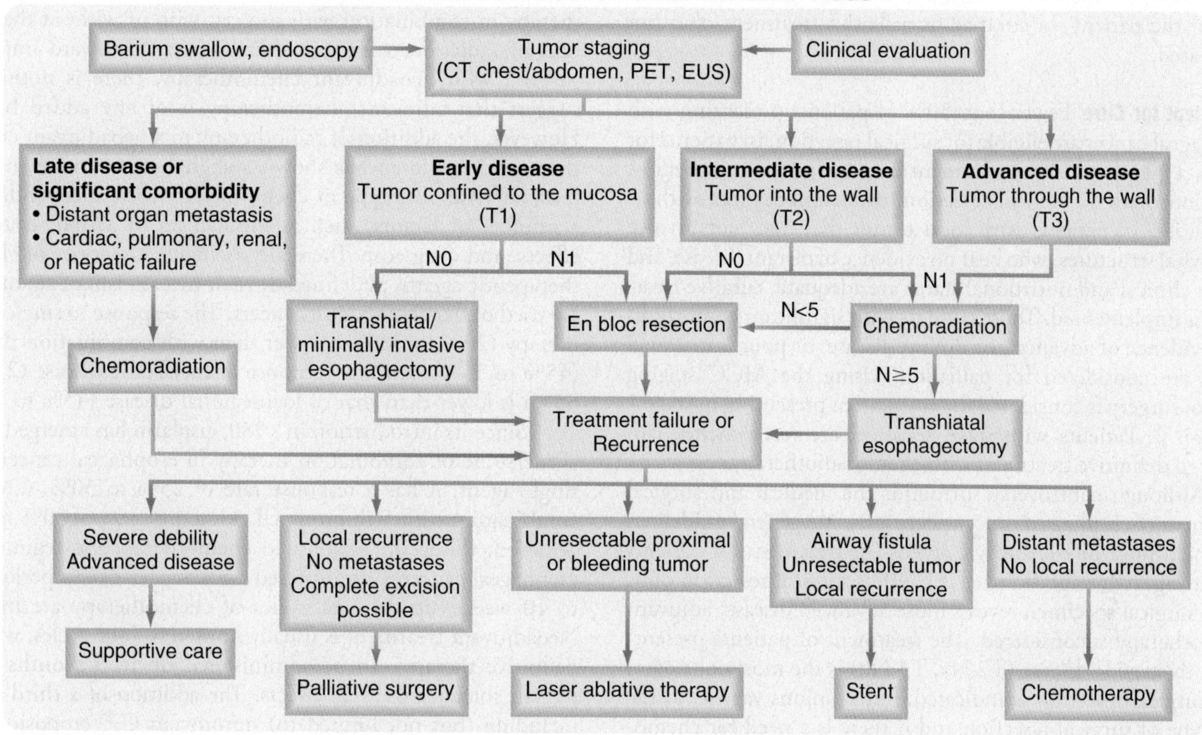


**FIGURE 43-54** Algorithm for the management of esophageal cancer.

versus 10.7%). One study has suggested that after neoadjuvant therapy, patients who have one positive lymph node have the same rate of 5-year survival as those who have all negative lymph nodes (34% versus 36%), whereas patients with two or more involved lymph nodes do considerably worse (6%). The study also suggested that the size of the involved lymph node significantly affects long-term survival; lymph nodes smaller than 4 mm carry a better prognosis than lymph nodes of greater size.[32] As more research is carried out, the best treatment for patients with positive local and regional lymph nodes will be clear. Until then, the crude guidelines that have been developed to date need to be interpreted judiciously, recognizing that it is often more than just science that motivates and guides the dogmas and decisions of physicians.

### Evidence of Distant Lymph Node or Systemic Disease

A lymph node that is more than one nodal basin away from the primary tumor is considered a distant lymph node. If a distant lymph node is involved with tumor, the patient is considered to have advanced disease. Patients presenting with involved distant lymph nodes or metastatic disease are treated with definitive chemoradiotherapy. If advanced disease is found at the time of surgery, resection is aborted and a feeding jejunostomy tube is placed. Palliative resection may be considered if a patient with complete obstruction desires alimentary continuity to facilitate eating.

### Condition of the Patient

It is well established that age, comorbidities, and nutritional status affect the ability of many patients to tolerate treatment for esophageal cancer. Although age alone is not a barrier to treatment, it may alter the choice of therapy in the presence of advanced disease. Patients older than 75 years have a higher operative risk and a shorter life expectancy, so aggressive surgical intervention is rarely indicated. Regardless of age, patients must be carefully evaluated for underlying cardiac, pulmonary, endocrinologic, hepatic, and renal conditions that can affect their ability to undergo surgical resection. Preoperative tests to assess cardiopulmonary status, including a pulmonary function test (PFT) and cardiac stress test, are imperative. There are no absolute contraindications to surgical resection but it is reserved for those in a reasonable state of health.

Many patients presenting with esophageal cancer have been nutritionally depleted for some time. More than a 10% weight loss is associated with a significant increase in operative morbidity and usually correlates well with the advanced nature of the disease. Patients presenting with a serum albumin level lower than 3.4 g/dL have an increased risk for surgical complications, including anastomotic breakdown. In patients who are otherwise fit and eligible to undergo surgical resection, efforts are directed toward improving nutritional status before surgery by placing a stent or feeding jejunostomy tube. Preoperative efforts attempting to improve nutrition will be rewarded.

### Treatment Intended to Be Curative or Palliative

Determining the appropriate treatment for a patient with esophageal cancer is multidimensional and complex. On evaluating the variables outlined in this section, the final decision is whether or not a curative or palliative treatment program is in the patient's best interest. To inform and help guide patients properly in this difficult decision making process, all consultants need to provide expert opinions, if indicated, before a surgical recommendation is made. Pulling all the pieces together—depth, location and type of tumor, lymph node and distant organ involvement, nutritional status, and underlying medical condition of the patient—a curative or palliative treatment plan can be created.

**Treatment for Cure** Fewer than 50% of patients presenting with esophageal cancer are eligible for surgical resection. In patients for whom a cure is possible, treatment may include chemotherapy, radiation therapy, surgical resection, or a combination of these modalities. In patients with local tumor that does not involve other vital structures, who bear no evidence of distant disease, and whose clinical and nutritional status are adequate, curative treatment is implemented. Those patients with significant comorbidities, evidence of advanced or distant disease, or poor nutritional status are considered for palliation. Using the AJCC staging system, surgery is considered for any patient presenting in stage 1 through 3. Patients with stage 4 cancer are recommended to undergo definitive treatment with chemoradiotherapy.

Although controversy surrounds the medical and surgical treatment of esophageal cancer, there are some general guidelines on which most physicians will agree. The treatment for patients presenting with stage I cancer, T1 N0, is surgical resection only. If the surgical specimen reveals more advanced disease, adjuvant chemotherapy is considered. The treatment of patients presenting with stage II disease (T2 Nx, T3 N0) is the most controversial. Surgical resection is indicated, but opinions vary as to the best type of surgical resection and if there is a need for chemotherapy. If chemotherapy is recommended, it is given in the neoadjuvant setting. Treatment of patients presenting with stage III disease (T3 N1, T4 N0) is also debated, but a little less so. Most physicians agree that multimodality therapy is needed, but the timing and type of surgical resection remain unresolved. Advocates of aggressive surgical resection (three-field en bloc esophagectomy, with a radical thoracic and abdominal lymphadenectomy) disagree with those who advocate multimodal therapy with neoadjuvant chemoradiotherapy followed by a more conservative surgical approach (transhiatal or transthoracic esophagectomy). Scientific evidence supporting the benefit of one over the other is lacking.

***Chemotherapy*** Although there is still no complete understanding of tumor biology, the concept that tumors begin in a particular location and spread by vascular and lymphatic channels is accepted. This may be an overly simplistic view of the true nature of malignancy but, nevertheless, it is the premise on which we have established management of esophageal cancer. In the earliest days of treatment, the only chance for cure was surgical excision of the primary tumor and regional tissues that might be involved. With the advent of chemotherapy, the management of cancer has changed dramatically, with surgery playing a less aggressive role. However, in the case of many cancers for which surgery is no longer a central theme, the chemotherapy available to treat those tumors is effective and can control and often eradicate local and distant tumors. Unfortunately, in esophageal and gastric tumors, this is not the case. Although some improvements have been made, chemotherapy for gastric and esophageal cancers remains poorly able to control local and distant disease. The best complete response rate for adenocarcinomas is 25% when chemotherapy is given in combination with radiation. Squamous cell cancers respond more favorably than adenocarcinomas but, without surgery or radiation therapy, chemotherapy is limited in its ability to achieve a cure.

Studies have shown that there is limited benefit to chemotherapy in combination with surgery, with or without the addition of radiation. Although there is a trend toward improved survival with neoadjuvant chemotherapy, there is nothing to suggest that adjuvant chemotherapy is of any added benefit. However, the addition of radiotherapy to a neoadjuvant chemotherapeutic regimen has shown a slight improvement in long-term survival. The type of chemotherapy used is dependent on a number of factors, such as mechanism of action, drug side effects, and drug cost. There are six major categories of chemotherapeutic agents, as defined by their mechanism of action, that are used to treat esophageal cancers. The response to single-agent therapy (20% to 30%) is lower than with combination therapy (45% to 55%), and the response of metastatic disease (25% to 35%) is lower than that of locoregional disease (45% to 75%).

Since its introduction in 1980, cisplatin has emerged as the cornerstone of combination therapy in esophageal cancer. As a single agent, it has a response rate of 25% to 30%. Given in combination with 5-fluorouracil, a response rate of 50% may be achieved; this is an established chemotherapeutic regimen for esophageal cancer. Administered once a week over a period of 2 to 10 weeks, up to eight cycles of chemotherapy are infused. Neoadjuvant treatment is usually limited to four cycles, whereas definitive therapy can be administered up to 3 months if the patient tolerates the side effects. The addition of a third agent, including (but not limited to) mitomycin C,[33] etoposide, and paclitaxel, is gaining favor and has resulted in some improvement in locoregional control and short-term survival. The use of new drugs and different combination therapy is encouraged, but patients need to be counseled about survival with established versus nonestablished therapy. There is a fine line between offering hope and taking advantage of the trusting naiveté of an emotionally fragile patient.

***Radiation Therapy*** Radiation therapy is used to control the tumor locally but is rarely administered alone. Given as definitive treatment, a total dose of 6000 to 6400 cGy in 180- to 200-cGy fractions is given 5 days a week for a period of 6 to 7 weeks. Studies have demonstrated that there is no survival benefit to neoadjuvant radiotherapy alone; however, in combination with chemotherapy, a trend toward improved survival is noted (Table 43-10). A neoadjuvant regimen that has shown some promise is induction cisplatin and paclitaxel followed by combination chemoradiotherapy with 5-fluorouracil, cisplatin, and paclitaxel and 4500 cGy of external beam radiation.[34] When followed by surgical resection, the 2-year survival approaches 76% for stage II or III esophageal adenocarcinomas. Neoadjuvant radiation must be limited to 4500 cGy to avoid the surgical morbidity associated with extensively radiated tissue beds. Injury to the airway and great vessels and poor tissue healing are associated with high-dose radiation. Preserving the gastric conduit for replacement of the esophagus is critical; this is considered as the radiation field is prepared. Eradication of the primary tumor is not necessary and is not the goal of neoadjuvant radiation. A balance between control of disease until the time of surgery and preservation of the gastric conduit and adjacent structures is critical, and often difficult to achieve.

**Surgical Resection** There are a number of esophageal resections used to treat esophageal cancer, and no one technique has established dominance. In contrast, with better understanding of

**Table 43-10 Compilation of Randomized Controlled Trials of Neoadjuvant Therapy Plus Surgery Versus Surgery Alone**

| STUDY (YEAR) | NO. OF PATIENTS: SURGERY VERSUS XRT + SURGERY | OPERATIVE MORTALITY (%): SURGERY VERSUS XRT – SURGERY | SURVIVAL (%): SURGERY VERSUS XRT + SURGERY |
|---|---|---|---|
| **5-yr Survival** | | | |
| Arnott et al (1998) | 86 vs 90 | 8 vs 10 | 16 vs 9 |
| Nygaard et al (1992) | 50 vs 58 | 12 vs 12 | 10 vs 21 |
| Wang et al (1989) | 102 vs 104 | 5 vs 5 | 37 vs 33 |
| Launois et al (1981) | 57 vs 67 | 11 vs 13 | 11 vs 10 |
| Gignoux et al (1987) | 106 vs 102 | 18 vs 24 | 10 vs 9 |
| **Total:** | 401 vs 421 | 11 vs 13 | 18 vs 17 |
| | **SURGERY VERSUS CRT + SURGERY** | **SURGERY VERSUS CRT + SURGERY** | **SURGERY VERSUS CRT + SURGERY** |
| **3-yr Survival** | | | |
| Nygaard et al (1992) | 38 vs 34 | 13 vs 24 | 11 vs 18 |
| Walsh et al (1996) | 55 vs 58 | 2 vs 7 | 7 vs 3 |
| Bosset et al (1997) | 139 vs 143 | 4 vs 13 | 41 vs 43 |
| **Total:** | 232 vs 235 | 5 vs 13 | 28 vs 37 |

Modified from Yau P, Jamieson GG: Adjuvant and neoadjuvant therapy for cancer of the esophagus. In Pearson FG (ed): Esophageal surgery, ed 2, Philadelphia, 2002, Churchill Livingstone, p 749, Table 47-1, 47-2.

*CRT,* Chemoradiotherapy; *XRT,* radiation therapy.

**Table 43-11 Factors Affecting Surgical Decision Making for Esophageal Cancer**

| TUMOR LOCATION | TYPE OF CONDUIT | SURGICAL APPROACH | ANASTOMOTIC LOCATION | ANASTOMOTIC TECHNIQUE | POSITION OF CONDUIT |
|---|---|---|---|---|---|
| Cervical<br>Upper thoracic<br>Midthoracic<br>Distal, cardia | THE<br>TTE<br>EBE<br>VSE<br>MIE | Cervical<br>Intrathoracic<br>Intra-abdominal (lower mediastinal) | Hand-sewn<br>Stapled | Gastric<br>Free jejunum<br>Supercharged jejunum<br>Colon<br>Forearm free graft | Posterior mediastinum<br>Pleural space<br>Substernal<br>Subcutaneous |

tumor biology, improved chemotherapy, and advanced technology, more surgical techniques are emerging. There are no prospective trials randomizing surgical resection options. All the data used to guide surgical therapy have come from retrospective reviews or clinical bias. A lack of patients and financial resources to perform randomized surgical trials results in training and institutional biases that drive the polarized surgical dogmas and individual preferences for particular surgical techniques. Several factors affect surgical decision making and subsequent operative and long-term outcomes (Table 43-11):

1. Location of the tumor
2. Surgical approach
3. Location of the anastomosis
4. Anastomotic technique
5. Type of replacement conduit
6. Position of the conduit

### *Location of the Tumor*

APPROACH TO CERVICAL TUMORS Most tumors of the upper esophagus above the level of the carina are squamous cell carcinomas. Surgical excision with immediate reconstruction significantly improves survival over radiation therapy alone for patients with upper esophageal tumors. Every attempt is made to stage these tumors properly because invasion into the trachea, vocal cords, or recurrent laryngeal nerves or positive surgical margins significantly alter outcomes. Tumors that do not invade the trachea, spine, larynx, or vessels are resected primarily. Tumors adjacent to the cricopharyngeus muscle or the larynx are treated with two to three cycles of chemotherapy and up to 3500 cGy of radiation therapy before surgical resection. To be sure that the tumor is resectable, surgery is initiated with endoscopy, bronchoscopy, and cervical exploration. Interval resection of tumor and esophagus with forearm free-graft reconstruction or transhiatal esophagectomy with a gastric pull-up may then be performed. Lesions that extend into the thoracic inlet are treated with a near-total esophageal resection through the transhiatal or transthoracic approach to ensure a safe and complete resection. Under these circumstances, a gastric conduit is used. In circumstances in which it is not available or offers inadequate length, alternative conduits are considered.

APPROACH TO THORACIC AND CARDIA TUMORS There are a variety of surgical resections for tumors of the thoracic esophagus and cardia. The transhiatal esophagectomy (THE), transthoracic esophagectomy (TTE), three-field en bloc esophagectomy (EBE), vagal-sparing esophagectomy (VSE), and minimally invasive esophagectomy (MIE) are all applied. They vary with regard to size and number of incisions, location of the anastomosis, extent of lymphadenectomy, need for a pyloroplasty, and preservation of the vagus nerves (Table 43-12). They each have

**Table 43-12 Comparison of Esophageal Resection Techniques**

| | EBE | TTE | THE | VSE | MIE |
|---|---|---|---|---|---|
| Incisions | Neck<br>Chest<br>Abdomen | Chest<br>Abdomen | Neck<br>Abdomen | Neck<br>Abdomen | Neck<br>(Chest)<br>(Abdomen) |
| Anastomosis | Neck | Chest | Neck | Neck | Neck |
| Lymphadenectomy | Radical thoracic, abdominal | Available thoracic, abdominal | Available lower mediastinal, abdominal | None | Available thoracic, abdominal |
| Pyloroplasty | Yes | Yes | Yes | No | Yes |
| Preservation of vagus nerves | No | No | No | Yes | No |

distinct advantages and disadvantages and the risks and benefits are still debated.

***Surgical Approach***

Transhiatal Esophagectomy THE has gained popularity in the past 25 years. It was developed to reduce the morbidity from respiratory failure and intrathoracic leak associated with transthoracic esophageal resections. The transhiatal resection requires two incisions, left neck and abdomen. The stomach and esophagus are mobilized through an upper midline abdominal incision, avoiding a thoracotomy. Mobilization of the esophagus is done blindly with manual manipulation through a widened hiatus. The stomach is tubularized and gently passed through the posterior mediastinum and a cervical esophagogastric anastomosis is performed. Accessible lymph nodes in the neck, lower chest, and abdomen are removed, but there is no additional attempt to perform an extensive lymphadenectomy.

There are several distinct advantages and disadvantages to THE. Advantages include a decreased anastomotic leak rate of 3% using the stapled technique,[35] less morbid cervical leak if a leak does occur, and mortality rate of 4% that compares favorably against the higher rates seen with the TTE and EBE. Reduced operative times, less blood loss, and fewer cardiorespiratory complications have all been reported with THE. Disadvantages include a higher rate of postoperative strictures, injury to great vessels, airway structures secondary to a blind transhiatal dissection, and inability to perform a complete lymph node dissection.

Despite these disadvantages, the literature has indicated that THE remains the safest esophageal resection.

Transthoracic Esophagectomy TTE was the first operation designed to resect the diseased esophagus with the intent of curing cancer. The procedure requires two incisions, right chest and abdomen. Surgery is initiated through an upper midline laparotomy incision. After the stomach and lower esophagus are mobilized, a feeding jejunostomy tube is placed and the patient is repositioned on the left side. A thoracotomy incision is made and the esophagus is mobilized. The esophagus is transected at the level of the azygos vein and an intrathoracic esophagogastric anastomosis is performed. No additional attempt is made to perform a radical lymphadenectomy or preserve an additional envelope of tissue around the tumor bed.

The risks and benefits of the transthoracic resection are well established. The overall morbidity and mortality rates are slightly higher than those seen with THE, but no more than seen with EBE. The mortality rate is just under 10%; the morbidity rate approaches 30% and includes pneumonia, effusions, respiratory failure, atrial fibrillation, and myocardial ischemia. Because of the improved blood supply to the midstomach, where the anastomosis is placed, the rate of anastomotic leak is the lowest of all esophageal resections and is 3% to 4% in most centers. When an anastomotic leak does occur, it may be difficult to control and can lead to an intrathoracic infection, sepsis, and death. Significant reflux may occur in patients who have undergone a transthoracic resection and, in the presence of Barrett's esophagus, may lead to the development of recurrent disease and metachronous cancers. Despite these shortcomings, advocates of the Ivor-Lewis TTE continue to demonstrate good operative and long-term results.

En Bloc Esophagectomy EBE is an aggressive resection that aims to achieve an R0 resection. The key components of the EBE that separate it from the other esophageal resections are the addition of a radical thoracic and abdominal lymphadenectomy and a wide local resection of tissues enveloping the tumor. It is the most extensive of all esophageal resections and requires three incisions—left neck, right chest, and abdomen. Surgery is initiated through a right thoracotomy incision. The healthy tissues surrounding the esophagus are mobilized so that the tumor bed is not disturbed. The venous and lymphatic vessels, including the azygos, hemiazygos, and intercostal veins, are ligated and divided and removed en bloc with the specimen. A radical thoracic lymphadenectomy is performed and all mediastinal lymph nodes (including the right paratracheal, subcarinal, paraesophageal, and right and left inferior pulmonary ligament nodes) and diaphragmatic lymph nodes, as well as the lymphatic tissues associated with the thoracic duct, are removed. An upper midline abdominal incision is made and the stomach is mobilized. A radical abdominal lymphadenectomy is performed that includes removal of paracardial, left gastric, portal, common hepatic, celiac, splenic, and lesser and greater curvature lymph nodes. The gastric conduit is brought up through the posterior mediastinal space and a cervical esophagogastric anastomosis is performed.

The benefits of EBE have been debated by many who prefer a conservative surgical approach. Advocates of EBE are committed to the concept that an aggressive R0 resection is essential to establish locoregional control and should be considered as the primary treatment modality for patients with esophageal cancer.[36] They have argued that chemotherapy alone is not effective in treating nodal disease and should be considered only for patients with more extensive disease found at the time of surgical resection. Retrospective reviews carried out in centers that advocate this approach have shown an increase in 5-year survival in patients with early-stage disease who undergo EBE as compared with THE. It has also been demonstrated that for patients with fewer than nine involved lymph nodes, EBE has an improved 2-year survival when compared with THE (40% versus 32%) but, if nine or more lymph nodes are involved, there is no added benefit to the en bloc resection.[37]

Although the advantages of EBE are disputed, the additional risks associated with this operation are not. In centers that perform this radical resection routinely, a mortality rate of 4.5% and a morbidity rate of 51% are noted.[36] Most postoperative complications are pulmonary. The anastomotic leak rate of 8% is consistent with a cervical esophagogastric anastomosis. Although there are no reports of an increase in graft failure, it is known to be a significant problem by surgeons who perform this surgery. EBE remains a significant approach to resection of esophageal cancer; however, it is performed in few centers and is avidly contested by those who do not perform radical resections routinely. To determine the real benefit of one esophageal resection over another, a prospective randomized trial is needed. With few patients, resources, and centers willing and able to support a radical resection, this trial will be difficult to initiate and complete. Improvements in chemotherapy and nonsurgical therapies are likely to render the radical and perhaps even more conservative surgical esophageal resections unnecessary, as they have in many other cancer arenas.

**Vagal-Sparing Esophagectomy** VSE has gained favor in a few centers in the United States. It is similar to the transhiatal resection facilitating a limited nodal dissection and is advocated for the treatment of intramucosal tumors. The technique varies from THE only in the method of removing the esophagus without severing the vagus nerves. The esophageal resection is performed by stripping the esophagus away from the vagus nerves, performing a highly selective vagotomy, and preserving the function of the pylorus so that a pyloroplasty is not needed. It can be done using minimally invasive techniques. Results have shown improved gastric function over esophageal resections that include a vagotomy and pyloroplasty.[10] Incomplete resection of the esophagus is a concern, especially if multiple biopsies have been performed and scarring or tethering to surrounding structures has occurred. The morbidity and mortality are otherwise comparable to those of THE.

**Minimally Invasive Esophagectomy** In the past 15 years, MIE has gained popularity. Thoracoscopy or transcervical mediastinoscopy are substituted for a thoracotomy, whereas laparoscopy is substituted for a laparotomy. Short-term outcomes have shown that the thoracoscopic-laparoscopic technique is safe and effective and offers comparable results to THE dissection, with the added benefits of less pain and a shorter hospital stay.[38] Although these minimally invasive approaches are not aimed at achieving a radical resection, one study has demonstrated the attempt of a hand-assisted, minimally invasive approach to a radical thoracic lymphadenectomy.[39] As these techniques are refined and taught in surgical training programs, learning curves will fade and long-term outcomes will be established.

***Location of the Anastomosis*** Although the location of the anastomosis is determined by the type of surgical resection performed, the success of the anastomosis is not. As with any gastrointestinal anastomosis, good blood supply and a tension-free repair will result in success. In esophageal surgery, this is often difficult to ensure. Patients who have comorbid conditions such as diabetes, hypertension, or history of tobacco abuse have compromised microvascular circulation that could affect the viability of the gastric conduit. In addition, radiation injury induces vascular changes that prevent proper tissue healing. An intrathoracic esophagogastric anastomosis has a slightly better chance of healing. The cervical gastroesophageal anastomosis, on the other hand, is fraught with the dangers of necrosis of the tip of the tubularized stomach because of compromised blood flow from compression of the conduit in the mediastinum. Anastomotic leaks that occur before 48 hours are caused by graft ischemia as a consequence of inadequate arterial blood supply to the graft. Leaks that occur from 7 to 9 days are caused by graft ischemia as a consequence of venous compromise. A reduction of cervical anastomotic leaks has occurred with newer anastomotic and reconstructive techniques.

***Anastomotic Technique*** There are two techniques for performing an anastomosis, hand-sewn and stapled. A hand-sewn anastomosis is performed using a single layer of interrupted 4-0 absorbable suture. The stapled anastomosis uses a linear stapling device to create the posterior layer and a hand-sewn or stapled technique to complete the anterior layer. The stapled technique has been shown to reduce the rate of postoperative strictures and cervical anastomotic leaks from 13% to 3%. If an intrathoracic anastomosis is required, an end-to-end anastomosis (EEA) may be accomplished by a hand-sewn technique or a stapled technique (using an EEA stapling device), with equivalent postoperative results.

***Replacement Conduits*** There are several methods for reestablishing gastrointestinal continuity after esophageal resection for cancer. In most cases, the stomach can be used and is the conduit of choice. Short interpositions can be accomplished with a free jejunal flap or free forearm graft. The vascularity of the free flap is maintained with a microvascular anastomosis to the internal mammary artery and vein or available cervical vessels. For longer segments, a supercharged jejunal (pedicle flap with an additional microvascular anastomosis) and colonic interposition are both good alternatives. Over time, long segments of jejunum or colon may assume a sigmoidal shape in the distal portions of the graft and result in obstructions that often require surgical revision. With the exception of the gastric pull-up, all conduits require an additional enteroenteric anastomosis, which increases the risk for leaks and subsequent morbidity.

***Conduit Position*** There are several routes along which the replacement graft may be placed—subcutaneously, substernally, in the right pleural space, or in the posterior mediastinum. The posterior mediastinal space is the shortest route between the stomach and cervical esophagus, but is often inaccessible. Patients undergoing resection of the esophagus with immediate reconstruction will have an opened posterior mediastinal space, which should be amenable to placement of any type of replacement conduit. A substernal route is preferred if there is evidence of fibrosis or tumor in the posterior mediastinum. It is a slightly longer route and there is a small decrease in function over the posterior mediastinal route but, overall, a conduit in the substernal position has good functional results. The subcutaneous route is also an option, although it is cosmetically unappealing and functionally challenged. It also requires a slightly longer conduit and is used only as a last resort. A gastric pull-up in the posterior mediastinal position has the best functional result, and every effort is made to preserve and use this successful combination.

**Treatment for Palliation** Palliative measures include chemotherapy, radiation therapy, photodynamic therapy, laser therapy, esophageal stenting, feeding gastrostomy or jejunostomy, and esophagectomy. These measures are aimed at reducing tumor burden or restoring nutritional access and should be considered in any patient who has no chance for cure or would not withstand the rigors of treatment for cure. Chemotherapy will treat systemic disease and help reduce the overall tumor burden. However, it usually needs to be given in combination with radiation therapy so that control of the local tumor is obtained. PDT is an alternative palliative treatment that provides relief from dysphagia for an average of 9.5 months.[40] Endoscopic laser therapy is an additional palliative measure that may be used. It is effective in restoring luminal patency, with low morbidity and mortality rates (<5%). Endoscopy with dilation and stent placement maintains enough patency of the lumen to handle swallowed saliva.[41] The patient is counseled for an esophagectomy before dilation because perforation occurs up to 10% of the time. A feeding tube may still be needed to restore nutritional access. The average survival after placement of a palliative stent is less than 6 months.

Many patients are interested in nontraditional treatment options, such as herbal medicines and supplements, acupuncture, and chelation therapy. Some, such as acupuncture, may offer some palliation to pain, whereas others, such as herbal remedies, help abate side effects from conventional medical treatment. There is limited scientific understanding of the many alternatives that are available, and their use must be encouraged with caution.

## UNUSUAL MALIGNANT ESOPHAGEAL TUMORS

Most malignant tumors in the esophagus are squamous cell carcinomas or adenocarcinomas. These two cell types account for 98% of all malignancies of the esophagus. The remaining 2% comprises a variety of unusual tumors that can arise from different layers and structures within the esophagus, including the mucosa, submucosa, muscularis propria, and adventitia. Among them, neuroendocrine tumors, carcinosarcomas, melanomas, and sarcomas are the most common. They each have distinct locations and characteristic patterns of spread. In general, epithelial tumors tend to be located in the mid and distal esophagus, whereas tumors arising from the deeper layers of the esophageal wall are more evenly distributed throughout. These tumors have varying biologic behavior, which is reflected in their metastatic patterns. Regardless of the cell type, these malignant tumors have the potential to spread through one of four mechanisms:

1. Intraesophageal spread
2. Wall penetration with invasion of adjacent structures
3. Lymphatic spread to regional and distant lymph nodes
4. Hematogenous spread

### Background

#### Neuroendocrine Tumors

Neuroendocrine tumors are small cell tumors that originate from the argyrophilic or argentaffinic cells of the esophageal mucosa or carcinoid tumors that arise from cells of the amine uptake and decarboxylation (APUD) system. Small cell tumors are the most common of the unusual malignant tumors found in the esophagus. Both types of tumors are found primarily in the distal esophagus and carry a poor prognosis.

#### Carcinosarcomas

Carcinosarcomas are rare entities that are composed of carcinomatous and sarcomatous elements. The exact cause is not yet elucidated, but a number of theories prevail:

1. Collision theory, whereby two separate tumors collide and become one
2. Stem cell theory, whereby both types of cells originate from the same stem cell, with dedifferentiation of the carcinomatous cells into sarcomatous cells
3. Theory that the sarcomatous portion represents reactive hyperplasia, not malignancy

These lesions are often polypoid, are found in the lower two thirds of the esophagus, and carry a prognosis similar to their individual elements.

#### Malignant Melanomas

Malignant melanomas arise from malignant transformation of melanocytes in the mucosa superficial to the lamina propria. Although uncommonly found in the esophagus, they account for 17% of all unusual esophageal tumors. They usually manifest as a polypoid, ulcerated, pigmented mass in the lower two thirds of the esophagus. Satellite lesions may also be present. More than 50% of patients present with metastatic disease at the time of diagnosis. They are most commonly found in the distal two thirds of the esophagus and carry a poor prognosis if there is evidence of disease outside the esophagus.

#### Sarcomas

Sarcomas are a heterogeneous group of tumors that include leiomyosarcomas and Kaposi's, sarcoma. They constitute less then 1% of all unusual tumors. Leiomyosarcomas are the most common and arise from the smooth muscle in the muscularis mucosa and muscularis propria. They are found with equal distribution within the esophagus.

### Symptoms and Diagnosis

These patients present with dysphagia and weight loss. Barium swallow and endoscopy are the primary diagnostic modalities and can identify an obstructing mass in the esophagus. Endoscopic biopsy is difficult and is associated with a poor diagnostic yield, but must be pursued when possible.

### Treatment

The rarity of these tumors and the lack of available information regarding treatment and survival make it difficult to establish educated therapeutic decisions. Surgical excision by esophageal resection is the treatment of choice for tumors that are clearly confined to the esophagus. The approach is guided by the location of the tumor. Adjuvant chemotherapy may be advocated for small cell tumors and atypical carcinoids. Unlike patients with other cancers of the esophagus, patients with esophageal leiomyosarcomas who have distant metastatic disease can experience long-term survival after resection if the following factors are noted:

1. Complete surgical resection
2. Early stage
3. Low grade
4. Polypoid growth pattern
5. Thoracic rather than cervical tumor

With improvements in medicine and technology, treatment of these tumors may change, and endoscopic resection with adjuvant chemotherapy may start to play a role in the overall management of these unusual tumors.

## CONCLUSION

History is a story that offers guidance to the future; science is a method that guides the integrity of our work. The history of esophageal surgery, its successes and failures, offers guidance to those whose practice is dedicated to understanding the function and dysfunction of the esophagus. The practice of surgical science guides our consciences to make safe and effective therapeutic decisions in our surgical practices. It is up to the esophageal surgeons of the 21st century to create public awareness, educate medical minds, and explore the details of this gastrointestinal territory that our surgical forefathers courageously placed on the map. It is in our best interest to let science determine the surgical principles of our time.

The challenges that lie ahead will fuel our curiosities and our quest for knowledge as we struggle to define the complexities that lurk within the esophagus. Let us learn from history and proceed confidently and courageously as well-educated surgeons dedicated to understanding this seemingly simple organ.

## SELECTED REFERENCES

Banki F, Mason RJ, DeMeester SR: Vagal-sparing esophagectomy: A more physiologic alternative. Ann Surg 236:324–335, 2002.

This was the first paper to describe the technique of vagal-sparing esophagectomy and document the physiologic outcomes in detail.

Gu Y, Swisher SG, Ajani JA, et al: The number of lymph nodes with metastasis predicts survival in patients with esophageal cancer or esophagogastric junction adenocarcinoma who receive preoperative chemoradiotherapy. Cancer 106:1017–1025, 2006.

This paper discusses the notion that in addition to location and response to neoadjuvant therapy, the number of lymph nodes may be one of the most significant predictors of outcome.

Orringer MB, Sloan H: Esophagectomy without thoracotomy. J Thorac Cardiovasc Surg 76:643–654, 1978.

This landmark paper was the first to describe the transhiatal esophagectomy and document the outcomes in detail.

Park W, Vaezi MF: Cause and pathogenesis of achalasia: The current understanding. Am J Gastroenterol 101:202–203, 2006.

This concise review of achalasia gives a thorough overview of the evolution of the cause and pathogenesis of this disease.

Yammamoto S, Kawahara K, Maekawa T: Minimally invasive esophagectomy for stage I and II esophageal cancer. Ann Thorac Surg 80:2070–2075, 2005.

This is one of the largest series of esophageal cancer patients undergoing a minimally invasive procedure to treat early-stage disease. It has become an important study, suggesting that minimally invasive surgery may be a viable option in these patients.

## REFERENCES

1. Orringer MB, Sloan H: Esophagectomy without thoracotomy. J Thorac Cardiovasc Surg 76:643–654, 1978.
2. Sadler TW: Digestive system. In Sadler TW, editor: Langman's medical embryology, ed 9, Philadelphia, 2004, Lippincott Williams & Wilkins.
3. Keck T, Rozsasi A, Grun PM: Surgical treatment of hypopharyngeal diverticulum (Zenker's diverticulum). Eur Arch Otorhinolaryngol 267:587–592, 2010.
4. Colombo-Benkmann M, Unruh V, Krieglstein C, et al: Cricopharyngeal myotomy in the treatment of Zenker's diverticulum. J Am Coll Surg 196:370–377, 2003.
5. Park W, Vaezi MF: Cause and pathogenesis of achalasia: The current understanding. Am J Gastroenterol 100:1404–1414, 2005.
6. Richter JE: Modern management of achalasia. Curr Treat Options Gastroenterol 8:275–283, 2005.
7. Moawad FJ, Wong RK: Modern management of achalasia. Curr Opin Gastroenterol 26:384–388, 2010.
8. Deb S, Deschamps C, Allen MS, et al: Laparoscopic esophageal myotomy for achalasia: Factors affecting functional results. Ann Thorac Surg 80:1191–1194, 2005.
9. St Peter SD, Swain JM: Achalasia: A comprehensive review. Surg Laparosc Endosc Percutan Tech 13:227–240, 2003.
10. Banki F, Mason RJ, DeMeester SR, et al: Vagal-sparing esophagectomy: A more physiologic alternative. Ann Surg 236:324–335, 2002.
11. Tutuian R, Castell DO: Review article: Oesophageal spasm—diagnosis and management. Aliment Pharmacol Ther 23:1393–1402, 2006.
12. Code CF, Schlegel JF, Kelley ML, Jr, et al: Hypertensive gastroesophageal sphincter. Proc Staff Meet Mayo Clin 35:391–399, 1960.
13. Blonski W, Vela M, Safder A, et al: Revised criterion for diagnosis of ineffective esophageal motility is associated with more frequent dysphagia and greater bolus transit abnormalities. Am J Gastroenterol 103:699–704, 2008.
14. Switzer-Taylor V, Schlup M, Lubcke R, et al: Barrett's esophagus: A retrospective analysis of 13 years surveillance. J Gastroenterol Hepatol 23:1362–1367, 2008.
15. Pera M: Epidemiology of esophageal cancer, especially adenocarcinoma of the esophagus and esophagogastric junction. Recent Results Cancer Res 155:1–14, 2000.
16. Babar M, Ennis D, Abdel-Latif M, et al: Differential molecular changes in patients with asymptomatic long-segment Barrett's esophagus treated by antireflux surgery or medical therapy. Am J Surg 199:137–143, 2010.

17. Rossi M, Barreca M, de Bortoli N, et al: Efficacy of Nissen fundoplication versus medical therapy in the regression of low-grade dysplasia in patients with Barrett esophagus: A prospective study. Ann Surg 243:58–63, 2006.
18. Stein HJ, Hutter J, Feith M, et al: Limited surgical resection and jejunal interposition for early adenocarcinoma of the distal esophagus. Semin Thorac Cardiovasc Surg 19:72–78, 2007.
19. Betalli P, Falchetti D, Giuliani S, et al: Caustic ingestion in children: Is endoscopy always indicated? The results of an Italian multicenter observational study. Gastrointest Endosc 68:434–439, 2008.
20. Reed MF, Mathisen DJ: Tracheoesophageal fistula. Chest Surg Clin N Am 13:271–289, 2003.
21. Islam S, Cavanaugh E, Honeke R, et al: Diagnosis of a proximal tracheoesophageal fistula using three-dimensional CT scan: a case report. J Pediatr Surg 39:100–102, 2004.
22. Tzifa KT, Maxwell EL, Chait P, et al: Endoscopic treatment of congenital H-Type and recurrent tracheoesophageal fistula with electrocautery and histoacryl glue. Int J Pediatr Otorhinolaryngol 70:925–930, 2006.
23. Altorjay A, Mucs M, Rull M, et al: Recurrent, nonmalignant tracheoesophageal fistulas and the need for surgical improvisation. Ann Thorac Surg 89:1789–1796, 2010.
24. Cassier PA, Blay JY: Molecular response prediction in gastrointestinal stromal tumors. Target Oncol 5:29–37, 2010.
25. Mutrie CJ, Donahue DM, Wain JC, et al: Esophageal leiomyoma: A 40-year experience. Ann Thorac Surg 79:1122–1125, 2005.
26. Kumbasar B: Carcinoma of esophagus: Radiologic diagnosis and staging. Eur J Radiol 42:170–180, 2002.
27. Sandha GS, Severin D, Postema E, et al: Is positron emission tomography useful in locoregional staging of esophageal cancer? Results of a multidisciplinary initiative comparing CT, positron emission tomography, and EUS. Gastrointest Endosc 67:402–409, 2008.
28. Krasna MJ, Reed CE, Nedzwiecki D, et al: CALGB 9380: A prospective trial of the feasibility of thoracoscopy/laparoscopy in staging esophageal cancer. Ann Thorac Surg 71:1073–1079, 2001.
29. Eguchi T, Nakanishi Y, Shimoda T, et al: Histopathological criteria for additional treatment after endoscopic mucosal resection for esophageal cancer: Analysis of 464 surgically resected cases. Mod Pathol 19:475–480, 2006.
30. Maish MS, DeMeester SR: Endoscopic mucosal resection as a staging technique to determine the depth of invasion of esophageal adenocarcinoma. Ann Thorac Surg 78:1777–1782, 2004.
31. Yamamoto S, Kawahara K, Maekawa T, et al: Minimally invasive esophagectomy for stage I and II esophageal cancer. Ann Thorac Surg 80:2070–2075, 2005.
32. Gu Y, Swisher SG, Ajani JA, et al: The number of lymph nodes with metastasis predicts survival in patients with esophageal or esophagogastric junction adenocarcinoma who receive preoperative chemoradiation. Cancer 106:1017–1025, 2006.
33. Geh JI, Bond SJ, Bentzen SM, et al: Systematic overview of preoperative (neoadjuvant) chemoradiotherapy trials in oesophageal cancer: Evidence of a radiation and chemotherapy dose response. Radiother Oncol 78:236–244, 2006.
34. Henry LR, Goldberg M, Scott W, et al: Induction cisplatin and paclitaxel followed by combination chemoradiotherapy with 5-fluorouracil, cisplatin, and paclitaxel before resection in localized esophageal cancer: A phase II report. Ann Surg Oncol 13:214–220, 2006.
35. Orringer MB, Marshall B, Iannettoni MD: Eliminating the cervical esophagogastric anastomotic leak with a side-to-side stapled anastomosis. J Thorac Cardiovasc Surg 119:277–288, 2000.
36. Portale G, Hagen JA, Peters JH, et al: Modern 5-year survival of resectable esophageal adenocarcinoma: Single-institution experience with 263 patients. J Am Coll Surg 202:588–596; discussion 596-588, 2006.
37. Yusuf TE, Harewood GC, Clain JE, et al: Clinical implications of the extent of invasion of T3 esophageal cancer by endoscopic ultrasound. J Gastroenterol Hepatol 20:1880–1885, 2005.
38. Luketich JD, Alvelo-Rivera M, Buenaventura PO, et al: Minimally invasive esophagectomy: outcomes in 222 patients. Ann Surg 238:486–494; discussion 494-485, 2003.
39. Suzuki Y, Urashima M, Ishibashi Y, et al: Hand-assisted laparoscopic and thoracoscopic surgery (HALTS) in radical esophagectomy with three-field lymphadenectomy for thoracic esophageal cancer. Eur J Surg Oncol 31:1166–1174, 2005.
40. Moghissi K, Dixon K: Photodynamic therapy (PDT) in esophageal cancer: A surgical view of its indications based on 14 years experience. Technol Cancer Res Treat 2:319–326, 2003.
41. Bona D, Laface L, Bonavina L, et al: Covered nitinol stents for the treatment of esophageal strictures and leaks. World J Gastroenterol 16:2260–2264, 2010.

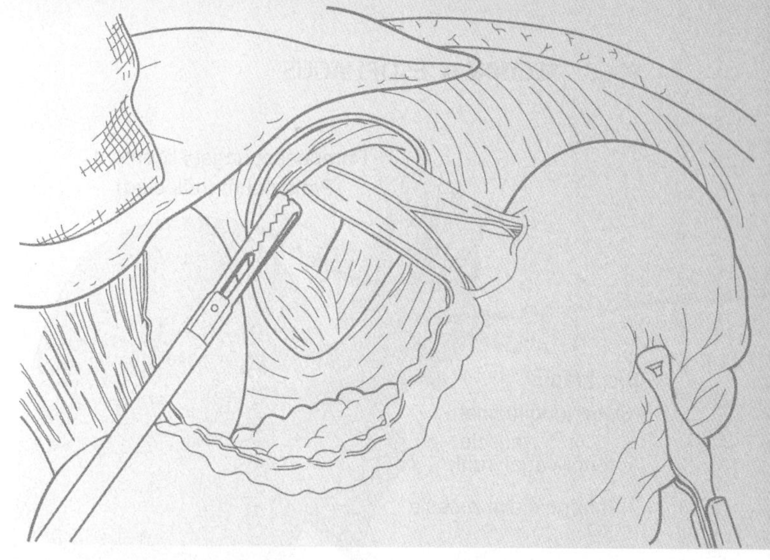

CHAPTER 44

# HIATAL HERNIA AND GASTROESOPHAGEAL REFLUX DISEASE

Rebecca P. Petersen, Carlos A. Pellegrini, and Brant K. Oelschlager



The role of operative treatment for gastroesophageal reflux and hiatal hernias changed dramatically during the 1990s. Once a relatively uncommon procedure, many antireflux operations and hiatal hernia repairs (mostly for paraesophageal hernias) are now performed in many centers around the world. The driving force behind increased surgical referral for treatment was the development of minimally invasive surgery. Although the techniques of antireflux operations have not changed, the approach to the operation has become more acceptable to the patient and referring physician because of the small incisions, relatively short hospital stay, and lack of associated perioperative pain when compared with open approaches. Thus, the surgeon must be familiar with all aspects of evaluating and treating both entities because he or she is ultimately responsible for the successful outcome of the patient.

## GASTROESOPHAGEAL REFLUX DISEASE

### Pathophysiology

The lower esophageal sphincter (LES) has the primary role of preventing reflux of the gastric contents into the esophagus. The sphincter is not a distinct anatomic structure but is a unique physiologic entity, located just cephalad to the gastroesophageal junction (GEJ). It is clearly identifiable as a zone of high pressure during manometric evaluation as the sensing device passes from the stomach into the esophagus.

Several factors contribute to the generation of this high-pressure zone. The first is the intrinsic musculature of the distal esophagus. These muscle fibers differ from those in other areas of the esophagus in that they are in a state of tonic contraction. They normally relax with initiation of a swallow and then return to a state of tonic contraction. The second contributing factor to LES pressure is the sling fibers of the cardia. These fibers are at the same anatomic depth as the circular muscle fibers of the esophagus but are oriented in a different direction. They run diagonally from the cardia-fundus junction to the lesser curve (Fig. 44-1). These fibers are responsible for a significant percentage of the lower esophageal high-pressure zone. The third contributing factor to the maintenance of the high-pressure zone in the distal esophagus is the diaphragm. As the esophagus passes from the chest to the abdomen, it is surrounded by the crura of the diaphragm. During inspiration, the anteroposterior diameter of the crural opening is decreased, compressing the esophagus and increasing the measured pressure at the LES. This concept is particularly important for the interpretation of esophageal manometry tracings. By convention, assess the LES pressure at mid or end expiration, thereby providing reliable, reproducible pressure measurements. The last component of the pressure generated at the lower esophageal high-pressure zone is the transmitted pressure of the abdominal cavity. The abdominal compartment has a relatively higher pressure than the thoracic cavity. A GEJ that is firmly anchored in the abdominal cavity will be exposed to a greater transmural pressure than one that is in the posterior mediastinum.

Gastroesophageal reflux may occur when the pressure of the high-pressure zone in the distal esophagus is too low to prevent gastric contents from entering the esophagus or when a sphincter with normal pressure undergoes spontaneous relaxation, not associated with a peristaltic wave in the body of the esophagus.[1] Other changes in the high-pressure zone, such as shortening, which occurs as part of cephalad displacement or as gastric distention from food or air, may also eliminate the barrier and result in reflux. Because even small changes in the high-pressure zone compromise its effectiveness, reflux episodes occur in normal people. The distinction between gastroesophageal reflux disease (GERD) and gastroesophageal reflux is a fine and important one and requires knowledge of associated symptoms, mucosal damage of the esophagus, total amount of acid exposure, and other factors.

GERD is often associated with a hiatal hernia. Although any type of hiatal hernia may give rise to an incompetent cardia, the most common is the type I hernia (Fig. 44-2*A*), also called a sliding hiatal hernia. A type I hernia is present when the GEJ is not maintained in the abdominal cavity by the phrenoesophageal ligament (membrane). Thus, the cardia migrates back and forth between the posterior mediastinum and peritoneal cavity. The phrenoesophageal ligament is a continuation of the endoabdominal fascia, which reflects onto the esophagus at the hiatus. It lies just superficial to the peritoneal reflection at the hiatus and continues into the mediastinum (Fig. 44-3). Although the presence of a small sliding hernia does not necessarily imply an incompetent cardia, the larger its size, the greater the risk for abnormal gastroesophageal reflux.

Hiatal hernias are classified by their anatomy into three types (I to III). Types II and III hiatal hernias are often referred

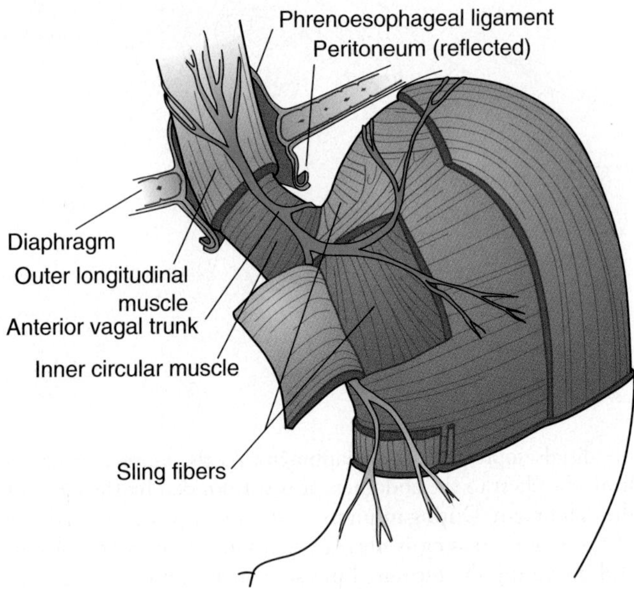


**FIGURE 44-1** Schematic drawing of the muscle layers of the esophagogastric region. The intrinsic muscle of the esophagus, diaphragm, and sling fibers contribute to the LES pressure. The circular muscle fibers of the esophagus are at the same depth as the sling fibers of the cardia.

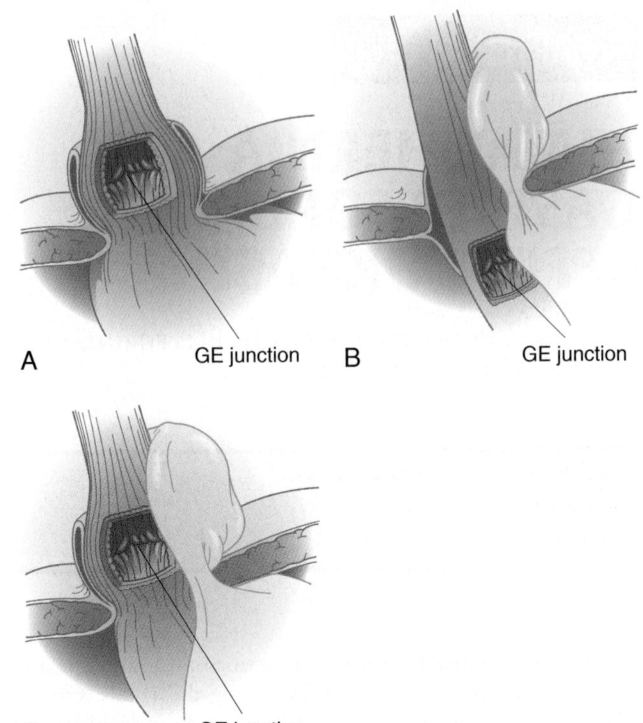


**FIGURE 44-2** The three types of hiatal hernia. **A,** Type I is also called a *sliding hernia.* **B,** Type II is known as a *rolling hernia.* **C,** Type III is referred to as a *mixed hernia. GE,* Gastroesophageal.

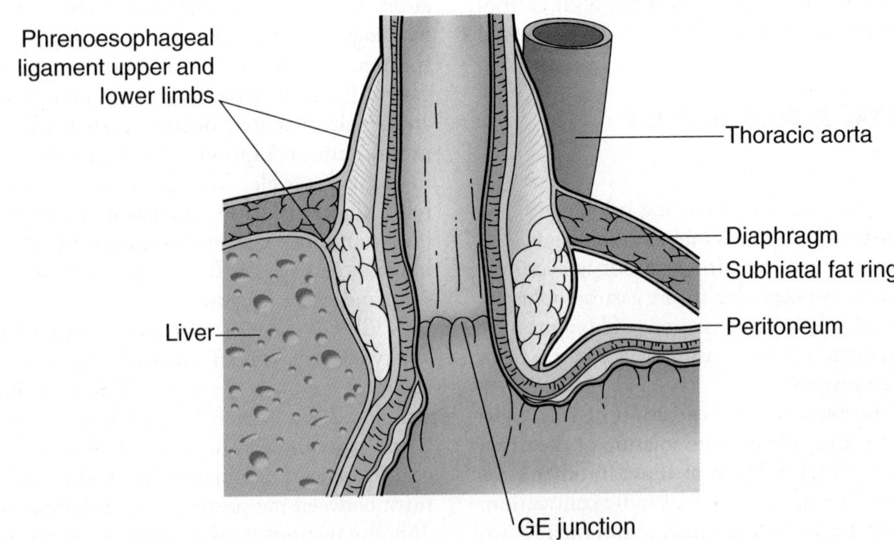


**FIGURE 44-3** Section of the GEJ demonstrates the relationship of the peritoneum to the phrenoesophageal membrane. The phrenoesophageal membrane continues as a separate structure into the posterior mediastinum. The parietal peritoneum continues as the visceral peritoneum as it reflects onto the stomach.

to as *paraesophageal hernias* and, although they may be associated with GERD, are also larger, more difficult hernias to treat and may be associated with acute or chronic obstructive symptoms. A type II hernia (see Fig. 44-2B), also called a rolling or paraesophageal hernia, occurs when the GEJ is anchored in the abdomen but the hiatal defect, which is usually large, provides space for viscera to migrate into the mediastinum. The relatively negative pressure in the thorax facilitates visceral migration. Usually, the fundus of the stomach migrates into the mediastinum; however, the colon and spleen are also occasionally identified. This is discussed in more detail later in this chapter ("Paraesophageal Hernias"). A type III hernia (see Fig. 44-2C) is a combination of the first two, in which the GEJ and fundus (or other viscera) are free to move into the mediastinum.

A hiatal hernia is neither necessary nor sufficient to make the diagnosis of GERD, and the presence of such a hernia does not constitute an indication for operative correction. The theoretical implications of a type I or III hiatal hernia being present is that the cardia and distal esophagus have the potential to be exposed to the negative pressure of the thoracic cavity. This would lower the pressure at the LES, thereby allowing reflux to occur more readily. Many patients with hiatal hernias do not have symptoms and do not require treatment.

## Clinical Presentation

The most common presentation of patients with GERD includes a long-standing history of heartburn and a shorter history of regurgitation. Heartburn, when typical, is a reliable symptom. Heartburn is confined to the epigastric and retrosternal areas. It is identified as a caustic or stinging sensation. It does not radiate to the back and is not characteristically described as a pressure sensation. It is best to ask the patient to describe in detail the sensation that he or she is experiencing. Sometimes, the symptoms will be more characteristic of peptic ulcer disease, cholelithiasis, or coronary artery disease.

The presence of regurgitation indicates progression of the disease. Some patients will be unable to bend over without experiencing the unpleasant event. A distinction between regurgitation of undigested and digested food needs to be made. Undigested food in the regurgitant is indicative of a different pathologic process, such as an esophageal diverticulum or achalasia.

In addition to heartburn and regurgitation, some patients suffer from dysphagia. Usually, dysphagia represents a mechanical obstruction and is more pronounced with solid food ingestion than with liquids. If dysphagia for liquids and solids occurs at the same time and is present with the same intensity, a neuromuscular disorder is suspected. When a patient is found to have dysphagia, peptic stricture of the distal esophagus is most likely to be the cause. However, tumor, diverticula, and motor disorders need to be excluded because this determination will affect the operative approach.

Other symptoms may be present in patients with gastroesophageal reflux. Most arise from the gastrointestinal tract; however, many patients will have symptoms involving the respiratory tract as well, called extraesophageal symptoms. The frequency of symptoms in more than 1000 patients evaluated at the gastrointestinal function laboratory of the University of Washington is shown in Table 44-1. Although many patients with gastrointestinal symptoms will also complain of extraesophageal symptoms, it is less common for a patient to present with only respiratory symptoms. This is discussed in detail at the end of this section.[2]

**Table 44-1 Prevalence of Symptoms in Gastroesophageal Reflux Disease***

| SYMPTOM | PREDOMINANCE (%) |
|---|---|
| Heartburn | 80 |
| Regurgitation | 54 |
| Abdominal pain | 29 |
| Cough | 27 |
| Dysphagia for solids | 23 |
| Hoarseness | 21 |
| Belching | 15 |
| Bloating | 15 |
| Aspiration | 14 |
| Wheezing | 7 |
| Globus | 4 |

*In more than 1000 patients evaluated. Symptoms reported occurred more frequently than once a week.

## Physical Examination

The physical examination of patients with GERD rarely contributes to confirmation of the diagnosis. In patients with advanced disease, several observations may help identify the source of the patient's discomfort. A patient who constantly drinks water during the interview is facilitating esophageal clearance, which may be indicative of continual reflux or distal obstruction. Other patients with advanced disease will sit leaning forward and carry out the interview with their lungs inflated to almost vital capacity. This is an attempt to keep the diaphragm flattened, the anteroposterior diameter of the hiatus narrowed, and thus the LES pressure elevated. Patients who have severe proximal reflux with regurgitation of gastric contents into their mouth may have erosion of their dentition (revealing yellow teeth caused by the loss of dentin), injected oropharyngeal mucosa, or signs of chronic sinusitis.

The physical examination may be helpful in determining the presence of other pathologic entities. The presence of abnormal supraclavicular lymph nodes in a patient with heartburn and dysphagia may suggest esophageal or gastric cancer. If the patient's retrosternal pain is reproducible with palpation, a somatic cause is likely. Short of these extreme presentations, the physical examination is generally not helpful in confirming or excluding gastroesophageal reflux as a pathologic entity.

## Preoperative Evaluation

The preoperative workup in a patient being considered for operative treatment will help confirm the diagnosis, exclude other pathologic entities, and direct the operative intervention.

### Endoscopy

Endoscopy is an essential step in the evaluation of patients with GERD who are being considered for operative intervention. The value of the study is its ability to exclude other diseases, especially a tumor, and to document the presence of peptic esophageal injury. The degree of injury can be measured using a scoring system such as the Savary-Miller interpretation (1 indicates erythema; 2, linear ulceration; 3, confluent ulceration; 4, stricture). The extreme of mucosal injury is Barrett's esophagus. Biopsy samples are taken to confirm the metaplastic transformation and to exclude dysplasia.

The endoscope has been used to grade the so-called flap valve.[3] This is interpreted on a retroflexed view of the GEJ. The flap valve is graded from 1 to 4, with 4 being a completely patulous junction, with the lumen of the esophagus in full view from the body of the stomach.

### Manometry

A significant amount of information about the function of the esophageal body and LES may be obtained from stationary esophageal manometry. This test will allow the surgeon to rule out primary motility disorders such as achalasia, which may mimic the symptoms of reflux and, in patients with GERD, will allow the surgeon to plan the operative procedure better by providing data about the ability of the esophagus to clear itself of ingested food. The manometry catheter is a flexible tube with pressure-sensing devices (water, perfused, or solid state) arranged at 5-cm intervals (Fig. 44-4). The upper esophageal sphincter (UES) is notoriously difficult to analyze because it migrates during the cervical phase of swallowing. Fortunately, the characteristics of the UES are infrequently relevant to clinical practice. The pertinent information to be gained from the manometry tracings concerns the function of the LES and the esophageal body.

The LES is analyzed for mean resting pressure. This may be determined in two ways, a station pull-through and a rapid pull-through. Most laboratories report the values recorded from the station pull-through. With this method, pressures are measured while the catheter is stagnant, with the radial ports at the high-pressure zone of the LES. Rapid pull-through measurements are obtained while the catheter is being pulled across the high-pressure zone at a rate of 1 cm/second. The latter measurements are usually higher than the station pull-through measurements because of the artifact of catheter movement. Normal pressures for a station pull-through at the LES range from 12 to 30 mm Hg. The sphincter generally relaxes to the pressure of the gastric baseline for several seconds when a swallow is initiated. Other information to be gained from the LES is the total length, intra-abdominal length, and location of the sphincter relative to the nares. The longer the high-pressure zone and the longer the intra-abdominal component, the greater is the barrier to reflux of gastric contents.

The esophageal body is assessed to determine the effectiveness of peristalsis. With the four channels located at 3, 8, 13, and 18 cm above the LES, the patient is given a series (at least 10) of 5-mL aliquots of water to swallow. Peristaltic activity is reported as the percentage of initiated swallows that are transmitted to each channel successfully. Normally, a patient has more than 80% peristalsis. The second characteristic of clinical importance is the amplitude of the peristaltic wave. The amplitude is simply the average of the pressures generated in the distal esophagus during effectively transmitted peristaltic waves. Ineffective esophageal motility is defined as less than 70% peristalsis or distal esophageal amplitudes lower than 30 mm Hg and is often associated with significant GERD.

High-resolution manometry is now being used to characterize esophageal function more accurately as compared with standard manometry. The specific advantage of high-resolution manometry is that it allows for effective continuous recording of motor activity along the entire length of the esophagus and yields a more complete and detailed picture of esophageal motility. A color-contour plot with time as the x-axis and esophageal length as the y-axis is produced by the recording device. Pressure is represented by a color scale (Fig. 44-5). This method also provides a more detailed analysis of the LES and is less likely to show a decrease in LES pressure with deglutition, sometimes referred to as *pseudorelaxation*.

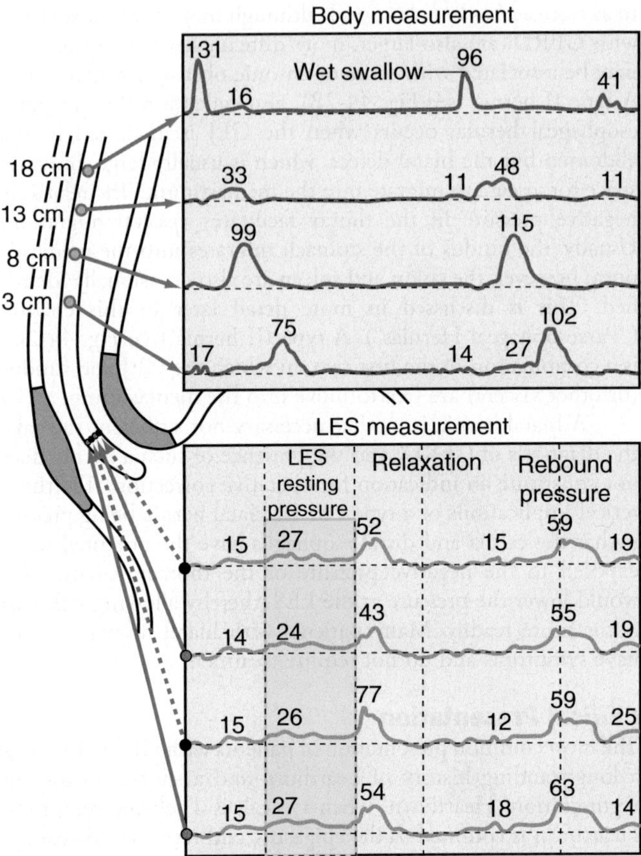


**FIGURE 44-4** Representative tracings from the body of the esophagus and the LES show the relative positions of the pressure-sensing channels during the study. Peristalsis is seen after a wet swallow in the body, whereas the LES is seen to relax to gastric baseline levels during the same interval.

### pH Monitoring

The gold standard for diagnosing and quantifying acid reflux is the 24-hour pH test. This study is performed by placing a thin catheter containing one or more solid-state electrodes in the esophagus. The electrodes are spaced 5 to 10 cm apart and are capable of sensing fluctuations in the pH between 2 and 7. The electrodes are connected to a data recorder that the patient wears for the period of observation. There is a digital clock displayed on the recorder. When the patient has an event (e.g., heartburn, chest pain, eructation), he or she records the event in a diary, noting the time on the recorder (Fig. 44-6).

A large amount of information may be gleaned from the study—total number of reflux episodes ($pH < 4$), longest episode

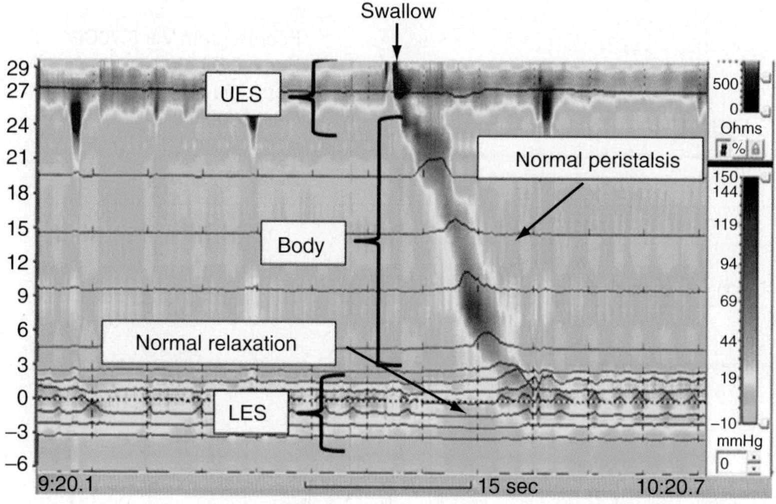


**FIGURE 44-5** High-resolution manometry—example of a normal swallow. Normal peristalsis is seen after a wet swallow in the body, whereas the LES relaxes during the same interval.

of reflux, number of episodes lasting longer than 5 minutes, extent of reflux in the upright position, and extent of reflux in the supine position. An overall score is obtained with the use of a formula that assigns a weight to each item according to its capacity to cause esophageal injury. This value, known as the DeMeester score, needs to be less than 14.7. A simpler way to determine whether abnormal reflux is occurring is to estimate the total percentage of time that the pH is below 4 in the proximal and distal channels. This is calculated by dividing how long the pH was lower than 4 by the total duration of the study and multiplying by 100. In the proximal esophagus (15 cm above the LES), acid exposure normally occurs less than 1% of the time; in the distal esophagus (5 cm above the LES), it normally occurs less than 4% of the time.

The patient's symptom diary needs to be correlated with episodes of reflux. The correlation of heartburn or chest pain with a decrease in the pH has significant clinical value because it helps confirm a cause and effect relationship. When interpreting these studies, it should be remembered that patients often do not maintain their normal activities and eating patterns when they have the catheter in place. Thus, their symptoms may not be as prevalent during the study period. If there is symptom correlation with low pH measurements, the suspicion of reflux-induced disease may be confirmed, even if the total acid exposure is normal.

Impedance pH testing is now being performed at specialized centers; this allows for further characterization of the refluxate as being acidic or nonacidic. Impedance monitoring detects reflux events based on the change in resistance to flow of an electrical current between electrodes, regardless of whether the refluxate is gas, liquid, or mixed. The intraluminal impedance increases with air and decreases with a liquid bolus. As compared with standard pH monitoring, impedance pH testing can distinguish between a true reflux event and ingestion of an acidic beverage by characterizing retrograde movement, as opposed to antegrade (normal swallow) along the esophagus. Also, another advantage is the ability of impedance pH testing to determine the proximal extent of reflux, which may be particularly useful for patients with extraesophageal symptoms such as cough, hoarseness, wheezing, or aspiration. One disadvantage, however, is that the automated analytic software tends to overestimate the number of reflux episodes, making it mandatory for all studies to be personally reviewed and edited manually, which can be time-consuming. Several studies have revealed that 30% to 40% of patients with persistent symptoms, despite maximal proton pump inhibitor (PPI) therapy with normal distal acid exposure as assessed by standard pH monitoring, have non–acid reflux events, with a high symptom correlation.[4,5] These persistent complaints tend to be regurgitation, chest pain, cough and, much less frequently heartburn. Currently, it remains unclear how impedance pH testing should be implemented in the clinical management of GERD. Until more research has been carried out, it should only be performed at specialized esophageal centers and in select patients. It tends to have the highest yield in patients with atypical symptoms of GERD or in patients with pulmonary symptoms thought to be related to or exacerbated by proximal esophageal reflux events.[6]

### Esophagography

The esophagogram provides valuable information in the evaluation of patients with symptoms of GERD when an operation is contemplated or when the symptoms do not respond as expected. Often, spontaneous reflux during the examination will be demonstrated. Although reflux may be induced in patients who do not have the disease, the occurrence of spontaneous reflux lends support to the diagnosis of abnormal gastroesophageal reflux. The true value of the study is to determine the external anatomy of the esophagus and proximal stomach. The presence and size of a hiatal hernia may be characterized (Fig. 44-7). Although this neither confirms nor refutes the presence of disease, it is extremely beneficial in planning the operation. A mediastinal GEJ that does not reduce into the peritoneal cavity during the study is a predictor of a more difficult operation that may require an esophageal lengthening procedure. Peptic esophageal strictures may also be found on an esophageal contrast study. The presence of a stricture will taint the interpretation of the 24-hour pH study, especially if it is tight enough to prevent reflux. Other anatomic abnormalities, such as diverticula, tumors, and unexpected paraesophageal hernias, will be discovered during esophagography. Esophagograms are being replaced by CT scans, which, when reconstructed, provide all

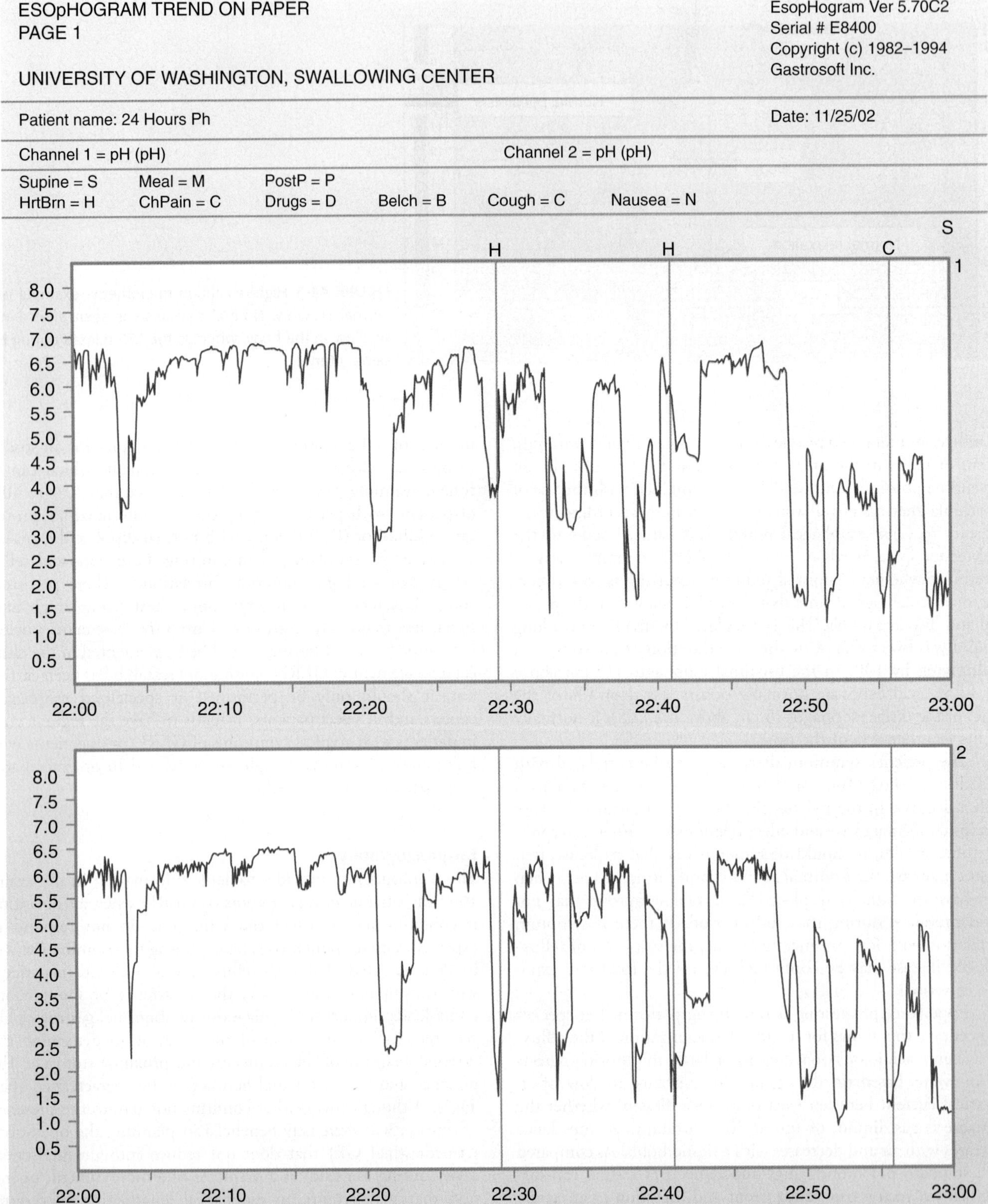


**FIGURE 44-6** Compressed tracing of a 24-hour pH study. Time is marked on the x-axis and pH is marked on the y-axis. Symptom events are marked along the top of the tracing. (Courtesy University of Washington Swallowing Center, Seattle.)

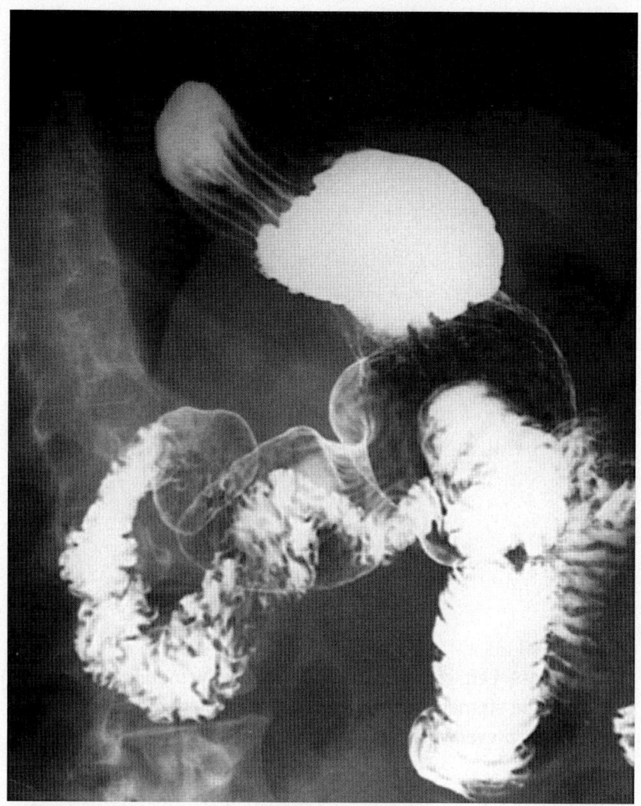

**FIGURE 44-7** Upper gastrointestinal contrast material study shows a large hiatal hernia with the rugal folds of the stomach clearly transgressing the shadow of the left hemidiaphragm.

the information of the esophagogram but have the benefit of providing information about the other adjacent organs.

### Other Tests

In unique circumstances, other diagnostic tests may be valuable. Occasionally, a patient will not be able to tolerate nasoesophageal intubation. A scintigraphic study to evaluate esophageal clearance and reflux may provide evidence of motility disorder and gastroesophageal reflux.[7] Gastric distention from delayed emptying may also be diagnosed with a scintigraphic study. Although this condition may contribute to reflux, it is not clear whether a gastric emptying procedure (pyloroplasty) needs to be added to an antireflux procedure in a patient with delayed gastric emptying.

Some patients have laryngeal symptoms of gastroesophageal reflux. Laryngoscopy and stroboscopic examinations help provide objective evidence of extraesophageal reflux; findings include inflammation of laryngeal mucosa, muscle tension abnormalities and, in severe cases, subglottic stenosis.

## Treatment and Outcome

### Medical Management

When a patient is first seen, a lengthy workup is not necessary if the history and examination are consistent with GERD. It would be prudent to check for chronic anemia in such a patient and to prescribe a 6-week course of acid suppression therapy. Most authors agree that a double dose of a PPI is the initial approach to medical management. Given in this manner, the use of medical therapy becomes in itself a diagnostic tool. If the symptoms persist after a trial of medical therapy, a more extensive evaluation, as described earlier, would be indicated. The medications available to treat acid reflux include antacids, motility agents, histamine 2 ($H_2$) blockers, and PPIs. Although lifestyle modification has been advocated before or as an adjunct to medical therapy, the efficacy of such changes in the treatment of esophagitis has not been proved.[8]

Pharmacologic treatment of GERD has been revolutionized by the advent of PPIs. This class of drugs is one of the most widely prescribed drugs worldwide and, in 2006, the expenditure on these drugs was approximately $24 billion.[9] These drugs act by irreversibly binding the proton pump in the parietal cells of the stomach, thus effectively stopping gastric acid production. The maximal effect occurs after approximately 4 days of therapy and the effects linger for the life of the parietal cell. Thus, the acid suppression will persist for 4 to 5 days after therapy has ended so the patient needs to be off therapy for 1 week before being evaluated with pH monitoring.

Compared with $H_2$ blockers, PPIs are more effective at healing esophageal ulceration secondary to acid exposure.[10] These medications are relatively expensive but are well tolerated. Side effects may include headache, abdominal pain, flatulence, constipation, and diarrhea. Recently, long-term side effects of PPI therapy have gained significant attention. Several studies have revealed an association between long-term PPI use and increased risk of nutritional deficiencies and infectious complications.[9] The results of these studies, however, need to be interpreted with caution, given that most were limited by small sample size and retrospective design. Larger studies have linked long-term use of PPIs to gastric polyp formation, usually occurring with more than 1 year of treatment. Most of these polyps are hyperplastic and do not appear to be malignant.

### Surgery

The indications for surgical therapy have changed since the advent of PPIs. Certainly, patients with evidence of severe esophageal injury (e.g., ulcer, stricture, Barrett's mucosa) and incomplete resolution of symptoms or relapses while on medical therapy are appropriate to consider for surgery. Other patients with a long duration of symptoms or those in whom symptoms persist at a young age are initially considered for surgery. In these patients, surgery is considered an alternative to medical therapy rather than a treatment of last resort.

Some patients have absolutely no response of their symptoms to the use of PPIs. They need to be scrutinized further before being offered surgical treatment, as opposed to being considered medical failures who would benefit from surgery. Because PPIs are so effective at decreasing the acid production of the stomach, the diagnosis of GERD in such patients is questionable and must be demonstrated with objective testing.

Since the application of minimally invasive techniques to the treatment of GERD, the cost of surgery has decreased. This has changed how surgical treatment is viewed. Considering the cost of PPI use and the cost of operative treatment with its accepted success rate, the length of time required for medical therapy to become more expensive than surgery is approximately 8 to 10 years.[11] This assumes that the patient uses the lowest dose of the medication. Therefore, in patients who have more than 8 years of life expectancy and are in need of lifelong therapy

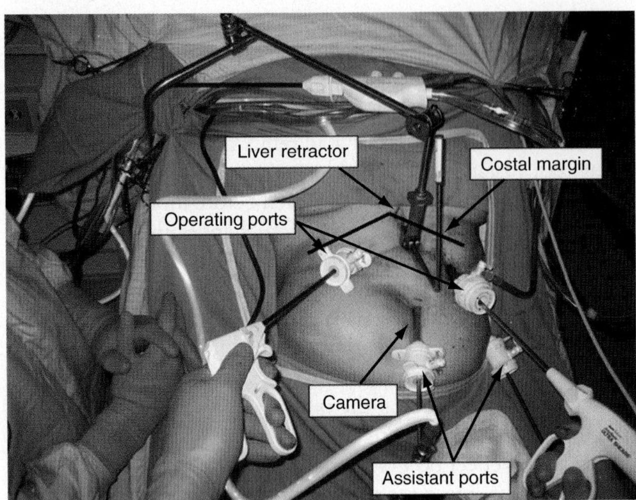


**FIGURE 44-8** Port placement for a laparoscopic approach to the hiatus. The surgeon operates through the two most cephalad ports (surgeon's right and left hand, SRH and SRL) and the assistant operates through the two closest caudad ports (assistant's right hand, ARH). *LR,* Liver retractor; *S,* videoendoscope.

because of a mechanically defective sphincter, surgical therapy may be considered the treatment of choice.

**360-Degree Wrap (Left Crus Approach)** The technique described here is the left crus approach to a 360-degree wrap (Nissen fundoplication), which is the procedure of choice for most patients. The left crus approach provides the advantage of a direct and early view of the short gastric vessels and spleen. After this obstacle is negotiated, there is little chance of injuring the spleen during the rest of the procedure.

The patient is placed in a low lithotomy position. The surgeon stands between the patient's legs, with the assistant on the left side of the patient. The four trocars and liver retractor are placed so that two equilateral triangles sharing a common medial angle are created. The surgeon operates through the two most cephalad ports. The assistant operates through the two closest caudad ports. The liver retractor is placed just left of the midline, in the subxiphoid region (Fig. 44-8).

With the assistant first retracting the greater curve and then the omentum, the left crus and greater curve are dissected by the surgeon. The short gastric vessels are taken early to mobilize the fundus (Fig. 44-9). With the fundus mobilized, the phrenoesophageal membrane over the left crus may be dissected until the crural fibers are identified. The entire length of the left crus is mobilized at this time (Fig. 44-10).

Right crural dissection is then performed by opening the lesser omentum and mobilizing this to the phrenoesophageal membrane on the right. Anterior and posterior dissection of the right crus will reveal the previously dissected left crus. Care is taken to preserve the anterior and posterior vagi during this mobilization (Fig. 44-11). Both will be contained by the wrap. A Penrose drain is placed around the esophagus to facilitate more proximal dissection and assist with creation of the wrap.

After the esophagus is mobilized, the crura are reapproximated posteriorly with heavy permanent sutures to allow the easy passage of a 52-Fr bougie (Fig. 44-12). The posterior aspect of the fundus is then passed behind the esophagus from left to right. The wrap is created over a length of 2.5 to 3 cm with three or four interrupted permanent sutures. This repair also allows the easy passage of a 52-Fr bougie (Fig. 44-13). With the bougie removed, the wrap is anchored to the esophagus and right crus at the hiatus. This helps prevent herniation and slipping. A similar suture is placed on the left (see Fig. 44-13, inset). The

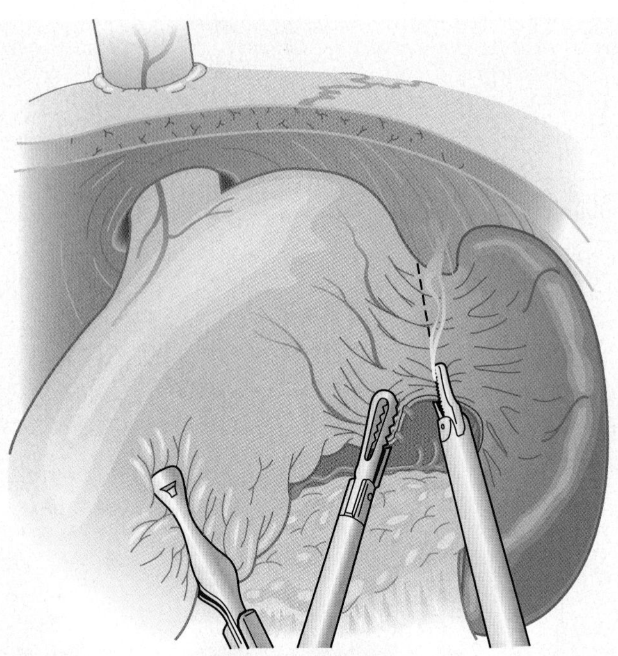

**FIGURE 44-9** Left crus approach shows early mobilization of the fundus of the stomach. The spleen is in plain view during dissection, which helps prevent injury.

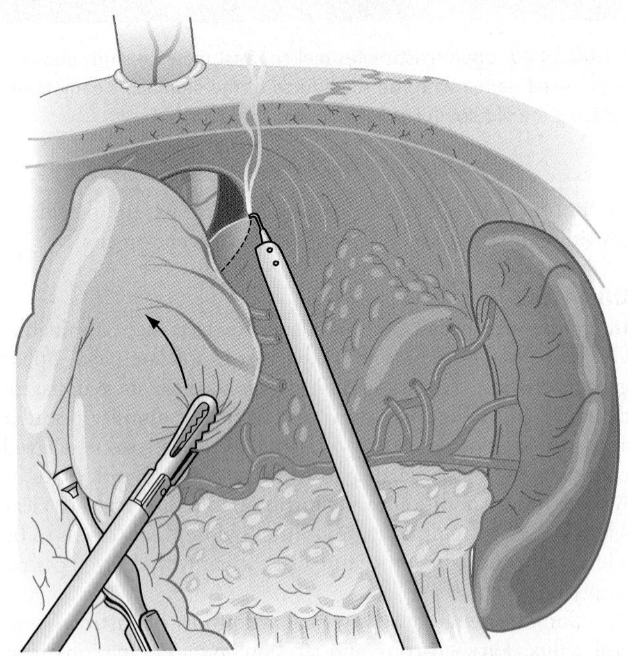

**FIGURE 44-10** After the fundus has been mobilized, the peritoneal reflection at the hiatus and phrenoesophageal membrane are incised anterior to the left crus to avoid injury to the esophagus and posterior vagus.

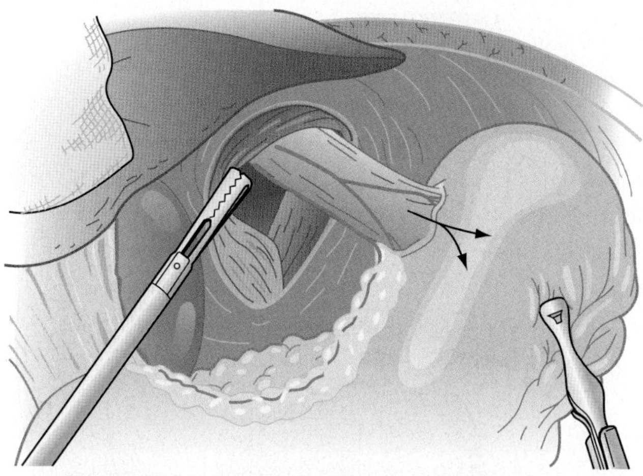

**FIGURE 44-11** Similar dissection of the right crus will complete the posterior and lateral exposure of the hiatus. As long as the dissection is performed along the crura, the likelihood of injury to adjacent structures is minimal.

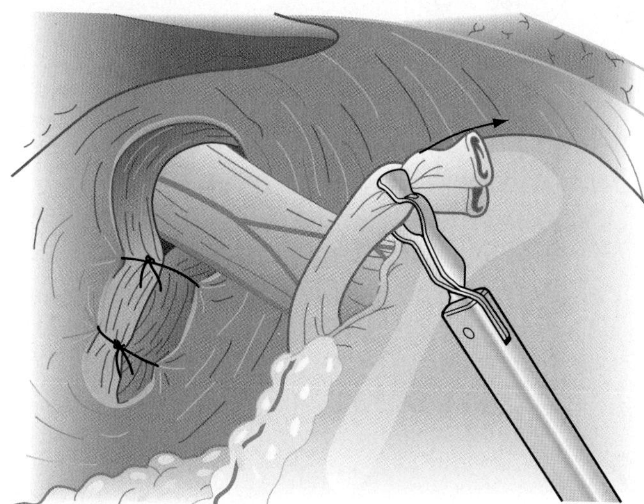

**FIGURE 44-12** Posterior crural closure is performed with heavy permanent suture. Note how the peritoneum and thus the phrenoesophageal membrane are incorporated into the closure. The exposure is facilitated by displacement of the esophagus to the left and anterior.

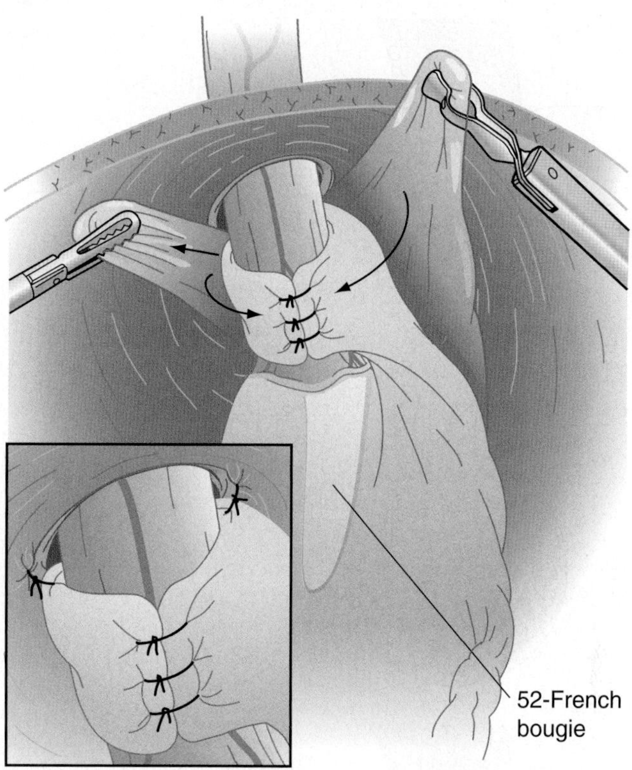


**FIGURE 44-13** The wrap is fashioned with fundus over a length of 2.5 to 3 cm. The bougie is placed after the first suture of wrap is secured to ensure a so-called floppy fundoplication. The wrap is secured to the diaphragm with right and left coronal sutures *(inset).*

wrap is anchored anteriorly and posteriorly to the crura with two additional sutures.

The wrap is inspected. The suture line lies just to the right of the middle of the esophagus. The posterior aspect of the wrap does not have redundant stomach, which would imply that the wrap was made too far inferior, possibly with the body instead of the fundus. There needs to be a gentle sweeping of the wrap toward the greater curvature (Fig. 44-14*A*). If it is angulated abruptly, there may be too much tension on the fundus. When all these steps are completed, the wrap is completed.

**Partial Fundoplication** When esophageal motility is poor, a partial fundoplication may be considered to prevent obstruction to bolus propagation in the esophagus. Although this was thought to be mandatory for all patients with ineffective esophageal motility (peristalsis <70% or distal esophageal amplitudes <30 mm Hg), this practice has been questioned. A recent randomized controlled trial conducted by Booth and colleagues[12] comparing laparoscopic Nissen with Toupet fundoplication, in which patients were stratified based on preoperative manometry, has revealed only minimal differences in regard to postoperative symptoms at 1 year. Interestingly, there was no difference in postoperative dysphagia between the effective and ineffective motility groups. Our experience is that a total fundoplication can be performed in most patients with ineffective esophageal motility, except perhaps those with absent peristalsis, without an increase in development of dysphagia.[13] Effective control of reflux with a total fundoplication usually improves premorbid dysphagia and often improves the esophageal motility. When needed, there are many types of partial fundoplications. Regardless of the type used, the initial dissection of the esophagus is the same.

If an anterior wrap procedure (e.g., Thal, Dor) is to be performed, there is no need to disrupt the posterior attachments of the esophagus (see Fig. 44-14*B*). The Dor and Thal fundoplications are created with the fundus folded over the anterior aspect of the esophagus. They are anchored to the hiatus and esophagus, as in the 360-degree wrap. The experience with these repairs is limited in patients being treated for gastroesophageal reflux. They are more commonly used in patients with achalasia after an anterior myotomy has been performed.

If a posterior wrap procedure (Toupet) is to be performed, the entire esophageal dissection is the same as for a 360-degree

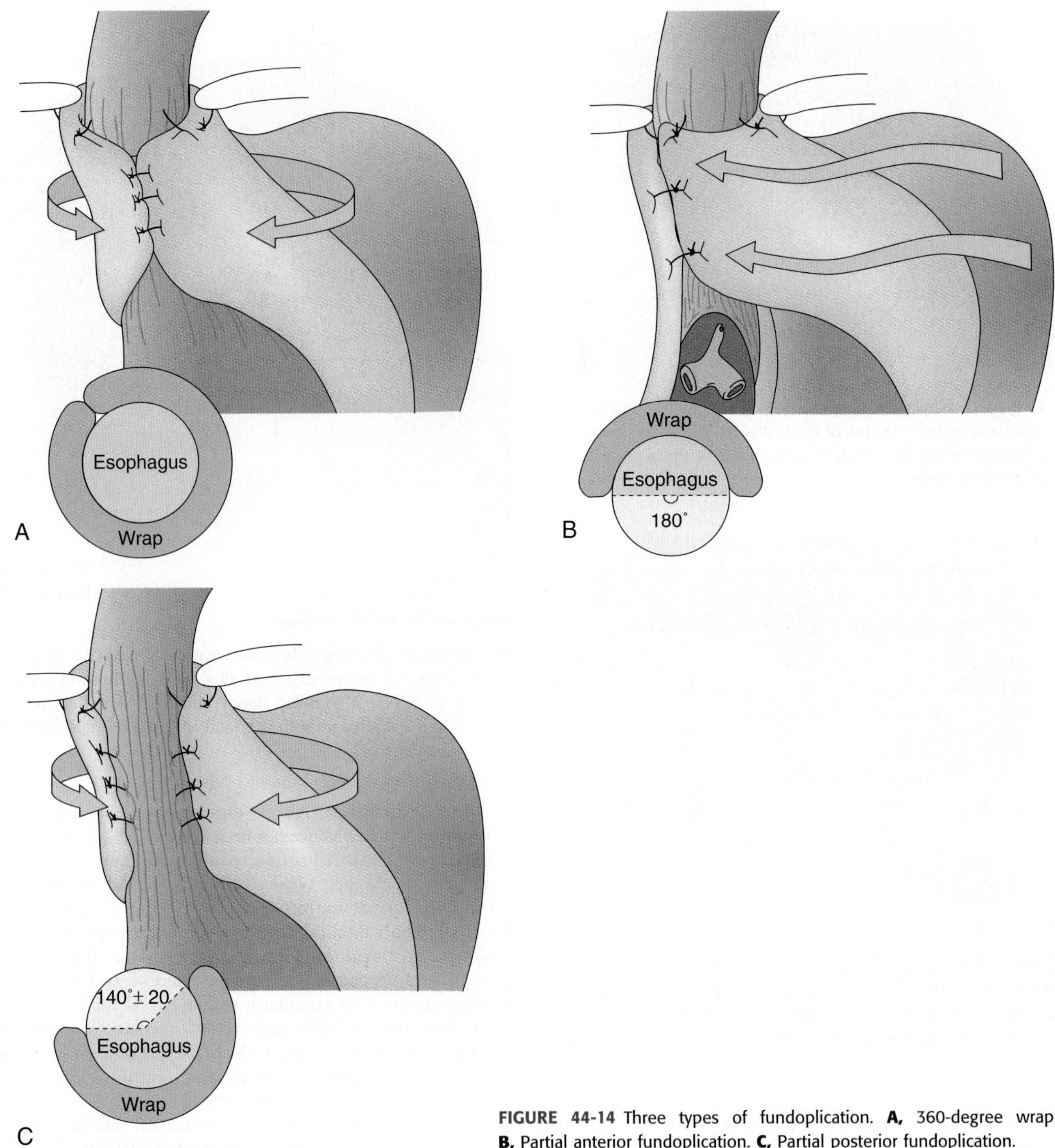


**FIGURE 44-14** Three types of fundoplication. **A,** 360-degree wrap. **B,** Partial anterior fundoplication. **C,** Partial posterior fundoplication.

wrap, and the crura are also reapproximated. The reconstruction of the posterior fundoplication is initiated by passing the posterior fundus behind the esophagus from left to right. The fundoplication is created by anchoring the posterior fundus to the crura and esophagus. The most cephalad sutures of the wrap incorporate all three structures (fundus, crus, esophagus). The wrap is anchored posteriorly to the crura with two or three sutures. The fundus is then sutured to the esophagus along the anterolateral aspects, creating a 220- to 250-degree wrap (see Fig. 44-14*C*).

**Outcomes** The results of operative intervention may be measured by relief of symptoms, improvement in acid exposure, complications, and failures. Several randomized trials with long-term follow-up have compared medical and surgical therapy for GERD (Table 44-2). Spechler and associates[14] have found that surgical therapy results in good symptom control after 10-year follow-up. Interestingly, 62% of patients in the surgical group were taking antisecretory medications at this time, although not necessarily for GERD because reflux symptoms did not change significantly when these patients stopped taking medications. In

**Table 44-2 Comparison of Surgery and Medical Therapies in Patients With Gastroesophageal Reflux Disease**

| STUDY (YEAR)* | ARMS | FOLLOW-UP (YR) | OUTCOME |
|---|---|---|---|
| Grant et al. (2008)[60] | PPI, $n$ = 179; ARS, $n$ = 178 | 1 | Reflux score: PPI, 73; ARS, 85; $P < .05$ |
| Lundell et al. (2009)[16] | Omeprazole, $n$ = 71; ARS, $n$ = 53 | 12 | Treatment failure: Omeprazole, 55%; ARS, 47%; $P = .022$ |
| Lundell et al. (2007)[15] | Omeprazole, $n$ = 119; ARS, $n$ = 99 | 7 | Treatment failure: Omeprazole, 53%; ARS, 33%; $P = .002$ |
| Mahon et al. (2005)[17] | PPI, $n$ = 108; ARS, $n$ = 109 | 1 | 12-mo GI well-being score: PPI, 35; ARS, 37; $P = 0.003$<br>3-mo DeMeester score: PPI, 17.7; ARS, 8.6; $P < .001$<br>3-mo % time pH < 4: PPI, 3.8; ARS, 1.4; $P = .002$ |
| Cookson et al. (2005)[11] | Omeprazole, $n$ = 50; ARS, $n$ = 50 | 1 | Cost-analysis: ARS broke even toward end of year 8, with cost differential between ARS and PPI therapy of ≈$1300 at year 5 |
| Spechler et al. (2001)[14] | PPI, $n$ = 91; ARS, $n$ = 38 | 10 | GRACI score: PPI, 83; ARS,79; $p = 0.07$ |

*ARS,* Antireflux surgery; *GRACI,* gastroesophageal reflux disease activity index.
*All studies were randomized controlled trials.

a separate randomized clinical trial by Lundell and coworkers,[15] in which patients with erosive esophagitis were followed for 7 years, surgical therapy resulted in 33% treatment failures as compared with 53% for medical therapy with omeprazole ($P$ = .002). Treatment failure in this study was a composite outcome variable, which was defined as a patient experiencing moderate or severe symptoms of heartburn, regurgitation, dysphagia, and/or odynophagia within 1 week of a clinic visit, recommencement of PPI therapy postoperatively, reoperation, or grade 2 esophagitis. Surgical intervention remained superior, even with dose escalation, in patients whose symptoms were not controlled by the initial dose of omeprazole. Moreover, the superiority of surgical intervention may have been even more pronounced because 34 patients, who were initially enrolled but had only a partial response to PPI therapy during the run-in period, were never randomized. Not unexpected however, the surgical patients experienced a higher frequency of obstructive symptoms (e.g., dysphagia, flatulence, inability to belch) as compared with the medically treated cohort. Recently, this same group has published their 12-year follow-up results and found that surgery still had fewer treatment failures compared with medical therapy; however, these results were based on fewer patients ($N$ = 71 with PPI [55%] versus $N$ = 53 with surgery [47%]; $P$ = .022).[16]

Another randomized trial with shorter follow-up also revealed that patients undergoing surgery compared to those receiving medical therapy had a significantly higher gastrointestinal well-being score at 12 months, in addition to a significantly lower 24-hour total percent acid contact time (pH < 4) and DeMeester Score at 3 months.[1] In regard to short- and long-term cost-effectiveness of laparoscopic Nissen fundoplication versus maintenance PPI therapy, Cookson and colleagues, in a subset analysis, found that surgery is cost-effective after 8 years of medical therapy.[11] Although more long-term follow-up studies are needed, antireflux procedures appear to provide an excellent alternative to medical therapy, with fairly durable results and few complications.

The experience with the laparoscopic approach for antireflux surgery has grown, especially because it makes surgery a more palatable alternative for patients. With this increased experience, reported results are better, especially in high-volume centers. For example, some groups have reported persistent control of GERD symptoms in 80% to 90% of patients and resumption of antisecretory medications in 10% to 20% of patients between 5 and 10 years after surgery.[18] Several long-term studies have been published that indicate excellent long-term results up to 10 years. A larger single-institution study following 100 patients undergoing laparoscopic fundoplication has found that 90% of patients remain symptom-free at 10 years.[19] We recently published our experience in a cohort of 288 patients undergoing laparoscopic fundoplication for whom the median follow-up was longer than 5 years. Most patients in this study had improved heartburn (90%) and regurgitation (92%).[2] These results confirm that a laparoscopic fundoplication can provide excellent durable relief of GERD.

## Endoscopic Therapy

Several endoscopic therapeutic approaches have been proposed for the treatment of GERD over the past decade. Endoscopic therapy continues to gain increasing interest because this treatment modality is theoretically less invasive than standard laparoscopic fundoplication. Several endoscopic treatments using varying techniques aimed at augmenting the LES have included radiofrequency energy (Mederi Therapeutics, Inc., Greenwich, CT), injection of inert biopolymers (Enteryx, Boston Scientific, Natick, Mass), creation of gastroplications (EndoCinch, Bard, Warwick, RI; EsophyX, EndoGastric Solutions, Redmond, Wash; Plicator, NDO Surgical, Mansfield, Mass), and other investigational devices, such as an artificial magnetic esophageal sphincter and implantation of an on-demand microstimulator in the LES.

Delivery of radiofrequency energy to the GEJ results in thermal coagulation necrosis and subsequent fibrosis, which may result in LES pressure augmentation and thus improvement of the antireflux barrier. Approximately 10,000 endoluminal radiofrequency treatments have been performed to date and there have been several studies reporting on its safety and efficacy.[20-22] Radiofrequency therapy has been shown in a recent, randomized, sham-controlled trial involving 36 patients to increase LES pressure at 12 months and reduce GERD symptoms, PPI use, and abnormal acid exposure.[20] Similar findings were found in a randomized controlled trial of 64 patients, published in 2003.[21] Patients in the radiofrequency arm at 6 and 12 months had decreased GERD symptoms and improved GERD quality of life score; however, there was no difference in medication use or esophageal acid exposure times when compared with patients in the sham arm. Although radiofrequency was one of the most widely used endoluminal therapies since its approval by the Food and Drug Administration in 2000 for the treatment of GERD, the device has not been available from 2006 to 2010, because the original producing company, Curon Medical, Inc. filed for bankruptcy in 2006 and was later acquired by Mederi Therapeutics, Inc.

One of the first endoluminal techniques used an endoscopic suturing device that re-created a fundoplication through endoscopic placement of suture to augment the cardiac flap valve. Since then, suturing device systems have resulted in improved short-term outcomes in regard to GERD symptoms, quality of life, and decreased medication usage compared with sham control procedures. Several studies have compared these devices to laparoscopic fundoplication and have shown variable results, with some demonstrating similar results and others showing inferior results in regard to symptom relief or medication usage.[21,23] In addition, some of the devices were associated with high re-intervention rates of up to 55% within 2 years.

Currently, there is only one available endoscopic suturing system (EsophyX), which consists of a flexible, multichannel endoluminal device that uses fasteners to construct a full-thickness valve at the GEJ during a single-device insertion. In a recently published study of 20 patients, it was shown to be associated with improved GERD symptoms and quality of life at 12 months, but there were no significant changes in LES pressures or total acid exposure from baseline.[24] However, 6 patients (30%) underwent subsequent laparoscopic surgery for persistent GERD symptoms, despite the addition of standard doses of PPIs.

In a larger multicenter study of 86 patients, most patients (>70%) had improvement in their GERD symptoms and quality of life at 12 months.[25] Of these patients, 81% discontinued daily PPI therapy. However, when the gold standard for objective measurement of the outcomes (pH monitoring) was used, only 37% of patients had normalization of esophageal acid exposure, a substantially lower number than would have been expected with laparoscopic Nissen fundoplication. With regard to serious adverse events, 2 patients experienced esophageal perforations during device insertion and 1 patient had significant intraluminal bleeding. Stratified analysis based on Hill grade classification revealed improved outcomes in patients with reconstructed, tight Hill grade I valves, suggesting a correlation between quality of anatomic reconstruction and improvement of clinical and physiologic outcome measures.

There are few studies that have directly compared the different endoscopic treatment modalities. One of these comparative studies evaluated the outcomes in 126 total patients undergoing a full-thickness plication of the gastric cardia or a radiofrequency treatment of the GEJ.[26] Patients were followed over a 4-year period, with a mean follow-up of 6 months, and both groups experienced a decrease in PPI use and in scores for voice symptoms and dysphagia. In addition, the radiofrequency group experienced decreased heartburn and cough whereas the full-thickness plication group had a significant reduction in regurgitation. A serious limitation to the study was the follow-up of only 51% patients. Based on these studies, endoscopic therapy for GERD is a feasible option for patients who are poor surgical candidates and who require more intensive therapy to control their symptoms, beyond that of standard medical therapies. However, until larger prospective comparison trials of standard laparoscopic fundoplication assessing long-term results are performed, endoscopic approaches should only be considered when laparoscopic approaches are contraindicated.

**Table 44-3 Complications in 400 Laparoscopic Antireflux Procedures**

| COMPLICATION | NO. OF PATIENTS (%) |
|---|---|
| Postoperative ileus | 28 (7) |
| Pneumothorax | 13 (3) |
| Urinary retention | 9 (2) |
| Dysphagia | 9 (2) |
| Other minor complications | 8 (2) |
| Liver trauma | 2 (0.5) |
| Acute herniation | 1 (0.25) |
| Perforated viscus | 1 (0.25) |
| Death | 1 (0.25) |
| **Total:** | **72 (17.25)** |

*Symptoms reported occurred more frequently than once a week.

## Complications

In general, complications have been reported in 3% to 10% of patients.[27] Many complications are minor and are related to surgical intervention in general (e.g., urinary retention, wound infection, venous thrombosis, ileus). Others are related specifically to the procedure or approach (e.g., splenic injury, hollow viscus perforation, dysphagia, pneumothorax). All complications in patients at the University of Washington are shown in Table 44-3. They may be divided into those identified at the time of the surgery and those identified in the postoperative period.

### *Operative Complications*

**Pneumothorax** Pneumothorax is one of the most common intraoperative complications, occurring in 5% to 8% of patients. The actual incidence of pneumothorax is unknown because routine postoperative chest radiographs are generally not obtained. Because the pneumothorax results from a violation of the pleural space by carbon dioxide, there is no need to evacuate the gas. Because carbon dioxide is absorbed rapidly and no underlying lung injury exists, the lung will reexpand without incident. If a pneumothorax is identified, the patient is maintained on oxygen therapy, and chest radiography is repeated 2 hours after the operation. The pneumothorax is resolved by this time.

***Gastric and Esophageal Injuries*** Gastric and esophageal injuries are far less common and usually result from overaggressive tissue manipulation or from passage of the bougie. Although usually reported as less than 1%, population-based studies have suggested that the incidence may be as high as 1.7% in inexperienced hands.[28] The injuries can be repaired with suture or an automatic stapler without sequelae if identified at the time of operation. If the injury is not seen at surgery, the patient will likely need a second operation to repair the viscus, unless the leak is small and contained.

***Splenic and Liver Injuries*** The incidence of splenic injury is about 2.3% in population-based studies, and major liver injury is rarely reported.[28] Splenic injury may result from dissection of the fundus and greater curvature. We prefer the left crus approach, which provides the advantage of a direct and early view of the short gastric vessels and spleen. Care must be taken during mobilization of the fundus to avoid excessive traction on the splenogastric ligament. In more than 2100 laparoscopic antireflux operations performed at the University of Washington, splenectomy has not been performed. Careful retraction of the left lobe of the liver will prevent significant lacerations and subcapsular hematomas. The use of a fixed retractor decreases the likelihood of liver injury.

***Postoperative Complications***

**Bloating** Early postoperative complaints of bloating may occur in up to 30% of patients; however, fewer than 4% of patients have the symptom after 2 months. There are at least three reasons for bloating. First, the patient may have more difficulty belching because of the wrap. Second, vagal trauma may contribute to delayed gastric emptying. Third, the patients will still have a tendency to swallow saliva (an unconscious effort to relieve symptoms of reflux) and, with it, a significant amount of air. Few patients require nasogastric tube decompression after the surgery.

***Dysphagia*** Postoperative dysphagia may occur in up to 20% of patients initially. A smaller percentage of patients require dilation for this problem.[2] Because the dissection of the hiatus and handling of the esophagus causes some edema, dysphagia caused by this is usually short-lived. When placing the wrap sutures, hematomas of the stomach or esophageal wall may result, resulting in dysphagia. If the wrap is too tight, the dysphagia is unlikely to resolve without dilation. The use of a graduated diet over the course of 4 to 6 weeks after the operation will limit the amount of dysphagia from the first two causes.

***Death*** Death is uncommon with this operation and is less than 0.5% in our experience.[2] Mortality does increase when age reaches 60 years, and patients older than 80 years have an 8.3% mortality rate.[28] This must be considered, along with the severity of GERD, when deciding to perform an antireflux procedure.

### Failures

Operative failures are patients who have persistent symptoms and physiologic evidence of continued acid exposure. The incidence is about 5% to 10%.[29] Most of these patients can be treated with acid suppression therapy, with good results. All patients who present with recurrent or persistent symptoms are evaluated with manometry and pH studies. If acid exposure is documented or if symptoms are severe, an esophagogram is obtained. The presence of an anatomic abnormality of the wrap, particularly a sizable herniation, is almost always best treated with surgery (Fig. 44-15*A*). If the esophagogram reveals good location of the wrap and absence of a recurrent hernia, an attempt may be made to treat the patient medically (see Fig. 44-15*B*). We have found, however, that in some cases, reoperation will relieve symptoms, even in patients with normal-appearing wraps on the esophagogram.

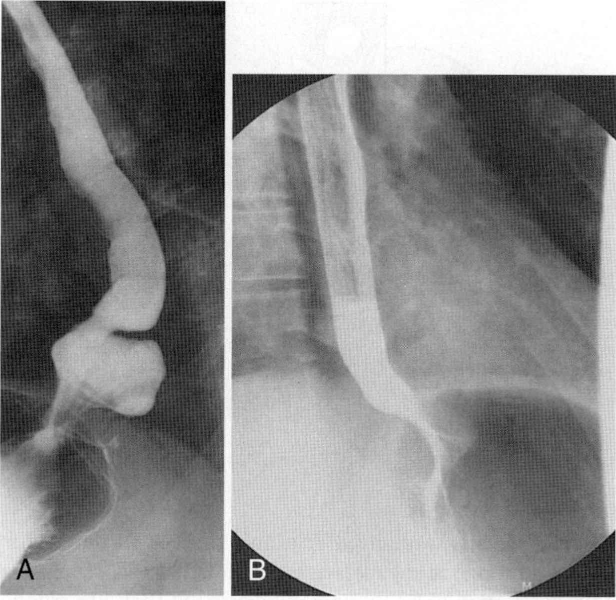


**FIGURE 44-15** Contrast material studies are invaluable for the assessment of persistent or recurrent postoperative symptoms. **A,** Patient with a herniated (into mediastinum) and slipped (wrap-around stomach) 360-degree fundoplication. **B,** Normal anatomic appearance of 360-degree wrap. Note the smooth tapering of the distal esophagus, the fluid level in the distal esophagus, and the air in the distended fundus above the wrap.

## Special Considerations

Within the purview of GERD, there are several entities that have received special attention. The surgeon needs to be aware of these variations and the considerations that arise from them.

### Strictures

Strictures pose a serious problem for the patient with GERD, although with better medical therapy, this is a fairly rare complication today. Dysphagia, a most troublesome symptom, often results from stricture formation. Furthermore, strictures are a manifestation of acute and chronic inflammation, which not only decreases the diameter of the esophagus but also shortens the esophagus, making operative intervention more difficult. The evaluation of these patients may be more difficult because the presence of a tight stricture may prevent reflux on the 24-hour pH study. The study would be ideally performed after dilation. Other causes of stricture (e.g., tumor, caustic injury) must be excluded before operative intervention. Strictures resulting from GERD are indicative of long-standing disease and may be associated with a shortened esophagus or Barrett's esophagus.

The most effective therapy for peptic stricture of the esophagus is an antireflux procedure. Although there is evidence to support effective symptom control with endoscopic dilation and PPI maintenance therapy, operative treatment results in fewer dilations per patient. Of 27 patients treated at the University of Washington for refractory peptic stricture, 21 proceeded with operative control of reflux. In these patients, the average number of dilations per patient was 2.8 preoperatively and 0.33 postoperatively. This compares favorably with the 6 patients who continued on medical therapy; they required an average of nine dilations per patient throughout the course of treatment.

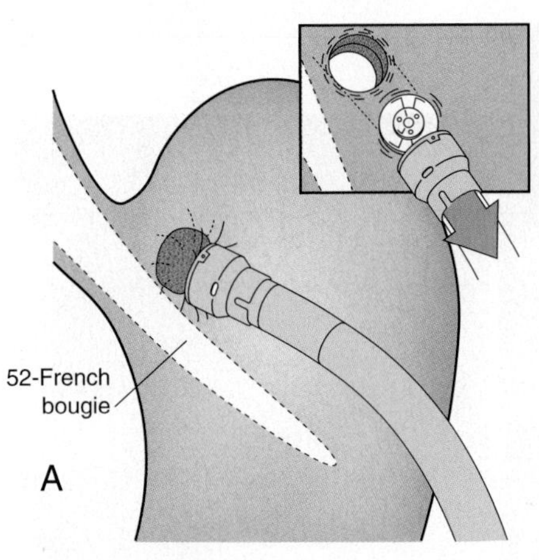


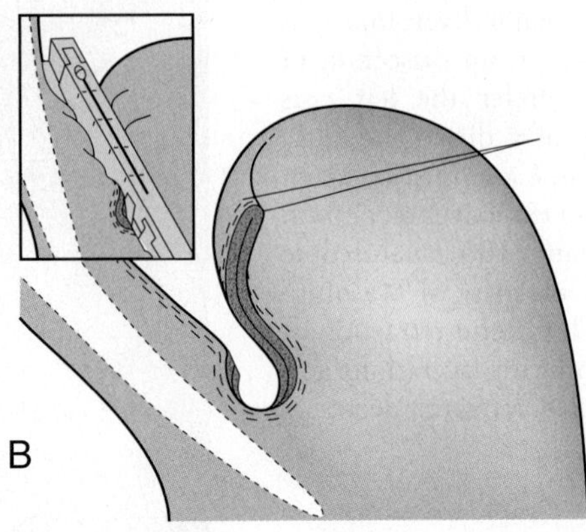


**FIGURE 44-16** Double-staple technique for esophageal lengthening. **A,** A circular stapling and cutting device is used to create a through and through opening of the cardia-fundus junction. **B,** A linear stapling and cutting device is then used to transect the remaining stomach toward the GEJ.

### Barrett's Esophagus

In some patients, prolonged acid and perhaps alkaline injury leads to a change in the esophageal mucosa from its usual squamous epithelium to a columnar configuration (Barrett's esophagus). The cells almost always extend proximally from the squamocolumnar junction in a contiguous pattern. If Barrett's esophagus is found, multiple biopsies are necessary to exclude dysplasia, which may indicate a tendency toward the development of adenocarcinoma. Although the incidence of adenocarcinoma in patients with Barrett's esophagus is about 40 times greater than that in the general population (Barrett's studies with increased incidence), the incidence of cancer in these patients is still very low.

Because Barrett's esophagus is the result of repeated injury of the mucosa by gastroesophageal reflux (of acid or bile), an antireflux procedure might be expected to decrease the rate of dysplasia and cancer. This issue is not resolved, however; the evidence in the literature is not conclusive.[20] Several studies have reported regression of intestinal metaplasia in 14% to 55% of patients after antireflux surgery.[30,31] Our experience at the University of Washington has supported this; we have seen regression in 55% of patients with short-segment Barrett's esophagus (<3 cm). Just as importantly, patients with Barrett's esophagus experienced excellent long-term clinical relief of GERD symptoms.[32] A more recent study by Rossi and associates[33] investigating the efficacy of surgery versus medical therapy in the regression of low-grade dysplasia in patients with Barrett's esophagus found laparoscopic Nissen fundoplication to be superior over high-dose PPIs. This was a prospective study in which 35 of 327 patients with Barrett's esophagus had low-grade dysplasia. At 18 months following therapy with high-dose PPIs or laparoscopic Nissen fundoplication, 12 of 19 patients (63%) in the medical arm and 15 of 16 (94%) in the surgery arm had regression from low-grade dysplasia to Barrett's esophagus ($P = .03$). Regardless of the impact of an antireflux procedure on the evolution of Barrett's esophagus, patients are examined endoscopically for surveillance of metaplasia after the operation is performed.

### Short Esophagus

As a result of repeated injury, the esophagus narrows (stricture) and shortens. The real challenge in these patients is in the operative approach.

By mobilizing the esophagus well into the mediastinum, a 2- to 3-cm segment of esophagus can usually be placed into the abdomen without tension. However, if this cannot be accomplished, a Collis gastroplasty may be performed. A double-staple technique may be used to create the neoesophagus (Fig. 44-16) after the dissection has been performed.

Unfortunately, postoperative physiologic testing on these patients has revealed an abnormal acid exposure in 50% of patients.[34] One reason for this is that the lengthening procedure often leaves parietal cells in the neoesophagus above the wrap. To deal with this problem, we have used single or bilateral vagotomy. Vagotomy, particularly when both vagi are divided and a thorough mediastinal mobilization has been completed, yields 3 to 4 cm of additional esophagus. In our study of 102 patients who underwent a redo laparoscopic antireflux surgery ($n = 50$) or paraesophageal hernia repair ($n = 52$), we performed a vagotomy in 30 patients (29%) to increase intra-abdominal esophageal length following extensive mediastinal mobilization.[35] We found no significant differences in regard to severity of abdominal pain, bloating, diarrhea or early satiety when comparing vagotomy patients with those patients who did not undergo a vagotomy.

### Extraesophageal Symptoms

A relatively new area of study in GERD is the involvement of the respiratory tract. Symptoms of hoarseness, laryngitis, cough, wheezing, and aspiration may occur when patients have high proximal reflux. Pulmonary fibrosis has also been associated with high gastroesophageal reflux. Several studies have shown a high incidence of GERD, from 66% to 94% in patients with idiopathic pulmonary fibrosis.[36]

About 30% of patients with typical symptoms of reflux have some type of extraesophageal symptom; however, about 10% of patients have only extraesophageal symptoms when they present for evaluation. Of the patients who present with primary laryngeal symptoms, fewer than 50% have typical manifestations of heartburn or regurgitation.[37] Unfortunately, standard diagnostic testing for GERD has diminished sensitivity and specificity in this group of patients. Often, the initial pH study shows abnormal acid exposure in the upper esophagus,[38] but this is not necessary for the diagnosis. The detection of acid in the pharynx on pH monitoring improves the diagnostic rates of laryngeal reflux. Furthermore, pharyngeal reflux is a better predictor of response to medical[39] and surgical therapy[40] than standard esophageal measurements. Still, the measurement of pharyngeal reflux has poor sensitivity, likely because the mechanism of extraesophageal disease is by vagal stimulation from esophageal acid exposure. The diagnosis may also be supported by a stroboscopic examination of the vocal cords showing evidence of inflammation and injury,[40] although these findings are too nonspecific by themselves to diagnose reliably reflux as the culprit. As noted, impedance pH testing may provide additional valuable data in this subset of patients in regard to extent of proximal reflux and whether these persistent atypical symptoms, with or without PPI therapy, are related to non–acid reflux events.

Medical and surgical therapies have been used to treat the extraesophageal manifestations of GERD. Resolution of symptoms, increased exercise, and cessation of corticosteroid use have all been observed. The rate of symptom response to therapy is less than that of heartburn and regurgitation (60% to 80%),[41] possibly because of the selection of patients. With further evaluation of this unique group of patients, selection criteria may improve the results of medical and operative intervention.

### Obesity

Obesity is a significant risk factor for the development of GERD. More than 30% of adults in the United States are obese (body mass index [BMI] >30) and this trend continues to rise, suggesting that the epidemic is going to get worse before it gets better. The increasing prevalence of GERD has paralleled that of obesity. Although the mechanism whereby obesity increases the risk of GERD remains unknown, several studies have shown an increased risk of recurrence in obese patients undergoing antireflux surgery.[42] In this subset of obese patients meeting surgical criteria, consideration should be given to performing a laparoscopic Roux-en-Y gastric bypass as opposed to a Nissen fundoplication to achieve a more durable response, in addition to providing benefits of weight loss and decreasing obesity-associated comorbidities.

## PARAESOPHAGEAL HERNIAS

Paraesophageal hernias, type II or III (see Fig. 44-2*B* and *C*), are less commonly encountered in surgical practice than GERD. The operative approach has varied considerably for several decades but the central issues have remained the same in the era of videoendoscopic surgery—the need to operate on asymptomatic patients, whether to use mesh for reinforcement, whether to add an antireflux procedure, whether to anchor the stomach to the abdominal wall, and the need to remove the hernia sac. The repair of a paraesophageal hernia is another procedure that is ideally suited for a laparoscopic approach.

The role of operative treatment for hiatal hernias changed dramatically during the 1990s. Once a relatively uncommon event, antireflux operations are now performed in large numbers at many centers around the world. The driving force behind increased surgical referral for treatment was the popularity of minimally invasive surgery. Although the techniques of antireflux operations have not changed, the approach to the surgery has become more palatable to the patient and referring physician. More and more surgeons are called on to treat GERD and paraesophageal hernias. Thus, the surgeon must be familiar with all aspects of evaluating and treating both entities because he or she is ultimately responsible for a successful outcome.

### Pathophysiology

The most common structure to herniate through the esophageal hiatus is the fundus of the stomach. Occasionally, the fundus of the stomach will rotate toward the right pleural cavity along the organoaxial axis defined by the phrenoesophageal membrane at the hiatus and the retroperitoneal attachment of the first portion of the duodenum. This results in what has been referred to as an *upside-down stomach*. Other structures that may be located in the hernia sac include the spleen, colon, and omentum. After repeated episodes of the viscera entering the hernia sac, adhesions between the wall of the sac and the structures may form, thus preventing the structures from returning to their position in the peritoneal cavity. The natural history of these large hernias is a matter of debate. Rarely, the herniated contents will become strangulated, causing an emergent condition that requires immediate operative intervention. Because of these risks, and early reports of Hill[43] and Skinner and Belsey,[44] for decades many have recommended repair of these hernias when detected, regardless of symptoms. More recent evidence, however, has suggested that the risk for acute strangulation is approximately 1%/year.[45] Therefore, we and many others recommend surgical intervention only for younger patients (<60 years) and those with significant symptoms.

### Clinical Presentation

The most common symptoms include intermittent dysphagia for solids, which results from episodes of acute gastric or esophageal obstruction, abdominal and chest pain secondary to visceral torsion; gastrointestinal bleeding from mucosal ischemia, and heartburn. This profile varies considerably from that of GERD. The symptoms are often nonspecific and do not lead the clinician to the diagnosis. Often, a diagnosis of paraesophageal hernia is made only after a contrast study or endoscopy is performed for proximal gastrointestinal tract complaints.

In the series of patients at the University of Washington, symptoms of heartburn were present in 50% of patients.[46] Episodic attacks of abdominal pain and dysphagia were also present in 50% of patients. Other symptoms occurred with varying frequency. Regurgitation is likely to occur in patients with large hiatal defects and a type III hernia, which allows the GEJ to migrate into the chest, thus promoting a pressure gradient and encouraging reflux. Episodic attacks of pain are thought to arise from transient distention and ischemia of the hernia contents. Spontaneous reduction provides relief. Dysphagia will occur if the GEJ is angled so that a food bolus may not enter the stomach after a swallow is initiated. Gastrointestinal bleeding is caused by ulceration of the mucosa at an area where the stomach folds back onto itself, and is often the cause of iron deficiency anemia. In cases of anemia in the setting of a paraesophageal hernia, especially without another source, repair of the hernia results in resolution of the anemia. Of patients presenting to the University of Washington, 34% were found to have a gastrointestinal source of blood loss.

### Preoperative Evaluation

The evaluation of patients with paraesophageal hernias is similar to that of patients undergoing workup for GERD. A contrast esophagogram in these patients, however, is the most important diagnostic test (Fig. 44-17). Endoscopy helps identify mucosal erosions as a source of gastrointestinal blood loss. Manometry is needed to determine the motor function of the esophageal body. pH testing can be avoided if an antireflux procedure is performed as part of the operative repair. However, if an

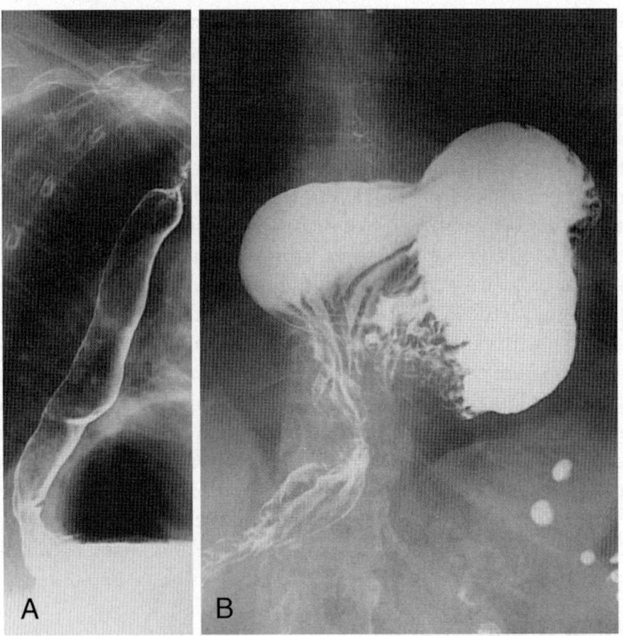


**FIGURE 44-17** Upper gastrointestinal contrast material study is essential for the evaluation of a paraesophageal hernia. **A,** Oblique view shows the stomach with an air-fluid level anterior to the esophagus and well into the mediastinum. **B,** Anteroposterior view of a patient with complete organoaxial volvulus, with the entire stomach in the mediastinum and the pylorus at the hiatus.

antireflux procedure is not planned, the extent of gastroesophageal reflux is evaluated.

In patients with large paraesophageal hernias, it may be difficult to complete the manometry and pH studies can be difficult. When the fundus of the stomach is angled so that the distal esophagus and GEJ may not be negotiated with the catheters, the studies may be incomplete. It is important to obtain some idea of the degree of peristalsis in the body of the esophagus before proceeding with the operation. This can be accomplished even if the stomach and distal esophagus cannot be cannulated.

## Treatment

After the introduction of laparoscopic techniques for the treatment of sliding hiatal hernias, their use in the repair of paraesophageal hernias naturally followed. Although technically more difficult, laparoscopic paraesophageal hernia repair is safe, feasible, and generally associated with less perioperative morbidity than open repair. Although it has been debated that there may be some differences in recurrence rates based on the surgical approach (laparotomy, thoracotomy, or laparoscopic), the recurrence rate seems to range from 8% to 27%[47,48] Although most of these recurrences are asymptomatic and found only on barium studies, they are of concern, and techniques to reduce recurrences are needed. As with other types of hernias, mesh has been used at the hiatus with the goal of reducing tension and reinforcing the repair by several surgeons. Unfortunately, synthetic mesh, which is used for most other hernia repairs, is associated with occasional esophageal erosion, ulceration, stricture, and dysphagia, limiting its practical use.[49,50] As a result of these complications associated with the use of synthetic mesh, biologic mesh has become an attractive alternative, with the idea that the temporary matrix would permit the patient's own tissue to replace the biomaterial and avoid complications previously described with permanent mesh. Several studies investigating the efficacy of biologic mesh in paraesophageal hernia repair have revealed low recurrence rates and few complications.[51-53] Most recently, a multi-institutional randomized clinical trial has revealed a significantly lower recurrence rate of 9% for biologic mesh reinforcement compared with 24% for primary repair ($P = .04$) without any mesh-associated complications. Unfortunately, at this time, we only have follow-up data at 6 months; further long-term follow-up is needed.

The operative approach through laparoscopy, our preferred approach, is similar to that of the gastroesophageal reflux procedures described earlier with respect to patient positioning and port placement. Several variations in the technique must be made to accommodate the unique operative findings in paraesophageal hernias.

The initial dissection for paraesophageal hernias begins with mobilization of the greater curve and fundus. Because the left crus is usually obscured by the lienogastric ligament and short gastric vessels, crural dissection may be hazardous at the beginning of the operation. By mobilizing the fundus and dividing the short gastric vessels with ultrasonic transection, the left crus may be exposed safely.

After the crural fibers are exposed on the left, the hernia sac will, by necessity, have been divided. At this point, the peritoneal sac may be divided anteriorly with minimal risk. Further dissection of the sac from its mediastinal attachments will free the stomach and allow it to be delivered into the peritoneal cavity. After the hernia contents are returned to the peritoneal cavity, the hernia sac must be transected circumferentially at the hiatus. The technically challenging aspect of the dissection is encountered during the posterior sac dissection. The esophagus and anterior vagus nerve are intimately associated with the sac posteriorly. Often, a lighted bougie is useful to identify the exact location of the esophagus. After the sac is freed at the hiatus, a concerted effort is made to remove as much of the hernia sac from the mediastinum as possible. It is unnecessary to remove the whole sac and, considering that the pleura, esophagus, and inferior pulmonary veins may be injured during the dissection, the desire to remove the entire sac must be tempered by the possible injury to vital structures.

After the dissection is completed, the crura are reapproximated with interrupted nonabsorbable suture, as with any antireflux procedure. Next, a 7- ×10-cm piece of biologic mesh is prepared by cutting it into a U-shaped configuration. The mesh is then strategically placed, with the U base overlying the posterior hiatal closure. It is then secured into place with several interrupted sutures between the mesh and diaphragm. An antireflux procedure is added to the procedure to prevent postoperative reflux after the extensive hiatal dissection. Although the need for an antireflux procedure is controversial, about 60% of patients with paraesophageal hernias have abnormal reflux and a hypotensive LES; thus, we consider a fundoplication to be appropriate.[54] The fundoplication will also act to seal the hiatus, preventing access by other viscera. As with fundoplication for GERD, the type of wrap is dictated by the preoperative manometry. Postoperative management of the patient is the same as for surgery performed for type I hernias and GERD.

## Outcome

Operative treatment of paraesophageal hernias is controls symptoms in 90% to 100% of patients.[46] In the past, paraesophageal hernias were repaired by thoracotomy or laparotomy, with a morbidity rate of about 20% and a mortality rate of 2%. With the popularization of minimally invasive techniques, most paraesophageal hernias are currently being repaired using a laparoscopic approach. The laparoscopic approach is associated with lower rates of morbidity, less pain, and faster recovery.[55] This may be even more important in this patient population because most patients with paraesophageal hernias are older and likely to have associated medical comorbidities.

Despite the approach used, what remains clear is that the anatomic recurrence of a hiatal hernia after these repairs is relatively high, even if many patients with a recurrence are minimally symptomatic or asymptomatic. In efforts to decrease the recurrence risk, one strategy has been to use mesh for reinforcement at the hiatus. Several comparison studies have been completed over the past decade investigating the use of permanent or biologic mesh in reducing recurrence risk in patients undergoing paraesophageal hernia repair. In general, recurrence rates have ranged from 0% to 9% in patients undergoing mesh placement; these rates were significantly lower than for patients undergoing primary repair (20% to 42%; Table 44-4).[49,51-53,56] The major weakness of these studies is the lack of long-term or complete follow-up. In addition, several of these studies did not have an established method for following symptoms such as dysphagia, which may be a potential side effect associated with the use of mesh. Only two retrospective studies have reported on mesh complications.[8] In a study of 54 patients, in which 35 underwent repair with Gore-Tex mesh, Zaninotto and colleagues[57] reported that 1 patient experienced mesh erosion requiring an esophagectomy. In another recent series of 138 patients with GERD undergoing hiatal hernia repair with polypropylene mesh, 14 patients (4.7%) experienced postoperative dysphagia.[58] It was not indicated whether the dysphagia was associated with the use of mesh. One patient did have a mesh-related complication and required reoperation for removal. In our randomized trial using biologic mesh, there were no clearly related mesh complications; although, again follow-up was limited.[52] It does appear, however, at least in the short term, that biologic mesh is safer as compared with permanent mesh. We currently recommend the use of biologic mesh for large hiatal hernia repairs.

## Strangulation

The clinical finding of persistent thoracic or epigastric pain, fever, or sepsis in a patient known to have a paraesophageal hernia is a surgical emergency. The mortality rate for ischemic stomach in the mediastinum is high. Although the consequences of this clinical situation are grave, it is a relatively rare occurrence in patients with paraesophageal hernias. Of 31 patients with complicated paraesophageal hernias, only 2 were found to have gastric necrosis and perforation.[59] Of the initial 42 patients operated on at the University of Washington, only 1 required an emergent repair. Interestingly, 11 patients were found to have gastric volvulus at the time of the operation. Thus, 25% of the patients had the potential to develop vascular compromise, but only 1 (2%) did. Emergent reduction of a paraesophageal hernia may be approached laparoscopically, but a low threshold for conversion is maintained.

## SUMMARY

Operative treatment of GERD and paraesophageal hernias has become more common in the era of laparoscopic procedures. Careful patient selection based on symptom assessment, response to medical therapy, and preoperative testing will optimize chances for successful surgical treatment. Scrupulous operative technique will allow for resolution of symptoms in almost all patients. Complications of the laparoscopic approach to these diseases are rare.

**Table 44-4 Comparison Studies of Biologic and Synthetic Mesh With No Mesh***

| STUDY (YEAR) | TYPE | ARMS | FOLLOW-UP (MO) | RECURRENCE |
|---|---|---|---|---|
| **Synthetic Mesh** | | | | |
| Frantzides et al. (2002)[56] | RCT | PTFE, $n$ = 36; no mesh, $n$ = 36 | 30 | PTFE, 0%; no mesh, 22%; $P = 0.006$ |
| Granderath et al. (2002)[49] | RCT | Polypropylene, $n$ = 50; no mesh, $n$ = 50 | 12 | Polypropylene, 8%; no mesh, 26%; $p < 0.001$ |
| Zaninotto et al. (2007)[58] | Retrospective | Gore-Tex, $n$ = 35; no mesh, $n$ = 19 | 71 | Gore-tex, 9%; no mesh, 42%; $P = 0.01$ |
| **Biologic Mesh** | | | | |
| Oelschlager et al. (2006)[52] | RCT | Surgisis, $n$ = 51; no mesh, $n$ = 57 | 6 | Surgisis, 9%; no mesh, 24%; $P = 0.04$ |
| Ringley et al. (2006)[53] | Retrospective | Alloderm, $n$ = 22; no mesh, $n$ = 22 | 7 | Alloderm, 0%; no mesh, 9%; $P < 0.05$ |
| Jacobs et al. (2007)[51] | Retrospective | Surgisis, $n$ = 127; no mesh, $n$ = 93 | 38 | Surgisis, 3%; no mesh, 20%; $p < 0.01$ |

*PTFE,* Polytetrafluoroethylene; *RCT,* randomized controlled trial.

*In patients undergoing paraesophageal hernia repair.

## SELECTED REFERENCES

Davis SS, Jr: Current controversies in paraesophageal hernia repair. Surg Clin North Am 88:959–978, 2008.

Excellent review of the current controversies in the surgical management of paraesophageal hernia repair.

Flum DR, Koepsell T, Heagerty P, et al: The nationwide frequency of major adverse outcomes in antireflux surgery and the role of surgeon experience, 1992-1997. J Am Coll Surg 195:611–618, 2002.

Population-based study reporting on the frequency of major outcomes in antireflux surgery.

Lundell L, Miettinen P, Myrvold HE, et al: Comparison of outcomes twelve years after antireflux surgery or omeprazole maintenance therapy for reflux esophagitis. Clin Gastroenterol Hepatol 7:1292–1298, 2009.

Long-term results of a large randomized trial comparing medical therapy with surgery for patients with GERD.

Oelschlager BK, Pellegrini CA, Hunter J, et al: Biologic prosthesis reduces recurrence after laparoscopic paraesophageal hernia repair: A multicenter, prospective, randomized trial. Ann Surg 244:481–490, 2006.

The only randomized study to date evaluating recurrence risk with the use of biologic mesh in paraesophageal hernia repair.

Oelschlager BK, Quiroga E, Parra JD, et al: Long-term outcomes after laparoscopic antireflux surgery. Am J Gastroenterol 103:280–287, 2008.

A large study reporting on long-term results of anitreflux surgery that also identifies preoperative predictors of outcome in a logistic regression model.

Smith CD: Antireflux surgery. Surg Clin North Am 88:943–958, 2008.

Comprehensive review of the diagnostic workup, patient selection criteria, surgical technique and postoperative management for patients with GERD.

Wileman SM, McCann S, Grant AM, et al: Medical versus surgical management for gastro-oesophageal reflux disease (GORD) in adults. Cochrane Database Syst Rev (3):CD003243, 2010.

Comprehensive review of major studies investigating whether medical or surgical management is the most clinically and cost-effective treatment for patients with GERD.

Wolf PS, Oelschlager BK: Laparoscopic paraesophageal hernia repair. Adv Surg 41:199–210, 2007.

A comprehensive review of the presentation, management, and controversies surrounding the repair of paraesophageal hernias.

## REFERENCES

1. Galmiche JP, Janssens J: The pathophysiology of gastro-oesophageal reflux disease: An overview. Scand J Gastroenterol Suppl 211:7–18, 1995.
2. Oelschlager BK, Quiroga E, Parra JD, et al: Long-term outcomes after laparoscopic antireflux surgery. Am J Gastroenterol 103:280–287, 2008.
3. Hill LD, Kozarek RA, Kraemer SJ, et al: The gastroesophageal flap valve: In vitro and in vivo observations. Gastrointest Endosc 44:541–547, 1996.
4. Mainie I, Tutuian R, Shay S, et al: Acid and non-acid reflux in patients with persistent symptoms despite acid suppressive therapy: A multicentre study using combined ambulatory impedance-pH monitoring. Gut 55:1398–1402, 2006.
5. Zerbib F, Roman S, Ropert A, et al: Esophageal pH-impedance monitoring and symptom analysis in GERD: A study in patients off and on therapy. Am J Gastroenterol 101:1956–1963, 2006.
6. Oelschlager BK, Quiroga E, Isch JA, et al: Gastroesophageal and pharyngeal reflux detection using impedance and 24-hour pH monitoring in asymptomatic subjects: Defining the normal environment. J Gastrointest Surg 10:54–62, 2006.
7. Stacher G, Bergmann H: Scintigraphic quantitation of gastrointestinal motor activity and transport: oesophagus and stomach. Eur J Nucl Med 19:815–823, 1992.
8. Finley K, Giannamore M, Bennett M, et al: Assessing the impact of lifestyle modification education on knowledge and behavior changes in gastroesophageal reflux disease patients on proton pump inhibitors. J Am Pharm Assoc (2003) 49:544–548, 2009.
9. Ali T, Roberts DN, Tierney WM: Long-term safety concerns with proton pump inhibitors. Am J Med 122:896–903, 2009.
10. Habu Y, Maeda K, Kusuda T, et al: "Proton-pump inhibitor-first" strategy versus "step-up" strategy for the acute treatment of reflux esophagitis: A cost-effectiveness analysis in Japan. J Gastroenterol 40:1029–1035, 2005.
11. Cookson R, Flood C, Koo B, et al: Short-term cost effectiveness and long-term cost analysis comparing laparoscopic Nissen fundoplication with proton-pump inhibitor maintenance for gastro-oesophageal reflux disease. Br J Surg 92:700–706, 2005.
12. Booth MI, Stratford J, Jones L, et al: Randomized clinical trial of laparoscopic total (Nissen) versus posterior partial (Toupet) fundoplication for gastro-oesophageal reflux disease based on preoperative oesophageal manometry. Br J Surg 95:57–63, 2008.
13. Oleynikov D, Eubanks TR, Oelschlager BK, et al: Total fundoplication is the operation of choice for patients with gastroesophageal reflux and defective peristalsis. Surg Endosc 16:909–913, 2002.
14. Spechler SJ, Lee E, Ahnen D, et al: Long-term outcome of medical and surgical therapies for gastroesophageal reflux disease: Follow-up of a randomized controlled trial. JAMA 285:2331–2338, 2001.
15. Lundell L, Miettinen P, Myrvold HE, et al: Seven-year follow-up of a randomized clinical trial comparing proton-pump inhibition with surgical therapy for reflux oesophagitis. Br J Surg 94:198–203, 2007.
16. Lundell L, Miettinen P, Myrvold HE, et al: Comparison of outcomes twelve years after antireflux surgery or omeprazole maintenance therapy for reflux esophagitis. Clin Gastroenterol Hepatol 7:1292–1298, 2009.
17. Mahon D, Rhodes M, Decadt B, et al: Randomized clinical trial of laparoscopic Nissen fundoplication compared with proton-pump inhibitors for treatment of chronic gastro-oesophageal reflux. Br J Surg 92:695–699, 2005.

18. Rice S, Watson DI, Lally CJ, et al: Laparoscopic anterior 180 degrees partial fundoplication: Five-year results and beyond. Arch Surg 141:271–275, 2006.
19. Dallemagne B, Weerts J, Markiewicz S, et al: Clinical results of laparoscopic fundoplication at ten years after surgery. Surg Endosc 20:159–165, 2006.
20. Aziz AM, El-Khayat HR, Sadek A, et al: A prospective randomized trial of sham, single-dose Stretta, and double-dose Stretta for the treatment of gastroesophageal reflux disease. Surg Endosc 24:818–825, 2010.
21. Corley DA, Katz P, Wo JM, et al: Improvement of gastroesophageal reflux symptoms after radiofrequency energy: A randomized, sham-controlled trial. Gastroenterology 125:668–676, 2003.
22. Reymunde A, Santiago N: Long-term results of radiofrequency energy delivery for the treatment of GERD: Sustained improvements in symptoms, quality of life, and drug use at 4-year follow-up. Gastrointest Endosc 65:361–366, 2007.
23. Chen D, Barber C, McLoughlin P, et al: Systematic review of endoscopic treatments for gastro-oesophageal reflux disease. Br J Surg 96:128–136, 2009.
24. Repici A, Fumagalli U, Malesci A, et al: Endoluminal fundoplication (ELF) for GERD using EsophyX: A 12-month follow-up in a single-center experience. J Gastrointest Surg 14:1–6, 2010.
25. Cadiere GB, Buset M, Muls V, et al: Antireflux transoral incisionless fundoplication using EsophyX: 12-month results of a prospective multicenter study. World J Surg 32:1676–1688, 2008.
26. Jeansonne LOt, White BC, Nguyen V, et al: Endoluminal full-thickness plication and radiofrequency treatments for GERD: An outcomes comparison. Arch Surg 144:19–24, 2009.
27. Cadiere GB, Himpens J, Rajan A, et al: Laparoscopic Nissen fundoplication: Laparoscopic dissection technique and results. Hepatogastroenterology 44:4–10, 1997.
28. Flum DR, Koepsell T, Heagerty P, et al: The nationwide frequency of major adverse outcomes in antireflux surgery and the role of surgeon experience, 1992-1997. J Am Coll Surg 195:611–618, 2002.
29. Lamb PJ, Myers JC, Jamieson GG, et al: Long-term outcomes of revisional surgery following laparoscopic fundoplication. Br J Surg 96:391–397, 2009.
30. Hofstetter WL, Peters JH, DeMeester TR, et al: Long-term outcome of antireflux surgery in patients with Barrett's esophagus. Ann Surg 234:532–538, 2001.
31. Kaufman JA, Houghland JE, Quiroga E, et al: Long-term outcomes of laparoscopic antireflux surgery for gastroesophageal reflux disease (GERD)–related airway disorder. Surg Endosc 20:1824–1830, 2006.
32. Oelschlager BK, Barreca M, Chang L, et al: Clinical and pathologic response of Barrett's esophagus to laparoscopic antireflux surgery. Ann Surg 238:458–464, 2003.
33. Rossi M, Barreca M, de Bortoli N, et al: Efficacy of Nissen fundoplication versus medical therapy in the regression of low-grade dysplasia in patients with Barrett esophagus: A prospective study. Ann Surg 243:58–63, 2006.
34. Jobe BA, Horvath KD, Swanstrom LL: Postoperative function following laparoscopic collis gastroplasty for shortened esophagus. Arch Surg 133:867–874, 1998.
35. Oelschlager BK, Yamamoto K, Woltman T, et al: Vagotomy during hiatal hernia repair: A benign esophageal lengthening procedure. J Gastrointest Surg 12:1155–1162, 2008.
36. Raghu G, Freudenberger TD, Yang S, et al: High prevalence of abnormal acid gastro-oesophageal reflux in idiopathic pulmonary fibrosis. Eur Respir J 27:136–142, 2006.
37. Koufman JA: The otolaryngologic manifestations of gastroesophageal reflux disease (GERD): A clinical investigation of 225 patients using ambulatory 24-hour pH monitoring and an experimental investigation of the role of acid and pepsin in the development of laryngeal injury. Laryngoscope 101:1–78, 1991.
38. Patti MG, Debas HT, Pellegrini CA: Clinical and functional characterization of high gastroesophageal reflux. Am J Surg 165:163–166, 1993.
39. Eubanks TR, Omelanczuk PE, Maronian N, et al: Pharyngeal pH monitoring in 222 patients with suspected laryngeal reflux. J Gastrointest Surg 5:183–190, 2001.
40. Oelschlager BK, Eubanks TR, Maronian N, et al: Laryngoscopy and pharyngeal pH are complementary in the diagnosis of gastroesophageal-laryngeal reflux. J Gastrointest Surg 6:189–194, 2002.
41. Oelschlager BK, Eubanks TR, Oleynikov D, et al: Symptomatic and physiologic outcomes after operative treatment for extraesophageal reflux. Surg Endosc 16:1032–1036, 2002.
42. Perez AR, Moncure AC, Rattner DW: Obesity adversely affects the outcome of antireflux operations. Surg Endosc 15:986–989, 2001.
43. Hill LD: Incarcerated paraesophageal hernia. A surgical emergency. Am J Surg 126:286–291, 1973.
44. Skinner DB, Belsey RH: Surgical management of esophageal reflux and hiatus hernia. Long-term results with 1030 patients. J Thorac Cardiovasc Surg 53:33–54, 1967.
45. Stylopoulos N, Gazelle GS, Rattner DW: Paraesophageal hernias: Operation or observation? Ann Surg 236:492–500; discussion 500–491, 2002.
46. Wolf PS, Oelschlager BK: Laparoscopic paraesophageal hernia repair. Adv Surg 41:199–210, 2007.
47. Mehta S, Boddy A, Rhodes M: Review of outcome after laparoscopic paraesophageal hiatal hernia repair. Surg Laparosc Endosc Percutan Tech 16:301–306, 2006.
48. Patel HJ, Tan BB, Yee J, et al: A 25-year experience with open primary transthoracic repair of paraesophageal hiatal hernia. J Thorac Cardiovasc Surg 127:843–849, 2004.
49. Granderath FA, Schweiger UM, Kamolz T, et al: Laparoscopic antireflux surgery with routine mesh-hiatoplasty in the treatment of gastroesophageal reflux disease. J Gastrointest Surg 6:347–353, 2002.
50. Tatum RP, Shalhub S, Oelschlager BK, et al: Complications of PTFE mesh at the diaphragmatic hiatus. J Gastrointest Surg 12:953–957, 2008.
51. Jacobs M, Gomez E, Plasencia G, et al: Use of surgisis mesh in laparoscopic repair of hiatal hernias. Surg Laparosc Endosc Percutan Tech 17:365–368, 2007.
52. Oelschlager BK, Pellegrini CA, Hunter J, et al: Biologic prosthesis reduces recurrence after laparoscopic paraesophageal hernia repair: A multicenter, prospective, randomized trial. Ann Surg 244:481–490, 2006.
53. Ringley CD, Bochkarev V, Ahmed SI, et al: Laparoscopic hiatal hernia repair with human acellular dermal matrix patch: our initial experience. Am J Surg 192:767–772, 2006.
54. Walther B, DeMeester TR, Lafontaine E, et al: Effect of paraesophageal hernia on sphincter function and its implication on surgical therapy. Am J Surg 147:111–116, 1984.

**55.** Karmali S, McFadden S, Mitchell P, et al: Primary laparoscopic and open repair of paraesophageal hernias: A comparison of short-term outcomes. Dis Esophagus 21:63–68, 2008.

**56.** Frantzides CT, Madan AK, Carlson MA, et al: A prospective, randomized trial of laparoscopic polytetrafluoroethylene (PTFE) patch repair vs simple cruroplasty for large hiatal hernia. Arch Surg 137:649–652, 2002.

**57.** Zaninotto G, Portale G, Costantini M, et al: Objective follow-up after laparoscopic repair of large type III hiatal hernia. Assessment of safety and durability. World J Surg 31:2177–2183, 2007.

**58.** Soricelli E, Basso N, Genco A, et al: Long-term results of hiatal hernia mesh repair and antireflux laparoscopic surgery. Surg Endosc 23:2499–2504, 2009.

**59.** Ozdemir IA, Burke WA, Ikins PM: Paraesophageal hernia. A life-threatening disease. Ann Thorac Surg 16:547–554, 1973.

**60.** Grant AM, Wileman SM, Ramsay CR, et al: Minimal access surgery compared with medical management for chronic gastro-oesophageal reflux disease: UK collaborative randomised trial. BMJ 337:a2664, 2008.

# SECTION X ABDOMEN

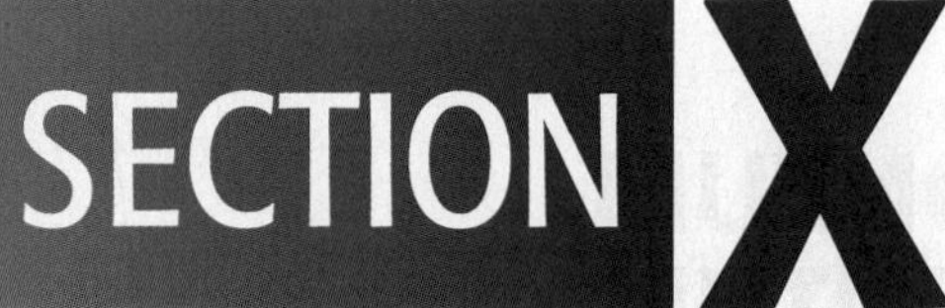

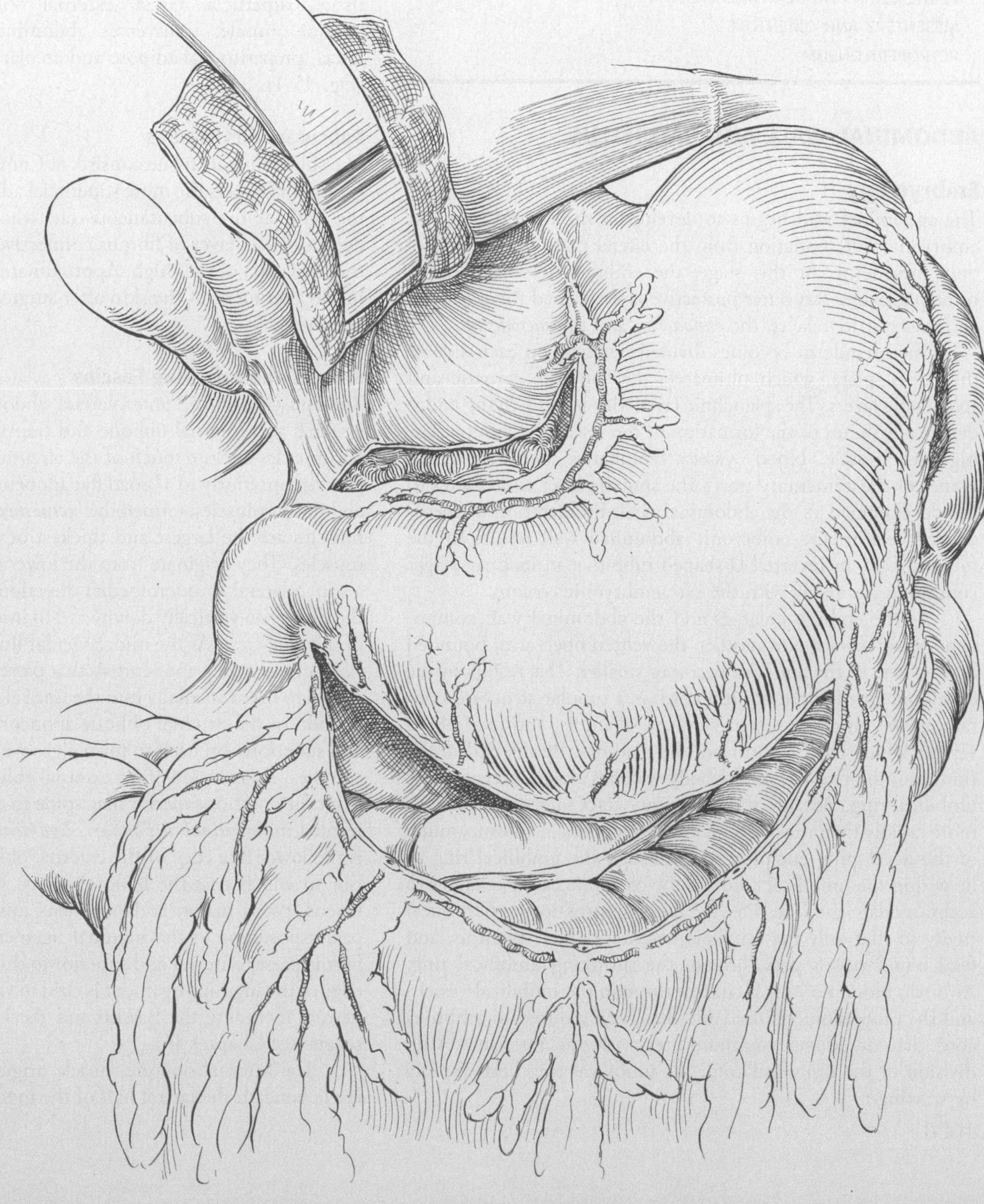

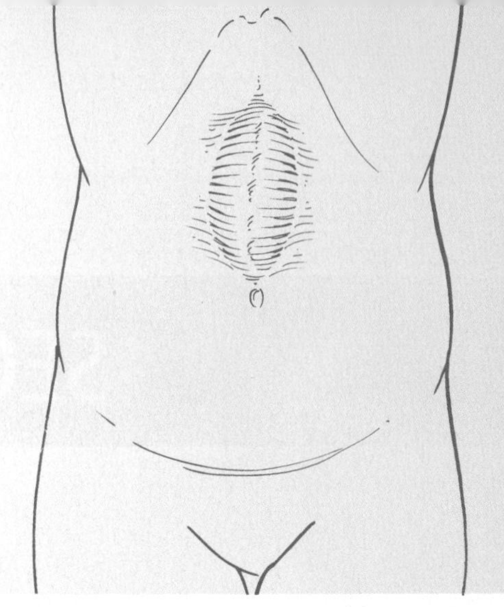

CHAPTER 45

# ABDOMINAL WALL, UMBILICUS, PERITONEUM, MESENTERIES, OMENTUM, AND RETROPERITONEUM

Richard H. Turnage and Brian Badgwell

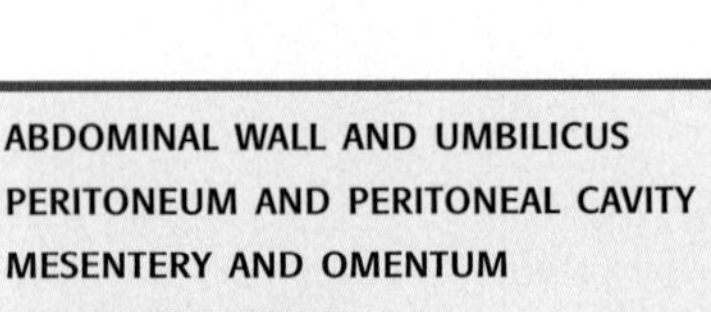



## ABDOMINAL WALL AND UMBILICUS

### Embryology

The abdominal wall begins to develop in the earliest stages of embryonic differentiation from the lateral plate of the embryonic mesoderm. At this stage, the embryo consists of three principal layers—an outer protective layer termed the *ectoderm,* an inner nutritive layer, the *endoderm,* and the *mesoderm.*

The mesoderm becomes divided by clefts on each side of the lateral plate, which ultimately develop into somatic and splanchnic layers. The splanchnic layer with its underlying endoderm contributes to the formation of the viscera by differentiating into muscle, blood vessels, lymphatics, and connective tissues of the alimentary tract. The somatic layer contributes to the development of the abdominal wall. Proliferation of mesodermal cells in the embryonic abdominal wall results in the formation of an inverted U-shaped tube that in its early stages communicates freely with the extraembryonic coelom.

As the embryo enlarges and the abdominal wall components grow toward one another, the ventral open area, bounded by the edge of the amnion, becomes smaller. This results in the development of the umbilical cord as a tubular structure containing the omphalomesenteric duct, allantois, and fetal blood vessels, which pass to and from the placenta. By the end of the third month of gestation, the body wall has closed, except at the umbilical ring. Because the alimentary tract increases in length more rapidly than the coelomic cavity increases in volume, much of the developing gut protrudes through the umbilical ring to lie within the umbilical cord. As the coelomic cavity enlarges to accommodate the intestine, the latter returns to the peritoneal cavity so that only the omphalomesenteric duct, allantois, and fetal blood vessels pass through the shrinking umbilical ring. At birth, blood no longer courses through the umbilical vessels, and the omphalomesenteric duct has been reduced to a fibrous cord that no longer communicates with the intestine. After division of the umbilical cord, the umbilical ring heals rapidly by scarring.

### Anatomy

There are nine layers to the abdominal wall—skin, subcutaneous tissue, superficial fascia, external oblique muscle, internal oblique muscle, transversus abdominis muscle, transversalis fascia, preperitoneal adipose and areolar tissue, and peritoneum (Fig. 45-1).

#### Subcutaneous Tissues

The subcutaneous tissue consists of Camper's and Scarpa's fascia. Camper's fascia is the more superficial adipose layer that contains the bulk of the subcutaneous fat, whereas Scarpa's fascia is a deeper denser layer of fibrous connective tissue contiguous with the fascia lata of the thigh. Approximation of Scarpa's fascia aids in the alignment of the skin after surgical incisions in the lower abdomen.

#### Muscle and Investing Fascias

The muscles of the anterolateral abdominal wall include the external and internal oblique and transversus abdominis. These flat muscles enclose much of the circumference of the torso and give rise anteriorly to a broad flat aponeurosis investing the rectus abdominis muscles, termed the *rectus sheath.* The external oblique muscles are the largest and thickest of the flat abdominal wall muscles. They originate from the lower seven ribs and course in a superolateral to inferomedial direction. The most posterior of the fibers run vertically downward to insert into the anterior half of the iliac crest. At the midclavicular line, the muscle fibers give rise to a flat strong aponeurosis that passes anteriorly to the rectus sheath to insert medially into the linea alba (Fig. 45-2). The lower portion of the external oblique aponeurosis is rolled posteriorly and superiorly on itself to form a groove on which the spermatic cord lies. This portion of the external oblique aponeurosis extends from the anterior superior iliac spine to the pubic tubercle and is termed the *inguinal* or *Poupart's ligament.* The inguinal ligament is the lower free edge of the external oblique aponeurosis posterior to which pass the femoral artery, vein, and nerve and the iliacus, psoas major, and pectineus muscles. A femoral hernia passes posterior to the inguinal ligament, whereas an inguinal hernia passes anterior and superior to this ligament. The shelving edge of the inguinal ligament is used in various repairs of inguinal hernia, including the Bassini and the Lichtenstein tension-free repair (see Chapter 46).

The internal oblique muscle originates from the iliopsoas fascia beneath the lateral half of the inguinal ligament, from the

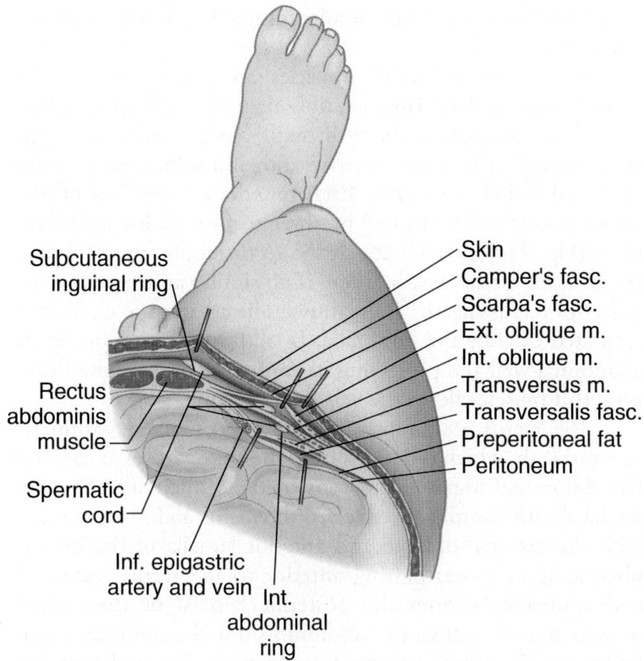


**FIGURE 45-1** The nine layers of the anterolateral abdominal wall. (From Thorek P: Anatomy in surgery, ed 2, Philadelphia, 1962, JB Lippincott, p 358.)

anterior two thirds of the iliac crest and lumbodorsal fascia. Its fibers course in a direction opposite to those of the external oblique—that is, inferolateral to superomedial. The uppermost fibers insert into the lower five ribs and their cartilages (Fig. 45-3; see Fig. 45-2*A*). The central fibers form an aponeurosis at the semilunar line, which, above the semicircular line (of Douglas), is divided into anterior and posterior lamellae that envelop the rectus abdominis muscle. Below the semicircular line, the aponeurosis of the internal oblique muscle courses anteriorly to the rectus abdominis muscle as part of the anterior rectus sheath. The lowermost fibers of the internal oblique muscle pursue an inferomedial course, paralleling that of the spermatic cord, to insert between the symphysis pubis and pubic tubercle. Some of the lower muscle fascicles accompany the spermatic cord into the scrotum as the cremasteric muscle.

The transversus abdominis muscle is the smallest of the muscles of the anterolateral abdominal wall. It arises from the lower six costal cartilages, spines of the lumbar vertebra, iliac crest, and iliopsoas fascia beneath the lateral third of the inguinal ligament. The fibers course transversely to give rise to a flat aponeurotic sheet that passes posterior to the rectus abdominis muscle above the semicircular line and anterior to the muscle below it (Fig. 45-4). The inferiormost fibers of the transversus abdominis originating from the iliopsoas fascia pass inferomedially along with the lower fibers of the internal oblique muscle. These fibers form the aponeurotic arch of the transversus

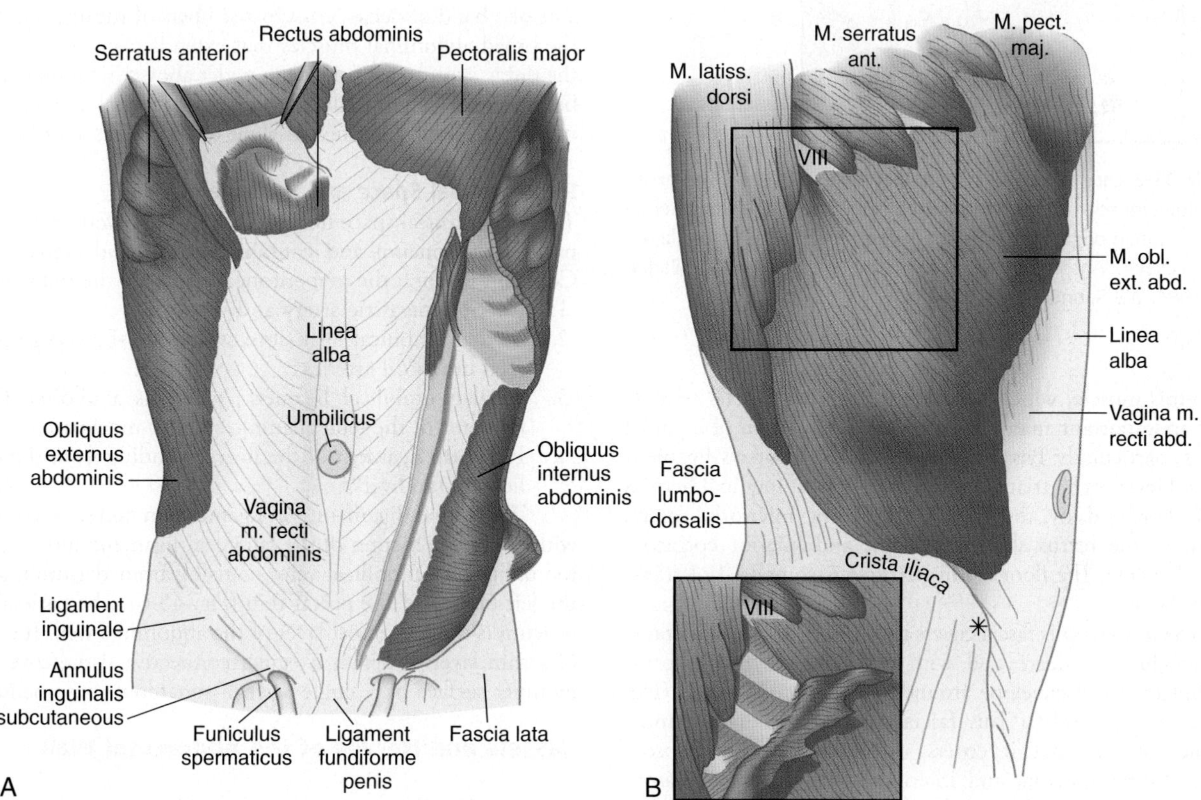


**FIGURE 45-2 A,** External oblique, internal oblique, and rectus abdominis muscles and anterior rectus sheath. **B,** Lateral view of the external oblique muscle and its aponeurosis as it enters the anterior rectus sheath. *Inset,* Origin of the external oblique muscle fibers from the lower ribs and their costal cartilages. (From McVay C: Anson and McVay's surgical anatomy, ed 6, Philadelphia, 1984, WB Saunders, pp 477–478).

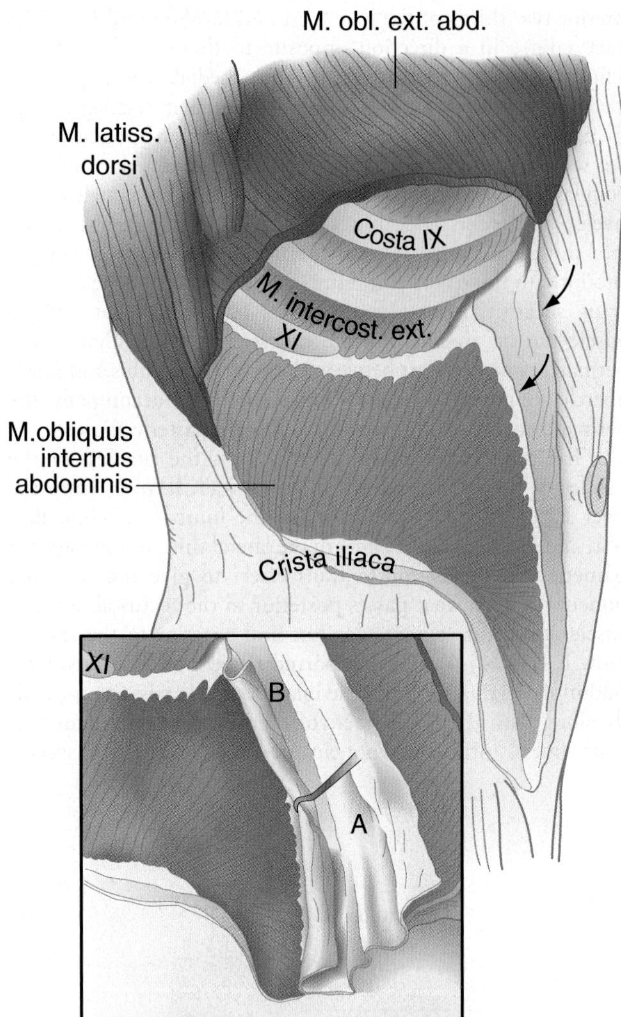


**FIGURE 45-3** Lateral view of the internal oblique muscle. The external oblique muscle has been removed to show the underlying internal oblique muscle originating from the lower ribs and costal cartilages. (From McVay C: Anson and McVay's surgical anatomy, ed 6, Philadelphia, 1984, WB Saunders, p 479.)

abdominis muscle, which lies superior to Hesselbach's triangle and is an important anatomic landmark in the repair of inguinal hernias, particularly Bassini's operation and Cooper's ligament repairs. Hesselbach's triangle is the site of direct inguinal hernias and is bordered by the inguinal ligament inferiorly, lateral margin of the rectus sheath medially, and inferior epigastric vessels laterally. The floor of this triangle is composed of transversalis fascia.

The transversalis fascia covers the deep surface of the transversus abdominis muscle and, with its various extensions, forms a complete fascial envelope around the abdominal cavity (Fig. 45-5; see Fig. 45-4*B*). This fascial layer is regionally named for the muscles that it covers—for example, the iliopsoas fascia, obturator fascia, and inferior fascia of the respiratory diaphragm. The transversalis fascia binds together the muscle and aponeurotic fascicles into a continuous layer and reinforces weak areas where the aponeurotic fibers are sparse. This layer is responsible for the structural integrity of the abdominal wall and, by definition, a hernia results from a defect in the transversalis fascia.

The rectus abdominis muscles are paired muscles that appear as long, flat triangular ribbons wider at their origin on the anterior surfaces of the fifth, sixth, and seventh costal cartilages and the xiphoid process than at their insertion on the pubic crest and pubic symphysis. Each muscle is composed of long parallel fascicles interrupted by three to five tendinous inscriptions (Fig. 45-5), which attach the rectus abdominis muscle to the anterior rectus sheath. There is no similar attachment to the posterior rectus sheath. These muscles lie adjacent to each other, separated only by the linea alba. In addition to supporting the abdominal wall and protecting its contents, contraction of these powerful muscles flexes the vertebral column.

The rectus abdominis muscles are contained within the rectus sheath, which is derived from the aponeuroses of the three flat abdominal muscles. Superior to the semicircular line, this fascial sheath completely envelops the rectus abdominis muscle, with the external oblique and anterior lamella of the internal oblique aponeuroses passing anterior to the rectus abdominis and aponeuroses from the posterior lamella of the internal oblique muscle, transversus abdominis muscle, and transversalis fascia passing posterior to the rectus muscle. Below the semicircular line, all these fascial layers pass anterior to the rectus abdominis muscle, except the transversalis fascia. In this location, the posterior aspect of the rectus abdominis muscle is covered only by transversalis fascia, preperitoneal areolar tissue, and peritoneum.

The rectus abdominis muscles are held closely in apposition near the anterior midline by the linea alba. The linea alba consists of a band of dense, crisscrossed fibers of the aponeuroses of the broad abdominal muscles that extends from the xiphoid to the pubic symphysis. It is much wider above the umbilicus than below, thus facilitating the placement of surgical incisions in the midline without entering the right or left rectus sheath.

### Preperitoneal Space and Peritoneum

The preperitoneal space lies between the transversalis fascia and parietal peritoneum and contains adipose and areolar tissue. Coursing through the preperitoneal space are the following:

1. Inferior epigastric artery and vein
2. Medial umbilical ligaments, which are the vestiges of the fetal umbilical arteries
3. Median umbilical ligament, which is a midline fibrous remnant of the fetal allantoic stalk or urachus
4. Falciform ligament of the liver, extending from the umbilicus to the liver

The round ligament, or ligamentum teres, is contained within the free margin of the falciform ligament and represents the obliterated umbilical vein, coursing from the umbilicus to the left branch of the portal vein (Fig. 45-6). The parietal peritoneum is the innermost layer of the abdominal wall. It consists of a thin layer of dense, irregular connective tissue covered on its inner surface by a single layer of squamous mesothelium.

## Vessels and Nerves of the Abdominal Wall

### Vascular Supply

The anterolateral abdominal wall receives its arterial supply from the last six intercostals and four lumbar arteries, superior and inferior epigastric arteries, and deep circumflex iliac arteries

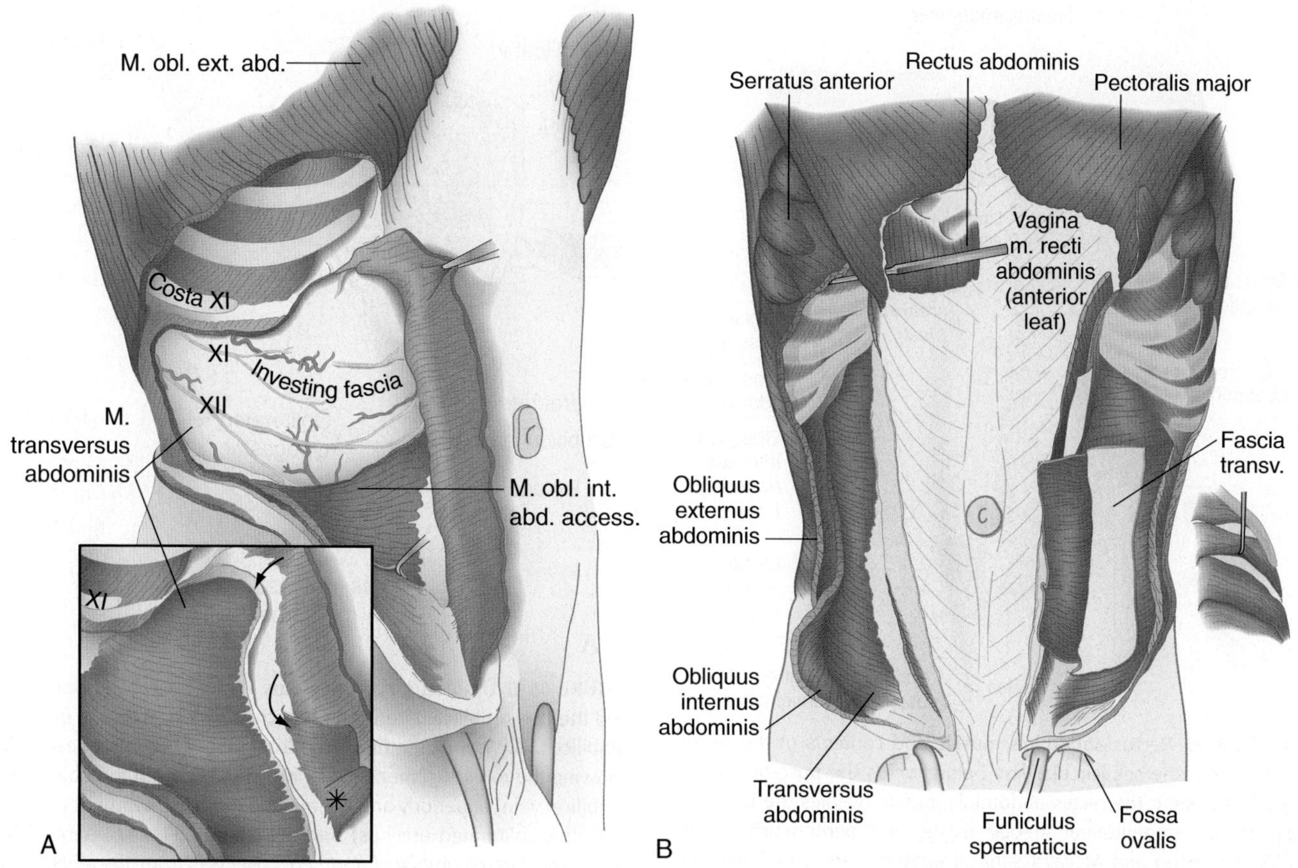


**FIGURE 45-4 A,** Anterolateral view of the investing fascia of the transversus abdominis muscle and the muscle itself with the fascia removed *(inset).* The external and internal oblique muscles have been removed. Also note the appearance of the intercostal nerves lying between the fascia of the transversus abdominis muscle and internal oblique muscle. **B,** Anterior view of the transversus abdominis muscle *(left)* and the transversalis fascia *(right).* Note that the transversalis fascia is shown by reflecting the overlying transversus abdominis muscle medially. (From McVay C: Anson and McVay's surgical anatomy, ed 6, Philadelphia, 1984, WB Saunders, pp 480–481.)

(Fig. 45-7). The trunks of the intercostal and lumbar arteries, together with the intercostal, iliohypogastric, and ilioinguinal nerves, course between the transversus abdominis and internal oblique muscles. The distalmost extensions of these vessels pierce the lateral margins of the rectus sheath at various levels and communicate freely with branches of the superior and inferior epigastric arteries. The superior epigastric artery, one of the terminal branches of the internal mammary artery, reaches the posterior surface of the rectus abdominis muscle through the costoxiphoid space in the diaphragm. It descends within the rectus sheath to anastomose with branches of the inferior epigastric artery. The inferior epigastric artery, derived from the external iliac artery just proximal to the inguinal ligament, courses through the preperitoneal areolar tissue to enter the lateral rectus sheath at the semilunar line of Douglas. The deep circumflex iliac artery, arising from the lateral aspect of the external iliac artery near the origin of the inferior epigastric artery, gives rise to an ascending branch, which penetrates the abdominal wall musculature just above the iliac crest, near the anterior superior iliac spine.

The venous drainage of the anterior abdominal wall follows a relatively simple pattern in which the superficial veins above the umbilicus empty into the superior vena cava by way of the internal mammary, intercostal, and long thoracic veins. The veins inferior to the umbilicus—the superficial epigastric, circumflex iliac, and pudendal veins—converge toward the saphenous opening in the groin to enter the saphenous vein and become a tributary to the inferior vena cava (Fig. 45-8). The numerous anastomoses between the infraumbilical and supraumbilical venous systems provide collateral pathways whereby venous return to the heart may bypass an obstruction of the superior or inferior vena cava. The paraumbilical vein, which passes from the left branch of the portal vein along the ligamentum teres to the umbilicus, provides important communication between the veins of the superficial abdominal wall and portal system in patients with portal venous obstruction. In this setting, portal blood flow is diverted away from the higher pressure portal system through the paraumbilical veins to the lower pressure veins of the anterior abdominal wall. The dilated superficial paraumbilical veins in this setting are termed *caput medusae.*

The lymphatic supply of the abdominal wall follows a pattern similar to the venous drainage. Those lymphatic vessels arising from the supraumbilical region drain into the axillary lymph nodes, whereas those arising from the infraumbilical region drain toward the superficial inguinal lymph nodes. The

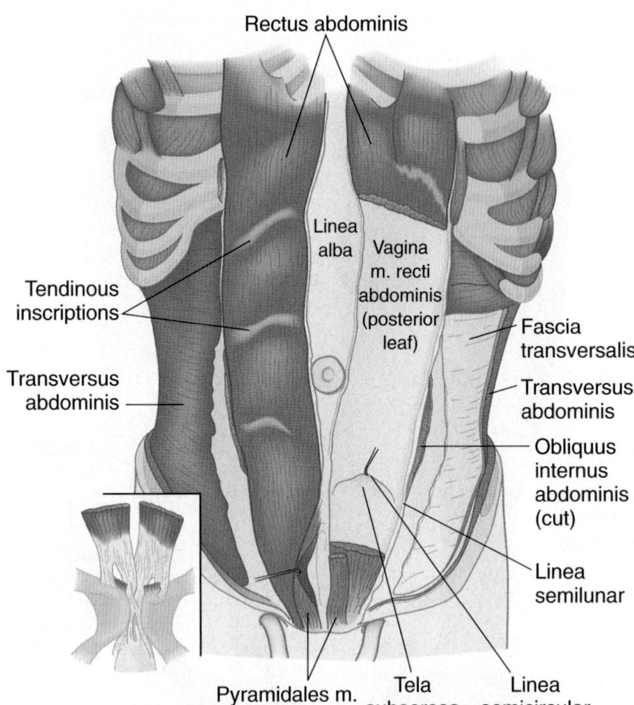


**FIGURE 45-5** Rectus abdominis muscle and contents of the rectus sheath. Note the semicircular line below which the posterior rectus sheath is absent; the rectus abdominis muscle overlies the transversalis fascia, preperitoneal areolar tissue, and peritoneum. (From McVay C: Anson and McVay's surgical anatomy, ed 6, Philadelphia, 1984, WB Saunders, p 482.)

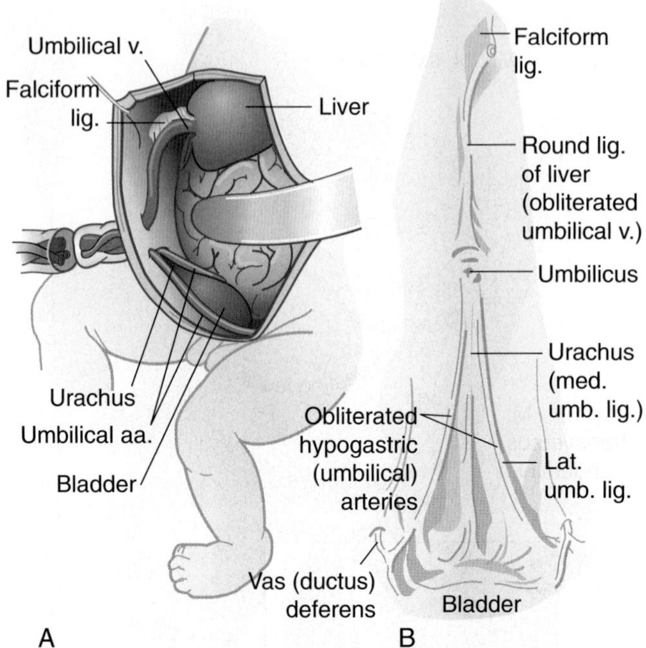


**FIGURE 45-6** Umbilicus. **A,** In the fetus, the umbilical vein superiorly and the two umbilical arteries and urachus inferiorly radiate from the umbilicus. **B,** View of the umbilicus from within the peritoneal cavity showing the round ligament of the liver (derived from the obliterated umbilical vein) superiorly and the median umbilical ligament (derived from the obliterated urachus) and medial umbilical ligaments (also called the *lateral umbilical ligaments*, derived from the obliterated umbilical arteries). (From Thorek P: Anatomy in surgery, ed 2, Philadelphia, 1962, JB Lippincott, p 375.)

lymphatic vessels from the liver course along the ligamentum teres to the umbilicus to communicate with the lymphatics of the anterior abdominal wall. It is from this pathway that carcinoma in the liver may spread to involve the anterior abdominal wall at the umbilicus (Sister Mary Joseph node [or nodule]).

## Innervation

The anterior rami of the thoracic nerves follow a curvilinear course forward in the intercostal spaces toward the midline of the body (see Fig. 45-7). The upper six thoracic nerves end near the sternum as anterior cutaneous sensory branches. Thoracic nerves 7 to 12 pass behind the costal cartilages and lower ribs to enter a plane between the internal oblique muscle and the transversus abdominis. The seventh and eighth nerves course slightly upward or horizontally to reach the epigastrium, whereas the lower nerves have an increasingly caudal trajectory. As these nerves course medially, they provide motor branches to the abdominal wall musculature. Medially, they perforate the rectus sheath to provide sensory innervation to the anterior abdominal wall. The anterior ramus of the 10th thoracic nerve reaches the skin at the level of the umbilicus and the 12th thoracic nerve innervates the skin of the hypogastrium.

The ilioinguinal and iliohypogastric nerves often arise in common from the anterior rami of the 12th thoracic and first lumbar nerves to provide sensory innervation to the hypogastrium and lower abdominal wall. The iliohypogastric nerve runs parallel to the 12th thoracic nerve to pierce the transversus abdominis muscle near the iliac crest. After coursing between

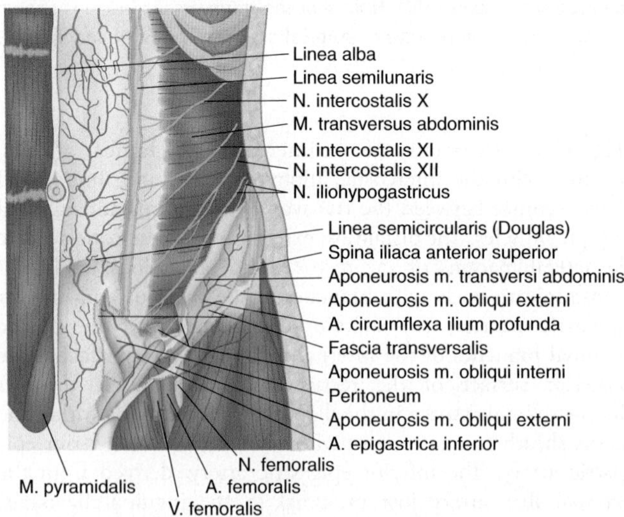


**FIGURE 45-7** Arteries and nerves of the anterolateral abdominal wall. (From McVay C: Anson and McVay's surgical anatomy, ed 6, Philadelphia, 1984, WB Saunders, p 501.)

the transversus abdominis muscle and internal oblique for a short distance, the nerve pierces the latter to travel under the external oblique fascia toward the external inguinal ring. It emerges through the superior crus of the external inguinal ring to provide sensory innervation to the anterior abdominal wall

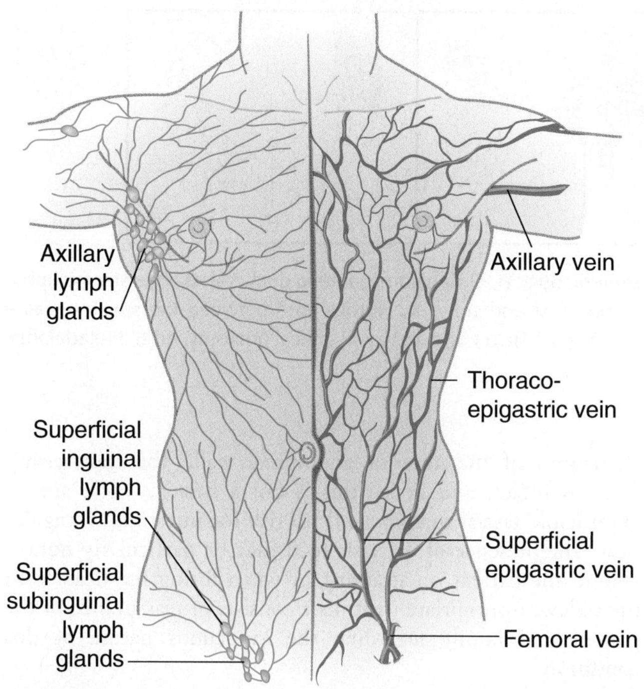


**FIGURE 45-8** Venous and lymphatic drainage of the anterolateral abdominal wall. (From Thorek P: Anatomy in surgery, ed 2, Philadelphia, 1962, JB Lippincott, p 345.)

in the hypogastrium. The ilioinguinal nerve courses parallel to the iliohypogastric nerve, but closer to the inguinal ligament. Unlike the iliohypogastric nerve, the ilioinguinal nerve courses with the spermatic cord to emerge from the external inguinal ring, with its terminal branches providing sensory innervation to the skin of the inguinal region and scrotum or labium. The ilioinguinal nerve, iliohypogastric nerve, and genital branch of the genitofemoral nerve are commonly encountered during the performance of inguinal herniorrhaphy.

## Abnormalities of the Abdominal Wall

These can be congenital or acquired.

### Congenital Abnormalities

**Umbilical Hernias** Umbilical hernias may be classified into three distinct forms:

1. Omphalocele and gastroschisis
2. Infantile umbilical hernia
3. Acquired umbilical hernia

***Omphalocele*** An omphalocele is a funnel-shaped defect in the central abdomen through which the viscera protrude into the base of the umbilical cord. It is caused by failure of the abdominal wall musculature to unite in the midline during fetal development. The umbilical vessels may be splayed over the viscera or pushed to one side. In larger defects, the liver and spleen may lie within the cord, along with a major portion of the bowel. There is no skin covering these defects, only peritoneum and, more superficially, amnion. Of infants who are born with an omphalocele, 50% to 60% will have concomitant congenital anomalies of the skeleton, gastrointestinal (GI) tract, and nervous, genitourinary, and cardiopulmonary systems.

***Gastroschisis*** Gastroschisis is another congenital defect of the abdominal wall in which the umbilical membrane has ruptured in utero, allowing the intestine to herniate outside the abdominal cavity. The defect is almost always to the right of the umbilical cord and the intestine is not covered with skin or amnion. Typically, the intestine has not undergone complete mesenteric rotation and fixation; hence, the infant is at risk for mesenteric volvulus, with resultant intestinal ischemia and necrosis. Concomitant congenital anomalies occur in about 10% of these patients. Both omphalocele and gastroschisis are discussed in greater detail in Chapter 67.

***Infantile Umbilical Hernia*** Infantile umbilical hernias appear within a few days or weeks after the stump of the umbilical cord has sloughed. It is caused by a weakness in the adhesion between the scarred remnants of the umbilical cord and umbilical ring. In contrast to omphalocele, the infantile umbilical hernia is covered by skin. Generally, these small hernias occur in the superior margin of the umbilical ring. They are easily reducible and become prominent when the infant cries. Most of these hernias resolve within the first 24 months of life, and complications such as strangulation are rare. Operative repair is indicated for those children in whom the hernia persists beyond the age of 3 or 4 years. This condition and its management are discussed further in Chapters 46 and 67.

***Acquired Umbilical Hernia*** In this condition, an umbilical hernia develops at a time remote from closure of the umbilical ring. This hernia occurs most commonly at the upper margin of the umbilicus and results from weakening of the cicatricial tissue that normally closes the umbilical ring. This may be caused by excessive stretching of the abdominal wall, which may occur with pregnancy, vigorous labor, or ascites. In contrast to infantile umbilical hernias, acquired umbilical hernias do not spontaneously resolve but gradually increase in size. The dense fibrous ring at the neck of this hernia makes strangulation of herniated intestine or omentum an important complication.

**Abnormalities Resulting from Persistence of the Omphalomesenteric Duct** During fetal development, the midgut communicates widely with the yolk sac through the vitelline or omphalomesenteric duct. As the abdominal wall components approximate one another, the omphalomesenteric duct narrows and comes to lie within the umbilical cord. Over time, communication between the yolk sac and intestine becomes obliterated and the intestine resides free within the peritoneal cavity. Persistence of part or all of the omphalomesenteric duct results in a variety of abnormalities related to the intestine and abdominal wall (Fig. 45-9).

Persistence of the intestinal end of the omphalomesenteric duct results in Meckel's diverticulum. These true diverticula arise from the antimesenteric border of the small intestine, most often the ileum. A Rule of 2s is often applied to these lesions in that they are found in approximately 2% of the population, are within 2 feet of the ileocecal valve, are often 2 inches in length, and contain two types of ectopic mucosa (gastric and pancreatic). Meckel's diverticula may be complicated by inflammation, perforation, hemorrhage, or obstruction. GI bleeding is caused by peptic ulceration of adjacent intestinal mucosa from hydrochloric acid secreted by ectopic parietal cells within the diverticulum. Intestinal obstruction associated with Meckel's diverticulum is usually caused by intussusception or volvulus

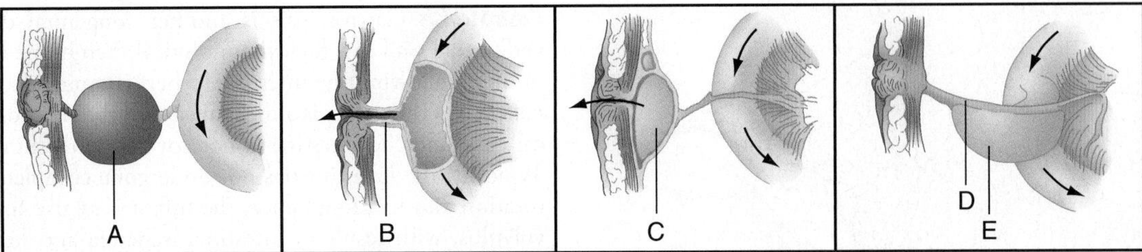


**FIGURE 45-9** Abnormalities resulting from persistence of the omphalomesenteric duct. **A,** Omphalomesenteric duct cyst. **B,** Persistent omphalomesenteric duct with an enterocutaneous fistula. **C,** Omphalomesenteric duct cyst and sinus. **D,** Fibrous cord between the small intestine and the posterior surface of the umbilicus. **E,** Meckel's diverticulum. (From McVay C: Anson and McVay's surgical anatomy, ed 6, Philadelphia, 1984, WB Saunders, p 576.)

around an abnormal fibrous connection between the diverticulum and posterior aspect of the umbilicus. These lesions are discussed in Chapter 50.

The omphalomesenteric duct may remain patent throughout its course, thus producing an enterocutaneous fistula between the distal small intestine and umbilicus. This condition presents with the passage of meconium and mucus from the umbilicus in the first few days of life. Because of the risk for mesenteric volvulus around a persistent omphalomesenteric duct, these lesions are promptly treated with laparotomy and excision of the fistulous tract. Persistence of the distal end of the omphalomesenteric duct results in an umbilical polyp, which is a small excrescence of omphalomesenteric ductal mucosa at the umbilicus. Such polyps resemble umbilical granulomas except that they do not disappear after silver nitrate cauterization. Their presence suggests that a persistent omphalomesenteric duct or umbilical sinus may be present, and hence they are most appropriately treated by excision of the mucosal remnant and underlying omphalomesenteric duct or umbilical sinus, if present. Umbilical sinuses result from the persistence of the distal omphalomesenteric duct. The morphology of the sinus tract can be delineated by a sinogram. Treatment involves excision of the sinus. Finally, the accumulation of mucus in a portion of a persistent omphalomesenteric duct may result in the formation of a cyst, which may be associated with the intestine or umbilicus by a fibrous band. Treatment consists of excision of the cyst and associated persistent omphalomesenteric duct.

**Abnormalities Resulting from Persistence of the Allantois** The allantois is the cranialmost component of the embryologic ventral cloaca. The intra-abdominal portion is termed the *urachus* and connects the urinary bladder with the umbilicus, whereas the extra-abdominal allantois is contained within the umbilical cord. At the end of gestation, the urachus is converted into a fibrous cord that courses between the extraperitoneal urinary bladder and umbilicus as the median umbilical ligament. Persistence of part or all of the urachus may result in the formation of a vesicocutaneous fistula, with the appearance of urine at the umbilicus, an extraperitoneal urachal cyst presenting as a lower abdominal mass, or an urachal sinus with the drainage of a small amount of mucus. Treatment is excision of the urachal remnant with closure of the bladder, if necessary.

## Acquired Abnormalities

**Diastasis Recti** Diastasis recti refers to a thinning of the linea alba in the epigastrium and is manifested as a smooth midline protrusion of the anterior abdominal wall. The transversalis fascia is intact, and hence this is not a hernia. There are no identifiable fascial margins and no risk for intestinal strangulation. The presence of diastasis recti may be particularly noticeable to the patient on straining or when lifting the head from the pillow. Appropriate treatment consists of reassurance of the patient and family regarding the innocuous nature of this condition.

**Anterior Abdominal Wall Hernias** Epigastric hernias occur at sites through which vessels and nerves perforate the linea alba to course into the subcutaneum. Through these openings, extraperitoneal areolar tissue and, at times, peritoneum may herniate into the subcutaneous tissue. Although these hernias are often small, they may produce significant localized pain and tenderness because of direct pressure of the hernia sac and its contents on the nerves emerging through the same fascial opening. Spigelian hernias occur through the fascia in the region of the semilunar line and present with localized pain and tenderness. The hernia sac is only rarely palpable because it is often small and tends to remain beneath the external oblique aponeurosis. Ultrasonography of the abdominal wall or computed tomography (CT) with thin cuts through the abdomen, after careful marking of the suspected site, should be diagnostic. Treatment consists of simple operative closure of the fascial defect. These hernias are discussed in Chapter 46.

**Rectus Sheath Hematoma** Rectus sheath hematoma is an uncommon condition characterized by acute abdominal pain and the appearance of an abdominal wall mass. It is more common in women than men and in older than younger individuals. A review of 126 patients with rectus sheath hematomas treated at the Mayo Clinic found that almost 70% were receiving anticoagulants at the time of diagnosis. A history of nonsurgical abdominal wall trauma or injury is common (48%), as is the presence of a cough (29%).[1] In young women, rectus sheath hematomas have been associated with pregnancy.

Patients with rectus sheath hematomas usually present with the sudden onset of abdominal pain, which may be severe and is often exacerbated by movements requiring contraction of the abdominal wall. Physical examination will demonstrate tenderness over the rectus sheath, often with voluntary guarding. An abdominal wall mass may be noted in some patients, 63% in the Mayo Clinic series.[1] Abdominal wall ecchymosis, including periumbilical ecchymosis (Cullen's sign) and blue discoloration in the flanks (Grey Turner's sign), may be present if there is a delay from the onset of symptoms to presentation. The pain and tenderness associated with this process may be severe enough to suggest peritonitis. In those cases in which the hematoma expands into the perivesical and preperitoneal spaces, the hematocrit level may fall, although hemodynamic instability is uncommon.

Ultrasonography or CT will confirm the presence of the hematoma and localize it to the abdominal wall in almost all cases. Usually, these patients may be managed successfully with rest and analgesics and, if necessary, blood transfusion. In the Mayo Clinic series, almost 90% of patients were managed successfully in this manner.[1] In general, coagulopathies are corrected, although continued anticoagulation of selected patients may be prudent, depending on the indications for anticoagulation and seriousness of the bleeding. Progression of the hematoma may necessitate angiographic embolization of the bleeding vessel or, uncommonly, operative evacuation of the hematoma and hemostasis.

## Malignancies of the Abdominal Wall

The most common primary malignancies of the abdominal wall are desmoid tumors and sarcomas. Although unusual, a variety of common cancers may metastasize through the bloodstream to the soft tissue of the abdominal wall, where it presents as a soft tissue mass. Metastatic melanoma, in particular, may present in this manner. Finally, transperitoneal seeding of the abdominal wall by intra-abdominal malignancies may complicate transabdominal biopsies or operative procedures.

### Desmoid Tumor

Desmoid tumor, also known as *fibromatosis* or *aggressive fibromatosis*, is an uncommon neoplasm that occurs sporadically or as part of an inherited syndrome, most notably, familial adenomatous polyposis (FAP) and Gardner's syndrome, an autosomal dominant syndrome of GI adenomatous polyps or adenocarcinoma, osteomas, and skin and soft tissue tumors. These tumors arise from fibroaponeurotic tissue and typically present as a slowly growing mass. Although they lack metastatic potential, they are locally aggressive and invasive, with a high propensity for recurrence.

Desmoid tumors are typically classified by location as extra-abdominal or extremity desmoids (i.e., those tumors occurring in the proximal extremities or limb girdle), abdominal wall tumors, and intra-abdominal desmoids, which involve the mesentery, pelvis, or bowel wall.

The frequency of desmoid tumors in the general population is 2.4 to 4.3 cases/million; this risk increases 1000-fold in patients with FAP.[2,3] The vast majority of desmoid tumors are sporadic, typically in young women during pregnancy or within a year of childbirth. Oral contraceptive use has also been associated with the occurrence of these tumors. These associations, combined with the detection of estrogen receptors within the tumor, suggest a regulatory role for estrogen in this disease.

Patients with a desmoid tumor present with an asymptomatic mass or with symptoms related to mass effect from the tumor. There is often a temporal association between the discovery of the tumor and an antecedent history of abdominal trauma or operation.[3] Imaging (CT or MRI) is necessary to delineate the extent of tumor involvement fully, but otherwise there is no need to perform staging for metastatic disease. On CT, a desmoid tumor appears as a homogeneous mass arising from the soft tissue of the abdominal wall (Fig. 45-10). A desmoid tumor will appear as a homogeneous and isointense mass compared with muscle on T1-weighted MRI images, whereas T2-weighted images demonstrate greater heterogeneity and a signal slightly less intense than fat.

Biopsy is required to establish the diagnosis. Core needle biopsy or incisional biopsy will demonstrate a tumor composed of bundles of spindle cells and an abundant fibrous stroma. The center of the tumor is often acellular, whereas the periphery contains most of the fibroblasts. The histology can be similar to that of a low-grade fibrosarcoma, but diagnosis is usually not difficult because the fibroblasts are highly differentiated and lack the mitotic activity found in malignancy. Immunohistochemistry can help clarify difficult diagnoses; the tumors typically stain positive for β-catenin, actin, and vimentin and stain negative for cytokeratin and S-100.

Resection of the tumor with a wide margin of normal tissue is currently considered the optimal treatment. Often, the extent of this resection will require abdominal wall reconstruction with local tissue flaps or mesh prostheses. The completeness of resection is an important prognostic factor; Stojadinovic and colleagues[4] have reported that 68% of desmoids tumors resected with a positive margin recur within 5 years, compared with none of the tumors in which the resection margin was free of disease.

Abdominal wall desmoids are responsive to radiation therapy, although the treatment effect is slow and may be progressive over several years. Radiotherapy alone is an acceptable treatment option for patients with unresectable desmoid tumors or tumors for which resection will be associated with high morbidity risks or major functional loss. A retrospective review from the M.D. Anderson Cancer Center has reported 10-year

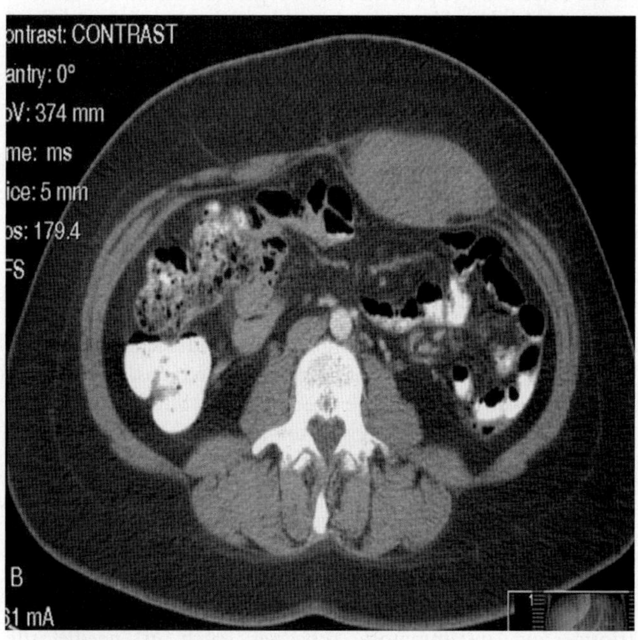


**FIGURE 45-10** CT scan of the abdomen demonstrating a desmoid tumor arising within the left rectus sheath. The tumor appears as a homogeneous soft tissue mass.

recurrence rates of 38% for surgery alone (27% for those with negative margins), 25% for combined surgery and radiation, and 24% for radiation therapy alone.[5] It was also concluded that radiation therapy can assuage the adverse effect of positive margins on local tumor recurrence. Similar large studies have reported local control rates of approximately 80% with radiotherapy alone, rates that are consistently equivalent or even superior to surgery alone.[6]

Adjuvant radiation therapy is controversial, with most centers reserving this modality for patients with positive margins, or close margins, because of critical structures. The use of neoadjuvant radiation therapy is less well accepted than adjuvant radiation therapy because of the slow response times, often 1 year or more, with the potential for making subsequent abdominal wall reconstruction more difficult, and few studies demonstrating a clear benefit.

Estrogen receptor antagonists, nonsteroidal anti-inflammatory drugs (NSAIDs), and systemic chemotherapy have been used successfully in the treatment of patients with locally advanced, recurrent or unresectable desmoid tumors. The use of these agents in an adjuvant or neoadjuvant setting is not well studied and they would be best used in the setting of a clinical trial.

The detection of estrogen receptors on desmoids tumors, as well as the association with pregnancy and oral contraceptives, provide some support for the use of antiestrogens, such as tamoxifen. Clinical improvement has been reported in 43% of patients receiving antiestrogens, although the response rate varies among studies. Tumor responses to antiestrogens are slow in onset but often last for several years.[7,8] Most reports of NSAID treatment use sulindac but indomethacin has also been used. A study using combination high-dose tamoxifen and sulindac recommended this regimen as initial treatment for FAP-associated desmoid tumors.[9]

Various cytotoxic chemotherapy regimens have been used in the treatment of patients with inoperable desmoids. Methotrexate with vinblastine, doxorubicin-based therapy, and ifosfamide-based regimens have been reported, with positive responses in 20% to 40% of patients.[7,10] For desmoids with rapid growth, medical oncologists may recommend therapies typically used for sarcomas, such as doxorubicin and dacarbazine. Recent reports have also suggested imatinib, a tyrosine kinase inhibitor, as another effective treatment option for patients with these tumors.[11]

### Abdominal Wall Sarcoma

Abdominal wall sarcoma are classified as truncal sarcoma—including the chest or abdominal wall—and account for 10% to 20% of sarcomas overall. In general, sarcomas are rare and abdominal wall sarcomas are exceedingly rare. Similar to desmoid tumors, these neoplasms most often present as a painless mass, although as many as one third of patients with abdominal wall sarcomas will have pain at the site of the tumor. Pertinent history, such as a history of retinoblastoma, FAP, neurofibromatosis, radiation therapy, or Li-Fraumeni syndrome, should be sought. The differential diagnosis includes many common conditions, such as lipomas, hematomas, ventral hernias, endometriosis, and inflammatory processes, such as needle site granulomas in diabetics. Histologic subtypes include liposarcoma, fibrosarcoma, leiomyosarcoma, rhabdomyosarcoma, and malignant fibrous histiocytoma.

Axial imaging with MRI or CT will provide important information regarding the location and extent of the tumor as well as involvement of contiguous structures. Chest CT should be included to rule out metastatic disease. Definitive diagnosis requires biopsy, which may be performed with a core needle or by incision. The accuracy of core needle biopsy is consistently reported as more than 90% and can be performed under CT guidance for deep lesions. If an incisional biopsy is performed, it is optimally done by the surgeon who will perform the definitive resection; it should be oriented in the same plane as the underlying muscle to minimize unnecessary tissue loss during the definitive procedure and facilitate reconstruction. No attempt is made to develop tissue flaps around the lesion, and hemostasis is meticulous to avoid dissemination of the tumor along the tissue planes by a postoperative hematoma.

Definitive treatment of abdominal wall sarcomas is resection with tumor-free margins, with most surgeons attempting to obtain at least a 2-cm margin around the tumor. Lymph node metastases are rare (2% to 3%). Reconstruction of the abdominal wall defect may be accomplished primarily, with myocutaneous flaps, or with prosthetic meshes, depending on the site and extent of resection. Response rates with radiation and chemotherapy are low.

Soft tissue sarcomas are discussed in greater detail in Chapter 33.

### Metastatic Disease

Metastases to the abdominal wall may occur by direct seeding of the abdominal wall during biopsy or resection of an intra-abdominal malignancy or by hematogenous spread of an advanced tumor. The risk of tumor implantation at the port site after laparoscopic colon resection for adenocarcinoma is 0.9% and has been shown in randomized controlled trials to be no different than the risk of tumor recurrence in the wound after open colon resections.[12] The most common tumors that metastasize to soft tissue are lung, colon, melanoma, and renal cell tumors. Although metastases to soft tissue are unusual, the abdominal wall is the site of such recurrence in approximately 20% of cases.[13] Similar to desmoids tumors or sarcomas, metastases to the abdominal wall present as a painless mass. Immunohistochemistry staining of the tumor may allow specific identification of the type of primary tumor and facilitate differentiation from primary sarcomas of the abdominal wall. The Sister Mary Joseph nodule is often described and seldom seen but represents a palpable nodule in the region of the umbilicus representing metastatic abdominal or pelvic cancer.

## Symptoms of Intra-Abdominal Disease Referred to the Abdominal Wall

Abdominal pain may be categorized as visceral, somatoparietal, and referred. Visceral pain is caused by stimulation of visceral nociceptors by inflammation, distention, or ischemia. The pain is dull in nature and poorly localized to the epigastrium, periumbilical regions, or hypogastrium, depending on the embryonic origin of the organ involved. Inflammation of the stomach, duodenum, and biliary tract (derivatives of the embryonic foregut) localizes visceral pain to the epigastrium. Stimulation of nociceptors in midgut-derived organs (small intestine, appendix, right colon) causes the sensation of pain in the periumbilical region, whereas inflammation or distention of hindgut-derived organs (left colon, rectum) causes hypogastric pain. The pain is felt in the midline because these organs transmit sympathetic sensory afferents to both sides of the spinal cord. The pain is poorly localized because the innervation of most viscera is multisegmental and contains fewer nerve receptors than highly sensitive organs such as the skin. The pain is often characterized as cramping, burning, or gnawing and may be accompanied by secondary autonomic effects such as sweating, restlessness, nausea, vomiting, perspiration, and pallor.

Somatoparietal pain arises from inflammation of the parietal peritoneum; it is more intense and more precisely localized than visceral pain. The nerve impulses mediating parietal pain travel within the somatosensory spinal nerves and reach the spinal cord in the peripheral nerves corresponding to the cutaneous dermatomes from the T6 to the L1 region. Lateralization of parietal pain is possible because only one side of the nervous system innervates a given part of the parietal peritoneum.

The difference between visceral and somatoparietal pain is well illustrated by the pain associated with acute appendicitis, in which the early, vague, periumbilical visceral pain is followed by the localized somatoparietal pain at McBurney's point. The visceral pain is produced by distention and inflammation of the appendix, whereas the localized somatoparietal pain in the right lower quadrant of the abdomen is caused by extension of the inflammation to the parietal peritoneum.

Referred pain is felt in anatomic regions remote from the diseased organ. This phenomenon is caused by convergence of visceral afferent neurons innervating an injured or inflamed organ with somatic afferent fibers arising from another anatomic region. This occurs within the spinal cord at the level of second-order neurons. Well-known examples of referred pain include shoulder pain on irritation of the diaphragm, scapular pain associated with acute biliary tract disease, and testicular or labial pain caused by retroperitoneal inflammation.

## PERITONEUM AND PERITONEAL CAVITY

### Anatomy

The peritoneum consists of a single sheet of simple squamous epithelium of mesodermal origin, termed *mesothelium,* lying on a thin connective tissue stroma. The surface area is 1.0 to 1.7 $m^2$, approximately that of the total body surface area. In males, the peritoneal cavity is sealed, whereas in females it is open to the exterior through the ostia of the fallopian tubes. The peritoneal membrane is divided into parietal and visceral components. The parietal peritoneum covers the anterior, lateral, and posterior abdominal wall surfaces and the inferior surface of the diaphragm and the pelvis. The visceral peritoneum covers most of the surface of the intraperitoneal organs (i.e., stomach, jejunum, ileum, transverse colon, liver, spleen) and the anterior aspect of the retroperitoneal organs (i.e., duodenum, left and right colon, pancreas, kidneys, adrenal glands).

The peritoneal cavity is subdivided into interconnected compartments or spaces by 11 ligaments and mesenteries. The peritoneal ligaments or mesenteries include the coronary, gastrohepatic, hepatoduodenal, falciform, gastrocolic, duodenocolic, gastrosplenic, splenorenal, and phrenicocolic ligaments and the transverse mesocolon and small bowel mesentery (Fig. 45-11). These structures partition the abdomen into nine potential spaces—right and left subphrenic, subhepatic, supramesenteric and inframesenteric, right and left paracolic gutters, pelvis, and lesser space. These ligaments, mesenteries, and peritoneal spaces direct the circulation of fluid in the peritoneal cavity and thus may be useful in predicting the route of spread of infectious and malignant diseases. For example, perforation of the duodenum from peptic ulcer disease may result in the movement of fluid (and the development of abscesses) in the subhepatic space, right paracolic gutter, and pelvis. The blood supply to the visceral peritoneum is derived from the splanchnic blood vessels, whereas the parietal peritoneum is supplied by branches of the intercostals, subcostal, lumbar, and iliac vessels. The innervation of the visceral and parietal peritoneum is discussed earlier.

### Physiology

The peritoneum is a bidirectional, semipermeable membrane that controls the amount of fluid in the peritoneal cavity, promotes the sequestration and removal of bacteria from the peritoneal cavity, and facilitates the migration of inflammatory cells from the microvasculature into the peritoneal cavity. Normally, the peritoneal cavity contains less than 100 mL of sterile serous

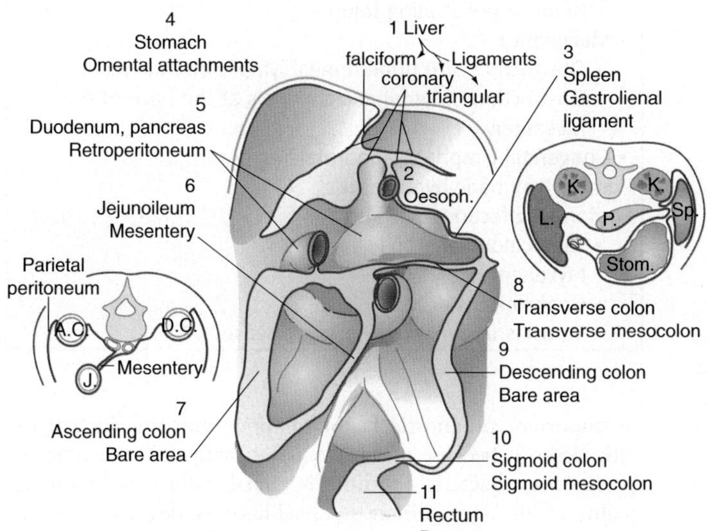


**FIGURE 45-11** Peritoneal ligaments and mesenteric reflections in the adult. These attachments partition the abdomen into nine potential spaces—right and left subphrenic, subhepatic, supramesenteric and inframesenteric spaces, right and left paracolic gutters, pelvis, and omental bursa *(inset, right).* (From McVay C: Anson and McVay's surgical anatomy, ed 6, Philadelphia, 1984, WB Saunders, p 589.)

fluid. Microvilli on the apical surface of the peritoneal mesothelium markedly increase the surface area and promote the rapid absorption of fluid from the peritoneal cavity into the lymphatics and portal and systemic circulations. The amount of fluid in the peritoneal cavity may increase to many liters in some diseases, such as cirrhosis, nephrotic syndrome, and peritoneal carcinomatosis.

The circulation of fluid in the peritoneal cavity is driven in part by the movement of the diaphragm. Intercellular pores in the peritoneum covering the inferior surface of the diaphragm (termed *stomata*) communicate with lymphatic pools in the diaphragm. Lymph flows from these diaphragmatic lymphatic channels through subpleural lymphatics to the regional lymph nodes and. Ultimately. the thoracic duct. Relaxation of the diaphragm during exhalation opens the stomata and the negative intrathoracic pressure draws fluid and particles, including bacteria, into the stomata. Contraction of the diaphragm during inhalation propels the lymph through the mediastinal lymphatic channels into the thoracic duct. It is postulated that this so-called *diaphragmatic pump* drives the movement of peritoneal fluid in a cephalad direction toward the diaphragm and into the thoracic lymphatic vessels. This circulatory pattern of peritoneal fluid toward the diaphragm and into the central lymphatic channels is consistent with the rapid appearance of sepsis in patients with generalized intra-abdominal infections, as well as the perihepatitis of Fitz-Hugh–Curtis syndrome in patients with acute salpingitis.

The peritoneum and peritoneal cavity respond to infection in five ways:

1. Bacteria are rapidly removed from the peritoneal cavity through the diaphragmatic stomata and lymphatics.
2. Peritoneal macrophages release proinflammatory mediators that promote the migration of leukocytes into the peritoneal cavity from the surrounding microvasculature.
3. Degranulation of peritoneal mast cells releases histamine and other vasoactive products, causing local vasodilation and the extravasation of protein-rich fluid containing complement and immunoglobulins into the peritoneal space.
4. Protein in the peritoneal fluid opsonizes bacteria, which, along with activation of the complement cascade, promotes neutrophil- and macrophage-mediated bacterial phagocytosis and destruction.
5. Bacteria become sequestered within fibrin matrices, thereby promoting abscess formation and limiting the generalized spread of the infection.

**BOX 45-1 Principal Causes of Ascites Formation Categorized According to Underlying Pathophysiology**

**Portal Hypertension**

Cirrhosis

Noncirrhotic

- Prehepatic portal venous obstruction
  - Chronic mesenteric venous thrombosis
  - Multiple hepatic metastases
- Posthepatic venous obstruction: Budd-Chiari syndrome

**Cardiac**

Congestive heart failure

Chronic pericardial tamponade

Constrictive pericarditis

**Malignancy**

Peritoneal carcinomatosis

- Primary peritoneal malignancies
  - Primary peritoneal mesothelioma
  - Serous carcinoma
- Metastatic carcinoma
  - Gastrointestinal carcinomas (e.g., gastric, colonic, pancreatic cancer)
  - Genitourinary carcinomas (e.g., ovarian cancer)

Retroperitoneal obstruction of lymphatic channels

- Lymphoma
- Lymph node metastases (e.g., testicular cancer, melanoma)

Obstruction of the lymphatic channels at the base of the mesentery

- Gastrointestinal carcinoid tumors

**Miscellaneous**

Bile ascites

- Iatrogenic after operations of the liver or biliary tract
- Traumatic after injuries to the liver or biliary tract

Pancreatic ascites

- Acute pancreatitis
- Pancreatic pseudocyst

Chylous ascites

- Disruptions of retroperitoneal lymphatic channels
  - Iatrogenic during retroperitoneal dissections: Retroperitoneal lymphadenectomy, abdominal aortic aneurysmorrhaphy
  - Blunt or penetrating trauma
- Malignancy
  - Obstruction of retroperitoneal lymphatic channels
  - Obstruction of lymphatic channels at the base of the mesentery
- Congenital lymphatic abnormalities

Primary lymphatic hypoplasia

Peritoneal infections

- Tuberculous peritonitis
- Myxedema
- Nephrotic syndrome
- Serositis in connective tissue disease

## Peritoneal Disorders

### Ascites

**Pathophysiology and Cause** Ascites is the pathologic accumulation of fluid in the peritoneal cavity. The principal causes of ascites formation and their pathophysiologic bases are listed in Box 45-1. Cirrhosis is the most common cause of ascites in the United States, accounting for approximately 85% of cases. Ascites is the most common complication of cirrhosis, with approximately 50% of compensated cirrhotic patients developing ascites within 10 years of diagnosis. The onset of ascites is an important prognostic factor for poor outcome in patients with cirrhosis because of its association with the occurrence of spontaneous bacterial peritonitis, renal failure, a worsened quality of life, and an increased likelihood of death within 2 to 5 years.

The two principal factors underlying the formation of ascites in cirrhotic patients are renal sodium and water retention and portal hypertension. Renal sodium retention is driven by activation of the renin-angiotensin-aldosterone and sympathetic nervous systems, which cause proximal and distal renal tubule sodium reabsorption. It is postulated that the abnormal release of nitric oxide within the splanchnic circulation causes vasodilation and a decrease in the effective circulating blood volume. Renin, aldosterone, and other hormones are generated as a counterregulatory mechanism to restore the effective circulating blood volume to normal. Portal hypertension is produced by postsinusoidal vascular obstruction from the deposition of collagen in the cirrhotic liver. Increased hydrostatic pressure within the hepatic sinusoids and splanchnic vasculature drives the extravasation of fluid from the microvasculature into the extracellular compartment. Ascites results when the capacity of the lymphatic system to return this fluid to the systemic circulation is overwhelmed. Some recent studies have reviewed the pathophysiology underlying fluid retention, hyponatremia, and ascites formation that characterizes patients with cirrhosis.[14,15]

Obstruction of the portal or hepatic venous blood flow in the absence of cirrhosis (e.g., portal vein thrombosis or Budd-Chiari syndrome, respectively) also causes ascites formation by increasing hydrostatic pressure within the splanchnic microvasculature. A similar pressure-based mechanism contributes to ascites formation in patients with heart failure, although the release of vasopressin and renin-angiotensin-aldosterone also promote sodium and water retention in these patients.

Patients with malignancies develop ascites by one of three mechanisms:

1. Multiple hepatic metastases cause portal hypertension by narrowing or occluding branches of the portal venous system.
2. Malignant cells scattered throughout the peritoneal cavity release protein-rich fluid into the peritoneal cavity, as in peritoneal carcinomatosis.
3. Obstruction of retroperitoneal lymphatics by a tumor, such as lymphoma, causes rupture of major lymphatic channels and the leakage of chyle into the peritoneal cavity.

Finally, ascites may result from the leakage of pancreatic juice, bile, or lymph into the peritoneal cavity after an iatrogenic or inflammatory disruption of a major pancreatic, bile, or lymphatic duct.

**Clinical Presentation and Diagnosis** The diagnosis of ascites is made on the basis of the medical history and appearance of the abdomen. Obviously, risk factors for hepatitis or cirrhosis are sought, as is evidence of cardiac or renal disease or malignancy. A full bulging abdomen with dullness of the flanks on percussion is suggestive of the presence of ascites. Approximately 1.5 liters of fluid must be present before dullness can be detected by percussion. Physical evidence of cirrhosis is also sought, such as palmar erythema, dilated abdominal wall collateral veins, and multiple spider angiomas. Patients with cardiac ascites have impressive jugular venous distention and other evidence of congestive heart failure.

***Ascitic Fluid Analysis*** Paracentesis with ascitic fluid analysis is the most rapid and cost-effective method of determining the cause of ascites and should be performed on patients with new-onset ascites. Another important indication for early paracentesis in a patient with ascites is the occurrence of signs and symptoms of infection, such as abdominal pain or tenderness, fever, encephalopathy, hypotension, renal failure, acidosis, and/or leukocytosis. Paracentesis can be performed safely in most patients, including those with cirrhosis and mild coagulopathy. It is usually performed in the lower abdomen, with the left lower quadrant preferred over the right. Ultrasound guidance may be useful in obese patients and in those with a history of laparotomy. Runyon[16] has suggested that only ongoing disseminated intravascular coagulation or clinically evident fibrinolysis is a contraindication to paracentesis in patients with ascites. In this study, no cases of hemoperitoneum, death, or infection after more than 229 paracenteses performed in 125 cirrhotic patients were reported; abdominal hematomas occurred in 2% of cases, with only 50% of these requiring blood transfusion.

Examination of the ascitic fluid begins with its gross appearance. Normal ascitic fluid is slightly yellow and transparent. The presence of more than 5000 leukocytes/mm$^3$ will cause the fluid to be cloudy, whereas ascitic fluid specimens with fewer than 1000 cells/mm$^3$ are almost clear. Blood in the ascitic fluid may be caused by a traumatic tap, in which case the fluid may be blood-streaked and will often clot unless immediately transferred to a tube containing an anticoagulant. Nontraumatic blood-tinged ascitic fluid does not clot because the required factors have been depleted by previous clotting in the peritoneal cavity. Lipid in the ascitic fluid, such as that which accompanies chylous ascites, causes the fluid to appear opalescent, ranging from cloudy to completely opaque. If placed in the refrigerator for 48 to 72 hours, the lipids usually layer out.

The most valuable laboratory tests on ascitic fluid are the cell count, differential, and determination of ascitic fluid albumin and total protein concentrations. The leukocyte count in uncomplicated cirrhotic ascites is usually less than 500 cells/mm$^3$, and approximately 50% of these cells are neutrophils. More than 250 neutrophils/mm$^3$ of ascitic fluid suggests an acute inflammatory process, the most common of which is spontaneous bacterial peritonitis. In this case, the total white blood cell and absolute neutrophil counts are elevated, with neutrophils accounting for more than 70% of the total cell count.

The serum-ascites albumin gradient (SAAG) is the most reliable method to categorize the various causes of ascites. The SAAG is calculated by measuring the albumin concentration of serum and ascitic fluid specimens and subtracting the ascitic fluid value from the serum value. If the SAAG is greater than or equal to 1.1 g/dL, the patient has portal hypertension; a SAAG of less than 1.1 g/dL is consistent with the absence of portal hypertension. Examples of high- and low-gradient causes of ascites are shown in Table 45-1. The accuracy of this measurement in predicting the presence or absence of portal hypertension is approximately 97%.[17]

**Treatment of Ascites in Cirrhotic Patients** The standard treatment protocol for patients with ascites caused by cirrhosis is a stepwise approach beginning with sodium restriction, diuretic therapy, and paracentesis.[14,15,18,19] The initial goal of medical therapy is to induce a state in which renal sodium excretion exceeds sodium intake, a situation that will reduce the extracellular volume and improve ascites. A reasonable dietary sodium restriction for most cirrhotic patients with ascites is 2 g/day. Patient compliance may be assessed by measuring the 24-hour urinary sodium excretion.

**Table 45-1 Classification of Ascites by Serum-Ascites Albumin Gradient**

| HIGH GRADIENT (≥1.1 g/dL) | LOW GRADIENT (<1.1 g/dL) |
|---|---|
| Cirrhosis | Peritoneal carcinomatosis |
| Alcoholic hepatitis | Tuberculous peritonitis |
| Cardiac failure | Pancreatic ascites |
| Massive liver metastases | Biliary ascites |
| Fulminant hepatic failure | Nephrotic syndrome |
| Budd-Chiari syndrome | Postoperative lymphatic leak |
| Portal vein thrombosis | Serositis in connective tissue diseases |
| Myxedema | |

From Runyon B: Ascites; spontaneous bacterial peritonitis. In Sleisenger MH, Feldman M, Friedman LS (eds): Sleisenger and Fordtran's gastrointestinal and liver disease: Pathophysiology, diagnosis, management, ed 7, Philadelphia, 2002, WB Saunders, p 1523.

Patients who are compliant with their dietary restriction and excrete more than 78 mmol/day of sodium in their urine lose weight. If the weight is increasing despite urinary sodium losses higher than 78 mmol/day, one can assume that the patient is consuming more sodium than is prescribed. Spironolactone and furosemide, when given in a dosing ratio of 100:40, will promote natriuresis while maintaining normokalemia. In general, spironolactone (100 mg/day) and furosemide (40 mg/day) are begun initially. If this regimen is ineffective in increasing urinary sodium excretion and decreasing body weight, the dosages of these drugs may be increased while maintaining the 100:40 ratio.

Large-volume paracentesis, in which more than 5 liters of ascites fluid is removed from the peritoneal cavity, may be useful for patients with ascites that has been unresponsive to sodium restriction and diuretic treatment; this occurs in less than 10% of patients. The IV infusion of albumin (6 to 8 g/liter of ascitic fluid removed) at the time of paracentesis will minimize the symptoms of intravascular volume depletion and renal insufficiency, which may accompany the removal of large volumes of ascitic fluid. The continuation of diuretics and salt restriction will prevent or delay the reaccumulation of ascites after paracentesis. Others have suggested that weekly albumin administration, independent of large-volume paracentesis, may be a useful adjunct to salt restriction and diuretic therapy in patients with refractory ascites. Transjugular intrahepatic portosystemic shunt and, ultimately, hepatic transplantation have been used to manage ascites refractory to simpler, less invasive options. These modalities are discussed in Chapter 54.

**Chylous Ascites** Chylous ascites is the collection of chyle in the peritoneal cavity and may result from one of three principal mechanisms:

1. Obstruction of major lymphatic channels at the base of the mesentery or the cisterna chyli, with exudation of chyle from dilated mesenteric lymphatics
2. Direct leakage of chyle through a lymphoperitoneal fistula caused by abnormal or injured retroperitoneal lymphatic vessels
3. Exudation of chyle through the walls of retroperitoneal megalymphatics, without a visible fistula or thoracic duct obstruction

In adults, the most common cause of chylous ascites is an intra-abdominal malignancy obstructing the lymphatic channels at the base of the mesentery or in the retroperitoneum. Lymphoma is the most common malignancy associated with chylous ascites, although chylous ascites has also been associated with ovarian, colon, renal, prostate, pancreatic, and gastric malignancies. Carcinoid tumors may cause chylous ascites by obstructing the lymphatics at the base of the mesentery through direct invasion and the dense fibrosis characteristic of this neoplasm. Chylous ascites may also result from injury of the retroperitoneal lymphatics during surgical procedures such as operations on the abdominal aorta and retroperitoneal lymph node dissections. Blunt and penetrating traumatic injuries are also important causes of chylous ascites, particularly in children. Chylous ascites in children may be caused by congenital lymphatic abnormalities, such as primary lymphatic hypoplasia, resulting in lower extremity lymphedema, chylothorax, and chylous ascites.

Patients with chylous ascites most often present with painless abdominal distention. Malnutrition and dyspnea occur in approximately 50% of cases. Paracentesis yields a characteristic milky fluid with a high protein and fat content. The SAAG will be less than 1.1 mg/dL and the triglyceride level will be higher than that of plasma, often two to eight times higher that of plasma. CT, lymphoscintigraphy, and lymphangiography may provide information regarding the site of obstruction, although the latter two modalities are rarely available.

Management of patients with chylous ascites includes the maintenance or improvement of nutrition, reduction in the rate of chyle formation, and correction of the underlying disease process. A low-fat, medium-chain triglyceride diet, combined with diuretics, has been used successfully to treat adults with chylous ascites complicating retroperitoneal lymph node dissections. It is postulated that reducing long-chain triglyceride intake will reduce the rate of chyle flow because their metabolites are transported through the splanchnic lymphatics as chylomicrons. In contrast, medium-chain triglycerides are directly absorbed by enterocytes and transported to the liver through the splanchnic blood vessels as free fatty acids and glycerol. Fasting with total parenteral nutrition, alone or in combination with somatostatin, has also been used successfully to manage patients with retroperitoneal lymphatic leak. Paracentesis may temporarily relieve the dyspnea and abdominal discomfort associated with chylous ascites; however, repeated paracentesis leads to hypoproteinemia and malnutrition. Experience with peritoneovenous shunts to treat chylous ascites has generally been disappointing. Surgical exploration of the abdomen and retroperitoneum is generally reserved for patients who fail to improve with nonoperative management. In some cases, the application of fibrin glue has been a beneficial adjunct to surgical exploration of the retroperitoneum.

**Peritonitis** Peritonitis is inflammation of the peritoneum and peritoneal cavity, usually caused by a localized or generalized infection. Primary peritonitis results from bacterial, chlamydial, fungal, or mycobacterial infection in the absence of perforation of the GI tract, whereas secondary peritonitis occurs in the setting of GI perforation. Frequent causes of secondary bacterial peritonitis include peptic ulcer disease, acute appendicitis, colonic diverticulitis, and pelvic inflammatory disease.

***Spontaneous Bacterial Peritonitis*** Spontaneous bacterial peritonitis (SBP) is defined as a bacterial infection of ascitic fluid in the absence of an intra-abdominal, surgically treatable source of infection. Although usually associated with cirrhosis, SBP may also occur in patients with nephrotic syndrome and, less commonly, congestive heart failure. It is extremely rare for patients with ascitic fluid containing a high protein concentration to develop SBP, such as those with peritoneal carcinomatosis. The most common pathogens in adults with SBP are the aerobic enteric flora *Escherichia coli* and *Klebsiella pneumoniae.* In children with nephrogenic or hepatogenic ascites, group A streptococcus, *Staphylococcus aureus,* and *Streptococcus pneumoniae* are common isolates.

Bacterial translocation from the GI tract is thought to be an important step in the pathogenesis of SBP. Impaired GI motility in cirrhotics is thought to alter normal gut microflora and impaired local and systemic immune function prevents the effective clearance of translocated bacteria from the mesenteric lymphatics and bloodstream. A low protein concentration in ascitic fluid prevents effective opsonization of bacteria and hence clearance by macrophages and neutrophils.

The diagnosis of SBP is made initially by demonstrating more than 250 neutrophils/mm$^3$ of ascitic fluid in a clinical setting consistent with this diagnosis—that is, abdominal pain, fever, or leukocytosis in a patient with low-protein ascites. It is unusual to document bacterascites on Gram staining of ascitic fluid, and delay of appropriate antibiotic management until the ascitic fluid cultures grow bacterial isolates risks the development of overwhelming infection and death. Bedside screening of ascitic fluid for leukocyte esterase, using colorimetric leukocyte esterase reagent strips, has been used to shorten the time from paracentesis to treatment, although its widespread use remains controversial.[20,21]

Broad-spectrum antibiotics, such as a third-generation cephalosporin, are started immediately in patients suspected of having ascitic fluid infection. These agents cover approximately 95% of the flora most commonly associated with SBP and are the antibiotics of choice for patients suspected to have SBP.[22,23] The spectrum of the antibiotic coverage may be narrowed once the results of antibiotic sensitivity tests are known. Repeat paracentesis with ascitic fluid analysis is not needed in the usual case, in which there is rapid improvement in response to antibiotic therapy. If the setting, symptoms, ascitic fluid analysis, or response to therapy are atypical, repeat paracentesis may be helpful for detecting secondary peritonitis. Multiple bacterial isolates, particularly of gram-negative enteric organisms, combined with a poor response to antibiotic therapy, suggest the presence of secondary peritonitis.

The immediate mortality risk caused by SBP is low, particularly if recognized and treated expeditiously. However, the development of other complications of hepatic failure, including GI hemorrhage or hepatorenal syndrome, contributes to the death of many of these patients during the hospitalization in which SBP is detected. The occurrence of SBP is an important landmark in the natural history of cirrhosis, with 1- and 2-year survival rates of approximately 30% and 20%, respectively. Several studies, including a randomized controlled trial, have shown that plasma expansion with albumin improves circulatory function and reduces the risk for hepatorenal syndrome and hospital mortality in patients with SBP.[24]

***Tuberculous Peritonitis*** Tuberculosis is common in impoverished areas of the world and is encountered with increasing frequency in the United States and other developed countries. Since 1985, the number of cases of tuberculosis in the United States and European nations has increased dramatically as the number of immigrants, refugees, and individuals with acquired immunodeficiency syndrome (AIDS) has increased. Others have described an association between peritoneal tuberculosis and alcoholic cirrhosis and chronic renal failure.[25] Peritoneal tuberculosis is the sixth most common site of extrapulmonary tuberculosis, after lymphatic, genitourinary, bone and joint, miliary, and meningeal. Most cases result from reactivation of latent peritoneal disease that had been previously established hematogenously from a primary pulmonary focus. Only approximately 17% of cases are associated with active pulmonary disease.

The illness often presents insidiously, with patients having had symptoms for several weeks to months at the time of presentation. Abdominal swelling caused by ascites formation is the most common symptom, occurring in more that 80% of cases. Similarly, most patients complain of a nonlocalized, vague abdominal pain. Constitutional symptoms such as low-grade fever and night sweats, weight loss, anorexia, and malaise are reported in approximately 60% of patients. The concomitant presence of other chronic conditions such as uremia, cirrhosis, and AIDS makes these symptoms difficult to interpret. Abdominal tenderness is present on palpation in approximately 50% of patients with peritoneal tuberculosis.[25] A positive tuberculin skin test is present in most cases, whereas only approximately 50% of these patients will have an abnormal chest radiograph. The ascitic fluid SAAG is less than 1.1 g/dL, consistent with a high protein concentration in the ascitic fluid. Microscopic examination of the ascites shows erythrocytes and an increased number of leukocytes, most of which are lymphocytes. Recently, measurement of ascitic fluid adenosine deaminase activity and polymerase chain reaction assays have been used as noninvasive and rapid tests for tuberculous peritonitis. Ascitic fluid adenosine deaminase activity, in particular, appears to be highly sensitive and specific for tuberculous peritonitis.

Abdominal imaging with ultrasound or CT may suggest the diagnosis but lacks the sensitivity and specificity to be diagnostic. Ultrasound may demonstrate the presence of echogenic material in the ascitic fluid, seen as fine mobile strands or particulate matter. CT will demonstrate the thickened and nodular mesentery with mesenteric lymphadenopathy and omental thickening.

The diagnosis is made by laparoscopy with directed biopsy of the peritoneum. In more than 90% of cases, laparoscopy demonstrates a number of whitish nodules (<5 mm) scattered over the visceral and parietal peritoneum; histologic examination demonstrates caseating granulomas. Multiple adhesions are commonly present between the abdominal organs and parietal peritoneum. The gross appearance of the peritoneal cavity is similar to that of peritoneal carcinomatosis, sarcoidosis, and Crohn's disease, thus reiterating the importance of biopsy. Blind percutaneous peritoneal biopsy has a much lower yield than directed biopsy, and laparotomy with peritoneal biopsy is reserved for cases in which laparoscopy has been nondiagnostic or cannot be safely performed. Microscopic examination of ascitic fluid for acid-fast bacilli identifies the organism in less than 3% of cases, and culture results are positive in less than 20% of cases. Furthermore, the diagnostic usefulness of mycobacterial cultures is further limited by the time it may take for the cultures to yield definitive information, up to 8 weeks.

Treatment of peritoneal tuberculosis consists of antituberculous drugs. Drug regimens useful in treating pulmonary tuberculosis are also effective for peritoneal disease, with isoniazid and rifampin daily for 9 months being a commonly used and effective regimen. The presence of associated alcoholic cirrhosis may complicate the use of these agents because of hepatotoxicity.

***Peritonitis Associated With Chronic Ambulatory Peritoneal Dialysis*** In the United States, approximately 8% of patients with chronic renal failure undergo peritoneal dialysis. Peritonitis is one of the most common complications of chronic ambulatory peritoneal dialysis, occurring with an incidence of approximately one episode every 1 to 3 years. A study of all patients undergoing peritoneal dialysis in Scotland between 1999 and 2002 found that one episode of peritonitis occurred in every 19.2 months of peritoneal dialysis. Importantly, refractory or recurrent peritonitis was the most common cause of technical failure, accounting for 43% of all cases of technique failure.[26]

Patients present with abdominal pain, fever, and cloudy peritoneal dialysate containing more than 100 leukocytes/mm$^3$, with more than 50% of the cells being neutrophils. Gram staining detects organisms only in approximately 10% to 40% of cases. Approximately 75% of infections are caused by gram-positive organisms, with *Staphylococcus epidermidis* accounting for 30% to 50% of cases. *S. aureus,* gram-negative bacilli, and fungi are also important causes of dialysis-associated peritonitis.[26]

Peritoneal dialysis–associated peritonitis is treated by the intraperitoneal administration of antibiotics, usually a first-generation cephalosporin. Overall, 75% of infections are cured by culture-directed antibiotic therapy. The cure rate for peritonitis caused by coagulase-negative staphylococcus is almost 90%, compared with the rates for peritonitis caused by *S. aureus,* gram-negative bacilli, or fungi of 66%, 56%, and 0%, respectively.[26] Recurrent or persistent peritonitis requires removal of the dialysis catheter and resumption of hemodialysis.

### Malignant Neoplasms of the Peritoneum

Primary malignancies of the peritoneum are rare; these include malignant mesothelioma, primary peritoneal carcinoma, and sarcomas (e.g., angiosarcoma). Most malignancies that involve the peritoneum are transperitoneal metastases originating from carcinomas of the GI tract (especially the stomach, colon, and pancreas), the genitourinary tract (usually, ovarian) or, more rarely, an extra-abdominal site (e.g., breast). When metastatic cancer deposits diffusely coat the visceral and parietal peritoneum, these peritoneal metastases are referred to as *carcinomatosis.*

**Pseudomyxoma Peritonei** Pseudomyxoma peritonei describes mucinous ascites arising from a ruptured ovarian or appendiceal adenocarcinoma. In this disease, the peritoneum becomes coated with a mucus-secreting tumor that fills the peritoneal cavity with tenacious semisolid mucus and large, loculated cystic masses. Although the term *pseudomyxoma peritonei* is often used to describe any condition with accumulation of intraperitoneal mucin or mucinous ascites, here we will focus on pseudomyxoma peritonei resulting from ruptured epithelial neoplasms of the appendix. The histology of appendiceal tumors is an important predictor of survival with adenomucinosis having the best survival rate (75% at 5 years) and peritoneal mucinous carcinomatosis the worst (14% at 5 years).[27]

Pseudomyxoma peritonei occurs most commonly in patients who are 40 and 50 years of age and occurs with equal frequency in men and women. Patients are often asymptomatic until late in the course of their disease. On presentation, they will often describe a global deterioration in their health long before the diagnosis is made. Symptoms of abdominal pain and distention and nonspecific complaints are common. Physical examination may reveal a new hernia, ascites, distended abdomen with nonshifting dullness and, occasionally, a palpable abdominal mass.

CT of the chest, abdomen, and pelvis may provide important information regarding the diagnosis and the ability to resect the tumor completely or perform an adequate cytoreduction. The latter is often limited by involvement of the small bowel or porta hepatis by tumor. Preoperative colonoscopy will differentiate a mucinous neoplasm of the appendix from that arising from the colon. Often, the diagnosis is made at laparotomy, when the surgeon is presented with a peritoneal cavity containing tenacious semisolid mucus and large, loculated cystic masses. If the surgeon is unprepared to perform a definitive procedure, the best approach is to establish the diagnosis by the least invasive procedure possible and relieve symptoms of intestinal obstruction, if present. The patient can then be referred to a center experienced in the management of these patients.

The treatment of patients with pseudomyxoma peritonei involves resection of as much of the tumor as possible (cytoreduction) and intraperitoneal heated chemotherapy (IPHC). Operative management includes omentectomy, stripping of involved peritoneum, resection of involved organs, and appendectomy, if not previously performed. There should be no residual tumor nodules larger than 2 mm in diameter after resection to facilitate penetration of the chemotherapy into any residual disease. Generally, a right hemicolectomy is performed for these tumors, although a review of 501 patients with mucinous tumors of the appendix has suggested that this is unnecessary if the resection margin at appendectomy is negative.[28] IPHC can be performed using an open technique, in which the abdomen is left open to ensure adequate chemotherapy distribution throughout the peritoneal cavity, or a closed technique, in which the abdomen is closed after inflow and outflow cannulas are placed. The latter allows for easier maintenance of hyperthermia (Fig. 45-12). There are many variations of surgical technique and chemotherapy administration but one commonly used technique has been reported extensively by Stewart and associates.[29]

Cytoreduction with IPHC is associated with improved survival for patients with pseudomyxoma peritonei when compared with historical controls. Prior to cytoreduction and IPHC, most studies reported long-term survival rates of 20% to 30% for patients with this disease undergoing serial debulking of the tumor with systemic chemotherapy. Gonzalez-Moreno and Sugarbaker[28] have reported 10-year survival rates of 55% in 501 patients undergoing cytoreduction and IPHC. Unfortunately, there are not likely to be any randomized controlled trials for

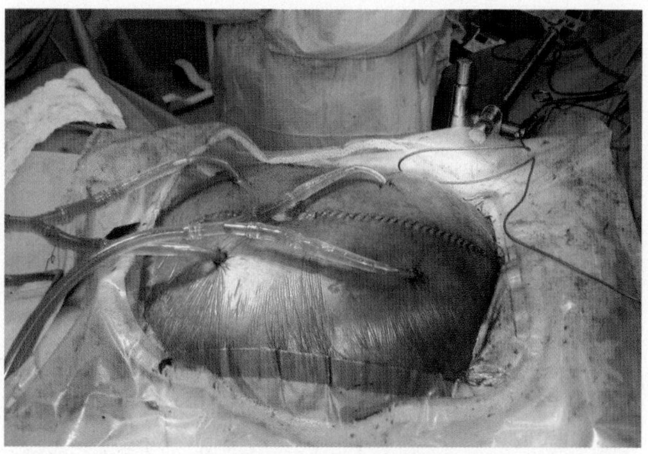

**FIGURE 45-12** Placement of peritoneal catheters during the performance of intraperitoneal hyperthermic chemotherapy using the closed technique for chemotherapy administration.

this technique, given the infrequency with which this disease is encountered. Furthermore, reported experiences are complicated by the use of various chemotherapy regimens, surgical techniques, and preoperative and intraoperative staging protocols.

At centers with experience in this technique, 30-day mortality rates are 2% to 3% with 25% to 35% of patients developing a complication. The most common postoperative complications are prolonged ileus and pulmonary complications, although bleeding, intra-abdominal infections, enterocutaneous fistula, pancreatitis, and bone marrow suppression have also been reported.

**Malignant Peritoneal Mesothelioma** The most common primary malignant peritoneal neoplasm is malignant mesothelioma, which results from malignant transformation of the simple squamoid epithelium covering the peritoneal cavity. Most patients are men, and their median age at presentation is in the 50s. As with mesothelioma of the pleura, most patients with peritoneal mesothelioma will have had exposure to asbestos.

Most patients present with abdominal pain and weight loss. Ascites is common and often intractable. The omentum may become diffusely involved with tumor and present as an epigastric mass. CT demonstrates mesenteric thickening, peritoneal studding, hemorrhage within the tumor, and ascites. At laparotomy, the ascitic fluid ranges from a serous transudate to a viscous fluid rich in mucopolysaccharides. The neoplasm tends to involve all peritoneal surfaces, producing masses and plaques of tumor that are hard and white. In contrast to pseudomyxoma peritonei, local invasion of intra-abdominal organs, such as the liver, intestine, bladder, and abdominal wall, can occur and encasement of bowel can create a malignant bowel obstruction. In some cases, it may be difficult to differentiate malignant peritoneal mesothelioma from diffuse peritoneal carcinomatosis arising from an intra-abdominal organ such as the stomach, pancreas, colon, or ovary. Careful examination of the pattern of spread and biopsy by histologic examination will often allow this distinction to be made. Furthermore, malignant peritoneal mesothelioma will generally remain confined to the abdomen, whereas advanced-stage intra-abdominal carcinomas frequently have pulmonary and other extra-abdominal metastases. Extension of the mesothelioma into one or both pleural cavities is more likely than hematogenous dissemination. Levy and colleagues[30] have reviewed the pathologic and radiographic features of peritoneal malignancies.

Complete surgical resection is usually not possible because of the extent of disease. Historically, operative management consisted of debulking of the tumor and enteroenterostomies to bypass areas of actual or impending intestinal obstruction. Unfortunately, systemic chemotherapy and abdominal radiation have been tried, without significant improvement in survival. Radiation therapy alone, whether using open-field techniques, intraperitoneal instillation of radioactive agents, or external-beam irradiation, has had limited success and substantial associated morbidity.

As with pseudomyxoma peritonei, combined-modality approaches using surgery and IPHC may offer substantial improvements compared to historical controls. There have been several retrospective series using this technique, with median survival rates of 30 to 60 months, and even 5-year survival rates of up to 50%. In light of these findings, and the rarity of the disease, a multi-institutional data registry from eight institutions was created, including 405 patients treated with cytoreductive surgery and perioperative intraperitoneal chemotherapy.[31] Chemotherapeutic regimens varied (cisplatin, mitomycin, and doxorubicin were most commonly used), as did the timing and administration of the chemotherapy. The morbidity rate was 46% and the mortality rate was 2%. Median survival was impressive at 53 months. Three- and 5-year survival rates were 60% and 47%, respectively, offering significant improvement over what was previously considered a preterminal condition.

## MESENTERY AND OMENTUM

### Embryology and Anatomy

The greater and lesser omenta are complex peritoneal folds that pass from the stomach to the liver, transverse colon, spleen, bile duct, pancreas, and diaphragm. They originate from the dorsal and ventral midline mesenteries of the embryonic gut. In the very early stages of development, the alimentary canal traverses the future coelomic cavity as a straight tube, suspended posteriorly by an uninterrupted dorsal mesentery and anteriorly by a ventral mesentery in the cranial portion of its extent. The embryonic stomach rotates 90 degrees on its longitudinal axis so that the lesser curvature faces to the right and the greater curvature to the left. Much of the embryonic ventral mesentery is resorbed; however, the portion extending from the fissure of the ligamentum venosum and porta hepatis to the proximal duodenum and lesser curvature of the stomach (gastrohepatic ligament) persists as the lesser omentum. The right border of the lesser omentum is a free edge that forms the anterior border of the opening into the lesser sac, termed the *foramen of Winslow.* Between the layers of the lesser omentum, and at its right border, are the common hepatic duct, portal vein, and hepatic artery.

The embryonic dorsal mesogastrium grows as a sheet of peritoneum extending from the greater curvature of the stomach over the anterior surface of the small intestine. After passing inferiorly almost to the pelvis, the peritoneal membrane turns up on itself to pass upward to a line of attachment on the transverse colon slightly above that of the transverse mesocolon. Fat is laid down in this omental apron and provides an insulating layer of protection of the abdominal viscera.

Early in its development, the small intestine elongates to form an anteriorly oriented intestinal loop, which then rotates counterclockwise so that the cecum and ascending colon move to the right side of the peritoneal cavity, and the descending colon assumes a vertical position on the left wall of the peritoneal cavity. The jejunum and ileum are supported by the peritoneum-covered dorsal mesentery carrying the mesenteric blood vessels and lymphatics. The posterior line of attachment of the mesentery extends obliquely from the duodenojejunal junction at the left side of the second lumbar vertebra toward the right iliac fossa to terminate anterior to the sacroiliac articulation.

### Physiology

The omentum and intestinal mesentery are rich in lymphatics and blood vessels. The omentum contains areas with high concentrations of macrophages, which may aid in the removal of foreign material and bacteria. Furthermore, the omentum becomes densely adherent to intraperitoneal sites of inflammation, often preventing diffuse peritonitis during cases of intestinal gangrene or perforation, such as acute diverticulitis or acute appendicitis.

## Diseases of the Omentum

### Omental Cysts

Omental cysts are unilocular or multilocular cysts containing serous fluid that are thought to arise from congenital or acquired obstruction of omental lymphatic channels. They are lined by a lymphatic endothelium similar to that of cystic lymphangiomas. These lesions are most common in children or young adults, in whom small cysts are usually asymptomatic and discovered incidentally; larger cysts present as a palpable abdominal mass. Uncomplicated cysts usually lie in the lower midabdomen and are freely movable, smooth, and nontender. Complications are more common in children and include torsion, infection, and rupture.

Plain radiographs of the abdomen may show a well-circumscribed soft tissue density in the midabdomen, and contrast studies of the intestine may show displacement of intestinal loops and extrinsic compression on adjacent bowel. Ultrasound or CT will show a fluid-filled, complex, cystic mass with internal septations. The differential diagnosis of these lesions includes cysts and solid tumors of the mesentery, peritoneum, and retroperitoneum, including desmoid tumors. Ultimately, the diagnosis is made by excision of the cyst and histologic examination of the wall. Local excision is curative; laparoscopic resection of these lesions has been reported.

### Omental Torsion and Infarction

Torsion of the greater omentum is defined as the axial twisting of the omentum along its long axis. If the twist is tight enough, or the venous obstruction is of sufficient duration, arterial inflow will become compromised, leading to infarction and necrosis. Omental torsion is classified as primary when no coexisting causative condition is identified or secondary when the torsion occurs in association with a causative condition such as a hernia, tumor, or adhesion. Primary omental torsion usually involves the right side of the omentum.

Omental torsion occurs twice as often in men as women and is most frequent in patients in their fourth or fifth decade of life. Patients present with the acute onset of severe abdominal pain localized to the right side of the abdomen in 80% of patients. Nausea and vomiting may be present but are not predominant findings. The patient's temperature is usually normal, and palpation of the abdomen demonstrates localized abdominal tenderness with guarding, suggesting peritonitis. A mass may be palpable if the involved omentum is sufficiently large.

The differential diagnosis includes any disease associated with right-sided abdominal pain and tenderness, most notably acute appendicitis, acute cholecystitis, and torsion of an ovarian cyst. CT often demonstrates an omental mass with signs of inflammation. Usually, the patient's clinical presentation justifies laparotomy or laparoscopy, at which time a segment of the omentum appears congested and acutely inflamed. Serosanguineous fluid is often present in the peritoneal cavity. Treatment consists of resection of the involved omentum and correction of any related condition.

### Omental Neoplasms

Primary malignancies of the omentum are extremely rare and are usually of soft tissue origin. Usually, the omentum is invaded by metastatic tumor that has spread transperitoneally from an intra-abdominal carcinoma.

### Omental Grafts and Transpositions

The arterial and venous blood supplies to the greater omentum are derived from omental branches of the right and left gastroepiploic arteries, which course along the greater curvature of the stomach. Division of the right or left gastroepiploic artery and vasa recta along the greater curvature of the stomach, with mobilization of the omentum from the transverse colon, allows the development of a vascularized omental pedicle flap. This graft may be used to cover chest and mediastinal wounds after chest wall resections and prevent the small intestine from entering the pelvis after abdominal perineal resection, thus preventing radiation enteritis during radiation therapy for rectal carcinoma. Finally, the formation of dense adhesions between the omentum and sites of perforation or inflammation facilitates its use as a patch for duodenal perforations from ulcer disease (termed a *Graham patch;* Fig. 45-13).

## Diseases of the Mesentery

### Mesenteric Cysts

The most common non-neoplastic mesenteric cysts are termed *mesothelial cysts,* based on the ultrastructure of the cells lining the cyst. The cysts contain chyle or a clear serous fluid and may occur in the mesentery of the small intestine (60%) or colon (40%). These cysts usually occur in adults, with a mean age of 45 years, and are twice as common in women as in men. Depending on the size of the cyst, patients may present with complaints of abdominal pain, fever, and emesis. A midabdominal mass may be palpable on examination of the abdomen. The diagnosis can usually be made preoperatively with ultrasonography or CT. Enucleation of the cyst at laparotomy is curative and can generally be accomplished because the mesenteric blood vessels and intestinal wall are usually not adherent to the cyst wall. Internal drainage of the cyst into the peritoneal cavity has also been successfully used in the treatment of very large cysts.

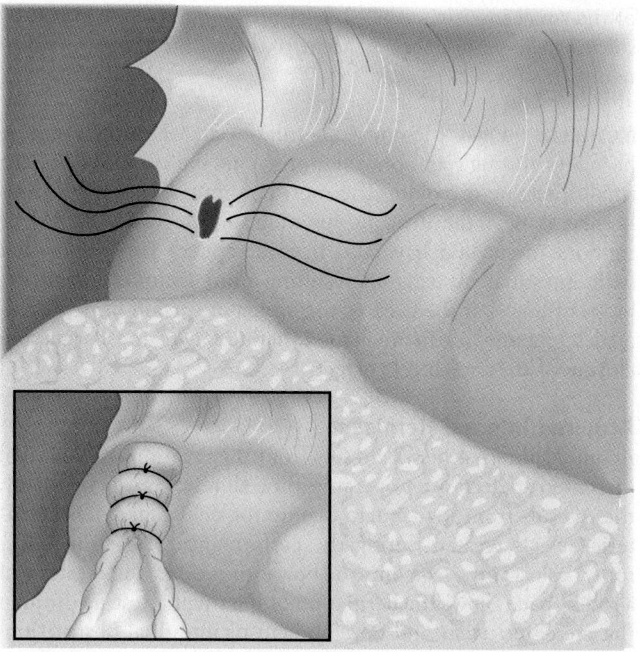

**FIGURE 45-13** Closure of a perforated duodenal ulcer with an omental (Graham) patch. (From Graham RR: The treatment of perforated duodenal ulcers. Surg Gynecol Obstet 64:235–238, 1937.)

Aspiration alone has a high rate of cyst recurrence. In those cases in which the cyst is not completely excised, the contents of the cyst and the internal architecture of the cyst wall must be carefully inspected and the cyst wall examined histologically to rule out a non-neoplastic cause.

### Acute Mesenteric Lymphadenitis

Acute mesenteric lymphadenitis is a syndrome of acute right lower quadrant abdominal pain associated with mesenteric lymph node enlargement and a normal appendix. Generally, the diagnosis is made on exploration of the abdomen of a patient suspected of having acute appendicitis at which time a normal appendix and enlarged mesenteric lymph nodes are discovered. This syndrome occurs most commonly in children and young adults, with equal frequency in males and females.

Numerous causative agents have been implicated in the pathobiology of acute mesenteric lymphadenitis, including viral, bacterial, parasitic, and fungal infections. *Yersinia enterocolitica* in particular has been associated with this syndrome in children. Culture and histologic examination of the enlarged lymph nodes, stool culture, and antibody titers have been used to identify causative agents but are not routinely used in the treatment of these patients.

The symptom complex associated with acute mesenteric lymphadenitis is similar to that of acute appendicitis; it includes the acute onset of periumbilical pain, which shifts to the right lower quadrant over time. Physical examination demonstrates right lower quadrant tenderness, with abdominal wall muscular rigidity and rebound tenderness. Nausea, vomiting, and anorexia may also be present but are not dominant symptoms. Generally, the patient's temperature and white blood cell count are normal or only slightly elevated.

The diagnosis is made at the time of operation for presumed acute appendicitis, at which time a normal-appearing appendix is found, with enlarged mesenteric lymph nodes. Excision of an enlarged lymph node with culture and nodal histology may provide information regarding the cause but is not routinely used.

### Sclerosing Mesenteritis

Sclerosing mesenteritis is a rare inflammatory disease of the mesentery characterized histologically by sclerosing fibrosis, fat necrosis with lipid-laden macrophages, chronic inflammation with germinal centers, and focal calcification. Early in the course of the disease, sclerosing mesenteritis has a loose myxomatous appearance that progresses to chronic inflammation and dense sclerosis. Grossly, this condition is characterized by marked thickening of the mesentery of the small intestine, with irregular areas of discoloration suggesting fat necrosis. There may also be multiple discrete nodules on the mesentery or the disease may appear as a single matted mass. The process most often involves the root of the small bowel mesentery and frequently encompasses the mesenteric vessels. It affects the small bowel by retraction and shortening of the mesentery without invasion. In advanced cases, mesenteric venous and lymphatic obstruction may be present. The mesocolon may also be affected but less frequently than the small bowel mesentery.[32]

Sclerosing mesenteritis is twice as common in men as women and usually occurs in the fifth decade of life. Most patients are asymptomatic and the diagnosis is discovered incidentally on imaging for an unrelated condition. When symptoms are present, abdominal pain or symptoms of intestinal obstruction with nausea, vomiting, and abdominal distention are most common. An abdominal mass is palpable in more than 50% of patients. Laboratory studies are usually normal, except that the erythrocyte sedimentation rate and C-reactive protein levels may be elevated.

The differential diagnosis of sclerosing mesenteritis includes a heterogenous group of conditions that alter the density of the mesenteric fat, including inflammatory and neoplastic causes. Differentiation from peritoneal carcinomatosis, carcinoid tumor, and mesenteric and retroperitoneal sarcomas is particularly important. The CT characteristics of sclerosing mesenteritis are well described[32,33] and include the following:

1. A fatty mass arising from the base of mesentery, which has well-delineated margins separating it from normal mesentery, a feature described as a *tumoral pseudocapsule*
2. The presence of normal adipose tissue surrounding mesenteric vessels, termed *fat ring sign*
3. The presence of normal mesenteric vessels coursing through the fatty mass, without evidence of vascular involvement or deviation
4. An intra-abdominal mass that displaces adjacent bowel loops without invading them

Laparotomy or laparoscopy with biopsy of the involved mesentery remains necessary for definitive diagnosis.

Most patients with mesenteric panniculitis experience spontaneous resolution of their symptoms. If patients do not improve, corticosteroids and other anti-inflammatory and immunosuppressive agents have been reported to be successful in improving the symptoms and radiographic findings. Operative management is indicated only for patients in whom there is confusion regarding the diagnosis and for treatment of intestinal obstruction.

## Intra-Abdominal (Internal) Hernias

### Internal Hernias Caused by Developmental Defects

There are three general mechanisms whereby developmental abnormalities result in the formation of internal hernias:

1. Abnormal retroperitoneal fixation of the mesentery resulting in anomalous positioning of the intestine (e.g., mesocolic or paraduodenal hernia)
2. Abnormally large internal foramina or fossae (e.g., foramen of Winslow, supravesical hernia)
3. Incomplete mesenteric surfaces with the presence of an abnormal opening through which the intestine herniates (e.g., mesenteric hernia)

The anatomic and radiographic features of acquired and congenital internal hernias have been reviewed by Martin and associates.[34]

**Mesocolic (Paraduodenal) Hernias** Mesocolic hernias are unusual congenital hernias in which the small intestine herniates behind the mesocolon. They result from abnormal rotation of the midgut and have been categorized as right or left. A right mesocolic hernia occurs when the prearterial limb of the midgut loop fails to rotate around the superior mesenteric artery. This results in most of the small intestine remaining to the right of the superior mesenteric artery. Normal counterclockwise rotation of the cecum and proximal colon into the right side of the abdomen and its fixation to the posterolateral peritoneum cause the small intestine to become trapped behind the mesentery of the right side of the colon. The ileocolic, right colic, and middle colic vessels lie within the anterior wall of the sac and the superior mesenteric artery courses along the medial border of the neck of the hernia (Fig. 45-14A).

Left mesocolic hernias are thought to be caused by in utero herniation of the small intestine between the inferior mesenteric vein and posterior parietal attachments of the descending mesocolon to the retroperitoneum. The inferior mesenteric artery and vein are integral components of the hernia sac (see Fig. 45-14*B*). Approximately 75% of mesocolic hernias occur on the left side.

Patients with paraduodenal hernias usually present with symptoms of acute or chronic small bowel obstruction. Barium radiographs will demonstrate displacement of the small intestine to the left or right side of the abdomen. CT with IV contrast may demonstrate displacement of the mesenteric vessels and evidence of intestinal obstruction, if present.

The operative treatment of patients with a right mesocolic hernia involves incision of the lateral peritoneal reflections along the right colon, with reflection of the right colon and cecum to the left. The entire gut then assumes a position simulating that of nonrotation of the prearterial and postarterial segments of the midgut. Opening the neck of the hernia will injure the superior mesenteric vessels and fails to free the herniated bowel (see Fig. 45-14*C*).

The operative treatment of patients with a left mesocolic hernia consists of incision of the peritoneal attachments and adhesions along the right side of the inferior mesenteric vein, with reduction of the herniated small intestine from beneath the inferior mesenteric vein. The vein is then allowed to return to its normal position on the left side of the base of the mesentery of the small intestine. The neck of the hernia may be closed by suturing the peritoneum adjacent to the vein to the retroperitoneum (see Fig. 45-14*D*).

**Mesenteric Hernias** Mesenteric hernias occur when the intestine herniates through an abnormal orifice in the mesentery of the small intestine or colon. The most common location for these hernias is near the ileocolic junction, although defects in the sigmoid mesocolon have also been described. Patients present with intestinal obstruction resulting from compression of the loops of bowel at the neck of the hernia or torsion of the herniated segment. Treatment involves reduction of the hernia and closure of the mesenteric defect.

### Acquired Internal Hernias

Acquired internal hernias result from the creation of abnormal mesenteric defects after operative procedures or trauma. Usually, these result from inadequate closure (or dehiscence of) mesenteric defects created during the performance of gastrojejunostomy, colostomy, ileostomy, or bowel resection. The creation of a small space allows the herniation of the small intestine through the mesenteric rent and development of intestinal obstruction. Internal hernias, including strangulated hernias, have been noted after the performance of operations for morbid obesity, especially Roux-en-Y gastric bypass. The treatment of these patients is operative reduction of the hernia and closure of the peritoneal defect.

## Malignancies of the Mesentery

Similar to the peritoneum and omentum, the most common neoplasm involving the mesentery is metastatic disease from an intra-abdominal adenocarcinoma. This may result from the direct invasion of the primary tumor (or its lymphatic metastases) into the mesentery or from the transperitoneal spread of the malignancy into the mesentery. Distortion and fixation of the mesentery by the tumor itself or by the resultant desmoplastic reaction, as in carcinoid tumors of the GI tract, may cause intestinal obstruction. The most common primary malignancy of the mesentery is a desmoid tumor.

### Mesenteric and Intra-Abdominal Desmoid Tumors

Mesenteric desmoids account for less than 10% of sporadic desmoid tumors although they are a particularly common tumor in patients with FAP. In this group of patients, 70% of the desmoid tumors are intra-abdominal, and 50% to 75% of these involve the mesentery.[2,3] The association between desmoid tumor and FAP is particularly strong in the subset of patients with Gardner's syndrome. Patients with FAP and a family history of desmoid tumors have a 25% chance of developing a desmoid tumor. Intra-abdominal desmoids are often found at the site of prior surgery. This is an important consideration in FAP patients undergoing abdominal colectomy. In one report, 12% of patients undergoing colectomy for FAP subsequently developed intra-abdominal or abdominal desmoid tumors.[35] Levy and coworkers[32] have reviewed the pathologic and radiographic findings of these uncommon tumors.

Intra-abdominal desmoids are more lethal than those that occur at other anatomic sites because of the possibility of bowel obstruction or ischemia. Resection is less frequently possible, involves greater risk to critical structures, and may be associated with causing more aggressive growth and progression in these

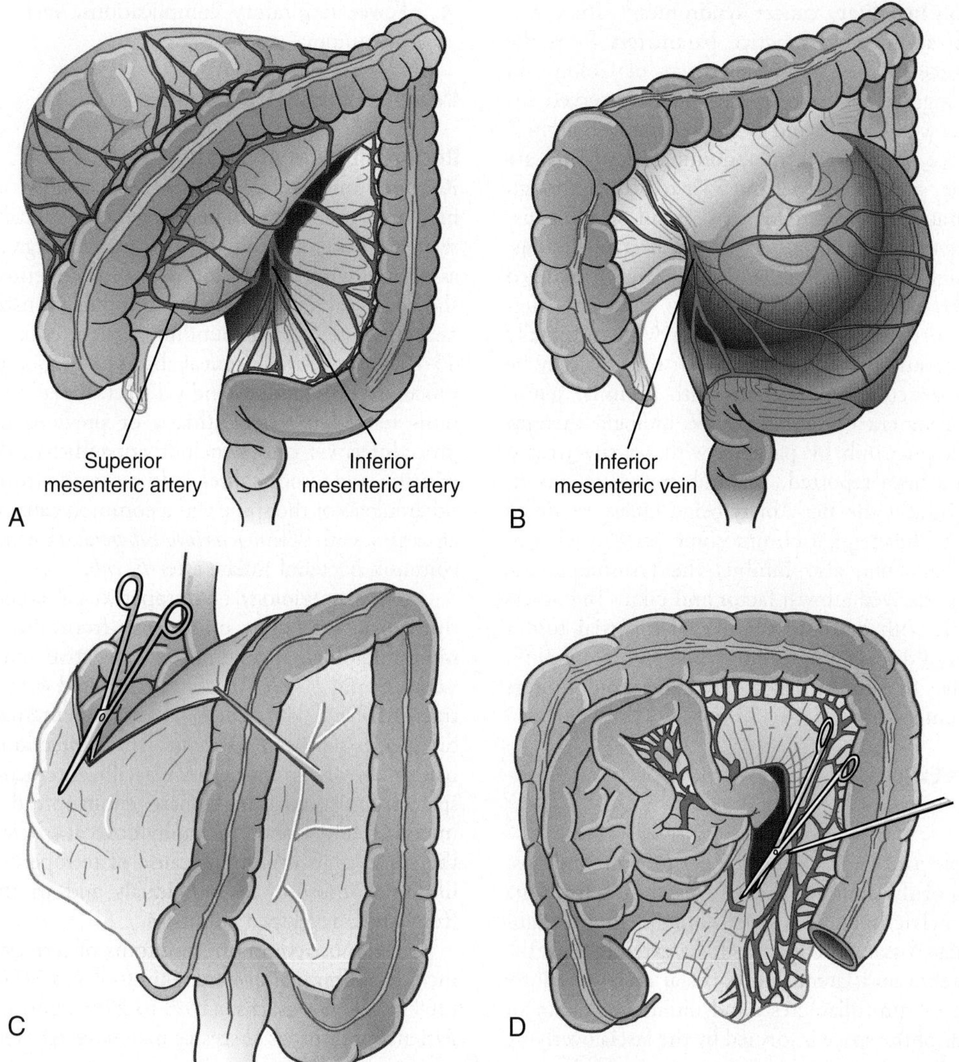


**FIGURE 45-14** **A,** Right mesocolic (paraduodenal) hernia. Note that the anterior wall of a right mesocolic hernia is the ascending mesocolon. The hernia orifice lies to the right of the midline and the superior mesenteric artery and ileocolic artery course along the anterior border of the hernia neck. **B,** Left mesocolic (paraduodenal) hernia. The hernia orifice is to the left of the midline and the herniated intestine lies behind the anterior wall of the descending mesocolon. **C,** A right mesocolic hernia is repaired by division of the lateral peritoneal attachments of the ascending colon, reflecting it toward the left side of the abdomen. The small and large intestine then assumes a position simulating that of nonrotation of the prearterial and postarterial segments of the midgut. Opening the neck of the hernia will injure the superior mesenteric vessels and fail to free the herniated bowel. **D,** A left mesocolic hernia is reduced by incising the hernia sac along an avascular plane immediately to the right of the inferior mesenteric vessels. (**A, B,** From Brigham RA, d'Avis JC: Paraduodenal hernia. In Nyhus LM, Condon RE [eds]: Hernia, ed 3, Philadelphia, 1989, JB Lippincott, pp 484–485; **C, D,** from Brigham R, Fallon WF, Saunders JR, et al: Paraduodenal hernia: Diagnosis and surgical management. Surgery 96:498–502, 1984.)

tumors. Intra-abdominal desmoids tumors are also more often multiple than those at other anatomic sites. Resection of mesenteric desmoids may require sacrifice of significant lengths of intestine, thus leaving the patient with an inadequate absorptive surface to maintain adequate nutrition. Finally, ureteral involvement of the tumor may require resection with reconstruction.

Although mesenteric desmoid tumors tend to be aggressive, there is considerable variability in their growth rate during the course of the disease. In fact, the biology of intra-abdominal desmoid tumors may be characterized by initial rapid growth followed by stability, or even regression.[35] Mesenteric desmoid tumors, by virtue of their relationship to vital structures and ability to infiltrate adjacent organs, may cause significant local complications requiring operative management, including intestinal obstruction, ischemia and perforation, hydronephrosis, and even aortic rupture. Despite these complications, the overall 10-year survival rate for patients with intra-abdominal desmoid tumors is 60% to 70%.[3,36]

Establishing the rate of growth can be helpful in determining the optimal treatment of intra-abdominal desmoid tumors. The American Society of Clinical Oncology and Society of Surgical Oncologists have reviewed the current role of risk-reducing surgery in common hereditary cancer syndromes.[37] These recommendations, in addition to practice parameters from the Standards Task Force of the American Society of Colon and Rectal Surgeons, suggest that surgery should be reserved for small tumors with a well-defined and clearly resectable margin.[38] Reported recurrence rates for intra-abdominal desmoids are higher than for other sites and range from 57% to 86%, although surgery can be curative in select patients.[36] Small bowel transplantation has been described for otherwise unresectable lesions.

Given the high likelihood of recurrence and prolonged survival, even in the setting of advanced disease, some have suggested that a trial of watchful waiting, along with minimally toxic agents such as sulindac and antiestrogen therapy, may be the best strategy, particularly in patients with minimal symptoms. In this nascent era of target-specific biologic therapy, clinical response to imatinib by patients with heavily treated desmoid tumor has been reported. Imatinib mesylate, specifically designed to inhibit the Bcr-Abl tyrosine kinase rendered constitutive by the Philadelphia chromosome translocation in chronic myeloid leukemia, also inhibits the tyrosine kinase receptor for platelet-derived growth factor and c-kit. The observation that patients with desmoid tumors have partial tumor response and arrest of disease progression while on oral imatinib offers an alternative to surgical resection of desmoid tumors arising in the mesentery.[11]

## RETROPERITONEUM

### Anatomy

The retroperitoneal space lies between the peritoneum and posterior parietal wall of the abdominal cavity, extending from the diaphragm to the pelvic floor. This space contains the contiguous lumbar and iliac fossae. The lumbar fossa extends from the 12th thoracic vertebra and lateral lumbocostal arch superiorly to the base of the sacrum, iliac crest, and iliolumbar ligament inferiorly. The floor of the space is formed by the fascia overlying the quadratus lumborum and psoas major muscles. This space contains varying amounts of fatty areolar tissue and the adrenal glands, kidneys, ascending and descending colons, and duodenum. It is also traversed by the ureter, renal vessels, gonadal vessels, inferior vena cava, and aorta. The iliac fossa is contiguous with the lumbar fossa superiorly, lateral and anterior preperitoneal spaces of the abdominal wall, and pelvis inferiorly. The iliacus muscle with its investing fascia is the floor of the iliac fossa, which contains the iliac vessels, ureter, genitofemoral nerve, gonadal vessels, and iliac lymph nodes.

### Operative Approaches

The aorta, vena cava, iliac vessels, kidneys, and adrenal glands may be approached operatively through the retroperitoneal space. Specific operative procedures performed through the retroperitoneum include extirpative procedures such as adrenalectomy and nephrectomy and aortic aneurysmorrhaphy and renal transplantation. The advantages to this approach over a transabdominal approach are as follows:

1. Less postoperative ileus, facilitating a more rapid resumption of diet and earlier discharge from the hospital
2. No intra-abdominal adhesions, thus reducing the likelihood of subsequent small bowel obstruction
3. Less intraoperative evaporative fluid losses, with less dramatic intravascular fluid shifts
4. Fewer respiratory complications, such as atelectasis and pneumonia

### Retroperitoneal Disorders

#### Retroperitoneal Abscesses

Retroperitoneal abscesses may be classified as primary if the infection results from hematogenous spread or secondary if related to an infection in an adjacent organ. The conditions associated with the development of retroperitoneal abscesses are shown in Table 45-2; the anatomic relationship of retroperitoneal abscesses to surrounding structures is shown in Figure 45-15. Most retroperitoneal abscesses originate as inflammatory processes in the kidney and GI tract. Renal causes include infections related to renal lithiasis or previous urologic operative procedures. GI causes include appendicitis, diverticulitis, pancreatitis, and Crohn's disease. In one series from an urban center, tuberculosis of the spine was a common cause of retroperitoneal abscesses, with *Mycobacterium tuberculosis* being the second most common bacterial isolate after *E. coli.*[39]

The bacteriology of retroperitoneal abscesses is related to the cause. Infections originating from the kidney are often monomicrobial, involving gram-negative rods such as *Proteus mirabilis* and *E. coli.* Abscesses associated with diseases of the GI tract involve *E. coli, Enterobacter* spp., enterococci, and anaerobic species such as *Bacteroides.* These infections are multimicrobial and involve gram-negative bacilli, enterococci, and anaerobic species. Infections from hematogenous spread are usually monomicrobial and related to staphylococcal species. Tuberculosis of the spine is an important cause of retroperitoneal abscesses in immunocompromised individuals and in those immigrating from underdeveloped countries.

The most common symptoms of retroperitoneal abscesses include abdominal or flank pain (60% to 75%), fever and chills (30% to 90%), malaise (10% to 22%), and weight loss (12%). Patients with psoas abscesses may have referred pain to the hip, groin, or knee. The duration of symptoms is usually longer than 1 week. Patients with retroperitoneal abscesses often have concurrent, chronic illnesses such as renal lithiasis, diabetes mellitus,

**Table 45-2 Cause and Relative Frequency of Retroperitoneal Abscesses***

| CAUSE | FREQUENCY (%) |
|---|---|
| Renal diseases | 47 |
| Gastrointestinal diseases, including diverticulitis, appendicitis, and Crohn's disease | 16 |
| Hematogenous spread from remote infections | 11 |
| Abscesses complicating operative procedures | 8 |
| Bone infections, including tuberculosis of the spine | 7 |
| Trauma | 4.5 |
| Malignancies | 4 |
| Miscellaneous causes | 3 |

*Data were from three retrospective reviews[40-42] of 134 patients treated between 1971 and 2001.

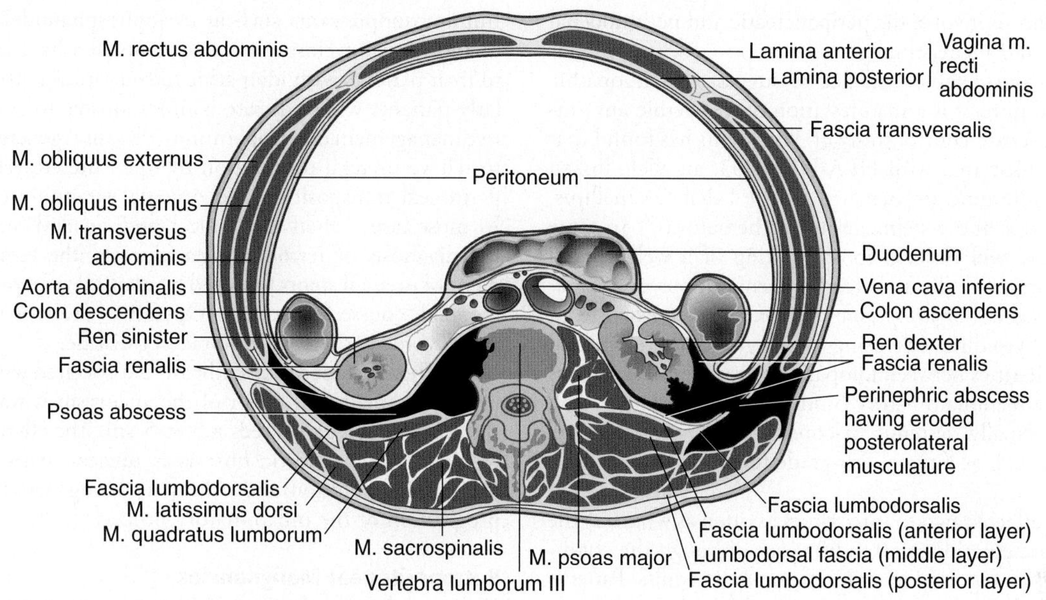


**FIGURE 45-15** Anatomic relationships of retroperitoneal abscesses to surrounding structures. A psoas abscess *(left)* and perinephric abscess are shown *(right)*. (From McVay C: Anson and McVay's surgical anatomy, ed 6, Philadelphia, 1984, WB Saunders, p 735.)

human immunodeficiency virus (HIV) infection, or malignancies. CT demonstrates a low-density mass in the retroperitoneum, with surrounding inflammation. Gas may be present in as many as one third of these lesions.[39] CT provides important information regarding the location of the abscess and its relationship to contiguous organs—hence, likely sources of the infection.

Treatment of retroperitoneal abscesses includes appropriate antibiotics and adequate drainage. Many reports have demonstrated the efficacy of CT-guided drainage in managing this aspect of treatment. Operative drainage through a retroperitoneal approach is indicated for lesions not amenable to percutaneous drainage or those that fail percutaneous drainage. The mortality rate for patients with retroperitoneal abscesses is related, in large part, to the presence of significant medical comorbidities.

### Retroperitoneal Hematomas

Retroperitoneal hematomas usually occur after blunt or penetrating injuries, in the setting of abdominal aortic or visceral artery aneurysms, or after acute or chronic anticoagulation or fibrinolytic therapy. The diagnosis and management of retroperitoneal hematomas occurring in the setting of trauma or aneurysmal rupture are considered in detail in Chapters 18, 62, and 64. Bleeding into the retroperitoneum may also complicate anticoagulant therapy for atrial fibrillation or deep venous thrombosis or arterial catheterization during cardiac catheterization and endovascular procedures. Retroperitoneal hematomas have also been described in patients undergoing fibrinolytic therapy for peripheral or coronary arterial thrombosis and in patients with bleeding diatheses, such as hemophilia.

Patients present with abdominal or flank pain, which may radiate into the groin, labia, or scrotum. Clinical evidence of acute blood loss may be present, depending on the volume of blood lost and the rapidity with which the patient bled. A palpable abdominal mass may be present, as well as physical evidence of ileus. As many as 20% to 30% of patients will develop evidence of a femoral neuropathy.[40] The complete blood count may provide evidence of subacute or chronic blood loss or platelet deficiency. The prothrombin and partial thromboplastin times may demonstrate a coagulopathy. Microscopic hematuria is a common finding on urinalysis. CT establishes the diagnosis by demonstrating a high-density mass in the retroperitoneum, with surrounding stranding in the retroperitoneal tissue planes. These findings are readily distinguishable from the low-density mass characteristic of retroperitoneal abscesses.

Patients who develop retroperitoneal hematomas as a result of anticoagulation are best managed by the restoration of circulating blood volume and correction of the underlying coagulopathy. In rare circumstances, arteriography with embolization of a bleeding artery or operative exploration is required to stop the bleeding.

### Retroperitoneal Fibrosis

Retroperitoneal fibrosis is characterized by chronic inflammation and fibrosis surrounding the abdominal aorta and iliac arteries, which extends laterally to envelop surrounding structures, especially the ureters. Seventy percent of cases are idiopathic (termed *Ormand disease*), whereas 30% are associated with various drugs (most notably, ergot alkaloids or dopaminergic agonists), infections, trauma, retroperitoneal hemorrhage or retroperitoneal operations, radiation therapy, or primary or metastatic neoplasms. Many idiopathic cases are associated with inflammatory abdominal aortic aneurysms; thus, idiopathic retroperitoneal fibrosis might best be categorized with inflammatory abdominal aortic aneurysms and perianeurysmal retroperitoneal fibrosis as a form of chronic periaortitis.[41] The fibrosis is usually confined to the central and paravertebral spaces between the renal arteries and sacrum and tends to encase the aorta, inferior vena cava, and ureters. The process usually begins at the level of the aortic bifurcation and spreads cephalad. In 15% of cases, the fibrotic process extends outside the retroperitoneum to involve the peripancreatic and periduodenal spaces, pelvis, and mediastinum.

There is considerable evidence to suggest that idiopathic retroperitoneal fibrosis is a manifestation of a systemic autoimmune disease. A case-control study of 35 patients has found that the disease is associated with HLA-DRB1*03, an allele linked to various autoimmune diseases such as type 1 diabetes mellitus, myasthenia gravis, and systemic lupus erythematosus.[42] In some patients, disease will develop in the setting of a well-defined systemic autoimmune disorder (e.g., systemic lupus erythematosus) or so-called *organ-specific autoimmune diseases* (e.g., Hashimoto's thyroiditis, sclerosing cholangitis). There are also histologic similarities between idiopathic retroperitoneal fibrosis and other systemic inflammatory conditions, such as large-vessel vasculitides.[41] Finally, systemic or constitutional symptoms are often present, such as fatigue, low-grade fever, weight loss, and myalgias.

Men are affected two to three times as often as women. The mean age at presentation is 50 to 60 years, although the condition has also been reported in children and older adults. Patients may present with localized symptoms of side, back, or abdominal pain or lower extremity edema. Scrotal swelling is common, as is the occurrence of a varicocele or hydrocele. In most patients, localized symptoms are preceded by or coexist with systemic or constitutional symptoms (see earlier). Laboratory tests may demonstrate azotemia and 80% to 100% of patients will have elevated concentrations of acute-phase reactants (e.g., erythrocyte sedimentation rate, C-reactive protein). The nonspecific nature of the clinical features of this disease contributes to the considerable delay between the onset of symptoms and the diagnosis. As such, ureteral involvement is present in 80% to 100% of cases.[41]

Evaluation of patients suspected to have retroperitoneal fibrosis should start with ultrasonography, which can define the retroperitoneal fibrosis as a hypoechoic or isoechoic mass that involves one or both of the ureters and document the presence of hydronephrosis. IV urography usually reveals the triad of medial deviation and extrinsic compression of the ureters with hydronephrosis. The most reliable imaging studies to detect retroperitoneal fibrosis are CT and MRI. Without IV contrast, the CT scan will demonstrate a homogenous fibrous plaque surrounding the lower abdominal aorta and the iliac arteries, which is usually isodense when compared with surrounding muscle. MRI of early benign retroperitoneal fibrosis may show areas of high signal intensity on T2-weighted images as a result of the abundant fluid content and hypercellularity associated with the acute inflammation. In the mature and quiescent stages of benign retroperitoneal fibrosis, the low signal intensity on T1- and T2-weighted images is similar to that of psoas muscle.

The primary goals of treatment for patients with idiopathic retroperitoneal fibrosis are to stop the progression of retroperitoneal inflammation and fibrosis, prevent or relieve ureteral obstruction, inhibit the systemic inflammatory response, and improve the constitutional manifestations of the disease. The mainstay of treatment has been the administration of corticosteroids, which suppress the synthesis of proinflammatory cytokines and inhibit collagen synthesis and maturation. This will often result in a prompt improvement in symptoms, reduction in the size of the retroperitoneal mass, and relief of ureteral obstruction. Unfortunately, the optimal dose and duration of treatment have not been not well established. Immunosuppressants such as cyclophosphamide, azathioprine, methotrexate, cyclosporine, and tamoxifen have also been used to treat patients with idiopathic retroperitoneal fibrosis, particularly patients whose disease is unresponsive to steroids. Operative management of retroperitoneal fibrosis is generally performed to relieve ureteral obstruction by open ureterolysis, with intraperitoneal transposition and omental wrapping of the ureters. In most cases, when the clinical findings and imaging suggest the diagnosis of retroperitoneal fibrosis, the temporary placement of ureteral stents followed by medical therapy is the recommended course of action. Operative ureterolysis would be reserved for patients with refractory disease.

When retroperitoneal fibrosis is associated with an abdominal aortic aneurysm, repair of the aneurysm is warranted when the aortic diameter exceeds 4.5 to 5 cm. The effect of aneurysm repair of the periaortic fibrosis is unclear, with some reports indicating resolution and others reporting persistence or even progression of the inflammatory process.

### Retroperitoneal Malignancies

Malignancies in the retroperitoneum may result from the following:

1. Extracapsular growth of a primary neoplasm of a retroperitoneal organ, such as the kidney, adrenal, colon, or pancreas
2. Development of a primary germ cell neoplasm from embryonic rest cells
3. Development of a primary malignancy of the retroperitoneal lymphatic system (e.g., lymphoma)
4. Metastases from a remote primary malignancy into a retroperitoneal lymph node (e.g., testicular cancer)
5. Development of a malignancy of the soft tissue of the retroperitoneum (e.g., sarcomas and desmoid tumors)

The most common primary malignancy of the retroperitoneum is a sarcoma.

**Retroperitoneal Sarcoma** Approximately 10,000 soft tissue sarcomas were diagnosed in the United States in 2009, of which 15% were usually retroperitoneal sarcomas.[43] The most common histologic subtypes are liposarcoma and leiomyosarcoma. Radiation is a known risk factor for the development of sarcomas, with radiation-associated sarcomas usually occurring approximately 10 years after exposure. Patients with von Recklinghausen's disease (neurofibromatosis type 1) can develop malignant transformation of neurofibromas into malignant peripheral nerve sheath tumors; patients with Li-Fraumeni syndrome and hereditary retinoblastoma also have an increased incidence of sarcoma.

Most patients with a retroperitoneal sarcoma present with an asymptomatic abdominal mass, often after the primary tumor has reached a considerable size. Abdominal pain is present in 50% of patients; less common symptoms include GI hemorrhage, early satiety, nausea and vomiting, weight loss, and lower extremity swelling. Symptoms related to nerve compression by the tumor, such as lower extremity paresthesia and paresis, have also been associated with retroperitoneal sarcoma.

CT and MRI provide important information regarding the size and precise location of the primary tumor and its relationship to major vascular structures (Fig. 45-16). These studies will also document the presence or absence of metastatic disease in the lung or liver. Usually, these imaging modalities will also

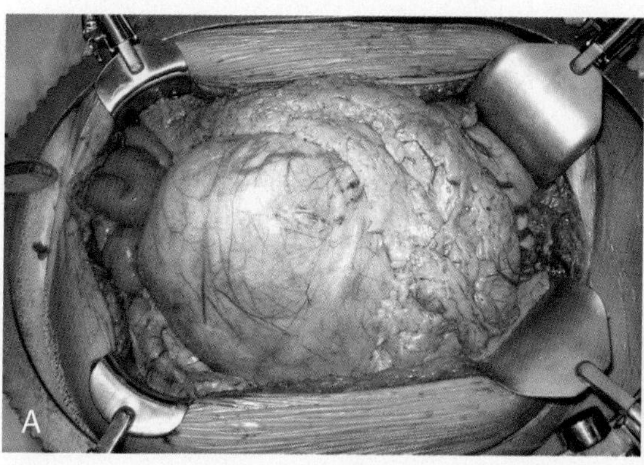


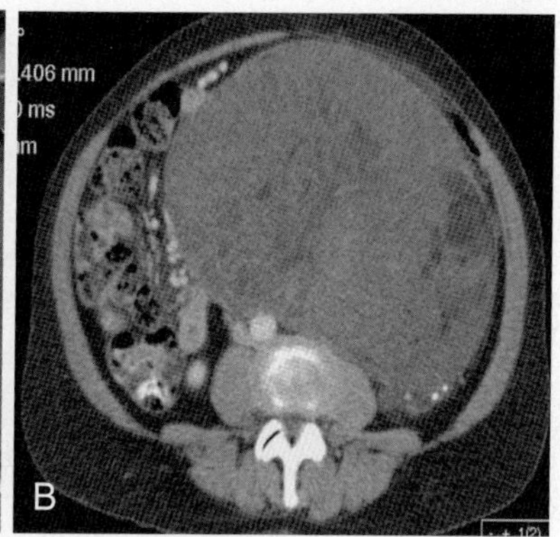


**FIGURE 45-16 A,** Intraoperative photograph of a large retroperitoneal sarcoma. **B,** CT scan of the same patient demonstrating the displacement of the aorta, inferior vena cava, and bowel to the right of the abdomen.

provide important diagnostic clues, thus obviating the need for image-guided biopsy in most cases.

Lymphoma, especially with bulky retroperitoneal adenopathy, may appear as a mass arising from the retroperitoneum. The presence of constitutional symptoms, including fevers, night sweats, and weight loss, may suggest the diagnosis of lymphoma. A careful search for other evidence of lymphadenopathy is warranted in these patients. The spread of testicular cancer to the retroperitoneal lymph nodes may also present as a large retroperitoneal mass. Hence, workup of male patients should include a testicular examination and serologic testing for α-fetoprotein and human chorionic gonadotropin. Finally, the local extension of tumors arising in the adrenal gland or pancreas may also be considered in the differential diagnosis of patients with large retroperitoneal tumors.

Prognostic staging is difficult for sarcomas because there are many histologic types of sarcomas, with variables grades and locations. The latest edition of the American Joint Commission on Cancer Staging System is notable in that it includes grade and depth to the fascia in addition to standard staging criteria, such as tumor size, nodal status, and distant metastasis.[44] Most retroperitoneal sarcomas are deep to the fascia and large, so grade is the main determinant of stage in nonmetastatic disease. Nodal disease had previously been classified as stage IV but is currently reassigned to stage III.

The goal of sarcoma treatment is complete en bloc resection of the tumor and any involved adjacent organs. Lymph node metastases by sarcoma are rare (<5%); therefore, lymphadenectomy is not required unless there is evidence of lymph node involvement. The main prognostic factors for patients with retroperitoneal sarcomas are the size of the tumor, histologic grade, and resection status.[45] The difficulty of obtaining resection margins free of tumor is related to the juxtaposition or invasion of the tumor and retroperitoneal structures, such as the aorta, inferior vena cava, intra-abdominal viscera (colon, duodenum, kidney, pancreas, spleen), and adjacent muscles (psoas, rectus abdominis, diaphragm). The kidney is the most commonly resected organ; recent series have reported multiorgan resection in approximately 50% of cases.[46] Thoracoabdominal incisions may be required for upper quadrant sarcomas, which does not appear to increase morbidity greatly. It can be difficult pathologically to determine a negative margin resulting from the large surface area and anatomic constraints of the tumor. Most experts in treating this disease consider the goal of surgery to be complete resection, defined by removal of all gross disease (macroscopically negative margin), with en bloc resection of adherent organs. Rates of resectability of the primary retroperitoneal sarcoma vary widely based on the extent of disease at presentation, surgeon's experience, and institution's referral pattern. A review of several large series has reported complete resectability rates of 50% to 67%.[47]

There is no difference in survival for patients who undergo incomplete resection when compared with those who are unresectable. Incomplete resection should only be undertaken for palliative purposes for all histologic types other than liposarcoma.[45] Incomplete resection of well-differentiated liposarcoma may prolong survival and has been shown to improve symptoms.[48] Local recurrence after surgery occurs in approximately 50% of patients and distant metastases occur in 20% to 30%. The 5-year survival rate is approximately 50%, although disease-specific death can occur after 5 years.[48]

In patients with recurrent disease, complete resection of recurrent tumor is beneficial. In a report by Lewis and colleagues[45] at the Memorial Sloan-Kettering Cancer Center, 35 of 61 patients with recurrent sarcoma underwent complete resection. This group of patients had a significantly higher survival rate than those undergoing incomplete resection (60% versus 18% 5-year disease-specific survival). Unlike extremity sarcoma, the role for external-beam radiation for local control after surgical resection is limited by the low tolerance for radiation injury of the surrounding normal tissue. Postoperative radiotherapy and combined postoperative and intraoperative radiotherapy has been shown to improve recurrence rates but has not been clearly shown to have an effect on survival. Preoperative radiotherapy has some theoretical benefits, but there have been no prospective randomized trials of preoperative radiotherapy. Neoadjuvant or adjuvant chemotherapy is unproven and most agents used for sarcoma therapy have significant toxicity.

## SELECTED REFERENCES

Fleshman J, Sargent DJ, Green E, et al: Laparoscopic colectomy for cancer is not inferior to open surgery based on 5-year data from the COST Study Group trial. Ann Surg 246:655–662, 2007.

This important paper defined the incidence of port site recurrence after laparoscopic colectomy for colon cancer and established the equivalency of laparoscopic and open colectomy for the treatment curable colon cancer.

Guillem JG, Wood WC, Moley JF, et al: ASCO/SSO review of current role of risk-reducing surgery in common hereditary cancer syndromes. J Clin Oncol 24:4642–4660, 2006.

This task force consensus statement outlines the current recommendations from the American Society of Clinical Oncology and Society of Surgical Oncology regarding surgery for desmoid tumors in patients with familial adenomatous polyposis.

Koulaouzidis A, Bhat S, Saeed AA: Spontaneous bacterial peritonitis. World J Gastroenterol 15:1042–1049, 2009.

This is a well-written and thorough review of the pathophysiology, bacteriology, and treatment of spontaneous bacterial peritonitis.

Martin LC, Merkle EM, Thompson WM: Review of internal hernias: Radiographic and clinical findings. AJR Am J Roentgenol 186:703–717, 2006.

This is a thorough and well-illustrated review of the types of congenital and acquired internal hernias.

Moller S, Henriksen JH, Bendtsen F: Ascites: Pathogenesis and therapeutic principles. Scand J Gastroenterol 44:902–911, 2009.

This is a well-written and thorough review of the pathophysiology of ascites formation in cirrhotics and the basic tenets of medical management.

Runyon BA, Montano AA, Akrividadis EA, et al: The serum-ascites albumin gradient is superior to the exudates-transudate concept in the differential diagnosis of ascites. Ann Intern Med 117:215–220, 1992.

This well-written paper established the use of serum-ascites albumin gradient in the elucidation of the pathophysiology of ascites formation.

Stewart JH, Shen P, Levine EA: Intraperitoneal hyperthermic chemotherapy for peritoneal surface malignancy: current status and future directions. Ann Surg Oncol 12:765–777, 2005.

This review covers the rationale, technical aspects, and outcomes for intraperitoneal hyperthermic chemotherapy for several malignancy types.

Thorek P: Anatomy in surgery, ed 2, Philadelphia, 1962, JB Lippincott.
McVay C: Anson and McVay's surgical anatomy, ed 6, Philadelphia, 1984, WB Saunders.

Thorek's and McVay's works are classic texts of anatomy, beautifully illustrated and written from a surgeon's perspective.

Vaglio A, Salvarani C, Buzio C: Retroperitoneal fibrosis. Lancet 367:241–251, 2006.

This is a well-written and thorough review of the pathophysiology, immunology, and clinical features of retroperitoneal fibrosis.

Willwerth BM, Zollinger RM, Izant RJ: Congenital mesocolic (paraduodenal) hernia: Embryologic basis of repair. Am J Surg 128:358–361, 1974.

This is a classic description of right and left mesocolic hernias. The authors suggest an embryologic basis for the occurrence of these hernias, as well as a clear description of their management.

## REFERENCES


1. Cherry WB, Mueller PS: Rectus sheath hematoma: Review of 126 cases at a single institution. Medicine (Baltimore) 85:105–110, 2006.
2. Gurbuz AK, Giardiello FM, Petersen GM, et al: Desmoid tumours in familial adenomatous polyposis. Gut 35:377–381, 1994.
3. Kulaylat MN, Karakousis CP, Keaney CM, et al: Desmoid tumour: A pleomorphic lesion. Eur J Surg Oncol 25:487–497, 1999.
4. Stojadinovic A, Hoos A, Karpoff HM, et al: Soft tissue tumors of the abdominal wall: Analysis of disease patterns and treatment. Arch Surg 136:70–79, 2001.
5. Ballo MT, Zagars GK, Pollack A, et al: Desmoid tumor: Prognostic factors and outcome after surgery, radiation therapy, or combined surgery and radiation therapy. J Clin Oncol 17:158–167, 1999.
6. Nuyttens JJ, Rust PF, Thomas CR, Jr, et al: Surgery versus radiation therapy for patients with aggressive fibromatosis or desmoid tumors: A comparative review of 22 articles. Cancer 88:1517–1523, 2000.
7. Janinis J, Patriki M, Vini L, et al: The pharmacological treatment of aggressive fibromatosis: A systematic review. Ann Oncol 14:181–190, 2003.
8. Clark SK, Neale KF, Landgrebe JC, et al: Desmoid tumours complicating familial adenomatous polyposis. Br J Surg 86:1185–1189, 1999.
9. Hansmann A, Adolph C, Vogel T, et al: High-dose tamoxifen and sulindac as first-line treatment for desmoid tumors. Cancer 100:612–620, 2004.
10. Azzarelli A, Gronchi A, Bertulli R, et al: Low-dose chemotherapy with methotrexate and vinblastine for patients with advanced aggressive fibromatosis. Cancer 92:1259–1264, 2001.
11. Heinrich MC, McArthur GA, Demetri GD, et al: Clinical and molecular studies of the effect of imatinib on advanced aggressive fibromatosis (desmoid tumor). J Clin Oncol 24:1195–1203, 2006.
12. Fleshman J, Sargent DJ, Green E, et al: Laparoscopic colectomy for cancer is not inferior to open surgery based on 5-year data from the COST Study Group trial. Ann Surg 246:655–662; discussion 662–654, 2007.
13. Plaza JA, Perez-Montiel D, Mayerson J, et al: Metastases to soft tissue: A review of 118 cases over a 30-year period. Cancer 112:193–203, 2008.
14. Kashani A, Landaverde C, Medici V, et al: Fluid retention in cirrhosis: Pathophysiology and management. QJM 101:71–85, 2008.
15. Moller S, Henriksen JH, Bendtsen F: Ascites: Pathogenesis and therapeutic principles. Scand J Gastroenterol 44:902–911, 2009.

16. Runyon BA: Paracentesis of ascitic fluid. A safe procedure. Arch Intern Med 146:2259–2261, 1986.
17. Runyon BA, Montano AA, Akriviadis EA, et al: The serum-ascites albumin gradient is superior to the exudate-transudate concept in the differential diagnosis of ascites. Ann Intern Med 117:215–220, 1992.
18. Gines P, Cardenas A, Arroyo V, et al: Management of cirrhosis and ascites. N Engl J Med 350:1646–1654, 2004.
19. Kuiper JJ, de Man RA, van Buuren HR: Review article: Management of ascites and associated complications in patients with cirrhosis. Aliment Pharmacol Ther 26(Suppl 2):183–193, 2007.
20. Koulaouzidis A, Leontiadis GI, Abdullah M, et al: Leucocyte esterase reagent strips for the diagnosis of spontaneous bacterial peritonitis: A systematic review. Eur J Gastroenterol Hepatol 20:1055–1060, 2008.
21. Nguyen-Khac E, Cadranel JF, Thevenot T, et al: Review article: The utility of reagent strips in the diagnosis of infected ascites in cirrhotic patients. Aliment Pharmacol Ther 28:282–288, 2008.
22. Chavez-Tapia NC, Soares-Weiser K, Brezis M, et al: Antibiotics for spontaneous bacterial peritonitis in cirrhotic patients. Cochrane Database Syst Rev (1):CD002232, 2009.
23. Koulaouzidis A, Bhat S, Saeed AA: Spontaneous bacterial peritonitis. World J Gastroenterol 15:1042–1049, 2009.
24. Fernandez J, Navasa M, Garcia-Pagan JC, et al: Effect of intravenous albumin on systemic and hepatic hemodynamics and vasoactive neurohormonal systems in patients with cirrhosis and spontaneous bacterial peritonitis. J Hepatol 41:384–390, 2004.
25. Sanai FM, Bzeizi KI: Systematic review: tuberculous peritonitis—presenting features, diagnostic strategies and treatment. Aliment Pharmacol Ther 22:685–700, 2005.
26. Kavanagh D, Prescott GJ, Mactier RA: Peritoneal dialysis-associated peritonitis in Scotland (1999–2002). Nephrol Dial Transplant 19:2584–2591, 2004.
27. Ronnett BM, Yan H, Kurman RJ, et al: Patients with pseudomyxoma peritonei associated with disseminated peritoneal adenomucinosis have a significantly more favorable prognosis than patients with peritoneal mucinous carcinomatosis. Cancer 92:85–91, 2001.
28. Gonzalez-Moreno S, Sugarbaker PH: Right hemicolectomy does not confer a survival advantage in patients with mucinous carcinoma of the appendix and peritoneal seeding. Br J Surg 91:304–311, 2004.
29. Stewart JH, Shen P, Levine EA: Intraperitoneal hyperthermic chemotherapy for peritoneal surface malignancy: current status and future directions. Ann Surg Oncol 12:765–777, 2005.
30. Levy AD, Arnaiz J, Shaw JC, et al: From the archives of the AFIP: primary peritoneal tumors: Imaging features with pathologic correlation. Radiographics 28:583–607; quiz 621–582, 2008.
31. Yan TD, Deraco M, Baratti D, et al: Cytoreductive surgery and hyperthermic intraperitoneal chemotherapy for malignant peritoneal mesothelioma: Multi-institutional experience. J Clin Oncol 27:6237–6242, 2009.
32. Levy AD, Rimola J, Mehrotra AK, et al: From the archives of the AFIP: Benign fibrous tumors and tumorlike lesions of the mesentery: radiologic-pathologic correlation. Radiographics 26:245–264, 2006.
33. Horton KM, Lawler LP, Fishman EK: CT findings in sclerosing mesenteritis (panniculitis): Spectrum of disease. Radiographics 23:1561–1567, 2003.
34. Martin LC, Merkle EM, Thompson WM: Review of internal hernias: Radiographic and clinical findings. AJR Am J Roentgenol 186:703–717, 2006.
35. Penna C, Tiret E, Parc R, et al: Operation and abdominal desmoid tumors in familial adenomatous polyposis. Surg Gynecol Obstet 177:263–268, 1993.
36. Smith AJ, Lewis JJ, Merchant NB, et al: Surgical management of intra-abdominal desmoid tumours. Br J Surg 87:608–613, 2000.
37. Guillem JG, Wood WC, Moley JF, et al: ASCO/SSO review of current role of risk-reducing surgery in common hereditary cancer syndromes. J Clin Oncol 24:4642–4660, 2006.
38. Church J, Simmang C: Practice parameters for the treatment of patients with dominantly inherited colorectal cancer (familial adenomatous polyposis and hereditary nonpolyposis colorectal cancer). Dis Colon Rectum 46:1001–1012, 2003.
39. Paley M, Sidhu PS, Evans RA, et al: Retroperitoneal collections—a cause and radiological implications. Clin Radiol 52:290–294, 1997.
40. Loor G, Bassiouny H, Valentin C, et al: Local and systemic consequences of large retroperitoneal clot burdens. World J Surg 33:1618–1625, 2009.
41. Vaglio A, Salvarani C, Buzio C: Retroperitoneal fibrosis. Lancet 367:241–251, 2006.
42. Martorana D, Vaglio A, Greco P, et al: Chronic periaortitis and HLA-DRB1*03: Another clue to an autoimmune origin. Arthritis Rheum 55:126–130, 2006.
43. Jemal A, Siegel R, Ward E, et al: Cancer statistics, 2009. CA Cancer J Clin 59:225–249, 2009.
44. Soft tissue sarcoma. In Edge SB, Byrd DR, Compton CC, et al, editors: AJCC cancer staging manual, ed 7, New York, 2010, Springer, pp 291–298.
45. Lewis JJ, Leung D, Woodruff JM, et al: Retroperitoneal soft-tissue sarcoma: Analysis of 500 patients treated and followed at a single institution. Ann Surg 228:355–365, 1998.
46. Russo P, Kim Y, Ravindran S, et al: Nephrectomy during operative management of retroperitoneal sarcoma. Ann Surg Oncol 4:421–424, 1997.
47. Mendenhall WM, Zlotecki RA, Hochwald SN, et al: Retroperitoneal soft tissue sarcoma. Cancer 104:669–675, 2005.
48. Shibata D, Lewis JJ, Leung DH, et al: Is there a role for incomplete resection in the management of retroperitoneal liposarcomas? J Am Coll Surg 193:373–379, 2001.

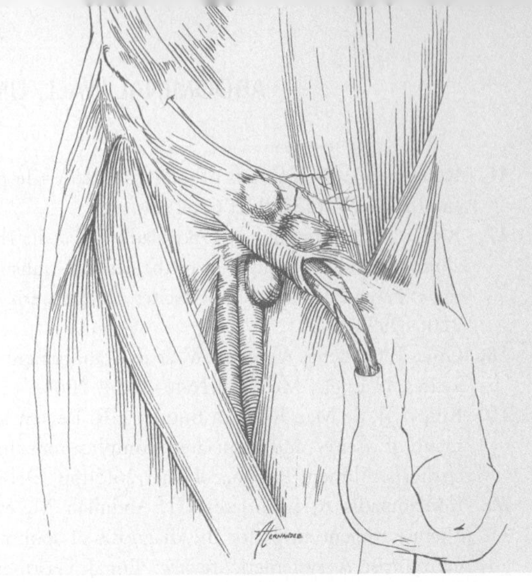

# CHAPTER 46

# HERNIAS

Mark A. Malangoni and Michael J. Rosen



More than 600,000 hernias are repaired annually in the United States, making hernia repair one of the most common operations performed by general surgeons. Despite the frequency of this procedure, no surgeon has ideal results, and complications such as postoperative pain, nerve injury, infection, and recurrence remain.

Hernia is derived from the Latin word for rupture. A hernia is defined as an abnormal protrusion of an organ or tissue through a defect in its surrounding walls. Although a hernia can occur at various sites of the body, these defects most commonly involve the abdominal wall, particularly the inguinal region. Abdominal wall hernias occur only at sites at which the aponeurosis and fascia are not covered by striated muscle (Box 46-1). These sites most commonly include the inguinal, femoral, and umbilical areas, linea alba, lower portion of the semilunar line, and sites of prior incisions (Fig. 46-1). The so-called neck or orifice of a hernia is located at the innermost musculoaponeurotic layer, whereas the hernia sac is lined by peritoneum and protrudes from the neck. There is no consistent relationship between the area of a hernia defect and the size of a hernia sac.

A hernia is reducible when its contents can be replaced within the surrounding musculature, and it is irreducible or incarcerated when it cannot be reduced. A strangulated hernia has compromised blood supply to its contents, which is a serious and potentially fatal complication. Strangulation occurs more often in large hernias that have small orifices. In this situation, the small neck of the hernia obstructs arterial blood flow, venous drainage, or both to the contents of the hernia sac. Adhesions between the contents of the hernia and peritoneal lining of the sac can provide a tethering point that entraps the hernia contents and predisposes to intestinal obstruction and strangulation. A more unusual type of strangulation is a Richter's hernia. In Richter's hernia, a small portion of the antimesenteric wall of the intestine is trapped within the hernia, and strangulation can occur without the presence of intestinal obstruction.

An external hernia protrudes through all layers of the abdominal wall, whereas an internal hernia is a protrusion of intestine through a defect in the peritoneal cavity. An interparietal hernia occurs when the hernia sac is contained within a musculoaponeurotic layer of the abdominal wall. In broad terms, most abdominal wall hernias can be separated into inguinal and ventral hernias. This chapter focuses on the specific aspects of each of these conditions individually.

## INGUINAL HERNIAS

Inguinal hernias are classified as direct or indirect. The sac of an indirect inguinal hernia passes from the internal inguinal ring obliquely toward the external inguinal ring and ultimately into the scrotum. In contrast, the sac of a direct inguinal hernia protrudes outward and forward and is medial to the internal inguinal ring and inferior epigastric vessels. As indirect hernias enlarge, it sometimes can be difficult to distinguish between indirect and direct inguinal hernias. This distinction is of little importance because the operative repair of these types of hernias is similar. A pantaloon-type hernia occurs when there is an indirect and direct hernia component.

### Incidence

Hernias are a common problem; however, their true incidence is unknown. It is estimated that 5% of the population will develop an abdominal wall hernia, but the prevalence may be even higher. About 75% of all hernias occur in the inguinal region. Two thirds of these are indirect and the remainder are direct inguinal hernias. Femoral hernias comprise only 3% of all groin hernias.

Men are 25 times more likely to have a groin hernia than women. An indirect inguinal hernia is the most common hernia, regardless of gender. In men, indirect hernias predominate over direct hernias at a ratio of 2 : 1. Direct hernias are uncommon in women. The female-to-male ratio in femoral and umbilical hernias, however, is about 10 : 1 and 2 : 1, respectively. Although femoral hernias occur more frequently in women than in men, inguinal hernias remain the most common hernia in women. Femoral hernias are rare in men. Ten percent of women and 50% of men who have a femoral hernia have or will develop an inguinal hernia.

Indirect inguinal and femoral hernias occur more commonly on the right side. This is attributed to a delay in atrophy of the processus vaginalis after the normal slower descent of the right testis to the scrotum during fetal development. The predominance of right-sided femoral hernias is thought to be caused by the tamponading effect of the sigmoid colon on the left femoral canal.

The prevalence of hernias increases with age, particularly for inguinal, umbilical, and femoral hernias. The likelihood of strangulation and need for hospitalization also increase with aging. Strangulation, the most common serious complication of a hernia, occurs in only 1% to 3% of groin hernias and is more common at the extremes of life. Most strangulated hernias are indirect inguinal hernias; however, femoral hernias have the highest rate of strangulation (15% to 20%) of all hernias and it is therefore recommended that all femoral hernias be repaired at the time of discovery.

**BOX 46-1 Primary Abdominal Wall Hernias**

**Groin**
Inguinal
- Indirect
- Direct
- Combined

Femoral

**Anterior**
Umbilical
Epigastric
Spigelian

**Pelvic**
Obturator
Sciatic
Perineal

**Posterior**
Lumbar
- Superior triangle
- Inferior triangle

## Anatomy of the Groin

The surgeon must have a comprehensive understanding of the anatomy of the groin to select and use various options for hernia repair properly. In addition, the relationships of muscles, aponeuroses, fascia, nerves, blood vessels, and spermatic cord structures in the inguinal region must be completely understood to obtain the lowest incidence of recurrence and avoid complications. These anatomic considerations must be understood from the anterior and posterior approaches because both are useful in different situations (Figs. 46-2 and 46-3).

From anterior to posterior, the groin anatomy includes the skin and subcutaneous tissues, below which are the superficial circumflex iliac, superficial epigastric, and external pudendal arteries and accompanying veins. These vessels arise from and drain to the proximal femoral artery and vein, respectively, and are directed superiorly. If encountered during operation, these vessels can be retracted or even divided when necessary.

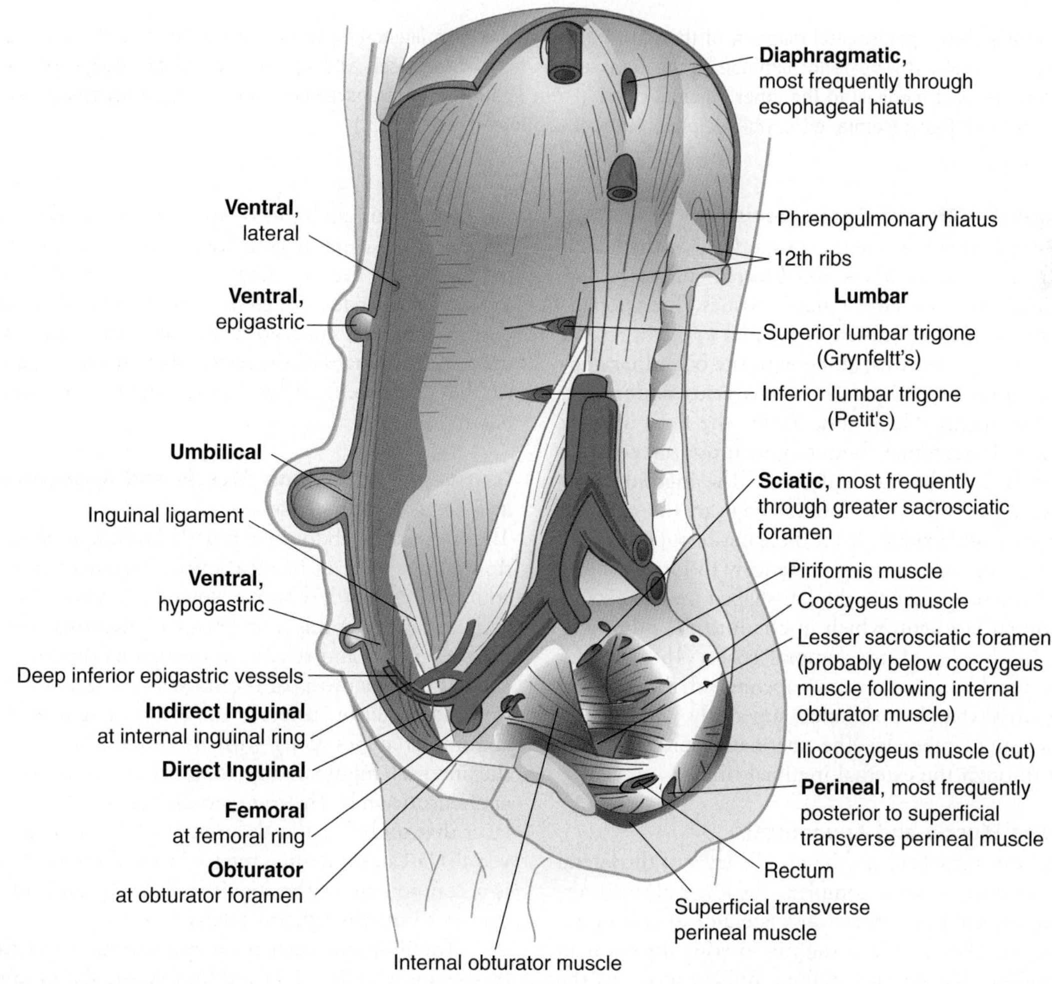


**FIGURE 46-1** Types of abdominal wall hernias. (From Dorland's illustrated medical dictionary, ed 31, Philadelphia, 2007, WB Saunders, Plate 21.)

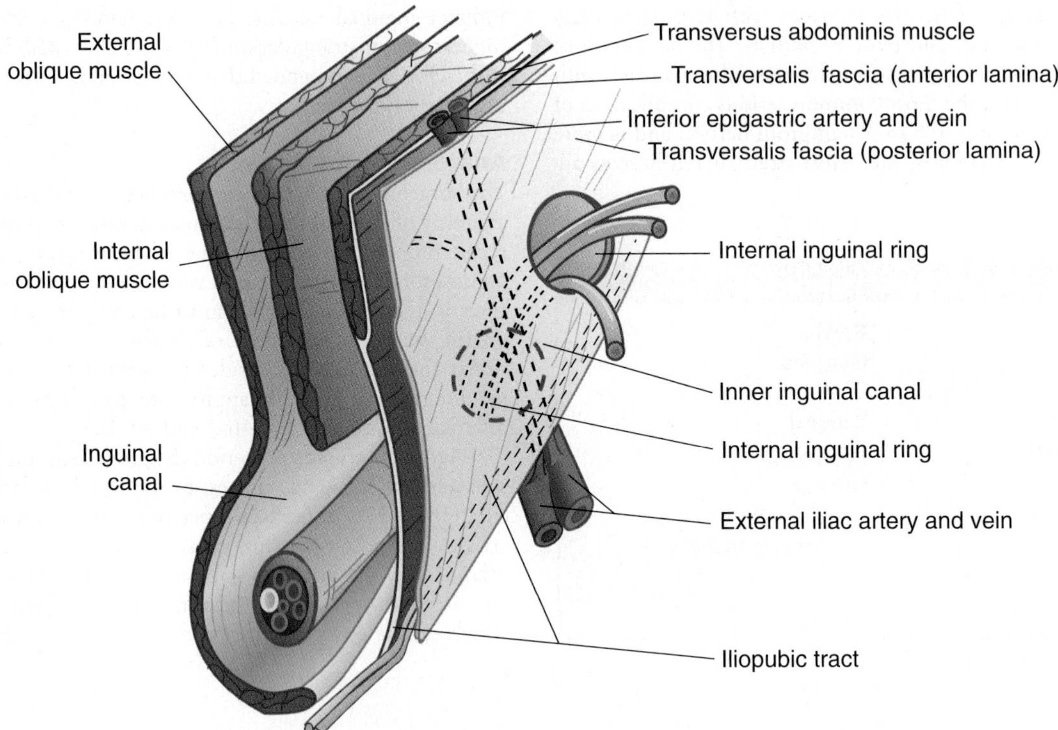


**FIGURE 46-2** Nyhus's classic parasagittal diagram of the right midinguinal region illustrating the muscular aponeurotic layers separated into anterior and posterior walls. The posterior laminae of the transversalis fascia have been added, with the inferior epigastric vessels coursing through the abdominal wall medially to the inner inguinal canal. (From Read RC: The transversalis and preperitoneal fasciae: A re-evaluation. In Nyhus LM, Condon RE [eds]: Hernia, ed 4, Philadelphia, 1995, JB Lippincott, pp 57–63.)

### External Oblique Muscle and Aponeurosis

The external oblique muscle is the most superficial of the lateral abdominal wall muscles; its fibers are directed inferiorly and medially and lie deep to the subcutaneous tissues. The aponeurosis of the external oblique muscle is formed by a superficial and deep layer. This aponeurosis, along with the bilaminar aponeuroses of the internal oblique and transversus abdominis, forms the anterior rectus sheath and, finally, the linea alba by linear decussation. The external oblique aponeurosis serves as the superficial boundary of the inguinal canal. The inguinal ligament (Poupart's ligament) is the inferior edge of the external oblique aponeurosis and extends from the anterior superior iliac spine to the pubic tubercle, turning posteriorly to form a shelving edge. The lacunar ligament is the fan-shaped medial expansion of the inguinal ligament, which inserts into the pubis and forms the medial border of the femoral space. The external (superficial) inguinal ring is an ovoid opening of the external oblique aponeurosis that is positioned superiorly and slightly laterally to the pubic tubercle. The spermatic cord exits the inguinal canal through the external inguinal ring.

### Internal Oblique Muscle and Aponeurosis

The internal oblique muscle forms the middle layer of the lateral abdominal musculoaponeurotic complex. The fibers of the internal oblique are directed superiorly and laterally in the upper abdomen; however, they run in a slightly inferior direction in the inguinal region. The internal oblique muscle serves as the cephalad (or superior) border of the inguinal canal. The medial aspect of the internal oblique aponeurosis fuses with fibers from the transversus abdominis aponeurosis to form a conjoined tendon. This structure actually is present in only 5% to 10% of patients and is most evident at the insertion of these muscles on the pubic tubercle. The cremasteric muscle fibers arise from the internal oblique, encompass the spermatic cord, and attach to the tunica vaginalis of the testis. These muscle fibers are essential to the cremasteric reflex but have little relevance to hernia repairs.

### Transversus Abdominis Muscle and Aponeurosis and Transversalis Fascia

The transversus abdominis muscle layer is oriented horizontally throughout most of its area; in the inguinal region, these fibers course in a slightly oblique downward direction. The strength and continuity of this muscle and aponeurosis are important for the prevention and treatment of inguinal hernia.

The aponeurosis of the transversus abdominis covers anterior and posterior surfaces. The lower margin of the transversus abdominis arches along with the internal oblique muscle over the internal inguinal ring to form the transversus abdominis aponeurotic arch. The transversalis fascia is the connective tissue layer that underlies the abdominal wall musculature. The transversalis fascia, sometimes referred to as the *endoabdominal fascia*, is a component of the inguinal floor. It tends to be denser in this area but still remains relatively thin.

The iliopubic tract is an aponeurotic band that is formed by the transversalis fascia and transversus abdominis aponeurosis and fascia. The iliopubic tract is located posterior to the inguinal ligament and crosses over the femoral vessels and inserts on

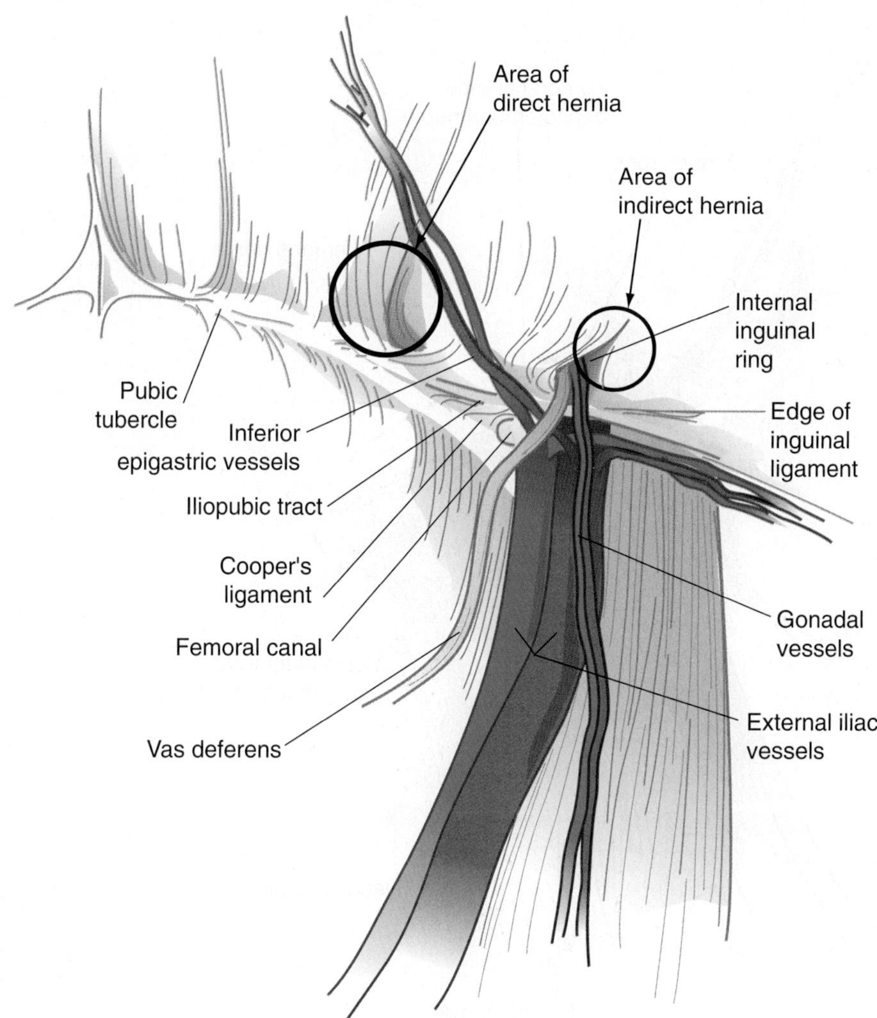


**FIGURE 46-3** Anatomy of the important preperitoneal structures in the right inguinal space. (From Talamini MA, Are C: Laparoscopic hernia repair. In Zuidema GD, Yeo CJ [eds]: Shackelford's surgery of the alimentary tract, ed 5, vol 5, Philadelphia, 2002, WB Saunders, p 140.)

the anterior superior iliac spine and inner lip of the wing of the ilium.

The inferior crus of the deep inguinal ring is comprised of the iliopubic tract; the superior crus of the deep ring is formed by the transversus abdominis aponeurotic arch. The lateral border of the internal ring is connected to the transversus abdominis muscle, which forms a shutter mechanism to limit the development of an indirect hernia.

The iliopubic tract is an extremely important structure in the repair of hernias from the anterior and posterior approaches. It comprises the inferior margin of most anterior repairs. The portion of the iliopubic tract lateral to the internal inguinal ring serves as the inferior border below which staples or tacks are not placed during a laparoscopic repair because the femoral, lateral femoral cutaneous, and genitofemoral nerves are located inferior to the iliopubic tract. Although it cannot always be visualized during posterior repairs, if the tacking device cannot be palpated on the anterior abdominal wall, one must assume it is below the iliopubic tract.

### Pectineal (Cooper's) Ligament

The pectineal (Cooper's) ligament is formed by the periosteum and aponeurotic tissues along the superior ramus of the pubis. This structure is posterior to the iliopubic tract and forms the posterior border of the femoral canal. In approximately 75% of patients, there will be a vessel that crosses the lateral border of Cooper's ligament that is a branch of the obturator artery. If this vessel is injured, troublesome bleeding can result. Cooper's ligament is an important landmark for open and laparoscopic repairs and is a useful anchoring structure, particularly in laparoscopic repairs.

### Inguinal Canal

The inguinal canal is about 4 cm in length and is located just cephalad to the inguinal ligament. The canal extends between the internal (deep) inguinal and external (superficial) inguinal rings. The inguinal canal contains the spermatic cord in men and the round ligament of the uterus in women.

The spermatic cord is composed of the cremasteric muscle fibers, testicular artery and accompanying veins, genital branch of the genitofemoral nerve, vas deferens, cremasteric vessels, lymphatics, and processus vaginalis. These structures enter the cord at the internal inguinal ring and vessels and vas deferens exit the external inguinal ring. The cremaster muscle arises from the lowermost fibers of the internal oblique muscle and encompasses the spermatic cord in the inguinal canal. The cremasteric

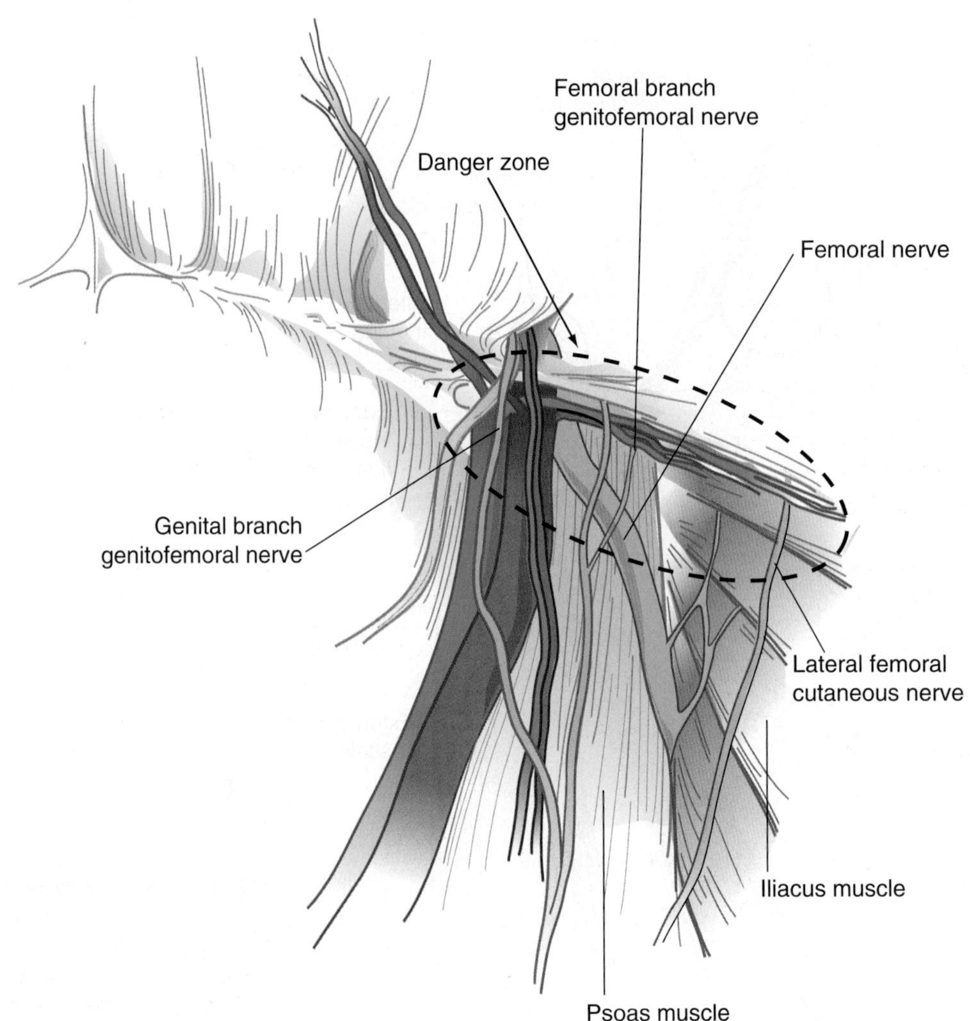


**FIGURE 46-4** Important nerves and their relationship to inguinal structures (right side is illustrated). (From Talamini MA, Are C: Laparoscopic hernia repair. In Zuidema GD, Yeo CJ [eds]: Shackelford's surgery of the alimentary tract, ed 5, vol 5, Philadelphia, 2002, WB Saunders, p 140.)

vessels are branches of the inferior epigastric vessels and pass through the posterior wall of the inguinal canal through their own foramen. These vessels supply the cremaster muscle and can be divided to expose the floor of the inguinal canal during hernia repair without damaging the testis.

The inguinal canal is bounded superficially by the external oblique aponeurosis. The internal oblique and transversus abdominis musculoaponeuroses form the cephalad wall of the inguinal canal. The inferior wall of the inguinal canal is formed by the inguinal ligament and lacunar ligament. The posterior wall, or floor of the inguinal canal, is formed by the aponeurosis of the transversus abdominis muscle and transversalis fascia.

Hesselbach's triangle refers to the margins of the floor of the inguinal canal. The inferior epigastric vessels serve as its superolateral border, the rectus sheath as medial border, and the inguinal ligament and pectineal ligament as the inferior border. Direct hernias occur within Hesselbach's triangle, whereas indirect inguinal hernias arise lateral to the triangle. It is not uncommon, however, for medium and large indirect inguinal hernias to involve the floor of the inguinal canal as they enlarge.

The iliohypogastric and ilioinguinal nerves and genital branch of the genitofemoral nerve are the important sensory nerves in the groin area (Fig. 46-4). The iliohypogastric and ilioinguinal nerves provide sensation to the skin of the groin, base of the penis, and ipsilateral upper medial thigh. The iliohypogastric and ilioinguinal nerves lie beneath the internal oblique muscle to a point just medial and superior to the anterior superior iliac spine, where they penetrate the internal oblique muscle and course beneath the external oblique aponeurosis. The main trunk of the iliohypogastric nerve runs on the anterior surface of the internal oblique muscle and aponeurosis medial and superior to the internal ring. The iliohypogastric nerve may provide an inguinal branch that joins the ilioinguinal nerve. The ilioinguinal nerve runs anterior to the spermatic cord in the inguinal canal and branches at the superficial inguinal ring. The genital branch of the genitofemoral nerve innervates the cremaster muscle and skin on the lateral side of the scrotum and labia. This nerve lies on the iliopubic tract and accompanies the cremaster vessels to form a neurovascular bundle.

### Preperitoneal Space

The preperitoneal space contains adipose tissue, lymphatics, blood vessels, and nerves. The nerves of the preperitoneal space of specific concern to the surgeon include the lateral femoral cutaneous nerve and genitofemoral nerve. The lateral femoral cutaneous nerve originates as a root of L2 and L3 and is occasionally a direct branch of the femoral nerve. This nerve courses along the anterior surface of the iliac muscle beneath the iliac fascia and passes under or through the lateral attachment of the inguinal ligament at the anterior superior iliac spine. This nerve runs beneath or occasionally through the iliopubic tract, lateral to the internal inguinal ring.

The genitofemoral nerve usually arises from the L2 or L1-L2 nerve roots. It divides into genital and femoral branches on the anterior surface of the psoas muscle. The genital branch enters the inguinal canal through the deep ring, whereas the femoral branch enters the femoral sheath lateral to the artery.

The inferior epigastric artery and vein are branches of the external iliac vessels and are important landmarks for laparoscopic hernia repair. These vessels course medial to the internal inguinal ring and eventually lie beneath the rectus abdominis muscle, immediately superficial to the transversalis fascia. The inferior epigastric vessels serve to define the types of inguinal hernia. Indirect inguinal hernias occur lateral to the inferior epigastric vessels, whereas direct hernias occur medial to these vessels.

The deep circumflex iliac artery and vein are located below the lateral portion of the iliopubic tract in the preperitoneal space. These vessels are branches of the inferior epigastric or external iliac artery and vein. It is important to dissect only above the iliopubic tract during a laparoscopic hernia repair to avoid injury to these vessels.

The vas deferens courses through the preperitoneal space from caudad to cephalad and medial to lateral to join the spermatic cord at the deep inguinal ring.

### Femoral Canal

The boundaries of the femoral canal are the iliopubic tract anteriorly, Cooper's ligament posteriorly, and the femoral vein laterally. The pubic tubercle forms the apex of the femoral canal triangle. This canal usually contains connective tissue and lymphatic tissue. A femoral hernia occurs through this space and is medial to the femoral vessels.

## Diagnosis

A bulge in the inguinal region is the main diagnostic finding in most groin hernias. There may be associated pain or vague discomfort in the region, but groin hernias are usually not extremely painful unless incarceration or strangulation has occurred. In the absence of physical findings, alternative causes for pain need to be considered. Occasionally, patients may experience paresthesias related to compression or irritation of the inguinal nerves by the hernia. Masses other than hernias can occur in the groin region. Physical examination alone often differentiates between a groin hernia and these masses (Box 46-2).

**BOX 46-2 Differential Diagnosis of Groin and Scrotal Masses**

Inguinal hernia
Hydrocele
Varicocele
Ectopic testis
Epididymitis
Testicular torsion
Lipoma
Hematoma
Sebaceous cyst
Hidradenitis of inguinal apocrine glands
Inguinal lymphadenopathy
Lymphoma
Metastatic neoplasm
Femoral hernia
Femoral lymphadenopathy
Femoral artery aneurysm or pseudoaneurysm

The inguinal region is examined with the patient in the supine and standing positions. The examiner visually inspects and palpates the inguinal region, looking for asymmetry, bulges, or a mass. Having the patient cough or perform a Valsalva maneuver can facilitate identification of a hernia. The examiner places a fingertip over the inguinal canal and repeats the examination. Finally, a fingertip is placed into the external inguinal ring by invaginating the scrotum to detect a small hernia. A bulge moving lateral to medial in the inguinal canal suggests an indirect hernia. If a bulge progresses from deep to superficial through the inguinal floor, a direct hernia is suspected. This distinction is not critical because repair is approached the same way, regardless of the type of hernia. A bulge identified below the inguinal ligament is consistent with a femoral hernia.

A bulge of the groin described by the patient that is not demonstrated on examination presents a dilemma. Having the patient stand or ambulate for a period of time may allow an undiagnosed hernia to become visible or palpable. If a hernia is strongly suspected, but undetectable, a repeat examination at another time may be helpful.

Ultrasonography also can aid in the diagnosis. There is a high degree of sensitivity and specificity for ultrasound in the detection of occult direct, indirect, and femoral hernias.[1] Other imaging modalities are less useful. Computed tomography (CT) of the abdomen and pelvis may be useful for the diagnosis of obscure and unusual hernias as well as atypical groin masses.[2] Occasionally, laparoscopy can be diagnostic and therapeutic for particularly challenging cases.

## Classification

There are numerous classification systems for groin hernias. One simple and widely used system is the Nyhus classification (Box 46-3). Although their purpose is to promote a common language and understanding for physician communication and to allow appropriate comparisons of therapeutic options, these classifications are incomplete and contentious. Most surgeons continue to describe hernias by their type, location, and volume of the hernia sac.

## Treatment

### Nonoperative Management

Most surgeons recommend operation on discovery of a symptomatic inguinal hernia because the natural history of a groin hernia is that of progressive enlargement and weakening, with a small potential for incarceration and strangulation. However, in patients with minimal symptoms, the clinician is often faced with balancing the risk for hernia-related complications such as incarceration and bowel strangulation, with the potential for complications in the short and long term. Fitzgibbons and

**BOX 46-3 Nyhus Classification of Groin Hernia**

**Type I**
Indirect inguinal hernia–internal inguinal ring normal (e.g., pediatric hernia)

**Type II**
Indirect inguinal hernia–internal inguinal ring dilated but posterior inguinal wall intact; inferior deep epigastric vessels not displaced

**Type III**
Posterior wall defect

- **A.** Direct inguinal hernia
- **B.** Indirect inguinal hernia–internal inguinal ring dilated, medially encroaching on or destroying the transversalis fascia of Hesselbach's triangle (e.g., scrotal, sliding, or pantaloon hernia)
- **C.** Femoral hernia

**Type IV**
Recurrent hernia

- **A.** Direct
- **B.** Indirect
- **C.** Femoral
- **D.** Combined

colleagues[3] have reported a prospective randomized trial of a watchful waiting strategy for men with asymptomatic or minimally symptomatic inguinal hernias. These investigators randomized more than 700 men to a watchful waiting or open tension-free hernia repair. At 2 years of follow-up, there were no deaths attributed to the study and the risk for hernia incarceration in the watchful waiting group was extremely low, 0.3% of study participants or 1.8 events/1000 patient-years. Almost 25% of patients assigned to watchful waiting crossed over to the surgical group, usually for pain related to the hernia that limited activity. Despite the seemingly high crossover rate, those patients, who later had surgery, did not have increased surgical site infections, longer operative times, or higher recurrence rates than those who were initially assigned to early repair. This study provides conclusive evidence that a strategy of watchful waiting is safe for older patients with asymptomatic or minimally symptomatic inguinal hernias and that even though almost 25% of patients eventually undergo repair, when they do, the operative risks and complication rates are no different than those of patients undergoing prophylactic repair. Watchful waiting also is a cost-effective management strategy for patients with no or minimal symptoms.

Patients electing nonoperative management can occasionally have symptomatic improvement with the use of a truss. This approach is more commonly used in Europe. Spring trusses are more versatile than elastic ones, although most information on their use has been anecdotal. Correct measurement and fitting are important. Hernia control has been reported in about 30% of patients. Complications associated with the use of a truss include testicular atrophy, ilioinguinal or femoral neuritis, and hernia incarceration.

It is generally agreed that nonoperative management is not used for femoral hernias because of the high incidence of associated complications, particularly strangulation.

## Operative Repair

**Anterior Repairs** Anterior repairs are the most common operative approach for inguinal hernias. Tension-free repairs are now standard and there are a variety of different types. Older tissue types of repair are rarely indicated, except for patients with simultaneous contamination or concomitant bowel resection, when placement of a mesh prosthesis may be contraindicated.

There are some technical aspects of the operation common to all anterior repairs. Open hernia repair is begun by making a transversely oriented linear or slightly curvilinear incision above the inguinal ligament and a fingerbreadth below the internal inguinal ring. The internal inguinal ring is located topographically at the midpoint between the anterior superior iliac spine and ipsilateral pubic tubercle. Dissection is continued through the subcutaneous tissues and Scarpa's fascia. The external oblique fascia and external inguinal ring are identified. The external oblique fascia is incised through the superficial inguinal ring to expose the inguinal canal. The genital branch of the genitofemoral nerve, as well as the ilioinguinal and iliohypogastric nerves, are identified and avoided or mobilized to prevent transection and entrapment. The spermatic cord is mobilized at the pubic tubercle by a combination of blunt and sharp dissection. Improper mobilization of the spermatic cord too lateral to the pubic tubercle can cause confusion in the identification of tissue planes and essential structures, and may result in injury to the spermatic core structures or disruption of the floor of the inguinal canal.

The cremasteric muscle of the mobilized spermatic cord is separated parallel to its fibers from the underlying cord structures. The cremasteric artery and vein, which join the cremaster muscle near the inguinal ring, can usually be avoided but may need to be cauterized or ligated and divided. When an indirect hernia is present, the hernia sac is located deep to the cremaster muscle and anterior and superior to the spermatic cord structures. Incising the cremaster muscle in a longitudinal direction and dividing it circumferentially near the internal inguinal ring help expose the indirect hernia sac. The hernia sac is carefully separated from adjacent cord structures and dissected to the level of the internal inguinal ring. The sac is opened and examined for visceral contents if it is large; however, this step is unnecessary in small hernias. The sac can be mobilized and placed within the preperitoneal space, or the neck of the sac can be ligated at the level of the internal ring and any excess sac excised. If a large hernia sac is present, it can be divided using electrocautery to facilitate ligation. It is not necessary to excise the distal portion of the sac. If the sac is broad-based, it may be easier to displace it into the peritoneal cavity rather than ligate it. Direct hernia sacs protrude through the floor of the inguinal canal and can be reduced below the transversalis fascia before repair. A lipoma of the cord actually represents retroperitoneal fat that has herniated through the deep inguinal ring; this should be suture-ligated and removed.

A sliding hernia presents a special challenge in handling the hernia sac. With a sliding hernia, a portion of the sac is composed of visceral peritoneum covering part of a retroperitoneal organ, usually the colon or bladder. In this situation, the grossly redundant portion of the sac (if present) is excised and the peritoneum reclosed. The organ and sac then can be reduced below the transversalis fascia, similar to the procedure for a direct hernia.

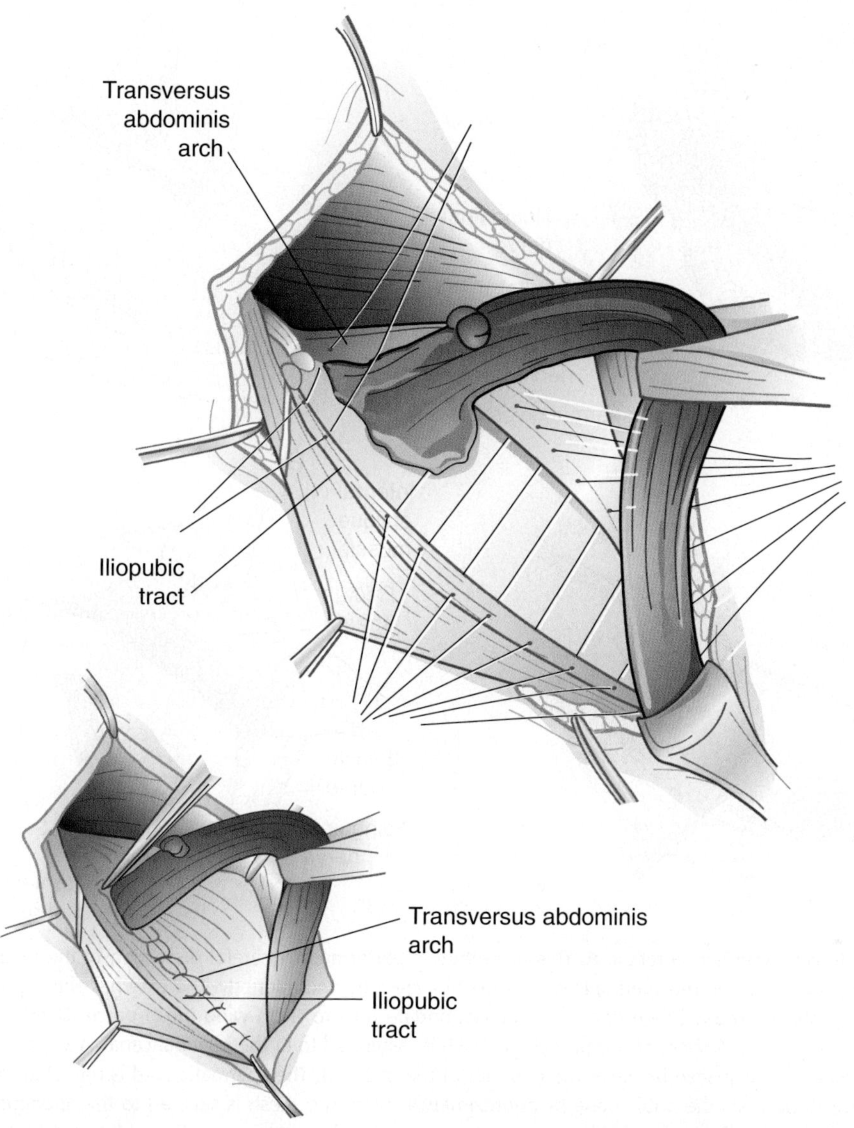


**FIGURE 46-5** Iliopubic tract repair. *Top,* Sutures lateral to the cord complete reconstruction of the deep inguinal ring. These sutures encompass the transversus abdominis arch above and the cremaster origin and iliopubic tract below. *Bottom,* The complete repair is ready for wound closure. The reconstruction of the deep ring should be snug but also loose enough to admit the tip of a hemostat. (From Condon RE: Anterior iliopubic tract repair. In Nyhus LM, Condon RE [eds]: Hernia, ed 2, Philadelphia, 1974, JB Lippincott, p 204.)

**Tissue Repairs** Although tissue repairs have largely been abandoned because of unacceptably high recurrence rates, they remain useful in certain situations. In strangulated hernias, for which bowel resection is necessary, mesh prostheses are contraindicated and a tissue repair is necessary. Available options for tissue repair include iliopubic tract, Shouldice, Bassini, and McVay repairs.

The iliopubic tract repair approximates the transversus abdominis aponeurotic arch to the iliopubic tract with the use of interrupted sutures (Fig. 46-5). The repair begins at the pubic tubercle and extends laterally past the internal inguinal ring. This repair was initially described using a relaxing incision (see later); however, many surgeons who use this repair do not perform a relaxing incision.

The Shouldice repair emphasizes a multilayer imbricated repair of the posterior wall of the inguinal canal with a continuous running suture technique. After completion of the dissection, the posterior wall of the inguinal canal is reconstructed by superimposing running suture lines progressing from deep to more superficial layers. The initial suture line secures the transversus abdominis aponeurotic arch to the iliopubic tract. Next, the internal oblique and transversus abdominis muscles and aponeuroses are sutured to the inguinal ligament. The Shouldice repair is associated with a very low recurrence rate and a high degree of patient satisfaction in highly selected patients.

The Bassini repair is performed by suturing the transversus abdominis and internal oblique musculoaponeurotic arches or conjoined tendon (when present) to the inguinal ligament. This once popular technique is the basic approach to nonanatomic hernia repairs and was the most popular type of repair done before the advent of tension-free repairs.

Cooper's ligament repair, also known as the McVay repair, has traditionally been popular for the correction of direct

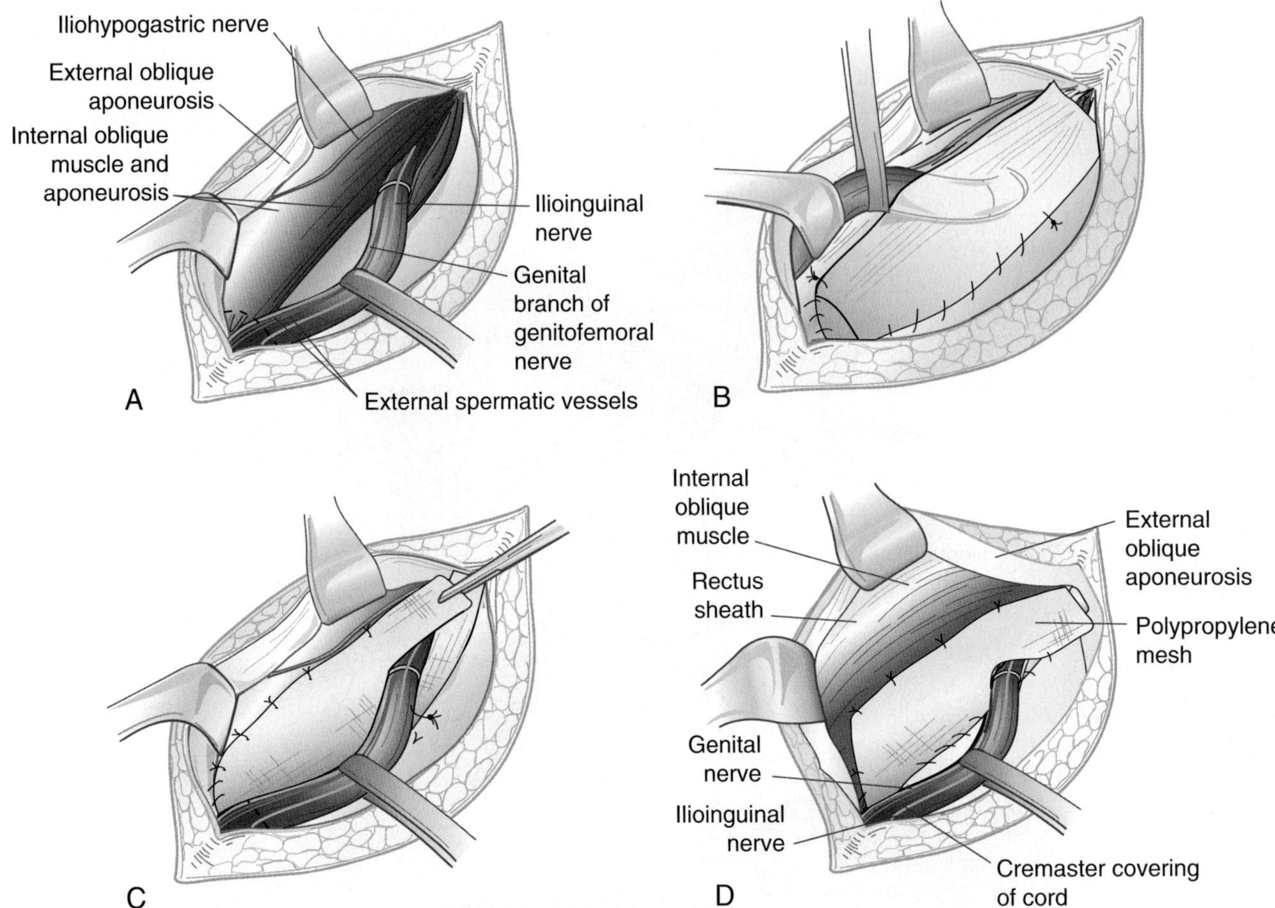


**FIGURE 46-6** Lichtenstein tension-free hernia repair. **A,** This procedure is performed by careful dissection of the inguinal canal. High ligation of an indirect hernia sac is performed and the spermatic cord structures are retracted inferiorly. The external oblique aponeurosis is separated from the underlying internal oblique muscle high enough to accommodate a 6- to 8-cm-wide mesh patch. Overlap of the internal oblique muscle edge by 2 to 3 cm is necessary. A sheet of polypropylene mesh is fashioned to fit the inguinal canal. A slit is made in the lateral aspect of the mesh and the spermatic cord is placed between the two tails of the mesh. **B,** The spermatic cord is retracted in the cephalad direction. The medial aspect of the mesh overlaps the pubic bone by approximately 2 cm. The mesh is secured to the aponeurotic tissue overlying the pubic tubercle using a running suture of nonabsorbable monofilament material. The suture is continued laterally by suturing the inferior edge of the mesh to the shelving edge of the inguinal ligament to a point just lateral to the internal inguinal ring. **C,** A second monofilament suture is placed at the level of the pubic tubercle and continued laterally by suturing the mesh to the internal oblique aponeurosis or muscle approximately 2 cm from the aponeurotic edge. **D,** The lower edges of the two tails are sutured to the shelving edge of the inguinal ligament to create a new internal ring made of mesh. The spermatic cord structures are placed within the inguinal canal overlying the mesh. The external oblique aponeurosis is closed over the spermatic cord. (From Arregui ME, Nagan RD [eds]: Inguinal hernia: Advances or controversies? Oxford, England, 1994, Radcliffe Medical.)

inguinal hernias, large indirect hernias, recurrent hernias, and femoral hernias. Interrupted nonabsorbable sutures are used to approximate the edge of the transversus abdominis aponeurosis to Cooper's ligament. When the medial aspect of the femoral canal is reached, a transition suture is placed to incorporate Cooper's ligament and the iliopubic tract. Lateral to this transition stitch, the transversus abdominis aponeurosis is secured to the iliopubic tract. An important principle of this repair is the need for a relaxing incision. This incision is made by reflecting the external oblique aponeurosis cephalad and medial to expose the anterior rectus sheath. An incision is then made in a curvilinear direction, beginning 1 cm above the pubic tubercle throughout the extent of the anterior sheath to near its lateral border. This relieves tension on the suture line and results in decreased postoperative pain and hernia recurrence. The fascial defect is covered by the body of the rectus muscle, which prevents herniation at the relaxing incision site. The McVay repair is particularly suited for strangulated femoral hernias because it provides obliteration of the femoral space without the use of mesh.

**Tension-Free Anterior Inguinal Hernia Repair** The tension-free repair has become the dominant method of inguinal hernia repair (Fig. 46-6). Recognizing that tension in a repair is the principal cause of recurrence, current practices in hernia management use a synthetic mesh prosthesis to bridge the defect, a concept popularized by Lichtenstein. There are several options for placement of mesh during anterior inguinal herniorrhaphy, including the Lichtenstein approach, plug and patch technique, and sandwich technique, with both an anterior and preperitoneal piece of mesh.

In the Lichtenstein repair,[4] a piece of prosthetic nonabsorbable mesh is fashioned to fit the canal. A slit is cut into the distal lateral edge of the mesh to accommodate the spermatic cord. There are various preformed, commercially available prostheses available for use. Monofilament nonabsorbable suture is used to secure the mesh, beginning at the pubic tubercle and running a length of suture in both directions toward the superior aspect above the internal inguinal ring to the level of the tails of the mesh. The mesh is sutured to the aponeurotic tissue overlying the pubic bone medially, continuing superiorly along the transversus abdominis or conjoined tendon. The inferolateral edge of the mesh is sutured to the iliopubic tract or shelving edge of the inguinal ligament to a point lateral to the internal inguinal ring. At this point, the tails created by the slit are sutured together around the spermatic cord, snugly forming a new internal inguinal ring. It is important to protect the ilioinguinal nerve and genital branch of the genitofemoral nerve from entrapment by placing them with the cord structures as they are passed through this newly fashioned internal inguinal ring or avoiding their enclosure in the repair.

Adapting the principles of tension-free repair, Gilbert[5] has reported using a cone-shaped plug of polypropylene mesh that when inserted into the internal inguinal ring, would deploy like an upside-down umbrella and occlude the hernia. This plug is sewn to the surrounding tissues and held in place by an additional overlying mesh patch. This patch may not need to be secured by sutures; however, to do so requires dissection to create a sufficient space between the external and internal oblique muscles for the patch to lie flat over the inguinal canal. This so-called plug and patch repair, an extension of Lichtenstein's original mesh repair, has now become the most commonly performed primary anterior inguinal hernia repair. Although this repair can be done without suture fixation by some experienced surgeons, most secure plug and patch with several monofilament nonabsorbable sutures, especially for very weak inguinal floors or large defects.

The sandwich technique involves a bilayered device, with three polypropylene components. An underlay patch provides a posterior repair similar to that of the laparoscopic approach, a connector functions similar to a plug, and an onlay patch covers the posterior inguinal floor. The use of interrupted fixating sutures is not mandatory, but most surgeons place three or four fixation sutures in this repair.

Another option for a tension-free mesh repair involves a preperitoneal approach using a self-expanding polypropylene patch.[6] A pocket is created in the preperitoneal space by blunt dissection and then a preformed mesh patch is inserted into the hernia defect, which expands to cover the direct, indirect, and femoral spaces. The patch lies parallel to the inguinal ligament. It can remain without suture fixation, or a tacking suture can be placed.

The Stoppa-Rives repair uses a subumbilical midline incision to place a large mesh prosthesis into the preperitoneal space.[7] Blunt dissection is used to create an extraperitoneal space that extends into the prevesical space, beyond the obturator foramen, and posterolateral to the pelvic brim. This technique has the advantage of distributing the natural intra-abdominal pressure across a broad area to retain the mesh in a proper location. The Stoppa-Rives technique is particularly useful for large, recurrent, or bilateral hernias.

**Preperitoneal Repair** The open preperitoneal approach is useful for the repair of recurrent inguinal hernias, sliding hernias, femoral hernias, and some strangulated hernias.[8] A transverse skin incision is made 2 cm above the internal inguinal ring and is directed to the medial border of the rectus sheath. The muscles of the anterior abdominal wall are incised transversely and the preperitoneal space is identified. If further exposure is needed, the anterior rectus sheath can be incised and the rectus muscle retracted medially. The preperitoneal tissues are retracted cephalad to visualize the posterior inguinal wall and the site of herniation. The inferior epigastric artery and veins are generally beneath the midportion of the posterior rectus sheath and usually do not need to be divided. This approach avoids mobilization of the spermatic cord and injury to the sensory nerves of the inguinal canal, which is particularly important for hernias previously repaired through an anterior approach. If the peritoneum is incised, it is sutured closed to avoid the evisceration of intraperitoneal contents into the operative field. The transversalis fascia and transversus abdominis aponeurosis are identified and sutured to the iliopubic tract with permanent sutures. Femoral hernias repaired by this approach require closure of the femoral canal by securing the repair to Cooper's ligament. A mesh prosthesis is frequently used to obliterate the defect in the femoral canal, particularly with large hernias.

**Laparoscopic Repair** Laparoscopic inguinal hernia repair is another method of tension-free mesh repair, based on a preperitoneal approach. The laparoscopic approach provides the mechanical advantage of placing a large piece of mesh behind the defect covering the myopectineal orifice and using the natural forces of the abdominal wall to support the mesh in place. Proponents have touted quicker recovery, less pain, better visualization of anatomy, usefulness for fixing all inguinal hernia defects, and decreased surgical site infections. Critics have emphasized longer operative times, technical challenges, risk of recurrence, and increased cost. Although controversy exists about the usefulness of laparoscopic repair for primary unilateral inguinal hernias, most agree that this approach has advantages for patients with bilateral or recurrent hernias.[9] Adopting practice guidelines for the performance of laparoscopic hernia repairs could help control costs.

When considering the laparoscopic approach for repair of inguinal hernias, the surgeon has several options. Initially, laparoscopic repairs involved placing a large piece of mesh in an intraperitoneal position, similar to a laparoscopic ventral hernia repair. This approach has been abandoned because of high recurrence rates and the drawbacks of intraperitoneal mesh. The most popular techniques include a totally extraperitoneal (TEP) and transabdominal preperitoneal (TAPP) approach. The main difference between these two techniques is the sequence of gaining access to the preperitoneal space. In the TEP approach, the dissection begins in the preperitoneal space using a balloon dissector. With the TAPP repair, the preperitoneal space is accessed after initially entering the peritoneal cavity. Each approach has its merits. Using the TEP approach, the preperitoneal dissection is quicker and the potential risk for intraperitoneal visceral damage is minimized. However, the use of dissection balloons

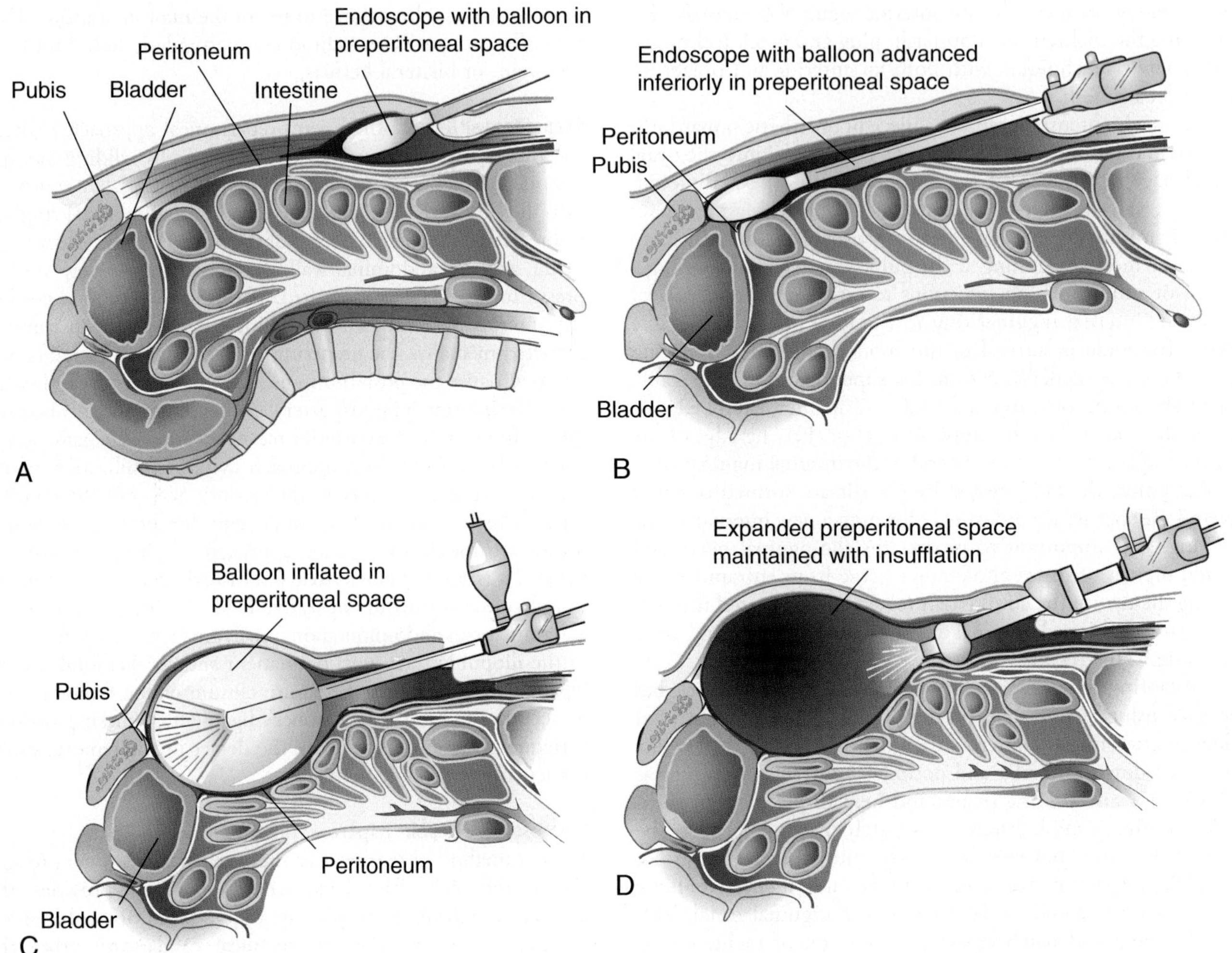


**FIGURE 46-7** TEP laparoscopic hernia repair. **A,** Access to the posterior rectus sheath is gained in the periumbilical region. A balloon dissector is placed on the anterior surface of the posterior rectus sheath. **B,** The balloon dissector is advanced to the posterior surface of the pubis in the preperitoneal space. **C,** The balloon is inflated, thereby creating an optical cavity. **D,** The optical cavity is insufflated by carbon dioxide and the posterior surface of the inguinal floor is dissected. (From Shadduck PP, Schwartz LB, Eubanks WS: Laparoscopic inguinal herniorrhaphy. In Pappas TN, Schwartz LB, Eubanks SE [eds]: Atlas of laparoscopic surgery, Philadelphia, 1996, Current Medicine.)

is costly, the working space is more limited, and it may not be possible to create a working space if the patient has had a prior preperitoneal operation. Also, if a large tear in the peritoneum is created during a TEP approach, the potential working space can become obliterated, necessitating conversion to a TAPP approach. For these reasons, knowledge of the transabdominal technique is essential when performing laparoscopic inguinal hernia repairs. The transabdominal approach allows identification of the groin anatomy before extensive dissection and disruption of natural tissue planes. The larger working space of the peritoneal cavity can make early experience with the laparoscopic approach easier.

There are no absolute contraindications to laparoscopic inguinal hernia repair other than the patient's inability to tolerate general anesthesia. Patients who have had extensive prior lower abdominal surgery can require significant adhesiolysis and may be best approached anteriorly. In particular, patients who have had a radical retropubic prostatectomy with the preperitoneal space previously dissected can make accurate and safe dissection challenging.

In the TEP approach, an infraumbilical incision is used. The anterior rectus sheath is incised, the ipsilateral rectus abdominis muscle is retracted laterally, and blunt dissection is used to create a space beneath the rectus. A dissecting balloon is inserted deep to the posterior rectus sheath, advanced to the pubic symphysis, and inflated under direct laparoscopic vision (Fig. 46-7). After it is opened, the space is insufflated and additional trocars are placed. A 30-degree laparoscope provides the best visualization of the inguinal region (see Fig. 46-3). The inferior epigastric vessels are identified along the lower portion of the rectus muscle and serve as a useful landmark. Cooper's ligament must be cleared from the pubic symphysis medially to the level of the external iliac vein. The iliopubic tract is also identified. Care must be taken to avoid injury to the femoral branch of the genitofemoral nerve and lateral femoral cutaneous nerve, which are located lateral to and below the iliopubic

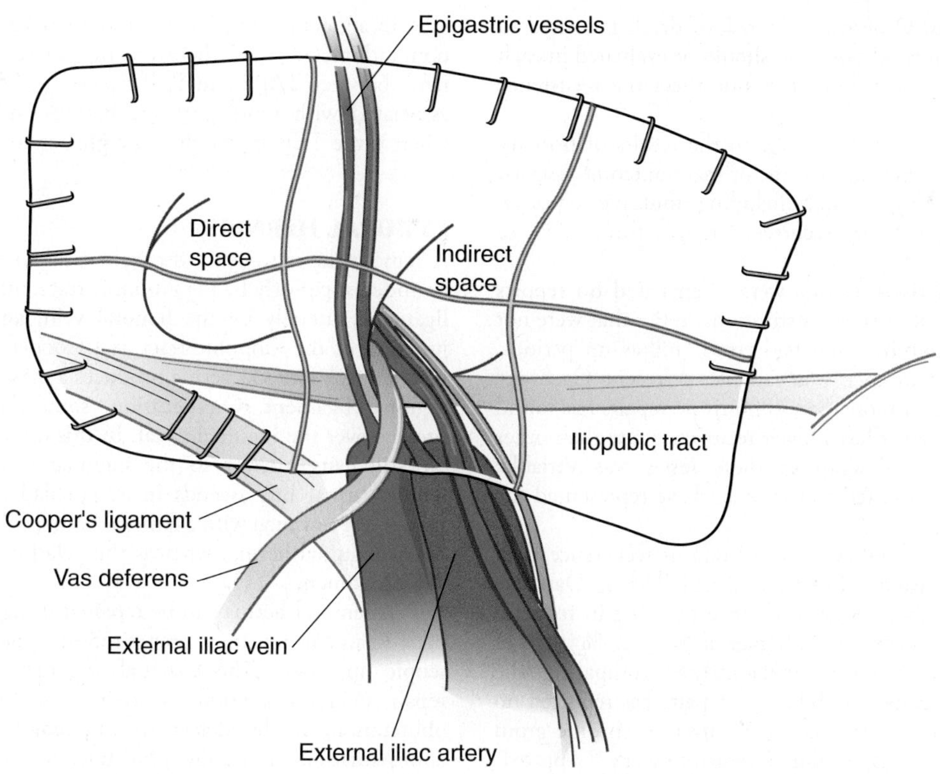


**FIGURE 46-8** Prosthetic mesh placement for TEP hernia repair. (From Corbitt J: Laparoscopic transabdominal transperitoneal patch hernia repair. In Ballantyne GH [ed]: Atlas of laparoscopic surgery, Philadelphia, 2000, WB Saunders, p 511.)

tract (see Fig. 46-4). Lateral dissection is carried out to the anterior superior iliac spine. Finally, the spermatic cord is skeletonized.

In the TAPP approach, an infraumbilical incision is used to gain access to the peritoneal cavity directly. Two 5-mm ports are placed lateral to the inferior epigastric vessels at the level of the umbilicus. A peritoneal flap is created high on the anterior abdominal wall, extending from the median umbilical fold to the anterior superior iliac spine. The remainder of the operation proceeds similar to a TEP procedure.

A direct hernia sac and associated preperitoneal fat are gently reduced by traction if not already reduced by balloon expansion of the peritoneal space. A small, indirect hernia sac is mobilized from the cord structures and reduced into the peritoneal cavity. A large sac may be difficult to reduce. In this case, the sac is divided with cautery near the internal inguinal ring, leaving the distal sac in situ. The proximal peritoneal sac is closed with a loop ligature to prevent pneumoperitoneum from occurring. After all hernias are reduced, a 12-×14-cm piece of polypropylene mesh is inserted through a trocar and unfolded. It covers the direct, indirect, and femoral spaces and rests over the cord structures. It is imperative that the peritoneum be dissected at least 4 cm off the cord structures to prevent the peritoneum from encroaching beneath the mesh, which can lead to recurrence. The mesh is carefully secured with a tacking stapler to Cooper's ligament from the pubic tubercle to the external iliac vein, anteriorly to the posterior rectus musculature and transversus abdominis aponeurotic arch at least 2 cm above the hernia defect, and laterally to the iliopubic tract. The mesh extends beyond the pubic symphysis and below the spermatic cord and peritoneum (Fig. 46-8). The mesh is not fixed in this area and tacks are not placed inferior to the iliopubic tract beyond the external iliac artery. Staples placed in this area may injure the femoral branch of the genitofemoral nerve or lateral femoral cutaneous nerve. Staples are also avoided in the so-called triangle of doom, bounded by the ductus deferens medially and spermatic vessels laterally, to avoid injury to the external iliac vessels and femoral nerve. As long as one can palpate the tip of the tacking device, these structures are not likely to be injured.

## Results of Hernia Repair

The true measure of success for the various types of hernia repair is based on the results. The best information on the results of hernia repair is available from large prospective randomized trials, meta-analyses of clinical trials, and two large national registries, the Danish Hernia Database and the Swedish Hernia Register. The Danish Hernia Database includes more than 98% of inguinal hernia repairs; the capture rate of the Swedish Hernia Register is approximately 80%.[10,11] In spite of the randomized nature of some trials, caution must be used when interpreting the results. Many of these patients were highly selected and most trials excluded recurrent hernias, obese individuals, and large inguinal hernias. Also, some follow-up results were completed by telephone interviews and not by physical examination. The national registries only collect information on operations, so the incidence of recurrence is lower than if all patients had been interviewed and examined.

The mortality of all types of repair is low and there are no significant differences reported among the various techniques. There is a greater mortality associated with the repair of strangulated hernias. Otherwise, the risk of death is related to individual comorbid conditions and should be evaluated in each patient. The type of anesthetic does not affect the recurrence rate.[11]

There are important differences in the results of primary hernia repair. Hernia recurrence is the primary outcome assessed by most studies. Large series, including multiple types of repairs, have suggested that recurrence ranges from 1.7% to 10%.[10-12]

The results of tissue repairs were often based on reports consisting of personal or single institutional series that were not prospective or randomized and had erratic follow-up periods. Not surprisingly, recurrence was variable. A recent Cochrane review of 16 studies of more than 4000 tissue repairs has found that the Shouldice repair has a lower recurrence rate than other nonmesh repairs.[13] Follow-up in these series was variable; patients were highly selected and may not have represented the population at large.

Tension-free repairs have a lower rate of recurrence than tissue repairs.[11,13,14] Results from the Danish Hernia Database have demonstrated that hernia recurrence resulting in reoperation following the Lichtenstein repair is only 25% that of nonmesh repairs.[10] A recent meta-analysis comparing the Lichtenstein, mesh plug, and bilayered repairs has reported no significant differences in the rate of recurrence, chronic groin pain, other complications, or time to return to work.[15] Approximately 50% of recurrences are found within 3 years after primary repair. Recurrence continues to occur after this time in nonmesh based repairs, but is uncommon with tension-free repairs. The bilayered repair was found to have a 20% hernia recurrence when used for large direct or recurrent hernias in one study.[16] These results demonstrate the limitations of a fixed mesh size in these circumstances.

An extensive systematic review of randomized controlled trials was published in 2002 by the European Union Hernia Trialists Collaboration.[17] The authors reported a meta-analysis of 4165 patients in 25 studies. Based on the available data, the laparoscopic repair resulted in a more rapid return to normal activity and decreased persistent postoperative pain. The recurrence rate for the laparoscopic repair was lower compared with open nonmesh repairs; however, open and laparoscopic mesh repairs had similar recurrence rates.

A prospective trial sponsored by the Veterans Administration randomized 1983 patients to undergo an open Lichtenstein repair or laparoscopic repair, of which 90% were TEP repairs.[12] Most surgeons in this study may have had a suboptimal experience with the laparoscopic approach; only 25 prior repairs were necessary to be eligible to enroll patients, which is consistent with the seemingly high conversion rate of 5%. Despite these factors, the investigators found a twofold higher incidence of recurrence after laparoscopic repair (10%) than open repair (5%). This difference in recurrence remained for primary hernias (10% laparoscopic versus 4% open); however, recurrent hernias repaired by the laparoscopic approach tended to have fewer rerecurrences (10% versus 14%). In another study by this group, surgeon inexperience with laparoscopy and surgeon age older than 45 years were both predictors of recurrence after laparoscopic repair.[15] What can be concluded from these results? This trial demonstrates that the laparoscopic repair of inguinal hernias may have a definite learning curve to achieve an acceptably low recurrence rate.

In a Cochrane review of more than 1000 patients in eight nonrandomized trials, there was no difference in hernia recurrence between TAPP and TEP repairs.[18] TAPP procedures were associated with more port site hernias and vascular injuries, whereas the TEP approach had a greater conversion rate.

## FEMORAL HERNIAS

A femoral hernia occurs through the femoral canal, which is bounded superiorly by the iliopubic tract, inferiorly by Cooper's ligament, laterally by the femoral vein, and medially by the junction of the iliopubic tract and Cooper's ligament (lacunar ligament). A femoral hernia produces a mass or bulge below the inguinal ligament. On occasion, some femoral hernias will present over the inguinal canal. In this case, the femoral hernia sac still exits inferior to the inguinal ligament through the femoral canal but ascends in a cephalad direction. Approximately 50% of men with a femoral hernia will have an associated direct inguinal hernia, whereas this relationship occurs in only 2% of women.

A femoral hernia can be repaired using the standard Cooper's ligament repair, a preperitoneal approach, or a laparoscopic approach. The essential elements of femoral hernia repair include dissection and reduction of the hernia sac and obliteration of the defect in the femoral canal, either by approximation of the iliopubic tract to Cooper's ligament or by placement of prosthetic mesh to obliterate the defect. The incidence of strangulation in femoral hernias is high; therefore, all femoral hernias should be repaired and incarcerated femoral hernias should have the hernia sac contents examined for viability. In patients with a compromised bowel, the Cooper's ligament approach is the preferred technique because mesh is contraindicated. When the incarcerated contents of a femoral hernia cannot be reduced, dividing the lacunar ligament can be helpful.

Femoral hernias were reported to occur in conjunction with inguinal hernias in 0.3% of patients in a large national hernia database of almost 35,000 patients.[19] The occurrence of a femoral hernia after repair of an inguinal hernia has been reported to be 15 times the normal expected rate. It is unclear whether this represents a femoral hernia overlooked at the prior operation or a propensity to develop a new hernia after inguinal hernia repair. Recurrence of femoral hernia after operation is only 2%. Recurrent femoral hernia repairs have a rerecurrence rate of about 10%.

## SPECIAL PROBLEMS

### Sliding Hernia

A sliding hernia occurs when an internal organ comprises a portion of the wall of the hernia sac. The most common viscus involved is the colon or urinary bladder. Most sliding hernias are a variant of indirect inguinal hernias, although femoral and direct sliding hernias can occur. The primary danger associated with a sliding hernia is the failure to recognize the visceral component of the hernia sac before injury to the bowel or bladder. The sliding hernia contents are reduced into the peritoneal cavity, and any excess hernia sac is ligated and divided. After reduction of the hernia, one of the techniques described earlier can be used for repair of the inguinal hernia.

## Recurrent Hernia

The repair of recurrent inguinal hernias is challenging, and results are associated with a higher incidence of secondary recurrence. Recurrent hernias almost always require placement of prosthetic mesh for successful repair. Recurrences after anterior hernia repair using mesh are best managed by a laparoscopic or open posterior approach, with placement of a second prosthesis.

## Strangulated Hernia

Repair of a suspected strangulated hernia is most easily done using a preperitoneal approach. (see earlier). With this exposure, the hernia sac contents can be directly visualized and their viability assessed through a single incision. The constricting ring is identified and can be incised to reduce the entrapped viscus with minimal danger to the surrounding organs, blood vessels, and nerves. If it is necessary to resect strangulated intestine, the peritoneum can be opened and resection done without the need for a second incision.

## Bilateral Hernias

The approach to repair of bilateral inguinal hernias is based on the extent of the hernia defect. Simultaneous repair of bilateral hernias has a similar recurrence rate to unilateral repair, regardless of whether the open or laparoscopic technique is used.[20] The use of a giant prosthetic reinforcement of the visceral sac (Stoppa repair)[7] or the laparoscopic repair is appropriate for simultaneous repair of bilateral inguinal hernias, although bilateral anterior repair through separate incisions can be used.

## Complications

There are a myriad of complications related to open and laparoscopic inguinal hernia repair (Table 46-1). Some are general complications that are related to underlying diseases and the effects of anesthesia. These vary by patient population and risk. In addition, there are technical complications that are directly related to the repair. Technical complications are affected by the experience of the surgeon and are more frequent after the repair of recurrent hernias. There is increased scarring and disturbed anatomy with hernia recurrence that can result in an inability to identify important structures at operation. This is the principal reason that we recommend using a different approach for recurrent hernias.

Although the overall complication rate from hernia repair has been estimated to be approximately 10%, many of these complications are transient and can be easily addressed. More serious complications from a large experience are listed in Table 46-1.

**Table 46-1 Complications After Open and Laparoscopic Inguinal Hernia Repair (%)**

| COMPLICATION | OPEN REPAIR (*N* = 994) | LAPAROSCOPIC REPAIR (*N* = 989) |
|---|---|---|
| Intraoperative complications | 1.9 | 4.8 |
| Postoperative complications | 19.4 | 24.6 |
| Urinary retention | 2.2 | 2.8 |
| Urinary tract infection | 0.4 | 1.0 |
| Orchitis | 1.1 | 1.4 |
| Surgical site infection | 1.4 | 1.0 |
| Neuralgia, pain | 3.6 | 4.2 |
| Life-threatening complications | 0.1 | 1.1 |
| Long-term complications | 17.4 | 18.0 |
| Seroma | 3.0 | 9.0 |
| Orchitis | 2.2 | 1.9 |
| Infection | 0.6 | 0.4 |
| Chronic pain | 14.3 | 9.8 |
| Recurrence | 4.9 | 10.1 |

From Neumayer L, Giobbie-Hurder A, Jonassen O, et al: Open mesh versus laparoscopic mesh repair of inguinal hernias. N Engl J Med 350:1819–1827, 2004.

### Surgical Site Infection

The risk for surgical site (wound) infection is estimated to be 1% to 2% after open inguinal hernia repair and less with laparoscopic repairs. These are clean operations, and the risk for infection is primarily influenced by associated patient diseases. Most would agree that there is no need to use routine antimicrobial prophylaxis for hernia repair.[17] Prospective randomized clinical trials have not supported the routine use of perioperative antimicrobial prophylaxis for inguinal hernia repair.[21] Patients who have significant underlying disease, as reflected by an American Society of Anesthesiology (ASA) score of 3 or more, receive perioperative antimicrobial prophylaxis with cefazolin, 1 to 2 g, given IV 30 to 60 minutes before the incision. Clindamycin, 600 mg IV, can be used for patients allergic to penicillin. Only a single dose of antibiotic is necessary. The placement of prosthetic mesh does not increase the risk for infection and does not affect the need for prophylaxis. Superficial surgical site infections are treated by opening the incision, local wound care, and healing by secondary intention. Some mesh infections will present as a chronic draining sinus that tracks to the mesh or occur with extruded mesh. Deep surgical site infections usually involve the prosthetic mesh, which should be explanted.

The risk for infection can be decreased by using proper operative technique, preoperative antiseptic skin preparation, and appropriate hair removal. There is an increased risk for infection for patients who have had prior hernia incision infections, chronic skin infections, or infection at a distant site. These infections are treated before elective surgery.

### Nerve Injuries and Chronic Pain Syndromes

Nerve injuries are an infrequent and underrecognized complication of inguinal hernia repair. Injury can occur from traction, electrocautery, transection, and entrapment. The use of prosthetic mesh can result in dysesthesias, which are usually temporary. The nerves most commonly affected during open hernia repair are the ilioinguinal, genital branch of the genitofemoral, and iliohypogastric nerves. During laparoscopic repair, the lateral femoral cutaneous and genitofemoral nerves are most often affected.[22] Rarely, the main trunk of the femoral nerve can be injured during open or laparoscopic inguinal hernia repair.

Transient neuralgias can occur and are usually self-limited and resolve within a few weeks after surgery. Persistent neuralgias usually result in pain and hyperesthesia in the area of distribution. Symptoms are often reproduced by palpation over the point of entrapment or hyperextension of the hip and may be relieved by flexion of the thigh. Transection of a sensory nerve usually results in an area of numbness corresponding to the distribution of the involved nerve.

With more attention to patient outcomes, chronic groin pain has replaced recurrence as the primary complication after open inguinal hernia repair. Several large series with systematic follow-up have reported pain rates ranging from 29% to 76%.[23,24] Strategies of routine nerve division in open surgery have not been associated with a reduction in chronic pain in mesh-based anterior repairs.[25] In contrast, routine ilioinguinal nerve division is associated with significantly more sensory disturbances. By operating in a remote area to the commonly injured nerves and judicious use of appropriately placed tacks, chronic groin pain intuitively is less common in laparoscopic repairs. Laparoscopic series and randomized controlled trials comparing laparoscopic and open repairs have reported significantly lower rates of chronic postoperative inguinal pain.

Various approaches to management of residual neuralgia have been described. Early symptoms are treated with anti-inflammatory agents, analgesics, and local anesthetic nerve blocks. Patients with nerve entrapment syndromes are best treated by repeat exploration with neurectomy and mesh removal through an anterior approach. Laparoscopic nerve injuries are minimized by not placing any tacks or staples below the lateral portion of the iliopubic tract. If nerve entrapment occurs, patients undergo reoperation to remove the offending tack or staple.

### Ischemic Orchitis and Testicular Atrophy

Ischemic orchitis usually occurs from thrombosis of the small veins of the pampiniform plexus within the spermatic cord. This results in venous congestion of the testis, which becomes swollen and tender 2 to 5 days after surgery. The process may continue for an additional 6 to 12 weeks and usually results in testicular atrophy. Ischemic orchitis also can be caused by ligation of the testicular artery. It is treated with anti-inflammatory agents and analgesics. Orchiectomy is rarely necessary.

The incidence of ischemic orchitis can be minimized by avoiding unnecessary dissection within the spermatic cord. The incidence increases with dissection of the distal portion of a large hernia sac and in patients who have anterior operations for hernia recurrence or for spermatic cord pathology. In these situations, the use of a posterior approach is preferred.

Testicular atrophy is a consequence of ischemic orchitis. It is more common after repair of recurrent hernias, particularly when an anterior approach is used. The incidence of ischemic orchitis increases by a factor of three or four with each subsequent hernia recurrence.

### Injury to the Vas Deferens and Viscera

Injury to the vas deferens and intra-abdominal viscera is unusual. Most of these injuries occur in patients with sliding inguinal hernias when there is failure to recognize the presence of intra-abdominal viscera in the hernia sac. With large hernias, the vas deferens can be displaced in an enlarged inguinal ring before its entry into the spermatic cord. In this situation, the vas deferens is identified and protected.

### Hernia Recurrence

Hernia recurrences are usually caused by technical factors, such as excessive tension on the repair, missed hernias, failure to include an adequate musculoaponeurotic margin in the repair, and improper mesh size and placement. Recurrence also can result from failure to close a patulous internal inguinal ring, the size of which is always assessed at the conclusion of the primary surgery. Other factors that can cause hernia recurrence are chronically elevated intra-abdominal pressure, a chronic cough, deep incisional infections, and poor collagen formation in the wound. Recurrences are more common in patients with direct hernias and usually involve the floor of the inguinal canal near the pubic tubercle, where suture line tension is greatest. The use of a relaxing incision when there is excessive tension at the time of primary hernia repair is helpful to reduce recurrence. A femoral hernia is found in approximately 10% of patients with an inguinal hernia recurrence and should always be investigated at surgery.[10]

Most recurrent hernias require the use of prosthetic mesh for successful repair.[26,27] Choosing a different approach (usually posterior) avoids dissection through scar tissue, improves visualization of the defect and reduction of the hernia, and decreases the incidence of complications, particularly ischemic orchitis and injury to the ilioinguinal nerve. Recurrences after initial prosthetic mesh repairs can be caused by displaced prostheses or the use of a prosthetic of inadequate size. Recurrences are best managed by placing a second prosthesis through a different approach.

A meta-analysis of 58 reports comparing synthetic mesh techniques to nonmesh repairs has demonstrated an almost 60% reduction in recurrence with the use of mesh.[17] This report concluded that there was no difference in the rate of hernia recurrence between laparoscopic and open approaches that used mesh. A recent meta-analysis of recurrent hernia repairs reported no difference between open and laparoscopic mesh repairs in rerecurrence or chronic groin pain.[28]

Recurrence is more common after repair of recurrent hernias and is directly related to the number of previous attempts at repair. Large population-based studies have reported a rerecurrence rate of 4% to 5% in the first 24 months, which increases to 7.5% at 5 years.[27,29] Tension-free and mesh-based repairs have the lowest rates of reoperation after recurrence and result in a reduction in recurrence of approximately 60% compared with more traditional repairs.[26]

There is a successive decrease in the time to hernia recurrence with each subsequent repair.[29] Rerecurrences are associated with increased operative times and a greater rate of complications.

### Quality of Life

The major quality indicators that have been assessed for hernia repair are postoperative pain and return to work. Tension-free and laparoscopic mesh-based approaches have been demonstrated to be less painful than nonmesh repairs. Laparoscopic repairs have the least amount of postoperative pain and have been shown to provide a marginal advantage in reducing time off work.[9]

## VENTRAL HERNIAS

A ventral hernia is defined by a protrusion through the anterior abdominal wall fascia. These defects can be categorized as spontaneous or acquired or by their location on the abdominal wall. Epigastric hernias occur from the xyphoid process to the umbilicus, umbilical hernias occur at the umbilicus, and hypogastric hernias are rare spontaneous hernias that occur below the umbilicus in the midline. Acquired hernias typically occur after surgical incisions and are therefore termed *incisional hernias.* Although not a true hernia, diastasis recti can present as a midline bulge. In this condition, the linea alba is stretched, resulting in bulging at the medial margins of the rectus muscles. Abdominal wall diastasis can occur at other sites in addition to the midline. There is no fascial ring or hernia sac and, unless significantly symptomatic, surgical correction is avoided.

## Incidence

Based on national operative statistics, incisional hernias account for 15% to 20% of all abdominal wall hernias; umbilical and epigastric hernias constitute 10% of hernias. Incisional hernias are twice as common in women as in men. As a result of the almost 4 million laparotomies performed annually in the United States and the 2% to 30% incidence of incisional hernia, almost 150,000 ventral hernia repairs are performed each year. Several technical and patient-related factors have been linked to the occurrence of incisional hernias. There is no conclusive evidence that demonstrates that the type of suture at the primary operation affects hernia formation.[30] Patient-related factors linked to ventral hernia formation include obesity, older age, male gender, sleep apnea, emphysema, and prostatism. It has been proposed that the same factors associated with destruction of the collagen in the lung result in poor wound healing, with increased hernia formation. Wound infection has been linked to hernia formation.

Whether the type of initial abdominal incision influences the incisional hernia rate remains controversial. As noted, the incidence of ventral herniation after midline laparotomy ranges from 3% to 20% and doubles if the operation is associated with a surgical site infection. A meta-analysis of 11 studies examining the incidence of ventral hernia formation after various types of abdominal incisions has concluded that the risk is 10.5% for midline, 7.5% for transverse, and 2.5% for paramedian incisions.[31] A recently published prospective randomized trial has reported no difference in hernia formation when comparing midline versus transverse incisions after 1 year, but noted a higher wound infection rate in the transverse incisions.[32] Given the likely similar rates of incisional hernia formation after transverse and midline incisions, the surgeon should plan the incision based on the operative exposure desired to complete the procedure safely.

Few data are available about the natural history of untreated ventral hernias. As noted, asymptomatic or minimally symptomatic inguinal hernias purposely observed over 2 years have a low incidence of complications.[3] Whether this paradigm applies for asymptomatic ventral or incisional hernias is unclear. Because there is no prospective cohort available to determine the natural history of untreated ventral hernias, most surgeons recommend that these hernias should be repaired when discovered.

## Anatomy

The anatomy of the anterior abdominal wall is straightforward and considerably easier to grasp than the anatomy of the inguinal area. However, a clear understanding of the blood supply and innervation of the abdomen is important when performing advanced abdominal wall reconstruction. The lateral musculature is composed of three layers, with the fascicles of each directed obliquely at different angles to create a strong envelope for the abdominal contents. Each of these muscles forms an aponeurosis that inserts into the linea alba, a midline structure joining both sides of the abdominal wall. The external oblique is the most superficial muscle of the lateral abdominal wall. Deep to the external oblique lies the internal oblique muscle. The fibers of the external oblique course in an inferomedial direction (like hands in pockets), whereas those of the internal oblique muscle run deep to and opposite the external oblique. The deepest muscular layer of the abdominal wall is the transversus abdominis muscle. Its fibers course in a horizontal direction. These three lateral muscles give rise to aponeurotic layers lateral to the rectus, which contribute to the anterior and posterior layers of the rectus sheath.

The medial extension of the external oblique aponeurosis forms the anterior layer of the rectus sheath. At the midline, the two anterior rectus sheaths form the tendinous linea alba. On either side of the linea alba are the rectus abdominis muscles, whose fibers are directed longitudinally and run the length of the anterior abdominal wall. Below each rectus muscle lies the posterior layer of the rectus sheath, which also contributes to the linea alba.

Another important anatomic structure of the anterior abdominal wall is the arcuate line, which is located 3 to 6 cm below the umbilicus. The arcuate line delineates the point below which the posterior rectus sheath is absent. Above the arcuate line, the aponeurosis of the internal oblique muscle contributes to the anterior and posterior rectus sheaths and the aponeurosis of the transversus abdominis muscle passes posterior to the rectus muscle to form the posterior rectus sheath. Below the arcuate line, the internal oblique and transversus abdominis aponeuroses pass completely anterior to the rectus muscle (Fig. 46-9). The rectus abdominis muscles are almost fused below the arcuate line with the transversalis fascia directly behind them.

The abdominal wall receives most of its innervation from intercostal nerves 7 through 12 and the first and second lumbar nerves. These rami provide innervation to the lateral abdominal muscles and the rectus muscle and overlying skin. The nerves traverse through the lateral abdominal wall between the transversus abdominus and internal oblique muscles, and penetrate the posterior rectus sheath just medial to the linea semilunaris.

The lateral abdominal muscles receive their blood supply from the lower three or four intercostal arteries, deep circumflex iliac artery, and lumbar arteries. The rectus abdominus has a more complex blood supply derived from the superior epigastric artery (a terminal branch of the internal mammary artery), inferior epigastric artery (a branch of the external iliac artery), and lower intercostal arteries. The superior and inferior epigastric arteries anastomose near the umbilicus. The periumbilical area provides critical perforator vessels that if preserved, can decrease skin flap necrosis during extensive skin undermining (Fig. 46-10).

## Diagnosis

The evaluation of abdominal wall hernias requires diligent physical examination. As with the inguinal region, the anterior abdominal wall is evaluated with the patient in standing and supine positions, and a Valsalva maneuver is also useful to demonstrate the site and size of a hernia. Imaging modalities may play a greater role in the diagnosis of more unusual hernias of the abdominal wall.

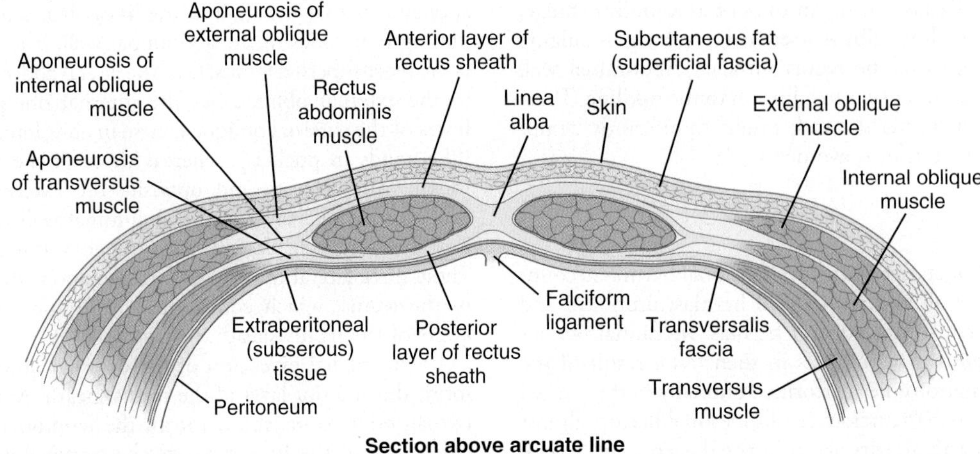


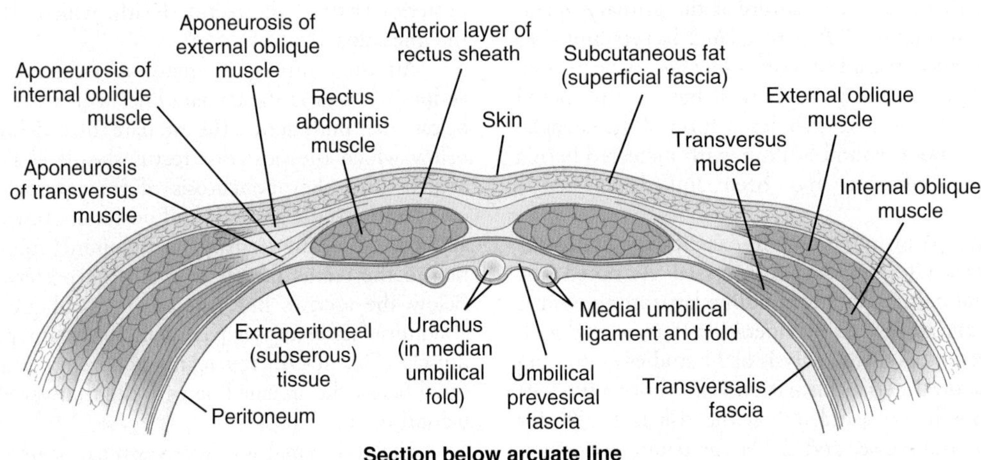


**FIGURE 46-9** Cross sections of the rectus abdominis muscle and aponeurosis above and below the arcuate line. (From Netter FT: Atlas of human anatomy, Summit, NJ, 1989, Ciba-Geigy, Plate 235.)

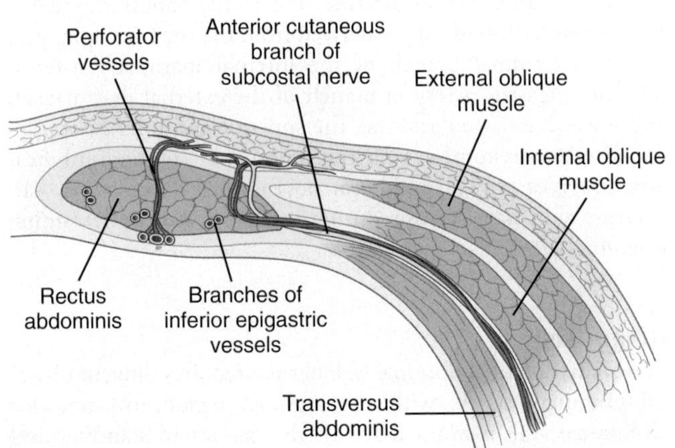


**FIGURE 46-10** Cross section of the lateral abdominal wall detailing location of intercostal neurovascular bundle travelling between the transversus abdominus and internal oblique muscles.

## Classification

### Umbilical Hernia

The umbilicus is formed by the umbilical ring of the linea alba. Intra-abdominally, the round ligament (ligamentum teres) and paraumbilical veins join into the umbilicus superiorly and the median umbilical ligament (obliterated urachus) enters inferiorly. Umbilical hernias in infants are congenital and are common. They close spontaneously in most cases by the age of 2 years. Those that persist after the age of 5 years are frequently repaired surgically, although complications related to these hernias in children are unusual. There is a strong predisposition toward the development of these hernias in individuals of African descent. In the United States, the incidence of umbilical hernia is eight times higher in African American than in white infants.

Umbilical hernias in adults are largely acquired. These hernias are more common in women and in patients with conditions that result in increased intra-abdominal pressure, such as pregnancy, obesity, ascites, or chronic abdominal distention. Umbilical hernia is more common in those who have only a single midline aponeurotic decussation compared with the normal decussation of fibers from all three lateral abdominal muscles. Strangulation is unusual in most patients; however, strangulation or rupture can occur in chronic ascitic conditions. Small asymptomatic umbilical hernias barely detectable on examination need not be repaired. Adults who have symptoms, a large hernia, incarceration, thinning of the overlying skin, or uncontrollable ascites should have hernia repair. Spontaneous rupture of umbilical hernias in patients with ascites can result in peritonitis and death.

Classically, repair was done using the vest over pants repair proposed by Mayo, which uses imbrication of the superior and inferior fascial edges. Because of increased tension on the repair and recurrence rates of almost 30% with long-term follow-up, however, the Mayo repair is rarely performed today. Instead, small defects are closed primarily after separation of the sac from the overlying umbilicus and surrounding fascia. Defects larger than 3 cm are closed using prosthetic mesh.[33] There are a number of techniques to place this mesh and no prospective data have conclusively found clear advantages of one technique over another. Options for mesh implantation include bridging the defect, placing a preperitoneal underlay of mesh reinforced with suture repair, and placing it laparoscopically. The laparoscopic technique requires general anesthesia and is reserved for large defects or recurrent umbilical hernias.[34] There is no universal consensus on the most appropriate method of umbilical hernia repair.

### Epigastric Hernia

Approximately 3% to 5% of the population has epigastric hernias. Epigastric hernias are two to three times more common in men. These hernias are located between the xiphoid process and umbilicus and are usually within 5 to 6 cm of the umbilicus. Like umbilical hernias, epigastric hernias are more common in individuals with a single aponeurotic decussation. The defects are small and often produce pain out of proportion to their size because of incarceration of preperitoneal fat. They are multiple in up to 20% of patients and approximately 80% are in the midline. Repair usually consists of excision of the incarcerated preperitoneal tissue and simple closure of the fascial defect, similar to that for umbilical hernias. Small defects can be repaired under local anesthesia. Uncommonly, these defects can be sizable, can contain omentum or other intra-abdominal viscera, and may require mesh repairs. Epigastric hernias are better repaired anteriorly because the defect is small and fat that has herniated from within the peritoneal cavity is difficult to reduce.

### Incisional Hernia

Of all hernias encountered, incisional hernias can be the most frustrating and difficult to treat. Incisional hernias occur as a result of excessive tension and inadequate healing of a previous incision, which may be associated with surgical site infection. These hernias enlarge over time, leading to pain, bowel obstruction, incarceration, and strangulation. Obesity, advanced age, malnutrition, ascites, pregnancy, and conditions that increase intra-abdominal pressure are factors that predispose to the development of an incisional hernia. Obesity can cause an incisional hernia to occur because of increased tension on the abdominal wall from the excessive bulk of a thick pannus and large omental mass. Chronic pulmonary disease and diabetes mellitus have also been recognized as risk factors for the development of incisional hernia. Medications such as corticosteroids and chemotherapeutic agents and surgical site infection can contribute to poor wound healing and increase the risk for developing an incisional hernia.

Large hernias can result in loss of abdominal domain, which occurs when the abdominal contents no longer reside in the abdominal cavity. These large abdominal wall defects also can result from the inability to close the abdomen primarily because of bowel edema, abdominal packing, peritonitis, and repeat laparotomy. With loss of domain, the natural rigidity of the abdominal wall becomes compromised and the abdominal musculature is often retracted. Respiratory dysfunction can occur because these large ventral defects cause paradoxical respiratory abdominal motion. Loss of abdominal domain can also result in bowel edema, stasis of the splanchnic venous system, urinary retention, and constipation. Return of displaced viscera to the abdominal cavity during repair may lead to increased abdominal pressure, abdominal compartment syndrome, and acute respiratory failure.

### Treatment: Operative Repair

Primary repair of incisional hernias can be done when the defect is small (≤2 to 3 cm in diameter) and there is viable surrounding tissue, or in cases in which the hernia was clearly a result of a technical error at the initial operation, such as a suture fracturing. Larger defects (>2 to 3 cm in diameter) have a high recurrence rate if closed primarily and are repaired with a prosthesis.[34] Recurrence rates vary between 10% and 50% and are typically reduced by more than 50% with the use of prosthetic mesh.[35] Prosthetic material may be placed as an onlay patch to buttress a tissue repair, interposed between the fascial defect, sandwiched between tissue planes, or put in a sublay position. Depending on its location, several important properties of the mesh must be considered.

### Prosthetic Materials for Ventral Hernia Repair

**Synthetic Materials** Various synthetic mesh products are available. Desirable characteristics of a synthetic mesh include being chemically inert, resistant to mechanical stress while maintaining compliance, sterilizable, noncarcinogenic, inciting minimal inflammatory reaction, and hypoallergenic. The ideal mesh has yet to be defined. When selecting the appropriate mesh, the surgeon must consider the position of the mesh, whether it will be in direct contact with the viscera, and the presence or risk of infection. Mesh constructs can be classified based on weight of the material, pore size, water angle (hydrophobic or hydrophilic), and whether there is an antiadhesive barrier present. When placing a mesh in the extraperitoneal position without the risk of bowel erosion, a macroporous unprotected mesh is appropriate. Both polypropylene and polyester mesh have been successfully placed in the extraperitoneal position. Polypropylene mesh is a hydrophobic macroporous mesh that allows for the ingrowth of native fibroblasts and incorporation into the surrounding fascia. It is semirigid, somewhat flexible, and porous. Placing polypropylene mesh in an intraperitoneal position directly apposed to the bowel is avoided because of unacceptable rates of enterocutaneous fistula formation.[36] Recently, lighter weight polypropylene mesh has been introduced to address some of the long-term complications of heavyweight polypropylene mesh. The definition of lightweight mesh was arbitrarily chosen at less than 50 $g/m^2$, with heavyweight mesh weighing more than 80 $g/m^2$. These lightweight mesh

**Table 46-2 Biologic Mesh for Abdominal Wall Reconstruction and Postharvesting Processing Techniques**

| PRODUCT | SOURCE | CROSS-LINKED | STERILIZATION METHOD |
|---|---|---|---|
| Alloderm (Lifecell, Branchburg, NJ) | Human dermis | No | Ionic |
| Allomax (Davol, Warwick, RI) | Human dermis | No | E beam |
| Flex HD (Ethicon, Sommerville, NJ) | Human dermis | No | Ethanol |
| Strattice (Lifecell, Branchburg, NJ) | Porcine dermis | No | Gamma irradiation |
| Permacol (Covidien, Norwalk, CT) | Porcine dermis | Yes | Ethanol |
| Collamend (Davol, Warwick, RI) | Porcine dermis | Yes | Ethanol |
| Xenmatrix (Davol, Warwick, RI) | Porcine dermis | No | Gamma irradiation |
| Surgimend (TEI Biosciences, Boston, MA) | Bovine fetal dermis | No | Ethanol |
| Veritas (Synovis, St. Paul, MN) | Bovine | No | |
| Periguard (Synovis, St. Paul, MN) | Bovine | Yes | |
| Surgisis (Cook, Bloomfield, IN) | Porcine intestine | No | Ethanol |

products often have an absorbable component of material that provides initial handling stability, typically composed of Vicryl (polyglactin 910) or Monocryl (poliglecaprone 25; Ethicon, Somerville, NJ).

Whether lightweight mesh results in improved patient outcomes is controversial. Two prospective randomized trials evaluating the incidence of postoperative pain after open inguinal hernia repair have shown mixed results.[37] In a randomized controlled trial evaluating lightweight versus heavy weight polypropylene mesh for ventral hernia repair, the recurrence rate was more than twice that in the lightweight group (17% versus 7% for heavyweight mesh), which approached statistical significance ($P = .052$).[38]

Polyester mesh is composed of polyethylene terephthalate and is a hydrophilic, heavyweight, macroporous mesh. This mesh has several different weaves that can yield a two-dimensional flat screen–like mesh and a three-dimensional multifilament weave. Unprotected polyester mesh should not be placed directly on the viscera because unacceptable rates of erosion and bowel obstruction have been reported.[36] When placed in the preperitoneal position in complex ventral hernia repairs, complication rates are low.[7,39]

When placing mesh in an intraperitoneal position, several options are available. A single sheet of mesh with both sides constructed to reduce adhesions, or a composite-type mesh with one side made to promote tissue ingrowth and the other to resist adhesion formation, are available. Single-sheet mesh is composed of expanded PTFE (polytetrafluoroethylene). This prosthetic has a visceral side that is microporous (3 μm) and an abdominal wall side that is macroporous (17 to 22 μm) and promotes tissue ingrowth. This product differs from other synthetic meshes in that it is flexible and smooth. Some fibroblast proliferation occurs through the pores, but PTFE is impermeable to fluid. Unlike polypropylene, PTFE is not incorporated into the native tissue. Encapsulation occurs slowly and infection can occur during the encapsulation process. When infected, PTFE almost always must be removed.

To promote better tissue integration, composite mesh was developed. This product combines the attributes of polypropylene and PTFE by layering the two substances on top of one another. The PTFE surface serves as a permanent protective interface against the bowel and the polypropylene side faces superficially, to be incorporated into the native fascial tissue. These materials have variable rates of contraction and, when placed together, can result in buckling of the mesh and visceral exposure to the polypropylene component. Recently, other composite meshes have been developed that combine a macroporous mesh with a temporary, absorbable antiadhesive barrier. Basic constructs of these mesh materials include heavyweight or lightweight polypropylene, or polyester. Absorbable barriers are typically composed of oxidized regenerated cellulose, omega-3 fatty acids, or collagen hydrogels. A number of small animal studies have validated the antiadhesive properties of these barriers, but currently no human trials exist evaluating the ability of these composite materials to resist adhesion formation.

**Biologic Materials** The newest development in prostheses for ventral hernia repair is nonsynthetic or natural tissue mesh. There are numerous biologic grafts available for abdominal wall reconstruction (Table 46-2). These products can be categorized based on the source material (e.g., human, porcine, bovine), postharvesting processing techniques (e.g., cross-linked, non–cross-linked) and sterilization techniques (e.g., gamma radiation, ethylene oxide gas sterilization, nonsterilized). These products are largely composed of acellular collagen and theoretically provide a matrix for neovascularization and native collagen deposition. These properties provide distinct advantages in infected or contaminated cases in which synthetic mesh is thought to be contraindicated. Ideal placement techniques are yet to be defined for these relatively new products; however, some general principles apply. These products function best when used as a fascial reinforcement rather than as a bridge or interposition repair.[40] Unfortunately, the long-term durability of biologic mesh is currently unknown. There are no data comparing the effectiveness of these natural tissue alternatives with that of synthetic mesh repairs.

### Operative Technique

**Ventral Hernias** It is generally agreed that all but the smallest incisional hernias can be repaired with mesh, and the surgeon has various options for placing the mesh. The onlay technique involves primary closure of the fascia defect and placement of a mesh over the anterior fascia. The major advantage of this approach is that the mesh is placed outside the abdominal cavity, avoiding direct interaction with the abdominal viscera. However, disadvantages include the large subcutaneous dissection, increased likelihood of seroma formation, superficial location of the mesh, which places it in jeopardy of contamination if the incision becomes infected, and the repair is usually under tension. Prospective analysis of this technique is not available, but a retrospective review has reported recurrence rates of 28%.[41] Interposition prosthetic repairs involve securing the mesh to the fascial edge without overlap. This results in a predictably high recurrence rate because the synthetic often pulls away from the fascial edge because of increased intra-abdominal pressure. A sublay or underlay technique involves placing the prosthetic below the fascial components. The mesh can be placed intraperitoneally, preperitoneally, or in the retrorectus (retromuscular) space. It is highly desirable to have the mesh placed beneath the fascia. With a wide overlap of mesh and fascia, the natural forces of the abdominal cavity act to hold the mesh in place and prevent migration. This can be accomplished using several techniques (Fig. 46-11).

***Intraperitoneal Mesh Placement*** After reopening the prior incision, and with the use of available dual-type mesh or composite mesh, the mesh can be placed in an intraperitoneal position at least 4 cm beyond the fascial margin and secured with interrupted mattress sutures. This technique requires raising subcutaneous flaps and the mesh may be in direct contact with the abdominal contents.

The laparoscopic approach for ventral hernia repair relies on the same principles as the retrorectus repair; however, the mesh is placed within the peritoneal cavity. This repair is useful, particularly for large defects. Trocars are placed as far laterally as feasible based on the size and location of the hernia. The hernia contents are reduced and adhesions are lysed. The surface area of the defect is measured, and a barrier-coated mesh is fashioned with at least 4 cm of overlap around the defect. The mesh is rolled, placed into the abdomen, and deployed. It is secured to the anterior abdominal wall with preplaced mattress sutures that are passed through separate incisions; tacking staples are placed between these sutures to secure the mesh 4 cm beyond the defect. The advantage of this approach is a quicker recovery time. There are fewer incisional complications with the laparoscopic approach because large incisions and subcutaneous undermining are avoided.

***Retromuscular Mesh Placement*** This technique involves placing prosthetic mesh in the extraperitoneal position in the preperitoneal space or retrorectus position. This technique was initially described by Stoppa.[7] A large piece of mesh is placed in the retromuscular space on top of the posterior rectus sheath or peritoneum. This space must be dissected laterally on both sides of the linea alba to a distance of 8 to 10 cm beyond the defect. The prosthetic mesh extends 5 to 6 cm beyond the superior and inferior borders of the defect. With smaller defects, the mesh does not need to be sutured because it is held in place by intra-abdominal pressure (Pascal's principle), allowing eventual incorporation into the surrounding tissues. Alternatively, in larger defects, the mesh can be secured laterally with several sutures. This approach avoids contact between the mesh and abdominal viscera and has been shown in long-term studies to have a respectable recurrence rate (14%) in large incisional hernias. The retrorectus space is bordered laterally by the linea semilunaris. In very large hernias or in those patients with atrophic rectus muscles, this might prevent adequate mesh overlap. Alternatively, the preperitoneal plane can be accessed by incising the posterior rectus sheath approximately 1 cm medial to the linea semilunaris. Once the preperitoneal space is accessed, the dissection can be carried laterally to the psoas muscle, if necessary.[42] Very large sheets of prosthetic mesh can be placed in this location with wide defect coverage. A retrospective review from the Mayo Clinic, with a median follow-up of 5 years, has documented a 5% overall hernia recurrence rate in 254 patients who underwent complex ventral hernia repair over a 13-year period.[43]

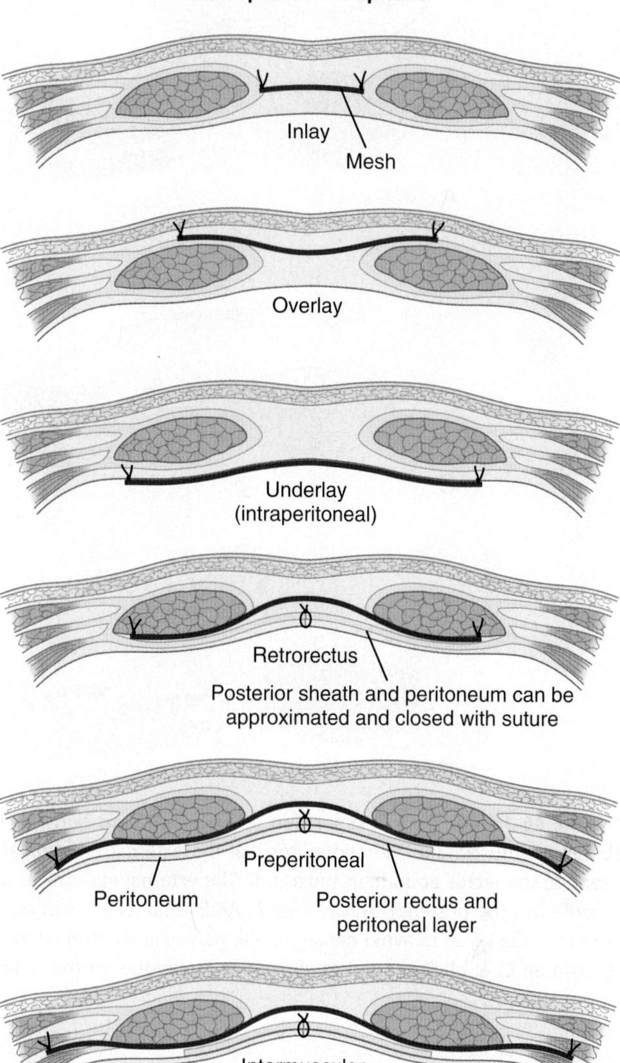


**FIGURE 46-11** Mesh placement options for abdominal wall reconstruction.

***Component Separation*** Another option for the repair of complex or large ventral defects is the component separation technique (Fig. 46-12). This involves separating the lateral muscular layers of the abdominal wall to allow their advancement. Primary

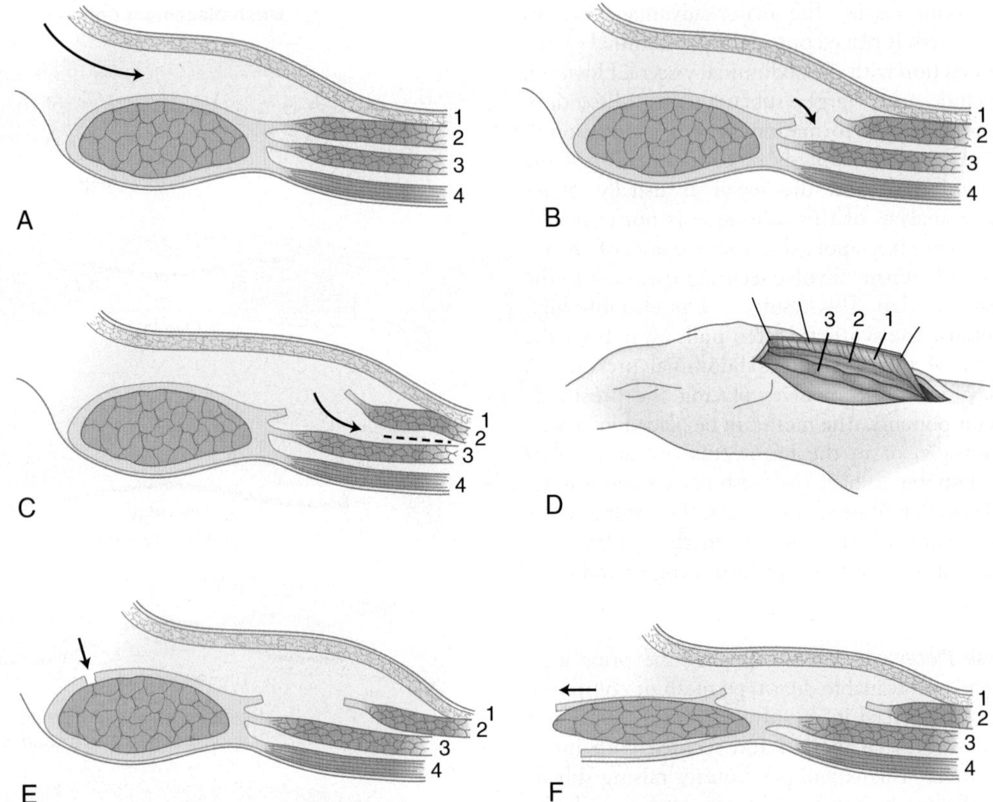


**FIGURE 46-12** Component separation technique. **A,** The skin and subcutaneous fat are dissected free from the anterior sheath of the rectus abdominis muscle and the aponeurosis of the external abdominal oblique muscle. **B,** The external abdominal oblique is incised 1 to 2 cm lateral to the rectus abdominis muscle. **C,** The external abdominal oblique is separated from the internal abdominal oblique. **D,** The dissection is carried to the posterior axillary line. **E,** Additional length can be achieved by incising the posterior rectus sheath above the arcuate line. **F,** Care must be taken to avoid damaging the nerves and blood supply that enter the rectus abdominis posteriorly. (deVries Reilingh TS, van Goor H, Rosman C, et al: Components separation technique for the repair of large abdominal wall hernias. J Am Coll Surg 196:32–37, 2003.)

fascial closure at the midline is often possible. The procedure is performed by raising large subcutaneous flaps above the external oblique fascia. These flaps are carried laterally past the linea semilunaris. This dissection itself can provide some advancement of the abdominal wall. Large perforating subcutaneous vessels can be preserved to prevent ischemic necrosis of the skin flaps. A relaxing incision is made 2 cm lateral to the linea semilunaris on the lateral external oblique aponeurosis from several centimeters above the costal margin to the pubis. The external oblique is then bluntly separated in the avascular plane, away from the internal oblique, allowing its advancement. Further relaxing incisions have been described to the aponeurotic layers of the internal oblique or transversus abdominis but this can result in problematic lateral bulges or herniation at this site. Additional release can be safely achieved by incising the posterior rectus sheath. These techniques, when applied to both sides of the abdominal wall, can yield up to 20 cm of mobilization. Although this technique often allows tension-free closure of these large defects, recurrence rates as low as 20% have been reported with the use of prosthetic reinforcement in large hernias.[44] It is important that patients understand that a lateral bulge can occur after releasing the external oblique aponeurosis. Recognizing the high recurrence rates with component separation alone, several authors have reported small series of biologic mesh reinforcement of these repairs.[40] To date, no randomized controlled trials have supported a lower recurrence rate with biologic prosthetic reinforcement. If a bioprosthetic is placed, it can be secured with an underlay or onlay technique. No comparative data exist demonstrating the superiority of either repair technique.[45]

***Endoscopic Component Separation*** One of the major limitations of open component separation is that large skin flaps are necessary to access the lateral abdominal wall musculature. Recognizing these limitations, innovative, minimally invasive approaches to component separation have been described.[46] The basic principle of a minimally invasive component separation is to gain direct access to the lateral abdominal wall without creating a lipocutaneous flap. Typically, this is performed by a direct cut down through a 1-cm incision off the tip of the 11th rib overlying the external oblique muscle (Fig. 46-13). The external oblique is split in the line of its fibers and a standard bilateral inguinal hernia balloon dissector is placed in between the external and internal oblique muscles, toward the pubis. Three laparoscopic trocars are placed in the space created and the dissection is carried from the pubis to several centimeters above the costal margin. The linea semilunaris is carefully identified and the external oblique is incised from beneath the muscle, at least

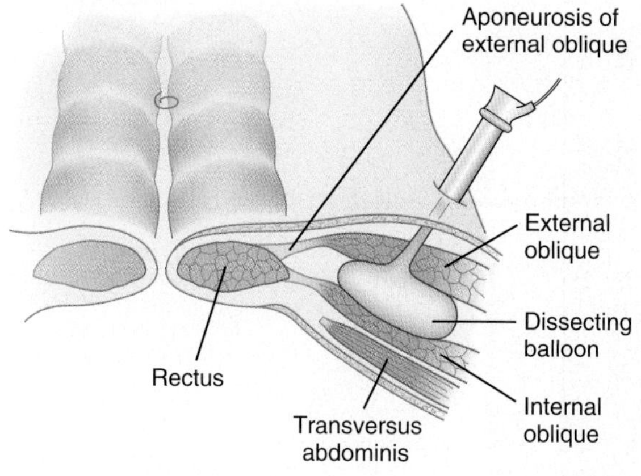


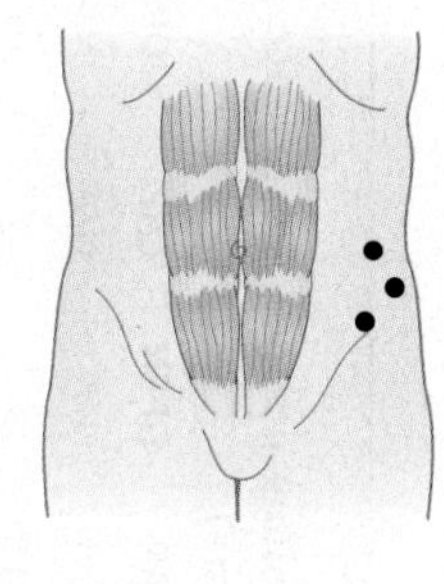

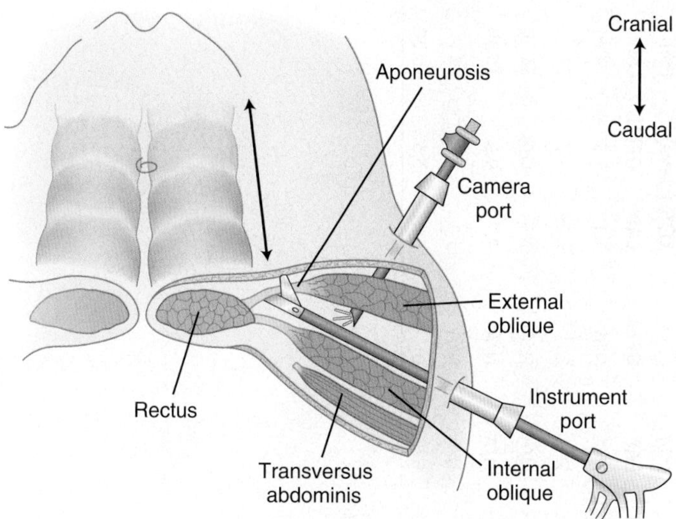


Cranial
Caudal

**FIGURE 46-13** Endoscopic component separation: port placement and surgical technique.

2 cm lateral to the linea semilunaris. The muscle is released from the pubis to several centimeters above the costal margin. This procedure is performed bilaterally. Synthetic or biologic mesh can be used to reinforce the repair of the midline closure. These relatively new techniques are feasible, but long-term data demonstrating equivalency to open techniques are lacking.

### Results of Incisional Hernia Repairs

Several prospective randomized trials have compared laparoscopic and open ventral hernia repairs (Table 46-3).[47-51] Although most of these studies were small, with fewer than 100 patients, the results tend to favor a laparoscopic approach. The incidences of postoperative complications and recurrence were less in hernias repaired laparoscopically. Several retrospective reports have demonstrated similar advantages for a laparoscopic approach. Based on the comparative trials listed in Table 46-3, laparoscopic incisional hernia repair results in fewer postoperative complications, lower infection rate, and decreased hernia recurrence.[42-48] Until an appropriately powered prospective randomized trial is performed, the ideal approach will largely be based on surgeon expertise and preference.

## UNUSUAL HERNIAS

There are a number of hernias that occur infrequently, of various types.

### Types

#### Spigelian Hernia

A spigelian hernia occurs through the spigelian fascia, which is composed of the aponeurotic layer between the rectus muscle medially and semilunar line laterally. Almost all spigelian hernias occur at or below the arcuate line. The absence of posterior rectus fascia may contribute to an inherent weakness in this area. These hernias are often interparietal, with the hernia sac dissecting posterior to the external oblique aponeurosis. Most spigelian hernias are small (1 to 2 cm in diameter) and develop during the fourth to seventh decades of life. Patients often present with localized pain in the area without a bulge because the hernia lies beneath the intact external oblique aponeurosis. Ultrasound or CT of the abdomen can be useful to establish the diagnosis.

A spigelian hernia is repaired because of the risk for incarceration associated with its relatively narrow neck. The hernia site is marked before operation. A transverse incision is made over the defect and carried through the external oblique aponeurosis. The hernia sac is opened, dissected free of the neck of the hernia, and excised or inverted. The defect is closed transversely by simple suture repair of the transversus abdominis and internal oblique muscles, followed by closure of the external oblique aponeurosis. Larger defects are repaired using a mesh prosthesis. Recurrence is uncommon.

**Table 46-3 Comparative Randomized Studies Between Open and Laparoscopic Ventral Hernia Repair**

| | No. of Patients | | Mesh Used | | Intraoperative Complications (%) | | LOS (days) | | Postoperative Complications (%) | | Follow-up (mo) | | Recurrence (%) | |
|---|---|---|---|---|---|---|---|---|---|---|---|---|---|---|
| STUDY (YEAR) | LAP | OPEN | LAP | OPEN | LAP | OPEN | LAP | OPEN | LAP | OPEN | LAP | OPEN | LAP | OPEN |
| McGreevy et al. (2003)[48] | 65 | 71 | ePTFE or polyester + collagen | PP | N/A | N/A | 1.1 | 1.5 | 7.70 | 21.10 | N/A | N/A | N/A | N/A |
| Lomanto et al. (2006)[49] | 50 | 50 | Polyester + collagen | ePTFE | 2 | 2 | 2.74 | 4.7 | 26 | 40 | 19.6 | 21 | 2 | 10 |
| Bingener et al. (2007)[50] | 127 | 233 | ePTFE, PP, or ePTFE | PP | N/A | N/A | N/A | N/A | 33.10 | 43.30 | 36 | 36 | 13 | 9 |
| Olmi et al. (2007)[47] | 85 | 85 | Polyester + collagen | PP | N/A | N/A | 2.7 | 9.9 | 16.50 | 29.40 | 24 | 24 | 2 | 4 |
| Pring et al. (2008)[59] | 31 | 27 | PTFE | PTFE | N/A | N/A | 1 | 1 | 33 | 49 | 28 | 28 | 3.30 | 4.20 |
| Asencio et al. (2009)[60] | 45 | 39 | PTFE or PP | PP | 6.70 | 0 | 3.46 | 3.33 | 5.20 | 33.30 | 12 | 12 | 9.70 | 7.90 |

*Lap,* Laparoscopic, *LOS,* length of stay; *PP,* polypropylene.

### Obturator Hernia

The obturator canal is formed by the union of the pubic bone and ischium. This canal is covered by a membrane pierced at the medial and superior border by the obturator nerve and vessels. Weakening of the obturator membrane may result in enlargement of the canal and formation of a hernia sac, which can lead to intestinal incarceration and strangulation. The patient can present with evidence of compression of the obturator nerve, which causes pain in the anteromedial aspect of the thigh (Howship-Romberg sign) that is relieved by thigh flexion. Almost 50% of patients with obturator hernia present with complete or partial bowel obstruction. An abdominal CT scan can establish the diagnosis, if necessary.

A posterior approach, open or laparoscopic, is preferred. This approach provides direct access to the hernia. After reduction of the hernia sac and contents, any preperitoneal fat within the obturator canal is reduced. If necessary, the obturator foramen is opened posterior to the nerve and vessels. The obturator nerve can be manipulated gently with a blunt nerve hook to facilitate reduction of the fat pad. The obturator foramen is repaired with prosthetic mesh, taking care to avoid injury to the obturator nerve and vessels. Patients with compromised bowel usually require laparotomy.

### Lumbar Hernia

Lumbar hernias can be congenital or acquired after an operation on the flank and occur in the lumbar region of the posterior abdominal wall. Hernias through the superior lumbar triangle (Grynfeltt's triangle) are more common. The superior lumbar triangle is bounded by the 12th rib, paraspinal muscles, and internal oblique muscle. Less common are hernias through the inferior lumbar triangle (Petit's triangle), which is bounded by the iliac crest, latissimus dorsi muscle, and external oblique muscle. Weakness of the lumbodorsal fascia through either of these areas results in progressive protrusion of extraperitoneal fat and a hernia sac. Lumbar hernias are not prone to incarceration. Small lumbar hernias are frequently asymptomatic. Larger hernias may be associated with back pain. CT is useful for diagnosis.

Both open and laparoscopic repairs are useful. Satisfactory suture repair is difficult because of the immobile bony margins of these defects. Repair is best done by placement of prosthetic mesh, which is sutured beyond the margins of the hernia. There is usually sufficient fascia over the bone to anchor the mesh.

### Interparietal Hernia

Interparietal hernias are rare and occur when the hernia sac lies between layers of the abdominal wall. These hernias most frequently occur in previous incisions. Spigelian hernias are almost always interparietal.

The correct preoperative diagnosis of interparietal hernia can be difficult. Many patients with complicated interparietal hernias present with intestinal obstruction. Abdominal CT can assist in the diagnosis. Large interparietal hernias usually require placement of prosthetic mesh for closure. When this cannot be done, the component separation technique may be useful to provide natural tissues to obliterate the defect.

### Sciatic Hernia

The greater sciatic foramen can be a site of hernia formation. These hernias are extremely unusual and difficult to diagnose and frequently are asymptomatic until intestinal obstruction occurs. In the absence of intestinal obstruction, the most common symptom is the presence of an uncomfortable or slowly enlarging mass in the gluteal or intragluteal area. Sciatic nerve pain can occur, but sciatic hernia is a rare cause of sciatic neuralgia.

A transperitoneal approach is preferred if bowel obstruction or strangulation is suspected. Hernia contents can usually be reduced with gentle traction. Prosthetic mesh repair is usually preferred. A transgluteal approach can be used if the diagnosis is certain and the hernia is reducible, but most surgeons are not familiar with this approach. With the patient prone, an incision is made from the posterior edge of the greater trochanter across the hernia mass. The gluteus maximus muscle is opened, and the sac is visualized. The muscle edges of the defect are reapproximated with interrupted sutures or the defect is obliterated with mesh.

### Perineal Hernia

Perineal hernias are caused by congenital or acquired defects and are quite uncommon. These hernias may also occur after abdominoperineal resection or perineal prostatectomy. The hernia sac protrudes through the pelvic diaphragm. Primary perineal hernias are rare, occur most commonly in older multiparous women, and can be quite large. Symptoms are usually related to protrusion of a mass through the defect that is worsened by sitting or standing. A bulge is frequently detected on bimanual rectal-vaginal examination.

Perineal hernias are generally repaired through a transabdominal approach or combined transabdominal and perineal approaches. After the sac contents are reduced, small defects may be closed with nonabsorbable suture, whereas large defects are repaired with prosthetic mesh.

### Loss of Domain Hernias

Loss of domain implies a massive hernia in which the herniated contents have resided for so long outside the abdominal cavity that they cannot simply be replaced into the peritoneal cavity. We typically classify loss of domain hernias into patients with and without preoperative contamination. Each group is then subcategorized into two groups. Patients with a small hernia defect and a massive hernia sac (e.g., large inguinoscrotal hernias) require restoration of peritoneal cavity domain, whereas patients with a large defect and a massive hernia sac (open abdomen with skin graft) require restoration of peritoneal domain and reconstruction of the abdominal wall.

Prior to repair of these complex defects, the patient must undergo careful preoperative evaluation. A clear understanding of the morbidity and mortality associated with these reconstructive procedures is critical. Weight reduction, smoking cessation, optimization of nutrition, and glucose control are all important aspects of complex abdominal wall reconstruction. Previously, methods to stretch the abdominal wall gradually were used to allow for the restoration of abdominal domain and closure. This was accomplished by insufflation of air into the abdominal cavity to create a progressive pneumoperitoneum. Repeated administrations of increasing volumes of air over 1 to 3 weeks allowed the muscles of the abdominal wall to become lax enough for primary closure of the defect. This technique is particularly suited for small defects and massive hernia sacs.[52] For large defects, we prefer a staged approach using expanded PTFE (ePTFE) dual mesh for patients with loss of abdominal domain and lateral retraction of the abdominal wall musculature. The initial stage involves reduction of the hernia and placement of a large sheet of ePTFE dual mesh secured to the fascial edges with a running suture. Subsequent stages involve serial elliptical excision of the mesh until the fascia can be approximated in the midline without tension. Finally, the mesh is completely excised and the fascia is reapproximated with component separation and a biologic underlay patch, if necessary.[53]

## Parastomal Hernia Repair

Parastomal hernia is a common complication of stoma creation. In fact, the creation of a stoma by strict definition is an abdominal wall hernia. The incidence of parastomal hernias is highest for colostomies and occurs in up to 50% of stomas. Fortunately, most patients remain asymptomatic and life-threatening complications, such as bowel obstruction and strangulation, are rare. Unlike midline incisional hernia repair, routine repair of parastomal hernias is not recommended. Surgical repair should be reserved for patients experiencing symptoms of bowel obstruction, problems with pouch fit, or cosmetic issues.

Three general approaches are available for parastomal hernia repair. These techniques include primary fascial repair, stoma relocation, and prosthetic repair. Primary fascial repair involves hernia reduction and primary fascial reapproximation through a peristomal incision. This technique carries a predictably high recurrence rate. The advantage of this approach is that the abdomen often is not entered, making the operation less complex. Because of the high recurrence rate with this technique, it should be reserved for patients who will not tolerate a laparotomy. Stoma relocation improves results; however, it requires a laparotomy and predisposes to another parastomal hernia in the future. To reduce the rate of recurrent herniation, some surgeons reinforce the repair with biologic mesh in a keyhole fashion around the new stoma site. Early results are promising but long-term outcomes have not yet been reported.[54] Prosthetic repairs of parastomal hernias can provide excellent long-term results with a lower rate of hernia recurrence, but a higher rate of prosthetic complications must be accepted.

Regardless of the technique, a permanent foreign body placed in apposition to the bowel can result in erosion, obstruction, and disastrous complications. Several approaches to prosthetic mesh placement have been described. The mesh can be placed as an onlay patch, intra-abdominally, or in the retrorectus position. When placing the mesh intraperitoneally, a keyhole is fashioned around the stoma site or placed as a flat sheet, lateralizing the stoma as it exits the abdomen, as described by Sugarbaker.[55] Several authors have described laparoscopic approaches to parastomal hernia repair, including keyhole and Sugarbaker-type repairs[56,57] (Fig. 46-14). All these series are small and have reported only short-term follow-up, limiting our ability to make clear recommendations for this difficult problem.

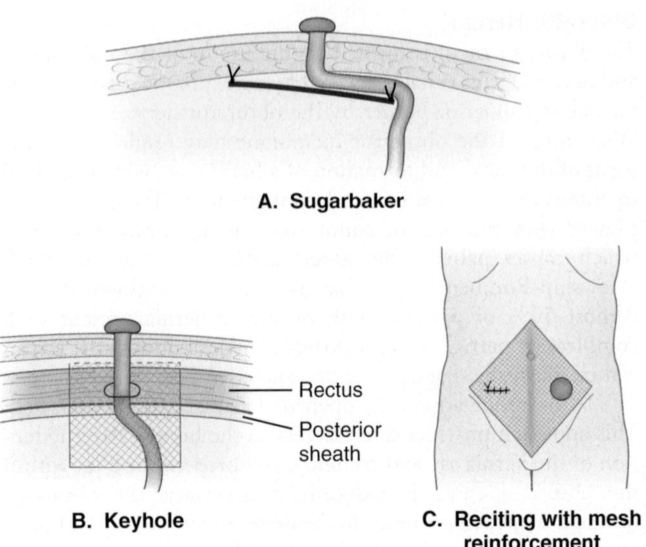


**FIGURE 46-14** Surgical approaches for parastomal hernia repair.

## Complications

### Mesh Infection

Mesh infections are serious complications that can be difficult to treat. If ePTFE becomes infected, it requires removal with the resultant morbidity of another defect, which often must be closed under tension, leading to inevitable recurrence. In open ventral hernia repair, incisional and mesh infections are not infrequent. Using the laparoscopic technique and placing a large piece of mesh without undermining large subcutaneous tissue flaps avoids wound complications. In a series of almost 1000 patients who had laparoscopic ventral hernia repair, mesh infections occurred in less than 1% of cases.[58] Perhaps the greatest advantage of the laparoscopic approach for repairing ventral hernias is this reduction in infectious complications. Two randomized controlled trials have compared laparoscopic and open ventral hernia repair.[59,60]

### Seromas

Seroma formation can occur after laparoscopic and open ventral hernia repair. In open ventral hernia repair, drains are often placed in an attempt to obliterate the dead space caused by the hernia and tissue dissection. These drains can cause mesh contamination and seromas can form after drain removal. With laparoscopic repair, the hernia sac is not resected and a seroma cavity will result. Most of these seromas will resolve over time as the mesh becomes incorporated on the hernia sac. Preoperative discussions with the patient describing the expectations of a temporary seroma are imperative before laparoscopic ventral hernia repair. We reserve aspiration for symptomatic or persistent seromas after 6 to 8 weeks.

### Enterotomy

Intestinal injury during adhesiolysis can be catastrophic. Management of an enterotomy during a hernia repair is controversial and depends on the segment of intestine injured (small versus large bowel) and amount of spillage. Options include aborting the hernia repair, using a primary tissue or biologic tissue repair, and performing a delayed repair using prosthetic mesh in 3 to 4 days. When there is gross contamination, the use of synthetic mesh is contraindicated.

## SELECTED REFERENCES

Anson BJ, McVay CB: Inguinal hernia: The anatomy of the region. Surg Gynecol Obstet 66:186–191, 1938.

Condon RE: Surgical anatomy of the transversus abdominis and transversalis fascia. Ann Surg 173:1–5, 1971.

Nyhus LM: An anatomic reappraisal of the posterior inguinal wall, with special consideration of the iliopubic tract and its relation to groin hernias. Surg Clin North Am 44:1305, 1960.

These three references are classic descriptions of the anatomy of the groin. All are well illustrated.

Bisgaard T, Bay-Nielsen M, Kehlet H: Re-recurrence after operation for recurrent inguinal hernia. A nationwide 8-year follow-up study on the role of type of repair. Ann Surg 247:707–711, 2008.

This long term population-based study provides useful information about the results of recurrent inguinal hernia repairs.

de Vries Reilingh TS, van Goor H, Charbon JA, et al: Repair of giant midline abdominal wall hernias: "Components separation technique" versus prosthetic repair: Interim analysis of a randomized controlled trial. World J Surg 31:756–763, 2007.

This is a prospective randomized trial evaluating outcomes of open ventral hernia repair with synthetic mesh versus component separation without reinforcement.

Forbes SS, Eskicioglu C, McLeod RS, et al: Meta-analysis of randomized controlled trials comparing open and laparoscopic ventral and incisional hernia repair with mesh. Br J Surg 96:851–858, 2009.

This is a meta-analysis evaluating eight prospective randomized trials comparing laparoscopic with open ventral hernia repair.

Itani KM, Hur K, Kim LT, et al: Veterans Affairs Ventral Incisional Hernia Investigators: Comparison of laparoscopic and open repair with mesh for the treatment of ventral incisional hernia: A randomized trial. Arch Surg 145:322–328, 2010.

This is a prospective randomized trial evaluating laparoscopic versus open ventral hernia repairs.

Neumayer L, Giobbie-Hurder A, Jonasson O, et al: Open mesh versus laparoscopic mesh repair of inguinal hernia. N Engl J Med 350:1819–1827, 2004.

Excellent prospective randomized trial comparing these two types of hernia repairs in Veterans Administration hospitals.

Zhao G, Gao P, Ma B, et al: Open mesh techniques for inguinal hernia repair: A meta-analysis of randomized controlled trials. Ann Surg 250:35–42, 2009.

Excellent meta-analysis of various techniques of tension-free repairs.

## REFERENCES


1. Bradley M, Morgan D, Pentlow B, et al: The groin hernia—an ultrasound diagnosis? Ann R Coll Surg Engl 85:178–180, 2003.
2. Della Santa V, Groebli Y: [Diagnosis of non-hernia groin masses.] Ann Chir 125:179–183, 2000.
3. Fitzgibbons RJ, Jr, Giobbie-Hurder A, Gibbs JO, et al: Watchful waiting vs repair of inguinal hernia in minimally symptomatic men: A randomized clinical trial. JAMA 295:285–292, 2006.
4. Lichtenstein IL, Shulman AG, Amid PK, et al: The tension-free hernioplasty. Am J Surg 157:188–193, 1989.
5. Gilbert AI: Sutureless repair of inguinal hernia. Am J Surg 163: 331–335, 1992.
6. Kugel RD: Minimally invasive, nonlaparoscopic, preperitoneal, and sutureless, inguinal herniorrhaphy. Am J Surg 178:298–302, 1999.
7. Stoppa RE: The treatment of complicated groin and incisional hernias. World J Surg 13:545–554, 1989.
8. Malangoni MA, Condon RE: Preperitoneal repair of acute incarcerated and strangulated hernias of the groin. Surg Gynecol Obstet 162:65–67, 1986.
9. Voyles CR, Hamilton BJ, Johnson WD, et al: Meta-analysis of laparoscopic inguinal hernia trials favors open hernia repair with preperitoneal mesh prosthesis. Am J Surg 184:6–10, 2002.
10. Bisgaard T, Bay-Nielsen M, Kehlet H: Re-recurrence after operation for recurrent inguinal hernia. A nationwide 8-year follow-up study on the role of type of repair. Ann Surg 247:707–711, 2008.
11. Nordin P, Haapaniemi S, van der Linden W, et al: Choice of anesthesia and risk of reoperation for recurrence in groin hernia repair. Ann Surg 240:187–192, 2004.
12. Neumayer L, Giobbie-Hurder A, Jonasson O, et al: Open mesh versus laparoscopic mesh repair of inguinal hernia. N Engl J Med 350:1819–1827, 2004.
13. Amato B, Moja L, Panico S, et al: Shouldice technique versus other open techniques for inguinal hernia repair. Cochrane Database Syst Rev (4):CD001543, 2009.
14. van Veen RN, Wijsmuller AR, Vrijland WW, et al: Long-term follow-up of a randomized clinical trial of non-mesh versus mesh repair of primary inguinal hernia. Br J Surg 94:506–510, 2007.
15. Zhao G, Gao P, Ma B, et al: Open mesh techniques for inguinal hernia repair: A meta-analysis of randomized controlled trials. Ann Surg 250:35–42, 2009.
16. Schroder DM, Lloyd LR, Boccaccio JE, et al: Inguinal hernia recurrence following preperitoneal Kugel patch repair. Am Surg 70:132–136, 2004.
17. EU Hernia Trialists Collaboration: Repair of groin hernia with synthetic mesh: Meta-analysis of randomized controlled trials. Ann Surg 235:322–332, 2002.
18. Wake BL, McCormack K, Fraser C, et al: Transabdominal preperitoneal (TAPP) vs totally extraperitoneal (TEP) laparoscopic techniques for inguinal hernia repair. Cochrane Database Syst Rev (1):CD004703, 2005.
19. Mikkelsen T, Bay-Nielsen M, Kehlet H: Risk of femoral hernia after inguinal herniorrhaphy. Br J Surg 89:486–488, 2002.
20. Kald A, Fridsten S, Nordin P, et al: Outcome of repair of bilateral groin hernias: A prospective evaluation of 1,487 patients. Eur J Surg 168:150–153, 2002.
21. Aufenacker TJ, van Geldere D, van Mesdag T, et al: The role of antibiotic prophylaxis in prevention of wound infection after Lichtenstein open mesh repair of primary inguinal hernia: A multicenter double-blind randomized controlled trial. Ann Surg 240:955–960, 2004.
22. Grant AM, Scott NW, O'Dwyer PJ: Five-year follow-up of a randomized trial to assess pain and numbness after laparoscopic or open repair of groin hernia. Br J Surg 91:1570–1574, 2004.
23. Nienhuijs SW, Boelens OB, Strobbe LJ: Pain after anterior mesh hernia repair. J Am Coll Surg 200:885–889, 2005.
24. Nienhuijs SW, van Oort I, Keemers-Gels ME, et al: Randomized trial comparing the Prolene Hernia System, mesh plug repair and

Lichtenstein method for open inguinal hernia repair. Br J Surg 92:33–38, 2005.

25. Picchio M, Palimento D, Attanasio U, et al: Randomized controlled trial of preservation or elective division of ilioinguinal nerve on open inguinal hernia repair with polypropylene mesh. Arch Surg 139:755–758, 2004.

26. Shulman AG, Amid PK, Lichtenstein IL: The "plug" repair of 1402 recurrent inguinal hernias. 20-year experience. Arch Surg 125:265–267, 1990.

27. Haapaniemi S, Gunnarsson U, Nordin P, et al: Reoperation after recurrent groin hernia repair. Ann Surg 234:122–126, 2001.

28. Karthikesalingam A, Markar SR, Holt PJ, et al: Meta-analysis of randomized controlled trials comparing laparoscopic with open mesh repair of recurrent inguinal hernia. Br J Surg 97:4–11, 2010.

29. Sevonius D, Gunnarsson U, Nordin P, et al: Repeated groin hernia recurrences. Ann Surg 249:516–518, 2009.

30. Rucinski J, Margolis M, Panagopoulos G, et al: Closure of the abdominal midline fascia: Meta-analysis delineates the optimal technique. Am Surg 67:421–426, 2001.

31. Carlson MA, Ludwig KA, Condon RE: Ventral hernia and other complications of 1000 midline incisions. South Med J 88:450–453, 1995.

32. Seiler CM, Deckert A, Diener MK, et al: Midline versus transverse incision in major abdominal surgery: A randomized, double-blind equivalence trial (POVATI: ISRCTN60734227). Ann Surg 249:913–920, 2009.

33. Luijendijk RW, Hop WC, van den Tol MP, et al: A comparison of suture repair with mesh repair for incisional hernia. N Engl J Med 343:392–398, 2000.

34. Wright BE, Beckerman J, Cohen M, et al: Is laparoscopic umbilical hernia repair with mesh a reasonable alternative to conventional repair? Am J Surg 184:505–508; discussion 508–509, 2002.

35. Anthony T, Bergen PC, Kim LT, et al: Factors affecting recurrence following incisional herniorrhaphy. World J Surg 24:95–100, 2000.

36. Leber GE, Garb JL, Alexander AI, et al: Long-term complications associated with prosthetic repair of incisional hernias. Arch Surg 133:378–382, 1998.

37. Koch A, Bringman S, Myrelid P, et al: Randomized clinical trial of groin hernia repair with titanium-coated lightweight mesh compared with standard polypropylene mesh. Br J Surg 95:1226–1231, 2008.

38. Conze J, Kingsnorth AN, Flament JB, et al: Randomized clinical trial comparing lightweight composite mesh with polyester or polypropylene mesh for incisional hernia repair. Br J Surg 92:1488–1493, 2005.

39. Rosen MJ: Polyester-based mesh for ventral hernia repair: Is it safe? Am J Surg 197:353–359, 2009.

40. Jin J, Rosen MJ, Blatnik J, et al: Use of acellular dermal matrix for complicated ventral hernia repair: Does technique affect outcomes? J Am Coll Surg 205:654–660, 2007.

41. de Vries Reilingh TS, van Geldere D, Langenhorst B, et al: Repair of large midline incisional hernias with polypropylene mesh: Comparison of three operative techniques. Hernia 8:56–59, 2004.

42. Novitsky YW, Porter JR, Rucho ZC, et al: Open preperitoneal retrofascial mesh repair for multiply recurrent ventral incisional hernias. J Am Coll Surg 203:283–289, 2006.

43. Iqbal CW, Pham TH, Joseph A, et al: Long-term outcome of 254 complex incisional hernia repairs using the modified Rives-Stoppa technique. World J Surg 31:2398–2404, 2007.

44. de Vries Reilingh TS, van Goor H, Charbon JA, et al: Repair of giant midline abdominal wall hernias: "Components separation technique" versus prosthetic repair: Interim analysis of a randomized controlled trial. World J Surg 31:756–763, 2007.

45. Ewart CJ, Lankford AB, Gamboa MG: Successful closure of abdominal wall hernias using the components separation technique. Ann Plast Surg 50:269–273, 2003.

46. Rosen MJ, Jin J, McGee MF, et al: Laparoscopic component separation in the single-stage treatment of infected abdominal wall prosthetic removal. Hernia 11:435–440, 2007.

47. Olmi S, Scaini A, Cesana GC, et al: Laparoscopic versus open incisional hernia repair: An open randomized controlled study. Surg Endosc 21:555–559, 2007.

48. McGreevy JM, Goodney PP, Birkmeyer CM, et al: A prospective study comparing the complication rates between laparoscopic and open ventral hernia repairs. Surg Endosc 17:1778–1780, 2003.

49. Lomanto D, Iyer SG, Shabbir A, et al: Laparoscopic versus open ventral hernia mesh repair: A prospective study. Surg Endosc 20:1030–1035, 2006.

50. Bingener J, Buck L, Richards M, et al: Long-term outcomes in laparoscopic vs open ventral hernia repair. Arch Surg 142:562–567, 2007.

51. DeMaria EJ, Moss JM, Sugerman HJ: Laparoscopic intraperitoneal polytetrafluoroethylene (PTFE) prosthetic patch repair of ventral hernia. Prospective comparison to open prefascial polypropylene mesh repair. Surg Endosc 14:326–329, 2000.

52. McAdory RS, Cobb WS, Carbonell AM: Progressive preoperative pneumoperitoneum for hernias with loss of domain. Am Surg 75:504–508, 2009.

53. Lipman J, Medalie D, Rosen MJ: Staged repair of massive incisional hernias with loss of abdominal domain: A novel approach. Am J Surg 195:84–88, 2008.

54. Taner T, Cima RR, Larson DW, et al: The use of human acellular dermal matrix for parastomal hernia repair in patients with inflammatory bowel disease: A novel technique to repair fascial defects. Dis Colon Rectum 52:349–354, 2009.

55. Sugarbaker PH: Peritoneal approach to prosthetic mesh repair of paraostomy hernias. Ann Surg 201:344–346, 1985.

56. Byers JM, Steinberg JB, Postier RG: Repair of parastomal hernias using polypropylene mesh. Arch Surg 127:1246–1247, 1992.

57. Janes A, Cengiz Y, Israelsson LA: Randomized clinical trial of the use of a prosthetic mesh to prevent parastomal hernia. Br J Surg 91:280–282, 2004.

58. Heniford BT, Park A, Ramshaw BJ, et al: Laparoscopic repair of ventral hernias: Nine years' experience with 850 consecutive hernias. Ann Surg 238:391–399; discussion 399–400, 2003.

59. Pring CM, Tran V, O'Rourke N, et al: Laparoscopic versus open ventral hernia repair: A randomized controlled trial. ANZ J Surg 78:903–906, 2008.

60. Asencio F, Aguilo J, Peiro S, et al: Open randomized clinical trial of laparoscopic versus open incisional hernia repair. Surg Endosc 23:1441–1448, 2009.

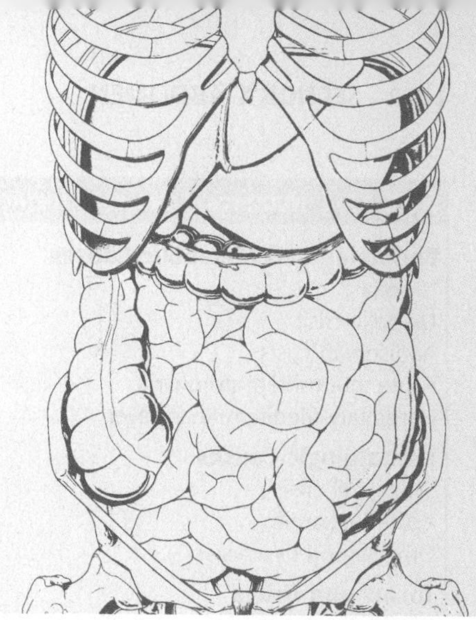

CHAPTER 47

# ACUTE ABDOMEN

Ronald A. Squires and Russell G. Postier



The term *acute abdomen* refers to signs and symptoms of abdominal pain and tenderness, a clinical presentation that often requires emergency surgical therapy. This challenging clinical scenario requires a thorough and expeditious workup to determine the need for operative intervention and initiate appropriate therapy. Many diseases, some of which are not surgical or even intra-abdominal,[1] can produce acute abdominal pain and tenderness. Therefore, every attempt should be made to make a correct diagnosis so that the therapy selected, often a laparoscopy or laparotomy, is appropriate.

The diagnoses associated with an acute abdomen vary according to age and gender.[2] Appendicitis is more common in younger individuals, whereas biliary disease, bowel obstruction, intestinal ischemia and infarction, and diverticulitis are more common in older adults. Most surgical diseases associated with an acute abdomen result from infection, obstruction, ischemia, or perforation.

Nonsurgical causes of an acute abdomen can be divided into three categories, endocrine and metabolic, hematologic, and toxins or drugs (Box 47-1).[3] Endocrine and metabolic causes include uremia, diabetic crisis, addisonian crisis, acute intermittent porphyria, acute hyperlipoproteinemia, and hereditary Mediterranean fever. Hematologic disorders include sickle cell crisis, acute leukemia, and other blood dyscrasias. Toxins and drugs causing an acute abdomen include lead and other heavy metal toxins, narcotic withdrawal, and black widow spider poisoning. It is important to consider these possibilities when evaluating a patient with acute abdominal pain.

Because of the potential surgical nature of the acute abdomen, an expeditious workup is necessary (Box 47-2). The workup proceeds in the usual order—history, physical examination, laboratory tests, and imaging studies. Although imaging studies have increased the accuracy with which the correct diagnosis can be made, the most important part of the evaluation remains a thorough history and careful physical examination. Laboratory and imaging studies are usually needed, but are directed by the findings on history and physical examination.

## ANATOMY AND PHYSIOLOGY

Abdominal pain is divided into visceral and parietal components. Visceral pain tends to be vague and poorly localized to the epigastrium, periumbilical region, or hypogastrium, depending on its origin from the primitive foregut, midgut, or hindgut (Fig. 47-1). It is usually the result of distention of a hollow viscus. Parietal pain corresponds to the segmental nerve roots innervating the peritoneum and tends to be sharper and better localized. Referred pain is pain perceived at a site distant from the source of stimulus. For example, irritation of the diaphragm may produce pain in the shoulder. Common referred pain sites and their accompanying sources are listed in Box 47-3. Determining whether the pain is visceral, parietal, or referred is important and can usually be done with a careful history.

Introduction of bacteria or irritating chemicals into the peritoneal cavity can cause an outpouring of fluid from the peritoneal membrane. The peritoneum responds to inflammation by increased blood flow, increased permeability, and formation of a fibrinous exudate on its surface. The bowel also develops local or generalized paralysis. The fibrinous surface and decreased intestinal movement cause adherence between the bowel and omentum or abdominal wall and help localize inflammation. As a result, an abscess may produce sharply localized pain, with normal bowel sounds and gastrointestinal function, whereas a diffuse process, such as a perforated duodenal ulcer, produces generalized abdominal pain, with a quiet abdomen. Peritonitis may affect the entire abdominal cavity or part of the visceral or parietal peritoneum.

Peritonitis is peritoneal inflammation of any cause. It is usually recognized on physical examination by severe tenderness to palpation, with or without rebound tenderness, and guarding. Peritonitis is usually secondary to an inflammatory insult, most often a gram-negative infection with an enteric organism or anaerobe. It can result from noninfectious inflammation; a common example is pancreatitis. Primary peritonitis occurs more commonly in children and is most often caused by *Pneumococcus* or hemolytic *Streptococcus* spp.[4] Adults with end-stage renal disease on peritoneal dialysis can develop infections of their peritoneal fluid, with the most common organisms being gram-positive cocci. Adults with ascites and cirrhosis can develop primary peritonitis and, in these cases, the organisms are usually *Escherichia coli* and *Klebsiella* spp.

**BOX 47-1 Nonsurgical Causes of the Acute Abdomen**

**Endocrine and Metabolic Causes**
Uremia
Diabetic crisis
Addisonian crisis
Acute intermittent porphyria
Hereditary Mediterranean fever

**Hematologic Causes**
Sickle cell crisis
Acute leukemia
Other blood dyscrasias

**Toxins and Drugs**
Lead poisoning
Other heavy metal poisoning
Narcotic withdrawal
Black widow spider poisoning

## HISTORY

A detailed and organized history is essential to formulating an accurate differential diagnosis and subsequent treatment regimen. Current technologic advances in imaging cannot and will never replace the need for a skilled clinician's bedside examination. The history must not only focus on the investigation of the pain complaints, but on past problems and associated symptoms as well. Questions should be open-ended whenever possible, and structured to disclose the onset, character, location, duration, radiation, and chronology of the pain experienced. It is tempting to ask questions about whether the pain is sharp or whether eating makes it worse. This specific yes or no style can facilitate the history taking by not allowing the patient to narrate, but it can miss vital details and potentially skew the response. A much better questioning style would be to determine how the pain feels to the patient or whether anything makes the pain better or worse. Often, additional information can be gained by observing how the patient describes the pain that is experienced. Pain identified with one finger is often more localized and typical of parietal innervation or peritoneal inflammation as compared with indicating the area of discomfort with the palm of the hand, which is more typical of the visceral discomfort of bowel or solid organ disease.

The intensity and severity of the pain are related to the underlying tissue damage. Sudden onset of excruciating pain suggests conditions such as intestinal perforation or arterial embolization with ischemia, although other conditions, such as biliary colic, can present suddenly as well. Pain that develops and worsens over several hours is typical of conditions of progressive inflammation or infection such as cholecystitis, colitis, and bowel obstruction. The history of progressive worsening versus intermittent episodes of pain can help differentiate infectious processes that worsen with time compared with the spasmodic colicky pain associated with bowel obstruction, biliary colic from cystic duct obstruction, or genitourinary obstruction (Figs. 47-2 to 47-4).

Equally as important as the character of the pain is its location and radiation. Tissue injury or inflammation can trigger visceral and somatic pain. Solid organ visceral pain in the abdomen is generalized in the quadrant of the involved organ, such as liver pain across the right upper quadrant of the abdomen.

**BOX 47-2 Surgical Acute Abdominal Conditions**

**Hemorrhage**
Solid organ trauma
Leaking or ruptured arterial aneurysm
Ruptured ectopic pregnancy
Bleeding gastrointestinal diverticulum
Arteriovenous malformation of gastrointestinal tract
Intestinal ulceration
Aortoduodenal fistula after aortic vascular graft
Hemorrhagic pancreatitis
Mallory-Weiss syndrome
Spontaneous rupture of spleen

**Infection**
Appendicitis
Cholecystitis
Meckel's diverticulitis
Hepatic abscess
Diverticular abscess
Psoas abscess

**Perforation**
Perforated gastrointestinal ulcer
Perforated gastrointestinal cancer
Boerhaave's syndrome
Perforated diverticulum

**Blockage**
Adhesion induction small/large bowel obstruction
Sigmoid volvulus
Cecal volvulus
Incarcerated hernias
Inflammatory bowel disease
Gastrointestinal malignancy
Intussusception

**Ischemia**
Buerger's disease
Mesenteric thrombosis/embolism
Ovarian torsion
Ischemic colitis
Testicular torsion
Strangulated hernias

**BOX 47-3 Locations and Causes of Referred Pain**

**Right Shoulder**
Liver
Gallbladder
Right hemidiaphragm

**Left Shoulder**
Heart
Tail of pancreas
Spleen
Left hemidiaphragm

**Scrotum and Testicles**
Ureter

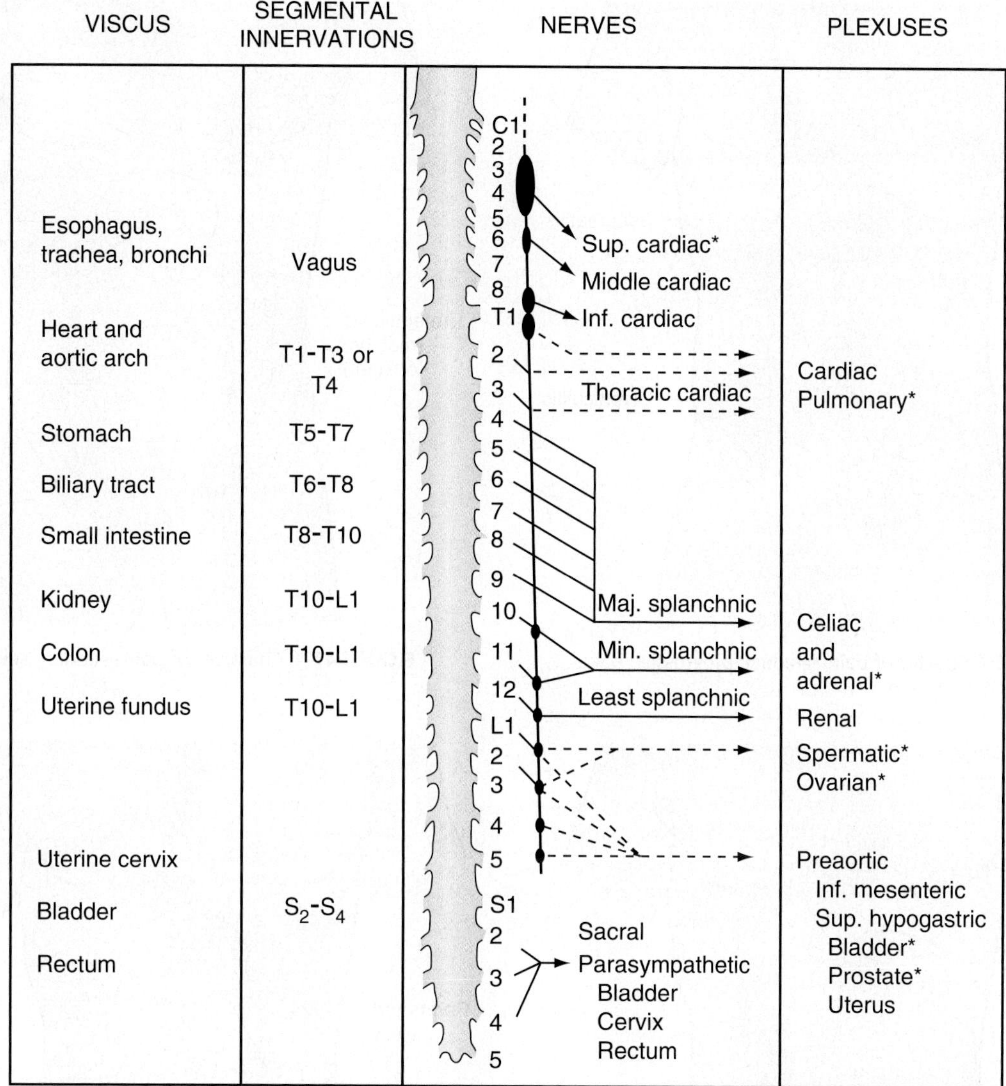


**FIGURE 47-1** Sensory innervation of the viscera. (From White JC, Sweet WH: Pain and the neurosurgeon, Springfield, Ill, 1969, Charles C Thomas, p 526.)

Small bowel pain is perceived as poorly localized periumbilical pain, whereas colon pain is centered between the umbilicus and pubis symphysis. As inflammation expands to involve the peritoneal surface, parietal nerve fibers from the spine allow for focal and intense sensation. This combination of innervation is responsible for the classic diffuse periumbilical pain of early appendicitis that later shifts to become an intense focal pain in the right lower abdomen at McBurney's point. If the physician focuses on the character of the current pain and does not thoroughly investigate its onset and progression, he or she will miss these strong historical clues (Figs. 47-5 and 47-6). Pain may also extend well beyond the diseased site. The liver shares some of its innervation with the diaphragm and may create referred pain to the right shoulder from the C3-C5 nerve roots. Genitourinary pain is another source of pain that commonly has a radiating pattern. Symptoms are primarily in the flank region, originating from the splanchnic nerves of T11-L1, but pain often radiates to the scrotum or labia via the hypogastric plexus of S2-S4.

Activities that exacerbate or relieve the pain are also important. Eating will often worsen the pain of bowel obstruction, biliary colic, pancreatitis, diverticulitis, or bowel perforation. Food can provide relief from the pain of nonperforated peptic ulcer disease or gastritis. Clinicians will often recognize that they are evaluating peritonitis while taking the history. Patients with peritoneal inflammation will avoid any activity that stretches or jostles the abdomen. They describe worsening of the pain with any sudden body movement and realize that there is less pain if their knees are flexed. The car ride to the hospital can be agonizing, with the patient feeling every bump along the way.

Associated symptoms can be important diagnostic clues. Nausea, vomiting, constipation, diarrhea, pruritis, melena, hematochezia, and/or hematuria can all be helpful symptoms if present and recognized. Vomiting may occur because of severe abdominal pain of any cause or as a result of mechanical bowel obstruction or ileus. Vomiting is more likely to precede the onset of significant abdominal pain in many medical conditions,

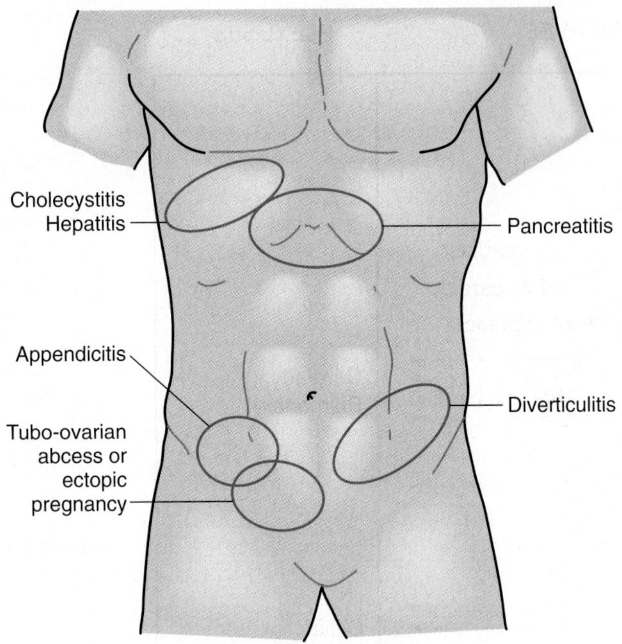


**FIGURE 47-2** Character of pain—gradual, progressive pain.

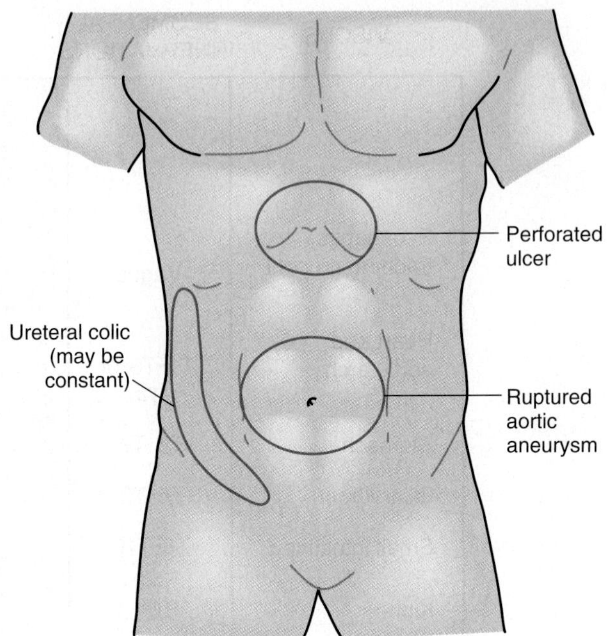


**FIGURE 47-4** Character of pain—sudden, severe pain.

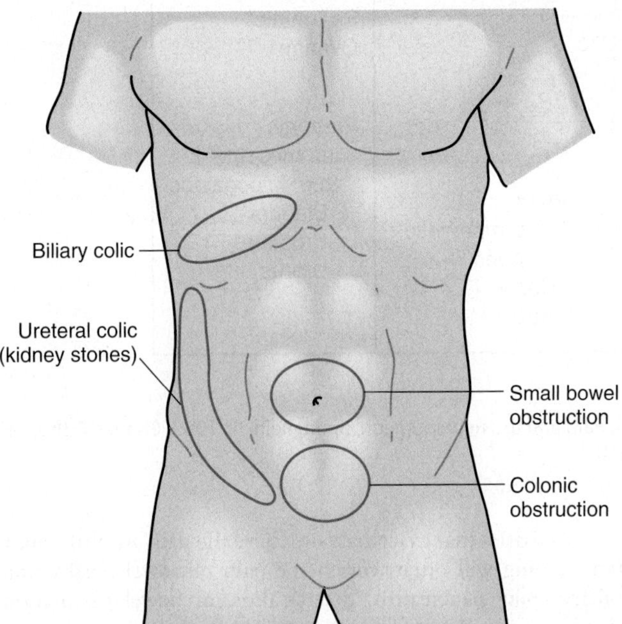


**FIGURE 47-3** Character of pain—colicky, crampy, intermittent pain.

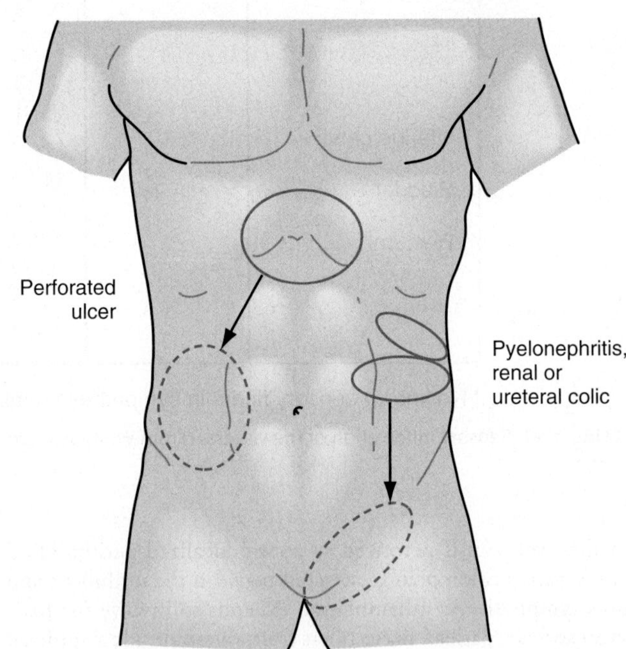


**FIGURE 47-5** Referred pain. *Solid circles* are primary or most intense sites of pain.

whereas the pain of an acute surgical abdomen presents first and stimulates vomiting via medullary efferent fibers that are triggered by visceral afferent pain fibers. Constipation or obstipation can be a result of mechanical obstruction or decreased peristalsis. It may represent the primary problem and require laxatives and prokinetic agents, or merely be a symptom of an underlying condition. A careful history should include whether the patient is continuing to pass any gas or stool from the rectum. A complete obstruction is more likely to be associated with subsequent bowel ischemia or perforation caused by the massive distention that can occur. Diarrhea is associated with several medical causes of acute abdomen, including infectious enteritis, inflammatory bowel disease or parasitic contamination. Bloody diarrhea can be seen in these conditions, as well as in colonic ischemia.

The past medical history could be more helpful than any other single part of the patient's evaluation. Previous illnesses or diagnoses can greatly increase or decrease the likelihood of certain conditions that would otherwise not be strongly considered. Patients may, for example, report that the current pain is similar to the kidney stone passage that they experienced a

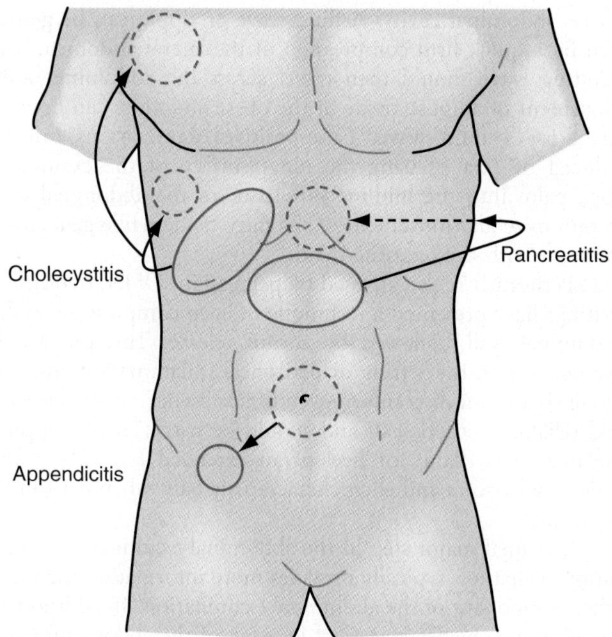


**FIGURE 47-6** Referred pain. *Solid circles* are primary or most intense sites of pain.

decade previously. On the other hand, a prior history of appendectomy, pelvic inflammatory disease, or cholecystectomy can significantly influence the differential diagnosis. During the abdominal examination, all scars on the abdomen should be accounted for by the medical history obtained.

A history of medications and the gynecologic history of female patient are also important. Medications can both create acute abdominal conditions or alternatively mask their symptoms. Although a thorough discussion of the impact of all medications is beyond the scope of this chapter, several common drug classes deserve mention. High-dose narcotic use can interfere with bowel activity and lead to obstipation and obstruction. Narcotics can also contribute to spasm of the sphincter of Oddi and exacerbate biliary or pancreatic pain. They can also suppress pain sensation and alter mental status, which can impair the ability to diagnose the condition accurately. Nonsteroidal anti-inflammatory drugs (NSAIDs) are associated with an increased risk of upper gastrointestinal inflammation and perforation; steroids can block protective gastric mucous production by chief cells and reduce the inflammatory reaction to infection, including advanced peritonitis. As a class, immunosuppressive agents increase a patient's risk of acquiring various bacterial or viral illnesses and also blunt the inflammatory response, diminishing the pain that is present and the overall physiologic response. Anticoagulants are more prevalent in our emergency patients as the population ages. These drugs may be the cause of gastrointestinal bleeds, retroperitoneal hemorrhages, or rectus sheath hematomas. They can also complicate the preoperative preparation of the patient and be the cause of substantial morbidity if their use goes unrecognized. Finally, recreational drugs can play a role in patients with an acute abdomen. Chronic alcoholism is strongly associated with coagulopathy and portal hypertension from liver impairment. Cocaine and methamphetamine can create an intense vasospastic reaction, which can create life-threatening hypertension and cardiac and intestinal ischemia.

Gynecologic health, specifically the menstrual history, is crucial in the evaluation of lower abdominal pain in a young woman. The likelihood of ectopic pregnancy, pelvic inflammatory disease, mittelschmerz, and/or severe endometriosis are all heavily influenced by the details of the gynecologic history.

Little has changed in the technique or goals of history taking since Dr. Zachary Cope first published his classic paper on the diagnosis of acute abdominal pain in 1921.[5] An exception is the application of computers to history taking, which has been extensively studied in Europe.[6-10] Data were collected by physicians on detailed standardized forms during history and physical examinations and entered into computers programmed with a medical database of diseases and their associated signs and symptoms. The computer-generated diagnosis, based on mathematical probabilities, was as much as 20% more accurate than physicians who didn't use computers to help arrive at a diagnosis. Statistically significant improvement was identified in regard to a timely laparotomy, shortened hospital stay, and reduced need for surgery and hospitalization. However, it should be noted that statistically significant improvements in accuracy and efficiency can be realized without computer assistance if similar standardized forms are used for data collection. This has also been observed in the settings of trauma and critical care.

## PHYSICAL EXAMINATION

An organized and thoughtful physical examination is critical to the development of an accurate differential diagnosis and the subsequent treatment algorithm. Despite newer technologies, including high-resolution computed tomography (CT) scanning, ultrasound, and magnetic resonance imaging (MRI), the physical examination remains a key part of a patient's evaluation and must not be minimized. Skilled clinicians will be able to develop a narrow and accurate differential diagnosis in most of their patients at the conclusion of the history and physical examination. Laboratory and imaging studies can then be used to confirm the suspicions further, reorder the proposed differential diagnosis or, less commonly, suggest unusual possibilities not yet considered.

The physical examination should always begin with a general inspection of the patient, to be followed by inspection of the abdomen itself. Patients with peritoneal irritation will experience worsened pain with any activity that moves or stretches the peritoneum. These patients will typically lie very still in bed during the evaluation and often maintain flexion of their knees and hips to reduce tension on the anterior abdominal wall. Disease states that cause pain without peritoneal irritation, such as ischemic bowel or ureteral or biliary colic, typically cause patients to shift and fidget in bed continually while trying to find a position that lessens their discomfort (Fig. 47-7). Other important clues such as pallor, cyanosis, and diaphoresis may also be observed during the general inspection.

Abdominal inspection should address the contour of the abdomen, including whether it appears distended or scaphoid or whether a localized mass effect is observed. Special attention should be paid to all scars present and, if surgical in nature, should correlate with the surgical history provided. Fascial hernias may be suspected and can be confirmed during palpation of the abdominal wall. Evidence of erythema or edema of skin may suggest cellulitis of the abdominal wall, whereas ecchymosis is sometimes observed with deeper necrotizing infections of the fascia or abdominal structures, such as the pancreas.

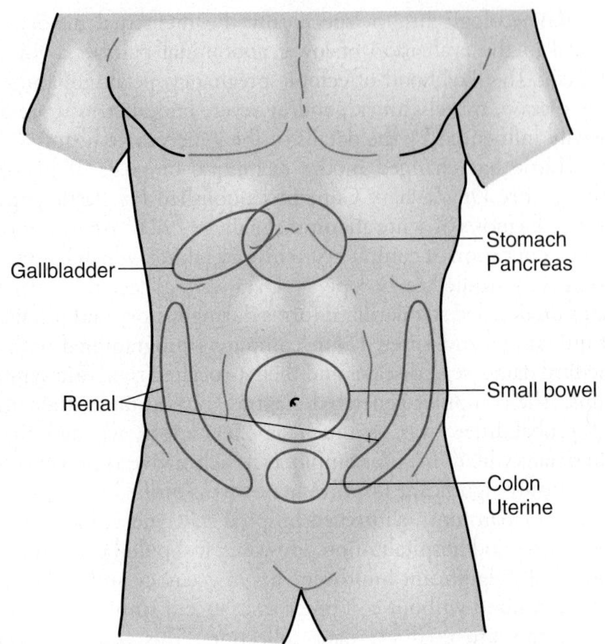


**FIGURE 47-7** Common locations for visceral pain.

Auscultation can provide useful information about the gastrointestinal tract and vascular system. Bowel sounds are typically evaluated for their quantity and quality. A quiet abdomen suggests an ileus, whereas hyperactive bowel sounds are found in enteritis and early ischemic intestine. The pitch and pattern of the sounds are also considered. Mechanical bowel obstruction is characterized by high-pitched tinkling sounds that tend to come in rushes and are associated with pain. Far away, echoing sounds are often present when significant luminal distention exists. Bruits heard within the abdomen reflect turbulent blood flow in the vascular system. These are most frequently encountered in the setting of high-grade arterial stenoses (70% to 95% but can also be heard if an arteriovenous fistula is present). The clinician can also perform a subtle test for the location and degree of pain during the auscultatory examination by varying the position and amount of pressure applied with the stethoscope. These data can then be compared with the findings during palpation and evaluated for consistency. Even though few patients will try to deceive their physician intentionally, some may exaggerate their pain complaints so as not to be disregarded or taken lightly.

Percussion is used to assess for gaseous distention of the bowel, free intra-abdominal air, degree of ascites, and/or presence of peritoneal inflammation. Hyperresonance, commonly termed *tympany to percussion,* is characteristic of underlying gas-filled loops of bowel. In the setting of bowel obstruction or ileus, this tympany is heard throughout all but the right upper quadrant, where the liver lies beneath the abdominal wall. If localized dullness to percussion is identified anywhere other than the right upper quadrant, an abdominal mass displacing the bowel should be considered. When liver dullness is lost and resonance is uniform throughout, free intra-abdominal air should be suspected. This air rises and collects beneath the anterior abdominal wall when the patient is in a supine position. Ascites is detected by looking for fluctuance of the abdominal cavity. A fluid wave or ripple can be generated by a quick firm compression of the lateral abdomen. The resulting wave should then travel across the abdominal wall. Movement of adipose tissue in the obese abdomen can be mistaken for a fluid wave. False-positive examinations can be reduced by first pressing the ulnar surface of the examiner's open palm into the midline soft tissue of the abdominal wall to minimize any movement of the fatty tissue while generating the wave with the opposite hand.

Peritonitis is also assessed by percussion. Older, traditional writings have presented a technique of deep compression of the abdominal wall, followed by abrupt release. This practice is excruciating in the setting of peritoneal inflammation and can create significant discomfort, even in its absence. More sensitive and reliable methods can and should be used. Firmly tapping the iliac crest, flank, or heel of an extended leg will jar the abdominal viscera and elicit characteristic pain when peritonitis is present.

The final major step in the abdominal examination is palpation. Palpation typically provides more information than any other component of the abdominal examination. In addition to revealing the severity and exact location of the abdominal pain, palpation can further confirm the presence of peritonitis and identify organomegaly or an abnormal mass lesion. Palpation should always begin gently and away from the reported area of pain. If considerable pain is induced at the outset of palpation, the patient is likely to guard voluntarily and will continue to do so, limiting the information obtained. Involuntary guarding, or abdominal wall muscle spasm, is a sign of peritonitis and must be distinguished from voluntary guarding. To accomplish this, the examiner applies consistent pressure to the abdominal wall, away from the point of maximal pain, while asking the patient to take a slow deep breath. In the setting of voluntary guarding, the abdominal muscles will relax during the act of inspiration; if involuntary, they remain spastic and tense.

Pain, when focal, suggests an early or well-localized disease process, whereas diffuse pain on palpation is present with extensive inflammation or a late presentation. If pain is diffuse, careful investigation should be carried out to determine where the pain is greatest. Even in the setting of extreme contamination from perforated peptic ulcers or colonic diverticula, the site of maximal tenderness often indicates the underlying source.

Numerous unique physical findings have come to be associated with specific disease conditions and are well described as examination signs (Table 47-1). Murphy's sign of acute cholecystitis results when inspiration during palpation of the right upper quadrant results in sudden worsening of pain because of descent of the liver and gallbladder toward the examiner's hand. Several signs help localize the site of underlying peritonitis, including obturator, psoas, and Rovsing's signs. Others, such as the Fothergill and Carnett signs, help distinguish intra-abdominal disease from that of the abdominal wall.

A digital rectal examination needs to be performed in all patients with acute abdominal pain, checking for the presence of a mass, pelvic pain, or intraluminal blood. A pelvic examination should be included for all women when evaluating pain located below the umbilicus. Gynecologic and adnexal processes are best characterized by a thorough speculum and bimanual evaluation.

**Table 47-1 Abdominal Examination Signs**

| SIGN | DESCRIPTION | DIAGNOSIS OR CONDITION |
|---|---|---|
| Aaron | Pain or pressure in epigastrium or anterior chest with persistent firm pressure applied to McBurney's point | Acute appendicitis |
| Bassler | Sharp pain created by compressing appendix between abdominal wall and iliacus | Chronic appendicitis |
| Blumberg | Transient abdominal wall rebound tenderness | Peritoneal inflammation |
| Carnett | Loss of abdominal tenderness when abdominal wall muscles are contracted | Intra-abdominal source of abdominal pain |
| Chandelier | Extreme lower abdominal and pelvic pain with movement of cervix | Pelvic inflammatory disease |
| Charcot | Intermittent right upper abdominal pain, jaundice, and fever | Choledocholithiasis |
| Claybrook | Accentuation of breath and cardiac sounds through abdominal wall | Ruptured abdominal viscus |
| Courvoisier | Palpable gallbladder in presence of jaundice | Periampullary tumor |
| Cruveihier | Varicose veins at umbilicus (caput medusa) | Portal hypertension |
| Cullen | Periumbilical bruising | Hemoperitoneum |
| Danforth | Shoulder pain on inspiration | Hemoperitoneum |
| Fothergill | Abdominal wall mass that does not cross midline and remains palpable when rectus contracted | Rectus muscle hematomas |
| Grey Turner | Local areas of discoloration around umbilicus and flanks | Acute hemorrhagic pancreatitis |
| Iliopsoas | Elevation and extension of leg against resistance creates pain | Apppendicitis with retrocecal abscess |
| Kehr | Left shoulder pain when supine and pressure placed on left upper abdomen | Hemoperitoneum (especially from splenic origin) |
| Mannkopf | Increased pulse when painful abdomen palpated | Absent if malingering |
| Murphy | Pain caused by inspiration while applying pressure to right upper abdomen | Acute cholecystitis |
| Obturator | Flexion and external rotation of right thigh while supine creates hypogastric pain | Pelvic abscess or inflammatory mass in pelvis |
| Ransohoff | Yellow discoloration of umbilical region | Ruptured common bile duct |
| Rovsing | Pain at McBurney's point when compressing the left lower abdomen | Acute appendicitis |
| Ten Horn | Pain caused by gentle traction of right testicle | Acute appendicitis |

**BOX 47-4 Laboratory Studies for the Acute Abdomen**

- Hemoglobin level
- White blood cell count with differential
- Electrolyte, blood urea nitrogen, creatinine levels
- Urinalysis
- Urine human chorionic gonadotropin level
- Amylase, lipase levels
- Total and direct bilirubin levels
- Alkaline phosphatase level
- Serum aminotransferase
- Serum lactate levels
- Stool for ova and parasites
- *C. dificile* culture and toxin assay

## EVALUATION AND DIAGNOSIS

### Laboratory Studies

A number of laboratory studies are considered routine in the evaluation of a patient with an acute abdomen (Box 47-4). They help confirm that inflammation or infection is present and also aid in the elimination of some of the most common nonsurgical conditions. A complete blood count with differential is valuable because most patients with an acute abdomen will have a leukocytosis or bandemia. Measurement of serum electrolyte, blood urea nitrogen, and creatinine levels will assist in evaluating the effect of factors such as vomiting or third space fluid losses. In addition, they may suggest an endocrine or metabolic diagnosis as the cause of the patient's problem. Serum amylase and lipase level determinations may suggest pancreatitis as the cause of the abdominal pain but can also be elevated in other disorders, such as small bowel infarction or duodenal ulcer perforation. Normal serum amylase and lipase levels do not exclude pancreatitis as a possible diagnosis caused by the effects of chronic inflammation on enzyme production and timing factors. Liver function tests, including determination of total and direct bilirubin, serum aminotransferase, and alkaline phosphatase levels are helpful in evaluating potential biliary tract causes of acute abdominal pain. Lactate levels and arterial blood gas determinations can be helpful in diagnosing intestinal ischemia or infarction. Urine testing, such as urinalysis, is helpful in the diagnosis of bacterial cystitis, pyelonephritis, and certain endocrine abnormalities, such as diabetes or renal parenchymal disease. Urine culture can confirm a suspected urinary tract infection and direct antibiotic therapy but cannot be done in time to be helpful in the evaluation of an acute abdomen. Urinary measurements of human chorionic gonadotropin level can suggest pregnancy as a confounding factor in the patient's presentation or aid in decision

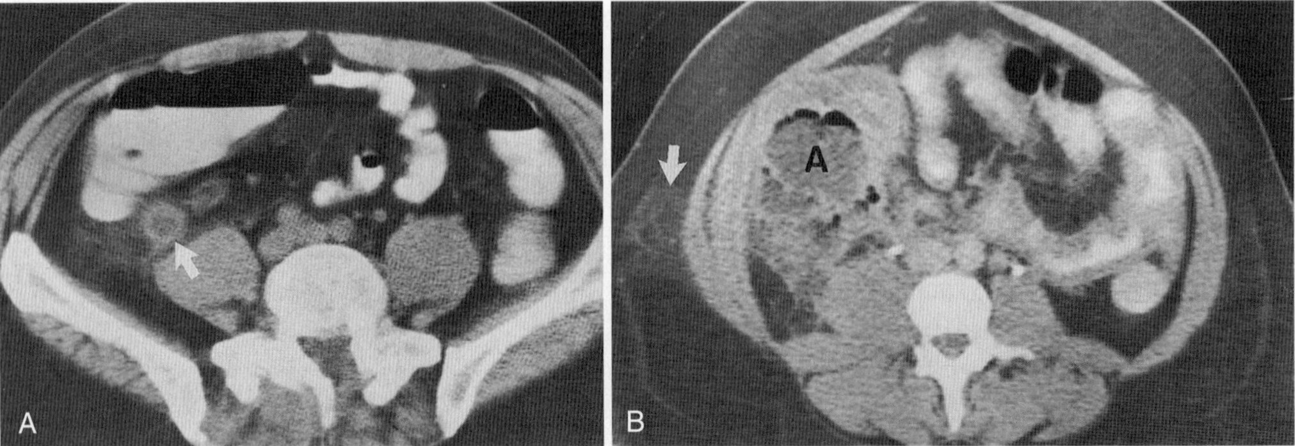

**FIGURE 47-8** Appendicitis. **A,** CT scan of uncomplicated appendicitis. A thick-walled, distended, retrocecal appendix *(arrow)* is seen with inflammatory change in the surrounding fat. **B,** CT scan of complicated appendicitis—a retrocecal appendiceal abscess (A) with an associated phlegmon posteriorly found in a 3-week postpartum, obese woman. Inflammatory change extends through the flank musculature into the subcutaneous fat *(arrow).*

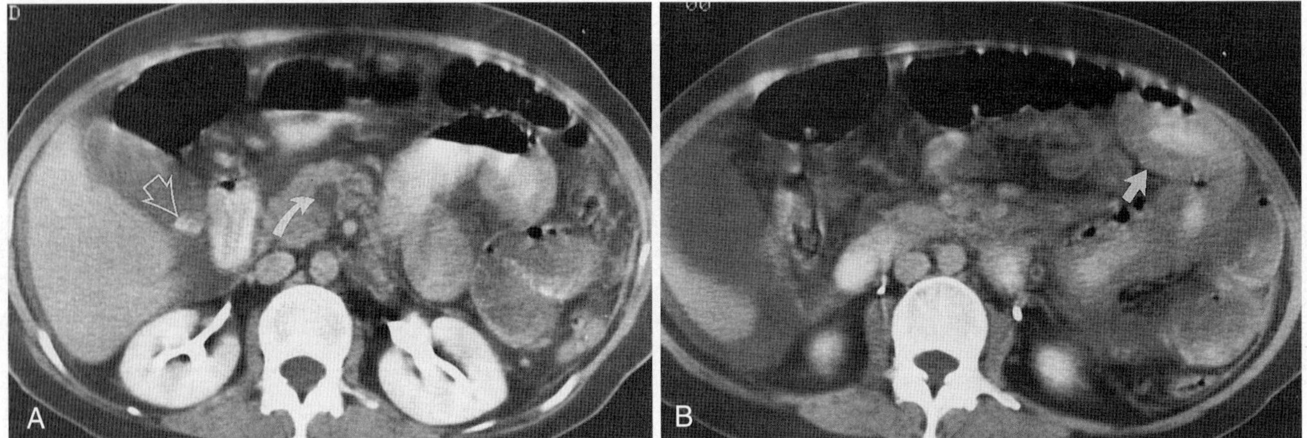

**FIGURE 47-9** Small bowel infarction associated with mesenteric venous thrombosis. **A,** Note the low-density thrombosed superior mesenteric vein *(solid arrow)* and incidental gallstones *(open arrow).* **B,** Thickening of proximal small bowel wall *(arrow)* coincided with several feet of infarcting small bowel at time of operation.

making regarding therapy. The fetus of a pregnant patient with an acute abdomen is best protected by providing the best care to the mother, including surgery, if indicated.[11] Stool testing for occult blood can be helpful in the evaluation of these patients but is nonspecific. Testing stool for ova and parasite evaluation, as well as culture and toxin assay for *Clostridium difficile,* can be helpful if diarrhea is a component of the patient's presentation.

## Imaging Studies

Improvements in imaging techniques, especially multidetector CT, have revolutionized diagnosis of the acute abdomen. The most difficult diagnostic dilemmas of the past—appendicitis in young women and ischemic bowel in older adults—can now be diagnosed with greater certainty and speed (Figs. 47-8 and 47-9).[12-14] This has resulted in more rapid operative correction of the problem, with less morbidity and mortality. Despite its usefulness, CT is not the only imaging technique available and is also not the first step in imaging for most patients. In addition, no imaging technique can replace a careful history and physical examination.

Plain radiographs continue to play a role in imaging for patients with acute abdominal pain. Upright chest radiographs can detect as little as 1 mL of air injected into the peritoneal cavity. Lateral decubitus abdominal radiographs can also detect pneumoperitoneum effectively in patients who cannot stand; as little as 5 to 10 mL of gas may be detected with this technique.[15] These studies are particularly helpful for patients suspected of having a perforated duodenal ulcer, because approximately 75% of these patients will have a large enough pneumoperitoneum to be visible (Fig. 47-10).[16] This obviates the need for further evaluation in most patients, allowing for laparotomy with little delay.

Plain films also show abnormal calcifications. Approximately 5% of appendicoliths, 10% of gallstones, and 90% of renal stones contain sufficient amounts of calcium to be radiopaque. Pancreatic calcifications seen in many patients with chronic pancreatitis are visible on plain films, as are the calcifications in abdominal aortic aneurysms, visceral artery aneurysm, and atherosclerosis in visceral vessels.

Upright and supine abdominal radiographs are helpful in identifying gastric outlet obstruction, and obstruction of the

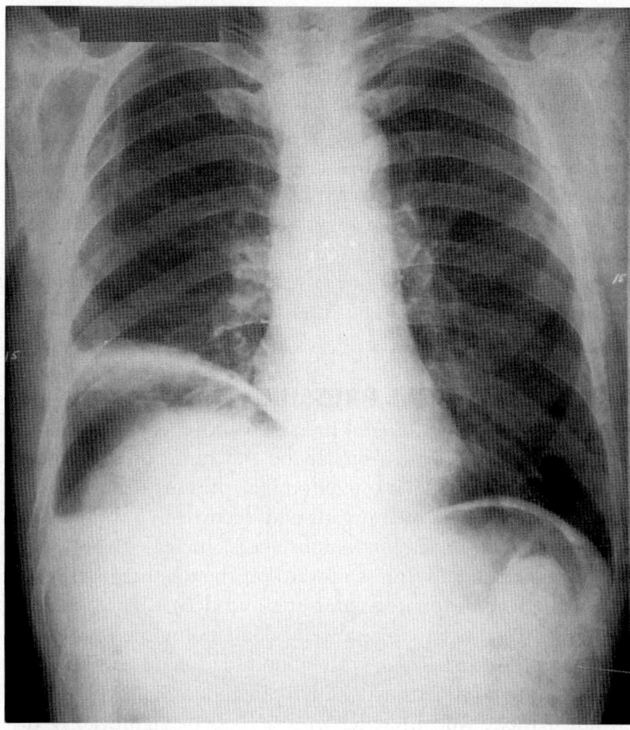

**FIGURE 47-10** Upright chest radiograph depicting moderate-sized pneumoperitoneum consistent with perforation of abdominal viscus.

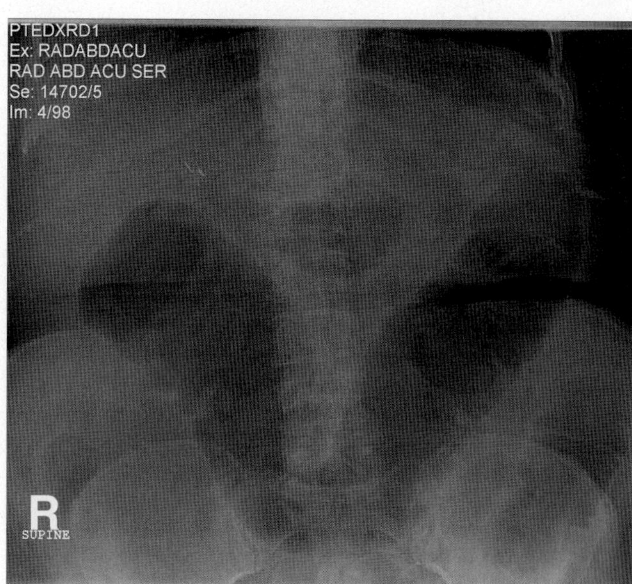


**FIGURE 47-11** Upright abdominal x-ray in a patient with an obstructing sigmoid adenocarcinoma. Note the haustral markings on the dilated transverse colon that distinguished this from small intestine.

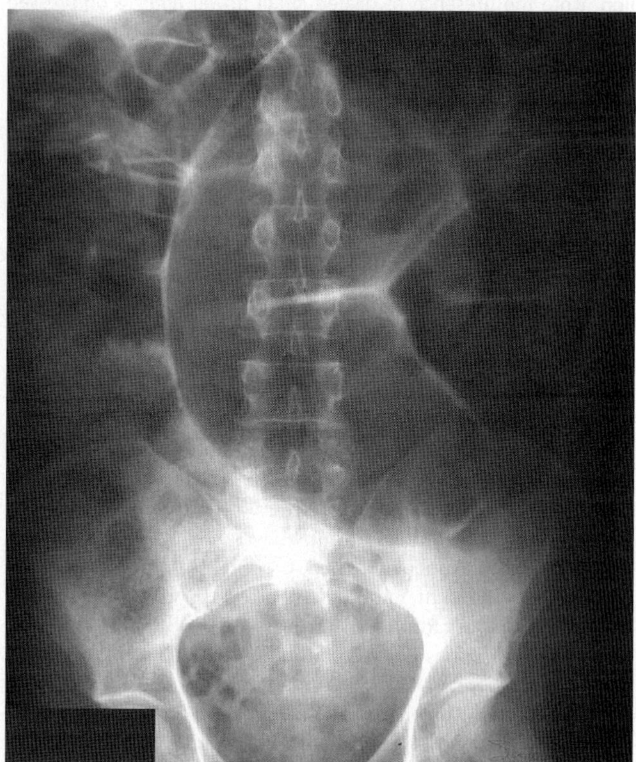

**FIGURE 47-12** Upright abdominal x-ray in a patient with a sigmoid colon volvulus. Note the characteristic appearance of a bent inner tube, with its apex in the right upper quadrant.

proximal, mid, or distal small bowel. They can also aid in determining whether a small bowel obstruction is complete or partial by the presence or absence of gas in the colon. Colonic gas can be differentiated from small intestinal gas by the presence of haustral markings caused bythe taenia coli present in the colonic wall. An obstructed colon appears as distended bowel with haustral markings (Fig. 47-11). Associated distention of small bowel may also be present, especially if the ileocecal valve is incompetent. Plain films can also suggest volvulus of the cecum or sigmoid colon. Cecal volvulus is identified by a distended loop of colon in a comma shape, with the concavity facing inferiorly and to the right. Sigmoid volvulus characteristically has the appearance of a bent inner tube, with its apex in the right upper quadrant (Fig. 47-12).

Abdominal ultrasonography is extremely accurate for detecting gallstones and assessing gallbladder wall thickness and presence of fluid around the gallbladder.[17] It is also helpful for determining the diameter of the extrahepatic and intrahepatic bile ducts. Its usefulness in detecting common bile duct stones is limited. Abdominal and transvaginal ultrasonography can aid in the detection of abnormalities of the ovaries, adnexa, and uterus. Ultrasound can also detect intraperitoneal fluid. The presence of abnormal amounts of intestinal air in most patients with an acute abdomen limits the ability of ultrasonography to evaluate the pancreas or other abdominal organs. There are important limits to the value of ultrasonography in the diagnosis of diseases that present as an acute abdomen. Ultrasound images are more difficult for most surgeons to interpret than plain radiographs and CT scans. Many hospitals have radiologic technologists available at all times to perform CT but this is often not the case with ultrasonography. As CT has become more widely available and less likely to be hindered by abdominal air, it is becoming the secondary imaging modality of choice in the patient with an acute abdomen, following plain abdominal radiography.

A number of studies have demonstrated the accuracy and usefulness of CT of the abdomen and pelvis in the evaluation of acute abdominal pain.[12-14] Many of the most common causes

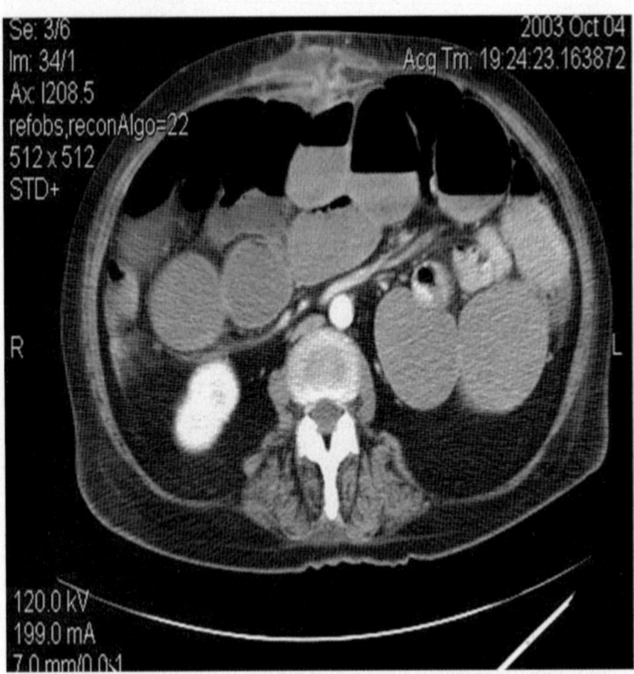


**FIGURE 47-13** CT scan of a patient with a partial small bowel obstruction. Note the presence of dilated small bowel and decompressed small bowel. The decompressed bowel contains air, indicating a partial obstruction.

of the acute abdomen are readily identified by CT scanning, as are their complications. A notable example is appendicitis. Plain films and even barium enemas add little to the diagnosis of appendicitis; however, a well-performed CT using oral, rectal, and IV contrast is highly accurate for evaluating this disease. It is equally important that an experienced radiologist, accustomed to reading abdominal CT scans, interprets the study to maximize the sensitivity and specificity of the exam. A prospective study from the Netherlands[15] has illustrated the variability of CT interpretation in the diagnosis of appendicitis. Three blinded groups of radiologists read CT scans of patients suspected of having appendicitis. All patients then underwent exploratory laparoscopy and 83% of patients were found to have appendicitis at surgery. Radiology group A was made up of radiology residents on call and trained in CT interpretation. Group B consisted of call staff radiologists; group C was composed of expert abdominal radiologists. For groups A, B, and C radiologists, the sensitivities of CT scanning for the diagnosis of acute appendicitis were 81%, 88%, and 95%, the specificities were 94%, 94%, and 100%, and the negative predictive values were 50%, 68%, and 81%, respectively. Differences between groups A and C were statistically significant. CT is also excellent for differentiating mechanical small bowel obstruction from paralytic ileus and can usually identify the transition point in mechanical obstruction (Fig. 47-13). Some of the most difficult diagnostic dilemmas, including acute intestinal ischemia and bowel injury following blunt abdominal trauma, can often be identified by this method.

Traumatic small bowel injuries can be a clinical diagnosis challenge. Associated abdominal wall, pelvic, or spinal injuries can be significant distracters that could compromise an otherwise careful history and physical examination. In addition, many patients suffering a blunt abdominal trauma will have altered mental states from coexisting closed head injuries or from intoxicating substances. When a bowel injury is suspected, optimal CT scanning uses oral and IV contrast agents. Zissin and colleagues[17] have reported an overall sensitivity of 64%, specificity of 97%, and accuracy of 82% when diagnosing small bowel injury following blunt trauma using dual-contrast CT scanning. Diagnostic clues include recognition of bowel wall thickening, identification of any gas outside the lumen of the intestine, and a moderate to large amount of intraperitoneal fluid without visible solid abdominal organ injury.

## INTRA-ABDOMINAL PRESSURE MONITORING

An elevated intra-abdominal pressure can be a symptom of an acute abdominal process or can be the cause of the process. Abnormally increased intra-abdominal pressures diminish the blood flow to abdominal organs and decrease venous return to the heart while increasing venous stasis. Increased pressure in the abdomen can also press upward on the diaphragm, thereby increasing peak inspiratory pressures and decreasing ventilatory efficiency. Risk of esophageal reflux and pulmonary aspiration has also been associated with abdominal hypertension. It is important to consider the possibility of abdominal hypertension in any patient who presents with a rigid or significantly distended abdomen.

Normal intra-abdominal pressure is considered to be 5 to 7 mm Hg for a relaxed individual of average body build lying in a supine position. Obesity and elevation of the head of the bed can increase the normal resting abdominal pressure. Morbid obesity has been shown to increase normal pressures by 4 to 8 mm Hg while elevation the head of the bed to 30 degrees raises the pressure by 5 mm Hg (average).[18] Pressures are most commonly measured via the bladder by a pressure transducer attached to a Foley catheter. Pressure readings are obtained at end-expiration following instillation of 50 mL of saline into an otherwise empty bladder. Abnormally elevated pressures are those higher than 11 mm Hg and are graded 1 to 4 by severity (Table 47-2). Abdominal hypertension grades 1 and 2 can usually be treated adequately with medical interventions focusing on maintaining euvolemia, gut decompression with a nasogastric tube and/or laxatives and enemas, withholding enteral feedings, catheter aspiration of ascitic fluid, abdominal wall relaxation, and judicious use of hypotonic IV fluids. Grades 3 and 4 often require surgical decompression via laparotomy with open packing of the abdomen if the severe hypertension and organ dysfunction do not respond promptly to aggressive medical intervention.

### Diagnostic Laparoscopy

A number of studies have confirmed the usefulness of diagnostic laparoscopy in patients with acute abdominal pain.[19-21] Purported advantages include a high sensitivity and specificity, the ability to treat a number of the conditions causing an acute abdomen laparoscopically, and decreased morbidity and mortality, length of stay, and overall hospital costs. It may be particularly helpful in the critically ill, intensive care patient, especially if a laparotomy can be avoided.[22] Diagnostic accuracy is high; the accuracy ranges from 90% to 100%, with the primary limitation being recognition of retroperitoneal processes. This compares favorably with other diagnostic studies showing superiority

**Table 47-2 Abdominal Hypertension**

| DEGREE OF HYPERTENSION | MESENTERIC PRESSURE | CO | CVP | PIP | GFR | PERFUSION | TREATMENT |
|---|---|---|---|---|---|---|---|
| Normal pressure | 5-7 mm Hg | ↔ | ↔ | ↔ | ↔ | ↔ | None |
| Grade 1 hypertension | 12-15 mm Hg | ↔ | ↔, ↑ | ↔, ↑ | ↓ | ↓ | Maintain euvolemia |
| Grade 2 hypertension | 16-20 mm Hg | ↓ | ↑* | ↑ | ↓ | ↓ | Nonsurgical decompression |
| Grade 3 hypertension | 21-25 mm Hg | ↓↓ | ↑↑* | ↑↑ | ↓↓ | ↓↓ | Surgical decompression |
| Grade 4 hypertension | >25 mm Hg | ↓↓↓ | ↑↑* | ↑↑ | ↓↓↓ | ↓↓↓ | Surgical decompression; reexplore |

*CO,* Cardiac output; *CVP,* central venous pressure; *GFR,* glomerular filtration rate; *PIP,* peak inspiratory pressure.
*Misleadingly elevated and not reflective of intravascular volume.

to peritoneal lavage, CT scanning, or ultrasound of the abdomen.[23] Because of advances in equipment and increased availability, this technique is being used more often in these patients.

## Differential Diagnosis

The differential diagnosis for acute abdominal pain is extensive. Conditions range from the mild and self-limited to the rapidly progressive and fatal. All patients must therefore be seen and evaluated immediately on presentation and reassessed at frequent intervals for changes in condition. Although many acute abdomen diagnoses will require surgical intervention for resolution, it is important to remember that many causes of acute abdominal pain are medical in nature (see Figs. 47-2 and 47-4).[24] Development of the differential diagnosis begins during the history and is further clarified during the physical examination. Refinements are then made with the assistance of laboratory analysis and imaging studies; typically, one or two diagnoses stand out. To be successful, this process requires a comprehensive knowledge of the medical and surgical conditions that create acute abdominal pain to allow individual disease features to be matched to patient demographics, symptoms, and signs.

Certain physical examination, laboratory, and radiographic findings are highly correlated with surgical disease (Box 47-5). At times, some patients will be too unstable to undergo comprehensive evaluations that require transportat to other departments, such as radiology. In this setting, peritoneal lavage can provide information that suggests pathology requiring surgical intervention. The lavage can be performed under local anesthesia at the patient's bedside. A small incision is made in the midline adjacent to the umbilicus and dissection is carried down to the peritoneal cavity. A small catheter or IV tubing is inserted and 1000 mL of saline is infused. A sample of fluid is allowed to siphon back out into the empty saline bag and is then analyzed for cellular or biochemical anomalies. This technique can provide sensitive evidence of hemorrhage or infection, as well as some types of solid or hollow organ injury.

Patients having emergency or life-threatening surgical disease are taken for immediate laparotomy; urgent diagnoses allow time for stabilization, hydration, and preoperative preparation, as needed. The remaining acute abdominal patients are grouped similarly to those with surgical conditions that sometimes require surgery, those with medical diseases, and those who as yet remain unclear. Hospitalized patients who do not go urgently to the operating room must be reassessed frequently, preferably by the same examiner, to recognize potentially serious changes in condition that could alter the diagnosis or suggest development of complications.

**BOX 47-5 Findings Associated With Surgical Disease in the Setting of Acute Abdominal Pain**

**Physical Examination and Laboratory Findings**
Abdominal compartment pressures >30 mm Hg
Worsening distention after gastric decompression
Involuntary guarding or rebound tenderness
Gastrointestinal hemorrhage requiring >4 U of blood without stabilization
Unexplained systemic sepsis
Signs of hypoperfusion (e.g., acidosis, pain out of proportion to examination findings, increasing liver function test results)

**Radiographic Findings**
Massive dilation of intestine
Progressive dilation of stationary loop of intestine (sentinel loop)
Pneumoperitoneum
Extravasation of contrast from bowel lumen
Vascular occlusion on angiography
Fat stranding, thickened bowel wall with systemic sepsis

**Diagnostic Peritoneal Lavage (1000 mL)**
>250 white blood cells/mL
>300,000 red blood cells/mL
Bilirubin level higher than plasma level (bile leak)
Particulate matter (stool)
Creatinine level higher than plasma level (urine leak)

Although the goal of every surgeon is to make the correct diagnosis preoperatively and plan the best possible surgical procedure prior to entering the operating suite, it must be emphasized that a clear diagnosis will not be able to be determined in every patient. Surgeons must always be willing to accept uncertainly and commit to abdominal exploration when examination findings warrant. Laboratory and imaging studies, although helpful, should never replace the bedside clinical judgment of an experienced surgeon. Patients are more likely to be seriously or fatally harmed by delaying surgical treatment to perform confirmatory tests than by misdiagnoses discovered at operation. Laparoscopy has proved to be a valuable tool when the diagnosis is unclear. The presence of surgical disease can be confirmed in all but the most hostile abdominal environments and, as surgeon experience grows, more conditions will also be able to be treated laparoscopically. Even when conversion to open technique is required, laparoscopic evaluation facilitates more accurate positioning of the laparotomy incision, thereby reducing its length.

## PREPARATION FOR EMERGENCY OPERATION

Patients with an acute abdomen vary greatly in their overall state of health when the decision to operate is made. Regardless of the severity of illness, all patients require some degree of preoperative preparation. IV access should be obtained and any fluid or electrolyte abnormalities corrected. Almost all patients will require antibiotic infusions. The bacteria common in acute abdominal emergencies are gram-negative enteric organisms and anaerobes. Antibiotic infusion should be initiated once a presumptive diagnosis has been made. Patients with generalized paralytic ileus, as manifested by absent or hypoactive bowel sounds, benefit from a nasogastric tube to decrease the likelihood of vomiting and aspiration. Foley catheter bladder drainage to assess urine output, a measure of adequacy of fluid resuscitation, is indicated for most patients. Preoperative urine output of 0.5 mL/kg/hr, along a with systolic blood pressure of at least 100 mm Hg and a heart rate of 100 beats/min or less, are indicative of an adequate intravascular volume. A common electrolyte abnormality requiring correction is hypokalemia. If significant potassium repletion is necessary, a central venous line is required. The ability to administer potassium through a peripheral line is limited by the potential development of phlebitis. Preoperative acidosis may respond to fluid repletion and IV bicarbonate infusion. Acidosis caused by intestinal ischemia or infarction may be refractory to preoperative therapy. Significant anemia is uncommon and preoperative blood transfusions are usually unnecessary. However, most patients should have their blood typed, cross-matched, and available at operation. There is an inherent uncertainty in the operation that will be required for these patients, so having cross-matched blood available avoids transfusion delay if unexpected intraoperative events occur. The need for preoperative stabilization of patients must be weighed against the increased morbidity and mortality associated with delay in the treatment of some of the surgical diseases that present as an acute abdomen. The underlying nature of the disease process, such as infarcted bowel, may require surgical correction before stabilization of the patient's vital signs and restoration of acid-base balance can occur. Deciding when the maximum benefit of preoperative therapy in these patients has been achieved requires good surgical judgment.

## ATYPICAL PATIENTS

### Pregnancy

Acute abdominal pain presenting in the pregnant patient creates several unique diagnostic and therapeutic challenges. Special emphasis must be placed on the possibility of gynecologic and surgical diseases when acute abdominal pain develops during pregnancy because of their frequency and morbidity if left unrecognized. Laparoscopy has had a major impact on the diagnosis and treatment of the gravid female with acute abdominal pain and is now routinely used for many clinical situations. Short-term follow-up has suggested equal or superior safety with the laparoscopic approach, but large series of long-term safety data are not available.[25-28] The greatest threat facing the pregnant patient with acute abdominal pain is the potential for delayed diagnosis. Delays in receiving surgical treatment have proven far

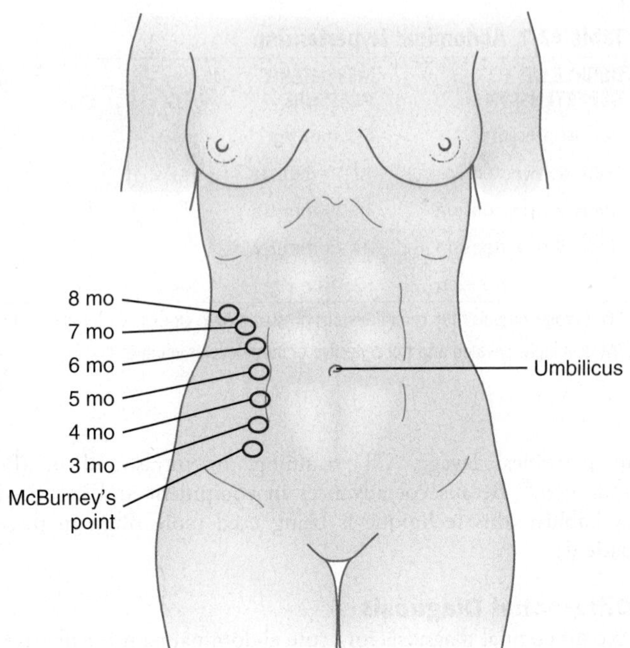


**FIGURE 47-14** Location of maternal normal appendix during fetal gestation.

more morbid than the surgery itself.[11,29] Delays occur for several reasons. Often, symptoms are attributed to the underlying pregnancy, including abdominal pains, nausea, vomiting, and anorexia. Pregnancy can also alter the presentation of some disease processes and make the physical examination more challenging because of the enlarged uterus in the pelvis. The appendix rises out of the pelvis to within a few centimeters of the right anterolateral costal margin late in the third trimester (Fig. 47-14).[30] Results of laboratory studies, such as white cell counts and other tests, are also altered in pregnancy, making recognition of disease more difficult. In addition, physicians may hesitate to perform typical imaging studies such as plain abdominal radiography or CT because of concern over radiation exposure to the developing fetus. The lack of radiologic information can take physicians out of their diagnostic routine and cause them to place extra emphasis on other modalities, such as monitoring vital signs and laboratory studies, which can confuse or underestimate the existing condition. Finally, physicians tend to be more conservative when treating pregnant patients. Surgery, especially in the pelvis, is associated with increased risks of spontaneous abortions in the first trimester and progressively increasing risk of preterm labor in the second and third trimesters. The overall risk attributed to surgery and anesthesia is estimated at 4% to 6%, but some have reported an incidence as high as 38%.[28,31,32] Perioperative risk is minimized by maintaining physiologic $O_2$ and $CO_2$ levels during surgery, avoiding episodes of hypotension, and minimally manipulating the uterus.

Appendicitis is the most common nonobstetric disease requiring surgery, occurring in 1 in 1500 pregnancies.[27,33] Its symptoms typically consist of right lateral abdominal pain, nausea, and anorexia, but so-called typical presentations account for only 50% to 60% of cases.[34] Fever is uncommon unless the appendix is perforated with abdominal sepsis. Symptoms can sometimes attributed to the underlying pregnancy and a high index of suspicion must be maintained. Laboratory studies can

**Table 47-3 Modified Alvarado Scoring System for Appendicitis**

| FEATURE | SCORE |
|---|---|
| **Symptoms** | |
| Right iliac fossa pain | 1 |
| Nausea, vomiting | 1 |
| Anorexia | 1 |
| **Signs** | |
| Right iliac fossa tenderness | 2 |
| Fever | 1 |
| Rebound tenderness | 1 |
| **Tests** | |
| WBC ≥10,000 | 2 |
| Left shift of neutrophils | 1 |
| Score ≥7 | Surgery recommended |

From Brown MA, Birchard KR, Semelka RC: Magnetic resonance evaluation of pregnant patients with acute abdominal pain. Semin Ultrasound CT MR 26:206–211, 2005.

also be misleading. Leukocytosis as high as 16,000 cells/mm$^3$ is common in pregnancy, and labor can increase the count to 21,000/mm$^3$. Many authors have suggested that a neutrophil shift more than 80% is suspicious for an acute inflammatory process, such as appendicitis; however, others have observed that only 75% of patients with proven appendicitis have a shift and as many as 50% of patients with a shift and pain are found to have a normal appendix.[11,28,35] Scoring systems have been advocated that assign numeric scores to certain symptoms, signs, and laboratory values to predict the likelihood of appendicitis.

Although systems such as the modified Alvarado scoring system (Table 47-3) help predict the need for surgical intervention, they have not been validated in a model of pregnancy.[34] Ultrasound has been relied on as the first imaging tool in many centers. Graded compression ultrasound has been shown to have a sensitivity of 86% in the nonpregnant patient.[27] In a case series of 42 pregnant women with suspected appendicitis, graded compression ultrasound was found to be 100% sensitive, 96% specific, and 98% accurate.[36] Three women were excluded from the analysis because of a technically inadequate examination because of advanced gestational age (>35 weeks). Helical CT scanning has been established as a valuable tool for evaluation of the nonpregnant patient and shows promise as a second-line study in pregnancy. Compared with traditional CT scans, helical CT can provide a much faster study, with radiation exposures to the fetus of approximately 300 mrad.[27] MRI is also beginning to play a role; it not only can demonstrate the normal appendix but it can also recognize an enlarged appendix, periappendiceal fluid, and inflammation.[37] Large prospective series documenting the success of MRI diagnosis of appendicitis are lacking; however, one study has documented successful evaluation of 10 of 12 pregnant women while avoiding radiation exposure.[38]

The added difficulties in evaluating the pregnant patient with right lower quadrant abdominal pain have resulted in a significantly higher negative appendectomy rate as compared with their nonpregnant peers. False-positive diagnoses leading to negative appendectomies occur in 15% to 35% of pregnant women presenting with lower abdominal pain.[28] Although this diagnostic error rate would be unacceptable in a typical young healthy woman, it is widely accepted because of the fetal mortality suffered when appendicitis progresses to perforation prior to surgery. Perioperative fetal loss associated with appendectomy for early appendicitis is 3% to 5%, whereas it increases to more than 20% in the setting of perforation.[39]

The second and third most common surgical diseases seen in pregnancy are biliary tract disorders and bowel obstructions. Surgery for biliary disease occurs in 1 to 6 in 10,000 pregnancies.[40] Symptoms of pain, nausea, and anorexia are the same as those in nonpregnant patients. Even though elevated estrogen levels should be more lithogenic, the incidence of disease is similar that for nongravid women.[27] With few exceptions, the evaluation and treatment during pregnancy are similar to that for all patients with biliary disease. Ultrasound is the diagnostic test of choice. The alkaline phosphatase level is elevated secondary to an elevated estrogen level and normal values must be adjusted. Nuclear scans of the biliary tract pose minimal risk to the fetus but a Foley catheter should be placed so that isotope cleared by the kidneys does not collect adjacent to the uterus.

Most surgeons try to treat simple biliary colic with conservative management in the first and third trimesters and plan elective laparoscopic cholecystectomy for the second trimester or the postpartum period to minimize fetal risk. Gallstone pancreatitis and acute cholecystitis should be managed more carefully. Gallstone pancreatitis has been associated with fetal loss as high as 60%.[41] If a woman does not respond quickly to conservative treatment with hydration, bowel rest, analgesia, and judicious use of antibiotics, surgical treatment should be performed.

Bowel obstructions are much less common, occurring in approximately 1 to 2 in 4000 deliveries; the underlying cause is adhesions in two thirds of cases. Volvulus is the second most common cause, occurring in 25% of cases compared with only 4% of the nonpregnant population.[28] Signs and symptoms are typical but must not be attributed to morning sickness. Colicky abdominal pain with rapid abdominal distention should suggest the diagnosis to the clinician. Three periods during gestation are associated with an increased risk of obstruction and correlate with rapid changes in uterine size. The first is from 16 to 20 weeks, when the uterus grows beyond the pelvis. The second is from 32 to 36 weeks, when the fetal head descends, and the third is in the early postpartum period. The evaluation should be the same as for any patient and there should be no hesitation to obtain abdominal x-rays if the situation warrants. As with other acute inflammatory processes in the abdomen, maternal and fetal morbidity are most affected by delayed definitive treatment.

## Critically Ill Patients

The critically ill patient with a potential acute abdomen is a difficult challenge for intensivists and surgeons. Many of the underlying diseases and treatments encountered in the intensive care unit (ICU) can predispose to acute abdominal disease. At the same time, unrecognized abdominal illness can be responsible for patients lingering in a critical state. Critically ill patients are often unable to appreciate symptoms to the same degree as their healthy peers because of nutritional or immune compromise, narcotic analgesia, or antibiotic use. Many of these patients have an altered mental status or are intubated and cannot provide detailed information to their providers.

Cardiopulmonary bypass (CPB) has been associated with several acute abdominal illnesses. Mesenteric ischemia, paralytic ileus, Ogilvie's syndrome, stress peptic ulceration, acute acalculous cholecystitis, and acute pancreatitis have all been linked to the low-flow state of CPB; their incidence appears to be linked to the duration of the cardiac procedure.[42,43] Vasoactive medications and ventilator support have also been linked to hypoperfusion and similar abdominal processes. When an acute abdominal complication occurs in an ICU patient, it has a dramatic effect on outcome. Gajic and associates[44] have studied 77 patients who experienced abdominal catastrophe while recovering in the medical ICU (MICU). Acute abdominal diagnoses included peptic ulcer, ischemic bowel, cholecystitis, bowel obstruction, and bowel inflammation. The APACHE III score on admission predicted an overall mortality of 31% in this group, yet they experienced an actual mortality of 63%. The development of a secondary acute abdominal illness doubled their observed mortality. Despite many of these patients having factors that could delay diagnosis, including antibiotics, analgesics, altered mental states, and intubations, 84% were still recognized as having abdominal pain, 95% as having abdominal tenderness, 73% as having abdominal distention, and 33% as having free intra-abdominal air. Intensivists should maintain a high index of suspicion for the development of intra-abdominal disease and consult with surgeons early to maximize recovery potential. Surgeons must then work to exclude the possibility of abdominal disease using all the methods described in this chapter, as well as bedside ultrasound, paracentesis, or minilaparoscopy so that early surgical intervention can be undertaken appropriately.

### Immunocompromised Patients

Immunocompromised patients have variable presentations with acute abdominal diseases. The variability is highly correlated to the degree of immunosuppression. There is no reliable test for determining the degree of immunosuppression experienced by a given patient so estimates are made by associations with certain disease states or medications. Mild to moderate compromise is experienced by older patients, malnourished individuals, diabetics, transplant recipients on routine maintenance therapy, cancer patients, renal failure patients, and HIV patients with CD4 counts higher than 200/mm$^3$. Although patients in this group have the same types of illnesses and infections as those who are immunocompetent, they still can present in an atypical fashion. Abdominal pain and systemic signs and symptoms are often linked to the development of inflammation. These patients may not be able to mount a full inflammatory response and therefore may experience less abdominal pain and have delayed development of fever and a blunted leukocytosis. Severely compromised patients would typically include transplant recipients having received immunosuppressant therapy for rejection in the past 2 months, cancer patients on chemotherapy, especially those with neutropenia, and HIV patients with CD4 counts lower than 200/mm$^3$. These patients present very late in their course, often with little or no pain, no fever, and vague constitutional symptoms, followed by an overwhelming systemic collapse.

Pseudomembranous colitis has traditionally been associated with recent broad-spectrum antibiotic use, although it is increasingly seen in immunocompromised patients with diseases such as lymphoma, leukemia, and AIDS.[45] Clinical manifestations commonly include diarrhea, dehydration, abdominal pain, fever, and leukocytosis; however, immunocompromised patients may fail to exhibit many of these findings because of their inability to mount a normal inflammatory response. Imaging studies such as abdominal CT become increasingly important in making early accurate diagnoses when presentations are atypical. Characteristic findings on CT scans that suggest pseudomembranous colitis include bowel wall thickening (mean thickness, 11 to 15 mm),[46] pancolonic distribution, and pericolonic standing. Other frequent findings include ascites, generalized mucosal enhancement, diffuse bowel dilation, and a double-halo sign, in which IV contrast enhances the mucosa and muscularis propria while edema in the submucosa creates an area of low attenuation in between (Table 47-4). These findings, when present, can greatly assist the clinician with forming the diagnosis of colitis. It is important to remember, however, that up to 14% of patients with proven pseudomembranous colitis will have had normal CT examinations and therefore the diagnosis should not be ruled out based solely on a negative scan.[47] In addition, these patients may suffer from atypical infections, including peritoneal tuberculosis, fungal infections, including aspergillus and endemic mycoses, or viral infections, including cytomegalovirus and Epstein-Barr virus (Box 47-6). When an

**Table 47-4 Frequency of Common CT Findings in Pseudo-Membranous Colitis**

| CT FINDINGS | FREQUENCY (%) |
|---|---|
| Bowel all thickening (>4 mm) | 86 |
| Pancolic distribution | 46 |
| Pericolic stranding | 45 |
| Ascites | 38 |
| Nodular/polypoid wall thickening | 38 |
| Mucosal enhancement | 18 |
| Bowel dilation | 14 |
| Accordion sign | 14 |

From Tsiotos GG, Mullany CJ, Zietlow S, et al: Abdominal complications following cardiac surgery. Am J Surg 167:553–557, 1994.

**BOX 47-6 Causes of Acute Abdominal Pain in the Immunocompromised Patient**

**Opportunistic Infections**

Endemic mycoses (e.g., coccidiomycosis, blastomycosis, histoplasmosis)
Tuberculin peritonitis
Aspirgillosis
Neutropenic colitis (typhlitis)
Pseudomembranous colitis
Cytomegalovirus colitis, gastritis, esophagitis, nephritis
Epstein-Barr virus
Hepatic abscess (fungal, pyogenic)

**Iatrogenic Conditions**

Graft-versus-host disease with hepatitis or enteritis
Peptic ulcer or perforation from steroid usage
Pancreatitis caused by steroids or azathioprine
Hepatic veno-occlusive disease (secondary to primary immunodeficiency or chemotherapy)
Nephrolithiasis caused by indinavir treatment of HIV

abdominal infection does occur, it is less likely to be walled off as a localized infection because of the lack of inflammatory reaction. All severely immunocompromised patients require prompt and thorough evaluation for any persistent abdominal complaints. All patients requiring hospitalization should receive a surgical consult to aid in timely diagnosis and treatment. High-resolution CT can be of great benefit in these patients, but a low threshold for laparoscopy or laparotomy should be maintained for those with equivocal diagnostic test results and persistent symptoms that remain unexplained.

### Morbidly Obese Patients

Morbid obesity creates numerous challenges to the accurate diagnosis of acute abdominal processes. Many authors have described alterations in the signs and symptoms of peritonitis in the morbidly obese. Findings of overt peritonitis are often late and usually ominous, leading to sepsis, organ failure, and death.[48] Abdominal sepsis is a more subtle diagnosis in this population and may only be associated with symptoms such as malaise, shoulder pain, hiccups, and shortness of breath.[49] Examination findings can also be difficult to interpret. Severe abdominal pain is not common and less specific findings such as tachycardia, tachypnea, pleural effusion, and fever may be the primary observation.[50] Appreciation of distention or intra-abdominal mass is also difficult because of the size and thickness of the abdominal wall.

Abdominal imaging is also adversely affected by obesity. Plain abdominal radiography can require multiple images to view the entire abdomen, and clarity is reduced. CT and MRI may be impossible to perform as a patient's girth or weight exceeds the size of the scanning aperture or weight limit of the mechanized bed. In these settings, a high index of suspicion and low threshold for surgical exploration must be maintained. Laparoscopy is a valuable tool in these patients. Specially designed trochars and hand-assist ports for the morbidly obese abdominal wall are now readily available and greatly facilitate minimally invasive exploration of the abdomen.

## ALGORITHMS IN THE ACUTE ABDOMEN

Algorithms can aid in the diagnosis of the patient with an acute abdomen. As noted, computer-assisted diagnosis has been shown to be more accurate than clinical judgment alone in a number of acute abdominal disease states. Algorithms are the basis for computer diagnosis and can be useful when making clinical decisions. The algorithms shown are helpful in acute abdomen patients and can allow for a focused workup and expeditious therapy (Figs. 47-15 to 47-20).

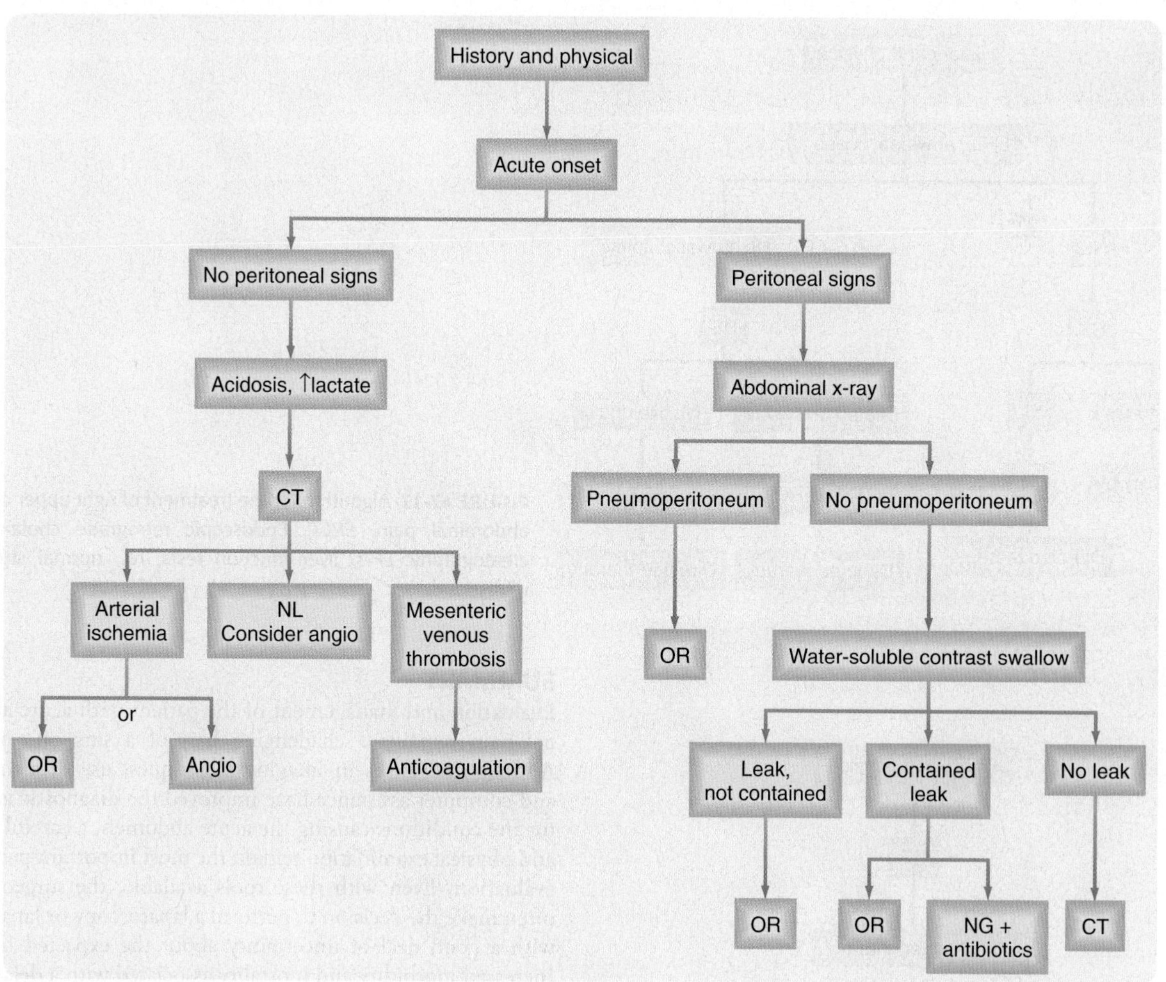


**FIGURE 47-15** Algorithm for the treatment of acute-onset, severe, generalized abdominal pain. *NG,* Nasogastric tube; *NL,* normal study; *OR,* operation.

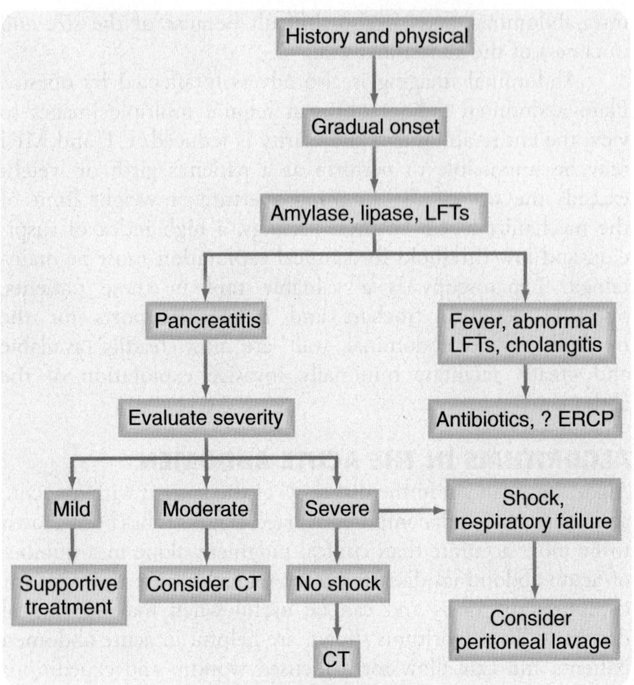


**FIGURE 47-16** Algorithm for the treatment of gradual-onset, severe, generalized abdominal pain. *ERCP,* Endoscopic retrograde cholangiopancreatography; *LFTs,* liver function tests.

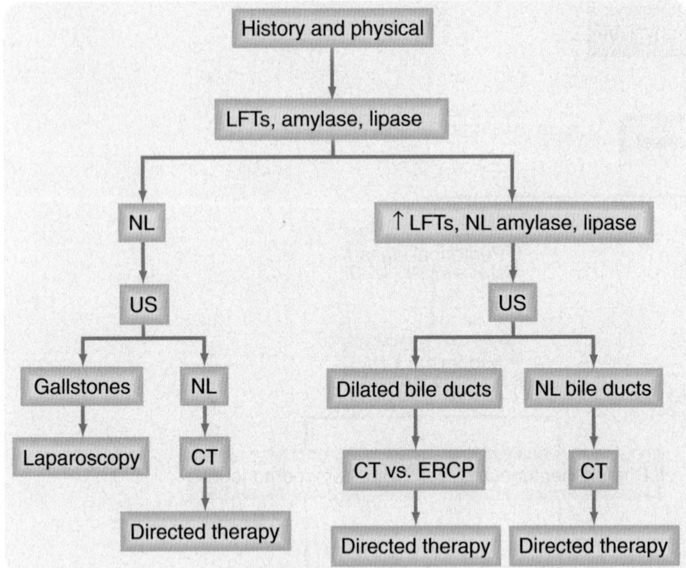


**FIGURE 47-17** Algorithm for the treatment of right upper quadrant abdominal pain. *ERCP,* Endoscopic retrograde cholangiopancreatography; *LFTs,* liver function tests; *NL,* normal study; *US,* ultrasound.

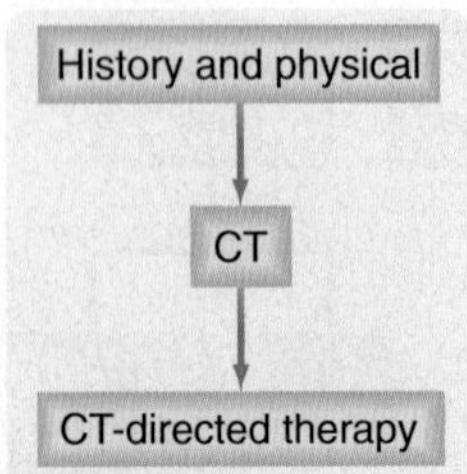


**FIGURE 47-18** Algorithm for the treatment of left upper quadrant abdominal pain.

## SUMMARY

Evaluation and management of the patient with acute abdominal pain remains a challenging part of a surgeon's practice. Although advances in imaging techniques, use of algorithms, and computer assistance have improved the diagnostic accuracy for the conditions causing the acute abdomen, a careful history and physical examination remain the most important part of the evaluation. Even with these tools available, the surgeon must often make the decision to perform a laparoscopy or laparotomy with a good deal of uncertainty about the expected findings. Increased morbidity and mortality associated with a delay in the treatment of many of the surgical causes of the acute abdomen argue for an aggressive and expeditious surgical approach.

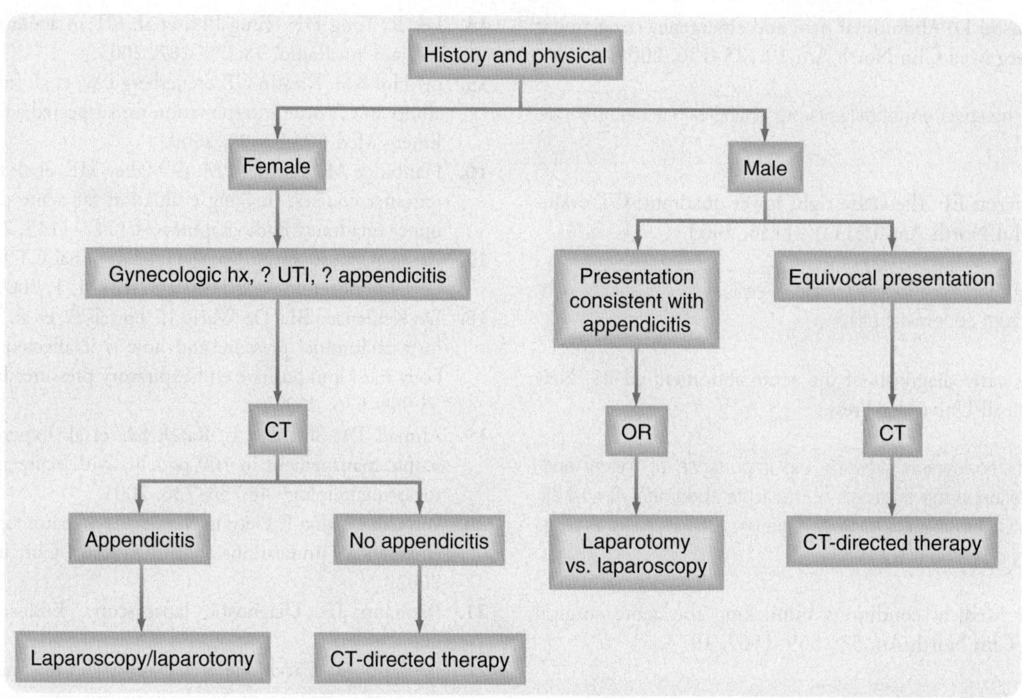


**FIGURE 47-19** Algorithm for the treatment of right lower quadrant abdominal pain. *hx,* History; *OR,* operation; *UTI,* urinary tract infection.

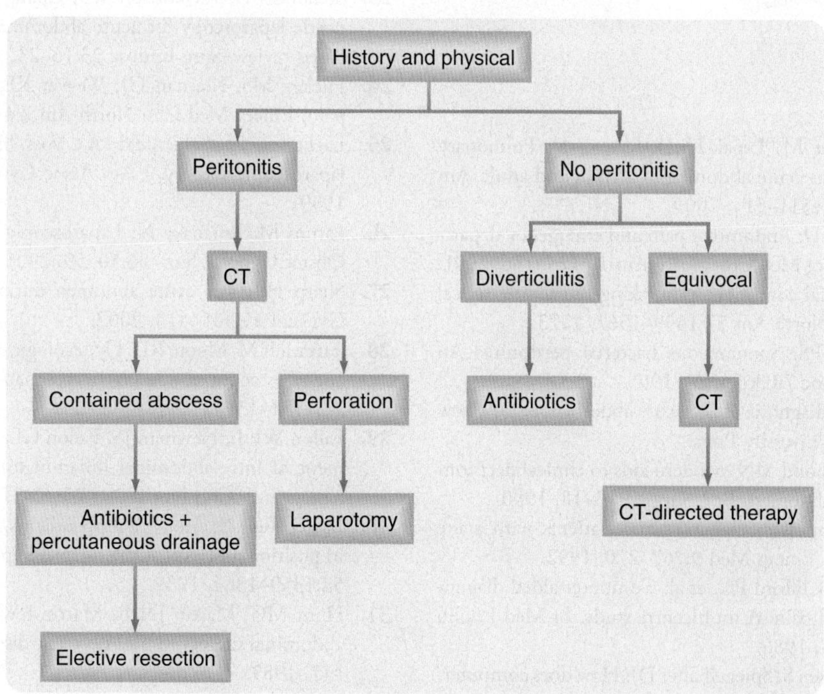


**FIGURE 47-20** Algorithm for the treatment of left lower quadrant abdominal pain.

## SELECTED REFERENCES


Ahmad TA, Shelbaya E, Razek SA, et al: Experience of laparoscopic management in 100 patients with acute abdomen. Hepatogastroenterology 48:733–736, 2001.


A description of the usefulness of laparoscopy in a large series of patients with acute abdomen. This is a good review of this important diagnostic and therapeutic tool.


Cademartiri F, Raaijmaker RHJM, Kuiper JW, et al: Multi-detector row CT angiography in patients with abdominal angina. Radiographics 24:969–984, 2004.


A good review of the computerized tomographic characteristics of acute mesenteric ischemia. This outlines the radiographic findings that have greatly assisted in the diagnosis of this otherwise difficult condition.

Graff LG, Robinson D: Abdominal pain and emergency department evaluation. Emerg Med Clin North Am 19:123–136, 2001.

Good review of the spectrum of patients presenting with acute abdominal pain.

Macari M, Balthazar EJ: The acute right lower quadrant: CT evaluation. Radiol Clin North Am 41:1117–1136, 2003.

A modern discussion of the role of CT in the evaluation of patients with right lower quadrant abdominal pain.

Silen W: Cope's early diagnosis of the acute abdomen, ed 21, New York, 2005, Oxford University Press.

This is a classic monograph stressing the importance of history and physical examination in the diagnosis of the acute abdomen. Almost all diseases presenting as an acute abdomen are presented. This is a must-read for the surgical resident.

Steinheber FU: Medical conditions mimicking the acute surgical abdomen. Med Clin North Am 57:1559–1567, 1973.

This classic article reviews the various medical conditions that can present as an acute abdomen. It is well written and remains pertinent to the evaluation of these patients.

## REFERENCES


1. Sethuraman U, Siadat M, Lepak-Hitch CA, et al: Pulmonary embolism presenting as acute abdomen in a child and adult. Am J Emerg Med 27:514 e511–515, 2009.
2. Graff LGT, Robinson D: Abdominal pain and emergency department evaluation. Emerg Med Clin North Am 19:123–136, 2001.
3. Steinheber FU: Medical conditions mimicking the acute surgical abdomen. Med Clin North Am 57:1559–1567, 1973.
4. Gilbert JA, Kamath PS: Spontaneous bacterial peritonitis: An update. Mayo Clin Proc 70:365–370, 1995.
5. Silen W: Cope's early diagnosis of the acute abdomen, ed 21, New York, 2005, Oxford University Press.
6. Paterson-Brown S, Vipond MN: Modern aids to clinical decision-making in the acute abdomen. Br J Surg 77:13–18, 1990.
7. de Dombal FT: Computers, diagnoses and patients with acute abdominal pain. Arch Emerg Med 9:267–270, 1992.
8. Adams ID, Chan M, Clifford PC, et al: Computer aided diagnosis of acute abdominal pain: A multicentre study. Br Med J (Clin Res Ed) 293:800–804, 1986.
9. Wellwood J, Johannessen S, Spiegelhalter DJ: How does computer-aided diagnosis improve the management of acute abdominal pain? Ann R Coll Surg Engl 74:40–46, 1992.
10. McAdam WA, Brock BM, Armitage T, et al: Twelve years' experience of computer-aided diagnosis in a district general hospital. Ann R Coll Surg Engl 72:140–146, 1990.
11. Kort B, Katz VL, Watson WJ: The effect of nonobstetric operation during pregnancy. Surg Gynecol Obstet 177:371–376, 1993.
12. Macari M, Balthazar EJ: The acute right lower quadrant: CT evaluation. Radiol Clin North Am 41:1117–1136, 2003.
13. Cademartiri F, Raaijmakers RH, Kuiper JW, et al: Multi-detector row CT angiography in patients with abdominal angina. Radiographics 24:969–984, 2004.
14. Lee R, Tung HK, Tung PH, et al: CT in acute mesenteric ischaemia. Clin Radiol 58:279–287, 2003.
15. in't Hof KH, Krestin GP, Steijerberg EW, et al: Interobserver variability in CT scan interpretation for suspected acute appendicitis. Emerg Med J 26:92–94, 2009.
16. Hanbidge AE, Buckler PM, O'Malley ME, et al: From the RSNA refresher courses: Imaging evaluation for acute pain in the right upper quadrant. Radiographics 24:1117–1135, 2004.
17. Zissin R, Osadchy A, Gayer G: Abdominal CT findings in small bowel perforation. Br J Radiol 82:162–171, 2009.
18. De Keulenaer BL, De Waele JJ, Powell B, et al: What is normal intra-abdominal pressure and how is it affected by positioning, body mass and positive end-expiratory pressure? Intens Care Med 35:969–976, 2009.
19. Ahmad TA, Shelbaya E, Razek SA, et al: Experience of laparoscopic management in 100 patients with acute abdomen. Hepatogastroenterology 48:733–736, 2001.
20. Perri SG, Altilia F, Pietrangeli F, et al: [Laparoscopy in abdominal emergencies. Indications and limitations.] Chir Ital 54:165–178, 2002.
21. Riemann JF: Diagnostic laparoscopy. Endoscopy 35:43–47, 2003.
22. Pecoraro AP, Cacchione RN, Sayad P, et al: The routine use of diagnostic laparoscopy in the intensive care unit. Surg Endosc 15:638–641, 2001.
23. Stefanidis D, Richardson WS, Chang L, et al: The role of diagnostic laparoscopy for acute abdominal conditions: an evidence-based review. Surg Endosc 23:16–23, 2009.
24. Hickey MS, Kiernan GJ, Weaver KE: Evaluation of abdominal pain. Emerg Med Clin North Am 7:437–452, 1989.
25. Lachman E, Schienfeld A, Voss E, et al: Pregnancy and laparoscopic surgery. J Am Assoc Gynecol Laparosc 6:347–351, 1999.
26. Fatum M, Rojansky N: Laparoscopic surgery during pregnancy. Obstet Gynecol Surv 56:50–59, 2001.
27. Sharp HT: The acute abdomen during pregnancy. Clin Obstet Gynecol 45:405–413, 2002.
28. Tarraza HM, Moore RD: Gynecologic causes of the acute abdomen and the acute abdomen in pregnancy. Surg Clin North Am 77:1371–1394, 1997.
29. Fallon WF Jr, Newman JS, Fallon GL, et al: The surgical management of intra-abdominal inflammatory conditions during pregnancy. Surg Clin North Am 75:15–31, 1995.
30. Baer J, Reis R, Arens R: Appendicitis in pregnancy with changes in position and axis of the normal appendix in pregnancy. JAMA 52:1359–1364, 1932.
31. Hunt MG, Martin JN Jr, Martin RW, et al: Perinatal aspects of abdominal surgery for nonobstetric disease. Am J Perinatol 6:412–417, 1989.
32. Kammerer WS: Nonobstetric surgery in pregnancy. Med Clin North Am 71:551–560, 1987.
33. Mazze RI, Kallen B: Appendectomy during pregnancy: A Swedish registry study of 778 cases. Obstet Gynecol 77:835–840, 1991.
34. Brown JJ, Wilson C, Coleman S, et al: Appendicitis in pregnancy: An ongoing diagnostic dilemma. Colorectal Dis 11:116–122, 2009.
35. Tamir IL, Bongard FS, Klein SR: Acute appendicitis in the pregnant patient. Am J Surg 160:571–575, 1990.
36. Lim HK, Bae SH, Seo GS: Diagnosis of acute appendicitis in pregnant women: Value of sonography. AJR Am J Roentgenol 159:539–542, 1992.

37. Brown MA, Birchard KR, Semelka RC: Magnetic resonance evaluation of pregnant patients with acute abdominal pain. Semin Ultrasound CT MR 26:206–211, 2005.
38. Cobben LP, Groot I, Haans L, et al: MRI for clinically suspected appendicitis during pregnancy. AJR Am J Roentgenol 183:671–675, 2004.
39. Mahmoodian S: Appendicitis complicating pregnancy. South Med J 85:19–24, 1992.
40. Lanzafame RJ: Laparoscopic cholecystectomy during pregnancy. Surgery 118:627–631, 1995.
41. Printen KJ, Ott RA: Cholecystectomy during pregnancy. Am Surg 44:432–434, 1978.
42. Tsiotos GG, Mullany CJ, Zietlow S, et al: Abdominal complications following cardiac surgery. Am J Surg 167:553–557, 1994.
43. Welling RE, Rath R, Albers JE, et al: Gastrointestinal complications after cardiac surgery. Arch Surg 121:1178–1180, 1986.
44. Gajic O, Urrutia LE, Sewani H, et al: Acute abdomen in the medical intensive care unit. Crit Care Med 30:1187–1190, 2002.
45. Ramachandran I, Sinha R, Rodgers P: Pseudomembranous colitis revisited: Spectrum of imaging findings. Clin Radiol 61:535–544, 2006.
46. Fishman EK, Kavuru M, Jones B, et al: Pseudomembranous colitis: CT evaluation of 26 cases. Radiology 180:57–60, 1991.
47. Kawamoto S, Horton KM, Fishman EK: Pseudomembranous colitis: Spectrum of imaging findings with clinical and pathologic correlation. Radiographics 19:887–897, 1999.
48. Mehran A, Liberman M, Rosenthal R, et al: Ruptured appendicitis after laparoscopic Roux-en-Y gastric bypass: Pitfalls in diagnosing a surgical abdomen in the morbidly obese. Obes Surg 13:938–940, 2003.
49. Byrne TK: Complications of surgery for obesity. Surg Clin North Am 85, 2001.
50. Hamilton EC, Sims TL, Hamilton TT, et al: Clinical predictors of leak after laparoscopic Roux-en-Y gastric bypass for morbid obesity. Surg Endosc 17:679–684, 2003.

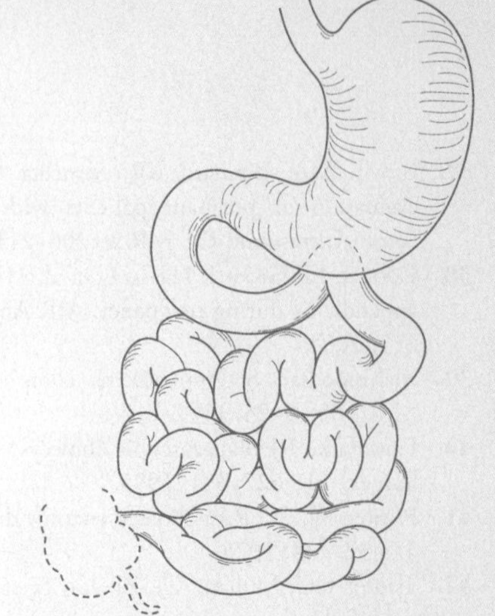

CHAPTER 48

# ACUTE GASTROINTESTINAL HEMORRHAGE

Ali Tavakkolizadeh and Stanley W. Ashley



Acute gastrointestinal (GI) hemorrhage is a common clinical problem with diverse manifestations. This bleeding may range from trivial to massive and can originate from almost any region of the GI tract, including the pancreas, liver, and biliary tree. Although no demographic group is spared, the annual incidence of approximately 170 cases/100,000 adults increases steadily with advancing age, and is slightly more common in men than women.[1] Furthermore, GI hemorrhage accounts for 1% to 2% of acute admissions, resulting in over 300,000 annual hospitalizations in the United States.[2] It is also a common complication in patients hospitalized for other illnesses, especially surgical patients. Although the total economic burden of GI hemorrhage has not been formally assessed, annual estimates have suggested that diverticular bleeding alone costs the health care system in excess of 1.3 billion dollars.[3]

Management of these patients is frequently multidisciplinary, involving emergency medicine, gastroenterology, intensive care, surgery, and interventional radiology. The importance of early surgical consultation in the care of these patients cannot be overemphasized.[4] In addition to aiding in the resuscitation of the unstable patient, in some settings the surgical endoscopist establishes the diagnosis and initiates therapy. Even when the gastroenterologist assumes this role, early collaboration with the surgeon permits the establishment of goals and limits for initial nonoperative therapy. Ultimately, 5% to 10% of patients hospitalized for bleeding require an operation intervention. Prompt surgical consultation permits more time for preoperative preparation and evaluation, as well as patient and family education, if urgent surgical intervention become necessary.[1]

Most patients with an acute GI hemorrhage stop bleeding spontaneously. This allows time for a more elective evaluation. However, in almost 15% of cases, major bleeding persists, requiring emergent resuscitation, evaluation, and treatment.[5] Improvements in the management of such patients, primarily by means of early endoscopy and directed therapy, have significantly reduced the length of hospitalization. Despite this, mortality remains more than 5% and is significantly higher in those initially hospitalized for other reasons. This discrepancy between therapeutic advances and outcomes is probably related to the aging of the population, with an increase in comorbidity. Today, the patient requiring operative intervention is both older and sicker than in the past.

Hemorrhage can originate from any region of the GI tract and is typically classified based on its location relative to the ligament of Treitz. Upper GI hemorrhage from proximal to the ligament of Treitz accounts for more than 80% of cases of acute bleeding.[1] Peptic ulcer disease and variceal hemorrhage are the most common causes. Most lower GI bleeding is from the colon, with diverticula and angiodysplasias accounting for most cases. In less than 5% of patients, the small intestine in responsible.[1] Obscure bleeding is defined as hemorrhage that persists or recurs after negative endoscopy. Occult bleeding is not apparent to patients until they present with symptoms related to the anemia. Determination of the site of bleeding is important for directing diagnostic interventions with minimal delay. However, attempts to localize the source should never precede appropriate resuscitative measures.

## APPROACH TO THE PATIENT

In patients with GI bleeding, several fundamental principles of initial evaluation and management must be followed. A well-defined and logical approach to the patient with GI hemorrhage is outlined in Figure 48-1. On presentation, a rapid initial assessment permits determination of the urgency of the situation. Resuscitation is initiated with stabilization of the patient's hemodynamic status and the establishment of a means for monitoring ongoing blood loss. A careful history and physical examination should provide clues to the cause and source of the bleeding and identify any complicating conditions or medications. Specific investigation should proceed to refine the diagnosis. Therapeutic measures are then initiated, bleeding is controlled, and recurrent hemorrhage is prevented.

### Initial Assessment

Adequacy of the patient's airway and breathing take first priority. Once these are ensured, the patient's hemodynamic status becomes the dominant concern and forms the basis for further management. The presentation of GI bleeding is variable, ranging from hemoccult-positive stool on rectal examination to exsanguinating hemorrhage. Initial evaluation should focus on rapid assessment of the magnitude of the preexisting deficits and of ongoing hemorrhage. Continuous reassessment of the patient's circulatory status determines the aggressiveness of subsequent evaluation and intervention. The history of the bleeding, its magnitude and frequency, should also provide some guidance.

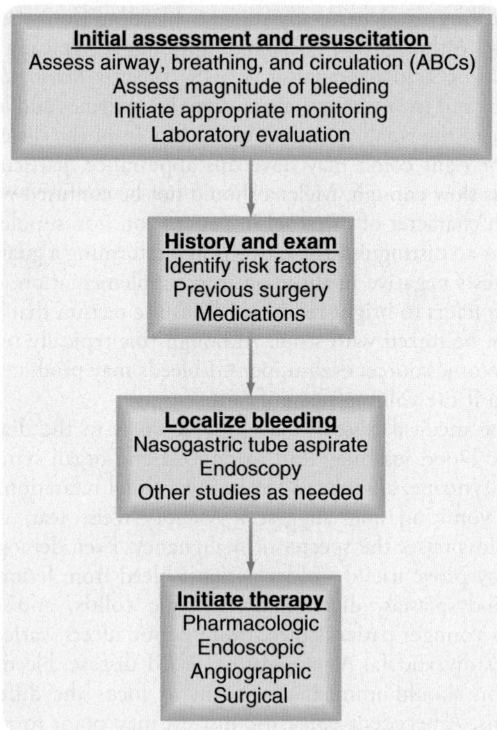


**FIGURE 48-1** General approach to the patient with acute GI hemorrhage.

The severity of the hemorrhage can be generally determined based on simple clinical parameters. Obtundation, agitation, and hypotension (systolic blood pressure <90 mm Hg in the supine position), associated with cool clammy extremities, are consistent with hemorrhagic shock and suggest a loss of more than 40% of the patients' blood volume. A resting heart rate over 100 beats/min, with a decreased pulse pressure, implies a 20% to 40% volume loss. In patients without shock, postural changes should be elicited by allowing the patient to sit up with his or her legs dangling for 5 minutes. A fall in blood pressure of more than 10 mm Hg or an elevation of the pulse of more than 20 beats/min again reflects at least a 20% blood loss. Patients with lesser degrees of bleeding may have no detectable alterations.

The hematocrit is not a useful parameter for assessing the degree of hemorrhage in the acute setting because the proportion of red blood cells and plasma initially lost is constant. The hematocrit level does not fall until plasma is redistributed into the intravascular space and resuscitation with crystalloid solution is begun. Similarly, the absence of tachycardia may be misleading; some patients with severe blood loss may actually have bradycardia secondary to vagal slowing of the heart. Hemodynamic signs are less reliable in older patients and patients taking beta blockers.

## Risk Stratification

Not all patients with GI bleeding require hospital admission or emergent evaluation. For example, the patient with a small amount of rectal bleeding that has ceased can generally be evaluated on an outpatient basis. Clearly, in many patients, the decision making is less straightforward. Others require admission and observation but may be further evaluated with endoscopy on a more *selective* basis. Several prognostic factors have been associated with adverse outcomes including the need for emergent operation and death (Box 48-1).[6] These factors should be considered during the initial assessment and resuscitation of patient with GI hemorrhage. For example, patients older than 60 years have higher mortality rates than their younger counterparts and should be evaluated more cautiously. This increased morbidity may be a reflection of concomitant disease. The deleterious effects of cardiac, renal, pulmonary, and hepatic comorbidity should all be considered when evaluating patient with GI bleeding. For example, one study has estimated that bleeding patients with significant renal disease have a mortality of almost 30%, which this increases to 65% in the presence of acute renal failure.[7] Other factors, including the magnitude of the initial hemorrhage, persistence or recurrence of the bleeding, and onset of bleeding during hospitalization for another illness also contributes to increased morbidity and mortality.

**BOX 48-1 Risk Factors for Morbidity and Mortality in Acute Gastrointestinal Hemorrhage**

- Age >60 yr
- Comorbid disease
  - Renal failure
  - Liver disease
  - Respiratory insufficiency
  - Cardiac disease
- Magnitude of the hemorrhage
  - Systolic blood pressure <100 mm Hg on presentation
  - Transfusion requirement
- Persistent or recurrent hemorrhage
- Onset of hemorrhage during hospitalization
- Need for surgery

Considerable effort has been devoted to the development of risk-scoring tools to facilitate patient triage. These scoring systems have been used to predict the risk of rebleeding and mortality, evaluate the need for intensive care unit admission (ICU), and determine the need for urgent endoscopy. Some scoring systems are nonspecific to GI bleeding (e.g., APACHE II scores) but can provide general information about the patient's condition and risk of adverse outcomes. There have also been attempts to develop disease specific scoring systems, such as the BLEED classification, that uses five criteria[8]: ongoing bleeding, systolic blood pressure less than 100 mm Hg, prothrombin time more than 1.2 times control, altered mental status, and unstable comorbid disease process that would require ICU admission. If any one of these criteria is present, the model predicts an approximately threefold increase in the risk of recurrent hemorrhage, need for surgical intervention, or death. Other systems take into account endoscopic findings that can improve on their predictive accuracy. Such scoring systems have been almost exclusively used in research studies, however, and until these have been prospectively validated for everyday clinical practice, they should only be applied in the context of clinical judgment.

## Resuscitation

The more severe the bleeding, the more aggressive the resuscitation. The single leading cause of morbidity and mortality in these patients is multiorgan failure related to inadequate initial or subsequent resuscitation. Intubation and ventilation should be initiated early if there is any question of respiratory compromise. In patients with evidence of hemodynamic instability or those in whom ongoing bleeding is suspected, two large-bore IV lines should be placed, preferably in the antecubital fossae. Unstable patients should receive a 2-liter bolus of crystalloid solution, usually lactated Ringer's, which most closely approximates the electrolyte composition of whole blood. The response to the fluid resuscitation should be noted. Blood should immediately be sent for type and crossmatch, hematocrit, platelet count, coagulation profile, routine chemistries, and liver function tests. A Foley catheter should also be inserted for assessment of end-organ perfusion. In older patients and patients with significant cardiac, pulmonary, or renal disease, placement of a central venous or pulmonary artery catheter should be considered for closer monitoring. The oxygen-carrying capacity of the blood can be maximized by administering supplemental oxygen. Frequently, these patients benefit from early admission to and management in the ICU.

The decision to transfuse blood depends on the response to the fluid challenge, age of the patient, whether concomitant cardiopulmonary disease is present, and whether the bleeding continues. The initial effects of crystalloid infusion and the patient's ongoing hemodynamic parameters should be the primary criteria. Once again, this process requires an element of clinical judgment. For example, a young healthy patient with estimated blood loss of 25% who responds to the fluid challenge with a normalization of hemodynamics may not need any blood products, whereas an older patient with a significant cardiac history and the same blood loss probably requires a transfusion. Although the hematocrit may take 12 to 24 hours to equilibrate fully, it is commonly used as one index of the need for blood replacement. In general, the hematocrit should be maintained above 30% in older adults and above 20% in young, otherwise healthy patients. Similarly, the propensity of the suspected lesion to continue bleeding or rebleed must play a role in this decision. For example, esophageal varices are likely to continue to bleed and transfusion might be considered earlier than if a Mallory-Weiss tear, which has a low rebleeding rate, is considered to be the culprit. In general, packed red blood cells are the preferred form of transfusion although whole blood, preferably warmed, may be used in scenarios of massive blood loss. Defects in coagulation and platelets should be replaced as they are detected and patients who require more than 10 U of blood should receive fresh-frozen plasma, platelets, and calcium empirically.

## History and Physical Examination

Once the severity of the bleeding is assessed and resuscitation initiated, attention is directed to the history and physical examination. The history helps make a preliminary assessment of the site and cause of bleeding and of significant medical conditions that could determine or alter the course of management.

Obviously, the characteristics of the bleeding provide important clues. The time of onset, volume, and frequency are important in estimating blood loss. Hematemesis, melena, and hematochezia are the most common manifestations of acute hemorrhage. Hematemesis is the vomiting of blood and is usually caused by bleeding from the upper GI tract although, rarely, bleeding from the nose or pharynx can be responsible. It may be bright red or older and therefore take on the appearance of coffee grounds. Melena, the passage of black, tarry, and foul-smelling stool, generally suggests bleeding from the upper GI tract. Although the melanotic appearance typically results from gastric acid degradation which converts hemoglobin to hematin, and from the actions of digestive enzymes and luminal bacteria in the small intestine, blood loss from the distal small bowel or right colon may have this appearance, particularly if transit is slow enough. Melena should not be confused with the greenish character of the stool in patients on iron supplements. One way to distinguish these two is by performing a guaiac test, which tests negative in those on iron supplementation. Hematochezia refers to bright red blood from the rectum that may or may not be mixed with stool. Although this typically reflects a distal colonic source, even upper GI bleeds may produce hematochezia if the volume is significant.

The medical history may provide clues to the diagnosis. Chronic blood loss may lead to non-GI end-organ symptoms, such as syncope, angina, and even myocardial infarction. Antecedent vomiting may suggest a Mallory-Weiss tear, whereas weight loss raises the specter of malignancy. Even demographic data may prove useful—older patients bleed from lesions such as angiodysplasias, diverticula, ischemic colitis, and cancer, whereas younger patients bleed from peptic ulcers, varices, and Meckel's diverticula. A past history of GI disease, bleeding, or operation should immediately begin to focus the differential diagnosis. Antecedent epigastric distress may point to a peptic ulcer, whereas previous aortic surgery suggests the possibility of aortoenteric fistula. A history of liver disease prompts a consideration of variceal bleeding. Medication use may also be revealing. A history of ingestion of salicylates, nonsteroidal anti-inflammatory drugs (NSAIDs), and/or selective serotonin-reuptake inhibitors (SSRIs) is common, particularly in older patients.[9] These medications are associated with GI mucosal erosions typically seen in the upper GI tract, but occasionally in the small bowel and colon. GI bleeding in the setting of anticoagulation therapy, warfarin or low-molecular-weight heparin, is still usually the result of GI pathology and should not be ascribed to the anticoagulation alone.[10]

The physical examination may also be revealing. The oropharynx and nose can occasionally simulate symptoms from a more distal source and should always be examined. Abdominal examination is only occasionally helpful but is important to exclude masses, splenomegaly, and adenopathy. Epigastric tenderness is suggestive, but not diagnostic, of gastritis or peptic ulceration. The stigmata of liver disease, including jaundice, ascites, palmar erythema, and caput medusae, may suggest bleeding related to varices, although these patients commonly bleed from other sources as well. Occasionally, the physical examination may reveal clues to more obscure diagnoses, such as the telangiectasias of Osler-Weber-Rendu syndrome or the pigmented lesions of the oral mucosa in Peutz-Jeghers syndrome. A rectal examination and anoscopy should be performed to exclude a low-lying rectal cancer or bleeding from hemorrhoids.

## Localization

Subsequent management of the patient with acute GI hemorrhage depends on localization of the site of the bleeding. An algorithm for the diagnosis of acute GI hemorrhage is shown in Figure 48-2.

Although melena is usually from the upper GI tract, it can be the result of bleeding from the small bowel and/or colon.

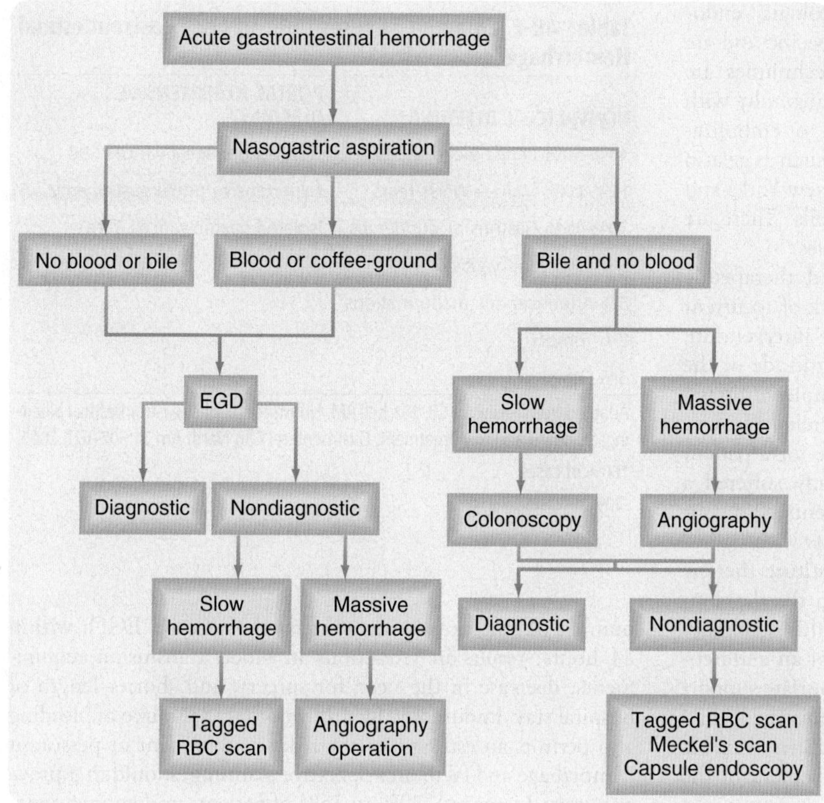


**FIGURE 48-2** Algorithm for the diagnosis of acute GI hemorrhage.

Similarly, hematochezia is sometimes the consequence of brisk upper GI bleeding. One approach to distinguishing these possibilities is the insertion of a nasogastric (NG) tube and examination of the aspirate. Although hematemesis is usually diagnostic of an upper GI bleed, the NG tube is still useful to assess the rate of ongoing bleeding and to begin to remove blood from the stomach to permit endoscopy. If the aspirate is positive, this effectively localizes the lesion. The presence of red blood or a coffee grounds appearance suggests an upper GI source. Testing for occult blood is rarely necessary. The return of bile from a gastric aspirate suggests that the duodenum has been sampled. Although a bilious, nonbloody, gastric aspirate generally excludes the upper GI tract, these findings can occasionally be misleading. One study found that only 6 of 10 yellow-green nasogastric aspirates actually tested positive for bile.[11] Similarly, almost 20% of patients with a clear aspirate are still bleeding from an upper GI source.[2] In patients with melena or even hematochezia from an upper lesion, the NG aspirate may be negative in the presence of significant duodenal bleeding and a competent pylorus preventing duodenogastric reflux. These considerations suggest that although the findings of the NG aspirate could be helpful, almost all patients with significant bleeding should undergo upper endoscopy.

Upper endoscopy under these circumstances is highly accurate for identifying an upper GI lesion and, if negative, for directing attention to a lower GI source. To maximize efficacy, early endoscopy should be performed within 24 hours, even in stable patients.[12] Early endoscopy with directed therapy has been shown to reduce resource use and transfusion requirements, and shorten hospital stay. The exact definition and timeline of an early endoscopy has been well studied and refined. Although there is little argument that in an unstable patient, an urgent endoscopy is often required, in those with overt sign of bleeding but who are stable, an endoscopy within 6 or 12 hours has not been shown to be of any additional benefit to endoscopies performed within 24 hours.[13,14]

Clinicians should be aware that esophagogastroduodenoscopy (EGD) in the urgent or emergent setting is associated with reduced accuracy, often because of poor visualization, and a significant increase in the incidence of complications, including aspiration, respiratory depression, and GI perforation, when compared with elective procedures. Airway protection is critical and may require endotracheal intubation if was not performed previously. Volume resuscitation should not be interrupted by the examination.

Subsequent evaluation depends on the results of the upper endoscopy and volume of the bleeding (Fig. 48-2). Angiography or even surgery may prove necessary for massive hemorrhage, precluding endoscopy, from the upper or lower GI tract. For slow or intermittent bleeding from the lower GI tract, colonoscopy is now the initial diagnostic maneuver of choice. When this is nondiagnostic, the tagged red blood cell (RBC) scan is usually used. For obscure bleeding, usually from the small bowel, capsule endoscopy has become the appropriate study. These diagnostic procedures are discussed subsequently in greater detail.

## Treatment

Depending on the source of the bleeding, a variety of therapeutic options are available. These include pharmacologic, endoscopic, angiographic, and surgical modalities. Pharmacologic, endoscopic, and surgical therapies are generally site-specific and are discussed in more detail later. Angiographic techniques are somewhat more generic and include selective angiography with infusion of a vasoconstrictor, typically vasopressin, or embolization. Embolic agents include temporary materials such as gelatin sponge (Gelfoam; Pharmacia & Upjohn, Pfizer, New York) and autologous clot or permanent devices such as coils. There are few data comparing the efficacy of these techniques.

For most patients, bleeding has ceased and therapeutic options are applied to prevent recurrence. The risk of recurrent bleeding, and therefore the need for preventative intervention, depends on the characteristics of the lesion, magnitude of the initial hemorrhage, and specific patient. For example, although the risk of recurrent diverticular hemorrhage is relatively low, elective colonic resection may still be appropriate for a patient with significant coronary disease who has already suffered a major bleed. For the approximately 15% of patients who continue to bleed, therapy is more urgent. In patients with hemodynamic instability, an appropriate goal is to institute therapy within 2 hours of presentation. This depends on the development of institution-specific protocols for the multidisciplinary management of these patients.[2] The availability of an endoscopist trained in techniques of hemostasis and appropriate support staff is critical. Similarly, angiographic expertise must be immediately accessible. Despite the relatively new modalities available for nonoperative control of bleeding, early involvement of the surgical team remains essential.

Traditional series demonstrated that the morbidity and mortality of surgery for GI bleeding increases significantly in patients who have lost more than 6 U of blood. This increase is particularly marked in older patients and those with major comorbidities, suggesting that intervention in these patients should be earlier than that for young healthy patients who might otherwise be better operative candidates. Although improvements in supportive care and directed therapy, particularly endoscopic, may have somewhat moderated this approach, surgical therapy should always be a serious consideration in the context of blood loss of this magnitude.

**Table 48-1 Common Causes of Upper Gastrointestinal Hemorrhage***

| NONVARICEAL BLEEDING* | PORTAL HYPERTENSIVE BLEEDING† |
|---|---|
| 30%-50% Peptic ulcer disease | Gastroesophageal varices >90 |
| 15%-20% Mallory-Weiss tears | Hypertensive portal gastropathy, <5 |
| 10%-15% Gastritis or duodenitis | Isolated gastric varices, rare |
| 5%-10% Esophagitis | |
| 5% Arteriovenous malformations | |
| 2% Tumors | |
| 5% Others | |

Adapted from Ferguson CB, Mitchell RM: Nonvariceal upper gastrointestinal bleeding: Standard and new treatment. Gastroenterol Clin North Am 34:607–621, 2005.

*80% of cases.

†20% of cases.

## ACUTE UPPER GI HEMORRHAGE

Upper GI bleeding refers to bleeding that arises from the GI tract proximal to the ligament of Treitz; it accounts for almost 80% of significant GI hemorrhage. The causes of upper GI bleeding are best categorized as nonvariceal sources or bleeding related to portal hypertension (Table 48-1). The nonvariceal causes account for approximately 80% of this bleeding, with peptic ulcer disease being the most common.[1] In the remaining 20% of patients, most of whom have cirrhosis, portal hypertension can lead to the development of gastroesophageal varices, isolated gastric varices, or hypertensive portal gastropathy, any of which can be the source of an acute upper GI bleed. Although patients with cirrhosis are at high risk of developing variceal bleeding, nonvariceal sources account for most upper GI bleeds, even in these patients.[2] However, because of greater morbidity and mortality of variceal bleeding, patients with cirrhosis should generally be assumed to have variceal bleeding; appropriate therapy should be initiated until an emergent endoscopy has demonstrated another cause for the hemorrhage.

The foundation for the diagnosis and management of patients with an upper GI bleed is an upper endoscopy. A number of studies have demonstrated that early EGD, within 24 hours, results in reductions in blood transfusion requirements, decrease in the need for surgery, and shorter length of hospital stay. Endoscopic identification of the source of bleeding also permits an estimate of the risk of subsequent or persistent hemorrhage and facilitates operative planning, should that prove necessary. In general, 20% to 35% of patients undergoing upper GI endoscopy will require a therapeutic endoscopic intervention, and 5% to 10% will eventually require surgery.[12]

As noted, it is somewhat surprising that studies have not shown any benefits in performing an endoscopy sooner (within 6 or 12 hours) than within 24 hours.[13,14] Although the best tool for localization of the bleeding source is an EGD, this intervention is associated with increased risk and poor visualization in the acute setting, which may offset some of its benefits. In 1% to 2% of patients with upper GI hemorrhage, the source cannot be identified because of the excessive blood impairing the visualization of the mucosal surface.[15] Aggressive lavage of the stomach with room temperature normal saline solution prior to the procedure can be helpful. Evidence has suggested that a single bolus injection of IV erythromycin, which stimulates gastric emptying, can significantly improve visualization.[16] If identification of the source is still not possible, angiography may be appropriate in the reasonably stable patient, although operative intervention should be seriously considered if the blood loss is extreme or the patient hemodynamically unstable. A tagged RBC scan is seldom necessary with a confirmed upper GI bleed and contrast studies are usually contraindicated because they will interfere with subsequent maneuvers.

### Specific Causes of Upper Gastrointestinal Hemorrhage

#### Nonvariceal Bleeding

**Peptic Ulcer Disease** Peptic ulcer disease (PUD) still represents the most frequent cause of upper GI hemorrhage, accounting for approximately 40% of all cases.[2] Approximately 10% to 15% of patients with PUD develop bleeding at some point in the course of their disease. Bleeding is the most frequent indication for operation and the principal cause for death in PUD. PUD is discussed in more detail in Chapter 49; this discussion focuses only on bleeding from ulcer disease.

The epidemiology of peptic ulcer continues to change. The incidence of uncomplicated peptic ulcer disease has declined dramatically. This change has been attributed to better medical therapy, including the use of proton pump inhibitors (PPIs) and regimens for the eradication of *Helicobacter pylori* (*H. pylori*). Despite this overall decline in ulcer frequency, the number of patients undergoing operation for ulcer-related complications had remained surprisingly stable until now. Recent reports, however, are documenting a decline in the rate of some, but not all, ulcer-related complications requiring surgical intervention. Although the need for surgery for perforated PUD has declined, the rate of bleeding PUD requiring surgical intervention has remained stable.[17] Some population-based studies in older patients have documented an increase in PUD bleeding requiring hospital admission.[18] Thus, when surgeries for upper GI hemorrhage are undertaken, they are now typically performed in the oldest and often the sickest patients.

Bleeding develops as a consequence of peptic acid erosion of the mucosal surface. Although chronic blood loss is common with any ulcer, significant bleeding typically results when there is involvement of an artery of the submucosa or, with penetration of the ulcer, an even larger vessel. Although duodenal ulcers are more common than gastric ulcers, gastric ulcers usually bleed; as a result, in most series, the relative proportions are almost equal. The most significant hemorrhage occurs when duodenal or gastric ulcers penetrate into branches of the gastroduodenal artery or left gastric arteries, respectively.

***Treatment*** Figure 48-3 outlines an approach to management. As noted, patients with clinical evidence of a GI bleed should receive an endoscopy within 24 hours and, while awaiting this procedure, they should be treated with a PPI. Although this approach has been shown to reduce the stigmata of a recent hemorrhage at index endoscopy, it has had no impact on clinical outcomes, such as transfusion requirement, mortality, or need for surgery. Nevertheless, it is believed to be a cost-effective intervention for those suspected of having an upper GI bleed.[19]

After the index endoscopy, treatment strategies depend on the appearance of the lesion at endoscopy. Endoscopic therapy is instituted if bleeding is active or, when bleeding has already stopped, if there is a significant risk of rebleeding. The ability to predict the risk of rebleeding permits prophylactic therapy, closer monitoring, and earlier detection of hemorrhage in high-risk patients. The Forrest classification was developed in an attempt to assess this risk based on endoscopic findings and stratify the patients into low-, intermediate-, and high-risk groups (Table 48-2). Endoscopic therapy is recommended in cases of active bleeding as well as those with a visible vessel (Forrest I to IIa). In case of an adherent clot (Forrest IIb), the clot is removed and the underlying lesion evaluated. Ulcers with a clean base or black spot, secondary to hematin deposition, are generally not treated endoscopically.

MEDICAL MANAGEMENT In cases of a confirmed peptic ulcer bleed, PPIs have been shown to reduce the risk of rebleeding and the need for surgical intervention. Therefore, patients with a suspected or confirmed bleeding ulcer should be started on a PPI.[20] Unlike perforated ulcers, which are generally associated with *H. pylori* infection, the association between *H. pylori*

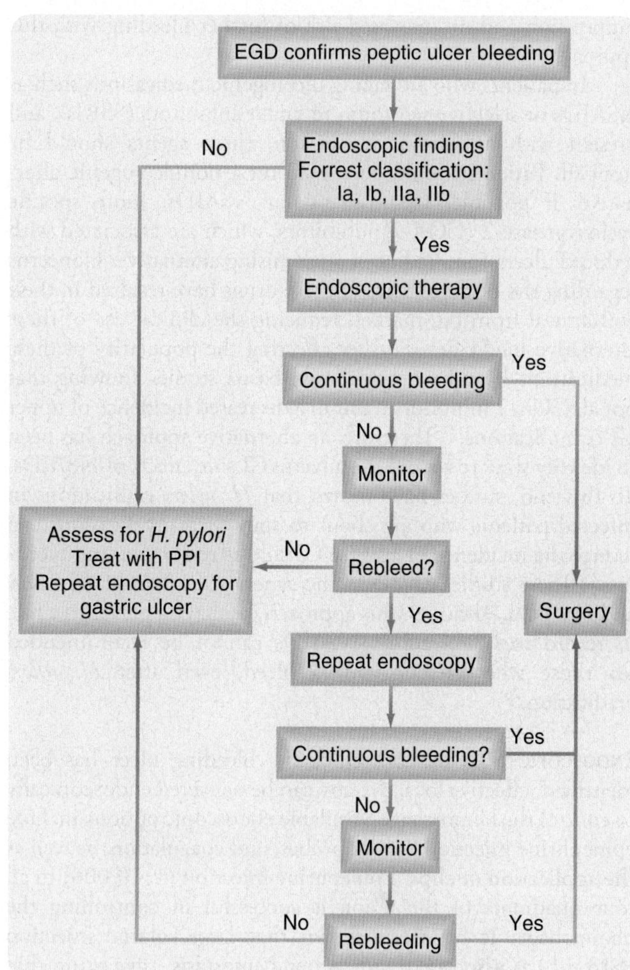


**FIGURE 48-3** Algorithm for the diagnosis and management of nonvariceal upper GI bleeding.

**Table 48-2 Forrest Classification for Endoscopic Findings and Rebleeding Risks in Peptic Ulcer Disease**

| **Classification** | | |
|---|---|---|
| **GRADE** | **DESCRIPTION** | **REBLEEDING RISK** |
| Ia | Active, pulsatile bleeding | High |
| Ib | Active, nonpulsatile bleeding | High |
| IIa | Nonbleeding visible vessel | High |
| IIb | Adherent clot | Intermediate |
| IIc | Ulcer with black spot | Low |
| III | Clean, nonbleeding ulcer bed | Low |

infection and bleeding is weaker. Only 60% to 70% of patients with a bleeding ulcer are *H. pylor*–positive.[21] This has generated some discussion about the importance of *H. pylori* treatment in patients with a bleeding peptic ulcer. Several studies and a large meta-analysis, however, have shown that *H. pylori* treatment and eradication, in patients who test positive for the infection, result in decreased rebleeding.[22] Importantly, once the *H. pylori* infection has been eradicated, there is no need for long-term acid suppression and no increased risk of further bleeding with this approach.[23]

In patients who are taking ulcerogenic medications such as NSAIDs or selective serotonin reuptake inhibitors (SSRIs), and present with a bleeding GI lesion, these agents should be stopped. Patients should be started on a nonulcerogenic alternative, if possible. In those taking NSAIDs, more specific cycloxygenase-2 (COX-2) inhibitors, which are associated with reduced ulceration, had been a promising alternative. Concerns regarding the cardiotoxicity of these drugs have resulted in their withdrawal from the market, reducing the clinical use of these alternative medicines. Further affecting the popularity of these medications have been population-based studies showing that not all COX-2 inhibitors result in a decreased incidence of upper GI complications.[24] Therefore, an alternative approach has been to identify ways to reduce the adverse GI side effects of NSAIDs. To this end, studies have shown that *H. pylori* eradications in infected patients who are about to start these medications can reduce the incidence of adverse GI side effects, including bleeding.[25] These studies highlight the synergistic effect of *H. pylori* and NSAIDs. Although this approach can have a preventive role in regard to GI bleeding, NSAIDs cannot be recommended for those who present with a bleed, even after *H. pylori* eradication.[26]

**Endoscopic Management** Once the bleeding ulcer has been identified, effective local therapy can be delivered endoscopically to control the hemorrhage. Available endoscopic options include epinephrine injection, heater probes, and coagulation, as well as the application of clips. Epinephrine injection (1 : 10,000) to all four quadrants of the lesion is successful in controlling the hemorrhage. It has been shown that large-volume injection (>13 mL) is associated with better hemostasis, suggesting that the endoscopic injection works in part by compressing the bleeding vessel and inducing tamponade.[27] Epinephrine injection alone is associated with a high rebleeding rate; standard practice is to provide combination therapy. This usually means the addition of thermal therapy to the injection. The sources of thermal energy can be heater probes, monopolar or bipolar electrocoagulation, or laser or argon plasma coagulation (APC). The most commonly used energy sources are electrocoagulation for bleeding ulcers and APC for superficial lesions. A combination of injection with thermal therapy achieves hemostasis in 90% of bleeding PUDs. The role of hemoclips is less clear; several studies have reported mixed results. Hemoclips (Fig. 48-4), which can be difficult to apply, may be particularly effective when dealing with a spurting vessel because they provide immediate control of hemorrhage.

Rebleeding of an ulcer is associated with a significant increase in mortality, and careful observation of patients at high risk of rebleeding, using criteria previously described, is important. In those who rebleed, the role of a second attempt at endoscopic control has been controversial but has been validated. For example, one study has demonstrated that a second attempt at endoscopic hemostasis is successful in 75% of patients.[28] Although this will fail in 25% of patients, who will then require emergent surgery, there does not appear to be any increase in morbidity or mortality with this treatment approach. Therefore, most clinicians would now encourage a second attempt at endoscopic control before subjecting the patient to surgery.

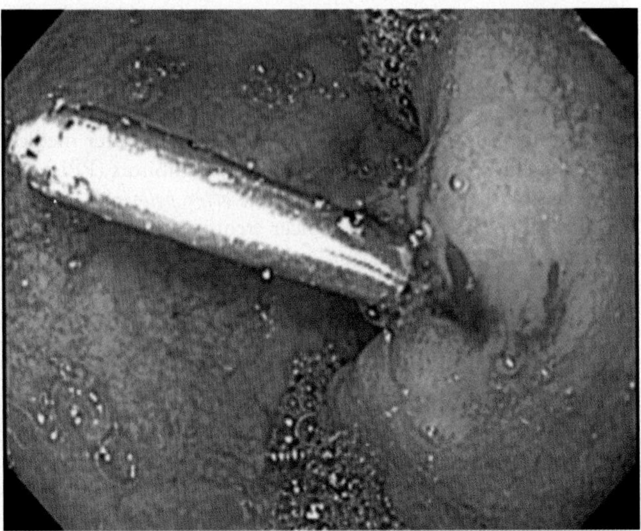

**FIGURE 48-4** Hemoclip that has been applied to a bleeding duodenal ulcer. (Courtesy Dr. Linda S. Lee, Brigham and Women's Hospital, Boston.)

**BOX 48-2 Indications for Surgery in Gastrointestinal Hemorrhage**

Hemodynamic instability despite vigorous resuscitation (>6 U transfusion)
Failure of endoscopic techniques to arrest hemorrhage
Recurrent hemorrhage after initial stabilization (with up to two attempts at obtaining endoscopic hemostasis)
Shock associated with recurrent hemorrhage
Continued slow bleeding with a transfusion requirement >3 U/day

**Surgical Management** Despite significant advances in endoscopic therapy, approximately 10% of patients with bleeding ulcers still require surgical intervention for effective hemostasis. Identifying patients who are likely to fail endoscopic therapy is difficult, however, and timing of surgery has been greatly debated. To assist in this decision making, several clinical and endoscopic parameters have been proposed that are thought to identify patients at high risk of failed endoscopic therapy. The clinical factors to consider are shock and a low hemoglobin level at presentation. At the time of endoscopy, although the Forrest classification is the most important indicator of rebleeding risk, the location and size of the ulcer are also significant. Ulcers larger than 2 cm, posterior duodenal ulcers, and gastric ulcers have a significantly higher risk of rebleeding.[29,30] Patients with these characteristics need closer monitoring and possibly earlier surgical intervention. Clearly, clinical judgment and local expertise must play a critical role in this decision.

Indications for surgery were traditionally based on the blood transfusion requirements. Increased blood transfusions are clearly associated with increased mortality. Although a less definitive criterion than it was formerly, most surgeons still consider an ongoing blood transfusion requirement in excess of 6 U an indication for surgical intervention, particularly in older patients, although an 8- to10-U loss may be more acceptable for younger patients. Current indications for surgery for peptic ulcer hemorrhage are summarized in Box 48-2. Secondary or relative indications include a rare blood type or difficult crossmatch, refusal of transfusion, shock on presentation, advanced age, severe comorbid disease, and a bleeding chronic gastric ulcer for which malignancy is a concern.

The first priority at operation should be control of the hemorrhage. Once this is accomplished, a decision must be made regarding the need for a definitive acid-reducing procedure. Each of these steps varies, depending on whether the lesion is a duodenal or gastric ulcer.

**Duodenal Ulcer.** The first step in surgery for a duodenal ulcer is exposure of the bleeding site. Because most of these lesions are in the duodenal bulb, longitudinal duodenotomy or duodenopyloromyotomy is performed. Hemorrhage can typically be controlled initially with pressure and then direct suture ligation with nonabsorbable suture. When ulcers are positioned anteriorly, four-quadrant suture ligation usually suffices. A posterior ulcer eroding into the pancreaticoduodenal or gastroduodenal artery may require suture ligation of the vessel proximal and distal to the ulcer, as well as placement of a U stich underneath the ulcer to control the pancreatic branches.

Once the bleeding has been addressed, a definitive acid-reducing operation should be considered. With the identification of the role of *H. pylori* infection in duodenal ulcer, the usefulness of such a procedure has been questioned, based on the argument that simple closure and subsequent treatment for infection should be sufficient to prevent recurrence. In contrast with a perforated ulcer, for which there is convincing evidence to support such an approach (see earlier), the evidence is weaker for a bleeding duodenal ulcer. Therefore, the controversy continues; the decision is probably best tailored based on the patient's clinical condition and surgeon's experience.

Historically, the choice among various operations was based on the hemodynamic condition of the patient and on whether there was a long-standing history of refractory ulcer disease. The various operations for PUD are discussed in greater detail in Chapter 49. Because the pylorus has often been opened longitudinally to control the bleeding, closure as a pyloroplasty, combined with truncal vagotomy, is the most frequently used operation for bleeding duodenal ulcer. There is some evidence to suggest that parietal cell vagotomy may represent a better therapy for a bleeding duodenal ulcer in the stable patient, although some of this benefit may be abrogated if the pylorus has been divided. Today, surgeon inexperience with this procedure may be the determining factor. In a patient who has a known history of refractory duodenal ulcer disease or who has failed more conservative surgery, antrectomy with truncal vagotomy may be more appropriate. However, this procedure is more complex and should be undertaken rarely in a hemodynamically unstable patient.

**Gastric Ulcer.** For a bleeding gastric ulcer, again, control of bleeding is the immediate priority. Although it may initially require gastrotomy and suture ligation, this alone is associated with a high risk of rebleeding of almost 30%. In addition, because of a 10% incidence of malignancy, gastric ulcer resection is generally indicated. Simple excision alone is associated with rebleeding in as many as 20% of patients so distal gastrectomy is generally preferred, although excision combined with vagotomy and pyloroplasty may be considered for the high-risk patient. Bleeding ulcers of the proximal stomach near the gastroesophageal junction are more difficult to manage. Proximal or near-total gastrectomy is associated with a particularly high mortality in the setting of acute hemorrhage. Options include distal gastrectomy combined with resection of a tongue of proximal stomach to include the ulcer, and vagotomy and pyloroplasty combined with wedge resection or simple oversewing of the ulcer.

**Mallory-Weiss Tears** Mallory-Weiss tears are mucosal and submucosal tears that occur near the gastroesophageal junction. These lesions usually develop in alcoholic patients after a period of intense retching and vomiting following binge drinking, but can occur in any patient who has a history of repeated emesis. The mechanism, proposed by Mallory and Weiss in 1929, is forceful contraction of the abdominal wall against an unrelaxed cardia, resulting in mucosal laceration of the cardia as a result of the increase intragastric pressure.

Such lesions account for 5% to 10% of cases of upper GI bleeding. They are usually diagnosed based on history. Endoscopy is frequently used to confirm the diagnosis. To avoid missing the diagnosis, it is important to perform a retroflexion maneuver and view the area just below the gastroesophageal junction. Most tears occur along the lesser curvature and less commonly on the greater curve. Supportive therapy is often all that is necessary because 90% of bleeding episodes are self-limited and the mucosa often heals within 72 hours.

In rare cases of severe ongoing bleeding, local endoscopic therapy with injection or electrocoagulation may be effective. Angiographic embolization, usually with an absorbable material such as a gelatin sponge, has been successfully used in cases of failed endoscopic therapy. If these maneuvers fail, high gastrotomy and suturing of the mucosal tear is indicated. It is important to rule out the diagnosis of variceal bleeding in cases of failed endoscopic therapy by a thorough examination of the gastroesophageal junction. Recurrent bleeding from a Mallory-Weiss tear is uncommon.

**Stress Gastritis** Stress-related gastritis is characterized by the appearance of multiple superficial erosions of the entire stomach, most commonly in the body. It is thought to result from the combination of acid and pepsin injury in the context of ischemia from hypoperfusion states, although NSAIDs produce a similar appearance. In the 1960s and 1970s, it was a commonly encountered lesion in critically ill patients, with significant morbidity and mortality from bleeding. These lesions are different from the solitary ulcerations, related to acid hypersecretion, that occur in patients with severe head injury (Cushing's ulcers). When stress ulceration is associated with major burns, these lesions are referred to as *Curling's ulcers*. In contrast with NSAID-associated lesions, significant hemorrhage from stress ulceration was a common phenomenon.

With improvements in the management of shock and sepsis, and the widespread use of acid suppressive therapy, significant bleeding from such lesions is rarely encountered. The overuse of acid suppressive therapy in this setting, however, has resulted in considerable cost and perhaps some risk to patients, with an increased incidence of nosocomial pneumonia secondary to gastric colonization. These issues have generated interest in identifying specific subgroups at high risk for stress gastritis to permit selective prophylactic therapy. The Canadian Critical Care Trials group has prospectively reviewed over 2200 patients admitted to the ICU and found an incidence of clinically significant bleeding in only 0.1% of patients considered at low risk

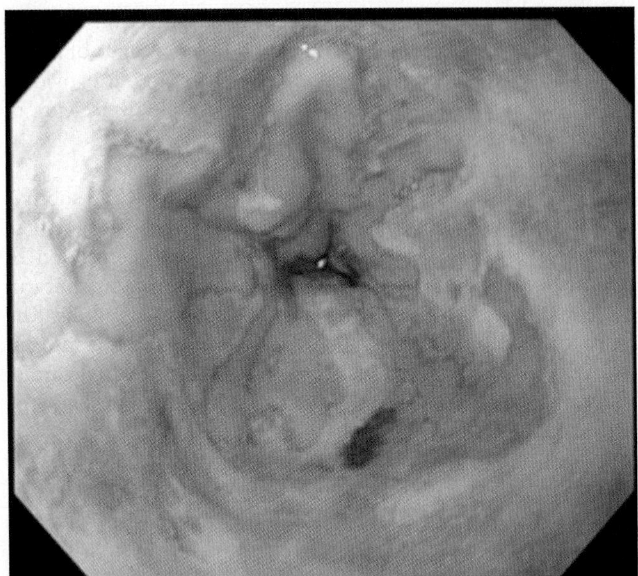

**FIGURE 48-5** Bleeding esophageal ulcer secondary to herpes esophagitis. (Courtesy Dr. Scott A. Hande, Brigham and Women's Hospital, Boston.)

of bleeding from stress-related gastritis.[31] Factors increasing the risk of hemorrhage from stress gastritis included ventilator dependence for longer than 48 hours and coagulopathy. For patients with these risk factors, clinically significant bleeding from stress-related gastritis occurred in 3.4%. Patients with these risk factors should be given prophylactic therapy with antacids, histamine-2 ($H_2$) receptor antagonists, PPIs, or sucralfate (Carafate). The primary prophylactic measure remains aggressive and appropriate resuscitation.

In those that develop significant bleeding, acid suppressive therapy is often successful in controlling the hemorrhage. In rare cases, when this fails, consideration should be given to administration of octreotide or vasopressin selectively via the left gastric artery, endoscopic therapy, or even angiographic embolization. Historically, such cases were seen more often and, at times, these patients underwent surgery. The surgical choices included vagotomy and pyloroplasty with oversewing of the hemorrhage, or near-total gastrectomy. These procedures carried mortality rates as high as 60%. Fortunately, they are seldom necessary today.

**Esophagitis** The esophagus is infrequently the source for significant hemorrhage. When it does occur, it is most commonly the result of esophagitis. Esophageal inflammation secondary to repeated exposure of the esophageal mucosa to the acidic gastric secretions in gastroesophageal reflux disease (GERD) leads to an inflammatory response that can result in chronic blood loss. Ulceration may accompany this but the superficial mucosal ulcerations generally do not bleed acutely and present as anemia or guaiac-positive stools. Various infectious agents may also cause esophagitis, particularly in the immunocompromised host (Fig. 48-5). With infection, hemorrhage can occasionally be massive. Other causes of esophageal bleeding include medications, Crohn's disease, and radiation.

Treatment typically includes acid suppressive therapy. Endoscopic control of the hemorrhage, usually with electrocoagulation or a heater probe, is often successful. In patients with

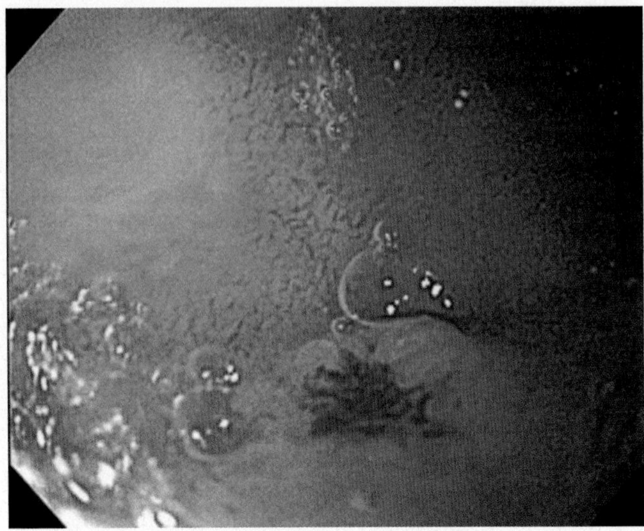

**FIGURE 48-6** Bleeding Dieulafoy's lesion of the stomach. (Courtesy Dr. Linda S. Lee, Brigham and Women's Hospital, Boston.)

an infectious cause, targeted therapy is appropriate. Surgery is seldom necessary.

**Dieulafoy's Lesion** Dieulafoy's lesions are vascular malformations found primarily along the lesser curve of the stomach within 6 cm of the gastroesophageal junction, although they can occur elsewhere in the GI tract (Fig. 48-6). They represent rupture of unusually large vessels (1 to 3 mm) found in the gastric submucosa. Erosion of the gastric mucosa overlying these vessels leads to hemorrhage. The mucosal defect is usually small (2 to 5 mm) and may be difficult to identify. Given the large size of the underlying artery, bleeding from a Dieulafoy's lesion can be massive.

Initial attempts at endoscopic control are often successful. Application of thermal or sclerosant therapy is effective in 80% to 100% of cases. In cases that fail endoscopic therapy, angiographic coil embolization can be successful. If these approaches are unsuccessful, surgical intervention may be necessary; because of difficulties in visualization and palpation of these lesions, prior endoscopic tattooing can facilitate the procedure. A gastrostomy is performed and attempts are made at identifying the bleeding source. The lesion can then be oversewn. In patients in whom the bleeding point is not identified, a partial gastrectomy may be necessary.

**Gastric Antral Vascular Ectasia** Also known as watermelon stomach, gastric antral vascular ectasia (GAVE) is characterized by a collection of dilated venules appearing as linear red streaks converging on the antrum in a longitudinal fashion, giving it the appearance of a watermelon. Acute severe hemorrhage is rare in GAVE and most patients present with persistent iron deficiency anemia from continued occult blood loss. Endoscopic therapy is indicated for persistent, transfusion-dependent bleeding and has been reportedly successful in up to 90% of patients. The preferred endoscopic therapy is APC (Fig. 48-7). Patients failing endoscopic therapy should be considered for antrectomy.

**Malignancy** Malignancies of the upper GI tract are usually associated with chronic anemia or hemoccult-positive stool rather than episodes of significant hemorrhage. On occasion,

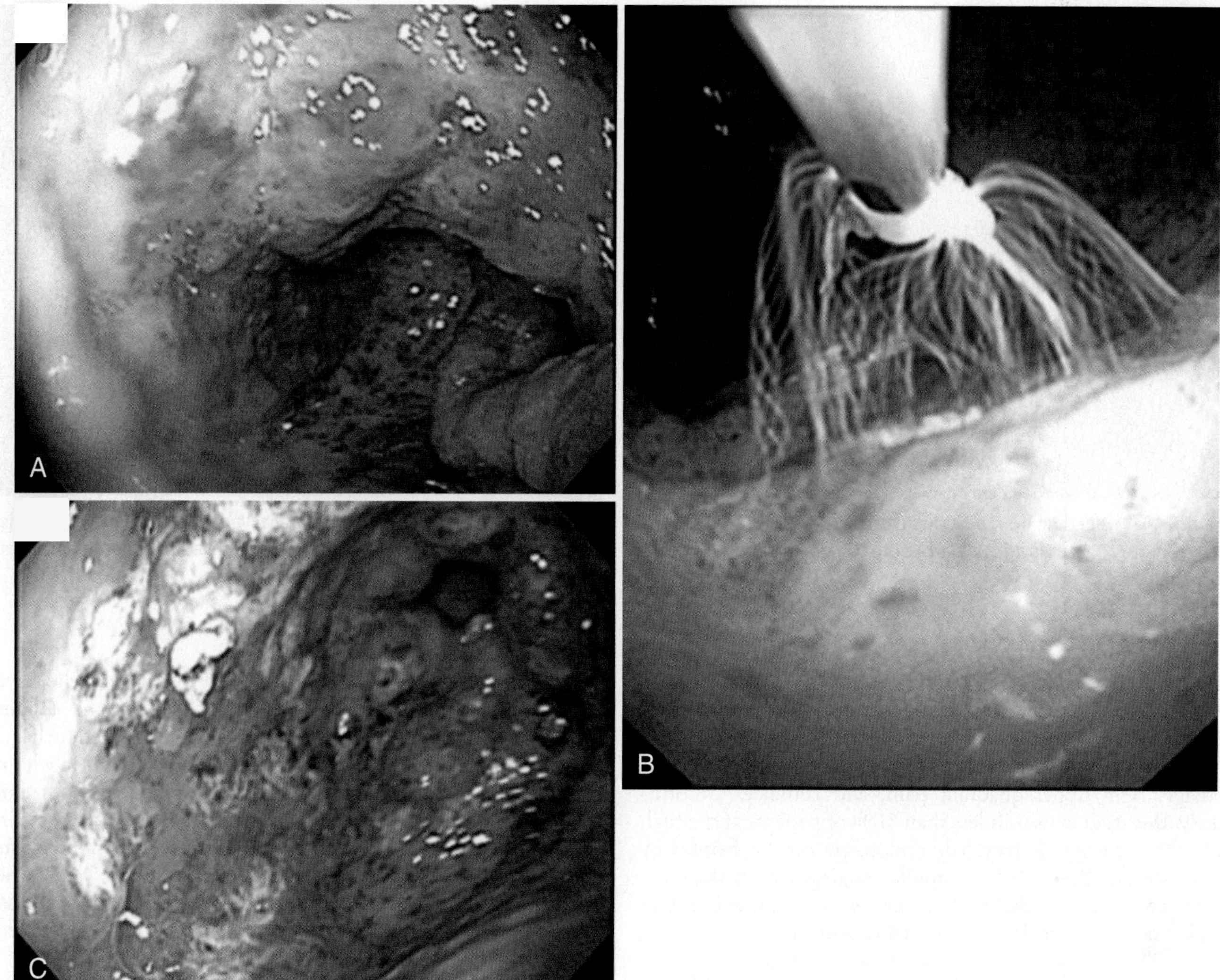


**FIGURE 48-7 A,** Gastric antral vascular ectasia (GAVE) can be seen in the gastric antrum, giving the stomach a watermelon appearance. **B,** APC therapy of a GAVE. **C,** Post-therapy appearance of the GAVE. (Courtesy Dr. David L. Carr-Locke, Brigham and Women's Hospital, Boston.)

malignancies will present as ulcerative lesions that bleed persistently. This is perhaps most characteristic of the GI stromal tumor (GIST), although it may occur with other lesions, including leiomyomas and lymphomas. Although endoscopic therapy is often successful in controlling these bleeds, the rebleeding rate is high; therefore, when a malignancy is diagnosed, surgical resection is indicated. The extent of resection is dependent on the specific lesion and whether the resection is believed to be curative or palliative. Palliative resections for control of bleeding usually entail wedge resections. Standard cancer surgeries are indicated, when possible, although this may depend on the hemodynamic stability of the patient.

**Aortoenteric Fistula** Primary aortoduodenal fistulas are rare lesions. They typically develop in the setting of a previous abdominal aortic aneurysm repair, although they may occur as a result of an inflammatory or infectious aortitis, and they may develop in up to 1% of aortic graft cases. Although the interval between surgery and hemorrhage can be days to years, the median interval is approximately 3 years. The sequence is thought to involve the development of a pseudoaneurysm at the proximal anastomotic suture line in the setting of an infection, with subsequent fistulization into the overlying duodenum.

This diagnosis should be considered in all bleeding patients with a known abdominal aortic aneurysm or a previous prosthetic aneurysm repair. Hemorrhage in this situation is often massive and fatal unless immediate surgical intervention is undertaken. Typically, patients with bleeding from an aortoenteric fistula will present first with a sentinel bleed. This is a self-limited episode that heralds the subsequent massive, and often fatal, hemorrhage. This should prompt urgent upper endoscopy because diagnosis at this stage can be lifesaving. Any evidence of bleeding in the distal duodenum (third or fourth portion) on EGD should be considered diagnostic. A computed tomography (CT) scan with IV contrast will demonstrate air around the graft (suggestive of an infection), possible pseudoaneurysm and, rarely, the presence of IV contrast in the duodenal lumen.

Therapy includes ligation of the aorta proximal to graft, removal of the infected prosthesis, and an extra-anatomic bypass. The defect in the duodenum is often small and can be repaired primarily. This is a complex and often morbid procedure.

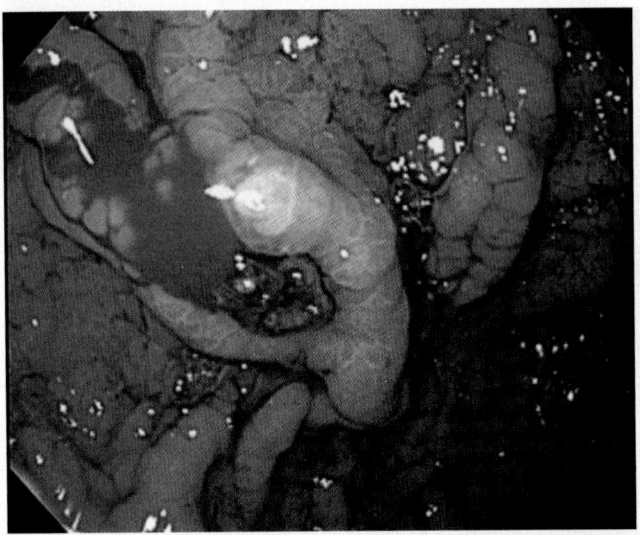

**FIGURE 48-8** Bleeding from a percutaneous endoscopic gastrostomy site. (Courtesy Dr. David L. Carr-Locke, Brigham and Women's Hospital, Boston.)

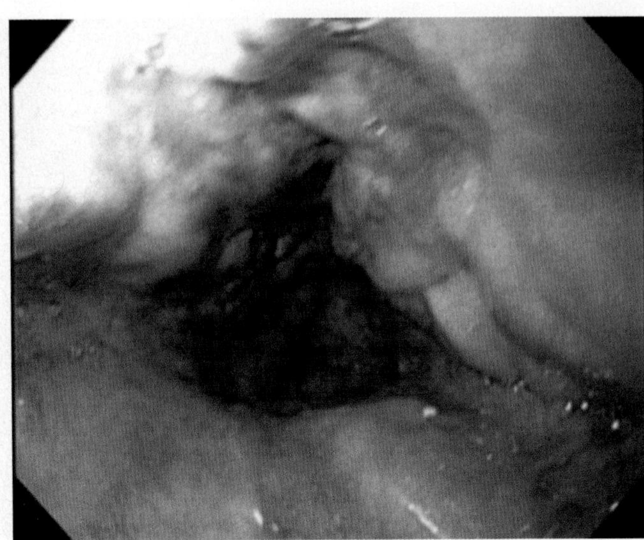

**FIGURE 48-9** Nonbleeding esophageal varices secondary to cirrhosis. (Courtesy Dr. David L. Carr-Locke, Brigham and Women's Hospital, Boston.)

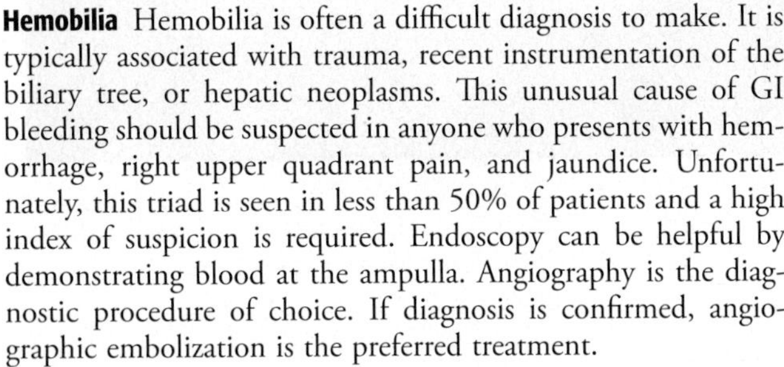

**Hemobilia** Hemobilia is often a difficult diagnosis to make. It is typically associated with trauma, recent instrumentation of the biliary tree, or hepatic neoplasms. This unusual cause of GI bleeding should be suspected in anyone who presents with hemorrhage, right upper quadrant pain, and jaundice. Unfortunately, this triad is seen in less than 50% of patients and a high index of suspicion is required. Endoscopy can be helpful by demonstrating blood at the ampulla. Angiography is the diagnostic procedure of choice. If diagnosis is confirmed, angiographic embolization is the preferred treatment.

**Hemosuccus Pancreaticus** Another rare cause of upper GI bleeding is bleeding from the pancreatic duct. This is often caused by erosion of a pancreatic pseudocyst into the splenic artery. It presents with abdominal pain and hematochezia. As with hemobilia, it is a difficult diagnosis to make and requires a high index of suspicion in patients with abdominal pain, blood loss, and a past history of pancreatitis. Angiography is diagnostic and permits embolization, which is often therapeutic. In patients amenable to a distal pancreatectomy, the procedure often results in cure.

**Iatrogenic Bleeding** Upper GI bleeding may follow a therapeutic or diagnostic procedure. As noted, hemobilia may be iatrogenic in nature, particularly following percutaneous transhepatic procedures. Another common cause of iatrogenic bleeding is endoscopic sphincterotomy; this can occur in up to 2% of cases. It is often mild and self-limited. Late hemorrhage usually occurs within the first 48 hours and may require injection of the area with epinephrine, which is usually successful. Surgical intervention is rarely required.

Percutaneous endoscopic gastrostomy (PEG) placement is an increasingly common procedure. Bleeding rates of up to 3% have been reported. Although most these cases reflect bleeding from the incision site, some are caused by bleeding from the gastric mucosa (Fig. 48-8). This can often be controlled endoscopically.

Upper GI bleeding can also be seen in patients who have recently undergone upper GI surgery. Any of the lesions described could be responsible for postoperative hemorrhage, and these possibilities should be considered. In patients in whom a resection and anastomosis have been performed, the source of the bleeding may be the suture line or staple line. In patients in whom this is persistent and intervention is needed, endoscopists are often concerned by the potential for suture or staple line disruption. However, it is safe to do this diagnostic or even therapeutic endoscopy, providing minimal insufflation is used and the procedure is done with care.[32]

### Bleeding Related to Portal Hypertension

Upper GI bleeding is a serious complication of portal hypertension, most often in the setting of cirrhosis. Cirrhosis and portal hypertension are covered in more detail in Chapter 54; only bleeding related to portal hypertension is discussed here.

Hemorrhage related to portal hypertension is usually the result of bleeding from varices. These dilated submucosal veins develop in response to the portal hypertension, providing a collateral pathway for decompression of the portal system into the systemic venous circulation. They are most common in the distal esophagus and can reach sizes of 1 to 2 cm. As they enlarge, the overlying mucosa becomes increasingly tenuous, excoriating with minimal trauma (Fig. 48-9).

Although these varices are most commonly seen in the esophagus, they may also develop in the stomach and hemorrhoidal plexus of the rectum. Portal hypertensive gastropathy, diffuse dilation of the mucosal and submucosal venous plexus of the stomach associated with overlying gastritis, is an incompletely understood entity in which the stomach acquires a snakeskin-like appearance, with cherry red spots. Unlike esophageal varices, it rarely causes major hemorrhage.

Gastroesophageal varices develop in approximately 30% of patients with cirrhosis and portal hypertension and 30% in this group develop variceal bleeding. Compared with nonvariceal bleeding, variceal hemorrhage is associated with an increased risk

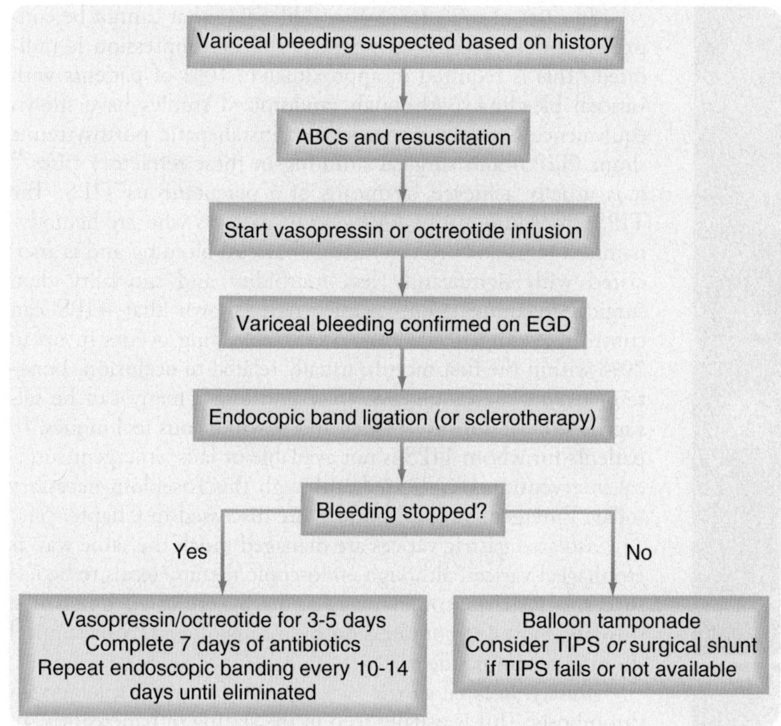


**FIGURE 48-10** Algorithm for diagnosis and management of GI hemorrhage related to portal hypertension.

of rebleeding, increased need for transfusions, longer hospital stay, and increased mortality. Hemorrhage is frequently massive, accompanied by hematemesis and hemodynamic instability. The hepatic functional reserve, estimated by Child's criteria (see Chapter 54), correlates closely with outcomes in these patients. Despite improvements in the medical management of these patients, the 6-week mortality rate following the first bleed is almost 20%.[33]

**Treatment** Figure 48-10 presents an algorithm for management. As with other causes of GI bleeding, adequate resuscitation is imperative. Fluid resuscitation in patients with cirrhosis is a delicate balance. These patients frequently have hyperaldosteronism associated with fluid retention and ascites. Animal studies have demonstrated that a rapid correction of fluid deficits and blood pressure increases the risk of further rebleeding from the varices.[34] Central venous pressure monitoring is indicated for most of these patients and early admission to an ICU should be considered. A low threshold for intubation is appropriate. Defects in coagulation are common and should be aggressively corrected. A significant percentage of patients with variceal bleeding have underlying sepsis, which may be associated with an aggravation in portal hypertension and lead to variceal bleeding. Studies have demonstrated that a 7-day course of a quinolone will lower the risk of rebleeding. Thus, patients with variceal bleeding should be given an empirical course of a broad-spectrum antibiotic.[35]

***Medical Management*** In patients with cirrhosis, pharmacologic therapy to reduce portal hypertension should be considered, even while preparing for emergent upper endoscopy. Vasopressin produces splanchnic vasoconstriction and has been shown to reduce bleeding significantly when compared with placebo. Unfortunately, this agent results in significant cardiac vasoconstriction, with resulting myocardial ischemia. Although vasopressin has been combined with nitroglycerin in clinical practice, somatostatin or its synthetic analogue, octreotide, is the vasoactive agent of choice.[36] Continuous IV infusion of these agents results in temporary control of bleeding and allows time for resuscitation and appropriate diagnostic and therapeutic maneuvers.

***Endoscopic Management*** Early EGD is critical to evaluate the source of bleeding because more than 50% of bleeding is cause by nonvariceal sources, including peptic ulcer, gastritis, and Mallory-Weiss tears. Studies have suggested that unlike peptic ulcer bleeding, an early endoscopy (within 15 hours of presentation) can affect survival in cases of variceal bleeding.[37]

Subsequent management is based on the endoscopic findings. If bleeding esophageal varices are identified, sclerotherapy and variceal banding have been shown to control hemorrhage effectively. Although sclerotherapy, which may use a variety of agents, is an easier procedure to perform, it is also associated with perforation, mediastinitis, and stricture. Banding seems to have a lower complication rate and, when expertise is available, should be the therapy of choice (Fig. 48-11). These endoscopic approaches, sometimes with up to three treatments over 24 hours, control the hemorrhage in up to 90% of patients with esophageal varices. Unfortunately, gastric varices are not managed effectively by endoscopic techniques.

***Other Management*** In patients for whom pharmacologic or endoscopic therapy fails to control the hemorrhage, balloon tamponade can be successful in temporizing the hemorrhage. The Sengstaken-Blakemore tube consists of a gastric tube with esophageal and gastric balloons. The gastric balloon is inflated and tension is applied on the gastroesophageal junction. If this does not control the hemorrhage, the esophageal balloon is also

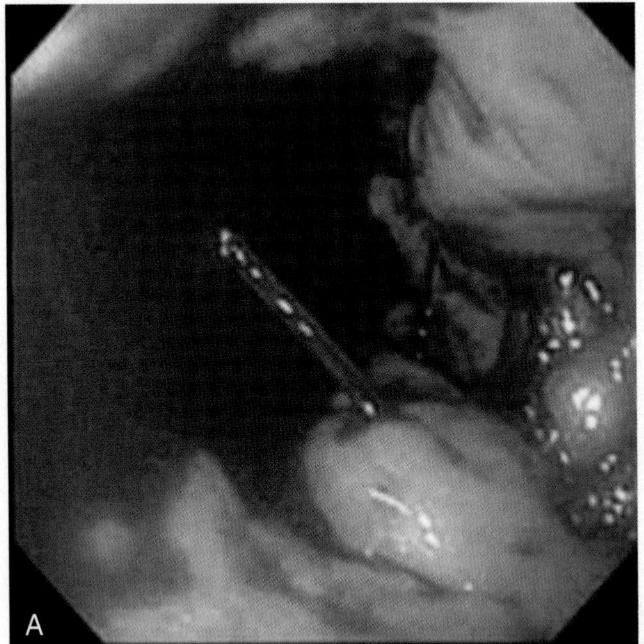


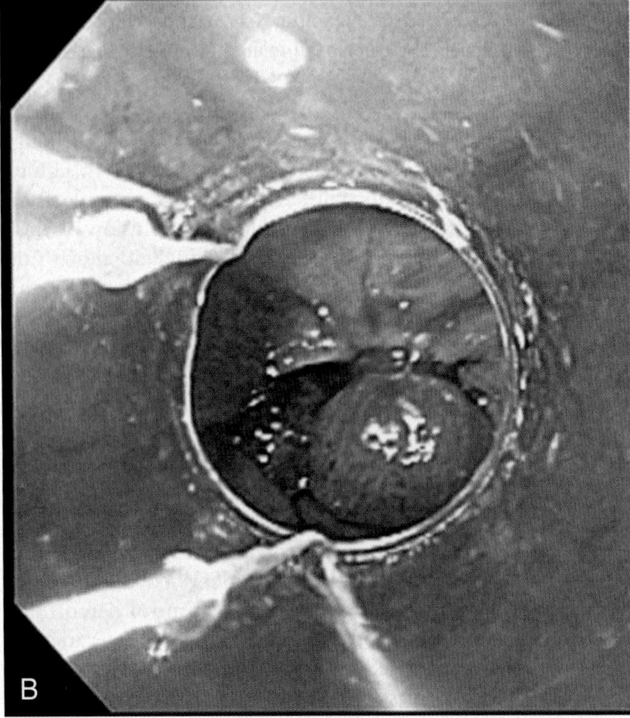


**FIGURE 48-11** **A,** Actively bleeding varices. **B,** Effective control after variceal banding. (Courtesy Dr. David L. Carr-Locke, Brigham and Women's Hospital, Boston.)

inflated, compressing the venous plexus between them. The Minnesota tube includes a proximal esophageal lumen for aspirating swallowed secretions. These tubes are associated with a high rate of complications related to aspiration and inappropriate placement, with esophageal perforation. Hemorrhage recurs on deflation in up to 50% of patients. Balloon tamponade is reserved for patients with massive hemorrhage to permit more definitive therapies.

In cases of refractory variceal bleeding that cannot be controlled endoscopically, emergent portal decompression is indicated. This is required in approximately 10% of patients with variceal bleeding.[33] Although randomized studies have shown equivalence between a transjugular intrahepatic portosystemic shunt (TIPS) and surgical shunting in these refractory cases,[38] it is usually achieved by means of a percutaneous TIPS. The TIPS procedure can be lifesaving in patients who are hemodynamically unstable from refractory variceal bleeding and is associated with significantly less morbidity and mortality than surgical decompression. Studies have shown that TIPS can control bleeding in 95% of cases. Rebleeding occurs in up to 20% within the first month, usually related to occlusion. Long-term patency rates are even lower, although many can be salvaged with careful surveillance and percutaneous techniques. In patients for whom TIPS is not available or fails, emergent surgical intervention is indicated, although this is seldom necessary today. Emergent surgical options are discussed in Chapter 54.

Isolated gastric varices are managed much the same way as esophageal varices, although endoscopic therapy tends to be less successful. Pharmacotherapy is primarily indicated but, when this fails, portal decompression by means of a TIPS or surgical shunt is recommended.[39]

Rarely, isolated gastric varices occur following splenic vein thrombosis. This is usually seen in the setting of pancreatitis. In these patients, central portal pressures are normal but left-sided hypertension, decompressed from the spleen to the short gastric vessels, produces the varices. This is best treated by performing a splenectomy. Although the risk of variceal bleeding was thought to be high in this group and splenectomy was routinely recommended, studies have suggested that the incidence of variceal bleeding is low (4% with a mean follow up of 34 months) and splenectomy should not be routinely undertaken.[40]

Unlike variceal hemorrhage, bleeding from portal hypertensive gastropathy is not amenable to endoscopic treatment because of the diffuse nature of the mucosal abnormalities. The underlying pathology involves elevated portal venous pressures, so pharmacologic therapy aimed at reducing portal venous pressure is indicated. If pharmacologic therapy fails to control acute bleeding, TIPS should be considered.

**Prevention of Rebleeding** Once the initial bleeding has been controlled, prevention of recurrent hemorrhage should be a priority. If no further treatment is undertaken, approximately 70% of patients will have a further bleed within 2 months. The risk of rebleeding is highest in the initial few hours to days following a first episode. Medical therapy to prevent recurrence includes a nonselective beta blocker, such as nadolol, and an antiulcer agent, such as a PPI or sucralfate. These are combined with endoscopic band ligation repeated every 10 to 14 days until all varices have been eradicated.

Although this aggressive approach results in a significant lowering of the rebleeding rate to less than 20%, it requires intensive medical follow-up and supervision.[41] In patients who are medically noncompliant or unable to tolerate such therapy, elective portal decompression should be considered if has not already been performed. The choice between TIPS and operative decompression in the stable patient depends on the residual liver function. In general, patients with poor liver reserve who are on the liver transplant list should be considered for TIPS. This procedure provides a temporizing measure and avoids postoperative scarring of the porta hepatis, which could complicate the transplantation procedure. Unfortunately, TIPS is associated with hepatic encephalopathy in up to 50% of patients within 1 year of the procedure.[42] Other shunt complications, such as thrombosis, can also occur in up to 30% of patients at 1 year. In those with good liver function who do not qualify for transplantation, surgical decompression is therefore preferred. This provides a more endurable long-term decompression, with a lower rate of hepatic encephalopathy. In those with good hepatic reserve, these advantages are thought to counterbalance the increased operative morbidity and mortality. The preferred elective shunt is a selective distal splenorenal shunt.

## ACUTE LOWER GASTROINTESTINAL HEMORRHAGE

When compared with upper GI hemorrhage, lower GI bleeding is a much less frequent reason for hospitalization—it is about 20% as common as bleeding from a location proximal to the ligament of Treitz. The incidence of lower GI bleeding, however, increases with age, and lower GI bleeding may be more common in older patients. In more than 95% of patients with lower GI bleeding, the source of hemorrhage is the colon. The small intestine is only occasionally responsible and, because these lesions are not typically diagnosed with the combination of upper and lower endoscopy, they will be considered later (see "Acute Gastrointestinal Hemorrhage from an Obscure Source"). In general, the incidence of lower GI bleeding increases with age and the cause is often age-related (Table 48-3). Specifically, vascular lesions and diverticular disease affect all age groups but have an increasing incidence in middle-aged and older adults. In the pediatric population, intussusception is most commonly responsible, whereas Meckel's diverticulum must be considered in the differential diagnosis in the young adult. The clinical presentation of lower GI bleeding ranges from severe hemorrhage with diverticular disease or vascular lesions to a minor inconvenience secondary to anal fissure or hemorrhoids.[3]

**Table 48-3 Differential Diagnosis of Lower Gastrointestinal Hemorrhage**

| COLONIC BLEEDING* | SMALL BOWEL BLEEDING† |
|---|---|
| 30%-40% Diverticular disease | Angiodysplasias |
| 5%-10% Ischemia | Erosions, ulcers (e.g., from potassium, NSAIDs) |
| 5%-15% Anorectal disease | Crohn's disease |
| 5%-10% Neoplasia | Radiation |
| 3%-8% Infectious colitis | Meckel's diverticulum |
| 3%-7% Postpolypectomy | Neoplasia |
| 3%-4% Inflammatory bowel disease | Aortoenteric fistula |
| 3% Angiodysplasia | |
| 1%-3% Radiation colitis, proctitis | |
| 1%-5% Other | |
| 10%-25% Unknown | |

Adapted from Strate LL: Lower gastrointestinal bleeding: Epidemiology and diagnosis. Gastroenterol Clin North Am 34:643–664, 2005.

*95% of cases.

†5% of cases.

### Diagnosis

Lower GI bleeding typically presents with hematochezia, which can range from bright red blood to old clots. If the bleeding is slower or from a more proximal source, lower GI bleeding often presents as melena. Hemorrhage from the lower GI tract tends to be less severe and more intermittent, and usually ceases more spontaneously than upper GI bleeding. When compared with upper GI bleeding, no diagnostic modality is as sensitive or specific as endoscopy for making an accurate diagnosis in lower GI bleeding. Diagnostic evaluation is further complicated by the observation that in up to 40% of patients with lower GI bleeding, more than one potential source for bleeding is identified. If more than one source is identified, it is critical to confirm the responsible lesion before initiating aggressive therapy. This approach may occasionally require a period of observation with several episodes of bleeding before a definitive diagnosis can be made. In up to 25% of patients with lower GI hemorrhage, the bleeding source is never accurately identified.

An algorithm for the evaluation of lower GI hemorrhage is shown in Figure 48-12. Once resuscitation has been initiated, the first step in the workup is to rule out anorectal bleeding with a digital rectal examination, anoscopy, and/or sigmoidoscopy. With significant bleeding, it is also important to eliminate an upper GI source. An NG aspirate that contains bile and no blood effectively rules out upper tract bleeding in most patients. However, when emergent surgery for life-threatening hemorrhage is being contemplated, preoperative or intraoperative EGD is usually appropriate. This is particularly relevant if blind subtotal colectomy for massive hemorrhage is being considered.

Subsequent evaluation depends on the magnitude of the hemorrhage. With major and/or persistent bleeding, the workup should progress depending on the patient's hemodynamic stability. The truly unstable patient who continues to bleed and requires ongoing aggressive resuscitation belongs in the operating room for expeditious diagnosis and surgical intervention. When hemorrhage is intermediate, resuscitation and hemodynamic stability permit a more directed evaluation and therapeutic intervention. Colonoscopy is the mainstay here because it allows visualization of the pathology and therapeutic intervention in colonic, rectal, and distal ileal sources of bleeding. The usual adjuncts to colonoscopy include a tagged RBC scan and angiography. If these modalities are not diagnostic, the source of the hemorrhage is considered obscure; such lesions and their evaluation are considered in the last section of this chapter.

### Colonoscopy

Colonoscopy is most appropriate in the setting of minimal to moderate bleeding; major hemorrhage interferes significantly with visualization and the diagnostic yield is low. In addition, in the unstable patient, sedation and manipulation may be associated with additional complications and can interfere with resuscitation. Although the blood is cathartic, gentle preparation with polyethylene glycol, orally or through an NG tube, can improve visualization. Findings may include an actively bleeding site, clot adherent to a focus of mucosa or diverticular orifice, or blood localized to a specific colonic segment, although this can be misleading because of retrograde peristalsis in the colon. Polyps, cancers, and inflammatory causes can frequently be seen. Unfortunately, angiodysplasias are often difficult to visualize, particularly in the unstable patient with mesenteric vascular

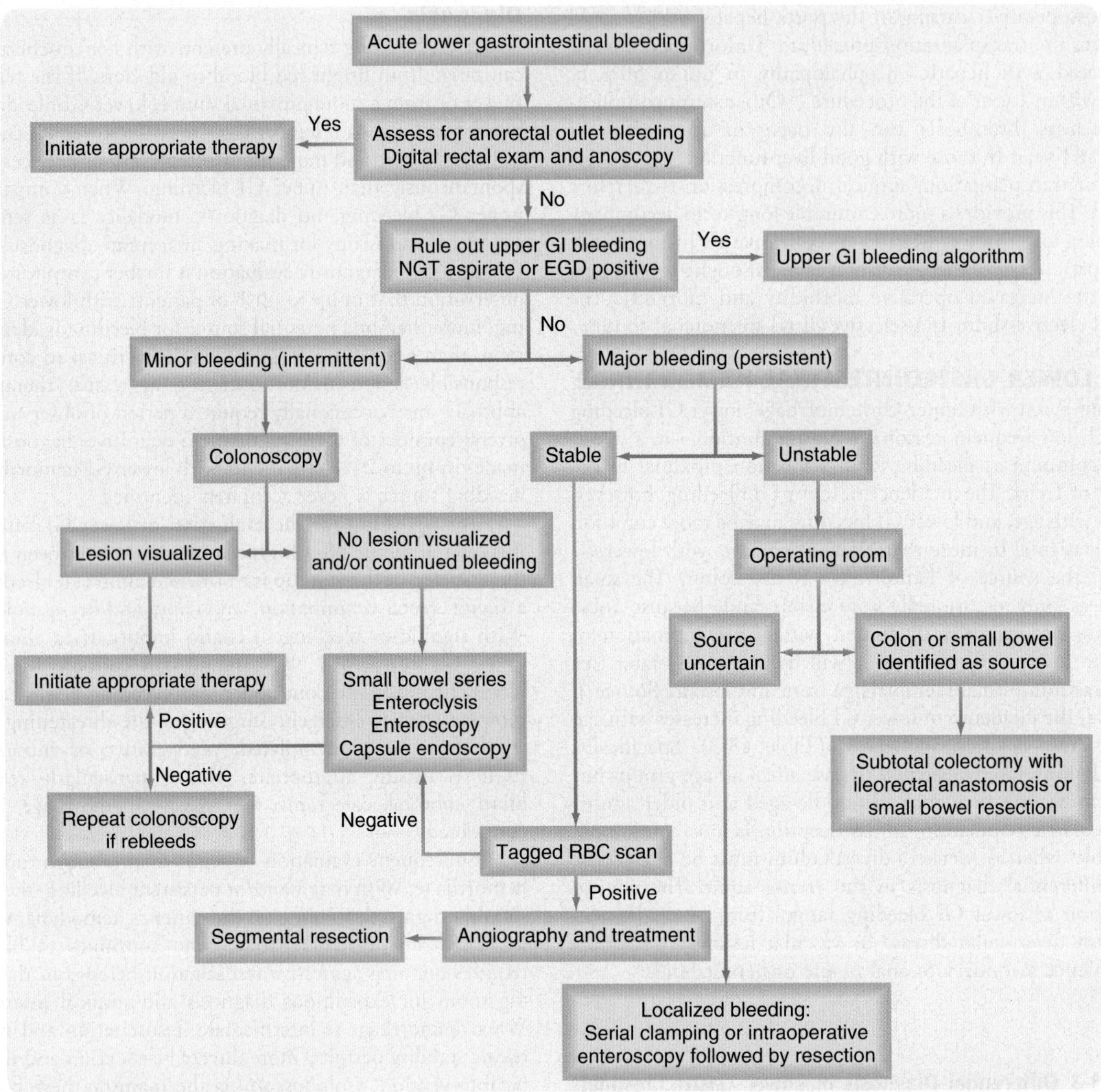


**FIGURE 48-12** Algorithm for diagnosis and management of lower GI hemorrhage. *NGT,* Nasogastric tube.

constriction. Diverticula are identified in most patients, whether or not they are the source of the hemorrhage. Despite these limitations, the diagnostic yield in experienced hands is reasonable. For example, some studies have reported that colonoscopy is successful in identifying the bleeding source in up to 95% of patients. Most of the bleeding is secondary to angiodysplasias or diverticuli.[43]

### Radionuclide Scanning

Radionuclide scanning with technetium-99m ($^{99m}$Tc–labeled RBC) is the most sensitive but least accurate method for localizing GI bleeding. With this technique, the patient's own red cells are labeled and reinjected. The labeled blood is extravasated into the GI tract lumen, creating a focus that can be detected scintigraphically. Initially, images are obtained frequently and then at 4-hour intervals, for up to 24 hours. The RBC scan can detect bleeding as slow as 0.1 mL/min and is reported to be more than 90% sensitive (Fig. 48-13).[3] Unfortunately, the spatial resolution is low and blood may move retrograde in the colon or distally in the small bowel. Reported accuracy of localization is in the range of only 40% to 60% and it is particularly inaccurate for distinguishing right-sided from left-sided colonic bleeding. The RBC scan is not usually used as a definitive study before surgery but instead as a guide to the usefulness of angiography; if the RBC scan is negative or only positive after several hours, angiography is unlikely to be revealing. Such an approach avoids the significant morbidity of angiography.

### Mesenteric Angiography

Selective angiography, using the superior or inferior mesenteric arteries, can detect hemorrhage in the range of 0.5 to 1.0 mL/min but is generally only used for the diagnosis of ongoing hemorrhage. It can be particularly useful in identifying the vascular patterns of angiodysplasias. It may also be used for localizing actively bleeding diverticula. In addition, it has therapeutic capabilities. Catheter-directed vasopressin infusion can provide temporary control of bleeding, permitting hemodynamic stabilization, although as many as 50% of patients will rebleed when

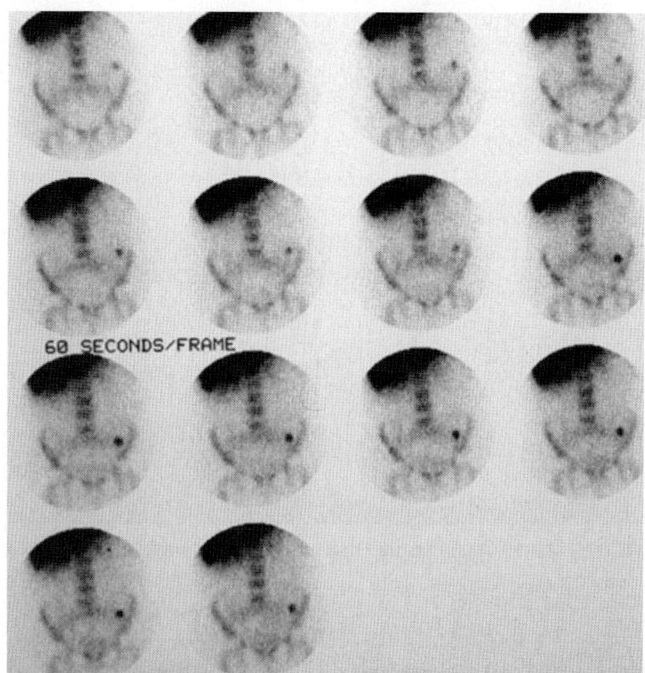


**FIGURE 48-13** Positive red blood cell scan localizing the bleeding to the left lower quadrant. (Courtesy Dr. Richard A. Baum, MD, Brigham and Women's Hospital, Boston.)

the medication is discontinued. It can also be used for embolization. Although the more limited collateral circulation of the colon has made this less appealing than in the upper GI tract, it has been have suggested that these techniques can be used safely in most patients. Typically, such therapy is reserved for patients whose underlying condition precludes surgical therapy. Unfortunately, angiography is associated with a significant risk of complications, including hematoma, arterial thrombosis, contrast reaction, and acute renal failure.

### Treatment

Therapeutic approaches with lower GI bleeding are clearly dependent on the lesion identified. The criteria for surgery, shown in Box 48-2, are similar to those for upper GI hemorrhage, although there is a stronger tendency to delay until the site is clearly localized.

## Specific Causes of Lower GI Bleeding

### Colonic Bleeding

**Diverticular Disease** In the United States, diverticula are the most common cause of significant lower GI bleeding. Some series have suggested that diverticula are responsible for up to 55% of cases.[3] In the past, diverticula were thought to be rare in patients younger than 40 years but is now an increasingly common diagnosis in this age group. Diverticulosis affects more than two thirds of the Western population who are in their 80s. Only 3% to 15% of individuals with diverticulosis experience any bleeding. Bleeding generally occurs at the neck of the diverticulum and is believed to be secondary to bleeding from the vasa recti as they penetrate through the submucosa. Of those that bleed, more than 75% stop spontaneously, although approximately 10% will rebleed within a year and almost 50% within 10 years.[3] Although diverticular disease is much more common on the left side, right-sided disease is responsible for more than 50% of the bleeding.

The best method of diagnosis and treatment is colonoscopy, although success is sometimes limited by the large amount of bleeding. If the bleeding diverticulum can be identified, epinephrine injection may control the bleeding. Electrocautery can also be used and, most recently, endoscopic clips have been successfully applied to control the hemorrhage. If bleeding ceases with these maneuvers or ceases spontaneously, expectant management may be appropriate; however, this requires clinical judgment based on the amount of the hemorrhage and any comorbidities, particularly cardiac disease.

If none of these maneuvers is successful or if hemorrhage recurs, angiography with embolization can be considered. Superselective embolization of the bleeding colonic vessel has gained popularity, with high success rates (>90%), although the risk of ischemic complications continues to be of concern.[44] Under these circumstances, colonic resection is indicated. Certainty of the site of bleeding is critical. Blind hemicolectomy is associated with rebleeding in more than 50% of patients, and operation based on RBC scan localization alone can result in recurrent hemorrhage in up to one third of patients.[45] Subtotal colectomy does not eliminate the risk of recurrent hemorrhage and, when compared with segmental resection, is accompanied by a significant increase in morbidity, particularly diarrhea in older patients, in whom the remaining rectum may never adapt. Mortality of emergent subtotal colectomy for bleeding is almost 30%.[45]

**Angiodysplasia** In some reports, hemorrhage secondary to these vascular lesions accounts for up to 40% of lower GI bleeding; however, most recent reports have noted the incidence to be much lower.[3] Angiodysplasias of the intestine, also referred to as *arteriovenous malformations* (AVMs), are distinct from hemangiomas and true congenital AVMS. They are thought to be acquired degenerative lesions secondary to progressive dilation of normal blood vessels within the submucosa of the intestine. Angiodysplasias have an equal gender distribution and are almost uniformly found in patients older than 50 years. These lesions are notably associated with aortic stenosis and renal failure, especially in older patients. The hemorrhage tends to arise from the right side of the colon, with the cecum being the most common location, although they can occur in the rest of the colon and small bowel. Most patients present with chronic bleeding but, in up to 15%, hemorrhage may be massive. Bleeding stops spontaneously in most cases, but approximately 50% will rebleed within 5 years.

These lesions can be diagnosed by colonoscopy or angiography. During colonoscopy, they appear as red stellate lesions with a surrounding rim of pale mucosa and can be treated with sclerotherapy or electrocautery. Angiography demonstrates dilated, slowly emptying veins and, sometimes, early venous filling. If these lesions are discovered incidentally, no further therapy is indicated. In acutely bleeding patients, they have been successfully treated with intra-arterial vasopressin, selective gel foam embolization, endoscopic electrocoagulation, or injection with sclerosing agents. If these measures fail, or bleeding recurs and the lesion has been localized, segmental resection, most commonly a right colectomy, is effective.

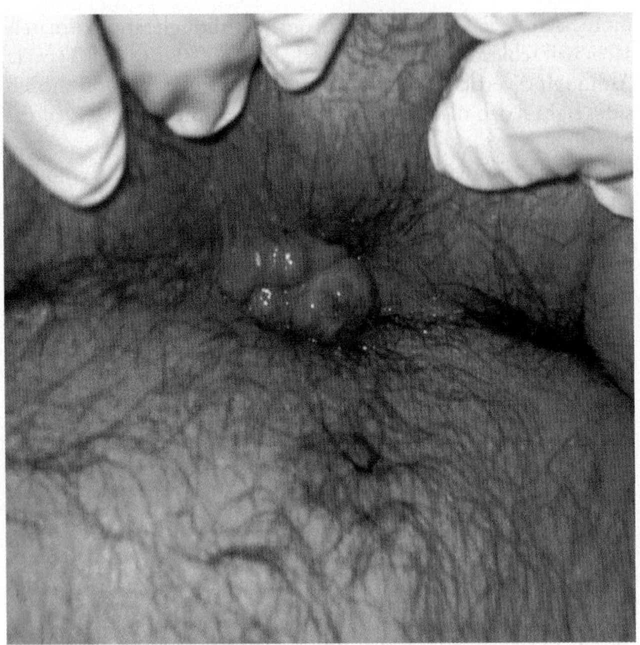

**FIGURE 48-14** Bleeding and prolapsed hemorrhoids.

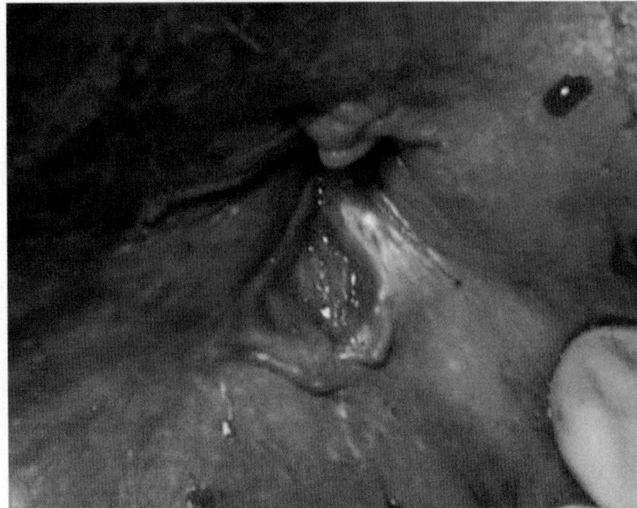

**FIGURE 48-15** Anal fissure that can be a source of lower GI bleeding.

**Neoplasia** Colorectal carcinoma is an uncommon cause of significant lower GI hemorrhage but is probably the most important one to rule out because more than 150,000 Americans are diagnosed annually with this type of cancer. The bleeding is usually painless, intermittent, and slow in nature and is frequently associated with iron deficiency anemia. Polyps can also bleed but the bleeding usually occurs after a polypectomy. Bleeding in the pediatric population is discussed in Chapter 67; juvenile polyps are the second most common cause of bleeding in patients younger than 20 years. Occasionally other colonic neoplasms, most notably GISTs, can be associated with massive hemorrhage. The best diagnostic tool is colonoscopy. If the bleeding is attributable to a polyp, it can be treated with endoscopic therapy.

**Anorectal Disease** The major causes of anorectal outlet bleeding are internal hemorrhoids, anal fissures, and colorectal neoplasia. Although hemorrhoids are the most common of these entities, they only account for 5% to 10% of all acute lower GI bleeding. In general, anorectal hemorrhage is low-volume bleeding that presents as bright red blood per rectum, which is seen in the toilet and on the toilet paper. Most hemorrhoidal bleeding arises from internal hemorrhoids; these are painless and often accompanied by prolapsing tissue that reduces spontaneously or has to be reduced manually by the patient (Fig. 48-14). Anal fissure, on the other hand, produces painful bleeding after a bowel movement; bleeding is only occasionally the main symptom in these patients (Fig. 48-15).

Because anorectal disease is common, a careful investigation to rule out all other sources of bleeding, especially malignancy, is imperative before lower GI bleeding can be attributed to such pathology. Anal fissure can be treated medically with stool-bulking agents (e.g., psyllium [Metamucil]), increased water intake, stool softeners, and topical nitroglycerin ointment or diltiazem to relieve sphincter spasm and promote healing. Internal hemorrhoids should be treated with bulking agents, increased dietary fiber, and adequate hydration. Office-based interventions, including rubber band ligation, injectable sclerosing agents, and infrared coagulation, have also been used. If these measures fail, surgical hemorrhoidectomy may be needed. Most anorectal bleeding is self-limited and responds to dietary and local measures.

**Colitis** Inflammation of the colon is caused by a number of disease processes, including inflammatory bowel disease (e.g., Crohn's disease, ulcerative colitis, indeterminate colitis), infectious colitis (0157:H7 *Escherichia coli,* cytomegalovirus [CMV], *Salmonella, Shigella,* and *Campylobacter* spp., and *Clostridium difficile*), radiation proctitis after treatment for pelvic malignancies, and ischemia.

Ulcerative colitis (UC) is more likely than Crohn's disease to present with GI bleeding. UC is a mucosal disease that starts distally in the rectum and progresses proximally to occasionally involve the entire colon. Patients can present with up to 20 bloody bowel movements daily. These are accompanied by crampy abdominal pain, tenesmus and, occasionally, abdominal pain. The diagnosis is secured by a careful history and flexible endoscopy with biopsy. Medical therapy with steroids, 5-aminosalicylic acid (ASA) compounds, immunomodulatory agents, and supportive care are the mainstays of treatment. Surgical therapy is rarely indicated in the acute setting unless the patient develops a toxic megacolon or hemorrhage refractory to medical management.

In contrast, Crohn's disease typically is associated with guaiac-positive diarrhea and mucus-filled bowel movements, but not with bright red blood. Crohn's disease can affect the entire GI tract. It is characterized by skip lesions, transmural thickening of the bowel wall, and granuloma formation. The diagnosis is made with endoscopy and contrast studies. Medical management consists of steroids, antibiotics, immunomodulators and ASA compounds. Because Crohn's disease is a relapsing and remitting disease, surgical therapy is used as a last resort. Massive colonic hemorrhage complicates ulcerative colitis in up to 15% of affected patients, whereas it only occurs in 1% of those with Crohn's colitis.[46]

Infectious colitis can cause bloody diarrhea. The diagnosis is usually established from the history and stool culture. *C. difficile* and CMV colitis deserve special attention. *C. difficile* colitis usually present with explosive, foul-smelling diarrhea in a patient with prior antibiotic use and/or hospitalization. Bloody bowel movements are not common but can be present, especially in severe cases in which there is associated mucosal sloughing. In North America, there has been an upsurge in the frequency and severity of *C. difficile*-associated colitis in the last 15 years. Treatment consists of stopping antibiotics, supportive care, and oral or IV metronidazole or oral vancomycin. CMV colitis should be suspected in any immunocompromised patient who presents with bloody diarrhea. Endoscopy with biopsy confirms the diagnosis; treatment is IV ganciclovir.

Radiation proctitis has become more common in the last 30 or 40 years as the use of radiation to treat rectal cancer, prostate cancer, and gynecologic malignancies has increased. Patients present with bright red blood per rectum, diarrhea, tenesmus, and crampy pelvic pain. Flexible endoscopy reveals the characteristic bleeding telangiectasias (Fig. 48-16). Treatment consists of antidiarrheals, hydrocortisone enemas, and endoscopic APC. In cases of persistent bleeding, ablation with 4% formalin solution usually works well.

**Mesenteric Ischemia** Mesenteric ischemia can be secondary to acute or chronic arterial or venous insufficiency. Predisposing factors include preexisting cardiovascular disease (e.g., atrial fibrillation, congestive heart failure, acute myocardial infarction), recent abdominal vascular surgery, hypercoagulable states, medications (e.g., vasopressors, digoxin), and vasculitis. Acute colonic ischemia is the most common form of mesenteric ischemia. It tends to occur in the watershed areas of the splenic flexure and rectosigmoid colon, but can be right-sided in up to 40% of patients. Patients present with abdominal pain and bloody diarrhea. CT will often show a thickened bowel wall. The diagnosis is generally confirmed with flexible endoscopy, which reveals edema, hemorrhage, and a demarcation between the normal and abnormal mucosa. Treatment focuses on supportive care consisting of bowel rest, IV antibiotics, cardiovascular support, and correction of the low-flow state. In 85% of cases, the ischemia is self-limited and resolves without incident, although some patients develop a colonic stricture. In the other 15% of cases, surgery is indicated because of progressive ischemia and gangrene. Marked leukocytosis, fever, a fluid requirement, tachycardia, acidosis, and peritonitis indicate a failure of the ischemia to resolve and the need for surgical intervention. During the surgery, resection of the ischemic intestine and creation of an end ostomy is indicated.[47]

## OBSCURE CAUSES OF ACUTE GASTROINTESTINAL HEMORRHAGE

Obscure GI hemorrhage is defined as bleeding that persists or recurs after an initial negative evaluation with an EGD and colonoscopy. Obscure bleeding can be further subdivided into obscure-occult or obscure-overt bleeding. Obscure-occult bleeding is characterized by iron deficiency anemia or guaiac-positive stools without visible bleeding. If initial upper and lower endoscopy fail to identify a source for obscure-occult bleeding and the patient has no systemic signs of disease, she or he is often treated with iron therapy and more than 80% resolve symptoms in less than 2 years. Obscure-overt bleeding is characterized by recurrent or persistent visible bleeding.[48]

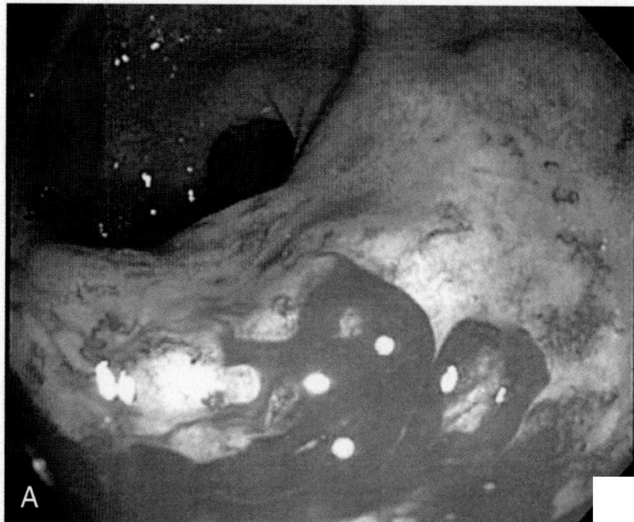


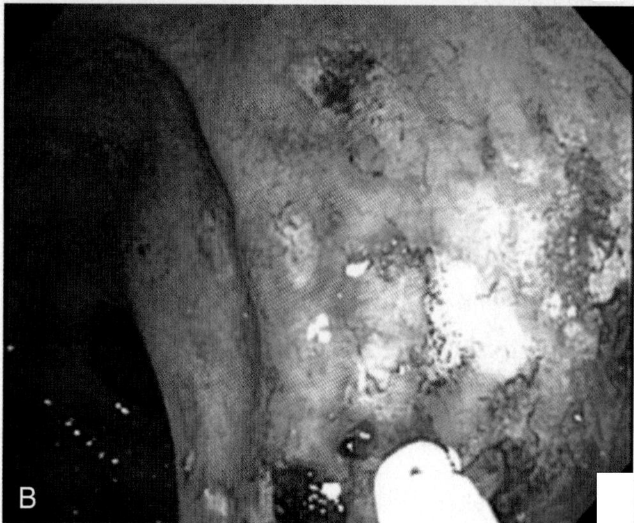


**FIGURE 48-16 A,** Rectal bleeding secondary to radiation damage. **B,** Effective control after application of argon plasma coagulation treatment. (Courtesy Dr. David L. Carr-Locke, Brigham and Women's Hospital, Boston.)

Obscure bleeding can be frustrating for the patient and physician and is especially true for obscure-overt bleeding ,which cannot be localized despite aggressive diagnostic measures. One study from a tertiary referral center has reported that the typical patient with obscure-overt bleeding suffers intermittent episodes of hemorrhage for 26 months, undergoes up to 20 diagnostic tests, and had receives an average of 20 U of blood before reaching a diagnosis.[49] Fortunately, obscure-overt bleeding is only responsible for about 1% of all cases of GI bleeding. The differential diagnosis of obscure-overt bleeding is long and varied (Box 48-3) and includes small bowel lesions not previously described. In a series of 200 patients with obscure bleeding, small bowel was identified as the source of bleeding in over 60% of cases. In these patients, small bowel ulcers and erosions secondary to Crohn's disease, Meckel's diverticulum, or NSAIDs was the most common cause.[50]

**BOX 48-3 Differential Diagnosis of Obscure Gastrointestinal Bleeding**

**Upper GI Bleeding**
Angiodysplasia
Peptic ulcer disease
Aortoenteric fistula
Neoplasia
HIV-related causes
Dieulafoy's lesion
Lymphoma
Sarcoidosis
Hemobilia
Hemosuccus pancreaticus
GAVE
Metastatic cancer

**Small Bowel Bleeding**
Crohn's disease
Meckel's diverticulum
Lymphoma
Radiation enteritis
Ischemia
HIV-related causes
Bacterial infection
Metastatic disease
Angiodysplasia
NSAID-induced erosions

**Colon Bleeding**
Colitis
- Ulcerative colitis
- Crohn's colitis
- Ischemic colitis
- Radiation colitis
- Infective colitis

Solitary rectal ulcer
Amyloidosis
Lymphoma
Endometriosis
Angiodysplasia
Neoplasia
HIV-related causes
Hemorrhoids

Adapted from McFadden DW: Occult and obscure sources of GI bleeding. In Cameron JL (ed): Current surgical therapy, ed 8, Philadelphia, 2004, Mosby, pp 117–121.

## Diagnosis

### Repeat Endoscopy

The cause of obscure-overt bleeding is often a common lesion that is missed on initial evaluation. Repeat upper and lower endoscopy are valuable tools for identifying missed lesions because up to 35% of patients will have the bleeding source identified on second-look endoscopy. Most of obscure GI hemorrhage is from a source distal to the ligament of Treitz. When repeat endoscopy fails to identify an obscure-overt bleeding source, investigation of the small bowel is warranted. This should proceed in an orderly fashion, depending on the degree of bleeding and the patient's hemodynamic status.

### Conventional Imaging

The next step is probably a tagged RBC scan, although its usefulness in this setting has not been established and, as discussed earlier, it may be misleading. Angiography may be more useful but usually requires significant ongoing hemorrhage. Provocative testing, which involves administering anticoagulants, fibrinolytics, or vasodilators to increase hemorrhage during angiography, has been used in small series with favorable results, but reluctance to induce uncontrolled hemorrhage has limited its use. Small bowel enteroclysis, which uses a tube to infuse barium, methylcellulose, and air directly into the small bowel, yields better images than simple small bowel follow-through. Because the yield has been reported to be very low and the test is poorly tolerated, it is now rarely used. It can identify gross lesions such as small bowel tumors, inflammatory conditions such as Crohn's disease, and small bowel ulcerations from NSAIDs and potassium supplementation. The limitation of small bowel radiography is that it cannot visualize angiodysplasias, the main cause of obscure small bowel hemorrhage.

In younger patients, usually younger than 30 years, part of the initial evaluation should be a Meckel's diverticulum scan. A Meckel's diverticulum with ectopic acid-secreting mucosa can ulcerate the small bowel and produce bleeding. This scan is performed by the administration of $^{99m}$Tc-pertechnetate that is taken up by the ectopic gastric mucosa in the diverticulum and localized with scintigraphy.

### Endoscopy

**Small Bowel Endoscopy** The hemodynamically stable patient should undergo small bowel enteroscopy. Usually performed with a pediatric colonoscope, it is referred to as *push endoscopy*. It can reach about 50 to 70 cm past the ligament of Treitz in most cases and permits endoscopic management of some lesions. Overall, push enteroscopy is successful in 40% of patients. Sonde pull endoscopy uses an enteroscope that passes passively into the very distal small bowel. A balloon on the end of the enteroscope permits normal small bowel peristalsis to carry the scope into the ileum; the mucosa is visualized as the scope is removed. This technique is cumbersome, does not permit intervention, and has largely been abandoned with the advent of capsule endoscopy.

Double-balloon endoscopy is another technique gaining in popularity. Although technically difficult, this approach is capable of providing a complete examination of the small bowel. In expert hands, double-balloon enteroscopy can identify a bleeding source in 77% of cases with occult bleeding, with the yield increasing to over 85% if the endoscopy is performed within 1 month of an overt bleeding episode.[50] The advantage of this technique is that as well as visualization, biopsies can be performed and therapeutic interventions undertaken.

**Video Capsule Endoscopy** Capsule endoscopy uses a small capsule with a video camera that is swallowed and acquires video images as it passes through the GI tract. This modality permits visualization of the entire GI tract, but offers no interventional capability. It is also time-consuming because someone has to watch the video to identify the bleeding source and a means to deal with the pathology then has to be developed. Despite this, capsule endoscopy is an excellent tool for the patient who is hemodynamically stable but continues to bleed. This technique has reported success rates as high as 90% in identifying a small bowel pathology. It is usually well tolerated, although it is contraindicated in patients with obstruction or a motility disorder.

**Intraoperative Endoscopy** Intraoperative enteroscopy should be reserved for patients who have transfusion-dependent obscure-overt bleeding in whom an exhaustive search has failed to identify a bleeding source. It typically uses a pediatric colonoscope introduced via the mouth or through an enterotomy in the small bowel made by the surgeon. In the latter case, a sterile colonoscope is passed onto the field, introduced into the small bowel, and passed bidirectionally, with the surgeon assisting to pass the bowel over the endoscope. Any suspicious areas are marked for possible resection or are dealt with endoscopically, if feasible. Because laparotomy has already been accomplished, it is usually preferable to resect the suspected areas.

### Treatment

Obscure GI hemorrhage requires a careful approach to diagnosis and management. Specific causes and their management are listed below. Up to 25% of cases of obscure lower GI hemorrhage remain without a diagnosis and 33% to 50% of patients will rebleed within 3 to 5 years.[48] Management strategies generally depend on the identification of a lesion. Iron replacement combined with intermittent transfusion is occasionally necessary, although this approach is not appealing.

## Specific Causes of Small Bowel Bleeding

### Angiodysplasias

Angiodysplasias are the most common cause of small intestinal bleeding, accounting for 40% of cases in older patients and 10% in younger patients. Most small intestinal vascular ectasias appear to occur in the jejunum, followed by the ileum and then the duodenum. The usual diagnostic tools are generally unsuccessful in identifying these lesions. Angiography is rarely positive. Instead, most small bowel vascular lesions require enteroscopy or capsule endoscopy for identification. In cases of severe hemorrhage requiring emergent operative intervention, intraoperative endoscopy may be helpful. Endoscope-directed segmental small bowel resection is the treatment of choice. Occasionally, these lesions may be diffuse; this may occur in hereditary hemorrhagic telangiectasia (Osler-Weber-Rendu syndrome), acute renal failure, or von Willebrand disease. In this situation, there has been limited experience with estrogen and progesterone treatment but it has been suggested that these agents may be of benefit.

### Neoplasia

Small bowel tumors are not very common, but can be sources of occult or frank GI bleeding. Bleeding typically results from erosion of the mucosa overlying the tumor. GISTs have the greatest propensity for bleeding. Small bowel tumors are typically diagnosed by small bowel contrast series or spiral CT scanning. Treatment involves surgical resection.

### Crohn's Disease

Patients with Crohn's disease may also present with small bowel bleeding in association with terminal ileitis. Bleeding is not generally significant nor is it usually the only presenting symptom. It is diagnosed by small bowel contrast series, and initial treatment is medical.

### Meckel's Diverticulum

Meckel's diverticulum is a true diverticulum in that it contains all layers of the small bowel wall. It is a congenital remnant of the omphalomesenteric duct, occurring in approximately 2% of the general population. Often, heterotopic tissue is present at the base of the diverticulum. Bleeding from a Meckel's diverticulum is usually from an ulcerative lesion on the ileal wall opposite the diverticulum, resulting from acid production by ectopic gastric mucosa. If nuclear medicine imaging is negative and bleeding is relatively brisk, angiography may be helpful in the diagnosis. Surgical management usually requires a segmental resection to incorporate the opposing ileal mucosa, which is typically the site of bleeding.

### Diverticula

Unlike a Meckel's diverticulum, small intestinal diverticula are false diverticula that do not involve all layers of the bowel. Bleeding from small bowel diverticula can present a diagnostic challenge. Capsule endoscopy or small intestinal contrast studies can confirm the diagnosis of diverticula and, in the absence of other sources of bleeding, it may be assumed that the diverticula are the source of bleeding. In cases of profuse bleeding, angiography or intraoperative endoscopy may be used to identify the bleeding source.

### SELECTED REFERENCES

Gralnek IM: Obscure-overt GI bleeding. Gastroenterology 128:1424–1430, 2005.

A concise discussion of the diagnostic approach to obscure bleeding, including the roles of small bowel fiberoptic and capsule endoscopy.

Rockey DC: Gastrointestinal bleeding. Gastroenterol Clin North Am 34:581–752, 2005.

A monograph covering all aspects of GI hemorrhage.

Sung JJ: Marshall and Warren Lecture 2009: Peptic ulcer bleeding: An expedition of 20 years from 1989-2009. J Gastroenterol Hepatol 25:229–233, 2010.

A review archiving the evolution of current endoscopic, pharmacologic, and surgical management of peptic ulcer bleeding. There is also a discussion of some of the present controversies.

Strate LL: Lower GI bleeding: Epidemiology and diagnosis. Gastroenterol Clin North Am 34:643–664, 2005.

A clear and concise review on the epidemiology of lower GI hemorrhage.

### REFERENCES

1. Peura DA, Lanza FL, Gostout CJ, et al: The American College of Gastroenterology Bleeding Registry: Preliminary findings. Am J Gastroenterol 92:924–928, 1997.

2. Rockey DC: Gastrointestinal bleeding. Gastroenterol Clin North Am 34:581–588, 2005.
3. Strate LL: Lower GI bleeding: Epidemiology and diagnosis. Gastroenterol Clin North Am 34:643–664, 2005.
4. Barkun A, Bardou M, Marshall JK: Consensus recommendations for managing patients with nonvariceal upper gastrointestinal bleeding. Ann Intern Med 139:843–857, 2003.
5. Dulai GS, Gralnek IM, Oei TT, et al: Utilization of health care resources for low-risk patients with acute, nonvariceal upper GI hemorrhage: An historical cohort study. Gastrointest Endosc 55:321–327, 2002.
6. Das A, Wong RC: Prediction of outcome of acute GI hemorrhage: A review of risk scores and predictive models. Gastrointest Endosc 60:85–93, 2004.
7. Lieberman D: Gastrointestinal bleeding: Initial management. Gastroenterol Clin North Am 22:723–736, 1993.
8. Kollef MH, O'Brien JD, Zuckerman GR, et al: BLEED: A classification tool to predict outcomes in patients with acute upper and lower gastrointestinal hemorrhage. Crit Care Med 25:1125–1132, 1997.
9. Tata LJ, Fortun PJ, Hubbard RB, et al: Does concurrent prescription of selective serotonin reuptake inhibitors and non-steroidal anti-inflammatory drugs substantially increase the risk of upper gastrointestinal bleeding? Aliment Pharmacol Ther 22:175–181, 2005.
10. Rubin TA, Murdoch M, Nelson DB: Acute GI bleeding in the setting of supratherapeutic international normalized ratio in patients taking warfarin: Endoscopic diagnosis, clinical management, and outcomes. Gastrointest Endosc 58:369–373, 2003.
11. Cuellar RE, Gavaler JS, Alexander JA, et al: Gastrointestinal tract hemorrhage. The value of a nasogastric aspirate. Arch Intern Med 150:1381–1384, 1990.
12. Cooper GS, Chak A, Way LE, et al: Early endoscopy in upper gastrointestinal hemorrhage: associations with recurrent bleeding, surgery, and length of hospital stay. Gastrointest Endosc 49:145–152, 1999.
13. Tsoi KK, Ma TK, Sung JJ: Endoscopy for upper gastrointestinal bleeding: How urgent is it? Nat Rev Gastroenterol Hepatol 6:463–469, 2009.
14. Sarin N, Monga N, Adams PC: Time to endoscopy and outcomes in upper gastrointestinal bleeding. Can J Gastroenterol 23:489–493, 2009.
15. Cheng CL, Lee CS, Liu NJ, et al: Overlooked lesions at emergency endoscopy for acute nonvariceal upper gastrointestinal bleeding. Endoscopy 34:527–530, 2002.
16. Frossard JL, Spahr L, Queneau PE, et al: Erythromycin intravenous bolus infusion in acute upper gastrointestinal bleeding: A randomized, controlled, double-blind trial. Gastroenterology 123:17–23, 2002.
17. Lassen A, Hallas J, Schaffalitzky de Muckadell OB: Complicated and uncomplicated peptic ulcers in a Danish county 1993-2002: A population-based cohort study. Am J Gastroenterol 101:945–953, 2006.
18. Higham J, Kang JY, Majeed A: Recent trends in admissions and mortality due to peptic ulcer in England: Increasing frequency of haemorrhage among older subjects. Gut 50:460–464, 2002.
19. Sung JJ: Marshall and Warren Lecture 2009: Peptic ulcer bleeding: An expedition of 20 years from 1989-2009. J Gastroenterol Hepatol 25:229–233, 2010.
20. Khuroo MS, Farahat KL, Kagevi IE: Treatment with proton pump inhibitors in acute non-variceal upper gastrointestinal bleeding: A meta-analysis. J Gastroenterol Hepatol 20:11–25, 2005.
21. Schilling D, Demel A, Nusse T, et al: *Helicobacter pylori* infection does not affect the early rebleeding rate in patients with peptic ulcer bleeding after successful endoscopic hemostasis: a prospective single-center trial. Endoscopy 35:393–396, 2003.
22. Gisbert JP, Khorrami S, Carballo F, et al: *H. pylori* eradication therapy vs. antisecretory non-eradication therapy (with or without long-term maintenance antisecretory therapy) for the prevention of recurrent bleeding from peptic ulcer. Cochrane Database Syst Rev CD004062, 2003.
23. Liu CC, Lee CL, Chan CC, et al: Maintenance treatment is not necessary after *Helicobacter pylori* eradication and healing of bleeding peptic ulcer: A 5-year prospective, randomized, controlled study. Arch Intern Med 163:2020–2024, 2003.
24. Hippisley-Cox J, Coupland C, Logan R: Risk of adverse gastrointestinal outcomes in patients taking cyclo-oxygenase-2 inhibitors or conventional non-steroidal anti-inflammatory drugs: Population-based nested case-control analysis. BMJ 331:1310–1316, 2005.
25. Chan FK, To KF, Wu JC, et al: Eradication of Helicobacter pylori and risk of peptic ulcers in patients starting long-term treatment with non-steroidal anti-inflammatory drugs: A randomised trial. Lancet 359:9–13, 2002.
26. Malfertheiner P, Megraud F, O'Morain C, et al: Current concepts in the management of Helicobacter pylori infection: The Maastricht III Consensus Report. Gut 56:772–781, 2007.
27. Lin HJ, Hsieh YH, Tseng GY, et al: A prospective, randomized trial of large- versus small-volume endoscopic injection of epinephrine for peptic ulcer bleeding. Gastrointest Endosc 55:615–619, 2002.
28. Lau JY, Sung JJ, Lam YH, et al: Endoscopic retreatment compared with surgery in patients with recurrent bleeding after initial endoscopic control of bleeding ulcers. N Engl J Med 340:751–756, 1999.
29. Guglielmi A, Ruzzenente A, Sandri M, et al: Risk assessment and prediction of rebleeding in bleeding gastroduodenal ulcer. Endoscopy 34:778–786, 2002.
30. Chung IK, Kim EJ, Lee MS, et al: Endoscopic factors predisposing to rebleeding following endoscopic hemostasis in bleeding peptic ulcers. Endoscopy 33:969–975, 2001.
31. Cook DJ, Fuller HD, Guyatt GH, et al: Risk factors for gastrointestinal bleeding in critically ill patients. Canadian Critical Care Trials Group. N Engl J Med 330:377–381, 1994.
32. Stiegmann GV: Endoscopic approaches to upper gastrointestinal bleeding. Am Surg 72:111–115, 2006.
33. Chalasani N, Kahi C, Francois F, et al: Improved patient survival after acute variceal bleeding: a multicenter, cohort study. Am J Gastroenterol 98:653–659, 2003.
34. Castaneda B, Morales J, Lionetti R, et al: Effects of blood volume restitution following a portal hypertensive-related bleeding in anesthetized cirrhotic rats. Hepatology 33:821–825, 2001.
35. Hou MC, Lin HC, Liu TT, et al: Antibiotic prophylaxis after endoscopic therapy prevents rebleeding in acute variceal hemorrhage: a randomized trial. Hepatology 39:746–753, 2004.
36. Corley DA, Cello JP, Adkisson W, et al: Octreotide for acute esophageal variceal bleeding: A meta-analysis. Gastroenterology 120:946–954, 2001.
37. Hsu YC, Chung CS, Tseng CH, et al: Delayed endoscopy as a risk factor for in-hospital mortality in cirrhotic patients with acute

variceal hemorrhage. J Gastroenterol Hepatol 24:1294–1299, 2009.

**38.** Henderson JM, Boyer TD, Kutner MH, et al: Distal splenorenal shunt versus transjugular intrahepatic portal systematic shunt for variceal bleeding: A randomized trial. Gastroenterology 130: 1643–1651, 2006.

**39.** Lo GH, Liang HL, Chen WC, et al: A prospective, randomized controlled trial of transjugular intrahepatic portosystemic shunt versus cyanoacrylate injection in the prevention of gastric variceal rebleeding. Endoscopy 39:679–685, 2007.

**40.** Heider TR, Azeem S, Galanko JA, et al: The natural history of pancreatitis-induced splenic vein thrombosis. Ann Surg 239: 876–880, 2004.

**41.** de la Pena J, Brullet E, Sanchez-Hernandez E, et al: Variceal ligation plus nadolol compared with ligation for prophylaxis of variceal rebleeding: A multicenter trial. Hepatology 41:572–578, 2005.

**42.** Riggio O, Angeloni S, Salvatori FM, et al: Incidence, natural history, and risk factors of hepatic encephalopathy after transjugular intrahepatic portosystemic shunt with polytetrafluoroethylene-covered stent grafts. Am J Gastroenterol 103:2738–2746, 2008.

**43.** Jensen DM, Machicado GA, Jutabha R, et al: Urgent colonoscopy for the diagnosis and treatment of severe diverticular hemorrhage. N Engl J Med 342:78–82, 2000.

**44.** Lipof T, Sardella WV, Bartus CM, et al: The efficacy and durability of super-selective embolization in the treatment of lower gastrointestinal bleeding. Dis Colon Rectum 51:301–305, 2008.

**45.** Bender JS, Wiencek RG, Bouwman DL: Morbidity and mortality following total abdominal colectomy for massive lower gastrointestinal bleeding. Am Surg 57:536–540, 1991.

**46.** Pardi DS, Loftus EV, Jr., Tremaine WJ, et al: Acute major gastrointestinal hemorrhage in inflammatory bowel disease. Gastrointest Endosc 49:153–157, 1999.

**47.** Walker AM, Bohn RL, Cali C, et al: Risk factors for colon ischemia. Am J Gastroenterol 99:1333–1337, 2004.

**48.** Gralnek IM: Obscure-overt gastrointestinal bleeding. Gastroenterology 128:1424–1430, 2005.

**49.** Szold A, Katz LB, Lewis BS: Surgical approach to occult gastrointestinal bleeding. Am J Surg 163:90–92; discussion 92–93, 1992.

**50.** Shinozaki S, Yamamoto H, Yano T, et al: Long-term outcome of patients with obscure gastrointestinal bleeding investigated by double-balloon endoscopy. Clin Gastroenterol Hepatol 8:151–158, 2010.

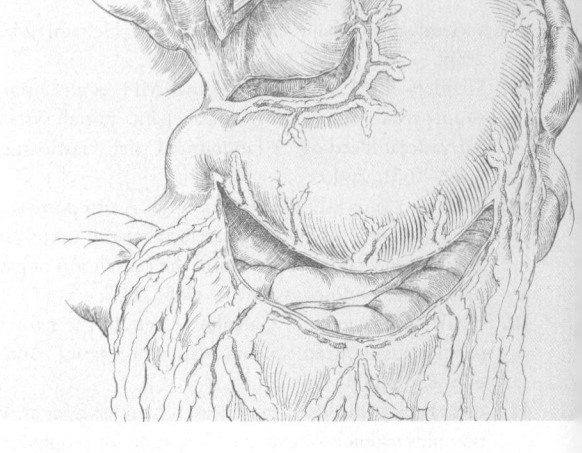

# CHAPTER 49

# STOMACH

David M. Mahvi and Seth B. Krantz



## ANATOMY

### Gross Anatomy

#### Divisions

The stomach begins as a dilation in the tubular embryonic foregut during the fifth week of gestation. By the seventh week, it descends, rotates, and further dilates with a disproportionate elongation of the greater curvature into its normal anatomic shape and position. Following birth, it is the most proximal abdominal organ of the alimentary tract. The most proximal region of the stomach is called the *cardia*, which attaches to the esophagus. Immediately proximal to the cardia is a physiologically competent lower esophageal sphincter. Distally, the pylorus connects the distal stomach (antrum) to the proximal duodenum. Although the stomach is fixed at the gastroesophageal (GE) junction and pylorus, its large midportion is mobile. The fundus represents the superiormost part of the stomach and is floppy and distensible. The stomach is bounded superiorly by the diaphragm and laterally by the spleen. The body of the stomach represents the largest portion and is also referred to as the *corpus*. The body also contains most of the parietal cells and is bounded on the right by the relatively straight lesser curvature and on the left by the longer greater curvature. At the angularis incisura, the lesser curvature abruptly angles to the right. It is here that the body of the stomach ends and the antrum begins. Another important anatomic angle (angle of His) is that formed by the fundus with the left margin of the esophagus (Fig. 49-1).

Most of the stomach resides within the upper abdomen. The left lateral segment of the liver covers a large portion of the stomach anteriorly. The diaphragm, chest, and abdominal wall bound the remainder of the stomach. Inferiorly, the stomach is attached to the transverse colon, spleen, caudate lobe of the liver, diaphragmatic crura, and retroperitoneal nerves and vessels. Superiorly, the GE junction is found about 2 to 3 cm below the diaphragmatic esophageal hiatus in the horizontal plane of the seventh chondrosternal articulation, a plane only slightly cephalad to that containing the pylorus. The gastrosplenic ligament attaches the proximal greater curvature to the spleen.

#### Blood Supply

The celiac artery provides most of the blood supply to the stomach (Fig. 49-2). There are four main arteries—the left and right gastric arteries along the lesser curvature and the left and right gastroepiploic arteries along the greater curvature. In addition, a substantial quantity of blood may be supplied to the proximal stomach by the inferior phrenic arteries and by the short gastric arteries from the spleen. The largest artery to the stomach is the left gastric artery, and it is not uncommon (15% to 20%) for an aberrant left hepatic artery to originate from it. Consequently, proximal ligation of the left gastric artery occasionally results in acute left-sided hepatic ischemia. The right gastric artery arises from the hepatic artery (or the gastroduodenal artery). The left gastroepiploic artery originates from the splenic artery and the right gastroepiploic originates from the gastroduodenal artery. The extensive anastomotic connection between these major vessels ensures that in most cases, the stomach will survive if three out of four arteries are ligated, provided that the arcades along the greater and lesser curvatures are not disturbed. In general, the veins of the stomach parallel the arteries. The left gastric (coronary) and right gastric veins usually drain into the portal vein. The right gastroepiploic vein drains into the superior mesenteric vein and the left gastroepiploic vein drains into the splenic vein.

#### Lymphatic Drainage

The lymphatic drainage of the stomach parallels the vasculature and drains into four zones of lymph nodes (Fig. 49-3). The superior gastric group drains lymph from the upper lesser curvature into the left gastric and paracardial nodes. The suprapyloric group of nodes drains the antral segment on the lesser curvature of the stomach into the right suprapancreatic nodes. The pancreaticolienal group of nodes drains lymph high on the greater curvature into the left gastroepiploic and splenic nodes. The inferior gastric and subpyloric group of nodes drains lymph along the right gastroepiploic vascular pedicle. All four zones of lymph nodes drain into the celiac group and into the thoracic duct. Although these lymph nodes drain different areas of the stomach, gastric cancers may metastasize to any of the four nodal groups, regardless of the cancer location. In addition, the extensive submucosal plexus of lymphatics accounts for the fact that there is frequently microscopic evidence of malignant cells several centimeters from gross disease.

### Innervation

As shown in Figure 49-4, the extrinsic innervation of the stomach is parasympathetic (via the vagus) and sympathetic (via the celiac plexus). The vagus nerve originates in the vagal nucleus in the floor of the fourth ventricle and traverses the neck in the carotid sheath to enter the mediastinum, where it divides into several branches around the esophagus. These branches coalesce above the esophageal hiatus to form the left and right vagus nerves. It is not uncommon to find more than two vagal trunks at the distal esophagus. At the GE junction, the ***l***eft vagus is ***a***nterior, and the ***r***ight vagus is ***p***osterior (LARP).

The left vagus gives off the hepatic branch to the liver and then continues along the lesser curvature as the anterior nerve of Latarjet. Although not shown, the so-called *criminal nerve of Grassi* is the first branch of the right or posterior vagus nerve; it is recognized as a potential cause of recurrent ulcers when left undivided. The right nerve gives a branch off to the celiac plexus and then continues posteriorly along the lesser curvature. A truncal vagotomy is performed above the celiac and hepatic branches of the vagi, whereas a selective vagotomy is performed below. A highly selective vagotomy is performed by dividing the crow's feet to the proximal stomach while preserving the innervation of the antral and pyloric parts of the stomach. Most (90%) of the vagal fibers are afferent, carrying stimuli from the gut to the brain. Efferent vagal fibers originate in the dorsal nucleus of the medulla and synapse with neurons in the myenteric and submucosal plexuses. These neurons use acetylcholine as their neurotransmitter and influence gastric motor function and gastric secretion. In contrast, the sympathetic nerve supply comes from T5 to T10, traveling in the splanchnic nerve to the

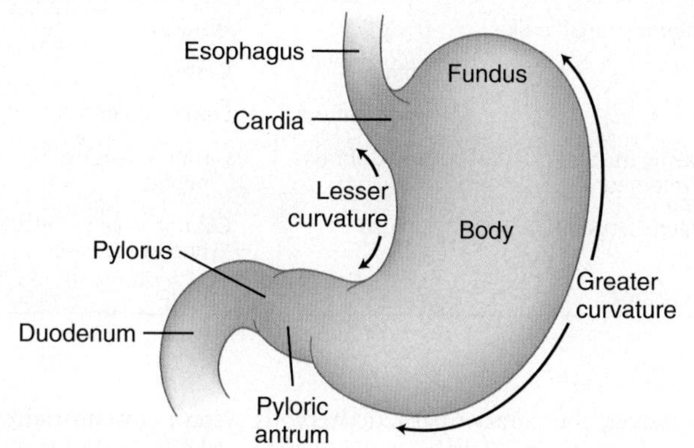


**FIGURE 49-1** Divisions of the stomach. (From Yeo C: Shackelford's surgery of the alimentary tract, ed 6, Philadelphia, 2007, WB Saunders.)

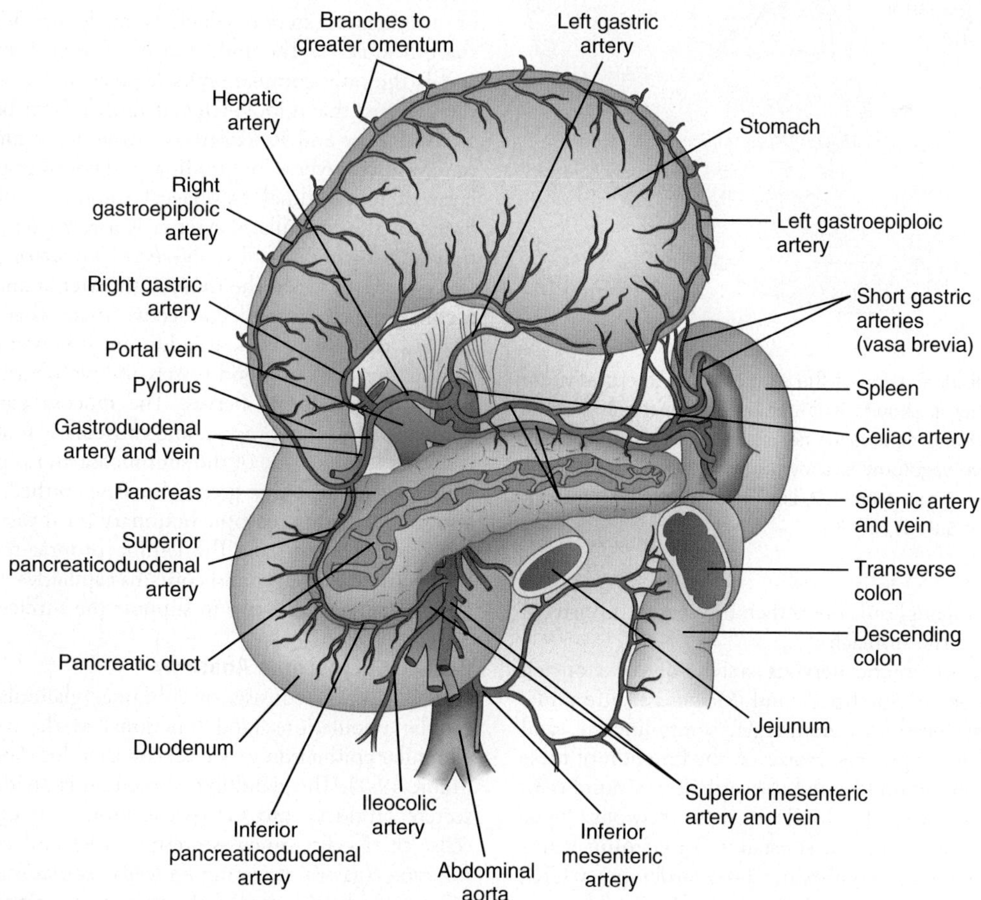


**FIGURE 49-2** Blood supply to the stomach and duodenum showing anatomic relationships to the spleen and pancreas. The stomach is reflected cephalad. (From Yeo C: Shackelford's surgery of the alimentary tract, ed 6, Philadelphia, 2007, WB Saunders.)

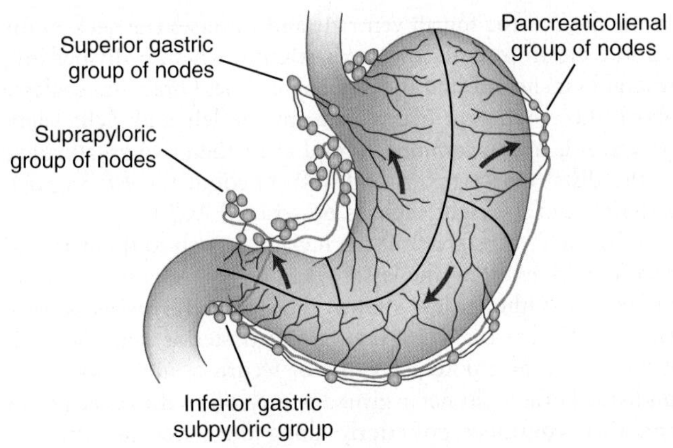


**FIGURE 49-3** Lymphatic drainage of the stomach.

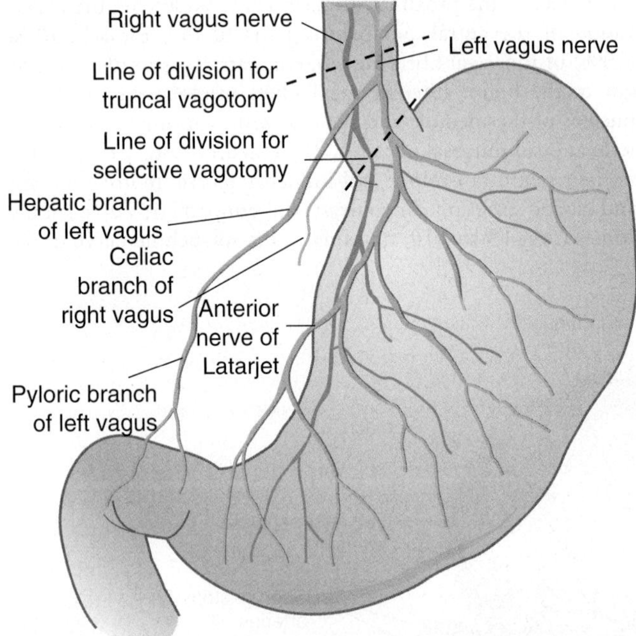


**FIGURE 49-4** Vagal innervation of the stomach. The line of division for truncal vagotomy is shown; it is above the hepatic and celiac branches of the left and right vagus nerves, respectively. The line of division for selective vagotomy is shown; this is below the hepatic and celiac branches. (From Mercer D, Liu T: Open truncal vagotomy. Oper Tech Gen Surg 5:8–85, 2003.)

celiac ganglion. Postganglionic fibers then travel with the arterial system to innervate the stomach.

The intrinsic or enteric nervous system of the stomach consists of neurons in Auerbach's and Meissner's autonomic plexuses. In these locations, cholinergic, serotoninergic, and peptidergic neurons are present. However, the function of these neurons remains poorly understood. Nevertheless, a number of neuropeptides have been localized to these neurons; these include acetylcholine, serotonin, substance P, calcitonin gene–related peptide (CGRP), bombesin, cholecystokinin (CCK), and somatostatin. Consequently, it is an oversimplification to think of the stomach as only containing parasympathetic (cholinergic input) and sympathetic (adrenergic input) supply.

**Table 49-1 Gastric Cell Types, Location, and Function**

| CELL TYPE | LOCATION | FUNCTION |
|---|---|---|
| Parietal | Body | Secretion of acid and intrinsic factor |
| Mucus | Body, antrum | Mucus |
| Chief | Body | Pepsin |
| Surface epithelial | Diffuse | Mucus, bicarbonate, prostaglandins (?) |
| Enterochromaffin-like | Body | Histamine |
| G | Antrum | Gastrin |
| D | Body, antrum | Somatostatin |
| Gastric mucosal interneurons | Body, antrum | Gastrin-releasing peptide |
| Enteric neurons | Diffuse | Calcitonin gene–related peptide, others |
| Endocrine | Body | Ghrelin |

Moreover, the parasympathetic nervous system contains adrenergic neurons and the sympathetic system also contains cholinergic neurons.

### Gastric Morphology

The stomach is covered by peritoneum, which forms the outer serosa of the stomach. Below it is the thicker muscularis propria, or muscularis externa, which is made up of three layers of smooth muscles. The middle layer of smooth muscle is circular and is the only complete muscle layer of the stomach wall. At the pylorus, this middle circular muscle layer becomes progressively thicker and functions as a true anatomic sphincter. The outer muscle layer is longitudinal and continuous with the outer layer of longitudinal esophageal smooth muscle. Within the layers of the muscularis externa is a rich plexus of autonomic nerves and ganglia, called *Auerbach's myenteric plexus*. The submucosa lies between the muscularis externa and mucosa and is a collagen-rich layer of connective tissue that is the strongest layer of the gastric wall. In addition, it contains the rich anastomotic network of blood vessels and lymphatics and Meissner's plexus of autonomic nerves. The mucosa consists of surface epithelium, lamina propria, and muscularis mucosae. The latter is on the luminal side of the submucosa and is probably responsible for the rugae that greatly increase epithelial surface area. It also marks the microscopic boundary for invasive and noninvasive gastric carcinoma. The lamina propria represents a small connective tissue layer and contains capillaries, vessels, lymphatics, and nerves necessary to support the surface epithelium.

### Gastric Microscopic Anatomy

Gastric mucosa consists of columnar glandular epithelia. The cellular populations (and functions) of the cells forming this glandular epithelium vary based on their location in the stomach (Table 49-1). The glandular epithelium is divided into cells that secrete products into the gastric lumen for digestion (parietal cells, chief cells, mucus-secreting cells) and cells that control function (gastrin-secreting G cells, somatostatin-secreting D cells) cells. In the cardia, the mucosa is arranged in branched glands and the pits are short. In the fundus and body, the glands are more tubular and the pits are longer. In the antrum, the

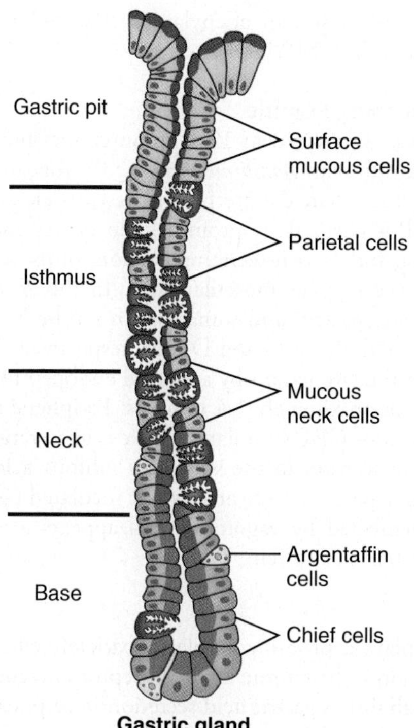


**FIGURE 49-5** Cells residing within a gastric gland. (From Yeo C: Shackelford's surgery of the alimentary tract, ed 6, Philadelphia, 2007, WB Saunders.)

glands are more branched. The luminal ends of the gastric glands and pits are lined with mucus-secreting surface epithelial cells, which extend down into the necks of the glands for variable distances. In the cardia, the glands are predominantly mucus-secreting. In the body, the glands are mostly lined from the neck to the base with parietal and chief cells (Fig. 49-5). There are a few parietal cells in the fundus and proximal antrum, but none in the cardia or prepyloric antrum. The endocrine G cells are present in greatest quantity in the antral glands.

## PHYSIOLOGY

The principal function of the stomach is to prepare ingested food for digestion and absorption as it is propulsed into the small intestine. The initial period of digestion requires that solid components of a meal be stored for several hours while they undergo a reduction in size and break down into their basic metabolic constituents.

Receptive relaxation of the proximal stomach enables the stomach to function as a storage organ. Receptive relaxation refers to the process whereby the proximal portion of the stomach relaxes in anticipation of food intake. This relaxation enables liquids to pass easily from the stomach along the lesser curvature, whereas the solid food settles along the greater curvature of the fundus. In contrast to liquids, emptying of solid food is facilitated by the antrum, which pumps solid food components into and through the pylorus. The antrum and pylorus function in a coordinated fashion, allowing entry of food components into the duodenum and also returning material to the proximal stomach until it is suitable for delivery into the duodenum.

In addition to storing food, the stomach begins digestion of a meal. Starches undergo enzymatic breakdown through the activity of salivary amylase. Peptic digestion metabolizes a meal into fats, proteins, and carbohydrates by breaking down cell walls. Although the duodenum and proximal small intestine are primarily responsible for digestion of a meal, the stomach facilitates this process.

### Regulation of Gastric Function

Gastric function is under neural (sympathetic and parasympathetic) and hormonal control (peptides or amines that interact with target cells in the stomach). An understanding of the roles of endocrine and neural regulation of digestion is critical to understanding gastric physiology. Abnormal secretion of gastrin and pepsin was thought to be the major causative factor in peptic ulcer disease (PUD). The discovery of *Helicobacter pylori (H. pylori)* and the effect of this organism on ulcer disease has rendered moot many of the theoretical rationales for acid hypersecretion. A general understanding of gastric physiology and the specific impact of peptides on acid secretion, however, is still critical to understanding the physiologic effects of gastric surgical procedures on digestion. We will initially focus here on peptide regulation of gastric function and then describe the interactions of these peptides with neural inputs in regard to acid secretion and gastric function.

### Gastric Peptides

#### Gastrin

Gastrin is produced by G cells located in the gastric antrum (see Table 49-1). It is synthesized as a prepropeptide and undergoes post-translational processing to produce biologically reactive gastrin peptides. Several molecular forms of gastrin exist. G-34 (big gastrin), G-17 (little gastrin), and G-14 (minigastrin) have been identified. However, 90% of antral gastrin is released as the 17–amino acid peptide, although G-34 predominates in the circulation because its metabolic half-life is longer than that of G-17. The pentapeptide sequence contained at the carboxyl terminus of gastrin is the biologically active component and is identical to that found on another gut peptide, CCK. CCK and gastrin differ by tyrosine sulfation sites. The release of gastrin is stimulated by food components in a meal, especially protein digestion products. Luminal acid inhibits the release of gastrin. In the antral location, somatostatin and gastrin release are functionally linked, and an inverse reciprocal relationship exists between these two peptides.[1]

Gastrin is the major hormonal regulator of the gastric phase of acid secretion following a meal. Histamine, released from enterochromaffin-like (ECL) cells, is also a potent stimulant of acid release from the parietal cell. Gastrin also has considerable trophic effects on the parietal cells and gastric ECL cells. Prolonged hypergastrinemia from any cause leads to mucosal hyperplasia and an increase in the number of ECL cells and, under some circumstances, is associated with the development of gastric carcinoid tumors.[2]

The detection of hypergastrinemia may suggest a pathologic state of acid hypersecretion but generally is the result of treatment with agents to lower acid secretion, such as proton pump inhibitors. Table 49-2 lists common causes of chronic hypergastrinemia. Hypergastrinemia that results from the administration of acid-lowering drugs is an appropriate response

**Table 49-2 Causes of Hypergastrinemia**

| ULCEROGENIC CAUSES | NONULCEROGENIC CAUSES |
|---|---|
| Antral G-cell hyperplasia or hyperfunction | Antisecretory agents (PPIs) |
| Retained excluded antrum | Atrophic gastritis |
| Zollinger-Ellison syndrome | Pernicious anemia |
| Gastric outlet obstruction | Acid-reducing procedure (vagotomy) |
| Short-gut syndrome | *Helicobacter pylori* infection<br>Chronic renal failure |

caused by loss of feedback inhibition of gastrin release by luminal acid. Lack of acid causes a reduction in somatostatin release, which in turn causes increased release of gastrin from antral G cells. Hypergastrinemia can also occur in the setting of pernicious anemia or uremia, or following surgical procedures such as vagotomy or retained gastric antrum after gastrectomy. In contrast, gastrin levels increase inappropriately in patients with gastrinoma (Zollinger-Ellison syndrome [ZES]). These gastrin-secreting tumors are not located in the antrum and secrete gastrin autonomously.

Gastrin initiates its biologic actions by activation of surface membrane receptors. These receptors are members of the classic G protein–coupled seven–transmembrane-spanning receptor family and are classified as type A or B CCK receptors. The gastrin or CCK-B receptor has high affinity for gastrin and CCK, whereas the type A CCK receptors have an affinity for sulfated CCK analogues and a low affinity for gastrin. Binding of gastrin with the CCK-B receptor has been associated with elevated intracellular calcium levels.

### Somatostatin

Somatostatin is produced by D cells and exists endogenously as the 14– or 28–amino acid peptide. The predominant molecular form in the stomach is somatostatin-14. It is produced by diffuse neuroendocrine cells located in the fundus and antrum. In these locations, D cell cytoplasmic extensions have direct contact with the parietal cells and G cells, where it presumably exerts its actions through paracrine effects on acid secretion and gastrin release.[3] Somatostatin is able to inhibit parietal cell acid secretion directly but can also indirectly inhibit acid secretion through inhibition of gastrin release and downregulation of histamine release from ECL cells. The principal stimulus for somatostatin release is antral acidification, whereas acetylcholine from vagal fibers inhibits its release.

Somatostatin receptors are also seven–transmembrane-spanning receptors. Binding of somatostatin with its receptors is coupled to one or more inhibitory guanine nucleotide–binding proteins. Parietal cell somatostatin receptors appear to be a single subunit of glycoproteins with a molecular weight of 99 kDa, with equal affinity for somatostatin-14 and somatostatin-28. Somatostatin can inhibit parietal cell secretion through G protein–dependent and G protein–independent mechanisms. However, the ability of somatostatin to exert its inhibitory actions on cellular function is primarily thought to be mediated through the inhibition of adenylate cyclase, with a resultant reduction in cyclic AMP levels.

### Gastrin-Releasing Peptide

Bombesin was discovered in 1970 in an extract prepared from skin of the amphibian *Bombina bombina* (European fire-bellied toad). Its mammalian counterpart is gastrin-releasing peptide (GRP). GRP is particularly prominent in nerves ending in the acid-secreting and gastrin-secreting portions of the stomach and is found in the circular muscular layer. In the antral mucosa, GRP stimulates gastrin and somatostatin release by binding to receptors located on the G and D cells, respectively. It is rapidly cleared from the circulation by a neutral endopeptidase and has a half-life of approximately 1.4 minutes. Peripheral administration of exogenous GRP stimulates gastric acid secretion, whereas central administration in the ventricles inhibits acid secretion. The inhibitory pathway activated is not mediated by a humoral factor, is unaffected by vagotomy, and appears to involve the sympathetic nervous system.

### Histamine

Histamine plays a prominent role in parietal cell stimulation. Administration of histamine 2 ($H_2$) receptor antagonists almost completely abolishes gastric acid secretion in response to gastrin and acetylcholine. This suggests that histamine may be a necessary intermediary of gastrin- and acetylcholine-stimulated acid secretion. Histamine is stored in the acidic granules of ECL cells and in resident mast cells. Its release is stimulated by gastrin, acetylcholine, and epinephrine following receptor-ligand interactions on ECL cells. In contrast, somatostatin inhibits gastrin-stimulated histamine release through interactions with somatostatin receptors located on the ECL cell. Thus, the ECL cell plays an essential role in parietal cell activation that possesses stimulatory and inhibitory feedback pathways that modulate the release of histamine and therefore acid secretion.

### Ghrelin

Ghrelin is a 28–amino acid peptide predominantly produced by endocrine cells of the oxyntic mucosa of the stomach, with substantially lower amounts from the bowel, pancreas, and other organs. Removal of the acid-producing part of the stomach decreases circulating ghrelin by 80%. Ghrelin appears to be under endocrine and metabolic control, has a diurnal rhythm, likely plays a major role in the neuroendocrine and metabolic responses to changes in nutritional status, and may be a major anabolic hormone.

In human volunteers, ghrelin administration enhances appetite and increases food intake. In patients who have undergone a gastric bypass, ghrelin levels are 77% lower than those of matched obese controls, a finding not seen after other forms of antiobesity surgery. Although the mechanism responsible for suppression of ghrelin levels after gastric bypass is unknown, this suggests that ghrelin may be responsive to the normal flow of nutrients across the stomach. Other studies have suggested that ghrelin leads to a switch toward glycolysis and away from fatty acid oxidation, which would favor fat deposition. It appears that ghrelin is upregulated in times of negative energy balance and downregulated in times of positive energy balance, although the precise role of ghrelin in energy metabolism remains unclear. Ghrelin may come to have a role in the treatment and prevention of obesity.

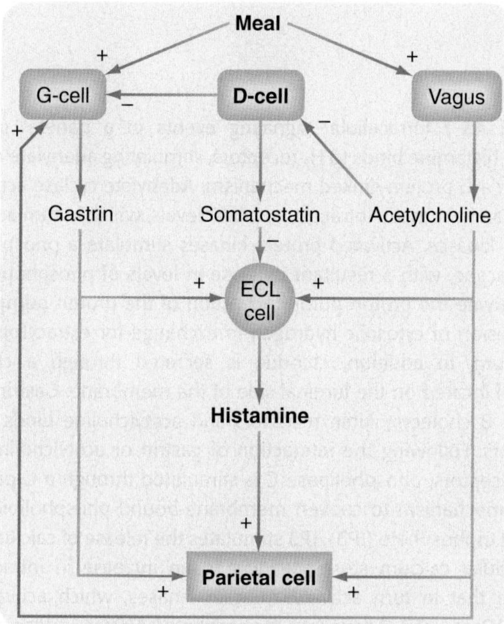


**FIGURE 49-6** Central role of the ECL cell in regulation of acid secretion by the parietal cell. As shown, ingestion of a meal stimulates vagal fibers to release acetylcholine (cephalic phase). Binding of acetylcholine to M3 receptors located on the ECL cell, parietal cell, and G cell results in the release of histamine, hydrochloric acid, and gastrin, respectively. Binding of acetylcholine to M3 receptors on D cells results in the inhibition of somatostatin release. Following a meal, G cells are also stimulated to release gastrin, which interacts with receptors located on ECL cells and parietal cells to cause the release of histamine and hydrochloric acid (gastric phase). Release of somatostatin from D cells decreases histamine release and gastrin release from ECL cells and G cells, respectively. In addition, somatostatin inhibits parietal cell acid secretion (not shown). The principal stimulus for the activation of D cells is antral luminal acidification (not shown). (From Yeo C: Shackelford's surgery of the alimentary tract, ed 6, Philadelphia, 2007, WB Saunders.)

## Gastric Acid Secretion

Gastric acid secretion by the parietal cell is regulated by three local stimuli—acetylcholine, gastrin, and histamine. These three stimuli account for basal and stimulated gastric acid secretion. Acetylcholine is the principal neurotransmitter modulating acid secretion and is released from the vagus and parasympathetic ganglion cells. Vagal fibers innervate not only parietal cells but also G cells and ECL cells to modulate release of their peptides. Gastrin has hormonal effects on the parietal cell and stimulates histamine release. Histamine has paracrine-like effects on the parietal cell and, as shown in Figure 49-6, plays a central role in the regulation of acid secretion by the parietal cell after its release from ECL cells. As depicted, somatostatin exerts inhibitory actions on gastric acid secretion. Release of somatostatin from antral D cells is stimulated in the presence of intraluminal acid to a pH of 3 or lower. After its release, somatostatin inhibits gastrin release through paracrine effects and also modifies histamine release from ECL cells. In some patients with PUD, this negative feedback response is defective. Consequently, the precise state of acid secretion by the parietal cell is dependent on the overall influence of the positive and negative stimuli.

In the absence of food, there is always a basal level of acid secretion that is approximately 10% of maximal acid output. Under basal conditions, 1 to 5 mmol/hr of hydrochloric acid is secreted, and this is reduced after vagotomy or $H_2$ receptor blockade. Thus, it appears likely that basal acid secretion is caused by a combination of cholinergic and histaminergic input.

### Stimulated Acid Secretion

**Cephalic Phase** Ingestion of food is the physiologic stimulus for acid secretion. Three phases of the acid secretory response to a meal have been described, cephalic, gastric, and intestinal. These three phases are interrelated and occur concurrently, not consecutively.

The cephalic phase originates with the sight, smell, thought, and/or taste of food, which stimulates neural centers in the cortex and hypothalamus. Although the exact mechanisms whereby senses stimulate acid secretion remain to be fully elucidated, it is hypothesized that several sites are stimulated in the brain. These higher centers transmit signals to the stomach by the vagus nerves, which release acetylcholine that in turn activates muscarinic receptors located on target cells. Acetylcholine directly increases acid secretion by the parietal cells and can inhibit and stimulate gastrin release, the net effect being a slight increase in gastrin levels. Although the intensity of the acid secretory response in the cephalic phase surpasses that of the other phases, it accounts for only 20% to 30% of the total volume of gastric acid produced in response to a meal because of the short duration of the cephalic phase.

**Gastric Phase** The gastric phase of acid secretion begins when food enters the gastric lumen. Digestion products of ingested food interact with microvilli of antral G cells to stimulate gastrin release. Food also stimulates acid secretion by causing mechanical distention of the stomach. Gastric distention activates stretch receptors in the stomach to elicit the long vagovagal reflex arc. It is abolished by proximal gastric vagotomy and is, at least in part, independent of changes in serum gastrin levels. However, antral distention also causes gastrin release in humans, a reflex that has been called the *pyloro-oxyntic reflex*. In humans, mechanical distention of the stomach accounts for about 30% to 40% of the maximal acid secretory response to a peptone meal, with the remainder caused by gastrin release. The entire gastric phase accounts for most (60% to 70%) of meal-stimulated acid output because it lasts until the stomach is empty.

**Intestinal Phase** The intestinal phase of gastric secretion remains poorly understood but appears to be initiated by entry of chyme into the small intestine. It occurs after gastric emptying and lasts as long as partially digested food components remain in the proximal small bowel. It accounts for only 10% of the acid secretory response to a meal and does not appear to be mediated by serum gastrin levels. It has been hypothesized that a distinct acid stimulatory peptide hormone (entero-oxyntin) released from small bowel mucosa may mediate the intestinal phase of acid secretion.

### Activation and Secretion by the Parietal Cell

The two second messengers principally involved in stimulation of acid secretion by parietal cells are intracellular cyclic AMP (cAMP) and calcium. Synthesis of these two messengers in turn

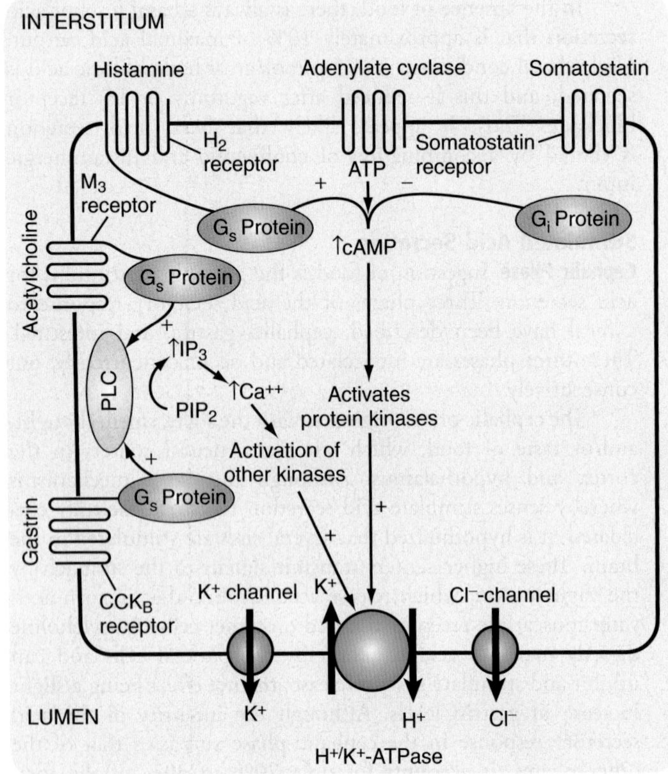


**FIGURE 49-7** Intracellular signaling events in a parietal cell. As shown, histamine binds to $H_2$ receptors, stimulating adenylate cyclase through a G protein–linked mechanism. Adenylate cyclase activation causes an increase in intracellular cAMP levels, which in turn activates protein kinases. Activated protein kinases stimulate a phosphorylation cascade, with a resultant increase in levels of phosphoproteins that activate the proton pump. Activation of the proton pump leads to extrusion of cytosolic hydrogen in exchange for extracytoplasmic potassium. In addition, chloride is secreted through a chloride channel located on the luminal side of the membrane. Gastrin binds to type B cholecystokinin receptors and acetylcholine binds to M3 receptors. Following the interaction of gastrin or acetylcholine with their receptors, phospholipase C is stimulated through a G protein–linked mechanism to convert membrane-bound phospholipids into inositol triphosphate (IP3). IP3 stimulates the release of calcium from intracellular calcium stores, leading to an increase in intracellular calcium that in turn activates protein kinases, which activate the $H^+,K^+$-ATPase. *ATP,* Adenosine triphosphate; *ATPase,* adenosine triphosphatase; *cAMP,* cyclic adenosine monophosphate; *Gi,* inhibitory guanine nucleotide protein; *Gs,*stimulatory guanine nucleotide protein; *PIP2,* phosphatidylinositol 4,5- diphosphate; *PLC,* phospholipase C. (From Yeo C: Shackelford's surgery of the alimentary tract, ed 6, Philadelphia, 2007, WB Saunders.)

activates protein kinases and phosphorylation cascades. The intracellular events following ligand binding to receptors on the parietal cell are shown in Figure 49-7. Histamine causes an increase in intracellular cAMP, which activates protein kinases to initiate a cascade of phosphorylation events that culminate in activation of $H^+$, $K^+$-ATPase. In contrast, acetylcholine and gastrin stimulate phospholipase C, which converts membrane-bound phospholipids into inositol triphosphate ($IP_3$) to mobilize calcium from intracellular stores. Increased intracellular calcium activates other protein kinases that ultimately activate $H^+$, $K^+$-ATPase in a similar fashion to initiate the secretion of hydrochloric acid.

$H^+$, $K^+$-ATPase is the final common pathway for gastric acid secretion by the parietal cell. It is composed of two subunits, a catalytic α-subunit (100 kDa) and a glycoprotein β-subunit (60 kDa). During the resting, or nonsecreting, state, gastric parietal cells store $H^+$, $K^+$-ATPase within intracellular tubulovesicular elements. Cellular relocation of the proton pump subunits through cytoskeletal rearrangements must occur in order for acid secretion to increase in response to stimulatory factors. The subsequent insertion and heterodimer assembly of the $H^+$, $K^+$-ATPase subunits into the microvilli of the secretory canaliculus causes an increase in gastric acid secretion. A KCl efflux pathway must exist to supply potassium to the extracytoplasmic side of the pump. Cytosolic hydrogen is secreted by $H^+$, $K^+$-ATPase in exchange for extracytoplasmic potassium (see Fig. 49-7), which is an electroneutral exchange and therefore does not contribute to the transmembrane potential difference across the parietal cell. Secretion of chloride is accomplished through a chloride channel moving chloride from the parietal cell cytoplasm to the gastric lumen. The secretion or exchange of hydrogen for potassium, however, does require energy in the form of

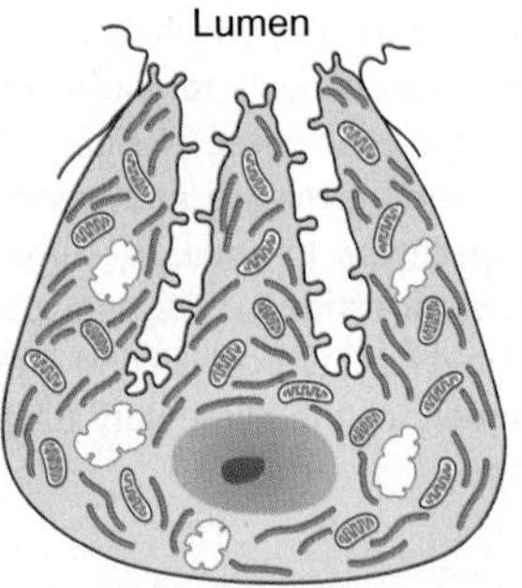


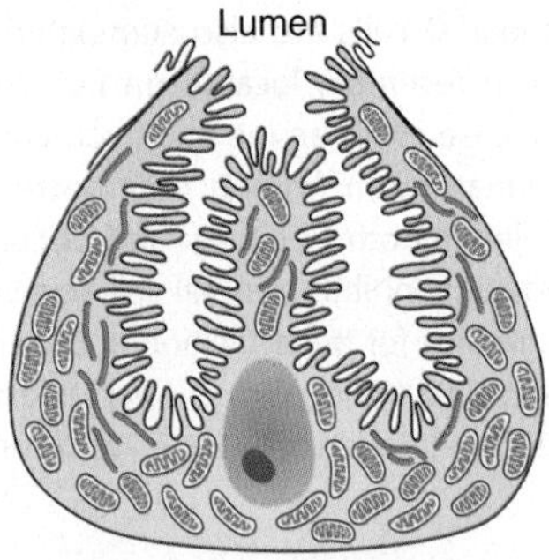


**Nonsecreting parietal cell** **Acid-secreting parietal cell**

**FIGURE 49-8** Diagrammatic representation of resting and stimulated parietal cells. Note the morphologic transformation between the nonsecreting parietal cell and stimulated parietal cell, with increases in secretory canalicular membrane surface area.

adenosine triphosphate (ATP) because hydrogen is being secreted against a gradient of more than a million-fold. Because of this large energy requirement, the parietal cell also has the largest mitochondrial content of any mammalian cell, with a mitochondrial compartment representing 34% of its cell volume. In response to a secretagogue, the parietal cell undergoes a conformational change, and a several-fold increase in the canalicular surface area occurs (Fig. 49-8). In contrast to stimulated acid secretion, cessation of acid secretion requires endocytosis of $H^+$, $K^+$-ATPase, with regeneration of cytoplasmic tubulovesicles containing the subunits, and this occurs through a tyrosine-based signal. The tyrosine-containing sequence is located on the cytoplasmic tail of the β-subunit and is highly homologous to the motif responsible for internalization of the transferrin receptor.

More than 1 billion parietal cells are found in the normal human stomach and are responsible for secreting about 20 mmol/hr of hydrochloric acid in response to a protein meal. Each individual parietal cell secretes 3.3 billion hydrogen ions/second, and there is a linear relationship between maximal acid output and parietal cell number. However, gastric acid secretory rates may be altered in patients with upper gastrointestinal (GI) disease. For example, gastric acid is often increased in patients with duodenal ulcer or gastrinoma, whereas it is decreased in patients with pernicious anemia, gastric atrophy, gastric ulcer, or gastric cancer. The lower secretory rates observed in gastric ulcer patients are typically for proximal gastric ulcers, whereas distal, antral, or prepyloric ulcers are associated with acid secretory rates similar to those in duodenal ulcer patients.

Gastric acid thus plays a critical role in the digestion of a meal. It is required to convert pepsinogen into pepsin, elicits the release of secretin from the duodenum, and limits colonization of the upper GI tract with bacteria.

## Pharmacologic Regulation

The diversity of mechanisms that stimulate acid secretion has resulted in the development of many site-specific drugs aimed at decreasing acid output by the parietal cell. The best-known site-specific antagonists are the group collectively known as the *$H_2$ receptor antagonists.* The most potent of the $H_2$ receptor antagonists is famotidine, followed by ranitidine, nizatidine, and cimetidine. The half-life for famotidine is 3 hours and approximately 1.5 hours for the others. All undergo hepatic metabolism, are excreted by the kidney, and do not differ much in bioavailability.

The newest class of antisecretory agents is the proton pump inhibitors (PPIs). These substituted benzimidazoles, of which omeprazole is a prime example, inhibit acid secretion more completely because of their irreversible inhibition of the proton pump. These PPIs are weak acids with a $pK_a$ of 4 and therefore become selectively localized in the secretory canaliculus of the parietal cell, which is the only structure in the body with a pH lower than 4. After oral administration, these agents are absorbed into the bloodstream as prodrugs and then selectively concentrate in the secretory canaliculus. At low pH, they become ionized and activated, with the formation of an active sulfur group. Because the proton pump is located on the luminal surface, the transmembrane pump proteins are also exposed to acid or low pH. The cysteine residues on the α-subunit form a covalent disulfate bond with activated benzimidazoles, which irreversibly inhibits the proton pump. Because of the covalent nature of this bond, these PPIs have more prolonged inhibition of gastric acid secretion than $H_2$ blockers. In order for recovery of acid secretion to occur, new protein pumps need to be synthesized. As a result, these agents have a longer duration of action than their plasma half-life, with the intragastric pH being maintained higher than 3 for 18 hours or longer.

One notable side effect of all antisecretory agents is the elevation of serum gastrin levels. Serum gastrin levels are higher after treatment with PPIs than with $H_2$ receptor antagonists. This effect is accompanied by hyperplasia of G cells and ECL cells when these agents are administered chronically. Chronic administration of omeprazole has been found to cause ECL hyperplasia that could progress to carcinoid tumors in rats.[3] This effect, however, was not specific for omeprazole and was reproduced by other agents that caused prolonged inhibition of acid secretion and resultant hypergastrinemia.

## Other Gastric Secretory Products

**Gastric Juice** Gastric juice is the result of secretion by the parietal cells, chief cells, and mucus cells, in addition to swallowed saliva and duodenal refluxate. The electrolyte composition of parietal and nonparietal gastric secretion varies with the rate of gastric secretion. Parietal cells secrete an electrolyte solution that is isotonic with plasma and contains 160 mmol/liter. The pH of this solution is 0.8. The lowest intraluminal pH commonly measured in the stomach is 2 because of dilution of the parietal cell secretion by other gastric secretions, which also contain sodium, potassium, and bicarbonate.

**Intrinsic Factor** Intrinsic factor is a 60-kDa mucoprotein secreted by the parietal cell that is essential for the absorption of vitamin $B_{12}$ in the terminal ileum. It is secreted in amounts that far exceed those necessary for vitamin $B_{12}$ absorption. In general, its secretion parallels that of gastric acid secretion, yet the secretory response is not necessarily linked to acid secretion. For example, PPIs do not block intrinsic factor secretion in humans nor do they alter the absorption of labeled vitamin $B_{12}$. Intrinsic factor deficiency can develop in the setting of pernicious anemia or in patients undergoing total gastrectomy, and both groups of patients require vitamin $B_{12}$ supplementation.

**Pepsinogen** Pepsinogens are proteolytic proenzymes with a molecular weight of 42,500 that are secreted by the glands of the gastroduodenal mucosa. Two types of pepsinogens are secreted. Group 1 pepsinogens are secreted by chief cells and by mucus neck cells located in the glands of the acid-secreting portion of the stomach. Group 2 pepsinogens are produced by surface epithelial cells throughout the acid-secreting portion of the stomach, antrum, and proximal duodenum. Consequently, group 1 pepsinogens are secreted by the same glands that secrete acid, whereas group 2 pepsinogens are secreted by acid-secreting and gastrin-secreting mucosa. In the presence of acid, both forms of pepsinogen are converted to pepsin by removal of a short amino-terminal peptide. Pepsins become inactivated at a pH higher than 5, although group 2 pepsinogens are active over a wider range of pH values than group 1 pepsinogens. As a result, group 2 pepsinogens may be involved in peptic digestion in the presence of increased gastric pH, which commonly occurs in the setting of stress or in patients with gastric ulcer.

**Mucus and Bicarbonate** Mucus and bicarbonate combine to neutralize gastric acid at the gastric mucosal surface. They are secreted by the surface mucus cells and mucus neck cells located in the acid-secreting and antral portions of the stomach. Mucus is a viscoelastic gel that contains approximately 85% water and 15% glycoproteins. It provides a mechanical barrier to injury by contributing to the unstirred layer of water found at the luminal surface of the gastric mucosa. It also acts as an impediment to ion movement from the lumen to the apical cell membrane and is relatively impermeable to pepsins. Mucus is in a constant state of flux because it is secreted continuously by mucosal cells on the one hand and solubilized by luminal pepsin on the other.

Mucus production is stimulated by vagal stimulation, cholinergic agonists, prostaglandins, and some bacterial toxins. In contrast, anticholinergic drugs and nonsteroidal anti-inflammatory drugs (NSAIDs) inhibit its secretion. *H. pylori,* on the other hand, secretes various proteases and lipases that break down mucin and impair the protective function of the mucus layer.

In the acid-secreting portion of the stomach, bicarbonate secretion is an active process, whereas in the antrum, active and passive secretion of bicarbonate occur. The magnitude of bicarbonate secretion, however, is considerably less than acid secretion. Although the luminal pH is 2, the pH observed at the surface epithelial cell is usually 7. The pH gradient found at the epithelial surface is a result of the unstirred layer of water in the mucus gel and of the continuous secretion of bicarbonate by the surface epithelial cells. Gastric cell surface pH remains higher than 5 until the luminal pH is less than 1.4. However, the luminal pH in duodenal ulcer patients is frequently less than 1.4, so the cell surface is exposed to a lower pH in these patients. This reduction in pH may reflect a reduction in gastric bicarbonate secretion and decreased duodenal bicarbonate secretion, and may explain why some duodenal ulcer patients have a higher relapse rate after treatment.

## Gastric Motility

Gastric motility is regulated by extrinsic and intrinsic neural mechanisms and by myogenic control. The extrinsic neural controls are mediated through parasympathetic (vagus) and sympathetic pathways, whereas the intrinsic controls involve the enteric nervous system (see earlier, "Anatomy"). In contrast, myogenic control resides in the excitatory membranes of the gastric smooth muscle cells.

### Fasting Gastric Motility

The electrical basis of gastric motility begins with the depolarization of pacemaker cells located in the midbody of the stomach, along the greater curvature. Once initiated, slow waves travel at 3 cycles/minute in a circumferential and antegrade fashion toward the pylorus. In addition to these slow waves, gastric smooth muscle cells are capable of producing action potentials, which are associated with larger changes in membrane potential than slow waves. In comparison to slow waves, which are not associated with gastric contractions, action potentials are associated with actual muscle contractions. During fasting, the stomach goes through a cyclical pattern of electrical activity composed of slow waves and electrical spikes, which has been termed the *myoelectric migrating complex* (MMC). Each cycle of the MMC lasts 90 to 120 minutes. The net effects of the MMC are frequent clearance of gastric contents during periods of fasting. The exact regulatory mechanisms of MMC activities are unknown, but these activities remain intact after vagal denervation.

### Postprandial Gastric Motility

Ingestion of a meal results in a decrease in the resting tone of the proximal stomach and fundus, referred to as *receptive relaxation* and *gastric accommodation*, respectively. Because these reflexes are mediated by the vagus nerves, interruption of vagal innervation to the proximal stomach, such as by truncal vagotomy or proximal gastric vagotomy, can eliminate these reflexes, with resultant early satiety and rapid emptying of ingested liquids. In addition to its storage function, the stomach is responsible for the mixing and grinding of ingested solid food particles. This activity involves repetitive forceful contractions of the mid and antral portions of the stomach, causing food particles to be propelled against a closed pylorus, with subsequent retropulsion of solids and liquids. The net effect is a thorough mixing of solids and liquids and sequential shearing of solid food particles to smaller than 1 mm.

The emptying of gastric contents is under the influence of well-coordinated neural and hormonal mediators. Systemic factors, such as anxiety, fear, depression, and exercise, can affect the rate of gastric motility and emptying. Additionally, the chemical and mechanical properties and temperature of the intraluminal contents can influence the rate of gastric emptying. In general, liquids empty more rapidly than solids and carbohydrates empty more readily than fats. An increase in the concentration or acidity of liquid meals causes a delay in gastric emptying. In addition, hot and cold liquids tend to empty at a slower rate than ambient temperature fluids. These responses to luminal stimuli are regulated by the enteric nervous system. Osmoreceptors and pH-sensitive receptors in the proximal small bowel have also been shown to be involved in the activation of feedback inhibition of gastric emptying. Inhibitory peptides proposed to be active in this setting include CCK, glucagon, vasoactive intestinal peptide, and gastric inhibitory polypeptide.

### Abnormal Gastric Motility

Symptoms of abnormal gastric motility are nausea, fullness, early satiety, abdominal pain, and discomfort. Although mechanical obstruction can and should be ruled out with upper endoscopy or radiographic contrast studies, objective evaluation of a patient with a suspected motility disorder can be accomplished with gamma scintigraphy, real-time ultrasound, and magnetic resonance imaging (MRI). Gastric motility disorders usually encountered in clinical practice are gastric dysmotility following vagotomy, delayed gastric emptying associated with diabetes mellitus, and gastric motility dysfunction related to *H. pylori* infection. Vagotomy results in loss of receptive relaxation and gastric accommodation in response to meal ingestion, with resultant early satiety, postprandial bloating, accelerated emptying of liquids, and delay in emptying of solids. Clinical manifestations of diabetic gastropathy, which can occur in insulin-dependent or insulin-independent patients, closely resemble the clinical picture of postvagotomy gastroparesis. Furthermore, structural changes have been identified in the vagus nerve of patients with diabetes, suggesting that a diabetic autonomic neuropathy may be responsible. However, the metabolic effects of diabetes have also been implicated. Specifically, hyperglycemia has been shown to cause a decrease in contractility of the gastric antrum, increase in pyloric contractility, and suppression of the migrating motor complex (MMC). Suppression of MMC activity is thought to be responsible for the accumulation of gastric bezoars seen in some diabetic patients. In contrast, hyperinsulinemia, which is often associated with non–insulin-dependent diabetes, may play a role in the gastroparesis seen in non–insulin-dependent diabetes because it also leads to suppression of MMC activity.[4]

*H. pylori*–infected patients with nonulcer dyspepsia have also been demonstrated to have impaired gastric emptying accompanied by a reduction in gastric compliance.[5] In rats, lipopolysaccharide derived from *H. pylori* causes a reduction in gastric emptying of a liquid meal for up to 12 hours by an unknown mechanism. Regardless of the cause of gastroparesis, treatment consists of prokinetic agents, such as metoclopramide and erythromycin, which have been shown to have some benefit, although the evidence is more compelling in diabetics.

### Gastric-Emptying Studies

There are a number of ways to assess gastric emptying. The saline load test is perhaps the simplest and is accomplished by instilling a known volume of saline into the stomach and aspirating the amount remaining at a certain time. Alternatively, fluoroscopic procedures can also provide information on gastric emptying and may reveal mechanical causes that could contribute to a delay, such as gastric outlet obstruction. However, computerized radionucleotide scans are more commonly used to assess gastric emptying. This can be done with radiolabeled liquids or with a radiolabeled solid meal. After a mechanical obstruction has been ruled out, gastric emptying studies using these radionucleotide scans can be particularly helpful for patients with gastric atony from an associated illness such as diabetes or in postgastrectomy patients.

### Gastric Barrier Function

Gastric barrier function depends on physiologic and anatomic factors. Blood flow plays a critical role in gastric mucosal defense by providing nutrients and delivering oxygen to ensure that the intracellular processes that underlie mucosal resistance to injury can proceed unabated. Decreased gastric mucosal blood flow has minimal effects on lesion production until it approaches 50% of normal. When blood flow is reduced by more than 75%, marked mucosal injury results, which is exacerbated in the presence of luminal acid. After damage occurs, injured surface epithelial cells are replaced rapidly by the migration of surface mucus cells located along the basement membranes. This process is referred to as *restitution* or *reconstitution*. It occurs within minutes and does not require cell division.

Exposure of the stomach to noxious agents causes a reduction in the potential difference across the gastric mucosa. In normal gastric mucosa, the potential difference across the mucosa is −30 to −50 mV and results from the active transport of chloride into the lumen and sodium into the blood by the activity of $Na^+$,$K^+$-ATPase. Damage disrupts the tight junctions between mucosal cells, causing the epithelium to become leaky to ions (i.e., $Na^+$ and $Cl^-$) and a resultant loss of the high transepithelial electrical resistance normally found in gastric mucosa. In addition, damaging agents such as NSAIDs or aspirin possess carboxyl groups that are nonionized at a low intragastric pH because they are weak acids. Consequently, they readily enter the cell membranes of gastric mucosal cells because they are now lipid-soluble, whereas they will not penetrate the cell membranes at neutral pH because they are ionized. On entry into the neutral pH environment found in the cytosol, they become reionized, will not exit the cell membrane, and are toxic to the mucosal cells.

## PEPTIC ULCER DISEASE

### Epidemiology

The estimated prevalence of PUD ranges from 5% to 15% in Western populations, with a lifetime incidence of almost 10%.[6] Although the incidence and hospitalization rate for PUD have been decreasing since the 1980s, it remains one of the most prevalent and costly GI diseases. Medical costs associated with PUD are an estimated $5.65 billion annually. An estimated 15,000 operations are performed each year on patients hospitalized with PUD. Significant progress has been made over the past 2 decades, with total admissions for PUD decreasing by almost 30%. Admissions for complications of ulcer disease have also been decreasing, which has led to a significant decrease in ulcer-related mortality, from 3.9% in 1993 to 2.7% in 2006.[7] Although overall mortality remains low, this still represents over 4000 deaths caused by PUD each year.

The role of surgery in the treatment of ulcer disease has also decreased, primarily caused by a marked decline in elective surgical therapy for chronic disease because the percentage of patients who require emergent surgery for complicated disease has remained constant, at 7% of hospitalized patients.[7] This represents over 11,000 surgical procedures annually.

Much of this decline in ulcer incidence and the need for hospitalization has stemmed from increased knowledge of ulcer pathogenesis. Specifically, the role of *H. pylori* has been defined and the risks of chronic NSAID use have been better elucidated. An increase in *H. pylori* eradication will hopefully result in a decrease of not just elective surgical procedures, but also a decline in complications and mortality from emergent complications.

### Pathogenesis

Peptic ulcers are caused by increased aggressive factors, decreased defensive factors, or both.[8] This in turn leads to mucosal damage and subsequent ulceration. Protective (or defensive) factors include mucosal bicarbonate secretion, mucus production, blood flow, growth factors, cell renewal, and endogenous prostaglandins. Damaging (or aggressive) factors include hydrochloric acid secretion, pepsins, ethanol ingestion, smoking, duodenal reflux of bile, ischemia, NSAIDs, hypoxia and, most notably, *H. pylori* infection.

#### *Helicobacter pylori* Infection

It is now believed that 90% of duodenal ulcers and approximately 75% of gastric ulcers are associated with *H. pylori* infection. When this organism is eradicated as part of ulcer treatment, ulcer recurrence is extremely rare. *H. pylori* is a spiral or helical gram-negative rod with four to six flagella that resides in gastric-type epithelium within or beneath the mucus layer. This location protects the bacteria from acid and antibiotics. Its shape and flagella aid its movement through the mucus layer and it produces enzymes that help it adapt to this hostile environment. Most notably, it is a potent producer of urease, which is capable of splitting urea into ammonia and bicarbonate, creating an alkaline microenvironment in the setting of an acidic gastric milieu. The secretion of this enzyme, however, facilitates detection of the organism. *H. pylori* is microaerophilic and can only live in gastric epithelium. Thus, it can also be found in heterotopic gastric mucosa in the proximal esophagus, Barrett's esophagus, gastric metaplasia in the duodenum, within a Meckel's diverticulum, and heterotopic gastric mucosa in the rectum.

The mechanisms responsible for *H. pylori*–induced GI injury remain to be fully elucidated, but three potential mechanisms have been proposed:

1. Production of toxic products that cause local tissue injury. Locally produced toxic mediators include

breakdown products from urease activity (e.g., ammonia), cytotoxins, a mucinase that degrades mucus and glycoproteins, phospholipases that damage epithelial cells and mucus cells, and platelet-activating factor, which is known to cause mucosal injury and thrombosis in the microcirculation.

2. Induction of a local mucosal immune response. *H. pylori* can also cause a local inflammatory reaction in the gastric mucosa, attracting neutrophils and monocytes, which then produce a number of proinflammatory cytokines and reactive oxygen metabolites.
3. Increased gastrin levels with a resultant increase in acid secretion. In patients with *H. pylori* infection, basal and stimulated gastrin levels are significantly increased, presumably secondary to a reduction in antral D cells because of infection with *H. pylori*. However, the association of acid secretion with *H. pylori* is not as straightforward. Although *H. pylori*–positive healthy volunteers had a small increase or no increase in acid secretion as compared with *H. pylori*–negative volunteers, *H. pylori*–infected patients with duodenal ulcers did have a marked increase in acid secretion.[9]

Peptic ulcers are also strongly associated with antral gastritis. Studies done before the *H. pylori* era have demonstrated that almost all peptic ulcer patients have histologic evidence of antral gastritis. It was later found that the only patients with gastric ulcers and no gastritis were those ingesting aspirin. It is now recognized that most cases of histologic gastritis are caused by *H. pylori* infection. Even 25% of patients with an NSAID-associated ulcer have evidence of a histologic antral gastritis, as opposed to 95% of those with non–NSAID-associated ulcers. In most cases, the infection tends to be confined initially to the antrum and results in antral inflammation. Other evidence supporting a causal role for *H. pylori* in histologic gastritis comes from two separate volunteer physicians who ingested inocula of *H. pylori* after first confirming normal gross and microscopic gastric mucosa. Both developed gastric *H. pylori* infection. Acute inflammation was observed histologically on days 5 and 10. By 2 weeks, it had been replaced by chronic inflammation with evidence of a mononuclear cell infiltration. These two reports provide documentation that *H. pylori* can cause histologic gastritis. However, histologic gastritis does not necessarily equate with symptoms of dyspepsia.

*H. pylori* infection usually occurs in childhood, and spontaneous remission is rare. There is an inverse relationship between infection and socioeconomic status. The reasons for this remain poorly understood but seem to be the result of factors such as sanitary conditions, familial clustering, and crowding. This likely explains why developing countries have a comparatively higher rate of *H. pylori* infection, especially in children.

A number of studies have demonstrated what appears to be a steady linear increase in the acquisition of *H. pylori* infection with age, especially in the United States and northern European nations. In the United States, *H. pylori* prevalence also varies among racial and ethnic groups.

*H. pylori* infection is associated with a number of common upper GI disorders, but most infected individuals are asymptomatic. Normal U.S. blood donors have an overall prevalence of about 20% to 55%. *H. pylori* infection is almost always present in the setting of active chronic gastritis and is present in most duodenal (>90%) and gastric (60% to 90%) ulcer patients. Noninfected gastric ulcer patients tend to be NSAID users. There is weaker association with nonulcer dyspepsia. In addition, most gastric cancer patients have current or past *H. pylori* infection. Although the association between *H. pylori* and cancer is strong, no causal relationship has been proven. *H. pylori*–induced chronic gastritis and intestinal metaplasia, however, are thought to play a role. There is also a strong association between +lymphoma and *H. pylori* infection. Regression of these lymphomas has been demonstrated after eradication of the organism.

Limited data are available to estimate the lifetime risk of PUD in patients with *H. pylori* infection. In a longitudinal study from Australia with a mean evaluation period of 18 years, 15% of *H. pylori*–positive subjects developed verified duodenal ulcer as compared with 3% of seronegative individuals. In a 10-year study of asymptomatic gastritis patients, 11% of patients with histologic gastritis developed PUD over a 10-year period, compared with only 1% of those without gastritis. Another factor implicating a causative role for *H. pylori* and ulcer formation is that eradication of *H. pylori* dramatically reduces ulcer recurrence. Many prospective trials have shown that patients with *H. pylori* infection and non-NSAID ulcer disease who have documented eradication of the organism almost never (<2%) develop recurrent ulcers.

### Nonsteroidal Anti-inflammatory Drugs

Hospitalizations for bleeding upper GI lesions have increased together with the increased use of NSAIDs. The risk for bleeding and ulceration is proportional to the daily dosage of NSAIDs. The risk also increases with age older than 60 years, patients having a prior GI event, or concurrent use of steroids or anticoagulants. Consequently, the ingestion of NSAIDs remains an important factor in ulcer pathogenesis, especially in regard to the development of complications and death. More than 3 million people in the United States use NSAIDs daily. When compared with the general population, NSAID users have a 2- to 10-fold increased risk for GI complications.

The risk for mucosal injury or ulceration is roughly proportional to the anti-inflammatory effect associated with each NSAID. In comparison to *H. pylori* ulcers, which are more frequently found in the duodenum, NSAID-induced ulcers are more often found in the stomach. *H. pylori* ulcers are also almost always associated with chronic active gastritis, whereas gastritis is not frequently found with an NSAID-induced ulcer, occurring only about 25% of the time. When NSAID use is discontinued, the ulcers usually do not recur.

### Acid

Acid plays an important but likely noncausative role in the formation of ulcers. In duodenal ulcers, there is a large overlap of acid levels between ulcer patients and normal subjects. Almost 70% of patients with duodenal ulcers have an acid output within the normal range. Acid levels alone provide little information and, as such, acid secretory testing is of little value in establishing a diagnosis of duodenal ulcer.

For types I and IV gastric ulcers, which are not associated with excessive acid secretion, acid acts as an important cofactor, exacerbating the underlying ulcer damage and attenuating the ability of the stomach to heal. For patients with type II or III gastric ulcers, gastric acid hypersecretion seems to be more common, and consequently they behave more like duodenal ulcers.

## Duodenal Ulcer

Duodenal ulcer is a disease with a number of causes. The only requirements are acid and pepsin secretion in combination with infection by *H. pylori* or ingestion of NSAIDs.

### Clinical Manifestations

**Abdominal Pain** Patients suffering from duodenal ulcer disease can present in various ways. The most common symptom associated with duodenal ulcer disease is midepigastric abdominal pain that is usually well localized. The pain is generally tolerable and frequently relieved by food. The pain may be episodic, seasonal in the spring and fall, and worse during periods of emotional stress. Many patients do not seek medical attention until they have had the disease for many years. When the pain becomes constant, this suggests that there is deeper penetration of the ulcer. Referral of pain to the back is usually a sign of penetration into the pancreas. Diffuse peritoneal irritation is usually a sign of free perforation.

### Diagnosis

History and physical examination are of limited value in distinguishing between gastric and duodenal ulceration. Routine laboratory studies include a complete blood count, liver chemistries, and serum creatinine, serum amylase, and calcium levels. A serum gastrin level should also be obtained in patients with ulcers that are refractory to medical therapy or require surgery. An upright chest radiograph is usually performed when ruling out perforation. The two principal means of diagnosing duodenal ulcers are upper GI radiography and fiberoptic endoscopy. Upper GI is less expensive, and most (90%) ulcers can be diagnosed accurately by this means. However, about 5% of ulcers that appear radiographically benign are malignant. *H. pylori* testing should also be done in all patients with suspected PUD.

***Helicobacter pylori* Testing** *H. pylori* can be diagnosed by mucosal biopsy, but noninvasive tests offer an effective screening tool and do not require an endoscopic procedure. Serology is the test of choice for initial diagnosis when endoscopy is not required. However, if endoscopy is to be performed, the rapid urease assay and histology are both excellent options.

***Serology*** There are various enzyme-linked immunosorbent assay (ELISA) laboratory-based tests available and some rapid office-based immunoassays. Serology has a 90% sensitivity and specificity rate. Antibody titers can remain high for 1 year or longer; consequently, this test cannot be used to assess eradication after therapy.

***Urea Breath Test*** The carbon-labeled urea breath test is based on the ability of *H. pylori* to hydrolyze urea. Its sensitivity and specificity are both higher than 95%. The urea breath test is less expensive than endoscopy and samples the entire stomach. False-negative results can occur if the test is done too soon after treatment, so it is usually best to perform this test 4 weeks after therapy is finished. The urea breath test is the method of choice to document eradication.

***Rapid Urease Assay*** A rapid urease test can detect urease in gastric biopsy specimens. Sensitivity is approximately 90% and specificity 98%, and the results are available within hours.

***Histology*** Endoscopy can also be performed with biopsy samples of gastric mucosa, followed by histologic visualization of *H. pylori* using routine hematoxylin and eosin stains or with special stains (e.g., silver, Giemsa, Genta stains) for improved visibility. Sensitivity is approximately 95% and specificity 99%. This test is widely available and affords the clinician the ability to assess the severity of gastritis and confirm the presence or absence of the organism.

***Culture*** Culturing of gastric mucosa obtained at endoscopy can also be performed to diagnose *H. pylori*. The sensitivity is approximately 80% and specificity 100%. However, it requires laboratory expertise, is not widely available and is relatively expensive, and diagnosis requires up to 3 to 5 days. Nevertheless, it provides the opportunity to perform antibiotic sensitivity testing on isolates, if needed.

**Upper Gastrointestinal Radiography** Diagnosis of duodenal ulcer by upper GI radiography requires the demonstration of barium within the ulcer crater, which is usually round or oval and may or may not be surrounded by edema. This study is useful to determine the location and depth of penetration of the ulcer and the extent of deformation from chronic fibrosis. A characteristic barium radiograph of a peptic ulcer is shown in Figure 49-9. The ability to detect ulcers on radiography requires the technical skills and abilities of the radiologist but is also dependent on the size and location of the ulcer. With single-contrast radiographic techniques, as many as 50% of duodenal ulcers may be missed, whereas with double-contrast studies, 80% to 90% of ulcer craters can be detected.

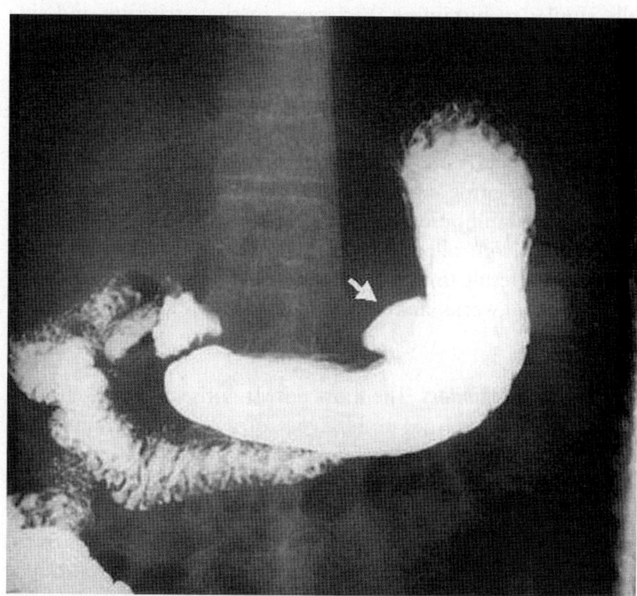

**FIGURE 49-9** There is a large benign-appearing gastric ulcer protruding medially from the lesser curvature of the stomach *(arrow)*, just above the gastric incisura. (Courtesy Dr. Agnes Guthrie, Department of Radiology, University of Texas Medical School, Houston.)

**Fiberoptic Endoscopy** Endoscopy is the most reliable method of diagnosing a duodenal ulcer. In addition to providing a visual diagnosis, endoscopy provides the ability to sample tissue for *H. pylori* testing and may also be used for therapeutic purposes in the setting of GI bleeding or obstruction

### Treatment

**Medical Management** Antiulcer drugs fall into three broad categories—those targeted against *H. pylori*, those that reduce acid levels by decreasing secretion or chemical neutralization, and those that increase the mucosal protective barrier. In patients with PUD and *H. pylori* infection, the focus of therapy is on eradication of the bacteria. In addition to medications, lifestyle changes, such as smoking cessation, discontinuing NSAIDs and aspirin, and avoiding coffee and alcohol, all help promote ulcer healing.

***Antacids*** Antacids are the oldest form of therapy for PUD. Antacids reduce gastric acidity by reacting with hydrochloric acid, forming a salt and thereby raising the gastric pH. Antacids differ greatly in their buffering ability, absorption, taste, and side effects. Magnesium antacids tend to be the best buffers but can cause significant diarrhea, whereas acids precipitated with phosphorus can occasionally result in hypophosphatemia and sometimes constipation. They are most effective when ingested 1 hour after a meal because they can be retained in the stomach and exert their buffering action for longer periods. If taken on an empty stomach, antacids are emptied rapidly and have only a transient buffering effect. Dosages of 200 to 1000 mmol/day produce minimal side effects and result in approximately 80% ulcer healing at 1 month. Although antacids may heal duodenal ulcers with an efficacy comparable to that observed with $H_2$ receptor antagonists, many patients have found large frequent doses to be unacceptable.

***$H_2$ Receptor Antagonists*** The $H_2$ receptor antagonists are structurally similar to histamine. Variations in ring structure and side chains cause differences in potency and side effects. Currently available $H_2$ receptor antagonists differ in their potency but only modestly in half-life and bioavailability. All undergo hepatic metabolism and are excreted by the kidney. Famotidine is the most potent and cimetidine is the weakest. Continuous IV infusion of $H_2$ receptor antagonists has been shown to produce more uniform acid inhibition than intermittent administration. Many randomized controlled trials have indicated that all $H_2$ receptor antagonists result in duodenal ulcer healing rates from 70% to 80% after 4 weeks and from 80% to 90% after 8 weeks of therapy.

***Proton Pump Inhibitors*** The most potent antisecretory agents are PPIs. These agents negate all types of acid secretion from all types of secretogogues. As a result, they provide a more complete and prolonged inhibition of acid secretion than $H_2$ receptor antagonists. $H_2$ receptor antagonists and PPIs are effective at night, but PPIs are more effective during the day. PPIs have a healing rate of 85% at 4 weeks and 96% at 8 weeks and produce more rapid healing of ulcers than standard $H_2$ receptor antagonists (14% advantage at 2 weeks and 9% advantage at 4 weeks). PPIs require an acidic environment within the gastric lumen to become activated; thus, using antacids or $H_2$ receptor antagonists in combination with PPIs could have deleterious effects by promoting an alkaline environment and thereby preventing activation of the PPIs. Consequently, antacids and $H_2$ receptor antagonists should not be used in combination with PPIs.

***Sucralfate*** Sucralfate is structurally related to heparin but does not have any anticoagulant effects. It has been shown to be effective in the treatment of ulcer disease, although its exact mechanism of action is not entirely understood. It is an aluminum salt of sulfated sucrose that dissociates under the acidic conditions in the stomach. It is hypothesized that the sucrose polymerizes and binds to protein in the ulcer crater to produce a protective coating that can last for up to 6 hours. It has also been suggested that it may bind and concentrate endogenous basic fibroblast growth factor, which appears to be important for mucosal healing. Duodenal ulcer healing after 4 to 6 weeks of treatment with sucralfate is superior to placebo and comparable that of $H_2$ receptor antagonists such as cimetidine.

***Treatment of* Helicobacter pylori *Infection*** Prior to the discovery of *H. pylori* infection as the causative agent in over 95% of duodenal peptic ulcers, the primary form of treatment was the reduction of acid in the stomach, with or without increasing the protective barrier with drugs such as sucralfate. After it became clear that increased acid secretion was an effect of *H. pylori* infection, there was a paradigm shift that saw PUD as an infectious disease, rather than a consequence of pathologic acid secretion. Accordingly, treatment philosophy has shifted to focus on eradication of the infectious agent.

Current therapy is twofold in its approach, combining antibiotics against *H. pylori* with antacid medications. The primary goal of the antacids is to promote short-term healing by reducing pathologic acid levels and improve symptoms. *H. pylori* eradication helps with initial healing, but its primary efficacy is in preventing recurrence. There have been numerous trials comparing eradication therapy with ulcer-healing drugs alone or no treatment. Eradication of *H. pylori* has shown recurrence rates as low as 2%, with initial healing as high as 90%. This compares with recurrence rates of up to 25% with ulcer-healing medications alone. One review has analyzed the results of these trials and further validated the role of antibiotics in the treatment of *H. pylori*–positive duodenal ulcers.[10] Both eradication therapy and ulcer-healing drugs alone have shown initial healing rates higher than 80%. Eradication therapy has resulted in long-term recurrence of less than 15%, in contrast to 64% recurrence in patients treated with only a short initial course of ulcer-healing drugs. Patients could achieve low recurrence rates similar to those of eradication therapy, but only if they were maintained on their antacid regiment long term, as opposed to a 1- or 2-week course of eradication therapy.

Given all these findings across multiple studies, and according to the recommendations of the American Gastroenterological Association, European *Helicobacter pylori* Study Group, and National Institutes of Health (NIH), the treatment of *H. pylori*–positive peptic duodenal ulcer disease is triple therapy aimed at the eradication of *H. pylori*, along with acid suppression (Box 49-1). This includes an antisecretory agent, now most commonly a PPI, although histamine antagonists are still used, along with two antibiotics, usually amoxicillin with clarithromycin or metronidazole, given for a 2-week course. Side effects, which are generally mild and resolve with cessation

**BOX 49-1 National Institutes of Health Consensus Panel Recommendations for *Helicobacter pylori* Treatment**

Patients with active PUD who are *H. pylori*-positive
- Use of NSAIDs should not alter treatment
- Document eradication in those with complications

Ulcer patients in remission who are *H. pylori*-positive, including patients on maintenance $H_2$ receptor antagonist therapy

*H. pylori*–positive patients with MALT lymphoma

Controversial issues in *H. pylori*–positive patients:
- First-degree relatives of gastric cancer patients
- Immigrants from countries with high prevalence of gastric cancer
- Individuals with gastric cancer precursor lesions (intestinal metaplasia)
- Non–ulcer dyspepsia patients who insist on eradication (benefit versus risk)
- Patients on long-term antisecretory therapy for reflux disease

**BOX 49-2 Surgical Treatment Recommendations for Complications Related to Peptic Duodenal Ulcer Disease**

Intractable: Parietal cell vagotomy ± antrectomy

Bleeding: Oversewing of bleeding vessel with treatment of *H. pylori*

Perforation: Patch closure with treatment of *H. pylori*

Obstruction: Rule out malignancy and gastrojejunostomy with treatment of *H. pylori*

of treatment, include diarrhea, nausea and vomiting, rash, and altered taste. For the 10% of patients with refractory disease, quadruple therapy with the addition of bismuth is recommended.

### Complicated Ulcer Disease

Ulcer disease was once very much the purview of the general surgeon, with ulcer surgery forming a major part of general surgery practice. With the shift in understanding of the disease from one primarily of aberrant acid physiology to one of infectious disease, this has changed significantly, with the overwhelming majority of ulcer patients being treated and cured medically. The surgeon's role now is primarily to treat the approximately 20% of patients who have a complication from their disease, which includes hemorrhage, perforation, and obstruction (Box 49-2). Frequently included in discussions of complicated ulcer disease is the intractable ulcer. Although intractable disease no doubt exists, its definition is nebulous and exactly when and what type of surgical intervention it requires remain primarily a matter of judgment.

For *H. pylori*–negative patients, an acid-reducing procedure should also be performed, such as truncal or parietal cell vagotomy.

**Hemorrhage** Upper GI bleeding remains a relatively common problem, with an annual incidence of approximately 1/1000.[11] Most nonvariceal bleeding (70%) is attributable to peptic ulcers. Most bleeding will stop spontaneously and requires no intervention; persistent bleeding, however, is associated with a 6% to 8% mortality.

The primary clinical criteria that predict persistent bleeding or rebleeding after initial cessation of bleeding, and thus increased mortality, are increased age, decreased hemoglobin (<10 g/dL) at presentation, shock, melena, and need for blood transfusion. Patients who meet any of these criteria should be considered as high risk.[11]

Almost all patients with an acute upper GI bleed should have endoscopy within 24 hours. Although the data are not conclusive, early endoscopy has been shown to be a cost-effective strategy by triaging patients to more rapid intervention, if warranted, and by identifying low-risk patients without the need for prolonged observation (and therefore earlier hospital discharge).

The initial approach to an upper GI bleed is similar to the approach to a trauma patient. Large-bore IV access, rapid restoration of intravascular volume with fluid and blood products as the clinical situation dictates, and close monitoring for signs of rebleeding are all essential to effective management of these patients. The role of nasogastric (NG) lavage remains an area of debate; however, it can be useful as a predictor of high-risk patients and as an aid for later endoscopic intervention. Patients with bright red blood on NG lavage, as opposed to clear or coffee ground lavage, are at much higher risk for persistent bleeding or rebleeding and warrant endoscopic intervention. Furthermore, the NG tube can be used to lavage the stomach and duodenum prior to endoscopy, removing clot and old blood that could obscure visualization of the source of bleeding. Given its relatively low risk and potential benefit, NG tube placement should be part of the treatment algorithm for these patients once appropriate intravascular access has been established and resuscitation begun.

Patients who are noted to have active bleeding, via an arterial jet or oozing, an adherent clot, or a visible vessel within the ulcer, are at high risk and intervention is required. Patients without active bleeding, no visible vessel, and a clean ulcer base are low risk and do not require further intervention. All patients undergoing endoscopic examination should be tested for their *H. pylori* status. For the high-risk patient requiring intervention, the best initial approach is endoscopic control, which results in primary hemostasis in approximately 90% of patients. The most common method of control is injection of a vasoconstrictor at the site of bleeding. However, with this method alone, primary hemostasis rates are high but up to 30% of patients have rebleeding. This has led to the development of new techniques, including use of a second vasoconstrictor or sclerosing agent, thermal coagulation, and placement of clips at the site of bleeding. A 2007 meta-analysis has compared the use of epinephrine alone to epinephrine plus any second technique.[12] A dual approach, when compared with epinephrine alone, showed better primary hemostasis, reduction in rebleeding rate, lower rate of surgery, and decreased mortality.

Importantly, both thermal coagulation and mechanical clips, in single-method comparisons with epinephrine, have shown significant superiority with respect to primary hemostasis and rebleeding. A meta-analysis comparing either of these two techniques alone to the use of dual methods has shown no significant difference, except in cases of active arterial bleeding, in which case use of a second method was superior. Although the cost and complications from epinephrine remain small, the use of dual methods does have slightly higher, although still less than 1%, complication rates (e.g., necrosis, perforation), than any single technique. Current 2003 guidelines for endoscopic control of bleeding advocate the use of epinephrine plus an additional method.[11] As more data become available, it may be demonstrated that thermal or mechanical treatment alone can be used for most patients. For patients who have rebleeding, repeat endoscopy does not increase their mortality and should be attempted prior to surgical intervention.

All high-risk patients should be placed in a monitored setting, preferably an intensive care unit, until all bleeding has stopped for 24 hours. As part of the 2003 consensus guidelines, all high-risk patients should be placed on an IV PPI, with an initial bolus followed by continuous infusion or intermittent dosing for up to 72 hours. When compared with a histamine blocker and placebo, the IV PPI showed lower rebleeding rates, lower rate of emergency surgery, and decreased mortality.[13] Patients deemed high risk based on clinical factors who are awaiting endoscopy should probably begin therapy, even prior to endoscopy.

Despite the use of PPIs and improved methods of endoscopic control, 5% to 10% of patients will have persistent bleeding that requires surgical intervention. The vessel most likely to be bleeding is the gastroduodenal artery because of erosion from a posterior ulcer. The duodenum is opened longitudinally, with the incision carried across the pylorus. The vessel is oversewn, with a three-point U stitch technique, which effectively ligates the main vessel along with any smaller branches. One must be careful to avoid incorporating the common bile duct into the stitch. The duodenotomy is closed transversely to avoid narrowing (Fig. 49-10).

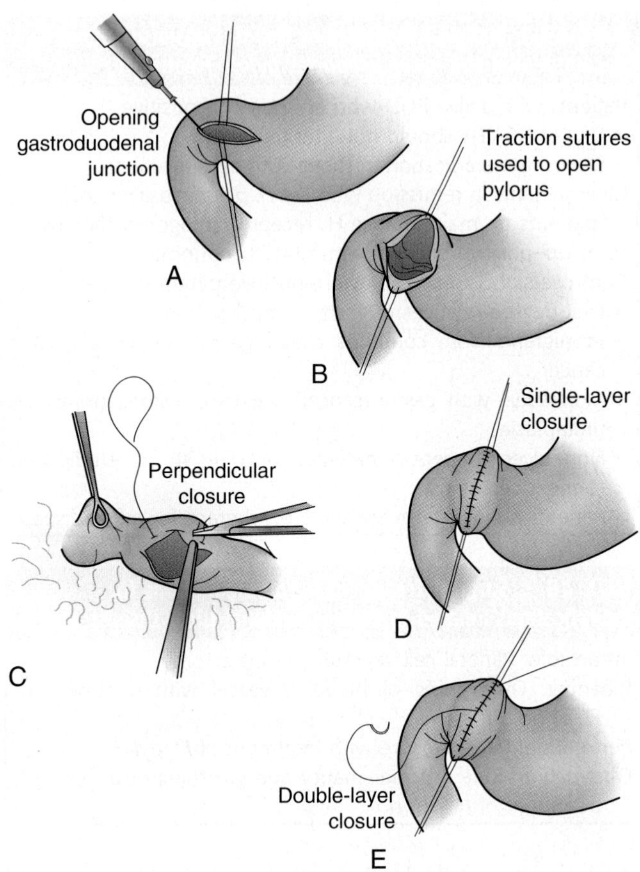


**FIGURE 49-10 A-E,** Heineke-Mikulicz pyloroplasty. (From Soreide JA, Soreide A: Pyloroplasty. Oper Tech Gen Surg 5:65–72, 2003.)

**Perforation** Patients with perforation typically complain of sudden onset, frequently severe epigastric pain. For many, it is their first symptom of ulcer disease. Patients will frequently have free air seen on the chest radiograph and, on examination, will have localized peritoneal signs. Patients with more widespread spillage will have diffuse peritonitis. For a small subset of patients, their perforations may seal spontaneously; however, operative intervention is required in almost all cases. Perforation has the highest mortality rate of any complication of ulcer disease, approaching 15%.

Perforation remains a surgical disease and conservative management means emergent surgical intervention. The perforation is usually in the first portion of the duodenum and can easily be accessed through an upper midline incision. Perforations smaller than 1 cm can generally be closed primarily and buttressed with well-vascularized omentum. For larger perforations, a Graham patch repair with a tongue of healthy omentum is performed. For very large perforations (>3 cm), control of the duodenal defect can be difficult. The defect should be closed by the application of healthy tissue, such as omentum or jejunal serosa , with placement of a duodenostomy tube and wide drainage. This likely will result in leakage of GI contents into the drain, but in most cases sepsis will resolve. An alternative in this difficult situation is antrectomy and a Billroth II reconstruction.

Perforations can also be treated laparoscopically. The results of two randomized controlled trials have shown that patients undergoing laparoscopic repair have, as expected, less pain and parenteral narcotic use. They also have an earlier time to discharge. There was no difference in pulmonary complications or abdominal septic complications. A meta-analysis of all studies comparing laparoscopic repair versus open repair, which included the randomized controlled trials, along with prospective and retrospective cohort studies, has shown overall similar outcomes, with longer operative times for laparoscopic repair.[14] However, these operating times have been decreasing in studies performed after 2001; in the most recent randomized controlled trial, laparoscopic repair was actually faster than open repair. The conversion rate ranged from 10% to 15% in most reports.

For patients who are known to be negative for *H. pylori*, are on chronic NSAIDs that they cannot discontinue, or have failed medical therapy in the past for their ulcer disease, an acid-reducing procedure can be added at the time of repair. The procedure must be based on the clinical situation and comfort of the surgeon.

After repair, the stomach is decompressed until bowel activity returns. Drains should be kept in place until the patients have eaten without a change in drain output or quality, which would suggest a leak. All *H. pylori*–positive patients should undergo eradication with appropriate triple-therapy regimens.

**Gastric Outlet Obstruction** Acute inflammation of the duodenum can lead to mechanical obstruction, with a functional gastric outlet obstruction manifested by delayed gastric emptying, anorexia, nausea, and vomiting. In cases of prolonged vomiting, patients may become dehydrated and develop a hypochloremic-hypokalemic metabolic alkalosis secondary to the loss of gastric juice rich in hydrogen and chloride. Chronic inflammation of the duodenum may lead to recurrent episodes of healing followed by repair and scarring, ultimately leading to fibrosis and stenosis of the duodenal lumen. In this situation, the obstruction is accompanied by painless vomiting of large volumes of gastric contents, with metabolic abnormalities similar to those seen in acute obstruction. The stomach can become massively dilated in this setting, and it rapidly loses its muscular tone. Marked weight loss and malnutrition are also common.

Gastric outlet obstruction from ulcer disease is now less common than obstruction from cancer. Cancer must be ruled out with endoscopy. Endoscopic dilation and *H. pylori* eradication are the mainstays of therapy. A study with an almost 5-year follow-up has shown that patients who have an identifiable cause (e.g., *H. pylori* infection) that could be treated, have good long-term results with endoscopic dilation, with a median of five dilations required, but no subsequent surgical therapy.[15] For patients with idiopathic duodenal ulcer disease causing gastric outlet obstruction, those treated with lifetime acid suppression also had good long-term results with endoscopic dilation. Patients with refractory obstruction are best managed with primary antrectomy and reconstruction along with vagotomy.

**Intractable Peptic Ulcer Disease** Intractability is defined as failure of an ulcer to heal after an initial trial of 8 to 12 weeks of therapy or if patients relapse after therapy has been discontinued. This is unusual for duodenal ulcer disease in the *H. pylori* era. Benign gastric ulcers that persist must be evaluated for malignancy. For any intractable ulcer, adequate duration of therapy, *H. pylori* eradication, and elimination of NSAID use must be confirmed. A serum gastrin level should also be determined in patients with ulcers refractory to medical therapy to rule out gastrinoma. Although rarely seen today, intractable duodenal ulcer should be treated with an acid-reducing operation. This can be a truncal or highly selective vagotomy, with or without an antrectomy.

**Surgical Procedures for Peptic Ulcers** Elective operative intervention has become rare as medical therapy has become more effective. The recognition of *H. pylori* and its eradication suggest that the intractability indication for surgery may apply only to patients in whom the organism cannot be eradicated or who cannot be taken off NSAIDs.

The goal of operative ulcer therapy is to reduce gastric acid secretion. This can be accomplished by removing vagal stimulation via vagotomy, gastrin-driven secretion by performing an antrectomy, or both. Vagotomy decreases peak acid output by approximately 50%, whereas vagotomy plus antrectomy decreases peak acid output by approximately 85%.

***Truncal Vagotomy*** As shown in Figure 49-4, truncal vagotomy is performed by division of the left and right vagus nerves above the hepatic and celiac branches, just above the GE junction. Truncal vagotomy is probably the most common operation performed for duodenal ulcer disease. Most surgeons use some form of drainage procedure in association with truncal vagotomy. The classic truncal vagotomy, in combination with a Heineke-Mikulicz pyloroplasty, is shown in Figure 49-10. When the duodenal bulb is scarred, a Finney pyloroplasty or Jaboulay gastroduodenostomy may be a useful alternative. In general, there is little difference in the side effects associated with the type of drainage procedure performed, although bile reflux may be more common after gastroenterostomy and diarrhea is more common after pyloroplasty. The incidence of dumping is the same for both.

***Highly Selective Vagotomy (Parietal Cell Vagotomy)*** The highly selective vagotomy is also called the *parietal cell vagotomy* or *proximal gastric vagotomy*. This procedure was developed after recognition that truncal vagotomy, in combination with a drainage procedure or gastric resection, adversely affects the pyloral antral pump function. A highly selective vagotomy divides only the vagus nerves supplying the acid-producing portion of the stomach within the corpus and fundus. This procedure preserves the vagal innervation of the gastric antrum so that there is no need for routine drainage procedures. Consequently, the incidence of postoperative complications is lower. In general, the nerves of Latarjet are identified anteriorly and posteriorly and the crow's feet innervating the fundus and body of the stomach are divided. These nerves are divided up until a point approximately 7 cm proximal to the pylorus or the area in the vicinity of the gastric antrum. Superiorly, division of these nerves is carried to a point at least 5 cm proximal to the GE junction on the esophagus (Fig. 49-11). Ideally, two or three branches to the antrum and pylorus should be preserved. The criminal nerve of Grassi represents a very proximal branch of the posterior trunk of the vagus, and great attention needs to be taken to avoid

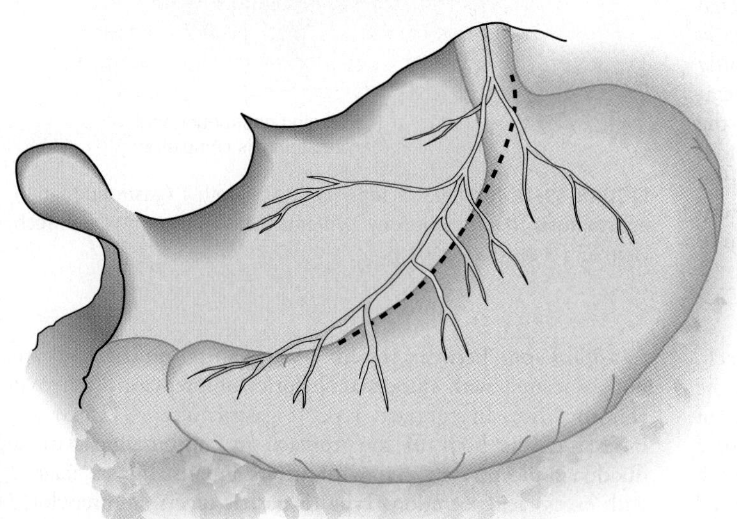

**FIGURE 49-11** Anterior view of the stomach and anterior nerve of Latarjet. Note the line of dissection for parietal cell or highly selective vagotomy *(dashed line).* The last major branches of the nerve are left intact and the dissection begins 7 cm from the pylorus. At the GE junction, the dissection is well away from the origin of the hepatic branches of the left vagus. (From Kelly KA, Teotia SS: Proximal gastric vagotomy. In Baker RJ, Fischer JE [eds]: Mastery of surgery, Philadelphia, 2001, Lippincott Williams & Wilkins.)

missing this branch in the division process because it is frequently cited as a predisposition for ulcer recurrence if left intact.

The recurrence rates after highly selective vagotomy are variable and depend on the skill of the surgeon and duration of follow-up. Lengthy longitudinal follow-up is necessary to evaluate the results of this procedure because of the reported increase in recurrent ulceration with time. Recurrence rates of 10% to 15% have been reported for this procedure when performed by a skilled surgeon. These are slightly higher than those reported after truncal vagotomy in combination with pyloroplasty; however, selective vagotomy has lower rates of postvagotomy dumping syndrome and diarrhea.

***Truncal Vagotomy and Antrectomy*** Antrectomy is generally not performed for duodenal ulcers and is more commonly done for gastric ulcers. Relative contraindications include cirrhosis, extensive scarring of the proximal duodenum that leaves a difficult or tenuous duodenal closure, and previous operations on the proximal duodenum, such as choledochoduodenostomy. When done in combination with truncal vagotomy, it is more effective at reducing acid secretion and recurrence than truncal vagotomy in combination with a drainage procedure or highly selective vagotomy. The recurrence rate for ulceration after truncal vagotomy and antrectomy is as low as 0% to 2%. However, this low recurrence rate needs to be balanced against the 20% rate of postgastrectomy and postvagotomy syndromes in patients undergoing antrectomy.

Antrectomy requires reconstruction of GI continuity that can be accomplished by a gastroduodenostomy (Billroth I procedure; Fig. 49-12) or gastrojejunostomy (Billroth II procedure; Fig. 49-13). For benign disease, gastroduodenostomy is generally favored because it avoids the problem of retained antrum syndrome, duodenal stump leak, and afferent loop obstruction associated with gastrojejunostomy after resection. If the duodenum is significantly scarred, gastroduodenostomy may be technically more difficult, necessitating gastrojejunostomy. If a gastrojejunostomy is performed, the loop of jejunum chosen for anastomosis is usually brought through the transverse mesocolon in a retrocolic fashion. The retrocolic anastomosis minimizes the length of the afferent limb and decreases the likelihood of twisting or kinking that could lead to afferent loop obstruction and predispose to the devastating complication of a duodenal stump leak. Although vagotomy and antrectomy are clearly effective at managing ulcerations, they are used infrequently today in the treatment of patients with PUD. In general, operations of lesser magnitude are performed more frequently in the *H. pylori* era. The overall mortality rate for antrectomy is approximately 2% but obviously is higher in patients with comorbid conditions, such as insulin-dependent diabetes or immunosuppression. Approximately 20% of patients develop some form of postgastrectomy or postvagotomy complications (see later).

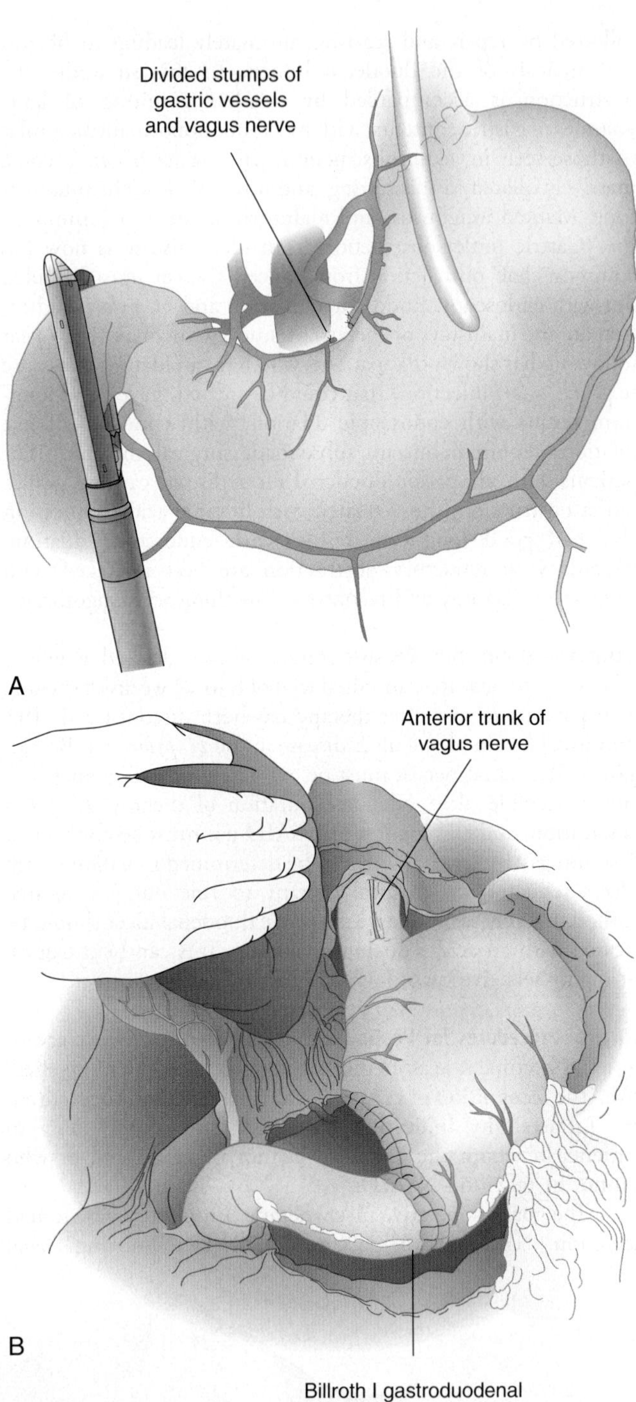


**FIGURE 49-12** Hemigastrectomy with a Billroth I (gastroduodenal) anastomosis. (From Dempsey D, Pathak A: Antrectomy. Oper Tech Gen Surg 5:86–100, 2003.)

## Gastric Ulcers

Gastric ulcers can occur at any location in the stomach, although they usually present on the lesser curvature, near the incisura, as shown in Table 49-3. Approximately 60% of ulcers are located in this location and are classified as type I gastric ulcers. These ulcers are generally not associated with excessive acid secretion and may occur with low to normal acid output. Most occur within 1.5 cm of the histologic transition zone between the fundic and antral mucosa and are not associated with duodenal, pyloric, or prepyloric mucosal abnormalities. In contrast, type II gastric ulcers (~15%) are located in the body of the stomach in combination with a duodenal ulcer. These types of ulcers are usually associated with excess acid secretion. Type III gastric ulcers are prepyloric ulcers and account for approximately 20% of the lesions. They

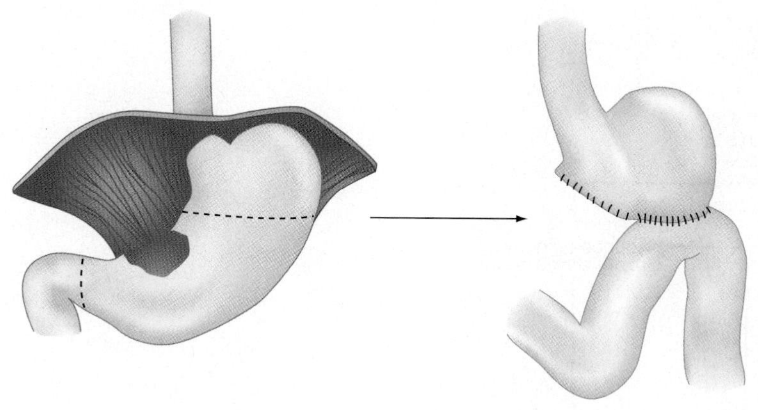

FIGURE 49-13 Subtotal gastrectomy with a Billroth II anastomosis.

**Table 49-3 Gastric Ulcer Types**

| TYPE | LOCATION | ACID LEVEL |
|---|---|---|
| I | Lesser curve at incisura | Low to normal |
| II | Gastric body with duodenal ulcer | Increased |
| III | Prepyloric | Increased |
| IV | High on lesser curve | Normal |
| V | Anywhere | Normal, NSAID-induced |

also behave like duodenal ulcers and are associated with hypersecretion of gastric acid. Type IV gastric ulcers occur high on the lesser curvature, near the GE junction. The incidence of type IV gastric ulcers is less than 10% and they are not associated with excessive acid secretion. Type V gastric ulcers can occur at any location and are associated with chronic NSAID use. Finally, some ulcers may appear on the greater curvature of the stomach, but the incidence is less than 5%.

Gastric ulcers rarely develop before the age of 40 years and the peak incidence occurs in those between the ages of 55 and 65 years. They are more likely to occur in those in a lower socioeconomic class and are slightly more common in the non-white than white population. The exact pathogenesis of a benign gastric ulcer remains unknown. Some conditions that may predispose to gastric ulceration are age older than 40, gender (female-to-male ratio of 2 : 1), ingestion of barrier-breaking drugs such as aspirin or NSAIDs, abnormalities in acid and pepsin secretion, gastric stasis from delayed gastric emptying, coexisting duodenal ulcer, duodenal gastric reflux of bile, gastritis, and infection with *H. pylori*. Some clinical conditions that may predispose to gastric ulceration include chronic alcohol intake, smoking, long-term corticosteroid therapy, infection, and intra-arterial therapy. With regard to acid and pepsin secretion, the presence of acid appears to be essential to the production of a gastric ulcer; however, the total secretory output appears to be less important. Nevertheless, it is noteworthy that rapid healing follows antacid therapy, antisecretory therapy, or vagotomy, even when the lesion-bearing portion of the stomach is left intact because in the presence of gastric mucosal damage, acid is ulcerogenic, even when present in normal or less than normal amounts.

### Clinical Manifestations

The clinical challenge of gastric ulcer management is the differentiation between gastric carcinoma and benign ulcer. Similar to duodenal ulcers, gastric ulcers are also characterized by recurrent episodes of quiescence and relapse. They also cause pain, bleeding, and obstruction and can perforate. On occasion, benign ulcers have also been found to result in spontaneous gastrocolic fistulas. Surgical intervention is required in 8% to 20% of patients who develop complications from their gastric ulcer disease. Hemorrhage occurs in approximately 35% to 40% of patients. Usually, patients who develop significant bleeding from their gastric ulcers are older, are less likely to stop bleeding spontaneously, and have higher morbidity and mortality rates than patients bleeding from a duodenal ulcer. Hemorrhage is most frequently observed in patients with types II and III gastric ulcers, and patients with type IV gastric ulcers may also present with life-threatening hemorrhage. The most frequent complication of gastric ulceration, however, is perforation. Most perforations occur along the anterior aspect of the lesser curvature. In general, older patients have increased rates of perforations and larger ulcers are associated with higher morbidity and mortality. Similar to duodenal ulcers, gastric outlet obstruction can also occur in patients with type II or III gastric ulcer. However, one must carefully differentiate between benign obstruction and obstruction secondary to antral carcinoma.

### Diagnosis and Treatment

The diagnosis and treatment of gastric ulceration generally mirror that for duodenal ulcer disease. The significant difference is the possibility of malignancy in a gastric ulcer. This critical difference demands that cancer be ruled out in acute and chronic presentations of gastric ulcer disease. Acid suppression and *H. pylori* eradication are both important aspects of any treatment.

As with duodenal ulcers, intractable nonhealing ulcers are becoming increasingly less common. It is important to ensure that adequate time has elapsed and appropriate therapy has been administered to allow healing of the ulcer to occur. This includes confirmation that *H. pylori* has been eradicated and that NSAIDs have been eliminated as a potential cause. The presentation of a nonhealing gastric ulcer in the *H. pylori* era should raise serious concerns about the presence of an underlying malignancy. These patients should undergo a thorough evaluation, with multiple biopsies, to exclude malignancy prior to any surgical intervention (Fig. 49-14). The approach for complicated gastric ulcer varies, depending on the type of ulcer and its association with

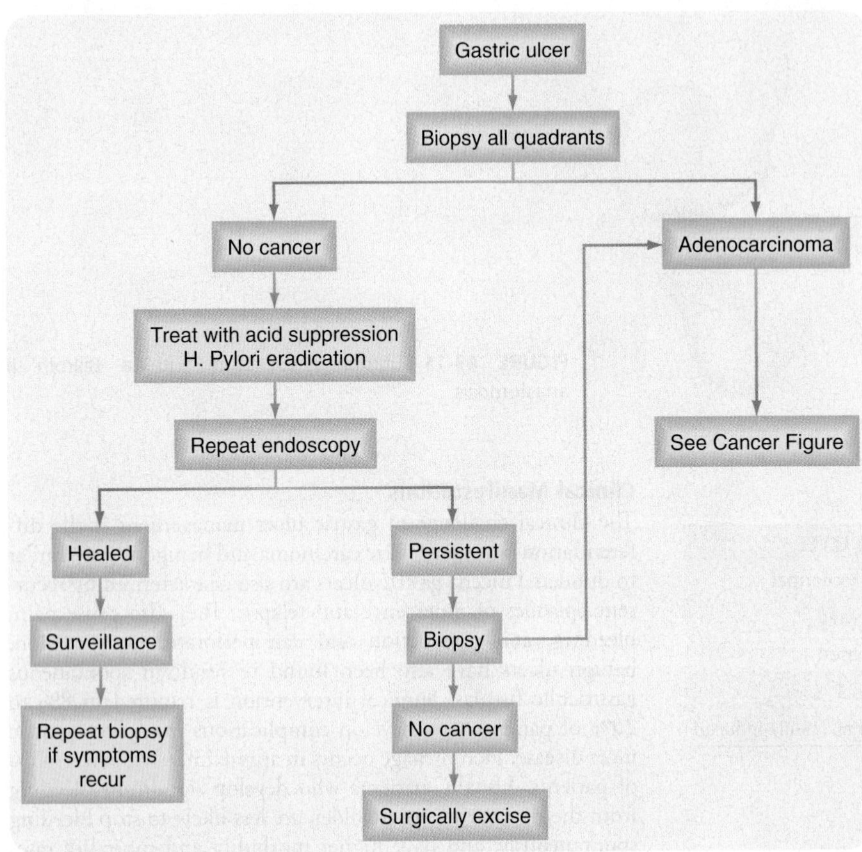


**FIGURE 49-14** Algorithm for evaluation, treatment, and surveillance of the patient with a gastric ulcer.

pathophysiologic acid levels. Type I and IV ulcers, which are not associated with increased acid levels, do not require acid-reducing vagotomy. Figure 49-15 provides an algorithm for managing complicated gastric ulcers.

**Type I Gastric Ulcer** For type I gastric ulcers, even with appropriate preoperative evaluation, malignancy remains a major concern, and excision of the ulcer is necessary. This is generally curative and allows more intense pathologic examination of the specimen. Distal gastrectomy without vagotomy can also be performed but has a morbidity of 3% to 5%, with mortality rates ranging from 1% to 2%. Recurrence is less than 5%. There is no evidence that gastrectomy is superior to resection of the ulcer alone.

**Type II or Type III Gastric Ulcers** Because types II and III gastric ulcers are associated with increased gastric acid levels, surgery for intractable disease should focus on acid reduction. A distal gastrectomy in combination with truncal vagotomy should be performed. It has been shown that patients undergoing highly selective vagotomy for type II or III gastric ulcers have a poorer outcome than those undergoing resection. However, there are still some who advocate performing a laparoscopic parietal cell vagotomy and reserve resection for those who develop ulcer recurrence.

**Type IV Gastric Ulcers** The type IV gastric ulcer presents a difficult management problem. Surgical treatment depends on ulcer size, distance from the GE junction, and degree of surrounding inflammation. Whenever possible, the ulcer should be excised. The preferred approach is to resect the ulcer without gastrectomy and the resultant morbidity of a small gastric remnant. At times, this is not possible, and a gastrectomy is necessary. The most aggressive approach is to perform a gastrectomy that includes a small portion of the esophageal wall and ulcer followed by a Roux-en-Y esophagogastrojejunostomy to restore intestinal continuity. For type IV gastric ulcers that are located 2 to 5 cm from the GE junction, a distal gastrectomy with a vertical extension of the resection to include the lesser curvature with the ulcer can be performed. After resection, bowel continuity is restored with an end-to-end gastroduodenostomy or gastrojejunostomy.

**Bleeding Gastric Ulcers** Treatment of bleeding gastric ulcers depends on their cause and location; however, the initial approach is similar to duodenal ulcers. Patients require resuscitation, monitoring, and endoscopic investigation. Up to 70% of gastric ulcers are *H. pylori*–positive, so an attempt should be made to control the bleeding endoscopically, with biopsy to rule out malignancy and testing of *H. pylori* status at that time. Patients whose bleeding can be controlled and who are *H. pylori*–positive should undergo treatment for their *H. pylori* infection. For bleeding that cannot be controlled, operative intervention again depends on the type of gastric ulcer. In all cases, the ulcer should ideally be excised with the addition of vagotomy dependent on ulcer type (e.g., type II or III ulcer or type IV ulcer in patients who cannot discontinue NSAIDS).

**Perforated Gastric Ulcer** For perforated type I gastric ulcers that occur in stable patients, distal gastrectomy with a Billroth I anastomosis is recommended. In unstable patients, simple

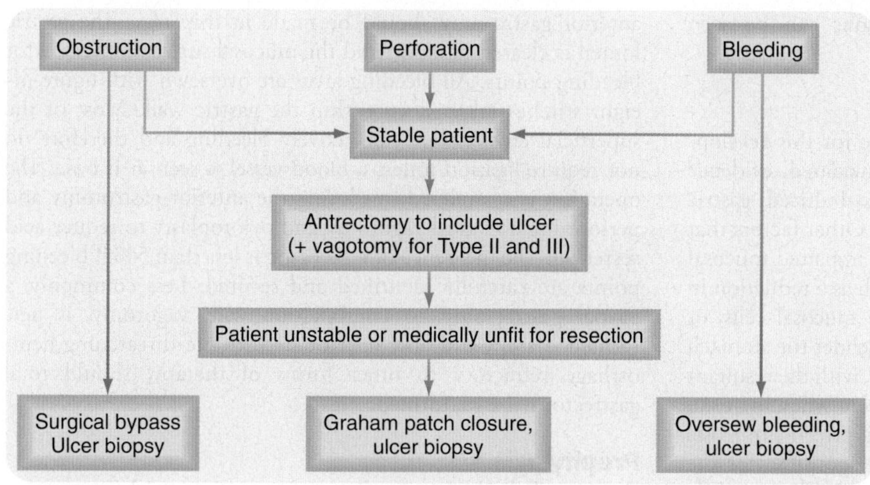


**FIGURE 49-15** Algorithm for the management of complicated gastric ulcer disease.

patching of the gastric ulcer with biopsy and treatment for *H. pylori*, if positive, is recommended. However, even if the biopsy is negative, the risk for malignancy still needs to be ruled out; therefore, documentation of healing is required with repeat endoscopy and biopsy. Adding vagotomy for perforated type I gastric ulcers is unlikely to be of any value. Because they behave like duodenal ulcers, types II and III gastric ulcers can be simply treated with patch closure, with or without truncal vagotomy and pyloroplasty, depending on the medical condition, hemodynamic status, and extent of peritonitis, followed by treatment for *H. pylori*–positive patients.

**Giant Gastric Ulcers** Giant gastric ulcers are defined as ulcers with a diameter of 2 cm or more. They are usually found on the lesser curvature and have a higher incidence of malignancy (10%) than smaller ones. It is not uncommon for these ulcers to penetrate into contiguous structures, such as the spleen, pancreas, liver, or transverse colon, and be falsely diagnosed as an unresectable malignancy, despite normal biopsy results. The incidence of malignancy ranges from 6% to 30% and increases with the size of the ulcer. Giant gastric ulcers have a high likelihood of developing complications (e.g., perforation or bleeding). Medical therapy heals 80% of these ulcers, although repeat endoscopy is indicated in 6 to 8 weeks. For complications or failure to heal, the operation of choice is gastrectomy including the ulcer bed, with vagotomy reserved for types II and III gastric ulcers. In the high-risk patient with significant underlying comorbid conditions, a local excision combined with vagotomy and pyloroplasty may be considered; otherwise, resection has the highest chance for successful outcome.

**Zollinger-Ellison Syndrome** ZES is a clinical triad consisting of gastric acid hypersecretion, severe PUD, and non–β-islet cell tumors of the pancreas. The islet cell tumor produces gastrin and thus PUD. Hypergastrinemia associated with ZES accounts for most, if not all, clinical symptoms experienced by patients. Abdominal pain and PUD are the hallmarks of the syndrome and typically occur in more than 80% of patients. Patients may also exhibit diarrhea, weight loss, steatorrhea, and esophagitis. Endoscopy frequently demonstrates prominent gastric rugal folds, reflecting the trophic effect of hypergastrinemia on the gastric fundus in addition to evidence of PUD.

Provocative tests are generally not required to establish the diagnosis of ZES because fasting and stimulated plasma gastrin levels are usually elevated. Most patients with gastrinoma have elevated fasting serum gastrin levels (>200 pg/mL), and values higher than 1000 pg/mL are diagnostic. In patients with equivocal gastrin levels, the most sensitive diagnostic test is the secretin stimulated gastrin level. Serum gastrin samples are measured before and after IV secretin (2 U/kg) administration at 5-minute intervals for 30 minutes. An increase in the serum gastrin level of greater than 200 pg/mL above basal levels is specific for gastrinoma versus other causes of hypergastrinemia, which do not demonstrate this response.

After diagnosis of gastrinoma, acid suppression therapy is initiated, preferably with a PPI. Medical management is indicated preoperatively and for patients with metastatic or unresectable gastrinoma. Localized gastrinoma should be resected.

## STRESS GASTRITIS

Stress gastritis, by definition, occurs after physical trauma, shock, sepsis, hemorrhage, or respiratory failure and may lead to life-threatening gastric bleeding. Stress gastritis is characterized by multiple superficial (nonulcerating) erosions that begin in the proximal or acid-secreting portion of the stomach and progress distally. They may also occur in the setting of central nervous system disease (Cushing's ulcer) or as a result of thermal burn injury involving more than 30% of the body surface area (Curling's ulcer).

Stress gastritis lesions typically change with time. They are considered early lesions if they appear within the first 24 hours. These early lesions are typically multiple and shallow, with discrete areas of erythema along with focal hemorrhage or an adherent clot. If the lesion erodes into the submucosa, which contains the blood supply, frank bleeding may result. On microscopy, these lesions appear as wedged-shaped mucosal hemorrhages with coagulation necrosis of the superficial mucosal cells. They are almost always seen in the fundus of the stomach and only rarely in the distal stomach. Acute stress gastritis can be classified as late if there is a tissue reaction or organization around a clot, or if an inflammatory exudate is present. This picture may be seen by microscopy 24 to 72 hours after injury. Late lesions appear identical to regenerating mucosa around a healing gastric ulcer. Both types of lesions can be seen endoscopically.

### Pathophysiology

Although the precise mechanisms responsible for the development of stress gastritis remain to be fully elucidated, evidence suggests a multifactorial cause. These stress-induced gastric lesions appear to require the presence of acid. Other factors that may predispose to their development include impaired mucosal defense mechanisms against luminal acid, such as a reduction in blood flow, mucus, bicarbonate secretion by mucosal cells, or endogenous prostaglandins. All these factors render the stomach more susceptible to damage from luminal acid, with the resultant hemorrhagic gastritis. Stress is considered present when hypoxia, sepsis, or organ failure occurs. When stress is present, mucosal ischemia is thought to be the main factor responsible for the breakdown of these normal defense mechanisms. There is little evidence to suggest that increased gastric acid secretion occurs in this situation. However, the presence of luminal acid appears to be a prerequisite for this form of gastritis to evolve. Moreover, complete neutralization of luminal acid or antisecretory therapy precludes the development of experimental stress gastritis.

### Presentation and Diagnosis

More than 50% of patients develop stress gastritis within 1 to 2 days after a traumatic event. The only clinical sign may be painless upper GI bleeding that may be delayed at onset. The bleeding is usually slow and intermittent and may be detected by only a few flecks of blood in the NG tube or an unexplained drop in the hemoglobin level. On occasion, there may be profound upper GI hemorrhage accompanied by hypotension and hematemesis. The stool is frequently guaiac-positive, although melena and hematochezia are rare. Endoscopy is required to confirm the diagnosis and differentiate stress gastritis from other sources of GI hemorrhage.

### Treatment

Any patient with upper GI bleeding requires prompt and definitive fluid resuscitation with correction of any coagulation or platelet abnormalities. Treatment of the underlying sepsis plays a major role in treating the underlying gastric erosions. More than 80% of patients who present with upper GI hemorrhage stop bleeding with only supportive care. There is little evidence to suggest that endoscopy with electrocautery or heater probe coagulation has any benefit in the therapy of bleeding from acute stress gastritis. However, some studies have suggested that acute bleeding can be effectively controlled by selective infusion of vasopressin into the splanchnic circulation through the left gastric artery. Vasopressin is administered by continuous infusion through the catheter at a rate of 0.2 to 0.4 IU/min for a maximum of 48 to 72 hours. If the patient has underlying cardiac or liver disease, vasopressin should not be used. Although vasopressin may decrease blood loss, it has not been shown to result in improved survival. Another angiographic technique that can be used is embolization of the left gastric artery if bleeding is identified on angiography. However, the extensive plexus of submucosal arterial vessels within the stomach makes this approach less appealing and not as successful.

Bleeding that recurs or persists, requiring more than 6 U of blood (3000 mL), is an indication for surgery. Because most of the lesions are in the proximal stomach or fundus, a long anterior gastrotomy should be made in this area. The gastric lumen is cleared of blood and the mucosal surface inspected for bleeding points. All bleeding areas are oversewn with figure-of-eight stitches taken deep within the gastric wall. Most of the superficial erosions are not actively bleeding and therefore do not require ligation unless a blood vessel is seen at it base. The operation is completed by closing the anterior gastrotomy and performing a truncal vagotomy and pyloroplasty to reduce acid secretion. The incidence of rebleeding is less than 5% if bleeding points are carefully identified and secured. Less commonly, a partial gastrectomy, in combination with vagotomy, is performed. Rarely, and only in patients with life-threatening hemorrhage refractory to other forms of therapy, should total gastrectomy be performed.

### Prophylaxis

Because of the high mortality rate in patients with acute stress gastritis who develop massive upper GI hemorrhage, high-risk patients should be treated prophylactically. Because mucosal ischemia may alter a number of mucosal defense mechanisms that enable the stomach to withstand luminal irritants and protect itself from injury, every effort should be made to correct any perfusion deficits secondary to shock. There appears to be no significant advantage of $H_2$ blockers over antacids. Most studies have demonstrated that it is easier to maintain a pH higher than 5 with antacids than with standard intermittent doses of $H_2$ receptor antagonists. However, it has been suggested that continuous infusions of $H_2$ receptor antagonists provide more consistent maintenance of intraluminal gastric pH than standard intermittent infusions.

Whether continuous infusion of $H_2$ receptor antagonists has a better clinical outcome or improves drug safety has yet to be determined. Nevertheless, $H_2$ receptor antagonists have approximately 97% efficacy when used as medical prophylaxis for stress gastritis.

Sucralfate (1 g every 6 hours) has also been used for stress gastritis prophylaxis. Similar to antacids and $H_2$ receptor antagonists, efficacy rates range from 90% to 97%. This form of prophylaxis has the added effect of allowing the stomach to maintain its normal pH and thus prevent bacterial overgrowth. This latter effect may be beneficial because it has been suggested that gastric luminal alkalinization predisposes the stomach to bacterial overgrowth and subsequent nosocomial pneumonia. Exogenous prostaglandins have also been used as stress gastritis prophylaxis agents, although their efficacy appears to be much less than that of other agents.

## POSTGASTRECTOMY SYNDROMES

Gastric surgery results in a number of physiologic derangements caused by loss of reservoir function, interruption of the pyloric sphincter mechanism, and vagal nerve transection. These physiologic changes usually cause no long-term symptoms. The GI and cardiovascular symptoms may result in disorders collectively referred to as *postgastrectomy syndromes*. Approximately 25% of patients who undergo surgery for PUD subsequently develop some degree of postgastrectomy syndrome, although this frequency is much lower in highly selective vagotomy. The physiologic changes are not specific to PUD and can occur after gastrectomy for resection of neoplasm. Fortunately, only approximately 1% of patients become permanently disabled from their symptoms.

### Dumping Syndrome

Dumping syndrome can be early (20 to 30 minutes after eating) or late (2 or 3 hours after a meal). Early dumping is more common, with more GI and fewer cardiovascular effects. GI symptoms include nausea and vomiting, a sense of epigastric fullness, cramping abdominal pain, and often explosive diarrhea. The cardiovascular symptoms include palpitations, tachycardia, diaphoresis, fainting, dizziness, flushing, and occasionally blurred vision. This symptom complex can develop after any operation on the stomach but is more common after partial gastrectomy with the Billroth II reconstruction. It is much less commonly observed following the Billroth I gastrectomy or after vagotomy and drainage procedures.

Dumping occurs because of the rapid passage of food of high osmolarity from the stomach into the small intestine. This occurs because gastrectomy, or any interruption of the pyloric sphincteric mechanism, prevents the stomach from preparing its contents and delivering them to the proximal bowel in the form of small particles in isotonic solution. The resultant hypertonic food bolus passes into the small intestine, which induces a rapid shift of extracellular fluid into the intestinal lumen to achieve isotonicity. After this shift of extracellular fluid, luminal distention occurs and induces the autonomic responses listed earlier.

The basic defect of late dumping is also rapid gastric emptying; however, it is related specifically to carbohydrates being delivered rapidly into the proximal intestine. When carbohydrates are delivered to the small intestine, they are quickly absorbed, resulting in hyperglycemia, which triggers the release of large amounts of insulin to control the rising blood sugar level. This results in an overcompensation so that a profound hypoglycemia occurs in response to the insulin. This activates the adrenal gland to release catecholamines, which results in diaphoresis, tremulousness, light-headedness, tachycardia, and confusion. The symptom complex is indistinguishable from insulin shock.

The symptoms associated with early dumping syndrome appear to be secondary to the release of several humoral agents, such as serotonin, bradykinin-like substances, neurotensin, and enteroglucagon. Dietary measures are usually sufficient to treat most patients. These include avoiding foods containing large amounts of sugar, frequent feeding of small meals rich in protein and fat, and separating liquids from solids during a meal.

In some patients without a response to dietary measures, long-acting octreotide agonists have ameliorated symptoms. These peptides not only inhibit gastric emptying but also affect small bowel motility so that intestinal transit of the ingested meal is prolonged. The side effects associated with administration of these synthetic peptides are relatively benign; however, they are somewhat expensive. Many operative procedures have been advocated for the surgical treatment of these patients. The paucity of patients treated for PUD with gastrectomy or vagotomy has made remedial procedures for dumping exceedingly rare.

### Metabolic Disturbances

The most common metabolic defect appearing after gastrectomy is anemia. Anemia is related to iron deficiency (more common) or impairment in vitamin $B_{12}$ metabolism. More than 30% of patients undergoing gastrectomy suffer from iron deficiency anemia. The exact cause remains to be fully understood but appears to be related to a combination of decreased iron intake, impaired iron absorption, and chronic blood loss. In general, the addition of iron supplements to the patient's diet corrects this metabolic problem.

Megaloblastic anemia from vitamin $B_{12}$ deficiency only rarely develops after partial gastrectomy, but is dependent on the amount of stomach removed. Vitamin deficiency occurs secondary to poor absorption of dietary $B_{12}$ because of the lack of intrinsic factor. If a patient develops a macrocytic anemia, serum vitamin $B_{12}$ levels should be determined and, if abnormal, treated with chronic $B_{12}$ therapy.

Both osteoporosis and osteomalacia have also been observed after gastric resection and appear to be caused by deficiencies in calcium. If fat malabsorption is also present, the calcium malabsorption is further aggravated because fatty acids bind calcium. The incidence of this problem also increases with the extent of gastric resection and is usually associated with a Billroth II gastrectomy. Bone disease generally develops approximately 4 to 5 years after surgery. Treatment of this disorder usually requires calcium supplements (1 to 2 g/day) in conjunction with vitamin D (500 to 5000 U daily).

### Afferent Loop Syndrome

Afferent loop syndrome occurs as a result of partial obstruction of the afferent limb, which is unable to empty its contents. After obstruction of the afferent limb, there is an accumulation of pancreatic and hepatobiliary secretions within the limb, resulting in its distention, which causes epigastric discomfort and cramping. The intraluminal pressure eventually increases enough to empty the contents of the afferent loop forcefully into the stomach, resulting in bilious vomiting that offers immediate relief of symptoms. If the obstruction has been present for a long time, it can also be aggravated by the development of the blind loop syndrome. In this situation, bacterial overgrowth occurs in the static loop and the bacteria bind with vitamin $B_{12}$ and deconjugated bile acids. This results in a systemic deficiency of vitamin $B_{12}$, with the development of megaloblastic anemia.

In contrast to the diagnosis of an acute bowel obstruction, the diagnosis of chronic afferent loop obstruction may be problematic. Failure to visualize the afferent limb on upper endoscopy is suggestive of the diagnosis. Radionuclide studies imaging the hepatobiliary tree have also been used with some success in diagnosing this syndrome. Normally, the radionuclide should pass into the stomach or distal small bowel after being excreted into the afferent limb. If it does not, the possibility of an afferent loop obstruction should be considered.

Surgical correction is indicated for this mechanical problem. A long afferent limb is usually the underlying problem, so treatment involves the elimination of this loop. Remedies include conversion of the Billroth II construction into a Billroth I anastomosis, enteroenterostomy below the stoma, and creation of a Roux-en-Y procedure. The Roux-en-Y reconstruction is a good combination of efficacy and ease, especially in the patient with a previous vagotomy. Marginal ulceration from the diversion of duodenal contents from the gastroenteric stoma is a potential complication of the Roux-en-Y conversion.

### Efferent Loop Obstruction

Obstruction of the efferent limb is usually rare. Efferent loop obstruction may occur at any time; however, more than 50% of cases do so within the first postoperative month. Establishing a diagnosis is difficult. Initial complaints may include left upper quadrant abdominal pain that is colicky in nature, bilious vomiting, and abdominal distention. The diagnosis is usually established by a GI contrast study of the stomach, with failure of barium to enter the efferent limb. Operative intervention is almost always necessary and consists of reducing the retroanastomotic hernia and closing the retroanastomotic space to prevent recurrence of this condition.

### Alkaline Reflux Gastritis

After gastrectomy, reflux of bile is common. In a small percentage of patients, this reflux is associated with severe epigastric abdominal pain accompanied by bilious vomiting and weight loss. Although the diagnosis can be made by taking a careful history, hepatobiliary iminodiacetic acid (HIDA) scans usually demonstrate biliary secretion into the stomach and even into the esophagus. Upper endoscopy demonstrates friable, beefy red mucosa.

Most patients suffering from alkaline reflux gastritis have had gastric resection performed with a Billroth II anastomosis. Although bile reflux appears to be the inciting event, a number of issues remain unanswered with respect to the role of bile in its pathogenesis. For example, many patients have reflux of bile into the stomach following gastrectomy without any symptoms. Moreover, there is no clear correlation between the volume or composition of bile and the subsequent development of alkaline reflux gastritis. Although it is clear the syndrome does exist, caution needs to be exercised to ensure that it is not overdiagnosed. After a diagnosis is made, therapy is directed at relief of symptoms. Unfortunately, most medical therapies that have been tried to treat alkaline reflux gastritis have not shown any consistent benefit. Thus, for patients with intractable symptoms, the surgical procedure of choice is conversion of the Billroth II anastomosis into a Roux-en-Y gastrojejunostomy, in which the Roux limb has been lengthened to more than 40 cm.

### Gastric Atony

After vagotomy, gastric emptying is delayed. This is true for truncal and selective vagotomies but not for a highly selective or parietal cell vagotomy. With selective or truncal vagotomy, patients lose their antral pump function and therefore have a reduction in the ability to empty solids. In contrast, emptying of liquids is accelerated because of loss of receptive relaxation in the proximal stomach, which regulates liquid emptying. Although most patients undergoing vagotomy and a drainage procedure manage to empty their stomach adequately, some patients have persistent gastric stasis that results in retention of food within the stomach for several hours. This may be accompanied by a feeling of fullness and, occasionally, abdominal pain. In still rarer cases, it may be associated with a functional gastric outlet obstruction.

The diagnosis of gastroparesis is confirmed by scintigraphic assessment of gastric emptying. However, other causes of delayed gastric emptying, such as diabetes mellitus, electrolyte imbalance, drug toxicity, and neuromuscular disorders, must also be excluded. In addition, a mechanical cause of gastric outlet obstruction, such as postoperative adhesions, afferent or efferent loop obstruction, and internal herniations, must be ruled out, and endoscopic examination of the stomach also needs to be performed to rule out any anastomotic obstructions.

In patients with a functional gastric outlet obstruction and documented gastroparesis, pharmacotherapy is generally used. The agents most commonly used are prokinetic agents such as metoclopramide and erythromycin. Metoclopramide exerts it prokinetic effects by acting as a dopamine antagonist and has cholinergic-enhancing effects because of facilitation of acetylcholine release from enteric cholinergic neurons. In contrast, erythromycin markedly accelerates gastric emptying by binding to motilin receptors on GI smooth muscle cells, where it acts as a motilin agonist. One of these two agents is usually sufficient to enhance gastric tone and improve gastric emptying. In rare cases of persistent gastric atomy refractory to medical management, gastrectomy may be required.

## GASTRIC CANCER

### Epidemiology and Risk Factors

#### Incidence

Gastric cancer is the 14th most common cancer and cause of cancer death in the United States, with an estimated 21,000 new cases/year and over 10,000 deaths.[16] The disease affects men disproportionately, with more than 60% of new cases occurring in men. It is a disease of older individuals, with peak incidence in the seventh decade of life. Among racial groups, the disease is more common and has a higher mortality in African Americans, Asian Americans, and Hispanics compared with whites.

Worldwide, gastric cancer is the fourth most common cancer and the second leading cause of cancer death. It is especially prevalent in East Asia and South America and has been increasing in developing countries, which now have almost two thirds of all distal gastric cancer cases. In contrast, rates have been decreasing in the United States (Fig. 49-16). Among developed countries, Japan and Korea have the highest rates of the disease. Gastric cancer is the most common cancer in Japan. As a result, gastric cancer screening in Japan was started in the 1970s and the mortality rate has dropped by 50% since that time. Although there has been an increase in proximal tumors in Japan, most are distal gastric cancers.

#### Risk Factors

The major risk factors for gastric cancer are discussed here; they include environmental and genetic factors (Box 49-3).

##### *Helicobacter pylori* Infection

In 1994, the international agency for research on cancer labeled *H. pylori* a definite carcinogen. A number of longitudinal prospective studies have demonstrated an association with the development of gastric cancer. The primary mechanism is thought to be the presence of chronic inflammation. Long-term infection with the bacteria leads to gastritis, primarily within the gastric body, with ventral gastric atrophy. In some patients, this progresses to intestinal metaplasia, dysplasia, and ultimately intestinal-type adenocarcinoma. A wide range of molecular alterations in intestinal metaplasia have been described and may affect the transformation into gastric cancer. These include overexpression of cyclooxygenase-2 and cyclin D2, *p53* mutations, microsatellite instability, decreased *p27* expression, and alterations in transcription factors such as CDX1 and CDX2. It is clear that intestinal metaplasia is a risk factor for the development of gastric carcinoma; however, not every patient with intestinal metaplasia develops invasive cancer. Host inflammatory responses play an important role in this process. Specifically,

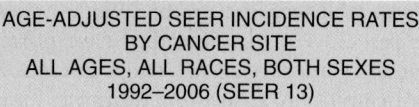


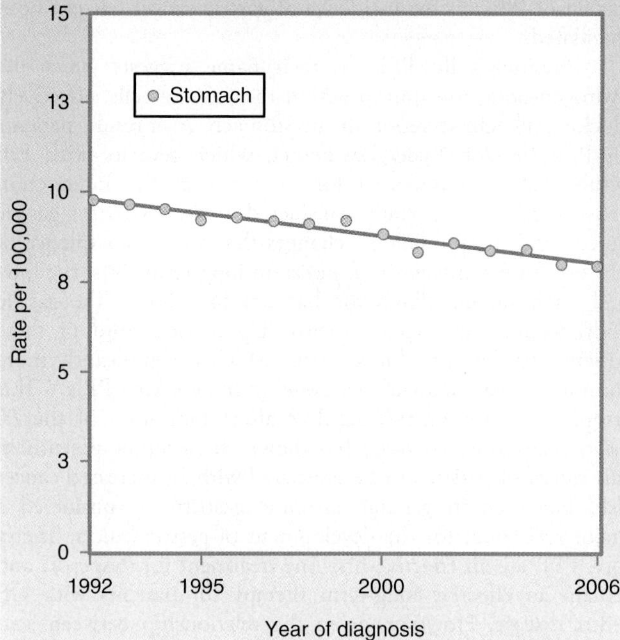


Cancer sites include invasive cases only unless otherwise noted.
Incidence source: SEER 13 areas (San Francisco, Connecticut, Detroit, Hawaii, Iowa, New Mexico, Seattle, Utah, Atlanta, San Jose-Monterey, Los Angeles, Alaska Native Registry and Rural Georgia).
Rates are per 100,000 and are age-adjusted to the 2000 US Std Population (19 age groups – Census P25-1130). Regression lines are calculated using the Joinpoint Regression Program Version 3.3.2, June 2008, National Cancer Institute.

**FIGURE 49-16** Age-adjusted incidence of gastric cancer, 1996-2006. (From National Cancer Institute, Surveillance Research Program: Fast Stats, 2009 (http://seer.cancer.gov/faststats. Accessed June 17, 2010.)

**BOX 49-3 Factors Associated With Increased Risk for Developing Stomach Cancer**

**Nutritional**
Low fat or protein consumption
Salted meat or fish
High nitrate consumption
High complex carbohydrate consumption

**Environmental**
Poor food preparation (smoked, salted)
Lack of refrigeration
Poor drinking water (e.g., contaminated well water)
Smoking

**Social**
Low social class

**Medical**
Prior gastric surgery
*H. pylori* infection
Gastric atrophy and gastritis
Adenomatous polyps

**Other**
Male gender

individuals with high levels of interleukin-1 expression are at increased risk of gastric cancer development.

Some regional variances in the development of cancer may be attributed to the prevalence and virulence of *H. pylori*. It is more common in poor areas with less sanitation; thus, infection rates remain high in developing countries, with a concomitant rise in gastric cancer incidence. The prevalence in more developed countries, in contrast, has been falling. The presence of the cytoxan-associated gene A *(cagA)* is associated with increased virulence and risk of gastric cancer. Countries with high levels of gastric cancer, such as Japan, have a much higher rate of *cagA*-positive *H. pylori* infection than in countries with lower rates of gastric cancer, such as the United States.

### Dietary Factors

High-salt foods, particularly those with salted or smoked meats that contain high levels of nitrate, along with low fruit and vegetable intake, are linked to an increased risk of gastric cancer. The mechanism is thought to be the conversion of nitrates in the food to N-nitroso compounds by bacteria in the stomach. Fresh fruits and vegetables contain ascorbic acid, which can remove the carcinogenic N-nitroso compounds and oxygen free radicals.

There is likely synergism between diet and *H. pylori* infection, with the bacteria increasing carcinogen production and inhibiting its removal. *H. pylori* has been shown to promote the growth of the bacteria that generate the carcinogenic N-nitroso compounds. At the same time, *H. pylori* can inhibit the secretion of ascorbic acid, thus preventing effective scavenging of oxygen free radicals and N-nitroso compounds. The increase in refrigeration over the past 70 years has likely contributed to the decrease in gastric cancer by reducing the amount of meat preserved by salting alone and allowing the increased storage and consumption of fresh fruits and vegetables.

### Hereditary Risk Factors and Cancer Genetics

Gastric cancer is associated with several rare inherited disorders. Hereditary diffuse gastric cancer is an inherited form of gastric cancer. Patients with this disorder, resulting from a gene mutation for the cell adhesion molecule E-cadherin, have an 80% lifetime incidence of developing gastric cancer. Prophylactic total gastrectomy should be considered for patients with this mutation. In familial adenomatous polyposis, approximately 85% of patients have fundic gland polyps, with up to 40% of these having some type of dysplasia and over 50% containing a somatic adenomatous polyposis coli mutation, which places these patients at risk of developing gastric cancer. These polyps, combined with the much higher frequency of potentially malignant duodenal polyps, warrant upper GI surveillance. The Li-Fraumeni syndrome is an autosomal dominant disorder caused by a mutation in the tumor suppressor *p53* gene. These patients are at risk for numerous malignancies, including gastric cancer. Hereditary nonpolyposis colorectal cancer, or Lynch syndrome, which accounts for 2% to 3% of all colon and rectal cancers and is associated with microsatellite instability, is also associated with an increased risk of gastric and ovarian cancers.

Several genetic alterations have been identified that are associated with gastric adenocarcinoma. These changes can be classified as the activation of oncogenes, inactivation of tumor suppressor genes, reduction of cellular adhesion, reactivation of telomerase, and presence of microsatellite instability. The *c-met* proto-oncogene is the receptor for the hepatocyte growth factor and is frequently overexpressed in gastric cancer, as are the k-*sam* and c-*erbB2* oncogenes. The inactivation of the tumor suppressor genes *p53* and *p16* has been reported in diffuse and intestinal-type cancers, whereas adenomatous polyposis coli gene mutations tend to be more frequent in intestinal-type gastric cancers. Also, a reduction or loss in the cell adhesion molecule E-cadherin can be found in approximately 50% of diffuse-type gastric cancers. Microsatellite instability can be found in approximately 20% to 30% of intestinal-type gastric cancers. Microsatellites are lengths of DNA in which a short (one to five nucleotide) motif is repeated several times. Microsatellite instability reflects a gain or loss of repeat units in a germline microsatellite allele, indicating the clonal expansion that is typical of a neoplasm.

### Other Risk Factors

Patients with pernicious anemia are at increased risk for developing gastric cancer. Achlorhydria is the defining feature of this condition; it occurs when chief and parietal cells are destroyed by an autoimmune reaction. The mucosa becomes very atrophic and develops antral and intestinal metaplasia. The relative risk for a patient with pernicious anemia developing gastric cancer is 2.1 to 5.6 of the general population.

**Polyps** Adenomatous polyps carry a distinct risk for the development of malignancy in the polyp. Mucosal atypia is frequent, and progression from dysplasia to carcinoma in situ has been observed. The risk for the development of carcinoma is approximately 10% to 20% and increases with increasing size of the polyp. Endoscopic removal is indicated for pedunculated lesions and is sufficient if the polyp is completely removed and there are no foci of invasive cancer on histologic examination. If the polyp is larger than 2 cm, is sessile, or has a proven focus of invasive carcinoma, operative excision is warranted.

Fundic gland polyps (Fig. 49-17) are benign lesions that are thought to result from glandular hyperplasia and decreased luminal flow. They are strongly associated with proton pump inhibitor use and occur in up to a third of patients by one year. Dysplasia, while common in patients whose polyps result from familial adenomatous polyposis, has only been described as individual case reports for patients whose polyps result from proton pump inhibitor therapy. As such, they do not require excision, regular surveillance, or cessation of therapy.

**Proton Pump Inhibitors** The use of PPIs has risen dramatically over the past 20 years because they have proven an effective treatment for patients with GI reflux disease. They are often prescribed empirically as first-line treatment for dyspepsia. The impact of PPIs on the incidence of gastric cancer has not been elucidated.

Physiologically, PPIs, as their name suggests, block the hydrogen-potassium pump within the parietal cells, effectively blocking all acid secretion in the stomach. As a result, patients on PPIs develop hypergastrinemia, which reverses with PPI withdrawal. The potential for cancer is at the intersection between *H. pylori,* already considered a carcinogen for gastric cancer, and the physiologic changes that are a consequence of PPI use. In patients with *H. pylori* on long-term PPIs, the low-acid environment allows the bacteria to colonize the gastric body, leading to corpus gastritis. Up to one third of these patients develop atrophic gastritis, which is significantly more common in patients with *H. pylori* who are taking PPIs.[17] This atrophic gastritis quickly resolves after eradication of the *H. pylori.* Currently, no study has shown the atrophic gastritis in this subset of patients to be associated with an increased cancer risk. However, in general, atrophic gastritis is considered a major risk factor for the development of gastric cancer. Therefore, PPIs are an effective first-line treatment for dyspepsia and remain an effective long-term therapy for patients with GE reflux disease. However, given the relationship between acid suppression, *H. pylori,* and the development of atrophic gastritis, a known risk factor for gastric cancer, in patients with persistent symptoms after initiation of therapy or who require long-term therapy, surveillance for and eradication of *H. pylori* is warranted.

## Pathology

Numerous pathologic classification schemes of gastric cancer have been proposed. The Borrmann classification system was developed in 1926; it remains useful today for the description of endoscopic findings. This system divides gastric carcinoma into five types, depending on the lesion's macroscopic appearance (Fig. 49-18). One type, linitis plastica, describes a diffusely infiltrating lesion involving the entire stomach. Other classification systems have been proposed, but the most useful and widely used system is the one proposed by Lauren in 1965. This system separates gastric adenocarcinoma into intestinal or diffuse types

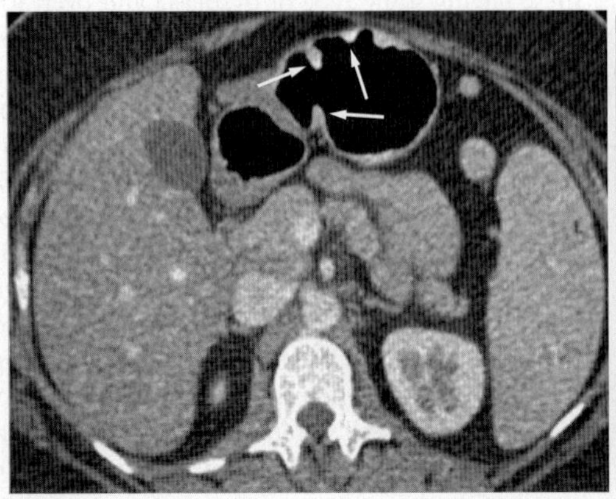

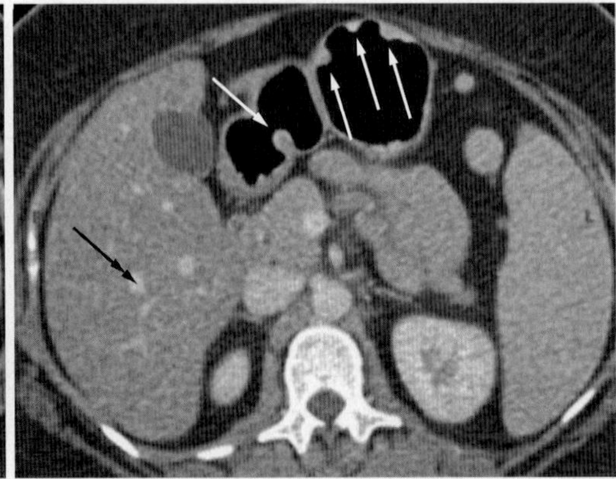

**FIGURE 49-17** CT scan of fundic gland polyps. (Courtesy Dr. David Bentrem, Department of Surgery, Northwestern University Feinberg School of Medicine, Chicago.)

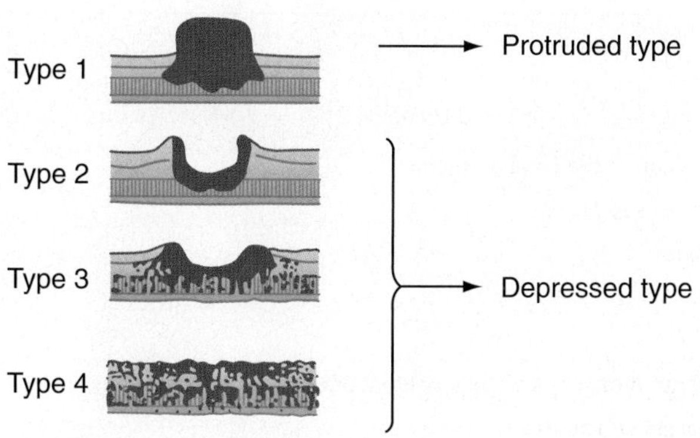


**FIGURE 49-18** Borrmann's pathologic classification of gastric cancer based on gross appearance. (From Iriyama K, Asakawa T, Koike H, et al: Is extensive lymphadenectomy necessary for surgical treatment of intramucosal carcinoma of the stomach? Arch Surg 124:30–311, 1989.)

**Table 49-4 Lauren Classification System**

| INTESTINAL | DIFFUSE |
|---|---|
| Environmental | Familial |
| Gastric atrophy, intestinal metaplasia | Blood type A |
| Men > women | Women > men |
| Increasing incidence with age | Younger age group |
| Gland formation | Poorly differentiated, signet ring cells |
| Hematogenous spread | Transmural,lymphatic spread |
| Microsatellite instability | Decreased E-cadherin |
| *APC* gene mutations | |
| *p53*, *p16* inactivation | *p53*, *p16* inactivation |

*APC*, Adenomatous polyposis coli.

based on histology, with both types having distinct pathology, epidemiology, and prognosis (Table 49-4).

The intestinal variant typically arises in the setting of a recognizable precancerous condition, such as gastric atrophy or intestinal metaplasia. Men are more commonly affected than women, and the incidence of the intestinal-type gastric adenocarcinoma increases with age. These cancers are typically well differentiated, with a tendency to form glands. Metastatic spread is generally hematogenous to distant organs. The intestinal type is also the dominant histology in areas in which gastric cancer is epidemic, suggesting an environmental cause.

The diffuse form of gastric adenocarcinoma consists of tiny clusters of small, uniform signet ring cells, is poorly differentiated, and lacks glands. It tends to spread submucosally, with less inflammatory infiltration than the intestinal type, with early metastatic spread via transmural extension and lymphatic invasion. It is generally not associated with chronic gastritis, is more common in women, and affects a slightly younger age group. The diffuse form also has an association with blood type A and familial occurrence, suggesting a genetic cause. Intraperitoneal metastases are frequent and, in general, the prognosis is less favorable than for patients with intestinal type cancers.

In 1990, the World Health Organization (WHO) recommended another classification system for gastric cancers based on morphologic features. In the WHO system, gastric cancer is divided into five main categories—adenocarcinoma, adenosquamous cell carcinoma, squamous cell carcinoma, undifferentiated carcinoma, and unclassified carcinoma. Adenocarcinomas are further subdivided into four types according to their growth pattern—papillary, tubular, mucinous, and signet ring. Each type is further subdivided by degree of differentiation. Although widely used, the WHO classification system offers little in terms of patient management, and there are a significant number of gastric cancers that do not fit into their categories. There is little evidence that any of the above classification systems can add to the prognostic information provided by the American Joint Cancer Commission (AJCC) tumor-node-metastasis (TNM) staging system.

## Diagnosis and Workup

### Signs and Symptoms

The symptoms of gastric cancer are generally nonspecific and contribute to its frequently advanced stage at the time of diagnosis. They include epigastric pain, early satiety, and weight loss. These symptoms are frequently mistaken for more common benign causes of dyspepsia including PUD and gastritis. The pain associated with gastric cancer tends to be constant, nonradiating, and is generally not relieved by eating. More advanced lesions may present with either obstruction or dysphagia depending on the location of the tumor. Some degree of GI bleeding is common, with up to 40% of patients having some form of anemia and up to 15% having frank hematemesis.

A complete history and physical examination should be performed, with special attention to any evidence of advanced disease. This includes metastatic nodal disease, supraclavicular (Virchow's) or periumbilical (Sister Mary Joseph's node), and evidence of intra-abdominal metastases such as hepatomegaly, jaundice, or ascites. Drop metastases to the ovaries (Krukenberg's tumor) may be detectable on pelvic examination and peritoneal metastases can be felt as a firm (Blummer's) shelf on rectal examination. A complete blood count, chemistry panel, including liver function tests, and coagulation studies should be carried out.

## Staging

Currently, the most widely use staging system is the AJCC TNM staging system. This is based on the depth of tumor invasion (T), number of involved lymph nodes (N), and presence or absence of metastatic disease (M; Table 49-5). Prior to 1997, N stage was determined by the anatomic location of the nodes with respect to the primary tumor, rather than the absolute number of nodes. This staging, based on anatomy, was intimately related to the D1 versus D2 anatomic lymphadenectomy debate (see later). The revised system does not differentiate among the locations of positive nodes. In the current staging system, a minimum of 15 nodes must be evaluated for accurate staging. Some have suggested that other factors be included in the T and N assessment, such as the location of the primary (cardia compared with distal tumors), because this may independently predict survival, and emphasis on the percentage of positive nodes (lymph node

**Table 49-5 TNM Classification of Carcinoma of the Stomach**

| **PRIMARY TUMOR (T)**† | | | |
|---|---|---|---|
| TX | Primary tumor cannot be assessed | | |
| T0 | No evidence of primary tumor | | |
| Tis | Carcinoma in situ; intraepithelial tumor without invasion of the lamina propria | | |
| T1 | Tumor invades lamina propria, muscularis mucosae, or submucosa | | |
| T1a | Tumor invades lamina propria or muscularis mucosae | | |
| T1b | Tumor invades submucosa | | |
| T2 | Tumor invades muscularis propria* | | |
| T3 | Tumor penetrates subserosal connective tissue without invasion of visceral peritoneum or adjacent structures†,‡ | | |
| T4 | Tumor invades serosa (visceral peritoneum) or adjacent structures†,‡ | | |
| T4a | Tumor invades serosa (visceral peritoneum) | | |
| T4b | Tumor invades adjacent structures | | |
| **REGIONAL LYMPH NODES (N)*** | | | |
| NX | Regional lymph node(s) cannot be assessed | | |
| N0 | No regional lymph node metastasis§ | | |
| N1 | Metastasis in 1-2 regional lymph nodes | | |
| N2 | Metastasis in 3-6 regional lymph nodes | | |
| N3 | Metastasis in 7 or more regional lymph nodes | | |
| N3a | Metastasis in 7-15 regional lymph nodes | | |
| N3b | Metastasis in 16 or more regional lymph nodes | | |
| **DISTANT METASTASIS (M)** | | | |
| M0 | No distant metastasis | | |
| M1 | Distant metastasis | | |
| **ANATOMIC STAGE** | **Prognostic Group** | | |
| 0 | Tis | N0 | M0 |
| IA | T1 | N0 | M0 |
| IB | T2<br>T1 | N0<br>N1 | M0<br>M0 |
| IIA | T3<br>T2<br>T1 | N0<br>N1<br>N2 | M0<br>M0<br>M0 |
| IIB | T4a<br>T3<br>T2<br>T1 | N0<br>N1<br>N2<br>N3 | M0<br>M0<br>M0<br>M0 |
| IIIA | T4a<br>T3<br>T2 | N1<br>N2<br>N3 | M0<br>M0<br>M0 |
| IIIB | T4b<br>T4b<br>T4a<br>T3 | N0<br>N1<br>N2<br>N3 | M0<br>M0<br>M0<br>M0 |
| IIIC | T4b<br>T4b<br>T4a | N2<br>N3<br>N3 | M0<br>M0<br>M0 |
| IV | Any T | Any N | M1 |

From Edge S, Byrd D, Compton C, et al (eds): AJCC cancer staging manual, ed 7, New York, 2010, Springer.

*A tumor may penetrate the muscularis propria with extension into the gastrocolic or gastrohepatic ligaments, or into the greater or lesser omentum, without perforation of the visceral peritoneum covering these structures. In this case, the tumor is classified T3. If there is perforation of the visceral peritoneum covering the gastric ligaments or the omentum, the tumor should be classified T4.

†The adjacent structures of the stomach include the spleen, transverse colon, liver, diaphragm, pancreas, abdominal wall, adrenal gland, kidney, small intestine, and retroperitoneum.

‡Intramural extension to the duodenum or esophagus is classified by the depth of the greatest invasion in any of these sites, including the stomach.

§A designation of pN0 should be used if all examined lymph nodes are negative, regardless of the total number removed and examined.

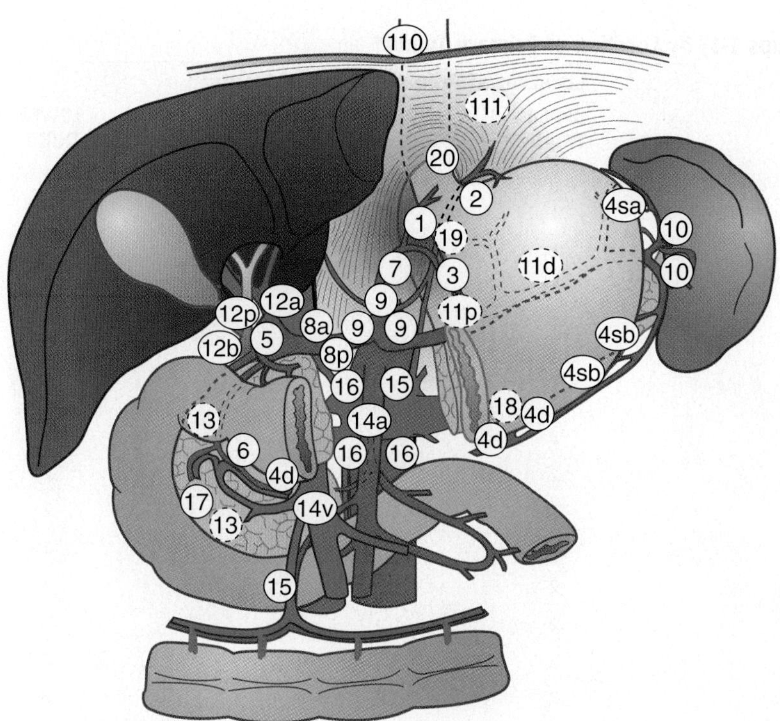


**FIGURE 49-19** Lymph node station numbers as defined by the Japanese Gastric Cancer Association. (From Japanese Gastric Cancer Association: Japanese Classification of Gastric Carcinoma, 2nd English edition. Gastric Cancer 1:10–24, 1998.)

ratio) rather than the number of positive nodes. However, the current AJCC staging system does not reflect these factors.

Although not part of the formal AJCC staging system, the term *R status,* first described by Hermanek in 1994, is used to describe tumor status after resection and is important for determining the adequacy of surgery. R0 describes a microscopically margin-negative resection, in which no gross or microscopic tumor remains in the tumor bed. R1 indicates removal of all macroscopic disease, but microscopic margins are positive for tumor. R2 indicates gross residual disease. Because the extent of resection can influence survival, some include this R designation to complement the TNM system. Long-term survival can be expected only after an R0 resection.

The AJCC system is not specific for nodal location, but the debate regarding lymphadenectomies for gastric cancer has continued. In the previous version of the Union Internationale Contre le Cancer (UICC) TNM system, N categories were defined by the location of lymph node metastases relative to the primary, with pN1 defined as positive nodes 3 cm or less from the primary and pN2 as more than 3 cm from the primary or nodal metastases along named blood vessels. The Japanese Classification for Gastric Carcinoma (JCGC) staging system was designed to describe the anatomic locations of nodes removed during gastrectomy. Sixteen distinct anatomic locations of lymph nodes are described, with the recommendation for nodal basin dissection dependent on the location of the primary (Fig. 49-19). The lymph node stations, or echelons, are numbered and further classified into groups of echelons corresponding to the location of the primary and reflect the likelihood of harboring metastases. The presence of metastasis to each lymph node group then determines the N classification. For example, metastasis to any of the group 1 lymph nodes in the absence of disease in more distant lymph node groups is classified as N1. This is represented graphically in Table 49-6. This system was not adopted by the AJCC. The AJCC pathologic staging system has been widely adopted in the United States.

### Staging Workup

The goal of any preoperative staging is twofold. The first is to gain information on prognosis to counsel the patient and family effectively. The second is to determine the extent of disease to determine the most appropriate course of therapy. The three main treatment paths are resection (with or without subsequent adjuvant therapy), neoadjuvant therapy followed by resection, or treatment of systemic disease without resection (Fig. 49-20).

The main modalities for staging gastric adenocarcinoma and thus guiding therapy are endoscopy, endoscopic ultrasound, cross-sectional imaging, such as computed tomography (CT), MRI, or positron emission tomography (PET), and diagnostic laparoscopy. Their roles are discussed here.

**Endoscopy and Endoscopic Ultrasound** Flexible endoscopy remains the essential tool for the diagnosis of gastric cancer. It allows visualization of the tumor, provides tissue for pathologic diagnosis, and can serve as a treatment for patients with obstruction or bleeding (Fig. 49-21). Increasingly, flexible endoscopy combined with ultrasound is being used to stage and risk-stratify patients with gastric cancer properly. Endoscopic ultrasound (EUS) is performed using a flexible endoscope with a 7.5-to 12-MHz ultrasound transducer. The stomach is filled with water to distend the stomach and the stomach wall is visualized as five alternating hypoechoic and hyperechoic layers (Fig. 49-22*A*). The mucosa and submucosa represent the first three layers (T1; see Fig. 49-22*B*). The fourth layer is the subserosa, invasion of which is a T2 tumor. The serosa is the fifth layer and tumor penetration of it is a T3 tumor (see Fig. 49-22*C*). The overall accuracy of EUS has been reported to be as high as 85% for T stage and 80% for N stage; however, these studies considered

**Table 49-6 Grouping of Regional Lymph Nodes (Groups 1-3) by Location of Primary Tumor***

| | | Location of Primary Tumor in Stomach | | |
|---|---|---|---|---|
| **LYMPH NODE STATION (NO.)** | **DESCRIPTION** | **UPPER THIRD** | **MIDDLE THIRD** | **LOWER THIRD** |
| 1 | Right paracardial | 1 | 1 | 2 |
| 2 | Left paracardial | 1 | 3 | M |
| 3 | Lesser curvature | 1 | 1 | 1 |
| 4sa | Short gastric | 1 | 3 | M |
| 4sb | Left gastroepiploic | 1 | 1 | 3 |
| 4d | Right gastroepiploic | 2 | 1 | 1 |
| 5 | Suprapyloric | 3 | 1 | 1 |
| 6 | Infrapyloric | 3 | 1 | 1 |
| 7 | Left gastric artery | 2 | 2 | 2 |
| 8a | Anterior comm. hepatic | 2 | 2 | 2 |
| 8p | Posterior comm. hepatic | 3 | 3 | 3 |
| 9 | Celiac artery | 2 | 2 | 2 |
| 10 | Splenic hilum | 2 | 3 | M |
| 11p | Proximal splenic | 2 | 2 | 2 |
| 11d | Distal splenic | 2 | 3 | M |
| 12a | Left hepatoduodenal | 3 | 2 | 2 |
| 12b, p | Posterior hepatoduodenal | 3 | 3 | 3 |
| 13 | Retropancreatic | M | 3 | 3 |
| 14v | Superior mesenteric vein | M | 3 | 2 |
| 14a | Superior mesenteric artery | M | M | M |
| 15 | Middle colic | M | M | M |
| 16al | Aortic hiatus | 3 | M | M |
| 16a2, b1 | Para-aortic, middle | M | 3 | 3 |
| 16b2 | Para-aortic, caudal | M | M | M |

*M,* Lymph nodes regarded as distant metastasis.

*According to the Japanese Classification of gastric carcinoma (Japanese Gastric Cancer Association: Japanese Classification of Gastric Carcinoma, 2nd English edition. Gastric Cancer 1:10–24, 1998).

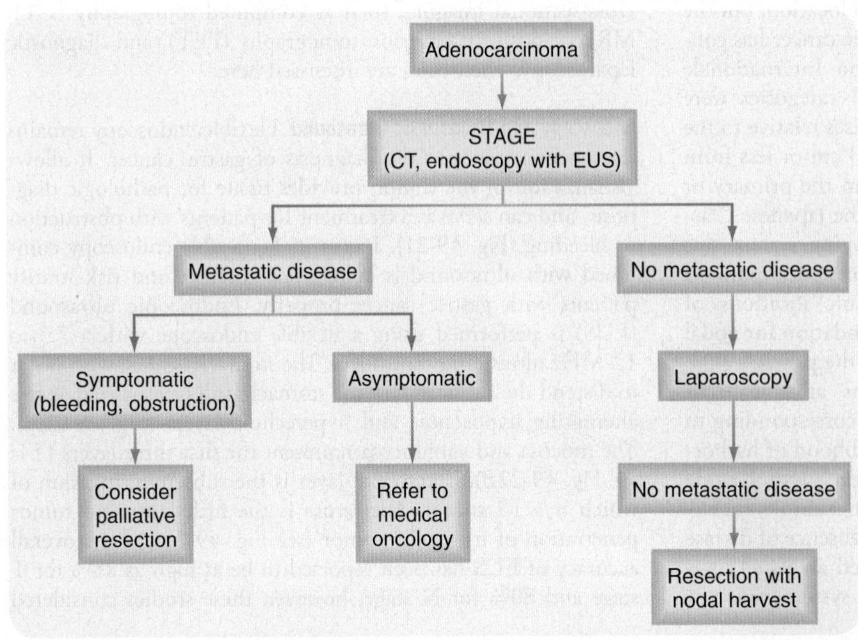


**FIGURE 49-20** General staging and treatment strategy for gastric adenocarcinoma.

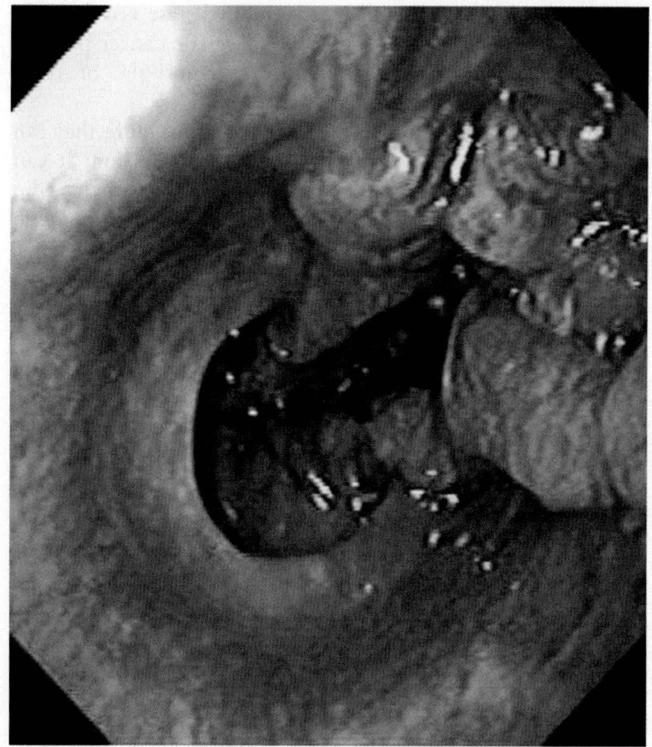

**FIGURE 49-21** Endoscopic view of intestinal-type adenocarcinoma of the gastric cardia. (Courtesy Dr. David Bentrem, Department of Surgery, Northwestern University Feinberg School of Medicine, Chicago.)

accuracy retrospectively, and not the predictive accuracy of EUS. A more recent, larger study[18] has shown lower accuracy of T and N stages. It considered the predictive accuracy of EUS for T and N stages and found them to be 57% and 50%, respectively. It showed improved accuracy, however, when T and N stages were grouped together to differentiate high-risk versus low-risk disease, defined by the presence of any serosal (T3/T4) involvement or any nodal disease (>N0). When this classification system was used, the positive predictive value of EUS to identify advanced disease was 76% and the negative predictive value to identify low-risk disease was 91% (Fig. 49-23).[18] From a prognostic and treatment standpoint, this classification may be more clinically relevant, because an EUS finding indicative of advanced disease strongly correlates with decreased resectability and poorer disease-specific survival.

Its role in the evaluation of metastatic disease is currently limited. In one study, however, a low-risk EUS had a 96% negative predictive value for the presence of metastatic disease. In the future, EUS may play a role in determining those patients who require further aggressive investigation of metastatic disease (e.g., laparoscopy) and those who do not.

As the accuracy of EUS improves, it will likely play an increasing role in determining treatment algorithms in gastric cancer, much as it does in rectal cancer. Currently, although its individual T and N stage accuracy may be lacking, it is has been shown to be a useful tool in differentiating between high-risk and low-risk patients, and that this differentiation correlates with prognosis.

**Computed Tomography** CT plays an important role in the evaluation of metastatic disease. CT remains the primary method for detection of intra-abdominal metastatic disease, with an overall

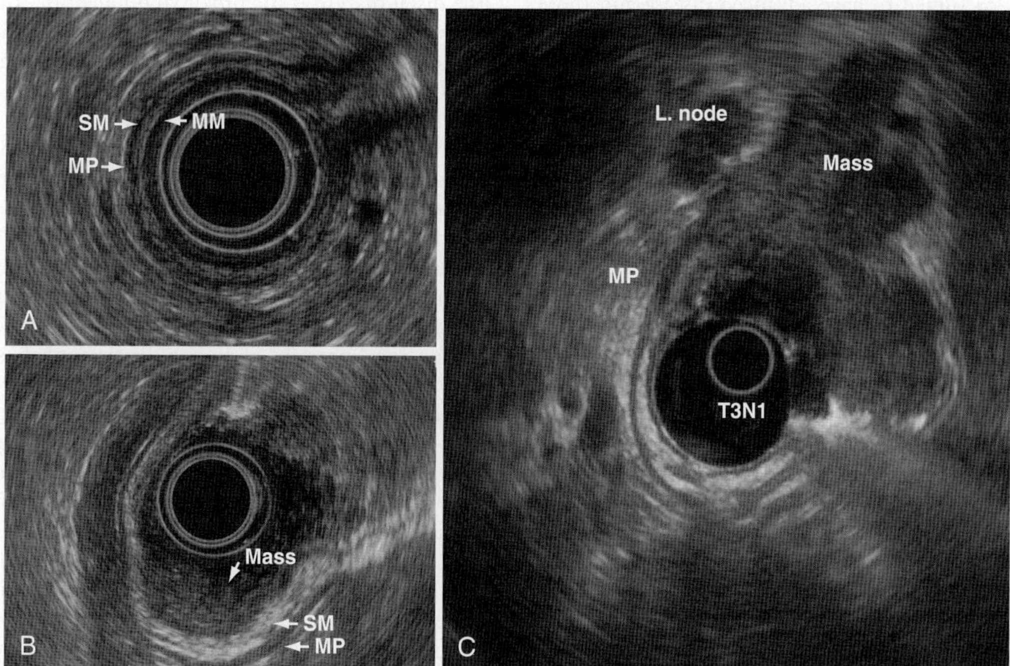


**FIGURE 49-22** Endoscopic ultrasound views of normal stomach **(A)**, T1 N0 gastric cancer **(B)**, and T3 N1 gastric cancer **(C)**. (Courtesy Dr. Rajesh Keswani, Division of Gastroenterology, Department of Medicine, Northwestern University Feinberg School of Medicine, Chicago.)

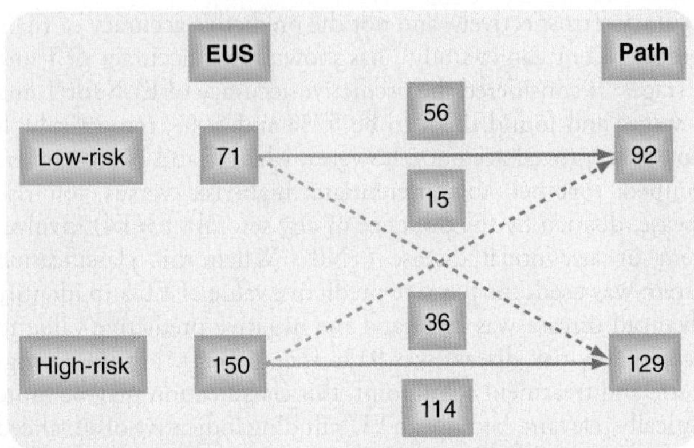


**FIGURE 49-23** Predictive accuracy of endoscopic ultrasound in gastric cancer. Of 71 patients identified as low risk (T1/2N0) on EUS, 56 were correctly staged and 15 were understaged. Of 150 patients identified as high risk (T3/4, any N, or any T, N+) on EUS, 114 were correctly staged and 36 were overstaged. (From Bentrem D, Gerdes H, Tang L, et al: Clinical correlation of endoscopic ultrasonography with pathologic stage and outcome in patients undergoing curative resection for gastric cancer. Ann Surg Oncol 14:1853–1859, 2007.)

detection rate of approximately 85%. The ability to image peritoneal metastases remains only 50%.

CT has also been used in locoregional staging. The accuracy of T and N stages as determined by CT is less accurate than EUS.[19] Although improved technology may increase the role for CT in locoregional evaluation and for neoadjuvant therapy, its primary role remains the evaluation of metastatic disease.

**Positron Emission Tomography** PET is not currently a primary staging modality for gastric cancer. Only 50% of gastric cancers are PET-avid, which limits its application. However, in PET-positive patients presumed to have advanced disease and those considered for neoadjuvant therapy, there may be a role for PET. PET response to neoadjuvant therapy strongly correlates with survival, with PET response seen within 14 days of treatment. PET may be an effective modality for monitoring response to these therapies, sparing unresponsive patients further toxic treatment.[20]

**Laparoscopy** Staging laparoscopy is an integral part of the standard workup for gastric cancer. The high rate of occult metastatic disease makes laparoscopy an attractive staging modality. In the late 1990s, two large studies evaluated laparoscopy as a staging modality for patients with gastric cancer.[21,22] Both studies demonstrated high rates of occult metastatic disease (37% and 23%, respectively) in patients undergoing staging laparoscopy for gastric cancer who were previously thought to have no metastatic disease as assessed by CT. The overall sensitivity of laparoscopy for detecting metastatic disease was higher than 95%. For patients who had metastatic disease, fewer than 15% went on to require palliative gastrectomy. As a result of these studies, staging laparoscopy has been advocated as part of the workup for gastric cancer to avoid unnecessary laparotomy in patients without a clear need for laparotomy.

As CT technology has improved, the need for staging laparoscopy has been reexamined. A 2007 study of 106 patients with gastric cancer showed, despite improved CT technology, that laparoscopy still has a role.[23] Unresectable disease not detected by prior imaging was found in 33% of gastric cancer patients undergoing staging laparoscopy. More than 75% of these patients had occult peritoneal or liver metastases.

Staging laparoscopy is a safe, low-risk procedure that can be planned as a single-stage procedure with resection; it can therefore be done with minimal added risk to patients who undergo laparotomy and with no additional risk for those who undergo an entirely laparoscopic resection. Meanwhile, there are many benefits of avoiding laparotomy, which include avoiding a delay in starting chemotherapy for patients with metastatic disease and limited life expectancy. Given the persistence of high rates of metastatic disease not detected by preoperative workup in a number of centers, even with improved imaging modalities, we believe that these benefits far outweigh the risk and that staging laparoscopy should be part of the workup for most patients with gastric cancer.

## Treatment

### Surgical Therapy

Complete resection of the gastric tumor with a wide margin of normal stomach remains the standard of care for resection with curative intent. The extent of resection depends on the location of the tumor in the stomach and size of the tumor. The standard technique is via a laparotomy; however, minimally invasive techniques, including laparoscopy and completely endoscopic resection for very early tumors, have proven effective methods of treatment.

For cancers of the distal stomach, including the body and antrum, a distal gastrectomy is the appropriate operation. The proximal stomach is transected at the level of the incisura at a margin of at least 6 cm, because studies have documented tumor spread as far as 5 cm laterally from the primary tumor. Frozen section analysis should be performed prior to reconstruction. The distal margin is the proximal duodenum. The possibility of recurrence in the tumor bed (duodenal suture line and surface of the pancreas) suggest a Billroth II reconstruction rather than a Billroth I, which will result in less risk of gastric outlet obstruction secondary to tumor recurrence.

For proximal lesions of the fundus or cardia, a total gastrectomy with a Roux-en-Y esophagojejunostomy or proximal gastrectomy is equivalent from an oncologic perspective. The postoperative anastomotic leak rate is higher for an esophagojejunostomy, but the margin will typically be larger than for a gastrojejunostomy. When a negative margin can be achieved, a gastrojejunostomy is performed. However, to construct a tension-free anastomosis to the distal esophagus, a Roux-en-Y esophagojejunostomy is usually required. A hand-sewn or stapled technique may be used.

Minimally invasive techniques have been used for many GI tumors. and gastric cancer is no exception. Several studies have shown good short-term and long-term outcomes for the laparoscopic approach. In a randomized controlled trial that compared open gastrectomy with laparoscopic-assisted gastrectomy, patients in the laparoscopic arm had similar perioperative morbidity and mortality, with shorter time to initiation of oral feeding (5.1 versus 7.4 days) and earlier discharge from the hospital (10.3 versus 14.5 days).[24] There was no difference in 5-year disease-free and overall survival. Importantly, the median lymph node count between the two groups was not significantly different; in both groups, the median count higher than 30, with at least 15 lymph nodes recommended for adequate oncologic staging. A large retrospective study of 250 patients has also shown similar short-term outcomes along with similar adequacy of lymphadenectomy.[25] Improvement in operating time for the laparoscopic group was also shown in this study, with mean operating time being only 10 minutes longer than open repair; this increased significantly over a learning curve of approximately 60 patients. Overall, laparoscopic gastrectomy has been shown to be a safe and effective treatment for gastric cancer. There does appear to be a learning curve; however, when performed by an experienced surgeon, it has equivalent oncologic outcomes, with less postoperative pain, earlier initiation of oral feeding, and earlier discharge from the hospital.

For early gastric cancer with limited penetration of the gastric wall and no evidence of lymph node metastases, purely endoscopic mucosal resection can be carried out. This has been widely practiced in Japan for decades and has been evaluated in the United States and Europe. There have been no randomized controlled trials comparing endoscopic mucosal resection with gastrectomy for early gastric cancer. Current practice is therefore based on nonrandomized prospective studies and retrospective reviews. The most significant advantage of endoscopic resection is avoiding the need for gastrectomy, whether by laparotomy or laparoscopy. The major disadvantage is incomplete resection because of tumor size or unrecognized lymph node metastases. To avoid undertreating patients, several studies have sought to identify risk factors for harboring lymph node metastases. A Japanese study of 1196 patients with intramucosal gastric cancer without known lymph node disease who underwent resection found, in multivariate analysis, that lymphatic vessel invasion, histologic ulceration of the tumor, and larger size (≥30 mm) were independent risk factors for regional lymph node metastasis. Patients without any of these risk factors had only a 0.36% chance of having lymph node metastases.[26] Based on these data, the general guidelines for endoscopic resection of early gastric cancer are as follows: (1) tumor limited to the mucosa; (2) no lymphovascular invasion; (3) tumor smaller than 2 cm; and (4) no ulceration. Findings of any of these on initial biopsy or during endoscopic resection is an indication for gastrectomy with lymph node dissection.

The basic principle for endoscopic mucosal resection involves elevating and encircling the diseased mucosa and then using a snare device to excise it. Perforation rates are low and bleeding rates are approximately 15%; these can generally be controlled without the need for further intervention (Fig. 49-24).

Long-term outcomes for properly selected patients are good. A 2007 multicenter retrospective review of 516 Korean patients showed complete resection in 77% of patients, 6% local recurrence rate for patients who had a complete resection, and no disease-specific mortality with 39-month median follow-up.[27] The data from the Japanese experience have shown similar rates of complete resection and recurrence.

Some authors have proposed expanding the eligibility criteria for endoscopic resection based on the results of several large studies of resected gastric cancer. A Japanese study of more than 5000 patients who underwent resection found that small tumors, regardless of ulcer status, and nonulcerated tumors, regardless of size, did not have associated lymph node disease.[28] It was also found that patients with submucosal invasion less than 500 µm

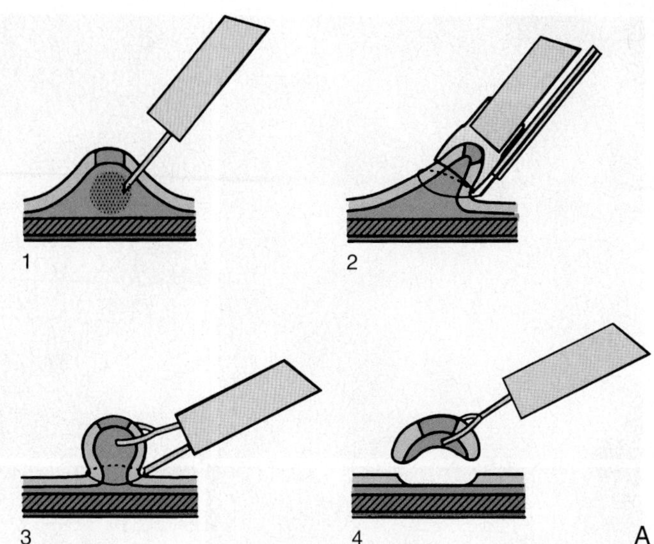


**FIGURE 49-24** Endoscopic mucosal resection (EMR). A, EMR by strip biopsy: saline is injected into the submucosal layer, and the area is elevated *(1)*. The top of the mound is pulled upward with forceps, and the snare is placed at the base of the lesion (*2* and *3*). Electrosurgical current is applied through the snare to resect the mucosa, and the lesion is removed *(4)*. (From Tanabe S, Koizumi W, Kokutou M, et al: Usefulness of endoscopic aspiration mucosectomy as compared with strip biopsy for the treatment of gastric mucosal cancer. Gastrointest Endosc 50:819–822, 1999.)

behaved similarly to patients who had completely intramucosal tumors. A later study of patients undergoing endoscopic mucosal resection showed similar results, with limited submucosal invasion having a low risk for lymph node metastases. Given these findings, the proposed extended criteria include all intramucosal tumors without ulceration, differentiated mucosal tumors smaller than 3 cm, regardless of ulceration status, and tumors with limited (SM1) submucosal invasion that were smaller than 3 cm and without ulceration.

In treating these larger tumors or those with SM1 invasion, standard endoscopic mucosal resection techniques are generally ineffective. Given the size and depth, physicians treating patients under this extended criteria have described an endoscopic submucosal resection technique. This involves marking the borders of the lesion using electrocautery. A submucosal injection of epinephrine with indigo carmine hydrodissects the lesion and an insulation-tipped knife is used to remove the lesion in a submucosal plane. Any bleeding is controlled with electrocautery (Fig. 49-25).

There are limited data on the outcomes of patients undergoing endoscopic mucosal resection or endoscopic submucosal resection with extended criteria. A review of 126 patients with mucosal cancer and 52 with submucosal cancer showed rates of lymph node metastases of 2% and 4%, respectively.[29] A similar study of patients undergoing endoscopic mucosal resection or endoscopic submucosal resection, including 73 for extended criteria, found 3 patients who met extended criteria and were lymph node–positive.[30] No patients with differentiated mucosal tumors without ulceration, regardless of size, had positive lymph nodes in either study.

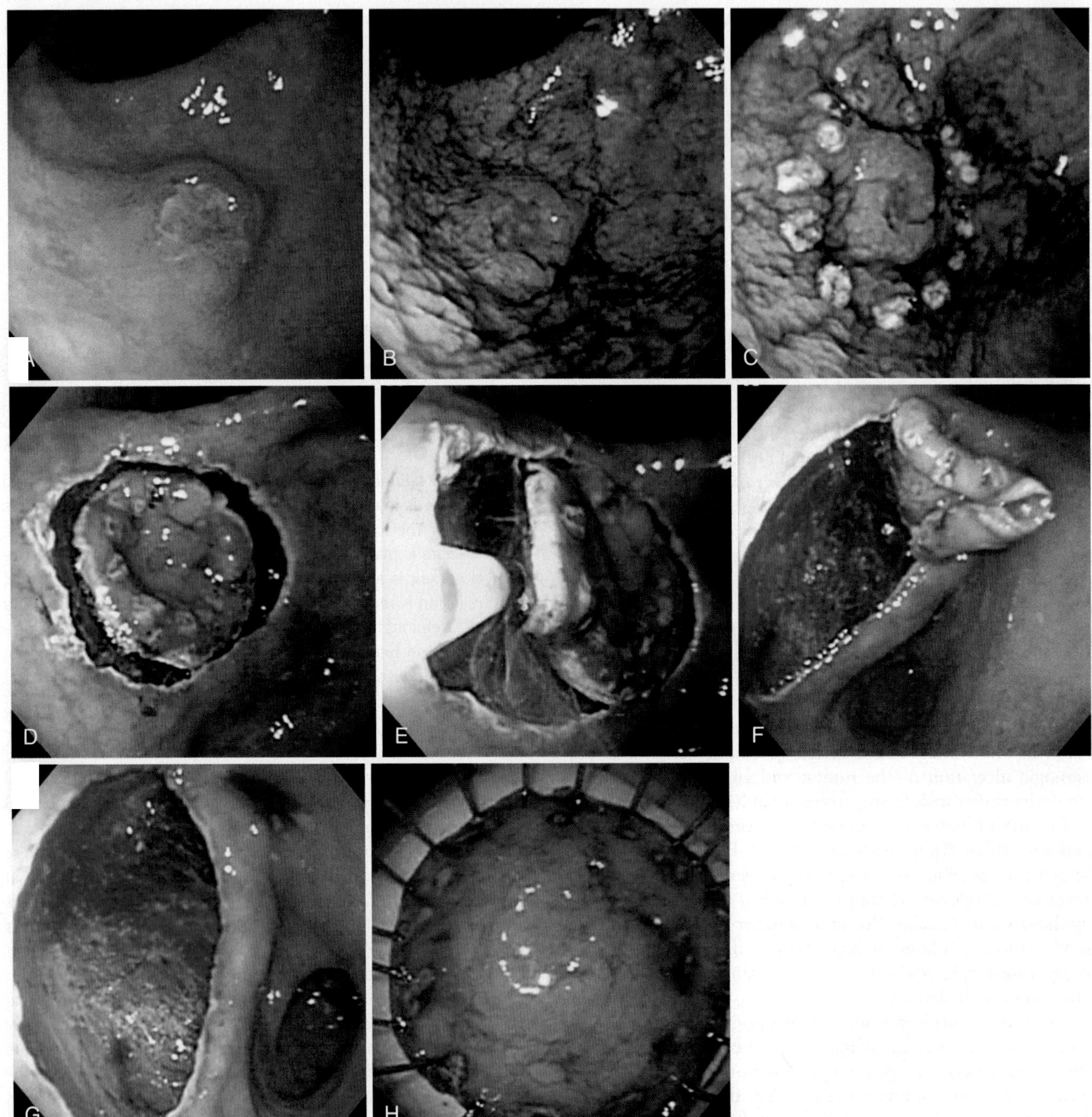


**FIGURE 49-25** Procedure of endoscopic submucosal dissection (ESD). **A,** A type IIa+IIc early gastric cancer was located at the lesser curvature side of the antrum. **B,** Indigo carmine dye was sprayed around the lesion to define the margin accurately. **C,** Marking dots were made circumferentially at approximately 5 mm lateral to the margin of the lesion. **D,** After a submucosal injection of saline with epinephrine mixed with indigocarmine, a circumferential mucosal incision was performed outside the marking dots to separate the lesion from the surrounding non-neoplastic mucosa. **E** and **F,** After an additional submucosal injection, the submucosal connective tissue just beneath the lesion was directly dissected using an electrosurgical knife instead of using a snare. **G,** The lesion was completely resected and the consequent artificial ulcer was seen. **H,** The resected specimen with a central early gastric cancer. (From Min B-H, Lee JH, Kim JJ et al: Clinical outcomes of endoscopic submucosal dissection (ESD) for treating early gastric cancer: Comparison with endoscopic mucosal resection after circumferential precutting (EMR-P). Digestive and liver disease. St Louis, 2009, Elsevier, pp 201–209.)

### Clinical Decision Making

Endoscopic therapy for gastric cancer is well established in Eastern countries. Endoscopic resection is a safe and effective technique for patients who meet the criteria and will continue to play an increasing role in the treatment of this disease. Although several larger studies of patients who underwent gastrectomy with lymphadenectomy have suggested that the eligibility could be safely expanded, two smaller studies of patients who underwent endoscopic resection under these criteria have shown a higher rate of lymph node disease. Given that all these patients had early gastric cancer, and were therefore potentially curable with gastrectomy and lymphadenectomy, undertreatment in this group is especially concerning. As a matter of standard practice, patients with tumors larger than 2 cm, with ulceration or with any submucosal invasion, should be referred for gastrectomy with lymph node dissection if not part of a clinical trial.

**Lymph Node Dissection** The extent of lymphadenectomy for gastric adenocarcinoma remains an area of ongoing debate. Historically, lymphadenectomy for gastric adenocarcinoma was defined by, and is still often discussed in terms of, the location of the nodes relative to the primary tumor. The extent of dissection ranges from the more local D1 lymphadenectomy involving only perigastric nodes to clearance of the celiac axis, with or without splenectomy, in an extended D2 dissection to complete clearance of the celiac axis and periaortic nodes in a superextended D3 lymphadenectomy.

Several randomized trials have compared the outcomes of patients undergoing D1 versus D2 dissection, unfortunately with conflicting results. Whether this is a result of different biology or of surgical technique is a matter of debate. The non-Japanese literature has historically shown that D2 lymphadenectomy, when compared with a D1 dissection, has increased surgical morbidity, without a benefit in survival.[31,32] In contrast, the Japanese have shown increased survival in patients undergoing a D2 dissection, with no increased or minimal increase in morbidity. One criticism of the Western data is that although randomized, the D2 group did not differentiate between patients who had a splenectomy and those who did not. Subsequent subgroup analysis of the D2 without splenectomy group has shown results similar to the Japanese studies, with increased survival and no significant increase in morbidity.

In 1997, the AJCC changed the TNM staging system so that N staging was defined not by the location of the nodes, but rather by the number of nodes. Along with this change was the recommendation that at least 15 lymph nodes be removed for adequate staging purposes. Several studies have examined the impact of this change with respect to prognosis and outcomes. In multivariate analyses, only the number of nodes, not the location, was a significant predictor of mortality. When the number of nodes was used for staging, there was more consistency in survival rates, providing higher quality prognostic information for patients within a given stage (Table 49-7).

The improvement in survival rates may be caused by stage migration. Patients who were previously understaged are now classified as having node-positive disease status, thus improving the prognosis of both groups. Regardless, better stage homogeneity and reducing understaging are critical to clinical decisions on prognosis and potential treatments.

Fifteen nodes has become a marker for adequate lymphadenectomy. The number of nodes removed is related to hospital volume and whether the hospital is a National Comprehensive Cancer Network–National Cancer Institute (NCCN-NCI) institution (Table 49-8).[33] However, even at high-volume and NCCN-NCI centers, the percentage of patients who have more than 15 lymph nodes examined is less than 50%. Overall, only 23.8% of the more than 3000 patients studied had more than 15 lymph nodes examined. There is clearly room for improvement, regardless of the type of institution.

How does one achieve an adequate 15–lymph node resection? Some argue that the studies cited indicate evidence that a formal D2 resection should be the standard. This is also a systems issue in a given institution that depends not only on the surgeon but also on the pathology department. For the practicing surgeon, the focus should be on achieving a wide enough lymph node dissection to stage the patient adequately. Given the predominance of D1 resection in the United States, and the overall failure to remove 15 lymph nodes consistently for analysis, simply clearing perigastric tissue is likely inadequate. There should be some attention to removing some fibrofatty tissue along named vessels. In a high-volume specialty center that can routinely perform a D2 resection without increased morbidity, wider resections are likely to be the more standard practice.

**Table 49-7 Median Survival According to Location of Positive Nodes (PN) Versus Number of PN**

| | Median Survival (mo) | | |
|---|---|---|---|
| SIZE | 1-6 PN | 7-15 PN | >15 PN |
| <3 cm (*n* = 402) | 38.8 (*n* = 311) | 20.8 (*n* = 82) | 9.5 (*n* = 9) |
| >3 cm (*n* = 233) | 35.5 (*n* = 81) | 19.7 (*n* = 96) | 12.5 (*n* = 56) |

Adapted from Karpeh MS, Leon L, Klimstra D, et al: Lymph node staging in gastric cancer: Is location more important than number? An analysis of 1038 patients. Ann Surg 232: 362–371, 2000.

**Table 49-8 Lymph Node Resection Rates in Gastric Cancer***

| VARIABLE | LYMPH NODES EXAMINED, MEDIAN NO. (INTERQUARTILE RANGE) | PATIENTS WITH AT LEAST 15 LYMPH NODES EXAMINED (%) |
|---|---|---|
| All hospitals | 7 (3-14) | 23.2 |
| Hospital type | | |
| NCCN-NCI | 12 (6-20) | 42.3 |
| Other academic | 8 (4-15) | 25.5 |
| Community | 6 (3-12) | 17.7 |
| Hospital volume | | |
| Highest | 10 (5-18) | 34.7 |
| High | 8 (4-14) | 22.2 |
| Moderate | 6 (2-13) | 17.8 |
| Low | 6 (3-12) | 16.8 |

From Bilimoria KY, Talamonti MS, Wayne JD, et al: Effect of hospital type and volume on lymph node evaluation for gastric and pancreatic cancer. Arch Surg 143:671–678, 2008.

*Stratified by hospital type and volume.

### Adjuvant and Neoadjuvant Therapy

Gastric cancer remains a biologically aggressive cancer, with high recurrence and mortality rates. A review of over 2000 patients who underwent R0 resection demonstrated recurrence rates of almost 30%, with most patients recurring within the first 2 years (mean, 21.8 months).[34] For patients with recurrence, the prognosis was almost uniformly fatal, with a mortality rate of 94% and a mean survival time after recurrence of only 8.7 months. Other large series have shown similar results.

Underlying these poor outcomes is the fact that the initial chemotherapy regimens for gastric cancer provide little benefit. Numerous primary studies and meta-analyses have shown inconclusive results. Overall, the survival for patients receiving adjuvant therapy was no better than surgery alone.

The Southwest Oncology Group (9008/INT-0116), however, has reported a randomized controlled trial of 556 patients who had undergone curative gastrectomy alone or gastrectomy combined with adjuvant 5-fluorouracil and radiotherapy.[35] This study demonstrated a significant benefit for adjuvant therapy for overall survival (41% versus 50%) and recurrence-free survival (41% versus 64%). As a result, adjuvant chemoradiation has become the standard of care for patients undergoing curative gastrectomy in the United States. Several authors have criticized these results, noting a high rate of inadequate lymphadenectomy (54% of patients underwent a D0 resection). Given these findings, it is possible that some of the benefit from radiation was clearance of residual disease in the perigastric nodal basin. Furthermore, only 64% of patients randomized to the treatment arm were able to complete therapy; 17% had to stop treatment because of toxic effects and 5% progressed while on treatment.

Given the relatively high rate of failure to complete treatment, there has been increased focus on combined perioperative treatment for gastric cancer, rather than postoperative adjuvant therapy. The most significant results are those of the MAGIC trial, a randomized controlled study of 503 patients with stage II or higher gastric cancer that compared perioperative chemotherapy with surgery alone.[36] The treatment group received three 3-week cycles of epirubicin, cisplatin, and a continuous infusion of 5-fluorouracil preoperatively and three additional cycles postoperatively. More than 90% of patients who started the preoperative chemotherapy were able to complete it; however, only 65% of these patients went on to receive postoperative chemotherapy and only 50% successfully completed both.

The treatment group had significantly better pathologic results and long-term outcomes. The chemotherapy group had a higher percentage of T1 and T2 tumors in the final specimens, along with a higher proportion of limited (N0 and N1) nodal disease when compared with the surgery arm alone. The rates of local recurrence, distant metastases, and 5-year overall survival were significantly improved in the chemotherapy group compared with the surgery-only group (14.4% versus 20.6%, 24.4% versus 36.8%, and 36.3% versus 23%, respectively).

Similar to the Southwest Oncology Group (9008/INT-0116; SWOG Inter 0116) study, MAGIC has been criticized for inadequate staging (no laparoscopy) and inadequacy of lymph node dissection. However, unlike the SWOG trial, in which over 50% of patients had a D0 resection, in the MAGIC trial most patients had a D2 resection, with 15% undergoing a D1 resection. Given the ongoing debate over D1 versus D2, and the shifting focus toward lymph node count rather than anatomic location, the lymphadenectomy in the MAGIC trial is generalizable to the entire population of patients with gastric cancer who undergo curative gastrectomy. Further strengthening the case for perioperative chemotherapy are the results of the French trial, FFCD 9703, which also studied combined neoadjuvant and adjuvant therapy. Here, the regimen was three preoperative cycles and three postoperative cycles of 5-fluorouracil and cisplatin, with a similar survival benefit for those who received chemotherapy (5-year survival 38% versus 24%).

One limitation of both studies is the lack of stratification. Although only patients with clinically resectable advanced gastric cancer were included (penetration through the submucosa), they were not further stratified according to stage or other prognostic factors. Other investigators have shown that factors such as serosal involvement or nodal positivity are independent, negative prognostic factors. Further studies examining which groups show the most benefit from these potentially toxic regimens will be essential. However, given the results of the MAGIC trial and FFCD 9703, patients with gastric cancer should be evaluated for preoperative systemic therapy.

### Palliative Therapy and Systemic Therapy

Patients with unresectable or metastatic gastric cancer represent almost 50% of patients with the disease and have only a 3- to 5-month median survival with the best supportive therapy. Palliative therapy for gastric cancer involves attempts to improve survival and palliation of the symptoms of advanced disease. Many patients with advanced disease are asymptomatic and palliation is focused on improvement in median survival. A significant subset of patients with unresectable gastric cancer, however, have debilitating symptoms and should be considered for surgical therapy, even in the setting of metastatic disease.

Chemotherapy does improve survival in patients with unresectable tumor. A 2006 meta-analysis has shown that triple therapy with 5-fluorouracil, cisplatin, and an anthracycline-based compound, generally epirubicin, was superior to single or double therapy (hazard ratio [HR], 0.77 and 0.83 for triple therapy versus without epirubicin and without cisplatin, respectively).[37] Adverse reactions are common, with up to 50% of patients having severe neutropenia or GI complaints.

Although clearly better than supportive care alone, results of systemic therapy treatments remain relatively poor. Investigators continue to evaluate new treatment regimens with less toxicity. Thus, there has been increased interest in directed therapies that specifically target cancer cells at the molecular level. These include the epidermal growth factor receptor (EGFR) inhibitor cetuximab and the human EGFR2 (HER2) antagonist trastuzumab (Herceptin), which is approved for HER2-positive breast cancer. HER2 positivity has been reported in 6% to 35% of gastric cancers. Results of a phase III trial were first presented in 2009, evaluating 3807 gastric cancer patients, of whom 22% were HER2-positive.[38] These 554 patients were randomized to receive capecitabine or 5-fluorouracil (5-FU) with cisplatin and herceptin or cisplatin alone. The herceptin group had a better median survival (13.5 versus 11.1 months) and overall response rate (47.3% versus 34.5%). Adverse events were not significantly different. These results again show a small but significant benefit, with no increase in adverse events.

Cetuximab has been evaluated as monotherapy and in phase II trials as part of combination therapy with FOLFIRI (5-FU, levofolinic acid, and irinotecan; FOLCETUX study) or doxatel and cisplatin (DOCETUX study).[39] In these limited efficacy trials, there was an increased overall response rate but no increase in overall survival. Phase III trials will be required to determine the role of cetuximab in gastric cancer more accurately.

### Complicated Gastric Cancer

Advanced gastric cancer represents a difficult challenge for the surgeon. Advanced disease is characterized by severe symptoms such as pain, obstruction, and/or bleeding. Determining the optimal treatment strategy for each patient can be complex and requires input and involvement of a multidisciplinary oncology team. The general approach for these problems is discussed here.

**Locally Advanced Gastric Cancer** Patients with advanced disease that is deemed unresectable because of adjacent organ involvement, generally the pancreas or spleen, or extensive nodal disease, including the para-aortic nodes, are particularly challenging. Data from two randomized controlled trials, the Dutch and British trials comparing D1 and D2 lymphadenectomy, including pancreaticosplenectomy as part of their D2 resection, have indicated that this multiorgan resection significantly increases morbidity and perioperative mortality.[31,32] As a result, multiorgan resection has generally been abandoned in patients with gastric cancer. However, in both these studies, multiorgan resection was performed regardless of tumor (T) status. In the British study, no patients had pathologically confirmed T4 disease, suggesting that most if not all the patients who had a multiorgan resection would have achieved an R0 resection, even without pancreaticosplenectomy. This is in contrast to the data from several retrospective studies, including a review of 1133 patients who underwent R0 resection at the Memorial Sloan Kettering Cancer Center. In that study, only male gender, depth of invasion, and nodal status were predictors of poor outcome on multivariate analysis.[40] Of the 268 patients who underwent an R0 multiorgan resection, the 5-year overall survival was 32%, with a median survival of 32 months.

Underlying all these studies, and the objective of performing multiorgan resection in general, is the desire to achieve an R0 resection. Patients with proven T4 disease who achieve an R0 resection have a clinically and statistically significant survival benefit over those undergoing only palliative resection, with the palliative resection group having survival rates similar to those for chemotherapy alone.

In an effort to increase the number of patients for whom an R0 resection can be achieved, several investigators have explored the role of neoadjuvant therapy in otherwise unresectable disease. A 2009 phase II trial by Sym and colleagues[41] treated 49 patients with clinically unresectable gastric cancer with cisplatin, docetaxel, and capecitabine and found an overall R0 resection rate of 63% compared with historical rates of 30% to 60%. Importantly, these patients were prospectively stratified according to which criteria made them unresectable—adjacent organ involvement, bulky para-aortic nodal disease, or limited peritoneal disease. For patients without peritoneal disease, the R0 resection rate was higher than 70%. Of all patients who achieved R0 resection, patients with adjacent organ involvement only had significantly better outcomes. At a median follow-up of 51 months, median progression-free and overall survival have yet to be reached, with a predicted 5-year overall survival of 54%. This small phase II trial demonstrated promising results, especially for patients with T4 disease, although these outcomes will need to be further validated in phase III studies.

All these data suggest that multiorgan resection is of benefit in properly selected patients. The difficulty is how to select these patients properly. The number of patients with clinical T4 disease who have true T4 disease on final pathology ranges from 14% to 38.5%, with CT having only a 50% positive predictive value for true T4 disease. As preoperative staging modalities improve in accuracy, so will the ability to select patients properly for various treatment modalities, including multiorgan resection. In the meantime, for those patients in whom an R0 resection can be performed, aggressive surgical therapy appears warranted. However, in patients who at the time of laparoscopy or laparotomy have clearly unresectable disease, and with no symptoms that would warrant resection, palliative resection should be avoided.

## Complications

Patients with unresectable disease can develop complications such as bleeding, perforation, and obstruction. Treatment should be focused on maximum palliation and minimal morbidity. For patients with bleeding, endoscopic measures (e.g., cautery, clipping, injection) should be considered first-line therapy and, similar to any acute GI hemorrhage, multiple attempts are reasonable in the hemodynamically stable patient. If endoscopy is unsuccessful, angiography with coil embolization is a reasonable but generally unsuccessful option. If the patient is unstable and other methods are unsuccessful, surgical intervention is warranted. The resection should be tailored to the clinical situation. For patients with a short expected survival, limited resection to grossly negative margins is indicated. Patients with more localized disease can be treated with more aggressive gastric resection.

For patients with a gastric outlet obstruction, several options are available. Endoscopic dilation and stent placement can provide good short-term palliation; however, tumor progression and stent migration limit the long-term efficacy. Chemoradiotherapy has shown overall response rates of up to 50% and may alleviate outlet obstruction. For patients predicted to have a longer survival (e.g., those without distant metastases or high-volume peritoneal disease), bypass with a gastrojejunostomy or palliative gastrectomy is a reasonable approach.

Perforation of gastric cancer requires surgical intervention. Primary closure of perforated, frequently necrotic, tumor is not generally possible. Given the relatively poor functional status and prognosis for many of these patients, closure with healthy omentum is a reasonable approach. If it can be done without excess morbidity, such as multiorgan resection, gastrectomy can also be performed.

Linitis plastica is a particularly aggressive form of the disease. These patients frequently have increased pain, obstruction, and poor gastric function. Symptom control and palliative chemoradiotherapy should be considered as the primary treatment. For patients with intractable symptoms not responding to other measures, a total gastrectomy can be performed.

## Outcomes

The overall mortality rate for gastric cancer is 3.7 deaths/100,000 people, a decline of 35% since 1992.[42] This incidence has been declining since 1930, is likely because of changes in diet, such as decreased sodium intake, changes in food storage and

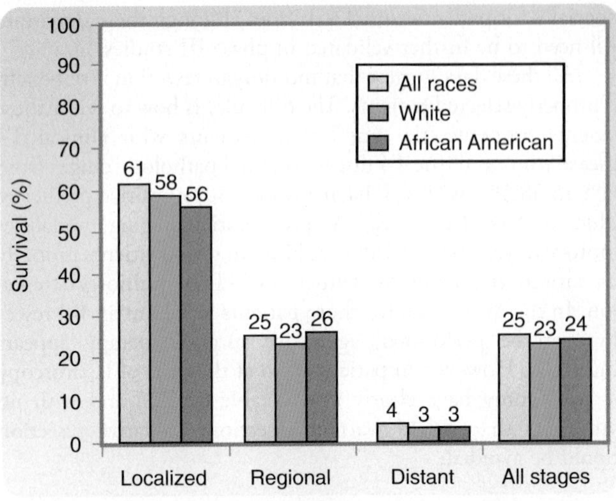


**FIGURE 49-26** Five-year relative survival rates in patients diagnosed with selected cancers by race and stage at diagnosis, United States, 1996-2004. (From Jemal A, Siegel R, Ward E, et al: Cancer statistics. CA Cancer J Clin 59:225–249, 2009.)

preparation, and decreased smoking. Nonetheless, the overall 5-year survival remains less than 25%. Many of these patients present at an advanced stage. For patients who undergo a potentially curative resection, overall 5-year survival rates range from of 24% to 57% and, for the subset with early gastric cancer, cure rates are higher than 80%. For patients who present with distant disease, long-term survival is only 4% (Fig. 49-26).[16] Unfortunately, over 63% of patients present with locally advanced or distant disease.

### Recurrence

Recurrence rates after gastrectomy remain high, from 40% to 80%, depending on the series. Most recurrences occur within the first 3 years. The locoregional failure rate ranges from 38% to 45%, whereas peritoneal dissemination as a component of failure occurs in 54% of patients in several series. Isolated distant metastases are uncommon because most patients with distant failure also have locoregional recurrence. The most common sites of locoregional recurrence are the gastric remnant at the anastomosis, in the gastric bed, and in the regional nodes. Hematogenous spread occurs to the liver, lung, and bone.

**Surveillance** Although all patients should be followed systematically, the evidence for how this should occur is not clear. Because most recurrences occur within the first 3 years, surveillance examinations are more frequent in the first several years. Follow-up should include a complete history and physical examination every 4 months for 1 year, then every 6 months for 2 years, and then annually thereafter. Laboratory tests, including complete blood counts and liver function tests, should be performed as clinically indicated. Many clinicians obtain chest x-rays and CT scans of the abdomen and pelvis routinely, whereas others obtain studies only when clinically suspicious of a recurrence. Annual endoscopy should be considered for patients who have undergone a subtotal gastrectomy.

## Gastric Lymphoma

### Epidemiology

The stomach is the most common site of lymphomas in the GI system. However, primary gastric lymphoma is still relatively uncommon, accounting for less than 15% of gastric malignancies and 2% of lymphomas. Patients often present with vague symptoms, such as epigastric pain, early satiety, and fatigue. Constitutional B symptoms are rare. Although overt bleeding is uncommon, more than 50% of patients present with anemia. Lymphomas occur in older patients, with the peak incidence in the sixth and seventh decades, and are more common in men (male-to-female ratio of 2 : 1). Gastric lymphomas, like carcinomas, usually occur in the gastric antrum but can arise from any part of the stomach. Patients are considered to have gastric lymphoma if the stomach is the exclusive or predominant site of disease.

### Pathology

In the management of gastric lymphomas, as in the management of nodal lymphomas, it is important to determine not only the stage of disease but also the subtype of lymphoma. There are a number of classification systems for lymphomas (Table 49-9). The most common gastric lymphoma is diffuse large B cell lymphoma (55%), followed by gastric MALT lymphoma (40%), Burkitt's lymphoma (3%), and mantle cell and follicular lymphomas (each <1%).

Diffuse, large B cell lymphomas are generally primary lesions; however, they may also occur from progression of less aggressive lymphomas, such as chronic lymphocytic leukemia–small lymphocytic lymphoma (CLL-SLL), follicular lymphoma, and MALT lymphoma. Immunodeficiencies and *H. pylori* infection are risk factors for the development of primary diffuse, large B cell lymphoma.

Burkitt's lymphomas of the stomach are associated with Epstein-Barr virus infections, as they are in other sites. Burkitt's lymphoma is very aggressive and tends to affect a younger population than other types of gastric lymphomas. Burkitt's lymphoma is usually found in the cardia or body of the stomach as opposed to the antrum.

### Evaluation

Endoscopy generally reveals nonspecific gastritis or gastric ulcerations. Occasionally, a submucosal growth pattern will render endoscopic biopsies nondiagnostic. Endoscopic ultrasound is useful to determine the depth of gastric wall invasion, specifically to identify patients at risk for perforation secondary to full-thickness involvement of the gastric wall. Evidence of distant disease should be sought through upper airway examination, bone marrow biopsy, and CT of the chest and abdomen to detect lymphadenopathy. Any enlarged lymph nodes should undergo biopsy. Histologic *H. pylori* testing should be performed and, if negative, confirmed by serology.

### Staging

The best staging system remains controversial. When possible, the TNM staging system should be used (using the criteria proposed for gastric carcinoma). Several other staging systems for primary gastric non-Hodgkin's lymphoma are available (Table 49-10).

**Table 49-9 Comparison of Gastrointestinal Lymphoma Classifications**

| WHO CLASSIFICATION | REAL | WORKING | LUKES-COLLINS | KLEL | RAPPAPORT |
|---|---|---|---|---|---|
| Extranodal marginal zone lymphoma (MALT lymphoma) | – | Small cleaved cell type | Small cleaved cell type | Immunocytoma | Well-differentiated lymphocytic |
| Follicular lymphoma | Follicular center lymphoma | Small cleaved cell type | Small cleaved cell type | Centroblastic-centrocytic, follicular and diffuse | Nodular, poorly differentiated lymphocytic |
| Mantle cell lymphoma | – | – | – | Centrocytic | Intermediately or poorly differentiated lymphocytic, diffuse or nodular |
| Diffuse, large, B cell lymphoma | Diffuse large B cell lymphoma | Large cleaved follicular center cell | Large cleaved follicular center cell | Centroblastic, B-immunoblastic | Diffuse mixed lymphocytic and histiocytic |
| Burkitt's lymphoma | Burkitt's lymphoma | Small noncleaved follicular center cell | Small noncleaved follicular center cell | Burkitt's lymphoma with intracytoplasmic immunoglobulin | Undifferentiated lymphoma, Burkitt's type |

**Table 49-10 Staging Systems for Primary Gastrointestinal Non-Hodgkin's Lymphoma**

| Stage | | | | |
|---|---|---|---|---|
| ANN ARBOR* | RAO ET AL† | MUSSHOFF‡ | DESCRIPTION | RELATIVE INCIDENCE (%) |
| IE | IE | IE | Tumor confined to GI tract | 26 |
| IIE | IIE | IIE | Tumor with spread to regional lymph nodes | 26 |
| IIE | IIIE | IIE | Tumor with nodal involvement beyond regional lymph nodes (para-aortic, iliac) | 17 |
| IIIE–IV | IVE | IIIE–IV | Tumor with spread to other intra-abdominal organs (liver, spleen) or beyond abdomen (chest, bone marrow) | 31 |

*Carbone PP, Kaplan HS, Musshoff K, et al: Report of the Committee on Hodgkin's Disease Staging Classification. Cancer Res 31:1860–1861, 1971.

†Rao AR, Kagan AR, Kagan AR, et al: Management of gastrointestinal lymphoma. Am J Clin Oncol 7:213–219, 1984.

‡Musshoff K: [Clinical staging classification of non-Hodgkin's lymphomas (author's trans, German)]. Strahlentherapie 153:218–221, 1977.

### Treatment

Most centers use a multimodality treatment program for patients with gastric lymphoma. The role of resection in gastric lymphoma remains controversial, and most patients are now treated with chemotherapy alone. The risk for perforation in patients treated with chemotherapy has been overstated in the past and is now approximately 5%. The most common chemotherapeutic combination is CHOP (cyclophosphamide, doxorubicin, vincristine, and prednisone). A prospective randomized study has evaluated several treatment strategies—surgical resection, resection plus radiation, resection plus chemotherapy, chemotherapy alone—in patients with early-stage (stage IE or IIE) disease.[43] The addition of chemotherapy was essential, with the surgery plus chemotherapy and chemotherapy-alone groups having significantly higher overall survival than the surgery-alone and surgery plus radiation groups. The addition of surgery to radiation therapy or chemotherapy did not improve outcomes. The primary role of surgery is for patients with limited gastric disease, patients with symptomatic recurrence of treatment failure, and those who develop complications, such as bleeding, gastric outlet obstruction, or perforation.

The diagnosis of lymphoma discovered unexpectedly at surgery can be confirmed by frozen section. Also, fresh tissue should be sent for fluorescence-activated cell sorting, immunohistochemistry, and genetic analysis. Consideration should be given to bone marrow aspiration at the time of surgery. If isolated stage IE or IIE lymphoma is encountered, surgical removal of all gross disease is ideal. Patients with disseminated lymphoma cannot be cured surgically, and the operation should focus on obtaining enough tissue for diagnosis and the repair of perforations.

## Mucosa-Associated Lymphoid Tissue Lymphomas

Numerous mucosal surfaces throughout the body have associated lymphoid tissue, including the lungs, small bowel, and stomach. In 1983, Isaacson and Wright noted that the histology of primary low-grade gastric B-cell lymphoma resembled that of mucosa-associated lymphoid tissue (MALT). From that initial finding, it has been determined that in the setting of prolonged inflammation, these rests of lymphoid tissue can progress to low-grade lymphomas. The MALT lymphoma concept has been extended beyond the stomach to include other extranodal low-grade B cell lymphomas of the salivary gland, lung, and thyroid. These organs lack native lymphoid tissue; thus, the lymphomas at these sites arise from MALT acquired as a result of chronic inflammation.

Gastric MALT lymphoma is usually preceded by *H. pylori*–associated gastritis. Evidence of *H. pylori* infection can be found in almost every case of gastric MALT lymphoma. Epidemiologic studies have also linked *H. pylori* infection with gastric lymphomas. Genetically, MALT lymphoma is characterized by the translocations t(1;14)(p22;q32) and t(11;18)(q21;q21), both of which result in impaired responsiveness to apoptotic signaling and increased nuclear factor-κB (NF-κB) activity. It has been suggested that the t(11;18)(q21;q21) and *BCL-10* nuclear expression may predict for nonresponsiveness to treatment by *H. pylori* eradication and lymphoma regression.

### Treatment

Given the strong association with *H. pylori* and the low-grade MALT lymphoma, there was interest in treating MALT lymphoma without chemotherapy. It has been suggested that early-stage MALT lymphomas and some cases of limited, diffuse, large B cell lymphoma may be effectively treated by *H. pylori* eradication alone. Successful eradication resulted in remission in more than 75% of cases. However, careful follow-up is necessary, with repeat endoscopy in 2 months to document clearance of the infection and biannual endoscopy for 3 years to document regression. Some patients continued to demonstrate the lymphoma clone after *H. pylori* eradication, suggesting that the lymphoma became dormant rather than disappearing.

The presence of transmural tumor extension, nodal involvement, transformation into a large cell phenotype, t(11;18), or nuclear *BCL-10* expression all predict failure after *H. pylori* eradication alone. Additionally, a small subset of MALT lymphoma patients is *H. pylori*–negative. In these patients, consideration should be given to surgical resection, radiation, and chemotherapy. The 5-year disease-free survival rate with multimodality treatment is higher than 95% in stage IE and 75% in stage IIE disease.

## Gastrointestinal Stromal Tumors

Gastrointestinal stromal tumors (GISTs) are the most common sarcomatous tumors of the GI tract. Originally thought to be a type of smooth muscle sarcoma, they are now known to be a distinct tumor derived from the interstitial cells of Cajal, an intestinal pacemaker cell. They can appear anywhere within the GI tract, although are usually found in the stomach (40% to 60%), small intestine (30%), and colon (15%). GISTs vary considerably in their presentation and clinical course, ranging from small benign tumors to massive lesions with necrosis, hemorrhage, and wide metastases. Their pathology, presentation, and management, as they relate to the stomach, are discussed here.

Gastric GISTs can present at any age, although most typically present in patients older than 50 years. They generally have an equal male-to-female ratio or a slight male predominance. They are rarely associated with familial syndromes such as GIST-paraganglioma syndrome (Carney triad), neurofibromatosis type I, and von Hippel-Lindau disease, but the overwhelming majority develop de novo. Most present symptomatically, typically with bleeding or vague abdominal pain or discomfort. Bleeding is generally in the form of melena or, less frequently, frank hematemesis. Tumor rupture with intra-abdominal hemorrhage is uncommon but, when it occurs, frequently requires emergent surgical intervention. Many patients remain asymptomatic and their tumors are discovered incidentally at the time of other surgery or, increasingly, during imaging performed for other indications.

**BOX 49-4 Suggested Guidelines for Assessing Malignant Potential of Gastric GISTs of Different Sizes and Mitotic Activity**

- Benign (no tumor-related mortality)
  No larger than 2 cm, no more than 5 mitoses/50 HPF
- Probably benign (<3% with progressive disease)
  >2 cm but ≤5 cm; no more than 5 mitoses/50 HPF
- Uncertain or low malignant potential
  No larger than 2 cm; >5 mitoses/50 HPF
- Low to moderate malignant potential (12%-15% tumor-related mortality)
  >10 cm; no more than 5 mitoses/HPF
  >2 cm but ≤5 cm; >5 mitoses/50 HPF
- High malignant potential (49%-86% tumor-related mortality)
  >5 cm but ≤10 cm; >5 mitoses/50 HPF
  >10 cm; >5 mitoses/50 HPF

From Miettinen M, Sobin L, Lasota J: Gastrointestinal stromal tumors of the stomach: A clinicopathologic, immunohistochemical, and molecular genetic study of 1765 cases with long-term follow-up. Am J Surg Pathol 29: 52–58, 2005.

Pathologically, GISTs have smooth muscle and neuroendocrine features, consistent with their origin from the interstitial cells of Cajal. They are now frequently identified by immunohistochemical staining for the *c-kit* proto-oncogene (CD117), found in more than 90% of these tumors, and for CD34, present in 80% of GISTs.[44] The mainstay of treatment is complete surgical resection. Depending on tumor size, this can include wide local excision, enucleation, sleeve gastrectomy, or total gastrectomy, with or without en bloc resection of adjacent organs.

Recurrence rates are approximately 40%, and most patients who recur demonstrate metastasis to the liver, with one third having only isolated local recurrence. Recurrence can occur as late as 20 years and long-term follow-up is warranted. Long-term disease-free survival is approximately 50%, with from 20% to 80% of patients dying of their disease.[45] Although there are no standard criteria that define benign versus malignant lesions, the most important risk factors for malignancy are tumor size larger than 10 cm and more than five mitoses/50 HPF. Based on a long-term follow-up study of 1700 patients with gastric GISTs, guidelines for assessing malignant potential based on the combination of these two factors have been developed (Box 49-4).[44]

### Adjuvant Therapy

Given the relatively high recurrence rates with increased disease-specific mortality for patients with larger lesions and increased mitotic rate, surgery alone for these patients appears inadequate. Adjuvant therapy, however, was not effective until the discovery of the tyrosine kinase inhibitor imatinib (Gleevec). Originally designed to treat chronic myelogenous leukemia, it has proven, in randomized controlled trials, to be an effective treatment modality for patients with metastatic disease or disease that carries a high risk for recurrence. In

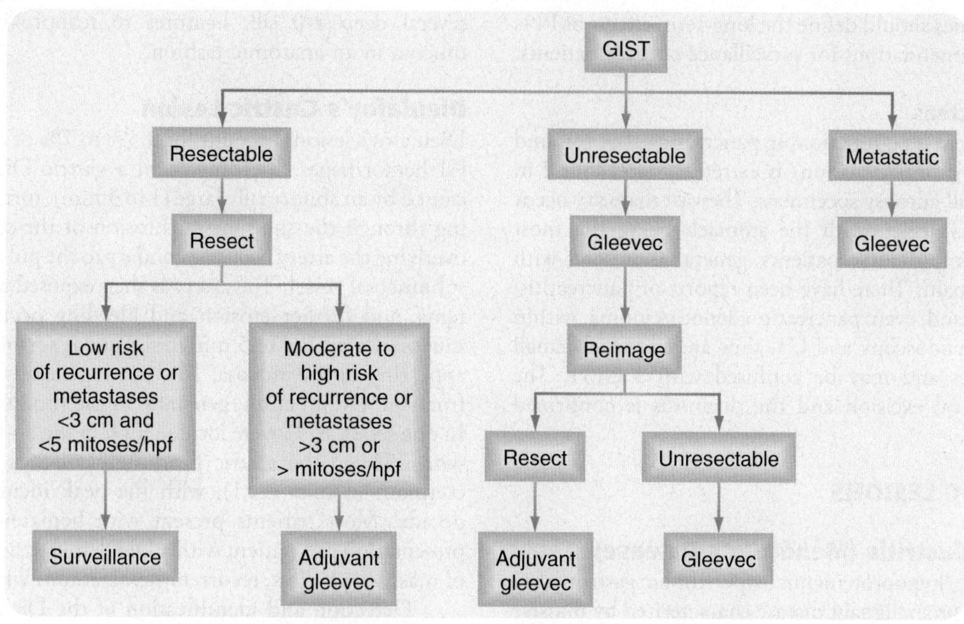


**FIGURE 49-27** Algorithm for the workup and treatment of GISTs.

patients with metastatic or unresectable disease, imatinib (400 mg daily) showed an overall 2-year survival of 70% compared with 25% for those on traditional chemotherapy.[46] In the adjuvant setting, patients with c-*kit* positive tumors 3 cm or larger who were completely resected and treated with imatinib for 1 year had a recurrence rate of 8% compared with 20% for untreated patients.[47] This was even more pronounced for patients with larger tumors. The side effects were generally mild, with less than 1% of patients having any grade 3 or 4 toxicities. Imatinib has also been reported to be successful in the neoadjuvant treatment of patients with nonmetastatic but unresectable disease, although this has not been evaluated in prospective randomized trials. Future trials will need to address whether longer treatment periods have better outcomes and further elucidate imatinib's role in the neoadjuvant setting. However, as a result of current trials, for patients with metastatic disease and those with resected primary disease at moderate risk of recurrence, indefinite treatment with imatinib has been approved by the U.S. Food and Drug Administration (FDA). Figure 49-27 presents an algorithm for using imatinib in the treatment of GISTs in the neoadjuvant, adjuvant, and palliative settings.

## Other Neoplasms

### Gastric Carcinoid

Overall, carcinoid tumors are a rare malignancy (0.49% of all malignancies) that arise from neuroendocrine precursor cells and can present at any site in the body. The most common location is the GI tract, encompassing almost 68% of all carcinoids. The most common sites in the GI tract are the small intestine, rectum, and appendix.

The stomach has historically been a rare site of GI carcinoid; however, a marked increase has been noted over the past several decades. Currently, it is the location of almost 8% of GI carcinoids, compared with 2% in 1950. They are also increasing as a percentage of all gastric tumors, increasing from 0.3% to 1.77% over the past 50 years.[48] There are three types, two of which are associated with low acid and increased gastrin secretion and derive from gastric ECL cells. Type I, the most common, is associated with chronic atrophic gastritis and has a benign prognosis. These tumors are generally small and have a overall 5-year survival of more than 95%. Type II is associated with ZES and multiple endocrine neoplasia type I. The prognosis is still good, with long-term survival from 70% to 90% and slightly higher levels of metastases. Type III tumors are sporadic lesions with few ECL cells. They have a more than 50% rate of metastatic spread and a 5-year survival of less than 35%. The combined 5-year overall survival for all localized gastric carcinoids is 63%.

The treatment for localized carcinoids is complete removal. For small pedunculated lesions, this can be accomplished endoscopically. Larger lesions may require wedge resection or partial gastrectomy. Patients with multiple gastric carcinoids may require total gastrectomy. For patients with recurrent or metastatic disease, somatostatin analogues can be used to decrease the burden of disease and treat carcinoid syndrome.

The incidence of gastric and small bowel carcinoid tumors has increased eightfold over the past 5 to 10 years. Although more endoscopies for GI complaints account for some of the increase, there also appears to be growth in development of the disease. Given the relationship among hypergastrinemia, low-acid states, and carcinoids, some authors have asked whether the use of PPIs is responsible. The profound gastric acid suppression noted with PPIs has resulted in hypergastrinemia and gastric carcinoid formation in in vivo animal studies. Although a direct causal link has not been shown in humans, database cohort studies have shown PPI use to be an independent risk factor for stomach and small bowel carcinoid development.[63] The clinical significance of this is unclear. With respect to small bowel carcinoids associated with PPI use, they tend to have a benign clinical course without any evidence of metastases, invasion of the muscle layer, or high mitotic rate. They can be treated successfully with local endoscopic excision, with a low recurrence rate. Ongoing studies should define the long-term effects of PPIs and provide recommendations for surveillance of these patients.

### Heterotopic Pancreas

Heterotopic pancreas (i.e., functioning pancreatic tissue is found in an abnormal anatomic location) is extremely rare, found in less than 0.2% of all autopsy specimens. The vast majority occur in the proximal GI tract, with the stomach being the most common site. Symptomatic patients generally present with vague abdominal pain. There have been reports of pancreatitis, islet cell tumors, and even pancreatic adenocarcinoma within these lesions. On endoscopy and CT, they are frequently small submucosal masses and may be confused with a GIST. The treatment is surgical excision and the diagnosis is confirmed pathologically.

## OTHER GASTRIC LESIONS

### Hypertrophic Gastritis (Ménétrier's Disease)

Ménétrier's disease (hypoproteinemic hypertrophic gastropathy) is a rare, acquired, premalignant disease characterized by massive gastric folds in the fundus and corpus of the stomach, giving the mucosa a cobblestone or cerebriform appearance. Histologic examination reveals foveolar hyperplasia (expansion of surface mucous cells), with absent parietal cells. The condition is associated with protein loss from the stomach, excessive mucus production, and hypochlorhydria or achlorhydria. The cause of Ménétrier's disease is unknown, but it has been associated with cytomegalovirus infection in children and *H. pylori* infection in adults. Also, increased levels of transforming growth factor-$\alpha$ has been noted in the gastric mucosa of patients with the disease. Patients often present with epigastric pain, vomiting, weight loss, anorexia, and peripheral edema. Typical gastric mucosal changes can be detected by radiographic or endoscopic examination. Biopsy should be performed to rule out gastric carcinoma or lymphoma. A chromium-labeled albumin test reveals increased GI protein loss and 24-hour pH monitoring reveals hypochlorhydria or achlorhydria,. Medical treatment has yielded inconsistent results; however, some benefit has been shown with the use of anticholinergic drugs, acid suppression, octreotide, and *H. pylori* eradication. Total gastrectomy should be performed in patients who continue to have massive protein loss despite optimal medical therapy or if dysplasia or carcinoma develops.

### Mallory-Weiss Tear

Mallory-Weiss tears are related to forceful vomiting, retching, coughing, or straining that results in disruption of the gastric mucosa high on the lesser curve at the GE junction. They account for 15% of acute upper GI hemorrhages and are rarely associated with massive bleeding. The overall mortality rate for the lesion is 3% to 4%, with the greatest risk for massive hemorrhage in alcoholic patients with preexisting portal hypertension. Most patients with active bleeding can be managed by endoscopic methods, such as multipolar electrocoagulation, epinephrine injection, endoscopic band ligation, or endoscopic hemoclipping. Angiographic intra-arterial infusion of vasopressin or transcatheter embolization may be of use in select high-risk cases. The need for operative intervention is rare. If surgery is required, the lesion at the GE junction is approached through an anterior gastrotomy and the bleeding site is oversewn with several deep 2-0 silk ligatures to reapproximate the gastric mucosa in an anatomic fashion.

### Dieulafoy's Gastric Lesion

Dieulafoy's lesions account for 0.3% to 7% of nonvariceal upper GI hemorrhages. Bleeding from a gastric Dieulafoy's lesion is caused by an abnormally large (1 to 3 mm), tortuous artery coursing through the submucosa. Erosion of the superficial mucosa overlying the artery occurs secondary to the pulsations of the large submucosal vessel. The artery is then exposed to the gastric contents, and further erosion and bleeding occur. Generally, the mucosal defect is 2 to 5 mm in size and is surrounded by normal-appearing gastric mucosa. The lesions generally occur 6 to 10 cm from the GE junction, generally in the fundus, near the cardia. In one series, 67% were located high in the body of the stomach, with 25% in the gastric fundus. Dieulafoy's lesions are more common in men (2 : 1), with the peak incidence in the fifth decade. Most patients present with hematemesis. The classic presentation of a patient with a Dieulafoy's lesion is sudden onset of massive, painless, recurrent hematemesis with hypotension.

Detection and identification of the Dieulafoy's lesion can be difficult. The diagnostic modality of choice is esophagogastroduodenoscopy, correctly identifying the lesion in 80% of patients. Because of the intermittent nature of the bleeding, repeated endoscopies may be needed to identify the lesion correctly. If the lesion can be identified endoscopically, attempts should be made to stop the bleeding using endoscopic modalities such as multipolar electrocoagulation, heater probe, noncontact laser photocoagulation, injection sclerotherapy, band ligation, or endoscopic hemoclipping. Angiography can be useful in cases in which endoscopy could not definitely identify the source. Angiographic findings may include a tortuous ectatic artery in the distribution of the left gastric artery, with accompanied contrast extravasation in the setting of acute bleeding. Gelfoam embolization has been reported to control bleeding successfully in patients with Dieulafoy's lesion, although the reported experience is limited.

Surgical therapy was once the only available treatment for Dieulafoy's lesion but is now reserved for patients in whom other modalities have failed. Surgical management consists of gastric wedge resection to include the offending vessel. The difficulty at the time of exploration is locating the lesion unless it is actively bleeding. The surgical procedure can be greatly facilitated by asking the endoscopist to tattoo the stomach when the lesion is identified. The traditional surgical approach has been through laparotomy with wide gastrotomy to identify the lesion with subsequent wide wedge resection. The lesion can also be approached laparoscopically, combined with intraoperative endoscopy. A wedge resection is performed with a linear stapling device using endoscopic transillumination to determine the resection margin.

### Gastric Varices

Gastric varices are broadly classified into two types, GE varices and isolated gastric varices. Isolated gastric varices are subclassified into type 1 varices, located in the fundus of the stomach; and type 2, isolated ectopic varices located anywhere in the stomach.

Gastric varices can develop secondary to portal hypertension, in conjunction with esophageal varices, or secondary to sinistral hypertension from splenic vein thrombosis. In generalized portal hypertension, the increased portal pressure is transmitted by the left gastric vein to esophageal varices and by the short and posterior gastric veins to the fundic plexus and cardia veins. Isolated gastric varices tend to occur secondary to splenic vein thrombosis. Splenic blood flows retrograde through the short and posterior gastric veins into the varices and then hepatopetally through the coronary vein into the portal vein. Left to right retrograde flow through the gastroepiploic vein to the superior mesenteric vein can explain the development of ectopic varices in the stomach.

The incidence of bleeding from gastric varices has been reported to be between 3% and 30% but, in most series, it is less than 10%. However, the incidence of bleeding can be as high as 78% in patients with splenic vein thrombosis and fundic varices. There are limited data on risk factors associated with hemorrhage in patients with gastric varices, although increasing size of the varices or a higher Child's status increases the risk for bleeding.

Gastric varices in the setting of splenic vein thrombosis are readily treated by splenectomy. Patients with bleeding gastric varices should have an imaging study to document splenic vein thrombosis before surgical intervention because gastric varices are more often associated with generalized portal hypertension.

Gastric varices in the setting of portal hypertension should be managed similarly to esophageal varices. The patient should be volume-resuscitated, with attention paid to the correction of abnormal coagulation profiles. Temporary tamponade can be attempted with a Sengstaken-Blakemore tube. Endoscopy serves as a diagnostic and therapeutic tool. Successful eradication of the esophageal varices through banding or sclerotherapy often results in obliteration of the gastric varices. Because gastric varices arise in the submucosa, a common complication associated with gastric variceal sclerotherapy is ulceration. A major problem with gastric varices is rebleeding, of which 50% is secondary to ulcers. Endoscopic variceal band ligation can achieve hemostasis in approximately 89% of patients; however, concerns about gastric perforations with this technique have tempered its use. Transjugular intrahepatic portosystemic shunting (TIPS) can be effective in controlling gastric variceal hemorrhage, with rebleeding rates of about 30%. A gastrorenal shunt between gastric varices and the left renal vein is present in 85% of patients with gastric varices. This spontaneous shunt decompresses the portal system and lessens the efficacy of TIPS. A balloon catheter can be inserted into the gastrorenal shunt through the left renal vein and the shunt occluded by inflating the balloon. A sclerosant (e.g., ethanolamine oleate) is then injected and left to remain until clots have formed in the varices. Balloon-occluded retrograde transvenous obliteration has been reported to have a high success rate (100%), with a low recurrence rate (0% to 5%). The major complication of this procedure is aggravation of esophageal varices secondary to a rise in portal pressure as a consequence of occluding the gastrorenal shunt. Also, ethanolamine oleate can cause hemolysis (treatable by haptoglobin administration), with subsequent renal damage.

## Gastric Volvulus

Gastric volvulus is an uncommon condition. Torsion occurs along the stomach's longitudinal axis (organoaxial) in about two thirds of cases and along the vertical axis (mesenteroaxial) in one third (Fig. 49-28). Usually, organoaxial gastric volvulus occurs acutely and is associated with a diaphragmatic defect, whereas mesenteroaxial volvulus is partial (<180 degrees), recurrent, and not associated with a diaphragmatic defect. In adults, the diaphragmatic defects are usually traumatic or paraesophageal hernias, whereas in children, congenital defects such as the foramen of Bochdalek or eventration are involved. The major symptoms at presentation are abdominal pain that is acute in onset, distention, vomiting, and upper GI hemorrhage. The sudden onset of constant and severe upper abdominal pain, recurrent retching with production of little vomitus, and the inability to pass an NG tube constitute Borchardt's triad. Plain films of the abdomen reveal a gas-filled viscus in the chest or upper abdomen. The diagnosis can be confirmed by barium contrast study or upper GI endoscopy. Acute volvulus is a surgical emergency. The stomach is reduced and uncoiled through a transabdominal approach. The diaphragmatic defect is repaired, with consideration given to a fundoplication in the setting of a paraesophageal hernia. In the unusual case in which strangulation has occurred (5% to 28%), the compromised segment of stomach is resected. Spontaneous volvulus, without an associated diaphragmatic defect, is treated by detorsion and fixation of the stomach by gastropexy or tube gastrostomy.

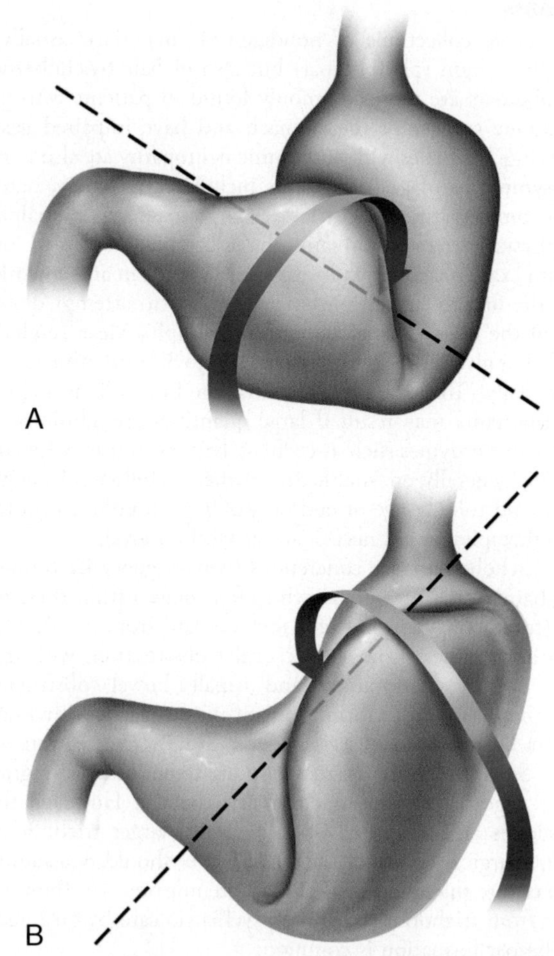


**FIGURE 49-28** Torsion of the stomach along the longitudinal axis (organoaxial) **(A)** and along the vertical axis (mesoaxial) **(B)**. (From White RR, Jacobs DO: Volvulus of the Stomach and Small Bowel. In Yeo CJ, Dempsey DT, Klein AS, et al [eds] Shackelford's surgery of the alimentary tract, ed 6, Philadelphia, 2007, Saunders.)

### Bezoars

Bezoars are collections of nondigestible materials, usually of vegetable origin (phytobezoar) but also of hair (trichobezoar). Phytobezoars are most commonly found in patients who have undergone surgery of the stomach and have impaired gastric emptying. Diabetics with autonomic neuropathy are also at risk. The symptoms of gastric bezoars include early satiety, nausea, pain, vomiting, and weight loss. A large mass may be palpable on physical examination and the diagnosis confirmed by a barium examination or endoscopy. In 1959, Dan and coworkers were the first to suggest enzymatic therapy to attempt dissolution of the bezoar. Papain, found in Adolph's Meat Tenderizer (AMT), is given in a dose of 1tsp in 150 to 300 mL water several times daily. The sodium concentration in AMT is high, so hypernatremia may result if large quantities are administered. Alternative enzymes such as cellulase have been used with some success. Generally, enzymatic débridement is followed by aggressive Ewald tube lavage or endoscopic fragmentation. Failure of these therapies would necessitate surgical removal.

Trichobezoars are concretions of hair, generally found in long-haired girls or women who often deny eating their own hair (trichophagy). Symptoms include pain from gastric ulceration and fullness from gastric outlet obstruction, with occasional gastric perforation and small bowel obstruction. Trichobezoars tend to form a cast of the stomach, with strands of hair having been observed as far distally as the transverse colon. Small trichobezoars may respond to endoscopic fragmentation, vigorous lavage, or enzymatic therapy. However, these techniques are of limited usefulness and larger trichobezoars require surgical removal. The small bowel should be examined to be ensure that additional bezoars are not present. Those who suffer from trichophagy require psychiatric care because recurrent bezoar formation is common.

### SELECTED REFERENCES

Barkun A, Bardou M, Marshall JK: Consensus recommendations for managing patients with nonvariceal upper gastrointestinal bleeding. Ann Intern Med 139:843–857, 2003.

An excellent overview of the prevalence of upper GI hemorrhage, along with an evidence-based assessment of various therapies. Recommendations are made with respect to the role of endoscopy, methods of endoscopic control, pharmacologic interventions, proper monitoring and triaging, risk factors for rebleeding, and which patients have increased mortality.

Bonenkamp JJ, Songun I, Hermans J, et al: Randomised comparison of morbidity after D1 and D2 dissection for gastric cancer in 996 Dutch patients. Lancet 345:745–748, 1995.

Cuschieri A, Weeden S, Fielding J, et al: Patient survival after D1 and D2 resections for gastric cancer: Long-term results of the MRC randomized surgical trial. Surgical Co-operative Group. Br J Cancer 79:1522–1530, 1999.

These two studies, both randomized controlled trials, were major challenges to the role of D2 lymphadenectomy in the non-Japanese population. They both showed increased morbidity without long-term survival benefit. They have been challenged on the grounds that patients in the D2 group were not stratified by whether they also underwent splenectomy, which later analysis showed as the major contributor to the increased operative morbidity.

Burke EC, Karpeh MS, Conlon KC, et al: Laparoscopy in the management of gastric adenocarcinoma. Ann Surg 225:262–267, 1997.

Lowy AM, Mansfield PF, Leach SD, et al: Laparoscopic staging for gastric cancer. Surgery 119:611–614, 1996.

These two trials were important in the implementation of staging laparoscopy as a standard for gastric cancer. They demonstrated high rates of occult metastatic disease (30% to 40%) and therefore avoided unnecessary laparotomy in a significant proportion of patients with gastric cancer.

Cunningham D, Allum WH, Stenning SP, et al: Perioperative chemotherapy versus surgery alone for resectable gastroesophageal cancer. N Engl J Med 355:11–20, 2006.

The second major study to show a benefit to chemotherapy in gastric cancer. These patients underwent neoadjuvant treatment and a much greater percentage were able to complete treatment than those who completed the adjuvant trial. More patients had adequate lymphadenectomy than in the SWOG Int 0116 trial.

DeMatteo RP, Lewis JJ, Leung D, et al: Two hundred gastrointestinal stromal tumors: Recurrence patterns and prognostic factors for survival. Ann Surg 231:51–58, 2000.

The first major cohort study to characterize the natural progression of patients with GIST. It demonstrated a relatively high rate of recurrence and subsequent metastases, which led to increased focus on the development of improved adjuvant therapies.

DeMatteo RP, Ballman KV, Antonescu CR, et al: Adjuvant imatinib mesylate after resection of localised, primary gastrointestinal stromal tumour: A randomised, double-blind, placebo-controlled trial. The Lancet 373:1097–1104, 2009.

This follow-up study to the use of imatinib for metastatic disease significantly broadened the indications for imatinib in GIST. It showed significantly less recurrence of patients who received imatinib than for those who did not; this was especially pronounced for patients at high risk of developing metastatic disease.

Ford AC, Delaney BC, Forman D, et al: Eradication therapy for peptic ulcer disease in Helicobacter pylori–positive patients. Cochrane Database Syst Rev (2):CD003840, 2006.

This meta-analysis definitively showed the benefit of *H. pylori* eradication in the treatment of ulcer disease. Although antiulcer medication showed good rates of initial healing, the recurrence rates for eradication therapy were significantly lower than for antiulcer therapy alone.

MacDonald JS, Smalley SR, Benedetti J, et al: Chemoradiotherapy after surgery compared with surgery alone for adenocarcinoma of the stomach or gastroesophageal junction. N Engl J Med 345:725–730, 2001.

One of the first studies to show a benefit of adjuvant therapy for the treatment of gastric cancer. This has become the standard of care in the United States as a result of this trial. It has been criticized for having inadequate surgery, with a very high D0 lymph node resection rate.

## REFERENCES


1. Saffouri B, Weir GC, Bitar KN, et al: Gastrin and somatostatin secretion by perfused rat stomach: functional linkage of antral peptides. Am J Physiol 238:G495–G501, 1980.
2. Queiroz DM, Mendes EN, Rocha GA, et al: Effect of *Helicobacter pylori* eradication on antral gastrin- and somatostatin-immunoreactive cell density and gastrin and somatostatin concentrations. Scand J Gastroenterol 28:858–864, 1993.
3. Mercer DW, Cross JM, Smith GS, et al: Protective action of gastrin-17 against alcohol-induced gastric injury in the rat: Role in mucosal defense. Am J Physiol 273:G365–G373, 1997.
4. Abrahamsson H: Gastrointestinal motility disorders in patients with diabetes mellitus. J Intern Med 237:403–409, 1995.
5. Saslow SB, Thumshirn M, Camilleri M, et al: Influence of *H. pylori* infection on gastric motor and sensory function in asymptomatic volunteers. Dig Dis Sci 43:258–264, 1998.
6. Aro P, Storskrubb T, Ronkainen J, et al: Peptic ulcer disease in a general adult population: The Kalixanda study: A random population-based study. Am J Epidemiol 163:1025–1034, 2006.
7. Wang YR, Richter JE, Dempsey DT: Trends and outcomes of hospitalizations for peptic ulcer disease in the United States, 1993 to 2006. Ann Surg 251:51–58, 2010.
8. Soll AH: Pathogenesis of peptic ulcer and implications for therapy. N Engl J Med 322:909–916, 1990.
9. Peterson WL, Barnett CC, Evans DJ, Jr, et al: Acid secretion and serum gastrin in normal subjects and patients with duodenal ulcer: The role of *Helicobacter pylori*. Am J Gastroenterol 88:2038–2043, 1993.
10. Ford AC, Delaney BC, Forman D, et al: Eradication therapy for peptic ulcer disease in *Helicobacter pylori* positive patients. Cochrane Database Syst Rev (2):CD003840, 2006.
11. Barkun A, Bardou M, Marshall JK: Consensus recommendations for managing patients with nonvariceal upper gastrointestinal bleeding. Ann Intern Med 139:843–857, 2003.
12. Vergara M, Calvet X, Gisbert JP: Epinephrine injection versus epinephrine injection and a second endoscopic method in high risk bleeding ulcers. Cochrane Database Syst Rev (2):CD005584, 2007.
13. Dorward S, Sreedharan A, Leontiadis GI, et al: Proton pump inhibitor treatment initiated prior to endoscopic diagnosis in upper gastrointestinal bleeding. Cochrane Database Syst Rev (4):CD005415, 2006.
14. Lunevicius R, Morkevicius M: Systematic review comparing laparoscopic and open repair for perforated peptic ulcer. Br J Surg 92:1195–1207, 2005.
15. Cherian PT, Cherian S, Singh P: Long-term follow-up of patients with gastric outlet obstruction related to peptic ulcer disease treated with endoscopic balloon dilatation and drug therapy. Gastrointest Endosc 66:491–497, 2007.
16. Jemal A, Siegel R, Ward E, et al: Cancer statistics, 2009. CA Cancer J Clin 59:225–249, 2009.
17. Kuipers EJ: Proton pump inhibitors and gastric neoplasia. Gut 55:1217–1221, 2006.
18. Bentrem D, Gerdes H, Tang L, et al: Clinical correlation of endoscopic ultrasonography with pathologic stage and outcome in patients undergoing curative resection for gastric cancer. Ann Surg Oncol 14:1853–1859, 2007.
19. Kim HJ, Kim AY, Oh ST, et al: Gastric cancer staging at multidetector row CT gastrography: Comparison of transverse and volumetric CT scanning. Radiology 236:879–885, 2005.
20. Podoloff DA, Ball DW, Ben-Josef E, et al: NCCN task force: Clinical utility of PET in various tumor types. J Natl Compr Canc Netw 7 Suppl 2:S1–26, 2009.
21. Burke EC, Karpeh MS, Conlon KC, et al: Laparoscopy in the management of gastric adenocarcinoma. Ann Surg 225:262–267, 1997.
22. Lowy AM, Mansfield PF, Leach SD, et al: Laparoscopic staging for gastric cancer. Surgery 119:611–614, 1996.
23. de Graaf GW, Ayantunde AA, Parsons SL, et al: The role of staging laparoscopy in oesophagogastric cancers. Eur J Surg Oncol 33:988–992, 2007.
24. Huscher CG, Mingoli A, Sgarzini G, et al: Laparoscopic versus open subtotal gastrectomy for distal gastric cancer: Five-year results of a randomized prospective trial. Ann Surg 241:232–237, 2005.
25. Lee SI, Choi YS, Park do J, et al: Comparative study of laparoscopy-assisted distal gastrectomy and open distal gastrectomy. J Am Coll Surg 202:874–880, 2006.
26. Yamao T, Shirao K, Ono H, et al: Risk factors for lymph node metastasis from intramucosal gastric carcinoma. Cancer 77:602–606, 1996.
27. Kim JJ, Lee JH, Jung H-Y, et al: EMR for early gastric cancer in Korea: A multicenter retrospective study. Gastrointestinal Endoscopy 66:693–700, 2007.
28. Gotoda T, Yanagisawa A, Sasako M, et al: Incidence of lymph node metastasis from early gastric cancer: Estimation with a large number of cases at two large centers. Gastric Cancer 3:219–225, 2000.
29. Jee YS, Hwang SH, Rao J, et al: Safety of extended endoscopic mucosal resection and endoscopic submucosal dissection following the Japanese Gastric Cancer Association treatment guidelines. Br J Surg 96:1157–1161, 2009.
30. Ishikawa S, Togashi A, Inoue M, et al: Indications for EMR/ESD in cases of early gastric cancer: Relationship between histological type, depth of wall invasion, and lymph node metastasis. Gastric Cancer 10:35–38, 2007.
31. Bonenkamp JJ, Songun I, Hermans J, et al: Randomised comparison of morbidity after D1 and D2 dissection for gastric cancer in 996 Dutch patients. Lancet 345:745–748, 1995.
32. Cuschieri A, Weeden S, Fielding J, et al: Patient survival after D1 and D2 resections for gastric cancer: Long-term results of the MRC randomized surgical trial. Surgical Co-operative Group. Br J Cancer 79:1522–1530, 1999.
33. Bilimoria KY, Talamonti MS, Wayne JD, et al: Effect of hospital type and volume on lymph node evaluation for gastric and pancreatic cancer. Arch Surg 143:671–678, 2008.
34. Yoo CH, Noh SH, Shin DW, et al: Recurrence following curative resection for gastric carcinoma. Br J Surg 87:236–242, 2000.
35. MacDonald JS, Smalley SR, Benedetti J, et al: Chemoradiotherapy after surgery compared with surgery alone for adenocarcinoma of the stomach or gastroesophageal junction. N Engl J Med 345:725–730, 2001.
36. Cunningham D, Allum WH, Stenning SP, et al: Perioperative chemotherapy versus surgery alone for resectable gastroesophageal cancer. N Engl J Med 355:11–20, 2006.

37. Wagner Ad, Grothe W, Haerting J, et al: Chemotherapy in advanced gastric cancer: A systematic review and meta-analysis based on aggregate data. J Clin Oncol 24:2903–2909, 2006.
38. Van Cutsem E, Kang Y, Chung H, et al: Efficacy results from the ToGA trial: A phase III study of trastuzumab added to standard chemotherapy (CT) in first-line human epidermal growth factor receptor 2 (HER2)–positive advanced gastric cancer (GC). J Clin Oncol 27, 2009.
39. Pinto C, Di Fabio F, Barone C, et al: Phase II study of cetuximab in combination with cisplatin and docetaxel in patients with untreated advanced gastric or gastro-oesophageal junction adenocarcinoma (DOCETUX study). Br J Cancer 101:1261–1268, 2009.
40. Martin RC, 2nd, Jaques DP, Brennan MF, et al: Extended local resection for advanced gastric cancer: Increased survival versus increased morbidity. Ann Surg 236:159–165, 2002.
41. Sym SJ, Chang HM, Ryu MH, et al: Neoadjuvant docetaxel, capecitabine and cisplatin (DXP) in patients with unresectable locally advanced or metastatic gastric cancer. Ann Surg Oncol 17:1024–1032, 2010.
42. National Cancer Institute, Surveillance Research Program: Fast Stats, 2009 (http://seer.cancer.gov/faststats).
43. Aviles A, Nambo MJ, Neri N, et al: The role of surgery in primary gastric lymphoma: Results of a controlled clinical trial. Ann Surg 240:44–50, 2004.
44. Miettinen M, Sobin LH, Lasota J: Gastrointestinal stromal tumors of the stomach: A clinicopathologic, immunohistochemical, and molecular genetic study of 1765 cases with long-term follow-up. Am J Surg Pathol 29:52–68, 2005.
45. DeMatteo RP, Lewis JJ, Leung D, et al: Two hundred gastrointestinal stromal tumors: Recurrence patterns and prognostic factors for survival. Ann Surg 231:51–58, 2000.
46. Blanke CD, Rankin C, Demetri GD, et al: Phase III randomized, intergroup trial assessing imatinib mesylate at two dose levels in patients with unresectable or metastatic gastrointestinal stromal tumors expressing the kit receptor tyrosine kinase: S0033. J Clin Oncol 26:626–632, 2008.
47. DeMatteo RP, Ballman KV, Antonescu CR, et al: Adjuvant imatinib mesylate after resection of localised, primary gastrointestinal stromal tumour: A randomised, double-blind, placebo-controlled trial. The Lancet 373:1097–1104, 2009.
48. Modlin IM, Lye KD, Kidd M: A 50-year analysis of 562 gastric carcinoids: Small tumor or larger problem? Am J Gastroenterol 99:23–32, 2004.

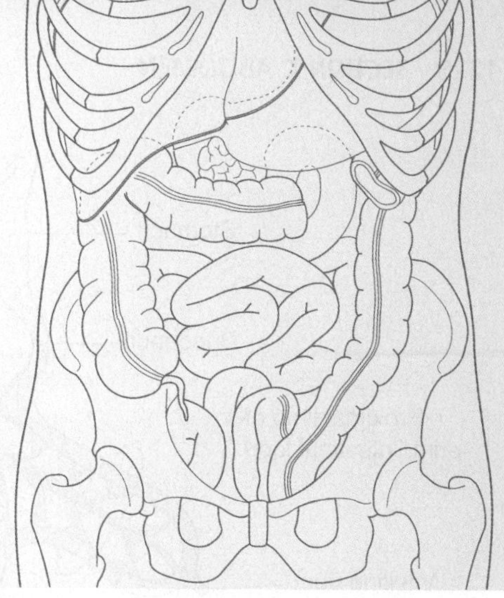

CHAPTER 50

# SMALL INTESTINE

Shaun McKenzie and B. Mark Evers



The small intestine is a marvel of complexity and efficiency. The primary role of the small intestine is the digestion and absorption of dietary components after they leave the stomach. This process depends on a multitude of structural, physiologic, endocrine, and chemical factors. Exocrine secretions from the liver and pancreas enable complete digestion of the foodstuffs. The enlarged surface area of the small intestinal mucosa then absorbs these nutrients. In addition to its role in digestion and absorption, the small bowel is the largest endocrine organ in the body and is one of the most important organs of immune function. Given its essential role and complexity, it is amazing that diseases of the small bowel are not more frequent. In this chapter, the normal anatomy and physiology of the small intestine are described, as well as disease processes involving the small bowel, which include obstruction, inflammatory diseases, neoplasms, diverticular disease, and miscellaneous disorders.

## EMBRYOLOGY

The primitive gut is formed during the fourth week of fetal human gestation.[1] The endodermal layer gives rise to the epithelial lining of the digestive tract and the splanchnic mesoderm surrounding the endoderm gives rise to the muscular connective tissue and all the other layers of the intestine. Except for the duodenum, which is a primitive foregut structure, the small intestine is derived from the midgut. During the fifth week of fetal development, when the intestinal length is rapidly increasing, herniation of the midgut occurs through the umbilicus (Fig. 50-1). This midgut loop has a cranial and caudal limb, with the cranial limb developing into the distal duodenum, jejunum, and proximal ilium and the caudal limb becoming the distal ilium and proximal two thirds of the transverse colon. The juncture of the cranial and caudal limbs is where the vitelline duct joins to the yolk sac. This duct structure normally becomes obliterated before birth; however, it can persist as a Meckel's diverticulum in approximately 2% of the population. This midgut herniation persists until about 10 weeks of fetal gestation, when the intestine returns to the abdominal cavity. After completing a 270-degree rotation from its initial starting point, the proximal jejunum reenters the abdomen and occupies the left side of the abdomen, with subsequent loops lying more to the right. The cecum enters last and is located temporarily in the right upper quadrant; however, with time, it descends to its normal position in the right lower quadrant. Congenital anomalies of gut malrotation and fixation can occur during this process.

The primitive small bowel is lined by a sheet of cuboidal cells until about the ninth week of gestation, when villi begin to form in the proximal intestine and then proceed in a caudal fashion until the entire small bowel, and even the colon, for a period of time, are lined by these finger-like projections. Crypt formation begins in the 10th to 12th weeks of gestation. The crypt layer of the small bowel is the site of continual cell renewal and proliferation. As the cells ascend the crypt-villous axis, proliferation ceases, and cells differentiate into one of the four main cell types: absorptive enterocytes, which compose about 95% of the intestinal cell population; goblet cells; Paneth cells; and enteroendocrine cells. Cells are eventually extruded into the intestinal lumen. Amazingly, this entire process of complete renewal of the intestinal lining occurs in less than 1 week in humans.

## ANATOMY

### Gross Anatomy

The entire small intestine, which extends from the pylorus to the cecum, measures 270 to 290 cm, with duodenal length estimated at approximately 20 cm, jejunal length at 100 to 110 cm, and ileal length at 150 to 160 cm. The jejunum begins at the duodenojejunal angle, which is supported by a peritoneal fold known as the *ligament of Treitz.* There is no obvious line of demarcation between the jejunum and the ileum; however, the jejunum is commonly considered to make up the proximal two fifths of the small intestine and the ileum makes up the remaining three fifths. The jejunum has a somewhat larger circumference, is thicker than the ileum, and can be identified at surgery by examining mesenteric vessels. In the jejunum, only one or two arcades send out long, straight vasa recta to the

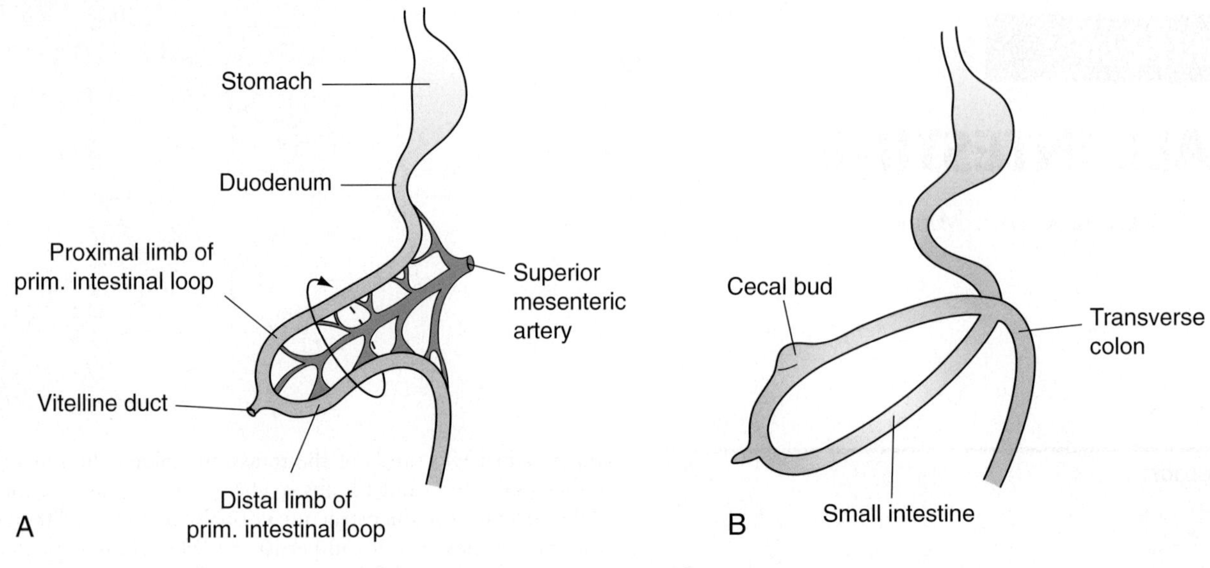


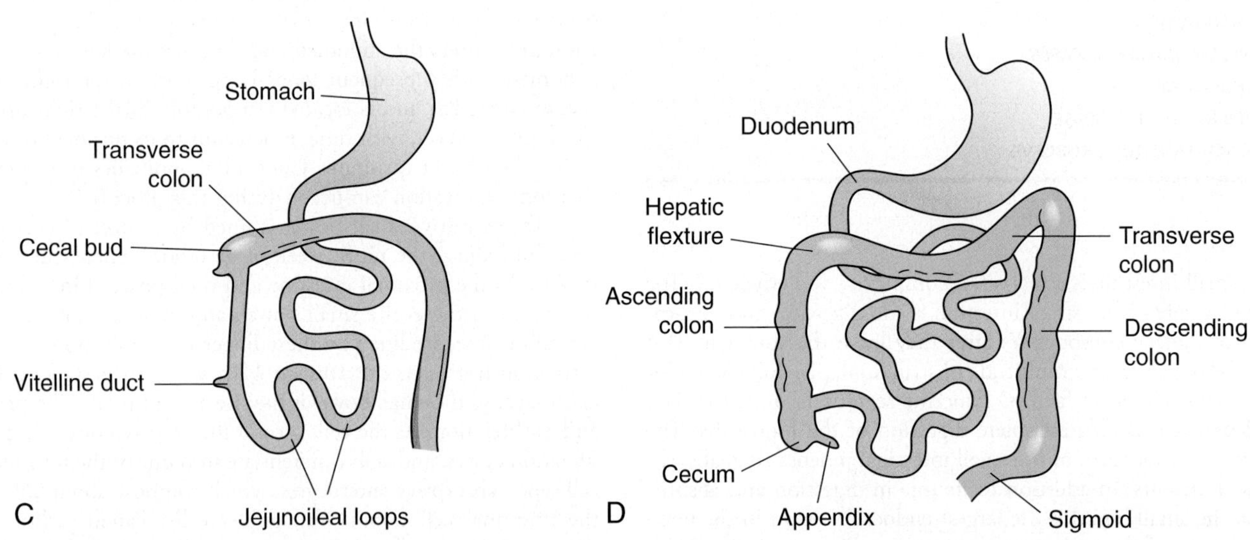


**FIGURE 50-1** Rotation of the intestine. **A,** The intestine after a 90-degree rotation around the axis of the superior mesenteric artery, the proximal loop on the right and the distal loop on the left. **B,** The intestinal loop after a further 180-degree rotation. The transverse colon passes in front of the duodenum. **C,** Position of the intestinal loops after reentry into the abdominal cavity. Note the elongation of the small intestine, with formation of the small intestine loops. **D,** Final position of the intestines after descent of the cecum into the right iliac fossa. (From Podolsky DK, Babyatshy MW: Growth and development of the gastrointestinal tract. In Yamada T [ed]: Textbook of gastroenterology, vol 2, Philadelphia, 1995, JB Lippincott.)

mesenteric border, whereas the blood supply to the ileum may have four or five separate arcades with shorter vasa recta (Fig. 50-2). The mucosa of the small bowel is characterized by transverse folds (plicae circulares), which are prominent in the distal duodenum and jejunum.

### Neurovascular-Lymphatic Supply

The small intestine is served by rich vascular, neural, and lymphatic supplies, all traversing through the mesentery. The base of the mesentery attaches to the posterior abdominal wall to the left of the second lumbar vertebra and passes obliquely to the right and inferiorly to the right sacroiliac joint. The blood supply of the small bowel, except for the proximal duodenum, which is supplied by branches of the celiac axis, comes entirely from the superior mesenteric artery (Fig. 50-3). The superior mesenteric artery courses anterior to the uncinate process of the pancreas and the third portion of the duodenum, where it divides to supply the pancreas, distal duodenum, entire small intestine, and ascending and transverse colons. There is an abundant collateral blood supply to the small bowel provided by vascular arcades coursing in the mesentery. Venous drainage of the small bowel parallels the arterial supply, with blood draining into the superior mesenteric vein, which joins the splenic vein behind the neck of the pancreas to form the portal vein.

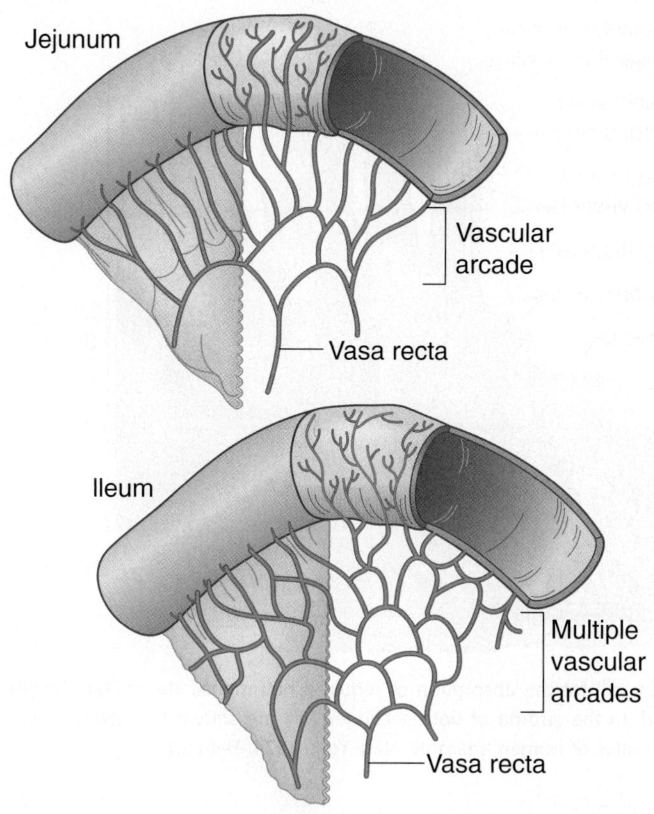


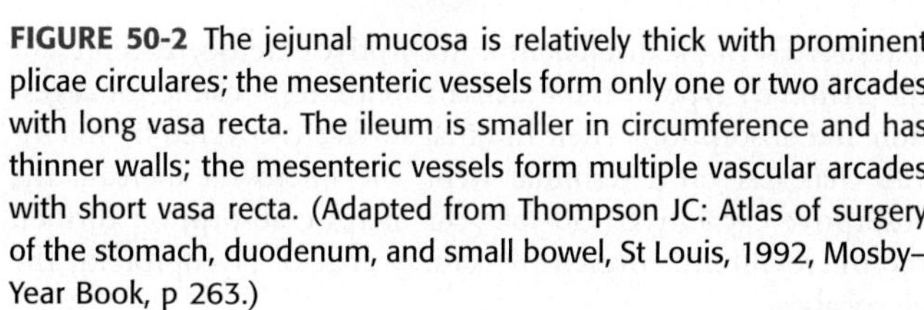


**FIGURE 50-2** The jejunal mucosa is relatively thick with prominent plicae circulares; the mesenteric vessels form only one or two arcades with long vasa recta. The ileum is smaller in circumference and has thinner walls; the mesenteric vessels form multiple vascular arcades with short vasa recta. (Adapted from Thompson JC: Atlas of surgery of the stomach, duodenum, and small bowel, St Louis, 1992, Mosby–Year Book, p 263.)

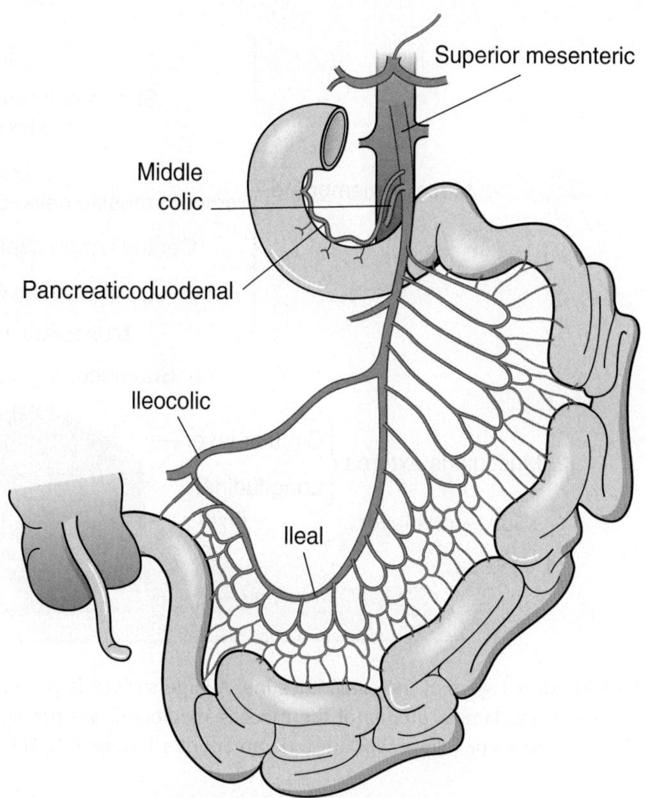


**FIGURE 50-3** Blood supply to the jejunoileum and distal duodenum is entirely from the superior mesenteric artery, which courses anterior to the third portion of the duodenum. The celiac artery supplies the proximal duodenum. (Adapted from Thompson JC: Atlas of surgery of the stomach, duodenum, and small bowel, St Louis, 1992, Mosby–Year Book, p 265.)

The innervation of the small bowel is provided by parasympathetic and sympathetic divisions of the autonomic nervous system, which in turn provide the efferent nerves to the small intestine. Parasympathetic fibers are derived from the vagus; they traverse the celiac ganglion and affect secretion, motility, and probably all phases of bowel activity. Vagal afferent fibers are present but apparently do not carry pain impulses. The sympathetic fibers come from three sets of splanchnic nerves and have their ganglion cells usually in a plexus around the base of the superior mesenteric artery. Motor impulses affect blood vessel motility and probably gut secretion and motility. Pain from the intestine is mediated through general visceral afferent fibers in the sympathetic system.

The lymphatics of the small intestine are noted in major deposits of lymphatic tissue, particularly in the Peyer patches of the distal small bowel. Lymphatic drainage proceeds from the mucosa through the wall of the bowel to a set of nodes adjacent to the bowel in the mesentery. Drainage continues to a group of regional nodes adjacent to the mesenteric arterial arcades and then to a group at the base of the superior mesentery vessels. From there, lymph flows into the cisterna chyli and then up the thoracic ducts, ultimately to empty into the venous system located in the neck. The lymphatic drainage of the small intestine constitutes a major route for transport of absorbed lipid into the circulation and similarly plays a major role in immune defense and also in the spread of cells arising from cancers of the gut.

## Microscopic Anatomy

The small bowel wall consists of four layers, the serosa, muscularis propria, submucosa, and mucosa (Fig. 50-4).

The serosa is the outermost layer of the small intestine and consists of visceral peritoneum, a single layer of flattened mesoepithelial cells that encircles the jejunoileum, and the anterior surface of the duodenum.

The muscularis propria consists of two muscle layers, a thin outer longitudinal layer and a thicker inner circular layer of smooth muscle. Ganglion cells from the myenteric (Auerbach) plexus are interposed between the muscle layers and send neural fibers into both layers, thus providing electrical continuity between the smooth muscle cells and permitting conduction through the muscle layer.

The submucosa consists of a layer of fibroelastic connective tissue containing blood vessels and nerves. It is the strongest component of the intestinal wall and therefore must be included in anastomotic sutures. It contains elaborate networks of lymphatics, arterioles, and venules and an extensive plexus of nerve fibers and ganglion cells (Meissner plexus). The nerves from the mucosa and submucosa muscle layers are interconnected by

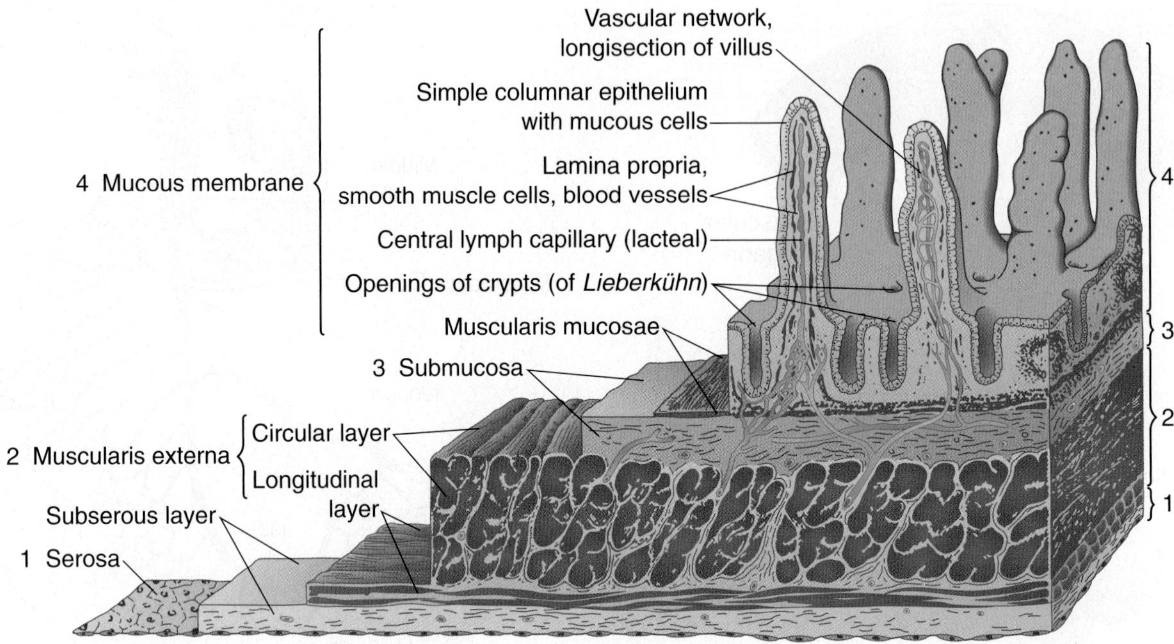


**FIGURE 50-4** Layers of the small intestine. A large surface is provided by villi for the absorption of required nutriments. The solitary lymph follicles in the lamina propria of the mucous membrane are not labeled. In the stroma of both sectioned villi are shown the central chyle (lacteal) vessels or villous capillaries. (From Sobotta J, Figge FHJ, Hild WJ: Atlas of human anatomy, New York, 1974, Hafner.)

small nerve fibers; cross connections between adrenergic and cholinergic elements have been described.

The mucosa can be divided into three layers, the muscularis mucosae, lamina propria, and epithelial layers (Fig. 50-5). The muscularis mucosae is a thin layer of muscle that separates the mucosa from the submucosa. The lamina propria is a connective tissue layer between the epithelial cells and muscularis mucosae that contains a variety of cells, including plasma cells, lymphocytes, mast cells, eosinophils, macrophages, fibroblasts, smooth muscle cells, and noncellular connective tissue. The lamina propria, the base on which the epithelial cells lie, serves a protective role in the intestine to combat microorganisms that penetrate the overlying epithelium, secondary to a rich supply of immune cells. Plasma cells actively synthesize immunoglobulins and other immune cells in the lamina propria and release various mediators (e.g., cytokines, arachidonic acid metabolites, histamines) that can modulate various cellular functions of the overlying epithelium. The epithelial layer is a continual sheet of epithelial cells covering the villi and lining the crypts. The main functions of the crypt epithelium are cell renewal and exocrine, endocrine, water, and ion secretion; the main functions of the villous epithelium are digestion and absorption. Four main cell types are contained in the mucosal layer: (1) goblet cells, which secrete mucus; (2) Paneth cells, which secrete lysozyme, tumor necrosis factor (TNF), and the cryptidins, which are homologues of leukocyte defensins thought to be related to the host mucosal defense system; (3) absorptive enterocytes; and (4) enteroendocrine cells, of which there are more than 10 distinct populations that produce the gastrointestinal hormones.

Microscopically, the mucosa is designed for maximal absorptive surface area, with villi protruding into the lumen. Villi are tallest in the distal duodenum and proximal jejunum and shortest in the distal ileum. Absorptive enterocytes represent the main cell type in the mucosa and are responsible for digestion and absorption. Their luminal surface is covered by microvilli that rest on a terminal web. The microvilli increase the absorptive capacity by 30-fold. To increase absorption further, the microvilli are covered by a fuzzy coat of glycoprotein, the glycocalyx.

## PHYSIOLOGY

### Digestion and Absorption

The complex process of digestion and eventual absorption of nutrients, water, electrolytes, and minerals is the main role of the small intestine. Liters of water and hundreds of grams of food are delivered to the small intestine daily and, with remarkable efficiency, almost all food is absorbed, except for indigestible cellulose. The stomach initiates the process of digestion with the breakdown of solids to particles 1 mm or smaller, which are then delivered to the duodenum, where pancreatic enzymes, bile, and brush border enzymes continue the process of digestion and eventual absorption through the small intestinal wall.[2] The small bowel is primarily responsible for the absorption of the dietary components (carbohydrates, proteins, and fats), as well as ions, vitamins, and water.

#### Carbohydrates

An adult consuming a normal Western diet will ingest 300 to 350 g of carbohydrates a day, with about 50% consumed as starch, 30% as sucrose, 6% as lactose, and the remainder as maltose, trehalose, glucose, fructose, sorbitol, cellulose, and pectins.[2] Dietary starch is a polysaccharide consisting of long chains of glucose molecules (Fig. 50-6). Amylose makes up

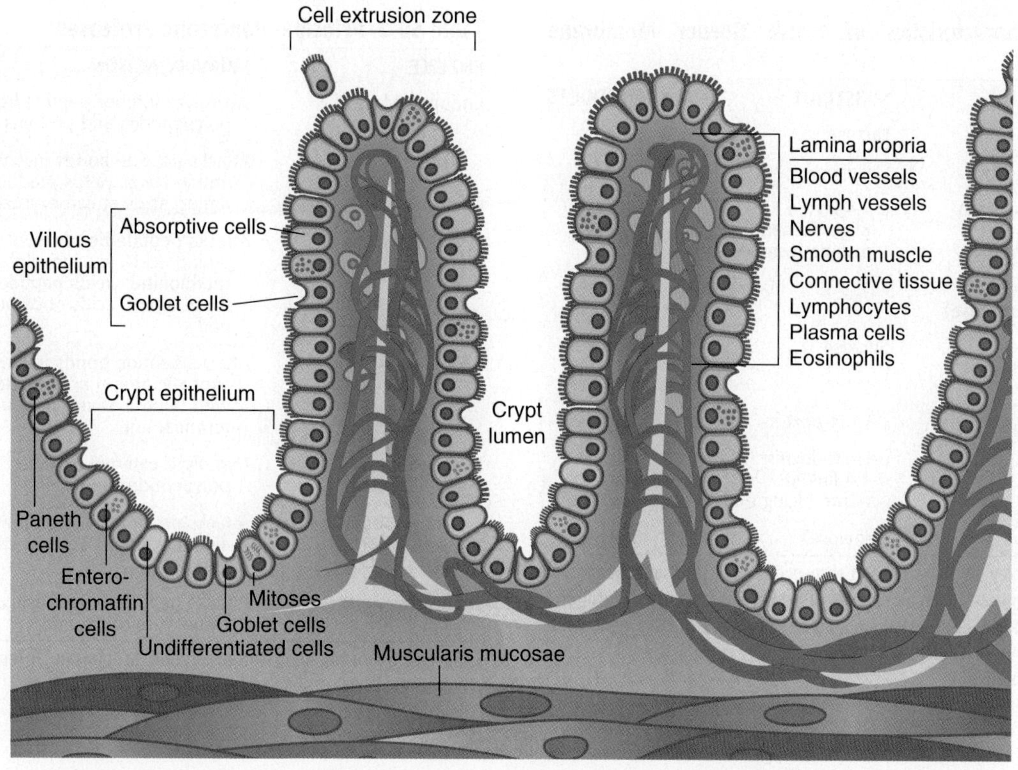


**FIGURE 50-5** Schematic diagram of the histologic organization of the small intestinal mucosa. (Adapted from Keljo DJ, Gariepy CE: Anatomy, histology, embryology, and developmental anomalies of the small and large intestine. In Feldman M, Scharschmidt BF, Sleisenger MH [eds]: Sleisenger & Fordtran's gastrointestinal and liver disease: Pathology, diagnosis, management, Philadelphia, 2002, WB Saunders, p 1646.)

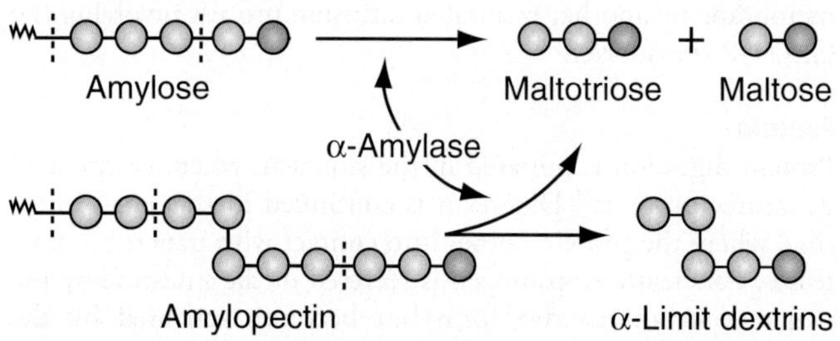


**FIGURE 50-6** Action of pancreatic α-amylase on linear (amylose) and branched (amylopectin) forms of starch to produce the breakdown products maltotriose, maltose, and dextrins. (Adapted from Alpers DH: Digestion and absorption of carbohydrates and proteins. In Johnson LR, Alpers DH, Christensen J, et al [eds]: Physiology of the gastrointestinal tract, ed 3, vol 2, New York, 1994, Raven Press, p 1727.)

about 20% of starch in the diet and is broken down at the α-1,4 bonds by salivary (i.e., ptyalin) and pancreatic amylases that convert amylose to maltotriose and maltose. Amylopectin, making up about 80% of dietary starch, has branching points every 25 molecules along the straight glucose chains; the α-1,6 glucose linkages in amylopectin produce the end products of amylase digestion—maltose, maltotriose, and the residual branch saccharides, the dextrins. In general, the starches are almost totally converted into maltose and other small glucose polymers before they have passed beyond the duodenum or upper jejunum. The remainder of carbohydrate digestion occurs as a result of brush border enzymes of the luminal surface.

The brush border of the small intestine contains the enzymes lactase, maltase, sucrase-isomaltase, and trehalase, which split the disaccharides, as well as other small glucose polymers, into their constituent monosaccharides (Table 50-1). Lactase hydrolyzes lactose into glucose and galactose. Maltase hydrolyzes maltose to produce glucose monomers. Sucrase-isomaltase is a complex of two subunits; sucrase hydrolyzes sucrose to yield glucose and fructose, and isomaltase hydrolyzes the α-1,6 bonds in α-limit dextrins to yield glucose. Glucose represents more than 80% of the final products of carbohydrate digestion, with galactose and fructose usually representing no more than 10% of the products of carbohydrate digestion.

The carbohydrates are absorbed in the form of monosaccharides. Transport of the released hexoses (glucose, galactose, and fructose) is by specific mechanisms involved in active transport. The major routes of absorption are by three membrane carrier systems—sodium glucose transporter 1 (SGLT-1), glucose transporter 5 (GLUT-5), and glucose transporter 2 (GLUT-2)[2] (Fig. 50-7). Glucose and galactose are absorbed by a carrier-mediated active transport mechanism, which involves the cotransport of $Na^+$ (SGLT-1 transporter). As $Na^+$ diffuses into the inside of the cell, it pulls the glucose or galactose along with it, thus providing the energy for transport of the monosaccharide. The exit of glucose from the cytosol into the intracellular space is predominantly by a $Na^+$-independent carrier (GLUT-2

**Table 50-1 Characteristics of Brush Border Membrane Carbohydrases**

| ENZYME | SUBSTRATE | PRODUCTS |
|---|---|---|
| Lactase | Lactose | Glucose |
| | Galactose | |
| Maltase (glucoamylase) | α-1,4-linked oligosaccharides, up to nine residues | Glucose |
| Sucrase-isomaltase (sucrose-α -dextrinase) | | |
| Sucrase | Sucrose | Glucose |
| | | Fructose |
| Isomaltase | α-Limit dextrin | Glucose |
| Both enzymes | α-Limit dextrin α-1,4-link at nonreducing end | Glucose |
| Trehalase | Trehalose | Glucose |

From Marsh MN, Riley SA: Digestion and absorption of nutrients and vitamins. In Feldman M, Sleisenger MH, Scharschmidt BF (eds): Sleisenger and Fordtran's gastrointestinal and liver disease: Pathophysiology, diagnosis, management, vol 2, Philadelphia, 1998, WB Saunders, p 1480.

**Table 50-2 Principal Pancreatic Proteases**

| ENZYME | PRIMARY ACTION |
|---|---|
| Endopeptidases | Hydrolyze interior peptide bonds of polypeptides and proteins |
| Trypsin | Attacks peptide bonds involving basic amino acids; yields products with basic amino acids at carboxyl-terminal end |
| Chymotrypsin | Attacks peptide bonds involving aromatic amino acids, leucine, glutamine, and methionine; yields peptide products with these amino acids at carboxyl-terminal end |
| Elastase | Attacks peptide bonds involving neutral aliphatic amino acids; yields products with neutral amino acids at carboxyl-terminal end |
| Exopeptidases | Hydrolyze external peptide bonds of polypeptides and protein |
| Carboxypeptidase A | Attacks peptides with aromatic and neutral aliphatic amino acids at carboxyl-terminal end |
| Carboxypeptidase B | Attacks peptides with basic amino acids at carboxyl-terminal end |

From Castro GA: Digestion and absorption. In Johnson LR (ed): Gastrointestinal physiology, St Louis, 1991, Mosby, pp 108-130.

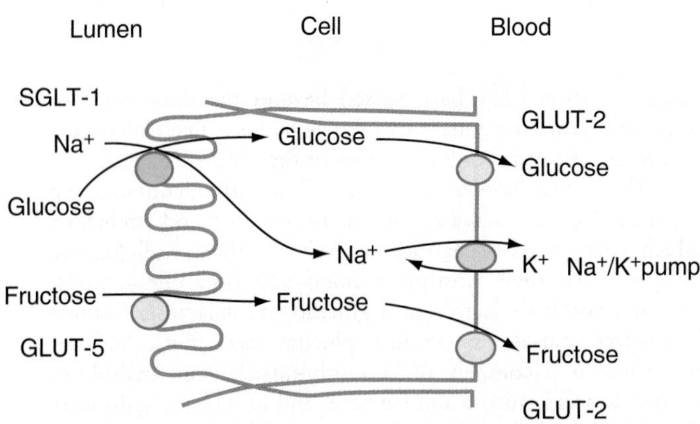


**FIGURE 50-7** Model for glucose, galactose, and fructose transport across the intestinal epithelium. Glucose and galactose are transported into the enterocyte across the brush border membrane by the $Na^+$ glucose cotransporter (SGLT-1) and then transported out across the basolateral membrane down their concentration gradients by GLUT-2. The low intracellular $Na^+$ driving uphill sugar transport across the brush border is maintained by the $Na^+$,$K^+$ pump on the basolateral membrane. Glucose and galactose therefore stimulate $Na^+$ absorption across the epithelium. Fructose is transported across the cell down the concentration gradient across the brush border and basolateral membranes. GLUT-5 is the brush border fructose transporter, whereas GLUT-2 handles fructose transport across the basolateral membrane. (From Wright EM, Hirayama BA, Loo DDF, et al: Intestinal sugar transport. In Johnson LR, Alpers DH, Christensen J, et al [eds]: Physiology of the gastrointestinal tract, ed 3, vol 2, New York, 1994, Raven Press, p 1752.)

transporter) located at the basolateral membrane. Fructose, the other significant monosaccharide, is absorbed from the intestinal lumen through a process of facilitated diffusion. The carrier involved in fructose absorption is GLUT-5, which is located in the apical membrane of the enterocyte. This transport process does not depend on $Na^+$ or energy. Fructose exits the basolateral membrane by another facilitated diffusion process involving the GLUT-2 transporter.

### Protein

Protein digestion is initiated in the stomach, where gastric acid denatures proteins.[2] Digestion is continued in the small intestine, where the protein comes into contact with pancreatic proteases. Pancreatic trypsinogen is secreted in the intestine by the pancreas in an inactive form but becomes activated by the enzyme enterokinase, a brush border enzyme in the duodenum. Activated trypsin then activates the other pancreatic proteolytic enzyme precursors. The endopeptidases, which include trypsin, chymotrypsin, and elastase, act on peptide bonds at the interior of the protein molecule, producing peptides that are substrates for the exopeptidases (carboxypeptidases), which serially remove a single amino acid from the carboxyl end of the peptide (Table 50-2). This results in splitting the complex proteins into dipeptides, tripeptides, and some larger proteins, which are absorbed from the intestinal lumen by an $Na^+$-mediated active transport mechanism and digested further by enzymes in the brush border and in the cytoplasm of the enterocytes (Fig. 50-8). These peptidase enzymes include aminopeptidases and several dipeptidases, which split the remaining larger polypeptides into tripeptides and dipeptides and some amino acids. The amino acids, dipeptides, and tripeptides are easily transported through the microvilli into the epithelial cells where, in the cytosol, additional peptidases hydrolyze the dipeptides and tripeptides into single amino acids; these then pass through the epithelial

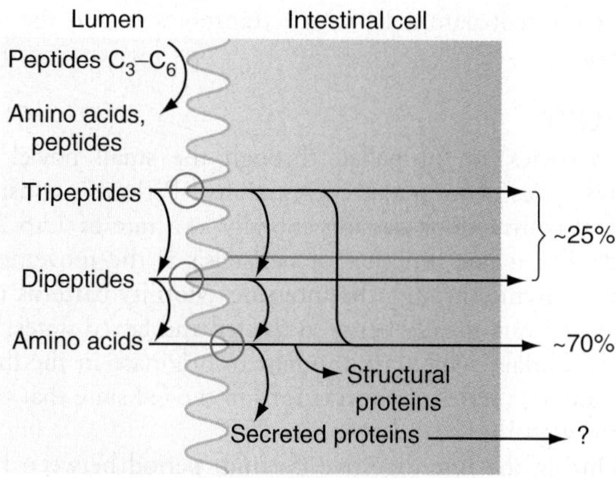


**FIGURE 50-8** Digestion and absorption of proteins. (Adapted from Alpers DH: Digestion and absorption of carbohydrates and proteins. In Johnson LR, Alpers DH, Christensen J, et al [eds]: Physiology of the gastrointestinal tract, ed 3, vol 2, New York, 1994, Raven Press, p 1733.)

cell membrane into the portal venous system. In normal humans, digestion and absorption of protein are usually 80% to 90% completed in the jejunum.

### Fats

**Emulsification** Most adults in North America consume 60 to 100 g/day of fat. Triglycerides, the most abundant fats, are composed of a glycerol nucleus and three fatty acids; small quantities of phospholipids, cholesterol, and cholesterol esters also are found in the normal diet. Essentially all fat digestion occurs in the small intestine, where the first step is the breakdown of fat globules into smaller sizes to facilitate further breakdown by water-soluble digestive enzymes, a process termed *emulsification.*[2] This process is facilitated by bile from the liver, which contains bile salts and the phospholipid lecithin. The polar parts of the bile salts and lecithin molecules are soluble in water, whereas the remaining portions are soluble in fat. Therefore, the fat-soluble portions dissolve in the surface layer of the fat globules and the polar portions, projecting outward, are soluble in the surrounding aqueous fluids. This arrangement renders the fat globules more accessible to fragmentation by agitation in the small intestine. Therefore, a major function of bile salts, and especially lecithin in the bile, is to allow the fat globules to be readily fragmented by agitation in the intestinal lumen. With the increase in surface area of the fat globules resulting from the action of the bile salts and lecithin, the fats can now be readily attacked by pancreatic lipase, the most crucial enzyme in the digestion of triglycerides, which splits triglycerides into free fatty acids and 2-monoglycerides.

**Micelle Formation** Fat digestion is further accelerated by bile salts, which, secondary to their amphipathic nature, can form micelles. Micelles are small spherical globules composed of 20 to 40 molecules of bile salts with a sterol nucleus that is highly fat-soluble and a hydrophilic polar group that projects outward. The mixed micelles thus formed are arrayed so that the insoluble lipid is surrounded by the bile salts oriented with their hydrophilic ends facing outward. Therefore, as quickly as the monoglycerides and free fatty acids are formed by lipolysis, they become dissolved in the central hydrophobic portion of the micelles, which then act to carry these products of fat hydrolysis to the brush borders of the epithelial cells, where absorption occurs.

**Intracellular Processing** The monoglycerides and free fatty acids, which are dissolved in the central lipid portion of the bile acid micelles, are absorbed through the brush border because of their highly lipid-soluble nature and simply diffuse into the interior of the cell.[2] After disaggregation of the micelle, bile salts remain within the intestinal lumen to enter into the formation of new micelles and act to carry more monoglycerides and fatty acids to the epithelial cells. The released fatty acids and monoglycerides in the cell re-form into new triglycerides. This re-formation of a triglyceride occurs in the cell through the interactions of intracellular enzymes that are associated with the endoplasmic reticulum.

The major pathway for resynthesis involves synthesis of triglycerides from 2-monoglycerides and coenzyme A (CoA)–activated fatty acids. Microsomal acyl-CoA lipase is necessary to synthesize acyl-CoA from the fatty acid before esterification. These reconstituted triglycerides then combine with cholesterol, phospholipids, and apoproteins to form chylomicrons, which consist of an inner core containing triglycerides and a membranous outer core of phospholipids and apoproteins. The chylomicrons pass from the epithelial cells into the lacteals, where they pass through the lymphatics into the venous system. From 80% to 90% of all fat absorbed from the gut is absorbed in this manner and transported to the blood by way of the thoracic lymph in the form of chylomicrons. Small quantities of short- to medium-chain fatty acids may be absorbed directly into the portal blood rather than being converted into triglycerides and absorbed into the lymphatics. These shorter chain fatty acids are more water-soluble, which allows for the direct diffusion into the bloodstream.

**Enterohepatic Circulation** The proximal intestine absorbs most of the dietary fat. Although the unconjugated bile acids are absorbed into the jejunum by passive diffusion, the conjugated bile acids that form micelles are absorbed in the ileum by active transport and are reabsorbed from the distal ileum. The bile acids then pass through the portal venous system to the liver for secretion as bile. The total bile salt pool in humans is 2 to 3 g; it recirculates about six times every 24 hours (the enterohepatic circulation of bile salts).[2] Almost all the bile salts are absorbed, with only about 0.5 g lost in the stool every day; this is replaced by resynthesis from cholesterol.

### Water, Electrolytes, and Vitamins

Eight to 10 liters of water/day enter the small intestine. Much of this is absorbed, with only approximately 500 mL or less leaving the ileum and entering the colon[2] (Fig. 50-9). Water may be absorbed by the process of simple diffusion. In addition, water may be drawn in and out of the cell through a process of osmotic pressure, resulting from active transport of sodium, glucose, or amino acids into cells.

Electrolytes can be absorbed in the small bowel by active transport or by coupling to organic solute.[2] $Na^+$ is absorbed by active transport through the basolateral membranes. $Cl^-$ is absorbed in the upper part of the small intestine by a process of passive diffusion. Large quantities of $HCO_3^-$ must be

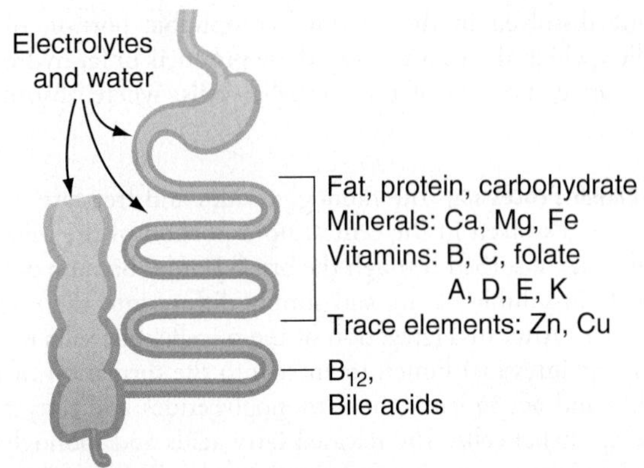


**FIGURE 50-9** Absorption of water and electrolytes in the small bowel and colon. (Adapted from Westergaard H: Short bowel syndrome. In Feldman M, Scharschmidt BF, Sleisenger MH [eds]: Sleisenger & Fordtran's gastrointestinal and liver disease: Pathology, diagnosis, management, Philadelphia, 2002, WB Saunders, p 1549.)

reabsorbed, which is accomplished in an indirect fashion. As the $Na^+$ is absorbed, $H^+$ is secreted into the lumen of the intestine. It then combines with $HCO_3^-$ to form carbonic acid, which then dissociates to form water and carbon dioxide. The water remains in the chyme, but the carbon dioxide is readily absorbed in the blood and is subsequently expired. Calcium is absorbed, particularly in the proximal intestine (duodenum and jejunum), by a process of active transport; absorption appears to be facilitated by an acid environment and is enhanced by vitamin D and parathyroid hormone. Iron is absorbed as a heme or nonheme component in the duodenum by an active process. Iron is then deposited within the cell as ferritin or transferred to the plasma bound to transferrin. The total absorption of iron is dependent on body stores of iron and the rate of erythropoiesis; any increase in erythropoiesis increases iron absorption. Potassium, magnesium, phosphate, and other ions also can be actively absorbed throughout the mucosa.

Vitamins are fat-soluble (e.g., vitamins A, D, E, and K) or water-soluble (e.g., ascorbic acid [vitamin C], biotin, nicotinic acid, folic acid, riboflavin, thiamine, pyridoxine [vitamin $B_6$], and cobalamin [vitamin $B_{12}$]).[2] The fat-soluble vitamins are carried in mixed micelles and transported in chylomicrons of lymph to the thoracic duct and into the venous system. The absorption of water-soluble vitamins appears to be more complex than originally thought. Vitamin C is absorbed by an active transport process that incorporates a sodium-coupled mechanism as well as a specific carrier system. Vitamin $B_6$ appears to be rapidly absorbed by simple diffusion into the proximal intestine. Thiamine (vitamin $B_1$) is rapidly absorbed in the jejunum by an active process similar to the sodium-coupled transport system for vitamin C. Riboflavin (vitamin $B_2$) is absorbed in the upper intestine by facilitated transport. The absorption of vitamin $B_{12}$ occurs primarily in the terminal ileum. Vitamin $B_{12}$ is derived from cobalamin, which is freed in the duodenum by pancreatic proteases. The cobalamin binds to intrinsic factor, which is secreted by the stomach, and is protected from proteolytic digestion. Specific receptors in the terminal ileum take up the cobalamin–intrinsic factor complex, probably by translocation. In the ileal enterocyte, free vitamin $B_{12}$ is bound to an ileal pool of transcobalamin II, which transports it into the portal circulation.

## MOTILITY

Food particles are propelled through the small bowel by a complex series of muscular contractions.[2] Peristalsis consists of intestinal contractions passing aborally at a rate of 1 to 2 cm/second. The major function of peristalsis is the movement of intestinal chyme through the intestine. Motility patterns in the small bowel vary greatly between the fed and fasted states. Pacesetter potentials, which are thought to originate in the duodenum, initiate a series of contractions in the fed state that propel food through the small bowel.

During the interdigestive (fasting) period between meals, the bowel is regularly swept by cyclical contractions that move aborally along the intestine every 75 to 90 minutes. These contractions are initiated by the migrating myoelectric complex (MMC), which is under the control of neural and humoral pathways. Extrinsic nerves to the small bowel are vagal and sympathetic. The vagal fibers have two functionally different effects; one is cholinergic and excitatory and the other is peptidergic and probably inhibitory. Sympathetic activity inhibits motor function, whereas parasympathetic activity stimulates it. Although intestinal hormones are known to affect small intestinal motility, the one peptide that has been clearly shown to function in this regard is motilin, which is found at its peak plasma level during phase III (intense bursts of myoelectrical activities resulting in regular, high-amplitude contractions) of MMCs.

## ENDOCRINE FUNCTION

### Gastrointestinal Hormones

The gastrointestinal hormones are distributed along the length of the small bowel in a spatially specific pattern. In fact, the small bowel is the largest endocrine organ in the body. Although often classified as hormones, these agents do not always function in a truly endocrine fashion (i.e., discharged into the bloodstream, where an action is produced at some distant site; Fig. 50-10). Sometimes, these peptides are discharged and act locally in a paracrine or autocrine manner. In addition, these peptides may serve as neurotransmitters (e.g., vasoactive intestinal peptide). The gastrointestinal hormones play a major role in pancreaticobiliary and intestinal secretion and motility. In addition, certain gastrointestinal hormones exert a trophic effect on normal and neoplastic intestinal mucosa and pancreas. The location, major stimulants of release, and primary effects of the more important gastrointestinal hormones are summarized in Table 50-3. In addition, the diagnostic and therapeutic uses of gastrointestinal hormones are listed in Table 50-4. Dockray[3] and Gariepy and Dickinson[4] have presented a more in-depth discussion of the structure, molecular biology, physiologic functions, and uses of these hormones.

### Receptors

The gastrointestinal hormones interact with their cell surface receptors to initiate a cascade of signaling events that eventually culminate in their physiologic effects. These hormones primarily signal through G protein–coupled receptors that traverse the plasma membrane seven times and represent the largest group of receptors found in the body. The heterotrimeric G proteins,

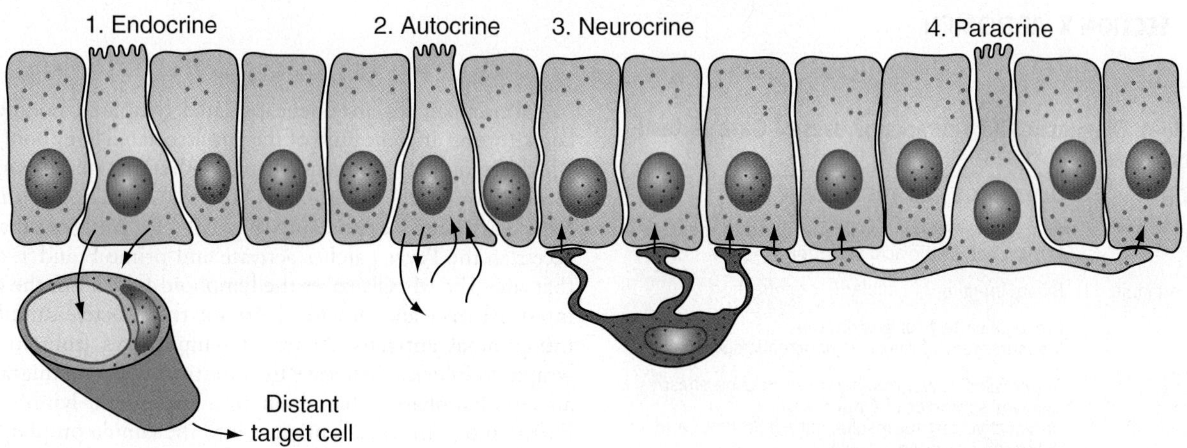


**FIGURE 50-10** Actions of intestinal hormones may be via endocrine, autocrine, neurocrine, or paracrine effects. (Adapted from Miller LJ: Gastrointestinal hormones and receptors. In Yamada T, Alpers DH, Laine L, et al [eds]: Textbook of gastroenterology, ed 3, vol 1, Philadelphia, 1999, Lippincott Williams & Wilkins, p 37.)

**Table 50-3 Gastrointestinal Hormones**

| HORMONE | LOCATION | MAJOR STIMULANTS OF PEPTIDE SECRETION | PRIMARY EFFECTS |
|---|---|---|---|
| Gastrin | Antrum, duodenum (G cells) | Peptides, amino acids, antral distention, vagal and adrenergic stimulation, gastrin-releasing peptide (bombesin) | Stimulates gastric acid and pepsinogen secretion<br>Stimulates gastric mucosal growth |
| Cholecystokinin | Duodenum, jejunum (I cells) | Fats, peptides, amino acids | Stimulates pancreatic enzyme secretion<br>Stimulates gallbladder contraction<br>Relaxes sphincter of Oddi<br>Inhibits gastric emptying |
| Secretin | Duodenum, jejunum (S cells) | Fatty acids, luminal acidity, bile salts | Stimulates release of water and bicarbonate from pancreatic ductal cells<br>Stimulates flow and alkalinity of bile<br>Inhibits gastric acid secretion and motility and inhibits gastrin release |
| Somatostatin | Pancreatic islets (D cells), antrum, duodenum | Gut: fat, protein, acid, other hormones (e.g., gastrin, cholecystokinin)<br>Pancreas: glucose, amino acids, cholecystokinin | Universal "off" switch:<br>Inhibits release of gastrointestinal hormones<br>Inhibits gastric acid secretion<br>Inhibits small bowel water and electrolyte secretion<br>Inhibits secretion of pancreatic hormones |
| Gastrin-releasing peptide (mammalian equivalent of bombesin) | Small bowel | Vagal stimulation | Universal "on" switch:<br>Stimulates release of all gastrointestinal hormones (except secretin)<br>Stimulates gastrointestinal secretion and motility<br>Stimulates gastric acid secretion and release of antral gastrin<br>Stimulates growth of intestinal mucosa and pancreas |
| Gastric inhibitory polypeptide | Duodenum, jejunum (K cells) | Glucose, fat, protein adrenergic stimulation | Inhibits gastric acid and pepsin secretion<br>Stimulates pancreatic insulin release in response to hyperglycemia |
| Motilin | Duodenum, jejunum | Gastric distention, fat | Stimulates upper gastrointestinal tract motility<br>May initiate the migrating motor complex |
| Vasoactive intestinal peptide | Neurons throughout the gastrointestinal tract | Vagal stimulation | Primarily functions as a neuropeptide<br>Potent vasodilator<br>Stimulates pancreatic and intestinal secretion<br>Inhibits gastric acid secretion |
| Neurotensin | Small bowel (N cells) | Fat | Stimulates growth of small and large bowel mucosa |
| Enteroglucagon | Small bowel (L cells) | Glucose, fat | Glucagon-like peptide-1:<br>Stimulates insulin release<br>Inhibits pancreatic glucagon release<br>Glucagon-like peptide 2:<br>Potent enterotrophic factor |
| Peptide YY | Distal small bowel, colon | Fatty acids, cholecystokinin | Inhibits gastric and pancreatic secretion<br>Inhibits gallbladder contraction |

**Table 50-4 Diagnostic and Therapeutic Uses of Gastrointestinal Hormones**

| HORMONE | DIAGNOSTIC AND THERAPEUTIC USES |
|---|---|
| Gastrin | Pentagastrin (gastrin analogue) used to measure maximal gastric acid secretion |
| Cholecystokinin | Biliary imaging of gallbladder contraction |
| Secretin | Provocative test for gastrinoma<br>Measurement of maximal pancreatic secretion |
| Glucagon | Suppresses bowel motility for endocrine spasm<br>Relieves sphincter of Oddi spasm<br>Provocative test for insulin, catecholamine, and growth hormone release |
| Somatostatin analogues | Treat carcinoid diarrhea and flushing<br>Decrease secretion from pancreatic and intestinal fistulas<br>Ameliorate symptoms associated with hormone-overproducing endocrine tumors<br>Treat esophageal variceal bleeding |

which are composed of α, β, and γ subunits, are the molecular switches for signal transduction. Agonist binding to the seven-transmembrane domain receptor is thought to cause a conformational change in the receptor that allows it to interact with the G proteins. Intracellular second messengers that can then be activated include cyclic adenosine monophosphate (cAMP), $Ca^{2+}$ cyclic guanosine monophosphate (cGMP), and inositol phosphate.

In addition to the gastrointestinal hormones, a number of other peptides and growth factors are located in the gastrointestinal mucosa, including epidermal growth factor, transforming growth factor-α and -β, insulin-like growth factor, fibroblast growth factor, and platelet-derived growth factor. These peptides play a role in cell growth and differentiation and act through tyrosine kinase receptors, which have a single membrane-spanning domain.

A third class of surface receptors, the ion channel–linked receptors, are found most commonly in cells of neuronal lineage and usually bind specific neurotransmitters. Examples include receptors for excitatory (acetylcholine and serotonin) and inhibitory (γ-aminobutyric acid, glycine) neurotransmitters. These receptors undergo a conformational change on binding of the mediator, which allows passage of ions across the cell membrane and results in changes in voltage potential.

## IMMUNE FUNCTION

During the course of a normal day, we ingest a number of bacteria, parasites, and viruses. The large surface area of the small bowel mucosa represents a potential major portal of entry for these pathogens; the small intestine serves as a major immunologic barrier in addition to its important role in digestion and endocrine function. As a result of constant antigenic exposure, the intestine possesses abundant lymphoid cells (e.g., B and T lymphocytes) and myeloid cells (e.g., macrophages, neutrophils, eosinophils, mast cells). To deal with the constant barrage of potential toxins and antigens, the gut has evolved into a highly organized and efficient mechanism for antigen processing, humoral immunity, and cellular immunity. The gut-associated lymphoid tissue is localized in three areas—Peyer patches, lamina propria lymphoid cells, and intraepithelial lymphocytes.

Peyer patches are unencapsulated lymphoid nodules that constitute an afferent limb of the gut-associated lymphoid tissue, which recognizes antigens through the specialized sampling mechanism of the microfold (M) cells contained within the follicle-associated epithelium (Fig. 50-11). Antigens that gain access to the Peyer patches activate and prime B and T cells in that site. The M cells cover the lymphoid follicles in the gastrointestinal tract and provide a site for the selective sampling of intraluminal antigens. Activated lymphocytes from intestinal lymphoid follicles then leave the intestinal tract and migrate into afferent lymphatics that drain into mesenteric lymph nodes. Furthermore, these cells migrate into the lamina propria. The B lymphocytes become surface immunoglobulin A (IgA)–bearing lymphoblasts, which serve a critically important role in mucosal immunity.

B lymphocytes and plasma cells, T lymphocytes, macrophages, dendritic cells, eosinophils, and mast cells are scattered throughout the connective tissue of the lamina propria. Approximately 60% of the lymphoid cells are T cells. These T lymphocytes are a heterogeneous group of cells and can differentiate into one of several types of T effector cells. Cytotoxic T effector cells damage the target cells directly. Helper T cells are effector cells that help mediate induction of other T cells or the induction of B cells to produce humoral antibodies. T suppressor cells perform just the opposite function. Approximately 40% of the lymphoid cells in the lamina propria are B cells, which are primarily derived from precursors in Peyer patches. These B cells and their progeny, plasma cells, are predominantly focused on IgA synthesis and, to a lesser extent, on IgM, IgG, and IgE synthesis.

The intraepithelial lymphocytes are located in the space between the epithelial cells that line the mucosal surface and lie close to the basement membrane. It is thought that most of the intraepithelial lymphocytes are T cells. On activation, the intraepithelial lymphocytes may acquire cytolytic functions that can contribute to epithelial cell death through apoptosis. These cells may be important in the immunosurveillance against abnormal epithelial cells.

As noted, one of the major protective immune mechanisms for the intestinal tract is the synthesis and secretion of IgA. The intestine contains more than 70% of the IgA-producing cells in the body. IgA is produced by plasma cells in the lamina propria and is secreted into the intestine, where it can bind antigens at the mucosal surface. The IgA antibody traverses the epithelial cell to the lumen by means of a protein carrier (the secretory component) that not only transports the IgA, but also protects it against the intracellular lysosomes. IgA does not activate complement and does not enhance cell-mediated opsonization or destruction of infectious organisms or antigens, which is in sharp contrast with the role of other immunoglobulins. Secretory IgA inhibits the adherence of bacteria to epithelial cells and prevents their colonization and multiplication. In addition, secretory IgA neutralizes bacterial toxins and viral activity and blocks the absorption of antigens from the gut.

## OBSTRUCTION

The description of patients presenting with small bowel obstruction dates back to the third or fourth century BC, when Praxagoras created an enterocutaneous fistula to relieve a bowel obstruction. Despite this success with operative therapy, the nonoperative management of these patients with attempted

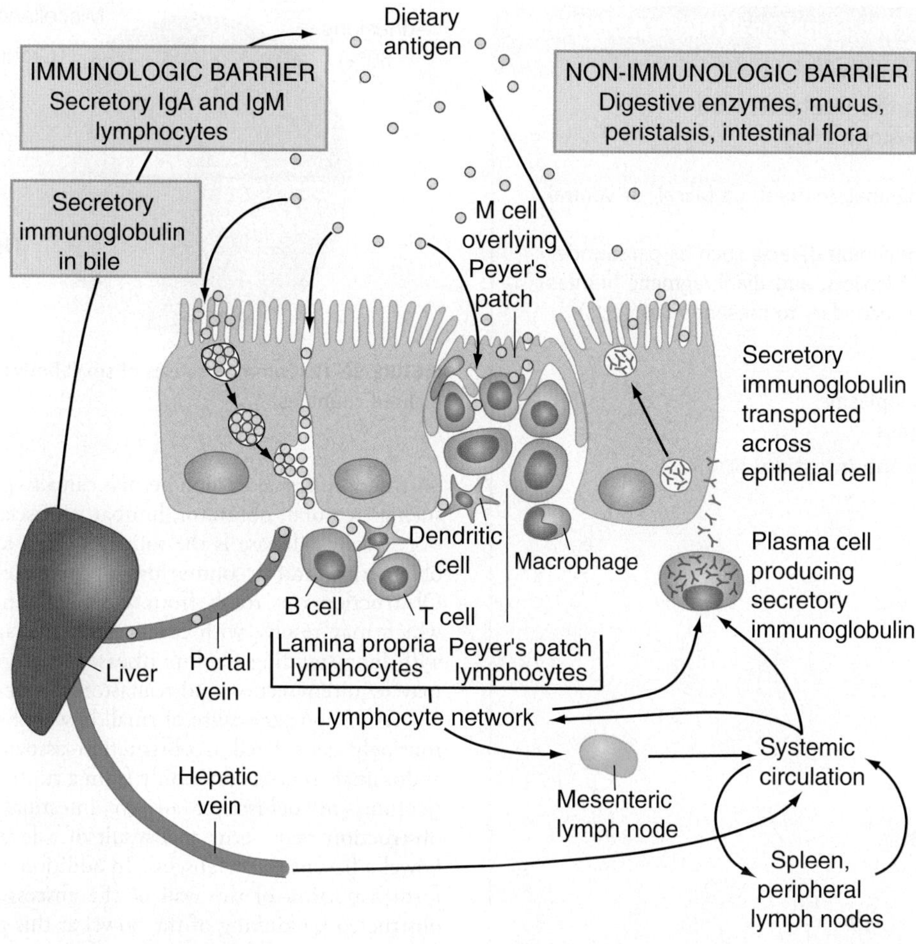


**FIGURE 50-11** Mucosal barrier of the gut. Antigens contact specialized microfold (M) cells overlying Peyer patches, which then process and present the antigen to the immune system. When B lymphocytes are stimulated by antigenic material, the cells develop into antibody-forming cells that secrete various types of immunoglobulins, the most important of which is IgA. (Adapted from Duerr RH, Shanahan F: Food allergy. In Targan SR, Shanahan F [eds]: Immunology and immunopathology of the liver and gastrointestinal tract, New York, 1990, Igaku-Shoin, p 510.)

reduction of hernias, laxatives, ingestion of heavy metals (e.g., lead, mercury), and leeches to remove toxic agents from the blood was the rule until the late 1800s, when antisepsis and aseptic surgical techniques made operative intervention safer and more acceptable. A better understanding of the pathophysiology of bowel obstruction and the use of isotonic fluid resuscitation, intestinal tube decompression, and antibiotics has greatly reduced the mortality rate for patients with a mechanical bowel obstruction. However, patients with a bowel obstruction still represent some of the most difficult and vexing problems that surgeons face with regard to correct diagnosis, optimal timing of therapy, and appropriate treatment. Ultimate clinical decisions regarding the management of these patients dictates a thorough history and workup and heightened awareness of potential complications.

## Causes

The causes of a small bowel obstruction can be divided into three categories (Box 50-1):

1. Obstruction arising from extraluminal causes (e.g., adhesions, hernias, carcinomas, abscesses)
2. Obstruction intrinsic to the bowel wall (e.g., primary tumors)
3. Intraluminal obturator obstruction (e.g., gallstones, enteroliths, foreign bodies, bezoars)

The causes of small bowel obstruction have changed dramatically since the 1900s.[5] At the turn of the 20th century, hernias accounted for more than 50% of mechanical intestinal obstructions. With the routine elective repair of hernias, this cause has dropped to the third most common cause of small bowel obstruction in industrialized countries. Adhesions secondary to previous surgery are now the most common cause of small bowel obstruction (Fig. 50-12).

Adhesions, particularly after pelvic operations (e.g., gynecologic procedures, appendectomy, colorectal resection), are responsible for more than 60% of all causes of bowel obstruction in the United States. This preponderance of lower abdominal procedures to produce adhesions that result in obstruction is thought to be caused by the fact that the bowel is more mobile in the pelvis and more tethered in the upper abdomen.

Malignant tumors account for approximately 20% of the cases of small bowel obstruction. Most of these tumors are metastatic lesions that obstruct the intestine secondary to

**BOX 50-1 Causes of Mechanical Small Intestinal Obstruction in Adults**

**Lesions Extrinsic to the Intestinal Wall**

Adhesions (usually postoperative)

Hernia

- External (e.g., inguinal, femoral, umbilical, or ventral hernias)
- Internal (e.g., congenital defects such as paraduodenal, foramen of Winslow, and diaphragmatic hernias or postoperative secondary to mesenteric defects)

Neoplastic

- Carcinomatosis
- Extraintestinal neoplasms

Intra-abdominal abscess

**Lesions Intrinsic to the Intestinal Wall**

**Congenital**

Malrotation

Duplications, cysts

**Inflammatory**

Crohn's disease

Infections

- Tuberculosis
- Actinomycosis
- Diverticulitis

**Neoplastic**

Primary neoplasms

Metastatic neoplasms

**Traumatic**

Hematoma

Ischemic stricture

**Miscellaneous**

Intussusception

Endometriosis

Radiation enteropathy/stricture

**Intraluminal, Obturator Obstruction**

Gallstone

Enterolith

Bezoar

Foreign body

Adapted from Tito WA, Sarr MG: Intestinal obstruction. In Zuidema GD (ed): Surgery of the alimentary tract, Philadelphia, 1996, WB Saunders, pp 375–416.

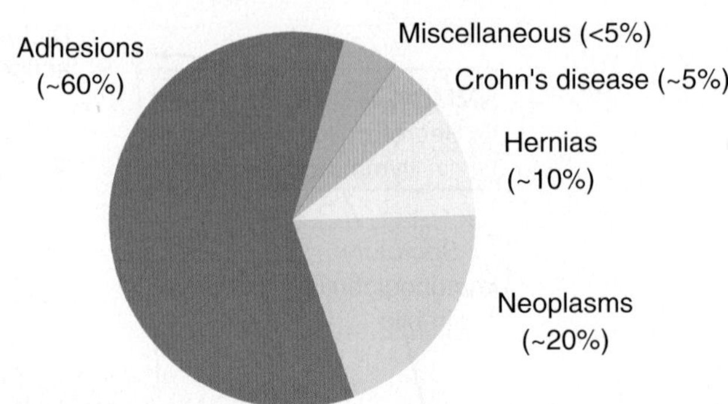


**FIGURE 50-12** Common causes of small bowel obstruction in industrialized countries.

peritoneal implants that have spread from an intra-abdominal primary tumor, such as ovarian, pancreatic, gastric, or colon cancer. Less often, malignant cells from distant sites, such as breast, lung, and melanoma, may metastasize hematogenously and account for peritoneal implants, resulting in an obstruction. Large intra-abdominal tumors may also cause small bowel obstruction through extrinsic compression of the bowel lumen. Primary colonic cancers, particularly those arising from the cecum and ascending colon, may present as a small bowel obstruction. Primary small bowel tumors can cause obstruction but are exceedingly rare.

Hernias are the third leading cause of intestinal obstruction and account for approximately 10% of all cases. Usually, these represent ventral or inguinal hernias. Internal hernias, generally related to prior abdominal surgery, can also result in small bowel obstruction. Less common hernias can also produce obstruction, such as femoral, obturator, lumbar, and sciatic hernias.

Crohn's disease is the fourth leading cause of small bowel obstruction and accounts for approximately 5% of all cases. Obstruction can result from acute inflammation and edema, which may resolve with conservative management. In patients with long-standing Crohn's disease, strictures can develop that may require resection and reanastomosis or strictureplasty.

An important cause of small bowel obstruction that is not routinely considered is obstruction associated with an intra-abdominal abscess, commonly from a ruptured appendix, diverticulum, or dehiscence of an intestinal anastomosis. The obstruction may occur as a result of a local ileus in the small bowel adjacent to the abscess. In addition, the small bowel can form a portion of the wall of the abscess cavity and become obstructed by kinking of the bowel at this point.

Miscellaneous causes of bowel obstruction account for 2% to 3% of all cases but should be considered in the differential diagnosis. These include intussusception of the bowel, which in the adult is usually secondary to a pathologic lead point, such as a polyp or tumor (Fig. 50-13), gallstones, which can enter the intestinal lumen by a cholecystenteric fistula and cause obstruction, enteroliths originating from jejunal diverticula, foreign bodies, and phytobezoars.

## Pathophysiology

Early in the course of an obstruction, intestinal motility and contractile activity increase in an effort to propel luminal contents past the obstructing point. The increase in peristalsis that occurs early in the course of bowel obstruction is present above and below the point of obstruction, thus accounting for the finding of diarrhea that may accompany partial or even complete small bowel obstruction in the early period. Later in the course of obstruction, the intestine becomes fatigued and dilates, with contractions becoming less frequent and less intense.

As the bowel dilates, water and electrolytes accumulate intraluminally and in the bowel wall itself. This massive third-space fluid loss accounts for the dehydration and hypovolemia. The metabolic effects of fluid loss depend on the site and duration of the obstruction. With a proximal obstruction, dehydration may be accompanied by hypochloremia, hypokalemia, and metabolic alkalosis associated with increased vomiting. Distal obstruction of the small bowel may result in large quantities of intestinal fluid into the bowel; however, abnormalities in serum electrolyte levels are usually less dramatic. Oliguria, azotemia,

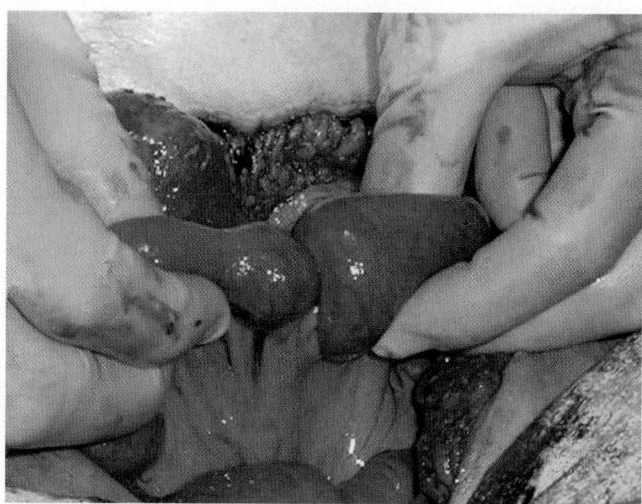

**FIGURE 50-13** Jejunojenunal intussusception in an adult patient. (Courtesy Dr. Steven Williams, Nampa, ID.)

and hemoconcentration can accompany the dehydration. Hypotension and shock can ensue. Other consequences of bowel obstruction include increased intra-abdominal pressure, decreased venous return, and elevation of the diaphragm, compromising ventilation. These factors can serve to potentiate the effects of hypovolemia further.

As the intraluminal pressure increases in the bowel, a decrease in mucosal blood flow can occur. These alterations are particularly noted in patients with a closed loop obstruction, in which greater intraluminal pressures are attained. A closed loop obstruction, produced commonly by a twist of the bowel, can progress to arterial occlusion and ischemia if left untreated and may potentially lead to bowel perforation and peritonitis.

In the absence of intestinal obstruction, the jejunum and proximal ileum are almost sterile. With obstruction, however, the flora of the small intestine changes dramatically, in both the type of organism (most commonly *Escherichia coli, Streptococcus faecalis,* and *Klebsiella* spp.) and the quantity, with organisms reaching concentrations of $10^9$ to $10^{10}$/mL. Studies have shown an increase in the number of indigenous bacteria translocating to mesenteric lymph nodes and even systemic organs. However, the overall importance of this bacterial translocation on the clinical course has not been entirely defined.

## Clinical Manifestations and Diagnosis

A thorough history and physical examination are critical to establishing the diagnosis and treatment of the patient with an intestinal obstruction. In most patients, a meticulous history and physical examination complemented by plain abdominal radiographs are all that is required to establish the diagnosis and devise a treatment plan. More sophisticated radiographic studies may be necessary in certain patients in whom the diagnosis and cause are uncertain. However, a computed tomography (CT) scan of the abdomen should not be the starting point in the workup of a patient with intestinal obstruction.

### History

The cardinal symptoms of intestinal obstruction include colicky abdominal pain, nausea, vomiting, abdominal distention, and a failure to pass flatus and feces (obstipation). These symptoms may vary with the site and duration of obstruction. The typical crampy abdominal pain associated with intestinal obstruction occurs in paroxysms at 4- to 5-minute intervals and occurs less frequently with distal obstruction. Nausea and vomiting are more common with a higher obstruction and may be the only symptoms in patients with gastric outlet or high intestinal obstruction. An obstruction located distally is associated with less emesis; the initial and most prominent symptom is the cramping abdominal pain. Abdominal distention occurs as the obstruction progresses and the proximal intestine becomes increasingly dilated. Obstipation is a later development. It must be reiterated that patients, particularly in the early stages of bowel obstruction, may relate a history of diarrhea that is secondary to increased peristalsis. Therefore, the important point to remember is that a complete bowel obstruction cannot be ruled out based on a history of loose bowel movements. The character of the vomitus is also important to obtain in the history. As the obstruction becomes more complete with bacterial overgrowth, the vomitus becomes more feculent, indicating a late and established intestinal obstruction.

### Physical Examination

The patient with intestinal obstruction may present with tachycardia and hypotension, demonstrating the severe dehydration that is present. Fever suggests the possibility of strangulation. Abdominal examination demonstrates a distended abdomen, with the amount of distention somewhat dependent on the level of obstruction. Previous surgical scars should be noted. Early in the course of bowel obstruction, peristaltic waves can be observed, particularly in thin patients, and auscultation of the abdomen may demonstrate hyperactive bowel sounds with audible rushes associated with vigorous peristalsis (borborygmi). Late in the obstructive course, minimal or no bowel sounds are noted. Mild abdominal tenderness may be present, with or without a palpable mass; however, localized tenderness, rebound, and guarding suggest peritonitis and the likelihood of strangulation. A careful examination must be performed to rule out incarcerated hernias in the groin, femoral triangle, and obturator foramen. A rectal examination should be performed to assess for intraluminal masses and to examine the stool for occult blood, which may be an indication of malignancy, intussusception, or infarction.

### Radiologic and Laboratory Studies

The diagnosis of intestinal obstruction is often immediately evident after a thorough history and physical examination. Therefore, plain radiographs usually confirm the clinical suspicion and define the site of obstruction more accurately. The accuracy of diagnosis of the small intestinal obstruction on plain abdominal radiographs is estimated to be approximately 60%, with an equivocal or a nonspecific diagnosis obtained in the remainder of cases. Characteristic findings on supine radiographs are dilated loops of small intestine, without evidence of colonic distention. Upright radiographs demonstrate multiple air-fluid levels, which often layer in a stepwise pattern (Fig. 50-14). Plain abdominal films may also demonstrate the cause of the obstruction (e.g., foreign bodies, gallstones; Fig. 50-15). In uncertain cases, or when one is unable to differentiate partial from complete obstruction, further diagnostic evaluation may be required.

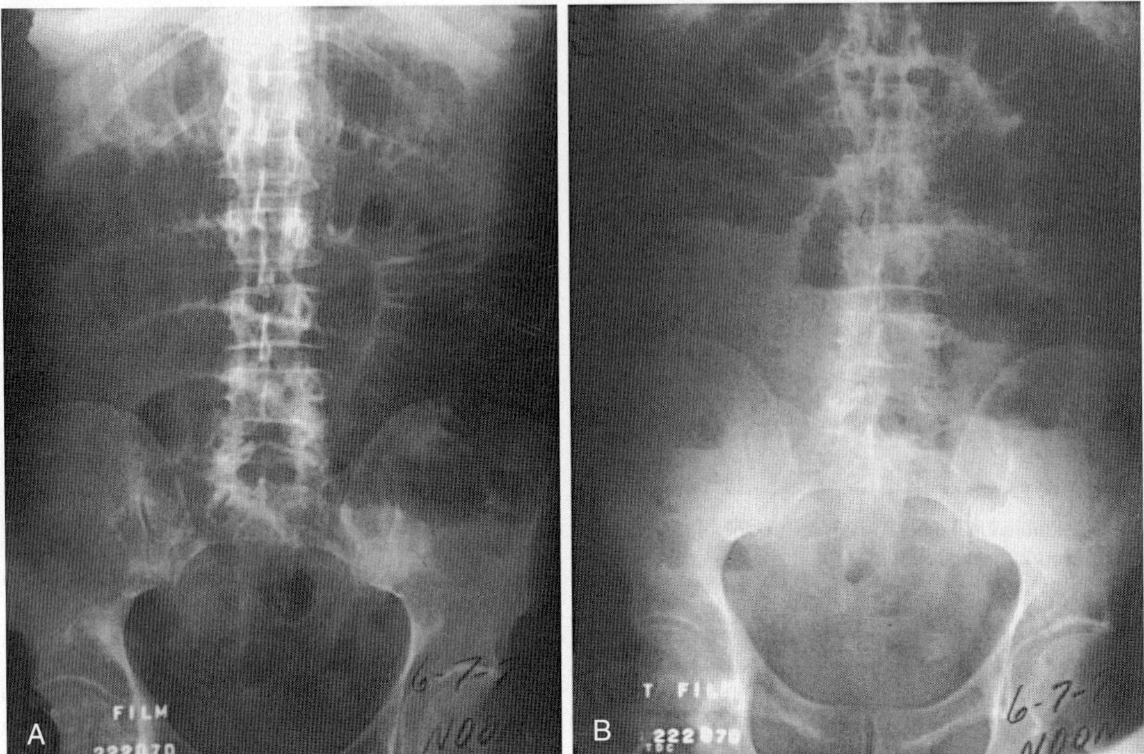


**FIGURE 50-14** Plain abdominal radiographs of a patient with a complete small bowel obstruction. **A,** Supine film shows dilated loops of small bowel in an orderly arrangement, without evidence of colonic gas. **B,** Upright film shows multiple, short air-fluid levels arranged in a stepwise pattern. (Courtesy Dr. Melvyn H. Schreiber, The University of Texas Medical Branch, Galveston, Tex.)

In the more complex patient in whom the diagnosis is not readily apparent, CT has proved to be beneficial (Fig. 50-16). CT is particularly sensitive for diagnosing complete or high-grade obstruction of the small bowel and for determining the location and cause of obstruction. The CT examination is less sensitive, however, in patients with partial small bowel obstruction.[6] In addition, CT is helpful if an extrinsic cause of bowel obstruction (e.g., abdominal tumors, inflammatory disease, or abscess) is suggested (Fig. 50-17). CT has also been described as useful for determining bowel strangulation. Unfortunately, CT findings associated with strangulation are those of irreversible ischemia and necrosis.

Barium studies have been a useful adjunct in certain patients with a presumed obstruction. In particular, enteroclysis, which involves the oral insertion of a tube into the duodenum to instill air and barium directly into the small intestine and to follow the movement fluoroscopically, has been helpful in the assessment of obstruction.[7] Enteroclysis has been advocated as the definitive study in patients for whom the diagnosis of low-grade, intermittent, small bowel obstruction is clinically uncertain. In addition, barium studies can precisely demonstrate the level of the obstruction as well as the cause of the obstruction in certain cases (Fig. 50-18). The main disadvantages of enteroclysis are the need for nasoenteric intubation, slow transit of contrast material in patients with a fluid-filled hypotonic small bowel, and enhanced expertise required by the radiologist to perform this procedure.

Ultrasound has been reported to be useful for pregnant patients because radiation exposure is a concern. Magnetic resonance imaging (MRI) has been described in patients with obstruction; however, it appears to be no better diagnostically than CT.

To summarize, plain abdominal radiographs are usually diagnostic of bowel obstruction in more than 60% of the cases, but further evaluation (possibly by CT or barium radiography) may be necessary in 20% to 30% of cases. CT examination is particularly useful in patients with a history of abdominal malignancy, postsurgical patients, and patients who have no history of abdominal surgery and present with symptoms of bowel obstruction. Barium studies are recommended for patients with a history of recurring obstruction or low-grade mechanical obstruction to define the obstructed segment and degree of obstruction precisely.

Laboratory tests are not helpful in the actual diagnosis of patients with small bowel obstruction but are extremely important in assessing the degree of dehydration. Patients with a bowel obstruction should routinely have laboratory measurements of serum sodium, chloride, potassium, bicarbonate, and creatinine levels. The serial determination of serum electrolyte levels should be performed to assess the adequacy of fluid resuscitation. Dehydration may result in hemoconcentration, as noted by an elevated hematocrit value. This should be monitored because fluid resuscitation results in a decrease in the hematocrit and some patients (e.g., those with intestinal malignancies) may require blood transfusions before surgery. In addition, the white blood cell count should be assessed. Leukocytosis may be found in patients with strangulation; however, an elevated white blood cell count does not necessarily denote strangulation. Conversely, the absence of leukocytosis does not eliminate strangulation as a possibility.

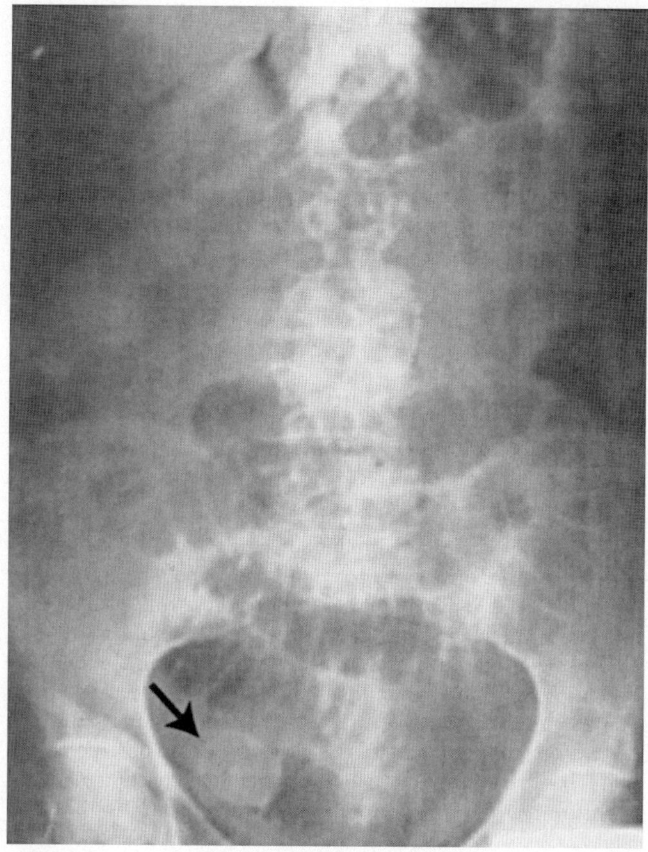

**FIGURE 50-15** Plain abdominal film shows complete bowel obstruction caused by a large radiopaque gallstone *(arrow)* obstructing the distal ileum.

## Simple Versus Strangulating Obstruction

Most patients with small bowel obstruction are classified as having simple obstructions that involve mechanical blockage of the flow of luminal contents without compromised viability of the intestinal wall. In contrast, strangulation obstruction, which usually involves a closed loop obstruction in which the vascular supply to a segment of intestine is compromised, can lead to intestinal infarction. Strangulation obstruction is associated with an increased morbidity and mortality risk, and therefore recognition of early strangulation is important. In differentiating from simple intestinal obstruction, classic signs of strangulation have been described; these include tachycardia, fever, leukocytosis, and a constant, noncramping abdominal pain. However, a number of studies have convincingly shown that no clinical parameters or laboratory measurements can accurately detect or exclude the presence of strangulation in all cases.

CT examination is useful only for detecting the late stages of irreversible ischemia (e.g., pneumatosis intestinalis, portal venous gas). Various serum determinations, including lactate dehydrogenase, amylase, alkaline phosphatase, and ammonia levels, have been assessed with no real benefit. Initial reports have described some limited success in discriminating strangulation by measuring serum D-lactate, creatine phosphokinase isoenzyme (particularly the BB isoenzyme), or intestinal fatty acid–binding protein; however, these are only investigational and cannot be widely applied to patients with obstruction. Finally, noninvasive determinations of mesenteric ischemia have been described using a superconducting quantum interference device (SQUID) magnetometer to detect mesenteric ischemia noninvasively. Intestinal ischemia is associated with changes in the basic electrical rhythm of the small intestine. This technique remains investigational and is not in widespread clinical use.

Thus, it is important to remember that bowel ischemia and strangulation cannot be reliably diagnosed or excluded preoperatively in all cases by any known clinical parameter, combination of parameters, or current laboratory and radiographic examinations.

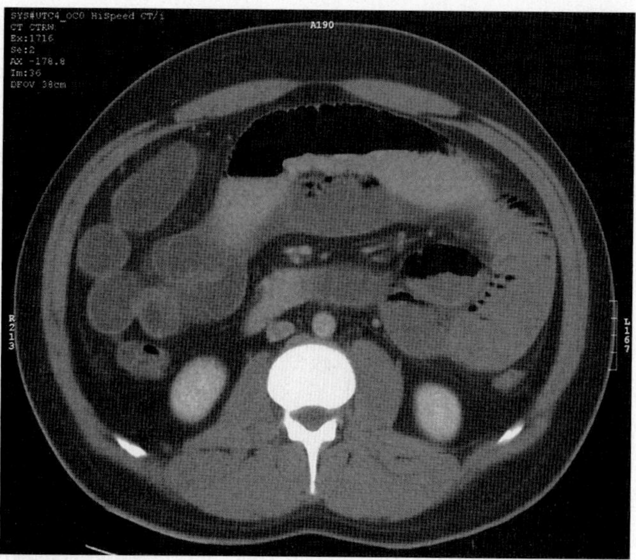

**FIGURE 50-16** CT scan through the midabdomen shows dilated small bowel loops filled with fluid and decompressed ascending and descending colon. These are typical CT findings in small bowel obstruction. (Courtesy Dr. Eric Walser, The University of Texas Medical Branch, Galveston, Tex.)

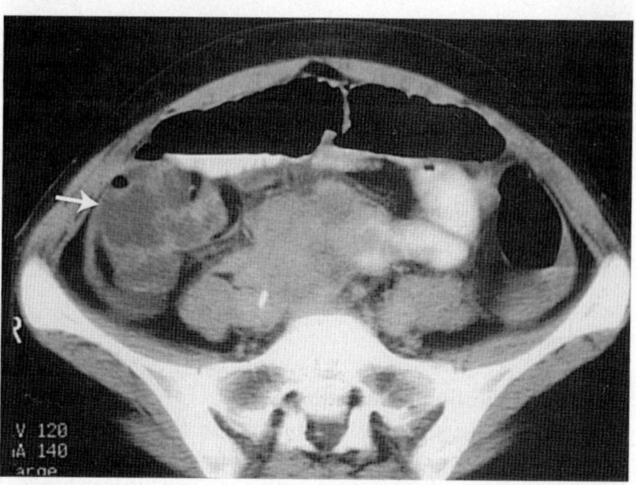


**FIGURE 50-17** CT scan of the abdomen of a patient with a mechanical bowel obstruction secondary to an abscess in the right lower quadrant *(arrow)*. Multiple dilated and fluid-filled loops of small bowel are noted. (Courtesy Dr. Melvyn H. Schreiber, The University of Texas Medical Branch, Galveston, Tex.)

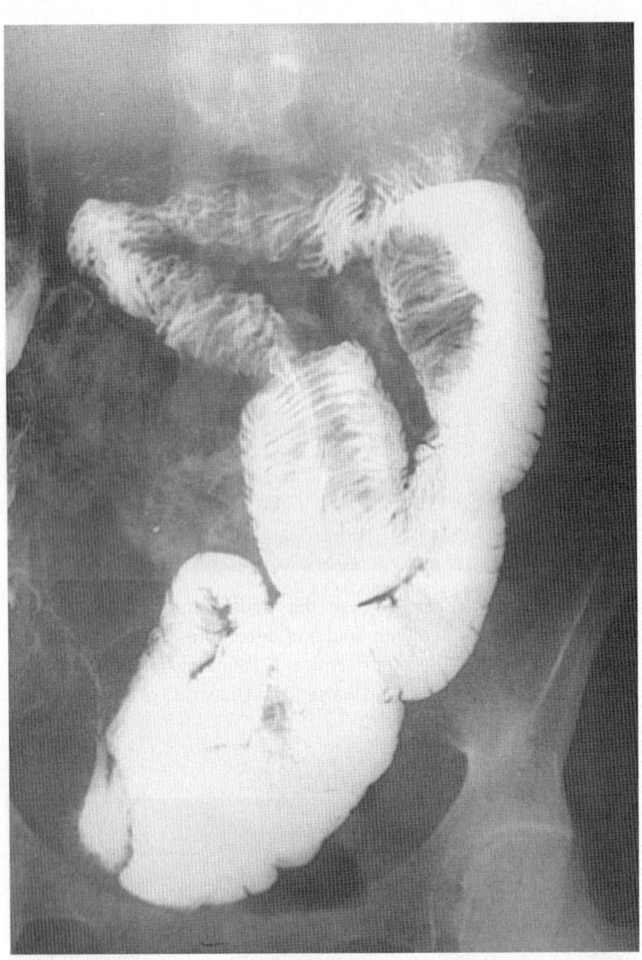

**FIGURE 50-18** Barium study demonstrates jejunojejunal intussusception. (Courtesy Dr. Melvyn H. Schreiber, The University of Texas Medical Branch, Galveston, Tex.)

## Treatment

### Fluid Resuscitation and Antibiotics

Patients with intestinal obstruction are usually dehydrated and depleted of sodium, chloride, and potassium, requiring aggressive IV replacement with an isotonic saline solution such as lactated Ringer's solution. Urine output should be monitored by the placement of a Foley catheter. After the patient has formed adequate urine, potassium chloride should be added to the infusion, if needed. Serial electrolyte level measurements, as well as hematocrit and white blood cell count, are performed to assess the adequacy of fluid repletion. Because of large fluid requirements, some patients, particularly older patients, may require central venous assessment and, in some cases, the placement of a Swan-Ganz catheter. Broad-spectrum antibiotics are given prophylactically by some surgeons based on the reported findings of bacterial translocation occurring even in simple mechanical obstructions. In addition, antibiotics are administered as a prophylaxis for possible resection or inadvertent enterotomy at surgery.

### Tube Decompression

In addition to IV fluid resuscitation, another important adjunct to the supportive care of patients with intestinal obstruction is nasogastric suction. Nasogastric suction with a Levin tube empties the stomach, reducing the hazard of pulmonary aspiration of vomitus and minimizing further intestinal distention from preoperatively swallowed air. The use of long intestinal tubes (e.g., Cantor or Baker tube) has been advocated by some. However, prospective randomized trials have demonstrated no significant differences with regard to the decompression achieved, success of nonoperative treatment, or morbidity rate after surgical intervention compared with the use of nasogastric tubes. Furthermore, the use of these long tubes has been associated with a significantly longer hospital stay, duration of postoperative ileus, and postoperative complications in some series. Therefore, it appears that long intestinal tubes offer no benefit in the preoperative setting over nasogastric tubes.

Patients with a partial intestinal obstruction may be treated conservatively with resuscitation and tube decompression alone. Resolution of symptoms and discharge without the need for surgery have been reported in 60% to 85% of patients with a partial obstruction.[5] Enteroclysis can assist in determining the degree of obstruction, with higher grade partial obstructions requiring earlier operative intervention. Although an initial trial of nonoperative management of most patients with partial small bowel obstruction is warranted, it should be emphasized that clinical deterioration of the patient or increasing small bowel distention on abdominal radiographs during tube decompression warrants prompt operative intervention. The decision to continue to treat a patient nonoperatively with a presumed bowel obstruction is based on clinical judgment and requires constant vigilance to ensure that the clinical course has not changed.

### Operative Management

In general, the patient with a complete small bowel obstruction requires operative intervention. A nonoperative approach to selected patients with complete small intestinal obstruction has been proposed by some, who argue that prolonged intubation is safe in these patients provided that no fever, tachycardia, tenderness, or leukocytosis is noted. Nevertheless, one must realize that nonoperative management of these patients is undertaken at a calculated risk of overlooking an underlying strangulation obstruction and delaying the treatment of intestinal strangulation until after the injury becomes irreversible. Retrospective studies have reported that a 12- to 24-hour delay of surgery in these patients is safe but that the incidence of strangulation and other complications increases significantly after this period.

The nature of the problem dictates the approach to management of the obstructed patient. Patients with intestinal obstruction secondary to an adhesive band may be treated with lysis of adhesions. Great care should be used in the gentle handling of the bowel to reduce serosal trauma and avoid unnecessary dissection and inadvertent enterotomies. Incarcerated hernias can be managed by manual reduction of the herniated segment of bowel and closure of the defect.

The treatment of patients with an obstruction and history of malignant tumors can be particularly challenging. In the terminal patient with widespread metastasis, nonoperative management, if successful, is usually the best course; however, only a small percentage of cases of complete obstruction can be successfully managed nonoperatively. In this case, a simple bypass of the obstructing lesion, by whatever means, may offer the best option rather than a long and complicated operation that might entail bowel resection.

An obstruction secondary to Crohn's disease will often resolve with conservative management if the obstruction is acute. If a chronic fibrotic stricture is the cause of the obstruction, a bowel resection or strictureplasty may be required.

Patients with an intra-abdominal abscess can present in a manner indistinguishable from those with mechanical bowel obstruction. CT is particularly useful in diagnosing the cause of the obstruction in these patients; percutaneous drainage of the abscess may be sufficient to relieve the obstruction.

Radiation enteropathy, as a complication of radiation therapy for pelvic malignancies, may cause bowel obstruction. Most cases can be treated nonoperatively with tube decompression and possibly corticosteroids, particularly during the acute setting. In the chronic setting, nonoperative management is rarely effective and will require laparotomy, with possible resection of the irradiated bowel or bypass of the affected area.

At the time of exploration, it can sometimes be difficult to evaluate bowel viability after the release of a strangulation. If intestinal viability is questionable, the bowel segment should be completely released and placed in a warm, saline-moistened sponge for 15 to 20 minutes and then reexamined. If normal color has returned and peristalsis is evident, it is safe to retain the bowel. A prospective controlled trial comparing clinical judgment with the use of a Doppler probe or the administration of fluorescein for the intraoperative discrimination of viability has found that the Doppler flow probe added little to the conventional clinical judgment of the surgeon. In difficult borderline cases, fluorescein fluorescence may supplement clinical judgment. Another approach to the assessment of bowel viability is the so-called *second-look laparotomy* 18 to 24 hours after the initial procedure. This decision should be made at the time of the initial operation. A second-look laparotomy is clearly indicated for a patient whose condition deteriorates after the initial operation.

Some studies have evaluated the efficacy of laparoscopic management of acute small bowel obstruction. The laparoscopic treatment of small bowel obstruction appears to be effective and leads to a shorter hospital stay in a highly selected group of patients.[8] Patients fitting the criteria for consideration of laparoscopic management include those with the following symptoms: (1) mild abdominal distention allowing adequate visualization; (2) proximal obstruction; (3) partial obstruction; and (4) anticipated single-band obstruction.

In particular, laparoscopic treatment has been found to be of greatest benefit in patients who have undergone less than three previous operations, were seen early after the onset of symptoms, and were thought to have adhesive bands as the cause. Currently, patients who have advanced, complete, or distal small bowel obstructions are not candidates for laparoscopic treatment. Unfortunately, most patients with obstruction are in this group. Similarly, patients with matted adhesions or carcinomatosis or those who remain distended after nasogastric intubation should be managed with conventional laparotomy. Therefore, the future role of laparoscopic procedures in the treatment of these patients remains to be defined.

## Management of Specific Problems

### Recurrent Intestinal Obstruction

All surgeons can readily (and most often painfully) remember the complicated patient with multiple previous abdominal operations and a frozen abdomen who presents with yet another bowel obstruction. An initial nonoperative trial is usually desirable and often safe. In those patients who do not respond conservatively, reoperation is required. This can often be a long and arduous procedure, with great care taken to prevent enterotomies. In these difficult patients, various surgical procedures and pharmacologic agents have been tried in an effort to prevent recurrent adhesions and obstruction.

External plication procedures have been described, in which the small intestine or its mesentery is sutured in large, gently curving loops. Common complications have included the development of fistulas, gross leakage, peritonitis, and death. For this reason, and because of the low overall success rate, these procedures have largely been abandoned. Several series have reported moderate success with internal fixation or stenting procedures using a long intestinal tube inserted through the nose, a gastrostomy, or even a jejunostomy and left in place for 2 weeks or longer. Complications associated with these tubes include prolonged drainage of bowel contents from the tube insertion site, intussusception, and difficult removal of the tube, which may require surgical reexploration.

Pharmacologic agents, including corticosteroids and other anti-inflammatory agents, cytotoxic drugs, and antihistamines, have been used with limited success. The use of anticoagulants, such as heparin, dextran solutions, dicumarol, and sodium citrate, has modified the extent of adhesion formation, but their side effects far outweigh their efficacy. Intraperitoneal instillation of various proteinases (e.g., trypsin, papain, pepsin), which cause enzymatic digestion of the extracellular protein matrix, has been unsuccessful. Hyaluronidase has been of questionable value and conflicting results have been obtained with fibrinolytic agents such as streptokinase, urokinase, and fibrinolytic snake venoms. In a prospective multicenter trial, the use of a hyaluronate-based, bioresorbable membrane reduced the incidence and severity of postoperative adhesion formation. Another study found that placement of this membrane reduced the severity, but not the incidence, of postoperative adhesion in patients undergoing a Hartmann procedure. Longer term, randomized studies will be required to determine the efficacy of this material to prevent adhesions and ultimately prevent bowel obstructions. This could represent a significant advance if the long-term incidence of obstruction is also shown to be reduced.

To date, the most effective means of limiting the number of adhesions is a good surgical technique, which includes the gentle handling of the bowel to reduce serosal trauma, avoidance of unnecessary dissection, exclusion of foreign material from the peritoneal cavity—the use of absorbable suture material when possible, the avoidance of excessive use of gauze sponges, and the removal of starch from gloves—adequate irrigation and removal of infectious and ischemic debris, and preservation and use of the omentum around the site of surgery or in the denuded pelvis.

### Acute Postoperative Obstruction

Small bowel obstruction that occurs in the immediate postoperative period presents a challenge in regard to diagnosis and treatment.[9] Diagnosis is often difficult because the primary symptoms of abdominal pain and nausea or emesis may be attributed to a postoperative ileus. Electrolyte deficiencies, particularly hypokalemia, can be a cause of ileus and should be corrected. Plain abdominal films are usually not helpful in distinguishing an ileus from obstruction. CT may be useful in this regard and, in particular, enteroclysis studies may be helpful in determining whether an obstruction exists and, if so, the level of the obstruction. More than 90% of early postoperative obstructions are partial and will resolve spontaneously, given ample time. Conservative management in the form of bowel rest, fluid resuscitation, electrolyte replacement, and parenteral nutrition, if necessary, is routinely successful. However, the development of complete obstruction or signs of strangulation mandates reoperative intervention. Postoperative bowel obstruction after laparoscopic surgery is more commonly associated with a definitive obstruction point such as a port site hernia or an internal hernia and should prompt a high index of suspicion for the need for operative intervention.

### Ileus

An ileus is defined as intestinal distention and the slowing or absence of passage of luminal contents without a demonstrable mechanical obstruction. An ileus can result from a number of causes, including drug induced, metabolic, neurogenic, and infectious factors (Box 50-2).

Pharmacologic agents that can produce an ileus include anticholinergic drugs, autonomic blockers, antihistamines, and various psychotropic agents, such as haloperidol and tricyclic antidepressants. One of the more common causes of drug-induced ileus in the operative patient is the use of opiates, such as morphine or meperidine. Metabolic causes of ileus are common and include hypokalemia, hyponatremia, and hypomagnesemia. Other metabolic causes include uremia, diabetic coma, and hypoparathyroidism. Neurogenic causes of an ileus include postoperative ileus, which occurs after abdominal operations. Spinal injury, retroperitoneal irritation, and orthopedic procedures on the spine or pelvis can result in an ileus. Finally, infections can result in an ileus; common infectious causes include pneumonia, peritonitis, and generalized sepsis from a nonabdominal source.

Patients often present in a manner similar to those with a mechanical small bowel obstruction. Abdominal distention, usually without the colicky abdominal pain, is the typical and most notable finding. Nausea and vomiting may occur but may also be absent. Patients with an ileus may continue to pass flatus and diarrhea, which may help distinguish these patients from those with a mechanical small bowel obstruction.

Radiologic studies may help distinguish ileus from small bowel obstruction. Plain abdominal radiographs may reveal distended small bowel as well as large bowel loops. In cases that are difficult to differentiate from obstruction, barium studies may be beneficial.

The treatment of an ileus is entirely supportive, with nasogastric decompression and IV fluids. The most effective treatment to correct the underlying condition may be aggressive treatment of the sepsis, correction of any metabolic or electrolyte abnormalities, and discontinuation of medications that may produce an ileus. Pharmacologic agents have been used but, for the most part, have been ineffective. Drugs that block sympathetic input (e.g., guanethidine) or stimulate parasympathetic activity (e.g., bethanechol, neostigmine) have been tried. In addition, hormonal manipulation, using cholecystokinin or motilin, has been evaluated, but the results have been inconsistent. IV erythromycin has been ineffective and cisapride, although apparently beneficial in stimulating gastric motility, does not appear to alter intestinal ileus.

**BOX 50-2 Causes of Ileus**

- After laparotomy
- Metabolic and electrolyte derangements (e.g., hypokalemia, hyponatremia, hypomagnesemia, uremia, diabetic coma)
- Drugs (e.g., opiates, psychotropic agents, anticholinergic agents)
- Intra-abdominal inflammation
- Retroperitoneal hemorrhage or inflammation
- Intestinal ischemia
- Systemic sepsis

Adapted from Turnage RH, Bergen PC: Intestinal obstruction and ileus. In Feldman M, Scharschmidt FG, Sleisenger MH (eds): Gastrointestinal and liver diseases: Pathophysiology, diagnosis, management, Philadelphia, 1998, WB Saunders, pp 1799–1810.

## INFLAMMATORY DISEASES

### Crohn's Disease

Crohn's disease is a chronic, transmural inflammatory disease of the gastrointestinal tract for which the cause is unknown. Crohn's disease can involve any part of the alimentary tract from the mouth to the anus but most commonly affects the small intestine and colon. The most common clinical manifestations are abdominal pain, diarrhea, and weight loss. Crohn's disease can be complicated by intestinal obstruction or localized perforation with fistula formation. Medical and surgical treatments are palliative; however, operative therapy can provide effective symptomatic relief for patients with complications from Crohn's disease and produces a reasonable long-term benefit.

#### History

The first documented case of Crohn's disease was described by Morgagni in 1761. In 1913, the Scottish surgeon Dalziel described nine cases of intestinal inflammatory disease. However, it is the landmark paper by Crohn and colleagues in 1932 that provided, in eloquent detail, the pathologic and clinical findings of this inflammatory disease in young adults.[10] This classic paper crystallized the description of this inflammatory condition. Although many different and sometimes misleading) terms have been used to describe this disease process, Crohn's disease has been universally accepted as its name.

#### Incidence and Epidemiology

Crohn's disease is the most common primary surgical disease of the small bowel, with an annual incidence of three to seven cases/100,000 of the general population; the incidence is highest in North America and Northern Europe.[11] Crohn's disease primarily attacks young adults in the second and third decades of life. However, a bimodal distribution is apparent, with a second smaller peak occurring in the sixth decade of life. Crohn's disease is more common in urban dwellers and, although earlier reports suggested a somewhat higher female predominance, the two genders are affected equally. The risk for developing Crohn's disease is about twice as high in smokers as in nonsmokers. Several studies have indicated an increased incidence of Crohn's disease in women using oral contraceptives; however, more recent studies have shown no differences. Although Crohn's disease is uncommon in African blacks, blacks in the United

States have rates similar to whites. Certain ethnic groups, particularly Jews, have a greater incidence of Crohn's disease than age- and gender-matched control subjects. There is a strong familial association, with the risk for developing Crohn's disease increased about 30-fold in siblings and 14- to 15-fold for all first-degree relatives. Other analyses supporting a genetic role for Crohn's disease have shown a concordance rate of 67% in monozygotic twins.

### Causes

The causes of Crohn's disease remain unknown. A number of potential causes have been proposed, with the most likely possibilities being infectious, immunologic, and genetic.[11,12] Other possibilities that have met with various levels of enthusiasm include environmental and dietary factors, smoking, and psychosocial factors. Although these latter factors may contribute to the overall disease process, it is unlikely that they represent the primary causative mechanism for Crohn's disease.

**Infectious Agents** Although a number of infectious agents have been proposed as potential causes of Crohn's disease, the two that have received the most attention are mycobacterial infections, particularly *Mycobacterium paratuberculosis,* and the measles virus. The existence of atypical mycobacteria as a cause for Crohn's disease was proposed by Dalziel in 1913. Subsequent studies using polymerase chain reaction (PCR) techniques have confirmed the presence of mycobacteria in intestinal samples of patients with Crohn's disease. Transplantation of tissue from patients with Crohn's disease has resulted in ileitis, but antimicrobial therapy directed against mycobacteria has not been effective in ameliorating the disease process.

**Immunologic Factors** Immunologic abnormalities that have been demonstrated in patients with Crohn's disease have included humoral and cell-mediated immune reactions directed against intestinal cells, suggesting an autoimmune phenomenon. Attention has focused on the role of cytokines, such as interleukin (IL)-1, IL-2, IL-8, and TNF-$\alpha$, as contributing factors in the intestinal inflammatory response. The role of the immune response remains controversial in Crohn's disease and may represent an effect of the disease process rather than an actual cause.

**Genetic Factors** Genetic factors play an important role in the pathogenesis of Crohn's disease because the single strongest risk factor for developing disease is having a first-degree relative with Crohn's disease. European and American studies have reported the presence of a locus on chromosome 16q, the *IBD1* locus.[13,14] Independent investigative groups have identified the *IBD1* locus as the *CARD15/NOD2* gene, a member of the CED4/APAF1 superfamily of apoptosis regulatory proteins, which mediates the innate immune response to microbial pathogens, leading to nuclear factor- κB (NF-κB) activation. Individuals with allelic variants of *CARD15/NOD2* have a 40-fold relative risk for Crohn's disease compared with the general population; the *IBD1* locus appears to be relatively specific for Crohn's disease and not ulcerative colitis. Other inflammatory bowel disease genomic regions include *IBD2* on chromosome 12q (observed more in ulcerative colitis) and *IBD3,* containing the major histocompatibility complex region located on chromosome 6p. Putative *IBD* loci have been identified on chromosomes 5q, 19p, 7q, and 3p.

Even with strong evidence for a genetic link to Crohn's disease, it is worth reiterating that there is a substantially less than 100% concordance rate between monozygotic twins, suggesting that simple mendelian inheritance cannot account for the pattern of occurrence. Therefore, it is likely that multiple causes (e.g., environmental factors) contribute to the cause and pathogenesis of this disease.

### Pathology

The most common sites of occurrence of Crohn's disease are the small intestine and colon. The involvement of the large and small intestine has been noted in about 55% of patients. Thirty percent of patients present with small bowel disease alone and, in 15%, the disease appears limited to the large intestine. The disease process is discontinuous and segmental. In patients with colonic disease, rectal sparing is characteristic of Crohn's disease and helps distinguish it from ulcerative colitis. Perirectal and perianal involvement occurs in about one third of patients with Crohn's disease, particularly those with colonic involvement. Crohn's disease can also involve the mouth, esophagus, stomach, duodenum, and appendix. Involvement of these sites can accompany disease in the small or large intestine, but in only rare cases have these locations been the only apparent sites of involvement.

**Gross Pathologic Features** At exploration, thickened grayish-pink or dull purple-red loops of bowel are noted, with areas of thick gray-white exudate or fibrosis of the serosa. Areas of diseased bowel separated by areas of grossly appearing normal bowel, called *skip areas,* are commonly encountered. A striking finding of Crohn's disease is extensive fat wrapping caused by the circumferential growth of the mesenteric fat around the bowel wall (Fig. 50-19). As the disease progresses, the bowel wall becomes increasingly thickened, firm, rubbery, and almost incompressible. The uninvolved proximal bowel may be dilated secondary

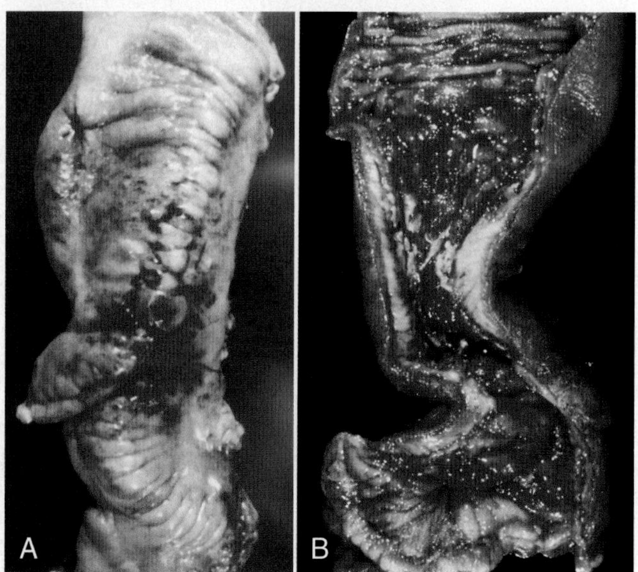


**FIGURE 50-19** Gross pathologic features of Crohn's disease. **A,** Serosal surface demonstrates extensive fat wrapping and inflammation. **B,** Resected specimen demonstrates marked fibrosis of the intestinal wall, stricture, and segmental mucosal inflammation. (Courtesy Dr. Mary R. Schwartz, Baylor College of Medicine, Houston.)

to obstruction of the diseased segment. Involved segments often are adherent to adjacent intestinal loops or other viscera, with internal fistulas common in these areas. The mesentery of the involved segment is usually thickened, with enlarged lymph nodes often noted.

On opening the bowel, the earliest gross pathologic lesion is a superficial aphthous ulcer noted in the mucosa. As the disease progresses, the ulceration becomes pronounced, and complete transmural inflammation results. The ulcers are characteristically linear and may coalesce to produce transverse sinuses with islands of normal mucosa in between, thus giving the characteristic cobblestone appearance.

**Microscopic Features** Mucosal and submucosal edema may be noted microscopically before any gross changes. A chronic inflammatory infiltrate appears in the mucosa and submucosa and extends transmurally. This inflammatory reaction is characterized by extensive edema, hyperemia, lymphangiectasia, an intense infiltration of mononuclear cells, and lymphoid hyperplasia. Characteristic histologic lesions of Crohn's disease are noncaseating granulomas with Langerhans' giant cells. Granulomas appear later in the course and are found in the wall of the bowel or in regional lymph nodes in 60% to 70% of patients (Fig. 50-20).

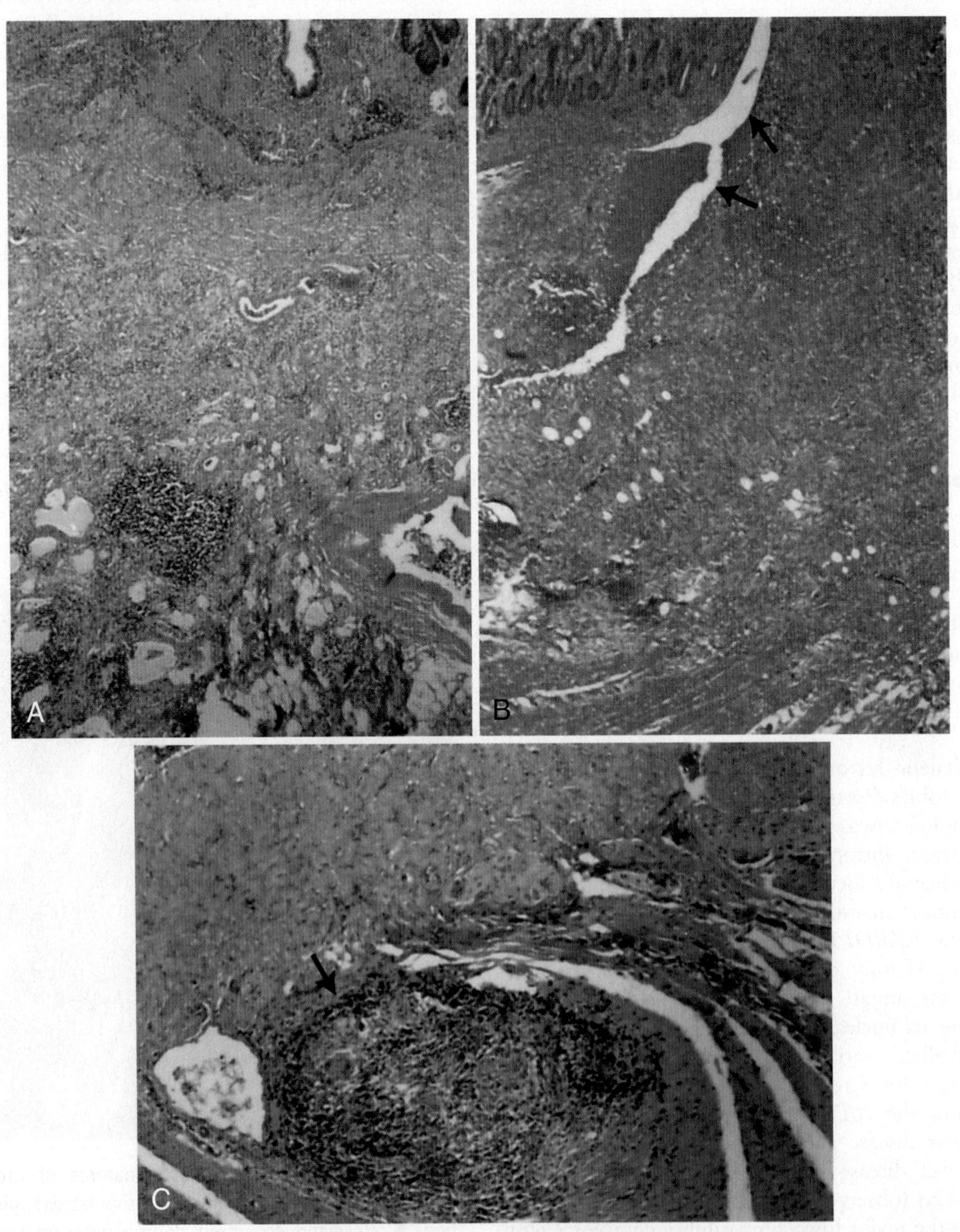


**FIGURE 50-20** Microscopic features of Crohn's disease. **A,** Transmural inflammation. **B,** Fissure ulcer *(arrows)*. **C,** Noncaseating granuloma located in the muscular layer of the small bowel *(arrow)*. (Courtesy Dr. Mary R. Schwartz, Baylor College of Medicine, Houston.)

**Clinical Manifestations**

Crohn's disease can occur at any age, but the typical patient is a young adult in the second or third decade of life. The onset of disease is often insidious, with a slow and protracted course. Characteristically, there are symptomatic periods of abdominal pain and diarrhea interspersed with asymptomatic periods of varying lengths. With time, the symptomatic periods gradually become more frequent, more severe, and longer lasting. The most common symptom is intermittent and colicky abdominal pain, most commonly noted in the lower abdomen. The pain, however, may be more severe and localized and may mimic the signs and symptoms of acute appendicitis. Diarrhea is the next most frequent symptom and is present, at least intermittently, in about 85% of patients. In contrast to ulcerative colitis, patients with Crohn's disease typically have fewer bowel movements, and the stools rarely contain mucus, pus, or blood. Systemic nonspecific symptoms include a low-grade fever, present in about one third of the patients, weight loss, loss of strength, and malaise.

Clinically, Crohn's disease is often classified based on its age of onset, behavior, and site of origin. The Vienna Classification (Table 50-5) divides all patients into 24 distinct categories based on symptom onset (before or after age 40), disease behavior (nonstricturing-nonpenetrating, stricturing, or penetrating), and disease site (terminal ileum, colon, ileocolon, upper gastrointestinal tract). This classification was developed to provide a reproducible staging of the disease to help predict remission and relapse and direct therapy. The main intestinal complications of Crohn's disease include obstruction and perforation. Obstruction can occur as a manifestation of an acute exacerbation of active disease or as the result of chronic fibrosing lesions, which eventually narrow the lumen of the bowel, producing partial or near-complete obstruction. Free perforations into the peritoneal cavity leading to a generalized peritonitis can occur in patients with Crohn's disease, but this presentation is rare. More commonly, fistulas occur between the sites of perforation and adjacent organs, such as loops of small and large intestine, urinary bladder, vagina, stomach, and sometimes the skin, usually at the site of a previous laparotomy. Localized abscesses can occur near the sites of perforation. Patients with Crohn's colitis may develop toxic megacolon and present with a marked colonic dilation, abdominal tenderness, fever, and leukocytosis. Bleeding is typically indolent and chronic, but occasionally massive GI bleeding can occur, particularly in duodenal Crohn's disease associated with chronic ulcer formation.

Long-standing Crohn's disease predisposes to cancer of the small intestine and colon.[15] The relative risk for adenocarcinoma of the small bowel in Crohn's disease is at least 100-fold greater than in matched control subjects. These carcinomas typically arise at sites of chronic disease and more commonly occur in the ileum. Most are not detected until the advanced stages, and prognosis is poor. Although this relative risk for small bowel cancer in Crohn's disease is high, the absolute risk is still small. Of greater concern is the development of colorectal cancer in patients with colonic involvement and a long duration of disease. Although the cancer risk is lower in Crohn's disease than in patients with extensive ulcerative colitis, evidence has indicated that with the same duration and anatomic extent of disease, the risk for cancer in Crohn's disease of the colon is at least as great as that in ulcerative colitis. Dysplasia is the putative precursor lesion for Crohn's-associated cancer. Although the dysplasia-carcinoma sequence has not been as extensively studied in Crohn's disease compared with ulcerative colitis, patients with long-standing Crohn's disease should have an equally aggressive colonoscopic surveillance regimen as patients with extensive ulcerative colitis. Extraintestinal cancer, such as squamous cell carcinoma of the vulva and anal canal and Hodgkin's and non-Hodgkin's lymphomas, may be more frequent in patients with Crohn's disease.

Perianal disease (fissure, fistula, stricture, or abscess) is common and occurs in 25% of patients with Crohn's disease limited to the small intestine, 41% of patients with ileocolitis, and 48% of patients with colonic involvement alone. Perianal disease may be the sole presenting feature in 5% of patients and may precede the onset of intestinal disease by months or even years. Crohn's disease should be suspected in any patient with multiple, chronic perianal fistulas.

Extraintestinal manifestations of Crohn's disease may be present in 30% of patients (Box 50-3). The most common symptoms are skin lesions, which include erythema nodosum

**Table 50-5 Vienna Classification of Crohn's Disease**

| | |
|---|---|
| Age at diagnosis (yr) | A1: <40<br>A2: ≥40 |
| Behavior | B1: Nonstricturing, nonpenetrating<br>B2: Stricturing<br>B3: Penetrating |
| Location | L1: Terminal ileum<br>L2: Colon<br>L3: Ileocolon<br>L4: Upper gastrointestinal tract |

**BOX 50-3 Extraintestinal Manifestations of Crohn's Disease**

Skin
- Erythema multiforme
- Erythema nodosum
- Pyoderma gangrenosum

Eyes
- Iritis
- Uveitis
- Conjunctivitis

Joints
- Peripheral arthritis
- Ankylosing spondylitis

Blood
- Anemia
- Thrombocytosis
- Phlebothrombosis
- Arterial thrombosis

Liver
- Nonspecific triaditis
- Sclerosing cholangitis

Kidney
- Nephrotic syndrome
- Amyloidosis

Pancreas
- Pancreatitis

General
- Amyloidosis

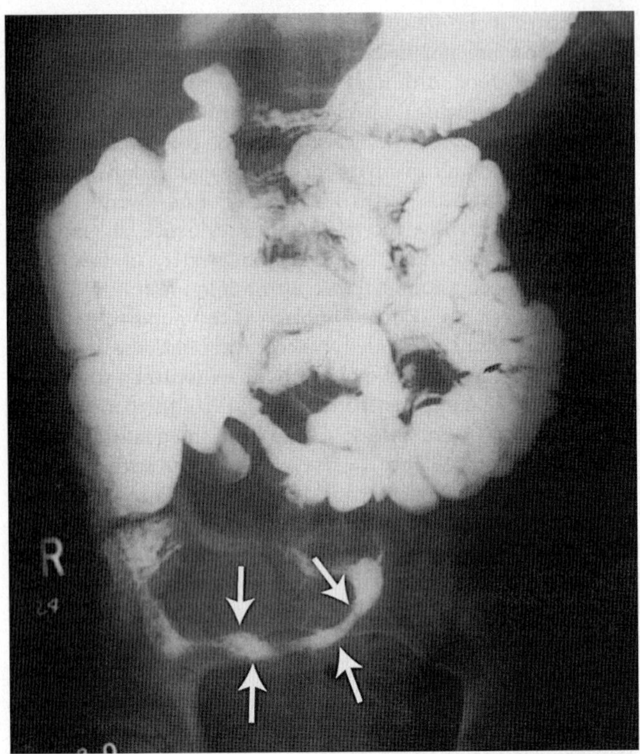


**FIGURE 50-21** Small bowel series in a patient with Crohn's disease demonstrates a narrowed distal ileum *(arrows)* secondary to chronic inflammation and fibrosis. (Courtesy Dr. Melvyn H. Schreiber, The University of Texas Medical Branch, Galveston, Tex.)

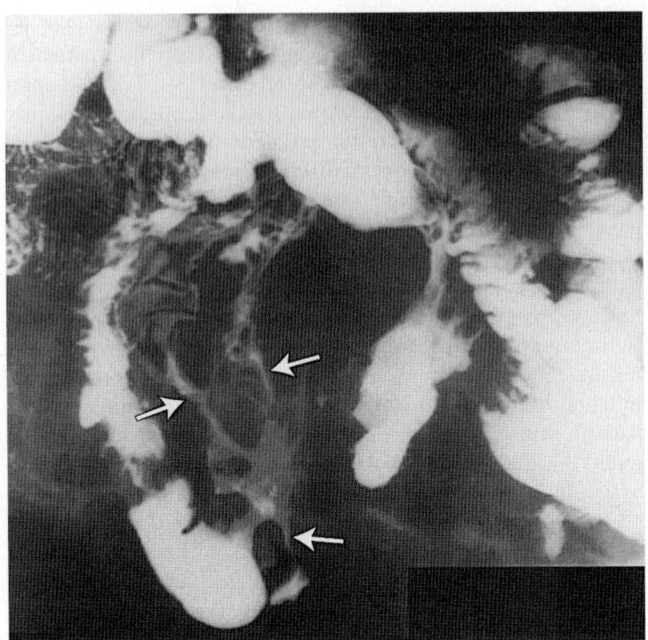

**FIGURE 50-22** Crohn's disease with multiple short fistulous tracts communicating between the distal loops of ileum and the proximal colon *(arrows).* (Courtesy Dr. Melvyn H. Schreiber, The University of Texas Medical Branch, Galveston, Tex; adapted from Evers BM, Townsend CM Jr, Thompson JC: Small intestine. In Schwartz SI [ed]: Principles of surgery, ed 7, New York, 1999, McGraw-Hill, p 1233.)

and pyoderma gangrenosum, arthritis and arthralgias, uveitis and iritis, hepatitis and pericholangitis, and aphthous stomatitis. In addition, amyloidosis, pancreatitis, and nephrotic syndrome may occur in these patients. These symptoms may precede, accompany, or appear independently of the underlying bowel disease.

## Diagnosis

A diagnosis of Crohn's disease should be considered in patients with chronic recurring episodes of abdominal pain, diarrhea, and weight loss. Typically, the diagnostic modalities most commonly used include barium contrast studies and endoscopy. Barium radiographic studies of the small bowel reveal a number of characteristic findings, including a cobblestone appearance of the mucosa composed of linear ulcers, transverse sinuses, and clefts. Long lengths of narrowed terminal ileum (Kantor's string sign) may be present in long-standing disease (Fig. 50-21). Segmental and irregular patterns of bowel involvement may be noted. Fistulas between adjacent bowel loops and organs may be apparent (Fig. 50-22).

CT may be useful in demonstrating the marked transmural thickening and it can also greatly aid in diagnosing extramural complications of Crohn's disease (Fig. 50-23). Ultrasonography has limited value in the evaluation of patients with Crohn's disease, but is useful in the assessment of undiagnosed right lower quadrant pain. When the colon is involved, sigmoidoscopy or colonoscopy may reveal characteristic aphthous ulcers with granularity and a normal-appearing surrounding mucosa. With more progressive and severe disease, the ulcerations involve

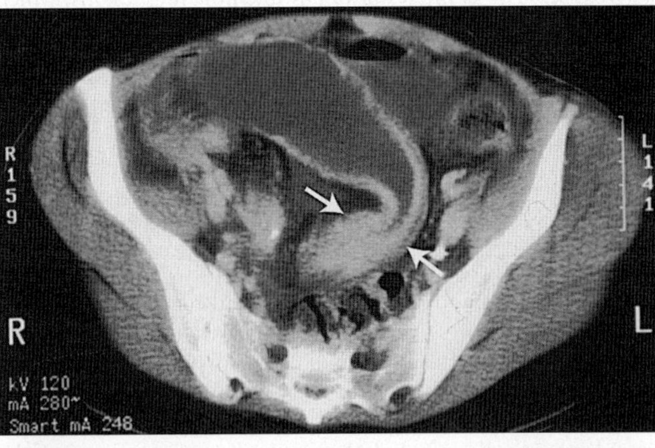


**FIGURE 50-23** CT scan of a patient with Crohn's disease demonstrates marked thickening of the bowel *(arrows)* with a high-grade partial small bowel obstruction and dilated proximal intestine. (Courtesy Dr. Melvyn H. Schreiber, The University of Texas Medical Branch, Galveston, Tex; adapted from Evers BM, Townsend CM Jr, Thompson JC: Small intestine. In Schwartz SI [ed]: Principles of surgery, ed 7, New York, 1999, McGraw-Hill, p 1233.)

more and more of the bowel lumen and may be difficult to distinguish from ulcerative colitis. However, the presence of discrete ulcers and cobblestoning, as well as the discontinuous segments of involved bowel, favors a diagnosis of Crohn's disease. Intubation of the ileocecal valve during colonoscopy allows examination and biopsy of the terminal ileum. Serologic markers may also be useful in the diagnosis of Crohn's disease. In particular, perinuclear antineutrophil cytoplasmic antibody (pANCA) and anti-*Saccharomyces cerevisiae* (ASCA) are two autoantibodies associated with inflammatory bowel disease. A large cohort study reported a specificity of 92% for Crohn's disease in patients who were ASCA-positive, pANCA-negative and of 98% for ulcerative colitis in patients who were ASCA-negative, pANCA-positive.

The differential diagnosis of Crohn's disease includes specific and nonspecific causes of intestinal inflammation. Bacterial inflammation, such as that caused by *Salmonella* and *Shigella,* intestinal tuberculosis, and protozoan infections, such as amebiasis, may present as an ileitis. In the immunocompromised host, rare infections, particularly mycobacterial and cytomegaloviral, have become more common and may cause ileitis. Acute distal ileitis may be a manifestation of early Crohn's disease, but it also may be unrelated, such as when it is caused by a bacteriologic agent (e.g., *Campylobacter, Yersinia*). Patients usually present in a similar fashion to those presenting with acute appendicitis with a sudden onset of right lower quadrant pain, nausea, vomiting, and fever. These entities normally resolve spontaneously and, when noted during surgery, no biopsy or resection should be performed.

In most cases, Crohn's disease of the colon can be readily distinguished from ulcerative colitis; however, in 5% to 10% of patients, the delineation between Crohn's and ulcerative colitis may be difficult, if not impossible, to make (Table 50-6). Ulcerative colitis almost always involves the rectum most severely, with lessening inflammation from the rectum to the ileocolic area. In contrast, Crohn's disease may be worse on the right side of the colon than on the left side, and sometimes the rectum is spared. Ulcerative colitis also demonstrates continuous involvement from rectum to proximal segments, whereas Crohn's disease is segmental. Although ulcerative colitis involves the mucosa of the large intestine, it does not extend deep into the wall of the bowel, as does Crohn's disease. Bleeding is a more common symptom in ulcerative colitis. Perianal involvement and rectovaginal fistulas are unusual in ulcerative colitis but are more common in Crohn's disease. Other endoscopic features of Crohn's disease are skip lesions, asymmetrical involvement of bowel, and the cobblestone appearance that results from ulcerations interspersed with islands of edematous mucosa.

**Table 50-6 Diagnosis of Crohn's Colitis Versus Ulcerative Colitis**

| PARAMETER | CROHN'S COLITIS | ULCERATIVE COLITIS |
|---|---|---|
| **Symptoms and Signs** | | |
| Diarrhea | Common | Common |
| Rectal bleeding | Less common | Almost always |
| Abdominal pain (cramps) | Moderate to severe | Mild to moderate |
| Palpable mass | At times | No (unless large cancer) |
| Anal complaints | Frequent (>50%) | Infrequent (<20%) |
| **Radiologic Findings** | | |
| Ileal disease | Common | Rare (backwash ileitis) |
| Nodularity, fuzziness | No | Yes |
| Distribution | Skip areas | Rectum extending upward and continuously |
| Ulcers | Linear, cobblestone, fissures | Collar-button |
| Toxic dilation | Rare | Uncommon |
| **Proctoscopic Findings** | | |
| Anal fissure, fistula, abscess | Common | Rare |
| Rectal sparing | Common (50%) | Rare (5%) |
| Granular mucosa | No | Yes |
| Ulceration | Linear, deep, scattered | Superficial, universal |

## Management

**Medical Therapy** There is no cure for Crohn's disease, so medical and surgical therapy are mainly palliative, directed toward relieving acute exacerbations or complications of the disease.[16,17] Drugs that have demonstrated efficacy in the induction and maintenance of remission include aminosalicylates (e.g., sulfasalazine, mesalamine), corticosteroids, immunosuppressive agents (e.g., azathioprine, 6-mercaptopurine, methotrexate), antibiotics, and infliximab (an anti–TNF-α antibody). Other innovative therapies based on selective molecular targets are currently being investigated.

***Aminosalicylate*** Sulfasalazine (Azulfidine), an aminosalicylate, is the most commonly prescribed drug for Crohn's disease. The active moiety of sulfasalazine is 5-aminosalicylic acid. Sulfasalazine is taken orally and has been shown in randomized controlled trials to be efficacious in patients with Crohn's disease. Although a clear benefit has been noted in patients with colonic involvement, the effectiveness of sulfasalazine alone in the treatment of Crohn's disease limited to the small bowel is controversial. In contrast to its use in ulcerative colitis, sulfasalazine has not been conclusively proven to maintain remission in Crohn's disease or to prevent recurrence after surgery. Newer sulfasalazine-like drugs (e.g., mesalamine) that provide for a slow release of 5-aminosalicylic acid during their passage through the small bowel and colon are being evaluated. Clinical trials have demonstrated efficacy of mesalamine at a dosage of 4 g/day without an increase in side effects. Despite a more predictable delivery to the small intestine and proximal colon as compared with sulfasalazine, mesalamine has not consistently been shown to induce remission in mild to moderate disease. Furthermore, although mesalamine has shown some efficacy as a postoperative maintenance strategy, its effectiveness after a medically induced remission has been questioned.[17] Studies are being conducted to evaluate even higher dosages. Nevertheless, given its reasonable side effect profile, mesalamine remains first-line therapy for Crohn's disease.

***Corticosteroids*** Corticosteroids, particularly prednisone, have been beneficial in the induction of remission in active Crohn's disease but are ineffective in maintaining remission in Crohn's disease. Newer corticosteroids have been evaluated, of which budesonide has been found to be the most promising. Budesonide has a high first-pass hepatic metabolism, which allows for targeted delivery to the intestine while mitigating the systemic effects of steroid therapy.[17] In one study, high-dose budesonide was more effective than placebo in achieving remission in patients with active Crohn's disease. Although the combination of sulfasalazine and corticosteroids may be used to maintain patients for short periods after resolution of an acute inflammatory exacerbation, the long-term use of these compounds, alone or in combination, has not been shown to be of benefit in preventing recurrence of disease. Given a relatively good response to mesalamine and its relative safety, budesonide may be considered as an alternative to mesalamine as first-line therapy for patients with active Crohn's disease.

***Antibiotics*** Certain antibiotics have also been found to be effective in the primary therapy of Crohn's disease.[18] The antibiotic used most is metronidazole, which has been shown in some studies to result in significant improvement in disease activity. Other antibiotics that have been used with varying success include ciprofloxacin, tetracycline, ampicillin, and clindamycin. Antibiotic therapy has a clear role in the septic complications associated with Crohn's disease and is beneficial in perianal disease. The mechanism of action of antibiotics in Crohn's disease is unclear, and side effects of these antibiotics preclude their long-term use. Therefore, antibiotics may play an adjunctive role in the treatment of Crohn's disease and, in selected patients, may be useful in treating perianal disease, enterocutaneous fistulas, or active colonic disease.

***Immunosuppressive Agents*** The immunosuppressive agents azathioprine and 6-mercaptopurine are effective in the treatment of Crohn's disease. Despite their potential toxicity, these drugs have proved to be relatively safe in these patients; the most common side effects include pancreatitis, hepatitis, fever, and rash. The most disconcerting implications of these immunosuppressants are bone marrow suppression and the potential for malignancy. Other immunosuppressive agents that have been used with some effectiveness include methotrexate, cyclosporine, and tacrolimus (FK-506). Tacrolimus inhibits the production of IL-2 by helper T cells and was found to be effective for fistula improvement, but not fistula remission, in patients with perianal Crohn's disease.

***Anticytokine and Cytokine Therapies*** The most promising therapy to emerge in recent years could be the introduction of immunomodulatory treatments using cytokines and anticytokines. Monoclonal antibodies to TNF-$\alpha$ have shown promise, with clinical trials demonstrating a rapid control of active Crohn's disease, tissue healing, and potential remission. A randomized controlled trial has demonstrated that infliximab, a chimeric monoclonal antibody to TNF-$\alpha$, is efficacious and safe in the treatment of moderate to severe Crohn's disease and resulted in fistula closure in 46% of patients compared with only 13% of patients receiving placebo.[19] Recently, randomized trials have confirmed that infliximab maintenance therapy is superior to episodic delivery based on exacerbations and potentiates the benefit of azathioprine maintenance therapy. Infliximab appears to have activity in the treatment of the extraintestinal manifestations of Crohn's disease as well.[16,17] Although highly effective in certain Crohn's patients with penetrating disease and extraintestinal disease, not every patient responds to infliximab. Also, there is an increased risk for tuberculosis reactivation, invasive fungal and other opportunistic infections, demyelinating central nervous system lesions, activation of latent multiple sclerosis, and exacerbating congestive heart disease.[20] Promising results have also been obtained using the anti-inflammatory cytokine IL-10. A multicenter randomized trial found that IL-10 demonstrated significant improvement in the clinical status in 46% of patients with Crohn's disease compared with 19% of placebo control subjects.

***Novel Therapies*** Other investigational therapeutic agents include IL-1 receptor antagonists, anti–IL-12, anti–IL-18, and anti–interferon-$\gamma$ antibodies, anti–adhesion molecule antibodies, and growth factors. Compounds are also being evaluated that block certain signaling pathways (e.g., NF-$\kappa$B, mitogen-activated protein [MAP] kinases, and proliferator-activated receptor-$\gamma$ [PPAR-$\gamma$]); in limited studies, some of these compounds have shown clinical improvements.[21] One trial has also been reported using natalizumab, a recombinant humanized monoclonal antibody against $\alpha_4$-integrin, with efficacy in reducing signs and symptoms of Crohn's disease that was at least similar to that of infliximab.

**Nutritional Therapy** Nutritional therapy in patients with Crohn's disease has been used with varying success. The use of chemically defined elemental diets has been shown in some studies to reduce disease activity, particularly in patients with disease localized to the small bowel. Liquid polymeric diets may be as effective as elemental feedings and are more acceptable to patients. With few exceptions, standard elemental diets have not been effective in the maintenance of remission in Crohn's disease. Total parenteral nutrition (TPN) has also been shown to be of use in patients with active Crohn's disease; however, complication rates exceed those for enteral nutrition. Although the primary role of nutritional therapy is questionable in patients with inflammatory bowel disease, there is definitely a secondary role for nutritional supplementation to replenish depleted nutrient stores, allowing intestinal protein synthesis and healing, and for preparing patients for operation.

**Smoking Cessation** Although the implications of tobacco abuse as a causative factor in the development of Crohn's disease has been difficult to prove, smoking clearly affects the disease course.[22] Smoking is associated with the late bimodal onset of disease and has been shown to increase the incidence of relapse and failure of maintenance therapy. It also appears to be associated with the severity of disease in a linear dose-response relationship. Therefore, smoking cessation therapy is an important component of medical therapy.

**Surgical Treatment** Although medical management is indicated during acute exacerbations of disease, most patients with chronic Crohn's disease require surgery at some time during the course of their illness. In patients with more than 20 years of disease, the cumulative probability of surgery was 78%. The indications for operation are limited to complications that include intestinal obstruction, intestinal perforation with fistula formation or abscess, free perforation, gastrointestinal bleeding, urologic complications, failure or intolerance of steroid therapy, cancer, and perianal disease.[23] Children with Crohn's disease and resulting systemic symptoms, such as growth retardation, may benefit from resection. The extraintestinal complications of Crohn's disease, although not primary indications for operation, often subside after resection of involved bowel, with the exception of ankylosing spondylitis and hepatic complications.

Operative therapy in patients with Crohn's disease should be specifically directed to the complication, and only the segment of bowel involved in the complicating process should be resected. Even if adjacent areas of bowel are clearly diseased, they should be ignored. Early in the history of the surgical therapy of Crohn's disease, surgeons tended to perform wider resections with the hope of cure or significant remission. However, repeated wide resections resulted in no greater remissions or cure and led to the short bowel syndrome, which is a devastating surgical complication. Frozen sections to determine microscopic disease are unreliable and are not recommended. It must be emphasized, therefore, that operative treatment of a complication be limited to that segment of bowel involved with the complication, and no attempt should be made to resect more bowel, even though grossly evident disease may be apparent.

The role of laparoscopic surgery for patients with Crohn's disease has been gaining acceptance as an alternative surgical approach. In appropriately selected patients, for example, those with localized abscesses, simple intra-abdominal fistulas, perianastomotic recurrent disease, and disease limited to the distal ileum, for which ileocecectomy is indicated, this technique appears feasible and safe. Randomized clinical trials have verified that laparoscopic surgery is safe and feasible in Crohn's disease, but studies with long-term follow-up have not demonstrated a clear advantage of laparoscopic surgery over traditional open techniques.[24] The potential for earlier recovery after laparoscopic resection has stimulated interest in extending the role of surgical resection in inducing remission; a randomized trial is currently under way comparing laparoscopic resection to infliximab as primary therapy for ileocolonic Crohn's disease.[25]

The decision to perform a primary anastomosis versus initial ostomy formation with delayed reconstruction can be a difficult one for those with Crohn's disease. Patients are often malnourished, on intensive immunosuppressive therapy, or present with some element of intra-abdominal sepsis. In general standard surgical principles should direct this decision. Patients with adequate nutrition and minimal intra-abdominal sepsis can safely undergo primary anastomosis at the initial operation, whereas malnourished and septic patients are best served by diversion, if possible. Although caution should be exercised when performing an anastomosis in the setting of high-dose immunosuppression, large series have confirmed that surgery while receiving perioperative infliximab or immunosuppressive therapy is safe for patients with Crohn's disease.[26]

## Specific Problems

**Acute Ileitis (Nonstricturing, Nonpenetrating)** Patients can present with acute abdominal pain localized to the right lower quadrant and signs and symptoms consistent with a diagnosis of acute appendicitis. At exploration, the appendix is found to be normal, but the terminal ileum is edematous and beefy red, with a thickened mesentery and enlarged lymph nodes. This condition, known as *acute ileitis*, is a self-limited disease. Acute ileitis may be a manifestation of early Crohn's disease but is most often unrelated. Bacteriologic agents such as *Campylobacter* or *Yersinia* may cause acute ileitis. Intestinal resection should not be performed. Although in the past the management of the appendix was controversial, it is clear now that in the absence of acute inflammatory involvement of the appendix or the cecum, appendectomy should be performed. This eliminates the appendix as a source of abdominal pain in the future.

**Stricturing Disease** Intestinal obstruction is the most common indication for surgical therapy in patients with Crohn's disease. Obstruction in these patients is often partial, and nonoperative management is initially indicated. The success of nonoperative management can often be predicted based on the chronicity of symptoms at the affected site. In patients for whom it is difficult to determine whether the site of obstruction is caused by an acute exacerbation or a chronically strictured segment, C-reactive protein levels may help identify acute inflammation and predict potential success of medical therapy. In case of a chronic strictured segment, medical therapy is rarely effective. Operative intervention is required for patients with complete obstruction and patients with partial obstruction whose condition does not resolve with nonoperative management. The treatment of choice of intestinal obstruction in patients with Crohn's disease is segmental resection of the involved segment with primary reanastomosis. This may involve segmental resection and primary anastomosis of a short segment of ileum if this is the site of the complication. More commonly, the cecum is involved contiguously with the terminal ileum, in which case resection of the involved terminal ileum and colon is required and the ileum is anastomosed to the ascending or transverse colon (Fig. 50-24).

In selected patients with obstruction caused by strictures (single or multiple), one option is to perform a strictureplasty that effectively widens the lumen but avoids intestinal resection. Strictureplasty is performed by making a longitudinal incision through the narrowed area of the intestine followed by closure in a transverse fashion in a manner similar to that for a Heineke-Mikulicz pyloroplasty (Fig. 50-25*A*). For longer diseased segments (>10 cm), the strictureplasty can be performed similar to a Finney pyloroplasty (see Fig. 50-25*B*) or a side-to-side isoperistaltic strictureplasty. Strictureplasty has the most application in patients in whom multiple short areas of narrowing are present over long segments of intestine, in those who have

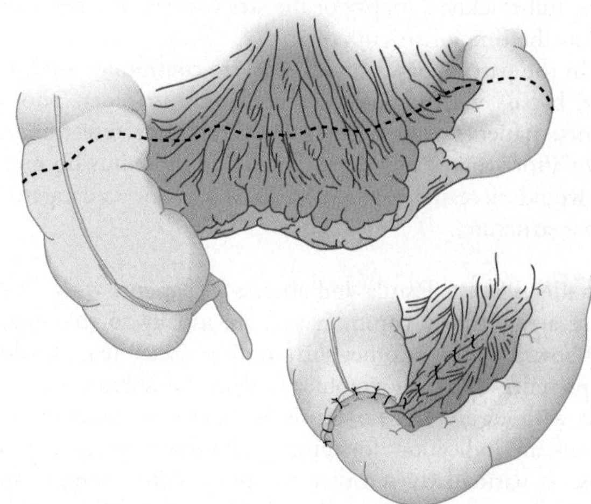

**FIGURE 50-24** Resection of the ileum, ileocecal valve, cecum, and ascending colon for Crohn's disease of the ileum. Intestinal continuity is restored by end-to-end anastomosis.

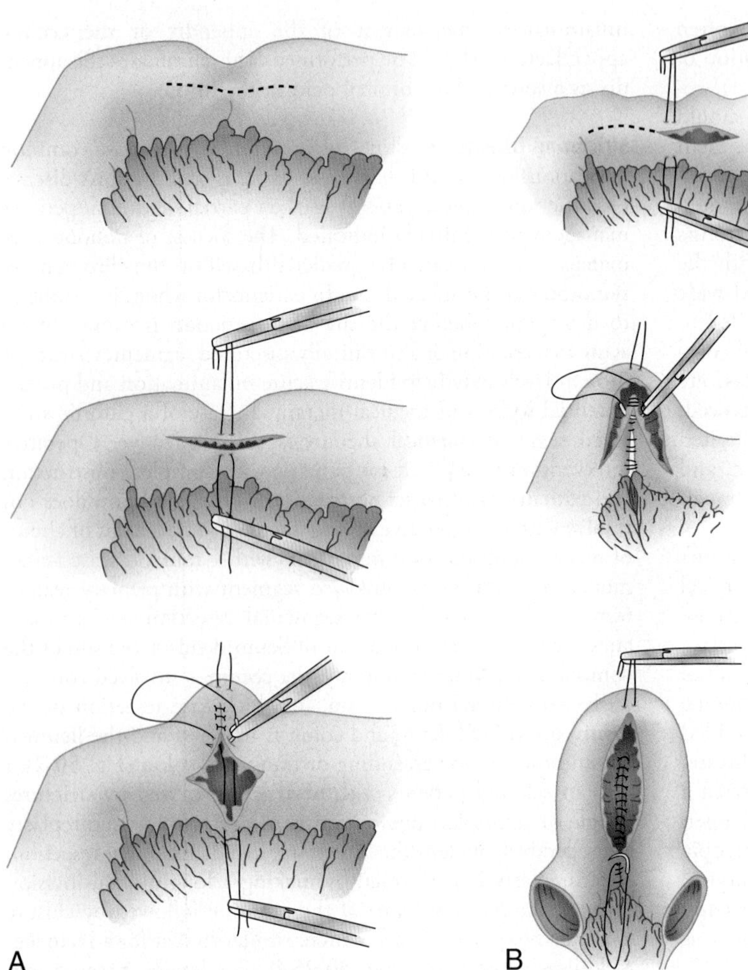


**FIGURE 50-25 A,** Technique of short strictureplasty in the manner of a Heineke-Mikulicz pyloroplasty. **B,** For longer diseased segments, strictureplasty may be performed in a manner similar to Finney pyloroplasty. (Adapted from Alexander-Williams J, Haynes IG: Up-to-date management of small-bowel Crohn's disease. In Mannick JA [ed]: Advances in surgery, St Louis, 1987, Mosby, pp 245–264.)

already had several previous resections of the small intestine, and when the areas of narrowing are caused by fibrous obstruction rather than acute inflammation. This procedure preserves intestine and is associated with complication and recurrence rates comparable to those of resection and reanastomosis. Given the concerns of carcinoma developing at chronically strictured segments, full-thickness biopsy of the stricture site has been advocated at the time of strictureplasty.[23]

In the past, bypass procedures were commonly used. Currently, bypass with exclusion is used only in older, poor-risk patients, patients who have had several prior resections and cannot afford to lose any more bowel, and those in whom resection would necessitate entering an abscess or endangering a normal structure.

**Penetrating Disease** Fistula and abscess in patients with Crohn's disease are relatively common and are usually to the adjacent small bowel, colon, or other surrounding viscera (e.g., bladder). The presence of a radiographically demonstrable enteroenteral fistula without any signs of sepsis or other complications is not in itself an indication for surgery. Furthermore, penetrating disease is particularly sensitive to anticytokine therapy, and a conservative, surgical approach to Crohn's related fistula is most appropriate. However, many of these patients will require eventual resection as the disease progresses and they have progressively worsening abdominal pain. Enterocutaneous fistulas may develop but are rarely spontaneous and are more likely to follow resection or drainage of intra-abdominal abscesses. Ideally, enterocutaneous fistulas should be managed by excising the fistula tract along with the diseased segment of intestine and performing a primary reanastomosis. If the fistula forms between two or more adjacent loops of diseased bowel, the involved segments should be excised. Alternatively, if the fistula involves an adjacent normal organ, such as the bladder or colon, only the segment of the diseased small bowel and fistulous tract should be resected, and the defect in the normal organ should simply be closed. Most patients with ileosigmoid fistulas do not necessarily require resection of the sigmoid because the disease is usually confined to the small bowel. However, if the segment of sigmoid is also found to have Crohn's disease, it should be resected along with the segment of diseased small bowel.

**Perforation** Penetrating disease in the form of perforation into the free peritoneal cavity occurs occasionally but is not common in patients with Crohn's disease. Typically, penetration presents with a localized abscess densely adherent to the diseased segment of bowel. In cases of free perforation, the segment of involved bowel should be resected and, in the presence of minimal contamination, a primary anastomosis should be performed. If generalized peritonitis is present, a safer option may be to perform enterostomies until the intra-abdominal sepsis is controlled and then return for restoration of intestinal continuity. Abscesses can be treated with percutaneous drainage and antibiotic and immunomodulatory therapy, although fistula or uncontrolled sepsis may ultimately develop requiring resection with or without primary anastomosis.

**Gastrointestinal Bleeding** Although anemia from chronic blood loss is common in patients with Crohn's disease, life-threatening gastrointestinal hemorrhage is rare. The incidence of hemorrhage is more common in patients with Crohn's disease involving the colon rather than the small bowel. As with the other complications, the segment involved should be resected and intestinal continuity restored. Arteriography may be useful to localize the bleeding before surgery. In cases of bleeding associated with duodenal disease, endoscopic intervention is usually successful. However, in cases of failure, duodenotomy with oversewing of the bleeding ulcerative area is indicated.[23]

**Urologic Complications** Genitourinary complications occur in 4% to 35% of patients with Crohn's disease. The most common urologic complication is ureteral obstruction, which is usually secondary to ileocolic disease with retroperitoneal abscess. Surgical treatment of the primary intestinal disease is adequate in most patients. In a few cases of long-standing inflammatory disease, periureteric fibrosis may be present and require ureterolysis.

**Cancer** Patients with long-standing Crohn's disease of the small bowel and, in particular, the colon have an increased incidence of cancer. The management of these patients is the same as that for any patient—resection of the cancer with appropriate margins and regional lymph nodes. Patients with cancer associated with Crohn's disease commonly have a worse prognosis than those who do not have Crohn's, based largely on the fact that the diagnosis in these patients is delayed.

**Colorectal Disease** The same principle applies to patients with Crohn's disease limited to the colon as to those with disease to the small bowel; that is, surgical resection should be limited to the segment producing the complications. Indications for surgery include a lack of response to medical management or complications of Crohn's colitis, which include obstruction, hemorrhage, perforation, and toxic megacolon. Depending on the diseased segments, procedures commonly include segmental colectomy with colocolonic anastomosis, subtotal colectomy with ileoproctostomy and, in patients with extensive perianal and rectal disease, total proctocolectomy with Brooke ileostomy. Patients with toxic megacolon should undergo colectomy, closure of the proximal rectum, and end ileostomy. Strictureplasty has limited usefulness in colonic Crohn's disease, and concerns of malignancy at an area of colonic obstruction should limit its application.

A particularly troubling problem after proctocolectomy in patients with Crohn's disease is delayed healing of the perineal wound. It has been found that 25% to 60% of perineal wounds are open 6 months after surgery. Persistent nonhealing wounds require excision with secondary closure. Large cavities or sinuses may be filled using well-vascularized pedicles of muscle (e.g., gracilis, semimembranosus, rectus abdominis) or omentum or by using an inferior gluteal myocutaneous graft.

Although controversial, continence-preserving operations, such as ileoanal pouch anastomoses or continent ileostomies (Kock pouch) that have been used in patients with ulcerative colitis, are not recommended for patients with Crohn's colitis because of the high rate of recurrence of Crohn's disease in the pouch, fistulas to the anastomosis, and peripouch abscesses.

**Perianal Disease** Diseases involving the perianal region include fissures and fistulas and are common in patients with Crohn's disease, particularly those with colonic involvement. The treatment of perianal disease should be conservative. Antibiotics and immunosuppressive agents (e.g., azathioprine, 6-mercaptopurine) have been used with varying success. Encouraging reports have been obtained using the TNF-$\alpha$ antibody infliximab and tacrolimus. Wide excision of abscesses or fistulas is not indicated, but more conservative interventions, including the liberal placement of drainage catheters and noncutting setons, are preferable. Definitive fistulotomy is indicated for most patients with superficial, low trans-sphincteric, and low intersphincteric fistulas, although one must recognize that some degree of anal stenosis may occur as a result of chronic inflammation. High trans-sphincteric, suprasphincteric, and extrasphincteric fistulas are usually treated with noncutting setons. Fissures are usually lateral, relatively painless, large, and indolent and often respond to conservative management. Abscesses should be drained, but large excisions of tissue should not be performed. Advancement flap closure of perineal fistulas may be required in certain cases. Selective construction of diverting stomas has good results when combined with optimal medical therapy to induce remission of inflammation. Proctectomy may be infrequently required in a subset of patients who have persistent and unremitting disease despite conservative medical and surgical therapy.

**Duodenal Disease** Crohn's disease of the duodenum occurs in 2% to 4% of patients with Crohn's disease. Operative intervention is uncommon. The primary indication for surgery in these patients is duodenal obstruction that does not respond to medical therapy. The use of gastrojejunostomy to bypass the disease rather than duodenal resection is the procedure of choice. Strictureplasties have been performed with success in selected patients and may avoid the marginal ulceration and diarrhea associated with gastrojejunostomy.

### Prognosis

Operations directed at Crohn's disease are not curative but often provide patients with significant symptomatic relief. High rates of recurrence are reported in most series.[23] It is important, however, to note how recurrence is defined in these studies. Endoscopic evidence of recurrence is detected in about 70% of patients within 1 year of surgery and in 85% by 3 years. Most of these recurrences are asymptomatic. If defined exclusively by the need for reoperation, however, recurrence rates are only 25% to 30% at 5 years and 40% to 50% at 20 years. To put this in perspective, after a first resection for Crohn's disease, about 45% of patients will ultimately require a second operation, of whom only 25% will require a third operation. Overall, almost 90% of those undergoing operation for Crohn's disease will never require more than one additional operation. Despite the risk for recurrence, many patients who have had surgery for Crohn's disease wish that they had had their operation sooner. Performed for proper indications, surgery almost invariably rehabilitates those disabled by Crohn's disease. The overwhelming majority of these patients report relief of symptoms after surgery, restoration of a feeling of well-being and the ability to eat normally, and a reduction in the need for medical therapy.

Standardized mortality rates in patients with Crohn's disease are increased in those patients whose disease began before the age of 20 years and in those who have had disease present for longer than 13 years. Long-term survival studies have suggested that patients with Crohn's disease have a death rate approximately two to three times higher than that in the general population. Gastrointestinal cancer remains the leading cause of disease-related death in patients with Crohn's disease; other causes of disease-related deaths include sepsis, thromboembolic complications, and electrolyte disorders.

## Typhoid Enteritis

Typhoid fever remains a significant problem in developing countries, most commonly in areas with contaminated water supplies and inadequate waste disposal. Children and young adults are most often affected. Improvements in sanitation have decreased the incidence of typhoid fever in industrialized countries; however, approximately 500 cases/year are still reported in the United States.

Typhoid enteritis is an acute systemic infection of several weeks' duration caused primarily by *Salmonella typhosa.* The pathologic events of typhoid fever are initiated in the intestinal tract after oral ingestion of the typhoid bacillus. These organisms penetrate the small bowel mucosa, making their way rapidly to the lymphatics and then systemically. Hyperplasia of the reticuloendothelial system, including lymph nodes, liver, and spleen, is characteristic of typhoid fever. Peyer patches in the small bowel become hyperplastic and may subsequently ulcerate, with complications of hemorrhage or perforation.

The diagnosis of typhoid fever is confirmed by isolating the organism from blood (positive in 90% of the patients during the first week of the illness), bone marrow, and stool cultures. In addition, the finding of high titers of agglutinins against O and H antigens is strongly suggestive of typhoid fever. Assays for the diagnosis of *S. typhosa* using the PCR assay have been developed but are still experimental.

Typhoid fever and uncomplicated typhoid enteritis are treated by antibiotic administration. Chloramphenicol, ampicillin, amoxicillin, and trimethoprim-sulfamethoxazole have all been used, with good results. In addition, short courses of third-generation cephalosporins have been used successfully to treat typhoid fever.

Complications requiring potential surgical intervention include hemorrhage and perforation. The incidence of hemorrhage was reported to be as high as 20% in some series but, with the availability of antibiotic treatment, this figure has decreased. When hemorrhage occurs, transfusion is indicated and usually suffices. Rarely, laparotomy must be performed for uncontrollable, life-threatening hemorrhage. Intestinal perforation through an ulcerated Peyer patch occurs in approximately 2% of cases. Typically, it is a single perforation in the terminal ileum, and simple closure of the perforation is the treatment of choice. With multiple perforations, which occur in about 25% of patients, resection with primary anastomosis or exteriorization of the intestinal loops may be required.

## Enteritis in the Immunocompromised Host

The AIDS epidemic, as well as the widespread use of immunosuppressive agents after organ transplantation, has resulted in a number of rare and exotic pathogens infecting the gastrointestinal tract. Almost all patients with AIDS have gastrointestinal symptoms during their illness, the most common of which is diarrhea. However, the surgeon may be asked to evaluate the immunocompromised patient with abdominal pain, an obvious acute abdomen, or gastrointestinal bleeding; a number of protozoal, bacterial, viral, and fungal organisms may be responsible.

### Protozoa

Protozoa (e.g., *Cryptosporidium, Isospora,* and *Microsporidium*) are the most frequent class of pathogens causing diarrhea in patients with AIDS. The small bowel is the most common site of infection. Diagnosis is usually established by acid-fast staining of the stool or duodenal secretions. Symptoms are most commonly related to diarrhea, which may be at times intractable. Current treatment regimens have not been entirely effective.

### Bacteria

Infections by enteric bacteria are more frequent and more virulent in HIV-infected individuals than in healthy hosts. *Salmonella, Shigella,* and *Campylobacter* are associated with higher rates of bacteremia and antibiotic resistance in the immunocompromised patient. The diagnosis of *Shigella* or *Salmonella* infection may be established by stool cultures. The diagnosis of *Campylobacter* infection, however, may be more difficult, with stool cultures often negative. These enteric infections manifest clinically with high fever, abdominal pain, and diarrhea that may be bloody. Abdominal pain may mimic an acute abdomen. Bacteremia should be treated by administration of parenteral antibiotics; ciprofloxacin is an attractive choice if the organisms are multiply resistant.

Diarrhea caused by *Clostridium difficile* is more common in patients with AIDS because of the increased antibiotic use in this population compared with healthy hosts. Diagnosis is by standard assays of stool for *C. difficile* enterotoxin. Treatment with metronidazole or vancomycin is usually effective.

### Mycobacteria

Mycobacterial infection is a frequent cause of intestinal disease in immunocompromised hosts. This can be secondary to *Mycobacterium tuberculosis* or *Mycobacterium avium* complex (MAC), which is an atypical mycobacterium related to the type that causes cervical adenitis (scrofula). The usual route of infection is by swallowed organisms that directly penetrate the intestinal mucosa. The luminal gastrointestinal tract is affected by MAC infection, with massive thickening of the proximal small intestine often noted (Fig. 50-26). Clinically, patients with MAC present with diarrhea, fever, anorexia, and progressive wasting.

The most frequent site of intestinal involvement of *M. tuberculosis* is the distal ileum and cecum, with 85% to 90% of patients demonstrating disease at this site. The gross appearance can be ulcerative, hypertrophic, or ulcerohypertrophic. The bowel wall appears thickened and an inflammatory mass often surrounds the ileocecal region. Acute inflammation is apparent, as well as strictures and even fistula formation. The serosal surface is normally covered with multiple tubercles, and mesenteric lymph nodes are frequently enlarged and thickened; on sectioning, caseous necrosis is noted. The mucosa is hyperemic, edematous and, in some cases, ulcerated. Histologically, the distinguishing lesion is a granuloma, with caseating granulomas

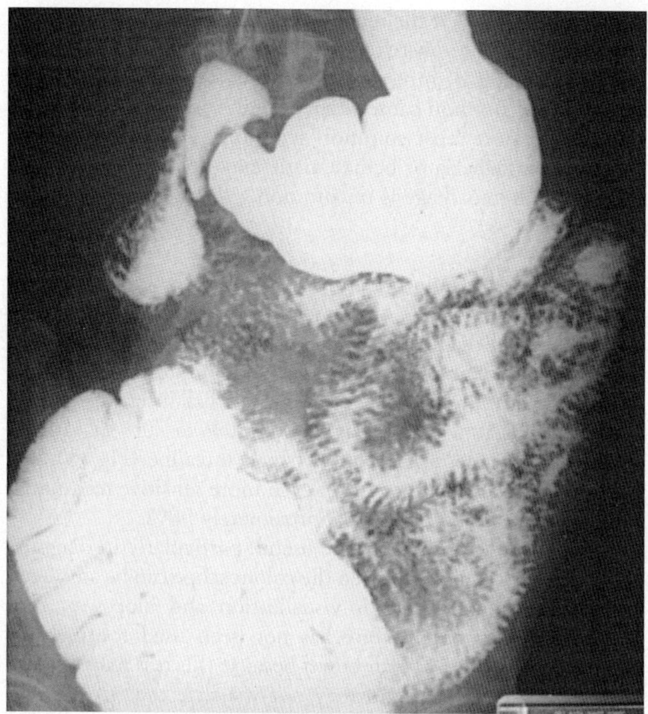

**FIGURE 50-26** Barium radiograph of a patient with AIDS shows thickened intestinal folds consistent with enteritis secondary to atypical mycobacterium. (Courtesy Dr. Melvyn H. Schreiber, The University of Texas Medical Branch, Galveston, Tex.)

found most commonly in the lymph nodes. Most patients complain of chronic abdominal pain, which may be nonspecific, weight loss, fever, and diarrhea.

The diagnosis of mycobacterial infection is made by identification of the organism in tissue by direct visualization with an acid-fast stain, culture of the excised tissue, or PCR assay. Radiographic examinations usually reveal a thickened mucosa with distorted mucosal folds and ulcerations. CT may be useful and shows a thickening of the ileocecal valve and cecum.

The treatment of *M. tuberculosis* is similar in the immunocompromised or nonimmunocompromised host. The organism is usually responsive to multidrug antimicrobial therapy. The therapy for MAC infection is evolving; drugs that have been successfully used in vivo and in vitro include amikacin, ciprofloxacin, cycloserine, and ethionamide. Clarithromycin has also been successfully used in combination with other agents. Surgical intervention may be required for intestinal tuberculosis, particularly *M. tuberculosis.* Obstruction and fistula formation are the leading indications for surgery; however, with current treatment, most fistulas now respond to medical management. Surgery may be necessary for ulcerative complications when free perforation, perforation with abscess, or massive hemorrhage occurs. The treatment is usually resection with anastomosis.

#### Viruses

Cytomegalovirus (CMV) is the most common viral cause of diarrhea in immunocompromised patients. Clinical manifestations include intermittent diarrhea accompanied by fever, weight loss, and abdominal pain. The manifestations of enteric CMV infection result from mucosal ischemic ulcerations, which account for the high rate of perforations noted with CMV. As a result of the diffuse ulcerating involvement of the intestine, patients may present with abdominal pain, peritonitis, or hematochezia. Diagnosis of CMV is made by demonstrating viral inclusions. The most characteristic form is an intranuclear inclusion, which is often surrounded by a halo, producing a so-called *owl's eye appearance.* There may also be cytoplasmic inclusions (Fig. 50-27). Cultures for CMV are usually positive when inclusion bodies are present, but these cultures are less sensitive and specific than histopathologic identification. Once diagnosed, the treatment for CMV is usually effective with ganciclovir. An alternative to ganciclovir is foscarnet, a pyrophosphate analogue that inhibits viral replication. Other less common viral infections have been reported and include adenovirus, rotavirus, and novel enteric viruses such as astrovirus and picornavirus.

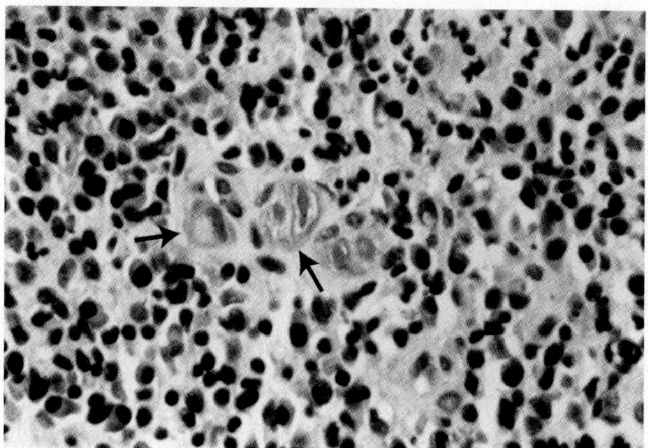

**FIGURE 50-27** Microscopic section of small bowel in a patient with AIDS who has cytomegalovirus enteritis. Multiple large cells with intranuclear and intracytoplasmic inclusions typical of cytomegalovirus are demonstrated *(arrows)*. (Courtesy Dr. Mary R. Schwartz, Baylor College of Medicine, Houston.)

#### Fungi

Fungal infections of the intestinal tract have been recognized in patients with AIDS. Gastrointestinal histoplasmosis occurs in the setting of systemic infection, often in association with pulmonary and hepatic disease. Diagnosis is made by fungal smear and culture of infected tissue or blood. The infection is most commonly treated by the administration of amphotericin B. Coccidioidomycosis of the intestinal tract is rare and, like histoplasmosis, occurs in the context of systemic infection.

## NEOPLASMS

### General Considerations

Small bowel neoplasms are exceedingly rare, despite the fact that the small bowel constitutes about 80% of the total length of the gastrointestinal tract and makes up more than 90% of the mucosal surface area. Only 5% of all gastrointestinal neoplasms and only 1% to 2% of all malignant tumors of the gastrointestinal tract occur in the small bowel. More than 5000 new cases of primary small intestinal cancer occur annually in the United States, equally distributed between men and women, with more than 1000 estimated cancer deaths. The reasons for this decreased incidence in cancer despite the rapidly proliferating mucosa are entirely speculative but may include such factors as the rapid transit of luminal contents, high turnover rate of small bowel epithelial cells, which may minimize carcinogenic exposure, alkalinity of small intestinal contents, high level of IgA in the intestinal wall, and low bacterial count of small intestine luminal contents.

The mean age at onset is approximately 59 years; the mean age of the presentation is 62 years for benign tumors and approximately 57 years for malignant lesions. Similar to other cancers, there appears to be a geographic distribution, with the highest cancer rates found among the Maori of New Zealand and ethnic Hawaiians. The incidence of small bowel cancer is particularly low in India, Romania, and other parts of Eastern Europe. Although the incidence of small bowel cancer is exceedingly small, as noted, there appears to be a disturbing trend of increased rates since the mid-1980s, possibly reflecting the spread of AIDS and increase in neoplasms, such as lymphomas, that occur in the immunocompromised host.

The incidence of small bowel neoplasia varies considerably, with benign lesions identified more often in autopsy series. In contrast, malignant neoplasms account for 75% of symptomatic lesions that lead to surgery. This reflects the fact that most benign neoplasms are asymptomatic and therefore are not found unless as an incidental finding. Leiomyomas and adenomas are the most frequent of the benign tumors. Benign lesions appear to be more common in the distal small bowel, but these numbers may be somewhat misleading because of the relatively short length of the duodenum. In fact, per unit area, duodenal tumors are most frequent. Depending on the series, adenocarcinoma or carcinoid tumor is the most common malignant neoplasm. Adenocarcinomas are more numerous in the proximal small bowel, whereas the other malignant lesions are more common in the distal intestine. Patients with Crohn's disease and familial adenomatous polyposis are at a higher risk for small bowel neoplasms than the general population. Although the molecular genetics of small bowel neoplasms have not been entirely characterized, similar to colorectal cancers, mutations of the *K-ras* gene are commonly found. Allelic losses, particularly involving tumor suppressor genes at chromosome locations 5q (the *APC* gene), 17q (the *p53* gene), and 18q (the *DCC* [***d***eleted in ***c***olon ***c***ancer] and *DPC4 [SMAD4]* genes), have been noted in some small bowel cancers.

Numerous risk factors and associated conditions have been described related to neoplasia of the small bowel. These include patients with familial adenomatous polyposis, hereditary nonpolyposis colorectal cancer (HNPCC), Peutz-Jeghers syndrome, Crohn's disease, gluten-sensitive enteropathy (i.e., celiac sprue), and biliary diversion (e.g., previous cholecystectomy). Controversial factors that may contribute to small bowel cancers include smoking, heavy alcohol consumption (>80 g/day of ethanol), and consumption of red meat or salt-cured foods.

## Clinical Manifestations

Symptoms associated with small bowel neoplasms are often vague and nonspecific and may include dyspepsia, anorexia, malaise, and dull abdominal pain, often intermittent and colicky. These symptoms may be present for months or years before surgery. Most patients with benign neoplasms remain asymptomatic, and the neoplasms are only discovered at autopsy or as incidental findings at laparotomy or upper gastrointestinal radiologic studies. Of the remainder, pain, most often related to obstruction, is the most frequent complaint. Usually, obstruction is the result of intussusception, and benign small tumors are the most common cause of this condition in adults. Hemorrhage is the next most common symptom. Bleeding is usually occult; hematochezia or hematemesis may occur, although life-threatening hemorrhage is uncommon.

## Diagnosis

Because of the insidious nature of many of the small bowel neoplasms, a high index of suspicion must be present for these neoplasms to be diagnosed. In most series, a correct preoperative diagnosis is made in only 20% to 50% of symptomatic patients. An upper gastrointestinal tract series with small intestinal follow-through yields an accurate diagnosis in 50% to 70% of patients with malignant neoplasms of the small intestine (Fig. 50-28). CT enteroclysis appears to be an even more sensitive technique, with a diagnostic accuracy of approximately 90%.[7]

Flexible endoscopy may be useful, particularly in diagnosing duodenal lesions, and often the colonoscope can be advanced into the terminal ileum for visualization and biopsy of ileal neoplasms. Push enteroscopy has not been used routinely to evaluate lesions in the small bowel because this test may take up to 8 hours to perform and may not visualize the entire small bowel. The use of swallowed radiotelemetry capsules (e.g., capsule endoscopy) that transmit images of the bowel wall may be of diagnostic value.

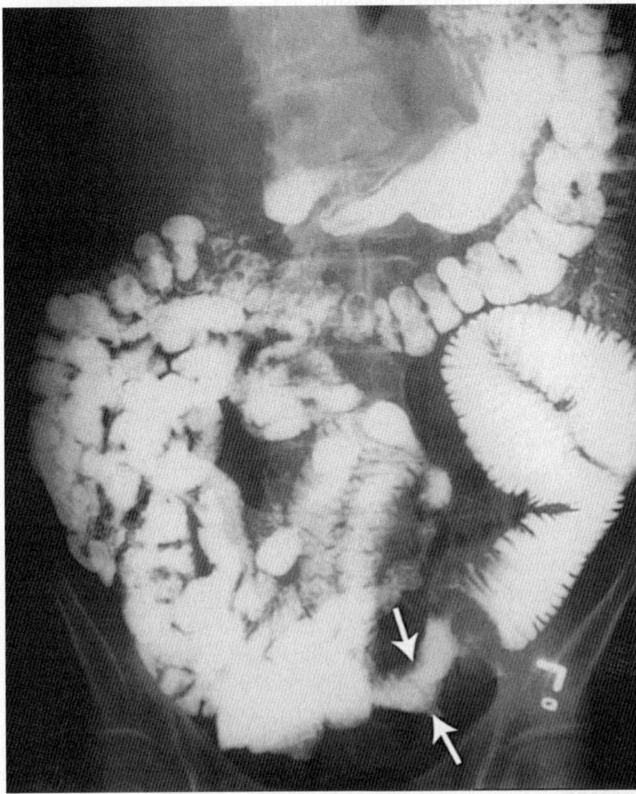

**FIGURE 50-28** Barium radiograph demonstrates a typical apple core lesion *(arrows)* caused by adenocarcinoma of the small bowel, producing a partial obstruction with dilated proximal bowel. (Courtesy Dr. Melvyn H. Schreiber, The University of Texas Medical Branch, Galveston, Tex.)

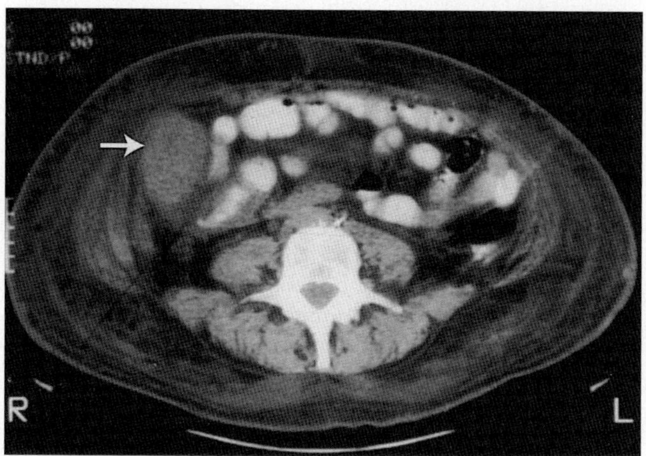


**FIGURE 50-29** CT scan of abdomen demonstrates a small bowel neoplasm *(arrow)*. (Courtesy Dr. Melvyn H. Schreiber, The University of Texas Medical Branch, Galveston, Tex.)

Plain films may confirm the presence of an obstruction; however, for the most part, they are useless in making a diagnosis of small bowel neoplasms. Angiography is of value in diagnosing and localizing tumors of vascular origin. CT of the abdomen can prove particularly useful in detecting extraluminal tumors, such as gastrointestinal stromal tumors (GISTs), and can provide helpful information regarding the staging of malignant cancers (Fig. 50-29). Ultrasonography has not proved to be effective in making the preoperative diagnosis of small bowel neoplasm. Despite sophisticated imaging and diagnostic modalities, diagnosis of a small bowel tumor is often achieved only at the time of surgical exploration, performed as an elective or emergency procedure.

## Benign Neoplasms

The most common benign neoplasms include benign GISTs, adenomas, and lipomas. Adenomas are the most common benign tumors reported in autopsy series, but GISTs are the most common benign small bowel lesions that produce symptoms. In general, when a benign tumor is identified at operation, resection is indicated because symptoms, if not the reason for operation, are likely to develop over time. At operation, a thorough search of the remainder of the small bowel is warranted because multiple tumors are not uncommon.

### Leiomyomas

Leiomyomas, benign tumors of smooth muscle origin, are the most common symptomatic benign neoplasms of the small bowel. As the origin of these tumors has become clearer, pathologists have shifted from designations such as leiomyoma or leiomyosarcoma to the term *stromal tumors* (i.e., GISTs).[27] Currently, these tumors are thought to arise from the interstitial cell of Cajal, an intestinal pacemaker cell of mesodermal descent. These tumors are made up of spindle (70%) and epithelioid (30%) cells, and benign GISTs are three to four times more common than malignant GISTs. Most (>90%) GISTs express CD117, the c-*kit* proto-oncogene protein that is a transmembrane receptor for the stem cell growth factor, and 70% to 80% express CD34, the human progenitor cell antigen. Less frequently, these tumors stain positive for actin and desmin. The incidence is equal in men and in women, and they are most frequently diagnosed in the fifth decade of life. Grossly, they are firm, gray-white lesions with a whorled appearance noted on cut surface; microscopic examination demonstrates well-differentiated smooth muscle cells. These tumors may grow intramurally and cause obstruction. Alternatively, the tumors demonstrate intramural and extramural growth, sometimes achieving considerable size and eventually outgrowing their blood supply, resulting in bleeding manifestations, which is the most common indication for surgery in patients with benign stromal tumors. Surgical resection is necessary for appropriate treatment. Mitotic counts higher than 2/50 high-power fields imply an increased risk for local recurrence.

### Adenomas

Adenomas account for approximately 15% of all benign small bowel tumors and are of three primary types: true adenomas, villous adenomas, and Brunner gland adenomas. Twenty percent of adenomas are found in the duodenum, 30% are found in the jejunum, and 50% are found in the ileum. Most of these lesions are asymptomatic, with most occurring singly and found incidentally at autopsy. The most common presenting symptoms are bleeding and obstruction. Villous adenomas of the small bowel are rare but do occur, are most commonly found in the duodenum, and may be associated with the familial polyposis syndrome. Both true and villous adenomas are thought to proceed along a similar adenoma-carcinoma sequence as colorectal adenomas and should be considered premalignant. Villous adenomas have a particular propensity for malignant degeneration and may be of relatively large size (>5 cm) in diameter. They are usually noted secondary to abdominal pain or bleeding; obstruction may also occur. The malignant potential of these lesions is reportedly between 35% and 55%. Treatment is determined by location and adenoma type. In the jejunum and ileum, the treatment of choice is segmental resection. Because of the potential morbidity associated with duodenal resection by pancreaticoduodenectomy or pancreas-preserving duodenectomy, the management of duodenal adenomas is different. For sporadic adenomas, endoscopic or open polypectomy can be performed if technically feasible. Although both these treatment strategies are associated with a recurrence rate of 30% to 50%, especially in adenomas larger than 3 cm, postpolypectomy surveillance remains possible.[28] Invasive changes or a recurrence after polypectomy necessitate more of a definitive resection, such as a pancreaticoduodenectomy.

Familial adenomas typically occur in the presence of familial adenomatous polyposis (FAP) syndrome and require a different algorithm. FAP-affected patients carry a 5% lifetime risk of developing duodenal adenocarcinoma, which represents the leading cause of cancer-related mortality in these kindreds. Typically, the adenoma burden is diffuse throughout the duodenum, making polypectomy impossible. To direct surveillance and treatment, patients are characterized by the Spigelman classification (Table 50-7). Screening endoscopy with a forward- and side-viewing endoscope is performed at regular intervals with biopsy of all suspicious, villous, or large (>3 cm) adenomas, in addition to random duodenal biopsies. Frequency of endoscopic screening is 1 to 3 years, depending on the Spigelman classification (I to III).[28] Endoscopic or surgical polypectomy can be performed on large adenomas. Ablative therapy in the form of argon beam coagulation or photodynamic therapy has been

**Table 50-7 Spigelman Classification for Duodenal Adenomatosis**

| | Points | | |
|---|---|---|---|
| **PARAMETER** | **1** | **2** | **3** |
| No. of polyps | 1-4 | 5-20 | >20 |
| Polyp size (mm) | 1-4 | 5-10 | >10 |
| Histology | Tubular | Tubulovillous | Villous |
| Degree of dysplasia | Mild | Moderate | Severe |

Stage 0, 0 points; stage 1, 1-4 points; stage 2, 5-6 points; stage 3, 7-8 points; stage 4, 9-12 points.

attempted for these patients, but with disappointing results. The presence of high-grade dysplasia, carcinoma in situ, or a Spigelman IV classification necessitates pancreaticoduodenectomy or pancreas-preserving duodenectomy.[28] Adenomas of the remaining small bowel also occur more frequently in FAP kindreds but are not as prevalent as the duodenal disease.

Brunner gland adenomas represent benign hyperplastic lesions arising from the Brunner glands of the proximal duodenum. These adenomas may produce symptoms mimicking those of peptic ulcer disease. Diagnosis can usually be accomplished by endoscopy and biopsy, and symptomatic lesions in an accessible region should be resected by simple excision. There is no malignant potential for Brunner gland adenomas and a radical resection should not be used.

### Lipomas

Lipomas, which are also included in the category of stromal tumors, are most common in the ileum and present as single intramural lesions located in the submucosa. They usually occur in the sixth and seventh decades of life and are more frequent in men. Less than one third of these tumors are symptomatic and, of these, the most common manifestations are obstruction and bleeding from superficial ulcerations. The treatment of choice for symptomatic lesions is excision. Lipomas do not have malignant potential and therefore, when found incidentally, should be removed only if the resection is simple.

### Peutz-Jeghers Syndrome

Hamartomas of the small bowel occur as part of the Peutz-Jeghers syndrome, an inherited syndrome of mucocutaneous melanotic pigmentation and gastrointestinal polyps. The pattern of inheritance is simple mendelian dominant, with a high degree of penetrance. The classic pigmented lesions are small, 1- to 2-mm, brown or black spots located in the circumoral region of the face, buccal mucosa, forearms, palms, soles, digits, and perianal area. The entire jejunum and ileum are the most usual portions of the gastrointestinal tract involved with these hamartomas; however, 50% of patients may also have rectal and colonic lesions, and 25% of patients have gastric lesions. The most common symptom is recurrent colicky abdominal pain, usually as a result of intermittent intussusception. Lower abdominal pain associated with a palpable mass has been reported to occur in one third of patients. Hemorrhage as a result of autoamputation of the polyps occurs less frequently and is most commonly manifested by anemia. Acute life-threatening hemorrhage is uncommon but may occur. Although once considered a purely benign disease, adenomatous changes have been reported in 3% to 6% of hamartomas. Extracolonic cancers are common, occurring in 50% to 90% of patients (small intestine, stomach, pancreas, ovary, lung, uterus, and breast). The small intestine represents the most frequent site for cancer, compared with that of the general population. The treatment of complications of Peutz-Jeghers syndrome is directed mainly at the complication of obstruction or persistent bleeding. Resection should be limited to the segment of bowel that is producing complications and usually involves a limited resection. Because of the widespread nature of intestinal involvement, cure is not possible, and extensive resections are not indicated.

### Hemangiomas

Hemangiomas are developmental malformations consisting of submucosal proliferation of blood vessels. They can occur at any level of the gastrointestinal tract; the jejunum is the most commonly affected small bowel segment. Hemangiomas account for 3% to 4% of all benign tumors of the small bowel and are multiple in 60% of patients. Hemangiomas of the small bowel may occur as part of an inherited disorder known as *Osler-Weber-Rendu disease*. In addition to the small bowel, hemangiomas may also be present in the lung, liver, and mucous membranes. Patients with Turner's syndrome are likely also to have cavernous hemangiomas of the intestine. The most common symptom of small bowel hemangiomas is intestinal bleeding. Angiography and $^{99m}$Tc–red blood cell scanning are the most useful diagnostic studies. If a hemangioma is localized preoperatively, resection of the involved segment of intestine is warranted. If not identified, intraoperative transillumination and palpation can be helpful

## Malignant Neoplasms

Recent population-based analyses have shown that the incidence of malignant neoplasms of the small intestine has increased steadily over the past 3 decades. This increase has mirrored the increase in diagnosis of small bowel carcinoids, which have surpassed adenocarcinoma as the primary cause of small bowel malignancy. Based on both the Surveillance, Epidemiology and End Result (SEER) program and National Cancer Data Base (NCDB), small bowel malignancies, in order of frequency, include carcinoid, adenocarcinoma, lymphoma, and GIST.[29] Surprisingly, treatment and outcome have changed little over the same time frame, which highlights the need for further investigation concerning the multidisciplinary management of these diseases.

In contrast to benign lesions, malignant neoplasms almost always produce symptoms, the most common of which are pain and weight loss. Obstruction develops in 15% to 35% of patients and, unlike the intussusception produced by benign lesions, is usually the result of tumor infiltration and adhesions. Diarrhea with tenesmus and passage of large amounts of mucus may occur. Gastrointestinal bleeding, manifested by anemia and guaiac-positive stools or occasionally by melena or hematochezia, occurs to varying degrees with malignant lesions and is more common with leiomyosarcomas. A palpable mass may be felt in 10% to 20% of patients and perforations develop in approximately 10%, usually secondary to lymphomas and sarcomas. Although presentation may be similar, each tumor type has a distinct biology that dictates management and prognosis.

### Carcinoid Tumors

Carcinoids of the small bowel arise from enterochromaffin cells (Kulchitsky cells), found in the crypts of Lieberkühn[30]; these cells are also known as *argentaffin cells* because of their staining by silver compounds. These tumors were first described by Lubarsch in 1888; in 1907, Oberndorfer coined the term *Karzinoide* to indicate the carcinoma-like appearance and the presumed lack of malignant potential. Carcinoid tumors have been reported in a number of organs, including most commonly the lungs, bronchi, and gastrointestinal tract. Most patients with small bowel carcinoids are in their fifth decade of life.

Carcinoids may be classified by the embryologic site of origin and secretory product. Carcinoid tumors may be derived from the foregut (respiratory tract, thymus), midgut (jejunum, ileum and right colon, stomach, proximal duodenum), and hindgut (distal colon, rectum). Foregut carcinoids characteristically produce low levels of serotonin (5-hydroxytryptamine) but may secrete 5-hydroxytryptophan (5-HTP) or adrenocorticotropic hormone. Midgut carcinoids are characterized by having high serotonin production. Hindgut carcinoids rarely produce serotonin but may produce other hormones, such as somatostatin and peptide YY. The gastrointestinal tract is the most common site for carcinoid tumors. After the appendix, the small intestine is the second most frequently affected site in the gastrointestinal tract. In the small intestine, carcinoids almost always occur within the last 2 feet of the ileum. Carcinoid tumors have a variable malignant potential and are composed of multipotential cells with the ability to secrete numerous humoral agents, the most prominent of which are serotonin and substance P (Table 50-8). In addition to these substances, carcinoid tumors have been found to secrete corticotropin, histamine, dopamine, neurotensin, prostaglandins, kinins, gastrin, somatostatin, pancreatic polypeptide, calcitonin, and neuron-specific enolase.

The primary importance of carcinoid tumors is the malignant potential of the tumors themselves. Although the carcinoid syndrome, which is characterized by episodic attacks of cutaneous flushing, bronchospasm, diarrhea, and vasomotor collapse, can occur and is dramatic in its most florid form, it occurs in only a small percentage of patients with malignant carcinoids.

**Table 50-8 Secretory Products of Carcinoid Tumors***

| AMINES | TACHYKININS | PEPTIDES | OTHER |
|---|---|---|---|
| 5-HT | Kallikrein | Pancreatic polypeptide (40%) | Prostaglandins |
| 5-HIAA (88%) | Substance P (32%) | Chromogranins (100%) | |
| 5-HTP | Neuropeptide K (67%) | Neurotensin (19%) | |
| Histamine | | HCG-α (28%) | |
| Dopamine | | HCG-β | |
| | | Motilin (14%) | |

*Values in parentheses represent percentage frequency.

*HCG,* Human chorionic gonadotropin; *5-HIAA,* 5-hydroxyindoleacetic acid; *5-HT,* 5-hydroxytryptamine; *5-HTP,* 5-hydroxytryptophan.

**Table 50-9 Distribution of Gastrointestinal Carcinoids: Incidence of Metastases and of Carcinoid Syndrome**

| SITE | CASES | AVERAGE METASTASIS (%) | CASES OF CARCINOID SYNDROME |
|---|---|---|---|
| Esophagus | 1 | | 0 |
| Stomach | 93 (2%) | 23 | 8 |
| Duodenum | 135 (4%) | 20 | 4 |
| Jejunoileum | 1032 (28%) | 34 | 91 |
| Meckel's diverticulum | 42 (1%) | 19 | 3 |
| Appendix | 1686 (45%) | 2 | 6 |
| Colon | 91 (2%) | 60 | 5 |
| Rectum | 592 (16%) | 18 | 1 |
| Ovary | 34 | 6 | 17 |
| Biliary tract | 10 | 30 | 0 |
| Pancreas | 2 | | 1 |
| **Total** | 3718 | | 136 |

Adapted from Cheek RC, Wilson H: Carcinoid tumors. Curr Probl Surg (Nov):4–31, 1970.

**Pathology** Carcinoid tumors may arise in organs derived from the foregut, midgut, and hindgut. Seventy percent to 80% of carcinoids are asymptomatic and found incidentally at the time of surgery. In the gastrointestinal tract, more than 90% of carcinoids are found in three sites—appendix (45%), ileum (28%), and rectum (16%; Table 50-9). The malignant potential (ability to metastasize) is related to location, size, depth of invasion, and growth pattern. Only approximately 3% of appendiceal carcinoids metastasize, but approximately 35% of ileal carcinoids are associated with metastasis. Most (≈75%) gastrointestinal carcinoids are smaller than 1 cm in diameter, and approximately 2% of these are associated with metastasis. In contrast, carcinoid tumors 1 to 2 cm in diameter and larger than 2 cm are associated with metastasis in 50% and 80% to 90% of cases, respectively.

Grossly, these tumors are small, firm submucosal nodules that are usually yellow on cut surface (Fig. 50-30). They may be as subtle as a small whitish plaque seen on the antimesenteric border of the small intestine. Typically, they are associated with a larger mesenteric mass caused by nodal disease and desmoplastic invasion of the mesentery, which is often mistaken for the primary tumor. They tend to grow very slowly but, after invasion of the serosa, the intense desmoplastic reaction produces mesenteric fibrosis, intestinal kinking, and intermittent obstruction. Small bowel carcinoids are multicentric in 20% to 30% of patients. This tendency to multicentricity exceeds that of any other malignant neoplasm of the gastrointestinal tract. Another unusual observation is the frequent coexistence of a second primary malignant neoplasm of a different histologic type. This is usually a synchronous adenocarcinoma (most commonly in the large intestine) that can occur in 10% to 20% of patients with carcinoid tumors. Carcinoid tumors are associated with multiple endocrine neoplasia type 1 in approximately 10% of cases.

**Clinical Manifestations** In the absence of carcinoid syndrome, symptoms of patients with carcinoid tumors of the small bowel

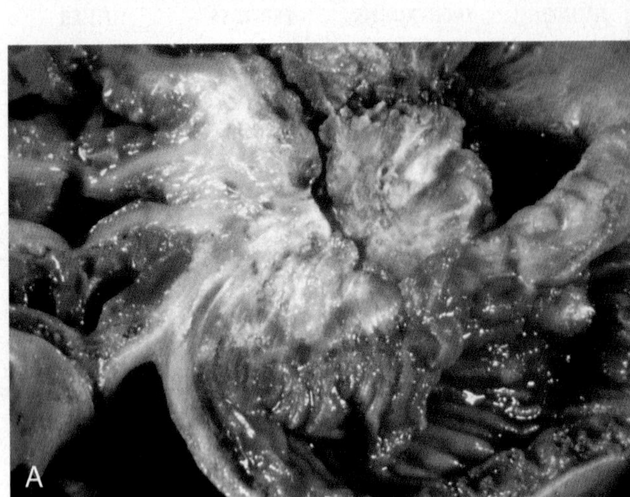


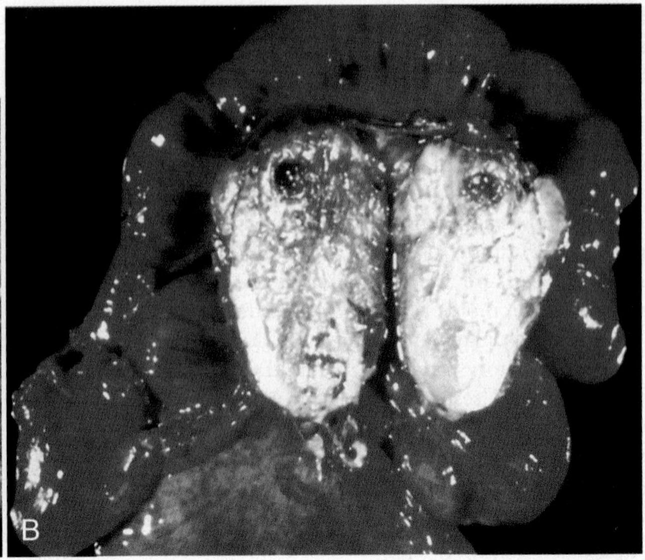


**FIGURE 50-30** Gross pathologic characteristics of carcinoid tumor. **A,** Carcinoid tumor of the distal ileum demonstrates the intense desmoplastic reaction and fibrosis of the bowel wall. **B,** Mesenteric metastases from a carcinoid tumor of the small bowel. (Adapted from Evers BM, Townsend CM Jr, Thompson JC: Small intestine. In Schwartz SI [ed]: Principles of surgery, ed 7, New York, 1999, McGraw-Hill, p 1245.)

are similar to those of patients with small bowel tumors of other histologic types. The most common symptoms include abdominal pain, which is variably associated with partial or complete small intestinal obstruction. Obstructive symptoms can be caused by intussusception but usually occur secondary to a local desmoplastic reaction, apparently produced by humoral agents elaborated by the tumor. Diarrhea and weight loss may also occur. The diarrhea is a result of a partial bowel obstruction rather than the secretory diarrhea noted in patients with the malignant carcinoid syndrome. As mesenteric and nodal extension progress, local venous engorgement and ultimately ischemia of the affected segment of intestine contribute to most symptoms and complications related to the tumor.

***Malignant Carcinoid Syndrome*** The malignant carcinoid syndrome is a relatively rare disease, occurring in fewer than 10% of patients with carcinoid tumors. The syndrome is usually associated with carcinoid tumors of the gastrointestinal tract, particularly from the small bowel, but carcinoids in other locations, such as the bronchus, pancreas, ovary, and testes, have also been described in association with the syndrome. Because of the first-pass metabolism of the vasoactive peptides responsible for carcinoid syndrome, hepatic metastasis or extra-abdominal disease is necessary to elicit the syndrome. The classic description of the carcinoid syndrome typically includes vasomotor, cardiac, and gastrointestinal manifestations. A number of humoral factors are produced by carcinoid tumors, but those considered to contribute to the carcinoid syndrome include serotonin, 5-HTP (a precursor of serotonin synthesis), histamine, dopamine, kallikrein, substance P, prostaglandin, and neuropeptide K. Most patients who exhibit malignant carcinoid syndrome have massive hepatic replacement by metastatic disease. However, tumors that bypass the liver, specifically ovarian and retroperitoneal carcinoids, may produce the syndrome in the absence of liver metastasis.

Common symptoms and signs include cutaneous flushing (80%), diarrhea (76%), hepatomegaly (71%), cardiac lesions, most commonly right heart valvular disease (41% to 70%), and asthma (25%). Cutaneous flushing in the carcinoid syndrome may be of four varieties:

1. Diffuse erythematous, which is short-lived and normally affects the face, neck, and upper chest
2. Violaceous, which is similar to a diffuse erythematous flush except that the attacks may be longer and patients may develop a permanent cyanotic flush, with watery eyes and injected conjunctivae
3. Prolonged flushes, which may last up to 2 to 3 days and involve the entire body, and may be associated with profuse lacrimation, hypotension, and facial edema and
4. A bright-red patchy flushing, typically seen with gastric carcinoids

The diarrhea associated with carcinoid syndrome is episodic (usually occurring after meals), watery, and often explosive. Increased circulating serotonin levels are thought to be the cause of the diarrhea because the serotonin antagonist methysergide effectively controls the symptom. Cardiac lesions of carcinoid tumors mainly involve the right side of the heart and are usually limited to the tricuspid and pulmonary valves. The three most common cardiac lesions are pulmonary stenosis (90%), tricuspid insufficiency (47%), and tricuspid stenosis (42%). Asthmatic attacks are usually observed during the flushing symptom, and serotonin and bradykinin have been implicated in this symptom. Malabsorption and pellagra (dementia, dermatitis, and diarrhea) are occasionally present and are thought to be caused by excessive diversion of dietary tryptophan.

**Diagnosis** The elevation of various humoral factors forms the basis for diagnostic tests in patients with carcinoid tumors and the carcinoid syndrome. Carcinoid tumors produce serotonin, which is then metabolized in the liver and the lung to the pharmacologically inactive 5-hydroxyindoleacetic acid (5-HIAA). Elevated urinary levels of 5-HIAA measured over 24 hours with high-performance liquid chromatography are highly specific, although not sensitive. A potentially useful marker of neuroendocrine tumors is the plasma concentration of chromogranin A, a protein made in the secretory granules, which is elevated in more than 80% of patients with carcinoid tumors. Although recent reports have proposed chromogranin A levels to be the test of choice for the diagnosis of carcinoid, the lack of specificity for this test limits its usefulness as a sole marker. It appears that the combination of 24-hour urine 5-HIAA and serum chromogranin A levels provides the best biochemical diagnostic accuracy. In terms of surveillance after resection or as a marker to monitor response to therapy, chromogranin A levels have proven efficacy over urine 5-HIAA levels. Plasma serotonin, substance P, neurotensin, neurokinin A, and neuropeptide K levels can be measured, but these peptides may not be elevated in all patients. Provocative tests using pentagastrin, calcium, or epinephrine may be used to reproduce the symptoms of carcinoid tumors. The administration of pentagastrin is the safest, most reliable, and most frequently used; however, with the accuracy of current diagnostic tests, there are relatively few indications today for provocative tests.

Carcinoid tumors of the small intestine are rarely diagnosed preoperatively. Barium radiographic studies of the small bowel may exhibit multiple filling defects as a result of kinking and fibrosis of the bowel (Fig. 50-31). There are a number of imaging techniques used to diagnose the extent and spread of carcinoid tumors. As CT technology has continued to progress, CT scanning has become the imaging modality of choice for identifying the site of disease and the presence of lymphatic or hematogenous metastases. CT angiography may be useful in cases associated with a large mesenteric process to identify encasement and pseudoaneurysm formation, typical of a malignant process in the mesentery. A novel imaging study that takes advantage of the fact that many of these tumors possess somatostatin receptors is somatostatin receptor scintigraphy using $^{111}$In-labeled pentetreotide. This scintigraphic localization study has shown encouraging results, with a higher reported sensitivity than conventional imaging techniques, such as CT, for delineating and localizing carcinoid tumors. In particular, somatostatin receptor scintigraphy is the test of choice to identify extra-abdominal metastatic disease or in cases in which the primary cannot be appreciated on CT scan. Although CT scanning and somatostatin receptor scintigraphy (SRS) are the predominant modalities for carcinoid tumor localization and staging, MRI is emerging as a potential adjunct to these current imaging techniques. When directly compared with CT or SRS, MRI has shown enhanced sensitivity for hepatic metastases evaluation. Unfortunately, MRI has not improved the ability to identify extrahepatic disease and remains constrained by institutional expertise. $^{18}$F-fluorodeoxyglucose positron emission tomography (FDG-PET) scanning, although important in the evaluation of other malignancies, has not proven beneficial for carcinoids. However, the addition of newer isotopes such as $^{11}$C–5-HTP and $^{18}$F-L-dihydroxyphenylalanine ($^{18}$F-DOPA) has dramatically improved the sensitivity of PET for neuroendocrine malignancies and, when fused with conventional CT scanning, may ultimately outperform the current accepted imaging modalities.[31]

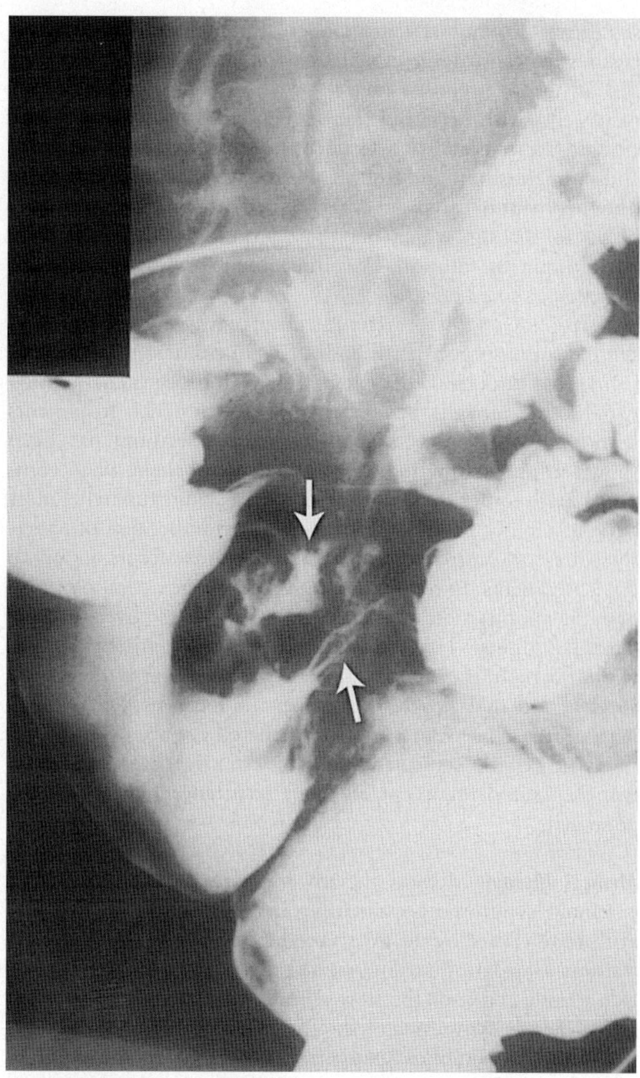

**FIGURE 50-31** Barium radiograph of a carcinoid tumor of the terminal ileum demonstrates fibrosis with multiple filling defects and high-grade partial obstruction *(arrows)*. (Courtesy Dr. Melvyn H. Schreiber, The University of Texas Medical Branch, Galveston, Tex.)

### Treatment

***Surgical Therapy*** The treatment of patients with small bowel carcinoid tumors is based on tumor size and site and presence or absence of metastatic disease.[30] For primary tumors smaller than 1 cm in diameter without evidence of regional lymph node metastasis, a segmental intestinal resection is adequate. For patients with lesions larger than 1 cm, with multiple tumors, or with regional lymph node metastasis, regardless of the size of the primary tumor, wide excision of bowel and mesentery is required. Lesions of the terminal ileum are best treated by right hemicolectomy. Small duodenal tumors can be excised locally; however, more extensive lesions may require pancreaticoduodenectomy. In addition to treatment of the primary tumor, it is important that the abdomen be thoroughly explored for multicentric lesions. In cases in which the mesenteric disease appears to involve a large portion of the mesentery, dissection of the tumor off the mesenteric vessels, with preservation of the blood supply to unaffected bowel, is appropriate, albeit technically demanding. Not only does removal of the mesenteric disease provide a significant survival advantage, but also mesenteric debulking ensures the most durable palliation for the patient.

Caution should be exerted in the anesthetic management of patients with carcinoid tumors because anesthesia may precipitate a carcinoid crisis characterized by hypotension, bronchospasm, flushing, and tachycardia predisposing to arrhythmias. The treatment of carcinoid crisis is IV octreotide given as a bolus of 50 to 100 μg, which may be continued as an infusion at 50 μg/hour. In addition, IV antihistamine and hydrocortisone may be of some benefit.

In patients with carcinoid tumors and widespread metastatic disease, surgery is still indicated. In contrast to metastases from other tumors, there is a definite role for surgical debulking, which often provides beneficial symptomatic relief. In patients with limited hepatic involvement, metastasectomy has been shown to provide the most durable survival benefit when compared with other treatment modalities. Unfortunately, most patients are not candidates for liver resection because of extensive disease; recurrence after metastasectomy occurs in up to 75% of patients. In these cases, transarterial chemoembolization or radioembolization has been shown to provide liver-directed control of disease. Furthermore, resection of the primary tumor, with or without mesenteric resection, has been shown to improve survival and slow progression of hepatic metastases in patients with unresectable disease. Although there have been some small series of hepatic transplantation for extensive liver metastases from carcinoid, unacceptably high recurrence rates limit this approach.

***Medical Therapy*** Medical therapy for patients with malignant carcinoid syndrome is primarily directed toward the relief of symptoms caused by the excess production of humoral factors.[30] Various long-acting analogues of somatostatin, such as octreotide (Sandostatin) or the slow-release formulation (Sandostatin LAR), relieve symptoms of the carcinoid syndrome (e.g., diarrhea, flushing) in most patients. In addition to the relief of symptoms using octreotide, tumor regression has been reported in some patients. A randomized controlled trial of 85 patients with unresectable metastatic midgut carcinoid compared treatment with Sandostatin LAR to placebo.[32] A significant improvement in progression-free survival was seen and was most pronounced in patients with a resected primary tumor and/or low hepatic burden.

Recently, second-generation right hemicolectomy somatostatin analogues have been developed to address the limitations of the current regimens. Pasireotide represents an important advance in current biologic therapy. With its broad somatostatin receptor inhibition and up to 40-fold increase in binding affinity, as compared with current somatostatin analogues, pasireotide my have a role as primary therapy or salvage therapy for patients who fail treatment on first-generation somatostatin therapy.[33] Interferon-α (IFN-α) has also been shown to provide symptomatic relief in patients with carcinoid syndrome. A clinical trial that evaluated the use of IFN-α in more than 100 patients with carcinoid syndrome identified decreases in urinary 5-HIAA levels in 42% of patients and tumor regression in 15%. However, the increased incidence of side effects (e.g., fever, fatigue, anorexia, weight loss) precludes the widespread use of this drug.

Serotonin receptor antagonists have been used with limited success. Methysergide is no longer used because of the increased incidence of retroperitoneal fibrosis. Ketanserin and cyproheptadine have been shown to provide some control of symptoms and other antagonists, such as ondansetron, may be even more effective.

Given the slow-growing nature of carcinoid, cytotoxic chemotherapy has had only limited success. The role of chemotherapy is confined predominantly to patients with metastatic disease who are symptomatic, unresponsive to other therapies, or have high tumor proliferation rates. The most frequent combination used is streptozotocin plus 5-fluorouracil or cyclophosphamide, which may result in some tumor regression in up to one third of the patients. The duration of response, however, is short-lived. The use of cisplatin and etoposide has shown some promise only in patients with well-differentiated carcinoids. Results using dacarbazine (DTIC) are conflicting.

In summary, the treatment of metastatic carcinoid tumors requires a multidisciplinary approach and combined modalities may be the best option, including surgical debulking, hepatic artery embolization or chemoembolization, and medical therapy. In addition, newer and more targeted therapies are being developed that may be useful in the future. Targeted therapy has progressed down four separate pathways. Given the hypervascular nature of carcinoids, antiangiogenesis therapy (e.g., bevacizumab) is being investigated in combination with cytotoxic and somatostatin therapy.[34] Based on the benefit of sunitinib seen in pancreatic neuroendocrine tumors, tyrosine kinase inhibitors have been evaluated as systemic therapy and as a liver-directed chemoembolization strategy for carcinoids as well. The PI3K-AKT-mTOR pathway has also recently emerged as a potential target for systemic therapy. Agents such as everolimus, an mTOR inhibitor, although initially developed as immunosuppressant therapy, have redefined themselves as potent antitumor agents and remain under active investigation for carcinoid disease. Perhaps the most promising targeted therapy to date is radiolabeled somatostatin analogue therapy. In a series of over 500 patients with gastrointestinal neuroendocrine tumors including carcinoid, [$^{177}$Lu-DOTA$^{0}$,Tyr$^{3}$]octreotate was well tolerated and provided significant improvements in response rates and overall survival when compared with historical controls.[35]

**Prognosis** Carcinoid tumors have the best prognosis of all small bowel tumors, whether the disease is localized or metastatic. Resection of a carcinoid tumor localized to its primary site approaches a 100% survival rate. Five-year survival rates are approximately 65% in patients with regional disease and 25% to 35% in those with distant metastasis. When widespread metastatic disease precludes cure, extensive resection for palliation is indicated. In fact, long-term palliation often can be obtained because these tumors are relatively slow-growing. A number of factors have been evaluated in an attempt to identify patients with carcinoid tumors who have a poor prognosis. Probably the most useful factor identified is an elevated level of chromogranin A, which was found to be an independent predictor of an adverse prognosis.

### Adenocarcinomas

Adenocarcinomas traditionally have constituted approximately 50% of the malignant tumors of the small bowel in most reported series, although the incidence has plateaued in recent years.[29] The peak incidence is in the seventh decade of life, and most series show a slight male predominance. Most of these

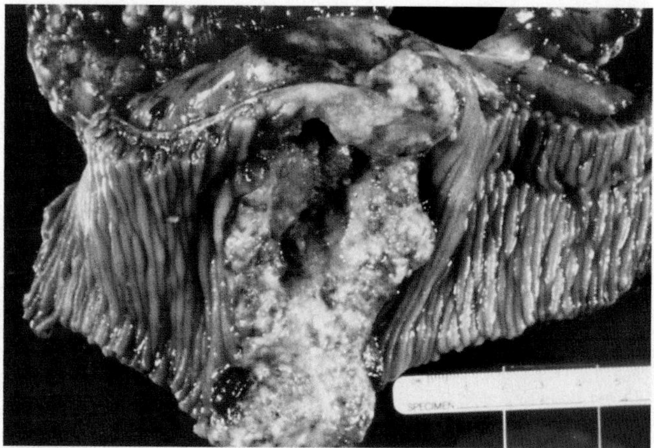

**FIGURE 50-32** Large circumferential mucinous adenocarcinoma of the jejunum. (Courtesy Dr. Mary R. Schwartz, Baylor College of Medicine, Houston.)

tumors are located in the duodenum and proximal jejunum (Fig. 50-32). Those arising in association with Crohn's disease tend to occur at a somewhat younger age, and more than 70% arise in the ileum. Tumors of the duodenum tend to present somewhat earlier than those in the most distal intestine, with symptoms of jaundice and chronic bleeding. Adenocarcinomas of the jejunum and ileum usually produce symptoms that may be more nonspecific and include vague abdominal pain and weight loss. Intestinal obstruction and chronic bleeding can also occur. Perforation is uncommon. As with adenocarcinomas in other organs, survival of patients with small bowel adenocarcinomas is related to the stage of disease at the time of diagnosis. Unfortunately, diagnosis is often delayed, and the disease is advanced at the time of surgery, secondary to various factors (e.g., vagueness of symptoms, absence of physical findings, lack of clinical suspicion because of the rarity of these lesions).

Treatment of small bowel adenocarcinoma is determined by location and stage. Duodenal adenocarcinomas are treated with pancreaticoduodenectomy or segmental resection if the tumor is in the third or fourth portion of the duodenum. Jejunal and ileal adenocarcinomas are treated with segmental resection with the associated mesentery (Fig. 50-33) or right colectomy for terminal ileal carcinomas. There is no standard adjuvant protocol for small bowel adenocarcinoma and adjuvant regimens are often dictated by location. Duodenal adenocarcinomas often receive a periampullary treatment protocol whereas midgut adenocarcinomas undergo a colorectal regimen. The prognosis of small bowel adenocarcinoma is poor, likely because of the delayed presentation and presence of advanced disease at diagnosis. Five-year survival rates are typically in the 15% to 20% range, although duodenal adenocarcinoma has a 5-year survival rate of 50%, probably because of the earlier symptom presentation and diagnosis.

### Lymphoma

Malignant lymphomas involve the small bowel primarily or as a manifestation of systemic disease. Primary gastrointestinal lymphomas, of which about one third occur in the small bowel, account for 5% of all lymphomas.[36] Lymphomas constitute 7% to 25% of small bowel malignant tumors in the adult; in children younger than 10 years, they are the most common

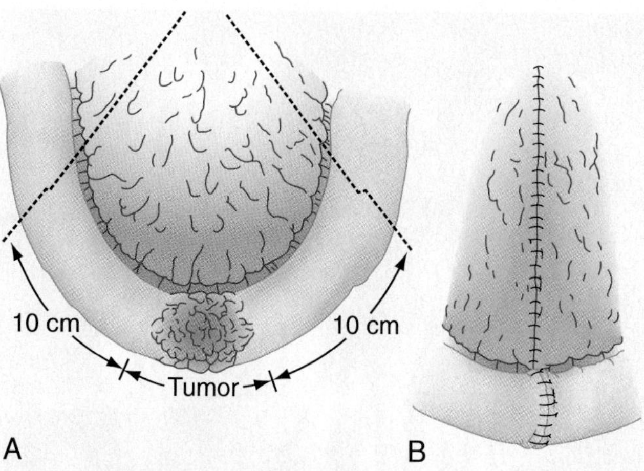


**FIGURE 50-33** Surgical management of carcinoma of the small bowel. **A,** Malignant tumors should be resected with a wide margin of normal bowel and a wedge of mesentery to remove the immediate draining lymph nodes. **B,** End-to-end anastomosis of the small bowel and repair of the mesentery. (Adapted from Thompson JC: Atlas of surgery of the stomach, duodenum, and small bowel, St Louis, Mosby–Year Book, 1992, p 299.)

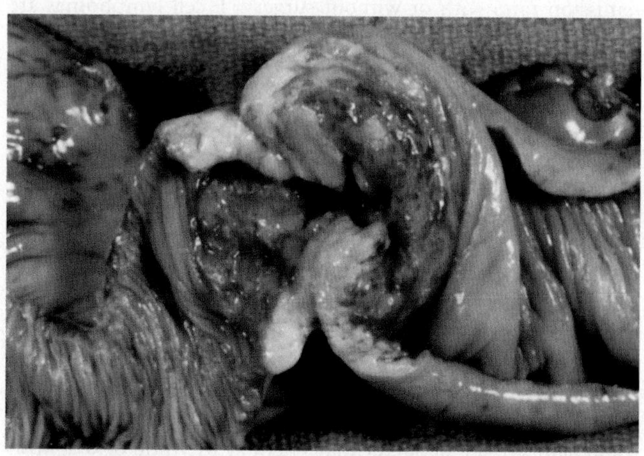

**FIGURE 50-34** Gross photograph of primary lymphoma of the ileum shows replacement of all layers of the bowel wall with tumor. (Courtesy Dr. Mary R. Schwartz, Baylor College of Medicine, Houston.)

intestinal neoplasm. Lymphomas are most commonly found in the ileum, where there is the greatest concentration of gut-associated lymphoid tissue. Increased risk for developing primary small bowel lymphomas has been reported in patients with celiac disease and immunodeficiency states (e.g., AIDS). Grossly, small intestine lymphomas are usually large, with most larger than 5 cm; they may extend beneath the mucosa (Fig. 50-34). Microscopically, there is often diffuse infiltration of the intestinal wall. Symptoms of small bowel lymphoma include pain, weight loss, nausea, vomiting, and change in bowel habits. Perforation may occur in up to 25% of patients (Fig. 50-35). Fever is uncommon and suggests systemic involvement.

The treatment of small bowel lymphoma remains controversial. Traditionally, a combination of surgery, chemotherapy and radiation were used for all small bowel tumors. However, in the absence of symptoms, small bowel lymphomas may

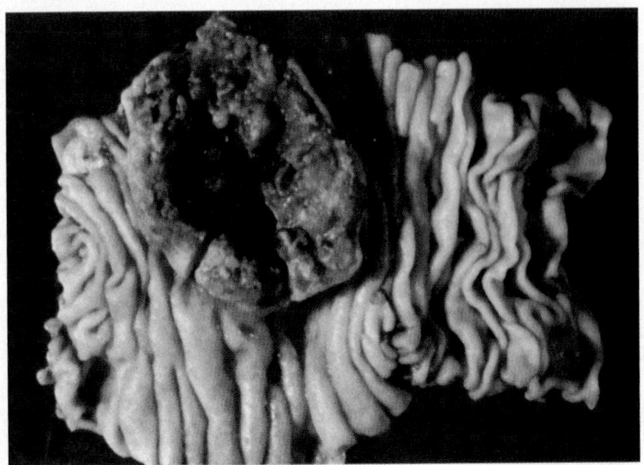

**FIGURE 50-35** Small bowel lymphoma presents as perforation and peritonitis. (Courtesy Dr. Mary R. Schwartz, Baylor College of Medicine, Houston.)

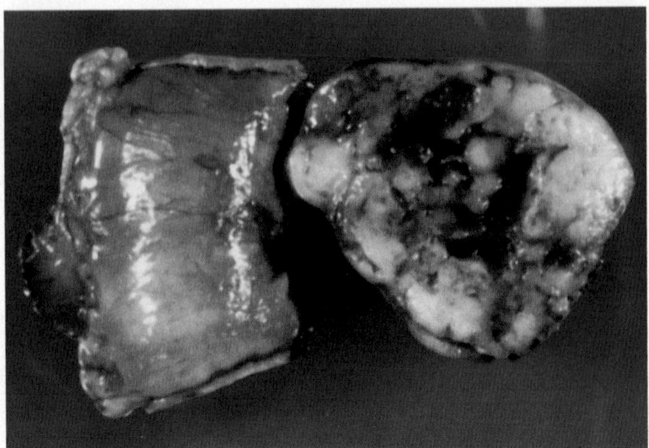

**FIGURE 50-36** Small bowel leiomyosarcoma (malignant gastrointestinal stromal tumor) with hemorrhagic necrosis. (Courtesy Dr. Mary R. Schwartz, Baylor College of Medicine, Houston.)

respond to chemotherapy without the need for surgery. This can typically be predicted by cell type because B cell lymphomas are more chemosensitive than T cell lymphomas and have high remission rates with or without surgery. T cell lymphomas are traditionally more resistant to therapy and will progress to symptoms of obstruction or perforation if not resected. Regardless of cell type, resection is indicated at any onset of symptoms because progression to life-threatening hemorrhage or perforation portends a dismal prognosis. Five-year survival of 50% to 60% can be expected and is dictated by response to systemic therapy rather than the success of surgical resection.

### Gastrointestinal Stromal Tumors

Malignant GISTs, or leomyosarcomas, arise from mesenchymal tissue and constitute about 20% of malignant neoplasms of the small bowel (Fig. 50-36). These tumors are more common in the jejunum and ileum, typically are diagnosed in the fifth and sixth decades of life, and occur with a slight male preponderance. Malignant GISTs are larger than 5 cm at the time of diagnosis in 80% of patients. GISTs mostly arise from the muscularis propria and generally grow extramurally. Most common indications for surgery include bleeding and obstruction, although free perforation may occur as a result of hemorrhagic necrosis in large tumor masses. Typically, GISTs tend to invade locally and spread by direct extension into adjacent tissues and hematogenously to the liver, lungs, and bone; lymphatic metastases are unusual. The most useful indicators of survival and the risk for metastasis include the size of the tumor at presentation, mitotic index, and evidence of tumor invasion into the lamina propria.

Treatment of GISTs continues to evolve and represents one of the first breakthroughs in signal transduction manipulation. Surgical management is straightforward, with segmental resection of the tumor containing segment to obtain negative margins. Wide resection of the mesentery with lymphadenectomy is not necessary. Until recently, adjuvant strategies for GIST were lacking and recurrence rates after resection were as high as 70%. However, the development of imatinib mesylate (Gleevec, formerly known as *STI571*) has altered previous treatment strategies. Imatinib mesylate is a tyrosine kinase inhibitor that blocks the unregulated mutant c-*kit* (CD117) tyrosine kinase and inhibits the BCR-ABL and platelet-derived growth factor (PDGF) tyrosine kinases. Previous randomized trials have verified its ability to control disease progression in patients with metastatic disease. However, a recent surgeon-initiated randomized trial has shown that 1 year of adjuvant imatinib mesylate, after complete resection of a GIST, significantly improved recurrence free survival.[37] Adjuvant imatinib mesylate is now the standard of care for malignant GISTs, especially with size larger than 5 cm, high mitotic rate, or small bowel location. Further trials have suggested that neoadjuvant imatinib mesylate may help determine which patients with locally advanced or metastatic GIST may benefit from aggressive resection.[38] Survival data are pending.

The prognosis of malignant GIST has traditionally been poor because of the high recurrence rate. However, in the era of tyrosine kinase modulation therapy, the impact of these new therapies on overall survival remains to be determined.

### Metastatic Neoplasms

Metastatic tumors involving the small bowel are much more common than primary neoplasms. The most common metastases to the small intestine are those arising from other intra-abdominal organs, including the uterine cervix, ovaries, kidneys, stomach, colon, and pancreas. Small intestinal involvement is by direct extension or implantation of tumor cells. Metastases from extra-abdominal tumors are rare but may be found in patients with adenocarcinoma of the breast and carcinoma of the lung. Cutaneous melanoma is the most common extra-abdominal source to involve the small intestine, with involvement of the small intestine noted in more than 50% of patients dying from malignant melanoma (Fig. 50-37). Common symptoms include anorexia, weight loss, anemia, bleeding, and partial bowel obstruction. Treatment is palliative resection to relieve symptoms or, occasionally, bypass if the metastatic tumor is extensive and not amenable to resection.

## DIVERTICULAR DISEASE

Diverticular disease of the small intestine is relatively common. It may present as true or false diverticula. A true diverticulum contains all layers of the intestinal wall and is usually congenital.

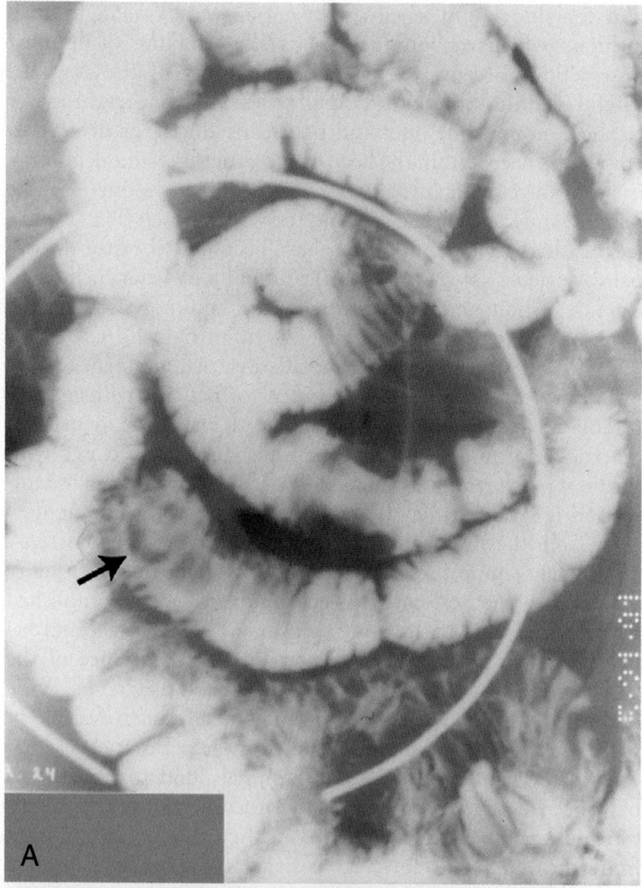


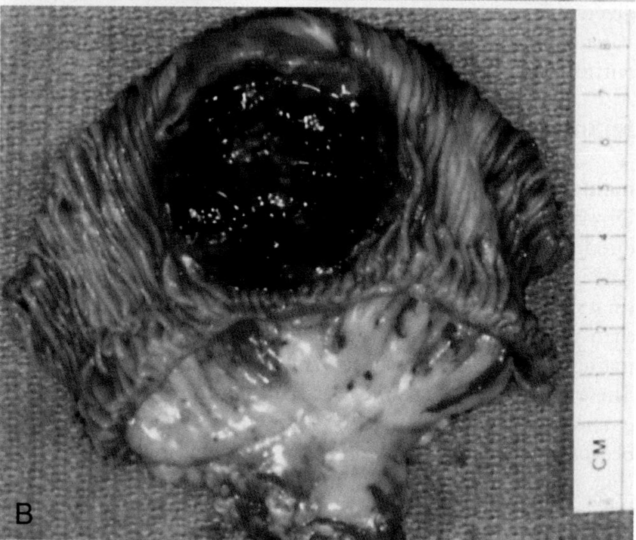


**FIGURE 50-37 A,** Barium radiograph shows target lesions consistent with metastatic melanoma of the small bowel *(arrow)*. **B,** Gross specimen demonstrating metastatic melanoma to the small bowel. (**A,** Courtesy Dr. Melvyn H. Schreiber, The University of Texas Medical Branch, Galveston, Tex; **B,** courtesy Dr. Mary R. Schwartz, Baylor College of Medicine, Houston.)

False diverticula consist of mucosa and submucosa protruding through a defect in the muscle coat and are usually acquired defects. Small bowel diverticula may occur in any portion of the small intestine. Duodenal diverticula are the most common acquired diverticula of the small bowel, and Meckel's

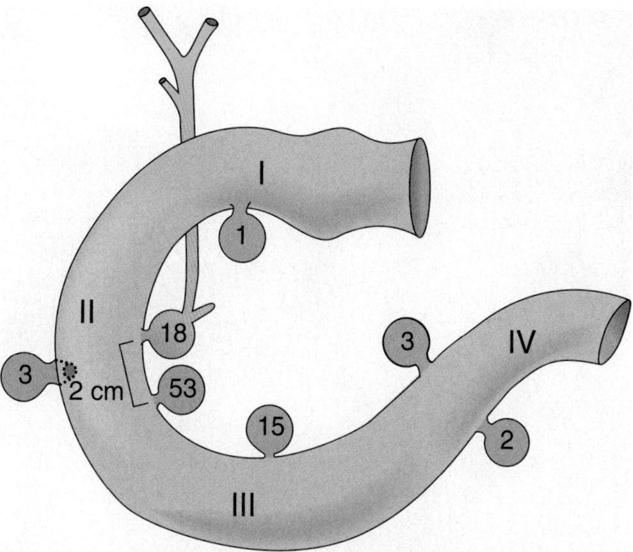


**FIGURE 50-38** Distribution of 95 duodenal diverticula within the four portions of the duodenum. (From Eggert A, Teichmann W, Wittmann DH: The pathologic implication of duodenal diverticula. Surg Gynecol Obstet 154:62–64, 1982.)

diverticulum is the most common true congenital diverticulum of the small bowel.

## Duodenal Diverticula

### Incidence and Cause

First described by Chomel, a French pathologist, in 1710, diverticula of the duodenum are relatively common, representing the second most common site for diverticulum formation after the colon. The incidence of duodenal diverticula varies, depending on the age of the patient and method of diagnosis. Upper gastrointestinal radiographic studies identify duodenal diverticula in 1% to 5% of all studies, whereas some autopsy series report the incidence as being as high as 15% to 20%. Duodenal diverticula occur twice as often in women as in men and are rare in patients younger than 40 years. They have been classified as congenital or acquired, true or false, and intraluminal or extraluminal. Two thirds to three fourths of duodenal diverticula are found in the periampullary region (within a 2-cm radius of the ampulla) and project from the medial wall of the duodenum (Fig. 50-38).

### Clinical Manifestations

The important thing to remember is that the overwhelming majority of duodenal diverticula are asymptomatic and are usually noted incidentally by an upper gastrointestinal series for an unrelated problem (Fig. 50-39). Diagnosis may also be obtained by upper gastrointestinal endoscopy or suggested by plain abdominal films showing an atypical gas bubble; CT can identify large diverticula. Less than 5% of duodenal diverticula will require surgery because of a complication of the diverticulum itself. Major complications of duodenal diverticula include obstruction of the biliary or pancreatic ducts that may contribute to cholangitis and pancreatitis, respectively, hemorrhage,

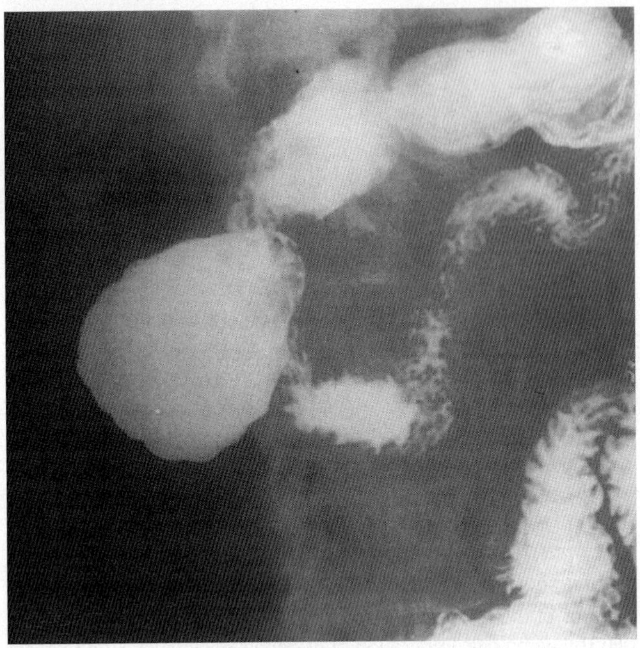

**FIGURE 50-39** Large diverticulum arises from the second portion of the duodenum. (Courtesy Dr. Melvyn H. Schreiber, The University of Texas Medical Branch, Galveston, Tex.)

perforation and, rarely, blind loop syndrome. Unfortunately, asymptomatic duodenal diverticula often present as an acute perforation that occurs during endoscopic misadventure.

Only those diverticula associated with the ampulla of Vater are significantly related to complications of cholangitis and pancreatitis. In these patients, the ampulla usually enters the duodenum at the superior margin of the diverticulum rather than through the diverticulum itself. The mechanism proposed for the increased incidence of complications of the biliary tract is the location of the perivaterian diverticulum, which may produce mechanical distortion of the common bile duct as it enters the duodenum, resulting in partial obstruction and stasis. Hemorrhage can be caused by inflammation, leading to erosion of a branch of the superior mesenteric artery. Perforation of duodenal diverticula has been described, but is rare. Finally, stasis of intestinal contents within a distended diverticulum can result in bacterial overgrowth, malabsorption, steatorrhea, and megaloblastic anemia (i.e., blind loop syndrome). Symptoms related to duodenal diverticula in the absence of any other demonstrable disease usually are nonspecific epigastric complaints that can be treated conservatively and may actually prove to be the result of another problem not related to the diverticulum itself.

### Treatment

As noted, most duodenal diverticula are asymptomatic and benign; when they are found incidentally, they should be left alone. Several operative procedures have been described for the treatment of the symptomatic duodenal diverticulum. The most common and effective treatment is diverticulectomy, which is most easily accomplished by performing a wide Kocher maneuver that exposes the duodenum. The diverticulum is then excised, and the duodenum is closed in a transverse or longitudinal fashion, whichever produces the least amount of luminal obstruction. Because of the close proximity of the ampulla, careful identification of the ampulla is essential to prevent injury to the common bile duct and pancreatic duct. For diverticula embedded deep within the head of the pancreas, a duodenotomy is performed, with invagination of the diverticulum into the lumen, which is then excised, and the wall is closed (Fig. 50-40*A* to *C*). Alternative methods that have been described for duodenal diverticula associated with the ampulla of Vater include an extended sphincteroplasty through the common wall of the ampulla in the diverticulum (see Fig. 50-40*D* to *F*).

The treatment of a perforated diverticulum may require procedures similar to those described for patients with massive trauma-related defects of the duodenal wall. The perforated diverticulum should be excised and the duodenum closed with a serosal patch from the jejunal loop. If the surrounding inflammation is severe, it may be necessary to divert the enteric flow away from the site of the perforation with a gastrojejunostomy or duodenojejunostomy. Interruption of duodenal continuity proximal to the perforated diverticulum may be accomplished by pyloric closure with suture or a row of staples. If the diverticulum is posterior and perforates into the substance of the pancreas, operative repair may be difficult and dangerous. Wide drainage with duodenal diversion may be all that is feasible in such cases. Great care should be taken if the perforation is adjacent to the papilla of Vater. Intraluminal duodenal diverticula have been described but are highly uncommon and, if symptomatic, can be completely excised if they arise at a site distant from the ampulla. However, if a symptomatic intraluminal diverticulum is encountered associated with the ampulla of Vater, subtotal resection of the diverticulum should be carried out to protect the entry of the biliary pancreatic ducts.

## Jejunal and Ileal Diverticula

### Incidence and Cause

Diverticula of the small bowel are much less common than duodenal diverticula, with an incidence ranging from 0.1% to 1.4% in autopsy series and 0.1% to 1.5% in upper gastrointestinal studies. Jejunal diverticula are more common and are larger than those in the ileum. These are false diverticula, occurring mainly in an older age group (after the sixth decade of life). These diverticula are multiple, usually protrude from the mesenteric border of the bowel, and may be overlooked at surgery because they are embedded within the small bowel mesentery (Fig. 50-41). The cause of jejunoileal diverticulosis is thought to be a motor dysfunction of the smooth muscle or the myenteric plexus, resulting in disordered contractions of the small bowel, generating increased intraluminal pressure, herniation of the mucosa and submucosa through the weakest portion of the bowel (i.e., the mesenteric side).

### Clinical Manifestations

Jejunoileal diverticula are usually found incidentally at laparotomy or during an upper gastrointestinal study (Fig. 50-42); the great majority remain asymptomatic. Acute complications such as intestinal obstruction, hemorrhage, or perforation can occur but are rare. Chronic symptomatology includes vague chronic abdominal pain, malabsorption, functional pseudo-obstruction, and chronic low-grade gastrointestinal hemorrhage. Acute

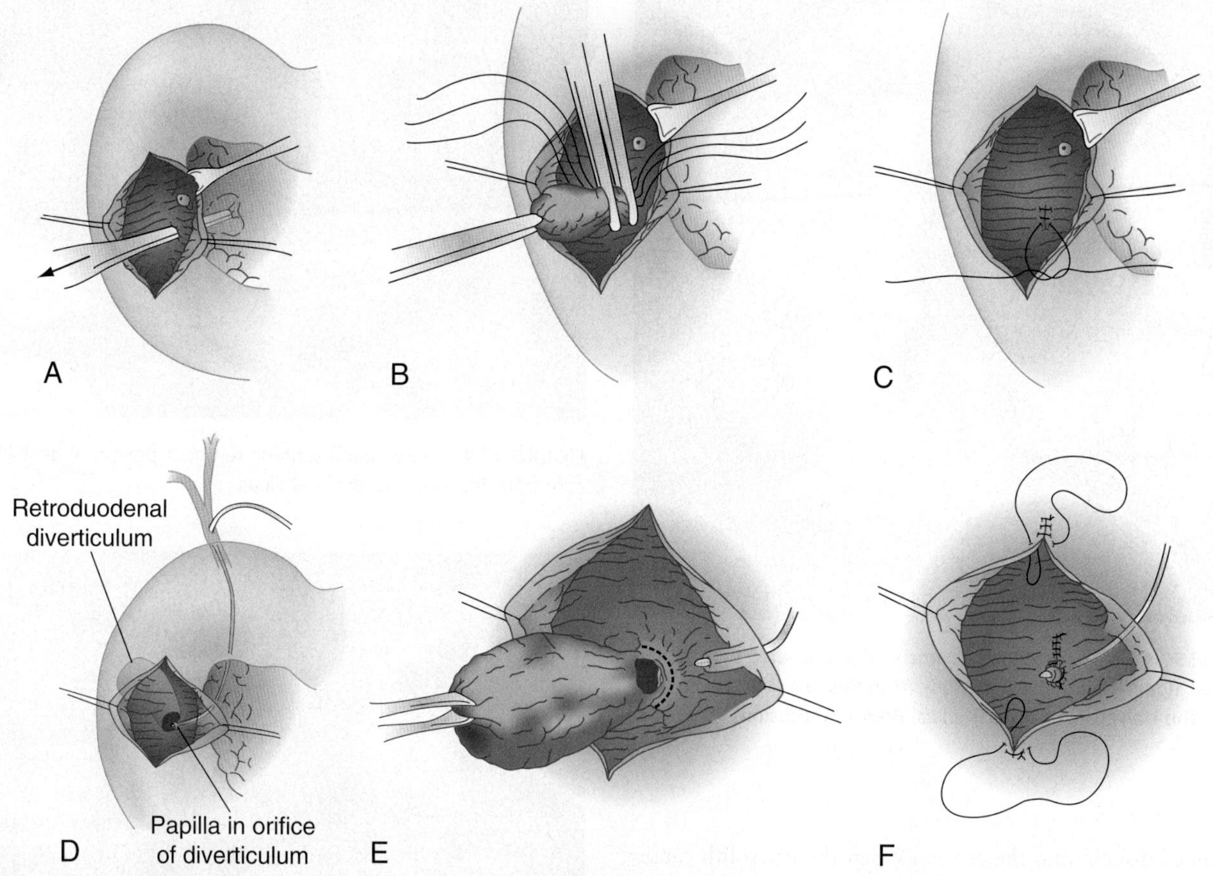


**FIGURE 50-40 A-C,** Treatment of a diverticulum protruding into the head of the pancreas. The duodenum is opened vertically. A clamp is used to invert the diverticulum into the lumen, where it is excised and the posterior wall defect is closed. **D-F,** Management of the unusual duodenal diverticula that arise in the periampullary location. A tube stent should be placed into the common bile duct and passed distally into the duodenum to facilitate identification and later dissection of the sphincter of Oddi. The diverticulum is inverted into the lumen of the duodenum. The round opening in the wall of the base of the diverticulum is the site at which the ampullary structures were freed by a circumferential incision. **E,** Line of division of the base of the diverticulum *(heavy broken line),* which is accomplished by free-hand dissection. After the diverticulum has been removed, the stent and enveloping papilla are protruded into the defect left by the division of the base of the diverticulum. The mucosa and muscle wall of the papilla are then sewn circumferentially to the wall of the duodenum. (Adapted from Thompson JC: Atlas of surgery of the stomach, duodenum, and small bowel. St Louis, 1992, Mosby–Year Book, pp 209–213.)

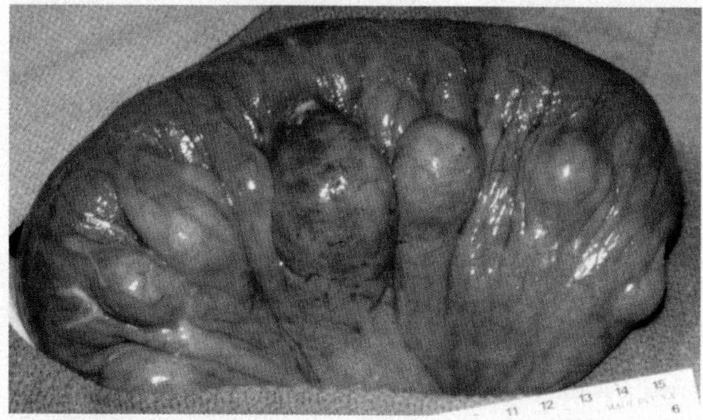

**FIGURE 50-41** Multiple large jejunal diverticula located in the mesentery in an older patient presenting with obstruction secondary to an enterolith. (Adapted from Evers BM, Townsend CM Jr, Thompson JC: Small intestine. In Schwartz SI [ed]: Principles of surgery, ed 7, New York, 1999, McGraw-Hill, p 1248.)

complications are diverticulitis, with or without abscess or perforation, gastrointestinal hemorrhage, and intestinal obstruction. Stasis of intestinal flow with bacterial overgrowth (blind loop syndrome), caused by the jejunal dyskinesia, may lead to deconjugation of bowel salts and uptake of vitamin $B_{12}$ by the bacterial flora, resulting in steatorrhea and megaloblastic anemia, with or without neuropathy.

### Treatment

For incidentally noted, asymptomatic jejunoileal diverticula, no treatment is required. Treatment of complications of obstruction, bleeding, and perforation is usually by intestinal resection and end-to-end anastomosis. Patients presenting with malabsorption secondary to the blind loop syndrome and bacterial overgrowth in the diverticulum can usually be given antibiotics. Obstruction may be caused by enteroliths that form in a jejunal diverticulum and are subsequently dislodged and obstruct the distal intestine. This condition may be treated by enterotomy and removal of the enterolith, or sometimes the enterolith can

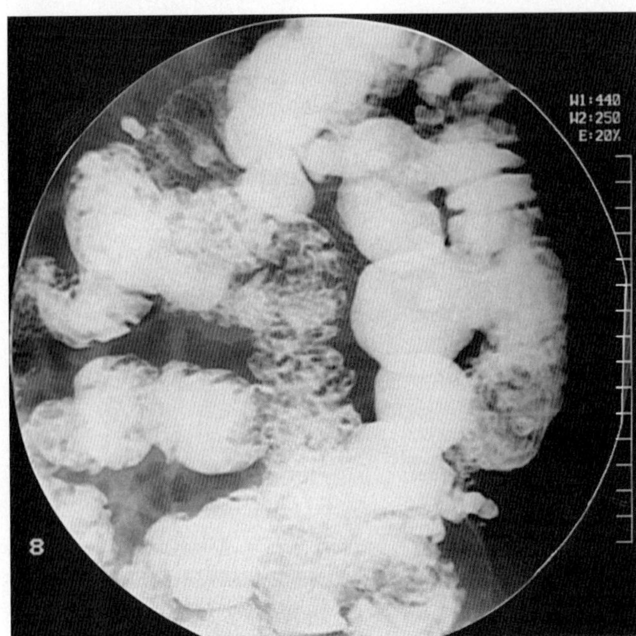


**FIGURE 50-42** Multiple jejunal diverticula demonstrated by a barium contrast upper gastrointestinal study. (Courtesy Dr. Melvyn H. Schreiber, The University of Texas Medical Branch, Galveston, Tex.)

be milked distally into the cecum. When the enterolith causes obstruction at the level of the diverticulum, bowel resection is necessary. When a perforation of a jejunoileal diverticulum is encountered, resection with reanastomosis is required because lesser procedures such as simple closure, excision, and invagination are associated with greater mortality and morbidity rates. In extreme cases, such as diffuse peritonitis, enterostomies may be required if judgment dictates that reanastomosis may be risky.

## Meckel's Diverticulum

### Incidence and Cause

Meckel's diverticulum is the most commonly encountered congenital anomaly of the small intestine, occurring in about 2% of the population. It was reported initially in 1598 by Hildanus and then described in detail by Johann Meckel in 1809. Meckel's diverticulum is located on the antimesenteric border of the ileum 45 to 60 cm proximal to the ileocecal valve and results from incomplete closure of the omphalomesenteric, or vitelline, duct. An equal incidence is found in men and women. Meckel's diverticulum may exist in different forms, ranging from a small bump that may be easily missed to a long projection that communicates with the umbilicus by a persistent fibrous cord (Fig. 50-43) or, much less commonly, a patent fistula. The usual manifestation is a relatively wide-mouthed diverticulum measuring about 5 cm in length, with a diameter of up to 2 cm (Fig. 50-44). Cells lining the vitelline duct are pluripotent; therefore, it is not uncommon to find heterotopic tissue within the Meckel diverticulum, the most common of which is gastric mucosa (present in 50% of all Meckel's diverticula). Pancreatic mucosa is encountered in about 5% of diverticula; less commonly, these diverticula may harbor colonic mucosa.

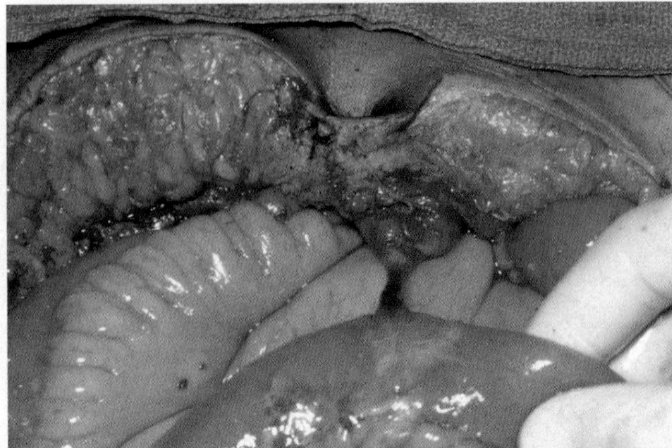

**FIGURE 50-43** Omphalomesenteric remnant persisting as a fibrous cord from the ileum to the umbilicus.

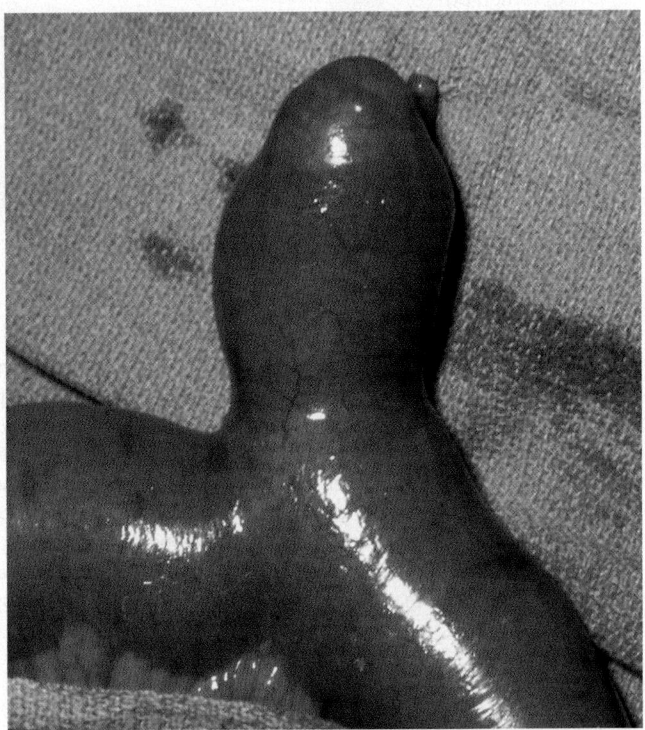

**FIGURE 50-44** Common presentation of a Meckel diverticulum projecting from the antimesenteric border of the ileum.

### Clinical Manifestations

Most Meckel's diverticula are entirely benign and are incidentally discovered during autopsy, laparotomy, or barium studies (Fig. 50-45). The most common clinical presentation of Meckel's diverticulum is gastrointestinal bleeding, which occurs in 25% to 50% of patients who present with complications; hemorrhage is the most common symptomatic presentation in children 2 years of age or younger. This complication may present as acute massive hemorrhage, anemia secondary to chronic bleeding, or a self-limiting recurrent episodic event. The usual source of the bleeding is a chronic acid-induced ulcer in the ileum adjacent to a Meckel's diverticulum that contains gastric mucosa.

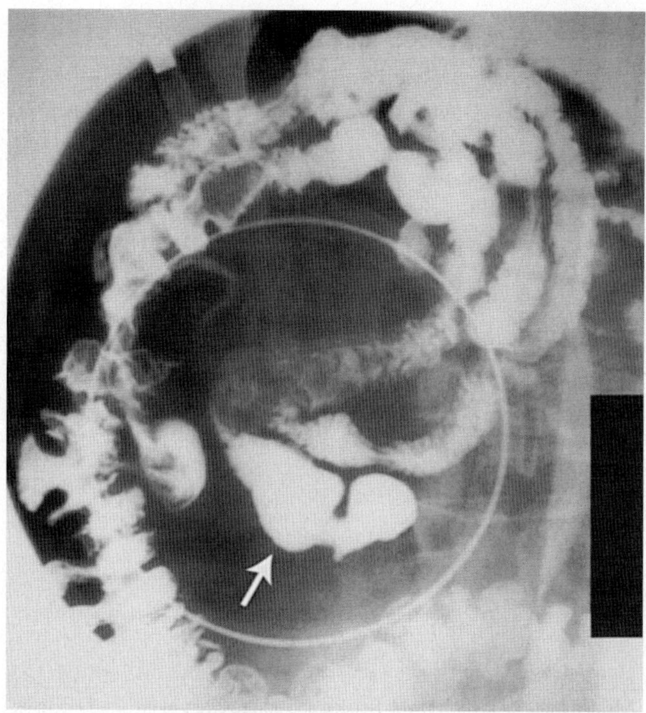

**FIGURE 50-45** Barium radiograph demonstrates an asymptomatic Meckel's diverticulum *(arrow)*. (Courtesy Dr. Melvyn H. Schreiber, The University of Texas Medical Branch, Galveston, Tex.)

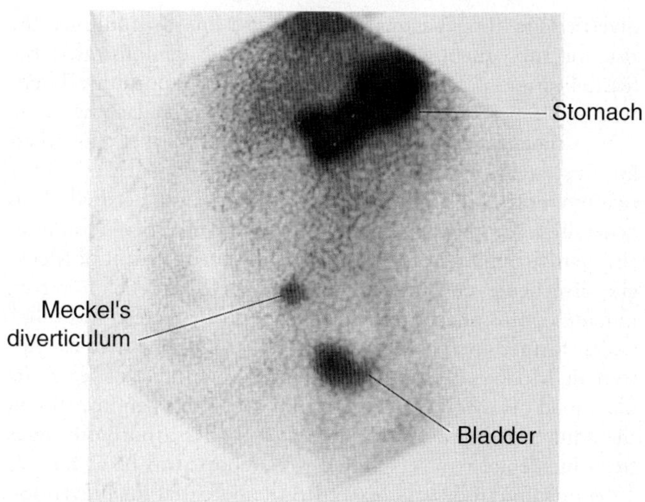


**FIGURE 50-46** $^{99m}$Tc-pertechnetate scintigram from a child demonstrates a Meckel's diverticulum clearly differentiated from the stomach and bladder. (Courtesy Dr. Melvyn H. Schreiber, The University of Texas Medical Branch, Galveston, Tex.)

Another common presenting symptom of Meckel's diverticulum is intestinal obstruction, which may occur as a result of a volvulus of the small bowel around a diverticulum associated with a fibrotic band attached to the abdominal wall, intussusception or, rarely, incarceration of the diverticulum in an inguinal hernia (Littre's hernia). Volvulus is usually an acute event and, if allowed to progress, may result in strangulation of the involved bowel. In intussusception, a broad-based diverticulum invaginates and then is carried forward by peristalsis. This may be ileoileal or ileocolic and present as acute obstruction associated with an urge to defecate, early vomiting and, occasionally, the passage of the classic currant jelly stool. A palpable mass may be present. Although reduction of an intussusception secondary to Meckel's diverticulum can sometimes be performed by barium enema, the patient should still undergo resection of the diverticulum to negate subsequent recurrence of the condition.

Diverticulitis accounts for 10% to 20% of symptomatic presentations. This complication is more common in adult patients. Meckel's diverticulitis, which is clinically indistinguishable from appendicitis, should be considered in the differential diagnosis of a patient with right lower quadrant pain. Progression of the diverticulitis may lead to perforation and peritonitis. It is important to remember that when the appendix is found to be normal during exploration for suspected appendicitis, the distal ileum should be inspected for the presence of an inflamed Meckel's diverticulum. Finally, much rarer complications of Meckel's diverticula include neoplasms, with the most common benign tumors reported as leiomyomas, angiomas, and lipomas. Malignant neoplasms include adenocarcinomas, which generally originate from the gastric mucosa, sarcoma, and carcinoid tumor.

### Diagnostic Studies

The diagnosis of Meckel's diverticulum may be difficult. Plain abdominal radiography, CT, and ultrasonography are rarely helpful. In children, the single most accurate diagnostic test for Meckel's diverticula is scintigraphy with sodium $^{99m}$Tc-pertechnetate. The $^{99m}$Tc-pertechnetate is preferentially taken up by the mucus-secreting cells of gastric mucosa and ectopic gastric tissue in the diverticulum (Fig. 50-46). The diagnostic sensitivity of this scan has been reported as high as 85%, with a specificity of 95% and an accuracy of 90% in the pediatric age group.

In adults, however, $^{99m}$Tc-pertechnetate scanning is less accurate because of the reduced prevalence of ectopic gastric mucosa within the diverticulum. The sensitivity and specificity can be improved by the use of pharmacologic agents such as pentagastrin and glucagon or histamine 2 ($H_2$) receptor antagonists (e.g., cimetidine). Pentagastrin indirectly increases the metabolism of mucus-producing cells, whereas glucagon inhibits peristaltic dilution and washout of intraluminal radionuclide. Cimetidine may be used to increase the sensitivity of scintigraphy by decreasing the peptic secretion, but not the radionuclide uptake, and retarding the release of pertechnetate from the diverticular lumen, thus resulting in higher radionuclide concentrations in the wall of the diverticulum. In adult patients, when nuclear medicine findings are normal, barium studies should be performed. In patients with acute hemorrhage, angiography is sometimes useful.

### Treatment

The treatment of a symptomatic Meckel's diverticulum should be prompt surgical intervention with resection of the diverticulum or resection of the segment of ileum bearing the diverticulum. Segmental intestinal resection is required for treatment of patients with bleeding because the bleeding site is usually in the ileum adjacent to the diverticulum. Resection of the diverticulum for nonbleeding Meckel's diverticula can be performed using a hand-sewn technique or stapling across the base of the diverticulum in a diagonal or transverse line to minimize the risk for subsequent stenosis. Reports have demonstrated the feasibility and safety of laparoscopic diverticulectomy. Long-term outcomes with this procedure, however, are lacking.

Although the treatment of complicated Meckel's diverticulum is straightforward, the optimal treatment of Meckel's diverticulum noted as an incidental finding is still debated. It is generally recommended that asymptomatic diverticula found in children during laparotomy be resected. The treatment of Meckel's diverticula encountered in the adult patient, however, remains controversial. In a landmark paper by Soltero and Bill,[39] which formed the basis of the surgical management of asymptomatic Meckel's diverticula in adults for a number of years, the likelihood of a Meckel's diverticulum becoming symptomatic in the adult patient was estimated as 2% or less; morbidity rates from incidental removal, which were reported to be as high as 12% in some studies, far exceeded the potential for prevention of disease. This study was criticized, however, because it was not a population-based analysis. An epidemiologic population-based study by Cullen and associates[40] has challenged the practice of ignoring an incidentally found Meckel's diverticulum. A 6.4% rate of development of complications from the Meckel's diverticulum was calculated to occur over a lifetime. This incidence of complications does not appear to peak during childhood, as originally thought. Therefore, the recommendation from this study was that an incidentally found Meckel's diverticulum be removed at any age up to 80 years as long as no additional conditions (e.g., peritonitis) make removal hazardous. The rates of short- and long-term postoperative complications from prophylactic removal were low (~2%), and death was related to the primary operation or the general health of the patient and not to the diverticulectomy. Zani and coworkers[41] have reviewed 244 articles evaluating the incidence and outcomes of Meckel's diverticulum, including autopsy, population, and surgical series. They identified a clear incidence of increased morbidity associated with incidental resection over no treatment and determined that more than 700 patients with incidental Meckel's diverticulum required resection to avoid one Meckel's related death. In short, treatment of incidental Meckel's diverticulum remains controversial, and conservative management of an incidental finding is a reasonable surgical approach.

## MISCELLANEOUS PROBLEMS

### Small Bowel Ulcerations

Ulcerations of the small bowel are relatively uncommon and may be attributed to Crohn's disease, typhoid fever, tuberculosis, lymphoma, and ulcers associated with gastrinoma (Table 50-10). Drug-induced ulcerations can occur and were, in the past, attributed to enteric-coated potassium chloride tablets and corticosteroids. In addition, ulcerations of the small intestine in which no causative agent can be identified have been described. It has been suggested that small bowel complications from nonsteroidal anti-inflammatory drugs (NSAIDs) may be more common than originally considered. NSAID-induced ulcers occur more commonly in the ileum, with single or multiple ulcerations noted. Complications necessitating operative intervention include bleeding, perforation, and obstruction. In addition to ulcerations, NSAIDs are known to induce an enteropathy characterized by increased intestinal permeability leading to protein loss and hypoalbuminemia, malabsorption, and anemia.

**Table 50-10 Causes of Small Intestine Ulceration**

| CAUSE | EXAMPLES |
|---|---|
| Infections | Tuberculosis, syphilis, cytomegalovirus, typhoid, parasites, *Strongyloides* hyperinfection, *Campylobacter, Yersinia* |
| Inflammatory | Crohn's disease, systemic lupus erythematosus, celiac disease, ulcerative enteritis |
| Ischemia | Mesenteric insufficiency |
| Idiopathic | Primary ulcer, Behçet's syndrome |
| Drug induced | Potassium, indomethacin, phenylbutazone, salicylates, antimetabolites |
| Radiation | Therapeutic, accidental |
| Vascular | Vasculitis, giant cell arteritis, amyloidosis (ischemic lesion), angiocentric lymphoma |
| Metabolic | Uremia |
| Hyperacidity | Zollinger-Ellison syndrome, Meckel's diverticulum, stomal ulceration |
| Neoplastic | Lymphoma, adenocarcinoma, melanoma |
| Toxic | Acute jejunitis (β-toxin–producing *Clostridium perfringens*), arsenic |
| Mucosal lesions | Lymphocytic enterocolitis |

Adapted from Rai R, Bayless TM: Isolated and diffuse ulcers of the small intestine. In Feldman M, Scharschmidt BF, Sleisenger MH (eds): Gastrointestinal and liver disease: Pathophysiology, diagnosis, management, Philadelphia, 1998, WB Saunders, pp 1771–1778.

Treatment of complications from small bowel ulcerations is segmental resection and intestinal reanastomosis.

### Ingested Foreign Bodies

Ingested foreign bodies, which can lead to subsequent perforation or obstruction of the gastrointestinal tract, are swallowed, usually accidentally, by children or adults. These include glass and metal fragments, pins, needles, toothpicks, fish bones, coins, whistles, toys, and broken razor blades (Fig. 50-47). Intentional ingestion of foreign bodies is sometimes seen in the prison population and those who are mentally unstable. For most patients, treatment is observation, which allows the safe passage of these objects through the intestinal tract. If the object is radiopaque, progress can be followed by serial abdominal films. Cathartic agents are contraindicated. Sharp pointed objects such as needles, razor blades, or fish bones may penetrate the bowel wall. If abdominal pain, tenderness, fever, or leukocytosis occurs, immediate laparotomy and surgical removal of the offending object are indicated. Laparotomy is also required for intestinal obstruction.

### Small Bowel Fistulas

Despite improvements in surgical nutrition and critical care, mortality from enterocutaneous fistulas remains high, 15% to 20% in recent reports.[42] Improvements in outcome are focused on prevention and, when fistulas occur, prompt recognition and intervention. Enterocutaneous fistulas are most commonly iatrogenic, with 75% to 85% of cases attributed to surgical misadventure (e.g., anastomotic leakage, injury of the bowel or blood supply, erosion by suction catheters, laceration of the bowel by wire mesh or retention suture). The remaining 15%

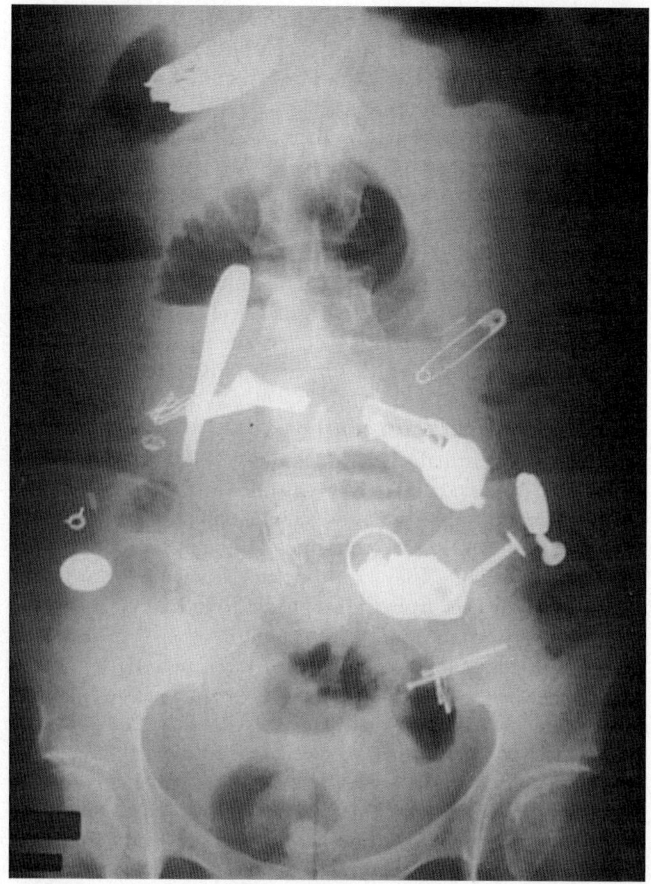

**FIGURE 50-47** Plain abdominal film demonstrates a number of ingested foreign bodies in a patient presenting with a small bowel obstruction. (Courtesy Dr. Melvyn H. Schreiber, The University of Texas Medical Branch, Galveston, Tex.)

to 20% of fistula occurrences are associated with predisposing conditions such as Crohn's disease, malignancy, radiation enteritis, diverticulitis, intra-abdominal sepsis, or trauma.

## Clinical Manifestations

Recognition of enterocutaneous fistulas is usually not difficult. The typical clinical presentation is that of a febrile postoperative patient with an erythematous wound. When a few skin sutures are removed, a purulent or bloody discharge is noted; leakage of enteric contents then occurs, sometimes immediately, but often within 1 or 2 days. The diagnosis rarely eludes the surgeon for long. Small bowel fistulas can also present with generalized peritonitis, although this is less common. Recently, the popularization of damage control laparotomy and staged management of the open abdomen has led to a more virulent form of small bowel fistula referred to as an *enteroatmospheric fistula*.[42] These patients typically present with an open segment of intestine exposed through a large fascial defect, without a surrounding epidermal margin.

Enterocutaneous fistulas are classified according to their location and volume of daily output. These factors dictate treatment and morbidity and mortality rates. Proximal fistulas are associated with higher output, greater fluid and electrolyte loss, and greater loss of digestive capacity. Distal fistulas tend to have lower output, making them easier to manage and more likely to close spontaneously. High-output fistulas are those that discharge 500 mL or more/24 hours. Factors that prevent the spontaneous closure of fistulas are shown in Box 50-4. Once a fistula is identified, management should focus on prompt resuscitation of the patient and consideration of potential factors that could prevent spontaneous closure. Successful management of patients with intestinal fistulas requires a coordinated staged approach that can be defined in three phases—stabilization, staging and supportive care, and definitive management.

**BOX 50-4 Factors Preventing Spontaneous Fistula Closure**

High output (>500 mL/24 hr)
Severe disruption of intestinal continuity (>50% of bowel circumference)
Active inflammatory bowel disease of bowel segment
Cancer
Radiation enteritis
Distal obstruction
Undrained abscess cavity
Foreign body in the fistula tract
Fistula tract <2.5 cm long
Epithelialization of fistula tract

## Treatment

**Stabilization** Historically, malnutrition and fluid losses were the leading causes of death in patients with small bowel fistula. However, with better nutritional supplementation and critical care support, sepsis has become the most common cause of death in affected patients. Nevertheless, the fluid losses and volume depletion associated with small bowel fistula cannot be marginalized. Therefore, prompt fluid resuscitation and electrolyte replacement should occur on recognition of a fistula. Sepsis control is critical and, in the early period, CT scanning may be invaluable in identifying undrained abscesses, complete distal obstructions, or generalized intra-abdominal sepsis with peritonitis. All infections should be adequately drained percutaneously or operatively, if necessary, along with appropriate antibiotic administration. Once sepsis is controlled and the patient is resuscitated, effluent control with skin protection and adequate nutrition are necessary. Fistula output is best controlled by intubation of the fistula tract with a drain. Protection of the skin around the fistulous opening is important to prevent excoriation and destruction of the skin. This is most easily accomplished by using a Stomahesive product with applications of zinc oxide, aluminum paste ointment, or karaya powder. The suction catheter can be brought out through the end of the Stomahesive bag, which is cut to just fit the fistulous opening. This will allow for collection and accurate measurement of the output. The use of TPN has been an important advance in the management of patients with enterocutaneous fistulas and significantly prevents the problems of malnutrition. Although its role in the maintenance of the patient after stabilization is less clear, TPN is valuable in the stabilization period to help minimize high-output fistula losses and for immediate nutritional repletion while the fistula is being delineated.

**Staging and Supportive Care** When sepsis has been controlled and nutritional therapy has been instituted, the fistula must be adequately staged. The combined use of fluoroscopic contrast studies, fistulography if necessary, and CT, along with the patient's clinical behavior, will characterize the anatomy and underlying pathology of the fistula. Some have advocated conservative management for up to 3 months to allow for spontaneous closure. However, others have shown that after sepsis is controlled, more than 90% of small intestinal fistulas that closed did so within 1 month. Fewer than 10% of the fistulas closed after 2 months and none closed spontaneously after 3 months. Therefore, a reasonable management plan would be to follow a conservative course for 4 to 6 weeks, at which time, if closure has not been obtained, surgical management should be considered. However, knowledge that spontaneous closure is unlikely should not prompt immediate reexploration at 8 weeks. In general, a period of 3 to 6 months is beneficial to allow the profound inflammatory response associated with intra-abdominal sepsis to subside completely and for the adhesion formation to stabilize. This period will provide a better opportunity for safe and successful operative intervention. Furthermore, as is the case with enteroatmospheric small bowel fistulas, it may take several months to stabilize the complex abdominal wound associated with the fistula.

Several adjuncts have been proposed to help assist in spontaneous fistula closure and management of the associated abdominal wound, although none are supported by vigorous level I data. Studies have suggested that bowel rest with TPN therapy improves fistula closure rates and time to closure, but this has recently been questioned. Although patients with high-output fistulas will benefit from TPN to help minimize fluid and protein losses, low-output fistulas can successfully be managed with enteral therapy while avoiding the known complications of enteral therapy. Dysmotility agents such as loperamide or codeine can also assist with attempts at enteral therapy. Furthermore, newer techniques, such as fistuloclysis, in which the distal limb of a proximal fistula is intubated and enteral therapy is delivered to the distal bowel, have proven effective. Several randomized trials have evaluated the role of octreotide in the management of fistulas. Although octreotide has been shown to decrease fistula output, which can be useful in the presence of a high output fistula, octreotide has not convincingly provided an improvement in spontaneous closure rates. Recently, vacuum devices have been added to the fistula armamentarium. Their use is controversial, but they are invaluable for enteroatmospheric fistulas to help contract the open abdominal wound around the associated fistula. Skin grafting up to the fistula has also been used in cases associated with an open abdomen, with a graft success rate of up to 80% in some series.[42,43]

**Definitive Management** Once the patient's nutritional, fluid, and wound care needs have been addressed, reoperative intervention will ultimately be necessary for some patients. Surgery is most easily accomplished by entering the previous abdominal wound, with great care taken to avoid further damage to adherent bowel. The preferred operation is fistula tract excision and segmental resection of the involved segment of intestine and reanastomosis. Simple closure of the fistula after removing the fistula tract almost always results in a recurrence of the fistula. If an unexpected abscess is encountered or if the bowel wall is rigid and distended over a long distance, thus making primary anastomosis unsafe, exteriorization of both ends of the intestine should be accomplished. Various bypass procedures have also been described as part of a staged approach in which exclusion of the segment containing the fistula is accomplished in the first reoperation and then another operation is required for resection of the involved segment and fistular tract. Although this may be necessary in extreme circumstances, this is certainly not the preferred surgical management.

In summary, enterocutaneous fistulas occur most commonly as a result of a previous operative procedure. Once identified, a three-phase approach of stabilization, staging and supportive care and, in some cases, definitive surgical intervention is necessary. Most of these fistulas heal spontaneously with 4 to 6 weeks of conservative management. If closure is not accomplished after this time, surgery is indicated.

## Pneumatosis Intestinalis

Pneumatosis intestinalis is an uncommon condition presenting as multiple gas-filled cysts of the gastrointestinal tract. The cysts may be located in the subserosa, submucosa and, rarely, muscularis layer and vary in size from microscopic to several centimeters in diameter. They can occur anywhere along the gastrointestinal tract, from the esophagus to the rectum; however, they are most common in the jejunum, followed by the ileocecal region and colon. Extraintestinal structures such as mesentery, peritoneum, and falciform ligament may also be involved. There is an equal incidence in males and females and the condition usually occurs in the fourth to seventh decades of life. Pneumatosis in neonates is usually associated with necrotizing enterocolitis. The cause of pneumatosis intestinalis has not been completely delineated. A number of theories have been proposed, of which the mechanical, mucosal damage, bacterial, and pulmonary hypotheses seem to be most promising.

Most cases of pneumatosis intestinalis are associated with chronic obstructive pulmonary disease or the immunocompromised state (e.g., AIDS, after transplantation, in association with leukemia, lymphoma, vasculitis, or collagen vascular disease, and in patients undergoing chemotherapy or taking corticosteroids). Other associated conditions include inflammatory, obstructive, or infectious conditions of the intestine, iatrogenic conditions such as endoscopy and jejunostomy placement, ischemia, and extraintestinal diseases, such as diabetes. Pneumatosis not associated with other lesions is referred to as *primary pneumatosis*.

Grossly, the cysts resemble cystic lymphangiomas or hydatid cysts. On histologic section, the involved portion has a honeycomb appearance. The cysts are thin-walled and break easily. Spontaneous rupture gives rise to pneumoperitoneum. Symptoms are nonspecific and, in pneumatosis associated with other disorders, the symptoms may be those of the associated disease. Symptoms in primary pneumatosis intestinalis, when present, usually include diarrhea, abdominal pain, abdominal distention, nausea, vomiting, weight loss, and mucus in stools. Hematochezia and constipation have also been described. Complications associated with pneumatosis intestinalis occur in about 3% of cases and include volvulus, intestinal obstruction, hemorrhage, and intestinal perforation. Usually, pneumoperitoneum occurs in these patients, generally in association with small bowel rather than large bowel pneumatosis. Peritonitis is unusual. In fact, pneumatosis intestinalis represents one of the few cases of sterile pneumoperitoneum and should be considered in the patient with free abdominal air but no evidence of peritonitis.

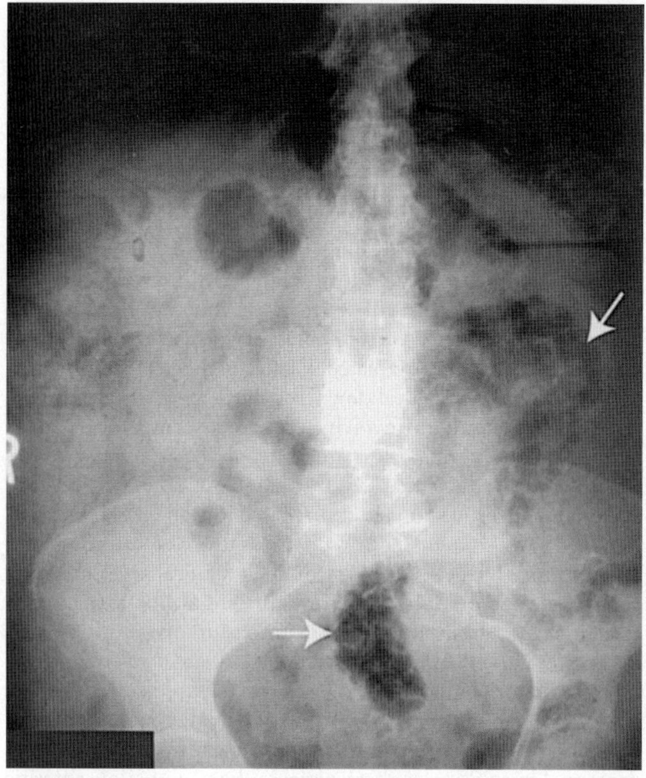

**FIGURE 50-48** Plain abdominal film demonstrates pneumatosis intestinalis *(arrows)*. (Courtesy Dr. Melvyn H. Schreiber, The University of Texas Medical Branch, Galveston, Tex.)

The diagnosis is usually made radiographically by plain abdominal or barium studies. On plain films, pneumatosis intestinalis appears as radiolucent areas within the bowel wall, which must be differentiated from luminal intestinal gas (Fig. 50-48). The radiolucency may be linear or curvilinear or appear as grape-like clusters or tiny bubbles. Alternatively, barium contrast or CT studies can be used to confirm the diagnosis. Visualization of intestinal cysts has also been described by ultrasound.

No treatment is necessary unless one of the very rare complications supervenes, such as rectal bleeding, cyst-induced volvulus, or tension pneumoperitoneum. Prognosis in most patients is that of the underlying disease. The important point is to recognize that pneumatosis intestinalis is a benign cause of pneumoperitoneum. Treatment should be directed at the underlying cause of the pneumatosis and surgical intervention should be predicated on the clinical course of the patient.

## Blind Loop Syndrome

Blind loop syndrome is a rare condition manifested by diarrhea, steatorrhea, megaloblastic anemia, weight loss, abdominal pain, and deficiencies of the fat-soluble vitamins (A, D, E, and K), as well as neurologic disorders. The underlying cause of this syndrome is bacterial overgrowth in stagnant areas of the small bowel produced by stricture, stenosis, fistulas, or diverticula (e.g., jejunoileal or Meckel's diverticulum). Under normal circumstances, the upper gastrointestinal tract contains fewer than $10^5$ bacteria/mL, mostly gram-positive aerobes and facultative anaerobes. However, with stasis, the number of bacteria increases with excessive proliferation of aerobic and anaerobic bacteria—bacteroides, anaerobic lactobacilli, coliforms, and enterococci are likely to be present in varying numbers. The bacteria compete for vitamin $B_{12}$, producing systemic deficiency of vitamin $B_{12}$ and megaloblastic anemia.

The syndrome can be confirmed by a series of laboratory investigations. Bacterial overgrowth can be diagnosed with cultures obtained through an intestinal tube or by indirect tests such as the $^{14}C$-xylose or $^{14}C$-cholylglycine breath tests. Excessive bacterial use of $^{14}C$ substrate leads to an increase in $^{14}C$-$CO_2$. After bacterial overgrowth and steatorrhea are confirmed, a Schilling test ($^{57}Co$-labeled vitamin $B_{12}$ absorption) may be performed, which should reveal a pattern of urinary excretion of vitamin $B_{12}$ resembling that of pernicious anemia, a urinary loss of 0% to 6% of vitamin $B_{12}$ compared with the normal of 7% to 25%). In patients with blind loop syndrome, vitamin $B_{12}$ excretion is not altered by the addition of intrinsic factor, but a course of a broad-spectrum antibiotic (e.g., tetracycline) should return vitamin $B_{12}$ absorption to normal.

Treatment of patients with blind loop syndrome includes parenteral vitamin $B_{12}$ therapy and a broad-spectrum antibiotic, usually tetracycline or amoxicillin-clavulanate potassium (Augmentin). An alternative choice is the combination of a cephalosporin (e.g., cephalexin [Keflex]) and metronidazole. If these agents are not effective, chloramphenicol may be used. For most patients, a single course of therapy (7 to 10 days) is sufficient and the patient may remain symptom-free for months. Prokinetic agents have been used without real success. Surgical correction of the condition causing stagnation and blind loop syndrome produces a permanent cure and is indicated for patients who require multiple rounds of antibiotics or are on continuous therapy.

## Radiation Enteritis

Radiation therapy is generally used as adjuvant therapy for various abdominal and pelvic cancers. In addition to tumor cells, however, other rapidly dividing cells in normal tissues may be affected by radiation. Surrounding normal tissue such as the small intestinal epithelium may sustain severe, acute, and chronic deleterious effects. The amount of radiation appears to correlate with the probability of developing radiation enteritis. Serious late complications are unusual if the total radiation dosage is less than 4000 cGy; morbidity risk increases with dosages exceeding 5000 cGy. Other factors, including previous abdominal surgeries, preexisting vascular disease, hypertension, diabetes, and adjuvant treatment with certain chemotherapeutic agents, such as 5-fluorouracil, doxorubicin, dactinomycin, and methotrexate, contribute to the development of enteritis after radiation treatments. A previous history of laparotomy increases the risk for enteritis, presumably because of adhesions that fix portions of the small bowel into the irradiated field. Radiation damage tends to be acute and self-limiting, with symptoms consisting mainly of diarrhea, abdominal pain, and malabsorption. The late effects of radiation injury are the result of damage to the small submucosal blood vessels, with a progressive obliterative arteritis and submucosal fibrosis, resulting eventually in thrombosis and vascular insufficiency[44] (Fig. 50-49). This injury may produce necrosis and perforation of the involved intestine but, more commonly, leads to stricture formation with symptoms of obstruction or small bowel fistulas.

Radiation enteritis may be minimized by adjusting ports and dosages of radiation to deliver optimal treatment specifically

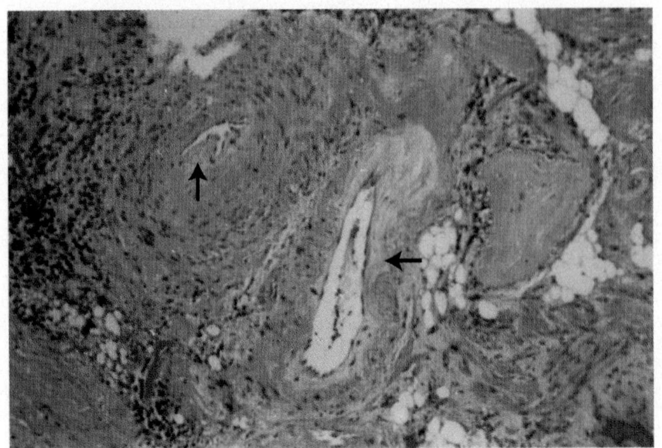

**FIGURE 50-49** Photomicrograph of the ileum of a patient with ulceration and stricture secondary to radiation enteritis. Note the obliterative arteritis, thickened arterial walls, and submucosal fibrosis *(arrows),* which are characteristic findings of chronic radiation injury. (Courtesy Dr. Mary R. Schwartz, Baylor College of Medicine, Houston.)

to the tumor and not to surrounding tissues. Placement of radiopaque markers, such as titanium clips, at the time of the original operation facilitates better targeting of the radiation treatment. Methods designed to exclude the small bowel from the irradiated field include reperitonealization, omental transposition, and placement of absorbable mesh slings.

A number of pharmacologic interventions have also been described to reduce the side effects of radiation enteritis. Sucralfate has been shown to be of value in preventing the diarrhea associated with abdominal radiation. Superoxide dismutase, a free radical scavenger, has been used successfully to reduce complications. Other compounds that have been evaluated include glutathione, antioxidants (e.g., vitamin A, vitamin E, beta-carotene), and histamine antagonists. The most effective radioprotectant agent appears to be amifostine (WR-2721), a sulfhydryl compound that is converted intracellularly to an active metabolite, WR-1065, which in turn binds to free radicals and protects the cell from radiation injury. Other agents that may prove useful in the prevention of the acute symptoms of acute radiation enteritis include glutamine-enriched enteral formulas and the hormones bombesin, growth hormone, glucagon-like peptide 2, and insulin-like growth factor 1 (IGF-1), which have demonstrated effectiveness in experimental studies in preventing or reducing symptoms associated with radiation enteritis.

The treatment of acute radiation enteritis is directed at controlling symptoms. Antispasmodics and analgesics may alleviate abdominal pain and cramping and diarrhea usually responds to opiates or other antidiarrheal agents. The use of corticosteroids for acute radiation enteritis is of uncertain value. Dietary manipulation, including oral elemental diets, has also been advocated to ameliorate the acute effects of radiation enteritis; however, results are conflicting.

Operative intervention may be required for a subgroup of patients with the chronic effects of radiation enteritis. This subgroup of patients represents only a small percentage (2% to 3%) of the total number of patients who have received abdominal or pelvic irradiation. Indications for operation include obstruction, fistula formation, perforation, and bleeding, with obstruction being the most common presentation. Operative procedures include a bypass or resection with reanastomosis. Advocates for bypass procedures contend that this procedure is safer and controls the symptoms better than resection. Advocates of resection contend that the high morbidity and mortality rates previously reported with resection and reanastomosis reflect inadequate resection and anastomosis of diseased intestine. In patients presenting with obstruction, extensive lysis of adhesions should be avoided. Obstruction caused by rigid, fixed intestinal loops in the pelvis is best bypassed. If resection and reanastomosis are planned, at least one end of the anastomosis should be from intestine outside the irradiated field. An incidence as high as 50% of anastomotic breakdown has been reported after resection and anastomosis involving diseased segments of bowel because of the poor healing qualities of the irradiated tissue. Macroscopic findings may not be accurate in evaluating the full extent of radiation damage. Frozen section and laser Doppler flowmetry techniques have been used to assist resection and anastomosis. However, reports of their clinical usefulness are conflicting. Perforation of the intestine should be treated with resection and anastomosis. When reanastomosis is thought to be unsafe, the ends should be exteriorized.

Radiation enteritis can be a relentless disease process. Almost 50% of patients who survive their first laparotomy for radiation bowel injury require further surgery for ongoing bowel damage. Up to 25% of these patients die of radiation enteritis and complications from its management.

## Short Bowel Syndrome

The short bowel syndrome results from a total small bowel length that is inadequate to support nutrition. Of these cases of short bowel syndrome, 75% occur from massive intestinal resection.[45] In the adult, mesenteric occlusion, midgut volvulus, and traumatic disruption of the superior mesenteric vessels are the most frequent causes. Multiple sequential resections, usually associated with recurrent Crohn's disease, account for 25% of patients. In neonates, the most common cause of short bowel syndrome is bowel resection secondary to necrotizing enterocolitis. The clinical hallmarks of short bowel syndrome include diarrhea, fluid and electrolyte deficiency, and malnutrition. Other complications include an increased incidence of gallstones caused by disruption of the enterohepatic circulation and of nephrolithiasis from hyperoxaluria. Specific nutrient deficiencies must be prevented and levels must be monitored closely; these nutrients include iron, magnesium, zinc, copper, and vitamins. The likelihood that a patient with short bowel syndrome will be permanently dependent on TPN is thought to be primarily influenced by the length, location, and health of the remaining intestine. In patients with short bowel syndrome, postabsorptive levels of plasma citrulline, a nonprotein amino acid produced by intestinal mucosa, may provide an indicator to differentiate transient from permanent intestinal failure.

The bowel has a remarkable capacity to adapt after small bowel resection; in many cases, this process of intestinal adaptation, termed *adaptive hyperplasia,* effectively prevents severe complications resulting from the markedly decreased surface area available for absorption and digestion. However, any adaptive mechanism can be overwhelmed, and adaptation can be inadequate if too much small bowel is lost. Although there is considerable individual variation, resection of up to 70% of the small bowel usually can be tolerated if the terminal ileum and ileocecal valve are preserved. Length alone, however, is not the only determining factor of complications related to small bowel resection. For example, if the distal two thirds of the ileum, including the ileocecal valve, is resected, significant abnormalities of absorption of bile salts and vitamin $B_{12}$ may occur, resulting in diarrhea and anemia, although only 25% of the total length of the small bowel has been removed. Proximal bowel resection is tolerated much better than distal resection because the ileum can adapt and increase its absorptive capacity more efficiently than the jejunum.

### Treatment

The most important issue to remember about short bowel syndrome is prevention. In patients with Crohn's disease, resections limited to the particular complication should be performed. In addition, during surgery for problems related to intestinal ischemia, the smallest possible resection should be performed and, if necessary, second-look operations should be carried out to allow the ischemic bowel to demarcate, thus potentially preventing unnecessary extensive resection of the bowel.

After massive small bowel resection, the treatment course may be divided into early and late phases. In its early phase, treatment is primarily directed at the control of diarrhea, replacement of fluid and electrolytes, and prompt institution of TPN. Volume losses may exceed 5 liters/day, and vigorous monitoring of intake and output with adequate replacement must be carried out. Diarrhea in this early phase can be caused by a multitude of sources. For example, hypergastrinemia and gastric hypersecretion occur after massive small bowel resection and greatly contribute to diarrhea after a massive small bowel resection. Acid hypersecretion can be managed by $H_2$ receptor antagonists or proton pump blockers, such as omeprazole. Diarrhea may also be caused by ileal resection, resulting in disruption of the enterohepatic circulation and excessive amounts of bile salts entering the colon. Cholestyramine may be beneficial when diarrhea is related to the cathartic effects of unabsorbed bile salts in the colon. In addition, the judicious use of agents that inhibit gut motility (e.g., codeine, diphenoxylate) may be helpful. The long-acting somatostatin analogue octreotide also appears to reduce the amount of diarrhea during the early phase of short bowel syndrome. Some studies have suggested that octreotide may inhibit gut adaptation; other studies, however, have not confirmed this deleterious effect of octreotide.

As soon as the patient has recovered from the acute phase, enteral nutrition should begin so that intestinal adaptation may be started early and proceed successfully.[46] The most common types of enteral diets are elemental (e.g., Vivonex, Flexical) and polymeric (e.g., Isocal, Ensure). Controversy exists regarding the optimal diet for these patients. Initially, a high-carbohydrate, high-protein diet is appropriate to maximize absorption. Milk products should be avoided and the diet should be begun at iso-osmolar concentrations, and with small amounts. As the gut adapts, the osmolality, volume, and caloric content can be increased. The provision of nutrients in their simplest forms is an important part of the treatment. Simple sugars, dipeptides, and tripeptides are rapidly absorbed from the intestinal tract. Reduction in dietary fat has long been considered to be important in the treatment of patients with short bowel syndrome. Supplementation of the diet with 100 g or more of fat, however, should be carried out, often requiring the use of medium-chain triglycerides, which are absorbed in the proximal bowel. Vitamins, especially fat-soluble vitamins, as well as calcium, magnesium, and zinc supplementation, should be provided. The roles of hormones administered systemically and glutamine administered enterally have been evaluated. The hormones neurotensin, bombesin, and glucagon-like peptide 2 (GLP-2) have demonstrated marked mucosal growth in various experimental studies and have been shown to prevent the gut atrophy associated with TPN in experimental studies; combination therapy appears more efficacious than single-agent administration. In addition, limited clinical studies using GLP-2 have shown improved intestinal absorption and nutritional status in patients with short bowel syndrome.

Two other hormones not derived from the gut that have been evaluated extensively in various experimental and limited clinical trials include growth hormone and IGF-1. In an uncontrolled clinical trial, Byrne and colleagues[47] used a combination of growth hormone, glutamine, and a modified diet and demonstrated a reduction in or elimination of TPN requirements in some refractory patients with severe short bowel syndrome and TPN dependence. However, in a double-blind, placebo-controlled randomized study, Scolapio and associates[48] demonstrated only modest improvements in electrolyte absorption but no improvements in small bowel morphology, stool losses, or macronutrient absorption using the combination of glutamine and growth hormone. Given the conflicting results in these studies, the potential efficacy of this treatment in TPN-dependent patients remains to be defined. The combination of various trophic hormones with glutamine and a modified diet may prove more efficacious in this difficult group of patients.

A number of surgical strategies have been attempted in patients who are chronically TPN- dependent, with limited success; these include procedures to delay intestinal transit time, methods to increase absorptive area, and small bowel transplantation. Methods to delay intestinal transit time include the construction of various valves and sphincters, with inconsistent results reported. Antiperistaltic segments of small intestine have been constructed to slow the transit, thus allowing additional contact time for nutrient and fluid absorption. Moderate successes have been described with this technique. Other procedures, including colonic interposition, recirculating loops of small bowel, and retrograde electrical pacing, have been tried but were found to be unsuccessful in humans and were largely abandoned. Surgical procedures to increase absorptive area include the intestinal tapering and lengthening procedure originally described by Bianchi.[49] This procedure improves intestinal function by correcting the dilation and ineffective peristalsis of the remaining intestine and by doubling the intestinal length while preserving the mucosal surface area. Although beneficial in selected patients, potential complications can include necrosis of divided segments and anastomotic leaks.

Intestinal transplantation has improved with the introduction of the immunosuppressive agent tacrolimus (FK506).[50] Intestinal transplantation procedures have included primarily isolated small intestinal grafts and combined liver–small intestinal grafts with a few more extensive cluster grafts in a large series reported from the International Intestinal Transplant Registry. Under tacrolimus treatment, 1-year graft and patient survival rates were 65% and 83%, respectively, for isolated bowel transplantation and 65% and 68% for liver–small bowel transplantation. Of the 86 survivors in this series, 78 had stopped TPN

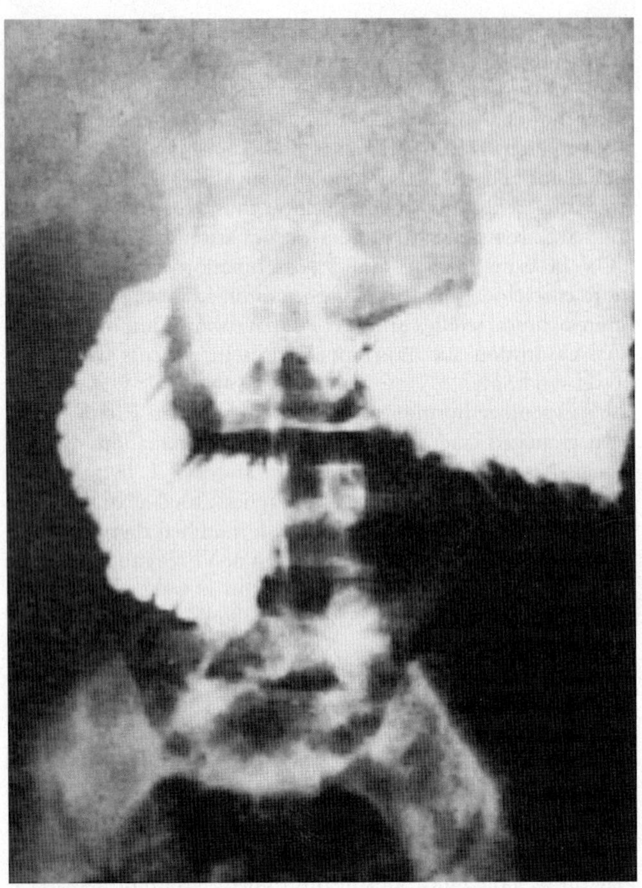

**FIGURE 50-50** Barium radiograph demonstrates obstruction of the third portion of the duodenum secondary to superior mesenteric artery compression as a consequence of burn injury. (Adapted from Reckler JM, Bruck HM, Munster AM, et al: Superior mesenteric artery syndrome as a consequence of burn injury. J Trauma 12:979–985, 1972.)

and were receiving oral nutrition. The largest experience in the United States has been at the University of Pittsburgh, where the reported patient survival rate was 72% at 1 year, 53% at 2 years, and 42% at 3 years. Currently, liver–small intestine transplantation has a survival rate similar to that of kidney and heart transplantation. The challenges of small bowel transplantation continue to be the need for better immunosuppression and earlier detection of rejection. An alternative to intestinal transplantation is mucosal stem cell transplantation, which involves transplanting enterocytes onto a biomatrix and achieving regeneration of intestinal mucosa. This procedure is, at best, preliminary but has shown some promise in experimental studies.

## Vascular Compression of the Duodenum

Vascular compression of the duodenum, also known as *superior mesenteric artery syndrome* or *Wilkie's syndrome*, is a rare condition characterized by compression of the third portion of the duodenum by the superior mesenteric artery as it passes over this portion of the duodenum. Symptoms include profound nausea and vomiting, abdominal distention, weight loss, and postprandial epigastric pain, which varies from intermittent to constant depending on the severity of the duodenal obstruction. Weight loss usually occurs before the onset of symptoms and contributes to the syndrome.

This syndrome is most commonly seen in young asthenic individuals, with women being more commonly affected than men. Predisposing factors for vascular compression of the duodenum, aside from weight loss, include supine immobilization, scoliosis, and placement of a body cast, sometimes called the *cast syndrome*. An association between vascular compression of the duodenum and peptic ulcer has been observed. Vascular compression of the duodenum has been reported in association with anorexia nervosa and after proctocolectomy and J-pouch anal anastomosis, resection of an arteriovenous malformation of the cervical cord, abdominal aortic aneurysm repair, and orthopedic procedures, usually spinal surgery. One report in the literature described a family with a preponderance of vascular compression of the duodenum.

Diagnosis of this condition is made by a barium upper gastrointestinal series (Fig. 50-50) or hypotonic duodenography, which demonstrates abrupt or near-total cessation of flow of barium from the duodenum to the jejunum. CT has been useful in certain cases. Treatment of this syndrome varies. Conservative measures are tried initially and have been increasingly successful as definitive treatment. The operative treatment of choice for vascular compression of the duodenum is duodenojejunostomy.

## SELECTED REFERENCES

Bianchi A: From the cradle to enteral autonomy: The role of autologous gastrointestinal reconstruction. Gastroenterology 130:S138–S146, 2006.

Concise review of the role for bowel-lengthening procedures as one operative strategy for the treatment of short gut syndrome. This review is written by one of the innovators of these techniques.

Crohn BB, Ginzburg L, Oppenheimer GD: Regional ileitis: A pathologic and clinical entity. JAMA 99:1323–1329, 1932.

This landmark paper succinctly crystallizes the clinical course, differential diagnosis, and pathologic findings of regional ileitis in young adults. Although other terms have been applied to this disease process, based on the descriptions in this classic paper, Crohn's disease has been universally accepted as the name.

Cullen JJ, Kelly KA, Moir CR, et al: Surgical management of Meckel's diverticulum: An epidemiologic, population-based study. Ann Surg 220:564–569, 1994.

This study, which was a carefully performed, epidemiologic, population-based analysis, challenges the prior dogma of selective resection of incidentally discovered Meckel's diverticula in the adult patient.

DeCosse JJ, Rhodes RS, Wentz WB, et al: The natural history and management of radiation-induced injury of the gastrointestinal tract. Ann Surg 170:369–384, 1969.

This report, presented at the annual meeting of the American Surgical Association in 1969, is a landmark article that clearly delineates the clinical features, complications, and management of patients with radiation enteritis.

Hayanga AJ, Bass-Wilkins K, Bulkley GB: Current management of small-bowel obstruction. Adv Surg 39:1–33, 2005.

This recent review nicely summarizes the current modalities for diagnosis and treatment of small bowel obstruction.

Korzenik JR, Podolsky DK: Evolving knowledge and therapy of inflammatory bowel disease. Nat Rev Drug Discov 5:197–209, 2006.

Succinct recent review which provides an up-to-date synopsis of current and emerging treatment for IBD.

Schecter WP, Hirshberg A, Chang DS, et al: Enteric fistulas: Principles of management. J Am Coll Surg 209:484–491, 2009.

This updated review provides a thorough synopsis of the current management guidelines for enterocutaneous fistulas and, in the era of damage control surgery and management of the open abdomen, characterizes the challenges associated with managing the recently appreciated phenomenon referred to as enteroatmospheric fistulae.

Woodside KJ, Townsend CM, Jr, Evers BM: Current management of gastrointestinal carcinoid tumors. J Gastrointest Surg 8:742–756, 2004.

Thorough overview of gastrointestinal carcinoid tumors and the current treatment strategies.

## REFERENCES


1. Moore KL, Persaud TVN: The digestive system. In Moore KL, Persaud TVN, editors: The developing human: Clinically oriented embryology, ed 8, PhiladelphiA, 2007, Elsevier, pp 255–286.
2. Chung DH, Evers BM: The digestive system. In O'Leary JP, editor: The physiologic basis of surgery, ed 3, PhiladelphiA, 2002, Lippincott Williams & Wilkins, pp 457–490.
3. Dockray GJ: Gastrointestinal hormones: Gastrin, cholecystokinin, somatostatin, and ghrelin. In Johnson LR, Barrett KE, Ghishan FK, editors: Physiology of the gastrointestinal tract, ed 4, San Diego, 2005, Elsevier, pp 91–120.
4. Gariepy CE, Dickinson CJ: Translation and posttranslation processing of gastrointestinal peptides. In Johnson LR, Barrett KE, Ghishan FK, editors: Physiology of the gastrointestinal tract, ed 4, San Diego, 2005, Elsevier, pp 31–62.
5. Hayanga AJ, Bass-Wilkins K, Bulkley GB: Current management of small-bowel obstruction. Adv Surg 39:1–33, 2005.
6. Mak SY, Roach SC, Sukumar SA: Small bowel obstruction: Computed tomography features and pitfalls. Curr Probl Diagn Radiol 35:65–74, 2006.
7. Schmidt S, Felley C, Meuwly JY, et al: CT enteroclysis: Technique and clinical applications. Eur Radiol 16:648–660, 2006.
8. Szomstein S, Lo Menzo E, Simpfendorfer C, et al: Laparoscopic lysis of adhesions. World J Surg 30:535–540, 2006.
9. Sajja SB, Schein M: Early postoperative small bowel obstruction. Br J Surg 91:683–691, 2004.
10. Crohn BB, Ginzburg L, Oppenheimer GD: Regional ileitis: A pathologic and clinical entity. JAMA 99:1323–1329, 1932.
11. Sartor RB: Mechanisms of disease: Pathogenesis of Crohn's disease and ulcerative colitis. Nat Clin Pract Gastroenterol Hepatol 3:390–407, 2006.
12. Hanauer SB: Inflammatory bowel disease: Epidemiology, pathogenesis, and therapeutic opportunities. Inflamm Bowel Dis 12(Suppl 1):S3–S9, 2006.
13. Gaya DR, Russell RK, Nimmo ER, et al: New genes in inflammatory bowel disease: Lessons for complex diseases? Lancet 367:1271–1284, 2006.
14. Ahmed FE: Role of genes, the environment and their interactions in the etiology of inflammatory bowel diseases. Expert Rev Mol Diagn 6:345–363, 2006.
15. Jess T, Gamborg M, Matzen P, et al: Increased risk of intestinal cancer in Crohn's disease: A meta-analysis of population-based cohort studies. Am J Gastroenterol 100:2724–2729, 2005.
16. Rutgeerts P, Vermeire S, Van Assche G: Biological therapies for inflammatory bowel diseases. Gastroenterology 136:1182–1197, 2009.
17. Cummings JR, Keshav S, Travis SP: Medical management of Crohn's disease. BMJ 336:1062–1066, 2008.
18. D'Haens GR, Vermeire S, Van Assche G, et al: Therapy of metronidazole with azathioprine to prevent postoperative recurrence of Crohn's disease: A controlled randomized trial. Gastroenterology 135:1123–1129, 2008.
19. Hommes DW, Oldenburg B, van Bodegraven AA, et al: Guidelines for treatment with infliximab for Crohn's disease. Neth J Med 64:219–229, 2006.
20. Bratcher JM, Korelitz BI: Toxicity of infliximab in the course of treatment of Crohn's disease. Expert Opin Drug Saf 5:9–16, 2006.
21. Korzenik JR, Podolsky DK: Evolving knowledge and therapy of inflammatory bowel disease. Nat Rev Drug Discov 5:197–209, 2006.
22. Mahid SS, Minor KS, Stevens PL, et al: The role of smoking in Crohn's disease as defined by clinical variables. Dig Dis Sci 52:2897–2903, 2007.
23. Gardiner KR, Dasari BV: Operative management of small bowel Crohn's disease. Surg Clin North Am 87:587–610, 2007.
24. Stocchi L, Milsom JW, Fazio VW: Long-term outcomes of laparoscopic versus open ileocolic resection for Crohn's disease: Follow-up of a prospective randomized trial. Surgery 144:622–627, 2008.
25. Eshuis EJ, Bemelman WA, van Bodegraven AA, et al: Laparoscopic ileocolic resection versus infliximab treatment of distal ileitis in Crohn's disease: A randomized multicenter trial (LIR!C-trial). BMC Surg 8:15, 2008.
26. Kunitake H, Hodin R, Shellito PC, et al: Perioperative treatment with infliximab in patients with Crohn's disease and ulcerative colitis is not associated with an increased rate of postoperative complications. J Gastrointest Surg 12:1730–1736, 2008.
27. Berman J, O'Leary TJ: Gastrointestinal stromal tumor workshop. Hum Pathol 32:578–582, 2001.
28. Johnson MD, Mackey R, Brown N, et al: Outcome based on management for duodenal adenomas: Sporadic versus familial disease. J Gastrointest Surg 14:229–235, 2010.
29. Bilimoria KY, Bentrem DJ, Wayne JD, et al: Small bowel cancer in the United States: Changes in epidemiology, treatment, and survival over the last 20 years. Ann Surg 249:63–71, 2009.
30. Woodside KJ, Townsend CM, Jr, Evers BM: Current management of gastrointestinal carcinoid tumors. J Gastrointest Surg 8:742–756, 2004.
31. Koopmans KP, Neels OC, Kema IP, et al: Improved staging of patients with carcinoid and islet cell tumors with $^{18}$F-dihydroxy-phenyl-alanine and $^{11}$C-5-hydroxy-tryptophan positron emission tomography. J Clin Oncol 26:1489–1495, 2008.

32. Rinke A, Muller HH, Schade-Brittinger C, et al: Placebo-controlled, double-blind, prospective, randomized study on the effect of octreotide LAR in the control of tumor growth in patients with metastatic neuroendocrine midgut tumors: A report from the PROMID Study Group. J Clin Oncol 27:4656–4663, 2009.
33. Modlin IM, Pavel M, Kidd M, et al: Review article: Somatostatin analogues in the treatment of gastroenteropancreatic neuroendocrine (carcinoid) tumours. Aliment Pharmacol Ther 31:169–188, 2010.
34. Capdevila J, Salazar R: Molecular targeted therapies in the treatment of gastroenteropancreatic neuroendocrine tumors. Target Oncol 4:287–296, 2009.
35. Kwekkeboom DJ, de Herder WW, Kam BL, et al: Treatment with the radiolabeled somatostatin analog [177 Lu-DOTA 0,Tyr3] octreotate: Toxicity, efficacy, and survival. J Clin Oncol 26:2124–2130, 2008.
36. Jackson LN, Evers BM: Gastrointestinal lymphomas. In Yeo CJ, editor: Shackelford's surgery of the alimentary tract, ed 6, PhiladelphiA, 2007, Elsevier, pp 1199–1212.
37. Dematteo RP, Ballman KV, Antonescu CR, et al: Adjuvant imatinib mesylate after resection of localised, primary gastrointestinal stromal tumour: A randomised, double-blind, placebo-controlled trial. Lancet 373:1097–1104, 2009.
38. Learn PA, Sicklick JK, DeMatteo RP: Randomized clinical trials in gastrointestinal stromal tumors. Surg Oncol Clin N Am 19:101–113, 2010.
39. Soltero MJ, Bill AH: The natural history of Meckel's diverticulum and its relation to incidental removal. A study of 202 cases of diseased Meckel's diverticulum found in King County, Washington, over a fifteen-year period. Am J Surg 132:168–173, 1976.
40. Cullen JJ, Kelly KA, Moir CR, et al: Surgical management of Meckel's diverticulum. An epidemiologiC, population-based study. Ann Surg 220:564–569, 1994.
41. Zani A, Eaton S, Rees CM, et al: Incidentally detected Meckel diverticulum: To resect or not to resect? Ann Surg 247:276–281, 2008.
42. Schecter WP, Hirshberg A, Chang DS, et al: Enteric fistulas: Principles of management. J Am Coll Surg 209:484–491, 2009.
43. Joyce MR, Dietz DW: Management of complex gastrointestinal fistula. Curr Probl Surg 46:384–430, 2009.
44. DeCosse JJ, Rhodes RS, Wentz WB, et al: The natural history and management of radiation induced injury of the gastrointestinal tract. Ann Surg 170:369–384, 1969.
45. Buchman AL: Etiology and initial management of short bowel syndrome. Gastroenterology 130:S5–S15, 2006.
46. Tappenden KA: Mechanisms of enteral nutrient-enhanced intestinal adaptation. Gastroenterology 130:S93–S99, 2006.
47. Byrne TA, Morrissey TB, Nattakom TV, et al: Growth hormone, glutamine, and a modified diet enhance nutrient absorption in patients with severe short bowel syndrome. JPEN J Parenter Enteral Nutr 19:296–302, 1995.
48. Scolapio JS, Camilleri M, Fleming CR, et al: Effect of growth hormone, glutamine, and diet on adaptation in short-bowel syndrome: A randomized, controlled study. Gastroenterology 113:1074–1081, 1997.
49. Bianchi A: From the cradle to enteral autonomy: The role of autologous gastrointestinal reconstruction. Gastroenterology 130:S138–S146, 2006.
50. Abu-Elmagd KM: Intestinal transplantation for short bowel syndrome and gastrointestinal failure: Current consensus, rewarding outcomes, and practical guidelines. Gastroenterology 130:S132–S137, 2006.

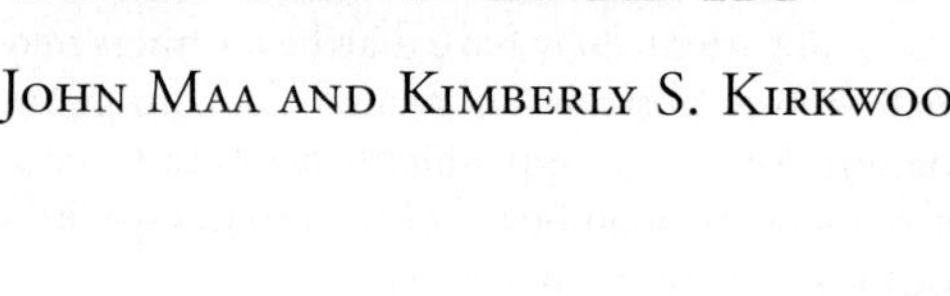

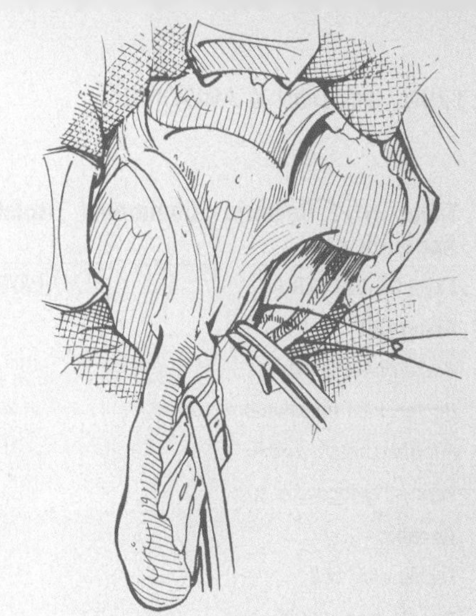

# CHAPTER 51

# THE APPENDIX

JOHN MAA AND KIMBERLY S. KIRKWOOD



Approximately 8% of those in Western countries have appendicitis at some time during their life, with a peak incidence between 10 and 30 years of age.[1] Acute appendicitis is the most common general surgical emergency, and early surgical intervention improves outcomes. The diagnosis of appendicitis can be elusive, and a high index of suspicion is important in preventing serious complications from this disease. *Worldwide, perforated appendicitis is the leading general surgical cause of death.*

## EMBRYOLOGY AND ANATOMY

The appendix, ileum, and ascending colon are all derived from the midgut. The appendix first appears at the eighth week of gestation as an outpouching of the cecum and gradually rotates to a more medial location as the gut rotates and the cecum becomes fixed in the right lower quadrant.

The appendiceal artery, a branch of the ileocolic artery, supplies the appendix. Histologic examination of the appendix indicates that goblet cells, which produce mucus, are scattered throughout the mucosa. The submucosa contains lymphoid follicles, leading to speculation that the appendix might have an important, as yet undefined, immune function early in development. The lymphatics drain into the anterior ileocolic lymph nodes. In adults, the appendix has no known function.

The length of the appendix varies from 2 to 20 cm, and the average length is 9 cm in adults. The base of the appendix is located at the convergence of the taeniae along the inferior aspect of the cecum and this anatomic relationship facilitates identification of the appendix at operation. The tip of the appendix may lie in various locations. The most common location is retrocecal but within the peritoneal cavity. It is pelvic in 30% and retroperitoneal in 7% of the population.[2] The varying location of the tip of the appendix likely explains the myriad of symptoms that are attributable to the inflamed appendix.

## APPENDICITIS

### Historical Perspective

In 1886, Reginald Fitz of Boston correctly identified the appendix as the primary cause of right lower quadrant inflammation. He coined the term *appendicitis* and recommended early surgical treatment of the disease. Richard Hall reported the first survival of a patient after removal of a perforated appendix, which focused attention on the surgical treatment of acute appendicitis. In 1889, Chester McBurney described characteristic migratory pain and localization of the pain along an oblique line from the anterior superior iliac spine to the umbilicus. McBurney described a right lower quadrant muscle-splitting incision for removal of the appendix in 1894. The mortality rate from appendicitis improved with the widespread use of broad-spectrum antibiotics in the 1940s. Advances have included improved preoperative diagnostic studies, interventional radiologic procedures to drain established periappendiceal abscesses, and the use of laparoscopy to confirm the diagnosis and exclude other causes of abdominal pain. Laparoscopic appendectomy was first reported by the gynecologist Kurt Semm in 1982 but has only gained widespread acceptance during the past decade. Other minimally invasive approaches to appendectomy have been reported, including transvaginal[3] and single-incision laparoscopic surgery (SILS)[4]; however, these have not as yet been widely adopted.

### Pathophysiology

Obstruction of the lumen is believed to be the major cause of acute appendicitis.[2] This may be caused by inspissated stool (fecalith or appendicolith), lymphoid hyperplasia, vegetable matter or seeds, parasites, or a neoplasm. The lumen of the appendix is small in relation to its length and this configuration may predispose to closed-loop obstruction. Obstruction of the appendiceal lumen contributes to bacterial overgrowth and continued secretion of mucus leads to intraluminal distention and increased wall pressure. Luminal distention produces the visceral pain sensation experienced by the patient as periumbilical pain. Subsequent impairment of lymphatic and venous drainage leads to mucosal ischemia. These findings in combination promote a localized inflammatory process that may progress to gangrene and perforation. Inflammation of the adjacent peritoneum gives rise to localized pain in the right lower quadrant. Although there is considerable variability, perforation typically occurs after at least 48 hours from the onset of symptoms and is accompanied by an abscess cavity walled off by the small intestine and omentum. Rarely, free perforation of the appendix into the peritoneal cavity occurs, which may be accompanied by peritonitis and septic shock and can be complicated by the subsequent formation of multiple intraperitoneal abscesses.

**Table 51-1 Bacteria Commonly Isolated in Perforated Appendicitis**

| TYPE OF BACTERIA | PATIENTS (%) |
|---|---|
| **Anaerobic** | |
| *Bacteroides fragilis* | 80 |
| *Bacteroides thetaiotaomicron* | 61 |
| *Bilophila wadsworthia* | 55 |
| *Peptostreptococcus* spp. | 46 |
| **Aerobic** | |
| *Escherichia coli* | 77 |
| *Streptococcus viridans* | 43 |
| Group D streptococcus | 27 |
| *Pseudomonas aeruginosa* | 18 |

Adapted from Bennion RS, Thompson JE: Appendicitis. In Fry DE (ed): Surgical infections, Boston, 1995, Little, Brown, pp 241–250.

## Bacteriology

The flora in the normal appendix is similar to that in the colon, with various facultative aerobic and anaerobic bacteria. The polymicrobial nature of perforated appendicitis is well established. *Escherichia coli, Streptococcus viridans,* and *Bacteroides* and *Pseudomonas* spp. are frequently isolated, and many other organisms may be cultured (Table 51-1). Among patients with an acute nonperforated appendicitis, cultures of peritoneal fluid are frequently negative and are of limited use. Among patients with perforated appendicitis, peritoneal fluid cultures are more likely to be positive, revealing colonic bacteria with predictable sensitivities. Because it is rare that the findings alter the selection or duration of antibiotic use, some have challenged the traditional practice of obtaining cultures.[5]

## Diagnosis

The differential diagnosis of appendicitis can include almost all causes of abdominal pain, as described in the classic treatise, *Cope's Early Diagnosis of the Acute Abdomen.*[6] A useful rule is never to place appendicitis lower than second in the differential diagnosis of acute abdominal pain in a previously healthy person.

### History

Appendicitis needs to be considered in the differential diagnosis of almost every patient with acute abdominal pain. Early diagnosis remains the most important clinical goal in patients with suspected appendicitis and can be made primarily on the basis of the history and physical examination in most cases. The typical presentation begins with periumbilical pain, caused by the activation of visceral afferent neurons, followed by anorexia and nausea. The pain then localizes to the right lower quadrant as the inflammatory process progresses to involve the parietal peritoneum overlying the appendix. This classic pattern of migratory pain is the most reliable symptom of acute appendicitis.[7] A bout of vomiting may occur, in contrast to the repeated bouts of vomiting that typically accompany viral gastroenteritis or small bowel obstruction. Fever ensues, followed by the development of leukocytosis. These clinical features may vary. For example, not all patients become anorexic. Consequently, the feeling of hunger in an adult patient with suspected appendicitis should not necessarily be a deterrent to surgical intervention. Occasional patients have urinary symptoms or microscopic hematuria, perhaps because of inflammation of periappendiceal tissues adjacent to the ureter or bladder, and this may be misleading. Although most patients with appendicitis develop an adynamic ileus and absent bowel movements on the day of presentation, occasional patients may have diarrhea. Others may present with small bowel obstruction related to contiguous regional inflammation. Therefore, appendicitis needs to be considered as a possible cause of small bowel obstruction, especially in patients without prior abdominal surgery.

### Physical Examination

Patients with acute appendicitis typically look ill and are lying still in bed. Low-grade fever is common (≈38° C). Examination of the abdomen usually reveals diminished bowel sounds and focal tenderness, with voluntary guarding. The exact location of the tenderness is directly over the appendix. Usually, this occurs at McBurney's point, located one third of the distance along a line drawn from the anterior superior iliac spine to the umbilicus; however, the normal appendix is mobile, so it may become inflamed at any point on a 360-degree circle around the base of the cecum. Thus, the site of maximal pain and tenderness can vary. Peritoneal irritation can be elicited on physical examination by the findings of voluntary and involuntary guarding, percussion, or rebound tenderness. Any movement, including coughing (Dunphy's sign), may cause increased pain. Other findings may include pain in the right lower quadrant during palpation of the left lower quadrant (Rovsing's sign), pain on internal rotation of the hip (obturator sign, suggesting a pelvic appendix), and pain on extension of the right hip (iliopsoas sign, typical of a retrocecal appendix).

Rectal and pelvic examinations are most likely to be negative. However, if the appendix is located within the pelvis, tenderness on abdominal examination may be minimal, whereas anterior tenderness may be elicited during rectal examination as the pelvic peritoneum is manipulated. Pelvic examination with cervical motion may also produce pain in this setting.

If the appendix perforates, abdominal pain becomes intense and more diffuse and abdominal muscular spasm increases, producing rigidity. The heart rate rises, with an elevation of temperature above 39° C. The patient may appear ill and require a brief period of fluid resuscitation and antibiotics before the induction of anesthesia. Occasionally, pain may improve somewhat after rupture of the appendix because of relief of visceral distension, although a true pain-free interval is uncommon.

### Laboratory Studies

The white blood cell count is elevated, with more than 75% neutrophils in most patients. A completely normal leukocyte count and differential is found in approximately 10% of patients with acute appendicitis. A high white blood cell count (>20,000/mL) suggests complicated appendicitis with gangrene or perforation. A urinalysis can also be helpful in excluding pyelonephritis or nephrolithiasis. Minimal pyuria, frequently seen in older women, does not exclude appendicitis from the differential diagnosis because the ureter may be irritated adjacent to the inflamed appendix. Although microscopic hematuria is common in appendicitis, gross hematuria is uncommon and may indicate the presence of a kidney stone. Other blood tests are generally not helpful and are not indicated for the typical patient with suspected appendicitis.

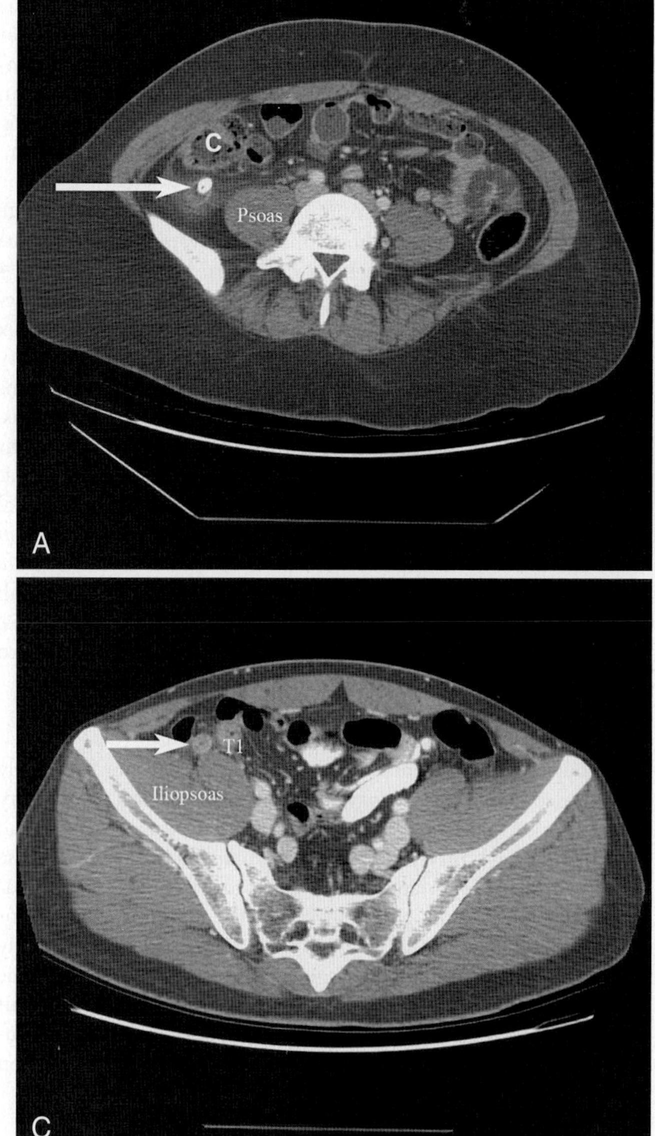


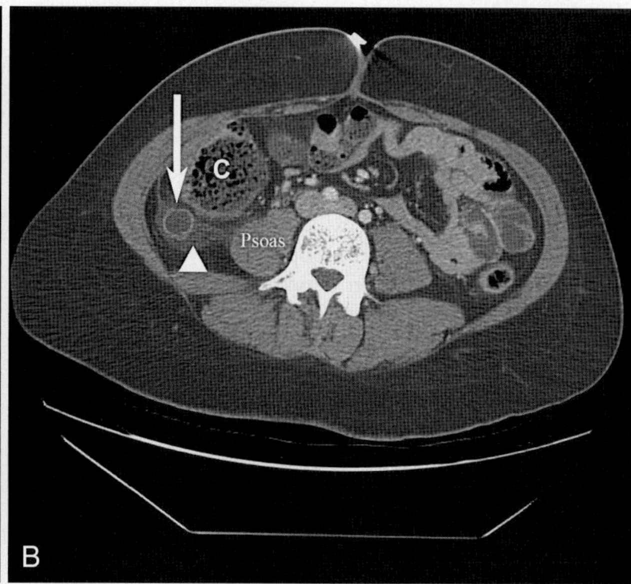


**FIGURE 51-1 A,** CT scan of the abdomen or pelvis in a patient with acute appendicitis may reveal an appendicolith *(arrow).* **B,** CT typically shows a distended appendix (*arrow*) with diffuse wall thickening and periappendiceal fluid *(arrowhead).* **C,** The appendix may be described as having mural stratification, referring to the layers of enhancement and edema within the wall *(arrow);* this may also be referred to as a target sign. *C,* Cecum; *TI,* terminal ileum.

## Radiographic Studies

Computed tomography (CT) is commonly used in the evaluation of adult patients with suspected acute appendicitis. Improved imaging techniques, including the use of 5-mm sections, have resulted in increased accuracy of CT scanning,[8] which has a sensitivity of approximately 90% and a specificity of 80% to 90% for the diagnosis of acute appendicitis in patients with abdominal pain. Results of a recent randomized study have suggested that the use of high-resolution multidetector CT (64-MDCT) with or without oral or rectal contrast results in more than 95% accuracy in the diagnosis of acute appendicitis.[9] In general, CT findings of appendicitis increase with the severity of the disease. Classic findings include a distended appendix more than 7 mm in diameter and circumferential wall thickening and enhancement, which may give the appearance of a halo or target (Fig. 51-1). As inflammation progresses, one may see periappendiceal fat stranding, edema, peritoneal fluid, phlegmon, or a periappendiceal abscess. CT detects appendicoliths in approximately 50% of patients with appendicitis and also in a small percentage of people without appendicitis. In patients with abdominal pain, the positive predictive value of the finding of an appendicolith on CT remains high (≈75%).

Should CT be used routinely in the diagnostic evaluation of patients with suspected appendicitis? We do not recommend it, but one study has found that liberal use of CT scans is probably warranted because this has been credited with a declining incidence of negative appendectomy (i.e., the fraction of pathologically normal appendices that are removed).[10] In the setting of typical right lower quadrant pain and tenderness with signs of inflammation in a young male patient, a CT scan is unnecessary, wastes valuable time, may be misinterpreted, and exposes the patient to risks for allergic contrast reaction, nephropathy, aspiration pneumonitis, and ionizing radiation. The latter carries increased risk in children in whom the rate of radiation-induced cancer has been estimated at 0.18% following an abdominal CT scan.[11] CT has proved most valuable for older patients in whom the differential diagnosis is lengthy, clinical findings may be confusing, and appendectomy carries increased risk.[12,13] In patients with atypical symptoms, CT scan may reduce the negative appendectomy rate. Liberal use of cross-sectional imaging seems most appropriate and, as always, the study needs to be performed only in settings in which it has a significant potential to alter management. Given the recent increased awareness of the risks of cumulative radiation exposure in young adults undergoing CT scanning,[14] it remains to be seen whether magnetic resonance imaging (MRI) will replace CT as the preferred modality for the evaluation of the appendix in younger patients.

The morbidity rate of perforated appendicitis far exceeds that of a negative appendectomy. Thus, the strategy has been to set a low enough threshold for removal of the appendix to minimize the cases of missed appendicitis. With increased use of CT, the frequency of negative explorations has declined in recent years, without an accompanying rise in the number of perforations. An analysis of more than 75,000 patients from 1999 to 2000 revealed a negative appendectomy rate of 6% in men and 13.4% in women.[12]

Among patients with abdominal pain, ultrasonography has a sensitivity of approximately 85% and a specificity of more than 90% for the diagnosis of acute appendicitis. Sonographic findings consistent with acute appendicitis include an appendix of 7 mm or more in anteroposterior diameter, a thick-walled, noncompressible luminal structure seen in cross section, referred to as a *target lesion*, or the presence of an appendicolith (Fig. 51-2). In more advanced cases, periappendiceal fluid or a mass may be found. Ultrasonography has the advantages of being a noninvasive modality requiring no patient preparation that also avoids exposure to ionizing radiation. Thus, it is commonly used in children and in pregnant patients with equivocal clinical findings suggestive of acute appendicitis. Ultrasonography has been shown to change the disposition of 59% of children with abdominal pain who had already been evaluated by the surgical team.[15] Disadvantages of ultrasonography include operator-dependent accuracy and difficulty interpreting the images by those other than the operator. Because performance of the study may require hands-on participation by the radiologist, ultrasonography may not be readily available at night or on weekends. Pelvic ultrasound can be especially useful in excluding pelvic pathology, such as tubo-ovarian abscess or ovarian torsion, which may mimic acute appendicitis.

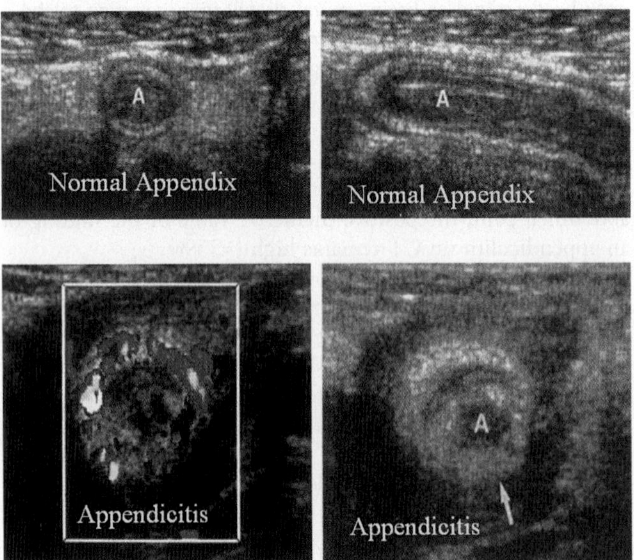


**FIGURE 51-2** Ultrasound of a normal appendix *(top)* illustrating the thin wall in coronal *(left)* and longitudinal *(right)* planes. In appendicitis, there is distention and wall thickening *(bottom, right),* and blood flow is increased, leading to the so-called *ring of fire appearance. A,* Appendix.

Although they are commonly obtained, the indiscriminate use of plain abdominal radiographs in the evaluation of patients with acute abdominal pain is unwarranted. In one study of 104 patients with acute onset of right lower quadrant pain, interpretation of plain x-rays changed the management of only six patients (6%) and, in one case, contributed to an unnecessary laparotomy.[16] A calcified appendicolith is visible on plain films in only 10% to 15% of patients with acute appendicitis. Although its presence strongly supports the diagnosis in a patient with abdominal pain, the low sensitivity of this test renders it of little value in preoperative decision making. Plain abdominal films may be useful for the detection of ureteral calculi, small bowel obstruction, or perforated ulcer, but such conditions are rarely confused with appendicitis. Failure of the appendix to fill during a barium enema has been associated with appendicitis, but this finding lacks sensitivity and specificity because up to 20% of normal appendices do not fill.

### Diagnostic Laparoscopy

Although most patients with appendicitis will be accurately diagnosed based on history, physical examination, laboratory studies and, if necessary, imaging studies, there are a small number in whom the diagnosis remains elusive. For these patients, diagnostic laparoscopy can provide a direct examination of the appendix and a survey of the abdominal cavity for other possible causes of pain. We use this technique primarily for women of childbearing age in whom preoperative pelvic ultrasound or CT fails to provide a diagnosis. Concerns about the possible adverse effects of a missed perforation and peritonitis on future fertility sometimes prompt earlier intervention in this patient population.

### Special Patient Populations

The diagnosis of appendicitis is particularly difficult in the very young and in older adults. It is in these groups that diagnosis is most often delayed and perforation occurs most frequently. Imaging studies are strongly considered here. Because of increasing concerns about radiation-induced cancers in children,[11] ultrasonography is the preferred initial imaging modality for this group. For older patients, CT offers the ability to detect the broader array of conditions, such as diverticulitis and malignancy, found in the differential diagnosis.

In infants, nonfocal findings such as lethargy, irritability, and anorexia may be present in the early stages of appendicitis, with vomiting, fever, and pain apparent as the disease progresses. Ultrasound is useful for the evaluation of appendicitis and other acute abdominal emergencies, such as pyloric stenosis, in infants.

In preschool-aged children, the differential diagnosis includes intussusception, Meckel's diverticulitis, and acute gastroenteritis. Intussusception may be distinguished by the colicky nature of the pain, with intervening pain-free periods, and the absence of peritonitis. Meckel's diverticulitis is relatively uncommon, but its presentation is similar to that of appendicitis, except that the pain and tenderness typically localize in the periumbilical region. Gastroenteritis can be difficult to distinguish from acute appendicitis in any age group. Typically, diarrhea and vomiting occur early and persistently in gastroenteritis, and focal abdominal tenderness and peritoneal signs are uncommon. Sonography should be used liberally. It is advisable to discuss the importance of reevaluation within 12 to 24 hours with the parents of a child suspected of having gastroenteritis if the child develops worsening abdominal pain or other signs of clinical deterioration, because misdiagnosed appendicitis remains high on the list of considerations.

In school-aged children, gastroenteritis often presents with abdominal pain and diarrhea, without fever or leukocytosis. The most common condition that mimics appendicitis in this population is mesenteric lymphadenitis, which may be caused by a wide variety of enteric infections.[17] Ultrasonography may be helpful for identifying enlarged lymph nodes in the region of the ileal mesentery in conjunction with thickening of the ileal wall and a normal appendix, in which case appendectomy may be avoided. MRI may be helpful to resolve ambiguous sonographic or clinical findings. It is important to remember that enlarged mesenteric lymph nodes may also be the result of acute appendicitis. Inflammatory bowel disease is also considered in children, particularly if there is a history of recurrent episodes of abdominal pain. Constipation and functional pain are common in this age group. Although constipation may be associated with relatively severe pain, there are no peritoneal signs, fever, or leukocytosis, and the diagnosis is supported by a recent history of hard stools. Functional pain is usually somewhat milder, recurrent, and self-limited.

In adults, it is important to consider other regional inflammatory conditions, such as pyelonephritis, colitis, and diverticulitis. The pain and tenderness of pyelonephritis are typically located in the flank and are accompanied by high fever and white blood cell count, as well as pyuria. Colitis is often accompanied by diarrhea and the location of the pain typically outlines the trajectory of the colon. In Crohn's colitis, diarrhea is uncommon, but there is often a pattern of recurrent symptoms. The onset of right-sided diverticulitis is typically insidious, worsening over a period of days, and involving a larger area of tenderness in the right lower abdomen than appendicitis. CT scan is helpful for identifying the inflamed diverticula and enhancement of cecal wall thickening that accompanies this diagnosis. The differential diagnosis for appendicitis in women of childbearing age is broad and accounts for the higher incidence of false-positive diagnoses in this group. Pelvic pathology that may mimic acute appendicitis includes pelvic inflammatory disease (PID), tubo-ovarian abscess, ruptured ovarian cyst or ovarian torsion, and ectopic pregnancy. These conditions are typically distinguished from acute appendicitis by the absence of gastrointestinal symptoms. Pelvic ultrasound is especially helpful for these patients because of its high sensitivity and specificity for the diagnosis of pelvic pathology. If a normal appendix is also seen, appendicitis is unlikely.

Appendicitis is the most common nonobstetric surgical disease of the abdomen during pregnancy. Diagnosis may be difficult because symptoms of nausea, vomiting, and anorexia, as well as elevated white blood cell count, are common during pregnancy. Moreover, the location of tenderness varies with gestation. After the fifth month of gestation, the appendix is shifted superiorly above the iliac crest and the appendiceal tip is rotated medially into the right upper quadrant by the gravid uterus. Ultrasound is helpful for establishing the diagnosis and location of the inflamed appendix. In cases in which ultrasound has been equivocal, MRI has been used successfully, thereby avoiding ionizing radiation exposure to the developing fetus. The main challenge is to recognize the possibility of appendicitis in pregnant patients and intervene promptly, because peritonitis significantly increases the rate of fetal loss (2.6% to 10.9% in one meta-analysis).[18] The challenge in the diagnosis is to balance this risk of perforation and risk of fetal demise and preterm labor from delayed diagnosis against the risk of a negative appendectomy. Laparoscopic appendectomy has been performed through the second trimester of pregnancy, although data are lacking comparing this approach to the open procedure.

Appendicitis in older patients can be difficult to diagnose because many patients delay seeking care and the presentation may be atypical. Fever is uncommon, the white blood cell count may be normal, and many older patients with appendicitis do not experience right lower quadrant pain. Approximately 50% of older patients are incorrectly diagnosed at the time of admission and they have a much higher rate of perforation at the time of surgery because of delays in operative intervention.[13] More than 50% of older patients with appendicitis are found to have perforated appendices, compared with fewer than 20% of younger patients. Diverticulitis and bowel obstruction are common misdiagnoses in older patients; the differential diagnosis also includes malignancies of the gastrointestinal tract and reproductive system, perforated ulcers, and cholecystitis. CT has become an invaluable tool for the evaluation of abdominal pain in older patients and its use has shortened preoperative hospital delays.[13]

### Diagnostic Algorithm

Patients for whom the diagnosis of appendicitis is being considered should have a surgical evaluation (Fig. 51-3). Early involvement of the surgical team in the diagnostic evaluation of these patients may improve diagnostic accuracy and help avoid expensive and unnecessary diagnostic studies.[19] Experienced clinicians accurately diagnose appendicitis based on a combination of history, physical examination, and laboratory studies approximately 80% of the time. We stratify patients based on their clinical findings starting with the extremes, which are easier to identify. Patients with a high probability of uncomplicated appendicitis undergo surgery. Patients suspected of having an appendiceal abscess undergo further imaging, typically ultrasonography for children or CT for adults. The next step in the evaluation of patients for whom the likelihood of appendicitis is believed to be low is determined by the probability and severity of alternate diagnoses under consideration. Some of these patients will be discharged with a planned follow-up visit or phone call the next day. Most older patients with abdominal pain undergo CT before discharge because of the high prevalence of surgical pathology in this patient population. The remaining patients are believed to have an intermediate probability of having appendicitis. Children and pregnant women in this category typically undergo abdominal ultrasonography. Women in their childbearing years may undergo pelvic ultrasonography, CT, or MRI, depending on the index of suspicion of pelvic pathology. Among patients who would otherwise be admitted to the hospital for observation, CT may reduce hospital costs by reducing length of stay. Following the completion of imaging studies, the patient is reexamined to determine

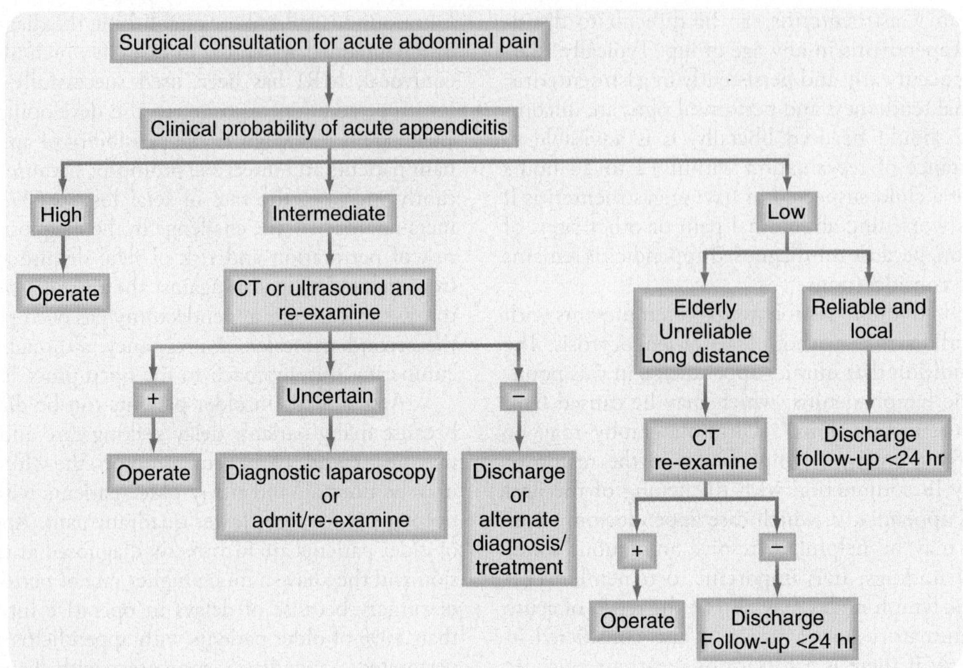


**FIGURE 51-3** Algorithm for the evaluation and management of patients with possible acute appendicitis based on surgical assessment of clinical probability of the diagnosis.

whether pain and tenderness have localized to the right lower quadrant. If the diagnosis remains uncertain at this point, patients undergo diagnostic laparoscopy, especially in fertile women, are admitted for observation and reexamination, or are discharged with follow-up the next day.

## Treatment

Most patients with acute appendicitis are managed by prompt surgical removal of the appendix. A brief period of resuscitation is usually sufficient to ensure the safe induction of general anesthesia. Preoperative antibiotics cover aerobic and anaerobic colonic flora. For patients with nonperforated appendicitis, a single preoperative dose of antibiotics reduces postoperative wound infections and intra-abdominal abscess formation.[20] Postoperative oral antibiotics do not reduce the incidence of infectious complications further in these patients.[21] For patients with perforated or gangrenous appendicitis, we continue postoperative IV antibiotics until the patient is afebrile.[22]

Several prospective randomized studies have compared laparoscopic and open appendectomy, and the overall differences in outcomes remain small. The percentage of appendectomies performed laparoscopically continues to increase.[23] Obese patients have less pain and shorter hospital stays after laparoscopic versus open appendectomy.[24] Patients with perforated appendicitis have lower rates of wound infections following laparoscopic removal of the appendix.[25] Patients treated laparoscopically have improved quality of life scores 2 weeks after surgery[26] and lower readmission rates. As compared with open appendectomy, the laparoscopic approach involves higher operating room costs, but these have been counterbalanced in some series by shorter lengths of stay. For patients in whom the diagnosis remains uncertain after the preoperative evaluation, diagnostic laparoscopy is useful because it allows the surgeon to examine the remainder of the abdomen, including the pelvis, for abnormalities. Our practice is to perform appendectomies laparoscopically for most patients, particularly fertile women, obese patients, and cases of diagnostic uncertainty. Extensive prior lower abdominal surgery with resultant adhesions precludes safe laparoscopic port placement in rare patients. Open appendectomy is usually easily performed through a transverse right lower quadrant incision (Davis-Rockey) or an oblique incision (McArthur-McBurney; Fig. 51-4). In patients with a large phlegmon or diagnostic uncertainty, a subumbilical midline incision may be used. For uncomplicated cases, we prefer a transverse, muscle-splitting incision lateral to the rectus abdominis muscle over McBurney's point. Local anesthetic, administered before the incision, reduces postoperative pain.[27]

After the peritoneum is entered, the inflamed appendix is identified by its firm consistency and delivered into the field. Particular attention is paid to gentle handling of the inflamed tissues to minimize the risk for rupture during the procedure. In difficult cases, enlarging the incision and working down the trajectory of the taeniae on the cecum will often facilitate localization and delivery of the appendix. The mesoappendix is divided between clamps and ties (see Fig. 51-4*A*). The base of the appendix is skeletonized at its junction with the cecum. A heavy absorbable tie is placed around the base of the appendix and the specimen is clamped and divided (see Fig. 51-4*B*). An absorbable purse-string suture or Z stitch is placed into the cecal wall (see Fig. 51-4*C*) and the appendiceal stump is inverted into a fold in the wall of the cecum (see Fig. 51-4*D*). Simple ligation and inversion probably have equivalent outcomes. If the base of the appendix and adjacent cecum are extensively indurated, an ileocecal resection is performed. The wound is closed primarily in most cases because the wound infection rate is less than 5%.

Laparoscopic appendectomy offers the advantage of diagnostic laparoscopy combined with the potential for shorter

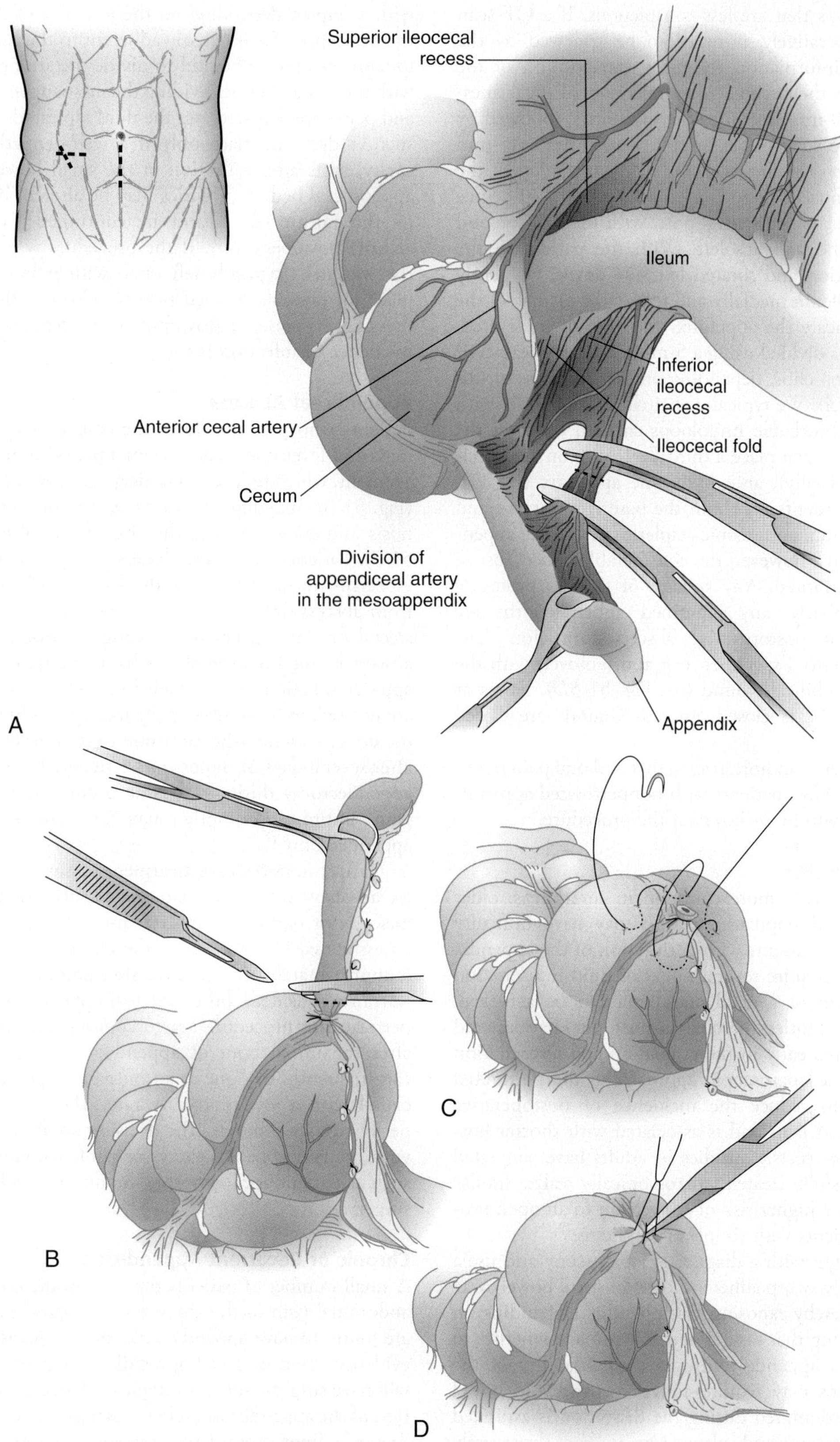


**FIGURE 51-4 A,** *Left,* Location of possible incisions for an open appendectomy. *Right,* Division of the mesoappendix. **B,** Ligation of the base and division of the appendix. **C,** Placement of purse-string suture or Z stitch. **D,** Inversion of the appendiceal stump. (From Ortega JM, Ricardo AE: Surgery of the appendix and colon. In Moody FG [ed]: Atlas of ambulatory surgery, Philadelphia, 1999, WB Saunders.)

recovery and incisions that are less conspicuous. If a CT scan was obtained preoperatively, it needs to be reviewed by the surgeon for useful information regarding the position of the appendix relative to the cecum. After injection of local anesthetic, we place a 10-mm port into the umbilicus, followed by a 5-mm port in the suprapubic midline region and a 5-mm port midway between the first two ports and to the left of the rectus abdominis muscle (Fig. 51-5). The 5-mm, 30-degree laparoscope is moved to the central port, with the surgeon and assistant both on the patient's left. With the patient in the Trendelenburg position and rotated left side down, we gently sweep the terminal ileum medially and follow the taeniae of the cecum caudad to locate the appendix, which is then elevated. The mesoappendix is divided using a 5-mm harmonic scalpel or Liga-Sure, or between clips, depending on the thickness of this tissue (see Fig. 51-5*A*). We typically encircle the appendix with one or two heavy absorbable Endoloops cinched down at the base of the appendix, then place a third Endoloop on the specimen side (≈1 cm distally), and divide the appendix (see Fig. 51-5*B* and *C*). In patients in whom the base is indurated and friable, we use a 30-mm endoscopic stapler to divide the appendix. For most patients, however, the considerable added cost of the stapler is unwarranted. Any spillage of fluid is promptly aspirated and, similarly, any identified appendicoliths are removed to prevent postoperative abscess formation. The appendix is placed into a specimen bag and removed with the port through the umbilical wound (see Fig. 51-5*D*). Fascia at the 10-mm trocar site is closed, and all wounds are closed primarily.

Patients are offered an unrestricted diet and oral pain medication after surgery. Most patients with nonperforated appendicitis are discharged within 24 hours of the procedure.

### Perforated Appendicitis

Perforated appendicitis is more common in rural areas, older adults, and uninsured populations, who may have difficulty getting access to care. Patients with perforation of the appendix may be very ill and require several hours of fluid resuscitation before safe induction of general anesthesia can be achieved. Broad-spectrum antibiotics directed against gut aerobes and anaerobes are initiated early in the evaluation and resuscitation phase. In children, a laparoscopic approach to the perforated appendix appears to reduce the incidence of postoperative wound infections and ileus and is associated with shorter hospital stays and lower costs.[28] Studies in adults have suggested that patients successfully treated laparoscopically realize similar benefits, albeit with a higher risk of conversion to an open procedure than for patients with simple appendicitis.[29]

We usually begin with a diagnostic laparoscopy and use a rolled gauze to gently sweep adherent loops of small bowel away from the cecum, thereby exposing the appendix. Depending on the ease of completing that task, a decision is made whether to convert to an open appendectomy. Extreme friability of the adjacent bowel loops may require conversion to avoid bowel injury. Any pus encountered during the dissection is aspirated and sent for Gram staining and culture. Oozing from the severely inflamed retroperitoneum is easily controlled with electrocautery or argon beam coagulation, if available. The inflamed indurated mesoappendix is divided using the LigaSure or harmonic scalpel. The taeniae of the cecum are followed onto the base of the appendix, and the stump is divided between Endoloops or with a stapler, depending on the integrity of the tissues. When the mesoappendix is densely adherent to the cecum or retroperitoneum, it may be helpful to divide the stump of the appendix with the stapler before dividing the mesoappendix. The abdomen and pelvis are irrigated and the fluid aspirated. We leave a closed suction drain in place only if a well-defined residual abscess cavity exists after reflection of the small bowel away from the appendiceal bed. Antibiotics may be altered, if necessary, based on the culture results and are continued until the patient is afebrile postoperatively. If the procedure was completed open, the wound is typically left open with nylon sutures laid into place for possible delayed primary closure after 3 to 5 days of dressing changes. Laparoscopic trocar sites are closed because the incidence of infection is low.

### Appendiceal Abscess

Patients who present late in the course of appendicitis with a mass and fever may benefit from a period of nonoperative management, which reduces complications and overall hospital stay[30] (Fig. 51-6). Imaging studies are useful for confirming the diagnosis and for evaluating the size of any abscess present (Fig. 51-7). Patients with large abscesses, larger than 4 to 6 cm, and especially those patients with abscess and high fever, benefit from abscess drainage. This may be accomplished via the transrectal or transvaginal route using ultrasound guidance if the abscess is suitably located[31] or by a percutaneous image-guided approach. Patients with smaller abscesses or phlegmon and who are not sick may be successfully managed initially with antibiotics alone. Patients who continue to have fever and leukocytosis after several days of nonoperative treatment are likely to require appendectomy during the same hospitalization, whereas those who improve promptly may be considered for interval appendectomy.[32]

After nonoperative treatment of suspected late appendicitis, adults who have not had one recently should undergo colonoscopy or barium enema because colon cancer is detected in an estimated 5% of cases.[33] The risk for recurrent appendicitis is approximately 15% to 25% after nonoperative treatment and warrants consideration of interval appendectomy. We typically perform this procedure laparoscopically approximately 6 weeks after the initial bout of appendicitis. Interval appendectomy can frequently be done as an outpatient procedure and is associated with a low morbidity rate. The procedure is routinely performed in children. The decision about whether to proceed with interval appendectomy for adult patients includes factors such as patient age, comorbid conditions, and prior abdominal surgery.

### Chronic or Recurrent Appendicitis

A small number of patients report episodic bouts of right lower abdominal pain in the absence of an acute febrile illness. Some are found to have appendicoliths on CT scans[34] or sonographic evidence of an enlarged appendiceal diameter[35]; most of these will have surgical and pathologic evidence of chronic inflammation of the appendix and relief of symptoms after appendectomy. These findings support the concept that appendicitis represents a spectrum of inflammatory changes that may, in rare cases, wax and wane.

The dilemma is more difficult when the report of pain is not accompanied by other clinical or radiographic findings. These patients fall into the category of those with chronic

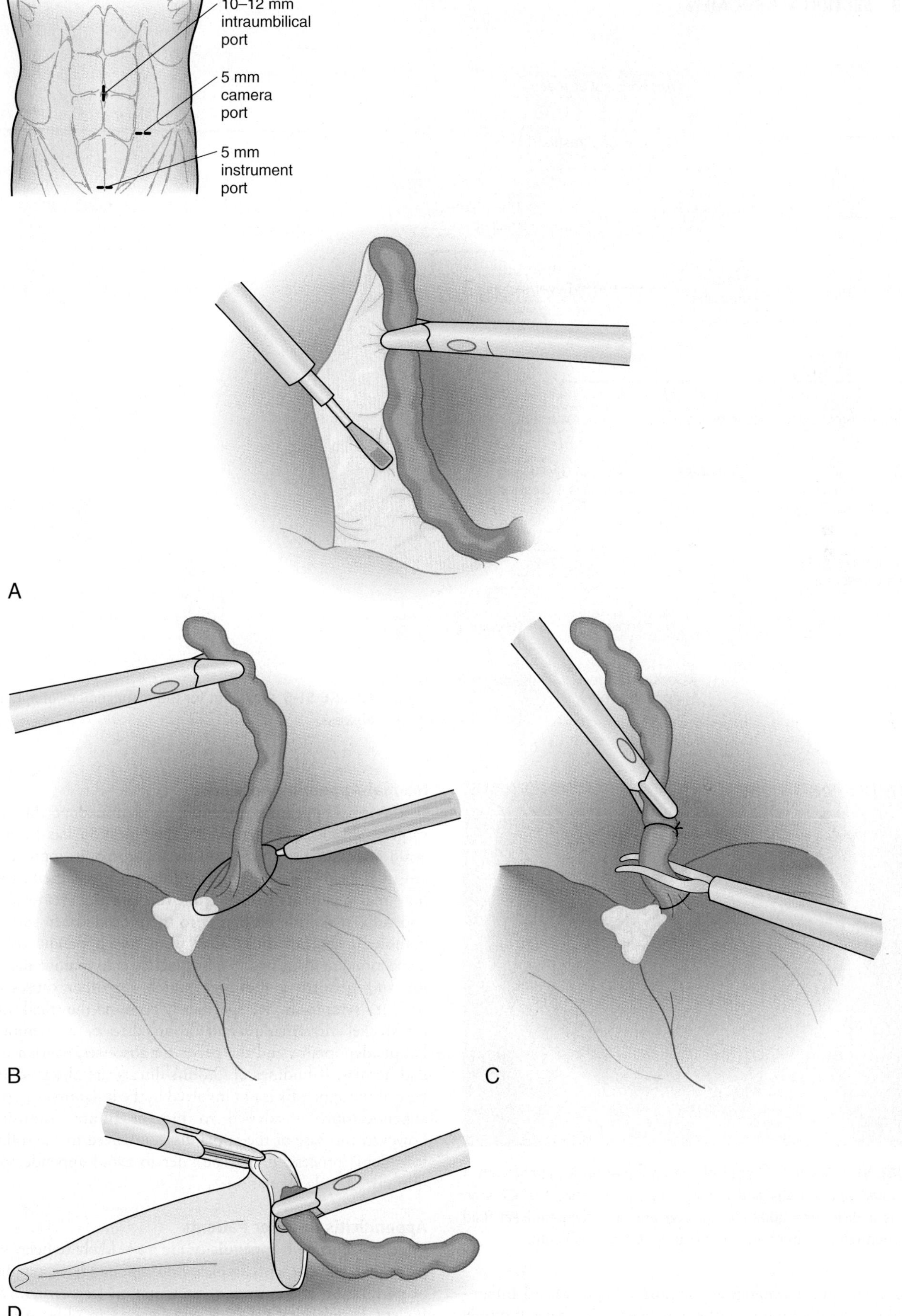


**FIGURE 51-5** **A,** *Upper left,* Location of port sites for laparoscopic appendectomy. *Right,* Division of the mesoappendix using the harmonic scalpel. **B,** Placement of an absorbable Endoloop encircling the base of the appendix. **C,** Division of the appendix between Endoloops. **D,** Placement of the appendix into a specimen bag before removal of the appendix with the umbilical port.

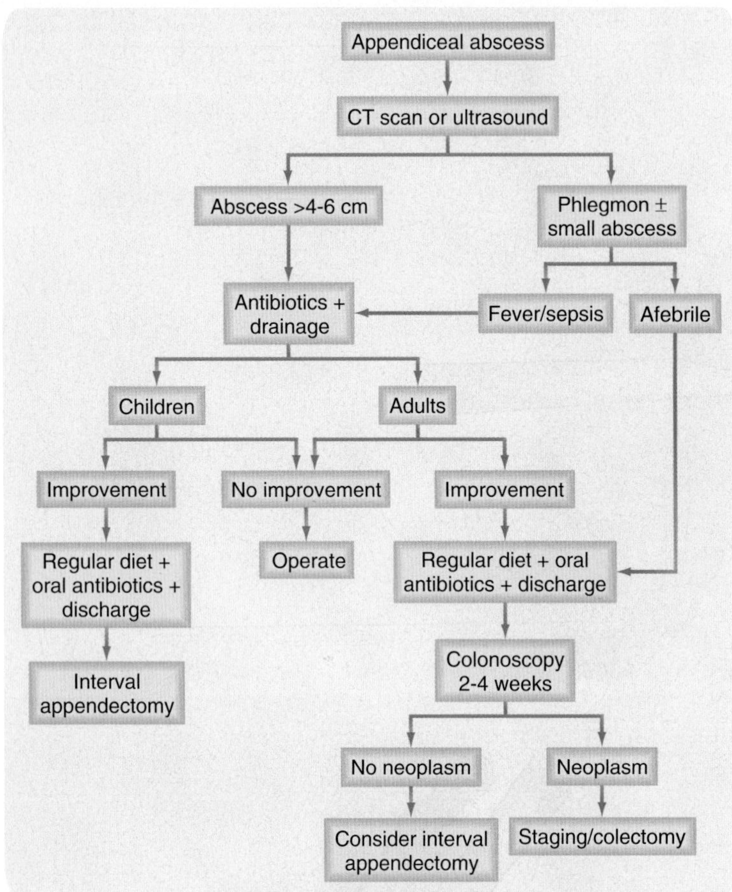


**FIGURE 51-6** Algorithm for the management of appendiceal abscess.

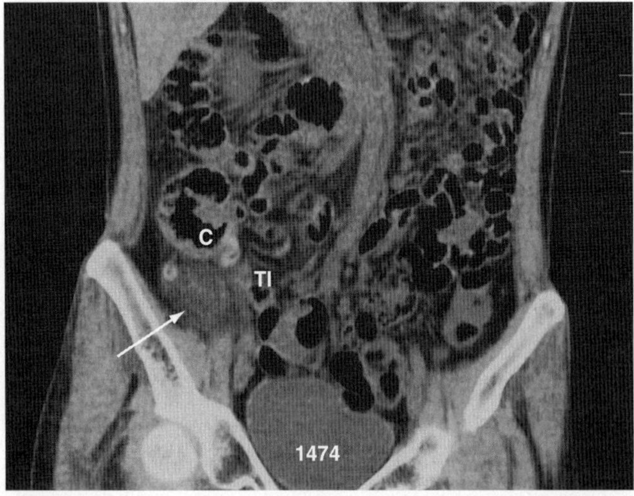


**FIGURE 51-7** Sagittal CT scan of the abdomen in a patient with A perforated appendicitis and periappendiceal abscess. The CT scan reveals a distended appendix *(arrow)* and a periappendiceal fluid collection with inflammation. *C,* Cecum; *TI,* terminal ileum.

abdominal pain; pathologically confirmed appendiceal inflammation is rarely found in these patients. We have typically sought evidence of appendiceal pathology before appendectomy for chronic pain using ultrasound, CT, or both, in combination with colonoscopy, to exclude other causes of pain.

## Normal-Appearing Appendix

If a normal-appearing appendix is identified at the time of surgery, should it be removed? This question has been raised again after the introduction of the laparoscopic approach; consensus is lacking on this point. Although it is difficult to know how many patients benefit from this practice, removal of the appendix adds little morbidity to the procedure. In some cases, pathologic abnormalities that were not apparent on visual inspection are identified.[36] Our practice is to remove the appendix and perform a thorough search for other causes of the patient's symptoms. We specifically examine the small intestine for Meckel's diverticulum and Crohn's disease, the mesentery for lymphadenopathy, and the pelvis for abscesses, ovarian torsion, and hernias. If findings of Crohn's disease are observed and the base of the appendix is not involved in the inflammatory process, appendectomy is advised to prevent future confusion. If, however, the base of the appendix is involved in the inflammatory ileitis process, it may be safer to avoid appendectomy to minimize fistula formation.

## Appendicitis in Older Patients

Older patients with appendicitis are more likely to delay seeking treatment, present with atypical findings, and have a higher rate of perforation at the time of presentation (see earlier, "Special Patient Populations"). CT is widely used in older patients to establish the diagnosis of appendicitis and to exclude neoplasms, diverticulitis, and other confounding conditions. Perforation and abscess formation are relatively common operative findings in older patients with appendicitis.[37] Older people have an increased incidence of cardiovascular, renal, and pulmonary complications after appendectomy. Analysis of a large administrative database has shown that the laparoscopic approach is associated with a shorter hospitalization and higher probability of discharge to home, rather than a skilled nursing facility, than open appendectomy for older patients with perforated or nonperforated appendicitis.[38] Following risk adjustment among groups, the benefits of laparoscopic appendectomy appear to be more pronounced for older patients than for their younger counterparts.[39]

### Treatment Algorithm

Our approach to the treatment of appendicitis is summarized in Figure 51-8. Patients are considered to have so-called *simple appendicitis* if the duration of symptoms is shorter than 48 hours or imaging studies reveal the absence of a large abscess or phlegmon. These patients typically undergo appendectomy. For patients with an atypical or long history and those who present during the recovery phase, imaging studies are obtained. CT is typically selected for nonpregnant women and ultrasound for pregnant women and children. Occasionally, these patients are found to have radiographic features of simple appendicitis and undergo appendectomy. More commonly, a phlegmon is found. An associated large abscess (>4 to 6 cm) is drained percutaneously, if it is located in the iliac fossa, or transrectally, if it is in the lower pelvis. Patients who are systemically ill are treated with antibiotics and bowel rest and reevaluated. If they do not improve, we perform an open appendectomy. Similarly, sick patients with a phlegmon or small abscess are treated with antibiotics and bowel rest and reevaluated for signs of improvement, as described earlier. Some present during the recovery phase from the acute illness and may be managed as outpatients. Adults who are managed nonoperatively during their initial presentation may undergo colonoscopy 2 to 4 weeks after their acute illness to exclude colitis or neoplasms. We typically remove the appendix in these patients 6 to 8 weeks after the initial presentation. The procedure is performed laparoscopically as an outpatient.

### Outcomes

The mortality rate after appendectomy is less than 1%. The morbidity of perforated appendicitis is higher than that of nonperforated cases and is related to increased rates of wound infection, intra-abdominal abscess formation, increased hospital stay, and delayed return to full activity.

Surgical site infections and deep space infections or abscesses are the most common complications seen after appendectomy. Approximately 5% of patients with uncomplicated appendicitis develop wound infections after open appendectomy. Laparoscopic appendectomy is associated with a lower incidence of wound infections; this difference is magnified in groups of patients with perforated appendicitis (14% versus 26%).[40] Patients with a fever and leukocytosis and a normal-appearing wound after appendectomy undergo CT or ultrasonography to exclude an intra-abdominal abscess. Similarly, if pus emanates from a fascial opening during wound inspection, an imaging study is performed to identify any undrained intra-abdominal fluid collections. In this situation, we place a percutaneous drain into the collection to divert the infected material away from the fascia and facilitate wound healing. For pelvic abscesses that are located in proximity to the rectum or vagina, we prefer ultrasound-guided transrectal or transvaginal drainage, thereby avoiding the discomfort of a percutaneous perineal drain.[31]

Small bowel obstruction occurs in less than 1% of patients after appendectomy for uncomplicated appendicitis and in 3% of patients with perforated appendicitis who are followed for 30 years.[41] Approximately 50% of these patients present with bowel obstruction during the first year.

The risk for infertility following appendectomy in childhood appears to be small. A history of simple or perforated appendicitis was sought in a large cohort of infertile patients and compared with the frequency of appendicitis in pregnant women; no significant differences were found.[42]

There are rare reports of appendicocutaneous or appendicovesical fistulas after appendectomy, typically for perforated appendicitis. Fistulas to the skin generally close after any local infection is treated. Fistulas to the bladder have been successfully diagnosed and treated laparoscopically.

## NEOPLASMS

Primary tumors of the appendix are rare. They are usually diagnosed after pathologic inspection of the appendix that was removed for suspected appendicitis. Although it was previously believed that carcinoid tumors were the most common appendiceal neoplasms, analysis of the Surveillance, Epidemiology, and End Results (SEER) database indicates that mucinous tumors of the appendix are more common.[12]

A mucocele of the appendix is the result of obstruction of the appendiceal orifice with distention of the appendix caused by intraluminal accumulation of mucoid material (Fig 51-9). A spectrum of histologic changes may be found in the mucosa of appendiceal mucoceles, ranging from benign epithelium to the invasive changes of mucinous adenocarcinoma.[43] Intact mucoceles smaller than 2 cm are almost always benign.[44] A retention cyst results from chronic obstruction of the proximal lumen, usually by fibrous tissue, which leads to a simple mucocele that is lined by flattened cuboidal epithelium and cured by appendectomy. Larger mucoceles are more likely to be neoplastic. Every effort is made to keep the mucocele intact during extraction, including placing the specimen in a bag or converting a laparoscopic procedure to an open procedure, if necessary.[44] The mesoappendix is removed with the appendix to determine lymph node status, but a right hemicolectomy is not indicated unless there is invasion of the base of the appendix by tumor.[45]

Mucoceles that have ruptured are more likely to be associated with the spread of epithelial cells within mucoid fluid throughout the peritoneal cavity, so-called *pseudomyxoma peritonei*, or mucinous carcinomatosis of appendiceal origin. The appendix is the most common source of mucoid fluid collections in the abdomen. Patients may present with appendicitis or in a subacute fashion, with increased abdominal girth from intraperitoneal accumulation of mucoid material. Preoperative imaging studies may reveal enlargement of the ovaries caused by entrapment of mucinous tumor cells within ovarian tissue or focal mucinous fluid collections in the pelvis, left paracolic gutter, subhepatic space, splenic hilum, and/or omentum. Appendiceal mucinous neoplasms have several unique characteristics of which the surgeon needs to be aware. Many patients have peritoneal dissemination of tumor cells at the time of diagnosis, but most of these neoplasms are noninvasive.[45] Nodal and liver

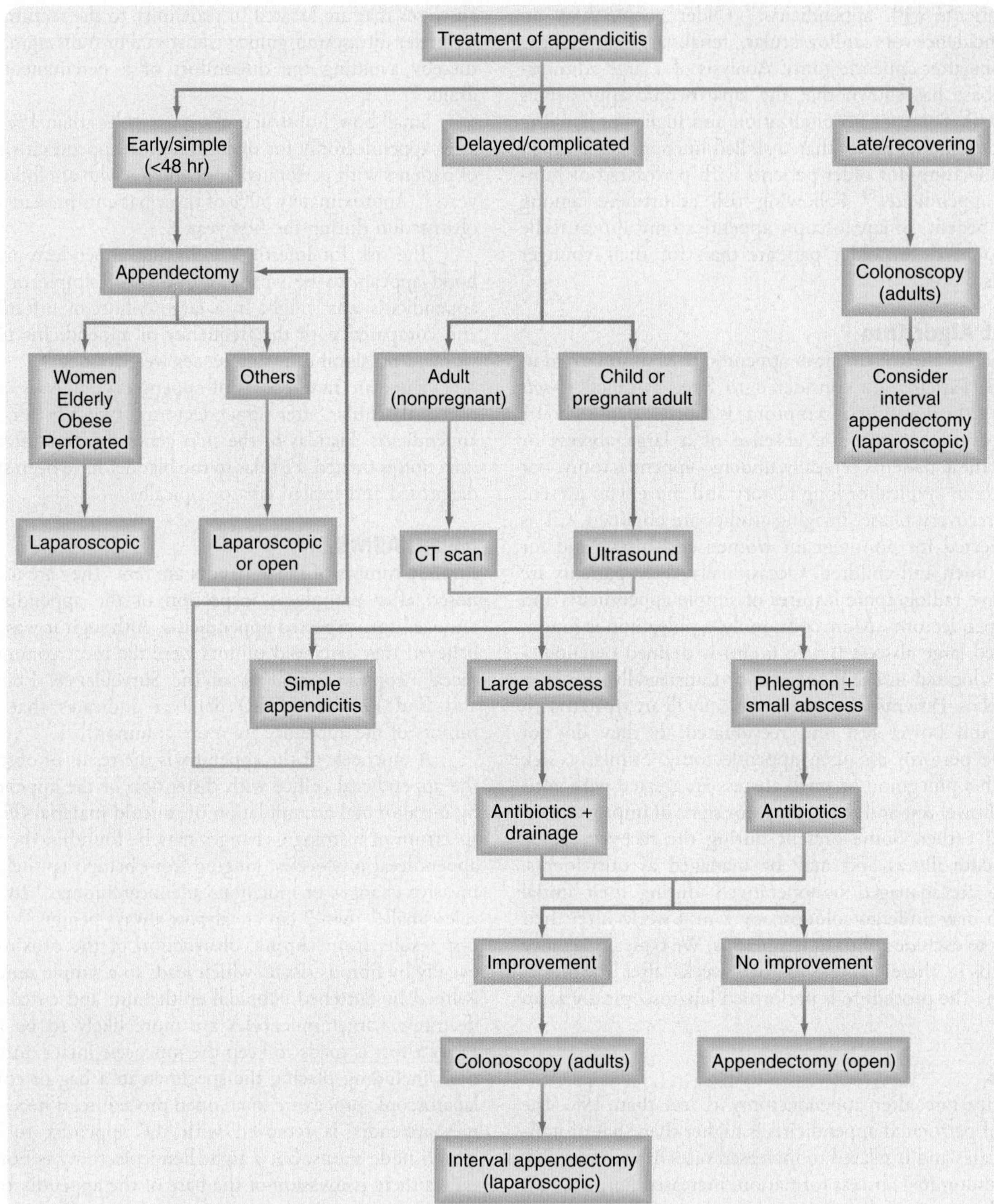


**FIGURE 51-8** Algorithm summarizing the treatment of acute appendicitis.

metastases are uncommon, whereas locoregional recurrence of mucinous tumors, which ultimately impair small bowel function, is typical. The bulk of the peritoneal tumor is an important prognostic factor that is independent of histologic grade.[43] An aggressive surgical approach involving extensive removal of the peritoneum and perioperative intraperitoneal chemotherapy may improve survival for these patients, especially if performed early in the course of this disease, before tumor cells become trapped in scar tissue surrounding the viscera.[45]

Appendiceal adenocarcinomas are diagnosed at a rate of 0.12 cases/1,000,000 annually and are found in less than 1% of appendectomy specimens. Most are discovered incidentally. The typical patient is older and the duration of symptoms is usually longer. A mild anemia may be present[46] but the diagnosis is not usually made preoperatively. The mucinous adenocarcinoma cell type is most common and has a better prognosis after resection than the colon or signet ring cell type, with 5-year survival rates approaching 50%.[12] Right hemicolectomy is recommended for noncarcinoid cancers larger than 1 cm.

Appendiceal carcinoids are neuroendocrine tumors that are usually of the enterochromaffin cell type. They frequently contain sustentacular cells that express S-100 protein.[47] Although they are classified as malignancies, most appendiceal carcinoids exhibit benign behavior patterns. These tumors tend to occur in

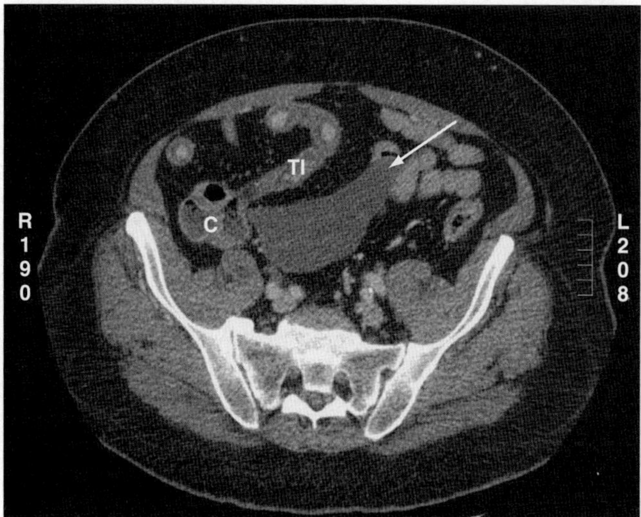


**FIGURE 51-9** CT scan of the abdomen in a patient with a benign 10-cm mucocele. The axial image shows a distended fluid-filled mass medial to the appendix *(arrow)*, without associated inflammation. *C*, Cecum; *TI*, terminal ileum.

patients in their 40s and most are localized to the appendix at the time of presentation.[12] For lesions smaller than 1 cm that are located in the tip of the appendix, appendectomy is curative almost 100% of the time.[12] Appendiceal carcinoids larger than 1 to 2 cm, involve the base of the appendix, or invade the mesoappendix may exhibit a more aggressive biologic behavior and warrant consideration of right hemicolectomy. A large population-based study has shown that goblet cell histology is associated with a particularly poor prognosis among carcinoids.[48] As with other neuroendocrine tumors, patients with appendiceal carcinoids may present with second primary tumors, especially of the gastrointestinal and genitourinary tracts, and this likelihood has been estimated at 18.2%.[49] Thus, these patients undergo colonoscopy and other screening procedures, as appropriate, based on the age of the patient and additional risk factors.

## SELECTED REFERENCES

Guller U, Hervey S, Purves H, et al: Laparoscopic versus open appendectomy: Outcomes comparison based on a large administrative database. Ann Surg 239:43–52, 2004.

Based on a representative large U.S. nationwide database, this was the first investigation that showed that laparoscopic appendectomy has significant advantages over the open approach with respect to length of hospital stay, rate of routine discharge, and postoperative in-hospital morbidity. The advantages of laparoscopy for the specific subset of older patients were addressed.

McGory ML, Maggard MA, Kang H, et al: Malignancies of the appendix: Beyond case series reports. Dis Colon Rectum 48:2264–2271, 2005.

Based on a review of the SEER database from 1973 to 2001, this study is one of the few population-based analyses of appendiceal carcinomas. It contains important epidemiologic information about the relative incidence of carcinoid and noncarcinoid appendiceal tumors. Surgical treatment recommendations are also discussed.

Prystowsky JB, Pugh CM, Nagle AP: Current problems in surgery. Appendicitis. Curr Probl Surg 42:688–742, 2005.

An eloquent and very readable review of the subject, this article offers a particularly thoughtful discussion of the pathophysiology of acute appendiceal inflammation.

Silen W: Cope's early diagnosis of the acute abdomen, ed 20, New York, 2000, Oxford University Press.

This short treatise provides a masterful account of the nuances of clinical presentations in patients with acute abdominal inflammatory processes.

Smith-Bindman R, Lipson J, Marcus R, et al: Radiation dose associated with common computed tomography examinations and the associated lifetime attributable risk of cancer. Arch Intern Med 169:2078–2086, 2009.

This study of 1119 patients undergoing 11 of the most commonly used types of diagnostic CT scans demonstrated that the dose of radiation delivered is widely variable, even within the same type of examination at different hospitals, and that radiation dosages delivered to patients were substantially higher than expected. It was estimated that the radiation that received by U.S. patients from CT scans will eventually result in 29,000 new cancer cases and 15,000 new cancer deaths each year at current levels of CT usage.

Walsh CA, Tang T, Walsh SR: Laparoscopic versus open appendicectomy in pregnancy: A systematic review. Int J Surg 6:339–344, 2008.

This review of 28 studies describing laparoscopic appendectomy between 1990 and 2007 characterizes the rates of fetal loss, entry-related injuries, preterm delivery, and other associated complications. It also highlights the relevant concerns for surgical intervention in the three trimesters of pregnancy.

## REFERENCES

1. Addiss DG, Shaffer N, Fowler BS, et al: The epidemiology of appendicitis and appendectomy in the United States. Am J Epidemiol 132:910–925, 1990.
2. Prystowsky JB, Pugh CM, Nagle AP: Current problems in surgery. Appendicitis. Curr Probl Surg 42:688–742, 2005.
3. Palanivelu C, Rajan PS, Rangarajan M, et al: Transvaginal endoscopic appendectomy in humans: A unique approach to NOTES—world's first report. Surg Endosc 22:1343–1347, 2008.
4. Chow A, Purkayastha S, Paraskeva P: Appendicectomy and cholecystectomy using single-incision laparoscopic surgery (SILS): The first UK experience. Surg Innov 16:211–217, 2009.
5. Gladman MA, Knowles CH, Gladman LJ, et al: Intra-operative culture in appendicitis: Traditional practice challenged. Ann R Coll Surg Engl 86:196–201, 2004.
6. Silen W: Cope's early diagnosis of the acute abdomen, ed 20, New York, 2000, Oxford University Press.
7. Lee SL, Ho HS: Acute appendicitis: Is there a difference between children and adults? Am Surg 72:409–413, 2006.

8. Weltman DI, Yu J, Krumenacker J, Jr, et al: Diagnosis of acute appendicitis: Comparison of 5- and 10-mm CT sections in the same patient. Radiology 216:172–177, 2000.
9. Anderson SW, Soto JA, Lucey BC, et al: Abdominal 64-MDCT for suspected appendicitis: The use of oral and IV contrast material versus IV contrast material only. AJR Am J Roentgenol 193:1282–1288, 2009.
10. Hawkins JD, Thirlby RC: The accuracy and role of cross-sectional imaging in the diagnosis of acute appendicitis. Adv Surg 43:13–22, 2009.
11. Brenner D, Elliston C, Hall E, et al: Estimated risks of radiation-induced fatal cancer from pediatric CT. AJR Am J Roentgenol 176:289–296, 2001.
12. McGory ML, Maggard MA, Kang H, et al: Malignancies of the appendix: Beyond case series reports. Dis Colon Rectum 48:2264–2271, 2005.
13. Storm-Dickerson TL, Horattas MC: What have we learned over the past 20 years about appendicitis in the elderly? Am J Surg 185:198–201, 2003.
14. Smith-Bindman R, Lipson J, Marcus R, et al: Radiation dose associated with common computed tomography examinations and the associated lifetime attributable risk of cancer. Arch Intern Med 169:2078–2086, 2009.
15. Kaiser S, Jorulf H, Soderman E, et al: Impact of radiologic imaging on the surgical decision-making process in suspected appendicitis in children. Acad Radiol 11:971–979, 2004.
16. Boleslawski E, Panis Y, Benoist S, et al: Plain abdominal radiography as a routine procedure for acute abdominal pain of the right lower quadrant: Prospective evaluation. World J Surg 23:262–264, 1999.
17. Macari M, Hines J, Balthazar E, et al: Mesenteric adenitis: CT diagnosis of primary versus secondary causes, incidence, and clinical significance in pediatric and adult patients. AJR Am J Roentgenol 178:853–858, 2002.
18. Cohen-Kerem R, Railton C, Oren D, et al: Pregnancy outcome following non-obstetric surgical intervention. Am J Surg 190:467–473, 2005.
19. Kosloske AM, Love CL, Rohrer JE, et al: The diagnosis of appendicitis in children: Outcomes of a strategy based on pediatric surgical evaluation. Pediatrics 113:29–34, 2004.
20. Andersen BR, Kallehave FL, Andersen HK: Antibiotics versus placebo for prevention of postoperative infection after appendicectomy. Cochrane Database Syst Rev (3):CD001439, 2005.
21. Taylor E, Berjis A, Bosch T, et al: The efficacy of postoperative oral antibiotics in appendicitis: A randomized prospective double-blinded study. Am Surg 70:858–862, 2004.
22. Mazuski JE, Sawyer RG, Nathens AB, et al: The Surgical Infection Society guidelines on antimicrobial therapy for intra-abdominal infections: Evidence for the recommendations. Surg Infect (Larchmt) 3:175–233, 2002.
23. Nguyen NT, Zainabadi K, Mavandadi S, et al: Trends in utilization and outcomes of laparoscopic versus open appendectomy. Am J Surg 188:813–820, 2004.
24. Enochsson L, Hellberg A, Rudberg C, et al: Laparoscopic vs open appendectomy in overweight patients. Surg Endosc 15:387–392, 2001.
25. Wei HB, Huang JL, Zheng ZH, et al: Laparoscopic versus open appendectomy: A prospective randomized comparison. Surg Endosc 24:266–269, 2010.
26. Katkhouda N, Mason RJ, Towfigh S, et al: Laparoscopic versus open appendectomy: A prospective randomized double-blind study. Ann Surg 242:439–448; discussion 448–450, 2005.
27. Lohsiriwat V, Lert-akyamanee N, Rushatamukayanunt W: Efficacy of pre-incisional bupivacaine infiltration on postoperative pain relief after appendectomy: Prospective double-blind randomized trial. World J Surg 28:947–950, 2004.
28. Aziz O, Athanasiou T, Tekkis PP, et al: Laparoscopic versus open appendectomy in children: A meta-analysis. Ann Surg 243:17–27, 2006.
29. Ball CG, Kortbeek JB, Kirkpatrick AW, et al: Laparoscopic appendectomy for complicated appendicitis: An evaluation of postoperative factors. Surg Endosc 18:969–973, 2004.
30. Brown CV, Abrishami M, Muller M, et al: Appendiceal abscess: Immediate operation or percutaneous drainage? Am Surg 69:829–832, 2003.
31. Sudakoff GS, Lundeen SJ, Otterson MF: Transrectal and transvaginal sonographic intervention of infected pelvic fluid collections: A complete approach. Ultrasound Q 21:175–185, 2005.
32. Nadler EP, Reblock KK, Vaughan KG, et al: Predictors of outcome for children with perforated appendicitis initially treated with non-operative management. Surg Infect (Larchmt) 5:349–356, 2004.
33. Lai HW, Loong CC, Chiu JH, et al: Interval appendectomy after conservative treatment of an appendiceal mass. World J Surg 30:352–357, 2006.
34. Giuliano V, Giuliano C, Pinto F, et al: Chronic appendicitis "syndrome" manifested by an appendicolith and thickened appendix presenting as chronic right lower abdominal pain in adults. Emerg Radiol 12:96–98, 2006.
35. Cobben LP, de Van Otterloo AM, Puylaert JB: Spontaneously resolving appendicitis: Frequency and natural history in 60 patients. Radiology 215:349–352, 2000.
36. Chiarugi M, Buccianti P, Decanini L, et al: "What you see is not what you get." A plea to remove a "normal" appendix during diagnostic laparoscopy. Acta Chir Belg 101:243–245, 2001.
37. Hui TT, Major KM, Avital I, et al: Outcome of elderly patients with appendicitis: Effect of computed tomography and laparoscopy. Arch Surg 137:995–998; discussion 999–1000, 2002.
38. Harrell AG, Lincourt AE, Novitsky YW, et al: Advantages of laparoscopic appendectomy in the elderly. Am Surg 72:474–480, 2006.
39. Guller U, Hervey S, Purves H, et al: Laparoscopic versus open appendectomy: Outcomes comparison based on a large administrative database. Ann Surg 239:43–52, 2004.
40. So JB, Chiong EC, Chiong E, et al: Laparoscopic appendectomy for perforated appendicitis. World J Surg 26:1485–1488, 2002.
41. Andersson RE: Small bowel obstruction after appendicectomy. Br J Surg 88:1387–1391, 2001.
42. Urbach DR, Marrett LD, Kung R, et al: Association of perforation of the appendix with female tubal infertility. Am J Epidemiol 153:566–571, 2001.
43. Misdraji J, Yantiss RK, Graeme-Cook FM, et al: Appendiceal mucinous neoplasms: A clinicopathologic analysis of 107 cases. Am J Surg Pathol 27:1089–1103, 2003.
44. Dhage-Ivatury S, Sugarbaker PH: Update on the surgical approach to mucocele of the appendix. J Am Coll Surg 202:680–684, 2006.
45. Sugarbaker PH: New standard of care for appendiceal epithelial neoplasms and pseudomyxoma peritonei syndrome? Lancet Oncol 7:69–76, 2006.

**46.** Todd RD, Sarosi GA, Nwariaku F, et al: Incidence and predictors of appendiceal tumors in elderly males presenting with signs and symptoms of acute appendicitis. Am J Surg 188:500–504, 2004.

**47.** Carr NJ, Sobin LH: Neuroendocrine tumors of the appendix. Semin Diagn Pathol 21:108–119, 2004.

**48.** McCusker ME, Cote TR, Clegg LX, et al: Primary malignant neoplasms of the appendix: A population-based study from the surveillance, epidemiology and end-results program, 1973-1998. Cancer 94:3307–3312, 2002.

**49.** Modlin IM, Lye KD, Kidd M: A 5-decade analysis of 13,715 carcinoid tumors. Cancer 97:934–959, 2003.

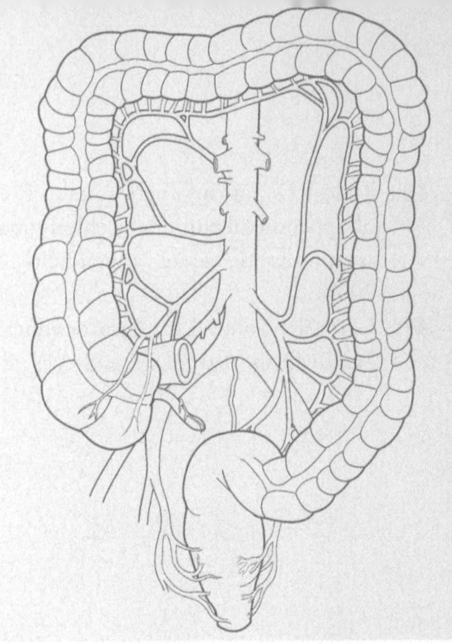

CHAPTER 52

# COLON AND RECTUM

Robert D. Fry, Najjia N. Mahmoud,
David J. Maron, and Joshua I.S. Bleier

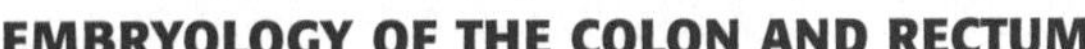



## EMBRYOLOGY OF THE COLON AND RECTUM

No comprehensive discussion of colorectal anatomy is complete without a thorough understanding of the genesis of the gastrointestinal (GI) tract. Knowledge of the developmental anatomy of the foregut, midgut, and hindgut establishes a context in which to consider mature structural and functional anatomic relationships.

The endodermal roof of the yolk sac gives rise to the primitive gut tube. At the beginning of the third week of development, the gut tube is divided into three regions—the midgut, which opens ventrally, positioned between the foregut in the head fold and the hindgut in the tail fold. Development progresses through the stages of physiologic herniation, return to the abdomen, and fixation. The acquisition of length and formation of dedicated blood and lymphatic supplies takes place during this time (Fig. 52-1).

Foregut-derived structures end at the second portion of the duodenum and rely on the celiac artery for blood supply. The midgut, extending from the duodenal ampulla to the distal transverse colon, is based on the superior mesenteric artery (SMA). The distal third of the transverse colon, descending colon, and rectum evolve from the hindgut fold and are supplied by the inferior mesenteric artery (IMA). Venous and lymphatic channels mirror their arterial counterparts and follow the same embryologic divisions. At the dentate line, endoderm-derived tissues fuse with the ectoderm-derived proctodeum, or ingrowth from the anal pit.

Distal rectal development is complex. The cloaca is a specialized area of the primitive distal rectum composed of endoderm- and ectoderm-derived tissues. This area is incorporated into the anal transition zone, which surrounds the dentate line in the adult. The cloaca exists in a continuum with the hindgut but, at approximately the sixth week, it begins to divide and differentiate into anterior urogenital and posterior anal and sphincter elements. Simultaneously, the urogenital and GI tracts are separated by caudal migration of the urogenital septum. During the 10th week of development, the external anal sphincter is formed from the posterior cloaca as the descent of the urogenital septum becomes complete. The internal anal sphincter is formed by the 12th week from enlarged circular muscle layers of the rectum.

## ANATOMY OF THE COLON, RECTUM, AND PELVIC FLOOR

The colon and rectum constitute a tube of variable diameter approximately 150 cm in length. The terminal ileum empties into the cecum through a thickened, nipple-shaped invagination, the ileocecal valve. The cecum is a capacious saclike segment of the proximal colon, with an average diameter of 7.5 cm and length of 10 cm. Although it is distensible, acute dilation of the cecum to a diameter more than 12 cm, which can be measured by a plain abdominal radiograph, can result in ischemic necrosis and perforation of the bowel wall. Surgical intervention may be required when this degree of cecal distention is caused by obstruction or pseudo-obstruction (Fig. 52-2).

The appendix extends from the cecum approximately 3 cm below the ileocecal valve as a blind-ending elongated tube, 8 to 10 cm in length. The proximal appendix is fairly constant in location, whereas the end can be located in a wide variety of positions relative to the cecum and terminal ileum. Most commonly, it is retrocecal (65%), followed by pelvic (31%), subcecal (2.3%), preileal (1.0%), and retroileal (0.4%). Clinically, the appendix is found at the convergence of the taeniae coli. Another clinical aid useful for detecting the location of the appendix through a small abdominal incision is the identification of the fold of Treves, the only antimesenteric epiploic appendage normally found on the small intestine, marking the junction of the ileum and cecum.

The ascending colon, approximately 15 cm in length, runs upward toward the liver on the right side; like the descending colon, the posterior surface is fixed against the retroperitoneum, whereas the lateral and anterior surfaces are true intraperitoneal structures. The white line of Toldt represents the fusion of the mesentery with the posterior peritoneum. This subtle peritoneal

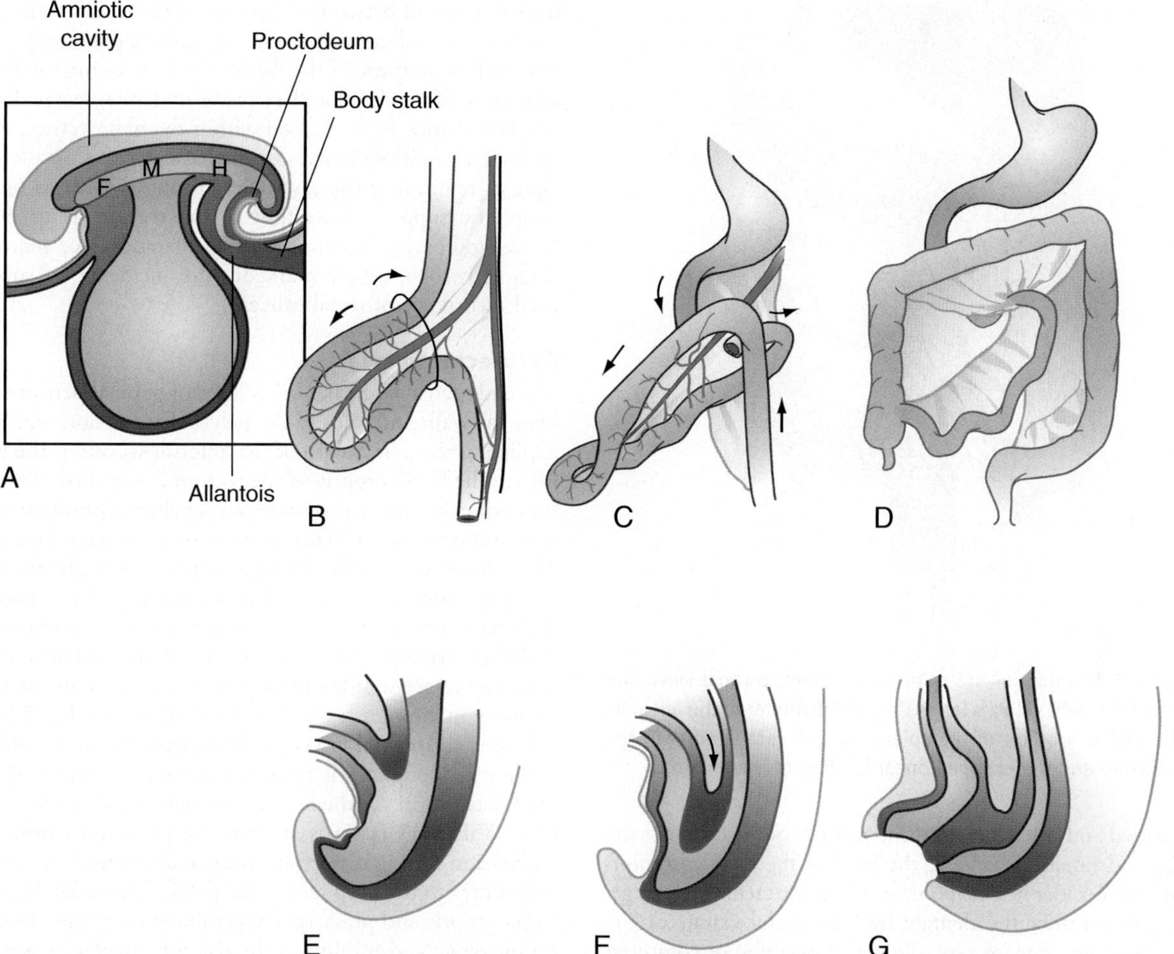


**FIGURE 52-1 A,** At the third week of development, the primitive tube can be divided into three regions—the foregut in the head fold, the hindgut with its ventral allantoic outgrowth in the smaller tail fold, and the midgut between these two portions. Stages of development of the midgut are physiologic herniation (**B**), return to the abdomen (**C**), and fixation (**D**). At the sixth week, the urogenital septum migrates caudally (**E**) and separates the intestinal and urogenital tracts (**F, G**). (From Corman ML [ed]: Colon and rectal surgery, ed 4, Philadelphia,1998, Lippincott-Raven, p 2.)

landmark serves as a guide for the surgeon for mobilizing the colon and mesentery from the retroperitoneum.

The transverse colon is approximately 45 cm in length. Hanging between fixed positions at the hepatic and splenic flexures, it is completely invested in visceral peritoneum. The nephrocolic ligament secures the hepatic flexure and directly overlies the right kidney, duodenum, and porta hepatis. The phrenocolic ligament lies ventral to the spleen and fixes the splenic flexure in the left upper quadrant. The angle of the splenic flexure is higher, more acute, and more deeply situated than that of the hepatic flexure. The splenic flexure is typically approached by dissecting the descending colon along the line of Toldt from below and then entering the lesser sac by reflecting the omentum from the transverse colon. This maneuver allows mobilization of the flexure to be achieved, with minimal traction required for exposure. Attached to the superior aspect of the transverse colon is the greater omentum, a fused double layer of visceral and parietal peritoneum (four total layers) that contains variable amounts of stored fat. Clinically, it is useful in preventing adhesions between surgical abdominal wounds and underlying bowel and is often used to cover intraperitoneal contents as incisions are closed. The omentum can be mobilized and placed between the rectum and vagina after repair of a high rectovaginal fistula, or used to fill the pelvic and perineal space left after excision of the rectum. The living tissue of the greater omentum makes a good patch in difficult situations, such as treatment of a perforated duodenum, when closure of inflamed and friable tissues is impossible or ill-advised.

The descending colon lies ventral to the left kidney and extends downward from the splenic flexure for approximately 25 cm. It is smaller in diameter than the ascending colon. At the level of the pelvic brim, there is a transition between the relatively thin-walled, fixed, descending colon and the thicker, mobile sigmoid colon. The sigmoid colon varies in length from 15 to 50 cm (average, 38 cm) and is very mobile. It is a small-diameter, muscular tube on a long floppy mesentery that often forms an omega loop in the pelvis. The mesosigmoid is frequently attached to the left pelvic sidewall, producing a small recess in the mesentery known as the *intersigmoid fossa*. This mesenteric fold is a surgical landmark for the underlying left ureter.

The rectum, along with the sigmoid colon, serves as a fecal reservoir. There is some controversy regarding the definition of

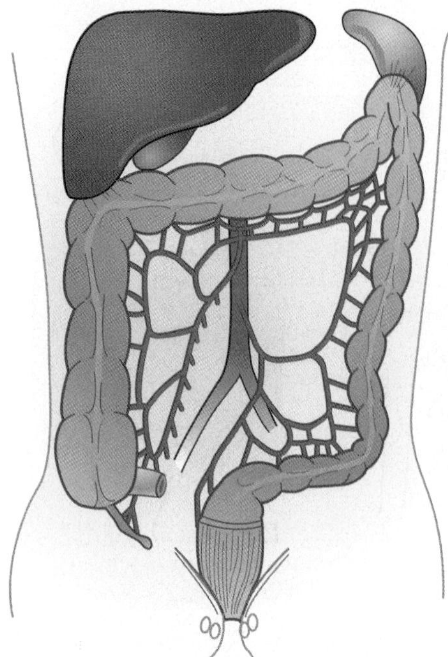

**FIGURE 52-2** Anatomy of the colon and rectum, coronal view. The diameter of the right colon is larger than the diameter of the left side. Note the higher location of the splenic flexure compared with the hepatic flexure and the extraperitoneal location of the rectum.

the proximal and distal extent of the rectum. Some consider the rectosigmoid junction to be at the level of the sacral promontory; others consider it to be point at which the taeniae converge. Anatomists consider the dentate line the distal extent of the rectum, whereas surgeons typically view this union of columnar and squamous epithelium as existing within the anal canal and consider the end of the rectum to be the proximal border of the anal sphincter complex. The rectum is 12 to 15 cm in length and lacks taeniae coli or epiploic appendices. It occupies the curve of the sacrum in the true pelvis and the posterior surface is almost completely extraperitoneal, in that it is adherent to presacral soft tissues and thus is outside the peritoneal cavity. The anterior surface of the proximal third of the rectum is covered by visceral peritoneum. The peritoneal reflection is 7 to 9 cm from the anal verge in men and 5 to 7.5 cm in women. This anterior peritonealized space is called the *pouch of Douglas*, pelvic cul-de-sac, or rectouterine pouch and may serve as the site of so-called *drop metastases* from visceral tumors. These peritoneal metastases can form a mass in the cul-de-sac (called *Bloomer's shelf*) that can be detected by a digital rectal examination.

The rectum possesses three involutions or curves, known as the *valves of Houston*. The middle valve folds to the left and the proximal and distal valves fold to the right. These valves are more properly called folds because they have no specific function as impediments to flow. They are lost after full surgical mobilization of the rectum, a maneuver that may provide approximately 5 cm of additional length to the rectum, greatly facilitating the surgeon's ability to fashion an anastomosis deep in the pelvis.

The posterior aspect of the rectum is invested with a thick, closely applied mesorectum. A thin layer of investing fascia (fascia propria) coats the mesorectum and represents a distinct layer from the presacral fascia against which it lies. During proctectomy for rectal cancer, mobilization and dissection of the rectum proceed between the presacral fascia and fascia propria. Total mesorectal excision is a well-described oncologic maneuver that makes good use of the tissue planes investing the rectum to achieve a relatively bloodless rectal and mesorectal dissection. The lymphatics are contained within the mesorectum, and total mesorectal excision adheres to the basic surgical oncologic principle of removal of the cancer in continuity with its blood and lymphatic supplies. Resection of the rectum using this technique, and based on a thorough understanding of anatomy, has been shown to reduce markedly the incidence of subsequent local recurrence of rectal cancer.

## Pararectal Fascia

The endopelvic fascia is a thick layer of parietal peritoneum that lines the walls and floor of the pelvis. The portion that is closely applied to the periosteum of the anterior sacrum is the presacral fascia. The fascia propria of the rectum is a thin condensation of the endopelvic fascia that forms an envelope around the mesorectum and continues distally to help form the lateral rectal stalks. The lateral rectal stalks or ligaments are actually anterolateral structures containing the middle rectal artery. The stalks reside in close proximity to the mixed autonomic nerves, containing sympathic and parasympathetic nerves, and division of these structures close to the pelvic sidewall may result in injury to these nerves, resulting in impotence and bladder dysfunction (Fig. 52-3).

The rectosacral fascia, or Waldeyer's fascia, is a thick condensation of endopelvic fascia connecting the presacral fascia to the fascia propria at the level of S4 that extends to the anorectal ring. Waldeyer's fascia is an important surgical landmark, and its division during dissection from an abdominal approach provides entry to the deep retrorectal pelvis. Dissection between the fascia propria and presacral fascia follows the principles of surgical oncology and minimizes the risk for vascular or neural injuries. Disruption of the presacral fascia may lead to injury of the basivertebral venous plexus, resulting in massive hemorrhage. Disrupting the fascia propria during an operation for rectal cancer may significantly increase the incidence of subsequent recurrence of cancer in the pelvis if mesorectum is then left behind.

## Pelvic Floor

The muscles of the pelvic floor, like those of the anal sphincter mechanism, arise from the primitive cloaca. The pelvic floor, or diaphragm, consists of the pubococcygeus, iliococcygeus, and puborectalis, a group of muscles that together form the levator ani. The pelvic diaphragm resides between the sacrum, obturator fascia, ischial spines, and pubis. It forms a strong floor that supports the pelvic organs and, with the external anal sphincter, regulates defecation. The levator hiatus is an opening between the decussating fibers of the pubococcygeus that allows egress of the anal canal, urethra, and dorsal vein in men and the anal canal, urethra, and vagina in women. The puborectalis is a strong, U-shaped sling of striated muscle coursing around the rectum just above the level of the anal sphincters. Relaxation of the puborectalis straightens the anorectal angle and permits descent of feces; contraction produces the opposite effect. The puborectalis is in a state of continual contraction, a factor vital to the maintenance of continence. Puborectalis dysfunction is an important cause of defecation disorders. The pubococcygeus and iliococcygeus most likely participate in continence by applying lateral pressure to narrow the levator hiatus (Figs. 52-4 and 52-5).

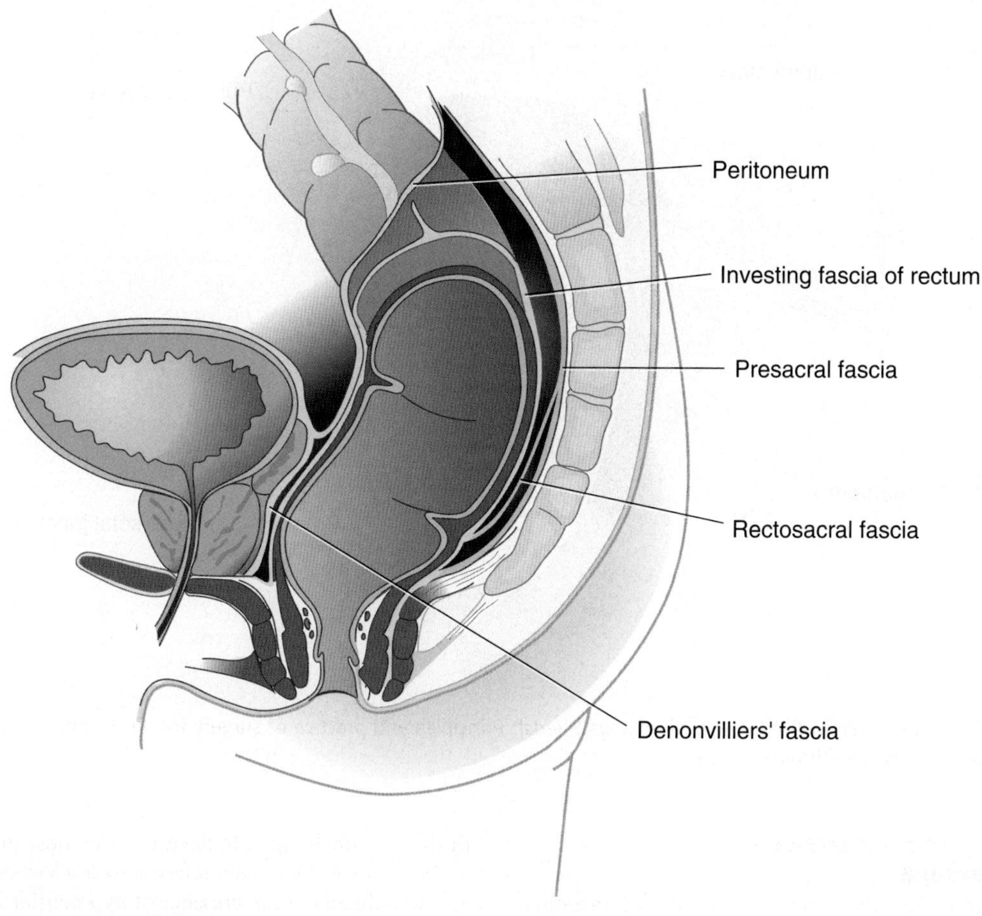


**FIGURE 52-3** Endopelvic fascia. (From Gordon PH, Nivatvongs S [eds]: Principles and practice of surgery for the colon, rectum and anus, ed 2, St Louis, 1999, Quality Medical Publishing, p 10.)

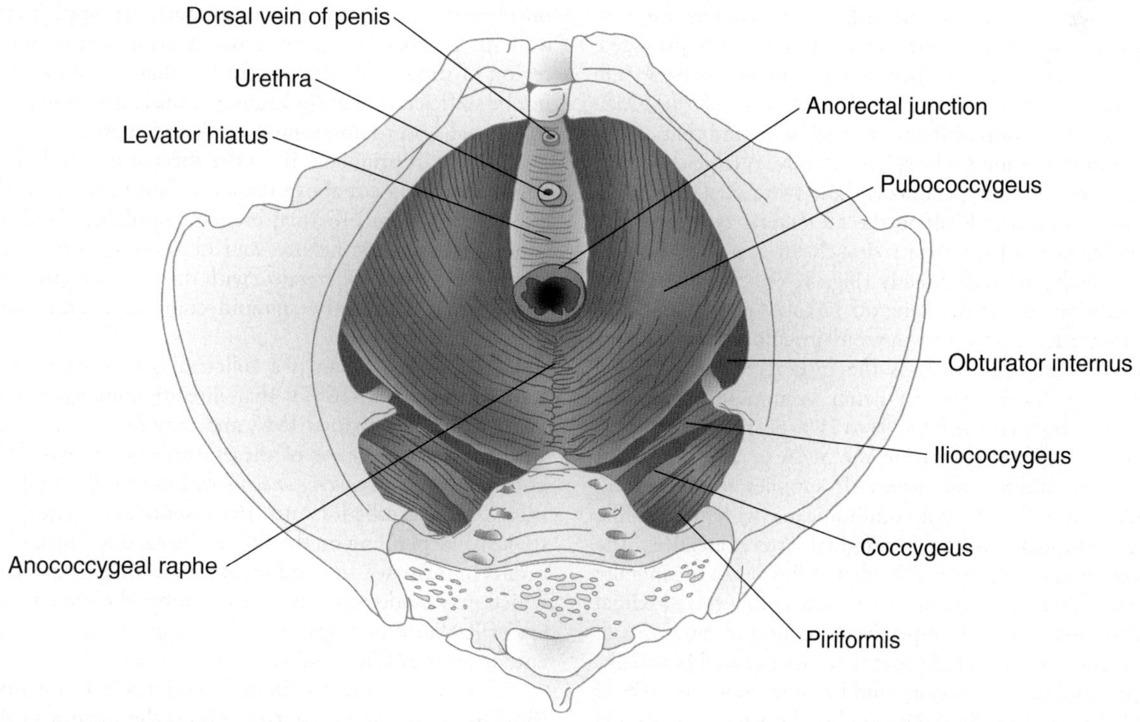


**FIGURE 52-4** Levator muscles. (From Gordon PH, Nivatvongs S [eds]: Principles and practice of surgery for the colon, rectum and anus, ed 2, St Louis, 1999, Quality Medical Publishing, p 18.)

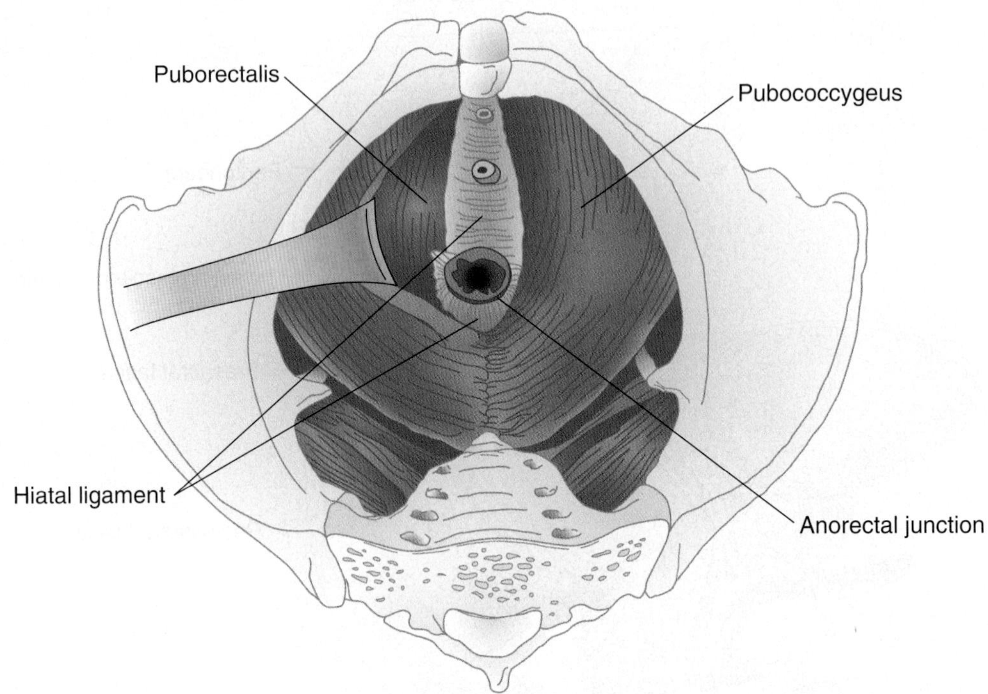


**FIGURE 52-5** Hiatal ligament. (From Gordon PH, Nivatvongs S [eds]: Principles and practice of surgery for the colon, rectum and anus, ed 2, St Louis, 1999, Quality Medical Publishing, p 18.)

## Arterial Supply and Venous and Lymphatic Drainage

Knowledge of the embryologic development of the intestinal tract provides an excellent foundation for understanding the anatomic blood supply. The foregut is supplied by the celiac artery, the midgut by the SMA, and the hindgut by the IMA (Figs. 52-6 and 52-7). Anatomic redundancy confers survival advantages and, in the intestinal tract, this feature is provided by extensive communication between the major arteries and collateral blood supply (Fig. 52-8). The territory of the SMA ends at the distal portion of the transverse colon and that of the IMA begins in the region of the splenic flexure. A large collateral vessel, the marginal artery, connects these two circulations and forms a continuous arcade along the mesenteric border of the colon. Vasa recta from this artery branch off at short intervals and supply the bowel wall directly (Fig. 52-9). The SMA supplies the entire small bowel, giving off 12 to 20 jejunal and ileal branches to the left and up to three main colonic branches to the right. The ileocolic artery is the most constant of these branches; it supplies the terminal ileum, cecum, and appendix. The right colic artery is absent in 2% to 18% of specimens; when present, it may arise directly from the SMA or as a branch of the ileocolic or middle colic artery. It supplies the ascending colon and hepatic flexure and communicates with the middle colic artery through collateral marginal artery arcades. The middle colic artery is a proximal branch of the SMA. It generally divides into right and left branches, which supply the proximal and distal transverse colon, respectively. Anatomic variations of the middle colic artery include complete absence in 4% to 20% and the presence of an accessory middle colic artery in 10% of specimens. The left branch of the middle colic artery may supply territory also supplied by the left colic artery through the collateral channel of the marginal artery. This collateral circulation in the area of the splenic flexure is the most inconsistent of the entire colon and has been referred to as a *watershed area*, vulnerable to ischemia in the presence of hypotension. In some studies, up to 50% of specimens were found to lack clearly identified arteries in a small segment of colon at the confluence of the blood supplies of the midgut and hindgut. These individuals rely on adjacent vasa recta in this area for arterial supply to the bowel wall. In practice, surgeons avoid making anastomoses in the region of the splenic flexure, fearing that the blood supply will not be sufficient to permit healing of the anastomosis, a situation that could lead to anastomotic leak and sepsis.

The IMA originates from the aorta at the level of L2 to L3, approximately 3 cm above the aortic bifurcation. The left colic artery is the most proximal branch, supplying the distal transverse colon, splenic flexure, and descending colon. Two to six sigmoid branches collateralize with the left colic artery and form arcades that supply the sigmoid colon and contribute to the marginal artery.

The arc of Riolan is a collateral artery, first described by Jean Riolan (1580-1657), that directly connects the proximal SMA with the proximal IMA and may serve as a vital conduit when one or the other of these arteries is occluded. It is also known as the *meandering mesenteric artery* and is highly variable in size. Flow can be forward (IMA stenosis) or retrograde (SMA stenosis), depending on the site of obstruction. Such obstruction results in increased size and tortuosity of this meandering artery, which may be detected by arteriography; the presence of a large arc of Riolan thus suggests occlusion of one of the major mesenteric arteries (Fig. 52-10).

The IMA terminates in the superior rectal (superior hemorrhoidal) artery, which courses behind the rectum in the mesorectum, branching and then entering the rectal submucosa. Here, the capillaries form a submucosal plexus in the distal

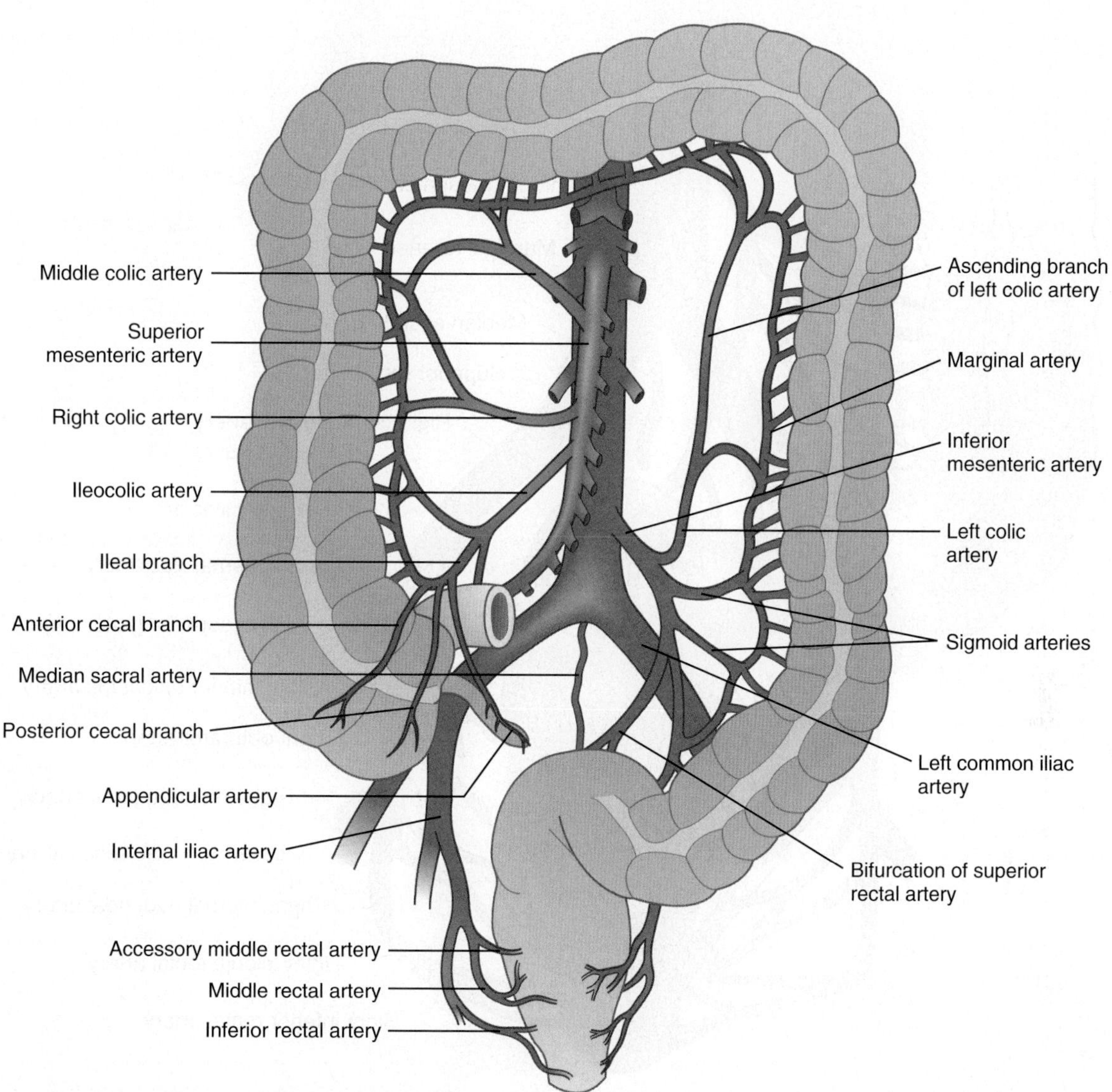


**FIGURE 52-6** Arterial supply of the colon. (From Gordon PH, Nivatvongs S [eds]: Principles and practice of surgery for the colon, rectum and anus, ed 2, St Louis, 1999, Quality Medical Publishing, p 23.)

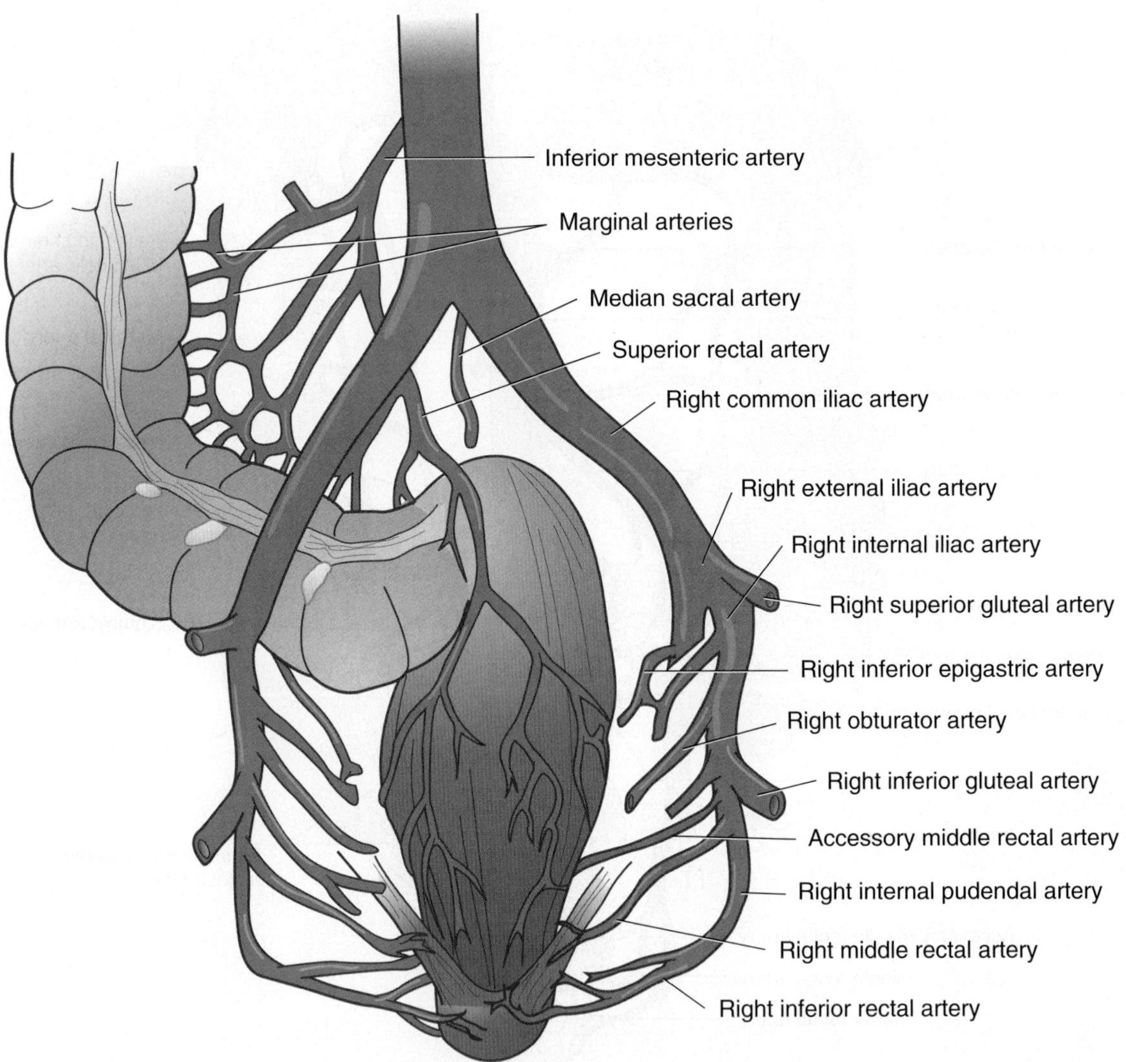


**FIGURE 52-7** Arterial supply of the rectum. (From Gordon PH, Nivatvongs S [eds]: Principles and practice of surgery for the colon, rectum and anus, ed 2, St Louis, 1999, Quality Medical Publishing, p 24.)

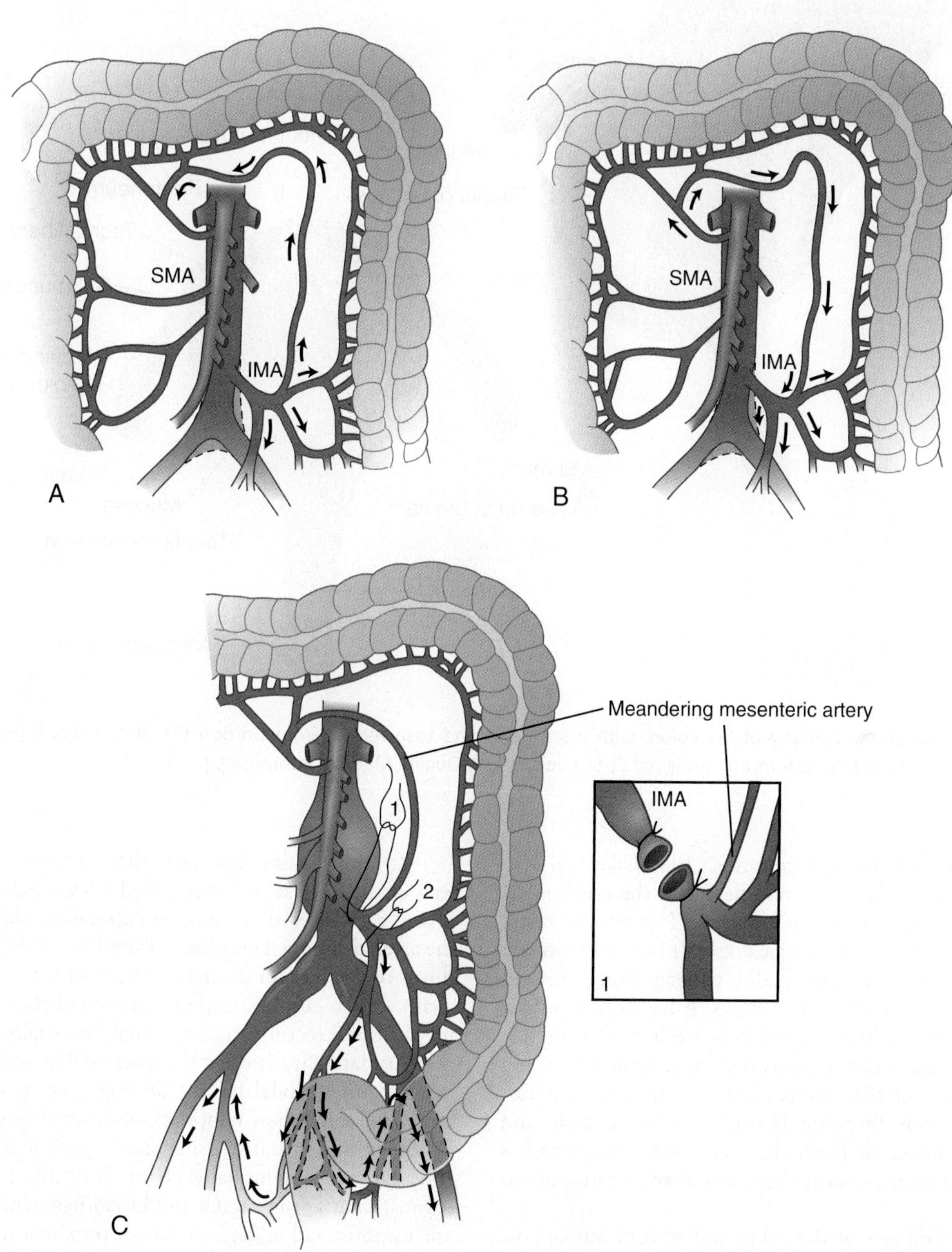


**FIGURE 52-8** Pathologic anatomy and occlusion of the SMA and IMA. **A,** Occlusion of SMA. **B,** Occlusion of the IMA. **C,** Ligating the IMA. 1, Correct location of ligation (see *inset*); 2, Incorrect location of ligation. (From Gordon PH, Nivatvongs S [eds]: Principles and practice of surgery for the colon, rectum and anus, ed 2, St Louis, 1999, Quality Medical Publishing, p 28.)

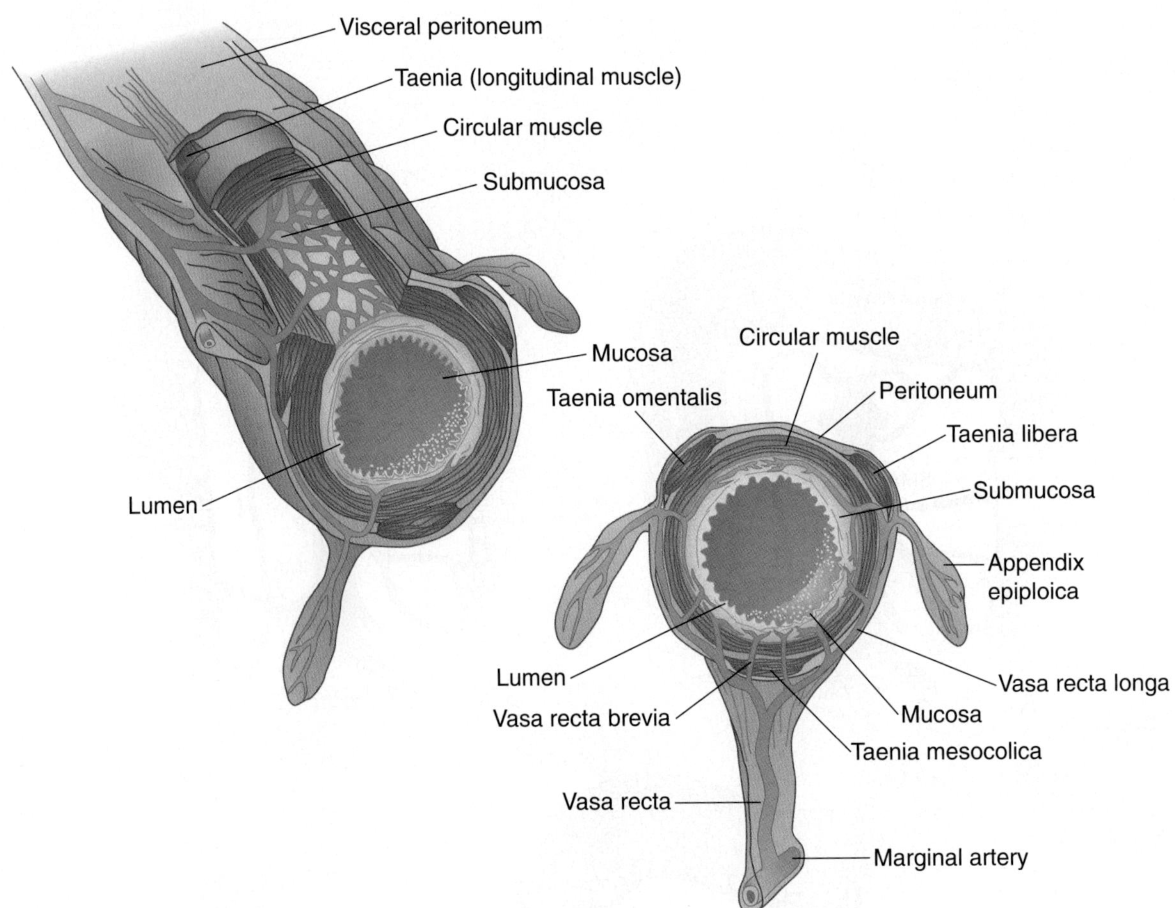


**FIGURE 52-9** Cross-sectional anatomy of the colon, with vasa brevia and vasa recta. (From Gordon PH, Nivatvongs S [eds]: Principles and practice of surgery for the colon, rectum and anus, ed 2, St Louis, 1999, Quality Medical Publishing, p 26.)

rectum at the level of the anal columns. The anal canal also receives arterial blood from the middle rectal (hemorrhoidal) and inferior rectal (hemorrhoidal) arteries. The middle rectal artery is a branch of the internal iliac artery. It is variable in size and enters the rectum anterolaterally, passing alongside and slightly anterior to the lateral rectal stalks. It has been reported to be absent in 40% to 80% of specimens studied. The inferior rectal artery is a branch of the pudendal artery, which itself is a more distal branch of the internal iliac. From the obturator canal, it traverses the obturator fascia, ischiorectal fossa, and external anal sphincter to reach the anal canal. This vessel is encountered during the perineal dissection of an abdominoperineal resection.

The venous drainage of the colon and rectum mirrors the arterial blood supply. Venous drainage from the right and proximal transverse colon empties into the superior mesenteric vein, which coalesces with the splenic vein to become the portal vein. The distal transverse colon, descending colon, sigmoid, and most of the rectum drain into the inferior mesenteric vein, which empties into the splenic vein to the left of the aorta. The anal canal is drained by the middle and inferior rectal veins into the internal iliac vein and subsequently the inferior vena cava. The bidirectional venous drainage of the anal canal accounts for differences in patterns of metastasis from tumors arising in this region (Fig. 52-11).

Lymphatic drainage also follows the arterial anatomy. The wall of the large bowel is supplied with a rich network of lymphatic capillaries that drain to extramural channels paralleling the arterial supply. Lymphatics from the colon and proximal two thirds of the rectum ultimately drain into the para-aortic nodal chain, which empties into the cisterna chyli. Lymphatics draining the distal rectum and anal canal may drain to the para-aortic nodes or laterally, through the internal iliac system, to the superficial inguinal nodal basin. Although the dentate line roughly marks the level where lymphatic drainage diverges, classic studies by Block and Enquist using dye injection demonstrated that spread through lymphatic channels occurs to adjacent pelvic organs, such as the vagina and broad ligament, when injections are administered as high as 10 cm proximal to the dentate line (Figs. 52-12 and 52-13).

Lymph nodes are commonly grouped into levels depending on their location. Epicolic nodes are located along the bowel wall and in the epiploic appendices. Nodes adjacent to the marginal artery are paracolic. Intermediate nodes are located along the main branches of the large blood vessels; primary nodes are located on the SMA or IMA. Lymph node invasion by metastatic cancer is an important prognostic factor for patients with colorectal cancer. Accurate pathologic assessment of lymph nodes is essential for accurate staging, which serves as a determinant for treatment of patients with colorectal cancer.

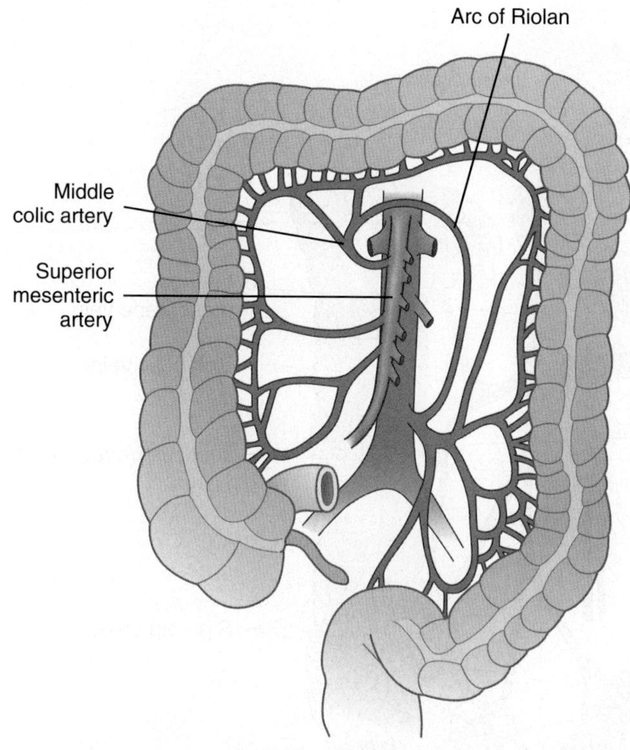


**FIGURE 52-10** Arc of Riolan. (From Gordon PH, Nivatvongs S [eds]: Principles and practice of surgery for the colon, rectum and anus, ed 2, St Louis, 1999, Quality Medical Publishing, p 27.)

### Nerves

Preganglionic sympathetic nerves from T6 to T12 synapse in preaortic ganglia. Postsympathetic fibers then course along blood vessels to reach the right and transverse colons. The right and transverse colon parasympathetic supply comes from the right vagus nerve. Parasympathetic fibers follow branches of the SMA to synapse in the wall of the bowel. The left colon and rectum receive sympathetic supply from the preganglionic lumbar splanchnics of L1 to L3. These synapse in the preaortic plexus located above the aortic bifurcation and the postganglionic elements follow the branches of the IMA and superior rectal artery to the left colon, sigmoid, and rectum. The lower rectum, pelvic floor, and anal canal receive postganglionic sympathetics from the pelvic plexus. The pelvic plexus is adherent to the pelvic sidewalls and is adjacent to the lateral stalks. It receives sympathetic branches from the presacral plexus, which condense at the sacral promontory into the left and right hypogastric nerves. These sympathetic nerves, which descend into the pelvis dorsal to the superior rectal artery, are responsible for delivery of semen to the posterior prostatic urethra. Failure to preserve at least one of the hypogastric nerves during rectal dissection results in ejaculatory dysfunction in males.

The pelvic parasympathetic nerves, or nervi erigentes, arise from S2 to S4. Preganglionic parasympathetic nerves merge with postganglionic sympathetics after the latter emerge from the sacral foramina. These nerve fibers, through the pelvic plexus, surround and innervate the prostate, urethra, seminal vesicles, urinary bladder, and muscles of the pelvic floor. Rectal dissection may disrupt the pelvic plexus and its subdivisions, resulting in neurogenic bladder and sexual dysfunction. Rates of bladder and erectile dysfunction after rectal surgery are as high as 45%. The degree and type of dysfunction are affected by the level of the neurologic injury. A high IMA ligation severing the hypogastric nerves near the sacral promontory results in sympathetic dysfunction characterized by retrograde ejaculation and bladder dysfunction. Injury to the mixed parasympathetic and sympathetic periprostatic plexus results in impotence and an atonic bladder.

## PHYSIOLOGY OF THE COLON

Generally speaking, the function of the colon is the recycling of nutrients, whereas the function of the rectum is the elimination of stool. The recycling of nutrients depends on the metabolic activity of the colonic flora, colonic motility, and mucosal absorption and secretion. Stool elimination involves dehydration of colonic contents and defecation.

### Recycling of Nutrients

During the digestive process, ingested nutrients are diluted within the intestinal lumen by biliopancreatic and GI secretions. The small intestine absorbs most ingested nutrients and some of the fluid and bile salts secreted into the lumen. However, the ileal effluent is still rich in water, electrolytes, and nutrients that resist digestion. The colon has the functional ability to recover these substances and avoid unnecessary losses of fluids, electrolytes, nitrogen, and energy. To accomplish this, the colon depends highly on its bacterial flora.

#### Colonic Flora

Nutrients are digested within the intestinal lumen with the aid of biliopancreatic and GI secretions. By the time the chyme reaches the terminal ileum, most of the nutrients have been absorbed, leaving a succus entericus composed of electrolyte-rich fluid, bile salts, and some proteins and starches that have resisted digestion. An enormous quantity of autochthonous flora, consisting of more than 400 bacterial species, resides in the large intestine. Large bowel contents may contain as many as $10^{11}$ to $10^{12}$ bacterial cells/g, contributing approximately 50% of fecal mass.[1] Most these colonic species are anaerobes. These bacteria feed on proteins sloughed from the bowel wall and undigested complex carbohydrates.

Colonic microflora provide several important functions to the host, including barrier functions that help maintain epithelial integrity, nutritive functions that utilize plant polysaccharides, and developmental functions that stimulate epithelial cell differentiation and angiogenesis and, finally, immune functions via the gut. Gut associated lymphoid tissue contributes to both innate and adaptive immunity.[1] Short-chain fatty acids (SCFAs) are produced by microbial breakdown and fermentation of dietary starches. These fatty acids are the principal source of nutrition for the colonocyte. *Bacteroides* species predominate throughout the colon, comprising two thirds of the total counts of the proximal colon and almost 70% of the bacteria in the rectum. *Escherichia, Klebsiella, Proteus, Lactobacillus,* and enterococci are the predominant species of facultative anaerobes.

#### Prebiotics and Probiotics

Probiotics can be defined as dietary supplements that contain live cultures of bacteria and yeast that are beneficial to colonic and host function. The two most widely used agents

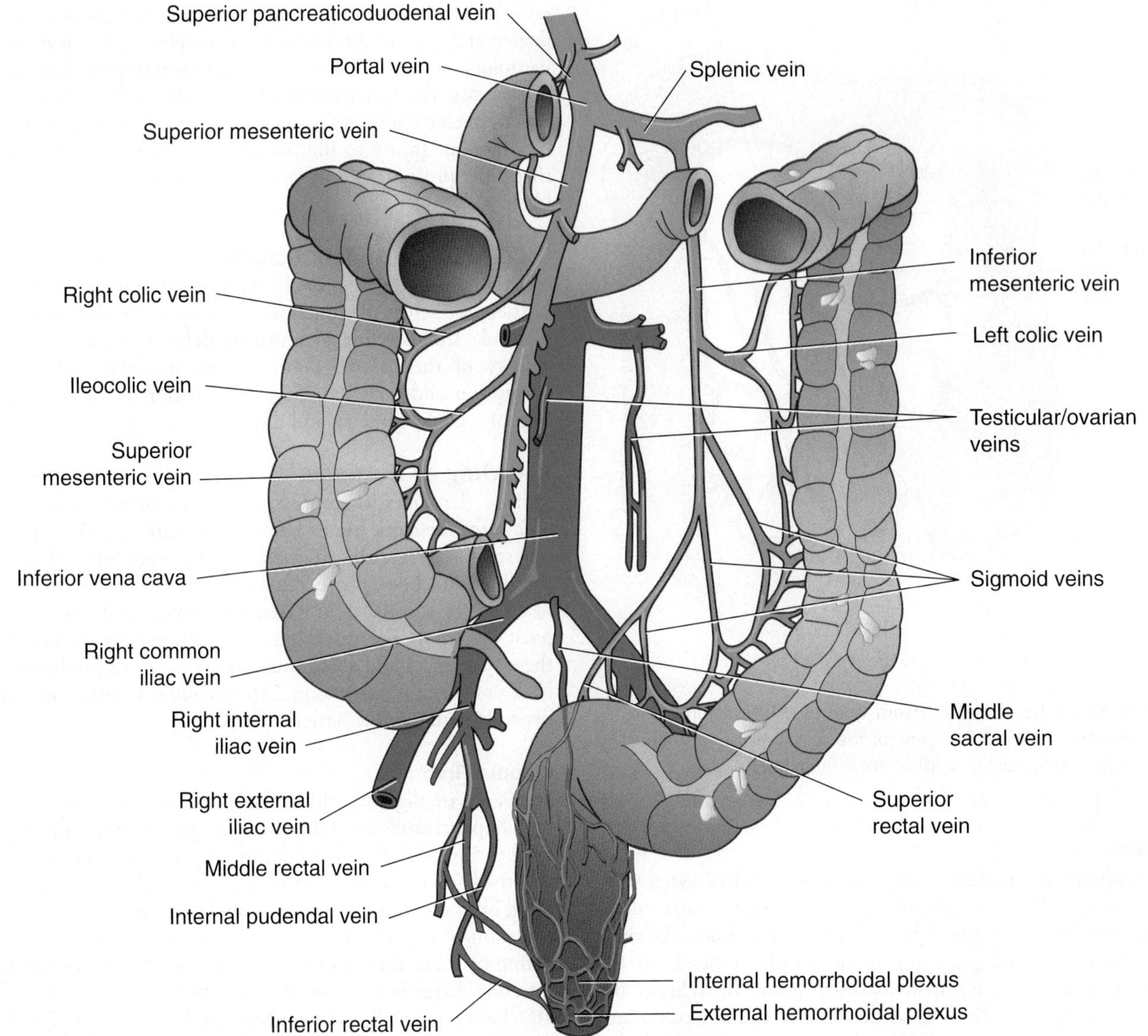


**FIGURE 52-11** Venous drainage of the colon and rectum. (From Gordon PH, Nivatvongs S [eds]: Principles and practice of surgery for the colon, rectum and anus, ed 2, St Louis, 1999, Quality Medical Publishing, p 30.)

are *Lactobacillus* and *Bifidobacterium*. Recent studies have indicated that probiotics may have widespread health benefits, including stimulation of immune function, anti-inflammatory effects, and suppression of enteropathogenic colonization.[2] In addition, they may increase the digestibility of dietary proteins, enhance absorption of amino acids, and play a protective or therapeutic role against *Clostridium difficile*–associated diarrhea.[3] The ultimate role of probiotics has not yet been determined. There is conflicting data in regard to whether they work more effectively as primary therapy or as prophylaxis against recurrent *C. difficile*–associated diarrhea. Indications for their use are evolving, but may include necrotizing enterocolitis in neonates, patients with HIV-AIDS, and neutropenic patients undergoing chemotherapy. Further research is needed, but the evidence for probiotic usage in various settings is encouraging.

Prebiotics are nondigestible oligosaccharides (e.g., inulin) that help the host by stimulating the growth of certain species of beneficial intestinal bacteria. There is a growing body of data suggesting health benefits; however, there is currently little evidence to guide recommendations for their use.

### Fermentation

Unlike most of the mucosal lining of the proximal GI tract, colonic mucosa does not receive its primary nutrition from the bloodstream. Instead, nutrient requirements are fulfilled from the colonic luminal contents. The primary energy source for the colonocyte is the SCFA butyrate. The manner in which this interaction occurs illustrates the essential symbiotic interaction between the colon and its resident bacterial flora.

The main source of energy for intestinal bacteria is dietary fiber, composed of complex carbohydrates (starches and nonstarch polysaccharides [NSPs]). This fiber is metabolized by the process of fermentation. Not all complex carbohydrates are fermented in the same manner, which underlies many of the dietary recommendations for bulking agents; lignin and

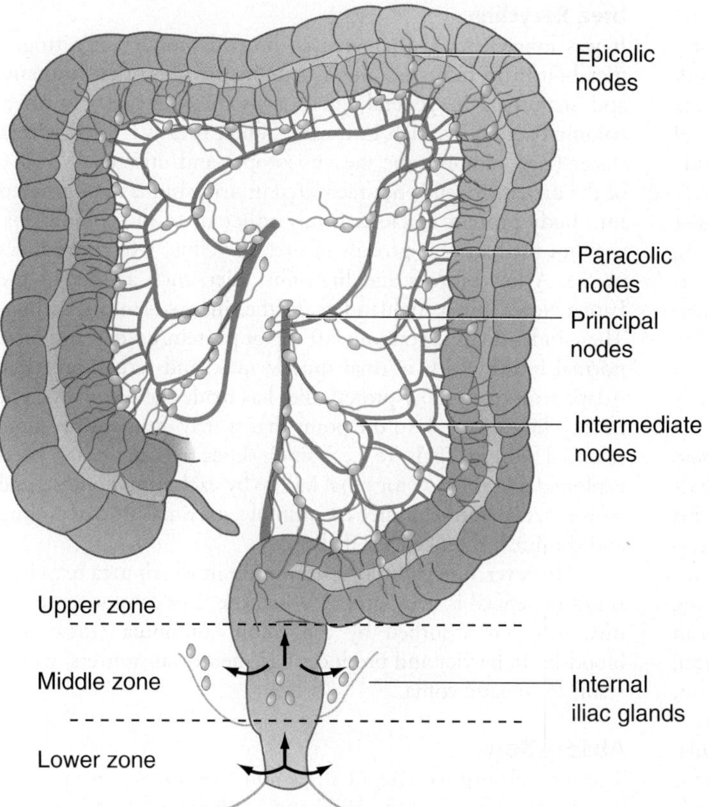


**FIGURE 52-12** Lymphatic drainage of the colon. (From Corman ML [ed]: Colon and rectal surgery, ed 4, Philadelphia,1998, Lippincott-Raven, p 21.)

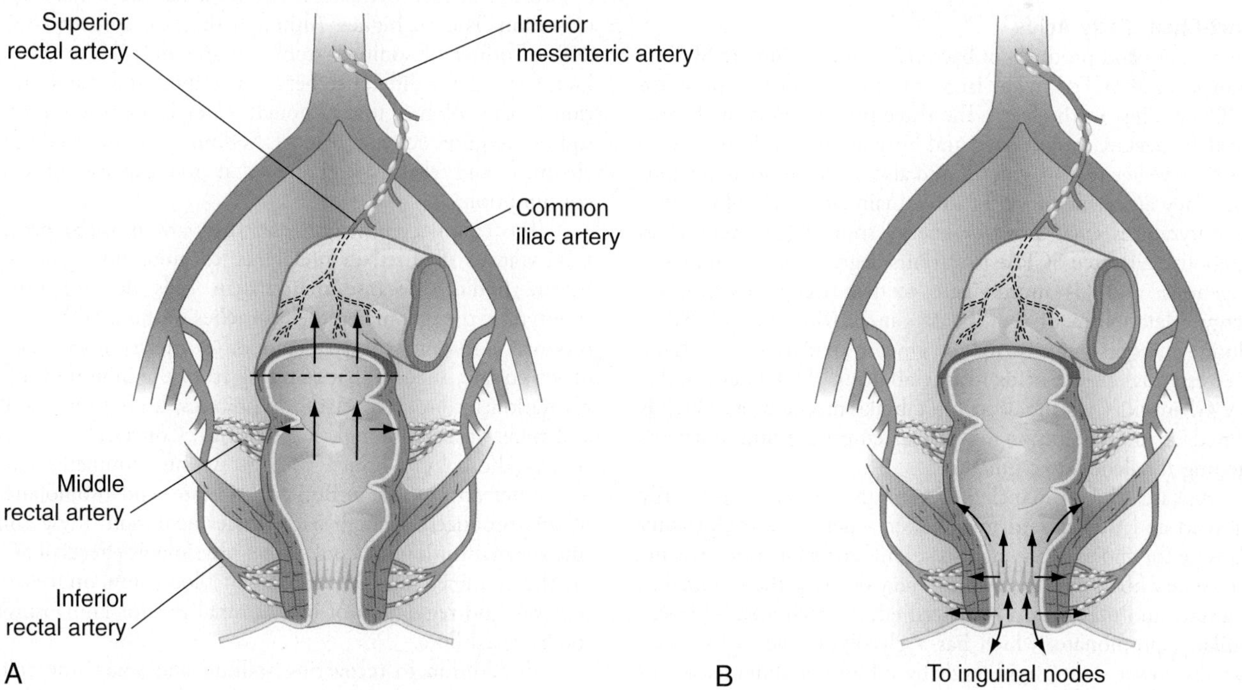


**FIGURE 52-13** Lymphatic drainage of the rectum (**A**) and anal canal (**B**). (From Gordon PH, Nivatvongs S [eds]: Principles and practice of surgery for the colon, rectum and anus, ed 2, St Louis, 1999, Quality Medical Publishing, p 32.)

psyllium are components of plants that are not fermented by human colonic flora. They are hydrophilic, thus leading to water resorption and stool bulking. Celluloses are partially fermented, whereas fruit pectins are completely metabolized by colonic bacteria. Diets high in nonfermentable NSPs contribute to stool bulk and increased transit time; highly fermentable NSPs provide minimal bulk, but enhanced colonocyte nutrition.

The end products of fermentation are SCFAs and gas—carbon dioxide, methane, and hydrogen. In addition to NSPs, colonic bacteria ferment poorly absorbed starches and proteins from the upper GI tract, known as *resistant starches*. Although highly variable from person to person, with daily variability dependent on diet, the gases produced by bacterial fermentation comprise approximately 50% to 75% of flatus, with the remainder consisting of swallowed air.

Protein fermentation, otherwise known as *putrefaction*, results in the formation of potentially toxic metabolites, including phenols, indoles, and amines. The production of these toxins is inhibited in many intestinal bacteria by the presence of alternate carbohydrate energy sources. This process becomes accentuated more distally in the colon as carbohydrate sources become scarcer. These deleterious end products of bacterial metabolism can lead to mucosal injury and reactive hyperproliferation, which have been hypothesized to promote carcinogenesis. Also, the presence of bulking agents decreases intracolonic pressures and may serve to prevent the formation of colonic diverticula. It can be seen, then, how providing adequate sources of various forms of dietary carbohydrates can serve positive roles in colonic health. These principles underlie the recommendations for dietary fiber, as do the evolving data on the helpful nature of probiotics and prebiotics.

### Short-Chain Fatty Acids

The primary end products of bacterial fermentation are SCFAs. Absorption of SCFAs in the large intestine is efficient; only 5% to 10% are lost in the feces. The three primary fatty acids produced are acetate, propionate, and butyrate in a ratio of 3 : 1 : 1. SCFAs have key roles in colonic and also overall human metabolism. They are metabolized in three main sites: (1) colonocytes use butyrate as their primary energy source; (2) hepatocytes metabolize all three SCFAs to various degrees for use in gluconeogenesis; and (3) muscle cells oxidize acetate to generate energy. Metabolism of the SCFAs can provide up to 70% of colonocyte energy needs, reduce glucose oxidation, and spare other essential amino acids for metabolism.[4] SCFAs also influence GI motility via the ileocolonic brake mechanism, which is defined as the inhibition of gastric emptying and nutrients reaching the ileocolonic junction.

Acetate, the principal SCFA in the colon, is primarily absorbed and transported to the liver, where it is the primary substrate for cholesterol synthesis. Nonabsorbable, nonfermentable dietary fiber, such as psyllium, may decrease the production of acetate and may have a beneficial effect on cholesterol levels. Similarly, propionate, which has a glycolytic role in the liver, may also lower serum lipid levels by inhibiting cholesterol synthesis. Butyrate is the primary energy source for colonic epithelial cells and may also play an important role in maintaining cellular health by arresting the proliferation of neoplastic colonocytes, while paradoxically being trophic for normal colonocytes. In addition, butyrate serves to regulate and stabilize cell adhesion molecules.

### Urea Recycling

It was long believed that urea is the end product of nitrogen metabolism in humans. This is true in the sense that humans, and mammals in general, do not produce urease. However, colonic bacteria are rich in urease. When urea is labeled with a tracer (e.g., radioisotope, heavy isotope) and injected IV, 10% of the urea nitrogen is not recovered in urine but is incorporated into body protein. Bacteria firmly adherent to the colonic epithelium mediate this process of urea recycling, which produces urease. A low-protein and high-fiber diet, such as that of the Papua New Guinea highlanders, further increases urea recycling. These individuals ingest only 10 mg of protein/kg/day and have normal health, with normal muscle mass and serum proteins. Adaptation to this low-protein diet has made the colon efficient in recycling nitrogen to the point that it may even absorb some essential amino acids (e.g., lysine). Urea recycling has been exploited as a therapy for renal failure by excluding nonessential amino acids from the diet to promote maximal urea recycling and diminish the need for dialysis.

However, one pathologic condition in which urea recycling is not beneficial is liver failure. When the liver cannot reuse the urea nitrogen absorbed by the colon, ammonia crosses the blood-brain barrier and produces false neurotransmitters, which result in hepatic coma.

## Absorption

The total absorptive area of the colon is estimated at approximately 900 $cm^2$. Between 1000 and 1500 mL of fluid is poured into the cecum by the daily ileal effluent. The total volume of water in stool is only 100 to 150 mL/day. This 10-fold reduction in water across the colon represents the most efficient site of absorption in the GI tract per surface area. The net absorption of sodium is even higher. Although the ileal effluent contains 200 mEq/liter of sodium, stool contains only 25 to 50 mEq/liter. One major difference between sodium and water absorption in the colon is that although water is absorbed passively, sodium requires active transport. Sodium is transported against chemical and electrical gradients at the expense of energy consumption.

The colonic epithelium can use various fuels; however, *n*-butyrate is oxidized in preference to glutamine, glucose, or ketone bodies. Because mammalian cells do not produce *n*-butyrate, the colonic epithelium relies on luminal bacteria to produce it through the fermentation of dietary fiber. The lack of *n*-butyrate, such as that resulting from the inhibition of fermentation by broad-spectrum antibiotics, leads to less sodium and water absorption and thus diarrhea. Conversely, the perfusion of the colonic lumen with *n*-butyrate stimulates sodium and water absorption. *n*-Butyrate, acetate, and propionate are SCFAs produced through bacterial fermentation; these constitute the main anions in stool. Other physiologic effects of SCFAs on the colon include stimulation of blood flow, mucosal cell renewal, and regulation of intraluminal pH for homeostasis of the bacterial flora.

In addition to recovering sodium and water, the colonic mucosa absorbs bile acids. The colon absorbs bile acids that escape absorption by the terminal ileum, thus making the colon part of the enterohepatic circulation. Bile acids are passively transported across the colonic epithelium by nonionic diffusion. When the colonic absorptive capacity is exceeded, colonic bacteria deconjugate bile acids. Deconjugated bile acids can then interfere with sodium and water absorption, leading to secretory, or choleretic, diarrhea. Choleretic diarrhea is seen early after right hemicolectomy as a transient phenomenon and more permanently after extensive ileal resection.

## Secretion

The physiologic role of colon secretion is demonstrated in patients with chronic renal failure. Uremic patients can remain normokalemic while ingesting a normal amount of potassium before requiring dialysis. This phenomenon is associated with a compensatory increase in colonic secretion and fecal excretion of potassium. This effect is blocked by spironolactone, which illustrates the effect of aldosterone on colonic potassium secretion. Potassium secretion requires both $Na^+,K^+$-ATPase and $Na^+$-$K^+$-$2Cl^-$ cotransport on the basolateral membrane and an apical potassium channel.

Many forms of colitis are associated with increased potassium secretion, such as inflammatory bowel disease (IBD), cholera, and shigellosis. In addition, some forms of colitis impair colonic absorption or produce secretion of chloride, such as collagenous and microscopic colitis and congenital chloridorrhea. Chloride is secreted by colonic epithelium at a basal rate, which is increased in pathologic conditions such as cystic fibrosis and secretory diarrhea. Secretion of chloride also requires the coupling of $Na^+,K^+$-ATPase and $Na^+$-$K^+$-$2Cl^-$ cotransport to exit passively through the apical membrane. Calcium and cyclic adenosine monophosphate both stimulate chloride secretion, whereas bicarbonate and SCFAs inhibit chloride secretion.

Colonic secretion of $H^+$ and bicarbonate is coupled to the absorption of $Na^+$ and $Cl^-$, respectively. It is through these exchangers that the colon is linked to systemic acid-base metabolism. The supply of $H^+$ and bicarbonate for these exchangers is maintained by the hydration of $CO_2$, catalyzed by colonic carbonic anhydrase. Changes in systemic pH induce changes in the activity of carbonic anhydrase, eliciting elimination of $H^+$ or bicarbonate as needed to bring the systemic pH back to normal.

## Motility

Colonic motility is a highly complex process, made difficult to investigate by a lack of standardized terminology and measurements. Additionally, movement through the colon is relatively slow compared with the proximal GI tract, and studies require prolonged observation.

Colonic motility patterns may be more simply divided into two primary patterns, segmental activity and propagated activity. Segmental activity consists of single contractions or rhythmic bursts of contractions. The purpose of these segmental contractions is to propel fecal matter distally via a directed pressure gradient toward the rectum in discrete distances and allow for mixing, which promotes optimal absorption. The second pattern is propagated activity, commonly classified on the basis of amplitude as low-amplitude or high-amplitude propagated contractions.[5] High-amplitude propagated contractions have been historically referred to as *mass movements*, or migrating motor complexes whose role is shifting large quantities of contents through the colon. These have an important role in defecation, with mass movements propelling larger volumes of fecal matter to the distal colon and emptying of the descending colon into the sigmoid colon and rectum. Little is known about low-amplitude propagated contractions, but they are associated with distention of the viscous and passage of flatus.

There seems to be a circadian rhythm to colonic motility, with maximum peaks of activity immediately after waking and after meals. Sleep is associated with a decrease in colonic motility.

Not surprisingly, food ingestion results in an increase of overall colonic motility for approximately 2 hours. This reflex is stimulated not only by gastric distention but also by the central nervous system (CNS), initiated by visualization of food. Additionally, meal composition affects colonic responses. Increased activity in response to carbohydrate meals is fairly short-lived, whereas fatty meals elicit longer term responses.

Ultimately, transit in the colon is controlled by the autonomic nervous system. Parasympathetic innervation reaches the colon through the vagus and pelvic nerves. The enteric nervous system in the colon is arranged in several plexuses—subserosal, myenteric (Auerbach), submucosal (Meissner), and mucosal plexuses. Sympathetic innervation originates in the superior and inferior mesenteric ganglia and reaches the colon via perivascular plexuses.

## Formation of Stool

The frequency of defecation is just as variable among individuals as is their perception of abnormal stool frequency. An individual who passes more than three loose stools daily is considered as having diarrhea, whereas fewer than three weekly stools is considered constipation. Any frequency within that range is considered normal, although many individuals will still seek medical attention for what they perceive as diarrhea or constipation. Many factors influence colonic transit rate. Colonic transit is longer in women than in men and longer in premenopausal than postmenopausal women. Conversely, colonic transit time is shortened in smokers. In normal subjects, supplementation with NSPs does not shorten colonic transit time, although it does increase fecal weight. In patients with idiopathic constipation, however, NSPs, in the form of psyllium seeds, shorten colonic transit time and increase stool weight.

## Defecation

Normal defecation requires adequate colonic transit time, stool consistency, and fecal continence. Fecal continence implies deferment of stool elimination, discrimination among gas, liquid, and solid stool, and selective elimination of gas without stool. There is some controversy regarding the actual role of the rectum under resting conditions. Some have proposed that the rectum is simply a conduit, which under resting conditions should be empty. If stool arrives at the rectum, the anorectal inhibitory reflex is triggered, forcing the subject to hold defecation by voluntary contraction of the external sphincter. However, any surgeon who performs routine rigid proctosigmoidoscopies in the office is well aware that a patient can have a rectum full of stool without any awareness. This leads to the opposing view, which regards the rectum as a reservoir. Just as stool triggers the anorectal inhibitory reflex, it also triggers a rectocolic reflex. This reflex allows continuous filling of the rectum with fecal material until the colon is emptied.

The mechanisms involved in fecal continence are not fully understood. A certain reservoir capacity is needed to achieve fecal continence. A stiff nondistensible rectum, such as in radiation proctitis, may produce incontinence, even when the sphincter muscles are competent. Some of the internal and external sphincter muscle fibers are necessary for adequate continence, although many patients have part of the sphincter severed during a fistulotomy and are still continent. Probably, the only factor needed for fecal continence is innervation of the sphincter. The motor nerve fibers, which produce contraction of the sphincter fibers, and also all the sensory innervation are important to empty the rectum adequately.

## BOWEL PREPARATION BEFORE SURGERY

Purging the feces and reducing the concentration of colonic intraluminal bacteria before operations on the colon have long been basic tenets of surgery. The normal, or autochthonous, microbial organisms in the colon comprise up to 90% of the dry weight of feces, reaching concentrations of up to $10^9$ organism/mL of feces. The anaerobic *Bacteroides* is the most common colonic microbe, whereas *Escherichia coli* is the most common aerobe. *Pseudomonas, Enterococcus, Proteus, Klebsiella,* and *Streptococcus* spp. are also present in large numbers.

The process of preparing the colon for an elective operation has traditionally involved two factors, purging the fecal contents (mechanical preparation) and administration of antibiotics effective against colonic bacteria. Tradition has held that an unprepared colon (i.e., one that contains intraluminal feces) poses an unacceptably high rate of failure of the anastomosis to heal. However, experience with primary repair of colonic injuries by trauma surgeons, along with reports from European surgeons describing elective operations conducted safely without the use of preoperative purging, have led to reconsideration of the true value of purging the colon before colonic surgery. Because the colonocytes receive nutrition from intraluminal free fatty acids produced by fermentation from colonic bacteria, there are concerns that purging may actually be detrimental to the healing of a colonic anastomosis. However, in the United States at present, the colon is generally cleansed in preparation for colonic operations. Effective cleansing is mandatory for adequate colonoscopy or the administration of contrast enema.

Although the use of preoperative parenteral antibiotics is well accepted and validated, the related issue of preoperative oral antibiotic use is controversial. A multiplicity of bowel preparation regimens and antibiotic combinations are in current use. A clear superiority of one over another has not been found; however, for some patients, certain bowel preparations may have adverse physiologic consequences. Knowledge of the history of bowel preparation practices, current controversies, and data is useful.

Mechanical bowel cleansing methods are used for colonoscopy and elective surgery. Complete bowel obstruction and free perforation are absolute contraindications to bowel preparation. For colonoscopy, properties of various preparations are judged by safety, patient tolerance, and efficacy or preparation quality. In the past, 4 to 5 days of clear liquids, along with laxatives such as senna, castor oil, and bisacodyl, whole bowel nasogastric irrigation, mannitol irrigation, and repeated enemas were some of the regimens used. Patient tolerance of these methods is poor and is associated with dehydration, electrolyte abnormalities, and severe abdominal cramping, and are generally not well tolerated by older or infirm patients.

In the 1980s, polyethylene glycol (PEG) solution, a nonabsorbed, sodium sulfate–based liquid, was developed as an oral mechanical bowel preparation. Patients are required to drink at least 2 to 4 liters of the solution, along with additional fluids. Abdominal cramping, nausea, and vomiting are common side effects of the preparation, and prophylactic antiemetics are often administered routinely. Sodium phosphate solution (Fleet's Phospho-soda) was developed in response to patient dissatisfaction with the large fluid volume required for PEG preparation and has been found in most trials to be a more tolerable preparation, with higher rates of patient satisfaction and compliance. The smaller volume (45 mL taken twice) seems to be the main benefit because the side effects are similar. Sodium phosphate pills (Visicol) were introduced as an alternative to liquids. The regimen consists of ingesting a total of 40 pills, with three pills taken every 15 minutes with 8 oz of fluid. Sodium phosphate, in liquid or pill form, has been linked more frequently than PEG to rare but serious electrolyte imbalances. In patients with impaired renal function, hyperphosphatemia, hypernatremia, hypokalemia, and hypocalcemia can occur. Thus, PEG is the recommended bowel preparation in patients with renal insufficiency, cirrhosis, ascites, or congestive heart failure. Investigation comparing the efficacy of mechanical bowel preparations has focused on comparisons between PEG and sodium phosphate solutions.

Cohen and colleagues have demonstrated a 90% excellent or good bowel preparation with sodium phosphate versus 70% with 4 liters of PEG. Frommer has found that sodium phosphate results in a cleaner bowel than PEG, with no difference in infectious complications. On the other hand, Poon and associates have found that there is no difference in bowel cleanliness when the volume of PEG is reduced to 2 liters and compared with 90 mL of sodium phosphate, and that the reduced volume enhances patient compliance. A Canadian study has found the use of sodium phosphate to be associated with increased patient compliance and an eightfold cost reduction when compared with PEG. Ultimately, patient comfort and economic factors may determine mechanical bowel preparation practices if the efficacy is similar.

For patients undergoing colonoscopy, the quality of the bowel preparation is essential for performing an accurate examination. For segmental resections, however, the necessity of mechanical bowel preparation has come under scrutiny. Zmora and coworkers, in a study comparing infectious complications in mechanically prepared bowel (PEG solution) versus unprepared bowel in patients undergoing segmental resection, found no differences in any type of infectious complication. Both groups received parenteral antibiotics. The study looked at left-sided anastomoses only and found that there was no significant difference between overall infection rates in unprepared (13.2%) versus prepared bowel (12.5%). Also, the wound infection rates in this study did not significantly differ, 6.6% in the prepared group and 10% in the unprepared group. Although studies of this type have been relatively small and significantly underpowered, they indicate the future possibility of avoiding the discomfort of bowel preparation and the small attendant risk for electrolyte irregularities and dehydration.

Antibiotic use in colorectal surgery is a well-established practice that reduces infectious complications. Elective colorectal cases are classified as clean-contaminated and, as such, benefit from routine single-dose administration of parenteral antibiotics 30 minutes before an incision. It has been shown that when operative times are prolonged, additional doses at 4-hour intervals reduce wound infection. When the operation is completed, postoperative administration of antibiotics for a clean-contaminated case, such as a routine segmental resection, does not reduce infectious complications further and may promote *C. difficile* colitis, *Candida* infection, and the emergence of bacterial antibiotic resistance. Polk and Lopez-Mayer showed a reduction in postoperative infection rates from 30% to 8% with the routine use of preoperative parenteral antibiotics; Gomez-Alonzo and colleagues repeated these results, showing a decrease from 39% to 9%. Antibiotics active against both aerobes and anaerobes are ideal; second- or third-generation cephalosporins alone, or a combination of a fluoroquinolone plus metronidazole or clindamycin, is typical. The use of additional oral antibiotics, theoretically to reduce the bacterial load further, is widely accepted, but not as well validated. In a survey of colon and rectal surgeons, 87% indicated that both oral and parenteral antibiotic usage is part of their routine preparation for elective colon operations. A typical preparation consists of erythromycin base (1 g) and neomycin (1 g) given in three preoperative doses the day before surgery. However, this regimen is associated with a high incidence of nausea and abdominal cramps, and some surgeons prefer to prescribe oral ciprofloxacin or metronidazole.

In studies comparing oral and parenteral antibiotics, a decrease in wound infection rate from 36% to 6.5% was seen with IV administration, whereas others comparing a combination of oral plus parenteral antibiotics, versus oral alone, found that the addition of IV antibiotics reduced infectious complications by half (22% to 11%). It is notable that there have been no prospective randomized trials examining this issue and that most retrospective reviews are poorly powered. Although it is clear that preoperative parenteral antibiotics reduce wound infection rates, oral antibiotics do not clearly benefit the patient by reducing wound infection or decreasing intra-abdominal abscess or leaks. The rate of intra-abdominal abscess is more dependent on technical factors affecting anastomotic integrity than on antibiotic prophylaxis.

## DIVERTICULAR DISEASE

A diverticulum is an abnormal sac or pouch protruding from the wall of a hollow organ, which is, for the purposes of this discussion, the colon. A true diverticulum is composed of all layers of the intestinal wall, whereas a false diverticulum, or pseudodiverticulum, lacks a portion of the normal bowel wall. The diverticula that commonly occur in the human colon are protrusions of mucosa through the muscular layers of the intestine. Because these mucosal herniations are devoid of the normal muscular layers, they are pseudodiverticula (Fig. 52-14).

*Diverticulosis* and *diverticular disease* are terms used to indicate the presence of colonic diverticula. Diverticulosis is a common condition of Western society and seems to be an unfortunate product of the Industrial Revolution. It is interesting that there seem to be no specimens of colonic diverticulosis in anatomic or medical museums in Europe that were archived before the Industrial Revolution. The process of roller-milling wheat flour was introduced in Europe approximately a quarter of a century earlier than the appearance of diverticulosis, which was initially observed in the first decade of the 20th century. It has been postulated that the decreased consumption of unprocessed cereals and increased consumption of sugar and meat by the general population are factors largely responsible for the appearance of diverticulosis. During the past 80 years or so, the amount of fiber consumed by individuals in North America and Western Europe has decreased, whereas the prevalence of diverticulosis has increased significantly. The formation of diverticula is also related to aging. Diverticula are rare in individuals younger than 30 years, but at least two thirds of Americans will have developed colonic diverticula by the age of 80 years.

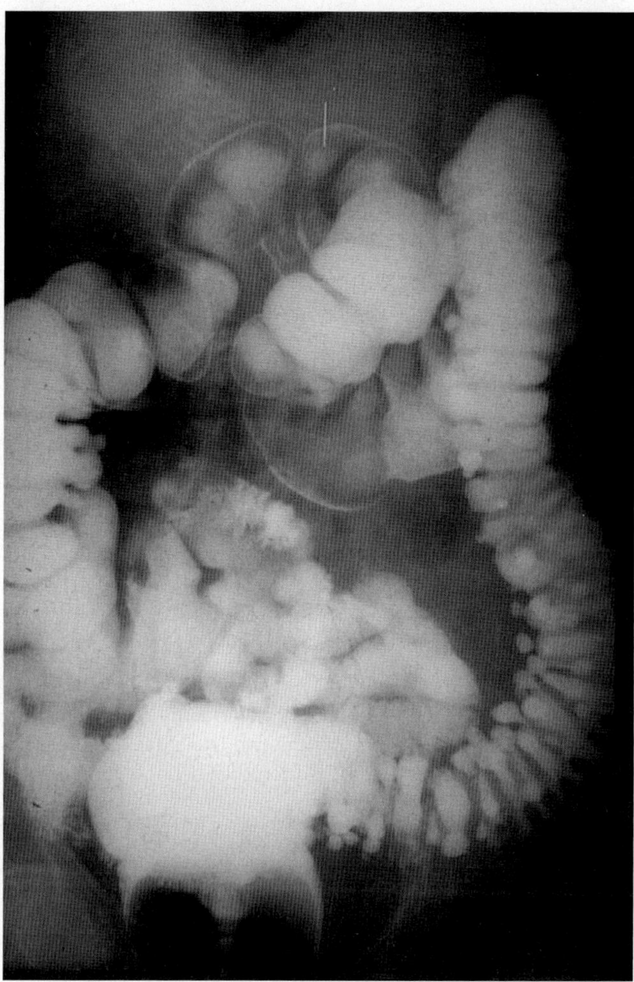

**FIGURE 52-14** X-ray of barium enema with extensive sigmoid diverticulosis.

Further evidence that a diet low in fiber and high in carbohydrates and meat contributes to the incidence of diverticulosis is the observation that diverticulosis is rare in sub-Saharan African blacks who consume a high-fiber diet; however, blacks in Johannesburg who consume a low-fiber diet have the same incidence of diverticulosis as South African whites.

### Pathogenesis

Diverticula are actually herniations of mucosa through the colon at sites of penetration of the muscular wall by arterioles. These sites are on the mesenteric side of the antimesenteric taeniae. In some cases, the arteriole penetrating the wall can be displaced over the dome of the diverticulum. This close relationship between the artery and diverticulum is responsible for the massive hemorrhage that can occasionally complicate diverticulosis (Fig. 52-15).

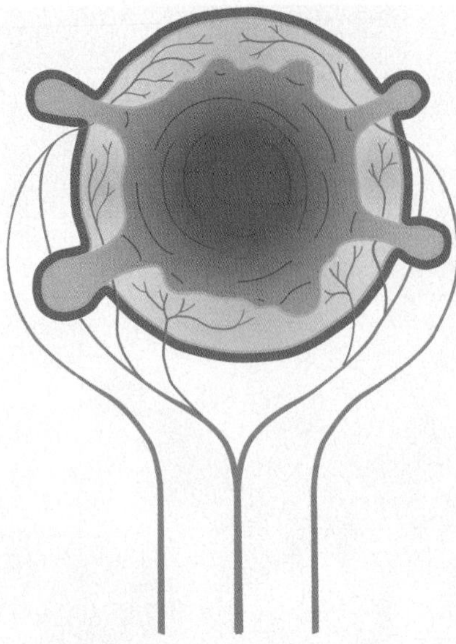

**FIGURE 52-15** Pathogenesis of diverticular disease. Diverticula are herniations of the mucosa through the points of entry of blood vessels across the muscular wall. Because the diverticula are formed only by the mucosa rather than by the entire wall of the intestine, they are called *false diverticula*. Note that the diverticula form only between the mesenteric taenia and each of the two lateral taeniae. Because there are no perforating vessels, diverticula do not form on the antimesenteric side of the colon.

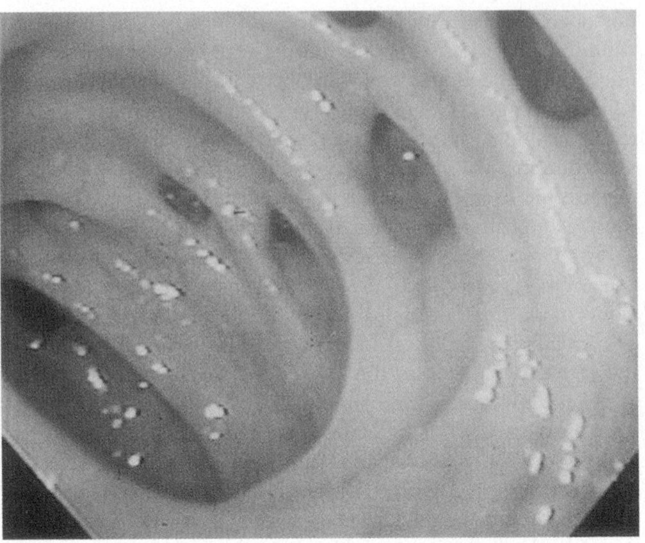

**FIGURE 52-16** Colonoscopic view of diverticula.

There is often a striking hypertrophy of the muscular layers of the colonic wall associated with diverticulosis. This thickening of the colonic wall, usually affecting the sigmoid colon, may precede the appearance of diverticula. Diverticula most commonly affect the sigmoid colon and are confined to the sigmoid in approximately 50% of patients with diverticulosis. The next most common area involved is the descending colon (≈40% of affected individuals), and the entire colon has diverticula in 5% to 10% of patients with diverticulosis. Even in patients with diverticula involving the entire colon, the muscular thickening characteristic of the disease is usually confined to the sigmoid (Fig. 52-16).

The sigmoid colon, the most common site of diverticula formation, is also the segment of colon with the smallest luminal diameter. If the colonic lumen contains a large volume of fiber, the contractile pressure required to propel the feces forward is low. In such circumstances, the colonic pressure in the sigmoid is only slightly higher than atmospheric pressure. However, with the decreased amount of fiber provided by today's typical dietary regimens, there is decreased colonic luminal content, requiring the generation of increased colonic pressures to propel the feces forward. Colonic pressures as high as 90 mm Hg can be generated by contraction of the narrow sigmoid colon. These high intraluminal pressures are thought to be responsible for the herniations of mucosa through the anatomically weak points in the colonic wall.

It has long been conjectured that factors contributing to diverticular disease, or at least diverticulitis, is the consumption of nuts, popcorn, and small seeds, such as are found in tomatoes, and patients with diverticular disease are often counseled to avoid these foods. However, a large prospective study of men without known diverticular disease has failed to detect an increase in the risk of diverticulosis or diverticular complications.[11]

## Diverticulitis

Diverticulitis is the result of a perforation of a colonic diverticulum. The term is somewhat of a misnomer because the disease is actually an extraluminal pericolic infection caused by the extravasation of feces through the perforated diverticulum. Peridiverticulitis would actually be the term that more appropriately describes the infectious process. Recognition that the infection is actually caused by a perforation of the colon, an event often controlled by the body's natural defenses, provides a basis for understanding the signs and symptoms of the disease and the rationale for determining appropriate diagnostic tests and treatment.[6,7] The sigmoid colon is the segment of large bowel with the highest incidence of diverticula and it is the most frequent site for involvement with diverticulitis. Patients with diverticulitis usually complain of left lower quadrant abdominal, pain that my radiate to the suprapubic area, left groin, or back. Alterations in bowel habits is a common complaint and fever, chills, and urinary urgency are common. This is an infectious inflammatory process and rectal bleeding is not usually associated with an attack of diverticulitis.

The physical findings are dependent on the site of perforation, amount of contamination, and presence or absence of secondary infection of adjacent organs. The most common physical finding is tenderness of the left lower abdomen. There may be voluntary guarding of the left abdominal musculature and a tender mass in the left lower abdomen is suggestive of a phlegmon or abscess. Abdominal wall distention may be detected if there is associated ileus or small bowel obstruction secondary to the inflammatory process. A rectal or vaginal examination may reveal a tender fluctuant mass typical of a pelvic abscess.

Sigmoid diverticulitis should be distinguished from cancer of the rectosigmoid, although it is seldom necessary to establish the distinction on an emergency basis. However, the surgical approach to diverticulitis is significantly different than that required for a perforated sigmoid cancer and, if urgent operation is indicated, an effort should be made to exclude the diagnosis of cancer. A limited sigmoidoscopic examination may at times be helpful in such circumstances. However, air should not be insufflated through the endoscope because of distention of the colon and the possibility that increased colonic pressure could force more bacteria through the perforation into the peritoneal cavity. The sigmoidoscope can seldom be advanced beyond 12 cm in a patient with diverticulitis, and the examination is usually only useful to exclude a cancer of the rectum as a cause of the symptoms.

The diagnosis of diverticulitis can often be presumed with a fair degree of reliability by a careful history and physical examination and it is reasonable to begin treatment with antibiotics on this evidence alone. However, if the diagnosis is in doubt, four diagnostic tests can be considered—computed tomography (CT) of the abdomen, magnetic resonance imaging (MRI), abdominal ultrasound, and water-soluble contrast enema. CT and MRI provide essentially the same information and advantages. There has been more experience with CT, which is considered by most surgeons to be the preferred test to confirm the suspected diagnosis of diverticulitis. It reliably reveals the location of the infection, extent of the inflammatory process, presence and location of an abscess, and sympathetic involvement of other organs, with secondary complications such as ureteral obstruction or a fistula to the bladder. In addition, an abscess detected by CT may often be drained by a percutaneous approach with the aid of CT guidance.

Ultrasound of the abdomen offers many of the advantages of CT, including the possibility of percutaneous drainage of an abscess with ultrasound guidance. The selection among CT, MRI, and ultrasound examinations varies considerably among institutions, but all three techniques have been shown to be useful in establishing the diagnosis of diverticulitis, especially when an abscess has complicated the disease.

The use of a contrast enema for the evaluation of a patient suspected of having diverticulitis has diminished considerably because of the advantages offered by the noninvasive tests described. An enema carries the risk of increasing the colonic pressure and causing further extravasation of feces through the perforated diverticulum. Some studies have shown an advantage of the contrast enema in distinguishing acute diverticulitis from perforated cancer, but many surgeons believe that the risk associated with a contrast enema outweighs the potential gain. If a contrast enema is used, the contrast should be water-soluble. Water-soluble contrast enemas do not carry the risk for barium fecal peritonitis, but there is still a considerable risk for extravasation of contrast material from the colon that could aggravate the infection and spread the extent of the peritonitis.

Diverticulitis obviously presents in a variety of ways with a broad spectrum of severity, from a single episode of mild self-limited disease, to repeated episodes that respond to antibiotics, to fulminant complicated disease characterized by life-threatening sepsis. Hinchey and associates have described a practical classification system that provides some organization of the broad clinical spectrum of the disease:

- Stage I: Pericolic or mesenteric abscess
- Stage II: Walled-off pelvic abscess
- Stage III: Generalized purulent peritonitis
- Stage IV: Generalized fecal peritonitis

Appropriate treatment obviously must be individualized based on the severity of the disease. The American Society of Colon and Rectal Surgeons has published practice guidelines for the treatment of diverticulitis.[8]

### Uncomplicated Diverticulitis

Uncomplicated diverticulitis, disease not associated with free intraperitoneal perforation, fistula formation, or obstruction, can often be treated with antibiotics on an outpatient basis. If the patient has significant pain characteristic of localized peritonitis, hospitalization and IV antibiotics are indicated.[9] The use of morphine should be avoided because of the increased intracolonic pressure associated with its use; meperidine has been reported to decrease intraluminal pressure and is a more appropriate analgesic.

Patients with uncomplicated diverticulitis usually respond promptly to antibiotic treatment, with marked improvement in symptoms within 48 hours. After the symptoms have subsided for at least 3 weeks, investigative studies should be conducted to establish the presence of diverticula and to exclude cancer, which can mimic diverticulitis. The preferred test is a colonoscopic examination, which can visualize the colonic lumen directly, even in the presence of numerous diverticula. A barium enema can demonstrate the extent of the diverticular disease, but a sigmoid cancer may be hidden by the numerous contrast-filled diverticula of the sigmoid colon, a fact that considerably diminishes the value of the contrast enema in the evaluation of the patient with diverticulosis (Fig. 52-17).

A first attack of uncomplicated diverticulitis that responds to antibiotic therapy is generally treated nonoperatively by the introduction of a high-fiber diet. A population-based study has demonstrated that only a small percentage (5.5%) of patients

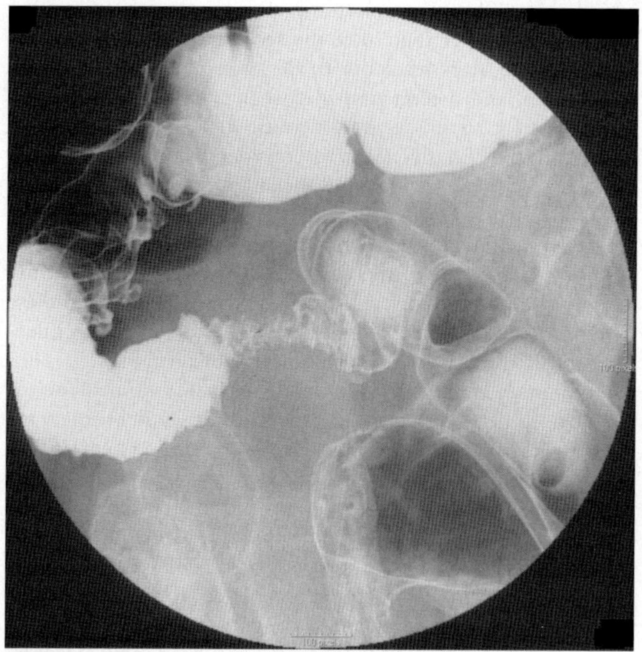

**FIGURE 52-17** X-ray of barium enema in a patient with a previous attack of diverticulitis. Note stricture in sigmoid colon. Colonoscopy was necessary to exclude cancer.

who recover from an initial episode of uncomplicated diverticulitis required subsequent emergency colectomy or colostomy.[10] The chances of a second attack of diverticulitis are relatively low, less than 25%. The management of patients younger than 45 years affected by an attack of uncomplicated diverticulitis is somewhat controversial. Many surgeons recommend an elective sigmoidectomy following recovery in younger patients because the natural history of diverticulitis in these individuals is not well understood, and there may be a high risk for recurrence of the disease over their expected longer life span. However, Vignati and coworkers studied 40 patients younger than 50 years who were hospitalized with diverticulitis and followed for up to 9 years. Two thirds of these patients did not require surgery during the follow-up period. These results are similar to the expectations for patients older than 50 years, and it was concluded that younger patients should be treated in the same manner as patients whose first attack of diverticulitis occurs after the age of 50 years.

If a patient suffers recurrent attacks of diverticulitis, surgical treatment should be considered. It has generally been recommended that sigmoidectomy be offered after two uncomplicated attacks of diverticulitis to prevent a future complicated episode that would require emergency operation or a colostomy. However, studies have thrown some doubt on this concept. It appears that the need for a colostomy to be fashioned is highest with the first attack of diverticulitis; the recommendation that sigmoidectomy be offered after two attacks on the basis of avoiding a colostomy in the future has to be reconsidered in light of newer evidence. Chapman and colleagues[12] have found that patients with more than two episodes of diverticulitis are not at increased risk for poor outcomes if they should subsequently develop complicated diverticulitis, and that morbidity and mortality are not significantly different between patients with multiple episodes of diverticulitis compared with those suffering only one or two prior attacks. Salem and associates[13] have determined that performing colectomy after the fourth episode of diverticulitis, rather than after the second episode, in patients older than 50 years results in 0.5% fewer deaths, 0.7% fewer colostomies, and a reduction in cost per patient. The recommendation for sigmoidectomy because of recurrent attacks of diverticulitis obviously needs to consider the patient's overall health and lifestyle, frequency of the attacks, and debility associated with each attack.

Diverticulitis in the immunocompromised host represents a special challenge for the surgeon. Selective sigmoidectomy after a single attack of diverticulitis should be considered in these patients because of their diminished ability to combat an infectious insult. There is some suggestion that medical therapy is less effective in these patients, resulting in an increased incidence of emergent surgery. Unfortunately, mortality rates after surgery are higher than those in patients whose immune system is not compromised.

A growing trend in elective surgery for diverticular disease has been the use of a laparoscopic approach. Most studies reveal a hospital length of stay 2 to 3 days shorter for patients undergoing sigmoidectomy by a laparoscopic approach when compared with patients receiving a standard midline incision. A hand-assisted laparoscopic approach has been advocated by some surgeons, who believe that this technique facilitates the division of fused tissue planes and the blunt disruption of fistula tracts.

### Complicated Diverticulitis

**Abscess** As noted, an abscess complicating diverticulitis is usually confined to the pelvis. Typically, patients with pelvic abscesses caused by diverticulitis have significant pain, fever, and leukocytosis. The abdominal, pelvic, or rectal examination may detect a tender, fluctuant mass and a CT scan, MRI, or ultrasound will confirm the diagnosis and location of the abscess. Unless the abscess is small (<2 cm in diameter), it should be drained, and the preferred method of drainage is a percutaneous route guided by CT or ultrasound. Occasionally, a pelvic abscess can be drained into the rectum through a transanal approach. These methods of drainage are highly preferable to a transabdominal approach by laparotomy, which risks spreading the contents of the abscess throughout the peritoneal cavity (Fig. 52-18).

Adequate drainage of the abscess, accompanied by the administration of IV antibiotics, usually results in a rapid clinical improvement. Although a fistula may result from the sigmoid colon at the insertion site of the percutaneous catheter that provided drainage, this can be easily handled at the time of elective surgery when the intense intra-abdominal infection has subsided.

Elective surgery should be offered after the patient has completely recovered from the infection, usually approximately 6 weeks after drainage of the abscess. At that time, it is generally feasible to excise the diseased sigmoid colon and fashion an anastomosis between the descending colon and rectum, thus avoiding a colostomy. It is essential to remove all the colon that is abnormally thickened and to incorporate rectum that is not inflamed or thickened into the distal component of the anastomosis. A major cause of recurrent diverticulitis after sigmoidectomy is failure to remove the entire abnormally thickened bowel that is associated with this disease completely. If the distal sigmoid colon is not resected, the rate of recurrent diverticulitis is unnecessarily elevated. Benn and coworkers have found the rate of recurrent diverticulitis to be 12% if the distal sigmoid is not resected compared with 6% if the anastomosis is to the top of the rectum. It is seldom necessary to mobilize the rectum further than 2 cm below the sacral promontory to

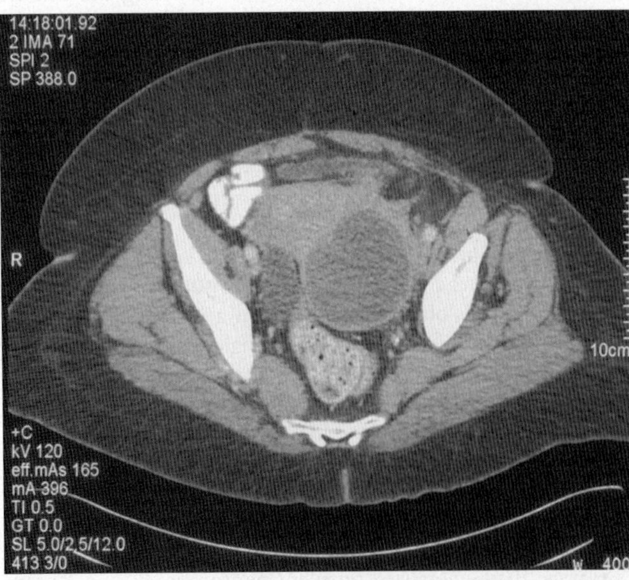


**FIGURE 52-18** CT scan of pelvis showing diverticulitis with abscess.

obtain normal bowel for a satisfactory anastomosis. Although diverticula may be present throughout the colon, it is not necessary to excise the entire colon in such circumstances; only the colon that is thickened and brittle (usually the entire sigmoid) needs to be resected.

**Fistula** A fistula between the sigmoid colon and skin, which may result from percutaneous drainage of an abscess, bladder, vagina, or small bowel is a relatively frequent complication of diverticulitis. Such a fistula commonly forms when an abscess is drained or necrotizes into an adjacent organ or onto the skin. The source of the infection—the perforated diverticulum—continues to supply the fistula, and cure will not be achieved until the source is eradicated by excising the diseased sigmoid colon. Diverticulitis is a more common cause of a fistula between the colon and bladder than Crohn's disease or cancer. Sigmoid-vesicular fistulas are more common in men than in women because the uterus prevents the sigmoid from adhering to the bladder. Women with sigmoid fistulas have usually had a prior hysterectomy.

Symptoms of a sigmoid-vesicular fistula include pneumaturia (passage of air from the urethra typically noted at the end of micturition), fecaluria, and recurring urinary tract infections. The fistula may cause significant urosepsis in men, with prostatic hypertrophy causing a relative obstruction of the distal urinary tract. The most reliable test to confirm the suspicion of a fistula between the intestine and bladder is CT, which may demonstrate air in the bladder (Fig. 52-19). A barium enema will fail to reveal a fistula 50% of the time, and an IV pyelogram is even less accurate. Cystoscopy usually reveals cystitis and bullous edema at the site of the fistula, but the test is helpful to exclude cancer (colon or bladder) as the cause of the fistula.

Initial treatment of any fistula caused by diverticulitis is to control the infection and reduce the associated inflammation. A fistula arising from the colon is rarely a cause for emergency surgery; in fact, the patient's condition is often improved when the abscess fistulizes and drains. Antibiotics should be administered to reduce the adjacent cellulitis and diagnostic steps should be taken to confirm the cause of the fistula before a definitive operation is undertaken. A colonoscopy should be done to examine the sigmoid mucosa and exclude colon cancer or Crohn's disease as the cause of the fistula. Every effort should be made to rule out cancer because the operation for a sigmoid-vesicular fistula secondary to sigmoid cancer requires en bloc excision of the involved organs, a more extensive operation than that required to interrupt the nonmalignant fistula and excise the diseased (but benign) sigmoid colon.

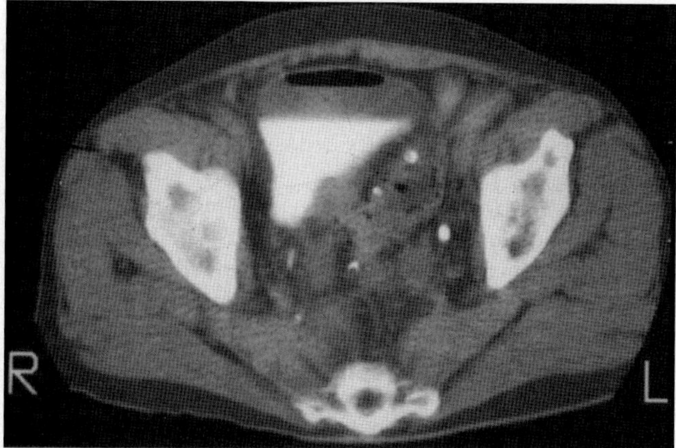


**FIGURE 52-19** CT scan of pelvis. The patient has diverticulitis, and air in the bladder indicates a fistula between the sigmoid and the bladder.

Fistulas caused by diverticulitis can usually be treated by a one-stage operation, taking down the fistula and excising the sigmoid colon, and then fashioning an anastomosis between the descending colon and rectum. The secondary organs involved, usually the bladder, will heal once the source of the infection, the sigmoid colon, is removed. The bladder defect is usually so small that no closure is necessary, and healing will occur if the bladder is drained with a Foley catheter or suprapubic cystostomy for 7 days after the operation. Larger bladder openings may require suture closure with absorbable (chromic) sutures combined with drainage. If there is significant inflammation in the abdomen and pelvis, despite a so-called *cooling-off period*, the use of ureteral stents placed preoperatively can facilitate identification of the ureters and minimize inadvertent ureteral injury. A technique of early identification of the ureter and proximal to distal dissection of the sigmoid colon facilitates the resection when a phlegmon caused by diverticulitis obliterates the normal anatomy.

**Generalized Peritonitis** Generalized peritonitis resulting from diverticulitis can have two causes: (1) a diverticulum perforates into the peritoneal cavity and the perforation is not sealed by the body's normal defenses; or (2) an abscess that is initially localized expands and suddenly bursts into the unprotected peritoneal cavity. In the former case, the peritoneal cavity is contaminated with feces; in the latter, contamination is from pus containing enteric bacteria. In either situation, the result is an overwhelming infection that requires immediate operative intervention. Fortunately, both these circumstances are relatively rare.

Patients with generalized peritonitis caused by a perforated diverticulum exhibit diffuse abdominal tenderness, with voluntary and involuntary guarding over the entire abdomen. Abdominal radiographs or CT scans may reveal intraperitoneal free air, but the absence of extraintestinal air does not exclude the diagnosis. Signs of generalized sepsis include an elevated white blood count, fever, tachycardia, and hypotension. Immediate celiotomy is mandatory to identify and excise the segment of colon containing the perforation. Under such circumstances, it is not safe to restore intestinal continuity because of the high likelihood that an intestinal anastomosis will not heal when fashioned in such a hostile and infectious environment. The proper surgical procedure in this situation is to resect the diseased sigmoid colon, construct a colostomy using noninflamed descending colon, and suture the divided end of the rectum closed. This procedure is called *Hartmann's operation*, after Henri Hartmann, the French surgeon who described this technique in 1921. Hartmann's operation, although initially described for the treatment of cancer, is the most common technique for emergency operations required for control of infection secondary to diverticulitis.

Eliminating the source of infection by excising the perforated sigmoid colon, establishing diversion of the feces with a colostomy, and controlling the peritoneal infection by irrigating the peritoneal cavity and administering IV antibiotics, along with appropriate generalized and nutritional support, should result in resolution of the infection. When the patient has recovered completely from the illness, usually after a period of at least 10 weeks, taking down the colostomy and fashioning an anastomosis between the descending colon and rectum will restore intestinal continuity.

There have been recent reports of successful treatment of acute complicated diverticulitis by laparoscopic lavage and IV antibiotics, without resecting the diseased segment.[15] Although these reports are intriguing, resection of the perforated segment seems the safest approach at this time.

**Obstruction** Intestinal obstruction associated with diverticular disease occurs in two circumstances. The first is relatively unusual and is caused by narrowing of the sigmoid because of the muscular hypertrophy of the bowel wall. This type of stricture rarely causes antegrade mechanical obstruction, but occasionally presents a diagnostic problem if a contrast study reveals a sigmoid stricture in an area containing numerous diverticula. It may be impossible for the radiologist to exclude a cancer as a cause of the stricture. In such cases, the stenosis may prevent the passage of a colonoscope for adequate evaluation, and sigmoidectomy may be the only remedy if cancer cannot be ruled out.

The more common type of intestinal obstruction is small bowel obstruction associated with the infectious and inflammatory aspect of diverticulitis. The small bowel may become adherent to the phlegmon or abscess, with obstruction caused by the infectious process. In such circumstances, the appropriate treatment is to pass a nasogastric tube to relieve the upper intestinal secretions while addressing the obstruction by treating the infection with antibiotics and percutaneous drainage of the abscess.

**Diverticular-Associated Colitis** Recently, attention has been drawn to a relatively unusual entity associated with diverticular disease that may mimic IBD. The entity is characterized by prolapse of the mucosa associated with diverticula, hyperplasia of the glands, and muscularization of the lamina propria. Erosions and hemosiderin deposition in the submucosa may suggest pathologic and endoscopic similarities to ulcerative colitis or Crohn's colitis. In severe cases, mucin depletion, chronic architectural distortion, cryptitis, and crypt abscesses may be detected.[16] This entity has been designated diverticular-associated colitis (DAC). Rectal sparing is a key finding to exclude ulcerative colitis, but the segmental nature of Crohn's colitis may at times confound the diagnosis.

In an attempt to classify and define DAC, Mulhall and colleagues[17] performed a systematic review of the literature and a review of patients from their own institution to define the clinical and pathologic features of DAC. Clinical features were characterized by tenesmus, hematochezia, diarrhea, and diarrhea. Endoscopic diagnosis included focal erythema submucosal ecchymosis, erosions, and ulcers. Pathologic findings were characterized by inflammation that could be consistent with ulcerative colitis or Crohn's disease in areas of diverticular disease. Once straightforward diverticulitis and IBD had been ruled out, 163 of 227 patients in the systematic review were thought to have DAC. Most of these patients were able to be treated medically; 25% of patients with DAC had recurrence, but more than 50% of these responded to subsequent medical therapy. Few patients ultimately required surgery. It was concluded that DAC is a distinct clinical entity that presents with segmental colitis and has a variety of clinical and pathologic features.

## COLONIC VOLVULUS

Volvulus describes the condition in which the bowel becomes twisted on its mesenteric axis, a situation that results in partial or complete obstruction of the bowel lumen and a variable degree of impairment of its blood supply. The condition usually affects the colon. Although colonic volvulus is relatively rare in the United States, ranking behind cancer and diverticulitis, it is responsible for approximately 4% of cases of large bowel obstruction. However, in the region known as the *volvulus belt*, an area extending along South America, Africa, the Middle East, India, and Russia, colonic volvulus is more common, and accounts for approximately 50% of all cases of colonic obstruction.

Any portion of the large bowel can torse if that segment is attached to a long and floppy mesentery that is fixed to the retroperitoneum by a narrow base of origin. However, the mesenteric anatomy is such that volvulus is most common in the sigmoid colon, with less frequent occurrences involving the right colon and terminal ileum (usually referred to as *cecal volvulus*), the cecum alone (the condition permitted by a highly mobile cecum, called a *cecal bascule*, that is mobile in a caudad to cephalad direction) and, most rarely, the transverse colon.

Sigmoid volvulus accounts for two thirds of all cases of colonic volvulus. The condition is permitted by an elongated segment of bowel accompanied by a lengthy mesentery with a narrow parietal attachment, a situation that allows the two ends of the mobile segment to come close together and twist around the narrow mesenteric base. Associated factors include chronic constipation and aging, with the average age of presentation being in the seventh to eighth decade of life. There is an increased incidence of the condition in institutionalized patients afflicted with neuropsychiatric conditions and treated with psychotropic drugs. These medications may predispose to volvulus by affecting intestinal motility. The increased incidence of volvulus in the so-called *volvulus belt countries* has been attributed to a diet high in fiber and vegetables.

Patients with sigmoid volvulus may present as acute or subacute intestinal obstruction, with signs and symptoms indistinguishable from those caused by cancer of the distal colon. There is usually a sudden onset of severe abdominal pain, vomiting, and obstipation. The abdomen is generally markedly distended and tympanitic, with the distention often more dramatic than would be associated with other causes of obstruction. There is always the possibility that the condition is associated with ischemia caused by mural ischemia resulting from the increased tension of the distended bowel wall, or by arterial occlusion caused by torsion of the mesenteric arterial supply. Therefore, severe abdominal pain, rebound tenderness, and tachycardia are ominous signs.

There may be a history of previous episodes of acute volvulus that spontaneously resolved. In this case, marked abdominal distention may occur with minimal tenderness.

Radiographic findings are often dramatic and enable prompt diagnosis and treatment (Fig. 52-20). Abdominal x-rays reveal a markedly dilated sigmoid colon that resembles a bent inner tube, with its apex in the right upper quadrant. An air-fluid level may be seen in the dilated loop of colon and gas is usually absent from the rectum. CT, although not necessary to establish the diagnosis, will typically reveal a characteristic mesenteric whorl (Fig. 52-21). A contrast enema typically demonstrates the point of obstruction with the pathognomonic

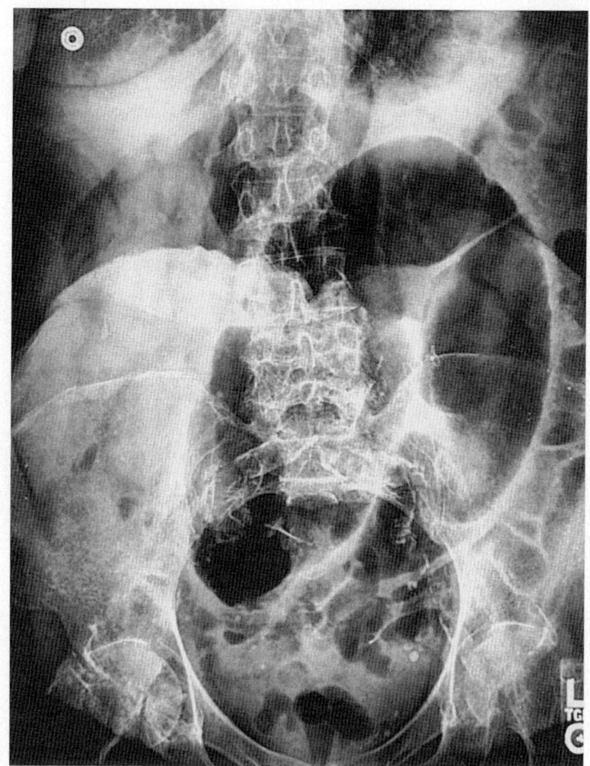

**FIGURE 52-20** Plain film of sigmoid volvulus. Note bent inner tube appearance.

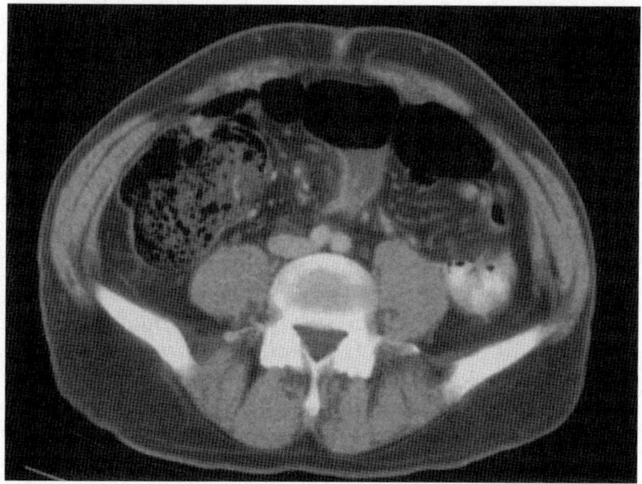

**FIGURE 52-21** Computed tomography scan of abdomen in patient with sigmoid volvulus. Note characteristic whorl in mesentery.

bird's beak deformity revealing the twist that obstructs the sigmoid lumen (Fig. 52-22).

Treatment of the sigmoid volvulus begins with appropriate resuscitation and, in most cases, involves nonoperative decompression. Decompression relieves the acute problem and allows resection as an elective procedure, which can be accomplished with reduced morbidity and mortality. Patients with signs of colonic necrosis are not eligible for nonoperative decompression.

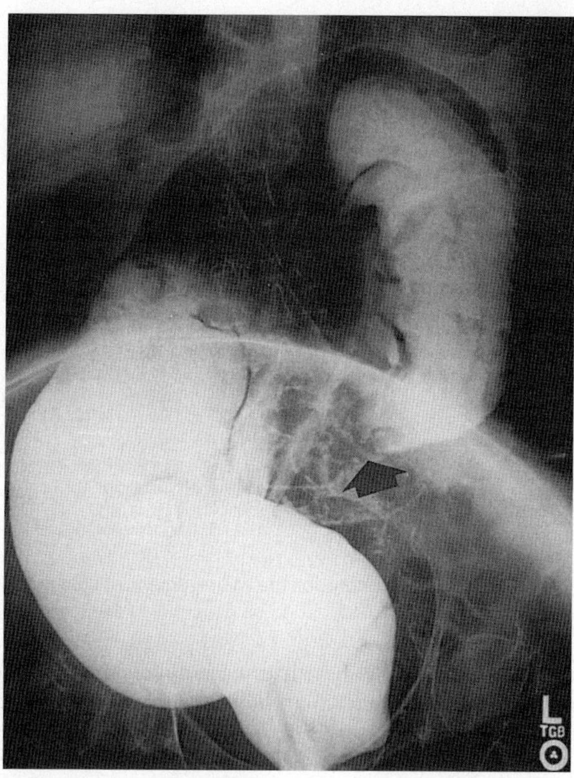

**FIGURE 52-22** X-ray of barium enema iof sigmoid volvulus. Contrast and air fill the rectum and distal sigmoid colon. The contrast stops abruptly at the point of torsion.

Decompression can be achieved by placement of a rectal tube through a rigid proctoscope, but more often a flexible sigmoidoscope is used. Decompression results in a sudden gush of gas and fluid, with a decrease in the abdominal distention. The reduction should be confirmed with an abdominal radiograph. The rectal tube should be taped to the thigh and left in place for 1 or 2 days to allow continued decompression and prevent immediate recurrence of the volvulus. The bowel can then be cleansed with cathartics and a complete colonoscopic examination performed. If detorsion of the volvulus cannot be accomplished with a rectal tube or flexible sigmoidoscope, laparotomy with resection of the sigmoid colon (Hartmann's operation) is required (Fig. 52-23).

Even if detorsion of the sigmoid is successful, elective sigmoid resection is indicated in most cases because of the extremely high recurrence rate, which approaches 70%. Colonoscopy should be performed before elective resection to exclude an associated neoplasm. The operation can be conducted through a small left lower quadrant incision or by a laparoscopic approach. Because the elongated colon and mesentery require almost no mobilization, resection with primary anastomosis is easily accomplished.

For patients with signs of colonic necrosis or in whom endoscopic detorsion has failed, the traditional treatment has been a sigmoid colectomy with closure of the rectum and end colostomy (Hartmann's procedure). Some surgeons have recently demonstrated, however, that resection with primary anastomosis, with or without protection from a proximal ostomy (transverse colostomy or ileostomy), may be accomplished in the acute

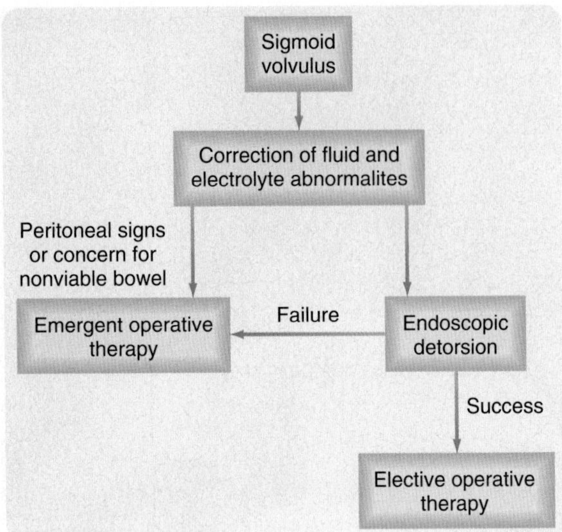


**FIGURE 52-23** Algorithm for the management of volvulus.

setting. For patients who have had successful endoscopic detorsion but have significant comorbidities, endoscopic colopexy may also be an option.

Although the term *cecal volvulus* is ingrained in the literature, true volvulus of the cecum probably never occurs. There is a well-recognized condition, a cecal bascule, in which the cecum folds in a cephalad direction anteriorly over a fixed ascending colon. Although gangrene may develop, this is exceedingly rare because there is no major vessel obstruction. The cecal bascule commonly causes intermittent bouts of abdominal pain because the mobile cecum permits intermittent episodes of isolated cecal obstruction that are spontaneously relieved as the cecum falls back into its normal position.

The condition commonly referred to as *cecal volvulus* is actually a cecocolic volvulus. It consists of an axial rotation of the terminal ileum, cecum, and ascending colon, with concomitant twisting of the associated mesentery. This is a relatively rare condition, accounting for less than 2% of all cases of adult intestinal obstruction and approximately 25% of all cases of colonic volvulus in the United States. Cecocolic volvulus is possible because of a lack of fixation of the cecum to the retroperitoneum. Studies on cadavers have shown that between 11% and 22% of people have a right colon that is sufficiently mobile to allow a volvulus to occur. Factors that have been implicated in causing a cecal volvulus include previous surgery, pregnancy, malrotation, and obstructing lesions of the left colon. Cecocolic volvulus is somewhat more common in women, whereas sigmoid volvulus occurs with equal frequency in men and women. Cecocolic volvulus affects a younger age group (most common in the late 50s) than sigmoid volvulus.

The typical presentation of patients with cecocolic volvulus is the sudden onset of abdominal pain and distention. In the early phases of a cecocolic volvulus, the pain is mild or moderate in intensity. If the condition is not relieved and ischemia occurs, the pain increases significantly. Physical examination may reveal asymmetrical distention of the abdomen, with a tympanitic mass palpable in the left upper quadrant or midabdomen. Plain radiographs of the abdomen reveal a dilated cecum that is usually displaced to the left side of the abdomen. The distended cecum

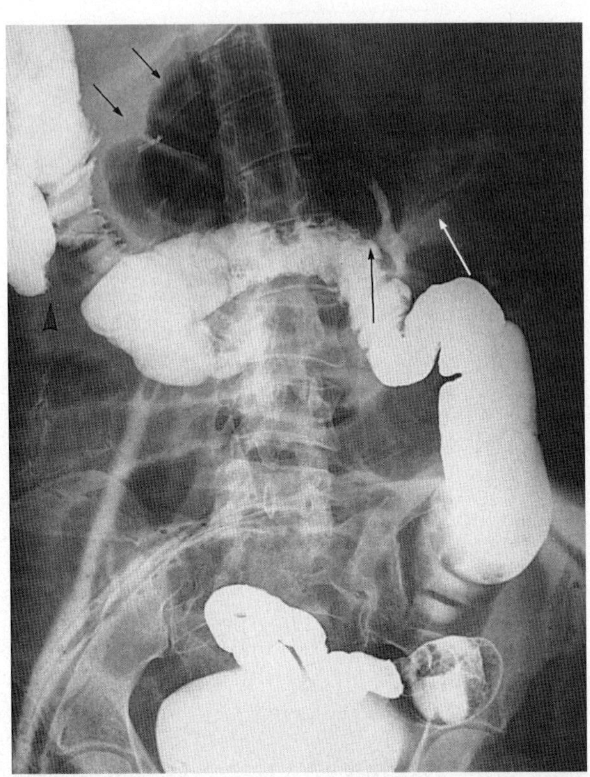

**FIGURE 52-24** X-ray of barium enema in a patient with cecal volvulus. The contrast stops abruptly at the proximal end of the hepatic flexure *(arrowhead)*. The dilated air-filled cecum crosses the midline of the abdomen toward the left upper quadrant *(arrows)*. (Courtesy Dr. Dina F. Caroline, Temple University Hospital, Philadelphia.)

generally assumes a gas-filled comma shape, the concavity of which faces inferiorly and to the right. Occasionally, the distended cecum appears as a circular shape with a narrow, triangular density pointing superiorly and to the right. Haustral markings in the distended loop indicate that the dilated bowel is colon. The torsion results in obstruction of the small bowel, and the radiographic pattern of dilated small intestine can cause diagnostic difficulty.

Although there have been reports of detorsion of cecocolic volvulus with a colonoscope, most cases require surgery to correct the volvulus and prevent ischemia. If ischemia has already occurred, an immediate operation is obviously required. Contrast enema can sometimes be helpful to confirm the diagnosis and exclude a carcinoma of the distal bowel as a precipitating cause of the volvulus (Fig. 52-24). Although there have been reports of endoscopic detorsion of cecal volvulus, the success rate is significantly lower than in sigmoid volvulus, and the procedure is associated with the risks of increasing distension because of insufflation of air during the procedure. Surgical intervention is therefore warranted in almost all cases of cecocolic volvulus.

Right colectomy is the procedure of choice. Primary anastomosis is usually preferred unless the volvulus has resulted in frankly gangrenous bowel, in which case resection of the gangrenous bowel with ileostomy is a safer approach. There have been many reports of correcting cecocolic volvulus with cecopexy, which should avoid the complication associated with an anastomosis. However, the procedure to provide fixation of the cecum is extensive and entails elevating and attaching a flap of peritoneum over the surface of the cecum and ascending colon. The recurrence rates are high with cecopexy, and right colectomy remains the procedure of choice for most surgeons.

Volvulus of the transverse colon is extremely rare and tends to be associated with other abnormalities, such as congenital bands, distal obstructing lesions, and pregnancy. Clinical features are indistinguishable from other causes of large bowel obstruction. Radiologic examination is not particularly useful because many cases are misdiagnosed as sigmoid volvulus. A contrast study may show a bird's beak deformity, indicating a volvulus. In such cases, colonoscopic reduction may result in detorsion and relief of obstruction. Elective resection should follow to prevent recurrence.

## LARGE BOWEL OBSTRUCTION AND PSEUDO-OBSTRUCTION

Large bowel obstruction can be classified as dynamic (mechanical) or adynamic (pseudo-obstruction). Mechanical obstruction is characterized by blockage of the large bowel (luminal, mural, or extramural), resulting in increased intestinal contractility as a physiologic response to relieve the obstruction. Pseudo-obstruction is characterized by the absence of intestinal contractility, often associated with decreased or absent motility of the small bowel and stomach.

Colorectal cancer is the single most common cause of large intestinal obstruction in the United States, whereas colonic volvulus is the more common cause in Russia, Eastern Europe, and Africa. Approximately 2% to 5% of patients with colorectal cancer in the United States present with complete obstruction. Intraluminal causes of colorectal obstruction include fecal impaction, inspissated barium, and foreign bodies. Intramural causes, in addition to carcinoma, include inflammation (e.g., diverticulitis, Crohn's disease, lymphogranuloma venereum, tuberculosis, schistosomiasis), Hirschsprung's disease (aganglionosis), ischemia, radiation, intussusception, and anastomotic stricture. Extraluminal causes include adhesions, the most common cause of small bowel obstruction, but rarely a cause of colonic obstruction, hernias, tumors in adjacent organs, abscesses, and volvulus.

The signs and symptoms of large bowel obstruction depend on the cause and location of the obstruction. Cancers arising in the rectum or left colon are more likely to obstruct than those arising in the more capacious proximal colon. Regardless of the cause of the blockage, the clinical manifestations of large bowel obstruction include the failure to pass stool and flatus associated with increasing abdominal distention and cramping abdominal pain.

The colon becomes distended as gas (approximately two thirds is swallowed air, and the remainder includes the products of bacterial fermentation), stool, and liquid accumulate proximal to the site of blockage. If the obstruction is the result of a segment of colon trapped by a hernia or by a volvulus, the blood supply can become compromised, or strangulated. The venous return is blocked initially, causing localized swelling that can, in turn, occlude the arterial supply with resultant ischemia that if uncorrected, can progress to necrosis or gangrene. The strangulation at first involves only the entrapped, or incarcerated, segment of bowel, but the colon proximal to that segment becomes progressively dilated because of the obstruction.

Another route to vascular compromise of the obstructed colon occurs if the bowel proximal to the point of obstruction distends to the extent that the intramural pressure within the intestinal wall exceeds the capillary pressure, depriving the bowel of adequate oxygenation. This route to ischemic necrosis can occur with mechanical obstruction and pseudo-obstruction.

A closed loop obstruction occurs when the proximal and distal parts of the bowel are occluded. A strangulated hernia or volvulus almost always leads to this condition. The more common form of closed loop obstruction, however, is seen when a cancer occludes the lumen of the colon in the presence of a competent ileocecal valve. In this situation, increasing colonic distention causes the pressure in the cecum to become so high that the vessels in the bowel wall are occluded, and necrosis and perforation can occur.

The treatment of large bowel obstruction obviously depends on the cause of the obstruction, and specific treatments are covered in the discussion of those entities (see later). However, some principles of diagnosis and treatment can be generalized. The obstruction needs to be relieved with some expediency before compromise of the blood supply results in ischemia and gangrene. The diagnosis should be established to guide appropriate treatment. History and physical examination provide important clues. The abdomen should be palpated for masses, the groins inspected for hernias, and a digital rectal examination performed to exclude rectal cancer. Plain films of the abdomen provide considerable information concerning the location of the obstruction and, in some situations, may be diagnostic of a volvulus. A CT scan may be helpful in revealing an inflammatory process, such as an abscess associated with diverticulitis. If a volvulus or distal sigmoid cancer is suspected, a water-soluble contrast enema may establish the diagnosis. Treatment options vary considerably, depending on the diagnosis, and it is helpful to establish the diagnosis before an operation to guide therapy properly. If the cause of the obstruction is a cancer of the distal or mid rectum, the preferred treatment is to relieve the obstruction by a loop colostomy and then treat the cancer with neoadjuvant chemoradiation, with the plan to resect the primary lesion at a later time. On the other hand, if the obstructing cancer is in the sigmoid colon, the surgical options include Hartmann's operation (sigmoidectomy with descending colostomy and closure of the rectal stump), sigmoidectomy with primary colorectal anastomosis (with or without intraoperative colonic lavage), and abdominal colectomy with ileorectal anastomosis.

Right-sided colonic obstruction, whether caused by cancer or the result of volvulus, is generally treated by resection and primary anastomosis of the ileum and transverse colon.

Pseudo-obstruction of the colon, also called *Ogilvie's syndrome*, after its description by Sir William Heneage Ogilvie in 1948, describes the condition of distention of the colon, with signs and symptoms of colonic obstruction, in the absence of an actual physical cause of the obstruction. Ogilvie described two patients with clinical features of colonic obstruction, despite a normal barium enema. Both patients underwent laparotomy for the condition; neither had mechanical obstruction, but both had unsuspected malignant disease involving the area of the celiac axis and semilunar ganglion. The cause of the dilation was attributed to the malignant infiltration of the sympathetic ganglia. Subsequently, there have been numerous descriptions of cases of colonic distention in the absence of mechanical obstruction and without malignant involvement of the visceral autonomic nerves. Very few cases of pseudo-obstruction have malignant infiltration of the autonomic nerves as the cause; in fact, the exact pathogenesis of the syndrome remains unknown, and it has been associated with a heterogeneous group of conditions.

Primary pseudo-obstruction is a motility disorder that is a familial visceral myopathy (hollow visceral myopathy syndrome) or a diffuse motility disorder involving the autonomic innervation of the intestinal wall. The latter may be modified by a disturbance of intestinal hormones or may be principally caused by disordered autonomic innervation.

Secondary pseudo-obstruction is more common and has been associated with neuroleptic medications, opiates, severe metabolic illness, myxedema, diabetes mellitus, uremia, hyperparathyroidism, lupus, scleroderma, Parkinson's disease, and traumatic retroperitoneal hematomas. One mechanism thought to play a role in the pathogenesis is sympathetic overactivity overriding the parasympathetic system. Indirect support for this theory has been derived from the success in treating the syndrome with neostigmine, a parasympathomimetic agent. Further support comes from reports of immediate resolution of the syndrome after administration of an epidural anesthetic that provides sympathetic blockade.

Pseudo-obstruction may present in an acute or chronic form. The acute variety usually affects patients with chronic renal, respiratory, cerebral, or cardiovascular disease. It generally involves only the colon, whereas the chronic form affects other parts of the GI tract, usually presents as bouts of subacute and partial intestinal obstruction, and tends to recur periodically.

Acute colonic pseudo-obstruction should be suspected when a medically ill patient suddenly develops abdominal distention. The abdomen is tympanitic, usually nontender, and bowel sounds are generally present. Plain abdominal radiographs reveal a distended colon, with the right and transverse segments tending to be most dramatically affected. The radiologic appearance is one of large bowel obstruction.

The most useful investigation is a water-soluble contrast enema, which should be performed in all patients in whom the diagnosis is suspected, provided their condition is stable enough to warrant the procedure (Figure 52-25). The contrast enema

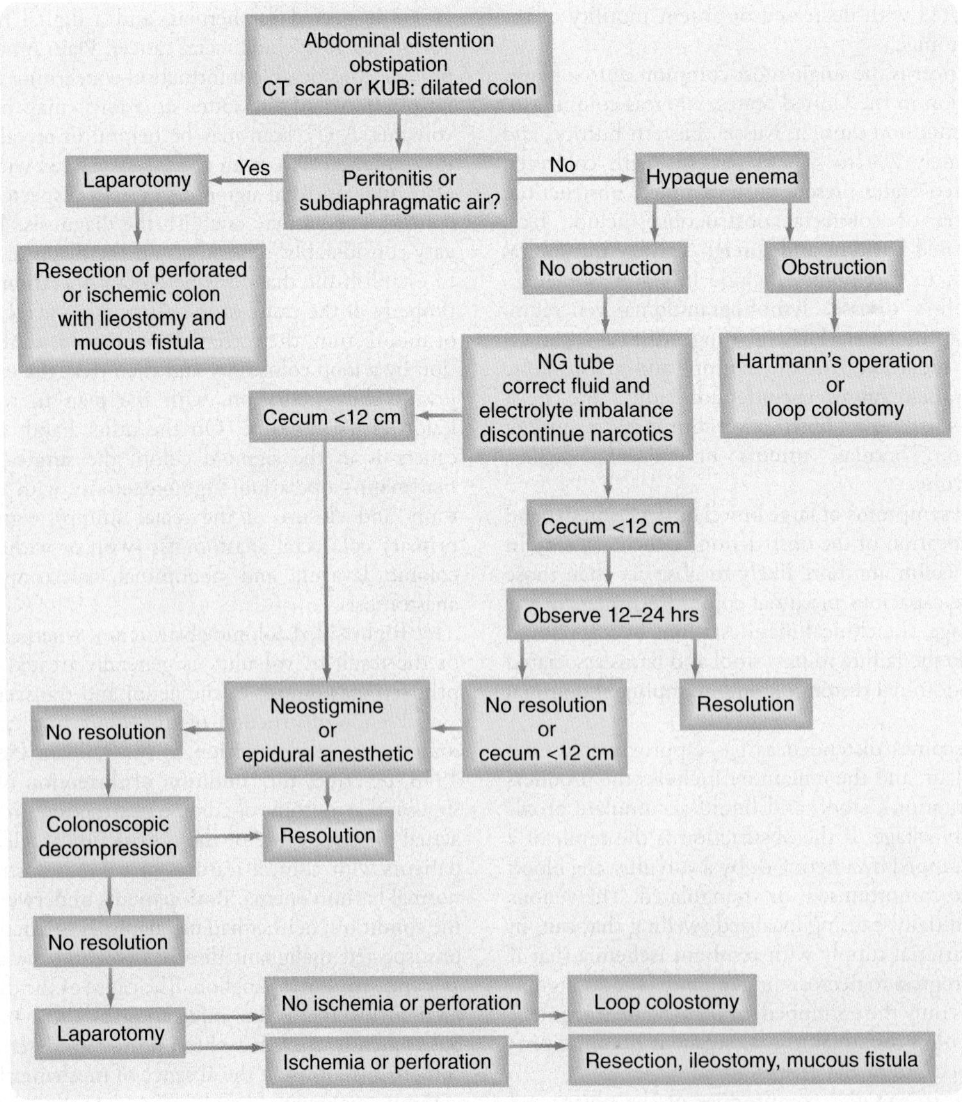


**FIGURE 52-25** Algorithm for Ogilvie's syndrome management.

can reliably differentiate between mechanical obstruction and pseudo-obstruction, a differentiation that is essential to guide appropriate therapy.

Colonoscopy is an alternative diagnostic investigation for pseudo-obstruction and has the attractive advantage that it can be used for treatment. However, colonoscopy runs the risk of distending the proximal colon even more, with insufflation of more air and, at present, the water-soluble contrast enema is generally the preferred initial test.

When the diagnosis of acute pseudo-obstruction is suspected, treatment should accompany the diagnostic evaluation. Initial treatment includes nasogastric decompression, replacement of extracellular fluid deficits, and correction of electrolyte abnormalities. All medications that inhibit bowel motility, such as opiates, should be discontinued. Patient response is monitored by serial abdominal examinations and radiography. Most patients improve with this regimen. Until the mid-1990s, the treatment generally used when the colonic distention failed to resolve with supportive measures was colonoscopic decompression. Although this approach was usually successful, it required skilled personnel and equipment and carried the risk for colonic perforation from instrument trauma and insufflation. In addition, the procedure often had to be repeated because of recurrence of the colonic distention.

Sympathetic blockade by epidural anesthesia has been shown to relieve colonic pseudo-obstruction successfully. However, at present, the trend has been to treat this condition with neostigmine, a parasympathomimetic agent. It is obviously imperative that mechanical obstruction be excluded by water-soluble contrast enema or colonoscopy before the administration of neostigmine because the subsequent high pressures generated in the colon against a distal obstruction could cause colonic perforation.

Neostigmine enhances parasympathetic activity by competing with acetylcholine for acetylcholinesterase binding sites. In the treatment of colonic pseudo-obstruction, 2.5 mg of neostigmine is given IV over 3 minutes. The resolution of the condition is indicated within less than 10 minutes of administration of the drug by the passage of stool and flatus by the patient. The recurrence rates following the administration of neostigmine appear to be far lower than those associated with colonoscopic decompression, with satisfactory decompression being achieved in approximately 90% of patients after a single administration of the medication.

A significant side effect of neostigmine is bradycardia, and all patients must be monitored by telemetry during administration of the drug. Atropine must be immediately available; patients with significant cardiac disease or asthma are not candidates for this treatment.

If treatment with neostigmine, an epidural anesthetic, or colonoscopic decompression is not successful, or if signs of peritonitis or intestinal perforation occur, laparotomy is required. In the absence of perforation or ischemia, a loop colostomy is indicated to vent the proximal and distal colon. Any areas of perforation or ischemia must be resected, which usually requires right colectomy, ileostomy and mucous fistula.

## INFLAMMATORY BOWEL DISEASE

The term *inflammatory bowel disease* is generally used to denote two diseases of unknown cause with similar general characteristics, ulcerative colitis and Crohn's disease. The distinction between the two entities can usually be established based on clinical and pathologic criteria, including history and physical examination, radiologic and endoscopic studies, gross appearance, and histology. However, in approximately 10% to 15% of patients with inflammatory disease confined to the colon, a clear distinction cannot be made, and the disease is labeled indeterminate colitis. The medical and surgical management of ulcerative colitis and Crohn's disease often differ significantly, so each entity is discussed separately here. A comparison of the characteristics of ulcerative colitis and Crohn's disease is presented in Table 52-1.

### Ulcerative Colitis

#### Epidemiology and Cause

Ulcerative colitis occurs more commonly in developed countries and is relatively unusual in Asia, Africa, and South America. There appears to be a seasonal variation in the activity of the disease, with onset and relapse occurring statistically more often between August and January. The incidence of the disease has remained relatively stable during the past 25 years, with new cases reported as 4 to 6 cases/100,000 white adults/year, with a prevalence from 40 to 100 cases/100,000. All ages are susceptible, but it more commonly affects patients younger than 30 years. A small secondary peak in the incidence occurs in the sixth decade. Both genders are equally affected, but the condition is more common in whites, Jews, and persons of northern European ancestry.

Although the cause of ulcerative colitis is unknown, its prevalence in industrialized countries and the increased incidence in individuals who migrate from low-risk to high-risk areas suggest an environmental influence. Speculation on the influence of dietary factors has included inadequate fiber intake, chemical food additives, refined sugars, and cow's milk. However, none of these have been demonstrated to play a definitive role. Infectious agents, including *C. difficile* and *Campylobacter jejuni,* have been implicated as playing a causative role in the pathogenesis, but such a role has not been confirmed.

Smoking appears to confer a protective effect against the development of ulcerative colitis, as well as providing a therapeutic influence; nicotine has been reported to induce remission in some cases. This is in contrast to Crohn's disease, which is more common in smokers and appears to be aggravated by the habit. Both ulcerative colitis and Crohn's disease are more common in women who use oral contraceptives compared with those who do not. Patients who have had an appendectomy appear to be at decreased risk for developing ulcerative colitis.

A family history of IBD is a significant risk factor. Several studies have demonstrated the existence of family aggregates with ulcerative colitis and a high degree of concordance in monozygotic twins. The genetic predisposition for ulcerative colitis is not inherited in a classic mendelian pattern, suggesting the influence of environmental factors on an individual's susceptibility. Two genetic abnormalities found to be associated with ulcerative colitis are variations in DNA repair genes and class II major histocompatibility complex genes. Patients with ulcerative colitis display specific alleles of group HLA and DR2 (HLA-DRB1), with an association between certain alleles and expression of the disease. The DR1501 allele is associated with a more benign course, whereas the DR1502 allele is associated with a more virulent form of the disease.

**Table 52-1 Comparisons of Ulcerative Colitis and Crohn's Colitis**

| | ULCERATIVE COLITIS | CROHN'S COLITIS |
|---|---|---|
| **Gross Appearance** | | |
| Thickened wall | 0 | 4+ |
| Thickened mesentery | 0 | 3+ |
| Serosal at fat wrapping | 0 | 4+ |
| Segmental disease | 0 | 4+ |
| **Microscopic Appearance** | | |
| Transmural | 0 | 4+ |
| Lymphoid aggregates | 0 | 4+ |
| Granulomas | 0 | 3+ |
| **Clinical Features** | | |
| Bleeding per rectum | 3+ | 1+ |
| Diarrhea | 3+ | 3+ |
| Obstructive symptoms | 1+ | 3+ |
| Anal or perianal disease | Rare | 4+ |
| Risk for cancer | 2+ | 3+ |
| Small bowel disease | 0 | 4+ |
| **Colonoscopic Features** | | |
| Distribution | Continuous | Discontinuous |
| Rectal disease | 4+ | 1+ |
| Friability | 4+ | 1+ |
| Aphthous ulcers | 0 | 4+ |
| Deep longitudinal ulcers | 0 | 4+ |
| Cobblestoning | 0 | 4+ |
| Pseudopolyps | 2+ | 2+ |
| **Operative Treatment** | | |
| Total proctocolectomy | Curative | Combined disease: colon + rectum |
| Segmental resection | Rare | Absence of anorectal disease |
| Ileal pouch | Preferred by most patients | Contraindicated |
| **Complications** | | |
| Postoperative recurrence | 0 | 4+ |
| Fistulas | Rare | 4+ |
| Sclerosing cholangitis | 1+ | Rare |
| Cholelithiasis | 0 | 2+ |
| Nephrolithiasis | 0 | 2+ |

Another theory of the cause of IBD concerns an altered immunologic response to external and host antigens. Although anticolon antibodies have been identified in blood and tissue of patients with IBD, there is little evidence that these play a pathogenic role. Other studies have shown that defective cell-mediated immunity, leukocyte chemotactic impairment, and abnormalities of antigen-specific helper and suppressor T cells may be involved in the pathogenesis.

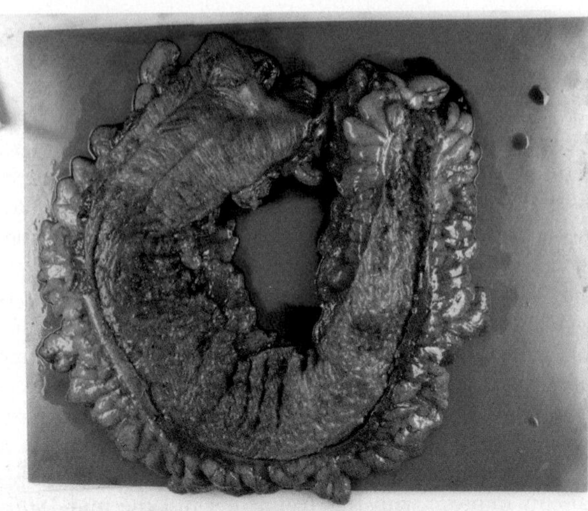

**FIGURE 52-26** Ulcerative colitis—macroscopic appearance of colitis extending continuously from the rectum *(upper right)* to the mid–ascending colon *(upper left)*. The proximal colon appears spared, with normal colonic folds. Most the colon exhibits erythema and granularity of the mucosal surface. (Courtesy Dr. Jeffrey P. Baliff, Thomas Jefferson University, Philadelphia.)

### Pathologic Features

**Gross Appearance** Ulcerative colitis is a disease in which the major pathologic process involves the mucosa and submucosa of the colon, with sparing of the muscularis. Despite the name, ulceration of the mucosa is not invariably present. In fact, the typical gross appearance of ulcerative colitis is hyperemic mucosa. Friable and granular mucosa is common in more severe cases, and ulceration may not be readily evident, especially early in the course of the disease. However, ulceration may appear and vary widely, from small superficial erosions to patchy ulceration of the full thickness of the mucosa (Fig. 52-26). The rectum is invariably involved with the inflammatory process. In fact, rectal involvement (proctitis) is the hallmark of the disease, and the diagnosis should be seriously questioned if the rectal mucosa is not affected. The mucosal inflammation extends in a continuous fashion for a variable distance into the more proximal colon. Pseudopolyps, or inflammatory polyps, represent regeneration of inflamed mucosa and are composed of a variable mixture of non-neoplastic colonic mucosa and inflamed lamina propria (Fig. 52-27).

As implied earlier, a diagnostic characteristic of ulcerative colitis is continuous uninterrupted inflammation of the colonic mucosa, beginning in the distal rectum and extending proximally to a variable distance. This is in contrast to Crohn's disease, in which normal segments of colon (skipped areas) may be interspersed between distinct segments of colonic inflammation. The entire colon, including the cecum and appendix, may be involved in ulcerative colitis. In contrast to Crohn's disease, ulcerative colitis does not involve the terminal ileum, except in cases of backwash ileitis, when the ileal mucosa may appear inflamed in the presence of extensive proximal colonic

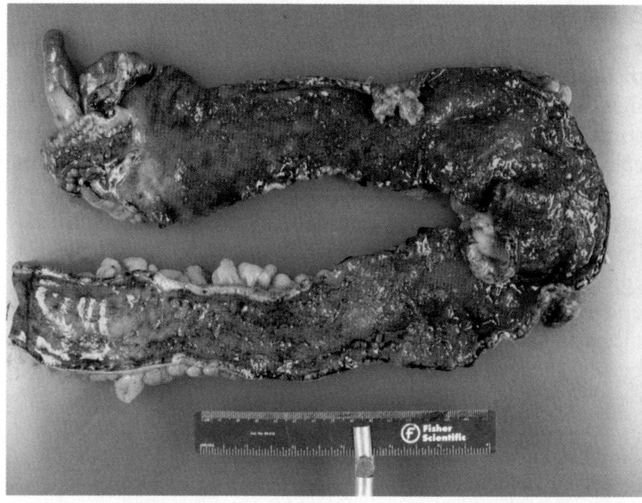

**FIGURE 52-27** Ulcerative colitis—macroscopic appearance of pancolitis. The entire length of the colonic mucosa exhibits prominent flattening, erythema, and friability, with focal areas of green-yellow exudate. There is a suggestion of linear ulcerations along the bowel axis. Overall, the colon is narrowed and shortened. The terminal ileum *(upper left)* is spared. (Courtesy Dr. Jeffrey P. Baliff, Thomas Jefferson University, Philadelphia.)

involvement. However, in such cases, contrast studies usually reveal the inflamed ileum to be dilated, in contrast to the frequently narrowed and contracted ileum characteristic of Crohn's disease.

Colonic strictures can occur in 5% to 12% of patients with chronic ulcerative colitis. Although these strictures are most often benign, caused by hypertrophy of the muscularis, cancer must be excluded as the cause of any colonic stricture occurring in the setting of ulcerative colitis. Three important features are suggestive of malignant strictures:

1. Appearance later in the course of ulcerative colitis (60% after 20 years versus 0% before 10 years)
2. Location proximal to the splenic flexure (86% malignant)
3. Large bowel obstruction caused by the stricture (Fig. 52-28)

**Histologic Appearance** The typical microscopic finding in ulcerative colitis is inflammation of the mucosa and submucosa. The most characteristic lesion is the crypt abscess, in which collections of neutrophils fill and expand the lumina of individual crypts of Lieberkühn (Fig. 52-29). Crypt abscesses, however, are not specific for ulcerative colitis and can be seen in Crohn's disease and infectious colitis. Hematochezia often results from the marked vascular congestion. Crypt branching may be seen in chronic ulcerative colitis and is an important characteristic. The number of goblet cells in the crypts is diminished, as is mucus production.

It has been stressed that the inflammatory process in ulcerative colitis spares the muscular coats of the colon, a characteristic that differentiates it from Crohn's disease—the latter is characterized by transmural inflammation, or involvement of all layers of the intestinal wall. However, in rare cases of severe inflammation characteristic of toxic megacolon in patients with ulcerative colitis, all layers of the colon may be involved, and

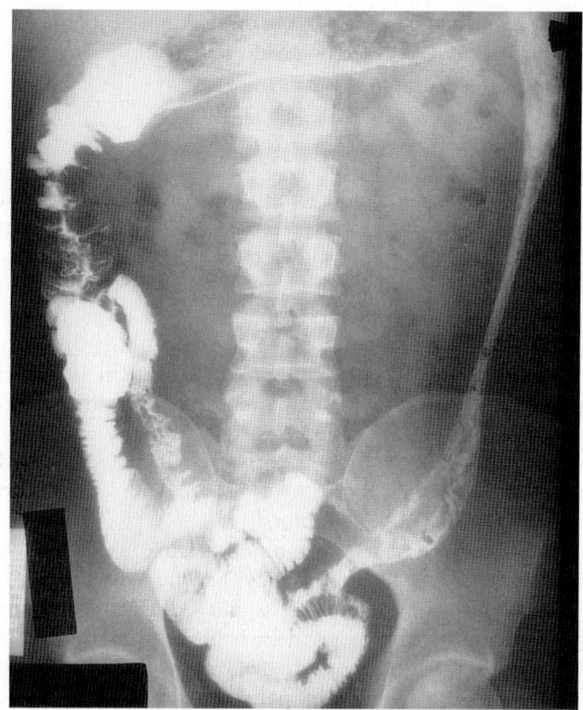

**FIGURE 52-28** X-ray of stricture in chronic ulcerative colitis. Colonoscopy revealed chronic inflammation, but no dysplasia or cancer.

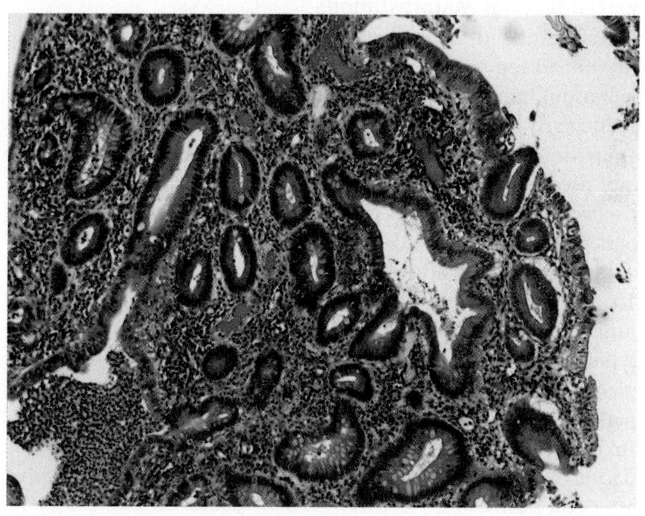

**FIGURE 52-29** Histologic section of active ulcerative colitis. There is glandular architectural distortion, manifested by irregular branching and orientation of glands relative to the surface. The lamina propria is expanded with inflammatory cells, and intraepithelial neutrophils are present. A crypt abscess is noted *(lower left)*. (Courtesy Dr. Jeffrey P. Baliff, Thomas Jefferson University, Philadelphia.)

perforation may occur if treatment is delayed. However, the inflammatory process in such cases is atypical and may be related to factors such as prolonged colonic distention with vascular compromise.

Numerous studies have demonstrated that antineutrophil cytoplasmic antibodies (ANCAs) with a perinuclear staining pattern (pANCA) are seen in up to 86% of patients with mucosal ulcerative colitis. The presence of pANCA has been used as a diagnostic test to help differentiate ulcerative colitis from Crohn's disease.

### Clinical Presentation

Ulcerative colitis and colonic Crohn's disease often have similar clinical presentations. Both may present with diarrhea and the passage of mucus. Patients with ulcerative colitis tend to have more urgency than those with Crohn's disease, likely because ulcerative colitis is invariable associated with distal proctitis. Rectal bleeding is also common in ulcerative colitis; although it may be present in patients with Crohn's disease, it is typically not as severe. Patients with acute-onset ulcerative colitis often complain of abdominal discomfort, but the pain is seldom as severe as that found in patients with Crohn's disease. A tender abdominal mass is suggestive of a phlegmon or abscess more commonly associated with Crohn's.

Perianal disease is an uncommon finding in patients with ulcerative disease, whereas it may be the only presenting symptom of Crohn's disease. It is interesting and seemingly paradoxical that rectal involvement is present in almost 100% of patients with ulcerative colitis, whereas anal involvement is rare. In contrast, patients with Crohn's disease may have normal rectal mucosa (so-called *rectal sparing*), although anal disease (e.g., fissures, fistulas, abscesses) is common.

### Extraintestinal Manifestations

Extraintestinal manifestations of ulcerative colitis include arthritis, ankylosing spondylitis, erythema nodosum, pyoderma gangrenosum, and primary sclerosing cholangitis (PSC). Arthritis, particularly of the knees, ankles, hips, and shoulders, occurs in approximately 20% of patients, typically in association with increased activity of the intestinal disease. Ankylosing spondylitis occurs in 3% to 5% of patients and is most prevalent in patients who are HLA-B27–positive or have a family history of ankylosing spondylitis. Erythema nodosum arises in 10% to 15% of patients with ulcerative colitis and often occurs in conjunction with peripheral arthropathy. Pyoderma gangrenosum typically presents on the pretibial region as an erythematous plaque that progresses into an ulcerated painful wound. Most patients who develop this condition have underlying active IBD. Arthritis, ankylosing spondylitis, erythema nodosum, and pyoderma gangrenosum typically improve or completely resolve after colectomy.

PSC occurs in 5% to 8% of patients with ulcerative colitis. Most patients with IBD who develop PSC are younger than 40 years and most are men. Genetics likely play a role because patients with ulcerative colitis who have the HLA-B8 or HLA-DR3 haplotype are 10 times more likely to develop PSC. Patients with PSC and ulcerative colitis typically have a more quiescent disease course; however, the risk for colon cancer in these patients is up to five times greater than in patients with ulcerative colitis alone. These tumors are more likely to arise proximal to the splenic flexure. PSC may be asymptomatic and diagnosed only by abnormal laboratory test results or it may present with symptoms of obstructive jaundice and abdominal pain. The disease is progressive and ultimately fatal unless liver transplantation is undertaken. Colectomy has no effect on the course of PSC.

### Diagnosis

Endoscopic examination of the colon and rectum is essential in the diagnosis of IBD. In the acute phase of the disease, proctosigmoidoscopy is often sufficient because the rectum is invariably inflamed in patients with ulcerative colitis. Complete colonoscopy offers little additional information in the acute setting and increases the risk for colonic perforation. The presence of diffuse, confluent, symmetrical disease from the dentate line proximally is consistent with ulcerative colitis; the mucosal appearance can vary from loss of the normal vessel pattern secondary to edema in the early stages of the disease to frank ulceration in more advanced disease. If the inflammation extends beyond the level of the sigmoidoscope, a full colonoscopy should be carried out after the disease is under control.

Conditions other than ulcerative colitis can present with similar symptoms of diarrhea and bleeding; it is important to identify these conditions because their treatment may be considerably different. Crohn's disease has features similar to those of ulcerative colitis; however, the rectum is spared in 40% of patients with Crohn's colitis, even in the presence of perianal disease. An upper GI radiograph with a small bowel follow-through should be obtained to rule out the possibility of small bowel involvement, a finding that would suggest Crohn's disease. Collagenous colitis is a condition that generally occurs in women older than 50 years. It typically presents with profuse watery diarrhea and is characterized histologically by marked thickening of the colonic subepithelial basement membrane. On endoscopic evaluation, the mucosa appears normal in most patients and the diagnosis is made by endoscopic biopsy. Treatment of collagenous colitis is typically medical.

In addition to multiple mucosal biopsy specimens from serial sites, stool samples should be sent to the laboratory to look for bacteria, ova, and parasites. Infectious conditions that mimic ulcerative colitis include colitis caused by *C. difficile, Entamoeba histolytica, C. jejuni,* and *Salmonella enteritidis.*

### Risk for Carcinoma

One of the most serious sequelae of mucosal ulcerative colitis is the development of colorectal carcinoma.[18] The most important risk factors include prolonged duration of the disease, pancolonic disease, continuously active disease, and severity of the inflammation. The cumulative risk for cancer increases with the duration of the disease, reaching 25% at 25 years, 35% at 30 years, 45% at 35 years, and 65% at 40 years. Patients with disease confined to the left side of the colon have a lower risk for developing carcinoma than patients with disease involving the entire colon. Carcinomas arising in ulcerative colitis tend to be poorly differentiated and highly aggressive tumors. As briefly noted, a colonic stricture in a patient with ulcerative colitis must be presumed carcinoma until proved otherwise. If malignancy cannot be ruled out by endoscopy, the presence of a stricture is an indication for operative intervention (Figs. 52-30 to 52-32).

There is considerable debate regarding the optimal method of surveillance colonoscopy in patients with ulcerative colitis. The American Cancer Society guidelines recommend surveillance colonoscopy every 1 to 2 years, beginning 8 years after the onset of pancolitis and 12 to 15 years after the onset of left-sided colitis. This strategy is based on the premise that a dysplastic lesion can be detected endoscopically before invasive carcinoma has developed (Fig. 52-33). Traditionally, 10 random biopsy

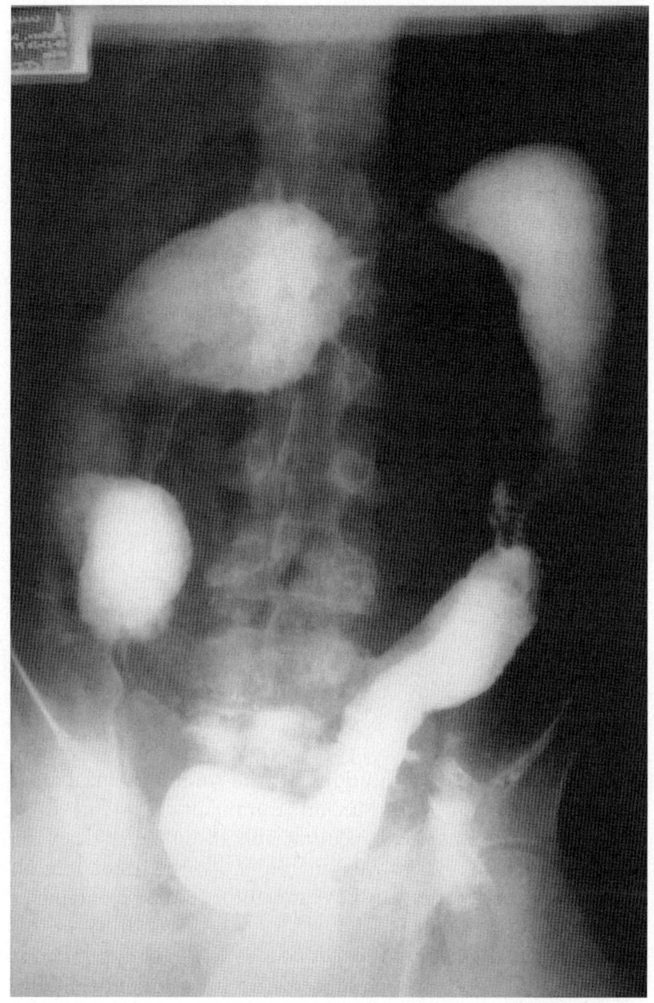

**FIGURE 52-30** X-ray of barium enema demonstrating stricture in transverse colon of patient with ulcerative colitis of 15 years' duration.

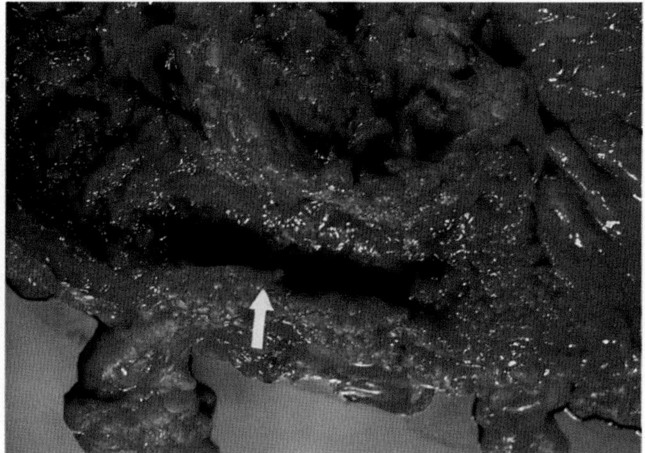

**FIGURE 52-31** Resected colon from patient in Figure 52-30, revealing the stricture *(arrow)* to be invasive cancer. The patient had liver metastases.

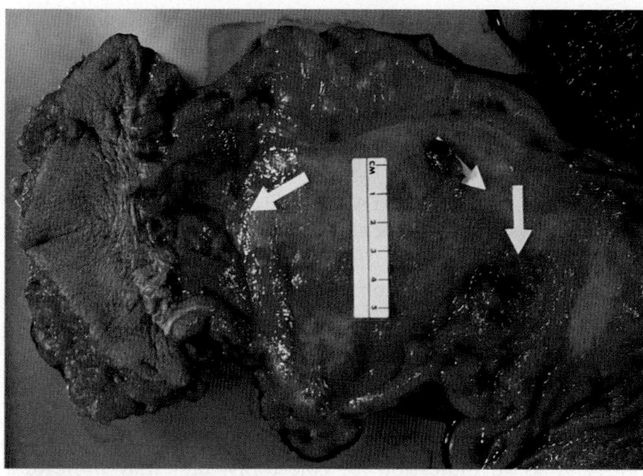

**FIGURE 52-32** Resected rectum from patient in Figure 52-30, showing invasive cancers in the rectum *(arrows).*

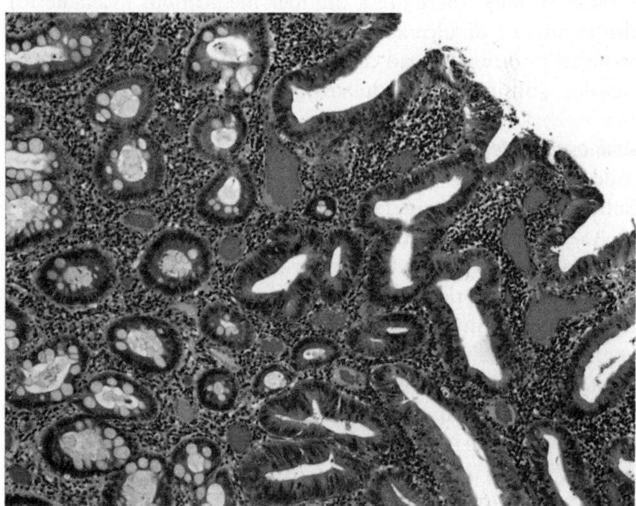

**FIGURE 52-33** Flat high-grade dysplasia arising in ulcerative colitis. Compared with the normal crypt epithelium *(left),* high-grade epithelial dysplasia exhibits an increased nuclear-to-cytoplasmic ratio, hyperchromaticity, and loss of polarity *(right).* (Courtesy Dr. Jeffrey P. Baliff, Thomas Jefferson University, Philadelphia.)

specimens were recommended; however, it has been suggested that at least 30 specimens be obtained.

The risk for cancer varies with the degree of dysplasia, with carcinoma found in 10% of colons displaying low-grade dysplasia, in 30% to 40% with high-grade dysplasia, and in more than 50% of colons with dysplasia associated with a lesion or mass (DALM). Neoplastic lesions of the colon of patients with ulcerative colitis can develop in DALM or in a coincidental adenoma, and approximately 25% of carcinomas in patients with ulcerative colitis are not associated with dysplasia elsewhere in the colon.

A meta-analysis of 10 prospective studies was performed to determine whether colonoscopic surveillance of dysplasia was a reasonable alternative to prophylactic colectomy.[19] Less than 3% of patients who had no dysplasia during the initial evaluation went on to develop evidence of dysplasia. In patients with high-grade dysplasia, however, 32% were found to have invasive carcinoma at the time of colectomy. These tumors tended to be of earlier stages when compared with tumors in patients in whom the diagnosis of cancer was made before colectomy. Other studies have shown no benefit to colonoscopic surveillance. Patients therefore need to be counseled about the potential for dysplasia so that they can take part in their management rationally. When high-grade dysplasia is found and has been confirmed by a second independent pathologist, proctocolectomy should be recommended. This is also true for patients who have DALM. If low-grade dysplasia is confirmed, strong consideration should also be given to proctocolectomy.

Flow cytometry of colonoscopic biopsies may also be useful for detecting dysplasia. A strong correlation between DNA aneuploidy and polyploidy and the presence of dysplasia has been found. Although the presence of these abnormalities should not serve as an indication for colectomy, they may indicate a need for more frequent colonoscopic surveillance.

### Treatment

**Medical Therapy** There are a number medications available for the treatment of ulcerative colitis. These medications can be grouped into three broad categories—aminosalicylates, corticosteroids, and immunomodulatory drugs.

***Aminosalicylates*** The most common therapy in the treatment of mild to moderate ulcerative colitis involves aminosalicylates. Sulfasalazine is composed of a molecule of 5-aminosalicylic acid (5-ASA) linked by a diazo bond to sulfapyridine. 5-ASA is released in the colon when bacterial azo reductases cleave the diazo bond; its actions involve blocking the cyclooxygenase and lipoxygenase pathways of arachidonic acid metabolism and scavenging free radicals in the colonic mucosa. Its usefulness is limited by toxicity, most of which is attributed to the sulfapyridine portion of the drug. Newer 5-ASA medications such as mesalamine (Asacol, Pentasa) have been developed that do not contain sulfapyridine, thereby minimizing side effects. Salicylates can be used in the treatment of active disease at higher doses and also play a role in maintaining remission at lower doses.

***Corticosteroids*** Corticosteroids are highly effective in the treatment of active ulcerative colitis and can be administered orally, IV, or topically through enemas. Steroids act to block phospholipase A2, thereby decreasing prostaglandins and leukotrienes. Side effects of steroid therapy, including hypertension, diabetes mellitus, osteoporosis, and increased susceptibility to infection, preclude long-term therapy with these medications. Hydrocortisone enemas delivered two or three times daily are often effective in the treatment of disease limited to the rectum and left side of the colon; these have the benefit of less absorption and therefore fewer systemic side effects. Newer steroid analogues have been developed that act locally in the colon and are then inactivated during first pass in the liver. Budesonide, a water-soluble analogue of hydrocortisone, has been shown to be as effective as prednisolone with far fewer side effects, including much less adrenal suppression.

***Immunomodulatory Medications*** Immunomodulatory medications are often used in the long-term management of patients with ulcerative colitis. 6-Mercaptopurine (6-MP), a purine analogue, and its precursor azathioprine act by causing chromosome breaks and inhibiting the proliferation of rapidly dividing cells such as lymphocytes (T cells more than B cells). Azathioprine and 6-MP are useful in inducing remission in patients who are refractory to 5-ASA, and their use allows steroids to be tapered or minimized in more than 50% of patients. Side effects of these medications include reversible bone marrow suppression and pancreatitis, and measurement of 6-MP metabolites has been proposed as a method to guide dosing to help avoid toxicity. Cyclosporine is an immunosuppressant used frequently in solid organ transplantation that inhibits interleukin-2 (IL-2) gene transcription, thereby reducing the activation of lymphocytes. Cyclosporine has serious potential side effects, including nephrotoxicity, hepatotoxicity, seizures, and lymphoproliferative disorders; it is typically reserved for use in acute severe ulcerative colitis and refractory Crohn's disease.

Infliximab is a monoclonal antibody directed against tumor necrosis factor-α (TNF-α) and its receptor, which neutralizes its biologic activity. It is given IV, typically at 6-week intervals following three loading doses. Infliximab has been shown to have a clinical response almost 70% of those treated and can induce remission of ulcerative colitis in a significant number of patients. Patients treated with infliximab also have a significantly lower risk of requiring surgical intervention. Potential side effects include an increased susceptibility to infection and the development of lymphoma.

**Indications for Surgery** Indications for the surgical management of mucosal ulcerative colitis include fulminant colitis with toxic megacolon, massive bleeding, intractable disease, and dysplasia or carcinoma (Box 52-1). Malnutrition and growth retardation may necessitate resection in pediatric and adolescent patients.

***Fulminant Colitis and Toxic Megacolon*** Patients with fulminant colitis typically present with high fever, severe abdominal pain, tenderness, tachycardia, and leukocytosis. These patients require hospitalization with IV hydration, nasogastric decompression, high-dose IV steroids if the patient is steroid-dependent, and broad-spectrum antibiotics. IV hyperalimentation may be useful, depending on the patient's nutritional status and length of illness before the fulminant episode. Patients should be closely monitored with serial abdominal examinations and leukocyte counts. Deterioration or lack of improvement within 48 to 72 hours of the initiation of medical treatment warrants an urgent procedure because the mortality rate is increased fourfold in patients with colonic perforation.

Toxic megacolon is a serious life-threatening condition that can occur in patients with ulcerative colitis, Crohn's colitis, and infectious colitides such as pseudomembranous colitis, in which the bacterial infiltration of the walls of the colon creates a dilation of the colon that progresses to the point of imminent perforation. This decompensation results in a necrotic thin-walled bowel in which pneumatosis can often be seen

**BOX 52-1 Ulcerative Colitis–Indications for Surgery**

Intractability
Dysplasia, carcinoma
Massive colonic bleeding
Toxic megacolon

radiographically. Although some patients with toxic megacolon have been successfully treated medically, a high rate of recurrence with subsequent urgent operation has been reported. Aggressive preoperative stabilization is required, using volume resuscitation with crystalloid solutions to prevent dehydration secondary to third-space fluid losses, stress-dose steroids for patients previously on steroid therapy, and broad-spectrum antibiotics.

Although a restorative proctocolectomy with ileal pouch–anal anastomosis (IPAA) as a single-stage procedure has been reported for toxic megacolon, proctectomy and anastomosis are generally ill advised in the acutely ill patient with an unprepared bowel. Total proctocolectomy in the urgent setting carries a prohibitively high mortality rate, and the leak rate from a primary anastomosis is unacceptably high. Whereas the goal in elective surgery is to remove all the colonic or dysplastic mucosa, the aim in emergent surgery is to rescue the patient from a life-threatening situation. A total abdominal colectomy with ileostomy and preservation of the rectum is therefore the preferred operation for this condition. This procedure can be expeditiously performed with relatively low morbidity and mortality, and it serves the main purpose of removing the diseased colon and avoiding a difficult and morbid pelvic dissection.

Preserving the rectum leaves the option of fashioning an ileorectal anastomosis in the future (Fig. 52-34). This is particularly important for patients in whom the diagnosis is unclear and a subsequent ileoanal pouch might be contraindicated (e.g., in Crohn's disease). Some controversy exists regarding management of the distal segment of bowel. The remaining rectum or rectosigmoid can be delivered as a mucous fistula placed subcutaneously, or closed as a Hartmann's pouch. Each management strategy has its proponents, but no randomized prospective trial

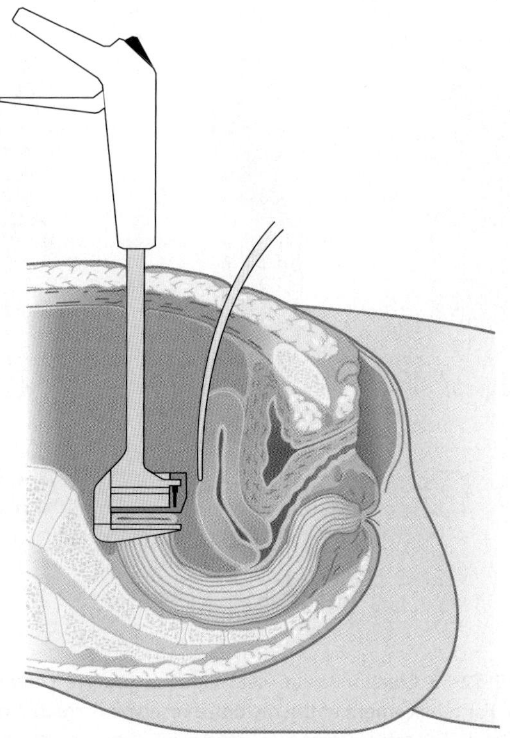

**FIGURE 52-34** Closure of rectal stump after resection of abdominal colon.

has been performed to date that has shown superiority of any of these options.

The blow-hole procedure was advocated in the past for treatment of patients with severe toxic megacolon in whom the distended colonic wall was so thin and fragile that any handling during the conduct of an operation would risk perforation of the colon, with massive peritoneal contamination. Currently, it is distinctly unusual that operative intervention is delayed to such a degree, but the operation may be advantageous in such dire circumstances. The technique consists of performing a skin level (blow-hole) transverse colostomy; sometimes the left colon is decompressed with a simultaneous, second, sigmoid skin level colostomy. Fashioning a loop ileostomy is an essential component of this operation. The operation was often rewarded with dramatic improvement in the patient's condition. After recovery from the acute illness, usually over a period of several months, the patient could then be treated with restorative proctocolectomy with IPAA or total proctocolectomy, depending on the circumstances.

***Massive Bleeding*** Massive hemorrhage from ulcerative colitis is an uncommon event, occurring in less than 5% of patients requiring operation. Patients obviously require resuscitation and stabilization before surgery, with replenishment of extracellular volume and transfusions, as needed. Subtotal colectomy is the procedure of choice and will usually suffice. However, if bleeding continues from the remaining rectal mucosa, emergency proctectomy may be required.

***Intractability*** Colitis with debilitating symptoms refractory to medical therapy is the most common indication for operative therapy. Patients with intractable disease have persistent symptoms such as crampy abdominal pain, frequent bowel movements, stool urgency, and anemia, which may result in deterioration of the patient's social and professional relationships. It has been demonstrated that patients' quality of life after surgery for ulcerative colitis is improved, regardless of the procedure performed. Complications of long-term steroid therapy, such as diabetes mellitus, avascular necrosis of the femoral head, cataracts, psychiatric problems, osteoporosis, and weight gain, are a frequent indication for surgical resection, even though the patient's symptoms may be controlled while on steroids. Elective surgery should also be considered for patients with significant extracolonic manifestations refractory to nonoperative measures.

***Dysplasia or Carcinoma*** The finding of dysplastic changes in the colon or carcinoma is an indication for surgical intervention (see earlier). The presence of cancer may influence the procedure selected or the sequence of staged procedures. It does not exclude the possibility of performing an ileoanal pouch, but the location and stage of the cancer must also be taken into consideration.

**Surgical Procedures** Elective surgical options for ulcerative colitis include total proctocolectomy with ileostomy, restorative proctocolectomy with IPAA, and total proctocolectomy with a continent ileal reservoir (Kock pouch). Segmental colectomy for ulcerative colitis, in contrast to Crohn's disease, has been shown to be an inadequate procedure for controlling disease. For example, in the case of colitis confined to the left side, a proctosigmoidectomy with an end-descending colostomy or coloanal anastomosis invariably results in the recurrence of disease in the remaining colon within a short time and is contraindicated.

In the past, abdominal colectomy with ileorectal anastomosis was advocated for patients with ulcerative colitis and rectal sparing. However, these patients are exceedingly rare. The inflammatory process typical of ulcerative colitis almost always involves the rectum, and an anastomosis of the ileum to the inflamed rectum invariably results in intractable diarrhea. Patients with true rectal sparing and left colitis most likely have Crohn's disease. In that situation, a segmental colectomy or subtotal colectomy with rectal anastomosis is an appropriate procedure.

***Total Proctocolectomy With End Ileostomy*** Total proctocolectomy has the advantage of removing all diseased mucosa, thereby preventing further inflammation and the potential for progression to dysplasia or carcinoma. The major disadvantage of this procedure is the need for a permanent ileostomy. In addition, despite improvements in bowel preparation, antibiotics, and surgical technique, a total proctocolectomy still has a fairly high morbidity rate. Most of the morbidity is related to perineal wound healing, adhesions, the ileostomy, and complications of pelvic dissection. Perineal wound problems may be reduced if an intersphincteric proctectomy is performed. This approach involves a dissection between the internal and external sphincters, preserving the external sphincter and levator ani for a more secure perineal wound closure.

Total proctocolectomy with end ileostomy was one of the earliest operations performed for ulcerative colitis and, despite advances in sphincter-saving procedures, continues to have a role. Older patients, those with poor sphincter function, and patients with carcinomas in the distal rectum may be candidates for this procedure. All patients should be marked for an ileostomy preoperatively in the sitting and standing positions. The preferred site of the stoma is within the body of the rectus abdominis muscle at the summit of the infraumbilical fat mound on the right side, away from bony prominences, the umbilicus, and the midline incision.

***Total Proctocolectomy With Continent Ileostomy*** The continent ileostomy was introduced by Kock in 1969 and became popular in the 1970s because it offered control of evacuations for patients with an ileostomy. A single-chambered reservoir is fashioned by suturing several limbs of ileum together after the antimesenteric border has been divided. The outflow tract is intussuscepted into the reservoir to create a valve that provides obstruction to the pouch contents (continence). As the pouch distends, pressure over the valve causes it close and retain stool, permitting patients to wear a simple bandage over a skin level stoma. Between two and four times daily, the patient introduces a tube through the valve to evacuate the pouch.

The major problem with the Kock pouch is the high complication rate necessitating reoperation in up to 50% of patients. The most common problem is a slipped valve, which occurs when the intussuscepted limb everts and the continent nipple is lost. This leads to the inability of the pouch to remain continent or the inability to intubate the pouch, leading to spontaneous emptying of the pouch as it overflows. Revision of the nipple valve corrects this problem. Other complications include inflammation of the ileal pouch mucosa (so-called *pouchitis*) in 15% to 30% of cases, fistula formation (10%), and stoma stricture (10%).

Since the introduction of restorative proctocolectomy and IPAA, the popularity of the continent ileostomy has declined, and it is now seldom used. High complication and reoperation rates have dampened enthusiasm among surgeons for the technique. Although ulcerative colitis patients in whom IPAA is contraindicated may be candidates, realistically, only a few centers presently offer the operation. The most common surgery related to continent ileostomies is revisional surgery. The Kock procedure should not be performed in obese patients, debilitated patients, or any patient with a physical or mental handicap that would prohibit safe catheterization of the reservoir. The procedure is contraindicated in patients with Crohn's disease because of the high incidence of its recurrence, causing failure of the pouch.

***Total Proctocolectomy With Ileal Pouch–Anal Anastomosis*** Restorative proctocolectomy with IPAA has become the most common definitive operation for the surgical treatment of ulcerative colitis. The procedure involves a near-total proctocolectomy, with preservation of the anal sphincter complex. A single-chambered pouch is fashioned from the distal 30 cm of the ileum (Fig. 52-35) and sutured to the anus using a double-stapled technique (Fig. 52-36). Alternatively, a hand-sewn anastomosis may be fashioned between the pouch and anus after stripping the distal rectal mucosa from the internal anal sphincter (mucosectomy; Fig. 52-37).

A critical consideration in restorative proctocolectomy is fashioning a tension-free anastomosis between the ileal reservoir and anal dentate line. Usually, there is sufficient mesenteric length for an ileal pouch, fashioned from the distal 30 cm of

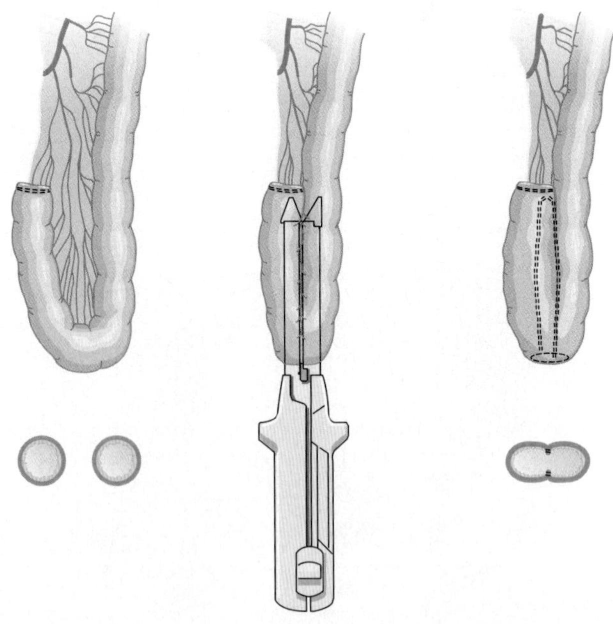

**FIGURE 52-35** Creation of an ileal J pouch using a cutting linear stapler. For replacement of the rectum, a reservoir is created from the distal ileum. The stapler joins two limbs of intestine with staples while dividing the intervening wall. The diameter of the pouch so created is twice as large as the original diameter of the ileum.

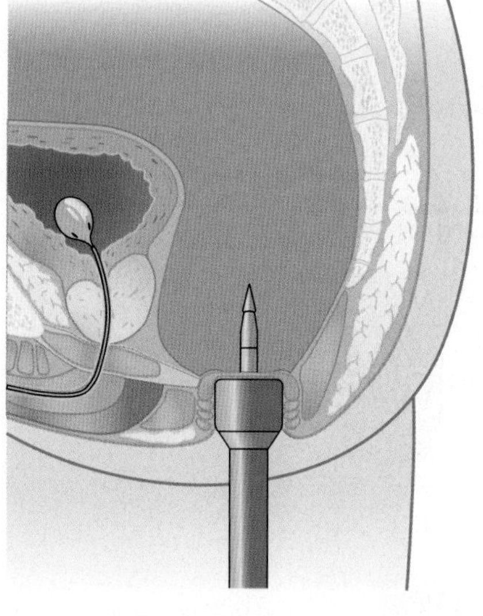

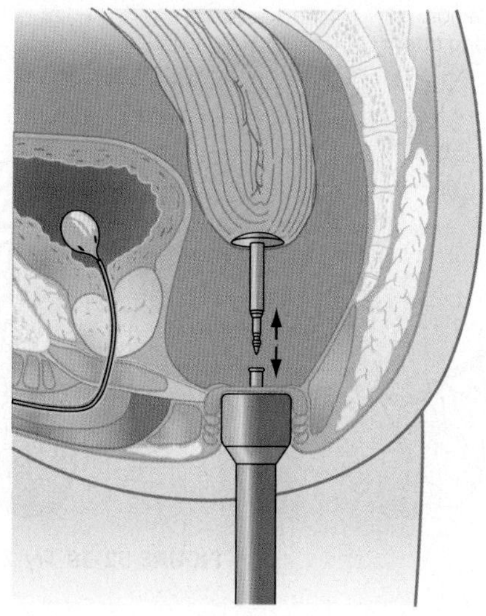

**FIGURE 52-36** Fashioning of stapled ileal pouch–anal anastomosis.

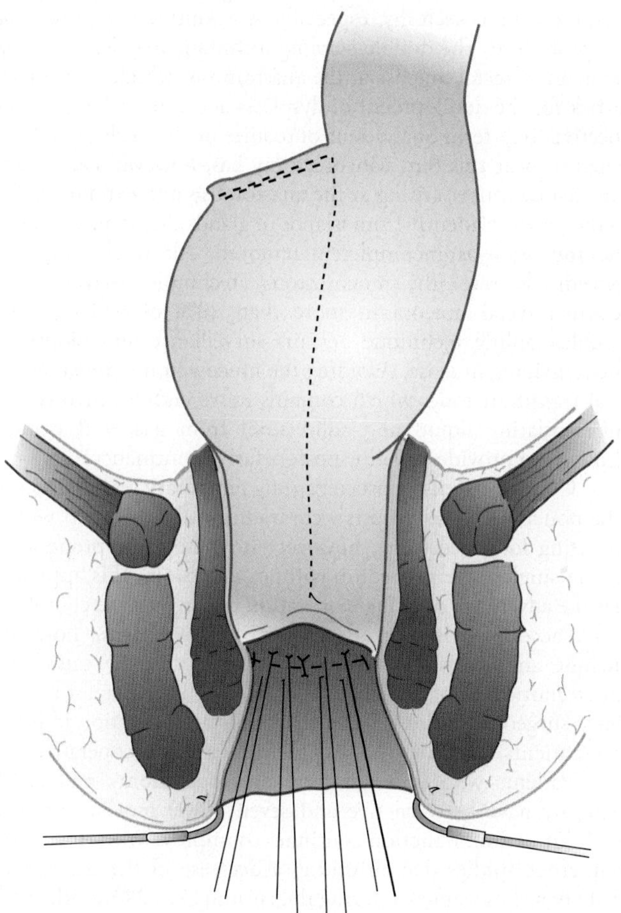

**FIGURE 52-37** Hand-sewn ileal pouch–anal anastomosis following anorectal mucosectomy.

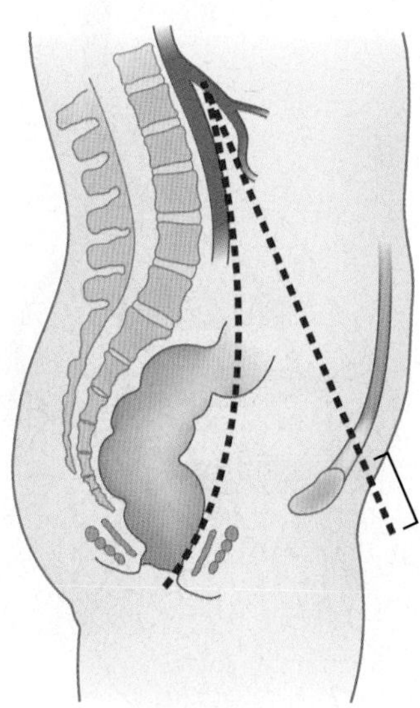

**FIGURE 52-38** Fry 1.

ileum, to reach the anus without unacceptable tension. However, occasionally, the anatomy will be such that specific maneuvers are required to allow the pouch to reach that level. It should be routine to mobilize the posterior attachment of the entire small bowel mesentery to the third portion of the duodenum, exposing the inferior portion of the head of the pancreas. An estimate of the ease of the pouch reaching the anus can be made by drawing the selected apex of the anticipated pouch over the symphysis pubis, with the expectation that it should extend 6 cm beyond the pubis to reach the anal canal easily (Fig. 52-38). This length may occasionally be obtained without further maneuvers, but generally an additional 2 to 5 cm of length will be necessary. To achieve this length, we usually divide the remnant of the ileocolic artery close to its origin from the SMA (Fig. 52-39). This is aided by transilluminating the mesentery to visualize the mesenteric arteries. The SMA will sustain the viability of the pouch after excision of the ileocolic artery. The apex of the pouch can be moved a few centimeters in either direction to determine the point that will reach the farthest. The peritoneum of the mesentery may be serially incised on its anterior and posterior surfaces; these relaxing incisions can confer an additional 1 or 2 cm of length and are especially beneficial if the mesentery has been thickened by adhesions from previous surgery (Fig. 52-40). These maneuvers will almost always suffice

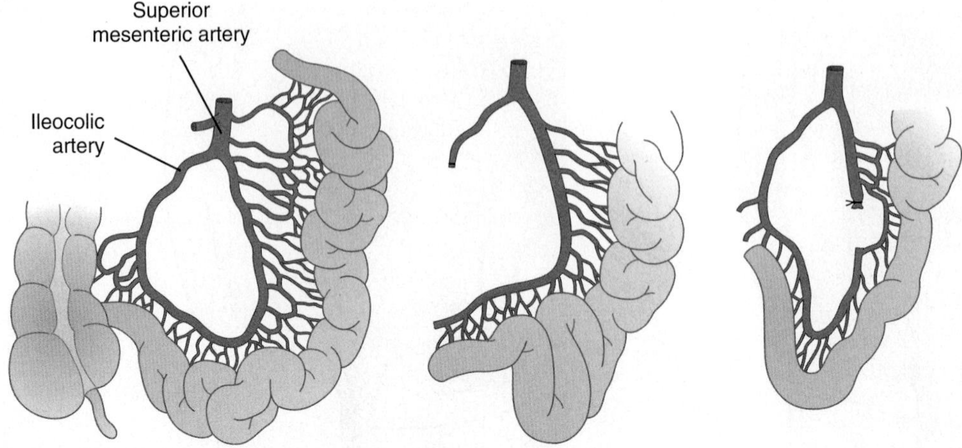


**FIGURE 52-39** Fry 2.

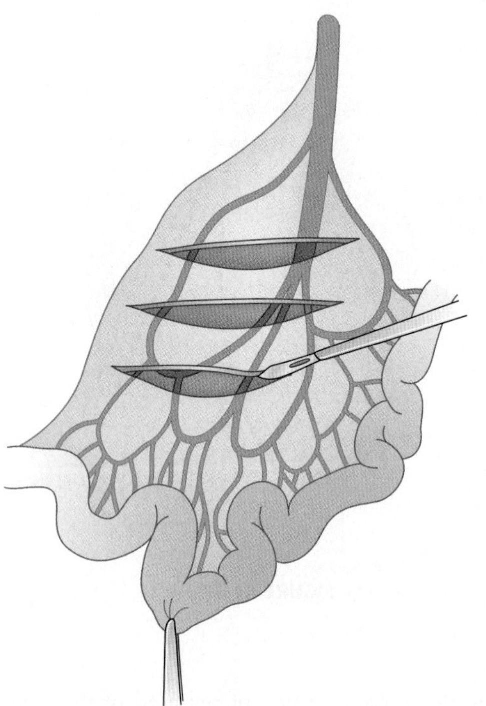

**FIGURE 52-40** Fry 3.

to provide adequate mesenteric length to fashion an anastomosis between the apex of the ileal pouch and anus.

In rare cases, the anatomy may be such that the ileal pouch will not extend to reach the anus. There have been reports of extending the small bowel mesentery with a saphenous vein interposition graft to the SMA, but this approach should only be used as a last resort.[20] Another alternative to be considered if the ileal pouch will not reach the anus, despite the maneuvers described, is to close the ileal enterotomy at the apex of the pouch, leave the pouch residing in the pelvis above the anus, and fashion a loop ileostomy proximal to the pouch. There have been several reports of successful ileal pouch anal anastomoses achieved several months later, when postoperative mesenteric lengthening permits adequate length for the pouch to reach the anus.

Some controversy exists concerning the advantages of performing a mucosectomy, especially as a routine component of the procedure. The double-stapling technique may leave a small remnant of rectal mucosa at the anastomosis, which in theory is at risk for the development of dysplasia and cancer. Large retrospective long-term analyses of outcomes of this technique have failed to bear this out. Mucosectomy has, however, been complicated by cancer arising at the anastomosis and extraluminally in the pelvis, evidently from islands of glands that remained after the mucosa was incompletely removed. Although cancer is exceedingly rare, the mucosectomy technique may conceal retained rectal mucosa in more than 20% of patients. The double-stapling technique permits surveillance and biopsy of the remaining mucosa. Avoiding the mucosectomy preserves the anal transition zone, which contains nerve endings involved in differentiating liquid and solid stool from gas, and is thus thought to provide superior postoperative continence.

Controversy also exists regarding temporary fecal diversion. The pouch and anastomosis were traditionally protected with a diverting loop ileostomy; however, there are some proponents of the single-stage procedure without diversion. This approach has the advantage of a single operation that avoids the complications accompanying an ileostomy. Disadvantages, however, include an increased risk for pelvic sepsis, usually caused by anastomotic leak of a pouch suture line or the anal anastomosis. Most surgeons routinely perform a two-stage operation in high-risk patients, particularly those taking steroids preoperatively.[21]

Patients who undergo total proctocolectomy and IPAA typically have between five and seven bowel movements in a 24-hour period. Function continues to improve with time, with numerous studies demonstrating a decrease in the number of daily bowel movements during the ensuing 3 to 24 months after reestablishment of continuity.

Restorative proctocolectomy and IPAA are associated with early and late complications. A common complication is small bowel obstruction, occurring in up to 27% of patients. Bowel obstruction after IPAA tends to be severe and requires surgery in almost 50% of cases. Another significant complication is pelvic sepsis. Anastomotic and pouch suture line leaks are devastating complications that can lead to pelvic abscess and seriously threaten the integrity and functionality of the pouch. Treatment of pelvic sepsis secondary to pouch leaks usually requires a diverting ileostomy and drainage of any abscesses. Delayed ileostomy closure after resolution of IPAA complications has no deleterious functional effects. A pouch–vaginal fistula is a specific form of pelvic sepsis that is difficult to manage and occurs in up to 7% of women. Persistence of the fistula after surgical closure (and often temporary diversion) usually signifies underlying Crohn's disease and may result in the loss of the pouch in a significant number of patients.

Inflammation of the mucosa of the ileal pouch, or pouchitis, occurs in 7% to 33% of patients with ulcerative colitis treated by IPAA. Pouchitis typically presents with increased stool frequency, fever, bleeding, cramps, and dehydration. The cause is unknown but may be related to bacterial overgrowth, mucosal ischemia, or other local factors. Episodes usually respond to rehydration and oral antibiotics, usually metronidazole or ciprofloxacin. Probiotics have been reported to provide dramatic resolution in some cases of pouchitis resistant to antibiotic therapy. The diagnosis of Crohn's disease must also be entertained in patients with significant pouchitis that does not respond to medical treatment.[22]

In some cases, the preoperative distinction between Crohn's disease and ulcerative colitis can be difficult, and the pathologist may label the disease indeterminate colitis. Patients with Crohn's disease are not candidates for IPAA because the high incidence of recurrent inflammation in the pouch can cause abscesses, fistulas, and loss of the reservoir. Patients with indeterminate colitis who undergo restorative proctocolectomy and IPAA who do not develop Crohn's disease have results that are more encouraging; patients with indeterminate colitis are generally considered candidates for IPAA if they understand that they are at increased risk for pouch complications related to underlying Crohn's disease.

**Summary of Elective Operations** A suggested algorithm for elective operations for patients with intractable mucosal ulcerative colitis is presented in Figure 52-41. Older patients or those with fecal incontinence should undergo a total proctocolectomy with an end ileostomy. Younger patients with no evidence of rectal dysplasia should undergo restorative proctocolectomy and IPAA with a double-stapled anastomosis and diverting loop ileostomy. Patients with confirmed rectal dysplasia should be treated with mucosectomy and a hand-sewn IPAA. Patients with significant debility who are poor operative candidates should undergo a total abdominal colectomy with a very low Hartmann closure and an end ileostomy.

### Postoperative Care

Postoperative care after restorative proctocolectomy with IPAA is similar to that for other major colorectal procedures. Nasogastric tubes are usually removed at the completion of the procedure, and liquid diets are offered to patients in the early recovery period. Diet is advanced with return of bowel function,

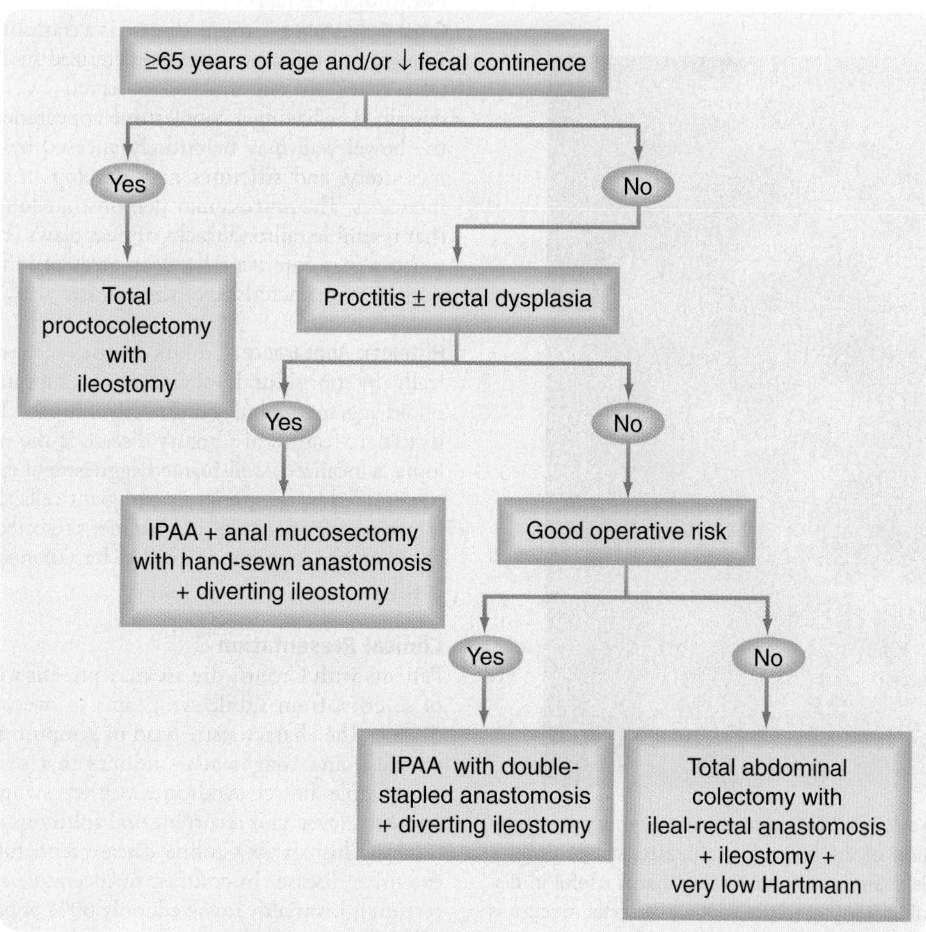


**FIGURE 52-41** Elective operations for ulcerative colitis.

as evidenced by ileostomy function. If a pelvic drain is used, it is typically removed after 48 to 72 hours. Bladder catheters are typically left in place for 3 to 4 days, depending on the difficulty of pelvic dissection. A contrast enema is performed approximately 10 weeks postoperatively to ensure an intact IPAA. If the enema shows a leak, the contrast examination is repeated in 6 weeks; almost 95% of anastomotic leaks heal in the absence of pelvic sepsis. If the radiograph shows no leak, the diverting ileostomy is closed.

## Crohn's Colitis

Originally described as regional ileitis, Crohn's disease is a nonspecific IBD that may affect any segment of the GI tract. Of patients with Crohn's disease, 15% have disease limited to the colon. The inflammatory process may affect the entire colon and mimic ulcerative colitis, or may affect only segments of the colon (Fig. 52-42). This section discusses Crohn's colitis; additional discussions of Crohn's disease are found elsewhere in this text.

### Epidemiology and Cause

A rapid increase in the incidence of Crohn's disease occurred between 1965 and 1980 and, since then, the incidence has increased at a slow pace. This is in contrast to the incidence of ulcerative colitis, which has been relatively constant over the same time period. The incidence of Crohn's disease varies between 1 and 10/100,000, depending on the geographic location, with the highest incidence in Scandinavian countries and Scotland, followed by England and North America. Similar to ulcerative colitis, there is a bimodal age distribution, with peaks between ages 15 and 30 years and a second smaller peak between 55 and 80 years of age. Crohn's disease is more common among patients of Jewish descent and occurs more frequently in urban residents.

The cause of Crohn's disease has not yet been determined. Three prevalent theories include response to a specific infectious agent, a defective mucosal barrier allowing an increased exposure to antigens, and an abnormal host response to dietary antigens. One infectious agent that has generated some interest is *Mycobacterium paratuberculosis,* which has been isolated in up to 65% of tissue samples from Crohn's patients. A statistically significant association between the onset of Crohn's disease and prior use of antibiotics has also been observed. Smoking appears to be a risk factor for Crohn's disease and, after intestinal resection, the risk of recurrence is greatly increased in smokers. Several studies have also shown an increased risk in patients taking oral contraceptives.

Advances in molecular biology have intensified the search for genetic factors and pathogenetic mechanisms in Crohn's disease. The *NOD2/CARD15* gene, located on chromosome 16, has been shown to be involved in the activation of nuclear factor-κB (NF-κB), a transcription factor that plays a significant role in Crohn's disease. Specific genotypes may also determine susceptibility, location, and behavior of Crohn's disease.[23]

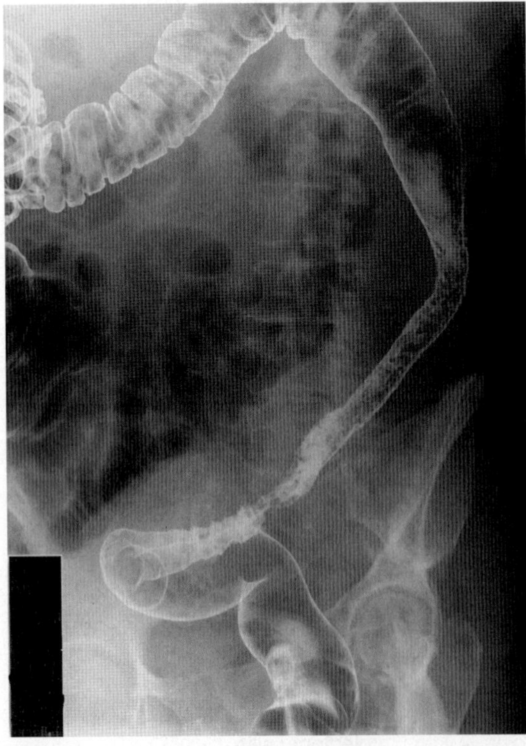

**FIGURE 52-42** Crohn's colitis. This barium enema x-ray demonstrates segmental inflammation of the left colon, characteristic of Crohn's disease. The rectum is spared, a clinical finding that is useful in distinguishing Crohn's colitis from ulcerative colitis. The rectal mucosa is almost always affected in patients with ulcerative colitis, whereas the pattern of colonic inflammation is variable in Crohn's colitis.

### Pathologic Features

**Gross Appearance** Crohn's disease is a transmural, predominantly submucosal inflammation characterized by a thickened colonic wall. The affected mucosa observed by endoscopy is often described as having a cobblestone appearance. In severe disease, the bowel wall may be entirely encased by creeping fat of the mesentery, and strictures may develop in the small and large intestines. The mucosa may demonstrate long, deep linear ulcers that resemble railroad tracks or bear claws (Fig. 52-43). Normal mucosa may intervene between areas of inflammation, causing skip areas characteristic of the disease.

**Histologic Appearance** Crohn's disease is characterized microscopically by transmural inflammation, submucosal edema, lymphoid aggregation and, ultimately, fibrosis. The pathognomonic histologic feature of Crohn's disease is the noncaseating granuloma, a localized, well-formed aggregate of epithelioid histocytes surrounded by lymphocytes and giant cells (Fig. 52-44). Granulomas are found in 50% of specimens resected in Crohn's disease; however, the number identified by colonoscopic biopsy is far smaller.

### Clinical Presentation

Patients with Crohn's disease may present with a wide spectrum of severity, from subtle symptoms to overwhelming fulminant disease. The characteristic triad of symptoms—abdominal pain, diarrhea, and weight loss—mimics that of viral gastroenteritis or irritable bowel syndrome. Other symptoms may include anorexia, fever, and recurrent oral aphthous ulcers. Patients with a family history of Crohn's disease tend to present with more extensive disease. In contrast to ulcerative colitis, in which the rectum is invariably involved, only 60% of patients with Crohn's colitis have rectal disease. Two thirds of patients with Crohn's colitis have involvement of the entire colon.

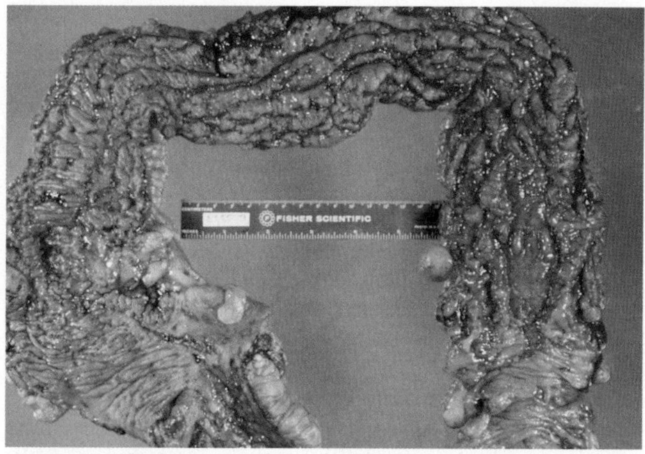


**FIGURE 52-43** Crohn's colitis. Linear ulceration of the mucosa, giving appearance of a railroad track or bear claw ulcers.

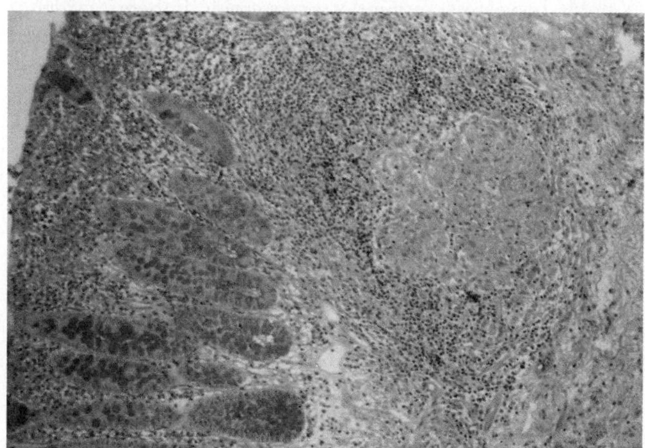

**FIGURE 52-44** Crohn's colitis with noncaseating granuloma.

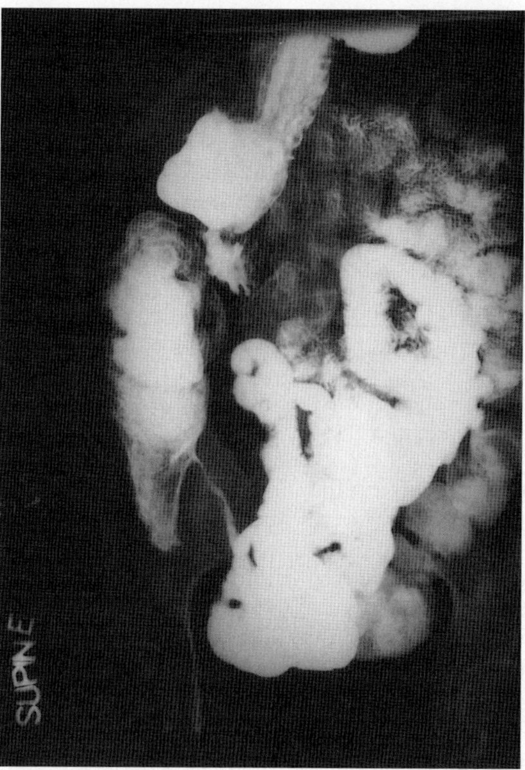


**FIGURE 52-45** Small bowel contrast study demonstrating string sign caused by inflammation and narrowing of the terminal ileum.

Anal disease, including anal fistulas, fissures, strictures, edematous skin tags, and erosion of the anoderm, occurs in up to 30% of patients with Crohn's disease of the terminal ileum and in more than 50% of patients with colonic disease. Anal disease in a patient with colitis suggests a diagnosis of Crohn's disease because primary anal disease is unusual in patients with ulcerative colitis.

## Diagnosis

The differential diagnosis of Crohn's colitis includes ulcerative colitis and various infectious agents. As for patients with ulcerative colitis, stool should be sent for culture and examined for ova and parasites. The diagnosis of Crohn's colitis is made by a combination of clinical, endoscopic, and radiologic features. Barium enema may not demonstrate any abnormalities in mild and early disease; colonoscopy is the more sensitive diagnostic modality. The disease is often patchy in distribution; however, some patients may have granular and friable mucosa in a continuous pattern involving the entire colon and rectum. Edema of the mucosa and aphthous ulcers are present in early Crohn's disease, with deep linear ulcers present in more severe disease and strictures more prevalent in chronic disease. It is at times difficult to distinguish Crohn's disease from ulcerative colitis, particularly if the rectum is involved. Biopsy samples should be obtained. However, unless a granuloma is identified, distinguishing between the two diseases may still be difficult.

An air-contrast enema may provide useful information in making the diagnosis and determining the extent of the disease. Characteristic radiologic findings in Crohn's colitis are skip lesions, contour defects, longitudinal and transverse ulcers, a cobblestone-like mucosal pattern, strictures, thickening of the haustral margin, and irregular nodular defects. A small bowel series or enteroclysis should be performed in all patients with suspected Crohn's disease or ulcerative colitis. Involvement of the small intestine strongly favors the diagnosis of Crohn's disease (Fig. 52-45). CT may demonstrate thickening of the colon, adenopathy, or intra-abdominal abscess.

## Treatment

**Medical Therapy** The medical treatment of Crohn's disease is similar to that of ulcerative colitis and includes aminosalicylates, steroids, and immunomodulatory medications (e.g., 6-MP, azathioprine, cyclosporine). One immunomodulatory drug that deserves mention in the treatment of Crohn's disease is infliximab, a monoclonal anti–TNF-α antibody designed to block the TNF-α receptor in an effort to decrease inflammation. Infliximab is given as an IV infusion to treat Crohn's disease in steroid-dependent or intractable patients and has also been shown to be of use in patients with chronic draining fistulas. Two thirds of patients with Crohn's disease and fistulas who were treated with infliximab demonstrate a significant decrease in the number of fistulas. Methotrexate has also been shown to be of

**BOX 52-2 Crohn's Colitis–Indications for Surgery**

Intractability
Intestinal obstruction
Intra-abdominal abscess
Fistulas
Fulminant colitis
Toxic megacolon
Massive bleeding
Cancer
Growth retardation

benefit in patients with colonic Crohn's disease who are steroid-dependent.

**Indications for Surgery** The indications for surgery in patients with Crohn's colitis are presented in Box 52-2. Operative treatment in Crohn's disease is intended to relieve symptoms when medical management has failed, correct complications, and prevent the development of cancer. It must be recognized that Crohn's disease is a pan-GI disease, and surgical intervention may therefore not cure the patient.

***Intractability*** Patients who fail to respond to optimal medical therapy for Crohn's disease and remain debilitated are often referred for surgical consultation. As with ulcerative colitis, this represents the most common indication for operative treatment for Crohn's disease.

***Intestinal Obstruction*** Intestinal obstruction in Crohn's disease may be caused by active inflammation, a fibrotic stricture from chronic disease, or an abscess or phlegmon causing a mass effect. Adhesions from previous abdominal operations must also be considered. Obstruction typically involves the small intestine, although large bowel obstruction from strictures may occur. Initial treatment includes bowel rest, nasogastric decompression, IV fluids, and anti-inflammatory medications, usually steroids. Obstruction caused by a stricture at a colonic anastomosis may be treated by endoscopic balloon dilation.

***Intra-Abdominal Abscess*** An intra-abdominal abscess in Crohn's disease is the result of intestinal perforation caused by transmural inflammation. An abscess is usually diagnosed by CT and can often be managed nonoperatively with CT-guided percutaneous drainage and antibiotics. If percutaneous drainage is not feasible or the patient does not respond to this therapy, laparotomy, drainage of the abscess, and resection of the involved bowel are indicated.

***Fistulas*** Fistulas may develop between the intestine and any other intra-abdominal organ, including the bladder, bowel, uterus, vagina, and stomach. Up to 35% of patients with Crohn's disease develop these fistulas, most of which involve the small intestine. Asymptomatic enteroenteric or enterocolic fistulas may not require operative therapy. A common fistula associated with Crohn's disease is an ileosigmoid fistula, which usually is caused by ileal disease with secondary involvement of the sigmoid. Symptomatic patients should undergo resection of the terminal ileum. When the inflammation in the sigmoid colon is minimal, the sigmoid defect can be primarily closed. Extensive inflammation in the sigmoid, however, also requires resection of the sigmoid colon. Colovesical and colovaginal fistulas require resection of the diseased bowel and closure of the bladder or vagina, with interposition of omentum between the bowel and contiguous organ.

Enterocutaneous fistulas in Crohn's disease may develop spontaneously, typically with ileal disease, or as the result of an early postoperative anastomotic breakdown. Patients are initially treated with bowel rest and drainage of any intra-abdominal abscess. Parenteral nutrition and medical treatment of the disease may result in spontaneous closure of the fistula; however, operative treatment is often necessary.

***Fulminant Colitis and Toxic Megacolon*** Patients with Crohn's disease may present with fulminant colitis in a fashion similar to patients with ulcerative colitis presenting with toxic megacolon. Fulminant colitis typically presents with high fever, severe abdominal pain, tenderness, tachycardia, and leukocytosis. Patients should be monitored in an intensive care unit and given IV fluids, bowel rest, antibiotics, and steroids. If there is evidence of clinical deterioration, or if there is no significant improvement within 48 to 72 hours, subtotal colectomy with an end ileostomy is indicated. Patients with toxic megacolon caused by Crohn's disease undergo surgical treatment similar to that for patients with toxic megacolon caused by ulcerative colitis. Because the pathologic process in Crohn's disease involves inflammation of the entire bowel wall, the colonic dilation characteristic of toxic megacolon may not occur in patients with Crohn's disease, but the toxicity of the colitis may be no less severe.

***Massive Bleeding*** Massive bleeding, although less common in Crohn's disease than in ulcerative colitis, has occurred in up to 13% of patients in some series. The terminal ileum represents the most common site of bleeding. If the disease involves the colon and spares the ileum, and the bleeding does not respond to medical therapy, flexible sigmoidoscopy or proctoscopy should be performed to rule out a rectal source. Appropriate operative treatment in the rare cases of colonic bleeding for Crohn's colitis is abdominal colectomy and ileostomy or ileorectal anastomosis if the rectum is not inflamed.

***Cancer*** The risk for development of carcinoma of the colon is not as high as the risk in long-standing, chronic ulcerative colitis, but it is present; therefore, patients with chronic active disease require periodic colonoscopic surveillance and biopsy.[14] The presence of high-grade dysplasia is an indication for colectomy. Patients who have undergone intestinal bypass for Crohn's disease have an increased risk for developing carcinoma; therefore, a bypassed segment of Crohn's disease should be resected, if possible.

***Extracolonic Manifestations*** Extraintestinal manifestations of Crohn's disease are similar to those associated with ulcerative colitis. With the exception of PSC, cirrhosis, and ankylosing spondylitis, most extracolonic manifestations of Crohn's disease improve after resection of the diseased bowel.

***Growth Retardation*** Young patients with Crohn's disease and ulcerative colitis may have impaired growth and mental development. Growth failure is often the result of prolonged inadequate caloric intake; therefore, nutritional support is an important component of care in these patients. Resection of severely diseased segments of bowel before puberty may help eliminate growth retardation and premature closure of bone epiphyses.

**Surgical Procedures** Because surgical intervention is not curative, medical therapy is the mainstay of treatment for Crohn's disease. Recurrence rates after surgery are high, and the risk continues with the passage of time. Therefore, an important principle in the surgical treatment of Crohn's disease is to resect only enough intestine to improve symptoms or correct complications. Intestine should be resected with the aim of obtaining margins free of disease by gross inspection. Frozen sections of the margins of resection are unnecessary because positive microscopic margins are not predictive of postoperative recurrence. Resection of grossly normal-appearing intestine may eventually lead to a short bowel syndrome, with insufficient absorptive surface to maintain nutrition. A suggested algorithm for elective operations for patients with intractable Crohn's disease is presented in Figure 52-46.

***Ileocecal Resection*** Ileocecal resection is indicated for patients with severe disease of the terminal ileum resulting in obstruction or perforation. It typically involves resection of approximately 6 to 12 inches of the terminal ileum and cecum, with an anastomosis created between the ileum and ascending colon. The terminal ileum is transected 2 cm proximal to the grossly apparent Crohn's disease. Stricturoplasty is not indicated for disease of the terminal ileum. In most series, the recurrence rate of Crohn's disease requiring reresection in patients who have undergone ileocolic resection, is approximately 50% in 10 years.

Occasionally, patients presenting with acute distal ileal disease (fever, right lower quadrant abdominal pain, leukocytosis) are misdiagnosed as having appendicitis. Traditional therapy for patients with terminal ileitis found at the time of surgery for appendicitis has been to perform an appendectomy when the cecum is normal, leave the ileum in place, and treat with medical therapy after surgery. A contradictory experience, however, has reported that 92% of patients found to have terminal ileitis at the time of surgery and who did not undergo resection require ileocolic resection for complications of Crohn's disease within 12 years.[24] Terminal ileitis may also be caused by *Yersinia enterocolitica* and *Campylobacter* spp., and distinguishing these processes from Crohn's disease intraoperatively may be difficult.

***Total Proctocolectomy With End Ileostomy*** Total proctocolectomy with end ileostomy involves removing all the abdominal colon, rectum, and anus and is indicated for patients with Crohn's disease involving the entire colon and rectum or when fecal incontinence is too severe to warrant preserving the rectum. Disadvantages of this procedure include delayed healing of the perineal wound and problems with malabsorption. Intersphincteric proctectomy decreases the incidence of perineal wound complications. Rapid small bowel transit and malabsorption of nutrients may occur more frequently after this procedure in patients with Crohn's disease as compared with patients with ulcerative colitis, because variable amounts of terminal ileum may be involved in the disease process.

***Total Abdominal Colectomy With Ileorectal Anastomosis or End Ileostomy*** Total abdominal colectomy with ileorectal anastomosis is indicated for patients with Crohn's colitis with sparing of the rectum and anus and offers the best functional result in patients who wish to maintain intestinal continuity. After this procedure, patients may expect to have between four and six bowel movements daily. The major disadvantage of the operation is the high likelihood of recurrence requiring completion proctectomy and ileostomy. Numerous studies have shown that approximately 50% of patients require proctectomy within 10 years. Patients who are poor operative candidates may best be served with a total abdominal colectomy and proximal proctectomy, with low Hartmann's closure and end ileostomy.

***Segmental Colon Resection*** Between 10% and 20% of patients with Crohn's colitis have disease limited to a segment of colon. Segmental colon resection may therefore be an option for patients with limited colonic disease associated with stricture or obstruction. It is contraindicated for patients with severe rectal or anal disease. As with total abdominal colectomy and ileorectal

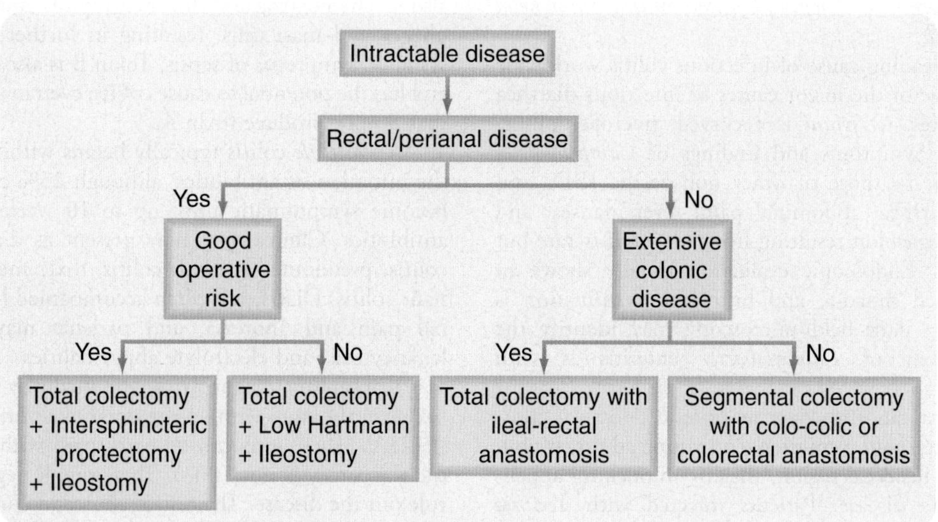


**FIGURE 52-46** Elective operations for Crohn's colitis.

anastomosis, the major disadvantage of segmental colon resection is the high rate of recurrence requiring subsequent operations. Within 5 years, recurrence rates range between 30% and 50%, with 60% of patients requiring reoperation by 10 years. Despite these high recurrence rates, segmental colectomy may be a good option for patients with limited disease who wish to avoid an ostomy.

**Postoperative Recurrence** A number of risk factors have been identified for recurrence of Crohn's disease after resection, including duration and severity of Crohn's disease before initial resection, smoking, and the presence of granulomas in the resected specimen. Longer disease-free resection margins and various types of anastomoses (i.e., end-to-side or side-to-side) have not been shown to affect recurrence rates. The reoperative rate for patients with Crohn's disease is 4% to 5%/year. In patients with Crohn's disease limited to the colon, total proctocolectomy has the lowest recurrence, with rates varying between 10% and 25%, depending on the length of follow-up.

Maintaining remission of Crohn's disease after resection remains an area of active investigation. Options include treatment with 5-ASA compounds, antibiotics, and the thiopurines azathioprine and 6-MP. A meta-analysis has demonstrated an 18% reduction in postoperative recurrence in patients treated with 4 g/day of 5-ASA. Metronidazole given for 3 months after surgery also has been shown to decrease recurrence; however, the side effects of long-term treatment with this medication preclude its routine use. In comparison with 5-ASA, azathioprine has been shown to have equal reduction in postoperative recurrence, with an increased benefit in patients who have undergone at least one previous resection.[25] Prophylaxis is typically begun within 2 weeks after surgery.

## INFECTIOUS COLITIS

Various forms of infectious enteritis are brought to the attention of the surgeon because they may present as an acute abdomen, masquerade as Crohn's disease or ulcerative colitis, result from standard treatment for a surgical procedure (prophylactic antibiotics for intestinal operations), or progress to the point that surgical treatment is required. The initial evaluation of a patient with diarrhea suspected of having IBD should include stool samples to be evaluated for *C. jejuni, Y. enterocolitica, Salmonella typhi,* and *C. difficile.*

*C. jejuni* is a leading cause of infectious colitis worldwide and has become one of the major causes of infectious diarrhea in the United States. *C. jejuni* is a curved, microaerophilic, gram-positive rod. Symptoms and findings of *Campylobacter* enteritis are similar to those of other nonspecific IBDs and include bloody diarrhea, abdominal pain, fever, nausea, and vomiting. Toxic megacolon resulting from *C. jejuni* is rare but has been reported. Endoscopic evaluation usually shows an edematous, inflamed mucosa, and histologic examination is usually nonspecific; dark field microscopy may identify the organism. Treatment of *Campylobacter* enteritis is with ciprofloxacin.

*Y. enterocolitica* can also cause an enteric infection, most commonly in infants, young children, and young adults. It typically occurs in the ileocecal region, thereby mimicking appendicitis and Crohn's disease. Patients infected with *Yersinia* typically present with bloody diarrhea and abdominal pain. Diagnosis is made by isolation of the bacteria from the stool. Radiographically, the terminal ileum may demonstrate a coarse, irregular, nodular mucosal pattern with ulcerations; however, because the disease is confined to the mucosa and submucosa, the characteristic string sign seen in Crohn's disease is absent. *Yersinia* enteritis will often resolve with supportive care alone; however, in more severe cases, patients should be treated with aminoglycosides or trimethoprim-sulfamethoxazole.

*S. typhi* causes an infectious enterocolitis in 16 million people worldwide annually and is the cause of typhoid fever. Invasion of the mucosa and submucosa of the small bowel and colon leads to an inflammatory reaction and release of an endotoxin from the bacterial cell. Severe septicemia may also occur if the organism enters the bloodstream. Toxic megacolon and intestinal perforation have been reported with *S. typhi* infection and, on rare occasions, patients may develop massive lower GI bleeding. Gangrenous cholecystitis has also been reported with typhoid fever. Diagnosis is based on culture of the organism from the stool or blood. Medical management includes treatment with fluoroquinolones or third-generation cephalosporins. Surgical intervention is warranted in cases of peritonitis secondary to perforation and generally requires resection of the affected bowel or diversion.

*C. difficile* is a gram-positive, spore-forming anaerobic microorganism related to the bacteria that cause tetanus and botulism. The organism has two forms, an active, infectious form that is difficult to culture and cannot survive in the environment for prolonged periods, and an inactive spore that can survive for long periods and can be often be found in hospitals, operating rooms, nursing homes, and extended care facilities. The spores can enter the intestinal tract and transform into the active form of the organism. Usually, the growth of the active organism is suppressed by the normal (autochthonous) bacteria of the colon, but antibiotics that suppress the colonic flora permit overgrowth of *C. difficile,* which releases toxins that cause diarrhea.

*C. difficile* produces two toxins (A and B), both of which are important in the pathogenesis of pseudomembranous colitis. Toxin A, the toxin that directly leads to the development of colitis, is released by the bacterium and binds to a colonocyte glycoprotein receptor. This leads to the destruction of the colonocyte and the release of inflammatory mediators. Toxin A is also a chemoattractant for neutrophils and activates macrophages and mast cells, resulting in further inflammation and systemic symptoms of sepsis. Toxin B is also a potent cytotoxin and has the potential to cause colitis, even in strains of *C. difficile* that do not produce toxin A.

*C. difficile* colitis typically begins within 4 to 9 days after the initiation of antibiotics, although 25% of patients may not become symptomatic until up to 10 weeks after a course of antibiotics. Clinically, it may present as diarrhea, self-limited colitis, pseudomembranous colitis, toxic megacolon, or fulminant colitis. Diarrhea is often accompanied by crampy abdominal pain and anorexia, and patients may also have fever, leukocytosis, and electrolyte abnormalities.

Laboratory diagnosis can be made by demonstrating the toxins in the stool with an enzyme-linked immunosorbent assay (ELISA). These tests can be performed within hours; however, their accuracy is not 100%. Therefore, a negative test does not rule out the disease. The test of choice to confirm the suspected diagnosis is the stool cytotoxin test, which has a high sensitivity (94% to 100%) and specificity (99%). A stool sample is filtered and added to cultured fibroblasts. A cytopathic effect that is neutralized by specific antiserum confirms the diagnosis. However, the test is expensive and requires overnight incubation and a tissue culture facility. If the diagnosis remains unclear, proctoscopy or flexible sigmoidoscopy may reveal inflamed mucosa covered by yellowish plaquelike membranes, or pseudomembranes. These are composed of a mixture of inflammatory cells, fibrin, and bacterial and cellular components and are seen in approximately 25% of patients with mild disease and 87% of patients with fulminant colitis.

Treatment should be tailored to the severity of the disease. For mild cases (patients without fever, abdominal pain, or leukocytosis), cessation of all antibiotics may be the only treatment necessary. Patients with more severe diarrhea or toxic symptoms should be treated by discontinuing the causative antibiotics and administering antibiotics directed against *C. difficile.* Vancomycin (oral) or metronidazole (oral or IV) are equally effective against the organism and improvement is usually seen within 3 days of initiating therapy. Treatment is generally continued for 10 days, but relapse occurs in approximately 25% of cases after cessation of treatment. Recurrence is treated with a repeated course of vancomycin or metronidazole.

There have been reports of patients with refractory *C. difficile* colitis in whom the pathologic bacteria cannot be eradicated with repeated and prolonged treatment by vancomycin or metronidazole, but in whom the symptoms of diarrhea and hematochezia persist but do not progress to a state of severe toxicity. Attempts to restore the normal colonic flora with a fecal transplant, usually with stool obtained from a family member, have been reported to be successful.[26] For obvious reasons, this treatment has not gained popular acceptance.

Severe cases of *C. difficile* colitis may progress to a fulminant disease and toxic megacolon. In such cases, abdominal colectomy with ileostomy is indicated. Unfortunately, the mortality rate associated with *C. difficile* colitis of such severity that colectomy is required is higher than 50%.

There have been reports of outbreaks of especially severe *C. difficile* colitis associated with a higher mortality rate than that expected with the usual strains. This strain has a defective gene, *TxcD,* which is associated with extremely high toxin production by the bacteria. Currently used diagnostic tests do not distinguish this strain from the usual strain, but it responds to treatment with metronidazole or vancomycin.

## COLONIC ISCHEMIA

Colonic ischemia (CI) is the most common form of intestinal ischemia. Most attacks are transient and resolve spontaneously; thus, the entity is often misdiagnosed or unrecognized. Although the cause of many cases of CI is obscure, aortic surgery, arteriosclerotic disease, and conditions causing transient hypotension have been implicated. Other factors associated with the disease include the use of oral contraceptives, cocaine abuse, hereditary coagulopathies, long distance running, and certain bacterial pathogens, including cytomegalovirus (CMV) and *E. coli* O157:H7.

As described earlier, the colon is supplied with arterial blood from the superior and inferior mesenteric arteries. There are collateral channels that may develop between these major mesenteric arteries; it is not unusual for the marginal artery or the arc of Riolan to provide collateral circulation adequate to sustain the left colon if the IMA has been gradually occluded by atherosclerosis. Actually, the IMA is frequently occluded in conditions requiring aortic surgery and, in such circumstances, transection of the IMA does not require reimplantation. However, in this situation, the left colon is dependent on collateral blood supply and transient hypotension at the time of the vascular procedure or immediately after surgery may result in ischemic injury to the vulnerable colonic mucosa.

The spectrum of CI includes transient ischemia, chronic ischemia, and gangrene. The disease is usually segmental in nature. If the ischemia is limited to the most vulnerable layer of the intestine, the mucosa, the disease may be transient and recovery may be complete. More significant ischemia involving the muscularis may result in scarring and a chronic stricture. Ischemia affecting the full thickness of the bowel wall may result in gangrene, with perforation and fecal peritonitis.

The signs and symptoms of CI include abdominal pain, hematochezia, and fever. These symptoms vary considerably, depending on the severity of the ischemia and length and thickness of the colon that is affected. Ischemia limited to a small segment of mucosa may cause cramping abdominal pain and passage of a small amount of blood; more significant mucosal ischemia may result in more severe abdominal pain and tenderness over the affected segment of colon, bacterial translocation, fever, leukocytosis, and acidosis. Compromise of blood supply to the full thickness of the colonic wall results in severe abdominal pain, fever, leukocytosis, acidosis, and signs of peritonitis.

Rapid and accurate diagnosis permits the institution of supportive measures or withdrawal of offending medications (e.g., oral contraceptives) that may halt the progression of the disease and prevent mucosal ischemia from progressing to transmural gangrene. Early diagnosis is obviously facilitated by a high suspicion for CI in the setting of mild to moderate abdominal pain, fever, and bloody diarrhea.

Radiologic investigation of CI usually begins with a plain film of the abdomen. The resulting picture is often nonspecific, but findings suggestive of CI include an ileus, an isolated segment of distended colon or, more specifically, thumbprinting—a sign caused by intestinal wall edema or submucosal hemorrhage. Free intraperitoneal air can result from gangrene causing intestinal perforation.

The use of a barium enema for the diagnosis of acute CI has become obsolete. The risk for perforation and barium peritonitis in this circumstance is unacceptable. Water-soluble contrast studies also carry a risk for perforation of the compromised intestine and should be avoided in the acute setting. However, contrast enemas are useful and acceptable for the detection and evaluation of a stricture that may have developed because of ischemia.

Flexible sigmoidoscopy provides the advantage of direct visualization of the colonic mucosa. Bacterial or viral cultures may be obtained and biopsies may be taken. Unfortunately, biopsies of the mucosa in this setting are typically nonspecific and uninformative. The segment of large bowel most prone to ischemia is the sigmoid. Cases of isolated ischemic proctitis have been reported but are rare. All segments of the colon may be involved, but it is rarely necessary to visualize the colon beyond the level of the splenic flexure to establish the diagnosis. The finding of hemorrhagic dusky mucosa is typical. Patches of inflammation may be interspersed with healthy-appearing mucosa. The major disadvantage of endoscopic diagnosis of CI is the inability to distinguish between mucosal and transmural gangrene.

CT with IV contrast is useful in such a situation. This modality also may permit visualization of the arterial supply to the entire intestine. Arteriography is not indicated unless it is believed that acute mesenteric ischemia involves the small intestine. Arteriography does not change the management or outcome of clinically apparent CI.

Treatment of CI depends on the presentation and severity of signs and symptoms (Fig. 52-47). Hospital admission, IV fluids, bowel rest, and general supportive measures until the patient is pain-free are usually adequate treatment for mucosal ischemia. Because loss of integrity of the mucosa may result in bacterial translocation, broad-spectrum antibiotics are generally advocated for the treatment of CI. Level I evidence for antibiotic treatment in humans is nonexistent, but antibiotics are associated with increased survival in rat models of CI.

There is a recognized risk for CI after abdominal aortic operations and this diagnosis must be considered when abdominal pain, fever, leukocytosis, or acidosis occurs after this type of surgery. Flexible sigmoidoscopy is indicated to establish the diagnosis. Monitoring of the patient includes serial abdominal examinations and frequent recording of vital signs, urine output, blood pH, and white blood cell count. Supportive measures are provided as described earlier. If transmural gangrene is suspected, immediate operation is indicated.

Surgical intervention for CI is relatively uncommon but, when it is indicated, the procedure of choice is partial or total colectomy with or without an end stoma (Box 52-3). Unlike mesenteric ischemia involving the small bowel, revascularization procedures to establish blood flow to the colon are not indicated. Indications for operation in CI are fairly straightforward. Colonic perforation is a clear indication for laparotomy and resection of the ischemic segment with end ileostomy or colostomy. Total CI is rare, but cases have been reported to mimic fulminant colitis or toxic megacolon. These require treatment by total colectomy and end ileostomy. Although rare, massive bleeding in the setting of acute ischemic colitis is a serious and life-threatening occurrence. Subtotal colectomy with an end ileostomy is usually indicated in this situation unless the specifically involved segment of colon can be accurately identified and resected.

Indications for surgery in subacute situations are uncommon. However, patients who remain symptomatic, with pain, bleeding, diarrhea, or recurrent bouts of sepsis for 2 to 3 weeks after presentation with no improvement, may require operation.

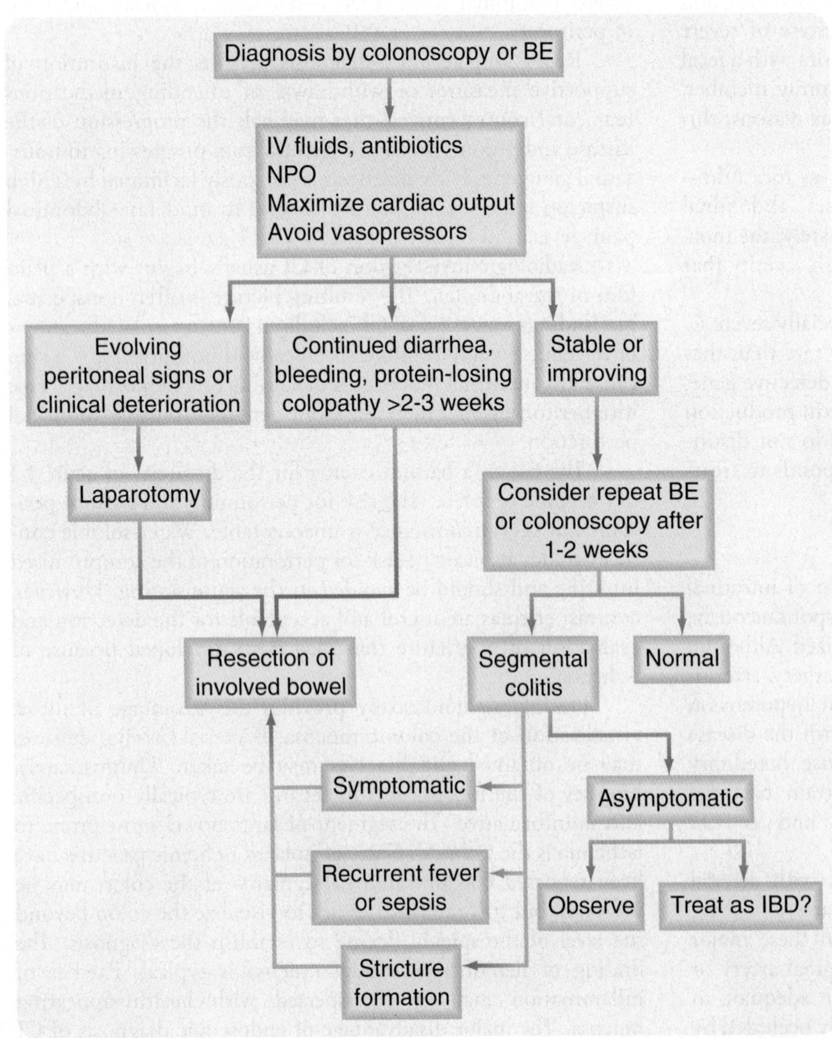


**FIGURE 52-47** Management of colonic ischemia. *BE,* Barium enema.

**BOX 52-3 Colonic Ischemia–Indications for Surgery**

**Acute Indications**

Peritoneal signs

Massive bleeding

Universal fulminant colitis, with or without toxic megacolon

**Subacute Indications**

Failure of an acute segmental ischemic colitis to respond within 2 to 3 wk, with continued symptoms or a protein-losing colopathy

Apparent healing but with recurrent bouts of sepsis

**Chronic Indications**

Symptomatic colon stricture

Symptomatic segmental ischemic colitis

Whether to fashion an anastomosis in this setting is unclear. The nature of this disease and potential for serious septic complications argues for creation of a stoma.

Chronic sequelae of CI include stricture formation and chronic segmental colitis. Strictures can be symptomatic, depending on their location and diameter. Strictures usually affect the sigmoid colon. Indications for treatment include obstructive symptoms, diagnostic uncertainty (suspicion of cancer as a cause of stricture), and impediment to endoscopic examination of suspected colonic lesions in the colon proximal to the stricture. Ischemic strictures have been successfully dilated by endoscopic techniques and stents. However, resection of the strictured segment with primary anastomosis is generally advocated for relatively healthy patients.

Patients with chronic segmental colitis typically have intermittent symptoms of pain and bleeding. Endoscopic examination reveals inflammation limited to a segment of colon, usually descending or sigmoid. Biopsy of the friable tissue is unrevealing but can rule out infectious causes. Frequently, colonoscopic examination of patients after a bout of CI reveals completely normal mucosa, testifying to the transient, intermittent nature of the attacks. It is extremely rare that attacks recur in an intermittent fashion that requires surgical intervention.

## NEOPLASIA

Adenocarcinoma of the colon and rectum is the third most common site of new cancer cases and deaths in men (following prostate and lung or bronchus cancer) and women (following breast and lung or bronchus cancer) in the United States. It was estimated that in 2009, there were 106,100 new cases of colon cancer (552,010 men and 54,090 women) and 40,870 new cases of rectal cancer (23,580 men and 17,290 women) diagnosed. In 2009, 49,920 Americans (25,240 men and 24,680 women) were predicted to die of colorectal cancer. The lifetime risk for developing colorectal cancer in the United States is 5.51% (1 in 18) for men and 5.10% (1 in 20) for women. The risk for developing invasive colorectal cancer increases with age, with more than 90% of new cases being diagnosed in patients older than 50 years. The incidence of colorectal cancer in men from 1998 to 2005 decreased at a rate of 2.8%/year and for women at a rate of 2.2%/year. The death rate for men and women decreased 4.3% annually over the period from 2002 to 2005. There has been a significant increase in 5-year survival rates over the last 30 years. The 5-year survival for colon cancer was 52% from 1975 to 1977, 59% from 1984 to 1986, and 65% from 1996 to 2004. The 5-year survival for Americans with rectal cancer was 49% from 1975 to 1977, 57% from 1984 to 1986, and 67% from 1996 to 2004.[27]

**Table 52-2 Familial Risk and Colon Cancer**

| FAMILIAL SETTING | APPROXIMATE LIFETIME RISK OF COLON CANCER |
|---|---|
| General U.S. population | 6% |
| One first-degree relative* with colon cancer | Two- to threefold increased |
| Two first-degree relatives* with colon cancer | Three- to fourfold increased |
| First-degree relative* with colon cancer diagnosed ≤50 yr | Three- to fourfold increased |
| One second- or third-degree relative†,‡ with colon cancer | 1.5-fold increased |
| Two second- or third-degree relatives†,‡ with colon cancer | Two- to threefold increased |
| One first-degree relative* with adenomatous polyp | Twofold increased |

From Burt RW: Colon cancer screening. Gastroenterology 119:837–853, 2000.

*First-degree relatives include parents, siblings, and children.

†Second-degree relatives include grandparents, aunts, and uncles.

‡Third-degree relatives include great-grandparents and cousins.

Colorectal cancer occurs in a hereditary, sporadic, or familial form. Hereditary forms of colorectal cancer have been extensively described and are characterized by family history, young age at onset, and the presence of other specific tumors and defects. Familial adenomatous polyposis (FAP) and hereditary nonpolyposis colorectal cancer (HNPCC) have been the subject of many investigations that have provided significant insights into the pathogenesis of colorectal cancer.

Sporadic colorectal cancer occurs in the absence of family history, generally affects an older population (60 to 80 years of age), and usually presents as an isolated colon or rectal lesion. Genetic mutations associated with the cancer are limited to the tumor itself, unlike hereditary disease, in which the specific mutation is present in all cells of the affected individual. Nevertheless, the genetics of colorectal cancer initiation and progression proceed along similar pathways in the hereditary and sporadic forms of the disease. Studies of the relatively rare inherited models of the disease have greatly enhanced the understanding of the genetics of the far more common sporadic form of the cancer.

The concept of familial colorectal cancer is relatively recent. Lifetime risk for colorectal cancer increases for members in families in which the index case is young (<50 years) and the relative is close (first-degree). The risk increases as the number of family members with colorectal cancer rises (Table 52-2). An individual who is a first-degree relative of a patient diagnosed with colorectal cancer before the age of 50 years is twice as likely as an individual in the general population to develop the cancer. This more subtle form of inheritance has been the subject of much investigation. Genetic polymorphisms, gene modifiers, and defects in tyrosine kinases have all been implicated in various forms of familial colorectal cancer.

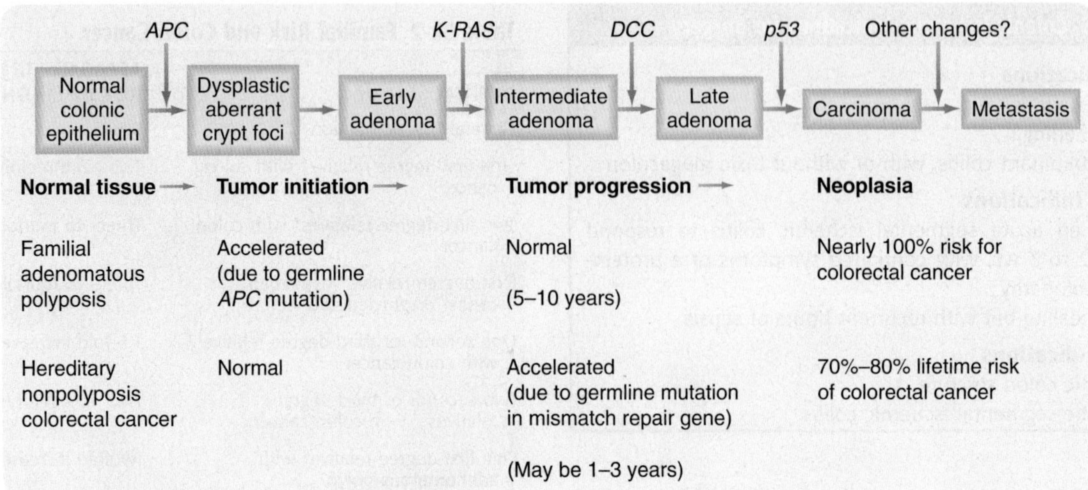


**FIGURE 52-48** Adenoma-carcinoma sequence in sporadic and hereditary colorectal cancer. (From Ivanovich JL, Read TE, Ciske DJ, et al: A practical approach to familial and hereditary colorectal cancer. Am J Med 107:68–77, 1999.)

## Colorectal Cancer Genetics

The field of colorectal cancer genetics was revolutionized in 1988 by the description of the genetic changes involved in the progression of a benign adenomatous polyp to invasive carcinoma. Since then, there has been an explosion of additional information about the molecular and genetic pathways that result in colorectal cancer. Tumor suppressor genes, DNA mismatch repair genes, and proto-oncogenes all contribute to colorectal neoplasia, in the sporadic and inherited forms. The Fearon-Vogelstein adenoma-carcinoma multistep model of colorectal neoplasia represents one of the best-known models of carcinogenesis (Fig. 52-48). This sequence of tumor progression involves damage to proto-oncogenes and tumor suppressor genes. The multistep carcinogenesis model can serve as a template to illustrate how certain early mutations produce accumulated defects resulting in neoplasia. The specific contributing mutations in genes such as adenomatous polyposis coli (APC) have been intensely studied. It is important to view this model and others as progressive and in flux while interconnected cell cycle control pathways and new functions for well-known genes are becoming recognized (Table 52-3).

**Table 52-3 Gene Mutations That Cause Colon Cancer**

| MUTATION TYPE | GENES INVOLVED | TYPE OF DISEASE CAUSED |
|---|---|---|
| Germline | *APC* | Familial adenomatous polyposis |
| | MMR | HNPCC (Lynch syndrome) |
| Somatic | Oncogenes:<br>*myc*<br>*ras*<br>*src*<br>*erbB* | Sporadic disease |
| | Tumor suppressor genes:<br>*TP53*<br>*DCC*<br>*APC* | |
| | MMR genes:<br>*bMSH2*<br>*bMLH1*<br>*bPMS1*<br>*bPMS2*<br>*bMSH6*<br>*bMSH3* | |
| Genetic polymorphism | *APC* | Familial colon cancer in Ashkenazi Jews |

*DCC*, Deleted in colorectal carcinoma.

## Specific Genes and Mutations

### Tumor Suppressor Genes

Tumor suppressor genes produce proteins that inhibit tumor formation by regulating mitotic activity and providing inhibitory cell cycle control. Tumor formation occurs when these inhibitory controls are deregulated by mutation. Point mutations, loss of heterozygosity (LOH), frame-shift mutations, and promoter hypermethylation are all types of genetic changes that can cause failure of a tumor suppressor gene. These genes are often referred to as *gatekeeper genes* because they provide cell cycle inhibition and regulatory control at specific checkpoints in cell division. The failure of regulation of normal cellular function by tumor suppressor genes is appropriately described by the term *loss of function.* Both alleles of the gene must be nonfunctional to initiate tumor formation.

The *APC* gene is a tumor suppressor gene located on chromosome 5q21. Its product is 2843 amino acids in length and forms a cytoplasmic complex with GSK-3β (a serine-threonine kinase), β-catenin, and axin. β-Catenin, a multifunctional protein, is a structural component of the epithelial cell adherens junctions and the actin cytoskeleton; it also binds in the cytoplasm to Tcf/LEF and is then transported into the nucleus, where it activates transcription of genes such as *c-myc* and others that regulate cellular growth and proliferation. APC therefore participates in cell cycle control by regulating the intracytoplasmic pool of β-catenin.

The Wnt signaling proteins are closely associated with the *APC*–β-catenin pathway. *APC* also influences cell cycle proliferation by regulating Wnt expression. Wnt gene products are extracellular signaling molecules that help regulate tissue development throughout the organism. The Wnt signaling proteins are closely associated with the *APC*–β-catenin pathway. Under normal conditions, reduced intracytoplasmic β-catenin levels inhibit Wnt expression. When APC is mutated, however, β-catenin levels rise and Wnt is activated. Overexpression of Wnt leads to activation of Wnt target genes such as cyclin D1 and *Myc,* which drive cell proliferation and tumor formation.

The earliest mutations in the adenoma-carcinoma sequence occur in the *APC* gene. The earliest phenotypic change present is known as *aberrant crypt formation* and the most consistent genetic aberrations within these cells are abnormally short proteins known as *APC* truncations. Most clinically relevant derangements in *APC* are truncation mutations created by inappropriate transcription of premature termination codons.

A germline *APC* truncation mutation is responsible for the autosomal dominant inherited disease, FAP. Thirty percent of cases of FAP are de novo germline mutations, thus presenting without a family history of the disease. FAP is rare, with an estimated incidence of 1 in 8000 of the U.S. population, occurring without gender predilection. It is typically characterized by more than 100 adenomatous polyps present in the colon and rectum. These polyps often number in the thousands and are almost always manifest by the late second or early third decade of life (Fig. 52-49). Because some of these polyps proceed through the adenoma-carcinoma sequence, most patients with FAP die of colon cancer by their fifth decade of life in the absence of surgical intervention. FAP is of great interest to those studying sporadic colorectal cancer because *APC* truncation mutations similar to those found in APC patients occur in 85% of sporadic colorectal cancers.

Most *APC* truncation mutations occur in the mutational cluster region of the gene, an area responsible for β-catenin binding. However, genotype-phenotype correlations exist with mutations in other regions of the gene. For example, mutations close to the 5′ end of the gene produce a short truncated protein that causes the syndrome known as *attenuated FAP* or (AFAP). These patients usually have far less than the hundreds of polyps usually associated with FAP, and the disease has a tendency to spare the rectum.

Classic FAP is characterized by truncation mutations occurring in the gene from codon 1250 to codon 1464. Mutations occurring further along the gene toward the 3′ end are rare and most likely result in a much attenuated phenotype or no detectable abnormality (Fig. 52-50).

The variability of the FAP phenotype is also demonstrated by the presence or absence of extraintestinal manifestations of disease. In the past, the term *Gardner's syndrome* was used to describe the coexpression of profuse colonic adenomatous polyps along with osteomas of the mandible and skull, desmoid tumors of the mesentery, and periampullary neoplasms.

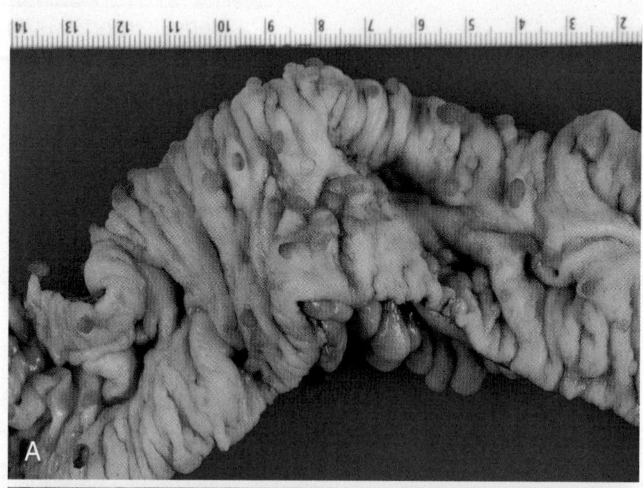


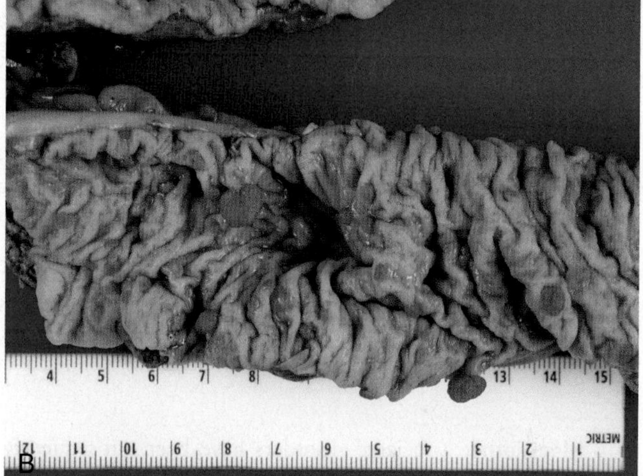


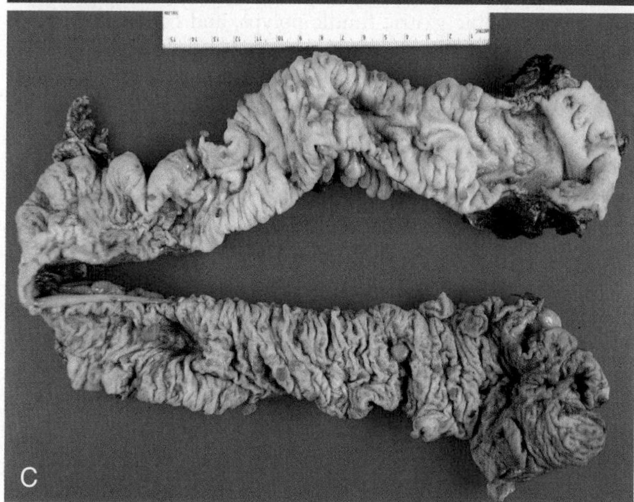


**FIGURE 52-49** Familial adenomatous polyposis, macroscopic appearance. The colonic mucosa exhibits numerous small polyps, both pedunculated and sessile. The entire colon contained hundreds of polyps. (Courtesy Dr. Jeffrey P. Baliff, Thomas Jefferson University, Philadelphia.)

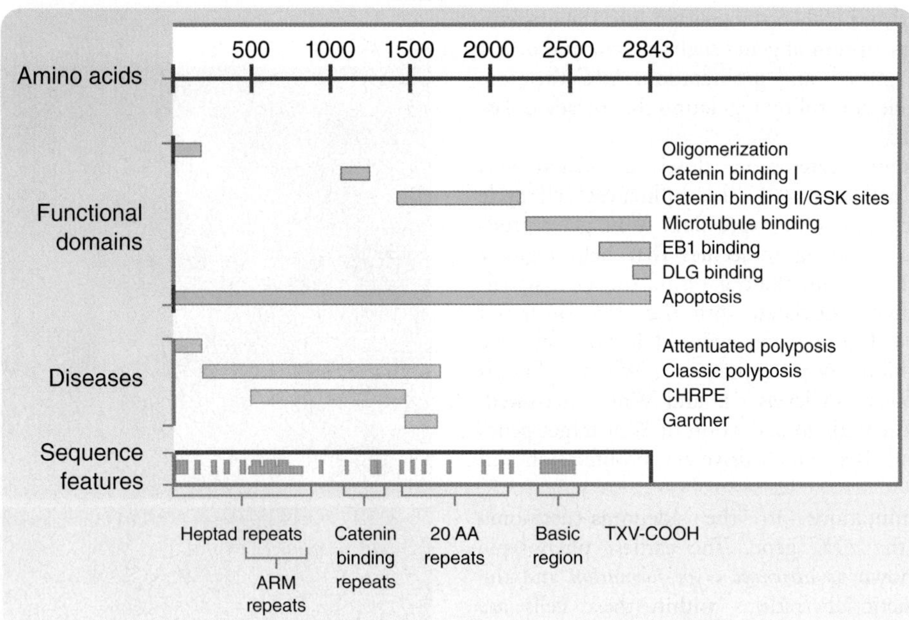


**FIGURE 52-50** Functional and pathogenic properties of APC. APC is a protein heterodimer 2843 amino acids in length. The figure depicts the functional domains of APC schematically as *blue bars* where regional mutations result in loss of protein binding, as described in the column on the right side of the figure. Mutations in these regions result in truncations that may affect cellular structure and cell signaling, such as the inability to bind catenins and interference with microtubule binding. Cellular processes such as apoptosis are affected by mutations occurring at many sites along the gene. Some mutational affects are unknown, such as those preventing EB1 and DLG binding (proteins with unclear functions). Diseases are similarly represented by *tan bars*. Mutations within the regions depicted result in the disease phenotypes described in the right column, including attenuated polyposis, classic polyposis, CHRPE, and Gardner's syndrome (extraintestinal manifestations of FAP). (From Kinzler KW, Vogelstein B: Lessons from hereditary colorectal cancer. Cell 87:159–170, 1996.)

Many other associated disorders have been subsequently described, including thyroid papillary tumors, medulloblastomas, hypertrophic gastric fundic polyps, and congenital hypertrophy of the retinal pigmented epithelium of the iris (CHRPE). The expression of extraintestinal manifestations of FAP is dependent on mutation location, with most of these signs seen only when the truncation occurs in a very small area of the mutational cluster region.

Another *APC* mutation implicated in approximately 25% of colorectal cancers afflicting Ashkenazi Jews is the I1307 point mutation caused by the substitution of a lysine for isoleucine at codon 1307. This was initially believed to be a genetic polymorphism, a substitution that does not affect the protein structure. However, it is now recognized as probably the most important cause of familial colorectal cancer in this population.

### *MYH* Mutations and *MYH*-Associated Polyposis

A number of families have been characterized with a phenotype resembling that of FAP or AFAP, but without a discoverable *APC* gene defect. In 2002, a report of a Welsh family ("family N") with apparent recessive inheritance of multiple colorectal polyps and a cancer was published. On analysis of tumor *APC*, frequent somatic mutations were found characterized by G:C to T:A substitutions typically caused by oxidative DNA damage. The authors found that those family members affected had two distinct mutations in the *MYH* gene, a gene responsible for base excision-repair and used to repair oxidative DNA damage. From several subsequent surveys of kindreds with familial colorectal cancer or polyp inheritance patterns, it has become clear that a number of *MYH* mutations exist, and may coexist in the same patient.[28] The mutation has been characterized in Northern European, Indian, and Pakistani populations, appears to affect the production of polyps and tumors by promoting *APC* defects, and is called *MYH*-associated polyposis (MAP). Although the proportion of colorectal cancers attributable to germline *MYH* mutations is unknown, all patients with biallelic *MYH* mutations are at increased risk for colorectal cancer. Greater numbers of polyps (100 to 1000), and even extracolonic manifestations such as duodenal adenomas, are associated with the presence of more than one germline *MYH* mutation in a single patient.

It is evident that the MAP phenotype is highly variable and that clinical management, for now, should follow guidelines previously established for FAP and AFAP. Surgery in carriers who have polyps is IPAA or ileorectal anastomosis, depending on the status of the rectum. Colonoscopic and duodenal surveillance every 1 or 2 years for those with biallelic mutations is warranted, given the uncertainty of the natural history of the disease.

It remains unclear whether heterozygotes are at increased risk for colorectal cancer; all offspring of those with the disease can be reasonably assured that they are heterozygotes unless they too have multiple polyps, an extremely unlikely event. However, it is certain that patients with MAP need to be distinguished from those with FAP or AFAP because it implies increased risk in siblings, rather than offspring. For those with biallelic mutations, spouses can also be tested in the unlikely event that both spouses possess a recessive *MYH* allele.

The most frequently mutated tumor suppressor gene in human neoplasia is *p53 (TP53),* located on chromosome 17p. Mutations in *p53* are present in 75% of colorectal cancers and occur rather late in the adenoma-carcinoma sequence. Under normal conditions, *p53* acts by inducing apoptosis in response to cellular damage or by causing $G_1$ cell cycle arrest, allowing DNA repair mechanisms to occur. One of the features of mutated *p53* is that it is unable to activate the *BAX* gene to induce apoptosis. For its role in regulating apoptosis, *p53* is known as the *guardian of the genome.* The minority of colon cancer patients who have intact *p53* in their tumors may possess a survival advantage. Studies have indicated that prognostic significance may be related to tumor *p53* status.

A number of genes on chromosome 18q are implicated in colorectal cancer, including *SMAD2, SMAD4,* and *DCC.* SMAD proteins are involved in the transforming growth factor-β (TGF-β) signal transduction pathway. *SMAD2* and *SMAD4* are mutated in 5% to 10% of sporadic colorectal cancers. *DCC* is encoded by a large gene and is involved in cell-cell or cell-matrix interactions. It is not clear how *DCC* is directly involved in colorectal neoplasia. *DPC4* is a gene adjacent to *DCC* and may be the tumor suppressor gene deleted in 18q mutations.

### Mismatch Repair Genes

Mismatch repair (MMR) genes are called *caretaker genes* because of their important role in policing the integrity of the genome and correcting DNA replication errors. MMR genes that undergo a loss of function contribute to carcinogenesis by accelerating tumor progression. Mutations in MMR genes (including *hMLH1, hMSH2, hMSH3, hPMS1, hPMS2,* and *hMSH6*) result in the HNPCC syndrome. Approximately 3% of colorectal cancers in the United States are caused by HNPCC. Mutations in MMR genes produce microsatellite instability. Microsatellites are repetitive sequences of DNA that appear to be randomly distributed throughout the genome. Stability of these sequences is a good measure of the general integrity of the genome. MMR gene mutations result in errors in S phase when DNA is newly synthesized and copied. Microsatellite instability exists in 10% to 15% of sporadic tumors and in 95% of tumors in patients with HNPCC. Even so, only 50% of patients diagnosed with HNPCC have readily identifiable MMR mutations.

### Oncogenes

Proto-oncogenes are genes that produce proteins that promote cellular growth and proliferation. Mutations in proto-oncogenes typically produce a gain of function and can be caused by mutation in only one of the two alleles. After mutation, the gene is called an *oncogene.* Overexpression of these growth-oriented genes contributes to the uncontrolled proliferation of cells associated with cancer. The products of oncogenes can be divided into categories. For example, growth factors (e.g., TGF-β, epidermal growth factor, insulin-like growth factor), growth factor receptors (e.g., *erbB2*), signal transducers (e.g., *src, abl, ras*), and nuclear proto-oncogenes and transcription factors *(myc)* are all oncogene products that appear to have a role in the development of colorectal neoplasia. The *ras* proto-oncogene is located on chromosome 12, and mutations are believed to occur early in the adenoma-carcinoma sequence. Mutated *ras* has been found to be present in aberrant crypt foci and adenomatous polyps. Activated *ras* leads to constitutive activity of the protein, which stimulates cellular growth. Of sporadic colon cancers, 50% possess *ras* mutations and trials of farnesyl transferase inhibitors, which block a step in *ras* post-translational modification, may hold therapeutic promise.

## Adenoma-Carcinoma Sequence

The adenoma-carcinoma sequence is recognized as the process through which most colorectal carcinomas develop. Clinical and epidemiologic observations have long been cited to support the hypothesis that colorectal carcinomas evolve through a progression of benign polyps to invasive carcinoma, and the elucidation of the genetic pathways to cancer described earlier has confirmed the validity of this hypothesis. However, before the molecular genesis of colorectal cancer was appreciated, there was considerable controversy about whether colorectal cancer arises de novo or evolves from a polyp that was initially a benign precursor. Although there have been a few documented cases of tiny colonic cancers arising de novo from normal mucosa, these are rare, and the validity of the adenoma-carcinoma sequence is now accepted by almost all authorities. The historical observations that led to the hypothesis are of interest because of the therapeutic implications implicit in an understanding of the adenoma-carcinoma sequence. Observations that provided support for the hypothesis include the following:

- Larger adenomas are found to harbor cancers more often than smaller ones, and the larger the polyp, the higher the risk for cancer. Although the cellular characteristics of the polyp are important, with villous adenomas carrying a higher risk than tubular adenomas, the size of the polyp is also important. The risk for cancer in a tubular adenoma smaller than 1 cm in diameter is less than 5%, whereas the risk for cancer in a tubular adenoma larger than 2 cm is 35%. A villous adenoma larger than 2 cm in size carries a 50% chance of containing a cancer.
- Residual benign adenomatous tissue is found in most invasive colorectal cancers, suggesting progression of the cancer from the remaining benign cells to the predominant malignant ones.
- Benign polyps have been observed to develop into cancers. There have been reports of the direct observation of benign polyps that were not removed progressing over time into malignancies.
- Colonic adenomas occur more frequently in patients who have colorectal cancer. Almost one third of all patients with colorectal cancer will also have a benign colorectal polyp.
- Patients who develop adenomas have an increased lifetime risk for developing colorectal cancer.
- Removal of polyps decreases the incidence of cancer. Patients with small adenomas have a 2.3 times increased risk for cancer after the polyp is removed, compared with an eightfold increased incidence of colorectal cancer in patients with polyps who do not undergo polypectomy.
- Populations with a high risk for colorectal cancer also have a high prevalence of colorectal polyps.
- Patients with FAP will develop colorectal cancer almost 100% of the time in the absence of surgical intervention. The adenomas that characterize this syndrome are histologically the same as sporadic adenomas.
- The peak incidence for the discovery of benign colorectal polyps is 50 years of age. The peak incidence for the development of colorectal cancer is 60 years of age. This suggests a

10-year time span for the progression of an adenomatous polyp to a cancer. It has been estimated that a polyp larger than 1 cm in diameter has a cancer risk of 2.5% in 5 years, 8% in 10 years, and 24% in 20 years.

These observations and studies by molecular biologists have documented that colonic mucosa progresses through stages to the eventual development of an invasive cancer. Colonic epithelial cells lose the normal progression to maturity and cell death and begin proliferating in an increasingly uncontrolled manner. With this uncontrolled proliferation, the cells accumulate on the surface of the bowel lumen as a polyp. With more proliferation and increasing cellular disorganization, the cells extend though the muscularis mucosae to become invasive carcinoma. Even at this advanced stage, the process of colorectal carcinogenesis generally follows an orderly sequence of invasion of the muscularis mucosae, pericolic tissue, lymph nodes and, finally, distant metastasis (Figs. 52-51 and 52-52).

## Colorectal Polyps

A colorectal polyp is any mass projecting into the lumen of the bowel above the surface of the intestinal epithelium. Polyps arising from the intestinal mucosa are generally classified by their gross appearance as pedunculated (with a stalk; Fig. 52-53) or sessile (flat, without a stalk; Fig. 52-54). They are further classified by their histologic appearance as tubular adenoma (with branched tubular glands), villous adenoma (with long finger-like projections of the surface epithelium; Fig. 52-55), or tubulovillous adenoma (with elements of both cellular patterns). The most common benign polyp is the tubular adenoma, constituting approximately 65% to 80% of all polyps removed. Approximately 10% to 25% of polyps are tubulovillous and 5% to 10% are villous adenomas. Tubular adenomas are most often pedunculated; villous adenomas are more commonly sessile. The degree of cellular atypia is variable across the span of polyps, but there is generally less atypia in tubular adenomas, and severe atypia or dysplasia (precancerous cellular change) is found more often in villous adenomas. The incidence of invasive carcinoma being found in a polyp is dependent on the size and histologic type of the polyp. As noted, there is less than a 5% incidence of carcinoma in an adenomatous polyp smaller than 1 cm in diameter, whereas there is a 50% chance that a villous adenoma larger than 2 cm in diameter will contain a cancer.

The treatment of an adenomatous or villous polyp is removal, usually by colonoscopy. The presence of any polypoid lesion is an indication for a complete colonoscopy and polypectomy, if feasible. Polyps on a stalk are often removed by a snare passed through the colonoscope, whereas sessile (flat) polyps present technical problems with this method because of the danger of perforation associated with the snare technique. Although it may be feasible to elevate the sessile polyp from the underlying muscularis with saline injection, permitting subsequent endoscopic excision, sessile lesions often require segmental colectomy for complete removal (Fig. 52-56).

As noted, adenomatous polyps should be considered precursors of cancer and, when cancer arises in a polyp, careful consideration needs to be given to ensure the adequacy of treatment. Invasive carcinoma describes the situation in which malignant cells have extended through the muscularis mucosae of the polyp, whether it is a lesion on a stalk or a sessile lesion. Carcinoma confined to the muscularis mucosae does not metastasize and the cellular abnormalities should be described as

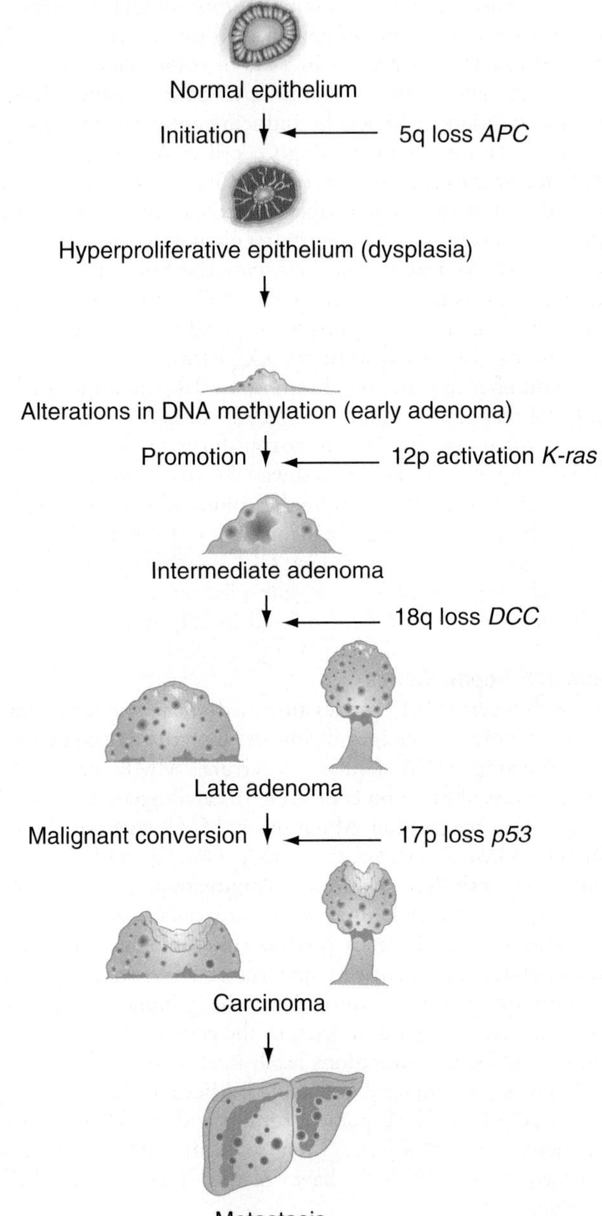


**FIGURE 52-51** Model of colorectal carcinogenesis. (Adapted from Corman ML [ed]: Colon and rectal surgery, ed 4, Philadelphia,1998, Lippincott-Raven, p 593.)

atypia. Complete excision of this type of polyp is adequate treatment.

If invasive carcinoma penetrates the muscularis mucosae, consideration of the risk for lymph node metastasis and local recurrence is required to determine whether a more extensive resection is required. Haggitt and colleagues have proposed a classification for polyps containing cancer according to the depth of invasion as follows (Fig. 52-57):

- Level 0: Carcinoma does not invade the muscularis mucosae (carcinoma-in-situ or intramucosal carcinoma).
- Level 1: Carcinoma invades through the muscularis mucosae into the submucosa but is limited to the head of the polyp.

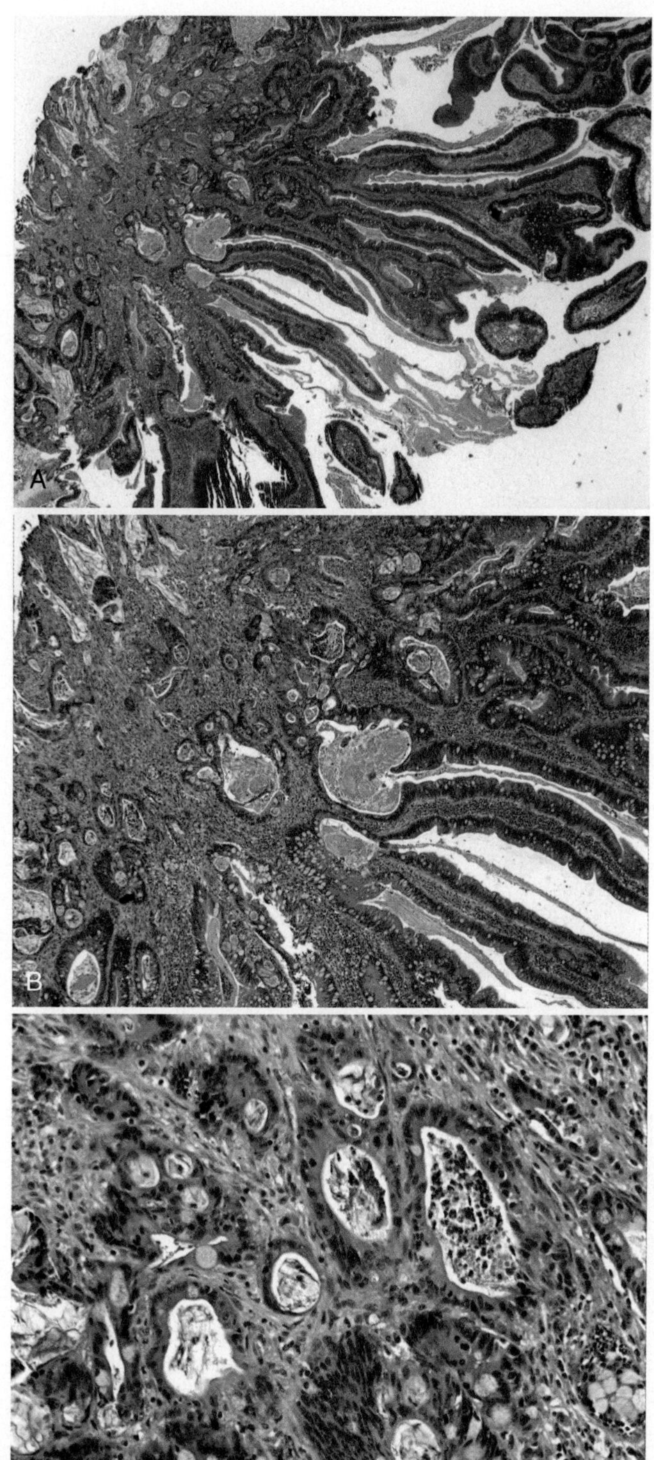


**FIGURE 52-52** Colon adenocarcinoma arising in an adenoma, microscopic appearance. **A,** Tubulovillous adenoma with finger-like projections *(right)* reveals a deeper area of infiltrating glands *(left).* **B,** Glands have penetrated the muscularis mucosa. **C,** On high power, neoplastic angulated glands with central dirty necrosis present within a desmoplastic stroma. (Courtesy Dr. Jeffrey P. Baliff, Thomas Jefferson University, Philadelphia.)

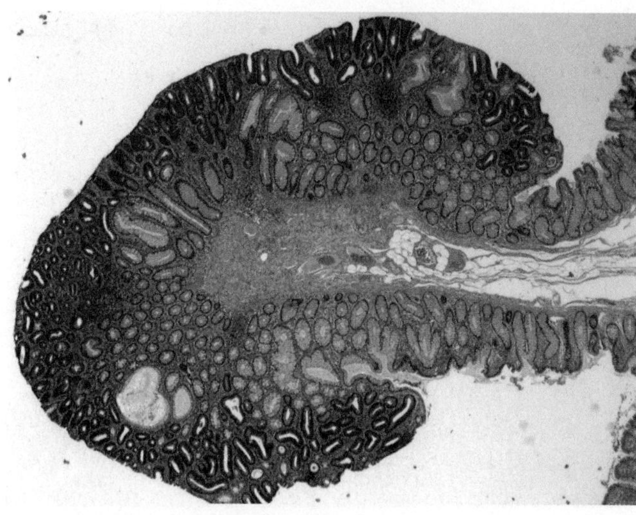

**FIGURE 52-53** Pedunculated adenomatous polyp, microscopic appearance. The head of the polyp is lined with dysplastic epithelium, whereas the stalk is lined with nondysplastic epithelium. (Courtesy Dr. Jeffrey P. Baliff, Thomas Jefferson University, Philadelphia.)

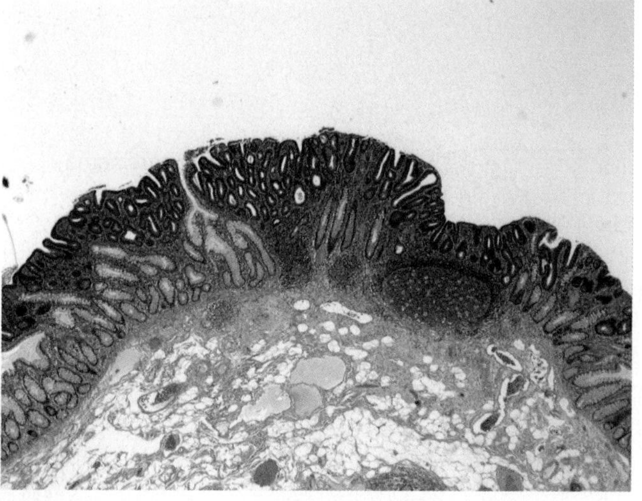

**FIGURE 52-54** Sessile adenomatous polyp, microscopic appearance. This tubular adenoma is called *sessile* because of its broad base, the preservation of the muscularis mucosae underneath, and the absence of a stalk. (Courtesy Dr. Jeffrey P. Baliff, Thomas Jefferson University, Philadelphia.)

- Level 2: Carcinoma invades the level of the neck of the polyp (junction between the head and stalk).
- Level 3: Carcinoma invades any part of the stalk.
- Level 4: Carcinoma invades into the submucosa of the bowel wall below the stalk of the polyp but above the muscularis propria.

By definition, all sessile polyps with invasive carcinoma are level 4 by Haggitt's criteria.

If a polyp contains a histologically poorly differentiated invasive carcinoma, or if there are cancer cells observed in the lymphovascular spaces, there is a more than a 10% chance of metastases and these lesions should be treated aggressively. A pedunculated polyp with invasion to levels 1, 2, and 3 has a low risk for lymph node metastasis or local recurrence and complete

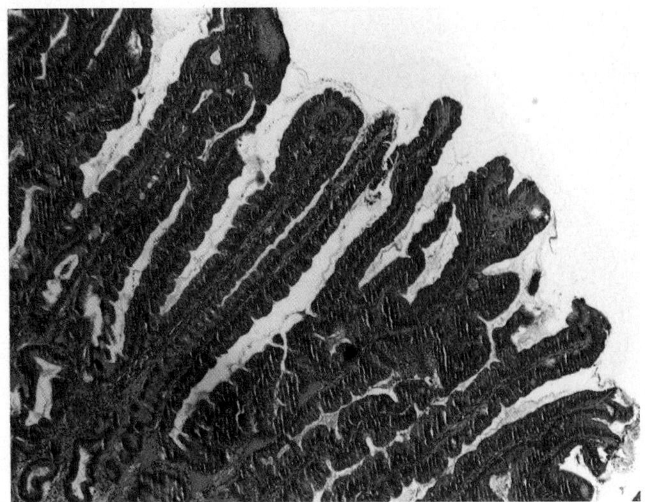

**FIGURE 52-55** Villous adenoma. This photomicrograph reveals the finger-like projections that give the appearance of villi. (Courtesy Dr. Jeffrey P. Baliff, Thomas Jefferson University, Philadelphia.)

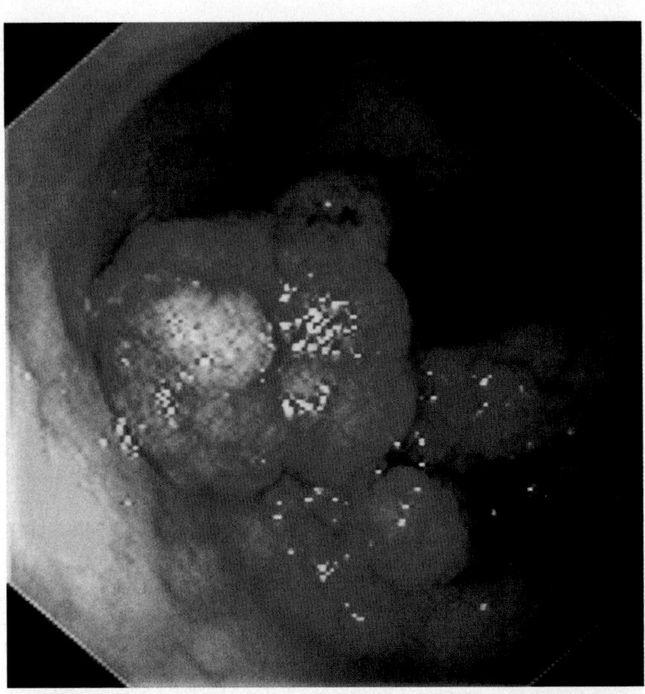

**FIGURE 52-56** Colonoscopic view of sessile polyp. This polyp proved to be a carcinoma after it was removed by segmental resection.

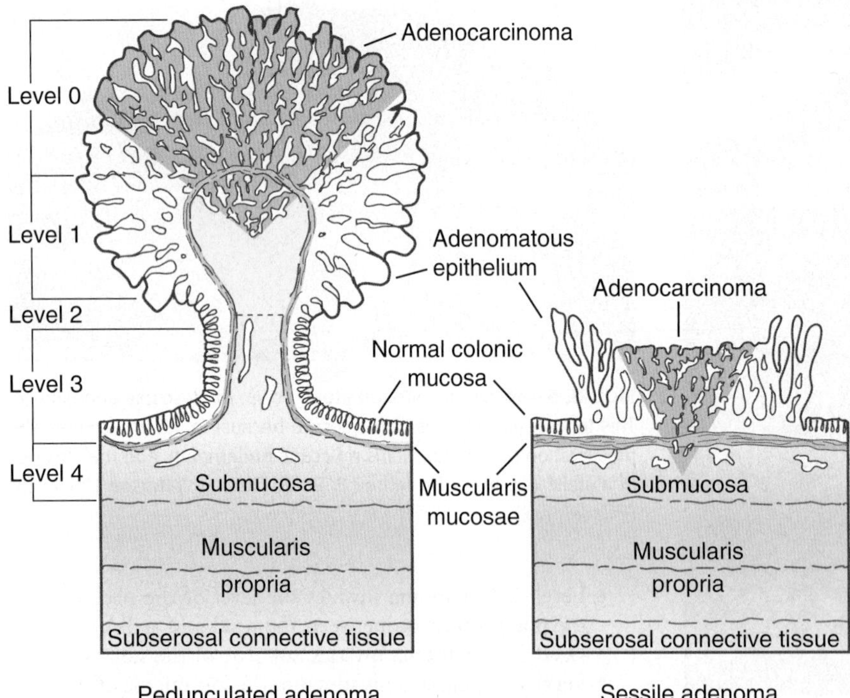


**FIGURE 52-57** Anatomic landmarks of pedunculated and sessile adenomas. (From Haggitt RC, Glotzbach RE, Soffer EE, et al: Prognostic factors in colorectal carcinoma arising in adenomas: Implications for lesions removed by endoscopic polypectomy. Gastroenterology 89:328–336, 1985.)

excision of the polyp is adequate if the poor prognostic factors mentioned earlier are absent. A sessile polyp containing invasive cancer has at least a 10% chance of metastasis to regional lymph nodes, but if the lesion is well or moderately differentiated, there is no lymphovascular invasion noted, and the lesion can be completely excised, the depth of invasion by the cancer may provide useful prognostic information. There is a high risk for lymph node and distant metastases associated with sessile cancers in the rectum, and these lesions should be treated aggressively.

Hyperplastic polyps are the most common colonic polyps but are usually small and composed of cells showing dysmaturation and hyperplasia. The small diminutive polyps have been regarded as benign in nature, with no neoplastic potential. The histologic appearance of these polyps is serrated (saw-toothed;

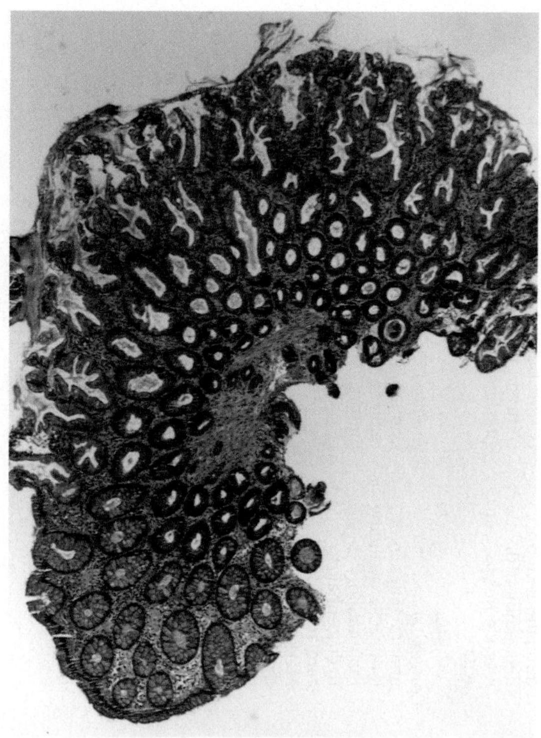

**FIGURE 52-58** Hyperplastic polyp. Elongated crypts reveal a serrated (saw-toothed) or star-shaped appearance. There is no epithelial dysplasia. (Courtesy Dr. Jeffrey P. Baliff, Thomas Jefferson University, Philadelphia.)

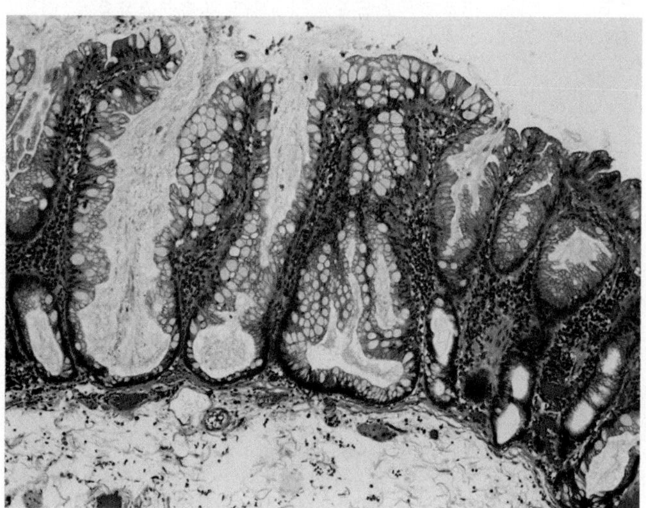

**FIGURE 52-59** Sessile serrated adenoma. This view shows basilar crypt dilation, epithelium proliferating in a serrated (saw-toothed) manner, and so-called *crypt architectural dysplasia* in the form of maloriented crypts, with one crypt extending horizontally. There is no cytologic dysplasia of the epithelium. (Courtesy Dr. Jeffrey P. Baliff, Thomas Jefferson University, Philadelphia.)

Figs. 52-58 and 52-59). Of these polyps, 90% are smaller than 3 mm in diameter, and these diminutive lesions are generally considered to have no malignant potential. However, adenomatous changes can be found in hyperplastic polyps, and therefore the polyps should be excised for histologic examination. These serrated adenomas have been observed to be associated with the development of cancers that predominate in the right side of the colon, more frequently in older women and smokers. They appear to be associated with the microsatellite instability characteristic of defects in DNA repair mechanisms.

## Hereditary Cancer Syndromes

Peutz-Jeghers syndrome is an autosomal dominant syndrome characterized by the combination of hamartomatous polyps of the intestinal tract and hyperpigmentation of the buccal mucosa, lips, and digits (Table 52-4). Germline defects in the tumor suppressor serine–threonine kinase 11 *(STK11)* gene are implicated in this rare autosomal dominant inherited disease. Although the syndrome was first described by Hutchinson in 1896, later separate descriptions by Peutz and then Jeghers in the 1940s brought recognition to the condition. The syndrome is associated with an increased (2% to 10%) risk for cancer of the intestinal tract, with cancers reported throughout the intestinal tract, from the stomach to the rectum. There is also an increased risk for extraintestinal malignancies, including cancer of the breast, ovary, cervix, fallopian tubes, thyroid, lung, gallbladder, bile ducts, pancreas, and testicles.

The polyps may cause bleeding or intestinal obstruction (from intussusception). If surgery is required for these symptoms, an attempt should be made to remove as many polyps as possible with the aid of intraoperative endoscopy and polypectomy. Any polyp that is larger than 1.5 cm should be removed if possible. It is reasonable to survey the colon endoscopically every 2 years, and patients should be screened periodically for malignancies of the breast, cervix, ovary, testicle, stomach, and pancreas.

Juvenile polyps are benign polyps composed of cystic dilations of glandular structures within the fibroblastic stroma of the lamina propria. They are relatively uncommon, yet may cause bleeding or intussusception. Therefore, the polyps should be treated by endoscopic removal.

Multiple polyposis coli is an autosomal dominant syndrome with high penetrance that carries an increased risk for both GI and extraintestinal cancer. The syndrome is usually discovered because of GI bleeding, intussusception, or hypoalbuminemia associated with protein loss through the intestine. The juvenile polyps in this syndrome are predominately hamartomas, but the hamartomas may contain adenomatous elements, and adenomatous polyps also are common. There is an increased cancer risk in afflicted individuals, with a malignant potential of at least 10% in patients with multiple juvenile polyps. Mutations in the tumor suppressor gene *SMAD4* are believed to cause up to 50% of reported cases.

In patients with relatively few juvenile polyps, endoscopic polypectomy should be carried out. However, patients with numerous polyps should be treated with abdominal colectomy, ileorectal anastomosis, and frequent endoscopic surveillance of the rectum. If the diffuse form of polyposis involves the rectal mucosa, consideration should be given to restorative proctocolectomy with IPAA.

FAP is the prototypical hereditary polyposis syndrome. The discovery of the gene responsible for the transmission of the disease, the *APC* gene, located on chromosome 5q21, lagged behind the first descriptions of cases of FAP by an entire century. In 1863, Virchow reported a 15-year-old boy with multiple colonic polyps. In 1882, Cripps described the occurrence of

**Table 52-4 Hereditary Cancer Syndromes**

| | Hereditary Adenomatous Polyposis Syndromes | | Hereditary Hamartomatous Polyposis Syndromes | | | |
|---|---|---|---|---|---|---|
| **HEREDITARY NONPOLYPOSIS COLON CANCER** | **FAMILIAL ADENOMATOUS POLYPOSIS (FAP)/ GARDNER'S SYNDROME** | **TURCOT'S SYNDROME** | **COWDEN'S DISEASE** | **FAMILIAL JUVENILE POLYPOSIS** | **PEUTZ-JEGHERS SYNDROME** | **RUVALCABA-MYHRE-SMITH SYNDROME (BANNAYAN-ZONANA SYNDROME)** |
| **GI Features** | | | | | | |
| Small number of colorectal polyps | Hundreds to thousands of colorectal polyps; duodenal adenomas and gastric polyps, usually fundic gland | Colorectal polyps, which may be few or resemble classic FAP | Polyps most commonly of colon and stomach | Juvenile polyps mostly in colon but throughout GI tract; defined by ≥10 juvenile polyps | Small number of polyps throughout GI tract but most common in small intestine | Hamartomatous GI polyps, usually lipomas, hemangiomas, or lymphangiomas |
| **Other Clinical Features** | | | | | | |
| Muir-Torre variant: sebaceous adenomas, keratoacanthomas, sebaceous epitheliomas, and basal cell epitheliomas | Osteomas, desmoid tumors, epidermoid cysts, and congenital hypertrophy of retinal epithelium | Brain tumors, including cerebellar medulloblastoma and glioblastomas | Mucocutaneous lesions, thyroid adenomas and goiter, fibroadenomas and fibrocystic disease of the breast, uterine leiomyomas, macrocephaly | Congenital abnormalities in at least 20%, including malrotation, hydrocephalus, cardiac lesions, Meckel's diverticulum, mesenteric lymphangioma | Pigmented lesions of skin; benign and malignant genital tumors | Dysmorphic facial features, macrocephaly, seizures, intellectual impairment, pigmented macules of shaft and glans of penis |
| **Malignancy Risk** | | | | | | |
| 70%-80% lifetime risk for colorectal cancer; 30%-60% lifetime risk for endometrial cancer; ↑ risk for ovarian cancer, gastric carcinoma, transitional cell carcinoma of the ureters and renal pelvis, small bowel cancer, and sebaceous carcinomas | Colorectal cancer risk approaches 100%; ↑ risk for periampullary malignancy, thyroid carcinoma, central nervous system tumors, hepatoblastoma | Colorectal carcinoma and brain tumors | 10% risk for thyroid cancer and up to 50% risk for adenocarcinoma of breast in affected women | 9% to 25% risk for colorectal cancer; ↑ risk for gastric, duodenal, and pancreatic cancer | ↑ risk for GI malignancy and pancreatic cancer and adenoma malignum of cervix; unknown risk for breast cancer | Malignant GI tumors identified but lifetime risk for malignancy unknown |

| | | | | | | |
|---|---|---|---|---|---|---|
| **Screening Recommendations** | | | | | | |
| Colonoscopy at age 20-25 yr; repeat every 1-3 yr; transvaginal ultrasound or endometrial aspirate at age 20-25 yr; repeat annually (expert opinion only) | Flexible procto-sigmoidoscopy at age 10-12 yr; repeat every 1-2 yr until age 35; after age 35 repeat every 3 yr; upper GI endoscopy every 1-3 yr starting when polyps first identified | Same as for FAP; also consider imaging of the brain | Annual physical examination with special attention to thyroid; mammography at age 30 or 5 yr before earliest breast cancer case in the family; routine colon cancer surveillance (expert opinion only) | Screening by age 12 yr if symptoms have not yet arisen; colonoscopy with multiple random biopsies every several years (expert opinion only) | Upper GI endoscopy, small bowel radiography, colonoscopy every 2 yr; pancreatic ultrasound and hemoglobin levels annually; gynecologic examination, cervical smear, pelvic ultrasound annually; clinical breast examination and mammography at age 25 yr; clinical testicular examination and testicular ultrasound in males with feminizing features (expert opinion only) | No known published recommendations |
| **Genetic Basis** | | | | | | |
| AD | AD | AD | AD | AD inheritance in some families | AD | AD |
| *MLH1* (chromosome 3p)<br>*MSH2* (chromosome 2p)<br>*MSH6/GTMP* (chromosome 2p) | *APC* (chromosome 5q) | *APC* mutations identified predominantly in families with cerebellar medullo-blastoma | *PTEN* (chromosome 10q) | Subset of families with mutation in *SMAD4 (DRC4)* (chromosome 10q) | *STK11* (chromosome 19p) | *PTEN* (chromosome 10q) in some |
| *PMS1* (chromosome 2q)<br>*PMS2* (chromosome 7q) | | *MLH1, PMS2* mutations identified in families with predominance of glioblastomas | | | | |
| **Genetic Testing** | | | | | | |
| Clinical testing of *MLH1* and *MSH2* genes available | Clinical testing of *APC* gene available | Clinical testing of *APC* and *MLH1* genes available | Research testing of *PTEN* gene available | Families being collected for research studies only | Research testing of *STK11* gene available | Research testing of *PTEN* gene available |

*AD,* Autosomal dominant; *GI,* gastrointestinal; ↑, increased.

numerous colonic polyps in multiple family members. In 1927, Cockayne demonstrated that FAP was genetically transmitted in an autosomal dominant fashion. Dukes was the first to establish some form of a familial tumor registry, which he reported with Lockhart-Mummery in 1930. Throughout the 20th century, many reports described various extraintestinal manifestations associated with FAP. In 1986, Lemuel Herrera demonstrated that the underlying genetic abnormality was a mutation in the *APC* gene.

The common expression of the syndrome is the invariable presence of multiple colonic polyps, frequent occurrence of gastric, duodenal, and periampullary polyps, and occasional association of extraintestinal manifestations, including epidermoid cysts, desmoid tumors in the abdomen, osteomas, and brain tumors. Gastric and duodenal polyps occur in approximately 50% of affected individuals. Most of the gastric polyps represent fundic gland hyperplasia, rather than adenomatous polyps, and have limited malignant potential. However, duodenal polyps are adenomatous in nature and should be considered premalignant. Patients with FAP have an increased risk for ampullary cancer. Adenomatous polyps and cancer have also been found in the jejunum and ileum of patients with FAP. Rare extraintestinal malignancies in FAP patients include cancers of the extrahepatic bile ducts, gallbladder, pancreas, adrenals, thyroid, and liver. An interesting marker for FAP is CHRPE, which can be detected by indirect ophthalmoscopy in approximately 75% of affected individuals.

The gene is expressed in 100% of patients with the mutation. Autosomal dominance results in expression in 50% of offspring. There is a negative family history in 10% to 20% of affected individuals, who apparently acquire the syndrome as the result of a spontaneous mutation. All patients with the defective gene will develop cancer of the colon if left untreated. The average age of discovery of a new patient with FAP is 29 years. The average age of a patient who is newly discovered to have colorectal cancer related to FAP is 39 years. Eponymous polyposis syndromes now recognized to belong to the general disorder of FAP include Gardner's syndrome (colonic polyps, epidermal inclusion cysts, osteomas) and Turcot's syndrome (colonic polyps, brain tumors).

Osteomas usually present as visible and palpable prominences in the skull, mandible, and tibia of individuals with FAP. They are almost always benign. Radiographs of the maxilla and mandible may reveal bone cysts, supernumerary and impacted molars, or congenitally absent teeth. Desmoid tumors can present in the retroperitoneum and abdominal wall of affected patients, usually after surgery. These tumors seldom metastasize but are often locally invasive; direct invasion of the mesenteric vessels, ureters, or walls of the small intestine can result in death.

Surgical treatment of patients with FAP is directed at removal of all affected colonic and rectal mucosa. Restorative proctocolectomy with IPAA has become the most commonly recommended operation. The procedure is usually accompanied by a distal rectal mucosectomy to ensure that all premalignant colonic mucosa is removed, and the IPAA is fashioned between the ileal pouch and dentate line of the anal canal. Patients who undergo this procedure for FAP have a better functional result than patients similarly treated for ulcerative colitis, in that the incidence of inflammation in the ileal pouch (pouchitis) is much lower in patients with FAP than in patients with ulcerative colitis.

An alternative approach, total abdominal colectomy with ileorectal anastomosis, was used extensively before the development of the technique of IPAA and has certain advantages. If an FAP patient has relatively few polyps in the rectum, consideration may be given to this option. The abdominal colon is resected and an anastomosis fashioned between the ileum and rectum. It is technically a simpler operation to perform and the pelvic dissection is avoided. This eliminates the potential complication of injury to the autonomic nerves that could result in impotence. In addition, there is theoretically less risk for anastomotic leak from the relatively simple ileorectal anastomosis fashioned in the peritoneal cavity, compared with the long suture (or staple) lines required to form the ileal pouch and then fashion the anastomosis between the ileal pouch and anus.

An additional argument in favor of abdominal colectomy and ileorectal anastomosis is the observation that sulindac and celecoxib have been observed to cause the regression of adenomatous polyps in some patients with FAP. The disadvantages are that the rectum remains at high risk for the formation of new precancerous polyps, a proctoscopic examination is required every 6 months to detect and destroy any new polyps, and there is a definite increased risk for cancer arising in the rectum with the passage of time.

It has been suggested that genetic testing may help make the decision between restorative proctocolectomy with IPAA and abdominal colectomy with ileorectal anastomosis. It has been observed that the risk for rectal cancer is almost three times higher in FAP patients with a mutation after codon 1250 than in patients with mutations before this codon. This may influence the decision to offer abdominal colectomy with ileorectal anastomosis to those whose mutation occurs proximal to codon 1250 if proctoscopic examination reveals no or few polyps in the rectum.

Patients who choose to be treated by abdominal colectomy with ileorectal anastomosis should realize that the risk for developing rectal cancer is real and has been shown to be 4%, 5.6%, 7.9%, and 25% at 5, 10, 15, and 20 years after the operation, respectively. Even though sulindac and celecoxib can produce partial regression of polyps, semiannual surveillance of the rectal mucosa is required, and approximately one third of patients treated by abdominal colectomy and ileorectal anastomosis develop florid polyposis of the rectum that will require proctectomy (and ileostomy or IPAA) within 20 years.

As noted, polyps of the stomach and duodenum are not uncommon in patients with FAP. The gastric polyps are usually hyperplastic and do not require surgical removal. However, the duodenal and ampullary polyps are generally neoplastic and require attention. A reasonable surveillance program is for upper GI surveillance every 2 years after the age of 30 years and endoscopic polypectomy, if possible, to remove all large adenomas from the duodenum. If numerous polyps are identified, the endoscopy obviously should be repeated with greater frequency. If an ampullary cancer is discovered at an early stage, pancreatoduodenectomy (Whipple procedure) is indicated.

The abdominal desmoid tumor can be an especially vexing and difficult extraintestinal manifestation of FAP. After surgical procedures, dense fibrous tissue forms in the mesentery of the small intestine or within the abdominal wall in some patients with FAP. If the mesentery is involved, the intestine can be tethered or invaded directly by the tumor. The locally invasive tumor can also encroach on the vascular supply to the intestine. Small desmoid tumors confined to the abdominal wall are appropriately treated by resection, but the surgical treatment of mesenteric desmoids is dangerous and generally futile. There have been sporadic reports of regression of desmoid tumors after treatment with sulindac, tamoxifen, low-dose methotrexate, radiation, and various types of chemotherapy. The initial treatment is usually with sulindac or tamoxifen.

The ability to identify the genetic mutation in most patients with FAP—although the mutation may not be identified in as many as 20% of patients with a well-documented, transmissible FAP syndrome—permits a method of screening family members at risk for inheriting the mutation. It is imperative that the *APC* mutation be clearly identified in the DNA of a family member known to have the disease. The DNA of other family members can then be analyzed directly, requiring only a venipuncture. If the analysis demonstrates noninheritance of a mutated *APC* gene, the individual can avoid annual endoscopic screening and should require only an occasional colonoscopy.

HNPCC is the most frequently occurring hereditary colorectal cancer syndrome in the United States and Western Europe. It accounts for approximately 3% of all cases of colorectal cancer and for approximately 15% of these cancers in patients with a family history of colorectal cancer. Dr. Alder S. Warthin, Chairman of Pathology at the University of Michigan, initially recognized this hereditary syndrome in 1985. Dr. Warthin's seamstress prophesied that she would die of cancer because of her strong family history of endometrial, gastric, and colon cancer. Dr. Warthin's investigations of her family's medical records revealed a pattern of autosomal dominant transmission of the cancer risk. This family (family G) has been further studied and characterized by Dr. Henry Lynch, who described the prominent features of the syndrome, including onset of cancer at a relative young age (mean, 44 years), proximal distribution (70% of cancers located in the right colon), predominance of mucinous or poorly differentiated (signet cell) adenocarcinoma, increased number of synchronous and metachronous cancers and, despite all these poor prognostic indicators, a relatively good outcome after surgery. Two hereditary syndromes were initially described. Lynch I syndrome is characterized by cancer of the proximal colon occurring at a relatively young age; Lynch II syndrome is characterized by families at risk for both colorectal and extracolonic cancers, including cancers of endometrial, ovarian, gastric, small intestinal, pancreatic, and ureteral and renal pelvic origin.

Before the genetic mechanisms underlying the Lynch syndromes were understood, the syndromes were defined by the Amsterdam Criteria, which required three criteria for the diagnosis:

1. Colorectal cancer in three family members (first-degree relatives)
2. Involvement of at least two generations
3. At least one affected individual being younger than 50 years at the time of diagnosis

These requirements were recognized as being too restrictive, and the modified Amsterdam Criteria expanded the cancers to be included to not only colorectal but also endometrial, ovarian, gastric, pancreatic, small intestinal, ureteral, and renal pelvic cancers. Further liberalization for identifying patients with HNPCC occurred with the introduction of the Bethesda criteria (Box 52-4).

**BOX 52-4 Clinical Criteria for Hereditary Nonpolyposis Colorectal Cancer**

**Amsterdam Criteria**

At least three relatives with colon cancer and all of the following:

- One affected person is a first-degree relative of the other two affected persons
- Two successive generations affected
- At least one case of colon cancer diagnosed before age 50 yr
- FAP excluded

**Modified Amsterdam Criteria**

Same as the Amsterdam criteria, except that cancer must be associated with HNPCC (colon, endometrium, small bowel, ureter, renal pelvis) instead of specifically colon cancer

**Bethesda Criteria**

The Amsterdam criteria or one of the following:

- Two cases of HNPCC-associated cancer in one patient, including synchronous or metachronous cancer
- Colon cancer and a first-degree relative with HNPCC-associated cancer and/or colonic adenoma (one case of cancer diagnosed before age 45 yr and adenoma diagnosed before age 40 yr)
- Colon or endometrial cancer diagnosed before age 45 yr
- Right-sided colon cancer that has an undifferentiated pattern (solid, cribriform) or signet-cell histopathologic characteristics diagnosed before age 45 yr
- Adenomas diagnosed before age 40 yr

Molecular biologists have demonstrated that the increased cancer risk in these syndromes is caused by malfunction of the DNA repair mechanism. Specific genes that have been shown to be responsible for the syndrome include *hMSH2* (located on chromosome 2p21), *hMLH1* (3p21), *hMSH6* (2p16-21), and *hPMS2* (7p21). A mutation in *hMSH2* has been shown to be responsible for the cancer prevalence in cancer family G. Mutations in *hMSH2* or *hMLH1* account for more than 90% of identifiable mutations in patients with HNPCC. The initially reported difference in the types of cancers in Lynch I and II syndromes cannot be accounted for by mutations in specific MMR genes. The cancer family syndrome involving *hMSH6* is characterized by an increased incidence of endometrial carcinoma.

The mainstay of the diagnosis of HNPCC is a detailed family history. Still, it should be remembered that as many as 20% of newly discovered cases of HNPCC are caused by spontaneous germline mutations, so a family history may not accurately reflect the genetic nature of the syndrome. Colorectal cancer, or an HNPCC-related cancer, arising in a person younger than 50 years should raise the suspicion of this syndrome. Genetic counseling and genetic testing can be offered. If the individual proves to have HNPCC by identification of a mutation in one of the known MMR genes, then other family members can be tested after obtaining genetic counseling. However, failure to identify a causative MMR gene mutation in a patient with a suggestive history does not exclude the diagnosis of HNPCC. In as many as 50% of patients with a family history

**Table 52-5 Screening Recommendations for Familial Adenomatous Polyposis and Hereditary Nonpolyposis Colorectal Cancer**

| LIFETIME CANCER RISK | SCREENING RECOMMENDATIONS |
|---|---|
| **FAP** | |
| Colorectal cancer, 100% | Colonoscopy annually, beginning age 10-12 yr |
| Duodenal or periampullary cancer, 5%-10% | Upper GI endoscopy every 1-3 yr, beginning age 20-25 yr |
| Pancreatic cancer, 2% | Possible periodic abdominal ultrasound |
| Thyroid cancer, 2% | Annual thyroid examination |
| Gastric cancer, <1% | Upper GI endoscopy as for duodenal and periampullary |
| Central nervous system cancer, <1% | Annual physical examination |
| **HNPCC** | |
| Colorectal cancer, 80% | Colonoscopy, every 2 yr beginning age 20 yr, annually after age 40 yr or 10 yr younger than earliest case in family |
| Endometrial cancer, 40%-60% | Pelvic examination, transvaginal ultrasound, endometrial aspirate every 1-2 yr, beginning age 25-35 yr |
| Upper urinary tract cancer, 4%-10% | Ultrasound and urinalysis every 1-2 yr; start at age 30-35 yr |
| Gallbladder and biliary cancer, 2%-18% | No recommendation |
| Central nervous system cancer, <5% | No recommendation |
| Small bowel cancer, <5% | No recommendation |

that clearly demonstrates HNPCC-type transmission of cancer susceptibility, DNA testing will fail to identify the causative gene.

The management of patients with HNPCC is somewhat controversial, but the need for close surveillance in patients known to carry the mutation is obvious. It is usually recommended that a program of surveillance colonoscopy should begin at the age of 20 years. Colonoscopy is repeated every 2 years until the age of 35 years, and then annually thereafter. In women, periodic vacuum curettage is begun at age 25 years, as are pelvic ultrasound and determination of CA-125 levels. Annual tests for occult blood in the urine should also be carried out because of the risk for ureteral and renal pelvic cancer (Table 52-5).

It has been shown that annual colonoscopy and removal of polyps, when found, will decrease the incidence of colon cancer in patients with HNPCC. However, there have been well-documented cases of invasive colon cancers occurring 1 year after a negative colonoscopy. It is obvious that the slow evolution from benign polyp to invasive cancer is not a feature of the pathogenesis in HNPCC patients, and this phenomenon of accelerated carcinogenesis mandates frequent (annual) colonoscopic examinations. Even with annual colonoscopic examinations, there is a documented risk for colon cancer but, when a cancer arises while the patient is under a vigorous surveillance program, the cancer stage is usually favorable (Fig. 52-60).

When colon cancer is detected in a patient with HNPCC, an abdominal colectomy–ileorectal anastomosis is the procedure of choice. If the patient is a woman with no further plans for childbearing, a prophylactic total abdominal hysterectomy and bilateral salpingo-oophorectomy are recommended. The rectum remains at risk for the development of cancer and annual proctoscopic examinations are mandatory after abdominal colectomy. Other forms of cancer associated with HNPCC are treated according to the same criteria as for nonhereditary cases. The role of prophylactic colectomy for patients with HNPCC has been considered in some cases, but this has not received universal acceptance. It is an interesting but well-documented fact that the prognosis is better for cancer patients with HNPCC than for non-HNPCC patients with cancer of the same stage.

## Sporadic Colon Cancer

It is important to recognize the increased risk for cancer in patients with hereditary cancer syndromes, but the most common form of colorectal cancer is sporadic in nature, without an associated strong family history.

Although the cause and pathogenesis of adenocarcinoma are similar throughout the large bowel, significant differences in the use of diagnostic and therapeutic modalities separate colonic from rectal cancers. This distinction is largely because of the confinement of the rectum by the bony pelvis. The limited mobility of the rectum allows MRI to generate better images and increases its sensitivity. In addition, the proximity of the rectum to the anus permits easy access of ultrasound probes for more accurate assessment of the extent of penetration of the bowel wall and the involvement of adjacent lymph nodes. The limited accessibility of the rectum, proximity to the anal sphincter, and close association with the autonomic nerves supplying the bladder and genitalia require special and unique consideration when planning treatment for cancer of the rectum. Therefore, colon and rectal adenocarcinomas are discussed separately.

The signs and symptoms of colon cancer are varied, nonspecific, and somewhat dependent on the location of the tumor in the colon, as well as the extent of constriction of the lumen caused by the cancer. In the past 4 decades, the incidence of cancer in the right colon has increased in comparison to cancer arising in the left colon and rectum. This is an important consideration, in that at least 50% of all colon cancers are located proximal to the area that can be visualized by the flexible sigmoidoscope. Colorectal cancers can bleed, causing red blood to appear in the stool (hematochezia). Bleeding from right-sided colon tumors can produce dark tarry stools (melena). Often, the bleeding is asymptomatic and detected only by anemia discovered by a routine hemoglobin determination. Iron deficiency anemia in any male or nonmenstruating female should lead to a search for a source of bleeding from the GI tract. Bleeding is often associated with colon cancer but, in approximately one third of patients with a proven colon cancer, the hemoglobin level is normal and the stool test results are negative for occult blood.

Cancers located in the left colon are often constrictive in nature. Patients with left-sided colon cancers may notice a change in bowel habit, most often reported as increasing constipation. Sigmoid cancers can mimic diverticulitis, presenting with pain, fever, and obstructive symptoms. At least 20% of patients with sigmoid cancer also have diverticular disease, making the correct diagnosis difficult at times. Sigmoid cancers

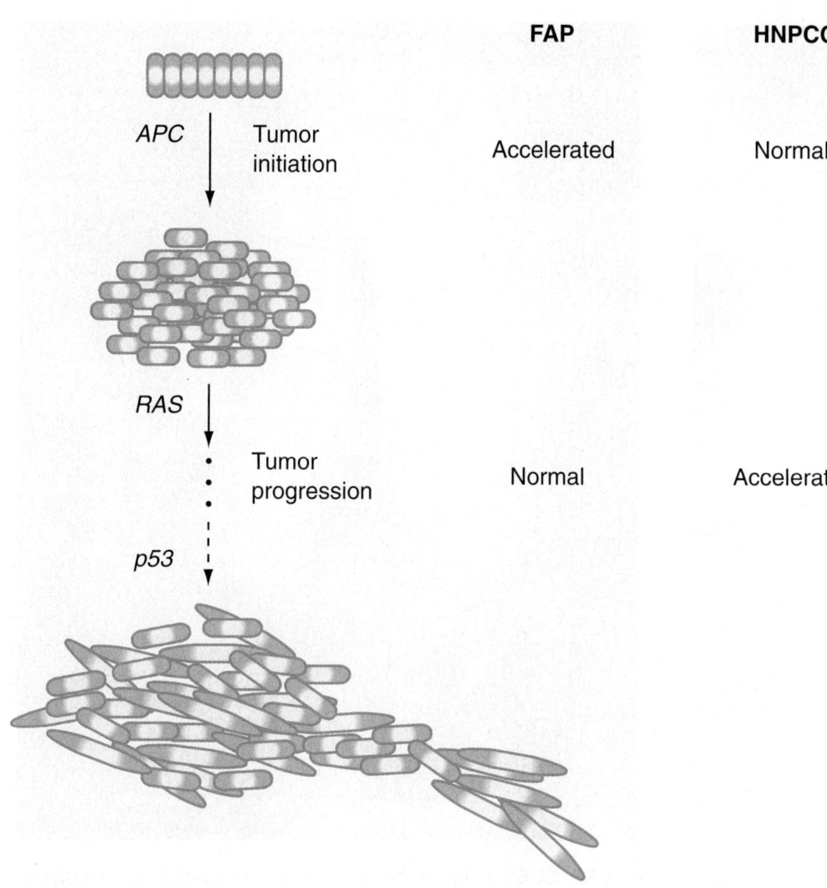


**FIGURE 52-60** Comparison of the development of cancer in FAP and HNPCC patients. (From Kinzler KW, Vogelstein B: Lessons from hereditary colorectal cancer. Cell 87:159–170, 1966.)

can also cause colovesical or colovaginal fistulas. Such fistulas are more commonly caused by diverticulitis, but it is imperative that the correct diagnosis be established because the treatment of colon cancer is substantially different than treatment of diverticulitis.

Cancers in the right colon more often present with melena, fatigue associated with anemia or, if the tumor is advanced, abdominal pain. Although obstructive symptoms are usually associated with cancers of the left colon, any advanced colorectal cancer can cause a change in bowel habits and intestinal obstruction (Figs. 52-61 and 52-62).

Colonoscopy is the gold standard for establishing the diagnosis of colon cancer. It permits biopsy of the tumor to verify the diagnosis while allowing inspection of the entire colon to exclude metachronous polyps or cancers; the incidence of a synchronous cancer is approximately 3%. Colonoscopy is generally performed even after a cancer is detected by barium enema to obtain a biopsy and to detect (and remove) small polyps that may be missed by the contrast study (Fig. 52-63).

In patients with tumors causing complete obstruction, the diagnosis is best established by resection of the tumor without the benefit of preoperative colonoscopy. A water-soluble contrast enema is often useful in such circumstances to establish the anatomic level of the obstruction. Primary anastomosis between the proximal colon and the colon distal to the tumor has been avoided in the past in the presence of obstruction because of a high risk for anastomotic leak associated with this approach. Thus, such patients were usually treated by resection of the segment of colon containing the obstructing cancer, suture closure of the distal sigmoid or rectum, and constructing a colostomy (Hartmann's operation). Intestinal continuity could be reestablished later, after the colon had been cleansed with purgatives, by taking down the colostomy and fashioning a colorectal anastomosis.

Alternatives to this approach have been to resect the segment of left colon containing the cancer and then cleanse the remaining colon with saline lavage by inserting a catheter through the appendix or ileum into the cecum and irrigating the contents from the colon. A primary anastomosis between the prepared colon and rectum can then be fashioned without the need for a temporary colostomy. A third approach occasionally used for obstructing cancers of the sigmoid colon is to resect the tumor and the entire colon proximal to the tumor and fashion an anastomosis between the ileum and distal sigmoid colon (subtotal colectomy and ileosigmoid anastomosis). This approach has the advantage of avoiding a temporary colostomy and eliminating the need to search for synchronous lesions in the colon proximal to the cancer. However, patients treated by this approach may have more frequent bowel movements.

More recently, endoscopic techniques have been developed that permit the placement of a stent introduced with the aid of a colonoscope that traverses the obstructed tumor and expands, re-creating a lumen, relieving the obstruction, and permitting a bowel preparation and elective operation with primary colorectal anastomosis.

The approaches discussed concern obstruction of the left colon. Complete obstruction of the right colon or cecum by cancer occurs less frequently. These patients present with signs and symptoms of a small bowel obstruction. If an obstruction of the proximal colon is suspected, a water-soluble contrast study

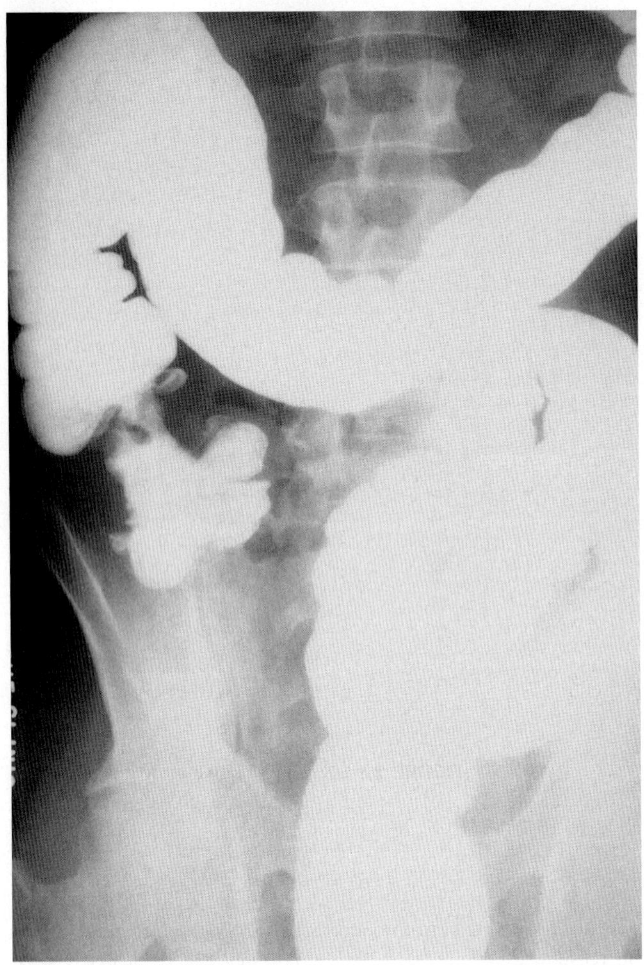

**FIGURE 52-61** X-ray of barium enema barium enema demonstrating apple core or napkin ring lesion caused by a constricting carcinoma.

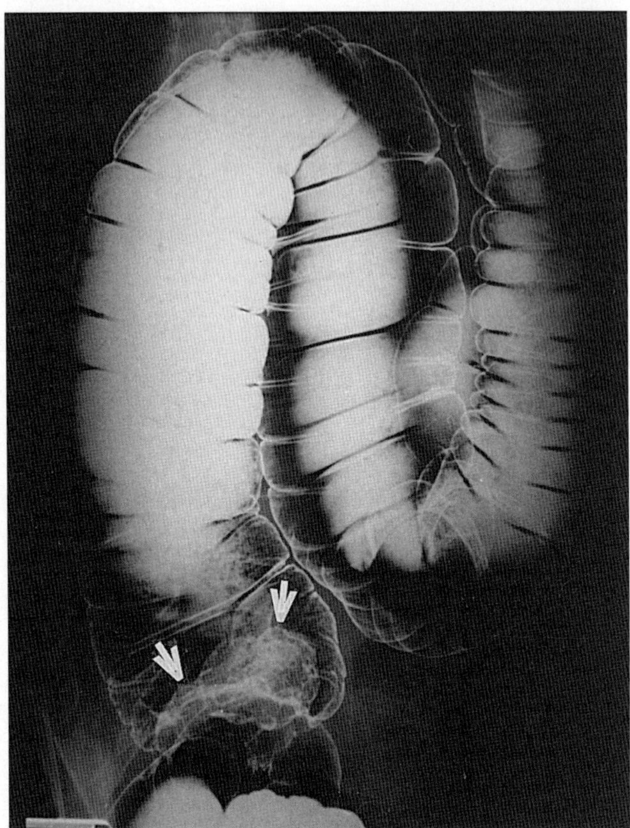

**FIGURE 52-62** X-ray of barium enema demonstrating a polypoid carcinoma arising in the cecum of a 35-year-old woman (*arrows*). (Courtesy Dr. Dina F. Caroline, Temple University Hospital, Philadelphia.)

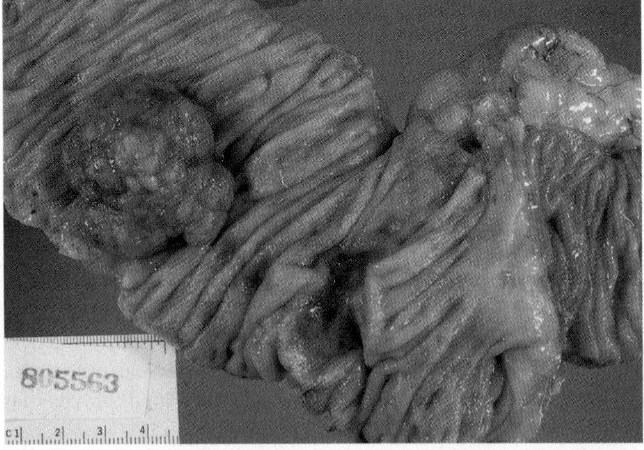


**FIGURE 52-63** Resected right colon containing large benign sessile polyp adjacent to an ulcerated carcinoma.

is useful to verify the diagnosis and evaluate the distal colon for the presence of a synchronous lesion. Obstructing cancer of the proximal colon is treated by right colectomy, with primary anastomosis between the ileum and transverse colon.

Patients with tumors that are not obstructing should undergo a thorough evaluation for metastatic disease. This includes a thorough physical examination, chest x-ray, liver function tests, and measurement of the carcinoembryonic antigen (CEA) level. Most surgeons now perform CT or MRI to inspect the liver more thoroughly for metastases and search for other intra-abdominal pathology.

The presence of hepatic metastatic disease does not preclude surgical excision of the primary tumor. Unless the hepatic metastatic disease is extensive, excising the primary cancer can provide excellent palliation. Bleeding and obstruction caused by the tumor can be avoided and, if the metastatic disease in the liver is resectable, the patient may yet be cured.

The objective of surgery for colon adenocarcinoma is the removal of the primary cancer with adequate margins, regional lymphadenectomy, and restoration of the continuity of the GI tract by anastomosis. The extent of resection is determined by the location of the cancer, its blood supply and draining lymphatic system, and presence or absence of direct extension into adjacent organs. It is important to resect the lymphatics, which parallel the arterial supply, to the greatest extent possible in an attempt to render the abdomen free of lymphatic metastases. If hepatic metastases are subsequently detected, they may still be resected for cure in some cases if the abdominal disease has been completely eradicated.

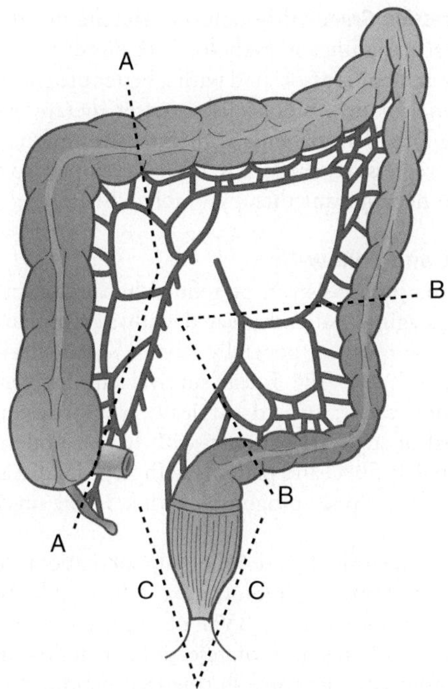


**FIGURE 52-64** Operative procedures for right-sided colon cancer, sigmoid diverticulitis, and low-lying rectal cancer. **A,** Right hemicolectomy involves resection of a few centimeters of terminal ileum and colon up to the division of the middle colic vessels into right and left segments. **B,** Sigmoidectomy consists of removing the colon between the partially retroperitoneal descending colon and the rectum. **C,** Abdominoperineal resection of the rectum is performed in a combined approach through the abdomen and through the perineum for the resection of the entire rectum and anus.

To restore the continuity of the GI tract, an anastomosis is fashioned with sutures or staples, joining the ends of the intestine (small or large). It is important that both segments of the intestine used for the anastomosis have an excellent blood supply and that there be no tension on the anastomosis. For lesions involving the cecum, ascending colon, and hepatic flexure, a right hemicolectomy is the procedure of choice. This involves removal of the bowel from 4 to 6 cm proximal to the ileocecal valve to the portion of the transverse colon supplied by the right branch of the middle colic artery (Fig. 52-64). An anastomosis is fashioned between the terminal ileum and transverse colon. An extended right hemicolectomy is the procedure of choice for most transverse colon lesions; this involves division of the right and middle colic arteries at their origin, with removal of the right and transverse colon supplied by these vessels. The anastomosis is fashioned between the terminal ileum and proximal left colon. A left hemicolectomy (resection from the splenic flexure to the rectosigmoid junction) is the procedure of choice for tumors of the descending colon, whereas a sigmoidectomy is appropriate for tumors of the sigmoid colon. Most surgeons prefer to avoid incorporating the proximal sigmoid colon into an anastomosis because of the often tenuous blood supply from the IMA and frequent involvement of the sigmoid colon with diverticular disease.

Abdominal colectomy (sometimes called *subtotal colectomy* or *total colectomy*) entails removal of the entire colon from the ileum to the rectum, with continuity restored by an ileorectal anastomosis. Because of loss of the absorptive and storage capacity of the colon, this procedure causes an increase in stool frequency. Patients younger than 60 years generally tolerate this well, with gradual adaptation of the small bowel mucosa, increased water absorption, and an acceptable stool frequency of one to three movements daily. In older individuals, however, abdominal colectomy may result in significant chronic diarrhea. Abdominal colectomy is indicated for patients with multiple primary tumors, for individuals with HNPCC, and occasionally for those with completely obstructing sigmoid cancers.

The chances that the patient has been cured by an operation performed to remove a colorectal cancer is dependent on several factors. These include technical aspects of the operation, such as the complete removal of all tumor, certain biologic properties of the cancer that are poorly understood, and stage of the disease.

Staging may be defined as the process whereby objective data are assembled to try to define the state of progression of the disease. Separate items of data are summated to provide a designated stage for an individual patient's disease, from which inferences may be drawn regarding the relative likelihood of residual disease and hence the chance of cure without further treatment and the advisability of considering further treatment. The ideal staging system would provide one ultimately important and simple item of information. Has the operation cured the patient, or will he or she die unless further intervention prevents it? Thus, there would be only two categories, those who are cured and those destined to die of their disease. Unfortunately, no current system even remotely approaches that goal. Still, every attempt should be made to assess the extent of the disease accurately to provide guidance for prognosis and need for further treatment.

### Staging

At present, the stage of the tumor is assessed by indicating the depth of penetration of the tumor into the bowel wall (T stage), the extent of lymph node involvement (N stage), and the presence or absence of distant metastases (M stage). The standard staging system was based on a system developed in 1932 by Dr. Cuthbert Dukes, a pathologist at St. Mark's Hospital in London that was later modified. The classification was developed for rectal cancer, but it was generally also used to describe the stage of colon cancer. The Dukes classification is simple to remember and is still frequently used. Dukes' stage A cancer is confined to the bowel wall. Stage B cancer penetrates the bowel wall, and stage C cancer indicates lymph node metastases. Kirklin and associates, from the Mayo Clinic, established a distinction between tumors that partially penetrated the muscularis propria (B1) and those that fully penetrated this layer (B2). Astler and Coller further separated the tumors that had invaded lymph nodes but did not penetrate the entire bowel wall (C1) from tumors that invaded lymph nodes and did penetrate the entire wall (C2). Turnbull and associates from the Cleveland Clinic added stage D for tumors with distant metastasis. All these modifications in various combinations are still in use and are often called the *modified Dukes classification*.

The classification in use by most hospitals in the United States was developed by the American Joint Committee on Cancer (AJCC) and approved by the International Union Against Cancer (UICC). This classification, known as the *TNM* (tumor, node, metastasis) *system*, combines clinical information obtained preoperatively with data obtained during surgery and after histologic examination of the specimen. There have been numerous and significant modifications in the system since its introduction in 1987; the seventh edition of the *AJCC Staging Manual* (2010) has taken into account survival and relapse data that refine the prognostic value of accurate staging of colorectal cancer.[19]

#### Rules for Classification

***Clinical Staging*** A clinical assessment of the stage of disease (cTNM) is based on evidence obtained by medical history, physical examination, and endoscopy. Examinations designed to detect metastatic disease (M) include chest x-rays, CT (including pelvis, abdomen, chest), MRI, and positron emission tomography (PET) or fused PET-CT scans. Clinical staging in patients with rectal cancer often determines whether preoperative adjuvant treatment is indicated. Modalities to assess the preoperative stage of rectal cancer include endorectal ultrasound (EUS), pelvic CT, and pelvic MRI, with or without an endorectal coil.

***Pathologic Staging*** The pathologic examination of the resected specimen (pTNM) provides a basis for prognosis and consideration of the need for further (adjuvant) treatment. Patients who were given a clinical stage (cTNM) prior to the initiation of preoperative adjuvant treatment, usually combined radiation and chemotherapy, will have a modified pathologic stage assessed after examination of the surgically resected specimen; that stage is indicated by the "y" prescript (ypTNM).

Cancer cells confined within the glandular basement membrane (intraepithelial) or lamina propria (intramucosal) with no extension through the muscularis mucosae are not associated with a risk of metastasis and are defined as in situ carcinoma –pTis.

Accumulated survival data reviewed by the AJCC have allowed for the provision of more accurate prognostic data with further stratification based on accuracy of staging. For example, it is now recognized that outcomes are different for tumors within the pT4 category based on extent of disease. T4 cancers that penetrate to the surface of the visceral peritoneum (pT4a) have a better prognosis than tumors that directly invade or adhere to other organs (pT4b), and the staging classification has been refined to reflect this. In addition, it is recognized that increasing numbers of involved lymph nodes are associated with a worsening prognosis, and the most recent classification system takes this into account.

The recent AJCC manual also recognizes prognostic factors in addition to serum CEA levels that should be ascertained. These include the following: tumor deposits—TDs, the number of satellite tumor deposits discontinuous from the edge of the cancer that are not associated with a residual lymph node; a tumor regression grade that permits the pathologic response to neoadjuvant therapy to be graded, the circumferential resection margin—CRM, the distance from the edge of tumor to the nearest dissected margin of the surgical resection; microsatellite instability (MSI); perineural invasion—PN, histologic cancerous invasion of the regional nerves); and KRAS mutation status. The KRAS mutation has been shown to be associated with lack of response to treatment with monoclonal antibodies directed against the epidermal growth factor receptor (EGFR) in patients with metastatic colorectal cancer.

***Tumor Regression Grade*** Although the data are not definitive, it appears that a significant pathologic response to preoperative adjuvant treatment is associated with a better prognosis. Patients with minimal or no residual disease after therapy may have a better prognosis than patients with extensive residual cancer. A four-point regression grade has been developed to assess the response to neoadjuvant therapy (Table 52-6).

### Treatment and Follow-Up

Although the prognosis can be refined by careful and accurate pathologic staging, patients treated with appropriate resection for stage I colon cancer generally have a 5-year survival rate of approximately 90%. The 5-year survival rate for patients with stage II colon cancer treated surgically is approximately 75%. The survival of stage III patients, with lymph node metastasis, is approximately 50%, and patients with stage IV disease (distant metastases) have a poor prognosis, with a 5-year survival of less than 5%.

Further treatment and follow-up of patients treated by segmental colectomy for colon cancer is directed by the stage of the disease. Approximately 85% of recurrences are detected within 2 years of the time of resection, so follow-up strategy should be especially intensive during that period.

A reasonable strategy to follow patients with stage I colon cancer is a colonoscopic examination 1 year after the operation to inspect the anastomosis but also to detect any new or missed polyps. The colonoscopy should be repeated annually if any polyps are detected and removed, until an examination reveals the absence of polyps. Then, a colonoscopy should be offered every 5 years unless a strong family history or other genetic risk factor is present, in which case more frequent endoscopic examinations are obviously indicated. A CEA level should be determined every 3 months during the first 2 years, even if the preoperative CEA level was normal. A rising CEA level requires further tests to search for metastatic disease, including a CT scan (or MRI) of the abdomen and chest, and possibly a PET scan. The goal of close follow-up testing is to detect early recurrence that is amenable to treatment. Isolated hepatic or pulmonary metastases are amenable to resection, with a 5-year survival rate of 20%. Multiple or unresectable metastases may respond to current chemotherapeutic agents.

Postoperative treatment of patients with stage II colon cancer is somewhat controversial. To date, no large randomized trial has shown a benefit from adjuvant chemotherapy for this rather heterogeneous group of patients. An attempt to stratify patients may identify a subset that would benefit from chemotherapy. The 5-year survival rate of patients with stage IIA disease is 85%, compared with 72% for stage IIB disease, which is actually worse than for patients with node-positive stage IIIA disease. The American Society of Clinical Oncology (ASCO) suggests a course of 5-flurouracil (5-FU)–based adjuvant chemotherapy for stage II patients with at least one poor prognostic indicator including insufficient lymph node sampling (<12 nodes resected with the specimen), T4 lesions, poorly differentiated histology, or bowel perforation. Whether oxaliplatin-based regimens should be used in stage II disease in addition to 5-FU–leucovorin is controversial, but current practice in most areas appears to favor the addition of oxaliplatin in early-stage disease. Further follow-up of stage II patients includes a CEA level every 3 months for 2 years, every 6 months for a total of 5 years, and

**Table 52-6 American Joint Committee on Cancer TNM Staging System for Colorectal Cancer**

| STAGE | FEATURES | | | | |
|---|---|---|---|---|---|
| **Primary Tumor (T)** | | | | | |
| TX | Primary tumor cannot be assessed | | | | |
| T0 | No evidence of primary tumor | | | | |
| Tis | Carcinoma in situ—intraepithelial or invasion of lamina propria* | | | | |
| T1 | Tumor invades submucosa | | | | |
| T2 | Tumor invades muscularis propria | | | | |
| T3 | Tumor invades through the muscularis propria into pericolorectal tissues | | | | |
| T4a | Tumor penetrates to the surface of the visceral peritoneum† | | | | |
| T4b | Tumor directly invades or is adherent to other organs or structures†,‡ | | | | |
| **Regional Lymph Nodes (N)** | | | | | |
| NX | Regional lymph nodes cannot be assessed | | | | |
| N0 | No regional lymph node metastasis | | | | |
| N1 | Metastasis in one to three regional lymph nodes | | | | |
| N1a | Metastasis in one regional lymph node | | | | |
| N1b | Metastasis in two or three regional lymph nodes | | | | |
| N1c | Tumor deposit(s) in the subserosa, mesentery, or nonperitonealized pericolic or perirectal tissues without regional nodal metastasis | | | | |
| N2 | Metastasis in four or more regional lymph nodes | | | | |
| N2a | Metastasis in four to six regional lymph nodes | | | | |
| N2b | Metastasis in seven or more regional lymph nodes | | | | |
| **Distant Metastasis (M)** | | | | | |
| M0 | No distant metastasis | | | | |
| M1 | Distant metastasis | | | | |
| M1a | Metastasis confined to one organ or site (e.g., liver, lung, ovary, nonregional node) | | | | |
| M1b | Metastases in more than one organ/site or the peritoneum | | | | |
| | **Stage Grouping** | | | | |
| **STAGE** | **T** | **N** | **M** | **DUKES§** | **MAC§** |
| 0 | Tis | N0 | M0 | — | — |
| I | T1 | N0 | M0 | A | A |
| | T2 | N0 | M0 | A | B1 |
| IIA | T3 | N0 | M0 | B | B2 |
| IIB | T4a | N0 | M0 | B | B2 |
| IIC | T4b | N0 | M0 | B | B3 |
| IIIA | T1-T2 | N1/N1c | M0 | C | C1 |
| | T1 | N2a | M0 | C | C1 |
| IIIB | T3-T4a | N1/N1c | M0 | C | C2 |
| | T2-T3 | N2a | M0 | C | C1/C2 |
| | T1-T2 | N2b | M0 | C | C1 |
| IIIC | T4a | N2a | M0 | C | C2 |
| | T3-T4a | N2b | M0 | C | C2 |
| | T4b | N1-N2 | M0 | C | C3 |
| IVA | Any T | Any N | M1a | — | — |
| IVB | Any T | Any N | M1b | — | — |

*Continued*

**Table 52-6 American Joint Committee on Cancer TNM Staging System for Colorectal Cancer—cont'd**

| STAGE | FEATURES |
|---|---|
| **Histologic Grade (G)** | |
| GX | Grade cannot be assessed |
| G1 | Well differentiated |
| G2 | Moderately differentiated |
| G3 | Poorly differentiated |
| G4 | Undifferentiated |
| **Residual Tumor (R)** | |
| R0 | Complete resection, margins histologically negative, no residual tumor left after resection (e.g., primary tumor, regional nodes) |
| R1 | Incomplete resection, margins histologically involved, microscopic tumor remains after resection of gross disease (primary tumor, regional nodes) |
| R2 | Incomplete resection, margins macroscopically involved or gross disease remains after resection (e.g., primary tumor, regional nodes, or liver metastasis) |

From Edge S, Byrd D, Compton C, et al (eds): AJCC cancer staging manual, ed 7, New York, 2010, Springer.

*This includes cancer cells confined within the glandular basement membrane (intraepithelial) or mucosal lamina propria (intramucosal), with no extension through the muscularis mucosae into the submucosa.

†Direct invasion in T4 includes invasion of other organs or other segments of the colorectum as a result of direct examination (e.g., invasion of the sigmoid colon by a carcinoma of the cecum) or, for cancers in a retroperitoneal or subperitoneal location, direct invasion of other organs or structures by extension beyond the muscularis propria (i.e., respectively, a tumor on the posterior wall of the descending colon invading the left kidney or lateral abdominal wall, or a mid or distal rectal cancer with invasion of prostate, seminal vesicles, cervix, or vagina).

‡Tumor that is adherent to other organs or structures, grossly, is classified as cT4b. However, if no tumor is present in the adhesion, microscopically, the classification should be pT1-4a, depending on the anatomic depth of wall invasion. The V and L classifications should be used to identify the presence or absence of vascular or lymphatic invasion whereas the PN site-specific factor should be used for perineural invasion.

§Dukes B is a composite of better (T3 N0 M0) and worse (T4 N0 M0) prognostic groups, as is Dukes C (any TN1 M0 and any T N2 M0). MAC is the modified Astler-Coller classification.

annual CT scans of the abdomen and chest for at least the first 3 years.

Patients with stage III disease clearly benefit from adjuvant chemotherapy. The addition of oxaliplatin to the 5-FU–leucovorin regimen (FOLFOX) has resulted in an improvement of disease-free survival rates at 3 years to 78% (compared with 73% with 5-FU–leucovorin alone). Irinotecan (Camptosar) has been investigated as an addition to 5-FU–based therapy in the adjuvant setting, based on its benefit against metastatic disease. Unfortunately, irinotecan has not demonstrated efficacy in the adjuvant setting and is not currently used for the treatment of stage III patients.

The method of delivery of the chemotherapeutic agents is evolving. Continuous infusion 5-FU is now generally considered to be superior to bolus infusions, with less toxicity. An oral fluoropyrimidine, capecitabine (Xeloda), has been shown to be at least equivalent to 5-FU IV and may have superior efficacy.

The treatment of stage IV patients depends on the location and extent of the metastases. Isolated hepatic or pulmonary lesions may be amenable to resection. Chemotherapy is indicated, with new agents complementing the 5-FU regimens that remain the keystone of therapy. The newest agents that have been shown to be effective for metastatic disease and are being studied in the adjuvant setting are the monoclonal antibodies bevacizumab (Avastin), cetuximab (Erbitux), and panitumumab (Vectibix). Cetuximab, a chimeric (mouse-human) monoclonal antibody, and panitumumab, a fully human monoclonal antibody, bind to and inhibit the EGFR, which is overexpressed in 60% to 80% of colorectal cancers and is associated with a shorter survival time. Cetuximab and panitumumab are effective only on tumors that do not have a mutation of the KRAS gene. Accordingly, genetic testing is now recommended to confirm the absence of KRAS mutations (indicating the presence of the KRAS wild-type gene) before recommending the use of these EGFR inhibitors.[23] These agents have shown clinical efficacy in patients with metastatic colorectal cancer, both as monotherapy and in combination with irinotecan and FOLFOX. Bevacizumab, a vascular endothelial growth factor inhibitor, has also improved survival when added to regimens that include irinotecan, 5-FU–leucovorin, or oxaliplatin.

## Rectal Cancer

Cancers arising in the distal 15 cm of the large bowel share many of the genetic, biologic, and morphologic characteristics of colon cancers. However, the unique anatomy of the rectum, with its retroperitoneal location in the narrow pelvis and proximity to the urogenital organs, autonomic nerves, and anal sphincters, makes surgical access relatively difficult. In addition, precise dissection in appropriate anatomic planes is essential because dissection medial to the endopelvic fascia investing the mesorectum may doom the patient to local recurrence of the disease, and dissection laterally to the avascular anatomic space risks injury to the mixed autonomic nerves, causing impotence in men and bladder dysfunction in men and women.[24]

Furthermore, the biologic properties of the rectum, combined with its anatomic distance from the small intestine afforded by its retroperitoneal pelvic location, provides an opportunity for treatment by radiation therapy that is not feasible for colon tumors. The large bowel can tolerate properly delivered radiation doses up to 6000 cGy, whereas such levels of radiation targeted at colon tumors would include small bowel in the treatment field. The small bowel cannot withstand radiation doses of this level without complications of radiation enteritis, including stricture, hemorrhage, and perforation.

The treatment of rectal cancer has changed significantly during the past 25 years; there is considerable controversy concerning the precise role of surgery, radiation therapy, and chemotherapy and the ideal timing of each modality with relation to the others. Although information from clinical trials has provided data supporting the multimodality treatment of rectal cancer, the criteria for patient selection remains controversial. However, some generalities can be made:

- Radiation therapy offers significant benefit to many patients with rectal cancer, and preoperative radiation is superior to postoperative radiation. Preoperative radiation (combined with chemotherapy) was generally reserved for locally advanced distal rectal cancers (within 10 cm of the anal verge, stage II or higher), but an analysis based on a cooperative 7-year trial of the National Research Council (NRC) of the United Kingdom and the National Cancer Institute of Canada (NCIC) has revealed that short-term preoperative radiation (25 Gy over 5 days) results in a significant reduction in the local recurrence rate and improved disease-free survival for all stages of rectal cancer.[29]
- Chemotherapy that has shown efficacy in the adjuvant setting in the treatment of colon cancer is also beneficial in the adjuvant setting for patients with rectal cancer. The combination of neoadjuvant (preoperative) radiation (usually, 4500 to 5040 cGy) with infusional 5-FU–leucovorin (and, more recently, with the addition of oxaliplatin) often results in dramatic reduction in tumor size (downstaging), and may result in apparently complete eradication of the tumor in up to 25% of cases.[30,31] Although interest has grown in using chemoradiation as the sole treatment for patients who have demonstrated a complete clinical response to chemoradiation, the ability to predict which patients actually have a complete response has been shown to be difficult. At least one series has shown that a complete clinical response occurs in only 10% of patients treated with neoadjuvant chemoradiation.[32] There is considerable interest in elucidating factors associated with complete eradication of rectal cancer by nonoperative treatment, and strategies and methods for predicting a complete clinical response have been attracting international interest.[33]
- Neoadjuvant chemoradiation may increase the ability of the surgeon to preserve continence by downstaging the cancer, in some cases shrinking tumor size to permit the achievement of a cancer-free margin at the distal extent of the resection, when a clear margin that would permit an anastomosis in the anal canal could not be achieved without such shrinkage.[34]
- The best course of neoadjuvant treatment has not yet been determined. In Europe, the short course of radiation (25 Gy), followed by extirpative surgery (low anterior resection or abdominal perineal resection), is the most common approach. In the United States, stage II or higher rectal cancers are more commonly treated with preoperative chemoradiation consisting of 4500 to 5040 cGy of radiation in conjunction with infusional 5-FU–based chemotherapy. The radiation is delivered over a period of 5 to 6 weeks, and surgery (low anterior resection or abdominal perineal resection) is done 6 to 10 weeks after completion of the radiation therapy. A diverting stoma (ileostomy or transverse colostomy) is usually fashioned (with irradiated rectum) to protect the anastomosis and the stoma is then closed 10 weeks later, when studies show satisfactory healing of the anastomosis. In Europe, a diverting stoma is not usually done, and the anastomotic leak rates appear low.
- Neoadjuvant therapy is not a substitute for a properly performed surgical procedure. As discussed later, dissection in the proper plane is essential to achieve adequate margins and remove the rectal lymphatics that may harbor metastases. A total mesorectal resection is appropriate for cancer of the mid and distal rectum, but the mesorectum can be divided below a cancer of the proximal rectum (>10 cm above the anus) to allow preservation of the distal rectum for the anastomosis. If a total mesorectal excision is performed and the anal sphincters are preserved, the anastomosis to establish continence will need to join the colon to the anus.

The most common symptom of rectal cancer is hematochezia. Unfortunately, this is often attributed to hemorrhoids, and the correct diagnosis is consequently delayed until the cancer has reached an advanced stage. Other symptoms include mucus discharge, tenesmus, and change in bowel habit.

The differential diagnosis of rectal cancer includes ulcerative colitis, Crohn's proctocolitis, radiation proctitis, and procidentia. Occasionally, so-called *hidden rectal prolapse* or internal intussusception of the sigmoid into the rectum can produce a solitary rectal ulcer that mimics an ulcerating cancer. It is thought that the chronic trauma from the recurrent intussusception results in ulceration of the rectal mucosa. Instead of a solitary rectal ulcer, this mucosal trauma from intussusception can sometimes produce the entity of colitis cystica profunda, a polypoid lesion characterized by the presence of benign columnar epithelium and mucous cysts residing deep to the muscularis mucosae. This histologic pattern can be confused with invasive adenocarcinoma, and it is obviously important to recognize this completely benign entity.

The preoperative assessment of patients with rectal cancer is similar to that described for patients with colon cancer, with some significant differences—the requirement for precise characterization of the cancer with respect to proximity to the anal sphincters and the extent of invasion, as determined by depth of penetration into the bowel wall and spread to adjacent lymph nodes. A complete colonoscopic examination should be done to exclude synchronous tumors in the colon, but the precise location of the rectal tumor is best determined by examination with a rigid proctosigmoidoscope. Rigid proctosigmoidoscopy should be done, even if the tumor has been diagnosed with a colonoscopic examination, because the flexible proctosigmoidoscope may not accurately measure the exact distance from the tumor

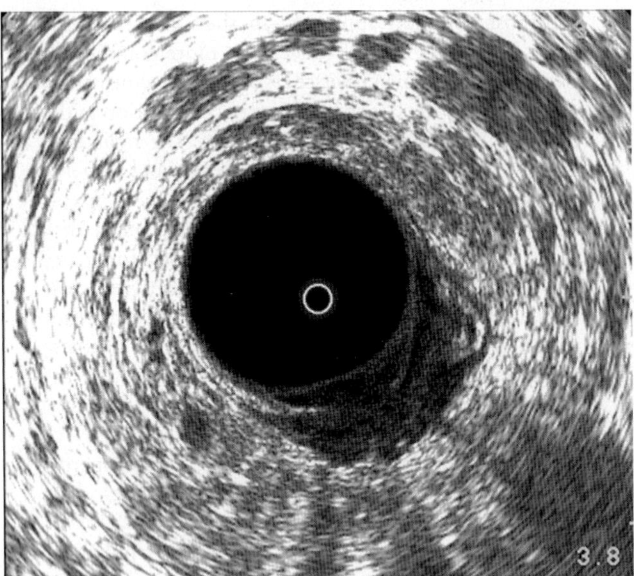


**FIGURE 52-65** Endorectal ultrasound of patient with T3 N1 rectal cancer. The cancer penetrates through all layers of the rectal wall, and an enlarged lymph node is clearly visible.

to the anal sphincter. The depth of penetration can be estimated by digital rectal examination (superficially invasive tumors are mobile, whereas the lesions become tethered and fixed with increasing depth of penetration), and EUS or MRI with endorectal coil can provide a fairly accurate assessment of the extent of invasion of the bowel wall (Fig. 52-65).[35]

Tumors located in the distal 3 to 5 cm of the rectum present the greatest challenge for the surgeon. Thorough and adequate assessment of tumors in this location is mandatory to select the proper treatment. If the tumor is confined to the submucosa (uT1, N0), excision by a transanal approach is an attractive option. In such circumstances, the incidence of lymphatic metastases is less than 8%, a factor that should be considered when contemplating the mortality and morbidity that would be associated with an abdominal perineal resection in a frail or older patient.[36] Cancers in this location that invade or penetrate the muscular wall of the rectum have a high incidence of local recurrence after transanal excision (>20%), and consideration should be given to treatment that is more aggressive than local excision. The preferred course of treatment requires consideration of many factors, including the patient's overall health and preferences. However, consideration should be given to more aggressive treatment for a T2 rectal cancer: chemoradiation or formal surgical excision (proctectomy with total mesorectal excision).

After the location and stage of the cancer have been determined, various options need to be considered for the optimal treatment of the rectal cancer. Other important considerations include the presence or absence of comorbid conditions and the patient's body habitus (an obese man with a narrow pelvis presents technical difficulties different than those in a thin woman with a wide pelvis). The appropriate operation should be tailored to eradicate the tumor while preserving function to the fullest extent possible. The following procedures are all useful in certain circumstances.

### Local Excision

Local excision of a rectal cancer may be appropriate for a small cancer in the distal rectum that has not penetrated into the muscularis. This is accomplished through a transanal approach, and usually involves excision of the full thickness of the rectal wall underlying the tumor. Local excisions do not allow complete removal of lymph nodes in the mesorectum, so operative staging is limited. In addition, definitive treatment of T1 rectal cancers by local excision has been shown to be associated with a three- to fivefold higher recurrence rate compared with similar stage cancers treated by radical surgical resection.[37] The operation is indicated for mobile tumors smaller than 4 cm in diameter, that involve less than 40% of the rectal wall circumference, and that are located within 6 cm of the anal verge. These tumors should be stage T1 (limited to the submucosa) or T2 (limited to the muscularis propria), well or moderately differentiated histologically, and with no vascular or lymphatic invasion. There should be no evidence of nodal disease on preoperative ultrasound or MRI. Adherence to these principles results in acceptable local recurrence rates compared with treatment by abdominal perineal resection. Local excision is also used for palliation of more advanced cancer in patients with severe comorbid disease, in whom extensive surgery carries a high risk for morbidity or mortality. Various technical approaches have been described to achieve transanal local excision, including use of a special proctoscope equipped with a magnifying camera (transanal endoscopic microsurgery), but all approaches require complete excision of the cancer, with adequate margins of normal tissue. Although many surgeons suture the rectal defect closed after the local excision, this is not mandatory because the operative site is below the peritoneal reflection. Unfortunately, as experience has accumulated with this approach, it has become clear that close follow-up is mandatory, in that approximately 8% of T1 lesions recur and the recurrence rate for T2 lesions has been shown in some series to exceed 20%. As noted, most clinicians believe that local excision is not adequate treatment for a T2 rectal cancer and further treatment is required, adjuvant radiation plus chemotherapy or radical excision (low anterior resection or abdominal perineal resection).

### Transanal Endoscopic Microsurgery

Transanal endoscopic microsurgery is an approach for the local excision of favorable rectal tumors (T1 cancers and sessile polyps) through a device designed to provide access to the mid and proximal rectum. The endosurgical device is a large (4-cm diameter) proctoscope through which four functions—carbon dioxide insufflation, water irrigation, suction, and monitoring of intrarectal pressure—are simultaneously regulated. The transanal microsurgery endoscope itself is closed and sealed, so that the rectum distends when carbon dioxide is insufflated into the system. This distention facilitates visualization afforded by binocular lenses attached to the system.

The endoscope is inserted through the anus and positioned to provide optimum visualization and access to the tumor. Positioning of the endoscope is critical for success of the operation, and the patient must be placed in the proper position on the operating table to permit it to be adequately secured in a stable position. Long operating instruments are then inserted through ports in the system and used to excise the tumor under direct vision. The advantages of the technique include excellent exposure to tumors in a difficult area of access. However, the technique is somewhat difficult to perfect, the equipment is expensive, and the number of lesions amenable to this approach is relatively small. The complications associated with the technique are the same as for standard transanal local excision—bleeding, urinary retention, perforation into the peritoneal cavity, and fecal soilage. The dilation of the anal sphincters by the large endoscope may be associated with subsequent fecal incontinence, but this appears to be a transient problem in most circumstances.

### Fulguration

The technique of fulguration, which eradicates the cancer by using an electrocautery device that destroys the tumor by creating a full-thickness eschar at the tumor site, requires extension of the eschar into the perirectal fat, thus destroying both the tumor and rectal wall. The procedure can be used only for lesions below the peritoneal reflection. Complications associated with this approach are postoperative fever and significant bleeding, which can occur as late as 10 days after the operation. Obviously, this technique cannot provide a specimen to assess the pathologic stage because the tumor and margins are disintegrated by fulguration. The procedure is reserved for patients with a prohibitive operative risk and limited life expectancy; it has largely been replaced by transanal excision, which provides the advantage of examination and more adequate staging of the specimen.

### Abdominal Perineal Resection

Complete excision of the rectum and anus, by concomitant dissection through the abdomen and perineum, with suture closure of the perineum and creation of a permanent colostomy, was first described by Ernest Miles, and is thus sometimes referred to as the *Miles procedure*. The rectum and sigmoid colon are mobilized through an abdominal incision. The pelvic dissection, done through the abdominal incision, mobilizes the mesorectum in continuity with the tumor-bearing rectum. The pelvic dissection is carried to the level of the levator ani muscles. The perineal portion of the operation excises the anus, anal sphincters, and distal rectum. Although there are different approaches to performing this operation, recent experience has shown that positioning the patient in the prone position for the perineal excision permits a more cylindrical specimen (wider margins of normal tissue) to be obtained, with a reduction in positive circumferential margins, which should reduce the incidence of local recurrence.[38] An abdominal perineal resection is indicated when the tumor involves the anal sphincters or is too close to the sphincters to obtain adequate margins, or in patients in whom sphincter-preserving surgery is not possible because of unfavorable body habitus or poor preoperative sphincter control. A well-fashioned colostomy will often provide a superior quality of life to coloanal anastomosis in an older patient or in a patient whose sphincter has been compromised by childbirth, radiation, or previous anorectal operations.[39]

### Low Anterior Resection

Resection of the rectum through an abdominal approach offers the advantage of removing the portion of bowel containing the cancer and the mesorectum completely, which contains the lymphatic channels that drain the tumor bed. The term *anterior resection* (an abbreviation for the more correct term, *anterior proctosigmoidectomy with colorectal anastomosis*) indicates resection of the proximal rectum or rectosigmoid above the peritoneal reflection. The term *low anterior resection* indicates that the operation entails resection of the rectum below the peritoneal reflection through an abdominal approach. The sigmoid colon is almost always included with the resected specimen because diverticulosis often involves the sigmoid, and the blood supply to the sigmoid is often not adequate to sustain an anastomosis if the IMA is transected. For cancers involving the lower half of the rectum, the entire mesorectum, which contains the lymph channels draining the tumor bed, should be excised in continuity with the rectum. This technique, total mesorectal excision, produces the complete resection of an intact package of the rectum and its adjacent mesorectum, enveloped within the visceral pelvic fascia with uninvolved circumferential margins. The use of the technique of total mesorectal excision has resulted in a significant increase in 5-year survival rates (50% to 75%), a decrease in local recurrence rates (30% to 5%), and a decrease in the incidence of impotence and bladder dysfunction (85% to <15%).

Intestinal continuity is reestablished by fashioning an anastomosis between the descending colon and rectum, which has been greatly facilitated by the introduction of the circular stapling device. After the colorectal anastomosis has been completed, it should be inspected with a proctoscope inserted through the anus. If there is concern about the integrity of the anastomosis, or if the patient has received high-dose preoperative chemoradiation, a temporary proximal colostomy or ileostomy should be made to permit complete healing of the anastomosis.[39,40] The stoma can be closed in approximately 10 weeks if proctoscopy and contrast studies verify the integrity of the anastomosis.

An end-to-end anastomosis between the descending colon and distal rectum or anus may result in significant alteration of bowel habits attributed to the loss of the normal rectal capacity (Fig. 52-66). Patients treated with this operation often experience frequent small bowel movements (low anterior resection syndrome or clustering). This problem can be addressed by fashioning a colonic J pouch as the proximal component of the anastomosis (Fig. 52-67).[41] As experience has accumulated with this approach, it appears that improvement in bowel function is significant for cancers located in the distal rectum but, if the anastomosis is created above 9 cm from the anal verge, there is little benefit of a J pouch compared with an end-to-end anastomosis. The limbs of the J pouch should be relatively short (6 cm) because patients with larger J pouches have a significant incidence of difficulty with evacuation. It is generally thought to be preferable to avoid using the sigmoid colon as the proximal component of a colorectal anastomosis, because the blood supply to the sigmoid from the IMA may be tenuous, and the presence of diverticular disease, common in the sigmoid colon, is often considered to be a risk factor for anastomotic leak. However, one study has demonstrated satisfactory results from fashioning the colonic J pouch from the sigmoid (instead of the descending) colon.[42]

In obese patients and in patients with a narrow pelvis, it may not be technically feasible to fashion a J pouch as the proximal component of the low pelvic anastomosis because the bulk of the pouch simply will not fit into the narrow pelvis. In such cases, a reservoir can be devised with a coloplasty. This technique provides a rectal reservoir by making an 8- to 10-cm colotomy 4 to 6 cm from the divided end of the colon. The

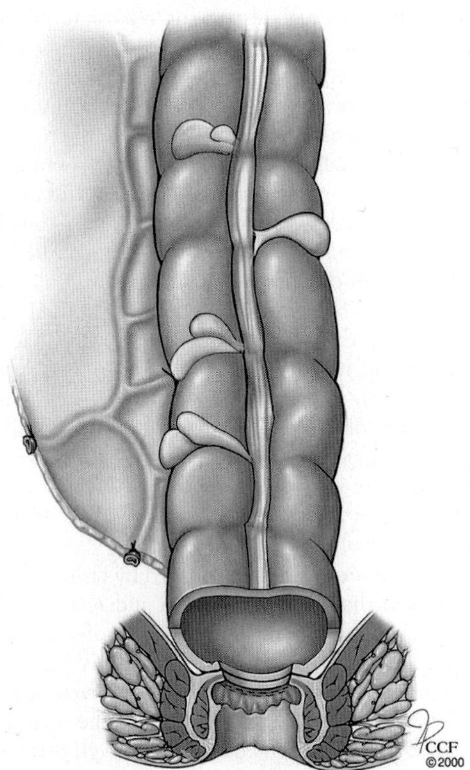


**FIGURE 52-66** Anastomosis between descending colon and anus, following complete resection of the rectum. The absence of the rectum often results in frequent small bowel movements, a phenomenon known as *clustering* or *low anterior resection syndrome*. (Courtesy Cleveland Clinic Foundation, Cleveland, 2000.)

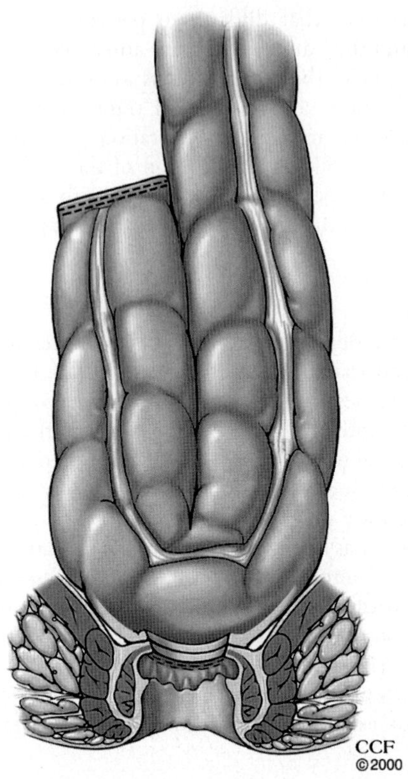


**FIGURE 52-67** J pouch fashioned from descending colon to form proximal portion of coloanal anastomosis. This increases its capacitance to decrease the frequency of bowel movements. (Courtesy Cleveland Clinic Foundation, Cleveland, 2000.)

colotomy is closed transversely to provide increased rectal space and capacitance (Figs. 52-68 and 52-69).[43]

### Sphincter-Sparing Abdominal Perineal Resection With Coloanal Anastomosis

Abdominal perineal resection is sometimes required because a cancer in the distal rectum cannot be resected with adequate margins while preserving the anal sphincter. However, the use of preoperative radiation and chemotherapy has been shown, in some cases, to shrink the tumor to an extent that acceptable margins can be achieved. If the anal sphincters do not need to be sacrificed to achieve adequate margins based on oncologic principles, a permanent stoma may be avoided with a sphincter-sparing abdominal perineal resection, with an anastomosis between the colon and anal canal.[44] This procedure has particular application for young patients with rectal tumors who have a favorable body habitus and good preoperative sphincter function. The operation can be conducted in a variety of ways, but all methods involve mobilizing the sigmoid colon and pelvic rectum through an abdominal approach, dissecting the rectal mucosa from the anal sphincters at the level of the dentate line, and completing the resection of the most distal rectum through the anal approach. An anastomosis is then fashioned between the descending colon and anus, often using a J pouch or coloplasty procedure described earlier for the low colorectal anastomosis. The anastomosis is made with sutures placed through a transanal approach by the surgeon in the perineal field.

## Colorectal Cancer Prevention and Screening

Cancer prevention can be divided into a discussion of primary and secondary prevention. Primary prevention is the identification of environmental factors responsible for cancer and subsequent modification of those factors to reduce risk (e.g., dietary modification, avoidance of environmental hazards, chemoprevention). Secondary prevention involves finding a precursor lesion or cancer at a stage at which metastasis and death can be prevented.

Cancer screening is the cornerstone of secondary prevention. Colorectal cancer is a preventable disease. An understanding of defined risk factors and screening options is essential for every health care physican. Our understanding of the natural history of colorectal cancer, precancerous conditions, patient risk factors, and efficacy of screening options is still in flux. Even so, achieving a basic facility with current evidence should be the goal.

Colorectal cancer is an ideal candidate for screening strategies for the following reasons:

1. It is a common and serious problem.
2. Precursor lesions exist.
3. It is slow growing.
4. Testing is available.

In 1993, the National Polyp Study Workgroup published a landmark study documenting a 76% to 90% reduction in colorectal cancer incidence compared with reference populations when adenomatous colon polyps are removed endoscopically. A

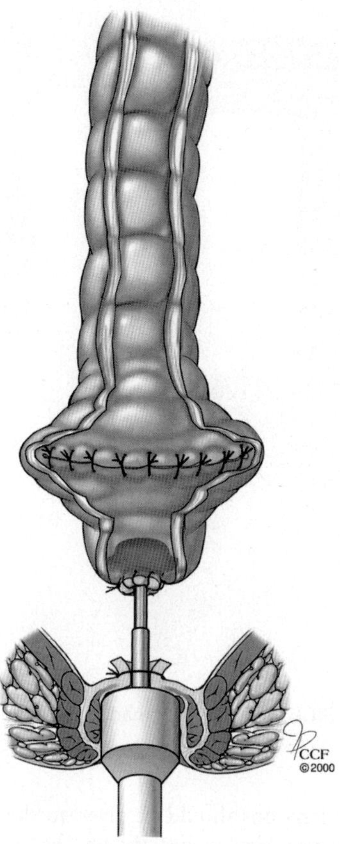


**FIGURE 52-68** A coloplasty is performed by making an 8- to 10-cm colotomy 4 to 6 cm from the cut end of the colon. The longitudinal colotomy is made between the taeniae on the antimesenteric side. It is closed transversely with absorbable sutures. An end-to-end stapled anastomosis then joins the colon to the distal rectum or anus. (Courtesy Cleveland Clinic Foundation, Cleveland, 2000.)

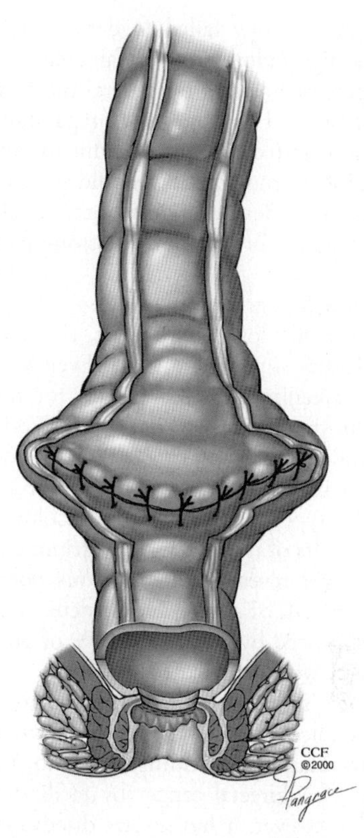


**FIGURE 52-69** The completed stapled coloplasty with anastomosis. (Courtesy Cleveland Clinic Foundation, Cleveland, 2000.)

year before this, Selby and Newcomb independently showed a 60% to 70% rectal cancer mortality reduction following sigmoidoscopy and polypectomy. Clearly, intervention results in mortality reduction.

Far more controversial is the choice of screening method. This area of prevention is rapidly changing, and updated recommendations are made frequently. Patients are risk-stratified with frequency and method of screening dictated by category (see Table 52-5). Most patients (70%) are of average risk; these patients have no personal or family history of colorectal cancer or polyps, and no predisposing conditions such as ulcerative colitis or Crohn's disease.

The most difficult risk category to define is the moderate-risk group. The American College of Gastroenterologists has stratified these patients into two groups. Patients with one first-degree relative with colorectal cancer diagnosed after age 60 years are twice as likely as an average-risk individual to develop colorectal cancer themselves. Furthermore, their risk for colorectal cancer at age 40 years is the same as the general population's risk at age 50 years. Therefore, these individuals are considered at moderately increased risk; screening recommendations are the same as for average-risk patients but should begin at age 40 years. Patients with a strong family history of colorectal cancer include those with multiple first-degree relatives with colorectal cancer or a single first-degree relative with cancer diagnosed before 60 years of age. Overall risk for developing cancer for this cohort is three to four times the average. Patients at high risk for developing colorectal cancer are those with a hereditary cancer syndrome such as FAP or HNPCC or with ulcerative or Crohn's colitis.

Perhaps the most frequently used, and least well understood, screening tool is fecal occult blood testing (FOBT). It has the advantages of being inexpensive, easy to use, and interpretable by primary care physicians. In randomized studies, annual use of FOBT alone with three consecutive stools produced a colorectal cancer-specific mortality reduction rate of 33%. Unfortunately, the false-negative rate using FOBT alone is unacceptably high. Only 30% to 50% of cancers were detectable in most series. A report from the Veterans Administration Study Group documented that only 24% of colorectal cancers produce a positive result. Only 7.0% of patients with polyps had a positive FOBT (compared with 6.4% of polyp-free patients). Thus, FOBT alone is not an adequate test for polyps or colorectal cancer in any risk group.

For average-risk individuals, combining FOBT with flexible sigmoidoscopy at 5-year intervals is deemed acceptable as a screening option. In 2001, the Veterans Administration Cooperative Study Group published the results of a large study (2885 patients) comparing FOBT and flexible sigmoidoscopy with colonoscopy. All patients underwent FOBT followed by full colonoscopy. The flexible sigmoidoscopy portion of the examination was carefully documented. Although sigmoidoscopy alone identified 70.3% of all cancers, the combination of FOBT and flexible sigmoidoscopy failed to detect 24% of proximal cancers. Flexible sigmoidoscopy is a valuable tool that can be used in an office-based setting by general physicians without a full bowel preparation. However, poor preparation, patient discomfort, and variable technique may limit its accuracy. Polyps detected by flexible sigmoidoscopy should prompt full colonoscopic examination. Flexible sigmoidoscopy alone or with FOBT is not adequate for those in the strong family history or high-risk group.

Double-contrast barium enema (DCBE) was once the diagnostic mainstay for lower GI disease. The advent of flexible fiberoptics has largely supplanted its use. Even so, it has retained a place in the screening armamentarium for the average-risk patient. In 2000, the National Polyp Study Work Group compared DCBE and colonoscopy in a prospective double-blinded trial in patients with a history of polyps. All 862 study subjects underwent both types of examination. Colonoscopists were blinded to the results of the antecedent barium enema. Of these colonoscopies, 45% revealed adenomatous polyps, compared with only 26% of DCBEs. The rate of detection on DCBE is significantly influenced by size. Only 48% of polyps 1.0 cm or larger in diameter were detected on DCBE.

Colonoscopy is considered the gold standard for screening. It is the test of choice for patients with greater than average risk and has the advantage of providing a way to intervene in the natural history of colorectal cancer by facilitating endoscopic polypectomy.[45] However, it has several disadvantages. It is the most morbid screening method. Colonic perforation (1/2000 to 2500 examinations), as well as significant bleeding (<1% of examinations), can occur. Colonoscopy requires a full bowel preparation accompanied by fasting, sedation, and a skilled endoscopist. Finally, colonoscopy is the most expensive screening test available. Even considering these limitations, the use of colonoscopy has become commonplace. It is the screening test recommended for average-risk individuals; indeed, it may be the most cost-effective test if administered once every 10 years, as recommended. For those with greater than average risk, colonoscopy is mandatory for initial screening and follow-up. Research has endeavored to establish reliable accuracy statistics for colonoscopy. Studies pairing back to back colonoscopies have demonstrated a 15% polyp miss rate. In the National Polyp Study Workgroup trial, colonoscopic examination revealed a 20% overall polyp miss rate. Clearly, the gold standard could be improved on, particularly for polyps smaller than 1.0 cm in diameter.

## INTESTINAL STOMAS

Occasionally, the intestinal tract needs to be interrupted and fused to the skin to divert bodily wastes, temporarily or permanently, for a variety of reasons. A stoma, or ostomy, is an artificial opening of the intestinal or urinary tract to the abdominal wall. The techniques of fashioning a stoma have been developed to provide a cure or palliation for benign or malignant diseases or to provide diversion of waste until conditions are attained that permit the restoration of normal intestinal continuity.

### Basic Types

A colostomy is an anastomosis fashioned between the colon and skin of the abdominal wall. Colostomies may be temporary or permanent, depending on the disease and conditions for which they are created. However, appropriate planning and careful technical considerations should be given to the creation of any colostomy, because history has shown that even colostomies intended to be temporary may prove to be permanent in a significant number of patients.[46]

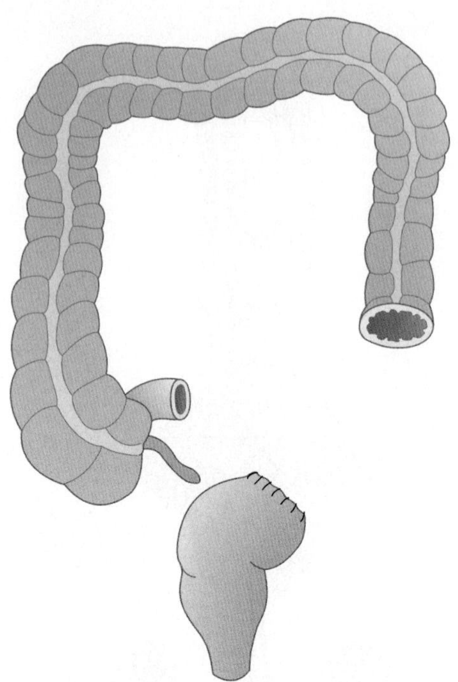

**FIGURE 52-70** Hartman's operation.

A colostomy may be indicated to divert colonic contents temporarily from a pathologic process in the distal colon or rectum, such as an obstructing rectal cancer or phlegmon of the sigmoid colon associated with diverticulitis. Such a colostomy is usually a loop colostomy using the transverse colon. Other circumstances are more appropriately treated by an end colostomy, in which the end of the sigmoid or, more commonly, descending colon is fused with the skin of the abdominal wall. An end colostomy is an essential component of an abdominal perineal proctectomy performed for rectal cancer. As noted, resection of the sigmoid colon with closure of the rectal stump and fashioning of a descending colon is usually referred to as *Hartmann's operation* (Fig 52-70). This may be a useful approach for patients with diverticulitis and some patients with rectal cancer.

An ileostomy is the union of the ileum to the skin of the abdominal wall. As described for colostomy, an ileostomy may also be fashioned as a loop or an end stoma. A temporary loop ileostomy may be fashioned to protect a distal anastomosis, such as a coloanal anastomosis in a patient who has received preoperative chemoradiation for rectal cancer, or to protect an ileal pouch anal anastomosis in a patient treated with restorative proctocolectomy for ulcerative colitis. An end ileostomy is required if the colon and rectum must be removed and the anal sphincter cannot be preserved. The most common indication for a permanent end ileostomy is Crohn's disease with severe involvement of the anorectum.

A urinary conduit is one method of compensating for the loss of or severe malfunction of the urinary bladder. Construction of a urinary conduit involves isolation of a segment of intestine, usually ileum, with restoration of the continuity of the remaining intestine. One end of the conduit is brought onto the abdominal wall as a stoma and the other end is closed. The ureters are implanted into the intestinal pouch, which serves as a conduit for the excretion of urine. Significant advances in techniques of bladder reconstruction have made the use of the ileal urinary conduit less frequent than in the past few decades.

## Physiologic Considerations and Practical Implications

### Colostomy

For practical purposes, the dominant physiologic properties of the proximal colon are the completion of digestion of complex carbohydrates by fermentation, retention of electrolytes, and absorption of water. The more distal colon participates to less of an extent in these processes and serves as a reservoir for the waste products of digestion pending elimination. The motility characteristics of the colon are segmentation and mass movements. The blood supply to the ascending and transverse colon is from the SMA, whereas the blood supply to the sigmoid colon is primarily from the IMA, although there is normally collateral communication between these arterial sources from the marginal artery. In some cases, the collateral communication via the marginal artery is not sufficient to sustain the sigmoid colon, so it is generally preferred to fashion a distal colostomy from the descending colon, which has a more reliable blood supply, than the sigmoid colon (especially if the IMA has been divided). In addition, the sigmoid colon is often afflicted with diverticulosis and the thickening of the colonic wall associated with that disease process, so the more pliable and capacious descending colon is the preferred choice for a left-sided colostomy.

The more proximal the site of the colon that is selected to fashion a colostomy, the more likely it is that the effluent will be liquid, noxious, and foul-smelling. Descending colostomies that pass formed feces are relatively easy to care for with a well-fitting enterostomal appliance, whereas transverse colostomies that expel significant amounts of feculent liquid are difficult to care for. Colostomies from the right colon are particularly troublesome, because there is a copious amount of liquid foul-smelling effluent that is difficult to contain with an appliance.

In addition, the motility characteristics of the colon are such that the more proximal the site of the colon selected to fashion a colostomy, the higher is the likelihood of prolapse through the stoma. This is distressing to the patient and makes maintenance of the stoma exceedingly difficult. As a general rule, with modern enterostomal techniques, it is much easier to care for an ileostomy than to care for a wet colostomy or a colostomy fashioned from the proximal colon.

Transverse colostomies, although at times very useful to protect a distal anastomosis or to divert colonic contents from a distal obstruction, should almost always be considered to be a temporary diversion to a transient problem. A transverse loop colostomy fashioned at skin level will completely divert the fecal stream for a period of at least 6 weeks but, with the passage of time and the natural maturation of the colostomy, the spur, or posterior wall of the colostomy, will retract and the stoma will no longer divert completely. In addition, the incidence of significant prolapse from a transverse loop colostomy is high and increases over time. Somewhat surprisingly, it is usually (but not always) the distal limb of the loop colostomy that prolapses through the stoma site.

### Ileostomy

The terminal ileum normally delivers up to 2 liters of succus entericus to the cecum during a 24- hour period. There is a remarkable adaptation following the construction of a stoma from the very distal ileum, in that after several weeks the absorptive capacity of the ileum increases to the extent that approximately 900 mL of effluent will be expected to be produced by the ileum during a 24-hour period. However, the intestinal adaptation cannot completely compensate for the loss of the absorptive capacity of the colon, and ileostomy patients need to recognize the need to increase their intake of fluid. Supplemental sodium chloride may often be necessary for ileostomates, although liberal addition of salt to the daily diet usually will suffice.

The ileal chyme is liquid and contains digestive substances that are normally inactivated in the colon. If the skin adjacent to the ileostomy is exposed to the effluent, significant erosion of the peristomal skin can occur. Therefore, the ileostomy is fashioned to protrude above the skin surface as a spigot that pours the ileal contents into an enterostomal appliance fitted to the abdominal skin at the base of the ileostomy so as to protect the skin from the corrosive properties of the ileal effluent.

## Logistic Considerations

If it is anticipated that the creation of a stoma, a colostomy or ileostomy, will be part of an operation, appropriate preparations should be made to optimize the outcome of the procedure. Preoperative consultation with an enterostomal therapist is helpful in most circumstances. This consultation provides the opportunity for education, counseling, and appropriate stoma site selection and marking. Such preparation significantly increases patient satisfaction and quality of life scores of patients who require permanent or temporary stomas.[47]

The preferred location of a stoma should be in an area of the anterior abdominal wall where there are no creases that could prohibit the satisfactory seal of the appliance to the peristomal skin. The stoma should be visible to the patient—not on the underside of a large panniculus in an obese individual—and easily accessible. Most surgeons think that it is desirable to bring the stoma through the rectus muscle, traversing an appropriately sized aperture (2 cm) that does not constrict the blood supply to the stoma but does not result in a peristomal hernia. In a normal-sized patient, the preferred site for stoma location is through the rectus muscle, slightly inferior to the umbilicus at the apex of the naturally occurring tissue mound of the abdomen (Fig. 52-71).

## Technical Considerations

### Colostomy

**End Descending Colostomy** As noted, it is generally preferable to use the descending colon, rather than the sigmoid colon, for the creation of a colostomy. The most common indication for an end descending colostomy is abdominal perineal resection for rectal cancer. In this case, we recommend dividing the IMA close to the aorta (for oncologic and anatomic reasons; see later). The sigmoid colon should be resected with the rectum, taking care to preserve the mesentery to the descending colon. The blood supply to the descending colon will be maintained through the collateral circulation from the marginal artery, and this collateral circulation is better maintained by dividing the IMA close to its

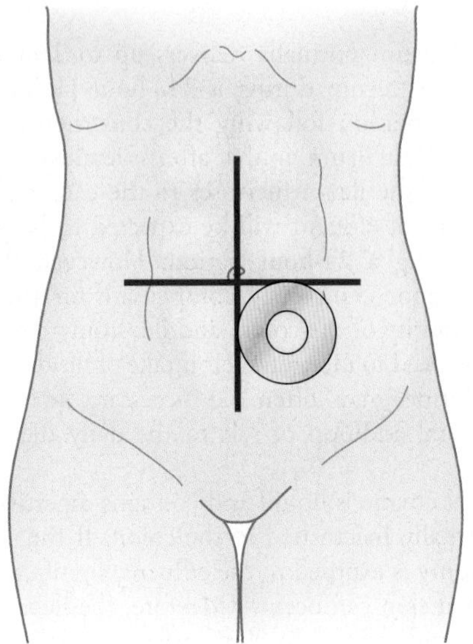

**FIGURE 52-71** Selecting a site.

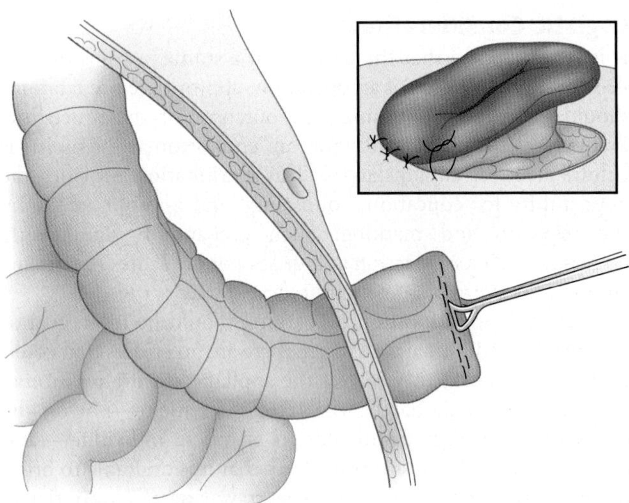

**FIGURE 52-72** End colostomy.

origin. The colon is the mobilized from the posterior abdominal wall and the prerenal (Gerota's) fascia in such a manner that the entire descending colon and its mesentery lie anterior to the small bowel (Fig. 52-72). Using this technique, there is no remaining lateral attachment of the colonic mesentery for the small intestine to twist around, and it is not necessary to approximate the mesentery of the descending colon to the lateral peritoneum to prevent an internal hernia.

The closed end of the descending colon is brought through an abdominal wall aperture created through the left rectus muscle at the site selected and marked prior to the operation. The colostomy is matured by approximating the wall of the colon to the skin with interrupted absorbable sutures. Some surgeons place the sutures in such a fashion to elevate the colostomy above skin level slightly, but this is not necessary with a descending colon because the effluent will be nonliquid and noncorrosive, and maintaining an appliance does not require eversion of the stoma.

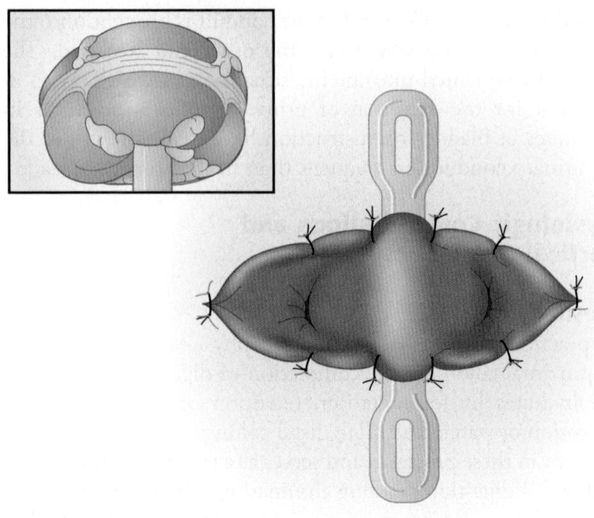

**FIGURE 52-73** Loop colostomy.

**Loop Colostomy** A loop colostomy may provide diversion from a distal obstruction (e.g., rectal cancer, diverticulitis) while simultaneously decompressing the limb of the colon leading to the obstruction. The most commonly performed type of loop colostomy is the transverse loop colostomy but, as noted, this stoma has the disadvantages of liquid effluent, eventual prolapse, and only temporary complete diversion. Although a loop transverse colostomy is certainly indicated in certain circumstances, consideration should be given to a loop ileostomy or loop descending colostomy. The former is easier to care for and maintain an appliance, and the latter's effluent is thicker, with less fluid loss and less chance of prolapse of the more distally placed colostomy. The technique of fashioning the descending loop colostomy is essentially the same as for the transverse loop colostomy; the transverse loop is often technically easier because it is mobile and more easily accessible in the midabdomen.

The transverse colon is brought through an abdominal wall aperture, usually selected in the midline well cephalad to the umbilicus, and well above a midline incision if the operation is conducted through such an incision. The exteriorized loop of colon is supported over a plastic stoma rod (Fig. 52-73). The antimesenteric surface of the colon is incised in a longitudinal incision and the edges of the resulting colostomy are sutured to the skin of the abdominal wall with absorbable sutures. The supporting rod is removed after the fifth postoperative day. This stoma will provide complete diversion of the feces and gas from the proximal colon while simultaneous venting the distal colon. However, after a period of approximately 6 weeks, the posterior wall of the stoma (the spur) will retract and feces from the proximal colon can spill over into the distal limb.

### Ileostomy

In forming an ileostomy, the ileum is brought through the abdominal wall at a site selected prior to the operation to ensure that the location is ideal for maintaining the seal of an appliance (i.e., away from natural abdominal wall creases, scars, hernias). A disc of skin is excised, the dissection is carried longitudinally through the center of the rectus muscle, and the posterior fascia is divided (Fig. 52-74). The abdominal wall aperture should be approximately 2.5 cm in diameter, thus admitting two fingers

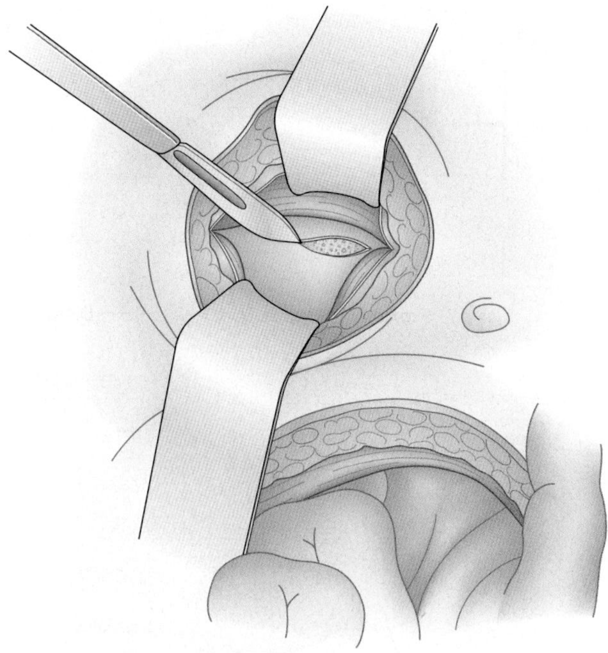

**FIGURE 52-74** Dividing fascia for ileostomy.

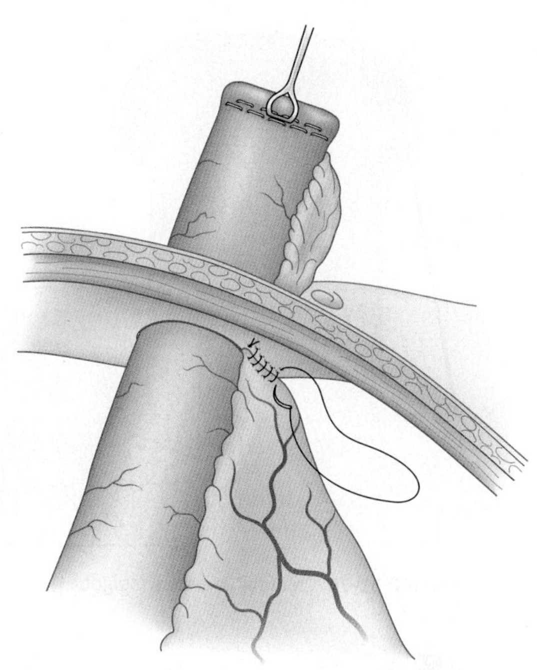

**FIGURE 52-76** Ileum brought through aperture.

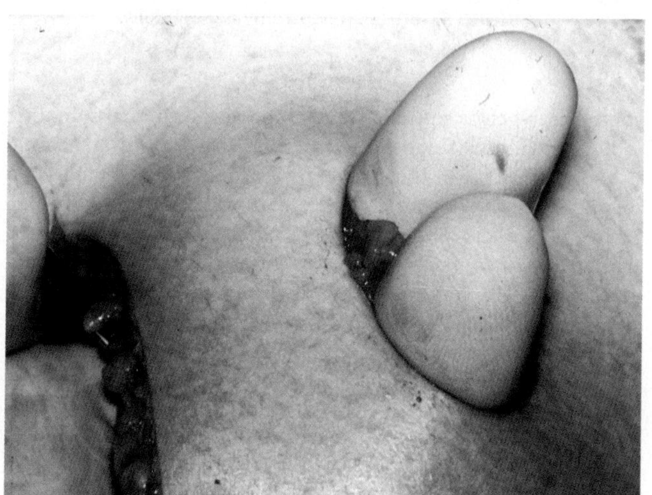

**FIGURE 52-75** Aperture for ileostomy.

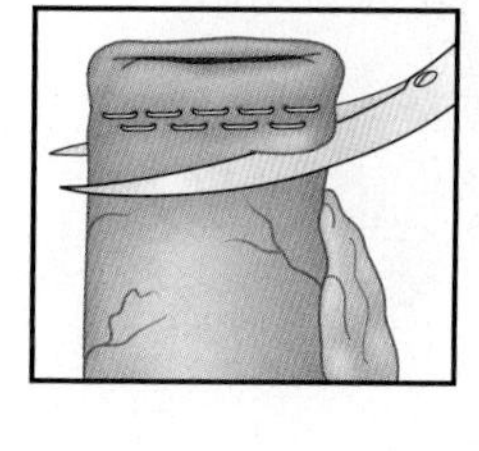

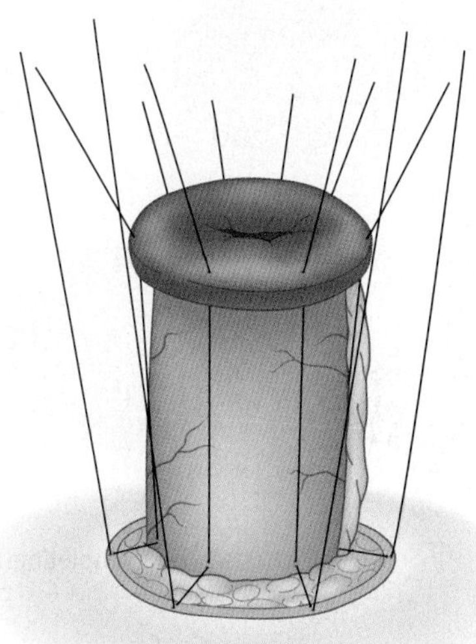

**FIGURE 52-77** Maturing ileostomy.

(Fig. 52-75). Sufficient length of well-vascularized ileum is brought through the abdominal wall to permit creation of a spigot that will protrude above skin level, allowing the ileal contents to pour into an appliance sealed to the adjacent skin (Fig. 52-76). The ileostomy is completed by approximating the full thickness of the divided wall of the ileum to the subcuticular tissue of the abdominal skin of the stoma site, placing sutures in so as to maintain the everted configuration of the stoma (Figs. 52-77 and 52-78).

Using these same principles, a loop ileostomy may be fashioned (Figs. 52-79 and 52-80). The loop ileostomy can be fashioned over an ileostomy rod, but a rod is not necessary to maintain the configuration of the stoma. Some surgeons prefer not to use a supporting rod because it may interfere with maintaining the seal of the appliance. If an ileostomy rod is used, it can be removed on the fifth postoperative day.

## PELVIC FLOOR DISORDERS AND CONSTIPATION

Disorders of the pelvic floor can be classified as primarily colorectal, urologic, or gynecologic. Often, problems requiring the attention of multiple specialists present in a synchronous fashion, a condition known as *complex prolapse*. Rectal prolapse (procidentia), enterocele, rectocele, and functional disorders of the muscles of the pelvic floor (anismus, levator spasm) are among the pelvic floor disorders treated by surgeons. A functional disorder is defined by the concurrent presence of normal anatomy and abnormal function. Surgeons are often consulted concerning functional disorders of the large bowel or pelvic floor. These problems do not usually require operative intervention; in fact, the surgical literature is replete with examples of failed operations to correct these problems. However, the signs and symptoms of these disorders mimic surgical diseases and

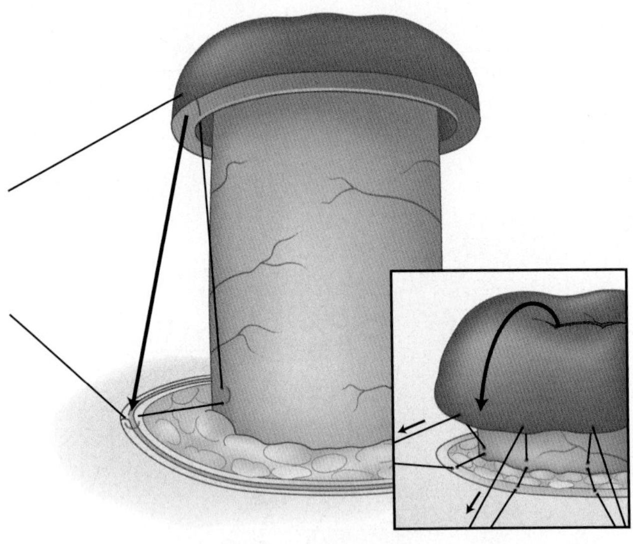
FIGURE 52-78 Creating ileostomy spigot.

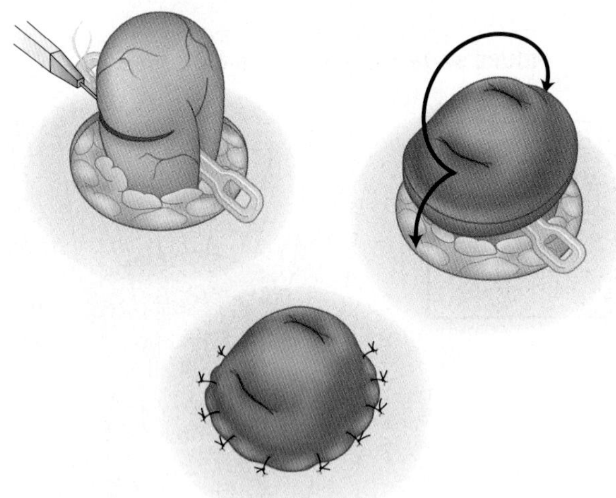
FIGURE 52-79 Completing loop ileostomy.

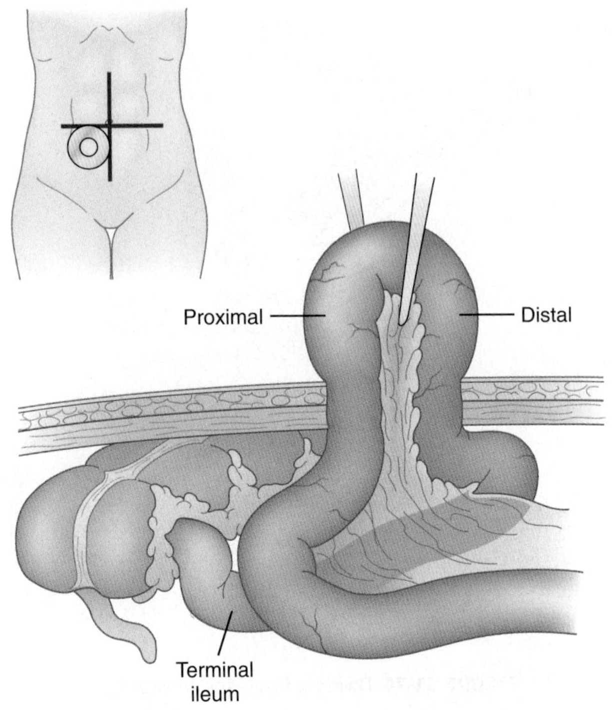

FIGURE 52-80 Loop ileostomy in continuity.

require proper recognition and treatment. Although chronic constipation is often considered an example of a functional problem, surgery is a consideration for some patients who fail medical management. The surgical evaluation and management of these disorders is discussed in this section.

## Diagnosis: Testing and Evaluation

### Anorectal Physiology Laboratory Testing

Anorectal physiology testing refers to the systematic evaluation of anal canal resting and squeeze pressures, anal reflexes, pudendal nerve conduction velocities, and electromyographic muscle fiber recruitment. Measurement of anal canal pressures (manometry) involves the use of water-filled balloons attached to catheters and transducers placed in the anal canal. The measurement of resting and squeeze pressures at various points in the anal canal reflects the strength, tone, and function of the internal and external sphincter. Normal resting and squeeze values are 40 to 80 mm Hg. Resting pressure reflects the function of the internal sphincter, whereas squeeze pressure measures external sphincter (voluntary muscle) contributions. Measurement of anal canal pressures is useful in the evaluation of conditions ranging from incontinence to obstructive defecation. Electromyographic recruitment refers to the motor unit potential of the puborectalis muscle and is compared for rest, squeeze, and push (simulated defecation). An increase in the recruitment of fibers during straining is pathognomonic for the syndrome of paradoxic puborectalis, or inappropriate puborectalis contraction. Pudendal nerve terminal motor latency (PNTML) times are measured with a special transducer attached to a glovelike apparatus designed to be worn on the finger and hand. A digital rectal examination is required, with application of the finger electrode to the right and left levator ani complex. Values between 1.8 and 2.2 milliseconds are normal. Prolonged values are seen in traumatic injuries of the vagina or anal canal (obstetric in cause), sacral nerve root damage, or chronic diseases such as diabetes.

### Defecography

Defecography is an extremely useful modality for determining the precise nature of various pelvic floor abnormalities. Barium paste is placed in the vagina and rectum after the patient ingests water-soluble contrast to opacify the small bowel. As the patient evacuates the rectal barium paste, abnormalities occurring during the act of defecation can be recorded with fluoroscopic videotaping. A vast amount of functional and anatomic information can be gathered from this test. The presence of multiple anatomic abnormalities, such as rectocele, enterocele, and vaginal vault prolapse, can be efficiently evaluated. Functional problems such as paradoxical puborectalis syndrome have characteristic defecographic patterns and can be evaluated in this way. Many contributing anatomic problems can be readily identified.

## Rectal Prolapse (Procidentia)

### Causes and Symptoms

Most information regarding how patients develop rectal prolapse is based on observation of the clinical characteristics of those suffering from this problem. The condition was documented in the Hippocratic Corpus and, since then, descriptions of causes and rectifying procedures have been numerous. However, two competing theories of rectal prolapse did evolve. In 1912, Alexis Moschcowitz proposed that a rectal prolapse was caused by a sliding herniation of the pouch of Douglas through the pelvic floor fascia into the anterior aspect of the rectum. His theory was based on the fact that the pelvic floor of prolapse patients is mobile and unsupported and on the observation that other adjacent structures can occasionally be seen alongside the rectal component of the prolapse. With the advent of defecography in 1968, however, Broden and Snellman were able to show convincingly that procidentia is basically a full-thickness rectal intussusception starting approximately 3 inches above the dentate line and extending beyond the anal verge. Both explanations take into consideration the weakness of the pelvic floor in rectal prolapse cases, the concept of herniation, and the observation that there are abnormal anatomic features that characterize this condition.

Women aged 50 years and older are six times as likely as men to present with rectal prolapse. The peak age of incidence is the seventh decade in women, whereas the relatively few men afflicted with the syndrome may develop prolapse at the age of 40 years or younger. One striking characteristic of young male patients is their tendency to have psychiatric disorders, and many are institutionalized. Young male patients with procidentia also tend to take constipating medications and report significant symptoms related to bowel function.

### Anatomy and Pathophysiology

Patients with prolapse are frequently found to have specific anatomic characteristics. Diastasis of the levator ani, abnormally deep cul-de-sac, redundant sigmoid colon, patulous anal sphincter, and loss of the rectal sacral attachments are commonly described.

Large case reviews aimed at elucidating other predisposing factors have supported several observations. Chronic or lifelong constipation with a component of straining is present in more than 50% of patients, and 15% experience diarrhea. Contrary to the common assumption that rectal prolapse is a consequence of multiparity, 35% of patients with rectal prolapse are nulliparous. Once a prolapse is apparent, fecal incontinence becomes a predominant symptomatic feature, occurring in 50% to 75% of cases. Proximal bilateral pudendal neuropathy is present in incontinent prolapse patients and is responsible for denervation atrophy of the external sphincter musculature. This finding is absent in normal controls. It is speculated that pudendal nerve damage is responsible for pelvic floor and anal sphincter weakening and may be the underlying cause of a spectrum of pelvic floor disorders. Pudendal nerve damage can result from direct trauma (e.g., obstetric injury), chronic diseases (e.g., diabetes), and neoplastic processes causing sacral nerve root damage.

Symptoms of prolapse progress as the prolapse develops. Often, the prolapse initially comes down with defecation or straining, only to reduce spontaneously afterward. Patients describe a mass or large lump that they may have to push back in after defecation (Fig. 52-81). The presenting complaint may be the concurrent fecal incontinence that results from the prolapse, or a sensation of chronic moisture and mucous drainage in the perineal area. Minimal or spontaneously reducible prolapses may progress to a chronically prolapsed rectum, requiring digital reduction. Chronically prolapsed rectal mucosa may become thickened or ulcerated and cause significant bleeding. Occasionally, the presentation of rectal prolapse can be dramatic when the prolapsed segment becomes incarcerated below the level of the anal sphincter. Emergent operative therapy is indicated in this situation.

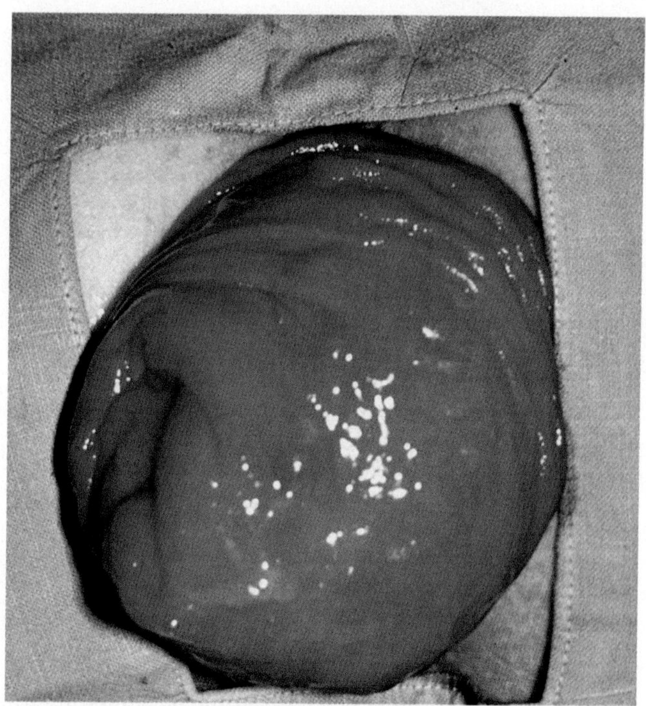

**FIGURE 52-81** Procidentia, or rectal prolapse. The entire rectum has protruded through the anal canal.

### Differential Diagnosis and Investigation

A common pitfall in the diagnosis of rectal prolapse is the potential for confusion with prolapsed incarcerated internal hemorrhoids. These conditions may be distinguished by close inspection of the direction of the prolapsed tissue folds. In the case of rectal prolapse, the folds are always concentric, whereas hemorrhoidal tissue develops radial invaginations defining the hemorrhoidal cushions. Prolapsed incarcerated hemorrhoids produce extreme pain and can be accompanied by fever and urinary retention. Unless incarcerated, rectal prolapse is easily reducible and painless.

Before operative intervention, a careful history, physical examination, and colonoscopy should be performed. Of patients with rectal prolapse, 35% complain of urinary incontinence and another 15% have a significant vaginal vault prolapse. These symptoms will require evaluation and potential multidisciplinary surgical intervention.

If the diagnosis is suspected from the history, but not detected on physical examination, confirmation can be obtained by asking the patient to produce the prolapse by straining while on a toilet. Inspection of the perineum with the patient in the sitting or squatting position is helpful for this purpose. In the event that the prolapse is still elusive, defecography (see earlier) may reveal the problem.

Although uncommon, a neoplasm may form the lead point for a rectal intussusception. For this reason, and because this age group has the highest incidence of colorectal neoplasia, colonoscopy or barium enema should precede an operation. A significant finding on colonoscopic inspection may change the operative approach.

Anal manometry and pudendal nerve terminal motor latency tests can be ordered preoperatively to evaluate symptoms of incontinence further. However, these test results rarely change the operative strategy. A finding of increased nerve conduction periods (nerve damage) may have postoperative prognostic significance for continence, although more studies are required to confirm this. Patients with evidence of nerve damage may have a higher rate of incontinence after surgical correction of the prolapse. Decreased anal squeeze or resting pressures are expected with this condition and may predate the actual development of the prolapse. Routine manometric studies for obvious prolapse are usually not done.

### Operative Repair

The number of procedures described in the literature, historically and in recent times, is breathtaking. More than 50 types of repair have been documented, most of historical interest only. Approaches have generally included anal encirclement, mucosal resection, perineal proctosigmoidectomy, anterior resection with or without rectopexy, rectopexy alone, and a host of procedures involving the use of synthetic mesh affixed to the presacral fascia. The apparent enthusiasm and ingenuity of surgeons in their quest to define the ideal prolapse operation only serves to highlight its elusiveness. Two predominant approaches, abdominal and perineal, are considered in the operative repair of rectal prolapse. The surgical approach is dictated by the comorbidities of the patient, surgeon's preference and experience, and patient age. It is generally believed that the perineal approach results in less perioperative morbidity and pain and a reduced length of hospital stay. These advantages have, until relatively recently, been considered to be offset by a higher recurrence rate but data are unclear on this point, however, and a properly executed perineal operation may yield the same good long-term results as an abdominal procedure. This point will be clarified by ongoing long-term studies. The advent of laparoscopic options may also provide advantages, but for now, recurrence data are scant.

**Ripstein Repair** The Ripstein repair has many advocates. It involves placement of a prosthetic mesh around the mobilized rectum, with attachment of the mesh to the presacral fascia below the sacral promontory. Recurrence rates for this procedure range from 2.3% to 5%. The bowel is mechanically prepared for this procedure with a polyethylene glycol or sodium phosphate solution. The procedure involves mobilizing the rectum on both sides posteriorly down to the coccyx. Division of the upper portion of the lateral rectal ligaments has been described, but some advocate leaving them wholly intact because the rates of postoperative constipation are 50% higher in patients with divided lateral stalks. After mobilization of the rectum, a 5-cm band of rectangular mesh is placed around its anterior aspect at the level of the peritoneal reflection, and both sides of the mesh are sutured with nonabsorbable suture to the presacral fascia, approximately 1 cm from the midline. Sutures are used to secure the mesh to the rectum anteriorly, and the rectum is pulled upward and posteriorly. Various materials have been recommended to secure the rectum, including autologous fascia lata, synthetic nonabsorbable products such as Marlex (Chevron Phillips Chemical, The Woodlands, Tex), Teflon (DuPont, Wilmington, Del), and absorbable prosthetics such as polyglycolic acid. The recurrence rates for all these materials are less than 10%, although follow-up times and evaluation criteria among studies have varied and strict comparisons cannot be made. Complications include large bowel obstruction, erosion of the mesh through the bowel, ureteric injury or fibrosis, small bowel obstruction, rectovaginal fistula, and fecal impaction. Postoperative morbidity rates are 20%, but most of these complications are minor. Although mesh rectopexy results in significant improvement in fecal incontinence (50%), no rectal prolapse operation should be advocated as a procedure to restore continence and patients, especially those with prolapse for longer than 2 years, should be warned of the possibility that incontinence could persist.

A significant complication of this operation is the incidence of new-onset or worsened constipation. Fifteen percent of patients experience constipation for the first time after Ripstein rectopexy, and at least 50% of those who are constipated preoperatively are made worse. Although some of these difficulties are attributed to complications of the procedure such as mesh stricture, obstruction at the level of the repair, or rectal dysfunction following lateral stalk division, a subset of patients will be found to have slow transit constipation characterizing a global motility disorder. Some advocate routine preoperative transit studies to select these patients out, but usually a good bowel habit history will suffice. The cause of any severe, unremitting postoperative defecation or obstruction problem should be investigated with a barium enema and perhaps with a small bowel study. Strictures, obstructions, adhesions, and fistulas may be identified by radiography.

Fiber, fluids, and stool softeners are useful in the management of functional constipation following rectal prolapse repairs of any type. Occasionally, mild laxatives such as milk of magnesia, magnesium citrate, or polyethylene glycol–based therapies may be necessary for short periods. Newer treatments for constipation involve oral administration of 5-$HT_4$ receptor agonists (e.g., tegaserod maleate) and may prove invaluable in the short-term treatment of this problem.

**Wells Procedure** The Wells procedure is an alternative mesh technique that reduces the incidence of rectal obstruction by eliminating the anterior placement of the mesh. The mesh is affixed to the posterior aspect of the rectal fascia propria and then to the presacral fascia as previously described. The Ivalon (polyvinyl alcohol) sponge is a method that at one point was popular among European surgeons, but has since fallen out of favor. The sponge is placed posteriorly in the deep pelvis in a manner similar to the Wells technique. In fact, Wells initially described this procedure. Although postoperative recurrence rate results have been as good as those involving synthetic nonabsorbable mesh, and reported evacuation disorders have been low, a disturbing feature of the Ivalon sponge is a high rate of pelvic abscess, necessitating sponge removal. Although polyvinyl alcohol is a sarcoma-producing carcinogen in rats, this effect has not been demonstrated in humans.

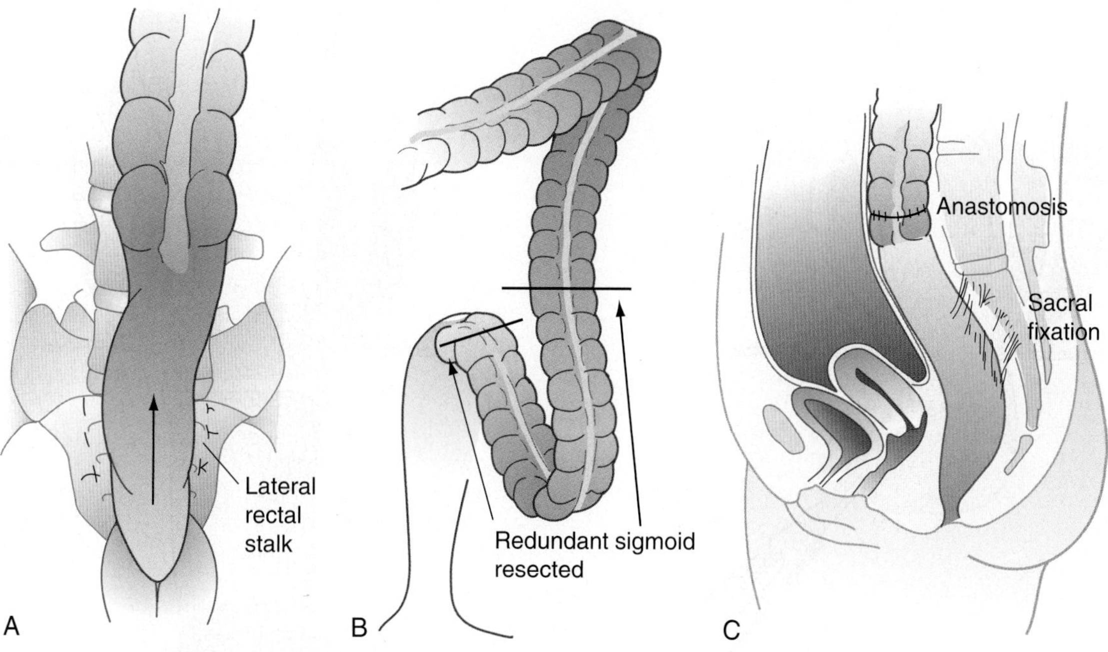


**FIGURE 52-82** Anterior resection with rectopexy, or the Frykman-Goldberg procedure, for rectal prolapse. **A,** After full mobilization by sharp dissection, the tissues lateral to the rectal wall are swept away laterally. **B,** Resection of the redundant sigmoid colon. **C,** Anastomosis is completed, and rectopexy sutures are placed. (From Gordon PH, Nivatvongs S [eds]: Principles and practice of surgery for the colon, rectum and anus, ed 2, St Louis, 1999, Quality Medical Publishing.)

**Resection Rectopexy** Resection rectopexy is a technique first described by Frykman and Goldberg in 1969 and popularized in the United States in the past 35 years (Fig. 52-82). Lack of artificial mesh, ease of operation, and reduction of redundant sigmoid colon are the principle advantages of the procedure. Recurrence rates are low, ranging from 2% to 5%, and major complication rates range from 0% to 20% and relate to obstruction or anastomotic leak. Basically, the sigmoid colon and rectum are mobilized to the level of the levatores. The lateral ligaments are divided, elevated from the deep pelvis, and sutured to the presacral fascia. The mesentery of the sigmoid colon is then divided, with preservation of the IMA, and a tension-free anastomosis is created. A revised version of this procedure involves preservation of the lateral stalks and unilateral fastening of the rectal mesentery to the sacrum at the level of the sacral promontory. Sigmoid resection is a unique and controversial feature of this procedure. It appears to reduce constipation by 50% in those who complain preoperatively of this symptom in some studies. Others have argued that sigmoidectomy is an inadequate operation for a chronic motility problem that affects the entire bowel and that those patients should be formally evaluated preoperatively and subtotal colectomy recommended if colonic inertia is detected. Interestingly, in patients who complain of incontinence before surgery, this symptom consistently improves in approximately 35%, even with the sigmoid resection. A variant of this procedure involves forgoing the sigmoid resection in those who report no history of constipation and whose predominant complaint is fecal incontinence.

**Perineal Proctosigmoidectomy and the Altemeier Procedure** Perineal proctosigmoidectomy was first introduced by Mikulicz in 1899 and remained the favored treatment for prolapse in Europe for many years. Miles advocated this procedure in the United Kingdom and it was promoted in the United States by Altemeier at the University of Cincinnati. As the abdominal approaches gained favor, principally because of the reduced recurrence rates, the perineal approach was increasingly reserved only for those with the highest operative risk. However, renewed interest in the technique has accompanied studies showing reduced recurrence rates, and a number of surgeons believe that strong consideration should be given to this technique when repairing prolapse in young men who have an increased risk for autonomic nerve injury resulting in impotence.

The Altemeier procedure combines a perineal proctosigmoidectomy with an anterior levatoroplasty (Fig. 52-83). The latter procedure is performed to correct the levator diastasis commonly associated with this condition. Theoretically, restoration of fecal continence is enhanced by this additional maneuver. As always, the large bowel is mechanically cleansed. The patient is placed in the prone jackknife position and a Foley catheter is placed. The rectal mucosa is serially grasped with Babcock or Allis clamps until a full-thickness prolapse is demonstrated. A full-thickness circumferential incision is made 1.5 cm proximal to the dentate line. The low peritoneal reflection can usually be incised anteriorly and the peritoneal cavity entered. The mesentery of the rectum and sigmoid colon is sequentially clamped and tied until no redundant bowel remains. The colon is transected at this point, and an anastomosis is fashioned between the colon and anal canal with sutures or staples.

Patients undergoing perineal proctosigmoidectomy are generally older and have significantly more comorbidities than those who are considered for abdominal repair. Complication rates are less than 10%, and recurrence rates have been reported as high as 16% although, as mentioned, some series have demonstrated significantly lower recurrence rates. Complications

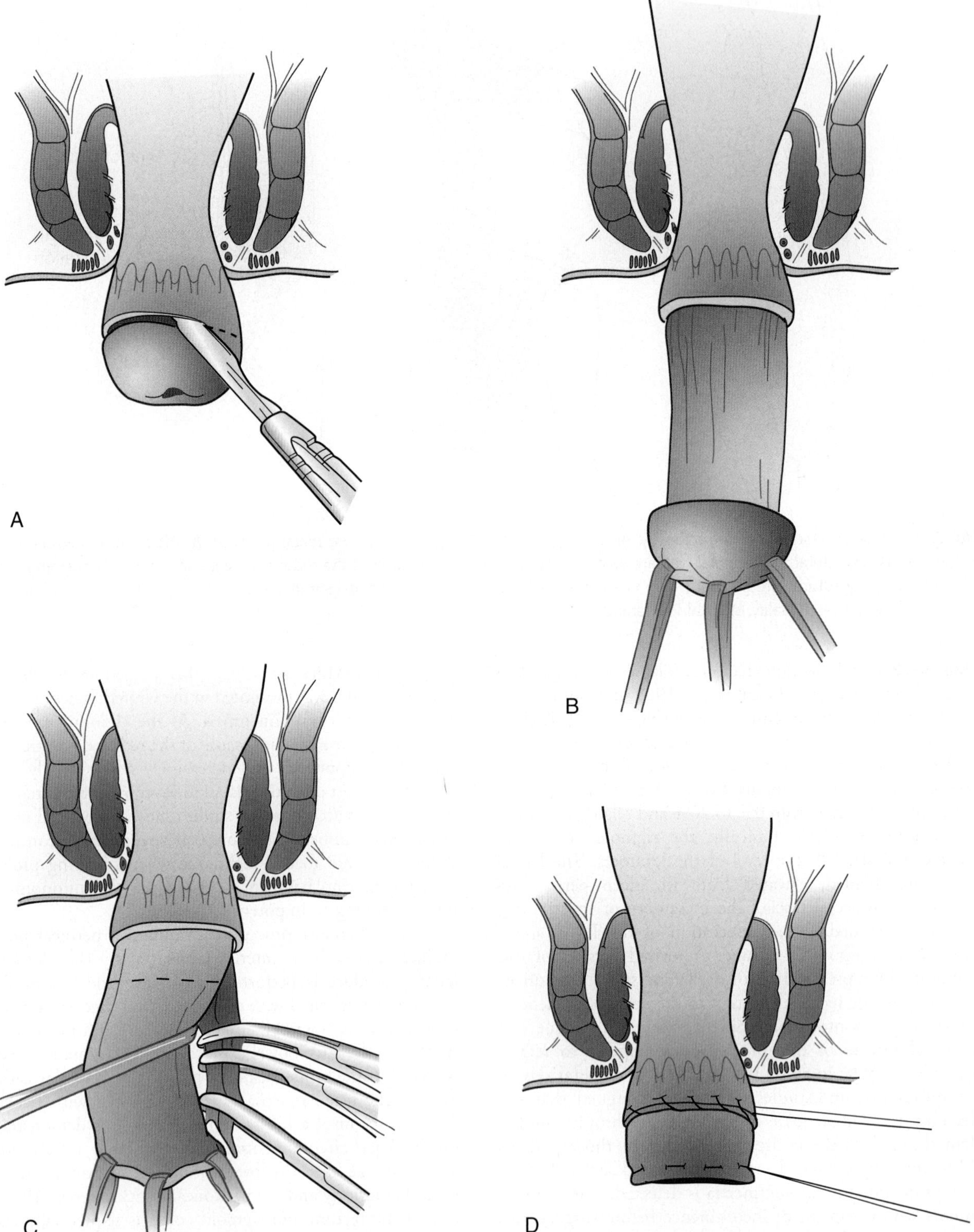


**FIGURE 52-83** Altemeier perineal rectosigmoidectomy. **A,** Circumferential incision of rectum proximal to dentate line. **B,** Delivery of redundant rectum and sigmoid colon. **C,** Ligation of blood supply to rectum. **D,** Placement of purse-string suture on proximal bowels and excision of redundant colon and rectum; whip stitch placed on rectal stump.

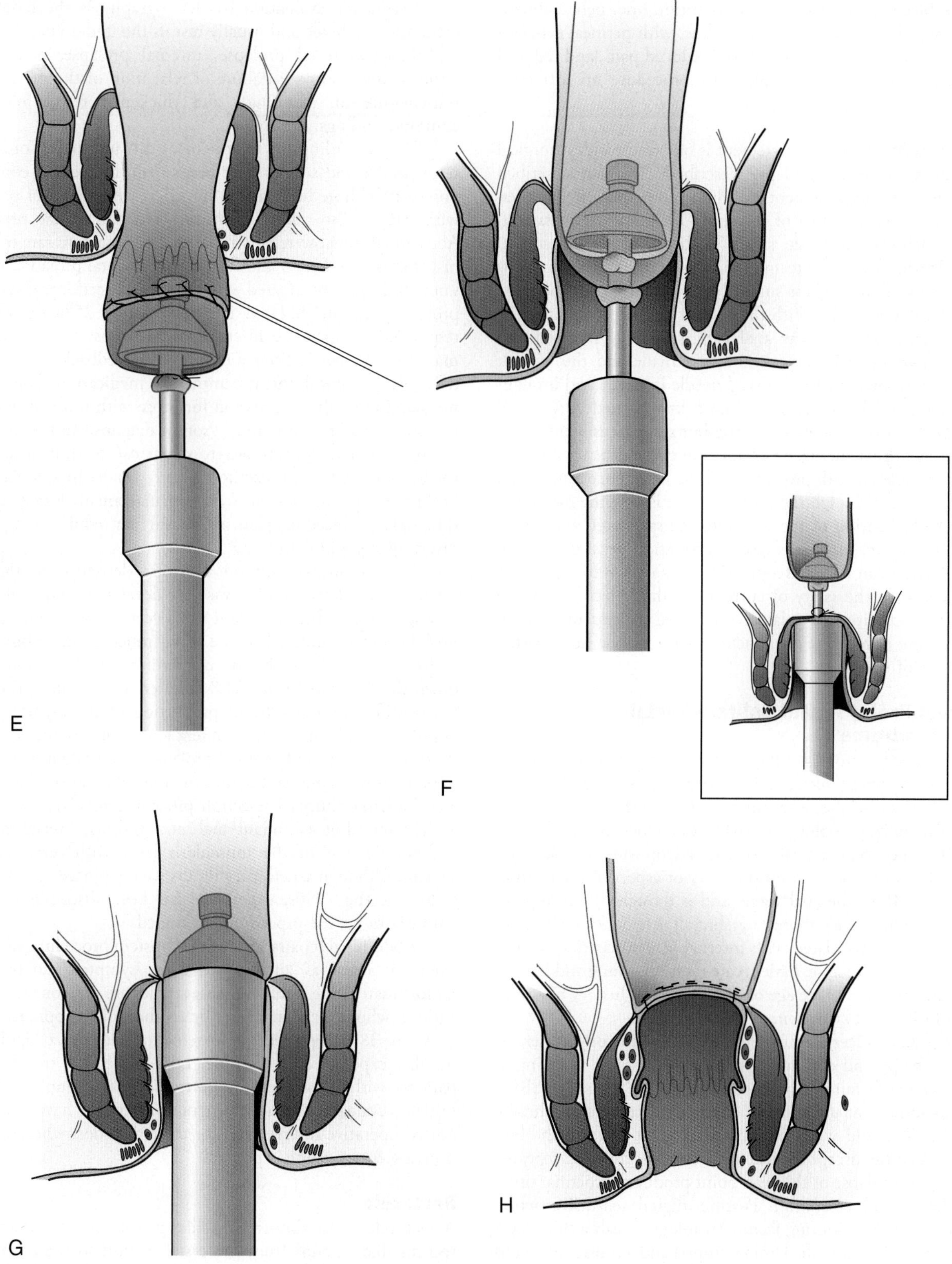


**FIGURE 52-83, cont'd E**, Proximal purse-string suture secured around central shaft. **F,** Proximal bowel advanced through anus and distal purse-string tied. **G,** Approximation of anvil to cartridge and activation of stapler. **H,** Completed anastomosis. (From Gordon PH, Nivatvongs S [eds]: Principles and practice of surgery for the colon, rectum and anus, ed 2, St Louis, 1999, Quality Medical Publishing.)

include bleeding from the staple or suture line, pelvic abscess and, rarely, dehiscence of the suture line, with perineal evisceration. Lack of an abdominal incision, reduced pain, and reduced length of hospitalization make this procedure an attractive option.

**Anal Encirclement** Anal encirclement is one of the oldest surgical techniques for rectal prolapse described. Thiersch described silver wire anal encirclement in 1891. Since then, it has been tried with a wide variety of materials, including stainless steel wire, nonabsorbable mesh, small Silastic bands, nylon suture, and polypropylene. This technique is reserved by most surgeons for patients of the highest surgical risk because it can be done under local anesthesia. With the patient in the prone jackknife or lithotomy position, the anal area is sterilely prepped and draped. Two small lateral incisions are made and the wire or suture is introduced with a curved needle into one and brought out the other. This is repeated, and a knot is tied and buried laterally. The orifice should be snug but should easily admit an index finger. Anal encirclement does not correct the fecal incontinence associated with prolapse, and the recurrence rate is high (>30%). Also, although the mortality rate is 0%, the morbidity rate is high. Erosion of the wire into the sphincter, anovaginal fistula formation, rectal prolapse incarceration, fecal impaction, and infection can occur. Reoperative rates of 7% to 59% have been reported. The safety of current anesthetic techniques and the low morbidity and relative functional success of perineal proctectomy have made anal encirclement, for the most part, a procedure of the past.

### Internal Prolapse and Solitary Rectal Ulcer Syndrome

Two areas of controversy related to rectal prolapse involve the treatment of solitary rectal ulcer syndrome (SRUS) and internal intussusception of the rectal mucosa. Although identified as an ulcer, the gross pathology of SRUS can range from a typical crater-like ulcer with a fibrinous central depression to a polypoid lesion. It is always located on the anterior aspect of the rectum, 4 to 12 cm from the anal verge, and is thought to correspond to the location of the puborectalis sling. It is frequently, although not exclusively, associated with internal intussusception or full-thickness rectal prolapse. Patients are typically young and female, however, with an average age of 25 years and a history of straining and difficult evacuation.

The rectal ulcer is usually found on proctoscopy or flexible sigmoidoscopy and commonly presents with rectal bleeding in the setting of straining or constipation. The cause of SRUS remains somewhat unclear, but speculation centers on chronic ischemia. The fold with the ulcer is thought to form the lead point of an intussusception into the anal canal. Chronic, repeated straining or prolapse of this lead point produces ischemia, tissue breakdown, and ulceration. Possible digital self-disimpaction may also be a contributing factor. Histology reveals a thick layer of fibrosis obliterating the lamina propria and a central fibrinous exudate. Other common pathologic findings include the presence of mucus-filled glands misplaced in the submucosa and lined with normal colonic epithelium (colitis cystica profunda). Differentiating SRUS from malignancy, infection, or Crohn's disease is important, but not difficult. The anterior location in the context of classic symptoms and pathologic findings is conclusive.

Diagnostic evaluation by defecography is the radiologic procedure of choice and usually reveals the underlying disorder. Full-thickness rectal prolapse, internal prolapse, paradoxical puborectalis syndrome (failure of relaxation of the pelvic floor musculature on straining), and thickened rectal folds are common findings.

Data regarding the treatment of this unusual disorder are retrospective and studies have been small, but several common observations have been made. In general, one third of patients with SRUS also suffer from full-thickness rectal prolapse. Abdominal prolapse repairs have resulted in a cure rate of 80% in patients with SRUS and full-thickness rectal prolapse. In the same study, patients treated with the same procedure for mucosal prolapse and SRUS fared far worse—only 25% of patients responded to operative intervention. In most studies, dietary management, pelvic floor retraining (biofeedback), and short-term use of topical anti-inflammatory medications containing mesalamine result in remission for those with internal prolapse or pelvic muscle dysfunction. Prompt diagnosis of the underlying problem and appropriate treatment can be difficult but are the keys to cure. Local excision usually results in a larger nonhealing wound and has no role in management. Rarely, symptoms of severe bleeding, pain, and spasm may require a temporary diverting sigmoid colostomy.

Internal intussusception was first described in the late 1960s, when defecography was first developed and came into widespread use. The condition is also called *internal* or *hidden prolapse* and is confined to the rectal mucosa and submucosa, which separates from the muscularis mucosae layer and slides down the anal canal (Fig. 52-84). Internal intussusception can be identified in a significant proportion of the asymptomatic population and appears to represent a normal variant. However, there are advocates of internal prolapse repair when it is found in patients who complain of dysfunctional defecation. The transanal Delorme mucosal resection procedure involves circumferential removal of redundant anal canal and distal rectal mucosa and imbrication of the muscularis layer with serial vertical sutures. Although satisfactory results were reported for this procedure in the 1990s, experience has been discouraging, and enthusiasm for the procedure has waned.

Abdominal repairs such as the Ripstein procedure have also been advocated as an alternative for symptomatic patients. Unfortunately, the results of these studies are not conclusive. Of patients who underwent repair by an abdominal approach, only 24% to 38% reported improvement, whereas a significant number experienced worsening. Like SRUS, the treatment of patients with incomplete or obstructed defecation should be initially evaluated with defecography. Studies have not supported operative intervention for these disorders when internal intussusception alone is present.

### Rectocele

A rectocele is an abnormal saclike projection of the anterior rectum that extends from the distal rectum to the distal anal canal. It usually begins just above the sphincter complex (Figs. 52-85 and 52-86). The cause of rectoceles is multifactorial. Stretching of the endopelvic fascia from antecedent pelvic floor injury, followed by chronic increased intra-abdominal pressure, causes an anterior full-thickness herniation of the rectum into the vagina. Rectal pressures are higher than those in the vagina; therefore, pressure tends to push the rectum anteriorly and

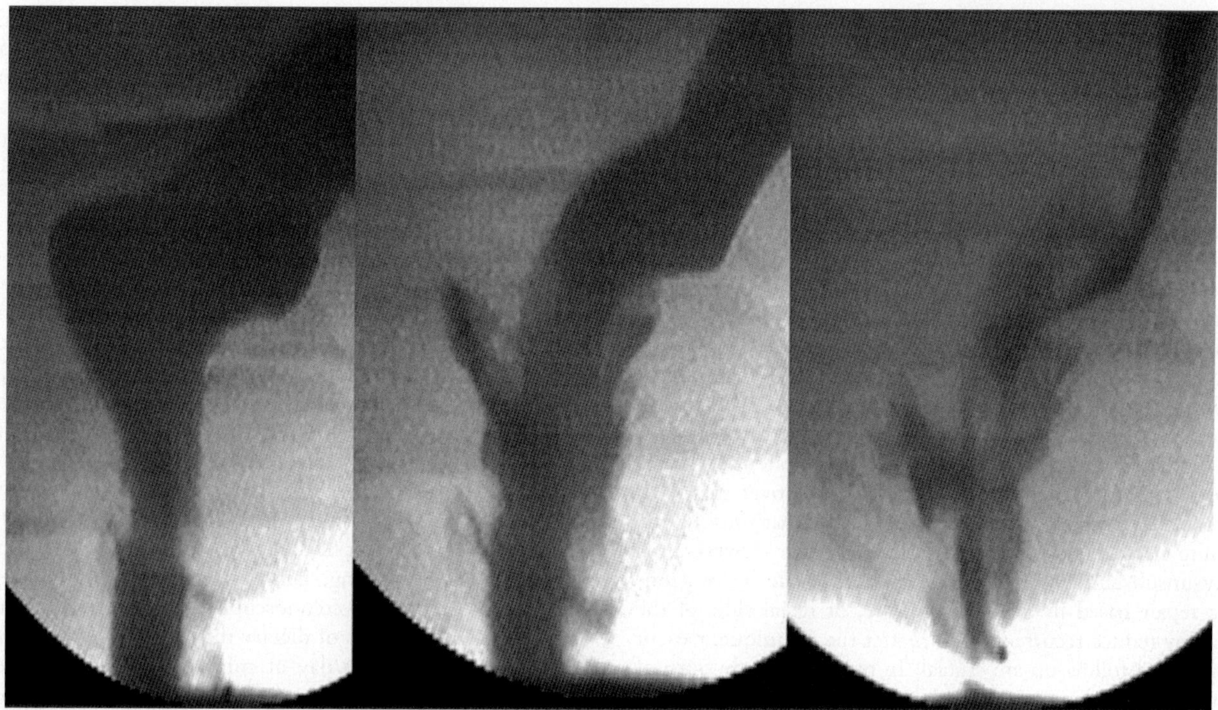

**FIGURE 52-84** Defecogram showing progression of internal intussusception.

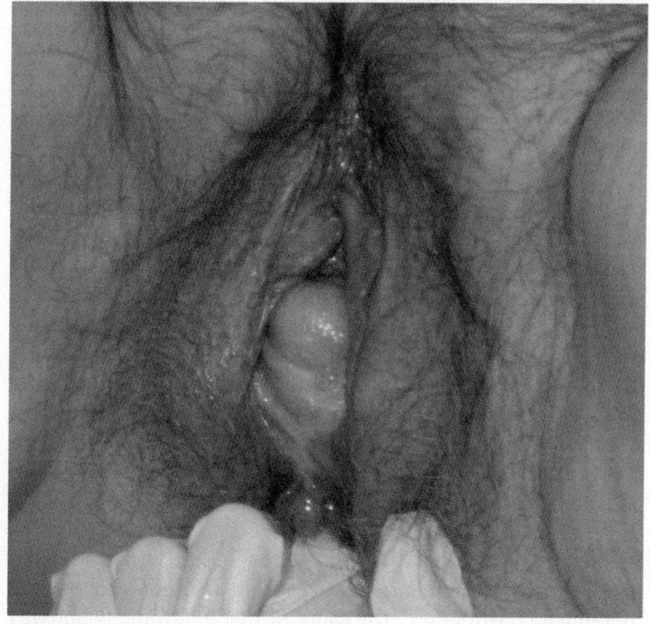

**FIGURE 52-85** Digital anorectal examination demonstrating anterior rectocele protruding from the vaginal introitus.

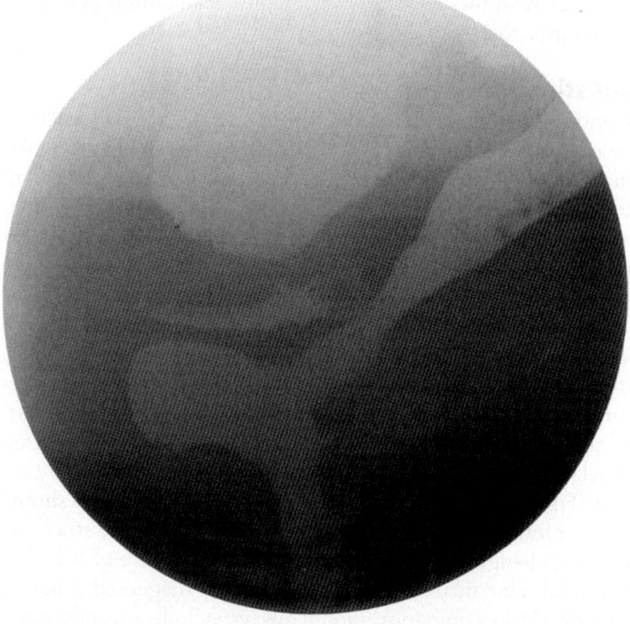

**FIGURE 52-86** Triple-contrast radiograph demonstrates large anterior rectocele. Contrast material is also in the vagina and small intestine.

stretch and shift the rectovaginal septum as well. The major symptom of rectocele is stool trapping, a form of obstructed defecation. Women commonly describe requiring vaginal pressure to reduce the bulge, effectively stenting the anterior rectum and enabling defecation.

Criteria for operative intervention include symptomatic stool trapping requiring digital evacuation or vaginal support and the presence of large protruding rectoceles that push vaginal mucosa beyond the introitus producing dryness, ulceration, and discomfort. Although small rectoceles are common, it is rare that a rectocele smaller than 2 cm is symptomatic.

There are two major operative approaches to rectoceles, transanal and transvaginal. Although the transvaginal approach has been criticized by surgeons because the repair is done on the low-pressure side of the rectovaginal septum, it does have certain distinct advantages. The bowel is fully prepared and the patient is placed in the lithotomy position. After the submucosal injection of lidocaine with 1% epinephrine, a swath of vagina is excised, starting at the vaginal introitus and carried to the apex of the vagina. The size of this segment is determined by the depth of the rectocele. The goal is to excise a full-thickness segment of vagina, dissect out and reduce an enterocele if one is found in the rectovaginal septum, and then obliterate the deep cul-de-sac by suturing the cut edges of the vagina closed, allowing the space to contract by fibrosis.

Alternatively, several approaches for the transanal correction of rectocele have been described. This technique was probably best described by Sullivan, who expected 80% of patients to have good to excellent results. An incision is made longitudinally in the rectum over the bulge above the sphincters. The incision's length varies with the size of the rectocele. The underlying vagina is exposed and imbricated to obliterate the sac and the rectum is separately imbricated and closed over that with absorbable sutures. Unfortunately, direct comparisons in the literature between these techniques are absent. However, the largely unsubstantiated argument has been made by surgeons that a repair based in the high-pressure, or rectal side, of the bulge may reduce recurrence. No matter the technique, patient selection and follow-up are crucial. In one study, only 54% of patients who underwent rectocele repair obtained relief from their symptoms of obstructive defecation. Paradoxical puborectalis syndrome was not ruled out and was responsible for continued problems. Postoperative biofeedback therapy is appropriate in these cases. Defecography evaluation is helpful to distinguish these problems before surgery.

## Constipation

Constipation is a symptom, and it is often used by patients to describe different problems. It occurs frequently in older populations; in one survey, 50% of women and 30% of men older than 65 years were affected. Although functional constipation appears to occur most often in older patients, a small subset of patients present at a young age with severe unremitting symptoms. These patients are evaluated differently (see later). Although most individuals describe constipation in terms of reduced stool frequency, up to 25% use the term to indicate straining, excessive pushing, or a feeling of incomplete defecation. Normal stool frequencies range from three times weekly to three times daily. The causes of constipation are numerous, but the evaluation of constipation is relatively straightforward and the indications for surgery are few (Fig. 52-87). The initial evaluation of constipation should elicit information regarding acuteness of symptoms, stool frequency, changes in stool form, presence or absence of blood in the stool, new medications, and any newly diagnosed illnesses. The physical examination should always include a rectal examination and proctoscopy. New-onset constipation can be divided into categories for further diagnostic consideration. These categories are depression or debilitation, new medications, endocrine conditions such as hypothyroidism, and obstructed defecation. For our purposes, we will focus on surgically correctable causes while recognizing that most constipation is chronic and functional and is rectified simply by the addition of fluid and fiber to the diet.

A patient whose symptoms include straining and incomplete defecation with a normal stool frequency should be evaluated for obstructive defecation. The best way to obtain the most information is through the physical examination and defecography. Symptomatic rectoceles are those that fail to empty completely on defecogram. Associated anatomic abnormalities (e.g., vaginal vault prolapse, enterocele) can be concurrently corrected. Anal manometry with electromyographic recruitment is an invaluable investigatory tool for the patient with normal anatomy and suspected paradoxical puborectalis syndrome. Biofeedback therapy is indicated in these cases. Occasionally, surgically correctable rectocele and functional defecatory disorders coexist. In this situation, biofeedback is usually initiated and rectocele repair is done subsequently.

The primary concern for the physician evaluating new-onset constipation is to rule out large bowel malignancy. A patient who presents with complaints of an acute change in bowel habits should be evaluated by colonoscopy in the absence of obvious causes such as narcotic usage. Suspect medications should be immediately stopped and reevaluation should take place shortly thereafter. No improvement or a guaiac-positive stool should lead to a colonoscopic examination. Barium enema is acceptable as well, but flexible sigmoidoscopy, even combined with stool guaiac testing, fails to detect 25% of right-sided malignancies. A normal colonoscopic examination is reassuring and should lead to trials of dietary therapy. Fluid intake should be increased to 2 liters/day at minimum, and fiber therapy should be instituted. Caffeinated beverages should be avoided. There are many other laxative-based strategies for the short-term treatment of functional constipation. Long-term failure to respond to these strategies necessitates further investigation.

### Transit Studies

Measurement of the colonic transit time is a valuable aid in the establishment of a diagnosis of slow-transit constipation, or colonic inertia. Although many different techniques exist to assess colonic transit times, two main goals of testing are to establish whole-gut and segmental transit values. A common and simple test has been devised by Martelli to do both. The patient is asked to refrain from the use of laxatives or constipating medications such as iron supplements for 3 to 4 days before the test. The patient ingests a capsule containing 20 radiopaque markers and an abdominal x-ray is obtained on each subsequent day for a total of 7 days, or until the markers are expelled. The capsules are quantified in three areas of the colon—right, left, and rectosigmoid. Normal subjects expel 80% of markers within 5 days after ingestion. Slow-transit constipation is diagnosed in patients who fail to meet these criteria.

**Slow-Transit Constipation: Colonic Inertia** It has been estimated that 2% of the population suffers from chronic, unremitting functional constipation. The cause of this syndrome is not well understood, but it has been suggested that most of the motility alterations in slow transit constipation might be of neuropathic origin, and there is some evidence suggesting that subtle alterations of the enteric nervous system, not evident to conventional histologic examination, may be present in these patients.[48] Most patients are female, with a mean age younger than 30 years. Most of them will report that they were constipated as children and that the constipation worsened during adolescence and early adulthood. Bowel movement frequency is widely variable and ranges from once or twice weekly to once every 2 to 3 weeks. Abdominal pain, bloating, and nausea accompany the constipation and make these patients miserable. Frequent use of over-the-counter laxatives and enemas characterize this group, and

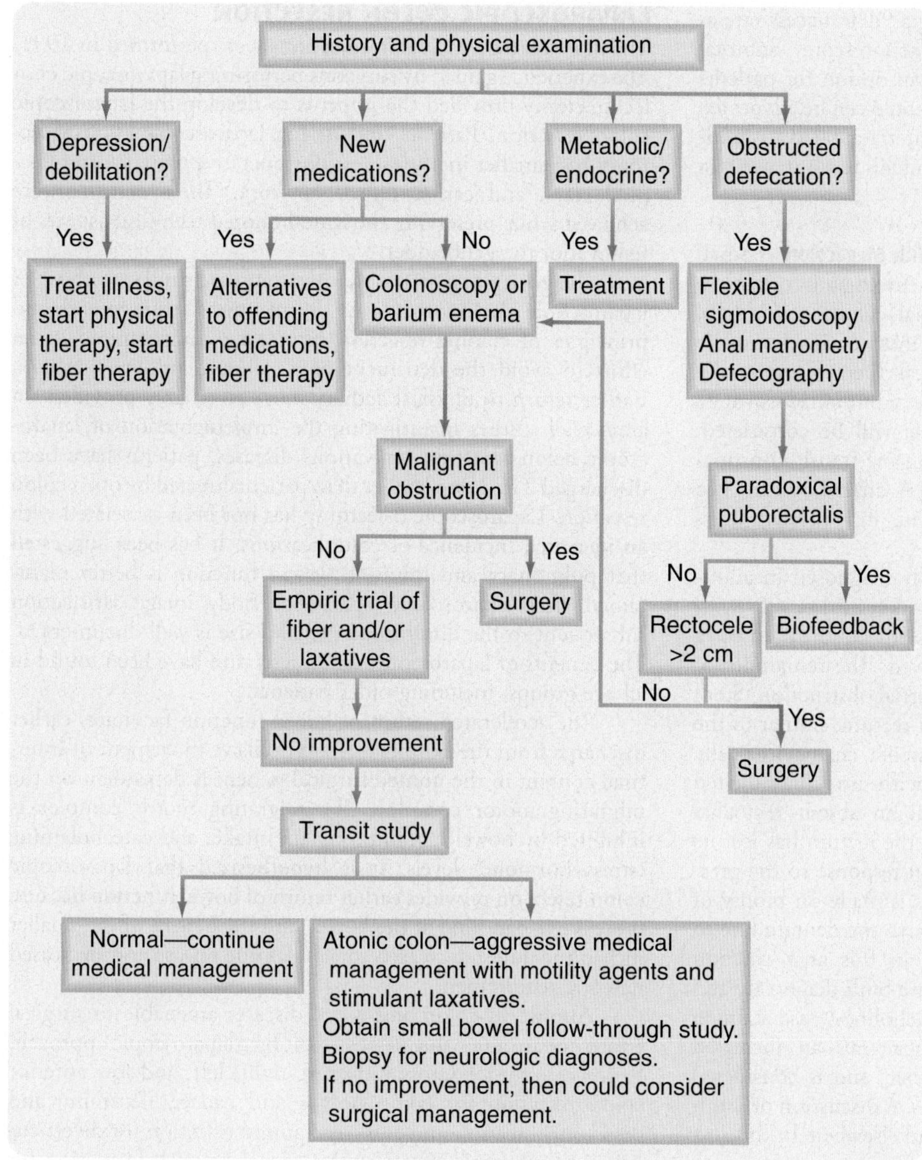


**FIGURE 52-87** Algorithm for management of patients with constipation.

concurrent psychiatric conditions such as depression are common. Although malignancy in this group is exceedingly rare, it should be ruled out. A barium enema is a useful initial examination; not only does it screen for large obvious lesions, but the morphology of the colon and presence of dilation can also be evaluated. A transit study is the next diagnostic step. Biopsies are usually not indicated unless a strong suspicion of neuropathic constipation is harbored. A loss of the argyrophil plexus, with a marked increase in Schwann cells indicating extrinsic damage to the myenteric plexus, may be found. This damage is thought to result from chronic laxative abuse. A delay in gastric emptying and small bowel follow-through has been noted in some patients, implying a global motility problem. This motility problem may be responsible for the mixed surgical outcomes reported.

An aggressive bowel regimen is always the first course of action after the diagnosis of slow-transit constipation. A combination of laxatives, fiber, and polyethylene glycol–based solutions can be helpful. A new class of laxative approved for short-term use is 5-$HT_4$ receptor agonists. These may prove beneficial and merit investigation.

Surgery for idiopathic colonic inertia is controversial. The most commonly described procedure is subtotal colectomy with ileorectal anastomosis. Traditionally, only patients with symptoms in the setting of megacolon or megarectum were considered for operative intervention, but now more patients with a normal-caliber colon and severe refractory constipation are being referred for surgery. The costs and inconvenience associated with medical therapy for severe chronic constipation are not inconsiderable. Intuitively, surgery may seem like an attractive option. However, the data concerning lasting cure are unclear. In most series that included more than 20 patients and had longer than 2-year follow-up, results ranged from 33% to 94% success rates (regular defecation without the use of laxatives). The wide range of results is concerning. It has been noted that often the symptoms of nausea, bloating, and abdominal pain can persist and be accompanied by incapacitating diarrhea. In effect, many patients trade one symptom complex for another. There have been only a few small prospective studies exercising strict selection criteria for surgery that includes normal defecography results and diffuse delay on transit study. These patients appear to fare best in follow-up, enjoying a 94% success rate as defined by good or excellent patient satisfaction scores. Subtotal colectomy with ileorectal anastomosis is an option for patients with normal-caliber colonic inertia, but should not be advocated as a perfect solution. Careful selection criteria applied to motivated, psychologically well-adjusted individuals result in the best long-term surgical results.

**Slow-Transit Constipation: Colonic Inertia With Megacolon** A small but important subset of constipation is neurologic in origin. In contrast to colonic inertia with a normal colon, as a group, 50% of these patients are male. Surgical intervention is usually indicated in these cases because medical therapy eventually fails. Among these entities, Chagas' disease, adult Hirschsprung's disease, and neuronal intestinal dysplasia will be considered. Commonly, all these causes present with slow-transit constipation in the presence of a dilated colon. A dilated rectum is a variable finding and is typically absent in Hirschsprung's disease.

Hirschsprung's disease is occasionally diagnosed in adulthood. These patients are typically young men in their 20s with lifelong evacuation complaints. Commonly, in these cases, a short, distal segment of rectum is involved. The remainder of the colon is dilated from chronic distal partial obstruction. Stool is characteristically absent from the distal rectum, similar to the physical finding in children. Barium enema characteristically demonstrates a narrow distal rectum with proximal dilated colon. Anal manometric findings reveal an absent rectoanal inhibitory reflex (RAIR), indicating that the rectum has lost its neurologically mediated ability to relax in response to the presence of a fecal load. Histologic diagnosis is made on biopsy of the distal rectal mucosa at least 3 cm above the dentate line to avoid the normal aganglionic segment in this area. Suction mucosal and superficial punch biopsies are both diagnostic and can be done in the office setting. Acetylcholinesterase staining of the submucosa and lamina propria reveals an increased number of large brown-stained nerve fibers and is considered 99% accurate in establishing the diagnosis. A discussion of surgical interventions for this problem is found elsewhere in this text (see Chapter 67, "Pediatric Surgery").

Megacolon is the most common complication of intestinal trypanosomiasis. The organism involved is *Trypanosoma cruzi,* a parasite endemic to South America. Nerve damage resulting from trypanosomiasis causes megacolon and megarectum. Fecal impaction and sigmoid volvulus are the most common complications. Subtotal colectomy for this problem results in a residual dyskinetic rectum; therefore, pull-through procedures with excision of the colon and rectum and creation of an ileal reservoir (ileal J pouch or Park's pouch) are preferable.

Neuronal intestinal dysplasia describes two distinct congenital defects of the intestinal mural ganglia. Type A is seen predominantly in children and consists of hypoplasia of the sympathetic innervation. Type B is present in children and adults and is characterized by dysplasia of the submucosal plexus, resulting in weak forward propulsion of stool. Histologically, hyperplasia and giant ganglia with seven to ten nerve cells are present. Acetylcholinesterase staining shows a dense plexus of parasympathetic fibers with increased activity. Laxative therapy in these individuals is usually a short-term strategy, and most patients fail treatment. Surgical resection with ileorectal anastomosis is the treatment of choice.

## LAPAROSCOPIC COLON RESECTION

The first laparoscopic colon resections were performed in 1991. The experience gained by surgeons performing laparoscopic cholecystectomy provided the impetus to develop the laparoscopic colon resection. Patients undergoing laparoscopic cholecystectomy had smaller incisions, less postoperative pain, shorter hospital stays, and earlier return to work. These benefits were achieved while preserving the time-honored technical aspects of removal of the gallbladder.

The goals of laparoscopic colectomy are similar to those of laparoscopic cholecystectomy. The technical requirements and principles of colonic resection cannot be compromised in an effort to avoid the detriment of a standard midline incision. Earlier return to physical activity must be reliably provided. In almost all studies investigating the implementation of laparoscopic colon resection for various diseases, patients have been discharged 2 to 3 days earlier than patients treated by open colon resection. Laparoscopic colectomy has not been associated with an increased incidence of complications. It has been suggested that pulmonary and immune system function is better maintained after laparoscopic operation. Body image satisfaction subsequent to the diminished incision size is well documented. The benefits of laparoscopic colon resection have been found in all age groups, including older patients.

The accelerated return of bowel function facilitates earlier discharge from the hospital. The propulsive movement of intestinal content in the nonfed surgical patient is dependent on the migrating motor complex. The migrating motor complex is inhibited by bowel handling, opiate intake, and catecholamine (stress hormone) levels. It is hypothesized that laparoscopic colon resection provides earlier return of bowel function because there is less handling of the bowel, and the benefit of the smaller incision includes decreased catecholamine release and decreased narcotic requirement.

Almost all colon and rectal diseases amenable to surgical treatment are amenable to treatment by a laparoscopic approach. Ileocecectomy for Crohn's disease, right, left, and low anterior colon resection for colon polyps and cancer, ileostomy and colostomy creation and closure, sigmoid resection for diverticulitis, and proctocolectomy with ileoanal J pouch formation for ulcerative colitis are all performed regularly at centers by colon and rectal surgeons who have advanced laparoscopic training. The indications for surgery are the same whether the approach is through a standard incision or by laparoscopic technique. The laparoscopic surgeon essentially performs a proven operation by a technique that reduces the length of the abdominal incision.

There are various nuances of the techniques used by laparoscopic surgeons. Laparoscopic techniques of colon resection invariably involve laparoscopic mobilization of the diseased colonic segments. The postoperative recovery benefit of laparoscopic colon resection is not altered if hand-assisted techniques are used or if bowel division and anastomosis are performed intracorporeally or extracorporeally.

In the first decade after the development of laparoscopic colectomy, there was a concern that laparoscopic colon resection for cancer might not achieve cure rates established by standard oncologic operations. These concerns seemed especially pertinent given a report from Europe in 1994 of a high rate of port site cancer recurrence. As experience has accumulated, port site recurrence appears equivalent to recurrence of cancer in the incision of patients treated by conventional operation.

If the operation is conducted correctly, proximal and distal resection margins and lymph node harvest are the same whether a laparoscopic or conventional incision approach is used. A landmark multi-institutional prospective randomized trial of patients undergoing curative colon cancer resection was reported in 2004,[49] and subsequent experience has confirmed the validity of laparoscopic colectomy as a viable oncologic operation.[50] These studies demonstrated noninferiority of laparoscopic colectomy when compared with operation conducted through a conventional midline incision. In the hands of experienced surgeons, laparoscopic colectomy has proven not only safe but also equally efficacious with regard to survival. The studies also demonstrated decreased pain medicine requirements and shorter hospital stay of patients in the laparoscopic group.

## Technical Considerations and Highlights

### Equipment

The performance of a laparoscopic colon resection requires instruments that will allow gentle handling of small and large bowel. We use 5-mm atraumatic Babcock graspers. A vessel sealant device permits the efficient division of vascularized structures within the abdomen. Although not commonly required, we have ready access to endoscopic loop ligature devices if vascular pedicles bleed after division.

### Positioning and Port Placement

Although there are many reported optimal patient and port positions, individual preferences determine practice. Some important constants exist. Foremost is the development and use of a standardized setup and operative routine. Efficiencies develop that are of benefit to the entire operative team if each operation is not performed as if it is the surgeon's first. In general, all ports should be separated by four fingerbreadths. Visualization is optimized by the placement of the camera port as far as possible from a hand-assist device. Use of a split-leg patient position allows the surgeon to stand between the patient's legs and enhances the ability to reach all quadrants of the abdomen.

### Conversion

At times, regardless of surgeon experience, the safe completion of an operation requires the need to make a larger incision. Many reasons for conversion exist, including adhesions from prior surgery, bleeding, obesity, inability to identify key structures (e.g., the ureter), and failure to move an operation to completion. We consider conversion not to be a technical shortcoming, but rather a necessary step to ensure an appropriate operation. Patients whose operations were converted from laparoscopic to open have not experienced adverse short- or long-term outcomes. Our advice is to convert early in an operation to minimize operating time. Part of the learning curve in laparoscopic colectomy is earlier recognition of the need to convert a laparoscopic procedure.

## Procedures

### Right Colon Resection

Our technique uses four ports, with a camera port created through an infraumbilical 10-mm incision. Two 5-mm ports are placed in the left lower quadrant. The first is two to three fingerbreadths superior and medial to the anterior superior iliac spine. The next is four fingerbreadths superior to this. Mobilization begins at the terminal ileum and proceeds to the hepatic flexure. The omentum is then taken off the transverse colon. The hepatic flexure attachments are divided with a tissue sealant device. Once mobilized, we generally create a window around the ileocolic pedicle toward its origin and divide the pedicle intracorporeally. A 3- to 5-cm inferior extension of the camera insertion site is created and a wound protector is placed in the wound. The terminal ileum, right colon, hepatic flexure, and transverse colon are delivered into the wound. Bowel division and stapled anastomosis are performed extracorporeally in standard fashion. The anastomosis is returned to the abdomen.

Figure 52-88 illustrates standard port placement. Figure 52-89 illustrates the mobilized right colon resected to excise an endoscopically unresectable polyp discovered at colonoscopy. It

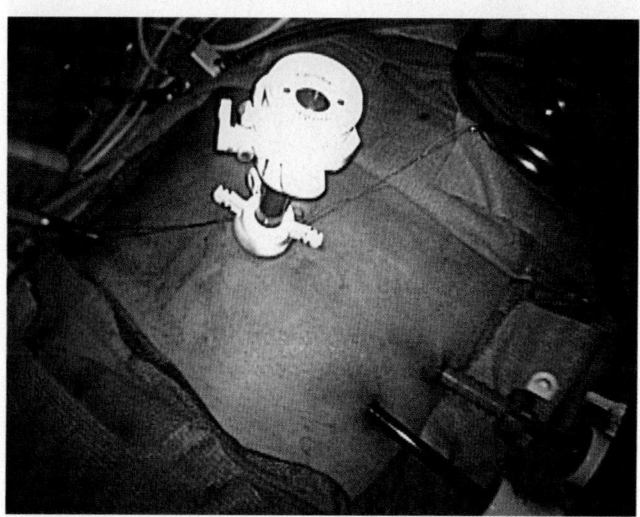

**FIGURE 52-88** Standard port placement for right colon resection.

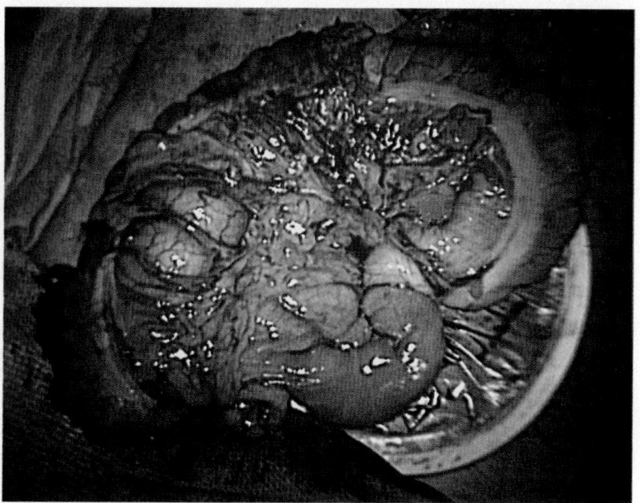

**FIGURE 52-89** Right colon, mobilized and delivered through a small midline wound. The right colon is being resected to excise an endoscopically unresectable polyp discovered at colonoscopy. It is helpful to note the ink tattoo that marked the location of the polyp.

is valuable to note the ink tattoo that marked the location of the polyp. Figure 52-90 represents ileocecal Crohn's disease, mobilized and then delivered through a 4-cm wound. Figure 52-91 represents a typical postoperative cosmetic result of a laparoscopic right colon resection.

### Hand-Assisted Laparoscopic Colon Resection

Even if a surgeon has the skills and desire to completely mobilize the colon and divide all vasculature intracorporeally, the specimen must be removed. Surgeons and device manufacturers have taken advantage of the need to make an incision of a few centimeters for specimen extraction. Hand-assist devices allow surgeons to place a single hand into a patient's abdomen through this wound while not losing pneumoperitoneum. Such techniques return the sense of touch to the surgeon, facilitating maneuvers such as finger fracture of a diverticular phlegmon off the pelvic sidewall, division of a colovesical fistula, and speeding of the division of vascular structures. Hand-assist devices lower the threshold for surgeons to attempt laparoscopic techniques. Figure 52-92 illustrates the division of a colovesical fistula that formed in response to diverticulitis. Recovery benefits are similar whether hand-assisted laparoscopic techniques are used or pure laparoscopic surgery is performed.

Clearly, there are a number of approaches to colectomy. Many surgeons perform a medial to lateral approach when the vascular pedicle is divided early in the operation. We believe that it is important for surgeons to be facile with all mobilization techniques.

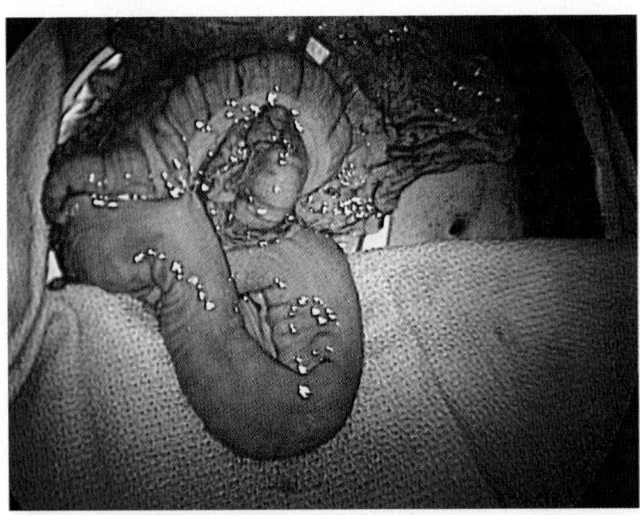

**FIGURE 52-90** Completed right colon resection with ileotransverse colon anastomosis. The exteriorized anastomosis is ready to be returned to the abdomen.

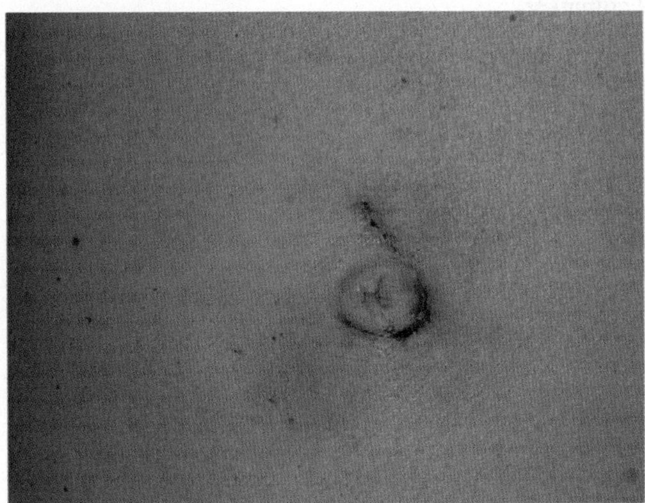

**FIGURE 52-91** Immediate postoperative cosmetic result after total abdominal colectomy.

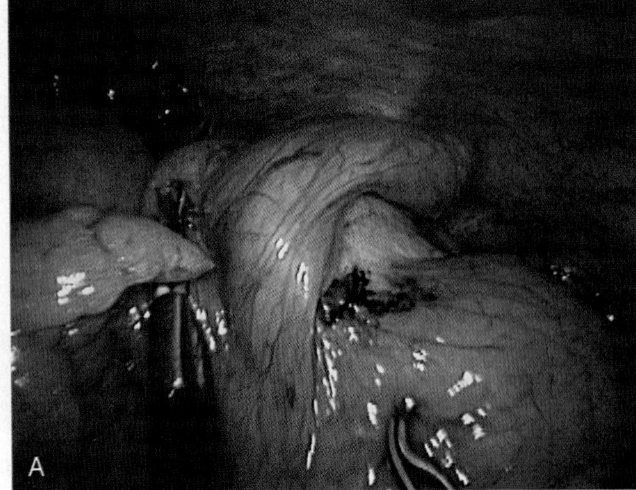


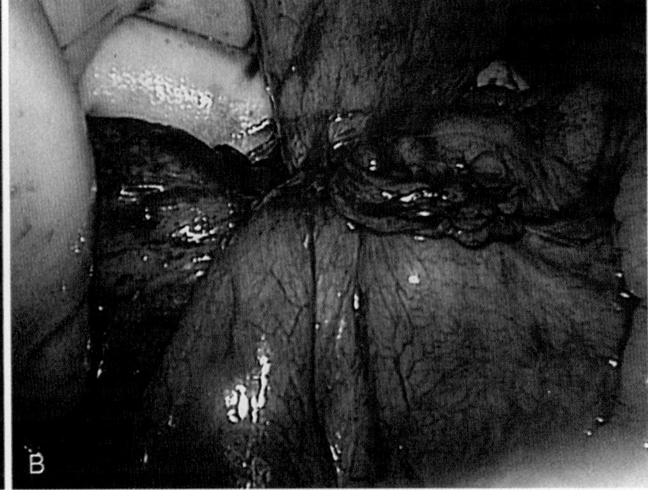


**FIGURE 52-92 A,** Laparoscopic identification of a colonic tattoo. The ink on the colon wall corresponds to the endoluminal location of a polyp. **B,** Hand-assisted division of a colovesical fistula.

## SELECTED REFERENCES


Clinical Outcomes of Surgical Therapy Study Group: A comparison of laparoscopically assisted and open colectomy for colon cancer. N Engl J Med 350:2050–2059, 2004.

A multi-institutional study demonstrating similar results for laparoscopically assisted colectomy and open colectomy performed for colon cancer.

Corman ML (ed): Colon and rectal surgery, ed 5, Philadelphia, 2005, Lippincott Williams & Wilkins.

A surgeon's view of the entire spectrum of colon and rectal surgery. Scattered throughout the text are 139 thumbnail biographical sketches of historical surgeons filled with fun factoids.

Dukes CE: The classification of cancer of the rectum. J Pathol Bacteriol 35:323–332, 1932.

A classification of rectal cancer that provided prognostic information based on the depth of penetration of the tumor and presence or absence of lymphatic metastases.

Gordon PL, Nivatvongs S (eds): Principles and practice of surgery for the colon, rectum, and anus, ed 3, London, 2007, Informa Healthcare.

This text provides excellent anatomic illustrations and detailed descriptions of all aspects of diseases of the colon, rectum, and anus. The discussion of anorectal abscesses and fistula-in-ano is particularly helpful.

Haggitt RC, Glotzbach RE, Soffer EE, et al: Prognostic factors in colorectal carcinomas arising in adenomas: Implications for lesions removed by endoscopic polypectomy. Gastroenterology 89:328–336, 1985.

Description of Haggitt's criteria, a classification for polyps with adenocarcinoma that assesses malignant potential according to the depth of invasion

Keighley MRB, Williams NS (eds): Surgery of the anus, rectum, and colon, ed 3, Philadelphia, 2008, Saunders Elsevier.

This comprehensive two-volume text has been expanded to include laparoscopic procedures and has added a number of contributers who are recognized authorities in their fields. Excellent illustrations accompany a lucid text.

Miles WE: Pathology of spread of cancer of rectum and its bearing on surgery of cancerous rectum. Surg Gynecol Obstet 52:350–359, 1931.

Classic article describing the lymphatic pathways whereby rectal cancer spreads, providing the rationale for abdominal perineal resection as a superior operation to perineal proctectomy.

Wolff BG, Fleshman JW, Beck DE, et al (eds): The ASCRS textbook of colon and rectal surgery, New York, 2007, Springer.

This text is sponsored by the American Society of Colon and Rectal Surgeons, with chapters written by recognized authorities in their field.

Vogelstein B, Fearon ER, Hamilton SR, et al: Genetic alterations during colorectal-tumor development. N Engl J Med 319:525–532, 1988.

An excellent description of the most common molecular pathways in the development of colorectal adenocarcinoma.


## REFERENCES


1. Pai R, Kang G: Microbes in the gut: A digestable account of host-symbiont interactions. Indian J Med Res 128:587–594, 2008.
2. Parkes GC, Sanderson JD, Whelan K: The mechanisms and efficacy of probiotics in the prevention of Clostridium difficile–associated diarrhoea. Lancet Infect Dis 9:237–244, 2009.
3. McFarland LV: Evidence-based review of probiotics for antibiotic-associated diarrhea and Clostridium difficile infections. Anaerobe 15:274–280, 2009.
4. Wong JM, de Souza R, Kendall CW, et al: Colonic health: fermentation and short-chain fatty acids. J Clin Gastroenterol 40:235–243, 2006.
5. Bassotti G, de Roberto G, Castellani D, et al: Normal aspects of colorectal motility and abnormalities in slow transit constipation. World J Gastroenterol 11:2691–2696, 2005.
6. Sheth AA, Longo W, Floch MH: Diverticular disease and diverticulitis. Am J Gastroenterol 103:1550–1556, 2008.
7. Janes SE, Meagher A, Frizelle FA: Management of diverticulitis. BMJ 332:271–275, 2006.
8. Rafferty J, Shellito P, Hyman NH, et al: Practice parameters for sigmoid diverticulitis. Dis Colon Rectum 49:939–944, 2006.
9. Rocco A, Compare D, Caruso F, et al: Treatment options for uncomplicated diverticular disease of the colon. J Clin Gastroenterol 43:803–808, 2009.
10. Anaya DA, Flum DR: Risk of emergency colectomy and colostomy in patients with diverticular disease. Arch Surg 140:681–685, 2005.
11. Strate LL, Liu YL, Syngal S, et al: Nut, corn, and popcorn consumption and the incidence of diverticular disease. JAMA 300:907–914, 2008.
12. Chapman JR, Dozois EJ, Wolff BG, et al: Diverticulitis: a progressive disease? Do multiple recurrences predict less favorable outcomes? Ann Surg 243:876–883, 2006.
13. Salem L, Veenstra DL, Sullivan SD, et al: The timing of elective colectomy in diverticulitis: a decision analysis. J Am Coll Surg 199:904–912, 2004.
14. Ouaissi M, Maggiori L, Alves A, et al: Colorectal cancer complicating inflammatory bowel disease: A comparative study of Crohn's disease vs ulcerative colitis in 34 patients. Colorectal Dis 13:684–688, 2011.
15. Alamili M, Gogenur I, Rosenberg J: Acute complicated diverticulitis managed by laparoscopic lavage. Dis Colon Rectum 52:1345–1349, 2009.
16. West AB: The pathology of diverticulitis. J Clin Gastroenterol 42:1137–1138, 2008.
17. Mulhall AM, Mahid SS, Petras RE, et al: Diverticular disease associated with inflammatory bowel disease-like colitis: A systematic review. Dis Colon Rectum 52:1072–1079, 2009.
18. Kiran RP, Khoury W, Church JM, et al: Colorectal cancer complicating inflammatory bowel disease: similarities and differences between Crohn's and ulcerative colitis based on three decades of experience. Ann Surg 252:330–335, 2010.

19. Edge SB, Byrd DR, Compton CC, et al (eds): AJCC cancer staging manual, ed 7, New York, 2010, Springer-Verlag.
20. Metcalf DR, Nivatvongs S, Sullivan TM, et al: A technique of extending small-bowel mesentery for ileal pouch-anal anastomosis: Report of a case. Dis Colon Rectum 51:363–364, 2008.
21. Remzi FH, Fazio VW, Gorgun E, et al: The outcome after restorative proctocolectomy with or without defunctioning ileostomy. Dis Colon Rectum 49:470–477, 2006.
22. Shen B, Fazio VW, Remzi FH, et al: Clinical approach to diseases of ileal pouch–anal anastomosis. Am J Gastroenterol 100:2796–2807, 2005.
23. Karapetis CS, Khambata-Ford S, Jonker DJ, et al: K-ras mutations and benefit from cetuximab in advanced colorectal cancer. N Engl J Med 359:1757–1765, 2008.
24. Schmidt CE, Bestmann B, Kuchler T, et al: Ten-year historic cohort of quality of life and sexuality in patients with rectal cancer. Dis Colon Rectum 48:483–492, 2005.
25. Ardizzone S, Maconi G, Sampietro GM, et al: Azathioprine and mesalamine for prevention of relapse after conservative surgery for Crohn's disease. Gastroenterology 127:730–740, 2004.
26. Silverman MS, Davis I, Pillai DR: Success of self-administered home fecal transplantation for chronic Clostridium difficile infection. Clin Gastroenterol Hepatol 8:471–473, 2010.
27. Jemal A, Siegel R, Xu J, et al: Cancer Statistics, 2010. CA Cancer J Clin 2010.
28. Sampson JR, Jones S, Dolwani S, et al: MutYH (MYH) and colorectal cancer. Biochem Soc Trans 33:679–683, 2005.
29. Stephens RJ, Thompson LC, Quirke P, et al: Impact of short-course preoperative radiotherapy for rectal cancer on patients' quality of life: Data From the Medical Research Council CR07/ National Cancer Institute of Canada Clinical Trials Group C016 randomized clinical trial. J Clin Oncol 28:4233–4239, 2010.
30. Guillem JG, Diaz-Gonzalez JA, Minsky BD, et al: cT3N0 rectal cancer: Potential overtreatment with preoperative chemoradiotherapy is warranted. J Clin Oncol 26:368–373, 2008.
31. Habr-Gama A, Perez RO, Nadalin W, et al: Long-term results of preoperative chemoradiation for distal rectal cancer correlation between final stage and survival. J Gastrointest Surg 9:90–99, 2005.
32. Nyasavajjala SM, Shaw AG, Khan AQ, et al: Neoadjuvant chemoradiotherapy and rectal cancer: Can the UK watch and wait with Brazil? Colorectal Dis 12:33–36, 2010.
33. O'Neill BD, Brown G, Heald RJ, et al: Non-operative treatment after neoadjuvant chemoradiotherapy for rectal cancer. Lancet Oncol 8:625–633, 2007.
34. Rengan R, Paty P, Wong WD, et al: Distal cT2N0 rectal cancer: Is there an alternative to abdominoperineal resection? J Clin Oncol 23:4905–4912, 2005.
35. Branagan G, Chave H, Fuller C, et al: Can magnetic resonance imaging predict circumferential margins and TNM stage in rectal cancer? Dis Colon Rectum 47:1317–1322, 2004.
36. Okabe S, Shia J, Nash G, et al: Lymph node metastasis in T1 adenocarcinoma of the colon and rectum. J Gastrointest Surg 8:1032–1039; discussion 1039-1040, 2004.
37. Bentrem DJ, Okabe S, Wong WD, et al: T1 adenocarcinoma of the rectum: Transanal excision or radical surgery? Ann Surg 242:472–477, 2005.
38. West NP, Finan PJ, Anderin C, et al: Evidence of the oncologic superiority of cylindrical abdominoperineal excision for low rectal cancer. J Clin Oncol 26:3517–3522, 2008.
39. Cornish JA, Tilney HS, Heriot AG, et al: A meta-analysis of quality of life for abdominoperineal excision of rectum versus anterior resection for rectal cancer. Ann Surg Oncol 14:2056–2068, 2007.
40. Matthiessen P, Hallbook O, Rutegard J, et al: Defunctioning stoma reduces symptomatic anastomotic leakage after low anterior resection of the rectum for cancer: A randomized multicenter trial. Ann Surg 246:207–214, 2007.
41. Ho YH: Techniques for restoring bowel continuity and function after rectal cancer surgery. World J Gastroenterol 12:6252–6260, 2006.
42. da Silva GM, Kaiser R, Borjesson L, et al: The effect of diverticular disease on the colonic J pouch. Colorectal Dis 6:171–175, 2004.
43. Remzi FH, Fazio VW, Gorgun E, et al: Quality of life, functional outcome, and complications of coloplasty pouch after low anterior resection. Dis Colon Rectum 48:735–743, 2005.
44. Rullier E, Laurent C, Bretagnol F, et al: Sphincter-saving resection for all rectal carcinomas: The end of the 2-cm distal rule. Ann Surg 241:465–469, 2005.
45. Baxter NN, Goldwasser MA, Paszat LF, et al: Association of colonoscopy and death from colorectal cancer. Ann Intern Med 150:1–8, 2009.
46. Francone TD, Saleem A, Read TA, et al: Ultimate fate of the leaking intestinal anastomosis: Does leak mean permanent stoma? J Gastrointest Surg 14:987–992, 2010.
47. American Society of Colon and Rectal Surgeons Committee Members; Wound Ostomy Continence Nurses Society Committee Members: ASCRS and WOCN joint position statement on the value of preoperative stoma marking for patients undergoing fecal ostomy surgery. J Wound Ostomy Continence Nurs 34:627–628, 2007.
48. Bassotti G, Villanacci V: Slow transit constipation: A functional disorder becomes an enteric neuropathy. World J Gastroenterol 12:4609–4613, 2006.
49. Clinical Outcomes of Surgical Therapy Study Group:A comparison of laparoscopically assisted and open colectomy for colon cancer. N Engl J Med 350:2050–2059, 2004.
50. Jayne DG, Thorpe HC, Copeland J, et al: Five-year follow-up of the Medical Research Council CLASICC trial of laparoscopically assisted versus open surgery for colorectal cancer. Br J Surg 97:1638–1645, 2010.

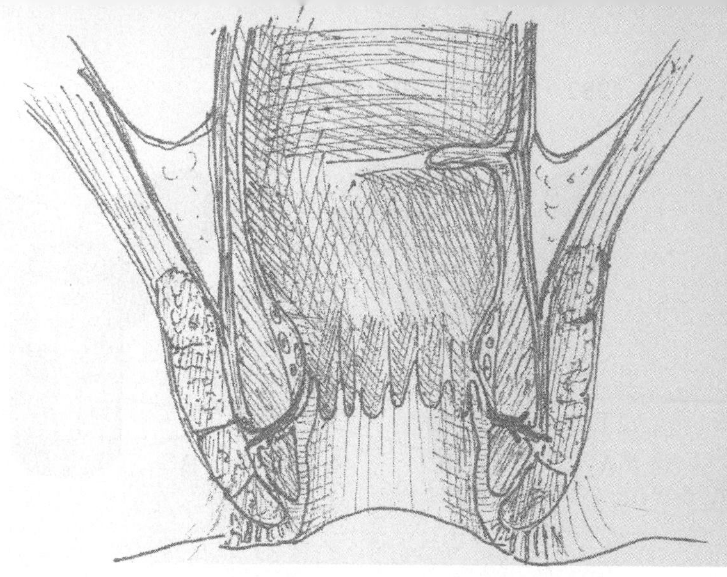

# CHAPTER 53

# ANUS

Heidi Nelson



## DISORDERS OF THE ANAL CANAL

The anal canal can be the site of rare lesions. Most conditions arising in this area, however, are common and benign but may be incapacitating and interfere with patients' daily quality of life. Moreover, these disorders are often misdiagnosed or maltreated, leading at times to disastrous consequences. A better knowledge of the functional anatomy of this portion of the gastrointestinal tract, as well as recent changes in our understanding of its physiology and that of the pelvic floor, should facilitate diagnosis and management of these ailments and result in more favorable outcomes.

### Anatomy

The anal canal, which extends for a distance of approximately 4 cm from the anorectal ring to the hairy skin of the anal verge, is the distalmost portion of the alimentary canal. Its lining, as well as its musculature, has important features that together with the pelvic floor structures, contribute significantly to the regulation of defecation and continence. Its borders include the coccyx posteriorly, ischiorectal fossa and its contents bilaterally, and perineal body and vagina in women and urethra in men anteriorly.

#### Anal Canal Musculature

The anal canal musculature, with its sphincteric apparatus, is the terminal muscular channel of the gastrointestinal tract and can be conceptualized as two tubular structures overlying each other. The inner component is the continuation of the smooth circular layer of the rectum forming the thickened and rounded internal sphincter, which ends 1.5 cm below the dentate line, slightly cephalad to the external sphincter (intersphincteric groove). The outer component is a continuous sheet of striated muscle constituting the pelvic floor, which is comprised of the levator ani muscle, puborectalis muscle, and external sphincter (Fig. 53-1). The latter is elliptical and engulfs the anal canal and internal sphincter, beyond which it terminates in a subcutaneous portion. The other two portions, the superficial and deep divisions, constitute a single muscular unit, which is continuous superiorly with the puborectalis and levator ani muscles. The external sphincter, bulbospongiosus, and transverse perineal muscles meet together centrally on the perineum and constitute the perineal body. The funnel-shaped configuration of the paired levator ani muscles form the major part of the pelvic floor and their fibers decussate medially with the contralateral side to fuse with the perineal body around the prostate or vagina.

The internal sphincter, which is innervated by the autonomic nervous system, is independent of voluntary control, whereas the external sphincter, which is supplied by the inferior rectal branch of the internal pudendal nerve and perineal branch of the fourth sacral nerve, is under voluntary control.

#### Anal Canal Lining

The epithelium that lines the anal canal incrementally transitions from normal, squamous, hair-bearing skin to gastrointestinal columnar epithelium in the short distance between the anal verge and top of the anal canal (Fig. 53-2). At the verge, the skin becomes anoderm, which is a modified squamous lining without skin appendages, such as hair. At the level of the dentate line, the squamous and columnar epithelium comingle; this is referred to as the anal transition zone. Finally, cephalad to the top of the anal canal, the lining becomes exclusively gastrointestinal columnar epithelium. These epithelial distinctions are helpful for understanding the basis and treatment of benign and malignant conditions. For example, fistulas developing from the condition of hidradenitis suppurativa can only arise from the appendages of skin, so this disorder can only occur below the dentate line, typically outside the anal verge. In contrast, fistulas that are derived from crypto glandular disease arise within the glands at the level of the dentate line and Crohn's fistulas typically arise in the gastrointestinal tract above the dentate line. These distinctions help differentiate the diagnoses. For cancer cases, the histology is the key to understanding the likely origin, behavior, and management of the disease. Squamous cell lesions that arise in the anal margin skin or anoderm are treated with wide excision as skin cancers (margin lesions) or with radiation chemotherapy (anal canal). Adenocarcinomas arising in the distal rectum or within the anal canal are usually treated with surgical removal of the rectum, with the adjunctive use of radiation and chemotherapy.

The lining also provides clues to the pattern of innervation or sensory perception and can help guide the appropriate surgical approach. External hemorrhoids below the dentate are sensitive to touch and therefore anesthesia (locoregional or general)

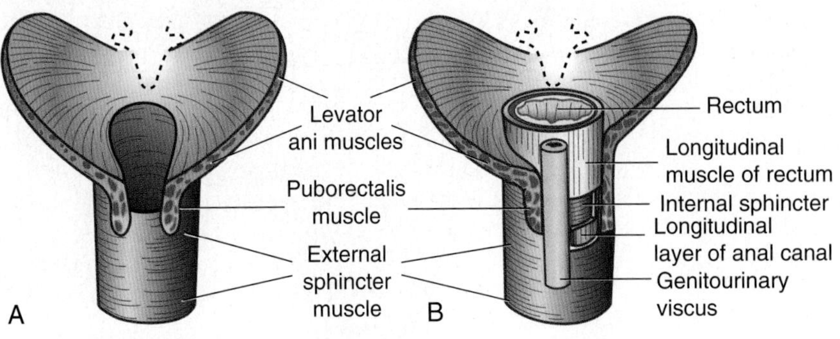


**FIGURE 53-1** The anal canal mechanism is comprised of two components, visceral and somatic, each of which is tubular. The visceral tube is enclosed by a skeletal muscle tube whereby continence is maintained. **A,** Diagrammatic representation of the skeletal muscle component. **B,** Composite arrangement after insertion of a simple visceral component. (From Parks AG, Gordon PH, Hardcastle JD: A classification of fistula-in-ano. Br J Surg 63:1–12, 1976.)

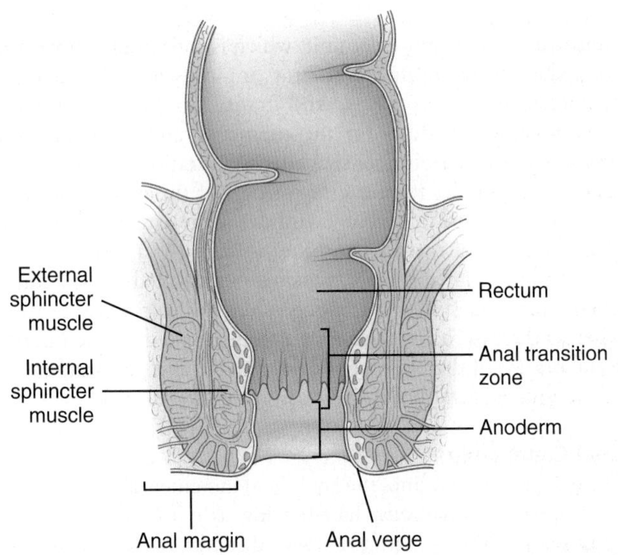


**FIGURE 53-2** The anal canal extends for a distance of 2 to 4 cm from the anal verge to the top of the anal canal musculature. The epithelium that lines the anal canal incrementally transitions from normal, squamous, hair-bearing skin to gastrointestinal columnar epithelium. Between the anal verge and dentate line, the lining is referred to as anoderm, and from the dentate line to the top of the anal canal it is referred to as the anal transition zone.

is required for surgical management. Internal hemorrhoids above the dentate can be manipulated without the need for anesthesia, in a manner analogous to the treatment of gastrointestinal polyps.

## Physiology

The physiology of the anal canal and pelvic floor is complex, but the advent of more sophisticated means to evaluate its functions (e.g., manometry, defecography, evacuability testing, electromyography) has improved our understanding of it. The principal function of the anal canal is the regulation of defecation and maintenance of continence. The ability to control defecation depends on the coordinated functions of the sensory and muscular activities of the anus, the compliance, tone, and evacuability of the rectum, the muscular activities of the pelvic floor, and the consistency, volume, and timing of the colonic fecal movements. Perturbations of any of the critical functions can result in fecal incontinence (Table 53-1).

The anal canal, which has a mean length of 4 cm, lengthens with squeezing of the external sphincter and shortens with straining. Resting pressure, or tone, which depends largely on the internal sphincter, averages 90 cm $H_2O$ and is lower in women and older patients than in men and younger patients. This high-pressure zone increases resistance to the passage of stool. Squeeze pressure, generated by contraction of the external anal sphincter and puborectalis muscle, more than doubles the intra–anal canal resting pressure. This maximal increase lasts for a minute, at the most; consequently, squeeze pressure serves only

**Table 53-1 Common Causes of Fecal Incontinence**

| CATEGORY | MECHANISM | COMMON CAUSES |
|---|---|---|
| Functional | Fecal impaction; dilated internal anal sphincter | Pelvic floor dyssynergia (difficulty relaxing sphincter when defecating), drug side effect, idiopathic, spinal cord injury |
| | Diarrhea; rapid transit and/or large volume | Irritable bowel syndrome; infectious and metabolic causes of diarrhea |
| | Cognitive, psychological; social indifference | Dementia, psychosis, willful soiling |
| Sphincter weakness | Sphincter muscle injury | Obstetric trauma, motor vehicle accident, foreign body trauma |
| | Pudendal nerve injury | Obstetric trauma, diabetic peripheral neuropathy, multiple sclerosis, idiopathic |
| | Central nervous system injury | Spina bifida, traumatic spinal cord injury, cerebrovascular accident, multiple sclerosis |
| Sensory loss | Afferent nerve injury: unable to detect rectal filling | Diabetic neuropathy, spinal cord injury, multiple sclerosis |

Adapted from Whitehead WE, Wald A, Norton NJ: Treatment options for fecal incontinence. Dis Colon Rectum 44:131–142, 2001.

to prevent leakage on presentation of the rectal content to the proximal anal canal at inappropriate times. The principal mechanism that provides continence is the pressure differential between the rectum (6 cm $H_2O$) and anal canal (90 cm $H_2O$). The anorectal angle is produced by the anterior pull of the puborectalis muscle as it encircles the rectum at the anorectal ring and contributes to fecal continence. This angle may act as a flap valve or have a sphincter-like function. Maneuvers that sharpen this angle augment continence, whereas those that straighten it favor defecation.

Anorectal sensation allows discrimination of the character of the enteric content—gas, liquids, or solids—and detection of the need to pass that content through sensory receptors located in the rectal muscular wall or pelvic floor musculature. The fact that such sensations persist after proctectomy and ileoanal anastomosis suggests that the receptors are situated in the pelvic floor. For the enteric content to reach the anal canal for discrimination, the internal sphincter must relax while the rectum distends and contracts, the rectal anal inhibitory reflex. This reflex involves inhibitory neurons of the myenteric plexus, which innervate the internal sphincter, and intramural nerves and neurotransmitters. Transient relaxation of the internal anal sphincter brings the rectal content into contact with the sensory mucosa of the proximal anal canal so that it can be recognized. Other factors important to continence include rectal compliance, tone, and capacity, rectal filling and emptying, and stool volume and consistency.

## Diagnostic Evaluation of the Anus

Systematic evaluation of anorectal disorders includes a careful history and physical examination of the anal canal area before elaborate laboratory testing.

### History

Important symptoms include bleeding, pain, discharge (mucoid, purulent, or fecal), and change in bowel habits. It is also paramount to know about associated illnesses, medications, family history, bleeding tendency, and exposure through travel or sexual contact.

Bleeding is a common presenting symptom of benign and malignant conditions of the anus and large bowel. Details regarding the type of bleeding can help differentiate between anorectal and large bowel disorders. Inquiry into the type of bleeding should include whether the blood is dark or bright red or associated with clots, whether it is mixed with the stool or separate, and whether it drips into the toilet bowl or only appears on the toilet paper. Blood that drips, is separate from stools, and is bright red is usually seen with bleeding internal hemorrhoids. Blood on toilet tissue may be associated with minor hemorrhoidal disease but also with anal fissure. Clots or melena indicate colonic or more proximal bleeding, respectively. Although a careful bleeding history may suggest a specific cause, consideration must always be given to proximal bowel evaluation to exclude the possibility of more serious conditions, such as cancer. This is particularly important when examination cannot confirm a bleeding source, when patients are at increased risk for cancer by age or family history, or when bleeding does not resolve promptly after treatment of the presumed source. When there is doubt, evaluate the proximal bowel.

Anorectal pain occurring during or immediately after stooling that is described as severe is usually associated with anal fissure. Pain that may or may not be related to stooling and is throbbing in nature is most often seen with an abscess or poorly draining fistula. Pain totally unrelated to stooling is likely to be associated with proctalgia fugax or levator ani syndrome, a condition characterized by painful episodes of short duration (<20 to 30 minutes); these often occur at night and are relieved by walking, warm baths, or other maneuvers. To ascertain change in bowel habits, it is necessary to establish the previous pattern of bowel habit by careful inquiry. Constipation may mean different conditions to different patients, and it is important to know whether the condition is of recent onset or chronic to determine the course of investigation.

### Physical Examination

The left lateral position, with the buttocks projecting slightly beyond the edge of the table, and the prone jackknife position are both suitable for evaluation of anal conditions. Inspection with good lighting should precede any other type of examination. Skin tags, excoriations, scars, and any changes in color or appearance of perianal skin are easily recognized. A patulous anus may indicate incontinence and possibly prolapse. Inspection while straining may help determine the presence of hemorrhoidal or rectal prolapse in multiparous women, and a protruding anus may be an indication of descending perineum syndrome. A careful and systematic digital examination with a well-lubricated index finger gradually inserted into the anal canal helps the examiner appreciate any mass, induration, or stricturing and assess the resting tone and strength of the squeeze pressure of the anal sphincter. In men, the prostate should be palpated; in women, the posterior vaginal wall should be pushed forward to detect rectocele.

After the preliminary evaluation has been completed, proctosigmoidoscopy after enema preparation enables satisfactory visualization of the anorectum. Early signs of mucosal inflammation include the loss of the vascular pattern with erythema, granularity, friability, and even ulcerations. Gross lesions, such as polyps or carcinoma, should be readily identifiable. Any suspicious area or mass should be sampled for biopsy, with the patient's permission, so that a precise histopathologic diagnosis can be established. On withdrawing the proctoscope, the anorectal area can be assessed for mucosal prolapse, hemorrhoids, fissure, polyps, and so forth. The anoscope can also be used for the same purpose; it optimizes the evaluation of lesions confined to the anus.

Other investigations may include barium enema, flexible sigmoidoscopy or colonoscopy, and stool examination, especially if infectious diarrhea or a sexually transmitted disease (STD) is suspected. Special studies, such as manometry, defecography, and electromyography, may help in the assessment of anorectal incontinence, constipation, or any other pelvic floor disorders. Ultrasonography and magnetic resonance imaging (MRI) have shown promise in the evaluation of anorectal suppurative processes. The indications and usefulness of these tests are discussed later under the specific disorders.

# PELVIC FLOOR DISORDERS

## Incontinence

A National Institutes of Health (NIH) State-of-the-Science Conference on the Prevention of Fecal and Urinary Incontinence in Adults was conducted in 2007.[1] Several important

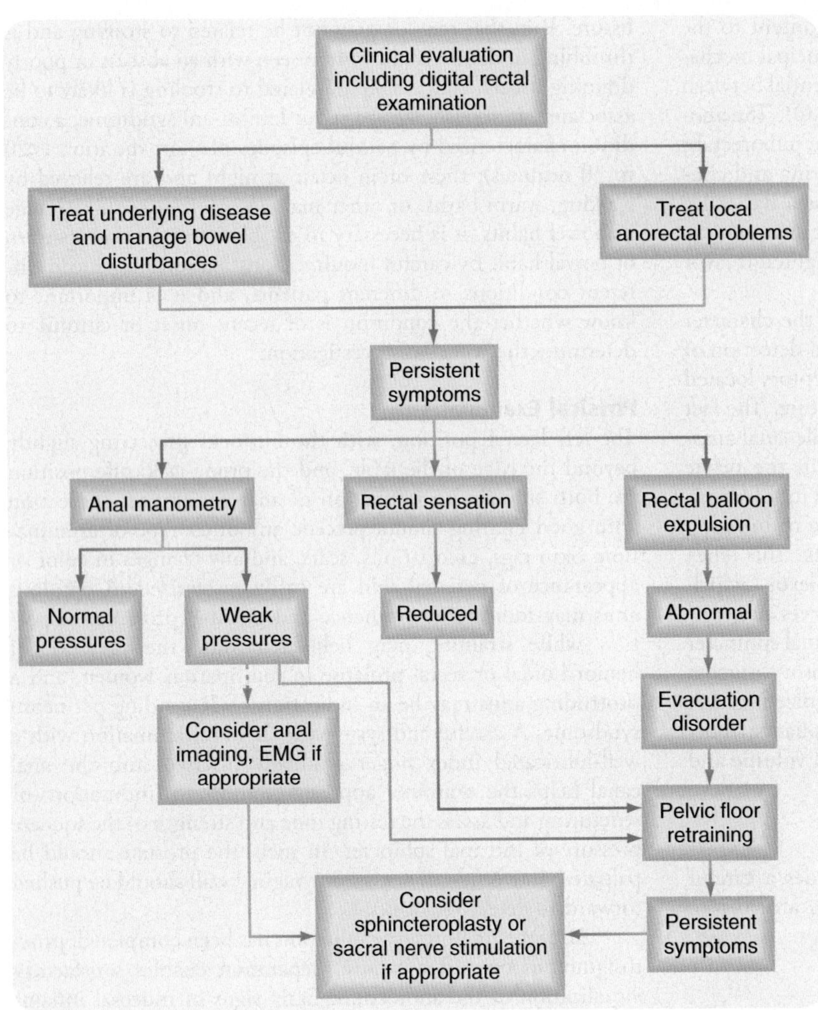


**FIGURE 53-3** Clinical evaluation of fecal incontinence. *EMG,* Electromyogram. (From Whitehead W, Bharucha AE: Diagnosis and treatment of pelvic floor disorders: What's new and what to do. Gastroenterology 138:1231–1235, 2010).

conclusions were reached, including that fecal and urinary incontinence will affect more than 25% of all U.S. adults during their lives. Fecal incontinence is now recognized as having serious effects, causing people to suffer physical discomfort, embarrassment, stigma, and social isolation. Furthermore, the panel concluded that financial costs and caregiver burden are substantial and may be underestimated because of underreporting.

### Clinical Evaluation

Determining the extent and nature of the problem should start by distinguishing true incontinence (i.e., complete loss of solid stools) from minor incontinence (i.e., occasional staining from seepage or urgency). Seepage of mucus from prolapsing hemorrhoids or from a large secretory villous polyp, urgency from colitis or proctitis, and overflow incontinence from fecal impaction may be confused with true incontinence. After true incontinence is established, the severity of the disability should be assessed by seeking information on control of flatus, liquid and solid stool, and effect on lifestyle and activities (see Table 53-1).[2]

Fecal incontinence is often multifactorial; defects in the sphincter may be the result of trauma from previous surgical procedures for hemorrhoids, fissures, or fistulas, forceful dilation of the anal canal, impalement injury, or obstetric injuries, either directly because of a tear or breakdown of episiotomy repair or indirectly from stretching of the pudendal nerve during labor, which may develop decades later. The NIH consensus panel concluded that for fecal incontinence, a routine episiotomy is the most preventable risk factor, but that additional risk factors include female gender, older age, and neurologic diseases, with contributions also from body mass, decreased activity, depression, and diabetes. The workup of fecal incontinence should include an evaluation of associated gastrointestinal disorders, such as diarrhea, which can aggravate disorders of continence (Fig. 53-3).[3] The physical examination should confirm a weak resting tone and squeeze pressure or a patulous anus and the presence of scars, defects, deformities, or keyhole abnormalities. Examination can also exclude the presence of prolapse, hemorrhoids, or other contributory or associated anorectal abnormalities. Endoscopy excludes the diagnoses of proctitis, fecal impaction, rectal polyps, and colitis cystica profunda.

Additional testing can be restricted to a few tests, depending on the extent of findings at examination.[4,5] Anal manometry confirms the extent of impairment of the internal and external sphincters by the resting and squeeze pressures, respectively. Manometry can also identify asymmetry, suggesting anatomic defects amenable to repair. Endoanal ultrasound has been recommended to detect occult defects and, in some centers with expertise, is considered more accurate than clinical or conventional methods of evaluation. Finally, electromyography of the

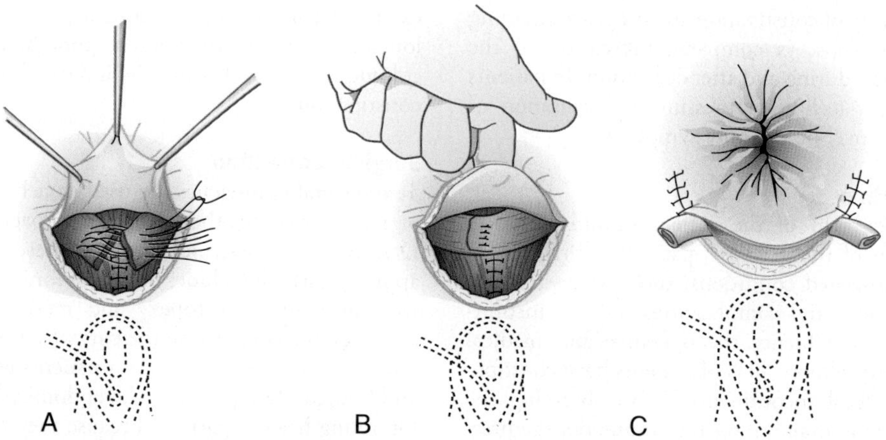


**FIGURE 53-4** Overlapping sphincteroplasty. **A,** A curvilinear incision is made midway between the anus and introitus, limited in its posterolateral extent to avoid pudendal nerve injury. The external sphincter ends are dissected, the scar excised when extensive, and the muscle ends reapproximated using overlapping suture technique. The levator ani muscles are also reapproximated. **B,** Tightness is judged by digital rectal examination. **C,** The wound edges are closed over drains, at times using a Y configuration to lengthen the perineal body. (Courtesy Mayo Foundation for Medical Education and Research, Rochester, Minn.)

pelvic floor can be used to differentiate between anatomic and neurogenic sources of incontinence, and pudendal nerve terminal motor latency testing can predict the likelihood of successful repair.

### Treatment

**Medical Management** Medical management is a preferred option for cases of mild incontinence and of generalized weakness in which reparable anatomic defects are not identified. A first-line approach includes the use of diet and medications to slow transit and increase stool consistency. Coupled with sphincter exercises, this may improve symptoms and restore normal function for mild cases.[4] Biofeedback training focuses on strengthening of the anal musculature and improving anorectal sensation and is reported with variable success rates of approximately 75% for at least modest reduction in incontinence frequency, with 50% accomplishing complete continence. A bowel management program has been a successful approach for patients with anorectal malfunctions, Hirschsprung's disease, and spina bifida.[6] Of note, medical management can also be considered complementary to surgical therapy and may be carried out before and/or after surgery to optimize surgical results.

**Surgical Repair** Surgical options range from the traditional approach of sphincter repair to the newer technique of sacral nerve stimulation and to the final step of colostomy creation. For discrete anatomic defects, the most common surgical approach is the direct overlapping sphincteroplasty, in which the separated muscular ends are dissected, reapproximated, and sutured (Fig. 53-4).[7] Fecal diversion is not typically required for these repairs unless there are extenuating circumstances. The overlapping sphincteroplasty is associated with low rates of morbidity and mortality and reasonable rates of success with good to excellent results achieved in 55% to 68% of patients.[4] Direct repair of anterior sphincter defects from obstetric injuries can be expected to restore fecal continence in 59% of patients. A study of 10-year outcomes after anal sphincter repair has suggested continued deterioration of function over time. For nonanatomic defects, postanal repair is advocated by some surgeons but reserved for highly select patients.

Highly specialized approaches to treating fecal incontinence include the dynamic graciloplasty, sacral nerve stimulation, and use of an artificial bowel sphincter. The transposition of the gracilis muscle is reserved for patients in whom the bulk of the anal sphincter is missing and requires total reconstruction. Sacral nerve stimulation, in contrast, is specifically designed for patients in whom the anal sphincter is intact but there is inadequate innervation. With proper patient selection, the success rates can be as high as 70%, at least in the short term. Finally, the complications associated with artificial sphincter include erosion, infection, and obstruction at defecation has limited enthusiasm for this approach.

## Prolapse of the Rectum

### Pathogenesis and Clinical Presentation

Prolapse of the rectum, or procidentia, is an uncommon problem of obscure cause characterized by full-thickness eversion of the rectal wall through the anus. The exact cause is unclear, but the disorder tends to predominate in women, those who strain excessively, and those with chronic mental disorders. The concept that rectal prolapse is the result of intussusception or infolding of the rectum or rectosigmoid has been strongly supported. As the intussusception progresses caudally, the intussusceptum gradually pulls the upper rectal wall away from its sacral and lateral moorings. With continued straining, the bowel continues to roll inside out until, initially, the mucocutaneous junction and eventually the rectal wall evert completely. This progressive phenomenon may explain why some patients have occult or hidden prolapse and why the sigmoid mesentery may elongate, the cul-de-sac may deepen, and the pelvic floor musculature may increasingly weaken. Such findings have been implicated as causative, but it is more likely that they are the result of the prolonged process of gradual prolapsing of the rectum.

The symptoms of early prolapse may be vague, including discomfort or a sensation of incomplete evacuation during defecation. A long history of constipation and excessive straining is common. When prolapse is complete, protrusion of the rectum is noted as a mass during and after defecation. In patients with occult prolapse, a feeling of pressure and sensation of incomplete evacuation may be the only symptoms.

### Preoperative Evaluation

The preoperative assessment of the patient should focus on establishing the extent of the prolapse, patient's overall health status, presence of associated conditions, such as constipation and pelvic floor disorders, and complications, such as incontinence. All these factors influence the operative and medical management. At history, almost 50% of patients have constipation and most have fecal incontinence.[8,9] By observing the patient while he or she is straining on the commode, the presence and extent of the prolapse can be verified. Complete prolapse demonstrates full-thickness rectal protrusion with concentric rings (Fig. 53-5). Frail older patients and those with high-risk comorbid conditions or limited life expectancy are ideally suited for perineal procedures. Younger patients, particularly those with constipation or evidence of pelvic floor defecating disorders, are best served with resection and fixation using open or laparoscopic approaches.

Complete lower gastrointestinal tract evaluations are performed as indicated. On endoscopy, redness of the anterior rectal mucosa or a solitary rectal ulcer 6 to 8 cm anteriorly may be present. A number of additional tests can be ordered but have limited value and are not typically required. Manometry documents the presence of sphincter damage but does not predict recovery. An abnormal pudendal nerve terminal motor latency predicts a high risk for postoperative anal incontinence but rarely influences the management. Defecography can demonstrate the extent of prolapse and transit studies can indicate the extent of constipation. Because a patient with significant prolongation in transit time may respond better to a more extensive colonic resection, this may be indicated for select patients with constipation.

### Surgical Correction

Two general approaches are used to achieve surgical correction of rectal prolapse, the perineal approach, which includes the Delorme and Altemeier procedures, and the abdominal approach, which includes but is not limited to anterior resection, with or without rectopexy and mesh fixation. The perineal approach is less taxing on the patient yet has a higher recurrence rate; thus, it is ideally suited for patients with high operative risk and limited life expectancy. An abdominal approach is preferred for young healthy patients because they can tolerate the procedure with low risk and are less likely to suffer a recurrence requiring reoperation.

**Perineal Procedures** The Delorme procedure is essentially a mucosal proctectomy and muscularis plicating procedure (Fig. 53-6). It is ideally applied to patients with up to 3 to 4 cm of prolapse, even though the mucosal tube resected can extend up to 15 cm. Even in frail older patients, the Delorme procedure is associated with low rates of mortality and major morbidity, approximately 1% and 14%, respectively.[9] Incontinence improves in as many as 69% of patients. Prolapse recurrence is not uncommon and is likely underestimated because this procedure is performed in patients with limited life expectancies and therefore short follow-up.

The Altemeier procedure is similar to the Delorme procedure, but rather than a mucosal resection, a full-thickness rectal resection is performed, starting 1 or 2 cm above the dentate line. The bowel and attendant mesentery are resected. Because the

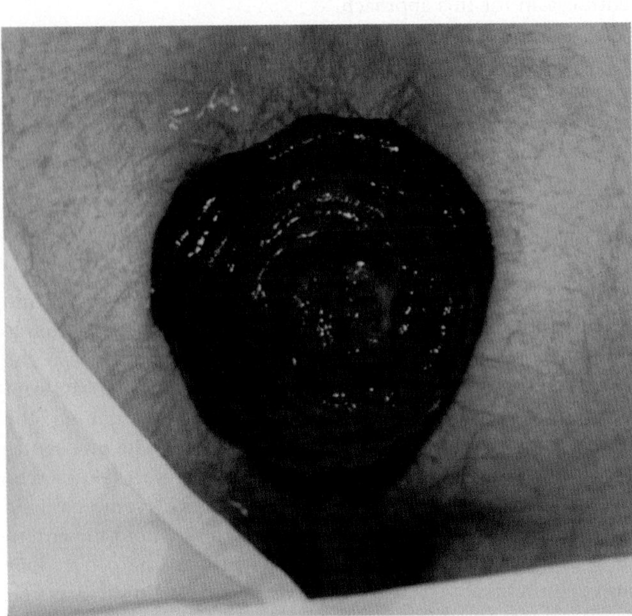

**FIGURE 53-5** Complete rectal prolapse. The everted rectal wall appears as a tubular mass made up of several concentric mucosal folds. (Courtesy Mayo Foundation for Medical Education and Research, Rochester, Minn.)

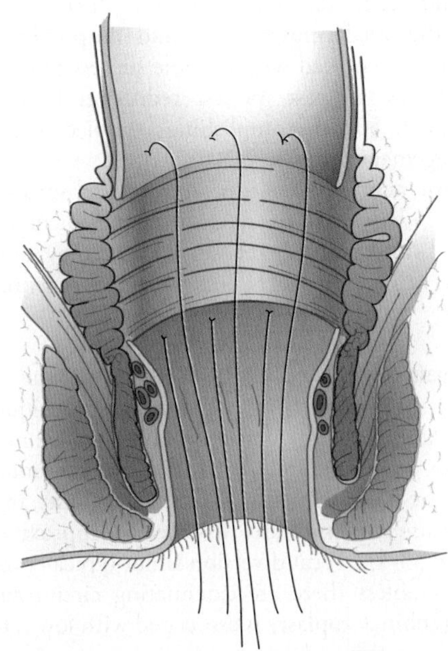

**FIGURE 53-6** Schematic representation of Delorme repair of complete rectal prolapse. Mucosal proctectomy is followed by muscular plication, anastomosing the proximal extent of the mucosal resection site to the distal mucosa, just proximal to the dentate. (Courtesy Mayo Foundation for Medical Education and Research, Rochester, Minn.)

pelvic cavity is entered, injury to the small bowel must be avoided. A full-thickness anastomosis is accomplished after the full extent of resection is completed. For patients with incontinence, a levatorplasty may be added to the resection. Results are similar to those described for the Delorme procedure.[8]

**Abdominal Procedures** The abdominal options include bowel resection and rectopexy, with or without mesh, performed alone or together. Complete mobilization of the rectum is required for the abdominal procedures; debate exists about whether the lateral stalks should be preserved.[10] Preservation of the stalks is thought to yield better functional results but a greater risk for recurrence. Although the entire rectum is mobilized to the level of the levatores, if resection and anastomosis are being performed, they should be performed high rather than low in the rectum, essentially an anterior resection. This minimizes the risk for anastomotic complications. Rectopexy is performed by securing the rectum to the presacral tissues. Resection with rectopexy is associated with low recurrence rates (0% to 9%) and can be performed safely, with morbidity and mortality rates commensurate with any large bowel resection. Constipation improves in up to 50% of patients and incontinence in most patients.

Rectopexy alone with mesh fixation is a well-described procedure, preferred by some centers. The risks for resection and anastomosis are avoided and recurrence rates are generally low. Complications can result, however, from the presence of a foreign body, and symptoms of constipation are often aggravated. The abdominal procedures can be performed through standard laparotomy or using laparoscopic techniques. Results have suggested that postoperative recovery is typically faster after laparoscopic resection with rectopexy. Furthermore, rates of morbidities, mortality, recurrence, and functional improvement are the same with laparoscopic and open techniques.

### Incontinence and Biofeedback

Because incontinence resulting from chronic stretching may or may not cause permanent pudendal nerve damage, many patients note improvement in continence after prolapse repair. The role of biofeedback for treating persistent postoperative incontinence or for preventing recurrent prolapse in patients with obvious pelvic floor dysfunction and a tendency toward excessive straining has not been well established. However, it can be beneficial to some patients and it is noninvasive, which encourages its use in select patients.

## Rectocele

### Clinical Evaluation

Patients with a rectocele present with a bulge or prolapse of the anterior rectal wall into the vagina. Symptoms attributable to a rectocele include the presentation of a vaginal bulge, inability to evacuate completely during defecation and, in most cases, the necessity to evacuate digitally through the vagina or through the rectum or perineum. The cause of rectoceles remains unclear; it is probably multifactorial because it is associated with a constellation of a number of pelvic floor disorders, including constipation, paradoxical muscular contraction, and neuropathies or anatomic disorders from childbirth.[11] Rectocele may coexist with other defecation disorders, such as slow-transit constipation or pelvic floor dysfunction, including pelvic organ prolapse, in which factors such as age, parity, obesity, constipation, pelvic surgery, and pulmonary and medical conditions may play a role. Associated disorders must be addressed to achieve resolution of all symptoms. A careful physical examination will reveal the size of the defect where the rectum prolapse extends to the vagina.

Defecography, which can demonstrate dynamic information on the process of rectal emptying, is the only test that is specifically diagnostic for a rectocele.[11] It is probably the most useful test for understanding the relevance of the rectocele in the defecation process, even though there is no exact correlation between any single test finding and results from surgery. Further colorectal evaluations and tests can be ordered, as appropriate, for other symptoms or coexisting disorders.

### Treatment

The optimization of bowel function through proper diet, fiber supplements, and good bowel habits is always appropriate as complementary therapy. Medical therapies, specifically biofeedback, have met with limited success, providing only partial relief in most patients but major relief in only a minority of patients.[12]

**Surgical Treatment** Patients with rectoceles should be considered for surgical correction if the rectocele is larger than 2 cm and the patient has to perform digitally assisted defecation.[13] Although gynecologic surgeons often perform a transvaginal repair, the defect between the vagina and rectum can be corrected using a transperineal approach, with or without mesh and including a levatorplasty, or using a transanal repair, with an anal mucosa flap and a plication technique without mesh. The repair should extend 7 to 10 cm above the anal canal. Symptomatic improvement can be anticipated in 73% to 79% of properly selected patients. Best results can be expected in patients who have a small rectocele, require digitally assisted evacuation, are without evidence of anismus, and can be repaired using a transperineal approach.

# COMMON BENIGN ANAL DISORDERS

## Hemorrhoids

### Clinical Presentation and Diagnostic Evaluation

Within the normal anal canal there are specialized, highly vascularized cushions forming discrete masses of thick submucosa containing blood vessels, smooth muscle, and elastic and connective tissue. They are located in the left lateral, right anterior, and right posterior quadrants of the canal to aid in anal continence. The term *hemorrhoids* should be restricted to clinical situations in which these cushions are abnormal and cause symptoms. The cause of hemorrhoids remains unknown. They may be no more than the downward sliding of anal cushions associated with gravity, straining, and irregular bowel habits. Hemorrhoids can be considered external or internal; the diagnosis is based on the history, physical examination, and endoscopy. External hemorrhoids are covered with anoderm and are distal to the dentate line; they may swell, causing discomfort and difficult hygiene, but cause severe pain only if actually thrombosed. Internal hemorrhoids cause painless, bright red bleeding or prolapse associated with defecation. Internal hemorrhoids are classified according to the extent of prolapse, which influences treatment options (Table 53-2). The patient may report dripping or even squirting of blood in the toilet bowl. Chronic occult

**Table 53-2 Internal Hemorrhoids: Grading and Management**

| GRADE | SYMPTOMS AND SIGNS | MANAGEMENT |
|---|---|---|
| First degree | Bleeding; no prolapse | Dietary modifications* |
| Second degree | Prolapse with spontaneous reduction | Rubber band ligation |
| | Bleeding, seepage | Coagulation<br>Dietary modifications |
| Third degree | Prolapse requiring digital reduction | Surgical hemorrhoidectomy |
| | Bleeding, seepage | Rubber band ligation<br>Dietary modifications |
| Fourth degree | Prolapsed, cannot be reduced | Surgical hemorrhoidectomy |
| | Strangulated | Urgent hemorrhoidectomy<br>Dietary modifications |

*Dietary modifications include increasing consumption of fiber, bran, or psyllium and water. Dietary modifications are always appropriate for the management of hemorrhoids, if not for acute care then for chronic management, and for prevention of recurrence after banding and/or surgery.

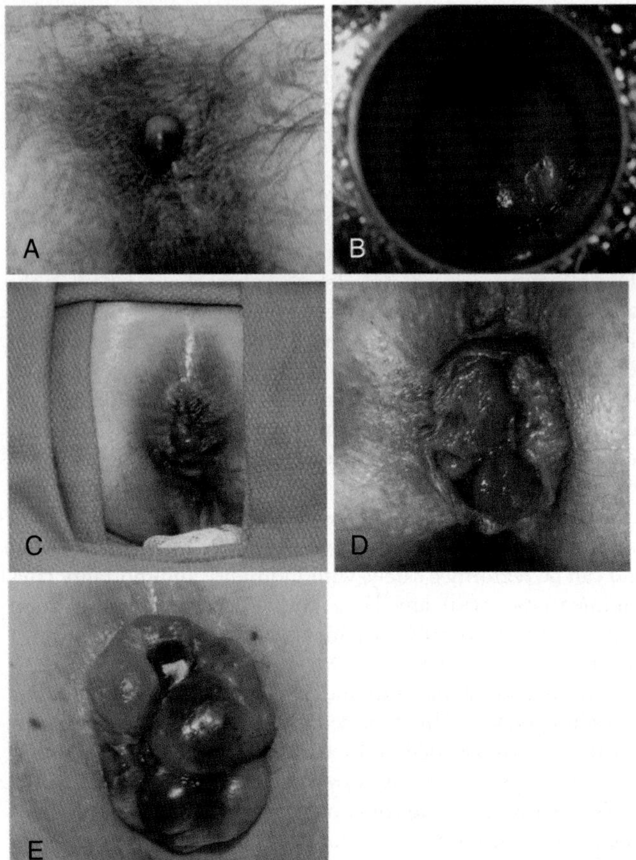


**FIGURE 53-7** Hemorrhoids. **A,** Thrombosed external. **B,** First-degree internal viewed through anoscope. **C,** Second-degree internal prolapsed, reduced spontaneously. **D,** Third-degree internal prolapsed, requiring manual reduction. **E,** Fourth-degree strangulated internal and thrombosed external. (Courtesy Mayo Foundation for Medical Education and Research, Rochester, Minn.)

bleeding leading to anemia is rare, and other causes of anemia must be excluded. Prolapse below the dentate line area can occur, especially with straining, and may lead to mucus and fecal leakage and pruritus. Pain is not usually associated with uncomplicated hemorrhoids but more often with fissure, abscess, or external hemorrhoidal thrombosis.

The physical examination should include inspection during straining, preferably on a commode, digital rectal examination, and anoscopy (Fig. 53-7). Digital examination enables assessment of internal and external hemorrhoidal disease and anal canal tone and exclusion of other lesions, especially low rectal or anal canal neoplasms. Because almost all anorectal symptoms are ascribed to hemorrhoids by patients, it is essential that other anorectal pathologies be considered and excluded. Anoscopy is the definitive examination, but a flexible proctosigmoidoscopy should always be added to exclude proximal inflammation or neoplasia. Colonoscopy or barium enema should be added if the hemorrhoidal disease is unimpressive, the history is somewhat uncharacteristic, or the patient is older than 40 years or has risk factors for colon cancer, such as a family history. Depending on the degree of disease, treatment falls into two main categories, nonsurgical and hemorrhoidectomy.

### Treatment

**Nonoperative Management** In many patients, hemorrhoidal symptoms can be ameliorated or relieved by simple measures, such as better local hygiene, avoidance of excessive straining, and better dietary habits supplemented by medication to keep stools soft, formed, and regular (see Table 53-2). A wide array of fiber supplements are now available over the counter. Symptoms of bleeding but not prolapse can be significantly reduced over a period of 30 to 45 days with the use of fiber supplements. Over-the-counter suppositories and anal salves, although popular, have never been tested for efficacy. Even though all patients should be counseled on dietary and fiber recommendations, patients with prolapse and internal plus external hemorrhoids benefit from additional interventions.

In the absence of symptomatic external hemorrhoids, second- and some third-degree internal hemorrhoids can be treated with office procedures that produce mucosal fixation. Although sclerotherapy, infrared coagulation, heater probe, and bipolar electrocoagulation have all been described, the simplest, most effective, and most widely applied office procedure is rubber band ligation. Rubber band ligation can be performed in the office without sedation through an anoscope, using a ligator (Fig. 53-8). Preferably, only one site should be banded each time. Because severe perineal sepsis and even deaths have been reported after rubber band ligation, patients should be instructed to return to the emergency department if delayed or undue pain, inability to void, or a fever develops. With one or more applications, symptoms are alleviated in 79% of patients.[14] Because of the risk for bleeding and sepsis, it is preferable that patients not be taking antiplatelet or blood-thinning medications and that subacute bacterial endocarditis prophylaxis is administered to patients at risk. Rubber band ligation should be avoided in immunodeficient patients.

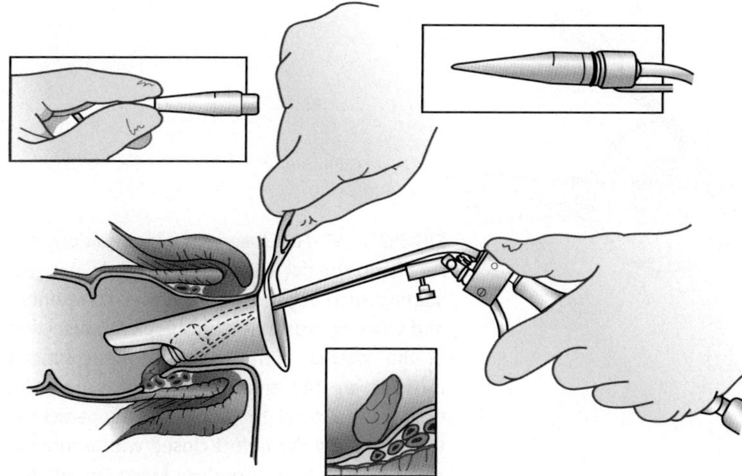

**FIGURE 53-8** The band is advanced onto the end of the ligator instrument using a conical attachment *(insets).* The hemorrhoid is identified at a level proximal to the dentate; this area is tested for sensation before banding. Occluding the suction port of the ligator instrument draws the hemorrhoid into the open end of the ligator, at which time the instrument is fired. The banded hemorrhoid typically sloughs off in 1 week. (Courtesy Mayo Foundation for Medical Education and Research, Rochester, Minn.)

**Surgical Treatment** Hemorrhoidectomy is the best means of curing hemorrhoidal disease and should be considered whenever patients fail to respond satisfactorily to repeated attempts at conservative measures, hemorrhoids are severely prolapsed and require manual reduction, hemorrhoids are complicated by strangulation or associated pathology, such as ulceration, fissure, or fistula, or hemorrhoids are associated with symptomatic external hemorrhoids or large anal tags. The choice of anesthesia should be individualized based on the patient's preference, build, and medical status. In most cases, local or regional anesthesia with mild sedation can be used effectively. For simple, thrombosed external hemorrhoids, excision in the office is best performed early in the course of the disease, during the period of maximum pain (Fig. 53-9). To remove complex internal or external hemorrhoids, an open or closed hemorrhoidectomy can be performed as an outpatient procedure.

Closed hemorrhoidectomy provides simultaneous excision of internal and external hemorrhoids (Fig. 53-10). Preoperative and intraoperative assessment determines the number and location of hemorrhoids requiring excision; typically, three bundles are identified in the right anterior, right posterior, and left lateral positions. Using a large operative scope retractor, such as the Fansler, ensures that sufficient anoderm is preserved to avoid the long-term complication of anal stenosis. Postoperative complications include fecal impaction, infection, urinary retention and, rarely, arterial bleeding. Patients typically recover sufficiently to return to work within 1 to 2 weeks. As an alternative to the closed technique, the surgical wounds can be left open to reduce postoperative pain, but at the expense of longer healing times.

Newer technology and techniques have been applied to the operative treatment of hemorrhoids, with the promise of less postoperative pain. The two main categories of these treatments involve the application of ultrasonic or controlled electrical energy, such as the Harmonic Scalpel (Soma, Bloomfield, Conn) and LigaSure (Covidien, Boulder, Colo) respectively, or a new operative approach to hemorrhoidal tissue excision. Both energy application modalities remove the excess hemorrhoidal tissue and coagulate or seal the blood vessels simultaneously, with minimal lateral thermal injury to nearby tissue. It is thought that the reduction in trauma to the surrounding anal canal mucosa and underlying anal sphincter will decrease postoperative edema and pain. Small single-institution reports have evaluated both

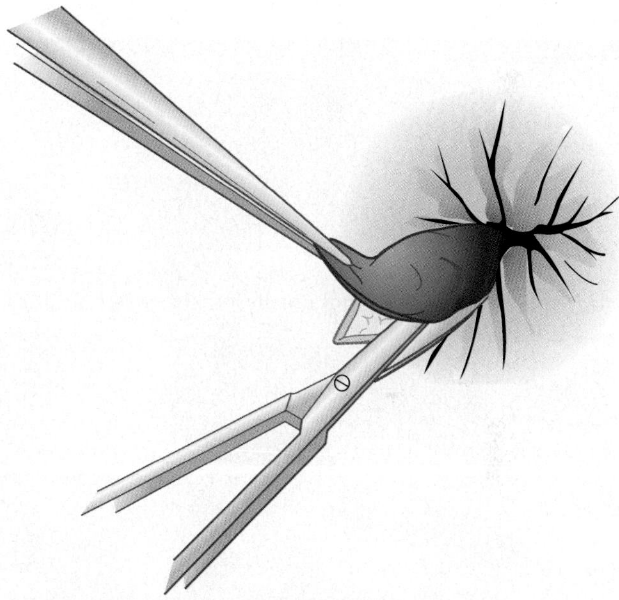

**FIGURE 53-9** Excision of thrombosed external hemorrhoid. The area is infiltrated with local anesthetic and the thrombosed hemorrhoid is excised sharply. The wound is left open. (Courtesy Mayo Foundation for Medical Education and Research, Rochester, Minn.)

these newer technologies compared with traditional excisional hemorrhoidectomy.[15] These studies all demonstrated decreased postoperative pain and analgesic use in the Harmonic Scalpel or Liga-Sure groups compared with traditional techniques, with similar short-term success rates.

Another operative technique developed to treat circumferential prolapsed and bleeding hemorrhoids was first described by Longo. Thus technique, commonly referred to as the stapled hemorrhoidectomy or stapled hemorrhoidopexy, excises a circumferential portion of the lower rectal and upper anal canal mucosa and submucosa and performs a reanastomosis with a circular stapling device. As a result, the prolapsed anal cushions are retracted and fixed into their normal anatomic positions within the anal canal. Stapled hemorrhoidectomy is performed

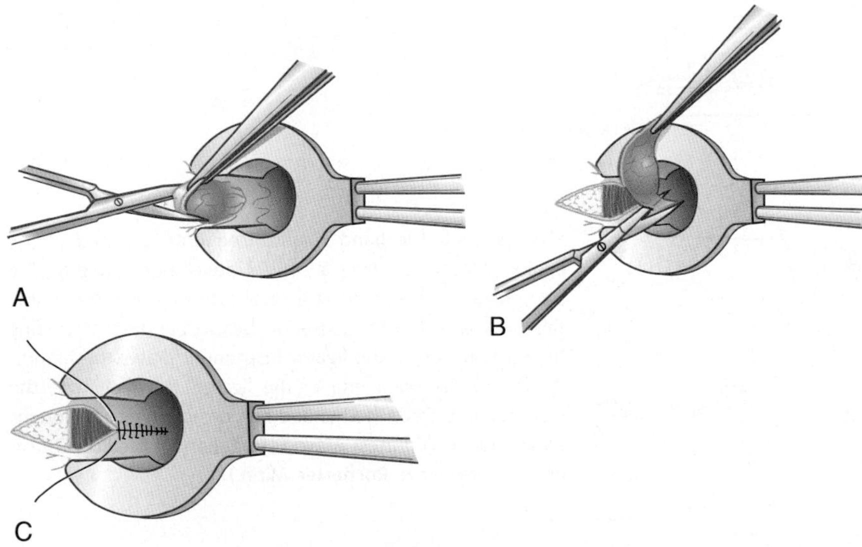


**FIGURE 53-10** Closed hemorrhoidectomy. **A,** Hemorrhoidal tissues are sharply excised, starting just beyond the external component and working proximally, finishing with resection of the internal component. **B,** The sphincter muscles are preserved by dissecting only the tissues superficial to them. **C,** The pedicle is transfixed and the defect closed with a running absorbable suture. (Courtesy Mayo Foundation for Medical Education and Research, Rochester, Minn.)

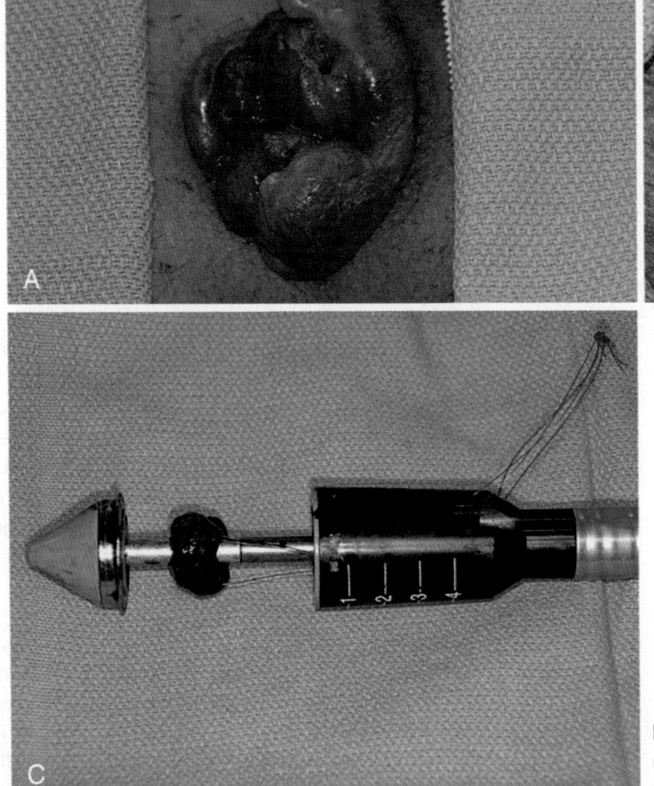


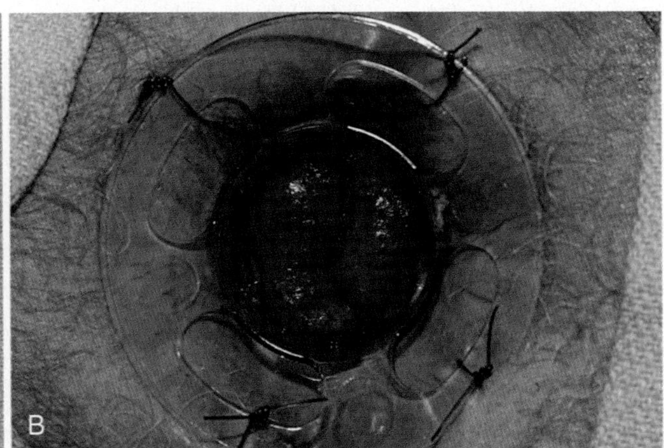


**FIGURE 53-11** **A,** Grade 4 hemorrhoid before reduction. **B,** Placement of stapling device obturator. **C,** Stapling device with circumferential excision of anal canal and hemorrhoid mucosa.

using a dedicated device, including an obturator and circular stapler (Fig. 53-11). To conduct the procedure, the hemorrhoidal tissue must first be reduced and the anal canal gently dilated to facilitate introduction of the stapler. A purse-string suture is placed 3 to 4 cm above the dentate line. Placement of this suture should incorporate all the redundant tissue circumferentially, with care being taken to avoid a full-thickness suture that would ensnare the vaginal wall in women. If the suture is placed too close to the dentate line, it could lead to severe and prolonged pain or urgency. If the suture is placed too far cephalad or does not include circumferential tissue incorporation, it will likely not resolve all symptoms.

A systematic review and meta-analysis of prospective randomized comparisons of stapled hemorrhoidopexy with

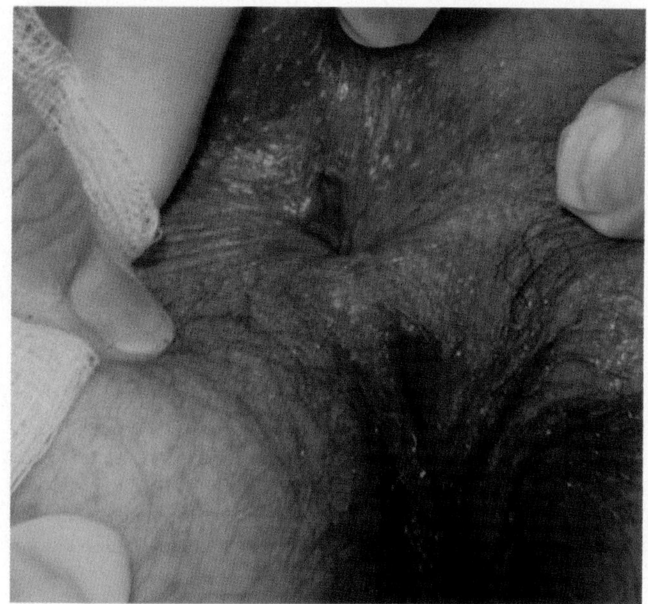

**FIGURE 53-12** Posterior anal fissure. (Courtesy Mayo Foundation for Medical Education and Research, Rochester, Minn.)

conventional hemorrhoidectomy has been conducted.[16] This review incorporated literature from 29 randomized clinical trials representing 2056 patients. It concluded that the stapled hemorrhoidopexy offers some short-term benefits over the conventional approach. The total incidence of complications was the same for both approaches but the stapled hemorrhoidopexy was associated with a higher rate of recurrent disease. Early reports of severe complications from stapled hemorrhoidopexy, including rectal perforation, rectovaginal fistulas, severe pelvic sepsis, and anastomotic dehiscence, appear to have abated as surgeons have gained experience with the technique.

## Anal Fissures

### Clinical Presentation and Diagnostic Evaluation

An anal fissure is a linear ulcer of the lower half of the anal canal, usually located in the posterior commissure in the midline (Fig. 53-12). Often misnamed as rectal fissures, these lesions actually involve just the anal tissues and are typically best seen by visually inspecting the anal verge with gentle separation of the gluteal cleft. Location may vary and an anterior midline fissure is seen more often in women, although most fissures in women and men are in the posterior midline. Characteristic associated findings include a sentinel pile or tag externally and an enlarged anal papilla internally. Fissures away from these two locations should raise the possibility of associated diseases, especially Crohn's disease, hidradenitis suppurativa, or an STD. Because it involves the highly sensitive squamous epithelium, fissure in ano is typically a painful condition. With defecation, the ulcer is stretched, causing pain and mild bleeding.

The diagnosis is secured by the history of pain and bleeding with defecation, especially if associated with prior constipation and confirmed by inspection after gently parting the posterior anus. Digital and proctoscopic examination may trigger severe pain, interfering with the ability to visualize the ulcer. An endoscopic examination should be performed, but it can be delayed 4 to 6 weeks until the pain is resolved with medical management or until surgery is performed for cases refractory to medical therapy.

### Pathogenesis

The exact cause of anal fissures is unknown but many factors appear likely, such as the passage of large hard stools, which may be the initiating factor, inappropriate diet, previous anal surgery, childbirth, and laxative abuse. Numerous authors have documented higher than normal resting anal canal pressures and reduced anal blood flow in the posterior midline. It is therefore believed that anal fissures are the result of anal sphincter hypertonia and subsequent mucosal ischemia. More information regarding the pathogenesis of anal fissures has led to the introduction of several new medical approaches.

### Treatment

The concept that hypertonia and reduced blood flow contribute to anal fissures has facilitated the development of several new therapies. According to this new understanding of the pathogenesis of anal fissures, the goal of therapy is to achieve internal sphincter relaxation without causing fecal incontinence. Toward this aim, several pharmacologic approaches have been introduced, including topical nitric oxide donors (e.g., nitroglycerin), calcium channel blockers (e.g., diltiazem, nifedipine), and botulinum injections. These agents have been compared with each other and with surgical outcomes; reviews of these comparisons have been published.[17,18]

Whether to start with medical or surgical therapy is a matter that now appears to be at the discretion of the patient and treating physician. As medical therapies evolve, it was assumed that all patients should be treated first with conservative medical treatment to avoid the risk of long-term fecal incontinence. However, this concept has been challenged by several prospective randomized trials comparing lateral internal sphincterotomy with medical therapies, including topical approaches (e.g., nitroglycerin) and botulinum. Patients who had lateral internal sphincterotomy were more satisfied, with more durable healing rates and no differences in complication rates, including long-term fecal incontinence. Based on these favorable trial results, it would seem reasonable for a patient and physician to select a medical or surgical approach that seems applicable to the presenting symptoms. For example, a patient with short-duration and mild symptoms might do well with a short course of topical therapy, with surgery reserved for failure to heal. In contrast, a patient who presents with a deep chronic fissure and severe pain would likely obtain the quickest relief from a lateral internal sphincterotomy, with botulinum reserved for refractory disease.

**Medical Management** Medical therapies for anal fissures are gaining in popularity, particularly for acute fissures—that is, those presenting within 3 to 6 weeks of symptom onset. The traditional first-line therapy for acute fissures was treatment with warm sitz baths and bran or bulking agents, with rates of fissure healing reported as 87%. Hydrocortisone and lidocaine were historically advocated as local topical therapies for acute fissures; however, prospective randomized evaluations have shown no benefit over sitz baths and bran. Because improving the dietary and bowel evacuation habits of patients is a good long-term strategy for reducing colon, rectal, and anal problems in general, and for reducing the risk for fissures specifically, counseling on proper diet and institution of commercial bulking agents (e.g., psyllium seeds) are always indicated.

Patients with chronic fissures should be started on the acute fissure regimen but are typically also started on other therapies simultaneously, including nitroglycerin or isosorbide dinitrate, theoretically producing reversible chemical sphincterotomy. For nitroglycerin, the limiting side effects are headaches and tachyphylaxis, which can be reduced by instructing the patient to rest lying down while applying the ointment. The topical application of diltiazem (2%) produces fewer side effects and similar efficacy as nitroglycerin. Fissure healing can be anticipated in approximately 70% of patients with chronic fissures using nitroglycerin or diltiazem.

The concept of reversible chemical sphincterotomy has also been applied to the technique of internal sphincter injection of botulinum toxin (Botox), a technique that transiently produces striated muscle denervation, leading to muscle paralysis and relaxation. It has been recommended as a nonsurgical treatment of fissures, with a low risk for complications. In the treatment of chronic anal fissure, such relaxation of the internal anal sphincter is thought to promote increased blood flow to the affected perianal skin, allowing the fissure to heal. The literature has documented a variable success rate, but 60% to 80% has been achieved. The most common side effect associated with botulinum toxin injections is temporary incontinence to flatus in up to 10% of patients, with rarely any events of temporary fecal incontinence. Unfortunately, there is no standardization in the administration of botulinum toxin regarding the appropriate dose, site of injection, or number or timing of injections, which may contribute to the variable success that has been reported. However, in patients who have not responded to standard dietary measures and medical therapy, such as topical nitroglycerin or calcium channel blockers, and who are at high risk for complications from surgery or wish to avoid surgery, botulinum injection may be a reasonable alternative treatment.

**Surgical Management** Patients with severe and chronic fissures and those who have been treated with and failed medical therapy can benefit from surgery. The most commonly performed procedure is the partial lateral internal sphincterotomy, which can be carried out using the closed or open (Fig. 53-13) technique, depending on surgeon preference, training, and experience. Although open sphincterotomy is more appealing from a training standpoint because the internal sphincter can be directly visualized and the extent of transection more readily quantitated, results from the literature do not support better healing rates and generally describe a greater frequency of complications. A recent prospective, randomized, controlled trial has examined the extent of internal sphincterotomy, with sphincterotomy up to the dentate line versus up to the level of the fissure apex.[19] The trial showed that sphincterotomy to the dentate line provided quicker relief of pain and faster healing of the fissure, but with significant postoperative alteration and fecal incontinence as compared with sphincterotomy just up to the fissure apex. Perfect continence was preserved in 89% to 98% of the patients evaluated. Healing at 4 weeks occurred in 87% to 96% of patients treated with surgery. The trial authors also pointed out that when carefully questioned, many patients may have mild incontinence prior to sphincterotomy and care should be exercised in these individuals so as not to further compromise sphincter function.

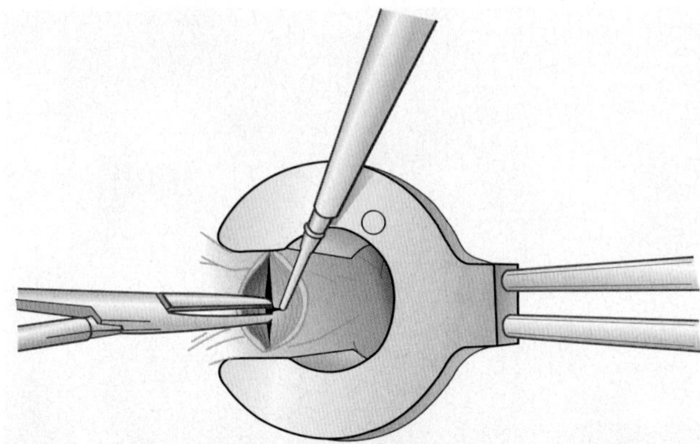

**FIGURE 53-13** Partial lateral internal sphincterotomy, closed technique. With an operating scope in place, a small transverse incision is made along the intersphincteric groove. The mucosa is elevated and the underlying internal sphincter is elevated and divided to release the tight band. (Courtesy Mayo Foundation for Medical Education and Research, Rochester, Minn.)

An alternate surgical approach is the anorectal advancement flap. The flap procedure is particularly attractive for patients with low anal pressures—that is, those who have failed previous sphincterotomy despite a postoperative lowering of anal pressure—and those with severe anal stenosis. The management of fissures in the setting of Crohn's disease is discussed later.

## Anorectal Suppuration

Although anorectal suppuration may have several causes, the most common is a nonspecific infection of cryptoglandular origin. Other causes are rare, except for Crohn's disease and hidradenitis suppurativa. The pathogenesis of abscesses and fistulas is usually the same, with the abscess representing the acute phase and the fistula the chronic sequela.[20]

### Abscess

Infection originates in the intersphincteric plane, most likely in one of the anal glands. This may result in a simple intersphincteric abscess or it may extend vertically upward or downward (Fig. 53-14), horizontally (Fig. 53-15), or circumferentially (Fig. 53-16), with varied clinical presentations.

**Clinical Presentations of Various Types of Abscesses** An intersphincteric abscess is limited to the primary site of origin and may be asymptomatic or result in severe throbbing pain that resembles the pain of a fissure. Pain persisting after adequate treatment of a coexisting fissure should raise suspicion of an underlying, unrecognized intersphincteric abscess. A perianal abscess results from the vertical downward spread of the intersphincteric infection to the anal margin and presents as a tender swelling, which can be misinterpreted as a thrombosed external hemorrhoid.

If the infection spreads vertically upward, an intermuscular abscess within the rectal wall or a supralevator abscess may develop, depending on which side of the longitudinal muscle the infection has tracked. These abscesses are difficult to diagnose because the patient may complain of vague discomfort and

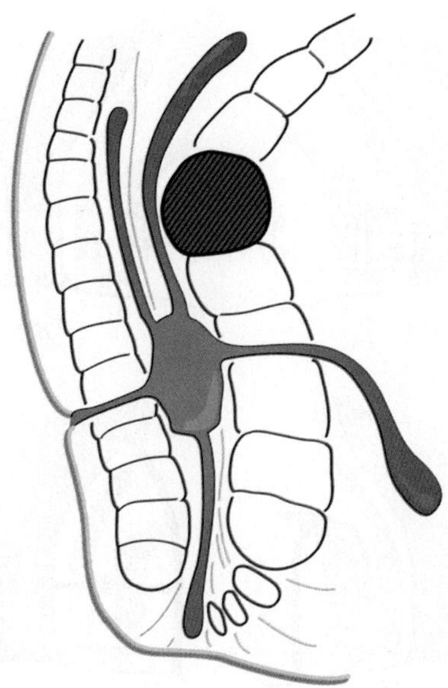

FIGURE 53-14 Various modes of spread from the primary locus in the intersphincteric zone of the midanal canal. The puborectalis muscle has been *cross-hatched* for easy recognition. (From Parks AG, Gordon PH, Hardcastle JD: A classification of fistula-in-ano. Br J Surg 63:1–12, 1976.)

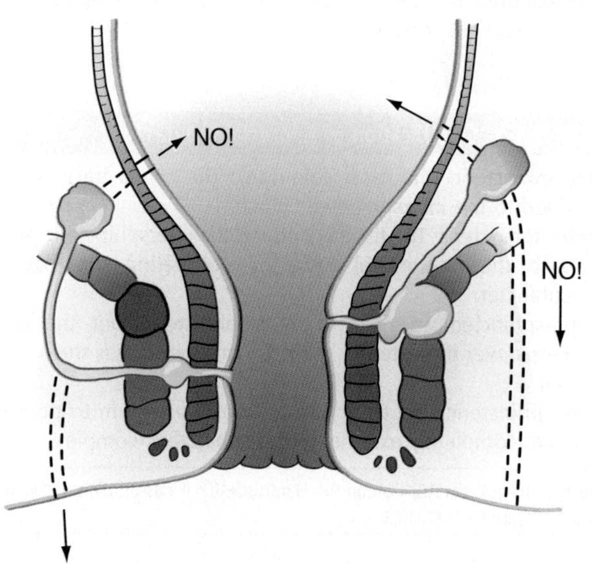


FIGURE 53-15 Two mechanisms whereby an acute pararectal abscess can form. It is essential that drainage be carried out in a way appropriate to the type of abscess. If incorrectly performed, a different extrasphincteric or suprasphincteric fistula may ensue. (From Parks AG, Gordon PH, Hardcastle JD: A classification of fistula-in-ano. Br J Surg 63:1–12, 1976.)

external manifestations are absent; the presence of rectal induration and swelling may be clearly established only with the aid of an examination under anesthesia.

Horizontal spread of infection may track across the internal sphincter into the anal canal or in the opposite direction across the external sphincter, into the ischiorectal fossa, to form an

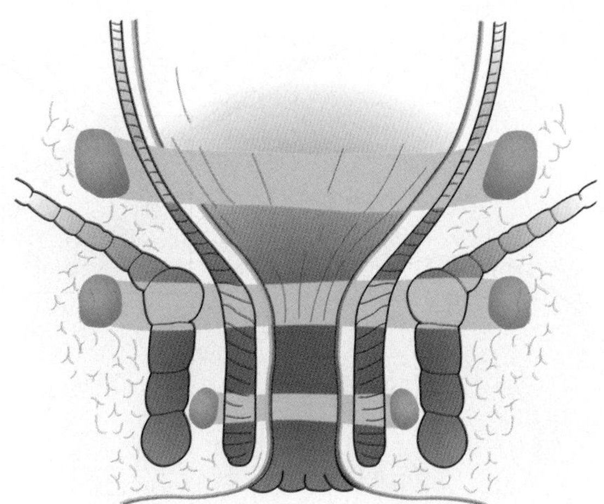

FIGURE 53-16 Three planes in which circumferential spread, or horseshoeing, can occur. (From Parks AG, Gordon PH, Hardcastle JD: A classification of fistula-in-ano. Br J Surg 63:1–12,1976.)

ischiorectal abscess. The abscess may be large, especially if neglected or treated only with antibiotics and allowed to expand to the roof of the fossa, or even through it into the supralevator space after traversing the levator ani muscle and downward to the perianal skin. The patient may complain of pain and fever before an erythematous mass is detectable. Ultimately, an obvious red fluctuant mass is visible. The infectious process may spread circumferentially from one side to the other of the intersphincteric space, supralevator space, or ischiorectal fossa, producing the complex horseshoe abscess.

**Treatment** Abscesses should be drained when diagnosed. Simple and superficial abscesses can most often be drained under local anesthesia in the office setting in patients who are otherwise healthy. Patients who manifest systemic symptoms, those who are immunocompromised for any reason (including AIDS, diabetes, cancer therapies, or chronic medical immunosuppression), and those with complex complicated abscesses are best treated in a hospital setting.

An intersphincteric abscess is drained by dividing the internal sphincter at the level of the abscess. For a perianal abscess, a simple skin incision is all that is necessary (Fig. 53-17). Intermuscular and supralevator abscesses, if not an ischiorectal abscess extension, need to be drained into the lower rectum and upper anal canal. An ischiorectal abscess requires immediate, wide local drainage through an appropriate cruciform incision through the skin and subcutaneous tissue overlying the infected space. At times, these abscesses are sufficiently deep that needle localization of the purulent material may be required to guide the surgeon for optimizing the skin incision site. The cavity should be gently examined digitally to break down loculations. Neglected abscesses can lead to devastating necrotizing infections of the perineum that can spread and become lethal. Failure of response to local treatment or recurrent abscesses may suggest inadequate drainage with residual pus, presence of a fistula, or immunoincompetence. Under these circumstances, antibiotics may be useful, together with examination under anesthesia after preliminary evaluation by computed tomography (CT) of the pelvis and perineum. For a horseshoe abscess, the deep postanal

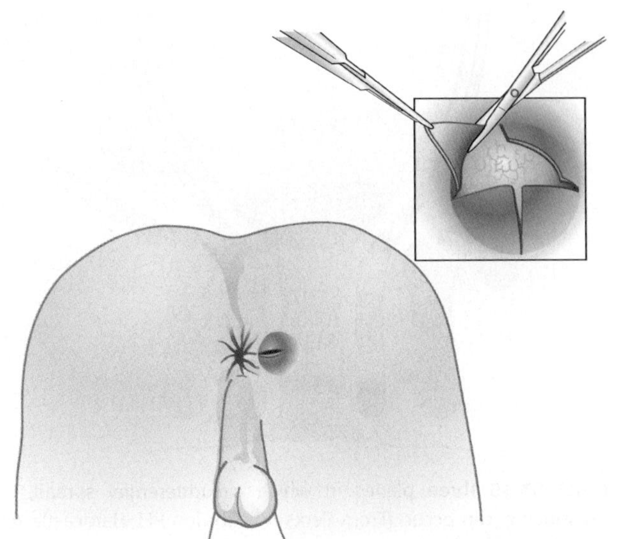

**FIGURE 53-17** Incision and drainage of an anorectal abscess. A cruciate incision is made and the wound is probed for loculations. The wound edges are kept open to facilitate proper drainage by excising the corners of the cruciate *(inset)* and packing the cavity. (Courtesy Mayo Foundation for Medical Education and Research, Rochester, Minn.)

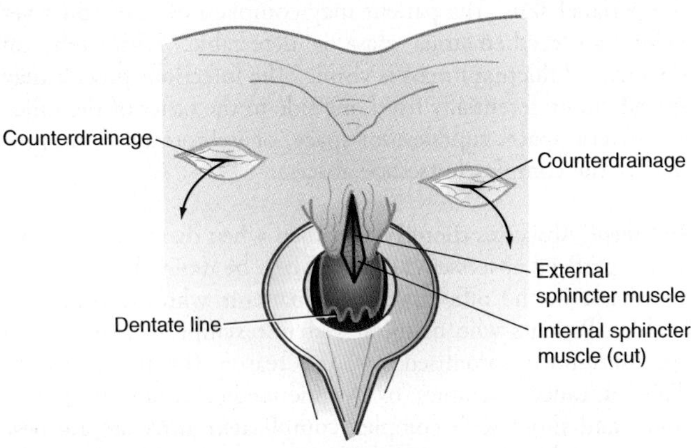


**FIGURE 53-18** Modification of Hanley's technique for incision and drainage of a horseshoe abscess. (From Gordon PH: Anorectal abscesses and fistula-in-ano. In Gordon PH, Nivatvongs S [eds]: Principles and practice of surgery for the colon, rectum, and anus, ed 2, St Louis, 1992, Quality Medical, p 232.)

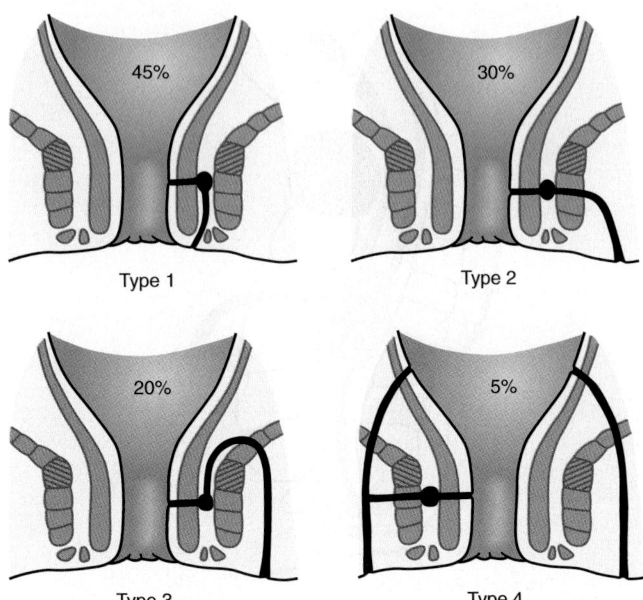


**FIGURE 53-19** Four main anatomic types of fistulas. The external sphincter mass is regarded as the keystone, and the prefixes trans-, supra-, and extra- refer to it. The puborectalis muscle has been *cross-hatched* for easy recognition. *Type 1,* Intersphincteric; *type 2,* trans-sphincteric; *type 3,* suprasphincteric; *type 4,* extrasphincteric. (From Parks AG, Gordon PH, Hardcastle JD: A classification of fistula-in-ano. Br J Surg 63:1–12, 1976.)

**BOX 53-1 Classification of Anorectal Fistulas**

Intersphincteric (the most common): The fistula track is confined to the intersphincteric plane.

Trans-sphincteric: The fistula connects the intersphincteric plane with the ischiorectal fossa by perforating the external sphincter.

Suprasphincteric: Similar to trans-sphincteric, but the track loops over the external sphincter and perforates the levator ani.

Extrasphincteric: The track passes from the rectum to perineal skin, completely external to the sphincteric complex.

Adapted from Parks AG, Gordon PH, Hardcastle JD: A classification of fistula-in-ano. Br J Surg 63:1–12, 1976.

space should be drained through a posterior midline incision extending from the subcutaneous portion of the external sphincter over the abscess to the tip of the coccyx, separating the superficial external sphincter and thus unroofing the postanal space and its ischioanal extension (Fig. 53-18). Para-anal incisions can be made and setons placed to drain the anterior extensions of a horseshoe abscess.

## Fistula in Ano

Anorectal sepsis can be complicated by a fistula in ano in approximately 25% of patients during the acute phase of sepsis or within 6 months thereafter.[21] Most fistulas are caused by sepsis originating in the anal canal glands at the dentate line. The path of a fistula is determined by the local anatomy; usually, they track in the fascial or fatty planes, especially the intersphincteric space between the internal and external sphincter into the ischiorectal fascia. In such cases, the track passes directly to the perineal skin. Circumferential spread may also occur in the ischiorectal fossa, with the track passing from one fossa to the contralateral one through the posterior rectum, a fistula known as the *horseshoe fistula*. Fistulas usually fall under four main anatomic categories, as described by Parks and colleagues[22] (Box 53-1; Fig. 53-19).

**Clinical Presentations** Intersphincteric fistulas are the most common anal fistulas, and in most cases, the infection passes directly downward to the anal margin. However, there are some variants of this type of fistula that are less common and more complex to treat. For instance, the track may travel upward in the rectal wall (higher track), with or without a perineal opening. Rarely, an intersphincteric fistula originates in the pelvis from the colon.[22] In trans-sphincteric fistulas, the track traverses the external sphincter to travel through the ischiorectal fossa and end at the perineal skin. If it passes through the muscle at a low level, it is uncomplicated and readily treatable; if, however, it penetrates the upper portion of the sphincter (high blind track), it constitutes a more difficult therapeutic dilemma. Indeed, it may be felt digitally through the wall of the rectum and may lead the surgeon to create an artificial connection with the rectum by forceful probing, a situation that can be difficult to correct. Suprasphincteric fistulas are rare, difficult to treat, and may be hazardous if dealt with by inexperienced surgeons.

The track may first travel upward in the intersphincteric plane before taking a lateral direction over the top of the puborectalis and finally downward through the ischiorectal fossa to the perineal skin. Because its trajectory is above all muscles of importance to continence, division of all external muscles results in incontinence. Moreover, the fistula may have an additional extension into the pelvis that runs parallel to the rectum (high blind track). In this instance, an indurated area can be palpated through the rectal wall. Finally, extrasphincteric fistula is rare, and its treatment is also hazardous. It travels from the perineal skin to the rectal wall above the levator ani that it pierces. The track is completely outside the sphincteric apparatus. Causes typically include trauma, either external or internal (e.g., fish bone piercing one wall of rectum), carcinoma, or Crohn's disease. Treatment is difficult, lengthy, and usually involves colostomy.

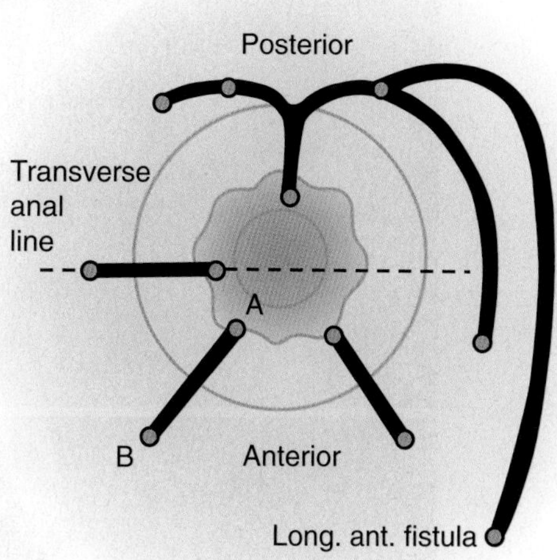


**FIGURE 53-20** The Goodsall rule. The usual relationship of primary and secondary fistula orifices is diagrammed. The internal (primary orifice) is marked A. The rule predicts that if a line is drawn transversely across the anus, an external opening (B) anterior to this line will lead to a straight radial tract, whereas an external opening that lies posterior to the line will lead to a curved tract and an internal opening in the posterior commissure. The long anterior fistula is an exception to the rule. (From Schrock TR: Benign and malignant disease of the anorectum. In Fromm O [ed]: Gastrointestinal surgery, New York, 1985, Churchill Livingstone, p 612.)

**Treatment** A fistula may first present as an acute abscess or, at times, simply as a draining sinus that may irritate the perineal skin. On examination, subcutaneous induration may be traced from the external opening to the anal canal. Digital examination may reveal a palpable nodule in the wall of the anal canal, an indication of the primary opening. A probe can be eased gently, not forcefully, from the external skin opening to the internal anal canal opening.

Management of fistula in ano should include the following steps:

1. Under anesthesia, palpation for induration, anoscopy for inspection, and gentle probing along the dentate line for internal openings allows accurate definition of the abnormal anatomy. The Goodsall rule (Fig. 53-20) is useful for anticipating the anatomy of simple fistulas. If the internal opening cannot be identified by direct probing, it should be identified by probing the external opening or by injecting a mixture of methylene blue and peroxide into the track using a pediatric feeding tube (Fig. 53-21*A*).
2. Drainage of primary intersphincteric infection in all types of fistulas, as well as the primary track across the external sphincter and secondary tracks within the anorectal fossa, is key. For superficial fistulas involving small quantities of sphincter muscle, primary fistulotomy is simple and definitive. For anterior fistulas in women and fistulas involving more than 25% to 50% of the bulk of sphincter muscles, seton placement should be preferred over primary fistulotomy (see Fig. 53-21*B* to *D*).
3. Close follow-up and careful nursing of the wound by a physician-nurse team involve sitz baths and wound dressing to ensure healing from the depth of the wound to the surface. A seton of monofilament nylon tied loosely around the fistulous track may be used to drain the trans-sphincteric track, traveling above the anal valves for a suprasphincteric fistula. The seton may be removed 2 to 3 months later, at which time the track may heal spontaneously. If not, the track may be divided because fibrosis may cause minimal separation of the cut ends. For more straightforward trans-sphincteric fistulas, a cutting seton can be placed at surgery and tightened in the office. This divides the track gradually over a few weeks and minimizes the sphincter defect and risk for significant fecal incontinence.

In rare circumstances, with complex, deep, or recurrent fistulas, alternatives to fistulotomy are preferred to avoid the complication of fecal incontinence. Currently, there are two therapies that use biologic material to promote the closure of fistulas without division of any sphincter muscle, injection of fibrin glue into the fistula track and insertion of a porcine small intestinal submucosa (SIS) plug. Both products are thought to promote healing of the track by providing a naturally derived extracellular matrix to act as scaffolding, allowing ingrowth of host tissue for incorporation and remodeling. Fibrin glue is a multicomponent system, with the primary agents being human pooled plasma fibrinogen and thrombin. Once prepared, the fibrin glue components are injected into the anal fistula track. Over a matter of minutes, the glue hardens and fills the entire

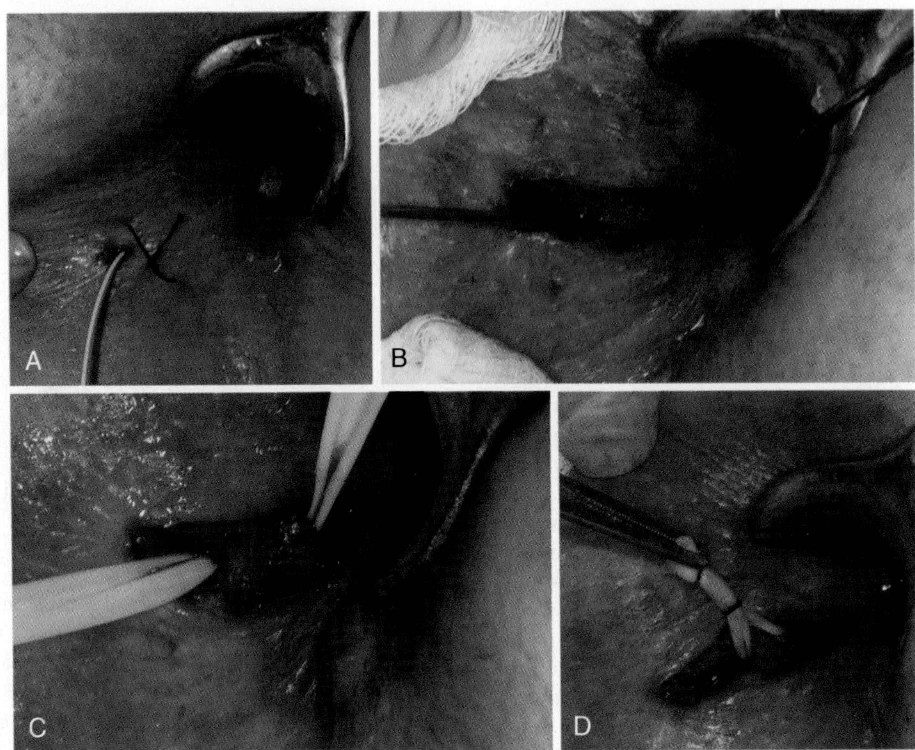


**FIGURE 53-21** Seton placement. **A,** If the primary opening cannot be identified by gentle probing along the dentate line, methylene blue plus peroxide injections may better delineate the internal fistula source. **B,** A probe is passed from the primary to the secondary openings and the skin is incised to reveal the tract and interposed sphincter muscle. **C,** An elastic cutting seton can be placed when generous muscle requires division. **D,** The seton is tightened in the operating room and again once or twice in the office to allow for fibrosis and gradual sphincter transection. (Courtesy Mayo Foundation for Medical Education and Research, Rochester, Minn.)

track. Initially, successful fistula closure rates of almost 70% were reported. A comprehensive review of the literature has reported that fibrin glue injection result in a broad range of successful fistula closure, from 14% to 60%.[20] This review included a randomized control trial of fibrin glue compared with standard treatment of fistulas; it demonstrated no difference in closure rate or patient satisfaction with the procedure. The only real difference was that fibrin glue patients returned to work earlier than the conventionally treated patients.

Based on this premise of providing scaffolding for tissue ingrowth, a biologically based product is now available, the Surgisis Fistula Plug (Cook Biotech, West Lafayette, Ind). This cone-shaped product is made of a porcine SIS. It is physically inserted into the fistula and then secured to the internal and external openings of the anal fistula with absorbable suture. Over time, tissue from the fistula wall will grow into the SIS plug and replace the matrix of the plug with new viable tissue that obliterates the fistula track. There has only been one recently published report of the use of an SIS plug in the treatment of benign anal fistulas.[23] In this small series, patients were treated with fibrin glue or an SIS plug. The 3-month fistula closure was 60% in the fibrin glue and 87% in the SIS plug group. Although the success rate of fistula closure for both these products is variable or relatively unknown because of their fairly recent clinical introduction, the benefit is that there is no permanent injury to the anal sphincter mechanism and therefore no risk for incontinence related to the treatment. If either modality fails to close the fistula, the patient has not been harmed.

Difficult and persistent high fistulas can be treated by advancement of a sliding flap made of mucosa, submucosa, and circular muscle to cover the internal opening. The Goodsall rule (see Fig. 53-20) is of little help in defining the anatomy of complex and recurrent fistulas. Diagnostic tests such as pelvic MRI and endorectal ultrasound and treatment by a specialist may be helpful here.

## Pilonidal Disease

Pilonidal infections and chronic pilonidal sinuses typically occur in the midline of the sacrococcygeal skin of young men. Although the exact pathogenesis of pilonidal disease remains elusive and controversial, hair seems to play a central role in the process of infection and perpetuation of granulation tissue in sinuses. This is consistent with the clinical observation that pilonidal patients are often hirsute and that pilonidal disease rarely occurs in those with less body hair. It is uncommon for pilonidal disease to be confused with clinical disorders such as anal fistulas, skin disorders, underlying malignancies, or true sacrococcygeal sinuses.

### Treatment

**Acute Management** Patients presenting acutely with new-onset disease may have a painful fluctuant abscess or a draining infected sinus. Both can be managed with simple office treatment, with more definitive procedures reserved for patients who suffer from a recurrence. Abscess can be drained in the office or emergency department using local anesthesia. Typically, the fluctuance extends to either side of the midline cleft, and incision and drainage down to the subcutaneous tissues off the midline provide for the best drainage and fastest healing. For abscesses and sinuses, hair should be removed from the wound and local skin should be shaved weekly to prevent the reintroduction of hair. Whereas short-term razor epilation is advised, long-term razor epilation is not advised; there is no proven efficacy in nonsurgical cases and, when performed as a long-term adjunct to surgery, it increases rates of recurrence.[24] Laser depilation can also be used to accomplish effective long-lasting, hair removal, especially if repeated.[25,26] Ideally, these patients should be seen weekly in the office for wound care until there is complete healing. Most do not require further care; those who do can be treated as described in the following section.

**Surgical Management** For patients who have recurring infections, definitive operative management is warranted. Numerous procedures have been described in the literature, ranging from simple incision and drainage to complex plastic flaps for cleft obliteration.

Comparative studies in this field are rare. Most reports have been limited to a single surgical approach, with only a few prospective randomized trials available in the current literature. In one comparative trial, the complex V-Y advancement flap was found not to be superior to simple primary suture methods.[27] In another trial, the Bascom cleft closure was found to offer more predictable healing than the Bascom simple surgery. The development of a classification scheme for pilonidal disease may help with future comparative studies because there are likely numerous patient factors that contribute to the causes and/or failures of a given procedure.

The simplest approach for chronic pilonidal disease is the ambulatory technique of midline excision and primary suture.[28] This approach was studied in 103 patients at a single institution, with excellent long-term follow-up. Patients with chronic disease or acute but not inflamed disease were treated with 3 days of preoperative oral antibiotics and the surgery was performed under local anesthesia. Methylene blue was injected into the sinus or pit, which stained the tissue to be excised. Suture closure included incorporation of the deep sacral fascia and a vacuum drain. Three patients experienced a recurrence; otherwise, wound healing occurred between 10 and 16 days postoperatively. For primary closure, the omission of wound drainage was associated with a higher frequency of minor and major wound infections and wound dehiscence.

An alternative to simple excision plus closure is marsupialization. In this procedure, the areas of midline pits and sinuses are removed and the wound reduced in size by suturing the wound edges to the fibrous base of the wound. This can reduce wound healing times and may be effective at removing extensive sinus tracts, but requires frequent office visits for meticulous wound care over several weeks. This approach is appealing because of its low rate of reinfection and wound breakdown.

Several more complicated approaches to pilonidal disease have been described, including rhomboid excision, Limberg flaps, and oblique excisions with bilateral gluteus maximus fascia advancement flaps, Bascom's cleft closure, and V-Y advancement flaps.[27] The Bascom closure and oblique excision are premised on the need to create an off-midline closure to facilitate healing. In most practices, the complex flap closures are reserved for patients with refractory disease for whom simple measures have failed.

## LESS COMMON BENIGN ANAL DISORDERS

### Rectovaginal Fistula

A rectovaginal fistula is a communication between the epithelial-lined surfaces of the rectum and vagina. Patients usually complain that they pass gas, mucus, blood, or stool through the vagina. Rectovaginal fistulas may be congenital or acquired through trauma, inflammatory bowel disease (IBD), irradiation, neoplasia, infection, or other rare causes. For fistulas associated with a history of trauma, anal manometry and endoanal ultrasound can determine the severity of underlying sphincter defect and help guide surgical therapy. Rectovaginal fistulas are classified as high or low, depending on whether they can be corrected transabdominally or transperineally, respectively.

#### Surgical Repair

Rectovaginal fistulas need not be corrected immediately; delay depends on the underlying disease, size of the fistula, presence of active inflammation, and severity of symptoms. Some fistulas may close spontaneously, whereas others, such as those associated with IBD, may heal with medical therapy alone. High rectovaginal fistulas require a transabdominal approach, whereas low rectovaginal fistulas can be approached transvaginally, transrectally, transperineally, trans-sphincterically, or transanally.

The most common surgical approaches to the low-lying fistula—typically, a true anovaginal fistula—are the endorectal advancement flap, sphincteroplasty, and transperineal procedures.[29] An endorectal advancement flap consists of a flap raised of rectal mucosa and underlying internal sphincter that is advanced to cover the primary fistula's opening in the rectum or anus after the fistula's opening has been excised and the underlying muscle reapproximated. The flap is best suited for the first attempt at repair or for patients without evidence of an underlying sphincter defect, and is accordingly associated with a healing rate of 50%. The transperineal repair excises the fistula tract completely and accomplishes a primary reapproximation of the internal, external, and levator muscles in discrete layers. Success rates are as high as 85% to 100% in patients with associated sphincter defects who have already failed other approaches.[29]

For high rectovaginal fistulas, a transabdominal approach is necessary. Whether a portion or the entire rectum is sacrificed depends on the nature and extent of the underlying disease. This approach involves mobilization of the rectovaginal septum, division of the fistula, and a layer closure of the rectal and vaginal defects. In some cases, no rectal resection is necessary, and a live pedicle of tissue may be interposed between the two anastomotic structures to supplement the repair. When rectal tissues are involved by severe irradiation changes, IBD, or neoplasia, rectal excision is required. Whenever possible, the sphincter apparatus can be preserved using a low anterior resection or coloanal anastomosis.[29] Whether the outcome of such procedures is favorable depends on the underlying disease, selection of patients, and the surgeon's experience and expertise.

In the setting of Crohn's disease, the low anovaginal fistula represents a unique challenge. Primary repair avoids the need for a permanent stoma and can be accomplished in up to 68% of patients using a variety of horizontal, linear, and sleeve advancement flaps.

**BOX 53-2 Organisms that Cause Sexually Transmitted Diseases**

**Bacterial**
*Neisseria gonorrhoeae*
*Treponema pallidum*
*Haemophilus ducreyi*
*Chlamydia species*
*Shigella flexneri*
*Campylobacter* spp.

**Viral**
Herpes simplex
Human papillomavirus
Molluscum contagiosum

**Parasitic**
*Entamoeba histolytica*
*Giardia lamblia*
*Cryptococcus* spp.
*Isospora belli*

## Sexually Transmitted Diseases and Acquired Immunodeficiency Syndrome

STDs, formerly referred to as venereal diseases, are exceeded in frequency only by the common cold and influenza. Multiple partners and anal-receptive intercourse increase the risk for STD transmission.[30] STDs can be bacterial, viral, or parasitic in origin (Box 53-2), and a variety of sexual practices may favor their development.

### Clinical Presentation

Patients with bacterial STDs may have no symptoms or may have symptoms of pruritus, bloody or mucopurulent rectal discharge, tenesmus, perineal or rectal pain, diarrhea, and fever. Depending on the causative agent, proctoscopy may reveal proctitis, discharge (mucopurulent in gonorrheal or *Campylobacter* spp. infection, bloody in chlamydial infection), anal ulcerations, and abscesses. The diagnosis is based on the clinical signs and physical examination, including endoscopy and cultures of stool or discharge specimens. Treatment is based on the causative agent.

Patients with viral STDs may complain of anorectal pain, discharge, bleeding, and pruritus. In molluscum contagiosum, the patient has painless dermal lesions that are flattened, round, and umbilicated. Endoscopy may reveal vesicles, ulcers, and diffuse friability, as in herpes, or anal warts, as in condylomata. The diagnosis is based on cultures, scrapings, or excisional biopsy. Herpes is best treated with acyclovir, whereas the other viral lesions are treated by destruction or excision.[30]

Patients with parasitic STDs have more systemic symptoms, such as fever, abdominal cramping, and bloody diarrhea. Ulcerations caused by *Entamoeba histolytica* are typically hourglass-shaped, whereas they are more diffuse when caused by *Giardia lamblia.* Diagnosis is based on biopsy specimens or scrapings and specific stains. *E. histolytica* and *G. lamblia* infections are treated with metronidazole and *Isospora belli* infection is managed with cotrimoxazole.

**Acquired Immunodeficiency Syndrome** Anorectal pathology is common in patients who are positive for HIV infection, affecting about one third of patients at some point in their disease. Anorectal pain, the presence of a mass, and bleeding per rectum are the most frequent presenting complaints. In a consecutive series of 260 HIV-positive patients, the most frequently occurring diseases were condylomata (42%), fistulas (34%), and fissures (32%).[31] For benign noninfectious disorders, fissures and ulcers are the most common presenting problems. This is uniquely different from HIV-negative patients, in whom the primary presenting diagnoses are hemorrhoids and skin tags.[32] When seeing patients with HIV, it is important to distinguish between anal fissures that are amenable to medical therapy or lateral internal sphincterotomy and anal ulcers that respond best to operative evaluation, biopsy, viral culture, débridement, and topical antiviral therapy. Herpes, cytomegalovirus, and *Chlamydia* spp. are the most typical infectious agents.

Neoplastic disorders in HIV-positive patients include condyloma, anal intraepithelial neoplasia, epidermoid carcinoma, and Kaposi's sarcoma; their incidence is higher in HIV-positive than HIV-negative patients.[31-33] Although therapies for anal condyloma are no different based on HIV status, the recurrence rates appear to be higher for HIV-positive than HIV-negative patients. For the management of in situ and invasive squamous cell carcinoma, it appears that the CD4 count and concomitant treatment with antiretroviral therapy are keys to success with local excision and radiation plus chemotherapy, respectively. Best-practice strategies for anorectal conditions complicating HIV are likely to evolve as more effective therapies to treat HIV-infected patients are developed.

Anal condyloma and human papilloma virus infections are considered as STDs. Because of their neoplastic potential, particularly in HIV patients, they are discussed later (see "Neoplastic Disorders").

## Hidradenitis Suppurativa

Hidradenitis suppurativa is a chronic inflammatory process affecting the apocrine glands of the perianal region characterized by abscesses and sinus formation. Although dermatologic studies have called into question the site of origin of hidradenitis, implicating occluding spongiform infundibulofolliculitis, a follicular disease, hidradenitis has traditionally been considered the result of keratotic debris plugging the apocrine gland. The plugging event is followed by bacterial proliferation, suppurative infection, gland rupture, and spread of inflammation to surrounding subcutaneous tissues. Numerous tracks and pits develop, and the tissues become fibrotic and thickened from the persistent inflammatory response. Various factors have been implicated in the development and perpetuation of hidradenitis, including the use of depilatories, close shaving, poor personal hygiene, tight-fitting and synthetic clothing, and antiperspirants. The most common bacterial organisms identified include *Streptococcus milleri, Staphylococcus aureus, Staphylococcus epidermidis,* and *Staphylococcus hominis.*

### Clinical Presentation

Clinically, patients may complain of burning, itching, and hyperhidrosis. Affected patients frequently have seborrheic skin and sometimes have involvement of other areas in which apocrine sweat glands are present, such as the axillae and mammary, inguinal, and genital regions. The affected areas have a purplish appearance, with drainage of watery pus. In advanced cases, numerous fistulous tracks are readily identified, and the

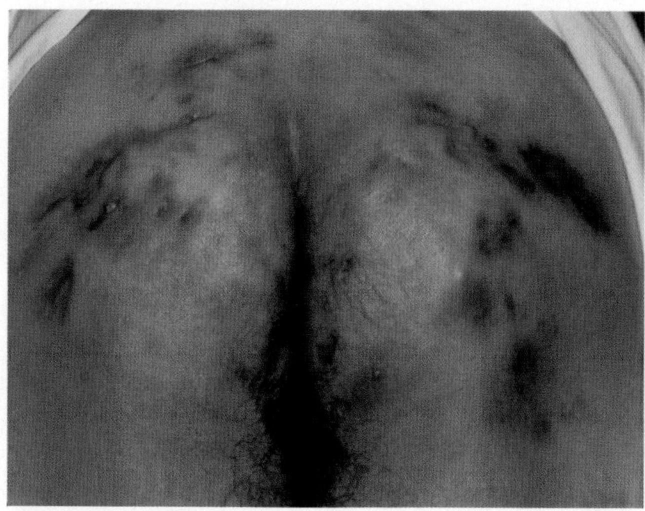

**FIGURE 53-22** Hidradenitis suppurativa. (Courtesy Mayo Foundation for Medical Education and Research, Rochester, Minn.)

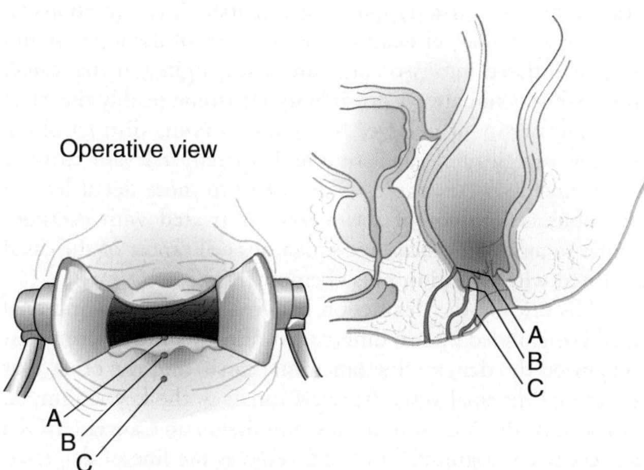


**FIGURE 53-23** Relationship of fistulous tracks in Crohn's disease, above dentate line (A), cryptoglandular abscess or fistula disease at dentate line (B), and hidradenitis suppurativa distal to dentate line (C). (From Culp CE: Chronic hidradenitis suppurativa of the anal canal: A surgical skin disease. Dis Colon Rectum 26:669–676, 1983.)

appearance is classic (Fig. 53-22). When the condition presents early and there are limited fistulous tracks around the anal and perianal tissues, hidradenitis must be differentiated from other types of fistulas, such as those arising from Crohn's disease or infected crypts. Fistulas from hidradenitis arise distal to the dentate line in the anal skin, allowing their differentiation from cryptoglandular fistulas, which communicate with the dentate line, and Crohn's disease, which may track to the anorectum proximal to the dentate line (Fig. 53-23).[34] Hidradenitis is more common in women and blacks; however, perianal hidradenitis is more common in men.

### Treatment

Perianal hidradenitis can present in one of several states, from early acute to late chronic and severe forms, and can present alone or with associated complications, such as severe anal fibrosis and incontinence, or even copresentation with squamous malignancies. To exclude the possibility of coexisting cancer, biopsies should be performed with liberal indications. For early limited disease, emphasis should be placed on incision and drainage of infections and prevention of recurrences. The role of oral antibiotic treatment, typically erythromycin, is not established but often recommended. Although not proved, frequent cleansing and warm water soaking, avoidance of tight-fitting and synthetic clothing, and avoidance of local chemical irritants may help prevent further disease or reduce the severity of active disease.

When hidradenitis sinus tracks are well established but relatively superficial, they can be unroofed or laid open.[34] Because these tracks are lined by epithelium, the floor of the track can be preserved; this facilitates rapid healing and minimizes scarring. For more extensive and deeper disease, wide excision may be required. Although wide excision is thought to be more effective for advanced cases, it is associated with recurrence rates of approximately 50% when both same-site and new-site disease are considered. In cases of aggressive wide excision, large wounds can be managed primarily, with delayed healing, flaps, or skin grafts. Wound closure can be tailored to the specific conditions of each patient. Skin grafting offers the advantage of early wound coverage, with a reduction in pain and time to complete healing, but requires compliance with delicate postoperative wound care. Healing by secondary intention requires less delicate wound care but takes 2 to 3 months for complete healing to be accomplished.

## Crohn's Disease of the Anorectum

### Clinical Presentation

Anal manifestations of Crohn's disease can be most devastating because of their painful nature and threat to the patient's continence. Almost 20% of patients with Crohn's disease will present with anal disease, including fissures, fistulas, or abscesses. Symptoms and signs of anal Crohn's disease may include pain, swelling, bleeding, soilage or frank incontinence, and fever. Pain may be caused by skin excoriation and maceration, hemorrhoids, fissures, or abscess and fistula disease (Fig. 53-24). Edematous purplish tags are characteristic of the disease. Bleeding may be from distal proctitis, fissures, hemorrhoids, or granulating fistulas. Soilage may result from prolapsing rectal mucosa, seepage of liquid stool, drainage from abscess, or poor continence. Poor continence may result from sphincter damage caused by the disease or aggressive surgery, anoperineal fistulas, rectovaginal fistulas, or loss of rectal compliance.

### Evaluation and Treatment

Early in the evaluation of a patient with Crohn's disease and new anal symptoms, it is key to establish whether the problem is likely related to the manifestation of Crohn's disease in the anus or is just coincident anal disease. Patients with Crohn's disease, especially quiescent disease, may present common anorectal conditions. It is important that the anorectal examination be conducted by a clinician familiar with both common conditions and the typical presentation of anal Crohn's disease, and that the examination be thorough (including endoscopy) and not painful. This may require anesthesia for diagnostic and therapeutic purposes. If the patient has no rectal or anal Crohn's disease that is obvious and has an otherwise normal-appearing anus but has a

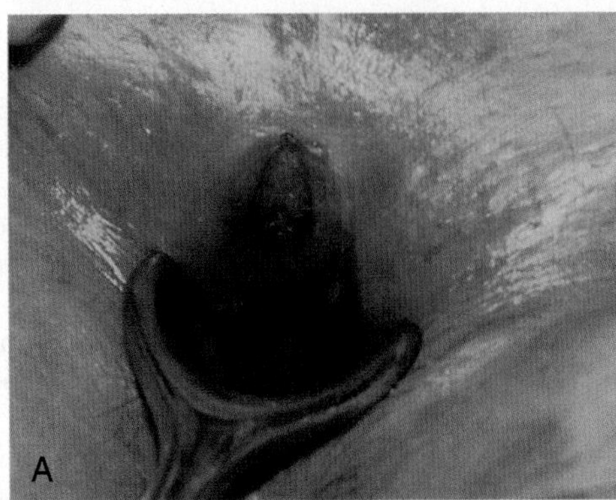


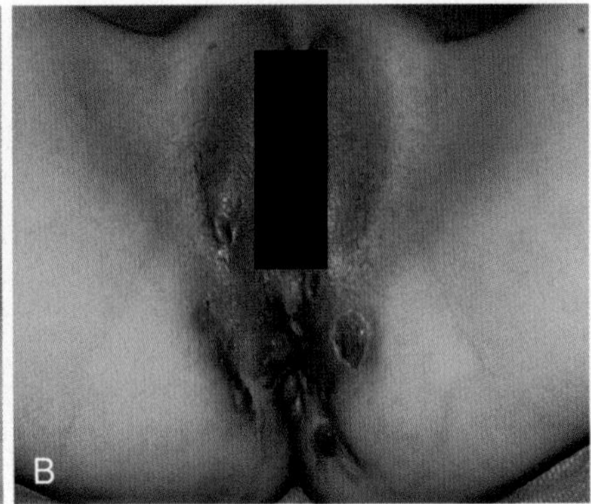


**FIGURE 53-24** Perineal Crohn's disease. **A,** Characteristic of Crohn's fissures are the shaggy edges, deep ulceration, and granulation tissue. **B,** Uncontrolled perianal Crohn's with multiple fistulas can present as a watering pot perineum. (Courtesy Mayo Foundation for Medical Education and Research, Rochester, Minn.)

simple fissure, fistula, or abscess, it may represent a non-Crohn's manifestation of these common conditions. In the absence of evidence of rectal or perianal Crohn's disease, these conditions may be best treated using standard approaches. Although caution is advised against aggressive approaches when treating a Crohn's patient with anorectal problems, undertreatment of symptomatic conditions is also discouraged.

When the clinician suspects the perianal involvement of Crohn's disease, a more complex treatment approach is required. For example, for Crohn's fissures which typically present as multiple, superficial, off-midline lesions, patients with lesions will typically respond to conservative measures with sitz baths, stool softeners, and oral analgesics. Those who have deeper ulcerations, such as true Crohn's ulcerations, may require medical treatment to control the disease. Sphincterotomy and fissurectomy should be avoided when perianal Crohn's disease is present. In the case of anorectal suppurative disease caused by underlying Crohn's disease, a combination of surgical and medical therapy is advised (Fig. 53-25).[35-37] For primary abscess, this should be drained under anesthesia; this allows an evaluation of the adjacent rectal tissue as well as adequate drainage of the infection. If a true fistula is present, a seton can be placed primarily at the time of the infection or secondarily when a fistula develops. In the presence of a mid to low fistula, local therapy and/or primary fistulotomy or seton placement can be complemented with the use of ciprofloxacin and metronidazole therapy. When the fistulas are more complex or severe, setons are required to maintain drainage while the patient receives infliximab or azathioprine and mercaptopurine. Patients with severe fistula should be prepared for the possibility of requiring diversion or even proctectomy at some point. Antibiotic treatment of Crohn's disease is associated with 48% complete healing and 24% advanced healing. For the more complex patients treated with azathioprine and mercaptopurine, 39% of patients can expect a complete response. The use of infliximab was associated with a 50% or greater reduction in the number of open fistulas in 68% of patients.

## NEOPLASTIC DISORDERS

Neoplasms of the anal area are rare and represent a wide spectrum of benign and malignant tumors (Box 53-3). Benign lesions may range from innocuous in situ Bowen's disease to clinically aggressive verrucous lesions; malignant lesions range from favorable early-stage squamous cell cancers of the anal margin to anal canal adenocarcinoma and melanoma. In all cases, it is essential to consider tumor location with reference to clear landmarks, such as anal verge, dentate line, and anorectal ring. For a number of reasons, the anatomy of the anus should be differentiated into two parts, the anal margin and anal canal. Although it is not always possible to determine readily the exact anatomic origin of a large, bulky anal tumor, distinguishing between margin and canal tumors is directly relevant to their management. For example, as described in more detail later, a squamous cell tumor of the margin is treated with excision, similar to any skin cancer, yet squamous cell cancer of the canal is treated with radiation plus chemotherapy.

Historically the distinction between anal margin and anal canal was clouded by two different working definitions, one that recognized the dentate line (anatomic canal) and the other that recognized the anal verge (surgical canal) as the key landmark. Fortunately, the American Joint Commission on Cancer (AJCC) has recently recognized[38] the anal verge as the line of demarcation between anal margin and anal canal tumors (see Fig. 53-2). This definition is the easiest to apply because most clinicians can readily determine the location of an anal tumor as inside or outside the anal verge using inspection alone—that is, without the aid of an anoscope or proctoscope. Differentiating tumors originating in the rectum, anal canal, and anal margin will always be difficult for tumors that are bulky and spill over from one location to another. In these cases, one has to consider the epicenter of the mass along with the histology. From a practical standpoint, most bulky adenocarcinomas of the distal rectum or proximal anal canal are going to receive the same treatment and bulky squamous cancers of the anal canal and margin will be treated in the same way, no matter the precise site of origin.

### Clinical Evaluation

Preoperative assessment should include a complete history and physical examination. The nature and duration of local anal symptoms, such as a mass, bleeding, and pruritus and distant manifestations, such as weight loss, should be documented. The perianal area should be closely inspected for skin alterations. Digital examination helps establish tumor location, tumor mobility or fixity, and integrity of the sphincter mechanism. Anoscopy or rigid proctosigmoidoscopy can verify the size and location of the tumor in relationship to the dentate line, anal

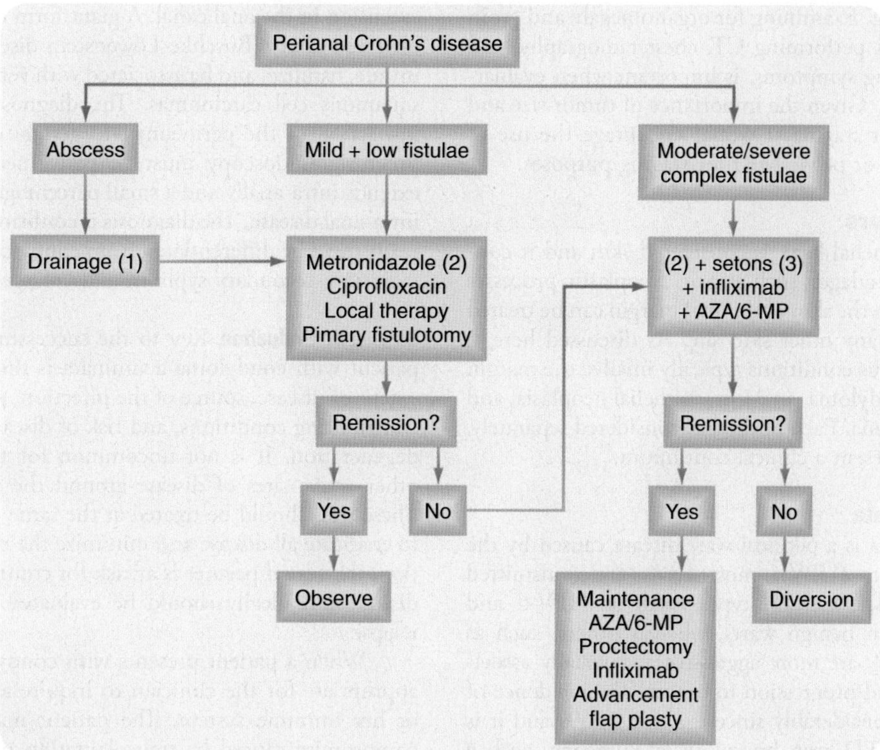


**FIGURE 53-25** Treatment algorithm for perianal fistulizing Crohn's disease. Primary abscesses require complete drainage. Fistulas are managed by a combination of surgical and medical therapy, with proctectomy and diversion reserved for severe and refractory cases. (From Rutgeerts P. Review article: Treatment of perianal fistulizing Crohn's disease. Aliment Pharmacol Ther 20:160–110, 2004.)

**BOX 53-3 Summary of Anal Tumors and Management**

**Anal Margin Tumors**

**Anal Intraepithelial Neoplasia**

Accurate lesion mapping
Focal excision or ablation
Imiquimod or 80% trichloroacetic acid
Close observation

**Bowen's Disease**

Accurate lesion mapping
Wide local excision for confluent disease, with flap repair as indicated
Exclude presence of locally invasive component or associated gynecologic malignancy

**Paget's Disease**

Accurate lesion mapping
Wide local excision with flap repair as indicated
Exclude underlying malignancy
APR and chemotherapy or radiation therapy if invasive adenocarcinoma present

**Basal Cell and Anal Margin Squamous Cell Carcinoma**

Local excision with clear margins
Radiation therapy for complex primary or recurrent lesions to avoid APR

**Verrucous Carcinoma**

Wide local excision; APR if extensive
Combined-modality therapy if transformation to squamous cell cancer has occurred

**Anal Canal Tumors**

**Epidermoid Cancer**

Local excision if favorable T1
Combined-modality, external beam radiation therapy plus 5-FU plus mitomycin
APR if incontinent or local treatment failure or recurrence after combined chemotherapy and radiation therapy
Triple-modality therapy in bulky T3 and T4 lesions (role of APR controversial)

**Adenocarcinoma**

APR with 5-FU and radiation therapy as indicated

**Melanoma**

APR or local excision to achieve an R0 resection

verge, or anorectal ring. Examining for organomegaly and groin adenopathy, as well as performing CT, chest radiography, and assessment of localizing symptoms, is important when evaluating a malignant lesion. Given the importance of tumor size and nodal involvement for staging, I would encourage the use of endorectal ultrasound or pelvic MRI for staging purposes.

## Anal Margin Tumors

The anal margin epithelial layer is considered skin and it contains typical skin appendages, such as hair. Neoplastic processes that exclusively involve the skin of the anal margin can be treated as for skin lesions at any other skin site. As discussed here, a number of precancerous conditions typically involve the margin and canal, such as condyloma, anal intraepithelial neoplasia, and squamous cell carcinoma. Each of these is considered separately, but they actually represent a clinical continuum.

### Condyloma Acuminata

Condyloma acuminata is a perineal wart disease caused by the human papillomavirus (HPV); most types are transmitted through sexual contact. Certain types, such as HPV-6 and HPV-11, are found in benign warts, whereas others, such as HPV-16 and HPV-18, are more aggressive and usually associated with dysplasia and progression to cancer. The incidence of HPV has increased considerably since the mid-1960s and it is the most common STD seen by colorectal surgeons, with a million new cases annually. Most patients with condyloma acuminata have a history of anal-receptive intercourse; the occurrence of anal HPV infection is strongly related to HIV-associated immunosuppression.

**Clinical Presentation** The usual symptoms include pruritus ani, bleeding, pain, discharge, and wetness. Examination reveals pinkish-white warts of varying sizes that may coalesce to form a mass, often foul-smelling (Fig. 53-26). Anoscopy may reveal extension in the anal canal. A giant form of the disease has been observed rarely (Buschke-Löwenstein disease). Such lesions can invade, fistulize, and be associated with verrucous carcinoma and squamous cell carcinomas. The diagnosis is based on direct inspection of the perineum and genital organs; anoscopy and proctosigmoidoscopy must be performed because the disease extends intra-anally and a small percentage of patients have only intra-anal disease. The diagnosis is confirmed histologically. Anal warts must be differentiated from condylomata molluscum contagiosum, secondary syphilis, and enlarged anal papillae.

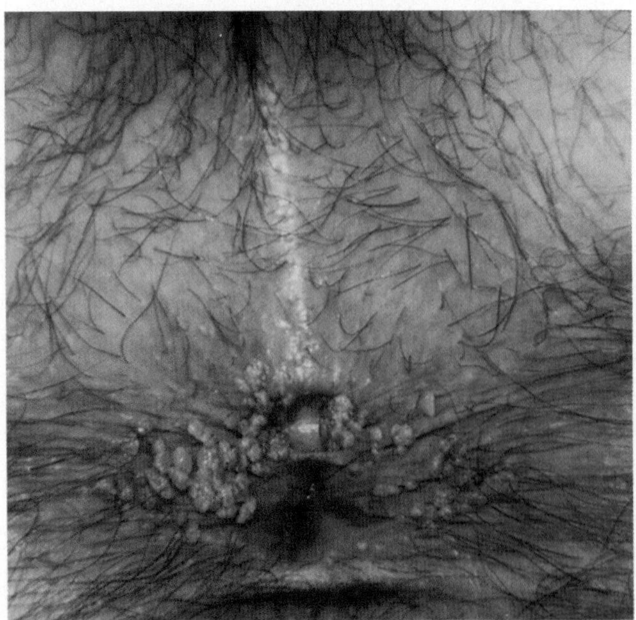

**FIGURE 53-26** Perianal condyloma acuminatum.

**Diagnostic Evaluation** Key to the successful management of the patient with condyloma acuminata is the establishment of the extent of disease, source of the infection, presence of underlying contributing conditions, and risk of disease for malignancy and degeneration. It is not uncommon for these patients to have other active sites of disease around the perineum or genitals. These sites should be treated at the same time as the anal warts to eradicate all disease and minimize the risk of relapse. In addition, the sexual partner is at risk for contracting or carrying the disease and ideally should be evaluated and treated to avoid relapse.

When a patient presents with condyloma acuminata, it is appropriate for the clinician to inquire about the status of his or her immune system. The patient may have immunologic compromise caused by transplantation medications, oncologic conditions and treatments, or HIV infection. This information can be important for the physician to understand contributing conditions and the risk for this being a premalignant condition. Although most condylomata are harmless benign lesions, some are indicative of more serious conditions such as anal intraepithelial neoplasia (AIN) or a more serious form of HPV infection. In the course of evaluating and treating a patient with condyloma acuminata, the patient should be asked about and tested for HIV, as appropriate, and tissue samples obtained for HPV and AIN evaluation. High-resolution anoscopy or colposcopy can help locate sites of high-risk lesions. The helpful algorithm shown in Figure 53-27 describes the incorporation of risk assessment into diagnostic and therapeutic strategies.[39]

**Treatment** Many treatments have been proposed and used, but none offers complete resolution of the disease process. Podophyllin, which is cytotoxic to condylomata but irritating to normal skin, must be applied to the warts. Its use should be limited to minimal disease and extra-anal warts and not repeated because of local complications and potential systemic toxicity. It requires no anesthesia and is inexpensive, but the results are often disappointing. Dichloroacetic acid (bichloracetic acid) can be used to destroy perianal and intra-anal warts, and is less irritating than podophyllin. The recurrence rate with both agents is much higher than with surgical excision. Early immunologic approaches to the treatment of perianal warts focused on the application of interferon injections. A more recent approach to immune therapy is the topical application of imiquimod, which creates an inflammatory response that eradicates the viral infection. The most common recommendation is for the topical application of imiquimod 5% cream three times weekly (6 to 10 hours) until visible inflammation is achieved.[40] This can be used as a primary treatment or as an adjunct after initial resection or ablation of condylomata and after HPV and AIN testing is complete.

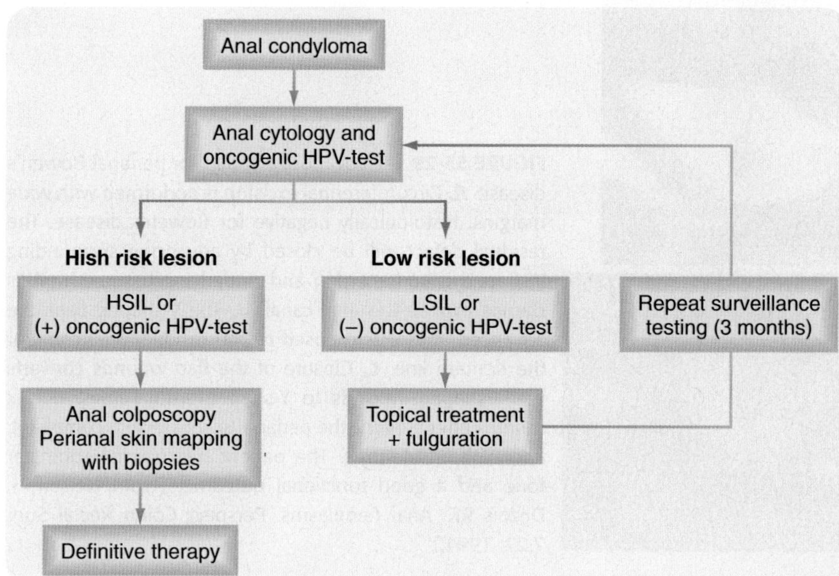


**FIGURE 53-27** Treatment algorithm for managing patients with anal condyloma. *HSIL,* high-grade squamous intraepithelial lesion; *LSIL,* low-grade intraepithelial lesion. (From Papaconsatntinou HT, Lee AJ, Simmang CL, et al. Screening methods for high-grade dysplasia in patients with anal condyloma. J Surg Res 127:8–13, 2005.)

Electrocauterization with a needle tip is effective and used extensively, often in combination with excision. Local, regional, or general anesthesia is necessary. Carbon dioxide laser can also be effective but is more expensive and offers no added benefits. With either technique, vapors should be aspirated. Excision with small scissors is preferred because it is precise, provides a tissue diagnosis, minimizes destruction of intervening skin, and can be used on larger lesions (Fig. 53-28). General or regional anesthesia is often necessary. No therapeutic option is completely satisfactory; they all are associated with a significant chance of recurrence. Combination of treatments may be valuable. Because recurrence is frequent, close follow-up of patients is recommended.

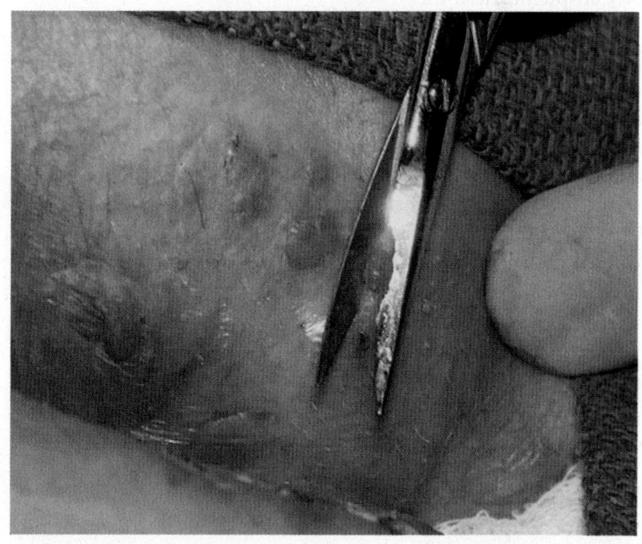

**FIGURE 53-28** Sharp excision of perianal condylomata is facilitated by raising the lesion by injecting a local anesthetic agent. (Courtesy Mayo Foundation for Medical Education and Research, Rochester, Minn.)

### Anal Intraepithelial Neoplasia

**Diagnostic Evaluation** A proper medical history, including a sexual history, should ascertain risks for exposure to or the known presence of HIV and HPV. Subtyping HPV will identify patients at high risk for cancer, including types 16, 18, 31, 33, 35, 39, 45, 51, and 52, and at low risk, types 6, 11, 42, 43, and 44.[41] Patients positive for HPV should be evaluated for other genital sites of viral involvement and should be considered for treatment with topical imidazoquinolones for perianal disease and in the future with antiviral vaccines. HIV patients should be treated and those with active disease followed closely. At least one long-term series of patients with immunosuppression has shown a heightened risk for the subsequent development of invasive anal squamous cell carcinoma during follow-up.[42]

**Treatment** In addition to diagnosing and treating underlying viral conditions, the neoplastic disease itself needs to be properly diagnosed with mapping and treated according to the extent and location of the disease. In situ lesions that are unifocal and visible can be managed with mapping and focal excision to achieve negative margins. The resulting defects can be of sufficient size to require wound closure with other than primary approximation; V-Y advancement flaps work well for most defects (Fig. 53-29). Multifocal disease can be mapped at multiple levels and in four quadrants. Perianal multifocal disease can be treated with imiquimod or 80% trichloroacetic acid. Multifocal anal canal disease is typically focally ablated. Imiquimod treatment has been associated with complete clinical and histologic clearance of AIN in some reports.[43] All cases are closely monitored for recurrence and for invasive disease. A management strategy for AIN observation proposed by Shepard considers the grade of AIN and immune status of the patient. Patients with AIN grade 1 or 2 and without immune compromise can be reviewed every 12 months in the absence of new or suspicious lesions. Patients with AIN grade 3 or with immunocompromise and AIN grade

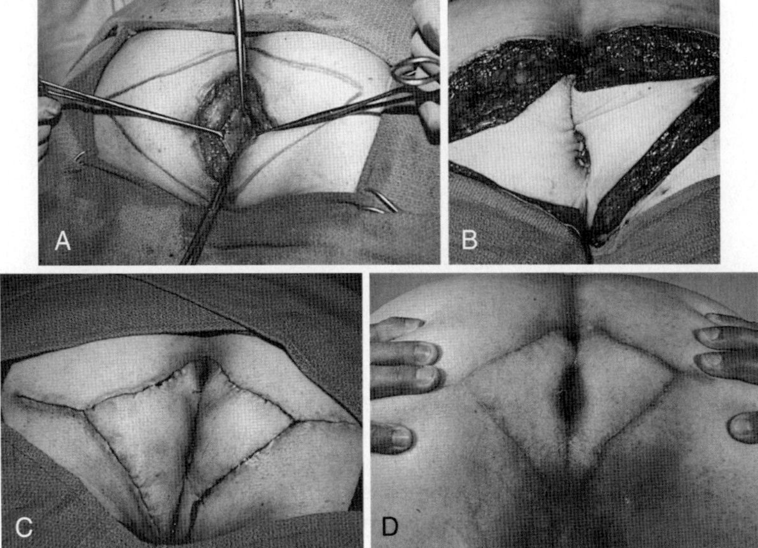


**FIGURE 53-29** V-Y advancement flap for perianal Bowen's disease. **A,** Circumferential excision is performed with wide margins, histologically negative for Bowen's disease. The residual defect will be closed by advancing surrounding V-shaped islands of skin and underlying tissue. The Allis clamps expose the anal canal. **B,** The V-shaped flaps are advanced and anastomosed to the residual anal canal at the dentate line. **C,** Closure of the flap wounds converts the V-shaped wounds to Y-shaped suture lines. **D,** Six months after surgery, the perianal scars are soft, compliant, and without stenosis. The patient has normal sphincter tone and a good functional outcome. (From Nelson H, Dozois RR: Anal neoplasms. Perspect Colon Rectal Surg 7:22, 1994.)

1 or 2 should be reviewed every 4 or 6 months and treated for any suspicious lesions.

### Bowen's Disease

The condition of anal squamous cell carcinoma in situ (Bowen's disease) was originally described by John T. Bowen in 1912 and redescribed as AIN in 1985.[44] The exact relationship between the two conditions has yet to be clarified; the histologies are the same and the clinical distinctions are challenging because these are rare conditions. From a historical perspective, Bowen's disease was described before the clinical recognition of HPV and before the outbreak of HIV; thus, the contribution of viral infections to the original Bowen's disease has not been established. Bowen's disease typically presented as a single confluent area of squamous cell carcinoma in situ managed with wide excision. AINIII has been more recently described in the setting of HIV and is diffuse, nonconfluent sites of dysplasia, not amenable to wide excision.

Patients with perianal Bowen's disease typically present with no symptoms or with minor complaints, such as burning or pruritus. Skin changes are variable (Fig. 53-30) and can show erythematous changes, thickening and fissuring, or brown-red plaques or even nodules. Such subtle physical findings can be difficult to differentiate from psoriasis, eczema, leukoplakia, and monilial infections. The description of AIN considers perianal and anal canal disease. It may be completely asymptomatic and detected during surgery for other conditions such as hemorrhoids, or as part of a screening program for high-risk individuals. Less important than the distinction of Bowen's and AIN are the points regarding diagnostic and therapeutic strategies that should be considered once the histology is confirmed. Confluent Bowen's disease is usually managed with wide local excision or, as more recently reported, with 16 weeks of topical 5-fluorouracil.[45]

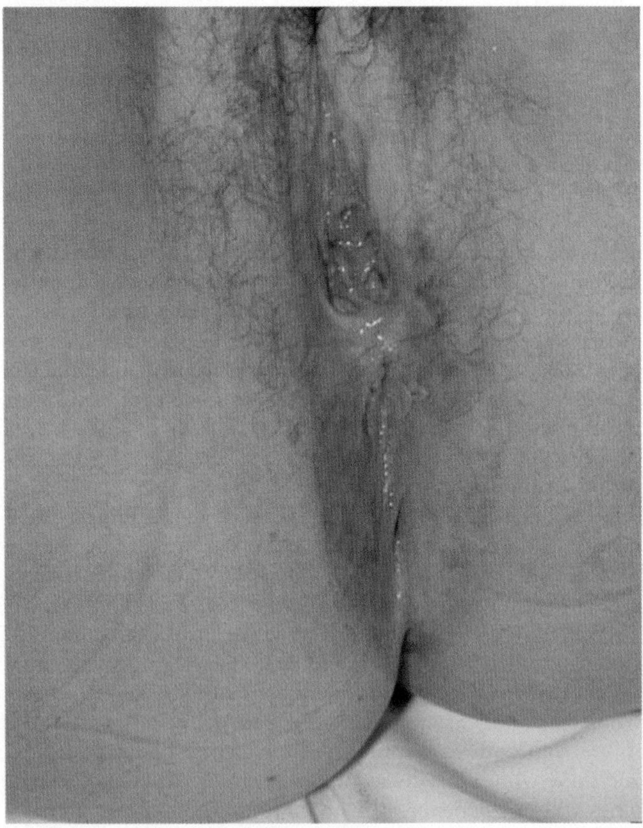

**FIGURE 53-30** Bowen's disease. (Courtesy Mayo Foundation for Medical Education and Research, Rochester, Minn.)

### Verrucous Carcinoma

Verrucous carcinoma, also referred to as giant condyloma acuminatum or Buschke-Löwenstein tumor, is poorly defined and best considered as an intermediate lesion, between condyloma acuminata and invasive squamous cell carcinomas, based on their common HPV cause.[45] The large wartlike lesions are soft and slow-growing. They may fistulize, become infected, and undergo malignant transformation.[46] Radical wide local excision or abdominal perineal resection (APR) is recommended. A poor prognosis can be expected for tumors progressing to invasive squamous cell carcinoma, although some may respond favorably to combined irradiation and chemotherapy.

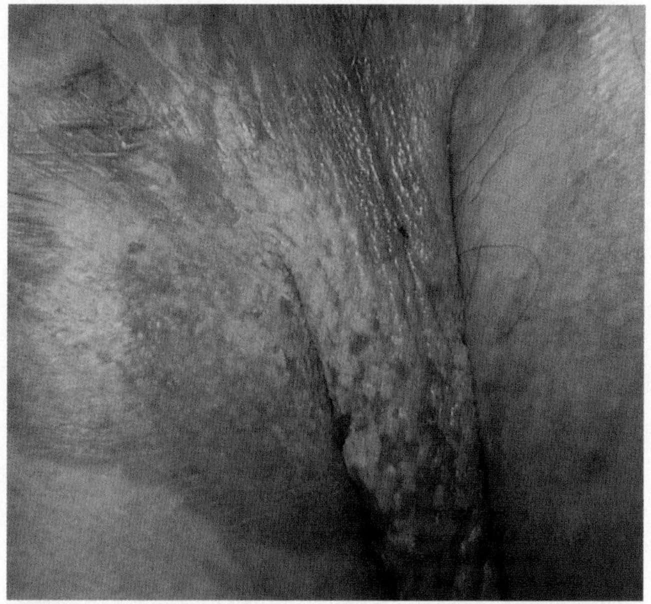

**FIGURE 53-31** Paget's disease. (Courtesy Mayo Foundation for Medical Education and Research, Rochester, Minn.)

### Squamous Cell Carcinoma

Although the oncologic behavior of squamous cell carcinoma resembles that of skin tumors elsewhere, the location of these lesions results in site-specific symptoms, such as a mass, chronic pruritus, bleeding, pain, and associated fistulas and condylomata.[46] Wide local excision is recommended for early anal margin squamous cell carcinoma, with excellent results. In one study, radiation therapy was applied in patients with anal margin tumors but 33% experienced long-term side effects.[47] Radiation is reserved for those who cannot be managed with local excision and/or those with recurrent disease wishing to avoid an abdominal perineal resection. Lymphadenectomy is indicated for those rare patients (<10%) presenting with evidence of regional lymph node metastases.

### Paget's Disease

Extramammary Paget's disease of the anus is a rare intraepithelial adenocarcinoma. The presence of intraepithelial adenocarcinoma in an area of squamous epithelium has led to speculation about the origin of Paget's cells. Various hypotheses have been proposed, including the possibility that they are derived from pluripotent epidermal stem cells, arise from apocrine or sweat glands, or are metastatic from underlying adenocarcinomas. Unlike Bowen's disease, Paget's disease is more common in older patients, is associated with an underlying carcinoma in 50% to 86% of patients, and has a poor prognosis.[46] The typical appearance of Paget's disease is that of well-demarcated eczematoid plaque, with whitish gray ulcerations or papillary lesions (Fig. 53-31). As is true for Bowen's disease, Paget's disease can have a variable and at times a subtle appearance and can be confused with other dermatologic conditions, such as hyperkeratosis, eczema, or lichen sclerosus et atrophicus. Histology demonstrates the presence of periodic acid–Schiff positive Paget cells, confirming the diagnosis.

Treatment is based on the local extent of the disease and presence or absence of underlying malignancies. More limited Paget's disease can be widely excised and the defect closed primarily or with V-Y advancement flaps. Biopsies of the proximal anal canal and distal anal skin margins can help map the extent of resection. Patients treated with repair of large perianal defects who have wide excision of Paget's disease experience acceptable functional results and quality of life similar to those for a normative population. An alternative to wide excision for patients without invasive cancer and who are poor operative candidates is a course of topical retinoic acid (0.025%), applied topically to the affected area until it generates discomfort and then applied every other day. Close observation is advised and biopsies for symptoms are recommended.[48] Patients with underlying rectal adenocarcinoma should undergo APR, whereas those with epidermoid anal canal cancer can be treated with combined radiation and chemotherapy. For patients with an invasive component, 5-year overall and disease-free survival rates of 59% and 64%, respectively, can be expected. Close follow-up is advised.

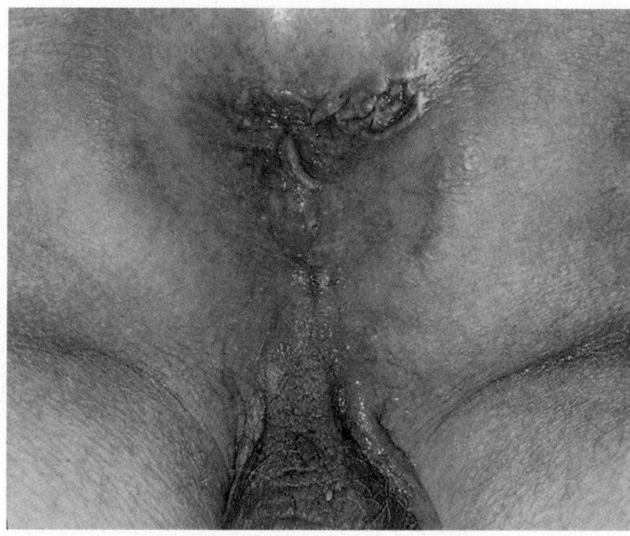

**FIGURE 53-32** Basal cell carcinoma of anal margin. (Courtesy Mayo Foundation for Medical Education and Research, Rochester, Minn.)

### Basal Cell Carcinoma

Basal cell carcinoma is a rare type of anal canal tumor. Macroscopically, these lesions have the same pearly borders, with central depression, as other basal cell cancers of the skin (Fig. 53-32). On occasion, it may be difficult to differentiate a cloacogenic (or basaloid) carcinoma arising in the transitional zone from a basal cell cancer arising in the anal skin. The distinction is crucial because of the dramatic behavioral difference and is based on location and histologic features.[45] Usually, these tumors can be treated adequately by wide local excision, reserving APR for extensive lesions.[46] Because almost one third of patients experience recurrence, close follow-up is indicated.

## Malignant Anal Canal Neoplasms

### Epidermoid Carcinoma

Tumors arising in the anal canal or in the transitional zone that have a squamous, basaloid, cloacogenic, or mucoepidermoid epithelium are similar in regard to clinical presentation, response to treatment, and prognosis[46] and are considered collectively. They typically present as a mass, sometimes with bleeding and pruritus (Fig. 53-33). At the time of diagnosis, almost 25% of these are superficial or in situ, half are smaller than 3 cm and the other half is larger. Approximately 71% have deep tumor penetration, 25% are node-positive, and 6% present with distant metastases.

AJCC staging for anal canal cancers is based on the depth and local infiltration of adjacent organs or structures (Fig. 53-34; Table 53-3).[38] The size of the primary tumor is considered the measure of its greatest dimension. A tumor that is 2 cm or smaller is designated T1, larger than 2 cm but not more than 5 cm is T2, and larger than 5 cm is T3. Any size tumor that invades a local structure is designated as T4.

In the past, treatment modalities included surgery alone or radiation therapy alone. Patients with tumors confined to epithelial or subepithelial tissue were treated by local excision and patients with more advanced lesions by APR. The introduction of multimodality therapy combining irradiation and chemotherapy promised to preserve continence, avoid colostomy, and offer similar survival advantage. In keeping with this concept, local excision alone remains an option for superficial, early-stage lesions, which have been associated with variable survivorship (61% to 87%; 100% in at least one study) if the lesion was smaller than 2 cm. Although some small superficial lesions can be treated with local excision, most patients are best treated with combined chemotherapy and irradiation.

Combined-modality therapy has evolved as the preferred alternative to radical surgery because, in theory, surgical mortality and morbidity are largely avoided, intestinal continuity is preserved, and survival compares favorably with that after surgery. Nigro and associates were the first to promote radiation therapy plus chemotherapy as definitive treatment for epidermoid anal canal malignancies. The current Nigro protocol includes external-beam radiation therapy to the pelvic tumor

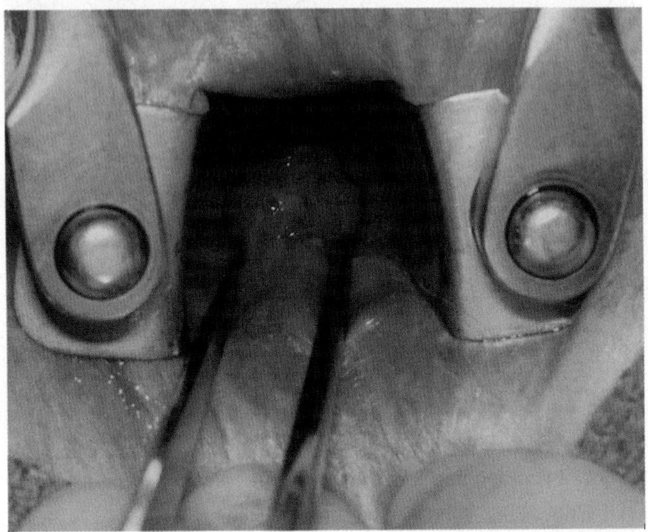

**FIGURE 53-33** Squamous cell carcinoma of anal canal. (Courtesy Mayo Foundation for Medical Education and Research, Rochester, Minn.)

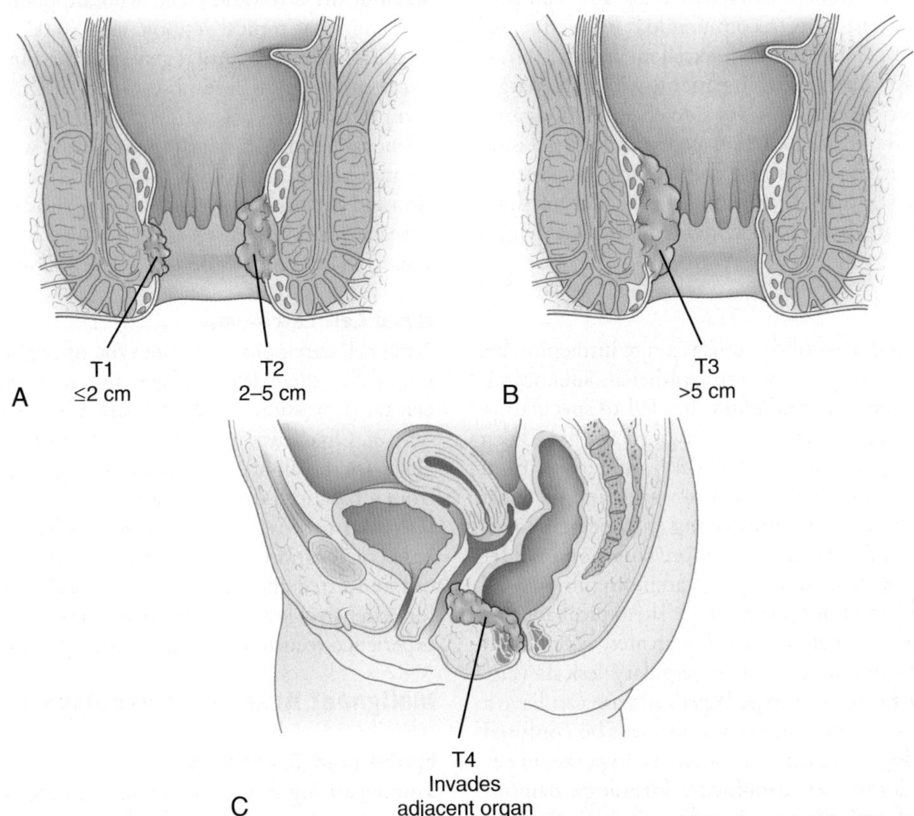


**FIGURE 53-34** Staging of primary tumors (T) of the anal canal. **A,** The greatest dimension of the T1 tumor is 2 cm or less and for T2 tumors is larger than 2 cm but not more than 5 cm. **B,** T3 tumors are larger than 5 cm. **C,** T4 tumors can be of any size. They invade adjacent organs or structures such as the vagina, urethra, or bladder.

**Table 53-3 TNM Staging Classifications for Anal Malignancies**

| | | | |
|---|---|---|---|
| **Primary Tumor (T)** | | | |
| Tx | Primary tumor cannot be assessed | | |
| T0 | No evidence of primary tumor | | |
| Tis | Carcinoma in situ (Bowen's disease, high-grade squamous intraepithelial lesion [HSIL], anal intraepithelial neoplasia II-III [AIN II-III]) | | |
| T1 | Tumor 2 cm or less in greatest dimension | | |
| T2 | Tumor more than 2 cm but not more than 5 cm in greatest dimension | | |
| T3 | Tumor more than 5 cm in greatest dimension | | |
| T4 | Tumor of any size that invades adjacent organ(s) (e.g., vagina, urethra, bladder*) | | |
| **Regional Lymph Nodes (N)** | | | |
| Nx | Regional lymph nodes cannot be assessed | | |
| N0 | No regional lymph node metastasis | | |
| N1 | Metastasis in perirectal lymph node(s) | | |
| N2 | Metastasis in unilateral internal iliac and/or inguinal lymph node(s) | | |
| N3 | Metastasis in perirectal and inguinal lymph nodes and/or bilateral internal iliac and/or inguinal lymph nodes | | |
| **Distant Metastasis (M)** | | | |
| M0 | No distant metastasis | | |
| M1 | Distant metastasis | | |
| **Stage Grouping** | | | |
| 0 | Tis | N0 | M0 |
| I | T1 | N0 | M0 |
| II | T2 | N0 | M0 |
| | T3 | N0 | M0 |
| IIIA | T1 | N1 | M0 |
| | T2 | N1 | M0 |
| | T3 | N1 | M0 |
| | T4 | N0 | M0 |
| IIIB | T4 | N1 | M0 |
| | Any T | N2 | M0 |
| | Any T | N3 | M0 |
| IV | Any T | Any N | M1 |

From Edge S, Byrd D, Compton C, et al (eds): AJCC cancer staging manual, ed 7, New York, 2010, Springer.

*Direct invasion of the rectal wall, perirectal skin, subcutaneous tissue, or the sphincter muscle(s) is not classified as T4.

and pelvic and inguinal nodes, to a total dose of 3000 cGy starting on day 1 using 15 fractions (200 cGy/day). Systemic chemotherapy includes 5-fluorouracil (5-FU), 1000 mg/m$^2$ for 24 hours as continuous infusion for 4 days, commencing on day 1 and again on day 28 (two cycles total). Mitomycin C is delivered as an IV bolus at 15 mg/m$^2$, starting on day 1 only. Many centers have modified the pelvic radiation doses, approximating the doses typically delivered in rectal cancer. Although some reports have described comparable results using radiation therapy alone, current studies support the continued use of 5-FU and mitomycin C. Although radiation plus chemotherapy has largely replaced the need for APR in anal canal cancers, there are still remain subsets of patients for whom APR may be considered appropriate as single-modality or combined-modality therapy. These groups would include patients who are already in need of a stoma for fecal incontinence, those for whom chemotherapy or radiation therapy is contraindicated, and those whose disease fails to resolve completely after radiation therapy plus chemotherapy. In patients treated with APR for persistent or locally recurrent disease, 5-year actuarial survival is reported at 57%.[49]

Despite high success rates with combination radiation and chemotherapy, some cases of locally advanced disease recur or fail to respond completely in the locoregional tumor bed. Whether patients with recurrent or persistent disease are treated with surgery or further radiation and chemotherapy hinges on their willingness and ability to undergo surgery. The standard treatment of surgical candidates is APR. From 50% to 57% of patients treated with salvage APR can expect a 5-year cure.[50] In contrast, only 27% of patients treated with salvage radiation and concurrent cisplatin-based chemotherapy can expect to be cured.

In those patients presenting with anal squamous cell carcinoma in the setting of HIV infection, standard treatments are not as well tolerated as for the general population. Historically, standard chemoradiation was associated with a 50% rate of severe acute hematologic toxicity. In the current era of HIV treatment, the consensus is that standard protocols for radiation and chemotherapy should be attempted, regardless of HIV status. In one study, 2-year survival rates for HIV-positive rates were the same as for HIV-negative patients, 77% and 75%, respectively.[51]

### Melanoma

Melanoma involving the anal canal is a rare tumor that can present as a mass, pain, or bleeding and/or can be amelanotic and identified during histopathologic examination of a hemorrhoidectomy specimen (Fig. 53-35). The overall outlook for patients with anal melanoma is poor with 5-year survival rates dependent on the extent of disease—32%, 17%, and 0%, for local, regional, and distant disease, respectively.[52] Although extent of disease correlates with long-term outcome, extent of surgery does not. Whether optimal results can be achieved with APR versus local excision remains an area of controversy. Nevertheless, achieving an R0 resection is key to achieving optimal 5-year survival rates, with 19% 5-year survival for R0 cases and 6% 5-year survival for cases with involved margins.

### Adenocarcinoma

True adenocarcinomas of the anal canal are thought to arise from the columnar epithelium of canal ducts, and are rare. For example, at a major cancer referral center, only 34 patients were diagnosed and treated with this condition over a 20-year period. Differentiating distal rectal cancer from true anal canal cancer may be difficult, but fortunately the treatment for both is the same. It is recommended that these patients be treated with multimodality therapy consisting of abdominal perineal excision, external beam radiation therapy, and chemotherapy. This approach is superior to local excision[53] and radiation therapy alone.

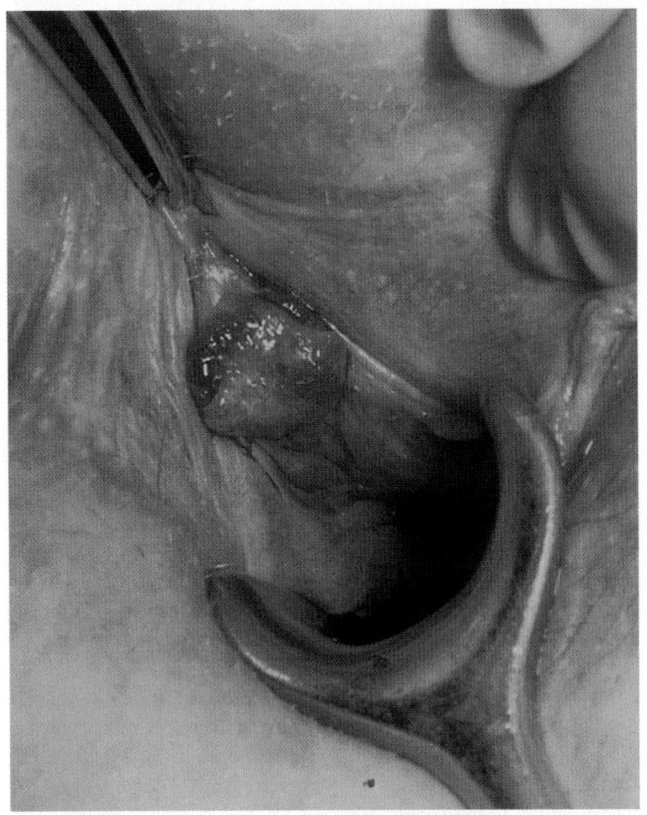

**FIGURE 53-35** Anal canal amelanotic melanoma. (Courtesy Mayo Foundation for Medical Education and Research, Rochester, Minn.)

## Other Tumors

Connective tissue sarcomas, such as leiomyosarcoma, rhabdomyosarcoma, and myoblastoma, are rare in the anal canal. Lymphoma of the anus is unusual. Carcinoid tumors can occasionally originate from anal canal endocrine cells and APR may be required, especially for those larger than 2 cm.

## SELECTED REFERENCES


Abbasakoor F, Boulos PB: Anal intraepithelial neoplasia. Br J Surg 92:277–290, 2005.

A comprehensive review of evolving diagnostic and treatment issues pertinent to anal intraepithelial neoplasia.

Billingham RP, Isler JT, Kimmins MH, et al: The diagnosis and management of common anorectal disorders. Curr Probl Surg 41:586–645, 2004.

An in-depth review of current diagnostic and therapeutic approaches to common conditions of the anus and distal rectum.

Czito BG, Willett CG: Current management of anal canal cancer. Curr Oncol Rep 11:186–192, 2009.

The multidisciplinary authorship of this publication uniquely offers an in-depth description of current practices in the management of anal cancer.

Hulme-Moir M, Bartolo DC: Hemorrhoids. Gastroenterol Clin North Am 30:183–197, 2001.

This article provides a well-referenced, comprehensive review of the classification, causes, anatomy, diagnosis, and treatment of hemorrhoids.

Nelson R: Nonsurgical therapy for anal fissure. Cochrane Database Syst Rev (4):CD003431, 2006.

An evidence-based review of best data on non-surgical approaches to chronic anal fissure.

Nelson R: Operative procedures for fissure in ano. Cochrane Database Syst Rev (2):CD002199, 2005.

An evidence-based review of the best data on five different surgical approaches to chronic anal fissure.

NIH state-of-the-science conference statement on prevention of fecal and urinary incontinence in adults. NIH Consens State Sci Statements 24:1–37, 2007.

Summary document from state-of-the-science conference conducted by the National Institutes of Health on the topic of fecal and urinary incontinence.

Parks AG, Gordon PH, Hardcastle JD: A classification of fistula-in-ano. Br J Surg 63:1–12, 1976.

A classic description of anorectal suppurative disease, this article includes the acute phase (abscesses) and chronic phase (fistulas). The anatomic descriptions, data, and classification schemes are still relevant today.

Ryan DP, Compton CC, Mayer RJ: Carcinoma of the anal canal. N Engl J Med 342:792–800, 2000.

A comprehensive review of the epidemiologic association, primary therapies, and expected outcomes for patients with carcinoma of the anal canal.


## REFERENCES


1. NIH state-of-the-science conference statement on prevention of fecal and urinary incontinence in adults. NIH Consens State Sci Statements 24:1–37, 2007.
2. Sagar PM, Pemberton JH: Anorectal and pelvic floor function. Relevance of continence, incontinence, and constipation. Gastroenterol Clin North Am 25:163–182, 1996.
3. Whitehead WE, Bharucha AE: Diagnosis and treatment of pelvic floor disorders: What's new and what to do. Gastroenterology 138:1231–1235, 2010.
4. Whitehead WE, Wald A, Norton NJ: Treatment options for fecal incontinence. Dis Colon Rectum 44:131–142, 2001.
5. Rudolph W, Galandiuk S: A practical guide to the diagnosis and management of fecal incontinence. Mayo Clin Proc 77:271–275, 2002.
6. Bischoff A, Levitt MA, Bauer C, et al: Treatment of fecal incontinence with a comprehensive bowel management program. J Pediatr Surg 44:1278–1283, 2009.

7. Galandiuk S, Roth LA, Greene QJ: Anal incontinence-sphincter ani repair: Indications, techniques, outcome. Langenbecks Arch Surg 394:425–433, 2009.
8. Kimmins MH, Evetts BK, Isler J, et al: The Altemeier repair: Outpatient treatment of rectal prolapse. Dis Colon Rectum 44:565–570, 2001.
9. Lechaux JP, Lechaux D, Perez M: Results of Delorme's procedure for rectal prolapse. Advantages of a modified technique. Dis Colon Rectum 38:301–307, 1995.
10. Bachoo P, Brazzelli M, Grant A: Surgery for complete rectal prolapse in adults. Cochrane Database Syst Rev (2):CD001758, 2000.
11. Goh JT, Tjandra JJ, Carey MP: How could management of rectoceles be optimized? ANZ J Surg 72:896–901, 2002.
12. Mimura T, Roy AJ, Storrie JB, et al: Treatment of impaired defecation associated with rectocele by behavorial retraining (biofeedback). Dis Colon Rectum 43:1267–1272, 2000.
13. Van Laarhoven CJ, Kamm MA, Bartram CI, et al: Relationship between anatomic and symptomatic long-term results after rectocele repair for impaired defecation. Dis Colon Rectum 42:204–210, 1999.
14. Bayer I, Myslovaty B, Picovsky BM: Rubber band ligation of hemorrhoids. Convenient and economic treatment. J Clin Gastroenterol 23:50–52, 1996.
15. Khan S, Pawlak SE, Eggenberger JC, et al: Surgical treatment of hemorrhoids: Prospective, randomized trial comparing closed excisional hemorrhoidectomy and the Harmonic Scalpel technique of excisional hemorrhoidectomy. Dis Colon Rectum 44:845–849, 2001.
16. Shao WJ, Li GC, Zhang ZH, et al: Systematic review and meta-analysis of randomized controlled trials comparing stapled haemorrhoidopexy with conventional haemorrhoidectomy. Br J Surg 95:147–160, 2008.
17. Nelson R: Operative procedures for fissure in ano. Cochrane Database Syst Rev (2):CD002199, 2005.
18. Nelson R: Nonsurgical therapy for anal fissure. Cochrane Database Syst Rev (4):CD003431, 2006.
19. Elsebae MM: A study of fecal incontinence in patients with chronic anal fissure: Prospective, randomized, controlled trial of the extent of internal anal sphincter division during lateral sphincterotomy. World J Surg 31:2052–2057, 2007.
20. Whiteford MH, Kilkenny J, 3rd, Hyman N, et al: Practice parameters for the treatment of perianal abscess and fistula-in-ano (revised). Dis Colon Rectum 48:1337–1342, 2005.
21. Henrichsen S, Christiansen J: Incidence of fistula-in-ano complicating anorectal sepsis: A prospective study. Br J Surg 73:371–372, 1986.
22. Parks AG, Gordon PH, Hardcastle JD: A classification of fistula-in-ano. Br J Surg 63:1–12, 1976.
23. Johnson EK, Gaw JU, Armstrong DN: Efficacy of anal fistula plug vs. fibrin glue in closure of anorectal fistulas. Dis Colon Rectum 49:371–376, 2006.
24. Petersen S, Wietelmann K, Evers T, et al: Long-term effects of postoperative razor epilation in pilonidal sinus disease. Dis Colon Rectum 52:131–134, 2009.
25. Lukish JR, Kindelan T, Marmon LM, et al: Laser epilation is a safe and effective therapy for teenagers with pilonidal disease. J Pediatr Surg 44:282–285, 2009.
26. Conroy FJ, Kandamany N, Mahaffey PJ: Laser depilation and hygiene: Preventing recurrent pilonidal sinus disease. J Plast Reconstr Aesthet Surg 61:1069–1072, 2008.
27. Nursal TZ, Ezer A, Caliskan K, et al: Prospective randomized controlled trial comparing V-Y advancement flap with primary suture methods in pilonidal disease. Am J Surg 199:170–177, 2010.
28. Tocchi A, Mazzoni G, Bononi M, et al: Outcome of chronic pilonidal disease treatment after ambulatory plain midline excision and primary suture. Am J Surg 196:28–33, 2008.
29. Saclarides TJ: Rectovaginal fistula. Surg Clin North Am 82:1261–1272, 2002.
30. El-Attar SM, Evans DV: Anal warts, sexually transmitted diseases, and anorectal conditions associated with human immunodeficiency virus. Prim Care 26:81–100, 1999.
31. Barrett WL, Callahan TD, Orkin BA: Perianal manifestations of human immunodeficiency virus infection: Experience with 260 patients. Dis Colon Rectum 41:606–611, 1998.
32. Nadal SR, Manzione CR, Galvao VM, et al: Perianal diseases in HIV-positive patients compared with a seronegative population. Dis Colon Rectum 42:649–654, 1999.
33. Place RJ, Gregorcyk SG, Huber PJ, et al: Outcome analysis of HIV-positive patients with anal squamous cell carcinoma. Dis Colon Rectum 44:506–512, 2001.
34. Culp CE: Chronic hidradenitis suppurativa of the anal canal. A surgical skin disease. Dis Colon Rectum 26:669–676, 1983.
35. Poupardin C, Lemann M, Gendre JP, et al: Efficacy of infliximab in Crohn's disease. Results of a retrospective multicenter study with a 15-month follow-up. Gastroenterol Clin Biol 30:247–252, 2006.
36. Schwartz DA, Pemberton JH, Sandborn WJ: Diagnosis and treatment of perianal fistulas in Crohn disease. Ann Intern Med 135:906–918, 2001.
37. Rutgeerts P: Review article: Treatment of perianal fistulizing Crohn's disease. Aliment Pharmacol Ther 20 (Suppl 4):106–110, 2004.
38. American Joint Committee on Cancer: AJCC cancer staging manual, ed 7, New York, 2010, Springer.
39. Papaconstantinou HT, Lee AJ, Simmang CL, et al: Screening methods for high-grade dysplasia in patients with anal condyloma. J Surg Res 127:8–13, 2005.
40. Schofer H: Evaluation of imiquimod for the therapy of external genital and anal warts in comparison with destructive therapies. Br J Dermatol 157 (2):52–55, 2007.
41. Chang GJ, Berry JM, Jay N, et al: Surgical treatment of high-grade anal squamous intraepithelial lesions: A prospective study. Dis Colon Rectum 45:453–458, 2002.
42. Scholefield JH, Castle MT, Watson NF: Malignant transformation of high-grade anal intraepithelial neoplasia. Br J Surg 92: 1133–1136, 2005.
43. Palefsky J: Human papillomavirus-related disease in people with HIV. Curr Opin HIV AIDS 4:52–56, 2009.
44. McCance DJ, Clarkson PK, Dyson JL, et al: Human papillomavirus types 6 and 16 in multifocal intraepithelial neoplasias of the female lower genital tract. Br J Obstet Gynaecol 92:1093–1100, 1985.
45. Graham BD, Jetmore AB, Foote JE, et al: Topical 5-fluorouracil in the management of extensive anal Bowen's disease: a preferred approach. Dis Colon Rectum 48:444–450, 2005.
46. Nelson H, Dozois RR: Anal neoplasms. Perspect Colon Rectal Surg 7:16–36, 1994.
47. Khanfir K, Ozsahin M, Bieri S, et al: Patterns of failure and outcome in patients with carcinoma of the anal margin. Ann Surg Oncol 15:1092–1098, 2008.

48. McCarter MD, Quan SH, Busam K, et al: Long-term outcome of perianal Paget's disease. Dis Colon Rectum 46:612–616, 2003.
49. Mariani P, Ghanneme A, De la Rochefordiere A, et al: Abdominoperineal resection for anal cancer. Dis Colon Rectum 51:1495–1501, 2008.
50. Pocard M, Tiret E, Nugent K, et al: Results of salvage abdominoperineal resection for anal cancer after radiotherapy. Dis Colon Rectum 41:1488–1493, 1998.
51. Gervaz P, Buchs N, Morel P: Diagnosis and management of anal cancer. Curr Gastroenterol Rep 10:502–506, 2008.
52. Podnos YD, Tsai NC, Smith D, et al: Factors affecting survival in patients with anal melanoma. Am Surg 72:917–920, 2006.
53. Chang GJ, Gonzalez RJ, Skibber JM, et al: A twenty-year experience with adenocarcinoma of the anal canal. Dis Colon Rectum 52:1375–1380, 2009.

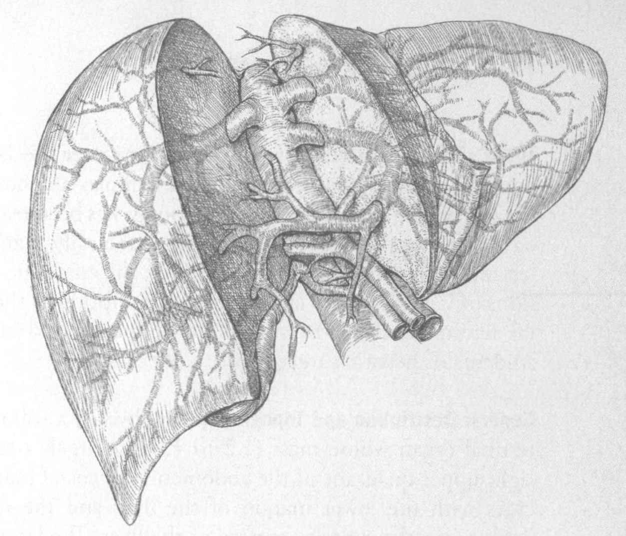

CHAPTER 54

# THE LIVER

Jason K. Sicklick, Michael D'Angelica, and Yuman Fong



## HISTORICAL PERSPECTIVE

The surface anatomy of the liver was described as early as 2000 years BC by the ancient Babylonians. Even Hippocrates understood and described the seriousness of liver injury. In 1654, Francis Glisson was the first physician to describe the essential anatomy of the blood vessels of the liver accurately. The beginnings of liver surgery are described as rudimentary excisions of eviscerated liver from penetrating trauma. The first documented case of a partial hepatectomy is credited to Berta, who amputated a portion of protruding liver in a patient with a self-inflicted stab wound in 1716.

In the late 1800s, the first gastrectomies and cholecystectomies were being performed in Europe. At that time, surgery on the liver was regarded as dangerous, if not impossible. In 1897, Elliot, in his report on liver surgery for trauma, said that the liver was so "friable, so full of gaping vessels and so evidently incapable of being sutured that it had always seemed impossible to successfully manage large wounds of its substance." European surgeons began to experiment with techniques of elective liver surgery on animals in the late 1800s. The credit for the first elective liver resection is a matter of debate and many surgeons have been given credit, but it certainly occurred during this time period.

The early 1900s saw some small but significant advances in liver surgery. Techniques for suturing major hepatic vessels and the use of cautery for small vessels were applied and reported. The most significant advance of that time was probably that of J. Hogarth Pringle. In 1908, he described digital compression of the hilar vessels to control hepatic bleeding from traumatic injuries. The modern era of hepatic surgery was ushered in by the development of a better understanding of liver anatomy and formal anatomic liver resection. Credit for the first anatomic liver resection is usually given to Lortat-Jacob, who performed a right hepatectomy in 1952 in France. Pack from New York and Quattelbaum from Georgia performed similar operations within the next year and were unlikely to have had any knowledge of Lortat-Jacob's report. Descriptions of the segmental nature of liver anatomy by Couinaud, Woodsmith, and Goldburne in 1957 opened the door even wider and introduced the modern era of liver surgery.

Despite these improvements, hepatic surgery was plagued by tremendous operative morbidity and mortality from the 1950s into the 1980s. Operative mortality rates in excess of 20% were common and usually related to massive hemorrhage. Many surgeons were reluctant to perform hepatic surgery because of these results and, understandably, many physicians were reluctant to refer patients for hepatectomy. With the courage of patients and their families, as well as the persistence of surgeons, safe hepatic surgery has now been realized. A complete list is not possible here, but courageous hepatic surgeons such as Blumgart, Bismuth, Longmire, Fortner, Schwartz, Starzl, and Ton deserve mention.

Advances in anesthesia, intensive care, antibiotics, and interventional radiologic techniques have also contributed tremendously to the safety of major hepatic surgery. Total hepatectomy with liver transplantation and live donor partial hepatectomy for transplantation are now performed routinely in specialized transplantation centers. Partial hepatectomy for a large number of indications is now performed throughout the world in specialized centers, with mortality rates of 5% or less. Partial hepatectomy performed on normal livers is now consistently performed, with mortality rates of 1% to 2%.

Safely performed open hepatic surgery and its liberal use in the management of a wide variety of diseases is now a reality. Moreover, minimally invasive approaches to liver surgery have been developed and are now being used in significant numbers. However, the learning curve remains steep and the indications for this technique are still being carefully defined. Thermal ablative techniques to treat hepatic tumors, including radiofrequency and microwave ablation, have exploded in popularity. Finally, techniques to improve the safety of liver resection further, such as portal vein embolization to induce preoperative hypertrophy of the future liver remnant (FLR), have been developed and are now being used.

## ANATOMY AND PHYSIOLOGY

### Anatomy

#### Gross Anatomy

A precise knowledge of the anatomy of the liver is an absolute prerequisite to performing surgery on the liver or biliary tree.

With the development of hepatic surgery over the last several decades, a greater appreciation for the complex anatomy beyond the misleading minimal external markings has been realized. The days of using the falciform ligament as the only marker of the left and right sides of the liver are over; the anatomic contributions of Couinaud (see later) and the description of the segmental nature of the liver should be embraced and studied by students of hepatic surgery.

**General Description and Topography** The liver is a solid gastrointestinal organ whose mass (1.2 to 1.6 kg) largely occupies the right upper quadrant of the abdomen. The costal margin coincides with the lower margin of the liver and the diaphragm drapes over the superior surface of the liver. The large majority of the right liver and most of the left liver is covered by the thoracic cage. The liver extends superiorly to the height of the fifth rib on the right and the sixth rib on the left. The posterior surface straddles the inferior vena cava (IVC). A wedge of liver extends to the left side of the abdomen. It crosses the epigastrium to lie above the anterior surface of the stomach and below the central and left portions of the diaphragm. The superior surface of the liver is convex and is molded to the diaphragm, whereas the inferior surface is mildly concave and extends to a sharp anterior border.

The liver is invested in peritoneum except for the gallbladder fossa, porta hepatis, and posterior aspect of the liver on either side of the IVC in two wedge-shaped areas. The region of liver to the right of the IVC is called the *bare area* of the liver.

The peritoneal duplications on the liver surface are referred to as ligaments. The diaphragmatic peritoneal duplications are referred to as the coronary ligaments whose lateral margins on either side are the right and left triangular ligaments. From the center of the coronary ligament emerges the falciform ligament, which extends anteriorly as a thin membrane connecting the liver surface to the diaphragm, abdominal wall, and umbilicus.

The ligamentum teres (the obliterated umbilical vein) runs along the inferior edge of the falciform ligament from the umbilicus to the umbilical fissure. The umbilical fissure is on the inferior surface of the left liver and contains the left portal pedicle. In early descriptions of hepatic anatomy, the falciform ligament, the most obvious surface marker of the liver, was used as the division of the right and left lobes of the liver. However, this description is inaccurate and of minimal usefulness to the hepatobiliary surgeon (see later for detailed segmental anatomy).

On the posterior surface of the left liver, running from the left portal vein in the porta hepatis toward the left hepatic vein and the IVC, is the ligamentum venosum (obliterated sinus venosus) which also runs in a fissure (Fig. 54-1). Hepatic arterial and portal venous blood enter the liver at the hilum and branch throughout the liver as a single portal pedicle unit, which also includes a bile duct. These portal triads are invested in a peritoneal sheath that invaginates at the hepatic hilum. Venous drainage is through the right, middle, and left hepatic veins that empty directly into the suprahepatic IVC.

**Normal Development and Embryology** The developing liver shares a common progenitor with the biliary tree and pancreas. During embryogenesis, signals are transmitted from the cardiac mesenchyme and septum transversum. The molecules regulating this (e.g., FGF, BMP, Wnt) have begun to be elucidated. The liver primordium begins to form in the third week of development as an outgrowth of endodermal epithelium, known as the *hepatic diverticulum* or liver bud, known as the *hepatic field*. The connection between the hepatic diverticulum and the future duodenum narrows to form the bile duct and an outpouching of the bile duct forms into the gallbladder and cystic duct. Hepatic

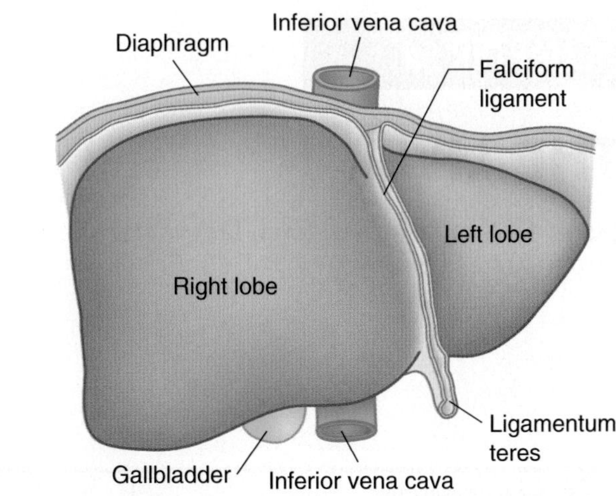


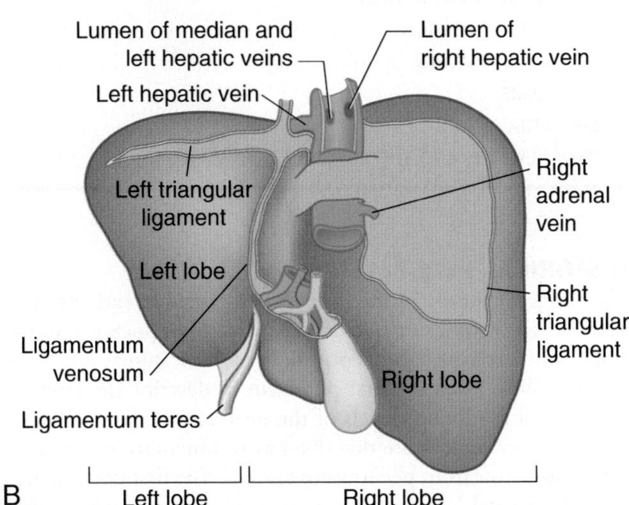


**FIGURE 54-1 A,** Historically, the liver was divided into right and left lobes by the external marking of the falciform ligament. On the inferior surface of the falciform ligament, the ligamentum teres can be seen entering the umbilical fissure. **B,** The posterior and inferior surface of the liver is shown. The liver embraces the IVC posteriorly in a groove. The lumens of the three major hepatic veins and right adrenal vein can be seen directly entering the IVC. The bare area, bounded by the right and left triangular ligaments, is illustrated. To the left of the IVC is the caudate lobe, which is bounded on its left side by a fissure containing the ligamentum venosum. The lesser omentum terminates along the edge of the ligamentum venosum and thus the caudate lobe lies within the lesser sac and the rest of the liver lies in the supracolic compartment. A layer of fibrous tissue can be seen bridging the right lobe to the caudate lobe posterior to the IVC, thus encircling it. This ligament of tissue must be divided on the right side when mobilizing the right liver off the IVC. (From Blumgart LH, Hann LE: Surgical and radiologic anatomy of the liver and biliary tract. In Blumgart LH, Fong Y [eds]: Surgery of the liver and biliary tract, London, 2000, WB Saunders, pp 3–34.)

cells develop cords and intermingle with the vitelline and umbilical veins to form hepatic sinusoids. Simultaneously, hematopoietic cells, Kupffer cells and connective tissue form from the mesoderm of the septum transversum. The mesoderm of the septum transversum connects the liver to the ventral abdominal wall and foregut. As the liver protrudes into the abdominal cavity, these structures are stretched into thin membranes, ultimately forming the falciform ligament and lesser omentum, respectively. The mesoderm on the surface of the developing liver differentiates into visceral peritoneum, except superiorly, where contact between the liver and mesoderm (future diaphragm) is maintained, forming a bare area devoid of visceral peritoneum (Fig. 54-2).

The primitive liver plays a central role in the fetal circulation. The vitelline veins carry blood from the yolk sac to the sinus venosus and ultimately form a network of veins around the foregut (future duodenum) that drain into the developing hepatic sinusoids. These vitelline veins eventually fuse to form the portal, superior mesenteric, and splenic veins. The sinus venosus, which empties into the fetal heart, becomes the hepatocardiac channel and then the hepatic veins and retrohepatic IVC. The umbilical veins, which are paired early on, carry oxygenated blood to the fetus. Initially, the umbilical veins drain into the sinus venosus but at week 5 of development, they begin to drain into the hepatic sinusoids. The right umbilical vein ultimately disappears and the left umbilical vein later drains directly into the hepatocardiac channel, bypassing the hepatic sinusoids through the ductus venosus. In the adult liver, the remnant of the left umbilical vein becomes the ligamentum teres, which runs in the falciform ligament into the umbilical fissure, and the remnant of the ductus venosus becomes the ligamentum venosus at the termination of the lesser omentum under the left liver (Fig. 54-3).

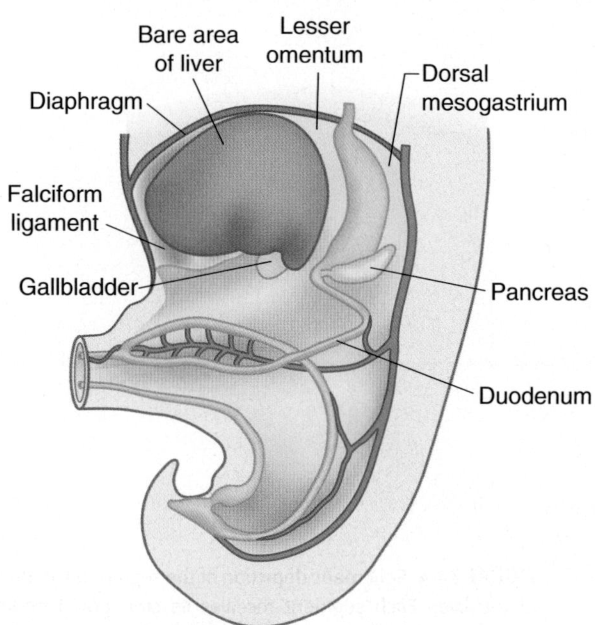


**FIGURE 54-2** An approximately 36-day-old embryo is shown. The extensions of the septum transversum can be seen developing as the liver protrudes into the abdominal cavity, stretching out and forming the lesser omentum and the falciform ligament. The liver is completely invested in visceral peritoneum, except for a portion next to the diaphragm known as the *bare area*. (From Sadler TW: Langman's medical embryology, ed 5, Baltimore, 1985, William & Wilkins.)

The fetal liver plays a very important role in hematopoiesis. In week 10 of gestation, the liver comprises 10% of the fetal body weight because of developing hepatic sinusoids and active hematopoiesis. During the last 2 months of intrauterine life, hepatic hematopoiesis decreases and the weight of the liver is decreased to 5% of the fetal body weight.

By week 12 of gestation, bile is formed in hepatocytes and secreted into the bile ductules of each hepatic lobule. Simultaneously, bile duct epithelial cells (cholangiocytes) develop along intrahepatic and extrahepatic bile ducts while the gallbladder completes its development. Together, this allows for the drainage of bile into the foregut.

The adult liver is a complex system of numerous cell types, including hepatocytes, cholangiocytes, neuroendocrine cells, hepatic progenitors (known as *oval cells*), myofibroblastic mesenchymal cells (known as *hepatic stellate cells* and portal myofibroblasts), resident macrophages (known as *Kupffer cells*), and vascular endothelial cells.

### Functional Anatomy

Historically, the liver was divided into left and right lobes by the obvious external landmark of the falciform ligament. Not only was this description oversimplified, but it was anatomically incorrect in relation to the blood supply to the liver. Later, a more accurate understanding of the lobar anatomy of the liver was developed. The liver is divided into right and left lobes determined by portal and hepatic vein branches.

Our understanding of functional liver anatomy has become more sophisticated. Briefly, a plane without any surface markings, known as the *portal fissure* or Cantlie's line, runs from the gallbladder to the left side of the IVC. This divides the liver into right and left lobes. The right lobe is further divided into anterior and posterior sectors. The left lobe is divided into a medial sector, also known as the *quadrate lobe*, that lies to the right of the falciform ligament and umbilical fissure and a lateral sector, also known as the *left lateral segment*, which lies to the left of these structures. This system, although anatomically more correct, is only sufficient for mobilization of the liver and simple hepatic resections. It does not describe the more intricate and functional segmental anatomy that is essential to understand before pursuing complex hepatobiliary surgery.

The functional anatomy of the liver (Figs. 54-4 and 54-5) is composed of eight segments, each supplied by a single portal triad (also called a *pedicle*) composed of a portal vein, hepatic artery, and bile duct. These segments are further organized into four sectors separated by scissurae containing the three main hepatic veins. The four sectors are even further organized into the right and left liver. The terms *right* liver and *left liver* are preferable to the terms *right lobe* and *left lobe* because there is no external mark that allows the identification of the right and left liver. This system was originally described in 1957 by Woodsmith and Goldburne, and by Couinaud. It defines hepatic anatomy because it is most relevant to surgery of the liver. The functional anatomy is more often seen as cross-sectional imaging (Fig. 54-6).

The main scissura contains the middle hepatic vein, which runs in an anteroposterior direction from the gallbladder fossa to the left side of the vena cava. It divides the liver into right and left hemilivers. The line of the main scissura is also known

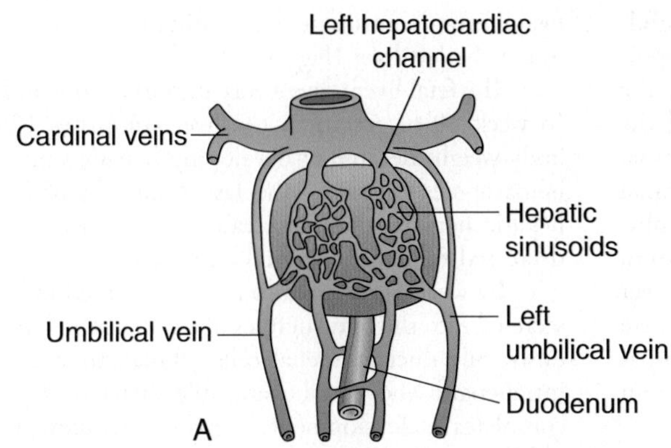


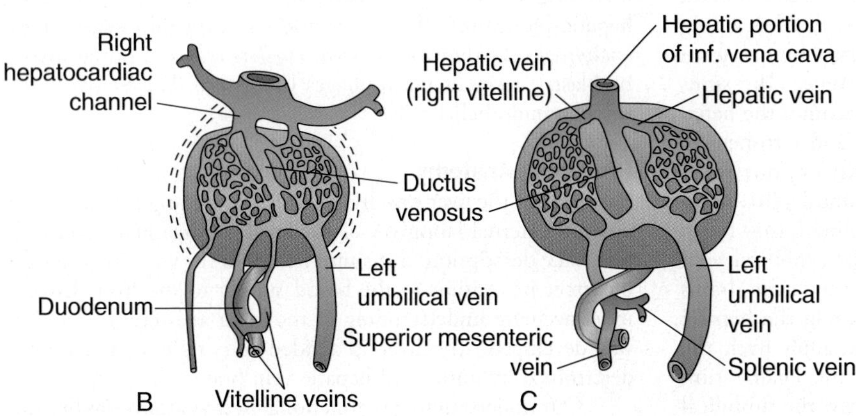


**FIGURE 54-3 A,** Umbilical and vitelline vein development of a 5-week-old embryo. The hepatic sinusoids have developed and, although there are channels that bypass these sinusoids, the vitelline and umbilical veins are beginning to drain into them. **B,** In the second month, the vitelline veins drain directly into the hepatic sinusoids. The ductus venosus has formed and accepts oxygenated blood from the left umbilical vein, bypasses the hepatic sinusoids, and directly enters the hepatocardiac channel. **C,** By the third month, the vitelline veins have formed into the portal system (splenic, superior mesenteric, and portal veins). The right umbilical vein has disappeared and the left umbilical vein (future ligamentum teres) drains into the sinus venosus, bypassing the hepatic sinusoids. Note the development of the IVC and hepatic veins. (From Sadler TW: Langman's medical embryology, ed 5, Baltimore, 1985, William & Wilkins.)

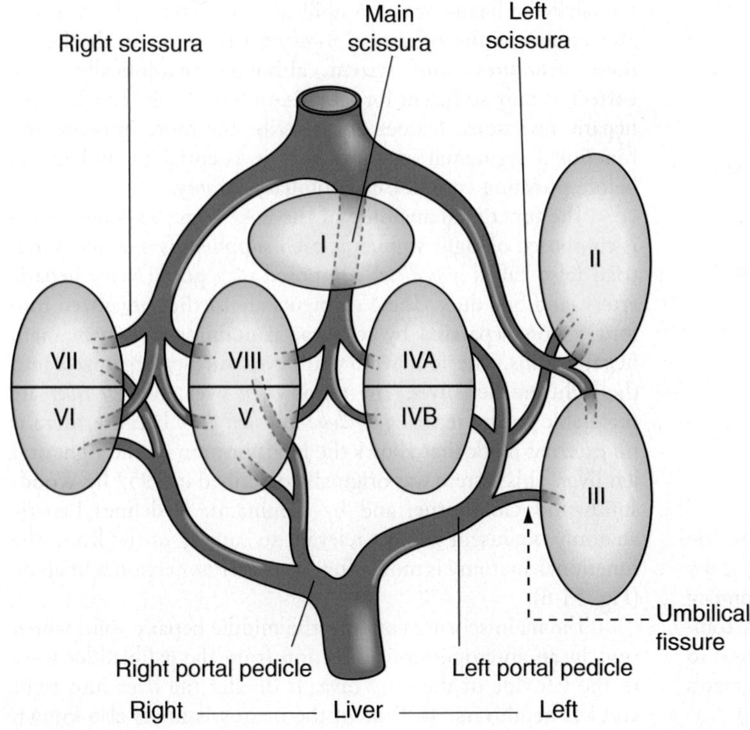


**FIGURE 54-4** Schematic depiction of the segmental anatomy of the liver. Each segment receives its own portal pedicle (triad of portal vein, hepatic artery, and bile duct). The eight segments are illustrated, and the four sectors, divided by the three main hepatic veins running in scissurae, are shown. The umbilical fissure (not a scissura) is shown to contain the left portal pedicle. (From Blumgart LH, Hann LE: Surgical and radiologic anatomy of the liver and biliary tract. In Blumgart LH, Fong Y [eds]: Surgery of the liver and biliary tract, London, 2000, WB Saunders, pp 3–34.)

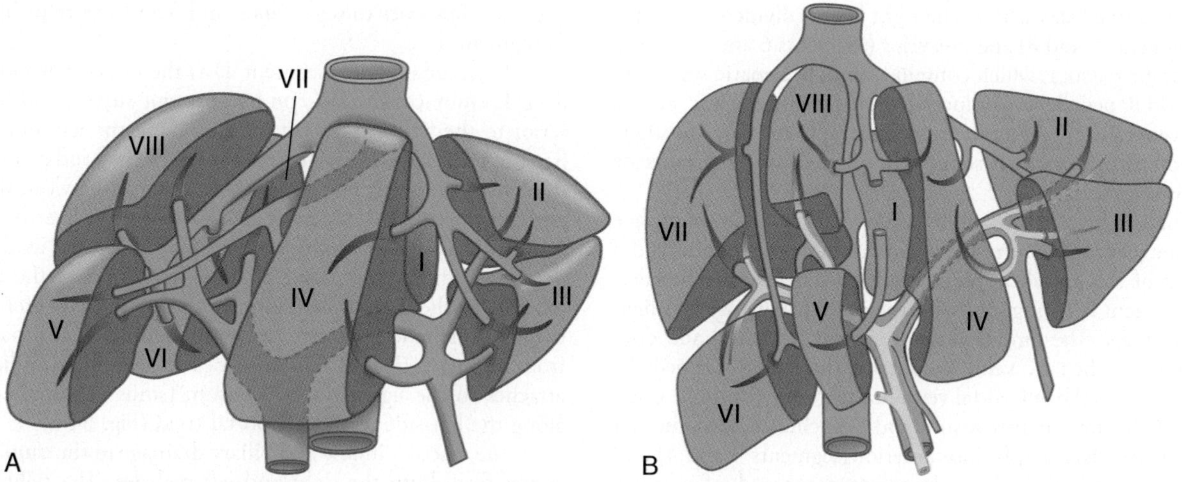


**FIGURE 54-5** Segmental anatomy of the liver. **A,** As seen at laparotomy in the anatomic position. **B,** In the ex vivo position. (From Blumgart LH, Hann LE: Surgical and radiologic anatomy of the liver and biliary tract. In Blumgart LH, Fong Y [eds]: Surgery of the liver and biliary tract, London, 2000, WB Saunders, pp 3–34.)

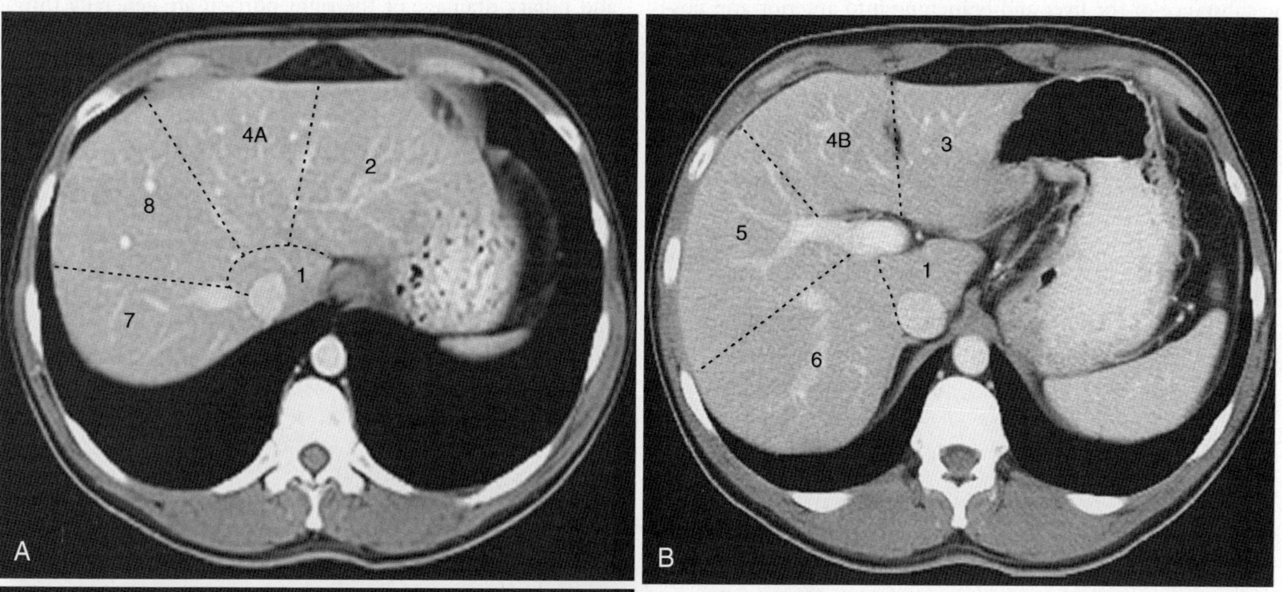


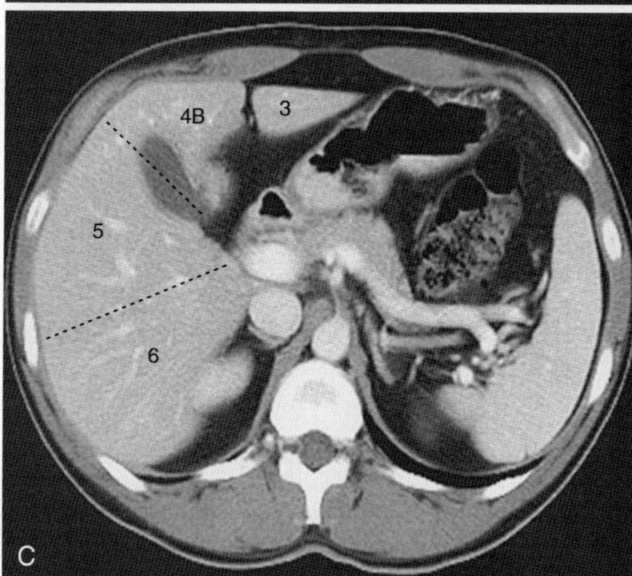


**FIGURE 54-6** Segmental anatomy of the liver is demonstrated at three levels on contrast-enhanced CT images. **A,** At the level of the hepatic veins, the caudate lobe (segment 1) is seen posteriorly embracing the vena cava. Segment 2 is separated from segment 4A by the left hepatic vein. Segment 4A is separated from segment 8 by the middle hepatic vein and segment 8 is separated from segment 7 by the right hepatic vein. **B,** At the level of the portal vein bifurcation, segment 3 is visible as it hangs inferiorly in its anatomic position and is separated from segment 4B by the umbilical fissure. Note that segment 2 is not visible at this level. Terminal branches of the middle hepatic vein separate segment 4B from segment 5 and terminal branches of the right hepatic vein separate segment 5 from segment 6. Note that Segments 4A, 8, and 7 are not visible at this level. Segment 1 is seen posterior to the portal vein and embracing the vena cava. **C,** Below the portal bifurcation, one can see the inferior tips of segments 3 and 4B. The terminal branches of the middle hepatic vein and the gallbladder mark the separation of segment 4B from segment 5. Segments 5 and 6 are separated by the distal branches of the right hepatic vein. Note how the right liver hangs well inferior to the left liver.

as Cantlie's line (see earlier). The right liver is divided into anterior (segments 5 and 8) and posterior (segments 6 and 7) sectors by the right scissura, which contains the right hepatic vein. The right portal pedicle is composed of the right hepatic artery, portal vein, and bile duct. It splits into right anterior and right posterior pedicles, which supply the segments of the anterior and posterior sectors.

The left liver has a visible fissure along its inferior surface called the *umbilical fissure*. The ligamentum teres, containing the remnant of the umbilical vein, runs into this fissure. The falciform ligament is contiguous with the umbilical fissure and ligamentum teres. The umbilical fissure is not a scissura and does not contain a hepatic vein; it contains the left portal pedicle, which contains the left portal vein, hepatic artery, and bile duct. This pedicle runs in this fissure and branches to feed the left liver. The left liver is split into anterior (segments 3 and 4) and posterior (segment 2, the only sector composed of a single segment) sectors by the left scissura. The left scissura runs posterior to the ligamentum teres and contains the left hepatic vein.

At the hilum of the liver, the right portal triad has a short extrahepatic course of approximately 1 to 1.5 cm before entering the substance of the liver and branching into anterior and posterior sectoral branches. The left portal triad, however, has a long extrahepatic course of up to 3 to 4 cm and runs transversely along the base of segment 4 in a peritoneal sheath, which is the upper end of the lesser omentum. This connective tissue is known as the *hilar plate* (Fig. 54-7). The continuation of the left portal triad runs anteriorly and caudally in the umbilical fissure and gives branches to segments 2 and 3 and recurrent branches to segment 4.

The caudate lobe (segment 1) is the dorsal portion of the liver. It embraces the IVC on its posterior surface and lies posterior to the left portal triad inferiorly and the left and middle hepatic veins superiorly. The main bulk of the caudate lobe is to the left of the IVC, but inferiorly it traverses between the IVC and left portal triad, where it fuses to the right liver (segments 6 and 7). This part of the caudate lobe is known as the *right portion* or the *caudate process*. The left portion of the caudate lobe lies in the lesser omental bursa and is covered anteriorly by the gastrohepatic ligament (lesser omentum) that separates it from segments 2 and 3 anteriorly. The gastrohepatic ligament attaches to the ligamentum venosum (sinus venosus remnant) along the left side of the left portal triad (Fig. 54-8).

The vascular inflow and biliary drainage to the caudate lobe comes from both the right and left pedicles. The right side of the caudate, the caudate process, largely derives its portal venous supply from the right portal vein or the bifurcation of the main portal vein. The left portion of the caudate derives its portal venous inflow from the left main portal vein. The arterial supply and biliary drainage of the right portion are generally through the right posterior pedicle system and the left portion through the left main pedicle. The hepatic venous drainage of the caudate is unique because a number of posterior small veins drain directly into the IVC.

The posterior edge of the left side of the caudate terminates as a fibrous component that attaches to the crura of the

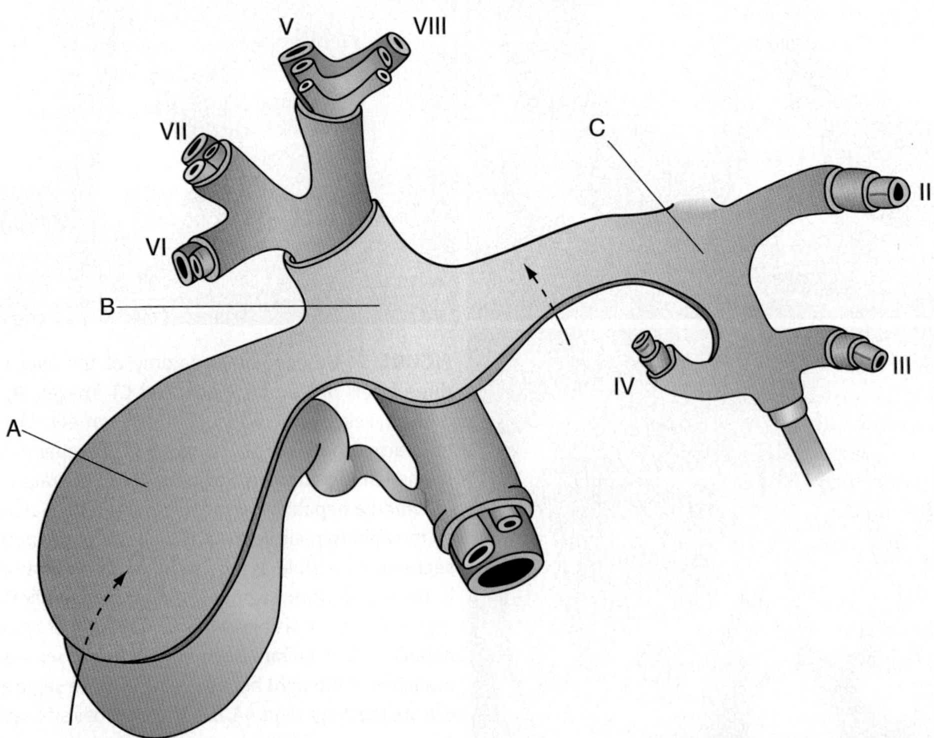


**FIGURE 54-7** The plate system. **A,** The cystic plate between the gallbladder and liver. **B,** The hilar plate at the biliary confluence at the base of segment IV. **C,** The umbilical plate above the umbilical portion of the portal vein. Shown are the plane of dissection of the cystic plate for cholecystectomy and the hilar plate for exposure of the hepatic duct confluence and main left hepatic duct *(arrows)*. (From Blumgart LH, Hann LE: Surgical and radiologic anatomy of the liver and biliary tract. In Blumgart LH, Fong Y [eds]: Surgery of the liver and biliary tract, London, 2000, WB Saunders, pp 3–34.)

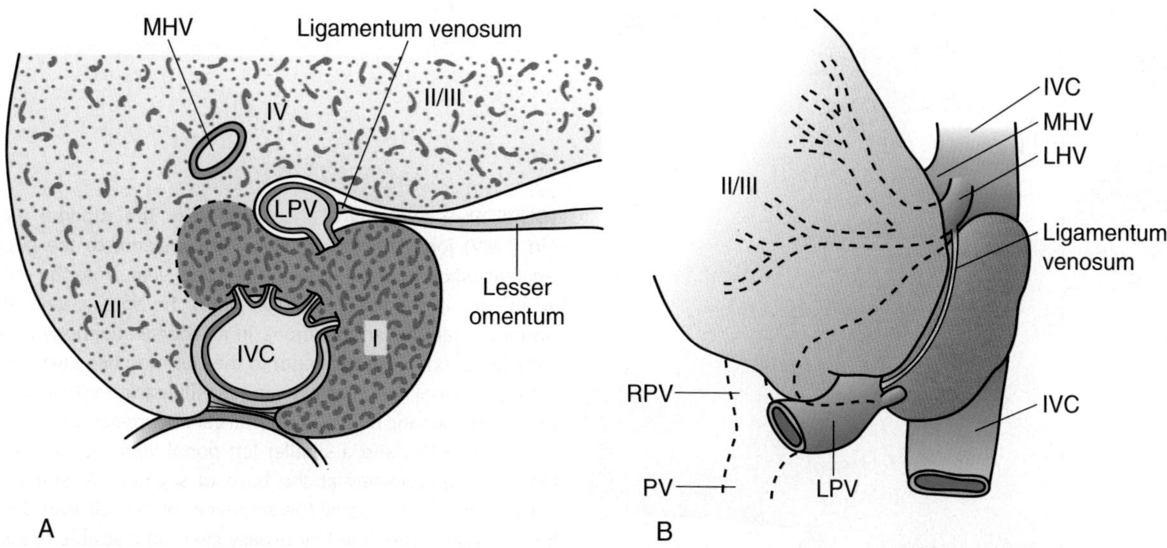


**FIGURE 54-8** Anatomy of the caudate lobe (segment I). **A,** Seen in cross section, most of the caudate is to the left of the IVC and lies posterior to the lesser omentum, which separates the caudate from segments II and III. The termination of the lesser omentum at the ligamentum venosum is demonstrated. The caudate lobe traverses to the right insinuating itself between the IVC and the left portal vein (LPV), where it attaches to the right liver. Note the proximity of the middle hepatic vein (MHV) to these structures. **B,** Segments II and III have been rotated to the patient's right, exposing the left side of the caudate. (From Blumgart LH, Hann LE: Surgical and radiologic anatomy of the liver and biliary tract. In Blumgart LH, Fong Y [eds]: Surgery of the liver and biliary tract, London, 2000, WB Saunders, pp 3–34.)

diaphragm and also runs posteriorly, wrapping behind the IVC and attaching to segment 7 of the right liver. In up to 50% of people, this fibrous component is composed partially or completely of liver parenchyma. Thus, liver tissue may completely encircle the IVC. This structure is known as the *caval ligament* and is important to recognize when mobilizing the right liver or the caudate lobe off the vena cava.

Anomalous development of the liver is uncommonly encountered. Complete absence of the left liver has been reported. A tongue of tissue extending inferiorly off the right liver has been described (Riedel's lobe). Rare cases of supradiaphragmatic liver in the absence of a hernia sac have been noted.

**Portal Vein** The portal vein provides approximately 75% of the hepatic blood inflow. Despite being postcapillary and largely deoxygenated, its high flow rate provides 50% to 70% of the liver's oxygen. The lack of valves in the portal venous system provides a system that can accommodate high flow at low pressure because of the low resistance. This allows for the measurement of portal venous pressure at any point along the system.

The portal vein forms behind the neck of the pancreas at the confluence of the superior mesenteric vein and the splenic vein at the level of the second lumbar vertebrae. The length of the main portal vein ranges from 5.5 to 8 cm and its diameter is usually approximately 1 cm. Cephalad to its formation behind the neck of the pancreas, the portal vein runs behind the first portion of the duodenum and into the hepatoduodenal ligament, where it runs along the right border of the lesser omentum, usually posterior to the common bile duct and proper hepatic artery.

The portal vein divides into main right and left branches at the hilum of the liver. The left branch of the portal vein runs transversely along the base of segment 4 and into the umbilical fissure, where it gives off branches to segments 2 and 3 and feedback branches to segment 4. The left portal vein also gives off posterior branches to the left side of the caudate lobe. The right portal vein has a short extrahepatic course; it usually enters the substance of the liver where it splits into anterior and posterior sectoral branches. These sectoral branches can occasionally be seen extrahepatically and can come off the main portal vein before its bifurcation. There is usually a small caudate process branch off the main right portal vein or at the right portal vein bifurcation, which comes off posteriorly to supply this portion of liver (Fig. 54-9).

There are a number of connections between the portal and systemic venous systems. Under conditions of high portal venous pressure, these portosystemic connections may enlarge secondarily to collateral flow. This concept is reviewed in more detail in later in the chapter, but the most significant portosystemic collateral locations are the following: (1) the submucosal veins of the proximal stomach and distal esophagus receive portal flow from the short gastric veins and the left gastric vein and can result in varices, with the potential for hemorrhage; (2) the umbilical and abdominal wall veins recanalize from flow through the umbilical vein in the ligamentum teres, resulting in caput medusae; (3) the superior hemorrhoidal plexus receives portal flow from inferior mesenteric vein tributaries and can form large hemorrhoids; and (4) other retroperitoneal communications yield collaterals that can make abdominal surgery hazardous.

The anatomy of the portal vein and its branches is relatively constant and has much less variation than the biliary ductal and hepatic arterial systems. The portal vein is rarely found anterior to the neck of the pancreas and duodenum. Entrance of the portal vein directly into the vena cava has also been described. Very rarely, a pulmonary vein may enter the portal vein. Finally, there may be a congenital absence of the left branch of the portal

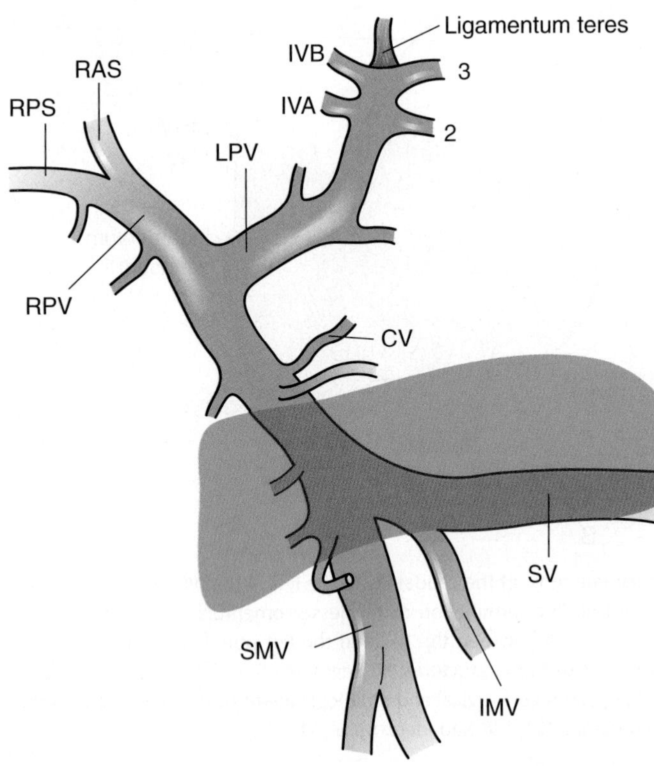


**FIGURE 54-9** Anatomy of the portal vein. The superior mesenteric vein (SMV) joins the splenic vein (SV) posterior to the neck of the pancreas *(shaded area)* to form the portal vein. Note the entrance of the inferior mesenteric vein (IMV) into the splenic vein, the most common anatomic arrangement. In its course superiorly in the edge of the lesser omentum posterior to the common bile duct and hepatic artery, the portal vein receives venous effluent from the coronary vein (CV). At the hepatic hilum, the portal vein bifurcates into a larger right portal vein (RPV) and a smaller left portal vein. The left portal vein (LPV) runs transversely at the base of segment IV and enters the umbilical fissure to supply the segments of the left liver. Just before the umbilical fissure, the LPV usually gives off a sizable branch to the caudate lobe. The RPV enters the substance of the liver and splits into right anterior sectoral (RAS) and right posterior sectoral (RPS) branches. It also gives off a posterior branch to the right side of the caudate lobe–caudate process. (From Blumgart LH, Hann LE: Surgical and radiologic anatomy of the liver and biliary tract. In Blumgart LH, Fong Y [eds]: Surgery of the liver and biliary tract, London, 2000, WB Saunders, pp 3–34.)

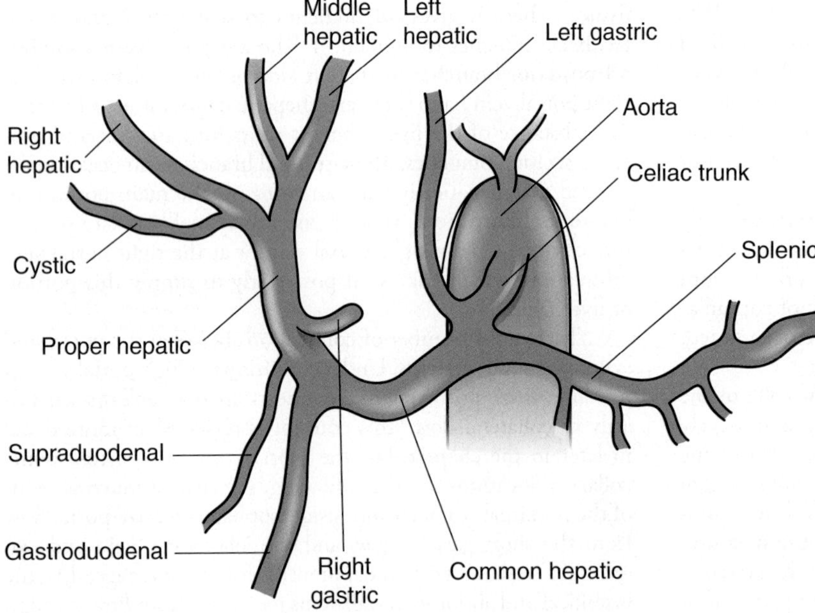


**FIGURE 54-10** Most common anatomy of the celiac axis and hepatic arterial system. The celiac axis, just below the diaphragmatic hiatus, trifurcates into the splenic, left gastric, and common hepatic arteries. The common hepatic artery heads to the right and turns superiorly toward the hilum. At the point of this turn, the gastroduodenal artery is given off and the proper hepatic artery is formed. The common hepatic artery gives off right and left hepatic arteries in the hilum. Note the middle hepatic artery off the proximal left hepatic artery, which goes on to supply segment IV. The cystic artery usually comes off the right hepatic artery within the triangle of Calot. (From Blumgart LH, Hann LE: Surgical and radiologic anatomy of the liver and biliary tract. In Blumgart LH, Fong Y [eds]: Surgery of the liver and biliary tract, London, 2000, WB Saunders, pp 3–34.)

vein. In this situation, the right branch courses through the right liver and curves around peripherally to supply the left liver, or the right anterior sectoral vein can arise from the left portal vein.

**Hepatic Artery** The hepatic artery, representing high-volume oxygenated systemic arterial flow, provides approximately 25% of the hepatic blood flow and 30% to 50% of its oxygenation. A number of smaller perihepatic arteries derived from the inferior phrenic and the gastroduodenal arteries also supply the liver. These vessels are important sources of collateral blood flow in case of occlusion of the main hepatic arterial inflow. In the case of ligation of the right or left hepatic artery, intrahepatic collaterals almost immediately provide for nutrient blood flow in most cases.

The common description of the arterial supply to the liver and biliary tree is only present approximately 60% of the time (Fig. 54-10). The celiac trunk originates directly off the aorta, just below the aortic diaphragmatic hiatus, and gives off three branches—the splenic artery, left gastric artery, and common hepatic artery. The common hepatic artery passes forward and to the right along the superior border of the pancreas and runs along the right side of the lesser omentum, where it ascends towards the hepatic hilum, lying anterior to the portal vein and to the left of the bile duct. At the point where the common hepatic artery begins to head superiorly towards the hepatic hilum, it gives off the gastroduodenal artery, followed by the supraduodenal artery and right gastric artery. The common hepatic artery beyond the takeoff of the gastroduodenal is called the *proper hepatic artery*; it divides into right and left hepatic arteries at the hilum. The left hepatic artery heads vertically towards the umbilical fissure to supply segments 2, 3, and 4. The left hepatic artery usually also gives off a middle hepatic artery branch that heads toward the right side of the umbilical fissure and supplies segment 4. The right hepatic artery usually runs posterior to the common hepatic bile duct and enters Calot's triangle, bordered by the cystic duct, common hepatic duct, and liver edge, where it gives off the cystic artery to supply the gallbladder and then continues into the substance of the right liver.

Unlike portal vein anatomy, hepatic arterial anatomy is extraordinarily variable (Fig. 54-11). An accessory vessel is described as an aberrant origin of a branch that is in addition to the normal branching pattern. A replaced vessel is described as an aberrant origin of a branch that substitutes for the lack of the normal branch. Usually, the hepatic artery originates off the celiac trunk. However, branches or the entire hepatic arterial system can originate off the superior mesenteric artery (SMA). The right and left hepatic arteries can also arise separately off the celiac axis. Replaced or accessory right hepatic arteries come off the SMA and are present approximately 11% to 21% of the time. Hepatic vessels replaced to the SMA run behind the head of the pancreas, posterior to the portal vein in the portacaval space. The right hepatic artery, in its usual branching pattern, can also course anterior to the common hepatic duct. A replaced or accessory left hepatic artery is present approximately 3.8% to 10% of the time, originates from the left gastric artery, and courses within the lesser omentum, heading toward the umbilical fissure. Other important variations include the origin of the gastroduodenal artery, which has been found to originate from the right hepatic artery and is occasionally duplicated. The anatomy of the cystic artery is also variable; knowledge of these variations is of particular importance in the performance of cholecystectomy (Fig. 54-12). An accessory cystic artery can originate from the proper hepatic artery or gastroduodenal artery, where it runs anterior to the bile duct. A single cystic artery can originate anywhere off the proper hepatic artery or gastroduodenal artery, or directly from the celiac axis. These variant cystic arteries can run anterior to the bile duct and are not necessarily present in the triangle of Calot. All these variations in hepatic arterial anatomy are of obvious importance during hepatic resection, hepatic arterial pump placement, cholecystectomy, and hepatic interventional radiologic procedures.

**Hepatic Veins** The three major hepatic veins drain from the superior-posterior surface of the liver directly into the IVC (see Figs. 54-4, 54-5, and 54-6). The right hepatic vein runs in the right scissura between the anterior and posterior sectors of the right liver and drains most of the right liver after a short (1-cm) extrahepatic course into the right side of the IVC. The left and middle hepatic veins usually join intrahepatically and enter the left side of the IVC as a single vessel, although they may drain separately. The left hepatic vein runs in the left scissura between segments 2 and 3 and drains segments 2 and 3; the middle hepatic vein runs in the portal scissura between segment 4 and the anterior sector of the right liver, comprised of segments 5 and 8, and drains segment 4 and some of the anterior sector of the right liver. The umbilical vein is an additional vein that runs under the falciform ligament, between the left and middle veins, and usually empties into the left hepatic vein. A number of small posterior venous branches from the right posterior sector and caudate lobe drain directly into the IVC. A substantial inferiorly located accessory right hepatic vein is commonly encountered. There is also often a venous tributary from the caudate lobe, which drains superiorly into the left hepatic vein.

**Biliary System** The intrahepatic bile ducts are the terminal branches of the right and left hepatic ductal branches that invaginate Glisson's capsule at the hilum, along with their corresponding portal vein and hepatic artery branches, forming the peritoneal covered portal triads also known as *portal pedicles.* Along these intrahepatic portal pedicles, the bile duct branches are usually superior to the portal vein, whereas the hepatic artery branches run inferiorly. The left hepatic bile duct drains segments 2, 3, and 4, which constitute the left liver. The intrahepatic ductal branches of the left liver join to form the main left duct at the base of the umbilical fissure, where the left hepatic duct courses transversely across the base of segment 4 to join the right hepatic duct at the hilum. In its transverse portion, the left hepatic duct drains one to three small branches from segment 4. The right hepatic duct drains the right liver and is formed by the joining of the anterior sectoral duct (draining segments 5 and 8) and the posterior sectoral duct (draining segments 6 and 7). The posterior sectoral duct runs in a horizontal and posterior direction; the anterior sectoral duct runs vertically. The main right hepatic duct bifurcates just above the right portal vein. The short right hepatic duct meets the longer left hepatic duct to form the confluence anterior to the right portal vein, constituting the common hepatic duct. The caudate lobe (segment 1) has its own biliary drainage, which is usually through right and left systems. However, in up to 15% of individuals, drainage is through the left system only and, in 5%, it is through the right system only.

The common hepatic duct drains inferiorly. Below the takeoff of the cystic duct, it is referred to as the common bile duct. The common bile duct usually measures 10 to 15 cm in length and is typically 6 mm in diameter. The common hepatic (bile) duct runs along the right side of the hepatoduodenal ligament (free edge of the lesser omentum) to the right of the hepatic artery and anterior to the portal vein. The common bile duct continues inferiorly behind the first portion of the duodenum and into the head of the pancreas in an inferior and slightly rightward direction. The intrapancreatic distal common bile duct then joins with the main pancreatic duct (of Wirsung), with or without a common channel, and enters the second portion of the duodenum through the major papilla of Vater. At the choledochoduodenal junction, a complex muscular complex known as the *sphincter of Oddi* regulates bile flow and prevents reflux of duodenal contents into the biliary tree. There are three major parts to this sphincter: (1) the sphincter choledochus, which is a circular muscle that regulates bile flow and the filling of the gallbladder; (2) the pancreatic sphincter, present to variable degrees, which surrounds the intraduodenal pancreatic

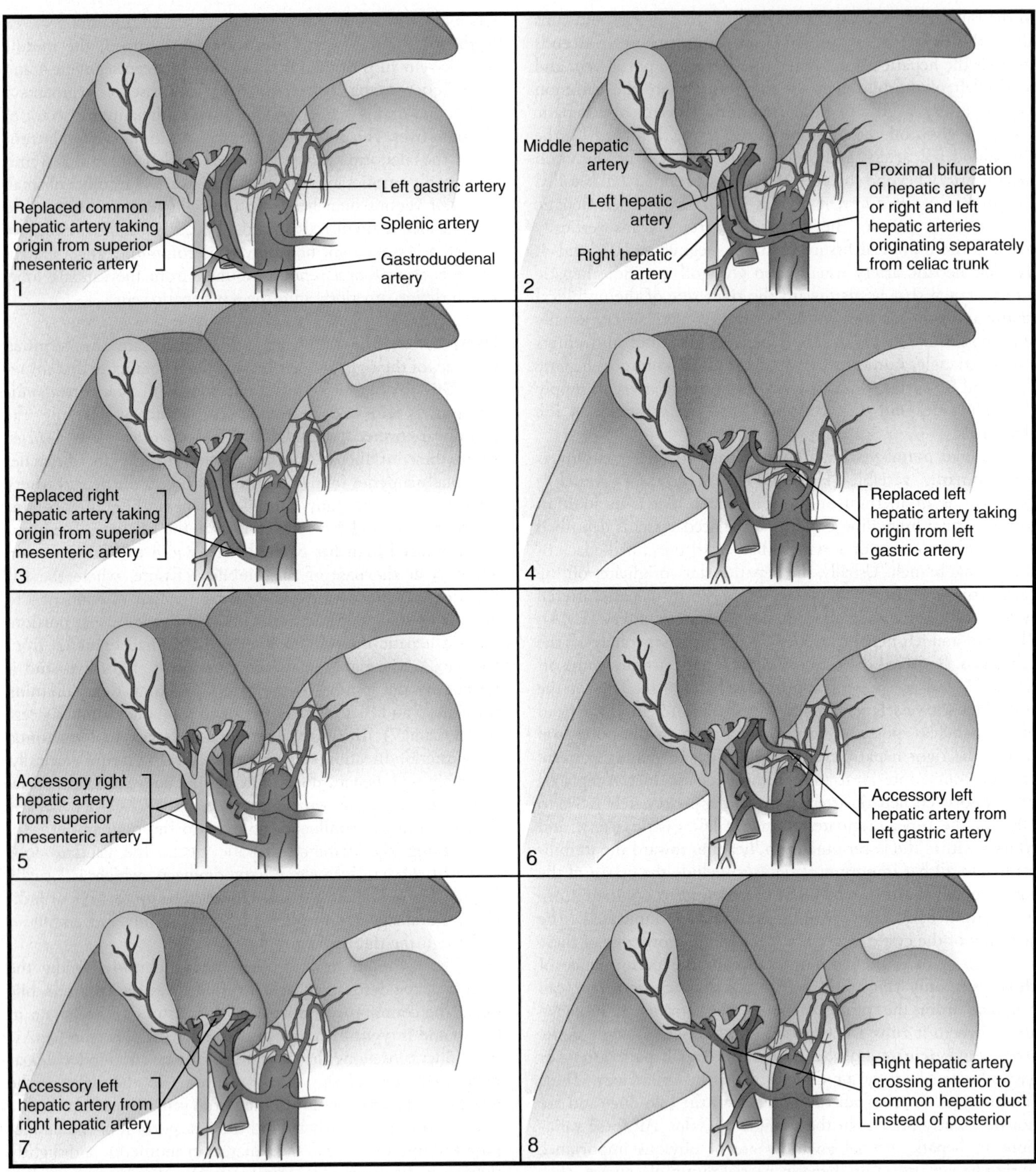


**FIGURE 54-11** Variable anatomy of the hepatic artery. The common hepatic artery can originate off the superior mesenteric artery instead of the celiac axis. A replaced or accessory right hepatic artery comes off the superior mesenteric artery and runs posterior to the head of the pancreas, to the right of the portal vein and behind the common bile duct into the hilum. A replaced or accessory left hepatic artery originates off the left gastric artery and runs through the lesser omentum into the umbilical fissure. (Netter illustration from www.netterimages.com. © Elsevier Inc. All rights reserved.)

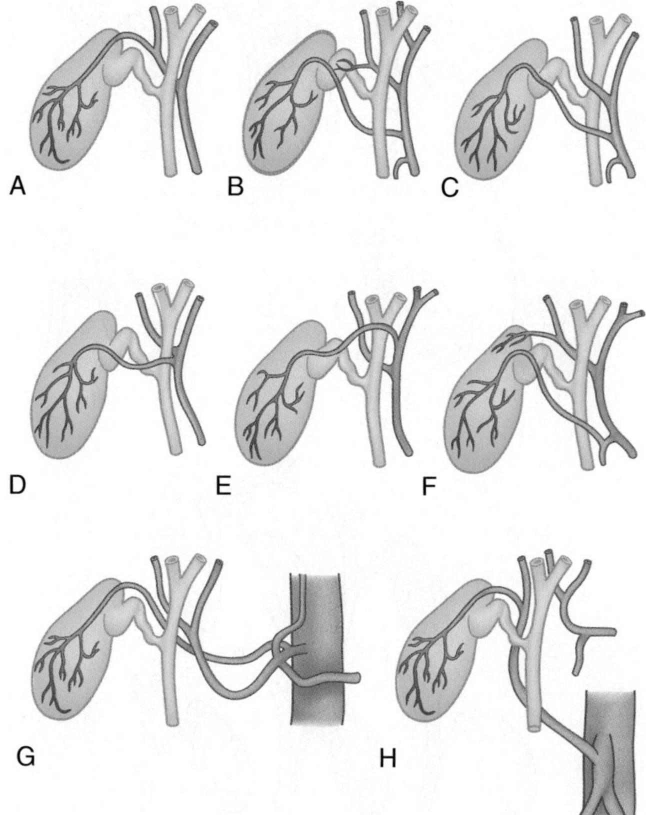


**FIGURE 54-12** Variations in the anatomy of the cystic artery. **A,** Most common anatomy. **B,** Double cystic artery, one off the proper hepatic artery. **C,** Origin off the proper hepatic artery and coursing anterior to the bile duct. **D,** Originating off the right hepatic artery and coursing anterior to the bile duct. **E,** Originating from the left hepatic artery and coursing anterior to the bile duct. **F,** Originating off the gastroduodenal artery. **G,** Originating off the celiac axis. **H,** Originating from a replaced right hepatic artery. (From Blumgart LH, Hann LE: Surgical and radiologic anatomy of the liver and biliary tract. In Blumgart LH, Fong Y [eds]: Surgery of the liver and biliary tract, London, 2000, WB Saunders, pp 3–34.)

duct; and (3) the sphincter ampullae, made up of longitudinal muscle, which prevents duodenal reflux.

The gallbladder is a biliary reservoir that lies against the inferior surface of segments 4 and 5 of the liver, usually making an impression against the liver. A peritoneal layer covers most of the gallbladder, except for the portion adherent to the liver. Here, the gallbladder adheres to the liver by a layer of fibroconnective tissue known as the *cystic plate*, an extension of the hilar plate (see Fig. 54-7). Variable in size, but usually about 10 cm long and 3 to 5 cm wide, the gallbladder is composed of a fundus, body, infundibulum, and neck, which ultimately empty into the cystic duct. The fundus usually projects just slightly beyond the liver edge anteriorly and, when folded on itself, is described as a Phrygian cap. Continuing toward the bile duct, the body of the gallbladder is usually in close proximity to the second portion of the duodenum and transverse colon. The infundibulum (or Hartmann's pouch) hangs forward along the free edge of the lesser omentum and can fold in front of the cystic duct. The portion of gallbladder between the infundibulum and cystic duct is referred to as the neck. The cystic duct is variable in its length, course, and insertion into the main biliary tree. The first portion of the cystic duct is usually tortuous and contains mucosal duplications, referred to as the folds of Heister, which regulate the filling and emptying of the gallbladder. Usually, the cystic duct joins the common hepatic duct to form the common bile duct.

Knowledge of the multiple and frequent variations in the anatomy of the biliary tree is absolutely essential for performing hepatobiliary procedures. Anomalies of the hepatic ductal confluence are common and are present approximately one third of the time. The most common anomalies of the biliary confluence involve variations in the insertion of the right sectoral ducts. Usually, this is the posterior sectoral duct. The confluence can be a trifurcation of the right anterior sectoral, right posterior sectoral, and left hepatic ducts. Either of the right sectoral ducts can drain into the left hepatic duct, common hepatic duct, cystic duct or, rarely, the gallbladder (Fig. 54-13).

Anomalies of the gallbladder itself are rare. Agenesis of the gallbladder, bilobar gallbladder with two ducts or a single duct, septations, and congenital diverticulum of the gallbladder have all been described. Anomalies of the position of the gallbladder are more common; these include an intrahepatic position or, rarely, located on the left side of the liver. The gallbladder can also have a long mesentery, which can predispose it to torsion.

The position and entry of the cystic duct into the main ductal system are also variable. Double cystic ducts draining a unilocular gallbladder and drainage into hepatic duct branches have been reported. Usually, the cystic duct joins the common hepatic duct at an angle, but can run parallel and enter it more distally. In the latter situation, the cystic duct can be fused to the hepatic duct along its parallel course by connective tissue. The cystic duct can also run a spiral course anteriorly or posteriorly and enter the left side of the common hepatic duct. Finally, the cystic duct can be very short or even absent (Fig. 54-14).

The supraduodenal and infrahilar bile duct are predominantly supplied by two axial vessels that run at 3- and 9-o'clock positions. These vessels are derived from the superior pancreaticoduodenal, right hepatic, cystic, gastroduodenal, and retroduodenal arteries. It has been estimated that only 2% of the arterial supply to this portion of the bile duct is segmental, arising directly off the proper hepatic artery. The bile duct and its bifurcation in the hilum derive their arterial blood supply from a rich network of multiple small branches from surrounding vessels. Similarly, the retropancreatic bile duct derives its arterial supply from the retroduodenal artery, which provides a rich network of multiple small branches (Fig. 54-15). Venous drainage of the bile duct parallels the arterial supply and drains into the portal venous system. The venous drainage of the gallbladder empties into the veins that drain the bile duct and does not flow directly into the portal vein.

**Nerves** The innervation of the liver and biliary tract is via sympathetic fibers originating from T7 through T10, as well as parasympathetic fibers from both vagal nerves. The sympathetic fibers pass through celiac ganglia before giving off postganglionic fibers to the liver and bile ducts. The right-sided celiac ganglia and right vagal nerve form an anterior hepatic plexus of nerves that runs along the hepatic artery. The left-sided celiac ganglia and left vagal nerve form a posterior hepatic plexus that runs

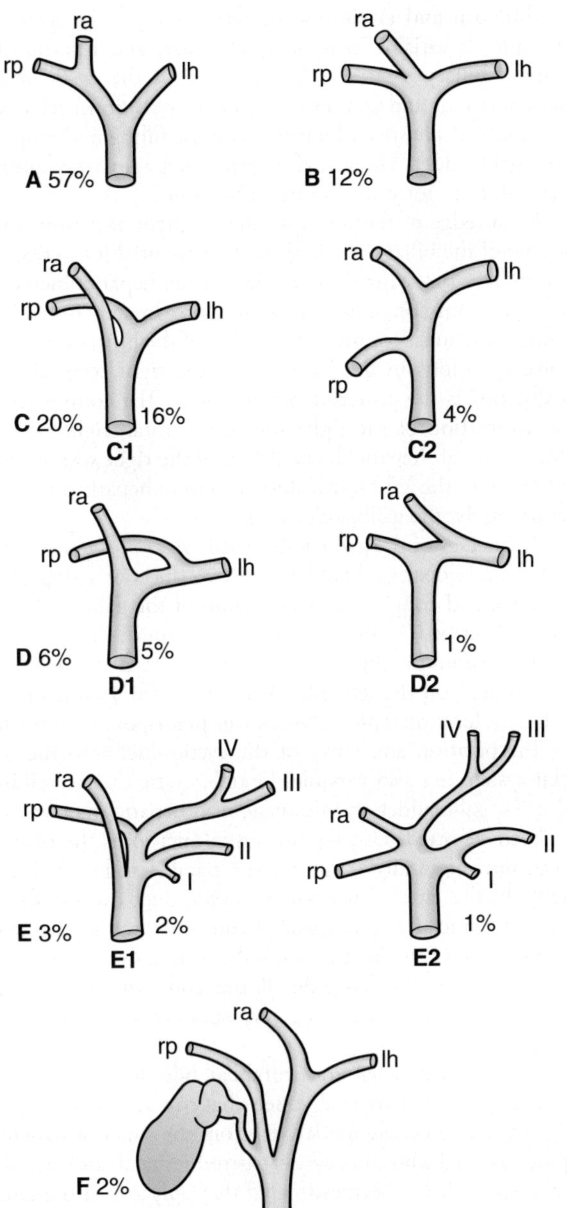


**FIGURE 54-13** Variations of the hepatic duct confluence. **A,** Most common anatomy. **B,** Trifurcation at the confluence. **C,** Either of the right sectoral ducts drains into the common hepatic duct. **D,** Either of the right sectoral ducts drain into the left hepatic duct. **E,** Absence of a hepatic duct confluence. **F,** Absence of right hepatic duct and drainage of right posterior sectoral duct into the cystic duct. (From Blumgart LH, Hann LE: Surgical and radiologic anatomy of the liver and biliary tract. In Blumgart LH, Fong Y [eds]: Surgery of the liver and biliary tract,. London, 2000, WB Saunders, pp 3–34.)

posterior to the bile duct and portal vein. The hepatic arteries are supplied by sympathetic fibers whereas the gallbladder and extrahepatic bile ducts receive innervation from sympathetic and parasympathetic fibers. The clinical significance of these nerves is still not well understood. Acute distention of the liver, and thus the liver capsule, can result in right upper quadrant pain, which may be referred to the right shoulder via phrenic nerve innervation of the diaphragmatic peritoneum.

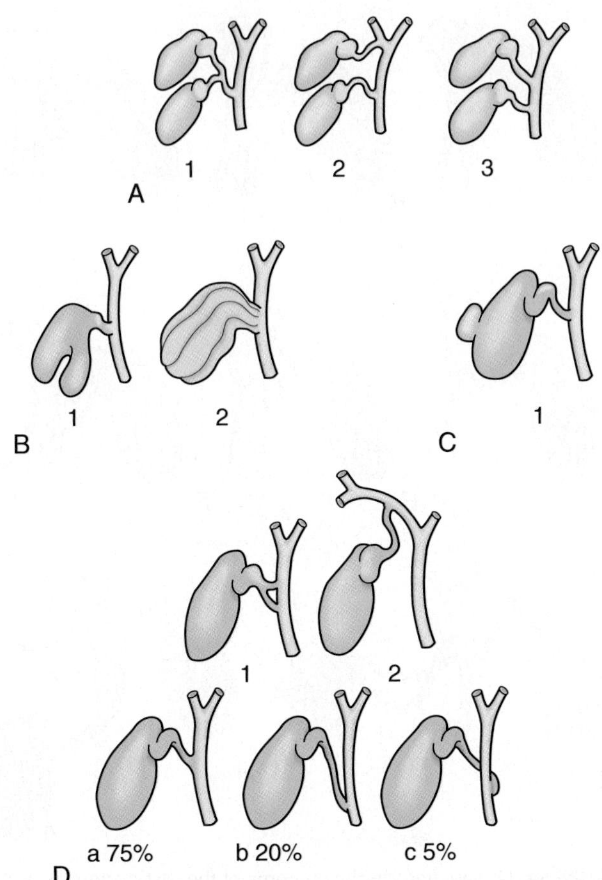


**FIGURE 54-14** Variations in the anatomy of the gallbladder and cystic duct. **A,** Bilobar gallbladder. **B,** Septations of the gallbladder. **C,** Diverticulum of the gallbladder. **D,** Variations in cystic duct anatomy. The three types of union of the cystic duct and common hepatic duct are illustrated. (From Blumgart LH, Hann LE: Surgical and radiologic anatomy of the liver and biliary tract. In Blumgart LH, Fong Y [eds]: Surgery of the liver and biliary tract, London, 2000, WB Saunders, pp 3–34.)

**Lymphatics** Most lymph node drainage from the liver is to the hepatoduodenal ligament. From here, lymphatic drainage usually continues along the hepatic artery to the celiac lymph nodes and then to the cisterna chyli. Lymphatic drainage can also follow the hepatic veins to lymph nodes in the area of the suprahepatic IVC and through the diaphragmatic hiatus. The lymphatic drainage of the gallbladder and most of the extrahepatic biliary tract is generally into the lymph nodes of the hepatoduodenal ligament. This drainage may follow along the hepatic artery to the celiac lymph nodes, but can also flow into lymph nodes behind the head of the pancreas or within the aortocaval groove.

### Microscopic Anatomy

**Functional Unit of the Liver** The organization of hepatic parenchyma into microscopic functional units has been described in a number of ways, referred to as an acinus or a lobule (Fig. 54-16). This was originally described by Rappaport and then modified by Matsumoto and Kawakami.[6] A lobule is made up of a central terminal hepatic venule surrounded by four to six

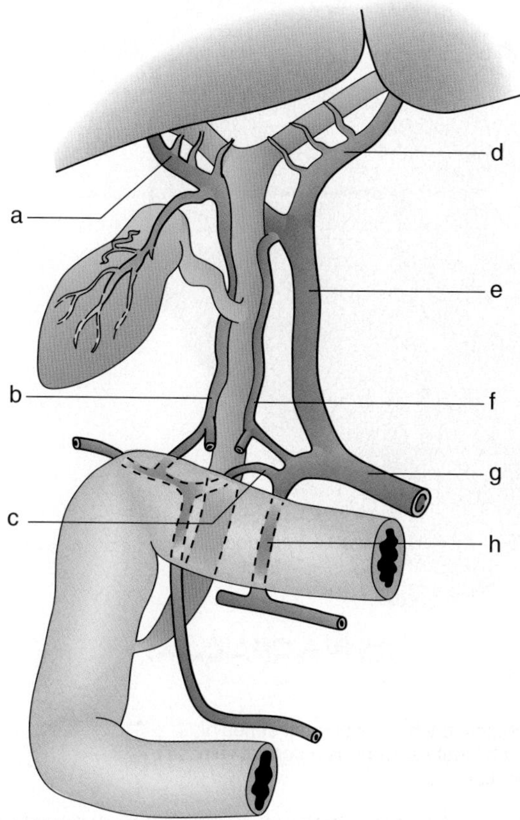


**FIGURE 54-15** The blood supply to the common bile duct and common hepatic duct is illustrated. **A,** Right hepatic artery. **B,** 9:00 artery. **C,** Retroduodenal artery. **D,** Left hepatic artery. **E,** Proper hepatic artery. **F,** 3:00 artery. **G,** Common hepatic artery. **H,** Gastroduodenal artery. (From Blumgart LH, Hann LE: Surgical and radiologic anatomy of the liver and biliary tract. In Blumgart LH, Fong Y [eds]: Surgery of the liver and biliary tract, London, 2000, WB Saunders, pp 3–34.)

terminal portal triads that form a polygonal unit. This unit is lined on its periphery between each terminal portal triad by terminal portal triad branches. In between the terminal portal triads and the central hepatic venule, hepatocytes are arranged in one cell–thick plates, surrounded on each side by endothelial-lined and blood-filled sinusoids. Blood flows from the terminal portal triad through the sinusoids into the terminal hepatic venule. Bile is formed within the hepatocytes and empties into terminal canaliculi, which form on the lateral walls of the intercellular hepatocyte. These ultimately coalesce into bile ducts and flow toward the portal triads. This functional hepatic unit provides a structural basis for the many metabolic and secretory functions of the liver.

Between the terminal portal triad and central hepatic venule are three zones that differ in their enzymatic makeup, as well as exposure to nutrients and oxygenated blood. There is debate about the shape of these zones and their relationship to the basic lobular unit but, in general, zones 1 through 3 splay out from the terminal portal triad toward the central hepatic venule. Zone 1 (periportal zone) is an environment rich in nutrients and oxygen. Zones 2 (intermediate zone) and 3 (perivenular zone) are exposed to environments that are poorer in oxygen and nutrients. The cells of the different zones differ enzymatically and respond differently to toxin exposure and hypoxia. This anatomic arrangement also explains the phenomenon of centrilobular necrosis from hypotension, because zone 3 is the most susceptible to decreases in oxygen delivery.

**Hepatic Microcirculation** Terminal portal venous and hepatic arterial branches directly supply the hepatic sinusoids with blood. The portal branches provide a constant-, but minimal flow into this low-volume system; the arterial branches provide the sinusoids with pulsatile-, but low-volume flow that enhances flow in the sinusoids. Hepatic arterial branches terminate in a plexus around the terminal bile ductules and provide nutrients. Arterial and portal vein flow vary inversely in the sinusoids and can be compensatory. Local control of blood flow in the sinusoids likely depends on arteriolar sphincters and contraction of the sinusoidal lining by endothelial cells and hepatic stellate cells or portal myofibroblasts. Blood within the sinusoids empties directly into terminal hepatic venules at the center of a functional lobule. This process results in the unidirectional flow of blood in the liver from zones 1 to 3.

The endothelium-lined sinusoids of the hepatic lobule represent the functional unit of the liver, where afferent blood flow is exposed to functional hepatic parenchyma prior to being drained into hepatic venules (Fig. 54-17). The hepatic sinusoids are 7 to 15 μm wide but can increase in size by up to 10-fold. This yields a low-resistance and low-pressure (generally, 2 to 3 mm Hg) system. The sinusoidal endothelial cells account for 15% to 20% of the total hepatic cell mass.

Sinusoidal endothelial cells are separated from hepatocytes by the space of Disse (perisinusoidal space). This is an extravascular fluid compartment into which hepatocytes project microvilli, which allows proteins and other plasma components from the sinusoids to be taken up by the hepatocytes. Within this space, the endothelial cells are specialized in that they lack intercellular junctions and a basement membrane but contain multiple large fenestrations. This arrangement provides for the maximal contact of hepatocyte membranes with this extravascular fluid compartment and blood in the sinusoidal space. Thus, this system permits bidirectional movement of solutes (high- and low-molecular-weight substances) into and out of hepatocytes, providing tremendous filtration potential. On the other hand, the fenestrations of the endothelial cells restrict movement of molecules between the sinusoids and hepatocytes and vary in response to exogenous and endogenous mediators.

Other cell types are found along the sinusoidal lining. Kupffer cells, derived from the macrophage-monocyte system, are irregularly-shaped cells that also line the sinusoids insinuating between endothelial cells. Kupffer cells are phagocytic, can migrate along sinusoids to areas of injury, and play a major role in the trapping of foreign substances and initiating inflammatory responses. Major histocompatibility complex II antigens are expressed on Kupffer cells, but do not confer efficient antigen presentation compared with macrophages elsewhere in the body. Other lymphoid cells also exist in hepatic parenchyma, such as natural killer (NK), natural killer T (NKT), CD4 T, and CD8 T cells. These provide the liver with an innate immune system. Hepatic stellate cells, previously known as *Ito cells*, are cells high in retinoid content (accounting for their phenotypic identification) found in the space of Disse. They have dendritic processes

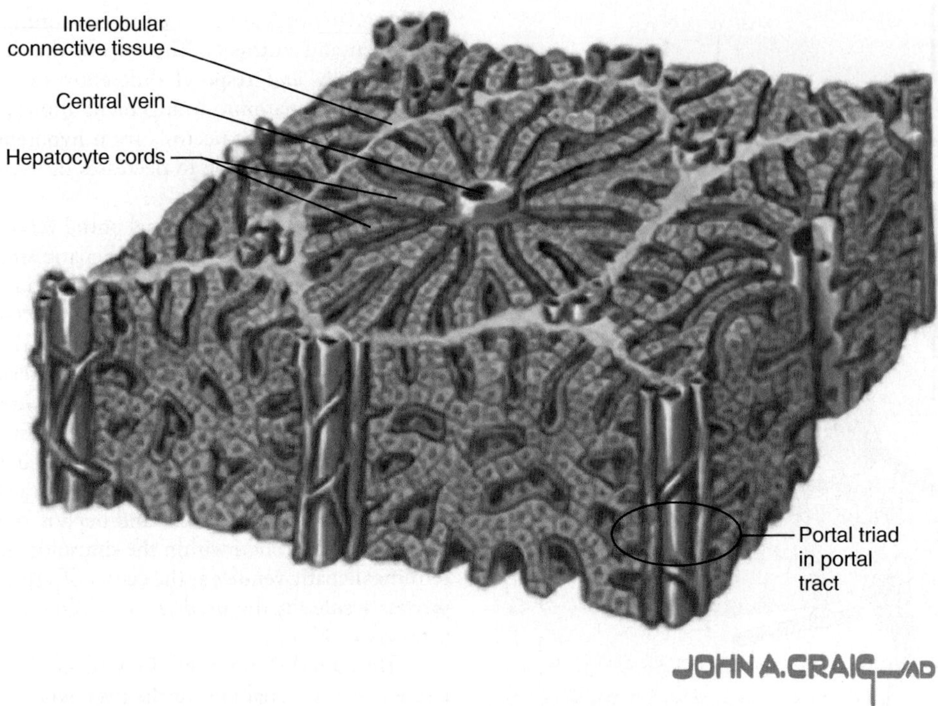


**FIGURE 54-16** Schematic illustration of a hepatic lobule seen as a three-dimensional polyhedral unit. The terminal portal triads (hepatic artery, portal vein, and bile duct) are at each corner and give off branches along the sides of the lobule. Hepatocytes are in single-cell sheets with sinusoids on either end aligned radially toward a central hepatic venule. (From Netter FH: Netter anatomy collection, Elsevier.)

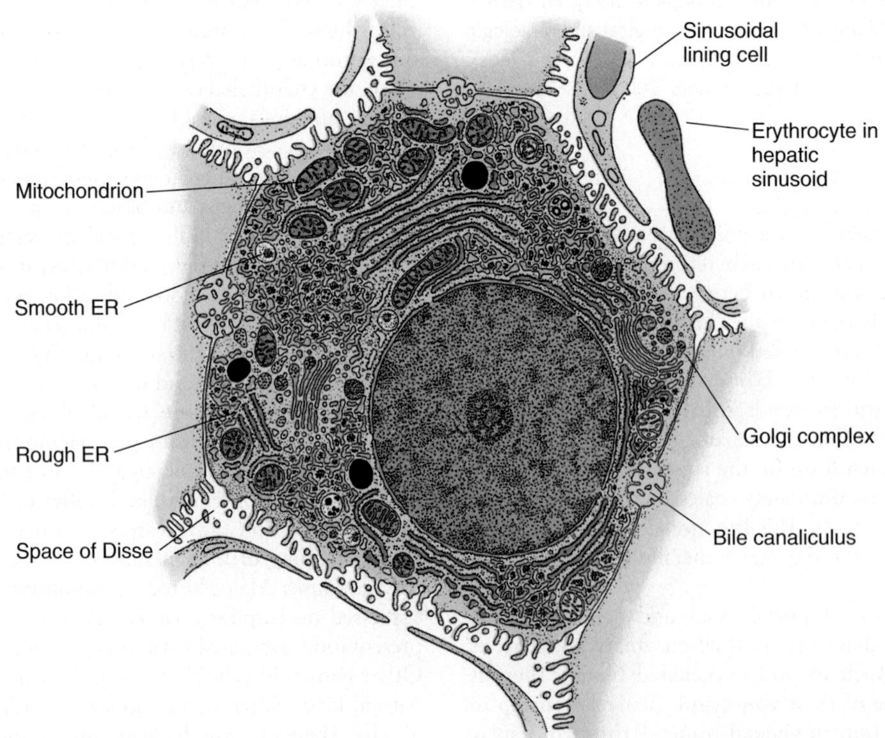


**FIGURE 54-17** A hepatocyte and its sinusoidal and lateral domains. ER, endoplasmic reticulum. (From Ross MH, Reith EJ, Romrell LJ. The liver. In Ross RH, Reith EJ, Romrell LJ: Histology: A Text and Atlas. Baltimore, Williams & Wilkins; 1989, pp 471–478.)

that contact hepatocyte microvilli and also wrap around endothelial cells. The major functions of these stellate cells include vitamin A storage and the synthesis of extracellular collagen and other extracellular matrix proteins. In acute and chronic hepatic liver injuries, hepatic stellate cells are activated to a myofibroblastic state associated with morphologic changes, cellular contractility, decreases in intracellular vitamin A, and production of extracellular matrix. Ultimately, stellate cells play a central role in the development and progression of hepatic fibrosis to cirrhosis and are the target for the development of antifibrotic treatments.

**Hepatocytes** Hepatocytes are complex multifunctional cells that make up 60% of the hepatic cellular mass and 80% of the cytoplasmic mass of the liver (see Fig. 54-17). Morphologically, the hepatocyte is a polyhedral cell with a central spherical nucleus. As noted, hepatocytes are arranged in single cell layer plates lined on either side by blood-filled sinusoids. Every hepatocyte has contact with adjacent hepatocytes, the biliary space (bile canaliculus), and the perisinusoidal space, enabling these cells to perform their broad range of functions. Among the many essential functions of the hepatocyte are the following: (1) uptake, storage and release of nutrients; (2) synthesis of glucose, fatty acids, lipids, and numerous plasma protein (including C-reactive protein and albumin); (3) production and secretion of bile for digestion of dietary fats; and (4) degradation and detoxification of toxins.

To carry out these functions, the plasma membrane of the hepatocyte is organized in a specific manner into three specific domains. The sinusoidal membrane is exposed to the space of Disse and has multiple microvilli that provide a surface specialized in the active transport of substances between the blood and hepatocytes. The lateral domain exists between neighboring hepatocytes and contains gap junctions that provide for intercellular communication. The canalicular membrane is a tube containing microvilli formed by two apposed hepatocytes. These bile canaliculi are sealed by zonula occludens (tight junctions), which prevent the escape of bile. The bile canaliculi form a ring around the hepatocyte that drains into small bile ducts known as *canals of Hering*, which empty into a bile duct at a portal triad. The canalicular membrane contains adenosine triphosphate (ATP)–dependent active transport systems that enable solutes to be secreted into the canalicular membrane against large concentration gradients.

The hepatocyte is one of the most diverse and metabolically active cells in the body, as reflected by its abundance of organelles. There are 1000 mitochondria/hepatocyte, occupying approximately 20% of the cell volume. Mitochondria generate energy (ATP) through oxidative phosphorylation and provide the energy for the metabolic demands of the hepatocyte. The hepatocyte mitochondria are also essential for fatty acid oxidation. The monoclonal antibody HepPar1 (hepatocyte paraffin-1) identifies a unique antigen on hepatocyte mitochondria and is widely used to identify hepatocytes or hepatocellular neoplasms on immunohistochemical examination.

An extensive system of interconnected membrane complexes made up of smooth and rough endoplasmic reticulum and the Golgi apparatus comprise what is known as the *hepatocyte microsomal fraction*. These complexes have a diverse range of functions, including the following: (1) synthesis of structural and secreted proteins; (2) metabolism of lipids and glucose; (3) production and metabolism of cholesterol; (4) glycosylation of secretory proteins; (5) bile formation and secretion; and (6) drug metabolism. Finally, hepatocytes also contain lysosomes, which are intracellular single-membrane vesicles that contain a number of enzymes. These vesicles store and degrade exogenous and endogenous substances. Coordination of these numerous organelles in the hepatocyte allows these cells to accomplish a large variety of functions.

## Functions

The unique anatomic arrangement of the liver described provides a remarkable landscape on which the multiple central and critical functions of this organ can be carried out. The liver is the center of metabolic homeostasis; it serves as the regulatory site for energy metabolism by coordinating the uptake, processing, and distribution of nutrients and their subsequent energy products. The liver also synthesizes a large number of proteins, enzymes, and vitamins that participate in a tremendously broad range of bodily functions. Finally, the liver detoxifies and eliminates many exogenous and endogenous substances, serving as the major filter of the human body. The following sections will summarize this broad range of functions.

### Energy

The liver is the critical intermediary between dietary sources of energy and the extrahepatic tissues that require this energy. The critical and central nature of the liver in regulating the body's energy metabolism is evidenced by the fact that despite accounting for only 4% of the total body weight, the liver consumes about 28% of the total body blood flow and 20% of the total oxygen consumed. The liver also uses about 20% of the total body caloric intake.

The liver receives dietary byproducts through the portal circulation and sorts, metabolizes, and distributes them into the systemic circulation. The liver also plays a major role in regulating endogenous sources of energy such as fatty acids and glycerol from adipose tissues and lactate, pyruvate, and certain amino acids from skeletal muscle. The two major sources of energy that the liver releases into the extrahepatic circulation are glucose and acetoacetate. Glucose is derived from the glycogenolysis of stored glycogen and from gluconeogenesis from lactate, pyruvate, glycerol, propionate, and alanine. Acetoacetate is derived from the β-oxidation of fatty acids. Also, storage lipids such as triacylglycerols and phospholipids are synthesized and stored as lipoproteins by the liver. These can be circulated systemically for uptake by peripheral tissues. These complex and essential functions are regulated by hormones, overall nutritional state of the organism, and requirements of obligate glucose-requiring tissues.

### Functional Heterogeneity

To add to the metabolic complexity of the liver, hepatocytes vary in their function, depending on their location within the lobule. This functional heterogeneity of hepatocytes is anatomically related to their location in the three zones of the lobule and is specifically related to the distance from the incoming portal triad. For example, cells located in the periportal zone (zone 1) are exposed to a high concentration of substrates. Thus, uptake of oxygen and solutes are greater here. A critically important function of hepatocytes, however, is their ability to change their metabolic functionality and be recruited to perform specific functions under varying physiologic conditions, regardless of anatomic location. Sinusoids in the periportal zone are narrower and more tortuous, facilitating increased uptake of substrate by the hepatocytes in this area. In contrast, sinusoids in zone 3 (perivenous) have larger fenestrations, allowing uptake of larger molecules. Thus, sinusoids are also variable in form and function.

Enzymatic makeup, plasma membrane proteins, and ultrastructure are also heterogenous among the hepatocyte population. This cellular protein variability can also be distinguished based on the hepatocyte location within the lobule. Glucose uptake and release, bile formation, and synthesis of albumin and fibrinogen take place in the periportal zone, whereas glucose catabolism, xenobiotic metabolism, and synthesis of $\alpha_1$-antitrypsin and α-fetoprotein (AFP) occur in the perivenous zone. Another example of enzymatic heterogeneity according to lobular zones is the location of the urea cycle enzymes in zone 3, adjacent to the terminal hepatic veins. The functional hepatocyte heterogeneity and its anatomic relationship to the lobular unit account for patterns of damage from metabolic or physiologic insults to the liver.

### Blood Flow

There is a dual blood supply to the liver that comes from the portal vein and hepatic artery. The portal vein provides approximately 75% of the blood flow to the liver, which is oxygen-poor but rich in nutrients. The hepatic artery provides the other 25% of the blood flow, which is oxygen- rich and represents systemic arterial blood flow. The large flow rate of the portal vein is still able to provide 50% to 70% of the afferent oxygenation to the liver. Overall, hepatic blood flow represents about 25% of the cardiac output, demonstrating its central role in whole body metabolism. Hepatic blood flow is decreased during exercise and increased after ingestion of food. Carbohydrates have the most profound effect on hepatic blood flow. Hepatic arterial pressure is representative of systemic arterial pressure. Portal pressure is generally 6 to 10 mm Hg and sinusoidal pressure is usually 2 to 4 mm Hg.

Hepatic blood flow is regulated by various factors. Differences in afferent and efferent vessel pressures, as well as muscular sphincters located at the inlet and outlet of the sinusoids, play a major role. Muscular sphincter tone is regulated by the autonomic nervous system, circulating hormones, bile salts, and metabolites. Specific endogenous factors known to affect hepatic blood flow include glucagon, histamine, bradykinin, prostaglandins, nitric oxide, and many gut hormones, including gastrin, secretin, and cholecystokinin. The sinusoids are also the primary regulators of hepatic blood flow through contraction and expansion of their endothelial cells, Kupffer cells, and hepatic stellate cells.

A one-way reciprocal relationship between hepatic artery and portal vein flow has been demonstrated. Increases in hepatic arterial flow accompany decreases in portal vein flow, but the opposite does not occur. Hepatic arterial compensation, however, cannot provide complete compensation to support hepatic parenchyma in total portal vein occlusion, which is likely the cause of ipsilateral atrophy in this case. Experimental evidence has suggested that the buildup of adenosine in the liver plays an important role in this hepatic arterial compensatory response.

**Table 54-1 Solute Concentrations of Hepatic Bile**

| SOLUTE | CONCENTRATION |
|---|---|
| $Na^+$ | 132-165 mEq/L |
| $K^+$ | 4.2-5.6 mEq/L |
| $Ca^{2+}$ | 1.2-4.8 mEq/L |
| $Mg^{2+}$ | 1.4-3.0 mEq/L |
| $Cl^-$ | 96-126 mEq/L |
| $HCO_3^-$ | 17-55 mEq/L |
| Bile acids | 3-45 mM |
| Phospholipid | 25-810 mg/dL |
| Cholesterol | 60-320 mg/dL |
| Protein | 300-3000 mg/L |

### Bile Formation

Bile production and secretion is one of the major functions of the liver. The physiologic role of bile is twofold. The first is to dispose of substances secreted into bile and the second is to provide enteric bile salts to aid in the digestion of fats. Bile is a substance containing organic and inorganic solutes produced by an active process of secretion and subsequent concentration of these solutes. The concentration of inorganic solutes in bile in the main biliary tree resembles that of plasma (Table 54-1). In the case of bile loss (e.g., from an external biliary fistula), the high concentrations of protein and electrolytes must be considered when replacing the losses. The osmolality of bile is approximately 300 mOsmol/kg and is accounted for by the inorganic solutes. The major organic solutes in bile are bile acids, bile pigments, cholesterol, and phospholipids.

The contents of bile are generally absorbed from the bloodstream through sinusoids into the hepatocyte through the sinusoidal membrane. Bile is initially secreted by hepatocytes into the canaliculi through specialized microvilli containing lateral membranes of the hepatocytes that form the canaliculi. Tight junctions along the canalicular membranes prevent leakage of bile in the normal state. This also provides a route for paracellular secretion of solutes and water into bile. The canaliculi coalesce into larger bile ductules containing biliary epithelium, which then form the intrahepatic and extrahepatic biliary tree. Thus, the liver, in part, serves as an epithelial structure that moves solutes from the blood to the bile and provides a route of secretion for bile into the intestines.

Approximately 1500 mL of bile are secreted daily and much of this (≈80%) is secreted by hepatocytes into canaliculi. Such canalicular bile flow is largely the result of water flow in response to active solute transport. Bile acids are transported from the sinusoidal blood into the hepatocyte by ATP-requiring active transport. Intracellular transport to the canalicular membrane is through bile acid–binding proteins that are transported by a vesicular system derived from the Golgi apparatus. The bile acids are then actively pumped into the canaliculus through an ATP-requiring active transport system. It is well recognized that bile flow has a linear association with bile acid secretion, known as *bile acid–dependent flow*. Because bile acids form micelles in the bile and do not provide osmotic potential, it is likely that flow related to bile acid secretion is secondary to ions that accompany the bile acids (counterions). Bile flow can also occur in the near-absence of bile acid secretion and is known as *bile acid–independent flow*. Experimental evidence has suggested that bile acid–independent flow is at least partially the result of biliary glutathione secretion.

Once bile has passed from the canaliculi to the biliary ductules and then to main bile ducts, bile undergoes further reabsorption and secretion. The epithelial cells of the biliary tract actively reabsorb and secrete water and electrolytes. Secretion is generally through a chloride channel activated by secretin, its most powerful activator, and its subsequent activation of cyclic adenosine monophosphate (cAMP) production. There is usually a net secretion of water and electrolytes, accounting for the other 20% of biliary secretion. Ultimately, bile becomes highly enriched in bicarbonate ions. Many organic substances such as glutathione are degraded in the biliary tree. It is important to note that many drugs can be secreted into the biliary tree in a highly concentrated form (e.g., ceftriaxone). The gallbladder acts as the reservoir of the biliary tree; its function is to store bile in the fasting state. The gallbladder reabsorbs water, concentrating stored bile, and secretes mucin. Contraction of the gallbladder is mediated hormonally, largely through cholecystokinin, in response to a meal, with the simultaneous relaxation of the sphincter of Oddi and release of bile into the duodenum.

### Enterohepatic Circulation

Bile salts are primarily produced in the liver and secreted to be used in the biliary tree and intestine. The primary bile salts cholic acid and chenodeoxycholic acid are produced in the liver from cholesterol and subsequently conjugated with glycine or taurine in the hepatocyte. Once secreted in the gut, the primary bile acids are modified by intestinal bacteria to form the secondary bile acids deoxycholic acid and lithocholic acid. Bile acids are reabsorbed passively into the jejunum and actively into the ileum. Thus, the bile acids reenter the portal venous system, and up to 90% of the bile acids are extracted by hepatocytes. Only a small fraction spills over into the systemic circulation because of efficient hepatic extraction, which accounts for low levels of plasma bile acids. After hepatic extraction, bile acids are recirculated into the canaliculi and back into the biliary tree, completing the circuit. A small amount of intestinal bile acids are not absorbed by the portal system and are excreted in the stool. Thus, the active secretion of bile salts from hepatocytes into bile and from ileal enterocytes into the portal vein is the engine behind the enterohepatic circulation.

The enterohepatic circulation is more than a unique mechanism for reusing physiologically valuable bile acids. This circulation of bile constitutes the major mechanism for eliminating excess cholesterol because cholesterol is consumed during the production of bile salts and is excreted in the feces by mixed micelles formed by organic biliary solutes. Bile salts also play a critical role in the absorption of dietary fats, fat-soluble vitamins (i.e., vitamins A, D, E, and K) and lipophilic drugs. Water movement from hepatocytes into bile and water absorption through the small bowel is also regulated by bile salts. The enterohepatic circulation is therefore central to a number of solubilization, transport, and regulatory functions.

### Bilirubin Metabolism

Bilirubin is the result of heme breakdown. An early phase of heme breakdown, accounting for 20% of bilirubin, is from hemoproteins (heme-containing enzymes) and occurs within 3 days of labeling with radioactive heme. A late phase of heme breakdown, accounting for 80% of bilirubin, is from senescent red blood cells. This occurs in approximately 110 days after administering radioactive labeled heme and is consistent with the life span of red blood cells. Heme is initially broken down into a green-colored biliverdin by heme oxygenase, which is then broken down into the orange-colored bilirubin by biliverdin reductase.

Circulating bilirubin is bound to albumin, which protects many organs from the potentially toxic effects of this compound. The bilirubin-albumin complex enters hepatic sinusoidal blood, where it enters the space of Disse through the large sinusoidal fenestrations. The bilirubin-albumin complex is disassociated in this space. Free bilirubin is internalized into the hepatocyte, where it is conjugated to glucuronic acid. Conjugated bilirubin is then secreted in an energy-dependent fashion into canalicular bile against a large concentration gradient. Bilirubin is secreted with bile into the gastrointestinal tract. Within the gastrointestinal tract, bilirubin is deconjugated by intestinal bacteria to a group of compounds known as *urobilinogens*. These urobilinogens are further oxidized and reabsorbed into the enterohepatic circulation and secreted into bile. A small percentage of the reabsorbed urobilinogens is excreted into urine. These oxidized urobilinogens account for the colored compounds that contribute to the yellow color of urine and the brown color of stool.

Bilirubin has long been known to be a toxic compound and is the agent responsible for neonatal encephalopathy and cochlear damage secondary to severe unconjugated hyperbilirubinemia (kernicterus). The binding of serum bilirubin to albumin protects the tissues from exposure to bilirubin. However, binding sites can be overwhelmed by increasing amounts of bilirubin or displaced by other binding agents (e.g., various drugs). The mechanism of bilirubin toxicity appears to be related to a number of its effects. Free bilirubin can uncouple oxidative phosphorylation, inhibit ATPases, decrease glucose metabolism, and inhibit a broad spectrum of protein kinase activities.

Portosystemic shunts, such as those seen with cirrhosis and portal hypertension, decrease the first-pass hepatic clearance of bilirubin, resulting in a mildly increased serum unconjugated hyperbilirubinemia. A number of disorders can result in an unconjugated serum hyperbilirubinemia, including neonatal hyperbilirubinemia (see earlier), an increased bilirubin load caused by hemolytic syndromes, and inherited enzymatic deficiencies such as Crigler-Najjar and Gilbert syndromes. Disorders presenting with serum conjugated hyperbilirubinemia include cholestasis, Dubin-Johnson, and Rotor syndromes.

### Carbohydrate Metabolism

The liver is the center of carbohydrate metabolism because it is the major regulator of storage and distribution of glucose to the peripheral tissues and, in particular, to glucose-dependent tissues such as the brain and erythrocytes. Both liver and muscle are capable of storing glucose in the form of glycogen, but only the liver can break down glycogen to provide glucose for systemic circulation. Glycogen that is broken down can only be used in muscle and is therefore not a source of systemically circulated glucose.

In the fed state, carbohydrate absorbed through the intestines (mostly glucose) is circulated systemically. Carbohydrates reaching the liver are rapidly converted to glycogen for storage. The liver contains up to 65 g of glycogen/kg of liver tissue.

Excess carbohydrate is mostly converted to fatty acids and stored in adipose tissue. In the postabsorptive state (between meals, nonfasting), there is no further systemic glucose coming directly from the gut and the liver becomes the primary source of circulating glucose by the breakdown of glycogen. This is crucial for the brain and erythrocytes, which rely on glucose for their metabolism. In the postabsorptive state, most other tissues begin to rely on fatty acids derived from adipose tissue as their primary fuel. Highly active muscle may deplete its own glycogen and depend on liver-derived glucose for its substrate in the postabsorptive state. After 48 hours of fasting, hepatic glycogen is depleted and the liver shifts from glycogenolysis to gluconeogenesis. The substrate for hepatic gluconeogenesis is mostly from amino acids (mainly alanine) derived from muscle breakdown, but they also comes from glycerol derived from adipose breakdown. During a prolonged fast, fatty acids from adipose breakdown are $\beta$-oxidized in the liver, which releases ketone bodies that then become the primary fuel for the brain.

Transition in and out of these various metabolic states and regulation of carbohydrate metabolism is mostly influenced by glucose concentration in sinusoidal blood and hormonal influences (e.g., insulin, catecholamines, glucagon). In the fasting state, during anaerobic metabolism, lactate is produced, largely from muscle. The liver uses this lactate, which is converted to pyruvate that enters into the gluconeogenic pathways to produce glucose. This cycle is known as the *Cori cycle.*

Derangements of carbohydrate metabolism are common in liver disease. Cirrhotics often demonstrate abnormal glucose tolerance. Its mechanism is not completely clear but is probably related to associated insulin resistance. This phenomenon is not caused by shunting of glucose containing blood away from the liver. Hypoglycemia is a distinctly uncommon entity in chronic liver disease because of the remarkable resilience of the liver and its metabolic function. Only with massive hepatocyte loss in fulminant hepatic failure does gluconeogenesis fail and hypoglycemia ensue.

### Lipid Metabolism

Fatty acids are synthesized in the liver during states of glucose excess, when the liver's ability to store glycogen has been exceeded. Adipocytes have a limited ability to synthesize fatty acids. Therefore, the liver is the predominant source of synthesized fatty acids, although they are largely stored in adipose tissue. During lipolysis, free fatty acids are transported to the liver, where they are metabolized. Fatty acids in the liver undergo esterification with glycerol to form triglycerides for storage or transportation, or they undergo $\beta$-oxidation, yielding energy in the form of ATP and ketone bodies. In general, this process is regulated by the nutritional state; starvation favors oxidation and the fed state favors esterification.

There is a constant cycling of fatty acids between the liver and adipose tissue that is under a delicate balance, which can easily be offset, resulting in fatty infiltration of the liver. A few factors influence this balance; for example, hepatic uptake of fatty acids is a function of plasma concentrations. Although there is no limit to the liver's ability to esterify fatty acids, its ability to dispose of or breakdown fatty acids is limited, as is its ability to secrete triglycerides in the form of lipoproteins. Therefore, conditions of increased circulating fatty acids can easily override the liver's ability to handle them, resulting in fatty accumulation in the liver. This is known as *steatosis* or, when associated with chronic inflammation in more advanced cases, steatohepatitis. A number of conditions have been associated with hepatic steatosis, such as diabetes, steroid use, starvation, obesity, and extensive administration of cytotoxic chemotherapeutic agents. Fatty liver associated with alcohol intake has a number of causes; it is related to increased lipolysis, reduced oxygenation, and augmented esterification of hepatic fatty acids, and may also be related to relative starvation in the chronic alcoholic.

### Protein Metabolism

The liver is also a central site for the metabolism of proteins and is involved in protein synthesis, catabolism of proteins into energy or storage forms, and managing excess amino acids and nitrogen waste. Ingested protein is broken down into amino acids that are circulated throughout the body, where they are used as the building blocks for proteins, enzymes, and hormones. Excess amino acids not used in peripheral tissues are generally handled by the liver, in which they are oxidized for energy—providing 50% of the liver's energy needs—or converted into glucose, ketone bodies, or fats. When amino acids are catabolized for energy production throughout the body, ammonia, glutamine, glutamate, and aspartate are produced. These products are largely processed in the liver, where the waste nitrogen is converted to urea via the urea cycle and the urea is generally excreted in the urine. Thus, the liver is central and critical to the body's nitrogen balance and amino acid metabolism.

Although the liver can catabolize most amino acids, yielding energy or other storable energy forms such as glucose or fats, notable exceptions are the branched-chain amino acids. Branched-chain amino acids cannot be catabolized in the liver and are mostly dealt with by muscle. It has been postulated that this may act as a so-called *safety net* that helps spare the liver some of the demands of protein and amino acid metabolism.

The liver also is the main site of synthesis for many proteins involved in such wide-ranging and critical functions as coagulation, transport, copper and iron binding, and protease inhibition. These proteins include ceruloplasmin, iron storage and binding proteins, and $\alpha_1$-antitrypsin. Albumin is made exclusively in the liver and is the predominant serum-binding protein. Hepatic insufficiency or specific genetic abnormalities can result in altered amounts and functions of these proteins, with wide-ranging pathologic effects.

The liver is also responsible for the so-called *acute-phase response*, a synthetic response by protein to trauma or infection. Its purpose is to restrict organ damage, maintain vital hepatic function, and control defense mechanisms. The response is incited by proinflammatory cytokines such as interleukin-1 (IL-1), IL-6, and tumor necrosis factor (TNF) which induce acute-phase protein gene expression in the liver. Some of the well-known hepatic acute-phase proteins are $\alpha_1$- $\alpha_2$-, and $\beta$-globulin, as well as C-reactive protein and serum amyloid A. An equally important part of this response is its termination. Anti-inflammatory cytokines such as IL-1 receptor antagonist, IL-4, and IL-10 appear to play important roles. The acute-phase response is usually completed in 24 to 48 hours but, in the context of ongoing injury, can be prolonged.

### Vitamin Metabolism

Along with the intestine, the liver is responsible for the metabolism of the fat-soluble vitamins A, D, E, and K. These vitamins are obtained exogenously and absorbed in the intestine. Their adequate intestinal absorption is critically dependent on adequate fatty acid micellization, which requires bile acids.

Vitamin A is from the retinoid family and is involved in normal vision, embryonic development, and adult gene regulation. Storage of vitamin A is solely in the liver and occurs in the hepatic stellate cells. Overingestion of vitamin A can result in hepatic toxicity. Vitamin D is involved in calcium and phosphorus homeostasis. One of vitamin D's activation steps (25-hydroxylation) occurs in the liver. Vitamin E is a potent antioxidant and protects membranes from lipid peroxidation and free radical formation. Finally, vitamin K is a critical cofactor in the post-translational γ-carboxylation of the hepatically synthesized coagulation factors II, VII, IX, and X, as well as protein C and protein S, the so-called *vitamin K–dependent cofactors*. Cholestasis syndromes can result in the inadequate absorption of these vitamins secondary to poor micellization in the intestine. The associated vitamin deficiency syndromes, such as metabolic bone disease (vitamin D deficiency), neurologic disorders (vitamin E deficiency), and coagulopathy (vitamin K deficiency) can subsequently occur.

The liver is also involved in the uptake, storage, and metabolism of a number of water-soluble vitamins, including thiamin, riboflavin, vitamin $B_6$, vitamin $B_{12}$, folate, biotin, and pantothenic acid. The liver is responsible for converting some of these water-soluble vitamins to active coenzymes, transforming some to storage metabolites and using some for enterohepatic circulation (e.g., vitamin $B_{12}$).

### Coagulation

The liver is responsible for synthesizing almost all the identified coagulation factors, as well as many of the fibrinolytic system components and several plasma regulatory proteins of coagulation and fibrinolysis. As noted, the liver is critical for the absorption of vitamin K, synthesizes the vitamin K–dependent coagulation factors, and contains the enzyme that activates these factors. Also, the reticuloendothelial system of the liver clears activated clotting factors, activated complexes of the coagulation and fibrinolytic systems, and the end products of fibrin degradation. Diseases of the liver are often associated with thrombocytopenia, qualitative platelet abnormalities, vitamin K deficiency with impaired modulation of vitamin K–dependent coagulation factors, and disseminated intravascular coagulation (DIC). It is no surprise that liver disease is firmly associated with coagulation disorders that are often challenging to deal with.

Warfarin, one of the most commonly dispensed anticoagulants, acts in the liver by blocking vitamin K–dependent activation of factors II, VII, IX, and X. Factor VII has the shortest half-life of the coagulation factors and its deficiency is manifested clinically as abnormalities of the measured prothrombin time (PT) or international normalized ratio (INR). Patients with hepatic synthetic dysfunction similarly have an abnormal PT.

### Metabolism of Drugs and Toxins (Xenobiotics)

The human body is exposed to an inordinate amount of foreign chemicals during a lifetime. This poses a challenge to our ability to detoxify and eliminate these potentially harmful chemicals. Many of these chemicals are not incorporated into cellular metabolism and are referred to as xenobiotics. The liver plays a central role in handling them through an enormously complex and numerous set of enzymes and reaction pathways, which are increasingly recognized as new chemicals are discovered.

Hepatic-based reactions to xenobiotics are broadly classified into phase I and II reactions. Phase I reactions, through oxidation, reduction, and hydrolysis, increase the polarity and thus water solubility of compounds. This in turn allows for easier excretion. It is important to realize that phase I reactions do not necessarily detoxify chemicals and may, in fact, create toxic metabolites. Phase I reactions occur in the cytochrome P450 (CYP) system. Phase II reactions generally act to create a less toxic or less active byproduct. This is generally accomplished through transferase reactions, in which a compound is usually coupled to a conjugate, rendering the xenobiotic more innocuous.

### Regeneration

The liver possesses the unique quality of adjusting its volume to the needs of the body. This is observed clinically in its regeneration after partial hepatectomy or after toxic liver injury. It is also seen in liver transplantation, in that donor liver size mismatches adjust to the new host. This quality is highly conserved evolutionarily because of the critical functions of the liver and the fact that the liver is the first line of exposure to ingested toxic agents.

Liver regeneration is a hyperplastic response of all cell types of the liver, in which the microscopic anatomy of the functional liver is maintained. Much information that we have about the regenerative response of the liver is based on experimental evidence in rodents. Normally quiescent hepatocytes rapidly enter the cell cycle after partial hepatectomy. Maximal hepatocyte DNA synthesis occurs 24 to 36 hours after partial hepatectomy and maximal DNA synthesis occurs in the other cell types by 48 to 72 hours later. Most of the increase in hepatic mass in rodents is seen by 3 days after partial hepatectomy and is usually almost complete after 7 days.

In the late 1960s, it was recognized that circulating factors were responsible, in part, for the regenerative response and, over the last 40 years, much research has focused on the humoral and genetic control of hepatic regeneration. The major circulating factors that have been identified, largely from rodent studies, are hepatocyte growth factor, epidermal growth factor, transforming growth factors, insulin, and glucagon and the cytokines TNF-α, IL-1, and IL-6. These factors, when infused into a normal host, do not result in hepatic growth, indicating that hepatocytes must be primed in some way before responding to these growth factors. Remarkable progress in the understanding of liver regeneration has been made because of the development of improved genetic and molecular biologic techniques. Hundreds of genes involved at all stages of regeneration have been identified by RNA microarray techniques. Also, numerous cytokine-dependent and growth factor–independent pathways have been further defined. A complete description is beyond the scope of this chapter, however, and many questions still remain.

## Future Developments

The study of the liver and its physiology continues to be a remarkable and exciting field. As the fields of molecular biology and genetic manipulation have exploded, so has the field of hepatology. Given the lack of alternative options to transplantation for patients with end-stage liver failure, tissue engineering and attempts to provide exogenous hepatic functional support continue to be studied. Liver repopulation with transplanted cells—hepatocytes or hepatic progenitor and stem cells—may also provide future options for patients with liver failure. Although the identification of specific and reliable markers for hepatic stem cells has been elusive, the concepts of liver progenitors and stem cells, and their potential usefulness for hepatic repopulation, have gained acceptance, making this an exciting area of research. Ongoing genetic comparisons of normal and diseased liver using new molecular biology and cell biology techniques will provide clues about the genetic regulation of liver diseases. Great strides have been made in the effectiveness of gene therapy and many groups continue to study liver-directed gene therapy strategies to treat acquired and inherited disorders. Ongoing molecular biology studies are researching hepatic cell cycle regulation, with implications for hepatocarcinogenesis. Research studies about the pathogenesis of hepatic fibrosis and, perhaps more exciting, reversing this process, are ongoing and likely to result in significant advances in the future.

## Assessment of Liver Function

A wide variety of tests are available to evaluate hepatic diseases. Screening for hepatic disease, assessing hepatic function, diagnosing specific disorders, and prognosticating are critical in the management of hepatic pathology. For the surgeon, assessment of hepatic function and estimating the ability of a hepatic remnant to be sufficient after liver resection are also of obvious importance. Unfortunately, most measures of hepatic disease are gross indicators and lack sensitivity, specificity, and accuracy. We have divided these hepatic function tests into three categories—routine screening, specific diagnostic, and quantitative tests.

### Routine Screening Tests

Screening blood tests are often used to determine whether there is pathology in the hepatobiliary system. Standard liver functions tests (LFTs) are generally not tests of function and are not always specific to hepatic pathology. Nonetheless, they are valuable as a general screening tool that can provide basic indications to recognize the presence of hepatic disease and yield clues about the cause of that disease. Total bilirubin, direct bilirubin (conjugated), and indirect bilirubin (unconjugated) levels can be affected by a number of processes related to bilirubin metabolism. Unconjugated hyperbilirubinemia can be a reflection of increased bilirubin production (e.g., hemolysis), drug effects, inherited enzymatic disorders, or physiologic jaundice of the newborn. Conjugated hyperbilirubinemia is generally a result of cholestasis or mechanical biliary obstruction, but can also be seen in some inherited disorders or hepatocellular disease.

The transaminases, alanine aminotransferase (ALT) and aspartate aminotransferase (AST), are the most common serum markers of hepatocellular necrosis, with subsequent leak of these intracellular enzymes into the circulation. AST is found in other organs such as the heart, muscle, and kidney, but ALT is liver-specific. However, the degree of elevation of these enzyme levels has never been shown to be of prognostic value. Alkaline phosphatase (ALP) is expressed in liver, bile ducts, bone, intestine, placenta, kidney, and leukocytes. Isoenzyme determinations can sometimes be helpful for distinguishing the source of an elevated ALP level. Elevations of ALP levels in hepatobiliary diseases are generally secondary to cholestasis or biliary obstruction. Such elevations are caused by increased production of this enzyme. The ALP level can also be increased in malignant disease of the liver. Gamma-glutamyl transpeptidase (GGT) is an enzyme in many organs in addition to the liver, such as the kidneys, seminal vesicles, spleen, pancreas, heart, and brain. Its level can be elevated in diseases affecting any of these tissues. It is also induced by alcohol intake and is elevated in biliary obstruction. Thus, it is also a nonspecific marker of liver disease but can be helpful in determining whether an elevated ALP is from hepatic pathology. 5′-Nucleotidase is also found in a wide variety of organs in addition to the liver, but increased levels are fairly specific to hepatic pathology. Like GGT, it can be helpful in determining whether an elevated ALP level is secondary to hepatic pathology.

Albumin is synthesized exclusively in the liver and can be used as a general measure of hepatic synthetic function. Because chronic malnutrition and acute injury or inflammation can decrease albumin synthesis, these factors must be taken into account when evaluating a low serum albumin level. Because of the remarkable protein synthetic capacity of the liver, hypoalbuminemia is a marker of severe liver disease. However, it lacks sensitivity and large decreases in hepatic function are required to be reflected in albumin levels. In general, it is most helpful in chronic liver disease.

Clotting factors are largely synthesized in the liver; abnormalities of coagulation can be a marker of hepatic synthetic dysfunction. Measurement of specific clotting factors, such as factors V and VII, have been used to evaluate hepatic function in the transplantation population. PT or INR is the best test to measure the effects of hepatic disease on clotting and is usually a marker of advanced chronic liver disease. Hepatic pathology can also affect clotting through intravascular coagulation and vitamin K malabsorption.

### Specific Diagnostic Tests

Once screening tests, along with clinical findings, have suggested liver disease, specific tests can be used to help elucidate the cause and guide treatment, if necessary. Hepatitis serologies are important to determine the presence of viral hepatitis. Autoimmune antibodies are used to diagnose primary biliary cirrhosis (e.g., antimitochondrial), primary sclerosing cholangitis (e.g., antineutrophil), and autoimmune hepatitis. $\alpha_1$-Antitrypsin and ceruloplasmin levels assist in the diagnosis of $\alpha_1$-antitrypsin deficiency and Wilson's disease, respectively. Tumor markers such as AFP and carcinoembryonic antigen (CEA) can be helpful in the diagnosis and management of primary and metastatic tumors of the liver.

In general, the LFTs discussed in this section are gross, nonspecific, and of little, if any, prognostic value. Many attempts have been made to formulate dynamic and quantitative tests of hepatic function based on the liver's ability to clear various exogenously administered substances. Despite many years of research, it still remains unclear whether these tests of hepatic function are any better than scoring systems derived from simple blood tests and clinical observations. For example, the aminopyrine breath test is based on CYP clearance of radiolabeled aminopyrine. A breath test measuring radiolabeled $CO_2$ as a breakdown product of aminopyrine is performed after administration at a specified time. The results largely depend on the functional hepatic mass, which is generally not depleted until end-stage liver disease has developed. There are varying results of studies comparing the aminopyrine breath test with standard LFTs and scoring systems; its main value appears to be prognosis in chronic liver disease, but it is clearly not an effective test to detect subclinical hepatic dysfunction.

Substances such as antipyrine and caffeine can evaluate liver function in a similar way, with similar results. The lidocaine clearance test yields similar information to the aminopyrine test because it is based on its clearance by the hepatic CYP test. Lidocaine clearance is dependent on blood flow and a complex distribution process, but measurement of one of its metabolites, monoethylglycinexylidide (MEGX), has greatly simplified the test. It has been shown to have some prognostic value in the transplantation population. The galactose elimination test is based on the liver's role in phosphorylating galactose and converting it to glucose. The rate at which galactose is eliminated from the bloodstream can be used as a measure of hepatic function. Problems related to this test are that the enzymes involved are genetically heterogeneous and considerable extrahepatic metabolism occurs. Also, multiple blood draws are necessary, which makes the test cumbersome. The value of this test is probably in assessing the prognosis of patients with chronic liver disease, rather than screening. Indocyanine green is a dye removed by the liver by a carrier-mediated process and excreted into bile. This dye is rapidly cleared from the bloodstream and is not metabolized. This is the only test that has been shown to have some prognostic ability in cirrhotic patients undergoing liver resection, although this is not universally demonstrated in studies nor is it universally accepted.

### Quantitative Tests

Finally, a large number of scoring systems based on clinical observation and standard blood tests have been proposed. The most commonly used system is Pugh's modification of the Child score (Table 54-2). Although all these systems are less than perfect and not universally accepted, the Child-Pugh score is commonly used for cirrhotic patients who require liver surgery. Mortality and survival rates after hepatectomy have been shown to correlate with this score, but are not always related to liver failure. Child-Pugh class B and C patients have higher perioperative mortality after any partial hepatectomy than Child-Pugh class A patients who can generally withstand a major hepatectomy.[1,2] The presence of portal hypertension has been shown to predict poor outcome after partial hepatectomy. The presence of portal hypertension in cirrhotic patients is usually manifested as thrombocytopenia, splenomegaly, and presence of intra-abdominal varices on imaging or at endoscopy. The best evidence for portal hypertension is a hepatic vein wedge pressure higher than 10 mm Hg, which has been shown to correlate strongly with postoperative liver failure.

**Table 54-2 Child-Pugh Classification**

| | No. of Points | | |
|---|---|---|---|
| **FACTOR** | **1** | **2** | **3** |
| Bilirubin (mg/dL) | <2 | 2-3 | >3 |
| Albumin (g/dL) | >3.5 | 2.8-3.5 | <2.8 |
| Prothrombin time (increased seconds) | 1-3 | 4-6 | >6 |
| Ascites | None | Slight | Moderate |
| Encephalopathy | None | Minimal | Advanced |

Class A, 5-6 points; class B, 7-9 points; class C, 10-15 points.

## PORTAL HYPERTENSION

At present, effective treatments for cirrhosis are nonexistent. As a result, its treatment has largely been focused on the treatment of portal hypertension and its complications. The major challenge for the hepatologist and/or surgeon who is treating patients with cirrhosis and end-stage liver disease is determining when definitive treatment (e.g., liver transplantation) rather than palliative treatment (e.g., interventions to prevent recurrent variceal hemorrhage) should be applied.

### Definition

As noted, the liver has a dual blood supply from the portal vein and hepatic artery. Hepatic blood flow averages 1500 mL/minute. This represents approximately 25% of the cardiac output. The portal vein contributes two thirds of the total hepatic blood flow, whereas hepatic arterial perfusion accounts for more than 50% of the liver's oxygen supply. The volume of portal venous flow is indirectly regulated by vasoconstriction and vasodilation of the splanchnic arterial bed. In contrast, hepatic arterioles respond to circulating catecholamines and sympathetic nervous stimulation; thus, hepatic arterial flow is regulated directly.

Portal hypertension is defined by a portal pressure higher than 5 mm Hg. However, higher pressures (8 to 10 mm Hg) are typically required to begin stimulating the development of portosystemic collateralization. Collateral vessels usually develop where the portal and systemic venous circulations are in close proximity (Fig. 54-18). The collateral network through the

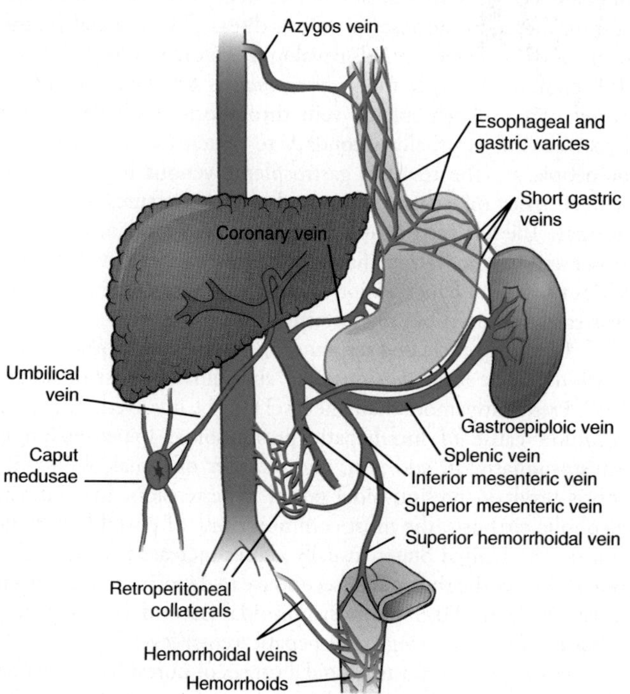


**FIGURE 54-18** Portosystemic collateral pathways develop where the portal venous and systemic venous systems are in close apposition. (From Rikkers LF: Portal hypertension. In Miller TA [ed]: Physiologic basis of modern surgical care, St Louis, 1988, Mosby, pp 417–428.)

coronary and short gastric veins to the azygos vein is clinically the most important because it results in formation of esophagogastric varices. However, other sites include a recanalized umbilical vein from the left portal vein to the epigastric venous system (caput medusae), retroperitoneal collateral vessels, and the hemorrhoidal venous plexus. In addition to extrahepatic collateral vessels, a significant fraction of portal venous flow passes through anatomic and physiologic (e.g., capillarization of hepatic sinusoids) intrahepatic shunts. As hepatic portal perfusion decreases, hepatic arterial flow generally increases (buffer response).[3]

## Pathophysiology

Portal hypertension usually occurs because of increased portal venous resistance that is prehepatic, intrahepatic, or posthepatic in location. Several factors may contribute to this, including the following: (1) increased passive resistance secondary to fibrosis and regenerative nodules; (2) increased hepatic vascular resistance caused by active vasoconstriction by norepinephrine, endothelin, and other humoral vasoconstrictors; (3) increased portal venous inflow secondary to a hyperdynamic systemic circulation and splanchnic hyperemia. The last one is a major contributor to the maintenance of portal hypertension as portal systemic collaterals develop. Unfortunately, the exact causes remain unknown, but splanchnic hormones, decreased sensitivity of the splanchnic vasculature to catecholamines, and increased production of nitrous oxide and prostacyclin may be involved. Understanding the pathophysiology of portal hypertension may have therapeutic implications because these factors may represent targets for treatment.

The most common cause of prehepatic portal hypertension is portal vein thrombosis. This accounts for approximately 50% of cases of portal hypertension in children. When the portal vein is thrombosed in the absence of liver disease, hepatopetal (to the liver) portal collateral vessels develop to restore portal perfusion. This combination is termed *cavernomatous transformation of the portal vein.* Isolated splenic vein thrombosis (left-sided portal hypertension) is usually secondary to pancreatic inflammation or neoplasm. The result is gastrosplenic venous hypertension, with superior mesenteric and portal venous pressures remaining normal. The left gastroepiploic vein becomes a major collateral vessel and gastric, rather than esophageal, varices develop. This variant of portal hypertension is important to recognize because it is easily reversed by splenectomy alone.

The site of increased resistance in intrahepatic portal hypertension may be at the presinusoidal, sinusoidal, or postsinusoidal level. Frequently, more than one level may be involved. The most common cause of intrahepatic presinusoidal hypertension is schistosomiasis. In addition, many causes of nonalcoholic cirrhosis result in presinusoidal portal hypertension. In contrast, alcoholic cirrhosis, the most common cause of portal hypertension in the United States, usually causes increased resistance to portal flow at the sinusoidal (secondary to deposition of collagen in the space of Disse) and postsinusoidal (secondary to regenerating nodules distorting small hepatic veins) levels.

Posthepatic or postsinusoidal causes of portal hypertension are rare; they include Budd-Chiari syndrome (hepatic vein thrombosis), constrictive pericarditis, and heart failure. Rarely, increased portal venous flow alone, secondary to massive splenomegaly (e.g., idiopathic portal hypertension) or a splanchnic arteriovenous fistula, causes portal hypertension.

## Assessment of Chronic Liver Disease and Portal Hypertension

The key aspects of assessing a patient with suspected chronic liver disease or complications of portal hypertension are the following: (1) diagnosis of the underlying liver disease; (2) estimation of functional hepatic reserve; (3) definition of portal venous anatomy and hepatic hemodynamic evaluation; and (4) identification of the site of upper gastrointestinal hemorrhage, if present. These diagnostic categories take on varying degrees of importance, depending on the clinical situation. For example, estimation of functional hepatic reserve is useful in determining the risk associated with therapeutic intervention and whether definitive (e.g., hepatic transplantation) or palliative (e.g., endoscopic variceal ligation or a shunt procedure) treatment is indicated.

## Variceal Hemorrhage

Bleeding from esophagogastric varices is the single most life-threatening complication of portal hypertension. It is responsible for approximately one third of all deaths in patients with cirrhosis. Approximately 50% of these deaths are caused by uncontrolled bleeding. The risk for death from bleeding is mainly related to the underlying hepatic functional reserve. Patients with extrahepatic portal venous obstruction and normal hepatic function rarely die of bleeding varices, whereas those with decompensated cirrhosis (e.g., Child-Pugh class C) may face a mortality rate in excess of 50%. Once controlled, the greatest risk for rebleeding from varices is within the first few days after the onset of hemorrhage; the risk declines rapidly between that point and 6 weeks. Subsequently, the risk returns to the prehemorrhage rate.

### Treatment

Therapy for portal hypertension and variceal bleeding has evolved over time and now encompasses a spectrum of treatment modalities, in which sequential therapies are often necessary.[4,5] Nonoperative treatments are generally preferred for acutely bleeding patients; they are often high operative risks because of decompensated hepatic function. However, only treatment associated with minimal morbidity and mortality should be considered for prophylaxis because approximately two thirds of patients with varices will never bleed.

Emergency treatment should be nonoperative whenever possible. Endoscopic treatment (e.g., sclerosis or ligation) has become the mainstay of nonoperative treatment of acute hemorrhage because bleeding can be controlled in more than 85% of patients. This allows for an interval of medical management for improvement of hepatic function, resolution of ascites and encephalopathy, and enhancement of nutrition before definitive treatment for prevention of recurrent bleeding is instituted. Pharmacotherapy can also be initiated and trials have suggested that it may be as effective as endoscopic treatment. Balloon tamponade, which is infrequently used, can be lifesaving in patients with exsanguinating hemorrhage when other nonoperative methods are not successful. A transjugular intrahepatic portosystemic shunt (TIPS) is another treatment option whereby a percutaneously connection is created within the liver, between the portal and systemic circulations, to reduce portal pressure in patients with complications related to portal hypertension. TIPS has replaced operative shunts for managing acute variceal bleeding when pharmacotherapy and endoscopic treatment fail to control bleeding. As a result, emergency surgical intervention in most centers is reserved for select patients who are not TIPS candidates.

**Pharmacotherapy** Medical therapy should be initiated at the onset of variceal bleeding. Because infections are common in patients with variceal bleeding, antibiotic prophylactic should be initiated. This has been shown to decrease the infection rate by over 50%, decrease rebleeding, and improve survival. Randomized trials have also shown that somatostatin, and its longer acting analogue octreotide, are as efficacious as endoscopic treatment for control of acute variceal bleeding. Because of the minimal adverse effects and ease of administration, octreotide is now commonly used as an adjunct to endoscopic therapy. In fact, the combination of octreotide and endoscopic therapy is more effective in controlling bleeding than octreotide alone and is the preferred treatment for most patients. In severe cases of hemorrhage, vasopressin can be used to diminish splanchnic blood flow. However, because of the adverse systemic effects of vasopressin, nitroglycerin should be simultaneously infused and then titrated to achieve blood pressure control.

**Variceal Tamponade** Controlled trials have demonstrated that balloon tamponade is as effective as pharmacotherapy and endoscopic therapy in controlling acute variceal bleeding. The major advantages of variceal tamponade using the Sengstaken-Blakemore tube are immediate cessation of bleeding in more than 85% of patients, as well as widespread availability of this device (Fig. 54-19). However, there are also significant disadvantages of balloon tamponade, including frequent recurrent hemorrhage in up to 50% of patients after balloon deflation, considerable discomfort for the patient, and a high incidence of serious complications when used incorrectly by an inexperienced health care provider.

**Interventional Approaches** In most institutions, TIPS has become the preferred treatment for acute variceal bleeding when pharmacotherapy and endoscopic treatment fail.

**Operative Approaches** Operative procedures are typically reserved for those situations in which TIPS is not indicated or is not available. Selection of the appropriate emergency operation should mainly be guided by the experience of the surgeon. Although nonoperative therapies are effective in most patients with acute variceal bleeding, an emergency operation should be promptly carried out when less invasive measures fail to control hemorrhage or are not indicated. The most common situations requiring urgent or emergency surgery are failure of acute endoscopic treatment, failure of long-term endoscopic therapy, hemorrhage from gastric varices or portal hypertensive gastropathy, and failure of TIPS placement.

Esophageal transection with a stapling device is rapid and relatively simple, but rebleeding rates after this procedure are high. Moreover, there is little evidence that operative mortality rates are lower than after surgical portal decompression.

A commonly performed shunt operation in the emergency setting is the portacaval shunt because it rapidly and effectively decompresses the portal venous circulation. Impressive results have been achieved by Orloff and colleagues,[6] but not by others, when an emergency portacaval shunt is used as routine therapy

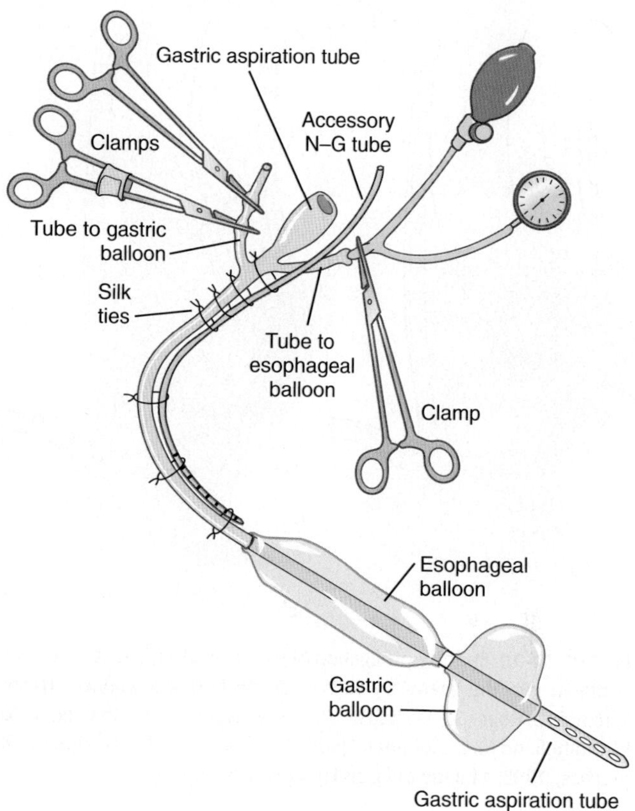


**FIGURE 54-19** Modified Sengstaken-Blakemore tube. Note the accessory nasogastric tube for suctioning of secretions above the esophageal balloon and the two clamps, one secured with tape, to prevent inadvertent decompression of the gastric balloon. (From Rikkers LF: Portal hypertension. In Goldsmith H [ed]: Practice of surgery, Philadelphia, 1981, Harper & Row, pp 1–37.)

for acute variceal bleeding. In patients who are not actively bleeding at the time of surgery and those in whom bleeding is temporarily controlled by pharmacotherapy or balloon tamponade, a more complex operation, such as the distal splenorenal shunt, may be appropriate. The major disadvantage of emergency surgery is that operative mortality rates exceed 25% in most reported series. Early postoperative mortality is usually related to the status of hepatic functional reserve rather than to the type of emergency operation selected.

### Prevention of Recurrent Variceal Hemorrhage

After a patient has bled from varices, the likelihood of a repeat episode exceeds 70%. Because most patients with variceal hemorrhage have chronic liver disease, the challenge of long-term management is prevention of recurrent bleeding and maintenance of satisfactory hepatic function. Options available for definitive treatment include pharmacotherapy, chronic endoscopic treatment, TIPS, shunt operations (e.g., nonselective, selective, partial), various nonshunt procedures, and liver transplantation. The most effective treatment regimen usually requires two or more of these therapies in sequence. In most centers, initial treatment consists of pharmacotherapy or endoscopic therapy with portal decompression by means of TIPS or an operative shunt reserved for failures of first-line treatment.

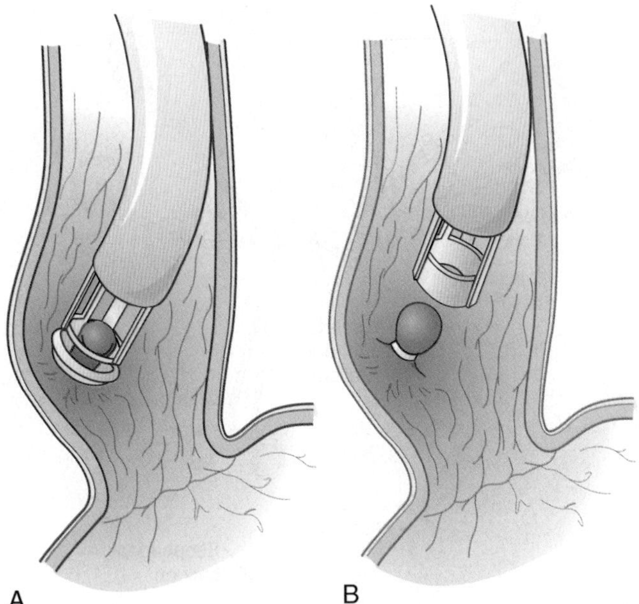


**FIGURE 54-20** Endoscopic ligation of esophageal varices. **A,** The varix is drawn into the ligator by suction. **B,** An O ring is applied. (From Turcotte JG, Roger SE, Eckhauser FE: Portal hypertension. In Greenfield LJ, Mulholland MW, Oldham KT [eds]: Surgery: Scientific principles and practice, 1993, Philadelphia, JB Lippincott, p 899.)

Hepatic transplantation is used for patients with end-stage liver disease.

**Pharmacotherapy** A meta-analysis of controlled trials of nonselective β-adrenergic blockade has shown that this treatment significantly decreases the likelihood of recurrent hemorrhage and demonstrates a trend toward decreased mortality.[7] The combination of a beta blocker and long-acting nitrate (e.g., isosorbide 5-mononitrate) has been shown to be more effective than variceal ligation.[8] Combination therapy is also more effective than beta blockade alone. Long-term pharmacotherapy should be used only in compliant patients who are observed closely by their physician.

**Endoscopic Therapy** Several controlled trials and a meta-analysis comparing endoscopic sclerotherapy to variceal ligation have shown a significant advantage to the latter technique. Complications are less frequent after variceal ligation, and fewer treatment sessions are required to eradicate varices (Fig. 54-20). Also, rebleeding and mortality rates appear to be lower following variceal ligation. The combination of variceal ligation and pharmacotherapy with nonselective beta blockade is more effective than variceal ligation alone.[9]

Several controlled trials comparing chronic endoscopic therapy to conventional medical management have been completed. Although fewer patients receiving endoscopic treatment than medical treatment experienced rebleeding in all the investigations, recurrent bleeding still occurred in approximately 50% of endoscopic therapy patients. Rebleeding is most frequent during the initial year. Rebleeding rate decreases by about 15% annually thereafter. Although a single episode of recurrent hemorrhage does not signify failure of therapy, uncontrolled hemorrhage, multiple major episodes of rebleeding, and hemorrhage from gastric varices and hypertensive gastropathy all require that endoscopic therapy be abandoned and another treatment modality substituted. Endoscopic treatment failure secondary to rebleeding occurs in as many as one third of patients. Thus, chronic endoscopic therapy is a rational initial treatment for many patients who bleed from esophageal varices, but subsequent treatment with TIPS, a shunt procedure, a nonshunt operation, or liver transplantation should be anticipated for a significant percentage of patients. Because of its relatively high failure rate, a course of chronic endoscopic therapy should not be undertaken for noncompliant patients and those living a long distance from advanced medical care.

**Interventional Therapy** TIPS is being increasingly used as a definitive treatment for patients who bleed from portal hypertension (Fig. 54-21). A major limitation of TIPS, however, is a high incidence (up to 50%) of shunt stenosis or shunt thrombosis within the first year. Shunt stenosis, which is usually secondary to neointimal hyperplasia, is more common than thrombosis and can often be resolved by balloon dilation of the TIPS or, in some cases, by placement of a second shunt. Total shunt occlusion occurs in 10% to 15% of patients. Shunt stenosis and shunt thrombosis are often followed by recurrent portal hypertensive bleeding. TIPS stenosis and occlusion may become less frequent as TIPS technology improves (e.g., covered stents).

TIPS has been compared with chronic endoscopic therapy in 11 randomized controlled trials. Fewer patients rebled after TIPS (19%) than following endoscopic treatment (47%), but encephalopathy was significantly more common in TIPS patients (34%). TIPS dysfunction developed in 50% of patients. The major advantage of TIPS is that it is a nonoperative approach. Thus, it would appear to be the ideal therapy when only short-term portal decompression is required. Liver transplantation candidates who fail endoscopic and/or pharmacotherapy are therefore well suited for TIPS followed by transplantation when a donor organ becomes available. As a result, the patient is protected from bleeding in the interim, and the transplantation procedure may be facilitated by the lower portal pressure. Another group of patients in whom TIPS may be advantageous includes those with advanced hepatic functional decompensation who are unlikely to survive long enough for the TIPS to malfunction. Because it functions as a side-to-side portosystemic shunt, TIPS is also effective for the treatment of medically intractable ascites.

**Surgical Therapy** Portosystemic shunts are clearly the most effective means of preventing recurrent hemorrhage in patients with portal hypertension. These procedures are effective because they all decompress the portal venous system to varying degrees by shunting portal flow into the lower pressure systemic venous system. However, diversion of portal blood, which contains hepatotropic hormones, nutrients, and cerebral toxins is also responsible for the adverse consequences of shunt operations—namely, portosystemic encephalopathy and accelerated hepatic failure. Depending on whether they completely decompress, compartmentalize, or partially decompress the portal venous circulation, portosystemic shunts can be classified as nonselective, selective, or partial. In addition to variceal decompression, selective and partial portosystemic shunts also aim to preserve

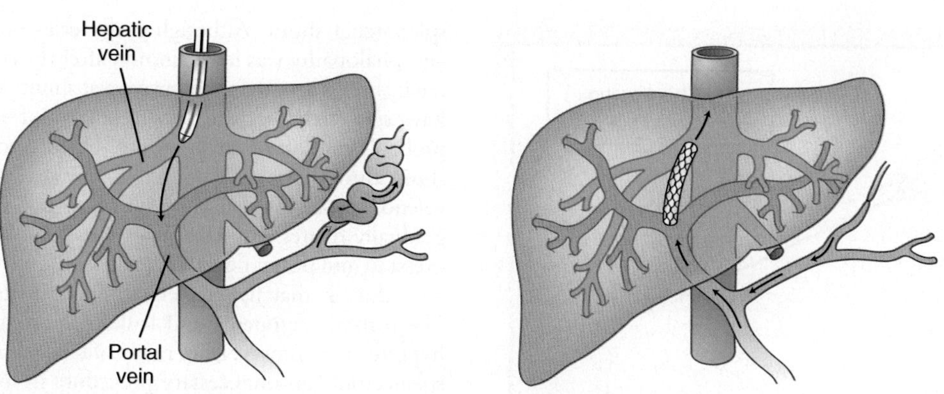


**FIGURE 54-21** Hepatocyte. Intracellular organelles are depicted. The endothelial-lined sinusoids on two sides of the cell are seen. In between the microvilli of the plasma membrane of the hepatocyte and the sinusoids, the extracellular fluid space of Disse is demonstrated. Along the lateral intercellular plasma membrane, bile canaliculi are formed by the apposing cells where microvilli extend into the canaliculus. Envisioning the cell in three dimensions, the bile canaliculi form a ring around each hepatocyte.

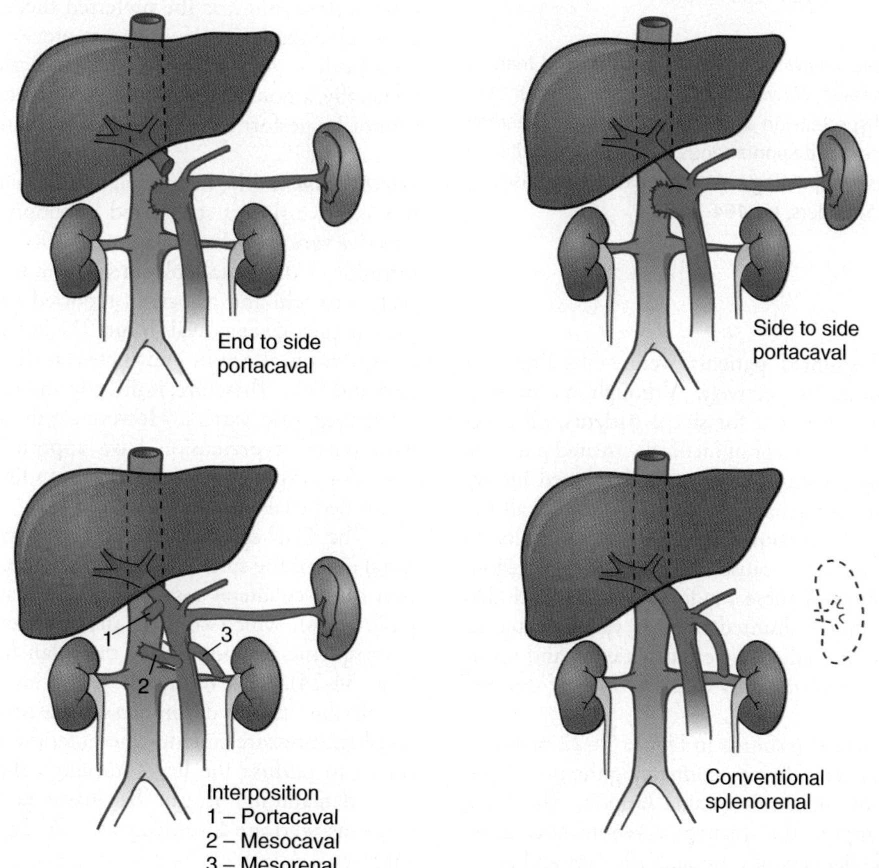


**FIGURE 54-22** Nonselective shunts completely divert portal blood flow away from the liver. (From Rikkers LF: Portal hypertension. In Moody FG, Carey LC, Scott Jones RS, et al [eds]: Surgical treatment of digestive disease, Chicago, 1986, Year Book Medical, pp 409–424.)

of hepatic portal perfusion and therefore prevent or minimize the adverse consequences of these procedures.

***Nonselective Shunts*** Commonly used nonselective shunts, all of which completely divert portal flow, include the end-to-side portacaval shunt (Eck fistula), side-to-side portacaval shunt, large-diameter interposition shunts, and conventional splenorenal shunt (Fig. 54-22). The end-to-side portacaval shunt is the prototype of nonselective shunts and is the only shunt procedure that has been compared with conventional medical treatment in randomized controlled trials. Figure 54-23 combines survival data from four controlled investigations of the therapeutic portacaval shunt, performed in patients with prior variceal hemorrhage. The most common causes of death in

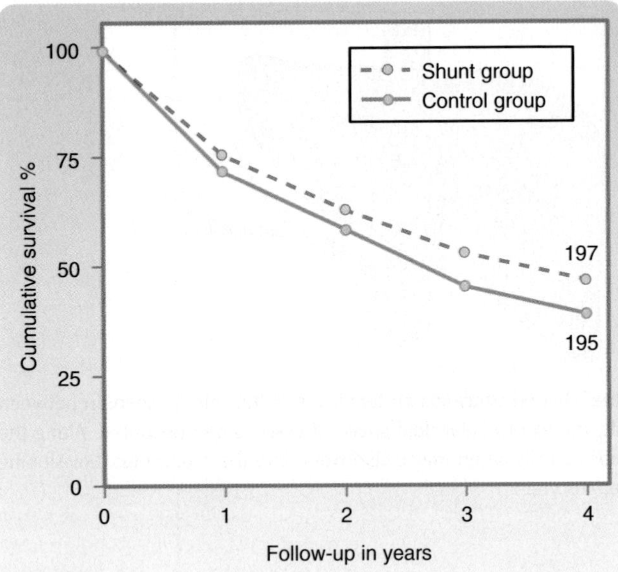


**FIGURE 54-23** Cumulative survival data from four controlled trials of the portacaval shunt versus conventional medical management. (From Boyer TD: Portal hypertension and its complications: Bleeding esophageal varices, ascites, and spontaneous bacterial peritonitis. In Zakim D, Boyer TD [eds]: Hepatology: A textbook of liver disease, Philadelphia, 1982, WB Saunders, pp 464–499.)

medically treated and shunted patients were rebleeding and accelerated hepatic failure, respectively. Although no survival advantage could be demonstrated for shunt patients, all these studies had a crossover bias in favor of medically treated patients, several of whom received a shunt when they developed intractable recurrent variceal hemorrhage. In addition, almost all the trial patients had alcoholic cirrhosis; therefore, these results do not necessarily apply to other causes of portal hypertension. Other important findings of these randomized trials included reliable control of bleeding in shunted patients, variceal rebleeding in more than 70% of medically treated patients, and spontaneous, often severe, encephalopathy in 20 to 40% of shunted patients.

All the other nonselective shunts in Figure 54-22 maintain continuity of the portal vein, thereby connecting the portal and systemic venous systems in a side-to-side fashion. Therefore, these procedures decompress the splanchnic venous circulation and intrahepatic sinusoidal network. Because the liver and intestines are both important contributors to ascites formation, side-to-side portosystemic shunts are the most effective shunt procedures for relieving ascites as well as preventing recurrent variceal bleeding. Because they completely divert portal flow, like the end-to-side portacaval shunt, however, side-to-side shunts also accelerate hepatic failure and lead to frequent postshunt encephalopathy.

The conventional splenorenal shunt consists of anastomosis of the proximal splenic vein to the renal vein. Splenectomy is also performed. Because the smaller proximal rather than the larger distal end of the splenic vein is used, shunt thrombosis is more common after this procedure than after the distal splenorenal shunt. Although early series noted that postshunt encephalopathy was less common after the conventional splenorenal shunt than after the portacaval shunt, subsequent analyses have suggested that this low frequency of encephalopathy was probably a result of restoration of hepatic portal perfusion after shunt thrombosis developed in many patients. A conventional splenorenal shunt that is of sufficient caliber to remain patent gradually dilates and eventually causes complete portal decompression and portal flow diversion. A purported advantage of the procedure is that hypersplenism is eliminated by splenectomy. The thrombocytopenia and leukopenia that accompany portal hypertension, however, are rarely of clinical significance, making splenectomy an unnecessary procedure in most patients.

In summary, nonselective shunts effectively decompress varices. Because of complete portal flow diversion, however, they are complicated by frequent postoperative encephalopathy and accelerated hepatic failure. Side-to-side nonselective shunts effectively relieve ascites and prevent variceal hemorrhage. Presently, nonselective shunts are only rarely indicated. TIPS, also a nonselective shunt, is the preferred therapy for most situations in which nonselective shunts were previously used (e.g., patients with both variceal bleeding and medically intractable ascites). Generally, a nonselective shunt is constructed only when a TIPS cannot be performed or when a TIPS fails.

***Selective Shunts*** The hemodynamic and clinical shortcomings of nonselective shunts stimulated development of the concept of selective variceal decompression. In 1967, Warren and colleagues introduced the distal splenorenal shunt and, in the following year, Inokuchi and associates reported their initial results with the left gastric vena caval shunt. The latter procedure consists of interposition of a vein graft between the left gastric (coronary) vein and IVC. Therefore, it directly and selectively decompresses esophagogastric varices. However, only a minority of patients with portal hypertension have appropriate anatomy for this operation; experience with it has been limited to Japan, and no controlled trials have been conducted.

The distal splenorenal shunt consists of anastomosis of the distal end of the splenic vein to the left renal vein and interruption of all collateral vessels (e.g., coronary vein and gastroepiploic veins), which connect the superior mesenteric vein and gastrosplenic components of the splanchnic venous circulation (Fig. 54-24). This results in separation of the portal venous circulation into a decompressed gastrosplenic venous circuit and high-pressure superior mesenteric venous system that continues to perfuse the liver. Although the procedure is technically demanding, it can be mastered by most well-trained surgeons who are knowledgeable in the principles of vascular surgery.

Not all patients are candidates for the distal splenorenal shunt. Because sinusoidal and mesenteric hypertension is maintained and important lymphatic pathways are transected during dissection of the left renal vein, the distal splenorenal shunt tends to aggravate rather than relieve ascites. Thus, patients with medically intractable ascites should not undergo this procedure. However, the larger population of patients who develop transient ascites after resuscitation from a variceal hemorrhage are candidates for a selective shunt. Another contraindication to a distal splenorenal shunt is prior splenectomy. A splenic vein diameter less than 7 mm is a relative contraindication to the procedure because the incidence of shunt thrombosis is high

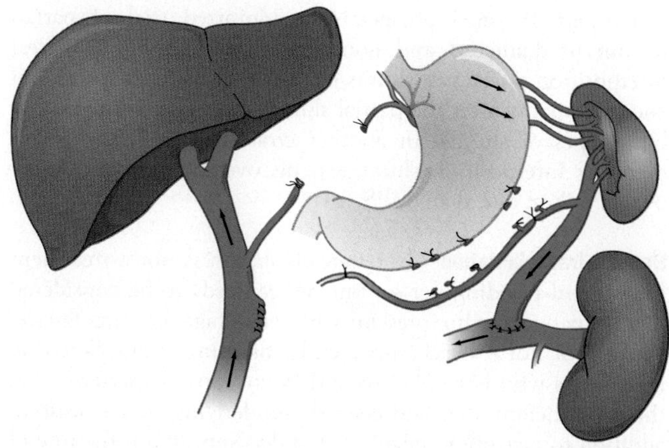

**FIGURE 54-24** The distal splenorenal shunt provides selective variceal decompression through the short gastric veins, spleen, and splenic vein to the left renal vein. Hepatic portal perfusion is maintained by interrupting the umbilical vein, coronary vein, gastroepiploic vein, and any other prominent collaterals. (From Salam AA: Distal splenorenal shunts: Hemodynamics of total versus selective shunting. In Baker RJ, Fischer JE [eds]: Mastery of surgery, ed 4, Philadelphia, 2001, Lippincott Williams & Wilkins, pp 1357–1366.)

when using a small-diameter vein. Although selective variceal decompression is a sound physiologic concept, the distal splenorenal shunt remains controversial after an extensive clinical experience spanning almost 40 years.

Although the distal splenorenal shunt results in portal flow preservation in more than 85% of patients during the early postoperative interval, the high-pressure mesenteric venous system gradually collateralizes to the low-pressure shunt, resulting in loss of portal flow in approximately 50% of patients by 1 year. The degree and duration of portal flow preservation depend on the cause of portal hypertension and the technical details of the operation, the extent to which mesenteric and gastrosplenic venous circulations are separated. Although portal flow is maintained in most patients with nonalcoholic cirrhosis and noncirrhotic portal hypertension (e.g., portal vein thrombosis), portal flow rapidly collateralizes to the shunt in patients with alcoholic cirrhosis.

Modification of the distal splenorenal shunt by purposeful or inadvertent omission of coronary vein ligation results in early loss of portal flow. Even when all major collateral vessels are interrupted, portal flow may be gradually diverted through a pancreatic collateral network (pancreatic siphon). This pathway can be discouraged by dissecting the full length of the splenic vein from the pancreas, splenopancreatic disconnection, which results in better preservation of hepatic portal perfusion, especially in patients with alcoholic cirrhosis. However, this extension of the procedure makes it technically more challenging and a significant disadvantage in an era when fewer shunts are being done because of increased use of endoscopic therapy, TIPS, and liver transplantation.

Six of the seven controlled comparisons of the distal splenorenal shunt to nonselective shunts have included predominantly alcoholic cirrhotic patients. None of these trials has demonstrated an advantage to either procedure with respect to long-term survival. Three of the studies found a lower frequency of encephalopathy after the distal splenorenal shunt, whereas the other trials showed no difference in the incidence of this postoperative complication. In contrast to survival, encephalopathy is a subjective end point that was assessed with various methods in the trials. Another important end point in comparing treatments for variceal hemorrhage was the effectiveness with which recurrent bleeding was prevented. In almost all uncontrolled and controlled series of the distal splenorenal shunt, this procedure was equivalent to nonselective shunts in preventing recurrent hemorrhage. Mainly because of these inconsistent results of the controlled trials, there is no consensus as to which shunting procedure is superior in patients with alcoholic cirrhosis. Because the quality of life (e.g., lower encephalopathy rate) was significantly better in the distal splenorenal shunt group in three of the trials, there appears to be an advantage to selective variceal decompression, even in this population.

Considerably less data are available regarding selective shunting in nonalcoholic cirrhosis and noncirrhotic portal hypertension. Because hepatic portal perfusion after the distal splenorenal shunt is better preserved in these disease categories, one might expect improved results. A single controlled trial in patients with schistosomiasis (presinusoidal portal hypertension) has demonstrated a lower frequency of encephalopathy after the distal splenorenal shunt than after a conventional splenorenal shunt (nonselective). Another large series from Emory University has shown that distal splenorenal shunt is associated with better survival in patients with nonalcoholic cirrhosis than in those with alcoholic cirrhosis. However, this has not been a consistent finding in all centers in which the distal splenorenal shunts have been performed.

Several controlled trials have also compared the distal splenorenal shunt with chronic endoscopic therapy. In these investigations, recurrent hemorrhage was more effectively prevented by selective shunting than by sclerotherapy. However, hepatic portal perfusion was maintained in a significantly higher fraction of patients undergoing sclerotherapy. Despite this hemodynamic advantage, encephalopathy rates were similar after both therapies.

The two North American trials were dissimilar with respect to the effect of these treatments on long-term survival. Sclerotherapy with surgical rescue for the one third of sclerotherapy failures resulted in significantly better survival than selective shunt alone, whereas 85% of sclerotherapy failures could be salvaged by surgery. In contrast, a similar investigation conducted in a sparsely populated area (Intermountain West and Plains) showed superior survival after the distal splenorenal shunt. Only 31% of sclerotherapy failures could be salvaged by surgery in this trial. The survival results of these two studies suggest that endoscopic therapy is a rational initial treatment for patients who bleed from varices if sclerotherapy failure is recognized and these patients promptly undergo surgery or TIPS. However, patients living in remote areas are less likely to be salvaged by shunt surgery when endoscopic treatment fails, and therefore a selective shunt may be preferable initial treatment for such patients.

In one nonrandomized comparison to TIPS, the distal splenorenal shunt had lower rates of recurrent bleeding, encephalopathy, and shunt thrombosis. Ascites was less prevalent after TIPS. A multicenter randomized trial comparing TIPS and the distal splenorenal shunt for the elective treatment of variceal bleeding in good-risk cirrhotic patients has shown generally equivalent results for these two procedures. Rebleeding rates were not significantly different between the distal splenorenal shunt (6%) and TIPS (11%), but this represents the lowest reported rate of rebleeding following TIPS. This was likely secondary to meticulous surveillance of TIPS patency by duplex ultrasound and angiography. Frequent re-intervention in TIPS patients (82% compared with 11% for distal splenorenal shunt patients) was necessary to achieve these results. In this trial, post-shunt encephalopathy and survival were similar after the two procedures.

***Partial Shunts*** The objectives of partial and selective shunts are the same: (1) effective decompression of varices; (2) preservation of hepatic portal perfusion; and (3) maintenance of some residual portal hypertension. Initial attempts at partial shunting consisted of small-diameter vein to vein anastomoses. In general, these thrombosed or dilated with time and thereby became nonselective shunts.

More recently, a small-diameter interposition portacaval shunt using a polytetrafluoroethylene (PTFE) graft, combined with ligation of the coronary vein and other collateral vessels, was described (Fig. 54-25). When the prosthetic graft is 10 mm or less in diameter, hepatic portal perfusion is preserved in most patients, at least during the early postoperative interval. Early experience with this small-diameter prosthetic shunt is that fewer than 15% of shunts have thrombosed, and most of these have been successfully opened by interventional radiologic techniques. A small prospective randomized trial of partial (8 mm in diameter) and nonselective (16 mm in diameter) interposition portacaval shunts has shown a lower frequency of encephalopathy after the partial shunt but similar survival after both types of shunts. In another controlled trial, the small-diameter interposition shunt was discovered to have a lower overall failure rate than TIPS.

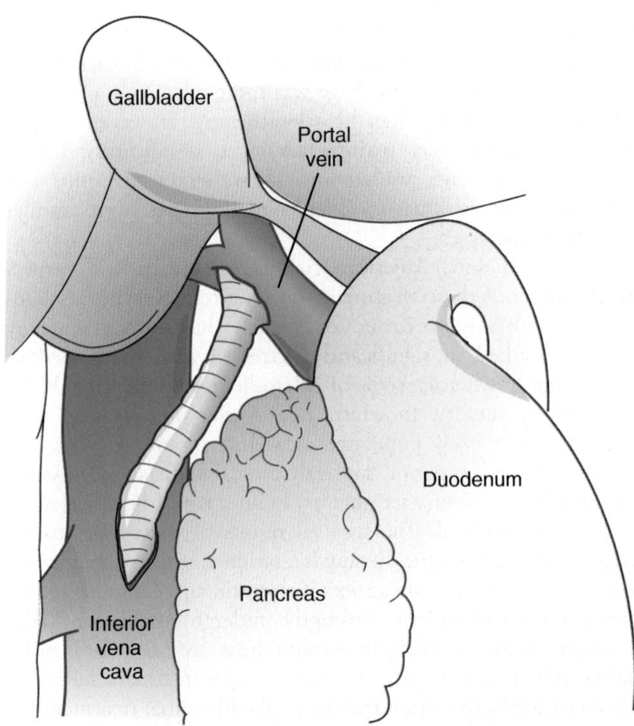


**FIGURE 54-25** A small-diameter (8 to 10 mm) interposition portacaval shunt partially decompresses the portal venous system and may preserve hepatic portal perfusion. (From Sarfeh IJ, Rypins EB, Mason GR: A systematic appraisal of portacaval H-graft diameters: Clinical and hemodynamic perspectives. Ann Surg 204:356–363, 1986.)

**Hepatic Transplantation** Liver transplantation is not a treatment for variceal bleeding per se, but rather needs to be considered for all patients who present with end-stage hepatic failure, whether or not it is accompanied by bleeding. Transplantation in patients who have bled secondary to portal hypertension is the only therapy that addresses the underlying liver disease in addition to providing reliable portal decompression. Because of economic factors and a limited supply of donor organs, liver transplantation is not available to all patients. Also, transplantation is not indicated for some of the more common causes of variceal bleeding, such as schistosomiasis (normal liver function) and active alcoholism (noncompliance).

There is accumulating evidence that variceal bleeders with well-compensated hepatic functional reserve (Child-Pugh class A and B+) are initially better served by nontransplantation strategies. The first-line treatment for such patients should be pharmacologic and endoscopic therapy. For those who fail first-line therapy, an operative shunt or TIPS can be performed. These can also be applied under circumstances in which pharmacologic or endoscopic treatment would be risky, such as patients with gastric varices and those geographically separated from tertiary medical care.

Patients with variceal bleeding who are transplantation candidates include nonalcoholic cirrhotic patients and abstinent alcoholic cirrhotic patients with limited hepatic functional reserve (Child-Pugh class B and C) or a poor quality of life secondary to their disease (e.g., encephalopathy, fatigue, bone pain). In these patients, the acute hemorrhage should be treated with endoscopic therapy and pharmacotherapy and the patient's transplantation candidacy immediately activated. If endoscopic treatment and pharmacotherapy are ineffective, a TIPS should be inserted as a short-term bridge to transplantation.

If a nontransplantation procedure (e.g., operative shunt or TIPS) is performed initially, these patients should be carefully assessed at regular intervals of 6 to 12 months. Hepatic transplantation should be considered when other complications of cirrhosis develop or hepatic functional decompensation is evident clinically or by careful assessment with quantitative LFTs.

### Algorithm for Management of Variceal Hemorrhage

In summary, an algorithm for definitive management of variceal hemorrhage is shown in Figure 54-26. Patients are first grouped according to their transplantation candidacy. This decision is based on a number of factors, including cause of portal hypertension, abstinence for alcoholic cirrhotic patients, presence or absence of other diseases, and physiologic rather than chronologic age. Transplantation candidates with decompensated hepatic function or a poor quality of life secondary to their liver disease should undergo transplantation as soon as possible.

Most future transplantation and nontransplantation candidates should undergo initial endoscopic treatment and/or pharmacotherapy unless they bleed from gastric varices or portal

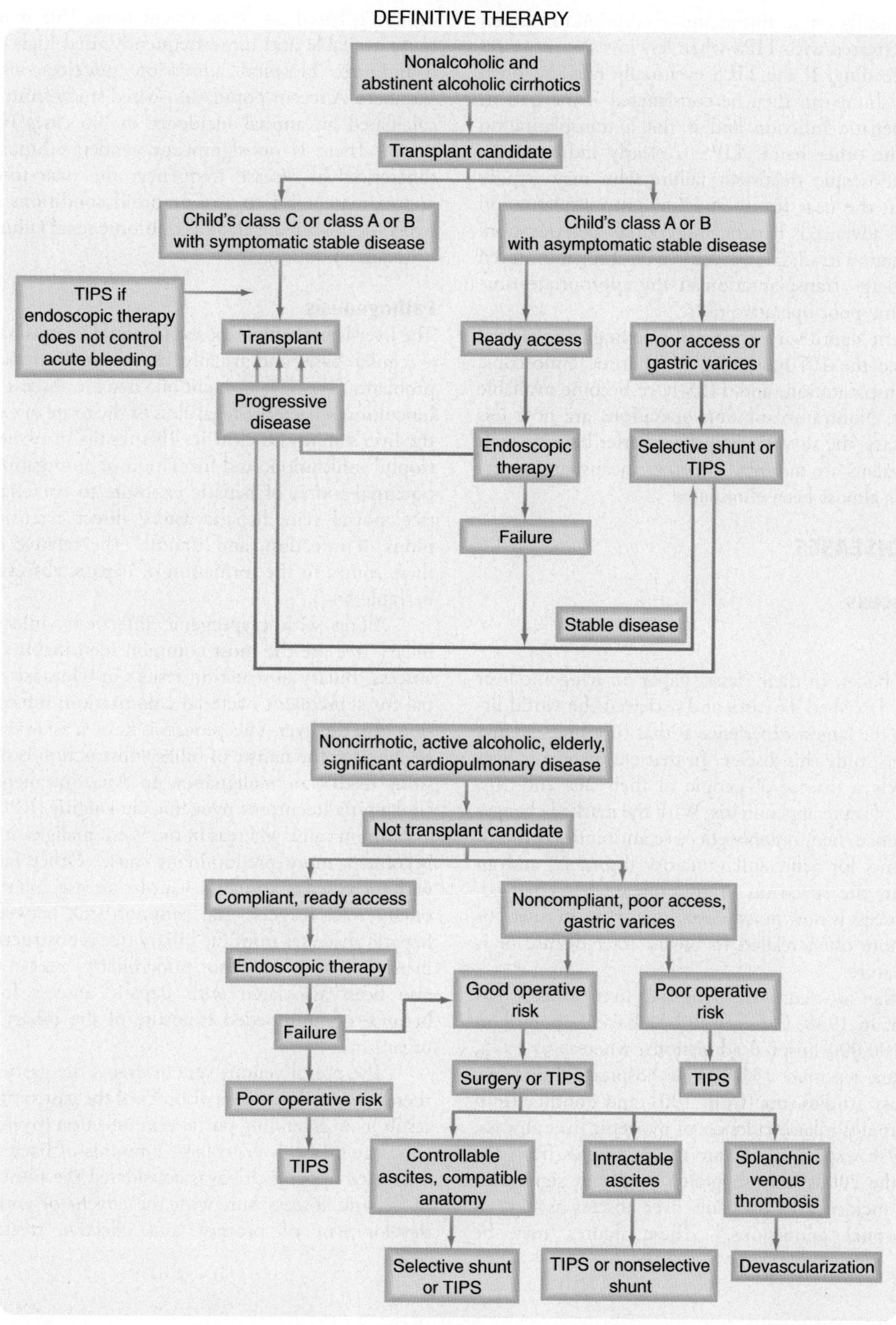


**FIGURE 54-26** Algorithm for definitive therapy of variceal hemorrhage (see text for details). (Adapted from Rikkers LF: Portal hypertension. In Levine BA, Copeland E, Howard R, et al [eds]: Current practice of surgery, vol 3, New York, 1995, Churchill Livingstone.)

hypertensive gastropathy or live in a remote geographic location and have limited access to emergency tertiary care. Patients who live in remote locations and those who fail endoscopic and drug therapy should receive a selective shunt or TIPS. A recent controlled trial has shown that if careful surveillance of TIPS patency and frequent TIPS re-interventions are done, these procedures are equally efficacious.

Until improvements in TIPS technology are fully realized, the distal splenorenal shunt is likely to remain a more durable long-term solution and a reasonable alternative for TIPS failure. However, a TIPS is more commonly done and few surgeons who are experienced in shunt surgery remain. Therefore, it is likely that operative shunts will play an even smaller role in the management of variceal bleeding in the future than they do now.

Patients with medically intractable ascites in addition to variceal bleeding are best treated with TIPS when less invasive measures fail to control bleeding. If the TIPS eventually fails, an open side-to-side type shunt can then be constructed if the patient has reasonable hepatic function and is not a transplantation candidate. On the other hand, TIPS is clearly indicated for patients with endoscopic treatment failure who may require transplantation in the near future and for nontransplantation candidates with advanced hepatic functional deterioration. Future transplantation candidates should be carefully monitored so that they undergo transplantation at the appropriate time before they become poor operative risks.

The treatment algorithm for variceal bleeding has changed considerably since the 1970s, during which time endoscopic therapy, liver transplantation, and TIPS have become available to these patients. Nontransplantation operations are now less frequently necessary, the survival results are better because high operative risk patients are managed by other means, and emergency surgery has almost been eliminated.

## INFECTIOUS DISEASES

### Pyogenic Abscess

#### Epidemiology

Ochsner and DeBakey, in their classic paper on pyogenic liver abscess in 1938, described 47 cases and reviewed the world literature. This was the largest experience at that time and the first serious attempt to study this disease. In that era, pyogenic liver abscess was largely a disease of people in their 20s and 30s, mostly the result of acute appendicitis. With the marked changes in medical care since then, notably effective antibiotics, prompt effective treatments for acute inflammatory disorders, and an aging population, the spectrum of this disease has changed. Pyogenic liver abscess is now mostly seen in patients in their 50s to 60s and is more often related to biliary tract disease or is cryptogenic in nature.

However, the incidence of pyogenic liver abscess has remained similar. In 1938, Ochsner and DeBakey reported an incidence of 8/100,000 hospital admissions, whereas in 1975, Pitt and Zuidema reported 13/100,000 hospital admissions. Two large autopsy studies, one from 1901 and another from 1960, have reported similar incidences of pyogenic liver abscess, 0.45% and 0.59% respectively. More recent studies from the 1980s through the 2000s have suggested small but significant increases in the incidence of pyogenic liver abscess as high as 22/100,000 hospital admissions.[10] These figures may be declining based on more recent data. This may reflect better, more available and more frequently used high quality imaging techniques. Hospital admission practices also affect these numbers. A recent population-based study from North America calculated an annual incidence of 3.6 cases/100,000 population.[11] There is no significant gender, ethnic, or geographic differences in disease frequency; the male-to-female ratio is approximately 1.5 to 1. Comorbid conditions associated with pyogenic abscess are cirrhosis, chronic renal failure, and a history of malignancy.

#### Pathogenesis

The liver is probably exposed to portal venous bacterial loads on a regular basis and usually clears this bacterial load without problems. The development of a hepatic abscess occurs when an inoculum of bacteria, regardless of the route of exposure, exceeds the liver's ability to clear it. This results in tissue invasion, neutrophil infiltration, and formation of an organized abscess. The potential routes of hepatic exposure to bacteria are the biliary tree, portal vein, hepatic artery, direct extension of a nearby nidus of infection, and trauma. The relative contribution of these routes to the formation of hepatic abscess is summarized in Table 54-3.

Along with cryptogenic infections, infections from the biliary tree are the most common identifiable cause of hepatic abscess. Biliary obstruction results in bile stasis with the potential for subsequent bacterial colonization, infection, and ascension into the liver. This process is known as *ascending suppurative cholangitis*. The nature of biliary obstruction is mostly related to stone disease or malignancy. In Asia, intrahepatic stones and cholangitis (recurrent pyogenic cholangitis [RPC]; see later) are a common cause whereas in the West, malignant obstruction has become a more predominant cause. Other factors associated with increased risk include Caroli's disease, biliary ascariasis, and biliary tract surgery. The common link between all causes of hepatic abscesses from the biliary tree is obstruction and bacteria in the biliary tract. Also, prior biliary-enteric anastomosis has also been associated with hepatic abscess formation, likely because of unimpeded exposure of the biliary tree to enteric organisms.

The portal venous system drains the gastrointestinal tract; therefore, any infectious disorder of the gastrointestinal tract can result in an ascending portal vein infection (pyelophlebitis), with exposure of the liver to large amounts of bacteria. Historically, untreated appendicitis was considered the most common cause of hepatic abscess but, with the advent of antibiotics and the development of prompt and effective treatment of acute

**Table 54-3 Pyogenic Abscesses Attributable to Specific Cause (%)**

| | | Cause | | | | | |
|---|---|---|---|---|---|---|---|
| YEAR OF REPORT | NO. OF PATIENTS | PORTAL VEIN | HEPATIC ARTERY | BILIARY TREE | DIRECT EXTENSION | TRAUMA | CRYPTOGENIC |
| 1927-1938: One study* | 622 | 42 | — | — | 17 | 4 | 20 |
| 1945-1982: Eight studies | 521 | 17 | 9 | 38 | 10 | 4 | 16 |
| 1970-1999: Eight studies | 1264 | 5 | 3 | 38 | 1 | 2 | 43 |

Ochsner A, DeBakey M, Murray S: Pyogenic abscess of the liver. Am J Surg 40:292–319, 1938.

*This is the classic study Ochsner-DeBakey that reviewed 286 previously reported cases and 47 new cases.

intra-abdominal infections, portal venous infections of the liver have become less frequent. The most common causes of pylephlebitis are diverticulitis, appendicitis, pancreatitis, inflammatory bowel disease, pelvic inflammatory disease, perforated viscus, and omphalitis in the newborn. Hepatic abscess has also been associated with colorectal malignancy.

Any systemic infection (e.g., endocarditis, pneumonia, osteomyelitis) can result in bacteremia and infection of the liver via the hepatic artery. Microabscess formation is a relatively common finding at autopsy in patients dying of sepsis, but these patients are generally not included in analyses of pyogenic liver abscess. Hepatic abscess from systemic infections may also reflect an altered immune response, such as in patients with malignancy, AIDS, or disorders of granulocyte function. Children with chronic granulomatous disease (CGD) are particularly susceptible.

Hepatic abscess can be the result of direct extension of an infectious process. Common examples include suppurative cholecystitis, subphrenic abscess, perinephric abscess, or even perforation of the bowel directly into the liver.

Penetrating and blunt trauma can also result in an intrahepatic hematoma or an area of necrotic liver, which can subsequently develop into an abscess. Bacteria may have been introduced from the trauma or the affected area may be seeded from systemic bacteremia. Hepatic abscesses associated with trauma can present in a delayed fashion up to several weeks after injury. Other mechanisms of iatrogenic hepatic necrosis such as hepatic artery embolization or, more recently, thermal ablative procedures can be complicated by abscess. This is an uncommon complication of these procedures but is seen more often when there has been a previous biliary-enteric anastomosis.

Usually, no cause for a hepatic abscess is found. Cryptogenic abscesses predominate in many series and are more common in some case reports. Possible explanations for cryptogenic hepatic abscess are undiagnosed abdominal pathology, resolved infectious process at the time of presentation, or host factors such as diabetes or malignancy rendering the liver more susceptible to transient hepatic artery or portal vein bacteremia. In patients with cryptogenic hepatic abscess, who have undergone computed tomography (CT) and ultrasonography, it has been argued whether a diligent search for a cause should ensue. In series evaluating colonoscopy and endoscopic retrograde cholangiopancreatography (ERCP) in patients with cryptogenic abscess, the yield has been low and often is only fruitful in patients with some objective finding that might have suggested a subclinical abnormality (e.g., mildly elevated bilirubin level). In general, these patients should undergo a thorough history, physical examination, and laboratory workup in search of abnormalities in the intestinal tract or biliary tree. Further invasive procedures or imaging studies should be based on clinical suspicions raised by this workup.

## Pathology and Microbiology

Most hepatic abscesses involve the right hemiliver, accounting for about 75% of cases. The explanation for this is not known, but preferential laminar blood flow to the right side has been postulated. The left liver is involved in approximately 20% of the cases; the caudate lobe is rarely involved (5%). Bilobar involvement with multiple abscesses is uncommon. Approximately 50% of hepatic abscesses are solitary. The size of hepatic abscesses can vary from less than 1 mm to 3 or 4 cm in diameter and can be multiloculated or a single cavity. At abdominal exploration, hepatic abscesses appear tan and are fluctuant to palpation, although deeper abscesses may not be visible and can be difficult to palpate. Surrounding inflammation can cause adhesions to local structures.

Studies of the microbiology of hepatic abscesses have had variable results, for a number of reasons. In early series, sterile abscesses were commonly reported but probably reflected inadequate culture techniques, whereas in modern series, few abscesses are sampled prior to the administration of antibiotics. Also, the heterogeneity of the routes of infection makes the microbiology variable. Abscesses from pyelophlebitis or cholangitis tend to be polymicrobial, with a high preponderance of gram-negative bacilli. Systemic infections, on the other hand, usually cause infection with a single organism.

Although the rate of sterility reported by Ochsner's review in 1938 was approximately 50%, series in the 1990s reported sterile abscess rates in approximately 10% to 20% of cases. Many hepatic abscesses are polymicrobial in nature and account for approximately 40% of cases. Some have suggested that solitary abscesses are more likely to be polymicrobial. Anaerobic organisms are involved approximately 40% to 60% of the time. The most common organisms cultured are *Escherichia coli* and *Klebsiella pneumoniae.* Other commonly encountered organisms are *Staphylococcus aureus, Enterococcus* sp., *Streptococcus viridans,* and *Bacteroides* spp. *Klebsiella* is frequently associated with gas-forming abscesses. *Enterococci* and *Streptococcus viridans* are generally found in polymicrobial abscesses whereas *Staphylococcal* infections are typically caused by single organism. Uncommonly encountered organisms (<10% of cultures) include species of *Pseudomonas, Proteus, Enterobacter, Citrobacter, Serratia,* beta-hemolytic streptococci, microaerophilic streptococci, *Fusobacterium, Clostridium,* and other rare anaerobes. Blood cultures are positive in approximately 50% to 60% of cases. Of note, highly resistant organisms in patients with indwelling biliary catheters, multiple episodes of cholangitis, and repeated use of antibiotics are being encountered as the use of these catheters becomes more common. Fungal and mycobacterial hepatic abscesses are rare and are almost always associated with immunosuppression, usually from chemotherapy.

## Clinical Features

The classic description of the presenting symptoms of hepatic abscess is fever, jaundice, and right upper quadrant pain, with tenderness to palpation. Unfortunately, this presentation is only present in 10% of cases. Fever, chills, and abdominal pain are the most common presenting symptoms but is a broad array of nonspecific symptoms can be present (Table 54-4). A study from Taiwan on 133 patients found fever in 96% of patients, chills in 80%, abdominal pain in 53%, and jaundice in 20%. Many of the symptoms, such as malaise or vomiting, were constitutional in nature. Involvement of the diaphragm may result in symptoms of cough or dyspnea. Rarely, patients can present with peritonitis secondary to rupture. Cases of rupture into the pleural space or pericardium have been reported but are distinctly uncommon. The duration of presenting symptoms is variable, ranging from an acute illness to a chronic presentation lasting months. It has been suggested that acute presentation is associated with identifiable abdominal pathology, whereas a chronic presentation is often associated with a cryptogenic

**Table 54-4 Pyogenic Abscesses With Noted Symptoms (%)**

| Year of Report | No. of Patients | Symptom | | | | | | | | |
|---|---|---|---|---|---|---|---|---|---|---|
| | | FEVER, CHILLS | NIGHT SWEATS | MALAISE | ANOREXIA, WEIGHT LOSS | NAUSEA, VOMITING | DIARRHEA | ABDOMINAL PAIN | CHEST PAIN | COUGH |
| 1927-1938: One study* | 333 | 94 | — | — | — | 33 | — | 92 | — | — |
| 1945-1982: Eight studies | 494 | 88 | 8 | 58 | 62 | 40 | 17 | 66 | 14 | 13 |
| 1970-1995: Ten studies | 1314 | 72 | 9 | 25 | 33 | 30 | 14 | 59 | 16 | 6 |

Ochsner A, DeBakey M, Murray S: Pyogenic abscess of the liver. Am J Surg 40:292–319, 1938.

*This is the classic study Ochsner/DeBakey that reviewed 286 previously reported cases and 47 new cases.

abscess. A rare complication specific to *Klebsiella* hepatic abscesses is endogenous endophthalmitis, occurring in approximately 3% of cases. This serious complication is more common in diabetics. Early diagnosis and treatment is the best chance to preserve visual function.

On physical examination, fever and right upper quadrant tenderness are the most common findings. Tenderness is present in 40% to 70% of patients. Also, jaundice is found in approximately 25% of cases and is often secondary to underlying biliary disease. Chest findings are often found in approximately 25% of patients and hepatomegaly is also commonly noted in approximately 50%. Ascites, splenomegaly and severe sepsis are uncommon signs of hepatic abscesses.

Nonspecific abnormalities of blood tests are common in pyogenic abscesses. Leukocytosis is present in 70% to 90% of patients and anemia is commonly encountered. Abnormalities of LFT results are generally present. The ALP level is mildly elevated in 80% of patients whereas total bilirubin is elevated 20% to 50% of the time. Transaminases are mildly elevated in approximately 60% of patients. Severe abnormalities of liver function are almost always associated with underlying biliary disease. Hypoalbuminemia or mild elevations of the PT and INR can be present and reflect a degree of chronicity. None of these blood tests specifically help diagnose a hepatic abscess. However, together they may suggest a liver abnormality that often leads to imaging studies.

The most essential element to establishing the diagnosis of hepatic abscess is radiographic imaging. Chest x-rays are abnormal approximately 50% of the time and findings generally reflect subdiaphragmatic pathology, such as an elevated right hemidiaphragm, right pleural effusion, or atelectasis. Occasionally, these can be left-sided findings in the case of an abscess involving the left liver. Plain abdominal x-rays, in rare cases, can be helpful. They can show air-fluid levels or portal venous gas (Fig. 54-27).

Ultrasound and CT are the mainstays of diagnostic modalities for hepatic abscess. Ultrasound usually demonstrates a round or oval area that is less echogenic than the surrounding liver. Ultrasound can reliably distinguish solid from cystic lesions. The limitations of ultrasound are in its ability to visualize lesions high up in the dome of the liver and that it is a user-dependent modality. The sensitivity of ultrasound in diagnosing hepatic abscess is 80% to 95%. CT demonstrates similar findings to ultrasound and lesions are of lower attenuation than surrounding hepatic parenchyma. High-quality CT scans can demonstrate very small abscesses and can more easily identify multiple small abscesses. The abscess wall usually has an intense enhancement on contrast-enhanced CT. The sensitivity of CT in diagnosing hepatic abscess is 95% to 100%. Both CT and ultrasound are useful in diagnosing other intra-abdominal pathologies, such as biliary disease (ultrasound) or inflammatory disorders such as appendicitis or diverticulitis (CT). Magnetic resonance imaging (MRI) can be helpful in distinguishing the cause of many hepatic masses and evaluating the biliary tree for pathology, but does not appear to have any distinct advantage over CT in diagnosing hepatic abscess.

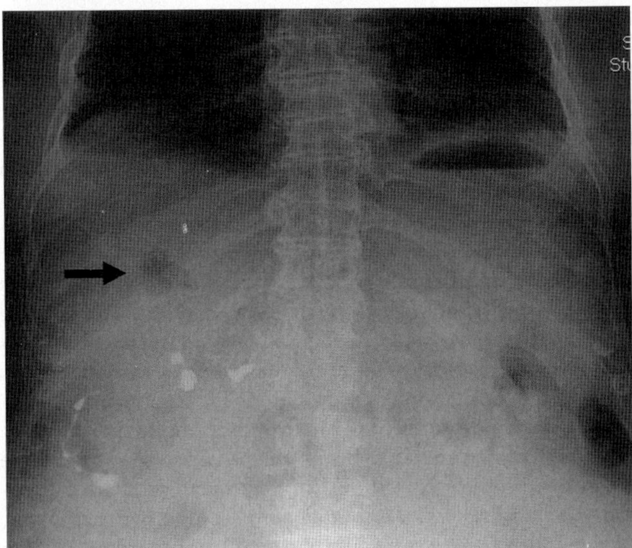

**FIGURE 54-27** Plain abdominal x-ray demonstrating an abnormal collection of air in the right upper quadrant consistent with a pyogenic hepatic abscess *(black arrow).*

### Differential Diagnosis

Differentiating pyogenic abscess from other cystic infective diseases of the liver such as amebic abscess or echinococcal cyst is important because of differences in treatment. Pyogenic abscess (see later) is largely treated by antibiotics and drainage. Amebic abscess is mainly treated by antibiotics, whereas echinococcal cysts often require surgical management. Fortunately, echinococcal cysts can usually be diagnosed by history and characteristic radiologic findings (see later). The presentations of amebic and pyogenic abscess, however, are more similar, with some notable exceptions that are critical in distinguishing the two (Table 54-5). Amebic abscesses generally occur in young Hispanic males whereas pyogenic abscess tends to occur in patients 50 to 60 years of age, with no predominant gender or race. Fever is common in both, but chills and symptoms of a severe acute bacteremia are more common in pyogenic abscess. Serologic tests for *Entamoeba histolytica* antibodies are almost always present in amebic abscesses but are uncommon in patients with pyogenic abscess. A recent study comparing 471 patients with amebic abscess to 106 patients with pyogenic abscess found age older than 50 years, pulmonary findings on physical examination, multiple abscesses, and low amebic serology titers to be independently predictive of pyogenic abscess. Occasionally, differentiating the two is not possible and diagnostic aspiration or a trial of antiamebic antibiotics may be necessary. Unfortunately, aspiration is only diagnostic in amebic abscess approximately 10% to 20% of the time.[12]

### Treatment

Before the availability of antibiotics and the routine use of drainage procedures, untreated hepatic pyogenic abscess was almost uniformly fatal. It was not until the classic review by Ochsner and DeBakey in 1938 (see earlier) that routine surgical drainage was used and dramatic reductions in mortality were noted. Open surgical drainage of pyogenic abscesses was the sole treatment (with the addition of antibiotics eventually) for hepatic abscess until the 1980s. Since then, less invasive percutaneous drainage techniques and IV antibiotics have been used. Laparotomy is generally reserved for failures of percutaneous drainage.

Once the diagnosis of pyogenic hepatic abscess is suspected, broad-spectrum IV antibiotics should be started immediately to control ongoing bacteremia and its associated complications. Blood cultures and cultures of the abscess from aspiration should be sent for aerobic and anaerobic cultures. In immunosuppressed patients, mycobacterial and fungal cultures of the aspirate should be considered. Patients who are at risk for amebic infections should have amebic serologies drawn. Until cultures have specifically identified the offending organism(s), broad-spectrum antibiotics covering gram-negative, gram-positive, and anaerobic organisms should be used. Combinations such as ampicillin, an aminoglycoside and metronidazole, or a third-generation cephalosporin with metronidazole are appropriate. The optimal duration of antibiotic treatment is not well defined and must be individualized, depending on the success of the drainage procedure. Antibiotics should certainly be continued while there is evidence of ongoing infection such as fever, chills, or leukocytosis. Beyond this, it is unclear how long to continue antibiotics, but recommendations are usually for 2 or more weeks.

Percutaneous drainage procedures for pyogenic hepatic abscesses was first reported in 1953, but did not gain widespread acceptance until the 1980s with the development of high-quality imaging and expertise in interventional radiologic techniques. Over the last 25 years, percutaneous catheter drainage has become the treatment of choice for most patients (Fig. 54-28). Success rates range from 66% to 90%.[11,13] The obvious advantages are the simplicity of treatment (usually at the time of radiologic diagnosis) and avoidance of general anesthesia and a laparotomy. Relative contraindications to percutaneous catheter drainage include the presence of ascites, coagulopathy, and proximity to vital structures. Percutaneous drainage of multiple abscesses is usually met with a higher failure rate, but reports have demonstrated a high enough success rate that percutaneous approaches should be made first, reserving surgery for failures. A retrospective study comparing surgical with percutaneous drainage for large abscesses (>5 cm) has shown a better success rate with surgical drainage. Despite this, two thirds of percutaneous treatments were successful and the overall morbidity and mortality rate were similar. There has never been a randomized prospective comparison between percutaneous and surgical therapy for hepatic abscess. However, case series have suggested that for most cases there are similar success and mortality rates. Modern series attempting to compare these two techniques retrospectively must be read with caution because most patients treated surgically have failed other less invasive techniques. In general, surgery should be reserved for patients who require surgical treatment of the primary pathology (e.g., appendicitis) or for those who have failed percutaneous techniques. It should be noted that laparoscopic drainage procedures have been reported with some success and this can be considered a reasonable option to pursue in select cases.[10]

Percutaneous aspiration without the placement of an indwelling drain has been investigated by a number of groups. Success rates are generally 60% to 90% and are somewhat similar to those for percutaneous catheter drainage.[13] Most patients, however, require more than one aspiration and 25% of patients require three or more aspirations. One randomized trial has evaluated percutaneous aspiration versus percutaneous catheter drainage. Success rates were 60% in the aspiration group and 100% in the catheter group. All but one patient in the aspiration group had a single aspiration. Another randomized trial of 64 patients has compared aspiration alone to catheter

**Table 54-5 Features of Amebic Versus Pyogenic Liver Abscess**

| CLINICAL FEATURES | AMEBIC ABSCESS | PYOGENIC ABSCESS |
|---|---|---|
| Age (yr) | 20-40 | >50 |
| Male-to-female ratio | ≥10 : 1 | 1.5 : 1 |
| Solitary versus multiple | Solitary 80%* | Solitary 50% |
| Location | Usually right liver | Usually right liver |
| Travel in endemic area | Yes | No |
| Diabetes | Uncommon (≈2%) | More common (≈27%) |
| Alcohol use | Common | Common |
| Jaundice | Uncommon | Common |
| Elevated bilirubin | Uncommon | Common |
| Elevated alkaline phosphatase | Common | Common |
| Positive blood culture | No | Common |
| Positive amebic serology | Yes | No |

*In acute amebic abscess, 50% are solitary.

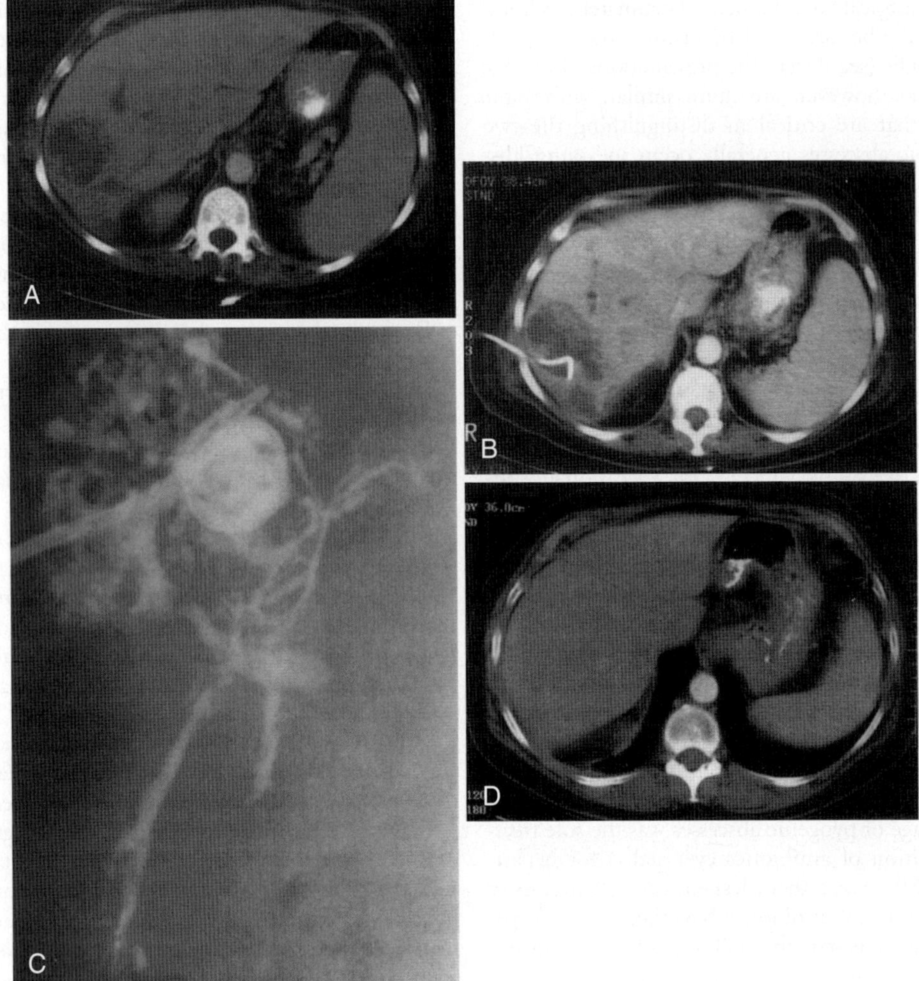

**FIGURE 54-28** **A,** CT scan demonstrating multiloculated hepatic abscess in the right liver. **B,** CT scan at the time of percutaneous drainage. **C,** Contrast study through the drainage catheter demonstrating typical irregular loculated type appearance, as well as communication with biliary tree. **D,** Follow-up CT scan 3 months after treatment demonstrating complete resolution of abscess. (From Brown KT, Getrajdman GI: Interventional radiologic techniques in the liver and biliary tract. In Blumgart LH, Fong Y [eds]: Surgery of the liver and biliary tract, London, 2000, WB Saunders, pp 575–594).

drainage. There were similar outcomes in terms of treatment success rate, hospital stay, antibiotic duration, and mortality. In the aspiration-only group, 40% required two aspirations and 20% required three aspirations. In general, catheter drainage remains the treatment of choice, although a trial of a single aspiration is reasonable to consider.

Some investigators have reported success with antibiotics alone. Most of these patients, however, have had a diagnostic aspiration and thus at least a partial drainage. Also, other series have reported that antibiotic treatment without drainage carries a prohibitively high mortality (59% to 100%). In patients who are not surgical candidates or who refuse any invasive procedure, an attempt at antibiotic treatment is reasonable. However, this is not recommended in other situations.

Liver resection is occasionally required for hepatic abscess. This may be required for an infected hepatic malignancy, hepatolithiasis, or intrahepatic biliary stricture. If hepatic destruction from infection is severe, some patients may benefit from resection.

### Outcomes

Mortality from pyogenic hepatic abscess has dramatically improved over the last 70 years. Prior to the routine use of surgical drainage, pyogenic abscess was uniformly fatal. With the routine use of surgical drainage and the use of IV antibiotics, mortality was reduced to approximately 50%, a figure that stayed relatively constant from 1945 until the early 1980s. Since then, the mortality has been reported from 10% to 20% and series from the 1990s have demonstrated a mortality rate under 10%.[13] The most recent series from Memorial Sloan-Kettering has reported a 3% mortality. A number of studies have analyzed factors predictive of a poor outcome in patients with hepatic pyogenic abscess. The presence of malignancy, factors associated with malignancy (e.g., jaundice, markedly elevated LFT results), and signs of sepsis appear to be a consistent marker of poor prognosis. Signs of chronic disease such as hypoalbuminemia are also often associated with a poor outcome. Finally, signs of severe infection such as marked leukocytosis, APACHE II (Acute Physiology and Chronic Health Evaluation II) scores, abscess rupture, bacteremia, and shock are also associated with mortality.

## Amebic Abscess

### Epidemiology

Amebiasis is largely a disease of tropical and developing countries but is also a significant problem in developed countries because of immigration and travel between countries. *E. histolytica* is endemic in Mexico, India, Africa, and parts of Central and South America. In 1995, the World Health Organization (WHO) estimated that 40 to 50 million people suffer from amebic colitis or amebic liver abscess worldwide, resulting in 40,000 to 100,000 deaths each year.[12] Prior to this, estimates of amebiasis were unreliable because *E. histolytica* (the pathogenic form) was not differentiated from *Entamoeba dispar* (nonpathogenic form). Male homosexuals with diarrhea, previously thought to harbor *E. histolytica,* were actually found to be infected with *E. dispar,* which requires no treatment. Epidemiologic studies specifically addressing *E. histolytica* infections have estimated that as many as 55% of those in endemic regions are infected, although less than 50% are symptomatic.

In contrast to pyogenic hepatic abscesses, patients with amebic liver abscesses tend to be Hispanic men, 20 to 40 years of age, with a history of travel to (or origination from) an endemic area. Poverty and cramped living conditions are associated with higher rates of infection. A male preponderance of more than 10 : 1 has been reported in almost all studies. For unclear reasons, menstruating women have a low incidence of invasive amebiasis and pregnancy appears to abrogate this resistance. Heavy alcohol consumption is commonly reported and may render the liver more susceptible to amebic infection. Patients with impaired host immunity also appear to be at higher risk of infection and have higher mortality rates. Patients with amebic liver abscess without a history of travel to an endemic area often have associated immunosuppression, such as HIV infection, malnutrition, chronic infection, or chronic steroid use.

### Pathogenesis

*E. histolytica* is a protozoan and exists as a trophozoite or a cyst. All other species in the genus *Entamoeba* are considered nonpathogenic and not all strains of *E. histolytica* are considered virulent. Ingestion of *E. histolytica* cysts through a fecal-oral route is the cause of amebiasis. Humans are the principle host and the main source of infection is human contact with a cyst-passing carrier. Contaminated water and vegetables are also routes of human infection. Once ingested, the cysts are not degraded in the stomach and pass to the intestines, where the trophozoite is released and passed on to the colon. In the colon, the trophozoite can invade mucosa resulting in disease.

It is thought that the trophozoites reach the liver through the portal venous system. There is no evidence for trophozoites passing through lymphatics. As implied by its name, *E. histolytica* trophozoites can lyse tissues through a complex set of events, including cell adherence, cell activation, and subsequent release of enzymes, resulting in necrosis. The principle mechanism is probably enzymatic cellular hydrolysis. Amebic liver abscesses are formed by progressing, localized hepatic necrosis producing a cavity containing acellular proteinaceous debris surrounded by a rim of invasive amebic trophozoites. Early development of an amebic liver abscess is associated with an accumulation of polymorphonuclear leukocytes, which are then lysed by the trophozoites.

Antiamebic antibodies develop rapidly in patients with invasive disease or an amebic hepatic abscess. Secretory immunoglobulin A (IgA) antibodies have been shown to inhibit adherence to colonic epithelium in vitro. However, the development of these antibodies does not halt the progression of disease. Interestingly, children who lack antiamebic IgG have innate resistance to invasive infection, suggesting an alternative immune-mediated response. There is now evidence that a cell-mediated helper T cell response is probably the major mechanism of resistance.

### Pathology

Hepatic amebic abscess is essentially the result of liquefaction necrosis of the liver producing a cavity full of blood and liquefied liver tissue. The appearance of this fluid is typically described as resembling anchovy sauce; the fluid is odorless unless secondary bacterial infection has taken place. The progressive hepatic necrosis continues until Glisson's capsule is reached because the capsule is resistant to hydrolysis by the amebae. Thus, amebic abscesses tend to abut the liver capsule. Because of the resistance of Glisson's capsule, the cavity is typically criss-crossed by portal triads protected by this peritoneal sheath. Early on, the formed cavity is ill-defined, with no real fibrous response around the edges. However, a chronic abscess can ultimately develop a fibrous capsule and may even calcify. Like pyogenic abscesses, amebic abscesses tend to occur mainly in the right liver.

### Clinical Features

Approximately 80% of patients with amebic liver abscess present with symptoms lasting from a few days to 4 weeks. The duration of symptoms has been found to be typically less than 10 days. The presenting clinical signs and symptoms are summarized in Table 54-6. The typical clinical picture is a patient 20 to 40 years of age who has recently traveled to an endemic area, with fever, chills, anorexia, right upper quadrant pain and tenderness, and hepatomegaly. The abdominal pain is typically constant, dull, and localized to the right upper quadrant. Although some studies report higher numbers, approximately 25% of patients have diarrhea despite an obligatory colonic infection. Synchronous hepatic abscess is found in one third of patients with active amebic colitis. Jaundice, as a result of a large abscess compressing the biliary tree, is not as rare as was once thought, with an average 22% of patients presenting with this feature worldwide. Weight loss and myalgias may occur when symptoms have been present for weeks. Pleuritic or right shoulder pain can occur if there is irritation of the right hemidiaphragm. Symptoms and tenderness may be epigastric or left-sided if the abscess is located in the left liver. Rupture into the peritoneum with peritonitis occurs infrequently; when it does occur, it is more often with left-sided abscesses. Rare cases of rupture into the pleural space, pericardium. and other intra-abdominal organs have also been reported.

Laboratory abnormalities are common in amebic abscess (see Table 54-6). Patients typically have a mild to moderate leukocytosis. without eosinophilia. Anemia is common. Mild abnormalities of LFT results, including albumin, PT-INR, ALP, AST, and bilirubin levels. are typical. The most common LFT abnormality is an elevated PT-INR level. Because more than

**Table 54-6 Signs, Symptoms, and Laboratory Findings in Amebic Liver Abscess***

| PARAMETER | AVERAGE | RANGE | NO. OF CASES REVIEWED |
|---|---|---|---|
| **Symptoms and Signs** | | | |
| Abdominal pain (%) | 92 | 73-100 | 1701 |
| Fever (%) | 90 | 72-100 | 2192 |
| Abdominal tenderness (%) | 78 | 40-100 | 1424 |
| Hepatomegaly (%) | 62 | 20-100 | 1539 |
| Anorexia (%) | 47 | 28-89 | 499 |
| Weight loss (%) | 39 | 11-83 | 871 |
| Diarrhea (%) | 23 | 12-40 | 1426 |
| Jaundice (%) | 22 | 5-50 | 1630 |
| **Laboratory Tests** | | | |
| Stool cysts, trophozoites (%) | 12 | 4-30 | 4908 |
| Amebae in cyst aspirate (%) | 42 | 30-76 | 1402 |
| Hemoglobin (g/dL) | 12.1 | 10.2-12.8 | 229 |
| Alkaline phosphatase (% >120 U/liter) | 76 | 65-91 | 589 |
| Total bilirubin (g/dL) | 1.4 | 0.8-2.4 | 509 |
| Albumin (g/dL) | 2.8 | 2.3-3.4 | 404 |
| AST (× upper limit normal) | 1.7 | 1.0-2.5 | 459 |

*In an extensive literature review.

70% of patients with amebic liver abscess do not have detectable amebae in their stool, the most useful laboratory evaluation is the measurement of circulating antiamebic antibodies, which are present in 90% to 95% of patients. A number of serologic tests have been devised over the years. An indirect hemagglutinin test was used extensively in the past and has a sensitivity of 90%. This test has largely been replaced by enzyme immunoassays (EIAs), which are simple, rapidly performed, and inexpensive. An EIA has a reported sensitivity of 99% and specificity higher than 90% in patients with hepatic abscess. Unfortunately, the presence of antibodies may reflect prior infection and interpretation can be difficult in endemic areas. Ongoing studies are focusing on identifying specific *E. histolytic* antigens in an attempt to identify acute infection.

Patients presenting acutely (symptoms <10 days) versus those with a chronic presentation (>2 weeks) differ clinically. Acute presentations are typically more dramatic with high fevers, chills, and significant abdominal tenderness. In the acute presentation, 50% of patients present with multiple lesions, whereas with the chronic presentation, more than 80% of patients have a single right-sided lesion. A more complicated course tends to ensue in the acute presentation, but response to therapy is similar in both groups.

Radiologic studies are a critical element in the diagnosis of amebic liver abscess. Plain chest radiographs are abnormal in approximately 50% of cases, usually demonstrating an elevated right diaphragm, pleural effusion, or atelectasis. Abdominal

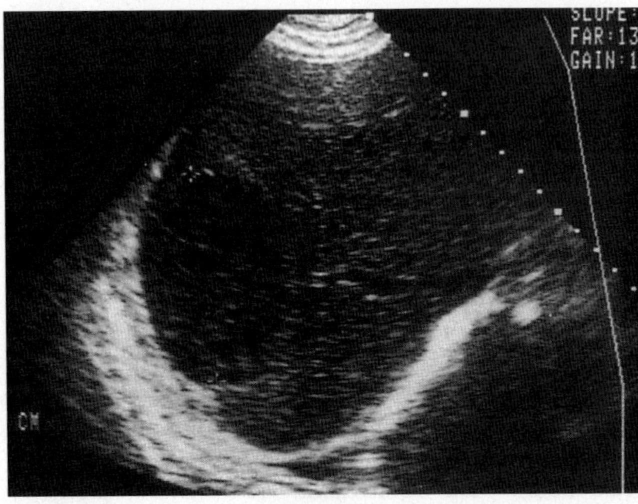


**FIGURE 54-29** Typical ultrasound of an amebic hepatic abscess. Note the peripheral location, rounded shape with poor rim, and internal echoes. (From Thomas PG, Ravindra KV: Amebiasis and biliary infection. In Blumgart LH, Fong Y [eds]: Surgery of the liver and biliary tract, London, 2000, WB Saunders, pp 1147–1166.)

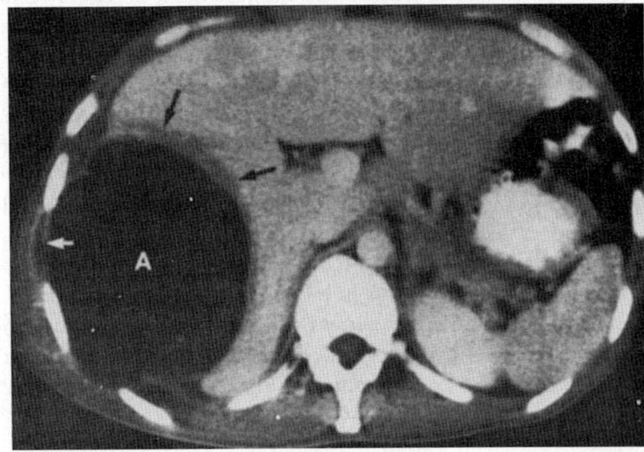


**FIGURE 54-30** CT scan of amebic abscess. The lesion is peripherally located and round. The rim is nonenhancing but shows peripheral edema *(black arrows)*. Note the extension into the intercostal space *(white arrow)*.

ultrasound has a reported accuracy of approximately 90% when combined with a typical history and clinical presentation. Typical findings on abdominal ultrasound are a rounded lesion abutting the liver capsule (see earlier) without significant rim echoes, interpreted as an abscess wall. The contents of the cavity are usually hypoechoic and nonhomogeneous (Fig. 54-29). These findings on ultrasound are found in 40% to 70% of cases. Abdominal CT scanning is probably more sensitive than ultrasound and is helpful in differentiating amebic from pyogenic abscess, with rim enhancement noted in the latter (Fig. 54-30). CT can also be helpful in identifying simple cysts and necrotic tumors. MRI of the liver has no distinct advantages over CT or ultrasound in typical cases, but may be helpful in differentiating atypical lesions. Nuclear medicine studies such as gallium scanning or $^{99m}$Tc liver scans can be helpful in differentiating pyogenic from amebic abscesses because the latter typically do not contain leukocytes and therefore do not light up on these scans.[14]

When the above-described workup is still not definitive and diagnostic uncertainty persists, two options should be considered. First, a therapeutic trial of antiamebic drugs can be used. If a rapid improvement occurs, this supports the diagnosis. In situations in which amebic serology is inconclusive and a therapeutic trial of antibiotics is deemed inappropriate or has failed to improve symptoms, the second option, a diagnostic aspiration, should be considered. A pyogenic abscess would have bacteria and leukocytes whereas an amebic abscess would contain the typical so-called *anchovy sauce*. Cultures of amebic abscess are usually negative and do not contain leukocytes. In patients for whom neoplasm or hydatid disease is in the differential diagnosis, aspiration should not be performed.

### Differential Diagnosis

The differential diagnosis of an amebic liver abscess can be broad and include diseases such as viral hepatitis, echinococcal disease, cholangitis, cholecystitis, or even other inflammatory abdominal disorders, such as appendicitis. Malignant lesions of the liver can also have similar presentations in atypical situations. Occasionally, primary pulmonary disorders must be considered. Usually, the most important distinction to be made is between pyogenic and amebic abscess. The essential elements of this distinction are summarized in Table 54-5 and in the earlier section on pyogenic abscess.

### Treatment

The mainstay of treatment for amebic abscesses is metronidazole (750 mg orally, three times daily for 10 days), which is curative in over 90% of patients. Clinical improvement is usually seen within 3 days. Other nitroimidazoles (e.g., secnidazole, tinidazole) are also as effective and are commonly used outside the United States. If response to metronidazole is poor or the drug is not tolerated, other agents can be used. Emetine hydrochloride is effective against invasive amebiasis, particularly in the liver, but requires intramuscular injections and has serious cardiac side effects. A more attractive option is chloroquine, but this is a less effective agent. After treatment of the liver abscess, it is recommended that luminal agents such as iodoquinol, paromomycin, and diloxanide furoate be administered to treat the carrier state.

Therapeutic needle aspiration of amebic abscesses has been proposed. Small randomized trials comparing metronidazole with or without aspiration have shown minor benefits with aspiration, but no major improvement to justify routine aspiration. In general, aspiration is recommended for diagnostic uncertainty (see earlier), failure to respond to metronidazole therapy in 3 to 5 days, or in abscesses thought to be at high risk for rupture. Abscesses larger than 5 cm in diameter and in the left liver are thought to be carry a higher risk of rupture, and aspiration should be considered.

### Outcomes

Although amebic liver abscesses usually respond rapidly to treatment, there are uncommon complications of which one must be aware. The most frequent complication of amebic abscess is rupture into the peritoneum, pleural cavity, or pericardium. The size of the abscess appears to be the most important risk factor for rupture and the overall incidence of rupture ranges from 3% to 17%. Most peritoneal ruptures tend to be contained by the diaphragm, abdominal wall, and/or omentum, but rupture can fistulize into a hollow viscus. A peritoneal rupture usually presents as abdominal pain, peritonitis, and a mass or generalized distention. Laparotomy was advocated in the past for this complication, but now many patients are treated successfully with percutaneous drainage. Laparotomy is indicated in cases of doubtful diagnosis, hollow viscous perforation, fistulization resulting in hemorrhage or sepsis, and failure of conservative therapy. Rupture into the pleural space usually results in a large and rapidly accumulated effusion that collapses the involved lung. Treatment consists of thoracentesis but, if secondary bacterial infection ensues, more aggressive surgical approaches may be necessary. Rupture can occur into the bronchi and is usually self-limited with postural drainage and bronchodilators. Rarely, a left-sided abscess may rupture into the pericardium and can present as an asymptomatic pericardial effusion or even tamponade. This must be treated with aspiration or drainage via a pericardial window. Other complications include compression of the biliary tree or IVC from a very large abscess and the development of a brain abscess.

The mortality for all patients with amebic liver abscess is approximately 5% and does not appear to be affected by the addition of aspiration to metronidazole therapy or by chronicity of symptoms. When an abscess ruptures, mortality ranges from 6% to as high as 50%. Factors independently associated with poor outcome are elevated serum bilirubin level (>3.5 mg/dL), encephalopathy, hypoalbuminemia (<2.0 g/dL), multiple abscess cavities, abscess volume larger than 500 mL, anemia, and diabetes. Although clinical improvement after adequate treatment with antiamebic agents is the rule, radiologic resolution of the abscess cavity is usually delayed. The average time to radiologic resolution is 3 to 9 months and, in some patients, can take years. Studies have shown that over 90% of the visible lesions disappear radiologically, but a small percentage of patients are left with a clinically irrelevant residual lesion.

## Hydatid Cyst

Hydatid disease or echinococcosis is a zoonosis that occurs primarily in sheep-grazing areas of the world, but is common worldwide because the dog is a definitive host. Echinococcosis is endemic in Mediterranean countries, the Middle East, Far East, South America, Australia, New Zealand, and East Africa. Humans contract the disease from dogs but there is no human to human transmission.[15,16]

There are three species that cause hydatid disease. *Echinococcus granulosus* is the most common and *Echinococcus multilocularis* and *Echinococcus ligartus* account for a small number of cases. Dogs are the definitive host of *E. granulosus;* the adult tapeworm is attached to the villi of the ileum. Up to thousands of ova are passed daily and deposited in the dog's feces. Sheep are the usual intermediate host, but humans are an accidental intermediate host. Humans are an end stage to the parasite. In the human duodenum, the parasitic embryo releases an oncosphere containing hooklets that penetrate the mucosa, allowing access to the bloodstream. In the blood, the oncosphere reaches the liver (most commonly) or lungs, where the parasite develops its larval stage—the hydatid cyst.

Three weeks after infection, a visible hydatid cyst develops, which then slowly grows in a spherical manner. A pericyst or fibrous capsule derived from host tissues develops around the hydatid cyst. The cyst wall itself has two layers, an outer gelatinous membrane (ectocyst) and an inner germinal membrane (endocyst). Brood capsules are small, intracystic cellular masses in which future worm heads develop into scoleces. In a definitive host, the scoleces develop into an adult tapeworm, but in the intermediate host they can only differentiate into a new hydatid cyst. Freed brood capsules and scoleces are found in the hydatid fluid and form the so-called *hydatid sand.* Daughter cysts are true replicas of the mother cyst. Hydatid cysts can die with degeneration of the membranes, development of cystic vacuoles, and calcification of the wall. Calcification of a hydatid cyst, however, does not always imply that the cyst is dead.

Hydatid cysts are diagnosed in equal numbers of men and women at an average age of about 45 years. Approximately 75% of hydatid cysts are located in the right liver and are solitary. The clinical presentation of a hydatid cyst is largely asymptomatic until complications occur. The most common presenting symptoms are abdominal pain, dyspepsia and vomiting. The most frequent sign is hepatomegaly. Jaundice and fever are each present in approximately 8% of patients. Bacterial superinfection of a hydatid cyst can occur and present like a pyogenic abscess. Rupture of the cyst into the biliary tree, bronchial tree, or free rupture into the peritoneal, pleural, or pericardial cavities can occur. Free ruptures can result in disseminated echinococcosis and/or a potentially fatal anaphylactic reaction. In cases of diagnostic uncertainty, a battery of serologic tests are available to evaluate antibody response, but all are plagued by low sensitivity and specificity.

Ultrasound is most commonly used worldwide for the diagnosis of echinococcosis because of its availability, affordability, and accuracy. A number of findings on ultrasound can be diagnostic but depend on the stage of the cyst at the time of the examination. A simple hydatid cyst is well circumscribed with budding signs on the cyst membrane and may contain free-floating hyperechogenic hydatid sand. A rosette appearance is seen when daughter cysts are present. The cyst can be filled with an amorphous mass, which can be diagnostically misleading. Calcifications in the wall of the cyst are highly suggestive of hydatid disease and can be helpful in the diagnosis (Fig. 54-31). Similar findings are seen on CT or MRI scans. These cross-sectional imaging studies can also evaluate extrahepatic disease and demonstrate detailed hepatic anatomic relationships to the cyst. In patients with suspected biliary involvement, ERCP or percutaneous transhepatic cholangiography (PTC) may be necessary.

The treatment of hepatic hydatid cysts is primarily surgical. In general, most cysts should be treated, but in older patients with small, asymptomatic, densely calcified cysts, conservative

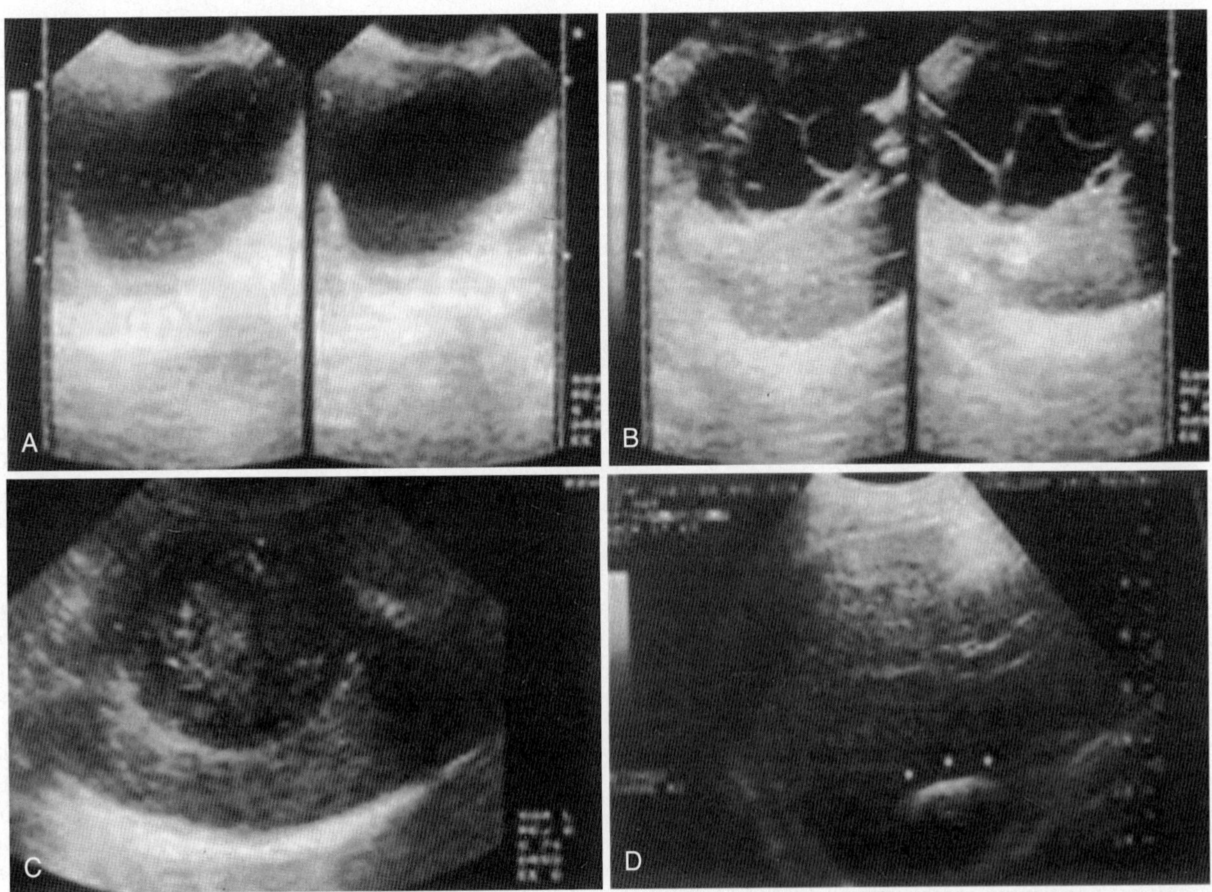


**FIGURE 54-31** Ultrasound demonstrating typical characteristics of a hydatid cyst at varying stages. **A,** Simple hydatid cyst with hydatid sand. **B,** Daughter and granddaughter cysts and typical rosette appearance. **C,** Hydatid cyst filled with amorphous mass giving a solid or semisolid appearance. **D,** Calcified cyst with eggshell appearance. (From Thomas PG, Ravindra KV: Amebiasis and biliary infection. In Blumgart LH, Fong Y [eds]: Surgery of the liver and biliary tract, London, 2000, WB Saunders, pp 1147–1166.)

management is appropriate. In preparation for an operation, preoperative steroids have been recommended, but are not universally used. The anesthesiologist should have epinephrine and steroids available in case of an anaphylactic reaction. A number of operations have been used but, in general, the abdomen is completely explored, the liver mobilized, and the cyst exposed. Packing off the abdomen is important because rupture can result in anaphylaxis and diffuse seeding. Usually, the cyst is then aspirated through a closed suction system and flushed with a scolicidal agent such as hypertonic saline. The cyst is then unroofed, which can then be followed by a number of possibilities, including excision (or pericystectomy), marsupialization procedures, leaving the cyst open, drainage of the cyst, omentoplasty, or partial hepatectomy to encompass the cyst. Total pericystectomy or formal partial hepatectomy can also be performed without entering the cyst (Fig. 54-32). Both radical (resection) and conservative (drainage and evacuation) surgical approaches appear to be equally effective at controlling disease, although a prospective comparison has never been performed. When bile duct communication is diagnosed preoperatively or at operation, it must be meticulously sought after. Simple suture repair is often sufficient, but major biliary repairs, approaches through the common bile duct, or postoperative ERCP may be necessary. Laparoscopic techniques for drainage and unroofing of cysts have been reported in a number of series, with encouraging results. Recurrence rates after surgical treatment range from 1% to 20% but are generally 5% or less in experienced centers.

In the past, percutaneous aspiration of hydatid cysts was contraindicated because of the risk of rupture and uncontrolled spillage. However, percutaneous aspiration and injection of scolicidal agents with high success rates in highly selected patients have reported. This technique is known as *PAIR* (puncture, aspiration, injection, and reaspiration) and has become more accepted in some centers. Two randomized trials, one comparing PAIR with surgery ($N = 50$) and one comparing PAIR with medical therapy have shown similar success rates. These trials were small and had significant methodologic problems, limiting the ability to draw firm conclusions.[17] Although surgery remains the treatment of choice, further prospective trials are clearly indicated to address this interesting and potentially useful technique. Treatment of echinococcosis with albendazole or mebendazole is effective at shrinking cysts in many patients with *E. granulosus,* but cyst disappearance occurs in well under 50% of patients. Preoperative treatment may decrease the risk of spillage and is a reasonable and safe practice.[15] Medical therapy without definitive resection or drainage should only be considered for widely disseminated disease or poor surgical candidates.

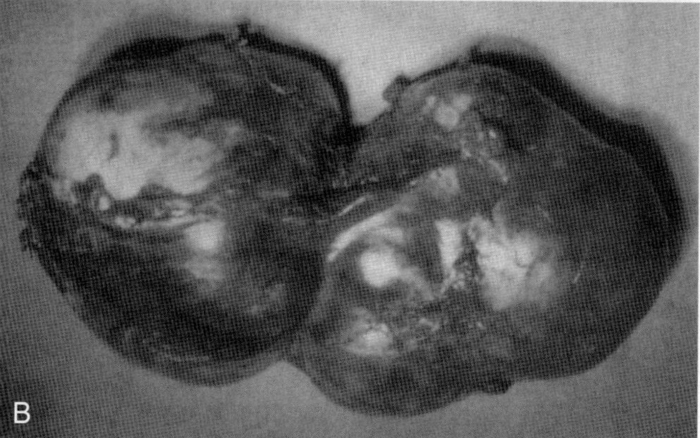


**FIGURE 54-32 A,** Peripheral hydatid cyst of the left liver. **B,** Intact specimen after pericystectomy. Note that the entire pericyst has been removed. (From Milicevic MN: Hydatid disease. In Blumgart LH, Fong Y [eds]: Surgery of the liver and biliary tract, London, 2000, WB Saunders, pp 1167–1204.)

### Recurrent Pyogenic Cholangitis

RPC is a syndrome of repeated attacks of cholangitis secondary to biliary stones and strictures that involve the extrahepatic and intrahepatic ducts. The condition has many names but is often referred to as Oriental cholangiohepatitis or hepatolithiasis. The disease is almost exclusively found in Asians and Asian medical centers. However, it is also seen in Asian immigrants throughout the world. Men and women are equally affected and, historically, the disease strikes at an early age (20 to 40 years) in patients from lower socioeconomic classes.[18]

The cause of RPC is unknown but is related to recurrent infection of biliary radicals with gut bacteria. Ultimately, stones and strictures develop in the biliary tree. but it is not known which occurs first. The stones are bilirubinate stones; in some patients, no stones are found and only biliary sludge is demonstrated. An association between RPC and *Clonorchis sinensis* and *Ascaris lumbricoides* infection has been noted, but a true causal relationship has never been proven.

Strictures can be found anywhere in the biliary tree, but usually involve the intrahepatic main hepatic ducts, most often the left hepatic duct. The gallbladder is only involved in approximately 20% of cases. Cirrhosis and liver failure are only seen in long-standing disease, usually after multiple operations. Other complications include choledochoduodenal fistulae and acute pancreatitis from common bile duct stones. An increased incidence of cholangiocarcinoma has been noted, but a causal relationship is difficult to prove.

The typical patient with RPC is a young Asian of a lower socioeconomic background who presents with repeated bouts of cholangitis. The symptoms and presentation are those of cholangitis. These include fever, right upper quadrant abdominal pain, and jaundice. Biliary obstruction is usually incomplete and therefore marked jaundice and pruritus are not common. There is usually leukocytosis and abnormal LFTs consistent with biliary obstruction. Evaluation of the anatomic distribution of disease is critical to formulating a sound therapeutic plan.

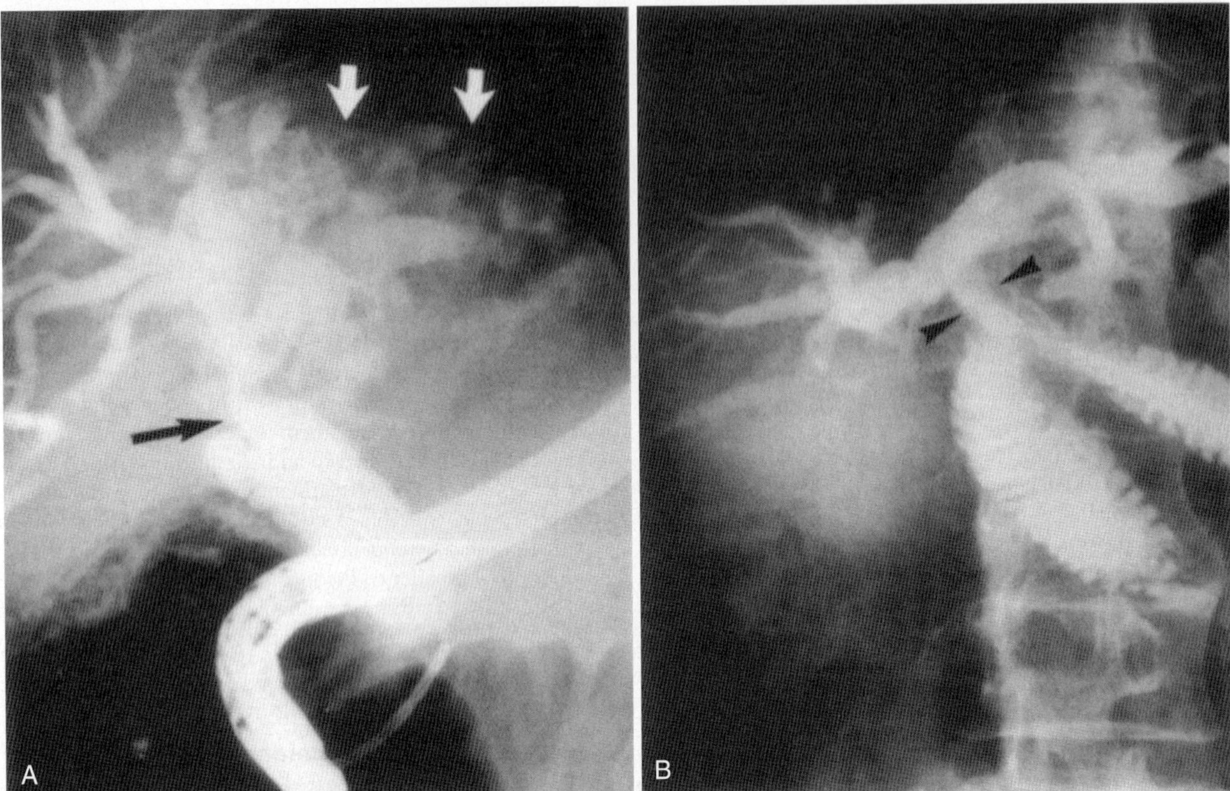

**FIGURE 54-33 A,** Cholangiogram of a patient with recurrent pyogenic cholangitis and a common hepatic duct stricture *(black arrow).* There are numerous stones inside dilated left ducts (white arrows). **B,** A hepaticojejunostomy to the segment III duct *(arrowheads)* has been performed and a flexible choledochoscope is shown passing through the anastomosis into the peripheral left ducts. All stones have been cleared. (From Fan ST, Wong J: Recurrent pyogenic cholangitis. In Blumgart LH, Fong Y [eds]: Surgery of the liver and biliary tract, London, 2000, WB Saunders, pp 1205–1225.)

A combination of ultrasound, CT, and direct cholangiography are often necessary to evaluate these patients. Direct cholangiography is performed endoscopically or transhepatically and is considered an important study complementing the cross-sectional imaging. Magnetic resonance cholangiopancreatography (MRCP) can combine cross-sectional imaging and cholangiography in one noninvasive test and may ultimately replace direct cholangiography.

In an acute presentation, most patients improve with conservative management, allowing time for radiologic studies and planning of a definitive operation, which is the treatment of choice. If intervention is necessary during the acute phase, it must focus on adequate decompression of the biliary tree through open common bile duct exploration or endoscopic papillotomy with stenting. Although nonoperative approaches such as percutaneous transhepatic cholangioscopic lithotomy (PTCSL) have been developed, surgical treatment remains the treatment of choice. PTCSL is generally used for poor-risk surgical patients and those who have failed surgical treatment. Stone clearance rates are high (>80%) and necessary for a successful long-term outcome. Unfortunately, stone recurrence is common and is mostly related to the presence of biliary strictures.[19]

The goal of operative approaches is to clear the biliary tree of stones and to bypass, resect, or enlarge strictures. Many cases only require exploration of the common bile duct, with or without hepaticojejunostomy. In complicated cases, providing permanent access to the biliary tree for interventional radiologic procedures by extending the end of the Roux-en-Y hepaticojejunostomy to the skin or subcutaneous space has been a successful approach (Fig. 54-33). Other potentially necessary procedures include stricturoplasty or partial hepatectomy. Partial hepatectomy is advocated for patients with intrahepatic strictures, hepatic atrophy, liver abscess, or suspicion of cholangiocarcinoma.[20]

In a large series from Asia, where surgery and hepatectomy are liberally applied, surgical mortality rates are 1%. Moreover, with aggressive treatment, there is almost a 100% stone clearance rate. Long-term outcome is excellent, with less than a 5% stone recurrence rate. Long-term survival is mostly related to the presence of cholangiocarcinom, which is found in approximately 10% of patients. Particularly complicated cases can have a higher rate of recurrent symptoms.

## NEOPLASMS

### Solid Benign Neoplasms

It is estimated that benign focal liver masses are present in approximately 10% to 20% of the population in developed countries. With the increasing use of rapidly improving radiologic examinations, these entities have been encountered more frequently. Familiarity with the clinical characteristics, natural history, imaging characteristics, and indications for surgery in these tumors is essential. Many benign lesions can be adequately characterized by modern imaging studies such as CT, ultrasound, and MRI. In unclear cases, serum tumor markers (e.g., AFP, CEA) and a search for a primary tumor in the case of suspected metastases should be carried out. A resection might be necessary to make a definitive diagnosis. Laparoscopic techniques for assessment, biopsy, and/or resection have become an important diagnostic technique as well.[21,22]

### Liver Cell Adenoma

Liver cell adenoma (LCA) is a relatively rare benign proliferation of hepatocytes in the context of a normal liver. It is predominantly found in young women (aged 20 to 40 years) and is often associated with steroid hormone use, such as chronic oral contraceptive pills (OCPs). The female-to-male ratio is approximately 11 : 1. LCAs are usually singular but multiple lesions have been reported in 12% to 30% of cases. The presence of 10 or more adenomata is termed *adenomatosis*. Interestingly, cases with multiple adenomata are not associated with OCP use and do not have as dramatic a female preponderance. Histologically, LCAs are composed of cords of benign hepatocytes containing increased glycogen and fat. Bile ductules are not observed histologically and the normal architecture of the liver is absent in these lesions. Hemorrhage and necrosis are commonly seen.[23] Molecular studies have recently identified genetic signatures associated with a higher risk of malignant transformation.[24]

Patients with LCA present with symptoms approximately 50% to 75% of the time. Upper abdominal pain is common and may be related to hemorrhage into the tumor or local compressive symptoms. The physical examination is usually unrevealing and tumor markers are normal. Dramatic presentations with free intraperitoneal rupture and bleeding can occur. CT usually demonstrates a well-circumscribed heterogenous mass that demonstrates early enhancement during the arterial phase. MRI scans of LCA have specific imaging characteristics, including a well-demarcated heterogenous mass containing fat or hemorrhage. Although, in the past, imaging studies lacked the accuracy to diagnose LCA, current imaging techniques can accurately identify most of these tumors.[25,26] Ultimately, however, resection may be necessary to secure a diagnosis in difficult cases.

The two major risks of LCA are rupture, with potentially life-threatening intraperitoneal hemorrhage, and malignant transformation. Quantifying the risk of rupture is difficult but has been estimated to be as high as 30% to 50% and may be related to size. Although there are numerous reports of transformation of LCA into hepatocellular carcinoma (HCC), the true risk of transformation is probably low.

Patients who present with acute hemorrhage need emergent attention. If possible, hepatic artery embolization is a helpful and usually effective temporizing maneuver. Once stabilized and appropriately resuscitated, a laparotomy and resection of the mass are required. Symptomatic masses should be similarly resected. Patients with asymptomatic LCAs on OCPs can be watched for regression after stopping the OCPs, although progression and rupture have been observed in this setting. Behavior of LCAs during pregnancy has been unpredictable and resection prior to a planned pregnancy is usually recommended. Overall, the surgeon must compare the risks of expectant management with serial imaging studies and AFP measurements against those of resection. Resection is usually recommended because of low mortality in experienced hands and the above-mentioned risks of observation. Margin status is not important in these resections and limited resections can be performed. The management of adenomatosis is controversial but large lesions should probably be resected because of the risk of rupture, whereas the risk of malignancy is low in lesions smaller than 5 cm.[27] Occasionally, liver transplantation is necessary for aggressive forms of adenomatosis.[28,29]

### Focal Nodular Hyperplasia

Focal nodular hyperplasia (FNH) is the second most common benign tumor of the liver and is predominantly discovered in young women. FNH is usually a small (<5 cm) nodular mass arising in a normal liver that involves the right and left liver equally. The mass is characterized by a central fibrous scar with radiating septae, although no central scar is seen in approximately 15% of cases (Fig. 54-34) Microscopically, FNH contains cords of benign-appearing hepatocytes divided by multiple fibrous septae originating from a central scar. Typical hepatic vascularity is not seen, but atypical biliary epithelium is found scattered throughout the lesion. The central scar often contains a large artery that branches out into multiple smaller arteries in a spoke wheel pattern.

The cause of FNH is not known, but the most common theory is that FNH is related to a developmental vascular malformation. Female hormones and OCPs have been implicated in the development and growth of FNH but the association is weak and difficult to prove. Occasional cases of resolution of symptoms after stopping OCPs have been reported. Nontypical forms of FNH have been described. Telangiectatic FNH, with or without atypia, and mixed hyperplastic-adenomatous FNH account for approximately 20% of cases. Although these may have risks of rupture or malignant degeneration, this remains unclear. These FNHs occur more frequently in men and are more difficult to characterize radiologically.

Most patients with FNH present as an incidental finding at laparotomy or, more commonly, on imaging studies. If symptoms are noted, they are most often vague abdominal pain, but

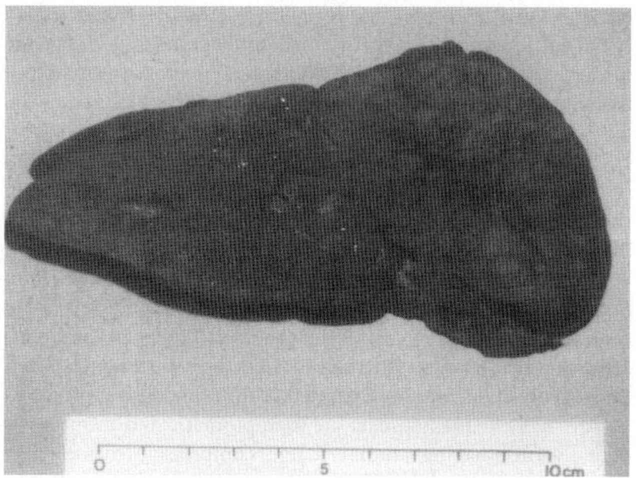


**FIGURE 54-34** Cross section of resected focal nodular hyperplasia (FNH). Note the well-defined central scar. (From Hugh TJ, Poston GJ: Benign liver tumors and masses. In Blumgart LH, Fong Y [eds]: Surgery of the liver and biliary tract, London, 2000, WB Saunders, pp 1397–1422.)

a variety of nonspecific symptoms have been described. It is often difficult to ascribe these reported symptoms to the presence of FNH and therefore other possible causes must be sought. Physical examination is usually unrevealing and mild abnormalities of liver function may be found. Serum AFP levels are normal.

With advances in hepatobiliary imaging, most cases of FNH can be diagnosed radiologically with reasonable certainty. Contrast-enhanced CT and MRI have become accurate methods of diagnosing FNH. These scans usually demonstrate a homogeneous mass with a central scar that rapidly enhances during the arterial phase of contrast administration. When no central scar is seen, however, radiologic diagnosis is difficult and differentiating from LCA or a malignant mass, especially fibrolamellar HCC, can sometimes be impossible. Occasionally, histologic confirmation is necessary and resection is recommended for definitive diagnosis. Fine-needle aspiration for the diagnosis of FNH has been recommended but is often unrevealing.

The natural history of FNH is not fully understood. However, most FNHs are benign and indolent tumors. Asymptomatic patients mostly remain for over long periods. Rupture, bleeding, and infarction are exceedingly rare and malignant degeneration of FNH has never been reported. The treatment of FNH, therefore, depends on diagnostic certainty and symptoms. Asymptomatic patients with typical radiologic features do not require treatment. If diagnostic uncertainty exists, resection may be necessary for histologic confirmation. Symptomatic patients should be thoroughly investigated to look for other pathology to explain the symptoms. Careful observation of symptomatic FNH with serial imaging is reasonable because symptoms may resolve in a significant number of cases. Patients with persistent symptomatic FNH or an enlarging mass should be considered for resection. Because FNH is a benign diagnosis, resection must be performed, with minimal morbidity and mortality.[30]

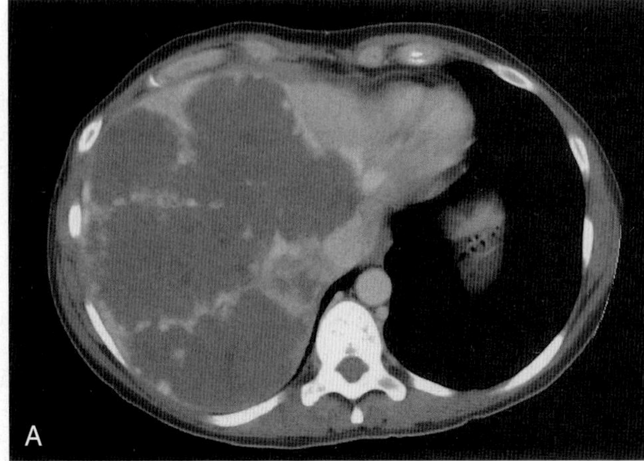


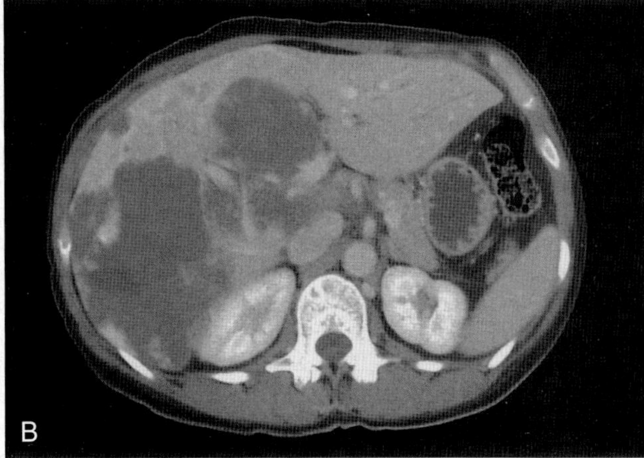


**FIGURE 54-35 A, B,** CT scans of a large cavernous hemangioma showing displacement of left and middle hepatic veins and abutment of the left portal vein. The mass was symptomatic and required an extended right hepatectomy to remove.

### Hemangioma

Hemangioma is the most common benign tumor of the liver. It occurs in women more than in men (3 : 1 ratio) and at a mean age of approximately 45 years. Small capillary hemangiomata are of no clinical significance, whereas larger cavernous hemangiomata more often come to the attention of the liver surgeon (Fig. 54-35). Cavernous hemangiomata have been associated with FNH and are also theorized to be congenital vascular malformations. The enlargement of hemangiomata is by ectasia rather than neoplasia. They are usually solitary, less than 5 cm in diameter, and occur with equal incidence in the right and left hemilivers. Lesions larger than 5 cm are arbitrarily called *giant hemangiomata.* Involution or thrombosis of hemangiomata can result in dense fibrotic masses that may be difficult to differentiate from malignancy. Microscopically, they are endothelium-lined, blood-filled spaces separated by thin fibrous septae.[31]

Usually, hemangiomata are asymptomatic and found incidentally on imaging studies. Large compressive masses may cause vague upper abdominal symptoms. Symptoms ascribed to a liver hemangioma, however, mandate a search for other pathology because, in approximately 50% of cases, an alternative cause of symptoms will be found. Rapid expansion or acute thrombosis can occasionally cause symptoms. Spontaneous rupture of liver hemangiomata is exceedingly rare. An associated syndrome of thrombocytopenia and consumptive coagulopathy known as *Kasabach-Merritt syndrome* is rare but well described.

LFTs and tumor markers are usually normal in liver hemangiomata. Radiologic investigation can make the diagnosis reliably in most cases. CT and MRI are usually sufficient if a typical peripheral nodular enhancement pattern is seen. Isotope-labeled red blood cell scans are an accurate test but are rarely necessary if high-quality CT and MRI are available. Percutaneous biopsy of a suspected hemangioma is potentially dangerous and inaccurate. Therefore, biopsy is not recommended.

The natural history of liver hemangioma is generally benign; it appears that most remain stable over long periods of time, with a low risk of rupture or hemorrhage. Growth and development of symptoms do occur, however, occasionally requiring resection. There has never been a report of malignant degeneration of a liver hemangioma. An asymptomatic patient with a secure diagnosis can therefore be simply observed. Symptomatic patients should undergo a thorough evaluation looking for alternative explanations for the symptoms, but are candidates for resection if no other cause is found. Rupture, significant change in size, and development of the Kasabach-Merritt syndrome are indications for resection. In rare cases of diagnostic uncertainty, resection may be necessary to make a definitive diagnosis. Resection of liver hemangiomata should be performed, with minimal morbidity and mortality. The preferred approach to resection is enucleation with arterial inflow control, but anatomic resections may be necessary in some cases. Surgery on large central hemangiomata can be associated with significant morbidity.

Liver hemangiomata in children are common, accounting for approximately 12% of all childhood hepatic tumors. They are usually multifocal and can involve other organs. Large hemangiomata in children can result in congestive heart failure secondary to arteriovenous shunting. Untreated symptomatic childhood hemangiomata are associated with a 70% mortality. On the other hand, almost all small capillary hemangiomata resolve. Symptomatic childhood hemangiomata may be treated with therapeutic embolization; medical therapy should be initiated for congestive heart failure. Radiation and chemotherapeutic agents have been used but experience has been limited. Resection may be necessary for symptomatic lesions or rupture.

### Other Benign Tumors

The vast majority of benign solid liver tumors are LCAs, FNHs, or hemangiomata, but there are other benign hepatic tumors. However, these are rare and can be difficult to differentiate from malignancy. Macroregenerative nodules, previously known as *adenomatous hyperplasia*, are single or multiple, well-circumscribed, bile-stained, bulging surface nodules that occur primarily in cirrhotics and result from the hyperplastic response to chronic liver injury. These lesions have malignant potential and can be difficult to distinguish from HCC. Nodular regenerative hyperplasia (NRH) is a benign diffuse micronodular (usually <2 cm) process associated with lymphoproliferative disorders, collagen-vascular diseases, and the use of steroids or chemotherapy. NRH has no malignant potential and is not associated with cirrhosis. Biopsy may be necessary to distinguish these focal nodules from malignancy.

Mesenchymal hamartomas are rare solitary tumors of childhood that account for 5% of pediatric liver tumors. They are usually large cystic masses found in the right liver that present as progressive, painless, abdominal distention. Resection of mesenchymal hamartomas may be necessary in the case of large lesions causing a mass effect.

Fatty tumors of the liver are rarely encountered, but can usually be distinguished by typical characteristics on CT or MRI scans. Fatty tumors of the liver include primary lipomas, myelolipomas (which contain hematopoietic tissue), angiolipomas (which contain blood vessels), and angiomyolipomas (which contain smooth muscle). Focal fatty change in the liver can be confused with a neoplastic process and is becoming more common with improved imaging and the increasing incidence of hepatic steatosis.

Benign fibrous tumors of the liver can become large and symptomatic, requiring resection. Inflammatory pseudotumors of the liver are localized masses of inflammatory cells that can mimic a neoplasm. The cause of these inflammatory lesions is unknown, but may be related to thrombosed vessels or old abscesses. Other extremely rare benign hepatic tumors include leiomyomas, myxomas, schwannomas, lymphangiomas, and teratomas.

Intrahepatic biliary cystadenomas or bile duct adenomas are rare, but can cause biliary symptoms. Biliary hamartomas or biliary hyperplasia are common and are often seen as small white surface lesions that can mimic small metastatic tumors at abdominal exploration. Adrenal and pancreatic rests have also been found in the liver.

## Primary Solid Malignant Neoplasms

### Hepatocellular Carcinoma

**Epidemiology** HCC is the most common primary malignancy of the liver and one of the most common malignancies worldwide, accounting for over 1 million deaths annually. The geographic distribution of HCC is clearly related to the incidence of hepatitis B (HBV) infection. The highest incidence of disease (>10 to 20 cases/100,000) is found in Southeast Asia and tropical Africa. The lowest incidence (1 to 3 cases/100,000) is found in Australia, North America, and Europe. In high-incidence areas, rates are variable. For example, Taiwan has an incidence of 150 cases/100,000 and Singapore has an incidence of 28 cases/100,000. Epidemiologic evidence strongly suggests that HCC is largely related to environmental factors; the incidence of HCC in immigrants eventually approaches that of the local population after several generations. An exception to this is that whites living in high-prevalence areas tend to have a low incidence of HCC. This is likely related to the continuation of the lifestyle and environment of their home country. It is probable that the variation in incidence rates among immigrants is related to HBV carrier rates. A significant rise in the incidence of HCC in the United States and other Western countries has been noted over the last 35 years. The explanation for this rising incidence is not understood, but the emergence of hepatitis C (HCV) infection and immigration patterns have been suggested.[32]

HCC is two to eight times more common in males compared with females in low- and high-incidence areas. Although sex hormones may play a minor role in the development of HCC, the higher incidence in males is probably related to higher rates of associated risk factors, such as HBV infection, cirrhosis, smoking, alcohol abuse, and higher hepatic DNA synthesis in cirrhosis. In general, the incidence of HCC increases with age, but a tendency to develop HCC earlier in high-incidence areas has been noted. For example, in Mozambique, 50% of patients with HCC were found to be younger than 30 years. This may be related to differing ages at infection and the natural histories of hepatitis B and C infections.

**Causative Factors** A large number of associations among hepatic viral infections, environmental exposure, alcohol use, smoking, genetic metabolic diseases, cirrhosis, oral contraceptives and development of HCC have been recognized. Overall, 75% to 80% of HCC cases are related to HBV (50% to 55%) or HBC (25% to 30%) infections. It is also clear from research that the development of HCC is a complex and multistep process that involves any number of these risk factors.[33,34]

Many years of research have documented a clear association between persistent HBV infection and the development of HCC. Studies have estimated relative risks of 5 to 100 for the development of HCC in HBV-infected individuals compared with noninfected individuals. Other evidence includes the following observations: (1) geographic areas high in HBV infection have high rates of HCC; (2) HBV infection precedes the development of HCC; (3) the sequence of HBV infection to cirrhosis to HCC is well documented; and (4) the HBV genome is found in the HCC genome. The HBV has no known oncogenes, but insertional mutagenesis into hepatocytes may be a contributing factor to the development of HCC. Another proposed mechanism is related to cirrhosis and chronic hepatic inflammation, which is present in 60% to 90% of patients with HBV infection and HCC. Cirrhosis, however, is not a prerequisite for the development of HBV-related HCC. It is important to note that the risk of HCC is not simply related to HBV exposure, but requires chronic infection (i.e., chronically positive HBV surface antigen). There is a higher risk of persistent infection (carrier state) when the infection is acquired at birth or during early childhood. Familial clustering of HCC is probably related to early vertical transmission of the virus and establishment of the chronic carrier state.

Hepatitis C has been discovered to be a major cause of chronic liver disease in Japan, Europe, and the United States, where there is a relatively low rate of HBV infection. Antibodies to the HCV are found in 76% of patients with HCC in Japan and Europe and in 36% of patients in the United States. HBV and HCV infection are both independent risk factors for the development of HCC but probably act synergistically when an individual is infected with both viruses. Although the natural history of HCV infection is not completely understood, it appears to be one of chronic infection, with a benign early course. However, the ultimate development of cirrhosis and HCC may ensue. Studies on the rates of progression to cirrhosis estimate a median time of 30 years, but differing progression rates yield a range of less than 20 to over 50 years. Factors associated with a more rapid progression include male gender, chronic alcohol use, and older age at the time of infection. HCV is an RNA virus that does not integrate into the host genome and therefore the pathogenesis of HCV-related HCC may be related to more chronic inflammation and cirrhosis than to direct carcinogenesis.[35]

The true relationship of cirrhosis and HCC is difficult to ascertain, and suggestions of causation remain speculative. Cirrhosis is not required for the development of HCC and hepatocarcinogenesis is not an inevitable result of cirrhosis. The relationship of cirrhosis and HCC is further complicated by the fact that they share common associations. Furthermore, some associations (e.g., HBV infection, hemochromatosis) are associated with higher risk of HCC, whereas others (e.g., alcohol, primary biliary cirrhosis) are associated with a lower risk of HCC. Research has demonstrated that cirrhotic livers with higher DNA replication rates are associated with the development of HCC.

Chronic alcohol abuse has been associated with an increased risk of HCC and there may be a synergistic effect with HBV and HCV infection. Alcohol causes cirrhosis, but has never been shown to be directly be carcinogenic in hepatocytes. Thus, alcohol likely acts as a cocarcinogen. Cigarette smoking has been linked to the development of HCC, but the evidence is not consistent and the contributing risk independent of viral hepatitis is likely small. Aflatoxin, produced by *Aspergillus* spp., is a powerful hepatotoxin. With chronic exposure, aflatoxin acts as a carcinogen and increases the risk of HCC. The offending fungi grow on grains, peanuts, and food products in tropical and subtropical regions. Ingestion of contaminated foods results in aflatoxin exposure. Levels of aflatoxin in these implicated foods are regulated in the United States.

Other chemicals have also been implicated as carcinogens related to HCC. These include nitrites, hydrocarbons, solvents, pesticide, and vinyl chloride. Thorotrast (colloidal thorium dioxide) is an angiographic medium that was used in the 1930s. It emits high levels of long-lasting radiation and has been associated with hepatic fibrosis, angiosarcoma, cholangiosarcoma, and HCC. Associations with inherited metabolic liver diseases such as hereditary hemochromatosis, $\alpha_1$-antitrypsin deficiency, and Wilson's disease have also been implicated as risk factors for HCC. Associations with hormonal manipulations, such as the use of OCPs, and anabolic steroids have been suggested but are weak and are probably better linked specifically to adenoma and well-differentiated HCC. Research has been focusing on relationships of HCC with diabetes, obesity, and nonalcoholic fatty liver disease.[32,36,37]

**Clinical Presentation** Most commonly, patients presenting with HCC are men 50 to 60 years of age who complain of right upper quadrant abdominal pain and weight loss, and have a palpable mass. In countries endemic for HBV, presentation at a younger age is common and probably related to childhood infection. Unfortunately, in unscreened populations, HCC tends to present at a later stage because of the lack of symptoms in early stages. Presentation at an advanced stage is often with vague right upper quadrant abdominal pain that sometimes radiates to the right shoulder. Nonspecific symptoms of advanced malignancy such as anorexia, nausea, lethargy, and weight loss are also common. Another common presentation of HCC is hepatic decompensation in a patient with known mild cirrhosis or even in patients with unrecognized cirrhosis.

HCC can rarely present as a rupture, with the sudden onset of abdominal pain followed by hypovolemic shock secondary to intraperitoneal bleeding. Other rare presentations include hepatic vein occlusion (Budd-Chiari syndrome), obstructive jaundice, hemobilia, and fever of unknown origin. Less than 1% of cases of HCC present with a paraneoplastic syndrome, usually hypercalcemia, hypoglycemia, and erythrocytosis. Small incidentally noted tumors have become a more common presentation because of the knowledge of specific risk factors, screening programs for diagnosed HBV or HCV infection, and increasing use of high-quality abdominal imaging.

**Diagnosis** Radiologic investigation is a critical part of the diagnosis of HCC. In the past, liver radioisotope scans and angiography were common methods of diagnosis, but ultrasound, CT, and MRI have replaced these studies. Ultrasound plays a significant role in screening and early detection of HCC, but definitive diagnosis and treatment planning rely on CT and/or MRI. Contrast-enhanced CT and MRI protocols aimed at diagnosing HCC take advantage of the hypervascularity of these tumors, and arterial phase images are critical to assess the extent of disease adequately. CT and MRI also evaluate the extent of disease in terms of peritoneal metastases, nodal metastases, and extent of vascular and biliary involvement. Detection of bland or tumor thrombus in the portal or hepatic venous system is also important and can be diagnosed with any of these modalities (Fig. 54-36).

AFP measurements can be helpful in the diagnosis of HCC. An AFP level higher than 20 ng/mL is noted in approximately 75% of documented cases of HCC. False-positive elevations of serum AFP levels can be seen in inflammatory disorders of the liver, such as chronic active viral hepatitis. The specificity and positive predictive values of AFP improve with higher cutoff

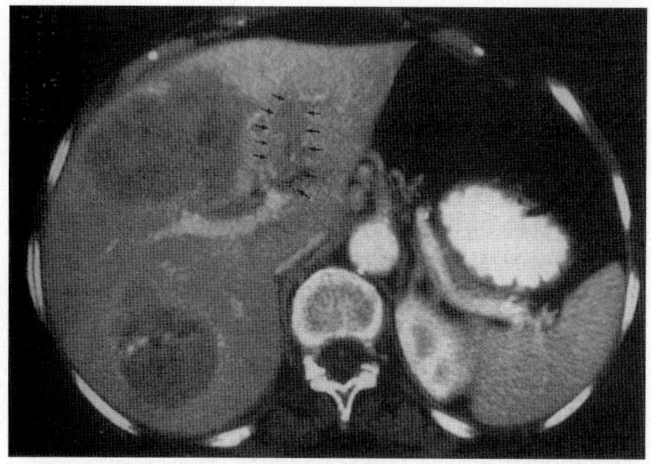

**FIGURE 54-36** Contrast-enhanced CT scan demonstrating multifocal hepatocellular carcinoma. The left portal vein is invaded and expanded by tumor. (From Roddie ME, Adam A: Computed tomography of the liver and biliary tree. In Blumgart LH, Fong Y [eds]: Surgery of the liver and biliary tract, London, 2000, WB Saunders, pp 309–340.)

levels (e.g., 400 ng/mL), but at the cost of sensitivity. With improvements in imaging technology and the ability to detect smaller tumors, AFP is largely used as an adjunctive test in patients with liver masses. AFP levels are particularly useful in monitoring treated patients for recurrence after normalization of levels.

At present, the diagnosis of HCC can be made according to the guidelines of the Barcelona-2000 European Association for the Study of the Liver (EASL) Conference[38] and to successive modifications of guidelines from the American Association for the Study of Liver Disease (AASLD).[39] Pathologic diagnoses of HCC are made according to the International Working Party criteria. For hepatic nodules from 1 to 2 cm in size, a triple-phase CT and MRI scan must show typical features of HCC—arterially enhancing mass with washout of contrast in delayed phases—to confirm the diagnosis. If atypical features appear on imaging, a biopsy should be obtained for histologic diagnosis. For hepatic nodules larger than 2 cm, a triple-phase CT or MRI scan is required if typical features of HCC are identified in combination with an AFP level higher than 200 ng/mL. If typical features appear on imaging, the diagnosis of HCC is confirmed. If atypical features are seen, then biopsy is required to confirm the histologic diagnosis.

Patients with appropriate risk factors and suggestive radiologic features, with or without an elevated AFP level, who are candidates for potentially curative surgical therapy do not require preoperative biopsy unless the diagnosis is in question. Percutaneous fine-needle aspiration of HCC does run a small risk of tumor cell spillage (estimated to be ≈1%) and rupture or bleeding, especially in cirrhotic livers and subcapsular tumors.

Once the diagnosis of HCC has been made, the patient must be staged to develop an appropriate treatment plan. Most patients with HCC have two diseases and survival is as much related to the tumor as it is to cirrhosis. Staging includes an extent of disease and extent of cirrhosis workup.

In assessing the extent of disease, the common sites of metastases must be considered. HCC largely metastasizes to the lung, bone, and peritoneum. Preoperative history should focus on symptoms referable to these areas. Extent of disease in the liver, including macrovascular invasion and the presence of multiple liver masses, must also be considered. Cross-sectional abdominal imaging, including arterial phase images (see earlier), yields information on the extent of disease in the liver, as well as peritoneal disease. A preoperative chest CT is mandatory because lung metastases are usually asymptomatic. Routine bone scans are not performed unless there are suggestive symptoms or signs.

Assessment of liver function is absolutely critical when considering treatment options for a patient with HCC. Liver resection is considered the treatment of choice for HCC and the risk of postoperative liver failure and/or death must be considered. This risk is related to the degree of cirrhosis, portal hypertension, amount of liver resected (functional liver reserve), and regenerative potential response. Other successful treatments are available for HCC, such as ablative techniques, embolization techniques, and liver transplantation. Therefore, a complete assessment of tumor and liver function must be carried out. A number of tests of liver function are available, generally divided into clinical assessment and functional tests, and there are many clinical assessment schemes (see earlier). However, Child-Pugh status is used most often. Child-Pugh class C patients are not candidates for resectional therapy whereas Child-Pugh class A patients can usually tolerate some extent of liver resection. Many consider Child-Pugh class B patients as candidates for operation, but they are generally borderline and therapy must be individualized.

Outside of scoring systems, it has been demonstrated that significant portal hypertension, regardless of biochemical assessments, is highly predictive of postoperative liver failure and death. Portal hypertension can be assessed directly through hepatic vein wedge pressures, but is usually obvious on high-quality imaging in the form of splenomegaly, a cirrhotic-appearing liver, and intra-abdominal varices. Blood work usually demonstrates marked cytopenias. Most typically, patients have thrombocytopenia. Functional tests of liver function have been well described but are not routinely used in most Western centers because the results of studies evaluating their predictive value have been mixed.

Staging laparoscopy has been used as a staging tool in HCC and spares about one in five patients a nontherapeutic laparotomy. Laparoscopy yields additional information about the extent of disease in the liver, extrahepatic disease, and cirrhosis. The yield of laparoscopy is dictated by the extent of disease and is only selectively used. The presence of clinically apparent cirrhosis, radiologic evidence of vascular invasion, or bilobar tumors increase the yield to 30%, whereas without these factors the yield is 5%.[40]

There are a number of staging systems for HCC but none have been shown to be particularly superior; they probably depend on the specific population being staged, as well as the cause of HCC in that particular patient population. The TNM staging system is not routinely used for HCC because it does not accurately predict survival; it does not take liver function into account. Moreover, the TNM staging system relies on pathology that is frequently unavailable preoperatively. The Okuda staging system is an older but simple and effective system that takes liver function and tumor-related factors into account. It adds up a single point for the presence of tumor involving more than 50% of the liver, presence of ascites, albumin level

**Table 54-7 Cancer of the Liver Italian Group Score***

| CLINICAL PARAMETERS | CUTOFF VALUES | POINTS |
|---|---|---|
| Child-Pugh class | A | 0 |
| | B | 1 |
| | C | 2 |
| Tumor morphology | Uninodular, <50% extension | 0 |
| | Multinodular, <50% extension | 1 |
| | Massive or extension >50% | 2 |
| AFP (ng/dL) | <400 | 0 |
| | >400 | 1 |
| Portal vein thrombosis | No | 0 |
| | Yes | 1 |

*Score ranges from 0 to 6; a score of 4 to 6 is generally considered advanced disease, whereas a score of 0 to 3 has the potential for long-term survival.

**BOX 54-1 Treatment Options for Hepatocellular Carcinoma**

**Surgical**
Resection
Orthotopic liver transplantation

**Ablative**
Ethanol (EtOH) injection
Acetic acid injection
Thermal ablation (cryotherapy, radiofrequency ablation, microwave)

**Transarterial**
Embolization
Chemoembolization
Radiotherapy

**Combination Transarterial and Ablative:**
**External Beam Radiation**
Systemic
Chemotherapy
Hormonal
Immunotherapy

less than 3 g/dL, and bilirubin level higher than 3 mg/dL. The Okuda staging system reliably distinguishes patients with a prohibitively poor prognosis from those with potential for long-term survival. The most well-validated staging system is the Cancer of the Liver Italian Program (CLIP), which was rigorously developed and has been prospectively validated (Table 54-7). An example of a scoring system that is probably population-specific is the Chinese University Prognostic Index (CUPI), which takes into account TNM stage, symptoms, ascites, and AFP, bilirubin, and ALP levels and appears to apply mainly to HBV-related HCC in China.

**Pathology** Histologically, HCC is graded as well, moderately, or poorly differentiated. The grade of HCC, however, has never been shown to predict outcome accurately. Grossly, the growth patterns of HCC have been classified in a number of ways. The most useful scheme divides HCC into three distinct growth patterns that have distinct relationships to outcome. The hanging type of HCC is connected to the liver by a small vascular stalk and is easily resected without sacrifice of a significant amount of adjacent non-neoplastic liver tissue. This type can grow to substantial size without involving much normal liver tissue. The pushing type of HCC is well demarcated and often contains a fibrous capsule. It is characterized by growth that displaces vascular structures rather than invading them. This type is usually resectable. The last type is called the *infiltrative type* of HCC, which tends to invade vascular structures, even at a small size. Resecting the infiltrative type is often possible, but positive histologic margins are common. Small tumors (<5 cm) usually do not fall into any of these groups and are often discussed as a separate entity.

Finally, HCC can present in a multifocal manner. Most HCC probably starts as a single tumor, but ultimately multiple satellite lesions can develop secondary to portal vein invasion and metastases. Multifocal tumors throughout the liver probably represent the end stage of HCC, with multiple metastases and multiple primary tumors.

**Treatment** There are a large number of treatment options for patients with HCC, reflecting the heterogeneity of this disease and the lack of a proven superior treatment, except complete resection (Box 54-1). Deciding on a treatment regimen for any one patient must take into consideration the stage of malignancy, condition of the patient and of the liver, and experience of the treating physician(s).

Complete excision of HCC by partial hepatectomy or by total hepatectomy and liver transplantation is the treatment of choice, when possible, because it has the highest chance of long-term survival. In general, however, only 10% to 20% of patients are considered to have resectable disease. Historically, mortality rates for partial hepatectomy have ranged from 1% to 20% but, if performed in healthy patients without advanced cirrhosis, most series have a mortality rate less than 5%. Advances in surgical technique have also allowed the development of limited segmental resections when appropriate, which preserves liver function and improves early postoperative recovery. Selection of the appropriate patient for resection is critical and must take into account the condition of the liver and extent of disease. Patients with Child-Pugh class B or C cirrhosis or portal hypertension do not tolerate resection. The volume of the FLR is also an important consideration and is associated with postoperative complications and mortality. Preoperative portal vein embolization is an effective strategy to increase the volume and function of the FLR and should be used liberally in patients with Child-Pugh class A cirrhosis with a small FLR (i.e., <30% to 40% of the total liver volume) who are being considered for a major resection. The overall postresection survival rates for HCC are 58% to 100% at 1 year, 28% to 88% at 3 years, 11% to 75% at 5 years, and 19% to 26% at 10 years. These results obviously depend on the stage of the tumor and degree of cirrhosis in each particular series. Together, they give a sense of the possibilities.

A variety of prognostic factors predictive of survival after resection have been identified, but none are universally agreed on . The most commonly cited negative prognostic factors are tumor size, cirrhosis, infiltrative growth pattern, vascular invasion, intrahepatic metastases, multifocal tumors, lymph node metastases, margin less than 1 cm, and lack of a capsule. The best outcomes are found in patients with single small tumors, but size alone should not contraindicate resection. Multifocal tumors and major vascular invasion are generally associated with a poor outcome but some groups advocate resection in highly select patients.[1,41]

Theoretically, orthotopic liver transplantation (OLT) is the ideal treatment for HCC because it addresses the liver dysfunction and cirrhosis, and the HCC. The limitations of transplantation are the need for chronic immunosuppression and the lack of organ donors. There has been growing interest in the use of partial hepatectomy from live donors, which addresses the latter point but remains a somewhat controversial approach. Early series of transplantation for HCC had high recurrence rates and relatively poor long-term survival, largely attributed to the fact that most of these patients were being transplanted for advanced disease. Refinements in patient selection—namely, patients with single tumors smaller than 5 cm, or no more than three tumors and 3 cm in size—have resulted in improved outcomes.[42] Long-term survival rates with more stringent selection criteria have ranged from 50% to 85%. Studies have begun to expand the indications for OLT without a major effect on long-term survival but likely an increase in overall recurrence rates. Comparing results of resection with transplantation is difficult and the two should be viewed as complementary rather than competitive.[43] Patients with advanced cirrhosis (Child class B and C) and early-stage HCC should be considered for transplantation whereas those with Child class A cirrhosis have similar results with transplantation and resection and should probably be resected.[44-46]

A number of other nonsurgical local ablative therapies are available for the treatment of small tumors. Percutaneous ethanol injection (PEI) is a useful technique for ablating small tumors. The tumor is killed by a combination of cellular dehydration, coagulative necrosis, and vascular thrombosis. Most tumors smaller than 2 cm can be ablated with a single application of PEI, but larger tumors may require multiple injections. Long-term survival after PEI for tumors smaller than 5 cm has been reported to range from 24% to 40%, but no randomized trials have compared PEI with resection. Percutaneous injection of acetic acid is a similar technique to PEI but has stronger necrotizing abilities, making it more useful in septated tumors.

Thermal ablative techniques that freeze or heat tumors to destroy them have become popular. Cryotherapy uses a specialized cryoprobe to freeze and thaw tumor and surrounding liver tissue, with resulting necrosis. Cryotherapy is usually performed at laparotomy or laparoscopically, but has been performed with percutaneous techniques. One advantage is that the ice ball formed is easily monitored with ultrasound. Disadvantages include a heat sink effect limiting the usefulness of freezing near major blood vessels and a relatively high complication rate of 8% to 41%. Reported 2-year survival rates for cryoablation of HCC range from 30% to 60%, but no comparative studies to resection have been carried out. Radiofrequency ablation (RFA) uses high-frequency alternating current to create heat around an inserted probe, resulting in temperatures higher than 60° C (140° F) and immediate cell death. Although initially limited to smaller tumors, improvements in technology have created RFA probes reportedly able to ablate tumors as large as 7 cm. Nonetheless, the efficacy of RFA for HCCs larger than 3 cm is limited because of increased local recurrence rates. RFA is also limited by the protective effect of blood vessels and does not ablate well in these areas. The procedure can easily be performed percutaneously, with low complication rates, and optimal guidance systems are being developed. Studies have suggested that RFA is superior to PEI for limited HCC for local tumor control but not survival. Recent data would also suggest that resection may be superior to RFA for small HCCs.[47] However, no long-term data for RFA of HCC exist.[48]

Transarterial therapy for HCC is based on the fact that most of the tumor's blood supply is from the hepatic artery. Hepatic arterial infusional chemotherapy using 5-fluorouracil (5-FU— based compounds, cisplatin, and doxorubicin has been studied in limited numbers. Response rates of 25% to 60% have been reported, but the requirement of a laparotomy to place the pump and associated hepatic toxicity limits the applicability of this approach to highly select patients.

Similarly, percutaneous transarterial embolization can induce ischemic necrosis in HCC, resulting in response rates as high as 50% (Fig. 54-37). Attempts to improve the efficacy of arterial embolization have included adding chemotherapeutic agents (chemoembolization) to the bland embolization particles and oils such as ethiodized oil (Ethiodol) that are selectively taken up by HCCs.[49] Randomized trials have not shown chemoembolization to be superior to bland embolization alone with regard to survival. However, a recent trial have suggested an improvement in local control.[50] Seven randomized trials have compared embolization or chemoembolization to conservative management. Two of these trials and a meta-analysis have confirmed an overall survival advantage from the embolization strategies.[51] The selection of appropriate candidates for embolization is important and treatment should generally be limited to patients with preserved liver function and asymptomatic multinodular tumors without vascular invasion. Poor selection will result in a higher incidence of treatment-induced liver failure, offsetting the potential benefits.

External beam radiation therapy (EBRT) has a limited role in the treatment of HCC, although occasional dramatic responses are seen. EBRT is limited by damage to normal liver parenchyma and to surrounding organs, but newer methods of conformal radiotherapy and breath-gated techniques are improving the usefulness of this treatment modality. Intra-arterial injections of iodine-131 with Ethiodol or yttrium-90 in glass microspheres have also been used to deliver localized radiation to HCCs, with reports of dramatic response rates. Transarterial radiotherapy is a potentially promising therapy for HCC as a primary or adjuvant therapy.

Systemic chemotherapy with a variety of agents (e.g., cisplatin, doxorubicin, etoposide, 5-FU, mitomycin C, amsacrine, mitoxantrone, picibanil, tamoxifen, uracil, VM-26) has been ineffective and has had a minimal role for the treatment of

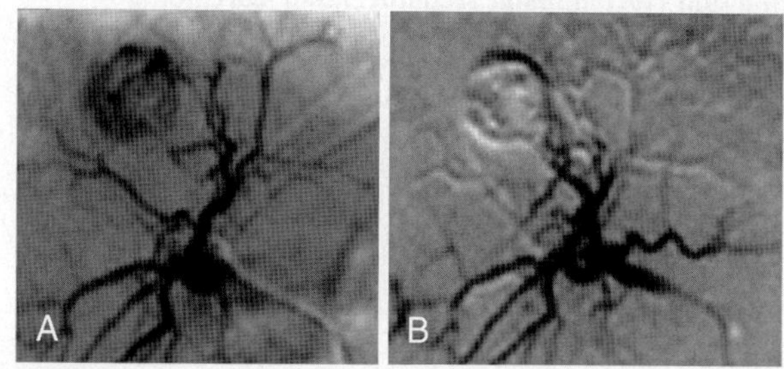


**FIGURE 54-37** Angiograms demonstrating hypervascular hepatocellular carcinoma before **(A)** and after **(B)** embolization.

HCC. Response rates are generally under 20% and of short duration. Systemic immunotherapy and hormonal therapy have been used in small numbers of patients with HCC, with some early promising results, but have not yet demonstrated superiority to standard regimens.

With the large number of available treatment strategies for HCC, it is no surprise that combinations of therapies and adjuvant or neoadjuvant strategies in conjunction with resection have been attempted. Two randomized trials have demonstrated a survival benefit to specific adjuvant strategies after resection of HCC. The first is the use of the retinoid polyprenoic acid and the second is transarterial iodine-131 Ethiodol treatment. Further studies and larger trials are awaited to confirm these promising strategies.

Most recently, sorafenib, a molecular targeted therapy that inhibits the serine-threonine kinases Raf-1 and B-raf, the receptor tyrosine kinase activity of vascular endothelial growth factor receptor (VEGFR) 1, 2, and 3, and platelet-derived growth factor-β (PDGF-β) was evaluated. Llovet and colleagues[52] have randomized 599 patients with advanced stage HCC and Child-Pugh level A cirrhosis to oral sorafenib or placebo. The median overall survival was 10.7 months in the sorafenib group and 7.9 months in the placebo group ($P < .001$), a difference of 2.8 months. The median time to radiologic progression was 5.5 months in the sorafenib group and 2.8 months in the placebo group ($P < .001$, a difference of 2.2 months. Neither group demonstrated any complete responses by radiologic criteria. Although the adverse event profile of sorafenib was similar to the placebo group, this and earlier studies have shown that sorafenib is best tolerated in patients with Child-Pugh class A cirrhosis.

**Distinct Variants of HCC** Fibrolamellar HCC is a variant of HCC with remarkably different clinical features, summarized in Table 54-8. This tumor generally occurs in younger patients without a history of cirrhosis. The tumor is usually well demarcated and encapsulated and may have a central fibrotic area. The central scar can make distinguishing this tumor from FNH difficult. Histologically, FHCC is composed of large polygonal tumor cells embedded in a fibrous stroma, forming lamellar structures (Fig. 54-38). FHCC does not produce AFP, but is associated with elevated neurotensin levels. In general, FHCC has a better prognosis than HCC, likely related to high resectability rates, lack of chronic liver disease, and a more indolent course. Long-term survival can be expected in approximately 50% to 75% of patients after complete resection, but recurrence is common and occurs in at least 80% of patients. The presence of lymph node metastases predicts a worse outcome. Resection of lymph node metastases and recurrent disease has been advocated because of a lack of alternative therapy and the possibility of long-term survival.

**Table 54-8 Comparison of Standard Hepatocellular Carcinoma and Fibrolamellar Hepatocellular Carcinoma**

| PARAMETER | HCC | FHCC |
|---|---|---|
| Male-to-female ratio | 2:1-8:1 | 1:1 |
| Median age (yr) | 55 | 25 |
| Tumor | Invasive | Well circumscribed |
| Resectability | <25% | 50%-75% |
| Cirrhosis | 90% | 5% |
| AFP-positive | 80% | 5% |
| Hepatitis B positive | 65% | 5% |

Rarely, HCC can present as a mixed hepatocellular-cholangiocellular tumor, with cellular differentiation of both types present. Whether this is two separate tumors growing into each other or mixed differentiation of the same tumor is not known. These mixed tumors tend to have a worse prognosis than standard HCC.

A clear cell variant of HCC also exists, in which the cells contain a clear cytoplasm. These tumors can resemble renal cell neoplasms. The clear cell variant may have a better prognosis than standard HCC, but this is a subject of debate. A pleomorphic or giant cell variant of HCC has also been reported. Cells in this type are multinucleated, pleomorphic, and large and likely originate from primary hepatic cells. Some HCCs show evidence of sarcomatoid differentiation and are referred to as a sarcomatoid variant or carcinosarcoma. These tumors tend not to produce AFP and have a higher incidence of metastases at presentation.

Childhood HCC is a distinct entity that comprises almost 25% of pediatric liver tumors, but rarely occurs in infancy. Viral hepatitis is associated with childhood HCC in Asia, but less so

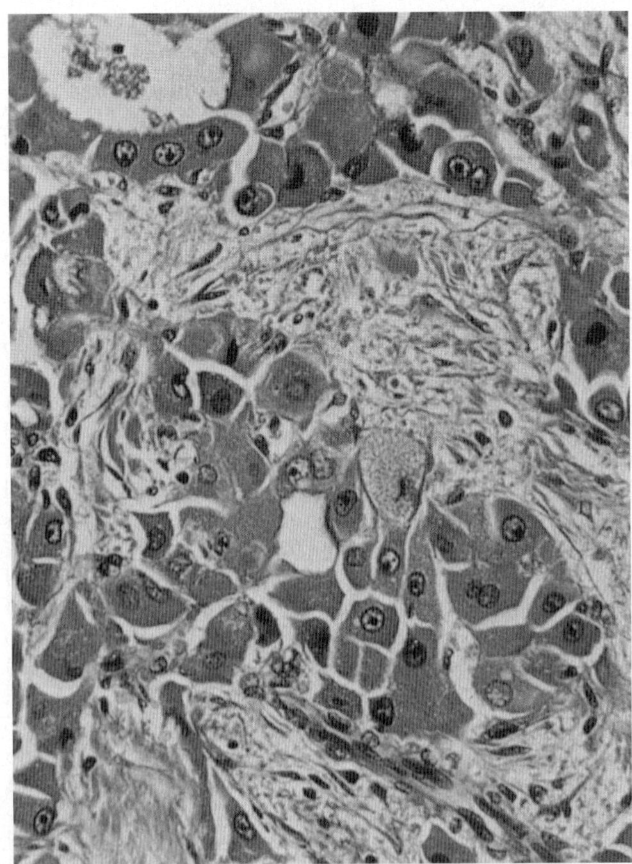

**FIGURE 54-38** FHCC. Abundant collagen is evident interconnecting clusters of cells. The cells are often in single-layer sheets. An acinus is present in the left upper field.

in the United States. Other inherited metabolic liver diseases (see earlier) are often associated with childhood HCC. As in adult HCC, complete resection is the only potentially curative treatment. There is a high incidence of multifocality, vascular invasion, and extrahepatic metastases, resulting in relatively poor long-term survival rates of 10% to 20%.

### Intrahepatic Cholangiocarcinoma

Cholangiocarcinoma is an uncommon neoplasm, with an incidence of 1 to 2/100,000 in the United States, and can develop anywhere along the biliary tree, from the ampulla of Vater to the peripheral intrahepatic bile ducts. Most of these tumors (40% to 60%) involve the biliary confluence (Klatskin's tumor), but approximately 10% emanate from intrahepatic ducts, presenting as a liver mass. Intrahepatic cholangiocarcinoma (IHC) is the second most common primary hepatic neoplasm and has also been referred to as peripheral cholangiocarcinoma or cholangiolar carcinoma. Studies on the incidence and natural history of IHC have been confused by the fact that many series include mixed hepatocellular-cholangiocarcinoma (see earlier). Also, it is likely that in the past, many of these tumors were mistaken for metastatic adenocarcinoma because biopsy is unable to differentiate the two.

Historically, the most common risk factors for the development of cholangiocarcinoma (all types) were primary sclerosing cholangitis, choledochal cyst disease, and RPC. Recent epidemiologic evidence has now linked IHC to HBV infection, HCV infection, HIV infection, cirrhosis and diabetes.[53-55] Increases in the diagnosis of IHC in the United States are likely related to better recognition of the disease and perhaps to the rise in HCV infections in the 1960s and 1970s.

The clinical presentation of IHC is similar to HCC. The most common symptoms are right upper abdominal pain and weight loss. Jaundice occurs in approximately 25% of patients. Patients have more been often presenting with incidentally found liver masses on cross-sectional imaging. Unlike HCC, the AFP level will be normal, although CEA or CA-19-9 levels can be elevated in some cases. Most often, a search for a primary tumor with endoscopy and imaging of the chest will be carried out and not yield any information. If a biopsy has been performed, it is often read as adenocarcinoma or adenocarcinoma of unknown primary. On CT and MRI, IHC is seen as a focal hepatic mass that may be associated with peripheral biliary dilation. The mass typically has peripheral or central enhancement on contrast-enhanced scans. Intrahepatic metastases, lymph node metastases, and growth along the biliary tree are often encountered.

Complete resection is the treatment of choice for IHC. Resectability rates generally range up to 60% and long-term survival in unresected patients is rare. If completely resected, 3-year survival rates range from 16% to 61% and 5-year survival rates range from 24% to 44%. Factors associated with a poor outcome include intrahepatic metastases, lymph node metastases, vascular invasion, and positive margins. There is little known about the effectiveness of radiation and chemotherapy for IHC because of the rarity of the disease. Thus, their application is not routine. Chemotherapy is largely considered ineffective for IHC but improvements in chemotherapy for other gastrointestinal tumors will hopefully translate into improved outcomes. Regional hepatic artery chemotherapy has been under study and may be a promising approach.

### Other Primary Malignant Neoplasms

Hepatoblastoma is the most common primary hepatic tumor of childhood. There are approximately 50 to 70 new cases/year in the United States. Rare cases of adult hepatoblastoma have been reported but, overall, the median age of presentation is 18 months and almost all cases occur before the age of 3 years. Hepatoblastoma has been associated with the familial polyposis syndrome. There are a number of histologic subtypes but, in general, the tumor is derived from fetal or embryonic hepatocytic progenitors and mesenchymal elements are often present. This tumor generally presents as an asymptomatic mass. Mild anemia and thrombocytosis are commonly found at presentation. Serum AFP levels are elevated in 85% to 90% of patients and can serve as useful marker for therapeutic response. Most studies have supported the use of chemotherapy followed by resection and survival appears to be dependent on complete resection. Chemotherapy can serve to downstage tumors, which facilitates resection. In patients without metastatic disease or the anaplastic variant, long-term survival rates of 60% to 70% can be expected with complete resection. Interestingly, 50% of patients with pulmonary metastases can be cured with resection of the hepatic tumor and chemotherapy and/or resection of the pulmonary metastases.

A variety of sarcomas can rarely present as primary liver tumors, but must always be considered metastatic lesions until proven otherwise. Angiosarcoma is probably the best- described primary hepatic sarcoma because of its well-known association with vinyl chloride or Thorotrast exposure. Angiosarcoma typically presents as multiple hepatic masses and can appear in childhood. Long-term survival is uncommon with primary hepatic angiosarcoma. Other sarcomas, including leiomyosarcoma, malignant fibrous histiocytoma, embryonic sarcoma, and primary hepatic rhabdoid tumors have been described but are rare. The latter two lesions are typically seen in the pediatric population.

Non-Hodgkin's lymphoma (NHL) can present primarily in the liver, with or without extrahepatic disease. Primary hepatic lymphoma should be treated in the same manner as lymphoma elsewhere in the body if the diagnosis can be made prior to a liver resection.

Primary hepatic neuroendocrine tumors or carcinoid tumors have been described but are probably extremely rare. Distinguishing the rare primary hepatic neuroendocrine tumor from a metastatic lesion can be difficult because the extrahepatic primary tumor can be radiologically occult for many years, and the liver is the most common site of metastases.

Malignant germ cell tumors of the liver including teratomas, choriocarcinomas, and yolk sac tumors are very rare and are principally described in the pediatric population.

Epithelioid hemangioendothelioma of the liver is a rare malignant vascular tumor that presents with multiple bilateral hepatic masses. Extrahepatic metastases occur in approximately 25% of patients and clinical behavior is unpredictable, with some patients having a prolonged indolent course. Most patients ultimately die of liver failure, but cases of successful transplantation have been reported.

## Metastatic Tumors

The most common malignant tumors of the liver are metastatic lesions. The liver is a common site of metastases from gastrointestinal tumors, presumably because of dissemination via the portal venous system. The most relevant metastatic tumor of the liver to the surgeon is colorectal cancer because of the well-documented potential for long-term survival after complete resection. However, a large number of other tumors commonly metastasize to the liver, including cancers of the upper gastrointestinal system (stomach, pancreas, biliary), genitourinary system (renal, prostate), neuroendocrine system, breast, eye (melanoma), skin (melanoma), soft tissue (retroperitoneal sarcoma), and gynecologic system (ovarian, endometrial, cervix). The large majority of metastatic liver tumors that present with concomitant extrahepatic disease will have unresectable liver disease or are not curable with resection, limiting the role of the surgeon to highly select cases. It is worth reemphasizing that metastatic adenocarcinoma to the liver of unknown primary is often a primary intrahepatic cholangiocarcinoma, and this diagnosis must always be kept in mind.

Traditionally, cancer spread to a distant site was considered a systemic disease in which locoregional therapies (i.e., surgery) were not effective. Some metastatic tumors to the liver and, in particular, metastatic colorectal cancer have been shown to be an exception to this rule. Over 35 years of clinical research has documented that metastatic colorectal cancer isolated in the liver can be resected, with the potential for long-term survival and cure.[56-58] Advances in systemic and regional chemotherapy have also broadened the number of patients eligible for surgical therapy and probably have improved long-term survival after resection.[59] Patient selection is the most important aspect of surgical therapy for metastatic disease in the liver and clinical follow-up of resected patients has identified those most and least likely to benefit. Although long-term survival is common and occurs in up to 50% to 60% of patients in current series, recurrence and chronic multimodal therapy are common, occurring in approximately 75% of patients. Therefore, realistic expectations and honest patient education is an important aspect of treatment. Tumors other than colorectal cancer presenting as isolated or limited hepatic metastases can also be resected for potential long-term survival, but data on these other tumors are sparse and less compelling than for colorectal cancer.

### Colorectal Metastases

There are over 50,000 cases of colorectal liver metastases a year in the United States. Most of these cases are associated with widespread disease and/or unresectable hepatic disease. It is estimated that approximately 5% to 10% of these patients are candidates for a potentially curative liver resection. With improved response rates to modern chemotherapy and advances in hepatic surgery, however, more patients are now candidates for hepatectomy than in the past; at present, up to 20% of patients may be candidates. In the distant past, patients with hepatic colorectal metastases generally presented with symptoms and signs of advanced malignancy such as pain, ascites, jaundice, weight loss, and a palpable mass. Presentation with these symptoms is a poor prognostic sign; few of these patients are candidates for therapy aside from chemotherapy or supportive care. This has led most physicians to follow patients with resected primary colorectal cancer carefully who are potential candidates for aggressive therapy with serial physical examinations, cross-sectional imaging studies, LFTs, and determination of CEA levels. Although not supported by randomized trials, clinical observations have indicated that patients who are carefully followed with these tests are those often found to have resectable metachronous disease and the greatest potential for long-term survival. In addition to these patients, some are found to have synchronous metastatic disease at the time of diagnosis of the primary colorectal cancer on preoperative imaging or at laparotomy.[57,58,60]

CEA is normally only secreted in utero, but is also secreted by most colorectal cancers. Although an elevated CEA level is not specific for recurrent colorectal cancer, a rising CEA level on serial examinations and a new solid mass on imaging studies are diagnostic of metastatic disease. Mild elevations in LFT results are common in metastatic colorectal cancer to the liver, but are not effective as a screening tool. The most common elevated test levels are those of ALP, GGT, and lactate dehydrogenase (LDH). Imaging of hepatic metastases is generally adequate with high-quality CT. Most physicians use thin-cut (5 mm), high-resolution, dynamic, contrast-enhanced helical scanning techniques. Timing with IV contrast should correspond to the portal venous phase to maximize hepatic parenchymal enhancement, which improves the disparity between parenchyma and tumor. Contrast-enhanced MRI can also be useful to characterize hepatic lesions of uncertain significance (see earlier).

Once a patient with colorectal liver metastases is considered a candidate for surgical therapy, a complete extent of disease workup must be performed. Colonoscopy should be performed if it has been longer than 1 year since the last examination to rule out local recurrence or metachronous colorectal lesions. Complete abdominal and pelvic cross-sectional imaging must also be performed. Chest CT is often performed, but is of low yield. Many studies have evaluated the added benefit of PET scans to detect occult extrahepatic disease. Approximately 25% of patients have a change in management based on PET scan findings but this is highly variable, depending on the quality of cross-sectional imaging, radiologic interpretation, and patient selection (Fig. 54-39). Staging laparoscopy prior to definitive laparotomy identifies approximately 50% of all unresectable patients. Overall, 10% of patients are spared a nontherapeutic laparotomy and the yield of laparoscopy correlates with the number of poor prognostic factors present, allowing it to be used on a selective basis.

To date, a prospective trial comparing surgery with no treatment or chemotherapy alone has not been performed, nor is this likely ever to be done. Therefore, the rationale for liver resection comes from retrospective comparisons of these treatment strategies. The surgeon must understand the natural history of colorectal liver metastases left untreated or treated with systemic chemotherapy to interpret survival data associated with hepatectomy appropriately. Before the 1980s, most hepatic metastases were left untreated. Two key studies retrospectively identified patients with isolated single hepatic metastases or multiple but resectable tumors who received no therapy. One study documented a 10% 3-year survival and the other a 2% 5-year survival for patients with limited and potentially resectable disease. It was clear from these studies that long-term survival is extremely rare without treatment and that survival is closely related to the extent of disease. In the past, 5-FU–based systemic chemotherapy was ineffective as sole therapy for hepatic colorectal metastases, with median survivals of approximately 12 months and response rates of 20% to 30%. Tremendous advances in systemic chemotherapy for metastatic colorectal cancer have now been achieved. Combination chemotherapy, including 5-FU with irinotecan or oxaliplatin combined with targeted

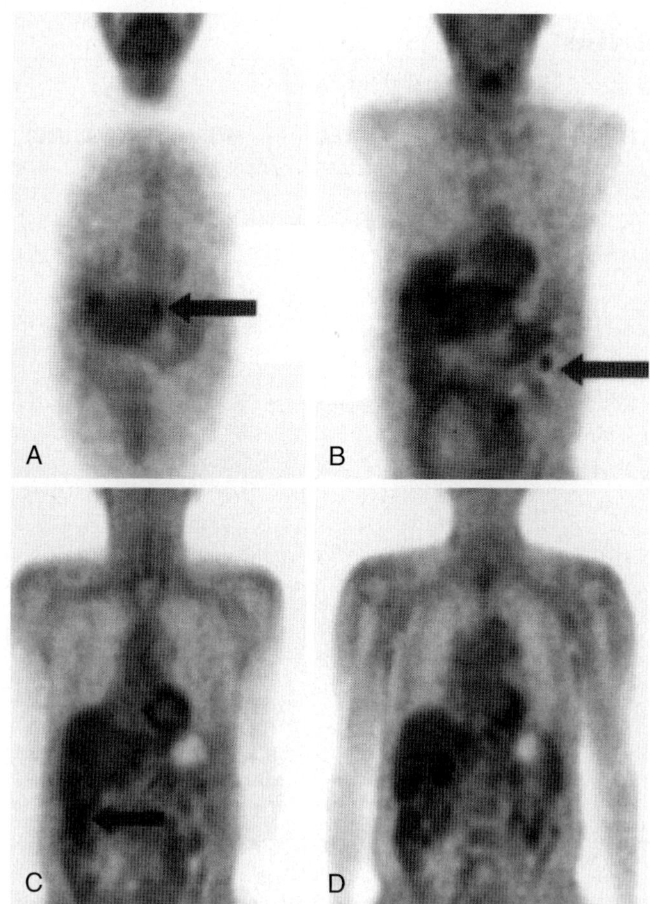


**FIGURE 54-39** Positron emission tomography scan in a patient diagnosed with colorectal cancer synchronously metastatic to the liver after resection of the colonic tumor. The scan demonstrates hypermetabolic activity throughout the liver, but also shows two areas in the left upper quadrant consistent with an omental lesion as well as an anastomotic recurrence. A recent CT scan demonstrated liver disease only. (From Akhurst T, Larson SM: The role of nuclear medicine in the diagnosis and management of hepatobiliary diseases. In Blumgart LH, Fong Y [eds]: Surgery of the liver and biliary tract, London, 2000, WB Saunders, pp 271–308.)

antiangiogenic antibodies such as bevacizumab (anti-VEGF antibody) or cetuximab (Erbitux; antiepidermal growth factor antibody) have now resulted in response rates of over 50% and median survivals of 20 months and longer for patients with advanced disease.[56] Although response rates and survival have improved, durable complete response and 5-year survival are rare with the administration of chemotherapy alone.

The sporadic partial hepatectomies performed for metastatic colorectal cancer prior to the 1980s were appropriately viewed with great skepticism. The high morbidity and mortality for liver surgery at that time, and the questionable rationale of resecting bloodborne metastases, were the major issues. Over the last 30 years, however, large series have demonstrated that liver surgery can now be practiced with acceptable safety and that patients with isolated and resectable hepatic metastases have the potential for long-term survival. Five-year survival rates range from 25% to 58%. There is also a clear trend toward longer survival in more recent series (Table 54-9). Perioperative mortality in experienced centers is consistently less than 5% and, in many series, has been less than 2%. Almost all demonstrate that almost 50% of patients undergoing a liver resection for metastatic colorectal cancer will survive 3 years and 20% will survive 10 years. Despite the low operative mortality, it must be stated that liver surgery is still associated with significant morbidity rates of 30% to 50%. Complications are most commonly bleeding, bile leak, abscess, and other generalized cardiorespiratory complications. With improvements in chemotherapy, a higher proportion of patients undergoing hepatectomy have been treated preoperatively. However, some studies have shown preoperative chemotherapy is associated with hepatic toxicity (steatohepatitis and sinusoidal obstructive syndrome) and higher rates of postoperative liver failure.

From these large series, we have learned much about prognostic factors, as well as which patients are most likely to benefit from a liver resection for hepatic colorectal metastases. Although not all studies agree, it has been found that poor prognostic factors include extrahepatic metastases, involved lymph nodes with the primary colorectal tumor, synchronous presentation (or shorter disease-free interval), larger number of tumors, bilobar involvement, CEA level elevation more than 200 ng/mL, size of largest hepatic tumor more than 5 cm, and involved histologic margins. In a series of 1001 liver resections from Memorial Sloan-Kettering Cancer Center (MSKCC), a multivariate analysis[61] identified five preoperative factors as the most influential on outcome—size larger than 5 cm, disease-free interval less than 1 year, more than one tumor, lymph node–positive primary, and CEA level higher than 200 ng/mL. Using these five factors, we have developed a risk score predictive of recurrence after liver resection (Table 54-10).

Traditionally, the presence of extrahepatic disease, four or more hepatic metastases, close margins, and the inability to resect all disease in the liver have been considered contraindications to hepatectomy. The only one of these historic contraindications that holds true today is the inability to resect all disease. Recent reports have shown that hepatectomy for four or more metastases is associated with an approximate 5-year survival of 33%, despite a high recurrence rate. Although the width of the closest margin has been shown to be associated with outcome, it is often confounded by its relationship to an overall poor prognostic tumor (i.e., multiple synchronous tumors). However, close or involved margins do not appear to preclude the possibility of long-term survival but patients with positive margins tend to fair poorly. Nonetheless, attempts at wide margins more than 1 cm are appropriate, when possible.[62] Resection of extrahepatic metastases that present simultaneously with liver metastases has recently been shown to be associated with long-term survival in highly select cases.[63] The sites that appear to be associated with the best outcomes in this situation are limited lung metastases, locoregional recurrences of the primary tumor, and portal lymph nodes. Patient selection is critical for this aggressive approach and generally requires preoperative chemotherapy to exclude progression and consideration of the overall bulk of metastatic disease.

Although long-term survival after liver resection for hepatic colorectal metastases is clearly possible, recurrence of disease is common. Overall, approximately 75% of patients recur, but in high-risk situations (e.g., four or more tumors, extrahepatic disease) recurrence rates approach 100%. Approximately 50%

**Table 54-9 Results of Hepatic Resection for Hepatic Colorectal Metastases***

| | | | Survival Rate (%) | | | |
|---|---|---|---|---|---|---|
| STUDY (YEAR) | NO. OF PATIENTS | OPERATIVE MORTALITY RATE (%) | 1 YEAR | 5 YEAR | 10 YEAR | MEDIAN SURVIVAL (MO) |
| Adson, 1984 | 141 | 2 | 82 | 25 | — | 24 |
| Hughes, 1986 | 607 | — | — | 33 | — | — |
| Schlag, 1990 | 122 | 4 | 85 | 30 | — | 32 |
| Doci, 1991 | 100 | 5 | — | 30 | — | 28 |
| Gayowski, 1994 | 204 | 0 | 91 | 32 | — | 33 |
| Scheele, 1995 | 469 | 4 | 83 | 33 | 20 | 40 |
| Fong, 1995 | 577 | 4 | 85 | 35 | — | 40 |
| Jenkins, 1997 | 131 | 4 | 81 | 25 | — | 33 |
| Rees, 1997 | 150 | 1 | 94 | 37 | — | |
| Jamison, 1997 | 280 | 4 | 84 | 27 | 20 | 33 |
| Fong, 1999 | 1001 | 3 | 89 | 37 | 22 | 42 |
| Minagawa, 2000 | 235 | 0 | — | 35 | 26 | 37 |
| Scheele, 2000 | 597 | — | — | 36 | — | 35 |
| Choti, 2002 | 226 | 1 | — | 40[†] | 26 | 46 |
| Abdalla, 2004 | 190 | — | — | 58 | — | Not reached |
| Nicoli, 2004 | 228 | 0.9 | | 16 | 9 | |
| Andres, 2008 | 210 | 0.5 | 95 | 40 | — | — |
| de Jong, 2009 | 243 | — | — | 47 | — | 36 |
| House, 2010 | 1600 | | | | | |
| 1985-1998 | 1037 | 2.5 | — | 35 | 16 | 43 |
| 1999-2004 | 563 | 0.5 | — | 43 | — | 64 |

*In selected series with more than 100 patients.

†The 5-year survival rate in the patients operated on in the most current time period in this study was 58%.

**Table 54-10 Clinical Risk Score and Survival in 1001 Patients Undergoing Liver Resection for Metastatic Colorectal Cancer***

| | Survival Rate (%) | | | |
|---|---|---|---|---|
| SCORE | 1 YEAR | 3 YEAR | 5 YEAR | MEDIAN SURVIVAL (MO) |
| 0 | 93 | 72 | 60 | 74 |
| 1 | 91 | 66 | 44 | 51 |
| 2 | 89 | 60 | 40 | 47 |
| 3 | 86 | 42 | 20 | 33 |
| 4 | 70 | 38 | 25 | 20 |
| 5 | 71 | 27 | 14 | 22 |

Adapted from Fong Y, Fortner J, Sun RL, et al: Clinical score for predicting recurrence after hepatic resection for metastatic colorectal cancer: Analysis of 1001 consecutive cases. Ann Surg 230:309–318, 1999.

*Each of the following five risk factors equals one point: node-positive primary, disease-free interval <12 months, >one tumor, size >5 cm, carcinoembryonic antigen level >200 ng/mL. Score is total number of points in an individual patient.

of recurrences are isolated to the liver and a small number of these patients (≈5% of all patients undergoing liver resection) are candidates for a second liver resection. These highly select patients, who undergo a second liver resection with complete removal of all disease, can expect further 5-year survival rates of 30% to 40%. Limited and isolated lung recurrences can also be resected, with the potential for further long-term survival. Furthermore, multiple lines of effective chemotherapy are now available, associated with prolongation of survival. Because of the potential for further effective therapeutic interventions after liver resection, patients eligible for such treatment should be followed with serial CEA level determinations and imaging studies to detect recurrences at an early, potentially treatable phase.

Adjuvant chemotherapy has been used in attempt to reduce recurrence and improve long-term survival. Prospective randomized clinical trials have shown a benefit to adjuvant hepatic intra-arterial chemotherapy but there has been a lack of prospective randomized trials that address the role of adjuvant systemic chemotherapy.

Recently, a randomized controlled trial was reported on this topic; the EORTC intergroup trial recruited 364 patients from multiple institutions randomized into two groups—182 patients were treated with surgery alone and 182 patients had surgery plus systemic chemotherapy.[64] Three cycles of systemic 5′-FU–folinic acid plus oxaliplatin (FOLFOX4) were administered preoperatively and postoperatively in the chemotherapy group. Among eligible patients after randomization, the progression-free survival of patients at 3 years was 28.1% in the group with surgery alone and 36.2% in the group with surgery plus chemotherapy ($P$ = .041). When analyzed by all patients, there was no significant difference in outcome. Although this trial provides evidence that perioperative systemic chemotherapy can delay recurrence of disease, there is little difference in the recurrences of these groups. Also, the benefit of adjuvant chemotherapy may be related to better selection of patients; on closer examination of the survival curve, the principal difference between the groups occurs at its initial measurement.

Another multicenter randomized trial by Portier and associates[65] has addressed the same question. This trial recruited 173 patients randomly assigned to a group who had hepatic resection alone (87 patients) and a second group (86 patients) who had hepatic resection plus systemic chemotherapy for 6 months after the operation (5-FU–folinic acid). Even though this chemotherapy regimen is no longer standard, the 5-year disease-free survival rate was 26.7% for patients who had surgery alone and 33.5% for patients who had surgery plus chemotherapy ($P$ = .028). As in the previous study, the difference in the progression-free survival was small between the two groups. In summary, there is level 1 clinical evidence that adjuvant systemic chemotherapy, when combined with liver resection, modestly improves progression-free survival in patients with colorectal liver metastases.

Neoadjuvant chemotherapy for resectable metastases is also a common strategy to treat occult systemic disease and can be helpful in selecting the small group of patients (<10%) that progress while on chemotherapy and have a poor outcome after hepatectomy. A prospective randomized study by the National Surgical Adjuvant Breast and Bowel Project (NSABP) has begun accruing patients to study the role of adjuvant chemotherapy in these patients.

A convincing argument for adjuvant therapy with the use of hepatic arterial infusion (HAI) chemotherapy can be made.[66,67] The rationale for adjuvant hepatic artery chemotherapy is based on the fact that liver metastases derive most of their blood supply from the hepatic artery. Regional infusion of chemotherapeutic agents such as fluorodeoxyuridine (FUDR) have hepatic extraction rates of 90%, providing high local concentrations with minimal systemic toxicity. Furthermore, approximately 50% of all recurrences after hepatectomy involve the liver, so controlling the liver is likely to affect long-term outcome. There is clearly a higher response rate for liver tumors with HAI therapy compared with systemic therapy. A trial from MSKCC comparing HAI therapy with systemic chemotherapy to systemic chemotherapy alone has demonstrated significantly lower recurrence rates (9% and 36%) and a survival advantage at 2 years (86% versus 72%).[68] Other trials have shown HAI therapy with FUDR to be more effective than hepatectomy alone, with significantly improved disease-free survival.

For patients with unresectable disease, preoperative systemic and HAI chemotherapy has been shown to convert some patients to resection candidates. A critical observation in these patients is that outcome after complete resection appears to be as good as those who were resectable at initial presentation. Strategies to extend the limits of liver resection have used parenchyma-preserving segmental resections, two-stage operations, and thermal ablative techniques, such as cryoablation or RFA. Most recently, microwave ablation is being studied as a treatment for these patients,[69] but there are no long-term results. Thus, multiple bilobar tumors can be extirpated by a combination of resection and ablation with preservation of sufficient hepatic parenchyma. In our series of patients with extensive hepatic disease treated with a combinations of resection and ablation, 3-year survival was 47%.[70]

In summary, the treatment of hepatic colorectal metastases is evolving at a rapid pace and improvements in hepatic surgery and chemotherapy have greatly improved prospects for patients. Chemotherapy has improved, but long-term survival with this modality alone is rare. Combinations of chemotherapy and complete resection of hepatic metastases are associated with long-term survival in up to 50% to 60% of patients. Long-term survival also appears to be possible in patients undergoing resection of extensive hepatic metastases and limited extrahepatic disease.[63] Complete resection of hepatic metastases appears to be a critically important treatment modality that is necessary for long-term survival.

### Neuroendocrine Metastases

Liver metastases from neuroendocrine tumors are common, but vary according to the primary tumor type. Examples of primary tumors that commonly metastasize to the liver are gastrinomas, glucagonomas, somatostatinomas, and nonfunctional neuroendocrine tumors. Insulinomas and carcinoid tumors metastasize to the liver less commonly.

There are two issues to consider when determining the appropriate therapy for metastatic neuroendocrine tumors. First, these are slow-growing, indolent tumors in which long-term survival is possible even in the absence of treatment. Thus, assessing the effects of any treatment is difficult. Second, these tumors often secrete functional neuropeptides that can create debilitating syndromes of hormonal excess so the goal of treatment is focused more often on quality of life rather than prolongation of life.

A number of effective nonsurgical therapies exist for neuroendocrine liver metastases. Long-acting somatostatin analogues are useful for alleviating hormonal symptoms and may have a cytostatic role as well. Liver tumors can also be treated by hepatic arterial embolization or thermoablative approaches. Combinations of these therapies can be effective in cytoreducing tumor loads and alleviating symptoms of hormonal excess.

Liver resection can play a role in patients whose tumor can be completely encompassed. Because these tumors are indolent, any therapy must be delivered with minimal morbidity. This has been the case in experienced hepatobiliary units.[71] Five-year survival rates in excess of 50% to 75% can be expected if a complete resection is accomplished. Retrospective comparisons have suggested that this survival is better than that in untreated patients, but selection bias accounts for at least some of this difference. Because of the rarity of this diagnosis, no prospective data exist. The other role of surgery is for those patients who have failed medical therapy and have recalcitrant symptoms of hormonal excess. If preoperative staging suggests that at least 90% of tumor can be removed without prohibitive operative risk, surgical cytoreduction is reasonable. Symptom improvement can be expected in most patients if adequate cytoreduction is achieved. Formal resections with wide margins are not necessary for neuroendocrine tumors and techniques such as enucleation or wedge resection are reasonable options. Thermoablative approaches such as cryoablation or RFA are also attractive alternatives in this type of cytoreductive surgery. Recently, laparoscopic RFA has been used, although long-term follow-up is not available.[72]

#### Noncolorectal, Non-Neuroendocrine Metastases

Other tumors can present as isolated liver metastases, but these are uncommon situations and therefore data for these situations are sparse.[73] There are many tumors that can present in this way, including breast, lung, melanoma, soft tissue sarcoma, Wilms', ocular melanoma, upper gastrointestinal (gastric, pancreas, esophagus, gallbladder), adrenocortical, urologic (bladder, renal cell, prostate, testicular), and gynecologic (uterine, cervix, ovarian) tumors. General principles that should be considered when dealing with these tumors as isolated liver metastases are similar to those for metastatic colorectal cancer. Prognosis tends to be dismal if there is extrahepatic disease, multiple tumors, large tumors, or a short disease-free interval and patients should be carefully selected for surgery based on these factors.

Although there have been rare reports of long-term survival after resection of isolated liver metastases from upper gastrointestinal tumor, in general, these patients have a dismal prognosis and liver resection is not recommended. In most series, liver resection for genitourinary tumors has the best prognosis and, in well-selected patients, liver resection should be considered. Breast tumor, melanoma, and sarcoma patients rarely present with isolated liver metastases and, with a long-disease free interval and/or long-term stability on chemotherapy, liver resection should be considered. In general, liver resection for metastatic noncolorectal, non-neuroendocrine tumors has to be considered cytoreductive and should only be used in the most favorable situations (see earlier). Liver resection can also be an effective therapy for symptomatic tumors in patients who have a reasonable life expectancy and no other effective therapy.

### Cystic Neoplasms

#### Simple Cyst

Simple cysts of the liver contain serous fluid, do not communicate with the biliary tree, and do not have septations. They are generally spherical or ovoid and can be as large as 20 cm. Large cysts can compress normal liver, inducing regional atrophy and sometimes compensatory contralateral hypertrophy. In 50% of cases, the cysts are singular. Histologically a single layer of cuboidal or columnar cells without atypia line these cysts. Simple cysts are generally regarded as congenital malformations.

Simple cysts are a relatively common finding in adults and are mostly asymptomatic incidental radiologic findings. Occasionally, a large cyst will cause symptoms. Although CT demonstrates anatomic relationships, ultrasound is a helpful test of choice to confirm a single, thin-walled simple cyst. Hydatid disease, cystadenoma, and metastatic neuroendocrine tumor are the most important differential diagnoses to consider. A thick or nodular wall raises the suspicion of a cystadenoma but can also represent hemorrhage within the cyst. The most common complication is intracystic bleeding but overall, complications are rare. The treatment of simple hepatic cysts is only indicated if they are symptomatic or there is diagnostic uncertainty. Because most cysts are asymptomatic, a thorough evaluation of the cause of the symptoms must be carried out before attributing them to the cyst. Nonsurgical treatment consists of aspiration and injection of a sclerosing agent. Few studies have documented long-term follow-up of sclerotherapy for hepatic cysts. Surgical therapy is achieved by fenestration, or unroofing the portion of the cyst that is extrahepatic. This can be performed at laparotomy with good long-term results or through laparoscopic approaches. The latter approach is favored, but long-term efficacy has not been well documented.[74]

#### Cystadenoma and Cystadenocarcinoma

Cystadenoma of the liver is a rare neoplasm that generally presents as a large cystic mass, usually 10 to 20 cm. The cyst has a globular external surface with multiple protruding cysts and locules of various sizes. The fluid contained in these cysts is usually mucinous. Microscopically, atypical cuboidal or columnar cells resting on a basement membrane, with ovarian-like stroma, line the cysts. The epithelium often forms polypoid or papillary projections.

Cystadenoma of the liver mainly affects woman older than 40 years. Although many cystadenomas are asymptomatic, symptoms can include abdominal pain, anorexia, nausea, and abdominal distention. The diagnosis is usually suspected by a combination of cross-sectional imaging (CT or MRI) and ultrasound. Ultrasound usually demonstrates a cystic structure with varying wall thickness, nodularity, septations, and fluid-filled locules. Importantly, contrast-enhanced CT demonstrates enhancement of the cyst wall and septae. Hydatid disease must always be considered in the differential diagnosis. Cystadenomas tend to grow slowly, but can eventually progress to their malignant counterpart, cystadenocarcinomas.

Cystadenocarcinoma is an extremely rare malignancy with little documentation of its natural history and outcome after resection. Malignant degeneration is typically suggested on imaging, with large projections and a markedly thickened wall. The treatment of cystadenoma or cystadenocarcinoma is complete excision, which can be done with an enucleation if there is no evidence of invasive malignancy. Incomplete resection risks recurrence and/or the development of cystadenocarcinoma.

#### Polycystic Liver Disease

Liver cysts are commonly seen in patients with the autosomal dominant inherited adult polycystic kidney disease. Histologically, the cysts are similar to simple cysts (see earlier). The main difference between the two entities is the number of cysts. When liver cysts are present in patients with adult polycystic kidney disease, they are always multiple in number. Also, there are usually numerous microscopic hepatic cysts, as well as the grossly visible macrocysts. Despite the large number of liver cysts, hepatic parenchyma and function are usually preserved. Liver cysts are always preceded by kidney cysts and their prevalence in adult polycystic kidney disease increases with age. In those younger than 20 years the prevalence of liver cysts is 0%, whereas in those older than 60 years it is 80%.

Liver cysts in patients with adult polycystic kidney disease are generally asymptomatic but, in a few patients, numerous large cysts may cause abdominal pain and distention. LFT results are almost always normal. Rare complications can occur; these include infection and intracystic bleeding. Ultrasound and CT reveal multiple simple cysts throughout the liver and kidneys. Treatment of polycystic liver disease is reserved for severe symptoms related to large cysts and complications. Treatment includes percutaneous aspiration with or without sclerotherapy, cyst fenestration (via laparotomy or laparoscopy), hepatic resection, and orthotopic liver transplantation. Liver transplantation is only used with progressive disease after fenestration or resection with liver or renal dysfunction. In the context of renal failure, a combined kidney and liver transplantation may be appropriate.

### Bile Duct Cysts

Bile duct cysts or choledochal cysts are congenital dilations of the biliary tree that are usually diagnosed in childhood but can present in adulthood. Because of the risk of malignancy and recurrent cholangitis, treatment is excision with reestablishment of biliary-enteric continuity. Most bile duct cysts involve the extrahepatic biliary tree but, in type IV cysts, there is involvement of the extrahepatic bile duct and intrahepatic ducts. In contrast, Caroli's disease (type V) is characterized by multiple intrahepatic cysts. Thus, bile duct cysts must be considered in the differential diagnosis of a patient with multiple hepatic cystic lesions. The intrahepatic lesions of type IV bile duct cysts and Caroli's disease are multifocal dilations of the segmental bile ducts separated by portions of normal-caliber bile ducts. Approximately 50% of cases of Caroli's disease are associated with congenital hepatic fibrosis; the cysts are diffusely located throughout the liver. In the other 50% of cases, the dilations may be confined to a portion of the liver, usually the left hemiliver. Recurrent bacterial cholangitis usually dominates the clinical course of these diseases and death generally ensues within 5 to 10 years without adequate treatment. When intrahepatic bile duct cysts are localized, hepatic resection, with or without biliary reconstruction, is the treatment of choice. Treatment of diffuse hepatic involvement is poor and, in complicated cases, the only probably effective treatment is transplantation.

## Principles of Hepatic Resection

Although liver resections were performed in the late 1800s, it was not until 1952 that Lortat-Jacob was given credit for the first true anatomic right hepatectomy. This event ushered in the modern era of hepatic surgery. However, early series were plagued by high morbidity and mortality, which were largely related to massive intraoperative blood loss. Series from the 1970s and 1980s often reported mortality rates in excess of 10%, often as high as 20%, especially for major resections. This high mortality limited the use of liver resection and there was reluctance to refer patients for such operations. Over the last 3 decades, a number of advances have improved perioperative outcomes dramatically for patients undergoing major hepatic surgery. The understanding that most blood loss during a liver resection comes from the hepatic veins has prompted surgeons to perform these operations with a low central venous pressure (CVP). We perform partial hepatectomy with a central line in place, the patient in a mild Trendelenburg position, and fluid restriction and venodilators if necessary to maintain a CVP lower than 5 mm Hg. The other major advance has been an improved understanding of the segmental anatomy of the liver, making intrahepatic dissection safer and more precise. There are numerous techniques to transect liver tissue and many methods to coagulate and control vessels. The most important concept, however, is that dividing liver tissue is a dissection done by a surgeon with complete understanding of the liver's vascular anatomy.

In experienced centers, perioperative mortality is routinely 5% or less and depends on a number of factors. The three most critical factors related to perioperative morbidity are blood loss, the amount of normal liver resected, and the condition of the liver itself (e.g., cirrhosis). A partial hepatectomy must be performed with these factors in mind to minimize morbidity. In a review of over 1800 liver resections over a 10-year period from MSKCC, the operative mortality was 3.1%.[75] The median blood loss was 600 mL and two thirds of patients did not require a red blood cell transfusion. Overall, postoperative morbidity was 45% but the median hospital stay was 8 days. Morbidity was mostly related to blood loss and the extent of resection. Minor resections were associated with a mortality of 1%. Most complications and deaths were seen in complex biliary tumors, cirrhotics with HCC, and extensive resections. Improving outcomes after partial hepatectomy continues and experienced hepatobiliary centers have reported mortality rates that approach 1% to 2%, with fewer patients now requiring perioperative blood transfusions. As a result of the increasing safety of hepatic surgery, liver resection has become the treatment of choice for a many malignant and benign hepatic conditions.

Bile leaks are a problem in cases requiring complex biliary reconstruction but can also occur in approximately 10% to 20% of hepatectomies without biliary reconstruction. Careful ligation of biliary radicals is of obvious importance in minimizing this complication. Because of the regenerative capacity of the liver, resections of up to 80% of normal noncirrhotic livers can be performed, with functional compensation within a few weeks. Because many resections encompass tumors and normal liver, the concept of functional liver parenchyma and FLR volume are important because there is often compensatory hypertrophy of normal liver when tumors occupy a significant amount of the liver volume. The risk of hepatic dysfunction is minimal if the reduction of functional liver parenchyma is less than 50% but begins to rise when this figure approaches 20% to 25%. Patients with cirrhosis have much higher rates of postoperative liver dysfunction because of impaired regenerative capacity and impaired primary liver function. Liver failure, extrahepatic multiorgan failure, and death are serious hazards to performing major liver resections in cirrhotics. In general, patients with Child class B or C cirrhosis or portal hypertension do not tolerate liver resections and patient selection is therefore critical. Ascites and infectious complications are also common problems after major liver resection. One strategy to minimize postoperative liver dysfunction and morbidity after major hepatectomy is to embolize the portal vein percutaneously on the side of the liver to be resected. In approximately 4 weeks, this induces atrophy of the liver parenchyma to be resected and hypertrophy of the FLR. In turn, this increases the relative volume of the FLR.

Techniques of liver resection differ according to the disease being treated. In benign hepatic diseases requiring resection, the indications for operation are usually symptoms or infection. Removal of normal liver should be kept to a minimum in these cases and techniques such as enucleation are appropriate, although a major resection is occasionally necessary. For malignant disease, a margin of normal tissue is important and formal anatomic resections yield the best results. Techniques such as wedge resection often result in higher rates of margin involvement and disease recurrence and should therefore be used carefully and sparingly.

Detailed knowledge of liver anatomy is essential to the practice of safe hepatic surgery (see earlier). Unfortunately, detailed and complicated descriptions of liver anatomy and common liver resections can be confusing to the student. A 2000 consensus conference conducted in Brisbane, Australia, with the assistance of the American Hepato-Pancreato-Biliary Association (AHPBA), has published guidelines for this terminology (Table 54-11; Fig. 54-40). In general, the term *lobectomy*

**Table 54-11 Nomenclature for Most Common Major Anatomic Hepatic Resections***

| SEGMENTS† | COUINAUD, 1957 | GOLDSMITH AND WOODBURNE, 1957 | BRISBANE, 2000 |
|---|---|---|---|
| V-VIII | Right hepatectomy | Right hepatic lobectomy | Right hemi-hepatectomy |
| IV-VIII‡ | Right lobectomy | Extended right hepatic lobectomy | Right trisectionectomy |
| II-IV | Left hepatectomy | Left hepatic lobectomy | Left hemi-hepatectomy |
| II, III | Left lobectomy | Left lateral segmentectomy | Left lateral sectionectomy |
| II, III, IV, V, VIII‡ | Extended left hepatectomy | Extended left lobectomy | Left trisectionectomy |

Adapted from the Terminology Committee of the International Hepato-Pancreatico-Biliary Association: The Brisbane 2000 terminology of liver anatomy and resections, 2000 (http://www.ahpba.org/assets/documents/Brisbane_Article.pdf).

*The original terminology is based on the anatomic descriptions of Couinaud and of Goldsmith and Woodburne.

†See Figure 54-31*A-E*.

‡Another common name for these operations is right or left trisegmentectomy.

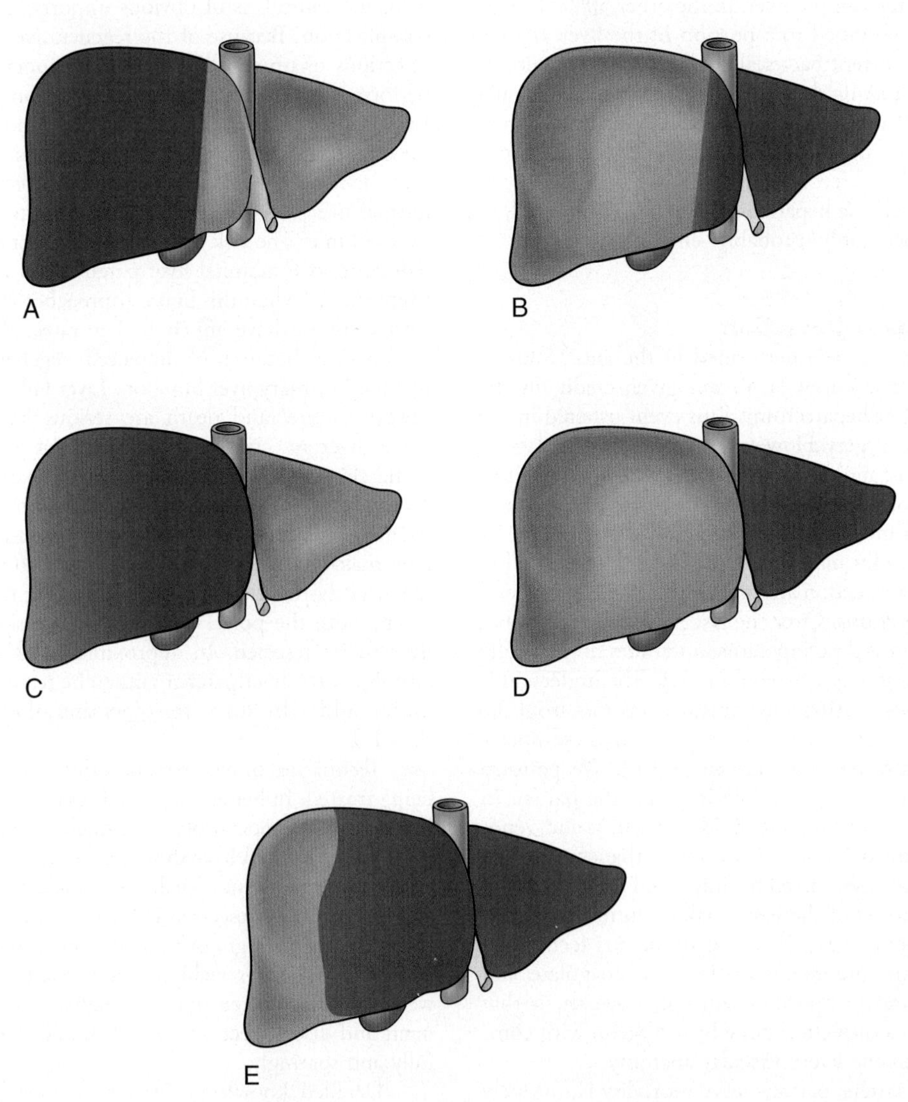


**FIGURE 54-40** Commonly performed major hepatic resections are indicated by the *shaded areas.* **A,** Right hepatectomy, right hepatic lobectomy, or right hemihepatectomy (segments V to VIII). **B,** Left hepatectomy, left hepatic lobectomy, or left hemihepatectomy (segments II to IV). **C,** Right lobectomy, extended right hepatic lobectomy, or right trisectionectomy (trisegmentectomy; segments IV to VIII). **D,** Left lobectomy, left lateral segmentectomy, or left lateral sectionectomy (segments II to III). **E,** Extended left hepatectomy, extended left lobectomy, or left trisectionectomy (trisegmentectomy; segments II to V, VIII). See Table 54-11. (From Blumgart LH, Jarnagin W, Fong Y: Liver resection for benign disease and for liver and biliary tumors. In Blumgart LH, Fong Y [eds]: Surgery of the liver and biliary tract, London, 2000, WB Saunders, pp 1639–1714.)

is not preferred because there are no external markings on the liver denoting a lobe. When in doubt, one should always revert back to the numeric segments of the liver if there is any confusion about the description of a liver resection. Recall that the right liver is comprised of segments 5 through 8 and *right hepatectomy* or *right hemihepatectomy* are appropriate terms for resection of these segments. Segments 2 through 4 comprise the left liver and *left hepatectomy* or *left hemihepatectomy* are appropriate terms for resection of these segments. A right hepatectomy can be extended further to the left to include segment 4 and a left hepatectomy can be extended further to the right to include segments 5 and 8. Terms such as *extended right-left hepatectomy, right-left trisectionectomy,* or *trisegmentectomy* are appropriate to describe these resections. Resection of segments 2 and 3 is a commonly performed sublobar resection and is often referred to as a left lateral segmentectomy or left lateral sectionectomy. Other common sublobar resections, such as that of the right posterior sector (segments 6 and 7) or the right anterior sector (segments 5 and 8), are referred to as a right posterior sectorectomy-sectionectomy and right anterior sectorectomy-sectionectomy, respectively. Single or bisegmental resections can always be simply referred to by a numeric description of the segments to be resected.

A detailed discussion of the techniques of liver resection is beyond the scope of this chapter and, in general, requires specialty training but general principles can be discussed. A liver resection must consider the disease to be treated and the goals of the operation, whether that be a margin negative resection of a malignancy or the removal of benign tissue to alleviate symptoms. The most basic steps can be distilled down to inflow control (portal vein, hepatic artery, bile duct), outflow control (hepatic veins), and parenchymal transection, with preservation of a liver remnant of adequate size with intact inflow, biliary drainage and venous outflow.

The most common approach to an anatomic resection, in the most common order, is mobilization of the liver to be resected, dissection of inflow and outflow structures, division of the inflow, division of the outflow, and parenchymal transection. Mobilization of the liver involves division of the right or left triangular ligaments, freeing up the liver from the diaphragm. Often, the liver must be mobilized completely off the vena cava, which it straddles, and this requires careful dissection and division of multiple retrohepatic caval venous branches. For major resections, the hepatic vein of the resected portion of liver is often encircled prior to the resection. There are various techniques to dissect, control, and divide inflow vessels. Classic inflow control is obtained by dissection of the liver hilum, with control of the portal vein and hepatic artery to the hemiliver to be resected. These can be suture-ligated or divided with vascular staplers. Unless tumor proximity mandates, we advocate dividing the bile duct within the liver substance to minimize absolutely contralateral biliary injuries related to anatomic anomalies. Inflow control can also be obtained by dissection of the intrahepatic inflow pedicle to the anatomic section of liver to be resected. Recall that the inflow structures invaginate peritoneum at the hepatic hilus and run intrahepatically as an invested pedicle of the three inflow structures. The inflow pedicles can be encircled by making flanking hepatotomies or by splitting parenchyma down to the pedicle of interest. The pedicle can usually be divided with a vascular stapler, but suture ligation is sometimes necessary. Typically, the hepatic vein is divided in its extrahepatic position, which can also usually be done with a vascular stapler.

The hepatic vein can also be divided within the substance of the liver during parenchymal transection. There are a number of methods of parenchymal transection, ranging from complex ultrasonic irrigators to radiofrequency energy coagulators to a simple clamp-crushing technique. In experienced hands, these can all be used effectively to minimize blood loss and it is important to develop a specific technique that one is comfortable performing. Ultimately, parenchymal transection is about dissecting intrahepatic anatomy, controlling vascular and biliary structures, minimizing blood loss, and avoiding injury to the future liver remnant.

## HEMOBILIA

A case of lethal hemobilia secondary to penetrating abdominal trauma was first described by Glisson in 1654. It was not until 1948 that Sandblom coined the term *hemobilia* in his seminal paper on the subject. Hemobilia is defined as bleeding into the biliary tree from an abnormal communication between a blood vessel and bile duct. It is a rare condition that is often difficult to distinguish from common causes of gastrointestinal bleeding. The most common causes of hemobilia are iatrogenic trauma, accidental trauma, gallstones, tumors, inflammatory disorders, and vascular disorders. Major hemobilia is relatively uncommon, whereas minor inconsequential hemobilia is a common consequence of gallstone disease or interventional radiologic hepatic procedures.

### Causes

The most common cause of hemobilia is iatrogenic trauma to the liver and biliary tree. Prior to the 1980s, the ratio of hemobilia attributed to accidental trauma compared with iatrogenic trauma was 2:1, but iatrogenic trauma is now regarded as the cause of hemobilia in 40% to 60% of cases. Percutaneous liver biopsy results in hemobilia in less than 1% of cases, but percutaneous transhepatic biliary drainage (PTBD) procedures have an incidence of 2% to 10%. Similarly, surgical exploration of the biliary tree can result in hemobilia from direct injury or arterial pseudoaneurysm. A number of cases of hemobilia following cholecystectomy have been reported. Hemobilia secondary to accidental trauma is more common with blunt than penetrating abdominal trauma and occurs with a reported incidence of 0.2% to 3%. Risk factors for the development of hemobilia following accidental trauma are central hepatic rupture with a cavity, the use of packs, and inadequate drainage. The gallbladder can be a source of bleeding from trauma, gallstones, or acalculous cholecystitis. Primary vascular pathology such as aneurysms, angiodysplasia, and hemangiomata are rare causes of hemobilia. Malignant tumors of the liver, biliary tree, gallbladder, and pancreas, as well as parasitic infections, hepatic abscesses, and cholangitis, are uncommon causes of hemobilia.

### Clinical Presentation

Portal venous bleeding into the biliary tree is rare and often self-limited unless the portal pressure is elevated. Minor hemobilia generally runs an uneventful asymptomatic clinical course. However, arterial hemobilia, the most common source, can be dramatic. Clinical sequelae of hemobilia are related to blood loss and the formation of potentially occlusive blood clots in the biliary tree. The classic triad of symptoms and signs of hemobilia are upper abdominal pain, upper gastrointestinal hemorrhage, and jaundice. In one report, all three were present in 22% of patients. The symptoms and signs of major hemobilia are melena (90% of cases), hematemesis (60% of cases), biliary colic (70% of cases), and jaundice (60% of cases). Upper gastrointestinal bleeding seen in conjunction with biliary symptoms must always raise the suspicion of hemobilia. One interesting aspect of hemobilia is the tendency for delayed presentations, up to weeks after the inciting causal event, as well as recurrent and brisk but limited bleeding over months and even years. Blood clots in the biliary tree can masquerade as stones if hemobilia goes unrecognized. These clots can cause cholangitis, pancreatitis, and cholecystitis.

## Diagnostic Workup

Once hemobilia is suspected, the first evaluation should be upper gastrointestinal endoscopy, which rules out other sources of hemorrhage and may visualize bleeding from the ampulla of Vater. However, upper endoscopy is only diagnostic of hemobilia in approximately 10% of cases. If upper endoscopy is diagnostic and conservative management is planned, no further studies are necessary. Ultrasound or CT may be helpful in demonstrating intrahepatic tumor or hematoma. Evidence of active bleeding into the biliary tree may be seen on contrast-enhanced CT in the form of pooling contrast, intraluminal clots, or biliary dilation. CT may also show risk factors associated with hemobilia, such as cavitating central lesions and aneurysms. Arterial angiography is now recognized as the test of choice when significant hemobilia is suspected and will reveal the source of bleeding in approximately 90% of cases. Cholangiography demonstrates blood clots in the biliary tree, which may appear as stringy defects or smaller spherical defects. The latter may be difficult to distinguish from stones.

## Treatment and Outcomes

The treatment of hemobilia must be focused on stopping the bleeding and relieving biliary obstruction. Most cases of minor hemobilia can be managed conservatively with correction of coagulopathy, adequate biliary drainage (only if necessary), and close observation. In a review of 171 reported cases from 1996 to 1999, 43% of cases were successfully managed conservatively. The first line of therapy for major hemobilia was transarterial embolization (TAE) and success rates of 80% to 100% were reported. Angiography with TAE is indicated for major hemobilia requiring blood transfusion (Fig. 54-41).

Surgery is indicated when conservative therapy and TAE have failed. It is important to note that surgical treatment of hemobilia is rarely necessary and, even in cases in which a laparotomy may be mandated for other reasons, TAE is still the therapy of choice for hemobilia because of its lower morbidity. Surgical approaches generally involve ligation of bleeding vessels, excision of aneurysms, or nonselective ligation of a main hepatic artery. Hepatic resection may be necessary for failed arterial ligation or for cases of severe trauma or tumor. Hemorrhage from the gallbladder or hemorrhagic cholecystitis mandates cholecystectomy. There have been isolated reports of successful management of hemobilia with endoscopic coagulation, somatostatin, and vasopressin. The management of hemobilia following PTBD

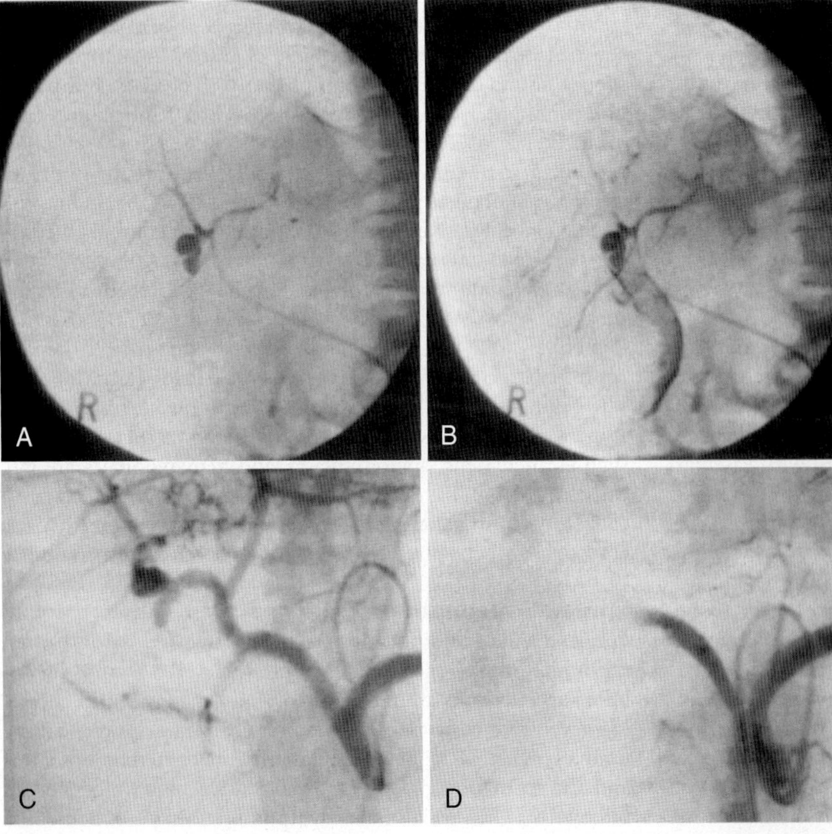


**FIGURE 54-41** Classic findings of hemobilia. After a complicated cholecystectomy, an iatrogenic pseudoaneurysm developed and ruptured into the biliary tree. Exsanguinating hemobilia ensued; the diagnosis was made by endoscopy and then treated by arterial embolization. **A,** Arteriogram demonstrating a pseudoaneurysm of the hepatic artery at the hilum. **B,** A few seconds later, the contrast is seen flowing down the hepatic duct, with evidence of clot in the biliary tree. The same aneurysm before **(C)** and after **(D)** successful embolization. (From Sandblom JP: Hemobilia and bilhemia. In Blumgart LH, Fong Y [eds]: Surgery of the liver and biliary tract, London, 2000, WB Saunders, pp 1319–1342.)

usually consists of removal of the catheter or replacement with larger catheters but may require TAE.

At the time of Sandblom's report from the early 1970s, the mortality for hemobilia was at least 25%. A report from 1987 noted a mortality of 12%. In a review of cases from 1996 through 1999, only four deaths were reported. There has clearly been a reduction in mortality from hemobilia, which is probably related to two factors. First, the incidence of minor self-limited hemobilia has increased secondary to the rising number of percutaneous hepatic procedures. Second, improvements in selective angiography and TAE have greatly improved the treatment of major hemobilia.

### Bilhemia

Bilhemia is an extremely rare condition in which bile flows into the bloodstream through the hepatic veins or portal vein branches. This flow occurs in the context of a high intrabiliary pressure exceeding that of the venous system. The cause can be gallstones eroding into the portal vein or accidental or iatrogenic trauma. The condition can be fatal secondary to embolization of large amounts of bile into the lungs. Usually, however, bile flow is low and the fistulae close spontaneously. The clinical presentation is that of rapidly increasing jaundice, marked direct hyperbilirubinemia without elevation of hepatocellular enzyme levels (e.g., AST, ALT), and septicemia. This diagnosis is best determined by ERCP. Treatment is directed at lowering intrabiliary pressures through stents or sphincterotomy.

## VIRAL HEPATITIS AND THE SURGEON

Epidemics of jaundice were noted in ancient civilizations and recorded by Hippocrates. During World War II these epidemics were called *catarrhal jaundice*. Over 28,000 cases were documented at that time. Epidemiologic studies in the 1940s documented the difference between bloodborne hepatitis (hepatitis B) and enteric hepatitis (hepatitis A). The most important discovery was that of the Australia antigen by Blumberg and coworkers in 1965. This antigen proved to be the hepatitis B surface antigen (HBsAg) and provided a means for differentiating the two types of hepatitis and characterizing the epidemiology of this disease. This discovery also led to the development of HBV vaccines based on this antigen, with obvious and profound effects worldwide. Further research led to the discovery of the delta virus (hepatitis D) and hepatitis C, explaining cases of non-A, non-B hepatitis. Hepatitis E has been found to be a unique enteral form of infectious hepatitis; the hepatitis G virus, discovered in 1995, is still being defined.

Viral hepatitis is a major health problem and is the most common cause of liver disease worldwide. Although fulminant acute hepatitis is uncommon, there are over 5 million people who suffer from chronic hepatitis. It is estimated that over 15,000 patients die each year of viral hepatitis in the United States alone. Viral hepatitis is not a surgical disease, but has important consequences for surgeons and surgical patients. For any surgeon performing hepatic surgery, the functional state of the liver is extremely important and patients with chronic viral hepatitis require special attention prior to any surgical intervention. Also, chronic viral hepatitis is a common cause of HCC. Finally, the risk of transmission from patient to surgeon and vice versa is an issue all surgeons should be familiar with.

### Definition

Viral hepatitis is an infection of the liver by one of six known viruses that have diverse genetic compositions and structures. HAV, HCV, HDV, HEV, and HGV have RNA genomes whereas HBV has a DNA genome that replicates through RNA intermediates. HAV and HEV are both responsible for forms of epidemic hepatitis and are transmitted via the fecal-oral route. HBV is the only one with the potential to integrate into host genomes, although this is not required for replication. HCV replicates in the cytoplasm of hepatocytes and has complex mechanisms of evading host immunity through hypervariable areas in its genome. HDV requires the presence of HBV coinfection for replication and infectivity and can alter the clinical course of HBV infection. HGV was discovered more recently and has similarities to HCV, but has no definitive association with clinical hepatitis.

### Diagnosis

Table 54-12 summarizes the serologic tests and their implications for HAV, HBV, and HCV. The diagnosis of HAV infection relies on the determination of antibodies to HAV. Both IgM and IgG antibodies are present early in the infection, but only IgG persists long term. HAV antigens and tests for HAV RNA have been developed, but are generally restricted to research laboratories.

HBV infection has been characterized by a number of antigens and antibodies (Fig. 54-42). HBsAg is the hallmark of the diagnosis of HBV infection and appears in the serum from 1 to 10 weeks after infection; it usually disappears in 4 to 6 months, but persistence in the serum implies chronic infection. Anti-HBs antibodies usually appear during a window period after the disappearance of HBsAg and indicate recovery after

**Table 54-12 Serologic Evaluation of the Most Common Viral Hepatitides**

| VIRUS | ANTIGEN NAME | INTERPRETATION | ANTIBODY NAME | INTERPRETATION |
|---|---|---|---|---|
| HAV | HAV antigen | Acute infection | Anti-HAV IgM | Acute infection |
| | | | Anti-HAV IgG | Immunity |
| HBV | HBsAg | Acute or chronic infection | Anti-HBs | Immunity |
| | HBeAg | HBV replication, infectivity | Anti-HBc | All phases of infection |
| | | | Anti-HBe | Late convalescence |
| HCV | None | – | Anti-HCV | Late convalescence or chronic infection |

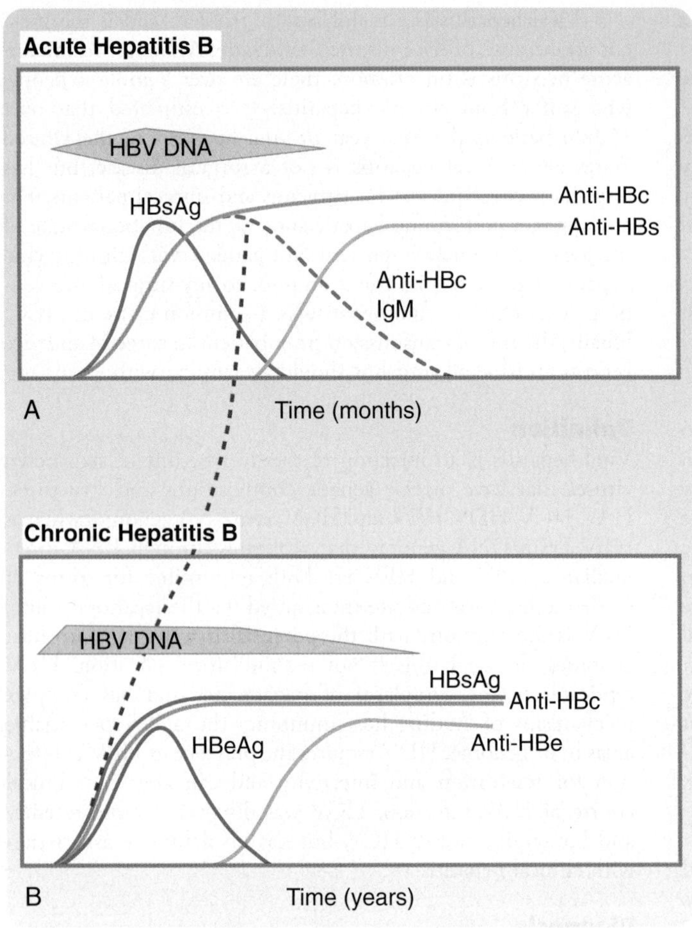


**FIGURE 54-42** Serologic makers in acute **(A)** and chronic HBV infection **(B).** (From Doo EC, Lian TJ: The hepatitis viruses. In Schiff ER, Sorrell MF, Maddrey WC [eds]: Schiff's diseases of the liver, Philadelphia, 1999, Lippincott-Raven, pp 725–744.)

HBV infection. Anti-HBs antibodies are also induced by the HBV vaccine. The hepatitis core antigen (HBcAg) is an intracellular antigen that is not detectable in serum. On the other hand, anti-HBc antibodies are detectable early on after infection and persist after recovery and in chronic infections. Hepatitis B e antigen (HBeAg) is a secretory protein that is a marker of HBV replication and infectivity. It is usually present early on and may persist for years in chronic infection, but generally disappears within months in the absence of chronic infection. Seroconversion to anti-HBe antibodies is usually associated with resolution of infection. It has also been shown that many patients who have seroconverted often have measurable HBV DNA, albeit at low levels. Quantification of HBV DNA in the serum has become the most accurate way of assessing HBV activity. Evidence has shown that many patients thought to have resolved acute HBV may have persistent viral infection and may be at risk for ongoing hepatitis or reactivation.

The diagnosis of HCV infection relies on the detection of antibodies to a number of HCV antigens. Current immunoassays are highly specific and sensitive. No specific HCV antigen tests exist, but there are a variety of quantitative and qualitative tests for HCV RNA, which have become important in confirming the diagnosis in unclear cases and assessing responses to therapy.

HDV coinfection of HBV-infected patients is best diagnosed by detection of HDV RNA, which can be measured in serum. The HDV antigen can be detected in liver specimens. HEV infection can be diagnosed by measurement of antibodies in serum or by detection of the virus or its components in feces, serum, or in the liver itself.

## Epidemiology and Transmission

The incidence of hepatitis A has fallen dramatically since the introduction of effective vaccines but vaccination is not routine in all countries. Hepatitis A is common in third-world countries, with seropositivity rates approaching 100% in some populations. Infection occurs in childhood and is facilitated by poor hygiene and sanitation. Infection rates are much lower in developed countries. In the United States, approximately 10% of children and 35% of adults have been infected with HAV. Despite vaccination availability, 6000 cases were reported in the U.S. in 2004, likely representing an estimated 60,000 cases nationwide. The primary route of HAV infection is the fecal-oral route. Most cases of HAV occur because of ingestion of contaminated water or food, and person to person contact. Parenteral transmission is possible, but uncommon. Sexual transmission has been documented in homosexual men.

Hepatitis B is a major worldwide health problem. There are over 300 million carriers and 250,000 associated deaths annually. The prevalence of HBV infection has considerable geographic variation. Low prevalence areas such as the United States and Western Europe have carrier rates of 0.1% to 2%. In these regions, transmission is generally through sexual intercourse or IV drug abuse (IVDA). Carrier rates in intermediate-prevalence areas such as Japan and Singapore range from 3% to 5%. In high prevalence areas such as Southeast Asia and sub-Saharan Africa, carrier rates range from 10% to 20%. Transmission in high-prevalence areas is largely perinatal and horizontal during childhood.

Transfusion-associated HBV was common in the 1960s and the risk has been estimated to be as high as 50% at that time. Currently, screening programs and limitation of blood donation to voluntary donors has decreased the risk of acquiring HBV from a blood transfusion to 1 in 63,000. Percutaneous transmission through the use of any contaminated needle is a major route of HBV infection and is common in IV drug abusers. Sexual transmission is common in low- prevalence countries and is estimated to account for approximately 30% of cases in the United States. There is a particularly high incidence in male homosexuals and heterosexuals with multiple sexual partners. Perinatal HBV infection accounts for less than 10% of cases in the United States but is common in endemic regions, with rates of transmission of 90% in some areas. Horizontal transmission among children is common and is probably related to minor breaks in the skin and mucous membranes. HBV is the most commonly transmitted virus among health care personnel and transmission is usually patient to patient or patient to worker. Needlestick risk has been related to HBeAg positivity. Rare cases of physician to patient transmission have been reported.

Hepatitis C is the most common cause of chronic liver disease in the United States, with an estimated prevalence of 1.8% accounting for 3.9 million infected people. New infections typically occurs at a younger age (20 to 39 years) and the most common risk factor is IVDA. Health care workers have higher carrier rates than the general public. Transmission among health care workers is usually related to needlestick incidents and the risk of transmission is higher than that of HBV and HIV. In the past, blood transfusion was the major cause of HCV infection, accounting for at least 85% of cases. Currently, less than 2% of acute infections are caused by transfusions and the risk of transfusion-associated transmission is estimated to be about 1 in 10,000. Although HCV has never been documented in semen, it is estimated that approximately 20% of HCV infections are caused by sexual transmission. Risk of sexual transmission appears to be related to the number of partners and presence of other sexually transmitted diseases. Monogamous sexual partners of HCV-infected people occasionally test positive for HCV in the absence of other risk factors, but this appears to be quite rare. Perinatal transmission has been documented, but is also rare as. No identifiable risk factors are found in 30% to 40% of HCV cases.

HDV infection occurs worldwide, with a variable distribution that parallels that of HBV infection. Approximately 5% of HBsAg-positive patients also harbor HDV infection. Transmission of HDV is parenteral and can only occur in patients previously infected with HBV.

HEV is endemic in Southeast and Central Asia and occurs with low frequency in other areas of the world. HEV outbreaks are usually large, affecting hundreds to thousands of people at once, and often follow large rains and flooding. There is a particularly high incidence and mortality in pregnant women. Transmission is fecal-oral and usually related to contaminated drinking water or food. Person to person and vertical transmission are rare.

## Pathogenesis and Clinical Presentation

The pathogenesis of hepatic injury from these viral infections is not completely understood. For all the viruses discussed in this section, hepatic inflammation appears to be caused by direct cytotoxicity or immune-related phenomena. A combination of these two mechanisms probably underlies the cause of hepatic damage.

Humans are the only host for HAV and no reservoir of infection has been identified. After oral intake, HAV can survive the acidic gastric pH, but the mechanism of hepatic uptake is not known. HAV infection results in acute inflammation of the liver and has no associated chronic sequelae. The most recent data suggest that hepatocyte damage is most likely an immunopathologic response rather than direct hepatotoxicity. Most children with HAV infection younger than 2 years are asymptomatic, whereas in pediatric patients older than 5 years, 80% will develop symptoms. Fulminant hepatitis develops in 1% to 5% of cases and mortality is generally under 1%.

Approximately 70% of patients with acute HBV infection have subclinical or anicteric hepatitis; the other 30% have icteric hepatitis. The incubation period for HBV ranges from 1 to 4 months. A prodromal serum sickness–like syndrome may develop, followed by a multitude of constitutional symptoms such as malaise, anorexia, and nausea. The constitutional symptoms last about 10 days and are followed by jaundice in 30% of patients. Clinical symptoms usually disappear within 3 months. Fulminant hepatic failure develops in 0.1 % to 0.5% of patients. Almost 80% of patients with fulminant HBV-related hepatitis will die unless liver transplantation is performed.

Risk of chronic HBV infection is related to immunocompetence and age. Immunocompetent adults have a risk of less than 5%, whereas 30% of children and 90% of infants will develop chronic disease. Most patients with chronic HBV infection are asymptomatic, but some may experience exacerbations of symptoms. Laboratory tests may be entirely normal in HBV carriers or mild elevations of ALT and AST levels may be the only findings. Progression to cirrhosis is marked by hepatic synthetic dysfunction and often cytopenias, related to hypersplenism. Extrahepatic manifestations of HBV infection, caused by circulating immune complexes, occur in approximately 10% to 20% of patients; these include polyarteritis nodosa, glomerulonephritis, essential mixed cryoglobulinemia, and papular acrodermatitis. The sequelae of chronic HBV infection range from none to cirrhosis, HCC, hepatic failure, and death. It has been noted that patients thought to have previously cleared their infections can have a reactivation, especially during a period of immunosuppression. In nonendemic areas the long-term risk appears to be low, but in endemic areas chronic HBV infection is a significant cause of morbidity and mortality.

Acute HCV infection generally presents with mild elevation of hepatocellular enzyme levels. In general, 80% of cases occur from 5 to 12 weeks after infection. Symptoms occur in less than 30% of patients and are usually so mild and nonspecific that they do not affect daily life. Jaundice occurs in less than 20% of patients and fulminant hepatic failure caused by HCV is extremely uncommon. Chronic HCV infection develops in approximately two thirds of patients; the other third appear to clear the infection. Most patients with chronic HCV infection are asymptomatic without evidence of overt liver disease and only present with mildly elevated hepatocellular enzyme levels. Despite this quiet clinical course, patients with chronic HCV infection are at risk for developing cirrhosis and HCC. Estimates place the risk of cirrhosis at 2% to 20% at a 20- to 30-year interval. The risk of developing HCC from that point has been estimated at 1% to 4%/year. Progression of liver damage can be variable and several factors appear to affect its rate. Factors associated with a more rapid progression include male gender, older age at infection, immunosuppression (e.g., HIV infection), coinfection with HBV, moderate alcohol intake, and obesity. Extrahepatic manifestations such as autoimmune disorders and lymphoma can occur with HCV infection and are likely related to circulating immune complexes.

The clinical presentation of HDV infection is related to a complex relationship between the degree of HBV and HDV infection. Simultaneous coinfection with high expression of HBV and HDV results in higher rates of acute fulminant hepatitis. Superinfection in a previous HBV carrier generally results in more rapidly progressive chronic liver damage. Some milder forms of acute HDV infection are associated with decreased expression of HDV and repression of HBV infection.

Hepatitis E has a different histologic picture than the other viral hepatitides in that a cholestatic type of hepatitis is seen in over 50% of patients. HEV is introduced orally and it is not known how the virus travels to the liver. The incubation period of HEV ranges from 2 to 9 weeks. The most common form of illness is acute icteric hepatitis; most series report jaundice in over 90% of patients. Asymptomatic forms of the disease occur and are probably more common than the icteric form, but the actual frequency is unknown. The disease is usually self-limited, but fulminant hepatic failure can occur in a small percentage of patients. Overall, the mortality rate is probably significantly less than 1%. Pregnant women tend to have a more severe clinical course; mortality rates range from 5% to 25%.

## Prevention

HAV prophylaxis has relies on sanitary measures and administration of serum immunoglobulin (Ig). The development of safe and effective HAV vaccines, however, has made the use of preexposure Ig unnecessary. Serum Ig is still the therapy of choice for postexposure prophylaxis and may be safely given, along with active immunization. In the United States, the Centers for Disease Control and Prevention has recommended universal vaccination of children based on the safety and efficacy of the vaccine in high-risk populations. Public health researchers are investigating vaccination schemes to eradicate HAV in high-risk populations throughout the world. However, cost-benefit analyses have not supported universal vaccination worldwide. Similarly, HEV prophylaxis has focused on sanitary measures, particularly strategies aimed at drinking water. Unfortunately, HEV Ig has not been successful in preexposure or postexposure prevention of HEV infection, whereas anti-HEV antibodies appear to be effective at attenuating the clinical syndrome. Vaccines for HEV infection have been developed and evaluated in clinical trials.

Remarkable advances have been made in the prevention of HBV infection. In the past, prevention of HBV infection was limited to passive immunization with Ig containing high titers of antibody to HBsAg. Currently, Ig immunization is only used in postexposure prophylaxis. HBsAg-containing vaccines have been developed, with good safety and efficacy profiles. These vaccines are used primarily for preexposure prophylaxis but can also be used in a postexposure setting along with Ig. HBV vaccination is recommended for high-risk groups such as health care workers. There are also programs for HBV vaccination to prevent perinatal transmission; currently, all children 11 or 12 years old should be vaccinated if this has not been done previously. HBV DNA-based vaccines have been developed, and a combined HBV and HAV vaccine was approved by the U.S. Food and Drug Administration (FDA) in 2001. Although no vaccine is available for HDV, effective HBV prevention prevents HDV infection.

The only effective preventive strategy for HCV infection relies on public health principles aimed at the major risk factors for transmission. Conventionally prepared anti-HCV Ig has been evaluated in a number of trials and has not been demonstrated to prevent transfusion-related non-A, non-B hepatitis. Screening of blood donors has rendered this issue irrelevant today. Unfortunately, because of various obstacles, a successful HCV vaccine has not been developed.

## Treatment

Treatment for HAV or HEV infection is supportive in nature and is generally aimed at correcting dehydration and providing adequate caloric intake. Although fatigue may mandate significant periods of rest, hospitalization is usually not necessary, except in cases of fulminant liver failure.

The treatment of HBV infection is largely aimed at patients with chronic active disease. The two approved therapies are interferon-α (IFN-α) and the nucleoside analogue lamivudine. IFN-α is an immunomodulatory agent with some antiviral properties that can induce a virologic response in 35% to 40% of patients. However, long-term benefit with IFN therapy has not been proven. Many nucleoside analogues for the treatment of HBV have been developed and probably work through inhibition of DNA synthesis. They have similar viral response rates to IFN-α, are inexpensive, are given orally, and have few side effects. On the other hand, nucleoside analogues o ften require long-term therapy (>1 year) and the development of resistant HBV mutants has been documented. Randomized trials have shown oral lamivudine to be effective at decreasing the risk of cirrhosis progression and HCC. Newer antiviral agents are in development and are likely to improve outcomes.

Over the last 20 years, tremendous advances in the treatment of HCV infection have occurred. A benefit for IFN-α in the treatment of non-A, non-B hepatitis was originally demonstrated in 1986, before the discovery of HCV. With current IFN-α treatment regimens, complete viral response, defined as sustained loss of serum viral RNA, occurs in 12% to 20% of patients. The addition of ribavirin to IFN-α has resulted in response rates of 35% to 45%. In the most recent trials, treatment with pegylated IFN-α and ribavirin for 48 weeks resulted in viral clearance in 55% of patients. The specific genotype appears to be predictive of response, with some types resulting in response rates of 80% and others of 45%. Relapse can occur but usually occurs with monotherapy and shortened courses of therapy. Because therapy with IFN-α has significant side effects, controversies such as indications for treatment, optimal doses, and duration of treatment are still being resolved.

## SELECTED REFERENCES

Blumgart LH: Surgery of the liver, biliary tract, and pancreas, ed 4, Philadelphia, 2008, Elsevier.

A comprehensive and clinical review of hepatobiliary anatomy. The text is specifically oriented toward surgery of the liver and biliary tree. It covers anatomy, pathophysiology, immunology, molecular biology, genetics, diagnosis, and treatment. In addition, it is accompanied by a DVD with detailed video clips of laparoscopic procedures, effectively allowing one to use it as an operative atlas.

Blumgart LH: Video atlas: Liver, biliary and pancreatic surgery, Philadelphia, 2011, Elsevier.

This video atlas includes an extensive library of narrated and captioned videos that present history, radiologic evidence, and operative procedures for hepatic and biliary surgery. It also includes laparoscopic approaches to liver resections.

El-Serag HB: Epidemiology of hepatocellular carcinoma in USA. Hepatol Res 37(Suppl 2):S88–S94, 2007.

A recent comprehensive and concise review of the subject.

Fong Y, Fortner J, Sun RL, et al: Clinical score for predicting recurrence after hepatic resection for metastatic colorectal cancer: Analysis of 1001 consecutive cases. Ann Surg 230:309–318, 1999.

At the time of publication, this was the largest single-institution series of liver resection for metastatic colorectal cancer. A very useful prognostic scoring system is presented and remains critically important in evaluating patients today.

Foster JH, Berman MM: Solid liver tumors. Philadelphia, 1977, WB Saunders.

A classic and comprehensive monograph that contains a complete history of liver surgery.

House MG, Ito H, Gonen M, et al: Survival after hepatic resection for metastatic colorectal cancer: Trends in outcomes for 1,600 patients during two decades at a single institution. J Am Coll Surg 210:744–752, 2010.

This study analyzes factors associated with differences in long-term outcomes after hepatic resection for metastatic colorectal cancer. Despite worse clinical and pathologic features, survival rates after hepatic resection for colorectal metastases have improved, which might be attributable to improvements in patient selection, operative management, and chemotherapy.

Jarnagin WR, Gonen M, Fong Y, et al: Improvement in perioperative outcome after hepatic resection: Analysis of 1,803 consecutive cases over the past decade. Ann Surg 236:397–406, 2002.

One of the largest series of hepatic resections that documents the remarkable improvement in perioperative outcomes.

Llovet JM, Ricci S, Mazzaferro V, et al: Sorafenib in advanced hepatocellular carcinoma. N Engl J Med 359:378–390, 2008.

The first randomized phase III clinical trial in patients with advanced hepatocellular carcinoma that showed a benefit of improved median survival and time to radiologic progression for patients treated with a chemotherapeutic agent as compared with patients who were given a placebo.

Ochsner A, DeBakey M, Murray S: Pyogenic abscess of the liver. Am J Surg 40:292–319, 1938.

A classic landmark study on pyogenic abscesses of the liver. This was the first serious attempt to study hepatic abscesses and ushered in the modern era of treatment.

Sandhu BS, Sanyal AJ: Management of ascites in cirrhosis. Clin Liver Dis 9:715–732, 2005.

This is an excellent, comprehensive, and practical review of the treatment of ascites in patients with cirrhosis.

Wright AS, Rikkers LF: Current management of portal hypertension. J Gastrointest Surg 9:992–1005, 2005.

This is a concise and fairly comprehensive review of the management of patients with variceal bleeding. Treatment of the acutely bleeding patient and prevention of rebleeding are discussed in detail.

## REFERENCES

1. Schiffman SC, Woodall CE, Kooby DA, et al: Factors associated with recurrence and survival following hepatectomy for large hepatocellular carcinoma: A multicenter analysis. J Surg Oncol 101:105–110, 2010.
2. Kusano T, Sasaki A, Kai S, et al: Predictors and prognostic significance of operative complications in patients with hepatocellular carcinoma who underwent hepatic resection. Eur J Surg Oncol 35:1179–1185, 2009.
3. Biernat J, Pawlik WW, Sendur R, et al: Role of afferent nerves and sensory peptides in the mediation of hepatic artery buffer response. J Physiol Pharmacol 56:133–145, 2005.
4. de Franchis R: Revising consensus in portal hypertension: Report of the Baveno V consensus workshop on methodology of diagnosis and therapy in portal hypertension. J Hepatol 53:762–768, 2010.
5. Garcia-Tsao G, Bosch J: Management of varices and variceal hemorrhage in cirrhosis. N Engl J Med 362:823–832, 2010.
6. Orloff MJ, Orloff MS, Orloff SL, et al: Three decades of experience with emergency portacaval shunt for acutely bleeding esophageal varices in 400 unselected patients with cirrhosis of the liver. J Am Coll Surg 180:257–272, 1995.
7. Bernard B, Lebrec D, Mathurin P, et al: Beta-adrenergic antagonists in the prevention of gastrointestinal rebleeding in patients with cirrhosis: A meta-analysis. Hepatology 25:63–70, 1997.
8. Villanueva C, Minana J, Ortiz J, et al: Endoscopic ligation compared with combined treatment with nadolol and isosorbide mononitrate to prevent recurrent variceal bleeding. N Engl J Med 345:647–655, 2001.
9. de la Pena J, Brullet E, Sanchez-Hernandez E, et al: Variceal ligation plus nadolol compared with ligation for prophylaxis of variceal rebleeding: A multicenter trial. Hepatology 41:572–578, 2005.

**10.** Fong Y, Wong J: Evolution in surgery: Influence of minimally invasive approaches on the hepatobiliary surgeon. Surg Infect (Larchmt) 10:399–406, 2009.

**11.** Meddings L, Myers RP, Hubbard J, et al: A population-based study of pyogenic liver abscesses in the United States: Incidence, mortality, and temporal trends. Am J Gastroenterol 105:117–124, 2010.

**12.** Salles JM, Salles MJ, Moraes LA, et al: Invasive amebiasis: An update on diagnosis and management. Expert Rev Anti Infect Ther 5:893–901, 2007.

**13.** Mezhir J, Fong Y, Jacks L, et al: Current management of pyogenic liver abscess: Surgery is now second-line treatment. J Am Coll Surg 975–983, 2010.

**14.** Benedetti NJ, Desser TS, Jeffrey RB: Imaging of hepatic infections. Ultrasound Q 24:267–278, 2008.

**15.** Dziri C, Haouet K, Fingerhut A, et al: Management of cystic echinococcosis complications and dissemination: Where is the evidence? World J Surg 33:1266–1273, 2009.

**16.** Agayev RM, Agayev BA: Hepatic hydatid disease: Surgical experience over 15 years. Hepatogastroenterology 55:1373–1379, 2008.

**17.** Nasseri Moghaddam S, Abrishami A, Malekzadeh R: Percutaneous needle aspiration, injection, and reaspiration with or without benzimidazole coverage for uncomplicated hepatic hydatid cysts. Cochrane Database Syst Rev CD003623, 2006.

**18.** Nguyen T, Powell A, Daugherty T: Recurrent pyogenic cholangitis. Dig Dis Sci 55:8–10, 2010.

**19.** Chen C, Huang M, Yang J, et al: Reappraisal of percutaneous transhepatic cholangioscopic lithotomy for primary hepatolithiasis. Surg Endosc 19:505–509, 2005.

**20.** Mori T, Sugiyama M, Atomi Y: Gallstone disease: Management of intrahepatic stones. Best Pract Res Clin Gastroenterol 20:1117–1137, 2006.

**21.** Buell JF, Cherqui D, Geller DA, et al: The international position on laparoscopic liver surgery: The Louisville Statement, 2008. Ann Surg 250:825–830, 2009.

**22.** Sasaki A, Nitta H, Otsuka K, et al: Ten-year experience of totally laparoscopic liver resection in a single institution. Br J Surg 96:274–279, 2009.

**23.** Huurman VA, Schaapherder AF: Management of ruptured hepatocellular adenoma. Dig Surg 27:56–60, 2010.

**24.** Rebouissou S, Bioulac-Sage P, Zucman-Rossi J: Molecular pathogenesis of focal nodular hyperplasia and hepatocellular adenoma. J Hepatol 48:163–170, 2008.

**25.** Curvo-Semedo L, Brito JB, Seco MF, et al: The hypointense liver lesion on T2-weighted MR images and what it means. Radiographics 30:e38, 2010.

**26.** Assy N, Nasser G, Djibre A, et al: Characteristics of common solid liver lesions and recommendations for diagnostic workup. World J Gastroenterol 15:3217–3227, 2009.

**27.** Deneve JL, Pawlik TM, Cunningham S, et al: Liver cell adenoma: A multicenter analysis of risk factors for rupture and malignancy. Ann Surg Oncol 16:640–648, 2009.

**28.** Wellen JR, Anderson CD, Doyle M, et al: The role of liver transplantation for hepatic adenomatosis in the pediatric population: Case report and review of the literature. Pediatr Transplant 14:E16–E19, 2010.

**29.** Vetelainen R, Erdogan D, de Graaf W, et al: Liver adenomatosis: Re-evaluation of a cause and management. Liver Int 28:499–508, 2008.

**30.** Koffron A, Geller D, Gamblin TC, et al: Laparoscopic liver surgery: Shifting the management of liver tumors. Hepatology 44:1694–1700, 2006.

**31.** Kamaya A, Maturen KE, Tye GA, et al: Hypervascular liver lesions. Semin Ultrasound CT MR 30:387–407, 2009.

**32.** El-Serag HB: Epidemiology of hepatocellular carcinoma in USA. Hepatol Res 37(Suppl 2):S88–S94, 2007.

**33.** Bartosch B, Thimme R, Blum HE, et al: Hepatitis C virus-induced hepatocarcinogenesis. J Hepatol 51:810–820, 2009.

**34.** Stefaniuk P, Cianciara J, Wiercinska-Drapalo A: Present and future possibilities for early diagnosis of hepatocellular carcinoma. World J Gastroenterol 16:418–424, 2010.

**35.** Tsai WL, Chung RT: Viral hepatocarcinogenesis. Oncogene 29:2309–2324, 2010.

**36.** Siegel AB, Zhu AX: Metabolic syndrome and hepatocellular carcinoma: Two growing epidemics with a potential link. Cancer 115:5651–5661, 2009.

**37.** Davila JA, Morgan RO, Shaib Y, et al: Diabetes increases the risk of hepatocellular carcinoma in the United States: A population-based case control study. Gut 54:533–539, 2005.

**38.** Bruix J, Sherman M, Llovet JM, et al: Clinical management of hepatocellular carcinoma. Conclusions of the Barcelona-2000 EASL conference. European Association for the Study of the Liver. J Hepatol 35:421–430, 2001.

**39.** Bruix J, Sherman M: Management of hepatocellular carcinoma. Hepatology 42:1208–1236, 2005.

**40.** Weitz J, D'Angelica M, Jarnagin W, et al: Selective use of diagnostic laparoscopy prior to planned hepatectomy for patients with hepatocellular carcinoma. Surgery 135:273–281, 2004.

**41.** Pawlik TM, Poon RT, Abdalla EK, et al: Critical appraisal of the clinical and pathologic predictors of survival after resection of large hepatocellular carcinoma. Arch Surg 140:450–457, 2005.

**42.** Mazzaferro V, Regalia E, Doci R, et al: Liver transplantation for the treatment of small hepatocellular carcinomas in patients with cirrhosis. N Engl J Med 334:693–699, 1996.

**43.** Llovet JM, Fuster J, Bruix J: Intention-to-treat analysis of surgical treatment for early hepatocellular carcinoma: resection versus transplantation. Hepatology 30:1434–1440, 1999.

**44.** Capussotti L, Ferrero A, Vigano L, et al: Liver resection for HCC with cirrhosis: Surgical perspectives out of EASL/AASLD guidelines. Eur J Surg Oncol 35:11–15, 2009.

**45.** Llovet JM, Schwartz M, Mazzaferro V: Resection and liver transplantation for hepatocellular carcinoma. Semin Liver Dis 25:181–200, 2005.

**46.** Facciuto ME, Rochon C, Pandey M, et al: Surgical dilemma: Liver resection or liver transplantation for hepatocellular carcinoma and cirrhosis. Intention-to-treat analysis in patients within and outwith Milan criteria. HPB (Oxford) 11:398–404, 2009.

**47.** Huang J, Yan L, Cheng Z, et al: A randomized trial comparing radiofrequency ablation and surgical resection for HCC conforming to the Milan criteria. Ann Surg 252:903–912, 2010.

**48.** Bruix J, Sala M, Llovet JM: Chemoembolization for hepatocellular carcinoma. Gastroenterology 127:S179–S188, 2004.

**49.** Mabed M, Esmaeel M, El-Khodary T, et al: A randomized controlled trial of transcatheter arterial chemoembolization with lipiodol, doxorubicin and cisplatin versus intravenous doxorubicin for patients with unresectable hepatocellular carcinoma. Eur J Cancer Care (Engl) 18:492–499, 2009.

**50.** Malagari K, Pomoni M, Kelekis A, et al: Prospective randomized comparison of chemoembolization with doxorubicin-eluting beads and bland embolization with BeadBlock for hepatocellular carcinoma. Cardiovasc Intervent Radiol 33:541–551, 2010.

**51.** Yopp AC, Jarnagin WR: Randomized clinical trials in hepatocellular carcinoma. Surg Oncol Clin N Am 19:151–162, 2010.

52. Llovet JM, Ricci S, Mazzaferro V, et al: Sorafenib in advanced hepatocellular carcinoma. N Engl J Med 359:378–390, 2008.
53. Jamal MM, Yoon EJ, Vega KJ, et al: Diabetes mellitus as a risk factor for gastrointestinal cancer among American veterans. World J Gastroenterol 15:5274–5278, 2009.
54. El-Serag HB, Engels EA, Landgren O, et al: Risk of hepatobiliary and pancreatic cancers after hepatitis C virus infection: A population-based study of U.S. veterans. Hepatology 49:116–123, 2009.
55. Endo I, Gonen M, Yopp AC, et al: Intrahepatic cholangiocarcinoma: Rising frequency, improved survival, and determinants of outcome after resection. Ann Surg 248:84–96, 2008.
56. Maithel SK, D'Angelica MI: An update on randomized clinical trials in advanced and metastatic colorectal carcinoma. Surg Oncol Clin N Am 19:163–181, 2010.
57. Carpizo DR, D'Angelica M: Liver resection for metastatic colorectal cancer in the presence of extrahepatic disease. Lancet Oncol 10:801–809, 2009.
58. Tomlinson JS, Jarnagin WR, DeMatteo RP, et al: Actual 10-year survival after resection of colorectal liver metastases defines cure. J Clin Oncol 25:4575–4580, 2007.
59. Poultsides GA, Servais EL, Saltz LB, et al: Outcome of primary tumor in patients with synchronous stage IV colorectal cancer receiving combination chemotherapy without surgery as initial treatment. J Clin Oncol 27:3379–3384, 2009.
60. Gold JS, Are C, Kornprat P, et al: Increased use of parenchymal-sparing surgery for bilateral liver metastases from colorectal cancer is associated with improved mortality without change in oncologic outcome: trends in treatment over time in 440 patients. Ann Surg 247:109–117, 2008.
61. Fong Y, Fortner J, Sun RL, et al: Clinical score for predicting recurrence after hepatic resection for metastatic colorectal cancer: Analysis of 1001 consecutive cases. Ann Surg 230:309–318, 1999.
62. Are C, Gonen M, Zazzali K, et al: The impact of margins on outcome after hepatic resection for colorectal metastasis. Ann Surg 246:295–300, 2007.
63. Carpizo DR, Are C, Jarnagin W, et al: Liver resection for metastatic colorectal cancer in patients with concurrent extrahepatic disease: Results in 127 patients treated at a single center. Ann Surg Oncol 16:2138–2146, 2009.
64. Nordlinger B, Sorbye H, Glimelius B, et al: Perioperative chemotherapy with FOLFOX4 and surgery versus surgery alone for resectable liver metastases from colorectal cancer (EORTC Intergroup trial 40983): A randomised controlled trial. Lancet 371:1007–1016, 2008.
65. Portier G, Elias D, Bouche O, et al: Multicenter randomized trial of adjuvant fluorouracil and folinic acid compared with surgery alone after resection of colorectal liver metastases: FFCD ACHBTH AURC 9002 trial. J Clin Oncol 24:4976–4982, 2006.
66. Kemeny N, Capanu M, D'Angelica M, et al: Phase I trial of adjuvant hepatic arterial infusion (HAI) with floxuridine (FUDR) and dexamethasone plus systemic oxaliplatin, 5-fluorouracil and leucovorin in patients with resected liver metastases from colorectal cancer. Ann Oncol 20:1236–1241, 2009.
67. Kemeny N, Jarnagin W, Gonen M, et al: Phase I/II study of hepatic arterial therapy with floxuridine and dexamethasone in combination with intravenous irinotecan as adjuvant treatment after resection of hepatic metastases from colorectal cancer. J Clin Oncol 21:3303–3309, 2003.
68. Kemeny N, Huang Y, Cohen AM, et al: Hepatic arterial infusion of chemotherapy after resection of hepatic metastases from colorectal cancer. N Engl J Med 341:2039–2048, 1999.
69. Martin RC, Scoggins CR, McMasters KM: Safety and efficacy of microwave ablation of hepatic tumors: A prospective review of a 5-year experience. Ann Surg Oncol 17:171–178, 2010.
70. Kemeny NE, Melendez FD, Capanu M, et al: Conversion to resectability using hepatic artery infusion plus systemic chemotherapy for the treatment of unresectable liver metastases from colorectal carcinoma. J Clin Oncol 27:3465–3471, 2009.
71. Que FG, Sarmiento JM, Nagorney DM: Hepatic surgery for metastatic gastrointestinal neuroendocrine tumors. Adv Exp Med Biol 574:43–56, 2006.
72. Mazzaglia PJ, Berber E, Milas M, et al: Laparoscopic radiofrequency ablation of neuroendocrine liver metastases: A 10-year experience evaluating predictors of survival. Surgery 142:10–19, 2007.
73. D'Angelica M, Jarnagin W, Dematteo R, et al: Staging laparoscopy for potentially resectable noncolorectal, nonneuroendocrine liver metastases. Ann Surg Oncol 9:204–209, 2002.
74. Mimatsu K, Oida T, Kawasaki A, et al: Long-term outcome of laparoscopic deroofing for symptomatic nonparasitic liver cysts. Hepatogastroenterology 56:850–853, 2009.
75. Jarnagin WR, Gonen M, Fong Y, et al: Improvement in perioperative outcome after hepatic resection: Analysis of 1,803 consecutive cases over the past decade. Ann Surg 236:397–406, 2002.

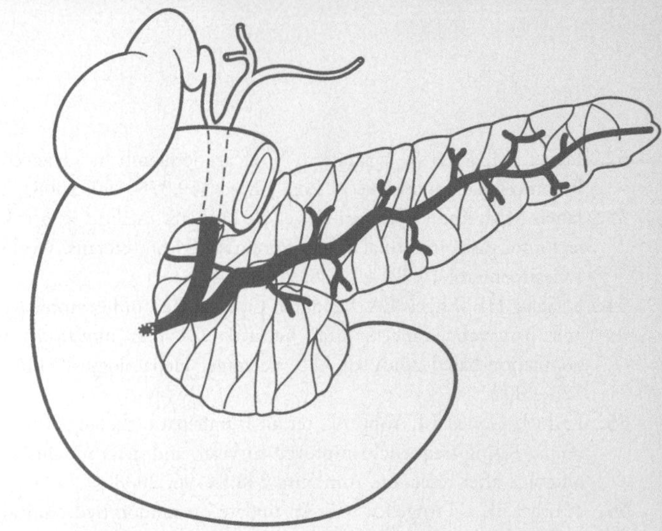

# CHAPTER 55

# BILIARY SYSTEM

Patrick G. Jackson and Steven R.T. Evans



## ANATOMY AND PHYSIOLOGY

Biliary anatomy is extremely variable, and precise knowledge of the normal and anatomic variants is critical to surgical intervention in the biliary tree. The distal common bile duct (CBD) inserts into the duodenum via the ampulla of Vater, passing through the sphincter of Oddi. Ascending from the duodenum, the common bile duct may join with the pancreatic duct in the wall of the duodenum, within the pancreas prior to insertion into the duodenal wall, or may enter the duodenum separately from the pancreatic duct (Fig. 55-1). The most inferior portion of the CBD is encompassed by the head of the pancreas. Superior to this portion, the common bile duct is divided into retroduodenal and supraduodenal segments. The insertion of the cystic duct marks the differentiation of the common hepatic duct above and the common bile duct below.

The cystic duct drains the gallbladder, which is divided into the neck, infundibulum with Hartmann's pouch, body, and fundus of the gallbladder. Roughly the size and shape of a common light bulb, the gallbladder holds 30 to 60 mL of bile as an extrahepatic reservoir. The gallbladder is attached to the inferior surface of the liver and is enveloped by liver for a variable portion of its circumference. Although some gallbladders are almost enveloped by liver parenchyma, others hang on a mesentery, predisposing to volvulus. The attachment of the gallbladder to the liver, known as the *gallbladder fossa*, identifies the separation of the left and right lobes of the liver (Fig. 55-2). Where the gallbladder attaches to the liver, Glisson's capsule does not form, and this common surface provides the venous and lymphatic drainage of the gallbladder. The cystic duct drains at an acute angle into the common bile duct and can range from 1 to 5 cm in length. There are a number of anatomic variations in insertion of the cystic duct, including into the right hepatic duct (Fig. 55-3). Within the neck of the gallbladder and cystic ducts lie folds of mucosa oriented in a spiral pattern, known as the spiral valves of Heister, which act to keep gallstones from entering the common bile duct, in spite of distention and intraluminal pressure. The dependent portion of Hartmann's pouch may overlie the common hepatic or right hepatic ducts, thus placing these structures at risk during the performance of a laparoscopic cholecystectomy.

Above the cystic duct lies the common hepatic duct, draining the left and right hepatic duct systems. The confluence of these structures lies at the hilar plate, which is an extension of Glisson's capsule. The absence of any vascular structures overlying the bile ducts at this location allows exposure of the bifurcation by incising this layer at the base of the segment IV, lifting the liver off these structures, known as lowering the hilar plate, and is generally used to expose the remainder of the extrahepatic biliary tree for resection or reconstruction.

### Vascular Anatomy

The segmental anatomy of the liver parenchyma is based on the vascular supply and drainage, and the biliary drainage is described by the corresponding vascular segment. The hepatic parenchyma is divided into lobes, each of which is divided into lobar segments (Fig. 55-4) to define the basic hepatic anatomic resections. The left lobe is comprised of medial and lateral segments. The right lobe is divided into posterior and anterior segments. Alternatively, the hepatic parenchyma can be divided into segments based on the specific hepatic venous drainage and portal inflow, allowing for a more precise description of anatomic pathology. In this classification system, as developed by Couinard,[1] the liver is composed of eight segments. Segment I refers to the caudate lobe. The left lobe of the liver, supplied by the left portal vein, constitutes segments II through IV. The left lobe is further subdivided by the falciform ligament, which separates segments II and III, also known as the left lateral segment, from segment IV. Within the left lateral segment, segment II lies superior to the insertion of the portal vein and segment III lies inferior to it. Segment IV is similarly divided into segments IVA, above, and segment IVB, below the portal vein insertion. The right portal vein supplies the right lobe of the liver and divides into the posterior and anterior sector. Each sector is then subdivided based on its relative location compared with the portal vein. Segment V is supplied by the inferior branch of the anterior sector and segment VIII is supplied by the superior branch. In the posterior sector, segment VI is supplied by the inferior branch and segment VII is supplied by the superior branch. There are three major hepatic veins that drain into the inferior vena cava, in addition to a number of small veins that drain directly from the right lobe. The right hepatic vein constitutes most of the venous drainage from the right lobe and generally lies in the intersegmental fissure between the anterior and

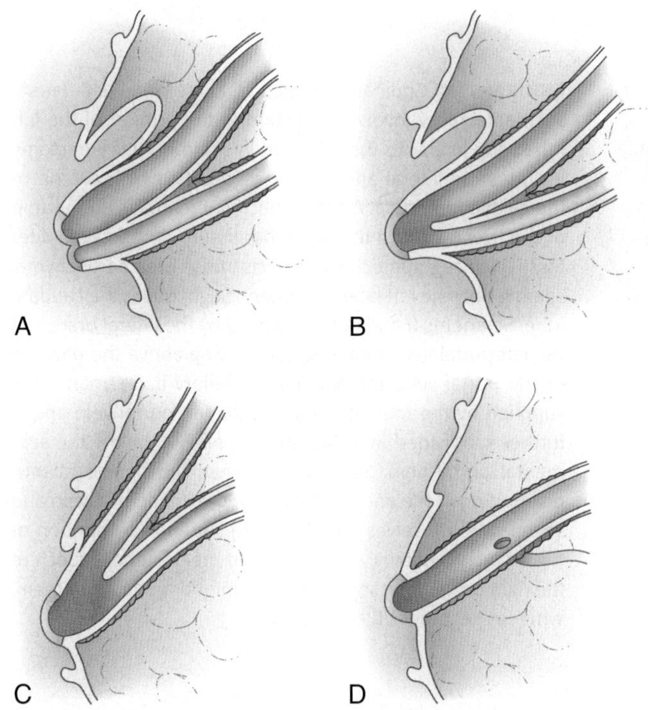


FIGURE 55-1 Patterns of biliary-pancreatic duct junction and insertion into the duodenal wall.

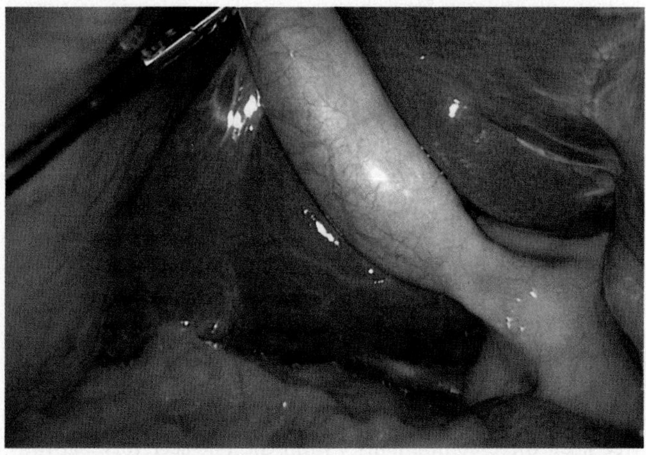

FIGURE 55-2 Laparoscopic photograph of the gallbladder in situ. The gallbladder is being suspended by the fundus to expose the infundibulum and porta hepatis.

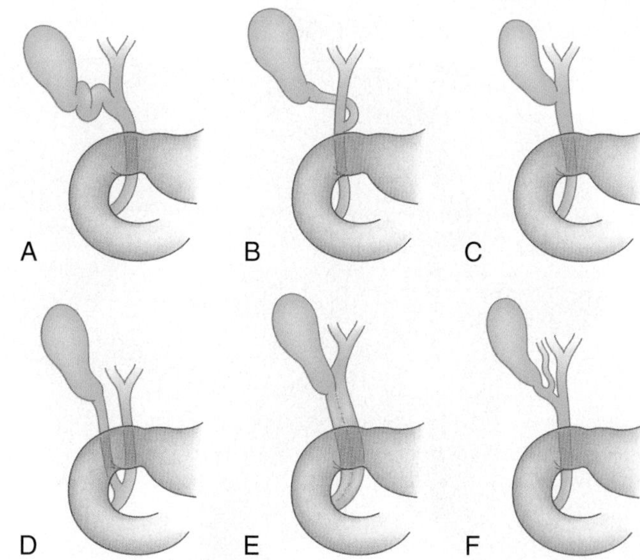


FIGURE 55-3 Variability in cystic duct anatomy. Knowledge of these variations is important to try to avoid inadvertent injury to the biliary tree during cholecystectomy.

posterior sectors of the right lobe. The middle hepatic vein drains the medial segment of the left lobe and a small amount of the medial portions of segments V and VIII. In most cases, the middle hepatic vein fuses with the left hepatic vein that drains the left lateral segment.

As opposed to the liver, where most perfusion comes from portal venous flow, the entire biliary tree is supplied solely by the arterial anatomy. This anatomic arrangement makes it particularly susceptible to ischemic injury at the intrahepatic and extrahepatic levels. The inferior bile duct, below the level of the duodenal bulb, receives its perfusion from tributaries of the posterosuperior pancreaticoduodenal and gastroduodenal arteries. The small branches coalesce to form the two vessels that run along the common bile duct at the 3 and 9 o'clock positions. With close dissection of the areolar tissue surrounding the bile duct, these vessels can be damaged, leaving the bile duct at risk for ischemic injury. The superior common bile duct, from the duodenal bulb to the cystic duct, and common hepatic ducts receive their blood supply from the right hepatic and cystic arteries. As the proper hepatic artery ascends on the anterior medial side of the porta, it divides into right and left hepatic arteries. In most cases, the right hepatic artery passes posterior to the common hepatic duct to supply the right lobe of the liver. After crossing the duct, the right hepatic artery passes through the triangle of Calot, bordered by the cystic duct, common hepatic duct, and edge of liver. In this triangle, the right hepatic artery gives off the cystic artery to the gallbladder and is at risk for injury during a cholecystectomy. An accessory or replaced right hepatic artery, when present, passes through the portocaval space and ascends to the right lobe along the lateral aspect of the common bile duct. A pulsatile structure on the most lateral aspect of the porta during a Pringle maneuver identifies this anomaly.

Normally, the cystic artery arises from the right hepatic artery, which can pass posterior or anterior to the common bile duct to supply the gallbladder. Similar to the variability of the cystic duct, the cystic artery may arise from the right hepatic, left hepatic, proper hepatic, common hepatic, gastroduodenal, or superior mesenteric artery. Although variable, the cystic artery generally lies superior to the cystic duct and is usually associated with a lymph node, known as Calot's node (Fig. 55-5). Because this node provides some of the lymphatic drainage of the gallbladder, it can be enlarged in the setting of gallbladder pathology, whether inflammatory or neoplastic.

Both within the liver and immediately outside the parenchyma, the bile ducts generally lie superior to the corresponding portal veins, which in turn are superior to the arterial supply (Fig. 55-6). Retaining a longer extrahepatic segment before

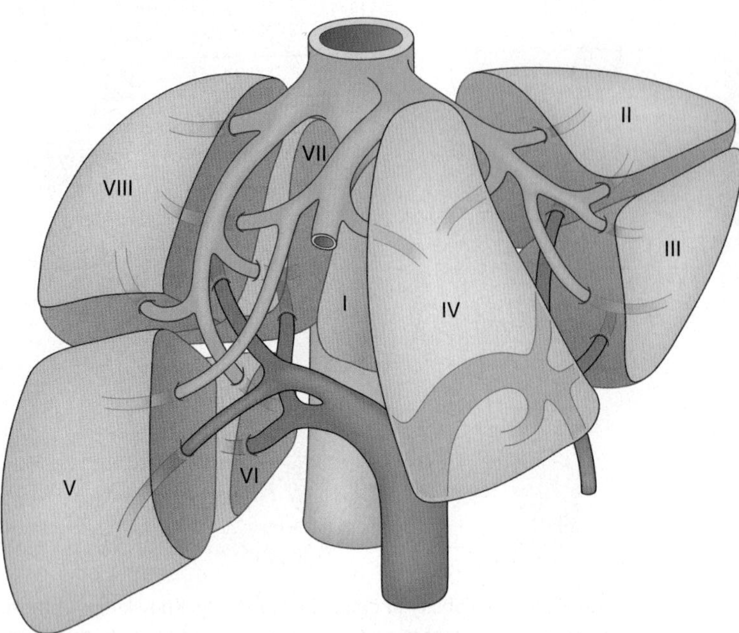


**FIGURE 55-4** Couinard segmental anatomy. A left lateral segmentectomy involves resection of the portion of the left lobe lying lateral to the falciform ligament. A left lobectomy includes the lateral and medial segments, which extend to the gallbladder fossa. A right lobectomy removes the portion of the liver lateral to the interlobar fissure at the gallbladder fossa. A trisegmentectomy resects most liver parenchyma, sparing only the left lateral segment. Segment I is the caudate lobe. Segments II and III are supplied by the lateral branch of the left portal vein, with segment II lying above the passage of the portal vein and segment III below it. Segment IV is supplied by the medial branch of the left portal vein and is further subdivided into IVA, above, and IVB, below the segmental portal vein. Segment V is supplied by the inferior distribution of the anterior branch of the right portal vein and segment VIII receives flow from the superior distribution of this branch. Similarly, with respect to the posterior branch of the right portal vein, segment VI lies inferior to the portal vein, whereas segment VII lies superior.

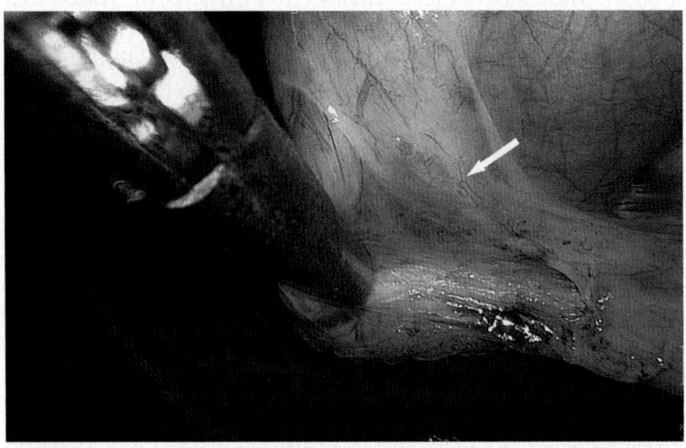

**FIGURE 55-5** Operative photograph of Calot's node. This node *(arrow)* is useful for identification of the common location of the cystic artery.

inserting into the liver, the left hepatic duct travels under the edge of segment IV before slipping superior and posterior to the left portal vein. During this transverse portion, it can receive a few subsegmental branches from segment IV. The left duct drains segments II, III, and IV, with the most distal branch draining segment IVa. Further superolateral, the ducts draining segment IVb arise, and further up the left duct are the ducts for segments II and III. These fused ducts can generally be found just posterior and lateral to the umbilical recess. The caudate lobe drains via smaller ducts that enter the right and left hepatic duct systems. The drainage of the right duct system includes segments V, VI, VII, and VIII and is substantially shorter than the left duct, bifurcating almost immediately. The fusion of two sectoral ducts, posterior and anterior, creates this short right hepatic duct. The anterior sectoral duct runs in a vertical direction to drain segments V and VIII, whereas the posterior sectoral duct follows a horizontal course to drain segments VI and VII.

## Physiology

Bile secretion from the hepatocyte serves two major roles in human physiology. First, because the liver is a major site of detoxification and cellular recycling, bile transport allows excretion of toxins and normal cellular metabolites. Second, bile salts have a critical role in the absorption of most lipids. Bile is secreted into bile canaliculi, which encircle each hepatocyte. Within the hepatic lobule, these canaliculi coalesce to form small bile ducts, eventually entering a portal triad. Four to six portal triads combine to create a hepatic lobule, the smallest functional unit of the liver, identified by its central terminal hepatic venule. On the opposite aspect from the canalicular surface of the hepatocyte lies the sinusoidal surface, which contacts the space of Disse. In this contact area, the hepatocyte is responsible for the absorption of circulating components of bile, an important step in the enterohepatic circulation of bile. Once absorbed and secreted into the bile canaliculi, the tight junctions in the biliary tree keep these components within the bile secretory pathway. The secretion of bile components into the biliary tree form a major stimulus to bile flow, and the volume of bile flow is an osmotic process. Because bile salts combine to form spherical pockets, known as micelles, the salts themselves provide no osmotic activity. Instead, the cations that are secreted into the biliary tree along with the bile salt anion provide the osmotic load to draw water into the duct and increase flow to keep bile electrochemically neutral. For this reason, bile maintains an osmolality approximately comparable to that of plasma.

Although some bile flow is bile salt–independent, serving to expel toxins and metabolites from the body, much of the flow is dependent on neural, humoral, and chemical stimuli. Vagal activity induces bile secretion, as does the gastrointestinal hormone secretin. Cholecystokinin (CCK), secreted by the intestinal mucosa, serves to induce biliary tree secretion and gallbladder wall contraction, thereby augmenting excretion of bile into the intestines.

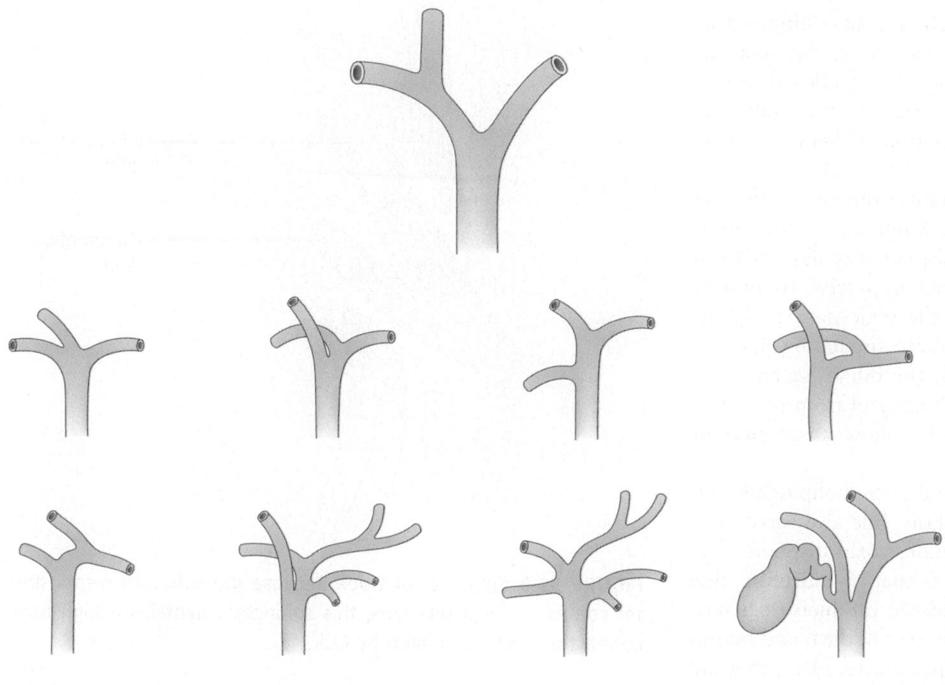

**FIGURE 55-6** Hepatic lobar segmental biliary anatomy.

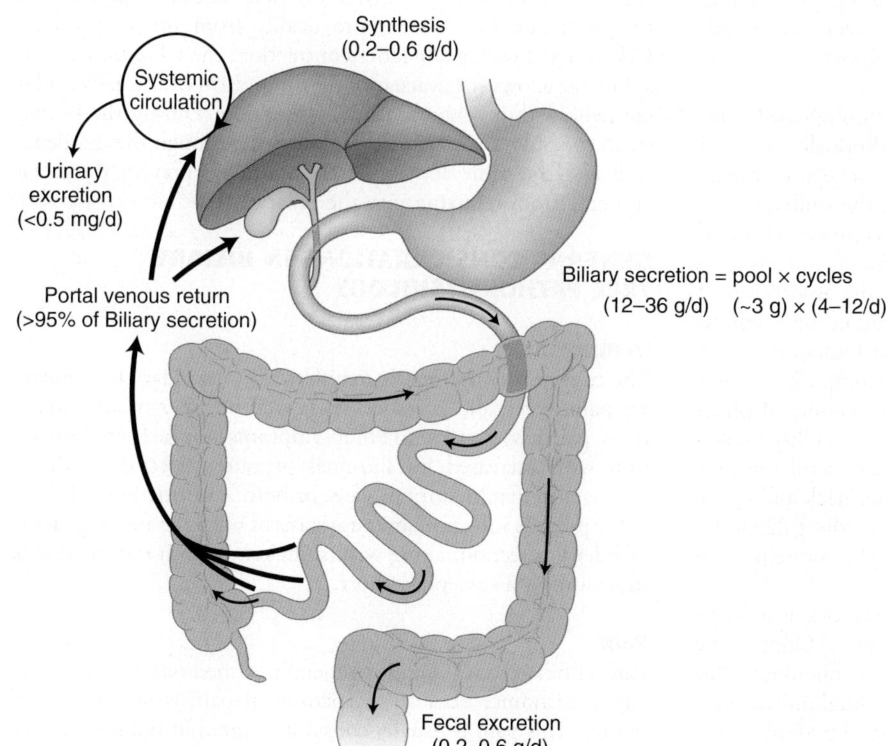


**FIGURE 55-7** Enterohepatic circulation.

Bile salts, such as cholic acid and deoxycholic acid, are originally created from cholesterol and secreted into bile canaliculi as cholic acid and its metabolite, deoxycholic acid. The liver actually makes only a small amount of the total bile salt pool used on a daily basis, because most bile salts are recycled after use in the intestinal lumen (Fig. 55-7). After passage into the intestinal tract and reabsorption by the terminal ileum, bile acids are transported back to the liver for recycling bound to albumin. Less than 5% of bile salts are lost each day in the stool. When sufficient quantities of bile salts reach the colonic lumen, the powerful detergent activity of the bile salts can cause inflammation and diarrhea.

The passage of bound bile salts through the space of Disse allows uptake into the hepatocyte in an efficient process that involves sodium cotransport and sodium-independent pathways. In the less specific sodium-independent pathway, a number of organic anions are transported, including unconjugated or indirect bilirubin. The transport of bile salts across the canalicular membrane remains the rate-limiting step in bile salt excretion. Given the vast differences in concentration of bile salts, the transport of bile up an extreme concentration gradient is adenosine triphosphate (ATP)–dependent.

In addition to bile salts, bile contains proteins, lipids, and pigments. The major lipid components of bile are phospholipids and cholesterol. These lipids not only dispose of cholesterol from low- and high-density lipoproteins, but also serve to protect hepatocytes and cholangiocytes from the toxic nature of bile. The sources of most biliary cholesterol are circulating lipoproteins and hepatic synthesis. Therefore, the biliary secretion of cholesterol actually serves to excrete cholesterol from the body. These lipids form micelles and thereby allow absorption of dietary lipids.

Although cholesterol, bile salts, and phospholipids play an important role in nutritional homeostasis, bile also serves as a major route of exogenous and endogenous toxin disposal. One such example of the disposal system is that of bilirubin. Bile pigments, such as bilirubin, are breakdown products of hemoglobin and myoglobin. These are transported in the blood bound to albumin and transported into the hepatocyte. Here, they are transferred into the endoplasmic reticulum and conjugated to form bilirubin glucuronides, also known as conjugated or direct bilirubin. It is the bile pigments that give the color to bile and, when converted to urobilinogen by bacterial enzymes in the intestines, give stool its characteristic color.

In the fasting state, secreted bile will pass through the biliary tree into the intestine and be reabsorbed. Additionally, bile will collect in the gallbladder, which serves as an extrahepatic storage site of secreted bile. To store bile secretions, the gallbladder is extremely efficient in water absorption and thus concentration of bile components. This absorption is an osmotic process performed via the active NaCl transport. With the absorption of NaCl and water across the gallbladder epithelium, the chemical composition of bile changes in the gallbladder lumen. Increases in cholesterol concentration, in addition to calcium, which is not as efficiently absorbed, then lead to decreased stability of phospholipid cholesterol vesicles. The reduced vesicle stability predisposes to nucleation of this stagnant pool of cholesterol and thus to cholesterol stone formation. The gallbladder neck and cystic duct also secrete glycoproteins to help protect the gallbladder from the detergent activity of bile. These glycoproteins also promote cholesterol crystallization.

The gallbladder fills through a retrograde mechanism. With an increase in the tonic activity of the sphincter of Oddi in the fasting state, pressure increases in the common bile duct. This increased pressure allows filling of the lower intraluminal pressure gallbladder, which is capable of storing up to 600 mL of the daily production of bile. The passage of fat, protein, and acid into the duodenum induces CCK secretion from duodenal epithelial cells. Cholecystokinin, as its name suggests, then causes gallbladder contraction, with intraluminal pressures up to 300 mm Hg. Vagal activity also induces gallbladder emptying, but is a less powerful stimulus to gallbladder contraction than CCK.

The distal portion of the bile duct passes through the sphincter of Oddi (Fig. 55-8). The musculature of this sphincter is independent from that of the duodenal intestinal wall and responds differently to neurohumoral controls. This muscular sphincter, which normally maintains high tonic and phasic activity, is inhibited by CCK. With CCK-induced relaxation of the sphincter, bile flows more readily from the biliary tree. Coordinated with gallbladder contraction, the relaxation of this sphincter allows for evacuation of up to 70% of the gallbladder contents within 2 hours of CCK secretion. During the fasting state, the oblique passage of the bile duct through the duodenal wall and the tonic activity of the sphincter prevent duodenal contents from refluxing into the biliary tree.

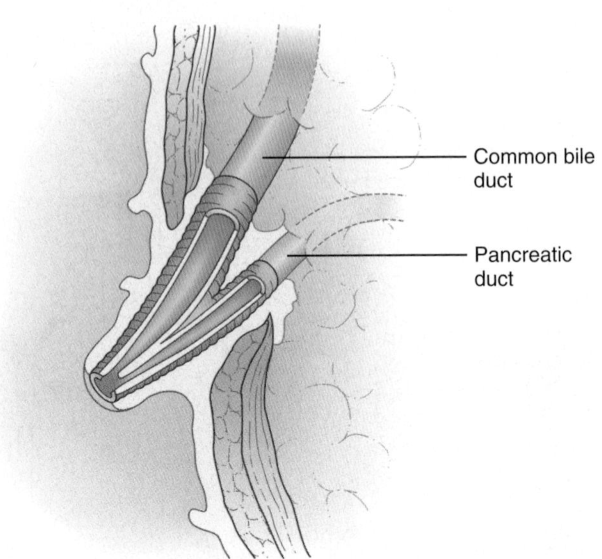


**FIGURE 55-8** Sphincter of Oddi. Because the sphincter responsible for control of most bile flow, this sphincter maintains a high tonic contraction, but is inhibited by CCK.

## GENERAL CONSIDERATIONS IN BILIARY TREE PATHOPHYSIOLOGY

### Symptoms

The common symptomatic manifestations of biliary tree disease are pain, fever, and jaundice. As is seen in other tubular structures, pain associated with other symptoms may be from obstruction with increased intraluminal pressure, infection with its associated inflammatory process, or both. Obstruction will generally precede infection, because stasis of bile is an inciting factor of biliary infection, along with sufficient quantity of infectious inoculum in a susceptible host.

#### Pain

Pain of biliary tract origin is generally termed *biliary colic,* actually a misnomer because the pattern of pain is not colicky in nature. This pain is usually constant, located in the right upper quadrant or epigastrium, and can be associated with meals. Right upper quadrant pain seen 1 hour or more after a meal is frequently caused by contraction of the gallbladder induced by CCK secretion. When the gallbladder lumen cannot fully empty because of a stone in the gallbladder neck, visceral pain fibers are activated, causing pain in the epigastrium or right upper quadrant. The same luminal obstruction of biliary colic, but associated with sufficient stasis, pressure, and bacterial inoculum, creates infection and thereby inflammation. With this infection and inflammation, the right upper quadrant pain of biliary colic will be accompanied by tenderness noted on palpation of the right upper quadrant. Specifically, the voluntary cessation of respiration when the examiner exerts constant pressure under the right costal margin, known as a Murphy's sign, suggests inflammation of the visceral and parietal peritoneal surfaces, and can be seen in diseases such as acute cholecystitis and hepatitis. Alternatively, biliary colic in the absence of infection and inflammation is not associated with any reproducible physical examination finding or systemic symptom.

#### Fever

Although biliary colic is not generally associated with other systemic manifestations, infection or inflammation in the gallbladder or biliary tree will usually cause fever. It can be seen in a number of inflammatory diseases, but fever associated with right upper quadrant pain is a hallmark of infectious process in the biliary tree. With immediate and direct access to the metabolically active hepatic parenchyma, infection of the gallbladder and biliary tree induces cytokine secretion and thereby direct systemic manifestations.

#### Jaundice

Jaundice, caused by elevation of the serum bilirubin level, can be demonstrated in the sclera, the frenulum of the tongue, or skin. Serum bilirubin levels over 2.5 mg/dL are necessary to detect scleral icterus routinely, and levels over 5 mg/dL will manifest as cutaneous jaundice. Failure to excrete bile from the liver into the intestines is a prerequisite of jaundice. Therefore, although both are associated with fever and pain, acute cholecystitis does not cause the jaundice seen in infection of the biliary tree, known as ascending cholangitis. The constellation of fever, right upper quadrant pain, and jaundice, known as Charcot's triad, suggests blockage of the biliary secretion from the liver, not just the gallbladder. With the addition of hypotension and altered mental status, known as Reynolds' pentad, patients will demonstrate the systemic manifestations of shock from biliary origin. Jaundice is generally divided into surgical, from obstruction, and medical, from a hepatocellular process.

### Laboratory Tests

Although termed *liver function tests,* the routine hepatic panel for most laboratories tests a number of aspects of metabolic and hepatic activity. The tests most useful for evaluation of biliary physiology include determination of levels of bilirubin, alkaline phosphatase, seen in any cholestatic process, and serum transaminases, suggesting evidence of hepatocellular injury. Bilirubin can be subdivided into the conjugated and unconjugated forms, thereby allowing delineation of cause based on cellular location of derangement. In other words, hyperbilirubinemia may be caused by increased synthesis of bilirubin, impaired hepatocyte uptake of unconjugated bilirubin, decreased intracellular conjugation, reduced intracellular transport and excretion of conjugated bilirubin, or obstruction of the biliary tree. Although an oversimplification of a complex process, derangements up to and including conjugation will manifest as elevated unconjugated bilirubin levels.

### Imaging Studies

#### Plain Films

Plain radiographs are of limited use in the overall evaluation of the biliary tree. Gallstones are not regularly seen by plain films and, even when seen, rarely change therapy. Therefore, the role of plain radiographs in the evaluation of possible biliary disease is limited to exclusion of other diagnoses, such as a duodenal ulcer with free air, small bowel obstruction, or right lower lobe pneumonia causing right upper quadrant pain.

#### Ultrasound

Transabdominal ultrasound is a sensitive, inexpensive, reliable, and reproducible test to evaluate most of the biliary tree, being able to separate patients with medical jaundice from those with surgical jaundice. Therefore, this modality is seen as the study of choice for the initial evaluation of jaundice or symptoms of biliary disease. The finding of a dilated common bile duct in the setting of jaundice suggests an obstruction of the duct from stones, usually associated with pain, or from a tumor, which is commonly painless (Fig. 55-9). Gallbladder diseases are regularly diagnosed by ultrasound, because its superficial location with no overlying bowel gas enables its evaluation by sound waves. Ultrasound has a high specificity and sensitivity for cholelithiasis, or gallstones. The density of gallstones allows crisp reverberation of the sound wave, showing an echogenic focus with a characteristic shadowing behind the stone (Fig. 55-10). Most gallstones, unless impacted, will move with positional changes in the patient. This feature allows their differentiation from gallbladder polyps, which are fixed, and from sludge which will move more slowly and does not have the sharp echogenic pattern of gallstones. Pathologic changes seen in many gallbladder diseases can be identified by ultrasound. For example, the gallbladder wall thickening and pericholecystic fluid seen in cholecystitis are visible by ultrasound (Fig. 55-11). Porcelain gallbladder, with its calcified wall, will appear as a curvilinear echogenic focus along the entire gallbladder wall, with posterior shadowing (Fig. 55-12). In addition to division of medical versus surgical jaundice, ultrasound can sometimes identify the cause of obstructive jaundice, showing common bile duct stones or even cholangiocarcinoma.

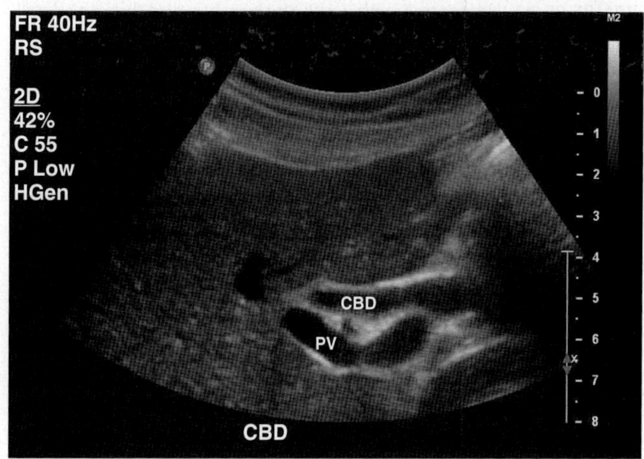


**FIGURE 55-9** Ultrasound of dilated biliary tree. The dilated CBD is dilated. As it travels parallel to the portal vein (PV), it is easy to identify. The depiction of the parallel stripes of duct and vein help ensure that the common duct diameter is not overestimated by a tangential view, which would artificially increase the anteroposterior diameter.

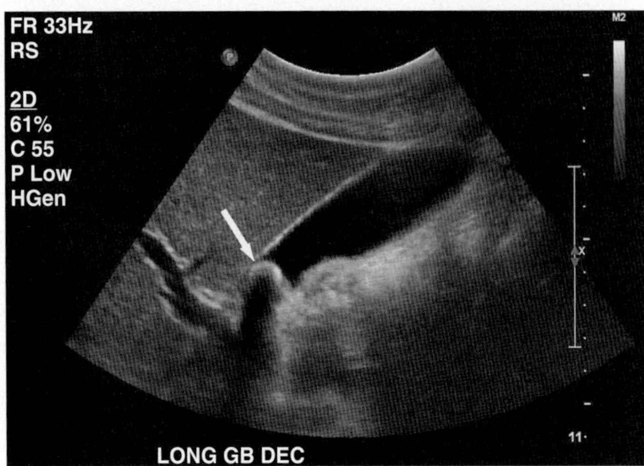


**FIGURE 55-10** Ultrasound of a gallstone in the gallbladder neck. The sharp echogenic wall of the gallstone *(arrow),* with the characteristic posterior shadowing stripe under the stone, help differentiate it from other intraluminal findings.

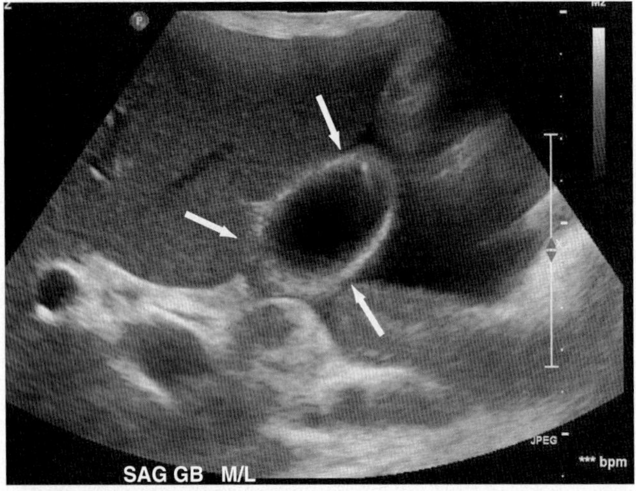


**FIGURE 55-11** Ultrasound with acute cholecystitis and thickened gallbladder wall *(arrows).*

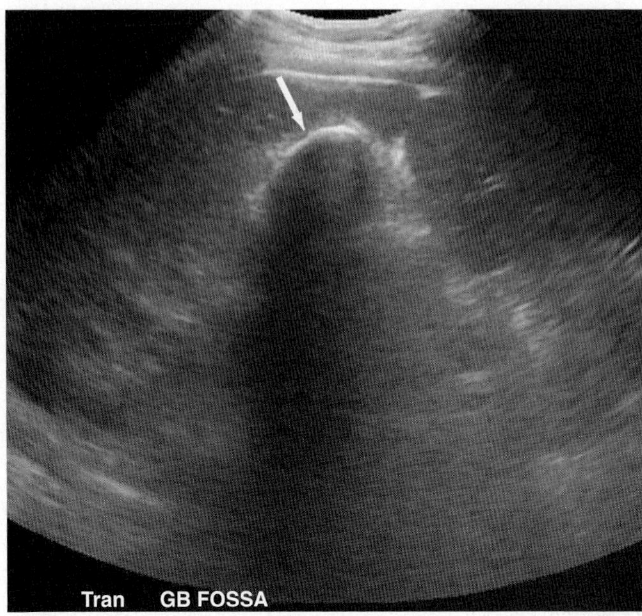


**FIGURE 55-12** Ultrasound of porcelain gallbladder. The curvilinear sharp echogenic focus *(arrow)* combined with substantial posterior shadowing help confirm this diagnosis.

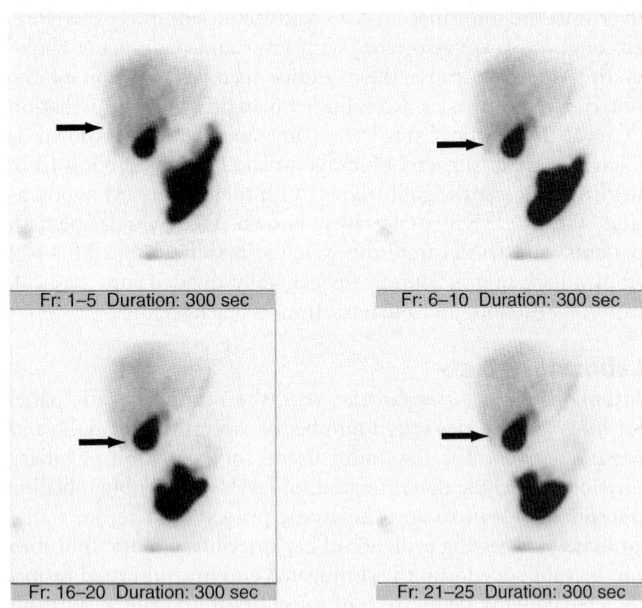


**FIGURE 55-13** HIDA scan showing filling of the gallbladder. With gallbladder filling *(arrows),* the diagnosis of acute cholecystitis is effectively eliminated.

### Hepatic Iminodiacetic Acid Scan

Although incapable of providing precise anatomic delineation of pathophysiology, biliary scintigraphy, also known as a hepatic iminodiacetic acid scan (HIDA) scan, can be used to evaluate the physiologic secretion of bile. The injection of an iminodiacetic acid, which is processed in the liver and secreted with bile, allows identification of bile flow. Therefore, the failure to fill the gallbladder 2 hours after injection demonstrates obstruction of the cystic duct, as seen in acute cholecystitis (Figs. 55-13 and 55-14). In addition, the scan will identify obstruction of the biliary tree and bile leaks, which may be useful in the postoperative setting. HIDA scans can also be used to determine gallbladder function, because the injection of CCK during a scan will document physiologic ejection of the gallbladder. This may be useful in patients with biliary tract pain but without stones, because some patients have pain from impaired emptying, known as biliary dyskinesia. As a nuclear medicine test, the test demonstrates physiologic flow, but does not provide fine anatomic detail, nor can it identify gallstones.

### Computed Tomography

Although ultrasound is clearly the first test of choice for delineation of biliary pathology, computed tomography (CT) provides superior anatomic information. Because most gallstones are radiographically isodense to bile, many will be indistinguishable from bile. However, because ultrasound is operator-dependent

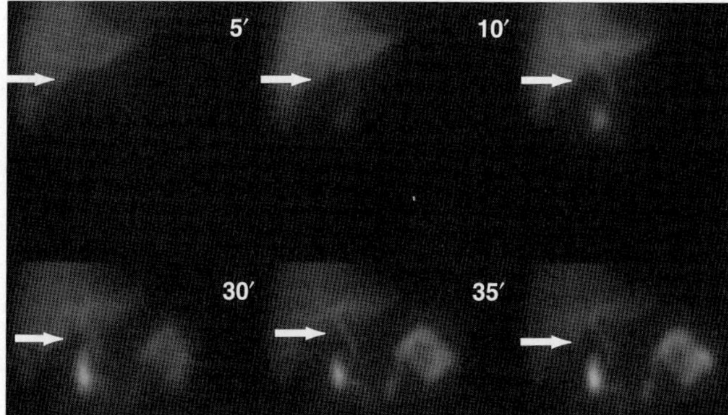


**FIGURE 55-14** HIDA scan showing nonfilling of the gallbladder. With no filling of the gallbladder *(arrows)* even on delayed images, HIDA confirms occlusion of the cystic duct, the characteristic feature of acute cholecystitis.

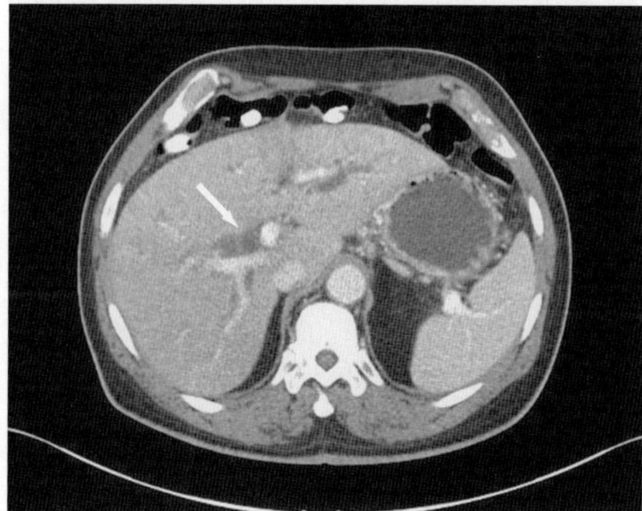

**FIGURE 55-15** CT scan showing dilated biliary tree *(arrow)* at the portal confluence. This dilation continued down to the head of the pancreas.

and provides no anatomic reconstruction of the biliary tree, CT can be used to identify the cause and site of biliary obstruction (Fig. 55-15). When performed for the evaluation of hepatic or pancreatic parenchyma or possible neoplastic processes, CT is invaluable in preoperative planning, and the use of arterial phase, portal venous phase, and delayed phase imaging, known as a triple-phase CT, has essentially replaced diagnostic angiography of the liver.

### Magnetic Resonance Imaging and Magnetic Resonance Cholangiopancreatography

Magnetic resonance imaging (MRI) uses the water in bile to delineate the biliary tree and thus provides superior anatomic definition of the intrahepatic and extrahepatic biliary tree and pancreas. Although management of most patients with biliary pathology does not require the fine detail of anatomic evaluation shown by cross-sectional imaging, MRI is noninvasive, requires no radiation exposure, and can prove extremely useful when

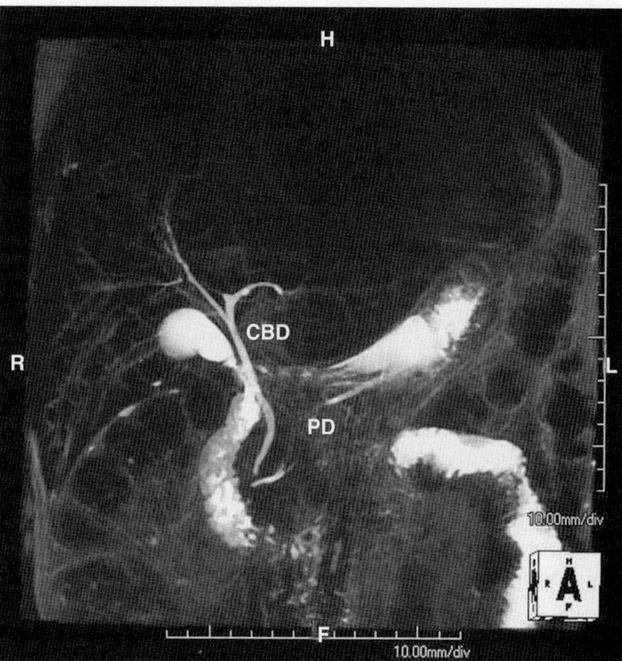


**FIGURE 55-16** Normal MRCP image. Note the normal CBD and pancreatic duct (PD).

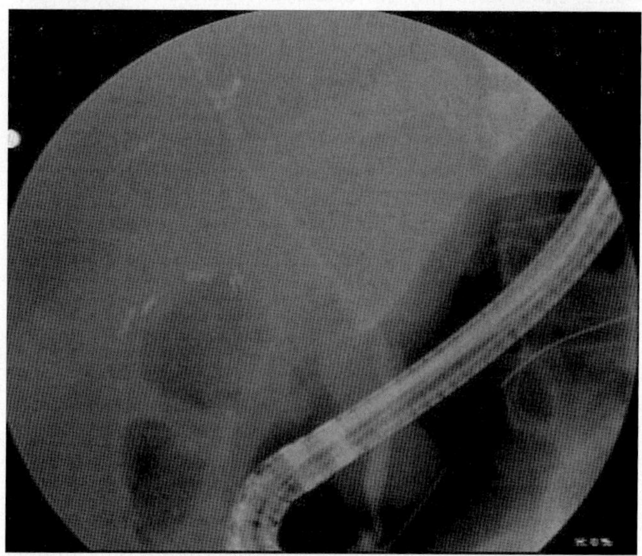

**FIGURE 55-17** Normal ERCP image.

planning resection of biliary or pancreatic neoplasms or management of complex biliary pathology. By using the water content of bile, a cholangiopancreatogram can be created (Fig. 55-16).

### Endoscopic Retrograde Cholangiopancreatography

Endoscopic retrograde cholangiopancreatography (ERCP) is an invasive test using endoscopy and fluoroscopy to inject contrast through the ampulla and image the biliary tree (Fig. 55-17). Although it does carry a complication rate of up to 10%, its usefulness lies in its ability to diagnose and treat many diseases of the biliary tree. For patients with malignant obstruction, ERCP can be used to provide tissue samples for diagnosis while also decompressing an obstruction, but does not stage patients accurately. Many benign diseases, such as choledocholithiasis, can be easily treated by endoscopic means. ERCP has also proven extremely useful in the diagnosis and treatment of complications of biliary surgery.

### Percutaneous Transhepatic Cholangiography

Interventional radiologic techniques can be used in the evaluation of biliary anatomy. Similar to ERCP, percutaneous transhepatic cholangiography (PTC) is an invasive procedure used to evaluate the biliary tree. A needle is passed directly into the liver to access one of the biliary radicals, and the tract is then used for insertion of transhepatic catheters. Useful for patients with intrahepatic biliary disease or in whom ERCP is not technically feasible, PTC can decompress biliary obstruction, stent obstructions nonoperatively, and provide anatomic information for biliary reconstruction.

### Intraoperative Cholangiography

Another imaging tool for the diagnosis of biliary tract abnormalities is the use of intraoperative cholangiography. With the injection catheter inserted via the cystic duct during a cholecystectomy or through another point in the biliary tree, intraoperative cholangiography can help delineate anomalous biliary anatomy, identify choledocholithiasis, or guide biliary reconstruction. Some surgeons advocate routine cholangiography during cholecystectomy. Advocates for routine cholangiography note that common duct injuries are less frequent when cholangiography is used routinely. However, because it adds operative time and fluoroscopic exposure to the operation, many surgeons use intraoperative cholangiography selectively during the performance of a cholecystectomy. Indications for the selective use of cholangiography include pain at the time of operative intervention, abnormal hepatic function panel, anomalous or confusing biliary anatomy, or inability to perform ERCP following cholecystectomy, dilated biliary tree, or any preoperative suspicion of choledocholithiasis (Box 55-1).

### Endoscopic Ultrasound

Although of limited use in the evaluation of gallbladder pathology or intrahepatic disease of the biliary tree, endoscopic ultrasound (EUS) is valuable in the assessment of distal common bile duct and ampulla. With the close apposition of the distal common bile duct and pancreas to the duodenum, sound waves generated by EUS provide detailed evaluation of the bile duct and ampulla and have proven most useful in assessing tumors for invasion into vascular structures. Echoendoscopes are subdivided into those that scan perpendicular to the long axis of the endoscope, known as radial echoendoscopes, and those that scan parallel, known as linear echoendoscopes. Radial echoendoscopes are most useful for providing a tomographic evaluation (Fig. 55-18), whereas linear echoendoscopes can guide interventions such as needle biopsies under real-time ultrasound guidance (Fig. 55-19).

**BOX 55-1 Indications for Selective Cholangiography**

- Pain at time of operation
- Abnormal hepatic function panel
- Anomalous or confusing biliary anatomy
- Inability to perform postoperative ERCP
- Dilated biliary tree
- Any suspicion of choledocholithiasis

### Fluorodeoxyglucose Positron Emission Tomography

Fluorodeoxyglucose positron emission tomography (FDG-PET) exploits the metabolic difference between a highly metabolically active tissue, such as a neoplasm, and normal tissue. With the injection of a radiolabeled glucose molecule, FDG-PET scans can differentiate benign and malignant lesions, detect recurrence, and identify metastatic disease. Unfortunately, FDG-PET is incapable of demonstrating carcinomatosis and, given the high metabolism of the immune system, is of limited value in the setting of infection or inflammation.

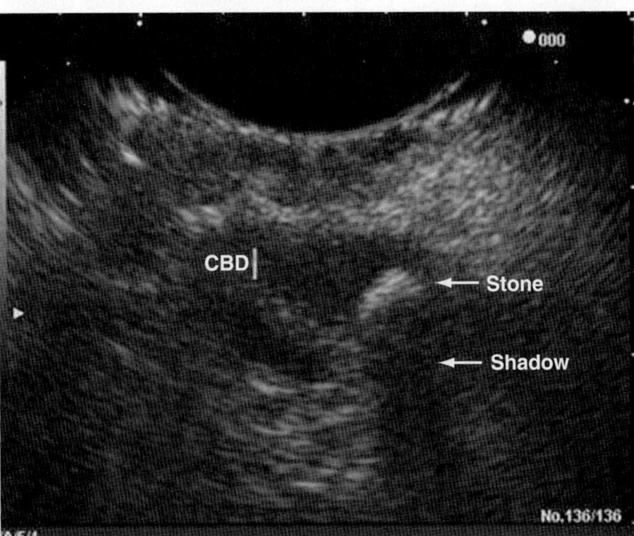


**FIGURE 55-18** Radial EUS showing choledocholithiasis in the distal CBD.

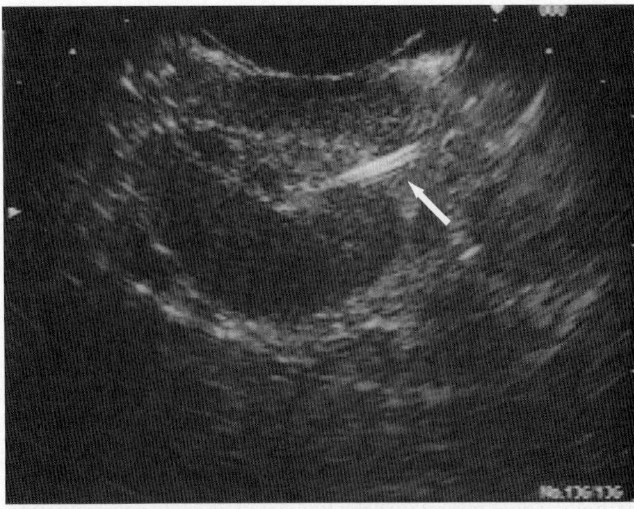

**FIGURE 55-19** Linear EUS with needle *(arrow)* biopsying a lymph node.

### Bacteriology

Without previous biliary intervention, most bile is considered sterile. However, with the presence of stones or obstruction, the likelihood of bacterial contamination increases. With nucleation of bile and gallstone formation, gallstones can provide a reservoir for bacteria, but the source of the bacteria is unclear. In that most bactibilia is caused by gram-negative aerobes, passage of bacteria upward from the duodenum into the biliary tree is a commonly held explanation for bacterial contamination. The most common types of bacteria found in biliary infections are Enterobacteriacae, such as *Escherichia coli, Klebsiella,* and *Enterobacter,* followed by *Enterococcus* spp. Stasis increases the likelihood of bacterial contamination of bile.

Prophylactic antibiotics should be used in most patients undergoing interventions in their biliary tree, such as ERCP or PTC. To cover the most common bacterial species, a first- or second-generation cephalosporin or fluoroquinolone should suffice. For those undergoing elective laparoscopic cholecystectomy for biliary colic, no antibiotic prophylaxis is necessary. However, antibiotics should be used for any patient with suspected or documented infection of the biliary tree, such as acute cholecystitis or ascending cholangitis, and should be chosen to cover gram-negative bacteria and anaerobes.

## BENIGN BILIARY DISEASE

### Calculous Biliary Disease

Gallstones can be subclassified into two major subtypes, depending on the principle solute that precipitates into a stone. More than 70% of gallstones in America are formed by precipitation of cholesterol and calcium, with pure cholesterol stones accounting for only a small (<10%) portion. Pigment stones, further subclassified as black or brown stones, are caused by precipitation of concentrated bile pigments, the breakdown products of hemoglobin. Four major factors explain most gallstone formation—supersaturation of secreted bile, concentration of bile in the gallbladder, crystal nucleation, and gallbladder dysmotility. High concentrations of cholesterol and lipid in bile secretion from the liver constitute one predisposing condition to cholesterol stone formation, whereas increased hemoglobin processing is seen in most patients with pigment stones. Once in the gallbladder, bile is concentrated further through the absorption of water and NaCl, increasing the concentrations of the bile solutes and calcium. With respect to cholesterol stones (Fig. 55-20), cholesterol precipitates out into crystals when the concentration in vesicles exceeds the solubility of cholesterol (Fig. 55-21).[2] This process of crystal formation is further accelerated by pronucleating agents, including glycoproteins and immunoglobulins. Finally, abnormal gallbladder motility can increase stasis in the gallbladder, allowing more time for solutes to precipitate in the gallbladder. Therefore, increased stone formation can be seen in conditions associated with impaired gallbladder emptying, such as prolonged fasting states, use of total parenteral nutrition, postvagotomy, and use of somatostatin analogues.

Pigment stones can be divided into black stones, as seen in hemolytic conditions and cirrhosis, or brown stones, which tend to be found in the bile ducts. The difference in color comes from incorporation of cholesterol into the brown stones. Because black pigment stones occur in hemolytic states from concentration of bilirubin, they are found almost exclusively in the gallbladder. Alternatively, brown stones occur within the biliary tree and suggest a disorder of biliary motility and associated bacterial infection.

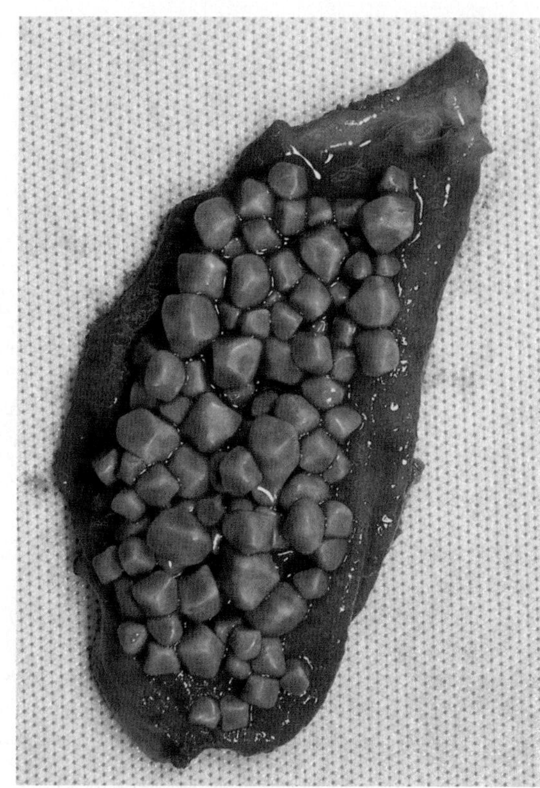

**FIGURE 55-20** Gallbladder, with characteristic yellow cholesterol stones.

#### Natural History

The vast majority of gallstones are asymptomatic, often being identified at time of abdominal imaging for other reasons or during laparotomy. To become symptomatic, the gallstone must obstruct a visceral structure, such as the cystic duct. Biliary colic, caused by temporary blockage of the cystic duct, tends to occur following a meal in which the secretion of CCK leads to gallbladder contraction. Stones that do not obstruct the cystic duct or pass through the entire biliary tree into the intestines without impaction do not cause symptoms. Only 20% to 30% of patients with asymptomatic stones will develop symptoms within 20 years and, because approximately 1% of patients with asymptomatic stones develop complications of their stones before onset of symptoms, prophylactic cholecystectomy is not warranted in asymptomatic patients.

Certain subsets of patients, however, constitute a higher risk pool, so prophylactic cholecystectomy should be considered. Among these are patients with hemolytic anemias, such as sickle cell anemia. These patients have an extremely high rate of pigment stone formation, and cholecystitis can precipitate a crisis. Patients with a calcified gallbladder wall, known as porcelain gallbladder, those with large (>2.5-cm) gallstones, and those with a long common channel of bile and pancreatic ducts all have a higher risk of gallbladder cancer and should consider

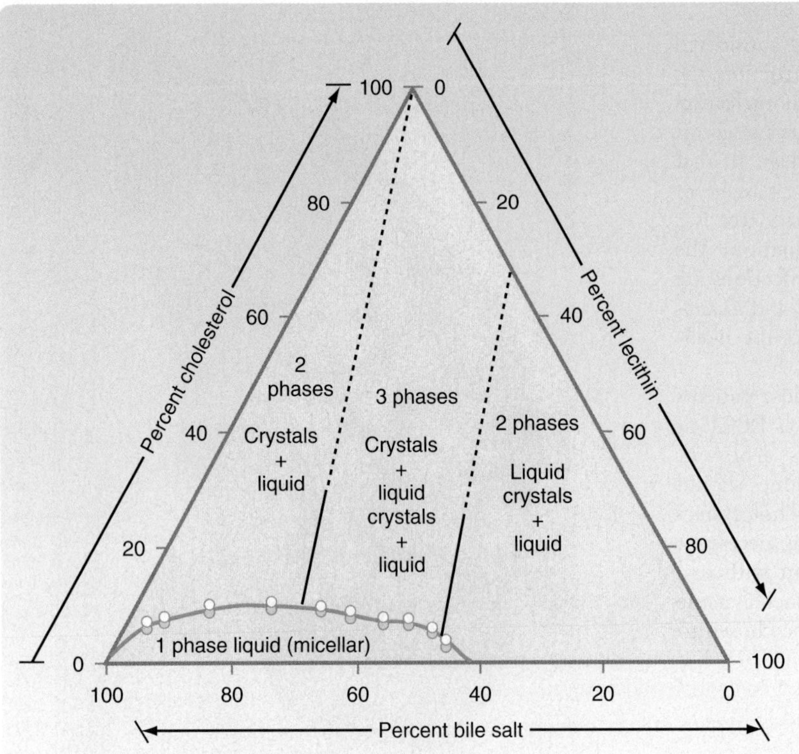


**FIGURE 55-21** Triangle of solubility. With the three major components of bile that determine cholesterol solubility and stability, each can be quantified by molar % to show a relative ratio to the other two. Cholesterol is completely soluble in only the small area in the left lower corner, where a clear micellar solution exists, below the *closed circles.* Just above this, in the area between the *open* and *closed circles,* cholesterol is supersaturated but stable, and thus only crystallized with stasis. In the remainder of the triangle, cholesterol is significantly supersaturated and unstable. In this region, crystals form immediately. (From Admirand WH, Small DM: The physicochemical basis of cholesterol gallstone formation in man J Clin Invest 47:1043–1052, 1968.)

cholecystectomy. Additionally, patients with asymptomatic gallstones undergoing bariatric surgery may also benefit from cholecystectomy. Not only does rapid weight loss favor stone formation but also, following gastric bypass, ERCP to remove common bile duct stones in ascending cholangitis is extremely challenging and usually unsuccessful. Finally, because severe infection can be life-threatening in the immunocompromised patient, some transplantation surgeons recommend prophylactic cholecystectomy prior to receipt of an organ transplant.

### Nonoperative Treatment of Cholelithiasis

Medical treatment of gallstones is generally unsuccessful and is used rarely. Options include dissolution with oral bile salt therapy, contact dissolution, which requires cannulation of the gallbladder and infusion of organic solvent, and extracorporeal shock wave lithotripsy. With the dissolution strategies, unacceptable recurrence rates of up to 50% limit their application to the most select group of patients. Extracorporeal shock wave lithotripsy has a lower recurrence rate, approximately 20%, and can be used in patients with single stones 0.5 to 2 cm in size. The widespread use, safety, and efficacy of laparoscopic cholecystectomy have relegated nonoperative therapy to patients for whom general anesthesia presents a prohibitively high risk.

## Chronic Cholecystitis

Recurrent attacks of biliary colic, which only temporarily occlude the cystic duct and do not cause acute cholecystitis, can cause some inflammation and scarring of the neck of the gallbladder and cystic duct. This process, called *chronic cholecystitis,* causes fibrosis as histologic evidence of repeated self-limited episodes of inflammation. The diagnosis of chronic cholecystitis lies along a continuum with biliary colic because it is results from recurrent attacks. Therefore, the presentation is that of symptomatic cholelithiasis, or biliary colic. Pain occurring after ingestion of a fatty meal, with the attendant increase in CCK secretion in response to duodenal intraluminal fat, is classic for biliary colic, although only 50% of patients will report an association with food. Pain from stones tends to locate in the epigastrium or right upper quadrant and may radiate around to the scapula. These attacks of pain generally last a few hours. Pain lasting longer than 24 hours or when associated with fever suggests acute cholecystitis. The pain of biliary colic, even in the absence of cholecystitis, may also cause other gastrointestinal symptoms such as bloating, nausea, or even vomiting.

Symptomatic stones constitute a different risk profile than the routine patient with asymptomatic stones, with a higher likelihood of complications from stones. Therefore, symptomatic cholelithiasis is an indication for cholecystectomy. To perform a cholecystectomy for symptomatic stones, one needs presence of symptoms and documentation of stones.

### Diagnosis

The diagnosis of symptomatic cholelithiasis, the clinical manifestation of chronic cholecystitis, relies on a history consistent with biliary tract disease. Transabdominal ultrasonography reliably documents the presence of cholelithiasis. Ultrasound can provide other important information, such as common bile duct dilation, gallbladder polyps, porcelain gallbladder, or evidence of hepatic parenchymal processes. Cholesterolosis, or the accumulation of cholesterol found in gallbladder mucosal macrophages, can also be seen (Fig. 55-22). Even in the absence of frank stones, so-called *sludge* found in the gallbladder on ultrasonography, with appropriate symptoms, is consistent with biliary colic.

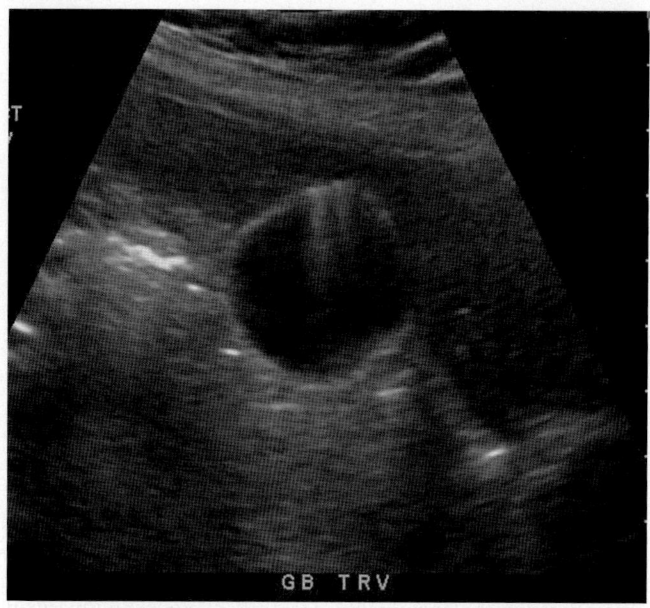


**FIGURE 55-22** Ultrasound of cholesterolosis.

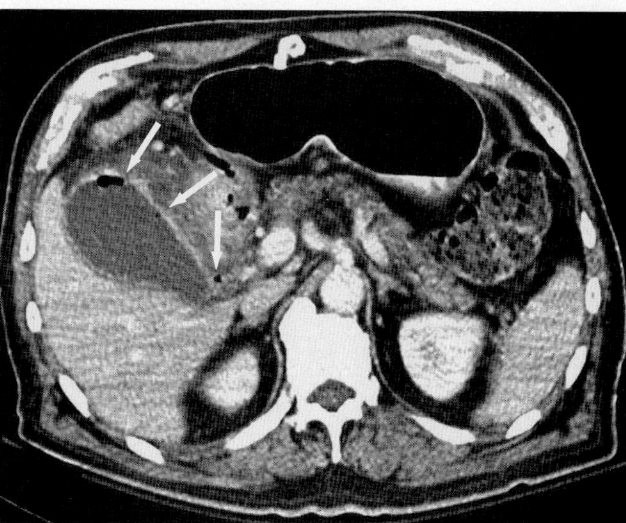

**FIGURE 55-23** CT scan of emphysematous cholecystitis. Significant pericholecystic inflammatory changes and air in the gallbladder wall *(arrows)* are signs of emphysematous cholecystitis.

### Treatment

Patients with sufficient symptoms from gallstones should undergo elective cholecystectomy. Cholecystectomy carries a low-risk profile but is not without complications, so an analysis of risks and benefits is important. Because patients with very mild symptoms have a low rate of complications from gallstones (1% to 3%/year), observation and dietary and lifestyle changes are appropriate in this population. Patients with more severe or recurrent symptoms have a higher rate of complications of the disease (7%/year), so elective laparoscopic cholecystectomy is warranted. In more than 90% of patients, cholecystectomy is curative, leaving them symptom-free.

## Acute Calculous Cholecystitis

Obstruction of the cystic duct from stone impaction eventually causes acute calculous cholecystitis. Temporary impaction, as seen with biliary colic, does not create inflammation as the obstruction resolves. If it does not resolve, however, inflammation ensues, with edema and subserosal hemorrhage, a process known as acute cholecystitis. Infection of the stagnant pool of bile is a secondary phenomenon; the primary pathophysiology is unresolved cystic duct obstruction. Without resolution of the obstruction, the gallbladder will progress to ischemia and necrosis. Eventually, acute cholecystitis becomes acute gangrenous cholecystitis and, when complicated by infection with a gas-forming organism, acute emphysematous cholecystitis (Fig. 55-23).

### Presentation

The inflammatory changes in the gallbladder wall manifest as fever, right upper quadrant pain, tenderness to palpation, and guarding in the right upper quadrant. This process will cause an arrest of inspiration with gentle pressure under the right costal margin, a finding known as Murphy's sign. Tenderness and a positive Murphy's sign help distinguish acute cholecystitis from biliary colic, in which there is no inflammatory process. Given that the common bile duct is not obstructed, profound jaundice in the setting of a picture of acute cholecystitis is rare and should raise the suspicion of cholangitis, with obstruction of the common bile duct, or Mirizzi syndrome, in which inflammation or a stone in the gallbladder neck leads to inflammation of the adjoining biliary system, with obstruction of the common hepatic duct. Mild elevations of alkaline phosphatase, bilirubin, and transaminase levels and a leukocytosis support the diagnosis of acute cholecystitis.

### Diagnosis

Transabdominal ultrasonography is a sensitive, inexpensive, and reliable tool for the diagnosis of acute cholecystitis, with a sensitivity of 85% and specificity of 95%. In addition to identifying gallstones, ultrasound can demonstrate pericholecystic fluid, gallbladder wall thickening, and even a sonographic Murphy's sign, documenting tenderness specifically over the gallbladder (Fig. 55-24). In most cases, an accurate history and physical examination, along with supporting laboratory studies and an ultrasound, make the diagnosis of acute cholecystitis. In atypical cases, a HIDA scan may be used to demonstrate obstruction of the cystic duct, which definitively diagnoses acute cholecystitis. Filling of the gallbladder during a HIDA scan essentially eliminates the diagnosis of cholecystitis. CT may show similar findings to ultrasound with pericholecystic fluid, gallbladder wall thickening, and emphysematous changes, but CT is less sensitive than ultrasound for the diagnosis of acute cholecystitis.

### Treatment

Although infection is a secondary event following stasis and inflammation, most cases of acute cholecystitis are complicated by superinfection of the inflamed gallbladder. Therefore, patients are given nothing by mouth and IV fluids and parenteral antibiotics are started. Given that gram-negative aerobes are the most common organisms found in acute cholecystitis, followed by anaerobes and gram-positive aerobes, broad-spectrum antibiotics are warranted. Parenteral narcotics are usually required to control the pain.

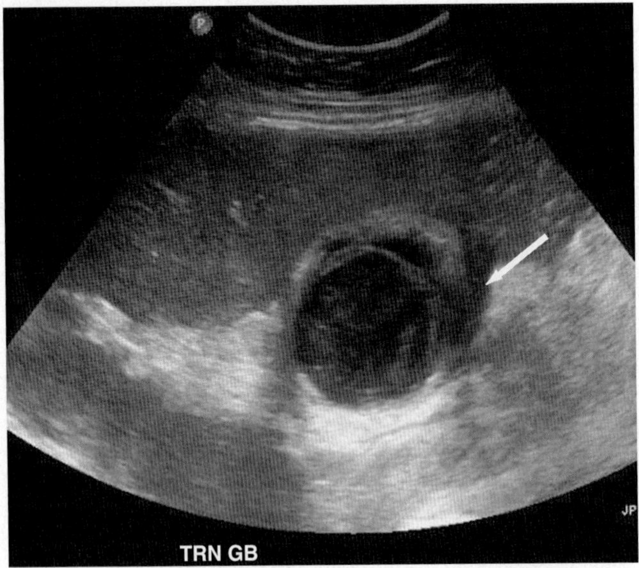


**FIGURE 55-24** Ultrasound of pericholecystic fluid. The thickened gallbladder wall with pericholecystic fluid *(arrow)* indicate acute cholecystitis.

Cholecystectomy, whether open or laparoscopic, is the treatment of choice for acute cholecystitis. The timing of operative intervention in acute cholecystitis has long been a source of debate. In the past, many surgeons advocated for delayed cholecystectomy, with patients managed nonoperatively during their initial hospitalization and discharged home with resolution of symptoms. An interval cholecystectomy was then performed at approximately 6 weeks following the initial episode. More recent studies have shown that when performed early in the disease process (within the first week), the operation can be performed laparoscopically with equivalent or improved morbidity, mortality, and length of stay, as well as a similar conversion rate to open cholecystectomy.[3] Additionally, approximately 20% of patients initially admitted for nonoperative management failed medical treatment prior to the planned interval cholecystectomy and required surgical intervention. Initial nonoperative therapy remains a viable option for patients who present in a delayed fashion and should be decided on an individual basis.

Given the inflammatory process occurring in the porta hepatis, early conversion to open cholecystectomy should be considered when delineation of anatomy is not clear or when progress cannot be made laparoscopically. With substantial inflammation, a partial cholecystectomy, transecting the gallbladder at the infundibulum with cauterization of the remaining mucosa, is acceptable to avoid injury to the common bile duct. Some patients present with acute cholecystitis but have a prohibitively high operative risk. For these patients, a percutaneously placed cholecystostomy tube should be considered. Frequently performed using ultrasound guidance under local anesthesia with some sedation, cholecystostomy can act as a temporizing measure by draining the infected bile. Percutaneous drainage allows improvement in symptoms and physiology, allowing for a delayed cholecystectomy, 3 to 6 months after medical optimization.

## Choledocholithiasis

Choledocholithiasis, or common bile duct stones, are classified by their point of origin, with primary common duct stones arising de novo in the bile duct and secondary common duct stones passing from the gallbladder into the bile duct. Primary choledocholithiasis is generally from brown pigment stones, which are a combination of precipitated bile pigments and cholesterol. Brown stones are more common in Asian populations and are associated with a bacterial infection of the bile duct. The bacteria secrete an enzyme that hydrolyzes bilirubin glucuronides to form free bilirubin, which then precipitates. Most common duct stones found in the United States are secondary, and are termed *retained common duct stones* when found within 2 years following cholecystectomy.

Many common duct stones are clinically silent and may be identified only during cholangiography, if performed routinely during cholecystectomy. Without pain or an abnormal liver function panel, a setting in which selective cholangiography is not performed, 1% to 2% of patients following cholecystectomy will present with a retained stone. When performed routinely, intraoperative cholangiography identifies choledocholithiasis in approximately 10% of asymptomatic patients, suggesting that most choledocholithiasis remains clinically silent.[4,5]

When not clinically silent, common duct stones may present with symptoms ranging from biliary colic to the clinical manifestations of obstructive jaundice, such as darkening of the urine, scleral icterus, and lightening of the stools. Jaundice with choledocholithiasis is more likely to be painful because the onset of obstruction is acute, causing rapid distention of the bile duct and activation of pain fibers. Fever, a common symptom, can be associated with right upper quadrant pain and jaundice, a constellation known as Charcot's triad. This triad suggests ascending cholangitis and, if untreated, may progress to septic shock. The addition of hypotension and mental status changes, both evidence of shock, to Charcot's triad is known as Reynolds pentad.

### Diagnosis

In the setting of choledocholithiasis, abnormalities of the hepatic function panel are common but neither sensitive nor specific and, with superinfection, leukocytosis may also be present. Ultrasound may show choledocholithiasis or only biliary ductal dilation. In patients with biliary pain, gallstones and jaundice, a dilated bile duct (>8 mm) is highly suggestive of choledocholithiasis, even if common duct stones are not documented ultrasonographically. Even without symptoms of biliary colic, a dilated bile duct in the presence of gallstones suggests choledocholithiasis.

ERCP is highly sensitive and specific for choledocholithiasis (Fig. 55-25) and can usually be therapeutic by clearing the duct of all stones in approximately 75% of patients during the first procedure and approximately 90% with repeat ERCP. During the endoscopic procedure, a sphincterotomy is performed with a balloon sweep and extraction of the stone, all of which have a complication rate of 5% to 8%. Indications for preoperative ERCP prior to cholecystectomy include cholangitis, biliary pancreatitis, limited surgeon experience with common duct exploration, and patients with multiple comorbidities.

Alternatively, magnetic resonance cholangiopancreatography (MRCP) is highly sensitive (>90%) with an almost 100%

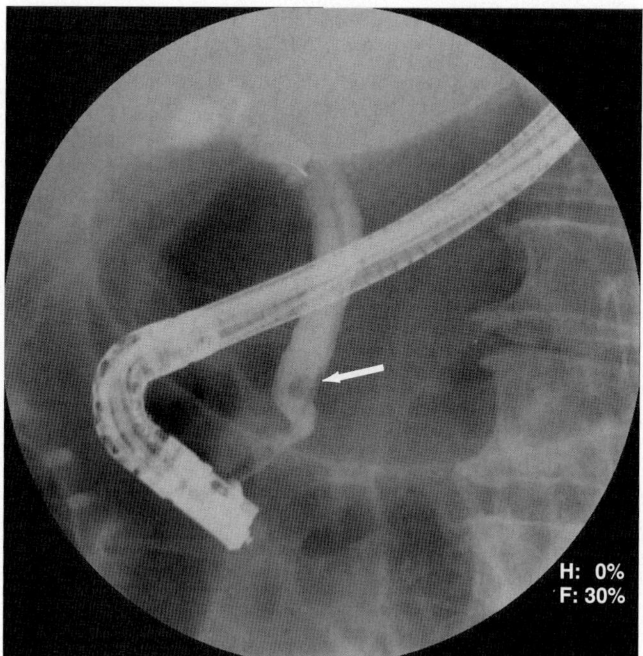


**FIGURE 55-25** ERCP with choledocholithiasis. With retrograde contrast injection, a filling defect noted within the lumen of the common bile duct *(arrow)* identifies choledocholithiasis. ERCP can also be used to remove the stone via sphincterotomy and balloons or baskets.

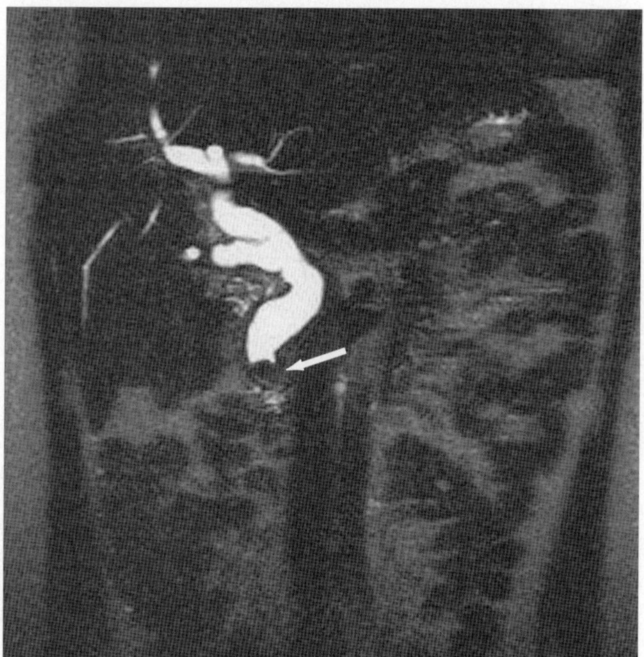

**FIGURE 55-26** MRCP with choledocholithiasis. The dilated common bile duct ends abruptly, with a convex intraluminal filling defect *(arrow)* consistent with choledocholithiasis.

specificity for the diagnosis of common duct stones (Fig. 55-26). As a noninvasive test, MRCP provides accurate imaging of the biliary tree but, in the setting of choledocholithiasis, does not provide a therapeutic solution. A clear cholangiogram by MRCP eliminates the need for ERCP. However, choledocholithiasis identified by MRCP requires intervention by some other method. With more surgeons becoming adept at laparoscopic common duct exploration, the inability of MRCP to remove common duct stones may prove less clinically relevant.

PTC can also be used to diagnose and treat choledocholithiasis. PTC is an invasive test with a complication rate similar to ERCP. Although requiring less skill, and at a lower cost, PTC is as effective in patients with a dilated biliary ductal system but less effective in the setting of a nondilated biliary tree.

Ultrasound should be used routinely for evaluation of the gallbladder and biliary tree, but the remaining studies should be chosen selectively based on the likelihood of finding common duct stones. Patients with highest risk, such as those with cholangitis or a dilated biliary tree, should undergo ERCP. Those with lower risk can undergo laparoscopic cholecystectomy with cholangiography, and possible laparoscopic common duct exploration, or MRCP, depending on the surgeon's expertise. Generally, choledocholithiasis identified but not removed during cholecystectomy mandates an ERCP for stone extraction.

### Treatment

**Endoscopic Retrograde Cholangiopancreatography** Endoscopic sphincterotomy with stone extraction is effective for the treatment of choledocholithiasis. When used in the preoperative setting, it can avoid an open procedure and, when unsuccessful at removing stones, will alter intraoperative decision making. Common reasons for endoscopic failure include large stones, intrahepatic stones, multiple stones, altered gastric or duodenal anatomy, impacted stones, and duodenal diverticula. Sphincterotomy with stone extraction does not eliminate the risk of recurrent biliary stone disease. When managed by ERCP and sphincterotomy, almost 50% of all patients have recurrent symptoms of biliary tract disease if not also treated by cholecystectomy.[6] More than one third of these patients eventually require cholecystectomy, suggesting that cholecystectomy should be offered to patients who present with choledocholithiasis. Interestingly, older patients (>70 years), have only a 15% rate of symptom recurrence, so cholecystectomy can be offered selectively to this patient population.

**Laparoscopic Common Bile Duct Exploration** At the time of cholecystectomy, an intraoperative cholangiogram will help identify choledocholithiasis. A laparoscopic common duct exploration can then be performed in an attempt to manage all calculous biliary tract disease in one setting, without the need for an additional anesthetic or procedure. Access to the common duct with a small-caliber cholangioscope is provided via the cystic duct or through a separate incision in the common duct itself. In the transcystic approach, the cystic duct is dilated and a flexible cholangioscope is passed down into the common bile duct. For the transcystic approach in the setting of a narrow cystic duct, the duct can be dilated with a flexible dilator passed over a wire, using a Seldinger technique. Given the angle of insertion of the cystic duct into the common bile duct, stones in the common hepatic duct above the cystic duct insertion are not accessible through the transcystic route. Other contraindications for the transcystic approach include a small, friable cystic duct, numerous (more than eight) stones in the common bile duct, and large stones (>1 cm), which would be difficult or impossible to extract through the cystic duct orifice. In any of these settings, a separate incision can be made in the common bile duct, with the only contraindication being that of a small common duct that may become strictured on closure.

**Open Common Bile Duct Exploration** With greater use of endoscopic and laparoscopic methods, the frequency of open common duct exploration has decreased. Open exploration should be used when endoscopic and laparoscopic means are not feasible for documented common duct stones, or when concomitant biliary drainage is required. Open exploration carries a low morbidity (8% to 15%) and mortality (1% to 2%), with a low rate of retained stones (5%). Impacted stones at the ampulla present a difficult problem for ERCP and common duct exploration. With unsuccessful attempts to remove an impacted stone in the setting of a nondilated biliary tree, a transduodenal sphincteroplasty can provide drainage. In a similar setting, but with a dilated biliary tree, drainage of the biliary tree through a separate choledochoenterostomy can be successful. The two options for drainage are that of a choledochoduodenostomy and Roux-en-Y choledochojejunostomy. Anastomosis to the duodenum can be performed rapidly with a single anastomosis (Fig. 55-27). This anatomic arrangement continues to allow endoscopic access to the entire biliary tree. The downside of this approach is that the bile duct distal to the anastomosis does not drain well and may collect debris that obstructs the anastomosis or the pancreatic duct, a process known as sump syndrome. Anastomosis to the jejunum in a Roux-en-Y arrangement provides excellent drainage of the biliary tree without a risk of sump syndrome, but does not allow future endoscopic evaluation of the biliary tree.

Intrahepatic stones, which are almost uniformly brown pigment stones, represent a different management challenge than secondary bile duct stones. Relatively uncommon in Western compared with Asian populations, these stones tend to occur specifically in patients with stasis of the biliary tree, such as those with strictures, parasites, choledochal cysts, or sclerosing cholangitis. Because these stones collect at sites above obstructions, the transhepatic approach to cholangiography is generally more successful. Percutaneous drainage catheters are left in place and upsized to perform percutaneous stone extraction. Long-term management of intrahepatic stones must be carefully tailored to the disease but frequently requires hepaticojejunostomy

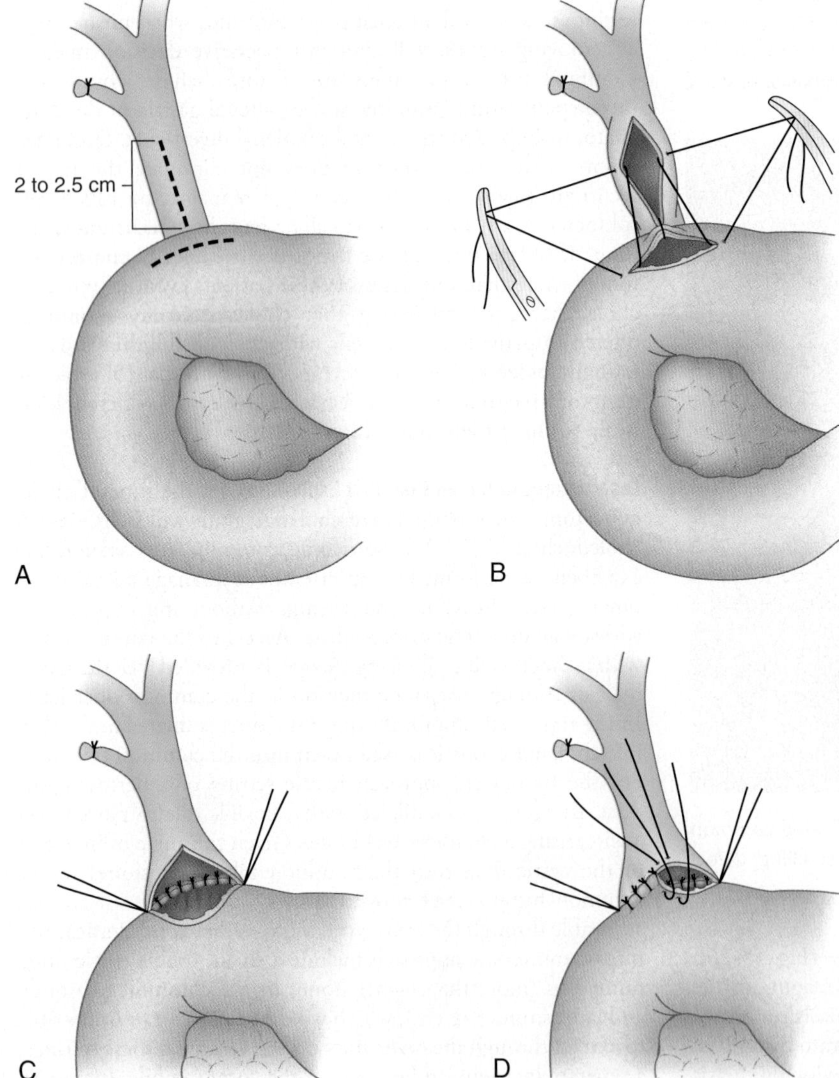


**FIGURE 55-27** Choledochoduodenostomy. In the setting of a dilated common bile duct with inability to clear all the stones from the distal duct, an anastomosis can be performed between the common bile duct and adjacent duodenum. Although maintaining the possibility of future endoscopic therapy, this arrangement risks sump syndrome in the undrained distal duct.

for better biliary drainage. Liberal use of choledochoscopy at the time of drainage procedure ensures removal of all current stones. This approach allows a stone clearance rate of more than 90%.

## Gallstone Pancreatitis

Pancreatitis can occur from the passage of a gallstone through the sphincter of Oddi and temporary blockage of the pancreatic exocrine secretions. A generally accepted pathophysiology involves temporary elevation of pancreatic ductal pressures causing a secondary inflammation of the pancreatic parenchyma. As opposed to the gallbladder, in which relief of the obstruction is accompanied by pain resolution, the symptoms in pancreatitis continue in spite of passage of the stone. With the diagnosis of pancreatitis in which the cause is unclear, ultrasound will help identify gallstones and may show choledocholithiasis or a dilated bile duct. Usually, the offending stone passes spontaneously but may still cause severe pancreatitis. In most cases of gallstone pancreatitis, the pathophysiology of pancreatitis is self-limited. If, by clinical assessment, the pancreatitis is severe, early ERCP to remove a stone that may not have passed is indicated and has been shown to reduce the morbidity of the episode of pancreatitis.[7] To prevent a future episode of gallstone pancreatitis, a laparoscopic cholecystectomy is warranted; this is generally recommended during the same hospitalization, just prior to discharge. Given the suspicion of choledocholithiasis, an intraoperative cholangiogram should be performed if the duct has not been previously cleared of stones by ERCP.

## Biliary Dyskinesia

Patients may present with classic symptoms of calculous biliary disease but have no ultrasonographic evidence of stones or sludge. In some of these cases, the dysfunction of the gallbladder creates pain, even in the absence of stones. These patients will have other diagnoses excluded by CT and upper endoscopy, and should undergo a CCK-stimulated HIDA scan, in which the radiolabeled iminodiacetic acid will collect in the gallbladder. The patient is given an IV dose of CCK and the percentage ejection of the gallbladder in response to CCK calculated. An ejection fraction less than one third at 20 minutes following CCK administration in patients without stones is considered diagnostic of dyskinesia, and should be managed with cholecystectomy. The symptoms of dyskinesia are fairly responsive to cholecystectomy, with more than 85% of patients showing improvement or resolution. In nonresponders, an ERCP with sphincterotomy may prove useful.

## Sphincter of Oddi Dysfunction

Sphincter of Oddi dysfunction, which manifests as biliary tract pain, with normal liver function tests and recurrent pancreatitis, may be caused by a structurally abnormal sphincter or histologically normal but functionally abnormal one. With injury to the sphincter from trauma, pancreatitis, gallstone passage, or congenital anomalies, inflammation and subsequent fibrosis lead to elevated sphincter pressure. Alternatively, patients may have elevated sphincter pressure in the absence of fibrosis, suggesting a spasm of the muscular component. This subset of patients may have evidence of altered motility elsewhere in the gastrointestinal tract. The diagnosis of sphincter of Oddi dysfunction should be suspected in patients with biliary pain and a common duct diameter more than 12 mm. The bile duct in these patients tends to increase in diameter in response to CCK, as does the pancreatic duct following secretin administration. Manometry has also been used to make the diagnosis, with sphincter pressure higher than 40 mm Hg predicting good response to therapy. Therapy consists of endoscopic sphincterotomy or transduodenal sphincteroplasty, with approximately equivalent results from the two approaches. In patients with objective evidence of sphincter of Oddi dysfunction, division of the sphincter will improve or resolve the pain in 60% to 80% of patients.

# Surgery for Calculous Biliary Disease

### Laparoscopic Cholecystectomy

Following the advent of laparoscopic surgery, with its accompanying smaller incisions, less pain, and shorter hospitalization, surgeons have performed an increasing number of laparoscopic cholecystectomies. Most cholecystectomies are performed for biliary colic, but the operation can be performed safely in the setting of acute inflammation. Acute cholecystitis carries longer operative times and a higher conversion rate to the open procedure than when laparoscopic cholecystectomy is performed in the elective setting. General anesthesia with muscle relaxation is required when performing a laparoscopic cholecystectomy,. Therefore, one contraindication to the procedure is the inability to tolerate general anesthesia. Others include end-stage liver disease with portal hypertension, precluding safe portal dissection, and coagulopathy. Because most pneumoperitoneum laparoscopy is performed using $CO_2$ and has a number of adverse physiologic effects, severe chronic obstructive pulmonary disease, with poor ability for gas exchange, and congestive heart failure are considered relative contraindications.

Patient preparation, induction of anesthesia, and sterile draping are performed as for an open cholecystectomy. Although use of a urinary catheter depends on the clinical setting, an orogastric tube is standard to decompress the stomach and help with exposure of the upper abdomen. Access to the peritoneal cavity and creation of pneumoperitoneum can be performed by the open or closed technique according to the expertise and discretion of the surgeon. The open technique involves making a small incision at the umbilicus, cutting down through the fascia of the abdominal wall, incising the peritoneum directly, and inserting a blunt trocar, known as a Hasson cannula. Alternatively, in the closed technique, an incision is made and a needle inserted into the peritoneal cavity to insufflate the abdomen prior to the placement of any trocars. Following the establishment of a $CO_2$ pneumoperitoneum, a brief exploration is performed and additional 5-mm ports are placed in the right anterior axillary line, right midclavicular line, and subxiphoid location (Fig. 55-28). The lateral port at the anterior axillary line is used to elevate the fundus of the gallbladder toward the right shoulder. This retraction provides exposure to the infundibulum and porta hepatis. The midclavicular trocar is used to grasp the gallbladder infundibulum, retracting it inferolaterally to open the triangle of Calot (Figs. 55-29 and 55-30). By distracting Hartmann's pouch laterally, the cystic duct no longer lies almost parallel to the common hepatic duct.

The dissection is then carried along the infundibulum on the anterior and posterior surfaces to expose the base of the gallbladder. This dissection will eventually clear all fibrofatty tissue from the triangle of Calot. Inferolateral traction of the infundibulum then allows documentation of two structures entering the gallbladder, the cystic duct and cystic artery. A

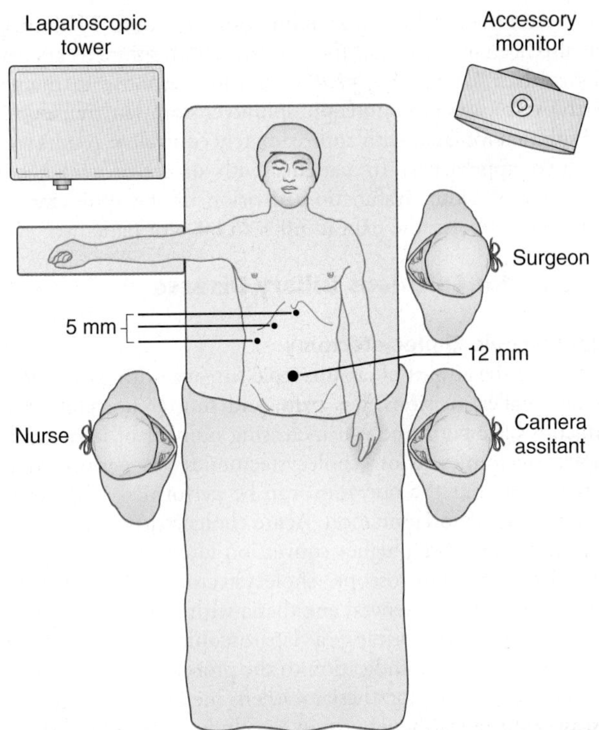


**FIGURE 55-28** Laparoscopic cholecystectomy ports. The assistant uses the periumbilical port to provide access for the camera and the most lateral port to elevate the fundus and expose the neck. The surgeon can then provide inferolateral traction on the infundibulum and open the critical view of safety.

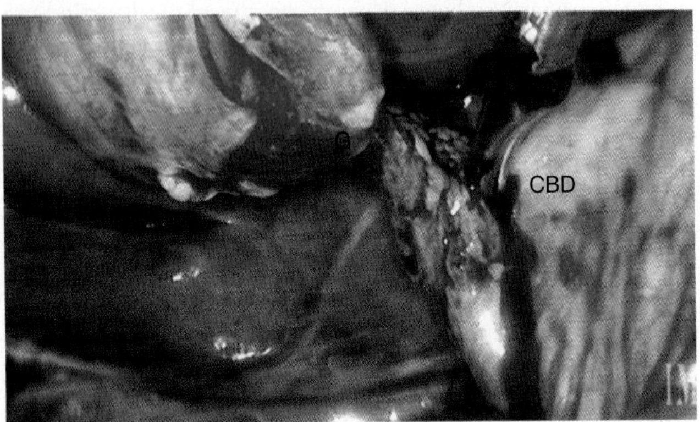


**FIGURE 55-29** Laparoscopic view of the porta and gallbladder infundibulum, without inferolateral traction on the infundibulum. Note that the gallbladder infundibulum (G) lies immediately adjacent to the CBD.

useful landmark for the cystic artery is the overlying lymph node, known as Calot's node. The view of the liver bed through the space between cystic duct and cystic artery and above the cystic artery is known as the critical view of safety, and minimizes the risk of inadvertent iatrogenic bile duct injury (Fig. 55-31).[8] With sufficient dissection, clips are placed on the cystic artery and cystic duct. If a cholangiography is performed, the cystic duct is only clipped adjacent to the gallbladder and the cystic duct incised, although not transected. A cholangiographic

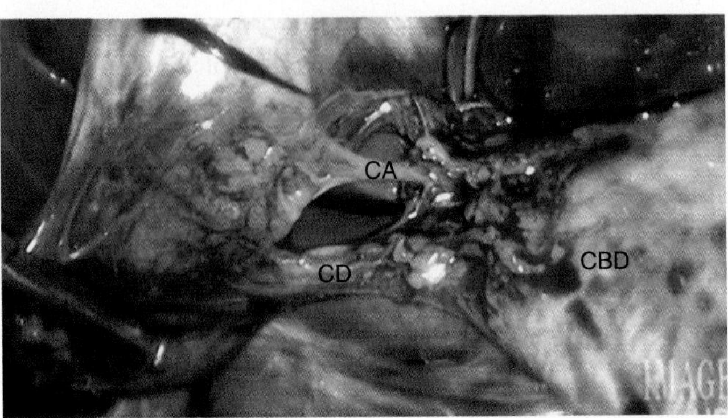


**FIGURE 55-30** Laparoscopic view of the same patient as in Figure 55-29, but with inferolateral traction on the infundibulum. Note the angular change to the cystic duct (CD) compared with the CBD. The dissecting tool indicates the location of the right hepatic artery. The key element to this view in minimizing CBD injury is the identification of the cystic artery (CA) and duct entering the gallbladder, with the inferior aspect of segment V of the liver identified in the space on either side of the artery and duct.

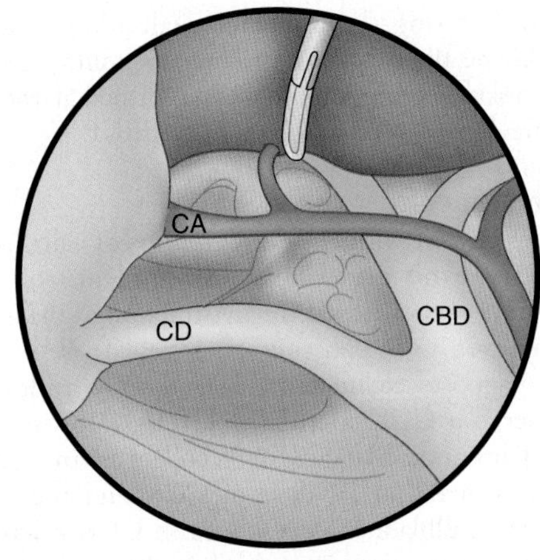


**FIGURE 55-31** An artist's representation of Figure 55-30, showing hidden anatomy.

catheter is then fed through the incised duct and fluoroscopic images obtained with injection of contrast into the cystic duct and biliary tree. On obtaining a normal cholangiogram or when cholangiography is not performed, the cystic duct is doubly clipped on the common duct side and transected. The previously clipped artery is also transected and the gallbladder dissected off the liver bed using electrocautery. Because the venous drainage of the gallbladder is directly into the liver bed through venules, excellent hemostasis must be achieved during this dissection. The cystic duct and cystic artery clips are inspected just prior to completion of the dissection of the fundic attachments, because the superior traction of the fundus has provided exposure to the porta and triangle of Calot. The gallbladder is then brought out of the abdominal cavity through the umbilical port. In the setting of acute cholecystitis, or if during dissection the gallbladder was entered, a plastic bag should be used for retrieval. Any stones that are spilled during a cholecystectomy should also be retrieved.

Opinion is sharply divided regarding the performance of selective versus routine cholangiography, with supportive data for each approach. Routine cholangiography will identify unsuspected stones in less than 10% of patients and the natural history of these asymptomatic stones suggests that they will remain asymptomatic. Iatrogenic bile duct injury occurs less often when cholangiography is performed routinely.[9,10] However, even when performed routinely, cholangiograms are frequently misinterpreted and thus do not adequately prevent an injury.[11] In many cases of laparoscopic cholecystectomy performed for biliary colic, a cholangiogram will not alter management. Also, it increases the operative time and adds fluoroscopic exposure. Indications for cholangiography in the selective setting include unexplained pain at the time of cholecystectomy, any suspicion of current or previous choledocholithiasis without preoperative duct clearance, any question of anatomic delineation during cholecystectomy, elevated preoperative liver enzyme levels, dilated common bile duct in preoperative imaging, and suspicion of intraoperative biliary injury. Although just as accurate as cholangiography for the identification of choledocholithiasis, laparoscopic ultrasonography is highly operator-dependent, requires additional instrumentation, and is not widely available.

### Open Cholecystectomy

As laparoscopic cholecystectomy has become the procedure of choice for the treatment of most gallbladder disease, experience with open cholecystectomy has drastically declined. Open cholecystectomy is generally performed following conversion from the laparoscopic approach or as a step during another operation, such as a pancreaticoduodenectomy. The open cholecystectomy can be performed through a midline or right subcostal incision. Retraction of segment IV provides exposure of the cystic duct and artery. With similar inferolateral traction to the gallbladder infundibulum, the cystic duct is taken out of alignment from the common duct for its identification and division. Early identification and ligation of the cystic artery limits the blood loss during the procedure, but may prove difficult because of inflammation. Another approach to the gallbladder infundibulum involves dissecting the fundus off the liver in a dome- down approach. Here, the attachments of the gallbladder are divided, allowing inferolateral traction of the entire gallbladder to open the triangle of Calot and identify the appropriate duct and artery. When performed for severe cholecystitis, the dissection of the gallbladder of the liver bed may be associated with substantial blood loss, but with removal of the infected gallbladder and packing of the area, the bleeding is usually well controlled.

### Laparoscopic Common Bile Duct Exploration

Given the risk of ascending cholangitis, gallstone pancreatitis, or cystic duct stump leak, all attempts must be made to remove known bile duct stones. Many factors are relevant to the decision regarding which approach to duct clearance should be used. The experience of the surgeon and/or endoscopist is important in determining if operative clearance or postoperative ERCP will be most effective, with lowest morbidity. Anatomic aspects such as duct size and stone size and number should be considered. As experience with laparoscopic surgery has grown, laparoscopic approaches to the bile duct clearance have become more prevalent. With a common bile duct stone identified fluoroscopically, the common duct can be irrigated and glucagon is given to relax the sphincter of Oddi. If this technique fails to flush the stone, a balloon catheter or wire basket can be passed under fluoroscopic guidance to attempt stone extraction. If still unsuccessful, flexible choledochoscopy is indicated. The two common laparoscopic approaches to explore the common bile duct for stone removal include the transcystic approach and via choledochotomy. In the transcystic approach, at the completion of the cholangiography, a wire is fed down the cystic duct into the common bile duct. Through a Seldinger technique or use of a balloon catheter, the cystic duct is gently dilated to allow passage of a flexible choledochoscope. Alternatively, a flexible ureteroscope can be used. To pass the fiberoptic scope through the duct system, a water irrigation system is attached and allowed to constantly infuse out the end of the scope. If available, the choledochoscopic image is projected onto a corner of the laparoscopic screen. With the surgeon feeding the choledochoscope into the cystic duct and the assistant adjusting the tip of the choledochoscope, keeping the lumen in the screen, the flexible choledochoscope is advanced to the distal bile duct. With identification of the offending stone, a wire basket is passed to ensnare the stone, withdrawing it and the choledochoscope together.

In the laparoscopic choledochotomy approach, a longitudinal incision is made in the common bile duct (i.e., below the cystic duct). To expose the CBD, two stay sutures are placed on either side of the planned choledochotomy (Fig. 55-32). The size of the incision should be at least as large as the diameter of the largest stone. The choledochoscope can then be fed down

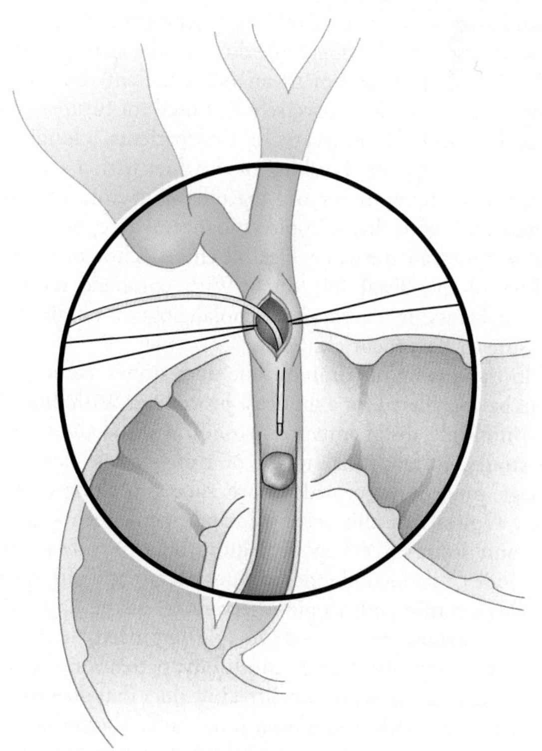

**FIGURE 55-32** Laparoscopic choledochotomy for common bile duct exploration.

into the distal bile duct and stone extraction performed as described earlier. At the completion of the exploration, a T tube should be placed via the choledochotomy and the bile duct closed using 4-0 absorbable sutures. Completion cholangiography via the T tube documents stone removal.

In addition to being technically easier, because it does not require fine laparoscopic suturing, the transcystic approach avoids a T tube. Contraindications to the transcystic approach include numerous (more than eight) stones, a stone larger than 1 cm, intrahepatic stones, and a cystic duct that does not allow dilation and choledochoscope passage. Given the need for suture closure of the incision in the bile duct, the only contraindication to the choledochotomy approach is that of a small-caliber bile duct (<6 mm), which could be strictured by closure. Both approaches are successful at stone removal, with most studies showing a 75% to 95% rate of stone clearance. This is comparable to that of laparoscopic cholecystectomy followed by postoperative ERCP, with the only difference being a shorter hospitalization and lower physician fees for patients undergoing common duct exploration, as the cholecystectomy and clearance of stones are performed in one setting by a single physician.[12]

### Open Common Bile Duct Exploration

With advanced laparoscopic, endoscopic, and percutaneous techniques, the use of open exploration of the bile duct has become less common. When open surgery is otherwise required, or previous surgery such as gastric bypass make other techniques unsuccessful, clearance of choledocholithiasis must be performed by the open approach. The exposure to the bile duct is through a midline or right upper quadrant incision. A Kocher maneuver must be performed to expose the distal bile duct. Gentle palpation of the distal bile duct will frequently find the offending stone, which may be milked backward. As in the laparoscopic approach, stay sutures are placed and a choledochotomy is performed in the supraduodenal bile duct. In the setting of dilated ducts with multiple stones in an older patient, the choledochotomy can be made transversely and used for future choledochoduodenostomy, if necessary. In most patients, a longitudinal incision is appropriate. Flushing of the duct with a soft rubber catheter will frequently remove the offending stone(s). Balloon catheters and, with fluoroscopic guidance, wire baskets may be useful to withdraw the stone. Flexible choledochoscopes are used to visualize the distal bile duct. With complete removal of stones, a T tube is placed and a cholangiogram obtained prior to closure to document clearance.

In the setting of common bile duct stones, some patients should be considered for a drainage procedure. With dilated bile ducts, multiple distal impacted stones, a distal duct stricture with stones, intrahepatic stones, or primary bile duct stones, drainage procedures provide more successful long-term outcomes. Options in this setting include choledochoduodenostomy and Roux-en-Y hepaticojejunostomy. A side-to-side or end-to side choledochoduodenostomy is a fast and safe approach that allows future endoscopic intervention of the upper biliary tree, if necessary. In the side-to-side approach, however, by leaving the distal bile duct in continuity, patients are at risk for sump syndrome, in which the distal bile duct that does not drain well may collect debris and even food stuffs. Occlusions of the ampulla, with subsequent pancreatitis, or anastomosis with cholangitis have been reported. An alternative to duodenostomy is that of a Roux-en-Y choledochojejunostomy. By using a 60-cm limb of jejunum for drainage, occlusion of the anastomosis by food debris is rare but endoscopic treatment of the hepatic duct is impossible.

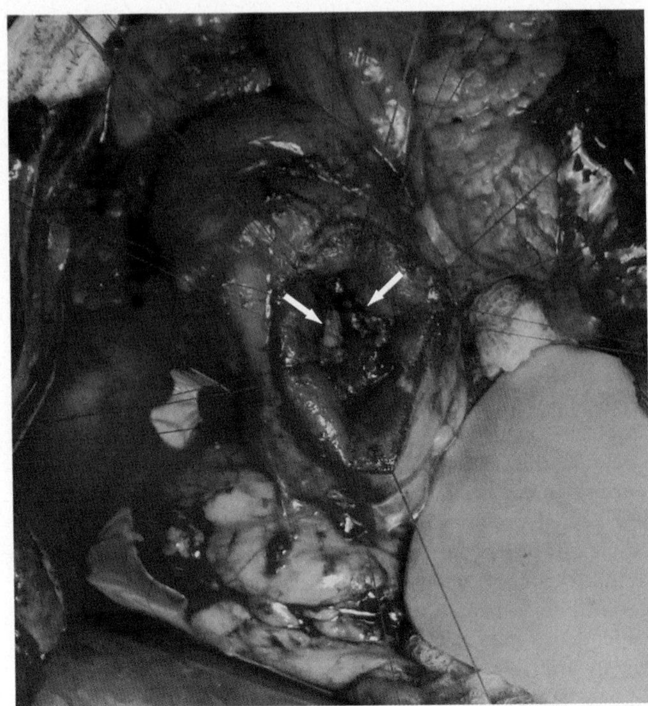

**FIGURE 55-33** Transduodenal sphincteroplasty. Note the generous opening of the distal common duct with sequential duct to mucosa approximation *(arrows).*

Impacted stones at the ampulla that cannot be removed via choledochotomy or several stones in a nondilated tree can be addressed by a transduodenal sphincteroplasty (Figs. 55-33 and 55-34). Having completed the Kocher maneuver, a longitudinal duodenotomy is made on the lateral wall. Compression of the lateral wall against the medial wall will allow palpation of the ampulla to plan placement of the duodenotomy appropriately. With identification of the ampulla, an incision is made at 11 o'clock and each wall elevated with stay sutures. The pancreatic duct usually enters at 5 o'clock on the ampulla and must be avoided. Sequential straight clamps are placed along the planned incision of the ampulla to guide visualization through hemostasis. With each step, the duodenal mucosa is sewn to the bile duct mucosa with absorbable 4-0 sutures. A 1.5-cm sphincterotomy is usually sufficient to allow stone removal and subsequent drainage. Closure of the longitudinal duodenotomy in transverse fashion avoids a future duodenal stricture.

## Postcholecystectomy Syndromes

### Bile Duct Injury

Although seen with any operation involving right upper quadrant dissection, injuries occurring during or following cholecystectomy account for more than 80% of all iatrogenic bile duct injuries. During laparoscopic or open cholecystectomy, injury to the common bile duct is an unusual but devastating complication. Inflammation in the porta, variable biliary anatomy, inappropriate exposure, aggressive attempts at hemostasis, and surgeon inexperience are commonly cited risk factors. Although

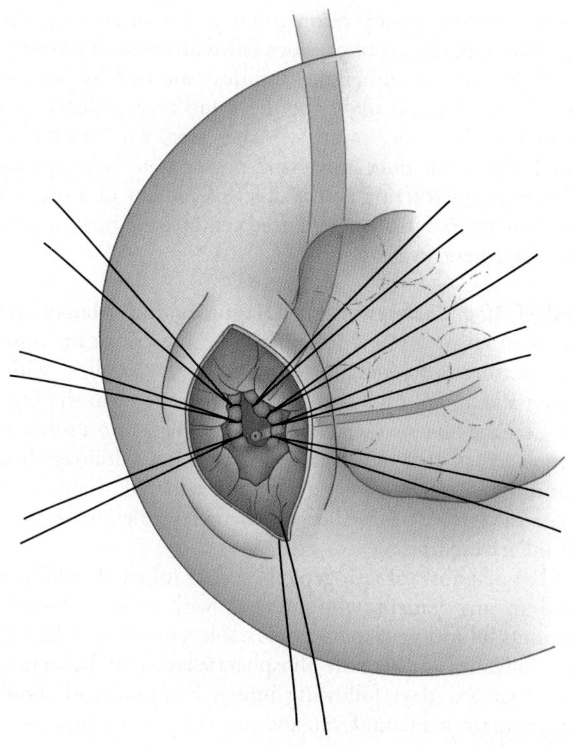

FIGURE 55-34 Transduodenal sphincteroplasty.

early reports suggested that surgical inexperience, performing less than 20 laparoscopic cholecystectomies, was highly correlated with bile duct injury, evidence has suggested that visual misperception accounts for 97% of iatrogenic biliary injuries and technical skill or knowledge accounts for only 3%.[13] With sufficient cephalad retraction of the gallbladder fundus, the cystic duct overlies the common hepatic duct, running in a parallel path. Without inferolateral traction of the gallbladder infundibulum to dissociate these structures, dissection of the apparent cystic duct may actually include the common hepatic duct, placing it in jeopardy. By retracting Hartmann's pouch inferolaterally, and opening the triangle of Calot, the cystic duct is displaced from the porta, no longer collinear with the hepatic duct. The use of a 30-degree laparoscope is useful to provide adequate visualization of the critical view of safety during laparoscopic cholecystectomy. Also, in many of these cases, a confirmation bias occurs, in which surgeons tend to rely on evidence that supports their perception while simultaneously discounting visual cues that suggest an alternative explanation. Confirmation bias helps explain why most bile duct injuries are identified in the postoperative setting, not intraoperatively.

The multifactorial nature of biliary injury highlights the concept that injury avoidance consists of many levels of protective mechanisms. Surgeon knowledge of biliary anatomy and aberrant anatomy, use of an angled laparoscope, appropriate and directed traction and countertraction on the gallbladder, sufficient suspicion of findings that discount the current perspective, and a low threshold for conversion to an open operation can help minimize the likelihood of biliary injury. Although the use of routine versus selective cholangiography is controversial, evidence has suggested that cholangiography does not completely avoid bile duct injury, but may reduce the incidence and extent of injury.[14] The original analysis of biliary reconstruction was

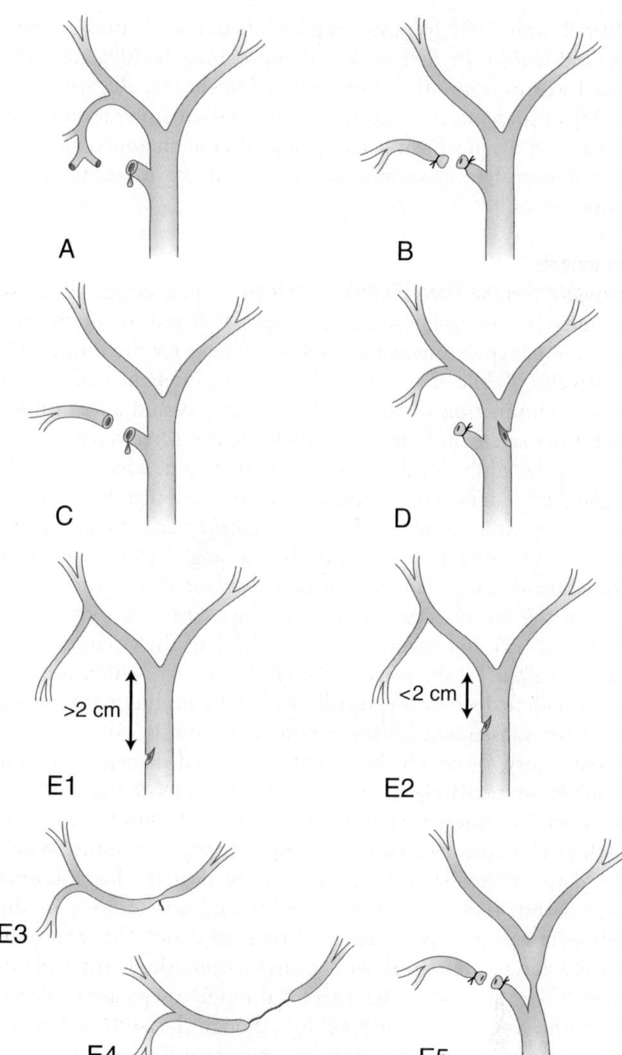


FIGURE 55-35 Strasberg classification of postoperative bile duct strictures.

based on the Bismuth classification, and has been modified by Strasberg. Classification of bile duct injuries is determined by location of injury and helps guide later surgical reconstruction (Fig. 55-35).[15] Among postoperative bile duct strictures, types E1 and E2 involve the common hepatic duct but not the bifurcation, with type E1 maintaining more than 2 cm of common hepatic duct below the bifurcation and type E2 being within 2 cm of the confluence. Type E3 strictures occur at the confluence preserving the extrahepatic ducts and, in type E4, the structuring process includes the extrahepatic biliary tree. Type E5 strictures involve aberrant right hepatic duct anatomy, with injury to the aberrant duct and common hepatic duct.

**Presentation** Bile duct injury may be identified intraoperatively but usually presents in the postoperative period. Leak of bile into the peritoneal cavity, with subsequent bile peritonitis, tends to present earlier than bile duct stricture and its associated jaundice. In the setting of bile leakage, patients may present with fever, increasing abdominal pain, jaundice, or bile leakage from an incision. Alternatively, injury to the bile duct that does not leak bile will usually present with jaundice, with or without pain.

Overall, only 10% of postoperative bile duct strictures are recognized within the first week and approximately 70% are diagnosed within 6 months of the original operation. Regardless of timing or presentation, adequate repair and subsequent outcome depend on diagnosis, sufficient delineation of anatomy, creation of a tension-free anastomosis, and liberal use of transanastomotic stents.[16,17]

#### Treatment

***Recognized at the Time of Cholecystectomy*** When suspected intraoperatively, conversion to an open operation and use of cholangiography help delineate management. Goals for the immediate treatment of bile duct injury include maintenance of ductal length, elimination of any bile leakage that would affect subsequent management, and creation of a tension-free repair.

In the adult, for ducts smaller than 3 mm, which by cholangiography drain only a single segment or subsegment of liver, simple ligation should suffice for management. Ducts larger than 3 mm usually drain more than a single segment of liver and thus, if transected, should be reimplanted into the biliary tree. If the injury occurs to a larger duct, but is not caused by electrocautery and involves less than 50% of the circumference of the wall, a T tube placed through the injury, which is effectively a choledochotomy, usually will allow healing without the need for subsequent biliary enteric anastomosis. Any cautery-based injury, in which the extent of thermal damage may not manifest immediately, or an injury involving more than 50% of the duct circumference requires resection of the injured segment with anastomosis to reestablish biliary enteric continuity. When the defect is smaller than 1 cm and not near the hepatic duct bifurcation, mobilization with end-to-end anastomosis of the bile duct can provide acceptable reconstruction. This approach should be accompanied with transanastomotic T tube placement. The tube should be inserted through a separate choledochotomy, and not exit the bile duct though the anastomosis. To ensure a tension-free anastomosis, a generous Kocher maneuver, mobilizing the duodenum and the head of the pancreas out of the retroperitoneum, is necessary.

Injuries adjacent to the bifurcation or involving more than a 1-cm defect between the ends of the bile duct require reanastomosis to the gastrointestinal tract. In this setting, the distal end is oversewn and the proximal end débrided to normal tissue. The choice of reconstruction depends on location and extent of injury, history of previous attempts at repair, and surgeon preference. Low injuries to the bile duct can be reimplanted into the duodenum, although the new choledochoduodenostomy anastomosis risks a duodenal fistula. Choledochoduodenostomy allows for endoscopic intervention if necessary, but the Roux-en-Y approach to reconstruction can be applied to injuries throughout the biliary tree. In addition, most injuries to the bile duct occur higher in the biliary tree, close to the hilum, thus not allowing for tension-free anastomosis to the duodenum. Therefore, in almost all cases of bile duct injury, a resection of the injured segment with mucosa to mucosa anastomosis using a Roux-en-Y jejunal limb is preferred. Transanastomotic stenting has been shown to improve anastomotic patency, with longer duration of stenting providing a more favorable outcome.

Because most bile duct injuries, and therefore most immediate repairs, occur at centers where biliary reconstruction is performed infrequently, most immediate repairs go unreported in the literature. However, the importance of surgical judgment and experience in biliary reconstruction cannot be overemphasized. Although reports of previous failed attempts at reconstruction have not documented injuries successfully managed immediately, they do highlight the value of experience in the treatment of bile duct injuries.[18] Therefore, when one is confronted with a bile duct injury and no surgeon with experience in biliary reconstruction is available, placement of a drain and immediate referral to an experienced center is the most appropriate management strategy.

***Identified After Cholecystectomy*** **Diagnosis and Management.** Patients suffering a bile duct injury who present in the postoperative setting are generally found to have jaundice, with an elevated alkaline phosphatase level, or leakage from the injured duct. Leakage may manifest as bilious drainage into a subhepatic drain placed at the time of operation or bilious drainage from a surgical incision. Without a site for external drainage, bile leakage can present as a biloma, whether sterile or infected, or with biliary ascites.

The diagnosis of iatrogenic bile duct injury should be suspected in any patient who presents with new or increasing symptoms following a laparoscopic cholecystectomy. Changes in serum bilirubin and alkaline phosphatase levels can be seen, even in the first few days following injury. Symptoms of shoulder pain, postprandial pain, fever, and malaise tend to improve after the first few days, because a laparoscopic cholecystectomy is generally well tolerated. Complaints that persist or increase over time should raise the suspicion of a bile duct injury.

Patients suspected of having an iatrogenic bile duct injury should undergo imaging to assess for a fluid collection and evaluate the biliary tree. Ultrasonography can achieve both these goals, but because percutaneous drainage may be required and anatomic delineation is valuable, cross-sectional imaging via CT will generally provide more useful data. Some surgeons advocate the use of radionucleotide scanning to confirm bile leakage, but with any documentation of a leak, CT will be necessary to plan management. Also, ischemia is a common cause of bile duct stricture. In the setting of a bile duct injury, 20% or more of patients will have concomitant unrecognized vascular injuries.[19]

In the delayed presentation of a bile duct injury, three major goals guide therapy (Box 55-2). First, control of infection with drainage of any fluid collections will minimize the inflammatory process. Inflammation in the porta hepatis leads to fibrosis, which only acts to increase stricture formation. Broad-spectrum antibiotics, decompression of the biliary tree,

**BOX 55-2 Goals of Therapy in Iatrogenic Bile Duct Injury**

1. Control of infection limiting inflammation
   - Parenteral antibiotics
   - Percutaneous drainage of periportal fluid collections
2. Clear and thorough delineation of entire biliary anatomy
   - MRCP/PTC
   - ERCP (especially if cystic duct stump leak suspected)
3. Re-establishment of biliary enteric continuity
   - Tension-free, mucosa-to-mucosa anastomosis
   - Roux-en-Y hepaticojejunostomy
   - Long-term transanastomotic stents if involving bifurcation or higher

and drainage, whether percutaneous or operative, of any fluid collections will achieve this goal. With control of sepsis, there is no urgency for biliary reconstruction. In fact, with time, resolution of the periportal inflammation helps with the execution of a durable reconstruction. Additionally, the retraction of an injured bile duct into the hilum of the liver, as well as inflammation in this region, make successful repair in the immediate postoperative setting unlikely. Therefore, although immediate reexploration to manage the injury as expeditiously as possible is tempting, successful-long term management of bile duct injuries identified postoperatively depends on clear and deliberate preoperative planning of the reconstruction.

A second goal of management is clear and thorough delineation of the biliary anatomy with cholangiography. Without preoperative cholangiography, any attempts at repair are unlikely to be successful. The cholangiogram must indicate the intrahepatic anatomy and bile duct bifurcation. For patients with bile duct continuity, ERCP may be possible, but PTC is generally more useful. PTC will demonstrate the intrahepatic biliary tree, identify the location of the injury, provide drainage of bile, and possibly even allow the leak to close (Fig. 55-36). Percutaneous biliary catheters can also be left in place during reconstruction to assist in dissection and provide drainage perioperatively. PTC can be combined with ERCP as necessary, depending on the site and extent of injury. Small bile leaks with bile duct continuity and cystic duct stump leaks can be successfully managed via endoscopic stenting and sphincterotomy.

The third goal of management is to reestablish durable biliary enteric drainage. Although a combination of percutaneous and endoscopic biliary dilations and stenting may establish continuity, surgical reconstruction has the highest patency rates. To achieve a successful and durable repair, the anastomosis must be performed between a minimally inflamed bile duct to intestines in a tension-free, mucosa to mucosa fashion. When the anastomosis is within 2 cm of the hepatic duct bifurcation, or involves intrahepatic ducts, long-term stenting appears to improve patency. If the bifurcation is involved, stenting of both right and left ducts should be performed. When the reconstruction involves the common bile duct or common hepatic duct more than 2 cm from the bifurcation, stenting is not necessary; therefore, a preoperatively placed transhepatic drain or intraoperatively placed T tube will provide adequate decompression in the immediate postoperative period.

At the time of operation, the adhesions of the duodenum and colon to the liver should be separated. The porta hepatis can be encircled with a Penrose drain. Although the bile duct should lie on the lateral border of the porta hepatis, the marked fibrosis and inflammatory process may make its identification difficult. Preoperatively placed percutaneous biliary drainage catheters can assist in the dissection. Also, clips placed at the previous operation may be identified. If necessary, a small-caliber needle attached to a syringe can be used to aspirate and identify the bile duct while avoiding inadvertent injury to a vascular structure (Fig. 55-37). Once identified, the distal end of the strictured segment is transected and oversewn. Once above the stricture, only a limited segment of bile duct (<5 mm) is dissected free. Any further dissection of normal duct risks vascular compromise of the segment to be used in the anastomosis. Preservation of as much normal biliary tree as possible remains a goal of the reconstruction. Next, the bile duct can be opened and the percutaneously placed catheters advanced through the incision. At this point, a wire can be used to exchange the catheters for long-term Silastic stents, if appropriate, or the catheters left in place for transanastomotic decompression. The mucosa-to-mucosa anastomosis can be created in an end-to-side fashion to the Roux-en-Y jejunal limb. In the setting of substantial inflammation at the bifurcation, another reconstruction option involves anastomosis of the Roux limb to the left hepatic duct. As noted, the left hepatic duct retains a substantial extraparenchymal length, allowing for an anastomosis in this portion of normal duct. Prior to using this section for drainage of the entire liver, cholangiography must confirm that the biliary bifurcation is widely patent,

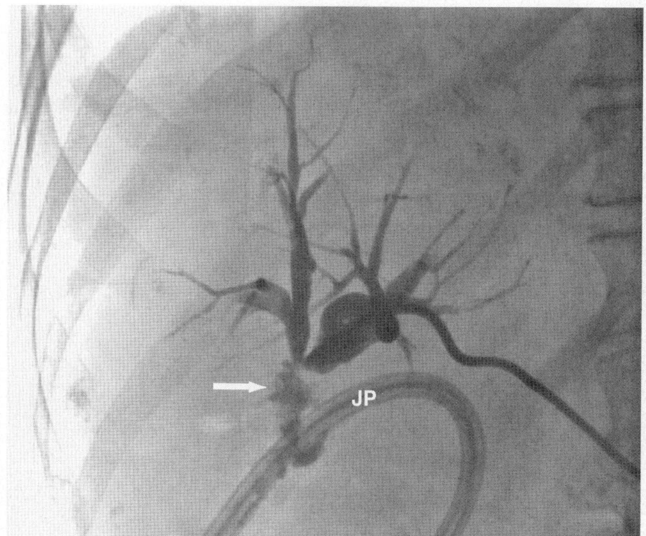


**FIGURE 55-36** Percutaneous transhepatic cholangiogram of bile duct injury. Note the contrast extravasation *(arrow)* and the Jackson-Pratt drain (JP) placed at the time of initial operation.

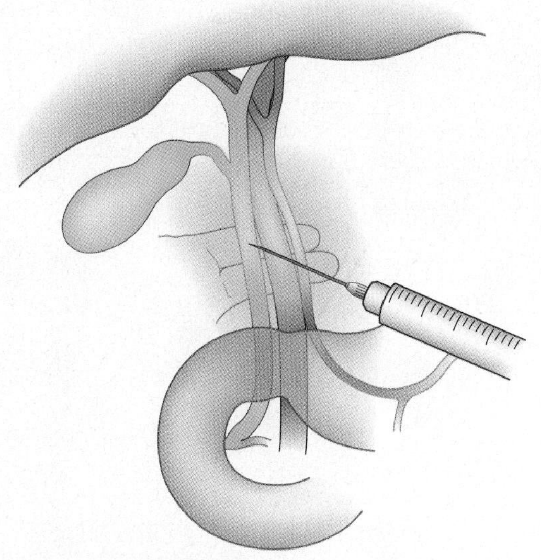

**FIGURE 55-37** Needle aspiration of porta used to identify the CBD in the setting of substantial inflammation.

thus ensuring drainage of the right lobe across the bifurcation to the left duct system.

**Interventional Radiologic and Endoscopic Techniques.** Although long-term patency rates are lower than those seen with surgical reconstruction, nonoperative techniques can be used. When the duct remains in continuity, transhepatic management of bile duct strictures can be performed using fluoroscopy, with sedation and local anesthesia. With percutaneous access to the biliary tree, a wire is used to traverse the stricture. Using balloon dilation techniques, the stricture is dilated and a catheter is left in place to decompress the system, allow healing, document resolution and, if necessary guide repeat dilations (Fig. 55-38). This approach is successful in up to 70% of patients.[20] Complications, although frequent, are generally limited, and include cholangitis, hemobilia, and bile leaks requiring repeat intervention. Endoscopic balloon dilation of bile duct strictures is generally reserved for those with primary bile duct strictures or patients who have undergone choledochoduodenostomy for reconstruction, because the Roux limb does not usually allow for endoscopic strategies. Therefore, series are limited, but results are encouraging, with 88% of patients responding to therapy and a complication rate of 8% from pancreatitis and cholangitis.

**Outcomes** Successful outcomes can be achieved in patients undergoing biliary enteric reconstruction following bile duct injury, with many series showing more than 90% of patients free of jaundice and cholangitis. High success rates are generally achieved when injuries are identified early and patients are referred immediately to experienced centers. In several studies, referral to centers performing complex biliary surgery routinely was associated with better long-term success.[21] In one study, reviewing the records of 85 patients, repair by the primary surgeon was only successful in 17% of patients and secondary repair by the primary surgeon was invariably unsuccessful. Alternatively, referral to a tertiary care biliary surgeon was associated with a success rate of 94% on the first attempt at repair. Independent factors associated with stricture recurrence include cholangitis prior to repair, primary repair within 3 weeks of the initial injury, and incomplete cholangiography. The number of attempts at repair is inversely correlated with the likelihood of a successful long-term outcome. In some studies, results were generally better if transanastomotic stents were used during reconstruction.[22] Chronic liver disease and hepatic fibrosis are associated with higher operative mortality and lower success rates.

Given variable definitions of success, and insufficient long-term follow-up, comparison of operative and nonoperative fluoroscopic and endoscopic management is difficult. Although there are no prospective randomized studies, surgical therapy generally reports longer follow-up with higher success rates, as defined by absence of symptoms, jaundice, or cholangitis. Two large retrospective reviews have been performed and both have shown higher success rates from surgical therapy, with lower morbidity and lower mortality following operative management compared with those for nonoperative strategies.

### Lost Stones

In the era of laparoscopic cholecystectomy, inadvertent opening of the gallbladder with spillage of stones is not infrequent, occurring in 20% to 40% of cholecystectomies. Risk factors for intraoperative perforation of the gallbladder include cholecystitis,

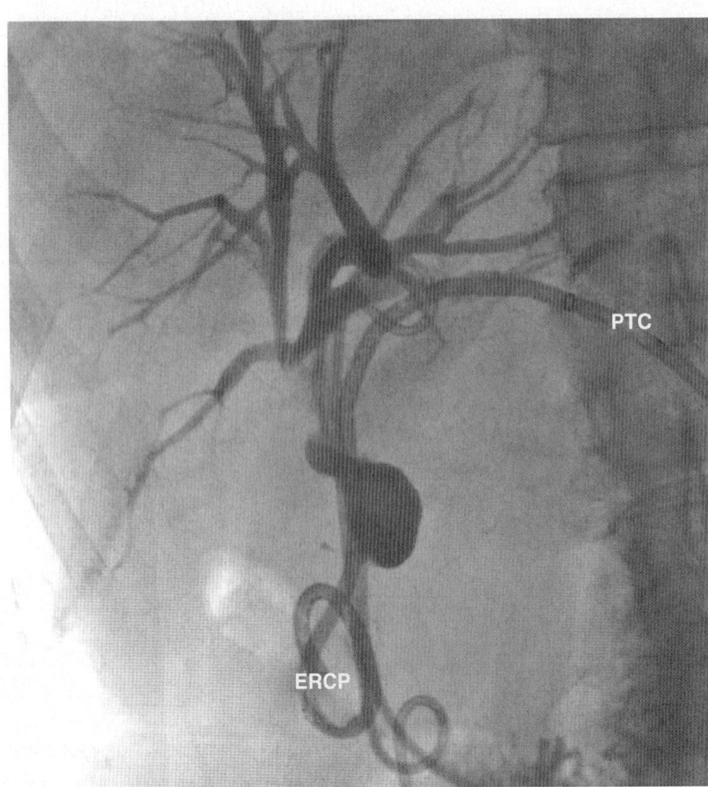


**FIGURE 55-38** PTC catheter (PTC) traversing common bile duct iatrogenic injury. This catheter was used to guide ERCP stenting (ERCP) in a poor operative candidate with iatrogenic injury but common bile duct continuity.

presence of pigmented stones, number of stones (>15), and performance of the operation by surgical resident. Unfortunately, stones lost during a cholecystectomy can have significant and even substantially delayed consequences, such as chronic abscess, fistula, wound infection, and bowel obstruction.[23] Most dropped stones settle into Morrison's pouch or the retrohepatic space along the abdominal wall, which may develop into a chronic abscess in this location. The likelihood of developing complications from lost stones is difficult to quantify, because surgeon documentation of gallbladder perforation is variable and a substantial delay frequently exists between cholecystectomy and complication from lost stones. Based on available studies, lost stones do not necessitate conversion to an open operation; treatment should include extensive irrigation, significant attempt to retrieve lost stones, a course of antibiotics, and documentation of the perforation in the operative notes.

### Postcholecystectomy Pain

Although unusual, pain similar to biliary colic may persist or recur following cholecystectomy. A thorough evaluation of the biliary tree should be undertaken following cholecystectomy if the pain recurs. Recurrence of pain, if associated with other system findings of jaundice, fever, or chills within days to weeks following cholecystectomy, raises the suspicion of a secondary choledocholithiasis or a bile leak. Other biliary tree phenomena may cause a similar picture, such as sphincter of Oddi dysfunction. Postoperative bile duct strictures, which usually present with jaundice, are generally identified within the first year following cholecystectomy and may present with pain or fever if only one lobar duct is obstructed. In the setting of a normal liver panel, other causes of right upper quadrant pain should be investigated.

### Retained Biliary Stones

Retained common bile duct stones, or secondary common duct stones, can be identified for up to 2 years following cholecystectomy. Secondary common duct stones, which by definition originate in the gallbladder and pass into the common duct, are usually cholesterol stones and frequently become symptomatic within weeks of a cholecystectomy. Patients will complain of sharp right upper quadrant pain, with jaundice. Fever, completing Charcot's triad, is also common. Hyperbilirubinemia and an elevated alkaline phosphatase level should raise the suspicion of a retained stone. Ultrasound may not show intrahepatic biliary ductal dilation if the stone does not fully occlude the duct or the obstruction is early. Endoscopic removal of these stones via a generous sphincterotomy is almost universally successful (Fig. 55-39).

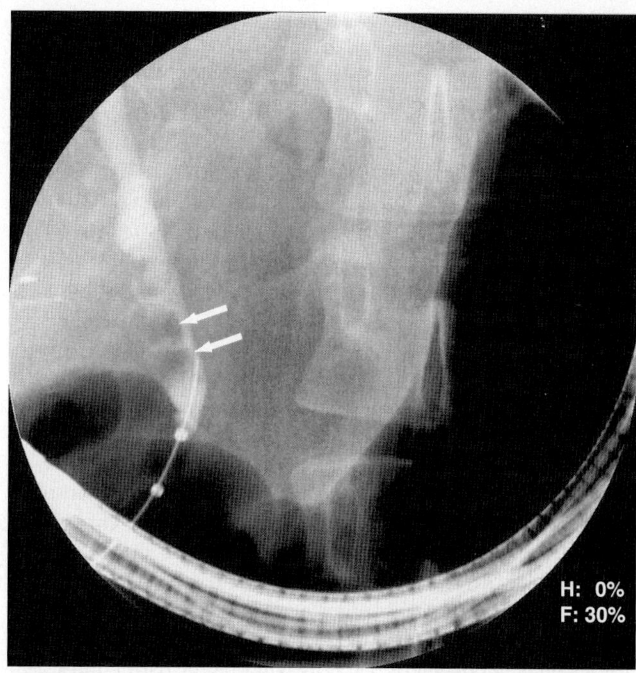


**FIGURE 55-39** ERCP showing multiple retained common bile duct stones *(arrows)*.

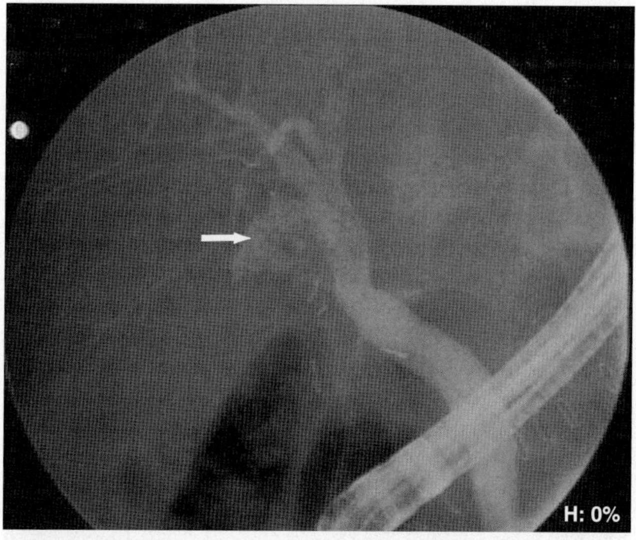


**FIGURE 55-40** ERCP showing cystic duct stump leak *(arrow)*.

### Biliary Leak

Following a cholecystectomy, patients may suffer a leak from the cystic duct or an unrecognized duct of Luschka. Fever, chills, right upper quadrant pain, jaundice, leakage of bile from an incision or into a drain, or persistent anorexia or bloating should raise the suspicion of a bile leak. Although it can be seen after any cholecystectomy, those performed for acute cholecystitis carry the greatest risk. With inflammation and fibrosis around an obstructed cystic duct, clips placed on the duct may not fully occlude it or may dislodge as the inflammatory process resolves. Patients will generally present within 1 week of cholecystectomy as the bile collects and becomes clinically manifest. On presentation, CT should be performed and will show ascites or a right upper quadrant fluid collection consistent with a biloma. Not only is reexploration in this setting unsuccessful, but it further complicates later reconstruction attempts that may be necessary. Endoscopic cholangiography should be performed, with percutaneous drainage of any fluid collections (Fig. 55-40). If the leak is from a cystic duct stump, sphincterotomy with stenting of the common duct will allow the leak to seal without need for surgical management. Reexploration in this setting is reserved for patients with evidence of septic shock or those in whom the leakage is not percutaneously accessible. If percutaneous drainage is not feasible because of overlying bowel, or the fluid is not localized and thus not amenable to percutaneous drainage, a laparoscopic washout of the abdomen and placement of subhepatic drains should be considered. No attempt should be made to fix the leak, because any such intervention is almost always unsuccessful and carries a risk of further injury to the biliary tree. Persistence of a bile leak after longer than 6 weeks should raise the suspicion of an unrecognized bile duct injury, thus mandating complete cholangiography by MRCP and repeat ERCP. Similar to common bile duct injuries, surgical treatment of a duct leak is most successful once the inflammatory process has resolved.

### Gallstone Ileus

A large stone in the dependent portion of the gallbladder may cause substantial inflammation and eventually fistulize into the adjacent duodenum. The stone may be of sufficient size to obstruct the small intestine. A mechanical small bowel obstruction from a gallstone passed through a spontaneous cholecystoenteric fistula is given the misnomer gallstone ileus. Most of these fistulae occur in older patients and may be caused by inflammation in the gallbladder or simply pressure necrosis.

**Presentation and Diagnosis** Patients will present with clinical evidence of a mechanical small bowel obstruction in the absence of surgical history or hernias. A history of symptoms referable to the biliary tree is variable. Although most patients will have constant pain from the obstruction, others can present with only episodic discomfort because the gallstone only intermittently obstructs the intestinal tract. The most common site of stone impaction is in the distal ileum, a few centimeters proximal to the ileocecal valve, where the caliber of the ileum decreases (Fig. 55-41). Plain radiographs demonstrate air-fluid levels consistent with a small bowel obstruction, although the offending stone may or may not be identified. Pneumobilia, which may only be identified by CT scan, is a ubiquitous finding, because the fistula that permitted a stone to pass into the duodenum allows air into the gallbladder and biliary tree (Fig. 55-42).

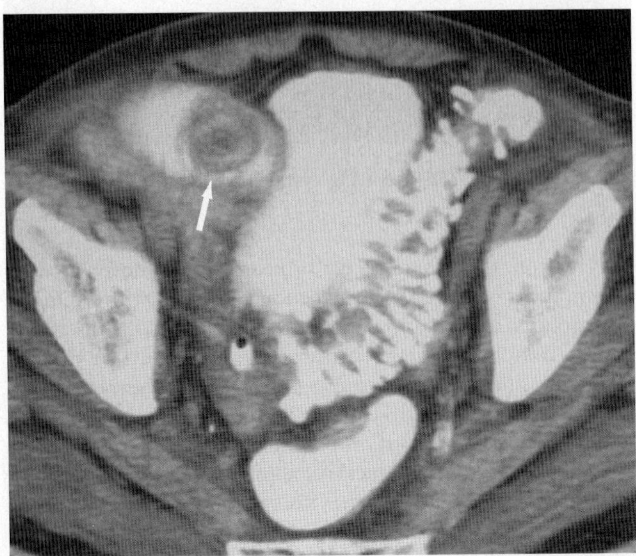

**FIGURE 55-41** CT scan of stone (arrow) obstructing distal ileum.

**Treatment** Exploration and enterotomy are required to relieve the obstruction. A longitudinal incision is made on the antimesenteric border of the ileum, a few centimeters proximal to the impacted stone. The stone can then be milked back through the enterotomy. The site of impaction is at risk for ischemia and pressure necrosis, with eventual perforation. Therefore, any suggestion of nonviability of this region should mandate resection. The remainder of the small intestine should be inspected, because approximately 10% of patients will have multiple large stones that have passed through the fistula. Although some surgeons advocate surgical treatment of the biliary enteric fistula at the same setting, the intense inflammatory process in the right upper quadrant may complicate the cholecystectomy and duodenal repair. In addition, because most of these patients are older, their overall physiologic status may not permit fistula repair in the emergent setting. One-stage repair should generally be performed in healthy patients without severe inflammatory changes in the right upper quadrant. Enterotomy with removal of the offending stone should suffice for patients with multiple comorbidities. A second operation can be considered to avoid the possibility of future biliary complications.

### Acute Cholangitis

Acute cholangitis is caused by an acute, ascending bacterial infection of the biliary tree caused by an obstruction. Although stones are a common cause, ascending cholangitis can be seen with any obstructing phenomenon, including malignancy. The two absolute requirements for the development of acute cholangitis are bacteria in the biliary tree and obstruction of flow, with increased intraluminal pressure. The source of bactibilia in patients with acute cholangitis is unclear, because culture of most bile is sterile. With obstruction from a stone, bactibilia can be identified in up to 90% of patients. The most common pathogens include *Klebsiella, E. coli, Enterobacter, Pseudomonas,* and *Citrobacter* spp.

The classic presentation of cholangitis is that of Charcot's triad, with fever, jaundice, and right upper quadrant pain. All three findings are seen in less than 50% of patients, with jaundice being the most variable. When the infection begins to manifest with shock, the two additional findings of mental status changes and hypotension join Charcot's triad to become

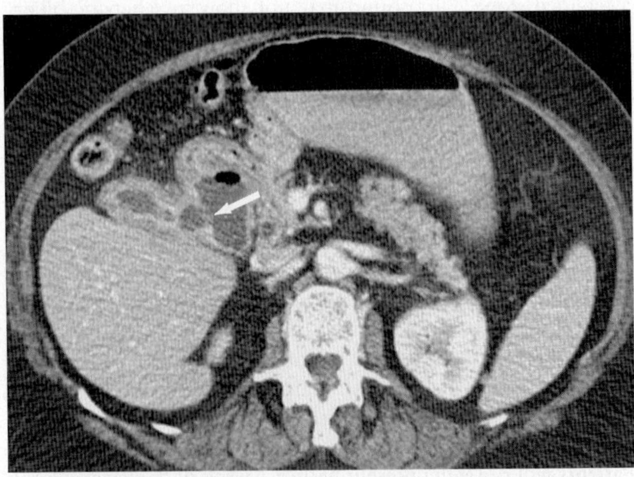

**FIGURE 55-42** CT scan of cholecystoduodenal fistula *(arrow)*.

Reynolds' pentad. With the acute obstruction of a visceral tubular structure, the pain can be severe but is not usually associated with abdominal tenderness.

**Diagnosis** As with any severe intra-abdominal infection, tachycardia and manifestations of shock are not uncommon. Leukocytosis with an abnormal liver panel is common. Hepatocellular injury from the infection and inflammation elevate serum transaminase levels, and alkaline phosphatase levels generally are significantly elevated. Ultrasound should be the first screening test and will commonly show dilation of the biliary tree. HIDA scans should be interpreted with caution, because infection of the biliary tree reduces the secretion of these agents into the biliary tree. CT can be helpful in identifying the site of obstruction, although not always the cause. Cholangiography via ERCP or PTC is critical not only to diagnosis but also therapy. These two modalities can usually identify the location and cause of obstruction, drain the biliary tree, allow for culture, and biopsy a lesion if necessary.

**Treatment** Acute cholangitis is a severe medical condition that can progress quickly to septic shock and death. Adequate hydration and IV antibiotics should be started immediately. Many patients will respond to medical therapy, so prompt diagnostic measures should be taken to identify the location and cause of obstruction. Others, however, will not respond to medical therapy and will progress to shock. These patients require emergent decompression of their biliary tree. Historically, this could only be achieved through a surgical route, with high morbidity and mortality. Endoscopic or percutaneous drainage achieve the same goal with less morbidity. Removal of the stone can be accomplished via endoscopic means, thus providing an advantage over percutaneous methods, which simply decompress the obstructed biliary tree. If endoscopic and percutaneous means are unavailable or unsuccessful, surgical drainage consists of common duct exploration with placement of a T tube. Given the unstable nature of the patient, definitive surgical treatment of the cause is deferred until the patient is stabilized, cholangitis treated, and the diagnosis confirmed.

### Recurrent Pyogenic Cholangitis

Recurrent pyogenic cholangitis is caused by cholangiohepatitis or intrahepatic stones and is usually found in East Asian populations. Biliary pathogens such as *Clonorchis sinensis* and *Ascaris lumbricoides* populate the biliary tree. These and other pathogens secrete an enzyme that hydrolyzes water-soluble bilirubin glucuronides to form free bilirubin, which then precipitates to form brown pigment stones. These stones may partially or fully obstruct the biliary tree, causing recurrent episodes of cholangitis and eventually abscesses or even cirrhosis. The chronicity of the infection and inflammation place these patients at risk for the development of cholangiocarcinoma. It is unclear whether the primary inciting event is infection causing inflammatory stricture or inflammatory stricture with subsequent infection of stagnant bile.

**Presentation** Recurrent pyogenic cholangitis tends to occur in the third to fourth decade of life, affecting men and women equally. The clinical presentation is that of cholangitis with fever, right upper quadrant pain, and jaundice. Because the infection, inflammation, and stones commonly present in a segmental or lobar pattern, the jaundice tends to be mild. Serum studies are similar to other causes of cholangitis, with a leukocytosis and elevated bilirubin and high alkaline phosphatase levels. Diagnosis is usually made by a combination of CT or MRCP with ERCP (Fig. 55-43). Lobar or segmental atrophy or hypertrophy may be seen in chronic cases.

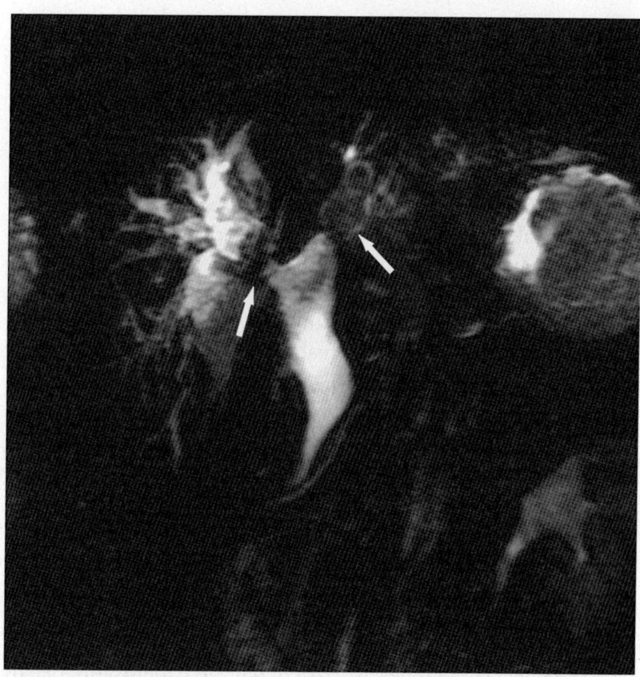

**FIGURE 55-43** MRCP of recurrent pyogenic cholangitis. Intraluminal filling defects from stones are noted in both lobes *(arrows)*.

**Treatment** In the setting of an acute attack, conservative treatment with parenteral antibiotics, IV fluids, and analgesics will usually suffice. Failure of this approach, with clinical deterioration, mandates biliary drainage via ERCP or percutaneous methods. Once the attack has subsided, a thorough investigation of biliary tree anatomy will help direct treatment. Definitive operative treatment is almost always required. The goals of surgical therapy are threefold: (1) remove all stones; (2) bypass, enlarge, or resect the strictures; and (3) provide adequate biliary drainage. The variability of presentation and location of disease has spurred the development of a number of operations to achieve these goals. The presence of intrahepatic strictures connotes a complicated case and may warrant resection, stricturoplasty, or hepaticocutaneous jejunostomy. When clearance of all stones is not possible, or future need for endoscopic therapy is anticipated, the terminal end of the Roux limb for a hepaticojejunostomy can be brought out as a stoma to provide easy access for choledochoscopy. Given the risk of cholangiocarcinoma, disease affecting predominantly one lobe should be resected in patients with adequate hepatic reserve.

## Noncalculous Biliary Disease

### Acute Acalculous Cholecystitis

Obstruction of the cystic duct in the absence of frank stones is known as acalculous cholecystitis. Although the exact pathophysiology is poorly understood, concentration of biliary solutes and stasis in the gallbladder clearly play important roles. Risk factors for the development of acalculous cholecystitis include older age, critical illness, burns, trauma, prolonged use of total parenteral nutrition, diabetes, and immunosuppression. The disease process is generally more fulminant than that of calculous cholecystitis and may progress to gangrene and perforation of the gallbladder.

The presentation of acalculous cholecystitis can be similar to that of calculous disease, with fever, anorexia, and right upper quadrant pain. Because many of these patients are critically ill, history may be impossible to obtain and the physical examination may be unreliable. The workup of fever in the intensive care patient may reveal a thickened gallbladder wall, with pericholecystic fluid (Fig. 55-44). HIDA scans may make the diagnosis but can have a false-positive rate of up to 40%.

Treatment of acalculous cholecystitis is similar to that for calculous cholecystitis, with cholecystectomy being therapeutic. Given the substantial inflammation and high risk of gallbladder gangrene, an open procedure is generally preferred. However, many of these patients are critically ill and would not tolerate the physiologic insult of a laparotomy, explaining why the mortality rate of cholecystectomy for acalculous cholecystitis is up to 40%. Accordingly, percutaneous drainage of the distended and inflamed gallbladder is carried out in patients unable to tolerate a laparotomy. The cholecystostomy tube used to drain the gallbladder can be placed by ultrasound or CT guidance. Approximately 90% of patients will improve with percutaneous drainage and the tube can eventually be removed. If follow-up imaging continues to demonstrate no stones, interval cholecystectomy is generally unnecessary.

### Primary Sclerosing Cholangitis

Primary sclerosing cholangitis (PSC) is an idiopathic, likely autoimmune process affecting the intrahepatic and extrahepatic biliary trees. Although the cause is unknown, it is associated with other autoimmune diseases, such as ulcerative colitis and Riedel's thyroiditis. As its name suggests, the disease causes inflammation and scarring in the biliary tree and must be distinguished from secondary sclerosing cholangitis, which involves a similar clinical picture but has an identifiable cause, such as malignancy, infection, or ischemia. The disease of PSC is characterized by progressive chronic cholestasis, and advances at an unpredictable rate to biliary cirrhosis and eventually death from liver failure. Although historically the diagnosis was only made in the late stages of disease, understanding of the disease, as well as increased frequency of liver function analyses and increased use of ERCP, have contributed to earlier diagnosis, frequently in the asymptomatic phase. The microscopic picture is one of inflammation, fibrosis, and cholestasis. In the absence of previous biliary manipulation, acute ascending cholangitis is uncommon in patients presenting with PSC.

**Clinical Presentation** The presentation of PSC is variable, but most patients present with fatigue, pruritus, and jaundice. This symptom complex spurs the physician to perform ERCP, although many patients have symptoms for 12 to 24 months before the diagnosis is made. The abnormalities seen on cholangiography confirm the diagnosis. Asymptomatic elevations of alkaline phosphatase levels can also occur and may be associated with evidence of hepatocellular injury and hyperbilirubinemia prior to clinical manifestations of symptoms. Abnormal liver function tests in a patient followed for inflammatory bowel disease should raise the suspicion of PSC. Elevation of perinuclear antineutrophil cytoplasmic antibodies (pANCAs) can be seen in 80% of patients. Disease severity does not correlate with pANCA titer.

ERCP is the preferred route for cholangiography and can demonstrate the characteristic multifocal, diffusely distributed dilations and strictures of the intrahepatic and extrahepatic biliary trees. The sequential stricturing, proximal dilation, and more proximal stricturing create a pattern described as beading. PTC is frequently unsuccessful because the proximal ducts are both fibrosed and generally not dilated. Other cholangiographic findings include multiple diverticulum-like outpouchings of the bile ducts and multiple short-segment strictures. MRCP can also be useful for diagnosis and monitoring of disease, but does not allow for interventions that may be necessary, such as brushing, balloon dilation, or stenting (Fig. 55-45). Liver biopsy tends to show an onion skin concentric periductal fibrosis. As the disease

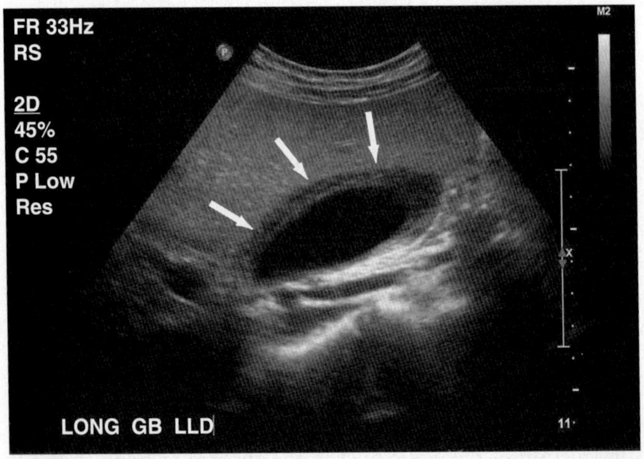

**FIGURE 55-44** Ultrasound of gallbladder with acute acalculous cholecystitis. The diffusely thickened gallbladder wall *(arrows)* is highly suggestive of cholecystitis.

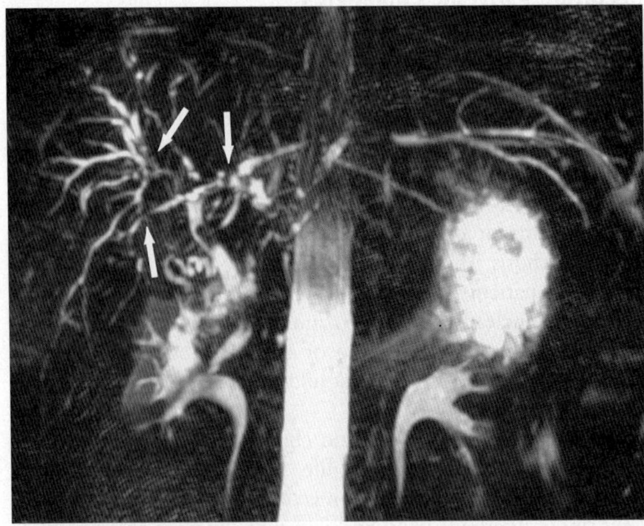

**FIGURE 55-45** MRCP showing primary sclerosing cholangitis. Note the multilevel strictures *(arrows)*.

progresses, periportal fibrosis occurs, progressing to bridging necrosis and eventually biliary cirrhosis. Unfortunately, PSC is associated with cholangiocarcinoma, and distinguishing the strictures of PSC fibrosis from those of cholangiocarcinoma can be challenging.

**Treatment** No specific effective medical therapy exists for the treatment of PSC. Although some experimental trials of ursodeoxycholic acid have shown improvement in liver function tests and histologic appearance compared with controls, this did not result in any significant clinical improvement when followed long term. Early in the disease, with mild symptoms, observation is a reasonable approach. Intervention must be specifically tailored to the pattern of disease and its clinical manifestations. Medical therapies are generally targeted to the underlying hepatobiliary disease process; these include choleretic agents such as ursodeoxycholic acid, immunosuppressive agents, and antifibrogenic agents such as colchicine. However, none of these agents has shown a consistent benefit. When performed in the symptomatic patient, endoscopic therapy, consisting of balloon dilation of the dominant strictures, has been shown to alleviate pruritus, reduce likelihood of cholangitis, and even prolong survival.

With the lack of effective, durable medical therapy in this progressive and ultimately fatal disease, an aggressive surgical approach is advocated. Options include biliary reconstructive procedures and liver transplantation. Although associated with ulcerative colitis, proctocolectomy does not appear to affect biliary disease progression or survival in patients with both ulcerative colitis and PSC. Biliary reconstruction is an option for patients with a dominant stricture at the hepatic bifurcation, for which resection of this region with long-term Silastic stenting can be performed. With increased success of orthotopic liver transplantation, the use of biliary reconstructive procedures has decreased.

Orthotopic liver transplantation appears to be the only lifesaving option for patients with progressive hepatic dysfunction from PSC. The survival rates for patients undergoing liver transplantation for PSC is approximately equivalent to those being transplanted for other noninfectious end-stage liver disease causes, with 5-year survival rates ranging from 75% to 85%.[24] Although the development of cholangiocarcinoma in a PSC liver is generally considered a contraindication to transplantation, some centers have shown excellent survival rates, up to 70% at 5 years, for patients with limited disease localized within the liver who undergo an extensive neoadjuvant protocol of chemotherapy and radiation followed by transplantation.[25] Because these results have not been reproduced elsewhere, the use of liver transplantation for the treatment of cholangiocarcinoma occurring in the setting of PSC is limited to experimental protocols. Following liver transplantation, many PSC patients develop strictures, raising the possibility of recurrence of disease in the donor liver. Biopsy may show identical findings as the original disease, but this is obviously complicated by the possibility of development of secondary sclerosing cholangitis from ischemia, infection, or rejection. Even with the development of strictures, disease progression does not usually follow the aggressive course for which PSC is known.

## Biliary Strictures

Benign strictures of the bile duct have a number of causes and generally affect the extrahepatic biliary tree, although cholangiohepatitis can create intrahepatic biliary strictures as well. Any inflammatory process occurring along the length of the common bile duct can cause a stricture. For example, the fibrotic inflammatory process of chronic pancreatitis can create a stricture of the intrapancreatic portion of the bile duct. The cholangiographic pattern of this stricture is that of a long (2 to 4 cm), smooth, gradually tapered narrowing affecting the distal common bile duct.

Strictures may occur in the middle portion of the common duct and are frequently associated with a process in the gallbladder. Any inflammatory process involving the gallbladder and cystic duct can secondarily inflame the common bile duct, causing an obstruction. Alternatively, a large stone in Hartmann's pouch can compress the adjacent bile duct and cause an apparent stricture. Both of these fall under the diagnosis of Mirizzi syndrome (Fig. 55-46). The prerequisites for this syndrome, characterized by gallbladder pathology causing obstructive jaundice, include a cystic duct that courses parallel to the common hepatic duct, an impacted stone in the gallbladder neck or cystic duct, and obstruction of the common hepatic duct caused by the stone or inflammatory response. The resultant inflammation can cause a cholecystocholedochal fistula. The treatment of Mirizzi syndrome is cholecystectomy, which may require repair of the common duct; when a large fistula exists, a choledochojejunostomy may be necessary.

Other strictures of the biliary tree include inflammatory strictures from long-standing choledocholithiasis, which tends to occur in the intrapancreatic portion of the bile duct, and stenosis of the sphincter of Oddi. ERCP with sphincterotomy, balloon dilation, and stent placement is generally regarded as primary treatment for benign bile duct strictures to make the diagnosis and potentially treat the process. Endoscopic and percutaneous therapy can provide long-term success in over 50% of patients. When unsuccessful, surgical management with anastomosis of the biliary tree to a Roux-en-Y jejunal limb has success rates of up to 90%.

## Biliary Cysts

Cysts of the biliary tree are rare, occurring in less than 1/100,000 patients, but are more common in those of Asian descent and are three to eight times more common in women than men.

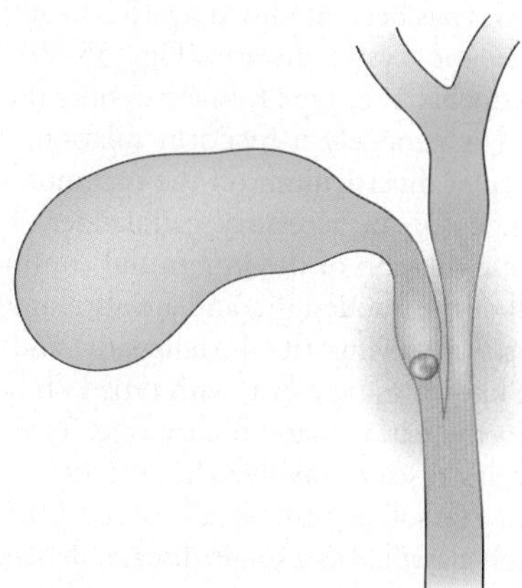

**FIGURE 55-46** Mirizzi syndrome. Obstruction of the bile duct from an inflammatory process is the hallmark of this syndrome; the cholecystocholedochal fistula may or may not be apparent.

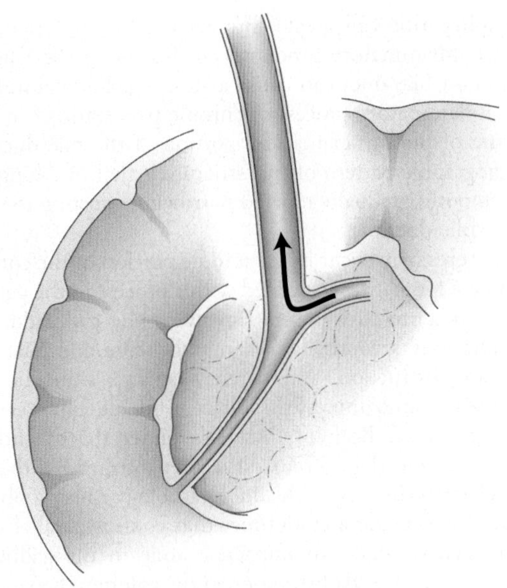

**FIGURE 55-47** Anomalous pancreaticobiliary junction. With fusion of the CBD and pancreatic ducts long before they pass through the duodenal wall, the pancreatic secretions can reflux into the CBD and may cause damage to the common duct through pressure or chemical injury.

Biliary cysts, known as choledochal cysts, are considered a premalignant condition requiring surgical intervention. They are commonly diagnosed in infancy, but many present in adulthood. Although not proven, the commonly accepted theory of their pathogenesis relies on the presence of an anomalous pancreaticobiliary junction (APBJ; Figs. 55-47 and 55-48).

With APBJ, the pancreatic duct and biliary tree fuse to form a common channel prior to passage through the duodenal wall; APBJ is seen in up to 90% of patients with choledochal cysts. The fused duct forms a long common channel, which allows pancreatic secretions to reflux into the biliary tree. Because the pancreatic duct has higher secretory pressures than the biliary tree, exocrine pancreatic secretions reflux up into the bile duct and can inflame and damage the biliary tree, resulting in cystic degeneration.

The original classification for choledochal cysts by Alonso-Lej and colleagues has been modified by Todani and associates to include intrahepatic cystic disease (Fig. 55-49).[26] The most common choledochal cyst, type I, involves only the extrahepatic biliary tree and is generally a fusiform dilation. Type II cysts appear as a saccular diverticulum off the common bile duct and may be mistaken for an accessory gallbladder. Type III cysts appear as a cystic dilation of the intramural common bile duct, within the wall of the duodenum, and are also known as choledochoceles. Cysts involving the intrahepatic and extrahepatic biliary tree are known as type IVa, with type IVb being multiple cysts limited to the extrahepatic biliary tree. Type V cysts, also known as Caroli's disease, involve the intrahepatic ducts only. Type V cysts may be solitary but usually occur diffusely in all segments. Although classified as a single disease, debate continues as to whether these constitute more than one pathologic entity.

**Presentation** The classic presentation of jaundice, right upper quadrant pain, and a palpable mass occurs rarely. Most patients have two of the three symptoms, with jaundice being the most consistent symptom prior to undergoing any diagnostic imaging. Other symptoms include nausea, pruritus, and weight loss. Long-standing disease can induce a chronic injury to the liver with cirrhosis. Cholangitis, pancreatitis, hepatic fibrosis, and malignancy have all been reported at the time of presentation. An unusual presentation is that of acute rupture of the cyst, with subsequent bile peritonitis.

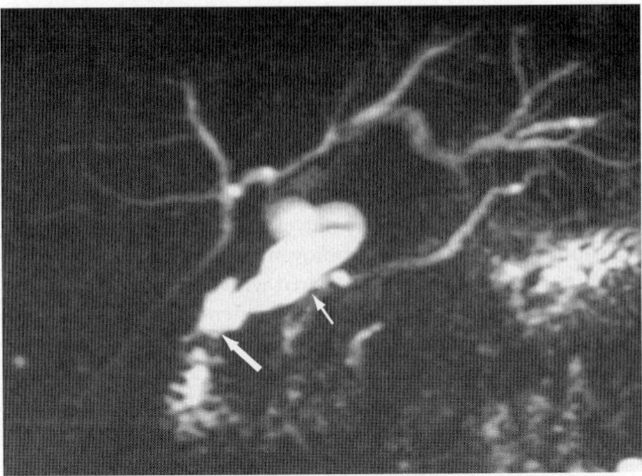

**FIGURE 55-48** MRCP showing anomalous pancreaticobiliary junction with long common channel. The pancreatic duct fuses with the CBD *(slender arrow)* and the common channel enters the duodenum *(bold arrow)*. Also noted in this illustration is the fusiform dilation of only the extrahepatic bile duct, as seen in a type I choledochal cyst.

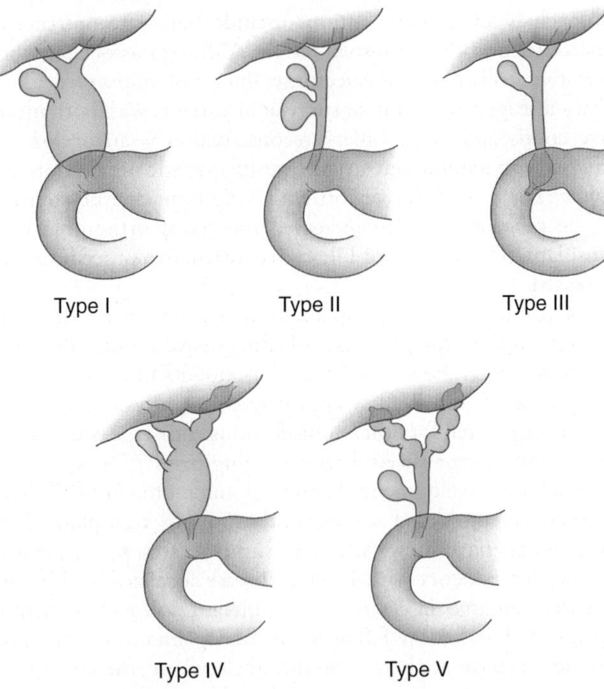


**FIGURE 55-49** Choledochal cyst classification.

Most cystic biliary lesions are originally identified and subsequently diagnosed by imaging, because the common presenting symptoms are nonspecific. With the current liberal use of CT, the diagnosis of a choledochal cyst is suspected, but further classified by MRCP. With a choledochal cyst, the upper biliary tree is difficult to fill and therefore evaluate by a retrograde route. Accordingly, MRCP helps create a complete cholangiogram. The distal bile duct is difficult to analyze by MRCP, so ERCP is more useful for defining the distal biliary tree and pancreatic duct–bile duct junction. Laboratory studies may identify cholestasis and jaundice. In late stages of disease, secondary hepatic injury and evidence of cirrhosis may be seen.

Because choledochal cysts are a premalignant condition, the original presentation of a choledochal cyst may be that of cholangiocarcinoma. The incidence of malignancy in patients with biliary cysts ranges from 10% to 30%. The pathogenesis appears to be one of a field defect, because the entire biliary tree is at risk, even in nondilated portions of the biliary tract, and complete excision of a benign choledochal cyst does not eliminate the risk of subsequent cholangiocarcinoma development. Malignant cyst degeneration is common and is thought to relate to chronic mucosal irritation from the refluxed pancreatic enzymes.

**Treatment** Surgical management of choledochal cysts consists of resection of the entire cyst and appropriate surgical reconstruction. Historically, enteric drainage of the cyst was performed without resection, but this approach is complicated by recurrent biliary stasis, infection, and development of malignancy. Type I cysts are treated by complete surgical excision, cholecystectomy, and Roux-en-Y hepaticojejunostomy. The proximal extent of resection should continue to the nondilated biliary tree and may require anastomosis to the left and right hepatic ducts. If there is substantial pericyst fibrosis, an intramural plane can be developed to excise the entire epithelium while leaving the fibrotic outer cyst wall in place. The distal duct is oversewn, with care not to injure the pancreatic duct. Type II cysts should be excised entirely and, in the presence of an APBJ, biliary enteric diversion by Roux-en-Y hepaticojejunostomy is appropriate. Type III cysts are uncommon and may be approached transduodenally. Because the pathogenesis of type III cysts is not clear, and may not involve APBJ, endoscopic drainage may suffice. In the setting of duodenal or biliary obstruction, transduodenal excision or sphincteroplasty can be performed. Surgical treatment of type IV cysts must be carefully individualized to the affected anatomy. Type IV cysts affecting only the extrahepatic bile ducts should be managed similarly to type I cysts, with excision and hepaticojejunostomy. Those with intrahepatic extension involving only one lobe can be treated with partial hepatectomy and reconstruction. Surgical treatment of Caroli's disease ranges from resection if the disease is unilobar to liver transplantation when diffuse disease is detected.

### Polypoid Lesions of the Gallbladder

Benign masses of the gallbladder are common, and consist of pseudotumors and adenomas. Pseudotumors are further divided into cholesterol polyps and adenomyomatosis. Cholesterol polyps appear as pedunculated echogenic lesions of the gallbladder, are usually smaller than 1 cm, and are frequently multiple. Alternatively, adenomyomatosis is seen as a sessile lesion, commonly in the fundus, with characteristic microcysts within the lesion, and frequently larger than 1 cm (Fig. 55-50). Adenomas are benign growths in the wall of the gallbladder that may be

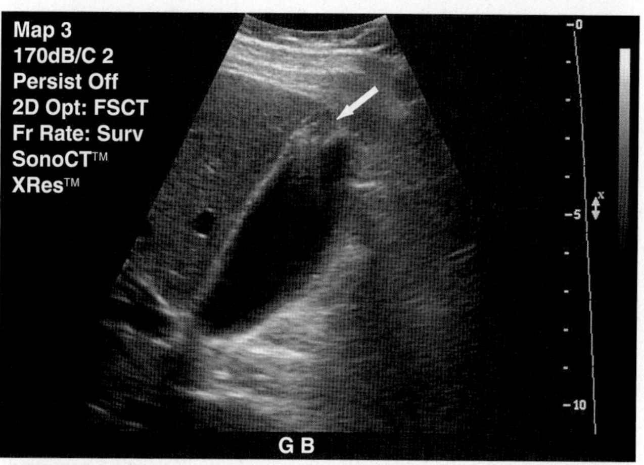


**FIGURE 55-50** Ultrasound of adenomyomatosis. Seen in the fundus of the gallbladder is a sessile thickening *(arrow)* with smaller microcysts within it, consistent with adenomyomatosis.

difficult to differentiate from adenocarcinoma preoperatively, because the only difference is that of transmural invasion, which can be challenging to detect by ultrasonography. Size larger than 10 mm is a risk factor for adenocarcinoma, along with growth, presence of gallstones, and patient age older than 60 years. The management of all symptomatic polypoid lesions of the gallbladder is laparoscopic cholecystectomy. Patients with a polypoid lesion and risk factors for adenocarcinoma or those suspected of having in situ or invasive cancer should undergo open cholecystectomy, because perforation during laparoscopy may spread tumor cells throughout the peritoneal cavity. Asymptomatic lesions smaller than 10 mm, with no other risk factors and no ultrasonographic features suggesting malignancy, can be observed with serial ultrasonography.

### Benign Biliary Masses

Benign intraluminal growths of the biliary tree are unusual, but mostly consist of adenomas. These lesions are soft fleshy growths occurring mostly in the periampullary bile duct arising from the glandular epithelium. The presentation is that of biliary obstruction, with jaundice and sometimes right upper quadrant pain. Treatment consists of complete resection with a small rim of normal epithelium, because incomplete excision of affected epithelium carries a high risk of recurrence. These lesions occur in the periampullary duct, so a transduodenal approach can be used.

Inflammatory lesions of the biliary tree, known as pseudotumors or benign fibrosing disease, may be mistaken for cholangiocarcinoma. When this process occurs following surgical intervention on the biliary tree, the masslike stricture may be the result of ischemia to the duct, with subsequent inflammation and fibrosis. Alternatively, pseudotumors may occur de novo; these commonly affect the extrahepatic biliary tree above the bifurcation.

## MALIGNANT BILIARY DISEASE

### Gallbladder Cancer

Gallbladder cancer is an aggressive malignancy and carries an extremely poor prognosis. Patients have no specific presenting symptoms and therefore presentation with late-stage disease is common. The poor prognosis corresponds to the high proportion of patients presenting with advanced disease. For patients with earlier stage disease, a more aggressive surgical approach is warranted.

### Incidence

Gallbladder cancer generally presents in the sixth and seventh decades of life and is two to three times more common in women than men. Ethnicity plays an important role in the development of gallbladder cancer, with the highest incidence in women from India and Pakistan. Among North American populations, Native Americans and immigrants from Latin America have the highest rates.

### Cause

Although not proven scientifically, the prevailing theory regarding gallbladder cancer focuses on chronic inflammation with subsequent cellular proliferation. Therefore, the presence of gallstones is considered to be the primary risk factor, and larger stones (>3 cm) carry an increased risk of cancer development. More than 80% of patients with gallbladder cancer have cholelithiasis, and gallbladder cancer is approximately 7 times more common in patients with gallstones than in those without stones. The type of stone does not correlate with incidence of gallbladder cancer. Other risk factors include entities that may also cause inflammation in the gallbladder wall, such as APBJ, choledochal cysts, and PSC.

Porcelain gallbladder and gallbladder polyps larger than 10 mm are additional risk factors for the development of cancer. Extensive calcification of the wall of the gallbladder can cause a brittle gallbladder wall, leading what is termed *porcelain gallbladder,* and carries a risk of cancer development.[27]

### Pathology and Staging

Gallbladder cancer is generally adenocarcinoma and pathologic specimens show the progression from dysplasia to carcinoma in situ to invasive carcinoma, as has been described for other carcinomas, and are staged using the standard TNM staging system (Table 55-1).[28] A small subset of gallbladder cancers are of the papillary subtype and carry a significantly better prognosis. These lesions tend to have an indolent course and are commonly limited to the gallbladder wall at the time of diagnosis (Fig. 55-51). Most gallbladder carcinomas, however, have systemic disease at the time of presentation, with nodal disease in 35% and distant metastases in 40%.

The draining nodal basin for gallbladder cancer includes the hepatoduodenal ligament. From there, affected lymph nodes may include periaortic nodes near the celiac axis or pancreaticoduodenal nodes around the superior mesenteric artery. Because the venous drainage of the gallbladder includes direct venous tributaries into the liver parenchyma, these tumors may spread directly into segment IV of the liver. Also, transperitoneal spread is common and can progress to carcinomatosis.

**Table 55-1 Staging for Gallbladder Cancer**

| **Primary Tumor (T)** | | | |
|---|---|---|---|
| Tx | Primary tumor cannot be assessed | | |
| T0 | No evidence of primary tumor | | |
| Tis | Carcinoma in situ | | |
| T1 | Tumor invades lamina propria or muscular layer | | |
| T1a | Tumor invades lamina propria | | |
| T1b | Tumor invades muscle layer | | |
| T2 | Tumor invades perimuscular connective tissue; no extension beyond serosa or into liver | | |
| T3 | Tumor perforates the serosa (visceral peritoneum) and/or directly invades the liver and/or one other adjacent organ or structure, such as the stomach, duodenum, colon, pancreas, omentum, or extrahepatic bile ducts | | |
| T4 | Tumor invades main portal vein or hepatic artery or invades two or more extrahepatic organs or structures | | |
| **Regional Lymph Nodes (N)** | | | |
| Nx | Regional lymph nodes cannot be assessed | | |
| N0 | No regional lymph node metastasis | | |
| N1 | Metastases to nodes along the cystic duct, common bile duct, hepatic artery, and/or portal vein | | |
| N2 | Metastases to periaortic, pericaval, superior mesenteric artery, and/or celiac artery lymph nodes | | |
| **Distant Metastasis (M)** | | | |
| M0 | No distant metastasis | | |
| M1 | Distant metastasis | | |
| **Anatomic Stage and Prognostic Groups** | | | |
| Stage 0 | Tis | N0 | M0 |
| Stage I | T1 | N0 | M0 |
| Stage II | T2 | N0 | M0 |
| Stage IIIA | T3 | N0 | M0 |
| Stage IIIB | T1-3 | N1 | M0 |
| Stage IVA | T4 | N0-1 | M0 |
| Stage IVB | Any T | N2 | M0 |
| | Any T | Any N | M1 |

From Edge SB, Byrd DR, Compton CC, et al (eds): AJCC cancer staging manual, ed 7, New York, 2010, Springer, pp 213–214.

### Clinical Presentation

Because 90% of gallbladder cancers originate in the fundus or body of the gallbladder, most do not produce symptoms until the disease is advanced (Fig. 55-52). Symptoms of acute cholecystitis, with obstruction of the neck of the gallbladder, may portend a better prognosis, because patients with these symptoms may present with earlier stages of disease. Weight loss, jaundice, or an abdominal mass are associated with later stages of disease. Some patients describe symptoms of chronic cholecystitis in which the pain has recently changed in quality or frequency. Other common symptoms include chronic epigastric pain, early satiety, and a sense of fullness.

### Diagnosis

Ultrasonography is generally the first examination used in the evaluation of right upper quadrant pain. Ultrasonographic findings of gallbladder cancer include an irregularly shaped lesion in

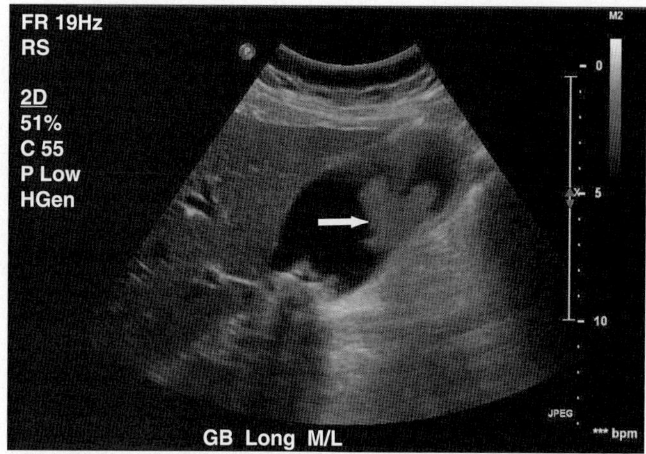


FIGURE 55-51 Ultrasound showing intraluminal polypoid gallbladder wall mass *(arrow)* but without extraluminal extension.

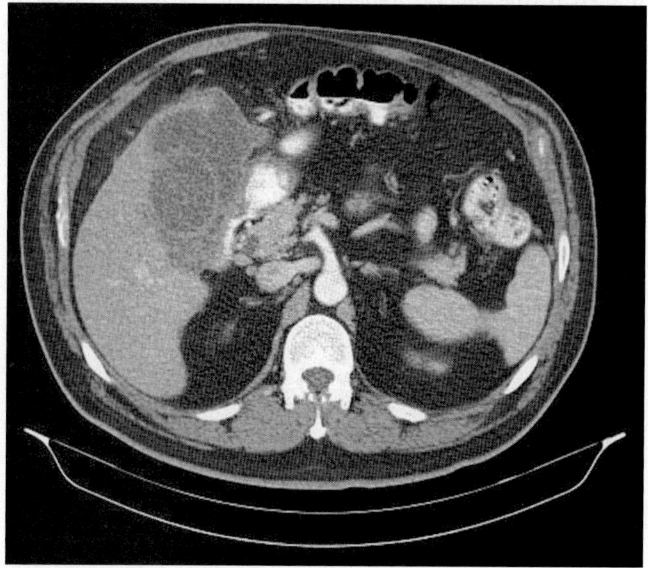

FIGURE 55-52 CT scan showing gallbladder cancer with invasion into the duodenum and liver parenchyma.

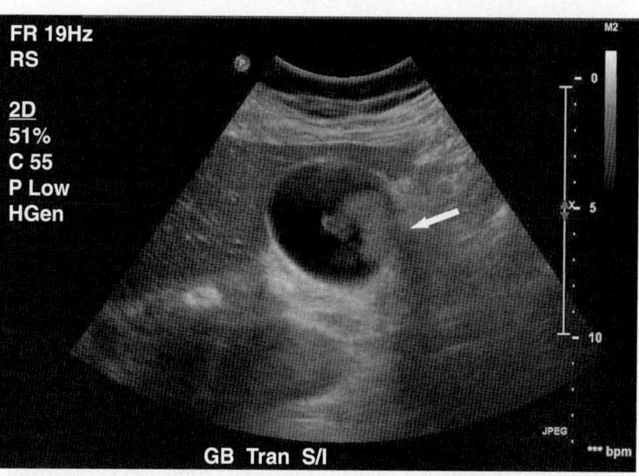


FIGURE 55-53 Ultrasound of gallbladder mass with loss of continuity of gallbladder wall *(arrow)*, suggesting extraluminal growth.

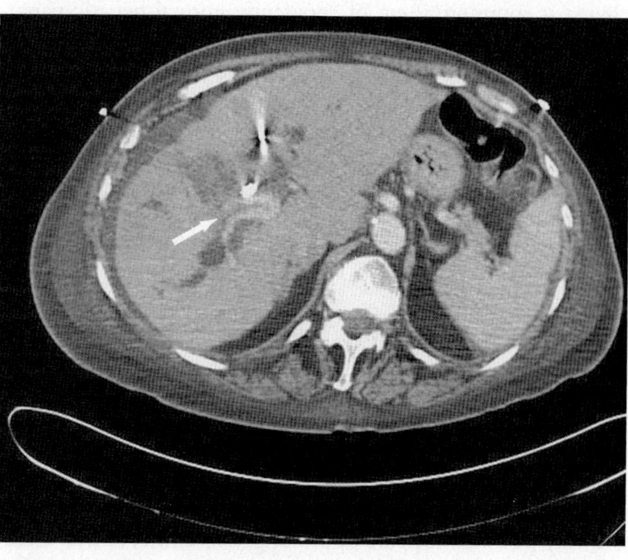

FIGURE 55-54 CT scan showing gallbladder mass with local invasion into portal vein *(arrow)*.

the subhepatic space, heterogeneous mass in the gallbladder lumen, and asymmetrically thickened gallbladder wall (Fig. 55-53). The finding of a polyp larger than 10 mm should raise the suspicion of gallbladder cancer.

CT can be useful in the staging and therefore treatment of gallbladder cancer. Although the sensitivity of CT for detection of direct extension into the liver is poor, CT can demonstrate peritoneal metastases, hepatic parenchymal metastases, lymphadenopathy, and adjacent vascular involvement (Fig. 55-54). Cholangiography can help delineate the location of obstruction in patients with gallbladder cancer, but most of these patients are incurable. Triphasic CT can be used to identify hepatic arterial or portal venous involvement. In the setting of unresectability (portal vein encasement or extensive hepatic involvement) or incurability (hepatic or peritoneal metastases), percutaneous methods for confirmatory tissue diagnosis should be used.

## Treatment

Resection of gallbladder cancer remains the only potential for cure. Patients with gallbladder cancer can be divided into four specific subgroups of presentation—patients with an incidental polyp on imaging, patients with an incidental finding of gallbladder cancer at time of or following cholecystectomy, patients suspected of having gallbladder cancer preoperatively, and patients with advanced disease at presentation.

### Patients With Incidental Findings

***Gallbladder Polyp*** Because gallbladder polyps larger than 10 mm carry an increased risk of malignancy, cholecystectomy is the treatment of choice, and should be performed via an open approach, because laparoscopic perforation in the setting of cancer may convert a potentially curable disease into an incurable one.

***Gallbladder Cancer Following Cholecystectomy*** With the finding of carcinoma following cholecystectomy, subsequent treatment depends on depth of penetration of the gallbladder wall and surgical margins. With T1a lesions, in which the carcinoma penetrates the lamina propria but does not invade the muscle layer, cholecystectomy should suffice for therapy. The likelihood of nodal disease in this setting is less than 3%. For those penetrating the muscularis but not the deeper connective tissue or serosa, classified as T1b lesions, cholecystectomy is sufficient as long as the margins are negative. With T1b lesions and perineural, lymphatic, or vascular invasion, the likelihood of nodal disease increases significantly and therefore an extended cholecystectomy is indicated. The extended cholecystectomy is directed at obtaining an R0 resection of the disease, including the draining lymph node basins. Therefore, removal of the pericholedochal, periportal, hepatoduodenal, right celiac, and posterior pancreaticoduodenal lymph nodes should be included. Resection of the cystic duct margin to uninvolved mucosa may require resection of the common bile duct with Roux-en-Y reconstruction. Because local extension into the hepatic parenchyma is common, 2 cm of apparently normal hepatic parenchyma from the gallbladder fossa is resected. Because port site recurrences have been reported for patients with even in situ disease, all port sites should also be excised. Management of patients with T2 lesions, in which the cancer extends past the muscularis but not beyond the serosa, a similar approach with radical cholecystectomy is indicated, because more than 40% of these patients have lymph node metastases and up to 25% have positive margins when treated with standard cholecystectomy alone.

**Patients Suspected of Having Gallbladder Cancer Preoperatively** Patients in whom preoperative evaluation suggests possibly resectable gallbladder cancer without metastatic disease should be offered an attempt at resection, even though survival is poor compared with those found incidentally. These patients tend to present with advanced locoregional disease and may require an extended liver resection. Because surgical intervention provides the only potential for cure or prolongation of life, radical resection should be considered for adequate operative candidates. The operation begins with a diagnostic laparoscopy to identify small-volume peritoneal or hepatic metastases that would preclude a resection, thereby avoiding an unnecessary operation. In the setting of metastatic disease, nonoperative strategies should be used to palliate symptoms. Radical resection in the setting of T3 and T4 lesions includes at least segments IVb and V, but more often requires a central hepatectomy, including all of segments IV, V, and VIII. If necessary to achieve R0 margin status, an extended right trisegmentectomy may be used. Direct extension of tumor into adjacent structures such as the hepatic flexure is not a contraindication to resection as long as negative margins can be obtained and all disease resected. Debulking without the possibility of complete resection has no role in the management of gallbladder cancer.

**Patients With Advanced Disease at Presentation** Many patients with gallbladder cancer will present with advanced disease, and therefore the goal of therapy is palliation of symptoms. Common symptoms requiring palliation include jaundice, pain, and intestinal obstruction. Jaundice can be managed by endoscopic biliary stenting and self-expanding endobiliary metal stents can provide a durable solution, with less need for repeated interventions than plastic stents. Pain is generally treated with oral narcotics, but may progress to require parenteral opioids in the hospice setting. Percutaneous neurolysis of the celiac ganglion can help with the palliation of pain. Intestinal obstruction is usually gastric outlet obstruction from local extension of tumor and is generally managed by an endoscopic duodenal wall stent. Unfortunately, neither chemotherapy nor radiation therapy have shown a survival benefit in the management of gallbladder cancer.

### Survival

Survival of patients diagnosed with gallbladder cancer is dependent on the stage of disease at presentation and whether surgical resection is performed. Independent factors affecting survival include T status, N status, histologic differentiation, and common bile duct involvement.[29] Advances in surgical management and extent of resection have led to improvements in survival, although most patients present with late-stage disease and are not candidates for resection. Patients with T1a lesions, limited to the mucosa and lamina propria, have an excellent prognosis. Complete resection of T1b lesions to negative margins also affords an excellent prognosis. Survival of patients with T2 lesions depends on nodal status and radical resection in this setting improves 5-year survival from approximately 20% to more than 60%. The 5-year survival of patients with T3 tumors is less than 20%, and patients with T4 lesions have a survival measured in months. Patients with metastatic disease at presentation have a median survival of 13 months. Because most patients with gallbladder cancer present with advanced disease, the overall survival of gallbladder cancer is less than 15%.

## Bile Duct Cancer

Cholangiocarcinoma is a rare disease entity that carries a dismal prognosis. Historically, evaluation and management of cholangiocarcinoma required arbitrary division of the bile duct into thirds based on the location of obstruction. Lesions of the middle third, however, are decidedly rare, so investigations have recently focused on perihilar and intrahepatic lesions, known as proximal lesions, versus those involving the periampullary region, known as distal disease. More than two thirds of all cholangiocarcinoma involve the proximal biliary tree near the bifurcation, known as Klatskin tumors (Table 55-2).

### Risk Factors

Although most patients with cholangiocarcinoma have no identifiable cause, the risk of development of cholangiocarcinoma appears to correlate with chronic inflammation in the biliary tree and compensatory cellular proliferation. Therefore, a number of predisposing disease states carry an increased risk of development of cholangiocarcinoma. Congenital lesions, such as choledochal cysts, predispose to the development of cholangiocarcinoma from exposure of the biliary epithelium to toxic pancreatic secretions. Cholangiocarcinoma is more prevalent in Southeast Asia, where infection with the liver flukes *Clonorchis sinensis* and *Opisthorchis viverrini* create chronic biliary inflammation, with obstructions and strictures. Recurrent pyogenic cholangitis is characterized by primary bile duct stone formation with infections and carries a risk of cholangiocarcinoma development. Finally, PSC with its autoimmune multifocal strictures of the intrahepatic and extrahepatic biliary trees, carries an increased

**Table 55-2 Staging for Intrahepatic Bile Duct Cancer**

| **Primary Tumor (T)** | | | |
|---|---|---|---|
| Tx | Primary tumor cannot be assessed | | |
| T0 | No evidence of primary tumor | | |
| Tis | Carcinoma in situ (intraductal tumor) | | |
| T1 | Solitary tumor without vascular invasion | | |
| T2a | Solitary tumor with vascular invasion | | |
| T2b | Multiple tumors, with or without vascular invasion | | |
| T3 | Tumor perforating the visceral peritoneum or involving local extrahepatic structures by direct extension | | |
| T4 | Tumor with periductal invasion | | |
| **Regional Lymph Nodes (N)** | | | |
| Nx | Regional lymph nodes cannot be assessed | | |
| N0 | No regional lymph node metastasis | | |
| N1 | Regional lymph node metastasis present | | |
| **Distant Metastasis (M)** | | | |
| M0 | No distant metastasis | | |
| M1 | Distant metastasis present | | |
| **Anatomic Stage and Prognostic Groups** | | | |
| Stage 0 | Tis | N0 | M0 |
| Stage I | T1 | N0 | M0 |
| Stage II | T2 | N0 | M0 |
| Stage III | T3 | N0 | M0 |
| Stage IVA | T4 | N0 | M0 |
| | Any T | N1 | M0 |
| Stage IVB | Any T | Any N | M1 |

From Edge SB, Byrd DR, Compton CC, et al (eds): AJCC cancer staging manual, ed 7, New York, 2010, Springer, pp 203–204.

**Table 55-3 Staging for Perihilar Bile Duct Cancer**

| **Primary Tumor (T)** | | | |
|---|---|---|---|
| Tx | Primary tumor cannot be assessed | | |
| T0 | No evidence of primary tumor | | |
| Tis | Carcinoma in situ | | |
| T1 | Tumor confined to the bile duct, with extension up to the muscular layer or fibrous tissue | | |
| T2a | Tumor invading beyond the wall of the bile duct to surrounding adipose tissue | | |
| T2b | Tumor invades the adjacent hepatic parenchyma | | |
| T3 | Tumor invades unilateral branches of the portal vein or hepatic artery | | |
| T4 | Tumor invading main portal vein or its branches bilaterally; or the common hepatic artery; or the second-order biliary radicals bilaterally; or unilateral second-order biliary radicals with contralateral portal vein or hepatic artery involvement | | |
| **Regional Lymph Nodes (N)** | | | |
| Nx | Regional lymph nodes cannot be assessed | | |
| N0 | No regional lymph node metastasis | | |
| N1 | Regional lymph node metastasis (including nodes along the cystic duct, common bile duct, hepatic artery, and portal vein) | | |
| N2 | Metastasis to periaortic, pericaval, superior mesenteric artery, and/or celiac artery lymph nodes | | |
| **Distant Metastasis (M)** | | | |
| M0 | No distant metastasis | | |
| M1 | Distant metastasis | | |
| **Anatomic Stage and Prognostic Groups** | | | |
| Stage 0 | Tis | N0 | M0 |
| Stage I | T1 | N0 | M0 |
| Stage II | T2a-b | N0 | M0 |
| Stage IIIA | T3 | N0 | M0 |
| Stage IIIB | T1-3 | N1 | M0 |
| Stage IVA | T4 | N0-1 | M0 |
| Stage IVB | Any T | N2 | M0 |
| | Any T | Any N | M1 |

From Edge SB, Byrd DR, Compton CC, et al (eds): AJCC cancer staging manual, ed 7, New York, 2010, Springer, p 221.

risk of cholangiocarcinoma. Although sporadic cases of cholangiocarcinoma tend to occur at the bifurcation, patients with PSC may have multifocal disease not amenable to resection. Medications and chemical carcinogens have been associated with the development of cholangiocarcinoma, including Thorotrast, oral contraceptives, asbestos, and cigarette smoke.

### Staging and Classification

The three distinct pathologic subtypes include sclerosing, nodular, and papillary cholangiocarcinoma. Sclerosing cholangiocarcinoma tends to occur in the proximal bile ducts, causing periductal fibrosis in a concentric pattern and a circumferential duct occlusion. The papillary and nodular subtypes tend to occur in distal cholangiocarcinomas and present with intraluminal growths. In the nodular subtype, a firm mass based in the duct wall can be seen growing into the duct lumen, whereas the more common papillary subtype appears as a polypoid lesion that is soft, with less periductal fibrosis and a better prognosis.

The staging of cholangiocarcinoma relies on the TNM staging system, but is slightly different based on anatomic location. The three staging subdivisions include intrahepatic (see Table 55-2), extrahepatic (Table 55-3), and distal bile duct (Table 55-4).[28] Similar to many adenocarcinomas, direct local invasion and local lymph node spread are common and portend a worse prognosis. Tumors confined to the bile duct (T1), and those extending outside the bile duct but not invading adjacent structures such as the hepatic artery or portal vein (T2), carry a significantly better prognosis than those invading any nearby structure. The two pathologic factors most influencing prognosis

**Table 55-4 Staging for Distal Bile Duct Cancer**

| | | | |
|---|---|---|---|
| **Primary Tumor (T)** | | | |
| Tx | Primary tumor cannot be assessed | | |
| T0 | No evidence of primary tumor | | |
| Tis | Carcinoma in situ | | |
| T1 | Tumor confined to the bile duct histologically | | |
| T2 | Tumor invades beyond the wall of the bile duct | | |
| T3 | Tumor invades the gallbladder, pancreas, duodenum, or other adjacent organs without involvement of the celiac axis or superior mesenteric artery | | |
| T4 | Tumor involves the celiac axis or superior mesenteric artery | | |
| **Regional Lymph Nodes (N)** | | | |
| N0 | No regional lymph node metastasis | | |
| N1 | Regional lymph node metastasis | | |
| **Distant Metastasis (M)** | | | |
| M0 | No distant metastasis | | |
| M1 | Distant metastasis | | |
| **Anatomic Stage and Prognostic Groups** | | | |
| Stage 0 | Tis | N0 | M0 |
| Stage IA | T1 | N0 | M0 |
| Stage IB | T2 | N0 | M0 |
| Stage IIA | T3 | N0 | M0 |
| Stage IIB | T1<br>T2<br>T3 | N1<br>N1<br>N1 | M0<br>M0<br>M0 |
| Stage III | T4 | Any N | M0 |
| Stage IV | Any T | Any N | M1 |

From Edge SB, Byrd DR, Compton CC, et al (eds): AJCC cancer staging manual, ed 7, New York, 2010, Springer, p 229.

following resection are complete (R0) resection to negative margins, and absence of lymph node metastases.

## Clinical Presentation

The presentation of cholangiocarcinoma depends on the site of origin and manifestations of biliary obstruction at that site. Painless jaundice is a common symptom, but patients with unilobar obstruction of a bile duct may proceed with unilateral lobar atrophy and subsequent contralateral lobar hypertrophy (Fig. 55-55). The resultant hepatic compensation can delay presentation until the later stages of disease. Therefore, cholangiocarcinoma causing obstruction at or below the hepatic bifurcation tends to present at earlier stages than intrahepatic cholangiocarcinoma. With obstruction of the biliary tree, the common manifestations of direct hyperbilirubinemia, such as pruritus, dark urine, and steatorrhea, can be seen. Cholangiocarcinomas tend to extend in a submucosal route, with associated perineural invasion, but constant pain on presentation suggests more advanced disease.

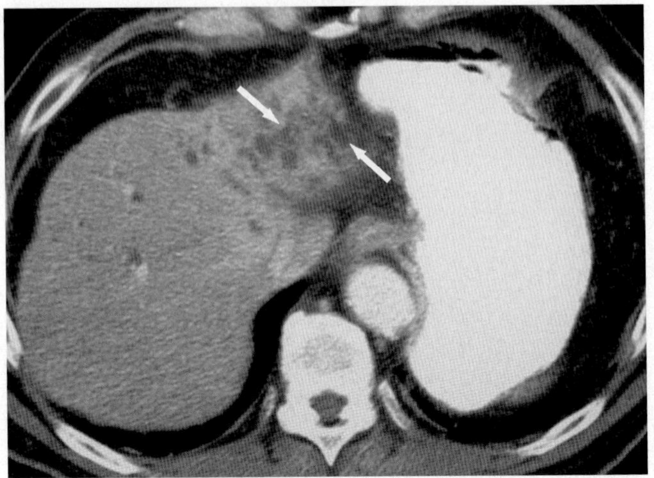

**FIGURE 55-55** CT scan of cholangiocarcinoma with left lobar atrophy caused by obstruction of the left duct. Noted in the atrophied left lobe are dilated biliary radicals *(arrows).*

## Diagnosis and Assessment of Resectability

At the time of presentation, most patients will have manifestations of obstructive jaundice with hyperbilirubinemia and an elevated alkaline phosphatase level. Other markers of hepatic function, such as prothrombin time and albumin level, are generally unaffected unless they occur later in the disease or the biliary obstruction is long-standing. Tumor markers, including carcinoembryonic antigen (CEA) and carbohydrate antigen 19-9 (CA19-9), are unreliable for diagnosing cholangiocarcinoma, but may be followed postoperatively in the surveillance of recurrence.

The radiologic evaluation of jaundice includes a right upper quadrant ultrasound, which may show intrahepatic biliary ductal dilation but does not usually identify the actual site of obstruction. With hilar cholangiocarcinomas, the gallbladder and visualized extrahepatic biliary tree are usually decompressed, whereas distal lesions will have extrahepatic biliary ductal dilation and gallbladder distention. Cross-sectional imaging by triphasic CT allows not only assessment of metastatic disease, but also evaluation of resectability. The location of the tumor can be identified and its relationship to vascular structures can also be assessed. Identification of aberrant anatomy and determination of segmental or lobar involvement by CT are helpful for preoperative planning.

Typically, CT alone is insufficient for the assessment of feasibility and appropriateness of resection. Cholangiography by MRCP, PTC, or ERCP helps determine the proximal extent of resection. Endoscopic cholangiography carries the additional risk of cholangitis by the introduction of enteric bacteria into an undrained portion of the biliary tree. Bilobar intrahepatic metastases or any extrahepatic disease are contraindications to resection, as is the involvement of bilateral secondary biliary radicals. Because complete (R0) resection is the only strategy that affords the possibility of cure, other contraindications to resection include encasement of the main portal vein (Fig. 55-56), bilateral hepatic lobar artery involvement, and lobar atrophy with involvement of the contralateral portal vein or biliary radicals. Involvement of unilobar vascular structures is managed with resection of the primary and affected lobe in continuity, and therefore is not a contraindication.

Tissue diagnosis prior to resection in operative patients is unnecessary. With obstructive jaundice, bile cytology and brushings are unreliable, and thus a negative cytology report does not exclude malignancy. Therefore, invasive attempts to establish a diagnosis prior to resection carry risk but do not alter subsequent management. Establishing a tissue diagnosis is only important when the patient is not a surgical candidate. However, preoperative biliary drainage may be useful in select cases. In patients with distal cholangiocarcinoma, preoperative biliary drainage increases the rate of infectious complications of resection, but is generally useful for those with preoperative hyperbilirubinemia (bilirubin level >10 mg/dL) and those with a prolonged time interval between presentation and resection. For patients with hilar cholangiocarcinoma, hepatic resection remains an important feature of their operative strategy. In the setting of complete biliary obstruction, hepatic resection carries an additional risk of bleeding, sepsis, and hepatic failure. In this setting, drainage of the obstructed but unaffected segments can enhance the postresection hypertrophy of the remaining liver,[30,31] but may increase perioperative infectious complications.[32]

### Treatment

**Operative Management** With the clinical suspicion of cholangiocarcinoma in adequate operative candidates without contraindications to resection, exploration should proceed, even in the absence of a confirmed tissue diagnosis. Between 7% and 15% of patients undergoing resection for suspected biliary malignancy will prove to have benign disease. Alternatively, more than 50% of patients undergoing exploration will have findings precluding resection, such as peritoneal metastases, hepatic metastases, or locally advanced lesions.

***Distal Cholangiocarcinoma*** Distal cholangiocarcinoma is managed by pancreaticoduodenectomy. Because these lesions tend to grow in a submucosal plane, a frozen section of the proximal bile duct margin helps ensure an R0 resection. An R0 resection remains one of the most important prognostic factors for this disease, with 5-year survival rates of up to 50% in node-negative patients with an R0 resection.

***Proximal Cholangiocarcinoma*** Surgical management of proximal cholangiocarcinoma involves resection of regional nodal tissue and en bloc resection of the common bile duct with hepatic parenchyma as necessary to achieve negative margins. The Bismuth-Corlette classification of the tumor by assessment of the involvement of biliary radicals helps with operative planning (Fig. 55-57).[33] Types I and II lesions are treated with common duct resection, cholecystectomy, and a 5- to 10-mm margin of resection. Type II lesions may also require partial hepatic resection, which commonly includes resection of the caudate lobe. Resection of the bile duct and nodal tissue requires skeletonization of the hepatic artery and portal vein. Reconstruction is performed using a Roux limb of jejunum. Types III and IV lesions may involve complex resection and reconstruction of the portal vein, hepatic artery, or both. With resection to secondary biliary radicals, transanastomotic stenting is used liberally to allow healing and even confirmation of anastomotic integrity.

A substantial improvement in long-term survival has correlated with the increasing use of hepatic resection to achieve negative margins. Negative margin status is the most important variable associated with outcome.[34] Five-year survival rates as high as 59% have been reported in selected series and, with vascular resection and reconstruction techniques, resectability rates have also increased.[35] Increases in the magnitude of the operation have also correlated with an expected increase in surgical mortality, from 2% to 4% to 3% to 11%.

**Palliation** In patients found to have unresectable or incurable disease preoperatively, all attempts to palliate their symptoms nonoperatively should be used. The goals of palliation should include relief of jaundice, alleviation of pain, and relief of duodenal obstruction, if necessary. Surgical palliation has not been shown to prolong survival or reduce complication rates, and thus

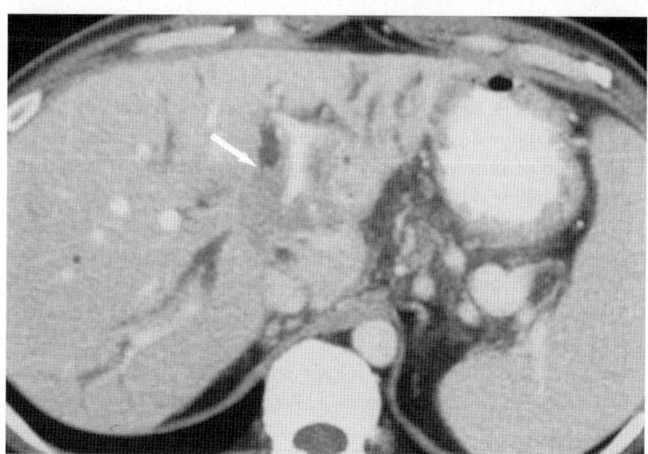

**FIGURE 55-56** CT scan of Klatskin tumor *(arrow)* encasing the main portal vein, consistent with unresectable disease.

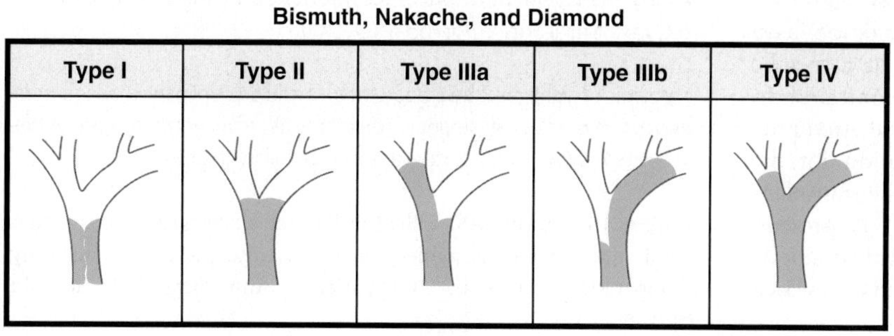

Bismuth, Nakache, and Diamond

Type I
Type II
Type IIIa
Type IIIb
Type IV

**FIGURE 55-57** Bismuth-Corlette classification of tumor involvement.

should be reserved for candidates found to be unresectable or metastatic at time of operation. Depending on the location of the biliary obstruction, endoscopic or percutaneous routes of drainage can be used, and placement of a self-expandable metallic wall stent provides a durable solution. When plastic stents are used, additional manipulation or placement of subsequent stents may be required. For distal cholangiocarcinomas, ERCP is the preferred route of nonoperative biliary drainage, whereas PTC is more useful for proximal lesions. Drainage of atrophic lobes with stents does not improve palliation of disease. Pain can be treated with oral narcotics. IV narcotics and even percutaneous destruction of the celiac plexus have shown some benefit. For distal cholangiocarcinomas, in which duodenal obstruction may occur, endoscopic duodenal stenting can relieve the obstruction in this preterminal condition.

**Medical Treatment** Chemotherapy has not been shown to improve survival in patients with cholangiocarcinoma. Additionally, radiation therapy has not been proven in a prospective fashion to affect survival. Therefore, neither chemotherapy nor radiation therapy are used routinely in the adjuvant or neoadjuvant setting. Although some retrospective studies have shown a small survival advantage with adjuvant radiation, prospective studies of adjuvant radiotherapy have shown no benefit in completely resected patients. Radiation therapy may provide a small survival advantage when used as an adjunct to resection when microscopic residual disease remains. Most studies have reported a clinical response rate of less than 10%. Even in the absence of supportive data, adjuvant chemoradiation is used routinely at many centers, but should be limited to patients with nodal disease, those with R1 resections, and those undergoing a clinical trial.

### Outcomes

Long-term survival is highly dependent on stage at presentation and whether surgical resection to negative margins is achieved. With the use of common duct resection with partial hepatectomy, negative margin rates have increased to over 75%. This has resulted in 5-year survival rates of 20% to 45% in most series. Although morbidity rates of 35% to 50% are common, mortality rates are generally low (<10%). In the setting of distal bile duct cancers, resection rates are generally higher, with approximately similar 5-year survival among patients undergoing R0 resections. Alternatively, because there is no reliable therapeutic alternative, the median survival of unresected patients ranges from 5 to 8 months.

Because negative margin status is easier to obtain by explanting the liver, some have advocated total hepatectomy with liver transplantation for treatment.[36] Unfortunately, initial experience with therapeutic transplantation was plagued by early mortality and high recurrence rates. Even the most aggressive and radical resections with multivisceral transplantation have not shown a survival advantage. Therefore, without a specific clinical trial, cholangiocarcinoma is considered a contraindication to transplantation. However, some centers have attempted neoadjuvant chemoradiation followed by exploration for the evaluation of resectability and metastases, and finally transplantation, with improved survival over resection alone.[37] At present, the role of transplantation in the management of cholangiocarcinoma is at best controversial, and should be limited to research protocols.

## METASTATIC AND OTHER TUMORS

Any primary or secondary tumor affecting the liver can cause biliary obstruction. The most common examples include portal nodal disease from adenocarcinomas such as hepatocellular carcinoma, pancreatic adenocarcinoma, and colorectal carcinoma. The metastatic nodes can compress the common bile duct at any point along its length. Lymphoma may affect the portal lymph node chain and, when isolated to periportal nodes, is notoriously difficult to differentiate from cholangiocarcinoma. Placement of temporary plastic stents to relieve the obstruction is usually the only therapeutic biliary intervention required, because these lymphomas will generally respond to chemotherapy and the obstruction will usually resolve.

Primary lesions of the liver or metastatic disease may obstruct the biliary tree from direct compression or extension, as seen in hepatocellular carcinoma, but this phenomenon does not create an intraluminal biliary growth. Rarely, tumor cells may actually pass into the biliary tree and embolize distally. As the exfoliated cellular mass grows, it may present with intraluminal biliary obstruction. Intrahepatic biliary cystadenomas or cystadenocarcinoma may obstruct the bile duct directly or by passage of the mucin that they produce.

## SELECTED REFERENCES

Endo I, Gonen M, Yopp AC, et al: Intrahepatic cholangiocarcinoma: Rising frequency, improved survival, and determinants of outcome after resection. Ann Surg 248:84–96, 2008.

This article documents the increase in hepatic resection, vascular reconstruction techniques, and outcomes for patients with cholangiocarcinoma.

Heimbach JK, Gores GJ, Haddock MG, et al: Predictors of disease recurrence following neoadjuvant chemoradiotherapy and liver transplantation for unresectable perihilar cholangiocarcinoma. Transplantation 82:1703–1707, 2006.

This article shows the impressive results seen in the management of cholangiocarcinoma when neoadjuvant chemoradiotherapy is combined with hepatic transplantation in an extremely tightly controlled trial.

Massarweh NN, Flum DR: Role of intraoperative cholangiography in avoiding bile duct injury. J Am Coll Surg 204:656–664, 2007.

This article summarizes the current debate regarding the role of cholangiography in minimizing rates of and damage from bile duct injury.

Nuzzo G, Giuliante F, Giovannini I, et al: Advantages of multidisciplinary management of bile duct injuries occurring during cholecystectomy. Am J Surg 195:763–769, 2008.

This article highlights the importance of multidisciplinary management and relative roles of surgery, percutaneous management, and endoscopic therapy in the coordinated care of biliary injuries.

Sicklick JK, Camp MS, Lillemoe KD, et al: Surgical management of bile duct injuries sustained during laparoscopic cholecystectomy: perioperative results in 200 patients. Ann Surg 241:786–792, 2005.

This article summarizes a large series of bile duct injuries and the strategies used in the repair.

Strasberg SM, Hertl M, Soper NJ: An analysis of the problem of biliary injury during laparoscopic cholecystectomy. J Am Coll Surg 180:101–125, 1995.

This article summarizes a large pool of data from biliary injuries sustained during laparoscopic cholecystectomy and creates a classification scheme for the injury patterns.

Todani T, Watanabe Y, Narusue M, et al: Congenital bile duct cysts: Classification, operative procedures, and review of thirty-seven cases including cancer arising from choledochal cyst. Am J Surg 134:263–269, 1977.

This is a classic article summarizing the classification system for choledochal cysts and the association with cancer.

Walsh RM, Henderson JM, Vogt DP, et al: Long-term outcome of biliary reconstruction for bile duct injuries from laparoscopic cholecystectomies. Surgery 142:450–456, 2007.

This article highlights the details of surgical management and the use of long-term stents in the care of biliary injuries.

Way LW, Stewart L, Gantert W, et al: Causes and prevention of laparoscopic bile duct injuries: Analysis of 252 cases from a human factors and cognitive psychology perspective. Ann Surg 237:460–469, 2003.

Prior to this article, most analyses of biliary injuries attributed the error to one of inexperience. By analyzing the human factors, this article notes the patterns of analysis, thereby explaining why even experienced hepatobiliary surgeons may injure a bile duct in the performance of this operation.

## REFERENCES

1. Couinard C: [Les envelopes vasculobiliares de foie ou capsule de Glisson: Leur interet dans la chirurgie vesiculaire, les resections hepatique et l'abord du hile du foie.] Lyon Chir 49:589–615, 1954.
2. Admirand WH, Small DM: The physicochemical basis of cholesterol gallstone formation in man. J Clin Invest 47:1043–1052, 1968.
3. Gurusamy K, Samraj K, Gluud C, et al: Meta-analysis of randomized controlled trials on the safety and effectiveness of early versus delayed laparoscopic cholecystectomy for acute cholecystitis. Br J Surg 97:141–150, 2010.
4. Petelin JB: Laparoscopic common bile duct exploration. Surg Endosc 17:1705–1715, 2003.
5. Horwood J, Akbar F, Davis K, et al: Prospective evaluation of a selective approach to cholangiography for suspected common bile duct stones. Ann R Coll Surg Engl 92:206–210, 2010.
6. Lee JK, Ryu JK, Park JK, et al: Roles of endoscopic sphincterotomy and cholecystectomy in acute biliary pancreatitis. Hepatogastroenterology 55:1981–1985, 2008.
7. van Santvoort HC, Besselink MG, de Vries AC, et al: Early endoscopic retrograde cholangiopancreatography in predicted severe acute biliary pancreatitis: A prospective multicenter study. Ann Surg 250:68–75, 2009.
8. Strasberg SM, Hertl M, Soper NJ: An analysis of the problem of biliary injury during laparoscopic cholecystectomy. J Am Coll Surg 180:101–125, 1995.
9. Ito K, Ito H, Tavakkolizadeh A, et al: Is ductal evaluation always necessary before or during surgery for biliary pancreatitis? Am J Surg 195:463–466, 2008.
10. Boerma D, Rauws EA, Keulemans YC, et al: Wait-and-see policy or laparoscopic cholecystectomy after endoscopic sphincterotomy for bile-duct stones: A randomised trial. Lancet 360:761–765, 2002.
11. Adamsen S, Hansen OH, Funch-Jensen P, et al: Bile duct injury during laparoscopic cholecystectomy: A prospective nationwide series. J Am Coll Surg 184:571–578, 1997.
12. Rogers SJ, Cello JP, Horn JK, et al: Prospective randomized trial of LC+LCBDE vs ERCP/S+LC for common bile duct stone disease. Arch Surg 145:28–33, 2010.
13. Way LW, Stewart L, Gantert W, et al: Causes and prevention of laparoscopic bile duct injuries: Analysis of 252 cases from a human factors and cognitive psychology perspective. Ann Surg 237:460–469, 2003.
14. Massarweh NN, Flum DR: Role of intraoperative cholangiography in avoiding bile duct injury. J Am Coll Surg 204:656–664, 2007.
15. Bismuth H, Majno PE: Biliary strictures: classification based on the principles of surgical treatment. World J Surg 25:1241–1244, 2001.
16. Lillemoe KD: Current management of bile duct injury. Br J Surg 95:403–405, 2008.
17. Sicklick JK, Camp MS, Lillemoe KD, et al: Surgical management of bile duct injuries sustained during laparoscopic cholecystectomy: Perioperative results in 200 patients. Ann Surg 241:786–792; discussion 793–785, 2005.
18. Nuzzo G, Giuliante F, Giovannini I, et al: Advantages of multidisciplinary management of bile duct injuries occurring during cholecystectomy. Am J Surg 195:763–769, 2008.
19. Schmidt SC, Langrehr JM, Hintze RE, et al: Long-term results and risk factors influencing outcome of major bile duct injuries following cholecystectomy. Br J Surg 92:76–82, 2005.
20. Misra S, Melton GB, Geschwind JF, et al: Percutaneous management of bile duct strictures and injuries associated with laparoscopic cholecystectomy: A decade of experience. J Am Coll Surg 198:218–226, 2004.
21. Goykhman Y, Kory I, Small R, et al: Long-term outcome and risk factors of failure after bile duct injury repair. J Gastrointest Surg 12:1412–1417, 2008.
22. Walsh RM, Henderson JM, Vogt DP, et al: Long-term outcome of biliary reconstruction for bile duct injuries from laparoscopic cholecystectomies. Surgery 142:450–456, 2007.
23. Zehetner J, Shamiyeh A, Wayand W: Lost gallstones in laparoscopic cholecystectomy: all possible complications. Am J Surg 193:73–78, 2007.
24. Mottershead M, Neuberger J: Transplantation in autoimmune liver diseases. World J Gastroenterol 14:3388–3395, 2008.
25. Rea DJ, Heimbach JK, Rosen CB, et al: Liver transplantation with neoadjuvant chemoradiation is more effective than resection for hilar cholangiocarcinoma. Ann Surg 242:451–458; discussion 458–461, 2005.
26. Todani T, Watanabe Y, Narusue M, et al: Congenital bile duct cysts: Classification, operative procedures, and review of thirty-seven cases including cancer arising from choledochal cyst. Am J Surg 134:263–269, 1977.

27. Stephen AE, Berger DL: Carcinoma in the porcelain gallbladder: A relationship revisited. Surgery 129:699–703, 2001.
28. Edge SB, Byrd DR, Compton CC, et al, editors: AJCC cancer staging manual, ed 7, New York, 2010, Springer.
29. D'Angelica M, Dalal KM, DeMatteo RP, et al: Analysis of the extent of resection for adenocarcinoma of the gallbladder. Ann Surg Oncol 16:806–816, 2009.
30. Ito F, Cho CS, Rikkers LF, et al: Hilar cholangiocarcinoma: Current management. Ann Surg 250:210–218, 2009.
31. Kennedy TJ, Yopp A, Qin Y, et al: Role of preoperative biliary drainage of liver remnant prior to extended liver resection for hilar cholangiocarcinoma. HPB (Oxford) 11:445–451, 2009.
32. Ferrero A, Lo Tesoriere R, Vigano L, et al: Preoperative biliary drainage increases infectious complications after hepatectomy for proximal bile duct tumor obstruction. World J Surg 33:318–325, 2009.
33. Bismuth H, Nakache R, Diamond T: Management strategies in resection for hilar cholangiocarcinoma. Ann Surg 215:31–38, 1992.
34. DeOliveira ML, Cunningham SC, Cameron JL, et al: Cholangiocarcinoma: Thirty-one-year experience with 564 patients at a single institution. Ann Surg 245:755–762, 2007.
35. Endo I, Gonen M, Yopp AC, et al: Intrahepatic cholangiocarcinoma: Rising frequency, improved survival, and determinants of outcome after resection. Ann Surg 248:84–96, 2008.
36. Alessiani M, Tzakis A, Todo S, et al: Assessment of five-year experience with abdominal organ cluster transplantation. J Am Coll Surg 180:1–9, 1995.
37. Heimbach JK, Gores GJ, Haddock MG, et al: Predictors of disease recurrence following neoadjuvant chemoradiotherapy and liver transplantation for unresectable perihilar cholangiocarcinoma. Transplantation 82:1703–1707, 2006.

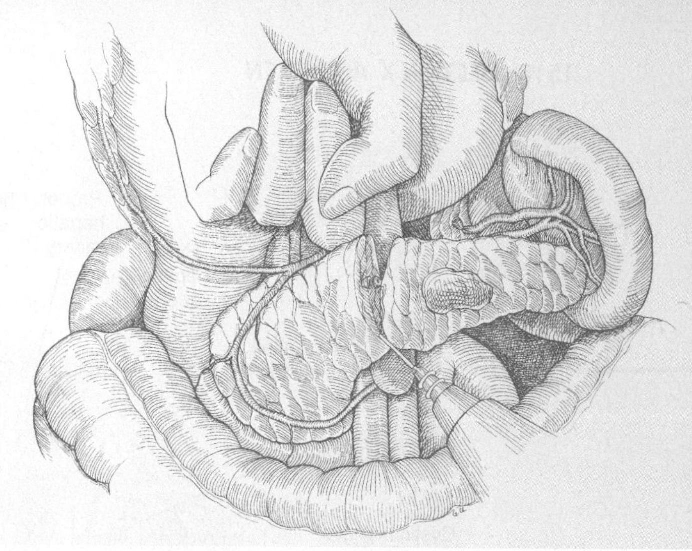

# CHAPTER 56

# EXOCRINE PANCREAS

Eric H. Jensen, Daniel Borja-Cacho,
Waddah B. Al-Refaie, and Selwyn M. Vickers



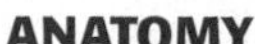

## ANATOMY

The average pancreas weighs between 75 and 125 g and measures 10 to 20 cm. It lies in the retroperitoneum just anterior to the first lumbar vertebrae and is anatomically divided into four portions, the head, neck, body and tail. The head lies to the right of midline within the C loop of the duodenum, immediately anterior to the vena cava at the confluence of the renal veins. The uncinate process extends from the head of the pancreas behind the superior mesenteric vein (SMV) and terminates adjacent to the superior mesenteric artery (SMA). The neck is the short segment of pancreas that immediately overlies the SMV. The body and tail of the pancreas then extend across the midline, anterior to Gerota's fascia and slightly cephalad, terminating within the splenic hilum (Fig. 56-1).

### Arterial Blood Supply

The pancreas is supplied by a complex arterial network arising from the celiac trunk and SMA. The head and uncinate process are supplied by the pancreaticoduodenal arteries (anterior and posterior), which arise from the hepatic artery via the gastroduodenal artery (GDA) superiorly and the SMA inferiorly. The neck, body, and tail receive arterial supply from the splenic arterial system. Several small branches originate from the length of the splenic artery, supplying arterial blood flow to the superior portion of the organ. The dorsal pancreatic artery arises from the splenic artery and courses posterior to the body of the gland to become the inferior pancreatic artery. The inferior pancreatic artery then runs along the inferior border of the pancreas, terminating at its tail.

### Venous Drainage

The venous drainage mimics the arterial supply, with blood flow from the head of the pancreas draining into the anterior and posterior pancreaticoduodenal veins. The posterior superior pancreaticoduodenal vein enters the SMV laterally at the superior border of the neck of the pancreas. The anterosuperior pancreaticoduodenal vein enters the right gastroepiploic vein just prior to its confluence with the SMV at the inferior border of the pancreas. The anterior and posteroinferior pancreaticoduodenal veins enter the SMV along the inferior border of the uncinate process. The remaining body and tail are drained via the splenic venous system.

## EMBRYOLOGY

The exocrine pancreas begins development during the fourth week of gestation. Pluripotent pancreatic epithelial stem cells give rise to exocrine and endocrine cell lines, as well as the intricate pancreatic ductal network. Initially, dorsal and ventral buds appear from the primitive duodenal endoderm (Fig. 56-2*A*). The dorsal bud typically appears first and ultimately develops into the superior head, neck, body, and tail of the mature pancreas. The ventral bud develops as part of the hepatic diverticulum and maintains communication with the biliary tree throughout development. The ventral bud will become the inferior part of the head and uncinate process of the gland. Between the fourth and eighth week, the ventral bud rotates posteriorly in a clockwise fashion to fuse with the dorsal bud (see Fig. 56-2*B*). At approximately 8 weeks' gestation, the dorsal and ventral buds are fused (see Fig. 56-2*C*).

The initiation of pancreas bud formation and differentiation of the ventral bud from the hepatic-biliary fates is dependent on the expression of pancreatic duodenal homeobox 1 (PDX1) protein and pancreas-specific transcription factor 1 (PTF1). In the absence of PDX1 expression in mice, pancreatic agenesis occurs, indicating its importance in the early phases of organogenesis. PTF1 expression is first detectable shortly after PDX1 in cells of the early endoderm, which will become the dorsal and ventral pancreas. By lineage analysis, 95% of acinar cells express PTF1. In PTF1 null mice, acini do not form. The notch signaling pathway is also critical to duct and acinar differentiation. In the absence of notch signaling, embryonic cells commit to endocrine lineage, suggesting that notch signaling is vital to exocrine differentiation. In addition to PDX1, PTF1, and notch signaling, complex interactions between mesenchymal growth factors such as transforming growth factor-β (TGF-β) and other signaling pathways, including hedgehog and Wnt, seem to play critical roles in pancreas development.[1] The precise interactions that lead to normal organogenesis continue to be defined. Table 56-1 summarizes the factors and pathways that affect pancreas development.

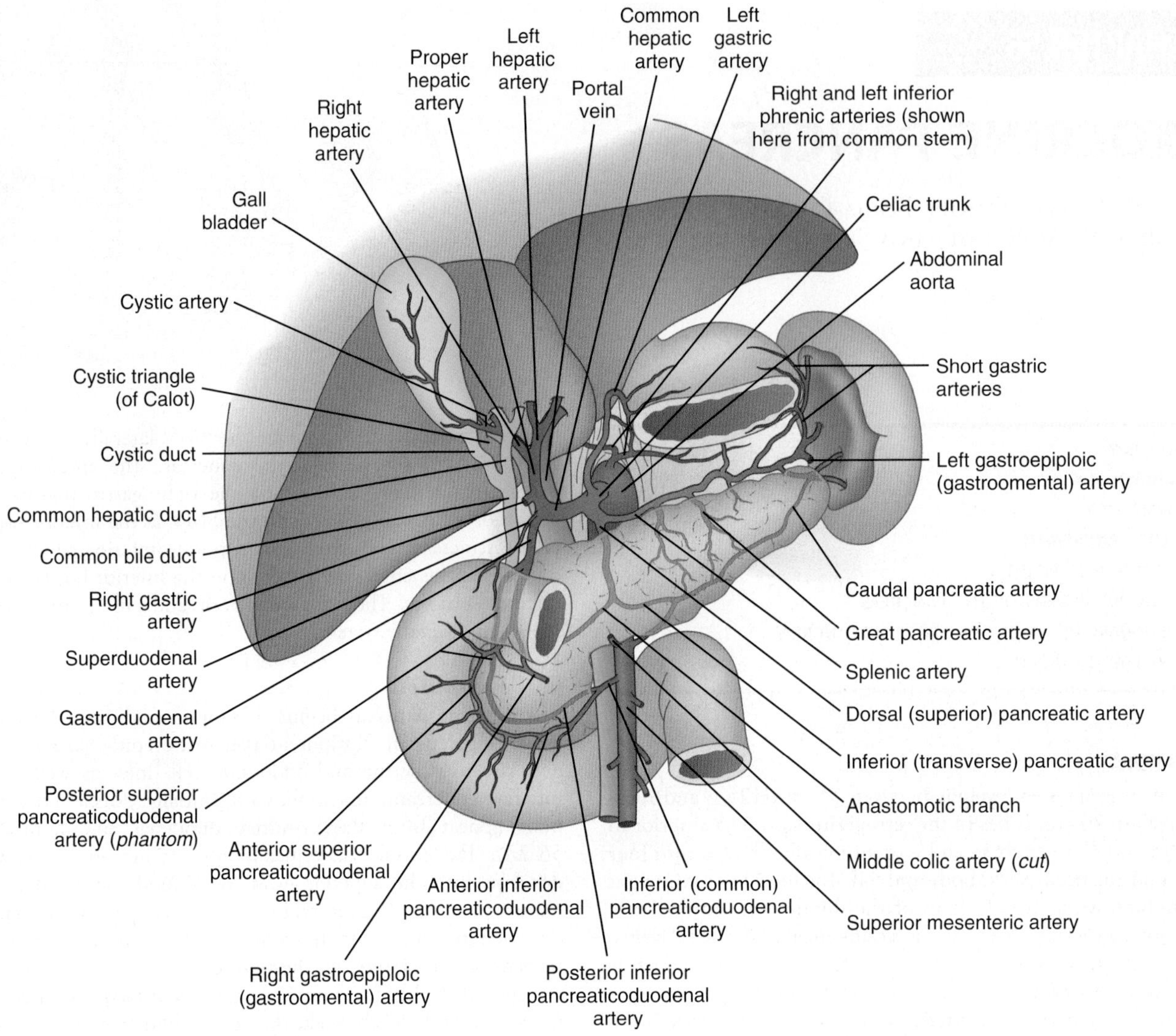

**FIGURE 56-1** Anatomy. (Netter illustration from www.netterimages.com. © Elsevier Inc. All rights reserved.)

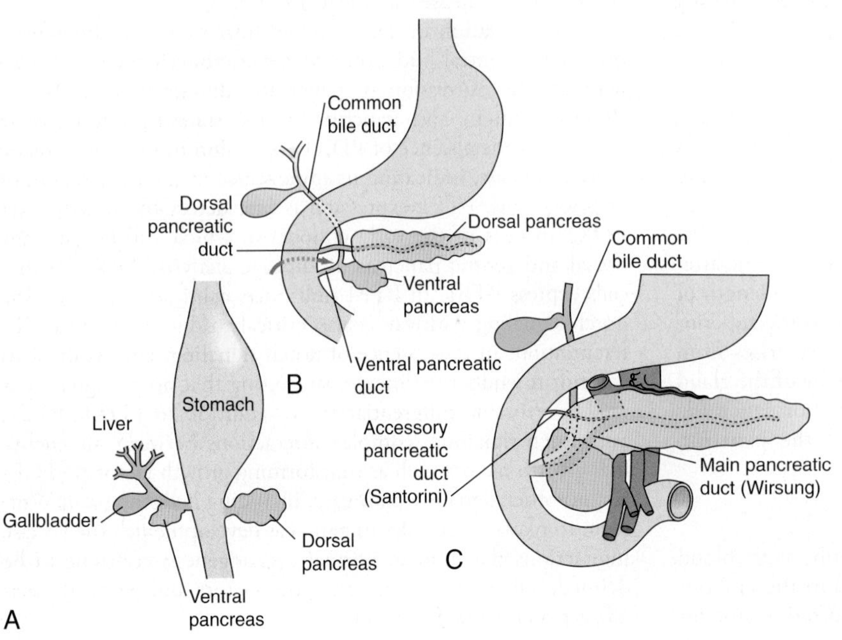


**FIGURE 56-2** Embryologic development of the pancreas.

**Table 56-1 Molecular Factors and Pathways Associated With Pancreatic Organogenesis**

| MUTATION | RELEVANCE |
|---|---|
| *PDX1* | Critical role in exocrine differentiation; knockout mice develop primitive pancreatic buds, but agenesis of the organ. |
| *PTF1* | Coexpression with *PDX1* determines progenitor cells to pancreatic fate. |
| Notch signaling pathway | Suppresses endocrine differentiation, promoting exocrine development. |
| Hedgehog signaling pathway | Inhibition of hedgehog in *PDX1*-positive cells leads to initiation of endoderm differentiation into pancreas lineage. |
| Wnt signaling pathway | Complex Wnt signaling is important in all aspects of pancreas development; lack of Wnt signaling results in absence of acinar tissue. |

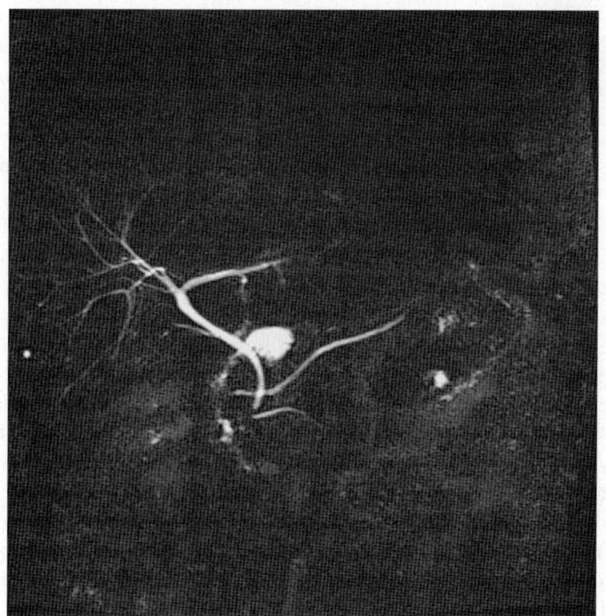

**FIGURE 56-3** MRCP showing pancreas divisum, with the dorsal pancreatic duct draining through the minor papilla and the ventral pancreatic duct joining the biliary tree draining through the major papilla.

### Pancreas Divisum

During normal organogenesis, the dorsal and ventral buds most commonly fuse to form a common duct, which enters the duodenum along with the common bile duct via the ampulla of Vater. Failure of the dorsal and ventral ducts to fuse during embryogenesis leads to pancreas divisum, a condition identified by a ventral pancreatic duct and common bile duct, which enter the duodenum via a major papilla, whereas a dorsal pancreatic duct enters through a minor papilla, which is slightly proximal (Fig. 56-3). Because most pancreatic exocrine secretions exit via the dorsal duct, pancreas divisum can lead to a condition of partial obstruction caused by a small minor papilla, leading to chronic backpressure in the duct. This relative outflow obstruction has been implicated in the development of relapsing acute or chronic pancreatitis. Although 10% of the population is affected by pancreas divisum, only rarely do affected individuals develop pancreatitis.

### Annular Pancreas

Annular pancreas results from aberrant migration of the ventral pancreas bud, which leads to circumferential or near-circumferential pancreas tissue surrounding the second portion of the duodenum. This abnormality may be associated with other congenital defects, including Down syndrome, malrotation, intestinal atresia, and cardiac malformations. If symptoms of obstruction occur, surgical bypass via duodenojejunostomy is performed.

### Ectopic Pancreas

Ectopic pancreas may arise anywhere along the primitive foregut, but is most common in the stomach, duodenum, and Meckel's diverticulum. Clinically, ectopic nodules may result in bowel obstruction caused by intussusception, bleeding, or ulceration. They can sometimes be found incidentally as firm yellow nodules that arise from the submucosa. Although there have been rare case reports of adenocarcinoma arising in ectopic pancreas tissue, resection is not necessary unless symptoms occur.

## PHYSIOLOGY

The human pancreas is a complex gland, with endocrine and exocrine functions. It is mainly composed of acinar cells (85% of the gland) and islets cells (2%) embedded in a complex extracellular matrix, which comprises 10% of the gland. The remaining 3% to 4% of the gland is comprised of the epithelial duct system and blood vessels.

### Major Components of Pancreatic Juice

The main function of the exocrine pancreas is to provide the vast majority of the enzymes needed for alimentary digestion. Acinar cells synthesize many enzymes (proteases) that digest food proteins such as trypsin, chymotrypsin, carboxypeptidase, and elastase. Under physiologic conditions, acinar cells synthesize these proteases as inactive proenzymes that are stored as intracellular zymogen granules. With stimulation of the pancreas, these proenzymes are secreted into the pancreatic duct and eventually the duodenal lumen. The duodenal mucosa synthesizes and secretes enterokinase, which is the critical enzyme in the enzymatic activation of trypsin from trypsinogen.[2] Trypsin also plays an important role in protein digestion by propagating pancreatic enzyme activation through autoactivation of trypsinogen and other proenzymes, such as chymotrypsinogen, procarboxypeptidase, and proelastase. Figure 56-4 summarizes the mechanisms of pancreatic exocrine secretion.

In addition to protease production, acinar cells also produce pancreatic amylase and lipase, also known as *glycerol ester hydrolase*, as active enzymes. With the exception of cellulose, pancreatic amylase hydrolyzes major polysaccharides into small oligosaccharides, which can be further digested by the oligosaccharidases present in the duodenal and jejunal epithelium. Pancreatic lipase hydrolyzes ingested fats into free fatty acids and 2-monoglycerides. In addition to pancreatic lipase, acinar cells produce other enzymes that digest fat, but they are secreted as proenzymes, like the proteases previously mentioned. These

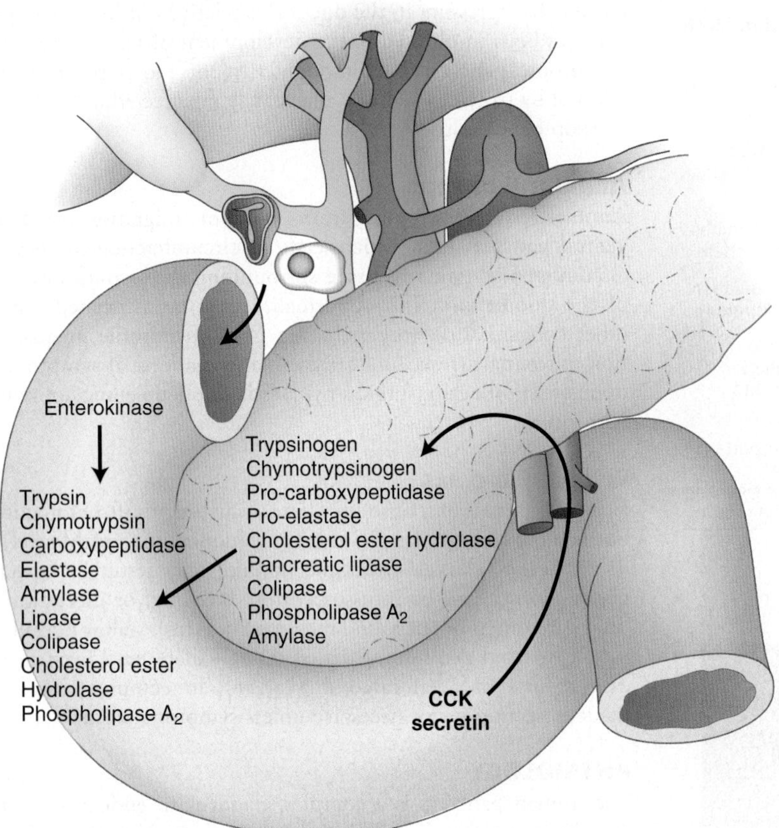


**FIGURE 56-4** Physiology of the secretion of pancreatic enzymes. The presence of peptides and fatty acids from food triggers the release of CCK. CCK induces the release of pancreatic enzymes into the duodenal lumen. Conversely, S cells located in the duodenum release secretin in response to the acidification of the duodenum. Secretin induces the secretion of $HCO_3^-$ from pancreatic cells into the duodenum.

include colipase, cholesterol ester hydrolase, and phospholipase A2. The main function of colipase is to increase the activity of pancreatic lipase. Cholesterol esters are cleaved by cholesterol ester hydrolase into free cholesterol and one fatty acid, phospholipase A2 hydrolyzes phospholipids, and pancreatic acinar cells also secrete deoxyribonuclease and ribonuclease. These are enzymes required for the hydrolysis of DNA and RNA, respectively.

Pancreatic enzymes are inactive inside acinar cells because they are synthesized and stored as inactive enzymes. In addition to this autoprotective mechanism, acinar cells synthesize pancreatic secretory trypsin inhibitor, which also protects acinar cells from autodigestion because it counteracts premature activation of trypsinogen inside acinar cells. Pancreatic secretory trypsin inhibitor is encoded by serine protease inhibitor Kazal type 1 *(SPINK-1)* gene. *SPINK-1* gene mutations are associated with the development of chronic pancreatitis, especially in childhood.

The primary function of pancreatic duct cells is to provide the water and electrolytes required to dilute and deliver the enzymes synthesized by acinar cells. Although the concentrations of sodium and potassium are similar to their respective concentration in plasma, the concentrations of bicarbonate and chloride vary significantly, according to the secretion phase.

The mechanism responsible of the secretion of bicarbonate was first described in 1988 based on in vitro studies. According to this model, extracellular $CO_2$ diffuses across the basolateral membrane of ductal cells. Once $CO_2$ is inside pancreatic duct cells, it is hydrated by intracellular carbonic anhydrase; as a result of this reaction, $HCO_3^-$ and $H^+$ are generated. The apical membrane of pancreatic duct cells contains an anion exchanger that secretes intracellular $HCO_3^-$ into the lumen of the cell and favors the exchange of luminal $Cl^-$ inside the ductal epithelium. Recent studies have shown that this exchanger interacts with the cystic fibrosis transmembrane conductance regulator (CFTR). This may correlate with the inability of patients with cystic fibrosis to secrete water and bicarbonate. Although the nature of this exchanger has not been completely elucidated, it is possible that this anion exchanger is an SLC26 family member. This family contains different anion exchangers that transport monovalent and divalent anions, such as $Cl^-$ and $HCO_3^-$. Some of these exchangers are known to interact with CFTR.

In addition to $HCO_3^-$, $CO_2$ hydration also generates $H^+$ ions, which are secreted by $Na^+$ and $H^+$ exchangers present in the basolateral membrane of ductal cells. These exchangers belong to the *SLC9* gene family. The main function of these exchangers is to maintain the intracellular pH within a physiologic range. In addition, the basolateral membrane of duct cells contains multiple $Na^+,K^+$-ATPases that provide the primary force that drives $HCO_3^-$ secretion; the $Na^+,K^+$-ATPase maintains the $Na^+$ gradient used to extrude $H^+$ as well. Finally, $K^+$ channels present in the basolateral membrane of acinar cells maintain the membrane potential to allow recirculation of $K^+$ ions brought by the $Na^+,K^+$ pump inside the cell. Figure 56-5 illustrates $HCO_3^-$ secretion inside pancreatic duct cells.

Once the $HCO_3^-$ secreted by pancreatic duct cells reaches the duodenal lumen, it neutralizes the hydrochloric acid secreted by parietal cells. Pancreatic enzymes are inactivated at a low pH; therefore, pancreatic bicarbonate provides an optimal pH for acinar cell enzyme function. The optimal pH for the function

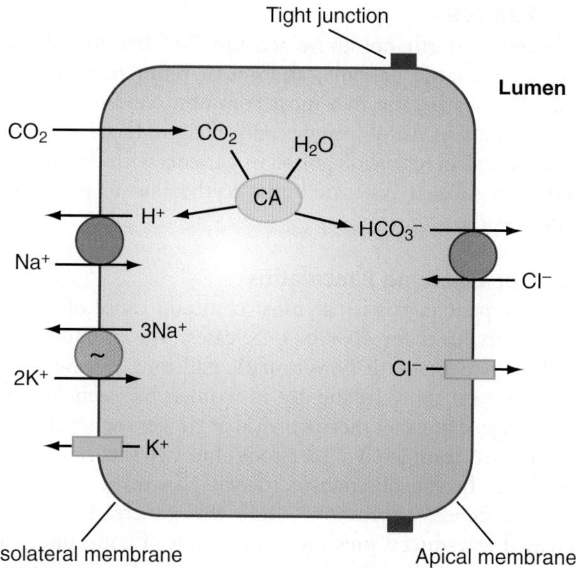


**FIGURE 56-5** Cellular mechanism proposed for $HCO_3^-$ secretion by pancreatic duct epithelium. (From Steward MC, Ishiguro H, Case RM: Mechanisms of bicarbonate secretion in the pancreatic duct. Annu Rev Physiol 67:377–409, 2005.)

of chymotrypsin and trypsin is from 8.0 to 9.0, for amylase the optimal pH is 7.0, and for lipase it is from 7.0 to 9.0.

### Phases and Regulation of Pancreatic Secretion

Pancreatic exocrine secretion occurs during the interdigestive state and after the ingestion of food, which is also known as the *digestive state*. The same phases of secretion that have been identified in the stomach during the digestive state have been also described in pancreatic secretion. The first phase is the cephalic phase, in which the pancreas is stimulated by the vagus nerve in response to the sight, smell, or taste of food. This phase is generally mediated by the release of acetylcholine at the terminal endings of postganglionic fibers. The main effect of acetylcholine is to induce acinar cell secretion of enzymes. This phase accounts for 20% to 25% of the daily secretion of pancreatic juice.

The second phase of pancreatic secretion is known as the *gastric phase*. It is mediated by vagovagal reflexes triggered by gastric distention after the ingestion of food. These reflexes induce acinar cell secretion. It accounts for 10% of the pancreatic juice produced daily.

The most important phase of pancreatic secretion is the intestinal phase, which accounts for 65% to 70% of the total secretion of pancreatic juice. It is mediated by secretin and cholecystokinin (CCK). Acidification of the duodenal lumen induces the release of secretin by S cells. Secretin was the first polypeptide hormone identified more than 100 years ago. It is the most important mediator of the secretion of water, bicarbonate, and other electrolytes into the duodenum. Secretin receptors are located in the basolateral membrane of all pancreatic duct cells but cannot be identified in other pancreatic components, such as islet cells, blood vessels, or extracellular matrix. Secretin receptors are members of the G protein–coupled receptor superfamily. The most important effect of secretin stimulation is an increase of intracellular cyclic adenosine monophosphate (cAMP), which activates the $HCO_3^-$-$Cl^-$ anion exchanger in the apical membrane of pancreatic duct cells. It also increases the activity of the enzyme carbonic anhydrase, the excretion of $H^+$ outside the duct cell, and the activity of the CFTR.

The presence of lipid, protein, and carbohydrates inside the duodenum induces the secretion of CCK-releasing factor and monitor peptide. Both peptides induce release of CCK by I cells present in the duodenal mucosa. Whereas secretin is the main mediator of the secretion of water and bicarbonate in the intestinal phase, CCK is the main mediator of the secretion of pancreatic enzymes. CCK exerts a number of effects:

1. It travels through the bloodstream and induces the release of pancreatic enzymes by acinar cells.
2. It induces local duodenal vagovagal reflexes that cause the release of acetylcholine, vasoactive intestinal peptide, and gastrin-releasing peptide, which promotes the release of pancreatic enzymes.
3. CCK induces the relaxation of the sphincter of Oddi. Also, it should be noted that CCK potentiates the effects of secretin, and vice versa.

## ACUTE PANCREATITIS

The incidence of acute pancreatitis (AP) has increased during the past 20 years. AP is responsible for more than 300,000 hospital admissions annually in the United States. Most patients develop a mild and self-limited course; however, 10% to 20% of patients have a rapidly progressive inflammatory response associated with prolonged length of hospital stay and significant morbidity and mortality. Patients with mild pancreatitis have a mortality rate of less than 1% but, in severe pancreatitis, this increases up to 10% to 30%.[3] The most common cause of death in this group of patients is multiorgan dysfunction syndrome. Mortality in pancreatitis has a bimodal distribution; in the first 2 weeks, also known as the *early phase*, the multiorgan dysfunction syndrome is the final result of an intense inflammatory cascade triggered initially by pancreatic inflammation. Mortality after 2 weeks, also known as the *late period*, is often caused by septic complications.[4]

### Pathophysiology

The exact mechanism whereby predisposing factors such as ethanol and gallstones produce pancreatitis is not completely known. Most researchers believe that AP is the final result of abnormal pancreatic enzyme activation inside acinar cells. Immunolocalization studies have shown that after 15 minutes of pancreatic injury, both zymogen granules and lysosomes colocalize inside the acinar cells. The fact that zymogen and lysosome colocalization occurs before amylase level elevation, pancreatic edema, and other markers of pancreatitis are evident suggests that colocalization is an early step in the pathophysiology and not a consequence of pancreatitis. In addition, the inflammatory response seen in AP can be prevented if acinar cells are pretreated with cathepsin B inhibitors. In vivo studies have also shown that cathepsin B knockout mice have a significant decrease in the severity of pancreatitis.[2]

Intra-acinar pancreatic enzyme activation induces autodigestion of normal pancreatic parenchyma. In response to this initial insult, acinar cells release proinflammatory cytokines, such as tumor necrosis factor-α (TNF-α), interleukins (IL)-1, -2, and -6, and anti-inflammatory mediators such as IL-10 and IL-1 receptor antagonist. These mediators do not initiate pancreatic injury but propagate the response locally and systemically. As a result, TNF-α, IL-1, and IL-7, neutrophils, and macrophages are recruited into the pancreatic parenchyma and cause the release of more TNF- α, IL-1, IL-6, reactive oxygen metabolites, prostaglandins, platelet-activating factor, and leukotrienes. The local inflammatory response further aggravates the pancreatitis because it increases the permeability and damages the microcirculation of the pancreas. In severe cases, the inflammatory response causes local hemorrhage and pancreatic necrosis. In addition, some of the inflammatory mediators released by neutrophils aggravate the pancreatic injury because they cause pancreatic enzyme activation.[5]

The inflammatory cascade is self-limited in approximately 80% to 90% of patients. However, in the remaining patients, a vicious cycle of recurring pancreatic injury and local and systemic inflammatory reaction persists. In a small number of patients, there is a massive release of inflammatory mediators to the systemic circulation. Active neutrophils mediate acute lung injury and induce the adult distress respiratory syndrome frequently seen in patients with severe pancreatitis. The mortality seen in the early phase of pancreatitis is the result of this persistent inflammatory response. A summary of the inflammatory cascade seen in AP is shown in Figure 56-6.

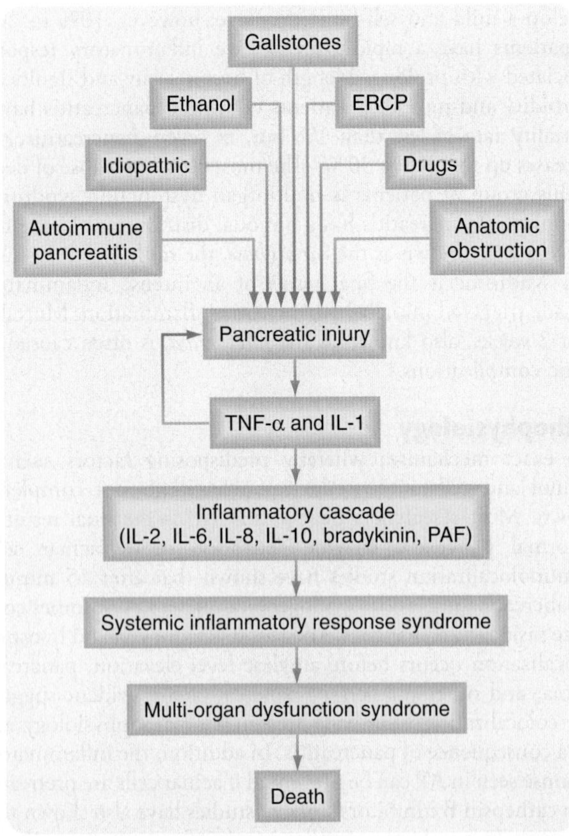


**FIGURE 56-6** Pathophysiology of severe acute pancreatitis. The local injury induces the release of TNF-α and IL-1. Both cytokines produce further pancreatic injury and amplify the inflammatory response by inducing the release of other inflammatory mediators, which cause distant organ injury. This abnormal inflammatory response is responsible for the mortality seen during the early phase of acute pancreatitis.

## Risk Factors

Gallstones and ethanol abuse account for 70% to 80% of AP cases. In pediatric patients, abdominal blunt trauma and systemic diseases are the two most common conditions that lead to pancreatitis. Autoimmune and drug-induced pancreatitis should be a differential diagnosis in patients with rheumatologic conditions such as systemic lupus erythematosus and Sjögren's syndrome.

### Biliary or Gallstone Pancreatitis

Gallstone pancreatitis is the most common cause of AP in the West. It accounts for 40% of U.S. cases. The overall incidence of AP in patients with symptomatic gallstone disease is 3% to 8%. It is seen more frequently in women between 50 and 70 years of age. The exact mechanism that triggers pancreatic injury has not been completely understood, but two theories have been proposed.[6] In the obstructive theory, pancreatic injury is the result of excessive pressure inside the pancreatic duct. This increased intraductal pressure is the result of continuous secretion of pancreatic juice in the presence of pancreatic duct obstruction. The second, or reflux, theory proposes that stones become impacted in the ampulla of Vater and form a common channel that allows bile salt reflux into the pancreas. Animal models have shown that bile salts cause direct acinar cell necrosis because they increase the concentration of calcium in the cytoplasm; however, this has never been proven in humans.[2]

### Alcohol-Induced Injury

Excessive ethanol consumption is the second most common cause of AP worldwide. It accounts for 35% of cases and is more prevalent in young men (30 to 45 years of age) than in women. However, only 5% to 10% of patients who drink alcohol develop AP. Factors that contribute to ethanol-induces pancreatitis include heavy ethanol abuse (>100 g/day for at least 5 years), smoking, and genetic predisposition. As compared with nonsmokers, the relative risk of alcohol-induced pancreatitis in smokers is 4.9.[7]

Alcohol has a number of deleterious effects in the pancreas. It triggers proinflammatory pathways such as nuclear factor κB (NF-κB), which increase the production of TNF-α and IL-1. It also increases the expression and activity of caspases. Caspases are proteases that mediate apoptosis. In addition, alcohol decreases pancreatic perfusion, induces sphincter of Oddi spasm, and obstructs pancreatic ducts through the precipitation of proteins inside the ducts.[8]

### Anatomic Obstruction

Abnormal flow of pancreatic juice into the duodenum can result in pancreatic injury. AP has been described in patients with pancreatic tumors, parasites, and congenital defects.

Pancreas divisum is an anatomic variation present in 10% of the population. Its association with AP is controversial. Patients with this variation have a 5% to 10% lifetime risk of developing AP caused by relative outflow obstruction through the minor papilla. Endoscopic retrograde cholangiopancreatography (ERCP) with minor papillotomy and stenting may be beneficial for such patients.

Infrequent anatomic obstructions that have been associated with AP include *Ascaris lumbricoides* infection and annular pancreas. Although pancreatic cancer is not uncommon, patients with pancreatic cancer usually do not develop AP.

#### Endoscopic Retrograde Cholangiopancreatography–Induced Pancreatitis

AP is the most common complication after ERCP, occurring in up to 5% of patients. AP occurs more frequently in patients who have undergone therapeutic procedures as compared with diagnostic procedures. It is also more common in patients who have had multiple attempts of cannulation, sphincter of Oddi dysfunction, and abnormal visualization of the secondary pancreatic ducts after contrast injection. The clinical course is mild in 90% to 95% of patients.[8]

#### Drug-Induced Pancreatitis

Up to 2% of AP cases are caused by medications. The most common agents include sulfonamides, metronidazole, erythromycin, tetracyclines, didanosine, thiazides, furosemide, 3-hydroxy-3-methylglutaryl-coenzyme A (HMG-CoA) reductase inhibitors (statins), azathioprine, 6-mercaptopurine, 5-aminosalicylic acid, sulfasalazine, valproic acid, and acetaminophen. More recently, antiretroviral agents used for the treatment of AIDS have been implicated in AP.

#### Metabolic Factors

Hypertriglyceridemia and hypercalcemia can also lead to pancreatic damage. Direct pancreatic injury can be induced by triglyceride metabolites. It is more common in patients with type I, II, or V hyperlipidemia. It should be suspected in patients with a triglyceride level higher than 1000 mg/dL. A triglyceride level higher than 2000 mg/dL confirms the diagnosis. Hypertriglyceridemia secondary to hypothyroidism, diabetes mellitus, and alcohol does not typically induce AP.

Hypercalcemia is postulated to induce pancreatic injury through the activation of trypsinogen to trypsin and intraductal precipitation of calcium, leading to ductal obstruction and subsequent attacks of pancreatitis. Approximately 1.5% to 13% of patients with primary hyperparathyroidism develop AP.[8]

#### Miscellaneous Conditions

Blunt and penetrating abdominal trauma can be associated with AP in 0.2% and 1% of cases, respectively. Prolonged intraoperative hypotension and excessive pancreatic manipulation during abdominal surgery can also result in AP. Pancreatic ischemia in association with acute pancreatic inflammation can develop after splenic artery embolization. Other rare causes include scorpion venom stings and perforated duodenal ulcers.

### Clinical Manifestations

The cardinal symptom of AP is epigastric and/or periumbilical pain that radiates to the back. Up to 90% of patients have nausea and/or vomiting that typically does not relieve the pain. The nature of the pain is constant; therefore, if the pain disappears or decreases, another diagnosis should be considered.

Dehydration, poor skin turgor, tachycardia, hypotension, and dry mucous membranes are commonly seen in patients with AP. Severely dehydrated and older patients may also develop mental status changes.

The physical examination of the abdomen varies according to the severity of the disease. With mild pancreatitis, the physical examination of the abdomen may be normal or reveal only mild epigastric tenderness. Significant abdominal distention, associated with generalized rebound and abdominal rigidity, is present in severe pancreatitis. Note the nature of the pain described by the patient may not correlate with the physical examination or the degree of pancreatic inflammation.

Rare findings include flank and periumbilical ecchymosis (Grey Turner and Cullen's signs, respectively). Both are indicative of retroperitoneal bleeding associated with severe pancreatitis. Patients with concomitant choledocholithiasis or significant edema in the head of the pancreas that compresses the intrapancreatic portion of the common bile duct can present with jaundice. Dullness to percussion and decreased breathing sounds in the left or, less commonly, in the right hemithorax suggest pleural effusion secondary to AP.

### Diagnosis

The cornerstone of the diagnosis of AP are the clinical findings plus an elevation of pancreatic enzyme levels in the plasma. A threefold or higher elevation of amylase and lipase levels confirms the diagnosis. Amylase's serum half-life is shorter as compared with lipase. In patients who do not present to the emergency department within the first 24 or 48 hours after the onset of symptoms, determination of lipase levels is a more sensitive indicator to establish the diagnosis. Lipase is also a more specific marker of AP because serum amylase levels can be elevated in a number of conditions, such as such as peptic ulcer disease, mesenteric ischemia, salpingitis, and macroamylasemia.

Patients with AP are typically hyperglycemic; they can also have leukocytosis and abnormal elevation of liver enzyme levels. The elevation of alanine aminotransferase levels in the serum in the context of AP confirmed by high pancreatic enzyme levels has a positive predictive value of 95% in the diagnosis of acute biliary pancreatitis.[6]

#### Imaging Studies

Although simple abdominal radiographs are not useful to diagnose pancreatitis, they can help rule out other conditions, such as perforated ulcer disease. Nonspecific findings in patients with AP include air-fluid levels suggestive of ileus, cutoff colon sign as a result of colonic spasm at the splenic flexure, and widening of the duodenal C loop caused by severe pancreatic head edema.

The usefulness of ultrasound to diagnose pancreatitis is limited by intra-abdominal fat and increased intestinal gas as a result of the ileus. Nevertheless, this test should always be ordered in patients with AP because of its high sensitivity (95%) in diagnosing gallstones. Combined elevation of liver transaminase and pancreatic enzyme levels, and the presence of gallstones on ultrasound, have an even higher sensitivity (97%) and specificity (100%) for diagnosing acute biliary pancreatitis.

Contrast-enhanced computed tomography (CT) is currently the best modality to evaluate the pancreas, especially if the study is performed using a multidetector CT scanner. The most valuable contrast phase to evaluate the pancreatic parenchyma is the portal venous phase (65 to 70 seconds after contrast injection), which allows evaluation of the viability of the pancreatic parenchyma amount of peripancreatic inflammation and presence of intra-abdominal free air or fluid collections. Noncontrast CT scanning may also be of value in the setting of renal failure by identifying fluid collections and/or extraluminal air.[9]

Abdominal magnetic resonance imaging (MRI) is also useful to evaluate the extent of necrosis, inflammation, and presence of free fluid. However, its cost and availability, and the fact that patients requiring imaging are critically ill and need to be in intensive care units, limit its applicability in the acute phase. Although magnetic resonance cholangiopancreatography (MRCP) is not indicated in the acute setting of AP, it has an important role in the evaluation of patients with unexplained or recurrent pancreatitis because it allows complete visualization of the biliary and pancreatic duct anatomy. In addition, IV administration of secretin increases pancreatic duct secretion, which causes a transient distention of the pancreatic duct. For example, secretin MRCP is useful in patients with AP and no evidence of a predisposing condition to rule out pancreas divisum, intraductal papillary mucinous neoplasm (IPMN), or the presence of a small tumor in the pancreatic duct.[9]

In the setting of gallstone pancreatitis, endoscopic ultrasound (EUS) may play an important role in the evaluation of persistent choledocholithiasis. Several studies have shown that routine ERCP for suspected gallstone pancreatitis reveals no evidence of persistent obstruction in most cases and may actually worsen symptoms because of manipulation of the gland. EUS has been proven to be sensitive for identifying choledocholithiasis; it allows for examination of the biliary tree and pancreas with no risk of worsening the pancreatitis. In patients in whom persistent choledocholithiasis is confirmed by EUS, ERCP can be used selectively as a therapeutic measure.

### Assessment of Severity of Disease

The earliest scoring system designed to evaluate the severity of AP was introduced by Ranson and colleagues in 1974.[10] It predicts the severity of the disease based on 11 parameters obtained at the time of admission and/or 48 hours later. The mortality rate of AP directly correlates with the number of parameters that are positive. Severe pancreatitis is diagnosed if three or more of the Ranson criteria are fulfilled. The main disadvantage is that it does not predict the severity of disease at the time of the admission because six parameters are only assessed after 48 hours of admission. Ranson's score has a low positive predictive value (50%) and high negative predictive value (90%). Therefore, it is mainly used to rule out severe pancreatitis or predict the risk of mortality.[11] The original scoring symptom designed to predict the severity of the disease and its modification for acute biliary pancreatitis are shown in Boxes 56-1 and 56-2.

AP severity can also be addressed using the Acute Physiology and Chronic Health Evaluation (APACHE II) score. Based on the patient's age, previous health status, and 12 routine physiologic measurements, APACHE II provides a general measure of the severity of disease. An APACHE II score of 8 or higher defines severe pancreatitis. The main advantage is that it can be used on admission and repeated at any time. However, it is complex, not specific for AP, and based on the patient's age, which easily upgrades the AP severity score. APACHE II has a positive predictive value of 43% and a negative predictive value of 89%.[11]

Using imaging characteristics, Balthazar and associates[12] have established the CT severity index. This index correlates CT findings with the patient's outcome. The CT severity index is shown in Table 56-2.

In 1992, the International Symposium on Acute Pancreatitis defined severe pancreatitis as the presence of local pancreatic complications (necrosis, abscess, or pseudocyst) or any evidence of organ failure. Severe pancreatitis is diagnosed if there is any evidence of organ failure or a local pancreatic complication (Box 56-3).

**BOX 56-1 Ranson's Prognostic Criteria for Nongallstone Pancreatitis**

At presentation
- Age >55 yr
- Blood glucose level >200 mg/dL
- WBC >16,000 cells/mm$^3$
- Lactate dehydrogenase level >350 IU/L
- Aspartate aminotransferase >250 IU/L

After 48 hours of admission
- Hematocrit*: Decrease >10%
- Serum calcium level <8 mg/dL
- Base deficit >4 mEq/L
- Blood urea nitrogen level†: Increase >5 mg/dL
- Fluid requirement >6 liters
- $Pao_2$ <60 mm Hg

Ranson score ≥3 defines severe pancreatitis.
*As compared with admission value.

**BOX 56-2 Ranson's Prognostic Criteria for Gallstone Pancreatitis**

At presentation
- Age >70 yr
- Blood glucose level >220 mg/dL
- WBC >18,000 cells/mm$^3$
- Lactate dehydrogenase level >400 IU/liter
- Aspartate aminotransferase level >250 IU/liter

After 48 hours of admission
- Hematocrit*: Decrease >10%
- Serum calcium level <8 mg/dL
- Base deficit >5 mEq/L
- Blood urea nitrogen level†: Increase >2 mg/dL
- Fluid requirement >4 liters
- $Pao_2$: Not available

Ranson score ≥3 defines severe pancreatitis.
*As compared with admission value.

C-reactive protein (CRP) is an inflammatory marker that peaks 48 to 72 hours after the onset of pancreatitis and correlates with the severity of the disease. A CRP level 150 mg/mL or higher defines severe pancreatitis. The major limitation is that it cannot be used on admission; the sensitivity of the assay decreases if CRP levels are measured within 48 hours after the onset of symptoms. In addition to CRP, a number of studies have shown other biochemical markers (e.g., serum levels of procalcitonin, IL-6, IL-1, elastase) that correlate with the severity of the disease. However, their main limitation is their cost and that they are not widely available.

### Treatment

Regardless of the cause or the severity of the disease, the cornerstone of the treatment of chronic pancreatitis is aggressive fluid resuscitation using isotonic crystalloid solution. The rate of administration should be individualized and adjusted based on age, comorbidities, vital signs, mental status, skin turgor, and urine output. Patients who do not respond to initial fluid

**Table 56-2 Computed Tomography Severity Index (CTSI) for Acute Pancreatitis**

| FEATURE | POINTS |
|---|---|
| **Pancreatic Inflammation** | |
| Normal pancreas | 0 |
| Focal or diffuse pancreatic enlargement | 1 |
| Intrinsic pancreatic alterations with peripancreatic fat inflammatory changes | 2 |
| Single fluid collection/or phlegmon | 3 |
| Two or more fluid collections or gas, in or adjacent to the pancreas | 4 |
| **Pancreatic Necrosis** | |
| None | 0 |
| ≤30% | 2 |
| 30%-50% | 4 |
| >50% | 6 |

CTSI, 0-3, mortality 3%, morbidity 8%; CTSI, 4-6, mortality 6%, morbidity 35%; CTSI, 7-10, mortality 17%, morbidity 92%.

**BOX 56-3 Atlanta's Criteria for Acute Pancreatitis**

**Organ Failure As Defined**

Shock (systolic blood pressure <90 mm Hg)

Pulmonary insufficiency ($Pao_2$ <60 mm Hg)

Renal failure (creatinine level >2 mg/dL after fluid resuscitation)

GI bleeding (>500 mL/24 hr)

**Systemic Complications**

Disseminated intravascular coagulation (platelet count ≤100,000)

Fibrinogen <1 gr/L

Fibrin split products >80 μg/dL

Metabolic disturbance (calcium level ≤7.5 mg/dL)

**Local Complications**

Necrosis

Abscess

Pseudocyst

Severe pancreatitis is defined by the presence of any evidence of organ failure or a local complication.

resuscitation or have significant renal, cardiac or respiratory comorbidities often require invasive monitoring with central venous access and a Foley catheter.

In addition to fluid resuscitation, patients with AP require continuous pulse oximetry because one of the most common systemic complications of AP is hypoxemia caused by the acute lung injury associated with this disease. Patients should receive supplementary oxygen to maintain arterial saturation above 95%.

It is also essential to provide effective analgesia. Narcotics are usually preferred, especially morphine. One of the physiologic effects described after systemic administration of morphine is an increase in tone in the sphincter of Oddi; however, there is no evidence that narcotics exert a negative impact in the outcome of patients with AP.

There is no proven benefit in treating AP with antiproteases (e.g., gabexate mesilate, aprotinin), platelet-activating factor inhibitors (e.g., lexipafant), or pancreatic secretion inhibitors.[3]

Nutritional support is vital in the treatment of AP. Oral feeding may be impossible because of persistent ileus, pain, or intubation. In addition, 20% of patients with severe AP develop recurrent pain shortly after the oral route has been restarted. The main options to provide this nutritional support are enteral feeding and total parenteral nutrition (TPN). Although there is no difference in the mortality rate between both types of nutrition, enteral nutrition is associated with less infectious complications and reduces the need for pancreatic surgery. Although TPN provides most nutritional requirements, it is associated with mucosal atrophy, decreased intestinal blood flow, increased risk of bacterial overgrowth in the small bowel, antegrade colonization with colonic bacteria, and increased bacterial translocation. In addition, patients with TPN have more central line infections and metabolic complications (e.g., hyperglycemia, electrolyte imbalance). Whenever possible, enteral nutrition should be used, rather than TPN.

Given the significant increase in mortality associated with septic complications in severe pancreatitis, a number of physicians advocated the use of prophylactic antibiotics in the 1970s. Recent meta-analyses and systematic reviews that have evaluated multiple randomized control trials have proven that prophylactic antibiotics do not decrease the frequency of surgical intervention, infected necrosis, or mortality in patients with severe pancreatitis. In addition, they are associated with gram-positive cocci infection such as by *Staphylococcus aureus*, and *Candida* infection, which is seen in 5% to 15% of patients.[13]

### Special Considerations

**Endoscopic Retrograde Cholangiopancreatography** Early ERCP, with or without sphincterotomy, was initially advocated to reduce the severity of pancreatitis because the obstructive theory of AP states that pancreatic injury is the result of pancreatic duct obstruction. However, three randomized trials have demonstrated that ERCP is only beneficial for patients with severe acute biliary pancreatitis. Routine use of ERCP is not indicated for patients with mild pancreatitis because the bile duct obstruction is usually transient and resolves within 48 hours after the onset of symptoms. In addition to severe acute biliary pancreatitis, ERCP is indicated for patients who develop cholangitis and those with persistent bile duct obstruction demonstrated by other imaging modalities, such as EUS. Finally, in older patients with poor performance status or severe comorbidities that preclude surgery, ERCP with sphincterotomy is a safe alternative to prevent recurrent biliary pancreatitis.

**Laparoscopic Cholecystectomy** In the absence of definitive treatment, 30% of patients with acute biliary pancreatitis will have recurrent disease. With the exception of older patients and those with poor performance status, laparoscopic cholecystectomy is indicated for all patients with mild acute biliary pancreatitis.[3] Studies have shown that early laparoscopic cholecystectomy, defined as laparoscopic cholecystectomy during the initial admission to the hospital, is a safe procedure that decreases recurrence of the disease.[6] Choledocolithiasis can be excluded via intraoperative cholangiography, ERCP, or laparoscopic common bile duct exploration.

For patients with severe pancreatitis, early surgery may increase the morbidity and length of stay.[14] Current recommendations suggest conservative treatment for at least 6 weeks before laparoscopic cholecystectomy is attempted in this setting. This approach has significantly decreased morbidity.[6]

## Complications

### Sterile and Infected Peripancreatic Fluid Collections

The presence of acute abdominal fluid during an episode of AP has been described in 30% to 57% of patients.[3] In contrast to pseudocysts and cystic neoplasias of the pancreas, fluid collections are not surrounded or encased by epithelium or fibrotic capsule. Treatment is supportive because most fluid collections will be spontaneously reabsorbed by the peritoneum. The presence of fever, elevated white blood cell (WBC) count, and abdominal pain suggest infection of this fluid and percutaneous aspiration is confirmatory. Percutaneous drainage and IV administration of antibiotics should be instituted if infection is present.

### Pancreatic Necrosis and Infected Necrosis

Pancreatic necrosis is the presence of nonviable pancreatic parenchyma or peripancreatic fat; it can present as a focal area or diffuse involvement of the gland. Contrast-enhanced CT is the most reliable technique to diagnose pancreatic necrosis. It is typically seen as areas of low attenuation (<40 to 50 HU) after the injection of IV contrast. Normal parenchyma usually has a density of 100 to 150 HU.[9] Up to 20% of patients with AP develop pancreatic necrosis. It is important to identify and provide proper treatment of this complication because most patients who develop multiorgan failure have necrotizing pancreatitis; pancreatic necrosis has been documented in up to 80% of the autopsies of patients who died after an episode of AP.[4]

The main complication of pancreatic necrosis is infection. The risk is directly related to the amount of necrosis; in patients with pancreatic necrosis involving less than 30% of the gland, the risk of infection is 22%. The risk is 37% for patients with pancreatic necrosis that involves 30% to 50% of the gland and up to 46% if more than 70% of the gland is affected.[4] This complication is associated with bacterial translocation usually involving enteric flora, such as gram-negative rods (e.g., *Escherichia coli*, *Klebsiella* and *Pseudomonas* spp.) and *Enterococcus* spp.

Infected pancreatic necrosis should be suspected in patients with prolonged fever, elevated WBC count, or progressive clinical deterioration. Evidence of air within the pancreatic necrosis seen on a CT scan confirms the diagnosis but is a rare finding. If infected necrosis is suspected, fine-needle aspiration (FNA) should be performed. A positive Gram stain and/or culture establish the diagnosis. Although positive cultures are confirmatory, a recent review has demonstrated that despite negative preoperative cultures, 42% of patients with so-called *persistent unwellness* will have infected necrosis.[15] Figure 56-7 illustrates the pathophysiology of pancreatic necrosis infection.

Once infection has been demonstrated, IV antibiotics should be given. Because of their penetration into the pancreas and spectrum coverage, carbapenems are the first option of treatment. Alternative therapy includes quinolones, metronidazole, third-generation cephalosporins, and piperacillin.

Definitive treatment for infected pancreatic necrosis is surgical débridement with necrosectomy, closed continuous irrigation, and open packaging (Fig. 56-8). The overall mortality rate after open necrosectomy is 25% to 30%.[15] Outcomes are time-dependent, with patients who undergo surgery in the first 14 days having a mortality rate of 75%; those who undergo surgery between 15 and 29 days and after 30 days have mortality rates of 45% and 8%, respectively.[16] As a result of the elevated morbidity and mortality rates with open débridement, endoscopic and laparoscopic techniques are being used more often. Both may ultimately provide similar outcomes, with hopes of reducing perioperative morbidity and mortality, although level 1 data are lacking.

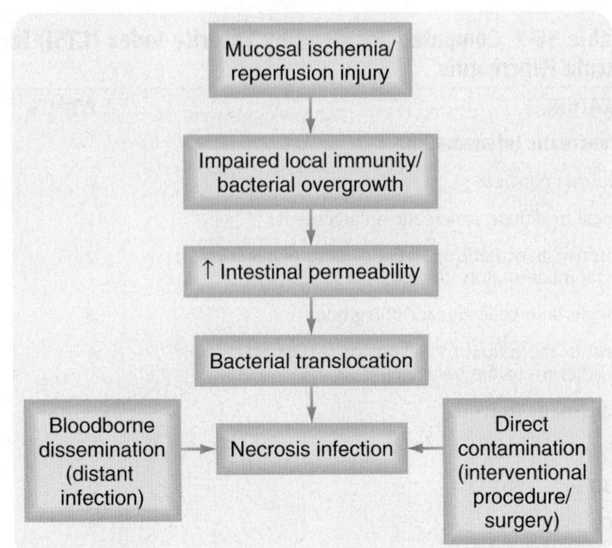


**FIGURE 56-7** Pathophysiology of pancreatic necrosis infection. The acute inflammatory injury that occurs during the first 48 to 72 hours causes mucosal ischemia and reperfusion injury. Both effects favor bacterial overgrowth because they alter local immunity. Mucosal ischemia also produces an increase in the permeability of intestinal cells, which is initiated 72 hours after the acute episode but typically peaks 1 week later. These transient episodes of bacteremia are associated with pancreatic necrosis infection. Less frequently, distant sources of infection such as pneumonia, vascular, or urinary tract infection associated with central lines and catheters are associated with bacteremia and pancreatic necrosis. Finally, local contamination after surgery or interventional procedures such as ERCP is responsible for necrosis infection.

### Pancreatic Pseudocysts

Pancreatic pseudocysts occur in 5% to 15% of patients who have peripancreatic fluid collections after AP. By definition, the capsule of a pseudocyst is composed of collagen and granulation tissue and it is not lined by epithelium.[17] The fibrotic reaction typically requires at least 4 to 8 weeks to develop. Figure 56-9 shows CT scans of a large pseudocyst arising in the tail of the pancreas.

Up to 50% of patients with pancreatic pseudocysts will develop symptoms. The presence of persistent pain, early satiety, nausea, weight loss, and elevated pancreatic enzyme levels in plasma suggest this diagnosis. The diagnosis is corroborated with by CT or MRI. EUS with FNA is indicated for patients in whom the diagnosis of pancreatic pseudocyst is not clear. Characteristic features of pancreatic pseudocysts include high amylase levels associated with the absence of mucin and low carcinoembryonic antigen (CEA) levels.

Observation is indicated for asymptomatic patients because spontaneous regression has been documented in up to 70% of cases; this is particularly true for patients with pseudocysts smaller than 4 cm in diameter, located in the tail, and no evidence of pancreatic duct obstruction or communication with the main pancreatic duct.[17] Invasive therapies are indicated for symptomatic patients or when the differentiation between a cystic neoplasm and pseudocyst is not possible. Because most patients are treated with decompressive procedures and not with resection, it is imperative to have a pathologic diagnosis. Surgical drainage has been the traditional approach for pancreatic pseudocysts. However, there is increasing evidence that transgastric and transduodenal endoscopic drainage are safe and effective approaches for patients with pancreatic pseudocysts in close contact (defined as <1 cm) with the stomach and duodenum, respectively. In addition, transpapillary drainage can be attempted in pancreatic pseudocysts communicating with the main pancreatic duct. For patients in whom a pancreatic duct stricture is associated with a pancreatic pseudocyst, endoscopic dilation and stent placement are indicated.

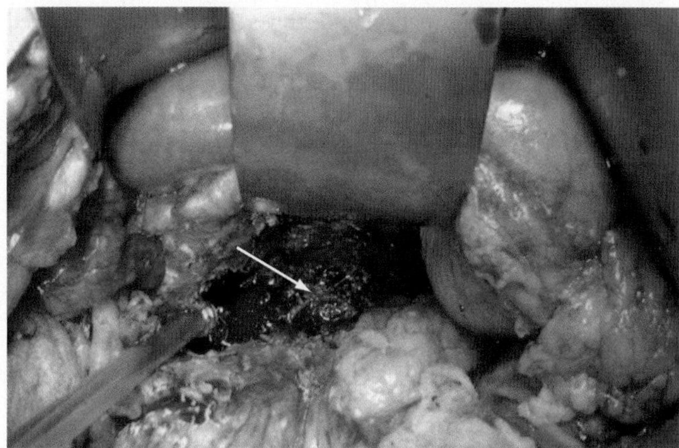

**FIGURE 56-8** Infected pancreatic necrosis. This 45-year-old man had severe ethanol-induced pancreatitis. Four weeks after the initial episode, the patient developed fever (39.5° C [103° F]), hypotension, and leukocytosis (19,000 cells/mm$^3$). The CT scan documented pancreatic necrosis involving 35% of the gland. After FNA, Gram staining documented the presence of gram-negative rods. The exploratory laparotomy indicated pancreatic necrosis involving mainly the body of the gland *(arrow)*. The patient was treated with necrosectomy, closed drainage, and IV meropenem. Final culture documented the presence of *Escherichia coli*. The patient was discharged home 56 days after the initial episode.

Surgical drainage is indicated for patients with pancreatic pseudocysts that cannot be treated with endoscopic techniques and patients who fail endoscopic treatment. Definitive treatment depends on the location of the cyst. Pancreatic pseudocysts closely attached to the stomach should be treated with a cystgastrostomy. In this procedure, an anterior gastrostomy is performed. Once the pseudocyst is located, it is drained through the posterior wall of the stomach using a linear stapler. The defect in the anterior wall of the stomach is closed in two layers. Pancreatic pseudocysts located in the head of the pancreas that are in close contact with the duodenum are treated with a cystoduodenostomy. Finally, some pseudocysts are not in contact with the stomach or duodenum. The surgical treatment for these patients is a Roux-en-Y cystojejunostomy. Surgical cyst enterostomy is successful in achieving immediate cyst drainage in over 90% of cases. Following initial resolution, recurrent pseudocyst formation may occur in up to 12% of cases during long-term follow-up, depending on the location of the cyst and underlying cause of the disease.[17]

Complications of pancreatic pseudocysts include bleeding and pancreaticopleural fistula secondary to vascular and pleural erosion, respectively, bile duct and duodenal obstruction, rupture into the abdominal cavity, and infection. Percutaneous drainage is only indicated for septic patients secondary to pseudocyst infection because it has a high incidence of external fistula.

### Pancreatic Ascites and Pancreaticopleural Fistulas

Although very rare, complete disruption of the pancreatic duct can lead to significant accumulation of, fluid. This condition should be suspected in patients who have an episode of AP, develop significant abdominal distention, and have free intraabdominal fluid. Diagnostic paracentesis typically demonstrates elevated amylase and lipase levels. Treatment consists of abdominal drainage combined with endoscopic placement of a

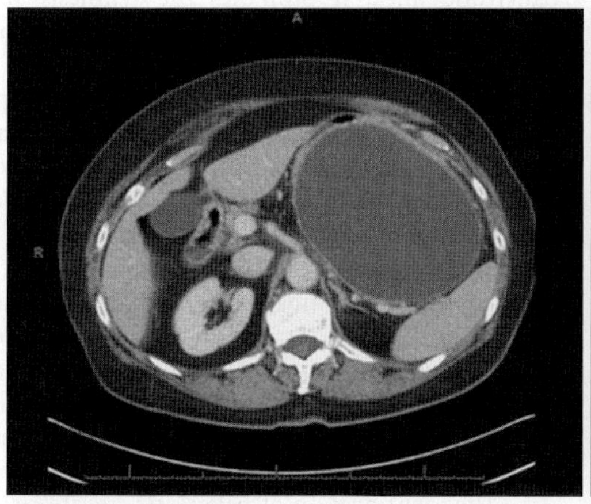

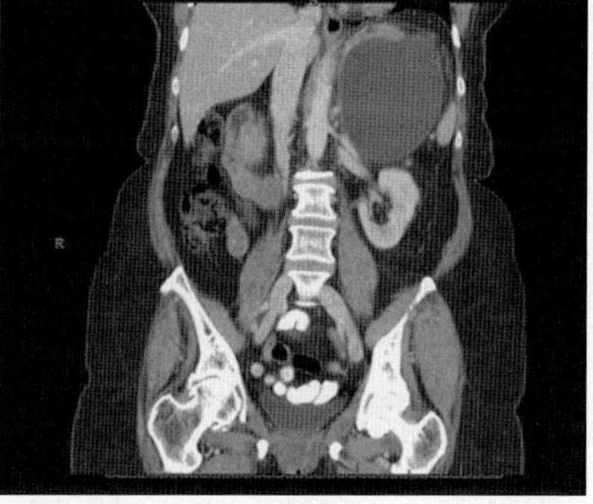

**FIGURE 56-9** CT scans showing a large pseudocyst arising in the tail of the pancreas.

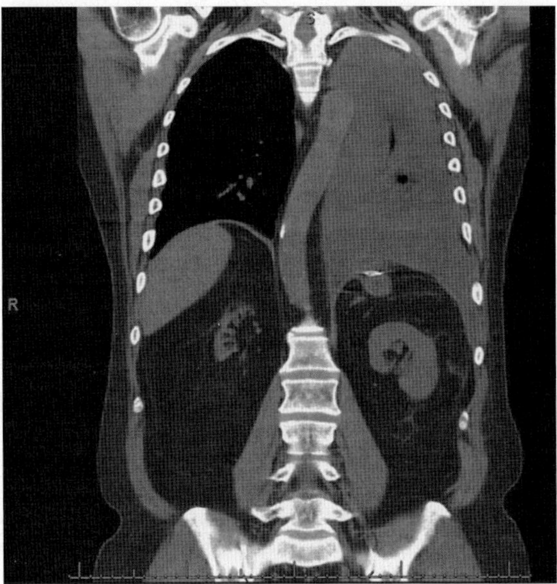

**FIGURE 56-10** Massive left pleural effusion secondary to a pancreaticopleural fistula.

pancreatic stent across the disruption. Failure of this therapy requires surgical treatment; it consists of distal resection and closure of the proximal stump.

Posterior pancreatic duct disruption into the pleural space has been described rarely. Symptoms that suggest this condition include dyspnea, abdominal pain, cough, and chest pain. The diagnosis is confirmed with chest x-ray, thoracentesis, and CT scan. Figure 56-10 demonstrates a large, left-sided pleural effusion caused by a pancreatic-pleural fistula. Amylase levels above 50,000 IU in the pleural fluid confirm the diagnosis. It is more common after alcoholic pancreatitis and, in 70% of patients, is associated with pancreatic pseudocysts. Initial treatment requires chest drainage, parenteral nutritional support, and administration of octreotide. Up to 60% of patients respond to this therapy. Persistent drainage should also be treated with endoscopic sphincterotomy and stent placement. Patients who do not respond to these measures require surgical treatment, similar to that described for pancreatic ascites.

### Vascular Complications

Acute pancreatitis is rarely associated with arterial vascular complications. The most common vessel affected is the splenic artery, but the superior mesenteric, cystic, and gastroduodenal arteries have also been found to be affected. It has been proposed that pancreatic elastase damages the vessels, leading to pseudoaneurysm formation. Spontaneous rupture results in massive bleeding. Clinical manifestations include sudden onset of abdominal pain, tachycardia, and hypotension. If possible, arterial embolization should be attempted to control the bleeding.[9] Refractory cases require ligation of the vessel affected. The mortality ranges from 28% to 56%.

Pancreatic inflammation can also produce vascular thrombosis; the vessel usually affected is the splenic vein but, in severe cases, it can extend into the portal venous system. Imaging demonstrates splenomegaly, gastric varices, and splenic vein occlusion. Thrombolytics have been described in the acute early phase; however, most patients can be managed with conservative treatment. Recurrent episodes of upper gastrointestinal bleeding caused by venous hypertension should be treated with splenectomy.

### Pancreatocutaneous Fistula

The frequency of pancreatic fistulas is low. Only 0.4% of patients develop this complication after an acute episode. However, the incidence of these complications increases in patients with other complications after AP—4.5% in patients with pancreatic pseudocysts (4.5%) and 40% in patients with infected necrosis after surgical débridement.[15] Treatment is conservative for most patients.

## CHRONIC PANCREATITIS

In contrast to AP, the histologic hallmark of chronic pancreatitis is the persistent inflammation and irreversible fibrosis associated with atrophy of the pancreatic parenchyma. These histologic features are associated with chronic pain and endocrine and exocrine insufficiency that significantly decrease the quality of life of these patients. Chronic pancreatitis affects between 3 and 10/100,000 persons.

### Risk Factors

The specific cause and frequency of each condition varies among countries, hospital population, and referral practice. In general, heavy alcohol consumption is the most common cause of chronic pancreatitis (70% to 80% of cases), especially in urban hospitals. Conditions such as chronic duct obstruction, trauma, pancreas divisum, cystic dystrophy of the duodenal wall, hyperparathyroidism, hypertriglyceridemia, autoimmune pancreatitis, tropical pancreatitis, and hereditary pancreatitis are rare and account for less than 10% of all cases. However, hereditary, chronic, and autoimmune pancreatitis are more common in referral centers. In up to 20% of patients, a clear cause cannot be documented and cases are considered to be idiopathic.[18]

### Alcohol Abuse

Prolonged alcohol abuse is the most important risk factor associated with chronic pancreatitis. The fact that only 3% to 7% of heavy drinkers develop chronic pancreatitis suggests that alcohol is only a cofactor and that other factors are required to develop this complication. Alcohol exerts multiple noxious effects in the pancreas—it increases the total protein concentration in the pancreatic juice, it promotes the synthesis and secretion of lithostathine by acinar cells, and increases glycoprotein 2 (GP2) secretion in pancreatic juice. These factors lead to protein precipitation and subsequent formation of protein plugs and eventually stones inside the pancreatic duct. As a result of the obstruction, acinar cells are no longer able to secrete pancreatic enzymes and are predisposed to autodigestion. In addition, several products of alcohol metabolism, such as fatty acid ethyl esters and reactive oxygen species, cause fragility of intra-acinar organelles such as zymogen granules and lysosomes, which leads to abnormal pancreatic enzyme activation inside acinar cells. Acetaldehyde, another alcohol metabolite, causes direct acinar injury. Chronic alcohol consumption is associated with enhanced NF-κβ activity, decreased perfusion in the microcirculation of the pancreas, and increased intracellular calcium levels.[18]

The identification of pancreatic stellate cells (PSCs) in the late 1990s is one of the most important discoveries in the pathophysiology of chronic pancreatitis.[19] PSCs are specialized quiescent fibroblasts found at the base of acinar cells. Once stimulated, PSCs differentiate into activated myofibroblasts, which synthesize proteins that form the extracellular matrix. Examples of these proteins include collagen I and III, fibronectin, laminin, and matrix metalloproteinases. PSCs have similar responses as hepatic stellate cells; chronic necrosis and inflammation (necroinflammation) induce the release of inflammatory mediators such as platelet-derived growth factor, TGF-β, TNF-α, IL-1, and IL-6 which are known to activate PSCs. Consequently, the synthesis of collagen and other components of pancreatic fibrosis is increased. It has been postulated that the chronic necroinflammation induced by ethanol activates PSCs and induces pancreatic fibrosis. Interestingly, it has also been shown that alcohol and some of its metabolites (e.g., acetaldehyde) cause direct activation of PSCs.

Although they only have been evaluated in preclinical studies, novel therapies that target the activation of PSCs are being investigated. It has been reported that antioxidants, angiotensin-converting enzyme inhibitors, peroxisome proliferator-activated receptor gamma (PPAR-γ) ligands, and vitamin A inhibit the activity of PSCs.

#### Smoking

Epidemiologic studies have shown that smoking increases the risk of alcohol-induced chronic pancreatitis. Active smokers develop chronic pancreatitis at a younger age as compared with nonsmokers. In addition, the risk of pancreatic calcifications and diabetes mellitus is increased in patients who smoke as compared with nonsmokers.

#### Gene Mutations

Under physiologic conditions, pancreatic enzyme activation is strictly controlled. Mutations in proteins that regulate this activation increase the risk of chronic pancreatitis. Mutations in the cationic trypsinogen gene (also known as *protease serine 1* [*PRSS1*] gene) are common in hereditary chronic pancreatitis. *PRSS1* is located in chromosome 7 and regulates trypsinogen production; mutations in this gene are associated with intra-acinar trypsinogen activation. *PRSS1* mutations have been documented in hereditary pancreatitis but are uncommon in other forms of chronic pancreatitis.

SPINK-1 is a peptide secreted by acinar cells that regulates the premature activation of trypsinogen. Because *SPINK1* mutations are present in 1% to 2% of healthy patients, but the prevalence of chronic pancreatitis is much lower, it has been hypothesized that *SPINK1* mutations are not enough to trigger pancreatic inflammation. However, they lower the threshold to develop it and influence the severity of the disease. *SPINK1* mutations are more prevalent in alcoholic, hereditary, and idiopathic pancreatitis.

The secretion of bicarbonate and chloride in respiratory and pancreatic secretions is regulated by the *CFTR* gene. *CFTR* mutations affect the normal secretion of bicarbonate, decrease pancreatic juice volume, and augment the concentration of pancreatic enzymes inside the pancreatic duct. Homozygous *CTFR* mutations result in cystic fibrosis; heterozygous mild mutations predispose to pancreatic exocrine insufficiency and chronic pancreatitis. The prevalence of *CFTR* gene mutations is higher in patients with alcoholic, idiopathic, and hereditary pancreatitis as compared with the general population.

### Types of Chronic Pancreatitis

#### Autoimmune Pancreatitis

Autoimmune pancreatitis is a chronic inflammatory disorder that involves the pancreas. At least two different histologic variants have been defined. Type 1 is the most common; it is characterized by dense, periductal lymphoplasmacytic infiltrates, storiform fibrosis, and obliterative venulitis. Plasmatic cells typically stain positive for immunoglobulin G4 (IgG4). In type 2, the pancreas is infiltrated by neutrophils, lymphocytes, and plasma cells that destroy and obliterate the epithelium in the pancreatic duct. Autoimmune pancreatitis is more common in men than women. Up to 80% of patients are older than 50 years. Patients with autoimmune pancreatitis can develop acute symptoms such as jaundice or AP, closely mimicking patients with pancreatic adenocarcinoma. However, most patients with chronic pancreatitis develop chronic abdominal discomfort associated with abnormal elevation of amylase and lipase levels.

#### Tropical Pancreatitis

Tropical pancreatitis is not common in the United States; it is more common in tropical areas within 30 degrees of the equator, particularly in India. Its pathophysiology has not been completely delineated but it has been associated with cassava ingestion and *SPINK1* mutations. Up to 45% to 50% of patients with tropical pancreatitis have *SPINK1* mutations.

#### Idiopathic Pancreatitis

In up to 10% to 20% of patients with chronic pancreatitis, a clear cause that predisposed to the disease is not evident. Future identification of genetic defects associated with chronic pancreatitis may allow for the identification of individuals at highest risk for development of this disease.

### Clinical Manifestations

Pain is the primary manifestation of chronic pancreatitis. Initially precipitated by oral intake, the intensity, frequency, and duration of pain gradually increase with worsening disease. Quality of life of these patients is significantly affected because of decreased oral intake, interference with daily activities, and dependence on narcotic pain medications. Nausea and vomiting are not common early on; however, they may appear as the disease progresses.

Pancreatic inflammation and fibrosis not only affect the pancreatic ducts, but also decrease the number and function of acinar cells. At least 90% of the gland needs to be dysfunctional before steatorrhea, diarrhea, and other symptoms of malabsorption develop. In severe cases, diseases associated with fat-soluble vitamin deficiency, such as bleeding, osteopenia, and osteoporosis, develop. Exocrine insufficiency occurs in 80% to 90% of patients with long-standing chronic pancreatitis.

Chronic pancreatitis also affects islet cell populations. As a result, 40% to 80% of patients will have clinical manifestations of diabetes mellitus. The prevalence depends on the predisposing condition and onset of symptoms. Diabetes mellitus typically occurs many years after the onset of abdominal pain and pancreatic exocrine insufficiency.

Jaundice or cholangitis occurs in 5% to 10% of patients because of fibrosis of the distal common bile duct. Extensive scarring in the head of the pancreas can also obstruct the duodenum, leading to severe nausea, vomiting, and abdominal pain.

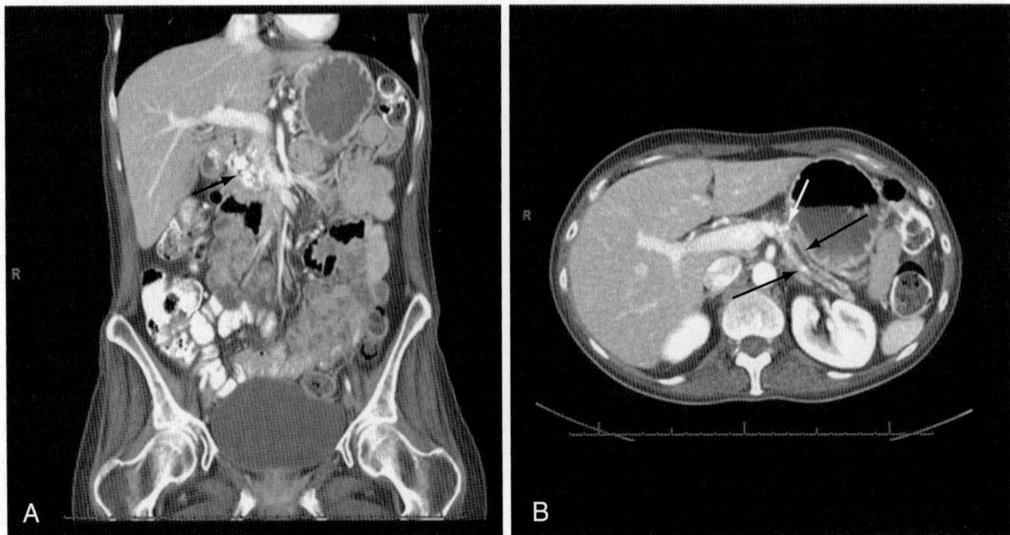


**FIGURE 56-11** Typical CT findings associated with chronic pancreatitis. Shown are pancreatic duct dilation *(long arrow)* and intrapancreatic calcifications, which are also typical of chronic pancreatitis *(small arrow).*

Upper gastrointestinal bleeding secondary to portal or splenic vein thrombosis is a rare manifestation of chronic pancreatitis.

## Diagnosis

### Imaging Studies

The diagnosis of chronic pancreatitis may be challenging early in the course of the disease because the correlation between symptoms and the structural changes seen on imaging studies is poor. The most common CT findings in chronic pancreatitis include dilated pancreatic duct (68%), parenchymal atrophy (54%), and pancreatic calcifications (50%; Fig. 56-11). Other findings include peripancreatic fluid, focal pancreatic enlargement, biliary duct dilation, and irregular pancreatic parenchyma contour. CT has a sensitivity of 56% to 95% and a specificity of 85% to 100% for the diagnosis of chronic pancreatitis. In addition to establishing the diagnosis, CT is particularly useful to assess complications, such as pancreatic duct disruption, pseudocysts, portal and splenic vein thrombosis, splenic, and pancreaticoduodenal artery pseudoaneurysms.

MRI is a reliable alternative to evaluate patients with chronic pancreatitis. The sensitivity for the diagnosis of pancreatic calcifications is lower, but MRI is useful to detect changes in the pancreatic parenchyma suggestive of chronic inflammation, such as changes in intensity, pancreatic atrophy, and irregularities in the contour. In addition, MRCP with secretin injection is particularly useful to evaluate intraductal strictures and pancreatic duct disruption.

Although ERCP was historically considered the gold standard for the diagnosis of chronic pancreatitis, the advent of secretin MRCP and EUS have significantly decreased its role as a diagnostic test. Current indications include patients for whom other diagnostic tests, including CT and MRCP, are contraindicated or have failed to corroborate the diagnosis. ERCP should be considered a therapeutic modalities in patients who develop pancreatic duct complications amenable to endoscopic therapy, such as stricture, stone, pseudocysts, and biliary stenosis.

EUS has emerged during the past 25 years as the most accurate technique to diagnose chronic pancreatitis in patients with minimal-change disease or in the early stages. Recently, a panel of endosonographers has defined the criteria required to diagnose chronic pancreatitis, known as the *Rosemont criteria* (Box 56-4). Histologic evidence of inflammation, atrophy, and fibrosis is the gold standard for the diagnosis of chronic pancreatitis; however, current evidence does not support the use of EUS-guided FNA or Tru-Cut biopsies to diagnose this disease.[20]

### Functional Tests

Measurement of the fecal elastase-1 level is the preferred noninvasive study to diagnose pancreatic exocrine insufficiency. It quantifies the amount of fecal elastase-1 using monoclonal or polyclonal anti–human elastase-1 antibodies. A fecal elastase-1 concentration above 200 μg/g feces is normal; a fecal elastase-1 concentration between 100 and 200 μg/g defines mild to moderate pancreatic insufficiency. Finally, a fecal elastase-1 concentration below 100 μg/g establishes the diagnosis of severe pancreatic exocrine insufficiency.

The fecal fat and weight estimation test measures the stool content of fat after a nutritional intake of 100 g of fat/day over 3 days. If the stool fat content exceeds 7 g/day, the diagnosis of steatorrhea is established.

## Treatment

### Medical Treatment

The main goal in the treatment of these patients is palliation of symptoms. Optimal treatment requires that a multidisciplinary team follow a systematized and well-structured therapeutic plan. Patient counseling is an important component because current evidence suggests that this disease is irreversible, but disease progression can be delayed if the predisposing condition is eradicated. Patients should be strongly encouraged to stop drinking and smoking.

Because most patients develop pain during the natural history of the disease, analgesic selection is a cornerstone of

**BOX 56-4 Rosemont Consensus-Based Endoscopic Ultrasound Features for Diagnosis of Chronic Pancreatitis**

**Parenchymal Features**

Major A criteria
- Hyperechoic foci with postacoustic shadowing

Major B criteria
- Honeycombing lobularity*

Minor criteria
- Hyperechoic, nonshadowing foci ≥3 mm in length and width
- Lobularity including three or more noncontiguous lobules in the body or tail
- Pancreatic cysts ≥2 mm in short axis
- At least three strands†

**Ductal Features**

Major A criteria
- Main pancreatic duct calculi‡

Minor criteria
- Irregular main pancreatic duct contour
- Dilated side branches§
- Main pancreatic duct dilation (≥3.5 mm in the body or ≥1.5 mm in the tail)
- Hyperechoic main pancreatic duct margin >50% of the main pancreatic duct in the body and tail*

**Diagnosis of Chronic Pancreatitis**

Consistent chronic pancreatitis
- One major A criteria + three or more minor criteria
- One major A criteria + major B criteria
- Two major A criteria

Suggestive of chronic pancreatitis¶
- One major A criteria + less than three minor
- Major B criteria + three or more minor criteria
- Five or more minor criteria

Indeterminate chronic pancreatitis¶
- 3-4 minor criteria in the absence of major
- Major B criteria + less than three minor criteria

Normal
- Fewer than three minor criteria

*Defined as lobularity that includes at least three contiguous lobules in the body or tail. It should be assessed in the body and tail.

†Strands are defined as hyperechoic lines ≥3 mm in length see in at least two different directions in the body or tail of the pancreas.

‡The presence of calculi in the main pancreatic duct, regardless of its the location, is the most predictive finding of chronic pancreatitis.

§Defined as at least three tubular anechoic structures, each one ≥1 mm in width, budding from the main pancreatic duct.

¶With suggestive and indeterminate chronic pancreatitis, the diagnosis needs to be confirmed with another imaging modality.

Adapted from Catalano MF, Sahai A, Levy M, et al: EUS-based criteria for the diagnosis of chronic pancreatitis: The Rosemont classification. Gastrointest Endosc 69:1251–1261, 2009.

treatment. Nonsteroidal anti-inflammatory drugs (NSAIDs) are the first line of treatment. Moderate to severe pain that does not respond to NSAIDs should be treated with tramadol or propoxyphene. Finally, patients with severe pain that does not respond to these recommendations should be treated with potent long-acting narcotics. It cannot be overemphasized that adjuvant measures to prevent addiction, depression, and poor quality of life should be considered for patients with severe pain who require narcotics. Alternative drugs useful in the treatment of other conditions associated with chronic pain, such as tricyclic antidepressants, selective serotonin reuptake inhibitors, combined serotonin and norepinephrine reuptake inhibitors, and $\alpha 2\delta$ inhibitors may also be considered.

There is no question about the digestive benefits of pancreatic enzyme replacement in patients with pancreatic exocrine insufficiency. However, it is controversial whether pancreatic enzyme replacement helps control the chronic pain seen in this condition. Therapeutic trials with pancreatic enzymes should last at least 6 weeks and should be given along with proton pump inhibitors because acid suppression improves the effects of uncoated pancreatic enzymes.[18]

### Interventional Therapy: Endoscopic Treatment

ERCP is the primary modality for treating symptomatic pancreatic duct obstruction with dilation and polyethylene stent placement. A number of sessions are usually required because of symptom recurrence. Note that the differential diagnosis of pancreatic duct strictures includes pancreatic cancer. Only after a thorough evaluation, which includes CT, MRCP, and/or EUS, has completely ruled out the possibility of malignancy should endoscopic treatment be considered. Surgical resection is indicated if any concern of malignancy exists.

Endoscopic stone extraction should be considered for patients with pain and pancreatic duct dilation secondary to stones. Extracorporeal shock wave lithotripsy followed by therapeutic ERCP may be required for the treatment of large impacted stones. The success rate varies from 44% to 77% for this technique.

Biliary obstruction caused by chronic pancreatitis occurs in 10% of patients and is best treated with surgical bypass. Temporary relief of the obstruction using plastic stents is indicated for patients with cholangitis or for those who are severely malnourished.

### Surgical Treatment

Several factors, including intractable pain, biliary, pancreatic duct or duodenal obstruction, pseudocyst or pseudoaneurysm formation, and theinability to rule out malignancy may prompt surgical intervention. The choice of surgical procedure depends on the symptoms requiring palliation and the presence or absence of pancreatic ductal dilation. In general, patients with a dilated pancreatic duct (defined as diameter >7 mm) require a decompressing procedure and patients with normal pancreatic duct require a resectional procedure. Several clinical scenarios that require surgical intervention are described here.

#### Pancreatic Duct Dilation Secondary to Duct Stones or Strictures

Pancreatic duct dilation is defined as a main pancreatic duct measuring at least 7 mm in diameter. Pancreatic duct dilation can be secondary to a single stone or stricture; however, it is often caused by multiple strictures and stones in the pancreatic duct. The pancreatic duct dilation observed in chronic pancreatitis is classically described as a chain of lakes, which reflects the presence of multiple dilations and stenosis. When accompanied by intractable pain, this condition is best treated with side-to-side Roux-en-Y pancreaticojejunostomy, also known as the *modified Puestow procedure*.

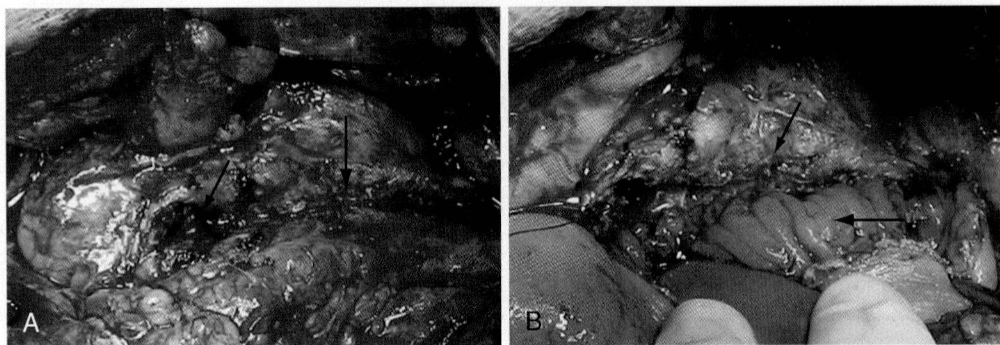

**FIGURE 56-12** Frey procedure, intraoperative photographs. **A,** Significant dilation of the main pancreatic duct at the level of the head *(short arrow)* and body of the pancreas *(large arrow)* after the anterior surface of the pancreas has been opened. **B,** Side-to-side anastomosis between the pancreatic duct *(short arrow)* and jejunum *(large arrow).*

The anterior surface of the pancreatic duct is opened and the anterior surface of the duct is completely unroofed. This tissue may be sent for frozen section to rule out underlying malignancy. The proximal extent of tissue resection is within 1 cm of the duodenum and the distal limit is within 1 to 2 cm of the end of the pancreas. After all stones are removed, a standard Roux-en-Y is used to create a two-layer lateral pancreaticojejunostomy. The main advantage offered by this procedure is parenchymal conservation, which preserves endocrine and exocrine function. The modified Puestow procedure provides palliation of pain in 80% of cases; however, 30% of cases will recur, usually after 3 to 5 years of surgery. Decompressive procedures temporarily relieve the ductal obstruction but, in most cases, they do not modify the natural history of the disease and chronic pancreatitis progresses. Other factors associated with recurrence include smoking and alcohol ingestion after surgery, failure to decompress the head and uncinate process properly, and length of the pancreaticojejunostomy.[21]

In 1987, Andersen and Frey[22] described the local resection of the pancreatic head with longitudinal pancreaticojejunostomy as an alternative procedure. The surgical approach is similar to the Puestow procedure; however, once the anterior surface of the pancreatic duct has been completely exposed, the anterior portion of the head of the pancreas is also resected, leaving a 1-cm rim of pancreatic tissue along the duodenal margin. Figure 56-12 shows intraoperative images of a Frey procedure. This procedure is also an alternative for patients with a dilated pancreatic duct secondary to a benign stricture in the head of the pancreas associated with severe inflammation, scarring, or portal hypertension surrounding the head of the pancreas that precludes a safe pancreaticoduodenectomy. The main disadvantage is the removal of pancreatic parenchyma. A recent study has demonstrated that 62% of patients are completely free of pain and 95% of patients have satisfactory pain control after this procedure. In the same series, 34% of patients developed endocrine or exocrine pancreatic insufficiency.[23]

**Pancreatic Duct Dilation Secondary to a Single Stricture and/or Stone** Occasionally, a single stricture that is proximal to the papilla produces pancreatic duct dilation. As an alternative to a Puestow or Frey procedure, a pancreaticoduodenectomy can be performed to relieve the obstruction. This procedure will be described later in the surgical treatment of pancreatic adenocarcinoma. It must be emphasized that this procedure is absolutely contraindicated if more than one obstruction is present in the duct. Single distal obstructions can occasionally be treated with a distal pancreatectomy. The main disadvantage of both procedures is that they can be associated with pancreatic insufficiency because normal parenchyma is removed.

**Focal Inflammatory Mass Without Significant Dilation of the Pancreatic Duct** In a small percentage of patients with chronic pancreatitis, a predominant mass in the head or, less commonly, in the tail of the pancreas without any evidence of pancreatic duct dilation is seen. Long-standing chronic pancreatitis is also a risk factor for developing pancreatic cancer; therefore, even in patients with a known history of chronic pancreatitis, finding a focal mass is concerning because it may represent an area of pancreatic adenocarcinoma that has developed in the setting of chronic pancreatitis. Resection is recommended for surgical candidates to avoid any error in diagnosis.

**Diffuse Glandular Involvement Without Dilation of the Pancreatic Duct** Decompressive procedures and local pancreatic resections are associated with an elevated failure rate in this group of patients. Patients who do not respond to medical and endoscopic therapies require surgical treatment. The most effective treatment to eliminate pain is total pancreatectomy. However, this procedure is invariably associated with diabetes mellitus. In contrast to type 1 diabetes mellitus, the severity and risk of hypoglycemia are increased in these patients.[24] In 1977, researchers at the University of Minnesota described islet autotransplantation after total pancreatectomy to prevent the effects of surgically induced diabetes. In the largest experience there, one third of patients who underwent this procedure were insulin-independent, an additional one third requires insulin intermittently, and the other third was fully dependent. According to this study, 90% had pain relief or reduction and 50% were able to discontinue narcotics. Similar results were demonstrated at the University of Cincinnati; up to two thirds of patients had complete or partial islet function, and 40% were insulin-independent. Narcotics were discontinued in 66% of patients.[25] Although preliminary results have been encouraging, routine implementation of this operative intervention has been controversial. Major limitations associated with this procedure include the cost and lack of islet processing facilities.

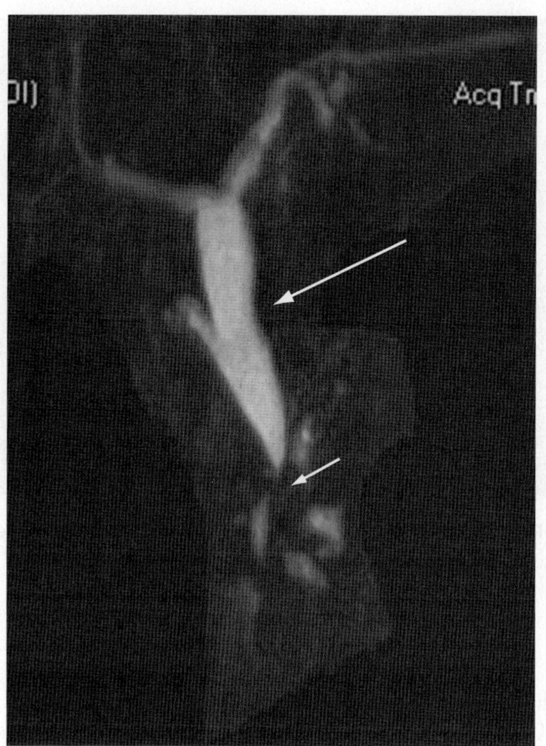


**FIGURE 56-13** Bile duct stricture secondary to chronic pancreatitis. This MRCP indicates common bile duct dilation *(large arrow)* secondary to a stricture at the level of the intrapancreatic portion of the common bile duct *(small arrow).*

**Biliary Strictures** Chronic scarring and fibrosis of the head of the pancreas result in external compression of the intrapancreatic portion of the common bile duct. Up to one third of patients with chronic pancreatitis develop radiologic evidence of bile duct dilation; however, significant biliary obstruction occurs in 6% of patients.[39] Biliary strictures typically appear as a long symmetrical narrowing that involves the intrapancreatic portion of the common bile duct in MRCP or ERCP (Fig. 56-13). IV fluid and antibiotic therapy and temporary bile duct decompression with plastic stents is indicated for patients who present with cholangitis. Pancreaticoduodenectomy is indicated for patients in whom malignancy cannot be excluded before surgery. A Roux-en-Y hepaticojejunostomy is an alternative treatment for patients without evidence of malignancy or significant scarring that precludes resection of the head of the pancreas.

**Duodenal Stenosis** Up to 1.2% of patients with chronic pancreatitis develop duodenal strictures.[39] Clinical manifestations include abdominal pain, nausea, vomiting, and significant weight loss. Differential diagnoses include other causes of gastric outlet obstruction secondary to upper gastrointestinal malignancies and gastroparesis. Severely malnourished patients require IV hydration, nutritional support, and gastric decompression with a nasogastric tube. Permanent treatment requires a gastrojejunostomy.

**Pancreatic Pseudocyst** Pancreatic pseudocysts develop more frequently in patients with chronic pancreatitis as compared with AP. Up to 30% to 40% of patients develop pseudocysts during the course of their disease. Only 10% of patients have spontaneous pancreatic pseudocyst regression. Spontaneous regression is less likely to occur in these patients because pancreatic pseudocysts arise more frequently in the setting of pancreatic duct obstruction. Indications for treatment include symptoms secondary to gastric, duodenal, or biliary compression or associated complications, such as bleeding, pancreaticopleural fistulas, rupture, or spontaneous bleedings. Alternative modalities in the treatment include endoscopic and surgical drainage (see earlier).

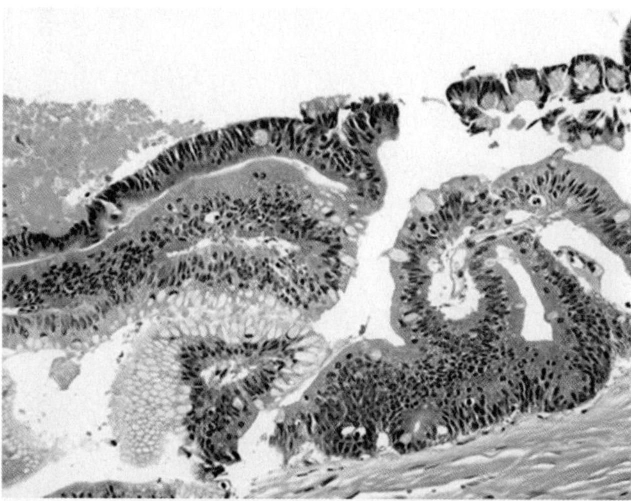

**FIGURE 56-14** Ovarian-like stroma is a histologic feature often seen in MCN.

## CYSTIC NEOPLASMS OF THE PANCREAS

Cystic tumors are the second most common exocrine pancreatic neoplasm, following only adenocarcinomas of the pancreas in incidence. Given the advances in modern cross-sectional imaging, the identification of cystic lesions of the pancreas is becoming common. Surgeons must be familiar with the characteristics and treatment of these lesions to determine individual management appropriately.

### Types of Cystic Neoplasms

#### Mucinous Cystic Neoplasm

In the 1970s, the clinicopathologic spectrums of mucinous and serous cystic tumors were described. Mucinous cystic neoplasms (MCNs) are the most common cystic neoplasms of the pancreas.[26] These tumors span the histologic spectrum from benign to invasive carcinomas. MCNs contain mucin-producing epithelium and are identified histologically by the presence of mucin-rich cells and ovarian-like stroma (Fig. 56-14). Estrogen and progesterone staining are positive in most cases. Frequently seen in young women, the mean age at presentation is in the fifth decade. Men are rarely affected. MCNs are typically found in the body and tail of the pancreas, but infrequently can occur elsewhere. Although incidental MCN is becoming increasingly common, up to 50% of patients present with vague abdominal pain. A history of pancreatitis may be found in up to 20% of patients, which explains the common misdiagnosis of pseudocyst.

The radiologic characteristic of an MCN on a CT scan is the presence of a solitary cyst, which may have fine septations

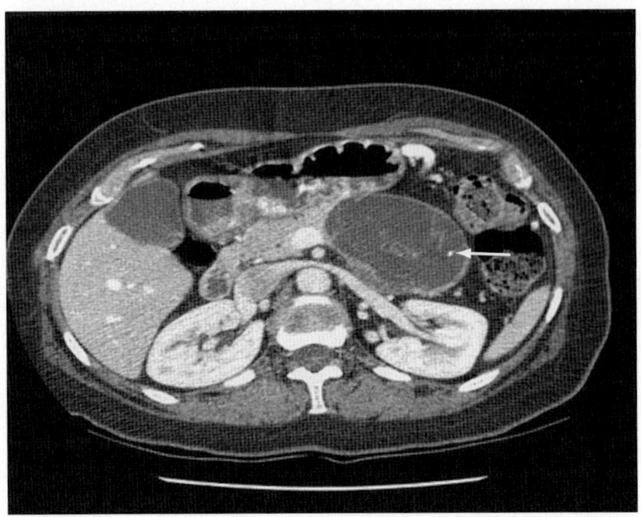

**FIGURE 56-15** CT scan of the tail of the pancreas mucinous cystic neoplasm showing a large multiloculated cyst in the absence of pancreatic ductal communication.

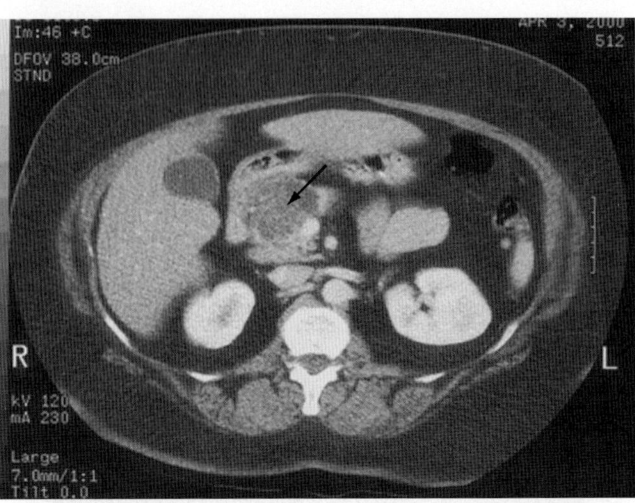


**FIGURE 56-17** CT scan of serous cyst neoplasm. The *arrow* depicts the sunburst appearance and central calcification.

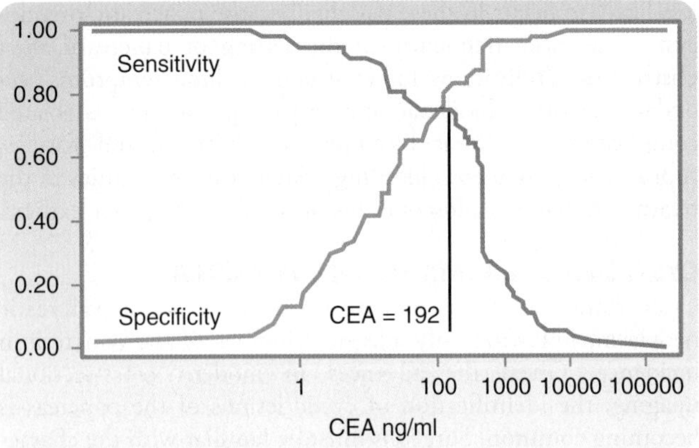


**FIGURE 56-16** Sensitivity and specificity curves of cyst fluid CEA concentrations (ng/mL; log scale) for differentiating between mucinous and nonmucinous cystic lesions. An optimal cutoff value of 192 ng/mL correlated with the crossover of the sensitivity and specificity curves. (From Brugge WR, Lewandrowski K, Lee-Lewandrowski E, et al: Diagnosis of pancreatic cystic neoplasms: A report of the cooperative pancreatic cyst study. Gastroenterology 126:1330–1336, 2004.)

and be surrounded by a rim of calcification (Fig. 56-15). Cross-sectional imaging may not be able to distinguish between benign and malignant MCNs; however, the presence of eggshell calcification, larger tumor size, or a mural nodule on cross-sectional imaging is suggestive of malignancy.

EUS and cyst fluid analyses play an important role in the diagnosis of MCN and other cystic neoplasms. FNA with cyst fluid analyses of MCNs demonstrate mucin-rich aspirate and high CEA levels (>192 ng/mL; log scale). Figure 56-16 illustrates the sensitivity and specificity of CEA in identifying mucinous neoplasms based on fine-needle fluid aspiration. Unlike pseudocysts, MCNs typically have low levels of cyst fluid amylase. These fluid analyses provide accurate diagnosis in up to 80% of cases.[27] Table 56-3 summarizes the distinguishing features of cystic neoplasms of the pancreas.[28]

Pancreatic resection is the standard treatment for MCNs, given the potential for malignant transformation. In the absence of invasive malignancy, resection is curative and no further surveillance is required. The prognosis of patients who undergo pancreatectomy for invasive MCNs is poor, although more favorable than that for ductal adenocarcinoma of the pancreas. Invasive MCNs exhibit slower growth, less frequent nodal involvement, and less aggressive clinical behavior compared with ductal adenocarcinoma; a 5-year survival of 50% to 60% can be expected following resection. Despite limited experience with invasive MCNs, most centers offer adjuvant systemic chemotherapy following surgical resection, especially when node-positive disease is present.

### Serous Cystic Neoplasm

Compared with MCNs, serous cystic neoplasms (SCNs) have a predilection for the head of the pancreas and occur in patients with a higher median age. Patients commonly present with vague abdominal pain and less frequently with weight loss and obstructive jaundice. On gross inspection, SCNs are large, well-circumscribed masses. Microscopic examination reveals multiloculated, glycogen-rich small cysts. Central calcification, with radiating septa giving the sunburst appearance, is a radiographic sign on CT in 10% to 20% of patients (Fig. 56-17). With the advent of EUS, these features can now be better delineated. Recently, differential cyst fluid protein expression was observed between SCNs and IPMNs, with accurate discrimination in 92% of patients.[29] Although serous cystic tumors are generally considered benign, pancreatectomy is suggested when the diagnosis of malignancy is uncertain, or in symptomatic serous cystadenomas. Patients with a tumor larger than 4 cm are more likely to be symptomatic and display a more rapid median growth rate than patients with tumors smaller than 4 cm. Thus, in select patients with large (>4 cm) or rapidly growing lesions, resection of an SCN is appropriate.

**Table 56-3 Defining Characteristics of Pseudocysts and Pancreatic Cystic Neoplasms**

| CHARACTERISTICS | PSEUDOCYST | SCN | MCN | IPMN |
|---|---|---|---|---|
| Epidemiology | | | | |
| Gender | F = M | F >> M (4:1) | F >>> M (10:1) | F = M |
| Age (years) | 40-60 | 60-70 | 50-60 | 60-70 |
| Imaging findings | | | | |
| Location | Evenly distributed | Evenly distributed | Head << body/tail | Head > diffuse > body/tail |
| Appearance | Round, thick-walled large cyst; gland atrophy ± calcification | Multiple small cysts separated by internal septations with central starburst calcifications | Thick-walled, septated macrocyst with smooth contour; ± solid component, egg-shell calcifications | Poorly demarcated, lobulated, polycystic mass with dilation of main or branch ducts |
| Communication with ducts | Yes | No | Very rare | Yes |
| Cyst fluid analysis | | | | |
| Cytology | Inflammatory cells | Scant glycogen-rich cells, with positive Periodic Acid Schiff stain | Sheets and clusters of columnar, mucin-containing cells | Tall, columnar mucin-containing cells |
| Mucin stain | Negative | Negative | Positive | Positive |
| Amylase | Very high | Low | Low | High |
| CEA | Low | Low | High | High |

*SCN,* Serous cystic neoplasm.

From Tran Cao HS, Kellogg B, Lowy AM, et al: Cystic neoplasms of the pancreas. Surg Oncol Clin N Am 19:267–295, 2010.

### Intraductal Papillary Mucinous Neoplasm

Several names have been given to IPMNs, such as mucin-secreting carcinoma, villous adenoma of the duct of Wirsung, diffuse intraductal papillary adenocarcinoma, intraductal cyst-adenoma, mucinous duct ectasia, and intraductal papillary mucinous tumor. First described by Ohashi, IPMNs of the pancreas typically present in the sixth to seventh decade of life. IPMNs encompass a wide spectrum of epithelial changes, including benign adenoma, borderline, carcinoma in situ, and invasive adenocarcinoma. Patients with invasive IPMNs tend to be 6.4 years older than patients with adenomas or borderline lesions. IPMNs appear to demonstrate no racial predilection, as shown by several studies of patients with different ethnic backgrounds.[30]

IPMNs are further characterized by the extent to which they involve the pancreatic ducts. Neoplasia that affects only the small side branches are termed *side branch* or *branch duct IPMNs,* whereas those that involve the main pancreatic duct are termed *main duct IPMNs.* Side branch IPMNs that extend into the main duct are termed *mixed-type IPMNs.*

**Side Branch Intraductal Papillary Mucinous Neoplasm** As the name implies, a side branch IPMN involves dilation of the pancreatic duct side branches that communicate with but do not involve the main pancreatic duct. Side branch IPMNs may be focal, involving a single side branch, or multifocal, with multiple cystic lesions throughout the length of the pancreas. Risk of malignant transformation has been described in side branch IPMNs and is directly related to the size of the cystic dilation. Other features that predict risk of malignancy include mural nodules or general thickening of the cyst wall. In addition, several clinical symptoms have been associated with elevated risk of malignancy, including jaundice, pain, and diabetes.[30,31] For asymptomatic lesions smaller than 3 cm, the risk of invasive malignancy is small, and therefore serial surveillance has been proposed.[32] A clinical decision tree for the management of side branch IPMN is shown in Figure 56-18. For individuals incidentally found to have small (<1 cm) IPMNs, surveillance with CT or MRI in 1 year is appropriate. For those with asymptomatic cysts between 1 and 3 cm, imaging at 6 months is appropriate, followed by annual evaluation if no change in size has occurred. Cysts larger than 3 cm warrant surgical resection because of the increased risk of malignancy. Any patient with symptoms or worrisome features related to side branch IPMNs (e.g., jaundice, mural nodule, dilated main pancreatic duct, pain, diabetes) should undergo surgical resection because the risk of malignancy in symptomatic patients is heightened. Overall, the risk of invasive malignancy in the setting of side branch IPMN is approximately 10% to 15%.

**Main Duct Intraductal Papillary Mucinous Neoplasm** In contrast to side branch IPMN, main duct IPMN indicates abnormal cystic dilation of the main pancreatic duct with columnar metaplasia and thick mucinous secretions, which can be seen oozing from a patulous papilla on endoscopic evaluation (Fig. 56-19). Involvement of the main pancreatic duct may be focal or diffuse; it is most relevant because of the significantly increased risk of malignant degeneration. Individuals with main duct IPMN have a 30% to 50% risk of harboring invasive pancreatic cancer at the time of presentation. Thus, surgical resection is the cornerstone of treatment. Figure 56-20 demonstrates main duct IPMN with dilation of the entire pancreatic duct.

Unlike patients with pancreatic ductal adenocarcinomas (PDACs), 50% of patients with IPMNs of the pancreas present with abdominal pain and up to 25% present with AP, which, not surprisingly, has led to the diagnosis of chronic pancreatitis

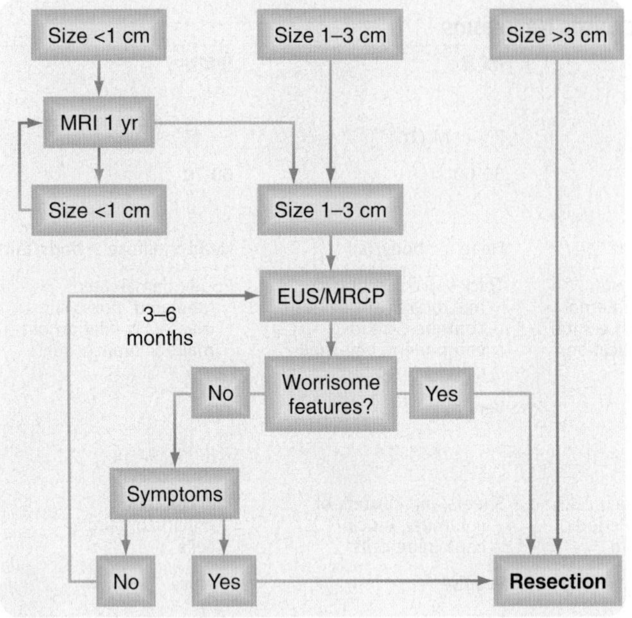

Size <1 cm
Size 1–3 cm
Size >3 cm
MRI 1 yr
Size <1 cm
Size 1–3 cm
EUS/MRCP
3–6 months
No
Worrisome features?
Yes
Symptoms
No
Yes
Resection

**FIGURE 56-18** Algorithm for the management of side branch IPMN.

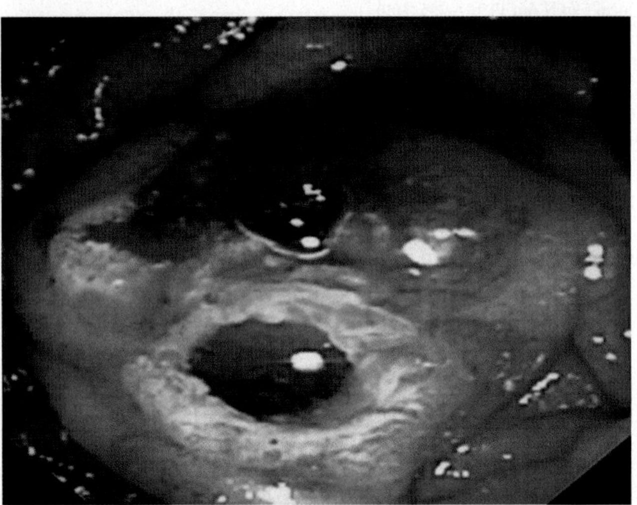

**FIGURE 56-19** Classic endoscopic view of IPMN showing viscous fluid oozing from a patulous ampulla of Vater.

in many series. Several investigators have studied clinical and pathologic markers as predictors of malignancy and found that jaundice, elevated serum alkaline phosphatase level, mural nodules, diabetes, and main pancreatic duct diameter of 7 mm or larger are strongly associated with invasive IPMNs.[30,31] On a molecular level, recent investigations using genomic array analysis of pancreatic cystic neoplasms have shown that IPMNs have several distinct cytogenetic alterations that separate it as an entity from ductal adenocarcinoma of the pancreas.

The radiographic features of IPMNs on pancreatic CT scans may include a dilated main pancreatic duct, cysts of varying sizes, and possibly mural nodules (Fig. 56-20). MRCP and EUS are important secondary diagnostic studies for the evaluation of patients with suspected IPMN. MRCP may allow

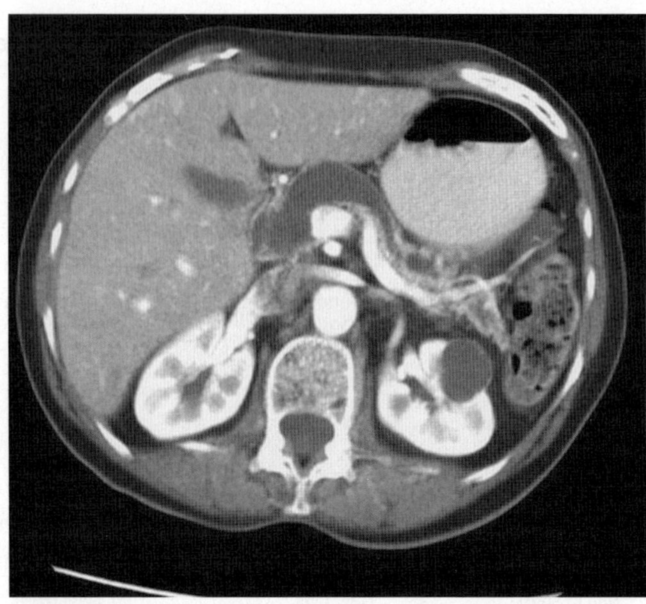

**FIGURE 56-20** Cross-sectional imaging of main duct IPMN throughout the entire pancreatic gland and a prominent ampulla of Vater.

for localization of mural nodules and pretreatment classification of suspected side branch or main duct types of IPMN. EUS can evaluate the pancreatic duct and assess the fluid and solid components of the neoplasm. Aspirated fluid is typically viscous and clear, and contains mucin. Cytology studies demonstrate mucin-rich fluid with variable cellularity; columnar mucinous cells with variable atypia may also be seen. As in MCNs and side branch IPMNs, fluid aspirates characteristically reveal an elevated CEA level (>192 ng/mL; log scale). It should be noted that this elevation of the CEA level is not predictive of invasive malignancy, only the presence of mucinous metaplasia.

**Mixed-Type Intraductal Papillary Mucinous Neoplasm** Mixed-type IPMN denotes a side branch IPMN that has extended to involve the main pancreatic duct to a varying degree. Concern for mixed-type IPMNs should be raised in individuals with side branch cysts who exhibit upstream dilation of the pancreatic duct, because this is an indication of main duct involvement. The biologic behavior of mixed-type IPMNs most closely resembles that for main duct IPMNs, with a significant risk of invasive malignancy at the time of presentation (30% to 50%). Like main duct IPMN, surgical resection is indicated for the treatment of mixed-type IPMN.

### Treatment: Surgical Resection for Intraductal Papillary Mucinous Neoplasm

Partial pancreatectomy is the primary treatment for main duct, symptomatic, and large branch-type IPMNs (>3 cm), or IPMNs with an invasive component; however, the optimal extent of pancreatic resection for some patients remains unknown. Many pancreatic surgeons recommend partial pancreatectomy with the knowledge that the disease is most often located in the head of the gland, even though ductal changes may extend to involve other parts of the pancreas.[33] Partial pancreatectomy also eliminates the risk of brittle diabetes, which accompanies total pancreatectomy. Although some investigators continue to advocate total pancreatectomy for the treatment of any IPMN, the evidence supporting this approach is decreasing with longer follow-up of patients treated by R0 and R1 partial pancreatectomy. It is appropriate to recommend partial pancreatectomy and discuss management of the pancreatic margin with the patient preoperatively, advising him or her them that approximately 15% of patients will require conversion to total pancreatectomy to achieve negative parenchymal resection margins. The surgical margins are assessed intraoperatively and additional margins are obtained for carcinomas in situ or invasive cancer.

Survival outcomes are significantly better in patients with IPMNs than in patients with PDACs. Sohn and associates[34] have analyzed a series of 136 patients with IPMNs; survival rates for patients with noninvasive IPMNs are 97% at 1 year, 94% at 2 years, and 77% at 5 years. When the group of patients with noninvasive IPMNs was analyzed further, no survival differences were found between patients with IPMNs and those with borderline IPMNs. On the contrary, there was a significant difference in survival rate between patients with noninvasive IPMNs and those with invasive IPMNs. The 1-, 3-, and 5-year survival rates for patients with invasive IPMNs were 72%, 58%, and 43%, respectively. Therefore, survival is clearly dependent on the invasive component of the lesion.

It is increasingly clear that not all patients with IPMNs require surgery. A recent consensus conference has recommended observation for patients with asymptomatic small (<3 cm) branch duct IPMNs that have no associated nodularity.[32] A plan for watchful surveillance with delayed intervention in these patients is reasonable because the risks for malignancy with small, asymptomatic branch duct tumors is low, most patients are older, and the time required to develop invasive malignancy may be longer than the patient's life expectancy.

## ADENOCARCINOMA OF THE EXOCRINE PANCREAS

### Epidemiology

In 2009, it was estimated that PDAC would affect approximately 42,470 individuals in the United States and 35,240 would die of the disease. Although it is the ninth most common cancer diagnosis, pancreatic cancer ranks fourth in cancer deaths each year. Despite significant advances in the treatment of other cancers, the prognosis of pancreatic cancer remains dismal. Overall, less than 5% of individuals will survive 5 years beyond their diagnosis. Men are affected slightly more commonly than women, with a 1.3 : 1 incidence ratio. African Americans have a slightly higher risk of developing pancreatic cancer and dying of their disease compared with whites. The risk of pancreatic cancer increases with age beyond the sixth decade; the mean age at diagnosis is 72 years.[35]

### Risk Factors

#### Environmental Risk Factors and Causes

Although the cause of pancreatic cancer remains unclear, several environmental risks have been associated with its increased incidence. The most notable risk factor is related to smoking. Several epidemiologic studies have shown an association with the amount and duration of smoking history with an elevated risk of pancreatic cancer. On average, smokers face a one- to threefold increase in risk for developing pancreatic cancer compared with nonsmokers. This risk seems to be a linear association, with pancreatic cancer incidence directly related to the number of pack-years smoked (packs/day × number of years smoking). As with other cancers, the risk of pancreatic cancer persists many years beyond smoking cessation. Over the years, there have been several other factors, including chronic pancreatitis, diabetes, and occupational exposure, which were thought to contribute to an elevated risk of pancreatic cancer; however, population data have been somewhat controversial. It is likely that these factors are associated with an elevated risk, but the magnitude of the risk is uncertain. Obesity has recently become the focus of investigation; several authors have found that obese patients may be up to three times more likely to develop pancreatic cancer than nonobese individuals. It remains unclear whether obesity itself or one of the comorbidities related to obesity is associated with the higher incidence of pancreatic cancer seen in this population.

#### Hereditary Risk Factors

A number of inheritable risk factors have been identified that are associated with elevated risk of developing pancreatic cancer. Table 56-4 summarizes several known gene mutations and their clinical significance.

**Table 56-4 Hereditary Risk Factors Associated With Development of Pancreatic Cancer**

| GENE | ASSOCIATED SYNDROME | CLINICAL SIGNIFICANCE |
|---|---|---|
| *PRSS1* | Familial pancreatitis | Mutation results in chronic pancreatitis and 40% lifetime risk of PDAC. |
| *STK11* | Peutz-Jeghers syndrome | Mutation results in >100-fold increase in risk of PDAC. |
| *CDKN2A* | Familial atypical mole and multiple melanoma syndrome | Mutation leads to increased risk of melanoma and >40-fold increase risk of PDAC. |
| *CTFR* | Cystic fibrosis | Thick secretions result in chronic pancreatitis and 30-fold increase in risk of PDAC. |
| *BRCA2* | Hereditary breast and ovarian cancer | Mutation results in elevated risk of breast and ovarian cancer and 10-fold increase in risk of PDAC. |
| *MLH1* | Lynch syndrome | Mismatch repair gene mutation leads to increased risk of colon cancer and eightfold increase in risk of PDAC. |
| *APC* | Familial adenomatous polyposis | Mutation results in polyposis coli and colon cancer with fourfold increase in risk of PDAC. |

**Familial Pancreatitis (*PRSS1* Gene Mutation)** It has long been noted that individuals with familial pancreatitis have an elevated risk of pancreatic cancer. Unlike sporadic chronic pancreatitis, this association is more uniformly accepted. Mutations in the cationic trypsinogen gene *(PRSS1)* lead to increased trypsin activity and chronic inflammatory conditions in the pancreas. Individuals with familial pancreatitis have a greater than 50-fold increase in their risk of developing pancreatic cancer compared with unaffected individuals.[36,37]

**Peutz-Jeghers Syndrome (*STK11* Gene Mutation)** Individuals with Peutz-Jeghers syndrome are distinguished by the development of gastrointestinal hamartomatous polyps and pigmented mucocutaneous lesions. The specific role of *STK11* is not defined, although it is thought to act as a tumor suppressor gene, with loss of heterozygosity leading to the development of gastrointestinal tumors. In addition to gastrointestinal cancers, individuals with Peutz-Jeghers syndrome are at a higher risk of lung, ovarian, breast, uterine, and testicular cancers. The risk of pancreatic cancer in the setting of Peutz-Jeghers syndrome is over 100 times greater than that in nonaffected individuals.[36,37]

**Cystic Fibrosis (*CFTR* Gene Mutation)** Although the cause remains unclear, those with cystic fibrosis (*CFTR* gene mutation) are up to 30 times more likely to develop pancreatic cancer than the general population. It is postulated that this elevated risk is caused by the chronic inflammatory condition of the pancreas resulting from a lifetime of thickened secretions and partial ductal obstruction.[36,37]

**Familial Atypical Mole and Multiple Melanoma Syndrome (*CDKN2A* Gene Mutation)** *CDKN2A* encodes for protein p16 which normally inhibits cell proliferation by binding to cyclin-dependent kinases (CDKs). Mutations of CDKN2A lead to uninhibited cell cycle activation and proliferation. Although most noted for its associated increased risk of melanoma, individuals with *CDKN2A* mutations have up to a 20-fold increase in risk for the development of pancreas cancer.[36,37]

**Hereditary Breast and Ovarian Cancer (*BRCA2* Gene Mutation)** Although germline *BRCA* mutations are most recognized because of their association with breast cancer, 10% of individuals from high-risk pancreatic cancer families (at least two first-degree relatives with pancreas cancer) have been found to have *BRCA2* mutations. Germline mutations of the *BRCA2* gene lead to an elevated risk forpancreatic cancer, which is up to 10 times that of the general population.[36,37]

**Lynch Syndrome (Mismatch Repair Gene Mutations)** Although most strongly associated with colon cancers caused by mutations in mismatch repair genes *(MLH1, MSH2, MSH6)*, Lynch syndrome also leads to an increased risk of pancreatic cancer. The microsatellite instability noted in colon cancer cells have also been seen in pancreatic cancer cells from individuals with Lynch syndrome, indicative of a common genetic cause. It is estimated that the risk of pancreatic cancer is increased eightfold in individuals with Lynch syndrome.[36,37]

**Familial Adenomatous Polyposis (*APC* Gene Mutation)** Familial adenomatous polyposis (FAP) results from mutation of the adenomatous polyposis coli gene *(APC)*, leading to the development of thousands of colonic polyps. It has been found that individuals affected by FAP are also significantly more likely to develop pancreas cancer, with a fourfold increase over that in the general population. These data remain observational because the cause of pancreatic cancer in this setting has not been defined.[36,37]

## Pathogenesis of Sporadic Pancreatic Cancer

Although there are several inherited forms of PDAC, most cases are sporadic. Like many other cancers, a sequential pathway has been observed in the development of PDAC from pancreatic intraepithelial neoplasia (PanIN) to invasive cancer. A number of tumor suppressor and oncogenes have been identified that play a significant role in the pathogenesis of PDAC, including *PDX1, KRAS2, CDKN2A/p16, P53,* and *DPC4 (SMAD4).*

### Genetic Progression of Pancreatic Intraepithelial Neoplasia to Invasive Pancreatic Ductal Adenocarcinoma

PanIN is defined histologically by progressive abnormality of the ductal epithelium from columnar metaplasia (PanIN-1A) through carcinoma in situ (PanIN-3). PanIN-1A is histologically characterized by the presence of columnar, mucin-producing ductal epithelium that maintains basally located homogeneous nuclei without atypia. The development of papillary architecture defines PanIN-1B, but is otherwise identical to PanIN-1A. PanIN-2 denotes the progression from simple papillary growth to evidence of nuclear atypia not seen in PanIN-1B. Enlarged nuclei with nuclear crowding and loss of polarity are present. Prominent nuclear abnormalities with complete loss of polarity and marked cytologic atypia are characteristic of PanIN-3 (carcinoma in situ). Clusters of abnormal cells can be usually seen within the duct lumen.

The *KRAS2* oncogene is activated in more than 95% of pancreatic cancers and is thought to be the initiating event in tumorigenesis. *KRAS2* is activated by point mutation (codons 12, 13, or 61), which causes constitutive activation and loss of regulation of mitogen-activated protein kinase cell signal transduction. Mutation of the *KRAS2* oncogene is one of the earliest genetic abnormalities identified in the progression of PanIN to PDAC and has been noted in 36% of PanIN-1 cases, 44% of PanIN-2, and 87% of PanIN-3.

*CDKN2A/p16, P53,* and *DPC4* are tumor suppressor genes that also appear to play critical roles in the development of PDAC. *CDKN2A* encodes a protein, p16, which binds to cyclin-dependent kinases (CDK4, CDK6), resulting in cell cycle arrest. Mutation of *CDKN2A* and loss of p16 leads to a loss of cell cycle regulation. Like *KRAS,* mutation of *CDKN2A* (loss of p16 expression) has been identified in 30% of PanIN-1, 55% of PanIN-2 and 71% of PanIN-3 cases. Approximately 90% of PDACs demonstrate loss of p16 function. Also, *p53* encodes for the protein p53, which regulates cell proliferation through cell cycle arrest and proapoptotic mechanisms. Although rare in PanIN, 79% of invasive PDACs demonstrate *p53* mutations, indicating its potential importance in the transition from noninvasive to invasive tumors. Similarly, *DPC4* mutations occur late in the pathway from PanIN to PDAC. Normally functioning as a downstream mediator related to TGF-β, loss of *DPC4* leads to decreased inhibition of cell growth and proliferation. Loss of *DPC4* function has been observed in 20% to 30% of PanIN-3 and localized cancers, whereas 78% of widely

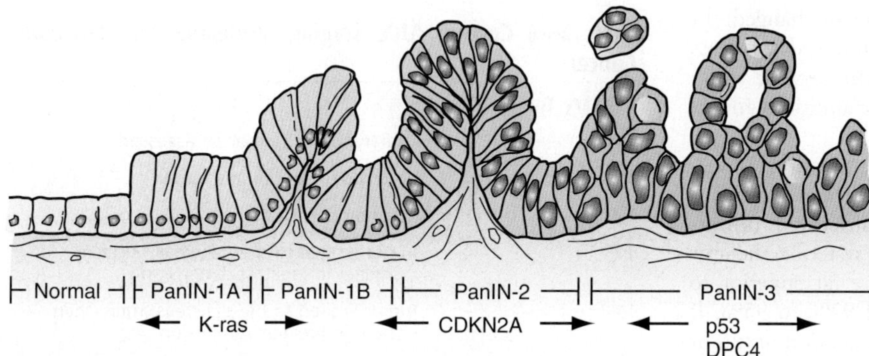


**FIGURE 56-21** Molecular genetic progression from PanIN to invasive ductal adenocarcinoma. (Adapted from Wilentz RE, Iacobuzio-Donahoe CA, Argani P, et al: Loss of expression of DPC4 in pancreatic intraepithelial neoplasia: Evidence that DPC4 inactivation occurs late in neoplastic progression. Cancer Res 60:2002–2006, 2000.)

**Table 56-5 Presenting Symptoms for Periampullary Tumors of the Pancreas**

| PRESENTING SYMPTOM | FREQUENCY (%) |
|---|---|
| Jaundice | 75 |
| Weight loss | 51 |
| Abdominal pain | 39 |
| Nausea/vomiting | 13 |
| Pruritis | 11 |
| Fever | 3 |
| Gastrointestinal bleeding | 1 |

metastatic tumors show loss of *DPC4.* Figure 56-21 demonstrates the molecular genetic alterations involved in the PanIN-PDAC pathway.

## Clinical Presentation

The defining presenting symptom for patients with PDACs in the periampullary region is jaundice. Although painless jaundice has frequently been described, a significant number of patients present with pain in addition to jaundice, typically arising in the epigastrium and radiating to the back. Weight loss is also common at the time of presentation, affecting more than 50% of individuals. For tumors of the body and tail of the pancreas, pain and weight loss become more common at presentation. In the largest single-institution experience reported to date, Winter and coworkers[38] have described 1423 pancreaticoduodenectomies for PDAC. Table 56-5 lists the most common presenting symptoms and their frequency. Except for jaundice, the physical examination is otherwise unremarkable for most patients with PDAC. A palpable distended gallbladder can be identified in approximately one third of patients with periampullary PDAC, an association first described by Courvoisier, a Swiss surgeon, in 1890. He noted that choledocholithiasis was commonly associated with a shrunken fibrotic gallbladder, whereas the slow progressive occlusion of by other causes, including tumors, was more likely to result in ectasia of the organ. Although not diagnostic in itself, Courvoisier's sign is familiar to medical students as a defining characteristic of PDACs. With widespread disease, a left supraclavicular node (Virchow's node) may be palpable. Similarly, periumbilical lymphadenopathy may be palpable (Sister Mary Joseph's node). In cases of peritoneal dissemination, perirectal tumor involvement may be palpable via digital rectal examination, referred to as *Blumer's shelf.*

## Diagnosis

### Laboratory Evaluation

Laboratory evaluation of patients presenting with suspected PDAC should include hepatic function evaluation, including a coagulation profile and nutritional assessment. An elevated bilirubin level is expected, but careful attention should be paid to nutritional values, including prealbumin and albumin levels if surgical intervention is to be considered. Individuals with malnutrition should be given preoperative nutritional supplementation. Several tumor markers may be appropriate at the initial evaluation, including CEA, carbohydrate antigen 19-9 (CA19-9), and α-fetoprotein. Of these, CA19-9 is most sensitive for pancreatic adenocarcinoma, with a sensitivity of approximately 79% and a specificity of 82%. A notable limitation of CA19-9 testing in the setting of periampullary tumors is the false elevation caused by biliary obstruction, which can be misleading. In addition, 10% to 15% of individuals do not develop elevation of the CA19-9 level, a finding that has been associated with blood Lewis antigen–negative status. Accepting these limitations, CA19-9 continues to be the most reliable tumor marker for pretreatment evaluation and post-treatment surveillance for pancreatic adenocarcinoma.

### Imaging Studies

Multidetector CT is the imaging study of choice for the evaluation of lesions arising in the pancreas. CT allows for an accurate determination of the level of biliary obstruction, the relationship of the tumor to critical vascular anatomy, and the presence of regional or metastatic disease. For suspected periampullary pathology, a three-phase (noncontrast, arterial, and portal venous) CT scan with 3-mm slices and coronal and three-dimensional reconstruction should be routine. Because of its widespread availability and excellent sensitivity (85%), CT has become the imaging modality of choice for the evaluation of suspected pancreatic cancer.

ERCP is frequently used in the assessment of the jaundiced patient because of its ability to perform a biopsy and palliate jaundice, if necessary. Although palliative biliary stenting remains routine for PDAC tumors resulting in jaundice, its usefulness is questionable for patients who are candidates for surgical resection. Preoperative biliary decompression may increase the rate of wound infection caused by bactibilia, although overall morbidity and mortality are unchanged. In modern medical practice, ERCP should be reserved for cases requiring therapeutic or palliative intervention because other imaging modalities provide superior diagnostic abilities without the invasiveness of ERCP.

EUS is becoming widely used for the evaluation of suspected pancreatic pathology. Perhaps its most important use is the ability to provide tissue diagnosis of suspected tumors through the use of FNA prior to initiating systemic therapy. FNA has a sensitivity and specificity that are far superior to brush cytology, with a diagnostic accuracy of 92% to 95%. It may also play a crucial role in the molecular evaluation of tumor samples from patients undergoing neoadjuvant therapy. Although the use of EUS is increasing for the evaluation of peritumoral vasculature and regional lymph node evaluation, it has not been shown to provide any significant benefit over CT alone in the absence of a need for tissue diagnosis. EUS may be beneficial for identifying small tumors that do not appear on CT scans and to delineate more clearly suspicious lesions smaller than 2 cm; it therefore plays an important complementary role.

For cases that require detailed assessment of luminal pancreatobiliary anatomy, MRCP should be considered. MRCP has become usefull for the investigation of cystic lesions of the pancreas, with sensitivity and specificity slightly superior to CT alone. MRCP also provides several advantages over ERCP, it is noninvasive, has no risk of inciting pancreatitis, and provides three-dimensional reconstruction of the ductal system.

**Biologic Imaging** $^{18}$F-fluorodeoxyglucose positron emission tomography (FDG-PET) in combination with CT scanning has been increasingly used in the evaluation of pancreatic cancer. The ability of FDG-PET to detect cancers is based on the principle that cells that are actively metabolizing will preferentially take up $^{18}$F-labeled glucose compared with surrounding normal tissues. Several studies have noted the potential benefits of FDG-PET with CT, including the ability to differentiate between benign and malignant pancreas tumors (autoimmune pancreatitis versus adenocarcinoma) and also to identify unsuspected pathology, which alters clinical planning in more than 10% of cases. False-positive findings are also possible, most notably because of inflammatory conditions, and the risk-benefit ratio of FDG-PET with CT has not yet been determined. Further studies will be necessary to clarify the role of FDG-PET with CT in the evaluation of pancreatic cancer before its routine use should be advocated.

## Staging

Pancreatic cancer staging is based on the American Joint Committee on Cancer (AJCC) tumor-node-metastasis (TNM) system (Table 56-6). Following biopsy confirmation, typically via EUS-FNA, accurate staging is accomplished by multidetector CT scanning of the abdomen and pelvis with three-phase contrast administration and three-dimensional reconstruction. Chest radiography is sufficient for the evaluation of potential pulmonary metastasis and should be followed by CT of the chest if any suspicious lesions are noted. Individuals with stages 1A to 2B tumors—tumor confined to the pancreas or peripancreatic tissue without evidence of celiac artery or SMA involvement and no evidence of metastasis—are considered potential candidates for surgical resection. Individuals with stage 3 (T4) disease involving the celiac artery or SMA or stage 4 (metastatic disease) are not candidates for immediate surgery.

**Table 56-6 Current AJCC Staging Guidelines for Pancreatic Cancer**

| **Primary Tumor (T)** | | | |
|---|---|---|---|
| TX | Primary tumor cannot be assessed | | |
| T0 | No evidence of primary tumor | | |
| Tis | Carcinoma in situ* | | |
| T1 | Tumor limited to the pancreas, 2 cm or smaller in greatest dimension | | |
| T2 | Tumor limited to the pancreas, more than 2 cm in greatest dimension | | |
| T3 | Tumor extends beyond the pancreas but without involvement of the celiac axis or superior mesenteric artery | | |
| T4 | Tumor involves the celiac axis or superior mesenteric artery (unresectable primary tumor) | | |
| **Regional Lymph Nodes (N)** | | | |
| NX | Regional lymph nodes cannot be assessed | | |
| N0 | No regional lymph node metastasis | | |
| N1 | Regional lymph node metastasis | | |
| **Distant Metastasis (M)** | | | |
| M0 | No distant metastasis | | |
| M1 | Distant metastasis | | |
| **Anatomic Stage–Prognostic Groups** | | | |
| Stage 0 | Tis | N0 | M0 |
| Stage IA | T1 | N0 | M0 |
| Stage IB | T2 | N0 | M0 |
| Stage IIA | T3 | N0 | M0 |
| Stage IIB | T1<br>T2<br>T3 | N1<br>N1<br>N1 | M0<br>M0<br>M0 |
| Stage III | T4 | Any N | M0 |
| Stage IV | Any T | Any N | M1 |

From Edge S, Byrd D, Compton C, et al (eds): AJCC cancer staging manual, ed 7, New York, 2010, Springer.

*This also includes the PanIN-3classification.

Following CT imaging, patients are classified into resectable, borderline resectable, or unresectable. Resectable tumors are defined as localized to the pancreas, with no evidence of SMV or portal vein involvement (i.e., no abutment, distortion, thrombus, or encasement) and a preserved fat plane surrounding the SMA and celiac artery branches, including the hepatic artery. Patients with imaging consistent with resectable disease should proceed with operative resection.

The appropriate definition of borderline resectable tumors continues to evolve. The National Comprehensive Cancer Network (NCCN) defines borderline resectable as tumors that exhibit one of the following characteristics: (1) severe unilateral or bilateral SMV-portal impingement; (2) less than 180-degree tumor abutment on the SMA; (3) abutment or encasement of hepatic artery, if reconstructible; and (4) SMV occlusion, if of a short segment, and reconstructible.[39] It should be noted that historically, many of these patients would be considered to have locally advanced, unresectable (T4) disease, and the benefit of arterial resection in the setting of significant vascular involvement remains to be determined. Complex procedures required for the extirpation of borderline tumors should be performed only by experienced surgeons, ideally in the setting of a clinical trial.

Unresectable tumors are those that exhibit metastasis, including lymph node metastasis outside the field of resection, ascites, or vascular involvement beyond what has been detailed here.

### Laparoscopy

Staging laparoscopy has been advocated by several authors as a means to reduce the frequency of nontherapeutic laparotomy for patients with unsuspected metastatic or locally advanced unresectable disease identified at the time of surgery. For patients who appear resectable on imaging studies alone, laparoscopy identifies additional unresectable disease in up to 30% of cases. Others have argued that with current imaging used properly, the benefit of additional laparoscopy only rarely alters surgical planning. Recently, there has been some consensus on a more selective use of laparoscopy for those at particularly high risk for occult disease, including those with large tumors (>3 cm), significantly elevated CA19-9 level (>100 U/mL), uncertain findings on CT, or body or tail tumors. It may be clinically prudent also to consider laparoscopy for patients with clinical indicators of widespread disease, including significant weight loss, malnutrition, or pain.[40] There are no level 1 data available to define the role of staging laparoscopy and therefore its use remains at the discretion of the surgeon.

## Treatment

Surgical resection remains the only potentially curative treatment of pancreas cancer.

### Surgery for Tumors of the Head of the Pancreas

For tumors involving the head of the pancreas, pancreaticoduodenectomy is the procedure of choice. Although first described in 1909 by Kausch, the technique became widely known after the first successful surgical resection was performed by Whipple and Parsons and presented to the American Surgical Association by Parsons in 1935. The first two attempts, in 1934, resulted in operative mortality but in 1935 a two-stage procedure, which included biliary decompression followed by pancreaticoduodenectomy, was successful. The initial operative description included ligation of the pancreas remnant without reanastomosis.

The first one-stage Whipple procedure was reported by Trimble and colleagues at Johns Hopkins University in 1941.[41] The modern Whipple procedure maintained a perioperative mortality of 25% and morbidity of well over 50% up until the late 1970s. The advent of improved outcomes for this complex procedure can be attributed to many surgeons and institutions. Most notable on this list of early and seminal leaders in regard to improved mortality and outcome are Cameron (Johns Hopkins Hospital, Baltimore), Tredi (Mannheim Clinic, Mannheim (Germany), Warshaw (Massachusetts General Hospital, Boston), and Brennan (Memorial Sloan Kettering Cancer Center, New York). Each surgeon and center performed more than 100 procedures without any deaths in the 1980s and 1990s.

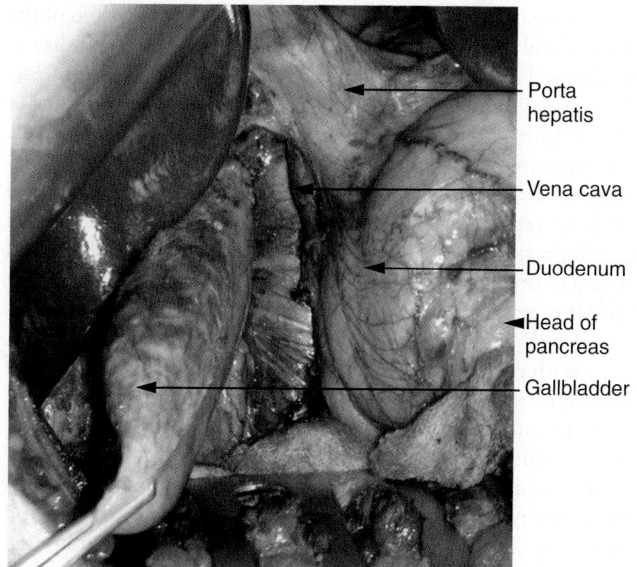


**FIGURE 56-22** Complete mobilization of the head of the pancreas is shown. The vena cava is visible posteriorly. The gallbladder has been freed from the gallbladder fossa.

**Surgical Technique** The modern pancreaticoduodenectomy begins with exploration of the peritoneal surfaces for evidence of metastatic disease, which would deem the patient inoperable. The right colon is then fully mobilized and reflected medially (Cattell-Braasch maneuver), exposing the infrapancreatic SMV. A Kocher maneuver is performed to the level of the left lateral border of the aorta, with attention to clearance of the lymphatic tissue overlying the great vessels. The transverse mesocolon is separated off the head of the pancreas. Figure 56-22 shows complete mobilization of the head of the pancreas and gallbladder. The lesser sac is entered via the gastrocolic ligament, sparing the gastroepiploic vessels. The right gastroepiploic vein is ligated at its confluence with the SMV, allowing the SMV to be dissected from the inferior border and posterior neck of the pancreas. The middle colic vein may also be sacrificed, if necessary, to allow adequate dissection at this level.

Once the infrapancreatic SMV is dissected and the head of the pancreas is fully mobilized, the gallbladder is removed and the common hepatic duct is circumferentially dissected. Division of the common hepatic duct allows for visualization of the suprapancreatic SMV. The duodenum is divided at least 2 cm distal to the pylorus using electrocautery or a blue load stapler. The hepatic artery is exposed proximally and distally and assessed for replacement or aberrant anatomy. The GDA and right gastric artery are visualized. Prior to division of the GDA, the vessel is temporarily occluded and blood flow through the distal common hepatic artery is ensured using a Doppler device. This maneuver is vital in patients with atherosclerosis of celiac origin to ensure that the hepatic blood supply is not dependent on collateral retrograde arterial flow from the SMA via the GDA. Once hepatic arterial flow is confirmed, the right gastric artery and GDA are ligated and divided. If flow in the hepatic artery is interrupted by occlusion of the GDA, resection may only proceed with preservation of the GDA or arterial resection and bypass, typically as an aortohepatic conduit.

The pancreas is then divided after four-point ligation of the inferior and superior pancreaticoduodenal arteries. Blunt dissection is used to separate the portal vein from the uncinate process. This dissection often includes ligation of a superior and inferior branch from the portal vein and SMV to the uncinate process. The jejunum is divided approximately 10 cm distal to the ligament of Treitz and the short mesenteric vessels are divided to allow for retromesenteric rotation of the jejunum and third and fourth portions of the duodenum. The head of the pancreas and attached small bowel are then retracted to the patient's right and the remaining portal vein and uncinate dissection is completed.

With the portal vein completely free, the gland is retracted further to the right to allow for complete visualization of the uncinate process and SMA. The retroperitoneal tissue is dissected from the SMA, allowing for complete removal of the caudate and periarterial lymphatic tissue. Figure 56-23*A* shows the anatomy following removal of the head of the pancreas and Figure 56-23*B* highlights complete clearance of periarterial tissue from the SMA. If portal venous or SMV tumor involvement is encountered, as shown in Figures 56-24*A* and *B*, venous resection should be performed. Resections that compromise less than 50% of the venous diameter can be closed primarily (see Fig. 56-24*C*); otherwise, segmental resection with primary anastomosis or interposition graft using internal jugular or femoral vein should be performed.

**Reconstruction** Prior to reconstruction, frozen section evaluation of the surgical margins is performed. Once negative margins are ensured, the proximal jejunum is brought through the transverse mesocolon or the retromesenteric defect in preparation for pancreaticojejunostomy and hepaticojejunostomy. The pancreaticojejunostomy is created in two layers, anterior and posterior, with a duct to mucosa anastomosis (Fig. 56-25). An internal pancreatic stent can be left in place for ducts smaller than 5 mm. The hepaticojejunostomy anastomosis is then created 6 to 8 cm downstream from the pancreaticojejunostomy in an end-to-side fashion. If the duct is smaller than 5 mm, it is spatulated to improve patency. Following this, an antecolic duodenojejunostomy is completed. External drains are selectively placed adjacent to the pancreaticojejunostomy and hepaticojejunostomy. Similarly, a feeding jejunostomy is placed in selected patients with significant preoperative malnutrition (albumin level <3.5 g/dL).

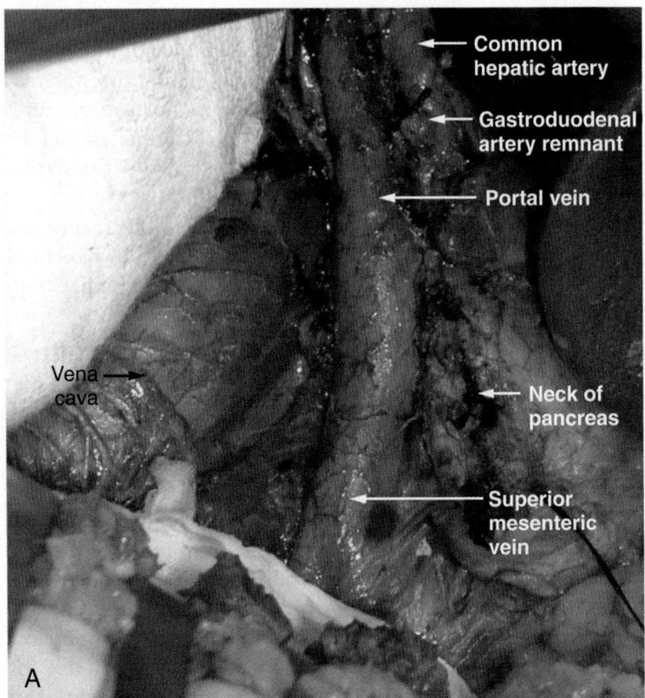


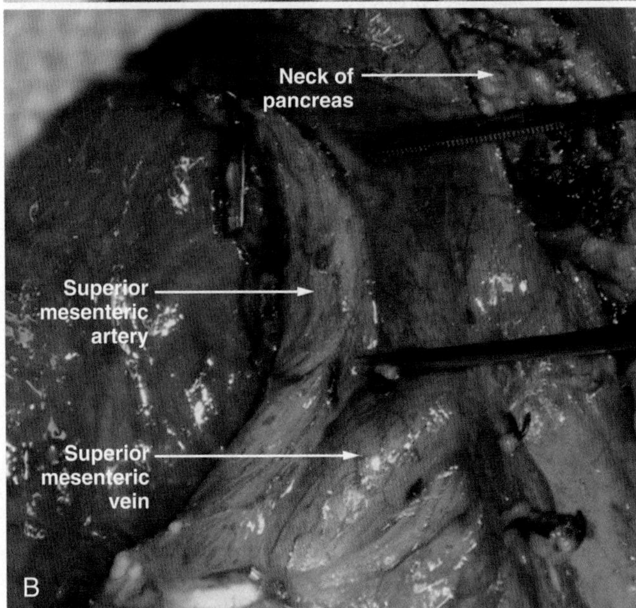


**FIGURE 56-23** **A,** Surgical anatomy following pancreaticoduodenectomy. The SMV, portal vein, hepatic artery, and vena cava are visualized. Complete lymphatic clearance is noted. **B,** SMA dissection illustrating complete clearance of periarterial lymphatic tissue.

## Surgery for Tumors of the Body and Tail of the Pancreas

Tumors arising in the body and tail of the pancreas are rarely resectable at the time of presentation, given the lack of symptoms with small tumors. Only 5% to 7% of individuals with body or tail PDACs will ultimately undergo surgery, and median survival is significantly shorter than PDACs of the pancreatic head because of the more advanced nature of resected tumors. Although tumor involvement of the splenic artery or vein does not preclude surgery, involvement of the celiac axis is a contraindication to resection. For resectable tumors, distal pancreatectomy and en bloc splenectomy should be performed. After inspection of the peritoneal surfaces, the gastrocolic and splenocolic ligaments and short gastric vessels are divided to expose the pancreas and spleen. The inferior border of the pancreas is dissected, exposing the retroperitoneal plane behind the gland. This anatomic plane can be used to mobilize the body and tail of the pancreas anterior to Gerota's fascia completely. At the superior border of the pancreas, the splenic artery is circumferentially dissected and divided at its origin from the celiac trunk. The splenic vein is carefully dissected from the posterior wall of the pancreas at its confluence with the SMV and divided. At this point, the distal pancreas and spleen are devascularized and the neck of the pancreas is divided. A medial to lateral dissection is completed and the spleen is detached from its posterior peritoneal attachments to allow en bloc removal of the specimen and

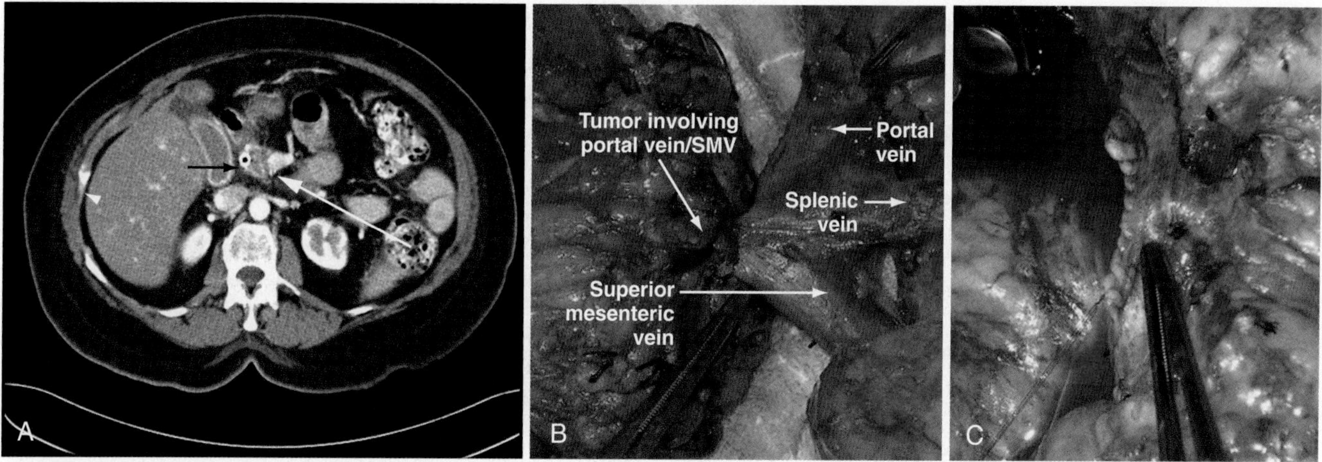


**FIGURE 56-24 A,** CT scan showing PDAC of the pancreatic head with involvement of portal vein–SMV confluence *(large arrow)*. A metal biliary stent is in place *(small arrow)*. **B,** Operative image demonstrating tumor involvement of the lateral aspect of the portal vein–SMV confluence. **C,** Primary closure of portal vein–SMV confluence following tumor removal with lateral vein resection.

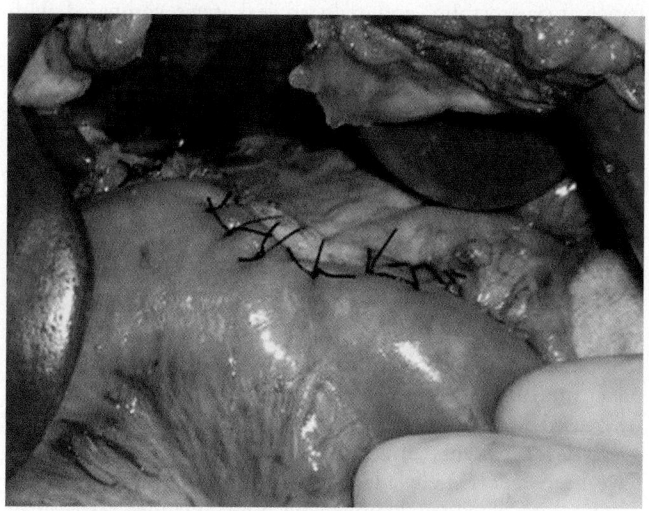

**FIGURE 56-25** Completed pancreaticojejunostomy.

surrounding lymph node basin. Several techniques may be used to close the pancreatic duct remnant, with the most common being direct suture ligation or use of a linear stapling device. Either technique is appropriate, with similar risk for the development of pancreatic fistula.

### Laparoscopic Distal Pancreatectomy

There has been growing interest in the use of minimally invasive surgery for the resection of tumors of the distal pancreas. Laparoscopic distal pancreatectomy (LDP) may offer advantages over open resection for select patients, with smaller incisions and shorter hospital stay. In a review of over 800 LDPs, Borja and colleagues[42] described an overall morbidity rate of 38% and hospital length of stay of 5 days, which compare favorably with large series following open pancreatectomy. Although LDP is increasingly used for benign conditions, its usefulness for the treatment of PDAC remains to be validated. There have been no randomized trials to evaluate LDP versus open resection, and few studies have reported outcomes of LDP for PDACs. Currently, LDP in the setting of PDACs should be considered experimental.

**Table 56-7 Morbidity Following Pancreaticoduodenectomy**

| COMPLICATION | FREQUENCY (%) |
|---|---|
| Delayed gastric emptying | 18 |
| Pancreas fistula | 12 |
| Wound infection | 7 |
| Intra-abdominal abscess | 6 |
| Cardiac events | 3 |
| Bile leak | 2 |
| Overall reoperation | 3 |

## Outcomes

### Perioperative Mortality: Long-Term Survival

Perioperative mortality has become a rare event following the Whipple procedure, occurring in less than 2% of cases at high-volume centers. Despite significant reduction in mortality, however, morbidity remains common, occurring after 30% to 50% of procedures.[38] Table 56-7 lists several of the most common postoperative morbidities and their frequencies.

Following surgical resection and adjuvant therapy for pancreatic cancer, the median survival is approximately 22 months, with 5-year survival of 15% to 20%. Most patients experience relapse of disease in the form of metastatic disease (85%) and, less commonly, local recurrence (40%). In the absence of surgical resection, those with locally advanced disease who receive palliative chemotherapy may survive 10 to 12 months, whereas those with metastases rarely survive beyond 6 months. The role of adjuvant chemotherapy and radiation is described later in this chapter.

**Table 56-8 ISGPF Classification of Pancreatic Fistulas**

| | Grade | | |
|---|---|---|---|
| **PARAMETER** | **A** | **B** | **C** |
| Clinical conditions | Well | Often well | Ill-appearing, bad |
| Specific treatment | No | Yes/no | Yes |
| US, CT scan (if obtained) | Negative | Negative/ positive | Positive |
| Persistent drainage (after 3 wk) | No | Usually yes | Yes |
| Reoperation | No | No | Yes |
| Death related to POPF | No | No | Possibly yes |
| Signs of infections | No | Yes | Yes |
| Sepsis | No | No | Yes |
| Readmission | No | Yes/no | Yes/no |

From Bassi C, Dervenis C, Butturini G, et al: Postoperative pancreatic fistula: An international study group (ISGPF) definition. Surgery 138:8–13, 2005.

*POPF*, Postoperative pancreatic fistula.

### Morbidity

The most common difficulty following pancreaticoduodenectomy is delayed gastric emptying, characterized by the need for prolonged nasogastric decompression and/or inability to tolerate oral intake. There are variable criteria used to define delayed gastric emptying precisely, but 10% to 50% of individuals have some alteration in food tolerance following Whipple surgery. The International Study Group of Pancreatic Surgery (ISGPS)[43] has suggested a uniform definition for delayed gastric emptying to allow for more rigorous investigation: "output via an intra-operatively placed drain (or percutaneous drain) of any measurable volume of drain fluid on or after postoperative day 3, with amylase >3 times normal serum value." This is frequently described following pancreaticoduodenectomy, occurring after 5% to 22% of surgeries. Perhaps the most predictive factor is the texture of the gland, with soft fatty glands at significantly higher risk of leak. Most fistulas are controlled by drainage catheters placed at the time of surgery and require no additional intervention. Rarely, uncontrolled fistulas require additional drain placement or operative exploration, sometimes mandating completion pancreatectomy to eliminate further abdominal contamination. The classification of pancreatic fistulas is given in Table 56-8.

Anastomotic leaks from the hepaticojejunostomy and duodenojejunostomy are rare, and occur after less than 5% of procedures. Infectious complications (e.g., intra-abdominal abscess, wound infection) are slightly more common and may require intervention with percutaneous drainage or open wound dressing changes.

Pancreatic endocrine and exocrine insufficiency can occur after pancreaticoduodenectomy, but the risk of these events is unpredictable. For individuals with a normal gland, pancreatic insufficiency is rare. However, for those with preexisting chronic pancreatitis, fibrosis of the gland, or insulin resistance, exogenous enzyme and insulin replacement are usually needed.

## Controversies

### Pylorus-Preserving Versus Non–Pylorus-Preserving Whipple Procedure

We have described the pylorus-preserving Whipple procedure, which is the operation of choice for a growing number of pancreatobiliary surgeons. It was initially proposed as a means to reduce postpancreatectomy dumping and bile reflux, which is common after a non–pylorus-preserving Whipple procedure. Although initial results were encouraging, there has been no trial to suggest the superiority of a pylorus-preserving over non–pylorus-preserving Whipple procedure. We prefer pylorus preservation when possible, but do not hesitate to proceed with a non–pylorus-preserving Whipple procedure in case of tumor involvement of the duodenum or concern for duodenal blood supply.

### Pancreaticojejunostomy Versus Pancreatogastrostomy

The pancreaticojejunostomy remains the Achilles' heel of the Whipple procedure because of the frequency of pancreatic fistula. Several studies have reported successful outcomes with pancreatogastrostomy and reduced leak rates compared with pancreaticojejunostomy, but this finding has not been reproducible in several randomized trials and most surgeons continue to prefer pancreaticojejunostomy.[44] In cases in which the pancreatic duct is not identified, invagination of the gland into the jejunal stump may also be performed.

### Extent of Lymphadenectomy

Given the fact that 75% to 80% of patients are found to have lymph node (LN) involvement at the time of the Whipple procedure and, overall, 80% to 85% of patients will experience tumor recurrence and cancer-related death, some have proposed that radical lymphadenectomy may improve outcomes. Regional pancreatectomy was first proposed by Fortner in 1973 and has been used widely in Japan, where significant improvements in survival for patients undergoing extended lymphadenectomy have been reported. In addition to peripancreatic, portal, and pyloric LN, extended lymphadenectomy includes retrieval of hilar and retroperitoneal LNs, extending from the celiac origin to the level of the inferior mesenteric artery and including all tissue between the renal hilum laterally. Several randomized control trials have since been completed, with no evidence to suggest improved survival following extended lymphadenectomy. In fact, more than one trial has shown increased morbidity associated with extended lymphadenectomy, including delayed gastric emptying, pancreatic fistula, and dumping.[45] In view of the current evidence, standard pancreaticoduodenectomy is the operation of choice for localized pancreatic adenocarcinoma.

### Laparoscopic Pancreaticoduodenectomy

The first laparoscopic pancreaticoduodenectomy was performed in 1994 by Gagner and Pomp. Since then, several case reports and small series have been published, which have demonstrated the feasibility of the minimally invasive approach. In the largest U.S. series to date, Kendrick and Cusati[46] have reported outcomes of 65 laparoscopic pancreaticoduodenectomies, with an overall morbidity rate of 42%—pancreatic fistula rate 18%, delayed gastric emptying 15%, bleeding 8%, wound infection 6%, reoperation 5%, and mortality of 1.5%. These results indicate that laparoscopic pancreaticoduodenectomy has similar short-term outcomes as the open approach. Given the complexity of the procedure and the fact that the major morbidities following pancreaticoduodenectomy are not related to the size of the incision, the laparoscopic Whipple procedure has not become widely adopted.

### Antecolic Versus Retrocolic Duodenojejunostomy

Delayed gastric emptying is a common occurrence following pancreaticoduodenectomy with an elusive cause. Emerging data suggest that creation of an antecolic duodenojejunostomy may improve gastric emptying compared with the retrocolic technique.

## Adjuvant Therapy for Pancreatic Cancer

### Chemotherapy and Radiation

Over the last 30 years, there have been conflicting reports regarding the survival benefit of adjuvant therapy following surgical resection of localized pancreatic cancer, particularly with regard to radiation therapy. Although the use of chemotherapy is widely accepted, the usefulness of radiation therapy has been increasingly questioned. In the United States, chemotherapy and radiation are still widely used, whereas European centers have stopped using radiation therapy as part of standard adjuvant therapy because of lack of evidence to support a survival benefit.

Several randomized trials have attempted to clarify the roles of chemotherapy and radiation as adjuvant treatment of pancreatic cancer following surgical resection. Table 56-9 summarizes the findings of several important trials. In 1974, the Gastrointestinal Tumor Study Group (GITSG) began a prospective randomized trial comparing adjuvant 5-fluorouracil (5-FU) and 4000-rad radiation with observation following curative resection.[47] The trial was terminated prematurely because of low accrual and the observation that the chemoradiation arm had a significant survival advantage. Over an 8-year period, only 49 patients were accrued and randomized (43 patients were included in the final analysis because of withdrawal of 5 individuals and misdiagnosis of 1). Median survival for the chemoradiation group was 20 months compared with 11 months for observation. Despite its limitations, this was the first randomized control trial that demonstrated an overall survival benefit following chemoradiation.

**Table 56-9 Summary of Clinical Trials Defining Role of Adjuvant Therapy Following Resection of Pancreatic Cancer**

| TRIAL | CONCLUSIONS |
|---|---|
| GITSG | Adjuvant chemoradiation with 5-FU and 40 Gy radiation therapy improves survival compared with observation alone. |
| ESPAC-1 | Adjuvant chemotherapy improves survival; chemoradiation is deleterious. |
| CONKO-001 | Adjuvant gemcitabine improves disease-free survival compared with observation. |
| RTOG 97-04 | Gemcitabine before and after 5-FU–based chemoradiation provides similar overall survival compared with 5-FU, but with significantly less toxicity. |
| ESPAC-3 | Adjuvant chemotherapy alone with gemcitabine provides similar overall survival as 5-FU, but with significantly less toxicity. |

The European Study Group for Pancreatic Cancer-1 (ESPAC-1) trial was a 2 × 2 factorial design that compared chemoradiotherapy alone (5-FU, 20 Gy over 2 weeks) versus chemotherapy alone (5-FU), versus chemoradiotherapy and chemotherapy versus observation.[48] At a median follow-up of 47 months, it was noted that the estimated 5-year survival for those who underwent chemoradiotherapy was significantly less than those who did not (10% versus 20%; $P = .05$). At the same time, those who received chemotherapy had a 5-year survival of 21% versus 8% for those who did not ($P < .009$). These findings led to the conclusion that although chemotherapy provided significant improvement in overall survival, the routine use of chemoradiation may be detrimental.

In 2007, the Charité Onkologie (CONKO-001) trial of 368 individuals enrolled over a 6-year period evaluated whether chemotherapy with gemcitabine (without radiation) could extend disease-free survival compared with observation.[49] Trial patients received six cycles of gemcitabine (days 1, 8, and 15 every 4 weeks for 6 months) and outcomes were compared with observation alone. Median disease-free survival was significantly improved in the gemcitabine group compared with observation (13.4 versus 6.9 months). There was a trend toward improved overall survival but this did not meet statistical significance (median, 22.1 versus 20.2 months). This trial established the use of adjuvant gemcitabine for the treatment of pancreatic cancer.

The Radiation Therapy Oncology Group (RTOG 97-04) trial compared 5-FU versus gemcitabine chemotherapy before and after 5-FU–based chemoradiation.[50] The purpose of the study was to determine whether gemcitabine provided a survival benefit over 5-FU in combination with 5-FU–based chemoradiation. It was noted that although overall survival was similar (20.5 months for gemcitabine versus 16.9 months for 5-FU; $P =$ NS), the treatment-related toxicity was significantly higher in the 5-FU group. These data have led to the use of gemcitabine as the first-line agent for adjuvant chemotherapy, with or without radiation.

The most recent international randomized controlled trial to be completed (ESPAC-3) was designed to evaluate overall survival comparing 5-FU (425 mg/m$^2$ IV bolus, given on days 1 to 5 every 28 days) versus gemcitabine (1000 mg/m$^2$ IV, days 1, 8, 15 every 4 weeks) following curative surgery. No observation arm was included because it was thought to be unethical, given the existing data suggesting a survival benefit of chemotherapy over observation alone. More than 1000 participants from 16 countries were randomized. Overall survival was similar between the groups (23.0 months for 5-FU, 23.6 months for gemcitabine), but gemcitabine was found to have less treatment-related toxicity, with fewer severe adverse events and better compliance. These results are currently awaiting publication, but support the continued use of gemcitabine as first-line treatment. A multicenter randomized trial evaluating the efficacy of albumin-bound paclitaxel and gemcitabine in the setting of metastatic disease is currently underway.

Current NCCN guidelines continue to recommend gemcitabine or 5-FU alone, or in combination with 5-FU– based chemoradiation, as adjuvant treatment following resection for PDAC. Given the overall poor prognosis, enrollment into clinical trials is encouraged.

### Role of Neoadjuvant Therapy

The administration of chemotherapy, with or without radiation, prior to planned surgical resection for pancreatic cancer is becoming increasingly common. The rationale for the neoadjuvant approach is multifaceted. Following surgical resection, approximately 25% of patients do not receive adjuvant therapy because of refusal, surgical complications, or an inability to recover physiologically. Giving therapy prior to surgery ensures that all patients will receive multimodality therapy and, by delivering therapy to an intact gland with an established blood supply, the efficacy of therapy may be maximized. In addition, by treating patients with measurable disease, response to therapy can be assessed more readily. Progression of disease during neoadjuvant treatment is indicative of aggressive tumor biology and may prevent these patients from undergoing extensive surgery, which is unlikely to provide any survival benefit. Finally, the administration of chemotherapy and radiation prior to surgery has been viewed as a physiologic stress test and helps select patients who would be unlikely to tolerate the major stress of surgical resection. Neoadjuvant therapy may provide improved patient selection, avoiding surgery for those who progress, but also improved negative margin rates and reduced LN metastasis. Despite all these benefits, no studies have shown an improvement in overall survival for patients who receive neoadjuvant chemotherapy and radiation.

In select patients, the role of neoadjuvant therapy is clearer, particularly those with significant venous or limited arterial involvement who are classified as borderline resectable. In these patients, where up-front surgical exploration has a significant risk of exposing patients to nontherapeutic laparotomy, the argument for neoadjuvant therapy is strengthened. For individuals with significant SMV–portal vein involvement (>180 degrees or short-segment encasement), or hepatic arterial or SMA abutment (<180 degrees) who have been traditionally considered unresectable, neoadjuvant therapy may play an important role in identifying the subset of patients most likely to derive benefit from aggressive multimodality therapy, including surgical resection with vascular reconstruction.[51] This type of aggressive treatment should be undertaken only by an experienced multidisciplinary team in the setting of a clinical trial.

## Palliative Therapy for Pancreatic Cancer

Given that 80% to 85% of those with pancreatic cancer have locally advanced or metastatic disease at the time of presentation, and are therefore not candidates for surgical resection, it is imperative that all surgeons be familiar with nonoperative and operative palliative options. In general, nonoperative management should be pursued whenever possible to expedite systemic therapy and optimize quality of life for these patients.

### Biliary Obstruction

Palliation of biliary obstruction is commonly required for patients who are not candidates for surgical resection. ERCP with metal stent placement provides excellent palliation of jaundice and, at high-volume university centers, successful biliary drainage is possible in more than 90% of cases. In patients for whom endoscopic palliation is impossible, percutaneous biliary drainage with subsequent internalization may be required. For patients who are found at laparotomy to have unresectable disease, or those for whom nonsurgical measures have failed, a surgical biliary-enteric bypass may be performed via Roux-en-Y hepaticojejunostomy, with excellent long-term patency.

### Gastric Outlet Obstruction

Approximately 20% of patients with locally advanced pancreatic cancer will develop gastric outlet obstruction. For those with metastatic disease or disease found to be unresectable based on imaging findings, who have symptoms of gastric outlet obstruction, endoscopic luminal stenting should be carried out. Palliative endoscopic stenting has excellent short-term results, with almost immediate improvement in oral intake, but is limited in its ability to provide long-term patency. For this reason, patients who are found to have unresectable cancer at the time of laparotomy may benefit from preventive gastrojejunostomy, with no increase in perioperative morbidity. For patients who require surgical intervention, a double bypass consisting of a Roux-en-Y hepaticojejunostomy and gastrojejunostomy may be performed.

### Pain Relief

Pain is a common component in the natural history of pancreatic cancer, affecting most patients with advanced disease. Palliation of pain is paramount for optimizing the quality of life for patients and should be a primary goal for physicians. The initial management of pain may include anti-inflammatories or long-acting opioids, taken orally or via a cutaneous patch. For patients with pain that is not well controlled, or who suffer side effects of narcotic use, celiac nerve block should be considered. The procedure involves injecting a combination of 3 mL of 0.25% bupivacaine and 10 mL of absolute alcohol into each celiac plexus. For cases that are found at exploration to be unresectable, this can be performed intraoperatively, as described by Lillemoe and coworkers.[52] For those with unresectable disease based on staging evaluation, who do not undergo surgical exploration, neurolysis can be achieved via EUS guidance, with pain relief expected in 80% of patients.[53] CT-guided percutaneous neurolysis may also be performed.

## PANCREATIC TRAUMA

Pancreatic injuries are uncommon. The mechanism of injury varies according to the age of the patient. The most common mechanism in pediatric patients is abdominal blunt trauma. Direct compression of the epigastrium against the vertebral column and a blunt object (handlebar) is typically seen after bicycle injuries. The most common segment of the pancreas affected is the body. Penetrating injuries into the abdomen are the most common injuries seen in adults.[54]

Isolated pancreatic injuries are not common. Up to 90% of patients present with associated hepatic, gastric, splenic, renal, colonic, or vascular lesions.[54] The diagnosis and therapy in unstable patients with severe retroperitoneal injuries, gunshot wounds, or penetrating injury into the abdomen are usually straightforward and do not require further evaluation. Hemodynamically stable patients represent a challenge because isolated pancreatic injures are normally associated with subtle or absent physical symptoms and signs. Undiagnosed pancreatic injuries are associated with significant complications, such as intra-abdominal abscess, fistula, or fluid collections in 60% of patients.[55] Pancreatic injuries should always be considered after epigastric compression during a car or bicycle accident.

**Table 56-10 American Association for the Surgery of Trauma Pancreatic Injury Grading**

| GRADE | | INJURY DESCRIPTION |
|---|---|---|
| I | Hematoma | Minor contusion without ductal injury |
| | Laceration | Superficial laceration without ductal injury |
| II | Hematoma | Major contusion without ductal injury or tissue loss |
| | Laceration | Major laceration without ductal injury or tissue loss |
| III | Laceration | Distal transaction or pancreatic parenchymal injury without ductal injury |
| IV | Laceration | Proximal transaction or pancreatic parenchymal injury involving the ampulla |
| V | Laceration | Massive disruption of the pancreatic head |

From Subramanian A, Dente CJ, Feliciano DV: The management of pancreatic trauma in the modern era. Surg Clin North Am 87:1515–1532, 2007.

The modality of choice to evaluate patients with abdominal trauma is CT scanning of the abdomen. Findings such as peripancreatic hematomas, free fluid in the lesser sack, or abnormal thickening of Gerota's fascia suggest pancreatic injury. Recent studies have shown that MRCP provides excellent visualization of the pancreatic duct, peripancreatic fluid contiguous to fractured segments of the pancreas, and hemorrhage after nonpenetrating trauma. Its main limitations include high cost, availability, and amount of time required to perform the study. Isolated pancreatic amylase level measurement is not recommended because up to 40% of patients with pancreatic duct transected have normal serum amylase levels. Serial quantification levels increase the sensitivity of the assay. Abnormal amylase level elevations require further imaging.

The most reliable test to demonstrate pancreatic duct integrity is ERCP. However, its applicability is frequently limited by the risk of inducing pancreatitis, availability, and severity of the trauma.

Pancreatic injuries are classified according to the system described by the American Association for the Surgery of Trauma (AAST; Table 56-10.) Definitive treatment is based on surgical findings. Major pancreatic resections have been described in stable patients with isolated pancreatic injury. However, pancreatic resections in unstable patients are associated with significant morbidity and mortality. Therefore, damage control surgery is indicated for complex injuries or unstable patients. Most pancreatic lesions can be temporarily controlled with drains. Once the physiologic insult has been controlled, definitive treatment should be considered, if indicated. Up to 75% of deaths occur within the 48 to 72 hours after trauma, and most are related to hypovolemic shock.[54]

## SELECTED REFERENCES


Abrams RA, Lowy AM, O'Reilly EM, et al: Combined modality treatment of resectable and borderline resectable pancreas cancer: Expert consensus statement. Ann Surg Oncol 16:1751–1756, 2009.

A consensus statement regarding recommending multimodality therapy to optimize outcomes for patients with resectable and borderline resectable pancreatic cancer.

Andersen DK, Frey CF: The evolution of the surgical treatment of chronic pancreatitis. Ann Surg 251:18–32, 2010.

A historical review of surgical techniques for the management of chronic pancreatitis.

Beger HG, Rau BM: Severe acute pancreatitis: Clinical course and management. World J Gastroenterol 13:5043–5051, 2007.

A review of the pathophysiology of acute pancreatitis and clinical management strategies.

Winter JM, Cameron JL, Campbell KA, et al: 1423 pancreaticoduodenectomies for pancreatic cancer: A single-institution experience. J Gastrointest Surg 10:1199–1210; discussion 1210–1191, 2006.

A historic review of the largest single institution pancreaticoduodenectomy experience.

Gittes GK: Developmental biology of the pancreas: a comprehensive review. Dev Biol 326:4–35, 2009.

A comprehensive review of pancreatic embryology and development.


## REFERENCES


1. Gittes GK: Developmental biology of the pancreas: a comprehensive review. Dev Biol 326:4–35, 2009.
2. Saluja AK, Lerch MM, Phillips PA, et al: Why does pancreatic overstimulation cause pancreatitis? Annu Rev Physiol 69:249–269, 2007.
3. Whitcomb DC: Clinical practice. Acute pancreatitis. N Engl J Med 354:2142–2150, 2006.
4. Beger HG, Rau BM: Severe acute pancreatitis: Clinical course and management. World J Gastroenterol 13:5043–5051, 2007.
5. Elfar M, Gaber LW, Sabek O, et al: The inflammatory cascade in acute pancreatitis: Relevance to clinical disease. Surg Clin North Am 87:1325–1340, 2007.
6. Larson SD, Nealon WH, Evers BM: Management of gallstone pancreatitis. Adv Surg 40:265–284, 2006.
7. Frossard JL, Steer ML, Pastor CM: Acute pancreatitis. Lancet 371:143–152, 2008.
8. Cappell MS: Acute pancreatitis: Cause, clinical presentation, diagnosis, and therapy. Med Clin North Am 92:889–923, 2008.
9. Saokar A, Rabinowitz CB, Sahani DV: Cross-sectional imaging in acute pancreatitis. Radiol Clin North Am 45:447–460, 2007.
10. Ranson JH, Rifkind KM, Roses DF, et al: Prognostic signs and the role of operative management in acute pancreatitis. Surg Gynecol Obstet 139:69–81, 1974.
11. Gravante G, Garcea G, Ong SL, et al: Prediction of mortality in acute pancreatitis: A systematic review of the published evidence. Pancreatology 9:601–614, 2009.
12. Balthazar EJ, Robinson DL, Megibow AJ, et al: Acute pancreatitis: Value of CT in establishing prognosis. Radiology 174:331–336, 1990.
13. Charbonney E, Nathens AB: Severe acute pancreatitis: A review. Surg Infect (Larchmt) 9:573–578, 2008.
14. Nealon WH, Bawduniak J, Walser EM: Appropriate timing of cholecystectomy in patients who present with moderate to severe gallstone-associated acute pancreatitis with peripancreatic fluid collections. Ann Surg 239:741–749, 2004.

15. Rodriguez JR, Razo AO, Targarona J, et al: Débridement and closed packing for sterile or infected necrotizing pancreatitis: Insights into indications and outcomes in 167 patients. Ann Surg 247:294–299, 2008.
16. Besselink MG, Verwer TJ, Schoenmaeckers EJ, et al: Timing of surgical intervention in necrotizing pancreatitis. Arch Surg 142:1194–1201, 2007.
17. Lerch MM, Stier A, Wahnschaffe U, et al: Pancreatic pseudocysts: Observation, endoscopic drainage, or resection? Dtsch Arztebl Int 106:614–621, 2009.
18. Witt H, Apte MV, Keim V, et al: Chronic pancreatitis: Challenges and advances in pathogenesis, genetics, diagnosis, and therapy. Gastroenterology 132:1557–1573, 2007.
19. Apte MV, Haber PS, Applegate TL, et al: Periacinar stellate-shaped cells in rat pancreas: Identification, isolation, and culture. Gut 43:128–133, 1998.
20. Catalano MF, Sahai A, Levy M, et al: EUS-based criteria for the diagnosis of chronic pancreatitis: The Rosemont classification. Gastrointest Endosc 69:1251–1261, 2009.
21. O'Neil SJ, Aranha GV: Lateral pancreaticojejunostomy for chronic pancreatitis. World J Surg 27:1196–1202, 2003.
22. Andersen DK, Frey CF: The evolution of the surgical treatment of chronic pancreatitis. Ann Surg 251:18–32, 2010.
23. Keck T, Wellner UF, Riediger H, et al: Long-term outcome after 92 duodenum-preserving pancreatic head resections for chronic pancreatitis: Comparison of Beger and Frey procedures. J Gastrointest Surg 14:549–556, 2010.
24. Heidt DG, Burant C, Simeone DM: Total pancreatectomy: Indications, operative technique, and postoperative sequelae. J Gastrointest Surg 11:209–216, 2007.
25. Blondet JJ, Carlson AM, Kobayashi T, et al: The role of total pancreatectomy and islet autotransplantation for chronic pancreatitis. Surg Clin North Am 87:1477–1501, 2007.
26. Compagno J, Oertel JE: Mucinous cystic neoplasms of the pancreas with overt and latent malignancy (cystadenocarcinoma and cystadenoma). A clinicopathologic study of 41 cases. Am J Clin Pathol 69:573–580, 1978.
27. Brugge WR, Lewandrowski K, Lee-Lewandrowski E, et al: Diagnosis of pancreatic cystic neoplasms: A report of the cooperative pancreatic cyst study. Gastroenterology 126:1330–1336, 2004.
28. Tran Cao HS, Kellogg B, Lowy AM, et al: Cystic neoplasms of the pancreas. Surg Oncol Clin N Am 19:267–295, 2010.
29. Allen PJ, Qin LX, Tang L, et al: Pancreatic cyst fluid protein expression profiling for discriminating between serous cystadenoma and intraductal papillary mucinous neoplasm. Ann Surg 250:754–760, 2009.
30. D'Angelica M, Brennan MF, Suriawinata AA, et al: Intraductal papillary mucinous neoplasms of the pancreas: An analysis of clinicopathologic features and outcome. Ann Surg 239:400–408, 2004.
31. Salvia R, Fernandez-del Castillo C, Bassi C, et al: Main-duct intraductal papillary mucinous neoplasms of the pancreas: Clinical predictors of malignancy and long-term survival following resection. Ann Surg 239:678–685; discussion 685–677, 2004.
32. Tanaka M, Chari S, Adsay V, et al: International consensus guidelines for management of intraductal papillary mucinous neoplasms and mucinous cystic neoplasms of the pancreas. Pancreatology 6:17–32, 2006.
33. Katz MH, Mortenson MM, Wang H, et al: Diagnosis and management of cystic neoplasms of the pancreas: An evidence-based approach. J Am Coll Surg 207:106–120, 2008.
34. Sohn TA, Yeo CJ, Cameron JL, et al: Intraductal papillary mucinous neoplasms of the pancreas: An updated experience. Ann Surg 239:788–797, 2004.
35. Altekruse SF, Kosary CL, Krapcho M, et al: SEER Cancer Statistics Review, 1975-2007, National Cancer Institute, 2010 (http://seer.cancer.gov/csr/1975_2007).
36. Landi S: Genetic predisposition and environmental risk factors to pancreatic cancer: A review of the literature. Mutat Res 681:299–307, 2009.
37. Klein AP, Hruban RH, Brune KA, et al: Familial pancreatic cancer. Cancer J 7:266–273, 2001.
38. Winter JM, Cameron JL, Campbell KA, et al: 1423 pancreaticoduodenectomies for pancreatic cancer: A single-institution experience. J Gastrointest Surg 10:1199–1210; discussion 1210–1191, 2006.
39. Benson AB, 3rd, Abrams TA, Ben-Josef E, et al: NCCN clinical practice guidelines in oncology: Hepatobiliary cancers. J Natl Compr Canc Netw 7:350–391, 2009.
40. Callery MP, Chang KJ, Fishman EK, et al: Pretreatment assessment of resectable and borderline resectable pancreatic cancer: Expert consensus statement. Ann Surg Oncol 16:1727–1733, 2009.
41. Trimble IR, Parsons JW, Sherman CP: A one-stage operation for the cure of carcinoma of the ampulla of Vater and the head of the pancreas. Surg Gynecol Obstet 73:711–722, 1941.
42. Borja-Cacho D, Al-Refaie WB, Vickers SM, et al: Laparoscopic distal pancreatectomy. J Am Coll Surg 209:758–765, 2009.
43. Bassi C, Dervenis C, Butturini G, et al: Postoperative pancreatic fistula: An international study group (ISGPF) definition. Surgery 138:8–13, 2005.
44. Wente MN, Shrikhande SV, Muller MW, et al: Pancreaticojejunostomy versus pancreaticogastrostomy: Systematic review and meta-analysis. Am J Surg 193:171–183, 2007.
45. Farnell MB, Aranha GV, Nimura Y, et al: The role of extended lymphadenectomy for adenocarcinoma of the head of the pancreas: Strength of the evidence. J Gastrointest Surg 12:651–656, 2008.
46. Kendrick ML, Cusati D: Total laparoscopic pancreaticoduodenectomy: Feasibility and outcome in an early experience. Arch Surg 145:19–23, 2010.
47. Kalser MH, Ellenberg SS: Pancreatic cancer. Adjuvant combined radiation and chemotherapy following curative resection. Arch Surg 120:899–903, 1985.
48. Neoptolemos JP, Stocken DD, Friess H, et al: A randomized trial of chemoradiotherapy and chemotherapy after resection of pancreatic cancer. N Engl J Med 350:1200–1210, 2004.
49. Oettle H, Post S, Neuhaus P, et al: Adjuvant chemotherapy with gemcitabine vs observation in patients undergoing curative-intent resection of pancreatic cancer: A randomized controlled trial. JAMA 297:267–277, 2007.
50. Regine WF, Winter KA, Abrams RA, et al: Fluorouracil vs gemcitabine chemotherapy before and after fluorouracil-based chemoradiation following resection of pancreatic adenocarcinoma: A randomized controlled trial. Jama 299:1019–1026, 2008.

**51.** Abrams RA, Lowy AM, O'Reilly EM, et al: Combined modality treatment of resectable and borderline resectable pancreas cancer: Expert consensus statement. Ann Surg Oncol 16:1751–1756, 2009.

**52.** Lillemoe KD, Cameron JL, Kaufman HS, et al: Chemical splanchnicectomy in patients with unresectable pancreatic cancer. A prospective randomized trial. Ann Surg 217:447–455, 1993.

**53.** Puli SR, Reddy JB, Bechtold ML, et al: EUS-guided celiac plexus neurolysis for pain due to chronic pancreatitis or pancreatic cancer pain: A meta-analysis and systematic review. Dig Dis Sci 54:2330–2337, 2009.

**54.** Stawicki SP, Schwab CW: Pancreatic trauma: Demographics, diagnosis, and management. Am Surg 74:1133–1145, 2008.

**55.** Subramanian A, Dente CJ, Feliciano DV: The management of pancreatic trauma in the modern era. Surg Clin North Am 87:1515–1532, 2007.

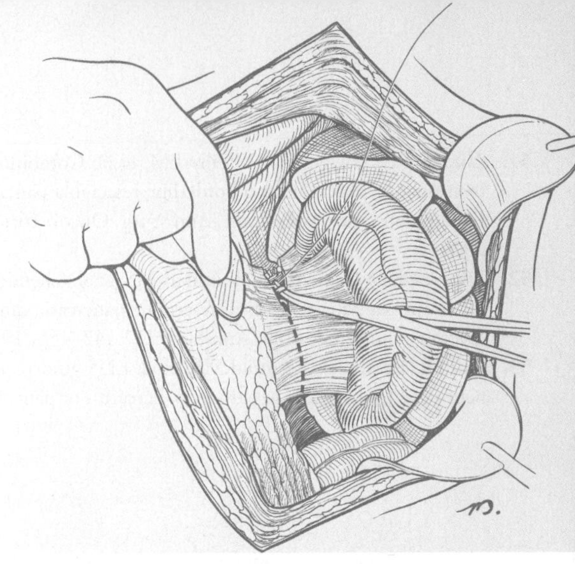

CHAPTER 57

# THE SPLEEN

Julie Shelton and Michael D. Holzman



## SPLENIC ANATOMY

The spleen is an 80- to 300-g organ that initially develops from mesenchymal cells in the dorsal mesogastrium during week 5 of embryogenesis and settles into the left uppermost aspect of the abdomen. Its superior surface is roofed by the diaphragm, separating it from the pleura. It should be noted, however, that the costodiaphragmatic recess extends to the inferiormost aspect of a normal-sized spleen. The spleen's visceral relationships include the greater curvature of the stomach, splenic flexure of the colon, apex of the left kidney, and tail of the pancreas (Fig. 57-1). It is protected by ribs 9, 10, and 11and is suspended in its location by multiple peritoneal reflections, the splenophrenic, gastrosplenic, splenorenal, and splenocolic ligaments. In patients without portal hypertension, the splenophrenic and splenocolic ligaments are relatively avascular. The gastrosplenic ligament carries the short gastric vessels in its superior aspect and the left gastroepiploic in its inferior aspect. The splenorenal ligament houses the splenic artery and vein, as well as the tail of the pancreas. The tail of the pancreas abuts the splenic hilum in 30% of individuals and is within 1 cm of the hilum in 70%.

The splenic artery, a branch of the celiac trunk, is a tortuous vessel that gives off multiple branches to the pancreas as it travels along its posterior aspect (Fig. 57-2). There are two typical arrays of the splenic artery—the magistral, which branches into terminal and polar arteries near the hilum of the spleen and the distributed, which, as the name implies, gives off its branches early and distant from the hilum. There is typically a superior polar artery, which sometimes communicates with the short gastric arteries, superior, middle, and inferior terminal arteries, and an inferior polar artery. Knowing these variable distributions is necessary when performing resections, especially a spleen-preserving procedure. Because of the variable nature of the splenic artery, one must be cautious when operating near this vessel and its tributaries.

The spleen is encased within a fibroelastic capsule. Trabeculae that compartmentalize the spleen pass from the splenic capsule. The spleen is also segmented by the divisions of the splenic vessels as they branch within the organ and merge with these trabeculae. The arterioles branch into even smaller vessels and leave these trabeculae to merge with the splenic pulp, where their adventitia is replaced by a covering of lymphatic tissue that continues until the vessels thin to capillaries. These lymphatic sheaths make up the white pulp of the spleen and are interspersed among the arteriolar branches as lymphatic follicles. The white pulp then interfaces with the red pulp at the marginal zone. It is in this marginal zone that the arterioles lose their lymphatic tissue and the vessels evolve into thin-walled splenic sinuses and sinusoids. The sinusoids then merge into venules, draining into veins that travel along the trabeculae to form splenic veins that mirror their arterial counterparts. The splenic vein leaves the splenic hilum, travels posteriorly to the pancreas, joining with pancreatic branches and often the inferior mesenteric vein to finally receive the superior mesenteric vein forming the portal vein.

## SPLENIC FUNCTION

During fetal development, the spleen has important hematopoietic functions, which include white and red blood cell production. This production is usurped by the bone marrow by the fifth month of gestation and, under normal conditions, the spleen has no significant hematopoietic function beyond this point. In certain pathologic conditions, such as myelodysplasia, the spleen may reacquire this function. Beyond hematopoiesis, the specialized vasculature in the spleen is directly related to its remaining functions, defense and cleansing. It is likely that the spleen's mechanical filtration contributes to control of infection by removing pathogens within cells (e.g., malaria) or circulating in the plasma. This filtration may be particularly important for removing microorganisms for which the host does not have a specific antibody (Box 57-1).

The immune functions of the spleen become obvious after splenectomy, when patients are noted to be significantly at risk for infection. The most serious sequela is overwhelming post-splenectomy infection (OPSI), with meningitis, pneumonia, or bacteremia.[1] Older studies have demonstrated that the risk of OPSI is greatest within the first 2 years after splenectomy but recent studies have confirmed that a lifelong risk remains. One third of cases occur more than 5 years after surgery, with the overall incidence reported to be 3.2% to 3.5%. For those who acquire OPSI, mortality is between 40% and 50%.[2] The risk is greatest in patients with thalassemia major and sickle cell disease. OPSI is typically caused by polysaccharide-encapsulated organisms, such as *Streptococcus pneumoniae, Neisseria meningitidis,*

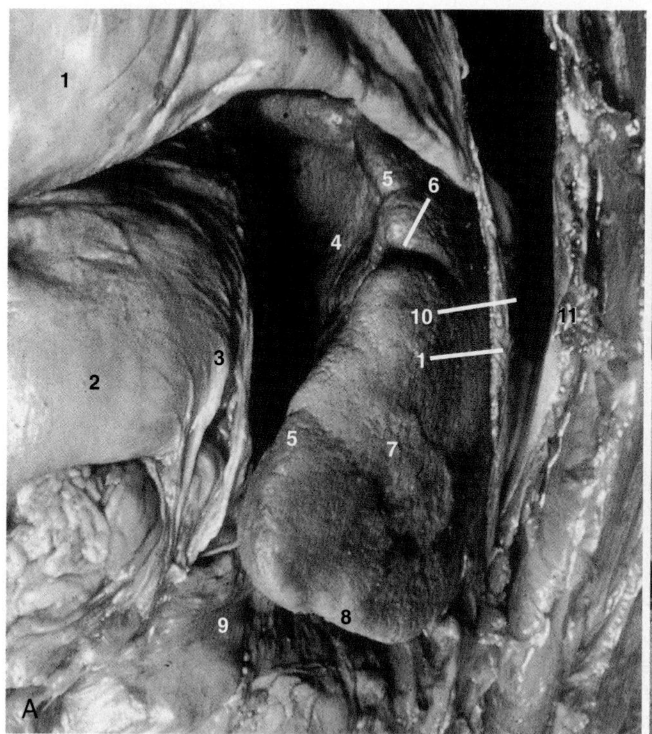


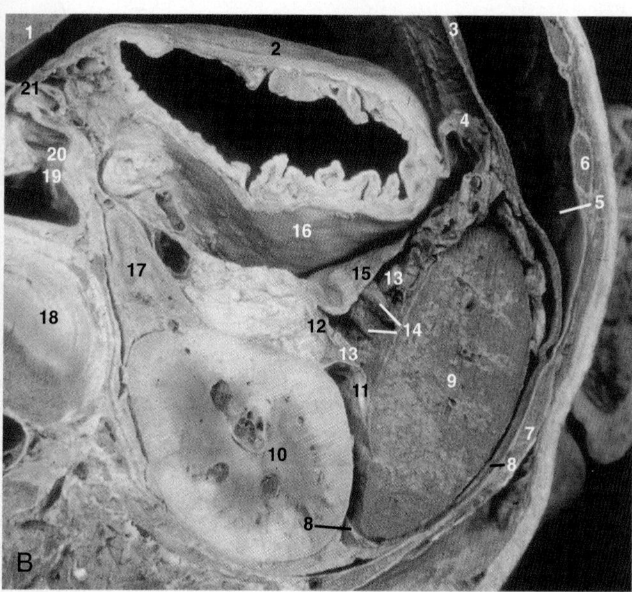


**FIGURE 57-1 A,** Spleen, from the front. (1) Diaphragm, (2) stomach, (3) gastrosplenic ligament, (4) gastric impression, (5) superior border, (6) notch, (7) diaphragmatic surface, (8) inferior border, (9) left colic flexure, (10) costodiaphragmatic recess, (11) thoracic wall. The left upper abdominal and lower anterior thoracic walls have been removed and part of the diaphragm (1) turned upward to show the spleen in its normal position, lying adjacent to the stomach (2) and colon (9), with the lower part against the kidney (**B,** 9 and 10). **B,** Spleen, in a transverse section of the left upper abdomen. (1) Left lobe of liver, (2) stomach, (3) diaphragm, (4) gastrosplenic ligament, (5) costodiaphragmatic recess of pleura, (6) ninth rib, (7) 10th rib, (8) peritoneum of greater sac, (9) spleen, (10) left kidney, (11) posterior layer of lienorenal ligament, (12) tail of pancreas, (13) splenic artery, (14) splenic vein, (15) anterior layer of lienorenal ligament, (16) lesser sac, (17) left suprarenal gland, (18) intervertebral disc, (19) abdominal aorta, (20) celiac trunk, (21) left gastric artery. The section is at the level of the disc (18) between the 12th thoracic and first lumbar vertebrae and is viewed from below looking toward the thorax. The spleen (9) lies against the diaphragm (3) and left kidney (10) but is separated from them by peritoneum of the greater sac (8). The peritoneum behind the stomach (2), forming part of the gastrosplenic (4) and ileorenal (15) ligaments, belongs to the lesser sac (16). (From McMinn RMH, Hutchings RT, Pegington J, Abrahams PH: Color atlas of human anatomy, ed 3, St Louis, 1993, Mosby-Year Book, pp 230–231.)

and *Haemophilus influenzae.* These and other organisms are identified and bound by antibodies and complement components in preparation for phagocytosis by macrophages in the spleen. After splenectomy, the antibodies continue to bind but digestion by splenic macrophages is no longer possible.

Asplenic patients have been noted to express similar postvaccination immunoglobulin G (IgG) antibody levels when comparing timing of pneumococcal vaccinations in postsplenectomy trauma patients; functional antibody levels, however, were lower.[3] Also, asplenic patients have been found to express subnormal IgM levels and their peripheral blood mononuclear cells exhibit a suppressed immunoglobulin response. The risk of developing OPSI or asplenic or hyposplenic overwhelming sepsis for reasons other than surgical removal of the spleen is linked to patient understanding of the risks of infection.[4] Registries that allow for long-term follow-up and periodic teaching of current recommendations should be considered for this high-risk population.[5,6]

Other factors involved in the immune response, such as properdin and tuftsin, opsonins produced in the spleen, exhibit reduced serum levels after splenectomy. Properdin, a globulin protein also known as *factor P*, initiates the alternate pathway of complement activation; this increases the destruction of bacteria, foreign, or otherwise abnormal cells. Tuftsin, a tetrapeptide, enhances the phagocytic activity of mononuclear phagocytes and polymorphonuclear leukocytes. Absence of a circulating mediator appears to result in suppressed neutrophil function. The spleen also plays a key role in cleaving tuftsin from the heavy chain of IgG; thus, circulating levels of tuftsin are subnormal in asplenic patients.

The filtration consists of two methods of blood flow within the spleen, the closed and open systems. In the closed system, blood flows directly from arteries to veins. In the open system, most of the spleen's blood flow occurs when blood flows through the arterioles and then trickles through a sievelike parenchyma made up of reticuloendothelial cells into the splenic sinuses before draining into the venous system (Fig. 57-3). The cellular elements are directed toward these reticuloendothelial cells, in which cellular cleansing processes take place. These include removal of senescent cells, cellular inclusion (e.g., red cell nucleoli), parasites, and sequestration of red cells (for maturation) and platelets (reservoir). The plasma is directed to the lymphoid tissue, where soluble antigens stimulate the production of antibodies.

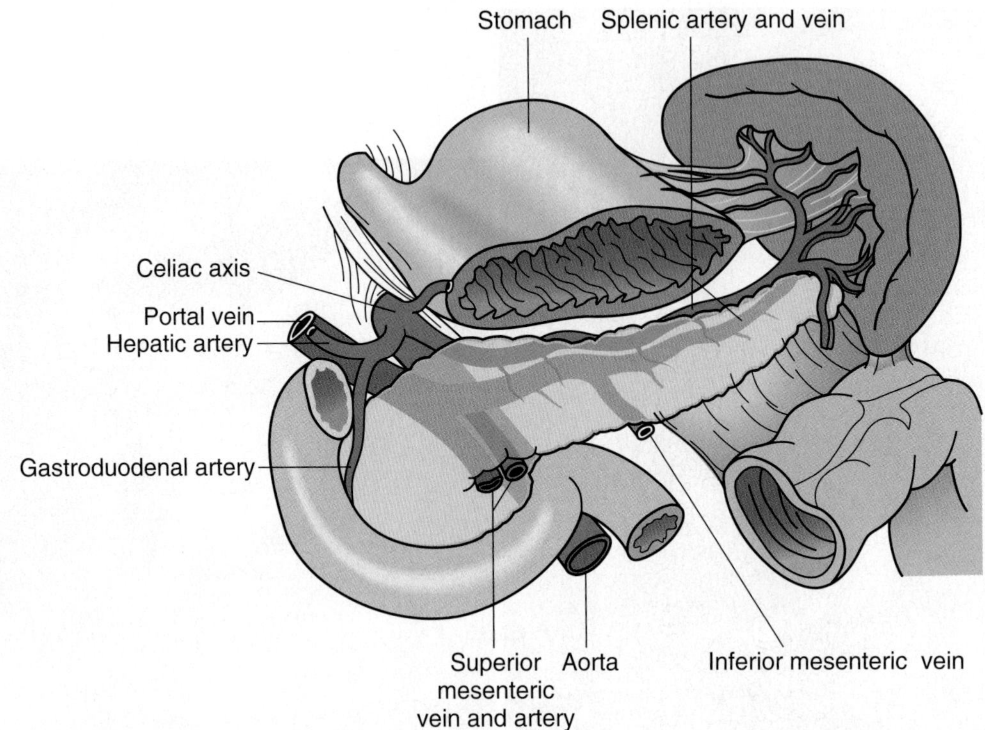


**FIGURE 57-2** Anatomic relationships of the splenic vasculature. (From Economou SG, Economou TS: Atlas of surgical techniques, Philadelphia, 1966, WB Saunders, p 562.)

**BOX 57-1 Biologic Substances Removed by the Spleen**

**Normal Subjects**
Red blood cell membrane
Red blood cell surface pits and craters
Howell-Jolly bodies
Heinz bodies
Pappenheimer bodies
Acanthocytes
Senescent red blood cells
Particulate antigen

**Patients With Disease**
Spherocytes (hereditary spherocytosis)
Sickle cells, hemoglobin C cells
Antibody-coated red blood cells
Antibody-coated platelets
Antibody-coated white blood cells

Adapted from Eichner ER: Splenic function: Normal, too much and too little. Am J Med 66:311–320, 1979.

Red cell morphology, and thus red cell function, is maintained by splenic filtration. Normal red blood cells are biconcave and deform easily. This plasticity allows passage through the microvasculature and optimizes the exchange of oxygen and carbon dioxide. Imperfect red cells with inclusions such as nucleoli, Howell-Jolly bodies (nuclear remnant), Heinz bodies (denatured hemoglobin), Pappenheimer bodies (iron granules), acanthocytes (spur cells), codocytes (target cells), and stippling cause these red blood cells to undergo cleansing in the spleen. Aged red blood cells with decreased plasticity (>120 days) become trapped and destroyed in the spleen.

Abnormal erythrocytes that result from sickle cell anemia, hereditary spherocytosis, thalassemia, or pyruvate kinase deficiency are also trapped and destroyed by the spleen. The overall effect is worsening anemia, splenomegaly, and sometimes autoinfarction of the spleen. Similarly, the spleen is involved in platelet destruction in immune thrombocytopenic purpura (ITP).

## SPLENECTOMY

Splenectomy may be performed for a number of reasons and conditions.

### Benign Hematologic Conditions

#### Immune Thrombocytopenic Purpura

ITP, classically known as *idiopathic thrombocytopenic purpura*, is characterized by a low platelet count despite normal bone marrow and the absence of other causes of thrombocytopenia that could be responsible for the finding. Autoantibodies are responsible for the disordered platelet destruction mediated by the overactivated platelet phagocytosis within the reticuloendothelial system. Within the bone marrow, normal (or sometimes increased) amounts of megakaryocytes are present. There persists, however, a relative bone marrow failure in that production cannot match destruction to compensate sufficiently.

The typical presentation of ITP is characterized by purpura, epistaxis, and gingival bleeding. Less commonly, gastrointestinal bleeding and hematuria are noted. Intracerebral hemorrhage is a rare but sometimes fatal presentation. The diagnosis of ITP involves the exclusion of other relatively common causes of

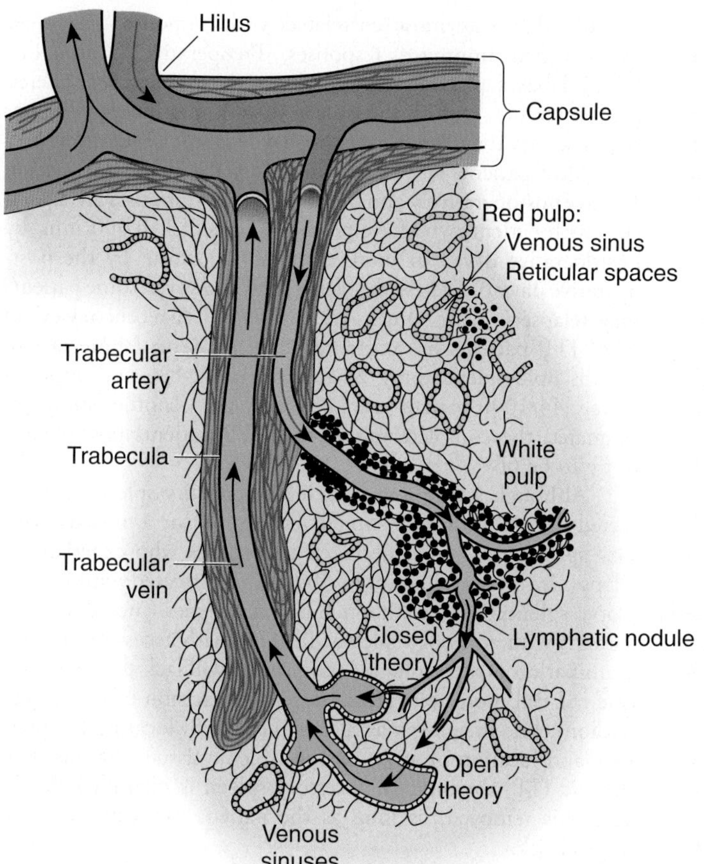


**FIGURE 57-3** Structure of the sinusoidal spleen showing the open and closed blood flow routes. (From Bellanti JA: Immunology: Basic brocesses. Philadelphia, 1979, WB Saunders.)

thrombocytopenia—pregnancy, drug-induced thrombocytopenia (e.g., heparin, quinidine, quinine, sulfonamides), viral infections, and hypersplenism (Box 57-2). Mild thrombocytopenia may be seen in approximately 6% to 8% of otherwise normal pregnancies and in up to 25% of women with preeclampsia. Drug-induced thrombocytopenia is thought to occur rarely, in approximately 20 to 40 cases/million users of common medications, such as trimethoprim-sulfonamide and quinine. Other medications, such as gold salts, have a higher incidence, almost 1% of users.[7] Viral infection (e.g., hepatitis C virus [HCV], HIV, rarely, Epstein-Barr virus [EBV]) can be responsible for thrombocytopenia independent of splenic sequestration. Once again, other processes must be ruled out but health care providers can be confident of these causative factors if platelet counts improve with successful treatment of the responsible infection. Bacterial infection, specifically *Helicobacter pylori,* has also been linked to infection-related thrombocytopenia that improves with eradication. Other causes are listed in Box 57-2; spurious laboratory values caused by platelet clumping or the presence of giant platelets should not be ignored.

ITP is predominantly a disease of young women; 72% of patients older than 10 years of age are women and 70% of affected women are younger than 40 years. ITP manifests somewhat differently in children—both genders are affected equally, onset is sudden, thrombocytopenia is severe, and complete spontaneous remissions are seen in approximately 80% of affected children. Girls older than 10 years with more chronic purpura are those in whom the disease seems to persist.

**BOX 57-2 Differential Diagnosis of Immune Thrombocytopenic Purpura**

**Falsely Low Platelet Count**

In vitro platelet clumping caused by ethylenediaminetetraacetic acid (EDTA)–dependent or cold-dependent agglutinins
Giant platelets

**Common Causes of Thrombocytopenia**

Pregnancy (gestational thrombocytopenia, preeclampsia)
Drug-induced thrombocytopenia (common drugs include heparin, quinidine, quinine, sulfonamides)
Viral infections, such as HIV, rubella, infectious mononucleosis
Hypersplenism caused by chronic liver disease

**Other Causes of Thrombocytopenia Mistaken for Immune Thrombocytopenic Purpura**

Myelodysplasia
Congenital thrombocytopenias
Thrombotic thrombocytopenic purpura and hemolytic-uremic syndrome
Chronic disseminated intravascular coagulation

**Thrombocytopenia associated with other disorders**

Autoimmune diseases, such as systemic lupus erythematosus
Lymphoproliferative disorders (chronic lymphocytic leukemia, non-Hodgkin's lymphoma)

Adapted from George JN, El-Harake MA, Raskob GE: Chronic idiopathic thrombocytopenic purpura. N Engl J Med 331:1207–1211, 1994.

Management of ITP depends primarily on the severity of the thrombocytopenia.[8] Asymptomatic patients with platelet counts higher than 50,000/mm$^3$ may be observed without further intervention. Platelet counts of 50,000/mm$^3$ and higher are rarely associated with clinical sequelae, even with invasive procedures. Patients with slightly lower platelet counts, between 30,000 and 50,000/mm$^3$, may always be observed but with more routine follow-up because they are at increased risk for progressing to severe thrombocytopenia. Initial medical treatment for patients with platelets counts less than 50,000/mm$^3$ and symptoms such as mucous membrane bleeding, high-risk conditions (e.g., active lifestyle, hypertension, peptic ulcer disease), or platelet counts less than 20,000 to 30,000/mm$^3$, even without symptoms, is glucocorticoid administration (typically, prednisone, 1 mg/kg body weight/day). Clinical response with increases in platelet levels to higher than 50,000/mm$^3$ is seen in up to two thirds of patients within 1 to 3 weeks of initiating treatment. Of patients treated with steroids, 25% will experience a complete response. Patients with platelet counts higher than 20,000/mm$^3$ who remain symptom-free, or who experience minor purpura as their only symptom, do not require hospitalization. Hospitalization may be required for patients whose platelets counts remain below 20,000/mm$^3$ with significant mucous membrane bleeding and is required for those who have life-threatening hemorrhage. Platelet transfusion is indicated only for those who experience severe hemorrhage. IV immunoglobulin is important for the treatment of acute bleeding, in pregnancy, or for patients being prepared for operation, including splenectomy. The usual dose is 1 g/kg body weight/day for 2 days. This dose usually increases the platelet count within 3 days; it also increases the efficacy of platelet transfusions.

Prior to the establishment of glucocorticoids as treatment for ITP in 1950, splenectomy was the treatment of choice.[8] For those two thirds of patients in whom glucocorticoids result in the normalization of platelet counts, no further treatment is necessary. For patients with severe thrombocytopenia, with counts less than 10,000/mm$^3$ for 6 weeks or longer, those with thrombocytopenia refractory to glucocorticoid treatment, or those who require toxic doses of steroid to achieve remission, the treatment of choice is to proceed to splenectomy. Splenectomy is also the treatment of choice for patients with incomplete response to glucocorticoid treatment and for pregnant women in the second trimester of pregnancy who have also failed steroid treatment or IV Ig therapy with platelet counts less than 10,000/mm$^3$ without symptoms or less than 30,000/mm$^3$ with bleeding problems. It is not necessary to proceed to splenectomy for patients who have platelet counts higher than 50,000/mm$^3$, have had ITP for longer than 6 months, are not experiencing bleeding symptoms, and who are not engaged in high-risk activities. A recent review of short-term and long-term failure of laparoscopic splenectomy has reported an overall approximate failure rate of 28% at 5 years after splenectomy.[9]

A systematic review of 436 published articles from 1966 to 2004 has reported that 72% of patients with ITP had a complete response to splenectomy. Relapse occurred in a median of 15% of patients (range, 1% to 51%), with a median follow-up of 33 months.[10]

In addition to relapse rates, predictors of successful splenectomy were examined. Of the variables in the multivariate model, age at the time of splenectomy was an independent variable that was most correlated with response.[10] Younger patients had improved responses. Preoperative indium-111 ($^{111}$In)–labeled platelet scintigraphy with platelets sequestered predominantly within the spleen had a significantly higher response rate than those noted to have hepatic sequestration.[11]

Most patients will exhibit improved platelet counts within 10 days postoperatively and durable platelet responses are associated with patients who have platelet counts of 150,000/mm$^3$ by postoperative day 3 or more than 500,000/mm$^3$ by the postoperative day 10. Even with splenectomy, however, some patients may relapse (~12%; range, 4% to 25%).[12] A recent review of 1223 ITP patients has estimated the long-term failure rate of laparoscopic splenectomy at approximately 8% and approximately 44/1000 patient-years of follow-up.[9] Another study has estimated the complete response of ITP patients postsplenectomy to be 66%.[10]

Although a thorough search for accessory spleens is completed during the initial surgery, evaluation for a missed accessory spleen must be undertaken in patients who experience a relapse. In their evaluation of 394 patients treated with laparoscopic splenectomy, Katkhouda and colleagues[12] noted 15% of patients with accessory spleens. In those with accessory spleens, examination of a peripheral blood smear will lack the characteristic red cell morphology resulting from excision of the spleen. Radionuclide imaging may also be helpful in locating the presence and location of any accessory splenic tissue. Patients with chronic ITP in whom an accessory spleen is identified should have this removed, as long as the patient can withstand the surgical risk.

Other treatment options for these patients include observation of stable nonbleeding patients with platelet counts higher than 30,000/mm$^3$, long-term glucocorticoid therapy, and treatment with azathioprine or cyclophosphamide. Recent evidence regarding thrombopoietin receptor agonists may offer a novel medical therapy for patients with no response to steroids, IV immunoglobulin therapy, or splenectomy.[13]

Other conditions linked to thrombocytopenia include thrombotic thrombocytopenic purpura, chronic disseminated intravascular coagulation, congenital thrombocytopenia, myelodysplasia, autoimmune disorders (e.g., systemic lupus erythematosus), and lymphoproliferative disorders (e.g., chronic lymphocytic leukemia, non-Hodgkin's lymphoma).

Approximately 10% to 20% of otherwise asymptomatic patients with HIV will develop ITP. Splenectomy is a safe treatment option for this cohort of patients and may actually delay HIV disease progression.[14,15]

### Hereditary Spherocytosis

Hereditary spherocytosis is an autosomal dominant disease affecting the production of spectrin, a red blood cell cytoskeletal protein. Loss of this protein causes red blood cells to lack their characteristic biconcave shape. This affects the red blood cells' deformability, because lack of this protein results in rigid erythrocytes that are small and sphere-shaped. Also, these cells have increased osmotic fragility and are more susceptible to trapping and destruction by the spleen. The resulting clinical features are anemia, occasionally with jaundice, and splenomegaly. Diagnosis is made by examination of a peripheral blood smear, increased reticulocyte count, increased osmotic fragility, and a negative Coombs' test.

The resultant anemia can be successfully treated with splenectomy, but normalization of the erythrocyte morphology does not occur. Splenectomy should be delayed until the age of 5 years to preserve immunologic function of the spleen and reduce the risk of OPSI. Just as with other hemolytic anemias, the presence of pigmented gallstones is common. The preoperative workup should include ultrasound evaluation; if gallstones are present, cholecystectomy may be performed at the same time as splenectomy.

Hereditary elliptocytosis, hereditary pyropoikilocytosis, hereditary xerocytosis, and hereditary hydrocytosis also result in anemia secondary to red blood cell membrane abnormalities. Splenectomy is indicated in cases of severe anemia with these conditions, except hereditary xerocytosis, which results in only mild anemia of limited clinical significance.

#### Hemolytic Anemia Caused by Erythrocyte Enzyme Deficiency

Pyruvate kinase deficiency and glucose-6-phosphate dehydrogenase (G6PD) deficiency are the predominant hereditary conditions associated with hemolytic anemia. Pyruvate kinase deficiency is an autosomal recessive disease that results in decreased red blood cell deformability and the formation of echinocytes, a type of spiculated red blood cell. This morphologic variant increases the likelihood that the cell will be trapped and destroyed by the spleen, which results in splenomegaly, hemolytic anemia, and associated transfusion requirements, which can be mitigated with splenectomy. Again, for reasons discussed earlier, splenectomy is delayed until 5 years of age.

In G6PD deficiency, however, splenectomy is rarely indicated. This X-linked condition is typically seen in people of African, Middle Eastern, or Mediterranean ancestry. Hemolytic anemia in these patients most often occurs after infection or exposure to certain foods, medications, or chemicals. Primary treatment, therefore, is avoidance of exacerbation of the condition.

#### Hemoglobinopathies

In addition to defects of cellular membranes or enzymes, hereditary anemias may also result from defects in hemoglobin molecules. Sickle cell disease and thalassemia are two disorders in which the hemoglobin molecules exhibit qualitative or quantitative defects. These lead to abnormally shaped erythrocytes, which may lead to splenic sequestration and subsequent destruction.

Sickle cell anemia results from a single amino acid substitution (valine for glutamic acid) in the sixth position of the β chain of hemoglobin A, which causes those hemoglobin chains, under reduced oxygen conditions, to become rigid and unable to deform within the microvasculature. This rigidity causes the red cells to assume the elongated crescent or sickle shape. Sickle cell disease results from homozygous inheritance of the defective hemoglobin (hemoglobin S) although sickling can also be seen when hemoglobin S is inherited along with other hemoglobin variants, such as hemoglobin C or sickle cell β-thalassemia. In African Americans, 8% are heterozygous for hemoglobin S (sickle cell trait) and approximately 0.5% are homozygous for hemoglobin S. During conditions of low oxygen tension, these hemoglobin S molecules crystallize, distorting the cell into a crescent shape. These misshapen cells are unable to pass through the microvasculature, which results in capillary occlusion, thrombosis, and ultimately microinfarction. This cascade of events frequently occurs in the spleen. These episodes of vaso-occlusion and progressive infarction result in autosplenectomy. The spleen, which is usually hypertrophied early in life, typically atrophies by adulthood, although splenomegaly may occasionally persist.

Other causes of hemolytic anemia are the thalassemias. These are inherited as autosomal dominant traits and result from a defect in hemoglobin synthesis that causes variable degrees of hemolytic anemia. Splenomegaly, hypersplenism, and splenic infarction, common in sickle cell disease, are also seen commonly in the thalassemias.

Hypersplenism and acute splenic sequestration are life-threatening disorders in children with thalassemia and sickle cell disease. In these conditions, there may be rapid splenic enlargement, which results in severe pain and may require multiple blood transfusions. Patients with acute splenic sequestration crisis present with severe anemia, splenomegaly, and an acute bone marrow response, with erythrocytosis. There may be a concurrent decrease in hemoglobin levels, abdominal pain, and circulatory collapse. Resuscitation with hydration and transfusion may be followed by splenectomy in these patients. Hypersplenism related to sickle cell disease is characterized by anemia, leukopenia, and thrombocytopenia requiring transfusions; transfusions may be reduced by performing splenectomy. Symptomatic massive splenomegaly that interferes with daily activities may also be improved by splenectomy. Finally, in children with sickle cell disease who exhibit growth delay or even weight loss because of increased metabolic rate and whole-body total protein turnover, splenectomy may relieve these symptoms.

Splenic abscesses may also be seen in patients with sickle cell anemia. These patients present with fever, abdominal pain, and a tender enlarged spleen. Most patients with splenic abscesses will have a leukocytosis, as well as thrombocytosis and Howell-Jolly bodies indicating a functional asplenia. *Salmonella* and *Enterobacter* spp. and other enteric organisms are commonly seen in those with a splenic abscess. These patients require resuscitation with hydration and transfusion and may require urgent splenectomy after stabilization.

### Malignancy

#### Lymphomas

**Hodgkin's Disease** Hodgkin's disease is a malignant lymphoma that usually affects young adults in their 20s and 30s. Rarely, patients present with constitutional symptoms such as night sweats, weight loss, and pruritus but, more typically, asymptomatic lymphadenopathy usually involving the cervical nodes. Hodgkin's disease is characterized histologically as lymphocyte-predominant, nodular-sclerosing, mixed cellularity, or lymphocyte-depleted. The disease is pathologically staged according to the Ann Arbor classification. Stage I is disease in a single lymphatic site. Stage II is disease in two or more lymphatic sites on the same side of the diaphragm. Stage III indicates disease on both sides of the diaphragm and includes splenic involvement. Stage IV disease is disease in which there is dissemination into extralymphatic sites such as liver, lung, or bone marrow. The addition of a subscript E to stage I, II, or III indicates single or contiguous extralymphatic spread; subscript S indicates splenic involvement. Patients who exhibit constitutional symptoms are denoted with a B (presence) and those without symptoms are denoted with an A (absence).

Historically, patients with Hodgkin's disease underwent a staging laparotomy that included splenectomy to provide pathologic staging information required to determine appropriate therapy. This was particularly common in stages I and II disease to rule out splenic or subdiaphragmatic involvement. In addition to splenectomy, the procedure involves splenic hilar lymphadenectomy, liver biopsy, retroperitoneal node biopsy, and biopsy of a hepatoduodenal node and oophoropexy in premenopausal women. Staging methods have evolved to include imaging techniques—computed tomography (CT), $^{18}$F-fluorodeoxyglucose positron emission tomography (FDG-PET), and lymphangiography—thus making invasive staging methods almost obsolete. Staging laparotomy remains appropriate for select patients, such as those with early clinical disease stages (IA or IIA) in whom abdominal staging will significantly alter therapeutic management. Early-stage Hodgkin's disease is often cured with radiation therapy alone. Laparotomy is no longer indicated for patients likely to relapse, those with evidence of intra-abdominal involvement on imaging, and those with B symptoms. These patients should receive systemic chemotherapy.

**Non-Hodgkin's Lymphomas** Splenomegaly or hypersplenism is a common occurrence during the course of non-Hodgkin's lymphoma (NHL). Splenectomy is indicated for NHL patients with massive splenomegaly leading to abdominal pain, early satiety, and fullness. It may also be indicated for patients who develop anemia, neutropenia, and thrombocytopenia associated with hypersplenism.

Splenectomy may also be instrumental in the diagnosis and staging of patients with isolated splenic disease. The most common primary splenic neoplasm is NHL. Less than 1% of patients present with splenomegaly without lymphadenopathy; however, 50% to 80% of patients with NHL have involvement of the spleen.[16] Patients with clinically isolated splenic disease are said to have malignant lymphoma with splenic involvement. Most patients have low-grade NHL, with frequent involvement of the splenic hilar lymph nodes, extrahilar nodes, bone marrow, or liver. Approximately 75% of these patients have clinically apparent hypersplenism. In patients with spleen-predominant features, survival is significantly improved after splenectomy compared with similar patients who did not undergo splenectomy.

### Leukemia

**Hairy Cell Leukemia** Hairy cell leukemia, a rare disease that accounts for approximately 2% of adult leukemias, is characterized by splenomegaly, pancytopenia, and neoplastic mononuclear cells in the peripheral blood and bone marrow. The cells that give the disease its name are B lymphocytes that have a ruffling of the cell membrane. This ruffling causes the cells to appear to have cytoplasmic projections under the light microscope. This disease affects older men who presents with palpable splenomegaly. Approximately 10% of patients require no treatment because of the indolent course of their disease. Treatment for cytopenias or splenomegaly typically begins with purine analogue chemotherapy.[17,18] For more refractory cancers, a second-line immunotherapy may be instituted. In others, however, the extent of splenomegaly or symptoms from hypersplenism, symptomatic anemia, infections from neutropenia, or hemorrhage from thrombocytopenia can lead to splenectomy. Most patients show improvement after the procedure, with a response lasting approximately 10 years after splenectomy, and some patients (≈40% to 60%) show normalization of blood counts after splenectomy.[19] Patients with diffusely involved bone marrow without massive splenomegaly are less responsive to splenectomy. Patients with hairy cell leukemia are also at a two- to threefold risk for developing other malignancies after their diagnosis of hairy cell leukemia. Most of these second malignancies are solid tumors, such as skin cancers, lung cancer, prostate cancer, and gastrointestinal adenocarcinomas. Hairy cell leukemia behaves like a chronic leukemia; many patients can achieve a clinical remission, with a normal or near-normal life span.

**Chronic Lymphocytic Leukemia** Chronic lymphocytic leukemia (CLL) is a clinically heterogeneous disease of B lymphocytes characterized by the progressive accumulation of relatively mature but functionally incompetent lymphocytes. CLL is seen with a slight predominance in men, mainly after the age of 50 years. CLL is staged according to the Rai system and correlates fairly well with survival. Low-risk CLL (formerly stage 0) involves bone marrow and blood lymphocytosis only, intermediate-risk CLL (formerly stages I and II) involves lymphocytosis and lymphadenopathy in any site or splenomegaly, hepatomegaly, or hepatosplenomegaly, and high-risk CLL (formerly stages III and IV) involves lymphocytosis and anemia or thrombocytopenia. The Rai system helps clinicians determine when therapy should be started. New molecular tests, such as that for ZAP-70, zeta-chain–associated protein 70 (an intracellular protein rarely found in normal B cells) are increasingly helpful for determining prognosis.[20] Medical treatment, consisting of nucleoside analogues or combination therapy, is indicated for symptomatic patients or those exhibiting evidence of rapid disease progression. Monoclonal antibodies are also used in the treatment of CLL.

Bone marrow transplantation currently offers the only known cure for CLL. Splenectomy is indicated for patients with refractory splenomegaly and pancytopenia, which results in improvements in blood counts in 60% to 70% of patients.[21]

**Chronic Myelogenous Leukemia** Chronic myelogenous leukemia (CML) is a myeloproliferative disorder that develops as a result of a neoplastic transformation of myeloid elements. CML is characterized by the progressive replacement of normal diploid elements of the bone marrow with mature-appearing neoplastic myeloid cells. Although CML can be asymptomatic at presentation, patients commonly present with fever, fatigue, malaise, effects of pancytopenia (infections, anemia, easy bruising), and occasionally splenomegaly. A chromosomal marker, the Philadelphia chromosome, is highly associated with CML and is caused by the fusion of fragments of chromosomes 9 and 22. This fusion results in expression of the bcr-abl gene product, a tyrosine kinase, which then accelerates cell division and inhibits DNA repair.

CML may occur in patients from childhood to old age. It usually presents with an asymptomatic chronic phase but may progress to an accelerated phase associated with fever, night sweats, and progressive splenomegaly. The accelerated phase may be asymptomatic, and may be detectable only by changes in peripheral blood or bone marrow. The accelerated phase may then progress to the blastic phase. This phase is also characterized by fever, night sweats, and splenomegaly but is also associated with anemia, infections, and bleeding.

The bcr-abl gene product is the target for therapy with tyrosine kinase inhibitors and other chemotherapeutic modalities. Bone marrow transplantation is an option but prognosis has improved dramatically with the advent of *recent* therapies, making transplantation less common. Studies evaluating the efficacy of newer therapies and combination therapies are ongoing. Symptomatic splenomegaly and hypersplenism in CML can be effectively treated with splenectomy, but there does not appear to be a survival benefit when performed during the early chronic phase.[22] Surgery is therefore reserved for patients with significant symptoms.

### Non-Hematologic Tumors of the Spleen

The spleen can also be the site of metastatic disease, seen in up to 7% of autopsies of cancer patients. The solid tumors that most frequently spread to the spleen are carcinomas of the breast, lung, and melanoma. Any primary malignancy, however, can metastasize to the spleen.[23] Metastases are often asymptomatic but may be associated with splenomegaly and even splenic rupture; thus, splenectomy may provide palliation for carefully chosen patients with symptomatic splenic metastases.

Primary tumors of the spleen are commonly vascular neoplasms and include benign and malignant variants. Hemangiomas are frequent findings in spleens removed for other reasons. Angiosarcomas (or hemangiosarcomas) of the spleen usually occur spontaneously, but have been linked to environmental exposures, such as thorium dioxide or monomeric vinyl chloride. Patients with angiosarcomas may present with splenomegaly, hemolytic anemia, ascites, pleural effusions, or even spontaneous splenic rupture. These tumors are aggressive and have a poor prognosis. Lymphangiomas, by contrast, are endothelium-lined cysts that come to attention because of splenomegaly secondary to cyst enlargement. These are usually benign tumors; however, lymphangiosarcoma has been found within lymphangiomas. Splenectomy is appropriate for the diagnosis, treatment, and/or palliation of these conditions.

## Miscellaneous Benign Conditions

### Splenic Cysts

Splenic cysts have been seen with increasing frequency since the advent of CT and ultrasound scanning. They are classified as true cysts, which can be parasitic or nonparasitic, or as pseudocysts. Tumors of the spleen may also appear to be cystic; these include lymphangiomas and cavernous hemangiomas (see earlier).[24] Primary true cysts of the spleen account for approximately 10% of all nonparasitic splenic cysts, whereas most nonparasitic cysts are pseudocysts secondary to trauma. True cysts are lined with a squamous epithelium and many are considered congenital. These epithelial cells are often positive for carbohydrate antigen 19-9 (CA19-9) and carcinoembryonic antigen (CEA) by immunohistochemistry. Patients with splenic epidermoid cysts may have elevated serum levels of one or both of these tumor markers. These cysts, however, are benign and apparently do not have malignant potential beyond that of the surrounding native tissue.

True splenic cysts are often asymptomatic and discovered incidentally. Patients may complain of abdominal fullness, early satiety, pleuritic chest pain, shortness of breath, and/or left shoulder or back pain. They may also experience renal symptoms from compression of the left kidney. On physical examination, an abdominal mass may be palpable. Rarely, splenic cysts present with acute symptoms related to rupture, hemorrhage, or infection. Diagnosis is best made by CT and operative intervention is indicated for those with symptomatic or large cysts. Total or partial splenectomy may provide appropriate treatment. Partial splenectomy has the advantage of preserving splenic function; 25% of the spleen appears to be sufficient to protect against pneumococcal pneumonia. Open and laparoscopic procedures allow total or partial splenectomy, cyst wall resection, or partial decapsulation.[24,25]

Most true splenic cysts are parasitic cysts and occur in areas of endemic hydatid disease (*Echinococcus* spp.). Radiographic imaging reveals cyst wall calcifications or daughter cysts and, although hydatid disease is uncommon in North America, this diagnosis must be excluded before invasive procedures are undertaken that might result in spillage of the cyst contents. Rupture of the cyst and expulsion of contents into the abdomen may precipitate anaphylactic shock and can also lead to intraperitoneal dissemination of the infection. Serologic testing is helpful for verifying the presence of these parasites. Splenectomy is the treatment of choice. As with hydatid cysts of the liver, the cysts may be sterilized by injection of a 3% sodium chloride solution, alcohol, or 0.5% silver nitrate. Even so, great care should be taken to avoid intraoperative rupture of the cyst.

Pseudocysts comprise the remaining 70% to 80% of nonparasitic splenic cysts. A history of prior trauma can typically be elicited. Pseudocysts of the spleen are not lined with epithelium. Radiologic imaging usually reveals a smooth, unilocular, thick-walled lesion, sometimes with focal calcifications. Asymptomatic, small (<4-cm) pseudocysts do not require treatment and may involute with time. Symptomatic pseudocysts present in a similar fashion as true splenic cysts; these are treated surgically with total or partial splenectomy, again remembering that partial splenectomy preserves splenic function. Percutaneous drainage has also been reported for splenic pseudocysts[26] although, in a recent case series, recurrence was common and subsequent complications were deemed too high.[27]

### Splenic Abscess

Splenic abscess is an unusual but potentially life threatening illness, with a 0.7% incidence in autopsy series.[28] The mortality rate for splenic abscess ranges from 15% to 20% in previously healthy patients, with single unilocular lesions, to 80% for multiple abscesses in immunocompromised patients. Illnesses and other factors that predispose to splenic abscess include malignancies, polycythemia vera, endocarditis, prior trauma, hemoglobinopathies, urinary tract infections, IV drug use, and AIDS.

Approximately 70% of splenic abscesses result from hematogenous spread of the infective organism from another location, as in endocarditis, osteomyelitis, and IV drug use. Spread may also occur in a contiguous fashion from local infections of the colon, kidney, or pancreas. Gram-positive cocci (commonly *Staphylococcus, Streptococcus,* or *Enterococcus* spp.) and gram-negative enteric organisms are typically involved. *Mycobacterium tuberculosis, Mycobacterium avium,* and *Actinomyces* spp. have also been found. Fungal abscesses (e.g., *Candida* spp.) also occur, typically in immunosuppressed patients.

Splenic abscesses present with nonspecific symptoms—vague abdominal pain, fever, peritonitis, and pleuritic chest pain. Splenomegaly is not typical. CT is the preferred method for diagnosis; however, the diagnosis can also be made with ultrasound.

Treatment of splenic abscesses depends on whether the abscess is unilocular or multilocular. In one third of adult patients, the abscess is multilocular. In one third of children, the abscess is unilocular. Unilocular abscesses are often amenable to percutaneous drainage, along with antibiotics,[29] with success rates reported at 75% to 90% for unilocular lesions. Multilocular lesions, however, are usually treated with splenectomy, drainage of the left upper quadrant, and antibiotics.[30] Laparoscopic splenectomy for abscess has been reported.[31]

### Wandering Spleen

Wandering spleen is a rare finding, seen in children and in women between the ages of 20 and 40 years. One of two causes is suspected. The first is theorized to result from a failure to form normal splenic peritoneal attachments that suspend the organ securely within its usual anatomic position. Failure to form these attachments is thought to arise from lack of fusion of the dorsal mesogastrium to the posterior abdominal wall during embryogenesis. The second theory surmises that in multiparous women, hormonal changes and abdominal laxity lead to an acquired defect in splenic attachments. In either case, without these attachments, the splenic pedicle is unusually long and prone to torsion.

Intermittent abdominal pain, splenomegaly resulting from venous congestion, or severe persistent pain are suggestive of wandering spleen and tension or intermittent torsion of the splenic pedicle. A mobile mass may be palpable on physical examination. CT, with IV contrast of the abdomen, provides confirmation of the diagnosis, with the spleen located outside its usual position. A noncontrasted spleen or whorled appearance of the vascular pedicle provides additional evidence for the condition and may be helpful in choosing splenopexy or splenectomy.[32]

## Other Considerations

### Splenic Trauma

See Chapter 18.

### Elective Laparoscopic Splenectomy

Laparoscopic splenectomy is now the preferred method for resecting the spleen. This technique was first described in 1991[33] and many studies have supported its use in terms of outcomes and patient safety.[12] Disadvantages of the laparoscopic technique are longer operating times and difficulty removing large organs; however, reduced hospital stay and more rapid postoperative recovery alleviate these limitations. Complications are typically linked to patients comorbidities.

Laparoscopic splenectomy has been reported for most splenic diseases and is the preferred method for most situations, barring trauma or cases of massive splenomegaly. When deciding whether to pursue laparoscopic methods for splenectomy, certain considerations should be taken into account, such as operative indication (e.g., benign or malignant disease), splenic size, and any potential contraindications to laparoscopy. Preoperative planning is aided by CT imaging especially regarding splenomegaly. Melman and Matthews[34] have noted that spleens measuring more than 22 cm in craniocaudal dimension, more than 19 cm in width, or more than 1600 g estimated weight will require hand-assisted laparoscopic procedures, if not open splenectomy. Laparoscopic splenectomy can be completed in approximately 90% of patients. The reported conversion to open splenectomy is between 0% and 20%. Most conversions are caused by intraoperative bleeding, lack of surgical experience, prohibitive adhesions,[35] massive splenomegaly,[22] and obesity.[1,15] As with other laparoscopic procedures, there is a learning curve and with increasing experience, conversion to open splenectomy declines.[3,36] Recently published guidelines regarding laparoscopic splenectomy reiterate the importance of indications for the procedure, preoperative imaging for determining size and volume and presence of accessory splenic tissue, choices regarding hand-assist techniques (early in cases of splenomegaly), contraindications (e.g., portal hypertension, major medical comorbidities), and splenic vaccinations.[37] Vaccinations for *N. meningitidis, S. pneumoniae,* and *H. influenzae* should be given 15 days prior to elective splenectomy or within 30 days of an emergent splenectomy to reduce the risk of OPSI (see earlier).

Postoperative recovery from laparoscopic splenectomy is rapid, as seen with laparoscopic cholecystectomy. The length of stay ranges from 1.8 to 6 days; shorter hospital stays are a major advantage of laparoscopic procedures.[16,17] A prospective randomized controlled trial comparing open and laparoscopic approaches was performed in patients with β-thalassemia major. This study reported a shorter median hospital stay in the laparoscopic patients but longer operative times and an increase in blood transfusions.[38] It is not known whether these results can be generalized to all patients with splenic disease. Several case series have also compared the laparoscopic with the open approach and consistently favored the laparoscopic approach, particularly in regard to earlier resumption of diet, decreased postoperative pain, and shorter hospital stay.[11]

Treatment outcomes are the primary concern when comparing these approaches. In published results to date, laparoscopic outcomes are equivalent to those of open splenectomy. In a review of laparoscopic splenectomy for malignant disease, Burch and associates[39] have reported that this patient population benefits from laparoscopic splenectomy, similar to those with benign disease. Katkhouda and coworkers[12] have reported that in the treatment of ITP, laparoscopic and open splenectomy results appear to be similar.

As noted, laparoscopic surgery needs careful consideration for special populations. Portal hypertension and its risk of operative hemorrhage prohibit laparoscopic splenectomy. Laparoscopic splenectomy during pregnancy for refractory thrombocytopenia carries an associated fetal mortality rate of 31%. There is scant literature regarding this rare patient population, although laparoscopic splenectomy can be performed during pregnancy.[37,40]

The laparoscopic technique may be performed with the patient in the supine or lateral position, or a combination. After induction of general anesthesia and endotracheal intubation, a nasogastric tube and urinary catheter are inserted. Standard antithrombotic precautions are taken. Patient positioning is crucial for the completion of a laparoscopic splenectomy. For all three positions, the patient is placed so that the kidney rest can be raised to maximize the space between the iliac crest and costal margin. The patient is positioned so that the table may be flexed to widen the working space. Finally, the patient is tilted in a reverse Trendelenburg position to facilitate retraction of the viscera caudally away from left upper quadrant.

In the supine position, the surgeon stands to the patient's left and the first assistant and camera assistant stand to the patient's right.[35] It may be easier for a right-handed surgeon to work from a position between the patient's legs, with the patient in a modified lithotomy position. The scrub nurse stands to the patient's left side, near the foot of the table. Alternatively, the patient may be placed in a 60-degree right lateral decubitus position using a beanbag and axillary roll. In this case, the patient's left arm is placed on an arm board or supported by a splint. With this approach, the surgeon and scrub nurse stand to the patient's right and the assistants stand to the patient's left. The spleen will thus be suspended from its diaphragmatic attachments, gravity retracts the stomach, omentum, and colon, and the splenic hilum will be under some degree of tension. For either approach, the video monitors are placed on either side of the table, at or above the level of the patient's shoulders.

Trocar access to the abdomen is gained and pneumoperitoneum is established to a pressure of 12 to 15 mm Hg. Three to five 2- to 12-mm-diameter ports are used, with the camera port at the umbilicus or offset between the umbilicus and costal margin. The other port sites are positioned as depicted in Figure 57-4.

The operation is begun with a thorough search of the abdominal cavity for the presence of accessory splenic tissue (Fig. 57-5); the stomach is retracted to the right side to facilitate examination of the gastrosplenic ligament. The splenocolic ligament, greater omentum, and phrenosplenic ligament are inspected next. The small and large bowel mesenteries, pelvis, and adnexal tissues are examined. Finally, the gastrosplenic ligament is opened and the tail of the pancreas is confirmed to be free of splenic tissue.

My preference has been to use the lateral decubitus approach. The initial dissection is begun by mobilizing the splenic flexure of the colon. Using sharp dissection, the splenocolic ligament is divided. The spleen can then be retraced cephalad; care should be taken not to rupture the splenic capsule during retraction. The lateral peritoneal attachments of the spleen are incised next, using scissors or ultrasonic shears. A 1-cm cuff of peritoneum is left along the lateral aspect of the spleen, which can then be grasped to facilitate medial retraction. The lesser sac is entered along the medial border of the spleen. Continuing the cephalad retraction, the short gastric vessels and main vascular pedicle can be identified. The tail of the pancreas is also visualized and care is taken to avoid it as it nears the splenic hilum. The short gastric vessels are divided. There are a number of options available currently available for this, including ultrasonic dissectors, hemoclips, bipolar devices, LigaSure (Covidien, Boulder, Colo), and endovascular stapling devices. Hemoclips are used minimally around the area of the splenic hilum to prevent interference with future use of a stapling device, which could lead to significant bleeding from improperly ligated hilar vessels.

After dividing the short gastric vessels, the splenic pedicle is carefully dissected from the medial and lateral aspects. After the artery and vein are dissected, the vessels are divided by application of endovascular staplers or suture ligatures. In the more prevalent distributed mode there are multiple vascular branches entering the spleen close to the hilum, so the dissection is carried out approximately 2 cm from the splenic capsule. Several branches may still be encountered, but these may be individually controlled more easily. A pedicle formed by the artery and vein that enters the hilum is known as the *magistral mode*. If this is seen, the pedicle is transected en bloc using a linear vascular stapler. The tail of the pancreas, which is within 1 cm of the splenic hilum in 75% of patients and touches the hilum in 30%, should be well visualized as the stapler is applied to avoid injury.

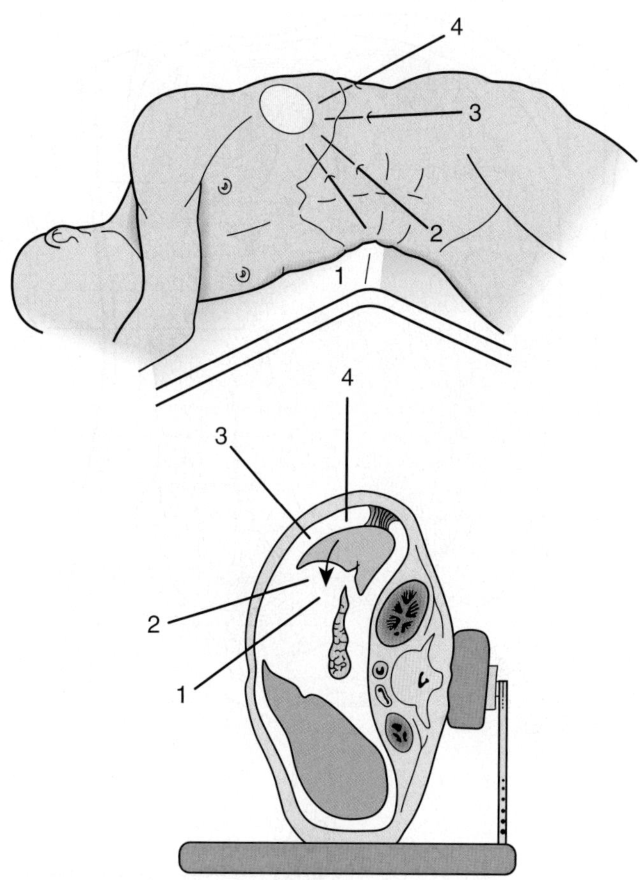


**FIGURE 57-4** Strict lateral position of the patient for laparoscopic splenectomy. The table is angulated, giving forced lateral flexion of the patient to open the costophrenic space. Trocars are inserted along the left costal margin more posteriorly. The spleen is hanged by its peritoneal attachments. The numbered lines show the position of laparoscopic ports. (From Gigot JF, Lengele B, Gianello P, et al: Present status of laparoscopic splenectomy for hematologic diseases: Certitudes and unresolved issues. Semin Laparosc Surg 5:147–167, 1998.)

The now-devascularized spleen is suspended only from a small cuff of avascular splenophrenic tissue at the superior pole. This tissue facilitates transfer of the spleen into a retrieval bag. To remove the detached spleen the puncture-resistant nylon bag is grasped by its drawstring, which can be drawn through a port, usually the epigastric or supraumbilical site. The bag is opened slightly, providing access to the still intra-abdominal spleen. The spleen is then morcellated with ring forceps or finger fracture and removed piecemeal (Fig. 57-6). In the rare cases requiring

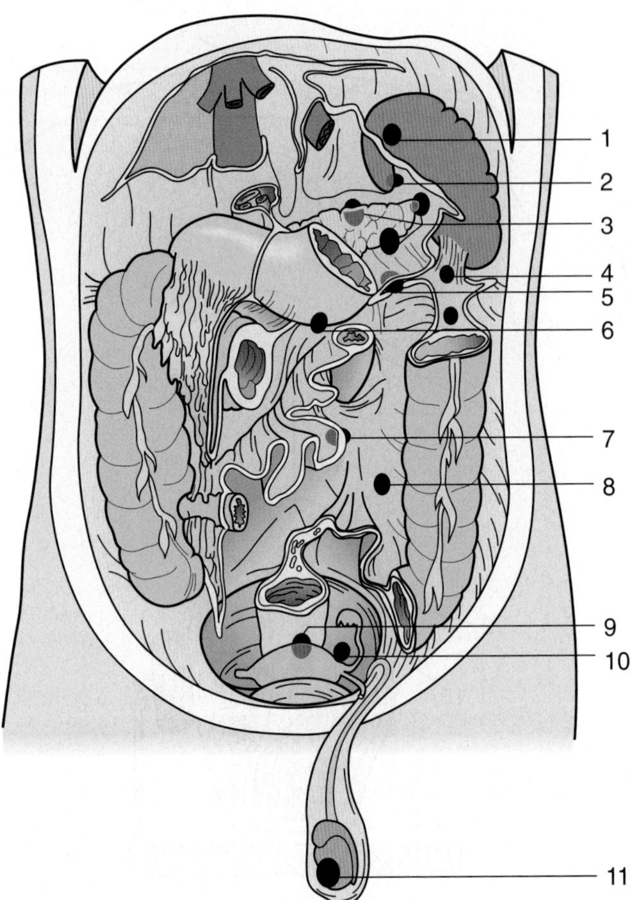


FIGURE 57-5 Usual location of accessory spleens. (1) Gastrosplenic ligament, (2) splenic hilum, (3) tail of the pancreas, (4) splenocolic ligament, (5) left transverse mesocolon, (6) greater omentum along the greater curvature of the stomach, (7) mesentery, (8) left mesocolon, (9) left ovary, (10) Douglas pouch, (11) left testis. (From Gigot JF, Lengele B, Gianello P, et al: Present status of laparoscopic splenectomy for hematologic diseases: Certitudes and unresolved issues. Semin Laparosc Surg 5:147–167, 1998.)

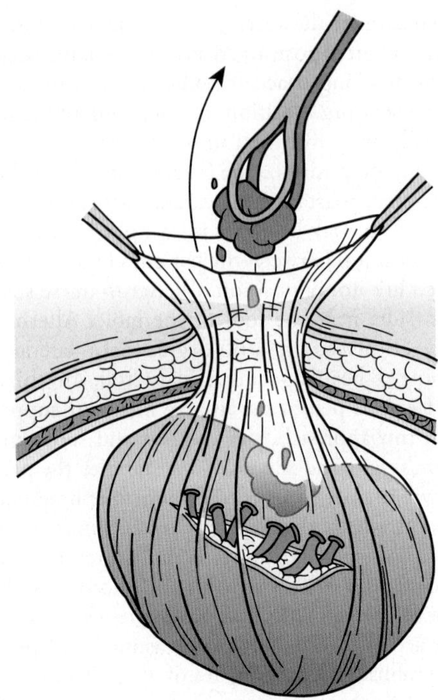

FIGURE 57-6 Extraction of the spleen within a heavy plastic bag, with instrumental morcellation of the organ with forceps. (From Gigot JF, Lengele B, Gianello P, et al: Present status of laparoscopic splenectomy for hematologic diseases: Certitudes and unresolved issues. Semin Laparosc Surg 5:147–167, 1998.)

pathologic examination of an intact spleen, an incision large enough to allow extraction of the spleen must be made. Care must be taken to avoid spillage of any splenic fragments into the abdominal cavity or wound. The laparoscope is then reinserted and the splenic bed assessed for hemostasis. Drains may be placed, if necessary. Pneumoperitoneum is then released and the fascia of all trocar ports larger than 5 mm are closed.

### Robotic Splenectomy

There have been few reports of splenic disease treated robotically and only one report specifically comparing laparoscopic with robotic splenectomy. In their retrospective report, Bodner and colleagues[41] compared operative times, hospital stay, and cost. They concluded that although the robotic procedure is feasible and safe for the patient, cost and operative times are both higher in the robotic group. In another study, Corcione and associates[42] evaluated the use of a robotic system in common general surgical procedures. Although they noted some benefits (e.g., availability of three-dimensional vision, greater dexterity with instruments), they reported concerns regarding the ability to control bleeding with only two instruments available; in these cases, they were required to convert to a traditional laparoscopic procedure. Overall, the addition of the robot to a straightforward procedure such as laparoscopic splenectomy is currently deemed unnecessary.

## LATE MORBIDITY AFTER SPLENECTOMY

Postsplenectomy thrombocytosis occurs particularly in patients with myeloproliferative disorders (e.g., CML, polycythemia vera, essential thrombocytosis), which can result in thrombosis of the mesenteric, portal, and renal veins and can be life-threatening because it can lead to hemorrhage and thromboembolism. The lifelong risk for deep venous thrombosis and pulmonary embolism has not been established but may be significant. Also, there have been case reports of acute myocardial infarction in postsplenectomy patients with thrombocytosis.

OPSI is the most common fatal late complication of splenectomy. Infection may occur at any time after splenectomy[1]; in one recent series, most infections occurred more than 2 years after splenectomy and 42% occurred more than 5 years after splenectomy, although the true incidence of OPSI has been difficult to determine because infection in postsplenectomy patients is likely to be underreported.

OPSI typically begins with a prodromal phase characterized by fever, rigors, and chills and other nonspecific symptoms, including sore throat, malaise, myalgias, diarrhea, and vomiting. Pneumonia and meningitis may be present. Many patients have no identifiable focal site of infection and present only with high-grade primary bacteremia. Progression of the illness is rapid, with the development of hypotension, disseminated intravascular coagulation, respiratory distress, coma, and death within hours of presentation. Despite antibiotics and intensive care, the mortality rate is between 50% and 70% for florid OPSI. Also, survivors often have a long and complicated hospital course with multiple sequelae, such as peripheral gangrene requiring amputation, deafness from meningitis, mastoid osteomyelitis, bacterial endocarditis, and cardiac valvular destruction.

The most frequently involved organism in OPSI is S. pneumoniae and is estimated to be responsible for between 50% and 90% of cases. Other organisms involved in OPSI include *H. influenzae, N. meningitidis, Streptococcus* and *Salmonella* spp., other pneumococcal organisms, and *Capnocytophaga canimorsus,* implicated in OPSI as a result of dog bites.

In an autopsy series by Pimpl and coworkers,[43] lethal pneumonia was identified twice as often in the postsplenectomy patients as in controls. Also, lethal sepsis with multiorgan failure was identified in 6.9% of postsplenectomy patients compared with 1.5% of autopsies on the controls. One intriguing observation is that the risk for OPSI is greater among patients who have received splenectomy for malignancy or hematologic conditions than for those who underwent splenectomy for trauma. The risk is also greater for young children (<4 years of age). The risk for fatal OPSI is estimated to be 1/300 to 350 patient-years follow-up for children and 1/800 to 1000 patient-years follow-up for adults. A review of selected reported splenectomy series of 7872 total cases, including children and adults, has revealed 270 episodes of sepsis (3.5%), with 169 septic fatalities (2.1%).[15] The incidence of nonfatal infection and sepsis is therefore likely to be significantly greater.

## PROPHYLACTIC TREATMENT OF SPLENECTOMIZED PATIENTS

### Immunization

Currently, the standard of care for postsplenectomy patients includes immunization with polyvalent pneumococcal vaccine (PPV23), *H. influenzae* type b conjugate, and meningococcal polysaccharide vaccine within 2 weeks of splenectomy if the patient did not receive these prior to surgery.[3] Despite this established standard, the literature reflects a diverse 11% to 75% postsplenectomy immunization rate. This may represent lack of understanding by patient and caregiver regarding the risk for postsplenectomy infection and sepsis.[44]

As noted, most cases of infection are caused by S. *pneumoniae, H. influenzae,* and *N. meningitides* and thus are potentially preventable if appropriate prophylactic vaccinations are given. There are reports of other, less common organisms as the cause of postsplenectomy infection.[2] Continued education of patients, families, and caregivers must stress the need for prompt medical attention if these patients show signs of infection.

Many cases of delayed OPSI have been in nonimmunized immunocompetent patients, before the current PPV23 that was introduced in 1983, which replaced the 14-valent vaccine licensed in 1977. PPV23 is composed of purified preparations of pneumococcal capsular polysaccharide antigens of 23 types of *S. pneumoniae* (25 mg each) that cause 88% of the bacteremic pneumococcal disease in the United States.

The relationship between antibody titer and protection from invasive disease has not been established. Most healthy adults show a twofold or greater rise in type-specific antibody within 2 to 3 weeks of vaccination. However, it has been clearly documented that after vaccination with PPV23, antibody levels decline after 5 to 10 years, and may fall to prevaccination levels. Even with vaccination, the development of a protective level of antibody against pneumococci is only about 50%. Currently available vaccines elicit a T cell–independent response and do not produce a sustained increase in antibody titers. Thus, the ability to define the need for revaccination based on serology continues to represent a clinical challenge.

Routine revaccination of immunocompetent persons is not recommended by the U.S. Centers for Disease Control and Prevention (CDC). Revaccination is, however, recommended for high-risk individuals. Candidates for revaccination with PPV23 include the following:

Persons who received the 14-valent vaccine who are at highest risk for fatal pneumococcal infection (e.g., asplenic patients):

- Adults at highest risk who received the 23-valent vaccine 6 years prior
- Adults at highest risk who have shown a rapid decline in pneumococcal antibody levels (e.g., patients with nephrotic syndrome, those with renal failure, transplant recipients)
- Children at highest risk (e.g., those with asplenia, nephritic syndrome, sickle cell anemia) who would be 10 years old at revaccination

Only one PPV23 revaccination dose is recommended for these high-risk individuals and it is administered 5 years after the initial dose. Rutherford and colleagues[45] have examined the efficacy and safety of pneumococcal revaccination after splenectomy for trauma. Of 45 patients offered revaccination 2 or more years after primary vaccination, 24 patients demonstrated a lack of understanding of the postsplenectomy state, confirming poor patient understanding of postsplenectomy risk. After revaccination, 48% of patients demonstrated at least a twofold increase in at least one titer (serotypes 6 and 23 pneumococcus).

The CDC has concluded that despite physician and patient education, pamphlets, and MedicAlert bracelets, patient retention regarding the risks of the postsplenectomy state is poor. They recommend that all splenectomy patients, including those with hereditary spherocytosis, be revaccinated and reeducated between 2 and 6 years after splenectomy. Recommendations include determination of pneumococcal antibody titers after immunization of every splenectomized patient because nonresponders to vaccination may be at high risk for OPSI. Subsequent follow-up of antibody titers is recommended at 3 to 5 years to evaluate for possible need for revaccination.

In an effort to improve host immunocompetence, partial splenic salvage or splenic autotransplantation has been considered because this may improve the humoral immune response to PPV23.[46] The difficulty with splenic salvage techniques is the lack of objective functional immune testing in humans. This is also true for patients who have undergone angiographic embolization for cessation of splenic hemorrhage in trauma. No studies are available regarding the risk of these patients for OPSI. Preclinical studies have examined the optimal site and amount of splenic tissue for autotransplantation. The most effective site of splenic autotransplantation was found to be the omental pouch, and approximately 50% of the spleen would be necessary for the prevention of pneumococcal sepsis. Although all efforts need to be made to preserve the spleen in trauma victims, the strategy of splenic autotransplantation seems to have limited applicability in humans.

Currently, it is suggested that educational intervention for patients who have undergone splenectomy is necessary; patients may require a number of instructional sessions. Communication with and educational efforts for primary care providers who assume medical care for asplenic patients is also extremely important because OPSI is preventable if appropriate precautions are taken. CDC immunization guidelines for 2010 have recommended the following for asplenic patients: tetanus (Td/Tdap), human papillomavirus (HPV), measles, mumps, rubella (MMR), varicella, zoster, influenza, pneumococcal polysaccharide, hepatitis A, hepatitis B, and meningococcal vaccines (see Table 57-1).

The 2006 recommendations of the Surgical Infection Society for patients 2 to 64 years of age are *H. influenzae* type B, meningococcal vaccine, and 23-valent pneumococcal vaccine.

**Table 57-1 Centers for Disease Control and Prevention Vaccine Recommendations for Asplenic Patients**

| VACCINE | RECOMMENDATION |
|---|---|
| Tetanus (Td/Tdap) | One dose every 10 years |
| Human papilloma virus (HPV) | Three doses for women through age 26 (0, 2, 6 mo) |
| Measles, mumps, rubella (MMR) | One or two doses |
| Varicella | Two doses (0, 4-8 wk) |
| Zoster | One dose |
| Influenza | One dose annually |
| Pneumococcal polysaccharide | One or two doses |
| Hepatitis A | Two doses (0, 6-12 mo or 0, 6-18 mo) |
| Hepatitis B | Three doses (0, 1-2 mo, 4-6 mo) |
| Meningococcal | One dose |

Several sources have reported that the conjugate pneumococcal vaccine is more effective in asplenic patients than the polysaccharide vaccine and should be given immediately postoperatively, as well as every 5 years to maintain efficacy. Shatz and associates[3] have evaluated antibody titers to pneumococcal vaccination in traumatic splenectomy patients randomized to receive the vaccine at 14 or 28 days postoperatively. Prior work by this group suggested that a delay in therapy might increase titer production; in the follow-up study, they determined that there was no statistically significant difference in antibody response between the two groups.

Despite lack of high-level evidence and because of the lifelong risk of OPSI, most recommend vaccines (*H. influenzae* type B, meningococcal vaccine, 23-valent pneumococcal vaccine) immediately for pneumococcal vaccination and at 14 days postoperatively or at least 2 weeks prior to elective splenectomy. Depending on patient reliability, these vaccinations may be given prior to hospital discharge for emergent splenectomy. The current recommendations are summarized in Figure 57-7.

## Antibiotics

Significant controversy still exists regarding antibiotic prophylaxis in postsplenectomy patients. The primary goal of this prophylaxis is to prevent OPSI, particularly that secondary to pneumococcal infection, which is reported to be the cause of OPSI in 50% to 90% of patients. However, OPSI secondary to penicillin-sensitive pneumococcal infection has been reported in children and adults receiving penicillin prophylaxis.

Regardless, prophylaxis with penicillin is routinely practiced in children, at least during the first 2 postsplenectomy years and some authors advocate this practice in adults, although evidence for this is scarce. Others recommend lifelong prophylaxis in adults and children. This length of treatment may be unacceptable to patients and there is evidence that there is no difference in the incidence of sepsis in postsplenectomy sickle cell patients when the antibiotic prophylaxis is ceased after 5 years.[47] Other studies have reported significant differences in the incidence of sepsis, with and without antibiotic prophylaxis.

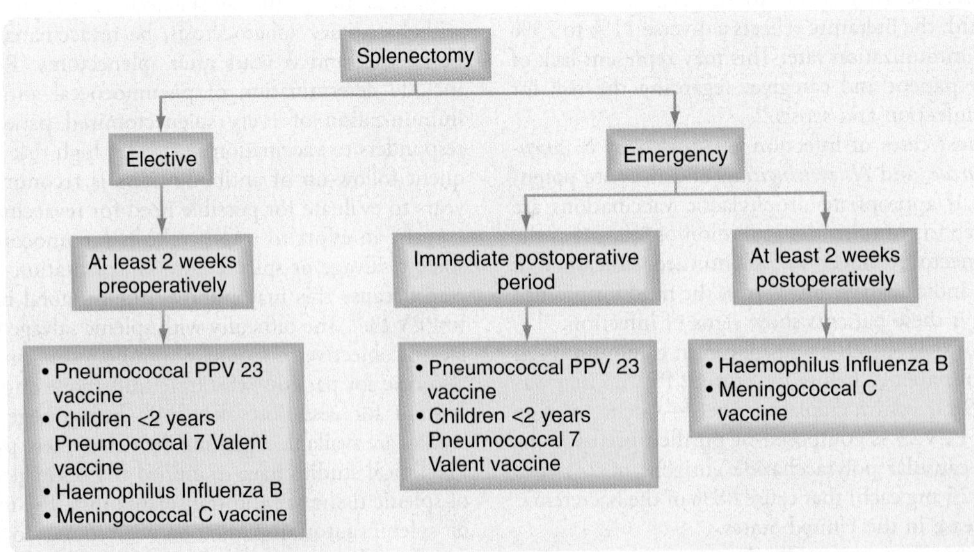


**FIGURE 57-7** Splenectomy immunoprophylaxis flow chart. (From Harji DP, Jaunoo SS, Mistry P, Nesargikar PN: Immunoprophylaxis in asplenic patients. Int J Surg 7:421–423, 2009.)

Again, OPSI has been reported in patients taking prophylactic medications and patients should be made aware that even with daily antibiotics, all infections may not be preventable.

A rational approach may be to provide a supply of oral antibiotics (standby antibiotics) to postsplenectomy adults, with instructions to begin taking the medication at the onset of a febrile illness or rigors if there is no access to immediate medical evaluation. There is evidence that the risk of OPSI is lowest in patients who exhibit the greatest understanding of the infectious risks of asplenia.[4] This highlights the importance of patient education, particularly at follow-up visits, to ensure compliance with antibiotic and vaccine prophylaxis.

Whether the patient elects to take antibiotic prophylaxis, and because of the risk of OPSI and the extreme level of associated mortality, any asplenic patient who presents with rigors or fever must be started immediately on aggressive empiric antibiotic coverage, even without culture data.

## SELECTED REFERENCES

George JN, Woolf SH, Raskob GE, et al: Idiopathic thrombocytopenic purpura: A practice guideline developed by explicit methods for the American Society of Hematology. Blood 88:3–40, 1996.

Comprehensive summary and practice guidelines for the treatment of ITP established by the American Society of Hematology; provides a comprehensive review of the current treatment recommendations and outcomes for pediatric and adult patients with ITP.

Gigot JF, Jamar F, Ferrant A, et al: Inadequate detection of accessory spleens and splenosis with laparoscopic splenectomy. A shortcoming of the laparoscopic approach in hematologic diseases. Surg Endosc 12:101–106, 1998.

Despite being over 10 years old, this article provides good technical tips for the surgeon. The article discusses numerous hematologic indications for splenectomy and their surgical outcome.

Habermalz B, Sauerland S, Decker G, et al: Laparoscopic splenectomy: The clinical practice guidelines of the European Association for Endoscopic Surgery (EAES). Surg Endosc 22:821–848, 2008.

Publications of an expert panel using a Delphi process to develop practice guidelines for laparoscopic splenectomy; Covers indications, preoperative evaluation, management, and operative and postoperative issues.

Katkhouda N, Hurwitz MB, Rivera RT, et al: Laparoscopic splenectomy: Outcome and efficacy in 103 consecutive patients. Ann Surg 228:568–578, 1998.

Large series of patients with long-term follow-up demonstrating the safety and efficacy of laparoscopic splenectomy. The discussion section provides an extensive review of previously published series and compares with versus laparoscopic splenectomy.

Spelman D, Buttery J, Daley A, et al: Guidelines for the prevention of sepsis in asplenic and hyposplenic patients. Intern Med J 38:349–356, 2008.

Reviews spectrum of causative organisms and recommended preventive strategies; consensus guidelines developed and discussed.

## REFERENCES

1. Horowitz J, Smith JL, Weber TK, et al: Postoperative complications after splenectomy for hematologic malignancies. Ann Surg 223:290–296, 1996.
2. Spelman D, Buttery J, Daley A, et al: Guidelines for the prevention of sepsis in asplenic and hyposplenic patients. Intern Med J 38:349–356, 2008.
3. Shatz DV, Schinsky MF, Pais LB, et al: Immune responses of splenectomized trauma patients to the 23-valent pneumococcal polysaccharide vaccine at 1 versus 7 versus 14 days after splenectomy. J Trauma 44:760–765, 1998.
4. El-Alfy MS, El-Sayed MH: Overwhelming postsplenectomy infection: Is quality of patient knowledge enough for prevention? Hematol J 5:77–80, 2004.
5. Spickett GP, Bullimore J, Wallis J, et al: Northern region asplenia register—analysis of first two years. J Clin Pathol 52:424–429, 1999.
6. Waghorn DJ: Overwhelming infection in asplenic patients: Current best practice preventive measures are not being followed. J Clin Pathol 54:214–218, 2001.
7. Aster RH, Bougie DW: Drug-induced immune thrombocytopenia. N Engl J Mede 357:580–587, 2007.
8. George JN, Woolf SH, Raskob GE, et al: Idiopathic thrombocytopenic purpura: A practice guideline developed by explicit methods for the American Society of Hematology. Blood 88:3–40, 1996.
9. Mikhael J, Northridge K, Lindquist K, et al: Short-term and long-term failure of laparoscopic splenectomy in adult immune thrombocytopenic purpura patients: A systematic review. Am J Hematol 84:743–748, 2009.
10. Kojouri K, Vesely SK, Terrell DR, et al: Splenectomy for adult patients with idiopathic thrombocytopenic purpura: A systematic review to assess long-term platelet count responses, prediction of response, and surgical complications. Blood 104:2623–2634, 2004.
11. Gigot JF, Jamar F, Ferrant A, et al: Inadequate detection of accessory spleens and splenosis with laparoscopic splenectomy. A shortcoming of the laparoscopic approach in hematologic diseases. Surg Endosc 12:101–106, 1998.
12. Katkhouda N, Hurwitz MB, Rivera RT, et al: Laparoscopic splenectomy: Outcome and efficacy in 103 consecutive patients. Ann Surg 228:568–578, 1998.
13. Kuter DJ, Bussel JB, Lyons RM, et al: Efficacy of romiplostim in patients with chronic immune thrombocytopenic purpura: A double-blind randomised controlled trial. Lancet 371:395–403, 2008.
14. Bernard NF, Chernoff DN, Tsoukas CM: Effect of splenectomy on T-cell subsets and plasma HIV viral titers in HIV-infected patients. J Hum Virol 1:338–345, 1998.
15. Hansen K, Singer DB: Asplenic-hyposplenic overwhelming sepsis: Postsplenectomy sepsis revisited. Pediatr Dev Pathol 4:105–121, 2001.
16. Morel P, Dupriez B, Gosselin B, et al: Role of early splenectomy in malignant lymphomas with prominent splenic involvement (primary lymphomas of the spleen). A study of 59 cases. Cancer 71:207–215, 1993.
17. Saven A, Burian C, Koziol JA, et al: Long-term follow-up of patients with hairy cell leukemia after cladribine treatment. Blood 92:1918–1926, 1998.
18. Forconi F, Sozzi E, Cencini E, et al: Hairy cell leukemias with unmutated IGHV genes define the minor subset refractory to

single-agent cladribine and with more aggressive behavior. Blood 114:4696–4702, 2009.

**19.** Goodman GR, Bethel KJ, Saven A: Hairy cell leukemia: An update. Curr Opin Hematol 10:258–266, 2003.

**20.** Chiorazzi N, Rai KR, Ferrarini M: Chronic lymphocytic leukemia. N Engl J Med 352:804–815, 2005.

**21.** Cusack JC, Jr, Seymour JF, Lerner S, et al: Role of splenectomy in chronic lymphocytic leukemia. J Am Coll Surg 185:237–243, 1997.

**22.** Friedman RL, Fallas MJ, Carroll BJ, et al: Laparoscopic splenectomy for ITP. The gold standard. Surg Endosc 10:991–995, 1996.

**23.** Morgenstern L, Rosenberg J, Geller SA: Tumors of the spleen. World J Surg 9:468–476, 1985.

**24.** Sardi A, Ojeda HF, King D, Jr: Laparoscopic resection of a benign true cyst of the spleen with the harmonic scalpel producing high levels of CA 19-9 and carcinoembryonic antigen. Am Surg 64:1149–1154, 1998.

**25.** Breitenstein S, Scholz T, Schafer M, et al: Laparoscopic partial splenectomy. J Am Coll Surg 204:179–181, 2007.

**26.** Pachter HL, Hofstetter SR, Elkowitz A, et al: Traumatic cysts of the spleen–the role of cystectomy and splenic preservation: Experience with seven consecutive patients. J Trauma 35:430–436, 1993.

**27.** Wu HM, Kortbeek JB: Management of splenic pseudocysts following trauma: A retrospective case series. Am J Surg 191:631–634, 2006.

**28.** Gadacz TR: Splenic abscess. World J Surg 9:410–415, 1985.

**29.** Gleich S, Wolin DA, Herbsman H: A review of percutaneous drainage in splenic abscess. Surg Gynecol Obstet 167:211–216, 1988.

**30.** Green BT: Splenic abscess: Report of six cases and review of the literature. Am Surg 67:80–85, 2001.

**31.** Carbonell AM, Kercher KW, Matthews BD, et al: Laparoscopic splenectomy for splenic abscess. Surg Laparosc Endosc Percutan Tech 14:289–291, 2004.

**32.** Sayeed S, Koniaris LG, Kovach SJ, et al: Torsion of a wandering spleen. Surgery 132:535–536, 2002.

**33.** Delaitre B, Maignien B: [Splenectomy by the laparoscopic approach. Report of a case.] Presse Med 20:2263, 1991.

**34.** Melman L, Matthews BD: Current trends in laparoscopic solid organ surgery: Spleen, adrenal, pancreas, and liver. Surg Clin North Am 88:1033–1046, vii, 2008.

**35.** Flowers JL, Lefor AT, Steers J, et al: Laparoscopic splenectomy in patients with hematologic diseases. Ann Surg 224:19–28, 1996.

**36.** Romanelli JR, Kelly JJ, Litwin DE: Hand-assisted laparoscopic surgery in the United States: An overview. Semin Laparosc Surg 8:96–103, 2001.

**37.** Habermalz B, Sauerland S, Decker G, et al: Laparoscopic splenectomy: The clinical practice guidelines of the European Association for Endoscopic Surgery (EAES). Surg Endosc 22:821–848, 2008.

**38.** Konstadoulakis MM, Lagoudianakis E, Antonakis PT, et al: Laparoscopic versus open splenectomy in patients with beta thalassemia major. J Laparoendosc Adv Surg Tech A 16:5–8, 2006.

**39.** Burch M, Misra M, Phillips EH: Splenic malignancy: A minimally invasive approach. Cancer J 11:36–42, 2005.

**40.** Gernsheimer T, McCrae KR: Immune thrombocytopenic purpura in pregnancy. Curr Opin Hematol 14:574–580, 2007.

**41.** Bodner J, Kafka-Ritsch R, Lucciarini P, et al: A critical comparison of robotic versus conventional laparoscopic splenectomies. World J Surg 29:982–985, 2005.

**42.** Corcione F, Esposito C, Cuccurullo D, et al: Advantages and limits of robot-assisted laparoscopic surgery: Preliminary experience. Surg Endosc 19:117–119, 2005.

**43.** Pimpl W, Dapunt O, Kaindl H, et al: Incidence of septic and thromboembolic-related deaths after splenectomy in adults. Br J Surg 76:517–521, 1989.

**44.** Brigden ML: Detection, education and management of the asplenic or hyposplenic patient. Am Fam Physician 63:499–506, 508, 2001.

**45.** Rutherford EJ, Livengood J, Higginbotham M, et al: Efficacy and safety of pneumococcal revaccination after splenectomy for trauma. J Trauma 39:448–452, 1995.

**46.** Leemans R, Harms G, Rijkers GT, et al: Spleen autotransplantation provides restoration of functional splenic lymphoid compartments and improves the humoral immune response to pneumococcal polysaccharide vaccine. Clin Exp Immunol 117: 596–604, 1999.

**47.** Falletta JM, Woods GM, Verter JI, et al: Discontinuing penicillin prophylaxis in children with sickle cell anemia. Prophylactic Penicillin Study II. J Pediatr 127:685–690, 1995.

# SECTION XI

# CHEST

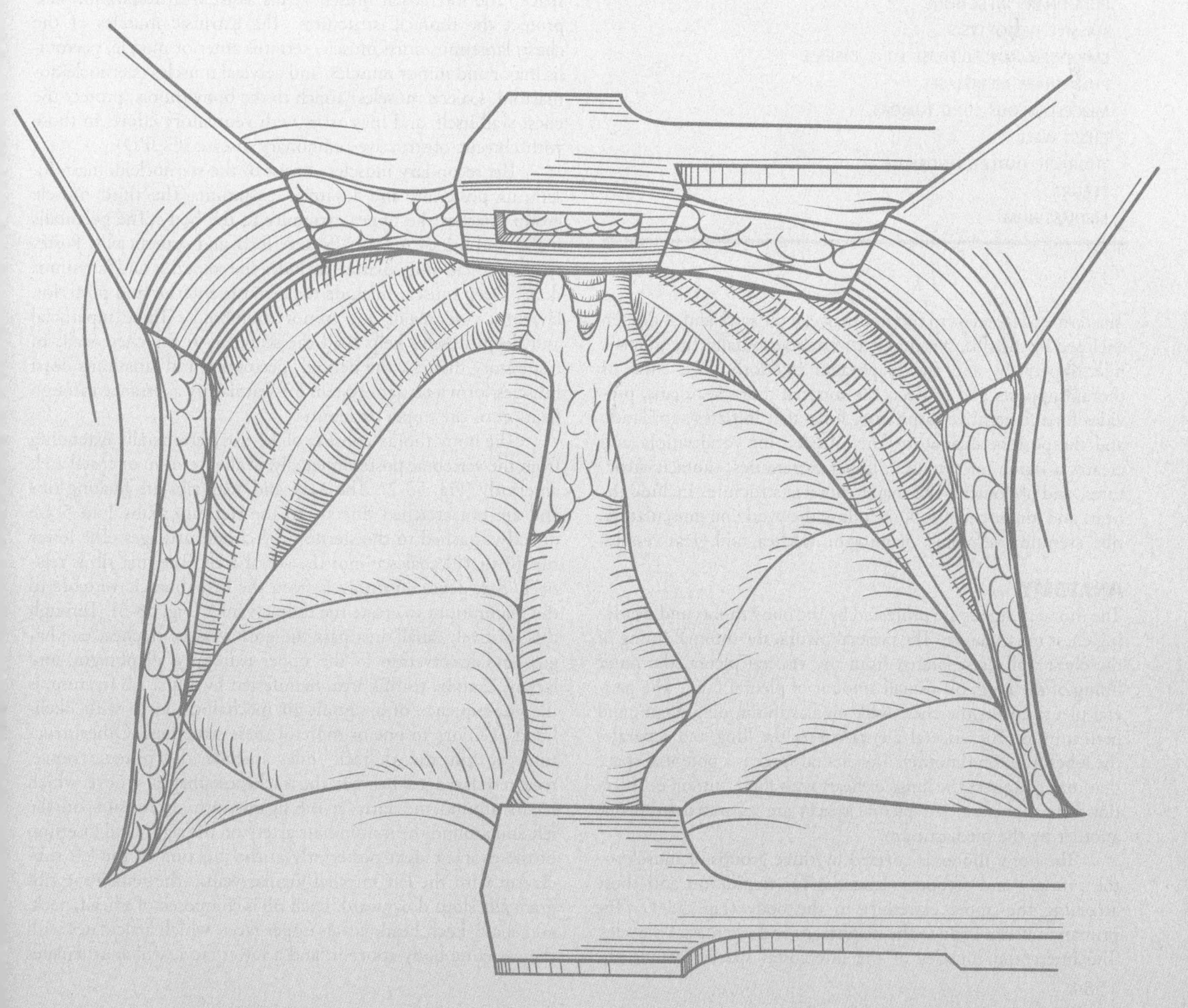

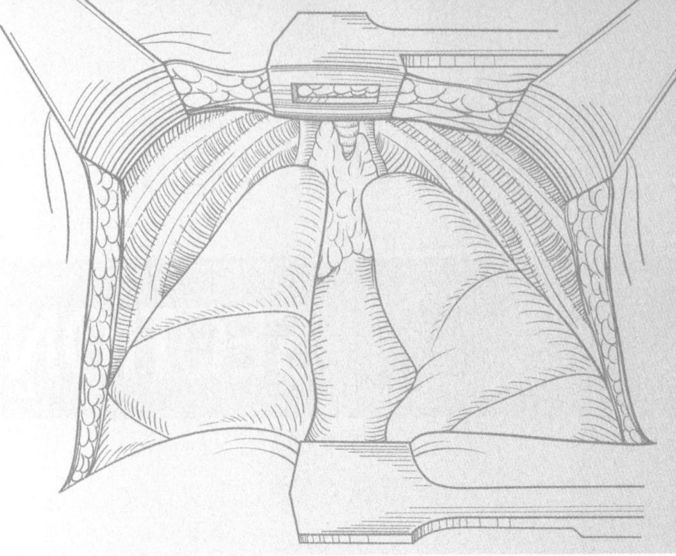

CHAPTER 58

# LUNG, CHEST WALL, PLEURA, AND MEDIASTINUM

Joe B. Putnam, Jr.



The term *thorax* refers to the area between the neck and abdomen enclosed by the ribs, sternum and vertebrae radially, the thoracic inlet superiorly, and the diaphragm inferiorly. The chest or thorax supports and protects the internal thoracic organs, provides for the negative inspiratory force that initiates ventilation and the positive expiratory force needed for vocalization, and creates a frame for the neck, upper extremities, thoracic structures, and abdomen. The major thoracic structures include the heart and lungs, chest wall, including the overlying musculature, ribs, sternum, vertebrae, diaphragm, trachea, and great vessels.

## ANATOMY

The thoracic organs are protected by the bony thorax and overlying chest musculature. The parietal pleura, the internal lining of the chest wall, is separated from the visceral pleura, the outer lining of the lung, by a small amount of pleural fluid. The parietal pleura covers the chest wall, mediastinum, diaphragm, and pericardium. The visceral pleura covers the lung and separates the lobes from one another. The pleural space is a potential space that may compress the lungs or heart with fluid, tumor, or infection. The right and left pleural spaces are separated from one another by the mediastinum.

The bony thorax is covered by three groups of muscles—the primary and secondary muscles for respiration and those attaching the upper extremity to the body (Fig. 58-1). The primary muscles include the diaphragm and intercostal muscles. The intercostal muscles of the intercostal spaces include the external, internal, and transverse or innermost muscles. Eleven intercostal spaces, each associated numerically with the rib superior to it, contain the intercostal bundles (vein, artery, and nerve) that travel along the lower edge of each rib. All intercostal spaces are wider anteriorly and each intercostal bundle falls away from the rib posteriorly to become more centrally located within each space. The intercostal muscle layers assist with respiration and protect the thoracic structures. The extrinsic muscles of the chest, latissimus dorsi muscle, serratus anterior muscle, pectoralis major and minor muscles, and cervical muscles (sternocleidomastoid, scalene muscles) attach to the bony thorax, protect the chest wall itself, and may assist with ventilatory efforts in those with chronic obstructive pulmonary disease (COPD).

The secondary muscles consist of the sternocleidomastoid, serratus posterior, and levatores costarum. The third muscle group attaches the upper extremity to the body. The pectoralis major and minor muscles lie anteriorly and superficially. Posterior superficial musculature includes the trapezius and latissimus dorsi. Deep muscles include the serratus anterior and posterior, levatores, and major and minor rhomboids. These superficial and deep muscles help hold the scapulae to the chest wall. In respiratory distress, the deltoid, pectoralis, and latissimus dorsi muscles form a tertiary system for ventilatory assistance through fixation of the upper extremities.

The bony thorax consists of 12 ribs peripherally extending from the vertebrae posteromedially, to the sternum or costal arch anteriorly (Fig. 58-2). The 11th and 12th ribs are floating ribs and are not attached directly to the sternum. Ribs 1 to 5 are directly attached to the sternum by costal cartilages. The lower ribs (6 to 10) coalesce into the costal arch. The first rib is relatively flat, dense, and travels from the first thoracic vertebra to the manubrium to create the thoracic inlet (Fig. 58-3). Through this relatively small area pass the great vessels, trachea, esophagus, and innervation to the upper extremity, diaphragm, and larynx. Trauma to this area, manifested by a first rib fracture, is the consequence of a significant mechanical force with likelihood of injury to one or more of these structures. Other structures within the thoracic inlet include the phrenic nerve, recurrent laryngeal nerve in the tracheoesophageal groove, which recurs around the aorta at the ligamentum arteriosum on the left and around the innominate artery on the right, and insertion of the thoracic duct posteriorly at the junction of the left subclavian with the left internal jugular veins. The remaining ribs gradually slope downward. Each rib is composed of a head, neck, and shaft. Each head has an upper facet, which articulates with the vertebral body above it, and a lower facet, which articulates

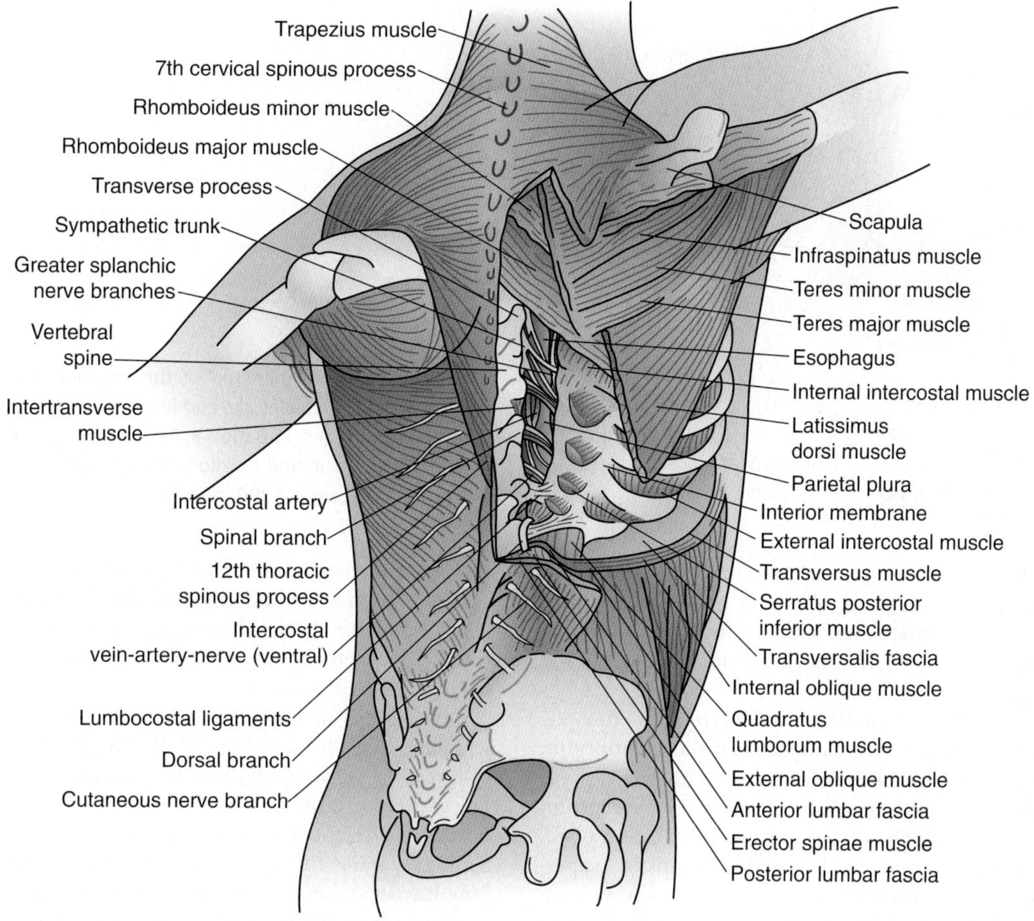


**FIGURE 58-1** Musculature of the chest wall. (From Ravitch MM, Steichen FM: Atlas of General Thoracic Surgery. Philadelphia, WB Saunders, 1988.)

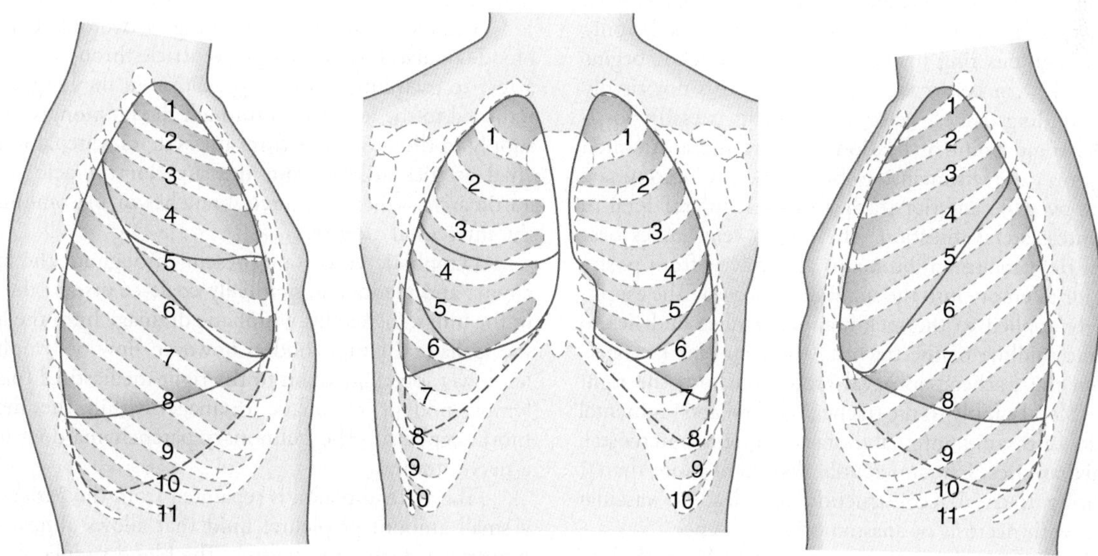


**FIGURE 58-2** The relationships of the lobes of the lung to the ribs and the pleural reflections with respiration. The topographic anatomy and the relationship of the fissures of the lobes to specific ribs in inspiration and expiration are important in evaluation of the routine posteroanterior and lateral chest film.

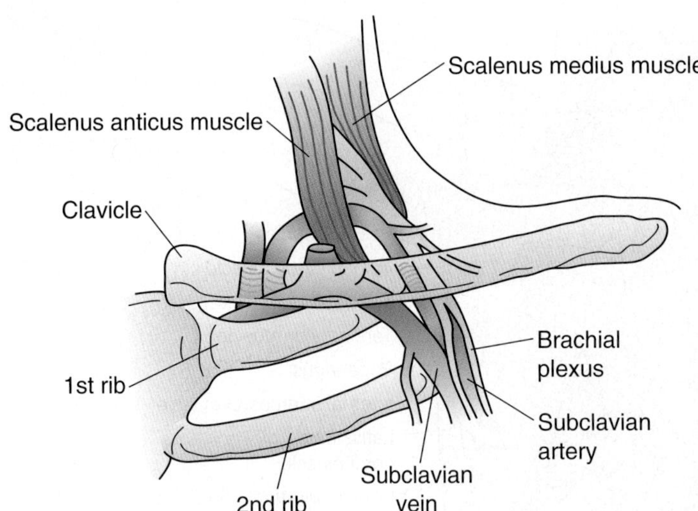


**FIGURE 58-3** Relationship of the neurovascular bundle to the scalenus muscles, clavicle, and first rib. (From Urschel HC: Thoracic outlet syndromes. In Baue AE, Geha AS, Hammond GL, et al [eds]: Glenn's Thoracic and Cardiovascular Surgery, ed 6, Stamford, CT, Appleton & Lange, 1996, p 567.)

with the corresponding thoracic vertebra to that rib, establishing the costovertebral joint. The neck of the rib has a tubercle with an articular facet; this articulates with the transverse process, creating the costotransverse joint and imparting strength to the posterior rib cage.

The sternum is flat, 15 to 20 cm in length, approximately 1.0 to 1.5 cm in thickness, and comprised of the manubrium, body, and xiphoid. The manubrium articulates with each clavicle and the first rib. The manubrium joins the body of the sternum at the angle of Louis, which corresponds to the anterior aspect of the junction of the second rib. The angle of Louis is a superficial anatomic landmark for the level of the carina. The anterior cartilaginous attachments of the true ribs to the sternum, along with intercostal muscles and the hemidiaphragms, allow for movement of the ribs with respiration.

The trachea in adults is approximately 12 cm in length, with 18 to 22 cartilaginous rings. The internal diameter is 2.3 cm laterally and 1.8 cm anteroposteriorly. The larynx ends with the inferior edge of cricoid cartilage. The cricoid is the only complete cartilaginous ring in the trachea. The trachea begins approximately 1.5 cm below the vocal cords and is not rigidly fixed to surrounding tissues. Vertical movement is easily possible. The most rigid point of fixation is where the aortic arch forms a sling over the left mainstem bronchus. The innominate artery crosses over the anterior trachea in a left inferolateral to high right anterolateral direction. The azygos vein arches over the proximal right mainstem bronchus as it travels from posterior to anterior to empty into the superior vena cava. The esophagus is closely applied to the membranous trachea and lies to the left of the midline of the trachea. The recurrent laryngeal nerves run in the tracheoesophageal groove on both the right and left. The blood supply to the trachea is lateral and segmental from the inferior thyroid, internal thoracic, supreme intercostal, and bronchial arteries. Circumferential dissection more than 1 to 2 cm during tracheal reconstruction may lead to vascular insufficiency, with necrosis or anastomotic dehiscence.

Lung development begins at approximately 21 to 28 days' gestation. The true alveolar stage, with air sacs surrounded on all sides by capillaries, occurs from approximately 7 months to term. Alveolar proliferation continues after birth. There are approximately 20 million alveoli at birth, which increase to approximately 300 million by age 10 years, with no more increase after that time. There are 23 generations of bronchi between the trachea and terminal alveoli. In the lung, 80% of its volume is air, 10% is blood, and approximately 10% is solid tissue. Alveoli make up approximately 50% of the entire lung volume.

The lungs are broadly divided into five lobes, with multiple segments in each lobe (Fig. 58-4). The right lung is composed of three lobes, the upper, middle, and lower. Two fissures separate these lobes. The major, or oblique, fissure separates the lower lobe from the upper and middle lobes. The minor or horizontal fissure separates the upper lobe from the middle lobe. The left lung has two lobes—the upper lobe and lower lobe. The lingula corresponds embryologically to the right middle lobe. A single oblique fissure separates the lobes.

The bronchopulmonary segments are divisions of each lobe that contain anatomically separate arterial, venous, and bronchial supplies. There are 10 bronchopulmonary segments on the right and eight bronchopulmonary segments on the left.

The blood supply of the lung is twofold. Unoxygenated blood circulates from the right ventricle through the pulmonary artery to each lung. After oxygenation in the lung, the blood is returned to the left atrium through the pulmonary veins. Blood supply to the bronchi is from the systemic circulation via bronchial arteries arising from the superior thoracic aorta or the aortic arch, either as discrete branches or in combination with the intercostal arteries.

Lymphatic vessels are present throughout the lung parenchyma and pleura and gradually coalesce toward the hilar areas of the lungs. Generally, lymphatic drainage from the lung affects the ipsilateral lymph nodes; however, flow of lymph from the left lower lobe may drain to the right mediastinal (paratracheal) lymph nodes. Lymphatic drainage within the mediastinum moves cephalad. The pulmonary parenchyma does not contain a nerve supply.

The visceral pleura is separated from the parietal pleura by a small amount of pleural fluid that allows almost frictionless movement during respiration. The blood supply of the parietal pleura comes from the systemic arteries and veins, including the posterior intercostal, internal mammary, anterior mediastinal, and superior phrenic arteries, and corresponding systemic veins. The blood supply of the visceral pleura is systemic and pulmonary. The lymphatic drainage of the parietal pleura is into

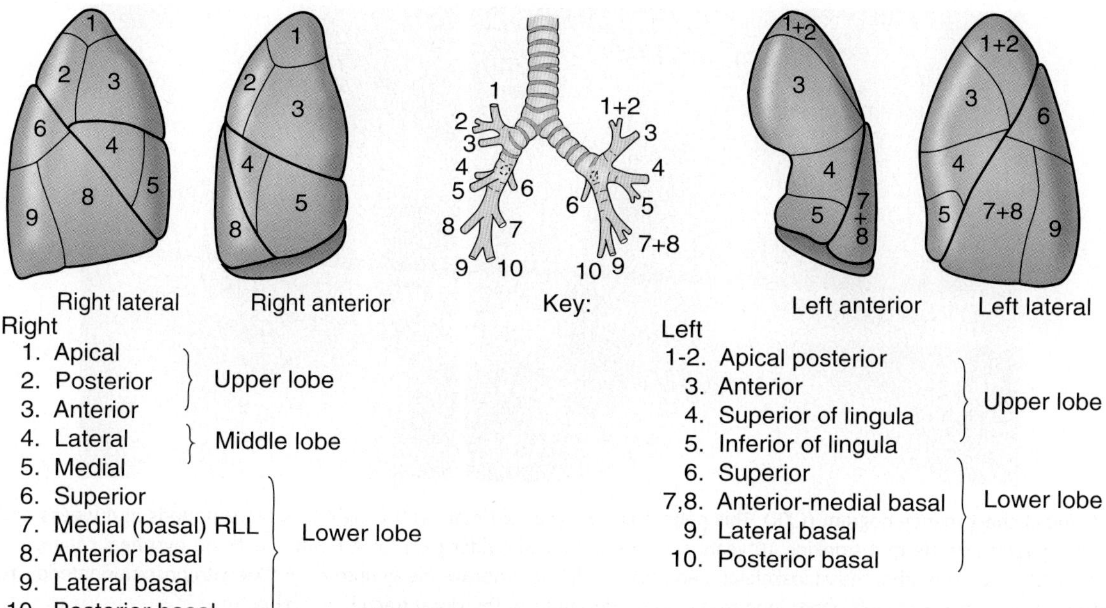


**FIGURE 58-4** Segments of the pulmonary lobes. (Adapted from Jackson CL, Huber JF: Correlated applied anatomy of the bronchial tree and lungs with a system of nomenclature. Dis Chest 9:319, 1943.)

regional lymph nodes, including the intercostal, mediastinal, and phrenic nodes. Visceral pleural lymphatics follow the superficial lung lymphatics and drain into the mediastinal lymph nodes. The parietal pleura underlying the ribs has rich nerve endings from the intercostal nerves. Generous local anesthesia is therefore necessary for chest tube insertion. The visceral pleura is innervated by vagal branches and the sympathetic system.

The anatomic boundaries of the mediastinum include the thoracic inlet superiorly, diaphragm inferiorly, sternum anteriorly, vertebral column posteriorly, and medially to the parietal pleura. Thoracic tumors that penetrate through the pleura (by definition) invade the mediastinum. Traditionally, the mediastinum can be divided into anterosuperior, middle, and posterior compartments. There no specific anatomic planes that define these areas. Fat and lymph nodes are found throughout the mediastinum.

The anterosuperior compartment includes the thymus gland. The right and left lobes of the thymus extend into the cervical areas; these portions of the thymus must be resected to provide for complete extirpation of the gland.

The middle mediastinum contains the heart, pericardium, great vessels, including the descending, transverse, and descending aorta, superior and inferior vena cava, pulmonary artery and veins, trachea and bronchi, and phrenic, vagus, and recurrent laryngeal nerves. The phrenic nerve enters the thorax through the thoracic inlet on the anterior aspect of the anterior scalene muscle.

The vagus nerve enters the thoracic inlet through the carotid sheath. It lies anterior to the subclavian and posterior to the innominate artery on the right. The right recurrent laryngeal nerve loops or recurs around the innominate artery to innervate the right vocal cord. The vagus nerve then continues posteriorly in the tracheoesophageal groove to innervate the trachea and continues down to innervate the esophagus. On the left side, the vagus nerves enters the thorax through the thoracic inlet and, as it exits the carotid sheath, moves along the anterior aspect of the aortic arch. The recurrent laryngeal nerve arises from the vagus nerve, loops around under the ligamentum arteriosum, continues superiorly under the aorta, and lies in the tracheoesophageal groove as it innervates the left recurrent laryngeal nerve. The left vagus continues posteriorly within the mediastinum posteriorly along the esophagus to innervate the trachea and esophagus.

The posterior mediastinum contains those structures between the heart and pericardium and trachea anteriorly, and the vertebral column and paravertebral spaces posteriorly. The posterior mediastinum contains the esophagus, descending aorta, azygos and hemiazygos veins, thoracic duct, sympathetic chain, and lymph nodes. The thoracic duct originates from the cisterna chyli in the abdomen. It enters the chest through the aortic hiatus in an anterolateral position, and travels superiorly just to the right of midline in the chest along the anterolateral surface of the vertebral column. At approximately the level of T5, it crosses over to the left and continues superiorly to empty, posteriorly, into the junction of the left jugular and subclavian veins.

The inferior border of the mediastinum is the diaphragm, which separates the abdominal contents from the thorax. Hernias through the esophageal hiatus (paraesophageal hernias), or through the foramen of Bochdalek (posteriorly) or the foramen of Morgagni (anteriorly), may be initially identified as a mediastinal mass.

Each spinal root exits the neural foramina of the vertebral body and bifurcates to form a branch to the intercostal nerve, to innervate the skin and intercostal musculature, and a branch to the sympathetic ganglion. Intercostal nerves innervate the skin and musculature of the intercostal muscles. The spinal root divides as it exits the neural foramina. One branch goes to the intercostal nerve and one lies in the posterior vertebral gutter to form the sympathetic ganglion. The thoracic sympathetic trunk is composed of several ganglia that lie along the ribs. The most superior ganglion is the stellate ganglion.

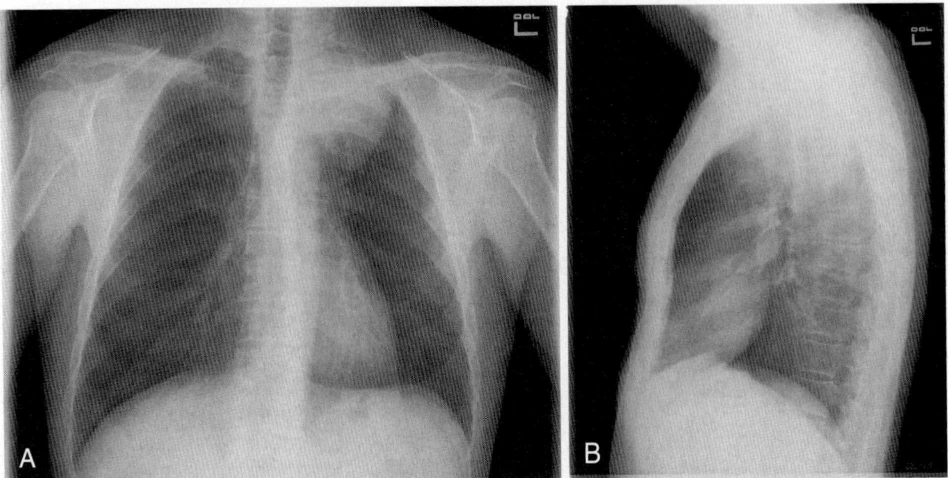


**FIGURE 58-5** Initial chest roentgenogram (CXR). This patient is a 67 year old man with weight loss of 10 pounds in 4 weeks and a 35 pack-year history of cigarette use. He quit smoking 10 years ago. He had left shoulder pain for 4 months with no dyspnea, cough, hemoptysis, or other symptoms. Massage and other musculoskeletal manipulation did not improve his symptoms. A CXR with posterior-anterior **(A)** and lateral views **(B)** demonstrates an 8.4 cm left upper lung mass. Some deviation of the distal trachea is noted.

## SELECTION OF PATIENTS FOR THORACIC OPERATIONS

The physiologic evaluation of the thoracic surgical patient must be individualized for each patient, but generally emphasizes pulmonary and cardiac function. The assessment of a patient's ability to tolerate lung resection from a cardiopulmonary standpoint is fundamental to patient selection for surgery. Patients with advanced pulmonary disease and severe pulmonary dysfunction may have a prohibitive risk, which may exist in more than one third of patients with otherwise resectable lung disease.[1]

Cigarette smoking is associated with up to a sixfold increase in the incidence of postoperative pulmonary complications after surgery.[2] If the patient is a smoker, he or she must stop smoking immediately. The physician must clearly communicate this message. Although there are few studies specific to pulmonary resection, there is evidence that preoperative smoking abstinence of 4 to 8 weeks' duration is necessary to reduce the incidence of complications. Ideally, patients are smoke-free for a minimum of 2 weeks and preferably 4 to 8 weeks before surgery,[3] although smoking cessation at any time is valuable.[4] Smoking cessation programs may be helpful for these patients, and they may need pharmacologic assistance. This combination may have increased efficacy in smoking cessation efforts over counseling alone.

Prior to the operation, and in the perioperative period, deep venous thrombosis prophylaxis is provided by subcutaneous heparin and/or by sequential compression stockings. Also, perioperative antibiotics are used to minimize complications from infections. Postoperative morbidity may also be minimized by adequate pain control to facilitate early ambulation. Routine use of a thoracic epidural catheter (or patient-controlled analgesia [PCA]) provides excellent pain control. Incentive spirometry assists in expanding the lung and reducing the incidence of pulmonary morbidity. Nasal bilevel positive airway pressure for patients with obstructive sleep apnea may delay or eliminate the need for intubation or reintubation after pulmonary resection. Early mobilization is essential to avoid most perioperative complications.

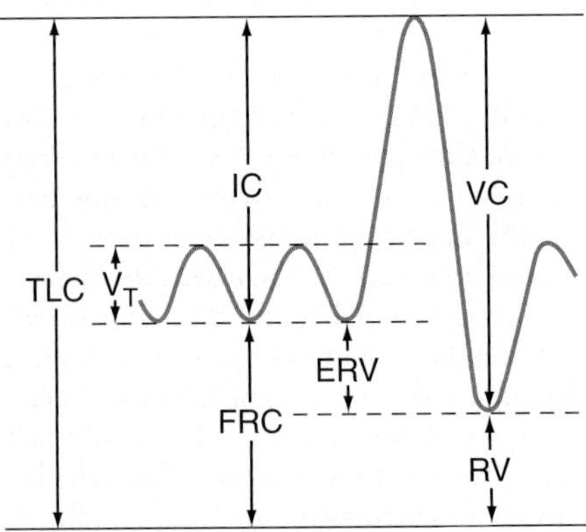


**FIGURE 58-6** Spirometry with subdivisions of lung volumes. *ERV,* Expiratory reserve volume; *FRC,* functional residual capacity, that is, lung volume at end-expiration; *IC,* inspiratory capacity; *RV,* residual volume, that is, lung volume after forced expiration from FRC; *TLC,* total lung capacity; *VC,* vital capacity, that is, the maximal volume of gas inspired from RV; *Vt,* tidal volume.

### Physiologic Evaluation

Before thoracic operations, patients may be evaluated by a combination of physiologic studies.[5] A plain chest roentgenogram is commonly obtained (Fig. 58-5). Spirometry measures the lung volumes (Fig. 58-6) and mechanical properties of lung elasticity, recoil, and compliance. Pulmonary function testing (Fig. 58-7) also evaluates gas exchange functions, such as DLCO (diffusion of carbon monoxide in the lung).

The predicted postoperative forced expiratory volume (FEV) in 1 second ($FEV_1$) is the most commonly used indicator of postoperative pulmonary reserve. Most patients with an $FEV_1$ in excess of 60% predicted will tolerate an anatomic lobectomy, depending on other evaluable factors. If the $FEV_1$ is less than 60% of predicted, further testing might be considered in an attempt to estimate postoperative $FEV_1$ (predicted postoperative $FEV_1$ [ppo-$FEV_1$]). The quantitative ventilation-perfusion lung

Section of Pulmonary Medicine
Pulmonary Function Report

| | | | |
|---|---|---|---|
| Last Name: | | First Name: | |
| Identification: | | | |
| Age: | 56 years | Room: | Out-patient |
| Sex: | Male | Race: | Caucasian |
| Height: | 65 inches | Physician: | |
| Weight: | 177 lbs | Operator: | |
| Date | | | |
| Time | | | |

| Spirometry | Pred | Pre BD | %Pred | Post BD | %Pred | %Chg |
|---|---|---|---|---|---|---|
| FVC..........[l] | 3.48 | 3.07 | 88 | 3.07 | 88 | 0 |
| $FEV_1$..........[l] | 2.83 | 2.23 | 79 | 2.26 | 80 | 1 |
| $FEV_1$/VC..........[%] | 80.81 | 72.26 | 89 | 69.78 | 86 | –3 |
| FEF 25–75..........[l/s] | 3.01 | 1.37 | 45 | 1.46 | 49 | 7 |
| PEF..........[l/s] | 7.57 | 6.43 | 85 | 7.10 | 94 | 10 |
| FIVC..........[l] | 3.48 | 3.09 | 89 | 3.24 | 93 | 5 |
| $FIV_1$..........[l] | | 3.09 | | 3.24 | | 5 |
| $FIV_1$/FVC..........[%] | | 100.00 | | 100.00 | | 0 |

| Lung Volumes | Pred | Measured | %Pred |
|---|---|---|---|
| SVC..........[l] | 3.48 | 3.04 | 87 |
| TLC..........[l] | 5.51 | 5.54 | 101 |
| RV..........[l] | 1.96 | 2.49 | 127 |
| RV/TLC..........[%] | 35.9 | 45.0 | 125 |
| FRC-Box..........[l] | 2.24 | 3.01 | 134 |

| Diffusion SB | Pred | Measured | %Pred |
|---|---|---|---|
| DLCO SB..........[ml/min/mm Hg] | 22.59 | 23.81 | 105 |
| DLCO Hb Corr[ml/min/mm Hg] | 22.6 | 24.2 | 107 |
| VA..........[l] | | 5.27 | |
| DLCO/VA..........[ml/min/mm Hg/l] | 3.93 | 4.52 | 115 |
| Hb..........[g/100ml] | | 14.1 | |

Interpretation
Spirometry reveals an isolated reduction in mid-expiratory flows consistent with an obstructive small airways defect. Increased residual volume (RV) is consistent with air trapping. Following the inhalation of a bronchodilator, there is no improvement of the obstructive airway defect. The diffusing capacity is normal.

**FIGURE 58-7** Pulmonary function report. The pulmonary function report provides complete spirometry data based on predicted values for height and weight. In this patient, the forced expiratory volume in 1 second ($FEV_1$) is 2.26 L after bronchodilators, which is 80% of predicted. The carbon monoxide diffusing capacity ($D_LCO$) is measured as 23.81 mL/min/mm Hg which is 105% of predicted. *FEF,* Forced expiratory flow; *$FIV_1$,* forced inspiratory volume in 1 second; *FIVC,* forced inspiratory vital capacity; *FRC,* functional reserve capacity; *FVC,* forced vital capacity; *HB,* hemoglobin; *PEF,* peak expiratory flow; *SB,* single breath; *SVC,* slow vital capacity; *TLC,* total lung capacity; *VA,* alveolar volume; *VC,* vital capacity.

scan is used to assist in the calculation of postoperative residual pulmonary function after resection. Patients with a ppo-$FEV_1$ of 35% to 40% should functionally tolerate the operation.

Quantitative radionucleotide perfusion scanning involves the injection of $^{99m}$Tc-radiolabeled albumin particles followed by the visual inspection of planar images (Fig. 58-8). Quantitative perfusion provides a measurement of the relative function of each lobe and lung, allowing a prediction of pulmonary function after lung resection:

$$\text{Ppo-FEV}_1 = \text{preoperative FEV}_1 \times (1 - \text{fraction of perfusion to region of planned resection})$$

A postoperative $FEV_1$ less than 30% predicted carries a greater postoperative risk for oxygen, and even ventilator dependence, but a decision to deny surgical resection to this group of patients must be considered on an individual basis because some will do better than expected with careful selection at experienced centers. Finally, in the immediate postoperative period, the objectively calculated ppo-$FEV_1$ will likely not be realized secondary to limited ambulation, pain, or other emotional or physical factors.

The carbon monoxide diffusing capacity (DLCO) can be measured by several methods, although the single-breath test is most commonly performed. The DLCO measures the rate at

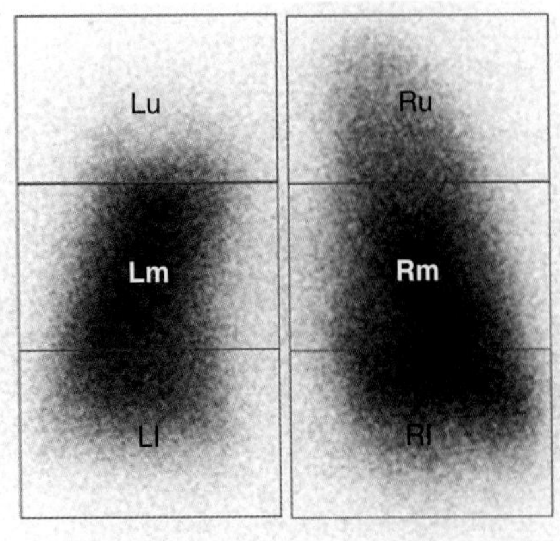


| | Left lung | | Right lung | |
|---|---|---|---|---|
| | % | Kct | % | Kct |
| Upper zone: | 4.7 | 22.66 | 9.5 | 46.27 |
| Middle Zone: | 24.0 | 116.91 | 28.3 | 138.05 |
| Lower zone: | 13.2 | 64.20 | 20.3 | 99.02 |
| Total lung: | 41.8 | 203.77 | 58.2 | 283.34 |

**FIGURE 58-8** The quantitative perfusion lung scan report provides the lung volume, and the perfusion to each lung. In a patient with a large Left hilar tumor, perfusion may be reduced in the involved left lung compared with the uninvolved right lung. The predicted post–left pneumonectomy right lung function can be obtained by multiplying the right lung percent perfusion (58.2%) by the observed best $FEV_1$ (2.26 L). The resulting value, 1.31 L, 46.5% predicted, is the predicated postoperative $FEV_1$ (following left pneumonectomy). This value suggests that a left pneumonectomy would be functionally tolerated.

which test molecules such as carbon monoxide move from the alveolar space to combine with hemoglobin in the red blood cells. The DLCO is determined by calculating the difference between inspired and expired samples of gas. DLCO levels less than 40% to 50% are associated with increased perioperative risk.[6]

The ratio of $FEV_1$ in 1 second to forced vital capacity ratio ($FEV_1$/FVC) describes the relationship between the $FEV_1$ and the functional lung volume. In obstructive disease, the ratio is low ($FEV_1$ is low and FVC is high); in restrictive disease, the ratio is approximately normal because both $FEV_1$ and FVC are reduced.

Flow-volume loops derived from spirometry describe the relationship between lung volume and air flow as the lung volume changes during a forced expiration and inspiration. The typical test consists of tidal breathing at rest, maximal inspiratory effort to total lung capacity, and maximal expiratory effort to residual volume, concluding with maximal inspiratory effort to total lung capacity.

## Cardiopulmonary Exercise Testing

Cardiopulmonary exercise testing (CPET) can be extremely useful for the evaluation of marginal candidates (ppo-$FEV_1$ or ppo-DLCO <50% predicted) or for patients who appear more disabled than expected from simple spirometry measurements. Formal CPET includes an exercise electrocardiogram (ECG), heart rate response to exercise, and measurements of minute ventilation and oxygen uptake/min. CPET allows a calculation of maximum oxygen consumption ($\dot{V}O_2$ max) and provides insight into overall cardiopulmonary function (the cardiopulmonary axis) that cannot be ascertained from other objective studies. CPET may identify clinically occult cardiac disease and provide a more accurate assessment of pulmonary function than spirometry and DLCO, which tend to overestimate functional loss after resection.

A patient's risk of perioperative morbidity and mortality may be stratified by $\dot{V}O_2$ max. Those with $\dot{V}O_2$ max above 20 mL/kg/min are not at increased risk for complications or death after resection of non–small cell lung cancer (NSCLC). A level below 15 mL/kg/min is associated with an increased risk, and $\dot{V}O_2$ max less than 10 mL/kg/min indicates very high risk, generally precluding operation.[7,8] Some have advocated stair climbing as a suitable measure of preoperative cardiopulmonary assessment.[9] Given the wide availability of more objective and standardized noninvasive tests for cardiopulmonary function, stair climbing performance should not be used as the sole criterion to determine physiologic suitability for lung cancer resection. In patients undergoing evaluation for lung volume reduction surgery or for lung transplantation, a 6-minute walk test is used for a measure of the cardiac and pulmonary reserve. Patients are told to walk as far and as fast as they can during this time period. Distances of more than 1000 feet suggest an uncomplicated course.

Measurement of diaphragm function by fluoroscopy, the sniff test, is needed to determine symmetry of effort and exclude paradoxical movement of the diaphragm. Paradoxical movement—elevation of one hemidiaphragm with active contraction or retraction of the other diaphragm—suggests paresis or paralysis. This finding may suggest a specific reason for breathlessness. Diaphragm plication may be therapeutic.

No single test result should be viewed as an absolute contraindication to surgical resection. Although the physiologic assessment for patients undergoing normal spirometry and minimal comorbidity is fairly straightforward, patients with marginal preoperative indices must be considered on an individual basis.

## Thoracic Incisions

The choice of incision depends on the operation, patient's underlying physiologic condition, and anticipated benefits and limitations of the planned approach.

Video-assisted thoracic surgery (VATS) and other minimally invasive techniques have been developed to treat most thoracic problems, including lung cancer, mediastinal tumors, pleural diseases, and parenchymal diseases, and diagnosis and staging of thoracic malignancies. Minimally invasive techniques appear to minimize pain and surgical trauma from the incisions, decrease hospitalization, and improve convalescence. Small incisions are made for the camera and other instruments, depending on the location of the tumor. The ribs are not spread. Improved lighting and optics create excellent exposure and visualization.

The posterior or posterolateral thoracotomy is used for operations on a single thorax, pulmonary resection, esophageal surgery or resection, or resection of portions of the chest wall. The patient is placed in a lateral decubitus position. An oblique incision is used posteriorly or a vertical axillary incision is made just anterior to the latissimus dorsi muscle.

The anterior or anterolateral thoracotomy is created by a curvilinear incision underneath the inferior border of the pectoralis major muscle at the inframammary fold. A median sternotomy is performed using a vertical incision from the sternal notch to the xiphoid. A sternal saw is then used to divide the sternum in the midline. With gentle retraction, the sternum can be spread approximately 8 to 10 cm to allow access to the mediastinum, heart, great vessels, and right and left thorax. The pleura can be opened on either side to explore the hemithorax. The sternum is usually closed with stainless steel wire.

The transverse sternotomy, or clamshell incision, is larger than a median sternotomy and more uncomfortable for the patient. This incision combines two anterior thoracotomy incisions in the inframammary fold with transverse division of the sternum at the fourth intercostal space. Both internal mammary arteries are ligated. This approach is ideal for accessing the right and left hilum, as well as providing additional exposure for large mediastinal tumors, bilateral hilar dissections, bilateral lung transplantation, or posterior-based metastases in both lungs.

## LUNG

### Congenital Lesions

Various congenital lung abnormalities can occur as a consequence of disturbed embryogenesis.[10] Bilateral agenesis of the lungs is fatal. Unilateral agenesis may occur more frequently on the left (≈70%) than on the right (≈30%), with more than a 2 : 1 male-to-female ratio.

Hypoplasia of the lungs may occur as a result of interference with the development of the alveolar system during the last 2 months of gestation. Bochdalek's hernia is the most frequent cause of hypoplasia. Conditions associated with hypoplasia of the lungs include oligohydramnios, prune belly syndrome (deficiency in the abdominal musculature, genitourinary abnormalities), scimitar syndrome (abnormal pulmonary vein draining into the inferior vena cava, demonstrated as a crescent along the right heart border on a cardiac angiogram), and dextrocardia. Isolated pulmonary hypoplasia is rare.

Hyaline membrane disease (or infant respiratory distress syndrome) is frequent in premature infants (24 to 28 weeks' gestation) and infants of diabetic mothers. At that point in gestation, infants have an immature surfactant system. Hyaline membrane disease develops in the alveoli, causing congestion and a grossly deep purple–appearing lung. Respiratory distress frequently ensues, requiring high concentrations of oxygen. Chest x-rays demonstrate a ground glass appearance from the interstitial edema. As needs for oxygen and ventilator pressure increase to counteract this interstitial edema, pneumothorax frequently occurs. Of these infants, 10% to 30% do not survive.

#### Cystic Lesions

Congenital cystic lesions generally occur secondary to separation of the pulmonary remnants from airway branchings. Clinically, about one third of patients are without symptoms, one third have cough, and one third have infection or, rarely, hemoptysis. Treatment may be antibiotics or, for more severe localized cases, resection. Any thoracic cystic lesion that enlarges on serial radiographs needs to be considered for resection.

A bronchogenic cyst arises from a tracheal or bronchial diverticulum (see later, "Mediastinal Cysts and Tumors"). This diverticulum becomes completely separated from the trachea and is frequently found as an asymptomatic mass on routine chest x-rays. Computed tomography (CT) of the chest demonstrates this abnormality as a homogeneous-type mass, well circumscribed, and adjacent to the trachea (Fig. 58-9). The bronchogenic cyst accounts for 10% of mediastinal masses in children and is located in the midmediastinum. Treatment consists of excision, even if the patient is asymptomatic, to confirm the diagnosis.

Cystic fibrosis is an autosomal recessive disorder found more commonly in whites. Approximately 20% of patients with cystic fibrosis survive to the age of 30 years. Lung failure is the most frequent cause of death in most patients. Excessively thick mucus leads to inspissation, recurrent infections, bronchitis, and bronchiectasis. Pneumothorax secondary to air trapping is also found. Fibrosis and cystic changes on pathologic examination are identified. A tension cyst may be a complication of cystic disease. A rapid increase in the size of the cyst may cause mechanical ventilation problems as well as mediastinal shift. Resection, usually lobectomy, corrects this problem. Pneumatoceles may develop as a result of childhood *Staphylococcus aureus* infection. They can be large and may cause mechanical complications, which may resolve completely as the pneumonia resolves. Resection may be needed.

#### Congenital Bronchopulmonary Malformations

Lobar emphysema[10] is the most commonly resected congenital cystic lesion (50%). The onset of rapidly progressive respiratory distress usually occurs from 4 to 5 days to several weeks after birth. It rarely occurs after 6 months of age. It predominantly affects the upper lobe. Bronchiolitis is probably the most common cause overall. Treatment is lobectomy.

Congenital cystic adenomatoid malformations are the second most commonly resected congenital cystic lesion. They are closely related to a hamartoma without cartilage. Terminal bronchioles proliferate, yielding the adenomatoid malformation. The lung has the appearance of Swiss cheese and feels like a large rubbery mass. With air trapping and overdistention, respiratory distress may occur, which is optimally relieved by lobectomy.

Pulmonary sequestration is an area of embryonic lung tissue, separate from the lung, which receives blood supply from an anomalous systemic artery from the aorta, not the pulmonary artery. This condition occurs secondary to an accessory lung bud caudal to the normal lung, but with a lack of absorption of primitive surrounding splanchnic vessels. During lung development, interlobar sequestration (75%) occurs early. Later, after the pleura forms, extralobar sequestration (ELS) occurs (25%), primarily on the left side (66%), and is completely enclosed by its own pleura. The ELS blood supply is usually from the thoracic or upper abdominal aorta to systemic (azygous or hemiazygous) veins. ELS is more common in males. Resection is recommended. Intralobar sequestration (ILS) mainly occurs within the lower lobes (>95%) and is equally distributed between the right and left lower lobes. ILS blood supply is from the descending thoracic aorta, which usually traverses the pulmonary ligament. Venous drainage is via the pulmonary veins. Ninety-five percent of the systemic blood supply to the pulmonary sequestration comes from the thoracic aorta.

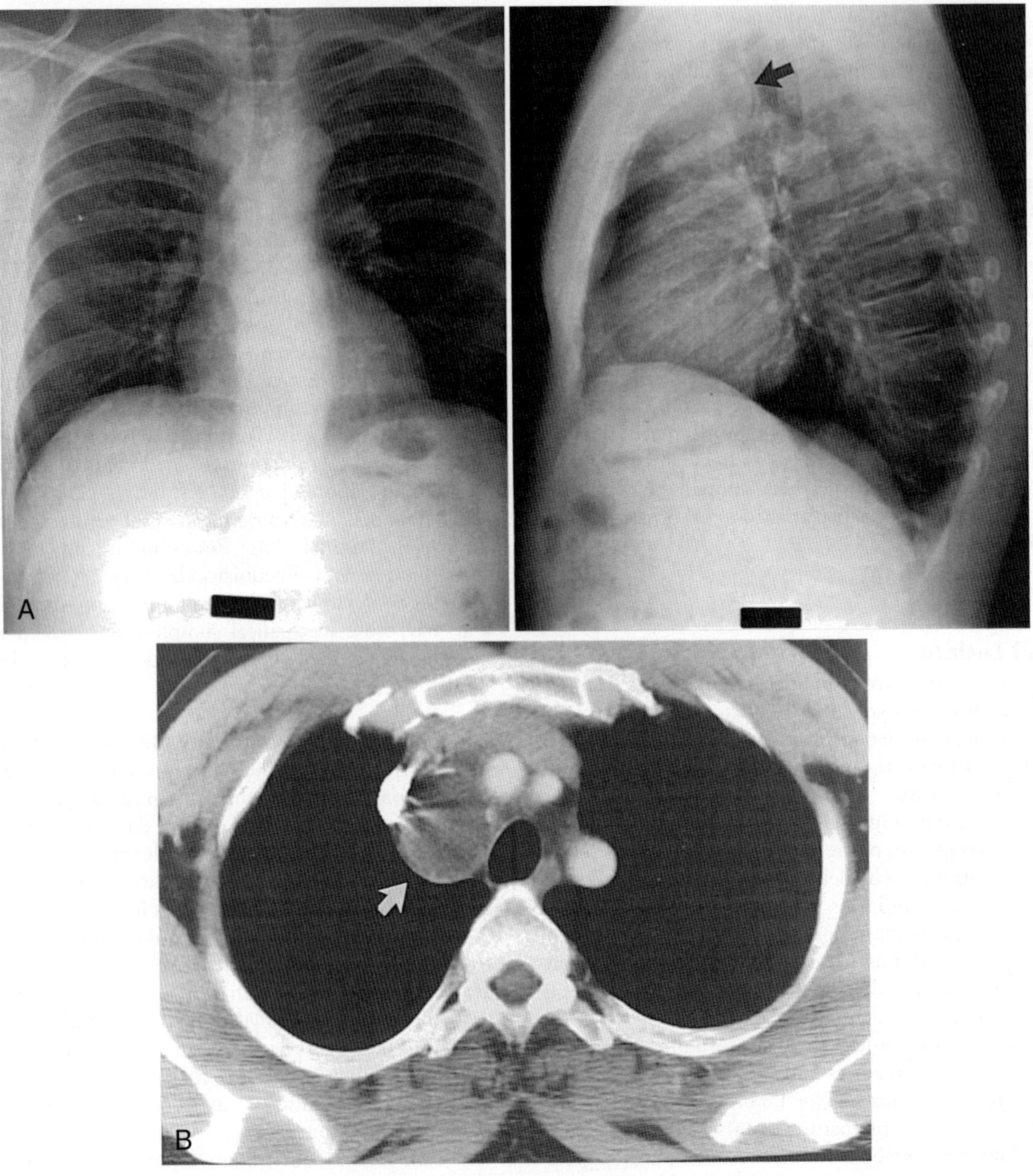

**FIGURE 58-9** Two chest roentgenograms **(A)** and a CT scan **(B)** of the chest of a patient with a bronchogenic cyst (*arrow*).

## Congenital Abnormalities of the Trachea and Bronchi

Esophageal atresia with tracheoesophageal fistula is the most frequent abnormality of the trachea in infants (see later, "Trachea") Bronchial atresia is the second most frequent congenital pulmonary lesion after tracheoesophageal fistula.[11] The lung tissue distal to the atresia expands and becomes emphysematous as a result of air entry through the pores of Kohn. With no exit for air or mucus because of this blind bronchial stump, emphysema from air trapping or development of a mucocele may develop. Chest x-rays may demonstrate hyperinflation of a lobe or segment. The oval density may be identified between the hyperinflated lung and hilum. The left upper lobe is the most frequently involved of all lobes within the lung. Diagnosis may be confirmed with bronchography or CT. The surgeon must rule out a mucous plug, adenoma, vascular compression, and sequestration.

Tracheal agenesis is a rare phenomenon and is fatal. The trachea is absent from the larynx to the carina, and bronchi communicate with the esophagus.

Tracheal stenosis is also rare and consists of generalized hypoplasia, a funnel-like trachea, and bronchial and segmental malformations. The right upper lobe bronchus may come from the trachea directly and may be associated with an aberrant left pulmonary artery (so-called *pulmonary artery sling*). Completely circular vascular rings are common. Repair is by incision of the trachea vertically and widening of the tracheal lumen.

Tracheomalacia can be identified by bronchoscopy. The surgeon will notice marked variation of the tracheal lumen with inspiration and expiration. The tracheal rings are ineffective in maintaining the lumen of the trachea and, with negative intrathoracic pressure, the trachea collapses. With the positive pressure exerted by exhalation, the trachea expands. Respiratory difficulty ensues from the intermittently collapsing trachea. Relief of the extrinsic compression is needed. Stent placement in adults or primary repair may be required. This condition may have a congenital predisposition but is most often seen in adults with COPD.

### Congenital Vascular Disorders

Congenital vascular disorders of the lungs may occur.[12] In Swyer-James-Macleod syndrome, there is an idiopathic hyperlucent lung. This problem develops from chronic pulmonary infections such as bronchiectasis. As the consolidation persists, decreased pulmonary artery blood supply may cause a so-called *autopneumonectomy* and hyperlucent lung.

Scimitar syndrome is associated with a hypoplastic right lung, with drainage of the pulmonary vein to the inferior vena cava. Usually, the anomaly is corrected using extracorporeal cardiopulmonary support. A patch from the pulmonary vein to the left atrium via an atrial septal defect corrects this problem.

Pulmonary arteriovenous malformations may exist as one or more pulmonary arteries to pulmonary vein connections, bypassing the pulmonary capillary bed. This connection results in a right-to-left shunt. Approximately one third of these patients have hereditary hemorrhagic telangiectasia (Osler-Weber-Rendu syndrome). Approximately 50% of the malformations are small (<1 cm) and tend to be multiple. Also, 50% are larger than 1 cm, usually smaller than 5 cm, and tend to be subpleural. These lesions need to be considered in the differential diagnosis of any patient with hemoptysis that is unexplained on the basis of bronchoscopy or routine imaging. Local resection or catheter embolization of these lesions can be curative.

A pulmonary vascular sling consists of an anomalous or aberrant left pulmonary artery, which causes airway obstruction and is associated with other anomalies. The aberrant left pulmonary artery arises from the right (main) pulmonary artery and courses between the trachea and esophagus to supply the left lung. More than 90% of patients have wheezing and stridor. Esophagoscopy will show the anomalous vessel anterior to the esophagus; bronchoscopy or bronchography will demonstrate the vessel posterior to the trachea. Surgical correction requires exploration of the left chest, division of the artery, and oversewing of the vessel as far as possible distally within the mediastinum. Reanastomosis to the main pulmonary artery is then performed.

Vascular rings[13] represent 7% of all congenital heart problems.[14] The most common vascular ring is a double aortic arch, which occurs in 60% of all cases. The right, or posterior, arch is the larger and gives rise to the right carotid and right subclavian arteries. The ring wraps around the trachea and esophagus. A posterior indentation is noted in the esophagus on barium swallow. Simple division corrects the anomaly. A right aortic arch with retroesophageal left subclavian artery and left ligamentum arteriosum occurs in approximately 25% to 30% of patients with vascular rings. Intracardiac defects occur with double aortic arch. Most of these infants require operation within the first weeks or months of life.

Most patients with vascular rings require only a careful history and barium swallow for diagnosis. Typically, one does not need bronchoscopy or esophagoscopy because it may be harmful; aortography adds little additional information. Repair is performed through the left chest. Division of the smaller arch, usually the left, is undertaken. The ligamentum is divided and the trachea and esophagus are freed from the surrounding tissues. When a retroesophageal right subclavian artery with left ligament occurs, the patient may complain of dysphagia, which is referred to as dysphagia lusoria. The differential diagnosis includes neuromotor diseases of the esophagus or stricture.

## LUNG CANCER

Lung cancer is a significant global health problem. In the United States in 2010, there were an estimated 222,550 new cases of cancer of the lung and bronchus.[15] Lung cancer is the most frequent cause of cancer death in men and women and accounts for 14.5% of all cancer diagnoses and 27.6% of all cancer deaths in the United States. Lung cancer deaths exceed the combined total deaths of breast, prostate, and colorectal cancer patients. Since 1987, more women have died of lung cancer than breast cancer. In men and women, changes in lung cancer incidence and the mortality rate probably reflect decreasing cigarette smoking over the previous 50 years and potentially earlier detection of smaller and asymptomatic lung cancers. However, smoking cessation in women has lagged behind smoking cessation in men, and the incidence of lung cancer in women continues to increase. African American men have the highest incidence and highest death rate from cancer of the lung and bronchus.

Cigarette smoking is unequivocally the most important risk factor in the development of lung cancer. Other environmental factors that may predispose to lung cancer include industrial substances such as asbestos, arsenic, chromium, or nickel, organic chemicals, radon, or iatrogenic radiation exposure, air pollution, and other factors, such as secondary smoke in nonsmokers.

Radon is the second leading cause of lung cancer in the United States and is associated with approximately 18,000 lung cancer deaths/year.[16] Radon is a natural radioactive gas released from the normal decay of uranium in the soil. Inhalation is associated with a health risk. Inexpensive test kits are available to determine the amount of radon present in a person's home.

Optimal treatment of lung cancer requires accurate diagnosis and clinical staging before treatment begins. The anatomic basis for staging (tumor, lymph nodes, metastases) includes the physical properties of the tumor and presence of regional or systemic metastases. The biologic basis for staging (molecular markers prognostic for survival, as well as indicators predictive for response to therapy) will be incorporated into staging systems of the future. Clinical trials are available for patient enrollment to better understand and evaluate various treatments.[17] The National Cancer Institute Clinical Trials Cooperative Group Program conducts clinical trials for patients with lung cancer and other malignancies throughout the United States.[18]

### Pathology

The pathology of lung cancer has been recently reviewed in detail.[19] Development of lung cancer follows a progression of histologic changes that results from smoking and includes the following: (1) proliferation of basal cells; (2) development of atypical nuclei with prominent nucleoli; (3) stratification; (4) development of squamous metaplasia; (5) carcinoma in situ; and (6) invasive carcinoma.

Adenocarcinoma (ACA) of the lung[20] is the most frequent histologic type and accounts for approximately 45% of all lung cancers. ACA of the lung develops from the mucus-producing cells of the bronchial epithelium. Microscopic features consist of cuboidal to columnar cells with adequate to abundant pink or vacuolated cytoplasm and some evidence of gland formation. Most of these tumors (75%) are peripherally located. ACA of the lung tends to metastasize earlier than squamous cell carcinoma (SCCA) of the lung and more frequently to the central nervous system (CNS). Bronchioloalveolar carcinoma (BAC) is a type of ACA but can sometimes be a more indolent disease. It is well differentiated and spreads along alveolar walls without invasion of stroma, blood vessels, or pleura. BAC may present as a solitary nodule, multiple nodules, or diffuse parenchymal infiltrates. Most ACAs, including those with a BAC component would be categorized as ACA, mixed subtype, because invasive components would be present.[21] BAC may require resection to confirm the diagnosis. A solitary focus is treated in a manner similar to ACA. Multifocal disease generally is not amenable to surgical resection.

SCCA of the lung occurs in approximately 30% of patients with lung cancer. Approximately two thirds of these tumors are centrally located and tend to expand against the bronchus, causing extrinsic compression. These tumors are prone to undergo central necrosis and cavitation. SCCA tends to metastasize later than ACA. Microscopically, keratinization, stratification, and intercellular bridge formation are exhibited. SCCA may be more readily detected on sputum cytology than ACA.

A diagnosis of large cell undifferentiated carcinoma may be made in approximately 10% of all lung tumors. Specific cytologic features of SCCA or ACA are lacking. These tumors tend to occur peripherally and may metastasize relatively early. Microscopically, these tumors show anaplastic pleomorphic cells, with vesicular or hyperchromatic nuclei and abundant cytoplasm. Neuroendocrine histopathology in ACA can also portend a poorer prognosis and is somewhat more common in the large cell variant.

Small cell lung cancer represents approximately 20% of all lung cancers; approximately 80% are centrally located. The disease is characterized by an aggressive tendency to metastasize. It often spreads early to mediastinal lymph nodes and distant sites, especially bone marrow and brain. Small cell lung cancer appears to arise in cells derived from the embryologic neural crest. Microscopically, these cells appear as sheets or clusters of cells, with dark nuclei and little cytoplasm. This oatlike appearance under the microscope gives the term *oat cell carcinoma* to this disease. Neurosecretory granules are evident on electron microscopy. This tumor is staged as limited stage (disease restricted to an ipsilateral hemithorax within a single radiation port) and extensive stage (obvious metastatic disease). These tumors are often advanced at presentation, with an aggressive tendency to metastasize. Chemoradiotherapy is generally used for treatment. Prophylactic cranial irradiation needs to be considered if the patient with limited- or extensive-stage disease responds well to first-line therapy. Complete responses may occur in approximately 30% of patients; however, the 5-year survival rate is only 5%. Patients with clinical early-stage disease (e.g., <3 cm in size, no nodal metastases, and no extrathoracic metastases) may be considered for surgical resection, followed by adjuvant systemic therapy. Preresection staging includes $^{18}$F-fluorodeoxyglucose positron emission tomography (FDG-PET), brain CT or magnetic resonance imaging (MRI), and mediastinoscopy. Mediastinal metastases on clinical staging suggest advanced disease best treated with chemoradiotherapy.

Lung cancers commonly metastasize to the pulmonary and mediastinal lymph nodes (lymphatic spread). Hematogenous spread of lung cancer is indiscriminate and almost all areas of the body are at risk. Metastases to the adrenal glands, brain, lung, and bone are common. ACA is more likely to metastasize to the CNS. Bone metastases are osteolytic. Extrathoracic metastases may occur without hilar nodes or mediastinal metastases.

## Screening

Patients with lung cancer often are seen with advanced-stage disease and symptoms at initial presentation. The pulmonary parenchyma does not contain nerve endings and tumors may grow undetected until symptoms of pain, hemoptysis, or obstructive pneumonia develop. With the increased use of CT in the United States, smaller asymptomatic lung cancers are being identified.

Screening for lung cancer reduces lung cancer mortality.[22] The National Lung Screening Trial (NLST) randomized participants to undergo three annual screenings with either low dose helical computed tomography or chest radiography; 53,454 patients were enrolled. Participants were between the ages of 55 and 74 years, and current or former heavy smokers (≥30 pack years of cigarette smoking at the beginning of the trial). Participants had no signs or symptoms of lung cancer on trial entry. Fewer lung cancer deaths occurred in the CT group ($n$ = 356) compared to the CXR group ($n$ = 443). The NLST demonstrated that low-dose helical CT screening in high-risk patients reduced the death rate from lung cancer by 20% (95% CI, 6.8-26.7; $p = 0.004$), and reduced all-cause mortality by 6.7% (95% CI, 1.2-13.6; $p = 0.02$). The study was closed early given the significant difference between the two arms.

At present, mass screening for early lung cancer detection in asymptomatic individuals is not recommended. However, patients with significant tobacco history, and falling within the eligibility characteristics of the NLST, may elect to undergo testing for early stage lung cancer on an individual basis based upon consultation and evaluation by their personal physicians—the shared-decision making model. Screening of asymptomatic patients may identify nonspecific findings causing unnecessary anxiety in the patient and family. Patients in areas of endemic histoplasmosis with a smoking history and a newly discovered pulmonary nodule can be particularly challenging. An update related to shared-decision making for testing for early lung cancer is not planned until the results of prospective clinical trials are available.

## Diagnosis

The diagnosis of lung cancer can be challenging.[23] Many benign conditions mimic lung cancer. Physical examination should focus on the cardiorespiratory system. In addition, the presence of supraclavicular lymph nodes, identified by careful examination of the cervical and supraclavicular lymph nodes, suggests advanced disease (N3 status for NSCLC) and therapy other than resection is recommended. Paraneoplastic syndromes are distant manifestations of lung cancer (not metastases) as revealed in extrathoracic nonmetastatic symptoms. The lung cancer affects these extrathoracic sites by producing one or more biologic or biochemical substances.

NSCLC typically occurs in patients who are 50 to 70 years of age who have a history of cigarette smoking. Patients develop symptoms based on the physical impact of tumor growth within the lung parenchyma. Symptoms such as cough, dyspnea, chest wall pain, and hemoptysis are related to the physical presence of the tumor and its interactions with the structures of the lung and chest wall.[24]

Pathologic confirmation of NSCLC can assist the patient and physician in discussions of risk and benefit for specific treatment options. Guidelines for management of the indeterminate (or solitary) pulmonary nodule (SPN) are available.[25] Under certain circumstances, a SPN may be deemed benign with adequate confidence in the absence of a pathologic diagnosis. SPNs that are entirely calcified or radiologically stable by CT of the chest for a minimum of 2 years are likely to be benign.[26,27] Review of old radiographs or other prior imaging studies will assist in evaluation of changes in the mass.

In patients with a clinically suspicious SPN and nondiagnostic fiberoptic bronchoscopy (FOB) and/or transthoracic needle aspiration (TTNA) studies, more invasive means for diagnosis are indicated. If histologic information is needed to assess risk and benefit for the patient, the least invasive strategy possible would be required. Newer techniques include navigational bronchoscopy[28] to match CT images of small peripheral lung nodules with guided real-time direction of small bronchoscopic catheters to improve access for biopsy. In a physiologically fit patient with a suspicious SPN nodule, nonanatomic or wedge resection provides diagnosis. Confirmation of NSCLC by the pathologist should be followed by definitive resection in the same setting. For an SPN in the absence of a cancer diagnosis that cannot be removed by wedge resection, a lobectomy can be considered for diagnosis (and treatment). A pneumonectomy is not performed without a cancer diagnosis.

Up to one third of patients with NSCLC have a pleural effusion at the time of presentation. Pleural fluid sampling with thoracentesis is required for cytologic examination.

Malignant pleural effusion (MPE; T4) represents a contraindication to resection; However, many pleural effusions in this setting may have a sympathetic or reactive cause.

Bronchoscopy is recommended before any planned pulmonary resection. The surgeon also will independently assess (via bronchoscopy) the endobronchial anatomy to exclude secondary endobronchial primary tumors and ensure that all known cancer will be encompassed by the planned pulmonary resection. When pneumonectomy or bronchoplastic resection is contemplated for a central tumor, the surgeon's assessment at bronchoscopy is critical to the determination of whether complete (R0) resection can be achieved.

TTNA guided by CT or fluoroscopy is particularly useful in the evaluation of peripheral lesions smaller than 3 cm in diameter, but is limited by a high rate of nondiagnostic examination. A nondiagnostic TTNA does not completely rule out malignancy; lung cancer can be excluded only in the presence of a specific benign alternative diagnosis. TTNA is not routinely recommended for the patient with good physiologic reserve and otherwise appropriate for surgery (e.g., stage I or II patients). If the patient does have hard palpable lymph nodes in the cervical or supraclavicular area, fine-needle aspiration (FNA) or biopsy may provide an accurate diagnosis of N3 disease. Otherwise, a superficial lymph node biopsy or a scalene node biopsy could be performed to obtain tissue for further evaluation.

## Staging

Staging is a description of the extent of the cancer based on similarities in survival for the group of patients with those characteristics. The staging system creates a shorthand description of the tumor, nodes, and metastatic characteristics of the patient to facilitate choice of optimal therapy and evaluate outcomes based on the clinical and pathologic stage. The American Joint Committee on Cancer (AJCC) and the International Union Against Cancer (UICC) have worked to establish and promulgate staging system guidelines. The current international staging system for NSCLC[29] provides the basis for specific patient stage groupings and is used for current treatment recommendations.

The clinician's responsibility is to ensure the highest possible degree of certainty of the clinical stage or extent of the disease and recommend therapy or a therapeutic combination of greatest efficacy. Optimal staging assists the clinician in providing the best recommendations for therapeutic interventions for the patient. The clinical stage is the physician's best and final estimate of the extent of disease based on all available information from invasive and noninvasive studies and prior to the initiation of definitive therapy. The pathologic stage is the determination of the physical extent of the disease based on histologic examination of the resected tissues, including the hilar and mediastinal lymph nodes.

### Evaluation of Stages

**T (Tumor) Stage** As the tumor size increases, survival decreases. Chest x-ray and CT of the chest and upper abdomen, including the liver and adrenals, are the most frequent diagnostic imaging studies performed in patients with lung cancer (Fig. 58-10). The chest x-ray provides information on the size, shape, density, and location of the primary tumor and its relationship to the mediastinal structures. CT of the chest provides more detail than the chest x-ray on tumor characteristics, and provides information on the relationship of the tumor to the mediastinum, chest wall, and diaphragm, as well as invasion into the vertebrae or mediastinal structures (clinical T4). MRI may complement CT in these patients (T4). MRI brain imaging may be reserved for patients with stage I or II cancer with new neurologic symptoms only (e.g., vertigo, headache), all patients with stage III or IV cancer,[30] and those with small cell carcinoma or superior sulcus tumors (Pancoast tumor), because these patient have a higher incidence of occult brain metastases.

**N (Nodal) Stage** Determination of metastases to mediastinal lymph nodes constitutes a critical point in staging and treatment recommendations.[30] Mediastinal lymph node metastases are present in 26% to 32% of patients at the time of diagnosis and initially assessed with chest CT. Lymph nodes may be enlarged normally from infection (e.g., histoplasmosis, previous bronchitis or pneumonia) or other inflammatory processes. Mediastinal adenopathy is most often defined as lymph nodes with a maximal transverse diameter more than 1 cm on axial tomographic images. In the absence of mediastinal nodes more than 1 cm in diameter, the likelihood of N2 or N3 disease is low. If mediastinal nodes more than 1 cm are identified, nodal tissue must be examined (e.g., by endoscopic bronchial ultrasound, cervical mediastinoscopy, esophageal ultrasound, VATS) for histologic evidence of metastases before definitive resection.

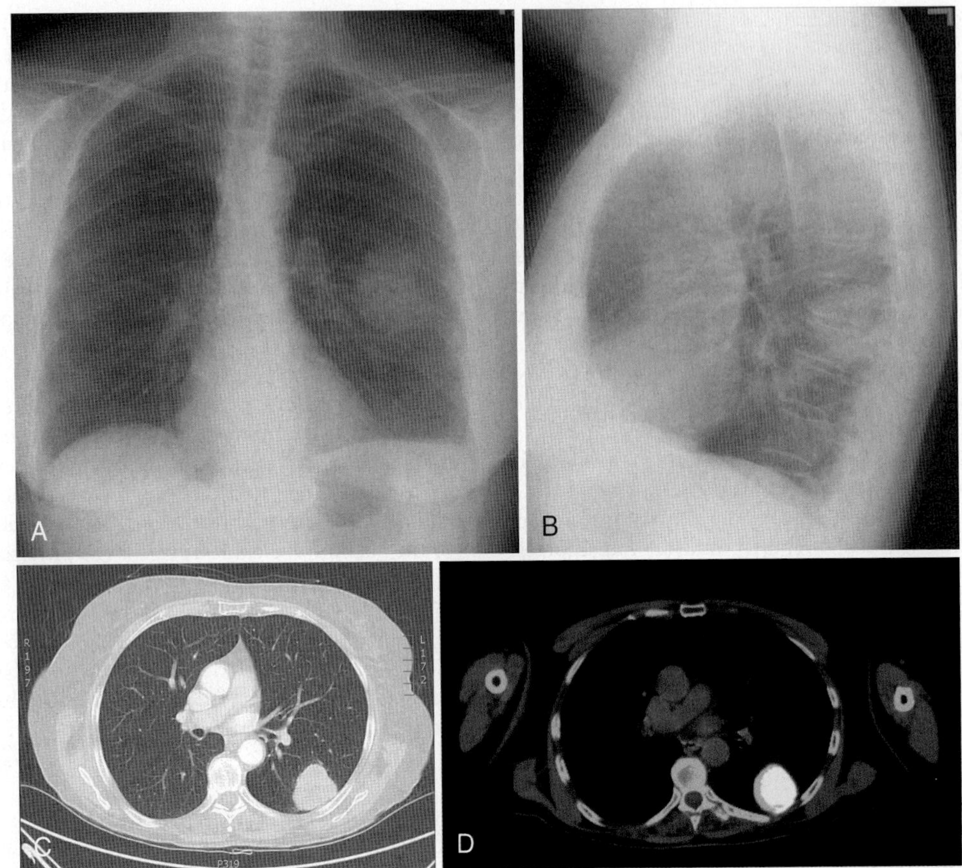


**FIGURE 58-10** Radiographic evaluation for any patient with known or suspected lung cancer includes a plain chest roentgenogram (posterior-anterior **(A)**; and lateral **(B)**. Other studies commonly performed include computed tomography (CT) of the chest **(C)**. Evaluation of the plain films and CT guides subsequent evaluations. FDG-PET with fused CT **(D)** provides the ability to correlate metabolic activity with physical findings. Although FDG-PET uses the increased metabolism in most neoplasms to create the FDG-PET image, other processes such as infection, inflammation, or sequelae of trauma or fractures can be identified as well. Sites of increased metabolism should be carefully evaluated for metastases.

CT has a reported sensitivity for mediastinal lymph node assessment in NSCLC of 57% to 79%, with a positive predictive value of just 56%.[30] No CT size criterion is entirely reliable for the determination of mediastinal lymph node involvement. Larger mediastinal lymph nodes are more likely to be associated with metastasis (>70%); however, normal-sized lymph nodes (<1 cm) have a 7% to 15% chance of containing metastases.

PET[31] may assist in evaluating the local extent and presence of known or occult metastases based on the differential increased metabolism of glucose by cancer cells compared with normal tissues (Fig 58-11). A PET scan is not a cancer-specific study because high cellular glucose metabolism is seen in inflammatory processes in addition to malignancy. Histologic confirmation of suspicious mediastinal lymph node involvement is indicated prior to final treatment decisions. Other areas of FDG uptake must be considered for the evaluation of histologic evidence of NSCLC. FDG-PET coupled with CT may yield increased sensitivity and specificity in determining the stage of patients with lung cancer before treatment interventions.[32] Reed and colleagues[33] have determined that PET and CT together are better than either one alone in determining a patient's suitability for resection. The negative predictive value of PET for mediastinal lymph node metastases from NSCLC was 87%.

Invasive staging includes cervical mediastinoscopy (CME) or mediastinotomy (Chamberlain's procedure), endoscopic bronchial ultrasound (EBUS), and esophageal ultrasound (EUS).[34] CME is traditionally indicated for patients with otherwise operable NSCLC with enlarged paratracheal or subcarinal lymph nodes, particularly if the cancer is proximal, pneumonectomy is planned, or the patient is at increased risk for the planned resection. CME is commonly performed for the biopsy of bilateral paratracheal (levels 2 and 4) and subcarinal (level 7) lymph nodes. A mediastinotomy is used to gain access to the mediastinum after resection of the second costosternal cartilage to evaluate the aortopulmonary window (level 5) or anterior mediastinum (level 6) lymph nodes. CME has a negative predictive value (NPV) above 90%, may be performed as an outpatient procedure, and is associated with a low rate of significant complications. When pathologic frozen section evaluation fails to demonstrate malignant nodal involvement, mediastinoscopy may be followed by resection under the same anesthetic. The use of CME, regardless of radiographic evidence of nodal involvement (routine mediastinoscopy), is not a cost-effective approach, and adds little to the accuracy of staging in patients with an adequate noninvasive preoperative evaluation.[35]

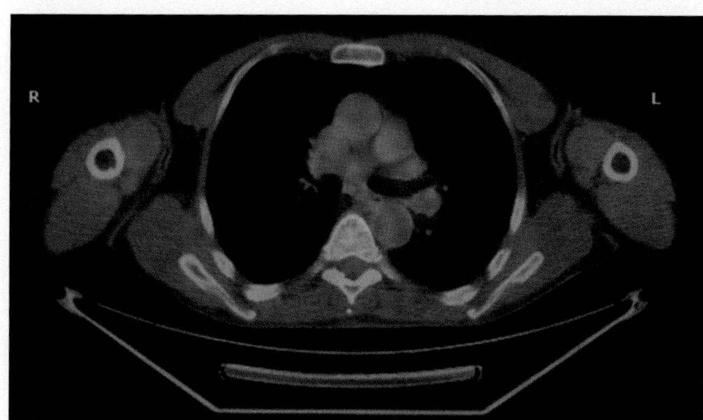


**FIGURE 58-11** A subcarinal LN has mild FDG uptake. Based on these findings, additional invasive staging is warranted to include bronchoscopy, and invasive staging of mediastinal lymph nodes. Endobronchial ultrasound with transtracheal needle aspiration can be performed with real-time ultrasound guidance to facilitate transtracheal needle placement. Other stations can be biopsied as well. If needed, cervical mediastinoscopy is performed with biopsy of high paratracheal (2R and 2 L), low paratracheal (4R and 4 L), pretracheal (3A), and subcarinal (7) lymph nodes. If left-sided aortopulmonary lymph nodes were FDG avid, Chamberlain's procedure (anterior mediastinotomy), or VATS with biopsy of aortopulmonary (AP) window lymph nodes, or hilar lymph nodes could also be performed. Additional evaluation of the patient would be warranted if the patient would be considered a surgical candidate.

Additional sampling techniques may be helpful.[30,34] EBUS may be more sensitive than mediastinoscopy. Combining EBUS and surgical staging may provide greater sensitivity for mediastinal nodal metastases than surgical staging alone and avoid unnecessary thoracotomies.[36] VATS techniques can evaluate enlarged level 5 or 6 lymph nodes, as well as enlarged level 8 or 9 or low-level 7 lymph nodes. EUS-guided aspiration can be easily used for transesophageal needles aspiration of subcarinal and left anteroposterior (AP) window lymph nodes.[30]

Extrathoracic or distant metastases (M1b) are common in lung cancer. Beyond a thorough history and physical examination, and standard staging techniques, additional evaluation for metastatic disease is indicated only for selected cases.[30] If metastatic disease is suspected based on imaging results, a tissue sample should be obtained for diagnosis to confirm the presence or absence of metastases.[34] Nodules in the contralateral lung are characterized as metastatic disease (M1a), as are MPE and pleural carcinomatosis.

Metastatic adrenal involvement is present in up to 7% of patients at presentation. The standard CT evaluation of the chest should also include evaluation of the upper abdomen to include the liver and adrenal glands. Indeterminate adrenal lesions on CT may be evaluated further with MRI or CT-guided percutaneous biopsy.

## Current American Joint Committee on Cancer Staging System

The International Association for the Study of Lung Cancer (IASLC) embarked on its lung cancer staging project to include all treatment and diagnostic groups, collect data for analysis, and reform future revisions.[37] The current AJCC descriptions for lung cancer staging reflect the impact of the IASLC lung cancer staging project.[38] The IASLC collected over 100,000 NSCLC cases treated between 1990 and 2000. Each patient had a minimum of 5 years of follow-up and all treatment modalities were included. Over 81,000 cases were submitted that were eligible for analysis, including 67,725 patients with NSCLC and 13,290 patients with small cell carcinoma. Survival was calculated by the Kaplan-Meier method. Prognostic groups were created using Cox regression analyses and results were internally and externally validated. Stage groupings were revised to reflect these analyses and internally and externally validated.[29] External validation was assessed against the Surveillance, Epidemiology and End Results (SEER) program database. The data collected were retrospective and an audit of the data was not performed; however, information was provided by credible centers, which facilitated data collection, and analysis of a large patient population. Future directions will most certainly include prospective data collection[39] and proteomic and genomic characteristics.

I have included the TNM definitions (Table 58-1), nodal characteristics (Box 58-1), and stage groupings of the TNM subsets with survival (Table 58-2). Other schematics have been created for the lymph node map[40] and T characteristics.[41]

The mediastinal and regional lymph node classification scheme is presented in Figure 58-12. This map presents a graphic representation of mediastinal and pulmonary lymph nodes in relation to other thoracic structures for optimal dissection and anatomic labeling by the surgeon.

**Tumor (T)** In the IASLC lung cancer staging project, over 18,000 patients had a T1 to T4 tumor with N0 lymph node dissection and R0 resection.[42] T1 was divided into T1a (≤2 cm) and T1b (>2 to 3 cm). T2 was divided into T2a (>3 to 5 cm) and T2b (>5 to 7 cm). T2c would have been more than 7 cm; however, these patients had a survival that was statistically similar to the survival of T3 patients. Lung cancers larger than 7 cm are categorized as T3.

Other T2 descriptors, such as visceral pleural invasion and partial atelectasis (less than the entire lung), could not be evaluated because of small number of patients and inconsistent data. In the current AJCC staging system, nodules in the same lobe were categorized as T3, nodules in a different lobe were categorized as T4, and a nodule in a contralateral lobe would be designated as M1a unless there was compelling evidence to suggest synchronous primary tumors.

T3 tumors may be characterized as a tumor with invasion into the pleura, pericardium, or diaphragm, an endobronchial tumor less than 2 cm from the carina, or an obstructing tumor causing atelectasis of the entire lung and, as noted, two nodules in the same lobe.

T4 tumors would involve the mediastinal structures such as the heart, great vessels, esophagus, and trachea, as well as the vertebral body or carina. Two nodules, one each in two separate ipsilateral lobes, would also be characterized as T4.

Pleural metastases, or MPE, was changed from T4 (in the AJCC sixth edition) to M1. Patients previously categorized as a clinical T4 based on an MPE, malignant pericardial effusions, or pleural nodules, are now categorized as clinical M1 based on poor survival more closely resembling patients with metastatic disease.

**Table 58-1 T, N, and M Descriptors for Lung Cancer Staging**

| | |
|---|---|
| **T (Primary Tumor)** | |
| TX | Primary tumor cannot be assessed, or tumor proven by the presence of malignant cells in sputum or bronchial washings but not visualized by imaging or bronchoscopy |
| T0 | No evidence of primary tumor |
| Tis | Carcinoma in situ |
| T1 | Tumor ≤3 cm in greatest dimension, surrounded by lung or visceral pleura, without bronchoscopic evidence of invasion more proximal than the lobar bronchus (i.e., not in the main bronchus)*<br>• T1a Tumor ≤2 cm in greatest dimension<br>• T1b Tumor >2 cm but ≤3 cm in greatest dimension |
| T2 | Tumor >3 cm but ≤7 cm or tumor with any of the following features‡<br>• Involves main bronchus, ≥2 cm distal to the carina<br>• Invades visceral pleura<br>• Associated with atelectasis or obstructive pneumonitis that extends to the hilar region but does not involve the entire lung<br>• T2a Tumor >3 cm but ≤5 cm in greatest dimension<br>• T2b Tumor >5 cm but ≤7 cm in greatest dimension |
| T3 | Tumor >7 cm or one that directly invades any of the following: chest wall (including superior sulcus tumors), diaphragm, phrenic nerve, mediastinal pleura, parietal pericardium; or<br>• Tumor in the main bronchus <2 cm distal to the carina* but without involvement of the carina; or<br>• Associated atelectasis or obstructive pneumonitis of the entire lung or<br>• Separate tumor nodule(s) in the same lobe |
| T4 | Tumor of any size that invades any of the following: mediastinum, heart, great vessels, trachea, recurrent laryngeal nerve, esophagus, vertebral body, carina; or<br>• Separate tumor nodule(s) in a different ipsilateral lobe |
| **N (Regional Lymph Nodes)** | |
| NX | Regional lymph nodes cannot be assessed |
| N0 | No regional lymph node metastasis |
| N1 | Metastasis in ipsilateral peribronchial and/or ipsilateral hilar lymph nodes and intrapulmonary nodes, including involvement by direct extension |
| N2 | Metastasis in ipsilateral mediastinal and/or subcarinal lymph node(s) |
| N3 | Metastasis in contralateral mediastinal, contralateral hilar, ipsilateral or contralateral scalene, or supraclavicular lymph node(s) |
| **M (Distant Metastasis)** | |
| MX | Distant metastasis cannot be assessed |
| M0 | No distant metastasis |
| M1 | Distant metastasis<br>• M1a Separate tumor nodule(s) in a contralateral lobe; tumor with pleural nodules or malignant pleural (or pericardial) effusion†<br>• M1b Distant metastasis |

Adapted from Goldstraw P, Crowley J, Chansky K, et al: The IASLC Lung Cancer Staging Project: Proposals for the revision of the TNM stage groupings in the forthcoming (seventh) edition of the TNM Classification of malignant tumours. J Thorac Oncol 2:706–714, 2007; and Edge SB, Byrd DR, Compton CC, et al: AJCC cancer staging manual, ed 7, New York, 2010, Springer.)

*The uncommon superficial spreading tumor of any size with its invasive component limited to the bronchial wall, which may extend proximally to the main bronchus, is also classified as T1.

†Most pleural (and pericardial) effusions with lung cancer are due to tumor. In a few patients, however, multiple cytopathologic examinations of pleural (pericardial) fluid are negative for tumor, and the fluid is nonbloody and is not an exudate. Where these elements and clinical judgment dictate that the effusion is not related to the tumor, the effusion should be excluded as a staging element and the patient should be classified as T1, T2, T3, or T4.

‡T2 tumors with these features are classified T2a if ≤5 cm or if size cannot be determined, and T2b if >5 cm but ≤7 cm.

**Lymph Nodes (N)** The nodal characteristic and designations did not change in the current AJCC guidelines.[43] Over 67,000 patients had T, N, and M characteristics as well as a description of histologic type and survival; 38,265 patients had clinical nodal and 28,371 had pathologic nodal staging information. Clinical staging studies included tests such as diagnostic imaging, CT, and mediastinoscopy. Thoracotomy for staging was excluded. PET was not widely used internationally in this cohort during this period. A new international lymph node map was proposed combining the integral aspects of the Japanese-Naruke and the North American–Mountain lymph node maps.[44] Of special note, the authors proposed radiographic regions for the location of specific mediastinal lymph nodes, particularly for integration with CT, to guide the radiologic staging of patients with NSCLC.

**Metastases (M)** Metastases were divided into M1a and M1b.[45] Patients with metastasis to the contralateral lung only were designated as M1a and metastases to regions outside the lung or pleura were designated as M1b. A second nodule in the nonprimary ipsilateral lobe, previously designated as M1, was changed to T4M0. In this situation, the patient received the benefit of the doubt approach because this might represent a second primary.

## Results of Treatment of Lung Cancer According to Stage

The choice of initial therapy, whether single modality or multimodality therapy, depends on the patient's clinical stage at presentation and availability of prospective protocols. However,

**BOX 58-1 Lymph Node Map Definitions**

**N2 Nodes***

1. Highest mediastinal nodes: Nodes lying above a horizontal line at the upper rim of the brachiocephalic (left innominate) vein where it ascends to the left, crossing in front of the trachea at its midline.
2. Upper paratracheal nodes: Nodes lying above a horizontal line drawn tangential to the upper margin of the aortic arch and below the inferior boundary of number 1 nodes.
3. Prevascular and retrotracheal nodes: Pretracheal and retrotracheal nodes may be designated 3A and 3P. Midline nodes are considered to be ipsilateral.
4. Lower paratracheal nodes: The lower paratracheal nodes on the right lie to the right of the midline of the trachea between a horizontal line drawn tangential to the upper margin of the aortic arch and a line extending across the right main bronchus at the upper margin of the upper lobe bronchus and contained within the mediastinal pleural envelope; the lower paratracheal nodes on the left lie to the left of the midline of the trachea between a horizontal line drawn tangential to the upper margin of the aortic arch and a line extending across the left main bronchus at the level of the upper margin of the left upper lobe bronchus, medial to the ligamentum arteriosum and contained within the mediastinal pleural envelope.

**Regional (N2) Lymph Node Classification**

5. Subaortic (aortopulmonary window): Subaortic nodes are lateral to the ligamentum arteriosum or the aorta or left pulmonary artery and proximal to the first branch of the left pulmonary artery and lie within the mediastinal pleural envelope.
6. Para-aortic nodes (ascending aorta or phrenic): Nodes lying anterior and lateral to the ascending aorta and the aortic arch or the innominate artery, beneath a line tangential to the upper margin of the aortic arch.
7. Subcarinal nodes: Nodes lying caudad to the carina of the trachea, but not associated with the lower lobe bronchi or arteries within the lung.
8. Paraesophageal nodes (below carina): Nodes lying adjacent to the wall of the esophagus and to the right or left of the midline, excluding subcarinal nodes.
9. Pulmonary ligament nodes: Nodes lying within the pulmonary ligament, including those in the posterior wall and lower part of the inferior pulmonary vein.

**N1 Nodes**[†]

10. Hilar nodes: The proximal lobar nodes, distal to the mediastinal pleural reflection and the nodes adjacent to the bronchus intermedius on the right; radiographically, the hilar shadow may be created by enlargement of both hilar and interlobar nodes.
11. Interlobar nodes: Nodes lying between the lobar bronchi.
12. Lobar nodes: Nodes adjacent to the distal lobar bronchi.
13. Segmental nodes: Nodes adjacent to segmental bronchi.
14. Subsegmental nodes: Nodes around the subsegmental bronchi.

From Mountain CF, Dresler CM: Regional lymph node classification for lung cancer staging. Chest 111:1718–1723, 1997.
*All N2 nodes (single-digit designator) lie within the mediastinal pleural envelope.
[†]All N1 nodes lie distal to the mediastinal pleural reflection and within the visceral pleura.

**Table 58-2 AJCC 7th Edition TNM Stage Groupings**

| | | | | 5-Year Survival (%) | |
|---|---|---|---|---|---|
| **STAGE** | **T** | **N** | **M** | **CLINICAL STAGE** | **PATHOLOGIC STAGE** |
| Occult cancer | TX | N0 | M0 | Not calculated | |
| 0 | Tis | N0 | M0 | Not calculated | |
| IA | T1a/b | N0 | M0 | 50 | 73 |
| IB | T2a | N0 | M0 | 43 | 58 |
| IIA | T2b<br>T1a/b; T2a | N0<br>N1 | M0<br>M0 | 36 | 46 |
| IIB | T2b<br>T3 | N1<br>N0 | M0<br>M0 | 25 | 36 |
| IIIA | Any T1; T2<br>T3<br>T4 | N2<br>N1/N2<br>N0/N1 | M0<br>M0<br>M0 | 19 | 24 |
| IIIB | T4<br>Any T | N2<br>N3 | M0<br>M0 | 7 | 9 |
| IV | Any T | Any N | M1a/b | 2 | 13 |

From Goldstraw P, Crowley J, Chansky K, et al: The IASLC Lung Cancer Staging Project: proposals for the revision of the TNM stage groupings in the forthcoming (seventh) edition of the TNM Classification of malignant tumours. J Thorac Oncol 2:706-714, 2007. Edge SB, Byrd DR, Compton CC, et al: AJCC Cancer Staging Manual, ed 7, New York, 2010, Springer.

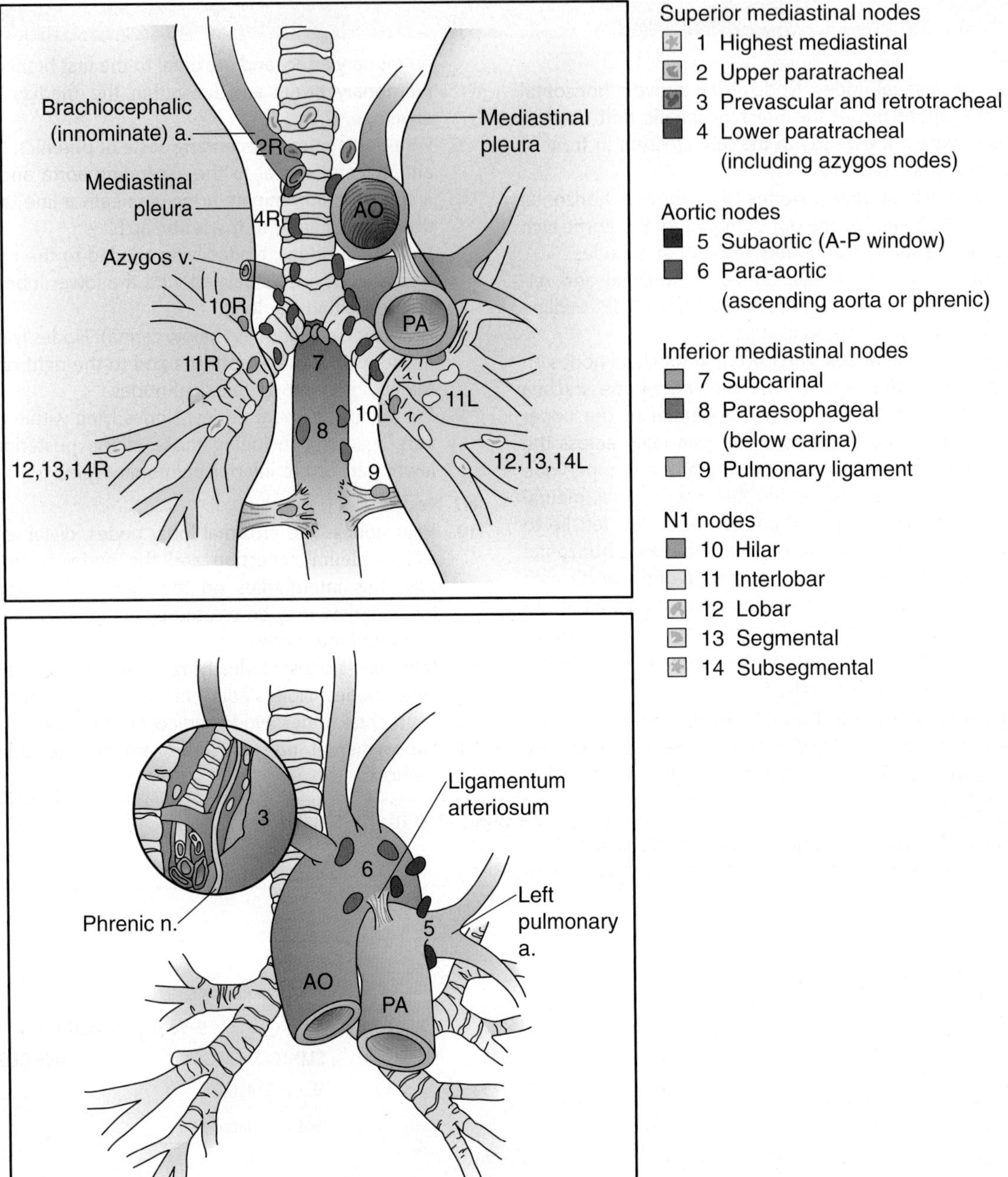


**FIGURE 58-12** Regional lymph node station location. AO, aorta; PA, pulmonary artery. (From Mountain CF, Libshitz HI, Hermes KE: Lung Cancer: A Handbook for Staging, Imaging, and Lymph Node Classification. Houston, 1999, Mountain, pp 1–71.)

treatment options may vary, even among different subsets of patients within the same clinical stage. Pretreatment staging remains the critical step before initiating therapy. With current efforts, 5-year survival rates by pathologic stage are 73% for stage IA, 58% for IB, 46% for IIA, 36% for IIB, 24% for IIIA, 9% for IIIB, and 13% for IV.[29] Treatment for lung cancer can be roughly grouped into three major categories:

1. Stages I and II tumors are contained within the lung and may be completely resected with surgery. Recently, stereotactic body radiation therapy has had good early results in selected patients not amenable to resection.[46]
2. Stage IV disease includes metastatic disease and is not typically treated by surgery, except for patients requiring surgical palliation. Systemic therapies for metastatic disease are common. Targeted therapies have provided carefully screened patients with excellent results.
3. Resectable stages IIIA and IIIB tumors are locally advanced tumors with metastasis to the ipsilateral mediastinal (N2) lymph nodes (stage IIIA) or involving mediastinal structures (T4N0M0). These tumors, by their advanced nature, may be mechanically removed with surgery; however, surgery does not consistently control the micrometastases

SURGICAL PATHOLOGY REPORT

DIAGNOSIS:
1) LYMPH NODE, 4R, EXCISION: FRAGMENTS OF LYMPH NODE, NEGATIVE FOR MALIGNANCY.
2) LYMPH NODE, 2R, EXCISION: FRAGMENTS OF LYMPH NODE, NEGATIVE FOR MALIGNANCY.
3) LYMPH NODE, PRE-CARINAL, EXCISION: FRAGMENTS OF LYMPH NODE, NEGATIVE FOR MALIGNANCY.
4) LYMPH NODE, LEVEL 4, EXCISION: FRAGMENTS OF LYMPH NODE, NEGATIVE FOR MALIGNANCY.
5) LYMPHNODE, LEVEL 2L, EXCISION: FRAGMENTS OF LYMPH NODE, NEGATIVE FOR MALIGNANCY.
6) LYMPH NODE, LEVEL 7, EXCISION: FRAGMENTS OF LYMPH NODE, NEGATIVE FOR MALIGNANCY.
7) LYMPH NODE, LEVEL 8, EXCISION: INVOLVED BY METASTATIC ADENOCARCINOMA.
8) LYMPH NODE, LEVEL 11, EXCISION: 1 LYMPH NODE, NEGATIVE FOR MALIGNANCY (0/1).
9) LYMPH NODE, LEVEL 10, EXCISION: FRAGMENTS OF LYMPH NODE, NEGATIVE FOR MALIGNANCY.
10) LUNG, LEFT LOWER LOBE, LOBECTOMY: POORLY-DIFFERENTIATED ADENOCARCINOMA, SIMILAR TO PREVIOUS (SEE S10-37167), PREDOMINANTLY SOLID TYPE, 4.9 CM IN GREATEST EXTENT, INVADING INTO VISCERAL PLEURA; RESECTION MARGINS NEGATIVE FOR MALIGNANCY; LARGE VESSEL INVASION PRESENT; CENTRIACINAR EMPHYSEMA.
11) LYMPH NODE, LEVEL 5, EXCISION: FRAGMENTS OF LYMPH NODE, NEGATIVE FOR MALIGNANCY.

COMMENT: These findings correspond to AJCC 7th Edition pathologic Stage IIIA (pT2a, pN2, pM n/a).

Lung Carcinoma Summary Findings

Specimen Type: lobectomy
Laterality: left
Tumor site: lower lobe
Tumor size: 4.9 x 4.1 x 3.8 cm
Tumor focality: unifocal
Histologic type: adenocarcinoma
Histologic Grade: poorly-differentiated
Visceral Pleura Invasion: present (confirmed with elastin stain)
Direct extension of tumor: limited to lung and visceral pleura
Venous (large vessel invasion): present
Arterial (large vessel invasion): negative
Lymphatic (small vessel invasion): negative
Treatment effect: n/a

Margins: 1.1 cm from parenchymal margin

Ancillary testing:
EGFR mutational analysis: yes
KRAS mutational analysis: yes
Other (specify): ALK
Pathologic staging (pTNM): IIIA
Primary tumor: pT2a
Regional lymph nodes: pN2
Distant metastasis: pM n/a

**FIGURE 58-13** Structured pathology report following left lower lobectomy. Lung Carcinoma Summary Findings are helpful in identifying factors critical for pathological staging, and which may influence survival subsequently. Today, ancillary testing for mutational analysis of EGFR, KRAS, and ALK is done routinely. Targeted agents exist, and others are being developed, for treatment of tumors with these characteristics.

that exist in the general area of the operation or systemically. Combinations of chemotherapy and radiotherapy are used for locally advanced disease or prior to resection.

Lung carcinoma should be resected when the local disease can be controlled, the patient's physical condition can tolerate the planned resection and reconstruction, and the anticipated operative mortality is less than the stage-specific 5-year survival. Conditions such as superior vena cava syndrome, tumor invasion across the mediastinum into the main pulmonary artery, N3 nodal metastases, malignant pleural or pericardial disease, and extrathoracic metastases carry greater risk than benefit for most patients. Some centers have had good results with resection and reconstruction of the trachea, atrium, great vessels, or other mediastinal or vertebral structures. These are complex operations requiring dedicated teams during the perioperative stage and multidisciplinary care. Patients with tracheoesophageal fistula from esophageal or lung carcinoma have a limited life expectancy. Palliative care should be considered.

### Local Therapy for Early-Stage Non–Small Cell Lung Cancer

Stages I and II NSCLC can be treated safely with surgery and mediastinal lymph node dissection alone and, in most patients, provides long-term survival.[47,48] Anatomic resection, lobectomy, with systematic mediastinal lymph node dissection and sampling, is the procedure of choice for lung cancer confined to one lobe (Fig. 58-13). The American College of Surgeons Oncology Group (ACOSOG) has defined a systematic sampling strategy for specific mediastinal lymph nodes.[49] At a minimum, nodal (not adipose) tissue from stations 2R, 4R, 7, 8, and 9 for right-sided cancers and stations 4 L, 5, 6, 7, 8, and 9 for left-sided cancers should be sampled. Mediastinal lymphadenectomy should include exploration and removal of lymph nodes from stations 2R, 4R, 7, 8, and 9 for right-sided cancers and stations 4 L, 5, 6, 7, 8 and 9 for left-sided cancers.

Lesser operations such as wedge resection or segmentectomy may be considered for patients at greater risk for lobectomy.[50] Prospective clinical trials are ongoing to evaluate the role of parenchyma-sparing surgery, such as wedge alone compared with lobectomy in select patients with small peripheral NSCLC. These prospective trials are evaluating the role of wedge resection with or without brachytherapy $^{131}$I threads, radiofrequency ablation, and wedge resection compared with stereotactic body radiation therapy.[51] Patients with NSCLC that invade into the chest wall may be resected with lobectomy with en bloc chest wall resection.

Other local control modalities include stereotactic body radiation therapy (SBRT).[46] Treatment with 54 Gy in three fractions appears to be well tolerated, with good early results. Prospective clinical trials (ACOSOG Z4099/RTOG 1021) are underway to evaluate high-risk patients (unable to tolerate a lobectomy) with early-stage NSCLC randomized between wedge resection and SBRT.

### Neoadjuvant and Adjuvant Therapy

Advanced-stage lung cancer, particularly with nodal spread, cannot typically be considered a disease effectively treated with a single modality. Survival following resection may be improved in select patients with adjuvant chemotherapy. The International Adjuvant Lung Trial (IALT)[52] enrolled 1867 patients with completely resected stages I to III NSCLC. These patients were randomized to observation or chemotherapy. Radiation therapy was at the discretion of the institution. The treatment group received one of four cisplatin-based doublet adjuvant regimens.[53] Survival was increased 5% in the adjuvant chemotherapy group. All patients staged IB to IIB were considered for adjuvant chemotherapy following resection.[47]

Surgery alone for stage IIIA (N2), IIIB, or IV lung cancer is infrequently performed; however, select patients may benefit from a multidisciplinary approach to treatment.[54] Resection for isolated brain metastasis is warranted for improvement in symptoms, quality of life, and survival rate. The primary lung tumor can then be treated according to T and N stage. Additional treatment beyond resection is needed.

Even with complete resection, patients with resectable NSCLC have poor survival. Preoperative therapy (induction or neoadjuvant) has been evaluated; preoperative paclitaxel and carboplatin followed by surgery was compared with surgery alone in patients with early-stage NSCLC. Median overall survival (OS) was 41 months in the surgery-only arm and 62 months in the preoperative chemotherapy arm (hazard ratio [HR], 0.79; 95% confidence interval [CI], 0.60 to 1.06; $P = .11$). Median progression free survival was 20 months for surgery alone and 33 months for preoperative chemotherapy (HR, 0.80; 95% CI, 0.61 to 1.04; $P = .10$). OS and progression-free survival (PFS) were both higher with preoperative chemotherapy, although the differences did not reach statistical significance.[55]

Induction chemoradiotherapy has been evaluated for the treatment of clinical stage IIIA (N2) NSCLC.[56] In one phase III trial, concurrent chemotherapy and radiotherapy followed by resection were compared with standard concurrent chemotherapy and definitive radiotherapy without resection. The median OS was similar in both groups (≈23 months). PFS was better in the surgery group (median, 12.8 versus 10.5 months; $P = .017$). The authors noted that pneumonectomy was associated with poor outcomes and OS was improved for patients undergoing induction chemoradiotherapy and lobectomy. In selected resectable stage IIIA NSCLC patients, induction chemoradiotherapy followed by resection is an alternative treatment to chemoradiotherapy alone.

Patients with local extension of lung cancer at the apex of the lung into the thoracic inlet may have shoulder and arm pain, Horner's syndrome, and occasionally paresthesia in the ulnar nerve distribution of the hand (fourth and fifth fingers; Fig. 58-14). Patients with all these characteristics may be classified as having Pancoast syndrome. Pain comes from the C8 and T1 nerve roots. Sympathetic nerve involvement may result in Horner's syndrome—miosis, ptosis, anhidrosis, and enophthalmos. Typically, the first, second, and third ribs are involved and require resection, but the bony spine and intraforaminal spaces can also be involved. MRI is necessary, in addition to CT, to plan the surgical procedure. Preoperative therapy includes chemoradiotherapy.[57,58]

### Treatment of Metastatic Disease

Metastatic disease (stage IV NSCLC) is usually incurable.[59] Performance and quality of life decline. Patients and families should be informed about the diagnosis and potential outcomes of treatment. Treatment decisions should be respectful of the patient's and family wishes and realistic expectations should be set and monitored during therapy.

Combination chemotherapy with platinum doublets has been well tolerated and associated with a modest improvement in survival rates.[53] The additional of bevacizumab (a monoclonal antibody to the vascular endothelial growth factor receptor) to paclitaxel and carboplatin has improved survival compared with patients treated with paclitaxel and carboplatin alone.[60] Induction chemotherapy followed by radiation appears to improve survival rate in patients with locally advanced unresectable lung cancer, as shown in prospective randomized studies.[61] In these studies, cisplatin-based combination chemotherapy improved survival. Additional strategies to identify the molecular characteristics of the tumor as part of the initial staging could also improve survival by creating better models for treatment of NSCLC. Advances in tumor biology have made available predictive markers of response to epidermal growth factor receptor (EGFR) mutations[62] and anaplastic lymphoma kinase (ALK), a chimeric protein originally identified in anaplastic large cell lymphoma) receptors.[63] These studies have focused efforts to target specific genetic mutations in specific lung cancers. Mutations in the *EGFR* gene strongly predict the response to EGFR inhibitors. Clinical trials have shown significant PFS in patients with metastatic NSCLC treated with gefitinib and platinum-based doublet chemotherapy compared with chemotherapy alone.[64,65] Targeted therapies in addition to, or alone, may limit toxicity and improve outcomes compared with current chemotherapeutic regimens.

Quality of life issues arise in patients with metastatic NSCLC. Dyspnea from MPE, superior vena cava syndrome, tracheoesophageal fistula, bone metastases, and pain occurs. Nutrition and hydration become significant issues. Palliation from symptoms may be accomplished, with good results.[66]

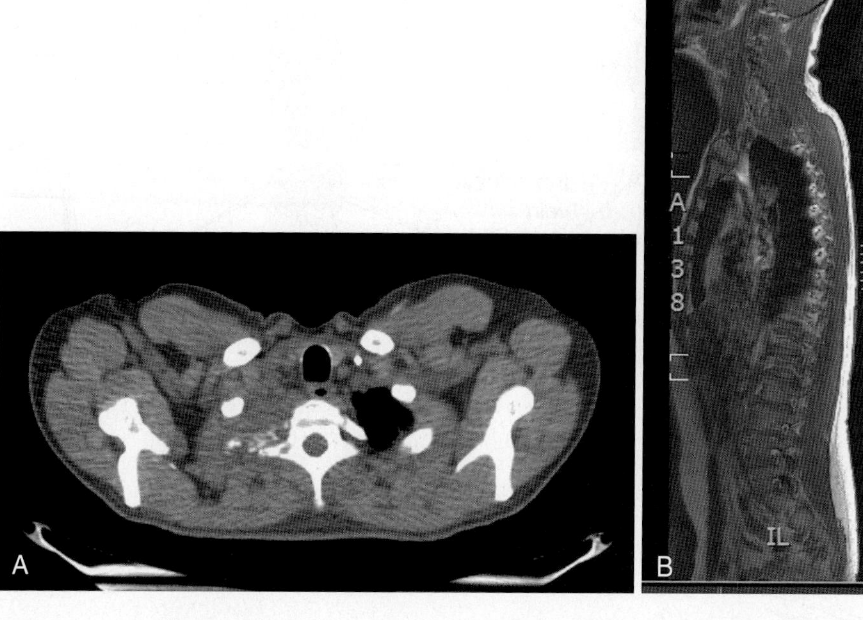


**FIGURE 58-14** The patient is a 50-year-old man with a right superior sulcus tumor. Diagnostic imaging revealed a right apical mass. Transthoracic biopsy was positive for poorly-differentiated adenocarcinoma (non-small cell lung carcinoma). Endobronchial ultrasound for mediastinal staging was negative. Induction chemoradiotherapy was given with 48 Gy in 24 fractions over one month with chemotherapy (carboplatin AUC of 5 + pemetrexed 500 mg/m$^2$). **A,** CT chest demonstrated the mass is present in the apex of the chest with complete destruction of the posterior aspect of the right second rib and cortical erosion of the right T2 vertebral body secondary to the mass. The patient is left hand dominant. **B,** The MRI of the thoracic spine demonstrates a medial right apical lung mass, consistent with a Pancoast tumor involving right lateral aspect of the T2 vertebral body, articular facet, and transverse process. There was also extension into the neural foramen and involvement of the nerve roots on the right at T1-2 and T2-3. There was no extension into the central canal or involvement of the spinal cord; CT head: no acute findings involving the brain. Complete resection was performed with a two surgeon team: Thoracic Surgery and Neurosurgery. The tumor was resected with right upper lobectomy en bloc with chest wall and a portion of the vertebral body. Spine stabilization was required.

## TRACHEA

The trachea's position can be up to 50% cervical, with hyperextension in the young patient. The location of the carina is at the level of the angle of Louis anteriorly and the T4 vertebra posteriorly. Stenosis of the trachea implies significant functional impairment. A normal 2-cm trachea has a 100% peak expiratory flow rate. A 10-mm opening provides an 80% peak expiratory flow rate. At 5 to 6 mm, only a 30% expiratory flow rate is obtained. Tracheostomy is one of the most commonly performed operations. Percutaneous tracheostomy is frequent,[67] although open procedures may be selected. Infection and inflammation are uncommon causes of tracheal obstruction.

Primary neoplasms of the trachea[68,69] include SCCA in approximately two thirds of patients and adenoid cystic carcinoma in other patients. SCCA may be focal, diffuse, or multiple. The physical appearance may be exophytic or ulcerative. One third of these primary tracheal tumors have extensive local spread or metastases at initial presentation. Adenoid cystic carcinoma (previously called *cylindroma*) has a propensity for intramural and perineural spread. In adenoid cystic carcinoma, negative margins are important. Margin evaluation with frozen section control is performed for stricture resection. Clinical features include dyspnea on exertion, wheezing, cough with or without hemoptysis, and recurrent pulmonary infections.

Involvement of the trachea from local extension from bronchogenic carcinoma may contraindicate resection. Involvement of the trachea caused by local extension of esophageal carcinoma may require palliative therapy or stenting.

### Tracheal Trauma

Penetrating injuries to the trachea are usually cervical; penetrating injuries that involve the mediastinal trachea are often lethal. Penetrating cervical injuries often involve the esophagus, and concurrent esophageal injury needs to be excluded by barium esophagography or esophagoscopy. Neck exploration may be required. Blunt trauma to the neck or trachea can produce lacerations, transections, or shattering injuries of the cervical and mediastinal trachea. Clinical features of a tracheal injury are suggested by subcutaneous air in the neck, respiratory distress, and hemoptysis. Diagnosis is made by bronchoscopy. Anesthetic management with a laryngeal mask airway may be helpful for initial examination for full visualization of the airway before endotracheal intubation. Primary repair of a tracheal injury may be accomplished with cervical exploration. Bronchial disruption may require thoracotomy. A right thoracotomy provides excellent visualization of the carina and proximal left mainstem bronchus.

Postintubation tracheal stenosis may occur because of laryngeal or tracheal irritation from an indwelling endotracheal tube. Low-pressure cuffs on the endotracheal tube have reduced pressure necrosis. Tracheal stenosis may present with dyspnea on exertion, stridor, or wheezing, which is easily noted, and perhaps

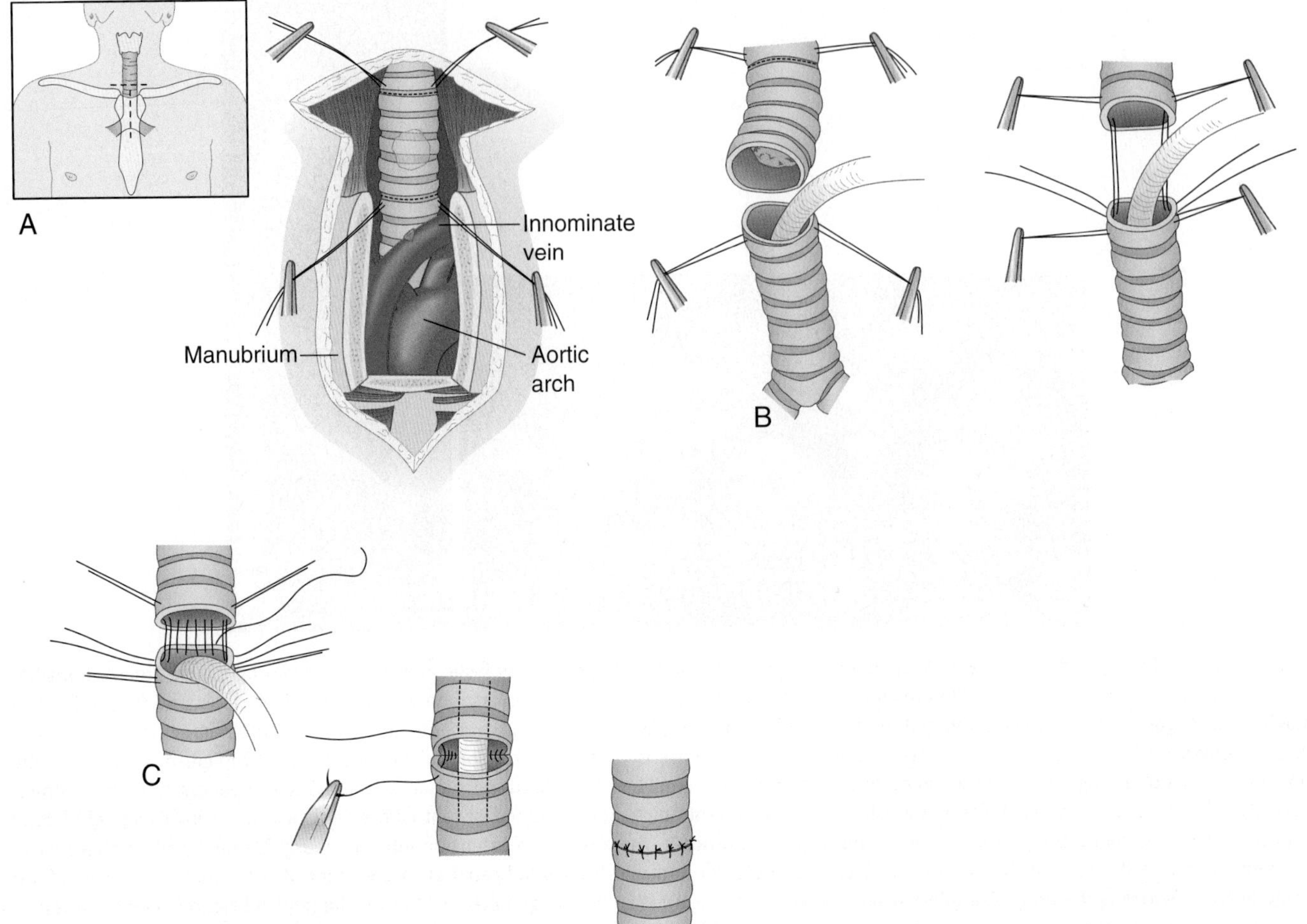


**FIGURE 58-15 A,** Exposure of the mid-trachea through a cervical and partial sternal-splitting incision. The extent of the resection has been marked by sutures. **B,** After distal division, a sterile, armored endotracheal tube is placed. After proximal resection, two mattress sutures are placed in the edges of the cartilaginous rings. A simple, running suture completes the membranous anastomosis. **C,** At this point, the original endotracheal tube is positioned in the distal trachea so that the anastomosis can be completed with interrupted, simple sutures between cartilaginous rings.

episodes of obstruction by small amounts of mucus. Emergency management of obstruction may include sedation, humidified air, or racemic epinephrine by nebulizer. In addition, dilation under general anesthesia may be helpful.

Acquired tracheoesophageal fistula is the result of prolonged intubation with erosion posteriorly. Repair involves separation of the trachea and esophagus, repair of the fistulous tract, and interposition of normal tissue, such as muscle, between the two structures.

Tracheoinnominate fistula may result from prolonged cuff erosion inferiorly and anteriorly in the trachea. An inappropriate low stoma may further increase the likelihood of direct erosion of the trachea by the innominate artery. The tip of the endotracheal tube may predispose to erosions or granulomas within the trachea. Tracheoinnominate fistula may present with sudden exsanguinating hemorrhage or with one or more previous sentinel hemorrhages. Investigation of these sentinel hemorrhage episodes is critical.

The surgical treatment of tracheal problems may be complex. General inhalational anesthesia is used and induction may take a long time if the stenosis is tight. The patient should be maintained spontaneously breathing, if possible. If the stenosis is less than 5 to 6 mm, dilation may be required with the rigid bronchoscope before passing the endotracheal tube. This may be performed with rigid bronchoscopy. If the stenosis is more than 5 to 6 mm, the endotracheal tube may be positioned to a point above the stricture for induction. Subglottic stenoses must be dilated for intubation. The endotracheal tube often goes alongside tumors.

The cervical approach is usually used for tumors of the upper half of the trachea, plus all benign tracheal stenoses, because these usually occur as a result of endotracheal tube placement. Occasionally, an upper sternal split may be needed (Fig. 58-15). The posterolateral thoracotomy (fourth interspace) is used for tumors of the lower half of the trachea, plus carinal reconstruction. Rigid bronchoscopy for diagnosis, biopsy, dilation, or morcellation of tumor, or other treatment modalities, such as laser treatment, may be required if the tumor cannot be immediately resected (Fig. 58-16).

In general, the maximal amount of trachea that can be resected is approximately 5 cm, but varies from person to person. Various techniques are used to mobilize the trachea to

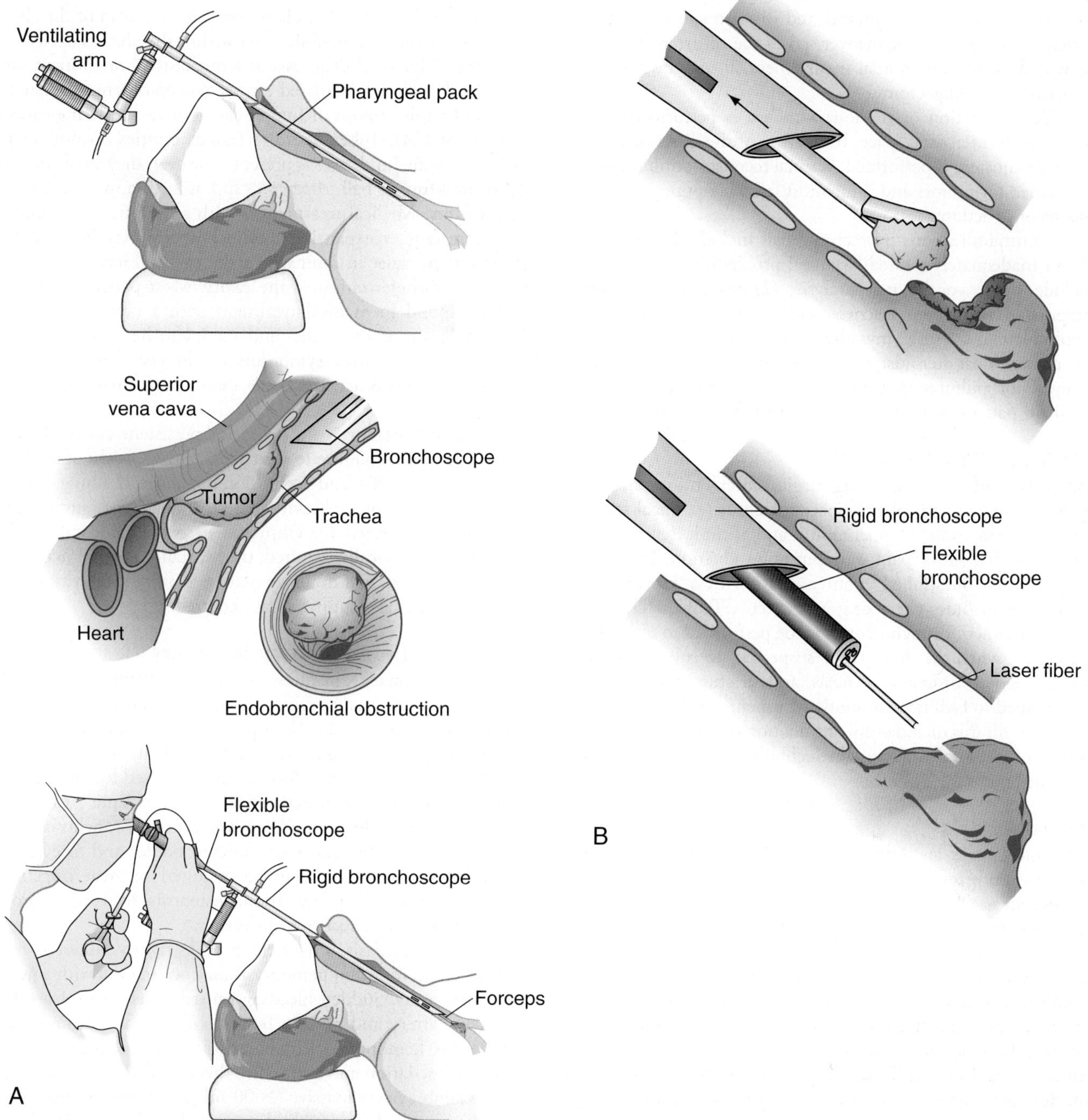


**FIGURE 58-16 A,** Proper technique for rigid bronchoscopy in a patient with a tracheal mass. *Top,* Pharyngeal packing is shown here and used to protect the esophagus. The surgeon should be cautious as this packing can move and may obstruct the larynx. Complete removal of the packing at the end of the operation is done. *Middle,* A nearly obstructing tumor is shown. *Bottom,* A flexible bronchoscope is placed into the rigid scope for the biopsy. This protects the airway. **B,** A technique for endoscopic resection of a tracheal mass with a rigid bronchoscope without (*top*) and with (*bottom*) use of the laser. (From Sugarbaker DJ, Mentzer SJ, Strauss G, Fried MP: Laser resection of endobronchial lesions: Use of the rigid and flexible bronchoscopes. Oper Tech Otolaryngol Head Neck Surg 3:93, 1992.)

create a repair without undue tension on the anastomosis. The anterior cervical approach, plus mobilization of the trachea and neck flexion, can allow for 4 to 5 cm of trachea resection. A suprahyoid release may allow for 1 cm of additional length. Mobilization of the right hilum, together with division of the pericardium around the right hilum, may allow for an additional 1.4 cm.

Stenosis of the subglottic larynx or cricoid stenosis is a challenging technical procedure. The recurrent nerves innervate the larynx just superior to the posterolateral cricoid on each side.

If the tracheal lesions only involve the anterior surface, the anterior cricoid can be removed and distal trachea beveled to match the defect. This maneuver spares the recurrent laryngeal nerves. With circumferential involvement, it may be necessary to perform a laryngectomy.

Reconstruction of the lower trachea is performed in the right fourth intercostal space. Intubation of the distal trachea or the left mainstem is performed. Carinal reconstruction is usually performed for tumors and is the most feasible option of alternative reconstructions.

Contraindications to trachea repair include the following: (1) an inadequately treated laryngeal problem, which does not include single vocal cord paralysis; (2) need for ventilatory support or permanent tracheostomy for patients with amyotrophic lateral sclerosis, myasthenia gravis, or quadriplegia; (3) use of high-dose steroids; and (4) inflamed or recent tracheostomy. Poor pulmonary reserve is not a contraindication for repair in patients who have been weaned from the ventilator.

## PULMONARY INFECTIONS

Pulmonary infections requiring surgical interventions are infrequent compared with pleural space infections. Clinical features are similar to those of pneumonia and include fever, cough, leukocytosis, pleuritic pain, and sputum production. The patient is specifically questioned about aspiration of a foreign body. Evaluation includes chest x-ray and often CT of the chest and upper abdomen. Bronchoscopy can be performed to clear secretions and, when the diagnosis is suspected, to rule out cancer, foreign bodies, bronchial stenosis, and stricture. Cultures may be obtained to facilitate antibiotic treatment. Medical treatment is optimized; this includes discontinuation of smoking and institution of postural drainage, bronchodilator medications, and oral antibiotics.

### Bronchiectasis

Bronchiectasis is an infection of the bronchial wall and surrounding lung of sufficient severity to cause destruction and dilation of the air passages. This condition has been decreasing in frequency and severity because of the use of antibiotics. There are numerous predisposing factors, including cystic fibrosis, $\alpha_1$-antitrypsin deficiency, immunodeficiency states, Kartagener's syndrome (sinusitis, bronchiectasis, situs inversus, and hypomotile cilia), and bronchial obstruction from foreign bodies, extrinsic lymph nodes that compress the bronchus, neoplasm, or mucus plug. The distribution is primarily in the basal segments of the lower lobes. Destructive changes and dilation of the bronchi accompany the infection. Massive hemoptysis is rare. Frequently, symptoms can be controlled with medical treatment, such as chronic antibiotic therapy and postural drainage. Disease limited to but involving one lobe is best treated surgically. If bilateral bronchiectasis exists, medical management continues.

### Lung Abscess

The incidence of lung abscess is decreasing in frequency as a result of the use of antibiotics. A lung abscess may occur from an infection behind a blocked bronchus. *Staphylococcus* bacteremia is frequently associated with lung abscess. Necrotizing pneumonia from *Klebsiella* spp. may rapidly destroy the involved lung, with minimal surrounding reaction. Rupture of a lung abscess may yield empyema and pneumothorax. Lung abscess may also be superimposed on structural abnormalities—for example, a bronchogenic cyst, sequestration, bleb, or tuberculous or fungal cavities. The chest x-ray and CT scan of the chest may demonstrate an air-fluid level within the abscess cavity.

The differential diagnosis of a mediastinal or thoracic air-fluid level includes loculated empyema, epiphrenic diverticulum, and a tuberculous or fungus cavity or cavitary lung cancer (usually SCCA). Tubercular and fungus cavities do not retain fluid, so no air-fluid level is present; however, they may contain debris or a fungus ball. *Aspergillus* spp. infection may present in this manner. Medical treatment is with antibiotics and pulmonary care (e.g., reexpansion). Bronchoscopy may be used for treatment to assist in drainage of the cavity directly via transbronchial catheterization of the cavity. Most patients (85% to 95%) respond to medical treatment with a rapid decrease in fluid, collapse of the walls, and complete healing in 3 to 4 months. Patients with symptoms for longer than 3 months before treatment or cavities larger than 4 to 6 cm are less likely to respond.

Surgical therapy is indicated for persistent cavity (≥2 cm and thick-walled), failure to clear sepsis after 8 weeks of medical therapy, hemoptysis, and excludsion of cancer. If a lung abscess ruptures into the pleural cavity, simple drainage may suffice, and the patient is treated for empyema or bronchopleural fistula. Lobectomy is typically required; the mortality rate is 1% to 5%. Occasionally, external drainage may be required for critically ill patients if pleural symphysis has occurred.

### Other Bronchopulmonary Disorders

Bronchopulmonary disorders caused by inflammatory lymph node disease are usually the result of tuberculosis or histoplasmosis. Lobar atelectasis, hemoptysis, or broncholithiasis can occur. Bronchial compressive disease usually occurs in the middle lobe. More than 20% of cases are caused by cancer. This condition results in repeated infection in the same area of the lung, which usually responds to antibiotics. Bronchoscopy is essential to rule out cancer and foreign bodies and to evaluate for stricture. Medical therapy is required to treat infection. Surgery is indicated to treat bronchostenosis, irreversible bronchiectasis, or severe recurrent infection.

Broncholithiasis is a calcified node tightly adherent to a bronchus. An innocent hemoptysis may occur, even with a negative chest x-ray. Sudden bleeding caused by erosion of a small bronchial artery and mucosa by a spicule in the calcified node causes this hemoptysis. Bright red bleeding occurs; it usually stops with sedation and antitussive therapy. This type of hemoptysis is almost never massive (≥600 mL in 24 hours). Bronchoscopy is possible during a bleeding episode to localize the site of the bleeding. Nasal or pharyngeal lesions, or hematemesis from a gastrointestinal (GI) source should be excluded.

Organizing pneumonia may replace lung parenchyma with scar tissue or persistent atelectasis or consolidation. If the shadow or mass persists over 6 to 8 weeks, resection is performed to exclude carcinoma. The differential diagnosis includes pneumonia, congenital abnormality, and aneurysm of the aorta.

### Mycobacterial Infections

Tuberculosis infects approximately 7% of patients exposed and develops in 5% to 10% of those patients infected. A primary infection develops. The exudative response progresses to caseous necrosis. Postprimary tuberculosis tends to occur in the apical and posterior segments of the upper lobes and superior segments of the lower lobes. Healing occurs with fibrosis and contracture. Extensive caseation with cavitation may occur early. Coalescing areas of caseous necrosis may form cavities. Frequently, there are incomplete septations and lobulations. Erosions of septations supplied by bronchial arteries cause hemoptysis, and may be secondarily infected.

Medical treatment is with isoniazid (INH), rifampin, ethambutol, streptomycin, or pyrazinamide.[70] Bronchoscopy may be required for patients not responding to medical treatment. Cancer should be excluded for a newly identified mass on chest x-ray, even with a positive tuberculosis skin test and acid-fast bacillus–positive sputum.

Surgical therapy may be considered when medical treatment fails and persistent tuberculosis-positive sputum remains, as well as when surgically correctable residua of tuberculosis may be of potential danger to the patient.[71,72] This is not the same treatment as for atypical mycobacteria; many of these patients remain clinically well, even with positive sputum. Indications for surgery include the following:

1. Open positive cavity after 3 to 6 months of chemotherapy, especially if resistant mycobacteria
2. Destroyed lung, atelectasis, bronchiectasis, bronchostenosis amenable to resection
3. Open negative cavities if thick-walled, slow response, or unreliable patient
4. Exclusion of cancer
5. Recurrent or persistent hemoptysis if more than 600 mL of blood is lost in 24 hours or less

Surgical options include resection, with preservation of good lung tissue. Surgical complications are doubled if the sputum is positive for *Mycobacterium tuberculosis* and decreased if the remaining lung tissue is fully expanded within the chest. Infectious complications include empyema, bronchopleural fistula, and endobronchial spread of the disease and are associated with a higher mortality rate. Tuberculosis infection of the pleural space without lung destruction is primarily treated medically.

Thoracoplasty or muscle flap interposition may be used to control postresection empyema space. Collapse therapy, with thoracoplasty or plombage, is rarely used to manage parenchymal disease alone.

## Fungal and Parasitic Infections

The surgical management of fungal infections includes diagnosis and treatment of complications of fungal disease. Frequently, cancer has to be excluded or other infectious or benign conditions confirmed. Medical treatment may be considered as initial treatment of fungal diseases in the lung and as part of the patient's overall management.

Immunocompromised patients suffer from *Aspergillus* spp. infection as the most frequent opportunistic infection, followed by *Candida* and *Nocardia* spp. and mucormycosis infections. Normal or immunocompetent patients may be affected by histoplasmosis, coccidioidomycosis, or blastomycosis. Both groups may be affected by actinomycosis and cryptococcosis. Although *Nocardia* and *Actinomyces* spp. are bacteria, they are usually discussed with fungal infections. Diagnosis is most often made by sputum examination using potassium hydroxide preparations (Fig. 58-17). Cultures are poor and may take some time for results to be obtained; Papanicolaou test cytology may be best. Silver methenamine stain is used for microscopic evaluation. Most infections are self-limited and do not require treatment. IV or oral antifungal agents may be used for treatment of these diseases.

Aspergillosis is an opportunistic infection, characterized by coarse fragmented septa and hyphae (see Fig. 58-17*A*). There are three types of aspergillosis—aspergilloma, invasive pulmonary aspergillosis, and allergic bronchopulmonary aspergillosis. Aspergilloma is the most common form of aspergillosis. The fungus colonizes an existing lung cavity, commonly a tuberculosis cavity. The chest x-ray may demonstrate a crescent radiolucency next to a rounded mass. Cavities may form because of destruction of the underlying pulmonary parenchyma and debris and hyphae may coalesce and form a fungus ball, which lies free in the cavity and can move with the patient's change in position. Invasion and destruction of parenchymal blood vessels occur in this cavity. Patients with aspergilloma fungus balls are at high risk for fatal hemorrhage, are treated aggressively, and undergo resection, when possible.[73] Involvement and destruction of parenchymal blood vessels occur. Prophylactic resection is controversial, although some recommend resection if isolated disease is present in low-risk patients. Surgery is indicated for treatment or massive or recurrent hemoptysis, or to rule out neoplasm.[74] The procedure of choice is lobectomy. The operation can be complex, with a significant inflammatory response within the hilum. Invasive aspergillosis occurs in immunocompromised patients and presents with chest pain, cough, and hemoptysis. The treatment is primarily medical, although lung biopsy may be necessary for diagnosis. Allergic aspergillosis is diagnosed by bronchoscopy and represents the allergic reaction to chronic colonization with the fungus. It is usually treated medically. Rarely, resection is performed for localized bronchiectasis.

Histoplasmosis is the most common of all U.S. fungal infections and is usually a serious systemic fungal disease.[75] *Histoplasma capsulatum* is endemic to the Mississippi and Ohio River Valleys, as well as portions of the southwestern United States. A high percentage of patients are affected, usually with a subclinical form of this disease. An inoculum, from the mycelial form found in soil, decaying materials, and bat or bird guano, can produce an acute pneumonic illness in immunocompetent hosts and usually resolves without specific treatment. The yeast form exists in macrophages or within the cytoplasm of the alveoli. Pathologic examination demonstrates granulomas (similar to tuberculosis) or caseating epithelioid granulomas. The lymphogenous reaction to *Histoplasma* causes mediastinal lymph node enlargement, middle lobe syndrome, bronchiectasis, esophageal traction diverticulum, broncholithiasis with hemoptysis, tracheoesophageal fistula, constrictive pericarditis, fibrosing mediastinitis with superior vena cava syndrome, or other problems relating to compression of mediastinal structures. In addition to the compressive symptoms, the lymphadenopathy caused by histoplasmosis may confound radiographic evaluation of the mediastinal lymph nodes in patients with lung cancer and may complicate lung resection.

Coccidioidomycosis is endemic to the Southwest and is localized in the soil. It is second only to histoplasmosis in frequency. Inhaling the organism results in a primary lung disease that is usually self-limited (see Fig. 58-17*B*). In endemic areas, coccidioidomycosis is a frequent cause of lung nodules, and resection may be required to rule out malignancy. Medical treatment is preferred. Surgery may be

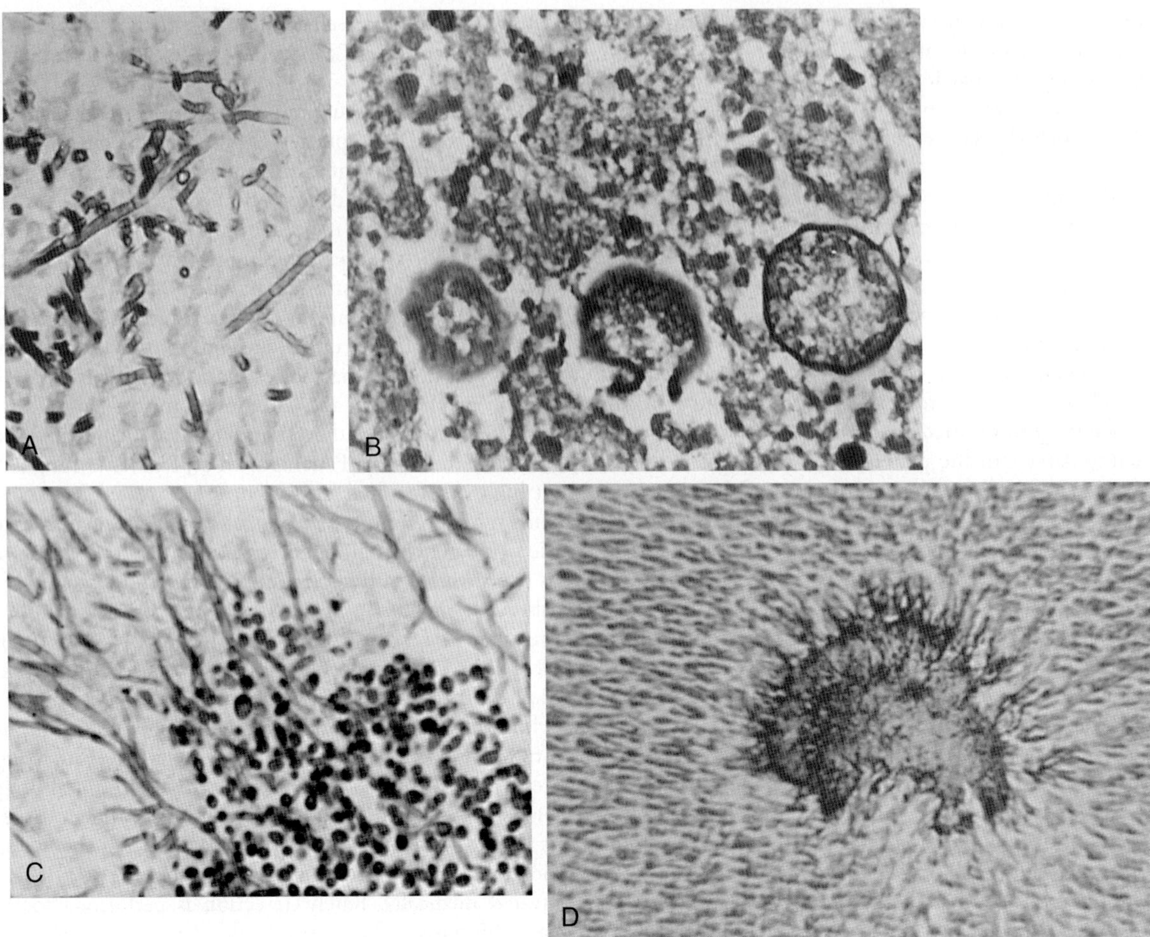

**FIGURE 58-17** **A,** The coarse, fragmented, septate mycelia of *Aspergillus fumigatus.* **B,** Microscopic section of a coccidioidal granuloma (x400) shows spherules packed with endospores. **C,** *Candida albicans* with both the mycelial and the yeast forms. **D,** Actinomycotic granule shows branching filaments of a microscopic colony of *Actinomyces israelii* (Gomori stain, x250). (**A** and **C,** from Takaro T: Thoracic mycotic infections. In Lewis' practice of surgery. New York, 1968, Hoeber Medical Division, Harper & Row. **B,** from Scott S, Takaro T: Thoracic mycotic and actinomycotic infections. In Shields TW [ed.]: General thoracic surgery, ed 4, Baltimore, 1994, Williams & Wilkins.)

considered for the treatment of cavitary disease or complications of cavitary disease.

Cryptococcosis the second most common lethal fungus, after histoplasmosis. Lungs are frequently involved. CNS involvement with meningitis is the most frequent cause of death. Any patient diagnosed with pulmonary cryptococcosis should undergo lumbar puncture to rule out CNS involvement. Surgery may be required for open lung biopsy for diagnosis or to exclude lung cancer.

Mucormycosis is a rare, opportunistic, rapidly progressive infection that occurs in immunocompromised patients, including those with diabetes. The appearance is that of a black mold; it has wide, nonseptate branching hyphae. The infection causes blood vessels to thrombose and lung tissue to infarct. Clinically, the rhinocerebral form occurs much more frequently than the pulmonary form of consolidation and cavities. Medical treatment is cessation of steroids and antineoplastic drugs; amphotericin and control of diabetes are initiatied. The disease is often too advanced for effective treatment. Aggressive surgical and medical treatment may improve what is usually a grave prognosis.

*Candida* is a small, thin-walled budding yeast that occurs in immunocompromised patients (see Fig. 58-17*C*). Lung involvement alone is rare. Surgery may be needed to confirm the diagnosis.

*Pneumocystis jiroveci* (formerly, *Pneumocystis carinii*) is an opportunistic infection that is positive on silver methenamine stain. Bronchoalveolar lavage obtains the diagnosis in more than 90% of patients. However, lung biopsy may be required to confirm the diagnosis.

Surgery may also be used to manage the sequelae and complications of parasitic infections. Infections with *Entamoeba histolytica* are usually confined to the right lower thorax and are related to extension from a liver abscess below the diaphragm via direct extension or lymphatics to the right thorax. Metronidazole (Flagyl) is usually effective, although metronidazole and tube drainage may be required for treatment of empyema. Open resection is infrequently required. Similarly, infection with *Echinococcus* spp. may occur. The hydatid cyst may rupture, flooding the lung or producing a severe hypersensitivity reaction. A lung abscess could occur with compression of the airway, great vessels, or esophagus. Surgery, if feasible, may include simple enucleation by cleavage of planes between the cyst and normal tissue. Aspiration and administration of hypertonic saline 10% may be done before enucleation. Positive pressure on the lung needs to be maintained until the cyst has been removed to prevent contamination, soilage, or hypersensitivity reaction. Nonoperative therapy for small, asymptomatic calcified cysts may be considered. Paragonimiasis is another common infection and cause of hemoptysis in Asia. In endemic areas, prevalence may reach 5%, and hemoptysis from paragonimiasis must be differentiated from tuberculosis or lung cancer.[76]

Actinomycosis is caused by a bacterium that is not found free in nature. It produces a chronic anaerobic endogenous infection deep within a wound. Sulfur granules draining from infected sinuses are microcolonies (see Fig. 58-17*D*). The cervicofacial form is the most common. The thoracic form usually occurs as a pulmonary parenchymal disease resembling cancer. Medical treatment is usually penicillin. Surgery may occasionally be required for radical excision of chest wall disease and empyema.

Nocardiosis is caused by an aerobic bacterium that is widely disseminated in soil and domestic animals; it was formerly rare, although its frequency is increasing in immunocompromised patients. Nocardiosis resembles actinomycosis in invading the chest wall and produces subcutaneous abscesses and sinuses draining sulfur granules. Surgery is performed to exclude cancer, obtain a diagnosis, or treat complications of the disease. Medical therapy may include sulfonamides.

## MASSIVE HEMOPTYSIS

Massive hemoptysis may be defined as more than 500 to 600 mL of blood loss from the lungs in 24 hours. However, the proximal airways may be occluded with as little as 150 mL of clotted blood, and even lower volume hemoptysis may be life-threatening.[77] The current mortality rate is approximately 13% and is related to drowning or suffocation rather than exsanguination. Diagnosis and treatment of massive hemoptysis typically include a chest x-ray and emergency rigid bronchoscopy. The major causes of massive hemoptysis are tuberculosis, bronchiectasis, and cancer. Flexible bronchoscopy is usually inadequate for treatment of hemoptysis, but may be considered for diagnosis, localization of the source of the bleeding, or observation if active bleeding has stopped.[78] Mortality is high with urgent or emergency resection.

Conservative management may consist simply of maintaining a functional and patent airway, bronchoscopy, clearing the airway of blood, cough suppression (with codeine), and monitoring until stabilized.

Angiographic catheterization for massive hemoptysis may be considered for patients with hemoptysis and inability to localize a bleeding site.[79] Risks include spinal cord ischemia and paralysis. Embolization with small particles of polyvinyl alcohol or other synthetic embolic materials occlude vessels at a peripheral level. Embolization may be repeated.

## EMPHYSEMA AND DIFFUSE LUNG DISEASE

### Emphysema

Emphysema is defined as dilation and destruction of the terminal air spaces. These air cavities are blebs, subpleural air spaces separated from the lung by a thin pleural covering, with only minor alveolar communications, or bullae, larger than a bleb, with some destruction of the underlying lung parenchyma. Bullous emphysema (Fig. 58-18) is congenital, without general lung disease, or is a complication of COPD, with more or less generalized lung disease. The challenge is to separate the disability related to the bullae from that caused by the chronic emphysema or chronic bronchitis. The DLCO is a good index of the state of severity of the generalized lung disease. On pulmonary angiography, bullae are vacant and do not contain vessels. The bullae may compress normal lung, with crowding of the relatively normal pulmonary vasculature. COPD may show abrupt narrowing and tapering of vessels. Surgical therapy includes resection of the bullae to leave functioning lung tissue. Simple removal of the bulla alone is required. Lobectomy is seldom indicated because good lung tissue is removed, which is frequently needed for independent function by patients with significant lung impairment.

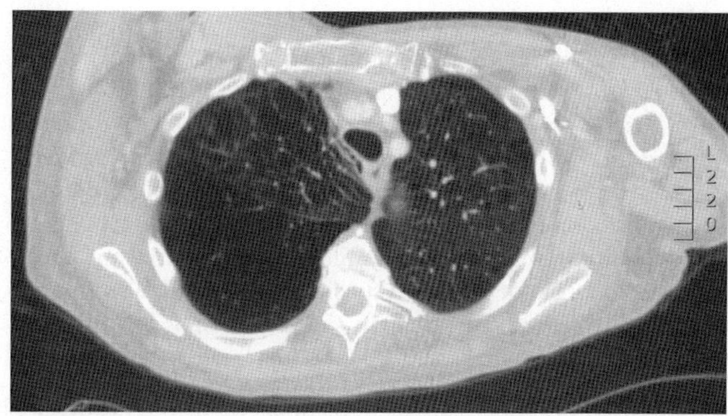

**FIGURE 58-18** Bullous emphysema. The patient is a chronic smoker (>100 pack/years) and developed emphysema which is progressing. The superior segment of the right lower lobe is completely destroyed and the resultant bullae is compressing functioning lung in the right upper lobe, and the basilar segments of the right lower lobe.

Treatment of emphysema is primarily medical, but there are surgical therapies. Although emphysema usually diffusely involves the lung, it may have a heterogenous distribution within the lung. These areas may be identified by CT and perfusion scanning. Often, the disease predominates in the upper lobes and superior segment of the lower lobes. Lung volume reduction surgery (LVRS) removes areas of greatest emphysematous involvement. The remaining lung tissue expands, with improved elastic recoil, improved aeration, and perfusion of the remaining lung, and improved chest wall mechanics. The National Emphysema Trial (NETT) has compared LVRS with best medical therapy. Patients with predominantly upper lobe emphysema and low exercise capacity had lower mortality with LVRS than medical therapy.[80] In patients with non–upper lobe emphysema and high exercise capacity, mortality was higher in the operative group. Long-term results have been favorable.[81] Endoscopic therapies have been developed, including airway bypass and one-way valves. These devices are still in the investigational stage.

Lung transplantation is performed for COPD, including $\alpha_1$-antitrypsin deficiency, pulmonary fibrosis, primary pulmonary hypertension, cystic fibrosis, and bronchiectasis.[82] The survival rates after lung transplantation (all lungs) are approximately 78% at 1 year, 56% at 5 years, and 30% at 10 years.[83] Chronic immunosuppression is required. Unilateral lung transplantation is more readily tolerated than bilateral lung transplantation; however, bilateral lung transplantation is more frequently performed and has a survival advantage after 1 year.

## Diffuse Lung Disease

The surgeon's role in diffuse lung disease is to obtain a diagnosis, typically by open lung biopsy after other methods (e.g., TTNA, bronchoscopy with transbronchial biopsy) have failed. The chest x-ray may demonstrate an alveolar pattern, fluffy with air bronchograms, or an interstitial pattern, ground glass or granular appearance, indicating a diffuse increase in interstitial tissue (Box 58-2). Patients may be mildly symptomatic and need biopsy to confirm or exclude a specific diagnosis before embarking on aggressive medical therapy, such as cyclophosphamide for Wegner's granulomatosis, or may be critically ill, in the intensive care unit, requiring mechanical ventilation.

Sarcoidosis affects the lungs in 90% of patients with this diagnosis, causing symptoms of dyspnea and dry cough. Foci of noncaseating epithelioid granulomas may be found in any part of the body. Insidious respiratory complaints without constitutional symptoms are seen in 40% to 50%, severe progressive pulmonary fibrosis may develop in 10% to 20%, and bilateral hilar mediastinal lymph nodes are involved in 60% to 80% of patients. Bronchoscopic lung biopsy is the initial diagnostic procedure. If required, mediastinal lymph nodes may be biopsied. Steroids may be used for treatment.

Lung biopsy may be required for progressive interstitial parenchymal changes for which no diagnosis can be obtained. Lung biopsies can be performed using minimally invasive techniques. Biopsies are sent for routine, fungal, and acid-fast bacillus culture. In immunocompromised patients, *Nocardia* cultures are considered. If possible, the surgeon should sample more than one area of the lung. One method is to resect the radiographically worst-appearing region and the most normal-appearing area. The normal-appearing lung may exhibit early-stage disease and may aid the pathologist in making the diagnosis. Frozen section is only used to confirm that adequate samples of the pathologic process were obtained. In the acute setting of a critically ill patient, an open lung biopsy is only performed when the results will significantly modify subsequent treatment, such as the initiation of protocol-based treatment for experimental antibiotics, or to withdraw futile care.

**BOX 58-2 Classification of Diffuse Lung Diseases**

**Infections (More Commonly Cause Focal Disease, Granuloma Formation)**

Viruses—especially influenza, cytomegalovirus

Bacteria—tuberculosis, all kinds of regular bacteria, Rocky Mountain spotted fever

Fungi—all types can cause diffuse disease

Parasites—Pneumocystis species infection, toxoplasmosis, paragonimiasis, among others

**Occupational Causes**

Mineral dusts

Chemical fumes—$NO_2$ (silo filler's disease), Cl, $NH_3$, $SO_2$, $CCl_4$, Br, HF, HCl, $HNO_3$, kerosene, acetylene

**Neoplastic Disease**

Lymphangitic spread

Hematogenous metastases

Leukemia, lymphoma, bronchioloalveolar cell cancer

**Congenital—Familial**

Niemann-Pick, Gaucher's, neurofibromatosis, and tuberous fibrosis

**Metabolic and Unknown**

Liver disease, uremia, inflammatory bowel disease

**Physical Agents**

Radiation, $O_2$ toxicity, thermal injury, blast injury

**Heart Failure and Multiple Pulmonary Emboli**

**Immunologic Causes**

**Hypersensitivity Pneumonia**

Inhaled antigens

Farmer's lung (actinomycosis)

Bagassosis (sugar cane)

Malt workers (Aspergillus species)

Byssinosis (cotton)

**Drug Reactions**

Hydralazine, busulfan, nitrofurantoin (Macrodantin), hexamethonium, methysergide, bleomycin

**Collagen Diseases**

Scleroderma, rheumatoid, systemic lupus erythematosus, dermatomyositis, Wegener's granulomatosis, Goodpasture's syndrome

**Other**

Sarcoidosis

Histiocytosis

Idiopathic hemosiderosis

Pulmonary alveolar proteinosis

Diffuse interstitial fibrosis, idiopathic pulmonary fibrosis

Desquamative interstitial pneumonia

Eosinophilic pneumonia (Note: some are caused by drugs, actinomycosis, and parasites)

Lymphangioleiomyomatosis

## Adult Respiratory Distress Syndrome

The adult respiratory distress syndrome is a complex biologic and clinical process. This acute deterioration of pulmonary function occurs exclusive of pulmonary edema, pneumonia, or exacerbation of COPD. Approximately 50,000 cases occur each year in the United States, with a mortality rate of 30% to 40%.

The initial clinical presentation of dyspnea, tachypnea, hypoxemia, and mild hypocapnia is nonspecific. A chest x-ray may show diffuse bilateral infiltrates secondary to increased interstitial fluid. Pathologically, vascular congestion occurs with alveolar collapse, edema, and inflammatory cell infiltration. The underlying mechanism is increased pulmonary capillary permeability, with extravasation of intravascular fluid and protein into the interstitium and alveoli. The leukocyte is the most prominent mediator of this injury. Stimuli such as sepsis activate the complement pathway, causing recruitment of leukocytes to the site of the infection. The lung releases potent mediators such as oxygen free radicals, arachidonic acid metabolites, and proteases. If the underlying disease is not controlled, these changes progress to vascular thrombosis, interstitial fibrosis, and hyaline membrane deposition in the alveoli. This process causes hypoxemia, pulmonary hypertension, $CO_2$ retention, secondary infections, and eventually right heart failure, hypoxia, and death. Other criteria include impaired oxygenation with the $PaO_2/FIO_2$ ratio less than 200. Also, pulmonary edema is present without cardiac failure, and the pulmonary capillary wedge pressure is less than 18 mm Hg (noncardiac pulmonary edema).

Treatment is supportive and directed to improve oxygenation. Maintaining the inspired oxygen concentration and positive end-expiratory pressure as low as possible to maintain adequate oxygenation and carbon dioxide exchange is helpful.[84] Tidal volumes are kept low.[85] Prone or rotational therapy does not improve outcomes of these patients.[86]

## PULMONARY METASTASES

Isolated pulmonary metastases represent a unique manifestation of systemic spread of a primary neoplasm. These patients, with metastases located only within the lungs, may be more amenable to local or local and systemic treatment options than other patients with multiorgan metastases.[87] Although primary tumors can be locally controlled with surgery or radiation, extraregional metastases are usually treated with systemic chemotherapy. Radiation therapy may be used to treat or palliate the local manifestations of metastatic disease, particularly when metastases occur within the bony skeleton and cause pain. Resection of solitary and multiple pulmonary metastases from sarcomas and various other primary neoplasms has been performed, with improved long-term survival rates in up to 40% of patients so treated. Therefore, isolated pulmonary metastases are treatable.

Certain clinical characteristics (prognostic indicators) may be used to select patients with more favorable disease-free and overall survival expectations. Patients who have complete resection of all metastases have associated longer survival than those whose metastases are unresectable. Long-term survival (>5 years) may be expected in approximately 20% to 30% of all patients with resectable pulmonary metastases. Optimal and more consistent survival statistics await improvements in local control, systemic therapy, and regional drug delivery to the lungs.

### Surgical Treatment

Predictors for improved survival rate have been studied retrospectively for various tumor types. These may allow the clinician to identify select patients who will optimally benefit from pulmonary metastasectomy. Patients should have pulmonary parenchymal nodules consistent with metastasis (or metastases), absence of uncontrolled or untreated extrathoracic metastases, control of the primary tumor, sufficient physiologic and pulmonary reserve to tolerate surgery, and probability of complete resection. Regardless of histology, patients with pulmonary metastases isolated to the lungs that are completely resected have improved survival rates when compared with patients with unresectable metastases. Resectability consistently correlates with improved post-thoracotomy survival rates for patients with pulmonary metastases. In one series of more than 5000 patients with metastases treated with resection, overall actuarial 5-year survival rate was 36%. Favorable clinical indicators included a disease-free interval longer than 3 years, an SPN, and germ cell histology.[88] Soft tissue sarcomas of all types predominantly metastasize to the lungs. CT usually underestimates the number of metastases by 50% to 100%.

Resection can be accomplished safely. Open or minimally invasive procedures may be used, with minimal mortality and morbidity. Patients with pulmonary metastases may also undergo multiple procedures for reresection of metastases, with prolonged survival expectations after complete resection. VATS procedures limit the ability of the surgeon to palpate the lung to identify occult metastases.[89] Follow-up with radiographic screening at regular intervals is recommended to exclude recurrence.

## MISCELLANEOUS LUNG TUMORS

Slow-growing lung tumors may arise from the epithelium, ducts, and glands of the bronchial tree and account for 1% to 2% of all lung neoplasms. Most are of low-grade malignant potential.

Carcinoid tumors (1% of lung neoplasms) arise from Kulchitsky (APUD [***a***mine ***p***recursor ***u***ptake ***d***ecarboxylase]) cells in bronchial epithelium. They have positive histologic reactions to silver staining and chromogranin. Special stains and tests can identify neurosecretory granules by electron microscopy. These typical carcinoid tumors (least malignant) are the most indolent of the spectrum of pulmonary neuroendocrine tumors, which include atypical carcinoid, large cell undifferentiated carcinoma, and small cell carcinoma (most malignant).[90] Histologic findings include less than 2 to 10 mitoses/10 high-power field (HPF). Peripheral tumors are usually without symptoms, although central tumors may produce endobronchial obstruction with cough, hemoptysis, recurrent infection or pneumonia, bronchiectasis, lung abscess, pain, or wheezing. Symptoms may persist for many years without diagnosis, particularly if only an endobronchial component partially obstructs the airway. Carcinoid syndrome (flushing, tachycardia, wheezing, and diarrhea) is not common and occurs with large tumors or extensive metastatic disease. Bronchoscopy is usually positive unless the nodule or mass is peripheral. Most carcinoids can be identified in this matter and, although they tend to bleed, biopsy can usually be performed safely.

Atypical carcinoids may have lymph node or vascular invasion with metastasis.[91] They are located in the mainstem bronchi (20%), lobar bronchi (70% to 75%), or peripheral bronchi (5% to 10%); they rarely occur in the trachea. Local invasion with involvement of peribronchial tissue occurs. At bronchoscopy, most carcinoids are sessile, although a few are polypoid. The histology is that of small uniform cells with oval nuclei and interlacing cords of vascular connective tissue stroma. Mitoses are infrequent but, occasionally, bizarre cells are noted. Atypical carcinoids are more pleomorphic and have more mitoses (>2 to 10 mitoses/HPF) than typical carcinoids. They have more prominent nucleoli but are more monotonous and have more cytoplasm than oat cell carcinoma. These tumors are more aggressive, with a 5-year survival rate of approximately 60%. They tend to metastasize to the liver, bone, or adrenal glands. Electron microscopy can be used to identify neurosecretory granules.

Surgical resection is standard, with complete removal of the tumor and as much preservation of lung as possible. Lobectomy is the most common procedure; endoscopic removal is performed only for rare polypoid tumors if thoracotomy is contraindicated. Survival rate is typically 85% at 5 to 10 years. Large cell neuroendocrine tumors and small cell cancers are not typically treated with surgery and may be best treated with combinations of chemotherapy and radiation; survival of these patients is poor.

Adenoid cystic carcinoma is a slow-growing malignancy involving the trachea and mainstem bronchi that is similar to salivary gland tumors.[92] Adenoid cystic carcinoma is more malignant than carcinoid tumors and has a slight female preponderance. The tumor typically involves the lower trachea, carina, and takeoff of the mainstem bronchi. Stridor is often the presenting symptom of adenoid cystic tumors because these tumors are most often found in the trachea and mainstem bronchi. One third of patients have tumors that have metastasized at the time of treatment. They typically have involvement of the perineural lymphatics, regional nodes, or liver, bone, or kidneys. The tumor arises from ducts in the submucosa and extends proximally and distally in that plane. Microscopic examination demonstrates cells with large nuclei, a small cytoplasm, and surrounding cystic spaces (pseudoacinar type); the medullary type has a Swiss cheese appearance. Treatment is wide en bloc resection, with conservation of as much lung tissue as possible.[93] Radiation treatment alone may be effective for patients not amenable to surgical resection.

Benign tumors of the lung account for less than 1% of all lung neoplasms and arise from mesodermal origins (Box 58-3). Hamartomas are the most frequent benign lung tumor; they consist of normal tissue elements found in an abnormal location. Hamartomas are manifested by overgrowth of cartilage, are typically identified at 40 to 60 years of age, and have a 2:1 male-to-female predominance. They are usually peripheral and slow-growing. The chest x-ray demonstrates a 2- to 3-cm mass that is sharply demarcated and frequently lobulated. It is usually not calcified, but the popcorn appearance on chest x-ray may provide the diagnosis of hamartoma. Cystic adenomatoid malformation may represent adenomatous hamartoma, which occur in infants as cysts or immature elements in the lung.

Very low-grade malignancies include hemangiopericytoma and pulmonary blastoma that arises from embryonic lung tissue. Treatment is resection. Tumorlets are epithelial proliferative lesions that may resemble oat cell carcinoma or carcinoid. These are typically incidental findings noted on examination of resected lung specimens. They rarely metastasize.

Primary sarcomas of the lung occur rarely. Resection, similar to lung carcinoma, is feasible for 50% to 60% of patients.[94] Prognosis of patients with leiomyosarcoma is excellent, with an approximately 50% survival rate at 5 years; all others have poor survival expectations.

Lymphoma of the lung usually occurs as disseminated lymphoma involving the lung. The disseminated lymphoma occurs in 40% of patients with Hodgkin's disease and 7% in those with non-Hodgkin's disease. Primary lymphoma of the lung is rare. The diagnosis is usually made at surgery. A thorough evaluation for other primary sites of lymphoma is carried out if primary pulmonary lymphoma is suspected preoperatively.

**BOX 58-3 Miscellaneous Lung Tumors**

**Hamartoma**

**Epithelial Origin Tumors**

Papilloma: Single or multiple, squamous epithelium, occurs in childhood, probably viral, may require bronchial resection but frequently recur

Polyp: Inflammatory-squamous metaplasia on a stalk; bronchial resection may be needed; these do not usually recur

**Mesodermal Origin Tumors**

Fibroma: Most frequent mesodermal tumor

Chondroma

Lipoma

Leiomyoma: Intrabronchial or peripheral; conservative resection

**Granular Cell Tumors**

Rhabdomyoma

Neuroma

Hemangioma: Subglottic larynx or upper trachea of infants; radiation therapy

Lymphangioma: Similar to cystic hygroma—upper airway obstruction in neonates

Hemangioendothelioma: Newborn lungs, often progressive and lethal

Lymphangiomyomatosis: Rare, slowly progressive—death from pulmonary insufficiency; fine, multinodular lesions, loss of parenchyma and honeycombing; usually women in their reproductive years

Arteriovenous fistula: Congenital, right-to-left shunt; cyanosis, dyspnea on exertion, clubbing, brain abscess; associated with hereditary hemorrhagic telangiectasia of lower lobes

**Inflammatory Tumors and Pseudotumors**

Plasma cell granuloma

Pseudolymphoma

Xanthoma

**Teratoma**

## CHEST WALL

### Pectus Excavatum

Pectus excavatum is the most common chest wall deformity, occurring in 1 of 400 children, with a male predominance (4:1).[95] More than 30% of patients have a family history of chest wall anomalies. Pectus excavatum refers to the sternal depression (depressed dorsally) caused by unequal growth rates or development of the lower ribs and costal cartilages, usually after the third rib. The sternum is not depressed equally or symmetrically, but is also rotated. This syndrome may be associated with other musculoskeletal abnormalities. Most patients are asymptomatic but some have decreased exercise capacity or pulmonary reserve. Patients are evaluated with plain chest x-ray, CT, pulmonary function studies, ventilation perfusion lung scans, and other physiologic studies.

Surgical repair of pectus excavatum can be accomplished by various techniques, including sternal osteotomy, osteotomy with posterior strut or other stabilization (e.g., a metal plate), removing the sternum and turning it over with stabilization, placement of a prosthesis to fill the defect, and placement of an internal (posterior) sternal support, which is more effective in younger patients. Open techniques typically reflect the overlying pectoralis major and rectus muscles. Involved costal cartilages are removed, leaving the perichondrium. The sternum is mobilized and stabilized. The muscles are reapproximated in the midline over the repair.

Pectus carinatum (also called *pigeon breast*) refers to the anterior protrusion of the sternum and costal cartilages and occurs with a male predominance (4:1). This condition is approximately five times less likely to occur than pectus excavatum.

Poland's syndrome is a rare nonfamilial disease of unknown cause that occurs in 1/30,000 births. Characteristics include absence of the pectoralis major muscle, absence or hypoplasia of the pectoralis minor muscle, absence of costal cartilages, hypoplasia of breast and subcutaneous tissue (including the nipple complex), and various hand anomalies.

**Table 58-3 Classification of Tumors of the Chest Wall**

| TYPE | BENIGN | MALIGNANT |
|---|---|---|
| **Bony Tissue** | | |
| Bone | Osteoid osteoma<br>Aneurysmal bone cyst | Osteosarcoma<br>Ewing's sarcoma |
| Cartilage | Enchondroma<br>Osteochondroma | Chondrosarcoma |
| Fibrous | Fibrous dysplasia | Malignant fibrous histiocytoma |
| Marrow | Eosinophilic granuloma | Plasmacytoma |
| Vascular | Hemangioma | Hemangiosarcoma |
| **Soft Tissue** | | |
| Adipose | Lipoma and variations | Liposarcoma |
| Muscle | Leiomyoma<br>Rhabdomyoma | Leiomyosarcoma<br>Rhabdomyosarcoma |
| Neural | Neurofibroma<br>Neurilemoma | Neurofibrosarcoma<br>Malignant schwannoma<br>Askin's tumor (primitive neuroectodermal tumor) |
| Fibrous | Desmoid | Fibrosarcoma |

Adapted from Faber LP, Somers J, Templeton AC: Chest wall tumors. Curr Probl Surg 32:661–747, 1995.

## Chest Wall Tumors

Chest wall tumors are rare.[96] The most frequent chest wall tumors are metastatic chest wall tumors related to metastasis to the chest wall from another primary tumors. Primary chest wall tumors are typically sarcomas of the chest wall (rib). Primary bone tumors can also occur in the ribs, scapula, and sternum (Table 58-3).

Clinical presentation of chest wall tumors can range from an enlarging painless mass to a painful and fungating mass. Pain can occur with periosteal invasion. Local tumor extension onto the lung or mediastinum can create associated symptoms. Evaluation requires diagnostic imaging such as chest radiography, CT, and FDG-PET. MRI is effective for tumors involving the thoracic inlet or upper chest that may involve the brachial plexus and for tumors that involve or abut the vertebral bodies. Histologic confirmation is required. A core needle biopsy is frequently effective. Excisional biopsy with minimal contamination of the surgical site may be required for a larger tumor. Consideration for future resection may dictate the size and location of the incisional biopsy. Resection and reconstruction with prosthesis or muscle flaps can be accomplished, with excellent results.[97] A multidisciplinary approach to the patient's therapeutic strategy will be complemented by a multispecialty team in the operating room.

### Bone Tumors

Benign bone tumors include fibrous dysplasia of the bone, which accounts for approximately 30% of these tumors. Chondromas account for 15% to 20% of benign chest wall lesions and arise from the anterior costochondral junction. Osteochondroma commonly occurs in young men as an asymptomatic tumor originating from the cortex of the rib. Eosinophilic granuloma is a benign component of malignant fibrous histiocytosis and primarily affects men. Skull and rib involvement are common; these appear as expansile lesions on radiographic evaluation. Excisional biopsy is indicated for solitary lesions and radiotherapy for multiple lesions. Aneurysmal bone cysts occur in the ribs that may be associated with previous trauma. Radiographic characteristics include a blowout lytic lesion (Fig. 58-19). Resection is recommended for diagnosis and relief of pain.

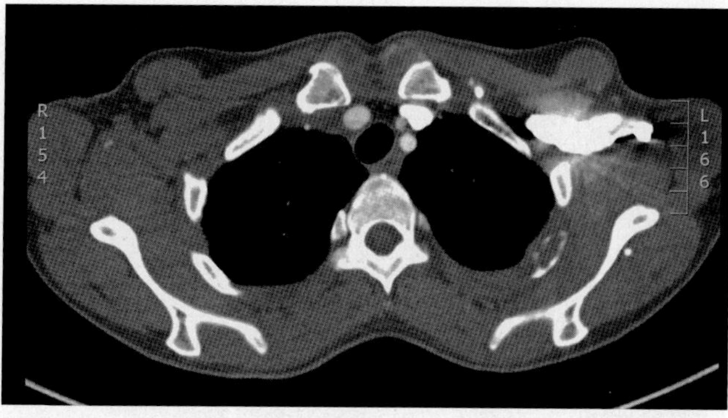

**FIGURE 58-19** Aneurysmal bone cyst.

Malignant bone tumors include chondrosarcoma as the most common malignant tumor of the chest wall, accounting for 20% of all bone tumors; these arise in the third and fourth decades. Radiographic characteristics include a poorly defined tumor mass that is destroying cortical bone. Resection with wide margins (3 to 5 cm) is the treatment of choice. Five-year survival is approximately 70% following complete resection. Osteosarcoma (osteogenic sarcoma) usually arises in the long bones of adolescents and young adults. Primary osteosarcomas in the chest account for 10% to 15% of malignant tumors. The tumor grows rapidly; radiographic features include a sunburst pattern on chest x-ray. Ewing's sarcoma commonly arises in bones of the pelvis, humerus, or femur of young men. It is the third most common malignant chest wall tumor (5% to 10%). Radiographic characteristics include an onion peel appearance, with periosteal elevation and bony remodeling. A 50% 5-year survival can be achieved with multimodality therapy. Solitary plasmacytoma is a rare tumor that occurs in older men as a painful solitary tumor arising from plasma cells. Multiple myeloma is the same tumor arising in more than one location. Radiographic characteristics include a diffuse, motheaten, or punched-out appearance of the bone. Systemic disease can be confirmed using serum protein electrophoresis, urinalysis (Bence Jones protein), and bone marrow aspiration. Complete resection of a solitary plasmacytoma is recommended.

### Soft Tissue Tumors

Soft tissue sarcomas are the most common malignant primary chest wall tumors.[98] Core needle or incisional biopsy is performed to establish the diagnosis (Fig. 58-20). Resection with wide local excision (3 to 5 cm) is required. These tumors should not be shelled out, despite the presence of a pseudocapsule. Complete resection is associated with excellent local control and prolonged survival. Combinations of chemotherapy and radiation therapy may be used as components of the multidisciplinary treatment plan.

### Metastatic Tumors

Metastatic neoplasms may involve the chest wall by direct extension, lymphatic metastasis, or hematogenous metastasis. Lung cancer and breast cancer can involve the chest wall by direct

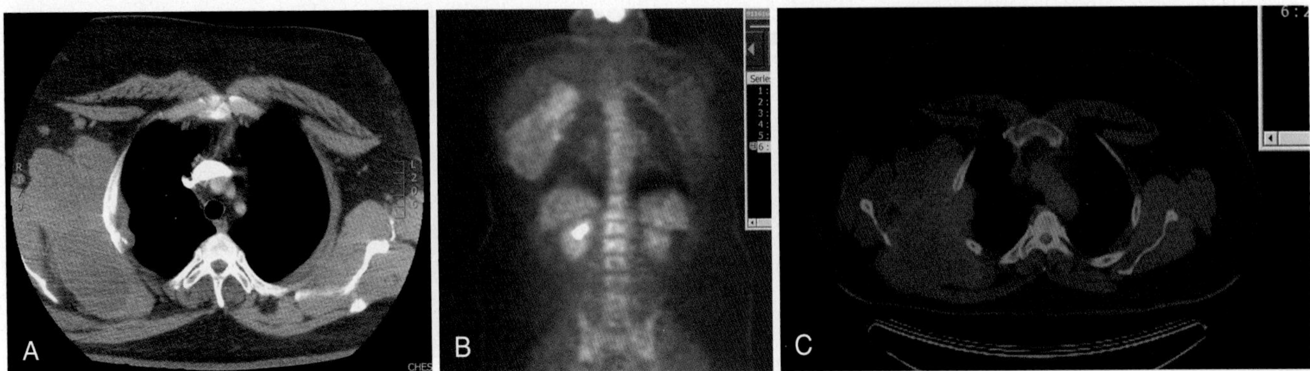

**FIGURE 58-20 A,** Primary chest wall tumor, desmoid tumor of the right lateral and posterior chest wall, is shown by computed tomography (CT). **B,** FDG-PET demonstrates mild FDG avidity. No sites of metastases were identified. **C,** A fused image of the CT and FDG-PET is shown. Resection of the tumor included chest wall musculature and chest wall. Reconstruction with prosthetic material, and muscle flap was required.

extension and, if identified, chest wall resection should be performed concurrently with resection of the primary neoplasm.

### Reconstruction

Reconstruction of the chest wall is dependent on the size, location, cosmetic, and functional impairment that results from resection. Prevention of flail chest and maintenance of physiologic stability requires careful judgment about the choice of prosthetic reconstruction, autologous tissue coverage available, including myocutaneous flaps, and free tissue flap transfer.

## Chest Wall Infections

Chest wall infections may occur after thoracic surgery, thoracic trauma, or other interventions. Inflammatory breast carcinoma is not an infection but may mimic a chest wall infection. Biopsy may be needed to confirm the diagnosis. Mondor's disease, thrombophlebitis of the superficial veins of the breast and anterior chest wall, is also not an infection. Ultrasound or biopsy may be necessary to confirm the diagnosis. Tietze's syndrome, or costochondritis, is usually self-limited and can be treated with nonsteroidal anti-inflammatory drugs (NSAIDs) and rest. Because of the limited blood supply to the cartilage, infection in this area may be difficult to diagnose. Débridement and reconstruction may be necessary. Sternal wound infections are complications following median sternotomy or cardiac surgery. Spontaneous primary chest wall infections can arise from various sources as a consequence of immunosuppression, drug-resistant organisms, including tuberculosis, or HIV infection.

## Chest Wall Trauma

Trauma to the chest wall is common. Plain chest radiography and chest CT are performed, often as part of the secondary survey in chest wall trauma. CT can identify rib, parenchymal, and other abnormalities. Blunt chest wall trauma commonly results in contusion of the chest wall tissues and underlying lung parenchyma. Supportive care is warranted.

Rib fractures are perhaps the most common traumatic injury sustained after blunt chest wall trauma. Symptoms include pain on inspiration and localized point tenderness. Plain films can confirm the diagnosis. Fractures of the first or second ribs may occur after significant trauma or high-velocity injury. Because of the size and thickness of the first rib, tremendous force is needed to fracture this rib. This traumatic event is associated with aortic disruption. Contusion or injury to underlying structures should be suspected with any rib fracture. Contusion of the lung parenchyma and/or injury to the spleen, liver, diaphragm, or kidney can occur. Treatment with analgesia and nerve blocks can be helpful. Flail chest may occur with multiple rib fractures; this results in an unstable chest wall that develops paradoxical motion during respiration (e.g., depression during the negative inspiratory phase and extrusion during the positive expiratory phase). Flail chest is often associated with an underlying pulmonary contusion and should be supported with pain relief, stabilization of the chest wall, or even mechanical ventilation.

Sternal injuries are uncommon and may result from blunt trauma to the anterior chest, typically from a steering wheel injury during a motor vehicle accident. An underlying cardiac injury must be considered, such as aortic disruption, cardiac contusion, pericardial effusion, or arrhythmia. Evaluation by heart rhythm monitoring, serial cardiac observations with modalities such as electrocardiography and enzyme level measurements, and echocardiography are used to exclude these injuries. Clavicular fractures may be associated with injury to the great vessels or the brachial plexus. Supportive care and stabilization are recommended.

# THORACIC OUTLET SYNDROME

Thoracic outlet syndrome (TOS) refers to compression of the subclavian vessels and nerves of the brachial plexus in the region of the thoracic inlet. Symptoms usually develop secondary to neural compromise; however, vascular and neurovascular symptoms have been reported.[99] The patient population most commonly affected by TOS is middle-aged women. The subclavian vessels and brachial plexus can be compressed at various locations as they pass between the thoracic inlet and upper extremities (Fig. 58-21). From medial to lateral, these anatomic regions are the interscalene triangle (artery and nerves), costoclavicular space (vein), and subcoracoid area (artery, vein, nerves).

## Diagnosis

The symptoms associated with TOS vary, depending on the anatomic structure that is compressed. In more than 90% of cases, neurogenic manifestations are reported. Symptoms of subclavian artery compression include fatigue, weakness, coldness, upper extremity claudication, thrombosis, and paresthesia.

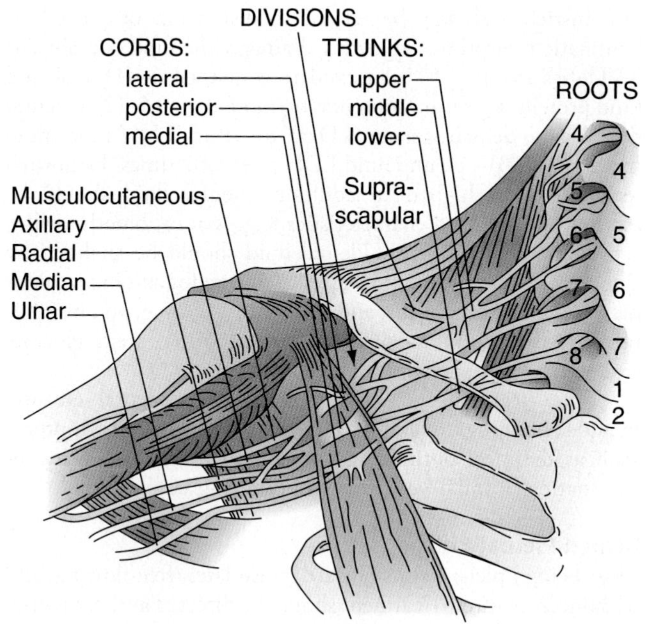


**FIGURE 58-21** Detailed view of brachial plexus. (From Urschel HC, Razzuk M: Upper plexus thoracic outlet syndrome: Optimal therapy. Ann Thorac Surg 63:935–939, 1997.)

Thrombosis with distal embolization rarely can occur, producing vasomotor symptoms (Raynaud's phenomenon) in the hand or ischemic changes. Venous compression results in edema, venous distention, collateral formation, and cyanosis of the affected limb. Venous TOS may be characterized by upper extremity edema, venous distention, or effort thrombosis, also known as Paget-Schroetter syndrome.

The diagnosis of neurogenic TOS is initially made clinically. Evaluation for TOS includes chest and cervical spine films.[100] A cervical rib or bony degenerative cervical spine changes may be present, and MRI or cervical myelography is sometimes helpful to rule out narrowing of the intervertebral foramina or cervical disc pathology. Doppler studies or vascular imaging (e.g., angiography, venography) may be indicated if the extent of vascular impairment cannot be determined clinically or if an aneurysm or venous thrombosis is suspected. Neurogenic TOS needs to be confirmed with nerve conduction studies to localize the area of slowing of nerve conduction and rule out other compression syndromes, such as carpal tunnel syndrome. Electromyelography or nerve conduction studies are helpful to rule out carpal tunnel syndrome. Patients with moderate to severe slowing of nerve conduction usually respond to nonoperative therapy. Vascular TOS must be confirmed with objective studies.

### Diagnostic Tests

Clinical maneuvers to evaluate a patient suspected of having TOS are performed to identify the loss or decrease of radial pulse or reproduce neurologic symptoms. A clear, objective validated definition for TOS is needed. Evocative tests may be used to a elicit patient's symptoms. These tests include the following:

**Adson (Scalene) Test** The patient inspires maximally and holds his or her breath while the neck is fully extended and the head is turned toward the affected side. This maneuver narrows the space between the scalenus anticus and medius, resulting in compression of the subclavian artery and brachial plexus. Decrease or loss of the ipsilateral radial pulse suggests compression.

**Halsted (Costoclavicular) Test** The patient is instructed to place the shoulders in a military position (drawn backward and downward) to narrow the costoclavicular space between the first rib and clavicle, thereby causing neurovascular compression. Reproduction of neurologic symptoms or decrease or loss of the ipsilateral radial pulse suggests compression.

**Wright (Hyperabduction) Test** The patient's arm is hyperabducted 180 degrees, which cause the neurovascular structures to be compressed in the subcoracoid region by the pectoralis tendon, head of the humerus, or coracoid process. Decrease or loss of the ipsilateral radial pulse suggests compression.

**Roos Test** The patient abducts the involved arm 90 degrees, with external rotation of the shoulder. Maintaining this body position, the modified Roos test is performed by opening and closing the hand rapidly for 3 minutes in an attempt to reproduce symptoms. Also, neurogenic compromise may be detected using provocative tests such as percussion of the nerve (Tinel's sign) or flexion of the elbow or wrist (Phalen's sign).

### Treatment

Results of treatment of TOS are variable because there are inconsistent objective criteria for the diagnosis of TOS other than clinical diagnosis. Initial management of TOS is nonoperative. Physical therapy is needed. Repetitive upper extremity mechanical work and muscular trauma are eliminated. Indications for surgery include failure of conservative management, progressive neurologic symptoms, prolonged ulnar or median nerve conduction velocities, narrowing or occlusion of the subclavian artery, and thrombosis of the axillary or subclavian vein. Objective agreed on outcome measures and clinical trials are needed to compare outcomes of surgery for TOS compared with no surgery.[101] Success rates with surgery only approach 70% at 5 years. Recurrent symptoms may prompt operation in up to one third of patients.

## PLEURA

### Pleural Effusions

The pleural space is a potential space normally defined by the small amount of pleural fluid separating the visceral and parietal pleura. Pleural space disorders, benign and malignant, can disrupt the balance of fluid production and absorption, leading to various pleural space problems, including increased mass effect from air, fluid, or tumor on the ipsilateral lung parenchyma and heart, infection, or dyspnea and pulmonary dysfunction. The causes of pleural effusions vary (Box 58-4).

The movement of fluid across the pleural membranes is governed by Starling's law of capillary exchange. The amount of pleural fluid is therefore controlled by a balance of oncotic and hydrostatic pressure within the pleural space and pleural capillaries. Under normal circumstances, the net pressure moves fluid from the parietal pleura into the pleural space. It is estimated that 5 to 10 liters of fluid are produced and transgress the pleural

**BOX 58-4 Pleural Effusions**

**Causes of Transudative Effusions**
Congestive heart failure
Cirrhosis
Nephrotic syndrome
Hypoalbuminemia
Fluid retention/overload
Pulmonary embolism
Lobar collapse
Meigs' syndrome

**Causes of Exudative Effusions**

**Malignant**
Primary lung, pleural, or metastatic carcinoma
Lymphoma
Mesothelioma

**Infectious**
Bacterial (parapneumonic) / Empyema
Tuberculosis
Fungal
Viral
Parasitic

**Collagen-Vascular Disease Related**
Rheumatoid arthritis
Wegener's granulomatosis
Systemic lupus erythematosus
Churg-Strauss syndrome

**Abdominal and Gastrointestinal Disease–Related**
Esophageal perforation
Subphrenic abscess
Pancreatitis, pancreatic pseudocyst
Meigs' syndrome

**Others**
Chylothorax
Uremia
Sarcoidosis
After coronary artery bypass grafting
Radiation / Trauma
Dressler's syndrome
Pulmonary embolism with infarction
Asbestosis related

space over a 24-hour period. However, the normal volume of pleural fluid is small. The balance of forces favors fluid resorption from the pleural cavity across the visceral pleura. However, under physiologic conditions, most pleural fluid is resorbed through lymphatics of the parietal pleura because protein that enters the pleural space cannot enter the relatively impermeable visceral pleura. The parietal pleura and its lymphatics have significant capacity for protein and fluid removal. A small imbalance of accumulation and absorption will lead to the development of a pleural effusion. These causative factors include increased hydrostatic pressure, increased negative intrapleural pressure, increased capillary permeability, decreased plasma oncotic pressure, and decreased or interrupted lymphatic drainage.

Pleural fluid is characterized as a transudate or exudate. Transudative effusions are protein-poor and result in change in the fluid balance in the pleural space. Exudative effusions are protein-rich and may be related to disruption of pleural or lymphatic resorption. Following drainage, the fluid is evaluated by Light's criteria.[102,103] An exudate is defined as (1) a pleural fluid protein–to–serum protein ratio more than 0.5, (2) a pleural fluid lactate dehydrogenase (LDH)–to–serum LDH ratio more than 0.6, or (3) a pleural fluid LDH level 1.67 times the normal serum level or higher. In addition, pleural fluid should be assessed for its visual characteristics (e.g., serous, bloody, milky, turbid, frankly purulent). Pleural fluid should be analyzed by cytology, cell counts, Gram staining, culture for aerobic, anaerobic, and fungal organisms, and tuberculosis testing, and by laboratory tests for simultaneous pleural and serum protein, glucose, and LDH levels and pH.

The treatment goals for patients with pleural effusion include obtaining a diagnosis, relieving or eliminating symptoms such as dyspnea, optimizing patient function, minimizing or eliminating hospitalization, and minimizing costs of care.

### Benign Pleural Effusions

Most benign pleural effusions are transudates, free-flowing, and without loculation. Treatment should be directed at the underlying cause, such as congestive heart failure, ascites, or malnutrition. Symptoms are typically dyspnea or cough. Pleural fluid can be identified on an upright chest radiograph; 300 mL of fluid causes blunting of the costophrenic angle. Clinical examination can detect 500 mL of fluid or more. Initial thoracentesis should achieve complete drainage for diagnosis and treatment. In addition, radiographic evidence of complete lung reexpansion should be sought. Failure of the lung to expand completely suggests a trapped lung, which may require decortication, particularly if symptoms such as dyspnea persist. Relief of symptoms with thoracentesis usually indicates the pleural effusion as the cause. Occasionally, symptoms are not relieved by thoracentesis and another diagnosis should be sought.

Recurrent effusions can occur, and repeat thoracenteses may be required. Alternative therapies such as chest tube insertion (tube thoracostomy) or thoracoscopic drainage, with or without mechanical and chemical pleurodesis, can be considered. Visceral and parietal pleural apposition are required to achieve pleurodesis. Drainage of the effusion can be diagnostic and therapeutic, as can video-assisted thoracoscopic drainage of effusions. Sclerosing agents can be placed to facilitate pleural symphysis. This pleurodesis is most effectively accomplished with a slurry of 5 g of talc in 100 mL of saline placed through the chest tube. Alternative sclerosants include doxycycline (300 to 500 mg). Pleural biopsies or wedge resection of the lung can be easily performed to facilitate diagnosis. Mechanical pleural abrasion or chemical pleurodesis with talc is typically used. The talc is insufflated within the hemithorax to cover all visceral pleural surfaces (e.g., talc poudrage). Pleurectomy is not commonly needed; however, persistent pleural effusions and trapped lung may not be amenable to more conservative measures. Decortication may be required.

### Malignant Pleural Effusion

Patients with known or previous malignancy can develop an MPE; 25% of MPEs will not have a histologic diagnosis of cancer within the fluid after two thoracenteses. Drainage is required for relief of dyspnea (Fig. 58-22).

MPE is an effusion with positive cytopathology. Not all pleural effusions associated with malignancy are caused by direct

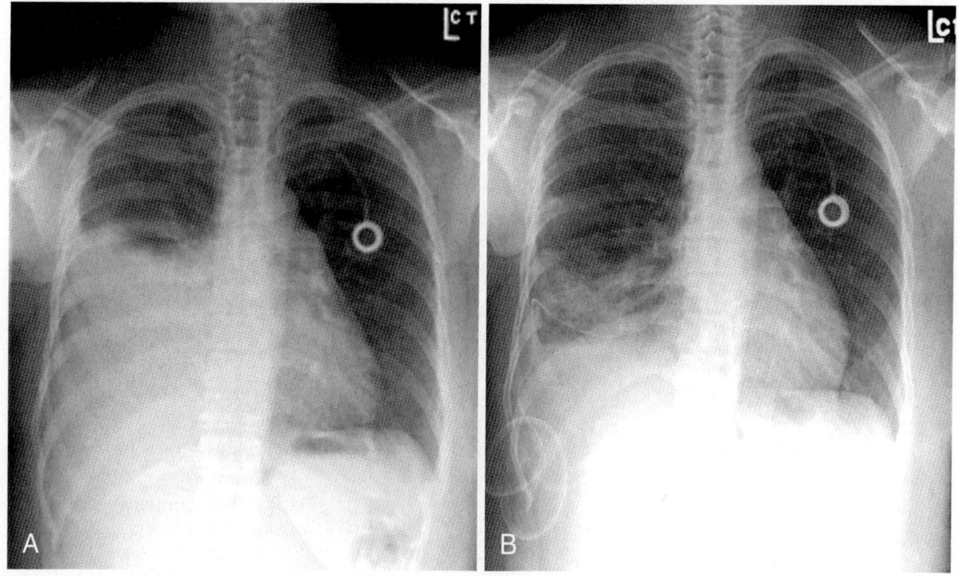


**FIGURE 58-22 A,** Malignant pleural effusion causing dyspnea. A chronic indwelling pleural catheter was placed as an outpatient to facilitate drainage at home to prevent dyspnea. Hospitalization was not required. **B,** Following drainage. A chronic indwelling pleural catheter is effective in patients with trapped lung. Every other day drainage reduces impairment of the contralateral lung and prevents mediastinal shift.

or metastatic pleural involvement. There are other mechanisms for their development (e.g., bronchial or lymphatic obstruction, hypoproteinemia, and sympathetic accumulation from infradiaphragmatic involvement). Although repeated cytologic evaluation of a pleural effusion achieves high positive and negative predictive values, limitations of this diagnostic procedure are important. After three thoracenteses, 70% to 80% of patients will have a cancer diagnosed. Thoracoscopy is diagnostic in 92% of patients.

A patient with an MPE has a limited life expectancy (median survival, 90 days).[104] Patients with breast cancer and an MPE have a median survival of approximately 5 months; those with lymphoma typically have a longer median survival.[105] Local treatment of malignant effusions does not affect the systemic disease process but may provide significant symptomatic relief. Complications of treatment include hemothorax, loculation of fluid, empyema, failure of pleurodesis, with recurrence of effusion, and lung entrapment caused by a nonexpansile lung. Open surgical pleurectomy and pleurodesis are reserved for patients who fail other therapies and who have a reasonably long life expectancy. A phase 3 study has demonstrated that a chronic indwelling pleural catheter is as effective as chest tube drainage with doxycycline pleurodesis.[106] Talc slurry is as effective as VATS with talc pleurodesis.[107] A treatment algorithm for MPE is shown in Figure 58-23.

## Empyema

Empyema is an infection of the pleural space and is commonly an exudate.[108] Empyemas progress from an acute phase with fluid that is thin and can be drained completely with a chest tube or small-bore catheter. This process typically worsens as the fluid becomes more turbid and thick and begins to loculate. Mucopurulent debris develops within the pleural space and compresses the underlying lung parenchyma. The organizing or chronic phase is reflected in more lung entrapment, with capillary ingrowth and creation of a pleural rind that traps the lung.

An empyema typically occurs following a reactive pleural effusion as a consequence of a lung infection.[109] These infections historically were the results of streptococcal or pneumococcal pneumonia; at present however, gram-negative and anaerobic organisms are common causes of empyema. Tuberculous empyema can also be identified. Empyema can follow trauma or thoracic surgery (from a residual pleural space or bronchopleural fistula), hematologic spread, rupture of a pulmonary or mediastinal abscess, or esophageal perforation.

Symptoms typically include constitutional symptoms of general malaise, fever, loss of appetite, and weight loss. Cough and dyspnea are common if lung infection is present. Evaluation includes a chest x-ray, posterior row anterior and lateral, and CT of the chest and upper abdomen.

Treatment of empyema depends on the extent of the disease and its location.[110] Complete and dependent drainage is required. Antibiotics and supportive care (e.g., fluids, nutrition, skin care) are commonly initiated. Use of fibrinolytic agents such as tissue plasminogen activator can be effective with mild loculations.

Simple dependent and complete drainage is required for a successful outcome. This drainage can be easily achieved with posterior rib resection and insertion of an empyema tube. The technique can be effectively used and can minimize operative time for patients who are critically ill or septic. Complete expansion of the lung may not be achieved at the time of surgery but, with time and drainage, the lung typically reexpands and the space closes. VATS decortication and thoracotomy, with débridement or formal decortication in later stage empyema, is reserved for treatment failures with persistent symptoms of dyspnea, loculations, or continued sepsis.[111]

Bronchopleural fistula following lobectomy or pneumonectomy will predispose to empyema. Management of bronchopleural fistula will require evaluation of the underlying cause of the fistula, drainage of the infection, and obliteration of the residual pleural space, with general supportive care. Chronic empyema with a residual pleural space can be treated with

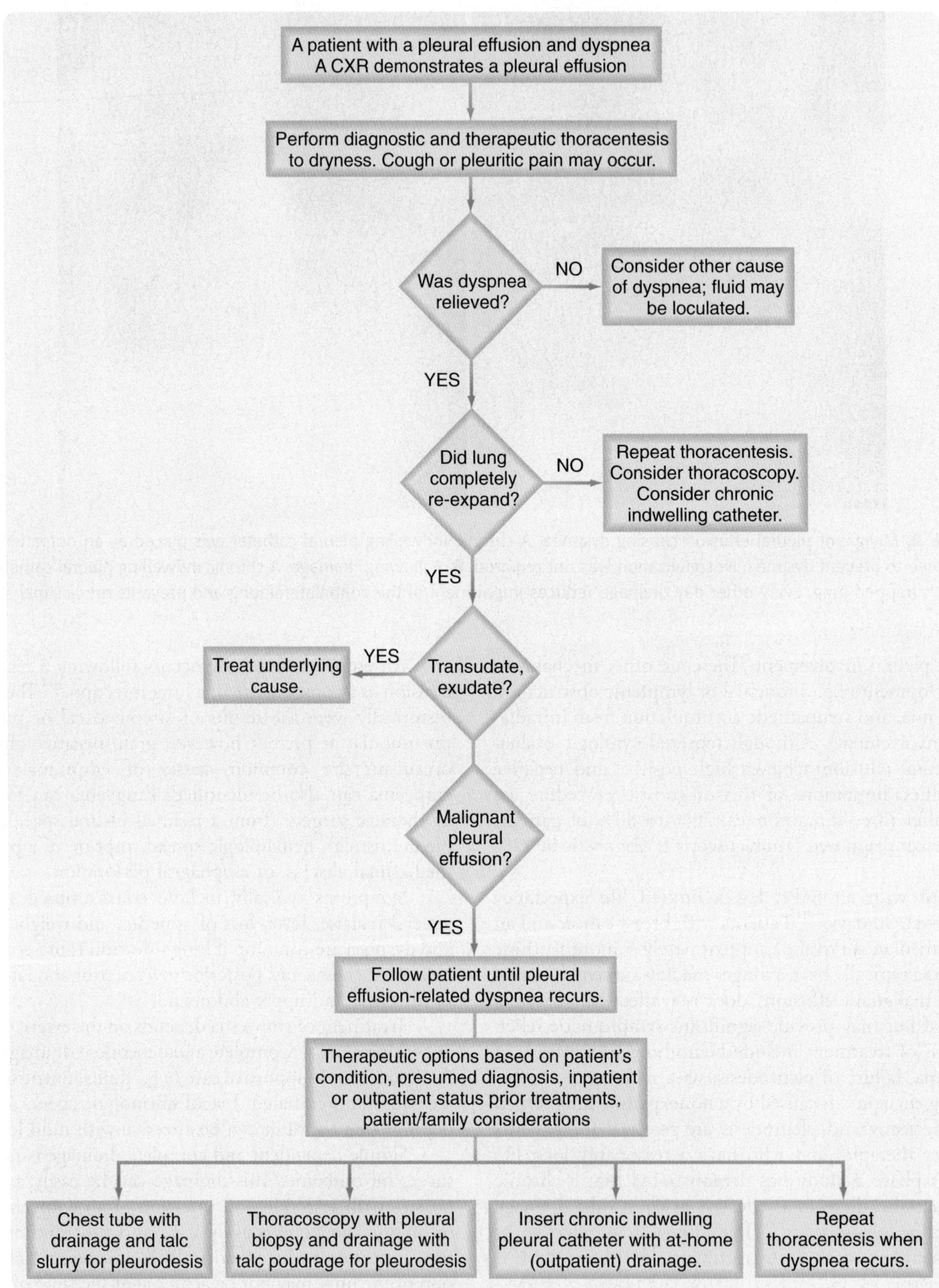
A patient with a pleural effusion and dyspnea
A CXR demonstrates a pleural effusion
Perform diagnostic and therapeutic thoracentesis
to dryness. Cough or pleuritic pain may occur.
Was dyspnea
relieved?
NO
Consider other cause
of dyspnea; fluid may
be loculated.
YES
Did lung
completely
re-expand?
NO
Repeat thoracentesis.
Consider thoracoscopy.
Consider chronic
indwelling catheter.
YES
Transudate,
exudate?
YES
Treat underlying
cause.
Malignant
pleural
effusion?
YES
Follow patient until pleural
effusion-related dyspnea recurs.
Therapeutic options based on patient's
condition, presumed diagnosis, inpatient
or outpatient status prior treatments,
patient/family considerations
Chest tube with
drainage and talc
slurry for pleurodesis
Thoracoscopy with pleural
biopsy and drainage with
talc poudrage for pleurodesis
Insert chronic indwelling
pleural catheter with at-home
(outpatient) drainage.
Repeat
thoracentesis when
dyspnea recurs.

**FIGURE 58-23** Algorithm to facilitate management of patients with pleural effusion.

drainage, gauze packing, or a skin flap (Eloesser flap), with eventual muscle transposition and skin closure. Lung resection or pleuropneumonectomy is rarelyrequired.[112]

## Chylothorax

Chylothorax occurs when chyle from the thoracic duct empties into the pleural space.[113] Chyle is a milky white fluid with a high concentration of triglycerides, chylomicrons, and white blood cells. It is nutritionally rich and depends on the nutritional and dietary status of the patient. It may be clear. Chylothorax has multiple causes (Box 58-5).

Symptoms from chylothorax are similar to those of any pleural fluid (e.g., dyspnea, cough). In addition, because of the nutritional consequences of chronic chyle leak (e.g., loss of fat, protein) and volume of the leak (0.5 to 3.0 liters/day), fluid and nutritional replacement and correction of the underlying

**BOX 58-5 Chylothorax**

**Traumatic (Chest and Neck)**
Blunt
Penetrating

**Iatrogenic**
Catheterization, particularly subclavian vein
Postsurgical
Excision of cervical/supraclavicular lymph nodes
Radical lymph node dissections of the neck or chest
Lung, esophageal, or mediastinal resection
Thoracic aneurysm repair
Sympathectomy
Congenital cardiovascular surgery

**Neoplasms**
Lymphoma, lung, esophageal, or mediastinal neoplasms
Metastatic carcinoma

**Infectious**
Tuberculous lymphadenosis
Mediastinitis
Ascending lymphangitis

**Other**
Lymphangioleiomyomatosis
Venous thrombosis

**Congenital**

**BOX 58-6 Pneumothorax**

**Spontaneous**
Primary
Secondary
- Chronic obstructive pulmonary disease (COPD)
- Bullous disease
- Cystic fibrosis
- *Pneumocystis*-related
- Congenital cysts
- Idiopathic pulmonary fibrosis (IPF)
- Pulmonary embolism

Catamenial
Neonatal

**Traumatic**
Penetrating
*Blunt*

**Iatrogenic**
Mechanical ventilation
Needle puncture: Thoracentesis, FNA lung nodule, central line insertion
Postsurgical

**Other**
Esophageal perforation

problem are necessary. Diagnosis may be made with thoracentesis or drainage of the fluid with a chest tube. Analysis of pleural fluid with chylomicrons confirms the diagnosis. Conservative measures such as a medium-chain triglyceride diet or total parenteral nutrition are used initially. If conservative measures fail, operative intervention may be considered between days 7 and 14. Commonly, ligation of the thoracic duct where it enters the chest through the diaphragmatic hiatus is achieved via a right thoracotomy or thoracoscopy. Placement of olive oil or ice cream by a nasogastric tube at the time of surgery may increase chyle drainage into the operative field and help identify the area of thoracic duct disruption. Percutaneous techniques with needle cannulation and duct occlusion have been proposed.[114]

## Pneumothorax

Pneumothorax is the accumulation of air within the pleural space. It may occur after trauma, surgery, needle aspiration, central line insertion, increased pressure from mechanical ventilation, or as a consequence of lung disease (e.g., COPD, cystic or pulmonary fibrosis) or other conditions (e.g., catamenial pneumothorax; Box 58-6). A primary spontaneous pneumothorax occurs as a consequence of subpleural blebs or some other pulmonary disease. Tension pneumothorax occurs when air continues to enter the pleural space without decompression. This problem results in positive intrathoracic pressure causing compression of the lung and mediastinum, shift of the mediastinum into the contralateral chest, and decrease in ventilation and venous return. Cardiopulmonary collapse and death ensue. Immediate decompression with needle or chest tube insertion is lifesaving.

Symptoms of pneumothorax include pain and dyspnea. Patients with spontaneous pneumothorax are usually tall, thin young men. Diagnostic imaging includes chest x-ray and occasionally CT. Apical blebs and bullae are common. CT should be reserved for patients with concern for other pulmonary diseases. Subcutaneous emphysema may or may not be present.

Treatment depends on size and symptoms. Smaller pneumothorax may be followed; this may resolve spontaneously, particularly those that occur after needle aspiration for lung biopsy. Progression in size of the pneumothorax requires intervention with drainage.

The initial spontaneous pneumothorax may be treated with small-bore drainage or chest tube insertion, with resolution of the air space and cessation of the air leak. A persistent air leak (>72 hours) or failure of the lung to expand fully suggests that additional intervention may be needed.

Operative intervention is recommended for patients who have a persistence or recurrence of a spontaneous pneumothorax or who develop a contralateral pneumothorax. High-risk professions (e.g., scuba diver, airplane pilots) should be avoided. Operative repair typically includes thoracoscopy to identify apical blebs, which are resected with endoscopic staplers. Mechanical abrasion of the parietal pleura is performed. Pleurodesis with talc in patients with malignancy or in older patients may be considered.

## Mesothelioma

Mesothelioma is a rare neoplasm that arises from mesothelial cells lining the parietal and visceral pleura and can present in a localized or diffuse manner. Pathology of pleural tumors has been recently reviewed.[115] Mesothelioma develops from the mesothelial cells that line the pleural cavity. Histologic subtypes include epithelial, sarcomatoid, and those of mixed histology.[116] Epithelial histology alone has the more favorable prognosis.

The localized variant, the solitary fibrous tumor of the pleura, is an uncommon benign neoplasm that usually presents as a well-defined, encapsulated tumor that is not associated with asbestos exposure. Historically, this was classified as a benign mesothelioma. Typically, the lesions are diagnosed as an asymptomatic mass on a chest radiograph. Complete surgical resection is the treatment of choice.

Diffuse malignant pleural mesothelioma presents as a locally aggressive tumor commonly associated with asbestos exposure (75%). A long latency period between asbestos exposure and the development of disease has been reported. Diagnostic imaging includes plain chest radiography, CT, and MRI. FDG-PET is useful to determine the extent of tumor invasion and for the evaluation of occult metastases, including mediastinal metastases. Echocardiography to determine cardiac involvement is also used. Diagnosis is made with pleural biopsy, which may include thoracentesis or pleural biopsy alone, or incisional biopsies via thoracoscopy or open techniques.

Survival for this disease is poor, from 4 to 12 months. Treatment includes chemotherapy, both standard and conformal radiation therapy, and extrapleural pneumonectomy. Combination therapy is commonly used. Extrapleural pneumonectomy and total pleurectomy are two commonly used surgical procedures.[117,118] Patients with epithelioid histology, negative margins, and negative mediastinal lymph nodes can achieve a 46% 5-year survival following extrapleural pneumonectomy with adjuvant chemoradiotherapy.[119] Other techniques include preoperative chemotherapy followed by extrapleural pneumonectomy and conformal radiotherapy for the pleural surface.[120] Even with treatment, survival remains poor. Improved therapies are needed.

## MEDIASTINUM

Mediastinal abnormalities may present as an asymptomatic mass identified on screening chest x-ray or with significant symptoms, including hypoxia, facial swelling, and acute respiratory distress. Symptoms are related to the involvement of the specific mediastinal structures. Diagnosis is needed to optimize treatment planning.[121] Cytology from FNA, core, or surgical biopsy may be needed for diagnosis and to determine optimal therapy. Simple observation of a mediastinal mass can rarely be justified. These lesions should be removed prophylactically to obtain a definitive diagnosis, achieve local control, and avoid future symptoms. If cancer is identified, adjuvant therapy given after complete resection may treat microscopic disease better than bulky disease.

Mediastinal masses differ between adults and children.[122] The most common mediastinal masses (Box 58-7) in adults are thymomas and thymic cysts (26.5%), neurogenic tumors (20.0%), thymomas (21%), other cysts (16.1%), germ cell tumors (13.8%), and lymphomas (12.7%). In a combined series of 718 children with mediastinal masses, neurogenic tumors (41.6%), germ cell tumors (13.5%), primary cysts (13.4%), and lymphomas (13.4%) were diagnosed most frequently. Pericardial cysts and thymomas are uncommon in children.

Malignant mediastinal neoplasms vary from 25% to 50% of mediastinal masses in adults. Lymphomas, thymomas, germ cell tumors, primary carcinomas, and neurogenic tumors are the most common. Primary carcinomas of the mediastinum constitute up to 10% of primary mediastinal masses and need to be differentiated from malignant thymomas, germ cell

**BOX 58-7 Classification of Primary Mediastinal Tumors and Cysts**

**Thymoma**
Benign
Malignant

**Lymphoma**
Hodgkin's disease
Lymphoblastic lymphoma
Large cell lymphoma

**Germ Cell Tumors**
Teratodermoid (Benign, malignant)
Seminoma
Nonseminoma
- Embryonal
- Choriocarcinoma
- Endodermal

**Primary Carcinomas**

**Mesenchymal Tumors**
Fibroma/fibrosarcoma
Lipoma/liposarcoma
Leiomyoma/leiomyosarcoma
Rhabdosarcoma
Xanthogranuloma
Myxoma
Mesothelioma
Hemangioma
Hemangioendothelioma
Hemangiopericytoma
Lymphangioma
Lymphangiomyoma
Lymphangiopericytoma

**Endocrine Tumors**
Intrathoracic thyroid
Parathyroid adenoma, carcinoma
Carcinoid

**Cysts**
Bronchogenic
Pericardial
Enteric
Thymic
Thoracic duct
Other

**Giant Lymph Node Hyperplasia**
Castleman's disease

**Chondroma**

**Extramedullary Hematopoiesis**

**Neurogenic Tumors**
Neurofibroma
Neurilemoma
Paraganglioma
Ganglioneuroma
Neuroblastoma
Chemodectoma
Neurosarcoma

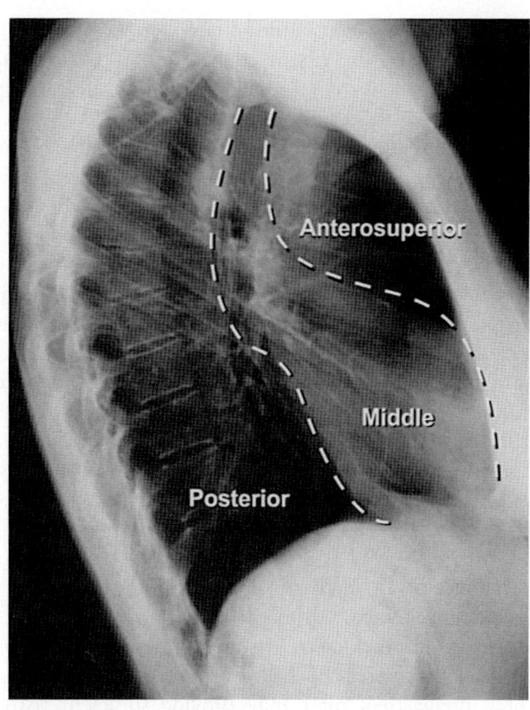


FIGURE 58-24 Lateral chest radiograph demonstrating the mediastinum divided into three anatomic subdivisions.

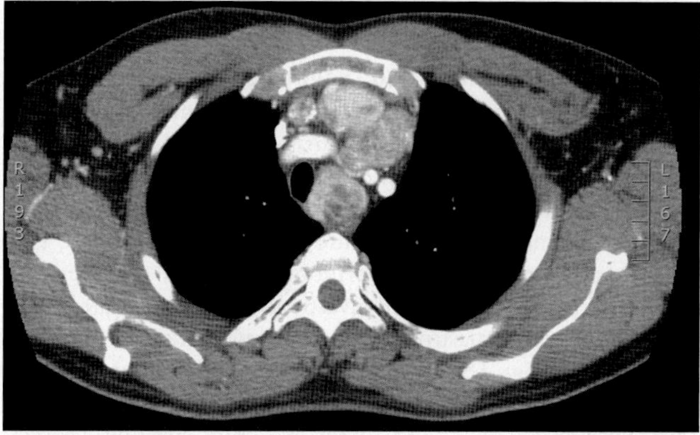

FIGURE 58-25 Thyroid carcinoma within the mediastinum. The tumor was resected via median sternotomy. No invasion was identified. A complete resection was accomplished.

tumors, carcinoid tumors, lymphomas, mediastinal extension of bronchogenic carcinomas, and metastatic tumors, which may have a similar appearance by light microscopy.

Many mediastinal lesions occur in characteristic sites within the mediastinum (Fig. 58-24). Approximately 50% of all mediastinal masses are located in the anterosuperior mediastinum, with the remainder divided between the posterior and middle mediastinum. In addition, the location of the mass explains some of the typical symptoms related to a mediastinal mass because of compression or invasion of adjacent mediastinal structures.

## Anatomy

### Anterosuperior Compartment

The anterosuperior compartment of the mediastinum borders the undersurface of the sternum ventrally, pericardium dorsally, and visceral pleura laterally, at the apposition of the pleura and pericardium. Tumors of the anterior mediastinum include thymomas, teratoma or germ cell tumors, a spectrum of lymphomas, including Hodgkin's disease, and thyroid goiter. In most cases, tissue (core biopsy) is required for diagnosis; FNA biopsy is usually inadequate.

Thymomas are usually the most frequent neoplasm of the anterior mediastinum; lymphomas are second. Germ cell neoplasms include benign and malignant teratomas, choriocarcinoma, seminoma, and embryonal cell neoplasm. Teratomas frequently occur in young adults. The gonads are the most common primary site, followed by the mediastinum. Most germ cell neoplasms are benign but 20% are malignant. Malignant teratomas may produce high serum levels of α-fetoprotein and carcinoembryonic antigen (CEA). Endocrine disease of the thyroid and parathyroid may occur in the anterior mediastinum as a result of their anatomic position in the adult (substernal goiter), or embryologic development (Fig. 58-25). Carcinoid tumors may be found within the thymus. Primary carcinomas of the mediastinum are often unresectable and respond poorly to treatment.

### Middle Compartment

The middle (or visceral) compartment extends from (and contains) the structures of the thoracic inlet (superiorly), the pericardium anteriorly, and the anterior surface of the vertebrae posteriorly. Lymphomas can occur in the middle mediastinum. Tumors of the heart and great vessels may be considered tumors of the middle compartment, as well as tumors of the trachea and mainstem bronchi and esophagus. Benign diseases such as pericardial cysts and bronchogenic cysts also occur here.

### Posterior or Paravertebral Sulci Compartment

The posterior compartment is bounded by the middle compartment anteriorly and the costophrenic angle laterally. Neurogenic tumors are usually the most common primary tumors of the mediastinum; approximately 25% of these tumors are malignant. They are located within the paravertebral sulcus and may erode the adjacent vertebra or rib. Schwannomas and neurilemmomas are the most common neurogenic tumors. Neurofibromas arise from the nerve sheath and fibers and occur in middle-aged patients. In children, ganglioneuroma is the most common neurogenic tumor. Frequently, the tumor attains a large size prior to the presentation of symptoms. Increased levels of catecholamines may produce symptoms. Surgical resection of these neurogenic tumors is usually the procedure of choice.

Embryologic development of the neural crest cells forms the basis of neuroendocrine tumors in the mediastinum; 1% of pheochromocytomas occur within the mediastinum. Chemodectomas or paragangliomas may arise from chemoreceptor tissues around the aorta and great vessels, including the carotid. Symptoms may result from catecholamine production and can be alleviated by surgical resection.

## Mediastinal Masses and Tumors

### Clinical Manifestations and Diagnosis

In adults, approximately one third of patients may develop symptoms from a mediastinal mass, including chest pain, dyspnea, and cough. The symptoms may vary widely and relate to size (fatigue, weight loss), location, extent of compression or invasion of mediastinal structures (superior vena cava syndrome), and production of hormones, markers, or other biochemicals (e.g., resulting in myasthenia gravis, fatigue, night sweats). Larger mediastinal tumors are more likely to produce symptoms; benign lesions are more often asymptomatic. Superior vena cava syndrome (obstruction of the superior vena cava, with head, neck, and upper extremity swelling), cough, hoarseness (from involvement of the recurrent laryngeal nerve), dyspnea from tumor volume or phrenic nerve paralysis, and/or dysphagia occur with compression or invasion of mediastinal structures. Other manifestations include Horner's syndrome and Pancoast syndrome.

Infections in the mediastinum are devastating. Because of the extensive, thin areolar planes between major structures, infections in a limited portion of the mediastinum may spread vertically or horizontally and become extensive. Synergistic aerobic and anaerobic infections from the perforated esophagus are particularly life-threatening. Treatment consists of surgical drainage and antibiotics.

Specific clinical syndromes may occur as a result of mediastinal tumors. Physical examination may reveal swelling of the head, neck, or upper extremities. Dyspnea may result from compression of the trachea, bronchus, or a portion of the lung parenchyma. Recurrent respiratory symptoms may occur for some time, until a chest x-ray is obtained and the abnormality identified. Postobstructive pneumonitis or infection of benign pericardial or enteric duplication cysts may produce fever or sepsis. Myasthenia gravis may result from thymomas. In addition, thymomas may result in autoimmune problems, such as hypogammaglobulinemia, red cell aplasia, and smooth muscle degeneration. Mediastinal Hodgkin's disease may produce an intermittent fever (Pel-Ebstein symptom). Patients with hypertension from pheochromocytoma, thyrotoxicosis from goiter, hypercalcemia from ectopic mediastinal parathyroid adenoma or carcinoma, or hypogammaglobulinemia should be evaluated carefully; mediastinal findings may affect subsequent therapeutic recommendations.

### Evaluation and Diagnostic Imaging

Diagnostic imaging typically includes a plain chest x-ray taken in two planes, posteroanterior and left lateral, which provides basic information about the location of the mass within the mediastinum. Given the known propensity of specific lesions to occur in the anterior, visceral (middle), or paravertebral sulcus (posterior), based on the anatomy and embryologic development of cervicothoracic organs, a differential diagnosis may be obtained.

A diaphragm fluoroscopy, or sniff test, is used to evaluate paradoxical motion of the diaphragm on rapid inspiration indicative of phrenic nerve paralysis. CT of the chest has replaced plain chest radiography as the diagnostic procedure of choice for mediastinal masses. MRI may enhance the diagnostic abilities of chest CT. Anterior mediastinal masses such as thymoma can be evaluated for the extent of compression or possible invasion into the pulmonary artery, innominate vein, or superior vena cava. Evaluation of the extent of invasion into the brachial plexus, great vessels, vertebral body, neural foramina, and spinal column may be easily accomplished with MRI.

Echocardiography and FDG-PET have been commonly used. High FDG uptake is more likely to correlate with invasion in thymic carcinomas and invasive thymomas.

Mediastinal tumors may secrete specific hormones or biologic markers. Parathyroid adenomas or functioning parathyroid carcinomas may secrete parathormone. Pheochromocytomas may secrete various catecholamines (in serum and urine), which might cause hypertension. Carcinomas may secrete CEA. Nonseminomatous germ cell neoplasms may secrete $\alpha$-fetoprotein or $\beta$-human chorionic gonadotropin ($\beta$-hCG). Skin tests for tuberculosis, histoplasmosis, and coccidioidomycosis may also yield positive results. Other diagnostic tests for mediastinal tuberculosis include sputum cytology, plain chest x-ray, and urine cytology.

**Histologic Diagnosis** A mediastinal mass cannot be treated until a diagnosis is obtained. Although radiographic diagnosis may suffice for mediastinal cysts, tissue for definitive diagnosis is needed for solid masses. FNA or needle biopsy with CT guidance of a mediastinal mass may provide sufficient tissue for diagnosis of thymic carcinoma or other defined neoplasms. For lymphomas in particular, and thymomas and neural tumors, larger amounts of tissue may be required for cellular analysis. In these patients, core needle biopsy, mediastinoscopy, or intrathoracic biopsy (via thoracoscopy or open thoracotomy) may be considered. Electron microscopy may be required for confirmation of specific histologies. For recurrent lymphomas following chemotherapy, an open technique for incisional biopsy is often required.

Median sternotomy provides a direct visual approach to the mediastinum and may be used for treatment of a wide range of mediastinal diseases. VATS and robotic techniques of resection are increasingly beings used for treatment of these noninvasive tumors. More extensive approaches include the transverse sternotomy or "clam-shell" incision. Anesthetic considerations should include avoidance of airway obstruction, awake-intubation, and avoidance of muscle paralytics or drugs such as fluoroquinolones with potential paralytic effects.

### Types of Mediastinal Cysts and Tumors

**Primary Cysts** Primary cysts of the mediastinum account for approximately 20% of mediastinal masses in most collected series. Cysts are characterized by the organ of origin and may be bronchogenic, pericardial, enteric, thymic, or of an unspecified nature. More than 75% of patients are asymptomatic, and these tumors rarely cause morbidity; however, with proximity to vital structures within the mediastinum and increasing size, the cyst may cause significant problems. A diagnosis for benign or malignant characteristics is needed. Benign cysts may be resected with minimally invasive techniques.

Bronchogenic cysts account most the primary cysts of the mediastinum (see Fig. 58-9). They originate as sequestrations from the ventral foregut, the antecedent of the tracheobronchial tree, and can be situated within the lung parenchyma or mediastinum. Bronchogenic cysts are usually located proximal to the trachea or bronchi and may be just posterior to the carina. A connection to the bronchus rarely exists; however, when it occurs, these cysts may become infected. Diagnostic imaging may reveal an air-fluid level within the mediastinum. Two thirds of bronchogenic cysts are asymptomatic. In infants, cysts cause severe respiratory compromise by compressing the trachea or the bronchus. Resection is recommended.

Pericardial cysts are second in frequency to bronchogenic cysts and occur in the cardiophrenic angle, mostly on the right (70%). These cysts may or may not communicate with the pericardium. Typically, clear fluid is encountered. The characteristics of pericardial cysts include location in the cardiophrenic angle, characteristic appearance, smooth borders, and attenuation approximating that of water for the cyst fluid. Needle aspiration and routine surveillance may be all that is needed. Resection may be used for diagnosis and to exclude malignant tumors.

Enteric cysts or duplication cysts arise from the primitive foregut, which develops into the upper division of the GI tract. These cysts are usually attached to the esophagus. Symptoms occur as size increases, with compression of the esophagus and dysphagia. Neuroenteric cysts are associated with anomalies of the vertebral column. Excision is recommended.

#### Primary Mediastinal Neoplasms

***Thymoma*** The pathology of thymoma has been recently reviewed.[123] Thymoma is the most common neoplasm of the anterosuperior compartment. The peak incidence is in the third through fifth decades, but may occur throughout adulthood. Thymoma is rare in the first 2 decades of life. On a radiograph, the thymoma may appear as a small, well-circumscribed mass or as a bulky lobulated mass confluent with adjacent mediastinal structures (Fig. 58-26). Symptoms at presentation would be related to local mass effects causing chest pain, dyspnea, hemoptysis, cough, and the superior vena cava syndrome or systemic syndromes caused by immunologic mechanisms. The most common syndrome is myasthenia gravis; others include pure red blood cell aplasia, pure white blood cell aplasia, aplastic anemia, Cushing's syndrome, hypogammaglobulinemia, hypergammaglobulinemia, dermatomyositis, systemic lupus erythematosus, progressive systemic sclerosis, hypercoagulopathy with thrombosis, rheumatoid arthritis, megaesophagus, and granulomatous myocarditis. Early surgical treatment of myasthenia gravis and small thymomas is often carried out. When thymectomy is performed early in the course of myasthenia gravis, a greater percentage of thymomas are benign.

Differentiation between benign and malignant disease is determined by the presence of gross invasion of adjacent structures, metastasis, or microscopic evidence of capsular invasion. Tumors smaller than 3 cm are frequently benign; however, determination of malignancy (invasion) can be challenging for patients with tumors from 3 to 5 cm in size. For tumors larger than 5 cm, a malignant process may be present.

Whenever possible, treatment for thymoma is excision, without removing or injuring vital structures.[124] Even with well-encapsulated thymomas, extended thymectomy with eradication of all accessible mediastinal fatty areolar tissue is performed to ensure removal of all ectopic thymic tissue and lower the risk of tumor recurrence. Protection and preservation of the phrenic nerves are integral components of thymectomy.

The perioperative management in patients with myasthenia gravis is extremely important to prevent complications. Anticholinesterase inhibitors are discontinued to decrease the amount of pulmonary secretions and prevent inadvertent cholinergic weakness. Plasmapheresis is used routinely within 72 hours of thymectomy. In most patients, plasmapheresis is effective in controlling generalized weakness.

Survival is based on stage. Stage I tumor is characterized as a well-encapsulated tumor, without evidence of gross or microscopic capsular invasion; stage II tumor exhibits pericapsular growth into adjacent fat or mediastinal pleura or microscopic invasion of the thymic capsule; stage III tumor invades adjacent organs; stage IVa tumor is characterized by intrathoracic metastases; and stage IVb tumor is characterized by extrathoracic metastases (uncommon). Complete resection (R0) is required and, for patients with stage I thymoma, resection alone is sufficient, without the need for adjuvant therapy. The use of adjuvant radiation therapy for stages II and III disease is common practice. Tumors larger than 5 cm, locally invasive tumors, unresectable tumors, and metastatic tumors are treated according to protocols that include chemotherapy followed by surgical exploration, with the goal of complete resection and postoperative (adjuvant) radiation therapy. Cisplatin-based regimens have excellent response rates.[125]

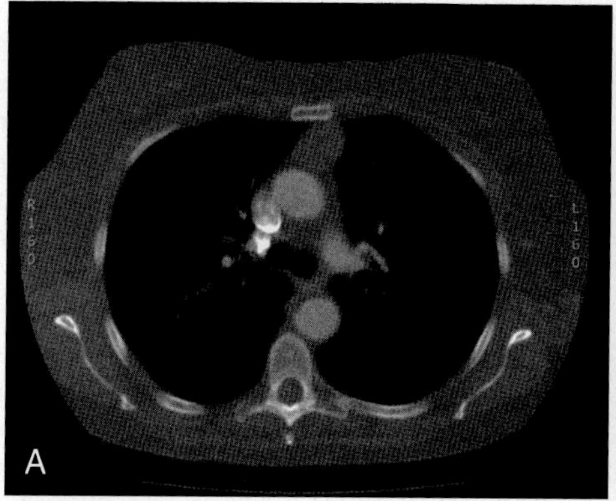


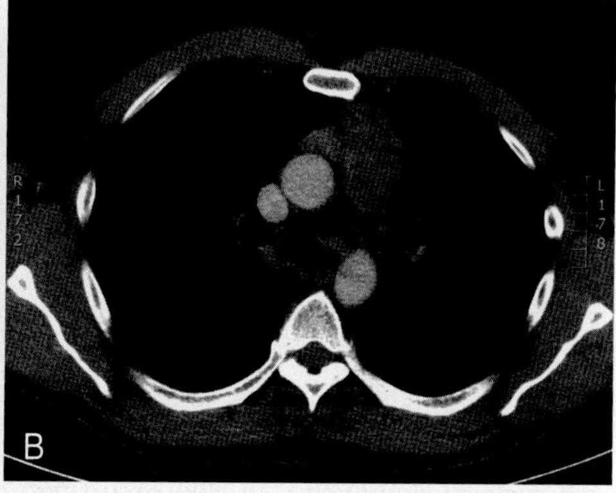


**FIGURE 58-26 A,** CT Chest in a patient with myasthenia gravis and thymoma. The thymoma is small with a plane of separation between the tumor and the pericardium. **B,** CT Chest in a patient with a larger mediastinal mass. The location, character, and size are noted. Transthoracic core needle biopsy was performed. Germ cell tumor markers were normal. Pathology demonstrated thymoma. Subsequently, a 6.5 cm thymoma was resected. There was no invasion of the pericardium. A complete resection (R0) was accomplished.

Invasive thymomas require radical resection of involved structures, which may include vascular reconstruction of the superior vena cava, innominate vein, or its branches.[126] Using this aggressive approach to obtain complete resection, a significant difference in 5-year survival rates has been seen in patients with stage III thymomas (94%) compared with those with incomplete resections (35%). Thymomas frequently recur and reoperation for recurrent disease has been recommended.

**Germ Cell Tumors** Germ cell tumors arise from primordial germ cells that fail to complete the migration from the urogenital ridge and rest in the mediastinum. The anterosuperior mediastinum is the most common extragonadal primary site of these tumors. Although these lesions are identical histologically to germ cell tumors originating in the gonads, they are not considered metastatic from primary gonadal tumors. The current recommendations for evaluating the testes of a patient with mediastinal germ cell tumor are careful physical examination and ultrasonography of the testes. Biopsy is reserved for positive findings. Blind biopsy or orchiectomy is contraindicated.

**Teratomas** Teratomas are the most common mediastinal germ cell neoplasms and are usually located in the anterosuperior mediastinum. They are composed of multiple tissue elements derived from the three primitive embryonic layers foreign to the area in which they occur. The peak incidence is in the second and third decades of life. There is no gender predisposition. Radiographic evidence of normal tissue (e.g., well-formed teeth or globular calcifications, a fatty mass) in an abnormal location can be considered specific. The teratodermoid (dermoid) cyst is the simplest form of a teratoma and composed of derivatives of the epidermal layer, including dermal and epidermal glands, hair, and sebaceous material. Teratomas are histologically more complex. The solid component of the tumor often contains well-differentiated elements of bone, cartilage, teeth, muscle, connective tissue, fibrous and lymphoid tissue, nerve, thymus, mucous and salivary glands, lung, liver, or pancreas. Malignant tumors are differentiated from benign tumors by the presence of primitive (embryonic) tissue or of malignant components. Immature teratomas contain combinations of mature epithelial and connective tissues, with immature areas of mesenchymal and neuroectodermal tissues. Teratomas with malignant components are divided into categories based on the elements present.

Diagnosis and therapy rely on surgical excision. For benign tumors that are so large or with involvement of adjacent mediastinal structures so that complete resection is impossible, partial resection can lead to the resolution of symptoms, frequently without relapse. For malignant teratomas, chemotherapy and radiation therapy, combined with surgical excision, are individualized for the type of malignant components contained in the tumors. The overall prognosis is poor for malignant teratomas

**Malignant Nonteratomatous Germ Cell Tumors** Malignant germ cell tumors occur predominantly in the anterosuperior mediastinum with a marked male predominance, usually occurring in the third and fourth decades of life.[127] Most patients have symptoms of chest pain, cough, dyspnea, and hemoptysis; the superior vena cava syndrome occurs commonly. A large anterior mediastinal mass is identified on diagnostic imaging. To determine intrathoracic spread of disease. CT and MRI are helpful to define the extent of disease and involvement of mediastinal structures. Serologic measurements of α-fetoprotein and β-hCG are useful for differentiating seminomas from nonseminomas tumors, assessing response to therapy, and diagnosing relapse or failure of therapy. Seminomas rarely produce β-hCG and never produce α-fetoprotein; in contrast, more than 90% of nonseminomas secrete one or both of these hormones. This differentiation is important because seminomas are radiosensitive and nonseminomas are relatively radiosensitive.

**Seminomas** Seminomas constitute 50% of malignant germ cell tumors; they usually remain intrathoracic. Symptoms are related to the mechanical effects of the tumor on adjacent mediastinal and pulmonary structures. The superior vena cava syndrome occurs in 10% to 20% of patients. These tumors are sensitive to irradiation and chemotherapy. Therapy is determined by the stage of the disease. Cytoreductive resection before chemotherapy or radiation therapy is unnecessary. Treatment consists of systemic and local therapy—chemotherapy with salvage surgery or combined chemoradiotherapy. Radiation therapy may be considered for early-stage disease, but is not recommended for regional disease. Platinum-based chemotherapy is common. Occasionally, excision is possible without injury to vital structures and can be recommended. When complete resection is possible, the use of adjuvant therapy is unnecessary. When excision is not possible, a biopsy sample of sufficient size to establish the diagnosis is obtained.

**Nonseminomatous Tumors** Malignant nonseminomatous germ cell tumors include choriocarcinomas, embryonal cell carcinomas, immature teratomas, teratomas with malignant components, and endodermal cell (yolk sac) tumors, which occur mostly in men in their third or fourth decade. Diagnostic imaging reveals a large anterior mediastinal mass with frequent extension to the lung, chest wall, and mediastinal structures. Nonseminomatous germ cell neoplasms are more aggressive tumors and more frequently disseminated at the time of diagnosis, they are rarely radiosensitive, and more than 90% produce β-hCG or α-fetoprotein. All patients with choriocarcinoma and some patients with embryonal cell tumors have elevated levels of β-HCG. The α-fetoprotein level is usually elevated in patients with embryonal cell carcinomas and yolk sac tumors. Mediastinal nonseminomas, but not testicular germ cell tumors, are associated with the development of rare hematologic malignancies, such as acute megakaryocytic leukemia, systemic mast cell disease, and malignant histiocytosis, as well as other hematologic abnormalities, including myelodysplastic syndrome and idiopathic thrombocytopenia refractory to treatment.

Currently, treatment of these nonseminomatous tumors is with cisplatin and etoposide-based regimens. Advanced disease, invasion into thoracic structures, and metastasis preclude surgical resection. Serum markers, α-fetoprotein or β-HCG, are followed to assess response to systemic treatment. If a complete serologic and radiologic response is achieved, patients are closely observed. If the disease progresses during therapy, salvage chemotherapy is initiated. Operative intervention may be required to establish a histologic diagnosis in patients without elevations in serum α-fetoprotein or β-HCG levels, for salvage resection after tissue, or for serologic response to therapy.[128] The pathology of the resected postchemotherapy specimen appears to be the most significant predictor of survival. The presence of residual disease after chemotherapy portends a poor prognosis and the need for additional chemotherapy. When tumor necrosis or a benign teratoma is found during surgical exploration after chemotherapy, an excellent or intermediate prognosis is conferred, respectively.

**Neurogenic Tumors** Neurogenic tumors are usually located in the posterior mediastinum and originate from the sympathetic ganglia (ganglioma, ganglioneuroblastoma, and neuroblastoma), intercostal nerves (neurofibroma, neurilemoma, and neurosarcoma), and paraganglia cells (paraganglioma). Although the peak incidence occurs in adults, neurogenic tumors make up a proportionally greater percentage of mediastinal masses in children. Most neurogenic tumors in adults are benign, but a greater percentage of neurogenic tumors are malignant in children.

The most common neurogenic tumor is the neurilemoma or schwannoma, which originates from perineural Schwann cells. They are benign, slow-growing neoplasms that frequently arise from a spinal nerve root, but can involve any thoracic nerve. These tumors are well circumscribed and have a defined capsule. They arise from the nerve sheath and compress the nerve fibers extrinsically. The peak incidence of these tumors is in the third through fifth decades of life, with men and women being equally affected.

Many of these tumors are asymptomatic. Symptoms such as pain occur from compression or invasion of intercostal nerve, bone, and chest wall, cough and dyspnea are caused by compression of the tracheobronchial tree, and Pancoast syndrome and Horner's syndrome result from involvement of the brachial and the cervical sympathetic chain. Approximately 10% of neurogenic tumors have extensions into the spinal column. They are termed *dumbbell tumors* because of their characteristic shape, with relatively large paraspinal and intraspinal portions connected by a narrow isthmus of tissue traversing the intervertebral foramen. Patients with paraspinal tumors should have an MRI scan to evaluate the presence and extent of the tumor and its relationship to the neural foramen and intraspinal space. During resection, the intraspinal component should be removed first via a posterior laminectomy. This approach minimizes the potential for spinal column hematoma, cord ischemia, and paralysis. A separate transthoracic approach is then needed for resection of the intrathoracic component.

Neuroblastomas originate from the sympathetic nervous system. The most common location for a neuroblastoma is in the retroperitoneum; however, 10% to 20% occur primarily in the mediastinum. These are highly invasive neoplasms that have frequently metastasized before diagnosis. Most of these tumors occur in children 4 years of age or younger. A 24-hour urine collection to measure catecholamine levels is obtained in children with a posterior mediastinal mass. Therapy is determined by the stage of the disease—stage I, surgical excision; stage II, excision and radiation therapy; stages III and IV, multimodality therapy using surgical debulking, radiation therapy, and multiagent chemotherapy as well as a second-look exploration to resect residual disease, when necessary. Chemotherapeutic agents include cisplatin, vincristine, doxorubicin, cyclophosphamide, and etoposide.

**Ganglion Tumors** Ganglioneuroblastomas are composed of mature and immature ganglion cells. Treatment ranges from surgical excision alone to various chemotherapeutic strategies, depending on histologic characteristics, age at diagnosis, and stage of disease. Ganglioneuromas are benign tumors originating from the sympathetic chain that are composed of ganglion cells and nerve fibers. These tumors typically present at an early age and are the most common neurogenic tumors occurring during childhood. The usual location is the paravertebral region. These tumors are well encapsulated and, when cross-sectioned, frequently exhibit areas of cystic degeneration. Surgical excision is curative.

**Paraganglioma (Pheochromocytoma)** Mediastinal paragangliomas are rare tumors, representing less than 1% of all mediastinal tumors and less than 2% of all pheochromocytomas. Although most are found in the paravertebral sulcus, an increasing number occur in the branchial arch structures, coronary and aortopulmonary paraganglia, atria, and islands of tissue in the pericardium. Although adrenal pheochromocytomas often produce epinephrine and norepinephrine, extra-adrenal paragangliomas rarely secrete epinephrine. Multiple paragangliomas will occur in 10% of patients. These tumors are more common in patients with multiple endocrine neoplasia syndrome, family history of disease, and Carney's syndrome (pulmonary chondroma, gastric leiomyosarcoma, and functioning extra-adrenal paraganglioma). In patients who have had excision of an adrenal pheochromocytoma and continue to have symptoms, a search for an extra-adrenal lesion is undertaken, with careful attention to the mediastinum. Tumor localization has improved through the use of CT and $^{131}$I-metaiodobenzylguanidine (MIBG) scintigraphy, particularly when the tumors are hormonally active. When appropriate, surgical resection is the optimal therapy. In patients with tumors involving the middle mediastinum, cardiopulmonary bypass may be necessary to enable resection. Preoperative embolization to reduce perioperative bleeding may be considered. Although 50% of tumors appear malignant morphologically, metastatic disease rarely develops.

**Lymphomas** Although the mediastinum is frequently involved in patients with lymphoma at some time during the course of their disease, it is infrequently the sole site of disease at the time of presentation. Hodgkin's and non-Hodgkin's lymphoma are distinct clinical entities with overlapping features. Patients usually have symptoms; chest pain, cough, dyspnea, hoarseness, and superior vena caval syndrome are the most common clinical manifestations. Nonspecific systemic symptoms of fever and chills, weight loss, and anorexia are frequently noted and are important in the staging of patients with Hodgkin's lymphoma. Symptoms characteristic of Hodgkin's lymphoma include chest pain after consumption of alcohol and the cyclic fevers first described by Pel and Ebstein.

Surgical excision of all disease is rarely possible, and the surgeon's primary role is to provide sufficient tissue for diagnosis and to assist in pathologic staging. A needle biopsy is often unsuccessful because larger tissue samples are needed to make a histologic diagnosis, particularly with nodular sclerosing lesions. Thoracoscopy, mediastinoscopy, or mediastinotomy and, rarely, thoracotomy or median sternotomy may be necessary to obtain sufficient tissue. The role of staging laparotomy has been minimized, and its only current indication is for patients with clinically limited disease who opt for limited treatment.

Patients with non-Hodgkin's lymphoma usually have symptoms because of involvement of adjacent mediastinal structures. Superior vena caval syndrome is relatively common. Lymphoblastic lymphoma occurs predominantly in children, adolescents, and young adults and represents 60% of cases of mediastinal non-Hodgkin's lymphoma.

After treatment of lymphomas, residual radiographic abnormalities within the mediastinum are commonly noted (64%-88%). CT cannot differentiate fibrosis or necrosis from residual tumor. FDG-PET has shown promise as a noninvasive way to detect active mediastinal disease and predict relapse in patients with lymphoma but tissue confirmation is required. Needle biopsy does not provide significant diagnostic material. Transthoracic incisional biopsy under general anesthesia is often needed given the significant fibrosis which remains after therapy.

## Endocrine Tumors

### Thyroid Tumors

Although substernal extension of a cervical goiter is common, totally intrathoracic thyroid tumors are rare and make up only 1% of all mediastinal masses in collected series. These tumors arise from heterotopic thyroid tissue, which occurs most commonly in the anterosuperior mediastinum but may also occur in the middle mediastinum between the trachea and esophagus as well as in the posterior mediastinum. Although there may be a demonstrable connection with the cervical gland (usually a fibrous connective tissue band), a true intrathoracic thyroid gland derives its blood supply from thoracic vessels. Substernal extensions of a cervical goiter can usually be excised using a cervical approach.

### Parathyroid Tumors

Although parathyroid glands may occur in the mediastinum in 10% of patients, they are usually accessible through the cervical incision. Most often, these adenomas are found in the anterosuperior mediastinum (80%) embedded in or near the superior pole of the thymus. This anatomic relationship is the result of the common embryogenesis of the inferior parathyroid glands from the third branchial cleft. The superior parathyroid glands and the lateral lobes of the thyroid gland are derived from the fourth branchial pouch. Because they migrate with the lateral lobes of the thyroid gland to a paraesophageal position, parathyroid adenomas can also be found in the posterior mediastinum.

Most frequently, the mediastinal parathyroid adenoma may be excised after a negative exploration of the cervical region, through the existing cervical incision. Usually, the vascular supply extends from cervical blood vessels. In patients with persistent hyperparathyroidism after cervical exploration if localization studies show residual parathyroid in the mediastinum, mediastinal exploration using a median sternotomy or thoracoscopy is indicated.

Parathyroid carcinomas have been reported and are usually hormonally active. Patients differ in clinical presentation in that they often have higher serum calcium levels and manifest more severe symptoms of hyperparathyroidism. When possible, resection is the optimal therapy.

### Neuroendocrine Tumors

Mediastinal neuroendocrine tumors, carcinoid tumors, arise from cells of Kulchitsky located in the thymus commonly occur in men in their 40s and 50s and are usually located in the anterosuperior mediastinum. These tumors are aggressive and 20% have metastatic spread to mediastinal and cervical lymph nodes, liver, bone, skin, and lungs and presentation. Over fifty percent of thymic neuroendocrine tumors are hormonally active, often associated with Cushing's syndrome because of production of adrenocorticotropic hormone, less frequently associated with multiple endocrine neoplasia syndromes, and only rarely associated with carcinoid syndrome (0.6%). If possible, resection is recommended; however, local invasion and metastasis often precludes complete excision. Adjuvant therapy is controversial, but irradiation should probably be added, particularly in patients with capsular invasion.

## SELECTED REFERENCES

Colice GL, Shafazand S, Griffin JP, et al: Physiologic evaluation of the patient with lung cancer being considered for resectional surgery: ACCP evidenced-based clinical practice guidelines (2nd edition). Chest 132:161S–177S, 2007.

National Comprehensive Cancer Network: NCCN Clinical Practice Guidelines in Oncology. Non-small cell lung cancer, 2011 (http://www.nccn.org/professionals/physician_gls/f_guidelines.asp).

Guidelines for diagnosis, treatment, and surveillance are published by various organizations based on evidence and consensus of experts. Two sets of recent guidelines for the management of non–small cell lung cancer have been published by the American College of Chest Physicians and the National Comprehensive Cancer Network.

The National Lung Screening Trial Research Team: Reduced lung-cancer mortality with low-dose computed tomographic screening. N Engl J Med 365:395–409, 2011.

Screening for lung cancer was evaluated by the National Lung Screening Trial. Fewer lung cancer–related deaths occurred in the CT-screened population compared with the chest x-ray–screened population.

Arriagada R, Bergman B, Dunant A, et al: Cisplatin-based adjuvant chemotherapy in patients with completely resected non–small-cell lung cancer. N Engl J Med 350:351–360, 2004.

Adjuvant therapy following complete resection of NSCLC has been shown to improve survival in selected patients. The International Lung Adjuvant Trial (IALT) proved that adjuvant platinum-based chemotherapy improved survival compared with no treatment.

Dresler CM, Olak J, Herndon JE 2nd, et al: Phase III intergroup study of talc poudrage vs talc slurry sclerosis for malignant pleural effusion. Chest 127:909–915, 2005.

A prospective randomized study evaluating chest tube with talc slurry versus VATS with talc poudrage. Both groups benefited from the intervention, neither was superior. VATS has the advantage of complete drainage, pleural biopsy, and direct placement of talc.

Goldstraw P, Crowley J, Chansky K, et al: The IASLC Lung Cancer Staging Project: Proposals for the revision of the TNM stage groupings in the forthcoming (seventh) edition of the TNM classification of malignant tumours. J Thorac Oncol 2:706–714, 2007.

Edge SB, Byrd DR, Compton CC, et al: AJCC cancer staging manual, ed 7, New York, 2010, Springer.

Pao W: Defining clinically relevant molecular subsets of lung cancer. Cancer Chemother Pharmacol 58(Suppl 1):S11–S15, 2006.

Staging for non–small cell lung carcinoma has changed significantly with the results of the International Association for the Study of Lung Cancer Staging Project. This data set was predominantly surgery-based but international in extent and internally and externally validated. These results have formed the basis for the AJCC and UICC staging systems. Future staging systems may evaluate the molecular characteristics of the tumor as prognostic (of survival) and predictive (of response) characteristics.

Fernando HC, Schuchert M, Landreneau R, et al: Approaching the high-risk patient: Sublobar resection, stereotactic body radiation therapy, or radiofrequency ablation. Ann Thorac Surg 89:S2123–S2127, 2010.

Timmerman R, Paulus R, Galvin J, et al: Stereotactic body radiation therapy for inoperable early stage lung cancer. JAMA 303:1070–1076, 2010.

New methods of local control of NSCLC are being studied. This recent review of local treatment options evaluated sublobar resection, stereotactic body radiation therapy, and radiofrequency. Clinical trials are underway to evaluate these treatment options prospectively.

Walsh GL, Davis BM, Swisher SG, et al: A single-institutional, multidisciplinary approach to primary sarcomas involving the chest wall requiring full-thickness resections. J Thorac Cardiovasc Surg 121:48–60, 2001.

One of the largest series on primary chest wall tumors.

## REFERENCES


1. Baser S, Shannon VR, Eapen GA, et al: Pulmonary dysfunction as a major cause of inoperability among patients with non-small-cell lung cancer. Clin Lung Cancer 7:344–349, 2006.
2. Bluman LG, Mosca L, Newman N, et al: Preoperative smoking habits and postoperative pulmonary complications. Chest 113:883–889, 1998.
3. Thomsen T, Villebro N, Moller AM: Interventions for preoperative smoking cessation. Cochrane Database Syst Rev (7):CD002294, 2010.
4. Mason DP, Subramanian S, Nowicki ER, et al: Impact of smoking cessation before resection of lung cancer: A Society of Thoracic Surgeons General Thoracic Surgery Database study. Ann Thorac Surg 88:362–370, 2009.
5. Colice GL, Shafazand S, Griffin JP, et al: Physiologic evaluation of the patient with lung cancer being considered for resectional surgery: ACCP evidenced-based clinical practice guidelines (2nd edition). Chest 132:161S–177S, 2007.
6. Poonyagariyagorn H, Mazzone PJ: Lung cancer: preoperative pulmonary evaluation of the lung resection candidate. Semin Respir Crit Care Med 29:271–284, 2008.
7. Beckles MA, Spiro SG, Colice GL, et al: The physiologic evaluation of patients with lung cancer being considered for resectional surgery. Chest 123:105S–114S, 2003.
8. Walsh GL, Morice RC, Putnam JB, Jr, et al: Resection of lung cancer is justified in high-risk patients selected by exercise oxygen consumption. Ann Thorac Surg 58:704–710, 1994.
9. Brunelli A, Sabbatini A, Xiume F, et al: Inability to perform maximal stair climbing test before lung resection: a propensity score analysis on early outcome. Eur J Cardiothorac Surg 27:367–372, 2005.
10. Mendeloff EN: Sequestrations, congenital cystic adenomatoid malformations, and congenital lobar emphysema. Semin Thorac Cardiovasc Surg 16:209–214, 2004.
11. Jaquiss RD: Management of pediatric tracheal stenosis and tracheomalacia. Semin Thorac Cardiovasc Surg 16:220–224, 2004.
12. Pegoli W, Mattei P, Colombani PM: Congenital intrathoracic vascular abnormalities in childhood. Chest Surg Clin North Am 3:529–546, 1993.
13. Maldonado JA, Henry T, Gutierrez FR: Congenital thoracic vascular anomalies. Radiol Clin North Am 48:85–115, 2010.
14. Bonnard A, Auber F, Fourcade L, et al: Vascular ring abnormalities: A retrospective study of 62 cases. J Pediatr Surg 38:539–543, 2003.
15. Jemal A, Siegel R, Xu J, et al: Cancer statistics, 2010. CA Cancer J Clin 60:277–300, 2010.
16. Field RW: Environmental factors in cancer: Radon. Rev Environ Health 25:23–31, 2010.
17. U.S. National Institutes of Health: 2011 (http://clinicaltrials.gov).
18. National Cancer Institute: NCI's clinical trials cooperative group program, 2011, (http://www.cancer.gov/cancertopics/factsheet/NCI/clinical-trials-cooperative-group).
19. Travis WD, Brambilla E, Muller-Hermelink HK, et al, editors: World Health Organization classification of tumours. Pathology and genetics of tumours of the lung, pleura, thymus, and heart. Lyon, France, 2004, IARC Press, pp 10–124.
20. Motoi N, Szoke J, Riely GJ, et al: Lung adenocarcinoma: Modification of the 2004 WHO mixed subtype to include the major histologic subtype suggests correlations between papillary and micropapillary adenocarcinoma subtypes, EGFR mutations and gene expression analysis. Am J Surg Pathol 32:810–827, 2008.
21. Travis WD, Garg K, Franklin WA, et al: Bronchioloalveolar carcinoma and lung adenocarcinoma: The clinical importance and research relevance of the 2004 World Health Organization pathologic criteria. J Thorac Oncol 1:S13–S19, 2006.
22. The National Lung Screening Trial Research Team: Reduced lung-cancer mortality with low-dose computed tomographic screening. N Engl J Med 365:395–409,2011.
23. Spiro SG, Gould MK, Colice GL: Initial evaluation of the patient with lung cancer: Symptoms, signs, laboratory tests, and paraneoplastic syndromes: ACCP evidenced-based clinical practice guidelines (2nd edition). Chest 132:149S–160S, 2007.
24. Alberts WM: Introduction: Diagnosis and management of lung cancer: ACCP evidence-based clinical practice guidelines (2nd Edition). Chest 132:20S–22S, 2007.
25. Gould MK, Fletcher J, Iannettoni MD, et al: Evaluation of patients with pulmonary nodules: when is it lung cancer?: ACCP evidence-based clinical practice guidelines (2nd edition). Chest 132:108S–130S, 2007.
26. Ost D, Fein AM, Feinsilver SH: Clinical practice. The solitary pulmonary nodule. N Engl J Med 348:2535–2542, 2003.

27. Tan BB, Flaherty KR, Kazerooni EA, et al: The solitary pulmonary nodule. Chest 123:89S–96S, 2003.
28. Makris D, Scherpereel A, Leroy S, et al: Electromagnetic navigation diagnostic bronchoscopy for small peripheral lung lesions. Eur Respir J 29:1187–1192, 2007.
29. Goldstraw P, Crowley J, Chansky K, et al: The IASLC Lung Cancer Staging Project: Proposals for the revision of the TNM stage groupings in the forthcoming (seventh) edition of the TNM Classification of malignant tumours. J Thorac Oncol 2:706–714, 2007.
30. Silvestri GA, Gould MK, Margolis ML, et al: Noninvasive staging of non-small cell lung cancer: ACCP evidenced-based clinical practice guidelines (2nd edition). Chest 132:178S–201S, 2007.
31. Juweid ME, Cheson BD: Positron-emission tomography and assessment of cancer therapy. N Engl J Med 354:496–507, 2006.
32. Fischer B, Lassen U, Mortensen J, et al: Preoperative staging of lung cancer with combined PET-CT. N Engl J Med 361:32–39, 2009.
33. Reed CE, Harpole DH, Posther KE, et al: Results of the American College of Surgeons Oncology Group Z0050 trial: The utility of positron emission tomography in staging potentially operable non–small cell lung cancer. J Thorac Cardiovasc Surg 126:1943–1951, 2003.
34. Detterbeck FC, Jantz MA, Wallace M, et al: Invasive mediastinal staging of lung cancer: ACCP evidence-based clinical practice guidelines (2nd edition). Chest 132:202S–220S, 2007.
35. Yap KK, Yap KS, Byrne AJ, et al: Positron emission tomography with selected mediastinoscopy compared with routine mediastinoscopy offers cost and clinical outcome benefits for preoperative staging of non–small cell lung cancer. Eur J Nucl Med Mol Imaging 32:1033–1040, 2005.
36. Annema JT, van Meerbeeck JP, Rintoul RC, et al: Mediastinoscopy vs endosonography for mediastinal nodal staging of lung cancer: A randomized trial. JAMA 304:2245–2252, 2010.
37. Shepherd FA, Crowley J, Van Houtte P, et al; International Association for the Study of Lung Cancer International Staging Committee and Participating Institutions: The International Association for the Study of Lung Cancer lung cancer staging project: Proposals regarding the clinical staging of small cell lung cancer in the forthcoming (seventh) edition of the tumor, node, metastasis classification for lung cancer. J Thorac Oncol 2:1067–1077, 2007.
38. Edge SB, Byrd DR, Compton CC, et al: AJCC cancer staging manual, ed 7, New York, 2010, Springer.
39. Giroux DJ, Rami-Porta R, Chansky K, et al: The IASLC Lung Cancer Staging Project: Data elements for the prospective project. J Thorac Oncol 4:679–683, 2009.
40. American Joint Committee on Cancer: AJCC 7th edition staging posters, 2011 (http://www.cancerstaging.org/staging/index.html).
41. Rice TW, Murthy SC, Mason DP, et al: A cancer staging primer: Lung. J Thorac Cardiovasc Surg 139:826–829, 2010.
42. Rami-Porta R, Ball D, Crowley J, et al: The IASLC Lung Cancer Staging Project: Proposals for the revision of the T descriptors in the forthcoming (seventh) edition of the TNM classification for lung cancer. J Thorac Oncol 2:593–602, 2007.
43. Rusch VW, Crowley J, Giroux DJ, et al: The IASLC Lung Cancer Staging Project: Proposals for the revision of the N descriptors in the forthcoming seventh edition of the TNM classification for lung cancer. J Thorac Oncol 2:603–612, 2007.
44. Rusch VW, Asamura H, Watanabe H, et al: The IASLC lung cancer staging project: A proposal for a new international lymph node map in the forthcoming seventh edition of the TNM classification for lung cancer. J Thorac Oncol 4:568–577, 2009.
45. Postmus PE, Brambilla E, Chansky K, et al: The IASLC Lung Cancer Staging Project: Proposals for revision of the M descriptors in the forthcoming (seventh) edition of the TNM classification of lung cancer. J Thorac Oncol 2:686–693, 2007.
46. Timmerman R, Paulus R, Galvin J, et al: Stereotactic body radiation therapy for inoperable early stage lung cancer. JAMA 303:1070–1076, 2010.
47. Scott WJ, Howington J, Feigenberg S, et al: Treatment of non-small cell lung cancer stage I and stage II: ACCP evidence-based clinical practice guidelines (2nd edition). Chest 132:234S–242S, 2007.
48. Kozower BD, Sheng S, O'Brien SM, et al: STS database risk models: Predictors of mortality and major morbidity for lung cancer resection. Ann Thorac Surg 90:875–881, 2010.
49. Darling GE, Allen MS, Decker PA, et al: Randomized trial of mediastinal lymph node sampling versus complete lymphadenectomy during pulmonary resection in the patient with N0 or N1 (less than hilar) non–small cell carcinoma: Results of the American College of Surgery Oncology Group Z0030 Trial. J Thorac Cardiovasc Surg 141:662–670, 2011.
50. Schuchert MJ, Pettiford BL, Keeley S, et al: Anatomic segmentectomy in the treatment of stage I non–small cell lung cancer. Ann Thorac Surg 84:926–932, 2007.
51. Fernando HC, Schuchert M, Landreneau R, et al: Approaching the high-risk patient: Sublobar resection, stereotactic body radiation therapy, or radiofrequency ablation. Ann Thorac Surg 89:S2123–S2127, 2010.
52. Arriagada R, Bergman B, Dunant A, et al: Cisplatin-based adjuvant chemotherapy in patients with completely resected non–small-cell lung cancer. N Engl J Med 350:351–360, 2004.
53. Schiller JH, Harrington D, Belani CP, et al: Comparison of four chemotherapy regimens for advanced non–small-cell lung cancer. N Engl J Med 346:92–98, 2002.
54. Robinson LA, Ruckdeschel JC, Wagner H Jr, et al: Treatment of non-small cell lung cancer-stage IIIA: ACCP evidence-based clinical practice guidelines (2nd edition). Chest 132:243S–265S, 2007.
55. Pisters KM, Vallieres E, Crowley JJ, et al: Surgery with or without preoperative paclitaxel and carboplatin in early-stage non-small-cell lung cancer: Southwest Oncology Group Trial S9900, an intergroup, randomized, phase III trial. J Clin Oncol 28:1843–1849, 2010.
56. Albain KS, Swann RS, Rusch VW, et al: Radiotherapy plus chemotherapy with or without surgical resection for stage III non-small-cell lung cancer: A phase III randomised controlled trial. Lancet 374:379–386, 2009.
57. Komaki R, Roth JA, Walsh GL, et al: Outcome predictors for 143 patients with superior sulcus tumors treated by multidisciplinary approach at the University of Texas M.D. Anderson Cancer Center. Int J Radiat Oncol Biol Phys 48:347–354, 2000.
58. Martinod E, D'Audiffret A, Thomas P, et al: Management of superior sulcus tumors: Experience with 139 cases treated by surgical resection. Ann Thorac Surg 73:1534–1539, 2002.
59. Socinski MA, Crowell R, Hensing TE, et al: Treatment of non–small cell lung cancer, stage IV: ACCP evidence-based clinical

practice guidelines (2nd edition). Chest 132:277S–289S, 2007.

**60.** Sandler A, Gray R, Perry MC, et al: Paclitaxel-carboplatin alone or with bevacizumab for non–small-cell lung cancer. N Engl J Med 355:2542–2550, 2006.

**61.** Jett JR, Schild SE, Keith RL, et al: Treatment of non-small cell lung cancer, stage IIIB: ACCP evidence-based clinical practice guidelines (2nd edition). Chest 132:266S–276S, 2007.

**62.** Pao W: Defining clinically relevant molecular subsets of lung cancer. Cancer Chemother Pharmacol 58(Suppl 1):S11–S15, 2006.

**63.** Pao W, Girard N: New driver mutations in non–small-cell lung cancer. Lancet Oncol 12:175–180, 2011.

**64.** Takeda K, Hida T, Sato T, et al: Randomized phase III trial of platinum-doublet chemotherapy followed by gefitinib compared with continued platinum-doublet chemotherapy in Japanese patients with advanced non-small-cell lung cancer: Results of a west Japan thoracic oncology group trial (WJTOG0203). J Clin Oncol 28:753–760, 2010.

**65.** Mitsudomi T, Morita S, Yatabe Y, et al: Gefitinib versus cisplatin plus docetaxel in patients with non-small-cell lung cancer harbouring mutations of the epidermal growth factor receptor (WJTOG3405): An open label, randomised phase 3 trial. Lancet Oncol 11:121–128, 2010.

**66.** Kvale PA, Selecky PA, Prakash UB: Palliative care in lung cancer: ACCP evidence-based clinical practice guidelines (2nd edition). Chest 132:368S–403S, 2007.

**67.** Kornblith LZ, Burlew CC, Moore EE, et al: One thousand bedside percutaneous tracheostomies in the surgical intensive care unit: Time to change the gold standard. J Am Coll Surg 212:163–170, 2011.

**68.** Honings J, Gaissert HA, Ruangchira-Urai R, et al: Pathologic characteristics of resected squamous cell carcinoma of the trachea: Prognostic factors based on an analysis of 59 cases. Virchows Arch 455:423–429, 2009.

**69.** Webb BD, Walsh GL, Roberts DB, et al: Primary tracheal malignant neoplasms: The University of Texas MD Anderson Cancer Center experience. J Am Coll Surg 202:237–246, 2006.

**70.** Blumberg HM, Burman WJ, Chaisson RE, et al: American Thoracic Society/Centers for Disease Control and Prevention/Infectious Diseases Society of America: Treatment of tuberculosis. Am J Respir Crit Care Med 167:603–662, 2003.

**71.** Pezzella AT, Fang W: Surgical aspects of thoracic tuberculosis: A contemporary review—part 1. Curr Probl Surg 45:675–758, 2008.

**72.** Sihoe AD, Shiraishi Y, Yew WW: The current role of thoracic surgery in tuberculosis management. Respirology 14:954–968, 2009.

**73.** Regnard JF, Icard P, Nicolosi M, et al: Aspergilloma: A series of 89 surgical cases. Ann Thorac Surg 69:898–903, 2000.

**74.** Domej W, Hermann J, Krause R, et al: [Lung cavities, mycetomas and hemoptysis.] Wien Med Wochenschr 157:466–472, 2007.

**75.** Hage CA, Wheat LJ, Loyd J, et al: Pulmonary histoplasmosis. Semin Respir Crit Care Med 29:151–165, 2008.

**76.** Jeon K, Koh WJ, Kim H, et al: Clinical features of recently diagnosed pulmonary paragonimiasis in Korea. Chest 128:1423–1430, 2005.

**77.** Dudha M, Lehrman S, Aronow WS, et al: Hemoptysis: Diagnosis and treatment. Compr Ther 35:139–149, 2009.

**78.** Shigemura N, Wan IY, Yu SC, et al: Multidisciplinary management of life-threatening massive hemoptysis: A 10-year experience. Ann Thorac Surg 87:849–853, 2009.

**79.** Chun JY, Morgan R, Belli AM: Radiological management of hemoptysis: A comprehensive review of diagnostic imaging and bronchial arterial embolization. Cardiovasc Intervent Radiol 33:240–250, 2010.

**80.** Fishman A, Martinez F, Naunheim K, et al: A randomized trial comparing lung-volume-reduction surgery with medical therapy for severe emphysema. N Engl J Med 348:2059–2073, 2003.

**81.** Sanchez PG, Kucharczuk JC, Su S, et al: National Emphysema Treatment Trial redux: Accentuating the positive. J Thorac Cardiovasc Surg 140:564–572, 2010.

**82.** Verleden GM, Dupont LJ, Van Raemdonck DE, et al: Lung transplantation: A 15-year single-center experience. Clin Transpl 121–130, 2007.

**83.** Hertz MI, Aurora P, Christie JD, et al: Scientific Registry of the International Society for Heart and Lung Transplantation: Introduction to the 2010 annual reports. J Heart Lung Transplant 29:1083–1088, 2010.

**84.** Malhotra A: Low-tidal-volume ventilation in the acute respiratory distress syndrome. N Engl J Med 357:1113–1120, 2007.

**85.** Briel M, Meade M, Mercat A, et al: Higher vs lower positive end-expiratory pressure in patients with acute lung injury and acute respiratory distress syndrome: Systematic review and meta-analysis. JAMA 303:865–873, 2010.

**86.** Taccone P, Pesenti A, Latini R, et al: Prone positioning in patients with moderate and severe acute respiratory distress syndrome: A randomized controlled trial. JAMA 302:1977–1984, 2009.

**87.** Sternberg DI, Sonett JR: Surgical therapy of lung metastases. Semin Oncol 34:186–196, 2007.

**88.** Pastorino U, Buyse M, Friedel G, et al: Long-term results of lung metastasectomy: Prognostic analyses based on 5206 cases. J Thorac Cardiovasc Surg 113:37–47, 1997.

**89.** Internullo E, Cassivi SD, Van Raemdonck D, et al: Pulmonary metastasectomy: A survey of current practice amongst members of the European Society of Thoracic Surgeons. J Thorac Oncol 3:1257–1266, 2008.

**90.** Detterbeck FC: Management of carcinoid tumors. Ann Thorac Surg 89:998–1005, 2010.

**91.** Davini F, Gonfiotti A, Comin C, et al: Typical and atypical carcinoid tumours: 20-year experience with 89 patients. J Cardiovasc Surg (Torino) 50:807–811, 2009.

**92.** Maziak DE, Todd TR, Keshavjee SH, et al: Adenoid cystic carcinoma of the airway: Thirty-two-year experience. J Thorac Cardiovasc Surg 112:1522–1531, 1996.

**93.** Gaissert HA, Grillo HC, Shadmehr MB, et al: Long-term survival after resection of primary adenoid cystic and squamous cell carcinoma of the trachea and carina. Ann Thorac Surg 78:1889–1896, 2004.

**94.** Blackmon SH, Rice DC, Correa AM, et al: Management of primary pulmonary artery sarcomas. Ann Thorac Surg 87:977–984, 2009.

**95.** Huddleston CB: Pectus excavatum. Semin Thorac Cardiovasc Surg 16:225–232, 2004.

**96.** Walsh GL, Davis BM, Swisher SG, et al: A single-institutional, multidisciplinary approach to primary sarcomas involving the chest wall requiring full-thickness resections. J Thorac Cardiovasc Surg 121:48–60, 2001.

**97.** Chang RR, Mehrara BJ, Hu QY, et al: Reconstruction of complex oncologic chest wall defects: A 10-year experience. Ann Plast Surg 52:471–479, 2004.

**98.** Gross JL, Younes RN, Haddad FJ, et al: Soft-tissue sarcomas of the chest wall: prognostic factors. Chest 127:902–908, 2005.

**99.** Sanders RJ, Hammond SL, Rao NM: Diagnosis of thoracic outlet syndrome. J Vasc Surg 46:601–604, 2007.

**100.** Demondion X, Herbinet P, Van Sint Jan S, et al: Imaging assessment of thoracic outlet syndrome. Radiographics 26:1735–1750, 2006.

**101.** Povlsen B, Belzberg A, Hansson T, et al: Treatment for thoracic outlet syndrome. Cochrane Database Syst Rev (1):CD007218, 2010.

**102.** Colice GL, Curtis A, Deslauriers J, et al: Medical and surgical treatment of parapneumonic effusions: An evidence-based guideline. Chest 118:1158–1171, 2000.

**103.** Light RW, Macgregor MI, Luchsinger PC, et al: Pleural effusions: The diagnostic separation of transudates and exudates. Ann Intern Med 77:507–513, 1972.

**104.** Putnam JB, Jr, Light RW, Rodriguez RM, et al: A randomized comparison of indwelling pleural catheter and doxycycline pleurodesis in the management of malignant pleural effusions. Cancer 86:1992–1999, 1999.

**105.** Heffner JE, Nietert PJ, Barbieri C: Pleural fluid pH as a predictor of survival for patients with malignant pleural effusions. Chest 117:79–86, 2000.

**106.** Warren WH, Kalimi R, Khodadadian LM, et al: Management of malignant pleural effusions using the pleurx catheter. Ann Thoracic Surg 85:1049–1055, 2008.

**107.** Dresler CM, Olak J, Herndon JE, 2nd, et al: Phase III intergroup study of talc poudrage vs talc slurry sclerosis for malignant pleural effusion. Chest 127:909–915, 2005.

**108.** Brims FJ, Lansley SM, Waterer GW, et al: Empyema thoracis: New insights into an old disease. Eur Respir Rev 19:220–228, 2010.

**109.** Light RW: Parapneumonic effusions and empyema. Proc Am Thorac Soc 3:75–80, 2006.

**110.** Molnar TF: Current surgical treatment of thoracic empyema in adults. Eur J Cardiothorac Surg 32:422–430, 2007.

**111.** Coote N, Kay E: Surgical versus non-surgical management of pleural empyema. Cochrane Database Syst Rev (4):CD001956, 2005.

**112.** Deschamps C, Bernard A, Nichols FC, 3rd, et al: Empyema and bronchopleural fistula after pneumonectomy: Factors affecting incidence. Ann Thorac Surg 72:243–247, 2001.

**113.** Nair SK, Petko M, Hayward MP: Aetiology and management of chylothorax in adults. Eur J Cardiothorac Surg 32:362–369, 2007.

**114.** Cope C: Management of chylothorax via percutaneous embolization. Curr Opin Pulm Med 10:311–314, 2004.

**115.** Churg A, Roggli V, Galateau-Salle F, et al: Tumours of the pleura. In Travis WD, Brambilla E, Muller-Hermelink HK, et al, editors: World Health Organization Classification of tumours. Pathology and genetics of tumours of the lung, pleura, thymus, and heart. Lyon, France, 2004, IARC Press, pp 128–136.

**116.** Travis WD: Sarcomatoid neoplasms of the lung and pleura. Arch Pathol Lab Med 134:1645–1658, 2010.

**117.** Teh E, Fiorentino F, Tan C, et al: A systematic review of lung-sparing extirpative surgery for pleural mesothelioma. J R Soc Med 104:69–80, 2011.

**118.** Cao CQ, Yan TD, Bannon PG, et al: A systematic review of extrapleural pneumonectomy for malignant pleural mesothelioma. J Thorac Oncol 5:1692–1703, 2010.

**119.** Sugarbaker DJ, Wolf AS: Surgery for malignant pleural mesothelioma. Expert Rev Respir Med 4:363–372, 2010.

**120.** Ahamad A, Stevens CW, Smythe WR, et al: Intensity-modulated radiation therapy: A novel approach to the management of malignant pleural mesothelioma. Int J Radiat Oncol Biol Phys 55:768–775, 2003.

**121.** Whitten CR, Khan S, Munneke GJ, et al: A diagnostic approach to mediastinal abnormalities. Radiographics 27:657–671, 2007.

**122.** Donahue JM, Nichols FC: Primary mediastinal tumors and cysts and diagnostic investigation of mediastinal masses. In Shields TW, LoCicero J III, Reed CE, et al, editors: General thoracic surgery, ed 7, Philadelphia, 2009, Lippincott Williams & Wilkins, pp 2195–2199.

**123.** Müller-Hermelink HK, Engel P, Kuo TT, et al: Tumours of the Thymus. In Travis WD, Brambilla E, Muller-Hermelink HK, et al, editors: World Health Organization Classification of tumours. Pathology and genetics of tumours of the lung, pleura, thymus, and heart. Lyon, France, 2004, IARC Press, pp 148–151.

**124.** Falkson CB, Bezjak A, Darling G, et al: The management of thymoma: A systematic review and practice guideline. J Thorac Oncol 4:911–919, 2009.

**125.** Kim ES, Putnam JB, Komaki R, et al: Phase II study of a multidisciplinary approach with induction chemotherapy, followed by surgical resection, radiation therapy, and consolidation chemotherapy for unresectable malignant thymomas: Final report. Lung Cancer 44:369–379, 2004.

**126.** Wright CD: Extended resections for thymic malignancies. J Thorac Oncol 5:S344–S347, 2010.

**127.** Kesler KA, Einhorn LH: Multimodality treatment of germ cell tumors of the mediastinum. Thorac Surg Clin 19:63–69, 2009.

**128.** Walsh GL, Taylor GD, Nesbitt JC, et al: Intensive chemotherapy and radical resections for primary nonseminomatous mediastinal germ cell tumors. Ann Thorac Surg 69:337–343, 2000.

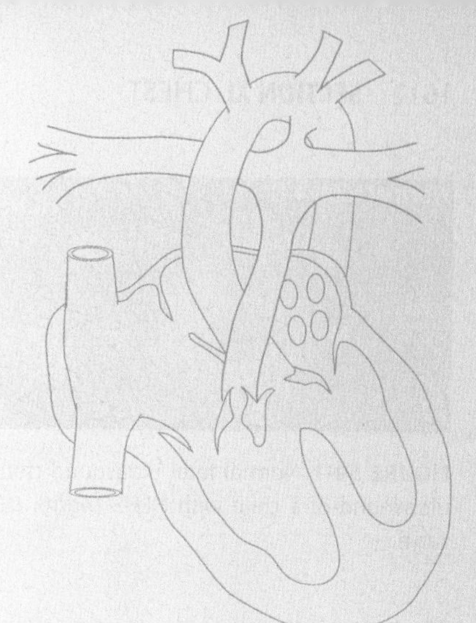

CHAPTER 59

# CONGENITAL HEART DISEASE

Charles D. Fraser, Jr., and Kathleen E. Carberry



This chapter is designed to provide medical students, general surgery residents, and practicing general surgeons with a working tool to aid in their understanding of the features of anatomy and physiology in patients presenting for general surgical procedures in the setting of repaired or unrepaired congenital cardiac lesions. The large scope and breadth of the evolving field of congenital heart surgery precludes an exhaustive treatise on all aspects of this specialty. Several excellent and thorough textbooks of congenital heart surgery will be referenced in this chapter, and the reader is encouraged to use them for additional in-depth understanding of the lesions to be reviewed. Today's practicing general surgeon needs to be well versed in the basics of cardiac anatomy, physiology, and specific derangements associated with the various known congenital cardiac lesions. Furthermore, there are few patients with complex congenital cardiac lesions who may be considered cured of their cardiac problem, even after successful reconstructive surgery. Thus, it is imperative that the general surgeon who needs to perform a noncardiac operation on such a patient be familiar with the specific issues of ongoing concern in those with congenital cardiac disease.

## HISTORY AND OTHER CONSIDERATIONS

The era of surgical treatment for congenital cardiac anomalies was initiated in November 1944, when Dr. Alfred Blalock and associates Vivien Thomas and Dr. Helen Taussig combined their unique talents and vision to treat a young child dying of cyanotic congenital heart disease (CHD).[1] This palliative operation involved the surgical creation of a systemic to pulmonary artery connection in the patient suffering from inadequate pulmonary blood flow. The procedure has since been recalled as miraculous and has carried the eponym of the Blalock-Taussig shunt (BT shunt) during the ensuing years, now more than 60 years later. The striking success of this simple concept and the reproducible nature of the operation in children suffering from otherwise fatal cardiac conditions has emboldened subsequent surgical innovators to venture inside the congenitally malformed heart. At first, a parent was asked to serve as a biologic oxygenator using the technique of controlled cross-circulation; soon thereafter, the mechanical, extracorporeal, heart-lung bypass pump was developed.[2,3] With the aid of this ability to support the patient's circulation during intracardiac exploration, surgeons have sequentially attacked almost every described congenital cardiac anomaly. The prospect of meaningful survival for patients born with otherwise devastating congenital cardiac lesions is now expected in most, if not all, cases.

As a result of this success story, there is now a large and growing population of adults with repaired or unrepaired CHD; estimates in the United States for 2005 placed the number of adult patients surviving with repaired or palliated congenital cardiac lesions at more than 1 million persons.[4] This reality has been associated with new challenges in the ongoing medical maintenance of such patients, with particular focus on the care of patients with congenital cardiac lesions presenting for surgery for noncardiac illnesses. The evolving subspecialty of adult CHD points to the unique needs of this population of patients.

### PATHWAYS FOR PRACTICING CONGENITAL HEART SURGERY

Before embarking on a review of the field, it is worthwhile to describe the setting in which patients with CHD seek and receive care in today's medical environment. With the development of sophisticated methods of fetal ultrasound, a large percentage of children requiring surgery for CHD are diagnosed during gestation (Fig. 59-1). Although not yet confirmed as affecting overall survival rates, a fetal diagnosis of complex CHD is of inordinate help to parents and the medical management team. This is particularly important in the setting of lesions dependent on persistent patency of the ductus arteriosus for postnatal survival. In these individuals, survival after delivery is predicated on the maintenance of ductal patency through the IV infusion of prostaglandin E1 (PGE1) initiated in the delivery suite, often through an umbilical vein catheter.

A growing number of congenital cardiac lesions is known to be associated with specific genetic mutations, many clearly inherited and some presumed to be sporadic. As such, a chromosomal analysis is frequently performed in those found to have major structural cardiac abnormalities; this analysis may be performed during gestation through an amniocentesis. The chromosomal evaluation is of benefit to the family when planning the risk of such an occurrence in future offspring. For the clinician, knowledge of chromosomal abnormalities in their patients, such as DiGeorge sequence, velocardiofacial syndrome, and

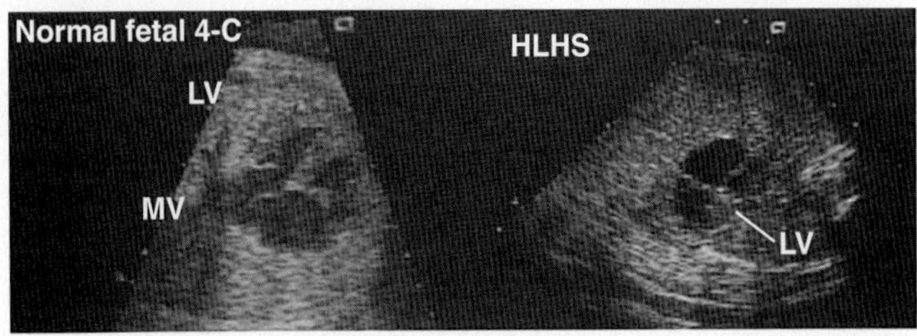


**FIGURE 59-1** Normal fetal ultrasound (four chamber; *left*) and fetal ultrasound of a child with HLHS *(right)*. *LV,* Left ventricle; *MV,* mitral valve.

Marfan syndrome, aids in the delivery of acute medical management.

In general terms, the timing of surgery for various congenital cardiac conditions depends on the presenting symptomatology and expectations for further associated complications. Children presenting with limited pulmonary blood flow or atretic pulmonary connections typically require surgery during the first few days of life and occasionally within hours of delivery. Lesions associated with excessive pulmonary blood flow result in early heart failure, which may manifest as poor feeding, tachypnea, or even respiratory failure. These patients are operated on during early infancy to ameliorate their symptoms and prevent the development of pulmonary vascular disease.

Preterm and low-birth-weight babies with CHD have been presenting for surgical consideration with more frequency. This treatment strategy requires thoughtful planning and coordination among the surgery, anesthesia, cardiology, intensive care, and neonatology teams. Recently, at our institution, the Texas Children's Hospital, we successfully operated on an 800-g baby with transposition of the great arteries (TGA).

The specialty of congenital heart surgery is now recognized as a subspecialty of cardiothoracic surgery. Congenital heart surgeons were previously certified in cardiothoracic surgery by the American Board of Thoracic Surgery (ABTS) and received additional fellowship training in the United States or abroad in congenital heart surgery. As of 2009, the ABTS offers a formal certification process for subspecialty training in Congenital Heart Surgery. At this time, there are 10 congenital cardiac surgery residency programs approved by the Accreditation Council for Graduate Medical Education. Most pediatric cardiac surgery is performed in large, multispecialty children's hospitals in association with formal programs focused on the care of these complex patients. The management team includes pediatric cardiac anesthesiologists, perfusionists, and nursing staff. Focused pediatric cardiac intensive care units have been developed to optimize the patients' opportunity for recovery.

Historically, pediatric cardiologists have provided the medical management of patients born with CHD. Pediatric cardiology is also evolving. With advances in catheter-based technology, lesions previously treated with surgery are now being addressed by interventional pediatric cardiologists. Examples include device closure of atrial and ventricular septal defects (VSDs), occlusion of patent ductus arteriosus (PDA), and dilation and stenting of stenotic vessels in the systemic and pulmonary circulation. For a more in-depth recent review of this specialty, see the excellent technical text by Mullins.[5]

The situation of care for adults with CHD is not as well organized as for children. This issue is of particular relevance to the general surgeon faced with operating on an adult patient with significant CHD. One overriding message needs to be clear to the general surgeon in this setting: it must be assumed that in patients with previously repaired congenital cardiac lesions, even without overt cardiac symptomatology, the potential for significant perioperative cardiorespiratory derangement exists. More simply stated, the presence of a surgical scar on the chest of a patient with known CHD does not suggest that the lesion has been cured. With this firmly in mind, the general surgeon may find it challenging to determine the best source for a qualified consult for such a patient. At present, many adult cardiologists are not adequately trained in CHD to be expected to provide competent consultation on adult patients with CHD.

On the other hand, pediatric cardiologists are not educated in adult medicine and cardiology; many feel uncomfortable providing consultation on adult patients with CHD. As noted, the subspecialty of adult CHD is still in a state of development but, at present, there are few physicans who have been educated specifically to care for these patients. This underscores the necessity of the practicing general surgeon to become familiar with the specific issues of concern for patients with CHD to ascertain that the patient's unique anatomic and physiologic issues have been evaluated properly. Adult patients with CHD who present for care in a center without a designated qualified specialist must be evaluated by a pediatric cardiologist in coordination with an adult cardiologist. Of equal importance, the anesthesiologists and intensivists caring for such a patient must have a working understanding of the complexities and nuances of the patient's cardiac condition.[6] The anesthetic management of patients with CHD undergoing general surgical procedures is complicated and can become disastrous if managed improperly.

## ANATOMY, TERMINOLOGY, AND DIAGNOSIS

### Anatomy and Terminology

One of the most intimidating aspects for the student of CHD is developing a level of comfort with the terminology used for describing specific lesions. To begin, a thorough and sound understanding of normal cardiac anatomy is mandatory. There are several excellent texts on this subject; in particular, the one edited by Wilcox and coworkers[7] is especially concise and clear. One difficulty that challenges proper understanding of anatomy is the frequent use of abbreviations and eponyms for various congenital lesions—for example, congenitally corrected transposition of the great arteries (ccTGA), ventricular inversion, and L-transposition all describe the same heart, but none provides a complete anatomic description. Unless otherwise clear to all involved in the care of these complicated patients, the anatomic description needs to be segmental and complete to avoid mistakes and misinterpretations of structure.

In describing congenital cardiac lesions, a segmental approach is used to determine the relationship of the various structural elements. The situs describes the relationship of sidedness—situs solitus (normal), situs inversus (reversed), or situs ambiguous (indeterminate). The cardiac elements described include (in sequence) the atria, ventricles, and great vessels. The relationship of the connections must be understood; connections are concordant (e.g., right atrium connecting to right ventricle) or discordant (e.g., right ventricle connecting to the aorta). The chamber sidedness must be clarified (e.g., a

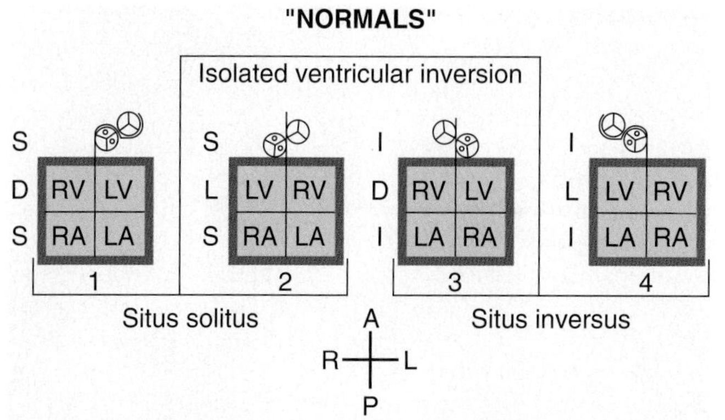

"NORMALS"

Isolated ventricular inversion

S D S — RV LV / RA LA — 1
S L S — LV RV / RA LA — 2
I D I — RV LV / LA RA — 3
I L I — LV RV / LA RA — 4

Situs solitus — Situs inversus

A, R, L, P

**FIGURE 59-2** Model depicting cardiac morphology for normal hearts—that is, hearts with atrioventricular concordance and ventriculoarterial concordance using Van Praagh nomenclature. The *vertical line* above the box denotes the position of the ventricular septum. (From Kirklin JW, Barratt-Boyes BG: General considerations: Anatomy, dimensions, and terminology. In Kirklin JW, Barratt-Boyes BG: Cardiac surgery, ed 2, New York, 1993, Churchill Livingstone.)

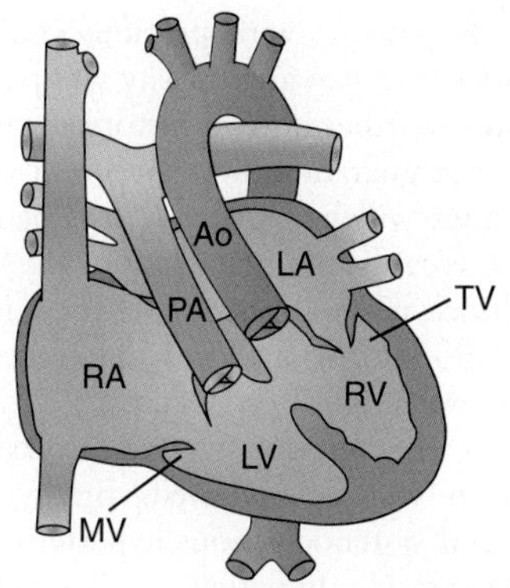


**FIGURE 59-3** Congenitally corrected transposition of the great arteries. Atrial situs solitus (normal) with atrioventricular discordance and ventriculoarterial discordance using Anderson nomenclature, S,L,L by Van Praagh classification. *Ao,* Aorta; LA, left atrium, *LV,* left ventricle; *MV,* mitral valve; *RA,* right atrium; *RV,* right ventricle; *TV,* tricuspid valve.

morphologic right atrium may be on the left side of the patient). The relationship and connections of the cardiac valves must then be assessed; connections may be normal, stenotic, atretic, or straddling. Of note to the general surgeon, abnormal sidedness of the cardiac structures is frequently associated with abnormal relationships of the thoracic and abdominal organs. A thorough assessment of the patient's anatomy is recommended before surgery.

There are two widely accepted and applied schools of cardiac morphologic description. The Van Praagh nomenclature uses abbreviations to describe the relationship of the atria, ventricular looping, and position of the aorta sequentially. The first letter describes the situs of the atrial chambers (and usually the abdominal organs): S for situs solitus (normal), I for situs inversus (reversed), or A for situs ambiguous (indeterminate). The second letter describes the relationship of the embryologic looping of the ventricles; D for dextro looping or right-handed topology (normal) or L (levo) for left-handed topology. The third and last letter describes the relationship of the aortic valve to the pulmonary valve, D for right-sided and L for left-sided (Fig. 59-2).

The Anderson nomenclature is more wordy and longer, but is perhaps simpler to understand. The descriptions are again of the sequential relationship of the structures. Starting with the atria, the connections and relationships are sequentially described. Thus, the atrial sidedness is described, followed by the sequence of connections to the ventricles and then great vessels. For example, atrial situs solitus (normal) with atrioventricular discordance (reversed) and ventriculoarterial discordance (reversed) describes the heart mentioned earlier as corrected transposition, or S,L,L by the Van Praagh classification (Fig. 59-3).

## Diagnosis

As with all aspects of surgery, there is a wide variety of highly sophisticated diagnostic tools available to examine cardiac structure and function. Despite the widespread availability and application of these tools, none has replaced or eliminated the necessity of a thorough history and physical examination. Most patients who have a history of CHD become very well informed about the specifics of their cardiac conditions, as do their parents. A detailed review of the patient's past medical history is absolutely mandatory. This includes, when possible, securing records from all previous diagnostic and procedural reports. It is disturbing how often an incorrect assumption is made about a patient's previous surgical history and anatomy, frequently in a setting in which a patient's old operative report or clinical summary could easily clarify the misunderstanding.

In adults with CHD, in particular, there are specific points of medical history that must be elucidated. A history of palpitations, syncope, and neurologic deficit must be further investigated. The incidence of significant dysrhythmias in certain categories of adults with CHD is high and, in many cases, warrants further investigation, including continuous monitoring (Holter), electrophysiologic study, and/or provocative testing.

### Physical Examination

A complete physical examination in a patient with previously repaired CHD will often yield information critical to the proper planning of a general surgical procedure. Patients need to be completely undressed and thoroughly examined. In many cyanotic patients, color changes may be prominent, particularly in the nail beds, lips, and mucous membranes. In other patients, cyanosis may be subtler, giving the patient a gray or even pale appearance. Previous surgical incisions need to be noted and reconciled with the known medical history. Thoracotomy incisions on either side may indicate a previous BT shunt using the turned-down, divided subclavian artery or with a prosthetic interposition graft, the so-called *modified BT shunt.* In patients with a left aortic arch, a left thoracotomy incision will be present if a previous coarctation repair has been carried out. Median sternotomy incisions or anterior thoracotomy incisions may indicate previous intracardiac or extracardiac surgery.

A complete vascular examination is often overlooked in patients with CHD. It is important to assess pulses and obtain blood pressure measurements in all four extremities. Patients who have an existing or have previously had a BT shunt often have diminished or absent pulses in the upper extremity corresponding to the previous shunt. This may also be true in the left upper extremity in patients with previous coarctation repairs, especially if a subclavian flap angioplasty was performed (Waldhausen procedure). Furthermore, a history of previous coarctation repair does not guarantee that the lower extremity pulses and blood pressures will be normal. Also, patients who have undergone previous cardiac catheterization may have chronically stenosed or occluded femoral vessels. All these issues may be of significance for monitoring and vascular access in a patient undergoing a general surgical procedure.

Later in this chapter, the Fontan procedure for single-ventricle palliation will be reviewed. Briefly, this operation results in significant systemic venous hypertension, often in the range of 12 to 15 mm Hg. In patients with a Fontan circulation, physical examination may reveal hepatic congestion, ascites, pedal edema, venous varicosities, and jugular venous distention. In some individuals, macronodular hepatic cirrhosis may be suspected on the basis of a firm fibrotic liver edge.

Entire textbooks have been dedicated to the physical examination of patients with cardiac disease and a thorough discussion of this issue, particularly the specifics of cardiac auscultation, is beyond our scope here. In general, however, the cardiac examination includes an assessment of the patient's rhythm, point of maximal impulse, and character of any auscultated murmurs. It must also be emphasized that the absence of a significant cardiac murmur does not rule out significant cardiac pathology.

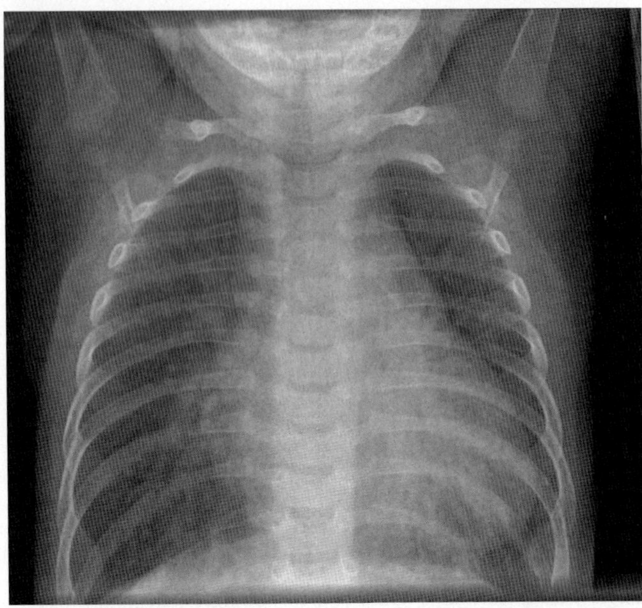

**FIGURE 59-4** Cardiomegaly and increased pulmonary vascular markings in a patient with complete atrioventricular canal defect.

### Diagnostic Tests

**Pulse Oximetry** Four-extremity pulse oximetry is an essential part of the clinical assessment of a patient with suspected CHD. In patients with ductal-dependent circulation to the lower body (severe aortic coarctation or aortic arch interruption), differential cyanosis may be presenting. This indicates the ejection of desaturated systemic venous blood through the patent ductus to the descending aorta contrasted with fully saturated pulmonary venous blood ejected to the ascending aorta and, thereby, the upper extremities. Baseline (room air) saturation must be documented in all patients for whom an operative intervention is anticipated to establish their normal range.

**Plain Radiography** Standard chest radiography with anteroposterior and lateral views is still an essential component of the assessment of a patient with CHD. Standard elements to be examined include a skeletal survey, assessment of the diaphragms and hepatic shadow, and location of the gastric bubble. The lung fields are assessed for pulmonary plethora (arterial or venous), air space disease, and presence of effusions. The cardiac silhouette may reveal much important information, such as a cardiothoracic ratio indicative of cardiomegaly or pericardial effusion, presence of atrial enlargement, presence or absence of the pulmonary artery shadow, and arch sidedness (Fig. 59-4).

**Electrocardiography** The electrocardiogram (ECG) is of significant importance in assessing patients with CHD. The rate and rhythm must be noted, including the presence or absence of P wave activity and axis. Many patients with CHD, especially those with complex conditions such as heterotaxy syndrome, may exhibit deranged or absent sinus node activity, giving rise to a predominant junctional rhythm, which may significantly compromise cardiac output. The QRS duration and axis yield important information concerning conduction delay and abnormal ventricular forces. For example, patients with atrioventricular canal defects are known to have left axis deviation. Furthermore, in patients undergoing repair of certain forms of CHD, there may be an early or late predisposition to malignant dysrhythmias. It is particularly important to elucidate a history of palpitations from a patient with repaired or unrepaired CHD; such a history may warrant further investigation with 24-hour continuous ECG monitoring (Holter).

**Echocardiography** Noninvasive imaging is well established as the primary diagnostic modality for structural cardiac disease. For most patients, excellent anatomic detail may be obtained using two-dimensional transthoracic imaging. Standard images include subcostal, suprasternal, parasternal, and subxiphoid views and are oriented in long and short axis directions. Furthermore, significant hemodynamic information may be inferred using echo Doppler blood flow velocities and interpreted using the modified Bernoulli formula (pressure gradient = $4V^2$, where V is echocardiographic velocity in m/sec). To assess the patient's cardiac lesion properly, segmental analysis of the cardiac structures, connections, and valves must be performed. A quantitative estimate of ejection fraction, shortening fraction, and valvular inflow velocity will aid in assessing cardiac function. For most patients with congenital cardiac disease, adequate diagnostic information is attainable through echocardiography in the hands of a qualified pediatric cardiologist.

**Magnetic Resonance Imaging and Computed Tomography** Cardiac magnetic resonance imaging (MRI) and computed tomography (CT) are adjuncts to echocardiography for noninvasive structural and functional assessment of the heart. MRI has been used with increasing frequency to provide anatomic detail in congenitally malformed hearts in which echocardiographic detail is lacking or unattainable. This modality has proved particularly useful for imaging the extracardiac great vessels and systemic and pulmonary venous connections, and for providing accurate estimates of cardiac function, especially right ventricular ejection fraction. CT may also be used for such imaging detail but has the potential detrimental association with significant radiation exposure.

**Cardiac Catheterization** Cardiac catheterization has long been considered the gold standard for diagnostic imaging of congenitally malformed hearts. With the current sophistication of echocardiography, this is no longer the case for most patients. Nonetheless, there are still circumstances in which diagnostic cardiac catheterization is necessary to obtain accurate anatomic detail. This may true for patients who have poor echocardiographic windows, although even this issue may be overcome using transesophageal echocardiography. More often, there are specifics of anatomic detail that neither echocardiography nor MRI can delineate, such as branch pulmonary artery (or segmental) stenoses, origin and course of aortopulmonary collateral vessels, and fistulous connections and intracardiac communications (septal defects) not clarified by other imaging modalities.

Usually, however, diagnostic cardiac catheterization is performed to obtain precise hemodynamic information needed to make an informed assessment of the consequences of the patient's cardiac lesions. Using oximetric measurements, pressure data, and thermodilution cardiac output determination, accurate assessment of the patient's hemodynamic profile is obtained. Measured or derived data include central venous pressure, atrial pressure, ventricular pressures (including end-diastolic pressure), shunt fraction (in the case of atrial or VSDs), pulmonary artery pressures, pulmonary capillary wedge pressure, systemic arterial pressure, and segmental oximetry of cardiac structures, including systemic and pulmonary venous return (Fig. 59-5). Thus, critical information is obtained about the presence and degree of shunting, systemic and pulmonary vascular resistance, and cardiopulmonary function. In certain clinical settings, these data are mandatory to a successful clinical management strategy. This may be particularly true for the adult patient with congenital cardiac disease requiring noncardiac surgery.

A thorough understanding of normal cardiorespiratory physiology is critical in interpreting data obtained by cardiac catheterization in the patient with CHD. Specifically, the normal pressure range, pulse waveforms, and oxygen saturations for the various cardiac chambers must be compared against data obtained in a deranged circulation. The various cardiac chambers have normal pulse waveforms. In the atria, there are characteristic waveforms—a wave corresponding to atrial contraction, c wave corresponding to atrioventricular valve closure, and v wave corresponding to atrial filling from venous return against the closed atrioventricular valve. Typical normal right atrial mean pressures range from 1 to 5 mm Hg and left atrial pressures range from 2 to 10 mm Hg. Right ventricular pressure tracings in normal hearts demonstrate a more gradual upstroke when compared with the left ventricle. Filling or end-diastolic pressures range between 2 and 10 mm Hg in normal hearts. The normal right ventricular systolic pressure ranges from 15 to 30 mm Hg (and thus pulmonary artery systolic pressure) and the left ventricular systolic pressure ranges from 90 to 110 mm Hg.

In normal hearts, there is a small, physiologically insignificant right-to-left shunt, which results from ventilation-perfusion mismatch in the lungs and coronary venous return directly to the left ventricle (thebesian venous return). This physiologic shunt represents less than 5% of the cardiac output and, in normal circumstances, does not produce detectable systemic arterial desaturation. Thus, significant systemic arterial desaturation represents a pathologic finding, consistent with pulmonary disease, intracardiac shunting, or both. As noted, the origin and degree of intracardiac shunting may be assessed by echo study. In certain circumstances, however, cardiac catheterization is necessary to measure cardiac oximetry, calculate shunt fraction, and

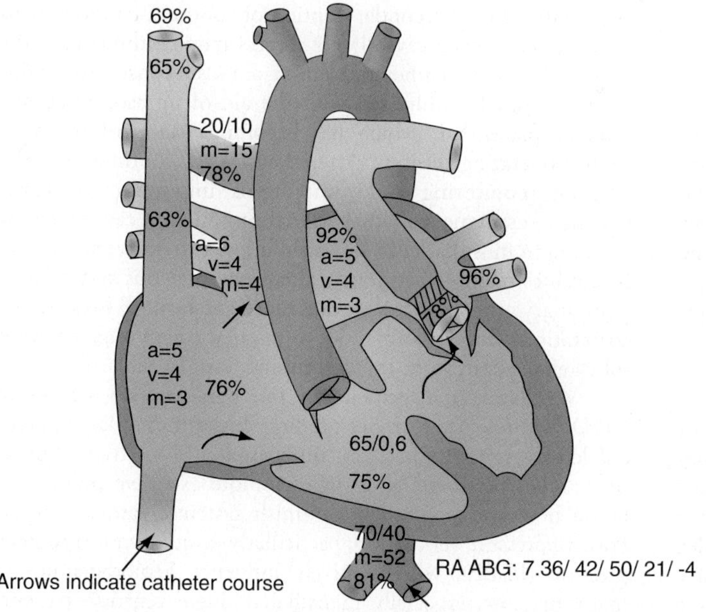


**FIGURE 59-5** Hemodynamic information obtained following cardiac catheterization.

derive systemic and pulmonary vascular resistance. Using a derivation of the Fick principle, the ratio of pulmonary blood flow (Qp) to systemic blood flow (Qs) flow can be determined as follows:

$$Qp/Qs = (Sa{O_2}\ sat - (\overline{M}{O_2}\ sat)/(\overline{P}{O_2}\ sat) - Pa{O_2}\ sat)$$

where $SaO_2$ sat is systemic arterial oxygen saturation, $\overline{M}O_2$ sat is mixed venous oxygen saturation, $\overline{P}O_2$ sat is pulmonary venous oxygen saturation, and $PaO_2$ sat is pulmonary arterial oxygen saturation.

Thus, in a patient with $\overline{M}$ sat of 60%, $\overline{P}O_2$ sat of 100%, $SaO_2$ sat of 100%, and $PaO_2$ sat of 80%,

$$Qp/Qs = (100 - 60)/(100 - 80) = 40/20 = 2:1$$

Calculating vascular resistances may also be extremely important in determining operability in the patient with CHD. In many settings, a precise measure of vascular resistance is unnecessary based on the clinical evidence. For example, in the small child with a large VSD seen on the echocardiogram, the clinical findings of tachypnea, cardiomegaly, and failure to thrive confirm a large left-to-right shunt and thereby infer acceptable pulmonary vascular resistance. In less clear circumstances, however, a precise calculation may be important in clinical decision making. The pulmonary vascular resistance may be calculated from cardiac catheterization data as follows:

Pulmonary vascular resistance (Rp) = (mean pulmonary artery pressure [in mm Hg] − mean left atrial pressure [in mm Hg])/(pulmonary blood flow [Qp, in liters/min/$m^2$])

In general, patients with an elevated Rp are further evaluated with pulmonary vasodilation—hyperventilation, hyperoxygenation, and inhaled nitric oxide—to determine whether the resistance is responsive. This information may be critical for patients who are otherwise marginal candidates.

Finally, it must be mentioned that cardiac catheterization has been evolving as the primary therapeutic method for a number of important structural cardiac defects. In many children's hospitals, including Texas Children's Hospital, most catheterizations now performed are for interventional procedures rather than diagnostic. This may be particularly pertinent to the general surgeon faced with treating a patient with a previous catheter-based correction of a cardiac defect. For example, the patient may have had an atrial or VSD closed with an occluder device in the past. This information may have important ramifications for infectious exposure and vascular access.

## PERIOPERATIVE CARE

Perioperative management of the patient with unrepaired or palliated congenital cardiac disease can be an extremely challenging proposition. Standard hemodynamic, respiratory, and pharmacologic manipulations appropriate for structurally normal hearts may be entirely inappropriate in settings of complex CHD. This is especially true in the operating room and intensive care settings. General rules include a thorough knowledge of the patient's intracardiac anatomy and expected physiology. It is certainly possible to make significant management errors based on incorrect physiologic expectations in the setting of incomplete understanding of the patient's anatomy. For example, in a patient with unrepaired tetralogy of Fallot (TOF) and associated significant right ventricular outflow tract obstruction (RVOTO), it is expected that the patient will exhibit some degree of systemic arterial desaturation. However, the patient with repaired tetralogy, with no residual intracardiac shunts, needs to be fully saturated. This is not an infrequent clinical scenario; a patient with a specific cardiac diagnosis, despite having undergone a successful correction, continues to be incorrectly presumed to have ongoing physiologic perturbation.

### Anesthesia Pitfalls

Providing physiologic anesthetic management can be challenging in patients with congenital cardiac disease, especially in situations such as chronic single-ventricle palliation, unrepaired CHD, chronic cyanosis, and residual intracardiac pathology. It is important to note that standard anesthetic management paradigms may be completely inappropriate and potentially disastrous in the setting of complex CHD. A thorough understanding of the patient's anatomy is mandatory, along with knowledge of the potential for unexpected response to anesthetic agents and ventilator settings. The field of pediatric and congenital cardiac anesthesia has evolved relative to this specific clinical need; the recent text by Andropoulos and colleagues is an excellent resource.[8]

Several points concerning anesthesia management merit discussion. The first is vascular access for intraoperative and postoperative management. In patients with complex CHD, especially those who have undergone previous complex surgical and catheterization procedures, obtaining appropriate vascular access may be challenging. Typically, a large-bore, multilumen central venous line is necessary for appropriate resuscitation and monitoring of right-sided filling pressures. In some patients, the placement of a thermodilution pulmonary artery catheter (oximetric) must be considered because one cannot presume that right-sided filling pressures correlate well with left heart volume or functional status (e.g., after a Fontan operation). Options for central access include percutaneous internal jugular or subclavian routes, with a secondary option of common femoral access to the inferior vena cava (IVC). Access may be difficult in the setting of previous catheterization or venous reconstruction; this situation may be addressed with the aid of ultrasound-guided catheter placement, which has become a standard in many cardiac operating theaters. Arterial access for continuous blood pressure monitoring and sampling is important for many patients. Percutaneous radial arterial cannulation can be readily achieved in most patients; however, upper extremity blood pressure values may be factitiously altered by previous systemic-to-pulmonary artery shunts, previous aortic arch surgery (especially coarctation), and abnormalities of vascular origin (e.g., aberrant subclavian origin from the descending aorta).

Ventilator management in the perioperative setting of CHD requires special understanding. In settings of large potential left-to-right shunts (e.g., unrepaired VSDs), hyperventilation and hyperoxygenation will promote excessive pulmonary blood flow and potentially diminish systemic cardiac output. Positive pressure ventilation, particularly positive end-expiratory pressure (PEEP), will negatively influence hemodynamics in many patients, especially in palliated single ventricle patients after the Fontan procedure. Early extubation in this population can be done to limit the deleterious effects of PEEP on the Fontan circulation. Early data have shown that this improves outcomes for these patients and reduces overall hospital costs.[9]

Finally, pharmacologic manipulation of systemic and pulmonary vascular resistance and cardiac performance is an important adjunct in the perioperative management of patients with CHD. In general, a low-dose infusion of epinephrine (0.05 μg/kg/min) with the addition of a phosphodiesterase inhibitor is an effective pharmacologic cocktail to promote cardiac inotropic state, lower systemic and pulmonary vascular resistance, and limit tachycardia. Other agents frequently used include dopamine, vasopressin, sodium nitroprusside, and nitroglycerin. Appropriate perioperative analgesia and sedation are also important aspects of the patient's management.[10]

### Neurologic Outcomes

With expectations of almost 100% survival following surgery for CHD, emphasis has been placed on the long-term neurologic outcomes and quality of life of these patients. The potential for neurologic insult in children following CHD arises from the nature of their disease (e.g., cyanotic defects, low cardiac output state, genetic syndromes, effects of cardiopulmonary bypass, circulatory arrest). There is also evidence to suggest that perhaps patients with CHD are genetically predisposed to neurologic insult. Recently, gestational age has been found to be an important factor to consider in the optimization of neurologic outcomes.[11]

## LESION OVERVIEW

### Defects Associated With Increased Pulmonary Blood Flow

#### Persistent Arterial Duct (Patent Ductus Arteriosus)

A persistent arterial duct or PDA is a frequently encountered congenital cardiac condition. The arterial duct is necessary during gestation to shunt right ventricular blood away from the unventilated pulmonary vasculature; ductal flow is from the pulmonary artery to the aorta during gestation. At delivery, after the first breath of the neonate, ductal flow reverses and becomes left to right in most individuals. Over the first several hours or days of postnatal life, the PDA closes spontaneously and is completely closed in most infants by 2 to 3 weeks of life.

In the absence of other congenital cardiac lesions—although a PDA may be present in association with other structural cardiac conditions and may sometimes be necessary for systemic or pulmonary blood flow—a PDA becomes pathologic related to its presence and degree of left-to-right shunting. The amount of shunting produced relates to the size and geometry of the duct and the pulmonary vascular resistance. A PDA may be responsible for a large Qp/Qs and result in pulmonary overcirculation, left heart volume overload, and congestive heart failure (CHF). A large unrestricted PDA will be associated with pulmonary hypertension; if left untreated, this will proceed to irreversible pulmonary vascular disease (Eisenmenger's syndrome), ultimately proceeding to pulmonary and right heart failure, only treatable by pulmonary transplantation. Even with a small, pressure-restrictive PDA, there is an ongoing risk for pulmonary congestion and left heart volume overloading; endocarditis is always of concern for even small PDAs. As such, closure is recommended for all PDAs.

The gold standard of therapy for closure of PDA is surgery, usually accomplished through a left thoracotomy using ductal division, ligation, or clipping (Fig. 59-6). This needs to be a low-risk procedure associated with minimal potential for persistence. Nonetheless, the invasive nature of this proven method has led to the development of alternative strategies for ductal occlusion. From a surgical perspective, many PDAs are

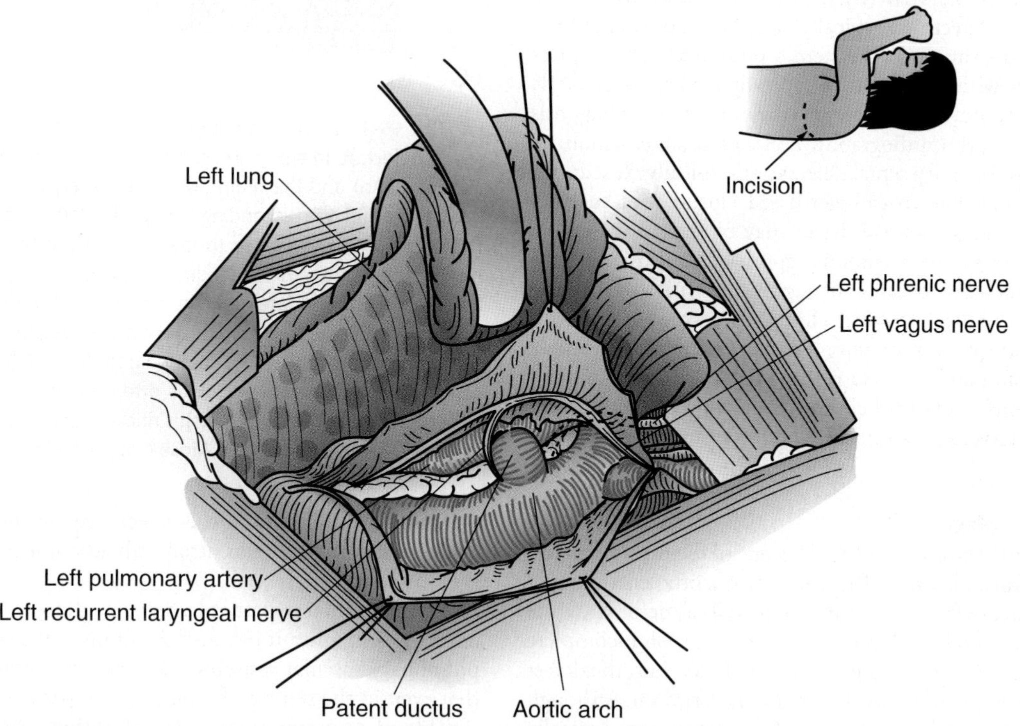


**FIGURE 59-6** Anatomic relationships of a patent ductus arteriosus, exposed from a left thoracotomy. (From Castaneda AR, Jones RA, Mayer JE Jr, Hanley FL: Patent ductus arteriosus. In Castaneda AR, Jones RA, Mayer JE Jr, Hanley FL: Cardiac surgery of the neonate and infant, Philadelphia, 1994, WB Saunders.)

amenable to thoracoscopic clipping through very small port incisions; robot-assisted PDA occlusion has been performed in many patients, with good results.[12] At present, however, most PDAs are occluded in the cardiac catheterization laboratory using occlusive devices. Even the repair of large defects in small babies has been successfully addressed. The long-term effects of the devices remaining in the vascular tree are as of yet not fully understood; however, successful device closure appears to be an extremely effective and durable therapy.[13]

A PDA in an adult patient can be challenging. As noted, a long-standing large PDA may be associated with pulmonary vascular disease. Clearly, a right-to-left shunt in a PDA is cause for significant concern and warrants further investigation. In adults with PDAs, the arterial wall may calcify, making an attempt at ligation or division hazardous. In these patients, ductal occlusion may require resection of the adjacent descending aorta with patch grafting or short-segment graft replacement (Dacron).

### Aortopulmonary Septal Defect (Aortopulmonary Window)

An aortopulmonary septal defect is a communication between the ascending aorta and, usually, the main pulmonary artery. This is a rare defect; it relates to the common embryologic origin of the arterial trunk and failure of complete separation into the aorta and pulmonary artery. Defects are classified by their location: type I is proximal, just above the aortic sinuses; type II is more distal on the ascending aorta and often involves the origin of the right pulmonary artery; and type III is more distal and associated with a separate origin of the right pulmonary artery from the aorta (Fig. 59-7). An aortopulmonary septal defect may occur in isolation or in association with other conditions, including interrupted aortic arch (IAA) and anomalous origin of a coronary artery. Defects are typically large and responsible for a large left-to-right shunt with systemic pulmonary artery pressures. Children with this problem typically present with CHF, failure to thrive, and frequent respiratory infections. Diagnosis may be made by echocardiography, MRI, or catheterization.

All aortopulmonary septal defects are surgically closed; this lesion is not amenable to catheter-based closure and such an attempt is hazardous. A small defect may be ligated through a thoracotomy or median sternotomy approach, but this method is not recommended because of significant risk for rupture or incomplete closure. Surgical closure is accomplished with cardiopulmonary bypass support. Options for closure include complete division and separate patch repairs of the great vessel defects or a sandwich type of closure, using a patch to construct a common intervening wall; both methods are effective (Fig. 59-8).

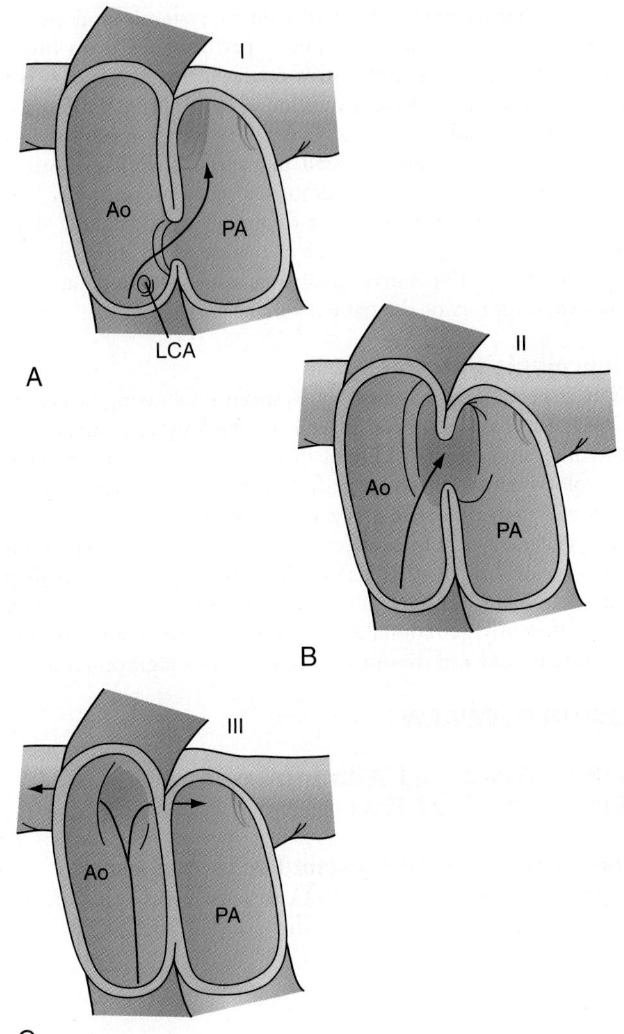


**FIGURE 59-7** Native anatomy and classification of aortopulmonary septal defect. **A,** In type I, the communication is between the ascending aorta (Ao) and the main pulmonary artery (PA) on the posterior medial wall of the ascending aorta. The left main coronary artery (LCA) orifice may be close to the defect. **B,** In type II, the defect is more cephalad on the ascending aorta. **C,** In type III, the defect is more posterior and lateral in the aorta. The communication is with the right pulmonary artery, which may be completely separate from the main pulmonary artery. (Adapted from Fraser CD: Aortopulmonary septal defects and patent ductus arteriosus. In Nichols DG, Ungerleider RM, Spevak PJ, et al [eds]: Critical heart disease in infants and children, Philadelphia, 2006, Mosby, pp 664–666.)

### Atrial Septal Defect

An isolated atrial septal defect (ASD) is one of the most common congenital cardiac lesions. The most frequently encountered ASD relates to a defect in the interatrial wall, as defined by the fossa ovalis. The defect develops as the result of incomplete closure of the embryologic patent foramen ovale; thus, the defect is a result of incomplete closure of the septum primum. Although the terminology can be confusing, these defects are typically termed *secundum atrial septal defects.* They present in a wide variety of configurations, ranging from single small defects to multiple fenestrations to complete absence of the septum primum. The confines of the defect may extend from the IVC orifice up to the superior atrial wall adjacent to the aortic root (Fig. 59-9).

The primary pathophysiologic derangement in ASDs relates to a significant left-to-right shunt in the setting of normal pulmonary vascular resistance. It must be emphasized, however, that even in the setting of a normal Rp, patients with ASDs are capable of transient right-to-left shunting, particularly during times of increased intrathoracic pressure. The effects of chronic, large left-to-right shunting (in some patients producing a Qp/Qs >3:1) include right heart volume overloading and

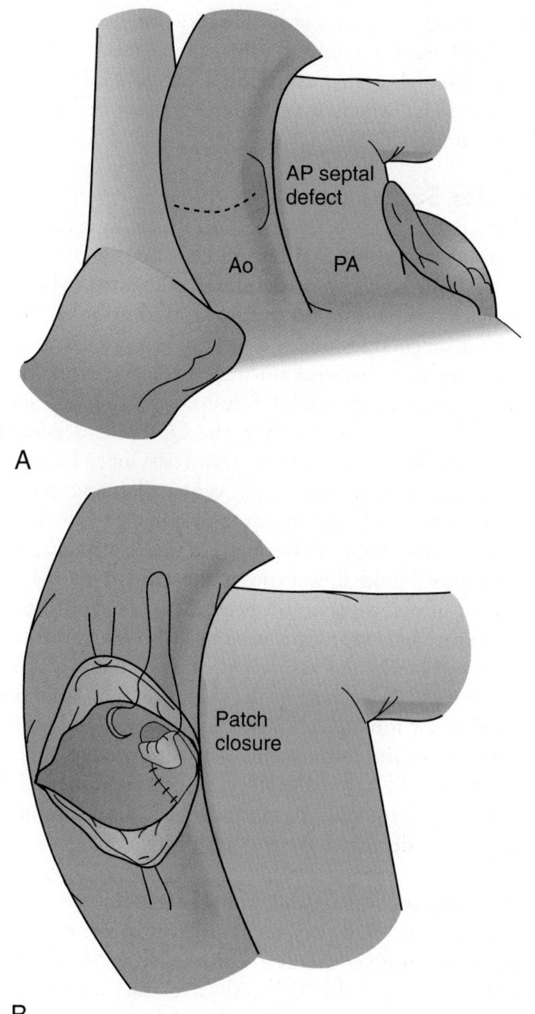


**FIGURE 59-8 A,** Surgical exposure of aortopulmonary (AP) septal defect includes a transverse incision in the ascending aorta (Ao). **B,** Aortopulmonary septal defect is closed by suturing a patch over the aortic side of the defect. *PA,* Pulmonary artery. (Adapted from Fraser CD: Aortopulmonary septal defects and patent ductus arteriosus. In Nichols DG, Ungerleider RM, Spevak PJ, et al [eds]: Critical heart disease in infants and children, Philadelphia, 2006, Mosby, pp 664–666.)

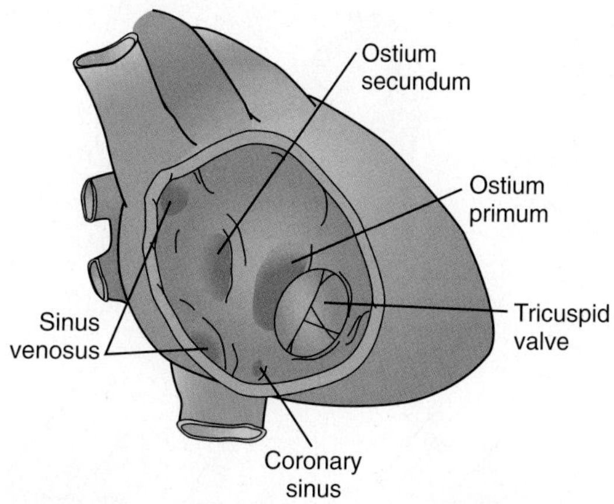


**FIGURE 59-9** Types of atrial septal defects as viewed through the right atrium—ostium secundum, ostium primum, and sinus venosus. (Adapted from Redmond JM, Lodge AJ: Atrial septal defects and ventricular septal defects. In Nichols DG, Ungerleider RM, Spevak PJ, et al [eds]: Critical heart disease in infants and children, Philadelphia, 2006, Mosby, p 580.)

enlargement. Most children are not overtly symptomatic but may exhibit some degree of exercise intolerance or frequent respiratory tract infection. Symptoms typically become more prevalent in adulthood and include dyspnea on exertion, palpitations and, ultimately, evidence of right heart failure. Pulmonary vascular disease is not a typical finding in secundum ASDs, but one may demonstrate an ASD in a patient with primary pulmonary hypertension. A rare form of presentation relates to the potential of right-to-left shunting at the atrial level; the ever-present risk for paradoxical embolus and cerebrovascular accident must be considered when recommending ASD closure.

Most centers recommend ASD closure before school age. The standard therapy for ASDs since the late 1950s has been surgical closure using cardiopulmonary bypass support. The defect is closed using direct suture closure, autologous pericardium, or prosthetic patch material (Fig. 59-10). This is an effective method, with a low associated perioperative risk, including the virtual absence of residual or recurrent defects, as noted in one study.[14] Minimally invasive techniques for ASD closure have also gained popularity.

The potential for closing defects using nonsurgical methods has led to the development of catheter-based therapies, which are now being widely applied to large numbers of patients worldwide for the treatment of ASD. The most commonly used device is the Amplatzer septal occluder (St. Jude Medical, St. Paul, Minn) device, of nitinol metal mesh, which is placed percutaneously and delivered with echocardiographic and fluoroscopic guidance. Early reports have indicated an acceptable procedure-related complication rate and successful closure rate.[15] It is clear, however, that the long-term effects of having such a device in mobile cardiac structures are not fully understood. Several recent reports have documented an alarming incidence of device erosion through the atrial wall and into the adjacent ascending aorta, as well as disruption of the conduction system.[16,17] A recent case of late severe endocarditis involving a previously placed Amplatzer ASD device has highlighted the need for ongoing observation of the long-term consequences of placing large prosthetic devices into the circulation.[18]

Sinus venosus atrial septal defects occur as the result of embryologic malalignment between the superior vena cava (SVC) or IVC. These defects are not associated with the ovale fossa and are frequently associated with partial anomalous pulmonary venous return. A superior sinus venosus ASD occurs high in the atrium, near the orifice of the SVC. This lesion is frequently associated with anomalous drainage of a portion of the right lung to the SVC. An inferior sinus venosus ASD is located low in the atrium, often extending into the IVC orifice. This lesion is typically associated with anomalous pulmonary venous drainage of the entire right lung to the IVC (potentially intrahepatic); pulmonary sequestration and an abnormal systemic artery perfusing the right lower lobe, with origin from the abdominal aorta, may also be present. In patients with total anomalous pulmonary venous return (TAPVR) to the IVC, the

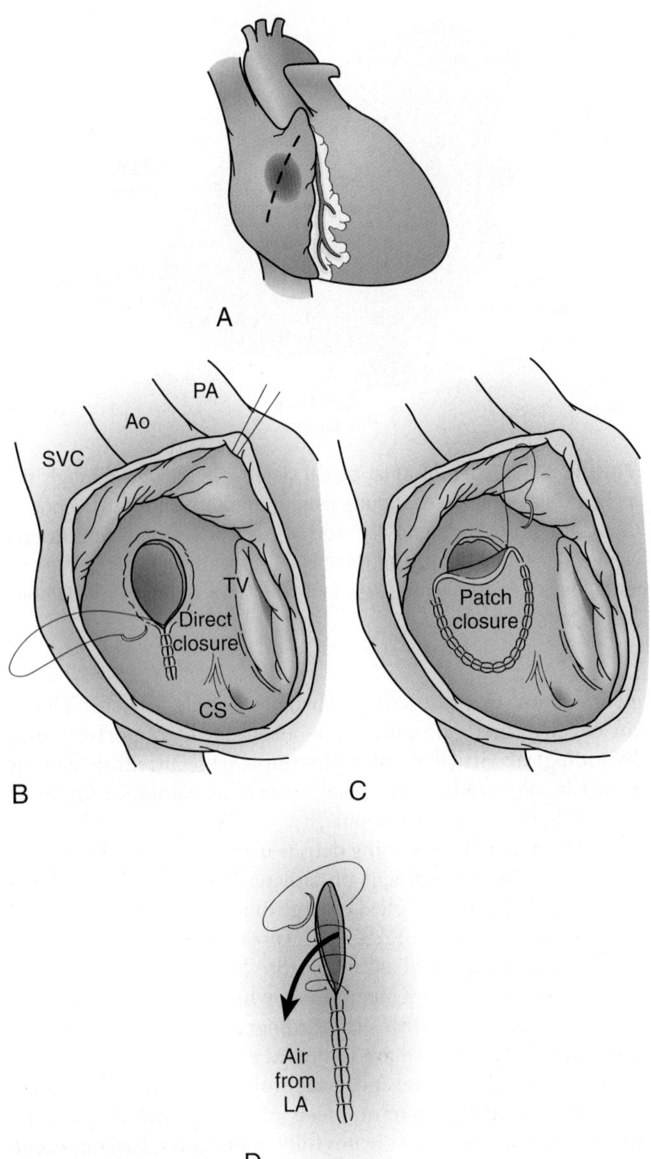


**FIGURE 59-10** Surgical closure for atrial septal defect. **A,** Right atriotomy. **B,** Direct suture closure. **C,** Patch closure. **D,** Deairing the left atrium (LA). *Ao,* Aorta; *CS,* coronary sinus; *PA,* pulmonary artery; *TV,* tricuspid valve. (Adapted from Redmond JM, Lodge AJ: Atrial septal defects and ventricular septal defects. In Nichols DG, Ungerleider RM, Spevak PJ, et al [eds]: Critical heart disease in infants and children, Philadelphia, 2006, Mosby, p 583.)

anomalous pulmonary vein may be readily obvious on a plain chest radiograph and has been described as appearing like a saber (scimitar syndrome), first described by Sabiston and Neill.[19]

Surgery for sinus venosus ASDs is recommended for the same pathophysiologic reasons as secundum ASDs. The repair is not amenable to catheter techniques, and surgery is more complicated than for an isolated secundum ASD. Superior sinus venosus defects with partial anomalous pulmonary venous return to the SVC may be treated with an intracardiac patch baffle; however, in the setting of high drainage of the anomalous pulmonary veins, an SVC translocation operation (Warden procedure) may be necessary.[20] Surgery for an inferior sinus venosus ASD with a scimitar vein can be more complicated, potentially involving the need for a patch baffle within the intrahepatic IVC, which may require periods of hypothermic circulatory arrest.

## Ventricular Septal Defect

A VSD is a pathologic communication involving a defect in the interventricular septum. Defects are classified in terms of their location and surrounding structures. Patients may be entirely asymptomatic, depending on the size and location of the VSD, along with associated lesions and pulmonary vascular resistance. In the setting of otherwise normal cardiac morphology and appropriate pulmonary vascular resistance, the net shunt in patients with VSD is left to right; the Qp/Qs is dependent on the size of the defect and pulmonary resistance. Large defects result in large shunts, high right ventricular and pulmonary artery pressures, and significant pulmonary overcirculation, CHF, and left heart volume overload. In these settings, unrestrictive pulmonary blood flow exposes the patient to the risk for pulmonary vascular disease and Eisenmenger's syndrome.

The ventricular septum can be best thought of in terms of the pathway of blood and associated cardiac anatomy. Thus, the right ventricular (RV) aspect of the septum has an inlet portion, midmuscular portion, apical, posterior, anterior, and outlet portions, and subaortic component. This knowledge aids in the classification of VSDs. Furthermore, defects are understood relative to their embryologic origins and have varying propensities for spontaneous decreases in size or closure.

### Perimembranous Ventricular Septal Defect

A perimembranous VSD occurs as a defect in the membranous portion of the interventricular septum; its associated margins include the annulus of the tricuspid valve, the muscular septum, and potentially the aortic annulus. The defects may be large and have associated prolapse of the noncoronary or right coronary aortic valve cusps. Perimembranous VSDs exhibit a potential for spontaneous closure, particularly small defects presenting early in childhood.

### Muscular Ventricular Septal Defect

Muscular VSDs occur in all aspects of the muscular interventricular septum. Margins of these defects are entirely muscle. The lesions may be isolated or involve multiple openings in the septum (so-called *Swiss cheese septum*). Small defects have great potential for regression or spontaneous closure.

### Subarterial (Supracristal or Outlet) Ventricular Septal Defect

Subarterial VSDs occur in association with the annulus of the aortic valve, pulmonary valve, or both. The defects are almost always associated with significant prolapse of the adjacent aortic valve cusp, usually the right coronary cusp, which may lead to significant cusp distortion, aortic valve insufficiency, and even cusp perforation. The only mechanism for spontaneous closure of these defects relates to the cusp prolapse and valve distortion and is generally not complete or a favorable arrangement. All these defects are surgically closed because of the ongoing risk for aortic valve injury (Fig. 59-11).

The indications for surgery to close VSDs relate to the size of the VSD, degree of shunting, and associated lesions. Thus,

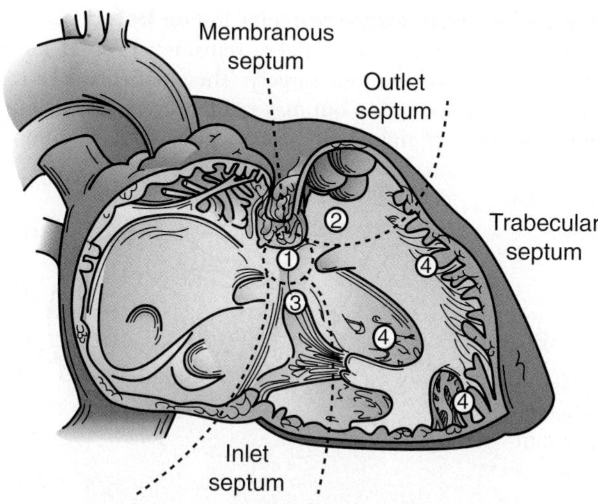


**FIGURE 59-11** Location of VSDs in the ventricular septum (view of the ventricular septum from the right side). 1, Perimembranous VSD; 2, subarterial VSD; 3, atrioventricular canal–type VSD; 4, muscular VSD. (From Tchervenkov CI, Shum-Tim D: Ventricular septal defect. In Baue AE, Geha AS, Hammond GL [eds]: Glenn's thoracic and cardiovascular surgery, ed 6, Stamford, Conn, 1996, Appleton & Lange.)

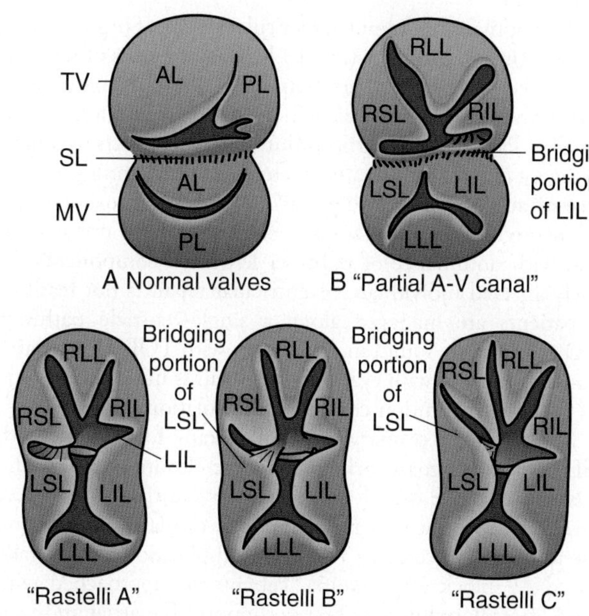


**FIGURE 59-12** Rastelli classification type A, B, or C. The difference in valve morphology in a normal **(A)**, partial **(B)**, and complete **(C)** canal defect is illustrated. *AL,* Anterior leaflet; *A-V,* atrioventricular; *MV,* mitral valve; *PL,* posterior leaflet; *RIL,* right inferior leaflet; *RLL,* right lateral leaflet; *RSL,* right superior leaflet; *TV,* tricuspid valve. (From Kirklin JW, Pacifico AD, Kirklin JK: The surgical treatment of atrioventricular canal defects. In Arciniegas E [ed]: Pediatric cardiac surgery. Chicago, 1985, Year Book Medical.)

small babies presenting with large VSDs, refractory heart failure, and large shunts undergo surgical closure of the defects in the newborn period, irrespective of age or size. Other defects are addressed based on the ongoing concerns of left-to-right shunting, aortic valve cusp distortion, and risk for endocarditis. Asymptomatic patients with evidence of significant shunts and cardiomegaly are proposed for surgical therapy. Prophylactic closure of small defects in asymptomatic patients with normal cardiac size and function is advocated by some surgeons because of the lifelong risk for endocarditis and comparatively low risk for surgery.

Although catheter-based therapies for some VSDs have been developed, particularly muscular defects, this mode of therapy is still not widely applicable to most VSDs.[21] The complex relationship of many defects, including close association with the aortic valve and cardiac conduction tissue, makes the existing technology less than ideal. At present, surgery remains the primary mode of therapy for VSD closure. Defects are approached with the aid of cardiopulmonary bypass support and may be closed with various materials, including autologous pericardium (our preference), Dacron, polytetrafluoroethylene (PTFE), and homograft material. Surgical closure of VSDs is a low-risk procedure with a high expectation of complete closure.[22] Challenging anatomic situations such as Swiss cheese septum or multiple apical muscular VSDs may be initially palliated by limiting pulmonary blood flow with a pulmonary artery band and deferring corrective surgery to later in life.

## Atrioventricular Septal Defect (Atrioventricular Canal Defect)

Atrioventricular septal defects (AVSDs) are a complex constellation of cardiac lesions involving deficiency of the atrial septum, ventricular septum, and atrioventricular valves. This lesion results from an embryologic maldevelopment involving the endocardial cushions; thus, the term *endocardial cushion defect* is often applied. AVSDs may be partial, involving no ventricular level component, intermediate or transitional, involving a small restrictive VSD, or complete, involving a large nonrestrictive VSD. The atrioventricular valve tissue is always abnormal in AVSD, although there is great individual variability in terms of the severity of the valvular malformation and thereby valve function. Complete AVSDs are frequently seen in patients with trisomy 21, but do occur in patients with normal chromosomes. The morphology of the septal defects in this condition is different than that previously discussed. The ASD in this defect is termed a *primum ASD* and is distinctly separate from the ovale fossa. There is displacement of the atrioventricular node and bundle of His to the inferior aspect of the primum defect and atrioventricular junction, a feature of critical importance during surgical repair. Patients with AVSD have an *inlet VSD,* which may extend into the subaortic region and have a component of septal malalignment. The chordal support of the atrioventricular valves has a variable relationship to the interventricular septum. The relationship of the chordal support and superior bridging component of the left atrioventricular (AV) valve have been used to classify complete AVSD, as described by Rastelli and associates[23]: type A with superior leaflet and chordal support committed to the left side of the ventricular septum; type B with straddling, shared chordal support; and type C with a floating left superior leaflet component and chordal support on the right side of the ventricular septum (Fig. 59-12).

Patients with complete AVSD typically present in infancy with large left-to-right shunts, cardiomegaly, and CHF. Without surgical treatment, patients exhibit severe failure to thrive, a susceptibility to severe respiratory infections, and potential for early development of pulmonary vascular disease. Surgical repair is recommended in infancy (usually before 6 months of life) but may be necessary in the newborn period for neonates with refractory heart failure, especially in association with aortic arch anomalies. Patients with partial or intermediate defects may have the surgery deferred until later in childhood, depending on the degree of atrial level shunting and presence of atrioventricular valve regurgitation. AVSD may also present in unbalanced forms, with dominance of right- or left-sided components. In severely affected individuals, biventricular repair is not feasible, and patients are managed along a single-ventricle pathway. AVSD may also be found in association with TOF; this combination is associated with cyanosis and repair is more challenging than for either condition considered in isolation.

Surgery is the primary mode of therapy for patients with AVSD. Operative goals include complete closure of ASDs and VSDs and effective use of available AV valve tissue to achieve valve competence. As noted, the inferiorly displaced conduction tissue must be protected to avoid the complication of surgically induced AV block (Fig. 59-13). Patients are approached with the aid of cardiopulmonary bypass support. The atrial and ventricular septal components are closed with a common patch (single-patch method) or separate patches (two-patch technique). We believe the two-patch method to be superior in preserving AV valve tissue (Fig. 59-14).[24] The critical component of the repair lies in the valve repair; typically, after suspending the valve tissue to the reconstructed septum, the line of coaptation between the superior and inferior leaflet components (cleft) is closed. However, care must be exercised to avoid valvular stenosis.

Perioperative care is predicated on an accurate and hemodynamically favorable repair. Patients with long-standing pulmonary overcirculation may have a potential for early perioperative pulmonary hypertensive crisis. This may require therapy, including continuous sedation, hyperventilation and, possibly, inhaled nitric oxide.

**Adult Patient With Atrioventricular Septal Defect**

A number of patients with partial or transitional AVSD survive well into adulthood without surgery. These patients have variable modes of presentation but may exhibit severe exercise intolerance, evidence of right heart dysfunction, some elevation of

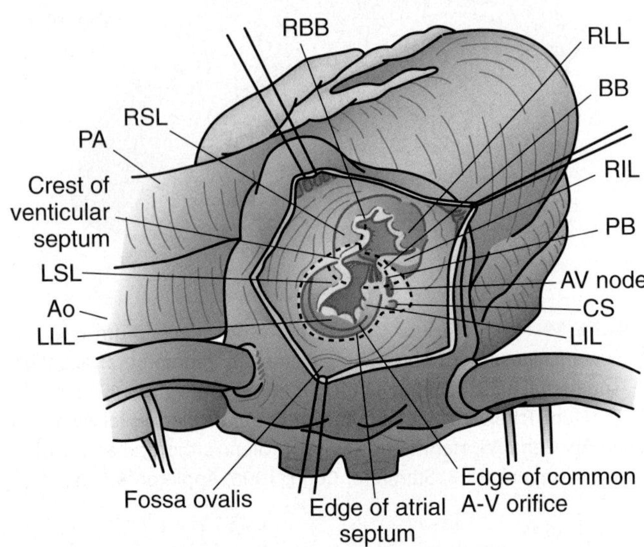


**FIGURE 59-13** Position of the conducting system in complete atrioventricular canal defect (CAVC). The anatomic relationships and morphology of the common atrioventricular (A-V) valve are shown. The view is through a right atriotomy. *Ao,* Aorta; *BB,* left bundle branch; *CS,* coronary sinus; *LIL,* left inferior leaflet; *LLL,* left lateral leaflet; *LSL,* left superior leaflet; *PA,* pulmonary artery; *PB,* penetrating bundle; *RBB,* right bundle branch; *RIL,* right inferior leaflet; *RLL,* right lateral leaflet; *RSL,* right superior leaflet. (From Bharati S, Lev M, Kirklin JW: Cardiac surgery and the conducting system, New York, 1983, Churchill Livingstone.)

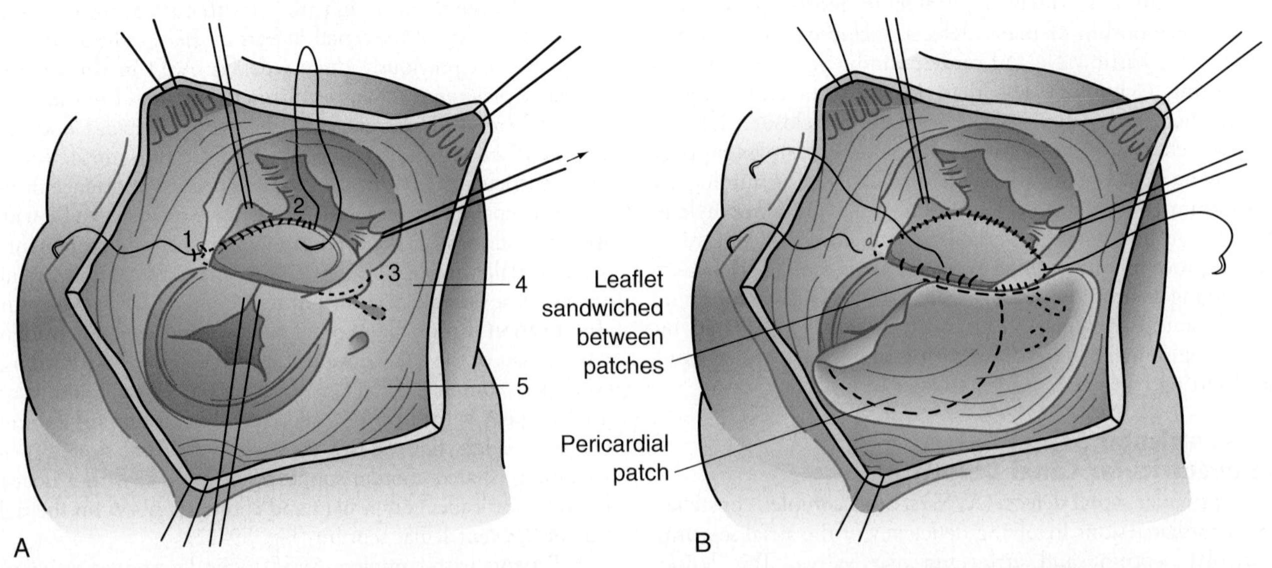


**FIGURE 59-14** Two-patch closure of complete atrioventricular canal defect. **A,** A ventricular septal patch is placed first and a separate patch is used to close the ASD component. **B,** Note the position of the coronary sinus and conducting system relative to the ASD patch suture line to avoid injury to the AV node. (From Kirklin JW, Barratt-Boyes BG: Cardiac surgery, New York, 1986, Churchill Livingstone.)

pulmonary vascular resistance and, possibly, atrial dysrhythmias, including atrial fibrillation. In such late-presenting patients, cardiac catheterization is often recommended to rule out occult coronary artery lesions and evaluate pulmonary vascular resistance. Nonetheless, in the absence of obvious surgical contraindication, surgery is recommended for adults with unrepaired AVSD to eliminate the chronic left-to-right shunt and repair the typically insufficient atrioventricular valves.

Other patients are now presenting well into adulthood with previously repaired AVSDs. These patients may have a widely disparate constellation of findings, including atrial and ventricular dysrhythmias, valvular insufficiency or stenosis, and right heart dysfunction. In many of them, secondary reparative surgery may become necessary. Furthermore, in the setting of a patient with remotely repaired AVSD requiring noncardiac surgery, it must be expected that there are potential ongoing hemodynamic concerns that will affect the perioperative course.

## Persistent Arterial Trunk (Truncus Arteriosus)

Truncus arteriosus or persistent arterial trunk results from failure of separation of the embryonic arterial trunk and semilunar valves. It is almost always associated with a large nonrestrictive VSD, is typically perimembranous, and is associated with varying degrees of truncal override of the interventricular septum, including 100% association of the trunk with the right ventricle. The condition is classified by the relationship of the origins of the pulmonary arteries: in type I truncus arteriosus, there is a demonstrable common main pulmonary artery with subsequent origins of the branch pulmonary arteries; in type II truncus arteriosus, the branch pulmonary arteries arise closely, but separately, from the trunk; and in type III arteriosus, the branch pulmonary arteries are widely separated in origin on the ascending aorta (Fig. 59-15).

In distinction to aortopulmonary septal defects, patients with truncus arteriosus have a single-outlet valve of highly variable morphology. The valve may have a normal appearance, with three well-formed and distinct cusps similar to those of a normal aortic valve. In other patients, the truncal valve may be severely malformed, with multiple cusps, dysmorphic leaflets, and abnormal commissural relationships. The truncal valve morphology and function have significant bearing on patient symptoms and the difficulty of surgery. Patients with truncus arteriosus frequently have coronary ostial abnormalities, including juxtacommissural origin and intramural course. There is an associated interruption of the aortic arch in as many as 25% of newborns presenting with truncus. Abnormalities of thymic genesis, T cell function, and calcium homeostasis may frequently be seen in this group of patients in association with a chromosome 22 deletion (DiGeorge syndrome).

Patients with truncus arteriosus present in the newborn period with unrestricted pulmonary blood flow and systemic pulmonary artery pressure. With the expected postnatal decrease in pulmonary vascular resistance, massive pulmonary overcirculation, and CHF, patients may exhibit a wide pulse pressure because of diastolic runoff of blood into the pulmonary vasculature. This situation will be further exacerbated in the setting of significant truncal valve insufficiency, resulting in poor systemic perfusion and cardiovascular collapse. Some infants can be initially managed with medical decongestive therapy (e.g., diuretics, angiotensin-converting enzyme inhibitors, and digoxin) and fortified nutritional support (through gastric intubation); however, this is a precarious arrangement. In the few

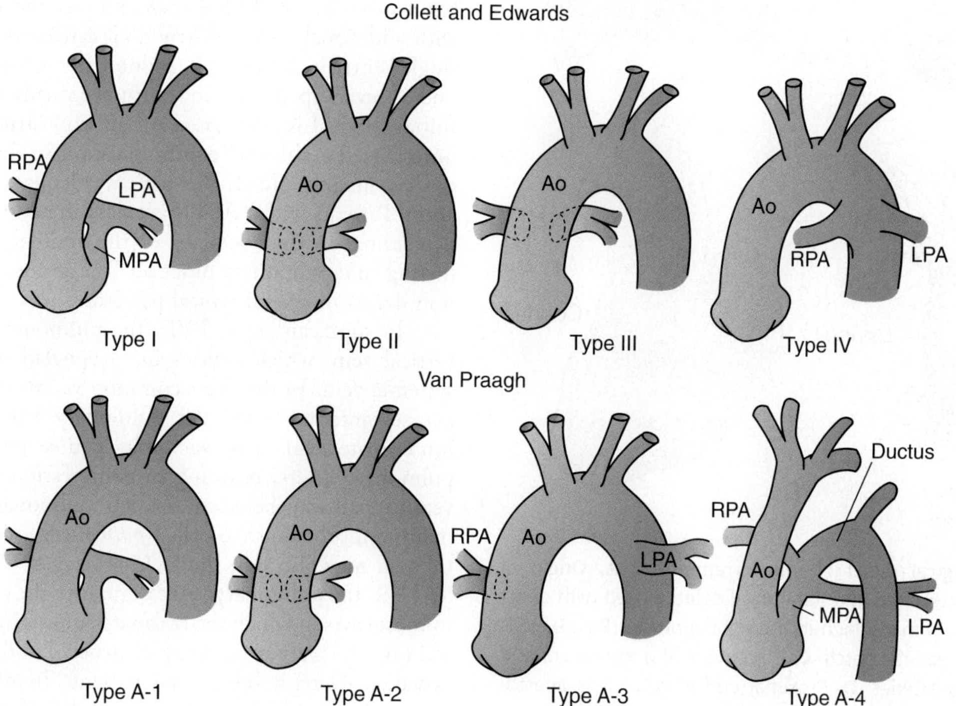


**FIGURE 59-15** Collett-Edwards and Van Praagh classification systems for persistent truncus arteriosus (see text for details). *Ao,* Aorta; *MPA,* main pulmonary artery; *LPA,* left pulmonary artery; *RPA,* right pulmonary artery. (Adapted from St Louis, JD: Persistent truncus arteriosus. In Nichols DG, Ungerleider RM, Spevak PJ, et al [eds]: Critical heart disease in infants and children, Philadelphia, 2006, Mosby, p 690.)

individuals who survive infancy, irreversible pulmonary vascular disease develops rapidly and patients become inoperable. In other patients, refractory CHF results in poor weight gain, respiratory insufficiency, and susceptibility to infection. In many newborns with unrepaired truncus arteriosus, the profound hemodynamic compromise places the patient at high risk for necrotizing enterocolitis (NEC). Patients with truncus arteriosus and IAA have ductal-dependent systemic blood flow. They are therefore dependent on IV PGE1 to maintain ductal patency until they undergo repair. Given these considerations, it is recommended that most newborn patients undergo repair in their first several weeks of life.

The surgical repair is performed on cardiopulmonary bypass support. Components of the repair include division of the common trunk and reconstruction of confluent central branch pulmonary arteries. The large VSD is closed with a patch, typically through a right ventriculotomy. In patients with abnormal, insufficient truncal valves, a valve repair may be necessary. It is unusual to have to replace the truncal valve at the initial operation; most valves can be at least partially repaired to provide the patient with an adequate aortic valve. Right ventricle–pulmonary artery continuity must then be established. Most surgeons prefer to interpose a valved conduit between the right ventriculotomy and pulmonary artery bifurcation (Fig. 59-16).

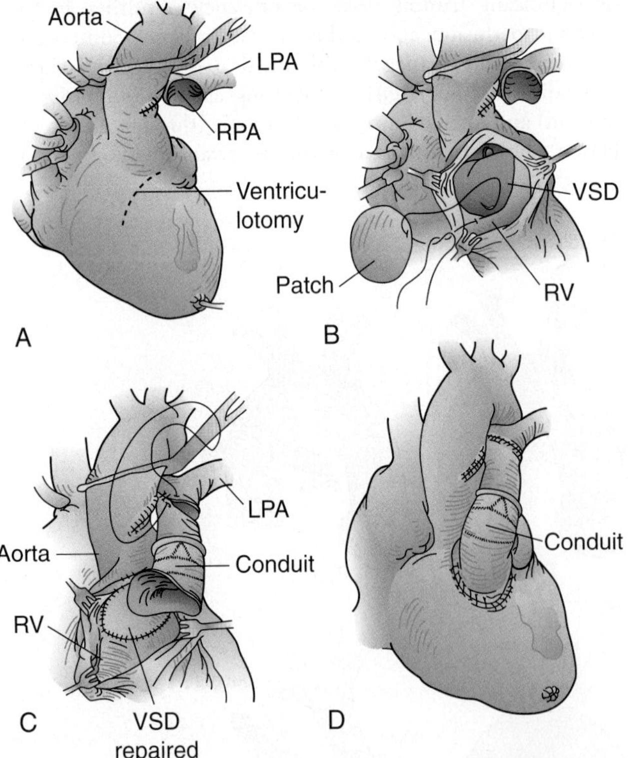


**FIGURE 59-16** Surgical repair of truncus arteriosus. **A,** Origin of truncus arteriosus is excised and the truncal defect closed with direct suture. The incision is made high in the right ventricle (RV). **B,** VSD is closed with a prosthetic patch. **C,** Placement of a valved conduit into the pulmonary arteries. **D,** Proximal end of conduit is anastomosed to the RV. *LPA,* Left pulmonary artery; *RPA,* right pulmonary artery. (From Wallace RB: Truncus arteriosus. In Sabiston DC Jr, Spencer FC [eds]: Gibbons surgery of the chest, ed 3, Philadelphia, 1976, WB Saunders.)

Conduit options are limited and include homograft (pulmonary artery or aorta, valved) or heterograft (bovine or porcine). Experience with a commercially available, glutaraldehyde-preserved, bovine jugular vein valved conduit (Contegra, Medtronic, Minneapolis) has been encouraging.[25] Successful truncus arteriosus repair in infants using a direct hooded anastomosis between the pulmonary artery bifurcation and right ventriculotomy has also been reported.[26] Unfortunately, no currently available option offers the patient the lifetime solution of a connection capable of somatic growth along with a competent, durable pulmonary valve. Thus, it is expected that all infants undergoing successful truncus repair will require multiple subsequent cardiac surgeries as they outgrow their current right ventricle–pulmonary artery conduit. Recent experience with a percutaneously delivered, catheter-mounted pulmonary valve has been encouraging as an interim solution for these patients in an effort to limit the number of required cardiac reoperations.[27]

A growing number of adults have been surviving after childhood truncus arteriosus repair. It is clear that all these patients require diligent longitudinal cardiology surveillance and that many will require reoperation. Issues of concern include late ventricular dysrhythmias, often related to surgical scarring from the previous right ventriculotomy, branch pulmonary artery stenosis, stenosis or insufficiency of the right ventricle–pulmonary artery conduit, truncal valve insufficiency, and right ventricular dysfunction.[28]

## Abnormalities of Venous Drainage

### Total Anomalous Pulmonary Venous Return

TAPVR results from embryonic failure of connection of the fetal pulmonary venous sinus to the left atrium. This fatal condition has a spectrum of clinical presentations and may be associated with additional complex structural cardiac disease, including a single ventricle. In TAPVR, pulmonary venous return may take one of several pathways to return eventually to the right heart. Initial survival is predicated on an unobstructed pathway and unrestricted atrial level communication so that sufficient intracardiac mixing affords the patient adequate systemic oxygenation. Patients with TAPVR are desaturated to varying degrees, depending on the adequacy of the anomalous pathway, atrial mixing, and pulmonary function. The abnormal venous connection drains in several typical patterns.

In supracardiac TAPVR, the pulmonary veins drain to a vertical vein, which courses in a cephalad direction to join a systemic vein. In the most common variation, the vertical vein courses anterior to the left pulmonary artery to join the left innominate vein. This vein may course posterior to the left pulmonary artery, resulting in compression of the pulmonary venous pathway between the left pulmonary artery and left mainstem bronchus (so-called *pulmonary artery vise*). The vertical vein may also join the SVC or azygos vein. In intracardiac TAPVR, the pulmonary veins drain into the coronary sinus and, in most cases in which the coronary sinus is intact, into the right atrium. This variant is rarely obstructed and may not be diagnosed until later in life in some patients. In infracardiac TAPVR, the vertical veins descend in a caudal direction through the diaphragm to join the embryologic ductus venosus, and then through the liver to join the IVC. This variation is almost always obstructed at some level (Fig. 59-17). In mixed TAPVR, the

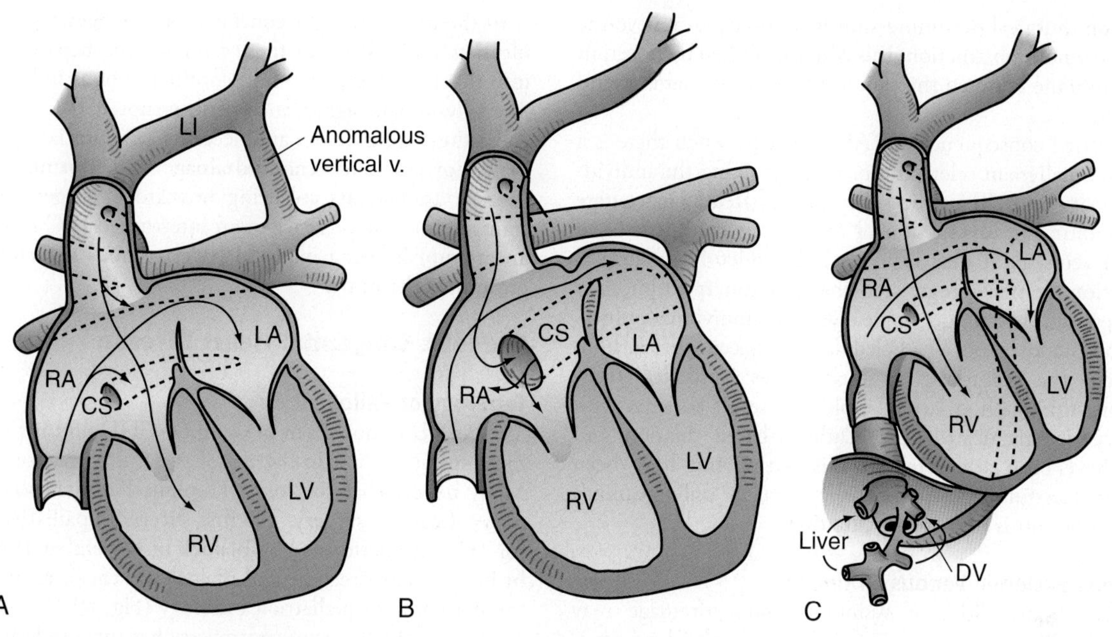


**FIGURE 59-17** Types of total anomalous pulmonary venous connection (TAPVC). **A,** Supracardiac type with a vertical vein joining the left innominate (LI) vein. **B,** Intracardiac type with connection to the coronary sinus. **C,** Infracardiac type with drainage through the diaphragm through an inferior connecting vein. *CS,* Coronary sinus; *DV,* ductus venosus; *LA,* left atrium; *LV,* left ventricle; *RA,* right atrium; *RV,* right ventricle. (From Hammon JW Jr, Bender HW Jr: Anomalous venous connections: Pulmonary and systemic. In Baue AE [ed]: Glenn's thoracic and cardiac surgery, ed 5, Norwalk, Conn, 1991, Appleton & Lange.)

pulmonary venous pathway drains in several pathways to reach the heart. Frequently, in mixed TAPVR, one or several pulmonary veins will connect to the SVC, with others draining to an infracardiac or supracardiac connection.

**Obstructed Total Anomalous Pulmonary Venous Return** Obstructed TAPVR is one of the few true surgical emergencies in congenital heart surgery. It is diagnosed with transthoracic echocardiographic evaluation when the condition is suspected. The condition occurs when one of the drainage patterns noted earlier is obstructed, resulting in severe pulmonary venous hypertension. Secondary effects include pulmonary edema, pulmonary artery hypertension, and profound hypoxemia. Interstitial pulmonary emphysema and frank pneumothorax may develop while attempting vigorous ventilatory support in profoundly desaturated children. Patients with obstructed TAPVR may present within hours of birth in extremis and will not respond to resuscitative efforts. The only useful therapy is rapid surgical repair, irrespective of the severity of the patient's preoperative status.

For other forms of TAPVR, elective surgical repair is recommended after the condition is diagnosed. On occasion, the diagnosis is not made until later in childhood in patients with an unobstructed vertical vein and widely patent atrial communication. These patients undergo elective repair to relieve the cyanosis, intracardiac mixing, and right heart volume overload.

Surgical repair of TAPVR requires cardiopulmonary bypass support; often, periods of profound hypothermia and circulatory arrest are necessary. The principles of repair include identification of the pulmonary venous confluence and individual pulmonary veins. An anastomosis is constructed between the venous confluence and left atrium using a superolateral[29] approach, with the heart reflected to the patient's right, or an incision directly through the interatrial septum and corresponding region of the posterior right atrial wall. The ASD and PDA that is typically present are closed as well (Fig. 59-18).

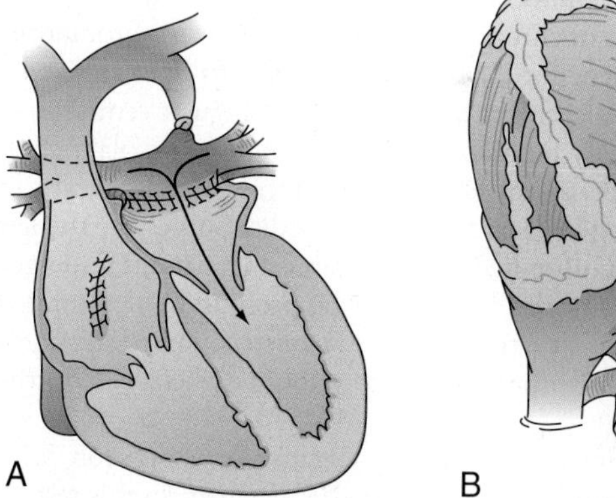

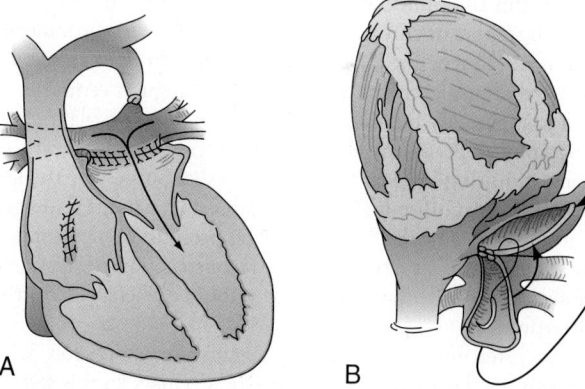


**FIGURE 59-18 A,** Repair of supracardiac total anomalous pulmonary venous connection (TAPVC) through a superior approach. **B,** Repair of infracardiac TAPVC. Elevating the apex of the heart to the right side exposes the left atrium and pulmonary confluence. Anastomosis is created as shown. (From Lupinetti FM, Kulik TJ, Beekman RH, et al: Correction of total anomalous pulmonary venous connection in infancy. J Thorac Cardiovasc Surg 106:880–885, 1993.)

**Cor Triatriatum** Cor triatriatum is a rare condition in which the pulmonary veins enter a chamber posterior to the left atrium with a small connection to the right or left atrium. These patients exhibit evidence of pulmonary hypertension and variable desaturation. Surgical decompression is necessary to relieve the pulmonary venous obstruction; this is accomplished by resection of the membrane between the pulmonary venous chamber and left atrium.

A dreaded consequence of TAPVR occurs when there is a progressive, malignant sclerosing process involving the individual pulmonary veins. This process may be initiated by inaccurate surgery resulting in obstruction of the venous confluence and individual veins, or it may progress independently of surgical manipulation. It may progress to intrapulmonary pulmonary venous stenoses. A technique to deal with the individual pulmonary venous stenoses uses a pedicled flap of adjacent pericardium to augment the pulmonary venous orifices (sutureless technique), but this method is not applicable to all patients with pulmonary venous obstruction. Catheter-based dilation and stenting have been attempted in this setting but have been largely unsuccessful. In the most severe cases, the only meaningful surgical option is lung transplantation.

### Anomalous Systemic Venous Drainage

Congenital abnormalities of systemic venous drainage may occur in isolation or in association with other significant structural cardiac defects. In the setting of an otherwise normal heart, the anomaly is frequently not of physiologic significance. The most common example is a persistent left SVC draining to the coronary sinus. In the absence of an intracardiac communication or unroofing of the coronary sinus, this is of anatomic significance only. In many cases, a persistent left SVC occurs, with absence of a communicating innominate vein. This becomes important in situations of mechanical occlusion, which may be seen with trauma or chronic venous intubation with thrombosis. It is not infrequent for a persistent left SVC to be incidentally discovered after placement of a left internal jugular central line, which is apparently found to track into the heart on plain chest radiography. A persistent left SVC becomes more significant in patients requiring intracardiac or extracardiac surgery. If the left SVC drains to an unroofed coronary sinus in a patient undergoing atrial septation, the patient will be profoundly desaturated after surgery. This situation requires reconstruction of the coronary sinus or some other method to reroute the left SVC to the right atrium.

An interrupted IVC usually occurs in association with other structural cardiac disease. The IVC drainage in this setting is to the azygos (azygos continuation) or hemiazygos vein and ultimately the SVC. In these patients, the hepatic veins drain into the atrium as a common confluence or as individual veins. The physiologic significance of interrupted IVC relates to the coexisting cardiac lesion and necessity of appreciating the abnormality of systemic venous drainage in performing corrective surgery. In patients requiring noncardiac surgery or catheter intervention, the presence of an interrupted IVC is noted when an attempt is being made to pass a venous catheter from the groin into the heart.

## Cyanotic Congenital Heart Disease

### Tetralogy of Fallot

TOF is a common form of cyanotic CHD and is probably the most studied lesion in the era of surgical correction for CHD. Many believe that the Johns Hopkins Hospital was the birthplace of cardiac surgery. The first successful palliative operation for TOF was performed by Blalock in November 1944, assisted by his laboratory technician.[1] Blalock was encouraged by Taussig, the matriarch of pediatric cardiology (Fig. 59-19). Until rather recently, some degree of controversy has surrounded the relative degree of contribution by these three individuals in bringing this historical event to fruition. In actuality, all three were significant participants in this momentous medical advance. While working at Vanderbilt Medical School, Blalock had charged his young and capable laboratory technician, Vivien Thomas, with the development of a surgical model of pulmonary hypertension. Thomas and Blalock developed a method of anastomosing the left subclavian artery to the divided left pulmonary artery in a canine model. Specifically, Thomas worked out the technical details, including crafting the necessary surgical instruments, and mastered the operation. This work did not produce the desired effect; in fact, canine pulmonary vascular resistance is almost infinitely low, and the animals did not develop a hypertensive pulmonary vasculature. Nonetheless, the technique was developed and published some 10 years in advance of the clinical application in 1944.

Blalock subsequently became the Chair of Surgery at Johns Hopkins. Taussig had, by that time, established a reputation as a meticulous diagnostician of complex congenital heart lesions. She had a large clinic of desperately ill children with disabling cyanosis, so-called *blue babies*. At her suggestion (and probably

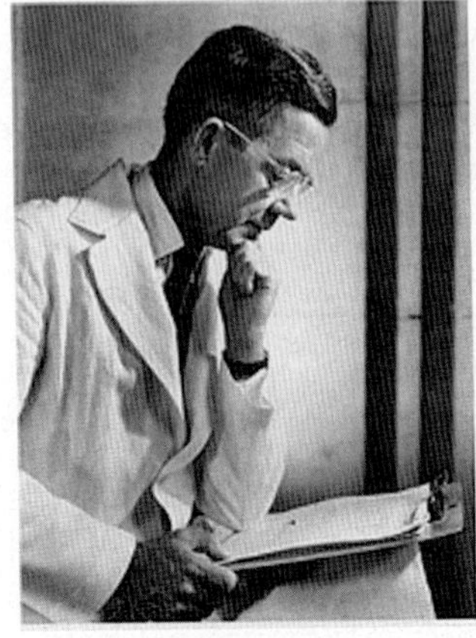
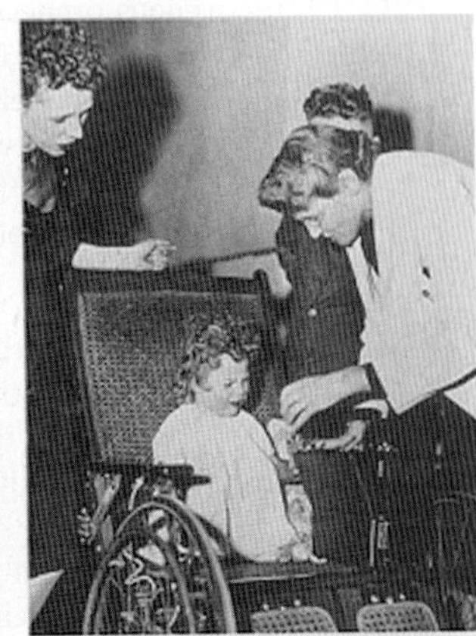
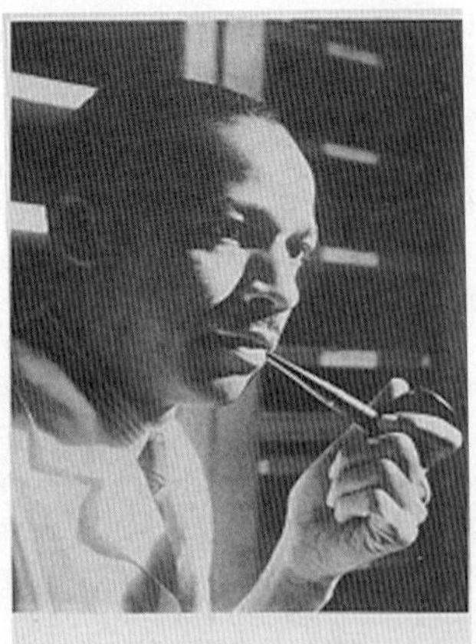

**FIGURE 59-19** Drs. Alfred Blalock, Helen Taussig, and Vivien Thomas.

her insistence), Blalock was convinced to attempt a surgical palliation for TOF by constructing the subclavian to pulmonary artery anastomosis in a human that had been perfected in the research laboratory (Fig. 59-20). Blalock performed the operation in conditions and with instruments that would be considered extremely crude by today's standards. Thomas stood immediately behind Blalock during that operation and many subsequent cases, providing instruction and encouragement. The clinical success was an earth-shattering event; literally hundreds of patients subsequently traveled to Johns Hopkins for surgical treatment and the era of cardiac surgery was ushered in. (These historic accounts are factual, the result of personal interviews with many of those in attendance at that event, including Drs. Vivien Thomas, Taussig, J. Alex Haller, and Denton Cooley.)

The historic account of the development of the BT shunt has relevance to the practice of congenital heart surgery today. First, it is important that the facts surrounding this achievement are acknowledged. Second, this remarkably simple concept still remains a frequently applied technique for children with inadequate pulmonary blood flow. Finally, over almost 75 years of treatment of TOF, thousands of patients have been successfully treated, but most are not cured; many require subsequent reoperative cardiac surgery, even after complete repair.

The anatomic hallmark of TOF is anterior malalignment of the infundibular septum, which leaves a deficiency in the subaortic region—a malalignment VSD. This is usually perimembranous, large, and pressure-nonrestrictive. The relative degree of malalignment influences the relationship of the aorta to the interventricular septum, producing varying degrees of aortic override. The deviated infundibular septum produces varying degrees of RVOTO. The path of pulmonary blood flow may be impeded at a number of levels, including the infundibulum, pulmonary valve and annulus, and main and branch pulmonary arteries. Secondary right ventricular hypertrophy occurs relative to the degree and duration of the obstruction and is progressive, contributing to the propensity for the lesion to worsen over time (Fig. 59-21).

The pathophysiology of TOF relates to shunting of desaturated, systemic venous blood through the VSD to mix with the systemic cardiac output. The greater the degree of obstruction to pulmonary blood flow, the larger the right-to-left shunt and thereby the worse the desaturation. There are several modes of presentation. Newborns with TOF and severe RVOTO may present soon after birth with profound cyanosis; some require PGE1 to maintain ductal patency for adequate oxygenation. The other end of the spectrum is in children with little infundibular obstruction and normal pulmonary valve and branch pulmonary arteries. These patients may have net left-to-right flow through the VSD, occasionally to the extent that they experience pulmonary overcirculation and CHF (so-called *pink TOF*). Most children present between these extremes; an initially mild to moderate degree of infundibular stenosis progresses over time to become severe with worsening desaturation. A TOF spell occurs when there is an acute change in the cardiac inotropic state, often in the setting of agitation and dehydration. The infundibular stenosis acutely worsens and patients become profoundly desaturated; this may be an extremely serious event, leading to brain damage or death. Acute treatment modalities include sedation, hydration, systemic afterload augmentation (α-adrenergic agonists), beta blockade to reduce the inotropic state, and even endotracheal intubation with supplemental inspired oxygen.

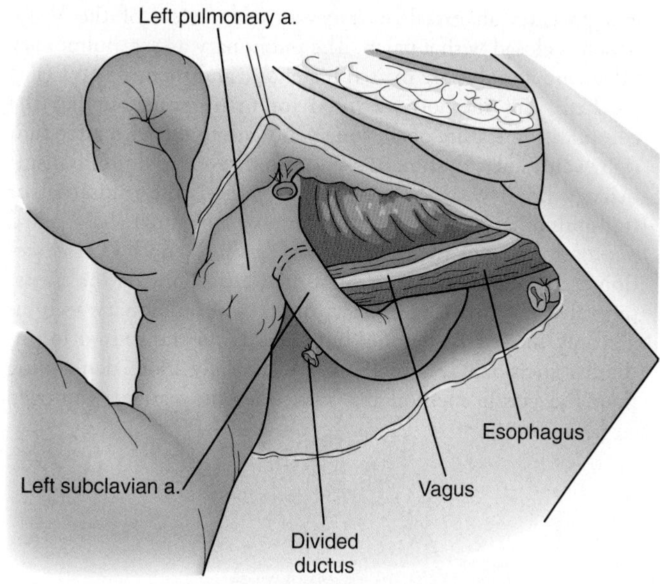


**FIGURE 59-20** Blalock-Taussig shunt.

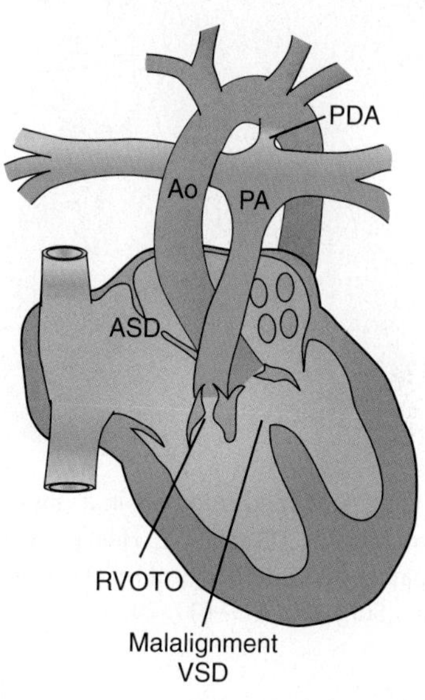


**FIGURE 59-21** Anatomy of tetralogy of Fallot. A malalignment VSD, aortic override, RVOTO, and subsequent right ventricular hypertrophy. *Ao,* Aorta; *PA,* pulmonary artery. (Adapted from Davis S: Tetralogy of Fallot with and without pulmonary atresia. In Nichols DG, Ungerleider RM, Spevak PJ, et al [eds]: Critical heart disease in infants and children, Philadelphia, 2006, Mosby, p 756.)

The natural history of untreated TOF is dismal, with most children succumbing to the ravages of progressive cyanosis before 10 years of age. Surgery remains the mainstay of therapy. Medical and catheter-based therapy may be used to temporize, but TOF is a surgical disease. The principles of surgical correction include patch closure of the VSD and relief of all levels of the RVOTO and pulmonary artery stenosis. The classic method of TOF repair uses a longitudinal incision through the RVOT;

this provides an excellent transventricular view of the VSD, which is closed with a patch. The pulmonary artery, pulmonary valve, and annulus are incised if stenotic and then the RVOT is patched. This method was used for many years but has the complicating feature of the long ventriculotomy, with attendant right ventricular dysfunction and often severe pulmonic insufficiency (Fig. 59-22). An alternate method, the transatrial or transpulmonary approach, first proposed by Imai, has gained popularity. In this method, the VSD closure and RVOT resection are accomplished through a right atriotomy via the tricuspid valve. The main pulmonary artery and pulmonary annulus are only incised if stenotic, but there is no transmural infundibular incision. This method is technically more demanding than the classic method but may offer the patient improved

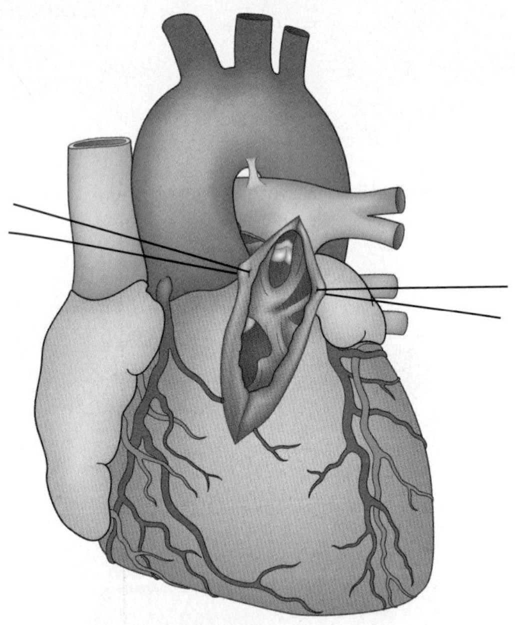

**FIGURE 59-22** Long right ventriculotomy in a classic transventricular approach. (From Morales DL, Zafar F, Heinle JS: Right ventricular infundibulum sparing (RVIS) tetralogy of Fallot repair: A review of over 300 patients. Ann Surg 250: 611–617, 2009.)

long-term RV function (Figs. 59-23 to Fig. 59-25). The approach has been further developed as an RV infundibulum-sparing (RVIS) strategy that focuses on minimizing the RV incision and preserving the pulmonary valve. The RVIS strategy includes an algorithm for optimal timing of the repair that considers the individual patient's weight, age, and overall clinical picture (Fig. 59-26). Midterm results with this approach have demonstrated preserved RV function.[30]

The long-term sequelae of TOF repair have been unfolding. It is clear that for most patients, successful childhood repair of TOF does not translate into a cure. As patients age after TOF repair, long-term complications may develop. Patients with long RVOT incisions (transannular) will by necessity have severe pulmonary insufficiency and a noncontractile infundibulum. Over time, the effects of chronic right heart volume overload include right ventricle dilation and decreased function, often with progressive tricuspid insufficiency and elevated central venous pressure. These patients may present with hepatomegaly, peripheral edema, and severe exercise intolerance. Dysrhythmias may frequently occur; patients with large right ventriculotomies develop endocardial scarring, which may be the substrate for ventricular tachycardia. Chronic right atrial dilation may ultimately lead to atrial dysrhythmias, including atrial tachycardia and fibrillation. Relative to these and other potential issues after TOF repair, patients require careful and lifelong medical follow-up. Many will need re-intervention; this is frequently the case in patients with chronic, severe pulmonary insufficiency, which is indicated when right ventricle dilation and dysfunction become significant. In these patients, placing a competent pulmonary valve will be necessary to relieve chronic right ventricle overload. These issues are of particular importance to the patient with repaired TOF presenting for noncardiac surgery. A careful assessment of the patient's cardiac anatomy and function is performed, including echocardiography, Holter monitoring and, on occasion, cardiac catheterization.

### Pulmonary Atresia and Intact Ventricular Septum

Pulmonary atresia with an intact ventricular septum (PA-IVS) presents with profound desaturation and ductal-dependent pulmonary blood flow in newborns. The cardiac morphology in this

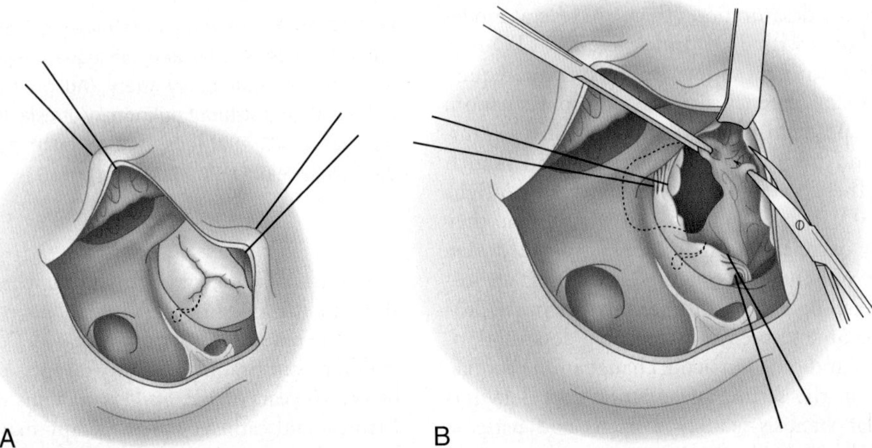


**FIGURE 59-23 A,** Surgeon's view through a transatrial incision in the transatrial/transpulmonary approach. **B,** RVOT muscle resection through the right atriotomy. (From Morales DL, Zafar F, Heinle JS: Right ventricular infundibulum sparing (RVIS) tetralogy of Fallot repair: A review of over 300 patients. Ann Surg 250:611–617, 2009.)

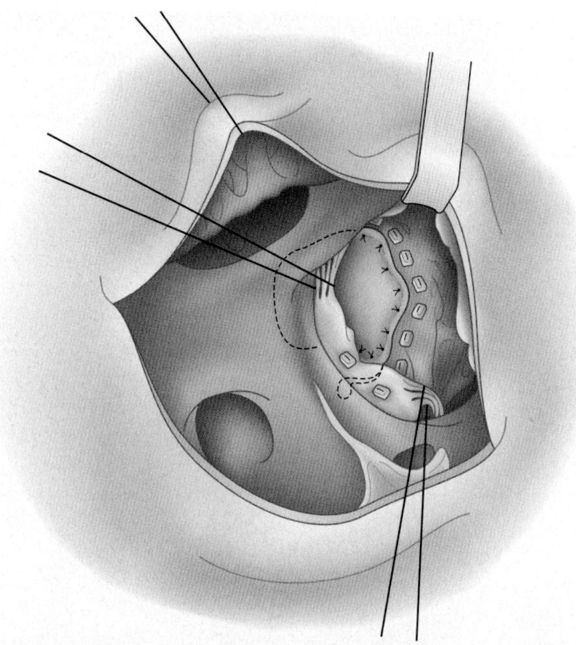

**FIGURE 59-24** VSD patch closure with pledgets around the defect and on to the tricuspid valve annulus to avoid the conduction system. (From Morales DL, Zafar F, Heinle JS: Right ventricular infundibulum sparing [RVIS] tetralogy of Fallot repair: A review of over 300 patients. Ann Surg 250:611–617, 2009.)

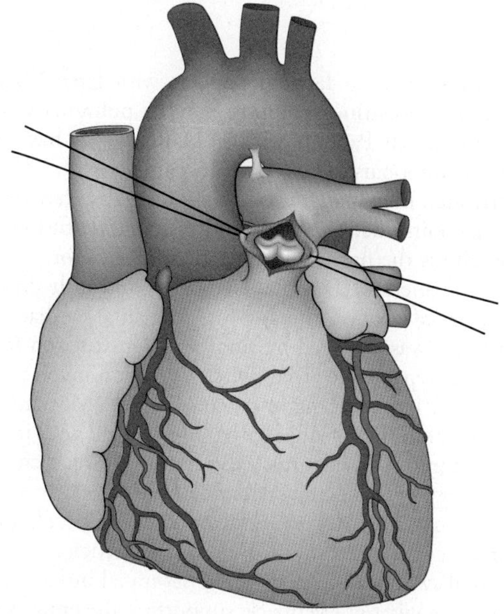

**FIGURE 59-25** Mini–transannular incision in the transatrial-transpulmonary approach. (From Morales DL, Zafar F, Heinle JS: Right ventricular infundibulum sparing [RVIS] tetralogy of Fallot repair: A review of over 300 patients. Ann Surg 250:611–617, 2009.)

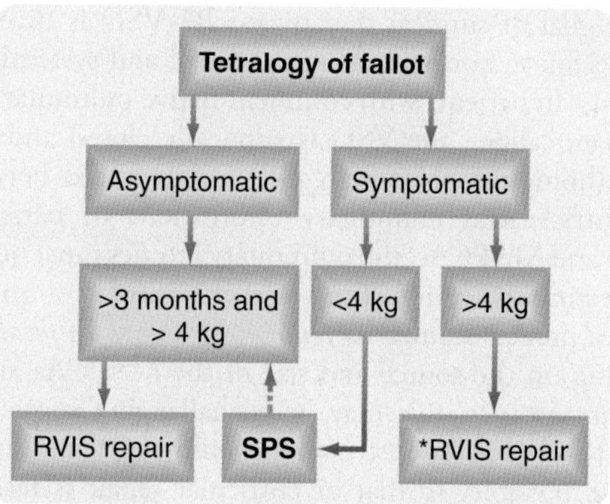


**FIGURE 59-26** Algorithm for the right ventricular infundibulum–sparing (RVIS) strategy. The goal of this strategy is to minimize the RV incision and preserve the pulmonary valve. It is an individualized approach that considers the patient's weight, age, and overall clinical picture. (From Morales DL, Zafar F, Heinle JS: Right ventricular infundibulum sparing [RVIS] tetralogy of Fallot repair: A review of over 300 patients. Ann Surg 250:611–617, 2009.)

condition varies widely. On the most severe end of the spectrum, patients have very small right ventricles, tiny tricuspid inlets, and often a right ventricle–dependent coronary circulation. In these cases, the right ventricle must remain hypertensive to provide flow to these segments of the coronary circulation. At the other end of the anatomic spectrum, patients have a relatively normal tricuspid valve and right ventricle. Most patients fall in between these extremes, with some degree of tricuspid valve and right ventricle underdevelopment.

Because patients are ductal-dependent at birth, an assessment must be made as to whether the right heart will be capable of ultimately supporting a biventricular circulation. If the coronary circulation is truly right ventricle–dependent, decompressing the right ventricle will result in coronary insufficiency. In these situations, a palliative BT shunt will be created in anticipation of promoting the patient down a single-ventricle pathway. In other patients, the atretic pulmonary valve must be opened with percutaneous balloon dilation or open surgical valvotomy. Over time, the hypertensive, often apparently underdeveloped right ventricle will improve in size and function and be capable of supporting all or a significant proportion of the cardiac output. At initial presentation, many patients have a large patent foramen ovale or ASD; in patients with a restrictive ASD and marginal right heart, an atrial septostomy (balloon) allows for atrial-level right-to-left shunting until the right ventricle improves. Ultimately, if the right ventricle is adequate, the ASD can be closed.

### Pulmonary Atresia With Ventricular Septal Defect

Pulmonary atresia (PA) with VSD (PA-VSD) is morphologically similar to TOF, with the exception of an atretic pulmonary valve. Patients may have confluent, normal-sized pulmonary arteries perfused by a PDA. In severe cases, the pulmonary arteries are discontinuous and the lungs are variably perfused by diminutive native branch pulmonary arteries and muscularized, collateral vessels originating from the descending aorta and brachiocephalic vessels. These major aortopulmonary collateral arteries (MAPCAs) have a propensity to develop severe stenoses as they are exposed to systemic arterial pressure. Many of these MAPCAs eventually occlude at an unpredictable rate during childhood. Because they may provide the only blood supply to some lung segments, patients will become progressively desaturated.

The goal of surgical therapy for PA-VSD is biventricular repair to achieve normal cardiac workload and systemic arterial saturations. In patients with confluent native pulmonary arteries of adequate caliber, the VSD is surgically closed and a valved conduit (homograft or heterograft) is interposed between the right ventricle and pulmonary bifurcation. In patients with PA-VSD and MAPCAs, the pulmonary arteries must be repaired by connecting the various lung segments into a common trunk through a process known as *pulmonary artery unifocalization.*[31] Depending on the source and size of the MAPCAs and native pulmonary arteries, this may be a challenging surgical procedure, but the goal is constructing a pulmonary tree as close to normal as possible, so that biventricular repair is feasible (see earlier).

The long-term issues of repair of PA-VSD are similar to those concerns described earlier for TOF. The addition of a right ventricle–pulmonary artery conduit guarantees the need for reoperation because no currently available conduit choice offers the potential for somatic growth or an indefinitely durable valve.

### Valvular Pulmonic Stenosis

Patients with isolated valvular pulmonary stenosis (PS) are almost always treated in infancy with a percutaneous balloon pulmonary valvotomy. The intermediate-term results of this treatment are good; however, all patients are left with significant pulmonary valve insufficiency and eventually require pulmonary valve replacement.

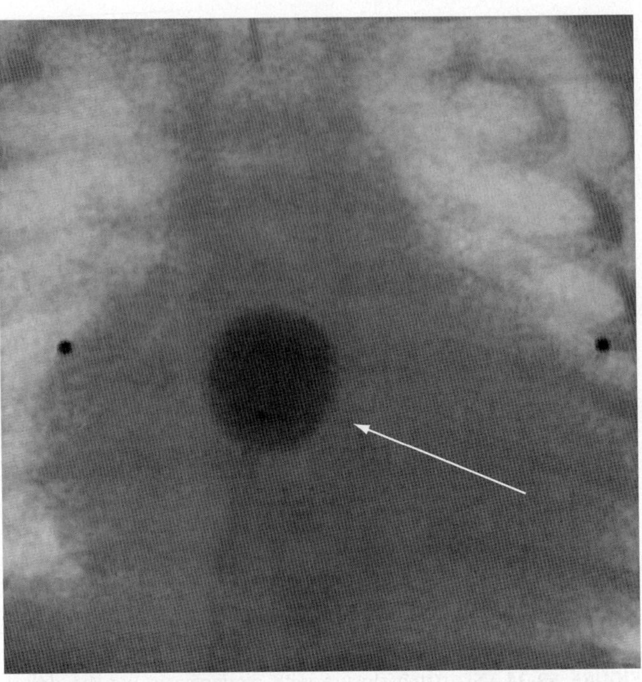

**FIGURE 59-27** Angiogram during balloon atrial septostomy. The *arrow* points to the inflated balloon catheter at the atrial septum. The interventional cardiologist will forcefully pull the balloon across the patent foramen ovale to create an open, unobstructed secundum atrial septal defect.

## Conotruncal Anomalies

### Transposition of the Great Arteries

TGA is a common cyanotic congenital cardiac lesion. In this section, our discussion relates only to TGA in which there are two good ventricles identified as being capable of independent function as the right and left ventricle. TGA is commonly referred to as D-TGA, in relationship to the typically normal D (dextro) ventricular looping that occurs in association with the discordant ventriculoarterial connection and normal atrioventricular connection. TGA occurs in the setting of an intact ventricular septum (TGA-IVS) or with associated VSD (TGA-VSD). In TGA-VSD, there may be associated aortic arch hypoplasia and coarctation. On the other extreme, there may be severe pulmonic and subpulmonic stenosis (left ventricular outflow tract obstruction [LVOTO]) or even pulmonary atresia (TGA-VSD with PA).

Patients with TGA-IVS typically present in the early newborn period with profound cyanosis, associated with normal perinatal PDA closure. In the absence of a significant ASD, the cyanosis will be severe and progress to death if left untreated. Administering IV PGE1 is almost uniformly successful in reestablishing ductal patency to improve the patient's arterial saturation by providing left-to-right shunting and improved pulmonary blood flow.

In most patients, a balloon atrial septostomy is performed (percutaneous through the umbilical vein or femoral vein) to allow atrial-level mixing (Fig. 59-27). This procedure is usually effective in allowing sufficient atrial-level mixing so that the patient is adequately saturated (70% to 80%).

Following the procedure, the prostaglandin infusion can be discontinued. In TGA with significant VSD, there is often sufficient shunting at the level of the VSD to promote adequate systemic saturation; in fact, in patients with large VSDs, the predominant presenting symptom may be pulmonary overcirculation and CHF. Patients with TGA-PA clearly have ductal-dependent pulmonary blood flow. In patients with TGA-VSD and aortic arch hypoplasia or coarctation, PGE1 may be necessary to maintain ductal patency and systemic perfusion. Echocardiography is the primary diagnostic modality for TGA.

The treatment of TGA has evolved significantly during the past 60 years of surgical therapy for congenital cardiac disease. Initial success was achieved by surgical reconstruction to create a physiologic repair. The atrial switch operation involves a series of intra-atrial baffles using a patch channel (Mustard procedure)[32] or infolding of the native atrial wall and interatrial septum (Senning procedure).[33] Both procedures achieve the same physiologic result; the systemic venous blood is redirected to the left ventricle (and thereby the pulmonary circulation) and the pulmonary venous blood to the right ventricle. After a successful atrial switch, patients are fully saturated but are left with their morphologic right ventricle supporting the entire systemic cardiac output. Unfortunately, in many (perhaps ultimately all) patients undergoing the atrial switch procedure, the right ventricle becomes dysfunctional over time, which is manifested by dilation, decreased ejection fraction, tricuspid insufficiency, and dysrhythmias. The observation of problems with the systemic right ventricle in patients after the atrial switch operation was the primary impetus behind the development and application of the arterial switch operation (ASO), which is now established as the surgical treatment of choice for patients with TGA. Currently, operative survival rates for the ASO have been approaching 100%.[34,35]

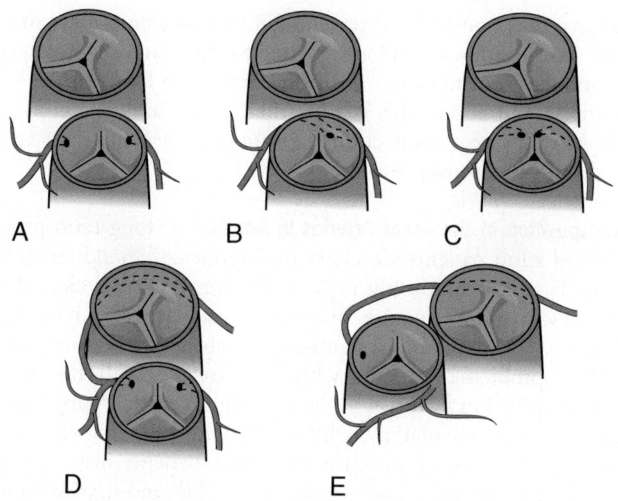


FIGURE 59-28 Five basic coronary artery configurations, as described by Yacoub and Radley-Smith. (Adapted from Mee R: The arterial switch operation. In Stark J, de Leval M [eds]: Surgery for congenital heart defects, ed 2, Philadelphia, 1994, WB Saunders, p 484.)

The ASO provides physiologic and anatomic correction of TGA by establishing ventriculoarterial concordance. The procedure involves transection and translocation of the malposed great vessels. The technically challenging requirement of the ASO relates to the translocation of the coronary arteries to the pulmonary root (the neoaorta). As noted, there are numerous possible branching patterns for the coronary arteries in TGA—some are easily transferred in the ASO, whereas others are more challenging (including single coronary ostium and intramural course; Fig. 59-28).[36] Nonetheless, precise surgical techniques have been described and successfully applied to all coronary branching patterns. Given this, and the known benefit of aligning the morphologic left ventricle with the systemic circulation, the ASO is offered to all patients with TGA irrespective of the coronary branching pattern. Thus, there is no need for precise anatomic definition before surgery; all patients will undergo the ASO.[34] In most patients undergoing this procedure, the pulmonary artery bifurcation is moved anterior to the reconstructed neoaorta to minimize the potential for pulmonary artery distortion and compression of the translocated coronary arteries, the maneuver of LeCompte (Fig. 59-29). Although there are inter-institutional biases in terms of nuances of treatment for TGA, the following surgical strategies are generally agreed on for this group of patients.

**Transposition of the Great Arteries–Intact Ventricular Septum** After balloon atrial septostomy (BAS) and weaning from PGE1, if possible, newborns with TGA-IVS undergo semielective ASO in the first few days to weeks of life. Rarely, patients present with profound desaturation refractory to BAS and PGE1; in this setting, an emergent ASO is indicated. We have found this to be necessary in one patient during the past decade in an experience involving more than 200 newborn ASOs. For other patients, the ASO needs to be performed in a timely but non-emergent setting. Even in the presence of adequate systemic saturation, the patient's morphologic left ventricle is functioning in a low-pressure work environment—supporting the

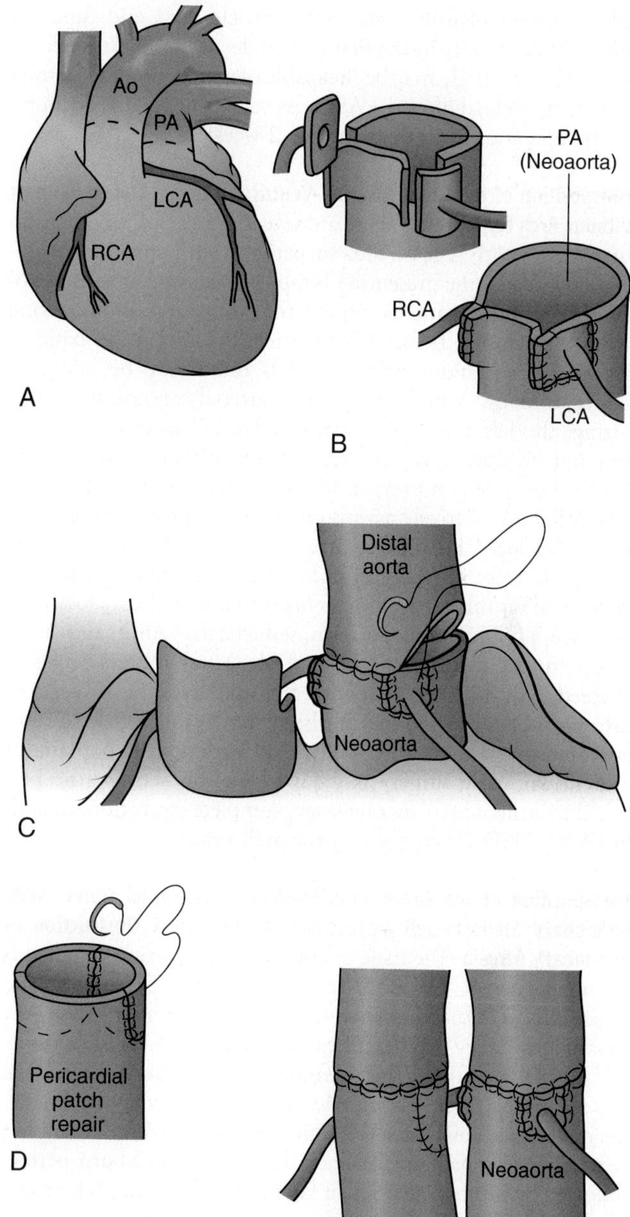


FIGURE 59-29 Arterial switch operation. **A,** The aorta (Ao) and pulmonary artery (PA) are transected above the sinuses of Valsalva. **B,** The coronaries are excised from the aorta and anastomosed to the pulmonary artery using a trapdoor technique. **C,** The distal aorta is brought behind the pulmonary artery (LeCompte maneuver) and anastomosed to the neoaorta. **D,** Separate pericardial patches are sutured to replace the excised coronary artery tissue from the aorta. **E,** Completed repair. *LCA,* Left coronary artery; *RCA,* right coronary artery. (Adapted from Karl TR, Kirshbom PM: Transposition of the great arteries and the arterial switch operation. In Nichols DG, Ungerleider RM, Spevak PJ, et al [eds]: Critical heart disease in infants and children, Philadelphia, 2006, Mosby, p 721.)

pulmonary circulation. Thus, left ventricle mass and function will involute rapidly in the first few weeks of life. By 6 weeks of life, the left ventricle may be incapable of supporting the normal systemic workload after the ASO. As such, the preferred timing for the operation is in the first 1 to 2 weeks of life.

**Transposition of the Great Arteries–Ventricular Septal Defect With or Without Arch Hypoplasia** There are several modes of presentation for patients with TGA-VSD. In patients with small, pressure-restrictive VSD, the presenting symptoms are similar to those of TGA-IVS. These patients require the ASO early in life, along with VSD closure before left ventricle involution. In patients with TGA and nonrestrictive VSD, there may be adequate mixing to allow reasonable systemic arterial saturation. In this setting, the left ventricle remains pressure-loaded and thereby does not involute; thus, the necessity of early promotion to the ASO is less time-compressed. Many newborns with TGA and a large VSD are relatively asymptomatic soon after birth; they go on to develop CHF in the first 1 to 2 months of life as the normal decrease in newborn pulmonary resistance occurs. Our preference for this group of patients is to follow them closely for evidence of CHF and perform semielective ASO and VSD closure in the first 4 to 6 weeks of life. Some centers prefer to proceed with this surgery sooner; this appears to be a matter of surgeon preference and has not been shown to affect long-term outcome. In patients with TGA-VSD with arch hypoplasia or coarctation, early surgery is required. In this setting, the preferred treatment involves one-stage, complete correction, including ASO, VSD closure, and aortic arch repair.

**Transposition of the Great Arteries–Ventricular Septal Defect With Pulmonary Stenosis–Left Ventricular Outflow Tract Obstruction or Pulmonary Atresia** The issue of concern in this group of patients is the degree of LVOTO. In patients with TGA-VSD and organic LVOTO, with a relatively normal pulmonary valve, the treatment strategy is as described earlier, with ASO, VSD closure, and LVOT resection. The situation becomes more complex in the setting of severe PS or PA. These patients may be ductal-dependent as newborns (PA) and require newborn complete correction or a palliative Blalock shunt in the newborn period, followed by biventricular repair later in infancy (our preference). The goal in these patients is to achieve biventricular repair to create an unobstructed connection between the morphologic left ventricle and systemic circulation. Several operations have been described and successfully used in this setting.

The Rastelli procedure involves an interventricular patch baffle, which commits the left ventricle to the aorta through the VSD. Typically, a right ventricle–pulmonary artery conduit is then placed to achieve pulmonary blood flow. Issues of concern include the potential for LVOTO (at or below the level of the VSD) and the certain need for future right ventricle–pulmonary artery conduit revision. The REV procedure is designed to minimize the potential of LVOT obstruction and to use all possible native tissue-tissue connections to limit the potential need for future surgery. This procedure involves resection of the muscular conus between the aorta and pulmonary roots, interventricular baffle of the left ventricle to the aorta, and translocation of the native main pulmonary artery to the right ventricle (by a LeCompte maneuver) without the use of an intervening conduit. The final option involves aortic root translocation, which includes resection of the entire native aortic root and coronary origins, resection of the intervening muscular conus, and posterior translocation of the aortic root to the surgically enlarged pulmonary root to achieve a direct connection between the left ventricle and aorta. The VSD is then closed and a conduit is placed or a direct connection is created between the right ventricle and pulmonary arteries.

**Transposition of the Great Arteries in Adults** The long-term prognosis of adult patients who have undergone childhood repair of TGA is still incompletely understood; however, it is clear that all these patients require lifelong surveillance and have the potential of developing significant anatomic and functional cardiac problems. Patients who were treated with the atrial switch operation have a morphologic right ventricle supporting their systemic circulation, which will predictably fail in many patients. Although fully saturated, these patients may present later in life with signs and symptoms of CHF and dysrhythmia. For severely affected individuals, the only realistic option may ultimately be in the form of cardiac transplantation.

The long-term issues related to the ASO are less well understood. Despite technical advances in reconstructive methods, there is still a troubling incidence of postoperative supravalvular and branch pulmonic stenosis. The neoaortic root may dilate in some patients undergoing the ASO, leading to neoaortic insufficiency and coronary artery distortion. The fate of the surgically translocated coronary ostia is unclear; there is clearly a risk for late, sudden cardiac death related to unsuspected coronary insufficiency noted elsewhere in this chapter. For the adult patient undergoing noncardiac surgery after previous surgery for complex congenital cardiac disease, including TGA, a high index of suspicion is warranted.

### Double-Outlet Right Ventricle

Double-outlet right ventricle (DORV) occurs when both great vessels are anatomically committed to the RV. This may be in association with a subaortic VSD, a noncommitted (remote) VSD, or a subpulmonary VSD (Taussig-Bing anomaly). As with other complex cardiac conditions, the goal of treatment relates to the presenting hemodynamic conditions and patient symptoms. The ultimate goal is to achieve a biventricular circulation when possible. Patients may present with severe cyanosis and require corrective or palliative therapy in the newborn period. Conversely, they may present with unrestricted pulmonary blood flow and develop CHF. The challenging issue of constructing a biventricular repair relates to achieving unobstructed outlets from the right and left ventricles. In patients with DORV with subaortic VSD and RVOTO, reconstruction is similar to that for TOF. More remote VSDs may require enlargement with interventricular tunnel repair. For the Taussig-Bing anomaly, the relationship of the VSD to the pulmonary artery makes the ASO the procedure of choice. These patients often have RVOTO and aortic arch hypoplasia, which require attention at the time of complete correction. For rare individuals, the relationship of the great vessels and complexity of the VSD preclude a biventricular repair, and the patient must be treated as if he or she has a functional single ventricle.

### Congenitally Corrected Transposition of the Great Arteries (L-Transposition)

ccTGA, or L-TGA, describes a constellation of conditions with the common feature of atrioventricular and ventriculoarterial discordance. This may be in association with VSD, pulmonic and subpulmonic stenosis, and displaced left AV valve (ebsteinoid left AV valve). In ccTGA, the morphologic mitral valve is right-sided and associated with the morphologic left ventricle; the morphologic tricuspid valve is associated with the morphologic right ventricle. Patients with this condition are physiologically corrected in that in the absence of ventricular-level shunting, they are fully saturated—hence, the term *corrected transposition.* The age and mode of patient presentation in this condition depend on the contribution of associated defects and the function of the morphologic right ventricle, which acts as the systemic ventricle. Controversy exists regarding the timing and mode of surgical treatment for patients presenting with various manifestations of ccTGA.

**Congenitally Corrected Transposition of the Great Arteries With Intact Ventricular Septum** Patients with ccTGA-IVS may be entirely asymptomatic throughout childhood and early adulthood. Frequently, the diagnosis is made incidentally. In other patients, the disease presents with symptoms of CHF in association with right ventricular dysfunction or left AV valve insufficiency. There is also a high incidence of complete heart block in patients with ccTGA, and the first manifestation may be this dysrhythmia, with associated symptoms.

Treatment for patients presenting with CHF is a challenging management scenario. For patients with ccTGA and preserved RV function, left AV valve repair or replacement may be considered. Unfortunately, in many of these patients, the valvular insufficiency may be more a manifestation of declining systemic RV function, with septal shift and annular dilation, rather than intrinsic valve pathology. In this setting, valve replacement will not correct the progression of RV dysfunction. For patients with systemic RV dysfunction, one option for treatment is through a complex reconstruction known as a *double switch* (Fig. 59-30). This procedure includes an atrial switch in combination with an arterial switch to align the morphologic left ventricle with the systemic circulation. In almost all patients with ccTGA-IVS and RV dysfunction (and in the absence of structural LVOTO), a period of left ventricle retraining will be required before the double-switch procedure. This relates to the fact that the left ventricle will have been functioning in the low-pressure pulmonary circulation and will be incapable of performing systemic work. Retraining or conditioning the left ventricle requires the surgical creation of PS by the placement of a pulmonary artery band. Most surgeons agree that the left ventricle must work at or very near systemic blood pressure for many months (we favor a minimum of 6 months) before the double-switch operation. The double switch is a technically challenging operation, with significant perioperative risk. Because of the small numbers of patients treated worldwide with this complicated surgical strategy, there are only limited data of the acute and midterm results.[37] An issue of concern centers on the long-term ability of the retrained left ventricle to function as the systemic ventricle. Nonetheless, patients with ccTGA and depressed RV function have a poor prognosis otherwise and, as such, the complexity and risk of the double-switch process appear justified. The only other surgical option for these patients is cardiac transplantation.

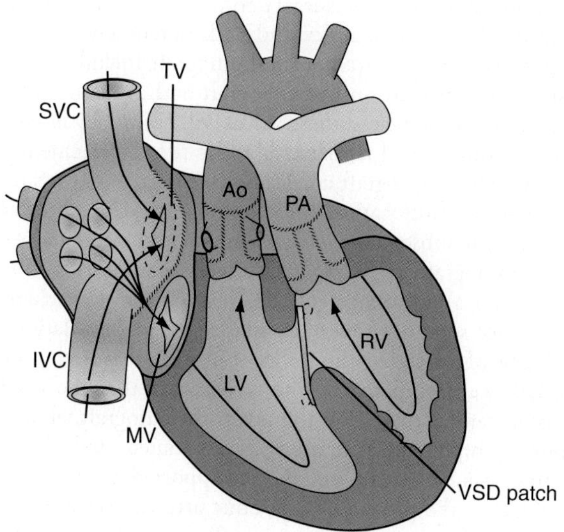


**FIGURE 59-30** Double-switch operation (Senning and arterial switch). *Ao,* Aorta; *LV,* left ventricle; *MV,* mitral valve; *PA,* pulmonary artery; *TV,* tricuspid valve. (Adapted from Karl TR, Cochrane AD: Congenitally corrected transposition of the great arteries. In Mavroudis C, Backer CL [eds]: Pediatric cardiac surgery. Philadelphia, 2003, Mosby, p 488.)

**Congenitally Corrected Transposition of the Great Arteries With Ventricular Septal Defect and Pulmonic Stenosis** Patients in this category are often well balanced and have mild cyanosis, with minimal symptoms in childhood, whereas others with more severe PS or pulmonary atresia present early in life with symptomatic cyanosis. Treatment for the overtly cyanotic infant with ccTGA-PS is initially palliative in the form of a Blalock shunt. The ultimate goal for all patients is a biventricular circulation, with normal arterial oxygen saturation. One option for these patients is to close the VSD surgically and place a conduit between the morphologic left ventricle and pulmonary arteries to relieve the pulmonary obstruction. This classic repair benefits the patient by separating the systemic and pulmonary circulations and allowing normal oxygen tension. The issue of concern in patients undergoing this repair is that the morphologic right ventricle must act independently as the systemic ventricle following repair. As noted, the ability of the right ventricle to support the systemic circulation may be of question over the long term in some patients. As such, an alternative strategy in these patients is to baffle the LV outflow to the aorta through the VSD, then perform an atrial switch to reroute the systemic and pulmonary venous return, and finally to place a conduit from the morphologic right ventricle to the pulmonary arteries. This option is a modification of the double-switch arrangement, affording the patient the benefit of a systemic left ventricle. Because the left ventricle has been working at systemic pressure before correction, a period of retraining is unnecessary.

Adult patients with ccTGA, with or without previous surgery, merit careful attention before any noncardiac operation. These patients may have various complex ongoing cardiac issues, including rhythm disturbance, ventricular dysfunction, and valvular insufficiency.

## Left Ventricular Outflow Tract Obstruction

LVOTO may present in isolation or in combination with other complex cardiac lesions. The physiologic consequences of severe LVOTO may be catastrophic, including diminished systemic cardiac output and tremendous LV pressure overload. Newborns with severe LVOTO may present in shock with diminished peripheral perfusion, cardiomegaly, and pulmonary congestion. There is a significant risk for NEC in these babies. In older patients, gradual onset of LVOTO may be initially asymptomatic, only to manifest over time as decreasing exercise tolerance and declining LV function. Patients with severe LVOTO and cardiomegaly are at high risk for myocardial ischemia and sudden cardiac death. The resting ECG will often demonstrate LV hypertrophy, with a strain pattern. If performed, an exercise stress test may demonstrate worrisome ST-segment depression and ventricular dysrhythmias. Echocardiography is the primary diagnostic tool for patients with LVOTO. In rare cases, diagnostic cardiac catheterization may be considered to delineate the level of obstruction.

### Valvular Aortic Stenosis

Congenital valvular aortic stenosis (AS) is a common cause of LVOTO. The degree of obstruction may range from mild in patients with a congenitally bicuspid aortic valve to severe in patients with critical AS with unidentifiable valve commissures and annular hypoplasia. Babies presenting with critical AS are often symptomatic early in the newborn period, presenting with shock and profoundly depressed ventricular function. Currently, these patients are almost all taken to the cardiac catheterization laboratory for balloon aortic valvotomy. This procedure may be lifesaving in relieving the AS and allowing for recovery of ventricular function. For most of the patients, however, the procedure is palliative, with a significant incidence of recurrence of AS or development of significant aortic insufficiency following the procedure. In patients with AS refractory to balloon dilation, an open aortic valvotomy may be necessary (Fig. 59-31). A surgical valvotomy, especially in small babies with adequate

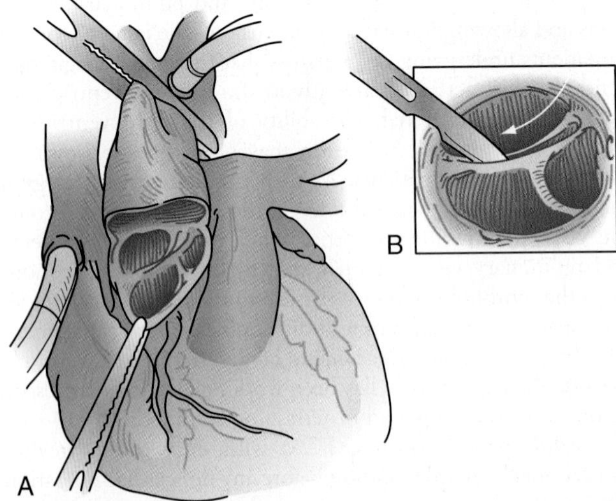


**FIGURE 59-31** Close-up of the aortic valve demonstrating a surgical valvectomy. **A,** The valve is bicuspid, with a prominent raphe in the anterior valve leaflet. **B,** The orifice is enlarged by incising the fused commissure between the two leaflets. (From Chang AC, Burke RP: Left ventricular outflow tract obstruction. In Chang AC, Hanley FL, Wernovsky G, Wessell DL [eds]: Pediatric cardiac intensive care. Baltimore, 1998, Williams & Wilkins.)

annular dimension, can be accomplished by an accurate incision down a rudimentary commissure or raphe to improve cusp mobility.

Recurrent AS after previous ballooning may be amenable to repeat dilation; however, when associated with significant aortic insufficiency, the patient will require surgery. Severe aortic insufficiency after previous balloon dilation is usually related to an avulsed cusp. In these cases, valve repair may be possible, but replacement may prove necessary. Recent published series have confirmed the usefulness of aortic valve repair procedures, which is a particularly attractive option for growing children.[38]

The decision to replace the aortic valve in growing children is clouded by the lack of an ideal aortic valve substitute—a valve capable of lifelong durability, appropriate somatic growth, easily implantable, and not requiring anticoagulation. Criteria for aortic valve replacement are beyond the scope of this chapter; however, severe valvular AS not amenable to catheter or open valvotomy is clearly an appropriate indication. Options for aortic valve replacement in children include a mechanical prosthesis, heterograft, homograft, and pulmonary autograft. A mechanical prosthesis may be considered in childhood; however, the valve size must be sufficient to provide adequate function as the patient grows. Most surgeons and cardiologists recommend therapeutic anticoagulation in children with a mechanical valve prosthesis, but this can be challenging and potentially dangerous in growing children and adolescents. As such, many surgeons believe the risk for such medical treatment outweighs the potential benefit of a theoretically durable valve.

Heterograft aortic valve prostheses historically have been associated with limited durability in children and are also not capable of somatic growth. Currently available heterograft prostheses have not undergone sufficient use in children to provide useful data concerning improved durability. Human cadaver aortic valves (aortic homograft) have been used extensively in children and young adults. These valves are usually implanted as a complete aortic root replacement, which require coronary ostial implantation. Thus, surgery to place an aortic homograft is considerably more complex and with potentially higher risk. The positive features of an aortic homograft include improved durability in comparison to heterograft and avoidance of anticoagulation. Nonetheless, these valves will eventually fail, necessitating a complicated reoperative aortic root replacement.

Pulmonary autograft aortic root replacement (Ross operation) involves translocation of the pulmonary valve to the aortic position with subsequent replacement of the pulmonary valve with a homograft or heterograft valved conduit (Fig. 59-32). The theoretical advantages of the Ross procedure include the potential for somatic growth, avoidance of anticoagulation, and possibility of extended durability. Enthusiasm for this procedure has been tempered by the recognition that the need for extension cardiac dissection to harvest the autograft, along with a more complex implantation, is associated with increased operative risk. Furthermore, the unsupported pulmonary root may dilate in the presence of systemic arterial pressure, leading to progressive autograft aortic insufficiency. This observation has led to various modifications of the implantation technique to support the aortic annulus and even the sinus segment. Given these considerations and the certain need for reoperation to replace the right ventricular–pulmonary artery conduit, great caution must be exercised in the application of the Ross operation.[39]

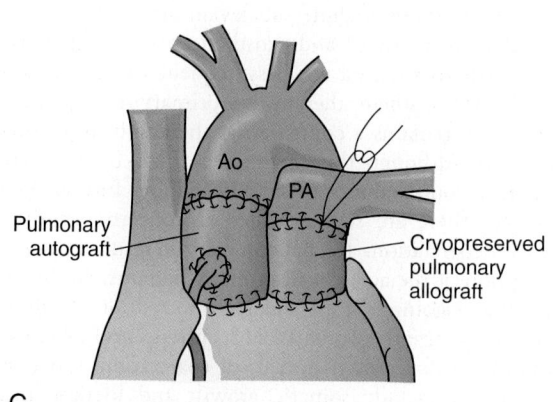

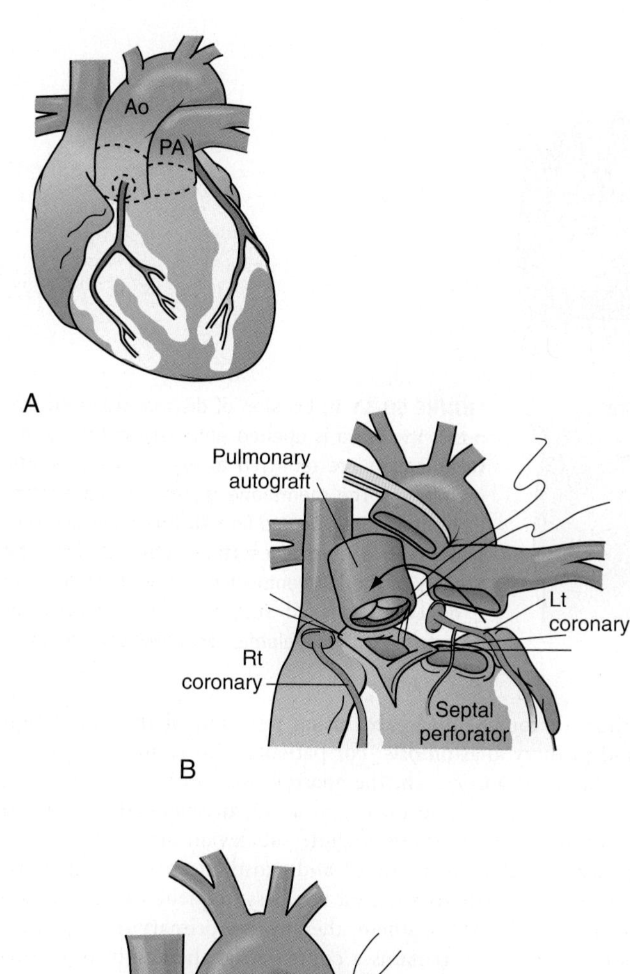


**FIGURE 59-32** Ross procedure. **A,** The great arteries are transected above the sinotubular ridge. The coronary arteries are excised using coronary artery buttons. **B,** The pulmonary autograft is excised from the right ventricular outflow tract and the proximal end of the autograft is anastomosed to the annulus. **C,** The coronary artery buttons are then anastomosed to the pulmonary autograft. *Ao,* Aorta; *PA,* pulmonary artery. (Adapted from St Louis JD, Jaggers J: Left ventricular outflow tract obstruction. In Nichols DG, Ungerleider RM, Spevak PJ, et al [eds]: Critical heart disease in infants and children, Philadelphia, 2006, Mosby, p 615.)

#### Fibromuscular Subaortic Stenosis

This condition is a progressive narrowing of the LVOT related to a dense fibrous membrane usually found in association with asymmetrical protrusion of the interventricular septum into the outflow tract. The membrane is often concentric and becomes densely adherent to the septum and mitral valve. The membrane progresses toward and eventually onto the undersurface of the aortic valve cusps, which leads to progressive LVOTO, aortic valve cusp retraction, and aortic insufficiency.

Echocardiography is the primary diagnostic tool when assessing the degree of obstruction and progression of subaortic stenosis. Unfortunately, it is not accurate for assessing subtle degrees of cusp extension.[40] Cardiac catheterization is rarely needed to diagnose this condition; balloon dilation is of no use in treating the LVOTO.

Surgery is the mainstay of treatment for subaortic stenosis but there is disagreement about surgical indications. Most surgeons believe that new onset of any degree of aortic insufficiency in association with a subaortic membrane, irrespective of the pressure gradient, is an indication for surgery. In other patients, an escalating LVOT gradient, associated LV hypertrophy, and appropriate anatomic substrate are acceptable indications for operation.

The surgical procedure for subaortic stenosis involves a transaortic resection of the subaortic membrane, including all attachments to the mitral valve, septum, and aortic valve cusps. A septal myectomy is performed, along with membrane resection, in most patients (Fig. 59-33). Complications include membrane recurrence, injury to the bundle of His, and iatrogenic VSD creation. Nonetheless, with careful technique, the risk for these complications is minimized.

#### Tunnel Subaortic Stenosis

This is a more severe form of LVOTO that is often associated with aortic annular hypoplasia and valvular aortic stenosis. In severe cases, the LVOTO is not amenable to subaortic resection alone. In this situation, an aortic root enlarging procedure may be necessary to relieve the obstruction (aortoventriculoplasty, or Konno procedure). This complex reconstruction generally is associated with the necessity of aortic valve replacement using one of the aforementioned options. It is also of note that all degrees of LVOTO may be seen in association with a number of left heart obstructive lesions (Shone's syndrome[41]), which may require extensive reconstruction.

### Aortic Arch Anomalies

#### Aortic Coarctation

Coarctation of the aorta is one of the most frequently encountered congenital cardiac lesions. This condition has a wide range of presentations, from the severely symptomatic newborn with CHF and depressed ventricular function to the adult with proximal hypertension and minimal symptoms. Coarctation is classified relative to its association with the ligamentum arteriosus and aortic arch. An infantile or preductal aortic coarctation is seen in combination with a large PDA, which may have predominantly right-to-left flow to the lower descending aorta. In this setting, the patient is ductal-dependent for systemic blood flow until the coarctation is repaired, and a PGE1 infusion must be maintained to prevent ductal closure. A periductal or juxtaductal coarctation occurs in the region of the ductal insertion and is distal to the aortic isthmus, which may be normal or hypoplastic (Fig. 59-34).

Aortic coarctation with or without aortic arch hypoplasia is frequently associated with intracardiac anomalies, including multiple left heart obstructive lesions (e.g., mitral stenosis, left ventricular hypoplasia or endocardial fibroelastosis, subaortic or aortic stenosis) known as Shone's syndrome.[41] Patients with large

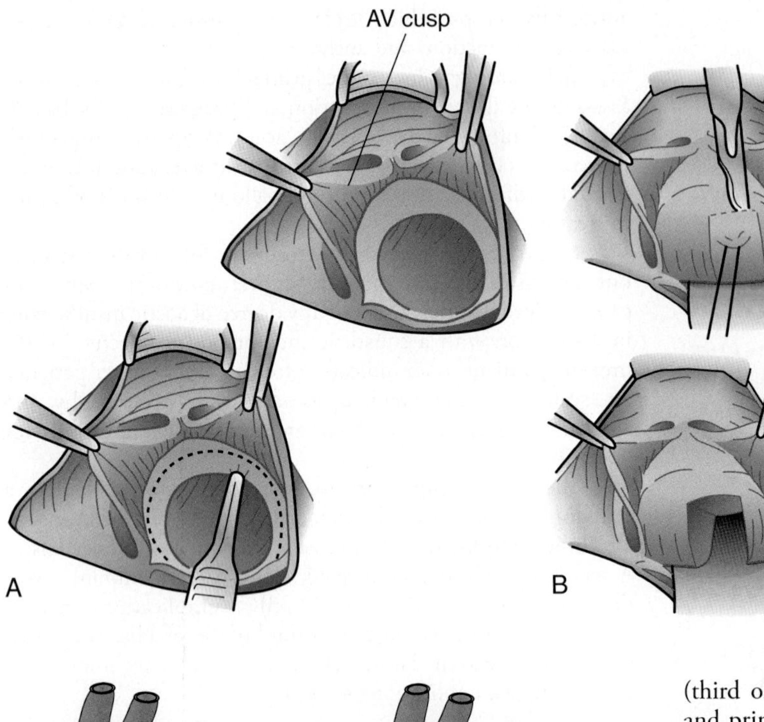


**FIGURE 59-33** **A,** Excision of discrete subaortic stenosis. The aorta is opened obliquely and the aortic valve leaflets are retracted to expose the subaortic membrane. The membrane is excised circumferentially along the *indicated line.* **B,** This is usually combined with a muscle resection. (From de Leval M: Surgery of the left ventricular outflow tract. In Stark J, de Leval M [eds]: Surgery for congenital heart defects, ed 2, Philadelphia, 1994, WB Saunders.)

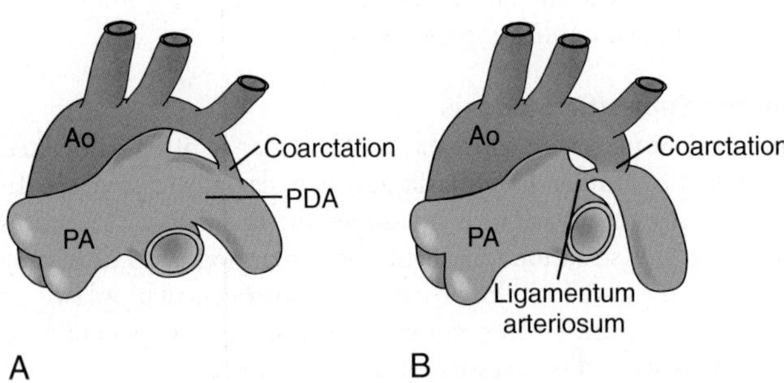


**FIGURE 59-34** Coarctation of the aorta (Ao). **A,** Infantile or preductal coarctation. **B,** Adult coarctation. *PA,* Pulmonary artery. (From Backer CL, Mavroudis C: Coarctation of the aorta. In Mavroudis C, Backer CL [eds]: Pediatric heart surgery. Philadelphia, 2003, Mosby, p 252.)

VSDs may present in infancy with severe aortic coarctation, with or without subaortic stenosis.

Aortic coarctation may be suspected on clinical examination by a significant upper-lower extremity blood pressure gradient and diminished or absent femoral and pedal pulses. In older patients with well-developed intercostal collateral arteries, a continuous murmur may be auscultated over the posterior thorax. Echocardiography is now the primary diagnostic modality for aortic coarctation. MRI and CT angiography may also be useful in some patients. In rare cases, cardiac catheterization is required to define the anatomy, but this modality is now used more frequently for treatment, including balloon dilation with or without stenting.

Treatment strategies for aortic coarctation have evolved significantly since the first successful surgical treatment almost 70 years ago. Newborns presenting with severe aortic coarctation with or without associated ductal-dependent systemic blood flow are best treated by surgery. Initial enthusiasm regarding balloon dilation in these patients has diminished as it has become clear that there is a high incidence of recurrent coarctation after neonatal dilation.[42] Most congenital cardiac surgeons perform isolated coarctation repair through a left thoracotomy incision (third or fourth interspace) using resection of the coarctation and primary anastomosis. For patients with relative hypoplasia of the distal aortic arch, the anastomosis can be brought along the lesser curve of the aortic arch using an extended end-to-end method. Other methods include subclavian artery flap aortoplasty (Waldhausen method) and prosthetic patch aortoplasty. These latter methods are used now less frequently than primary repair (Fig. 59-35). Catheter therapy as a primary treatment for aortic coarctation remains a controversial therapy in most surgeons' opinions. Although this methodology has been widely applied, its true comparability to surgery requires further prospective study. There are several issues of concern regarding angioplasty for coarctation. The balloon dilation results in transmural disruption of the aortic wall in many patients, and there is an acute and ongoing risk for aneurysm formation. To limit this risk and minimize the potential of recurrence, off-label use of stents has been done for treatment of coarctation. Obvious issues of concern include somatic growth and lifetime risk potential of a metal device in the descending aorta.

Another issue of controversy surrounds the concomitant treatment of coarctation and significant intracardiac pathology. Several series have now demonstrated superior outcomes for simultaneous therapy in selected groups of patients, including neonates with large VSDs and coarctation with arch hypoplasia. Our approach to this has included one-stage complete repair of intracardiac defects along with aortic arch advancement through median sternotomy on cardiopulmonary bypass.

### Interrupted Aortic Arch

IAA results from lack of proper fusion and involution of the fetal aortic arches. This is a fatal condition without treatment, and IAA is frequently associated with serious intracardiac pathology. IAA is classified based on the level of the interruption. Type A is distal to the left subclavian artery; type B occurs between left subclavian and common carotid arteries; and type C occurs proximal to the left subclavian artery (Fig. 59-36). There is a frequent finding of an aberrant right subclavian artery (retroesophageal) from the descending aorta. Survival for patients with

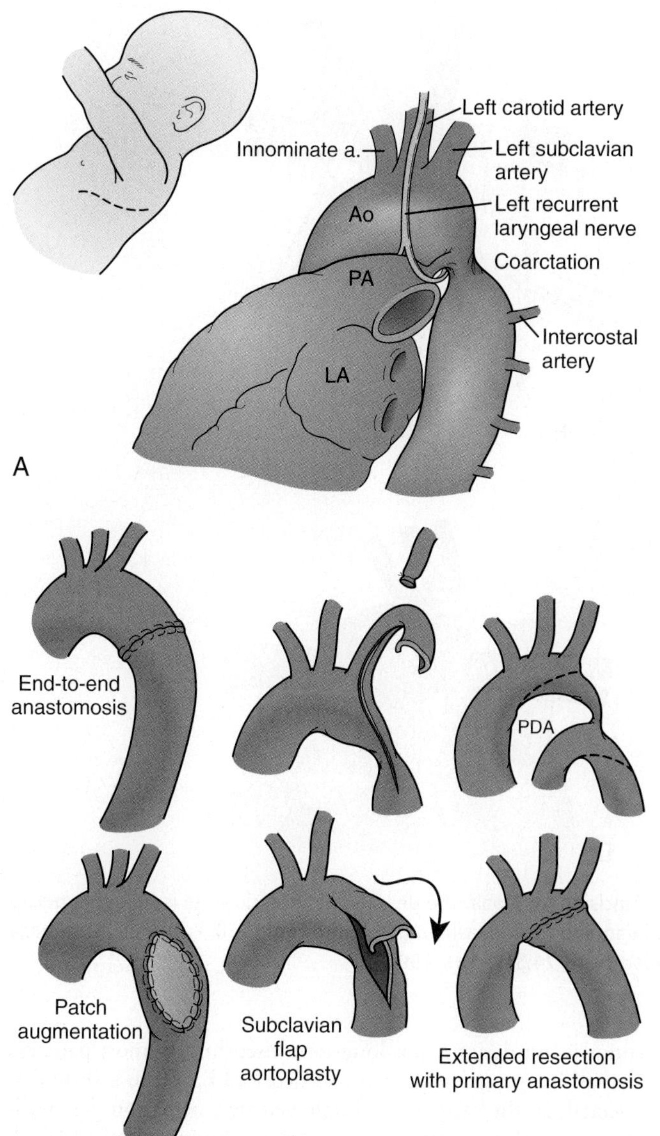


**FIGURE 59-35** Surgical repair for aortic coarctation. **A,** Surgical incision and anatomic orientation. **B,** Four different methods are shown: end-to-end anastomosis; patch augmentation; subclavian flap aortoplasty; and extended resection with primary anastomosis. *Ao,* Aorta; *LA,* left atrium; *PA,* pulmonary artery. (Adapted from Hastings LA, Nichols DG: Coarctation of the aorta and interrupted aortic arch. In Nichols DG, Ungerleider RM, Spevak PJ, et al [eds]: Critical heart disease in infants and children, Philadelphia, 2006, Mosby, p 635.)

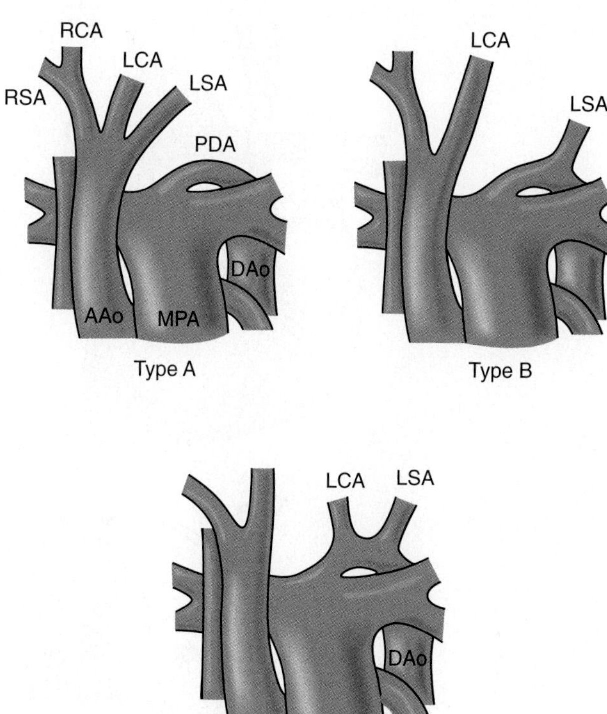


**FIGURE 59-36** Classification of interrupted aortic arch. *AAo,* Ascending aorta; *DAo,* descending aorta; *LCA,* left common carotid artery; *LSA,* left subclavian artery; *MPA,* main pulmonary artery; *RCA,* right common carotid artery; *RSA,* right subclavian artery. (Adapted from Monro JL: Interruption of aortic arch. In Stark J, de Leval M [eds]: Surgery for congenital heart defects, ed 2, Philadelphia, 1994, WB Saunders, p 299.)

IAA is initially predicated on ductal patency; thus, a PGE1 infusion is required to stabilize the patient. Diagnosis is confirmed by echocardiography; other methods, including cardiac catheterization, are needed infrequently.

IAA requires surgical treatment in the newborn period, which typically involves simultaneous repair of intracardiac lesions (Fig. 59-37). Repair may be accomplished with the aid of an aortic arch augmentation patch, although researchers at Texas Children's Hospital have recently reported a series confirming that a primary tissue-tissue repair can be performed in most patients and minimizes the potential for recurrent aortic arch obstruction.[43]

## SINGLE VENTRICLE

Single-ventricle physiology is a frequently encountered form of congenital cardiac disease. Patients may present as newborns with inadequate pulmonary blood flow, excessive pulmonary blood flow, or balanced circulations. The single ventricle may be of right, left, or indeterminate morphology. Surgical treatment is required to provide adequate systemic oxygen delivery while protecting the pulmonary vasculature. The function of the single ventricle must be preserved to afford the patient the best possible long-term outcome.

The rapid evolution of successful palliation for patients with various forms of single ventricle since the late 1970s has led to a large and growing population of adults with single ventricle. For most of these patients, lifelong cardiac attention is needed and the potential for subsequent cardiac reoperation is high. Patients in this category who present for noncardiac surgery may be especially difficult to manage.

An exhaustive discussion of the various forms of single ventricle is well beyond the scope of this chapter. As such, this discussion will be limited to common forms of single right and left ventricles to provide examples of the surgical management strategies for a single ventricle.

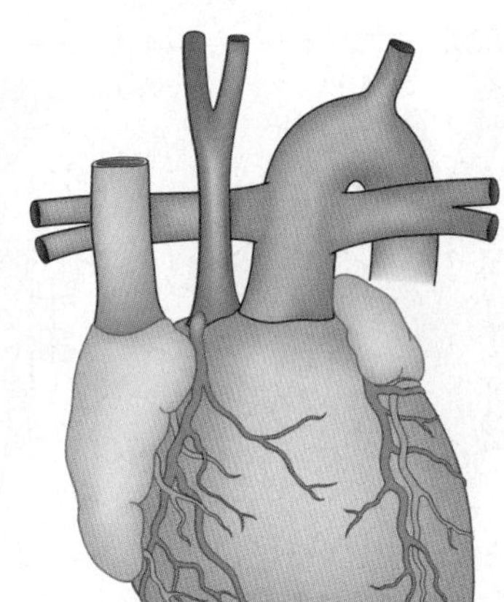


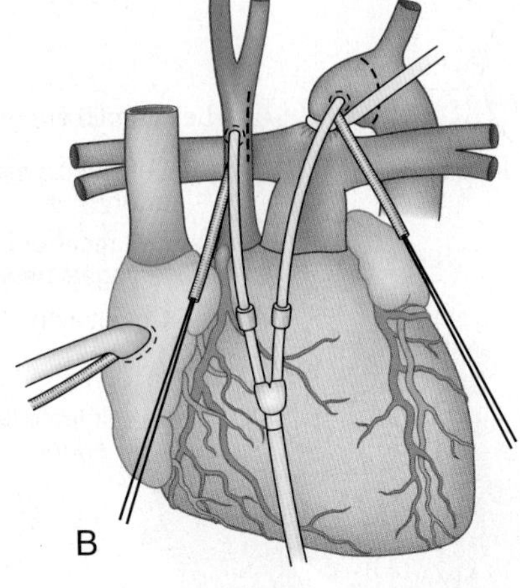


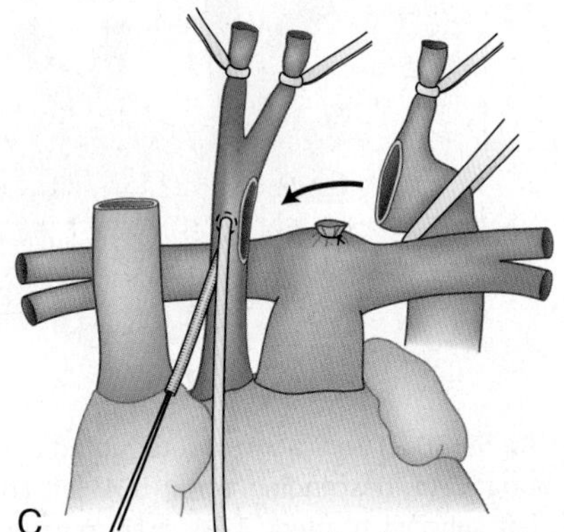


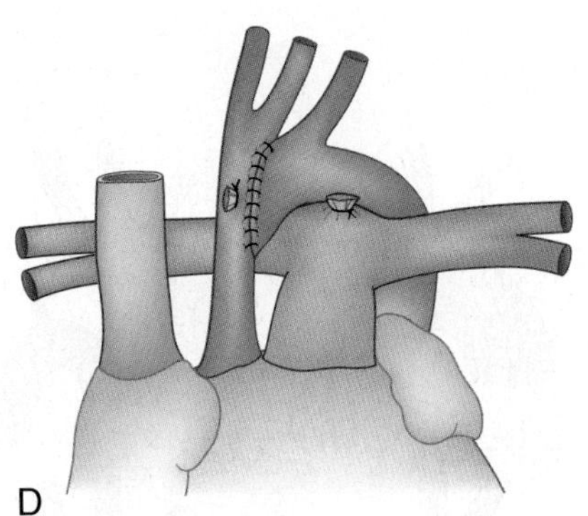


**FIGURE 59-37** **A,** Type B interrupted aortic arch. **B,** Cannulation and site of incision for repair. The descending thoracic aorta is brought upward into the mediastinum **(C)** and then anastomosed to the ascending aorta in an end-to-side fashion **(D).** (From Hirooka K, Fraser CD: One-stage neonatal repair of complex aortic arch obstruction or interruption. Tex Heart Inst J 24:317–321, 1997.)

## Tricuspid Atresia

Tricuspid atresia (TA) is the template of a single-ventricle lesion for which most of our current palliative strategies were developed. Patients with TA have a single morphologic left ventricle and may have normally related or transposed great vessels (Fig. 59-38). They may present with excessive pulmonary blood flow and require pulmonary artery banding early in infancy to relieve pulmonary overcirculation and CHF. Conversely, patients may have PS or pulmonary atresia and require creation of a Blalock shunt to provide adequate pulmonary blood flow and systemic oxygenation.

As noted, the initial palliative goals in patients with TA include adequate systemic oxygenation, protection of ventricular function, and adequate pulmonary arterial growth. Patients with ductal-dependent pulmonary blood flow require a Blalock shunt in the newborn period. Our preference is to construct the shunt to the morphologic right pulmonary artery through a right thoracotomy. This allows shunt flow to be governed by the size of the subclavian artery. Furthermore, the right pulmonary artery is typically longer and runs in a more horizontal plane in comparison to the left pulmonary artery. This facilitates avoiding distortion of a lobar branch. The goal of the shunt is to protect the pulmonary arteries, promote adequate pulmonary artery development, and support systemic arterial oxygenation for the first 4 to 6 months of life until the next planned stage of palliation (see later discussion of Glenn and Fontan operations). The shunt is not designed for long-term use; thus, in most patients, a small interposition graft (expanded PTFE, 3.0 to 4.0 mm) is selected. In the early era of single-ventricle palliation, less well-controlled shunts were constructed, including classic Blalock (divided native subclavian artery to branch pulmonary artery), Pott's (side to side left pulmonary artery to descending aorta), and Waterston (side to side right pulmonary artery to ascending aorta) shunts (Fig. 59-39). These native tissue-tissue connections are capable of somatic growth but have the confounding risks for pulmonary overcirculation, pulmonary artery hypertension (potentially irreversible), and branch pulmonary artery distortion with hypoplasia. During the early stages of development of single-ventricle palliation, many patients were treated with these poorly controlled shunts. Thus, there are now significant numbers of adult patients presenting with complications of these palliations, including chronic cardiac volume overload and decreased ventricular function, severe pulmonary artery distortion or isolation, pulmonary vascular disease, and profound cyanosis. These patients may present for surgery for noncardiac illness and are extremely difficult to manage.

## Hypoplastic Left Heart Syndrome

Hypoplastic left heart syndrome (HLHS) is the prototypical single right ventricle. Patients with this condition present with inadequate left heart structures ranging from mitral and aortic stenosis with left ventricular hypoplasia to almost complete

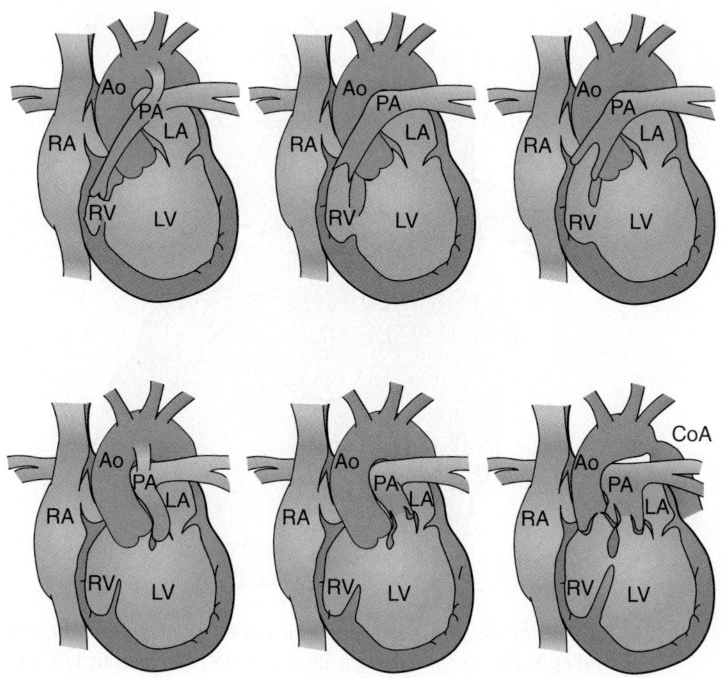


**FIGURE 59-38** Anatomy of the various types of tricuspid atresia. *Top,* Normally related great vessels. *Bottom,* D-Transposition of the great vessels. *Ao,* Aorta; *CoA,* coarctation of the aorta; *LA,* left atrium; *LV,* left ventricle; *PA,* pulmonary artery; *RA,* right atrium; *RV,* right ventricle. (Adapted from Lok JM, Spevak PJ, Nichols DG: Tricuspid atresia. In Nichols DG, Ungerleider RM, Spevak PJ, et al [eds]: Critical heart disease in infants and children, Philadelphia, 2006, Mosby, pp 800–801.)

absence of the left heart structures with aortic and mitral atresia (AA-MA). In the case of AA-MA, the ascending aorta is typically small (1 to 2 mm) and is perfused through retrograde aortic arch flow provided by the PDA. In HLHS, ductal closure results in rapid cardiovascular collapse, with profound systemic hypoperfusion and hypoxia, followed quickly by death. Therefore, patients diagnosed in the antenatal period must be born in a facility qualified to institute appropriate medical management immediately, including the establishment of suitable vascular access (umbilical artery catheter) and institution of IV PGE1 to maintain ductal patency. Patients undiagnosed at birth will typically have an early grace period of a few hours but, with the initiation of ductal closure, these children become critically ill and require aggressive resuscitation for survival. Without treatment, HLHS is a uniformly fatal condition. This fact is extremely poignant given that most children with HLHS are otherwise normal (Fig. 59-40).

After delivery, medical treatment is directed at maintaining ductal patency and balancing systemic and pulmonary blood flow. Balancing the circulations will become increasingly challenging with the normal decline in neonatal pulmonary vascular resistance (PVR), resulting in massive pulmonary overcirculation. As the overcirculation progresses, babies become tachypneic and may exhibit decreased systemic perfusion. NEC is a significant risk in these children and, if there is any question of visceral malperfusion, many centers avoid enteral nutrition in an effort to minimize this potential. Other medical maneuvers include deliberate hypoventilation, low inspired oxygen concentration, and additional carbon dioxide in an attempt to increase PVR and thereby limit pulmonary flow. These options are of limited use in newborns with HLHS; over days to weeks, the children become progressively ill, with pulmonary congestion and marginal systemic cardiac output. Patients fortunate enough to be maintained have the potential of developing increased PVR as they age, and there is a known association with advanced age (>30 days) and increased operative mortality.

Surgery in the newborn period is the only realistic option for long-term survival in babies born with HLHS. Currently, outcomes for surgical palliation of HLHS have come to be synonymous with the reputation of the treating center and surgeons. As with TA, patients with HLHS require a staged palliative approach. The first stage is, in all centers' experiences, the most challenging and risk-laden. The various first-stage options are described in the following sections.

### Neonatal Cardiac Transplantation

Transplantation is a theoretically attractive option in babies with HLHS that replaces the malformed heart with a structurally normal one. Dr. Leonard Bailey has been an influential champion of this approach and was the first to report exciting results with transplantation in newborns with HLHS.[44] Furthermore, although there is an ever-present risk for rejection and infection in transplanted children, long-term meaningful survival is possible and the quality of life of the recipients is good. Clearly, the option of cardiac transplantation is limited by the small numbers of suitable donor hearts and, for most children with HLHS, waiting for a donor graft is unsuccessful. This has led most centers, including Texas Children's Hospital, to abandon cardiac transplantation as the primary mode of therapy for most neonates with HLHS.

### Norwood Reconstruction

After initial work and success at Boston Children's Hospital, Norwood and colleagues at the Children's Hospital of Philadelphia gained international attention for developing and implementing a reconstructive technique to palliate newborns with HLHS; this methodology now carries the widely used eponym of the Norwood procedure.[45] This was gradually refined as experience accrued. The most common method involves surgical connection of the divided main pulmonary artery to the reconstructed aortic arch. In almost all children with HLHS, there is associated aortic arch hypoplasia, with coarctation. As such, a

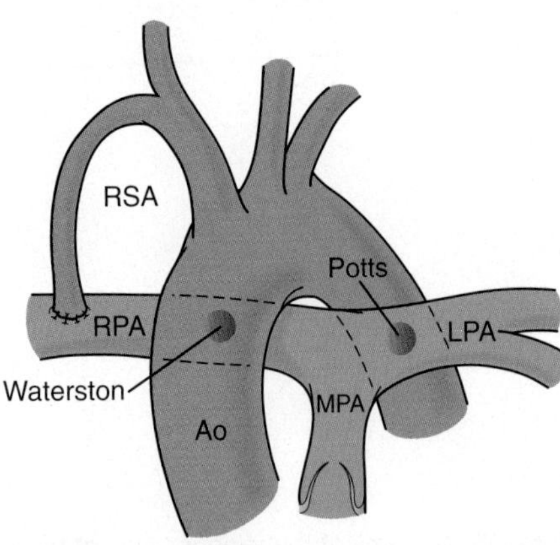


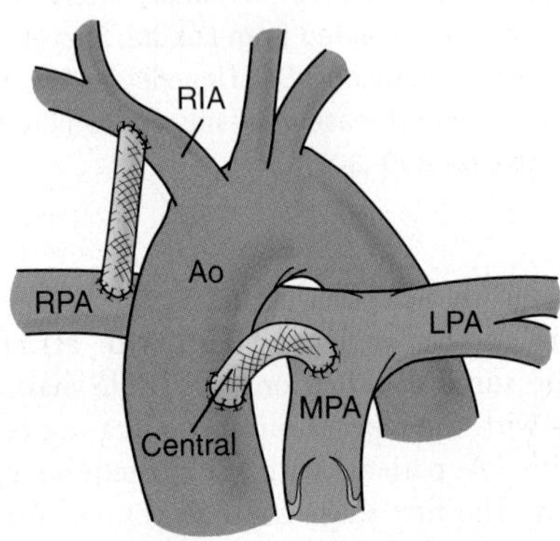


**FIGURE 59-39** Systemic to pulmonary artery shunts. *Ao,* Aorta; *MPA,* main pulmonary artery; *LPA,* left pulmonary artery; *RIA;* right innominate artery; *RPA,* right pulmonary artery; *RSA,* right subclavian artery. (Adapted from Marino BS, Wernovsky G, Greeley WJ: Single-ventricle lesions. In Nichols DG, Ungerleider RM, Spevak PJ, et al [eds]: Critical heart disease in infants and children, Philadelphia, 2006, Mosby, p 793.)

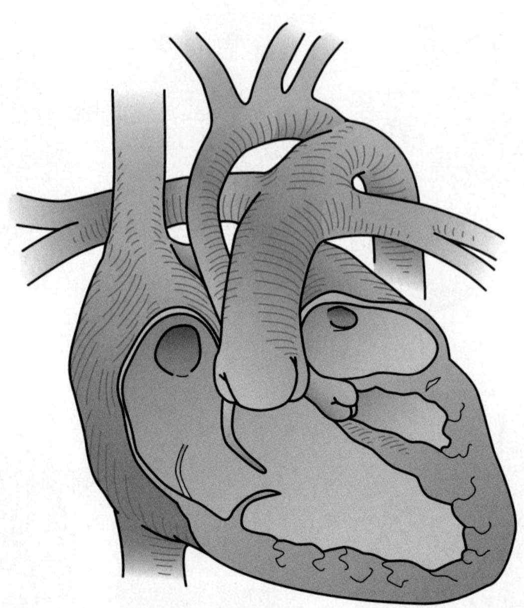

**FIGURE 59-40** Anatomy of hypoplastic left heart syndrome. The tiny ascending aorta is seen arising from a markedly hypoplastic left ventricle. The ductus arteriosus is large, providing forward flow to the systemic circuit. The right ventricle is hypertrophied and the pulmonary artery is enlarged. (From Wernovsky G, Bove EL: Single ventricle lesions. In Chang AC, Hanley FL, Wernovsky G, Wessell DL [eds]: Pediatric cardiac intensive care, Baltimore, 1998, Williams & Wilkins.)

critical feature of the operation is to reconstruct the aortic arch to provide unrestricted systemic blood flow. Most surgeons use some form of prosthetic material, usually pulmonary artery homograft patching. Some have reported accomplishing the arch reconstruction without the necessity of additional material. After reconstructing the aortic arch, the divided main pulmonary artery is anastomosed to the arch and small ascending aorta to create a neoaortic confluence providing systemic output from the right ventricle. The challenging feature of the reconstruction involves the accurate connection of this often miniscule ascending aorta to the confluence of the arch and main pulmonary artery stump. The opportunity for torsion and thereby coronary insufficiency is high. The final element of the classic Norwood reconstruction is the creation of a controlled source of pulmonary blood flow in the form of a modified BT shunt (Fig. 59-41).

## Sano Modification of Norwood's Operation

Achieving survival after the Norwood operation is a challenging proposition, involving innumerable technical and medical details. At best, after a Norwood procedure, the patient is fragile, with a delicate balance between systemic and pulmonary blood flow. This fact and the observation of widely disparate outcomes for the procedure have led to a number of important advances in the treatment of these children. One issue relates to the difficulty of balancing the systemic to pulmonary artery shunt, which lowers diastolic blood pressure (and thereby coronary perfusion pressure) and volume loads the heart. Sano and associates[46] from Okayama University in Japan were the first to report a series of babies undergoing a successful Norwood procedure, but with the modification of a right ventricle to pulmonary artery (RV-PA) conduit rather than a Blalock shunt. The theoretical advantage of this approach is the increase in diastolic pressure, creating a physiology more akin to a banded circulation rather than shunted. Early reports with this method were encouraging, although patients appeared to become more rapidly desaturated as they aged when compared with the shunted patients. The long-term effects of the right ventriculotomy on cardiac function are as of yet unknown. In a recently published report, patients undergoing the Norwood operation were randomized to receive an RV-PA shunt or modified Blalock-Taussig shunt. Twelve months after randomization, transplantation-free survival was higher in the RV-PA shunt group, as was the rate of unplanned re-interventions and complications.[47]

## Hybrid Procedure

The notion of a combined therapy between interventional cardiology and surgery for the first-stage palliation of HLHS has achieved significant attention. The idea is to minimize the risk of the first operation by banding the branch pulmonary arteries and delivering a stent into the ductus to maintain patency. This

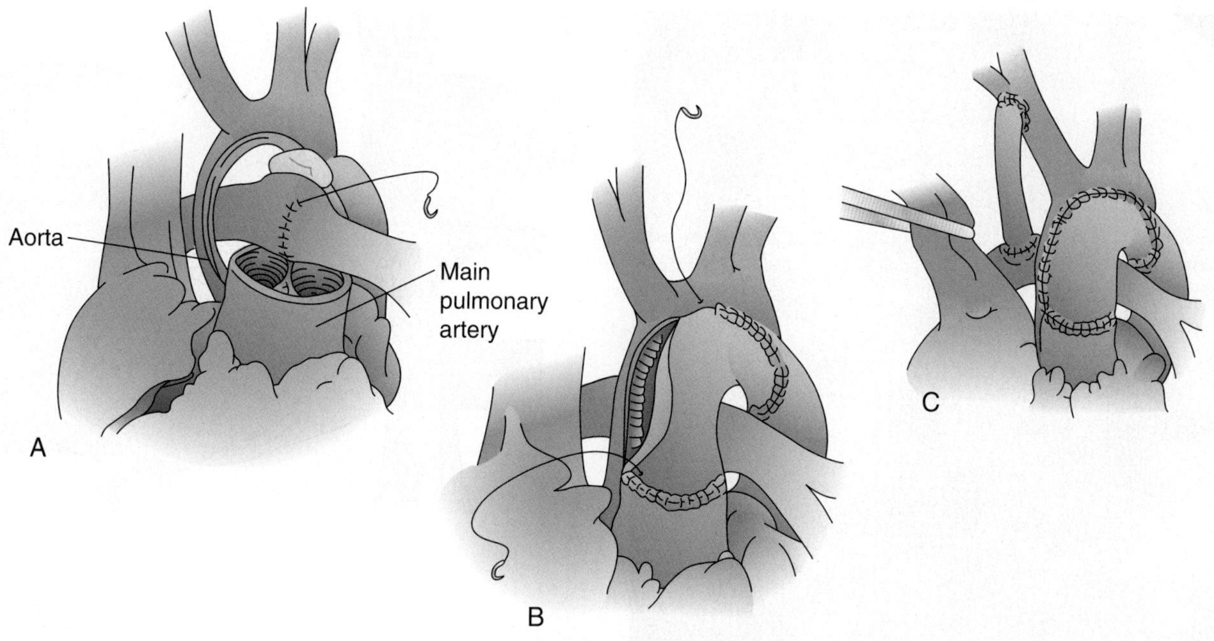


**FIGURE 59-41** Norwood procedure for first-stage palliation of hypoplastic left heart syndrome. **A,** The main pulmonary artery (MPA) is divided proximal to the bifurcation, the ductus arteriosus is ligated and divided, and the aortic arch is opened from the level of the transected MPA to a point distal to the ductal insertion in the descending aorta. **B,** A segment of homograft is cut to an appropriate size and shape. This is sutured into place, creating an unobstructed outflow from the right ventricle to the pulmonary artery and aorta. **C,** PTFE tube graft is placed from the innominate artery to the right pulmonary artery. The atrial septectomy is done while the patient is under circulatory arrest as well. (From Castaneda AR, Jonas RA, Mayer JE, Hanley FL: Hypoplastic left heart syndrome. In Castaneda AR, Jonas RA, Mayer JE, Hanley FL Cardiac surgery of the neonate and infant, Philadelphia, 1994, WB Saunders.)

hybrid arrangement is designed to allow newborn survival so that a more complete reconstruction may be performed later in infancy in a larger child. There appears to be a significant learning curve with this approach, as with any new procedure, and the incidence of complications warrants further study. Recent data have shown that the prevalence of NEC following the hybrid procedure is significant and comparable to reports following the Norwood procedure.[48] In addition to this, concerning features include the effect of the banding on long-term pulmonary artery growth, the fact that cardiac perfusion is still retrograde through the aortic arch, and the risk profile of the more extensive reconstruction later in life. The true place for this mode of therapy is currently unclear, but it represents an important direction of advancement to optimize the opportunity of survival for these children.

### Fontan Operation

The long-term goal of single-ventricle palliation is to optimize ventricular function and promote systemic oxygen delivery. As noted earlier, patients with a single ventricle who are shunted or banded have ongoing concerns, including systemic desaturation, continued intracardiac mixing, and chronic cardiac volume overload. The current strategy for addressing these concerns uses a direct connection between the branch pulmonary arteries and systemic venous return, as initially proposed by Fontan in the early 1970s.[49] The Fontan operation is now the treatment of choice for children born with all varieties of single ventricle and, in suitable patients, provides acceptable long-term palliation. It must be recognized, however, that the Fontan circulation is not normal and even in the best of circumstances results in significant alteration in normal cardiorespiratory physiology.

The Fontan circulation is established by connecting the systemic venous return directly into isolated branch pulmonary arteries without an intervening power source. Thus, blood flow in the Fontan circuit is passive, being promoted only by the pressure differential between the systemic venous system and pulmonary venous atrium. As such, an impediment to flow in the systemic to pulmonary pathway will result in a poor Fontan outcome. Established criteria for creating an effective Fontan circulation include the ability to connect the systemic venous return surgically to the pulmonary arteries in an unobstructed manner, normal pulmonary artery architecture and resistance, normal pulmonary venous drainage and low left atrial pressure, absence of significant AV valve regurgitation, good ventricular function (and thereby low ventricular end-diastolic pressure), an unobstructed systemic arterial outlet, and good aortic valve function. Compromise of any of these elements may compromise the quality of the Fontan circulation.

The Fontan operation has undergone several technical modifications in the almost 40 years of successful application to patients with single-ventricle physiology. Many patients underwent an atriopulmonary connection in which the open right atrial appendage was directly anastomosed to the pulmonary artery bifurcation with surgical closure of the ASD. Many of these patients are now presenting with extreme dilation of the right atrium, with resulting sluggish flow, hepatic congestion, and atrial dysrhythmias (Fig. 59-42). Today, the most widely practiced modification of the Fontan operation is the total cavopulmonary connection (TCPC). First described by DeLeval, this

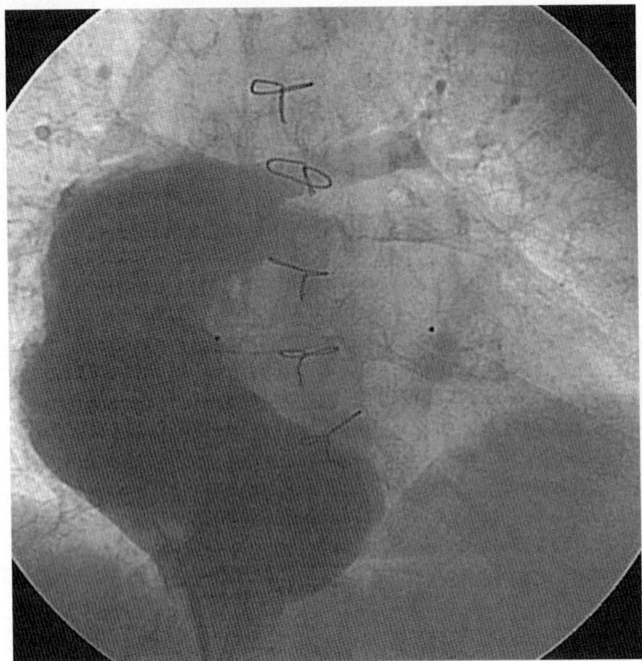

**FIGURE 59-42** Angiogram of a dilated right atrium in a patient with an atriopulmonary Fontan connection.

operation involves connection of the divided SVC to the superior and inferior aspects of the right pulmonary artery (typically somewhat offset), along with the creation of a channel to direct the IVC flow into the pulmonary arteries. The channel may be created using a surgically created lateral tunnel in the right atrium (Fig. 59-43) or interposing a conduit between the IVC and pulmonary arteries (extracardiac Fontan; Fig. 59-44).

The change from a volume-loaded circulation in shunted or banded single-ventricle patients to a Fontan circulation results in acute volume unloading of the systemic ventricle. In the chronic overloaded heart, this acute change may be poorly tolerated, with resultant diastolic dysfunction and decreased ventricular compliance. To deal with this problem, patients with a single ventricle typically undergo an intervening stage of palliation in the form of a bidirectional, superior cavopulmonary anastomosis (Glenn shunt). The bidirectional Glenn shunt is constructed by anastomosing the cephalad end of the divided SVC to the superior aspect of the right pulmonary artery (Fig. 59-45). Other sources of pulmonary blood flow are typically eliminated, and thus the heart is volume-unloaded; however, systemic cardiac output is maintained because the IVC return is preserved. After the Glenn shunt, the patients are not fully saturated; typically, patients run saturations of about 80%. Over time, the unloaded ventricle remodels and the patient is promoted to reoperation and completion of the Fontan circulation.

Note that perioperative care of the Fontan patient can be challenging. The acute changes in cardiac volume loading may negatively affect cardiac output. Even in patients with supposedly ideal Fontan connections, the central venous pressure acutely rises to 12 to 15 mm Hg. Consequences of this increased venous pressure include pleural effusions, hepatic congestion, and ascites. In marginal Fontan candidates, some surgeons routinely place an intentional leak, or fenestration; the goal here is

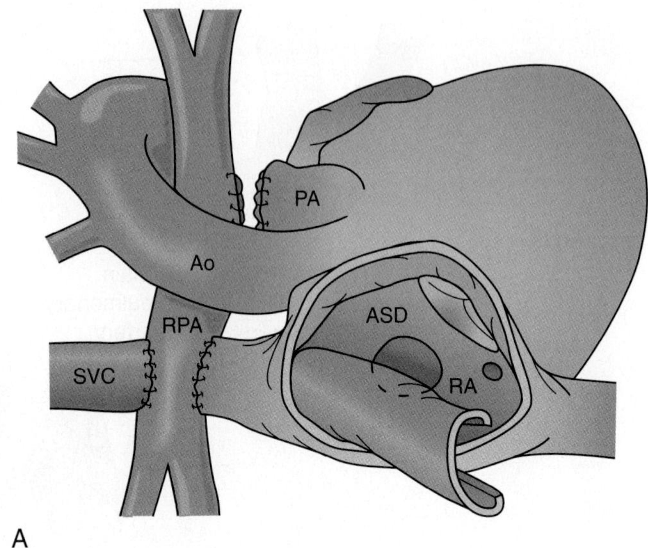


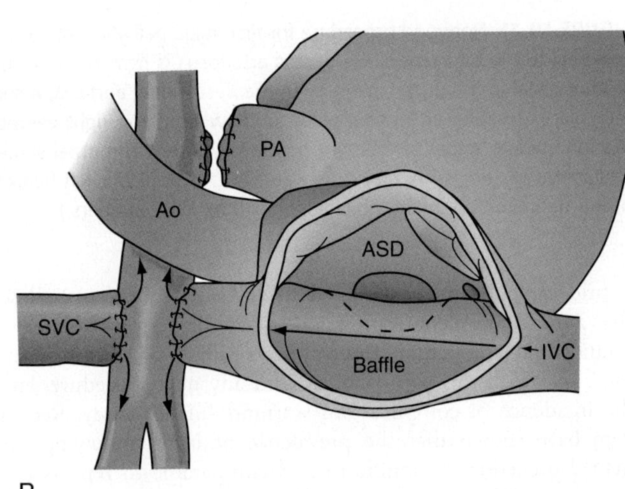


**FIGURE 59-43 A, B,** Lateral tunnel Fontan procedure. *Ao,* Aorta; *PA,* pulmonary artery; *RA,* right atrium; *RPA,* right pulmonary artery; (Adapted from Lok JM, Spevak PJ, Nichols DG: Tricuspid atresia. In Nichols DG, Ungerleider RM, Spevak PJ, et al [eds]: Critical heart disease in infants and children, Philadelphia, 2006, Mosby, p 813.)

to preserve systemic ventricular volume loading and decrease systemic venous congestion at the expense of some degree of desaturation caused by the right-to-left shunting. The practice of routine fenestration following the Fontan operation has been examined and some early data have shown that excellent outcomes can be achieved with highly selective application of a fenestration, which mitigates the risks associated with such a procedure, including hypoxia and systemic embolism.[50] Any impediment to passive pulmonary blood flow will inhibit Fontan flow and result in right heart failure. Positive-pressure ventilation, especially elevated levels of PEEP, will impede pulmonary blood flow in the Fontan patient. Conversely, early extubation and effective spontaneous ventilation will improve pulmonary blood flow in the Fontan patient. Recent data have suggested that early extubation in the operating room for patients

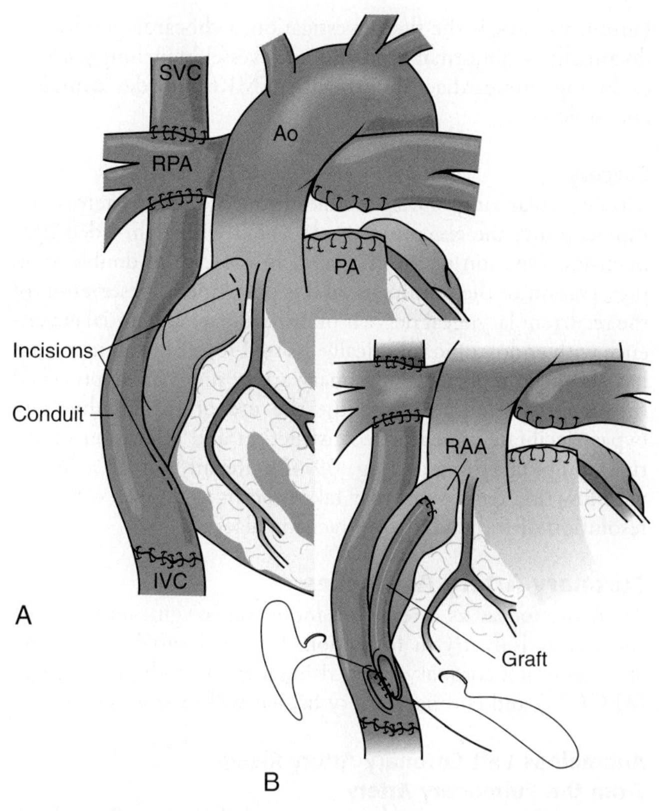


**FIGURE 59-44 A,** Extracardiac Fontan procedure. **B,** Creation of a fenestration in an extracardiac Fontan procedure using a graft between the extracardiac conduit and right atrial appendage (RAA). *Ao,* Aorta; *PA,* pulmonary artery; *RPA,* right pulmonary artery. (Adapted from Lok JM, Spevak PJ, Nichols DG: Tricuspid atresia. In Nichols DG, Ungerleider RM, Spevak PJ, et al [eds]: Critical heart disease in infants and children, Philadelphia, 2006, Mosby, p 814.)

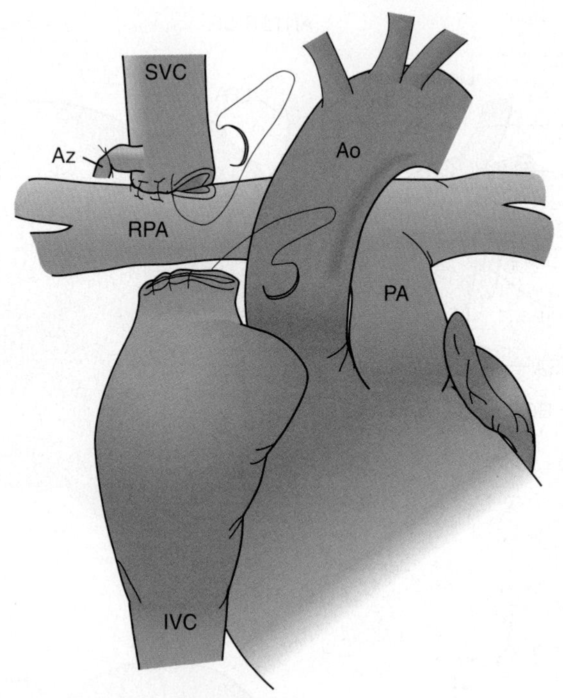


**FIGURE 59-45** Bidirectional Glenn shunt. *Ao,* Aorta; *Az,* azygos vein; *PA,* pulmonary artery; *RPA,* right pulmonary artery. (Adapted from Lok JM, Spevak PJ, Nichols DG: Tricuspid atresia. In Nichols DG, Ungerleider RM, Spevak PJ, et al [eds]: Critical heart disease in infants and children, Philadelphia, 2006, Mosby, p 809.)

following the Fontan procedure improves hemodynamics, decreases the length of stay for patients, and decreases hospital costs.[9]

The chronic complications of living with a Fontan circulation are still unfolding, but include chronic hepatic congestion and cirrhosis, protein-losing enteropathy, atrial dysrhythmias, and venous stasis disease. Management of patients with failing Fontan circulations is especially challenging. These patients are at high risk for severe cardiac compromise while undergoing general anesthesia with positive-pressure ventilation or any procedure involving large fluid shifts, including abdominal surgery. Patients with chronic hepatic congestion may develop a coagulopathy related to a decrease in factor production.

## MISCELLANEOUS ANOMALIES

### Vascular Rings and Pulmonary Artery Slings

#### Vascular Rings

Vascular rings are abnormalities of the aortic arch and its branches, compressing the trachea, esophagus, or both. The ring may be complete or partial. A pulmonary artery sling occurs when the left pulmonary artery arises from the right pulmonary artery, passing leftward between the trachea and the esophagus. The trachea may be compressed, the cartilage may be soft, or there may be intrinsic stenosis of the trachea in the form of complete cartilage rings. Categorization of the defects is useful for description:

**Complete Vascular Rings**

- Double arch: Equal arches or left or right arch dominant (Fig. 59-46)
- Right arch: Left ligamentum arteriosus from anomalous left subclavian artery
- Right arch: Mirror image branching, with left ligamentum from descending aorta

**Partial Vascular Rings**

- Left arch: Aberrant right subclavian artery
- Left arch: Innominate artery compression

#### Pulmonary Artery Slings

The double aortic arch is the most common form of complete ring. Two arches arise from the ascending aorta, forming a true ring. The left arch is usually smaller. The right arch–left ligamentum complex is formed from persistence of the right fourth arch and regression of the left fourth arch. The anomalously arising left subclavian artery is often associated with a diverticulum at its base (Kommerell's diverticulum). In partial rings, the most common form is an aberrant right subclavian artery arising distal to the left subclavian artery with a left arch. The right subclavian artery passes behind the esophagus from left to right. Innominate artery compression arises from a more posterior and leftward origin of the innominate artery from a left arch, leading to anterior compression of the trachea.

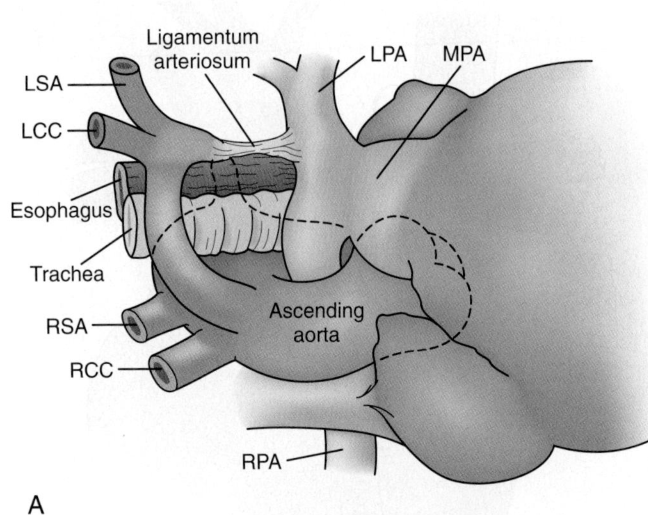


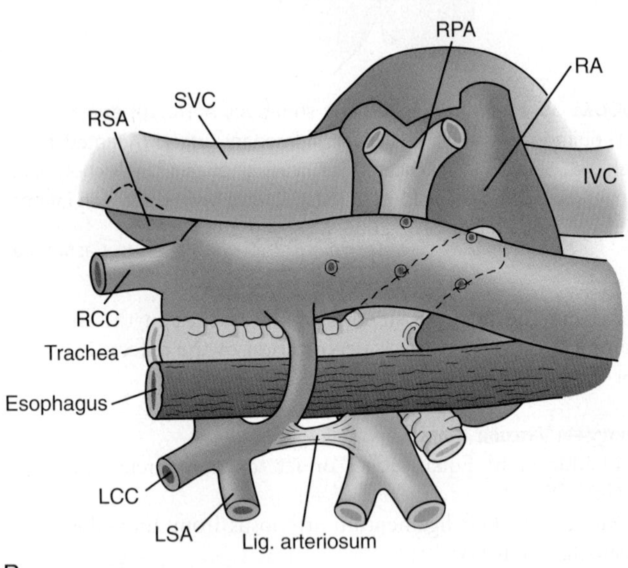


**FIGURE 59-46** Double aortic arch, posterior **(A)** and superior **(B)** views. *LCC,* Left common carotid artery; *LPA,* left pulmonary artery; *LSA,* left subclavian artery; *MPA,* main pulmonary artery; *RA,* right atrium; *RCC,* right common carotid artery; *RSA,* right subclavian artery. (Adapted from Jonas RA: Comprehensive surgical management of congenital heart disease. New York, 2004, Oxford University Press, p 499.)

### Diagnosis and Indications for Intervention

Symptoms reflect the degree of tracheal and esophageal compression, as well as the presence of coexistent tracheomalacia or stenosis from complete rings. Upper respiratory symptoms predominate, with a characteristic brassy cough, recurrent respiratory infections, failure to thrive, and sometimes esophageal motility problems. In children, documentation of a ring is an indication for surgery. Older patients are often asymptomatic. Initially, diagnosis is made by a high index of suspicion and the barium swallow is the first investigation. Echocardiography can document an abnormal head and neck vessel branching pattern, excluding intracardiac abnormalities. MRI provides complete anatomic detail.

### Surgery

Most vascular rings are accessible through a left posterolateral thoracotomy; the exception is a left arch with right-sided ligamentum. Division of the ring and, in the case of double arch, preservation of the dominant arch is performed. Preservation of the recurrent laryngeal nerve is of importance. The initial experience with endoscopic robotically assisted repair of vascular rings has also been reported. Pulmonary artery slings are approached through the midline; currently, the use of cardiopulmonary bypass facilitates tracheal reconstruction and relocation of the right pulmonary artery (Fig. 59-47). Repair can be achieved with low risk. Symptoms may take months to resolve, with slow resolution of the underlying tracheomalacia.

## Coronary Artery Anomalies

Anomalies occur as a result of anomalous origin, termination, courses, and aneurysm formation. Of these variables, only an anomalous left coronary artery rising from the pulmonary artery (ALCAPA) and coronary artery fistulas will be discussed here.

### Anomalous Left Coronary Artery Rising From the Pulmonary Artery

An ALCAPA is a rare lesion often lethal in early infancy. Untreated, the mortality rate approaches 90%.

**Anatomy and Pathophysiology** Developmentally, failure of the normal connection of the left coronary artery bud to the aorta results in an abnormal connection to the pulmonary artery. The abnormal origin can be situated in the main pulmonary artery or proximal branches. Associated abnormalities are rare but important to recognize because lowering of the pulmonary artery pressure by PDA ligation or closure of a VSD can be fatal if the ALCAPA is not noted. In utero, with equal pulmonary arterial and aortic pressures, satisfactory perfusion of the ALCAPA can occur. After birth, the pulmonary artery pressure falls and left coronary artery perfusion decreases. Ischemia causes impaired ventricular function and myocardial infarcts and leads to left ventricular dilation. Papillary muscle dysfunction causes mitral regurgitation. Early coronary collateral development may prevent ongoing infarction.

**Diagnosis and Indications for Intervention** ALCAPA is suspected in any infant with mitral regurgitation, ventricular dysfunction, or dilated cardiomyopathy. Infants present with a low cardiac output and systemic heart failure. Feeding may also precipitate sudden death and angina in infants. Sudden death has been described in older children. The ECG may reflect ischemic changes. The echocardiogram is usually diagnostic. However, because this diagnosis is often confused with dilated cardiomyopathy, there is an argument in favor of catheterizing all patients with dilated cardiomyopathy in whom the coronary artery anatomy cannot be clearly defined on echocardiography. Secondary findings of dilated cardiac chambers and segmental wall motion abnormalities together with mitral regurgitation prompt a search for an ALCAPA. Diagnosis of an ALCAPA is an indication for intervention.

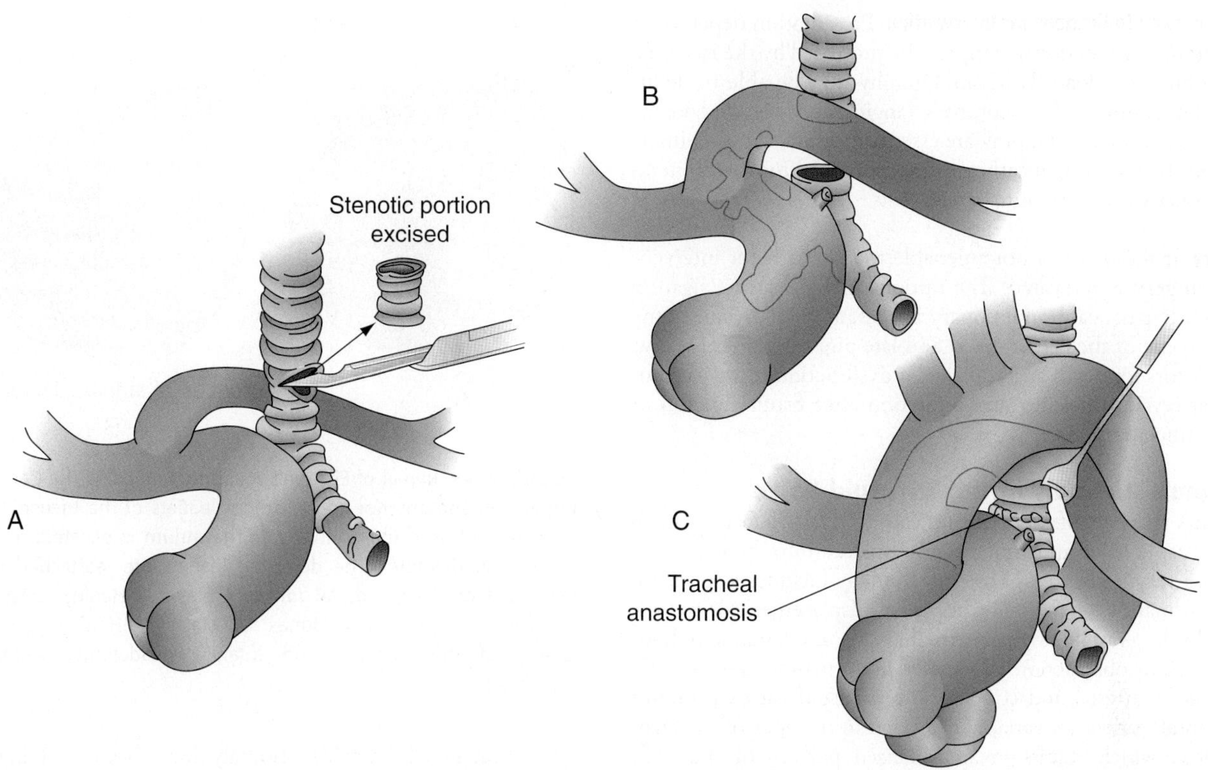


**FIGURE 59-47** Method for the management of a pulmonary artery sling with associated tracheal stenosis, using cardiopulmonary bypass. **A,** Tracheal resection of the involved segment. **B,** Anterior translocation of the left pulmonary artery after transection of the trachea. **C,** Direct anastomosis of the trachea. (From Castaneda AR, Jonas RA, Mayer JE, Hanley FL: Vascular rings, slings, and tracheal anomalies. In Castaneda AR, Jonas RA, Mayer JE, Hanley FL: Cardiac surgery of the neonate and infant, Philadelphia, 1994, WB Saunders.)

**Surgery** A degree of ventricular dysfunction is usually present. Preoperative inotropic support and optimization of hemodynamics may be required before surgical intervention. Severe cardiomyopathy may, rarely, necessitate cardiac transplantation. Current experience indicates that creation of a dual coronary system is safe and reproducible and offers the best opportunity for recovery of function.[51] Operative considerations include optimal myocardial protection and prevention of left heart distention. Direct reimplantation of the ALCAPA into the ascending aorta is currently the procedure of choice (Fig. 59-48). Sometimes, limited mobility of the coronary artery will preclude reimplantation, and a surgically created aorta–pulmonary artery–coronary artery tunnel is created, the Takeuchi procedure. Ligation of the ALCAPA is not recommended.

Postoperative management is directed toward maintaining adequate coronary perfusion and cardiac output. Mechanical support of the heart may be temporarily required. Mitral regurgitation usually improves and valve replacement is rarely necessary. Current intervention has a low operative mortality. Risks for nonsurvival relate to preoperative ventricular dysfunction and cardiogenic shock. The Takeuchi repair is associated with tunnel complications such as obstruction, leak, aortic valve damage, and RVOTO in the long term.

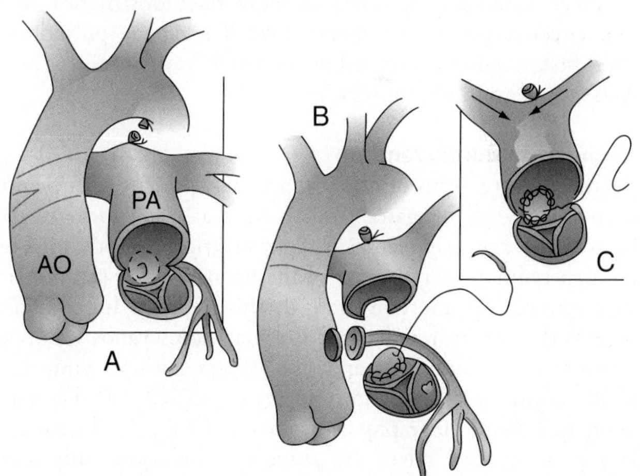


**FIGURE 59-48** Direct reimplantation of ALCAPA. **A,** Excision of ALCAPA from the pulmonary artery (PA). **B,** Aortic reimplantation of the coronary ostium into the aorta. **C,** Reconstruction of the PA with autologous pericardium. *AO,* Aorta. (From Vouhe PR, Tamisier D, Sidi D, et al: Anomalous left coronary artery from the pulmonary artery: Results of isolated aortic reimplantation. Ann Thorac Surg 54:621–626, 1992.)

## Coronary Arteriovenous Fistula and Aneurysms

Isolated coronary artery fistula is more rare than ALCAPA. Drainage of coronary artery fistula is reported to terminate more commonly in the right side of the heart or pulmonary artery than in the left side of the heart. A shunt from the high-pressure coronary artery system into a low-pressure cardiac chamber may result in coronary steal and some degree of cardiac volume overload. Coronary artery aneurysms are associated with Kawasaki disease.

**Diagnosis and Indications for Intervention** Presentation depends on the amount of functional compromise produced by the ischemia and volume overload. Echocardiography may be able to delineate the anomaly, but coronary angiography is diagnostic. Details of coronary anatomy are essential for determining intervention. Interventional catheterization is useful for the obliteration of fistulas and terminal aneurysms.

**Surgery** If the lesion is not amenable to transcatheter intervention, surgery is indicated. The options include suture ligation without bypass, cardiopulmonary bypass, and aneurysmectomy with closure of the fistula. Early and late mortality rates are low. Risk factors for death and ventricular dysfunction relate to coronary artery insufficiency and infarction after fistula ligation or aneurysmectomy.[52]

## Ebstein's Anomaly of the Tricuspid Valve

Ebstein's anomaly of the tricuspid valve is a rare defect in which the tricuspid valve attachments are displaced into the right ventricle to varying degrees. Ebstein's anomaly includes a spectrum of abnormalities involving a degree of displacement of the tricuspid valve, variable right ventricular size, and variable pulmonary outflow obstruction. Associated abnormalities are an ASD, pulmonary atresia, and ccTGA. The tricuspid valve's posterior and septal leaflets are variably displaced to the apex of the right ventricle, which results in an atrialized portion of the right ventricle. The anterior leaflet remains large and sail-like. The major hemodynamic issue is tricuspid incompetence with decreased pulmonary blood flow and, if an ASD is present, right-to-left shunting causing cyanosis. Long-standing tricuspid incompetence leads to volume overload of an abnormal right ventricle. Variable pulmonary outflow tract obstruction will limit effective pulmonary blood flow. If adequate pulmonary blood flow requires continued ductal patency, the need for neonatal intervention is almost certain.

### Diagnosis and Intervention

The more severe forms of Ebstein's anomaly present with cyanosis in infancy. Ill neonates tend to have a severe form of the disease, with a grossly inefficient right ventricle compounded by the high pulmonary resistance of the neonate or by pulmonary valve atresia. The mortality rate in this group is high. Older patients present in heart failure and may have cyanosis. Supraventricular dysrhythmias and the pre-excitation syndrome, Wolff-Parkinson-White syndrome, are associated with Ebstein's anomaly. Echocardiography is diagnostic. Critically ill neonates have poor survival rates, and surgery is indicated only after stabilization with PGE1 and controlled ventilation. In the older patient, cyanosis and heart failure are indications to intervene, although earlier intervention in the asymptomatic patient, before excessive right ventricular dilation, has now been more actively pursued.

### Surgery

In critically ill neonates, after stabilization, palliation with a systemic-to-pulmonary artery shunt may be required. The Starnes operation has allowed salvage in previously hopeless cases. This consists of patch closure of the tricuspid orifice, atrial septectomy, and a systemic-to-pulmonary artery shunt. In patients with less severe forms of this disease, tricuspid valve repair or replacement is also an option.[53] Surgical techniques for the treatment of Ebstein's anomaly have been evolving and outcomes are improving for this challenging group of patients (Fig. 59-49).[54]

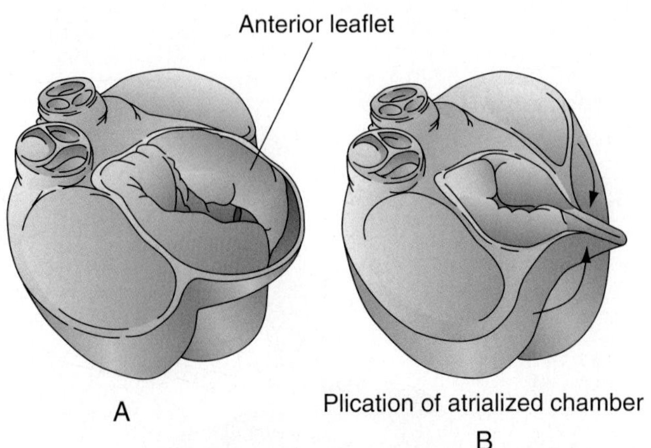


**FIGURE 59-49** Repair of Ebstein's malformation using the Carpentier method. **A,** The anterior and posterior leaflets of the tricuspid valve are detached from the annulus. **B,** The atrium is plicated, reducing the annular diameter. The detached leaflets are reattached to the annulus. (From Castaneda AR, Jonas RA, Mayer JE, Hanley FL: Ebstein's anomaly. In Castaneda AR, Jonas RA, Mayer JE, Hanley FL: Cardiac surgery of the neonate and infant, Philadelphia, 1994, WB Saunders.)

## Mitral Valve Anomalies

Most abnormalities of the mitral valve are associated with other complex lesions (e.g., Shone's complex). More commonly, mitral disease in children is inflammatory in nature—that is, rheumatic disease or infective endocarditis. It may also be associated with collagen vascular disease and Marfan syndrome.

### Mitral Stenosis

Mitral stenosis is caused by obstruction at a supravalvular, valvular, or subvalvular level, singly or in combination. Supravalvular stenosis is caused by a ring of fibrous tissue above the annulus of the mitral valve or attached to the proximal leaflets. Valvular stenosis involves the leaflets, with commissural fusion occurring with or without hypoplasia of the valve ring. Hypoplasia of the mitral valve is often associated with left ventricular hypoplasia. Frequently, the leaflets and subvalvular apparatus are also dysplastic. Fusion of the leaflets can lead to an accessory orifice and produce mitral stenosis at a purely valvular level (so-called *double-orifice mitral valve*). Three types of subvalvular stenosis have been recognized—parachute mitral valve, hammock valve, and absence of one or both papillary muscles. Mitral regurgitation is a result of secondary annular dilation, congenital isolated clefts of the valve, and prolapse of the leaflets from abnormal chordae or papillary muscle insertion.

Echocardiography is diagnostic. Intervention includes balloon valvuloplasty, particularly for selected forms of rheumatic mitral stenosis, and surgical intervention. Intervention is timed to avoid irreversible sequelae related to chronic volume overload or pulmonary hypertension. Surgical intervention is aimed at preserving the mitral valve and valvuloplasty techniques have a valuable place in children. Prosthetic valves are the least desirable option. Bioprosthetic or tissue valves need to be avoided in children. Supra-annular placement of the prosthesis may be necessary. Repeat placement is ensured.

## SUMMARY

This chapter provides a basic overview of the major congenital cardiac lesions and a framework for the diagnosis and treatment of these conditions. It must be emphasized that for most patients, the diagnosis of CHD, whether surgically treated or not, carries lifelong implications. For patients with CHD presenting for noncardiac surgery, a thorough understanding of the patient's unique anatomy and physiology is mandatory in deriving a rational management strategy. The reader is directed to several excellent texts on CHD for a more thorough review of each of the lesions reviewed in this chapter.

## SELECTED REFERENCES

Bailey LL, Nehlsen-Cannarella SL, Doroshow RW, et al: Cardiac allotransplantation in newborns as therapy for hypoplastic left heart syndrome. N Engl J Med 315:949–951, 1986.

This classic reference describes the first report of cardiac transplantation in newborns with HLHS. Although limited in its applicability because of limited donor organs, neonatal cardiac transplantation has provided children born with HLHS a new option for survival.

Blalock A, Taussig HB: The surgical treatment of malformations of the heart in which there is pulmonary stenosis or pulmonary atresia. JAMA 128:189–202, 1945.

This landmark article describes the surgical procedure that commenced the era of elective cardiac surgery. The study reported the initial experience with palliative surgical treatment of patients with pulmonary stenosis or pulmonary atresia using the Blalock-Taussig shunt.

Fontan F, Baudet E: Surgical repair of tricuspid atresia. Thorax 26:240–248, 1971.

This article represents a milestone in the evolution of surgical management of patients with single ventricle physiology. It described the first corrective operation for patients with tricuspid atresia. Although previous palliations, provided by various systemic-pulmonary artery shunts, improved patients' clinical condition, systemic blood was still a mixture of oxygenated and deoxygenated blood. The Fontan operation redirected superior and inferior vena cava blood flow to the lungs so that only oxygenated blood returned to the heart and subsequently to the systemic circulation.

Kirklin JW, Dushane JW, Patrick RT, et al: Intracardiac surgery with the aid of a mechanical pump-oxygenator system (gibbon type): Report of eight cases. Mayo Clin Proc 30:201–206, 1955.

This is landmark article demonstrated that open repairs of congenital cardiac defects using mechanical pump oxygenator systems could be performed with minimal risk to the patient.

Mustard W: Successful two-stage correction of transposition of the great vessels. Surgery 55:469–472, 1964.

This clasic reference describes one of the initial surgical approaches to the treatment of D-TGA. Although the arterial switch operation is now the surgical treatment of choice for D-TGA, there are many adult congenital patients who have been palliated with the Mustard operation. Understanding the operation and resulting physiology is critical to general surgery management strategies for noncardiac operations.

Nichols DG, Ungerleider RM, Spevak PJ, et al, editors: Critical heart disease in infants and children, ed 2, Philadelphia, 2006, Mosby.

This text provides a comprehensive and current review of heart disease in infants and children. It contains numerous surgical drawings and diagnostic images to supplement the didactic material.

Norwood WI, Lang P, Casteneda AR, Campbell DN: Experience with operations for hypoplastic left heart syndrome. J Thorac Cardiovasc Surg 82:511–519, 1981.

In this landmark article, Norwood and others reported the outcomes of what was then a new reconstructive surgical technique to palliate newborns with hypoplastic left heart syndrome. Until the Norwood operation, the only option for survival of patients with HLHS was cardiac transplantation. At most centers today, the Norwood operation is the primary mode of therapy for most neonates with HLHS.

Senning A: Surgical correction of transposition of the great vessels. Surgery 45:966–980, 1959.

This classic reference describes the initial surgical approach to management of D-TGA. Although the arterial switch operation is currently the surgical treatment of choice for D-TGA, there are many adult congenital patients in the community who have had the Senning operation. Understanding the operation and resulting physiology is critical to general surgery management strategies for noncardiac operations.

Warden HE, Cohen M, Read RC, Lillehei CW: Controlled cross circulation for open intracardiac surgery: Physiologic studies and results of creation and closure of ventricular septal defects. J Thorac Surg 28:331–341, 1954.

This landmark article described the technique of cross circulation to facilitate cardiopulmonary bypass and intracardiac repair of congenital heart lesions. Lillehei and colleagues documented the successful use of cross-circulation to correct defects such as ventricular septal defect.

Wilcox B, Cook A, Anderson R: Surgical anatomy of the heart, ed 3, Cambridge, England, 2004, Cambridge University Press.

This text provides an excellent reference manual for understanding the complex anatomy of the heart. It contains color photographs and diagrams and is an invaluable resource for any student of cardiac surgery.

## REFERENCES

1. Blalock A, Taussig HB: The surgical treatment of malformations of the heart in which there is pulmonary stenosis or pulmonary atresia. JAMA 128:189–202, 1945.
2. Warden HE, Cohen M, Read RC, et al: Controlled cross circulation for open intracardiac surgery: Physiologic studies and results of creation and closure of ventricular septal defects. J Thorac Surg 28:331–341, 1954.
3. Kirklin JW, Dushane JW, Patrick RT, et al: Intracardiac surgery with the aid of a mechanical pump-oxygenator system (gibbon

type): Report of eight cases. Proc Staff Meet Mayo Clin 30:201–206, 1955.

4. Williams RG, Pearson GD, Barst RJ, et al: Report of the National Heart, Lung, and Blood Institute Working Group on research in adult congenital heart disease. J Am Coll Cardiol 47:701–707, 2006.
5. Mullins CE: Cardiac catheterization in congenital heart disease: Pediatric and adult, Malden, Mass, 2006, Blackwell Futura.
6. Cannesson M, Earing MG, Collange V, et al: Anesthesia for noncardiac surgery in adults with congenital heart disease. Anesthesiology 111:432–440, 2009.
7. Wilcox BR, Cook AC, Anderson RH: Surgical anatomy of the heart, ed 3, Cambridge, England, 2004, Cambridge University Press.
8. Andropoulos DB, Stayer SA, Russell IA, et al: Anesthesia for congenital heart disease, ed 2, Hoboken, NJ, 2010, Wiley-Blackwell.
9. Morales DL, Carberry KE, Heinle JS, et al: Extubation in the operating room after Fontan's procedure: Effect on practice and outcomes. Ann Thorac Surg 86:576–581, 2008.
10. Perioperative management of patients with congenital heart disease. In Nichols DG, Ungerleider R, Spevak PJ, et al, editors: Critical heart disease in infants and children, ed 2, Philadelphia, 2006, Mosby.
11. Licht DJ, Shera DM, Clancy RR, et al: Brain maturation is delayed in infants with complex congenital heart defects. J Thorac Cardiovasc Surg 137:529–536, 2009.
12. Suematsu Y, Mora BN, Mihaljevic T, et al: Totally endoscopic robotic-assisted repair of patent ductus arteriosus and vascular ring in children. Ann Thorac Surg 80:2309–2313, 2005.
13. Thanopoulos BV, Eleftherakis N, Tzannos K, et al: Further experience with catheter closure of patent ductus arteriosus using the new Amplatzer duct occluder in children. Am J Cardiol 105:1005–1009, 2010.
14. Hopkins RA, Bert AA, Buchholz B, et al: Surgical patch closure of atrial septal defects. Ann Thorac Surg 77:2144–2149, 2004.
15. Knepp MD, Rocchini AP, Lloyd TR, et al: Long-term follow up of secundum atrial septal defect closure with the amplatzer septal occluder. Congenit Heart Dis 5:32–37, 2010.
16. Clark JB, Chowdhury D, Pauliks LB, et al: Resolution of heart block after surgical removal of an amplatzer device. Ann Thorac Surg 89:1631–1633, 2010.
17. Piatkowski R, Kochanowski J, Scislo P, et al: Dislocation of Amplatzer septal occluder device after closure of secundum atrial septal defect. J Am Soc Echocardiogr 23:1007, e1–e2, 2010.
18. Slesnick TC, Nugent AW, Fraser CD, Jr, et al: Images in cardiovascular medicine. Incomplete endothelialization and late development of acute bacterial endocarditis after implantation of an Amplatzer septal occluder device. Circulation 117:e326–e327, 2008.
19. Neill CA, Ferencz C, Sabiston DC, et al: The familial occurrence of hypoplastic right lung with systemic arterial supply and venous drainage "scimitar syndrome." Bull Johns Hopkins Hosp 107:1–21, 1960.
20. DiBardino DJ, McKenzie ED, Heinle JS, et al: The Warden procedure for partially anomalous pulmonary venous connection to the superior caval vein. Cardiol Young 14:64–67, 2004.
21. Crossland DS, Wilkinson JL, Cochrane AD, et al: Initial results of primary device closure of large muscular ventricular septal defects in early infancy using perventricular access. Catheter Cardiovasc Interv 72:386–391, 2008.
22. Scully BB, Morales DL, Zafar F, et al: Current expectations for surgical repair of isolated ventricular septal defects. Ann Thorac Surg 89:544–549, 2010.
23. Rastelli GC, Weidman WH, Kirklin JW: Surgical repair of the partial form of persistent common atrioventricular canal, with special reference to the problem of mitral valve incompetence. Circulation 31(Suppl 1):31–35, 1965.
24. Bakhtiary F, Takacs J, Cho MY, et al: Long-term results after repair of complete atrioventricular septal defect with two-patch technique. Ann Thorac Surg 89:1239–1243, 2010.
25. Morales DL, Braud BE, Gunter KS, et al: Encouraging results for the Contegra conduit in the problematic right ventricle-to-pulmonary artery connection. J Thorac Cardiovasc Surg 132:665–671, 2006.
26. Chen JM, Glickstein JS, Davies RR, et al: The effect of repair technique on postoperative right-sided obstruction in patients with truncus arteriosus. J Thorac Cardiovasc Surg 129:559–568, 2005.
27. Vezmar M, Chaturvedi R, Lee KJ, et al: Percutaneous pulmonary valve implantation in the young: 2-year follow-up. JACC Cardiovasc Interv 3:439–448, 2010.
28. Tlaskal T, Chaloupecky V, Hucin B, et al: Long-term results after correction of persistent truncus arteriosus in 83 patients. Eur J Cardiothorac Surg 37:1278–1284, 2010.
29. Fraser CDJ: "Lateral" approach to surgical repair of total anomalous pulmonary venous return. Oper Tech Thor Cardiovasc Surg 11:275–285, 2006.
30. Morales DL, Zafar F, Heinle JS, et al: Right ventricular infundibulum sparing (RVIS) tetralogy of Fallot repair: A review of over 300 patients. Ann Surg 250:611–617, 2009.
31. Davies B, Mussa S, Davies P, et al: Unifocalization of major aortopulmonary collateral arteries in pulmonary atresia with ventricular septal defect is essential to achieve excellent outcomes irrespective of native pulmonary artery morphology. J Thorac Cardiovasc Surg 138:1269–1275, e1261, 2009.
32. Mustard WT: Successful two-stage correction of transposition of the great vessels. Surgery 55:469–472, 1964.
33. Senning A: Surgical correction of transposition of the great vessels. Surgery 45:966–980, 1959.
34. Dibardino DJ, Allison AE, Vaughn WK, et al: Current expectations for newborns undergoing the arterial switch operation. Ann Surg 239:588–596, 2004.
35. Angeli E, Formigari R, Pace Napoleone C, et al: Long-term coronary artery outcome after arterial switch operation for transposition of the great arteries. Eur J Cardiothorac Surg 38:714–720, 2010.
36. Yacoub MH, Radley-Smith R: Anatomy of the coronary arteries in transposition of the great arteries and methods for their transfer in anatomical correction. Thorax 33:418–424, 1978.
37. Ly M, Belli E, Leobon B, et al: Results of the double switch operation for congenitally corrected transposition of the great arteries. Eur J Cardiothorac Surg 35:879–883, 2009.
38. Bacha EA, McElhinney DB, Guleserian KJ, et al: Surgical aortic valvuloplasty in children and adolescents with aortic regurgitation: Acute and intermediate effects on aortic valve function and left ventricular dimensions. J Thorac Cardiovasc Surg 135:552–559, 2008.
39. Shinkawa T, Bove EL, Hirsch JC, et al: Intermediate-term results of the Ross procedure in neonates and infants. Ann Thorac Surg 89:1827–1832, 2010.

40. Booth JH, Bryant R, Powers SC, et al: Transthoracic echocardiography does not reliably predict involvement of the aortic valve in patients with a discrete subaortic shelf. Cardiol Young 20:284–289, 2010.
41. Shone JD, Sellers RD, Anderson RC, et al: The developmental complex of "parachute mitral valve," supravalvular ring of left atrium, subaortic stenosis, and coarctation of aorta. Am J Cardiol 11:714–725, 1963.
42. Cowley CG, Orsmond GS, Feola P, et al: Long-term, randomized comparison of balloon angioplasty and surgery for native coarctation of the aorta in childhood. Circulation 111:3453–3456, 2005.
43. Morales DL, Scully PT, Braud BE, et al: Interrupted aortic arch repair: Aortic arch advancement without a patch minimizes arch reinterventions. Ann Thorac Surg 82:1577–1583; discussion 1583–1574, 2006.
44. Bailey LL, Nehlsen-Cannarella SL, Doroshow RW, et al: Cardiac allotransplantation in newborns as therapy for hypoplastic left heart syndrome. N Engl J Med 315:949–951, 1986.
45. Norwood WI, Lang P, Casteneda AR, et al: Experience with operations for hypoplastic left heart syndrome. J Thorac Cardiovasc Surg 82:511–519, 1981.
46. Sano S, Ishino K, Kado H, et al: Outcome of right ventricle-to-pulmonary artery shunt in first-stage palliation of hypoplastic left heart syndrome: A multi-institutional study. Ann Thorac Surg 78:1951–1957, 2004.
47. Ohye RG, Sleeper LA, Mahony L, et al: Comparison of shunt types in the Norwood procedure for single-ventricle lesions. N Engl J Med 362:1980–1992, 2010.
48. Luce WA, Schwartz RM, Beauseau W, et al: Necrotizing enterocolitis in neonates undergoing the hybrid approach to complex congenital heart disease. Pediatr Crit Care Med 12:46–51, 2011.
49. Fontan F, Baudet E: Surgical repair of tricuspid atresia. Thorax 26:240–248, 1971.
50. Salazar JD, Zafar F, Siddiqui K, et al: Fenestration during Fontan palliation: Now the exception instead of the rule. J Thorac Cardiovasc Surg 140:129–136, 2010.
51. Alsoufi B, Sallehuddin A, Bulbul Z, et al: Surgical strategy to establish a dual-coronary system for the management of anomalous left coronary artery origin from the pulmonary artery. Ann Thorac Surg 86:170–176, 2008.
52. Valente AM, Lock JE, Gauvreau K, et al: Predictors of long-term adverse outcomes in patients with congenital coronary artery fistulae. Circ Cardiovasc Interv 3:134–139, 2010.
53. Starnes VA, Pitlick PT, Bernstein D, et al: Ebstein's anomaly appearing in the neonate. A new surgical approach. J Thorac Cardiovasc Surg 101:1082–1087, 1991.
54. Brown ML, Dearani JA, Danielson GK, et al: The outcomes of operations for 539 patients with Ebstein anomaly. J Thorac Cardiovasc Surg 135:1120–1136, 1136, e1121–1127, 2008.

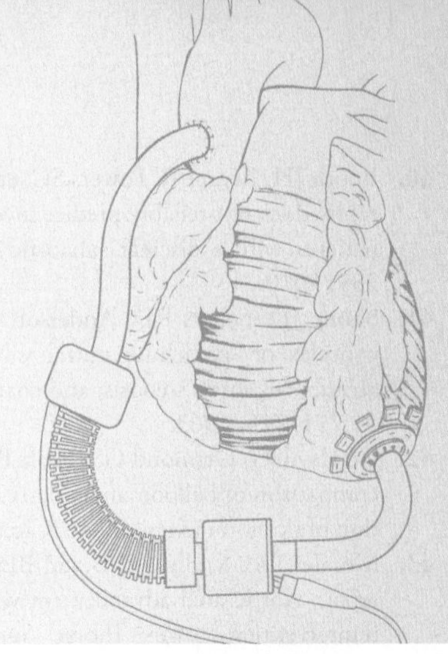

CHAPTER 60

# ACQUIRED HEART DISEASE: CORONARY INSUFFICIENCY

Raja R. Gopaldas, Danny Chu, and Faisal G. Bakaeen



Cardiovascular disease is the leading cause of death in the United States. Coronary artery disease, which is responsible for more than 50% of all cardiovascular disease–related deaths, was expected to account for more than $80 billion in direct costs in 2010. In the United States, approximately 1 million people sustain an acute myocardial infarction (MI) every year because of atherosclerotic coronary disease. Although recent advances in percutaneous intervention have reduced the number of referrals for surgical intervention, coronary artery bypass grafting (CABG) still remains one of the most effective treatments for coronary artery disease and is the most commonly performed open cardiac procedure in the United States.

## CORONARY ARTERY ANATOMY AND PHYSIOLOGY

### Anatomic Considerations

The coronary arteries are the predominant blood supply conduits to the heart. The coronary arteries arise from the sinuses of Valsalva, which are elastic saccular bulges of the aortic root. The coronary arteries are the first arterial branches of the aorta and usually two are present. They are designated as right and left according to the embryologic chamber that they predominantly supply. The left coronary artery (LCA) arises from the left coronary sinus, which is located posteromedially, whereas the right coronary artery (RCA) arises from the right coronary sinus, which is located anteromedially. The LCA, also called the *left main coronary artery*, averages approximately 2 to 3 cm in length and courses in a left posterolateral direction, winding behind the main pulmonary artery trunk and then splitting into the left anterior descending (LAD) and left circumflex arteries. The LAD courses in an anterolateral direction to the left of the pulmonary trunk and runs anteriorly over the interventricular septum. The diagonal branches of the LAD supply the anterolateral wall of the left ventricle. The LAD is considered the most important surgical vessel because it supplies more than 50% of the left ventricular mass and most of the interventricular septum. The LAD has several septal perforating branches that supply the interventricular septum from the anterior aspect. The LAD extends over the interventricular septum up to the apex of the heart, where it may form an anastomosis with the posterior descending artery (PDA), which is typically a branch of the right coronary system (Fig. 60-1).

The circumflex artery passes through the atrioventricular groove (AV) and follows a clockwise course. Where the circumflex artery courses through the AV groove, it gives off branches in a perpendicular fashion that extend toward, but do not quite reach, the apex of the heart. These branches are designated the obtuse marginal braches and are designated numerically from proximal to distal. The circumflex coronary artery usually terminates as the left posterolateral branch after taking a perpendicular turn toward the apex.

The term *ramus intermedius* is used to designate a dominant epicardial coronary vessel that arises from the occasional trifurcation of the left main coronary artery. The ramus typically emerges from under the left atrial appendage, which is used as a landmark for identifying this branch and courses over the anterolateral wall of the left ventricle. This branch can be intramyocardial and difficult to locate at times.

The RCA supplies most of the right ventricle, as well as the posterior part of the left ventricle. The RCA emerges from its ostium in the right coronary sinus, passes deep in the right AV groove, and then proceeds over the anterior surface of the heart. At the superior end of the acute margin of the heart, the RCA turns posteriorly toward the crux and usually bifurcates into the PDA over the posterior interventricular sulcus and right posterolateral artery. The RCA also supplies multiple right ventricular branches (acute marginal branches). Occasionally, the PDA arises from both the RCA and LCA and the circulation is considered to be codominant. The AV node artery arises from the RCA in approximately 90% of patients. The sinoatrial node artery arises from the proximal RCA in 50% of patients. Other prominent branches arising from the RCA include the acute marginal artery and anterior ventricular branches. Although the source of the PDA is often used clinically to define dominance

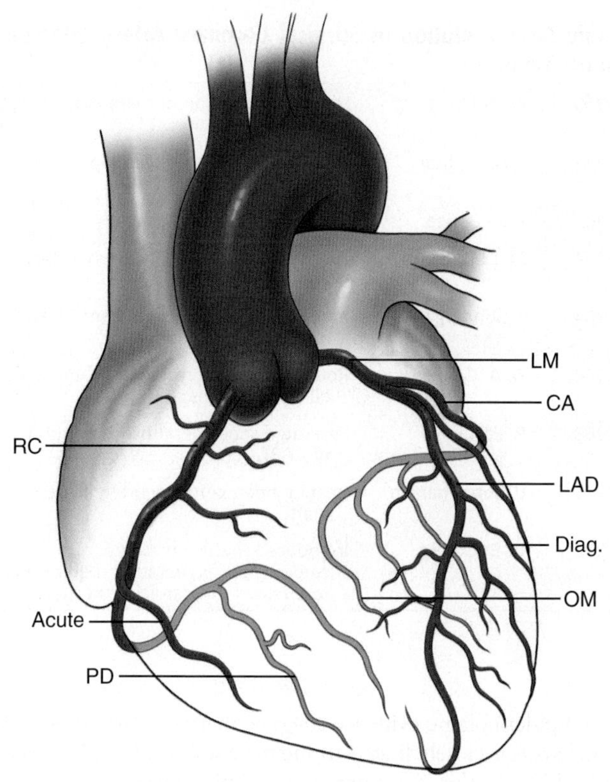


**FIGURE 60-1** Anatomy of normal coronary artery vasculature.

**Table 60-1 Anatomic Architecture of Coronary Arteries**

| NAMED VESSELS | BRANCHES |
|---|---|
| Left main coronary artery | Left anterior descending<br>Circumflex coronary<br>Ramus intermedius |
| Left anterior descending | Diagonal arteries<br>Septal perforators |
| Circumflex coronary artery | Obtuse marginal branches<br>Left posterolateral artery |
| Right coronary artery | Acute marginal artery<br>Posterior descending artery<br>Right posterolateral artery |

of circulation in the heart, anatomists define it according to where the sinoatrial node artery arises. Table 60-1 summarizes the hierarchy of the coronary artery anatomy.

All the epicardial conductance vessels and septal perforators from the LAD give rise to a multitude of branches, termed *resistance vessels,* which traverse perpendicularly into the ventricular wall. These vessels play a crucial role in oxygen and nutrient exchange with the myocardium by forming a rich plexus capillary network. The rich capillary plexus offers a low-resistance sink to allow for unimpeded increase of arterial blood flow when oxygen demand rises. This is important because the myocardial vascular bed extracts oxygen at its full capacity, even in low-demand circumstances, thereby allowing no margin for further oxygen extraction when demand is high.

An intricate network of veins drains the coronary circulation and the venous circulation can be divided into three systems—the coronary sinus and its tributaries, the anterior right ventricular veins, and the thebesian veins. The coronary sinus predominantly drains the left ventricle and receives 85% of coronary venous blood. It lies within the posterior AV groove and empties into the right atrium. The anterior right ventricular veins travel across the right ventricular surface to the right AV groove, where they enter directly into the right atrium or form the small cardiac vein, which enters into the right atrium directly or joins the coronary sinus just proximal to its orifice. The thebesian veins are small venous tributaries that drain directly into the cardiac chambers and exit primarily into the right atrium and right ventricle. Understanding the anatomy of the coronary sinus is essential for placing the retrograde cardioplegia cannula during cardiopulmonary bypass.

**BOX 60-1 Unique Features of Coronary Blood Flow**

- Autoregulated over wide pressure ranges
- Blood flow: 0.7 to 0.9 mL/g of myocardium per minute
- 75% oxygen extraction
- Coronary sinus blood is the most deoxygenated blood in the body
- 4 to 7 fold increase in flow with increased demand
- 60% blood flow occurs during diastole
- Flow limited oxygen supply

## Physiology and Regulation of Coronary Blood Flow

Aortic pressure is a driving force in the maintenance of myocardial perfusion. During resting conditions, coronary blood flow is maintained at a fairly constant level over a wide range of aortic perfusion pressures (70 to 180 mm Hg) through the process of autoregulation.

Because the myocardium has a high rate of energy use, normal coronary blood flow averages 225 mL/min (0.7 to 0.9 mL/g of myocardium/min) and delivers 0.1 mL/g/min of oxygen to the myocardium. Under normal conditions, more than 75% of the delivered oxygen is extracted in the coronary capillary bed, so any additional oxygen demand can only be met by increasing the flow rate. This highlights the importance of unobstructed coronary blood flow for proper myocardial function. Box 60-1 summarizes the unique features of coronary blood flow.

In response to increased load, such as that caused by strenuous exercise, the healthy heart can increase myocardial blood flow fourfold to sevenfold. Increased blood flow occurs through several mechanisms. Local metabolic neurohumoral factors cause coronary vasodilation when stress and metabolic demand increase, thereby lowering the coronary vascular resistance. This results in increased delivery of oxygen-rich blood, mimicking the phenomenon of reactive hyperemia. When a transient occlusion to the coronary artery is released (e.g., during the performance of a beating heart operation), blood flow immediately rises to exceed the normal baseline flow and then gradually returns to its baseline level. The autoregulatory mechanism responsible is guided by several metabolic factors, including $CO_2$, $O_2$ tension, hydrogen ions, lactate, potassium ions, and adenosine. Of these, adenosine is one of the leading candidates in the autoregulatory mechanism. Adenosine, a potent vasodilator and a degradation product of adenosine triphosphate (ATP), accumulates in the interstitial space and relaxes vascular smooth muscle. This results in vasomotor relaxation, coronary vasodilation, and increased blood flow. Another substance that plays an important role is nitric oxide (NO), which is produced by the endothelium. Without the endothelium, coronary arteries do not autoregulate, suggesting that the mechanism for vasodilation and reactive hyperemia is endothelium-dependent.

Extravascular compression of the coronaries during systole also plays an important role in the regulation of blood flow. During systole, the intracavitary pressures generated in the left ventricular wall exceed intracoronary pressure and blood flow is impeded. Hence, approximately 60% of the coronary blood flow occurs during diastole. During exercise. increased heart rate and reduced diastolic time can compromise flow time but this can be offset by vasodilatory mechanisms of the coronary vessels. Buildup of atherosclerotic plaques and fixed coronary occlusion significantly impair coronary blood compensatory mechanisms during increased heart rates. This forms the basis for exercise-induced stress tests, in which increased activity or exercise unmasks underlying coronary disease.

## HISTORY OF CORONARY ARTERY BYPASS SURGERY

One of the first attempts at myocardial revascularization was made by Dr. Arthur Vineberg from Canada. He operated on a series of patients who presented with symptoms of myocardial ischemia and implanted the left internal mammary artery into the myocardium by creating a pocket. The operation did not entail a direct anastomosis to any coronary vessel and was performed on a beating heart through a left anterolateral thoracotomy. Dr. Michael DeBakey performed a successful aortocoronary saphenous vein graft in 1964. Dr. Mason Sones, who is credited with inventing cardiac catheterization, helped establish coronary artery bypass surgery as a planned and consistent therapy in patients with angiographically documented coronary artery disease.

The development of the heart-lung machine and demonstration of successful clinical use by Dr. John Heysham Gibbon in the 1950s and the advancement of cardioplegia techniques in later years by Dr. Gerald Buckberg allowed surgeons to perform coronary anastomosis on an arrested (nonbeating) heart with a relatively bloodless field, thus increasing the safety and accuracy of the coronary bypass. In the 1990s, the advent of devices that could atraumatically stabilize the heart provided another pathway for the development of off-pump techniques of myocardial revascularization. Today, an armamentarium of techniques, ranging from conventional on-pump CABG to minimally invasive robotic and percutaneous approaches, is available to manage coronary artery disease. Table 60-2 summarizes the timeline of major historical events in the development of surgery for myocardial revascularization.

**Table 60-2 Evolution of Surgical Coronary Artery Interventions: Timeline**

| | | |
|---|---|---|
| 1950 | A. Vineberg | Direct implantation of mammary artery into myocardium |
| 1953 | J. H. Gibbon | First successful use of cardiopulmonary bypass machine |
| 1962 | F. M. Sones | Successful cine-angiography |
| 1964 | M. E. DeBakey | First successful coronary artery bypass grafting |
| 1964 | T. Sondergaard | Introduced routine use of cardioplegia for myocardial protection |
| 1964 | D. A. Cooley | Routine use of normothermic arrest for all cardiac cases |
| 1968 | R. Favoloro | First large series demonstrating success of CABG |
| 1973 | V. Subramanian | Beating heart coronary artery bypass graft |
| 1979 | G. Buckberg | Introduced the use of blood cardioplegia as preferred method for to arrested myocardial protection |

## ATHEROSCLEROTIC CORONARY ARTERY DISEASE

Coronary atherosclerosis is a process that begins early in the patient's life. Epicardial conductance vessels are the most susceptible and intramyocardial arteries, the least. Risk factors for atherosclerosis include elevated plasma levels of total cholesterol and low-density lipoprotein cholesterol (LDLc), cigarette smoking, hypertension, diabetes mellitus, advanced age, low plasma levels of high-density lipoprotein cholesterol (HDLc), and a family history of premature coronary artery disease.

Epidemiologic evidence suggests that coronary artery atherosclerosis is closely linked to the metabolism of lipids, specifically LDLc. The development of lipid-lowering drugs has resulted in a significant reduction in mortality. In one observational study of patients who received statin therapy and were known to have coronary artery disease (CAD), statin treatment was associated with improved survival in all age groups.[1] The greatest survival benefit was found in those patients in the highest quartile of plasma levels of high-sensitivity C-reactive protein (hs-CRP), a biomarker of inflammation and CAD.[2] Animal and human studies have demonstrated that statin therapy also modifies the lipid composition within plaques by lowering the amount of LDLc and stabilizing the plaque through various mechanisms, including reduction in macrophage accumulation, collagen degradation, reduction in smooth muscle cell protease expression, and decrease in tissue factor expression.

### Pathogenesis

The primary cause of atherosclerotic coronary disease is endothelial injury induced by an inflammatory wall response and lipid deposition. There is evidence that an inflammatory response is involved in all stages of the disease, from early lipid deposition to plaque formation, plaque rupture, and coronary artery thrombosis. Vulnerable or high-risk plaques that are prone to rupture are characterized by the following:

1. A large, eccentric, soft lipid core
2. A thin fibrous cap
3. Inflammation within the cap and adventitia
4. Increased plaque neovascularity
5. Evidence of outward or positive vessel remodeling

Thinner fibrous caps are at a higher risk for rupture, probably because of an imbalance between the synthesis and degradation of the extracellular matrix in the fibrous cap that results in an overall decrease in the collagen and matrix components (Fig. 60-2). Increased matrix breakdown caused by matrix degradation by an inflammatory cell-mediated metalloproteinase or

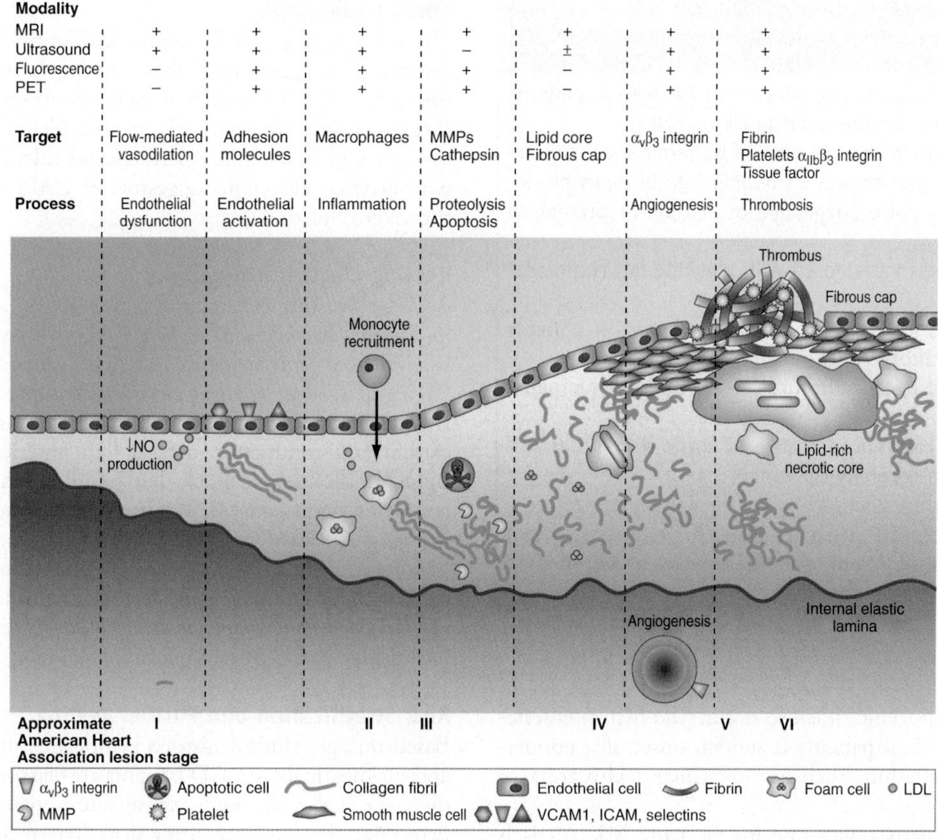


**FIGURE 60-2** Components of atherosclerotic plaque. Thinning of the fibrous cap eventually results in plaque rupture with extrusion of highly thrombogenic lipid laden material into the coronary artery. This causes an acute occlusion of the coronary artery resulting in myocardial infarction. (Adapted from Choudhury RP, Fuster V, Fayad ZA. Molecular, cellular and functional imaging of atherothrombosis. Nature Rev Drug Discov 3:913–925, 2004.)

reduced production of extracellular matrix results in thinner fibrous caps. Not all plaque ruptures are symptomatic; whether they are is dependent on the thrombogenicity of the plaque's components. Tissue factor within the lipid core of the plaque, secreted by activated macrophages, is one of the most potent thrombogenic stimuli. Rupture of a vulnerable plaque may be spontaneous or caused by extreme physical activity, severe emotional distress, exposure to drugs, cold exposure, or acute infection.

### Fixed Coronary Obstructions

More than 90% of patients with symptomatic ischemic heart disease have advanced coronary atherosclerosis caused by a fixed obstruction. Atherosclerotic plaques of the coronary arteries are concentric (25%) or eccentric (75%). Eccentric lesions compromise only a portion of the lumen; through vascular remodeling, the arterial lumen may remain patent until late in the disease process. The impact of an arterial stenosis on coronary blood flow can be appreciated in the context of Poiseuille's law. Reductions in luminal diameter up to 60% have minimal impact on flow but when the cross-sectional area of the vessel has decreased by 75% or more, coronary blood flow is significantly compromised. Clinically, this loss of flow often coincides with the onset of exertional angina. A 90% reduction in luminal diameter results in resting angina.

## CLINICAL MANIFESTATIONS AND DIAGNOSIS OF CORONARY ARTERY DISEASE

### Clinical Presentation

The most common presenting symptom of CAD is angina. It may be accompanied by dyspnea or mistaken for a gastrointestinal disturbance. The symptoms typically are exacerbated or incited by effort but subsequently resolve with rest. Unstable angina encompasses resting angina, new-onset angina, and accelerated angina and is usually indicative of severe ischemia and impending MI. However, not all cases of angina are necessarily indicative of CAD, because disease processes from other systems can closely mimic those of angina. Approximately 15% of patients with CAD do not present with angina.

The term *acute coronary syndrome* (ACS) has evolved to refer to a constellation of clinical symptoms that represent myocardial ischemia. It encompasses both ST-segment elevation MI (STEMI) and non–ST-segment elevation MI (NSTEMI). MI often presents as crushing chest pain that may be associated with nausea, diaphoresis, anxiety, and dyspnea. Symptoms of hypoperfusion may also include dizziness, fatigue, and vomiting. Heart rate and blood pressure may be initially normal, but both increase in response to the duration and severity of pain. Loss of blood pressure is indicative of cardiogenic shock and indicates a poorer prognosis. At least 40% of the ventricular mass must

**BOX 60-2 Sequelae of Coronary Artery Disease: Clinical Manifestations**

Abnormal neck vein pulsations, which may be seen in patients with second- or third-degree heart block or CHF:

- Bradycardia—a subtle presentation of ischemia involving the right coronary territories and a possible sign of heart block
- Weak or thready pulse suggestive of ectopic or premature ventricular beats
- Third heart sound that is noted with elevated left ventricular filling pressures/CHF
- Fourth heart sound, which is commonly heard in patients with acute and chronic CAD
- Mitral regurgitant heart murmurs caused by ischemic papillary muscles
- Ejection systolic murmur indicative of aortic stenosis, which can contribute to coronary ischemia
- Holosystolic murmurs caused by ventricular septal rupture
- Manifestations of CHF, such as rales, hepatomegaly, right upper abdominal quadrant tenderness, ascites, and marked peripheral and presacral edema

be involved for cardiogenic shock to occur. The first manifestation of CAD in 40% of patients is sudden onset of a nonperfusing ventricular rhythm, such as ventricular tachycardia or fibrillation.

The prehospital mortality rate for an acute MI (AMI) is approximately 50%. Of those patients who reach the hospital, another 25% die during the hospital stay and another 25% die in the first year afterward.[3,4] Mechanical complications of MI include acute ventricular septal defect (VSD), papillary muscle rupture, and free ventricular rupture. They usually occur approximately 7 to 10 days after the initial MI.

## Physical Examination

Some clinical findings are generic and are related to the systemic manifestations of atherosclerosis. Eye examination may reveal a copper wire sign, retinal hematoma or thrombosis secondary to vascular occlusive disease, and hypertension. Corneal arcus and xanthelasma are features noticed in cases of hypercholesterolemia. Other clinical manifestations are caused by sequelae of CAD, as noted in Box 60-2.

A thorough vascular evaluation is essential for any patient who presents with coronary disease because atherosclerosis is a systemic process. In addition, if surgery is being planned, the extremities should be evaluated for any previous surgical scars or fractures that could potentially preclude vein harvest.

## Diagnostic Testing

### Biochemical Studies

Patients suspected of having an ACS should undergo appropriate blood testing. Levels of creatinine kinase muscle and brain subunits (CK-MB) and troponin T or I should be assessed at least 6 to 12 hours apart. Additional laboratory tests include a complete blood count (CBC), comprehensive metabolic panel, and lipid profile (total cholesterol, triglycerides, LDLc, HDLc). Elevated brain natriuretic peptide (BNP) and CRP levels suggest a worse outcome.

### Chest Radiography

The chest radiograph is helpful in identifying causes of chest discomfort or pain other than CAD. Chest radiography does not detect CAD directly; it only identifies sequelae, such as cardiomegaly, pulmonary edema, and pleural effusions, that are indicative of heart failure. Evidence of calcification in the coronary arteries, although suggestive of CAD, is not reflective of the severity of the disease.

### Resting Electrocardiography

A 12-lead resting electrocardiogram (ECG) should be obtained in patients suspected of having CAD or its sequelae. The ECG is evaluated for evidence of left ventricular hypertrophy, ST-segment depression or elevation, ectopic beats, or Q waves. In addition, arrhythmias (atrial fibrillation or ventricular tachycardia) and conduction defects (left anterior fascicular block, right bundle branch block, left bundle branch block) are suggestive of CAD and MI. Persistent ST-segment elevation or an evolving Q wave is consistent with myocardial injury and ongoing ischemia. Fifty percent of patients have normal electrocardiographic results despite having significant CAD, and 50% of ECGs obtained during chest pain at rest will be normal, indicating the inaccurate nature of the test.

### Risk Stratification and Further Testing

Based on age, clinical history, symptomatology, physical signs, and diagnostic tests, CAD patients are classified as low, intermediate, or high risk. Such stratification enables the clinician to determine the intensity of medical therapy and timing of coronary angiography.

Low- to intermediate-risk patients treated early and with a conservative strategy may undergo stress testing for further risk stratification. The choice to conduct stress testing depends on the patient's resting ECG and ability to perform exercise.

An exercise stress ECG is helpful in unmasking underlying CAD and is a more reliable screening test than a resting ECG in patients older than 40 years. The Bruce protocol is the most commonly used standardized treadmill exercise protocol. The protocol involves five 3-minute bouts of treadmill exercise, each designed to elicit greater myocardial oxygen demand than the last, to determine the patient's ischemic threshold. A typical protocol requires the patient to expend about 12 metabolic equivalents (METs) of energy to ensure a complete test. A positive exercise ECG may show progressive flattening of the ST segment or ST-segment depression as exercise progresses. During the recovery phase, ST depression may persist, with downsloping segments and T wave inversion. Additional findings associated with an adverse prognosis and the presence of multivessel occlusive disease include a duration of symptom-limited exercise of less than 6 METs, the failure of systolic blood pressure to increase to more than 120 mm Hg, and the appearance of ventricular arrhythmias. For detection of CAD, the sensitivity and specificity of an exercise ECG approach 70% and 80%, respectively (Box 60-3).

Conditions that preclude accurate interpretation of the stress ECG include digoxin therapy, widespread resting ST-segment depression (≥1 mm), left ventricular hypertrophy, left bundle branch block, and other conduction abnormalities. For patients with these conditions and those unable to exercise, a pharmacologic stress test with an imaging modality using a radionuclide agent such as thallium or sestamibi, multiple-gated

**BOX 60-3 Stress Tests to Identify Coronary Artery Disease**

**Exercise Stress ECG***
- Bruce protocol (vide infra)
- Five 3 minute bouts of treadmill exercise
- Determines the ischemic threshold
- 12 metabolic equivalents of energy expenditure needed for complete test
- Low cost and short duration
- Highly sensitive in multivessel disease

Limitations:
- Suboptimal sensitivity
- Low detection rate of one-vessel disease;
- Nondiagnostic with abnormal baseline ECG
- Poor specificity in premenopausal women
- Many cannot accomplish the 12 mets for a complete test or an appropriate heart rate response

**Exercise/Pharmacologic SPECT Perfusion Imaging**
- Simultaneous evaluation of perfusion and function
- Higher sensitivity and specificity than exercise ECG
- Quantitative image analysis

Limitations:
- Long procedure time with $99^{m}$Tc
- Higher cost
- Radiation exposure
- Poor-quality images in obese patients

**Exercise/Pharmacologic Stress Echocardiography**
- Higher sensitivity and specificity than exercise ECG
- Comparable value with dobutamine stress
- Short examination time
- Identification of structural cardiac abnormalities
- Simultaneous evaluation of perfusion with contrast agents
- No radiation

Limitations:
- Decreased sensitivity for detection of one-vessel disease or mild stenosis
- Highly operator dependent
- No quantitative image analysis
- Poor imaging in some patients
- Infarct zone poorly defined

*Commonly known as the treadmill test.

acquisition [MUGA] scanning, or positron emission tomography (PET) should be considered. Echocardiography may be considered as an alternative. Pharmacologic stress agents include adenosine, dobutamine, and dipyridamole.

### Echocardiography

Many patients undergoing CABG also undergo transthoracic echocardiography by the evaluating cardiology team to estimate ventricular wall abnormalities and the ejection fraction. Common indications for a resting echocardiogram include heart murmurs and a suspicion of a structural problem, such as aortic stenosis or insufficiency, hypertrophic cardiomyopathy, mitral valve stenosis or regurgitation, and congestive heart failure. Ventricular dilation and wall thinning are other features noted on the echocardiogram in patients with chronic ischemic CAD or prior infarcts.

### Multidetector Computed Tomography

Multidetector computed tomography (MDCT), one of the most recent imaging modalities, allows imaging of the coronary arteries, especially of coronary artery bypass grafts. Studies have indicated that the sensitivity and specificity MDCT approach or exceed those of other noninvasive methods of visualizing the coronary artery anatomy.[5] MDCT is especially useful for imaging proximal CAD and coronary artery bypass grafts. More recent technology improves on conventional MDCT by adding more arrays to the imaging process; 128-slice MDCT arrays are currently available. These scanners can acquire myocardial images within 1 second while exposing the patient to less radiation than traditional scanners. Although it is still preferable that patients have relatively low heart rates during imaging (to reduce artifact), the technology has significantly advanced and produces images on par with those generated by the gold standard, conventional angiography.[6]

### Magnetic Resonance Imaging and Gadolinium Magnetic Resonance Imaging

Myocardial first-pass perfusion magnetic resonance imaging (MRI) has been considered a good alternative to nuclear cardiac ischemia and viability testing. However, the procedure has not gained widespread popularity because special training and expertise are required to perform this type of imaging and interpret the results.

### Cardiac Catheterization and Intervention

Cardiac catheterization remains the gold standard for evaluating the anatomy of the coronary arteries. High-quality coronary angiography is essential for identifying CAD and assessing its extent and severity.

Cardiac catheterization is commonly performed by inserting a short, self-sealing vascular sheath into either femoral artery. Vascular access may also be obtained via a brachial or radial artery. Angiography is done by using hollow preshaped catheters (5 or 6 Fr), which are placed under fluoroscopic guidance retrograde through the aorta into the ostia of the coronary arteries and coronary bypass grafts. A solution of radiographic contrast material is injected through the catheter to opacify the lumen. Images are recorded in rapid succession onto film or in a digital format. The surgeon typically uses the coronary angiography images to determine the number and location of coronary targets where bypass anastomoses are to be constructed (Figs. 60-3, 60-4, and 60-5).

Other information obtained from cardiac catheterization includes coronary and aortic calcification, ventricular function, and, if ventriculography is performed, mitral regurgitation. Injection of contrast into the aortic root provides useful root and ascending aortic images when indicated.

Right heart catheterization is used to measure central venous, right atrial, right ventricular, pulmonary artery, and pulmonary wedge pressures, as well as cardiac output. It can also be used to identify intracardiac shunts, assess arrhythmias, and initiate temporary cardiac pacing. Preoperative right heart catheterization is used selectively and is generally not necessary unless right ventricular dysfunction or pulmonary vascular disease is suspected.

Percutaneous coronary intervention (PCI) techniques in current use include balloon dilation, stent-supported dilation, atherectomy, and plaque ablation with a variety of devices,

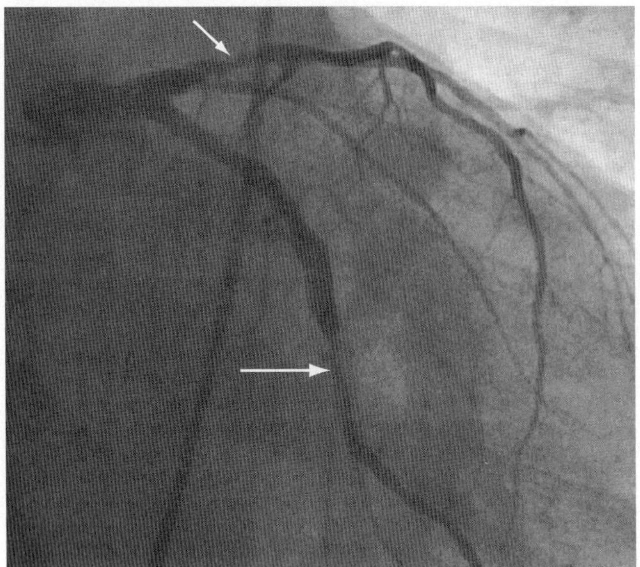

**FIGURE 60-3** Left coronary angiogram demonstrating hemodynamically severe lesions in the left anterior descending artery *(small arrow)* and the circumflex artery *(large arrow).*

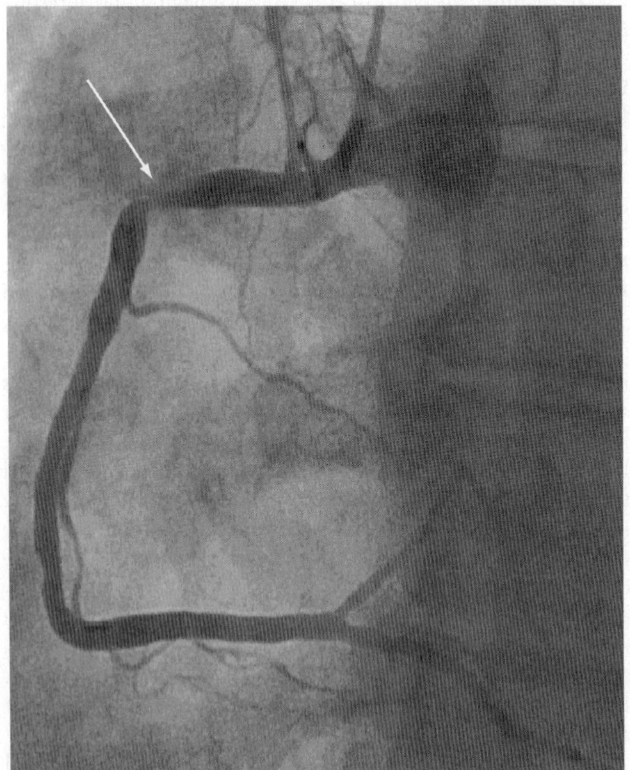

**FIGURE 60-4** Right coronary angiogram demonstrating hemodynamically significant lesions *(arrow).* The right coronary artery terminates as a posterior descending artery in the right dominant system.

thrombectomy with aspiration devices, specialized imaging, and physiologic assessment with intracoronary devices.

Coronary artery stents were the first substantial breakthrough in the prevention of restenosis after angioplasty. Although stent recoil or compression are not completely insignificant problems, the greatest cause of lumen loss in stented coronary arteries is neointimal hyperplasia. This is the principal mechanism of in-stent stenosis and results from inappropriate cell proliferation—hence, the advent of cytotoxic drug-eluting stents.

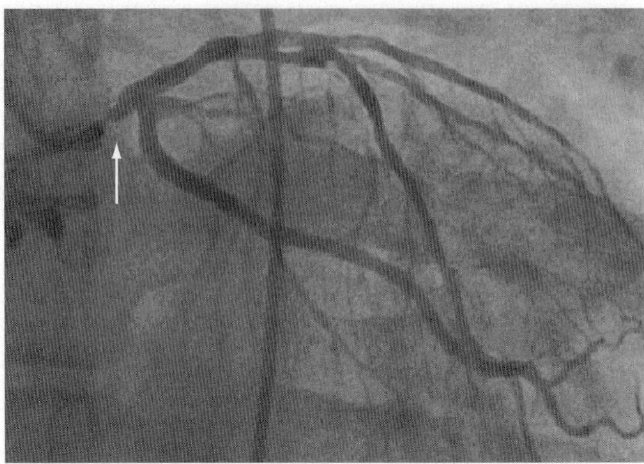

**FIGURE 60-5** Coronary angiogram demonstrating critical left main coronary artery stenosis *(arrow).*

**BOX 60-4 Indications for Coronary Artery Revascularization**

1. Angina unresponsive to medical therapy
2. Unstable angina
3. Congestive heart failure with viable myocardium
4. Cardiogenic shock
5. Left main stenosis >50%
6. Left main equivalent disease–a combination of hemodynamically significant lesions involving the proximal circumflex and LAD territory
7. Concomitant triple-vessel CAD, EF <50%, and diabetes
8. Acute coronary occlusion after failed PCI
9. Mechanical complication of acute MI

## INDICATIONS FOR CORONARY ARTERY REVASCULARIZATION

Box 60-4 summarizes the indications for myocardial revascularization. The first four indications are managed preferably by PCI, whereas indications 5 through 7 are managed preferably by surgical revascularization. The last two indications constitute surgical emergency. Although this stratification is broad and provides a bird's eye view of the management approach, each patient should be risk-stratified before an appropriate strategy is initiated. When possible, proper risk stratification is absolutely essential to determine the balance of risks and benefits of medical management, PCI, and CABG.

### Chronic Stable Angina

Cardiovascular risk reduction strategy is essential to treating patients with chronic stable angina. In the 2007 focused update of the 2002 American Heart Association (AHA)/American College of Cardiology (ACC) guidelines[7] for managing chronic stable angina, cardiovascular risk reduction strategies included smoking cessation, blood pressure control, lipid-lowering regimens, physical activity, antiplatelet agents, angiotensin-converting enzyme (ACE) inhibitors, weight control, diabetes management, and influenza vaccination. Such risk reduction strategies should be used for all patients, irrespective of the type of intervention planned on the coronary artery.

### Coronary Artery Bypass Grafting Versus Medical Management

In the 1970s and 1980s, several prospective randomized clinical trials evaluated the survival benefit of CABG in patients with chronic stable angina. The most influential of these trials were the Veterans Administration Study of Chronic Stable Angina (VA Study), European Coronary Surgery Study (ECAS), and Coronary Artery Surgery Study (CASS). These studies have shown that CABG has significant benefits, resulting in the widespread use of CABG to treat patients with CAD. They also helped identify specific categories of patients with angina who were most likely to benefit from CABG—namely, patients with left main CAD, one-, two-, or three-vessel disease with proximal LAD involvement, and three-vessel disease with impaired left ventricular function.

In the current practice of medicine, the results of these trials should be viewed with caution because of advancements in modalities and therapeutics not available at the time. Many patients were not on aspirin or beta blockers, and most patients did not receive an internal thoracic artery (ITA) graft. Calcium channel blockers, ACE inhibitors, and lipid-lowering agents were not available. In addition, women and young patients were excluded from most of the trials. Nonetheless, modern comparative studies have shown a persistent advantage of revascularization over optimal medical management, especially in higher risk patients with more severe coronary disease.

### Percutaneous Coronary Intervention Versus Medical Management

In the 1980s, PCI was introduced as an alternative to CABG. Although the short-term symptomatic success rate for PCI approaches 85% to 90%, the usefulness of PCI remains controversial for patients with angina whose symptoms are adequately controlled with medical therapy.[8,9] The main results of the VA Clinical Outcomes Utilizing Revascularization and Aggressive druG Evaluation (COURAGE) trial revealed no significant differences in the primary end point of all-cause mortality or nonfatal MI, or in the major secondary end points, during a median 4.6-year follow-up period in patients with stable CAD who were randomly assigned to receive optimal medical therapy (OMT), with or without PCI.[10]

### Coronary Artery Bypass Grafting Versus Percutaneous Coronary Intervention

**Pre–Stent Era** One of the first large-scale, prospective, randomized studies of PCI and CABG was the Bypass Angioplasty Revascularization Investigation (BARI) trial reported in 1996.[11] Patients with multivessel disease were randomly assigned to CABG or PCI and followed up for a mean of 5.4 years. In the short term, the incidence of MI was higher in the CABG group (4.6% versus 2.1%), but stroke rates were similar (0.8% versus 0.2%, CABG versus PCI). Five years after treatment, the survival rate was 89.3% for the CABG cohort and 86.3% for the PCI cohort ($P$ = .19). Of the PCI patients, however, 54% required additional revascularization procedures, whereas only 8% of the CABG patients required repeat revascularization. Thus, although PCI did not compromise the 5-year survival rate in patients with multivessel disease, subsequent revascularization, including CABG, was required more often. Among the diabetic patients, the 5-year survival rate for the CABG patients was markedly greater (80.6% versus 65.5%).

**Bare Metal Stent Era** In the 1990s, coronary stents were introduced to address the problematic occurrence of restenosis after PCI. Six randomized trials have compared PCI with stenting and CABG.[12-14] Except for the Angina With Extremely Serious Operative Mortality Evaluation (AWESOME) trial, these trials enrolled patients who were relatively low risk and had no serious comorbidities, normal ventricular function, and mostly two-vessel CAD that was amenable to both PCI and CABG. All these trials showed similar survival rates but there were higher revascularization rates in patients with bare metal stents. A meta-analysis of four randomized trials has shown that PCI with stenting is associated with a long-term safety profile similar to that of CABG. However, as a result of persistently lower repeat revascularization rates in the CABG patients, overall major adverse cardiac and cerebrovascular event rates were significantly lower in the CABG group at 5 years.[15] Although these randomized studies are often used to demonstrate survival equivalence of CABG and PCI in patients with multivessel CAD, the studies were underpowered, the patients were low-risk, and the follow-up was too short. In contradistinction, a large New York State registry study has demonstrated that patients with double- or triple-vessel disease derive a greater survival benefit from CABG than from PCI with stenting.[16] Analysis of this large database of more than 50,000 patients found that during the 3-year follow-up, repeat revascularization was 11 times higher in the percutaneous transluminal coronary angioplasty (PTCA) group (37% versus 3.3% CABG). Furthermore, 3-year mortality was significantly higher in the PTCA group.

**Drug-Eluting Stent Era** The proponents of drug-eluting stent (DES) implantation claim that improved technology has made the results of randomized controlled trials (RCTs) favoring CABG obsolete. However, in patients with multivessel disease, PCI with DES can produce survival rates equivalent to those associated with CABG only if the reduction in restenosis rate translates into reduced mortality. Additionally, no mortality benefit of DES compared with bare metal stents has been demonstrated; in a meta-analysis of 11 RCTs of PCI with DES versus bare metal stents, none of the trials found a mortality benefit for DES.[17]

The Synergy between PCI with Taxus and Cardiac Surgery (SYNTAX) trial compared PCI and CABG for patients with previously untreated three-vessel or left main CAD. At 12 months, major adverse cardiac or cerebrovascular events were significantly more frequent in the PCI group (17.8% versus 12.4%). This finding was attributed primarily to the greater use of imaging surveillance in the CABG group (13.5% versus 5.9%). Although the trial found similar rates of death and MI, stroke was significantly more likely to occur in CABG patients (2.2% versus 0.6%). Nevertheless, the study findings suggested that CABG remains a favorable option in the care of patients with three-vessel or left main CAD.

It is likely that the use of a DES, or any stent, does not confer a mortality benefit because subsequent coronary events are often related to the progression of disease in arteries other than the stented artery or in other segments of the stented artery. In contrast, CABG treats the stenosis present at the time of surgery and any additional stenoses that develop proximal to the bypass graft in the future.

Finally, one must remember that CABG has a long track record, with studies reporting over 2 decades of follow-up, whereas reports on DES performance are short- to midterm studies. This is an important limitation on comparisons of the durability and cost-effectiveness of the two procedures. Reports of early thrombosis of a DES have dictated the use of a dual antiplatelet regimen for at least 1 year after stent deployment. Clopidogrel is usually used in conjunction with aspirin, but there are other more potent antiplatelet agents on the horizon. The increased risk of bleeding and additional cost of dual antiplatelet therapy are important limitations of treatment with DES.

In summary, compared with PCI, CABG confers superior long-term survival in patients with specific anatomic lesions (e.g., multivessel disease, left main CAD, one- and two-vessel disease with proximal LAD obstruction) and is associated with fewer subsequent interventions.

## Acute Coronary Syndrome

### Unstable Angina and Non–ST-Segment Elevation Myocardial Infarction

Patients who present with unstable angina (UA) or NSTEMI may have associated symptoms that confer a high short-term risk of death that necessitates invasive intervention. Two treatment pathways are used for treating UA-NSTEMI patients: the early invasive strategy and an initial conservative strategy. Patients treated with an invasive strategy generally undergo coronary angiography within 4 to 24 hours of admission.[2] Estimating the risk of an adverse outcome is paramount for determining which strategy is best for an individual patient. High-risk patients who benefit from invasive therapy include those with recurrent angina, ischemia at rest, low-level activity despite intensive medical therapy, elevated levels of cardiac biomarkers (troponins), new ST-segment depression, signs or symptoms of congestive heart failure or of new or worsening mitral regurgitation, findings from noninvasive testing that suggest high risk, hemodynamic instability, sustained ventricular tachycardia, PCI within the previous 6 months, prior CABG, and reduced left ventricular function (<40%).

According to the AHA/ACC/American Association for Thoracic Surgery (AATS) guidelines, UA-NSTEMI and features associated with high short-term risk of death or nonfatal MI indicate revascularization of the presumed culprit artery. These indications are similar to those for coronary revascularization in patients with chronic stable angina.[18]

### Adjunctive Therapy to Percutaneous Coronary Intervention

To minimize the complications of acute coronary occlusion and restenosis after PCI with stenting, current catheter-based revascularization now includes adjuvant (i.e., in addition to aspirin) use of platelet GP IIb/IIIa receptor inhibitors and adenosine diphosphate (ADP) receptor inhibitors (thienopyridines) such as clopidogrel. Antiplatelet therapy has been shown to reduce the risk of cardiac events in patients who present with acute coronary syndrome. However, all effective antiplatelet therapies also increase the risk of bleeding.

For patients who received clopidogrel on admission in anticipation of PCI but who did not undergo it, it is preferred to wait for 5 days for the effect to wear off before proceeding with CABG unless the patient is unstable and requires urgent CABG.

## ST-Segment Elevation Myocardial Infarction–Acute Myocardial Infarction

### Percutaneous Coronary Intervention Versus Medical Management for Acute Myocardial Infarction

In general, PCI has a survival advantage over thrombolytics as an initial treatment for STEMI-AMI, and the use of delayed PCI as an adjunct to therapy, including therapy with thrombolytics, does not affect survival. In the Global Use of Strategies to Open Occluded Coronary Arteries in Acute Coronary Syndromes (GUSTO) IIb trial,[19] the 30-day rate of the composite end point of death, nonfatal MI, and nonfatal disabling stroke was 9.6% for PCI patients and 13.7% for recipients of thrombolytics.

Prospective observational data collected from the Second National Registry of Myocardial Infarction between June 1994 and March 1998 included a cohort of 27,080 consecutive patients with AMI associated with ST-segment elevation or left bundle branch block. These patients were all treated with primary angioplasty; the study revealed that the adjusted odds of mortality were significantly higher (62% versus 41%) for patients with door to balloon times longer than 2 hours. The longer the door to balloon time, the higher the mortality risk, emphasizing that door to balloon time has a significant impact on the outcomes for patients with AMI.[20]

On the basis of this evidence, PCI facilities have been required to establish a target door to balloon time of no longer than 90 minutes. Depending on the available facilities in a particular region, it is the responsibility of emergency medical services (EMS) personnel to determine whether that goal can be achieved by transferring the patient to a PCI-capable facility. If this cannot be accomplished, a medical management strategy should be considered, with the goal being a door to needle time of 30 minutes or less.[21]

### Role of Coronary Artery Bypass Grafting

Although an increasing number of patients undergo catheterization early after AMI, the initial treatment is directed by the interventionalist, which has significantly diminished the role of emergency CABG. In general, patients who undergo CABG early after AMI are sicker and efforts to improve myocardial function are typically refractory to medical therapy. These patients typically have a higher incidence of comorbidities and are more likely to require intra-aortic balloon pump (IABP) insertion. The optimal timing of CABG after AMI is not well established. A review of California Discharge Data has identified 9476 patients who were hospitalized for AMI and subsequently underwent CABG. Of these, 4676 (49%) were in the early CABG group and 4800 (51%) were in the late CABG group. The mortality rate was highest among patients who underwent CABG on day 0 (8.2%) and declined to a nadir of 3.0% among patients who underwent CABG on day 3. The mean time to CABG was 3.2 days. Early CABG was an independent predictor of mortality, suggesting that CABG may best be deferred for 3 or more days after admission for AMI in nonurgent cases.[22]

The SHOCK (Should We Emergently Revascularize Occluded Coronaries for Cardiogenic Shock) trial has shown the survival advantage of emergency revascularization versus initial medical stabilization in patients in whom cardiogenic shock developed after AMI. A subanalysis that compared the effects of PCI and CABG on 30-day and 1-year survival showed that survival rates were similar at both time points. Among SHOCK trial patients randomly assigned to undergo emergency revascularization, those treated with CABG had a greater prevalence of diabetes and worse coronary disease than those treated with PCI. However, survival rates were similar.[23]

In patients with AMI, CABG is usually performed in conjunction with an operation to treat a specific complication, such as refractory postinfarction angina, papillary muscle rupture with mitral regurgitation, and infarction ventricular septal defect. The rationale for urgent or emergent surgery is often based on high early mortality risk because of mechanical complications.

### Preoperative Evaluation

The success of coronary artery revascularization depends on proper workup and patient selection. Comorbidities that affect CABG outcomes and that are typically incorporated into risk models include age, gender, urgency of the procedure, ejection fraction, need for mechanical circulatory support, MI, smoking status, use of immunosuppressive drugs, prior coronary interventions, and presence of hypertension, diabetes, peripheral vascular disease, and cerebrovascular disease. In addition, the severity of angina, as designated by the Canadian Cardiovascular Society (CCS) classification of anginas and New York Heart Association (NYHA) classification for congestive heart failure are important risk variables.

The following are essential components of a preoperative workup for CABG patients:

1. Detailed history and physical examination, including conduit evaluation
2. Review of medications, including ACE inhibitors, beta blockers, antiplatelet agents, and anticoagulants
3. Carotid duplex ultrasonography in patients who have clinical bruit or are at high risk for cerebrovascular disease
4. Cardiac echocardiography to evaluate ventricular function and the structural integrity of valves and chambers
5. Cardiac viability study in high-risk or reoperation surgical candidates and in patients with suspected end-stage cardiac disease with depressed ejection fraction
6. Cardiac catheterization to delineate the coronary anatomy
7. Chest radiography
8. Coagulation and platelet profile, comprehensive metabolic panel, and CBC

Depending on the findings of these tests, patients may need additional workup. In emergency circumstances, several of these tests may be skipped so that immediate revascularization can be performed.

## Technique of Myocardial Revascularization: Conventional On-Pump Cardiopulmonary Bypass

### Positioning and Draping

General anesthesia with a single-lumen endotracheal tube is the anesthetic technique of choice. Isoflurane is the preferred inhalation anesthetic for cardiac surgery. After anesthetic induction and placement of necessary access and monitoring lines, the patient is positioned supine, with the roll underneath the shoulder blades. The arms are tucked beside the patient with appropriate padding to minimize the chance of any nerve injury. A warming blanket is typically placed underneath the patient to assist in rewarming after controlled hypothermia during cardiopulmonary bypass. The entire chest, abdomen, and lower extremities are prepped. Circumferential prepping of the lower extremities is important, because the leg may have to be maneuvered during harvesting of the saphenous vein conduit. If radial artery harvesting is being contemplated, the arm also has to be circumferentially prepped and positioned 90 degrees from the bedside on an arm board. Because most patients have a multilumen central line in the internal jugular vein or a Swan-Ganz catheter, the anesthesiologist must have continuous access to the central line in the internal jugular vein or a Swan-Ganz catheter, but without compromising the domain of the surgeon. Anchor points on the drapes are designated appropriately to allow for cardiopulmonary bypass circuit lines to be secured without compromising sterility.

## Cardiopulmonary Bypass

Cardiopulmonary bypass (CPB) is the establishment of artificial oxygenation and perfusion of the human body by diverting all returning venous blood from the body to the heart-lung machine and returning the oxygenated blood in a controlled, pressurized manner. In essence, most blood flow to the heart and lungs is bypassed. Establishing CPB is a critical step for any major cardiac procedure and allows complete control of the operation.

The basic components of an extracorporeal heart pump circuit are venous cannulas to drain the returning venous blood, venous reservoir that collects blood by gravity, oxygenator and heat exchanger, perfusion pump, blood filter in the arterial line, and arterial cannula (Fig. 60-6). The blood conduits are designed to minimize turbulence, cavitation, and changes in blood flow velocity, which are detrimental to the integrity of component blood cells. Because the circuit contains a dead space created by the tubing and pump, a certain volume of nonblood solution is necessary to prime the pump and tubing. The priming solution consists of a balanced salt solution and often a starch solution. Homologous blood or fresh-frozen plasma (FFP) may be added if the patient is anemic or if a bleeding problem is anticipated. The circuit has multiple access ports or sites to obtain blood samples for laboratory studies and to infuse blood, blood products, crystalloids, or drugs.

Supplemental components include a cardiotomy suction system to collect undiluted or clean blood from open cardiac chambers and the surgical field. This blood is filtered, de-aired, and returned to the bypass pump. Diluted field blood and blood that has mixed with inflammatory cytokines or fat is collected through a separate device that concentrates washed red cells before returning them directly to the patient.

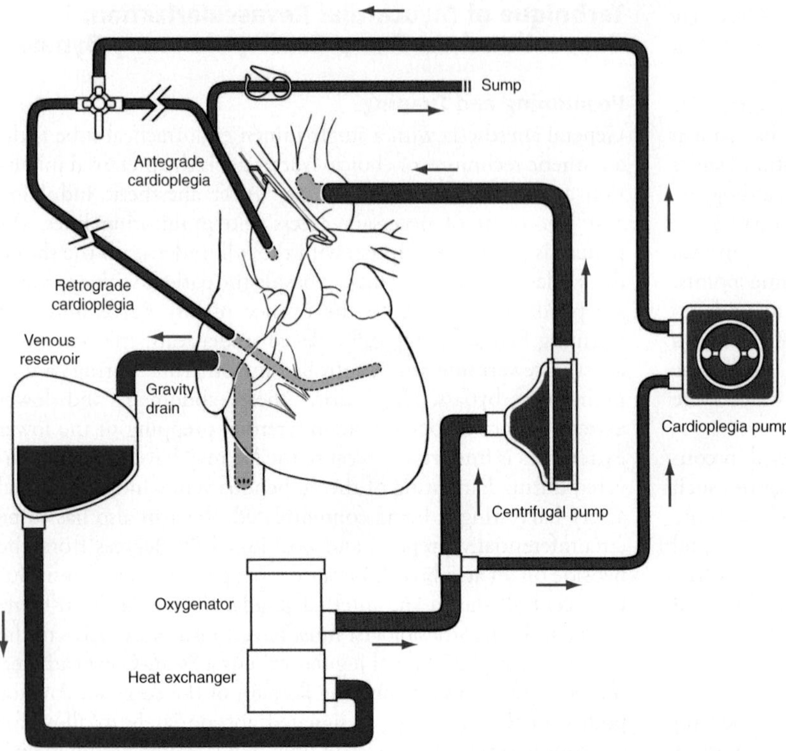


**FIGURE 60-6** Schematic of total cardiopulmonary bypass circuit. All returning venous blood is siphoned into a venous reservoir and is oxygenated and temperature regulated before being pumped back through a centrifugal pump into the arterial circulation. The common site for inflow into the patient is the ascending aorta, but alternate sites include the femoral arteries or the right axillary artery in special circumstances (vide infra). A parallel circuit derives oxygenated blood that is mixed with cold (4° C) cardioplegia in the ratio 4:1 and administered in an antegrade or retrograde fashion to accomplish cardiac arrest. Antegrade cardioplegia is administered into the aortic root and retrograde through the coronary sinus. During the administration of retrograde cardioplegia, the efflux of blood from the coronary ostium is siphoned off via the sump drain. The sump drain, a return parallel circuit connected to the venous reservoir (not shown), also helps to keep the heart decompressed during the arrest phase.

A cardioplegia infusion device consists of a separate pump, reservoir, and heat exchanger. It is used to deliver cold, potassium-enriched blood or crystalloid solutions into the coronary circulation to arrest and protect the heart.

Use of CPB requires suppression of the clotting cascade with heparin because the surgical wound and components of the bypass pump are powerful stimuli for thrombus formation. A strict anticoagulation protocol should be enforced before cardiopulmonary bypass is initiated. The pump prime is premixed with 4U/mL heparin and the patient is systemically heparinized with 300 U/kg before cannulation. An activated clotting time (ACT) obtained approximately 3 minutes after the injection of heparin should be more than 400 seconds before cannulation is begun and should be maintained for more than 450 seconds throughout CPB, with intermittent doses given as needed during the operation.

The usual pumps are roller head pumps, which consist of circumferential tubing that is compressed by a roller on the outside, thereby forcing blood in one direction. This pump mechanism is associated with higher rates of hemolysis than centrifugal pumps, so roller head pumps are used only in cardiotomy suction and cardioplegia pumps. The main systemic pump is a centrifugal pump that consists of a vortex polyurethane-embedded magnetic cone housed in a conical chamber. The vortex spins at approximately 2000 to 5000 rpm, thereby generating centrifugal force to pump blood. Because the flow is entirely caused by a nonturbulent vortex generated by a finless cone, this mechanism is almost atraumatic to the blood cells and is therefore associated with less hemolysis than the roller head pump mechanism (Fig. 60-7).

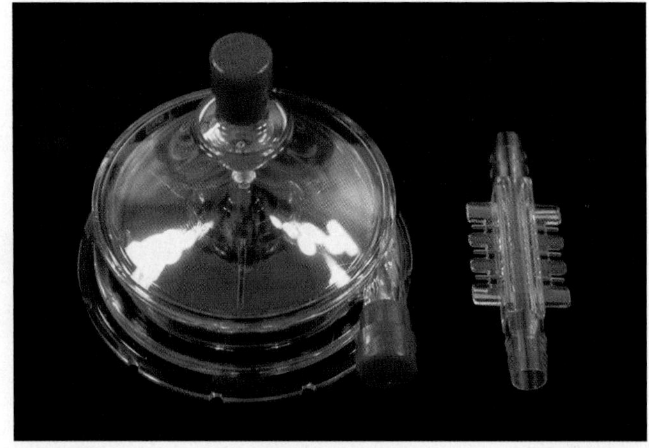

**FIGURE 60-7** Main centrifugal pump used in most cardiopulmonary bypass circuits. The entire unit is sterile molded and contains a finless cone that spins at 2000 to 5000 rpm generating a powerful yet nonturbulent vortex. A flowmeter (shown) must be used with these pumps as the ultimate volume of flow depends on outflow resistance rather than rpm. The conventional roller head pumps are still being used for the auxiliary circuits such as cardiotomy suction and cardioplegia circuits.

## Neurologic Protection During Cardiopulmonary Bypass

The incidence of stroke after CPB is approximately 2.5%, but neurocognitive deficits are more frequent. Thus, several steps should be taken during CPB to minimize the risk of neurologic insult, including maintaining adequate cerebral perfusion, minimizing fat microemboli by eliminating the unnecessary use of cardiotomy suction, minimizing aortic manipulation by using single-clamp techniques when feasible, and instituting moderate hypothermia.

The oxygen consumption of a patient on CPB at normal temperatures averages 80 to 125 mL/min/m$^2$, similar to that of an anesthetized adult not on bypass. However, with the use of hypothermia, the oxygen consumption is markedly lower and the flow rate can be reduced to less than 2.2 L/min/m$^2$. This is because the mean oxygen consumption of the body decreases by 50% for every 10° C decrease in body temperature. Below 28° C, a flow rate of 1.6 L/min/m$^2$ may be safe for as long as 2 hours. Significant disadvantages of using systemic hypothermia to accommodate lower flow rates include the extra time required to rewarm the patient and associated changes in the reactivity of blood elements, particularly platelets. These changes may result in a greater propensity for bleeding once the patient has been rewarmed.

## Median Sternotomy

The most common approach for performing coronary artery bypass is a median sternotomy, although anterolateral thoracotomy is used in certain circumstances. A traditional sternotomy incision commences at the midpoint of the manubrium and is carried down to the xiphoid. The sternum is split through the middle with a sternal saw. It is essential that gentle upward force and a backward tilt be applied to the saw to prevent it from engaging the lung or soft tissues in the anterior mediastinum. Once the sternotomy is completed, the periosteum of the posterior table is cauterized, and a passive hemostatic agent such as bone wax or a reconstituted mixture of vancomycin may be used to prevent bleeding from the marrow. The most important consideration during the sternotomy is staying in the midline, because the most common cause of sternal dehiscence is an off-midline sternotomy and the consequent technically suboptimal closure. Other potential problems associated with the sternotomy include indirect injury to the liver and direct injury to the heart, innominate vein, and lungs.

### Conduit Choice and Harvesting

***Left Internal Mammary Artery*** In a seminal study from the Cleveland Clinic, Loop and colleagues[24] have shown improved 10-year survival in patients who received a left internal mammary artery (LIMA) graft; patients who received an SVG had 1.6 times the risk of death than patients who received a LIMA graft. The long-term patency rate of the LIMA graft has been shown to be approximately 95% and 90% at 10 and 20 years, respectively. The best patency rates are achieved when the LIMA is used as an in situ pedicled graft and is anastomosed to the LAD.

***Bilateral Internal Mammary Artery*** Although currently available data are weak, it has been suggested that the use of bilateral internal mammary artery (BIMA) grafts improves survival and significantly reduces the need for reopration without increasing mortality. However, compared with saphenous vein grafts (SVGs), BIMA grafts are associated with a higher (twofold) incidence of deep sternal wound infection and a 30- to 45-minute prolongation of surgery. These grafts are best used by experienced surgeons in younger, nondiabetic, nonobese patients. Four major studies that tilted the balance in favor of BIMA were the Cleveland Clinic studies (1999 and 2004), in which

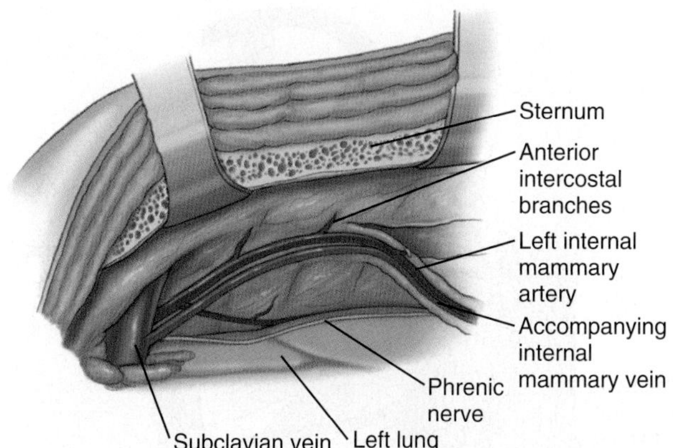


**FIGURE 60-8** Surgeons view of the left internal mammary artery as it is being harvested. A mammary retractor is used to elevate the left hemithorax to provide adequate visualization. The mammary artery is dissected away from the chest wall as a pedicle with its accompanying venae comitatantes. Low-voltage electrocautery with no-touch technique is crucial for the atraumatic harvest of this most important conduit. Understanding the relation to the phrenic nerve and subclavian veins is important to prevent injury to these structures during the harvest of the left internal mammary artery.

propensity scores were used to match SIMA and BIMA graft recipients; the Oxford meta-analysis (2001), and a retrospective study from Japan (2001). Skeletonization of the ITA grafts may reduce the wound complication rate.

The mammary artery is harvested after the sternotomy is completed. A specially designed mammary retractor is used to elevate the appropriate hemithorax, typically the left for harvesting the LIMA. Adequately exposing the undersurface of the sternum is essential for successful harvest of the mammary artery (Fig. 60-8). The artery may be harvested as a pedicle that includes the two venae comitantes and surrounding soft tissue from the level of the subclavian vein to the level of the bifurcation of the artery into the superior epigastric and musculophrenic branches. The alternative method of harvesting is the skeletonized harvest, in which only the internal mammary artery is dissected away from the chest wall.

The basic principle of harvesting the mammary artery relies exclusively on the no-touch technique, using low-voltage electrocautery, and clipping the anterior intercostal branches. Care must be taken during the harvest to identify the course of the phrenic nerves and avoid injuring them. This is particularly important while harvesting the right internal mammary artery, because the phrenic nerve is more closely related to it at the level of the second or third intercostal space. The mammary artery is a fragile vessel, and direct handling or undue traction should be avoided because it may cause traumatic dissection of the vessel. The distal end of the mammary artery should be divided only after the patient is fully heparinized to avoid thrombosis of the conduit. Once the mammary artery is divided, the distal end is spatulated appropriately to fashion the anastomosis.

***Greater Saphenous Vein*** Grafts made from this vein have a patency rate of 90% at 1 year (BARI).[25] Beyond 5 years after surgery, graft atherosclerosis develops in a substantial number of these grafts and, by 10 years, only 60% to 70% of grafts are patent, and 50% of those have angiographic evidence of atherosclerosis.

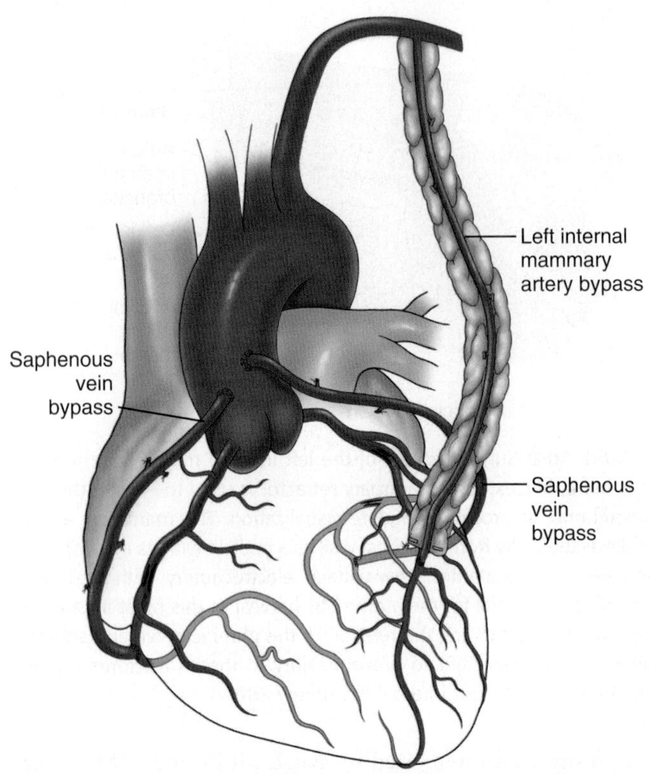


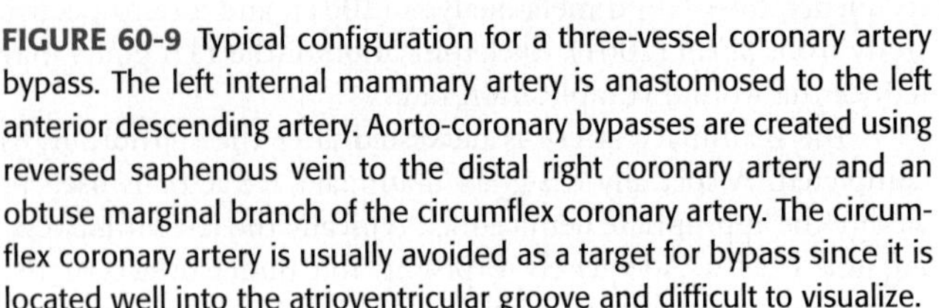

**FIGURE 60-9** Typical configuration for a three-vessel coronary artery bypass. The left internal mammary artery is anastomosed to the left anterior descending artery. Aorto-coronary bypasses are created using reversed saphenous vein to the distal right coronary artery and an obtuse marginal branch of the circumflex coronary artery. The circumflex coronary artery is usually avoided as a target for bypass since it is located well into the atrioventricular groove and difficult to visualize.

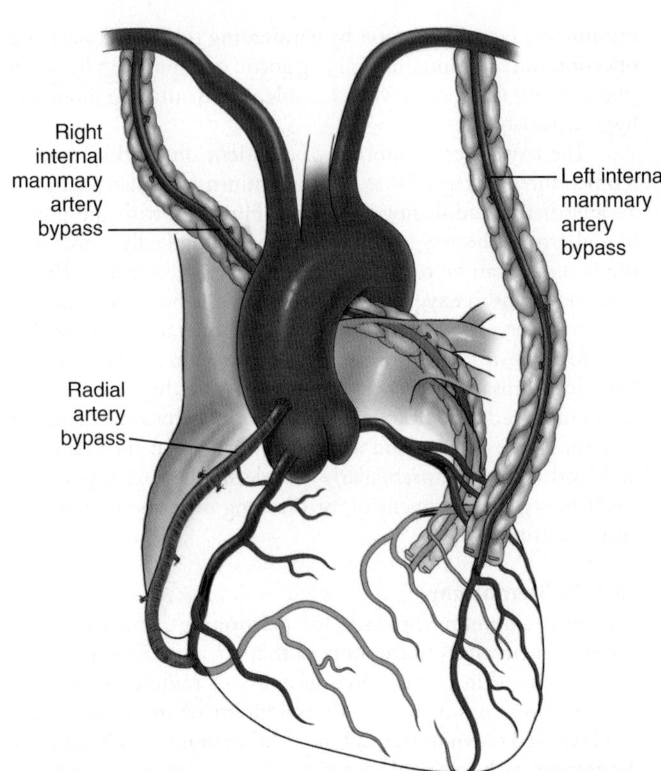


**FIGURE 60-10** Total arterial revascularization using bilateral mammary artery and radial artery conduits. The right internal artery mammary artery, bypassed to an obtuse marginal branch, is routed behind the aorta and the pulmonary artery through the transverse sinus.

While the sternotomy is being done, a separate team begins harvesting saphenous or radial artery conduits. Saphenous vein harvesting can be performed by open or endoscopic techniques. The conventional method of open vein harvesting involves making a long incision along the entire length of the harvested vein. Alternatively, a bridging technique can be used in which multiple 1- to 2-inch incisions are made, with intact bridges of skin between them. The most common complications associated with long open incisions are pain, slow wound healing, and dehiscence, which is compounded by the fact that a significant number of CABG patients have diabetes or peripheral vascular disease. The use of endoscopic or bridging techniques significantly alleviates, but does not entirely eliminate, these problems. There are some centers that avoid endoscopic vein harvesting entirely on the assumption that the technique is too traumatic to the vein itself, may be associated with intimal trauma, and may impair the long-term patency of the conduit. However, recent studies have shown reduced graft patency in endoscopically harvested veins. These reports were based on post hoc analysis of data from trials designed to address other aspects of coronary revascularization.[26] Once the vein is extracted and the branches are ligated, the graft is soaked in heparinized solution while waiting to be implanted. The veins are typically used in a reversed fashion and hence may not require valvotomy. A typical configuration of a three-vessel coronary artery bypass graft is shown in Figure 60-9.

Alternative conduits may be needed in patients who have had previous coronary bypass, peripheral vascular surgery with the use of of vein conduits, or lower extremity amputations, and those who have unusable saphenous vein conduits because of severe varicosities of the saphenous vein. Other manifestations of venous insufficiency or disease may also pose problems. In addition, patients who have severely calcified ascending aortas may not be amenable to a vein-based aortocoronary bypass because anastomosis to the ascending aorta is complicated. In these cases, alternative bypass strategies include total arterial revascularization with bilateral mammary artery pedicles (Fig. 60-10). In addition, the mammary artery may be used as the main conduit from which further arterial conduits may be Christmas-treed in an off-pump setup so that any aortic manipulation is avoided.

### Other Conduits

***Radial Artery*** At 1 year, radial artery conduits have an occlusion rate of approximately 10%, and another 15% have diffuse angiographic narrowing (string sign), which indicates a bad graft. It is of interest that inducible ischemia is uncommon in myocardial territories supplied by grafts with a string sign, so the patency of these grafts may improve over time as the native vessel stenosis progresses. At 5 years, the patency rate is 80% to 85%. Radial grafts are more likely than SVGs to become occluded or have a diffuse spasm when grafted to a coronary artery that is not severely stenotic because of competitive flow in the native coronary vessel, resulting in a retrograde stagnation point in the conduit.

**Gastroepiploic Artery** Bergsma and associates,[27] in 1998, used gastroepiploic artery (GEA) grafts in conjunction with BIMA grafts for total arterial revascularization and reported one of the best results for the GEA conduit. At 5 years, the rate of freedom from angina was 86% and the GEA graft patency rate was 90%. The GEA conduit is sensitive to competitive flow and is best used as a pedicled graft because free grafts have not done well.

### Cannulation for Cardiopulmonary Bypass

Cannulation for establishing CPB commences after conduit harvest and preparation is completed, the pericardium is opened, and the thymus is divided along the embryologic fusion plane. The patient is fully heparinized at a dose of 3 mg/kg. A purse string is created on the anterior surface of the distal ascending aorta at the cannulation site. The aortic purse string should involve only a partial thickness of the aorta, incorporating the adventitia and media but entirely avoiding the intimal layer. It is essential that the cannulation site be free of calcified plaques or atheroma to minimize the chance of embolization and cannulation site bleeding. Manual palpation, the commonly practiced method of assessment, is unreliable. Doppler transesophageal or epiaortic ultrasound guidance should be used whenever aortic disease is suspected. Also, the presence of calcium elsewhere in the ascending aorta may preclude safe clamp application. Although cannulating the aorta may be a simple task, loss of control of the aortic cannulation site or inadvertent dissection could lead to a disastrous situation.

With a sharp scalpel, the adventitia is teased and a full-thickness stab incision is made. The aortic cannula is inserted with the outflow bevel aimed toward the aortic arch. Tourniquet snares are used to secure the cannula in position and are tied. After the cannula is de-aired, it is connected to the arterial line of the cardiopulmonary bypass circuit. Alternate sites of arterial cannulation include the femoral artery and right axillary artery, which are used in reoperations or cases in which concomitant complex aortic and arch reconstruction may be required. Axillary artery cannulation is usually achieved via an 8-mm graft anastomosed end-to-side to the axillary artery.

For venous cannulation, a purse string is then placed around the right atrial appendage. The tip of this appendage is amputated and a dual-stage venous cannula is inserted and positioned with the tip at the level of the diaphragm. The basket of the dual-stage cannula should rest in the main chamber of the right atrium to capture drainage from the superior vena cava (SVC) into the right atrium (Figs. 60-11 and 60-12).

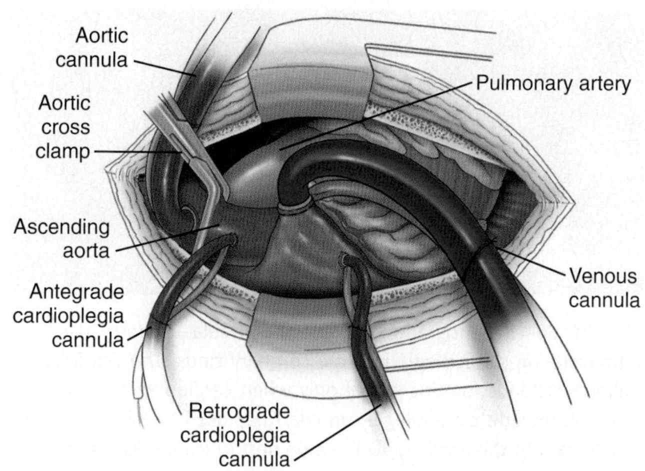


**FIGURE 60-11** Surgeon's view of the heart after cannulation. The cross clamp isolates the aortic root and coronary vessels from the rest of the systemic circulation. This allows administration of cardioplegia in a closed circuit and prevents the systemic blood from washing the cardioplegia out of the coronary system during the arrest phase. Application of the cross clamp prevents active blood flow through the coronary arteries and thus allows the surgeon to perform the distal anastomoses in a bloodless field.

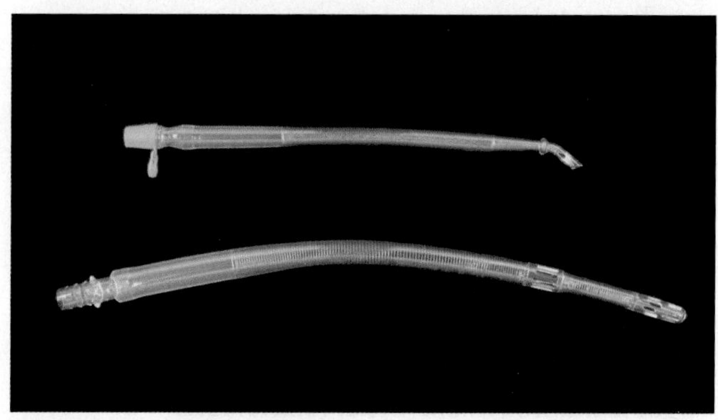

**FIGURE 60-12** Aortic cannula *(top):* The specially designed tip is angulated to allow laminar flow of blood into the aortic arch. Dual-stage venous cannula *(bottom):* The first stage is the fenestrated basket that usually rests at the level of the hepatic veins and captures all venous return from the inferior vena cava. The second-stage basket is located such that it remains within the right atrium and captures venous return from the superior vena cava, azygos vein, coronary sinus and direct collateral drainage into the right atrium. The venous drainage is a passive siphon aided by gravity.

### Cardiac Arrest and Myocardial Protection

The initiation of cardiopulmonary bypass allows the heart to be stopped. To achieve cardiac arrest, a large dose of potassium solution (cardioplegia) is injected into the coronary vessels. This requires the coronary blood flow to be completely isolated from the systemic circulation, which is done by applying a cross clamp to the ascending aorta proximal to the aortic cannula.

There are several different delivery options for cardioplegia solutions. One involves taking a balanced approach; the cardioplegic solution is administered antegrade through the ascending aorta proximal to the cross clamp and then retrograde through a coronary sinus catheter inserted through a purse-string suture placed in the right atrium using special cannulas (Fig. 60-13). The extensive collateralization among the coronary veins and arteries and paucity of valves in the coronary vein system ensure a relatively homogeneous distribution of cardioplegia when the retrograde approach is used. Patients with high-grade proximal lesions, especially those with suboptimal collateral vessels, may benefit from the application of both techniques. After the initial administration of cardioplegia, additional doses are usually administered every 15 to 20 minutes.

An antegrade cardioplegia line with a Y-connector to the circuit is inserted into the ascending aorta. This is to allow

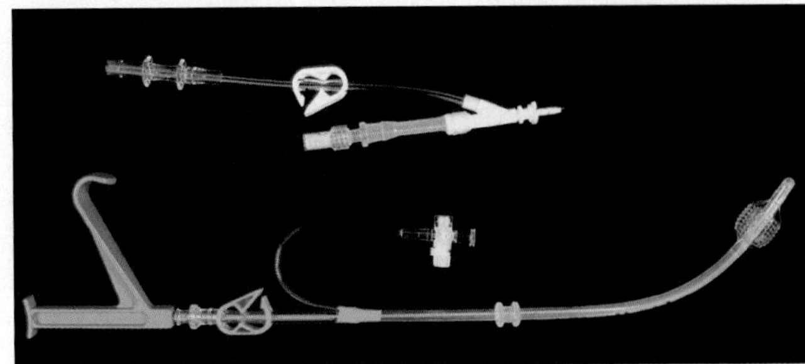

**FIGURE 60-13** Retrograde cardioplegia cannula *(bottom)* used for administering cardioplegia into the coronary sinus. The self-inflating balloon distends forming a seal only when cardioplegia is administered. Antegrade cardioplegia cannula *(top)* used to administer cardioplegia into the aortic root. The side port functions as a sump.

administration of antegrade cardioplegia and also to sump and decompress the ascending aorta while retrograde cardioplegia is administered into the coronary sinus. The sump drain also functions to keep the coronary arteries free of any blood, thus providing the surgeon with a bloodless field in which to fashion the distal anastomoses. The sump drain also performs the important function of decompressing the left ventricle while the heart is arrested (see Figs. 60-6 and 60-11).

The most important task for ensuring myocardial protection is establishing complete diastolic arrest with an unloaded heart. In this state, the myocardial consumption of ATP is extremely low and allows maximal preservation of myocytes. In a conventional CABG with total CPB, the decompression of the ventricle by off-loading, systemic cooling, topical cooling, and diastolic arrest of the heart with potassium cardioplegia serves to decrease myocardial oxygen consumption. Approximately 40% of the myocardial metabolic demand is eliminated when total CPB is established before diastolic arrest or cooling are instituted.

### Target Identification and Distal Anastomosis

Once successful diastolic arrest of the heart is accomplished, the target coronary arteries to be bypassed are identified. Some of the epicardial conductance vessels are intramyocardial and therefore may not be directly visible. Once a target vessel is identified, it is opened with a sharp blade. Typically arteriotomy is approximately 5 mm long. The conduit, which is prepared and spatulated, is then grafted in an end to side fashion with running 7-0 Prolene suture. This component of the operation is technically the most challenging and requires precision. The flow and integrity of each vein conduit is tested by flushing it with cold blood or cardioplegia mix. The LIMA to LDA anastomosis is usually the last one to be performed (Fig. 60-14) because it is best to avoid manipulating the heart once this anastomosis is completed in case avulsion of the LIMA conduit occurs. Bypassing the PDA and obtuse marginal (OM) targets requires the apex of heart to be lifted out of the pericardium.

Typically, a single segment of conduit is anastomosed to each planned distal target. Occasionally, a single conduit can be used to supply blood to two targets, which is known as a *sequential anastomosis*. This is a good technique to use when there is a shortage of available vein conduits or when the target vessels are small; in these cases, using this technique ensures a higher rate of blood flow through the vein conduit, reducing the risk of graft thrombosis (Fig. 60-15).

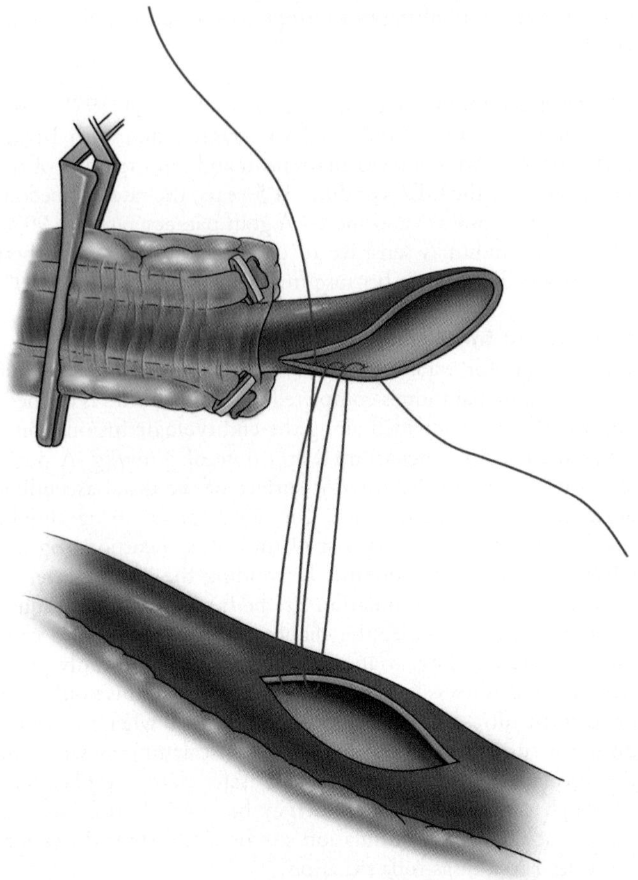

**FIGURE 60-14** Technique of constructing the distal anastomoses: left internal mammary artery to left anterior descending artery—magnified surgeon's view. A 5-mm longitudinal arteriotomy is made on the coronary artery to be bypassed. The distal end of the left internal mammary artery is spatulated to an appropriate size match. 7-0 Prolene suture is used to create the anastomosis with a parachuting technique.

As the last distal anastomosis is being completed, the patient is warmed back to physiologic temperature. The cross clamp is released after the final dose of warm cardioplegia is administered, which helps in scavenging the accumulated free radicals in the myocardium. A partial clamp is then applied to the ascending aorta and the proximal anastomoses are constructed in an end to side fashion with running 5-0 Prolene sutures. If there are concerns about the quality of the aorta, use of a partial clamp is typically avoided in favor of a single-clamp technique. The latter approach involves constructing the proximal anastomoses on an arrested heart, as for the distal anastomoses.

In patients in whom the ascending aorta is calcified or a free mammary artery pedicle needs to be used, a branching pattern of proximal anastomosis is used. This conserves vein length to a certain extent but also minimizes the number of aortotomies, especially if the ascending aorta is short or a concomitant aortic procedure has been performed. The ascending aorta is allowed to de-air as the aortic clamp is released, after which the vein grafts are de-aired.

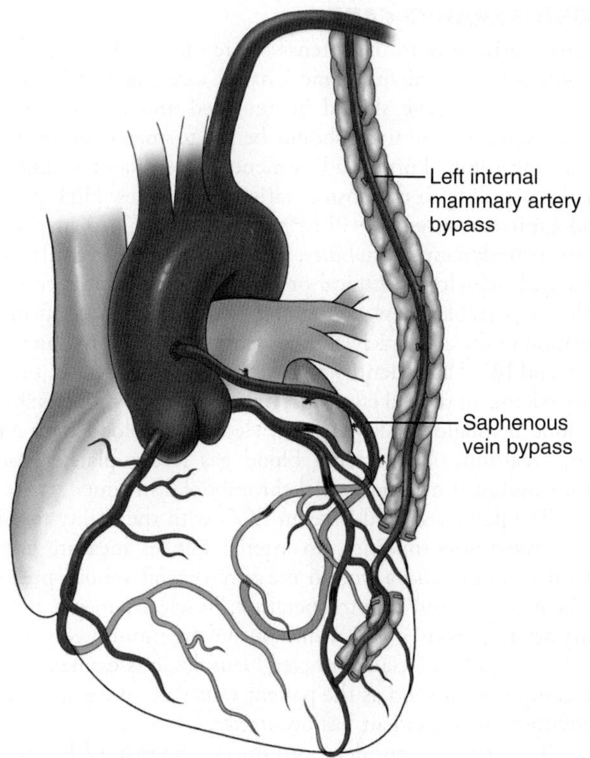


**FIGURE 60-15** Alternate configuration for a three-vessel coronary artery bypass. The left internal mammary artery is anastomosed sequentially to a diagonal branch and to the distal left anterior descending artery. Aortocoronary bypasses using reversed saphenous vein in sequential configuration to left posterolateral and an obtuse marginal branch of the circumflex coronary artery. The ideal configuration depends on the extent and distribution of the coronary blockages.

### Weaning from Cardiopulmonary Bypass

Weaning commences once a set of physiologic parameters has been ensured, as follows:

1. Resumption of rhythmic electromechanical activity
2. Attainment of physiologic temperature >36.5°C
3. Availability of adequate reserve blood volume
4. Restoration of normal systemic potassium levels
5. Resumption of ventilation with an acceptable arterial blood gas

A few other actions that may be considered at this point are placing temporary pacing wires and inserting an IABP, if needed. Typically, the cardiopulmonary bypass flows are progressively decreased as the following parameters are closely observed:

1. Data from the Swan-Ganz catheter
2. Direct visual observations of cardiac function and chamber volume
3. The transesophageal echocardiogram

Most patients usually have a transient systemic inflammatory response, causing vasodilation that becomes more pronounced as they are warmed. Thus, administration of intravascular fluids to restore volume deficit or vasoconstrictive pressors may be needed to maintain systemic blood pressure. Inotropic agents may be used if ventricular function is not adequate. Weaning from cardiopulmonary bypass is the primary responsibility of the surgeon and requires dynamic communication between the perfusionist and anesthesiologist.

Once weaning from cardiopulmonary bypass is accomplished, the venous cannula is removed and the purse string is tied down. Once it is confirmed that the heart is providing satisfactory perfusion, protamine is administered. Close monitoring is needed because adverse reactions to protamine range from transient hypotension to fatal anaphylaxis. Such reactions necessitate the resumption of cardiopulmonary bypass.

**BOX 60-5 Major Steps in On-Pump Coronary Artery Bypass Grafting**

- Induction of anesthesia and establishment of intraoperative monitoring adjuncts
- Positioning and draping
- Median sternotomy or appropriate approach
- Harvest and evaluation of blood conduits
- Heparinization and cannulation for cardiopulmonary bypass
- Establishment of cardiopulmonary bypass
- Myocardial arrest and protection
- Identification of target vessels and construction of distal anastomoses
- Restoration of myocardial electromechanical activity
- Creation of proximal anastomoses
- Weaning from cardiopulmonary bypass
- Evaluate and establish necessary adjuncts–inotropes, IABP, pacing wires
- Reversal of anticoagulation and establishing hemostasis
- Evaluate surgical sites and establish surgical drainage
- Closure of sternotomy

### Hemostasis

As protamine is being administered, hemostasis is expeditiously accomplished. As the patient rewarms, blood vessels that had been hemostatic may dilate and rebleed. Persistent bleeding should alert the surgeon to the following possible causes:

1. Aspects of surgical technique
2. Platelet dysfunction
3. Inadequate protamine reversal
4. Hypothermia

The administration of blood and blood products may be necessary.

### Sternal Closure and Completion of Surgery

Chest tube and temporary pacing wires should be checked for appropriate positioning. The sternum is approximated with stainless steel wires. The soft tissues and skin are closed in layers with absorbable sutures. Box 60-5 outlines all the major steps of an on-pump coronary artery bypass graft operation.

## ADJUNCTS TO CABG

### Transesophageal Echocardiography

Using transesophageal echocardiography (TEE) enables the assessment of ventricular wall motion abnormalities and the detection of any chamber or valve anomalies that may change the strategy of the operation. Some TEE findings that may affect the conduct of the operation are an incidentally discovered large patent foramen ovale (PFO) or fibroelastoma of the valves. New-onset or worsening mitral regurgitation after CABG suggests inferior wall ischemia and may indicate reevaluation of the bypass grafts or valve repair or replacement. Also, TEE helps in assessing ejection fraction and the volume status of the heart after surgery.

### Inotropes and Pharmacotherapy

Cardioplegic arrest causes transient myocardial ischemia and lactic acid accumulation. After perfusion is reestablished, the ventricles are stiffer and require higher filling pressures to maintain adequate stroke volume. Also, CPB may cause significant third spacing and vasodilation. Thus, epinephrine as an inotropic agent is ideal to maintain adequate contractility in the initial recovery phase and during separation from cardiopulmonary bypass. Alpha agonists such as norepinephrine, phenylephrine, and vasopressin may be used to counteract the effects of inflammatory vasodilation. In patients with depressed myocardial function, such as left or right heart failure, dobutamine or a phosphodiesterase inhibitor such as milrinone may be required to enhance myocardial contractility and decrease afterload or pulmonary vascular resistance. Because hypotension is a common side effect of these drugs, the systemic volume must be adequate and an alpha agonist may be required. Calcium channel blockers or nitroglycerin may be needed in patients with preexisting hypertension. It is essential to maintain a mean arterial pressure (MAP) higher than 60 mm Hg in the initial postoperative period, but hypertension should be avoided because it puts stress on a myocardium that is trying to recover and increases the risk of bleeding from anastomotic suture lines. Blood pressure management requires a thorough understanding of physiologic and pharmacologic principles. It is a balancing act geared toward maintaining adequate systemic pressure, cardiac output, and peripheral perfusion while minimizing myocardial stress. Urine output is the most reliable indicator of peripheral organ perfusion.

### Intra-Aortic Balloon Pump

For patients who have profound myocardial dysfunction and are unresponsive to volume resuscitation and significant pharmacologic therapy, IABP support may be indicated. The IABP is a special Silastic balloon with a capacity of 40 to 60 mL that is positioned in the descending aorta just beyond the origin of the left subclavian artery. The balloon is designed to be actively inflated and deflated during each cardiac cycle; its timing is controlled by a specially designed computer with input from an arterial line tracing or ECG. Intra-aortic balloon counterpulsation has the unique benefit of decreasing myocardial work and oxygen consumption while increasing coronary perfusion. The balloon is actively deflated just before systolic contraction begins, thereby decreasing left ventricular (LV) impedance and assisting in the ejection of blood. The balloon then actively inflates at the time of aortic valve closure—that is, it is timed to occur at the dicrotic notch of the arterial line tracing. This increases the diastolic perfusion pressure and improves coronary blood flow, both of which decrease the time-tension index and increase the diastolic pressure-time index, thereby increasing the myocardial oxygen supply-to-demand ratio. The use of IABP is absolutely contraindicated in patients with aortic regurgitation and aortic dissection. It is relatively contraindicated in patients with peripheral vascular disease or aortic aneurysm.

## POSTOPERATIVE CARE

Postoperative care in the intensive care unit (ICU) begins with a thorough physical and hemodynamic assessment. Mediastinal chest tube drainage should be recorded and assessed hourly. Initial ventilator settings should be set to match those in the operating room. Further adjustments in ventilator settings are made according to the postoperative blood gases. High positive end-expiratory pressure (PEEP) should be avoided in patients with hemodynamic instability. The ideal mode of ventilation is that with which the surgical or intensive care team is comfortable. A portable chest radiograph is obtained to confirm the position of the endotracheal tube, central lines, Swan-Ganz catheter, and IABP and identify a pneumothorax, atelectasis, pulmonary edema, or pleural effusions. Initial laboratory studies should include hemoglobin, hematocrit, electrolyte, blood urea nitrogen, creatinine, and arterial blood gas levels, platelet count, prothrombin time, and partial thromboplastin time.

The patient should have an ECG with the ability to assess ST-T wave abnormalities, an arterial line to measure arterial blood pressure, and a line to measure central venous pressure, pulse oximetry and core temperature. In select patients, pulmonary artery pressures and cardiac output are monitored continuously using a Swan-Ganz catheter. Neurologic assessment should be completed as soon as the patient wakes up to ensure that no cerebrovascular accident has occurred.

The primary considerations during the first 12 hours after the operation should be the maintenance of adequate blood pressure, cardiac output, correction of coagulation defects, correction of electrolytes, stabilization of intravascular volume, and normalization of the peripheral vascular resistance. This often involves the administration of crystalloid solutions, blood or blood products, inotropic agents, calcium, and vasodilators or vasoconstrictors.

Some of the goals in the postoperative period are as follows:

1. Avoidance of marked elevations in blood pressure
2. Maintaining adequate perfusion pressure (60 to 80 mm Hg)
3. Maintaining core body temperature higher than 36.5° C by warming the patient with forced hot air blankets
4. Maintaining adequate cardiac output and a cardiac index of 2.2 liters/min/$m^2$
5. Keeping mixed venous oxygenation at 60%
6. Reducing afterload, as appropriate, to minimize myocardial work
7. Volume resuscitation with crystalloid or blood products, as necessary
8. Maintaining hemoglobin higher than 8 g/dL, or higher than 10 g/dL in older patients or those with severe cerebrovascular disease
9. Maintaining homeostatic pH. Metabolic acidosis may be caused by hypoperfusion from low cardiac output, poor resuscitation, hypovolemia, or end-organ ischemia from embolism.
10. Monitoring neurologic and peripheral vascular status
11. Maintaining a sinus or perfusing rhythm at a rate of 70 to 100 beats/min
12. Monitoring and treating postoperative cardiac arrhythmias

13. Ensuring adequate pain control to minimize fluctuations in blood pressure and myocardial stress
14. Keeping blood sugar levels below 180 mg/dL. Insulin infusion based on standardized regimens should be initiated if needed.

### Pulmonary Care

It is desirable to initiate the process of ventilator weaning as soon as the patient awakens, is hemodynamically stable with minimal chest tube drainage, and can maintain a satisfactory spontaneous tidal volume and respiratory rate. Coughing and deep breathing exercises with appropriate sternal precautions are essential for postoperative recovery. Suboptimal postoperative pulmonary function may require additional therapy, including the use of bronchodilators, mucolytics, and chest physical therapy. Although β-adrenergic bronchodilators and N-acetyl cysteine are useful adjuncts, they have the capacity to induce atrial fibrillation.

After extubation, it is important to provide the patient with sufficient pain relief to minimize emotional distress, poor coughing, and the reluctance to begin ambulation. Unrelieved pain can also be a source of tachycardia, hypertension, myocardial ischemia, atelectasis, hypoxia and pneumonia.

### Discharge from the Intensive Care Unit

Before the patient leaves the ICU, unnecessary lines and catheters should be removed. Chest tubes are removed at approximately 48 hours when the combined drainage is less than 200 mL per shift and the chest x-ray reveals no effusion. Removal of temporary atrial and ventricular pacing wires is often deferred to the third postoperative day.

## Outcomes

### Hospital Mortality

Seven core variables—emergency of operation, age, prior heart surgery, gender, left ventricular ejection fraction (LVEF), percentage stenosis of left main, number of major coronaries with more than 70% stenosis—have the greatest impact on CABG mortality. Other variables are important but have minimal impact when added to these core variables; these include recent MI (<1 week), angina severity, ventricular arrhythmia, congestive heart failure (CHF), mitral regurgitation (MR), diabetes, peripheral vascular disease (PVD), renal insufficiency, and creatinine level.

In cardiac surgery, operative mortality has traditionally included 30-day and in-hospital mortality. The mortality figure for CABG is 1% to 3% in most modern series. Risk-adjusted outcomes have become the gold standard when reporting and comparing cardiac surgery outcomes. The Society of Thoracic Surgeons (STS) database is the largest and most authoritative voluntary national database to date. The STS has developed a risk calculator that estimates morbidity and mortality for a given patient risk profile. The observed-to-expected mortality (O/E) ratio for a given surgeon or institution can then be determined.

### Long-Term Survival

Survival after CABG is related to cardiac and noncardiac comorbidities. Risk factors for atherosclerosis, particularly cigarette smoking, hypercholesterolemia, hypertension, and diabetes, are associated with decreased survival.

In no longitudinal study has CABG obliterated the negative impact of abnormal LV function on late survival. Incomplete revascularization is associated with decreased survival, whereas complete revascularization, the use of the LIMA and, in some studies, the use of BIMA are associated with improved survival.

The CASS has documented overall survival of 96%, 90%, 74%, 56%, and 45% at 1, 5, 10, 15, and 18 postoperative years, respectively.[28] These figures are inferior to those for the age-matched U.S. population and inferior to modern series of patients receiving single or bilateral mammary grafts.

### Morbidity

**Tamponade** Pericardial tamponade is caused by the formation of pericardial clot and compression of the heart. The condition should be suspected if the patient exhibits evidence of low cardiac output, hypotension in the setting of tachycardia, and elevated central venous pressure (CVP). The quantity of mediastinal drainage is unreliable in predicting tamponade, although an abrupt decline in mediastinal chest tube drainage should raise the suspicion for tamponade caused by absence of an exit path for the blood. Widening of the mediastinum on chest x-ray and evidence of a pericardial effusion by echocardiography should confirm the diagnosis.

If a Swan-Ganz catheter is in place and right and left heart pressures are monitored, the CVP and pulmonary capillary wedge pressure are usually elevated and equal. The earliest manifestation of tamponade is an acute drop in mixed venous oxygen saturation. After the diagnosis is made, the patient should be returned to the operating room for evacuation of the clot and relief of the compression. If the patient's condition is rapidly deteriorating, the sternotomy incision may have to be opened at the bedside.

**Postoperative Bleeding** The combination of heparinization, hypothermia, CPB, and protamine reversal is associated with increased risk for bleeding after CABG. Bleeding after CABG requiring transfusion or reoperation to stop the bleeding is associated with a significant increase in morbidity and mortality. A minority of patients having cardiac procedures (15% to 20%) consume more than 80% of the blood products transfused at operation. Blood must be viewed as a scarce resource that carries significant risks and unproven benefits. There is a high-risk subset of patients who require multiple preventive measures to reduce the chance of postoperative bleeding. Nine variables stand out as important indicators of risk (Box 60-6).

**BOX 60-6 Risk Factors for Postoperative Bleeding**

- Advanced age
- Low preoperative red blood cell volume (preoperative anemia or small body size)
- Preoperative antiplatelet or antithrombotic drugs
- Reoperative or complex procedures
- Emergency operations
- Noncardiac patient comorbidities
- Renal failure
- Chronic obstructive pulmonary disease
- Congestive heart failure

Available evidence-based blood conservation techniques include the following:

1. Drugs that increase preoperative blood volume (e.g., erythropoietin) or decrease postoperative bleeding (e.g., epsilon aminocaproic acid). Aprotinin is currently banned in the United States because some studies have shown increased mortality, stroke, and renal failure when administered to cardiac surgery patients.
2. Intraoperative blood salvage and blood-sparing interventions
3. Interventions that protect the patient's own blood from the stress of operation (e.g., autologous predonation, normovolemic hemodilution)
4. Institution-specific blood transfusion algorithms supplemented with point of care testing

Despite efforts at blood conservation to limit perioperative bleeding and blood transfusions, 2% to 3% of patients will require reexploration for bleeding and as many as 20% will have excessive bleeding and blood transfusion after operation. Bleeding more than 500 mL in the first hour or persistent bleeding more than 200 mL/hour for 4 hours is an indication for mediastinal exploration. Exploration is also indicated if a large hemothorax is identified on chest x-ray or pericardial tamponade occurs. Usually, a specific bleeding site is not identified. Box 60-7 summarizes the common causes of immediate postoperative bleeding.

### Neurologic Complications

There are two types of neurologic deficit after CABG—type I deficit, in which there is a focal neurologic deficit, and type II deficit, which manifests as nonspecific encephalopathy. In a 1996 multi-institutional prospective study, adverse outcomes in 6% of patients, evenly distributed between the two types of deficit, were identified. Mortality was 20% for type I, which is twice the mortality for type II deficit. Age (especially older than 70 years) and hypertension are consistent risk factors for both types. History of previous neurologic abnormality, diabetes, and atherosclerosis of the aorta are risk factors for type I. Significant atherosclerosis of the ascending aorta mandates a surgical approach that will minimize the possibility of atherosclerotic emboli. Patients with concomitant carotid stenosis are at a higher risk for neurologic complications. One approach involves a staged procedure in which the more symptomatic and more critical vascular bed is addressed first. Otherwise, a combined approach may be used, but with increased overall risk.

**BOX 60-7 Causes of Immediate Postoperative Bleeding**

Surgical
- Conduit
- Anastomoses
- Cannulation sites
- Mammary bed
- Thymic veins
- Pericardial edge
- Sternal wire sites

Platelet dysfunction
Inadequate protamine reversal
Hypothermia

### Mediastinitis

The incidence of deep sternal wound infection is 1% to 4% in CABG patients. Risk factors include obesity, reoperation, diabetes, and duration and complexity of operation. BIMA use can increase the risk of sternal wound complications in high-risk patients. The use of perioperative antibiotics and a strict protocol aimed at controlling the blood glucose level to less than 180 mg/dL by continuous IV insulin has been shown to reduce the incidence of mediastinitis significantly. Early débridement and muscle flap closure improve outcome. More recently, good outcomes have also been reported with the use of wound VACs after adequate débridement.[29]

### Renal Dysfunction

Mangano and coworkers[30] have reported an incidence of postoperative renal dysfunction (PRD) in 7.7% of patients, with mortality rates of 0.9%, 19%, and 63% in patients without PRD, patients with PRD but without need for dialysis, and patients who required dialysis, respectively. The latter figure was confirmed in a large Veterans Admistration (VA) study.[31]

## Medical Adjuncts for Postoperative Management

The following drugs are considered essential components in the postoperative management of CABG patients:

1. Aspirin, 81 to 325 mg orally or rectally, is begun on the same day after CABG, unless the patient is bleeding from platelet dysfunction. This is a quality of care index and has been shown to be of long-term benefit in graft patency.
2. Beta blockers should begin after all inotropes have been weaned. The goal is to maintain a heart rate of 60 to 80 beats/min with adequate mean perfusion pressures.
3. Afterload reduction is important in all patients with a low ejection fraction (EF). Afterload reduction is commenced after all inotropes are weaned and adequate beta blockade is achieved. ACE inhibitors are first-line drugs for afterload reduction. Creatinine levels should be monitored.
4. For antiarrhythmic treatment, amiodarone is used in many cardiac centers as a prophylactic or treatment against atrial fibrillation. This drug should be used with caution in patients with preexisting interstitial lung disease or those who take concurrent warfarin. A prolonged Q-T interval is a contraindication.
5. Furosemide, a diuretic, is begun on the first postoperative day; the goal is to maintain a negative fluid balance. Chest x-ray, creatinine levels, physical examination, and input-output charts help guide the dose of furosemide.

# ALTERNATIVE METHODS FOR MYOCARDIAL REVASCULARIZATION

## Cardiopulmonary Bypass With Hypothermic Fibrillatory Arrest

Hypothermic fibrillatory arrest is a good on-pump alternative to conventional cardioplegic arrest and avoids the use of the aortic cross clamp. Although cardioplegic arrest offers maximal myocardial protection while allowing a stable immobile target for the surgeon to perform the distal anastomoses, not all patients are amenable to cardioplegia-based arrest. In patients with an extensively calcified aorta, cross clamp application may be precarious and associated with a higher incidence of stroke.

In these cases, a hypothermic fibrillatory arrest strategy may be used in which aortic manipulation is minimized. Once cardiopulmonary bypass is initiated, the patient is cooled to 28° C. The heart typically begins fibrillating at approximately 32° C. A left ventricular sump is usually introduced through the right superior pulmonary vein to ensure LV decompression. Handling the distal and proximal targets is similar to off-pump CABG (OPCAB) techniques because the coronaries are still fully perfused while the anastomoses are being performed. Vessel loops or occluders may be needed. In patients with extensive aortic calcification, there may not be any room for placing an aortic canula or proximal vein graft on the ascending aorta. In these cases, the right axillary artery may be used for arterial perfusion and the saphenous vein can be anastomosed to the innominate artery if it is free of disease, or a total arterial vascularization approach should be considered with the use of one or both mammary arteries.

Once the anastomoses are completed, the patient is rewarmed to physiologic temperature and the heart is defibrillated into sinus rhythm. The use of hypothermic fibrillatory arrest is contraindicated in patients with significant aortic valve incompetence because the ventricle would distend with the regurgitant blood once fibrillation sets in and no stroke volume is generated. Increased ventricular wall tension and energy consumption could lead to myocardial ischemia.

## On-Pump Beating Heart Bypass

On-pump beating heart bypass is a selective strategy used for patients who have a very low EF and have suffered a fresh MI. The logic behind this approach is that the myocardium is severely compromised and would tolerate further ischemic compromise poorly. Despite currently available techniques for myocardial protection, there is always a certain degree of ischemia associated with cardioplegic arrest. This is especially true in patients with severe coronary disease and a stunned myocardium, in whom uniform protection of the ventricle with cardioplegia may be difficult to achieve and an on-pump beating heart strategy can be considered. The coronaries continue to be perfused, and exposure and handling of the anastomoses are similar to those for OPCAB. The use of CPB offloads the ventricle and offers a safety margin to manipulate the heart and visualize all the targets that need to be bypassed. Use of IABP should be considered for most of these patients because their hemodynamics is precarious to begin with.

## Off-Pump Coronary Artery Bypass Grafting

Cardiopulmonary bypass is associated with a systemic inflammatory response caused by contact of blood components with the surface of the bypass circuit. This has been shown to contribute to postoperative bleeding, neurocognitive dysfunction, thromboembolism, fluid retention, and reversible organ dysfunction. OPCAB eliminates the use of a cardiopulmonary bypass circuit and can potentially reduce some pump-associated complications. An initial wave of enthusiasm was tempered by the number of OPCAB cases in the United States stabilizing at 20% for the last several years. This is because of the added technical complexity of OPCAB and mixed reports regarding its outcomes.

Puskas and colleagues[32] have compared in-hospital major adverse cardiac events (MACEs) and long-term survival after OPCAB versus on-pump CABG in 12,812 consecutive isolated CABG patients from 1997 to 2006. OPCAB was associated with a significant reduction in operative mortality, stroke, and MACEs. OPCAB, however, did not offer a long-term survival advantage. The same group and others have also demonstrated the unique benefit of OPCAB in women and higher risk patients.[33] Using nationwide data in a cohort of 63,000 patients, Chu and associates[34] have shown that traditional on-pump CABG and OPCAB have similar rates of in-hospital mortality (3.0% versus 3.2%) and postoperative stroke (1.8% versus 1.7%). However, OPCAB patients had longer hospital stays and higher hospital costs than on-pump CABG patients.

In view of persistent controversy surrounding the benefits of OPCAB, the multicenter VA Randomized On/Off Bypass (ROOBY) trial was initiated.[35] Patients scheduled for surgical revascularization were randomly assigned to undergo on-pump CABG or OPCAB. The proportion of patients with fewer grafts completed than originally planned was higher with off-pump than with on-pump CABG. Follow-up angiograms demonstrated that the overall rate of graft patency was lower in the OPCAB group than in the on-pump group (82.6% versus 87.8%). There were no treatment-based differences in neuropsychological outcomes or short-term use of major resources. The study concluded that at 1 year of follow-up, patients in the off-pump group had worse composite outcomes and poorer graft patency than patients in the on-pump group.

The primary benefit from OPCAB is presumably believed to arise from the neuroprotective effect caused by the absence of aortic manipulation. Patel and associates[36] have studied 2327 consecutive patients and divided them into three groups—on-pump, off-pump with aortic manipulation (aorta used as source of graft inflow), and off-pump without aortic manipulation (pedicle-based inflow). In this study, CPB was a risk factor for focal neurologic deficit, but there were no differences in focal deficits between the OPCAB surgery patients with or without aortic manipulation. Although this study also supported the concept that CPB may be associated with more neurologic events, it did not appear to be related to aortic manipulation as defined by the investigators. Hammon and coworkers,[37] in a randomized trial, have demonstrated that surgical technique is important in determining cognitive outcome after CABG. All patients in their study underwent an 11-part neuropsychologic examination preoperatively and at 1 week, 6 weeks, and 6 months postoperatively. Neuropsychological examinations were carried out on 107 patients with no postoperative neurologic deficits at all four testing periods. At 6 months, 26% of 27 multiple aortic cross clamp patients had neuropsychological deficits, 27% of 26 off-pump CABG patients had neuropsychological deficits, and only 9% of 54 single aortic cross clamp patients had neuropsychological deficits ($P = .067$ versus multiple aortic cross clamp and off-pump CABG). The results suggest that CPB is not the most important factor in determining outcome and, when carefully performed with single cross clamp and minimal aortic manipulation, is equal or may be superior to off-pump operation. It was inferred that mild hypothermia in on-pump surgery is additionally neuroprotective, which is a benefit not possible with OPCAB.

The technique and operative strategy for OPCAB differ significantly from on-pump CABG. Certain adjuncts are needed to provide adequate exposure of the coronary vessels. Because the heart is fully contractile and maintaining systemic perfusion, the manipulation should proceed in a planned and systematic manner. Both the pleural spaces are opened to allow the heart to rotate into either side to visualize the targets, especially the lateral and inferior wall. The more critical areas of the myocardium are revascularized first, which minimizes ischemic time, improves myocardial reserve, and permits more complex manipulation of the heart for the other targets. Mammary artery–based pedicles are typically approached first because these do not require a proximal anastomosis, thus providing immediate coronary blood flow to the bypassed vessel.

Once the target vessel is selected, a small area of the coronary artery is exposed proximal and distal to the planned area of anastomosis to allow placement of vessel loops or bulldog clamps for proximal and distal control. A coronary occluder may also be used. Two stabilizers are used to stabilize the myocardium (Fig. 60-16). The fork-octopus has a suction padded tip with two limbs that straddles the coronary artery target and is attached to a multifunctional versatile arm. The fork is positioned so that the limbs straddle the coronary target and suction is applied, which attaches the device to the myocardium while the arm is secured in position. The other device consists of a suction cup that is applied to the apex of the heart and used to lift it out of the chest to visualize the posterior aspect. A sling attached to the posterior pericardium allows the heart to be elevated out and enhances visualization of the posterior targets.

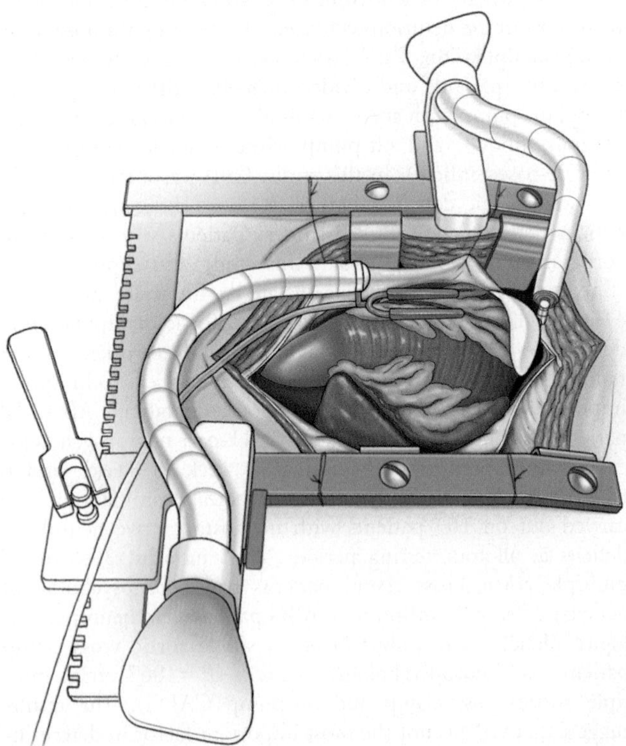

**FIGURE 60-16** Off-pump coronary artery bypass requires the use of vacuum assisted multi-articulating arms to position and stabilize the myocardium. This minimizes the movement of the heart thereby allowing the surgeon to feasibly perform the distal anastomoses. Here the stabilizer is positioned in preparation for creating a bypass to the left anterior descending artery.

Full heparinization is not needed; generally, 50% of the usual dose is used. Success of the operation requires coordinated efforts between the surgeon and anesthesiologist so that adequate systemic perfusion is maintained throughout the operation while allowing a comfortable milieu in which the surgeon can operate. Short-acting beta blockers to slow the heart rate and alpha constrictors to maintain systemic perfusion pressures are important adjuncts for this.

The management of the postoperative course of off-pump coronary bypass is significantly different compared with patients who undergo conventional coronary bypass grafting, primarily because of the reduced inflammatory effects, which are more prominent in CPB patients. These patients do not manifest the vasodilatory response or massive fluid shifts seen with CPB. Rather, these patients behave more like those who have undergone a major general surgery operation and require early deep venous thrombosis (DVT) and stress ulcer prophylaxis and balanced postoperative fluid management. In our practice, all patients who undergo off-pump coronary artery bypass are placed on aspirin and clopidogrel (Plavix) on the day of surgery.

## Minimally Invasive Direct Coronary Artery Bypass

Minimally Invasive Direct Coronary Artery Bypass (MIDCAB) describes any technique of coronary artery bypass that uses a minimally invasive approach, such as an anterolateral thoracotomy (Fig. 60-17), ministernotomy, or subxiphoid approach, without the use of a robot. Most MIDCABs are performed on the beating heart and involve vascularization of the anterior wall. A meta-analysis of all published outcome studies of MIDCAB grafting performed from January 1995 through October 2007 has revealed early and late (>30 days) death rates of 1.3% and 3.2%, respectively. Of the grafts that were studied angiographically immediately after surgery, 4.2% were occluded and 6.6% had a significant stenosis (50% to 99%). At 6-month follow-up,

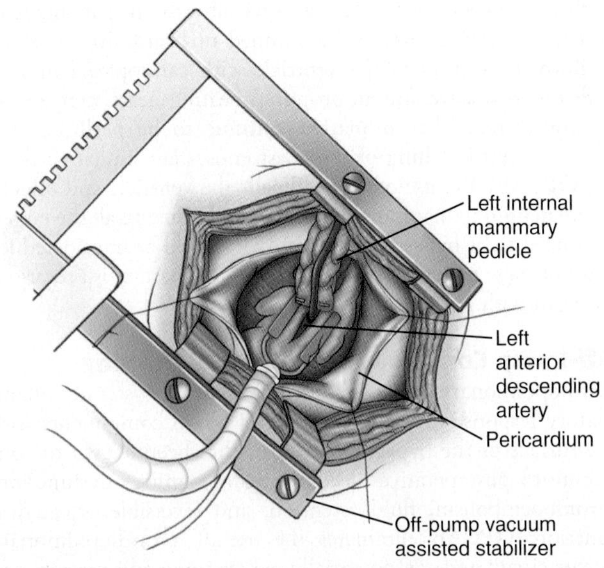


**FIGURE 60-17** Left thoracotomy approach for performing off-pump left internal mammary to left anterior descending bypass. This is commonly used in the minimally invasive direct coronary artery bypass approach (MIDCAB). Multiarticulating stabilizers are essential for this technique.

3.6% were occluded and 7.2% had significant stenosis.[38] Long-term follow-up results and further randomized, prospective, clinical trials comparing MIDCABs with standard revascularization procedures in large patient cohorts are needed. Although MIDCAB offers several advantages, such as the avoidance of sternotomy and CPB, it is subject to the same limitations of OPCAB in addition to its own technical challenges and limited revascularization territory.

### Robotics: Totally Endoscopic Coronary Artery Bypass

Rapid advances in technology have led to the application of robotic CABG. Robotically assisted microsurgical systems have the theoretical advantage of enhancing surgical dexterity and minimizing the invasive nature of conventional coronary artery surgery. The da Vinci system (Intuitive Surgical, Mountain View, Calif) is the most commonly used. It consists of three major components—the surgeon-device interface module, computer controller, and specific patient interface instrumentation. It allows real-time surgical manipulation of tissue, advanced dexterity in multiple degrees of freedom, and optical magnification of the operative field, all through minimal access ports. The technology has seen significant use in valve repair operations and other surgical specialties as well.

In a multicenter totally endoscopic coronary artery bypass (TECAB) trial, 98 patients requiring LAD revascularization were enrolled at 12 centers.[39] The procedure was performed with femorofemoral CPB, endoaortic balloon occlusion, and thoracoscopy. All aspects of the procedure were performed with the robotic system, from internal mammary artery harvest to coronary anastomosis. Robotic TECAB was accomplished with no mortality and low morbidity; the angiographic patency and reintervention rates were suboptimal but encouraging.

Oehlinger and colleagues[40] have demonstrated the feasibility of this procedure in the largest single-center series, 2001 to 2007, that was performed in 100 patients All patients received LIMA grafts to the LAD artery using the da Vinci system. There was no perioperative mortality. For the entire patient series, 5-year postoperative survival, freedom from angina, and freedom from major adverse cardiac and cerebral events were 100%, 91%, and 89%, respectively. The learning curve for operative times and improvements in clinical outcome continued, even at 100 procedures, although the curve was steep during the early experience.

Current limitations of robotic TECAB include its lack of applicability to all patients, prolonged operating room time, limited applicability to access all vessels, cost, and limited training opportunities. However, over time, the use of robotic surgery is likely to be more of a niche for a subset of surgeons tailored to a specific patient population.

### Transmyocardial Laser Revascularization

Patients with chronic severe angina refractory to medical therapy who cannot be completely revascularized with percutaneous catheter intervention or CABG present clinical challenges. Transmyocardial laser revascularization (TMLR), either as sole therapy or as an adjunct to CABG surgery, may be appropriate for some of these patients. The STS Evidence-Based Workforce has reviewed available evidence and recommends the use of TMLR for patients with an EF greater than 0.30 and CCS class III or IV angina that is refractory to maximal medical therapy.[41] These patients should have reversible ischemia of the LV free wall and CAD corresponding to the regions of myocardial ischemia. In all regions of the myocardium, the coronary disease must not be amenable to CABG or PCI.

TMLR uses a high-energy laser beam to create myocardial transmural channels that were originally thought to provide direct access to oxygenated blood in the LV cavity. This is no longer considered the mechanism whereby TMLR causes a reduction in symptoms of ischemic heart disease. Although some local neovascularization has been documented, the magnitude of changes does not account for any substantive increases in myocardial perfusion. One mechanism that has been proposed relates to a local effect on cardiac neuronal signaling. It has been hypothesized that local tissue injury by TMLR damages ventricular sensory neurons and autonomic efferent axons, which leads to local cardiac denervation and anginal relief. Regardless of the mechanism, TMLR therapy is associated with a reproducible improvement in symptoms. Patients undergoing TMLR show a persistent improvement in angina class using the CCS classification.[8] This improvement is achieved in 60% to 80% of patients within 6 months after the operation.

### Hybrid Procedures

It is generally accepted that the LIMA to LAD anastomosis is the single most important component of CABG that confers long-term benefit unmatched by any other intervention. State of the art PCIs with drug-eluting stents have produced competitive outcomes compared to vein grafts to non-LAD targets. This has led to an integrated approach to coronary revascularization, termed the *hybrid procedure.* The hybrid procedure consists of a minimally invasive LIMA to LAD anastomosis in conjunction with PCI to non–LAD-obstructed coronary arteries.

This approach has met with initial success, but many potential pitfalls exist. The procedural costs may be greater than those of either CABG alone or DES implantation alone. The timing and staging of the procedures is uncertain and limited data are available on long-term outcomes.

## REOPERATION FOR CORONARY ARTERY DISEASE

Within 5 years, 15% of CABG patients experience a recurrence of symptoms, typically angina. This increases to approximately 40% within 10 years. Recurrent symptoms almost always indicate progression of disease in the native coronary circulation or graft disease. In most cases, the indications to proceed with coronary angiography, PCI with or without stenting, or repeat CABG are the same as for the first operation. Patients who are considered candidates for reoperative CABG are usually older, have more diffuse CAD, and have diminished ventricular function. Factors that increase the risk for reoperation include the absence of an ITA graft, younger age at the time of primary surgery, prior incomplete revascularization, congestive heart failure, and NYHA Class III or IV angina.

Technical aspects of reoperative CABG differ significantly from those of the primary procedure. Reentry into the chest and dissection of the old grafts can sometimes be challenging. Preparation for femoral cannulation for femorofemoral bypass or axillary cannulation should be considered with preemptive availability of blood products. Redo sternotomy is typically completed with an oscillating saw or after dissecting the heart away from the sternum via a subxiphoid approach. Injury to the right ventricle or to the aorta or vein grafts is of potential concern. A poorly placed LIMA graft from the prior operation is also at risk during the sternotomy. If a cardiac or vascular injury is identified, an assistant holds the sternum together to tamponade further bleeding, and expeditious cannulation of alternate sites is begun with the institution of cardiopulmonary bypass. Preoperative CT scans are helpful in planning the operation.

Once the sternotomy is completed, the rest of the adherent cardiac structures are dissected away from the underside of the sternum to allow placement of a sternal retractor. No retractor should be placed unless the heart is adequately dissected away; this will result in disruption of the aorta or right ventricle, which may be difficult to control.

The next steps are geared toward establishing sites for cannulation. The right atrium and aorta are dissected first; then, the rest of the heart is dissected away from the pericardium, which may be performed on CPB. The areas of previous cannulation and vein grafts are the most adherent regions, whereas the diaphragmatic aspect is least adherent and provides a good starting point to gain entry into the correct plane.

Manipulation of the old grafts should be kept to a minimum to avoid distal coronary bed microembolization. Isolation of the LIMA pedicle is often necessary and should be carefully performed, with the ability to start bypass rapidly if an inadvertent injury were to occur (Fig. 60-18). The rest of the operation proceeds in a similar fashion to primary CABG and can be performed on or off pump. In some cases, the surgery could be accomplished through a left anterolateral thoracotomy approach. Typically, this is used in patients who had previous mediastinitis or multiple sternotomies, or when an extensive area of the heart is adherent to the sternum, precluding a safe entry. The vein

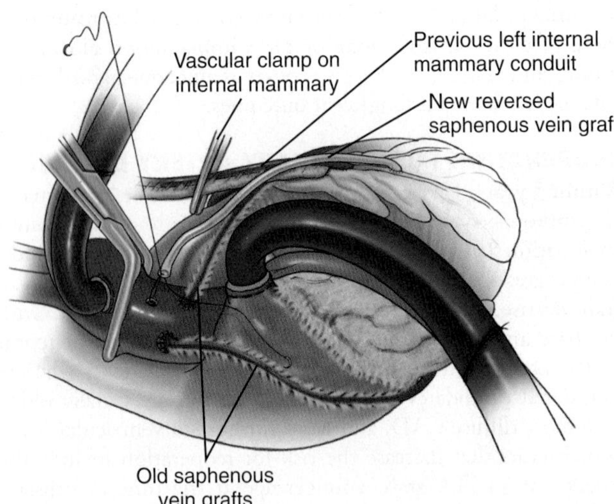


**FIGURE 60-18** Redo coronary artery bypass graft. The cannulation is very similar to a first time coronary artery bypass operation in most cases. However, identification of coronary targets are much more difficult due to scarring. The course of the prior grafts is useful in identifying the targets. In addition to clamping the aorta above the previous vein grafts, the left internal mammary pedicle should be dissected and clamped separately if feasible. A single-clamp technique is preferred as it avoids the tedious and potentially dangerous dissection around the proximal aorta that may be needed to place a partial side-biting clamp.

conduit is anastomosed to the descending aortas in these cases (Fig. 60-19).

To summarize, some of the unique difficulties that could be encountered in redo CABG are as follows:

1. Injury to heart during sternotomy
2. Injury to mammary pedicle
3. Limited space on ascending aorta for placement of new grafts
4. Inability to identify distal targets because of scars and adhesions
5. Availability of conduits
6. Increased risk of perioperative MI because atheroembolic embolization from diseased vein grafts and diffuse coronary disease preclude optimal cardioplegia
7. Increased bleeding because of higher inflammatory response and more raw surface
8. Injury to pulmonary artery during cross-clamping of the aorta

In most published series, the mortality rate of reoperative CABG exceeds that of primary CABG; in some series, it has been reported to be as high as 10%. Also, overall patient survival and freedom from angina over time are diminished.

## MECHANICAL COMPLICATIONS OF CORONARY ARTERY DISEASE

### Left Ventricular Aneurysm

The incidence of ventricular aneurysm after AMI has been declining because of early interventional therapies. Of left ventricular aneurysms, 90% are the result of a transmural MI secondary to an acute occlusion of the LAD. Patients may develop an aneurysm (pseudoaneurysm) as early as 48 hours after infarction, but most patients develop one within weeks. Approximately two thirds of patients who develop ventricular aneurysms remain asymptomatic.

The 10-year survival rate is 90% for asymptomatic patients and 50% for symptomatic patients. The most common causes of death are arrhythmias (>40%), CHF (>30%), and recurrent MI (>10%). The risk for thromboembolism is low and long-term anticoagulation is not recommended unless there is a mural thrombus. The diagnosis is usually made by echocardiography. Thallium imaging or PET is useful for detecting the extent of the aneurysm and viability of adjacent regions.

Surgery for left ventricular aneurysm is indicated if the patient is scheduled to undergo CABG for symptomatic coronary artery disease, there is contained rupture or evidence of a false aneurysm, or the patient experiences a thromboembolic event despite anticoagulation. The 5-year survival rate after surgery has been reported to range between 60% and 80%. In general, surgical repair or resection in conjunction with CABG results in angina relief and resolution of heart failure symptoms for most patients. *Surgical ventricular restoration* is a technical term that describes the surgical resection of the aneurysm with reconstruction of the native ventricular geometric shape. This is ideally performed with CPB, without cardioplegic arrest, as long as the aortic valve is competent. The aneurysm is usually recognized by the paradoxical movement of the walls compared with the rest of the viable LV myocardium. The aneurysm is opened and a purse-string Fontan stitch is placed at the junction of the viable and nonviable myocardium, which can be manually

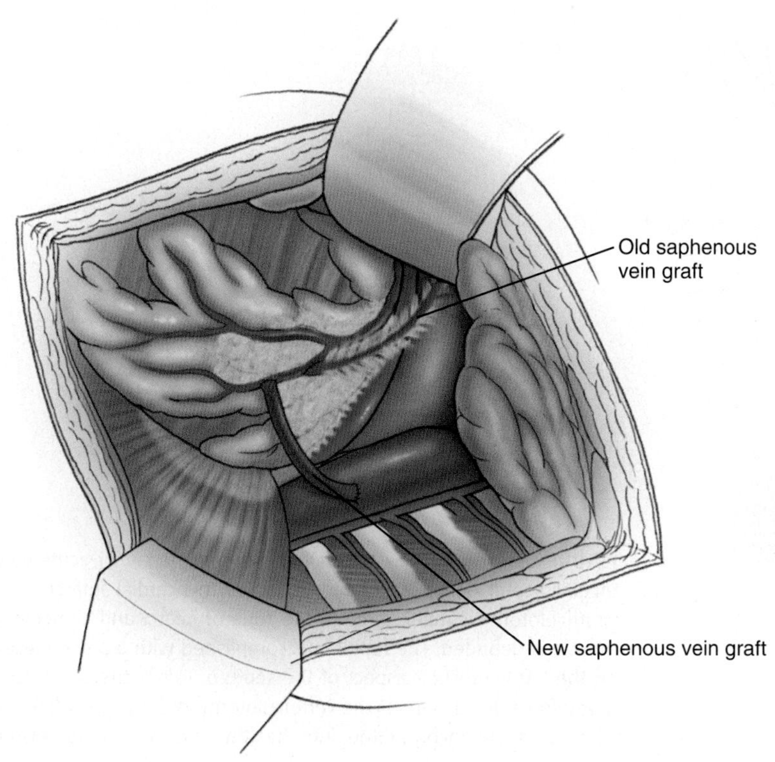


**FIGURE 60-19** Left thoracotomy approach for recurrent coronary artery disease. This approach avoids the hazards of a difficult redo sternotomy and is used as an alternative in some cases. New saphenous vein graft: descending thoracic aorta to obtuse marginal bypass.

palpated on the beating heart. A Dacron or bovine pericardial patch is used to exclude the aneurysm and the aneurysm is closed over the patch.

Two potentially acute complications that require surgical intervention are postinfarction ventricular septal defect and postinfarction mitral regurgitation caused by papillary muscle rupture.

### Ventricular Septal Defect

This occurs in less than 1% of patients and is associated with an acute LAD occlusion. The defect is more common in men (3:2) and typically presents within 2 to 4 days of the infarction. However, a VSD that occurs in the first 6 weeks after an infarct is still considered acute. The VSD is usually located in the anterior or apical aspect of the ventricular septum. A posterior VSD occurs in approximately 25% of patients caused by an inferior wall MI from occlusion of the RCA system or a distal branch LCA. A full-thickness infarct is a prerequisite for a VSD to occur. A new, loud, systolic cardiac murmur after an MI suggests the diagnosis; an echocardiogram is effective for determining the size and character of the VSD, as well as the degree of left to right shunting. Right heart catheterization typically shows an increase in oxygen saturation levels in the right ventricle and pulmonary artery. The defect is usually approximately 1 to 2 cm in size.

After the diagnosis is established, patients should undergo immediate left heart catheterization to characterize the degree of CAD, magnitude of LV dysfunction, and presence of mitral valve insufficiency. Approximately 60% of patients with an infarction VSD have significant CAD in an unrelated vessel. The mortality rate in the untreated patient is high, with 25% of patients dying within 24 hours from refractory heart failure. Patient survival rates at 1 week, 1 month, and longer than 1 year are 50%, 20%, and less than 3%, respectively.

Patients who are considered candidates for surgery should be managed early with closure of the defect and concomitant CABG. In the absence of refractory heart failure and hemodynamic instability, the survival rate may be as high as 75%. The infarct exclusion technique is used to repair the VSD and is technically one of the most challenging procedures. The left ventricle is opened longitudinally on the infarct and the defect is evaluated. Multiple VSDs may be present and necrotic myocardium is débrided to viable tissue. A prosthetic Dacron patch or bovine pericardium is then sutured to the LV side of the septal defect and brought out through the ventriculotomy, where it is incorporated with the closure (Fig. 60-20). In this method, the posterior aspect of the patch is thus anchored to the remnant viable septum and the anterior aspect is incorporated with the free ventricular wall, forming the neointerventricular septum. Felt strips are used to buttress the closure.

### Mitral Regurgitation

Approximately 40% of patients who sustain an AMI develop chronic ischemic mitral regurgitation (IMR) detectable by color-flow Doppler echocardiography. In 3% to 4% of cases, the degree of mitral regurgitation is moderate or severe.

The cause of chronic IMR is ischemic papillary muscle dysfunction and LV dilation associated with mitral annular dilation and restriction of the posterior leaflet. The operation for chronic IMR is usually performed on an elective basis. It consists of complete myocardial revascularization and mitral valve repair with the use of an annuloplasty ring.

Acute IMR may occur as a result of papillary muscle necrosis and rupture caused by occlusion of the overlying epicardial

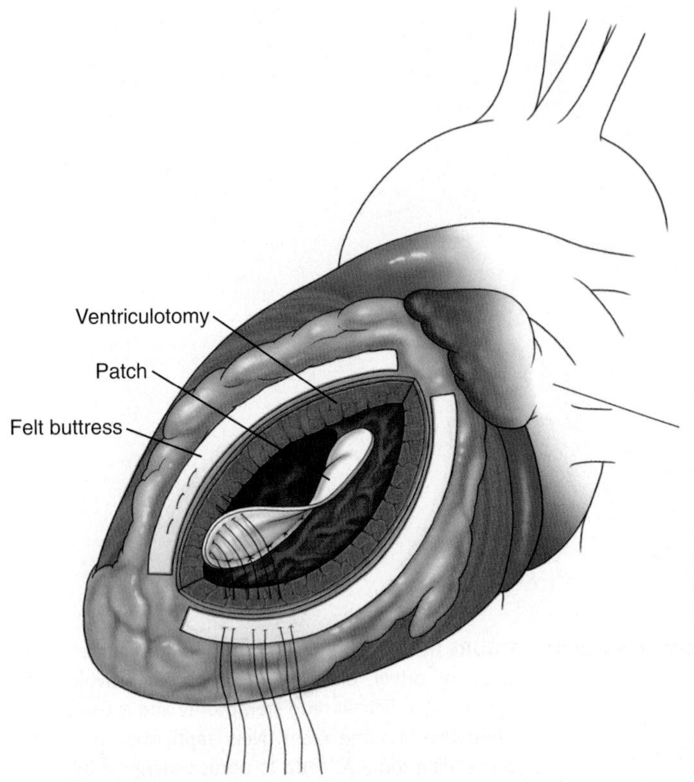


**FIGURE 60-20** Infarct exclusion technique for repair of acute ventricular septal defect secondary to acute myocardial infarction. A ventriculotomy is made through the zone of infarct and all necrotic muscle is débrided. The repair is accomplished with a patch placed on the left ventricular aspect of the septum. Felt buttress are used to reinforce the closure of the ventriculotomy and it is essential that all sutures are incorporated into healthy myocardium to ensure durability of the repair.

arteries that give rise to the penetrating vessels that supply the papillary muscles. The posterior papillary muscle is involved three to six times more often than the anterior muscle (Fig. 60-21), and either the entire trunk of the muscle or one of the heads to which chordae attach may rupture partially or totally.

In most cases, prompt surgical intervention provides the best chance for survival. Predictors of in-hospital death include CHF, renal insufficiency, and multivessel CAD. Emergent surgical treatment usually involves mitral valve replacement and concomitant CABG. The hospital mortality rate may be as high as 50% in the acute setting. Mitral repair should not be attempted in the acute setting because it may not be feasible in papillary muscle rupture; it requires prolonging the cross clamp time (compared with replacement), which is not ideal in an acute setting. Operations on patients with acute mechanical complications from MI are challenging; the surgeon has to anticipate and be prepared for placing an LV assist device if failure to wean off CPB develops (Fig. 60-22).

## CORONARY ARTERY BYPASS GRAFTING AND SPECIAL PATIENT POPULATIONS

### Patients With Diabetes

Mortality and morbidity rates after CABG are higher in diabetic patients than in the general population. The BARI trial demonstrated the benefits of CABG in diabetics with multivessel disease over any other treatment modality

### Older Patients

Approximately 10% of patients who undergo CABG are older than 80 years. Older age is an independent predictor of surgical morbidity and mortality and a nonroutine discharge status.[42] CABG should not be denied to patients based on age alone,

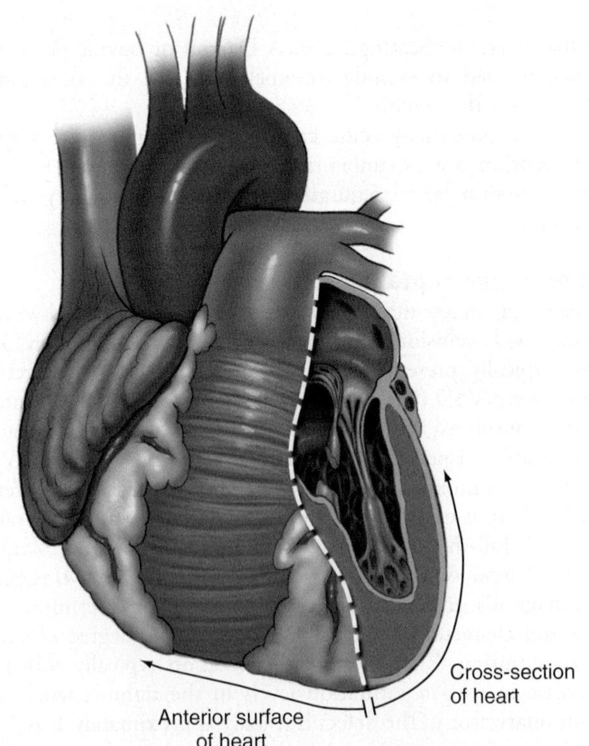


**FIGURE 60-21** Mechanical complication of acute myocardial infarction: Acute papillary muscle rupture (shown here) and acute ventricular septal defect are two sequelae in patient who suffer from extensive zones of infarct. Acute papillary muscle rupture results in acute mitral regurgitation that manifests as cardiogenic shock and immediate pulmonary decompensation. If the patient is a surgical candidate, mitral valve replacement is the only option.

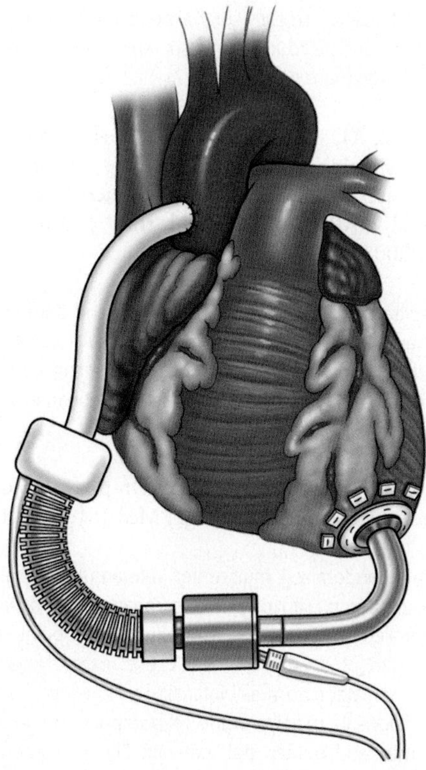

**FIGURE 60-22** The axial flow left ventricular assist device is used as temporary mechanical support or a bridge to transplant for patient in end-stage cardiomyopathy due to coronary artery disease not amenable to bypass surgery. The inflow of blood into the pump is from the apex of the left ventricle. The blood is then pumped into the ascending aorta via specially designed grafts that are incorporated with the pump. The axial flow pumps are less bulky and relatively easy to implant. They have only a single moving part, which is the axial impeller.

although it should be considered in the risk stratification. Appropriate arrangements should be made beforehand with the expectation that only one in five patients will be able to go home without additional support.

### Women

Although women in every age group have a lower incidence of CAD than men, CAD is still the leading cause of death in women in the United States. Historically, serious manifestations and associated complications of CAD in women were considered uncommon. Examination of the STS database in two separate studies has revealed that the operative mortality rate is higher in women—3.15% versus 2.61% in men.[43,44]

With evolving strategies, studies have been designed to evaluate specific aspects of coronary artery bypass that would benefit women. OPCAB has demonstrated favorable outcomes in women. A recent review of 42,477 patients in the STS National Cardiac Database has revealed that women have a significantly greater adjusted risk of death, prolonged ventilation, and longer length of stay than men in on-pump CABG. In contrast, among OPCAB cases, women had a lower risk of reexploration than men and a similar risk for death, MI, and prolonged ventilation and hospital stay.[45]

### Patients With Renal Disease

Renal insufficiency is also an independent risk factor for survival after CABG. A preoperative serum creatinine level higher 1.4 to 2.5 mg/dL is independently associated with a twofold increase in mortality.[46] In one retrospective study[47] of 59,576 patients who underwent CABG or PCI, a survival benefit with CABG in patients with a serum creatinine level higher than 2.5 mg/dL was demonstrated. The 1-, 2-, and 3-year survival rates were 84.1%, 77.4%, and 65.9%, respectively, for CABG compared with 70.8%, 51.9%, and 46.1% for PCI. This effect was more dramatic in diabetic patients. Long-term survival is also affected by the presence of preoperative renal dysfunction, especially if the creatinine clearance is less than 30 mL/min.[48] Although CABG in patients with renal insufficiency and failure is associated with increased morbidity and mortality, CABG is associated with better survival when compared with PCI.

### Obese Patients

The incidence of postoperative renal failure, prolonged ventilation, and sternal wound infection are significantly higher in obese patients. Extremes of weight are risk factors for CABG mortality.

Increasing evidence has suggested that obesity and renal insufficiency are associated with increased systemic inflammation, thrombogenicity, and endothelial dysfunction. Obese patients with preoperative renal insufficiency had higher rates of postoperative MI and low cardiac output syndrome and increased hospital stay than nonobese patients with preoperative renal insufficiency in a single-institution retrospective study of 10,000 patients.

## ACKNOWLEDGMENTS

We would like to acknowledge Scott Weldon and Michael DeLaflor for graphic services, Johnny Airheart for photographic support, Dr. Chinnapapu Muthusamy for assistance with review questions, and Dr. Stephen N. Palmer for organizing the references and editing the review questions.

## SELECTED REFERENCES

Chu D, Bakaeen FG, Dao TK, et al: On-pump versus off-pump coronary artery bypass grafting in a cohort of 63,000 patients. Ann Thorac Surg 87:1820–1826, 2009.

This study was a nationwide comparison of on-pump versus off-pump coronary artery bypass grafting in the United States. The study highlighted the fact that OPCAB does not produce lower postoperative mortality or stroke rates than conventional on-pump CABG. OPCAB was associated with longer hospital stays and higher hospital costs.

Edwards FH, Carey JS, Grover FL, et al: Impact of gender on coronary bypass operative mortality. Ann Thorac Surg 66:125–131, 1998.

This study analyzed the outcomes of more than 300,000 patients from the STS database and used multivariate analysis and risk model stratification to compare the outcomes of female patients. Female gender was demonstrated to be an independent predictor of higher mortality in low- to moderate-risk patients but not in high-risk patients.

Gopaldas RR, Chu D, Dao TK, et al: Predictors of surgical mortality and discharge status after coronary artery bypass grafting in patients 80 years and older. Am J Surg 198:633–638, 2009.

This study was a nationwide comparison of octogenarians with younger patients who underwent CABG. Although the mortality for this subset of older patients was acceptable at 7%, only 21% of these patients were routinely discharged home. The remaining patients required further specialized care, such as home health services and rehabilitation services.

Influence of diabetes on 5-year mortality and morbidity in a randomized trial comparing CABG and PTCA in patients with multivessel disease: The Bypass Angioplasty Revascularization Investigation (BARI). Circulation 96:1761–1769, 1997.

Follow-up results from the initial randomized trial established that patients with treated diabetes mellitus who were assigned to undergo CABG had a striking reduction in mortality compared with PTCA. This benefit was attributed predominantly to the left internal mammary artery conduit.

Loop FD, Lytle BW, Cosgrove DM, et al: Influence of the internal-mammary-artery graft on 10-year survival and other cardiac events. N Engl J Med 314:1–6, 1986.

This study was a retrospective study that evaluated 5931 patients operated at a single institution and compared the outcomes of patients who had a mammary artery graft with those who had only vein grafts for CABG. The findings of this landmark study established the superiority of the internal mammary artery compared to any other conduit. Over a 10-year period, patients who had only vein grafts had a 1.6 times higher risk of mortality compared with those who had mammary grafts.

Lopes RD, Hafley GE, Allen KB, et al: Endoscopic versus open vein-graft harvesting in coronary-artery bypass surgery. N Engl J Med 361:235–244, 2009.

This retrospective study evaluated the effects of endoscopic vein harvesting on the rate of vein graft failure and on clinical outcomes. Endoscopic vein harvesting was shown to be independently associated with vein graft failure and adverse clinical outcomes compared with open vein harvesting.

Parisi AF, Khuri S, Deupree RH, et al: Medical compared with surgical management of unstable angina: 5-year mortality and morbidity in the Veterans Administration Study. Circulation 80:1176–1189, 1989.

This multicenter VA prospective randomized trial compared surgical and medical management and established the principle of survival superiority of surgical intervention for triple-vessel coronary disease over medical management.

Peduzzi P, Kamina A, Detre K: Twenty-two-year follow-up in the VA Cooperative Study of Coronary Artery Bypass Surgery for Stable Angina. Am J Cardiol 81:1393–1399, 1998.

This study evaluated the 22-year results of initial coronary artery bypass surgery with saphenous vein grafts compared with initial medical therapy on survival, incidence of myocardial infarction, reoperation, and symptomatic status in 686 patients with stable angina who participated in the Veterans Affairs Cooperative Study of Coronary Artery Bypass Surgery. This trial provided strong evidence that initial bypass surgery did not improve survival for low-risk patients and did not reduce the overall risk of myocardial infarction. The early survival benefit with surgery in high-risk patients did not translate to long-term survival rates that became comparable in both treatment groups.

Serruys PW, Ong AT, van Herwerden LA, et al: Five-year outcomes after coronary stenting versus bypass surgery for the treatment of multivessel disease: The final analysis of the Arterial Revascularization Therapies Study (ARTS) randomized trial. J Am Coll Cardiol 46:575–581, 2005.

The final results of the ARTS were summarized and demonstrated that the overall major adverse cardiac and cerebrovascular events was higher in patients who underwent coronary artery stenting compared with CABG. This was driven by the increased need for repeat revascularization in the stent group.

Shroyer AL, Grover FL, Hattler B, et al: On-pump versus off-pump coronary-artery bypass surgery. N Engl J Med 361:1827–1837, 2009.

This study was a randomized, multicenter, Veterans Affairs trial comparing conventional on-pump with off-pump coronary artery bypass grafting. The study enrolled 2203 patients. The primary end point of the study was a composite of death from any cause, repeat revascularization procedure, or nonfatal myocardial infarction within 1 year after surgery. At 1 year of follow-up, patients in the off-pump group had worse composite outcomes and poorer graft patency. The presumed benefit of lower neuropsychological outcomes was not demonstrated in off-pump CABG patients.

White HD, Assmann SF, Sanborn TA, et al: Comparison of percutaneous coronary intervention and coronary artery bypass grafting after acute myocardial infarction complicated by cardiogenic shock: Results from the Should We Emergently Revascularize Occluded Coronaries for Cardiogenic Shock (SHOCK) trial. Circulation 112:1992–2001, 2005.

This randomized trial was designed to compare surgery with percutaneous coronary intervention in patients who presented with cardiogeneic shock. The trial evaluated 30-day and 1-year mortality and demonstrated comparable results between the two groups, although patients who underwent CABG had a higher prevalence of diabetes and worse coronary artery disease.

## REFERENCES

1. Allen Maycock CA, Muhlestein JB, Horne BD, et al: Statin therapy is associated with reduced mortality across all age groups of individuals with significant coronary disease, including very elderly patients. J Am Coll Cardiol 40:1777–1785, 2002.
2. de Winter RJ, Windhausen F, Cornel JH, et al: Early invasive versus selectively invasive management for acute coronary syndromes. N Engl J Med 353:1095–1104, 2005.
3. Solomon SD, Zelenkofske S, McMurray JJ, et al: Sudden death in patients with myocardial infarction and left ventricular dysfunction, heart failure, or both. N Engl J Med 352:2581–2588, 2005.
4. Boersma E, Mercado N, Poldermans D, et al: Acute myocardial infarction. Lancet 361:847–858, 2003.
5. Stein PD, Beemath A, Kayali F, et al: Multidetector computed tomography for the diagnosis of coronary artery disease: a systematic review. Am J Med 119:203–216, 2006.

6. Lell M, Hinkmann F, Anders K, et al: High-pitch electrocardiogram-triggered computed tomography of the chest: initial results. Invest Radiol 44:728–733, 2009.
7. Fraker TD Jr, Fihn SD, Gibbons RJ, et al: 2007 chronic angina focused update of the ACC/AHA 2002 guidelines for the management of patients with chronic stable angina: A report of the American College of Cardiology/American Heart Association Task Force on Practice Guidelines Writing Group to develop the focused update of the 2002 guidelines for the management of patients with chronic stable angina. J Am Coll Cardiol 50:2264–2274, 2007.
8. Parisi AF, Khuri S, Deupree RH, et al: Medical compared with surgical management of unstable angina: 5-year mortality and morbidity in the Veterans Administration Study. Circulation 80:1176–1189, 1989.
9. Coronary angioplasty versus medical therapy for angina: The second Randomised Intervention Treatment of Angina (RITA-2) trial. RITA-2 trial participants. Lancet 350:461–468, 1997.
10. Boden WE, O'Rourke RA, Teo KK, et al: Impact of optimal medical therapy with or without percutaneous coronary intervention on long-term cardiovascular end points in patients with stable coronary artery disease (from the COURAGE Trial). Am J Cardiol 104:1–4, 2009.
11. Influence of diabetes on 5-year mortality and morbidity in a randomized trial comparing CABG and PTCA in patients with multivessel disease: The Bypass Angioplasty Revascularization Investigation (BARI). Circulation 96:1761–1769, 1997.
12. Goy JJ, Kaufmann U, Goy-Eggenberger D, et al: A prospective randomized trial comparing stenting to internal mammary artery grafting for proximal, isolated de novo left anterior coronary artery stenosis: The SIMA trial. Stenting vs Internal Mammary Artery. Mayo Clin Proc 75:1116–1123, 2000.
13. Rodriguez A, Bernardi V, Navia J, et al: Argentine randomized study: coronary angioplasty with stenting versus coronary bypass surgery in patients with multiple-vessel disease (ERACI II): 30-day and one-year follow-up results. ERACI II Investigators. J Am Coll Cardiol 37:51–58, 2001.
14. Serruys PW, Unger F, Sousa JE, et al: Comparison of coronary-artery bypass surgery and stenting for the treatment of multivessel disease. N Engl J Med 344:1117–1124, 2001.
15. Daemen J, Boersma E, Flather M, et al: Long-term safety and efficacy of percutaneous coronary intervention with stenting and coronary artery bypass surgery for multivessel coronary artery disease: A meta-analysis with 5-year patient-level data from the ARTS, ERACI-II, MASS-II, and SoS trials. Circulation 118:1146–1154, 2008.
16. Serruys PW, Ong AT, van Herwerden LA, et al: Five-year outcomes after coronary stenting versus bypass surgery for the treatment of multivessel disease: The final analysis of the Arterial Revascularization Therapies Study (ARTS) randomized trial. J Am Coll Cardiol 46:575–581, 2005.
17. Babapulle MN, Joseph L, Belisle P, et al: A hierarchical Bayesian meta-analysis of randomised clinical trials of drug-eluting stents. Lancet 364:583–591, 2004.
18. ACC/AHA 2007 Guidelines for the Management of Patients With Unstable Angina/Non-ST-Elevation Myocardial Infarction: Executive Summary: A Report of the American College of Cardiology/American Heart Association Task Force on Practice Guidelines (Writing Committee to Revise the 2002 Guidelines for the Management of Patients With Unstable Angina/Non-ST-Elevation Myocardial Infarction): Developed in Collaboration with the American College of Emergency Physicians, the Society for Cardiovascular Angiography and Interventions, and the Society of Thoracic Surgeons: Endorsed by the American Association of Cardiovascular and Pulmonary Rehabilitation and the Society for Academic Emergency Medicine. Circulation 116:803–877, 2007.
19. Berger PB, Ellis SG, Holmes DR Jr, et al: Relationship between delay in performing direct coronary angioplasty and early clinical outcome in patients with acute myocardial infarction: Results from the global use of strategies to open occluded arteries in Acute Coronary Syndromes (GUSTO-IIb) trial. Circulation 100:14–20, 1999.
20. Cannon CP, Gibson CM, Lambrew CT, et al: Relationship of symptom-onset-to-balloon time and door-to-balloon time with mortality in patients undergoing angioplasty for acute myocardial infarction. JAMA 283:2941–2947, 2000.
21. Antman EM, Hand M, Armstrong PW, et al: 2007 Focused Update of the ACC/AHA 2004 Guidelines for the Management of Patients With ST-Elevation Myocardial Infarction: A report of the American College of Cardiology/American Heart Association Task Force on Practice Guidelines: Developed in collaboration With the Canadian Cardiovascular Society endorsed by the American Academy of Family Physicians: 2007 Writing Group to Review New Evidence and Update the ACC/AHA 2004 Guidelines for the Management of Patients With ST-Elevation Myocardial Infarction, Writing on Behalf of the 2004 Writing Committee. Circulation 117:296–329, 2008.
22. Weiss ES, Chang DD, Joyce DL, et al: Optimal timing of coronary artery bypass after acute myocardial infarction: A review of California discharge data. J Thorac Cardiovasc Surg 135:503–511, 511.e1–e3, 2008.
23. White HD, Assmann SF, Sanborn TA, et al: Comparison of percutaneous coronary intervention and coronary artery bypass grafting after acute myocardial infarction complicated by cardiogenic shock: Results from the Should We Emergently Revascularize Occluded Coronaries for Cardiogenic Shock (SHOCK) trial. Circulation 112:1992–2001, 2005.
24. Loop FD, Lytle BW, Cosgrove DM, et al: Influence of the internal-mammary-artery graft on 10-year survival and other cardiac events. N Engl J Med 314:1–6, 1986.
25. Holmes DR Jr, Kim LJ, Brooks MM, et al: The effect of coronary artery bypass grafting on specific causes of long-term mortality in the Bypass Angioplasty Revascularization Investigation. J Thorac Cardiovasc Surg 134:38–46, 46.e1, 2007.
26. Lopes RD, Hafley GE, Allen KB, et al: Endoscopic versus open vein-graft harvesting in coronary-artery bypass surgery. N Engl J Med 361:235–244, 2009.
27. Bergsma TM, Grandjean JG, Voors AA, et al: Low recurrence of angina pectoris after coronary artery bypass graft surgery with bilateral internal thoracic and right gastroepiploic arteries. Circulation 97:2402–2405, 1998.
28. Myers WO, Blackstone EH, Davis K, et al: CASS Registry long-term surgical survival. Coronary Artery Surgery Study. J Am Coll Cardiol 33:488–498, 1999.
29. Cowan KN, Teague L, Sue SC, et al: Vacuum-assisted wound closure of deep sternal infections in high-risk patients after cardiac surgery. Ann Thorac Surg 80:2205–2212, 2005.
30. Mangano CM, Diamondstone LS, Ramsay JG, et al: Renal dysfunction after myocardial revascularization: Risk factors, adverse outcomes, and hospital resource utilization. The Multicenter

Study of Perioperative Ischemia Research Group. Ann Intern Med 128:194–203, 1998.

**31.** Peduzzi P, Kamina A, Detre K: Twenty-two-year follow-up in the VA Cooperative Study of Coronary Artery Bypass Surgery for Stable Angina. Am J Cardiol 81:1393–1399, 1998.

**32.** Puskas JD, Kilgo PD, Lattouf OM, et al: Off-pump coronary bypass provides reduced mortality and morbidity and equivalent 10-year survival. Ann Thorac Surg 86:1139–1146, 2008.

**33.** Puskas JD, Thourani VH, Kilgo P, et al: Off-pump coronary artery bypass disproportionately benefits high-risk patients. Ann Thorac Surg 88:1142–1147, 2009.

**34.** Chu D, Bakaeen FG, Dao TK, et al: On-pump versus off-pump coronary artery bypass grafting in a cohort of 63,000 patients. Ann Thorac Surg 87:1820–1827, 2009.

**35.** Shroyer AL, Grover FL, Hattler B, et al: On-pump versus off-pump coronary-artery bypass surgery. N Engl J Med 361:1827–1837, 2009.

**36.** Patel NC, Deodhar AP, Grayson AD, et al: Neurological outcomes in coronary surgery: Independent effect of avoiding cardiopulmonary bypass. Ann Thorac Surg 74:400–406, 2002.

**37.** Hammon JW, Stump DA, Butterworth JF, et al: Coronary artery bypass grafting with single cross-clamp results in fewer persistent neuropsychological deficits than multiple clamp or off-pump coronary artery bypass grafting. Ann Thorac Surg 84:1174–1179, 2007.

**38.** Kettering K: Minimally invasive direct coronary artery bypass grafting: A meta-analysis. J Cardiovasc Surg (Torino) 49:793–800, 2008.

**39.** Bonatti J, Schachner T, Bonaros N, et al: Effectiveness and safety of total endoscopic left internal mammary artery bypass graft to the left anterior descending artery. Am J Cardiol 104:1684–1688, 2009.

**40.** Oehlinger A, Bonaros N, Schachner T, et al: Robotic endoscopic left internal mammary artery harvesting: What have we learned after 100 cases? Ann Thorac Surg 83:1030–1034, 2007.

**41.** Bridges CR, Horvath KA, Nugent WC, et al: The Society of Thoracic Surgeons practice guideline series: Transmyocardial laser revascularization. Ann Thorac Surg 77:1494–1502, 2004.

**42.** Gopaldas RR, Chu D, Dao TK, et al: Predictors of surgical mortality and discharge status after coronary artery bypass grafting in patients 80 years and older. Am J Surg 198:633–638, 2009.

**43.** Edwards FH, Carey JS, Grover FL, et al: Impact of gender on coronary bypass operative mortality. Ann Thorac Surg 66:125–131, 1998.

**44.** Hartz RS, Rao AV, Plomondon ME, et al: Effects of race, with or without gender, on operative mortality after coronary artery bypass grafting: A study using The Society of Thoracic Surgeons National Database. Ann Thorac Surg 71:512–520, 2001.

**45.** Puskas JD, Edwards FH, Pappas PA, et al: Off-pump techniques benefit men and women and narrow the disparity in mortality after coronary bypass grafting. Ann Thorac Surg 84:1447–1456, 2007.

**46.** Litmathe J, Kurt M, Feindt P, et al: The impact of pre- and postoperative renal dysfunction on outcome of patients undergoing coronary artery bypass grafting (CABG). Thorac Cardiovasc Surg 57:460–463, 2009.

**47.** Szczech LA, Reddan DN, Owen WF, et al: Differential survival after coronary revascularization procedures among patients with renal insufficiency. Kidney Int 60:292–299, 2001.

**48.** van Straten AH, Soliman Hamad MA, van Zundert AA, et al: Preoperative renal function as a predictor of survival after coronary artery bypass grafting: Comparison with a matched general population. J Thorac Cardiovasc Surg 138:971–976, 2009.

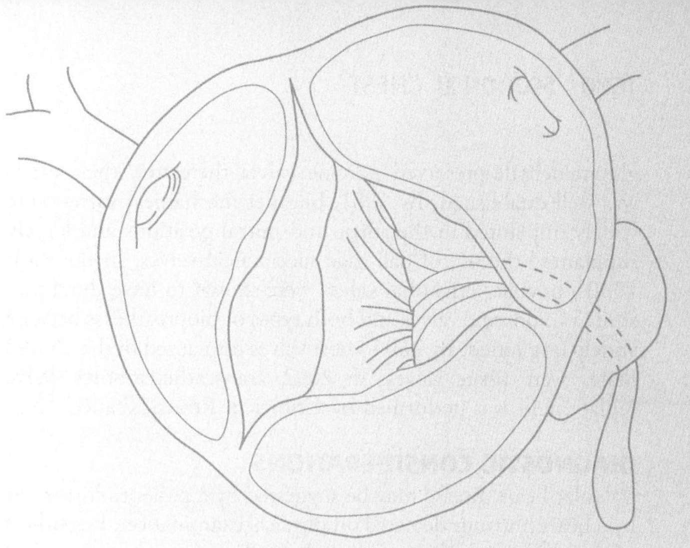

CHAPTER 61

# ACQUIRED HEART DISEASE: VALVULAR

David A. Fullerton and Alden H. Harken



Stenotic or regurgitant cardiac valves create hemodynamic demands on one or both ventricles of the heart. The compensatory mechanisms of the ventricles permit the heart to tolerate these lesions for varying periods of time, sometimes years, before surgical intervention is required. Ultimately, however, significant valvular lesions produce systolic and/or diastolic ventricular dysfunction, leading to heart failure. As a general rule, surgery for stenotic valve lesions may be deferred until the patient develops symptoms. Regurgitant valve lesions, however, may produce significant ventricular dysfunction before symptoms develop; therefore, surgery in patients who do not have symptoms may be indicated. Among the heart's valves, the aortic and mitral valves are the most likely to acquire disease; therefore, this chapter focuses on diseases of the aortic and mitral valves.

## HISTORICAL PERSPECTIVE

Heart failure from mitral stenosis was well recognized by the late 19th century, and efforts at surgical correction began well before the heart-lung machine was available.[1] In 1897, Samways suggested (but never acted on) the possibility of dilating the stenotic mitral valve. Based on his postmortem studies of rheumatic heart disease in London, Brunton in 1902 proposed surgical intervention for mitral stenosis by passing a dilator through the wall of the left ventricle retrograde into the mitral valve orifice. His proposal was shunned by London physicians, and Brunton never tried this maneuver. The concept, however, was applied 20 years later in Boston when the first report of successful surgical correction of mitral stenosis appeared in 1923. Cutler and Levine reported successful relief of mitral stenosis by incision of the valve with a knife introduced through an apical left ventriculotomy. In 1925, Soutter performed the first successful closed mitral commissurotomy at the London Hospital by introducing his index finger through the left atrial appendage. Despite Soutter's success, he received no more patient referrals, and another 20 years elapsed before the procedure became widespread. In June 1948, Bailey in Philadelphia and Harken in Boston each performed a successful closed mitral commissurotomy. Thereafter, it became widely used to treat mitral stenosis.

By the mid-1970s, the closed technique was supplanted by open mitral commissurotomy. Although closed mitral commissurotomy achieved good palliation of mitral stenosis for its era, open mitral commissurotomy offered several advantages. First, the valvuloplasty could be performed under direct vision. The primary reason for failure of closed mitral commissurotomy was residual stenosis, not restenosis. In up to 75% of patients, the subvalvular apparatus of the mitral valve contributes significantly to the stenosis. The open technique permitted precise and maximal division of fused commissures, as well as fused chordae. In addition, calcium could be sharply débrided from the valve, and any residual mitral insufficiency could be corrected at the time of operation. Finally, the closed technique had the disadvantage of potentially dislodging a left atrial thrombus, resulting in intraoperative embolization and stroke. Today, however, open mitral commissurotomy is rarely performed; it was supplanted by balloon mitral valvuloplasty by the mid-1990s.

Surgical attempts to correct aortic stenosis also began in the early 20th century.[1] In 1912, Tuffier, in Paris, unsuccessfully attempted transaortic digital dilation of a stenotic aortic valve. In Charleston, South Carolina, in 1948, Smithy performed the first successful aortic valvotomy in a 21-year-old woman from Ohio. Smithy died later that same year of aortic stenosis at the age of 34 years. Three years later, in Philadelphia, Bailey reported successful aortic valvotomy by insertion of a mechanical dilator across the stenotic valve of patients to open fused commissures. In 1952, Hufnagel and Harvey at Georgetown University placed the first prosthetic ball valve into the descending aorta of a patient with aortic insufficiency. Surgery on the aortic valve under direct vision required the development of cardiopulmonary bypass by Gibbon in 1954. In 1955, Swann performed the first successful aortic valvotomy using hypothermia and inflow occlusion. Initially, open aortic valve operations were limited to aortic valve commissurotomy and débridement of calcified aortic valve leaflets. Harken, in Boston, in 1960, and Starr, in Portland, Oregon, in 1963, however, reported replacement of the aortic valve with a prosthesis. In 1962, Ross in London successfully performed orthotopic homograft valve replacement. In 1967, Ross performed the first pulmonary autograft procedure (Ross procedure) for correction of aortic stenosis. In the mid-1960s, stent-mounted porcine aortic valves were implanted, but these formaldehyde-fixed valves degenerated rapidly. In 1974, Carpentier, in Paris, reported superior longevity of the glutaraldehyde-preserved porcine valve; thereafter, their usage was well established. By 1981, bileaflet mechanical valves were widely implanted in the aortic and mitral positions and largely supplanted the use of ball cage mechanical valves. In the mid-1990s, bovine pericardial valves were shown to have durability similar to porcine valves and both types of bioprostheses became widely implanted. By 2004, most valves implanted in the United States were tissue valves. In 2002, transcatheter aortic valve replacement was performed by Cribier in Rouen, France.

## DIAGNOSTIC CONSIDERATIONS

Valvular heart disease may be suggested by a patient's history or by a heart murmur detected on physical examination. Regardless of the valve lesion in question, echocardiography should be used to assess the severity of the stenosis, regurgitation, or both. Information available from the echocardiogram includes definition of valve anatomy, assessment of ventricular contractile function, determination of the magnitude of valve regurgitation using color flow Doppler imaging, and determination of the severity of valve stenosis.

Transthoracic echocardiography is noninvasive and may provide the necessary information. If more information is needed, transesophageal echocardiography may provide better definition of aortic and mitral valve anatomy; it is also a more sensitive imaging modality for the detection of mitral regurgitation.

Although most valve lesions may be accurately diagnosed by echocardiography, cardiac catheterization may be necessary to confirm the diagnosis or to provide additional information pertaining to ventricular function. Before surgery, it may be appropriate to exclude the presence of coronary artery disease. Mitral or aortic valve areas may be determined at cardiac catheterization using the Gorlin formula,[2] which permits calculation of the valve area, as follows:

$$\text{Valve area} = \text{flow across the valve}/(C \times [\sqrt{\text{mean transvalvular gradient}}])$$

where C is an empirical constant, 44.5 for the aortic valve and 38 for the mitral valve.

## MITRAL VALVE

### Surgical Anatomy of the Mitral Valve

The normal function of the mitral valve is dependent on coordinated interaction of the mitral valve apparatus, which includes the mitral valve annulus, valve leaflets, valve chordae tendineae, and left ventricular papillary muscles. The normal mitral valve has two leaflets, the anterior (or aortic) and posterior or (mural) leaflet. Two papillary muscles arise from the left ventricular wall, the posterior (or posteromedial) and anterior (or anterolateral). Each leaflet of the mitral valve is connected to each of the papillary muscles by tendons, the chordae tendineae.

The leaflets are suspended from the mitral annulus, a collagenous structure that encircles the orifice between the left atrium and ventricle. Although the two leaflets have approximately the same surface area, they have different shapes (Fig. 61-1). The anterior leaflet is rectangular. Its base is attached to the mitral annulus anteriorly and the width of the base is approximately one third the circumference of the mitral annulus.

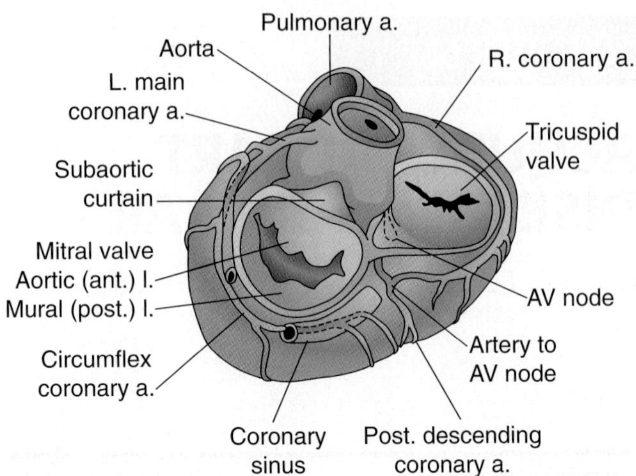


**FIGURE 61-1** Anatomy of the mitral valve as it relates to other cardiac structures. Important surgical landmarks include the relationship of the mitral valve to the aortic valve, circumflex coronary artery, and atrioventricular (AV) node. (From Buchanan SA, Tribble CG: Reoperative mitral replacement. In Kaiser LR, Kron IL, Spray TL [eds]: Mastery of cardiothoracic surgery. Philadelphia, 1998, Lippincott-Raven, p 351.)

This attachment of the anterior leaflet to the mitral annulus extends to the aortic annulus through fibrous tissue, providing fibrous continuity between the aortic and mitral valves; the left ventricular side of the anterior leaflet of the mitral valve is visible immediately as the surgeon looks down through the aortic valve into the left ventricle. The posterior leaflet is rectangular and its attachment to the mitral annulus extends for approximately two thirds of the circumference of the mitral annulus. The two leaflets are separated by two distinct commissures.

There are three important surgical landmarks (see Fig. 61-1). First, the circumflex coronary artery runs along the epicardial surface of the heart overlying the posterior mitral annulus. Only millimeters of left atrial muscle separate the artery from the annulus, making it susceptible to injury during mitral valve surgery. Second, the aortic valve is in close approximation to the anterior leaflet of the mitral valve (aortomitral continuity). The noncoronary leaflet of the aortic valve is therefore susceptible to injury during mitral surgery. Third, the atrioventricular node is located deep to the posteromedial commissure of the mitral valve.

### Mitral Stenosis

#### Causes

Rheumatic fever is the principal cause of mitral stenosis, and approximately two thirds of patients with rheumatic mitral stenosis are female. Rheumatic fever usually occurs in childhood or adolescence (mean age, 8 to 12 years) and creates an inflammatory infiltration of the myocardium and valves. Perhaps because the disease afflicts young people and many years pass before symptoms are manifest, a prior history of rheumatic fever is often difficult to confirm. As the mitral valve heals after acute rheumatic fever, the mitral apparatus may become deformed slowly and the patient typically remains asymptomatic for at least 10 years. Symptoms most commonly appear during the patient's third or fourth decade of life. Healing of the inflammation from rheumatic fever ultimately causes the cusps and commissures of the mitral valve to thicken and fuse, with concomitant fusion and shortening of the chordae tendineae. The structure of the valve apparatus then calcifies and narrows, becoming funnel-shaped. Such thickening and fusion of the valve not only creates stenosis but also often prevent complete closure of the valve. Of all patients with rheumatic mitral valve disease, approximately 50% have combined mitral stenosis and mitral regurgitation.

Other causes of mitral stenosis that are far less common than rheumatic fever include malignant carcinoid, systemic lupus erythematosus, and rheumatoid arthritis. Rarely, congenital malformation of the valve may cause mitral stenosis, and congenital mitral stenosis is almost never an isolated congenital cardiac lesion.

## Pathophysiology

The cross-sectional area of the normal mitral valve is 4 to 6 $cm^2$. A mitral valve area of 2 $cm^2$ is considered moderate mitral stenosis and an area of 1 $cm^2$ is considered severe mitral stenosis. Under normal conditions, there is no pressure gradient across the mitral valve and the left atrial pressure is usually less than 15 mm Hg. As the mitral valve becomes more narrowed, an increasing pressure gradient is required to move the blood across the mitral valve from the left atrium into the left ventricle during diastole; a transvalvular gradient of 10 mm Hg indicates severe mitral stenosis. The significance of the transvalvular gradient is that left atrial pressure progressively increases as the mitral valve becomes more stenotic. In turn, the increased left atrial pressure is transmitted retrograde into the pulmonary veins, pulmonary capillaries, and ultimately pulmonary arteries. A left atrial pressure of approximately 25 mm Hg increases pulmonary capillary pressure enough to produce pulmonary edema.

The severity of obstruction across the valve is determined by the transvalvular gradient and flow rate across the valve. The flow rate is a function of cardiac output and heart rate; because flow across the mitral valve occurs during diastole and diastole is shortened as heart rate increases, a faster heart rate at any given cardiac output increases the transvalvular gradient and raises left atrial pressure. The contribution of the atrial contraction (kick) to cardiac output is particularly important in mitral stenosis; it accomplishes as much as 30% of the transvalvular gradient. Thus, the onset of symptoms is generally associated with exertional activities or loss of the atrial kick with the onset of atrial fibrillation.

To maintain adequate left ventricular filling across a 1-$cm^2$ valve, for example, a pressure gradient of 20 mm Hg is required. A normal left ventricular end-diastolic pressure of 5 mm Hg results in a left atrial pressure of 25 mm Hg. Left atrial pressure rises further if flow rate across the valve increases (increased cardiac output), transit time across the valve is shortened (decreased diastolic time), or atrial kick is lost (atrial fibrillation).

Pulmonary hypertension is an important component of the pathophysiology of mitral stenosis and, when severe, may dominate the clinical picture. At least three pathophysiologic mechanisms contribute to the pulmonary hypertension seen in long-standing mitral valvular disease: (1) increased left atrial pressure transmitted retrograde into the arterial circulation; (2) vascular remodeling of the pulmonary vasculature in response to chronic obstruction to pulmonary venous drainage (fixed component); and (3) pulmonary arterial vasoconstriction (reactive component).

## Diagnosis

**Symptoms** Dyspnea is the principal symptom of mitral stenosis. Dyspnea is typically brought on with exertion or is associated with the abrupt onset of atrial fibrillation. The increased cardiac output or heart rate with exertion or the loss of atrial kick and tachycardia with atrial fibrillation result in an increased transvalvular gradient. This in turn increases left atrial pressure and the pulmonary veins and capillaries become engorged, producing the sensation of dyspnea and promoting pulmonary edema. If the left atrium enlargement is sufficient to compress surrounding structures, the patient may complain of dysphagia or hoarseness. Marked elevation in left atrial pressure may produce hemoptysis.

**Physical Examination** The left ventricle is typically normal in size and the apex is therefore not displaced. The murmur of mitral stenosis is best heard at the apex. It is a low-pitched, rumbling diastolic murmur that decreases with inspiration and increases during expiration; it may be markedly decreased by the Valsalva maneuver. An opening snap precedes the murmur, is heard at the apex, and represents the completed excursion of the mitral valve leaflets. If the mitral leaflets are stiff or calcified, an opening snap may not be heard. In patients with pulmonary hypertension, signs of elevated right ventricular and central venous pressure may dominate the clinical picture. Physical findings, such as distended neck veins, hepatomegaly, ascites, and peripheral edema, combined with a loud pulmonary valve component of the second heart sound ($P_2$) heard on cardiac auscultation, suggest significant pulmonary hypertension.

### Diagnostic Tests

***Chest Radiography*** Several findings may be noted on the chest radiograph. The cardiac silhouette may be normal in size, but the left atrium is enlarged. The enlarged left atrium may be seen as a double density behind the right atrium on the poster anterior projection or it may be seen to displace the left mainstem bronchus superiorly. On the lateral projection, the enlarged left atrium may displace the esophagus posteriorly. Calcification of the mitral leaflets or the mitral annulus may be seen. Pulmonary venous hypertension should be suspected when the pulmonary arteries are enlarged and there is cephalization of pulmonary blood flow.

***Echocardiography*** Echocardiography is the principal modality used to confirm the diagnosis. Using the echocardiogram, the mitral valve area may be determined by two mechanisms. First, the mitral valve area may be determined directly from the echocardiogram by planimetry. Second, measurement of the velocity of blood flow across the valve by Doppler echocardiography permits calculation of the transvalvular gradient. Because the transvalvular gradient persists longer with greater stenosis of the valve, the time required for the transvalvular gradient to decline may be measured; this is referred to as the pressure half-time. The mitral valve area may then be calculated using the following formula:

$$\text{Mitral valve area} = 220/(\text{pressure half-time})$$

***Cardiac Catheterization*** Although rarely necessary, mitral stenosis may also be diagnosed by cardiac catheterization. However, before undergoing surgical correction of mitral stenosis, cardiac catheterization and coronary angiography should be considered in patients with a history of angina and in those who are older than approximately 50 years to exclude occlusive coronary artery disease. At the time of cardiac catheterization, left atrial pressure may be determined directly (by transatrial puncture) or inferred from pulmonary capillary wedge pressure. Simultaneous measurement of the left ventricular diastolic pressure permits calculation of the transvalvular gradient; a transvalvular gradient higher than 10 mm Hg is consistent with significant mitral stenosis. Using the Gorlin formula, the mitral valve area (MVA) may be calculated as follows:

$$MVA = F/(38 \times [\sqrt{\Delta P}])$$

where $\Delta P$ is the mean diastolic transvalvular gradient (in mm Hg), F is the mean diastolic mitral flow in milliliters per second (derived from the measured cardiac output and determination of diastolic duration), and 38 is a constant.

### Natural History

Currently, the natural history of mitral stenosis is impossible to know precisely because of successful surgical intervention. Data collected from the era before widespread surgery for mitral stenosis, however, have indicated that after diagnosis, the mean survival of patients with asymptomatic mitral stenosis was 15 to 20 years; on the other hand, patients with symptoms had a mean survival of only 2 to 7 years.[3] Left atrial distention predisposes to atrial fibrillation and its associated intra-atrial thrombus formation. Up to 20% of patients with mitral stenosis and atrial fibrillation may sustain systemic embolization, especially strokes.

### Treatment

The symptom-free patient in sinus rhythm requires only prophylaxis against bacterial endocarditis. When symptoms appear, medical treatment of mitral stenosis includes diuretics to lower left atrial pressure and efforts to maintain sinus rhythm with beta-blocking agents or calcium channel blocking agents. Digoxin may be helpful in controlling ventricular rate in patients who do go into atrial fibrillation. Patients in atrial fibrillation may require chronic anticoagulation with warfarin (Coumadin) therapy to lower the risk for systemic embolization.

Mechanical intervention for mitral stenosis should be considered when patients develop symptoms, evidence of pulmonary hypertension appears, or the mitral valve area is reduced to approximately 1 cm$^2$. Other conditions that should prompt surgical consideration include systemic embolization, worsening pulmonary hypertension, and endocarditis. The options for mechanical intervention for mitral stenosis include balloon mitral valvuloplasty, open surgical mitral valvuloplasty (commissurotomy), and mitral valve replacement.

**Balloon Mitral Valvuloplasty** First performed in 1984, balloon mitral valvuloplasty has become the treatment of choice for select patients with mitral stenosis.[4] Echocardiography may be used to determine patients considered to be good candidates, including those with pliable valve leaflets but without significant valvular calcification or deformation of the chordae tendineae. Contraindications to this procedure include the presence of moderate mitral regurgitation, thickening and calcification of the mitral leaflets, and scarring and calcification of the subvalvular apparatus.[5] Performed in the cardiac catheterization suite under fluoroscopic guidance, the technique entails advancement of one or two balloon catheters across the interatrial septum and inflation of the balloon within the stenotic mitral valve.

Balloon mitral valvuloplasty has provided good short-term and intermediate-term results in appropriately selected patients. Balloon inflation should increase the mitral valve area to approximately 2 cm$^2$. This increase in mitral valve area is usually associated with a significant decline in left atrial pressure and transvalvular gradient and with at least a 20% increase in cardiac output. The mortality rate associated with balloon mitral valvuloplasty is 0.5% to 2%. Other risks associated with this procedure include systemic embolism, cardiac perforation, and creation of mitral regurgitation; the risk of each of these complications is approximately 1% to 2%. Increased pulmonary vascular resistance has been shown to decline after successful balloon valvuloplasty. Approximately 10% of patients are left with a residual interatrial septal defect. Three years after balloon valvuloplasty, at least 66% of patients are free of subsequent intervention. In appropriately selected patients, the results of balloon valvuloplasty compare favorably with those of surgical valvuloplasty.[6]

**Open Mitral Commissurotomy** Open surgical valvuloplasty (commissurotomy) is not commonly performed and has largely been supplanted by balloon mitral valvuloplasty. However, the procedure permits careful examination of the mitral valve and chordae tendineae under direct visualization and removal of left atrial thrombus. Left atrial thrombus typically originates in the left atrial appendage; this open procedure permits surgical closure of the orifice of the appendage from within the left atrium, thereby reducing the risk for subsequent embolization. The surgeon may then sharply divide fused commissures and leaflets, mobilize scarred chordae, and débride calcification. Furthermore, reconstruction of the valve may eliminate preexistent mitral regurgitation. The presence of significant mitral regurgitation, however, should prompt consideration of mitral valve replacement.

The mortality rate associated with open mitral valvuloplasty is less than 2%.[6] When performed in appropriately selected patients, the freedom from subsequent mitral valve intervention is approximately 75% at 5 years. Nonetheless, because of less procedure-related morbidity, balloon valvuloplasty is the procedure of choice.

**Mitral Valve Replacement** The mitral valve should be replaced when valvuloplasty is precluded by dense calcification of the leaflets or subvalvular apparatus or because of concomitant mitral regurgitation. Regardless of whether a tissue or mechanical prosthesis is implanted, efforts should be made to preserve the continuity between the left ventricular apex and mitral annulus provided by the chordae tendineae. This may be accomplished by preservation of the chordae tendineae at the time of mitral valve replacement.

The contribution of the mitral apparatus to overall left ventricular function is now well appreciated.[7] A mechanical advantage is afforded the left ventricle by the connection of its apex (via the papillary muscles) to the mitral annulus through the chordae tendineae; elimination of this connection by removal of the entire mitral apparatus leads to loss of left ventricular function. Convincing data have demonstrated that preservation of at least some of the chordae tendineae at the time of mitral valve replacement results in better long-term left ventricular function than mitral valve replacement with chordal separation. Therefore, if mitral valve replacement is required, efforts should be made to preserve the posterior and, in some cases, anterior leaflets of the native mitral valve.

The operative mortality rate associated with mitral valve replacement for mitral stenosis is 2% to 10%.[8] Operative mortality is increased with advanced age and the presence of coronary disease. Pulmonary hypertension typically resolves after valve replacement, but several weeks or months may be required. The 5-year survival rate after replacement is 70% to 90%.[6,9]

## Mitral Regurgitation

### Causes

Competency of the mitral valve requires an intact mitral valve apparatus. Abnormalities of any component of the mitral valve apparatus may produce mitral regurgitation—the mitral leaflets, chordae tendineae, mitral valve annulus, or papillary muscles. Worldwide, rheumatic fever remains the most common cause of mitral regurgitation; it results in deformity and retraction of the leaflets and shortening of the chordae. The leaflets may be perforated by trauma or infective endocarditis. Calcification of the mitral annulus may result in annular rigidity and prevent valve closure, and mitral annular dilation resultant to left ventricular dilation may similarly preclude leaflet apposition during systole.

Chordal rupture may result from trauma, endocarditis, rheumatic fever, or diseases of collagen formation; chordae to the posterior leaflet rupture more frequently than those to the anterior leaflet. Mitral valve prolapse is found in approximately 2% of the U.S. population and up to 5% of patients with mitral valve prolapse develop mitral regurgitation secondary to chordal elongation or rupture. Coronary artery disease may cause infarction of the papillary muscle, resulting in mitral regurgitation. Infarction in the distribution of the anterior descending coronary artery may necrose the anterolateral papillary muscle, whereas the posteromedial muscle may infarct if blood flow through the posterior descending coronary artery is interrupted. Mitral regurgitation caused by myocardial infarction typically presents as a new murmur several days after infarction.

### Pathophysiology

The regurgitant mitral valve offers an alternative route whereby blood may exit the left ventricle. During isovolumetric contraction and systole, blood is preferentially ejected into the low-pressure left atrium. The volume of the regurgitant flow (regurgitant fraction) is dependent on the size of the regurgitant orifice and pressure gradient between the left ventricle and left atrium.

Increased left ventricular afterload or decreased forward left ventricular stroke volume increases left ventricular pressure and thereby increases the pressure gradient between the left ventricle and atrium. The mitral valve annulus is enlarged by dilation of the left ventricle. Therefore, the size of the regurgitant orifice is increased by diminished left ventricular contractility, increased left ventricular preload, and increased afterload. Because the valve leaks during systole, the volume of regurgitant flow also increases as heart rate (number of systoles per minute) increases.

The compensatory mechanism whereby the left ventricle adapts to maintain an adequate systemic blood flow (forward cardiac output) is volume overload; it must pump the combined volume of systemic and regurgitant flows (Fig. 61-2). Volume overload leads to cardiac dilation as well as left ventricular hypertrophy. Because the left ventricle ejects into the reduced resistance of the left atrium, parameters of systolic function (ejection fraction) are increased in mitral regurgitation. As with aortic insufficiency, however, the left ventricle ultimately fails with chronic volume overload. Normal parameters of systolic function indicate significant contractile dysfunction of the left ventricle. An ejection fraction less than 40% in the setting of mitral regurgitation indicates significant left ventricular contractile dysfunction.

As in mitral stenosis, left atrial hypertension results from mitral regurgitation. This pressure is transmitted retrograde into the pulmonary circulation and, if high enough, produces pulmonary hypertension. The magnitude of the left atrial pressure is a function of the compliance of the left atrium. Normal or low compliance of the left atrium, such as that which may occur in acute mitral regurgitation, results in a relatively rapid rise in left atrial pressure. On the other hand, chronic left atrial volume overload that develops slowly may create significant enlargement of a compliant left atrium with relatively low left atrial pressure.

### Diagnosis

**Symptoms** The symptoms of mitral regurgitation are those of heart failure—shortness of breath, dyspnea on exertion, orthopnea, pulmonary edema, and diminished exercise tolerance. Symptoms are determined by the degree of mitral regurgitation, rate of its progression, degree of pulmonary hypertension, and magnitude of left ventricular contractile dysfunction. For example, patients with mild mitral regurgitation may remain symptom-free for most of their lives. At the other extreme, patients with acute, severe mitral regurgitation, such as that which may occur with endocarditis or a ruptured chordae tendineae, may have pulmonary edema and require urgent surgery. The onset of atrial fibrillation impairs the patient's functional status, but not to the same degree as with mitral stenosis. With chronic moderate to severe mitral regurgitation, patients may be symptom-free for long periods. Lack of symptoms, however, may be deceiving because the contractile function of the left ventricle may be slowly deteriorating from volume overload. When symptoms occur, left ventricular contractile dysfunction may be irreversible.

**Physical Examination** On cardiac auscultation, a holosystolic murmur is heard best at the apex and radiates to the axilla and left scapular region. The pulmonary examination may be significant for rales and bronchospasm caused by increased pulmonary interstitial fluid. Mitral valve pathology should be considered in the differential diagnosis of patients with adult-onset asthma.

#### Diagnostic Tests

***Electrocardiography*** The electrocardiogram is notable for left atrial enlargement and, frequently, atrial fibrillation.

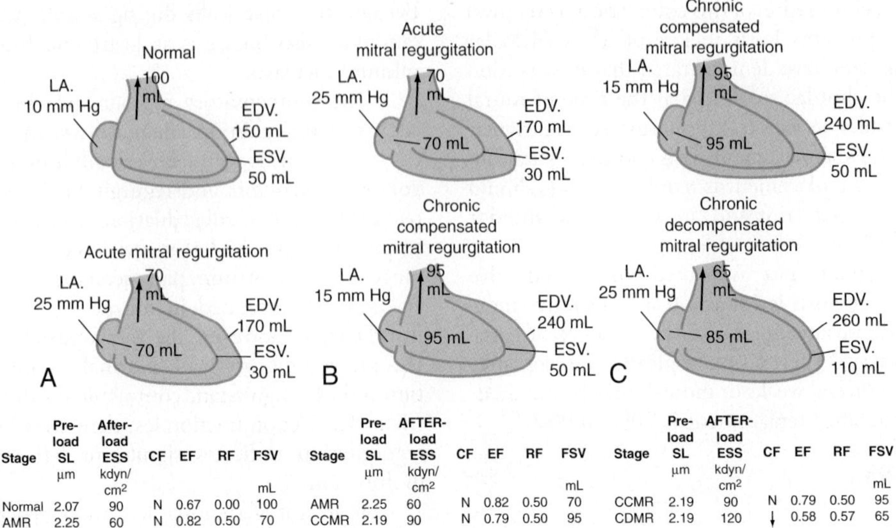


| Stage | Preload SL µm | Afterload ESS kdyn/cm² | CF | EF | RF | FSV mL |
|---|---|---|---|---|---|---|
| Normal | 2.07 | 90 | N | 0.67 | 0.00 | 100 |
| AMR | 2.25 | 60 | N | 0.82 | 0.50 | 70 |

| Stage | Preload SL µm | AFTERload ESS kdyn/cm² | CF | EF | RF | FSV mL |
|---|---|---|---|---|---|---|
| AMR | 2.25 | 60 | N | 0.82 | 0.50 | 70 |
| CCMR | 2.19 | 90 | N | 0.79 | 0.50 | 95 |

| Stage | Preload SL µm | AFTERload ESS kdyn/cm² | CF | EF | RF | FSV mL |
|---|---|---|---|---|---|---|
| CCMR | 2.19 | 90 | N | 0.79 | 0.50 | 95 |
| CDMR | 2.19 | 120 | ↓ | 0.58 | 0.57 | 65 |

**FIGURE 61-2** Pathophysiology and compensation for acute and chronic mitral regurgitation. **A,** With acute mitral regurgitation, end-diastolic volume (EDV) increases from 150 to 170 mL. Because the left ventricle ejects blood into both the aorta and the left atrium (LA), end-systolic volume (ESV) decreases from 50 to 30 mL. The ejection fraction therefore increases acutely but, because a significant percentage is ejected into the LA, the volume of blood flow into the aorta (forward stroke volume, FSV) decreases from 100 to 70 mL. The regurgitant volume into the LA increases LA pressure. **B,** Myocardial compensation for chronic mitral regurgitation includes eccentric left ventricular hypertrophy. Left ventricular EDV increases from 170 to 240 mL. The larger ventricle results in an increased total stroke volume as well as FSV. Enlargement of the LA increases in capacitance, which accommodates the regurgitant volume at a lower pressure. The left ventricular ejection fraction is supernormal. **C,** Ultimately, the heart decompensates, and the contractile force (CF) of the left ventricle declines; the end-systolic volume increases from 50 to 110 mL. FSV declines. The left ventricle dilates, which further compromises the ability of the mitral valve apparatus to close; the regurgitant volume increases. The ejection fraction remains above normal until contractile function declines further. *EF,* Ejection fraction; *ESS,* end-systolic stress; *RF,* regurgitant fraction; *SL,* sarcomere length. (From Carabello BA: Mitral regurgitation: Basic pathophysiologic principles. Mod Concepts Cardiovasc Dis 57:53, 1988.)

***Chest Radiography*** The chest radiograph may be significant for cardiomegaly and left atrial enlargement. Pulmonary venous hypertension may manifest as cephalization of pulmonary blood flow and pulmonary edema.

***Echocardiography*** The diagnosis is confirmed by echocardiography. Transesophageal echocardiography is particularly effective for providing an anatomic explanation for the regurgitation, such as perforated leaflets, poor leaflet coaptation, or ruptured chordae. Doppler echocardiography reveals a high-velocity jet of regurgitant blood flow into the left atrium during systole.

By convention, the determination of the severity of mitral regurgitation is semiquantitative. The severity of the regurgitation is gauged as a function of the distance from the mitral annulus that the jet can be visualized (e.g., into the pulmonary veins) and the width of the regurgitant jet. The regurgitation is scored subjectively on a scale from 1 (mild) to 4 (severe). The chronicity of the regurgitation may be inferred from the size of the left atrium; an enlarged left atrium suggests chronic mitral regurgitation. Contrast ventriculography, performed at cardiac catheterization, may similarly demonstrate mitral regurgitation during systole.

### Natural History

The natural history of the disease is variable, determined by the cause of mitral regurgitation, regurgitant volume, and magnitude of left ventricular systolic dysfunction. Patients with mild mitral regurgitation typically remain symptom-free for years and rarely go on to develop severe mitral regurgitation. As is the situation with most valve diseases, the natural history of mitral regurgitation is obscure because surgical intervention has effectively altered this history. In the presurgical era, however, approximately 80% of patients with severe mitral regurgitation survived 5 years and 60% survived 10 years.[10,11] Patients with combined mitral stenosis and regurgitation had a worse prognosis, with a 5-year survival rate of only 67%.

### Treatment

The cornerstone of medical management is diuresis and afterload reduction with angiotensin-converting enzyme (ACE) inhibitors. The importance of afterload reduction cannot be overemphasized. Because blood leaving the left ventricle travels the path of least resistance, lowering systemic vascular resistance increases systemic cardiac output. In the setting of heart failure from acute mitral regurgitation, IV vasodilators (nitroprusside) may be needed. When a patient is stabilized, conversion to oral ACE inhibitors may be achieved. Diuretics function not only to relieve pulmonary edema, but also to reduce left ventricular diameter. The size of the mitral annulus is thereby diminished and the regurgitant fraction reduced.

The indications for surgical intervention include symptoms that persist despite medical management, severe mitral regurgitation in the presence of an identified structural abnormality,

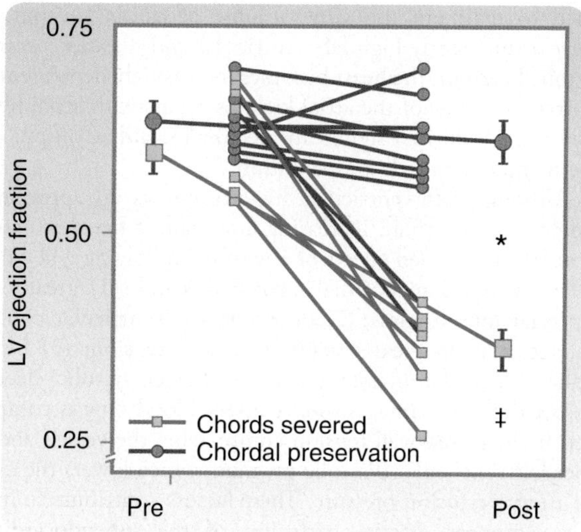


**FIGURE 61-3** Postoperative ejection fraction after mitral valve replacement with *(circles)* and without *(squares)* preservation of the chordae tendineae. The ejection fraction decreases significantly without chords severed but is preserved with choral preservation. (From Roseate JD, Carabello BA, Ushere BW, et al: Mitral valve replacement with and without chordal preservation in patients with chronic mitral regurgitation. Circulation 86:1718–1726, 1992.)

such as a ruptured chorda tendinea, development of pulmonary hypertension, or evidence of deteriorating left ventricular contractile function as determined by echocardiography or contrast ventriculography.

Asymptomatic left ventricular dysfunction may develop insidiously. It may therefore be helpful to follow up closely with serial echocardiograms. Two parameters of left ventricular function are useful in making the decision regarding timing of surgery—ejection fraction (EF) and end-systolic diameter (ESD). Because mitral regurgitation lowers the total impedance against left ventricular ejection, the EF should be supernormal in the presence of normal myocardial contractile function. An EF less than 60% suggests myocardial dysfunction and operative mortality begins to increase.[12] The other useful parameter of left ventricular function is the left ventricular ESD. ESD is less preload-dependent than EF and the information it provides is complementary. When the left ventricular ESD exceeds 45 mm, the prognosis after surgery is worse.[13] Even in the absence of symptoms, therefore, patients should be referred for surgery when the left ventricular EF is less than 60% or when the left ventricular ESD is more than 45 mm.[14]

In those cases, there are two surgical options, mitral valve repair or replacement. When possible, the valve should be repaired. The final decision about which of these options to use is made intraoperatively after valve inspection. Mitral valve repair has several advantages over replacement. First, left ventricular function is better preserved after repair[15,16]; valve repair preserves the continuity between the mitral annulus and ventricular papillary muscle provided by the chordae tendineae, thus providing the left ventricle a mechanical advantage and optimizing its function. When the chordae tendineae are sacrificed during a mitral valve replacement, the postoperative ejection fraction typically decreases (Fig. 61-3). Therefore, even when mitral valve replacement is necessary for mitral regurgitation, the chordae tendineae should be preserved, if possible.[17]

Second, mitral valve replacement subjects the patient to the risks associated with the valve prosthesis, such as thromboembolism and risk for prosthetic valve endocarditis. Bioprosthetic valves may ultimately experience structural deterioration and mechanical prosthetic valves obligate the patient to lifelong anticoagulation with warfarin. After mitral valve repair, patients in sinus rhythm do not require long-term warfarin therapy.

Third, the operative mortality rate associated with mitral valve repair (0 % to 2%) is less than that for replacement (4% to 8%).[6] Long-term survival also appears to be better with repair. These outcomes likely derive from the superior left ventricular function after mitral repair than after replacement.

The operative risks of mitral repair or replacement are increased in the setting of significant left ventricular dysfunction. However, current surgical series have demonstrated excellent results with mitral valve repair, even in patients with severe heart failure and a left ventricular EF below 20%.[18] The functional status of such patients has been significantly improved and the need for hospital admission for treatment of heart failure has been markedly decreased. Preservation of the mitral apparatus at the time of repair is essential to achieve those results.

## AORTIC VALVE

### Surgical Anatomy of the Aortic Valve

The normal aortic valve is composed of three thin pliable leaflets, or cusps, attached to the heart at the junction of the aorta and left ventricle. The leaflets are attached in the three sinuses of Valsalva of the proximal aorta and join together in three commissures, which create the shape of a coronet. Because the coronary arteries arise from two of the three sinuses of Valsalva, the aortic leaflets are named after their respective sinuses as the left coronary leaflet, right coronary leaflet, and noncoronary leaflet. There are two important surgical landmarks. First, the commissure between the left and noncoronary leaflets is positioned over the anterior leaflet of the mitral valve. Second, the commissure between the noncoronary and right coronary leaflets is positioned over the left bundle of His. Injury to this conduction bundle during aortic valve surgery may create heart block (Fig. 61-4).

### Aortic Stenosis

#### Causes

Acquired aortic stenosis usually results from calcification of the aortic valve associated with advanced age. Although the process is usually idiopathic,[19] rheumatic fever may affect the aortic valve in a process similar to that of the mitral valve. In rheumatoid aortic stenosis, inflammation produces adhesions and fusion of the commissures and leaflets, with thickening and calcification. Retraction of the leaflets often makes these valves regurgitant and stenotic. The inflammatory process of rheumatic fever rarely involves the aortic valve alone; it usually involves the mitral valve as well. In idiopathic degenerative or senile aortic stenosis, grossly normal leaflets become calcified as a result of normal leaflet stress at the flexion points, causing leaflet immobility. This calcification may extend down onto the anterior mitral valve leaflet or upward along the aorta, occasionally causing coronary ostial stenosis.

Congenital valvular abnormalities may be clinically significant immediately after birth, as with unicuspid and dome-shaped valves. Patients born with a congenitally bicuspid aortic valve are uncommonly symptomatic in childhood but are prone to develop aortic stenosis early in adulthood. The bicuspid valve produces turbulent flow across the leaflets, leading to fibrosis, calcification, and stiffening. Patients with a bicuspid aortic valve are prone to develop aortic stenosis at an earlier age (fifth and sixth decades of life) than those with a tricuspid valve (seventh, eighth, and ninth decades; Fig. 61-5).

## Pathophysiology

In acquired aortic stenosis, there is a chronic progressive narrowing of the aortic valve. As the valve narrows, the appropriate compensatory response of the left ventricle is hypertrophy. As the ventricle hypertrophies, it becomes stiffer as its compliance decreases; a higher left ventricular end-diastolic pressure is needed to maintain the same volume of cardiac output. To achieve a sufficiently high left ventricular end-diastolic pressure (diastolic loading), the heart becomes increasingly dependent on the atrial kick; loss of the atrial kick, as occurs with atrial fibrillation, may result in a significant decline in cardiac output and acute hemodynamic decompensation.

Although left ventricular hypertrophy is an appropriate biologic response to an increasing afterload, it has detrimental effects. The combined effects of any of the following will culminate in increased myocardial oxygen demand: (1) greater left ventricular muscle mass; (2) decreased left ventricular compliance, resulting in greater ventricular wall tension; (3) higher systolic ventricular pressure; and (4) longer systolic ejection time. At the same time, coronary artery blood flow is compromised by increased wall tension compressing the vessels and by higher left ventricular diastolic pressure, which lowers the coronary artery perfusion pressure. These factors contribute to inadequate coronary arterial perfusion of the subendocardium, leading to chronic ischemia. In turn, chronic ischemia leads to cell death and fibrosis.

Left ventricular hypertrophy may allow the heart to achieve a normal cardiac output under resting conditions.[20] To do so, however, a pressure gradient across the valve is required and, as the aortic valve area becomes smaller, the gradient across the valve from left ventricle to aorta increases. This relationship of flow across the valve, valve area, and transvalvular pressure gradient is expressed in the Gorlin formula,[2] as follows:

$$AVA = F/(44.5 \times [\sqrt{\Delta P}])$$

where ΔP is the mean pressure gradient across the valve, F is aortic valve flow, equal to cardiac output (in mL/min) divided by systolic ejection period (in sec/min), AVA is the aortic valve area (in $cm^2$), and C is an empirical orifice constant, 44.5.

For quick calculations, this simplifies to the following:

$$AVA = \text{cardiac output}/(\sqrt{\text{mean pressure gradient}})$$

The relationship of flow across the aortic valve and transvalvular pressure gradient is shown in Figure 61-6. As the valve area decreases to 1 $cm^2$, there is little change in the transvalvular gradient needed to generate the same flow and patients

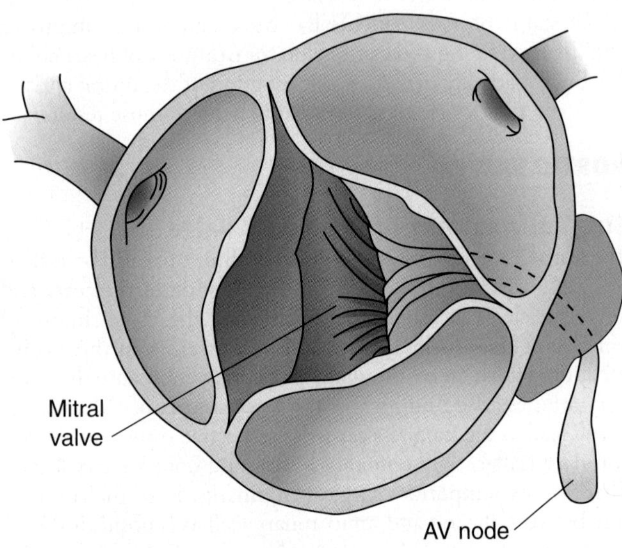


**FIGURE 61-4** Surgical anatomy of the aortic valve. The commissure between the noncoronary and left coronary leaflets lies anterior to the left bundle of the His. Injury to this conduction tissue during aortic valve surgery may result in heart block. *AV,* Atrioventricular.

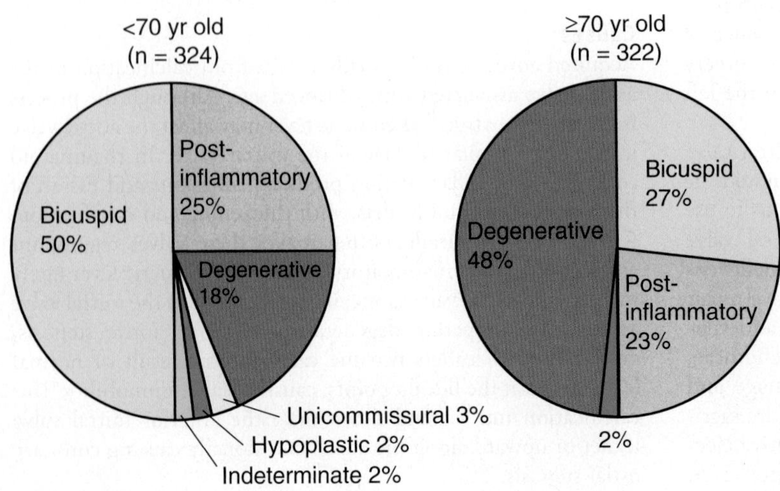


**FIGURE 61-5** Causes of aortic stenosis as a function of age. (From Passik CS, Ackermann DM, Pluth JR, Edwards WD: Temporal changes in the causes of aortic stenosis: A surgical pathologic study of 646 cases. Mayo Clin Proc 62;119–123, 1987.)

frequently experience no symptoms. With a valve area of 0.8 $cm^2$, patients invariably develop symptoms.

## Diagnosis

**Symptoms** The classic symptoms of aortic stenosis are angina, syncope, and heart failure. Patients may not develop symptoms until the aortic valve area is approximately 1 $cm^2$; this usually requires years. When this degree of stenosis has been reached, however, it may quickly narrow further, with rapid onset of symptoms and, occasionally, sudden death.

**Physical Examination** Auscultation of the chest in patients with aortic stenosis reveals a systolic murmur best heard at the base of the heart that radiates into the carotid arteries; it may be difficult to distinguish the murmur of aortic stenosis from a bruit in the carotid artery. This murmur is associated with a slow prolonged rise in the arterial pulse, called *pulsus parvus et tardus*. The murmur of severe aortic stenosis is soft and high-pitched and is often described as a seagull murmur.

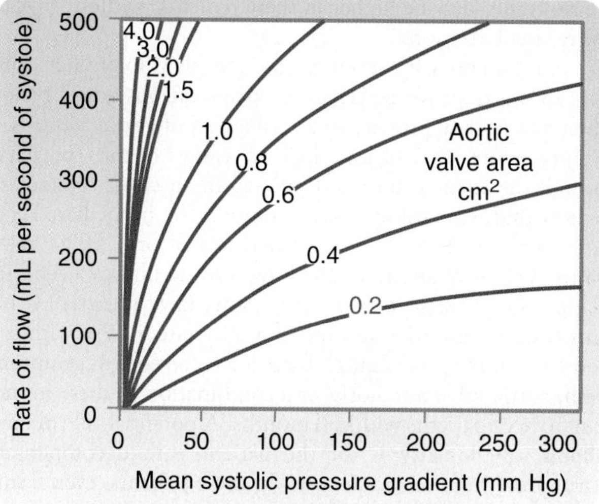


**FIGURE 61-6** Relationship between the mean systolic pressure gradient across the aortic valve and rate of flow across the aortic valve per second of systole, as predicted by the Gorlin formula. As the valve area is reduced to approximately 0.7 $cm^2$, little increase in flow is achieved, despite marked increases in mean gradient, thus defining critical aortic stenosis. (From Hurst JW, Logue RB, Schlant RC, Wenger NK [eds]: Hurst's The heart: Arteries and veins, ed 3, New York, 1974, McGraw-Hill, p 811.)

### Diagnostic Tests

***Electrocardiography*** The electrocardiogram is notable for left ventricular hypertrophy in 85% of patients and evidence of left atrial enlargement in 80% of patients. T wave inversion and ST-segment depression are common.

***Chest Radiography*** The cardiac silhouette on the chest radiograph is usually normal but may reveal poststenotic dilation of the ascending aorta or calcification of the aortic valve. Patients with symptoms of heart failure may have visible evidence of pulmonary edema.

***Echocardiography*** The severity of aortic stenosis may be accurately estimated by echocardiography. The peak transvalvular gradient may be calculated from velocity of blood traversing the valve by the following formula:

$$\text{Gradient} = 4V^2$$

where V is the maximal measured blood velocity (in m/sec) across the valve. Echocardiographic determination of the velocity across the valve may also be used to calculate the aortic valve area using the continuity equation (Fig. 61-7).[21]

***Cardiac Catheterization*** If the degree of aortic stenosis cannot be determined by echocardiography, cardiac catheterization may be necessary for diagnosis. After measuring left ventricular pressure, a catheter may be pulled back from the left ventricle to the aorta to determine the transvalvular pressure gradient. Patients with angina or who are older than approximately 50 years may require coronary angiography before aortic valve surgery to exclude coronary artery disease.

## Natural History

The natural history of aortic stenosis was reported by Ross and Braunwald.[22] Patient survival is not diminished until patients develop symptoms, associated with a reduction in the aortic valve area from the normal 3 to 4 $cm^2$ to less than 1 $cm^2$. Once symptoms develop, patient survival is limited. The three principal symptoms of aortic stenosis are angina, syncope, and heart failure (Fig. 61-8). Angina is usually the earliest symptom; the mean survival of a patient with aortic stenosis and angina is 4.7 years. Once a patient experiences syncope, survival is typically less than 3 years. Patients with symptoms of heart failure have a mean survival of 1 to 2 years. Heart failure is the presenting symptom in almost one third of patients.

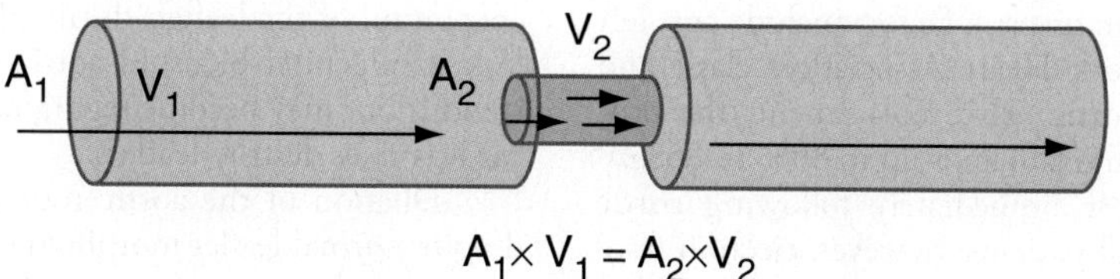


**FIGURE 61-7** Determination of aortic valve area using the continuity equation. For blood flow ($A_1 \times V_1$) to remain constant when it reaches a stenosis ($A_2$), velocity must increase to $V_2$. Determination of the increased velocity $V_2$ by Doppler ultrasound permits calculation of the aortic valve gradient and solution of the equation for $A_2$. *A,* Area; *V,* velocity. (From Carabello BA: Aortic stenosis. In Crawford MH [ed]: Current diagnosis and treatment in cardiology, Norwalk, Conn, 1995, Appleton & Lange, p 87.)

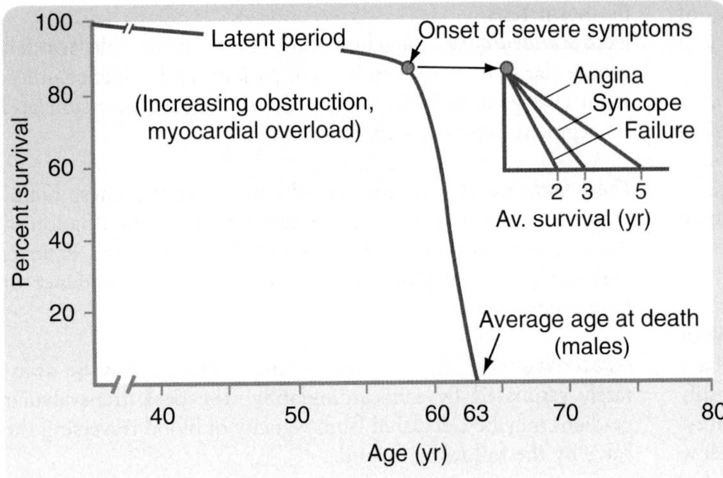


**FIGURE 61-8** Natural history of medically treated aortic stenosis. (From Ross J Jr, Braunwald E: Aortic stenosis. Circulation 38:61–67, 1968.)

### Treatment

Aortic stenosis is a mechanical obstruction to flow from the left ventricle. The only effective therapy is aortic valve replacement. The existence of symptoms is an indication for valve replacement. The issue of aortic valve replacement in patients with aortic stenosis who do not have symptoms is less clear. A small number of symptom-free patients do develop symptoms precipitously and then experience sudden death. Investigators agree, however, that in patients with aortic stenosis without symptoms, survival is excellent.[23-25] The risk for sudden death in symptom-free patients with severe aortic stenosis with a transvalvular gradient of 50 mm Hg or higher or a valve area of less than 0.5 $cm^2$ is approximately 4%/year.[26] In one study of 113 symptom-free patients with critical aortic stenosis, 38 developed symptoms within 2 years. There were no sudden cardiac deaths in 118 patient-years of follow-up.[25] To identify better those symptom-free patients likely to develop symptoms, a group of 123 adults (mean age, 63 years) with asymptomatic aortic stenosis with an initial mean transvalvular gradient of 30 mm Hg were followed prospectively. During 2.5 years of follow-up, there were no sudden deaths. However, aortic stenosis is a progressive disease. Among symptom-free patients with an initial transvalvular velocity of more than 4 m/sec (severe aortic stenosis), only 21% were alive and free of valve replacement at 2 years of follow-up.[26] It may therefore be appropriate to consider aortic valve surgery in patients with symptomatic and asymptomatic disease who have evidence of left ventricular decompensation or a transvalvular gradient of more than 4 m/sec.

In patients with good ventricular function, aortic valve replacement is associated with an operative mortality rate of 2% to 8%.[27] Independent perioperative risk factors include age, left ventricular function, New York Heart Association class, and pulmonary function. After aortic valve replacement, the projected 10-year age-matched survival rate is up to 80% to 85%.[28] Symptoms are relieved almost immediately following aortic valve replacement in almost all patients; however, ejection fraction and resolution of ventricular hypertrophy may require months to improve. Surgical mortality increases exponentially with decreasing left ventricular ejection fraction. Aortic valve replacement in patients with significant heart failure carries a mortality rate of up to 24%. In patients with aortic stenosis and coronary artery disease, valve replacement and myocardial revascularization should be performed concurrently. Perioperative mortality may be higher in these patients, without myocardial revascularization.

For patients with severe aortic stenosis who are not candidates for aortic valve replacement, percutaneous aortic balloon valvuloplasty may provide some palliation of aortic stenosis. In this procedure, one or two balloon catheters may be passed through the aortic orifice and inflated in an effort to crack the calcium that is retarding leaflet motion. The immediate results show an increase in the aortic valve area of only 50%, with a 3% to 10% mortality rate. The long-term results are even more disappointing: 30% to 35% of patients have recurrent symptoms within 6 months, and the mortality rate is 60% within 18 months after the procedure.[29] There is a recurrence of symptoms, death, aortic valve restenosis, or a combination of these in more than 50% of patients within 6 months. A potential role of aortic balloon valvuloplasty is for the patient with decompensated heart failure from aortic stenosis. In these patients, even a small improvement in the size of the aortic valve orifice may sufficiently improve the patient's cardiac output and acute condition to lower the operative risks of aortic valve replacement significantly.

## Aortic Insufficiency

### Causes

Aortic insufficiency may result from disease of the valve leaflets or aortic root. Rheumatic fever may affect the leaflets by shortening the distance from the leaflet-free edge to the aortic annulus rather than by leading to commissural fusion. This prevents coaptation of the leaflets during diastole and results in a central leak. Congenital bicuspid aortic valves typically lead to aortic stenosis but may become regurgitant if a leaflet prolapses. Endocarditis may destroy leaflets.

Dilation of the aortic root produces aortic regurgitation, despite normal leaflet morphology, by precluding leaflet coaptation. The most common of these conditions is annuloaortic ectasia, an idiopathic dilation of the aortic root and annulus; as the sinuses of Valsalva and the proximal aorta dilate, diastolic coaptation of the leaflets is precluded, resulting in valvular insufficiency. Similarly, myxoid degeneration of the aortic root may lead to dilation of the root, as seen in Marfan syndrome,

Ehlers-Danlos syndrome, and cystic medial necrosis. Those conditions may lead to leaflet redundancy, progressive prolapse, and regurgitation. Trauma or dissection of the aortic wall may produce aortic regurgitation if it leads to loss of commissural suspension and leaflet prolapse.

### Pathophysiology

The aortic valve leaks during diastole, which lowers diastolic pressure and widens the pulse pressure. Because coronary blood flow occurs primarily in diastole, the lower diastolic blood pressure lowers coronary perfusion pressure. Unlike aortic stenosis, in which the pathologic process is left ventricular pressure overload, the pathophysiology of aortic insufficiency derives from left ventricular volume overload. The increased left ventricular end-diastolic volume (preload) results from filling through the mitral valve and incompetent aortic valve. Patients with chronic aortic insufficiency may have the greatest left ventricular end-diastolic volume of any form of heart disease. Because left ventricular compliance is often increased, however, left ventricular end-diastolic pressure may or may not be elevated. With left ventricular dilation, normal forward stroke volume and ejection fraction may be maintained by increased left ventricular end-diastolic and end-systolic volumes. According to the law of Laplace, this left ventricular dilation increases the left ventricular wall tension required to develop systolic pressure. Such increased wall stress not only increases myocardial oxygen demand but also initiates left ventricular hypertrophy and increases left ventricular wall mass. Ultimately, myocardial fibrosis occurs.

With well-compensated aortic insufficiency, exercise may be tolerated because peripheral vascular resistance declines, lowering the left ventricular afterload and increasing effective forward flow. At the same time, heart rate increases, which shortens diastolic time, thereby decreasing the regurgitant flow. Because the ventricle ultimately decompensates, however, the left ventricular end-diastolic volume increases, even without an increase in aortic regurgitant volume. The end-systolic volume increases as the forward stroke volume declines because ventricular emptying is impaired—the ventricle fails.

In severe aortic regurgitation, increased myocardial oxygen demand exceeds myocardial oxygen supply, causing ischemia despite normal coronary arteries. Increased left ventricular mass and wall tension occur concurrently with low diastolic pressures (low coronary perfusion pressure). Consequently, and particularly with exercise when the diastolic period shortens, coronary blood flow may not meet demand.

### Diagnosis

**Symptoms** The compensatory mechanisms of aortic regurgitation may permit patients to remain symptom-free for long periods. When these compensatory mechanisms begin to fail, however, left ventricular dysfunction becomes manifest, and patients experience symptoms of heart failure. Symptoms, generally the result of an elevation in left atrial pressure, include dyspnea on exertion, orthopnea, and paroxysmal nocturnal dyspnea. Nocturnal angina may occur as a result of a slow heart rate and an exceedingly low diastolic pressure, with resultant poor coronary flow.

**Physical Examination** The physical examination of patients with aortic regurgitation is distinctive because of the wide pulse pressure. The peripheral pulses rise and fall abruptly (Corrigan's, or water hammer, pulse), the head may bob with each systole (de Musset's sign), and the capillaries pulsate visibly (Quincke's sign). Auscultation reveals a high-frequency, decrescendo, diastolic regurgitant murmur. A middle to late diastolic rumble may be heard (Austin-Flint murmur); this represents rapid antegrade flow across the mitral valve that closes prematurely as a result of rapid ventricular filling secondary to the aortic regurgitation.

#### Diagnostic Tests

***Chest Radiography*** The chest radiograph typically reveals an enlarged cardiac silhouette, with an enlarged left atrial shadow and chronic aortic regurgitation. With acute aortic regurgitation, however, the cardiac size may not be enlarged.

***Electrocardiography*** The electrocardiogram is usually nonspecific, but may reveal left ventricular hypertrophy and left atrial enlargement.

***Echocardiography*** Doppler echocardiography is the most accurate noninvasive technique to confirm the diagnosis of aortic regurgitation and determine the severity of aortic insufficiency. As with mitral regurgitation, the severity is graded semiquantitatively as mild, moderate, or severe.

***Cardiac Catheterization*** The severity of the aortic regurgitation may be visualized angiographically at cardiac catheterization. As with echocardiography, the severity is graded subjectively from mild to severe.

### Natural History

Because of the compensatory mechanisms discussed earlier, patients with chronic aortic regurgitation may be symptom-free for long periods of time. Patients with mild to moderate aortic regurgitation are typically symptom-free and have an excellent long-term prognosis; the 10-year survival rate after diagnosis is approximately 85% to 95%. With more severe aortic regurgitation, symptoms can be expected to develop. Once symptoms of heart failure occur, survival is markedly decreased; almost 50% of patients with heart failure die within 2 years.

### Treatment

Medical therapy for aortic regurgitation is based on a combination of afterload reduction and diuretics. Afterload reduction with nifedipine has been shown to delay the need for aortic valve replacement. Chronic use of ACE inhibitors is more common for afterload reduction.

Patients with symptomatic aortic insufficiency require surgical therapy because their prognosis, when treated medically, is only a few years. Optimal timing of surgical intervention in patients with or without symptoms, however, may be a difficult clinical decision.[30] Some patients may be successfully managed with diuretics and afterload reduction for long periods. Unfortunately, significant irreversible left ventricular systolic dysfunction may develop insidiously and before clinical evidence of congestive heart failure.

Therefore, symptom-free patients should be carefully followed with serial echocardiography for evidence of systolic dysfunction, increasing end-systolic left ventricular diameter, and/or decreasing left ventricular ejection fraction. Aortic valve replacement must be performed before the left ventricle has irreversibly dilated. An end-systolic dimension more than 55 mm estimated by echocardiography has been associated with irreversible left ventricular dysfunction, even after aortic valve replacement,[14] and aortic valve replacement should be performed before the ventricular dimension exceeds this diameter. In addition, the use of the end-systolic volume value may help in determining management for these symptom-free patients. When end-systolic volume is less that 30 mL/m$^2$, prognosis after surgical therapy is excellent. Progressive systolic dysfunction with end-systolic volumes greater than 90 mL/m$^2$ have poor intermediate short-term and long-term results. When left ventricular dysfunction is noted in patients with diminished ejection fraction, even despite good exercise tolerance, elective operation is recommended. Persistent medical management of these patients will severely jeopardize surgical outcome and ultimate prognosis.

The mortality rate associated with aortic valve replacement for aortic insufficiency is approximately 4% to 6%.[14] Long-term survival is a function of preoperative left ventricular function; early and late results are improved when surgical intervention precedes left ventricular decompensation.

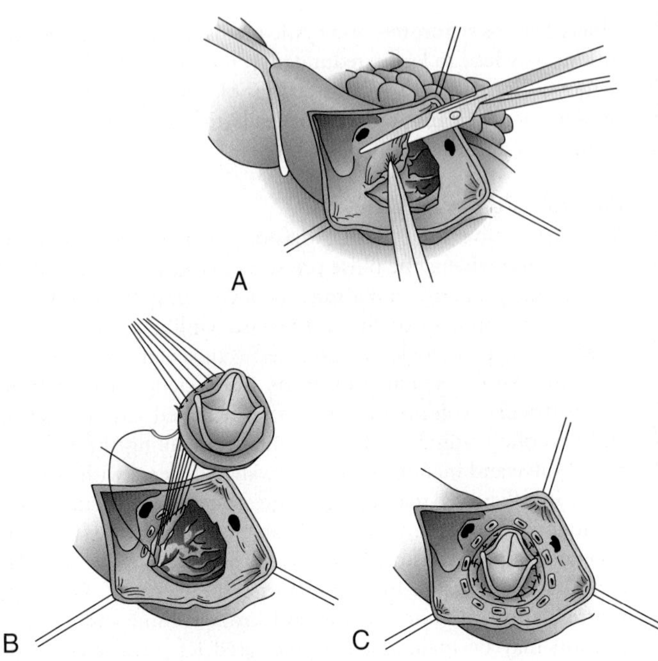


**FIGURE 61-9** Aortic valve replacement. **A,** The diseased leaflets are excised and the prosthetic valve is sewn in place with interrupted pledgeted mattress stitches **(B, C).** (From Albertucci M, Karp RB: Prosthetic valve replacement. In Al Zaibag M, Duran CMG [eds]: Valvular heart disease. New York, 1994, Marcel Dekker, p 615.)

## OPERATIVE TECHNIQUES

### Aortic Valve Replacement

The standard incision for an aortic valve replacement is a median sternotomy. Once the incision has been made, the patient is connected to the cardiopulmonary bypass circuit by cannulation of the distal ascending aorta and right atrium. Myocardial protection is achieved by topical myocardial cooling and cardioplegia. Most surgeons use moderate systemic hypothermia (28° to 32° C) during the procedure.

After the heart fibrillates and the aortic cross clamp has been applied, a transverse aortotomy is performed approximately 4 cm distal to the origin of the right coronary artery. The aortotomy is extended to the left and right, thus exposing the aortic valve (Fig. 61-9). The native aortic valve leaflets are excised, taking great care to remove any particles of calcium. Once the leaflets have been removed, an appropriately sized prosthetic valve is sewn in place. The aortotomy is closed, cardiac function is resumed, and the patient is weaned from cardiopulmonary bypass.

### Mitral Valve Replacement and Repair

The standard incision for mitral valve replacement is a median sternotomy, although a right thoracotomy may sometimes be appropriate for reoperation. The patient is connected to the arterial limb of the cardiopulmonary bypass circuit by cannulation of the distal ascending aorta. Venous drainage for the cardiopulmonary bypass is established by cannulation of the superior and inferior vena cava (bicaval cannulation). Myocardial protection is achieved by topical myocardial cooling and cardioplegia. Most surgeons use moderate systemic hypothermia (28° to 32° C) during the procedure.

Surgical exposure of the mitral valve may be difficult but may be achieved by using several different incisions on the heart. The most common incision used to expose the valve is a left atriotomy made in the right lateral wall of the left atrium, just anterior to the left pulmonary veins. An alternative surgical approach to the mitral valve is through an incision in the right atrium, followed by an incision through the interatrial septum, which provides excellent exposure to the left atrium and mitral valve.

Once the mitral valve has been exposed, it must be carefully examined to determine whether it may be repaired or must be replaced. If the valve must be replaced, efforts should be made to preserve the native mitral valve apparatus to preserve the mechanical continuity between the mitral valve annulus and left ventricular apex. This may usually be accomplished by imbricating the leaflets of the mitral valve with sutures and placing an appropriately sized prosthetic valve within the annulus of the native valve (Fig. 61-10).

If the valve is reparable, various surgical techniques may used to restore valve competency. In most cases, an incompetent portion of one or both of the mitral valve leaflets must be resected, and the leaflet then reapproximated (Fig. 61-11). At the time of mitral valve repair, the specific pathology responsible for the regurgitation is addressed. For example, a common cause of mitral regurgitation is a ruptured chorda tendinea. At the time of surgery, the prolapsed or flail leaflet subtended by the ruptured chorda tendinea is resected, the leaflet is primarily reapproximated, and the circumference of the mitral annulus is reduced by use of an annuloplasty ring. The adequacy of the repair is judged under direct vision by filling the left ventricle with saline under modest pressure. After the patient has been weaned from cardiopulmonary bypass, a final determination about the competency of the repair is made using intraoperative transesophageal echocardiography. The durability of a given mitral valve repair is largely dependent on the pathology responsible for the regurgitation. In most series, however, the failure rate of mitral valvuloplasty for mitral regurgitation is less than 1%/year. The mitral annulus is invariably dilated in surgical

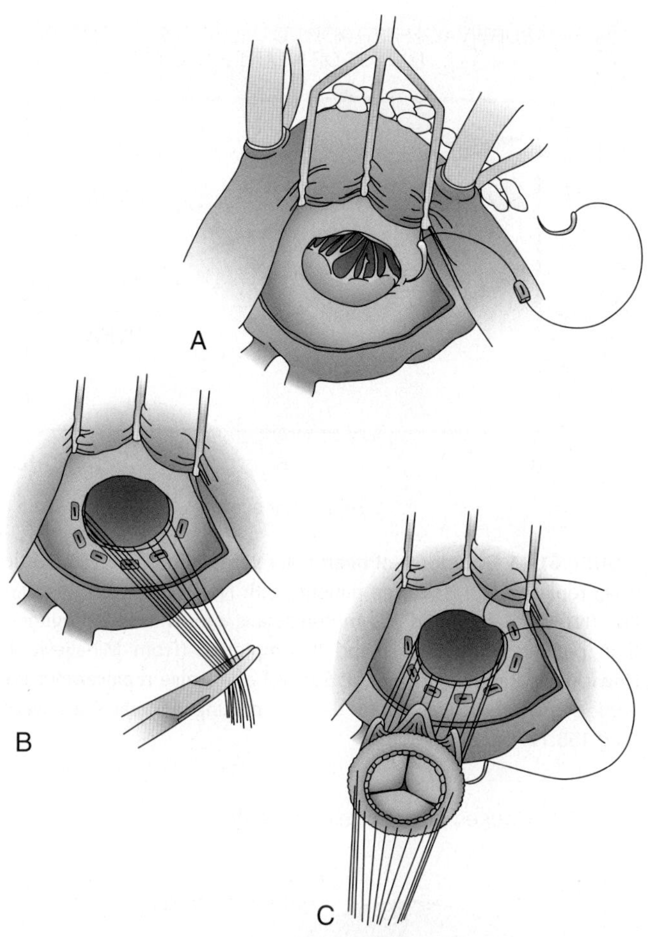


**FIGURE 61-10 A-C,** Mitral valve replacement with preservation of the posterior leaflet. This preserves the annular-apical connection by means of the chordae tendineae. (From Albertucci M, Karp RB: Prosthetic valve replacement. In Al Zaibag M, Duran CMG [eds]: Valvular heart disease. New York, 1994, Marcel Dekker, p 613.)

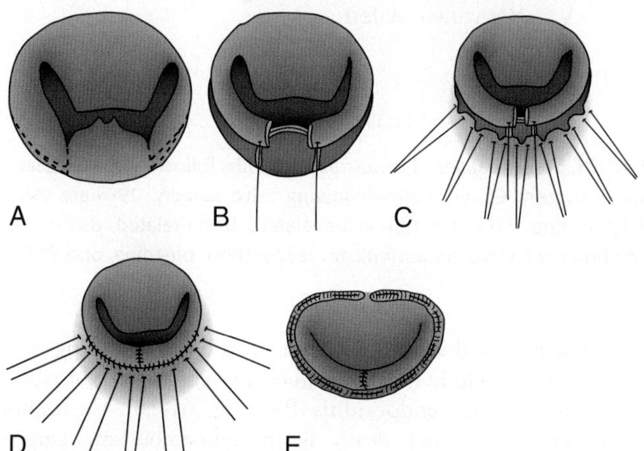


**FIGURE 61-11 A-E,** Mitral valve repair. In this example, the specific pathology is a flail posterior leaflet. It is repaired by resection of the flail segment, reapproximation of the leaflet, and reduction of the mitral annulus circumference using an annuloplasty ring. (From Perier P, Clausnizer B, Mistarz K: Carpentier "sliding leaflet" technique for repair of mitral valve: Early results. Ann Thorac Surg 57:383–386, 1994.)

cases of mitral regurgitation, contributing to poor coaptation of the anterior and posterior mitral valve leaflets during systole. To return the enlarged mitral annular diameter to normal and reinforce the leaflet repair, an annuloplasty ring is then sewn to the perimeter of the mitral annulus.

## SURGICAL OUTCOMES

According to the Society of Thoracic Surgeons (STS) National Cardiac Surgery Database, approximately 100,000 valve operations are performed in the United States annually.[31] The operative mortality rate for valve replacement surgery is influenced by several variables, including which valve is replaced, whether coronary bypass surgery is performed at the same operation, and other patient-specific factors.

The operative mortality rate in the STS database for isolated aortic valve replacement is approximately 3.2%. On the other hand, the operative mortality rate for mitral valve replacement is 5.7% compared with 1.6% operative mortality for mitral valve repair.[32,33] Other databases, including the New York State Department of Health Cardiac Surgery Reporting System and Department of Veteran Affairs Cardiac Surgery database, have found similar mortality rates for cardiac valve operations.[34]

## CHOICE OF PROSTHETIC VALVES

For replacement of the aortic or mitral valve, there are two principal choices of cardiac valve prostheses, mechanical and bioprosthetic. Bioprosthetic valves are porcine or bovine pericardial valves. The hemodynamic performance of the valves is similar. The operative risks associated with cardiac valve replacement are not associated with the choice of prosthesis.

The choice of prosthetic valve must be patient-specific. Mechanical valves have excellent durability and will perform indefinitely, without structural deterioration. However, because they are thrombogenic, mechanical valves obligate the patient to lifelong anticoagulation (warfarin). Hence, the patient with a mechanical valve incurs the risks of chronic anticoagulation. Bioprosthetic valves do not require anticoagulation, but will undergo structural deterioration. The durability of a bioprosthetic valve is inversely related to the patient's age when the valve is implanted. If a bioprosthetic valve structurally deteriorates, the patient will require reoperation and valve rereplacement. It is important to recognize that approximately 80% of all aortic and mitral valve replacements in the United States are performed in patients older than 60 years. The patient's age should be considered because it may be dangerous to commit a geriatric patient to chronic anticoagulation.

The 10-year survival for patients following aortic valve replacement ranges from 40% to 75%, with an average in the literature of approximately 50%.[35] In most published series, the type of prosthesis does not affect survival (Fig. 61-12). Instead, other patient-specific factors, such as age at operation and the presence or absence of coronary artery disease, do have an effect on survival following valve replacement. Perhaps the strongest patient-specific risk factor is the presence of significant heart failure, especially in patients with aortic stenosis (Fig. 61-13). Regardless of the type of prosthetic valve implanted, approximately one third of patients die of valve-related causes. An important consideration for the choice of valve for any patient is therefore how the individual patient may be affected by valve-related morbidity or mortality.

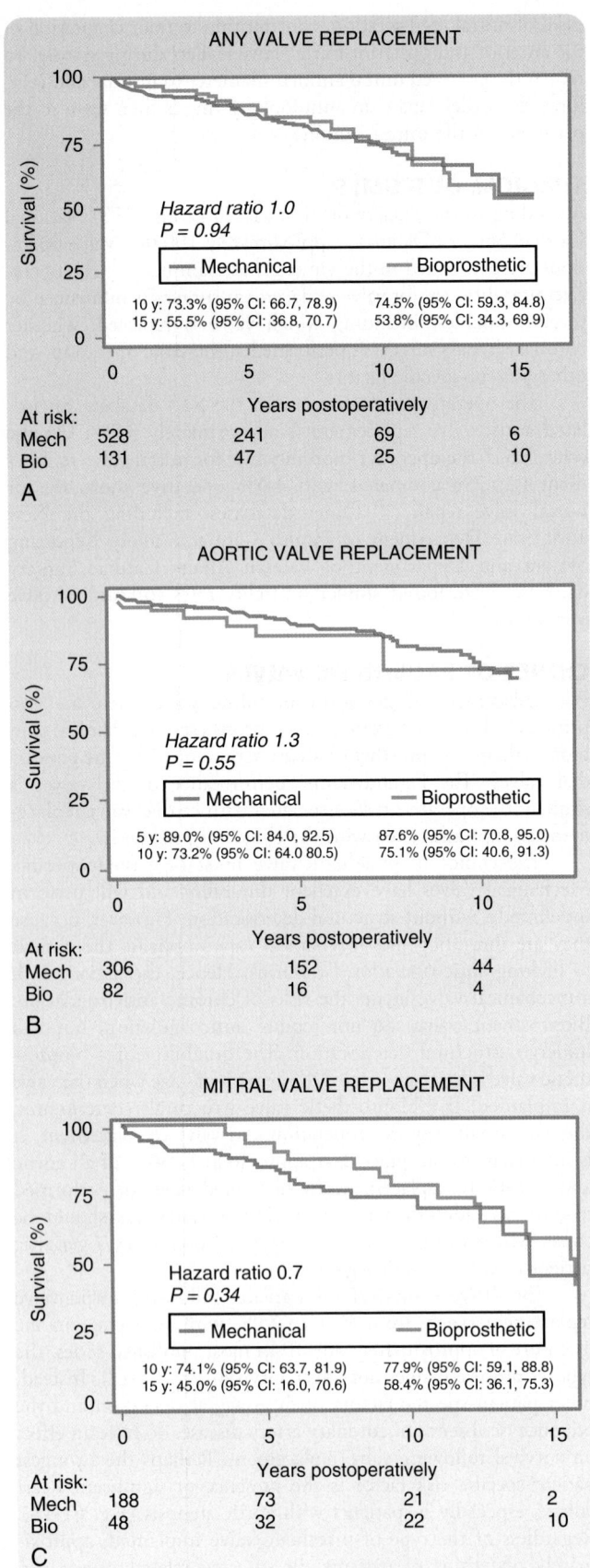

ANY VALVE REPLACEMENT

Hazard ratio 1.0
P = 0.94
Mechanical — Bioprosthetic
10 y: 73.3% (95% CI: 66.7, 78.9) 74.5% (95% CI: 59.3, 84.8)
15 y: 55.5% (95% CI: 36.8, 70.7) 53.8% (95% CI: 34.3, 69.9)
Survival (%)
Years postoperatively
At risk:
Mech 528 241 69 6
Bio 131 47 25 10
A

AORTIC VALVE REPLACEMENT

Hazard ratio 1.3
P = 0.55
Mechanical — Bioprosthetic
5 y: 89.0% (95% CI: 84.0, 92.5) 87.6% (95% CI: 70.8, 95.0)
10 y: 73.2% (95% CI: 64.0 80.5) 75.1% (95% CI: 40.6, 91.3)
Survival (%)
Years postoperatively
At risk:
Mech 306 152 44
Bio 82 16 4
B

MITRAL VALVE REPLACEMENT

Hazard ratio 0.7
P = 0.34
Mechanical — Bioprosthetic
10 y: 74.1% (95% CI: 63.7, 81.9) 77.9% (95% CI: 59.1, 88.8)
15 y: 45.0% (95% CI: 16.0, 70.6) 58.4% (95% CI: 36.1, 75.3)
Survival (%)
Years postoperatively
At risk:
Mech 188 73 21 2
Bio 48 32 22 10
C

**FIGURE 61-12** Survival following aortic valve replacement is no different between mechanical and bioprosthetic valves. (From Kulik A, Bedard P, Lam BK, et al: Mechanical versus bioprosthetic valve replacement in middle-aged patients. Eur J Cardiothorac Surg 30:485–491, 2006.)

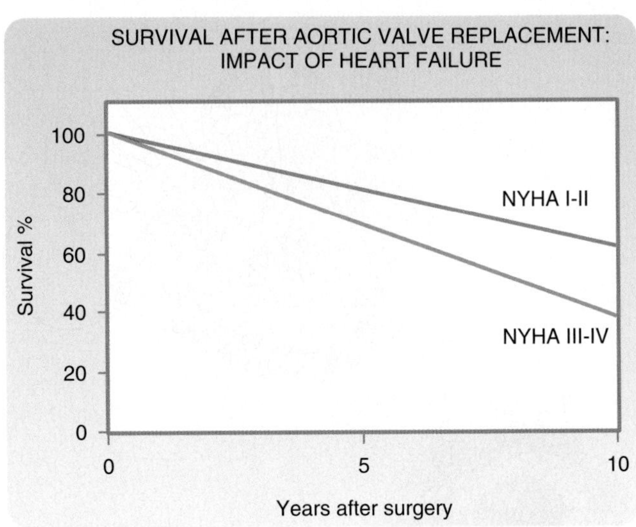


**FIGURE 61-13** Symptoms of heart failure are an indication for aortic valve replacement. However, patients with New York Heart Association (NYHA) Class III and IV symptoms have a much worse prognosis than patients with Class I and II symptoms. (From Mihaljevic T, Nowicki ER, Rajeswaran J, et al: Survival after valve replacement for aortic stenosis: Implications for decision making. J Thorac Cardiovasc Surg 135:1270–1278, 2008.)

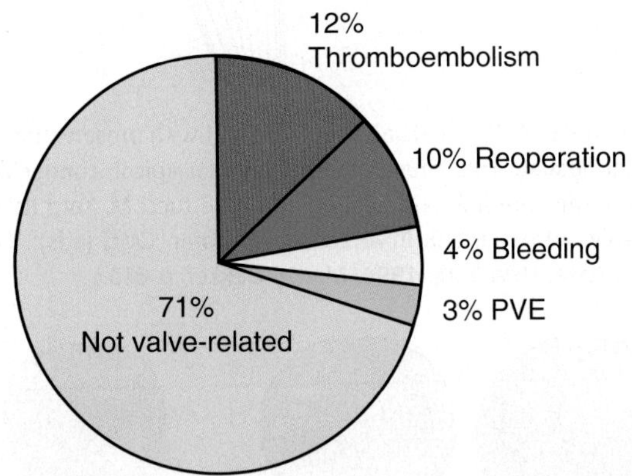


**FIGURE 61-14** Causes of valve-related deaths following valve replacement surgery. Of all deaths following valve surgery, 29% are valve-related and 71% are not valve-related. Valve-related deaths are attributable to thromboembolism, reoperation, bleeding, and PVE.

The principal causes of valve-related death following valve implantation include thromboembolism, reoperation, bleeding, and prosthetic valve endocarditis (PVE; Fig. 61-14). The leading cause of valve-related death is thromboembolism. Largely because mechanical valves are thrombogenic, the risk of thromboembolism is greater with mechanical valves. At 10 years following aortic valve replacement, the risk of thromboembolism is 20% for mechanical valves[36] and 9% for bioprosthetic valves.[37]

The risk of PVE is no different between mechanical and tissue valves. It is approximately 4%, spread over the patient's lifetime. However, if PVE does occur, it is associated with a 50% mortality rate.[38]

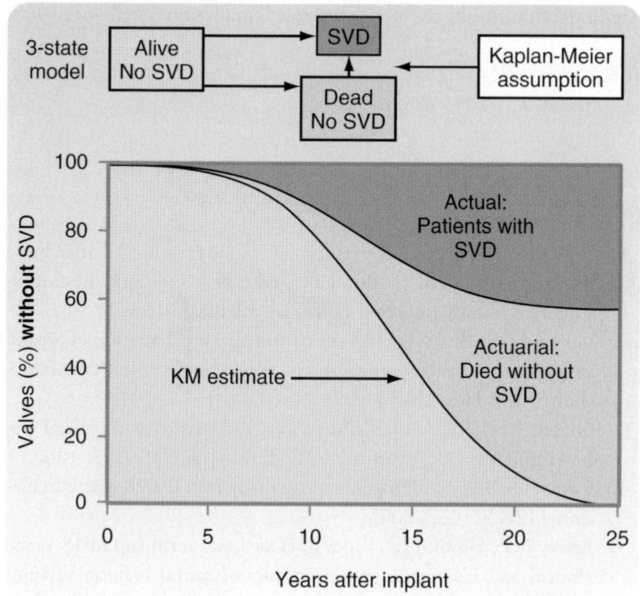


**FIGURE 61-15** Actuarial analysis may overestimate the incidence of structural valve deterioration (SVD). Kaplan-Meier methodology uses the assumption that patients who died before SVD would eventually have had SVD. The group of patients in the group is labeled as having virtual SVD. (From Grunkemeier GL, Wu YX: Interpretation of nonfatal events after cardiac surgery: Actual versus actuarial reporting. J Thorac Cardiovasc Surg 122:216–219, 2001.)

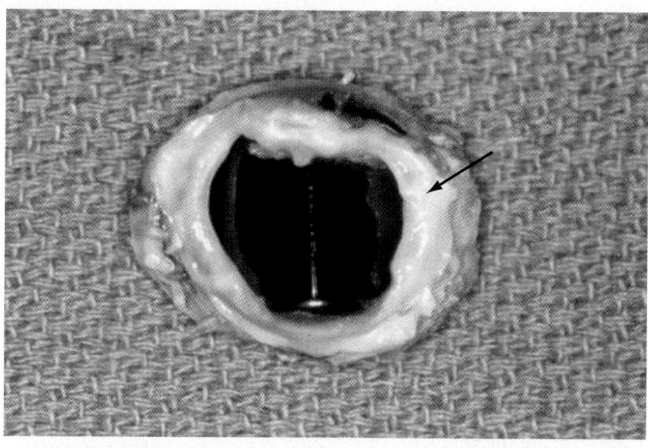

**FIGURE 61-16** Although mechanical valves will not fail structurally, the ingrowth of scar tissue (pannus) may cause a mechanical to become dysfunctional. In this photograph of an explanted mechanical valve, pannus is indicated by the *arrow.*

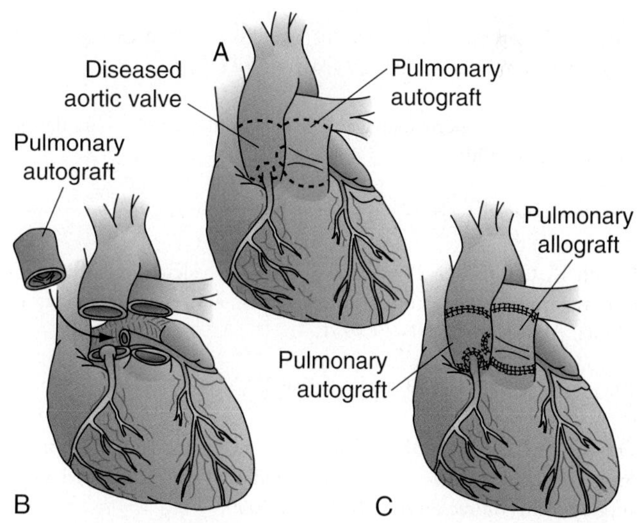


**FIGURE 61-17 A-C,** Pulmonary autograft (Ross) procedure. The diseased aortic valve and proximal aortic root are excised. The pulmonary valve and main pulmonary artery (autograft) are excised, and the autograft is used to replace the aortic root. The coronary artery buttons are reimplanted into the pulmonary root. A pulmonary homograft is then used to reconstruct the right ventricular outflow tract. (From Kouchoukos NT, Davila-Roman VG, Spray TL, et al: Replacement of the aortic root with a pulmonary autograft in children and young adults with aortic-valve disease. N Engl J Med 330:1–6, 1994.)

The choice of prosthetic valve must consider the risks of anticoagulation (mechanical valve) and the likelihood and risks of reoperation for structural valve deterioration (bioprosthetic valve). The risk of bleeding complications from chronic anticoagulation is from 1% to 2%/ year; 4% of valve-related deaths result from bleeding (see Fig. 61-14). Bioprosthetic valves are indicated for patients with contraindications to anticoagulation because of their occupation or coexistent medical conditions. Similarly, patients who are medically noncompliant or whose level of anticoagulation may not be closely monitored should not receive mechanical valves. Of valve-related deaths, 10% result from reoperation, which moves some patients and physicians away from bioprosthetic valves. However, recent data have demonstrated that actuarial statistical methodology may overestimate the incidence of structural valve deterioration. Therefore, some authorities recommend the use of actual rather than actuarial statistical methodology (Fig. 61-15). Unfortunately, valve reoperation may not be completely avoided with the use of a mechanical valve. Although a mechanical valve will not fail structurally, it may become dysfunctional for other reasons. The primary cause of such dysfunction is the ingrowth of scar tissue into the mechanism of the valve, causing the valve to become stenotic or regurgitant (Fig. 61-16). To help balance the risks of anticoagulation and valve reoperation, a joint task force from the American Heart Association and American College of Cardiology (AHA/ACC) has provided guidelines regarding the choice of valve. The task force recommended that tissue valves be placed in the aortic position in patients older than 65 years and in the mitral position in patients older than 70 years.[14]

An alternative treatment of aortic valve disease in young patients is the pulmonary autograft procedure (Ross procedure). Initially performed by Ross in 1967, the procedure has gained wider acceptance during the past 2 decades. The procedure is particularly applicable for children and young adults; it is not commonly performed in older adults. The procedure entails use of the patient's own pulmonary root as an autograft to replace the diseased aortic valve and root. A cryopreserved pulmonary homograft is then used to replace the patient's pulmonary root (Fig. 61-17). Although it is a technically demanding procedure, the operative mortality rate associated with the

Ross procedure is 5% or less, no different from that associated with isolated aortic valve replacement when performed by experienced surgeons. Intermediate-term data have suggested excellent function of the pulmonary autograft; the need for autograft reoperation is low within the first postoperative decade. The durability of the pulmonary homograft is satisfactory; 80% of patients are free of homograft dysfunction at 16 years. Chronic anticoagulation is not required, and the risk of valve-related complications is extremely low.[39]

## SELECTED REFERENCES

Bonow RO, Carabello BA, Chatterjee K, et al: 2008 focused update incorporated into the ACC/AHA 2006 guidelines for the management of patients with valvular heart disease: A report of the American College of Cardiology/American Heart Association Task Force on Practice Guidelines (writing committee to revise the 1998 guidelines for the management of patients with valvular heart disease). Endorsed by the Society of Cardiovascular Anesthesiologists, Society for Cardiovascular Angiography and Interventions, and Society of Thoracic Surgeons. J Am Coll Cardiol 52:e1–e142, 2008.

This is an outstanding reference that addresses almost all aspects of valvular heart disease, including indications for surgery.

Carabello BA: Modern management of mitral stenosis. Circulation 112:432–437, 2005.

This is a concise review of the management of mitral stenosis.

Gorlin R, Gorlin SG: Hydraulic formula for calculation of area of stenotic mitral valve, other cardiac valves, and central circulatory shunts. Am Heart J 41:1–29,1951.

This study provided the ability to determine valve orifice sizes.

O'Brien SM, Shahian DM, Filardo G, et al: The Society of Thoracic Surgeons 2008 cardiac surgery risk models: Part 2—isolated valve surgery. Ann Thorac Surg 88:S23-S42, 2009.

This is a useful compilation of data from the largest cardiac surgical database in the world.

Olesen KH: The natural history of 271 patients with mitral stenosis under medical treatment. Br Heart J 24:349–357, 1962.

This study provided the natural history of medically treated mitral stenosis.

Song JK, Kim MJ, Yun SC, et al: Long-term outcomes of percutaneous mitral balloon valvuloplasty versus open cardiac surgery. J Thorac Cardiovasc Surg 139:103–110, 2010.

This study confirmed the role of balloon mitral valvuloplasty as the treatment for mitral stenosis.

Stewart RL, Chan KL: Management of asymptomatic severe aortic stenosis. Curr Cardiol Rev 5:29–35, 2009.

This is a comprehensive review of the management of asymptomatic aortic stenosis.

Ross J, Jr, Braunwald E: Aortic stenosis. Circulation 38:61–67, 1968.

This is the classic study that provided the natural history of aortic stenosis. It continues to guide therapy today.

## REFERENCES

1. Westaby S, Bosher C: Development of surgery for valvular heart disease. In Westaby S, Bosher C, editors: Landmarks in cardiac surgery, Oxford, England, 2000, Isis Medical Media.
2. Gorlin R, Gorlin SG: Hydraulic formula for calculation of area of stenotic mitral valve, other cardiac valves, and central circulatory shunts. Am Heart J 41:1–29, 1951.
3. Olesen KH: The natural history of 271 patients with mitral stenosis under medical treatment. Br Heart J 24:349–357, 1962.
4. Carabello BA: Modern management of mitral stenosis. Circulation 112:432–437, 2005.
5. Fawzy ME, Shoukri M, Fadel B, et al: Long-term (up to 18 years) clinical and echocardiographic results of mitral balloon valvuloplasty in 531 consecutive patients and predictors of outcome. Cardiology 113:213–221, 2009.
6. Song JK, Kim MJ, Yun SC, et al: Long-term outcomes of percutaneous mitral balloon valvuloplasty versus open cardiac surgery. J Thorac Cardiovasc Surg 139:103–110, 2010.
7. Solomon NA, Pranav SK, Naik D, et al: Importance of preservation of chordal apparatus in mitral valve replacement. Expert Rev Cardiovasc Ther 4:253–261, 2006.
8. Gammie JS, Sheng S, Griffith BP, et al: Trends in mitral valve surgery in the United States: Results from the Society of Thoracic Surgeons Adult Cardiac Surgery Database. Ann Thorac Surg 87:1431–1437, 2009.
9. Ruel M, Kulik A, Lam BK, et al: Long-term outcomes of valve replacement with modern prostheses in young adults. Eur J Cardiothorac Surg 27:425–433, 2005.
10. Rapaport E: Natural history of aortic and mitral valve disease. Am J Cardiol 35:221–227, 1975.
11. Buja P, Tatantini G, Del Bianco F, et al: Ischemic mitral regurgitation on the threshold of a solution: From paradoxes to unifying concepts. Circulation 112:745–758, 2005.
12. Heikkinen J, Biencari F, Satta J, et al: Quality of life after mitral valve repair. J Heart Valve Dis 14:722–726, 2005.
13. Bonow RO, Cheitlin MD, Crawford MH, Douglas PS: Task Force 3: Valvular heart disease. J Am Coll Cardiol 45:1334–1340, 2005.
14. Bonow RO, Carabello BA, Chatterjee K, et al: 2008 focused update incorporated into the ACC/AHA 2006 guidelines for the management of patients with valvular heart disease: A report of the American College of Cardiology/American Heart Association Task Force on Practice Guidelines (writing committee to revise the 1998 guidelines for the management of patients with valvular heart disease). Endorsed by the Society of Cardiovascular Anesthesiologists, Society for Cardiovascular Angiography and Interventions, and Society of Thoracic Surgeons. J Am Coll Cardiol 52:e1–e142, 2008.
15. Adams DH, Anyanwu A: Pitfalls and limitations in measuring and interpreting the outcomes of mitral valve repair. J Thorac Cardiovasc Surg 13:523–529, 2006.
16. Borger MA, Adam A, Murphy PM, et al: Chronic ischemic mitral regurgitation: repair, replace or rethink? Ann Thorac Surg 81: 1153–1161, 2006.

17. Muthialu N, Varma SK, Ramanathan S, et al: Effect of chordal preservation on left ventricular function. Asian Cardiovasc Thorac Ann 13:233–237, 2005.
18. De Bonis M, Lapenna E, La Canna G, et al: Mitral valve repair for functional mitral regurgitation in end-stage dilated cardiomyopathy: Role of the "edge-to-edge" technique. Circulation 112:I402–I408, 2005.
19. Rahimtoola SH: The year in valvular heart disease. J Am Coll Cardiol 47:427–439, 2006.
20. Anselmi A, Lotrionte M, Biondi-Zoccai GG, et al: Left ventricular hypertrophy, apoptosis, and progression to heart failure in severe aortic stenosis. Eur Heart J 26:2747, 2005.
21. Schroeder RA, Mark JB: Is the valve OK or not? Immediate evaluation of a replaced aortic valve. Anesth Analg 101:1288–1291, 2005.
22. Ross J, Jr, Braunwald E: Aortic stenosis. Circulation 38:61–67, 1968.
23. Carabello BA, Paulus WJ: Aortic stenosis. Lancet 373:956–966, 2009.
24. Fullerton DA: Aortic valve replacement. In Kaiser LR, Kron IL, Spray TL, editors: Mastery of cardiothoracic surgery, ed 2, Philadelphia, 2007, Lippincott Williams & Wilkins.
25. Awais M, Bach DS: Exercise stress testing in asymptomatic severe aortic stenosis. J Heart Valve Dis 18:235–238, 2009.
26. Baumgartner H, Otto CM: Aortic stenosis severity: Do we need a new concept? J Am Coll Cardiol 54:1012–1013, 2009.
27. Stewart RL, Chan KL: Management of asymptomatic severe aortic stenosis. Curr Cardiol Rev 5:29–35, 2009.
28. Puvimanasinghe JP, Takkenberg JJ, Edwards MB, et al: Comparison of outcomes after aortic valve replacement with a mechanical valve or a bioprosthesis using microsimulation. Heart 90:1172–1178, 2004.
29. Andrus BW, O'Rourke DJ.: Percutaneous and surgical treatment of aortic stenosis. Expert Rev Cardiovasc Ther 4:203–920, 2006.
30. Stout KK, Verrier ED: Acute valvular regurgitation. Circulation 119:3232–3241, 2009.
31. O'Brien SM, Shahian DM, Filardo G, et al: The Society of Thoracic Surgeons 2008 cardiac surgery risk models: Part 2—isolated valve surgery. Ann Thorac Surg 88:S23-S42, 2009.
32. Welke KF, Peterson ED, Vaughan-Sarrazin MS, et al: Comparison of cardiac surgery volumes and mortality rates between the Society of Thoracic Surgeons and Medicare databases from 1993 through 2001. Ann Thorac Surg 84:1538–1546, 2007.
33. Rankin JS, Burrichter CA, Walton-Shirley MK, et al: Trends in mitral valve surgery: A single practice experience. J Heart Valve Dis 18:359–366, 2009.
34. Hannan EL, Samadashvili Z, Lahey SJ, et al: Aortic valve replacement for patients with severe aortic stenosis: Risk factors and their impact on 30-month mortality. Ann Thorac Surg 87:1741–1749, 2009.
35. Kulik A, Bédard P, Lam BK, et al: Mechanical versus bioprosthetic valve replacement in middle-aged patients. Eur J Cardiothorac Surg 30:485–491, 2006.
36. Takahashi T, Hasegawa Y, Ohshima K, et al: Long-term follow-up after aortic valve replacement with a small aortic prosthesis. Ann Thorac Cardiovasc Surg 11:245–248, 2005.
37. Mistiaen W, Van Cauwelaert P, Muylaert P, et al: Thromboembolic events after aortic valve replacement in elderly patients with a Carpentier-Edwards Perimount pericardial bioprosthesis. J Thorac Cardiovasc Surg 127:1166–1170, 2004.
38. Mahesh B, Angelini G, Caputo M, et al: Prosthetic valve endocarditis. Ann Thorac Surg 80:1151–1158, 2005.
39. Takkenberg JJ, Klieverik LM, Schoof PH, et al: The Ross procedure: a systematic review and meta-analysis. Circulation 119:222–228, 2009.

# SECTION XII

## VASCULAR

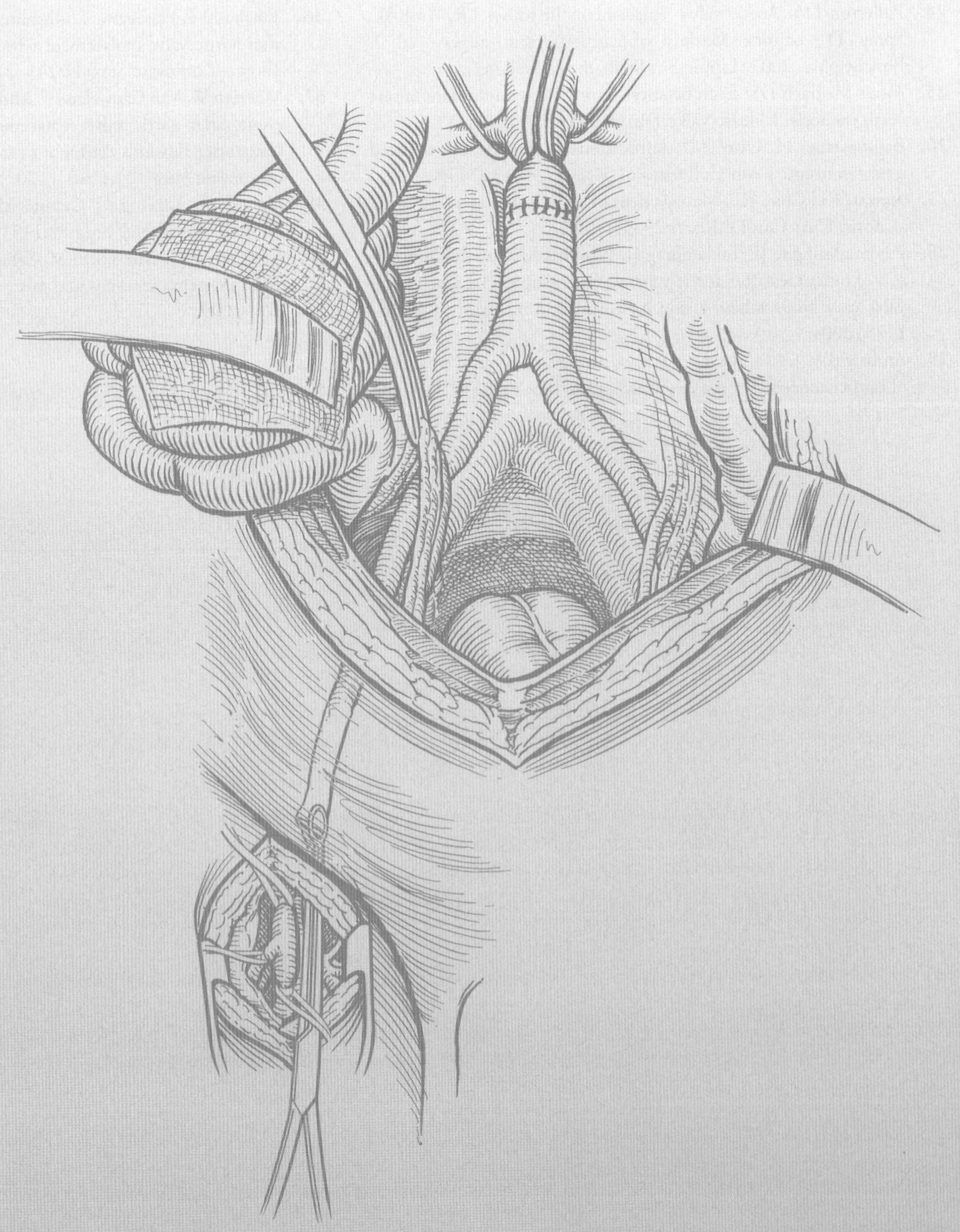

CHAPTER 62

# THE AORTA

Margaret C. Tracci and Kenneth J. Cherry, Jr.



A discussion of the aorta is a broad topic, encompassing the diagnosis and treatment of aneurysms, occlusive disease, and dissections of the abdominal and thoracic aorta. In the past 2 decades, endovascular therapy has offered a frequently less morbid approach to each of these disease entities. The rapid adoption of endovascular techniques and technologies has clearly revolutionized the management of aortic disease. Endovascular repair of abdominal aortic aneurysms (EVAR) is performed much more frequently now than is open repair. Endovascular repair of thoracic aortic aneurysms (TEVAR) is now the recommended first treatment option. The new Trans-Atlantic Inner-Society Consensus guidelines (TASC III) will recommend endovascular therapy as the first option for almost all degrees of aortoiliac occlusive disease (AIOD).

We have tried to make this chapter relevant to general surgery residents training in the second decade of the 21st century, with particular attention to the fact that with the rise of endovascular therapy, the use of open reconstructive techniques for the thoracic and abdominal aorta has declined noticeably. Nationwide, surgical and vascular surgical residents now obtain far less experience in the open surgical treatment of the aorta. Only a few centers still offer rich experience in open aortic surgery and, in particular, the most complex cases. Yet, mastery of aortic surgery remains a necessity. Dense calcium, involvement of visceral vessels, infections, trauma, small arteries, and failed endografts may and do lead to the necessity of a formal open reconstruction. The training necessary to acquire mastery of aortic surgery is changing. We hope that these changes will allow not only the maintenance of current standards with regard to the surgeon's skill set and outcomes, but will also permit future generations to continue to drive advances in state of the art vascular surgery.

## ANEURYSMAL DISEASE

Aneurysms, defined as an increase in size of more than 50% of the normal arterial diameter, may occur anywhere in the aorta, from the aortic root to the bifurcation. Although most nonruptured aneurysms are asymptomatic, a number of risk factors for the development, expansion, and rupture of an abdominal aortic aneurysms (AAA) have been identified (Table 62-1). Risk factors for developing an AAA include age, male gender, family history, tobacco use, hypertension, hyperlipidemia, and height. Aneurysm development is also associated with the presence of connective tissue disorders, such as Marfan syndrome, and of concurrent aneurysmal or atherosclerotic disease.[1-11] Aneurysmal enlargement of the aorta is associated with factors that result in weakening of the arterial wall and increased local hemodynamic forces. These may include heritable conditions such as Marfan syndrome, familial thoracic aortic aneurysm and dissection (TAAD), and vascular-type Ehlers-Danlos syndrome, as well as less well-defined entities that contribute to the significantly elevated incidence in patients with a family history of aneurysm. Factors that contribute to the degradation of collagen and elastin are also associated with aneurysmal disease; research in this area has focused on the role of matrix metalloproteinases (MMPs) and other mediators of tissue enzyme function. The immune response has also been implicated in the pathophysiology of aneurysm formation.[12]

### Diagnosis

An abdominal aneurysm may be detected on physical examination as a palpable pulsatile mass, most commonly supraumbilical and in the midline. The location may, however, be variable, because aortic tortuosity may render the palpable mass lateral and/or infraumbilical. The sensitivity of physical examination is, as one might expect, dependent on aneurysm size and patient habitus.[1]

The detection and characterization of aneurysms may be greatly aided by modern imaging techniques. Ultrasound examination has been demonstrated to afford excellent sensitivity and specificity (Fig. 62-1).[1] Ultrasound may be limited by patient habitus or bowel gas, but because it avoids the complications associated with invasive testing, radiation, and contrast media, is an excellent choice for screening. It must also be noted that ultrasound is not an ideal method for detecting rupture, because ultrasound cannot image all portions of the aortic wall and the nonfasting status of emergently examined patients may further preclude ideal image acquisition. It has been estimated that ultrasound may fail to detect up to 50% of aneurysm ruptures.

Computed tomography (CT) provides excellent imaging of AAA, with greater reproducibility of diameter measurements than ultrasound.[1] CT, particularly with the adjunctive use of iodinated contrast to carry out CT angiography (CTA), provides a wealth of anatomic information, detects vessel calcification, thrombus, and concurrent arterial occlusive disease, and permits

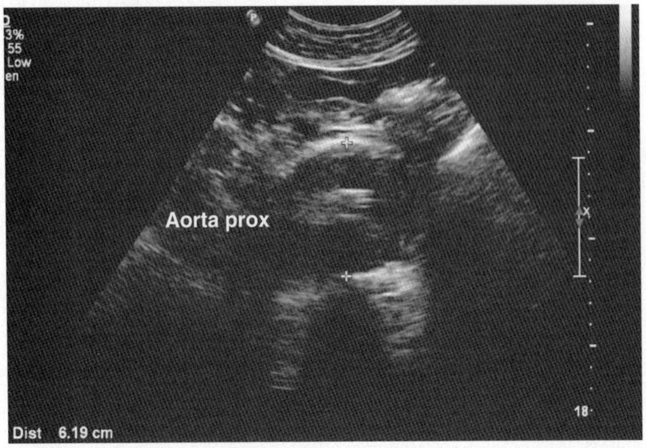

**FIGURE 62-1** Gray scale cross-sectional ultrasound image of an infrarenal aortic aneurysm measuring 6.19 cm in maximal anteroposterior diameter.

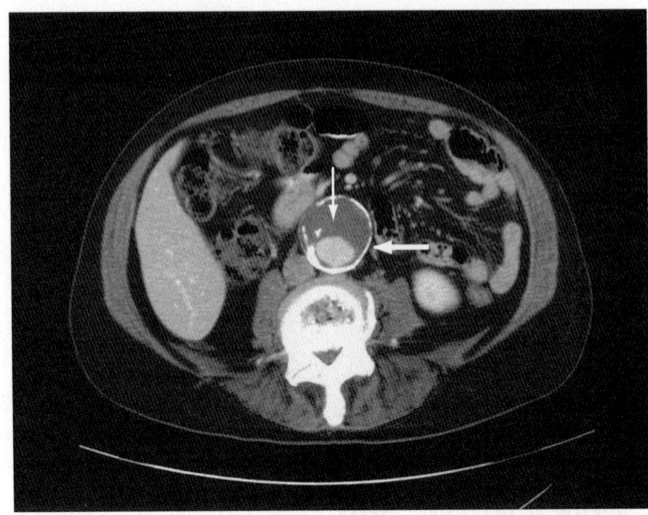

**FIGURE 62-2** CTA axial plane image of an infrarenal abdominal aortic aneurysm demonstrating aortic wall calcification *(solid arrow)* and intraluminal thrombus *(thin arrow)*.

**Table 62-1 Risk Factors for Aneurysm Development, Expansion, and Rupture**

| SYMPTOM | RISK FACTORS |
|---|---|
| AAA development | Tobacco use |
| | Hypercholesterolemia |
| | Hypertension |
| | Male gender |
| | Family history (male predominance) |
| AAA expansion | Advanced age |
| | Severe cardiac disease |
| | Previous stroke |
| | Tobacco use |
| | Cardiac or renal transplant |
| AAA rupture | Female gender |
| | ↓ $FEV_1$ |
| | Larger initial AA diameter |
| | Higher mean blood pressure |
| | Current tobacco use (length of time smoking ≫ amount) |
| | Cardiac or renal transplantation |
| | Critical wall stress–wall strength relationship |

Adapted from Chaikof EL, Brewster DC, Dalman RL, et al: The care of patients with an abdominal aortic aneurysm: The Society for Vascular Surgery practice guidelines. J Vasc Surg 50:S2–S49, 2009.

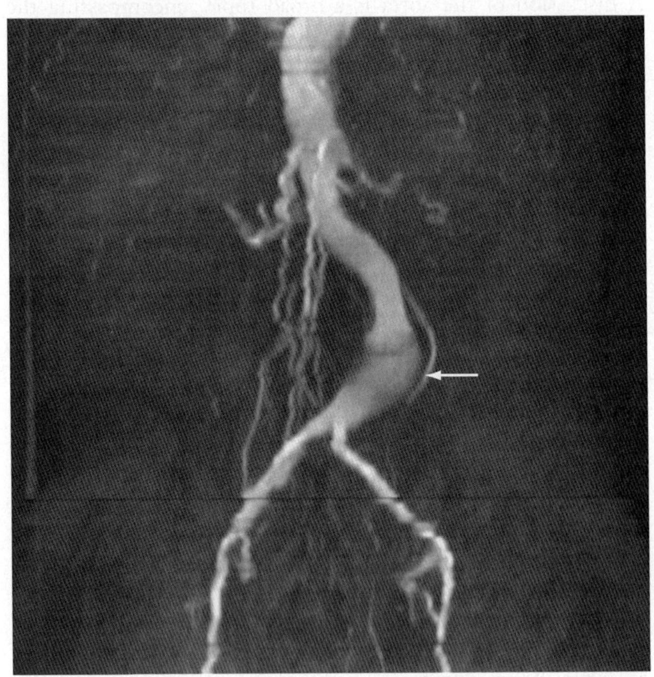

**FIGURE 62-3** MRA coronal view of an infrarenal aneurysm *(solid arrow)*.

multiplanar and three-dimensional reconstruction and analysis for operative planning (Fig. 62-2). Drawbacks include substantial radiation exposure, particularly in the setting of serial examinations, and the use of iodinated contrast media in a population with a high incidence of comorbid kidney disease.

Magnetic resonance imaging (MRI) and magnetic resonance angiography (MRA) are, like CT, sensitive for the detection of AAA (Fig. 62-3). Unlike CT, MRI does not demonstrate aortic wall calcification, which may be important in operative planning. Although the study does not require the use of iodinated contrast, MRA uses gadolinium, which has been associated with the development of nephrogenic systemic fibrosis in patients with a low glomerular filtration rate (GFR). The ability to acquire dynamic images throughout the cardiac cycle may ultimately prove clinically useful.[13]

## Risk of Rupture

Guidelines for surveillance and treatment of AAA are based on data regarding risk factors for rupture. Published risk factors for rupture include chronic obstructive pulmonary disease (COPD), current tobacco use, larger initial AAA diameter, female gender, cardiac or renal transplantation, and certain patterns of wall stress.[1,14-23] The most widely adopted surrogate for rupture risk is maximal cross-sectional aneurysm diameter (Table 62-2).

**Table 62-2 Estimated Annual Rupture Risk**

| AAA DIAMETER (cm) | RUPTURE RISK (%/yr) |
|---|---|
| <4 | 0 |
| 4-5 | 0.5-5 |
| 5-6 | 3-15 |
| 6-7 | 10-20 |
| 7-8 | 20-40 |
| >8 | 30-50 |

Adapted from Brewster DC, Cronenwett JL, Hallett JW Jr, et al: Guidelines for the treatment of abdominal aortic aneurysms. Report of a subcommittee of the Joint Council of the American Association for Vascular Surgery and Society for Vascular Surgery. J Vasc Surg 37:1106–1117, 2003.

In addition, despite a relative paucity of natural history data regarding growth rate and rupture, most clinicians incorporate into practice the concept of rate of enlargement as a risk factor for rupture. In this case, a rate of growth of more than 5 to 7 mm/6 months or more than 1 cm/year has been widely adopted as an indication for repair, independent of aneurysm size. It is important to note that size is an imperfect predictor of rupture risk, because autopsy studies have discovered evidence of rupture in up to 12% of aneurysms less than 5 cm in diameter.[24] There are a number of investigational models that have attempted to quantify rupture risk based on calculations of wall stress or the combination of multiple factors thought to contribute to increased wall stress and/or decreased strength.

## Screening and Surveillance Recommendations

Screening recommendations for AAA are based on the sensitivity and specificity of ultrasound screening, detection yield of screening based on various risk factor selection criteria, and cost. A major recent compilation of evidence-based recommendations for screening and surveillance of abdominal aortic aneurysms has been provided by practice guidelines developed by the Clinical Practice Council of the Society for Vascular Surgery (SVS).[1] The SVS committee charged with reviewing available data regarding screening made a strong recommendation for one-time screening of all men aged 65 years or older or men 55 or older with a family history of AAA. Screening of women is also strongly recommended for those aged 65 years or older with a family history of AAA or a personal smoking history. The evidence basis of these recommendations was deemed to be strong in the former case and moderate in the latter. The U.S. Preventive Services Task Force has issued a more limited recommendation for one-time screening of men between 65 and 75 years of age who have a personal smoking history.[25] It is important to note that payer policies regarding reimbursement may not track of these recommendations. Medicare, for example, as a result of the Screening Abdominal Aortic Aneurysms Very Efficiently (SAAVE) Act, covers screening for select populations (men with a personal smoking history and men or women with a family history of AAA), but only as a part of the initial welcome to Medicare physical examination.

Once an aneurysm has been detected, the SVS Clinical Practice Council recommends further screening intervals as follows, based on aneurysm size (maximum external aortic diameter) and associated risk of rupture[1]:

- Less than 2.6 cm: No further screening recommended
- 2.6 to 2.9 cm: Reexamination at 5 years
- 3.0 to 3.4 cm: Reexamination at 3 years
- 3.5 to 4.4 cm: Reexamination at 12 months
- 4.5 to 5.4 cm: Reexamination at 6 months

## Treatment

### Medical Therapy

Once an aneurysm has been diagnosed, a number of measures may be taken to optimize the patient's medical regimen and potentially minimize the rate of aneurysm expansion and rate of rupture. As noted, current tobacco use has been associated with an increased rate of aneurysm expansion. Smoking cessation may also yield benefits with regard to perioperative morbidity and mortality in the event that the aneurysm ultimately requires repair. Control of blood pressure and rate of increase of left ventricular pressure (dP/dT) has been proposed as being important in minimizing wall stress that may contribute to aneurysm expansion or rupture. However, studies of beta blockade with propranolol to accomplish both these goals failed to show an effect on aneurysm expansion. More recently, angiotensin-converting enzyme inhibitors (ACEIs), angiotensin receptor blockers (ARBs), statins, and antibiotics (e.g., doxycycline) have been associated with a decreased rate of expansion.[26]

### Surgical Treatment

Surgical treatment is generally recommended for aneurysms larger than 5.5 cm in maximal diameter, those demonstrating more than a 5-mm growth in 6 months or more than 1 cm in 1 year, and aneurysms with a saccular rather than the typical fusiform anatomy. However, significant gender differences in the natural history of AAA have emerged, with research suggesting that although women develop aneurysms somewhat less frequently than men, aneurysm prevalence increases sharply with age in women. In addition, there is evidence that aneurysms in women exhibit more rapid growth and rupture at smaller sizes (average diameter of 5 cm in female versus 6 cm in male patients).[27]

**Preoperative Evaluation** The preoperative evaluation of patients with AAA comprises operative planning as well as the identification and management of important medical comorbidities, such as coronary artery disease (CAD), renal insufficiency, peripheral arterial occlusive disease, diabetes, and obstructive lung disease. Because CAD is the primary cause of mortality following open or endovascular repair of AAA, much attention has been focused on the preoperative evaluation and management of comorbid CAD. The guiding principles in this evaluation have traditionally been the identification of information that will alter management and the institution of therapy that will improve cardiac-related mortality. In 2007, the American College of Cardiology/American Heart Association (ACC/AHA) published guidelines regarding the preoperative cardiac evaluation of patients undergoing noncardiac vascular surgery.[28] These guidelines stratify patients according to the presence or absence of symptomatic cardiac disease, presence of significant clinical risk factors (e.g., mild angina, prior myocardial infarction [MI], compensated congestive heart failure [CHF], diabetes mellitus, renal insufficiency), and the level, quantified as metabolic equivalent (MET), of the patient's functional capacity. All patients should be assessed with a resting electrocardiogram (ECG). Echocardiography may be used to evaluate the cardiac function of those with a history of heart failure or current dyspnea. The decision to proceed with noninvasive testing in patients without symptoms of active cardiac disease should be based on patient functional capacity and the presence of three or more significant additional risk factors. Coronary angiography should be considered for patients with evidence of active cardiac disease based on screening questions or evidence of ischemia on noninvasive stress testing. Adjunctive medical therapy may also serve to reduce the risk of perioperative cardiac events. Perioperative beta blockade, statin use, and aspirin use are widely accepted; there is also evidence to support the use of other antihypertensives during this period (Fig. 62-4).[1]

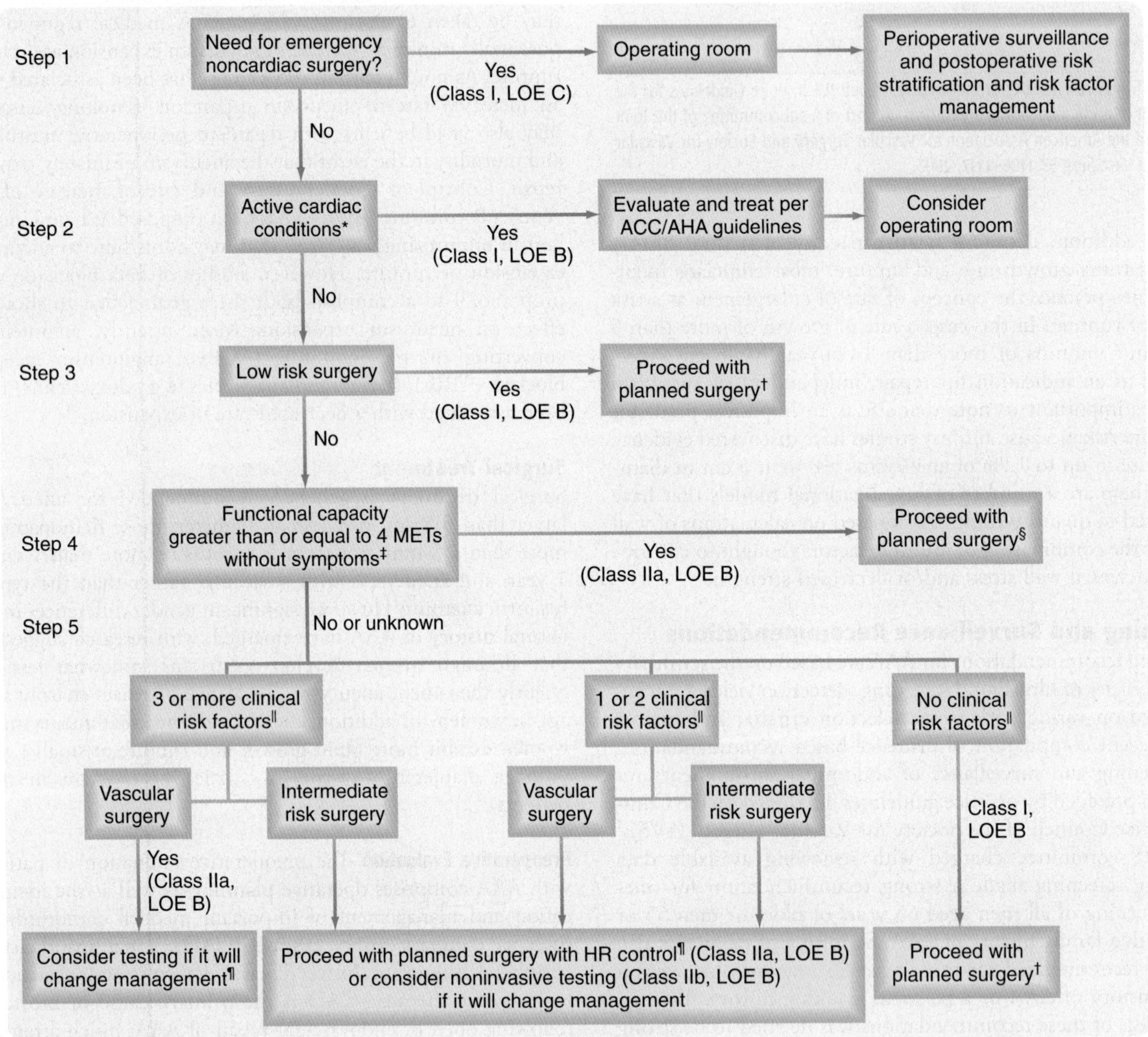


*See Table 2 for active clinical conditions.
†See Class III recommendations in Section 5.2.3, Noninvasive Stress Testing.
‡See Table 3 for estimated MET level equivalent.
§Noninvasive testing may be considered before surgery in specific patients with risk factors if it will change management.
||Clinical risk factors include ischemic heart disease, compensated or prior heart failure, diabetes mellitus, renal insufficiency, and cerebrovascular disease.
¶Consider perioperative beta blockade (see Table 12) for populations in which this has been shown to reduce cardiac morbidity/mortality.
ACC/AHA indicates American College of Cardiology/American Heart Association; HR, heart rate, LOE, level of evidence; and MET, metabolic equivalent.

**FIGURE 62-4** Cardiac evaluation and care algorithm for noncardiac surgery based on active clinical conditions, known cardiovascular disease, or cardiac risk factors for patients 50 years of age or older. (From Fleisher LA, Beckman JA, Brown KA, et al: ACC/AHA 2007 guidelines on perioperative cardiovascular evaluation and care for noncardiac surgery: A report of the American College of Cardiology/American Heart Association Task Force on Practice Guidelines [Writing Committee to Revise the 2002 Guidelines on Perioperative Cardiovascular Evaluation for Noncardiac Surgery]: Developed in collaboration with the American Society of Echocardiography, American Society of Nuclear Cardiology, Heart Rhythm Society, Society of Cardiovascular Anesthesiologists, Society for Cardiovascular Angiography and Interventions, Society for Vascular Medicine and Biology, and Society for Vascular Surgery. Circulation 116:e418–e499, 2007.)

Renal insufficiency related to renovascular or medical renal disease is a well-established risk factor for morbidity and mortality following AAA repair. Coexisting renal artery occlusive disease may be present in 20% to 38% of patients with AAA.[29] Also, open and endovascular repair of AAA may result in further deterioration in the renal function of patients with preexisting renal disease. Concurrent repair of clinically significant renal occlusive disease is appropriate at the time of open or endovascular aneurysm repair. Various strategies for intraoperative renal protection have been proposed. Current recommendations include adequate hydration, perioperative discontinuation of ACEIs and ARBs, and avoidance of hypotension. There is mixed evidence regarding the benefits of antioxidants (e.g., mannitol, ascorbic acid, vitamin E, N-acetylcysteine, allopurinol) and there are some data supporting the beneficial effects of infused fenoldopam.[30,31] When suprarenal clamp placement is necessary, we endorse the use of cold saline perfusion of the kidneys, preclamp administration of furosemide (Lasix) and mannitol, and selective use of fenoldopam. An additional consideration, particularly in patients with preexisting renal dysfunction, is contrast-induced nephropathy (CIN) associated with the administration of iodinated contrast agents for CT imaging or angiography. Current data support IV hydration with sodium bicarbonate or normal saline and possibly the use of antioxidants, such as ascorbic acid or N-acetylcysteine. When EVAR is contemplated, carbon dioxide may be used as an imaging agent to alleviate or minimize the need for iodinated agents, because the rate of CIN is related to the amount of agent administered, age, and prior renal function.

Data are mixed with regard to the impact of pulmonary disease, particularly COPD, on mortality following AAA repair. However, there is evidence that optimal management of comorbid COPD may improve morbidity and mortality.[32] We support obtaining a preoperative pulmonary function assessment, including arterial blood gases, to assess risk and guide management in the perioperative period. Patients with poor pulmonary function must be made aware of the increased risk that they will require prolonged ventilatory support postoperatively and the attendant possibility that tracheostomy will be required during this period. Smoking cessation prior to surgery may be beneficial; this can be aided by counseling and a variety of pharmacologic therapies. Although several studies have suggested that initiating smoking cessation less than 2 weeks before surgery may actually be associated with worse outcomes, a recent meta-analysis has suggested that smoking cessation at any period of time within 8 weeks of surgery is not associated with a higher rate of overall complications or pulmonary complications postoperatively.[33]

The preoperative evaluation should also include chest radiography, complete blood count, blood chemistries, coagulation studies, and urinalysis. The chest radiograph may demonstrate evidence of infection, thoracic aortic pathology, or malignancy, all of which should be thoroughly investigated prior to AAA repair. The use of various anticoagulant agents is common in patients with AAA and management is tailored according to the indication for use. Vitamin K antagonists should be stopped 5 to 7 days prior to surgery and bridging anticoagulation provided, if indicated, using low-molecular-weight or unfractionated heparin. Thienopyridines are typically stopped 7 to 10 days prior to surgery, although patients on thienopyridine therapy for drug-eluting coronary stents necessitate careful consideration of the merits of delaying surgery until therapy is discontinued in light of the additional bleeding risk associated with these drugs. Aspirin is typically continued perioperatively because it may confer some degree of benefit with regard to cardiac complications in the perioperative period.

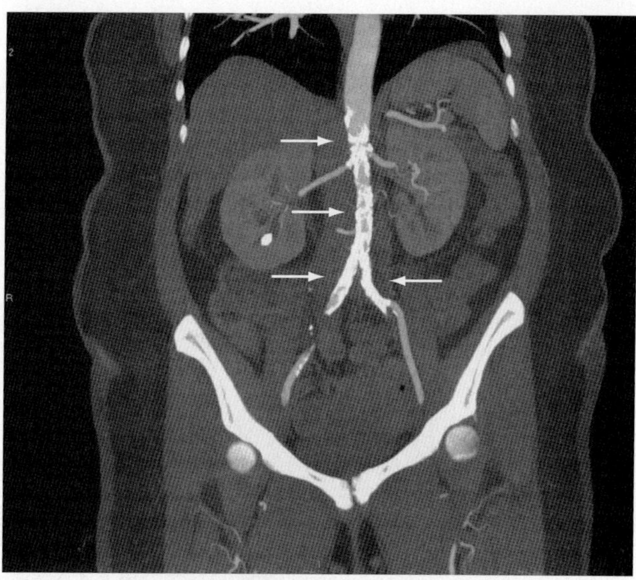

**FIGURE 62-5** Coronal reconstruction of a CTA demonstrating heavy calcification *(solid arrows),* extending from above the renal arteries distally through both common iliac arteries.

Careful evaluation of preoperative imaging is crucial when planning repair. Anatomic variations such as a retroaortic renal vein, variant inferior vena cava, or horseshoe kidney may significantly affect the selection of surgical approach and, if not appreciated preoperatively, can lead to disastrous complications. CT affords the additional advantage of demonstrating vascular calcification, thus permitting the surgeon to assess the feasibility of clamping the aorta and iliac arteries at various levels (Fig. 62-5). Occlusion balloons may be substituted for arterial clamp placement, most frequently at the iliac arteries, should severe calcification render clamp placement untenable. Finally, the size and patency of branch vessels, such as the inferior mesenteric, accessory renal, iliac, and lumbar arteries, can be assessed and may further contribute to preoperative planning.

### Technique of Open Surgical Repair of Abdominal Aortic Aneurysms

Open surgical repair of AAAs may be accomplished by a transperitoneal or retroperitoneal approach. The choice of technique may be guided by technical advantages and disadvantages afforded by each, as well as by surgeon experience and preference. Transperitoneal repair via a midline laparotomy incision is the most widely used approach to the usual infrarenal aneurysm and offers a rapid exposure, excellent access to renal and iliac vessels, and the ability to examine the abdominal contents fully. Adjunctive measures to improve exposure at or above the level of the renal arteries may include ligation and division of the tributaries (gonadal, lumbar, and adrenal) of the left renal vein, if the vein is to be preserved, or division of the proximal left renal vein itself. Although data are mixed regarding the effect of left renal vein ligation on postoperative renal function, it is essential that these tributaries be preserved to provide collateral outflow if renal vein ligation is planned. Alternatively, repair of the left renal vein following ligation has been reported.

The infrarenal transperitoneal repair begins with the administration of perioperative antibiotic, typically a first-generation cephalosporin, and scrupulous skin preparation from the nipples to the thighs. If treating a ruptured aneurysm, skin preparation and draping are accomplished prior to the induction of general anesthesia to permit rapid exposure and control if induction incites hemodynamic collapse. The patient is draped and a generous midline laparotomy incision is made from the xiphoid to just above the pubis. Extension of this incision along the xiphoid may facilitate supraceliac exposure, if necessary. If repair is elective and preoperative imaging has demonstrated iliac disease necessitating extension of a bifurcated graft to the femoral artery on one or both sides, the femoral artery dissection should be accomplished prior to laparotomy (Fig. 62-6).

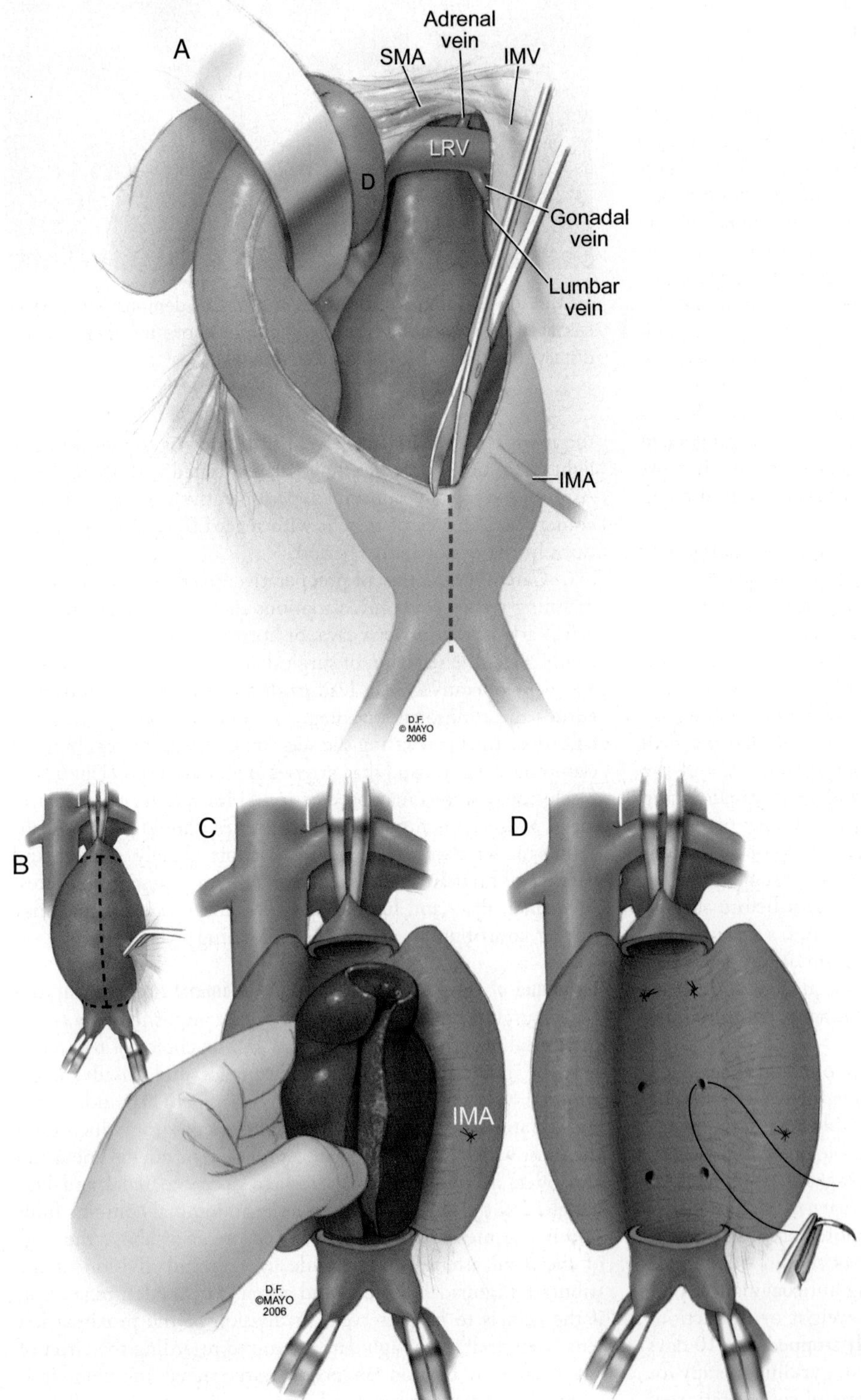


**FIGURE 62-6** Technique of open operative repair of an infrarenal abdominal aortic aneurysm using a straight tube graft (H) or a bifurcated aortoiliac or aortofemoral (I) configuration. Note the attention to closure of the aneurysm sac over the completed repair, with additional closure of retroperitoneal tissues to exclude the duodenum fully (J). (Courtesy Mayo Foundation for Medical Education and Research.)

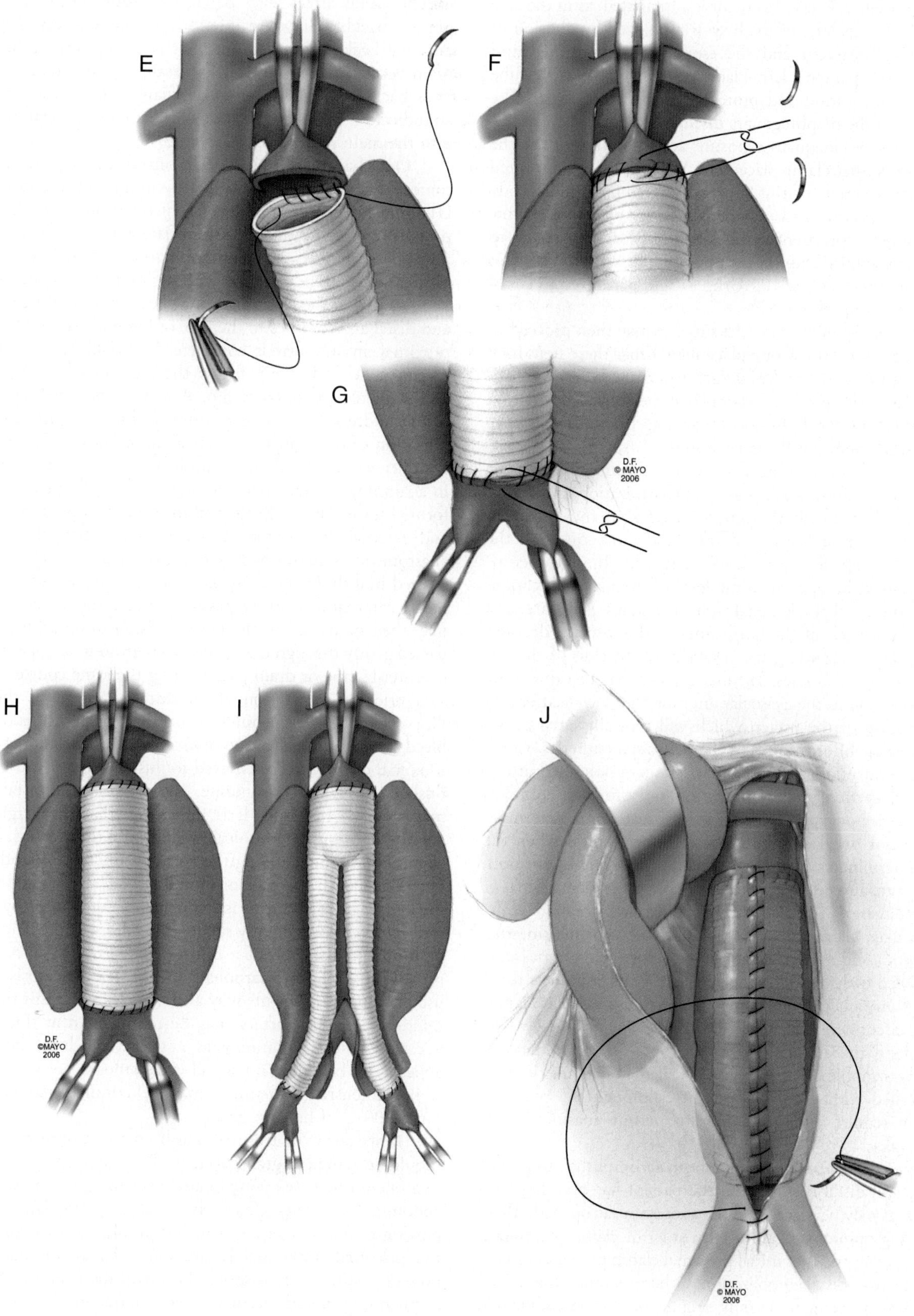


**FIGURE 62-6, cont'd.**

If supraceliac clamp placement is anticipated, as in the case of rupture, the left lobe of the liver is mobilized by division of the triangular ligament and the esophagus is identified and reflected to the patient's left. Placement of a nasogastric tube facilitates identification and protection of the esophagus. The crural fibers of the diaphragm are divided proximal to the celiac artery to provide adequate exposure and mobilization of the aorta for supraceliac clamp placement. When treating a ruptured aneurysm, placement of this supraceliac clamp should greatly facilitate resuscitation and provide a measure of hemodynamic stability. Surgeon preference guides the decision with regard to IV heparin administration in rupture. Typical systemic heparin administration consists of 100 U/kg IV and permitted to circulate prior to clamp placement.

In the setting of rupture, the surgeon may then proceed to with iliac dissection and clamp placement. Once these steps have been accomplished, the neck of the aneurysm may be approached. In some cases, the proximal clamp may be moved down to a suprarenal or infrarenal position at this stage, permitting perfusion of visceral and, ideally, renal vessels.

Elective repair permits controlled exposure of the iliac arteries and aneurysm neck prior to heparinization and clamp placement. Exposure of the infrarenal neck of the aneurysm requires careful mobilization of the duodenum, distal to the ligament of Treitz, to the patient's right side. The retroperitoneum may then be opened to the level of the iliac bifurcation. Mobilization of the left renal vein facilitates exposure and control of the neck of the aneurysm. At this time, a decision should be made regarding the necessity of division of the left renal vein or its tributaries. The iliac arteries may be exposed by careful dissection in the avascular anterior plane, with attention to preservation of the ureter, which will typically cross at the level of the iliac bifurcation, and the pelvic sympathetics, which cross the bifurcation and proximal left common iliac artery. Extensive dissection of the bifurcation and proximal common iliac arteries is not typically necessary, because clamp placement in the mid or distal common iliacs is more typical when the aneurysm terminates at or is proximal to the aortic bifurcation, permitting repair with a simple tube graft. When aneurysmal or occlusive disease of the iliac arteries requires replacement of the common iliac, clamps may be placed at the proximal internal (hypogastric) and external iliac arteries. Soft iliac arteries may be controlled with vessel loops placed in a Potts fashion or using a Rumel tourniquet. However, we prefer to use vascular clamps to avoid circumferential dissection of the iliac arteries, where possible, and the attendant risk of venous injury, which can lead to catastrophic bleeding. Severely calcified iliac arteries may be controlled with occlusive balloons, although the proximal ends may require endarterectomy to permit anastomosis or oversewing.

Once adequate dissection has been accomplished to permit proximal and distal control, and the patient has been heparinized, clamps may be placed and the aneurysm sac opened. There are differing opinions regarding the order of clamp placement, with some believing that initial proximal clamp placement minimizes the risk of distal embolization. Others maintain that initial distal clamp placement permits staging of the hemodynamic effect of clamp placement. The sac should be opened just below the aneurysm neck and the opening extended along the right side of the anterior surface of the aneurysm, leaving the orifice of the inferior mesenteric artery in situ. Lumbar arteries and the middle sacral artery may be ligated from within the sac to prevent backbleeding. An inferior mesenteric artery with brisk pulsatile backbleeding or one that is chronically occluded, as often occurs in aneurysms, may be safely oversewn at its origin. Poor backbleeding suggests inadequate collateralization and is an indication for reimplantation of the inferior mesenteric artery into the main graft or left iliac limb.

Once backbleeding has been controlled, the proximal anastomosis may be addressed, typically in an end-to-end running fashion using nonabsorbable monofilament sutures such as polypropylene (Prolene) and an appropriately sized woven or knitted polyester graft. An aneurysm terminating at or before the aortic bifurcation may be repaired with a simple tube graft, whereas involvement of the iliac vessels may necessitate a bifurcated graft and distal anastomoses to the iliac or femoral arteries. Once the proximal anastomosis is complete, it should be examined by placing a second clamp below the anastomosis and carefully removing the proximal clamp. Any areas of bleeding may be readily addressed with repair sutures at this time, prior to immobilization of the graft by the distal anastomosis. If a tube graft is sufficient, the distal anastomosis may similarly be completed in a running fashion. Iliac anastomoses may frequently be performed at the level of the iliac bifurcation, incorporating internal and external iliac arteries as a common orifice. If an emoral anastomosis is performed, a retroperitoneal tunnel should be created bluntly in the avascular anatomic plane anterior to the native external iliac artery, passing beneath the ureter. The limb may then be passed to the groin incision using a blunt clamp passed gently through the tunnel from groin to retroperitoneum or a sterile tape or drain passed along the same course.

Prior to completion of the distal anastomosis, the distal iliac or femoral vessels should sequentially be permitted to backbleed to flush out any thrombus or atherosclerotic debris, the proximal clamp briefly removed to flush the graft, and the graft flushed with heparinized saline. The proximal and distal clamps may then be removed. It is imperative that the surgical and anesthesia teams communicate well during this process, because clamping and unclamping the aorta produces profound hemodynamic effects. The patient should be well resuscitated prior to unclamping, because this is frequently accompanied by significant hypotension. Slightly staging the release of the iliac arteries or limbs, in the case of a bifurcated graft, may alleviate this somewhat. Sodium bicarbonate to counteract acidosis and the use of vasopressor agents may also be required at this time. The inferior mesenteric artery may be reimplanted at this time, if necessary, most commonly as a Carrel patch. If hemostasis appears to be adequate at all anastomoses and the patient is normotensive, protamine may be administered at 0.5 to 1 mg/100 U of heparin given.

Once aortic replacement has been accomplished, attention should be turned to graft coverage. The aneurysm sac and retroperitoneum may be approximated over the graft to exclude the abdominal contents effectively and, in particular, the third portion of the duodenum, which typically rests just anterior to the proximal, infrarenal suture line. The abdominal and, if present, groin incisions should be closed meticulously. Hernias, as previously noted, occur relatively frequently following open aneurysmorrhaphy. Wound breakdown, particularly at the groin, can be costly and difficult for the patient and significantly increases the risk of catastrophic graft infection. We do not routinely drain groin incisions.

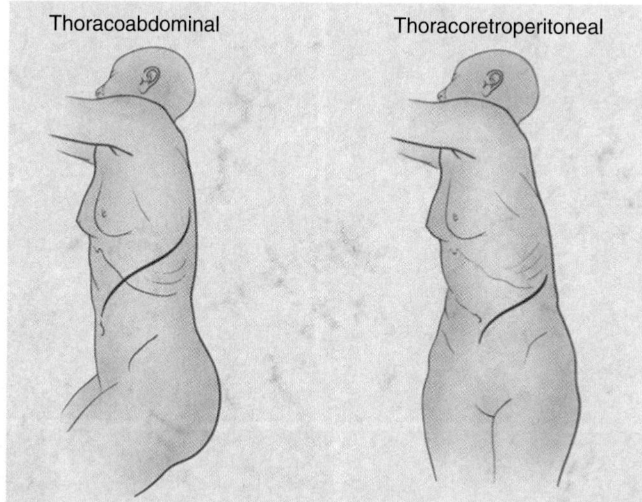


**FIGURE 62-7** Patient positioning and incision for thoracoabdominal and thoracoretroperitoneal exposures. Note the open configuration of the hips in the latter, facilitating bilateral access to the iliac and femoral arteries.

The retroperitoneal approach is thought by some to reduce physiologic stress on the patient and to result in fewer postoperative pulmonary complications, as well as a reduction in postoperative ileus.[34] Both approaches are associated with a significant rate of wound healing complications. Midline incisions for AAA repair were complicated by radiographically apparent abdominal wall defects in approximately 20% of cases in a recent series, although clinically significant hernias are less frequent. Persistent postoperative pain, flank wall laxity, and hernia have been described as complicating retroperitoneal repair and some investigators have reported more frequent occurrence of these complications using the retroperitoneal technique. With regard to operative exposure, the retroperitoneal approach does afford greater access to the visceral segment of the abdominal aorta and may be aided, if required, by thoracic extension of the incision and exposure with or without division of the diaphragm.

A retroperitoneal aortic exposure may be accomplished with the patient in a modified right lateral decubitus position, with the thorax rotated but the hips relatively flat to permit access to both groins (Fig. 62-7). A curvilinear incision is made from the costal margin to below the umbilicus, depending on the extent of exposure required and patient habitus. The retroperitoneal plane may be entered at the lateral border of the rectus sheath. The rectus abdominus may be reflected medially or laterally. Some surgeons prefer lateral reflection, because this may result in less difficulty with postoperative body wall laxity. Care is taken to avoid entering the peritoneum. Much of the initial portion of this dissection may be carried out bluntly, with the aid of a tonsil sponge on a ring or Kelly forceps. The abdominal contents, enveloped in peritoneum, may be swept medially. The ureter will be visualized and swept medially. The left kidney may be elevated or left in situ, although we generally prefer to medialize the kidney, which also serves to mobilize the left renal vein. The gonadal tributary, however, must generally be identified, ligated, and divided. Proximally, the spleen is carefully mobilized within its peritoneal covering to expose the underside of the diaphragm. The fibers of the left crus of the diaphragm, when divided, expose the supraceliac and visceral portions of the aorta. The left renal artery should be readily accessible and the celiac and superior mesenteric arteries may be mobilized by careful dissection. The right renal artery is frequently difficult to isolate prior to aortotomy. Distally, the iliacs are carefully exposed in the avascular plane by gently mobilizing overlying structures, including the ureters. Again, the full exposure of the right iliac is typically more difficult by this approach, depending on patient habitus. The extensive exposure of the supraceliac and visceral portions of the aorta permit full access and nuanced decision making regarding clamp placement, which may be suprarenal, supramesenteric, or supraceliac. Visceral and renal vessels may be controlled by clamp placement, vessel loops or, after aortotomy, use of occlusion balloons, with great care taken in handling to avoid dissection or embolization. Occlusive disease or aneurysmal involvement of renal or visceral vessels may be readily addressed by this approach. According to patient indications and surgeon preference, cardiopulmonary bypass may be used as an adjunct; this provides the ability to perfuse the renal and visceral vessels actively if a complex or prolonged reconstruction is anticipated.

Once adequate exposure has been achieved, proximal and distal clamps may be placed. As in the transperitoneal approach, repair is typically accomplished by endoaneurysmorrhaphy using end-to-end proximal and distal anastomoses to replace the diseased portion of the aorta as an interposition. Once again, the aneurysm thrombus is removed at the time of aortotomy and lumbar arteries are ligated within the sac. The same principles of backbleeding and flushing of the graft prior to completion of the distal anastomosis apply. This approach also permits a variety of approaches to reconstruction of the juxtarenal, pararenal, and paravisceral aorta. Branch vessels may be incorporated together by careful beveling of the graft, reimplanted individually as Carrel patches, or reconstructed using short bypass grafts. When treating thoracoabdominal aneurysms, the incision may be extended into the chest at the appropriate rib space and the diaphragm circumferentially divided to afford enough exposure to extend the repair to almost any level of the descending aorta. The rib may be circumferentially dissected and divided posteriorly to improve thoracic exposure further, as needed. When hemostasis is achieved, the sac may, again, be closed over the graft, although the retroperitoneally placed graft is not as vulnerable to erosion and aortoduodenal fistula as that placed transperitoneally (Fig. 62-8).

Medial visceral rotation, introduced by Mattox for trauma and adapted to aortic reconstruction by Stoney, is a third technique that may, through an abdominal incision, afford exposure of the entire abdominal aorta. This technique is may be used for type IV or high paravisceral aneurysms and is best suited for who are not obese or asthenic, with narrow costal margins extending to the iliac crest.

***Postoperative Management*** In the immediate postoperative period, patients are typically admitted to an intensive care unit, with continuous cardiopulmonary monitoring. Adequate pain control, appropriate resuscitation, adequate oxygenation, and heart rate control all serve to minimize the risk of a postoperative MI. Epidural anesthesia and patient-controlled analgesia are both excellent options for postoperative pain management; the former may actually decrease postoperative complications.[35] The use of appropriate prophylaxis for deep venous thrombosis is

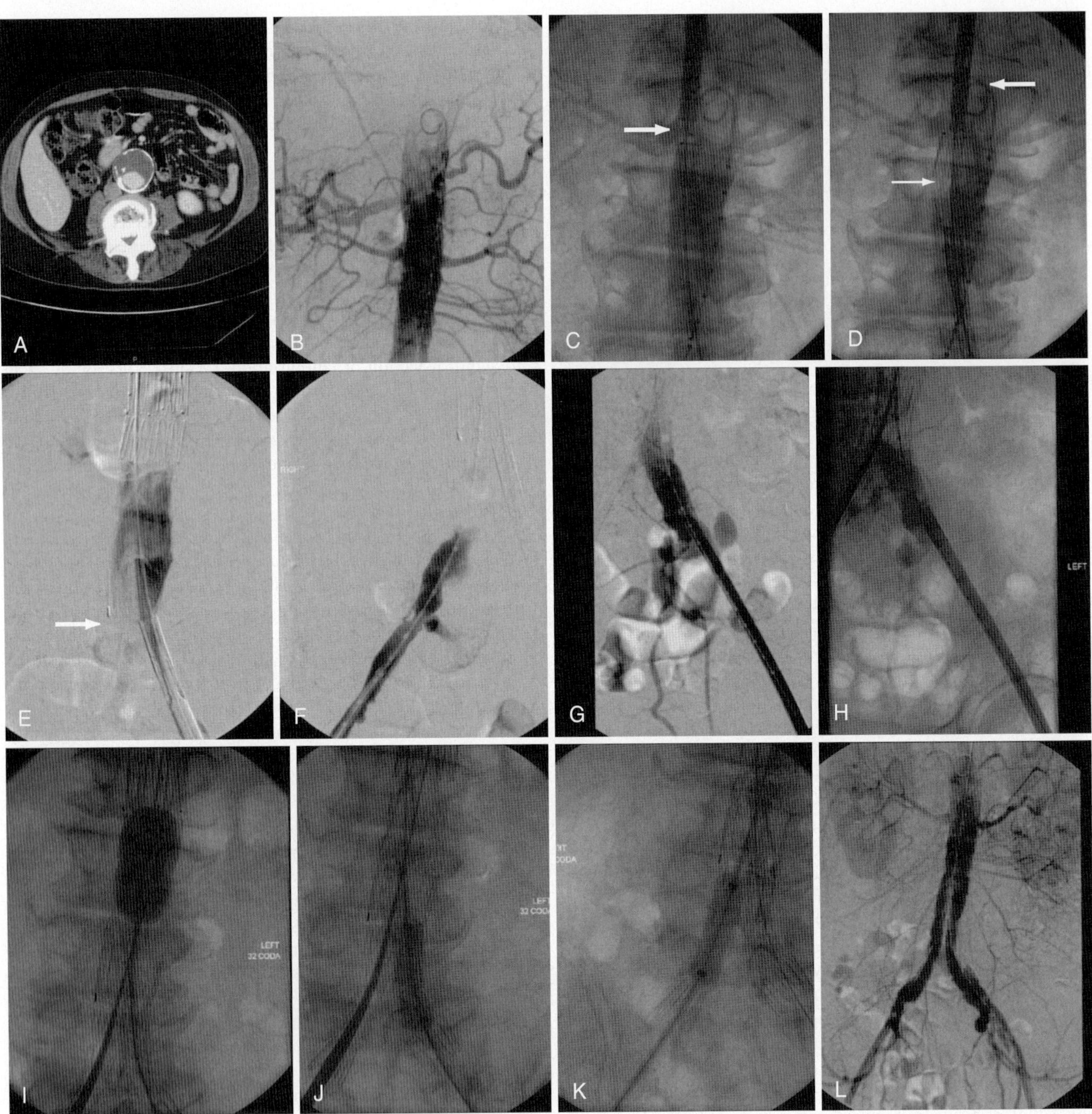


**FIGURE 62-8** Technique of EVAR. **A,** Initial aortogram profiling the renal arteries. **B,** Device has been advanced over a stiff wire to the level of the renal arteries. Note radiopaque markers indicating the beginning of fabric coverage *(solid arrow)*. **D,** Device sheath withdrawn, permitting partial opening of the proximal graft *(thin arrow)*. Note that the top cap continues to constrain the suprarenal fixation wires *(solid arrow)*. **E,** The contralateral iliac limb gate *(thick arrow)* has been cannulated; contrast is introduced using a rim catheter to confirm successful cannulation prior to placement of iliac extension. **F-H,** Angiography of both iliac arteries with marker catheters in place to permit deployment of iliac extensions, with preservation of both internal iliac arteries. **I-K,** Balloon molding of the proximal graft, overlap segments of the main graft and iliac limbs, and the distal seal zones of the iliac limbs to facilitate proximal, distal, and intercomponent seals. **L,** Completion aortogram demonstrating successful exclusion of the aneurysm and no evidence of endoleak, which would manifest as continued contrast filling of the aneurysm sac.

important and is not precluded by the use of an epidural catheter. Attention to early mobilization and patient nutrition are also essential to recovery.

Although late events following open surgical repair are relatively rare, a program of surveillance is typical to detect these complications as the formation of anastomotic or para-anastomotic aneurysms, which may occur up to 20% of the time at 15 years postrepair.[36,37] We typically image patients with CT initially and then at 5-year intervals following repair. Ultrasound may also be used for surveillance, but is operator-dependent and lacks the sensitivity of CT for detecting anastomotic or para-anastomotic changes.

**Endovascular Repair** Endovascular repair of an AAA was first reported by Parodi and colleagues in 1991[38] and has been widely adopted since the first U.S. Food and Drug Administration (FDA)–approved devices for EVAR, the AneuRx (Medtronic, Minneapolis) and Ancure (Guidant, Menlo Park, Calif) became available in 1999. Driven by lower rates of early morbidity and mortality, EVAR has largely supplanted open surgical repair of infrarenal aortic aneurysms in patients with favorable anatomy. Several anatomic considerations guide patient suitability for EVAR, including the anatomy of the aneurysm neck (size, length, shape, and angulation) and the iliac arteries (caliber, tortuosity, and aneurysmal involvement). The features of currently available devices, as summarized in their approved indications for use (IFU), are shown in Table 62-3. Most available devices are modular bifurcated grafts consisting of an aortic main body to be used with a variable number of iliac or aortic extension components. Aortouni-iliac devices are also available and may be used, generally in conjunction with femoral-femoral bypass grafting, primarily or to salvage a failed bifurcated device.

Although early morbidity and mortality rates are lower with EVAR, there is overall a higher rate of re-intervention after endovascular than open aneurysm repair and, after 2 years, no significant difference in the overall mortality rate.[1] In addition, the new technology has brought an entirely new set of complications. Endoleak is the most common complication following EVAR. Type I endoleak is defined as failure to seal completely at the proximal (type IA) or distal (type IB) seal zones. In general, a type I endoleak represents a failure to exclude the aneurysm fully and should be addressed at the time of detection. More aggressive balloon inflation within the seal zone, placement of additional graft components, and placement of balloon-expandable stents are among the most common endovascular therapies for type I endoleak. Type II endoleaks are the most common form and represent continued filling of the aneurysm sac by lumbar branches or the inferior mesenteric artery. Further treatment is indicated if a persistent type II endoleak is accompanied by an increase in sac size. Treatment may include embolization of feeding branches by selective catheterization or direct sac puncture or laparoscopic ligation of these vessels. Type III endoleaks represent failure of an individual component or of the seal between components of a modular graft system. As with type I leaks, all type III endoleaks should be treated, typically by relining the offending area with new graft components. Type IV endoleaks represent seepage through porous graft material and are typically self-limiting, resolving when procedural anticoagulation is reversed. Finally, an entity known as *endotension* is sometimes considered a fifth type of endoleak. This represents persistent growth of the aneurysm sac in the absence of a detectable leak. It has been proposed that this phenomenon is caused by the passage of serous ultrafiltrate across an excessively porous fabric or, as some believe, by the existence of an undetected endoleak of one of the prior types.

Device migration, intraprocedurally or over time, may occur. In the EVAR setting, migration may be facilitated by unfavorable aneurysm neck anatomy. Manufacturers have attempted to address this issue by various mechanisms, including increased radial force, use of barbs or suprarenal fixation, or use of anatomic fixation at the aortic bifurcation. Device failure resulting from fracture of metallic components or fabric failure may also occur. The iliac limbs of these devices are also subject to thrombosis and occlusion, possibly at a higher rate than bifurcated grafts placed during open surgical repair.[39]

It is recommended that contrast CT surveillance be conducted at 1, 6, and 12 months after graft implantation and annually thereafter. Concern over accumulated lifetime radiation exposure and use of nephrotoxic contrast agents has driven investigation into the role of duplex ultrasonography in graft surveillance. In general, lengthened imaging intervals or the substitution of ultrasound for CT is reserved for patients in whom no endoleak has been detected at procedure or during initial follow-up. Implantable sensor technology has been approved by the FDA to monitor pressure within the aneurysm sac. As this technology develops, it may ultimately augment or even supplant routine CT for postoperative aneurysm surveillance.

In 2006, the Agency for Health Research and Quality (AHRQ) published a comparison of EVAR and open surgical repair for AAA that concluded that "EVAR has shorter length of stay, lower 30-day morbidity and mortality, but does not improve quality of life beyond 3 months or survival beyond 2 years."[40] These advantages, although limited, have been sufficient to make EVAR more frequently performed in recent years than open surgical repair for aneurysms with suitable anatomy.[41]

**Thoracic and Thoracoabdominal Aortic Aneurysms** Aneurysms of the descending thoracic aorta may be classified as type A, B, or C, depending on whether the aneurysm involves the proximal, mid, or distal third of the descending aorta, respectively (Fig. 62-9). Thoracoabdominal aneurysms (TAAs) are typically distinguished according to the Crawford classification system (Fig 62-10). As with aneurysms of the abdominal aorta, rupture risk is closely associated with aneurysm size and, to a lesser extent, female gender. Current guidelines recommend repair of the descending thoracic aorta at 5.5 cm.

***Open Repair of Thoracic and Thoracoabdominal Aneurysms*** The level of entry into the thoracic cavity for the repair of thoracic or thoracoabdominal aneurysms is guided by the proximal extent of the aneurysm, with incision at the fifth or sixth interspace providing excellent exposure of the proximal descending aorta, the eighth or ninth interspace the mid-descending, and the 10th or 11th interspace the infradiaphragmatic portion of the aorta. The use of cardiopulmonary bypass combined with the selective use of distal aortic and visceral perfusion and hypothermic circulatory arrest have yielded exemplary results in experienced hands.[42]

**Table 62-3 Endovascular Repair Devices: Indications for Use**

| DEVICE (MANUFACTURER) | STENT OR GRAFT MATERIAL | SHEATH OR DEVICE DIAMETER (MAIN BODY) | AORTIC DIAMETER* (MM) | ILIAC DIAMETER (MM) | MAXIMUM ANGULATION | MINIMUM NECK LENGTH | OTHER |
|---|---|---|---|---|---|---|---|
| AneuRX (Medtronic) | Nitinol, polyester | 21 Fr | 20-28 (graft) | 12-24 (graft) | 45-degree neck | 15 mm | Initial FDA approval 1999<br>No suprarenal fixation or barbs<br>Sheath not required |
| Talent (Medtronic) | Nitinol, polyester | 22 Fr | 18-32 (aorta)<br>22-36 (graft) | 8-22 (iliac)<br>8-24 (graft) | 60-degree neck | 10 mm | Suprarenal fixation stent<br>Tapered and flared limbs available<br>Uni-iliac Talent Converter device available |
| Endurant (Medtronic) | Nitinol, polyester | 18 Fr, 20 Fr | 19-32 (aorta)<br>23-36 (graft) | 8-25 (iliac)<br>10-28 (graft) | 60-degree neck | 10 mm | Barbed suprarenal fixation stent<br>Like Talent, approved for 10-mm neck<br>Thin fabric, low delivery profile |
| Zenith (Cook Medical) | Stainless steel, polyester | 18 Fr, 20 Fr, 22 Fr | 18-32 (aorta)<br>22-36 (graft) | 7.5-20 (iliac)<br>9-24 (graft) | 60-degree neck | 15 mm | Barbed suprarenal fixation stent<br>Tapered limb configurations available<br>Zenith Renu aortouni-iliac graft available<br>Graft sizing based on outer diameter |
| Excluder (WL Gore) | Nitinol, ePTFE | 18 Fr, 20 Fr | 19-29 (aorta)<br>23-31 (graft) | 8-13.5 (ipsilateral graft)<br>12-14.5 (ipsilateral graft)<br>8-18.5 (contra-lateral graft)<br>12-20 (contra-lateral graft)<br>10-20 (extender) | 60-degree neck | 15 mm | Available ipsilateral limb sizes vary with size of primary graft<br>Contralateral limb components may be used as iliac extenders<br>Proximal nitinol anchors |
| Powerlink (Endologix) | Cobalt-chromium, ePTFE | 19 Fr, 21 Fr | 18-32 (aorta)<br>22, 25, 28 (graft)<br>25, 28, 34 (aortic cuff) | 10-23 (iliac)<br>13-16 (graft)<br>16-25 (extensions) | 60-degree neck, 90-degree iliac | 15 mm | Anatomic fixation on aortic bifurcation<br>Seal achieved with suprarenal or infrarenal proximal aortic cuff<br>IntuiTrak system avoids need to cannulate contralateral gate |
| AFX (Endologix) | Cobalt-chromium, ePTFE | 17 Fr | 18-32 (aorta)<br>22, 25, 28 (graft)<br>25, 28, 34 (aortic cuff) | 10-23 (iliac)<br>13-16 (graft)<br>16-25 (extensions) | 60-degree neck, 90-degree iliac | 15 mm | Similar to Powerlink in design<br>Multiple limb configurations<br>Low profile delivery system for bifurcated graft and proximal cuff |

*Recommended methods of vessel sizing and guidelines for graft oversizing vary by device.

***Endovascular Management of Thoracic and Thoracoabdominal Aneurysms*** In 2005, the FDA approved the GORE TAG Thoracic Endoprosthesis (WL Gore, Flagstaff, Ariz) for the treatment of dTA-A. Since then, open surgical therapy of aneurysms of the descending thoracic aorta (dTAA) has largely been supplanted by TEVAR for anatomically suitable lesions.[43]

As with abdominal aortic endografts, initial and subsequent studies have demonstrated a significantly lower rate of short-term morbidity and mortality than with open repair. Unlike EVAR, TEVAR appears to offer a significant, long-term aneurysm-related mortality advantage.[44] The most frequent complications of thoracic endovascular aneurysm repair are related to injuries to femoral or iliac access vessels. Because the French sizes of the delivery devices for thoracic endografts may be considerably larger than those required for EVAR, many surgeons have developed a distinctly conservative approach to device access, performing femoral cutdowns or placing iliac or aortic conduits to prevent injury. Because of the passage of endovascular wires, catheters, and other devices through the aortic arch, TEVAR carries the additional risk of embolic

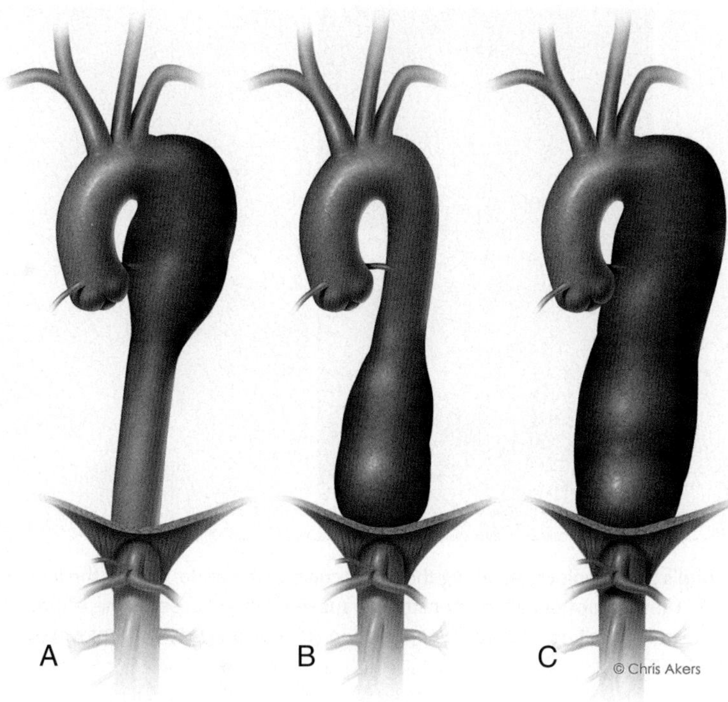


**FIGURE 62-9** Classification, descending thoracic aortic aneurysm. **A,** Type A, distal to the left subclavian artery to the sixth intercostal space. **B,** Type B, sixth intercostal space to above the diaphragm (12th intercostal space). **C,** Type C, entire descending thoracic aorta, distal to the left subclavian artery to above the diaphragm (12th intercostal space). (Courtesy Chris Akers, 2006.)

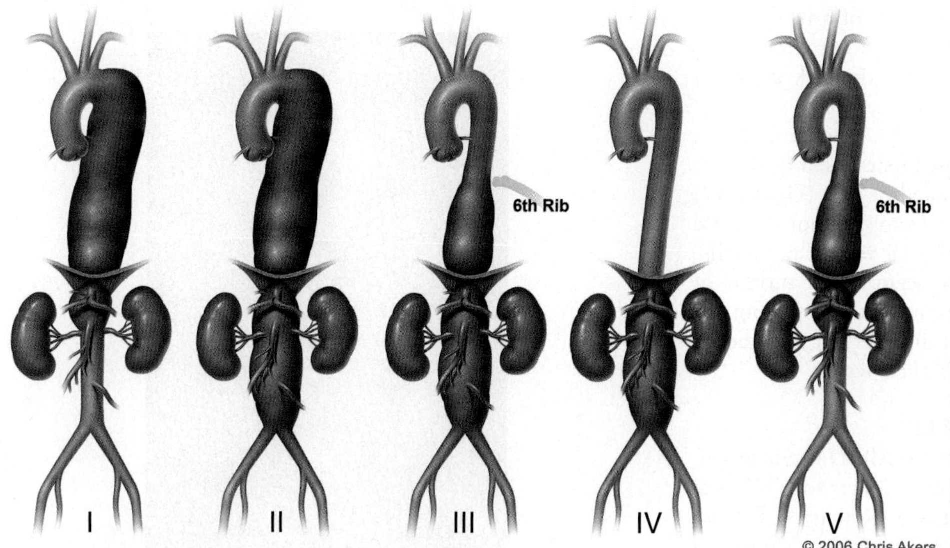


**FIGURE 62-10** Normal thoracoabdominal aorta aneurysm classification—extent I, distal to the left subclavian artery to above the renal arteries; extent II, distal to the left subclavian artery to below the renal arteries; extent III, from the sixth intercostal space to below the renal arteries; extent IV, from the 12th intercostal space to the iliac bifurcation (total abdominal aortic aneurysm); extent V, below the sixth intercostal space to just above the renal arteries (modified Crawford classification). (Courtesy Chris Akers, 2006.)

stroke.[45] TEVAR has, however, consistently yielded lower rates of early mortality and common postoperative complications than open repair, with Bavaria and associates[46] reporting perioperative mortality rates of 2.1% versus 11.7%, spinal cord ischemia rates of 3% versus 14%, respiratory failure rates of 4% versus 20%, and renal insufficiency rates of 1% versus 13% in low-risk patients following endovascular and open repair, respectively.

Several anatomic considerations guide patient selection for TEVAR. As with EVAR, the size and configuration of the proximal aneurysm neck must suit the configuration and capabilities of available grafts. Commercially available thoracic endograft diameters currently range from 21 to 46 mm, creating limitations in patients with large proximal necks or small-caliber aortas. Tapered configurations are also available. The radius of the aortic arch and proximal descending aorta can also challenge device conformability and may result in a bird's beak deformity on deployment and, potentially, device collapse, with consequent compromise of the aortic lumen (Fig. 62-11). In addition, coverage of one or more supra-aortic vessels may be required to achieve an adequate proximal landing and seal zone for the graft, necessitating decisions regarding extra-anatomic reconstruction. Usually, the left subclavian artery origin is covered. Justifications for reconstruction of the subclavian

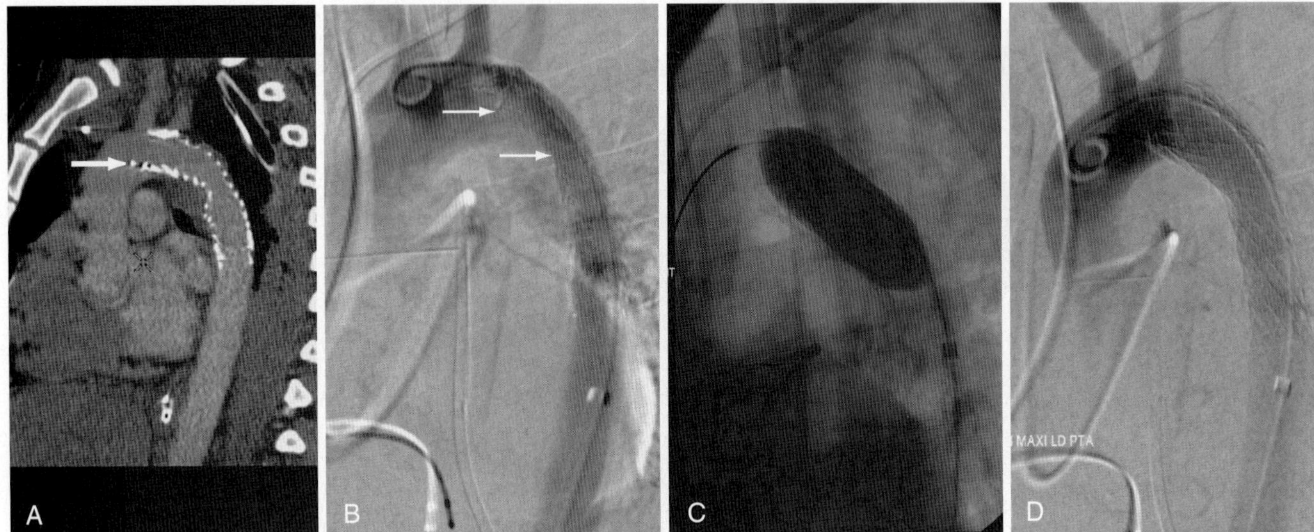


**FIGURE 62-11** **A,** CT scan demonstrating thoracic endograft with bird's beak deployment along the lesser curve of the aorta, leaving the leading edge of the endograft projecting into the lumen *(solid arrow).* **B,** Thoracic aortogram demonstrating subsequent collapse of the endograft caused by pressure on the protruding proximal portion of the endograft, resulting in distal hypoperfusion *(thin arrows).* **C, D,** Deployment of a balloon-expandable Palmaz stent to reopen the proximal graft.

artery, generally by carotid-subclavian artery bypass or subclavian artery transposition, include prevention of arm claudication, preservation of flow to a dominant left vertebral artery and, perhaps most importantly, maximization of collateral spinal cord perfusion.

Currently, endovascular therapy for TAAs is limited to a few centers with access to investigational fenestrated devices or experience creating customized fenestrated devices (Fig. 62-12) or using debranching (antegrade grafts from the thoracic aorta or retrograde iliac grafts to the renovisceral vessels, permitting stent graft coverage of the perivisceral segment) or snorkel or chimney techniques (use of covered stents extending from the branch vessels beyond the proximal or distal extent of an aortic stent-graft) to maintain perfusion to branch vessels.[47,48]

## AORTOILIAC OCCLUSIVE DISEASE

In 1950, the first aortic reconstruction for AIOD (Leriche syndrome) was performed by Jacques Oudot in France. This was done via a retroperitoneal approach using a homograft. Following the investigational and clinical work of Arthur Vorhees at Columbia University, prosthetic grafts of Vinyon B and nylon were used for the reconstruction of aortic occlusive and aneurysmal disease. Both these materials had significant problems associated with their use. Wylie introduced aortoiliac endarterectomy to the United States in 1952 and that technique was the most commonly used during the 1950s. In 1958, DeBakey introduced Dacron grafts and aortofemoral grafting with Dacron became the most widely used technique for open reconstruction, although aortoiliac endarterectomy was still performed at certain centers, notably San Francisco, Boston, and Portland, Oregon. It is still useful for patients with aortoiliac disease confined to the aorta and common iliac arteries, especially those with small aortas and iliac arteries, for whom endovascular repair may not be optimal. Axillofemoral artery grafting and femorofemoral artery grafting were introduced to provide inflow procedures for

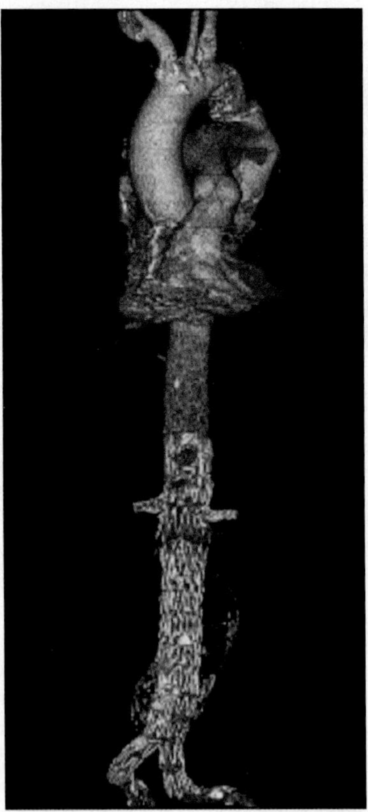

**FIGURE 62-12** CT reconstruction demonstrating successful placement of an endovascular graft with fenestrations at the level of the renal arteries, permitting renal stent placement and use of a proximal seal zone above the renal arteries, with preservation of renal perfusion. (Courtesy Dr. Gilbert R. Upchurch, Jr.)

poor risk patients and patients with unilateral iliac disease, respectively.

Endovascular repair for occlusive disease of the aorta and iliac arteries was introduced in the 1990s. The use of kissing stents, and the size of the common iliac arteries especially, has allowed this modality to work extremely well for most patients with aortoiliac occlusive disease. The Trans Atlantic Inter-Society Consensus document on management of peripheral arterial disease (TASC I) was published in January 2000.[49,50]

These guidelines were developed to help in the rational choice of an open or endovascular approach to aortoiliac disease in particular patients. At present, endovascular treatment is the treatment of choice for type A lesions (see Table 63-6). It is also the most commonly used modality for type B. For type C lesions with more extensive disease of the external iliacs or bilateral occlusions of the common iliacs, surgical treatment has been recommended more often. For type D lesions—that is, extensive disease of the common and external iliac arteries—surgery has been the treatment of choice. Nonetheless, a number of authors have documented good success with endovascular treatment even for TASC C and TASC D lesions.[51-53]

The next iteration of the TASC recommendation is expected soon; endovascular treatment will likely be that the recommended first-line treatment for all patients. However, it is difficult to imagine endovascular therapy to be as good or as long lasting for AIOD for these very extensive lesions, especially in young patients. Women especially, and men with very small aortas and iliac arteries, may not be well treated by endovascular methods. It is also hard to imagine its usefulness for juxtarenal aortic occlusions, with its so-called *dunce's cap* of chronic thrombus extending upward between the renal arteries, without a disproportionate increase in renal failure.

Concomitant with the change in TASC definitions has been a marked increase in the use of endovascular techniques in comparison to open techniques. This increase corresponds to improvements in the delivery systems and stents used, as well as to improved skill sets of vascular radiologists, cardiologists, and vascular surgeons. Upchurch and coworkers[54] documented an increase of 850% in endovascular usage by 2000, with a concomitant 16% decrease in open cases. There was a 34% increase in treated disease, without an increase in the prevalence of the disease. These trends have continued and amplified; endovascular repair for AIOD is performed much more commonly than open repair.

The typical indications for AIOD were claudication, rest pain, and threatened limb viability, manifested by tissue loss, nonhealing ulcers, and/or frank gangrene. Rest pain and threatened limb viability implied extensive disease of the deep femoral artery or of the femoropopliteal segments, in addition to the aortoiliac disease. The advent of endovascular techniques has, as noted, broadened the indications, with mild claudication being treated much more frequently than in the past. There is certainly more justification for stenting short-segment iliac stenoses than for performing aortofemoral bypass grafting (AFBG).

Nonetheless, open surgery remains the gold standard for long term patency. Chiu and colleagues[55] have performed a meta-analysis of AFBG, iliofemoral bypass grafting (IFBG), and aortoiliac endarterectomy. Their analysis yielded 29 studies, including 5738 patients for AFBG, 11 studies of 778 patients for iliofemoral bypass grafting, and 11 studies of 1490 patients for endarterectomy. Operative mortality was 4.1% for AFBG, 2.7 for IFB, and 2.7% for aortoiliac endarterectomy. Morbidity rates were 16%, 18.9%, and 12.5%, respectively. Five-year primary patency rates were 86.3%, 85.3%, and 88.3%, respectively. This meta-analysis was published in 2009 and shows that formal aortic reconstruction is still the procedure of choice in terms of long-term patency. That durability may be more appealing to younger healthier patients than return trips for further endovascular intervention. Similarly, an earlier meta-analysis covering the years 1970 to 1996 showed constant patency rates for aortic bifurcation grafts and declining mortality and morbidity over time; mortality after 1975 was 3.3%.[56]

Axillofemoral artery bypass grafting is reserved for extremely poor-risk patients with rest pain or tissue loss. Its suspect patency makes it a poor choice for claudicants. It is used as one of the mainstays of reconstruction for infected aortic grafts or aorta enteric fistulas. This modality is offered to a different, more high-risk group than AFBG. Hertzer and coworkers[57] have reported a 12% mortality, compared with 5.6% for femorofemoral grafting and 2.3% for aortic reconstruction. Within that latter group, mortality was only 1.2% for AFBG, but 5.6% for aortoiliac endarterectomy or aortoiliac grafting.

Unilateral external iliac occlusive disease not amenable to endovascular therapy, or having failed endovascular therapy, is probably better treated, if possible, by iliofemoral artery grafting than femorofemoral grafting. Ricco and Probst[58] have compared these two operative methods in 143 patients. Primary 5-year patency for iliofemoral grafting was 92.7% versus 73.2% for femorofemoral grafting.

As in all vascular beds, endovascular repair of the aortoiliac segments requires much more re-intervention than its open counterpart, but the mortality is lower. At some aortic centers there is no difference in mortality but, on average, open mortality is approximately 4%. in an elegant paper, Hertzer's group[57] has reported a mortality rate of 2.3% for direct aortic reconstructions. Both Hertzer and Reed and coworkers[59] have found increased limb occlusion in patients with small arteries, especially women. Primary assisted and secondary patency rates for endovascular repair almost equal the primary patency rates of open reconstruction, and this has been the rationale for the widespread application of endovascular techniques for most patients with AIOD, accepting a repeat intervention as a necessary component of treatment.

A number of authors have written about the endovascular treatment of TASC C and D lesions, as well as aortic occlusion. Klonaris and colleagues[60] have recommended primary stenting for all aortic occlusive disease, including occlusion. Their study, however, did not include juxtarenal aortic occlusions as opposed to more distal aortic obstruction.

Jongkind and associates[53] have reviewed all published articles of patients undergoing endovascular treatment of TASC C and D lesions from 2000 to 2009. There were 1711 patients identified. Technical success was achieved in 86% to 100% of those studies. Clinical symptoms were improved in 83% to 6.7% and complication rates varied, from 3% to 45%. Primary patency rates ranged from 60% to 86% and secondary patency rates from 80% to 98%.

Higashiura and coworkers[52] have reported technical success in 99% of their 125 TASC D and D patients. Complications were significantly higher than for their TASC A and B patients (9% versus 3%). Their 5-year patency was 83%, among the highest reported.

Ye and colleagues[51] have performed a meta-analysis of TASC C and D patients undergoing endovascular reconstruction. TASC C patients had a 93.7% technical success rate and a 1-year primary patency rate of 89.6%. TASC D patients had 90.1% technical success and 87.3% had a 1-year patency. Indes and associates,[61] in a review of the Nationwide Inpatient Sample for 4119 patients, found endovascular procedures were associated with lower cost, lower complication rates, and shorter length of stay. Mortality was not different statistically, 1.8% for endovascular and 2.5% for open repair.

There is a third option for aortic reconstruction—laparoscopic aortic surgery. Its greatest proponents have been in Europe, particularly France, and Québec. This has not gained widespread popularity in the United States.[62]

## Presentation and Evaluation

Patients with AIOD may present with claudication, a much more likely presentation for AIOD than rest pain or tissue loss. Rest pain or tissue loss, as noted, indicates disease of the deep femoral artery or femoropopliteal segments in addition to the aorta and iliac segments. Historically, physical examination has been accurate in these patients. A decreased femoral pulse is indicative of at least common femoral disease or more proximal aortoiliac disease. With the advent of the obesity epidemic in the United States, physical examination of femoral pulses is not as accurate as it once was. Consequently, vascular laboratory examination is of even more importance than in the past. Determination of wave patterns and ankle-brachial index (ABI) is necessary to localize the disease to aortoiliac segments, femoropopliteal segments, or both. This is also vital in identifying the contribution of AIOD to patients with multiple diseases contributing to their lower extremity problems, including neurogenic claudication, spinal stenosis, and hip arthritis, alone or in combination with arterial disease.

With a tentative diagnosis of aortoiliac occlusive disease, the most commonly used modality to visualize the arteries is CTA. There are some patients in whom the calcium load is so great that MRA or conventional arteriography is necessary to determine whether areas of calcific involvement are highly stenotic. Surgeons for whom endovascular treatment is uniformly their first choice may proceed directly to conventional arteriography, with planned endovascular intervention at the same time.

As with all vascular patients, cardiac risk is the highest at operation. Consequently, most authors recommend that all these patients undergo cardiac function evaluation by stress testing. Patients with their myocardium at risk are usually treated by cardiologists or cardiac surgeons prior to embarking on an aortic reconstruction in an elective situation. Hertzer and associates[57] have shown a marked decrease in cardiac mortality when patients underwent preoperative cardiac evaluation and treatment.

As endovascular techniques gain wider acceptance, the most common indication for formal aortic reconstruction may be claudication or severe ischemia in the setting of failed multiple attempts at endovascular repair. These occluded stents make the operation more complex, often with the need for suprarenal aortic clamping and more extended profundaplasties.

## Treatment

### Technique of Open Reconstruction

**Aortofemoral Bypass Grafting** For AFBG, the patient is prepped from the nipples to the knees (Fig. 62-13). If concomitant distal bypass grafting will be necessary, the patient is prepped to the toes. This would be done for tissue loss with multilevel disease only. Epidural catheters may be used to alleviate postoperative pain. Bilateral groin incisions are made. These are usually done

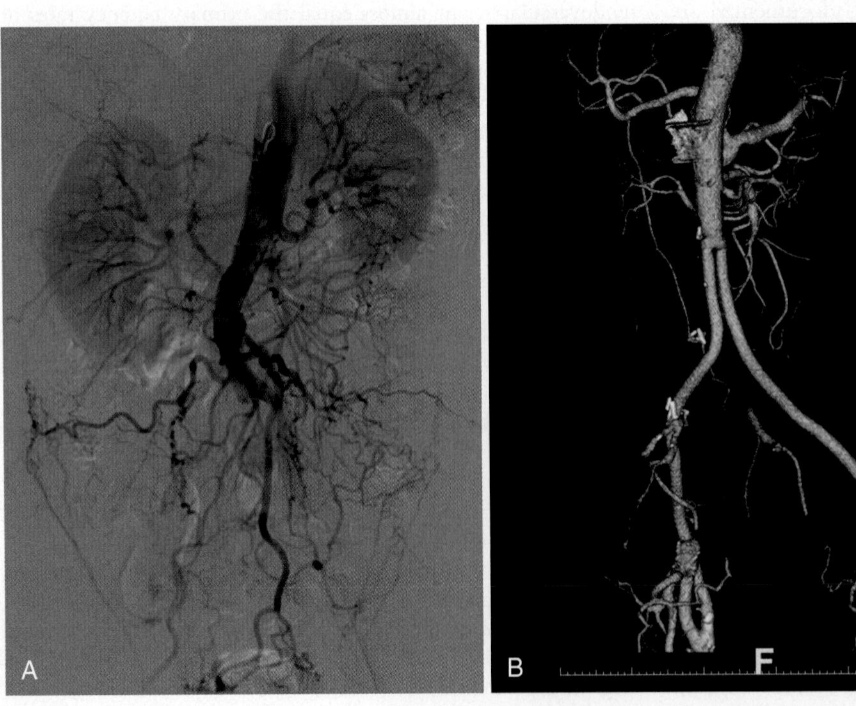


**FIGURE 62-13 A,** Preoperative aortogram demonstrating occlusion of the distal aorta and iliacs with extensive collateralization. **B,** Postoperative three-dimensional CT reconstruction demonstrating revascularization using an aortofemoral bypass graft.

in a vertical or slight curvilinear fashion. The common, superficial, and deep femoral arteries are dissected free. These need to be dissected distally to where they are soft and suitable for anastomosis. Most surgeons use a midline incision for the aortic exposure, although a transverse incision or retroperitoneal approach can be used. We favor a standard midline with infracolic exposure. The abdominal contents are mobilized so that the retroperitoneum can be entered. If the mobilized viscera can be kept inside the abdominal cavity, rather than being placed on the abdominal wall, the patient's gastrointestinal functional recovery usually occurs sooner. The retroperitoneum is entered. Care is taken to stay to the patient's right of the inferior mesenteric vein to avoid violating the left mesocolon. The aorta is dissected free below the renal arteries. The surgeon needs to remember that this disease extends from the renal arteries and not from the level of the lower lying renal vein. The vein may be mobilized by division and ligation of its tributaries. In general, the exposure required for occlusive disease is less than what is necessary for aneurysmal disease. The aorta is exposed down to the level of the inferior mesenteric artery. Retroperitoneal tunnels are made, connecting this wound with the groin wounds. On the left side, a counterincision in the gutter lateral to the white line of Toldt may be necessary. The tunnels should be made posterior to the ureters. We prefer to create the left tunnel posterior to the inferior mesenteric artery as well to allow the left limb of the graft to be isolated from the gastrointestinal tract by the left mesocolon following completion of reconstruction. The patient is heparinized.

Control of the aorta and distal aorta is obtained below the renal arteries. The aorta is divided. Distally, a portion of the aorta is resected on an angular bias and the distal aorta is oversewn. That area of excision should be done proximal to the inferior mesenteric artery. This allows comfortable placement of an end-to-end graft. An appropriately chosen graft is fashioned to fit and is sewn to the end of the proximal aorta using running 3-0 or 4-0 permanent sutures. If one extremity has been less symptomatic that the other, that side is reconstructed first, because it is less used to ischemia. The graft is brought through the tunnel into the groin and control of the femoral arteries is obtained. An arteriotomy is made running, from the common femoral artery down to the appropriate level. In many cases, this would be down to a point on the deep femoral artery. If endarterectomy of the common and deep femoral arteries is necessary, it is undertaken at this point. The graft is fashioned to fit and is sewn end to side using running 4-0 or 5-0 permanent sutures. Appropriate backbleeding and forward bleeding are allowed prior to that. The opposite is done in a similar manner. When flow is restored to the limbs, it is restored first to the common, then to the deep, and finally to the superficial femoral artery.

In general, end-to-end anastomoses are performed. These may lessen the chance of aortoenteric fistula. They have better flow characteristics than end-to-side proximal anastomoses. If the patient has bilateral external iliac artery occlusions, a proximal end-to-side aortic anastomosis or formal reconstruction of one of the internal iliac arteries is necessary to ensure continued blood flood to the pelvis.

The retroperitoneum should be carefully closed in layers to exclude the graft from the gastrointestinal tract. If there is insufficient tissue, an omental flap should be created and placed over the graft to isolate it from the duodenum.

**Axillofemoral Bypass Grafting** Axillobifemoral bypass grafting (Fig. 62-14) was introduced in the 1960s to provide inflow to patients who were poor physiologic candidates for aortic reconstruction. Its use has been extended to patients having aortic graft infections or otherwise hostile abdomens for whom an in-line aortic reconstruction is considered too hazardous.

The patient is prepped from the shoulders down to the knees. It is our practice to extend the upper extremity on the side on which the graft is to be based by 90 degrees. This will prevent the graft from being too taut when the patient moves the extremity. Reports of pseudoaneurysms and ruptures secondary to short grafts have been published. A transverse incision is made in the deltopectoral groove. The axillary artery is exposed as medially as possible. The more medial the anastomosis, the less excursion of the graft with use of the upper extremity. The pectoralis minor tendon may be incised to facilitate this exposure. If the tendon is not incised, the tunnel should be posterior to the tendon and then brought to the midaxillary line. In general, the right side is chosen, if possible, because the right subclavian artery is less prone to atherosclerotic disease than the left. Furthermore, if a later formal aortic reconstruction is planned, a right axillofemoral graft is much less a hindrance than one on the left, especially if a retroperitoneal approach is planned. Bilateral groin incisions are made. If the tunnel connecting the ipsilateral groin incision to the axillary incision can be created without a counterincision, this should be done. If not, a counterincision can be made in the patient's flank. The counterincision seems to be prone to infection and we try to avoid its use. Grafting is then done in the usual manner. The long portion of the graft should be at least 8 mm in diameter, preferably 10 or 12 mm, to prevent a functional aortic stenosis. Mortality rates are higher for these patients than for those having aortic reconstruction, ranging from 10% to 15%. This is because this is a much sicker patient population. Five-year primary patency rates vary greatly but an approximately 50% failure rate can be expected over the course of 5 years.

**Femorofemoral Artery Bypass Grafting** The femoral arteries are exposed in the standard manner. Most surgeons now use a bucket handle approach rather than trying to create a completely antegrade sigmoid-shaped reconstruction. This is done superior to the pubis at the subcutaneous level. Expanded polytetrafluoroethylene (ePTFE) or polyester can be used. Grafts of at least 7 or 8 mm are usually preferred. However, the patency rate has not been nearly as good as was first expected, ranging from 60% to 80% at 5 years. See Figure 62-15.

**Iliofemoral Artery Bypass Grafting** In-line reconstruction of isolated external iliac artery lesions is preferable to femorofemoral artery grafting if the patient's physiology and anatomy will allow. A flank incision is made and the retroperitoneal plane is developed. The proximal anastomosis is performed to the common iliac artery or to the distal aorta, as necessary, and then brought out through that tunnel into the groin. Patency rates at 5 years are in the 90% range. See Figure 62-16.

**Aortoiliac Endarterectomy** This operation is usually done through a midline incision. In distinction to exposure for aortic grafting, for endarterectomy, the aorta, common iliac arteries, and origins of the internal and external iliac arteries all need to be circumferentially exposed. In addition to clamping the aorta and iliac

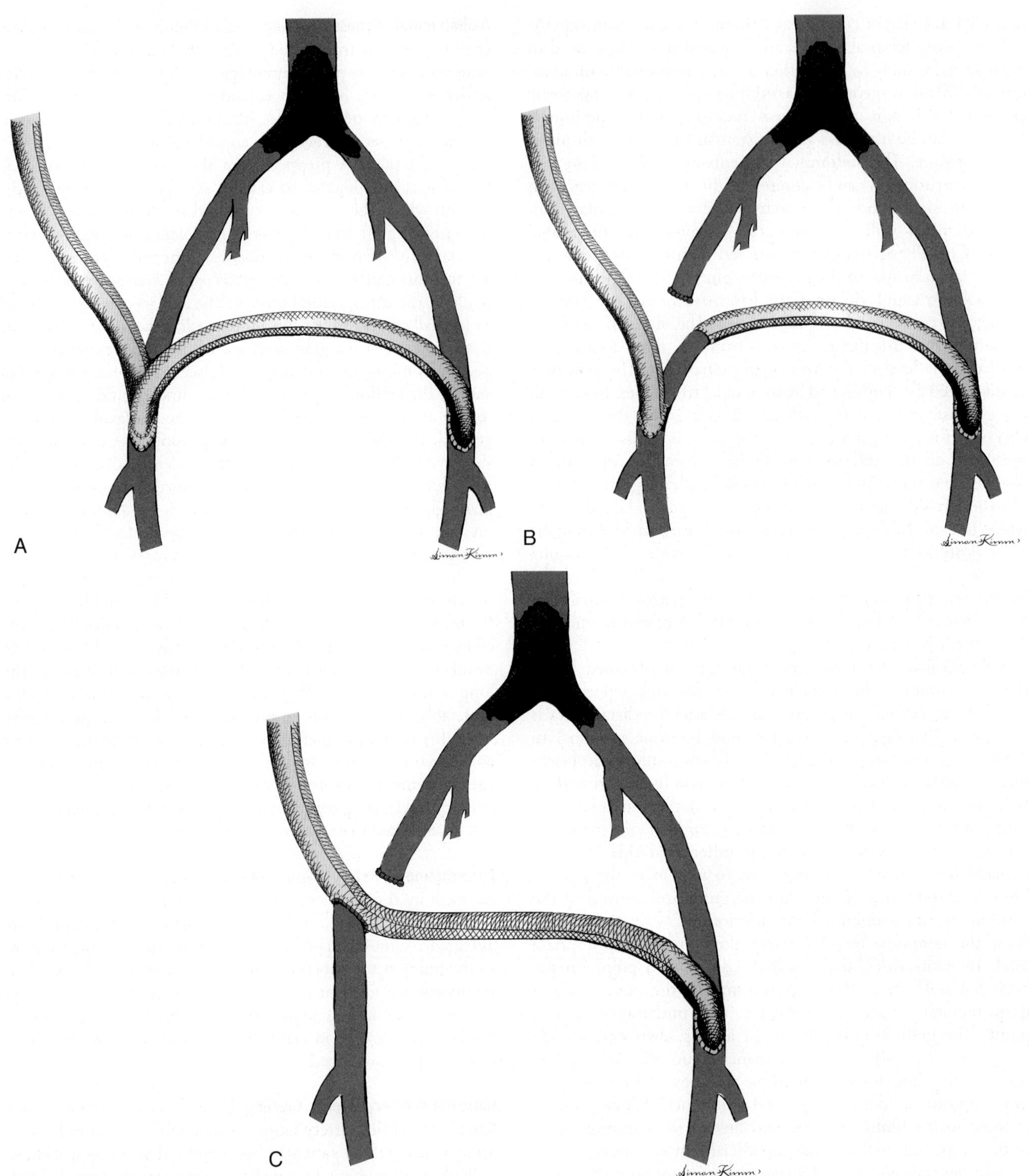


**FIGURE 62-14** Three configurations of axillobifemoral bypass grafts. All three are shown with a right-sided axillofemoral graft component. **A,** The most comment configuration. **B, C,** Modifications described by Blaisdell and associates **(B)** and Rutherford and Rainer **(C),** designed to prevent competitive inflow from a patent ipsilateral iliac system. (From Cronenwett J, Johnston KW [eds]: Rutherford's vascular surgery, ed 7, Philadelphia, 2011, Elsevier.)

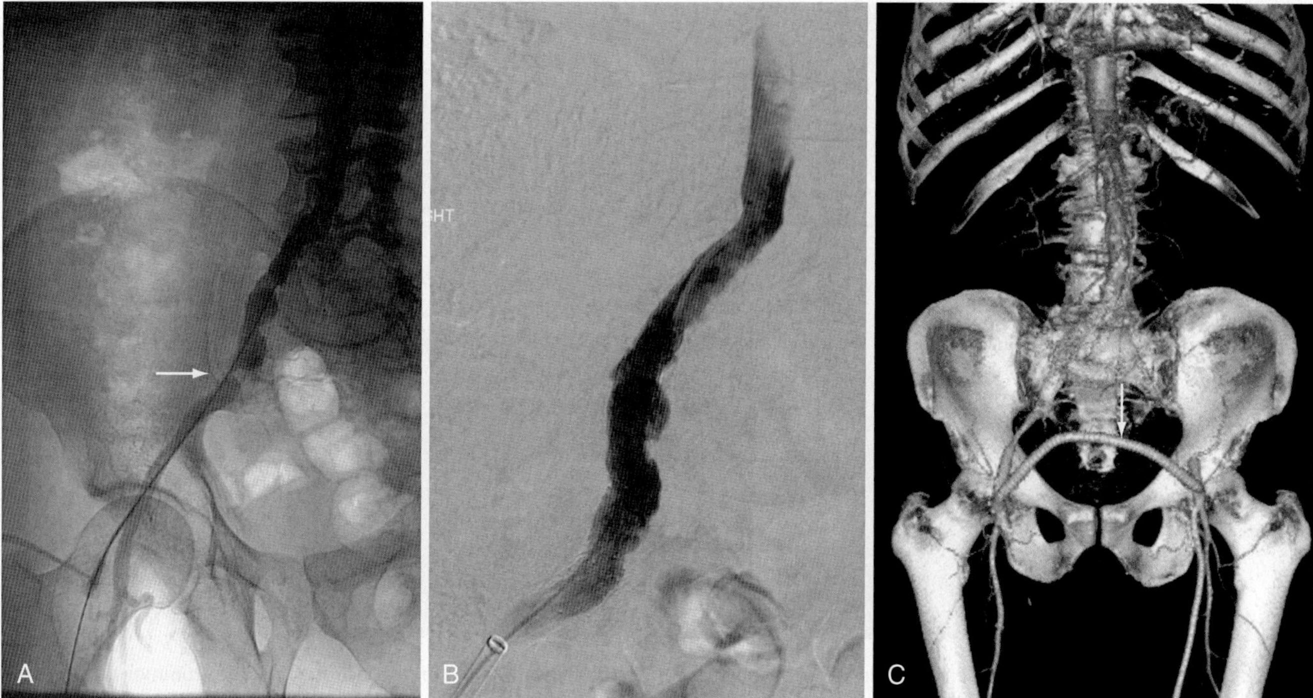


**FIGURE 62-15 A,** Preoperative angiogram demonstrating occlusion of the left iliac system in severe focal atherosclerotic disease of the right iliac artery *(solid arrow).* **B,** Magnified view of the right iliac system following angioplasty and stent placement to establish adequate inflow for femorofemoral bypass graft. **C,** Three-dimensional CT reconstruction demonstrating completed right to left femorofemoral bypass grafting *(solid arrow).*

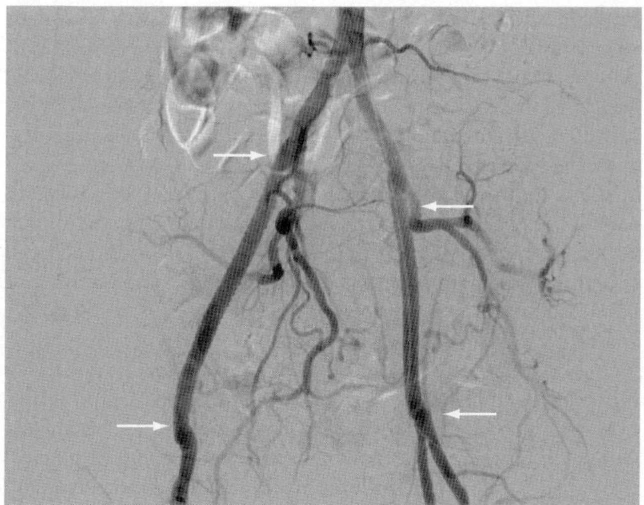

**FIGURE 62-16** Arteriogram demonstrating iliofemoral bypasses extending from the bilateral common iliac to common femoral arteries *(thin arrows).*

arteries, it is also best to clamp the lumbar arteries with small clamps to prevent annoying backbleeding, which impedes accurate endarterectomy. The patient is heparinized. Control is obtained of the aorta and iliac arteries. A vertical aortotomy is made. Using an elevator, an endarterectomy of the aorta is performed down to the origins of the common iliacs. At this point, transverse incisions (our preference) or vertical incisions may be made at the distal common iliac arteries. The endarterectomy plane is begun here. There may be a tongue of atherosclerosis extending into the origin of the external and internal iliac arteries. These are elevated. A stripper such as a Wylie stripper is used. Usually, this is passed in a retrograde manner. In some patients with deep pelvises, passing in an antegrade manner might be more advantageous. An appropriately sized stripper is picked and the endarterectomy of the iliac artery is completed. The atherosclerotic plaque from the aorta and iliac arteries may be brought out as a single specimen if retrograde iliac endarterectomy has been performed The arterial incisions are closed primarily with fine permanent sutures after appropriate flushing and ascertainment of good end points. Interestingly enough, when flow is restored, the aorta remains essentially the same size and the common iliac arteries balloon up, much like pantaloons. The retroperitoneum and abdomen are then closed in a standard manner. See Figure 62-17.

## Complications of Aortic Surgery

A number of complications may arise following operations to repair the aorta, whether for aneurysmal or occlusive disease.[63] These may be site-specific complications, such as wound infection or hematoma, also commonly seen with endograft approaches. Of more concern and major morbidity are intra-abdominal and systemic complications. Cardiac ischemia is the most frequent complication of open aortic surgery and, even with an experienced surgeon, one can expect that 50% of deaths related to aortic reconstruction will be attributable to the heart. Only a minority of patients with occlusive disease have normal coronary arteries. Stress testing, cardiac angiography, and coronary intervention (catheter-based or, more rarely, open) have reduced mortality rates for direct aortic operations. Some

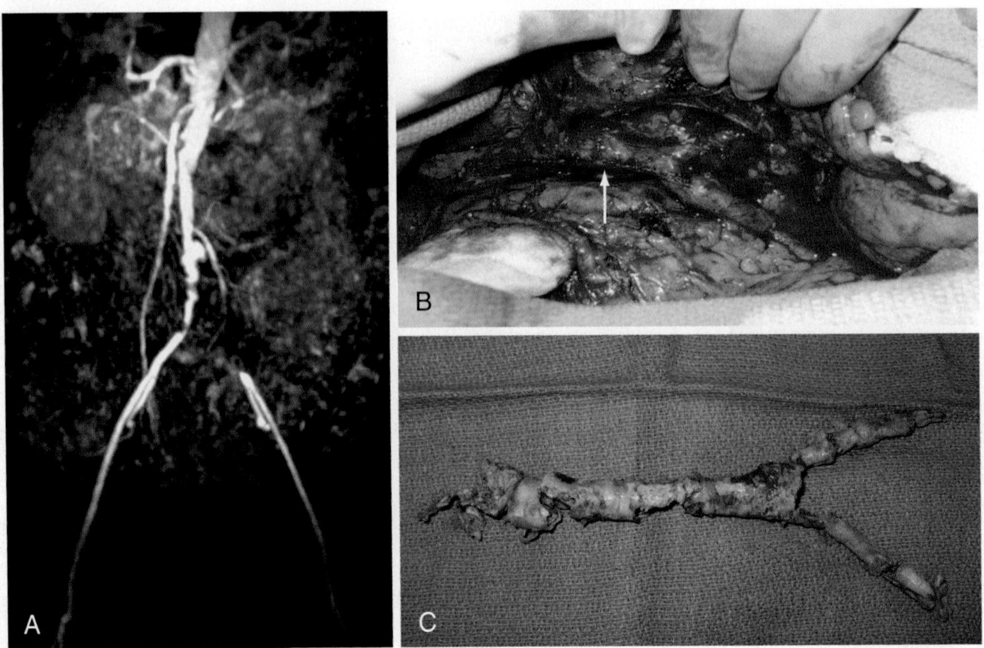


**FIGURE 62-17** **A,** Preoperative MRA demonstrating severe atherosclerotic disease involving the infrarenal aorta and both common iliac arteries. **B,** Intraoperative photograph of completed aortoiliac endarterectomy showing suture line of primary closure *(solid arrow)*. **C,** Photograph of intact specimen demonstrating contiguous near-occlusive plaque.

specialty centers with aggressive heart evaluation management protocols have reported mortality rates in the range of 1% to 2.5%.[57]

Renal insufficiency is a common complication and may result from embolization from clamping, prolonged ischemia with suprarenal clamping, intrinsic renal artery disease, hypovolemia, or hypoperfusion. It is exacerbated by paravisceral aortic repair and intraoperative complications. It most probably relates directly to the patient's preoperative renal and cardiac status. Accurate assessment of the patient's anatomy and a precise preoperative plan for clamping site and sequence are necessary to minimize the incidence of perioperative renal insufficiency.

Pulmonary dysfunction is a frequent and serious complication. This is also more prevalent with proximal and paravisceral aortic procedures. Transverse abdominal incisions, epidural analgesia, and retroperitoneal approaches may mitigate against pulmonary complications.

Limb thrombosis can occur. It is associated with female gender, younger patients, and extra-anatomic bypass grafting. It may be expected in 5% to 10% of patients.[57,59]

Anastomotic pseudoaneurysms are a relatively frequent complication of aortic surgery. This may be a sterile process or the result of infection. These pseudoaneurysms usually occur at the femoral anastomosis rather than at the iliac and aortic anastomoses, which may reflect the higher rate of wound complications and graft infection in this region and the more clinically apparent nature of degeneration at the femoral site. Anastomotic pseudoaneurysms may result from degeneration of the suture line. True aneurysms tend to be para-anastomotic in nature, forming in the aorta proximal to the iliac or femoral arteries distal to an aortic graft. True aneurysms occur more frequently in patients treated for aneurysmal than occlusive disease. Hypertension, COPD, smoking, hyperlipidemia, suture type, technical failures, and postoperative wound complications may be associated with this phenomenon.

Detection of anastomotic pseudoaneurysms in the iliac or aortic position is highly reliant on imaging. Prospective studies using routine imaging of arterial grafts in a variety of anatomic positions have demonstrated higher rates of anastomotic pseudoaneurysm than those relying on clinical detection. For example, routine surveillance with ultrasound has demonstrated intra-abdominal anastomotic pseudoaneurysms in 10% of patients and 6.3% of aortic anastomoses following abdominal aortic graft placement at a mean interval of 12 years from operation.[34] CT and MRI provide excellent visualization of pseudoaneurysms and aneurysmal degeneration of the para-anastomotic area (Fig. 62-18).

Although some anastomotic pseudoaneurysms are sterile, it is prudent to begin evaluation and treatment with a presumption of infection. Diagnosis should include history (e.g., fever, chills, malaise, weight loss), physical examination (e.g., erythema, fluctuant mass, induration, drainage, or tenderness to palpation), and laboratory evaluation (complete blood count, blood and fluid cultures, C-reactive protein level, or erythrocyte sedimentation rate. With regard to imaging, ultrasound may demonstrate the pseudoaneurysm itself as well as perigraft fluid suggestive of infection. CT and MRI may characterize these findings more completely (Fig. 62-19). The use of nuclear medicine modalities such as $^{111}$In- or $^{99m}$Tc-tagged white blood cell scans has greatly improved the surgeon's ability to evaluate for infection in a noninvasive manner (Fig. 62-20). It must be remembered that although positive cultures are definitive, many organisms common in graft infections are fastidious and may yield multiple negative culture results, despite clear clinical evidence of infection. If diagnostic investigation yields evidence of infection, thorough débridement of infected material accompanied by in situ or extra-anatomic arterial reconstruction are mainstays of management. Some recent data have supported the use of endovascular therapies for treating lesions demonstrated to be sterile.[64] In any event, expeditious treatment is appropriate for a large, enlarging, or symptomatic lesion. It is important to note that although graft infection occurs more commonly following open surgery, endovascular graft infections have also been reported.[65]

**Surgical Treatment of Anastomotic Pseudoaneurysms** Surgical management of anastomotic pseudoaneurysm is dictated by the presence or absence of infection, the nature of presentation, and surgeon experience and preference. In an uninfected field, débridement and interposition grafting may suffice. Extensive infection should be treated as a graft infection by removal of the entire affected graft with débridement of all infected or devitalized tissue, traditionally accompanied by extra-anatomic reconstruction. Staging this process by performing the extra-anatomic bypass and then proceeding to débridement or permitting a recovery interval of up to several days has greatly improved the historically substantial morbidity and mortality rates associated with primary graft resection followed by reconstruction.[66] Further investigation has suggested that in cases of infection limited to a single limb of the graft, satisfactory results may be achieved by limiting resection to the involved limb or limb segment, followed by in situ or extra-anatomic reconstruction and, according to surgeon preference, combined with sterile antibiotic irrigation of the field through operatively placed drains.[67] However, recurrent graft infection, graft thrombosis, and the almost invariably fatal complication of aortic stump infection or disruption still contribute to significant morbidity, mortality, and limb loss following this operation. Thorough débridement, layered closure, and vascularized pedicle flap coverage of the aortic stump are considered of paramount importance for avoiding the latter complication.

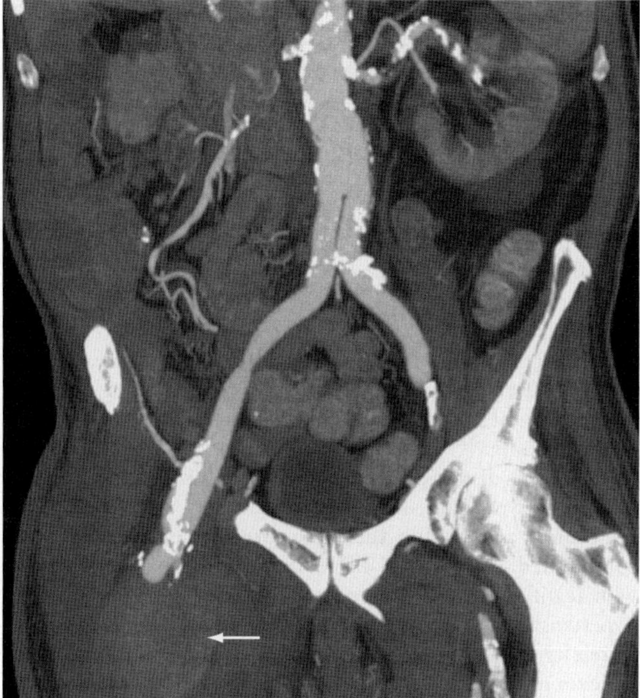

**FIGURE 62-18** CT demonstrating large anastomotic pseudoaneurysm arising at the right femoral anastomosis of an aortofemoral graft.

In situ reconstruction may be accomplished by using a rifampin-soaked or silver-coated polyester graft, cryopreserved arterial allograft, or saphenofemoral vein allograft.[67-70] The first of these is the most expeditious, but yields a higher rate of reinfection and poor results in grossly purulent operative fields. Those expousing its use tend to embrace to use of adjuncts such as wrapping the new graft and anastomoses in vascularized pedicle flaps, antibiotic irrigation therapy, or creation of clean retroperitoneal tunnels. The neoaortoiliac system (NAIS) venous autograft reconstruction described by Clagett is a lengthy procedure that places significant demands on the patient and operative team, but yields the lowest reported rate of reinfection. Reported results using cryopreserved arterial allograft for in situ reconstruction have been mixed, but generally reflect an intermediate rate of reinfection.[71] Endovascular treatment of anastomotic disruptions is generally limited to cases without evidence of infection. It may use covered stent exclusion of the

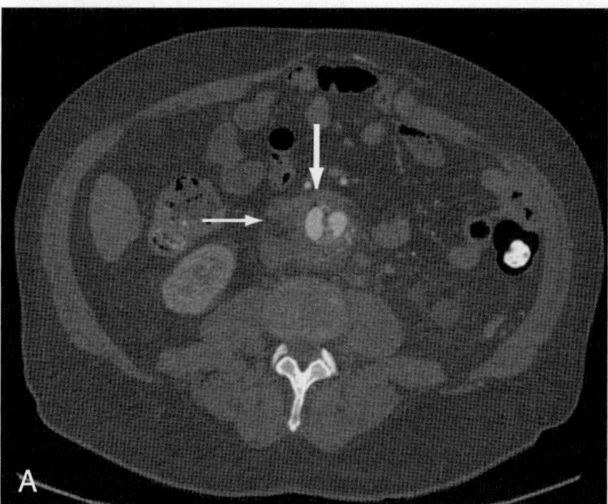


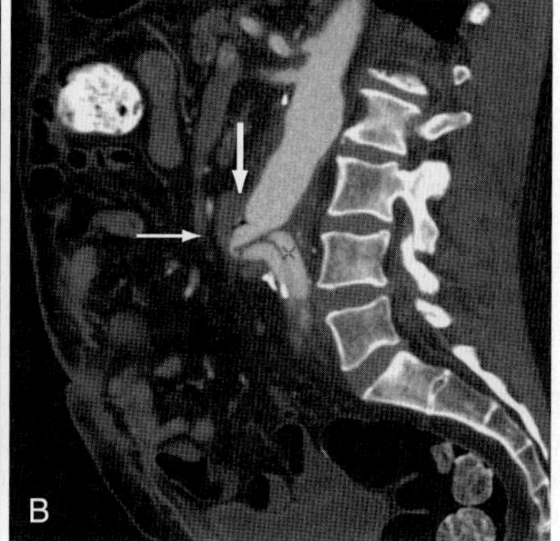


**FIGURE 62-19** Axial **(A)** and sagittal **(B)** CT views of an infected aortofemoral graft following repair of an infrarenal aneurysm. Foci of gas *(thick arrows)* and extensive inflammation *(thin arrows)* are visible surrounding the graft. Of note, the tortuosity of the limbs of this graft represent a technical error.

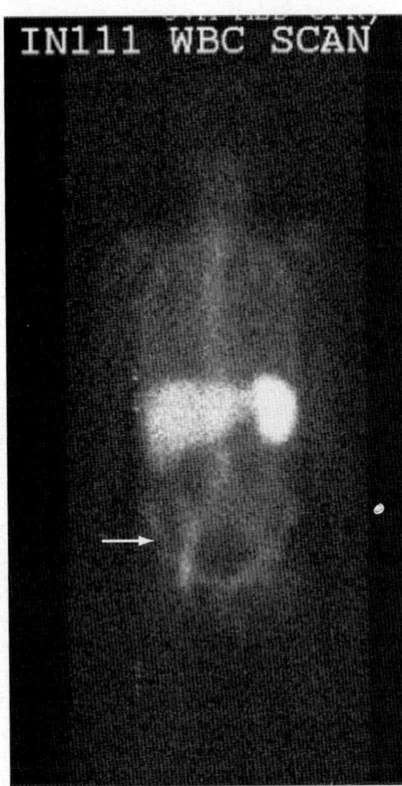


**FIGURE 62-20** $^{111}$In-tagged white blood cell scan images at 20 hours delay demonstrate abnormal uptake in the region of the right limb of an aortofemoral graft *(solid arrow)*.

pseudoaneurysm or embolization of the pseudoaneurysm, generally using coils or occlusion devices.

Aortoenteric fistula (AEF) represents the most severe manifestation of aortic graft infection. It rarely occurs as a primary process, generally because of erosion of an untreated aneurysm into the duodenum. Usually, the lesion is at the point of contact of the third portion of the duodenum with the proximal graft anastomosis. AEF has been reported in association with aortic stent-graft placement. This complication generally presents with herald upper or lower gastrointestinal bleeding which, if left untreated, may be followed by exsanguinating hemorrhage. AEF should be suspected when gastrointestinal bleeding develops in a patient with a history of abdominal aortic surgery or endograft. Although endoscopy may confirm the diagnosis, CT is a more sensitive diagnostic study for demonstrating an erosion or frank exposure of the graft, usually in the duodenum. The placement of endovascular grafts in the setting of an infected pseudoaneurysm, graft infection, primary aortic infection, or AEF is perhaps best viewed as a temporizing measure and is attended by high rates of re-intervention, morbidity, and mortality.[72]

## AORTIC DISSECTION

Aortic dissection occurs when a tear in the intimal layer of the vessel permits blood to create a false channel within the aortic wall, typically between the media and adventitia. The aorta is divided into true and false lumens, separated by a septum referred to as the *dissection flap*. A number of conditions, including connective tissue disorders such as Marfan syndrome, hypertension, and pregnancy are associated with the development of aortic dissection, as are activities such as cocaine abuse and power weight lifting.[73]

A number of important distinctions must be made once the diagnosis of aortic dissection has been made. The DeBakey and Stanford classifications systems define dissections based on anatomic extent. DeBakey type I (involving both the ascending and thoracoabdominal aorta) and type II (limited to the ascending aorta) dissections correspond to the Stanford type A (any involvement of the ascending aorta), whereas the DeBakey type III a (confined to the descending thoracic aorta) and type IIIb (involving the descending thoracic and abdominal aorta) correspond with the Stanford type B (not involving the ascending aorta; Figs. 62-21 and 22).

Type A dissection typically presents acutely with chest or back pain, commonly described as ripping or tearing in nature. This may be accompanied by profound hypotension, particularly in the setting of pericardial tamponade or disruption of the aortic valve, and distal hypoperfusion, as seen in type B dissections. Distal pulse deficits or other evidence of malperfusion in a patient presenting with sudden-onset, severe chest or back pain should immediately prompt evaluation for aortic dissection. CT and echocardiography can both not only diagnose dissection, but can rapidly assess the status of the proximal aorta, permitting the critical distinction between type A and type B lesions. Acute type A dissection is generally considered a surgical emergency. Repair necessitates the use of adjuncts such as cardiopulmonary bypass and hypothermic circulatory arrest and, on occasion, replacement of the aortic valve in addition to replacement of the ascending aorta.[43]

Type B dissection is further characterized as acute (≤14 days from symptoms onset) or chronic (>14 days from initial symptoms) and, within these categories, as uncomplicated or complicated. Acute type B dissections will also frequently present with tearing chest or back pain, often in the setting of severe hypertension. Malperfusion of the spine, renal, visceral, or lower extremity vessels may complicate the presentation. Rarely, patients may present with frank rupture. Anatomically, type B dissections generally originate from a primary tear in the proximal descending thoracic aorta, just distal to the origin of the left subclavian artery. Extension is typically antegrade, extending as far as the iliac arteries, although retrograde extension may occur. Fenestrations or openings in the dissection flap may permit communication between true and false lumens at intervals along the length of the dissection.

Penetrating atherosclerotic ulcer (PAU) and intramural hematoma (IMH) are also considered to be variants of aortic dissection. PAU represents focal intimal ulceration of the aorta within a region of preexisting atherosclerotic disease. These lesions may eventually extend into the media and evolve into a true dissection. IMH occurs when intramural thrombus is found without evidence of associated intimal disruption, possibly as a result of disrupted vasa vasorum within the aortic wall. Similar to PAU, IMH may evolve into dissection if a frank intimal tear develops.[74]

CT remains the mainstay of diagnostic imaging because it provides excellent anatomic data, the ability to localize the entry tear and fenestrations, assessment of branch vessel patency, and detection of extravasation of contrast consistent with rupture (Fig. 62-23). Recently, ECG gated techniques have enabled the acquisition of motion-free images of the proximal aorta. CT is widely available and excellent studies may be obtained rapidly

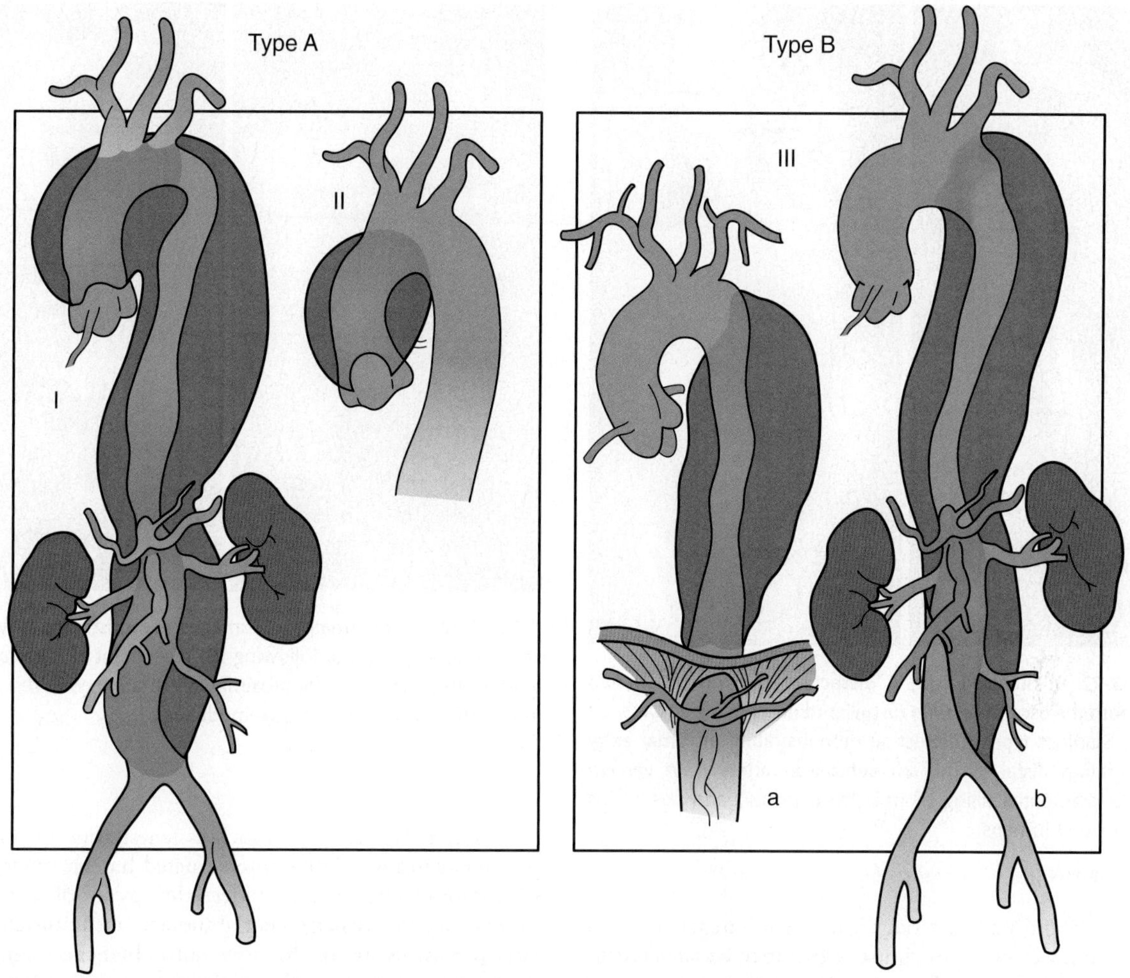


**FIGURE 62-21** Classification systems for aortic dissection. Stanford type A corresponds to DeBakey type I (involving the ascending and descending aorta) and type II (involving the ascending aorta). Stanford type B corresponds to DeBakey type III (origin of the dissection distal to the left subclavian artery and involving the descending aorta only or the descending and abdominal aorta).

with modern multidetector helical scanners, often in a few minutes.[43] As in abdominal aortic imaging, the effect of iodinated contrast on renal function remains the principal drawback of CT.

MRI scabs are substantially more time-consuming to obtain and may be limited by patient factors, such as the presence of metallic debris or medical implants that preclude its use. ECG gating of contrast-enhanced MRI can provide exceptional motion-free images of the proximal aorta. In addition, unlike contrasted CT, MRI permits appreciation of the direction of blood flow, as well as the calculation of values such as peak flow and velocity.

Catheter angiography provides excellent information about aortic and branch anatomy and involvement, the ability to visualize dissection flap anatomy and fenestrations, particularly with the adjunct of intravascular ultrasound (IVUS), and the ability to evaluate dissection physiology by measuring true and false lumen pressures and pressure differentials across fenestrations. In addition, angiography permits intervention on the coronary vessels, aorta, and branch vessels at the same setting.

The treatment of type B dissection is evolving, particularly since the advent of endovascular therapy. Traditionally, intensive medical management has been the mainstay of therapy for uncomplicated dissection whereas dissections complicated by rupture, aneurysmal expansion, and evidence of malperfusion or, according to some sources, intractable pain, have been managed surgically.[75] Aortic branch vessels to the lower extremities, viscera, and spine may originate from a true or false lumen. Malperfusion may result from dynamic compression of the true lumen by the false thrombosis of one or both lumens, or static obstruction caused by extension of the dissection into the branch vessel. It may present as new-onset renal dysfunction, abdominal pain and mesenteric ischemia, lower extremity ischemia, or neurologic dysfunction ranging from paresthesia to paraplegia.

Open surgical therapy for type B dissection may consist of replacement of the descending aorta or fenestration of the abdominal aorta to address visceral or limb malperfusion. Whereas replacement addresses the risk of further aortic enlargement or rupture within the replaced segment of aorta, fenestration addresses malperfusion exclusively. This procedure, which is rarely performed, involves creating a transverse (if an interposition graft is anticipated) or longitudinal aortotomy in the dissected but nonaneurysmal paravisceral aorta to excise a portion of the dissection flap to permit perfusion of

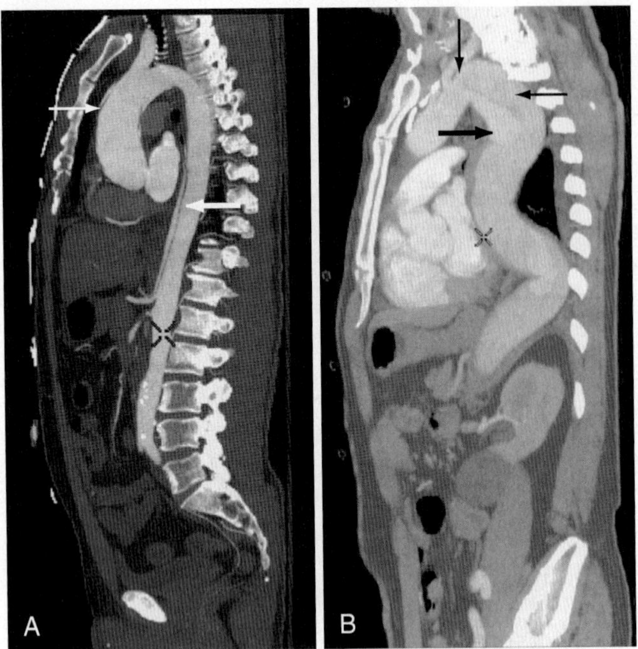


**FIGURE 62-22 A,** Stanford type A dissection with dissection flap visible in both the ascending *(thin arrow)* and descending aorta *(solid arrow)*. **B,** Stanford type B dissection demonstrating proximal entry tear fenestration distal to the left subclavian artery *(thin vertical arrow)* and differential filling of true *(solid arrow)* and false *(thin horizontal arrow)* lumens.

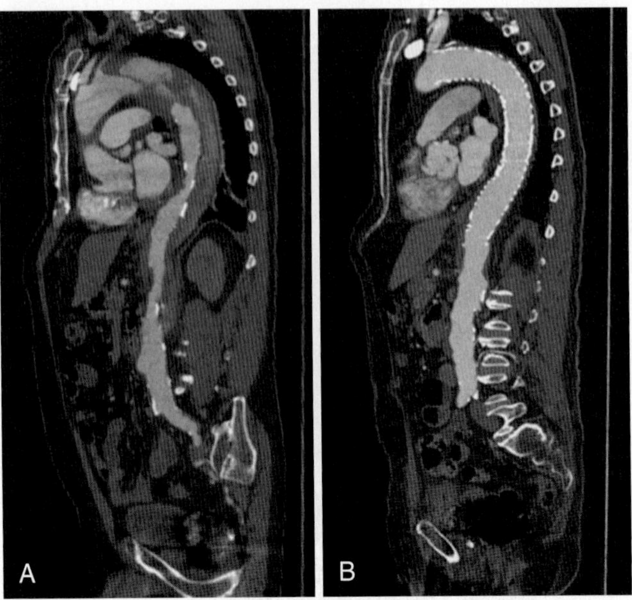


**FIGURE 62-23** Reformatted CT images demonstrating a type B dissection prior to **(A)** and following **(B)** placement of a thoracic endograft. Note coverage of the proximal fenestration, with resulting false lumen thrombosis and aortic remodeling.

the mesenteric and renal arteries or, in the infrarenal aorta, to reperfuse the lower limbs. A similar effect may be achieved in an endovascular fashion by traversing the dissection flap at the level of the desired fenestration and using an angioplasty balloon to enlarge the opening. Angioplasty may be used alone or with subsequent stent placement within the fenestration.[76]

Historically, open surgical therapy for complicated type B dissection has been associated with high rates of morbidity and mortality. A review of data from the International Registry of Acute Aortic Dissection (IRAD) yielded a 29.3% overall rate of in-hospital mortality among patients treated surgically for acute, complicated type B dissection, whereas Panneton and colleagues reported a 43% rate of operative mortality for emergency open surgical fenestration. Of the patients in the IRAD report, 69% were treated with replacement of the descending aorta, 28% with partial or complete replacement of the aortic arch, and 9% with surgical fenestration. Surgical or endovascular approaches to revascularizing malperfused branch territories were used in 20% and 9% of patients, respectively.[76,77]

In 1999, Dake and associates[78] reported the placement of endovascular stent-grafts for acute aortic dissection as an alternative to traditional surgical therapy. The principle of endovascular stent-graft therapy is coverage of the entry tear, depressurizing the false lumen, expansion of the true lumen and, ideally, complete thrombosis of the false lumen, generally within the first several months post-treatment. False lumen thrombosis may then initiate aortic remodeling, with an increase in the diameter of the true lumen, a decrease in the diameter of the false lumen and, in some cases, a decrease in overall aortic diameter (Fig. 62-24).

Adjunctive techniques such as fenestration or direct stent placement to restore flow to obstructed branch vessels are also important components of modern therapy for dissection. As in the endovascular management of thoracic aortic aneurysms, cervical reconstruction of the supra-aortic branches may facilitate coverage of portions of the aortic arch to achieve an adequate proximal seal zone for the device.

In the setting of chronic dissection, progressive thickening of the intimal flap has generally occurred. Distal reentry fenestrations are well established, rendering false lumen thrombosis more difficult to induce than in acute dissection and probably decreasing the overall occurrence of favorable remodeling.[74]

Procedural complications of endovascular stent-graft therapy for dissection generally correlate with those of TEVAR. There are, however, several complications primarily specific to the treatment of dissection, including retrograde dissection (converting a type B into a type A dissection), worsening of malperfusion, and continued false lumen filling, with an inability to induce thrombosis.

At the present time, there is a general consensus that medical therapy remains the standard of care for acute, uncomplicated type B dissection. However, interest in the potential for aortic remodeling and the prevention of aneurysmal dilation over time has prompted investigation of early stent-grafting versus medical therapy in this population. Although an early analysis of results has failed to show a survival advantage at 2 years, the study was noted to be underpowered at this point. These early findings demonstrated aortic remodeling in 91% of stent graft patients versus 19% of patients randomized to medical therapy, which supports the hope of many physicians that this therapy may ultimately provide a survival advantage over time, and that this trial may aid in identifying subgroups of patients most likely to benefit.[79]

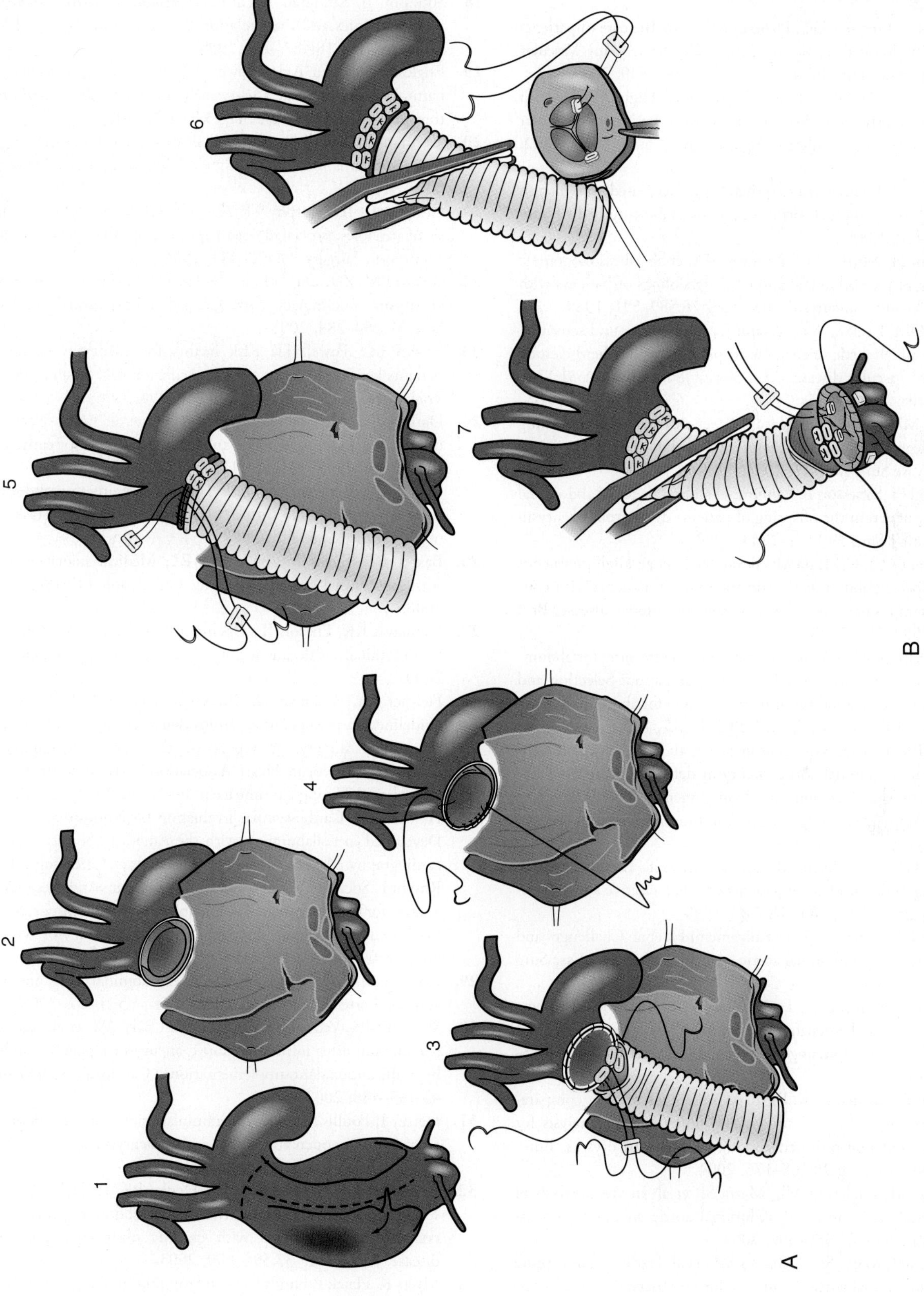


**FIGURE 62-24** **A,** Ascending aorta dissection repair. Under circulatory arrest, the ascending aorta and transverse arch are opened, exposing the dissection *(1, 2)*. The false lumen is obliterated *(3)*. The graft is sutured to the transverse arch in an open distal anastomosis *(4)*. **B,** The distal anastomosis is reinforced *(5)*. The aortic valve is resuspended *(6)*. The proximal anastomosis is constructed *(7)*.

## REFERENCES


1. Chaikof EL, Brewster DC, Dalman RL, et al: The care of patients with an abdominal aortic aneurysm: The Society for Vascular Surgery practice guidelines. J Vasc Surg 50:S2–S49, 2009.
2. Allardice JT, Allwright GJ, Wafula JM, et al: High prevalence of abdominal aortic aneurysm in men with peripheral vascular disease: screening by ultrasonography. Br J Surg 75:240–242, 1988.
3. O'Kelly TJ, Heather BP: General practice-based population screening for abdominal aortic aneurysms: A pilot study. Br J Surg 76:479–480, 1989.
4. Bengtsson H, Norrgard O, Angquist KA, et al: Ultrasonographic screening of the abdominal aorta among siblings of patients with abdominal aortic aneurysms. Br J Surg 76:589–591, 1989.
5. Shapira OM, Pasik S, Wassermann JP, et al: Ultrasound screening for abdominal aortic aneurysms in patients with atherosclerotic peripheral vascular disease. J Cardiovasc Surg (Torino) 31:170–172, 1990.
6. Webster MW, Ferrell RE, St Jean PL, et al: Ultrasound screening of first-degree relatives of patients with an abdominal aortic aneurysm. J Vasc Surg 13:9–13, 1991.
7. Bengtsson H, Sonesson B, Lanne T, et al: Prevalence of abdominal aortic aneurysm in the offspring of patients dying from aneurysm rupture. Br J Surg 79:1142–1143, 1992.
8. MacSweeney ST, O'Meara M, Alexander C, et al: High prevalence of unsuspected abdominal aortic aneurysm in patients with confirmed symptomatic peripheral or cerebral arterial disease. Br J Surg 80:582–584, 1993.
9. Lindholt JS, Juul S, Henneberg EW, et al: Is screening for abdominal aortic aneurysm acceptable to the population? Selection and recruitment to hospital-based mass screening for abdominal aortic aneurysm. J Public Health Med 20:211–217, 1998.
10. Lederle FA, Johnson GR, Wilson SE, et al: Prevalence and associations of abdominal aortic aneurysm detected through screening. Aneurysm Detection and Management (ADAM) Veterans Affairs Cooperative Study Group. Ann Intern Med 126:441–449, 1997.
11. van der Gra-af Y, Akkersdijk GJ, Hak E, et al: Results of aortic screening in the brothers of patients who had elective aortic aneurysm repair. Br J Surg 85:778–780, 1998.
12. Wassef M, Upchurch GR, Jr, Kuivaniemi H, et al: Challenges and opportunities in abdominal aortic aneurysm research. J Vasc Surg 45:192–198, 2007.
13. Engellau L, Albrechtsson U, Dahlstrom N, et al: Measurements before endovascular repair of abdominal aortic aneurysms. MR imaging with MRA vs. angiography and CT. Acta Radiol 44:177–184, 2003.
14. Venkatasubramaniam AK, Fagan MJ, Mehta T, et al: A comparative study of aortic wall stress using finite element analysis for ruptured and non-ruptured abdominal aortic aneurysms. Eur J Vasc Endovasc Surg 28:168–176, 2004.
15. Fillinger MF, Raghavan ML, Marra SP, et al: In vivo analysis of mechanical wall stress and abdominal aortic aneurysm rupture risk. J Vasc Surg 36:589–597, 2002.
16. Fillinger MF, Marra SP, Raghavan ML, et al: Prediction of rupture risk in abdominal aortic aneurysm during observation: wall stress versus diameter. J Vasc Surg 37:724–732, 2003.
17. Hall AJ, Busse EF, McCarville DJ, et al: Aortic wall tension as a predictive factor for abdominal aortic aneurysm rupture: Improving the selection of patients for abdominal aortic aneurysm repair. Ann Vasc Surg 14:152–157, 2000.
18. Sonesson B, Sandgren T, Lanne T: Abdominal aortic aneurysm wall mechanics and their relation to risk of rupture. Eur J Vasc Endovasc Surg 18:487–493, 1999.
19. Englesbe MJ, Wu AH, Clowes AW, et al: The prevalence and natural history of aortic aneurysms in heart and abdominal organ transplant patients. J Vasc Surg 37:27–31, 2003.
20. Norman PE, Powell JT: Abdominal aortic aneurysm: The prognosis in women is worse than in men. Circulation 115:2865–2869, 2007.
21. Cronenwett JL, Murphy TF, Zelenock GB, et al: Actuarial analysis of variables associated with rupture of small abdominal aortic aneurysms. Surgery 98:472–483, 1985.
22. Brown PM, Zelt DT, Sobolev B: The risk of rupture in untreated aneurysms: The impact of size, gender, and expansion rate. J Vasc Surg 37:280–284, 2003.
23. Brown LC, Powell JT: Risk factors for aneurysm rupture in patients kept under ultrasound surveillance. UK Small Aneurysm Trial Participants. Ann Surg 230:289–296, 1999.
24. Darling RC, Messina CR, Brewster DC, et al: Autopsy study of unoperated abdominal aortic aneurysms. The case for early resection. Circulation 56:II161–II164, 1977.
25. U.S. Preventive Services Task Force: Screening for abdominal aortic aneurysm, 2005 (http://www.uspreventiveservicestaskforce.org/uspstf/uspsaneu.htm).
26. Baxter BT, Terrin MC, Dalman RL: Medical management of small abdominal aortic aneurysms. Circulation 117:1883–1889, 2008.
27. Hannawa KK, Eliason JL, Upchurch GR, Jr: Gender differences in abdominal aortic aneurysms. Vascular 17(Suppl 1):S30–S39, 2009.
28. Fleisher LA, Beckman JA, Brown KA, et al: ACC/AHA 2007 guidelines on perioperative cardiovascular evaluation and care for noncardiac surgery: A report of the American College of Cardiology/American Heart Association Task Force on Practice Guidelines (Writing Committee to Revise the 2002 Guidelines on Perioperative Cardiovascular Evaluation for Noncardiac Surgery): Developed in collaboration with the American Society of Echocardiography, American Society of Nuclear Cardiology, Heart Rhythm Society, Society of Cardiovascular Anesthesiologists, Society for Cardiovascular Angiography and Interventions, Society for Vascular Medicine and Biology, and Society for Vascular Surgery. Circulation 116:e418–e499, 2007.
29. Corriere M, Edwards M, Hansen KJ: Abdominal aortic aneurysm and renal artery stenosis. Vasc Dis Manage 5:16–21, 2008.
30. Wijnen MH, Vader HL, Van Den Wall Bake AW, et al: Can renal dysfunction after infra-renal aortic aneurysm repair be modified by multi-antioxidant supplementation? J Cardiovasc Surg (Torino) 43:483–488, 2002.
31. Hersey P, Poullis M: Does the administration of mannitol prevent renal failure in open abdominal aortic aneurysm surgery? Interact Cardiovasc Thorac Surg 7:906–909, 2008.
32. Upchurch GR, Jr, Proctor MC, Henke PK, et al: Predictors of severe morbidity and death after elective abdominal aortic aneurysmectomy in patients with chronic obstructive pulmonary disease. J Vasc Surg 37:594–599, 2003.
33. Myers K, Hajek P, Hinds C, et al: Stopping smoking shortly before surgery and postoperative complications: A systematic review and meta-analysis. Arch Intern Med 171:983–989, 2011.
34. Sicard GA, Toursarkissian B: Midline versus retroperitoneal approach for abdominal aortic aneurysm surgery. In Calligaro KD, Dougherty MJ, Holllier LH, editors: Diagnosis and

treatment of aortic and peripheral arterial aneurysms, Philadelphia, 1999, WB Saunders, pp 135–148.

35. Nishimori M, Ballantyne JC, Low JH: Epidural pain relief versus systemic opioid-based pain relief for abdominal aortic surgery. Cochrane Database Syst Rev (3):CD005059, 2006.
36. Edwards JM, Teefey SA, Zierler RE, et al: Intra-abdominal para-anastomotic aneurysms after aortic bypass grafting. J Vasc Surg 15:344–350, 1992.
37. Ylonen K, Biancari F, Leo E, et al: Predictors of development of anastomotic femoral pseudoaneurysms after aortobifemoral reconstruction for abdominal aortic aneurysm. Am J Surg 187:83–87, 2004.
38. Parodi JC, Palmaz JC, Barone HD: Transfemoral intraluminal graft implantation for abdominal aortic aneurysms. Ann Vasc Surg 5:491–499, 1991.
39. Greenhalgh RM, Brown LC, Powell JT, et al: Endovascular versus open repair of abdominal aortic aneurysm. N Engl J Med 362: 1863–1871, 2010.
40. Wilt TJ, Lederle FA, Macdonald R, et al: Comparison of endovascular and open surgical repairs for abdominal aortic aneurysm. Evid Rep Technol Assess (Full Rep) 144:1–113, 2006.
41. Dimick JB, Upchurch GR, Jr: Endovascular technology, hospital volume, and mortality with abdominal aortic aneurysm surgery. J Vasc Surg 47:1150–1154, 2008.
42. Kouchoukos NT, Masetti P, Murphy SF: Hypothermic cardiopulmonary bypass and circulatory arrest in the management of extensive thoracic and thoracoabdominal aortic aneurysms. Semin Thorac Cardiovasc Surg 15:333–339, 2003.
43. Hiratzka LF, Bakris GL, Beckman JA, et al: 2010 ACCF/AHA/AATS/ACR/ASA/ SCA/SCAI/SIR/STS/SVM guidelines for the diagnosis and management of patients with Thoracic Aortic Disease: A report of the American College of Cardiology Foundation/American Heart Association Task Force on Practice Guidelines, American Association for Thoracic Surgery, American College of Radiology, American Stroke Association, Society of Cardiovascular Anesthesiologists, Society for Cardiovascular Angiography and Interventions, Society of Interventional Radiology, Society of Thoracic Surgeons, and Society for Vascular Medicine. Circulation 121:e266–e369, 2010.
44. Makaroun MS, Dillavou ED, Wheatley GH, et al: Five-year results of endovascular treatment with the Gore TAG device compared with open repair of thoracic aortic aneurysms. J Vasc Surg 47:912–918, 2008.
45. Gutsche JT, Cheung AT, McGarvey ML, et al: Risk factors for perioperative stroke after thoracic endovascular aortic repair. Ann Thorac Surg 84:1195–1200, 2007.
46. Bavaria JE, Appoo JJ, Makaroun MS, et al: Endovascular stent grafting versus open surgical repair of descending thoracic aortic aneurysms in low-risk patients: A multicenter comparative trial. J Thorac Cardiovasc Surg 133:369–377, 2007.
47. Greenberg R, Eagleton M, Mastracci T: Branched endografts for thoracoabdominal aneurysms. J Thorac Cardiovasc Surg 140: S171–S178, 2010.
48. Duwayri Y, Jim J, Sanchez L: Alternative techniques to abdominal debranching. Vasc Dis Manage 7:E210–E213, 2010.
49. Norgren L, Hiatt WR, Dormandy JA, et al: Inter-society consensus for the management of peripheral arterial disease (TASC II). J Vasc Surg 45(Suppl):S5–S67, 2007.
50. Dormandy JA, Rutherford RB: Management of peripheral arterial disease (PAD). TASC Working Group. TransAtlantic Inter-Society Consensus (TASC). J Vasc Surg 31:S1–S296, 2000.
51. Liu CW, Ye W, Ricco JB, et al: Early and late outcomes of percutarreous treatment of TransAtlantic Inter-Society Consensus class C and D aorto-iliac lesions. J Vasc Surg 53:1728–1737, 2011.
52. Higashiura W, Ichihashi S, Itoh H, et al: Long-term outcomes for systematic primary stent placement in complex iliac artery occlusive disease classified according to Trans-Atlantic Inter-Society Consensus (TASC)-II. J Vasc Surg 53:992–999, 2011.
53. Jongkind V, Akkersdijk GJ, Yeung KK, et al: A systematic review of endovascular treatment of extensive aortoiliac occlusive disease. J Vasc Surg 52:1376–1383, 2010.
54. Upchurch GR, Dimick JB, Wainess RM, et al: Diffusion of new technology in health care: The case of aorto-iliac occlusive disease. Surgery 136:812–818, 2004.
55. Chiu KW, Davies RS, Nightingale PG, et al: Review of direct anatomical open surgical management of atherosclerotic aorto-iliac occlusive disease. Eur J Vasc Endovasc Surg 39:460–471, 2010.
56. de Vries SO, Hunink MG: Results of aortic bifurcation grafts for aortoiliac occlusive disease: A meta-analysis. J Vasc Surg 26:558–569, 1997.
57. Hertzer NR, Bena JF, Karafa MT: A personal experience with direct reconstruction and extra-anatomic bypass for aortoiliofemoral occlusive disease. J Vasc Surg 45:527–535, 2007.
58. Ricco JB, Probst H: Long-term results of a multicenter randomized study on direct versus crossover bypass for unilateral iliac artery occlusive disease. J Vasc Surg 47:45–53, 2008.
59. Reed AB, Conte MS, Donaldson MC, et al: The impact of patient age and aortic size on the results of aortobifemoral bypass grafting. J Vasc Surg 37:1219–1225, 2003.
60. Klonaris C, Katsargyris A, Tsekouras N, et al: Primary stenting for aortic lesions: From single stenoses to total aortoiliac occlusions. J Vasc Surg 47:310–317, 2008.
61. Indes JE, Mandawat A, Tuggle CT, et al: Endovascular procedures for aorto-iliac occlusive disease are associated with superior short-term clinical and economic outcomes compared with open surgery in the inpatient population. J Vasc Surg 52:1173–1179, 2010.
62. Cau J, Ricco JB, Corpataux JM: Laparoscopic aortic surgery: Techniques and results. J Vasc Surg 48:37S–44S, 2008.
63. Cherry KJ: Complications following reconstructions of the pararenal aorta and its branches. In Towne JB, Hollier LH, editors: Complications in vascular surgery, ed 2, New York, 2004, Marcel Dekker, pp 275–287.
64. Sachdev U, Baril DT, Morrissey NJ, et al: Endovascular repair of para-anastomotic aortic aneurysms. J Vasc Surg 46:636–641, 2007.
65. Heyer KS, Modi P, Morasch MD, et al: Secondary infections of thoracic and abdominal aortic endografts. J Vasc Interv Radiol 20:173–179, 2009.
66. Reilly LM, Stoney RJ, Goldstone J, et al: Improved management of aortic graft infection: The influence of operation sequence and staging. J Vasc Surg 5:421–431, 1987.
67. Oderich GS, Bower TC, Cherry KJ, Jr, et al: Evolution from axillofemoral to in situ prosthetic reconstruction for the treatment of aortic graft infections at a single center. J Vasc Surg 43:1166–1174, 2006.
68. Clagett GP, Bowers BL, Lopez-Viego MA, et al: Creation of a neo-aortoiliac system from lower extremity deep and superficial veins. Ann Surg 218:239–248, 1993.
69. Batt M, Magne JL, Alric P, et al: In situ revascularization with silver-coated polyester grafts to treat aortic infection: Early and midterm results. J Vasc Surg 38:983–989, 2003.

70. Noel AA, Gloviczki P, Cherry KJ, Jr, et al: Abdominal aortic reconstruction in infected fields: Early results of the United States cryopreserved aortic allograft registry. J Vasc Surg 35:847–852, 2002.
71. Brown KE, Heyer K, Rodriguez H, et al: Arterial reconstruction with cryopreserved human allografts in the setting of infection: A single-center experience with midterm follow-up. J Vasc Surg 49:660–666, 2009.
72. Lonn L, Dias N, Veith Schroeder T, et al: Is EVAR the treatment of choice for aortoenteric fistula? J Cardiovasc Surg (Torino) 51:319–327, 2010.
73. Cherry KJ, Dake MD: Aortic dissection. In Hallett JW, Mills JL, Earnshaw JJ, et al, editors: Comprehensive vascular and endovascular surgery, ed 2, Philadelphia, 2009, Mosby, pp 517–531.
74. Swee W, Dake MD: Endovascular management of thoracic dissections. Circulation 117:1460–1473, 2008.
75. Estrera AL, Miller CC, 3rd, Safi HJ, et al: Outcomes of medical management of acute type B aortic dissection. Circulation 114: 1384–1389, 2006.
76. Panneton JM, Teh SH, Cherry KJ, Jr, et al: Aortic fenestration for acute or chronic aortic dissection: An uncommon but effective procedure. J Vasc Surg 32:711–721, 2000.
77. Trimarchi S, Nienaber CA, Rampoldi V, et al: Role and results of surgery in acute type B aortic dissection: insights from the International Registry of Acute Aortic Dissection (IRAD). Circulation 114:1357–1364, 2006.
78. Dake MD, Kato N, Mitchell RS, et al: Endovascular stent-graft placement for the treatment of acute aortic dissection. N Engl J Med 340:1546–1552, 1999.
79. Nienaber CA, Rousseau H, Eggebrecht H, et al: Randomized comparison of strategies for type B aortic dissection: the INvestigation of STEnt Grafts in Aortic Dissection (INSTEAD) trial. Circulation 120:2519–2528, 2009.

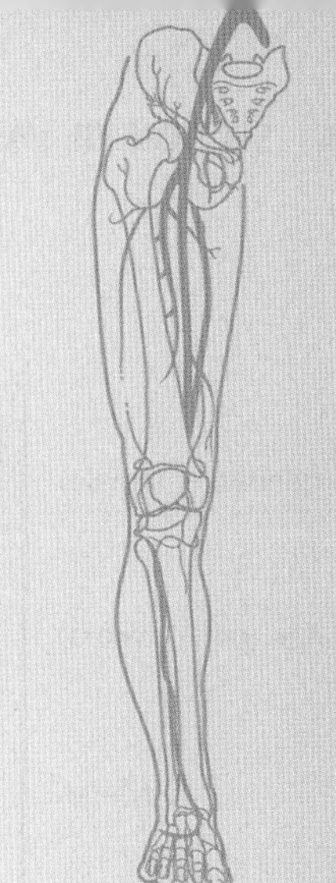

CHAPTER 63

# PERIPHERAL ARTERIAL OCCLUSIVE DISEASE

Michael B. Silva, Jr., Lori Choi, and Charlie C. Cheng



The specialty of vascular surgery has matured dramatically over the past decade. With the advent of new devices and techniques and the expansion of catheter and guidewire skills, the management of almost all vascular pathologic processes has been undergoing a process of reevaluation. Surgeons have traditionally been called on to make diagnoses and manage patients with emergent, urgent, and elective vascular surgical conditions. Although other medical disciplines are participating in this process to a greater degree, the surgeon with advanced open skills and complete facility with endovascular techniques is ideally suited to manage these patients. As our population ages and the prevalence of vascular disease increases, along with the growing awareness of potential therapeutic benefits by an educated populace, it is incumbent on the vascular specialist to be facile with a widening set of tools and techniques—medical, surgical, and endovascular—to meet the needs of our patients.

This chapter will cover epidemiology, basic science, diagnostic workup, and medical treatment of peripheral vascular disease. Treatments of acute and chronic limb ischemia, open and endovascular, will be discussed. Management of the diabetic foot, with an emphasis on amputations, is included. Less common causes of limb ischemia are presented for completion. The rapidly changing treatment paradigm of carotid stenosis is discussed, as well as that of renovascular hypertension. Management of peripheral and splanchnic aneurysms will be reviewed. Finally, arteriovenous (AV) access for the patient with end-stage renal disease (ESRD) is presented in detail because this remains an important component of contemporary general and vascular surgical practice.

## EPIDEMIOLOGY

*Peripheral artery occlusive disease* (PAOD), commonly referred to as *peripheral arterial disease* (PAD) or *peripheral vascular disease* (PVD), refers to the obstruction or deterioration of arteries other than those supplying the heart and within the brain. There are a number of pathologic processes that manifest their effects on the arterial circulation.

The common denominator among these processes is the impairment of circulation and resultant ischemia to the end organ involved. Highly prevalent in our society, arterial occlusive disease, in its myriad iterations, constitutes the leading overall cause of death. In addition to death from myocardial infarction or stroke, significant disability and loss of function from PAD result in an enormous cost in impaired quality of life for our aging population and a direct financial cost to our health care system.

The incidence of symptomatic PAD increases with age, from approximately 0.3%/year for men aged 40 to 55 years to approximately 1%/year for men older than 75 years. In the United States, PAD affects 12% to 20% of Americans aged 65 years and older.

PAD is more prevalent in nonwhite populations, and this is not completely explained by an increased incidence of comorbid diseases.[1] An ankle-brachial index (ABI) less than 0.90 is almost twice as common in non-Hispanic blacks than whites. Risk is increased in smokers and in patients with hypertension (HTN), dyslipidemia, hypercoagulable states, renal insufficiency, and diabetes mellitus (DM) (Fig. 63-1). The prevalence of PAD is strikingly higher in a younger diabetic population, affecting one in three diabetics older than 50 years. Diagnosis is critical, because people with PAD have a risk of heart attack or stroke four to five times higher than the age-matched population (Fig. 63-2). The risk of PAD also increases in individuals who older than 50 years, male, obese, or with a family history of vascular disease, heart attack, or stroke. Other risk factors that are being studied include levels of various inflammatory mediators, such as C-reactive protein and homocysteine.

## BASIC SCIENCE OF VASCULAR DISEASE

### Vascular Wall Microanatomy

The arterial wall consists of three concentric layers:

1. The innermost layer is the intima. This is structurally a tube of endothelial cells in which the long axis of each cell is oriented longitudinally. The cells are aligned in a single layer and interface with the blood, providing metabolic

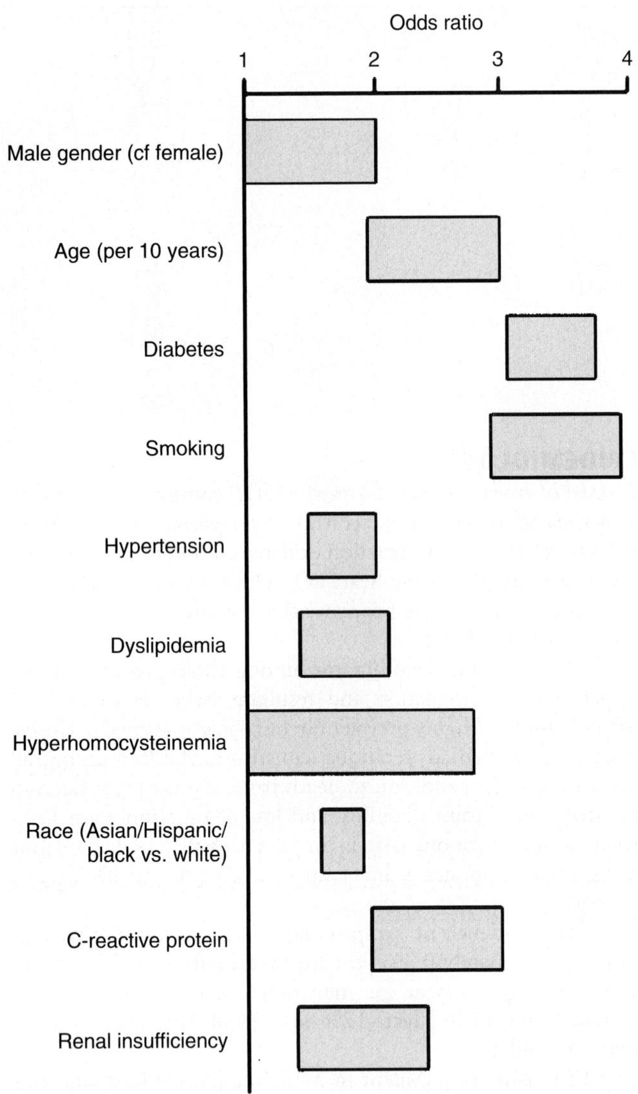


**FIGURE 63-1** Risk factors for symptomatic peripheral arterial disease.

reactivity and signaling via transport of mediators through their internal cellular architecture. The intima is separated from the media by the internal elastic membrane.

2. The media is the major structural support for the artery. It is composed predominantly of circumferentially arranged smooth muscle cells, collagen, elastin, and proteoglycans. Proteoglycans are formed of disaccharides bound to protein; they serve as binding or cement material in the interstitial spaces. The blood supply for the inner part of the media is by direct diffusion through the intima whereas the outer part is supplied by smaller penetrating arteries, known as *vasa vasorum*. The media is separated from the outermost layer, the adventitia, by the external elastic membrane.
3. The adventitia contains fibroblasts, collagen, and elastic tissue and is the strength layer of the artery.

## Atherosclerosis

Atherosclerosis is the most common pathology associated with PAD. There are a number of terms used to describe this process that are similar and yet distinct in spelling and meaning, and are often confused. The principle root, *athera,* is from the Greek word meaning gruel; an atheroma can be translated literally as a lump of gruel. Atherosclerosis is a hardening of an artery specifically caused by an atheromatous plaque. The term *atherogenic* is used for substances or processes that cause atherosclerosis. *Arteriosclerosis* is a general term describing any hardening (and loss of elasticity) of medium or large arteries (from the Greek *arteria,* meaning artery, and *sclerosis,* meaning hardening); arteriolosclerosis is any hardening (and loss of elasticity) of arterioles (small arteries).

A number of causative factors have been identified for atherosclerosis. Hyperlipidemia, hypercholesterolemia, hypertension, diabetes mellitus, and exposure to infectious agents or toxins such as from cigarette smoking are all important and independent risk factors. The common mechanism is thought to be endothelial cell injury, smooth muscle cell proliferation, inflammatory reactivity, and plaque deposition.

There are several components found in atherosclerotic plaque—lipids, smooth muscle cells, connective tissue and inflammatory cells, often macrophages. Lipid accumulation is central to the process and distinguishes atheromas from other arteriopathies. In advanced plaques, calcification is seen and erosive areas or ulcerations can occur, exposing the contents of the plaque to circulating prothrombotic cells. There is an important correlation between plaque morphology and clinical sequelae. The plaque's lipid core may become a necrotic mix of amorphous extracellular lipid, proteins, and prothrombotic factors covered by a layer of smooth muscle cells and connective tissue of variable thickness, the fibrous cap. If the thin fibrous cap ruptures and the contents of the lipid core are exposed to circulating humoral factors, the body, perceiving the ulceration as an injury, may lay down platelets and initiate clot formation. In this manner, a relatively low-grade, hemodynamically insignificant narrowing can precipitate an acute thrombosis and result in a dramatically significant ischemic event, such as a myocardial infarction.

Plaque morphology can be evaluated by ultrasound and magnetic resonance imaging. The heterogenous plaque with a thin fibrous cap or ulceration, often described as unstable or vulnerable, is more likely to be virulent in nature, with an increased risk for embolization of particulate and thrombotic potential. Ischemia, therefore, can result from a number of possible plaque behaviors, such as encroachment on the lumen (stenosis or narrowing) with hypoperfusion, stagnation, and thrombosis; rupture of the fibrous cap inducing thrombus formation in the lumen, with outright occlusion; and embolization of thrombotic debris into the downstream circulation.

Although atherosclerosis is a systemic disorder, there is an interestingly predictable pattern of distribution of atheromatous plaques throughout the arterial tree that is likely a result of consistent hemodynamic stresses associated with human anatomic design. Plaques tend to occur at bifurcations or bends associated with repetitive external stresses. Areas at which shear stress increases from disturbances in flow or turbulence, with lateralizing vectors and eddy formation, are prone to atheromatous degeneration. The infrarenal abdominal aorta, iliac bifurcations, carotid bifurcations, superficial femoral arteries as they exit at Hunter's canal, and ostia of the coronary, renal, and mesenteric arteries, are all common sites of plaque formation. Conversely, the upper extremity arteries and common carotid,

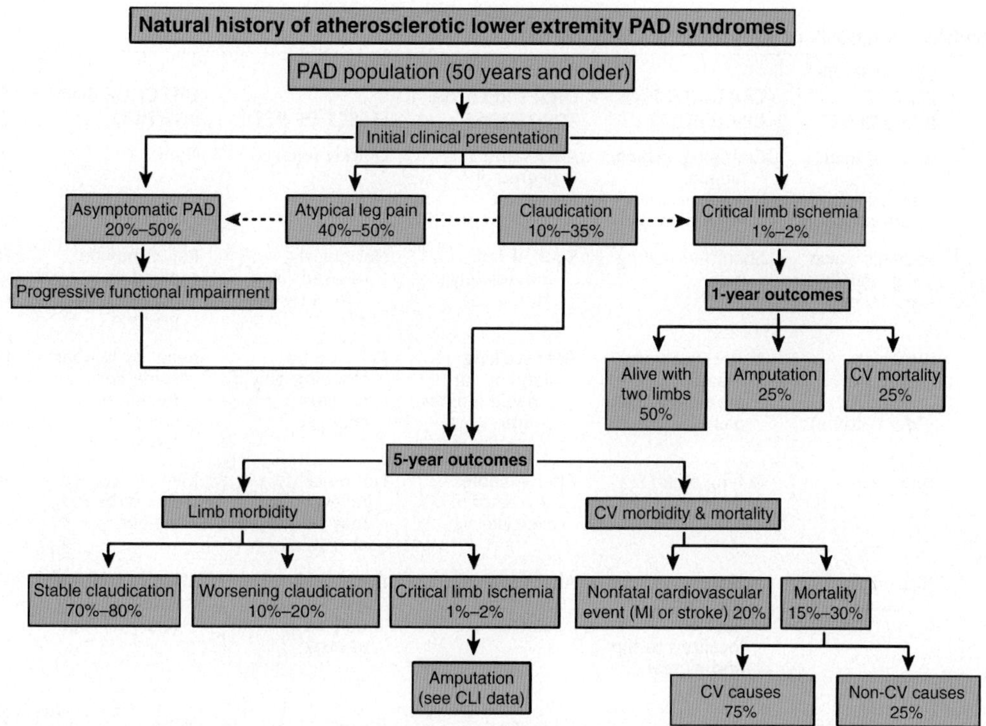


**FIGURE 63-2** Outcomes of atherosclerotic peripheral arterial disease at 5 years. (From Hirsch AT, Haskal ZJ, Hertzer NR, et al; American Association for Vascular Surgery/Society for Vascular Surgery; Society for Cardiovascular Angiography and Interventions; Society for Vascular Medicine and Biology; Society of Interventional Radiology; ACC/AHA Task Force on Practice Guidelines: ACC/AHA Guidelines for the Management of Patients with Peripheral Arterial Disease [lower extremity, renal, mesenteric, and abdominal aortic]: A collaborative report from the American Associations for Vascular Surgery/Society for Vascular Surgery, Society for Cardiovascular Angiography and Interventions, Society for Vascular Medicine and Biology, Society of Interventional Radiology, and the ACC/AHA Task Force on Practice Guidelines [writing committee to develop guidelines for the management of patients with peripheral arterial disease]—summary of recommendations. J Vasc Interv Radiol 17:1383–1397, 2006.)

renal, and mesenteric arteries, beyond their origins, are often much less involved.

## EVALUATING AND TREATING THE PATIENT WITH PERIPHERAL ARTERIAL DISEASE

Patients are typically referred to the vascular specialist to clarify a diagnosis and determine a strategy for treatment. The process involves clinical assessment, establishing the particulars of the patient's medical history and performing a physical examination, diagnostic studies to clarify and localize the problem and potentially elucidate the functional severity of the condition, and ultimately balancing the severity of the patient's condition with the potential risks and benefits of therapeutic intervention.

### History and Physical Examination

Rapidly advancing technology in imaging and endovascular therapies epitomize the cutting edge, the "high-tech" side of vascular surgery, but the foundation of this field is profoundly "low-tech." The history and physical examination process can often identify the location and relative severity of the patient's vascular disease accurately.

The most common presenting symptom in lower extremity vascular disease is pain. Characterizing the pain—location, precipitating, aggravating, and relieving factors, frequency, duration, and evolution—can allow one to diagnose or exclude most arterial and venous diseases with a high degree of sensitivity, even before examining the patient. Clarifying the nature of the pain as a starting point allows one to segregate patients into two broad categories of presentation for PAD, chronic arterial insufficiency and acute arterial occlusion.

### Chronic Arterial Insufficiency

The clinical presentation ranges from asymptomatic to gangrenous tissue loss. Intermittent claudication is a common presentation in the outpatient setting, and usually signifies mild to moderate vascular occlusive disease. Classically, pain occurs with activity or ambulation and is relieved with rest. Because of the frequency of superficial femoral arterial disease, the usual location of the pain is in the calf, but claudication may also involve the thighs or the buttocks because the arterial disease may be located in the aorto-iliac segment. The arterial disease is usually one level above the symptomatic muscle group. The differential diagnosis of leg pain is broad and the treatment modalities are equally disparate. Table 63-1 outlines an approach to the differential diagnosis of claudication.

Patients who are limited in ambulation because of arthritis, severe lung disease, or heart failure, or who are diabetic with neuropathy, may not experience leg pain and may present initially with advanced disease. Worsening perfusion leads to critical limb ischemia (CLI), which may be manifested by rest pain.

**Table 63-1 Differential Diagnosis of Intermittent Claudication**

| CONDITION | LOCATION OF PAIN OR DISCOMFORT | CHARACTERISTIC DISCOMFORT | ONSET RELATIVE TO EXERCISE | EFFECT OF REST | EFFECT OF BODY POSITION | OTHER CHARACTERISTICS |
|---|---|---|---|---|---|---|
| Intermittent claudication | Buttock, thigh, or calf muscles and rarely the foot | Cramping, aching, fatigue, weakness, or frank pain | After same degree of exercise | Quickly relieved | None | Reproducible |
| Nerve root compression (e.g., herniated disc) | Radiates down leg, usually posteriorly | Sharp lancinating pain | Soon, if not immediately after onset | Not quickly relieved (also often present at rest) | Relief may be aided by adjusting back position | History of back problems |
| Spinal stenosis | Hip, thigh, buttocks (follows dermatome) | Motor weakness more prominent than pain | After walking or standing for variable lengths of time | Relieved by stopping only if position changed | Relief by lumbar spine flexion (sitting or stooping forward) | Frequent history of back problems, provoked by intra-abdominal pressure |
| Arthritic, inflammatory process | Foot, arch | Aching pain | After variable degree of exercise | Not quickly relieved (and may be present at rest) | May be relieved by not bearing weight | Variable, may relate to activity level |
| Hip arthritis | Hip, thigh, buttocks | Aching discomfort, usually localized to hip and gluteal region | After variable degree of exercise | Not quickly relieved (and may be present at rest) | More comfortable sitting, weight taken off legs | Variable, may relate to activity level, weather changes |
| Symptomatic Baker's cyst | Behind knee, down calf | Swelling, soreness, tenderness | With exercise | Present at rest | None | Not intermittent |
| Venous claudication | Entire leg, but usually worse in thigh and groin | Tight, bursting pain | After walking | Subsides slowly | Relief speeded by elevation | History of iliofemoral deep vein thrombosis, signs of venous congestion, edma |
| Chronic compartment syndrome | Calf muscles | Tight, bursting pain | After much exercise (e.g., jogging) | Subsides very slowly | Relief speeded by elevation | Typically occurs in heavily muscled athletes |

Adapted from Dormandy JA, Rutherford RB: Management of peripheral arterial disease (PAD). TASC Working Group. TransAtlantic Inter-Society Consensus (TASC). J Vasc Surg 31:S1–S296, 2000.

This is described as pain that occurs at rest; it may wake the patient from sleep. CLI patients present also with tissue loss with ulceration or nonhealing wounds of the foot. This usually in the dorsum of the foot, relieved with dangling the leg over the edge of the bed. Patient may also have tissue loss with ulcerations or nonhealing wounds of the foot (Table 63-2).

Initial evaluation must include a detailed medical history of comorbid conditions. In addition to coronary artery disease (CAD), carotid artery stenosis (CAS), and prior stroke, risk factors for atherosclerosis (e.g., diabetes, hypertension, dyslipidemia, tobacco abuse, hyperhomocysteinemia) should be queried and their level of optimization understood. Because medical management is a cornerstone of vascular therapy, a review of the patient's medications is imperative, with attention to the potential need for antiplatelet agents, beta blockers, angiotensin-converting enzyme (ACE) inhibitors, and statins as a matter of course. Previous exposure to heparin, protamine, and NPH insulin (neutral protamine Hagedorn)[2] should be noted. Allergies to contrast agents or iodine should be documented.

The surgical history and physical examination include details of surgical incisions as indicative of prior surgical intervention. Many patients will have undergone coronary artery bypass grafting; the presence of a left internal mammary–left anterior descending coronary graft and previous great saphenous vein harvest can change the surgical plan for peripheral revascularization. Frequent or recent coronary catheterization (or peripheral angiograms) can suggest challenging groin access with significant scar tissue. Procedure reports should be reviewed for

**Table 63-2 Clinical Classification of Peripheral Arterial Disease: Fontaine and Rutherford Systems**

| Fontaine Classification | | Rutherford Classification | |
|---|---|---|---|
| STAGE | CLINICAL | GRADE | CLINICAL |
| I | Asymptomatic | 0 | Asymptomatic |
| IIa | Mild claudication | 1 | Mild claudication |
| IIb | Moderate to severe claudication | 2<br>3 | Moderate claudication<br>Severe claudication |
| III | Ischemic rest pain | 4 | Ischemic rest pain |
| IV | Ulceration or gangrene | 5<br>6 | Minor tissue loss<br>Major tissue loss |

details of access closure or incidental findings of peripheral artery stenoses. Previous surgery, whether neck, abdominal, spine, joint, or vascular operations, can affect decision making and efforts to gain the details of these are important. A family history of a first-degree relative with abdominal aortic aneurysm, stroke, or early myocardial infarction should be sought.

A vascular review of symptoms documents the presence or absence of transient ischemic attack or stroke, such as unilateral weakness or sensory deficit, difficulty with speech or swallowing, word-finding difficulties or memory changes, dizziness, drop attacks, blurry vision, arm fatigue, weight loss or pain after eating, renal insufficiency or poorly controlled hypertension, impotence, claudication, rest pain, or tissue loss. As for all patients, a detailed understanding of the patient's functional status helps delineate goals of therapy and perioperative risk. Patients who are limited in their activities of daily living by their vascular disease or other comorbidities cannot provide an accurate picture of their cardiac function and will likely require further cardiac workup. History of tobacco abuse must be documented, as well as all clinical efforts for encouraging smoking cessation.

The physical examination begins with vital signs, which often reveals hypertension and tachycardia. Blood pressure in both arms should be documented. The presence or absence of carotid bruits, cardiac murmurs, abdominal, flank, or groin bruits should be noted. The abdomen should be palpated for the aortic pulsation. Incision scars should be noted. Bilateral carotid, radial, ulnar, femoral, popliteal, dorsalis pedis (DP), and posterior tibial (PT) pulses should be palpated and characterized. If pulses are not palpable, a continuous wave Doppler can be used to check for signals. Common physical findings of PAD include hair loss and dry shiny skin with nail hypertrophy. In CLI, the classic findings of dependent rubor and pallor with elevation of the limb can be observed. In cases of severe rest pain, patients may have peripheral edema because they are unable to take their legs from the dependent position without pain. The feet should be meticulously inspected for wounds and signs of skin breakdown. A neurologic examination documenting equivalent strength and sensation in the limbs and cranial nerves should be performed.

Routine laboratory work should include a complete blood count, chemistry (to evaluate renal function and glucose), and a lipid panel. An albumin level can be helpful in delineating the adequacy of a patient's nutritional status, if this is in question. The hemoglobin A1c (HbA1c) level indicates the patient's level of glycemic control over the previous 120 days.

A baseline electrocardiogram should be obtained. Any previous cardiac testing, including echocardiography, stress echocardiography, dobutamine-adenosine sestamibi scan, and coronary catheterization, should be reviewed and documented.

## Physiologic Testing and Imaging

The vascular laboratory is a powerful tool in the armamentarium of the surgeon. Noninvasive testing confirms and localizes disease, provides end points to demonstrate improvement following intervention, enables long-term follow-up of bypass grafts and percutaneous interventions, and can detect silent disease recurrence. Tests commonly performed in the laboratory include the ABI, with multisegmental pressures, waveforms, and toe-brachial index (TBI), pulse volume recording (PVR), photoplethysmyography (PPG), and arterial duplex examination.

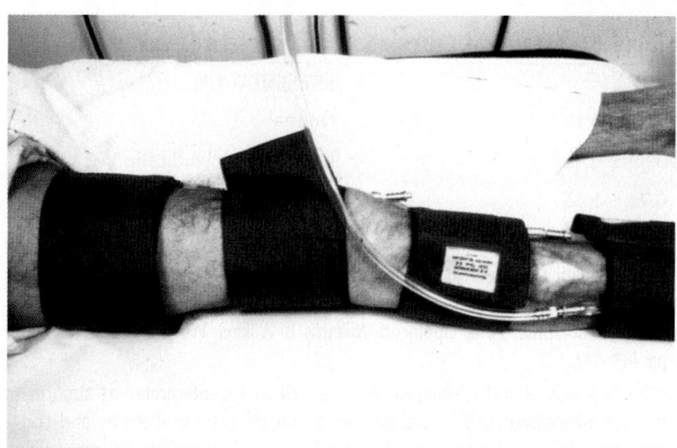

**FIGURE 63-3** Segmental pressure is measured with the same technique as ankle pressure, but with cuffs placed at the upper part of the thigh, lower part of the thigh, below the knee, and ankle. (From Kohler TR, Sumner DS: Vascular laboratory: Arterial physiologic assessment. In Cronenwett JL, Johnston W [eds]: Rutherford's vascular surgery, ed 7, Philadelphia, 2010, Saunders.)

The vascular laboratory represents one of the last arenas in which a nonimaging indirect measure of physiology is still widely used as a diagnostic tool.

Regardless of plans for intervention, it is recommended that asymptomatic patients at risk for PAD and those with symptoms undergo ABI testing. This examination can be performed simply with a manual blood pressure cuff at the ankle and a continuous wave Doppler probe. With the patient in a supine position, after several minutes of rest to allow limb pressure to return to baseline, the cuff is inflated at the ankle, with the Doppler probe held at the location of the distal DP or PT signal. The systolic pressure is recorded as the pressure in the cuff when the Doppler signal returns. This process can be performed with multiple cuffs allowing for segmental pressure determination (Fig. 63-3), which is helpful in localizing the level of the obstructing lesion. The ABI for a limb is calculated using the higher of the two ankle pressures divided by the higher of the two brachial pressures (Tables 63-3 and 63-4). Patients with an ABI of 0.90 or less have a three- to sixfold increased risk of cardiovascular mortality.

Continuous wave Doppler analog waveforms can be obtained along with the segmental pressures. PPG uses an infrared light-emitting source and a photosensor; it is based on the principle that red light is decreased with increased blood flow in tissues to generate a pressure and waveform within the digit. The data generated from these studies should include bilateral brachial artery, high thigh, low thigh, calf, DP, PT, and toe pressures with waveforms (Fig. 63-4). A decrease in pressure of 20 to 30 mm Hg between adjacent segments is indicative of a significant lesion. The normal Doppler arterial waveform demonstrates triphasic flow with a sharp systolic upstroke, reversal of flow in early diastole from vessel compliance, and low-amplitude forward flow throughout diastole. With obstructive disease, the initial feature lost is the reversal of the flow component, leading to multiphasic (previously called *biphasic*) flow. Severe disease

## Table 63-3 Clinical Correlation of Different Levels of ABI*

| ABI | PRESENTATION |
|---|---|
| 1.11 ± 0.10 | Normal |
| 0.59 ± 0.15 | Intermittent claudication |
| 0.26 ± 0.13 | Ischemic rest pain |
| 0.05 ± 0.08 | Tissue loss |

From Moneta GL, Zaccardi MJ, Olmsted KA: Lower extremity arterial occlusive disease. In Zierler RE, editor: Strandness's duplex scanning in vascular disorders, ed 4, Philadelphia, 2010, Lippincott Williams & Wilkins, Wolters Kluwer Health, pp 133–147.

*The diagnosis of PAD is given to ABI <0.9. ABI >1.3 is interpreted as abnormal because of incompressible tibial arteries, frequently seen in diabetes and end-stage renal failure. Example: The ABI is calculated using the higher of the two ankle pressures (as indicative of limb perfusion), and the higher brachial pressure (as indicative of systemic pressure). In this example, the left and right ABI values are both 0.30.

## Table 63-4 Calculation of ABI

| PARAMETER | RIGHT | LEFT |
|---|---|---|
| Brachial blood pressure | 150 mm Hg | 100 mm Hg |
| Dorsalis pedis | 50 mm Hg | 25 mm Hg |
| Posterior tibia | 25 mm Hg | 50 mm Hg |
| ABI | 0.30 | 0.30 |

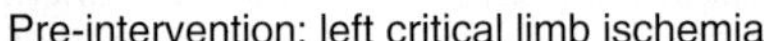


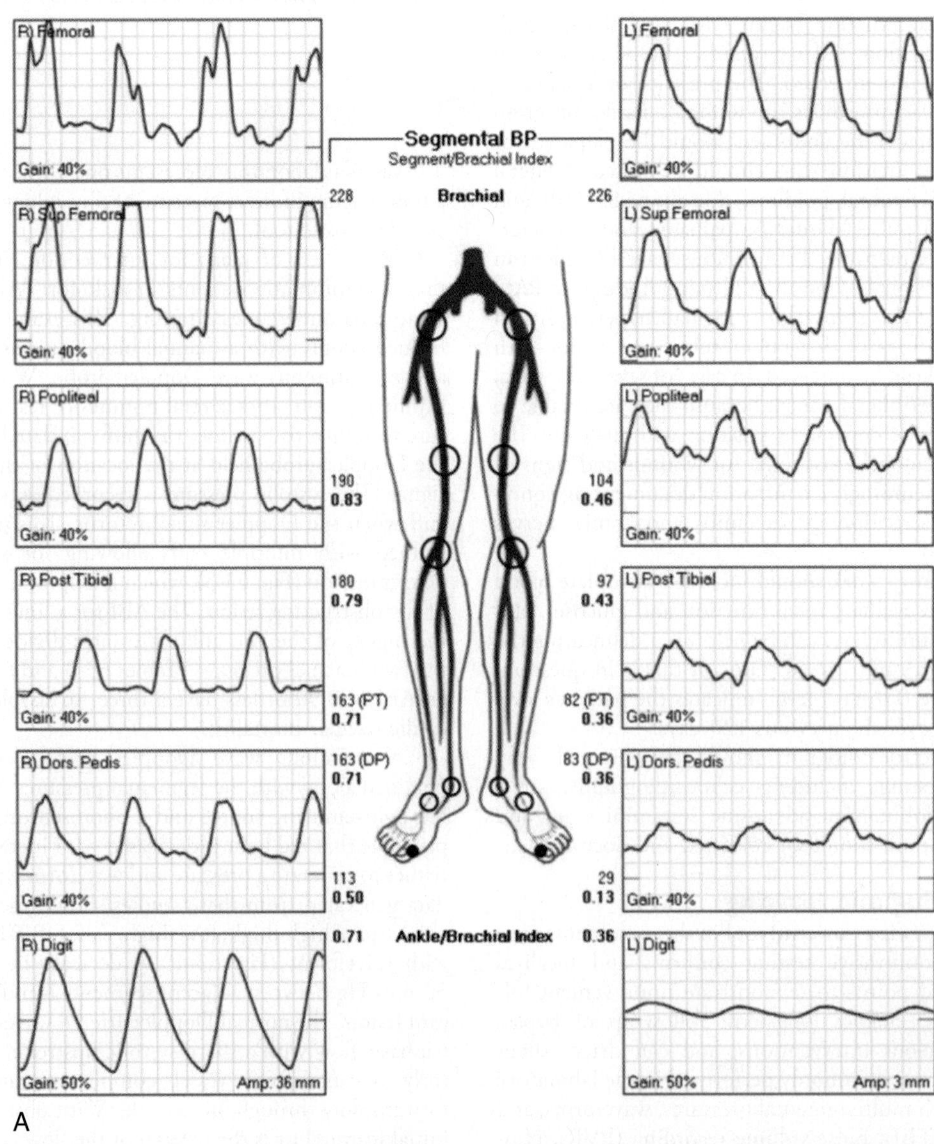


**FIGURE 63-4 A,** Patient with severe left leg claudication and diabetes. Segmental pressures demonstrate left ileofemoral obstruction.

leads to blunting of the arterial waveform, with decreased amplitude and decreased slope of the upstroke. With worsening symptoms, there is increased diastolic flow, resulting in monophasic flow. A change in waveform can be interpreted, along with a change in pressure, as indicative of disease at that level. Limitations of ABI and segmental pressure determinations include mural calcification, such as seen in DM and ESRD, leading to elevated pressures that do not accurately reflect intra-arterial perfusion pressure. With a noncompressible vessel, a TBI higher than 0.70 with an absolute digit pressure higher than 50 mm Hg, with a normal waveform, is indicative of preserved flow because digit arteries are relatively resistant to the intramural calcification. The high thigh pressure cannot always distinguish among common iliac, external iliac or common femoral disease. A proximal stenosis can decrease flow to the extent that accuracy is lost when interpreting gradients downstream.

Symptomatic patients with palpable distal pulses or a normal resting ABI should undergo exercise testing with measurement of the postexercise ABI. The decrease in peripheral vascular resistance that occurs with exercise-induced vasodilation will increase the drop in pressure seen across a stenotic lesion. Patients undergo resting ABI testing, followed by treadmill exercise until symptoms occur; repeat ABI testing may then reveal a decrease in ankle pressure of 20 mm Hg or a decrease in the ABI of 0.20. These changes, or a failure of the ABI to return to preexercise baseline within 3 minutes, are interpreted as a positive result.

Arterial duplex ultrasonography provides B mode (gray scale) imaging, pulsed Doppler spectral waveforms, and color flow data for analysis and, in experienced hands, can provide sensitive and specific information about the abdominal aorta and visceral, renal, iliac, and distal limb vessels. Peak systolic velocities (PSVs) and end-diastolic velocities are recorded. Waveforms are generated and analyzed. Color flow is useful for demonstrating patent vessels in very low-flow states and for distinguishing antegrade from retrograde flow. As in continuous flow Doppler analysis, a change in waveform from triphasic to monophasic, or an increase in PSV followed by a drop in velocity, indicates a hemodynamically significant lesion. A ratio of the PSV within the stenosis to the PSV of the proximal normal segment of 2.0 or more correlates with a stenosis of 50% or more. Visualization of intra-abdominal segments requires the

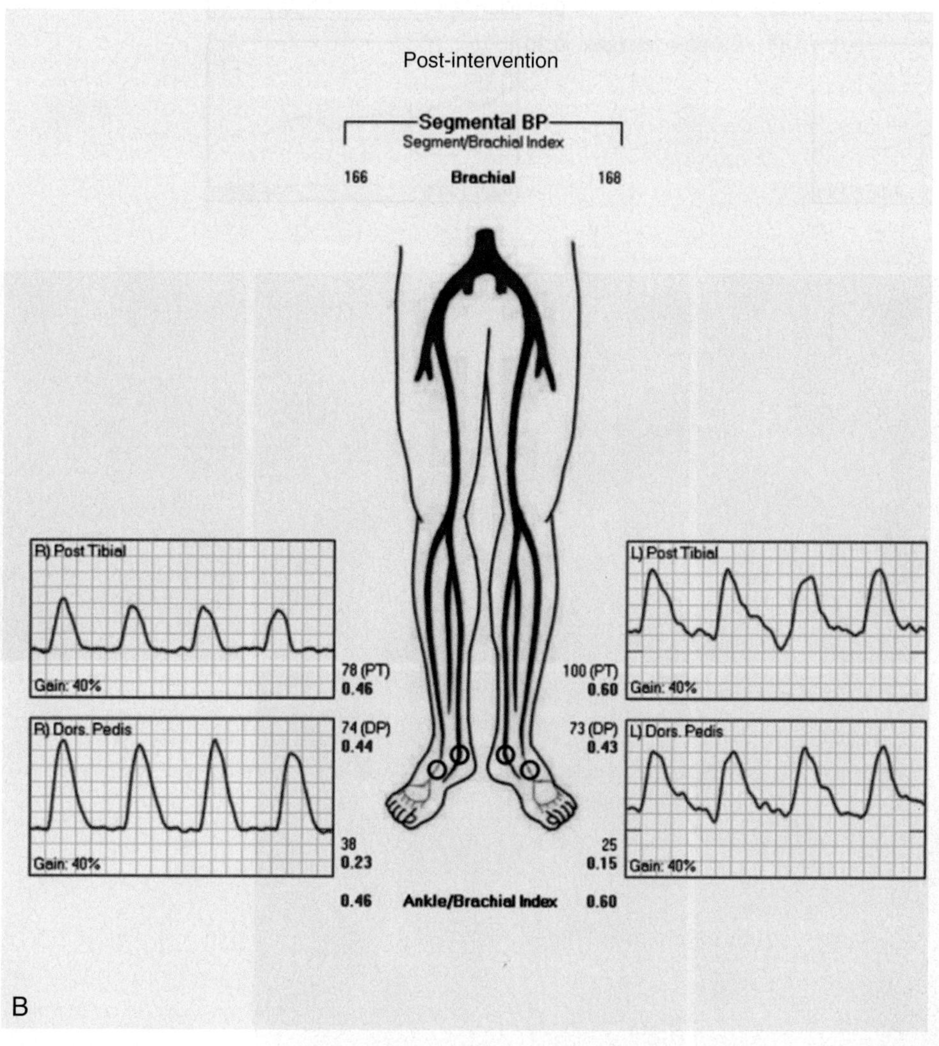


**FIGURE 63-4, cont'd B,** Following left ileofemoral bypass and common iliac artery stent placement, the ABI is significantly improved and the patient is asymptomatic.

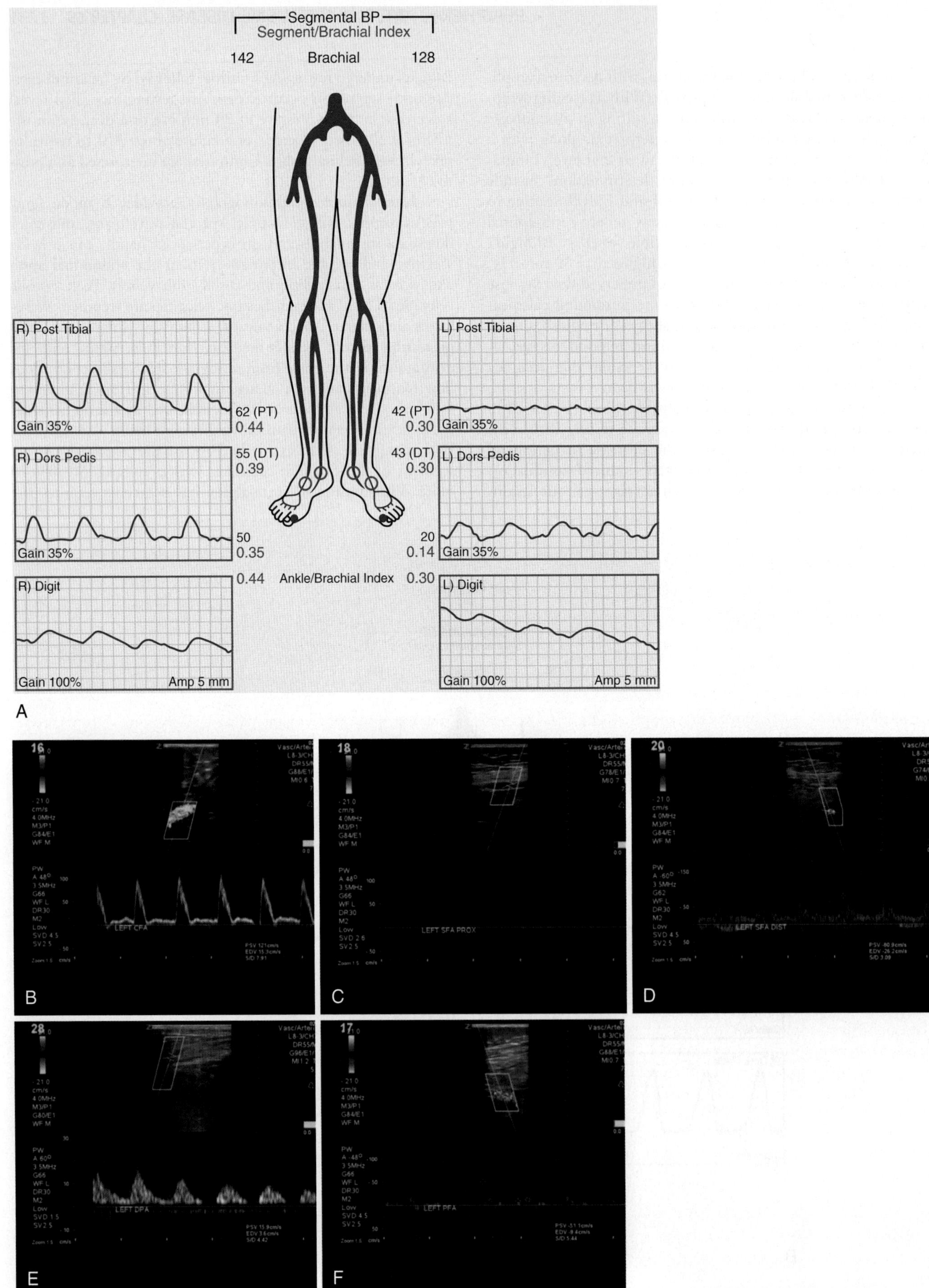


**FIGURE 63-5** Arterial duplex scanning, left critical limb ischemia. Although both ABIs are abnormal **(A)**, the right limb waveforms are multiphasic and the left-sided waveforms are monophasic. Arterial duplex images show normal left CFA **(B)** and no flow in the proximal SFA **(C)**; however, flow in the distal SFA **(D)** and dorsalis pedis arteries **(E)** is present because of collateral flow from the profunda femoris **(F)**.

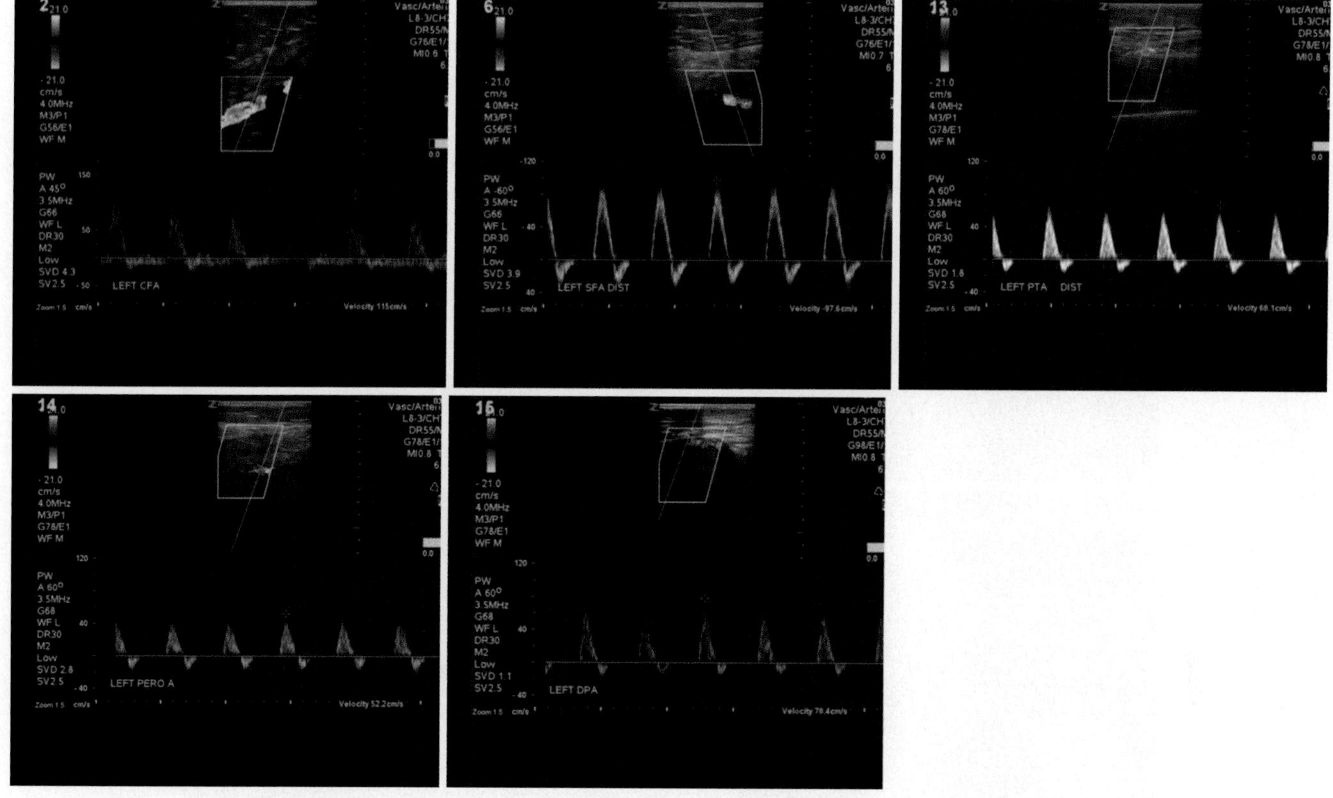


**FIGURE 63-6** Postintervention on the same patient as Figure 63-5 shows intact flow throughout SFA and improved distal flow.

patient to be fasting prior to the examination to eliminate bowel gas; studies can be limited by body habitus. Severe calcification of the distal vessels can impede imaging of flow (Figs. 63-5 and 63-6).

## Imaging Studies

When intervention is planned, further imaging to delineate the location and nature of disease is needed. The gold standard for these purposes has been angiography. Because of the invasive nature of this test, with attendant risks of complications, imaging was previously reserved as a preoperative study for patients determined to be operative candidates because of the severity of their disease and their suitability for surgery. This algorithm has changed somewhat in contemporary practice. Most angiography is therapeutic rather than diagnostic, with lesions that are deemed amenable for endovascular intervention addressed in the same setting as the initial angiogram. Alternatively, computed tomography angiography (CTA) or magnetic resonance angiography (MRA) may enable the acquisition of the same vascular roadmap prior to a planned intervention.

**Angiography** Access is usually via the contralateral common femoral or left brachial artery. A complete diagnostic study is performed in four steps: (1) abdominal aortography, with a multiside hole catheter placed at the level of the diaphragm, imaging the abdominal aorta, celiac artery, superior mesenteric artery (SMA), inferior mesenteric artery (IMA), and aortic bifurcation; (2) pelvic angiography with a multiside hole catheter at the aortic bifurcation, imaging the bilateral common iliac, hypogastric, and external iliac arteries, common femoral arteries, and proximal superficial femoral (SFA) and profunda femoris artery (Fig. 63-7). (3) The contralateral common femoral artery is then selected using an end-hole catheter, and images of the contralateral SFA, profunda, popliteal, tibial, and pedal vessels are obtained in one to three low-bolus runs. (4) The access sheath is then pulled back to the level of the distal ipsilateral external iliac artery to image the ipsilateral limb. Trans-stenotic pressure gradients and multiplanar images can clarify the significance of an ambiguous lesion. Complete assessment of the aortic and iliac inflow and bilateral lower extremities requires 75 to 100 mL of contrast.

Risks of diagnostic angiography and all endovascular procedures include groin hematoma, retroperitoneal bleeding, pseudoaneurysm, and arterial dissection. Even a small amount of bleeding after brachial artery access can cause symptomatic brachial sheath hematoma and neural compromise requiring exploration and evacuation. These risks are reduced by the routine use of ultrasound-guided access and micropuncture techniques.

The risk of contrast nephropathy is limited by prudent use of contrast, selective catheterization, which decreases the volume of the contrast bolus required to opacify the vessels, and use of lower ionic load or iso-osmolar contrast agents. Patients are counseled to increase oral hydration in preparation for and following arteriography. Metformin and ACE inhibitors, as well as diuretics, are held prior to the procedure and for 48 hours postprocedure. There is some evidence for preoperative medication with acetylcysteine, 1200 mg PO twice daily, before and after arteriography, as well as IV fluid hydration using half-normal saline with 1.5 ampules of sodium bicarbonate or D5W

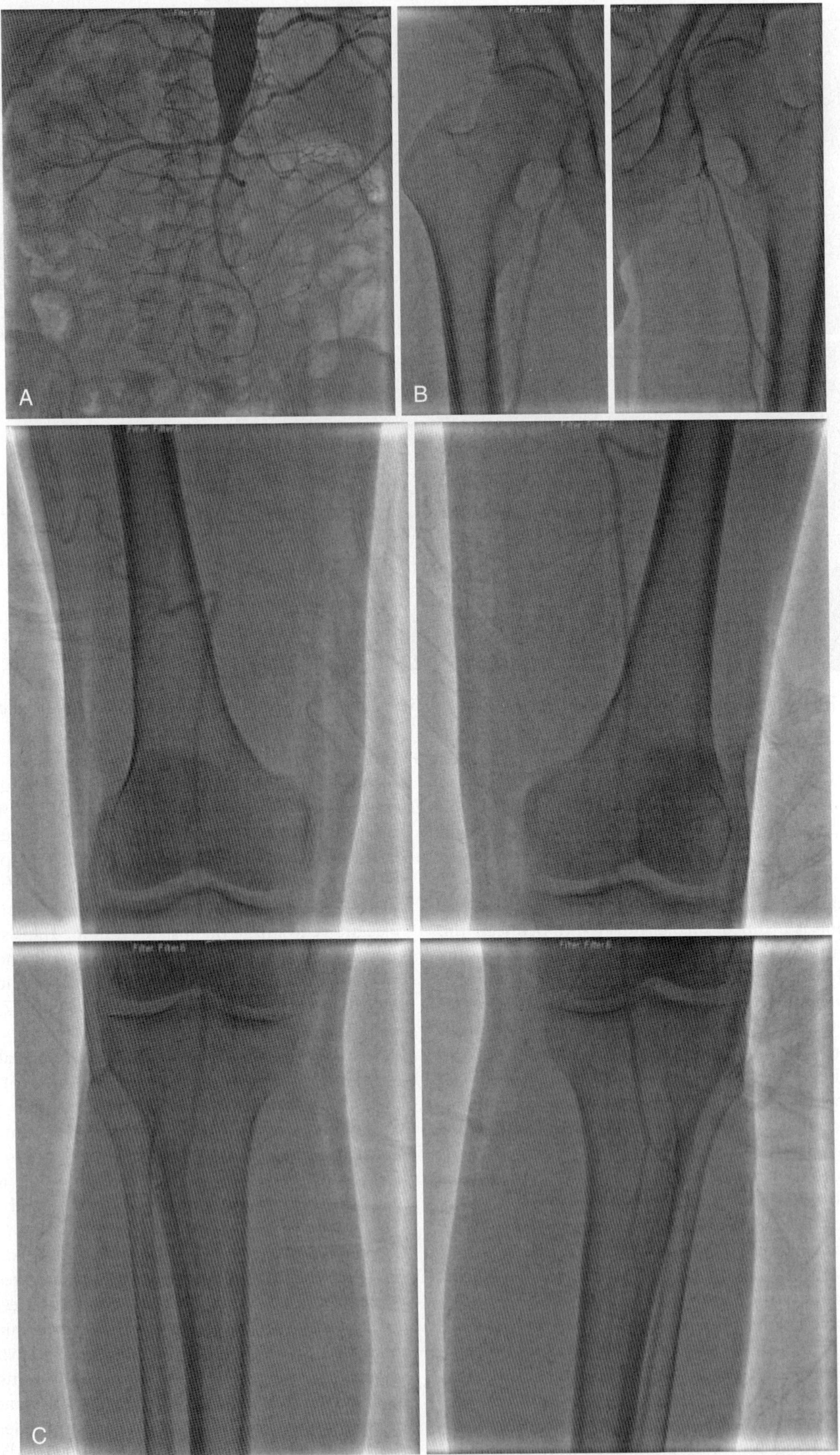

**FIGURE 63-7** Aortogram with bilateral lower extremity runoff, nonsubtracted. **A,** Occluded aorta with left renal artery occlusion. **B,** Reconstitution of bilateral common femoral arteries, flush SFA occlusions. **C,** Reconstitution of right above-knee popliteal artery, left SFA. Below the knee, proximal bilateral tibial flow appears intact.

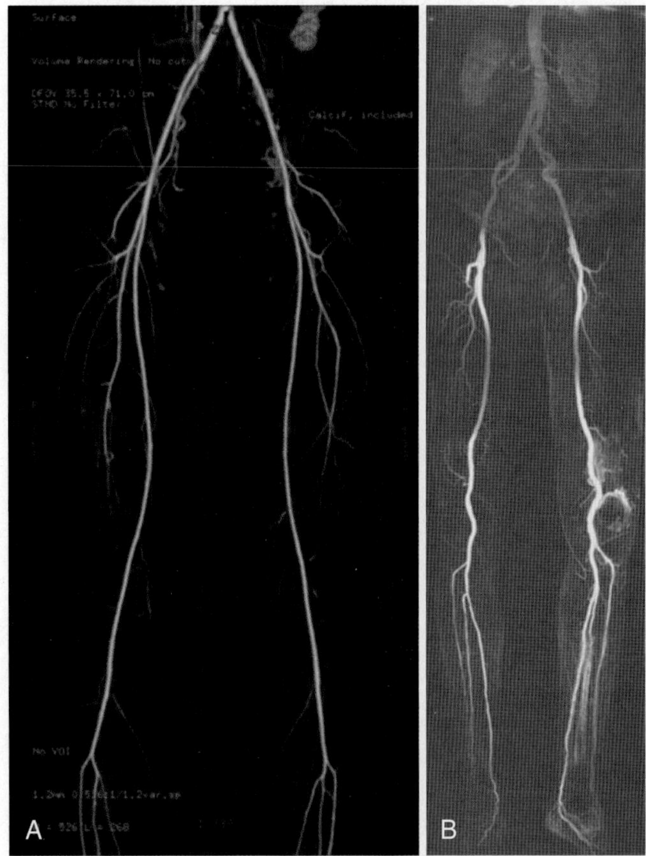


**FIGURE 63-8 A,** CTA scan with volume rendering demonstrates normal common iliac, external iliac, common femoral, deep and superficial femoral, popliteal and proximal tibial arteries. **B,** MRA scan demonstrating distal tibial disease. (Courtesy Dr. Douglas Hughes, University of Texas Medical Branch at Galveston [UTMB], Department of Radiology.)

with three ampules of sodium bicarbonate. Patients with a history of contrast allergy should be premedicated according to institutional guidelines with steroids and histamine blockers (e.g., diphenhydramine).

Risk of radiation exposure for diagnostic procedures is limited but, with the growing complexity of endovascular interventions, cumulative exposure is a potential concern for the patient and for the physician exposed during the therapeutic procedure. Monitoring is essential and routine.

***Computed Tomography Angiography*** The widespread use of multidetector row CT scanners has improved the speed, volume coverage, and slice thickness of images so that a single contrast bolus can be imaged as it passes through the arterial system. One advantage of CTA (Fig 63-8*A*) is the depiction of the entire vessel, with the ability to appreciate thrombus and calcification; arteriography typically characterizes only the lumen of the artery. Thin slices of 0.625 mm allows for three-dimensional reconstructions and multiplanar reformatting that is not routinely achieved with conventional arteriography. CTA disadvantages are similar to those of arteriography, with the potential for complications from the use of iodinated contrast agents and significant accumulation of radiation exposure.

***Magnetic Resonance Angiography*** Advocates of contrast-enhanced MRA with gadolinium (see Fig. 63-8*B*) report a high sensitivity and specificity of this modality for demonstrating the degree of stenosis and lesion length, and even superiority in identifying distal target vessels when compared with conventional arteriography.[3] Disadvantages of MRA technology include the need for patient cooperation, patient discomfort, longer studies, expense, contraindications with certain metallic implants, and renal toxicity reported with use of the contrast agent, Gadolinium. Its use is contraindicated in renal disease because of the risk of nephrogenic systemic fibrosis. This is a rare complication associated with the administration of gadolinium-based agents to patients with renal failure or renal insufficiency having a glomerular filtration rate 30 mL/min or lower.[4] Patients develop fibrosed nodules of the skin, eyes, and joints. Severe contracture limiting movement or involvement of the heart, liver, and lungs has been described.

***Carbon Dioxide Angiography*** Angiography using $CO_2$ as a contrast medium can be helpful in patients with severe chronic renal insufficiency. $CO_2$ temporarily displaces the blood in the artery being imaged. $CO_2$ rapidly dissolves, but 3 to 5 minutes must be allowed to pass between injections. The limitations to use of this contrast agent include poor detail, especially for distal vessels. The bolus may cause significant patient discomfort. Sequelae of $CO_2$ embolus, with gas trapping leading to mesenteric ischemia, have been described. $CO_2$ is not used for arch or cerebral arteriography.

**Intravascular Ultrasound** With improvements in high-frequency smaller transducers, the use of catheter-based intravascular ultrasound IVUS (Fig. 63-9) has increased. IVUS provides a transverse, 360-degree image of the lumen of the vessel to be imaged throughout its length and provides qualitative data about the wall anatomy. It has been used in peripheral interventions for opening chronic total occlusions (CTOs) and has been instrumental in the endovascular treatment of aortic dissection. As a diagnostic tool, adjuncts such as color flow Doppler enable the delineation between flow and thrombus, whereas virtual histology, in which color is assigned to plaque components of fibrous, fibrofatty, calcified, and necrotic lipid core densities, has been shown to correlate well with actual histology in assessment of coronary[5] and carotid arteries disease.[6] The use of IVUS, however, increases the length of procedures and its expense limits its applicability.

## Treatment

### Medical Treatment

Despite the aging of our population and increasing numbers of people afflicted by atherosclerotic arterial disease, morbidity from myocardial infarction and stroke is decreasing. This is likely secondary to advances in medical management and increasing awareness by affected individuals about the availability of medications that can limit the progression of the disease process. The American Heart Association (AHA) has published guidelines for risk modification that have grown increasingly aggressive in efforts to treat this important public health concern. In contemporary surgical practice, lipid modification, antiplatelet and antihypertensive control, and smoking cessation strategies are all becoming standard management issues for the patient with

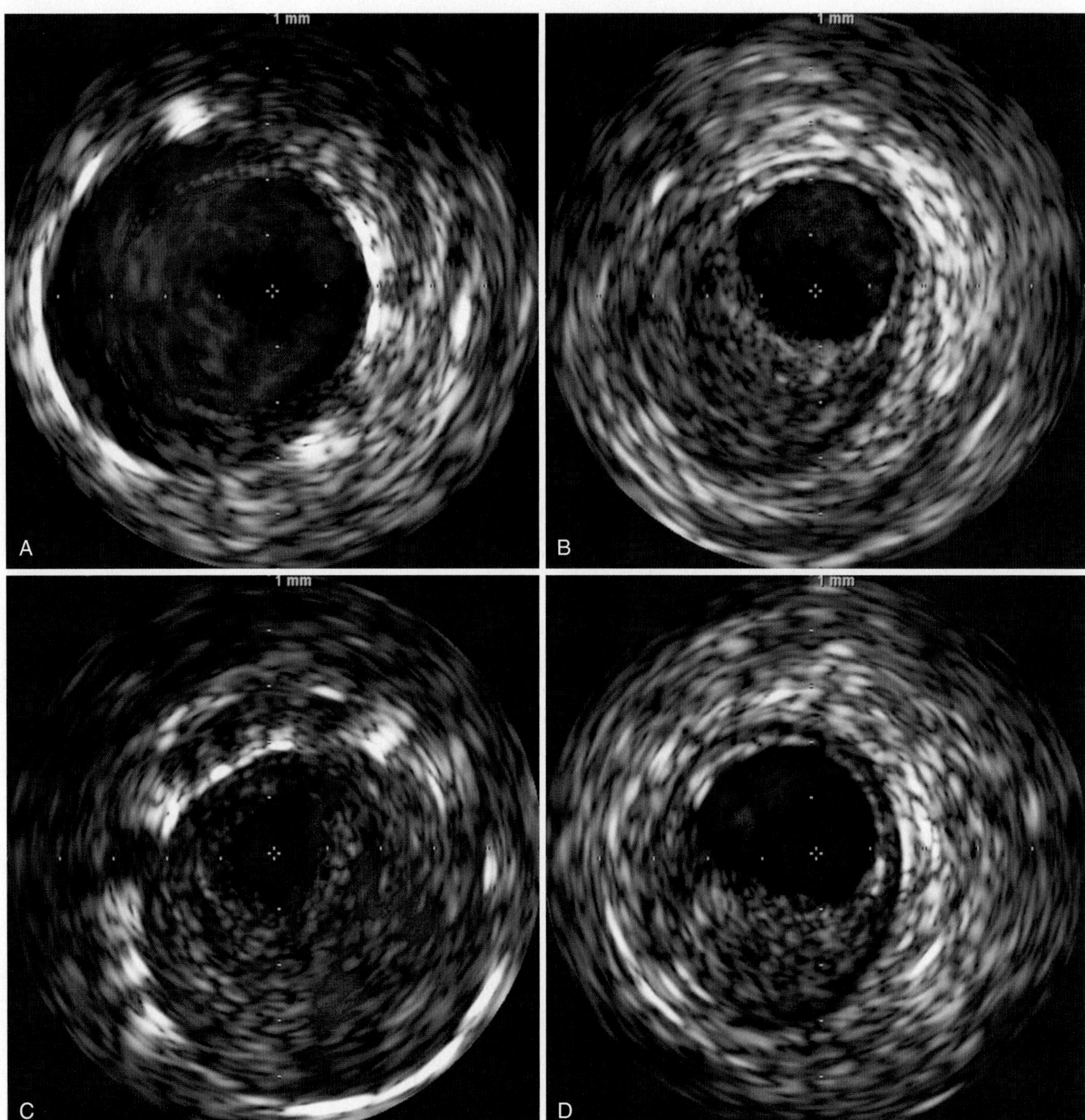


**FIGURE 63-9** Intravascular ultrasound. Counterclockwise from left corner: patent common iliac artery stent **(A)**; common iliac artery stent thrombosis **(B)**; external iliac artery plaque **(C)**; external iliac artery plaque **(D)**. (Courtesy Dr. Syed Gilani, University of Texas Medical Branch at Galveston [UTMB], Department of Cardiology.)

vascular disease. Table 63-5 summarizes the AHA guidelines for risk factor modification.

Risk factors contributing to PAD are the same as those for atherosclerosis:

- Smoking. Tobacco use in any form is the single most important modifiable cause of PVD internationally. Smokers have up to a tenfold increase in relative risk for PVD in a dose-related effect. Exposure to secondhand smoke from environmental exposure has also been shown to promote changes in endothelium, the precursor to atherosclerosis.
- Dyslipidemia. Decreased high-density lipoprotein (HDL) cholesterol and elevations of total cholesterol, low-density lipoprotein (LDL) cholesterol, and triglyceride (TG) levels have been correlated with accelerated PAD. Correction of dyslipidemia by diet and/or medication is associated with a major improvement in short-term rates of heart attack and stroke. This

**Table 63-5 Medical Therapy for Peripheral Arterial Disease**

| DISORDER | RECOMMENDED PHARMACOLOGIC AGENT | PURPOSE OF CARDIOVASCULAR RISK REDUCTION | CLASS OF RECOMMENDATIONS | LEVEL OF EVIDENCE | COMMENTS |
|---|---|---|---|---|---|
| Dyslipidemia | Statin | Statin therapy, with target LDL <100 mg/dL | I | B | |
| | | Statin therapy, with target LDL <70 mg/dL | II | B | High-risk patients with multiple and/or poorly controlled risk factors: DM, continued tobacco abuse, metabolic syndrome (TG ≥ 200 mg/dL + HDL ≤40 mg/dL + non-HDL ≥130 mg/dL), acute coronary syndrome |
| | Gemfibrozil | May be useful in PAD pts with low HDL, normal LDL, high TG | II | C | Gemfibrozil reduces risk of nonfatal MI or cardiovascular death by 22% in CAD patients with low HDL; effects on PAD unknown |
| Hypertension | | 140/90 mm Hg in nondiabetics, 130/80 mm Hg in DM and CRI | I | A | Reduces risk of MI, CHF, cardiovascular death and stroke |
| | Beta blocker | Effective, not contraindicated | I | A | Reduces risk of MI and death in CAD patients; does not impair walking distance |
| | ACE inhibitors | Reasonable in symptomatic PAD to decrease risk of cardiovascular events. | IIa | B | In patients with symptomatic PAD, ramipril reduces risk of MI, stroke, or vascular death by ≈25% |
| | | May be used in asymptomatic PAD to decrease risk of cardiovascular events | IIb | C | No evidence for efficacy of ACE inhibitors in patients with asymptomatic PAD |
| Diabetes | | Proper foot care; skin lesions, ulcerations should be addressed urgently in all diabetic patients with lower extremity PAD | I | B | |
| | | HbA1c <7% | IIa | C | Can be effective to reduce microvascular complications, potentially improve cardiovascular outcome |
| Atherosclerosis | ASA | 75-325 mg PO qd reduces risk of MI, stroke and vascular death | I | A | Reduces risk of events by 26% to 32% |
| | Clopidogrel | 75 mg PO qd, effective alternative to ASA to reduce risk of MI, stroke, vascular death | I | B | Reduces risk of events by 23.8% |
| Smoking | | Clinicians to advise smoking cessation, offer medical therapy | I | B | Physician's advice with frequent follow-up: 1-year success rate, 5% Without physician's interventions: 1-year success rate, 0.1%. With nicotine replacement: 1-year success rate,16% With buproprion: 1-year success rate, 30% |

Hirsch AT, Haskal ZJ, Hertzer NR, et al: ACC/AHA 2005 Practice Guidelines for the management of patients with peripheral arterial disease (lower extremity, renal, mesenteric, and abdominal aortic): a collaborative report from the American Association for Vascular Surgery/Society for Vascular Surgery, Society for Cardiovascular Angiography and Interventions, Society for Vascular Medicine and Biology, Society of Interventional Radiology, and the ACC/AHA Task Force on Practice Guidelines (Writing Committee to Develop Guidelines for the Management of Patients With Peripheral Arterial Disease): endorsed by the American Association of Cardiovascular and Pulmonary Rehabilitation; National Heart, Lung, and Blood Institute; Society for Vascular Nursing; TransAtlantic Inter-Society Consensus; and Vascular Disease Foundation. Circulation 113:e463–e654, 2006.

*CHF,* Congestive heart failure; *CRI,* chronic renal insufficiency; *MI,* myocardial infarction.

benefit is gained even though current evidence does not demonstrate a major reversal of peripheral and/or coronary atherosclerosis

- Hypertension. Elevated blood pressure is correlated with an increased risk of developing PAD and associated coronary and cerebrovascular events (e.g., heart attack, stroke).
- Diabetes mellitus. The presence of DM involves a two- to fourfold increased risk of PVD by causing endothelial and smooth muscle cell dysfunction in peripheral arteries. Diabetics account for up to 70% of nontraumatic amputations performed, and a known diabetic who smokes has an approximately 30% risk of amputation within 5 years.

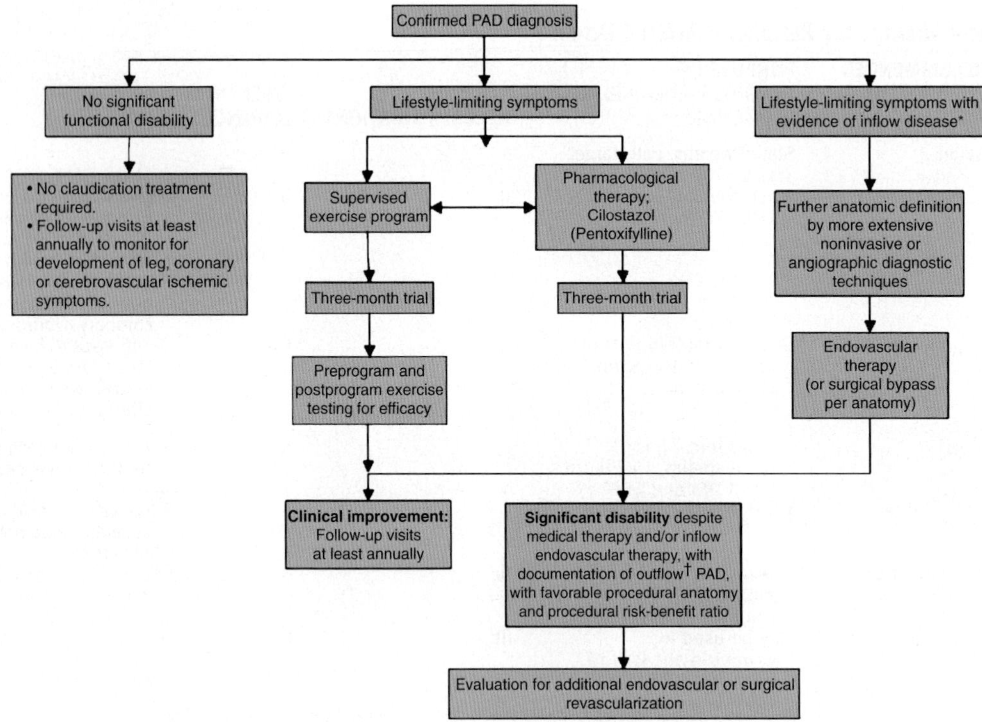


**FIGURE 63-10** Intermittent claudication treatment algorithm. (From Norgren L, Hiatt WR, Dormandy JA, et al: Inter-Society Consensus for the Management of Peripheral Arterial Disease [TASC II]. J Vasc Surg 45[Suppl]:S5–S67, 2007.)

## Revascularization: Surgical Treatment

**Intermittent Claudication** Patients with intermittent claudication (IC) are treated by risk factor modification to decrease their risk of myocardial infarction (MI) and cerebral vascular accident (CVA). A trial of cilostazol and supervised exercise is recommended; these therapies, combined with risk factor modification (particularly smoking cessation), have been shown to improve walking distance. Patients are reassured that they are at limited risk of limb loss, approximately 2% to 3% at 5 years. Although significant disability may occur as a result of IC, symptoms remain stable because of the development of collateral flow, or perhaps alterations in gait that favor nonischemic muscle groups.[7] However, 25% of IC patients will see deterioration in their clinical course, usually during the first year after diagnosis; the best predictor of this decline is the initial ABI. Patients with an initial ABI of less than 0.50 have a hazard ratio of more than 2 compared with patients with an ABI higher than 0.50. IC patients with an initial ankle pressure of 40 to 60 mm Hg have an annual limb loss rate of 8.5%.

Patients who present initially with low ankle pressures or absent femoral pulses, or patients who return with unabated, severe, lifestyle-limiting symptoms that have not adequately responded to nonoperative measures, are considered for intervention (Fig. 63-10).

**Critical Limb Ischemia** Patient who present initially with rest pain, or who progress from claudication to rest pain, undergo the same detailed history and physical examination with risk factor modification as patients presenting with milder disease. However, because rest pain is associated with a significant risk of limb loss without intervention, patients are immediately offered imaging and revascularization if prohibitive perioperative risk does not preclude this.

Similarly, patients who present with nonhealing wounds of the feet, dry gangrene, or necrotizing infection are offered an expeditious workup to plan a revascularization that will reestablish in-line blood flow to the foot. In case of tissue loss with infection, an immediate decision regarding the need for operative débridement or amputation prior to revascularization must be made. In case of severe sepsis with hemodynamic instability or evidence of multisystem organ failure, patients may require amputation prior to revascularization. However, if a patient with systemic toxicity from the infection responds rapidly to administration of IV antibiotics, revascularization prior to débridement may minimize tissue loss. See Figure 63-11.

**Diabetic Foot** PVD is common among patients with diabetes (Fig. 63-12). IC is twice as common among diabetic patients than among nondiabetic patients. An increase in $HgbA_{1C}$ by 1% can result in more than a 25% risk of PAD. Major amputation rates are five to ten times higher in diabetics than nondiabetics. Because of these causal relations, the American Diabetes Association recommends ABI screening every 5 years in patients with diabetes.[8]

The care of diabetic patients should start with preventive measures, and it is important to avoid infections in patients with insensate feet because of neuropathy. These patients need to wear properly fitted shoes at all times for protection. Orthotic inserts should be used to distribute weight evenly to avoid pressure on the metatarsal heads of the foot.

Diabetic patients may be unaware of the presence of infections or ulcerative lesions because of peripheral neuropathy and

CLI confirmed

Candidate for revascularization → Imaging (Duplex, angiography, MRA, CTA) → Revascularization as appropriate

Not candidate for revascularization → Stable pain and lesion → Medical treatment (nonoperative)

Not candidate for revascularization → Not-tolerable pain, spreading infection → Amputation

**FIGURE 63-11** Algorithm for treatment of the CLI patient. (From Norgren L, Hiatt WR, Dormandy JA, et al: Inter-Society Consensus for the Management of Peripheral Arterial Disease [TASC II]. J Vasc Surg 45[Suppl]:S5–S67, 2007.)

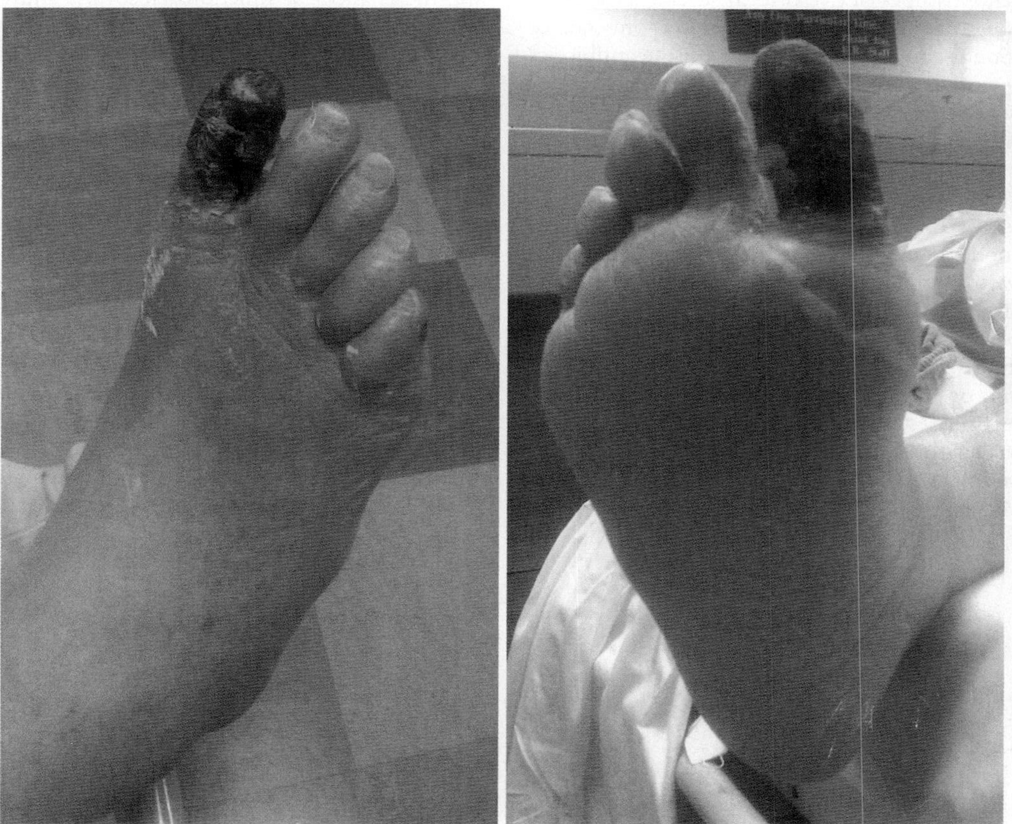

**FIGURE 63-12** Diabetic patient who presented with chronic dry gangrene of the right great toe, with dependent rubor of the forefoot.

a decreased ability to sense pain. In this population, infections can progress rapidly, with significant tissue damage from a combination of delayed presentation and compromised immune function.

On presentation, a careful physical examination is important to plan for appropriate treatment. The overlying cellulitis is assessed, and any possible underlying abscess is examined by palpation for crepitus or detection of drainage of purulent fluid. Cellulitis should not be confused with dependent rubor caused by severe ischemia in patients with PAD. The presence of an abscess requires immediate drainage prior to revascularization.

The status of arterial circulation is documented. The presence or absence of lower extremity pulses in the common femoral, popliteal, and pedal arteries is examined. The pulses may be difficult to palpate because of swelling from foot infection; noninvasive arterial ultrasound can be useful in assessing the extent of arterial disease.

Insulin-dependent diabetic patients may have calcified walls of the medium and small arteries that can falsely elevate the segmental pressures of the leg. In this situation, digital pressures of the toes can be accurately measured and a pressure higher than 30 mm Hg is predictive of healing after local amputation and debridement.

Plain x-rays with multiple views of the foot can assist in assessing the extent of foot infection. Gas in soft tissue signifies deep tissue infection and the need for urgent surgical débridement. Advanced osteomyelitis can be detected; however, plain films may not show early bone infection. Magnetic resonance imaging (MRI) of the foot is a sensitive imaging modality for detecting soft tissue infection and early osteomyelitis.

Routine laboratory work is sent and evaluated for subtle signs of sepsis. Sudden worsening of glycemic control or a rise in creatinine level is seen frequently, often without leukocytosis.

In infections with only cellulitis and no underlying soft tissue involvement, patients are treated with IV antibiotic therapy. If the cellulitis does not resolve in several days, there may not be adequate antibiotic coverage and the presence of deep tissue infection is considered. The choice of the antibiotics used and the foot need to be reevaluated; reimaging the foot may be necessary.

The cause of persistent cellulitis and nonhealing infection is usually underlying deep infection or osteomyelitis. Other patients may present with gangrene, open joint or exposed bone, or abscess. In these patients, surgical débridement is required in addition to antibiotic therapy. Small open wounds can be treated with simple débridement, but often there is deep tissue involvement that is not visible on the surface. To remove all nonviable tissue and wide drainage, amputation may be required. If there is extensive infection of the foot with gas, calf pain, or systemic sepsis, the patient may require amputation as an initial therapy. After surgical débridement, patients are treated with aggressive wound care using dressing changes and continued, broad-spectrum antibiotic therapy until intraoperative culture sensitivities are finalized and allow for the use of targeted antimicrobials. Wounds are evaluated closely for persistent infection that may require additional surgical intervention. In patients with adequate arterial circulation, the wound can be closed secondarily after resolution of the infection.

All patients with evidence of concomitant arterial occlusive disease are considered for lower extremity revascularization with open bypass surgery or endovascular stenting or angioplasty to optimize wound healing and limb salvage.

### Lower Extremity Amputations

Amputation, unfortunately, in the minds of most surgeons and their patients, represents a failure of therapy or care. Consent for this operation, regardless of the level, is usually imbued with an emotional gravity that few other, even more complex, dangerous, life-altering procedures carry. Not infrequently, amputations in the vascular patient are prone to breakdown and the need for revision is common, thereby prolonging the patient's time in the hospital, lengthening the recovery process, decreasing the chances of functional recovery, and contributing to a high rate of depression. It is therefore incumbent on the surgeon to ensure that all steps are taken to minimize the risks of local and systemic complications.[9]

The perioperative mortality rate for below-knee amputation (BKA ) is 5% to 10% and that of above-knee amputation (AKA) even higher, 10% to 15%, testifying to the limited reserves of patient facing these procedures.[10] Wound healing in BKA is poor; almost one third of patients require débridement or healing by secondary intention or conversion to AKA (Fig. 63-13). Despite optimistic preoperative counseling, functional recovery with ambulation is poor for AKA patients.[11]

The determination of the appropriate level for amputation has been studied extensively (Table 63-6). In an effort to preserve limb length and decrease the metabolic demands of ambulation, toe and transmetatarsal amputations (TMAs) are usually attempted. Aside from clinical judgment, segmental arterial pressures, Doppler waveforms, and toe pressures have been studied. Diabetes, combined with a toe pressure of lower than

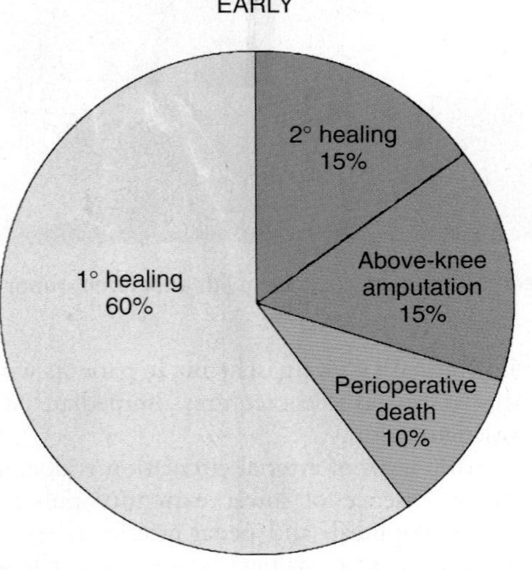


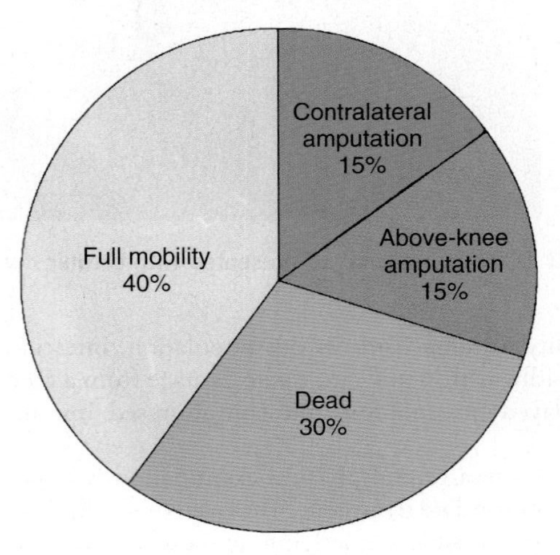


**FIGURE 63-13** Early and 2-year outcomes of the BKA patient. (From Norgren L, Hiatt WR, Dormandy JA, et al: Inter-Society Consensus for the Management of Peripheral Arterial Disease [TASC II]. J Vasc Surg 45[Suppl]:S5–S67, 2007.)

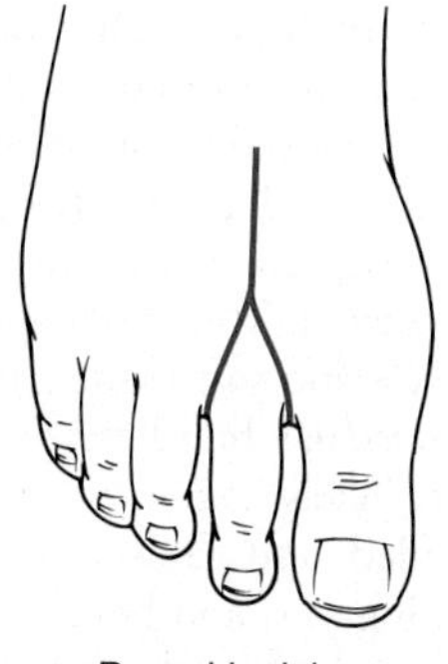


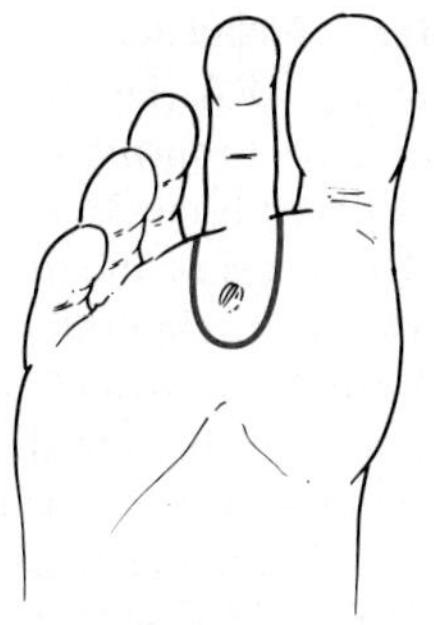


**FIGURE 63-14** Surgical approach to ray amputation. (From Eidt JF, Kalapatapu VR: Techniques and results. In Cronenwett JL, Johnston W [eds]: Rutherford's vascular surgery, ed 7, Philadelphia, 2010, Saunders, pp 1772–1790.)

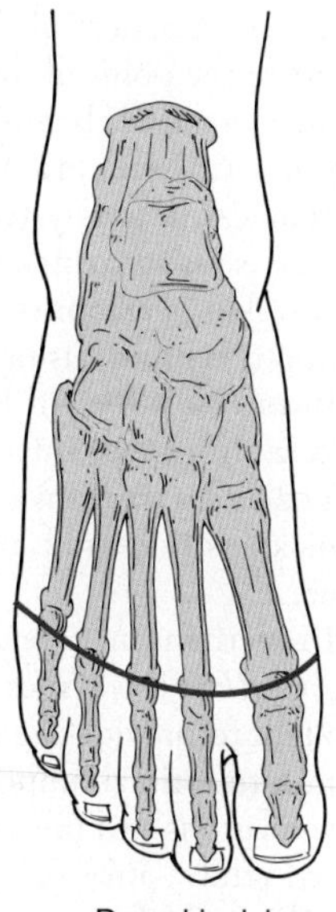


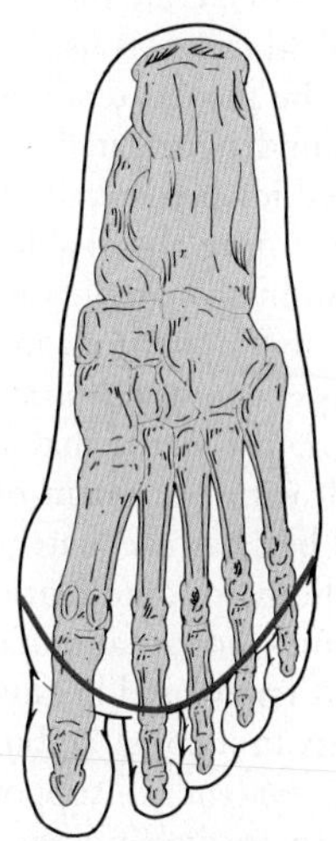


**FIGURE 63-15** Surgical approach to transmetatarsal amputation. (From Eidt JF, Kalapatapu VR: Techniques and results. In Cronenwett JL, Johnston W [eds]: Rutherford's vascular surgery, ed 7, Philadelphia, 2010, Saunders, pp 1772–1790.)

**Table 63-6 Prediction of Wound Healing by Vascular Studies**

| | | Wound Healing (%) | | | |
|---|---|---|---|---|---|
| **STUDY** | **THRESHOLD (MM HG)** | **BELOW THRESHOLD** | **ABOVE THRESHOLD** | **SENSITIVITY (%)** | **SPECIFICITY (%)** |
| SPP | 40 | 10 | 69 | 72 | 88 |
| $tcPo_2$ | 30 | 14 | 63 | 60 | 87 |
| TBP | 30 | 12 | 67 | 63 | 90 |
| ABP | 80 | 11 | 45 | 74 | 70 |

*ABP,* Ankle blood pressure; *SPP,* skin perfusion pressure; *TBP,* toe blood pressure; *$tcPo_2$,* transcutaneous oxygen pressure.

30 mm Hg, has been correlated with failure of healing minor amputations. Transcutaneous $O_2$ pressure ($TcPo_2$) measurement, easily obtained via a small sensor placed on the skin in the area of proposed amputation, has an accuracy of higher than 87% for predicting wound healing. A reading higher than 40 mm Hg is associated with successful healing, whereas $TcPo_2$ less than 20 mm Hg is associated with failure. Absolute ankle pressure higher than 60 mm Hg has been shown to predict the healing of BKAs with an accuracy of 50% to 90%.[12]

**Ray Amputation** For ray amputation, a tennis racquet incision around the base of the affected toe is made. For first toe amputations, the handle of the racquet is oriented along the medial aspect of the metatarsal head; for the fifth toe, it is oriented laterally. For toes 2 to 4, the incision is along the dorsal midline (Fig. 63-14). Neighboring digital vessels are carefully preserved as the soft tissues are divided. The extensor tendons are divided under tension and permitted to retract. The bone is divided proximal to the metatarsal head. If sesamoid bones are encountered, these are removed. Plantar soft tissue is divided; flexor tendons are similarly allowed to retract after being divided under tension. Soft tissue is closed over the metatarsal head with absorbable sutures. Minimal handling of the skin prevents ischemic trauma. The skin is approximated without tension or left open for closure by secondary intention.

The great toe and first metatarsal bone are important for normal gait because weight is transferred from the posterolateral foot during heel strike toward the medial toes, and the transfer of weight forward occurs principally through force transmitted during push off through the first metatarsal and great toe. Because of the significant rate of repeat ulceration and need for revision in up to 60% of patients requiring a great toe ray amputation, some have advocated proceeding directly to TMA in these patients.

Partial TMA can be performed when two digits are involved and the foot is deemed salvageable. However, multiple ray amputations will narrow the foot, resulting in instability and change in gait that may lead to repeat ulceration, wound breakdown, and the need for revision.

**Transmetatarsal Amputation** A curvilear incision is made above the metatarsal heads, with an intentionally longer flap fashioned on the plantar surface (Fig. 63-15). Soft tissues anterior to the bone are divided, including the tendons of the extensor muscles.

Digital arteries are suture-ligated as needed. A periosteal elevator is applied to elevate the soft tissues just to the point of division. An oscillating saw is used to divide the metatarsals behind their heads. The plantar tendons and plantar soft tissues are divided. The wound is irrigated using a mechanical lavage system and inspected for hemostasis. The soft tissue is reapproximated over the bone using absorbable sutures. The skin is reapproximated, with minimal manipulation and without tension, using interrupted nylon vertical mattress sutures. Non–weight-bearing status is encouraged for at least 4 weeks. In case of infection, a guillotine procedure may be performed and a vacuum dressing applied, with placement of a split-thickness skin graft after the wound bed has adequately granulated.

Alternative, more proximal TMA incisions include the Lisfranc and Chopart amputations (Fig. 63-16). The Symes amputation is rarely used because it is thought to provide the patient with less functional ambulation than a transtibial amputation. There is evidence to support multiple revisions and preservation of length in diabetic patients. In one study, 56% of patients failed to heal their initial TMA; of these, 9 of 41 underwent major amputation; 32 underwent midfoot amputations and achieved functional ambulation. Toe pressure higher than 50 mm Hg had a positive predictive value (PPV) of 91% for determining healing of TMA-midfoot amputations.[13]

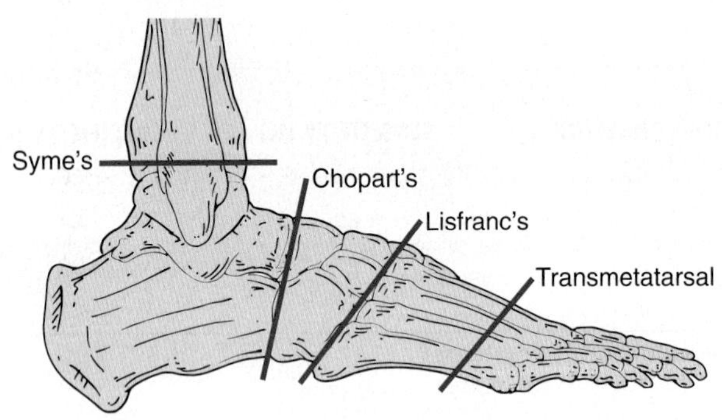


**FIGURE 63-16** Alternative distal amputation approaches. (From Eidt JF, Kalapatapu VR: Techniques and results. In Cronenwett JL, Johnston W [eds]: Rutherford's vascular surgery, ed 7, Philadelphia, 2010, Saunders, pp 1772–1790.)

**Below-Knee Amputation** There are multiple skin incisions described for BKA (Fig. 63-17). The most common is the long posterior flap. A tourniquet may be used to decrease blood loss, which can be substantial, even in the vascular patient. Approximately 10 cm below the tibial tuberosity, an anterior incision of two thirds of the circumference is created. The great saphenous vein is ligated and divided. All muscle and soft tissue structures anterior to the tibia are divided. Vascular bundles are suture-ligated with care because they are likely extremely calcified. Nerves are tied under tension, divided, and allowed to retract. The tibia is divided with an oscillating saw, and beveled anteriorly. The fibula is divided approximately 2 cm proximal to the tibia after detaching the anterior, lateral, and posterior compartment muscles. The posterior flap incision is created with the length approximately one third the circumference of the leg. The muscle flap is created just deep to the tibia, including the soleus and gastrocnemius muscles. After irrigation and inspection for hemostasis, the fascia is reapproximated using interrupted absorbable sutures. The skin is reapproximated using monofilament vertical mattress sutures or staples. A dressing of gauze wrap and Ace bandage is applied. A splint is created or a well-padded knee immobilizer is applied to prevent knee contracture.

In case of severe necrotizing foot infection, emergent guillotine transtibial amputation can be performed just proximal to the ankle, followed by formal revision. Two small studies have documented improved overall infection rates with staged BKA.[14-16]

Cryoamputation or physiologic amputation has been described to isolate the infected or acutely ischemic limb and prevent it from causing systemic effects in an already critically ill individual.[17]

**Above-Knee Amputation** In general, the longer the stump, the better. A fishmouth incision is created (Fig. 63-18). The great saphenous vein is ligated and divided. The sartorius, rectus femoris, and vastus lateralis are divided. The femoral artery and vein are separately suture-ligated and divided. Laterally, the vastus lateralis and intermedius are divided. The periosteal elevator is used to clear the femur at the level of the skin; the bone is divided using a pneumatic saw and beveled anteriorly. The profunda femoris artery and vein, or their branches, are ligated

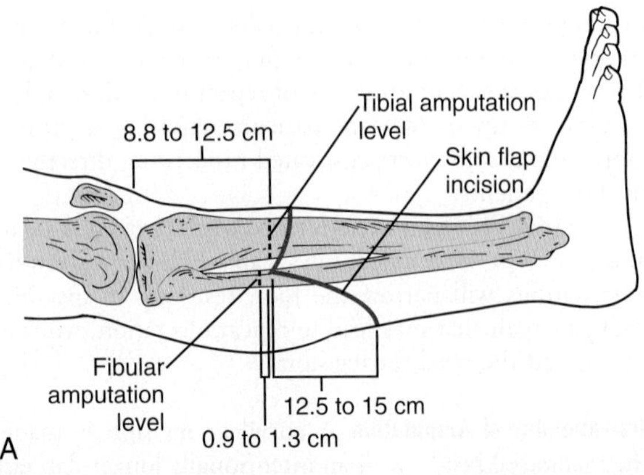


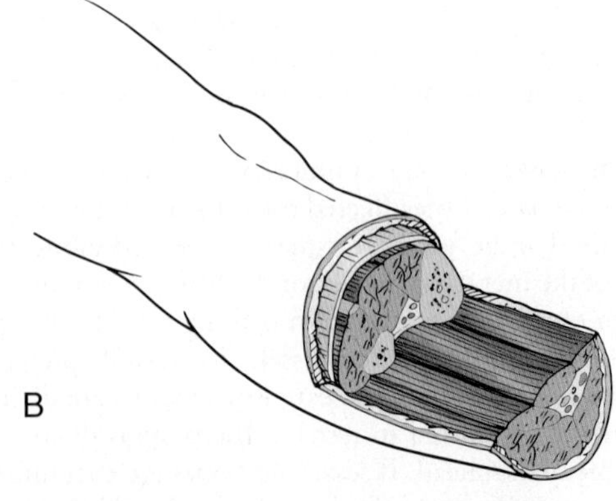


**FIGURE 63-17** Surgical approach to posterior flap for BKA. (From Eidt JF, Kalapatapu VR: Techniques and results. In Cronenwett JL, Johnston W [eds]: Rutherford's vascular surgery, ed 7, Philadelphia, 2010, Saunders, pp 1772–1790.)

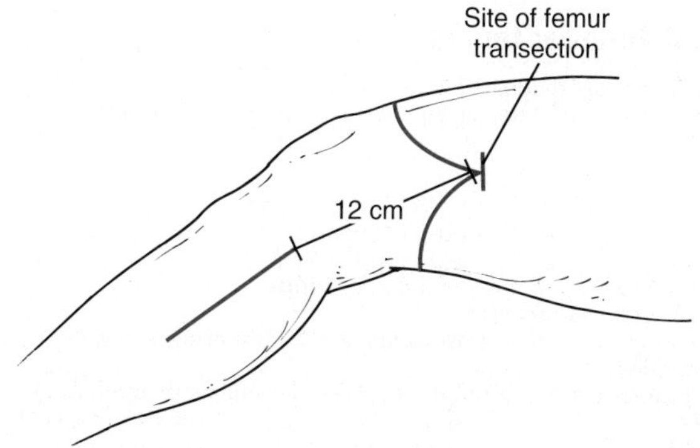


**FIGURE 63-18** Surgical approach to fishmouth incision for transfemoral (AKA) amputation. (From Eidt JF, Kalapatapu VR: Techniques and results. In Cronenwett JL, Johnston W [eds]: Rutherford's vascular surgery, ed 7, Philadelphia, 2010, Saunders, pp 1772–1790.)

and divided. The sciatic nerve is cut under tension and allowed to retract. After irrigation and inspection of hemostasis, the fascia of the muscles is approximated over the bone, using absorbable interrupted sutures, and the skin is closed.

Complications of AKA include hip contracture; this, as well as poor rates of ambulation, are related to unopposed action of the hip flexors. Preservation of adductor function is improved with myodesis; the length of the adductor magnus may be preserved and anchored to the lateral aspect of the femur via drill holes.[18]

Trans-knee amputations may be used as an alternative to AKA in younger patients for improved functional capability.

## Surgical Revascularization Procedures

There are fewer areas in medicine today in which treatment algorithms are changing more rapidly than in arterial occlusive disease. Currently, the decision for revascularization is based on the risks for the surgical intervention balanced against the expected benefits, including the durability of the treatment and options for further intervention if there is recurrence of symptoms. Rapid advances in endovascular techniques and devices have made the therapeutic decision making process increasingly complex; opinions about which therapies should be used first are varied. In an effort to characterize patients and their lesions and provide guidance about open versus endovascular alternatives, the Trans-Atlantic Inter-Society Document on Management of Peripheral Arterial Disease (TASC) was written and published in January 2000. As practice patterns matured, a second TASC II document was released later in the decade, in 2007. These documents provided classifications of aortoiliac and femoropopliteal disease and strategies for their treatment. (Tables 63-7 and 63-8). TASC II recommendations state the following[8]:

> Endovascular therapy is the treatment of choice for type A lesions and surgery is the treatment of choice for type D lesions. Endovascular treatment is the preferred treatment for type B lesions and surgery is the preferred treatment for good-risk patients with type C lesions. The patient's comorbidities, fully informed patient preference, and the local operator's long-term success rates must be considered when making treatment recommendations for type B and type C lesions.

Arguably, as long as endovascular intervention does not negatively affect a patient's option to have an open surgery in the event of restenosis or reocclusion, endovascular intervention can be attempted for even complex lesions.

### Open Surgical Management

***Aortoiliac Disease*** Most patients with aortoiliac occlusive disease are treated with endovascular management. When the extent of disease or involvement of the common femoral arteries necessitates an open approach, patients typically undergo aortobifemoral bypass with a prosthetic graft via the transabdominal or retroperitoneal approach (Fig. 63-19). Preoperative imaging should delineate the target vessels, usually the common femoral or profunda femoris arteries. Proximal anastomoses can be performed in end-to-end or end-to-side configuration. For patients with occlusive disease, the end-to-side configuration is more commonly used because it may preserve perfusion to the pelvis via the diseased but patent iliacs and lumbar collaterals. Arguments for end-to-end anastomosis include improved flow dynamics and the potential for decreased friction between the overlying bowel and graft. In the past, it was common practice to cut the body of the graft to leave minimal redundancy; however, it has become more popular to leave a longer segment of graft, body and limbs, to increase the ease of endovascular approaches in the future. Minimal dissection in the area of the left common iliac artery is performed to protect the nervi erigentes and avoid the complication of retrograde ejaculation. It is usual practice to close the retroperitoneum over the graft to protect it from friction from the overlying bowel.

Alternative inflow sources include the thoracic aorta, axillary artery, and contralateral femoral artery if disease is unilateral.

***Lower Extremity Occlusive Disease*** Patients with significant lesions involving the common femoral artery and origin of the profunda artery are usually best served with open groin exploration, common femoral artery endarterectomy, and profundaplasty or ileofemoral bypass. If concomitant iliac artery or superficial femoral artery (SFA) disease is present, patients may undergo combination procedures with iliac stent placement via open femoral access and/or SFA revascularization by femoropopliteal bypass or SFA stenting.

All bypass procedures are performed with the patient under general, spinal, or epidural anesthesia. A radial arterial catheter is generally used for continuous arterial blood pressure monitoring. All patients receive prophylactic antibiotic treatment.

Vascular control is achieved with minimal force or traction. Heparin, 100 to 150 U/kg, is given for anticoagulation during periods of vascular occlusion. Anastomoses are constructed with care using small, evenly placed bites to include all layers of the vessel wall. Intraoperative completion arteriography is performed in all small, distal tibial vessel bypasses, as well as larger arterial bypasses, such as femoropopliteal bypass, to assess technical adequacy and outflow. The anastomoses, graft, and runoff vessels are carefully examined in multiple planes and any defects corrected prior to closure.

**Conduits.** The two main graft types used for lower extremity bypasses are the great saphenous veins and polytetrafluoroethylene (PTFE) grafts. The greater saphenous veins should be used preferentially in all bypasses, especially in those reconstructions using below-knee popliteal and small tibial arteries as the distal

**Table 63-7 TransAtlantic Inter-Society Consensus (TASC) Classification of Aortoiliac Lesions**

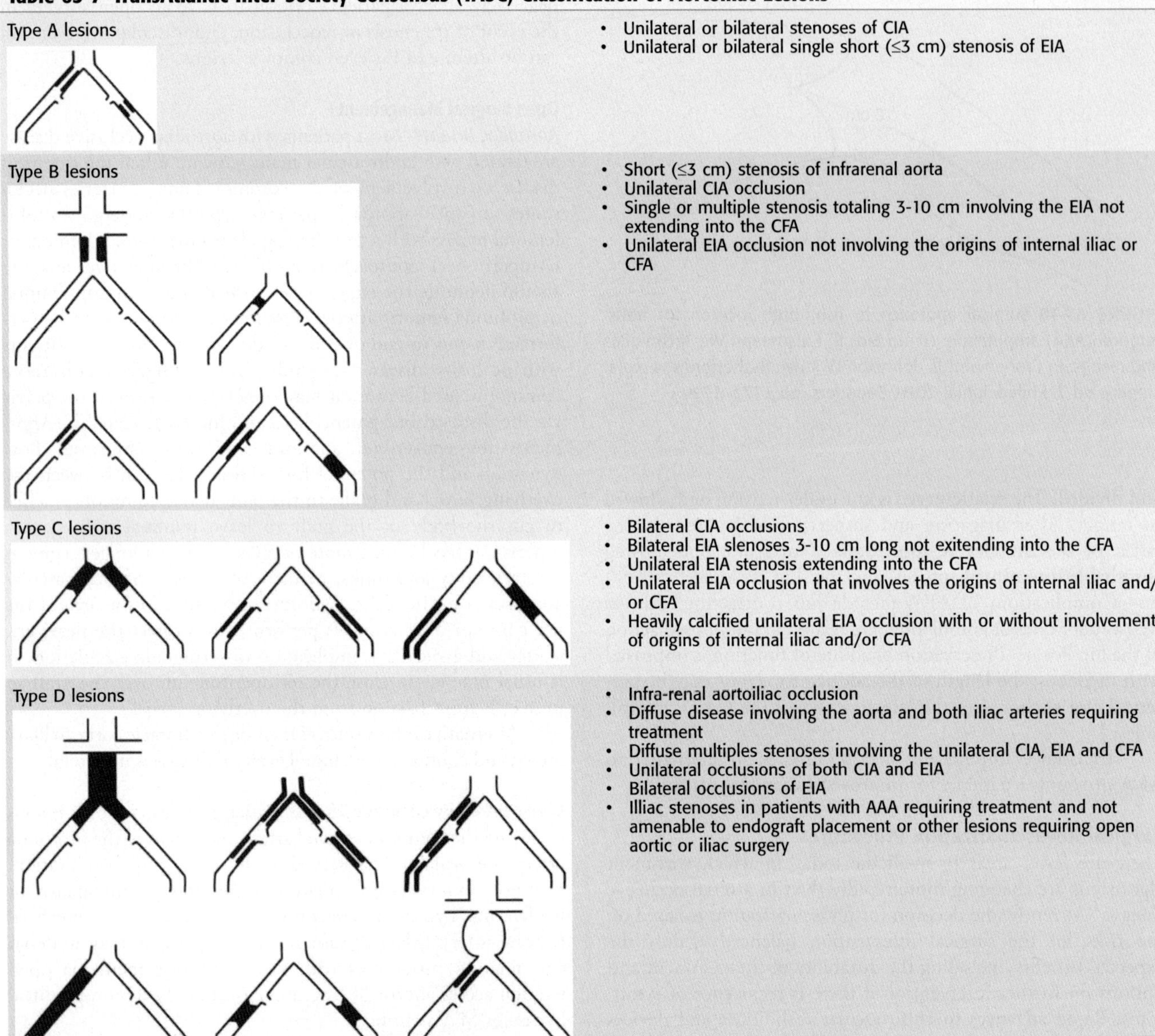

| | |
| --- | --- |
| Type A lesions | • Unilateral or bilateral stenoses of CIA<br>• Unilateral or bilateral single short (≤3 cm) stenosis of EIA |
| Type B lesions | • Short (≤3 cm) stenosis of infrarenal aorta<br>• Unilateral CIA occlusion<br>• Single or multiple stenosis totaling 3-10 cm involving the EIA not extending into the CFA<br>• Unilateral EIA occlusion not involving the origins of internal iliac or CFA |
| Type C lesions | • Bilateral CIA occlusions<br>• Bilateral EIA slenoses 3-10 cm long not exitending into the CFA<br>• Unilateral EIA stenosis extending into the CFA<br>• Unilateral EIA occlusion that involves the origins of internal iliac and/or CFA<br>• Heavily calcified unilateral EIA occlusion with or without involvement of origins of internal iliac and/or CFA |
| Type D lesions | • Infra-renal aortoiliac occlusion<br>• Diffuse disease involving the aorta and both iliac arteries requiring treatment<br>• Diffuse multiples stenoses involving the unilateral CIA, EIA and CFA<br>• Unilateral occlusions of both CIA and EIA<br>• Bilateral occlusions of EIA<br>• Illiac stenoses in patients with AAA requiring treatment and not amenable to endograft placement or other lesions requiring open aortic or iliac surgery |

From Norgren L, Hiatt WR, Dormandy JA, et al: Inter-Society Consensus for the Management of Peripheral Arterial Disease (TASC II). J Vasc Surg 45 (Suppl S):S5–S67, 2007.
*AAA,* Abdominal aortic aneurysm; *CFA,* common femoral artery; *CIA,* common iliac artery; *EIA,* external iliac artery.

target vessels. PTFE grafts can be used for bypasses to above-knee popliteal arterial segments with satisfactory patency rates.

To date, the disappointing patency rates for prosthetic grafts in below-knee and tibial bypasses have discouraged their use. Recently, a new PTFE graft with heparin coating on the luminal surface has been shown to be more resistant to thrombosis. Although these grafts may have an advantage over non–heparin-coated grafts, an adequately sized (4 mm or larger) saphenous vein remains preferable to synthetic conduits because of its innate antithrombotic properties.

The great saphenous vein can be placed in situ or reversed because of the presence of valves. The advantage of the reversed saphenous vein graft is that the valves do not need to be rendered incompetent with the use of a valvulotome. For the in situ vein graft, there is better size match—larger thigh vein for the common femoral artery and smaller leg vein for the tibial artery. Neither of these configurations has been shown to be superior and surgeons use both, depending on their personal preference.

In the absence of a usable great saphenous vein, the cephalic and basilic veins from the upper extremities, as well as the small saphenous vein of the leg, should be evaluated. However, these veins have thinner walls and may have diseased segments that appear normal on external inspection. Furthermore, when several veins are joined to form a composite graft to achieve adequate length, there is the potential for technical complications and reduced overall patency. There is some evidence that the use of a vein patch with a prosthetic femorodistal bypass

**Table 63-8 TransAtlantic Inter-Society Consensus (TASC) Classification of Femoropopliteal Lesions**

| Lesion type | Criteria |
|---|---|
| Type A lesions 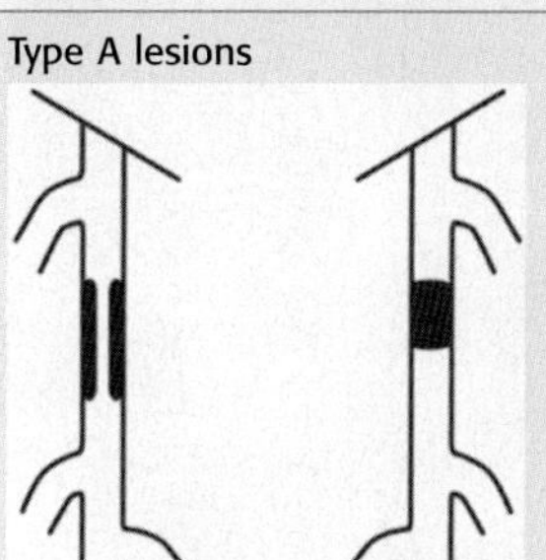 | • Single stenosis ≤10 cm in length<br>• Single occlusion ≤5 cm in length |
| 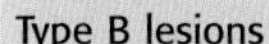 Type B lesions 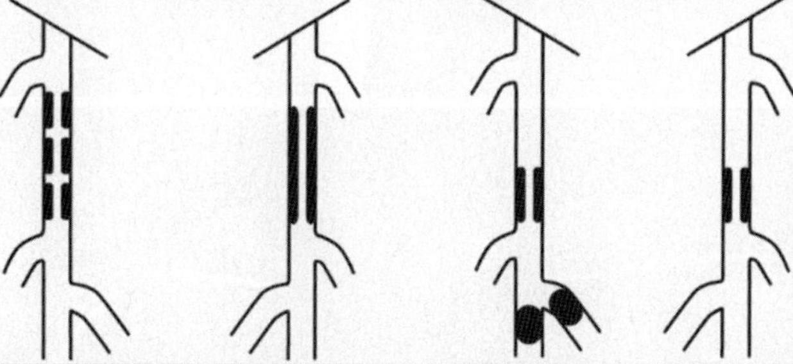 | • Multiple lesions (stenoses or occlusions), each ≤5 cm<br>• Single stenosis or occlusion ≤15 cm not involving the intra geniculate popliteal artery<br>• Single or multiple lesions in the absence of continuous tibial vessels to improve inflow for a distal bypass<br>• Heavily calcified occlusion ≤5 cm in length<br>• Single popliteal stenosis |
| Type C lesions 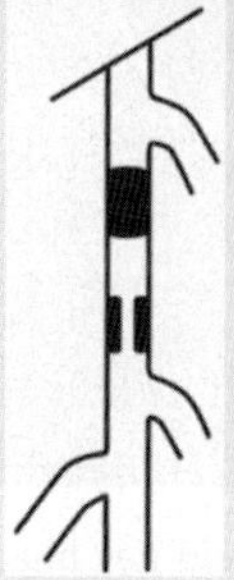 | • Multiple stenoses or occlusions totaling >15 cm with or without heavy calcification<br>• Recurrent stenoses or occlusions that need treatment after two endovascular interventions |
| 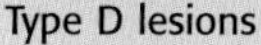 Type D lesions 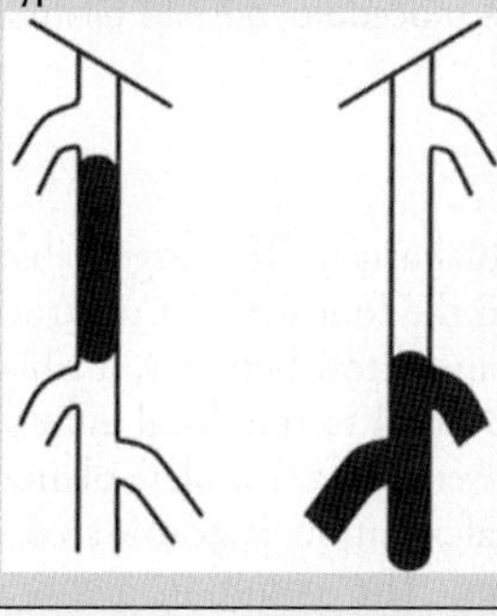 | • Chronic total occlusions of CFA or SFA (>20 cm, involving the popliteal artery)<br>• Chronic total occlusions of popliteal artery and proximal bifurcation vessels |

From Norgren L, Hiatt WR, Dormandy JA, et al: Inter-Society Consensus for the Management of Peripheral Arterial Disease (TASC II). J Vasc Surg 45 (Suppl S):S5–S67, 2007.
*CFA,* Common femoral artery; *SFA,* superficial femoral artery.

improves patency. Other conduits include cryopreserved arteries and veins, which have been shown to be more resistant to infection in the setting of gross infection.

For endarterectomy patch angioplasty, there are prosthetic patches of PTFE or Dacron. Bovine pericardial patches are also available. Alternatively, an endarterectomized segment of the native occluded SFA can be used for common femoral or profunda artery patch angioplasty, or as a short-segment bypass conduit.

**Femoropopliteal Bypass.** The femoropopliteal bypass is used in patients with superficial femoral and popliteal arterial occlusion with a popliteal artery segment distal to the occlusion that is patent, with luminal continuity with any tibial arterial branches.

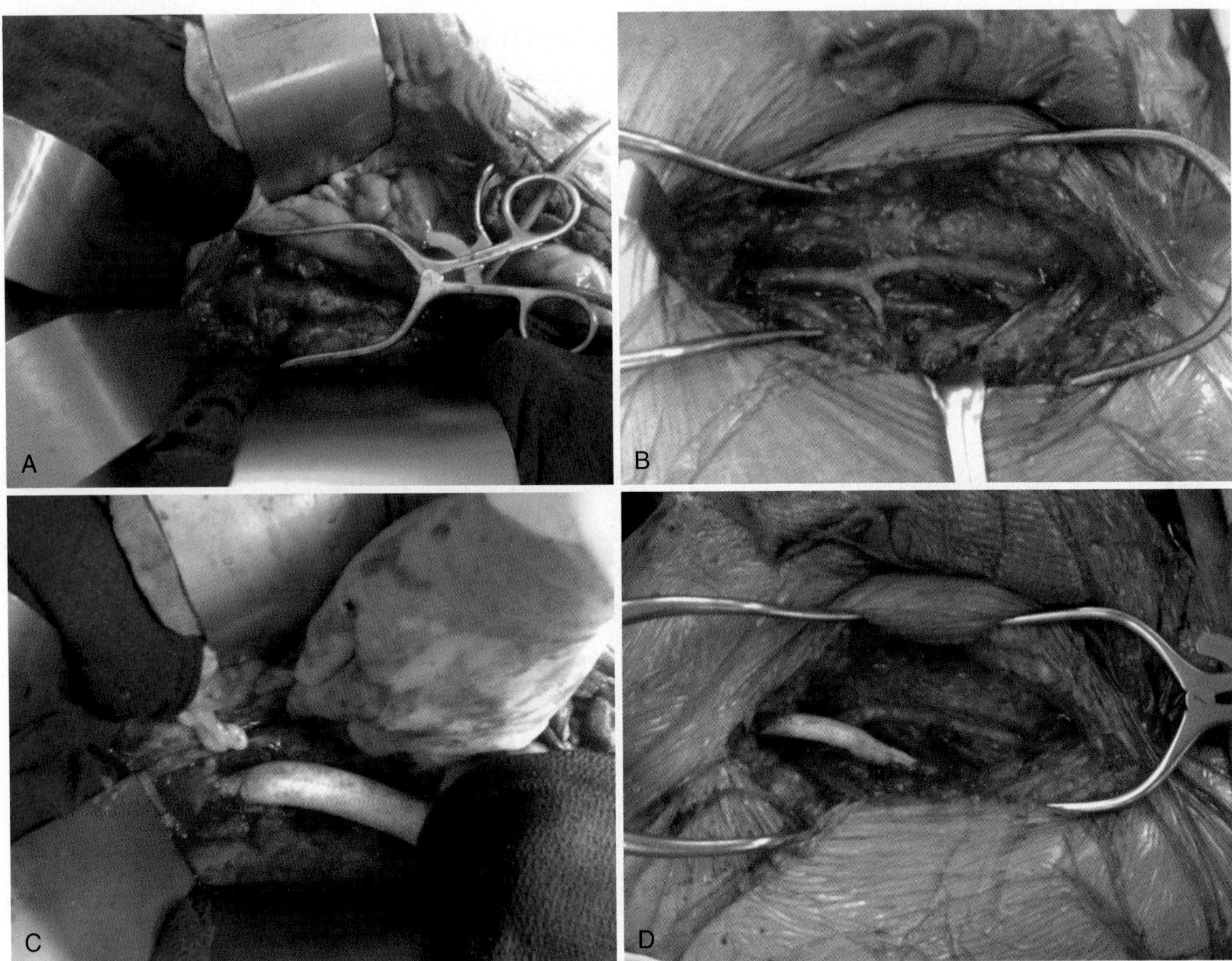


**FIGURE 63-19** The patient from Figure 63-7 underwent aortobifemoral bypass. **A,** Note bilateral renal arteries. The left renal vein has been divided. **B,** Exposure of the right common femoral, profunda, and superficial femoral arteries. **C,** End-to-side aortic anastamosis using PTFE bifurcated graft. **D,** End-to-side profunda anastamosis. The patient had palpable distal pulses at the close of the procedure, despite bilateral SFA occlusions, caused by long-term occlusion and excellent collateral flow.

Bypasses can be performed even if one or more of the tibial arteries is occluded in the leg.

A longitudinal groin incision is used to access the common femoral artery. The popliteal artery is exposed medially from the thigh or the leg. In above-knee popliteal bypasses, an incision is made proximal to the knee for exposure of the artery near the adductor hiatus, or Hunter's, canal, distal to the occlusive disease. In below-knee popliteal bypass, the popliteal space is accessed. The more superficial popliteal vein is retracted with a Silastic loop to assist with dissection of the underlying popliteal artery. If the saphenous vein is to be used, skin incisions are placed directly over the vein. A single long or multiple smaller skip incisions can be used. Alternatively, endoscopic vein harvesting can be performed. The graft is tunneled and placed in the anatomic space, under the sartorius muscle, unless an in situ saphenous vein graft is used.

INFRAPOPLITEAL BYPASS. The infrapopliteal bypass is used for arteries beyond the popliteal artery when there is arterial disease that involves the popliteal or proximal tibial artery. The target tibial artery will have luminal continuity to the foot without obstruction. With femoropopliteal and infrapopliteal bypasses, a tibial artery with stenosis of less than 50% distal to the distal anastomosis is acceptable, and neither the absence of a complete plantar arch nor the presence of vascular calcification is considered a contraindication to revascularization. The common femoral artery is generally used as the inflow for these bypasses. Shorter bypasses are preferred because of improved patency, so the SFA or popliteal artery may provide inflow if there is no proximal arterial disease. Bypasses to the arteries near the ankle or the foot can be performed if there is no patent artery more proximally.

Exposure of the posterior tibial artery is via a medial calf incision. The soleus muscle attachments to the tibia are taken down to expose the posterior tibial artery. Division of the overlying tibial veins exposes the tibial peroneal trunk. Further separation of the soleus muscle from the tibia provides access to terminal branches, the peroneal and posterior tibial arteries. For bypass to the anterior tibial artery, an additional anterolateral

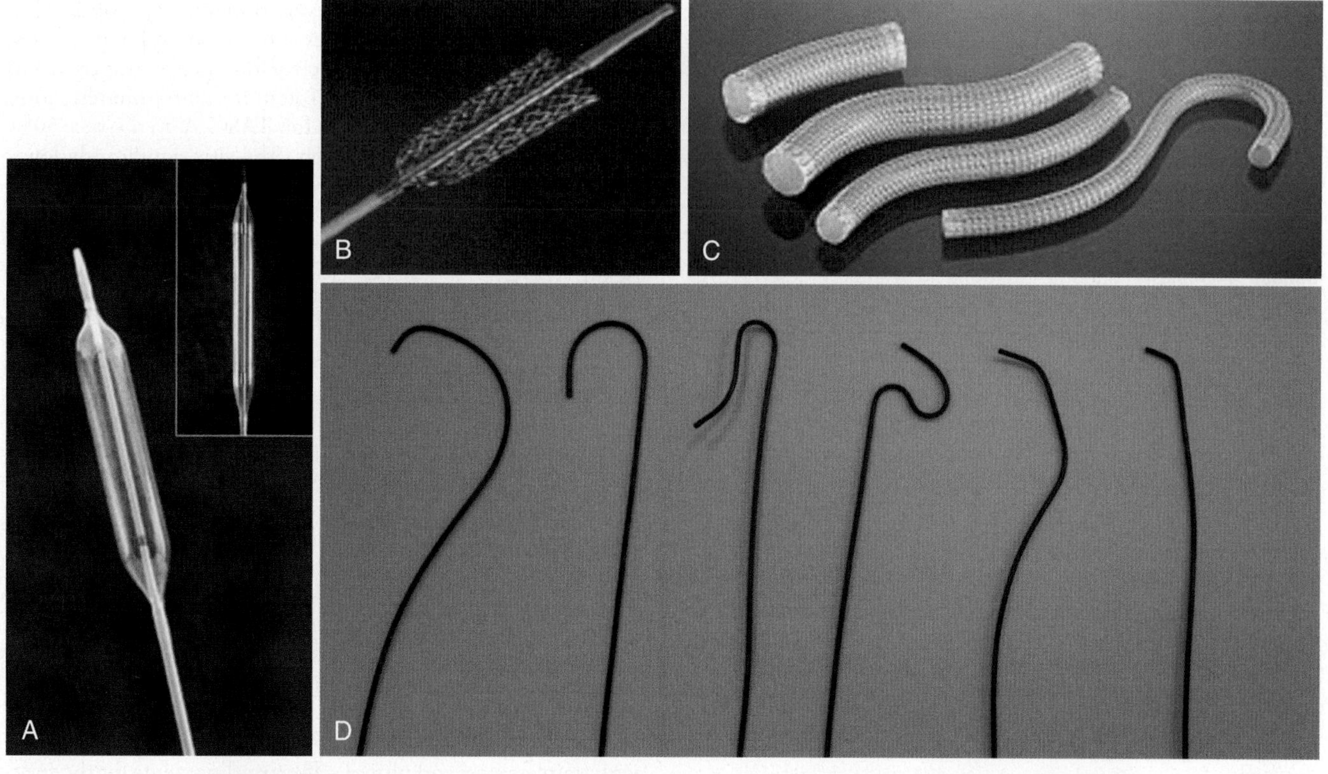


**FIGURE 63-20** Clockwise from left: balloon **(A)**; bare metal stent **(B)**; stent graft **(C)**; catheters **(D)**.

incision in the leg is made, midway between the tibia and fibula. Separation of the anterior tibial muscle and the extensor longus muscle exposes the neurovascular bundle. Further posterior dissection allows access to the interosseous membrane, and an incision is made to allow for tunneling of the bypass graft. Exposure of the peroneal artery can be made via a medial incision, laterally by fibulectomy, or posteriorly by mobilization of the Achilles tendon.

**Complications** Complications of surgery include superficial and deep wound infections, including those that involve the graft itself. One of the dreaded complications of aortic bypass is aortoduodenal fistula, which has high mortality rates. The treatment is extra-anatomic bypass and graft removal, with débridement of the retroperitoneal tissues. Alternatives to extra-anatomic bypass grafting are in situ bypass using bilateral superficial femoral veins, cryopreserved aortoiliac arteries, or antibiotic-soaked Decron graft as conduit. In case of severe sepsis, an endograft system can be placed as a temporizing measure, with endograft and graft explantation when the patient is more stable. Other complications include groin hematoma, lymphatic leak or lymphocele, femoral nerve entrapment, limb swelling, and knee contracture.

## Endovascular Management

Endovascular techniques require familiarity with a variety of devices such as wires of varying lengths, thicknesses, and flexibility with hydrophobic or hydrophilic coatings, catheters with differing curves to negotiate angles with varying degrees of flexibility, sheaths to provide scaffolding support, balloons to dilate lesions, and bare metal and covered stents to provide continuous outward radial force, prevent arterial recoil, and manage occlusive disease or dissections (Fig. 63-20).

There are a multitude of endovascular devices and techniques available to the surgeon to treat PAD and aneurysmal disease but little consensus about the best choice. The following are all viable alternatives to reestablish continuity of blood flow; each method has its enthusiastic proponents.

**Subintimal Angioplasty** First described in 1987,[19,20] the subintimal angioplasty technique involves use of a wire to create an arterial dissection purposely, beginning at the proximal segment of the arterial occlusion. Using this plane, a chronic total occlusion (CTO) can be circumvented. Once the wire has passed beyond the lesion, it reenters the true arterial lumen. The false lumen is treated with balloon angioplasty to increase its diameter. Although technical success rates have been favorable, long-term patency and limb salvage rates have not been impressive. Even in more recent reviews, the same pattern of results prevails. In a review of 472 patients treated for principally TASC C and D lesions, 63% of patients presented with critical limb ischemia and the remaining with disabling claudication.[21] Stenotic lesions were not included. Technical success was 87%, with 73% of failures caused by an inability to reenter the true lumen. The median follow-up was 12.4 months (range, 0 to 48 months). The mean increase in ABI was 0.27, from 0.50 ± 0.16 to 0.77 ± 0.23. The primary patency rates were disappointing 45%, 30%, and 25% at 12, 24, and 36 months, respectively. Patency was higher in limbs treated for claudication, whereas reduced patency was significantly associated with femorotibial occlusions and critical limb ischemia. At 3 years, primary patency was 30% for claudication and 21% for critical limb ischemia. Bare metal stents were used in 20.3% of successful cases, but stent use was not associated with improved patency. Limb salvage for CLI was a respectable 88% at 12 months, 81% at 24 months, and 75% at 36 months. Claudication was improved in 96.8% of limbs and sustained in 67% at 36 months. Overall, the results of subintimal angioplasty as a stand-alone procedure for critical limb ischemia have been underwhelming; adjuncts such as stents and stent grafts often are used to increase patency.

**Balloon Angioplasty** Balloon angioplasty, originally described in 1974, first requires crossing the arterial lesion transluminally with a guidewire and then inflating a balloon advanced over the wire at the location of the lesion. The treatment is considered successful if the residual stenosis is less than 30% or there is no pressure gradient across the area treated.

Clark and colleagues[22] have reported a multicenter experience with angioplasty in the STAR registry. The authors evaluated angioplasty of femoropopliteal lesions in 219 limbs of 205 patients. Patients were followed prospectively with clinical outcomes as well as objective testing using angiography and/or duplex ultrasound. The primary patencies at 12, 24, and 36 months for all limbs were 87%, 80%, and 69%, respectively. At 48 and 60 months, it was 55%. A negative predictor of long-term patency was found to be poor tibial runoff, specifically single tibial vessel runoff with 50% to 99% stenosis or occlusion. Diabetes or renal failure was also associated with lower patency.

Dorros and associates[23] have studied the feasibility of angioplasty in tibioperoneal vessels in a nonrandomized series of 312 patients with 417 vessels and 657 lesions. Overall technical success was 92% (98% in stenotic and 77% in occlusive lesions); 13 patients required stenting for intimal flap or dissection refractory to prolonged inflation. Success was higher in patients with claudication. More specifically, claudication was relieved in 98% of patients with stenoses and in 86% presenting with occlusions. Resolution of critical limb ischemia was noted in 98% when stenotic lesions were treated and in 77% of patients with occlusions.

In a subsequent report, the same authors evaluated their 5-year experience for the same patients, but focused on those with critical limb ischemia.[24] There were 284 limbs in 235 patients with 529 lesions in the tibioperoneal vessels; 167 (59%) limbs required concomitant dilation of the inflow lesions to access the distal vessels. Follow-up was obtained in 215 (97%) of successfully treated patients; 8% of the limbs required bypass surgery and 9% required amputation, yielding an overall limb salvage rate of 91% at 5 years. As expected, Fontaine class III patients had significantly less bypass surgeries and amputations compared with class IV patients.

Giles and coworkers[25] have reported similar results in a recent series of infrapopliteal lesions causing critical limb ischemia. In their series of 176 limbs in 163 patients, 76% of patients presented with tissue loss and 15% had rest pain. All lesions were evenly distributed in the four TASC classes. The technical success was 93%, with 58% requiring concomitant dilation of the femoropopliteal lesions and 8% requiring adjunctive stenting, usually for residual stenosis. Similar to the results described earlier, the success rate was higher for less severe lesions (100% for TASC A to C; 75% for TASC D; $P < .0001$). Dorros and colleagues,[23] however, did not describe their lesions using the TASC classification. Follow-up was performed at 2 weeks, every 3 months for 1 year, and every 6 months thereafter. Measurement of patency used duplex ultrasound and angiography, when indicated, and followed Society for Vascular Surgery (SVS) standard criteria for patency. At 1 year, freedom from restenosis, re-intervention, or amputation for TASC A to D was 50%, 39%, 53%, and 14%, respectively. This was significantly lower for TASC D lesions and was predicted by univariate and multivariate analyses to have a lower rate. Primary patency at 1 year for TASC A to D was 53%, 58%, 67%, and 37%, respectively. Again, TASC D was a predictor of lower rate by multivariate analysis. Limb salvage at 1 year was 84%, with TASC D lesion as a predictor for limb loss.

Kudo and associates[26] have published a 10-year experience of angioplasty for critical limb ischemia. There were 138 limbs in 111 patients, and the most distal lesions treated were 33% in the iliac, 30% in the femoropopliteal, and 37% in the below-knee group. of these lesions, 91% were TASC C and D. Reporting standards followed SVS criteria. Follow-up intervals and the studies used were similar to the report by Giles and coworkers.[25] Using Kaplan-Meier analysis, the primary patency and limb salvage rates for the femoropopliteal and below-knee groups at 3 years were 59.4% and 92.7% and 23.5% and 77.3%, respectively. Significant independent risk factors for outcomes included multiple segment, more distal, and TASC D lesions.

**Stenting** Sabeti and colleagues[27,28] have reported their experience with stainless steel and nitinol self-expanding stents for the treatment of femoropopliteal diseases in a retrospectively reviewed nonrandomized study. In their studies, 175 consecutive patients presented with claudication (150 patients) and critical limb ischemia (25 patients). Stents were placed electively following balloon angioplasty failure caused by residual stenosis or flow-limiting dissection. This resulted in 123 patients receiving stainless steel stents and 52 receiving nitinol stents. The choice of stents was at the discretion of the interventionist. The length of the lesions treated ranged from 5 to 6 cm. Duplex ultrasound with angiographic confirmation was used for follow-up. The cumulative patency rates at 6, 12, and 24 months were 85%, 75%, and 69%, respectively, for nitinol stenting versus 78%, 54%, and 34%, respectively, for stainless steel stenting. The authors noted significantly improved primary patency rates for nitinol stents.

The same authors also reported their early experience with long lesions, at least 10 cm, in the femoropopliteal segment. Only nitinol stents were used and placed after primary failure of balloon angioplasty, as described earlier. The median length of the stented segments was 16 cm. The median follow-up was 8 months, with in-stent restenosis noted in 40% of patients. The overall cumulative freedom from restenosis at 6 and 12 months was 79% and 54%, respectively. This was not affected by stent length or the number of stents used. However, patency was decreased in diabetics.

They later randomly assigned 104 patients with stenotic or occlusive SFA lesions to undergo primary stenting (51 patients) or angioplasty (53 patients), with optional stenting (32% receiving stents).[29,30] The mean length of the lesions was 13.2 cm for the stent group and 12.7 cm for the angioplasty group. At 6 months, the rate of restenosis was 24% in the stent group and 43% in the angioplasty group. At 12 months, the rates were 37% and 63%, respectively. These results were sustained at 2 years. In a subsequent report of the same patient group, the authors noted a restenosis rate of 45.7% for the stent group versus 69.2% for the angioplasty group. During this period, re-intervention was also lower in the primary stenting group (37% versus 53.8%).

Vogel and associates[31] have also reported their results of primary stenting. There were 41 patients with femoropopliteal disease; 37 had TASC B lesions and 4 had TASC D lesions. The mean lesion length was 6.69 cm. Primary patency rates using Kaplan-Meier analysis at 6 months, 1-year, and 2-year were 95%, 84%, and 84%, respectively. The limb salvage rate during a similar period was 92%, 89%, and 89%, respectively. The lesions treated in this study were shorter than those reported by Sabeti and coworkers.[27,28]

Midterm results were reported by Mewissen.[32] There were 122 patients with femoropopliteal lesions in 137 limbs. Of these, 125 limbs presented with TASC B and C.[33] Primary patency rates at 6, 12, 18, and 24 months were 92%, 76%, 66%, and 60%, respectively.

Ferreira and colleagues[34] have noted similar favorable results in a long-term study of long femoropopliteal lesions. In this report of 59 patients with 74 lesions, there were 16% lesions in TASC C and 61% in TASC D. The mean lesion length was 19 cm; the mean follow-up was 2.4 years. The primary patency rates estimated by Kaplan-Meier at 1, 2, 3, 4, and 4.8 years were 90%, 78%, 74%, 69%, and 69%, respectively. In another recent study, Baril and associates[33] also noted the sustained results of using a nitinol stent. The study retrospectively reviewed 125 patients with 108 TASC B and 32 TASC C lesions. The mean follow-up period was 12.7 months; 41 limbs experienced restenosis or occlusion at 8 months. Freedom from restenosis or occlusion at 12 months for the entire cohort was 58.9% and 47.9% at 24 months. There was no difference between TASC B and C lesions.

With advances in technology, angioplasty and stenting of infrapopliteal lesions are gaining acceptance. Kickuth and coworkers[35] have recently reported their initial experience with a low-profile, self-expanding nitinol stent. They treated 35 patients, 19 with lifestyle-limiting claudication and 16 with critical limb ischemia. Selective stenting was performed after failed balloon angioplasty caused by residual stenosis, elastic recoil, or flow-limiting dissections. Stent placement was performed in 22 patients with distal popliteal artery lesions and in 13 with tibioperoneal artery lesions. Technical success was achieved in all patients. Follow-up studies were performed with duplex ultrasound and angiography. The 6-month primary patency rate was 82%. The authors noted the feasibility of treating infrapopliteal lesions with the new nitinol stent.

A recent meta-analysis was reported by Mwipatayi and colleagues[36] comparing balloon angioplasty with stenting for the treatment of femoropopliteal lesions. A systemic review of the literature was performed on reports published between September 2000 and January 2007. The search included studies that reported long-term results of at least 1 year. Seven randomized controlled trials (RCTs) comparing angioplasty with stenting were used for this meta-analysis, a total of 934 patients; 482 patients were treated with stenting and the rest (452) with balloon angioplasty. For the stent group, the 1-year primary patency rates varied from 63% to 90% and 2-year primary patency ranged from 46% to 87%. In the angioplasty group, the maximal vessel length treated was 30.2 cm with a mean of 4.3 cm. In the stent group, the maximal length was 32 cm with a mean of 4.6 cm. The use of stents did not improve the patency rate at 1 year. However, limitations include length of follow-up, various stents used, and inconsistent use of optimal medical therapy.

Ihnat and associates[37] have recently evaluated the effect of lesion severity on patency after stenting of femoropopliteal segment. There were 95 patients treated (109 limbs); 71 patients (65%) were treated for claudication and 38 (35%) for CLI. The average lesion length was 15.7 cm. The type of lesions according to TASC classification was 39% A, 14% B, 29% C, and 18% D. The average runoff score was 4.6. The overall 36-month primary patency rate was 52%. The rate of limb salvage was 75% in patients with CLI. Decreased patency rates were noted in TASC D lesions and limbs with poor initial runoff score.

**Stent Graft** One of the most widely used stent grafts (Fig. 63-21) in the treatment of chronic lower extremity ischemia is the Viabahn endoprosthesis (Gore Medical, Flagstaff, Ariz). It is constructed with an expanded polytetrafluoroethylene (ePTFE) liner attached to an external nitinol stent. The inner surface is bonded with heparin. This stent graft is extremity flexible, allowing it to conform closely to the anatomy of the SFA.

Railo and coworkers[38] first reported preliminary results in 15 patients with femoropopliteal lesions. The clinical presentation varied from claudication to acute leg ischemia, as well as one ruptured popliteal artery aneurysm. Primary patency rates at 1, 12, and 24 months were 100%, 93%, and 84%, respectively. There was no limb loss during the follow-up period.

Jahnke and colleagues[39] have reported their midterm experience in 52 patients with medium- or long-segment occlusions and stenoses of the femoropopliteal artery. The technical success was 100%; the mean length of the covered segments was 10.9 cm ± 5.13. There was initial hemodynamic improvement, with the ABI increasing from 0.54 ± 0.12 to 0.89 ± 0.14. The mean follow-up duration was 23.8 months. Patients were followed with DU and the primary patency rates at 12 and 24 months were 78.4% and 74.1%, respectively. The length of implanted stent graft did not affect the primary patency rates.

In a 6-year experience, Fischer and associates[40] evaluated outcomes for 57 patients treated for stenoses (13%) or occlusions (87%) of the SFA. The average length of treated lesions was 10.7 cm; 10% suffered early thrombosis of the graft within 30 days. The mean follow-up was 55 months (range, 8 to 78 months). The primary patency rates for 30 days and 1, 3, and 5 years were 90%, 67%, 57%, and 45%, respectively. In an earlier long-term study, Bleyn and coworkers[41] treated 67 patients with a mean lesion length of 14.3 cm. The 5-year primary patency rate was 47%.

The most recent results were reported by Shaikh and colleagues.[42] They reported a series of 81 patients with 98 SFAs using 167 stent grafts; 80% of the interventions were for TASC C and D lesions. The 1-year primary patency was 96%. In their second group, 43 patients were randomized to stent graft or SilverHawk (ev3 Endovascular, Plymouth, Minn) atherectomy interventions; 23 patients were treated with Viabahn in 29 SFAs and 20 patients were treated with atherectomy in 23 SFAs. The technical success rate was 100% in both groups. There were significantly more complications in the atherectomy group (5 patients [21%]) than Viabahn (0 patients). The 1-year primary patency rate was 90% for Viabahn and 57% for SilverHawk atherectomy.

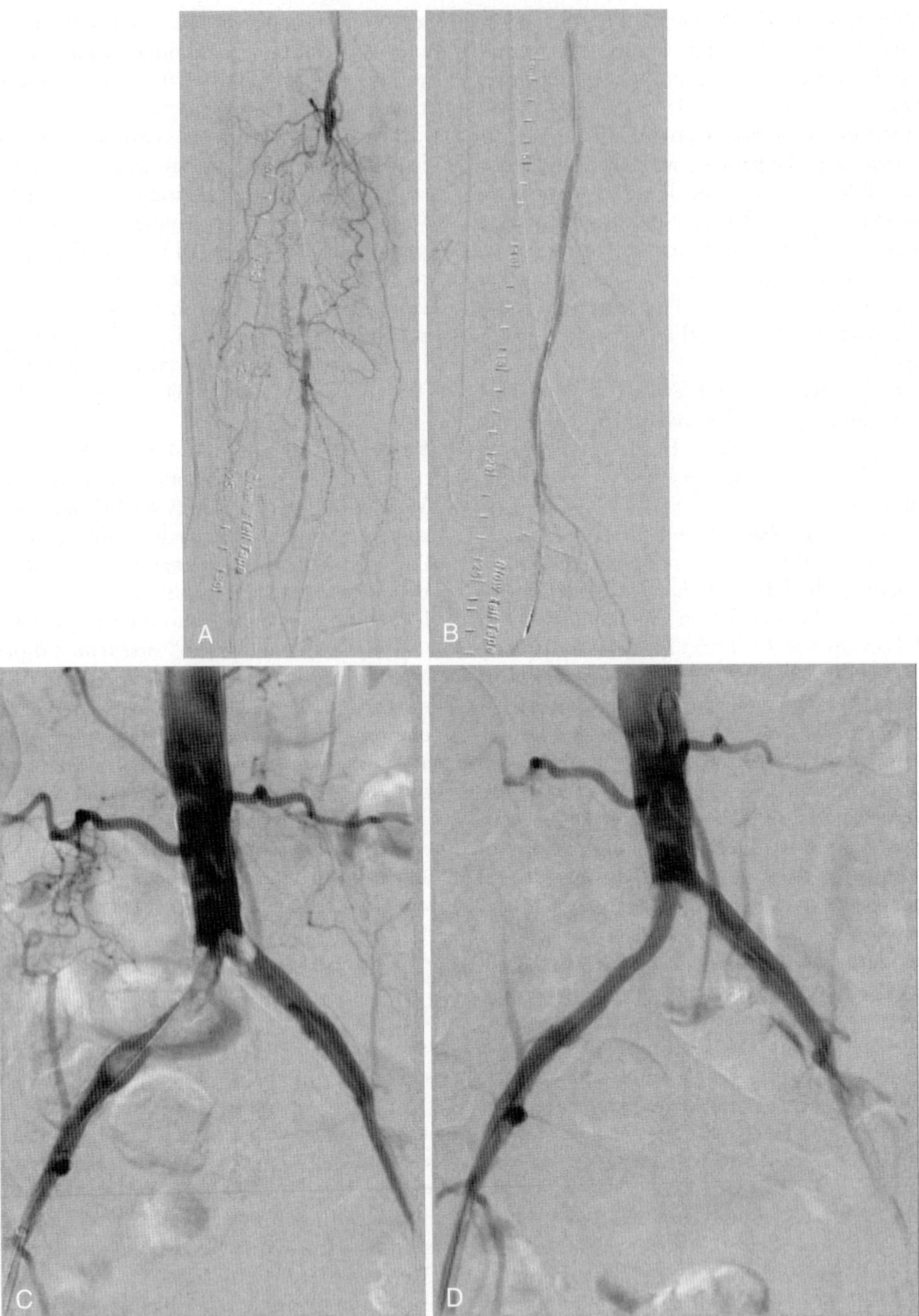

**FIGURE 63-21** **A,** Distal superficial femoral to proximal popliteal artery occlusion. **B,** Completion angiogram following recanalization and stent placement. **C,** Bilateral common iliac artery thrombus, acute. **D,** Successful treatment with stent graft. Flow was restored without distal embolization.

Comparison of Viabahn treatment with different modalities has been reported by others as well. Saxon and associates[43] have compared stent graft with percutaneous transluminal angioplasty (PTA) alone in a multicenter, prospective randomized study. The stent graft group had 97 patients and the PTA had 100. The stent graft group had a significantly higher technical success rate (95% versus 66%; *P* <.0001). Follow-up at 1 year using duplex ultrasound showed that the primary patency rate was 65% for stent graft and 40% for PTA alone. This improvement was noted for lesions at least 3 cm long.

In a prospective randomized study, Kedora and coworkers[44] compared Viabahn with above-knee surgical bypass with synthetic graft material; 86 patients with 100 limbs were randomized to 50 limbs each for the stent graft and bypass. The mean length of artery stented was 25.6 cm. ABIs and DU were used for follow-up at 3, 6, 9, and 12 months. The primary patency at 3, 6, 9, and 12 months were 84%, 82%, 75.6%, and 73.5% for stent grafts, respectively. For bypass, it was 90%, 81.8%, 79.7%, and 74.2%, respectively. The authors also noted similar re-intervention and secondary patency rates.

**Other Variations of Balloon Angioplasty** These include cutting balloon angioplasty and cryoplasty.

***Cutting Balloon*** The cutting balloon was originally designed for use in the coronary artery for lesions resistant to compliant balloon angioplasty or in-stent restenotic lesions. The balloon features three or four atherotomes, or microsurgical blades, mounted longitudinally on the surface of a noncompliant balloon. The blades score the lesion and dilate the vessels with less force than conventional balloon angioplasty.

***Cryoplasty*** The PolarCath Peripheral Dilatation System (Boston Scientific, Natick, Mass) provides mechanical dilation and cryotherapy through the use of nitrous oxide. The gas is used to fill the angioplasty balloon and to cool its surface to −10° C. As the balloon is inflated, it exerts mechanical and biologic effects. The cooling is purported to promote apoptosis, which reduces excess thickening from intimal hyperplasia of smooth muscle cells after angioplasty, and should result in reduced restenosis.

***Atherectomy*** Endovascular atherectomy allows the physical removal of atherosclerotic plaque material from the blood vessel, with a theoretical benefit of removing the obstructing plaque rather than merely displacing it, as with angioplasty and stenting. Excisional atherectomy catheters remove and collect the atheroma, whereas ablative devices fragment the atheroma into small particles. Rotational cutters turn at speeds up to 8000 rpm, shaving the atherosclerotic plaque material from the luminal surface of the arterial wall and collecting it in a storage chamber. Small case series have reported technical success of 87% with the need for adjunct procedures such as balloon angioplasty or stenting in 20% to 63%.[45-47] Postprocedure ABI improved by 0.24 to 0.36. The 1-year patency rates range from 22% to 84% with limb salvage rates of 62% to 86%. Some studies reported decreased patency when the target lesion was restenotic,[46] whereas others did not.[45] Another study reported that treatment of multiple vessels did not influence patency or limb salvage and adjunctive therapy did not improve results.[48]

An example of ablative atherectomy includes the laser atherectomy, a cold-tipped laser that delivers bursts of ultraviolet xenon energy in short pulse durations. Its reported key feature is the ability to debulk tissue without damaging surrounding tissue, minimizing restenosis. When compared with balloon angioplasty alone, no difference was reported in 1-year patency or technical success.[49] The largest trial was the LACI (Laser Angioplasty for Critical Limb Ischemia) phase 2 study that involved 14 sites in the United States and Germany.[50] There were 145 patients with 155 limbs and 423 lesions—41% SFA, 15% popliteal, 41% infrapopliteal, and 70% a combination of stenoses. Technical success was achieved in 86% of limbs, with most lesions in TASC C and D. Limb salvage at 6 months was 93%. Similar results were achieved by a five-center registry in Belgium; Bosiers and colleagues[51] presented outcomes of 48 patients with 51 limbs in Rutherford category 4, 5, or 6 who were poor candidates for bypass surgery. The limb salvage at 6 months was 90.5%.

### Acute Limb Ischemia

A popular pneumonic for describing the presentation of an acutely ischemic leg is referred to as the five(or six) Ps, depending on one's willingness to include ***p***oikilothermia. ***P***ain, ***p***allor, ***p***ulselessness, ***p***aresthesias, and ***p***aralysis are often cited as indicative of acute arterial ischemia. These symptoms and findings, however, are often variable in degree and not necessarily predictive of the extent of disease or degree of ischemia. A similar presentation may be seen in the setting of blunt or penetrating trauma, in which the native, nondiseased blood supply is suddenly interrupted. It is the acuity of the insult that leads to this constellation of symptoms; the chronically ischemic limb may have become so over a duration of time that allowed collateral flow to develop. The patient with acute ischemia may have less developed collateral circulation and less tolerance to prolonged ischemia.

The cause of acute limb ischemia is usually thromboembolism in the intervention-naïve patient. The source of the embolism can be the heart, in which case atrial fibrillation is a commonly observed comorbidity. Alternative embolic sources include the valvular leaflets, and the aorta and iliac arteries may house thrombus, with or without concurrent aneurysmal disease. Patients presenting with a surgical history of previous bypass or stent placement may have an acute occlusion from graft or stent failure, or may have disease progression. This history and the location of the occlusive lesion will affect surgical decision making. Acute limb ischemia constitutes a surgical emergency. As in most cases of vascular disease, there are endovascular and open surgical methods for addressing the problem.

As in all cases, a detailed history and physical examination are needed for a clinical diagnosis of the severity of disease:

- Category I limbs are viable and not immediately threatened.
- Category IIa limbs are threatened but salvageable if treated.
- Category IIb limbs are salvageable if treated as an emergency.
- Category III limbs have irreversible ischemia and are not salvageable.

Therefore, patients whose limbs are viable and do not appear immediately threatened (category I), as well as those threatened but salvageable without paralysis, but with mild sensory changes (category IIa), are potential candidates for thrombolytic therapy. Patients with threatened limbs with more significant neurologic changes (category IIb) require a more urgent intervention and may best be served with an operative intervention. Patients with irreversible ischemia and a nonsalvageable limb usually require primary amputation (Fig. 63-22).

Patients with viable or minimally threatened limbs are candidates for thrombolytic therapy. They must have no contraindication to thrombolysis, which would include an active bleeding diathesis, recent gastrointestinal bleeding (less than 10 days), intracranial or spinal surgery, or intracranial trauma within the previous 3 months. Also, patients with a recent cerebral vascular accident, within 2 months, represent an absolute contraindication to thrombolysis. Relative major contraindications include major nonvascular surgery or trauma within the previous 10 days, uncontrolled hypertension, puncture of noncompressible vessels, intracranial tumors, and recent eye surgery. Minor contraindications to thrombolysis include hepatic failure, bacterial endocarditis, pregnancy, and diabetic hemorrhagic retinopathy.

An alternative to thrombolysis is open thrombectomy. Patients are begun on heparin on presentation. Proximal and distal control on the femoral versus below-knee popliteal artery

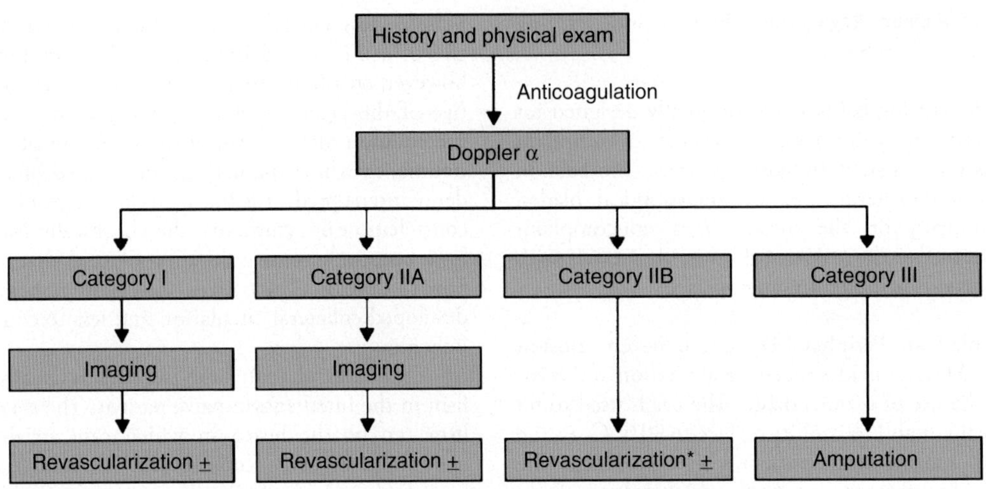


**FIGURE 63-22** Algorithm for the treatment of acute limb ischemia.

is obtained. A longitudinal arteriotomy is created and the thrombectomy balloon is passed proximally and distally with care until excellent forward bleeding and reasonable back bleeding are seen. Fluoroscopy can be used to assist in the thrombectomy procedure, with contrast used in the embolectomy balloon and within the artery. Once the clot is successfully removed, the artery is flushed proximally and distally with heparinized saline before replacing the clamps. Patch angioplasty should be considered to avoid narrowing the artery. Completion angiography is helpful for confirming removal of most of the thrombus and identifying a culprit lesion. Four-compartment fasciotomy may be necessary, depending on the duration of ischemic insult.

Complications of open thrombectomy include intimal damage and dissection. Complications of thrombolysis include bleeding, which in minor cases is from the arterial access, venipuncture site(s), or Foley catheter, but can be severe and lead to hemothorax, gastrointestinal bleeding, and symptomatic intracranial hemorrhage.

If no culprit lesion is found, the patient should undergo a hypercoagulable workup. Oral anticoagulation should be considered.

## OTHER CAUSES OF ACUTE AND CHRONIC LIMB ISCHEMIA

### Nonatherosclerotic Arteriopathies

Other causes of arterial occlusive disease, although far less common than atherosclerosis in the West, should be considered for patients who do not fit the risk factor profile outlined earlier.

Episodic digital ischemia was first described by Maurice Raynaud in 1862. Raynaud's phenomenon is characterized by recurrent episodic vasospasm of the digits precipitated by a stimulus such as environmental cold or emotional stress, manifesting as tricolor changes—white, blue, and red. It initially produces pallor from cold exposure and vasoconstriction, subsequent cyanosis from hypoxia, and then rubor from the hyperemic response associated with rewarming. The digits return to normal 10 to 15 minutes after removal of the stimulus, and the fingers remain normal between ischemic episodes. Fingers of both hands are usually involved, extending to the metacarpophalangeal joint, with sparing of the thumb. The lower extremities are rarely involved. The clinical spectrum is broad, ranging from milder forms managed by avoidance to cold to more severe symptoms of ulceration and tissue loss from vascular occlusions beyond vasospasm. Secondary Raynaud's phenomenon can be associated with various connective tissue diseases such as scleroderma or exposure to drugs, toxins, or repetitive trauma.

The prevalence of Raynaud's syndrome (RS) varies with climate, approaching 20% to 25% in cool damp regions such as Scandinavia and the Pacific Northwest. It usually occurs in young women, with a median age of onset of 14 years, and rarely after the age of 40 years. In these patients, 25% have a family history of RS in a first-degree relative.

The evaluation of patients for RS should include complete blood cell count determination of erythrocyte sedimentation rate, antinuclear antibody titer, and rheumatoid factor. Routine vascular laboratory testing with digital photoplethysmography and digital blood pressures can help distinguish patients with obstructive disease from those with an abnormal vasoconstrictive response. A digital hypothermic cold challenge test has been described, with an overall sensitivity and accuracy of approximately 90%.

The hallmark of conservative treatment is the avoidance of cold and emotional stimuli. All patients with RS should refrain from tobacco use. The most widely used pharmacologic agents are calcium channel blockers. Patients with digital ulcers can usually be healed with aggressive local wound care and débridement. Surgical intervention is reserved for patients with proximal atherosclerotic or aneurysmal disease in an effort to eliminate any embolic source or potential physical impediment to perfusion.

### Buerger's Disease

Thromboangiitis obliterans, or Buerger's disease, predominately affects young male smokers in their 30s, presenting with distal limb ischemia and localized digital gangrene. There is an increasing incidence in women that likely parallels changes in smoking patterns. There is an increased incidence in patients of Eastern European or Japanese heritage. Diagnostic hallmarks include age of onset before 45 years, exposure to tobacco, absence of arterial lesions proximal to the knee or elbow, and absence of other atherosclerotic risk factors.

Thromboangiitis obliterans is a polyarteritis nodosa (PAN) vasculitis, with surgical specimens showing involvement of arteries and veins. Occlusive lesions are seen typically in small and medium-sized arteries. It usually occurs in the distal portions of the upper and lower extremities distal to the elbow and knee. Patients frequently have rest pain, ulceration and, often, digital gangrene. Objective confirmation can be obtained with four-limb digital plethysmography, showing obstructive arterial waveforms in all digits. Arteriography typically reveals extensively diseased infrageniculate vessels and diffuse plantar arterial occlusions. The reconstitution of distal arterial segments is provided by tortuous, pathognomonic, corkscrew collaterals.

Treatment requires absolute tobacco cessation, which often results in clinical remission. Finger ulcers can frequently be healed with aggressive local wound care. Up to one third of patients with lower extremity disease will eventually require major amputation. Distal arterial bypass or endovascular intervention should be considered when anatomically feasible for CLI, but the distal to proximal pattern of disease progression often precludes successful surgical revascularization. Currently, there is no effective pharmacologic treatment.

## Vasculitis

The term *vasculitis* refers to a primary inflammatory process involving blood vessels with resultant transmural injury, necrosis, and obstruction or obliteration of the lumen. Vessels of any size and location can be affected. A useful classification system for vasculitis may be based on the size of the vessels involved by the inflammatory process—large-, medium-, or small-vessel vasculitis.

### Large-Vessel Vasculitis

The large vessel vasculitides includes giant cell arteritis (GCA), also referred to as temporal arteritis, and Takayasu's arteritis. Although both vasculitides can affect the aorta and its major branches, GCA primarily involves the extracranial branches of the carotid artery. GCA usually occurs in older patients, whereas Takayasu's arteritis afflicts younger female patients, with a higher prevalence in those of Asian or Eastern European heritage. Both conditions are associated with the development of aneurysms of the thoracic and abdominal aorta and the progression of occlusive disease in the carotid, upper extremity, visceral, and renal arteries.

**Giant Cell Arteritis (Temporal Arteritis)** GCA usually occurs in patients older than 55 years. It is two to three times more common in women than men. The average annual incidence is 18 cases/100,000 in older women. It primarily affects branches of the external carotid artery, although it may involve any large artery of the body. Patients may describe a history of a febrile myalgic process, with aching and stiffness of the hip, back, and shoulders lasting 4 weeks or more. Constitutional symptoms include headaches, malaise, anorexia, and weight loss. A characteristic presentation is severe pain over the temporal artery, with tenderness and nodularity of the artery that is frequently bilateral. Up to 20% of patients may development permanent unilateral blindness, with one third of them progressing to contralateral blindness within an additional week's time.

Treatment should be prompt, consisting of high-dose corticosteroids. Patients suspected of having GCA should undergo temporal artery biopsy prior to the initiation of steroid therapy. Bilateral sequential temporal artery biopsies may be needed. The erythrocyte sedimentation rate is elevated in 75% of patients, although the C-reactive protein level may be a more sensitive indicator.

Early initiation of steroid therapy can result in prevention of blindness and restoration of pulses. Revascularization is rarely needed because of the collateral vessels that develop; it is relatively contraindicated during the acute phase of GCA.

**Takayasu's Disease** Takayasu's disease most commonly occurs in young, Asian female patients ranging in age from 3 to 35 years (85%). Patients present initially with fever, anorexia, and myalgia, followed by a second stage of multiple arterial occlusive symptoms, depending on the location of disease involvement.

The disease frequently affects the aorta, its major branches, and the pulmonary artery. Lesions are usually stenotic, but may also present as aneurysmal degeneration. Four patterns of cardiovascular manifestations have been described. Type I is localized to the arch and the arch vessels. Type II involves the descending thoracic and abdominal aorta. Type III involves the arch vessels and abdominal aorta and its branches. Type IV involves the pulmonary arteries.

Patients are best treated with conservative medical management. Surgical or endovascular intervention is used for symptomatic stenotic disease but is only undertaken when the active inflammatory process has been brought under control.

### Medium-Vessel Vasculitis

**Polyarteritis Nodosa** PAN is a disseminated disease with transmural arterial necrosis of the medium-sized arteries. It occurs typically in the fourth to sixth decade and is more common in men than women by a 2:1 margin. The arteries of the kidney, liver, heart, and gastrointestinal tract are commonly affected. It is characterized by the formation of multiple visceral aneurysms, with attendant risk of rupture. Alternatively, the inflammatory process of PAN may lead to arterial occlusions, manifesting as enteric perforation, gastrointestinal bleeding, or appendicitis.

The use of immunosuppressive therapy has greatly improved the 5-year survival from15% to 80%. Patients with mild symptoms can be treated with steroid therapy alone. However, patients with poor prognostic indicators such as renal insufficiency require immunosuppressive therapy in addition to steroids.

**Kawasaki's Disease** Kawasaki's disease (KD) is an acute vasculitis with a predilection for involving the coronary arteries in children younger than 5 years, with a peak incidence at 1 year of age. Boys are affected more commonly than girls. The distinguishing feature of advanced KD is the formation of diffuse fusiform and saccular coronary artery aneurysms. Systemic arteritis can also occur, commonly affecting the iliac arteries in addition to the coronaries.

Death may result from acute myocardial infarction or arrhythmia following thrombosis of a coronary artery aneurysm. Alternatively, aneurysm rupture may occur. Treatment with aspirin and immune globulin therapy has decreased the mortality over the past 2 decades and reduced the incidence of coronary artery aneurysmal degeneration. If refractory, more complete immunosuppressive therapy should be considered.

**Behçet's Disease** Behçet's disease (BD) commonly manifests as iritis associated with oral and genital mucocutaneous ulcerations. It primarily affects patients from the Mediterranean area and Japan. The vasculitis component of BD involves the venous and arterial systems. Venous thrombosis is the most common vascular disorder with BD. Arterial lesions, although less frequent, are associated with a higher incidence of mortality. Aortic aneurysmal degeneration and rupture in these patients is the usual cause of mortality.

Patients with BD and venous thrombosis are managed with lifelong oral anticoagulation. Immunosuppressive therapy is used for nonarterial symptoms, such as mucocutaneous lesions and eye disease. Traditional aneurysm repair with interposition grafting has been associated with a high incidence of thrombosis and anastomotic pseudoaneurysms. Endovascular aneurysm repair is emerging as the treatment of choice.

**Cogan's Syndrome** Cogan's syndrome (CS) is a rare disease consisting of interstitial keratitis and vestibuloauditory symptoms. It may occasionally consist of aortitis, with subsequent aortic valvular insufficiency. CS commonly affects young patients in their third decade. High-dose steroid therapy can be used to reverse visual and auditory complications. Surgical intervention may be needed for aortic valve replacement, mesenteric revascularization, or thoracoabdominal aortic aneurysm repair.

### Small-Vessel Vasculitis

**Antineutrophil Cytoplasmic Antibody–Associated Vasculitides** The major forms of small-vessel vasculitis are associated with the presence of antineutrophil cytoplasmic antibodies (ANCAs), autoantibodies formed against enzymes found in primary granules of neutrophils. ANCA-associated vasculitides (AAVs) include Wegener's granulomatosis (WG), microscopic polyangiitis (MPA), and Churg-Strauss syndrome (CSS), and often have circulating ANCAs. WG is the most common form. The overall incidence of AAVs in the population is 10 to 20 per million/year, affecting men and women equally, with a peak onset in the 60s. Patients present with constitutional symptoms that include fever and weight loss. WG is characterized by renal and respiratory tract involvement. MPA is characterized by rapid progressive glomerulonephritis in almost all patients. CSS is characterized by allergic rhinitis and asthma, eosinophilic infiltrative disease, and small-vessel vasculitis. Diagnostic testing should include assessment for inflammatory markers and for liver and renal function, as well as assays for ANCAs, antinuclear antibodies, and rheumatoid factor. Small-vessel vasculitis can be documented by microscopic examinations of biopsy specimens from affected tissues, such as skin and kidney. Treatment involves three stages using corticosteroids and immunosuppressive therapy—induction of remission, maintenance of remission, and treatment of relapses.

**Vasculitis Associated With Connective Tissue Diseases** Vasculitis is frequently associated with scleroderma, rheumatoid arthritis, and systemic lupus erythematous. Scleroderma is characterized by small-vessel occlusion within the arterioles of the skin, gastrointestinal tract, kidneys, lung, and heart. Rheumatoid arthritis typically involves digital arteries and small vessels of the vasa nervorum. Lupus patients commonly have Raynaud's syndrome, but may also have atherosclerosis of large vessels. Treatment consists of steroid and immunosuppressive therapies.

## Heritable Arteriopathies

### Cystic Medial Necrosis

Cystic medial necrosis, formerly known as medial degeneration, is associated with collagen vascular disorders, Ehlers-Danlos and Marfan's syndromes, with elastolysis degrading aortic medial collagen and elastin. Aortic dissection is the result. Although also seen in normal aging, cystic medial necrosis is accelerated by hypertension and atherosclerosis.

### Pseudoxanthoma Elasticum

Pseudoxanthoma elasticum is an inherited diseased, with most patients demonstrating an autosomal recessive inheritance. The prevalence is 1 in 70,000 to 160,000. Patients present with baggy skin and yellow-orange cutaneous papules in intertriginous areas. Symptoms may include intermittent claudication, angina, and abdominal pain caused by involvement of cerebral, coronary, visceral, and peripheral vessels. Arterial disease can be seen in young patients (20s to 30s) without risk factors for atherosclerosis. Digital plethysmography shows abnormal pulse waveforms from loss of the elastic recoil of vessels. Arterial stenosis and occlusion with extensive calcification can be seen radiographically. Surgical and endovascular management options are the same as for atherosclerotic occlusive disease.

### Arteria Magna Syndrome

Arteria magna syndrome is a disease characterized by arterial elongation, dilation, and tortuosity. It occurs in younger patients with no evidence of atherosclerosis, with a familial incidence in first-degree relatives. There is a propensity for arterial aneurysm formation in multiple sites. Arteriograms show characteristic arterial widening and tortuosity, slow arterial flow velocity, and multiple aneurysms. The low-velocity arterial flow makes arteriography difficult to perform, requiring a large volume of contrast and multiple injections with delayed timing. These patients should be screened annually for the development of aneurysms in the aorta, iliac, femoral, and popliteal arteries. Symptomatic aneurysms or those whose diameters are 2 to 2.5 times that of the parent arteries should be repaired. Complications of arterial occlusions are almost always caused by thrombosis or embolization. A number of surgical interventions are often needed for aneurysms at multiple sites.

## Congenital Conditions Affecting the Arteries

### Persistent Sciatic Artery

The sciatic artery in the embryo is a vessel that arises from the umbilical artery and supplies the lower extremity. During development, this artery is replaced by the femoral artery from the external iliac artery, and the remnants of the sciatic artery remain as the inferior gluteal artery, distal popliteal artery, and peroneal artery. Rarely, this sciatic artery persists as a large artery that is located in the posterior thigh, exiting the pelvis to continue as the popliteal artery. The superficial femoral artery may coexist or be hypoplastic or absent. Occasionally, this may be detected in an individual with an absent femoral pulse, but palpable distal pulses. However, the persistent sciatic artery usually is not detected until patients are in their 50s and symptoms typical of peripheral vascular disease develop. Up to 25% of patients may present with pulsatile buttock masses caused by aneurysmal degeneration. Surgical intervention is indicated for ischemic and aneurysmal complications. Options included arterial ligation, endovascular coiling for occlusion of an isolated aneurysm, and iliopopliteal or femoropopliteal bypasses.

### Popliteal Entrapment Syndromes

This syndrome is based on an anomalous anatomic relationship between the popliteal artery and surrounding gastrocnemius muscle that may occur during embryonic development. The most common variant (50%) is the medial location of the popliteal artery to the normally placed medial head of the gastrocnemius muscle. The second most common variant (25%) is the medial location of the popliteal artery to the abnormally attached medial head of the gastrocnemius muscle. In other variants, the normally located popliteal artery may be compressed by muscle slips of the medial head of the gastrocnemius muscle or fibrous bands. Symptoms are caused by obstruction of the popliteal artery with gastrocnemius contraction. The typical patient is a younger man (younger than 30 years; 90%) without risk factors for PVD; 20% of patients have the disorder bilaterally. Popliteal entrapment syndrome should be suspected in younger patients with calf claudication.

Diagnosis with noninvasive arterial duplex and photoplethysmography is difficult and findings are nonspecific. Arteriography may be nonspecific. MRI is the diagnostic modality of choice because it will show the anomalous relationships between the popliteal artery and gastrocnemius muscle. Treatment is indicated for symptomatic patients and requires surgical intervention. Removal of the medial gastrocnemius head may be sufficient for patients with minimal arterial disease. Patients with arterial stenosis or aneurysmal degeneration should be treated with arterial bypass using autogenous veins.

### Adventitial Cystic Disease

Adventitial cystic disease is another rare condition that should be considered in younger patients with claudication. The arterial stenosis is caused by compression of the lumen from synovial-like cysts in the subadventitial layer of the arterial wall. It is commonly located in the popliteal artery, but may also be found in the iliac and femoral arteries. Patients present in their 40s, and 80% are men. Diagnosis may be made with ultrasonography, CT, or MRI. Arteriography may show a scimitar sign, with luminal compression by the cyst. The artery is normally placed, with no signs of atherosclerotic disease. Treatment with CT- or ultrasound- guided needle aspiration may be used for small cysts, although there may be a 10% rate of recurrence. Arterial bypass with an autogenous vein is used for patients with large cysts causing arterial compression or occlusion.

## Peripheral Artery Aneurysms

### Femoral and Popliteal Artery Aneurysms

Femoral and popliteal artery aneurysms account for more than 90% of peripheral aneurysms, with popliteal artery aneurysms being the most common, 70%. However, they are still relatively uncommon. The estimated incidence of femoral and popliteal aneurysms is approximately 7/100,000 men and 1/100,000 women. Femoral aneurysms usually involve the common femoral artery, but may occasionally extend or be limited to the superficial femoral artery in the midthigh. Femoral and popliteal aneurysms are commonly associated with other aneurysms, with approximately 80% of patients having multiple aneurysms. In patients with common femoral aneurysms, 90% have an aortoiliac aneurysm and 60% have bilateral femoral aneurysms. In patients with popliteal aneurysms, 70% have an aortoiliac aneurysm and 50% have bilateral popliteal aneurysms. Femoral and popliteal aneurysms show a high incidence of thromboembolic complications, which can result in limb loss.

The diagnosis of femoral and popliteal aneurysms is suspected in patients with widened pulses that are easily palpated. These aneurysms should be considered in patients presenting with foot embolization or acute limb ischemia. CT and ultrasonography can accurately diagnose the femoral and popliteal aneurysms. Ultrasonography should be used for patients with aortoiliac aneurysms to search for these peripheral aneurysms. Arteriography is important for visualization of the aneurysms and runoff to plan for surgical intervention.

Femoral and popliteal aneurysms should be considered for treatment when the diagnosis is made. Because of the high incidence of thromboembolic events, these aneurysms are repaired, regardless of size. Even small aneurysms can cause ischemic limb complications. Surgical intervention of the femoral aneurysms consists of resection of the aneurysms with interposition grafts. Treatment of the popliteal aneurysms usually involves bypass using autogenous veins, with exclusion of the aneurysm to prevent embolization. Patients with ischemic limbs from embolic complications may require thrombolytic therapy to establish arterial outflow prior to bypass surgery. Endovascular repair with covered stents is emerging as the treatment of choice for popliteal aneurysms (Fig. 63-23).

## Evaluating the Success of Revascularization Procedures

Although there is a lack of consensus about the best endovascular modality to use for most patients, there is certainly a need for routine follow-up and close involvement of all patients treated for claudication and CLI. The ultimate success of any intervention performed, endovascular or open surgical bypass, can be improved by a continued relationship with the patient and regular examination. Smoking cessation counseling and adjuvant techniques such as medications and nicotine replacement are used routinely to help patients with this important aspect of their treatment. Lifelong administration of oral antiplatelet agents (81 mg aspirin daily and 75 mg clopidogrel daily) and aggressive lipid modification in all patients who have had a vascular intervention is routine.

Duplex arterial ultrasound has gained wide acceptance as the modality of choice for surgical bypass graft surveillance, and it is has become the standard for following patients treated with endovascular therapy. Contemporary practice guidelines include a baseline duplex ultrasonography (DU) scan before intervention, another following the intervention to document improvement (the timing of this scan varies from 1 day to 2 weeks following the intervention), and then additional scans at 3 and 6 month postprocedure to assess for continued efficacy. DU is then performed at 6-month intervals thereafter. Evaluation of continued subjective clinical improvement and determining ABIs are essential and simple adjunctive measures that should be performed at each visit. Most studies discussed earlier used

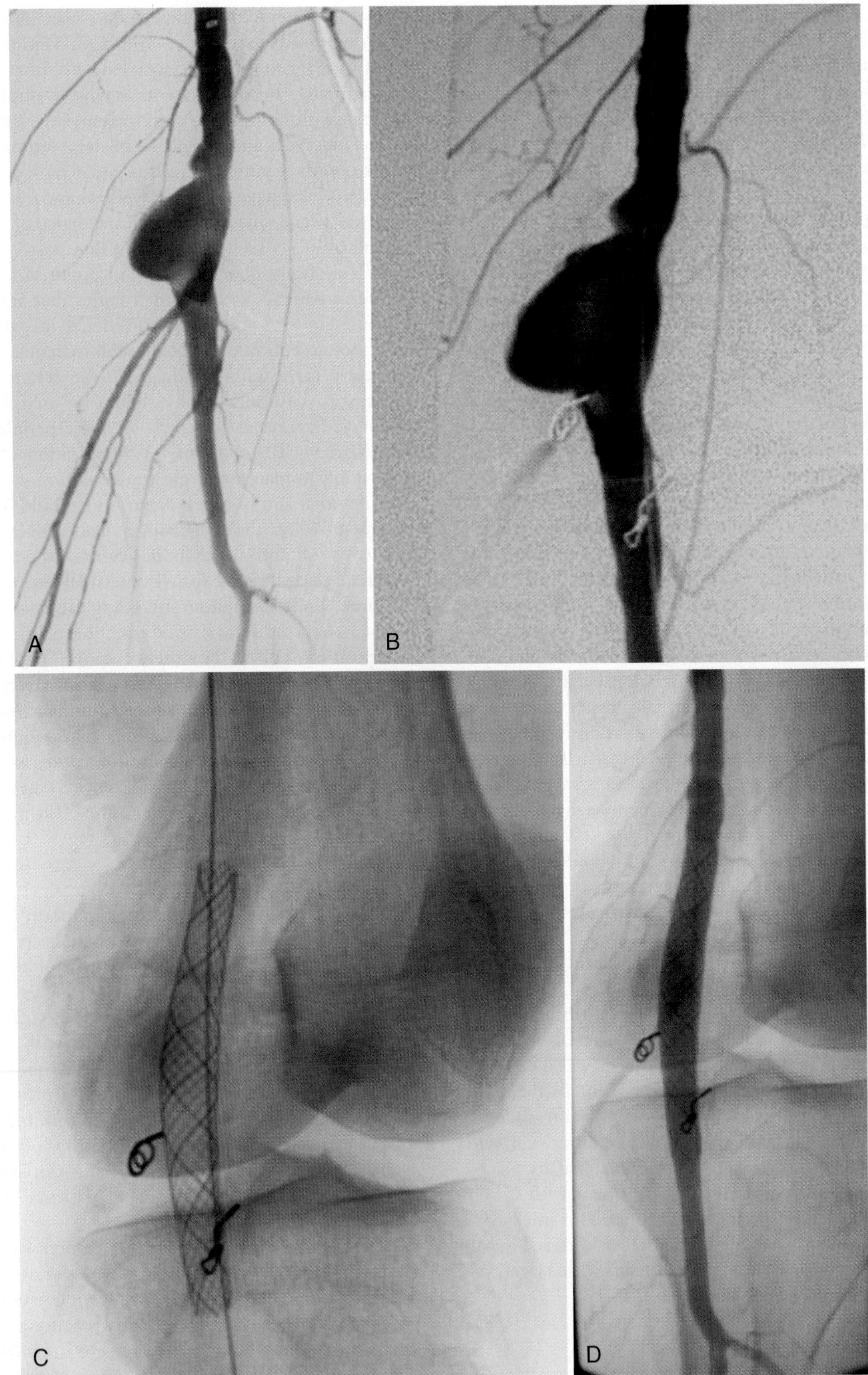


**FIGURE 63-23 A,** Popliteal aneurysm. **B,** Collateral feeding branches treated with coil embolization. **C,** Stent placement to exclude flow into aneurysm sac. **D,** Completion angiogram showing successful repair.

DU as their method of imaging follow-up. Although very early studies and coronary trials used routine postprocedure contrast angiography (at 6 months and 1 year), the ready availability, lower risk, and proven sensitivity and specificity of DU have made it the preferred method of follow-up over contrast angiography. Once a problem has been identified, routine surveillance with DU and selective angiography have become the standard for open and endovascular intervention.

The benefit of graft surveillance using DU in lower extremity bypass has been established. Reports from Idu and colleagues[52] and Buth and associates[53] have shown that all vein grafts progress to occlusion when stenosis of more than 70% diameter reduction was detected by ultrasound surveillance. Buth and coworkers further established the duplex criteria needed to identify high-risk lesions—peak systolic velocity (PSV) at the site of the lesion exceeding 300 to 350 cm/sec or a velocity ratio exceeding 3.5 or 4. The ratio is calculated using the PSV at the site of the lesion divided by the PSV of a normal graft segment proximal to the lesion.

Using these duplex criteria, Mills and colleagues[54] studied the natural history of autogenous infrainguinal vein grafts with intermediate and critical stenosis. A PSV higher than 300 cm/sec or velocity ratio more than 4 was used to detect critical stenosis. In grafts with the unrevised critical stenosis, almost 80% progressed to occlusion, all within 4 months of ultrasound detection. For grafts with intermediate stenosis, the occlusion rate was no different from grafts without stenosis, and serial surveillance was safe and effective.

Calligaro and associates[55,56] have established the usefulness of surveillance in prosthetic grafts; 85 prosthetic bypasses in 59 patients were studied in a graft surveillance protocol. There were 35 femoropopliteal, 16 femorotibial, 15 iliofemoral, 13 axillofemoral, and 6 femorofemoral bypasses. The benefit of duplex ultrasound was compared with other noninvasive studies such as changes in symptoms or pulses and ABI. Follow-up was performed 1 week and every 3 months after the initial bypass or after graft revision, for a mean of 11 months. Duplex ultrasound was able to predict 81% of graft failures versus 24% using nonultrasound findings. In the presence of a normal study, the likelihood of a graft failure was 7% using duplex criteria versus 21% with nonultrasound studies.

In a recent report, Carter and coworkers[57] studied the natural history of stenosis in the lower extremity bypass graft with duplex surveillance. There were 212 infrainguinal lower limb grafts in 197 patients. Duplex ultrasound studies were performed at 0, 1, 3, 6, 12, and 18 months after surgery, and 56.2% of grafts remained patent during this period. It was noted that prosthetic grafts and femorocrural bypasses tended to occlude without any prior documented stenosis. In this study, 40.5% of salvage procedures were performed at the 6-month time point. In contrast, vein grafts were more likely to develop progressive stenosis prior to occlusion. The authors concluded that surveillance is a valid method for detecting high-risk lesions in vein grafts, but failed in prosthetic and femorocrural grafts. This is in contrast to the findings by Calligaro and colleagues,[55,56] who found surveillance of prosthetic femorotibial grafts to be beneficial.

In a recent retrospective analysis, Tinder and associates[58] found other factors that enhanced the efficacy of DU surveillance. There were 353 infrainguinal vein bypasses performed in 329 patients. Factors predictive of stenosis detected during surveillance included non-single-segment saphenous vein conduits, warfarin drug therapy, and redo bypass grafting. Factors not predictive of graft revision were procedure indication, postoperative ABI level, statin drug therapy, and vein conduit orientation. Another predictive factor was abnormal initial duplex velocities (PSV of 180 to 300 cm/sec or velocity ratio of 2 to 3.5). Of these grafts, 40% had earlier revision and a lower 3-year assisted primary patency rate. In a report by Passman and coworkers,[59] normal initial duplex velocities were not predictive of long-term patency; 31% of grafts had abnormal duplex results first detected more than 6 months after surgery.

Lesion characteristics detected during ultrasound surveillance may also be used to determine the type of re-intervention needed. Gonsalves and colleagues[60] noted factors based on temporal and duplex data. PTA is recommended for short (<2 cm) stenoses in good-caliber veins (≥3.5 mm) found more than 3 months after the bypass procedure. Direct surgical repair or replacement is recommended for early (<3 months) and/or long-segment stenoses in small-caliber veins.

Hagino and associates[61] have also found other lesion characteristics to be of useful predictive value. Grafts treated for early lesions continued to have high failure rates, regardless of modality used, compared with late lesions. Lesions located at the anastomoses were better treated by surgical revision, although patency was no different from those treated with endovascular means. Endovascular therapy was recommended for focal late-appearing lesions involving the midgraft.

Although the use of DU in endovascular follow-up is intuitive and consistent with the usefulness observed in the management of surgical bypass, few large studies have looked at its ability to predict failure and impact on long-term results. Tielbeek and coworkers[62] used DU surveillance, clinical examination, and ABI on femoropopliteal lesions successfully treated with endovascular interventions. Impending failure was diagnosed with a PSV ratio more than 2.5. Failure was diagnosed as occlusion or recurrent stenosis requiring intervention for severe symptoms. Treatment failure was predicted by DU, with a sensitivity of 86% and a specificity of 75%. Interestingly, ABI decrease was even more predictive, with a sensitivity of 93% and specificity of 90%.

In another study, by Spijkerboer and colleagues,[63] 34 femoropopliteal segments were treated with PTA. The PSV ratio was determined with DU before PTA, 1 day and 1 year after PTA. Segments with residual stenosis detected on day 1 after PTA all occluded within the year. In those segments with good initial ultrasound results after PTA, there was deterioration in 30%. This suggests the need for more frequent routine DU follow-up.

CLI is often a hallmark of the beginning of the end game in the battle for survival in patients with diffuse atherosclerotic disease. With a known 5-year survival of less than 50%, this population is extremely disadvantaged. The surgeon's best chance for helping this group of patients lies in providing the least invasive intervention that will provide pain relief, tissue healing, and limb salvage. Close follow-up with appropriate counseling is essential, as is intensive medical management with repeat interventions performed as clinical conditions warrant. These measures offer the best strategy for limb salvage and improved mortality for patients with vascular disease. However, the final determinant of success is the patient's perception of enhancement in the quality of his or her remaining years of life.

## RENAL ARTERY DISEASE

Renovascular hypertension occurs as a consequence of decreased blood flow through a stenotic renal artery. The renin-angiotensin system is a potent regulator of blood pressure. Renin is an enzyme produced in the juxtaglomerular cells of the afferent arterioles of the kidney. It is released into the bloodstream in response to reduced renal blood flow. Once systemic, renin acts on a plasma substrate to produce angiotensin I. Angiotensin I is converted to angiotensin II in the pulmonary circulation by angiotensin-converting enzyme (ACE). Angiotensin II, in addition to being a potent vasoconstrictor of smooth muscle in the arterial walls, stimulates the secretion of aldosterone from the adrenal cortex. Aldosterone enhances sodium absorption in the renal tubules, with an attendant increase in water retention and overall volume expansion. ACE inhibitors, which prevent the conversion of angiotensin I to the vasoactive angiotensin II, are a commonly used class of antihypertensive drugs.

In patients with unilateral renal artery stenosis (RAS), renin is elaborated and the blood pressure rises in response to arterial constriction and volume retention. The opposite unaffected kidney may successfully respond by excreting the excess intravascular volume. This condition, of elevated renin levels in the presence of unilateral renal artery stenosis and the contralateral kidney producing compensatory euvolemia, is known as *renin-dependent hypertension.* In patients with bilateral RAS, renin levels rise and volume expands and is maintained. Elevated renin levels may initiate a negative feedback response from the afferent arteriole endothelium, with a resultant normal or decreased serum renin level but a persistent expansion of intracellular and intravascular volume. Thus, bilateral RAS results in what is referred to as *volume-dependent hypertension.* The natural history of RAS is a progressive decline in renal function and worsening hypertension refractory to medical management, presumably from a combination of ischemia and repetitive embolization.[64-70] Atherosclerosis is the most common cause of renal artery stenosis, and renal atrophy has been observed in patients with atherosclerotic renal disease and progression of stenoses.[68,70] Hypertension directly attributable to RAS is identified in less than 5% of all patients treated for hypertension. However, the prevalence of RAS increases in certain populations, such as patients with atherosclerotic peripheral or coronary artery disease, young patients presenting with hypertension, and patients with a combination of hypertension refractory to medical management and concomitant renal insufficiency. Renal insufficiency and ischemic nephropathy can be a direct result of renal artery stenoses. As many as 40% of patients with ESRD requiring dialysis have been found to have a significant RAS when evaluated with duplex ultrasound.[71-73]

### Diagnosis

The diagnosis of RAS can be made by DU examination of the renal arteries. DU combines direct visualization of the renal arteries (B mode) with hemodynamic measurements in the renal arteries (Doppler-derived velocity). Furthermore, ultrasonography allows direct measurement of renal size. The procedure identifies the abdominal aorta at the level of the renal arteries and records blood velocity at this site, followed by identification and measurement of blood velocity in the renal arteries. Other measurements include those of renal parenchymal velocities from the upper, middle, and lower poles of the kidneys, as well as renal size. The important parameter is the ratio of velocity in the renal artery to that of the aorta. If the ratio is more than 3.5, this is likely to be associated with a stenosis of more than 60%. If the renal artery velocity is more than 180 cm/sec, this is also considered abnormal. The test is limited by the experience of the operator and by patient habitus, being more difficult in obese patients, and bowel gas. Thus, Doppler ultrasonography of the kidneys is best performed in the early morning, after fasting. Reported sensitivity and specificity range from 90% to 95% and 60% to 90%, respectively. In one study, if renal arteriograms were obtained on all patients with a positive Doppler ultrasound, a 2.7% false-positive rate was found. A further use of Doppler ultrasonography may be in predicting which patients would benefit from revascularization. The renal resistive index (RRI) is obtained from Doppler ultrasonography. It can be expressed by the following:

$$\text{RRI} = 1 - \frac{\text{End-diastolic velocity}}{\text{Maximal systolic velocity}} \times 100$$

RRI has been predictive in determining the response of blood pressure to revascularization. An RRI higher than 0.80 has identified patients with RAS in whom angioplasty or surgery did not improve blood pressure or renal function. Finally, the presence of asymmetrical kidney size may be a clue to underlying RAS and renal ischemia.

#### Magnetic Resonance Angiography

This technique can be used for the diagnosis of proximal (and thus largely atherosclerotic) RAS. Gadolinium is used as a contrast agent for patients with a glomerular filtration rate of >30 mL/min. Reconstructions of images are used to obtain detailed views of the renal arteries. Limitations include the high cost, limited availability, and substantial expertise needed to analyze images. Results for CT angiography are similar, again with the disadvantage of requiring contrast material, with the attendant risk of nephropathy.

Other imaging studies in addition to MRA, such as contrast angiography, may also be diagnostic, but are associated with increased cost and morbidity. In practice, however, many renal artery stenotic lesions are discovered incidentally during studies performed for other reasons.

Serologic renin measurements of blood obtained by venous sampling were once commonly used to validate the significance of an identified renal artery stenosis. These required that a catheter be inserted into the venous system and blood samples obtained from each renal vein and the vena cava. In patients with unilateral RAS, a renin ratio of the affected kidney to the opposite kidney of 1.5 or higher is highly suggestive of the stenosis functionally activating the renin system. In a large series, an abnormal ratio was 92% predictive of curability with revascularization; however, 65% of patients with nonlateralizing renin ratios also had curable disease. In an effort to improve the sensitivity and specificity of the test, the renal–systemic renin index has been used. This allows determination of the functional significance of bilateral lesions. The index is obtained by subtracting the systemic (infrarenal vena cava). Plasma renin activity (PRA) from the PRA levels in the renal veins and dividing by the systemic PRA. An index above 0.24 indicates excessive renin production from that kidney, whereas lower levels are indicative of renin suppression. However, given the invasive nature of these tests and the low specificity, renal vein renin sampling is usually reserved for diagnostic dilemmas.

### Treatment

Difficult to control hypertension (e.g., patient taking three or more antihypertensive medications) or decreased renal function and a hemodynamically significant stenosis are the most commonly used indications for intervention.

### Open Renal Artery Bypass

Open renal artery bypass is rarely performed as an isolated procedure with the advent of renal artery stenting. Surgical procedures used to correct renal artery stenosis included aortorenal bypass with vein grafts, arterial autografts (for children) or prosthetic grafts, aortorenal endarterectomy, hepatic artery–renal artery bypass, gastroduodenal-renal artery bypass, and splenic artery–renal artery bypass. These procedures, although durable and revered by surgeons, are obviously maximally invasive and can be associated with significant morbidity. They have been almost universally supplanted by angioplasty and stenting procedures.

### Renal Artery Stenting

**Value, Limitations, and Techniques** Percutaneous therapy for renovascular occlusive disease has become the preferred alternative to open renal revascularization. In the appropriately selected patient, angioplasty and stenting of renal artery stenoses have been shown to be safe and effective options for severe hypertension and ischemic nephropathy. Catheter-based treatment, especially when performed with lower profile systems, can be performed with minimal morbidity and a reliably high degree of initial technical success. The long-term beneficial effects on blood pressure control and renal function have been debated but appear to be valid.

Renal angioplasty was first performed in 1978 by Gruntzig and colleagues,[74] and there have been many series demonstrating the success of this interventional procedure. With the advent of the stent, durability, efficacy and ultimately acceptance of catheter-based management of renal artery lesions have increased. Stents were initially used for cases of immediate technical failure such as residual anatomic stenoses more than 30%, residual pressure gradients or postangioplasty dissections, or recurrent stenoses following prior angioplasty. Routine stenting of renal artery stenoses (as an adjunct to balloon angioplasty), especially when treating ostial lesions, has become an accepted practice. The incidence of recurrent stenosis has been shown to be significantly decreased with angioplasty and stent placement versus angioplasty alone.[75-77]

Although the number of patients completely cured of renovascular hypertension following renal artery stenting has been reported to be as low as 5% or less,[77-79] up to 80% of patients treated demonstrate measurable improvement in blood pressure control.[76-85] Henry and associates[83] have reported a series of 210 patients with chronic hypertension and a diastolic blood pressure higher than 90 mm Hg who underwent renal artery angioplasty and stenting. A favorable response was seen in 80% of patients, with 35% reported as cured of hypertension. In this study, a hypertensive cure was defined as diastolic blood pressure less than 90 mm Hg achieved without the administration of antihypertensive medications. In another series of patients treated with stenting for RAS associated with hypertension, impaired renal function, or both, only 4.2% achieved a complete cure, but an additional 79% benefited from an improvement in hypertensive control.[78] A meta-analysis of 14 studies involving renal angioplasty and stenting has found an overall 20% cure rate for hypertension, with 49% of patients experiencing an improvement in hypertensive control.[76] This meta-analysis recognized the variability among reporting criteria for a cure among the different renal angioplasty and stent series. With numerous series showing a benefit from angioplasty and stenting, there have also been several randomized and controlled series that suggest a lower efficacy for catheter-based management in the treatment of renovascular hypertension.[86-88]

Improvement in serum creatinine level may be seen in approximately 30% of patients following renal angioplasty and stenting.[83] However, a higher percentage of patients demonstrate a clinical benefit of creatinine stabilization when renal artery stents are placed for ischemic nephropathy.[78,89,90] Rundback and coworkers[91] have reported a series of 45 patients with azotemia who received a renal stent for treatment of a renal stenosis. A clinical benefit was defined as improvement or stabilization of creatinine levels. Life table analysis demonstrated a benefit at 12, 24, and 36 months in 72%, 62%, and 54% of patients, respectively. In patients with significant RAS and a solitary functioning kidney, renal artery stenting has been shown to be a safe alternative to surgery.[92] Bush and colleagues[93] have reported a series of 27 patients, each with a solitary functioning kidney and azotemia, who underwent endovascular treatment of their significant RAS. An improvement or stabilization of renal function was seen in 74% of patients.

There is variability among series in terms of renal stent patency rates. The reported incidence of recurrent stenoses of renal stents has ranged as low as 1.5%[94] to as high as 25%[95] at 6 months. Several series of renal artery stenting have shown a patency of up to 5 years by life table analysis. Rodriquez-Lopez and associates[80] have performed a life table analysis of 108 patients undergoing renal angioplasty and primary stent placement and found 74% primary and 85% secondary patency rates. A larger series of patients with renal artery stents placed for failed angioplasty, recurrent stenosis, dissection, or ostial lesions was reported by Henry and colleagues.[83] This series demonstrated a 79% primary and 98% secondary patency at 5 years by life table analysis. Blum and coworkers[96] have reported a 92% secondary patency at 5 years among patients with renal artery stents placed for angioplasty failures.

Duplex surveillance is accurate for identifying recurrent renal artery stenosis.[97,98] The stenosis within a stent is most often caused by myointimal hyperplasia. Treatment usually consists of repeat angioplasty and, occasionally, a new stent is required. Bax and colleagues[99] have reported a series of 15 patients with 20 stents with recurrent stenoses; 18 stents were successfully treated with angioplasty alone and only two required the placement of a second stent. The 1-year success rate of the repeat interventions was 75%. Balloon-expandable covered stents may be helpful for recurrent in-stent restenosis in the future.

The morbidity and mortality of a major operative procedure can be avoided with endovascular treatment of renal artery stenoses. Mackrell and associates[100] have reported their experience with 165 patients who underwent endovascular or surgical intervention for RAS. They noted a shift from open surgical revascularization of RAS to endovascular treatment. Comparing endovascular treatment with surgical renal revascularization and combined aortic and renal revascularization, all had excellent technical success rates, but the surgical group had a significantly higher morbidity (5.6% versus 15% and 23%, respectively) and mortality rate (0% versus 9.1% and 8.1%).

With combined aortic and renal open reconstructions, the complexity of surgery is increased. Endovascular repair has become popular for the treatment of abdominal aortic aneurysms with suitable aortic anatomy. A RAS in the presence of an abdominal aortic aneurysm can be treated before or after the aortic endograft is placed. A benefit to placing the renal stent before the endograft is to allow the stent to serve as a radiopaque marker for the origin of the renal artery. This may help in positioning and placement of the endograft below the renal arteries. One must be cautious not to entrap the endograft or the delivery system on the stent if it protrudes out into the aortic lumen.

The technical success of renal artery stent placement is high in most of the series, with technical failures usually caused by poor positioning or deployment of the stent. Access to the renal artery is an important consideration for renal artery stenting. The angulation of the renal arteries relative to the aorta and the short distance of the renal artery beyond the stenosis for secure guidewire placement can make renal stenting from a femoral artery access point challenging. A brachial or axillary approach is sometimes required to overcome the angulation of the renal artery or avoid significant aortic and iliac pathology. Radial artery access with angioplasty and stenting of the renal artery has been described.[101-104]

One early technical limitation of renal artery stenting was the large size of the 0.035-inch guidewire–based balloons and stents. These platforms required a 7 or 8 Fr sheath, and tracking the stent into an angulated renal artery was difficult or sometimes not possible from a femoral approach. Miniaturization of balloons and stents was first shown to be safe and effective in coronary use[105,106] and, in some cases, resulted in shorter procedural times and use of less contrast.[107] The required guiding sheath size is reduced with the use of lower profile balloons and stents that use 0.014- and 0.018-inch guidewire platforms. The lower profile angioplasty balloons and stents have a better ability to negotiate difficult angles. These factors have led to the routine use of 0.014-inch systems for RAS. The following is a stepwise guide to our preferred technique for renal artery angioplasty and stenting using the lower profile angioplasty balloons and stents.

**Renal Angioplasty and Stent Procedure** See Figure 63-24.

***Renal Artery Access and Guide Sheath Positioning*** Arterial access, femoral or brachial, is an important initial decision that has been made easier with the lower profile balloon, stent, and sheath systems. Retrograde common femoral access is the first choice, usually secondary to table and patient positioning constraints. Brachial access is used only in certain circumstances, such as severe aortoiliac occlusive disease, aortic aneurysms, and extreme caudal renal artery angulation. In most cases, an anteroposterior (AP) aortogram is first obtained, with a pigtail catheter in the suprarenal position. Oblique angulation is sometimes required to visualize the renal origins better. To limit contrast, a selective catheterization can be made without the aortogram if one has been previously obtained. Alternative contrast agents, such as carbon dioxide and gadolinium, have been successfully used in renal angiography and renal artery interventions.[108-116] Most renal arteries can be accessed simply with an angled catheter (Glidecath, Boston Scientific); however, some will require a more complex-shaped catheter such as a cobra, shepherd's hook, or Simmons catheter. A selective renal angiogram is then obtained with hand injections of contrast or careful power injections. All phases of the renal circulation are visualized, including the arterial, parenchymal, and venous phases.

A 0.035-inch guidewire (Glidewire, Terumo Medical, Elkton, Md) is then positioned in the tertiary renal branches. Maintaining guidewire position and stability become difficult because of the relatively short length of renal artery. A 6 French guide sheath (Pinnacle, Terumo Medical, Eikton, MD) is advanced into the proximal renal artery. Using a 4 or 5 Fr glide catheter to help maintain guidewire crossing of the renal stenosis, a 0.035-inch guidewire is then exchanged for a 0.014- inch guidewire (Spartacore Guidewire, Abbott Vascular, Temecula, Calif).

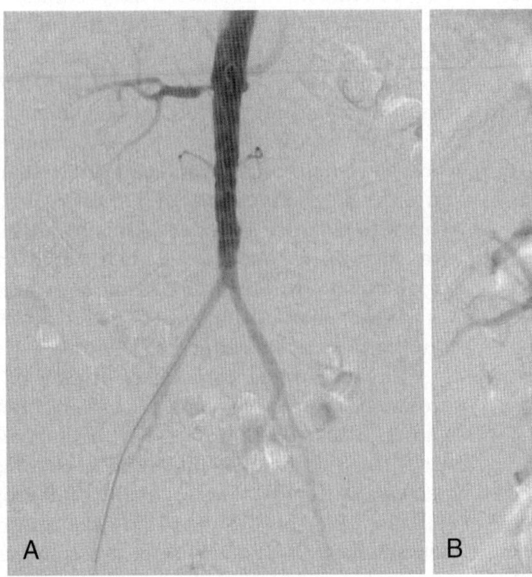


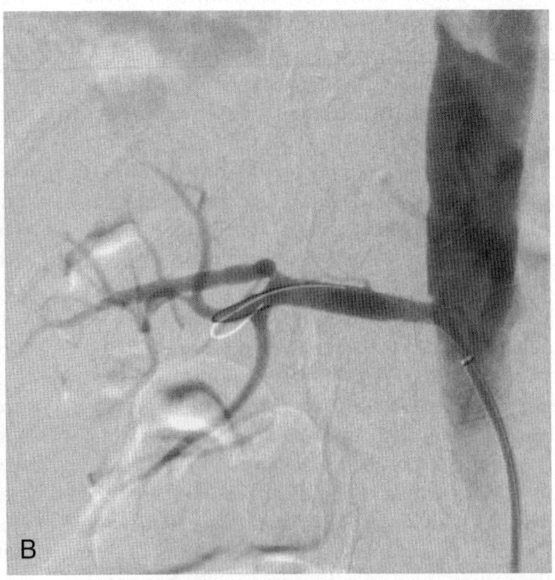


**FIGURE 63-24** Renal artery stent. **A,** Right renal artery stenosis. **B,** Lesion improved following stent placement.

***Renal Angioplasty*** The patient receives a systemic IV bolus of heparin (100 U/kg) after initial sheath placement. Prior to angioplasty, contrast is injected through the sheath and the image intensifier angle is adjusted for optimal visualization of the proximal renal artery. Over the 0.014-inch guidewire, an angioplasty balloon is advanced across the stenosis. The balloon should be approximately the size of the native normal renal artery beyond the stenosis, not a segment with poststenotic dilation. Typically, the initial angioplasty is performed with a 4-mm semicompliant balloon (CrossSail, Guidant, Santa Clara, CA or Gazelle, Boston Scientific, Natick, MA). The compliant nature of the balloon gives a range of diameters above and below 4 mm, depending on the inflation pressure. While the balloon is inflated, a saved image is obtained to compare the size of the angioplasty balloon with the native artery. This comparison will be taken into account when deciding whether a larger angioplasty balloon is needed and what size stent to choose.

***Stent Placement*** A postangioplasty angiogram is then performed and the renal artery is assessed for residual stenosis or significant dissection. If present, a stent is placed. All renal artery lesions involving the origin will require a stent. A balloon-expandable stent (Niroyal, Boston Scientific/Medi-Tech; or Palmaz Genesis, Cordis, Miami) from a low-profile 0.014- and 0.018-inch system is used (0.018-inch balloons and stents can also be delivered over a 0.014-inch guidewire). With 0.035-inch-based systems, the guide sheath was often advanced across the renal stenosis to protect the balloon-mounted stent as it crossed the lesion. With lower profile systems, this is rarely necessary. Contrast may be puffed through the sheath positioned in the aorta near the ostium of the renal artery to confirm proper positioning of the renal stent. The stent is deployed by expanding the angioplasty balloon to its predetermined deployment pressure. Higher pressures may be required to expand the stent further. However, the rated burst pressure should not be exceeded. (Always read the accompanying package insert for the deployment and rated burst pressures.)

***Completion Angiography*** Prior to removal of the guidewire and sheath, a completion angiogram with a flush catheter in the aorta is obtained. This presents an interesting question: How can a good quality completion study be obtained to include the renal artery origin without losing guidewire access? This can easily be done using a tandem wire technique. The sheath is withdrawn into the infrarenal aorta while maintaining guidewire position across the stented segment of renal artery. A second guidewire is advanced into the aorta; a 4 French pigtail catheter is placed over this wire and through the same sheath in the suprarenal position to obtain good detail of the renal artery origin.

**Technical Tips**

1. The renal arteries often originate anteriorly or posteriorly, and the initial diagnostic evaluation of the renal artery origins may be improved with oblique image intensifier views.
2. Catheter selection for initial access to the renal artery will depend on the patient's anatomy. Although most branch vessels can be accessed with just an angled Glidecath, a formed catheter such as a cobra or Simmons catheter may be required.
3. Arterial perforation is possible with inadvertent guidewire advancement into the renal parenchyma; thus, one should be very conscious of the tip of the wire throughout the entire procedure.
4. The saved image of the fully expanded initial angioplasty balloon will help estimate the native artery diameter and optimal stent size.
5. Care must be taken not to overdilate and risk rupture of the renal artery.
6. Stents placed for ostial lesions should extend into the aorta by approximately 2 mm.
7. Always read the package insert for the balloon and stent system for sheath and guidewire compatibility, balloon compliance, and the nominal deployment and rated burst pressures.

Renal artery stenting may be an effective treatment of renovascular hypertension and ischemic nephropathy that avoids the morbidity and mortality of open surgical treatment. The role of renal stents following angioplasty can be debated; however, there is good evidence for stenting all ostial lesions. A more traditional approach to stenting may be used for nonostial stenosis, with the stent reserved for angioplasty failures. Lesions caused by fibromuscular dysplasia usually do not require adjuvant stenting because they respond well to primary angioplasty. The technical success of renal stenting is high, with most technical failures caused by imprecise stent placement. Using a lower profile 0.014- or 0.018-inch platform for percutaneous renal artery interventions will reduce the sheath size necessary for access and has replaced the more cumbersome 0.035-inch platforms.

## SPLANCHNIC ANEURYSMS: SPLENIC, MESENTERIC, AND RENAL ARTERY ANEURYMS

The most common splanchnic artery aneurysm (Fig. 63-25) is the splenic artery aneurysm, accounting for 60% of all splanchnic artery aneurysms. However, it is still rare, with an incidence of 0.78% in patients undergoing abdominal arteriography; it is found incidentally in 0.1% to 10% of autopsies. Splenic aneurysms are more common in women than men, with a ratio of 4 : 1. Pregnancy is associated with up to 50% of all ruptures. The overall mortality from rupture is approximately 25%. However, rupture during pregnancy is associated with high maternal (80%) and fetal (90%) mortality. The most common risk factors associated with splenic aneurysms are female gender, history of multiple pregnancies, and portal hypertension.

Splenic aneurysms are commonly diagnosed incidentally during arteriographic and CT studies performed for other indications. A signet ring calcification in the left upper quadrant may be seen on plain abdominal radiographs. Ultrasonography, CT, and MRI are useful for aneurysm surveillance in asymptomatic patients.

Patients with splenic aneurysms may report a history of left upper quadrant or epigastric pain. The term *double rupture* has been used to describe these aneurysms, but is relatively rare. There is initial contained bleeding in the lesser sac, followed by free hemorrhage into the peritoneal cavity, causing hypovolemic shock. Treatment should be considered in aneurysms larger than 2 cm in diameter. Because of the high mortality rate, treatment is warranted for pregnant women and those of childbearing age. Simple ligation or excision of the aneurysm is preferred to

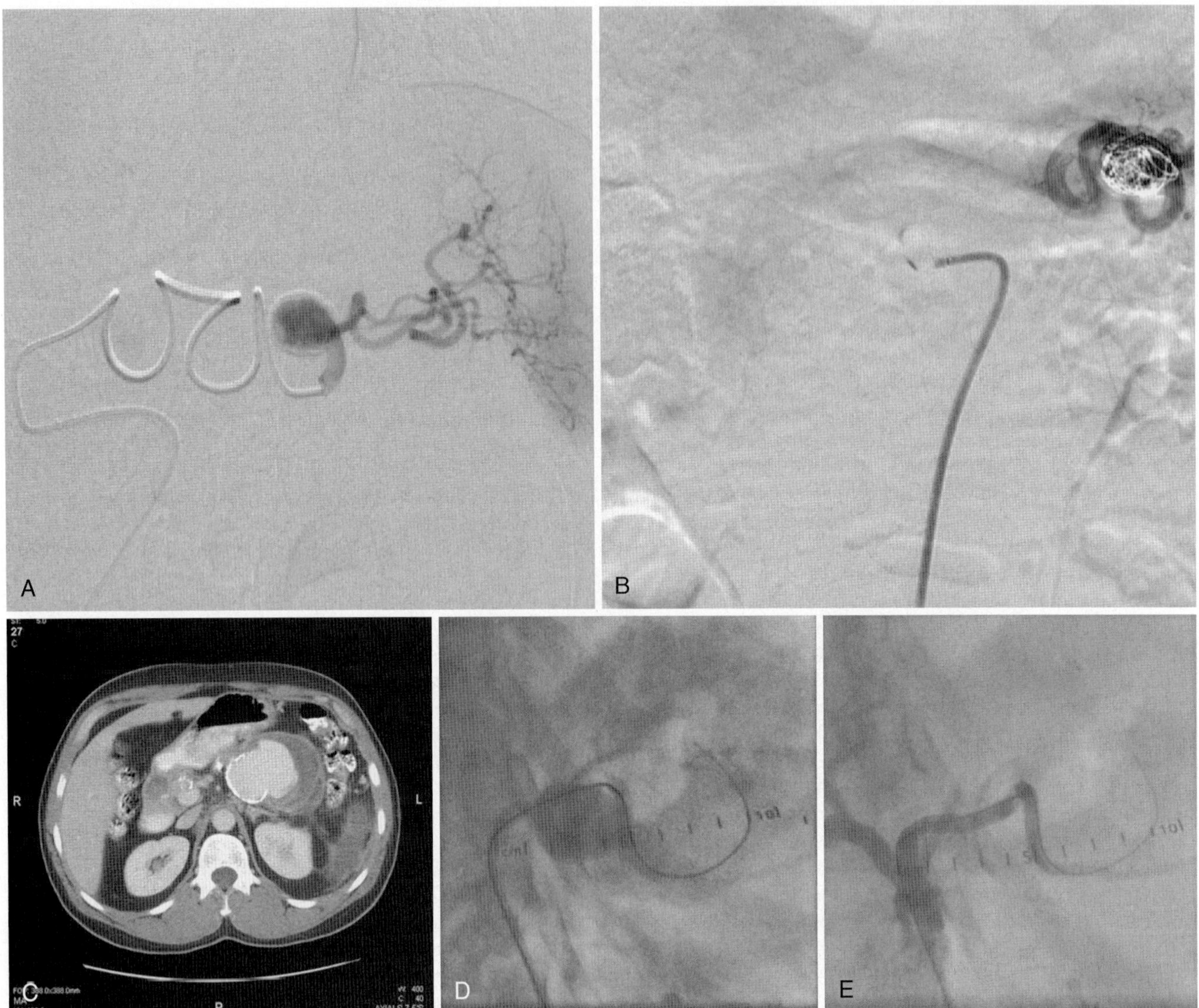


**FIGURE 63-25** **A,** Splenic artery aneurysm. **B,** Same aneurysm after treatment with coil embolization. **C,** CT scan demonstrating ruptured splenic aneurysm. **D,** Arteriogram demonstrates sac with wire passing through aneurysm into intact distal artery. **E,** Flow into sac excluded with stent graft.

splenectomy. Endovascular repair is emerging as the treatment of choice, with embolization or exclusion with a covered stent.

Hepatic aneurysms are the second most common splanchnic aneurysms, accounting for 20%. These are usually discovered incidentally. Management recommendations are for immediate repair in symptomatic patients or when pseudoaneurysm is suspected, such as those lesions related to iatrogenic injury; otherwise, asymptomatic aneurysms are repaired when the diameter is greater than 2 cm. Surgical approach depends on the location of the lesion and options include ligation of common hepatic artery lesions, open aneurysmorrhaphy or aneurysmectomy with reconstruction. In favorable anatomy, endovascular exclusion can be successful using either covered stents or coil embolization.

Superior mesenteric artery (SMA) aneurysms account for 5.5% of splanchnic aneurysms; the majority are mycotic and symptomatic, presenting with abdominal pain, nausea, vomiting or gastrointestinal bleeding. Due to the high mortality risk associated with rupture or intestinal ischemia, SMA aneurysms are repaired regardless of size. Surgical options, which depend on patient factors as well as the anatomy, include ligation, open aneurysmorrhaphy or resection, endovascular repair using either covered stent grafts or coil embolization.

Celiac axis aneurysms are rarer still and constitute 5% of all splanchnic aneurysms. These are associated with infection, trauma and dissection as well as degenerative disease. Similar to splenic lesions, these may initially present with rupture into the lesser sac with epigastric pain and hypotension, followed by shock due to free rupture into the abdominal cavity. Due to high mortality, all symptomatic lesions are repaired immediately as well as asymptomatic lesions greater than 1.5 cm in diameter. Ligation may be well tolerated. Open or endovascular intervention should be selected based on patient anatomy.

The true incidence of renal artery aneurysms is difficult to estimate, ranging from 0.09–0.9% based on autopsy studies or radiographic series. Pathogenic contributors include fibromuscular dysplasia, atherosclerotic disease and trauma. The majority of true aneurysms is saccular and often occurs at the main renal artery bifurcation, complicating surgical repair. 10% bilaterality is seen. Fibromuscular dysplasia (FMD), particularly medial dysplasia, is known to cause multiple stenosis with post-stenotic dilation, effecting the "string of beads" appearance on imaging. The majority are asymptomatic; symptomatic patients present with rupture. Indications for repair include symptomatic lesions, lesions greater than 2 cm, or lesions in women of childbearing age. Options for repair depend upon the location of the lesion. FMD is treated with balloon angioplasty alone. The rare aneurysm that occurs along the straight portion of the artery can be treated either with coil embolization or stent placement or both. Aneurysms that occur at major branch points, in which one of the branches cannot be sacrificed, require open repair. The complexity of this approach varies from simple aneurysmorrhaphy, to resection with reconstruction with inflow from the aorta, or the hepatic, splenic or iliac arteries, to explantation of the kidney for back table repair, to nephrectomy.

## CAROTID ARTERY DISEASE

Stroke is the third leading cause of death and is the leading cause of serious disability in the United States. There are about 700,000 strokes/ year with almost 175,000 deaths (25%) occurring within 1 year after the stroke. Approximately 85% of strokes have an ischemic cause, with 15% caused by primary hemorrhage, such as intraparenchymal bleeding from hypertension. Of the ischemic stokes, 20% to 30% are secondary to emboli from atherosclerotic cerebrovascular disease. In patients with greater than 50% stenosis, 20% of patients were shown to have embolic events in transcranial Doppler (TCD) studies. The incidence and frequency increase with increased stenosis and recent symptomatic neurologic events. The most common location for atherosclerosis in the cerebrovascular circulation is the carotid bifurcation; thus, many strokes are preventable with carotid intervention.

### Pathophysiology

The development of atherosclerotic plaque in the extracranial arteries is the leading cause of ischemic stroke in North America and Europe. It accounts for approximately 90% of extracranial cerebrovascular disease, with the remaining 10% caused by disease processes such as fibromuscular dysplasia and arteritis. Usually, atherosclerotic lesions occur at the proximal internal carotid artery (ICA) and carotid bifurcation along the wall opposite the origin of the external carotid artery (ECA). The enlargement of carotid bifurcation at the carotid bulb creates a well-defined region of low wall shear stress, flow separation, and loss of unidirectional flow. In this region of low shear stress with sluggish flow, there is prolonged exposure and interaction of plasma lipids and vessel walls, which may account for the localized plaque at the carotid bulb. In contrast, regions with high shear stress, such as the inner border of the carotid sinus, are usually free of atherosclerosis. After the development of a hemodynamically significant stenosis, the atherosclerotic plaque may cause stroke by one of the three principal mechanisms—embolization of atherosclerotic particle, thrombotic occlusion, or hypoperfusion.

### Clinical Presentation

Symptoms of carotid artery disease include transient ischemic attacks (TIAs), amaurosis fugax, and/or stroke. A TIA is defined as a brief acute loss of focal cerebral function, generally less than 24 hours in duration. There is no persistent deficit after each TIA, but there are often multiple attacks. The loss of function can be localized to a region of brain that is supplied by one vascular system, such as the right or left carotid artery. Most TIAs are brief, lasting 2 to 15 minutes, and are rapid in onset. Symptoms include unilateral motor and sensory loss, aphasia (difficulty finding words), or dysarthria (difficulty speaking because of motor dysfunction). Motor function loss may present as weakness, paralysis, dysarthria, or clumsiness of the upper and/or lower extremities and/or face that is contralateral to the affected carotid artery. Sensory function loss may present as numbness or paresthesia of the contralateral upper and/or lower extremities and/or face. Aphasia occurs when the speech center, usually located in the dominant hemisphere, is affected. If the neurologic deficit lasts longer than 24 hours, but there is return of full neurologic function with 48 to 72 hours, it is termed a *reversible ischemic neurologic deficit* (RIND). A patient with persistent neurologic deficit is considered to have a stroke. In contrast, fleeting episodes lasting only a few seconds are usually not considered to be TIAs.

Amaurosis fugax is the transient unilateral loss of vision. It is caused by an embolus to the ophthalmic artery, the first branch of the internal carotid artery. Patients describe the event as a shade descending or ascending over the entire eye, half of the eye, or a quadrant of one eye. The location of the affected visual field depends on whether the embolization is to the superior or inferior retinal artery. If the entire retinal artery is transiently affected, the patient may complain of complete loss of vision in one eye. Similar to TIAs, most incidents of amaurosis fugax are sudden in onset and last for minutes. However, there may be occasional patients with permanent blindness.

A patient may also be asymptomatic when diagnosed with hemodynamically significant carotid artery disease. An audible carotid bruit may be heard in the neck during routine physical examination. It should be noted that severe carotid disease may not have an audible bruit due to markedly reduced blood flow. A screening carotid duplex using ultrasound should be performed in asymptomatic patients with bruits or high-risk patients without bruits.

### Diagnosis

Once a patient is diagnosed with TIA, amaurosis fugax, or stroke, expedient workup with confirmation of carotid artery disease and treatment are needed because the risk of a stroke is greatest within the first 3 months after the initial event. This risk returns to baseline at approximately 6 months. The most useful test for the diagnosis of extracranial carotid artery disease is duplex ultrasound. Carotid duplex ultrasonography (Fig. 63-26) allows for accurate indirect determination of the severity of the carotid stenosis by measuring velocity. As the stenosis increases and the lumen narrows, there is an increase in the blood velocity to maintain distal flow. Many studies have confirmed the correlation of increased velocity with severity of disease. CT and MRA (Fig. 63-27) can also be used to determine the degree of carotid stenosis at the bifurcation. In addition, they are useful for studying potential tandem lesions that may be present in the proximal supra-aortic trunk or intracranial vessels and to assess the configuration of the aortic arch. These studies are also useful for confirmation of duplex findings and planning intervention with a carotid endarterectomy or stenting. Contrast arteriography (Fig. 63-28) is occasionally performed. It is most useful for patients with negative duplex studies or for whom a noninvasive study is in disagreement with the clinical presentation. In addition to similar findings on CTA and MRA, contrast arteriography can be used to identify intracranial vascular disease or unusual nonatherosclerotic arteriopathies, such as fibromuscular dysplasia.

| RIGHT | cm/s (S) | cm/s (D) | Percent | Plaque |
|---|---|---|---|---|
| ECA | 266 | 0 | | |
| DICA | 56 | 24 | | |
| MICA | 80 | 28 | | |
| PICA | 867 | 443 | | |
| DCCA | 56 | 11 | | |
| MCCA | 62 | 8 | | |
| PCCA | 77 | 12 | | |
| SUBCL | 155 | 0 | | |

**Max ICA Stenosis** 80-99%
**ICA/CCA Ratio** 11.3

| LEFT | cm/s (S) | cm/s (D) | Percent | Plaque |
|---|---|---|---|---|
| ECA | 249 | 0 | | |
| DICA | 97 | 28 | | |
| MICA | 83 | 31 | | |
| PICA | 149 | 37 | 50-79% | |
| DCCA | 147 | 36 | | |
| MCCA | 101 | 27 | | |
| PCCA | 103 | 20 | | |
| SUBCL | 176 | 0 | | |

**Max ICA Stenosis** 50-79%
**ICA/CCA Ratio** 1.0

A

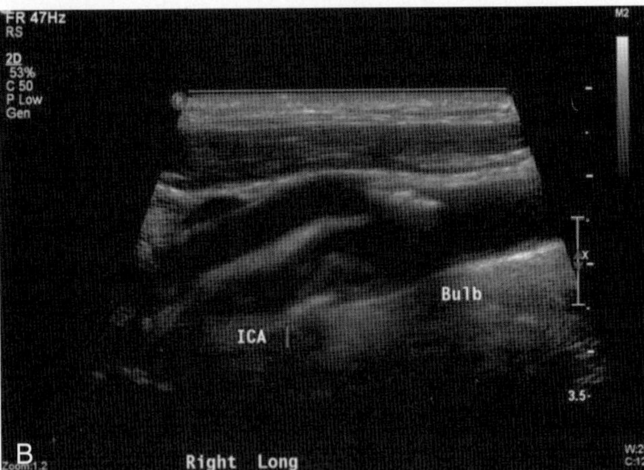


**FIGURE 63-26 A,** Carotid duplex velocities demonstrating severe right internal carotid artery stenosis. **B,** Soft plaque is seen within the right ICA on gray scale imaging.

## Treatment

### Carotid Endarterectomy

**Indications** Carotid endarterectomy (CEA) is the removal of the atherosclerotic plaque from the carotid bifurcation. In the North American Symptomatic Carotid Endarterectomy Trial (NASCET), the effectiveness of CEA was evaluated for symptomatic patients with carotid artery stenosis ranging from 30% to 99% in the United States and Canada. Patients with TIA, amaurosis fugax, or nondisabling stroke were randomized to best medical therapy or CEA. In the first study of patients with 70% stenosis or greater, CEA reduced the incidence of ipsilateral stroke from 26% to 9% at 2 years. The incidence of a major or fatal ipsilateral stroke was 13.1% for the medical group and 2.5% for the surgical group. In a subsequent report, the results of patients with symptomatic mild (30% to 49%) and moderate (50% to 69%) ipsilateral stroke were reported. The 5-year risk of ipsilateral stroke in patients with moderate stenosis was 22.2% for the medical group and 15.7% for the surgical group. For patients with mild stenosis, the risk of ipsilateral stroke was equivalent for the medical and surgical groups. The NASCET outcome showed that symptomatic patients with severe stenosis (70% to 99%) gained substantial benefit from surgical intervention over a brief period of less than 2 years. The results also favored surgery in symptomatic patients with 50% to 69% stenosis. It should be noted that best medical therapy at the time of NASCET trial did not include clopidogrel (Plavix) or statin anticholesterol agents, both of which have been shown to decrease the risk of stroke.

CEA has also been shown to be effective in asymptomatic patients. The Asymptomatic Carotid Atherosclerosis Study (ACAS) randomized asymptomatic patients with 60% to 99% stenosis to best medical treatment or CEA. The 5-year risk of ipsilateral stroke and any perioperative stroke or death was 11% for the medical group and 5.1% for the surgical group. The perioperative complication rate was low, 2.3%, with approximately 50% of the risk associated with mandatory preoperative contrast

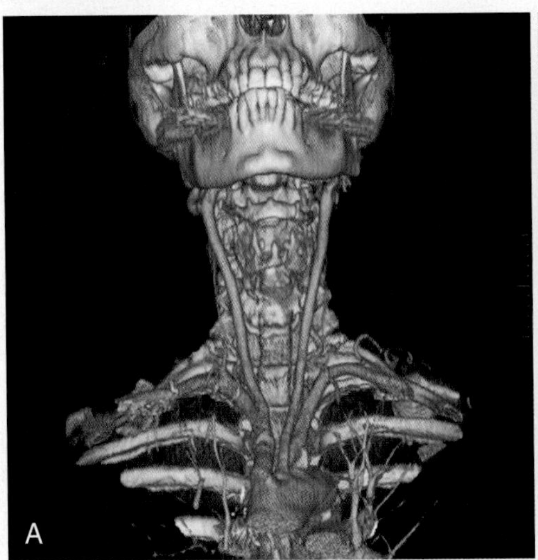


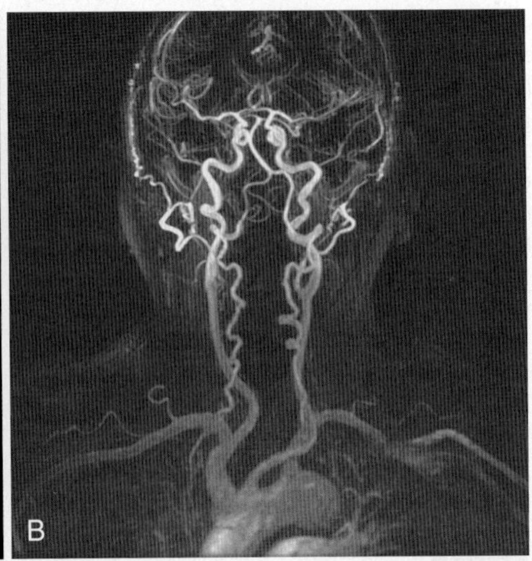


**FIGURE 63-27 A,** Arch and cervical carotid CTA reconstruction. **B,** Arch, cervical, and intracranial MRA scans with gadolinium. (Courtesy Dr. Douglas Hughes, University of Texas Medical Branch at Galveston [UTMB], Department of Radiology.)

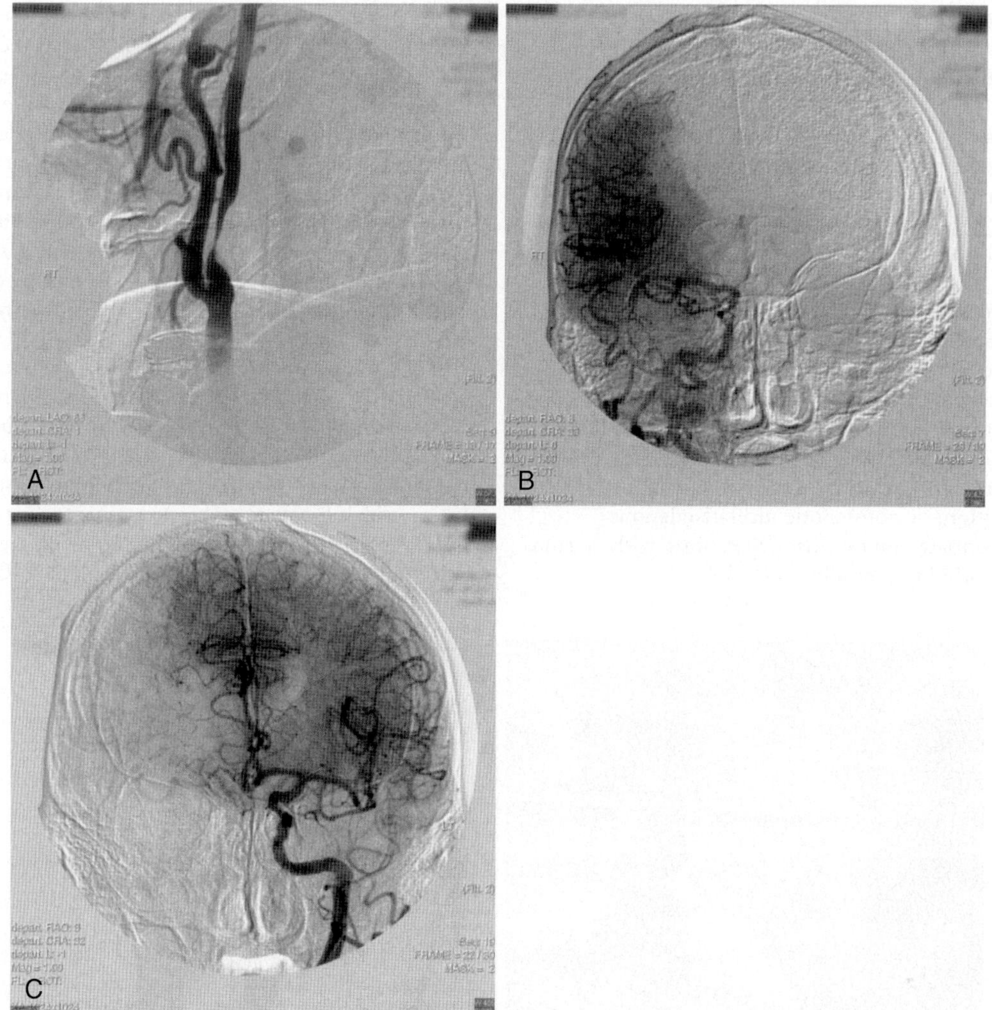


**FIGURE 63-28** Same patient as in Figure 63-26. **A,** Severe right ICA stenosis, correlating with carotid duplex findings. **B,** Intracerebral AP angiogram of right CCA injections demonstrates no filling of the anterior circulation. **C,** Injection of the left ICA demonstrates filling of the right anterior circulation.

arteriography for patients randomized to CEA. Therefore, the actual surgical complication rate was only 1.5%. The largest trial was the Asymptomatic Carotid Surgery Trial (ACST), with equal randomization of 3120 patients to CEA or medical treatment. The results were similar, with a 5-year stroke risk of 11.8% in the medical group and 5.4% for the surgical group. The perioperative complication was also low, 3.1%.

The results of landmark studies of CEA have confirmed that surgery provides better protection from ipsilateral stroke in patients with symptomatic or asymptomatic disease. The Stroke Council of the American Heart Association convened a consensus conference on the indications for CEA. The recommendation recognized four categories: (1) proven—the strongest indication, usually supported by results of prospective, randomized trials; (2) acceptable but not proven—a good indication for operation supported by promising but not scientifically certain data; (3) uncertain—data insufficient to define the risk-benefit ratio; and (4) proven inappropriate—current data adequate to show that the risk of surgery outweighs any benefits. The recommendations are further classified for patients with symptomatic or asymptomatic carotid disease.

For symptomatic good-risk patients treated by a surgeon whose surgical morbidity and mortality rate is less than 6%, the indications for CEA are as follows:

#### *Proven Indications*

- One or more TIAs in the last 6 months and carotid stenosis ≥70%
- Mild stroke with carotid stenosis ≥70%

#### *Acceptable But Not Proven Indications*

- TIAs in the past 6 months and stenosis of 50% to 69%
- Progressive stroke and stenosis ≥70%
- Mild or moderate stroke in the past 6 months and stenosis of 50% to 69%
- Carotid endarterectomy ipsilateral to TIAs and stenosis ≥70%, combined with required coronary bypass grafting

#### *Uncertain Indications*

- TIAs with stenosis ≤50%
- Mild stroke with stenosis ≤50%
- Symptomatic acute carotid thrombosis

***Proven Inappropriate Indications***

- Moderate stroke with stenosis ≤50%, not receiving aspirin
- Single TIA, stenosis ≤50%, not receiving aspirin
- High-risk patient with multiple TIAs, stenosis ≤50%, not receiving aspirin
- High-risk patient, mild or moderate stroke, stenosis ≤50%, not receiving aspirin
- Global ischemic symptoms with stenosis ≤50%
- Acute internal carotid dissection, asymptomatic, receiving heparin

For asymptomatic good-risk patients treated by a surgeon whose surgical morbidity and mortality rates are each less than 3%, the indications for CEA are as follows:

- Proven indications: Stenosis ≥60%
- Acceptable but not proven indications: None defined
- Uncertain indications: High-risk patient or surgeon with a morbidity-mortality rate greater than 3%, combined carotid-coronary operation, or nonstenotic ulcerative lesions
- Proven inappropriate indications: Operations with a combined stroke morbidity-mortality rate ≥5%

**Technique** See Figure 63-29. The patient is positioned supine on a shoulder roll, with the neck extended and the head turned to the contralateral side. A longitudinal incision is placed parallel and along the anterior border of the sternocleidomastoid muscle. Alternatively, an oblique incision can be made along the skin lines of the neck. The longitudinal incision may provide better exposure, whereas the oblique incision may result in a more cosmetic scar when healed. With the longitudinal exposure, the incision can be extended proximally to the sternal notch or distally to the mastoid process for exposure of the proximal common or distal ICA, respectively. The platysma is divided. The sternocleidomastoid muscle is mobilized away from the carotid sheath and retracted posteriorly. The internal jugular vein may be exposed along the anterior border until the large common facial vein is identified. The common facial vein is devided; the carotid bifurcation is usually located underneath. The internal jugular vein may be mobilized laterally to provide exposure to the carotid bifurcation. The vagus nerve (cranial nerve X) is found posterolateral to the common carotid artery (CCA) in the carotid sheath. Therefore, dissection of the CCA is performed

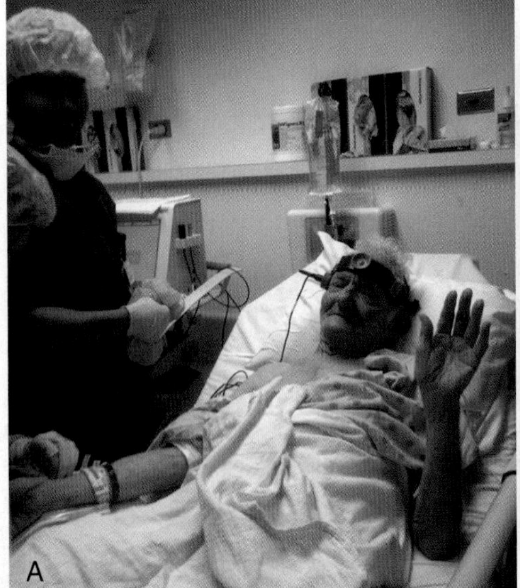


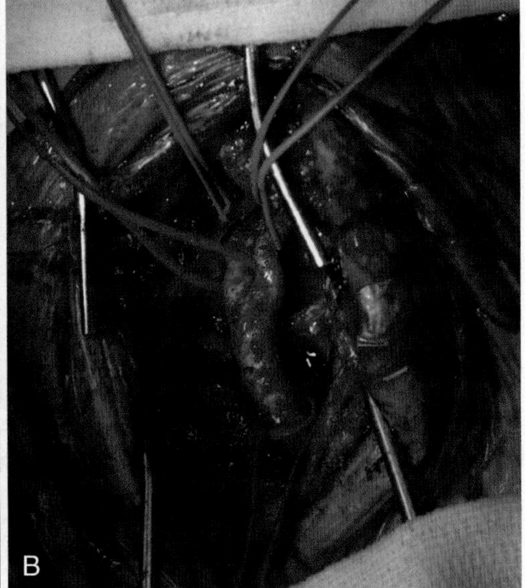


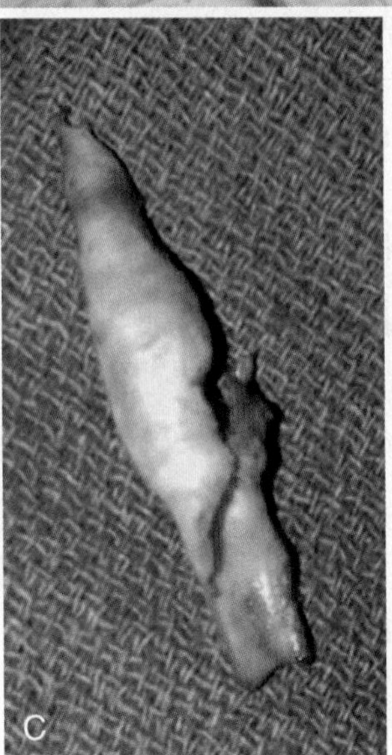


**FIGURE 63-29 A,** Patient preparing for carotid endarterectomy with intraoperative transcranial duplex monitoring. **B,** Carotid exposure with hypoglossal nerve at top of incision. **C,** Carotid plaque with calcified and friable components.

anteriorly to avoid nerve injury. However, care must still be exercised to identify the occasional anomalous anterior course of the vagus nerve and the presence of a rare nonrecurrent laryngeal nerve that branches directly from the vagus to innervate the vocal cord. The nonrecurrent laryngeal nerve usually occurs on the right side of the neck.

Meticulous dissection of the carotid artery is necessary to avoid embolization. Movement of the carotid bulb should be minimized; the initial dissection should be limited to the normal ICA and ECA distal to the diseased segment and the CCA proximal to the diseased segment. During mobilization of the ICA superiorly, the hypoglossal nerve (cranial nerve XII) needs to be identified and protected. Dissection near the carotid bifurcation and carotid body may cause reflex bradycardia and hypotension. This can be prevented with the injection of 1% lidocaine into the carotid body.

Occasionally, there may be patients with a high carotid bifurcation or an extensive lesion, and maximum exposure of the ICA may be needed. There are several techniques that can be used to provide this exposure. The skin incision is first extended all the way superiorly to the mastoid process and the sternocleidomastoid muscle is mobilized to its tendinous insertion on the mastoid process. At this level of dissection, the spinal accessory nerve (cranial nerve XI) is identified and protected. Addition exposure of the ICA can be achieved with the division of the posterior belly of the digastric muscle. If further exposure of the ICA superiorly is necessary, the styloid process can be transected and the mandible displaced anteriorly. At this level of dissection, the glossopharyngeal nerve (cranial nerve IX) crosses the ICA near the base of the skull. Injury to this nerve can be avoided by dissecting close to the anterior surface of this artery. When retracting the wound superiorly, care should also be exercised to avoid other nerve injuries. There can be temporary compression injury to the greater auricular nerve laterally and the marginal mandibular branch of the facial nerve medially.

Once the carotid arteries are fully exposed, vessel loops are placed around the arteries and heparin is given for full anticoagulation. To avoid embolization, the ICA is clamped first, followed by control of the CCA and ECA. The CCA is opened and a longitudinal arteriotomy is extended through the plaque into the normal ICA distally. If a shunt is to be used, it is inserted at this time. The decision whether to shunt can be made using electroencephalographic or back-pressure criteria. Using back-pressure criteria, an arterial pressure transducer is setup. A 22-gauge needle bent at a 45-degree angle is carefully inserted into the CCA, with the distal needle in the lumen of the ICA. The pressure of the ICA is measured with the ECA and CCA clamped. If the back pressure is a mean arterial pressure of 65 mm Hg or higher, there is adequate collateral cerebral circulation and a shunt can be avoided. Alternative methods of cerebral blood flow evaluation include intermittent neurologic checks on the awake patient undergoing CEA with local anesthesia only, or transcranial duplex or electroencephalographic monitoring of the patient undergoing CEA under general anesthesia.

The endarterectomy is started in the CCA. The optimal plan for endarterectomy is the plane between the inner and outer medial layers. This results in the removal of the intima, plaque and a portion of the media. The remaining arterial wall thus consists of the adventitia and residual media. The plaque is divided proximally in the CCA and the endarterectomy is extended distally into the carotid bulb. The vessel loop around the ECA is loosened and endarterectomy of the ECA is performed by simple eversion. Removal of the plaque is continued distally into the ICA. Endarterectomy of the distal ICA is feathered to its transition to the normal distal intima. If the distal plaque cannot be feathered, the residual intima is sharply transected and secured in place using tacking sutures. After completion of the endarterectomy, the residual wall is copiously irrigated with heparinized saline solution and any remaining debris or medial fibers are removed to prevent embolization. The ICA, ECA, and CCA are allowed to back-bleed.

The arteriotomy is closed using a patch. There is evidence showing that patch angioplasty has better results with a reduced risk of restenosis, especially in female patients, patients with small ICAs, and patients who continue to smoke. Once the arteriotomy is completed, flow is first established to the ECA with release of clamps to the ECA and CCA. After several heartbeats to flush debris out the ECA, flow is then reestablished into the ICA.

If desired, heparin reversal is given with protamine.

**Postoperative Care** At the completion of the endarterectomy, a gross neurologic examination of the patients is performed in the operating room. If no deficit is found, the patient is transferred to the recovery room. Patients are monitored closely during the postoperative period. Although they were formerly cared for in the intensive care unit routinely, most patients now can be transferred to a regular room if they are neurologically intact and hemodynamically normal in the postanesthesia care unit. Usually, patients are discharged safely the next day. Important factors to be monitored are the patient's neurologic status, blood pressure, and incision, to evaluate for hematoma.

If, at the completion of the procedure, there is neurologic deficit, the patency of the ICA is evaluated with noninvasive carotid duplex. Initial flap or occlusion of the ICA on duplex requires immediate reoperation. If the ICA is patent, an arteriography is performed to detect possible clots or defects. Any lesion is treated with reoperation. If there is no lesion on the arteriogram in a patent ICA, the patient is treated conservatively with anticoagulation, antiplatelet agents, or both. However, if the patient continues to have repeated or worsening neurologic events, immediate reoperation may be needed.

Blood pressure monitoring and control during the postoperative period are of paramount importance to prevent stroke. Immediately after carotid endarterectomy, 20% of patients may have significant hypertension and 30% may have hypotension. Up to 9% of these patients were found to have neurologic deficits, whereas there was no neurologic morbidity in normotensive patients. In addition, blood pressure fluctuation has adverse effects on myocardial function. Systolic blood pressure should be kept below 140 mm Hg for normotensive patients and below 160 mm Hg for chronically hypertensive patients. Diastolic pressure is maintained below 100 mm Hg. Hypertension should be treated immediately; sodium nitroprusside can be used. Hypotension is initially treated with fluid to correct the volume deficit; if refractory, vasoconstrictors can be initiated.

The use of antiplatelet therapy and intraoperative heparin anticoagulation can cause wound hematoma after endarterectomy; the incidence of reoperation for hematoma drainage is less than 1%. Usually, there is diffuse ooze from the wound, rather than bleeding from the suture line. A large hematoma may cause compression on the ICA and adjacent cranial nerves and wound infection. If there is airway compromise, the incision needs to be opened at the bedside for drainage of the hematoma. The incidence may be decreased with the routine use of a silastic drain.

It is not unusual for patients to complain of headache after carotid endarterectomy; they may complain of these symptoms at approximately 3 to 5 days postoperatively. This is likely caused by reperfusion syndrome from dysfunction in the cerebral circulation autoregulation once the blood flow is restored after endarterectomy. It is usually self-limiting and resolves spontaneously. However, if there is associated neurologic deficit, CT should be performed.

**Complications** Stroke is the most feared complication of carotid endarterectomy; it occurs in 1% to 3% of patients, depending on the indication for the surgery. Causes include embolization from a friable or ulcerated plaque during carotid dissection, inadequate cerebral perfusion during endarterectomy, thrombosis from a flap or technical error, and reperfusion syndrome. Most of the reported low rates of stroke are from specialized centers, and a more realistic complication rate from the community data for combined stroke morbidity and mortality ranges from 6% to 20%. The Stroke Council of the American Heart Association has set standards for upper acceptable limits of stroke and death as a function of indications for endarterectomy. For patients with asymptomatic carotid disease, the combined operative stroke morbidity and mortality should not be more than 3%; for TIA, 5%; for history of previous stroke, 7%; and for recurrent carotid stenosis, 10%.

Injury to the cranial nerves can cause postoperative morbidity. The incidence has been found to be approximately 16%; incidence increases to 39% if further evaluation was performed by a speech pathologist. Only 60% of these patients are symptomatic and most of these symptoms are temporary. After 6 weeks, the incidence was between 1% to 4%. Dysfunction of the superior laryngeal and recurrent laryngeal nerves is the most common cranial nerve injury encountered. This is likely caused by retraction injury or direct trauma by forceps during surgery, which can lead to paralysis of the vocal cord in the paramedian position, resulting in hoarseness and loss of an effective cough mechanism. Unilateral injury can be asymptomatic but can cause air way obstruction if there is bilateral injury. If staged bilateral carotid endarterectomy is planned, routine direct visualization of the vocal cord by laryngoscopy is recommended after the first endarterectomy. Staged surgery is delayed if there is cord paralysis. Wound retraction can also cause injury to the hypoglossal nerve during superior exposure for high carotid bifurcation. This is manifested by tongue deviation to the ipsilateral side, but can occasionally cause speech impairment and mastication problem.

### Carotid Angioplasty and Stent Procedure

Many randomized trials have shown that carotid endarterectomy is effective in preventing stroke in symptomatic and asymptomatic patients with significant internal carotid stenosis. It has been accepted that CEA is the gold standard of treatment for these patients. However, there remain a group of patients that has been identified as high risk for CEA. Carotid angioplasty and stenting (CAS) has emerged as a safe and effective alternative to CEA for patients with indications for carotid intervention. Over the past decade, CAS has seen a rapid evolution in technique and technology with the introduction of self-expanding nitinol stents, smaller delivery systems, and embolic protection devices (EPD).

Early single-center studies performed from 1990 to 1999 showed significantly higher rates of stroke and death for CAS than for CEA in 30-day outcomes for symptomatic patients. The risk of major stroke or death was 3.9% after CAS and 2.2% after CEA, and the risk of any stroke or death was 7.8% for CAS and 4% for CEA. During these studies, most CAS procedures were performed without an EPD. When early studies were designed to randomize patients between CAS and CEA, many had to be terminated prematurely because of inferior results with CAS. These studies showed that patients with unprotected CAS without EPD had a higher stroke rate than with CEA and protected CAS, and that unprotected CAS was not equivalent to CEA. The Stenting and Angioplasty with Protection in Patients at High Risk for Endarterectomy (SAPPHIRE) trial was the first randomized study to show the benefits of using EPD in CAS, and that protected CAS was not inferior to CEA in high risk patients. Most recently, in 2010, preliminary results from the Carotid Revascularization Endarterectomy vs. Stent Trial (CREST) became available. This was the first multicenter prospective, randomized clinical trial funded by the National Institutes of Health to compare the safety and efficacy of CAS and CEA in symptomatic and asymptomatic patients. Preliminary end points were any clinical stroke, myocardial infarction, or death and any ipsilateral stroke over the entire follow-up period. There were 2502 patients (asymptomatic, 47%; symptomatic 53%), with a median follow-up period of 2.5 years. In regard to the primary composite end point, there was no difference between CAS and CEA (7.2% for CAS versus 6.8% for CEA; $P = .51$). There was a statistically significant difference in 30-day stroke rate, 4.1% for CAS and 2.3% for CEA. The risk of myocardial infarction was significantly lower for CAS, 1.1%, compared with CEA, 2.3%. At median follow-up of 2.5 years, there was no difference in stroke rate between CAS and CEA.

The latest data from CREST have shown similar composite outcomes between the two procedures, which led the investigators to conclude that both CAS and CEA had similar composite outcomes, with differences in periprocedural stroke and myocardial infarction. It is likely that there will be more demand from the public for this less invasive modality for the treatment of high-grade carotid disease. Of note, carotid angioplasty and stenting procedures performed during the second half of this 10-year trial had a significantly lower incidence of complications as compared with those CAS procedures performed during the first half of the study. These findings indicate improvements in device design and operator experience over time and suggest that future results may continue to improve with this technique.

**Indications and Contraindications** CAS is currently indicated for symptomatic high-risk patients. Indications for symptomatic patients with high-grade carotid stenosis were outlined in the consensus conference of the Stroke Council of the American Heart Association (see earlier). At the time of this printing, The Centers for Medicine and Medicaid Services continue to deny coverage for carotid stent procedures for asymptomatic patients as well as symptomatic patients who are deemed good-risk candidates for CEA.

There is a group of patients that are considered high risk for open surgical CEA. They can be grouped into two main categories, those with anatomic or physiologic conditions. High-risk anatomic conditions include the following: (1) restenosis after previous CEA caused by association with higher risk of cranial nerve injury; (2) "hostile" neck from previous neck radiation, radial neck dissection, permanent tracheostomy, or frozen neck; (3) high or low lesions above C2 or below the clavicle, respectively; and (4) other carotid lesions, including tandem lesions within the same carotid artery and contralateral high-grade ICA disease. High-risk physiologic conditions include the following: (1) class III or IV angina or congestive heart failure; (2) severe chronic obstructive pulmonary disease (forced expiratory volume ≤1 or the need for home oxygen); and (3) cardiac disease necessitating open heart surgery within 4 weeks.

Contraindications for CAS include coils or kinking of the common or internal carotid artery, and excessive calcification of the carotid disease. Difficult access because of iliac disease and a tortuous and calcified arch, or tandem common carotid stenoses, may also contribute to difficulties in stent delivery.

### Technique

***Carotid Artery Access and Guide Sheath Positioning*** Just as in CEA, patients are medically optimized with anti-hypertensives, statins, and smoking cessation. Patients who have not been taking clopidogrel are given an oral leading dose of 600 mg, and then maintained on 75 mg by mouth daily. Retrograde common femoral artery access is usually the first choice, primarily secondary to table and patient positioning constraints. Brachial access is used only in certain circumstances, such as severe aortoiliac occlusive disease. The patient receives a systemic IV bolus of heparin (≈100 U/kg) after initial sheath placement. In most cases, diagnostic arteriography and the intervention are performed at separate times. A diagnostic arch aortography with four-vessel extracranial and bilateral cerebral arteriography is first performed for the evaluation of the carotid disease, cerebral circulation, and procedural planning. The aortogram is obtained with a pigtail catheter in the ascending aorta in left anterior oblique angulation. The bilateral common carotid arteries are then catheterized for arteriograms of the ICA and cerebral circulation. The subclavian arteries are catheterized for the evaluation of vertebral arteries. After the diagnostic arteriography, the patient is discharged on the same day.

For patients requiring treatment, the intervention is performed at a later time. Based on the diagnostic arteriogram, appropriately shaped catheters and sheaths are chosen. To limit contrast, a selective catheterization can be made based on a previous arch aortogram. Most common carotid arteries can be accessed simply with an angled catheter (e.g., Glidecath); however, some will require a more complex-shaped catheter, such as a cobra, shepherd's hook, or Simmons catheter. Selective carotid angiography is then performed with careful hand injections of contrast. A 0.035-inch guidewire (e.g., Glidewire) is positioned in the ECA and catheterized by the angled catheter. An angiogram is used to confirm the location of the ECA. A stiff wire is then placed in this artery and the catheter and short groin sheath are removed and exchanged for a long 6 Fr sheath. The tip of the sheath is advanced to the distal common carotid artery. The stiff wire is removed from the patient.

***Placement of Embolic Protection Device*** With the long sheath near the carotid bulb, a careful angiogram with hand injection is obtained to determine the anatomy of the disease and location of the ICA. The wire with the EPD is advanced across the disease and into the distal ICA, just prior to the horizontal petrous segment. The EPD is deployed. Flow through the EPD and its apposition to the wall is evaluated.

***Carotid Stent Placement*** An angiogram is then obtained, noting the location of the carotid disease. The stent is advanced carefully across the disease and it is deployed from the ICA into the CCA, covering the ECA origin (Fig. 63-30). Prestenting angioplasty is not routinely performed unless necessary to create a space needed for placement of the stent in near-occlusive lesions. The self-expanding nitinol stent is typically 8 to 10 mm in diameter by 30 mm in length. It is sized to the largest portion of the vessel, usually the distal CCA. A small stent that does not oppose the carotid wall may become a nidus for thrombus formation. Current stents are designed to be used in small delivery systems using a rapid exchange or monorail platform.

***Carotid Angioplasty*** After stenting, poststenting angioplasty is performed. The patient receives 0.5 mg of atropine intravenously immediately prior to angioplasty to blunt the effect of pressure from the balloon on the carotid bulb. An angioplasty balloon is advanced over the 0.014-inch guidewire across the location of the narrowest area of the stent. The balloon should approximate the size of the native normal internal carotid artery beyond the stenosis, not a segment with poststenotic dilation. Typically, the initial angioplasty is performed with a 5-mm semicompliant balloon. The balloon is inflated slowly until apposition is achieved and then deflated slowly. Transcranial Doppler may be used to monitor for embolic debris. Experience with this procedure has shown that the greatest number of emboli are released with balloon deflation.

***Completion Angiogram*** Prior to removal of the guidewire and sheath, a completion angiogram is obtained to confirm adequate resolution of the carotid disease and to ensure flow through the ICA. Spasm of the ICA distal to the stent can be treated with vasodilators such as nitroglycerin or papaverine. However, most spasms resolve with removal of the EPD. Once the EPD is removed, another angiogram is obtained to confirm vasodilation of the vessel and flow. A closure device is then used to close the arteriotomy. If a patient has neurologic functional changes, a cerebral angiogram is obtained and compared with previous diagnostic angiograms. Nonvisualization of cerebral arteries after stenting, but that were previously seen on a diagnostic angiogram, is of concern for an embolic event and an intervention must be carried out (Fig. 63-31).

Neurologic deficits that occur as a result of stent placement are not the same as those that occur with carotid surgery.[117] Rather than an immediate intraprocedural event, a substantial number of the periprocedural events that occur with CAS occur hours to days after the procedure. In one study, 26% of the periprocedural neurologic events occurred more than 1 day (and up to 14 days) after the procedure, and after patient discharge.[118] In another study, 71% of the periprocedural deficits (10 of 14) after carotid stent placement in 111 patients occurred after the procedure was completed, rather than during the procedure.[119] This presents logistic challenges if intracranial thrombolysis ever

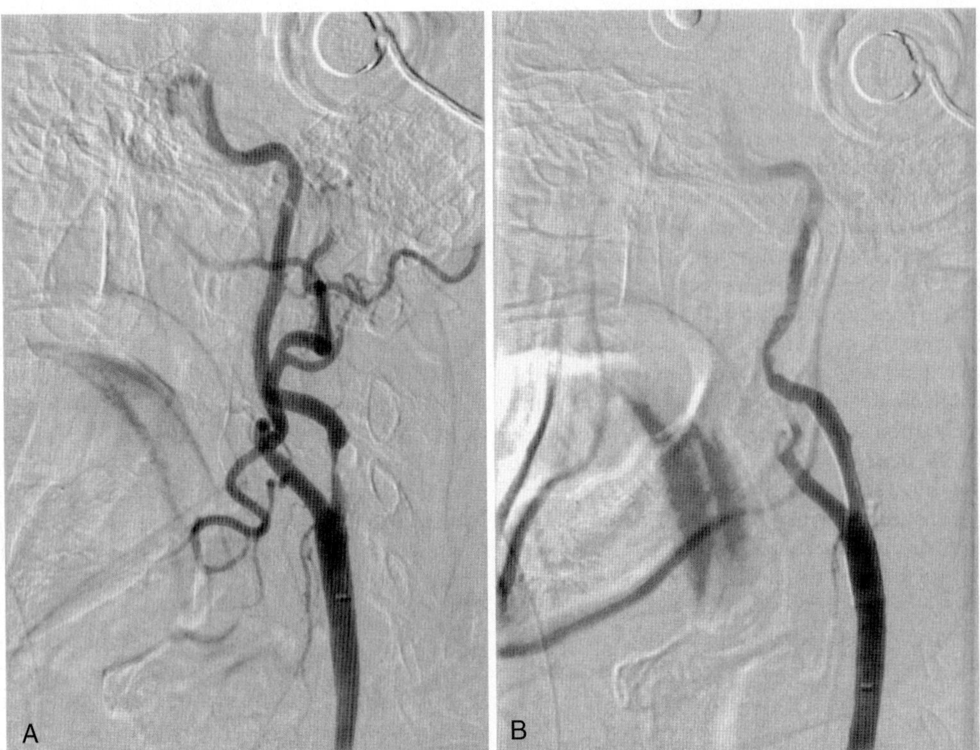


**FIGURE 63-30** Carotid stent. **A,** Severe ICA stenosis. **B,** Improved flow following ICA stent placement.

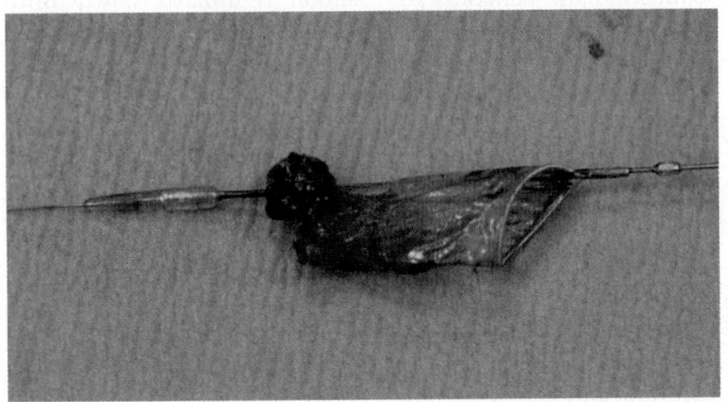

**FIGURE 63-31** Embolic protection device; filter with acute thrombus.

becomes the standard method for managing this problem, because it often occurs after catheters and intra-arterial access devices have been removed; in some cases, the patient may already have been discharged. The patient would have to return and be treated in a timely manner. The site at which the carotid stent was placed would require repeat instrumentation (crossing with guidewires and catheters), with the attendant added risk of additional embolization.

***Conclusions*** The CREST trial demonstrated a significant learning curve with CAS. In carotid angioplasty and stenting, patient selection is the key to early success. Patients who are good stent candidates because of high medical comorbidities may not always have favorable anatomy for stent placement and will likely have an elevated risk of periprocedural complications, even from a percutaneous procedure. Some patients with complex anatomy but who are otherwise good candidates for CAS may have to be treated by alternative means if seen early in the program's development, while the physican is accumulating experience. The best early candidates for CAS are patients with focal recurrent stenosis. Performance of CAS requires excellent imaging; the procedure is facilitated by the use of a floating radiolucent table. Specific equipment and tools for carotid arteriography, balloon angioplasty, and stent placement differ somewhat from those used for other vascular beds. The components for carotid intervention must be determined, understood, requested, and assembled before proceeding. There is growing consensus that CAS may be an effective alternative treatment for high-grade carotid artery disease that avoids the morbidity and mortality of open surgical treatment. Outside of clinical trials, it is currently indicated for symptomatic high-risk patients. With the results from CREST recently published, it is likely that approved indications will be expanded to include normal-risk, high-grade symptomatic and asymptomatic patients. Vascular surgeons have traditionally assumed a leadership role in the management of carotid disease. If we are to continue to provide our patients with the full breadth of therapeutic alternatives, it is imperative that we develop the necessary skills to perform safe and effective carotid angioplasty and stenting procedures while maintaining our open surgical expertise with carotid endarterectomy. Further rigorous scientific investigation will allow us to elucidate the subtle characteristics of patients and their lesions that may better inform our recommendations for one of these two competing treatment options.

## DIALYSIS ACCESS

### Dialysis Outcomes Quality Initiative (DOQI) Guidelines

Three types of access are commonly placed for hemodialysis: (1) autogenous fistula (AF); (2) prosthetic bridging graft (BG); and (3) indwelling central venous catheter. The ideal access delivers a flow rate sufficient for effective dialysis, is easily cannulated, has a long life, and has a low complication rate.

### Dialysis Outcome Quality Initiative Guidelines

Currently, autogenous fistulas are preferred to prosthetic grafts and central venous catheters because of their higher primary patency rates and lower frequency of stenosis, thrombosis, and infection.[134,135] Previously, prosthetic conduit was often used for the initial hemodialysis access. Justification for a preference for prosthetic grafts included technical ease of procedure, avoidance of prolonged maturation times, ease of cannulation, differences in reimbursement, and disbelief in the superiority of autogenous fistulas.[136] The reluctance to perform native fistulas was also fueled by the wide range of reported rates of patency and maturation to a functional access with traditional single-incision direct arteriovenous fistulas, such as the wrist radiocephalic fistula. Maturation rates of arteriovenous fistulas range from 25% to 90%.[123,137-139]

The U.S. Renal Data System (USRDS), which accumulates and reviews data from the nation's dialysis centers, reported in 1995 that the frequency of native AF construction in the United States was less than 30% of total access procedures performed, with some regions having AF placement rates less than 10%.[121] In 1996, the DOQI Vascular Access Work Group met at the request of the National Kidney Foundation to address all aspects of current medical and surgical issues associated with hemodialysis and publish a set of practice guidelines.

To attain the goals recommended by DOQI, surgeons are expected to increase their rates of autogenous arteriovenous fistulas to at least 50% of all new permanent hemodialysis accesses constructed. An important objective of DOQI is to have a prevalence of autogenous fistulas in 40% of all hemodialysis patients.

### Nomenclature

In 2002, the Committee on Reporting Standards for Arterio-Venous Accesses of the Society for Vascular Surgery and the American Association for Vascular Surgery published standardized definitions related to arteriovenous access procedures and recommended reporting standards for patency and complications.[145] *Autogenous* refers to the native vein. An autogenous AV access is an access created by a connection between an artery and vein, and the vein serves as the access site for needle cannulation. A transposition is an access performed with a transposed vein. The peripheral portion of the vein is moved from its original position, usually through a superficial subcutaneous tunnel, and connected to the artery. The more central venous segment in a transposed access is left in its anatomic position. In contrast, the term *translocated* is used to describe an access constructed from a segment of vein that has been completely mobilized, disconnected proximally and distally, and placed in a location remote from its origin. The recommended nomenclature for the autogenous transposition procedures can be found in Table 63-9.

**Table 63-9 Recommended Nomenclature for Transposition Access Procedures**

| RECOMMENDED NOMENCLATURE | TRADITIONAL NOMENCLATURE |
|---|---|
| Forearm | |
| Autogenous radial-basilic forearm transposition | Superficial venous transposition in the forearm, basilic vein to radial artery |
| Autogenous ulnar-basilic forearm transposition | Superficial venous transposition in the forearm, basilic vein to ulnar artery |
| Autogenous radial-cephalic forearm transposition | Superficial venous transposition in the forearm, cephalic vein to radial artery |
| Autogenous brachial-cephalic forearm transposition | Superficial venous transposition in the forearm, cephalic vein to brachial artery |
| Upper arm | |
| Autogenous brachial-basilic upper arm transposition | Basilic vein transposition |
| Lower extremity | |
| Autogenous femoral-greater saphenous looped access transposition | Greater saphenous vein end-to-side to femoral artery fistula |

Adapted from Sidawy AN, Gray R, Besarab A: Recommended standards for reports dealing with arteriovenous hemodialysis accesses. J Vasc Surg 35:603–810, 2002.

Configuration descriptors provide information about the anastomotic connection and course of the conduit. An access has a direct or indirect configuration. A direct access describes the connection between native artery and vein and involves such configurations as end-to-side, side-to-side, and end-to-end anastamoses.[145] In an indirect access, an autogenous or prosthetic graft is interposed between the native artery and vein. Additional descriptors may be used, such as transposed, translocated, straight, and looped.

*Primary patency* refers to the interval from the time of access placement to the intervention designed to maintain or reestablish patency or access thrombosis, or the time of measurement of patency. *Assisted primary patency* refers to the interval from the time of access placement until access thrombosis or the time of measurement or patency, including interventions designed to maintain the function of a patent access. *Secondary patency* refers to the interval from the time of access placement until access abandonment or thrombosis, or the time of patency measurement, including interventions to reestablish function in a thrombosed access.[145]

### Superficial Venous System of the Upper Extremity

An understanding of the venous anatomy of the upper extremity is essential for the planning of permanent hemodialysis access. Although there is an anatomic commonality among patients that represents a starting point for inspection, anatomic variations and segmental venous stenoses and occlusions from previous medical or surgical interventions are important to identify by thorough preoperative assessment.

### Cephalic Vein

The cephalic vein arises from the radial aspect of the veins draining the dorsum of the hand and travels around the radial border of the forearm. On the proximal aspect of the volar forearm, the median cubital vein arises. This vein communicates with the deep veins in the forearm and then crosses the antecubital fossa to join the basilic vein. As it crosses the elbow, the cephalic vein is found in an anatomic groove between the brachioradialis and biceps muscles. The cephalic vein travels superficially to the musculocutaneous nerve and then ascends in the groove along the lateral border of the biceps muscle. In the upper third of the arm, the cephalic vein passes between the pectoralis major and deltoid muscles, crosses the axillary artery, and joins the axillary vein just below the clavicle. The accessory cephalic vein arises from the ulnar side of the dorsum of the hand or the posterior aspect of the forearm and usually joins the cephalic vein below the elbow.

### Basilic Vein

The basilic vein originates on the ulnar aspect of the dorsum of the hand and travels in the subcutaneous space up the ulnar side of the forearm, shifting from the posterior surface distally toward a more anterior orientation below the elbow. The median antecubital vein joins the basilic vein in the antecubital fossa and then travels in the groove between the biceps and pronator teres muscles to cross the brachial artery. In this region, the vein is crossed anteriorly and posteriorly by branches of the median cutaneous nerve. As it courses proximately along the medial border of the biceps muscle, the basilic vein descends below the deep fascia to travel parallel to the brachial artery and vein. The union of the basilic and brachial veins in the axilla forms the axillary vein.

### Median Antebrachial Vein

The median antebrachial vein drains the palmar surface of the hand and is located on the ulnar side of the anterior forearm. In the proximal forearm, it joins the basilic vein or median antecubital vein.

## Initial Evaluation for New Access

The first step in establishing hemodialysis access is to select the best available site, based on optimal arterial inflow and venous outflow, observing the preference of an AF over a BG, forearm over upper arm, and nondominant over dominant upper extremity. Visual inspection and physical examination of the upper extremity are performed but may be inadequate to assess certain factors, especially vein size, quality, and adequacy of central venous outflow. For this reason, duplex ultrasound scanning is used for all patients.

The examination is initiated at the wrist of the nondominant upper extremity and a tourniquet is placed at the midforearm. After dilation of the superficial veins by gentle tapping and stroking, the veins are insonated with a 5- or 7-MHz scanning probe. They are evaluated for diameter, compressibility, and continuity with upper arm veins. Patency of the deep system and continuity with patent axillary and subclavian veins are also verified. Central venous stenosis or thrombosis precludes use of that arm.

The largest diameter superficial vein of good quality is mapped with skin markings. Suitability criteria for access include the following:

1. Target vein diameter more than 2.5 mm for an AF and more than 4.0 mm for a BG
2. Continuity with the deep and central system
3. Absence of stenoses

When favorable venous anatomy is found, the arterial system is then evaluated for target artery diameter and patency of the palmar arch. Reduced pressure measurements, compared with the other arm or abnormal Doppler waveforms, indicate proximal arterial stenosis and preclude use of that arm for access unless the problem is successfully addressed. The basic requirements are as follows:

1. An arterial luminal diameter greater than 2.0 mm
2. Absence of obliterating calcification
3. Palmar arch patency

Evaluation of central venous outflow stenosis or occlusion is an integral part of the duplex ultrasound examination. Central venous stenosis usually results from previous use of central catheters, especially in the subclavian vein.[124]

If a unilateral central vein problem is found, the contralateral extremity becomes the preferred choice regardless of the issue of extremity dominance. If bilateral central vein problems exist but are amenable to endovascular treatment, this should be attempted on the least diseased side.

If a subsequent duplex scan confirms effective treatment of the central vein problem, this arm can be selected for access. If not, the patient requires a nonstandard complex access solution (see later).

Anticipated duration of dialysis determines the type of catheter access selected.

1. Patients expected to require dialysis for less than 3 weeks are candidates for noncuffed central venous catheter access for dialysis; these dual-lumen catheters may be placed at the bedside without fluoroscopic guidance.
2. For patients expected to require dialysis longer than 3 weeks, cuffed tunneled catheters are placed.
3. For patients undergoing placement of an AF who require immediate dialysis, a cuffed tunneled catheter is placed concurrently, typically in the contralateral internal jugular vein, to provide access while the AF matures.

The internal jugular vein is preferred over the subclavian vein; the contralateral deep venous system is accessed when possible to avoid catheter obstruction of venous outflow or catheter-induced venous stenosis during the period of AF maturation. Duplex scans aid in the selection of a patent normal vein for catheter placement. Femoral catheters can also be used on a temporary basis if the deep central venous system of the upper extremity is intractably compromised.

## Central Venous Catheters

A cuffed central venous catheter is placed in all patients requiring immediate dialysis following AF formation so that adequate maturation time (6 to 12 weeks) can be provided before cannulation of the AF. Because a BG can generally be used within 3 weeks, temporary noncuffed catheters can be used in this group.

The contralateral internal jugular vein is the preferred site, if available, because it limits ipsilateral venous outflow obstruction and would not be associated with the development of subclavian vein stenosis. Alternate sites may be used:

1. Ipsilateral internal jugular vein. This choice poses some risk of venous outflow obstruction because the catheter physically rests across the confluence of the internal jugular vein and the now high-flow subclavian vein, but has the benefit of limiting subclavian vein stenosis.
2. Contralateral subclavian vein. Perhaps there would be less outflow obstruction but greater potential for negative long-term sequelae if stenosis results.
3. Ipsilateral subclavian vein. This is the least attractive alternative, with potential for outflow obstruction and stenosis.

The routine use of upper extremity duplex ultrasound imaging for access planning identifies many patients who have veins suitable for AF formation but that are too deep for successful cannulation or that are too remote from the optimal arterial inflow to allow direct anastomosis without tension. Superficial venous transposition in the forearm increases AF rates in these patients.[125] This technique involves extensive dissection of a vein identified by duplex scan as being suitable in diameter, with ligation of side branches and transposition to a subcutaneous tunnel along the volar aspect of the forearm, bringing the vein to the inflow artery. This position is optimal for comfortable arm positioning during dialysis.

## Types of Venous Transpositions

### Upper Arm Venous Transposition

The basilic vein in the upper arm is often a good conduit for dialysis access because of its relatively large size and location in the deeper tissue planes. The traumatic consequences of repeated venipunctures observed in more superficial veins are not seen in the basilic vein because of its deeper position. Classically, the brachiobasilic transposition was regarded as a secondary option after a failed forearm fistula or graft.[146] The creation of an access using the proximal basilic vein was devised on the basis of the theoretical benefits of using a superficial vein spared repeated venipunctures and with a relatively large diameter and length. As with all venous transpositions, only one anastomosis is required, and anatomic continuity with the axillary vein is maintained. The transposition of the basilic vein to the brachial artery was described by Dagher in 1976. Four years after the original description of 24 brachiobasilic fistulas, the 5-year follow-up of a series of 90 fistulas was reported, with a 73.5% patency rate. The long-term patency remained good; a 70% functional patency rate at 8 years in 176 fistulas was reported.[147]

In certain patient subgroups, such as those with small cephalic veins, peripheral vascular disease, and diabetes, the maturation rate of the radiocephalic fistula has been poor. The brachiobasilic transposition has been a good second option for these patients. Hakaim and associates[137] have reported on the superior fistula maturation in brachiobasilic transpositions (73%) compared with primary radiocephalic arteriovenous fistulas (30%). When the forearm cephalic vein is not suitable for access creation, the basilic vein in the forearm and upper arm are excellent secondary options.[148] Ascher and coworkers[149] have reviewed their experience using arm veins to create brachiocephalic and brachiobasilic arteriovenous fistulas. They found no significant difference between primary patency rates at 1 year (72% for brachiocephalic versus 70% for brachiobasilic). Because of excellent patency with these fistulas, this group proposed an algorithm for the placement of arteriovenous fistulas. If a radiocephalic fistula is not feasible, a brachiocephalic fistula should first be attempted. If the brachiocephalic fistula fails or is not possible, a brachiobasilic fistula should be placed before an arteriovenous graft. In an attempt to maximize the autogenous fistula rate, we favor a similar algorithm, with the addition of the superficial venous transposition of the forearm before performance of the brachial artery–based fistulas—that is, radiocephalic fistula, followed by forearm basilic venous transposition, followed by brachiocephalic fistula, followed by brachiobasilic fistula.

Long-term patency with translocated brachiobasilic fistulas that have matured has been good, with reported primary patency rates as high as 90% at 1 year and 86% at 2 years.[150] In 2000, a series of 74 arteriovenous fistulas constructed using transposed basilic vein was reported by Murphy and colleagues.[151] Successful needle cannulation for hemodialysis was accomplished in 50 fistulas (68%) and the cumulative secondary patency rate was 73% at 1 year, 53% at 2 years, and 43% at 3 years. In 2003, Taghizadeh and associates[152] reported a series of 75 brachiobasilic transpositions performed over 5 years, with a mean follow-up of 14 months. In their series, 92% of fistulas matured to allow hemodialysis access. The cumulative patency was 66% at 1 year, 52% at 2 years, and 43% at 3 years. Overall, complications developed in 55% of fistulas; these included thrombosis (33%), stenosis (11%), local infection (6%), arm edema (5%), hemorrhage (3%), aneurysm (1%), and steal syndrome (1%).

The overall patency rate for autogenous brachial-basilic transpositions is superior to that of polytetrafluoroethylene (PTFE) upper arm dialysis grafts. A review of all basilic vein transpositions and brachial PTFE arteriovenous fistulas created over a 5-year period has demonstrated a statistically significant difference in primary patency rate at 1 year (90% versus 70%; $P<.01$) and 2 years (86% versus 49%; $P<.001$).[150] In this study, complications occurred approximately twice as frequently with the PTFE grafts than with the venous transpositions. Another comparison between brachial-basilic transpositions and PTFE upper arm grafts has shown significant better patency rate at 2 years with venous transpositions (70% versus 46% for PTFE grafts).[153]

### Forearm Venous Transpositions

The radiocephalic fistula, performed through a single incision, was initially described in 1966 by Brescia and coworkers.[154] This primary arteriovenous fistula was a dramatic improvement over the other, less durable modes of hemodialysis access available at the time and soon became the preferred approach to long-term dialysis access. The hemodialysis population has changed, and the dialysis patient who has a suitable vein in close proximity to the radial artery is becoming uncommon. Therefore, venous transposition procedures in the forearm have become important for enabling these patients to have a primary arteriovenous fistula.

Physical examination and visual inspection alone identify suitable arteries and veins in the upper extremity poorly. Duplex ultrasound examination allows a more thorough evaluation of the superficial venous system, increasing the number of patients who can have a forearm fistula.[125] The duplex scan can identify veins in the forearm that may have been spared repeated venipunctures because of their deeper subcutaneous location. The size of these veins may be suitable for arteriovenous creation but, if left in situ, their position in the deeper subcutaneous tissues and their anatomic position on the forearm make needle cannulation for hemodialysis technically more difficult. These usable veins on the posterior aspect of the forearm, such as the basilic vein, if not transposed, require uncomfortable and awkward positioning of the arm for dialysis. Therefore, once identified by duplex scanning, these veins are mobilized and transposed to a more favorable location on the forearm through a superficial subcutaneous plane.

To increase the number of primary autogenous fistulas, Silva and colleagues,[125] in 1997, described the routine use of duplex scanning for preoperative access planning for superficial venous transposition of forearm veins for autogenous hemodialysis access. They reported a series of 89 patients in whom arteries and veins were identified with duplex scanning as suitable for primary arteriovenous fistulas. After the superficial venous transposition procedure, 91% of the fistulas matured, to be used for hemodialysis access. The primary patency rate was 84% at 1 year and 69% at 2 years. (The beneficial impact of a preoperative duplex ultrasound assessments was reported in 1998.[123]) This group demonstrated a dramatic improvement in their autogenous fistula rate with the institution of the protocol of routine use of duplex scanning for preoperative access planning. Their autogenous fistula rate was 14% before the institution of the protocol and 63% after the protocol was established. Table 63-10 demonstrates the three general areas in which the superficial veins are found and the rates at which they were used in the study. Note that the minority (15%) of the transpositions were accomplished through a single incision, with the artery and vein in close proximity. Approximately 50% of transposed veins arose from the volar surface of the forearm and a third were harvested from the dorsal aspect of the forearm.

### Lower Extremity Venous Transpositions

The upper extremity is the preferred site for hemodialysis access, with the lower extremity generally being reserved for use once upper extremity options have been exhausted. If the extremity is not suitable for fistula creation, a prosthetic graft can be placed. However, there is a concern about increased thrombosis and infection rates in thigh hemodialysis grafts, which have been reported as high as 55% and 35%, respectively. Tashjian and associates,[155] reviewing their experience with 73 femoral artery–based hemodialysis grafts, found a primary patency rate of 71% and a secondary patency rate of 83% at 1 year. The infection rate in this series was 22%.

Venous transpositions in the lower extremity using the greater saphenous vein (GSV) and superficial femoral vein (SFV) have been described.[135,156] The use of translocated GSVs and SFVs in the leg have theoretical benefits similar to those of venous translocations in the upper extremity. The venous conduits are long and generally of good caliber, and are less prone to infection than prosthetic grafts. Importantly, only one anastomosis is required, because the more central venous segment maintains its native connection with the common femoral vein.

The SFV, part of the deep venous system, has a diameter in the range of 6 to 10 mm, has relatively thick walls, and has been used for a wide variety of vascular reconstructions.[157] Gradman and coworkers have reported a retrospective analysis of 25 patients who underwent arteriovenous construction using SFVs. Of these patients, 18 underwent SFV transposition and 7 were given a composite loop fistula of SFV and PTFE. The cumulative primary fistula patency rate was 78% at 6 months and 73% at 1 year. The cumulative secondary patency rate was 91% at 5 months and 86% at 1 year. There were no fistula infections, but the rate of major wound complications was 28%. Eight patients required secondary procedures for symptomatic steal syndrome and 1 patient ultimately needed an above-knee amputation after the development of ipsilateral compartment syndrome.[156]

The saphenous vein has been used for arterial reconstructions in almost all vascular beds and in the construction of arteriovenous access in the upper and lower extremities. The GSV has been used to create an autogenous fistula in the upper thigh in a looped configuration and an arterial anastomosis with the common femoral artery or SFA.[158-160] Although described more than 30 years ago, this configuration is seldom used.[35] Illig and coworkers,[161] noting that the incidence of infection can be as high as 40% in traditional saphenous vein harvest, have used an endoscopic vein harvest technique in combination with the creation of a transposed saphenous vein arteriovenous fistula.

**Table 63-10 Superficial Venous Transpositions of the Forearm**

| TRANSPOSITION PERFORMED | % OF TOTAL |
|---|---|
| Type A | 15 |
| Artery and vein in immediate proximity | |
| Single incision | |
| Superficial subcutaneous transposition only | |
| Type B | 33 |
| Dorsally located vein transposed to volar surface artery | |
| Separate incisions | |
| Superficial subcutaneous transposition | |
| Type C | 52 |
| Volar vein transposed to mid forearm volar surface | |
| Separate incisions | |
| Superficial subcutaneous transposition | |

From Silva MB Jr, Hobson RW 2nd, Pappas PJ, et al: Vein transposition in the forearm for autogenous hemodialysis access. J Vasc Surg 26:981–986, 1997.

## Techniques of Venous Transposition

### Patient Assessment and Selection of Optimal Site

The patient evaluation and preoperative assessment are the most important steps in the establishment of durable hemodialysis access. First, the best available site is selected, based on optimal arterial inflow and venous outflow,. According to DOQI guidelines, the preference is for an autogenous fistula over a prosthetic graft, the forearm over the upper arm, and the nondominant arm over the dominant arm.

Preference for the nondominant arm relates to convenience for the patient, allowing the dominant arm to be used for activity during dialysis. When duplex ultrasound surveillance identifies a suitable vein and artery in the nondominant forearm, an AF constructed between them becomes the procedure of choice. Duplex ultrasonography to select the optimal anastomotic site. If the radial or ulnar arteries are disadvantaged, a suitable vein in the forearm may be dissected and looped back to the brachial artery in the antecubital space. All autogenous forearm possibilities are exhausted before proceeding to autogenous upper arm alternatives, because this maximizes future possible sites.

Absence of suitable veins in both forearms necessitates construction of the access in the upper arm. Again, duplex ultrasonography is valuable in identifying a superficial (preferred) or deep (second-choice) arm vein that can be transposed to a volar subcutaneous location for creation of an AF with the brachial artery. The dominant upper arm is used if the arteries and veins in the nondominant upper arm are unsuitable.

If there are no suitable veins for an AF, outflow through the deeper venous system in the arm is examined to identify a possible site of placement of a prosthetic BG. A looped BG configuration is used in the nondominant forearm when an appropriate antecubital vein and brachial artery are present.

The dominant forearm is the next site of choice. If both forearms are unsuitable, the nondominant upper arm, followed by the dominant upper arm, are the next options for curved brachial artery to axillary vein BGs.

Duplex ultrasonography is used to identify and mark the best possible location for the anastomosis and to confirm adequate central venous runoff. When possible, avoid placement of prosthetic BGs in patients who are significantly immunocompromised because of the significant risk of infection and the complexities involved with removal of the BG and restoration of prograde arterial flow.[126]

### Superficial Venous Transposition of the Forearm

The superficial venous transposition of the forearm is performed using local 1% lidocaine infusion supplemented with IV sedation. Lidocaine with epinephrine is avoided because of its vasoconstrictive properties. The entire arm is prepared in a sterile fashion and the procedure is performed by the surgeon and assistant in the seated position.

Once the skin and subcutaneous tissue overlying the vein have been properly anesthetized, a longitudinal incision is made directly over the cephalic or basilic vein, beginning at the distal extent of the previously mapped and marked vein. The incision proceeds toward the antecubital fossa for a distance of at least 15 cm. A 3-0 silk suture ligature is used to ligate the portion of vein remaining in its distal bed and the vein is transected at the wrist. The vein is dissected free from its surrounding tissue so that it may be completely transposed to a superficial tunnel in the midportion of the volar aspect of the forearm. Most venous branches along the length of the vein are ligated and divided; however, those that will not interfere with transposition are left intact to maximize outflow. Heparinized saline is flushed through the open end of the vein with digital compression for occlusion of outflow at the antecubital fossa; this results in substantial dilation of the freed segment of vein. The vein is wrapped in a heparin- and saline-soaked sponge and attention is then turned to the arterial dissection.

The segment of artery that has been preoperatively identified as suitable for inflow is exposed. Usually, the radial artery is identified between the brachial radialis and flexor carpi radialis tendons. The superficial branch of the radial nerve is located lateral to the radial artery, and this nerve is separated from the radial artery by the brachial radialis muscle. The nerve is sensory at this level and care must be taken not to injure it. Concomitant veins run parallel to the artery on either side. These should be carefully dissected free from the artery, facilitating identification of the numerous small arterial branches. Although there are usually no arterial branches on the anterior aspect of the artery, several paired arterial branches usually leave the radial artery on each side, and they must be addressed. These may be ligated, with the ligature placed approximately 2 mm away from the radial artery to avoid impingement once dilation has occurred. Vessel loops are placed proximally and distally along the artery for vascular control.

A tunneling instrument is passed through the subcutaneous tissues to develop a superficial tunnel. The vein is marked along its length with a sterile marking pen to facilitate passage through the tunnel without twisting or kinking. Once the vein has been passed through the subcutaneous tunnel and hemostasis has been ensured, the patient is typically given 3000 U of heparin IV, and a 1- to 2-mm arteriotomy is made with a no. 11 scalpel blade on the volar surface of the artery. The arteriotomy is extended to approximately 15 to 20 mm with fine Potts scissors. With an 18-gauge angiocatheter, the artery is heparinized locally by injection of heparinized saline distally and then proximally while the vessel loops are simultaneously opened.

An end-to-side anastomosis is performed with 7-0 polypropylene or Gore-Tex PTFE suture (Gore Medical). Before completion of the anastomosis, vascular dilators are used to size the vein and radial artery. This step has the benefit of allowing enlargement of blood vessels in spasm from vessel loops and manipulation.

After the anastomosis is constructed, it is essential that a thrill be felt within the vein. Absence of a thrill indicates a probable technical or anatomic defect and requires further investigation, with exploration of the anastomosis. Wounds are closed with a running subcuticular absorbable stitch. Care is taken to maintain strict atraumatic technique during handling of the skin edges to limit wound complications. Adhesive strips or tape applied directly to the skin are not used.

### Superficial Venous Transposition of the Arm

The transposition of the cephalic or basilic vein is performed with local anesthesia using 1% lidocaine and IV sedation or regional anesthesia using an interscalene nerve block. The entire arm and ipsilateral axilla and shoulder are prepared in a sterile fashion. For the cephalic vein transposition, the vein is found in an anatomic groove between the brachioradialis and biceps muscles. It travels superficially to the musculocutaneous nerve and then ascends in the groove along the lateral border of the biceps muscle. A longitudinal incision over the cephalic vein is used for exposure. For the basilic vein transposition, the vein is identified anterior to the medial epicondyle of the humerus and, through a longitudinal incision along the medial aspect of the upper arm to the axilla, the basilic vein is exposed. The median cutaneous nerve is close to the basilic vein and should be preserved.

All venous branches are ligated and divided. The cephalic vein is mobilized for at least 15 cm. The basilic vein is mobilized to its junction with the brachial vein. The brachial artery can be exposed through the same incision or through a separate incision. Vessel loops are loosely encircled around the brachial artery proximally and distally.

Next, the cephalic or basilic vein is divided near the antecubital fossa and flushed and distended with heparinized saline.

A sterile marking pen is used to mark the vein along its entire length to help avoid twisting during passage through the subcutaneous tunnel created anteriorly between the axilla and antecubital fossa. Approximately 3000 U of IV heparin is administered and proximal and distal control of the brachial artery is obtained with the vessel loops. An end-to-side anastomosis with the brachial artery is constructed with 6-0 polypropylene sutures. After completion of the anastomosis, the fistula is inspected for a thrill. If a thrill is not present, a technical or structural problem is suspected that will require correction. The subcutaneous tissues and skin are closed with absorbable suture.

### Follow-Up

Adequate arterialization of the vein usually occurs within 8 to 12 weeks. Hand exercises are advocated to encourage fistula maturation.

The AF access is studied by duplex ultrasound approximately 6 weeks after placement to assess maturation and to mark sites most suitable for initial cannulation by the dialysis center staff. For a new AF, dialysis should be initiated through a 16- or 17-gauge needle and for longer sessions at minimal rates of flow.

At least three successful hemodialysis sessions should be accomplished before removing the central venous catheter. If flow rates are insufficient for successful dialysis or if follow-up duplex ultrasonography identifies a problem in the access, the access is considered a failure and the patient is referred for evaluation and treatment (see below).

## Patients With Failing or Failed Access

For patients with a failing or failed access, the first step is a thorough duplex ultrasound evaluation of the access and underlying arterial and venous anatomy to ascertain the cause of failure, correctability, or salvage and alternative sites. In particular, patients with a prosthetic BG should be evaluated for graft salvage and for the identification of a possible site for placement of a new AF in case the BG salvage is not successful.

Patients with a failing dialysis catheter typically present with suboptimal flow on dialysis or, less commonly, upper extremity swelling secondary to pericatheter deep vein thrombosis. A duplex ultrasound scan can easily identify the latter, in which case endovascular treatment to reestablish deep venous outflow following catheter removal is considered. Subsequent imaging is directed at assessing the efficacy of treatment and identifying an alternative insertion site.

In patients with poor catheter flow rates but no evidence of central venous compromise, transcatheter thrombolytic therapy has been effective. Tissue plasminogen activator (TPA) instilled directly through the catheter access port and allowed to dwell for some period of time has been effective.

Catheters compromised by malpositioning of the tip or encapsulation in a fibrin sheath can be treated endovascularly.[131] If catheter salvage is unsuccessful, the catheter is exchanged. Over the wire techniques may be used for noncuffed catheters but can be challenging, with cuffed catheters having exit sites remote from the insertion site. This technique may result in similarly poor flow rates if the problem is a suboptimal subcutaneous tunnel, either acutely angled or compromised by proximity to the clavicle. Usually, a new percutaneous placement is performed at the site identified as optimal by duplex ultrasound scans.

Information available from duplex ultrasound examination of a threatened or failed AF or BG is essential for directing treatment. Results with salvaging fistulas or grafts that have thrombosed are significantly worse than with those that are patent but have an identifiable stenosis. Thrombolytic therapy and surgical thrombectomy have poor 6-month primary efficacy rates.[132] Nonetheless, the value of sustaining each access site in today's dialysis population usually warrants an attempt at salvage.

Thrombolysis and surgical thrombectomy are aimed at removing clot as a prerequisite to identifying the underlying anatomic anomaly. Post-thrombectomy access imaging in the surgical suite is imperative. Appropriate adjunctive management of the offending lesion follows—first with endovascular options, if warranted, and surgical revision if the former prove unsuccessful.

Prospective monitoring of the access for hemodynamically significant stenoses, when combined with correction, improves patency and decreases the incidence of thrombosis. A number of techniques have been proposed to monitor for stenoses, including the following:

1. Intra-access flow
2. Static or dynamic venous pressure measurements
3. Measurements of recirculation using urea concentration or dilution techniques
4. Observation for changes in characteristics of pulse or thrill in the access
5. Prolongation of bleeding after needle withdrawal

Most of these techniques suggest increasing resistance at the venous anastomosis, which is the most common site of myointimal hyperplastic problems.

DOQI guidelines suggest that persistent abnormalities in any of these parameters mandate venography. Comprehensive duplex scan can also serve as the initial examination. The decision to proceed with endovascular or surgical treatment is determined by the type of lesion identified and the physician's experience.

In modern vascular practice, endovascular balloon dilation of venous outflow stenoses in a BG or segmental stenoses in an AF is the initial choice of treatment. This must eliminate the hemodynamically significant stenosis and restore normal flow for it to be considered a success (Fig. 63-32).

Postprocedure evaluation by duplex ultrasound scan at 1 month to assess efficacy is recommended. Repeated angioplasty may be performed if indicated. In our practice, two failures of endovascular treatment for the same lesion within a 3-month period prompt open surgical intervention.

Surgical revision can be guided by the duplex scan and by subsequent contrast studies obtained during attempted endovascular revision. Surgical revision is focused on eliminating the causative lesion and preserving the maximal usable segment of vein for future use.

Recalcitrant stenoses in an AF can be treated by patch angioplasty or segmental resection and interposition of a translocated reversed segment of vein or, frequently, by mobilization of the matured vein and primary repair. Arterial or venous stenoses near or involving the anastomosis can be treated with patch angioplasty or, alternatively, with mobilization and formation of a new arteriovenous connection.

For focal defects in a BG, such as midgraft stenosis or pseudoaneurysm, direct excision and interposition of a new

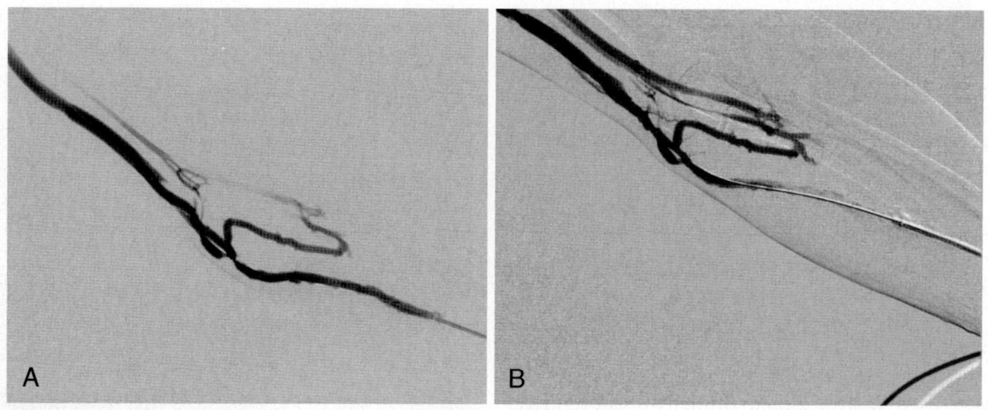


**FIGURE 63-32** Endovascular-assisted arteriovenous fistula (AVF) maturation. **A,** Severe stenosis of radiobasilic AVF. **B,** After balloon angioplasty, flow improved and the patient was able to undergo dialysis within 2 weeks using the AVF.

segment may be indicated. The BG venous outflow lesion resistant to endovascular treatment may be treated with surgical patch angioplasty or a jump graft to a segment of uninvolved vein with good outflow.

Any failed or failing graft that undergoes successful revision and salvage is reassessed at 1 month by duplex ultrasound examination. To achieve the reported 60% 1-year success rates following endovascular or surgical intervention, further intervention is typically required.[133]

## Secondary Interventions in Autogenous Fistulas

Few published series have focused on re-intervention of failing or nonmaturing autogenous arteriovenous fistulas, and most of those that have been reported focused on the traditional radiocephalic arteriovenous fistula. Recognizing this, Hingorani and colleagues[162] have reviewed their experience with salvage procedures in the management of nonfunctioning or nonmaturing arteriovenous fistulas, which included fistulas based in the upper arm. The distribution of fistulas that required salvage procedures were 37% radiocephalic, 47% brachiocephalic, and 16% brachiobasilic. In 46 patients (49 fistulas ), 75 procedures, both open and endovascular, were performed; 17 patients underwent 26 balloon angioplasties and 20 patients had vein patch angioplasty. The group performed 12 fistula revisions to a more proximal level and 4 vein interposition grafts. Although the total number of subsequent procedures required for percutaneously treated fistulas was higher than that for open repair, there was no statistical difference between primary patency rates. It was concluded that salvage procedures may allow maturation and extend the life span of arteriovenous fistulas for hemodialysis.

The beneficial effects of secondary interventions on the maturation and maintenance of autogenous arteriovenous fistulas has been demonstrated by Berman and Gentile.[163] They placed 170 autogenous fistulas in 163 patients—115 brachiocephalic, 47 radiocephalic, and 8 brachiobasilic. Secondary procedures for failure to mature were required in 9 patients and for failure of previously functioning fistulas in 6 patients. A functional access was achieved in 90% of patients; these researchers demonstrated a 10% improvement in accomplishing or maintaining functional autogenous access through secondary procedures.

In a series of arm cephalic and basilic vein arteriovenous fistulas that encompassed 109 brachiocephalic and 63 brachiobasilic arteriovenous fistulas, Ascher and asociates[149] reported thrombosis in 12% and 6%, respectively (no statistical difference). No thrombosed fistula in either group was treated with thrombolysis or thrombectomy. In the brachiocephalic group, 15 secondary interventions were performed—6 balloon angioplasties, 5 patch angioplasties, 2 superficial elevation procedures, and 1 extension to the jugular vein for subclavian vein thrombosis. There were 7 secondary interventions in the brachiobasilic group, 5 balloon angioplasties and 2 patch angioplasties.

In the series of 89 patients with superficial venous transposition of forearm veins after duplex mapping for establishment of hemodialysis access, Silva and coworkers[125] reported a total of 18 failed fistulas. With surgical revision, 4 were successfully salvaged and 6 were converted to ipsilateral prosthetic grafts (3 forearm, 3 upper arm). Additionally, access was established on the other arm in 5 patients (3 autogenous fistulas, 2 prosthetic grafts).

## Complex Access

Complex access solutions are required when all upper extremity access sites have been exhausted or when extensive central venous obliteration is not responsive to endovascular treatment. If the central venous system is patent, placement of a cuffed catheter is the simplest alternative.

In patients with refractory central subclavian vein occlusion and a patent ipsilateral internal jugular vein, the jugular vein turndown procedure may be performed.[127] The cephalad portion of the jugular vein at the angle of the mandible is divided; after mobilization, the jugular vein is anastomosed to the patent axillary vein segment, just proximal to the subclavian occlusion, to provide runoff for the upper arm. Resection of the central portion of the clavicle may be performed to facilitate a favorable anatomic lie of the vein graft. Other nonstandard access configurations, such as axillary artery to axillary vein body wall prosthetic grafts (loop configuration if ipsilateral, crossover or collar graft if contralateral), may be considered.[128] Axillary arterial to right atrial BGs and axillary arterial to arterial prosthetic configurations have been used when extensive central venous obliteration is encountered, but these options are compromised by their potential for increased morbidity.[129,130]

If upper extremity options are unsatisfactory and the superior central venous system is occluded, lower extremity access options can be used. Transposition of the saphenous vein in a loop configuration to the superficial femoral artery or common femoral artery has been performed. Alternatively, a prosthetic BG can be placed in a loop configuration from the common femoral vein to the superficial femoral or common femoral artery. A prosthetic BG can also be created from one femoral artery to a contralateral femoral vein and tunneled subcutaneously across the lower anterior abdominal wall. With a percutaneous approach to the femoral vein, a cuffed catheter can be tunneled into the anterior thigh. In patients with lower extremity venous thrombosis, a translumbar approach to the inferior vena cava has been used with a lateral tunnel for the cuffed catheter.

### Vascular Access Complications

Infection is the second leading cause of death in dialysis patients, causing 10% of deaths, exceeded only by cardiovascular disease. Most of the systemic infections are directly related to infections from vascular access. The increased rate of infection in dialysis patients is caused by immunodeficiency and poor wound healing associated with chronic renal failure. *Staphylococcus aureus* is the most common cause of infection, and the use of aseptic technique is the best way to prevent bacterial colonization and vascular access site infection. Infection of an autogenous arteriovenous fistula is rare; it can be treated with appropriate antibiotics and local wound care, with drainage of abscess. Infection of a prosthetic arteriovenous graft is more common and is caused by contamination from skin flora during implantation or direct inoculation of the graft by an access needle from inadequately prepped skin. Treatment is with excision of the prosthetic material. The use of perioperative antibiotics has been shown to be effective in reducing infections. Cephalosporins can significantly decrease postoperative wound infections and vancomycin can reduce graft infections.

The most common complication of vascular access is thrombosis of the venous fistula or prosthetic graft. The cause of most graft failures is the development of intimal hyperplasia at the venous anastomosis and/or venous outflow tract. This can account for 85% of graft failures, with 55% of thromboses caused by venous anastomosis and 30% caused by venous outflow occlusion or long-segment stenosis. For venous fistula, the specific offending location is not as clear. The lesion can be located at the arterial anastomosis or within the fistula. Flow in the vascular access can be restored with open surgical thrombectomy or endovascular thrombolysis and angioplasty. Venous outflow or anastomotic lesions need to be treated to prevent a high graft failure rate of 70% at 6 months. An improved patency rate of more than 70% at 6 months can be achieved with surgical anastomotic revision or endovascular stenting.

Aneurysmal degeneration of fistula can develop over time. These massively dilated venous segments can involve the skin, placing the patient at risk of significant bleeding. The low resistance of the enlarged fistula can lead to steal syndrome (see later). Treatment is with interposition grafts and removal of the infected portion (Fig. 63-33).

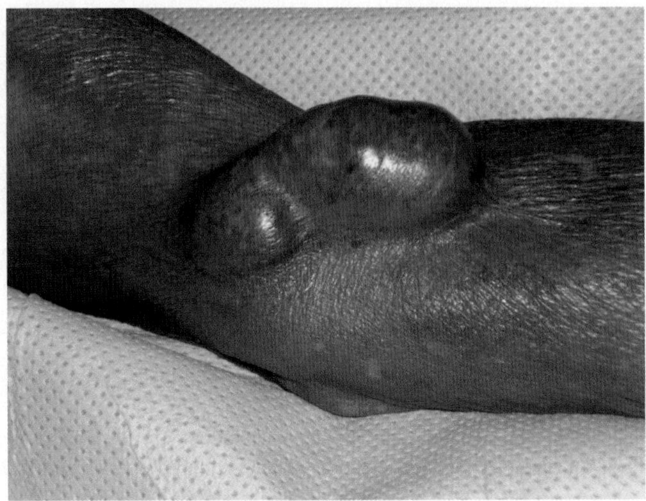

**FIGURE 63-33** Fistula aneurysm without evidence of skin involvement.

Arterial insufficiency, or steal syndrome, can develop in patients with vascular access. The creation of this access results in a low-resistance circulation that shunts arterial inflow into this low-pressure venous outflow. In addition, the flow in the artery distal to the access origin may become retrograde and is no longer antegrade. The effect is that the vascular access steals arterial flow, which may compromise distal limb perfusion. This physiologic steal phenomenon can be demonstrated in 75% to 90% of patients; however, only 1% to 6% are symptomatic. Symptoms may include a cold and painful hand or foot; with significant flow compromise, patients may develop tissue loss in their fingers or toes (Fig. 63-34). In patients with forearm vascular access using radial artery as inflow, such as radiocephalic or radiobasilic fistulas, ligation of the artery just distal to the fistula restores flow in the palmar arch. In patients with vascular access in the upper arm, the distal revascularization with interval ligation (DRIL) procedure is used to revascularize the distal limb while preserving the vascular access. The procedure is a bypass from the inflow artery proximal to the access to the artery distal to the access. The arterial segment between the vascular access and distal anastomosis of the bypass is ligated to prevent steal. The low-pressure zone around the access origin may shunt blood flow from the bypass into the access rather than restoring distal flow. An autogenous conduit should be used for this bypass if possible.

## CONCLUSION

Ultimately, the goals of DOQI are to minimize the deep effects on the ESRD patient's quality of life that hemodialysis dependence entails. Increasing rates of autogenous arteriovenous access increase patency rates, decrease complications and therefore decrease the number of unplanned interventions and hospitalizations that this population is required to endure. This vision cannot be realized with traditional arteriovenous access alone. Early referral to vascular surgery, institutional strategies of preoperative noninvasive vascular assessments and use of venous transposition procedures can be effective in increasing autogenous access in the dialysis population. A system of prospective monitoring for the development of hemodynamically significant stenosis can improve long-term assisted patency. A multidisciplinary approach involving the nephrologist, vascular surgeon and hemodialysis center nurses, as well as the patient and the patient's social support system, is required to optimize the care of this complex patient population.

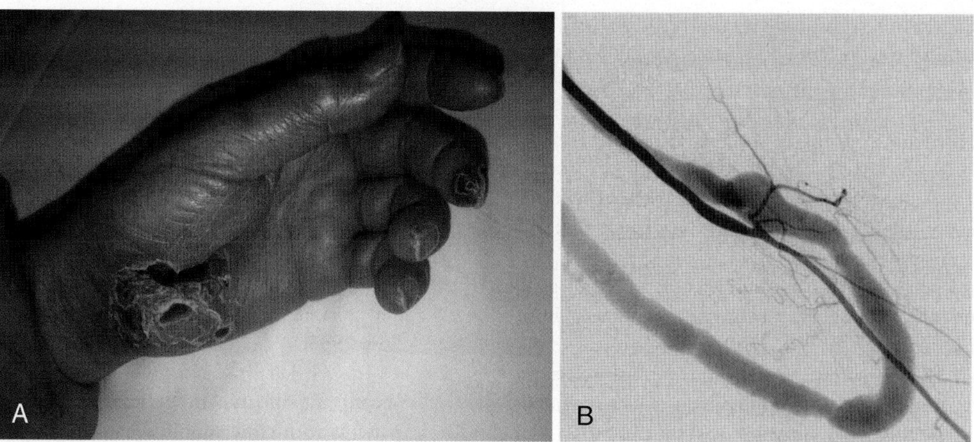


**FIGURE 63-34 A,** Patient with tissue loss of the hand because of steal. He underwent arterial duplex and angiography before distal revascularization and interval ligation **(B)**, with immediate symptomatic improvement.

## SELECTED REFERENCES

Hirsch AT, Haskal ZJ, Hertzer NR, et al: ACC/AHA 2005 Practice Guidelines for the management of patients with peripheral arterial disease (lower extremity, renal, mesenteric, and abdominal aortic): a collaborative report from the American Association for Vascular Surgery/Society for Vascular Surgery, Society for Cardiovascular Angiography and Interventions, Society for Vascular Medicine and Biology, Society of Interventional Radiology, and the ACC/AHA Task Force on Practice Guidelines (Writing Committee to Develop Guidelines for the Management of Patients With Peripheral Arterial Disease): endorsed by the American Association of Cardiovascular and Pulmonary Rehabilitation; National Heart, Lung, and Blood Institute; Society for Vascular Nursing; TransAtlantic Inter-Society Consensus; and Vascular Disease Foundation. Circulation 113:e463–e654, 2006.

AHA/ACC guidelines is a consensus document describing targets for medical management of vascular disease, including current thoughts on prevention.

Brott TG, Hobson RW, 2nd, Howard G, et al: Stenting versus endarterectomy for treatment of carotid-artery stenosis. N Engl J Med 363:11–23, 2010.

CREST—The definitive randomized prospective trial comparing carotid stenting and carotid endarterectomy; it lasted over 10 years and producing the best results from both therapies ever reported in such a trial. Results from carotid stenting were dramatically improved during the second half of the trial as compared with the first half, suggesting the evolutionary nature of endovascular procedures and an identifiable learning curve for new technologies.

Barnett HJ, Taylor DW, Eliasziw M, et al: Benefit of carotid endarterectomy in patients with symptomatic moderate or severe stenosis. North American Symptomatic Carotid Endarterectomy Trial Collaborators. N Engl J Med 339:1415–1425, 1998.

NASCET was a randomized prospective trial confirming the superiority of carotid endarterectomy over medical management for patients with high-grade symptomatic carotid disease.

Endarterectomy for asymptomatic carotid artery stenosis. Executive Committee for the Asymptomatic Carotid Atherosclerosis Study. JAMA 273:1421–1428, 1995.

ACAS was a randomized prospective trial confirming the superiority of Carotid Endarterectomy over medical management for the treatment of asymptomatic carotid disease.

Adam DJ, Beard JD, Cleveland T, et al: Bypass versus angioplasty in severe ischaemia of the leg (BASIL): Multicentre, randomised controlled trial. Lancet 366:1925–1934, 2005.

A randomized trial that showed in patients with severe limb ischemia due to infra-inguinal disease and who are suitable for surgery and angioplasty, a bypass-surgery-first and a balloon-angioplasty-first strategy are associated with broadly similar outcomes in terms of amputation-free survival, and in the short-term, surgery was more expensive than angioplasty.

CAPRIE Steering Committee: A randomized, blinded, trial of clopidogrel versus aspirin in patients at risk of ischemic events (CAPRIE). Lancet 348:1329–1339, 1996.

A blinded randomized trial that showed clopidogrel to be more effective and safer than aspirin in reducing the combined risk of ischemic stroke, myocardial infarction, or vascular deaths in patients with atherosclerosis.

Norgren L, Hiatt WR, Dormandy JA, et al: Inter-Society Consensus for the Management of Peripheral Arterial Disease (TASC II). J Vasc Surg 45(Suppl):S5–S67, 2007.

This consensus document describes an approach for choosing open revascularization versus endovascular therapy for patients based on lesion characteristics.

## REFERENCES

1. Criqui MH, Vargas V, Denenberg JO, et al: Ethnicity and peripheral arterial disease: The San Diego Population Study. Circulation 112:2703–2707, 2005.

2. Stewart WJ, McSweeney SM, Kellett MA, et al: Increased risk of severe protamine reactions in NPH insulin-dependent diabetics undergoing cardiac catheterization. Circulation 70:788–792, 1984.
3. Kreitner KF, Kalden P, Neufang A, et al: Diabetes and peripheral arterial occlusive disease: Prospective comparison of contrast-enhanced three-dimensional MR angiography with conventional digital subtraction angiography. AJR Am J Roentgenol 174:171–179, 2000.
4. Sam AD, 2nd, Morasch MD, Collins J, et al: Safety of gadolinium contrast angiography in patients with chronic renal insufficiency. J Vasc Surg 38:313–318, 2003.
5. Nair A, Kuban BD, Tuzcu EM, et al: Coronary plaque classification with intravascular ultrasound radiofrequency data analysis. Circulation 106:2200–2206, 2002.
6. Diethrich EB, Pauliina Margolis M, Reid DB, et al: Virtual histology intravascular ultrasound assessment of carotid artery disease: The Carotid Artery Plaque Virtual Histology Evaluation (CAPITAL) study. J Endovasc Ther 14:676–686, 2007.
7. McDermott MM, Criqui MH, Greenland P, et al: Leg strength in peripheral arterial disease: Associations with disease severity and lower-extremity performance. J Vasc Surg 39:523–530, 2004.
8. Norgren L, Hiatt WR, Dormandy JA, et al: Inter-Society Consensus for the Management of Peripheral Arterial Disease (TASC II). J Vasc Surg 45(Suppl):S5-S67, 2007.
9. Nehler MR, Hiatt WR, Taylor LM, Jr: Is revascularization and limb salvage always the best treatment for critical limb ischemia? J Vasc Surg 37:704–708, 2003.
10. Feinglass J, Pearce WH, Martin GJ, et al: Postoperative and late survival outcomes after major amputation: Findings from the Department of Veterans Affairs National Surgical Quality Improvement Program. Surgery 130:21–29, 2001.
11. Houghton AD, Taylor PR, Thurlow S, et al: Success rates for rehabilitation of vascular amputees: Implications for preoperative assessment and amputation level. Br J Surg 79:753–755, 1992.
12. Taylor SM, Kalbaugh CA, Blackhurst DW, et al: Preoperative clinical factors predict postoperative functional outcomes after major lower limb amputation: An analysis of 553 consecutive patients. J Vasc Surg 42:227–235, 2005.
13. Stone PA, Back MR, Armstrong PA, et al: Midfoot amputations expand limb salvage rates for diabetic foot infections. Ann Vasc Surg 19:805–811, 2005.
14. Tisi PV, Callam MJ: Type of incision for below-knee amputation. Cochrane Database Syst Rev (1):CD003749, 2004.
15. Desai Y, Robbs JV, Keenan JP: Staged below-knee amputations for septic peripheral lesions due to ischaemia. Br J Surg 73:392–394, 1986.
16. Fisher DF, Jr, Clagett GP, Fry RE, et al: One-stage versus two-stage amputation for wet gangrene of the lower extremity: A randomized study. J Vasc Surg 8:428–433, 1988.
17. Winburn GB, Wood MC, Hawkins ML, et al: Current role of cryoamputation. Am J Surg 162:647–650, 1991.
18. Pinzur MS, Gottschalk FA, Pinto MA, et al: Controversies in lower-extremity amputation. J Bone Joint Surg Am 89:1118–1127, 2007.
19. Bolia A, Brennan J, Bell PR: Recanalisation of femoro-popliteal occlusions: Improving success rate by subintimal recanalisation. Clin Radiol 40:325, 1989.
20. Bolia A, Sayers RD, Thompson MM, et al: Subintimal and intraluminal recanalisation of occluded crural arteries by percutaneous balloon angioplasty. Eur J Vasc Surg 8:214–219, 1994.
21. Scott EC, Biuckians A, Light RE, et al: Subintimal angioplasty: Our experience in the treatment of 506 infrainguinal arterial occlusions. J Vasc Surg 48:878–884, 2008.
22. Clark TW, Groffsky JL, Soulen MC: Predictors of long-term patency after femoropopliteal angioplasty: results from the STAR registry. J Vasc Interv Radiol 12:923–933, 2001.
23. Dorros G, Jaff MR, Murphy KJ, et al: The acute outcome of tibioperoneal vessel angioplasty in 417 cases with claudication and critical limb ischemia. Cathet Cardiovasc Diagn 45:251–256, 1998.
24. Dorros G, Jaff MR, Dorros AM, et al: Tibioperoneal (outflow lesion) angioplasty can be used as primary treatment in 235 patients with critical limb ischemia: Five-year follow-up. Circulation 104:2057–2062, 2001.
25. Giles KA, Pomposelli FB, Spence TL, et al: Infrapopliteal angioplasty for critical limb ischemia: Relation of TransAtlantic Inter-Society Consensus class to outcome in 176 limbs. J Vasc Surg 48:128–136, 2008.
26. Kudo T, Chandra FA, Ahn SS: The effectiveness of percutaneous transluminal angioplasty for the treatment of critical limb ischemia: A 10-year experience. J Vasc Surg 41:423–435, 2005.
27. Sabeti S, Schillinger M, Amighi J, et al: Primary patency of femoropopliteal arteries treated with nitinol versus stainless steel self-expanding stents: Propensity score-adjusted analysis. Radiology 232:516–521, 2004.
28. Schillinger M, Sabeti S, Loewe C, et al: Balloon angioplasty versus implantation of nitinol stents in the superficial femoral artery. N Engl J Med 354:1879–1888, 2006.
29. Sabeti S, Mlekusch W, Amighi J, et al: Primary patency of long-segment self-expanding nitinol stents in the femoropopliteal arteries. J Endovasc Ther 12:6–12, 2005.
30. Schillinger M, Sabeti S, Dick P, et al: Sustained benefit at 2 years of primary femoropopliteal stenting compared with balloon angioplasty with optional stenting. Circulation 115:2745–2749, 2007.
31. Vogel TR, Shindelman LE, Nackman GB, et al: Efficacious use of nitinol stents in the femoral and popliteal arteries. J Vasc Surg 38:1178–1184, 2003.
32. Mewissen MW: Self-expanding nitinol stents in the femoropopliteal segment: technique and mid-term results. Tech Vasc Interv Radiol 7:2–5, 2004.
33. Baril DT, Marone LK, Kim J, et al: Outcomes of endovascular interventions for TASC II B and C femoropopliteal lesions. J Vasc Surg 48:627–633, 2008.
34. Ferreira M, Lanziotti L, Monteiro M, et al: Superficial femoral artery recanalization with self-expanding nitinol stents: Long-term follow-up results. Eur J Vasc Endovasc Surg 34:702–708, 2007.
35. Kickuth R, Keo HH, Triller J, et al: Initial clinical experience with the 4-F self-expanding XPERT stent system for infrapopliteal treatment of patients with severe claudication and critical limb ischemia. J Vasc Interv Radiol 18:703–708, 2007.
36. Mwipatayi BP, Hockings A, Hofmann M, et al: Balloon angioplasty compared with stenting for treatment of femoropopliteal occlusive disease: A meta-analysis. J Vasc Surg 47:461–469, 2008.
37. Ihnat DM, Duong ST, Taylor ZC, et al: Contemporary outcomes after superficial femoral artery angioplasty and stenting:

The influence of TASC classification and runoff score. J Vasc Surg 47:967–974, 2008.

38. Railo M, Roth WD, Edgren J, et al: Preliminary results with endoluminal femoropopliteal thrupass. Ann Chir Gynaecol 90:15–18, 2001.
39. Jahnke T, Andresen R, Muller-Hulsbeck S, et al: Hemobahn stent-grafts for treatment of femoropopliteal arterial obstructions: Midterm results of a prospective trial. J Vasc Interv Radiol 14:41–51, 2003.
40. Fischer M, Schwabe C, Schulte KL: Value of the hemobahn/viabahn endoprosthesis in the treatment of long chronic lesions of the superficial femoral artery: 6 years of experience. J Endovasc Ther 13:281–290, 2006.
41. Bleyn J, Schol F, Vanhandenhove I, et al: Endovascular reconstruction of the superficial femoral artery. In Becquemin JP, Alimi YS, Watelet J, et al, editors: Controversies and updates in Vascular cardiac surgery, ed 14, Torino, Italy, 2004, Edizioni Minerva Medica, pp 87–91.
42. Shaikh F, DjelMami-hani M, Solis J, et al: Percutaneous endovascular treatment of SFA disease using the Gore Viabahn endoprosthesis. Do the procedure success and 1-year follow-up data make this the treatment of choice? Endovasc Today Feb 2007:4–8, 2007.
43. Saxon RR, Dake MD, Volgelzang RL, et al: Randomized, multicenter study comparing expanded polytetrafluoroethylene-covered endoprosthesis placement with percutaneous transluminal angioplasty in the treatment of superficial femoral artery occlusive disease. J Vasc Interv Radiol 19:823–832, 2008.
44. Kedora J, Hohmann S, Garrett W, et al: Randomized comparison of percutaneous Viabahn stent grafts vs prosthetic femoral-popliteal bypass in the treatment of superficial femoral arterial occlusive disease. J Vasc Surg 45:10–16; discussion 16, 2007.
45. Zeller T, Rastan A, Schwarzwalder U, et al: Percutaneous peripheral atherectomy of femoropopliteal stenoses using a new-generation device: Six-month results from a single-center experience. J Endovasc Ther 11:676–685, 2004.
46. Keeling WB, Shames ML, Stone PA, et al: Plaque excision with the Silverhawk catheter: Early results in patients with claudication or critical limb ischemia. J Vasc Surg 45:25–31, 2007.
47. Yancey AE, Minion DJ, Rodriguez C, et al: Peripheral atherectomy in TransAtlantic InterSociety Consensus type C femoropopliteal lesions for limb salvage. J Vasc Surg 44:503–509, 2006.
48. Sarac TP, Altinel O, Bannazadeh M, et al: Midterm outcome predictors for lower extremity atherectomy procedures. J Vasc Surg 48:885–890; discussion 890, 2008.
49. Scheinert D, Laird JR, Jr, Schroder M, et al: Excimer laser-assisted recanalization of long, chronic superficial femoral artery occlusions. J Endovasc Ther 8:156–166, 2001.
50. Laird JR, Zeller T, Gray BH, et al: Limb salvage following laser-assisted angioplasty for critical limb ischemia: Results of the LACI multicenter trial. J Endovasc Ther 13:1–11, 2006.
51. Bosiers M, Peeters P, Elst FV, et al: Excimer laser assisted angioplasty for critical limb ischemia: Results of the LACI Belgium Study. Eur J Vasc Endovasc Surg 29:613–619, 2005.
52. Idu MM, Blankenstein JD, de Gier P, et al: Impact of a color-flow duplex surveillance program on infrainguinal vein graft patency: A five-year experience. J Vasc Surg 17:42–52, 1993.
53. Buth J, Disselhoff B, Sommeling C, et al: Color-flow duplex criteria for grading stenosis in infrainguinal vein grafts. J Vasc Surg 14:716–726, 1991.
54. Mills JL, Sr, Wixon CL, James DC, et al: The natural history of intermediate and critical vein graft stenosis: Recommendations for continued surveillance or repair. J Vasc Surg 33:273–278, 2001.
55. Calligaro KD, Musser DJ, Chen AY, et al: Duplex ultrasonography to diagnose failing arterial prosthetic grafts. Surgery 120:455–459, 1996.
56. Calligaro KD, Doerr K, McAffee-Bennett S, et al: Should duplex ultrasonography be performed for surveillance of femoropopliteal and femorotibial arterial prosthetic bypasses? Ann Vasc Surg 15:520–524, 2001.
57. Carter A, Murphy MO, Halka AT, et al: The natural history of stenoses within lower limb arterial bypass grafts using a graft surveillance program. Ann Vasc Surg 21:695–703, 2007.
58. Tinder CN, Chavanpun JP, Bandyk DF, et al: Efficacy of duplex ultrasound surveillance after infrainguinal vein bypass may be enhanced by identification of characteristics predictive of graft stenosis development. J Vasc Surg 48:613–618, 2008.
59. Passman MA, Moneta GL, Nehler MR, et al: Do normal early color-flow duplex surveillance examination results of infrainguinal vein grafts preclude the need for late graft revision? J Vasc Surg 22:476–481, 1995.
60. Gonsalves C, Bandyk DF, Avino AJ, et al: Duplex features of vein graft stenosis and the success of percutaneous transluminal angioplasty. J Endovasc Surg 6:66–72, 1999.
61. Hagino RT, Sheehan MK, Jung I, et al: Target lesion characteristics in failing vein grafts predict the success of endovascular and open revision. J Vasc Surg 46:1167–1172, 2007.
62. Tielbeek AV, Rietjens E, Buth J, et al: The value of duplex surveillance after endovascular intervention for femoropopliteal obstructive disease. Eur J Vasc Endovasc Surg 12:145–150, 1996.
63. Spijkerboer AM, Nass PC, de Valois JC, et al: Evaluation of femoropopliteal arteries with duplex ultrasound after angioplasty. Can we predict results at one year? Eur J Vasc Endovasc Surg 12:418–423, 1996.
64. Strandness DE Jr: Natural history of renal artery stenosis. Am J Kidney Dis 24:630–635, 1994.
65. Zierler RE, Bergelin RO, Davidson RC, et al: A prospective study of disease progression in patients with atherosclerotic renal artery stenosis. Am J Hypertens 9:1055–1061, 1996.
66. Zierler RE, Bergelin RO, Isaacson JA, et al: Natural history of atherosclerotic renal artery stenosis: A prospective study with duplex ultrasonography. J Vasc Surg 19:250–257, 1994.
67. Tullis MJ, Zierler RE, Caps MT, et al: Clinical evidence of contralateral renal parenchymal injury in patients with unilateral atherosclerotic renal artery stenosis. Ann Vasc Surg 12:122–127, 1998.
68. Guzman RP, Zierler RE, Isaacson JA, et al: Renal atrophy and arterial stenosis. A prospective study with duplex ultrasound. Hypertension 23:346–350, 1994.
69. Caps MT, Perissinotto C, Zierler RE, et al: Prospective study of atherosclerotic disease progression in the renal artery. Circulation 98:2866–2872, 1998.
70. Caps MT, Zierler RE, Polissar NL, et al: Risk of atrophy in kidneys with atherosclerotic renal artery stenosis. Kidney Int 53:735–742, 1998.
71. Mailloux LU, Napolitano B, Bellucci AG, et al: Renal vascular disease causing end-stage renal disease, incidence, clinical correlates, and outcomes: A 20-year clinical experience. Am J Kidney Dis 24:622–629, 1994.

72. van Ampting JM, Penne EL, Beek FJ, et al: Prevalence of atherosclerotic renal artery stenosis in patients starting dialysis. Nephrol Dial Transplant 18:1147–1151, 2003.
73. Appel RG, Bleyer AJ, Reavis S, et al: Renovascular disease in older patients beginning renal replacement therapy. Kidney Int 48:171–176, 1995.
74. Gruntzig A, Kuhlmann U, Vetter W, et al: Treatment of renovascular hypertension with percutaneous transluminal dilation of a renal-artery stenosis. Lancet 1:801–802, 1978.
75. Boisclair C, Therasse E, Oliva VL, et al: Treatment of renal angioplasty failure by percutaneous renal artery stenting with Palmaz stents: Midterm technical and clinical results. AJR Am J Roentgenol 168:245–251, 1997.
76. Leertouwer TC, Gussenhoven EJ, Bosch JL, et al: Stent placement for renal arterial stenosis: Where do we stand? A meta-analysis. Radiology 216:78–85, 2000.
77. van de Ven PJ, Kaatee R, Beutler JJ, et al: Arterial stenting and balloon angioplasty in ostial atherosclerotic renovascular disease: A randomised trial. Lancet 353:282–286, 1999.
78. Gill KS, Fowler RC: Atherosclerotic renal arterial stenosis: Clinical outcomes of stent placement for hypertension and renal failure. Radiology 226:821–826, 2003.
79. Klow NE, Paulsen D, Vatne K, et al: Percutaneous transluminal renal artery angioplasty using the coaxial technique. Ten years of experience from 591 procedures in 419 patients. Acta Radiol 39:594–603, 1998.
80. Rodriguez-Lopez JA, Werner A, Ray LI, et al: Renal artery stenosis treated with stent deployment: Indications, technique, and outcome for 108 patients. J Vasc Surg 29:617–624, 1999.
81. Bonelli FS, McKusick MA, Textor SC, et al: Renal artery angioplasty: Technical results and clinical outcome in 320 patients. Mayo Clin Proc 70:1041–1052, 1995.
82. Ramsay LE, Waller PC: Blood pressure response to percutaneous transluminal angioplasty for renovascular hypertension: An overview of published series. BMJ 300:569–572, 1990.
83. Henry M, Amor M, Henry I, et al: Stents in the treatment of renal artery stenosis: Long-term follow-up. J Endovasc Surg 6:42–51, 1999.
84. Dorros G, Jaff M, Mathiak L, et al: Four-year follow-up of Palmaz-Schatz stent revascularization as treatment for atherosclerotic renal artery stenosis. Circulation 98:642–647, 1998.
85. Bush RL, Najibi S, MacDonald MJ, et al: Endovascular revascularization of renal artery stenosis: Technical and clinical results. J Vasc Surg 33:1041–1049, 2001.
86. Webster J, Marshall F, Abdalla M, et al: Randomised comparison of percutaneous angioplasty vs continued medical therapy for hypertensive patients with atheromatous renal artery stenosis. Scottish and Newcastle Renal Artery Stenosis Collaborative Group. J Hum Hypertens 12:329–335, 1998.
87. van Jaarsveld BC, Krijnen P, Pieterman H, et al: The effect of balloon angioplasty on hypertension in atherosclerotic renal-artery stenosis. Dutch Renal Artery Stenosis Intervention Cooperative Study Group. N Engl J Med 342:1007–1014, 2000.
88. Plouin PF, Chatellier G, Darne B, et al: Blood pressure outcome of angioplasty in atherosclerotic renal artery stenosis: a randomized trial. Essai Multicentrique Medicaments vs Angioplastie (EMMA) Study Group. Hypertension 31:823–829, 1998.
89. Rocha-Singh KJ, Ahuja RK, Sung CH, et al: Long-term renal function preservation after renal artery stenting in patients with progressive ischemic nephropathy. Catheter Cardiovasc Interv 57:135–141, 2002.
90. Rundback JH, Manoni T, Rozenblit GN, et al: Balloon angioplasty or stent placement in patients with azotemic renovascular disease: A retrospective comparison of clinical outcomes. Heart Dis 1:121–125, 1999.
91. Rundback JH, Gray RJ, Rozenblit G, et al: Renal artery stent placement for the management of ischemic nephropathy. J Vasc Interv Radiol 9:413–420, 1998.
92. Shannon HM, Gillespie IN, Moss JG: Salvage of the solitary kidney by insertion of a renal artery stent. AJR Am J Roentgenol 171:217–222, 1998.
93. Bush RL, Martin LG, Lin PH, et al: Endovascular revascularization of renal artery stenosis in the solitary functioning kidney. Ann Vasc Surg 15:60–66, 2001.
94. Henry M, Amor M, Henry I, et al: Stent placement in the renal artery: Three-year experience with the Palmaz stent. J Vasc Interv Radiol 7:343–350, 1996.
95. Dorros G, Jaff M, Jain A, et al: Follow-up of primary Palmaz-Schatz stent placement for atherosclerotic renal artery stenosis. Am J Cardiol 75:1051–1055, 1995.
96. Blum U, Krumme B, Flugel P, et al: Treatment of ostial renal-artery stenoses with vascular endoprostheses after unsuccessful balloon angioplasty. N Engl J Med 336:459–465, 1997.
97. Zeller T, Frank U, Muller C, et al: [Duplex ultrasound for follow-up examination after stent-angioplasty of ostial renal artery stenoses.] Ultraschall Med 23:315–319, 2002.
98. Bakker J, Beutler JJ, Elgersma OE, et al: Duplex ultrasonography in assessing restenosis of renal artery stents. Cardiovasc Intervent Radiol 22:475–480, 1999.
99. Bax L, Mali WP, Van De Ven PJ, et al: Repeated intervention for in-stent restenosis of the renal arteries. J Vasc Interv Radiol 13:1219–1224, 2002.
100. Mackrell PJ, Langan EM, 3rd, Sullivan TM, et al: Management of renal artery stenosis: Effects of a shift from surgical to percutaneous therapy on indications and outcomes. Ann Vasc Surg 17:54–59, 2003.
101. Scheinert D, Braunlich S, Nonnast-Daniel B, et al: Transradial approach for renal artery stenting. Catheter Cardiovasc Interv 54:442–447, 2001.
102. Braunlich S, Ludwig J, Scheinert D: Transradial renal artery angioplasty and stenting. J Invasive Cardiol 14:147–149, 2002.
103. Galli M, Tarantino F, Mameli S, et al: Transradial approach for renal percutaneous transluminal angioplasty and stenting: A feasibility pilot study. J Invasive Cardiol 14:386–390, 2002.
104. Kessel DO, Robertson I, Taylor EJ, et al: Renal stenting from the radial artery: a novel approach. Cardiovasc Intervent Radiol 26:146–149, 2003.
105. Schobel WA, Mauser M: Miniaturization of the equipment for percutaneous coronary interventions: A prospective study in 1200 patients. J Invasive Cardiol 15:6–11, 2003.
106. Schobel WA, Spyridopoulos I, Hoffmeister HM, et al: Percutaneous coronary interventions using a new 5 French guiding catheter: Results of a prospective study. Catheter Cardiovasc Interv 53:308–312, 2001.
107. Rakhit RD, Matter C, Windecker S, et al: Five French versus 6 French PCI: A case control study of efficacy, safety and outcome. J Invasive Cardiol 14:670–674, 2002.
108. Hawkins IF, Jr, Wilcox CS, Kerns SR, et al: $CO_2$ digital angiography: A safer contrast agent for renal vascular imaging? Am J Kidney Dis 24:685–694, 1994.

109. Spinosa DJ, Matsumoto AH, Angle JF, et al: Renal insufficiency: Usefulness of gadodiamide-enhanced renal angiography to supplement $CO_2$-enhanced renal angiography for diagnosis and percutaneous treatment. Radiology 210:663–672, 1999.
110. Caridi JG, Stavropoulos SW, Hawkins IF, Jr.: Carbon dioxide digital subtraction angiography for renal artery stent placement. J Vasc Interv Radiol 10:635–640, 1999.
111. Caridi JG, Stavropoulos SW, Hawkins IF Jr: $CO_2$ digital subtraction angiography for renal artery angioplasty in high-risk patients. AJR Am J Roentgenol 173:1551–1556, 1999.
112. Beese RC, Bees NR, Belli AM: Renal angiography using carbon dioxide. Br J Radiol 73:3–6, 2000.
113. Spinosa DJ, Matsumoto AH, Angle JF, et al: Safety of $CO_2$- and gadodiamide-enhanced angiography for the evaluation and percutaneous treatment of renal artery stenosis in patients with chronic renal insufficiency. AJR Am J Roentgenol 176:1305–1311, 2001.
114. Spinosa DJ, Angle JF, Hagspiel KD, et al: Feasibility of gadodiamide compared with dilute iodinated contrast material for imaging of the abdominal aorta and renal arteries. J Vasc Interv Radiol 11:733–737, 2000.
115. Spinosa DJ, Angle JF, Hartwell GD, et al: Gadolinium-based contrast agents in angiography and interventional radiology. Radiol Clin North Am 40:693–710, 2002.
116. Ailawadi G, Stanley JC, Williams DM, et al: Gadolinium as a nonnephrotoxic contrast agent for catheter-based arteriographic evaluation of renal arteries in patients with azotemia. J Vasc Surg 37:346–352, 2003.
117. Sheehan MK, Baker WH, Littooy FN, et al: Timing of postcarotid complications: A guide to safe discharge planning. J Vasc Surg 34:13–16, 2001.
118. Wholey MH, Tan WA, Toursarkissian B, et al: Management of neurological complications of carotid artery stenting. J Endovasc Ther 8:341–353, 2001.
119. Qureshi AI, Luft AR, Janardhan V, et al: Identification of patients at risk for periprocedural neurological deficits associated with carotid angioplasty and stenting. Stroke 31:376–382, 2000.
120. Kherlakian GM, Roedersheimer LR, Arbaugh JJ, et al: Comparison of autogenous fistula versus expanded polytetrafluoroethylene graft fistula for angioaccess in hemodialysis. Am J Surg 152:238–243, 1986.
121. U.S. Renal Data System: USRDS 1995 Annual Data Report. Am J Kidney Dis 26:S12–S166, 1995.
122. NKF-DOQI clinical practice guidelines for vascular access. Am J Kidney Dis 30:S150–S191, 1997.
123. Silva MB, Jr, Hobson RW, 2nd, Pappas PJ, et al: A strategy for increasing use of autogenous hemodialysis access procedures: Impact of preoperative noninvasive evaluation. J Vasc Surg 27:302–307, 1998.
124. Khanna S, Sniderman K, Simons M, et al: Superior vena cava stenosis associated with hemodialysis catheters. Am J Kidney Dis 21:278–281, 1993.
125. Silva MB Jr, Hobson RW, 2nd, Pappas PJ, et al: Vein transposition in the forearm for autogenous hemodialysis access. J Vasc Surg 26:981–986, 1997.
126. Curi MA, Pappas PJ, Silva MB, Jr, et al: Hemodialysis access:Influence of the human immunodeficiency virus on patency and infection rates. J Vasc Surg 29:608–616, 1999.
127. Puskas JD, Gertler JP: Internal jugular to axillary vein bypass for subclavian vein thrombosis in the setting of brachial arteriovenous fistula. J Vasc Surg 19:939–942, 1994.
128. McCann RL: Axillary grafts for difficult hemodialysis access. J Vasc Surg 24:457–461, 1996.
129. Scholz H, Zanow J, Petzod M, et al: Arterioarterial interposition as angioaccess for hemodialysis. In Henry ML, editor: Vascular access for hemodialysis VI, Chicago, 1999, Gore & Associates and Precept Press.
130. El-Sabrout RA, Duncan JM: Right atrial bypass grafting for central venous obstruction associated with dialysis access: Another treatment option. J Vasc Surg 29:472–478, 1999.
131. Schwab SJ, Beathard G: The hemodialysis catheter conundrum: Hate living with them, but can't live without them. Kidney Int 56:1–17, 1999.
132. Marston WA, Criado E, Jaques PF, et al: Prospective randomized comparison of surgical versus endovascular management of thrombosed dialysis access grafts. J Vasc Surg 26:373–380, 1997.
133. Valji K, Bookstein JJ, Roberts AC, et al: Pulse-spray pharmacomechanical thrombolysis of thrombosed hemodialysis access grafts: Long-term experience and comparison of original and current techniques. AJR Am J Roentgenol 164:1495–1500, 1995.
134. III. NKF-K/DOQI Clinical Practice Guidelines for Vascular Access: Update 2000. Am J Kidney Dis 37:S137-S181, 2001.
135. Lok CE, Oliver MJ: Overcoming barriers to arteriovenous fistula creation and use. Semin Dial 16:189–196, 2003.
136. Huber TS, Ozaki CK, Flynn TC, et al: Prospective validation of an algorithm to maximize native arteriovenous fistulas for chronic hemodialysis access. J Vasc Surg 36:452–459, 2002.
137. Hakaim AG, Nalbandian M, Scott T: Superior maturation and patency of primary brachiocephalic and transposed basilic vein arteriovenous fistulas in patients with diabetes. J Vasc Surg 27:154–157, 1998.
138. Mendes RR, Farber MA, Marston WA, et al: Prediction of wrist arteriovenous fistula maturation with preoperative vein mapping with ultrasonography. J Vasc Surg 36:460–463, 2002.
139. Palder SB, Kirkman RL, Whittemore AD, et al: Vascular access for hemodialysis. Patency rates and results of revision. Ann Surg 202:235–239, 1985.
140. Kinnaert P, Vereerstraeten P, Toussaint C, et al: Nine years' experience with internal arteriovenous fistulas for haemodialysis: A study of some factors influencing the results. Br J Surg 64: 242–246, 1977.
141. Limet RR, Lejeune GN: Evaluation of 110 subcutaneous arteriovenous fistulas in 100 chronically hemodialysed patients. J Cardiovasc Surg (Torino) 15:573–576, 1974.
142. Rohr MS, Browder W, Frentz GD, et al: Arteriovenous fistulas for long-term dialysis. Factors that influence fistula survival. Arch Surg 113:153–155, 1978.
143. Ascher E, Gade P, Hingorani A, et al: Changes in the practice of angioaccess surgery: Impact of dialysis outcome and quality initiative recommendations. J Vasc Surg 31:84–92, 2000.
144. Miller A, Holzenbein TJ, Gottlieb MN, et al: Strategies to increase the use of autogenous arteriovenous fistula in end-stage renal disease. Ann Vasc Surg 11:397–405, 1997.
145. Sidawy AN, Gray R, Besarab A, et al: Recommended standards for reports dealing with arteriovenous hemodialysis accesses. J Vasc Surg 35:603–610, 2002.
146. LoGerfo FW, Menzoian JO, Kumaki DJ, et al: Transposed basilic vein-brachial arteriovenous fistula. A reliable secondary-access procedure. Arch Surg 113:1008–1010, 1978.

**147.** Dagher FJ: The upper arm AV hemoaccess: Long term follow-up. J Cardiovasc Surg (Torino) 27:447–449, 1986.

**148.** Gormus N, Ozergin U, Durgut K, et al: Comparison of autologous basilic vein transpositions between forearm and upper arm regions. Ann Vasc Surg 17:522–525, 2003.

**149.** Ascher E, Hingoran A, Gunduz Y, et al: The value and limitations of the arm cephalic and basilic vein for arteriovenous access. Ann Vasc Surg 15:89–97, 2001.

**150.** Coburn MC, Carney WI, Jr: Comparison of basilic vein and polytetrafluoroethylene for brachial arteriovenous fistula. J Vasc Surg 20:896–902, 1994.

**151.** Murphy GJ, White SA, Knight AJ, et al: Long-term results of arteriovenous fistulas using transposed autologous basilic vein. Br J Surg 87:819–823, 2000.

**152.** Taghizadeh A, Dasgupta P, Khan MS, et al: Long-term outcomes of brachiobasilic transposition fistula for haemodialysis. Eur J Vasc Endovasc Surg 26:670–672, 2003.

**153.** Matsuura JH, Rosenthal D, Clark M, et al: Transposed basilic vein versus polytetrafluorethylene for brachial-axillary arteriovenous fistulas. Am J Surg 176:219–221, 1998.

**154.** Brescia MJ, Cimino JE, Appel K, et al: Chronic hemodialysis using venipuncture and a surgically created arteriovenous fistula. N Engl J Med 275:1089–1092, 1966.

**155.** Tashjian DB, Lipkowitz GS, Madden RL, et al: Safety and efficacy of femoral-based hemodialysis access grafts. J Vasc Surg 35:691–693, 2002.

**156.** Gradman WS, Cohen W, Haji-Aghaii M: Arteriovenous fistula construction in the thigh with transposed superficial femoral vein: Our initial experience. J Vasc Surg 33:968–975, 2001.

**157.** Huber TS, Ozaki CK, Flynn TC, et al: Use of superficial femoral vein for hemodialysis arteriovenous access. J Vasc Surg 31:1038–1041, 2000.

**158.** May J, Tiller D, Johnson J, et al: Saphenous-vein arteriovenous fistula in regular dialysis treatment. N Engl J Med 280:770, 1969.

**159.** Kinnaert P, Vereerstraeten P, Toussaint C, et al: Saphenous vein loop fistula in the thigh for maintenance hemodialysis. World J Surg 3:95–98, 132–133, 1979.

**160.** Gorski TF, Nguyen HQ, Gorski YC, et al: Lower-extremity saphenous vein transposition arteriovenous fistula: An alternative for hemodialysis access in AIDS patients. Am Surg 64:338–340, 1998.

**161.** Illig KA, Orloff M, Lyden SP, et al: Transposed saphenous vein arteriovenous fistula revisited: New technology for an old idea. Cardiovasc Surg 10:212–215, 2002.

**162.** Hingorani A, Ascher E, Kallakuri S, et al: Impact of reintervention for failing upper-extremity arteriovenous autogenous access for hemodialysis. J Vasc Surg 34:1004–1009, 2001.

**163.** Berman SS, Gentile AT: Impact of secondary procedures in autogenous arteriovenous fistula maturation and maintenance. J Vasc Surg 34:866–871, 2001.

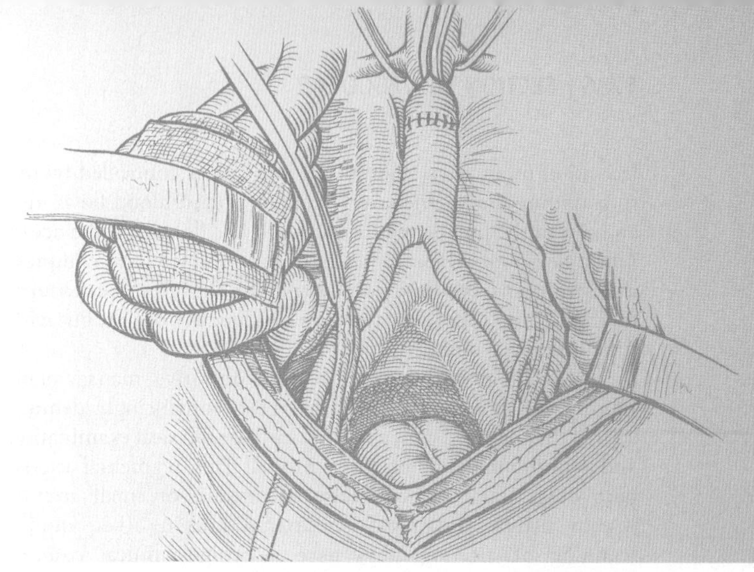

CHAPTER 64

# VASCULAR TRAUMA

Michael J. Sise and Steven R. Shackford



Vascular trauma remains one of the most significant challenges in the management of injured patients. The advent of trauma systems and improved prehospital care have resulted in an increasing number of patients with what were previously fatal vascular injuries arriving at trauma centers still alive, but in immediate danger of death.[1,2] Vascular trauma is not always obvious and timely recognition may be difficult in patients with multiple injuries.[3] The time urgency and high-risk potential in managing these injuries requires an organized approach to deliver appropriate care in a timely fashion. Because so much is at stake, this is a high-risk clinical environment requiring systematic planning, preparation, and the use of practice guidelines for successful early recognition and effective treatment.

This chapter reviews the pathophysiology, clinical presentation, diagnostic workup, management, and outcome of vascular injuries. The educational objectives of this review include the following:

- Elucidate the mechanisms of vessel injury and resulting clinical manifestations.
- Provide an organized approach to assess injured patients rapidly for the presence of vascular injuries in the neck, torso, and extremities.
- Present management guidelines to help decide which treatment options best apply and how to implement them effectively.
- Articulate the clinically important sequelae of vascular injuries and their appropriate management to maximize functional recovery.

## GENERAL APPROACH TO VASCULAR TRAUMA

### Mechanism of Injury

Vascular injury can be produced by a blunt or penetrating mechanism. Penetrating injury tends to be more discrete or focal, whereas blunt injury is more diffuse, with injury not only to the vascular structures but also to the bone, muscle, and nerves. The diffuseness of the blunt injury not only affects the major vascular conduit, but also disrupts smaller vessels that would normally provide collateral flow. As a result, ischemia is worsened or exaggerated. Penetrating injury is generally classified as low velocity (<2500 ft/sec; e.g., stab wound, fragment injury, handgun wound) or high velocity (>2500 ft/sec; e.g., military rifle wound).[4] High-velocity weapons produce significantly more tissue damage than low-velocity weapons for three main reasons[5,6]:

- Energy imparted—energy equals the mass of the projectile multiplied by the velocity squared.
- Tract cavitation—the missile creates a rapidly expanding and rapidly contracting cavity that can reach a size equal to 30 times the diameter of the projectile, at right angles to the missile tract, which stretches and tears the adjacent tissue.
- Lead splatter—fragments of the deteriorating projectile become missiles themselves.

Trauma to a blood vessel (artery or vein) can produce hemorrhage, thrombosis, or spasm, alone or in combination, depending on the magnitude of the force applied to the vessel and on the degree of injury. Hemorrhage is produced when all of the layers, the intima, media, and adventitia, are disrupted or lacerated. If the bleeding is controlled locally, a hematoma is produced, which may or may not be pulsatile. If bleeding is not controlled, exsanguination can occur. Thrombosis occurs if there is damage to the intima exposing the underlying media and causing local thrombus formation, which may propagate and occlude the lumen or embolize distally. In addition, the injured intima can prolapse into the lumen as a result of blood flow dissecting under it, producing partial or complete obstruction. Trauma to surrounding bony structures may cause external compression of the vessel, interrupting flow and producing thrombosis. Spasm occurs if there is external trauma to the vessel, such as stretching or contusion, which can stimulate the release of mediators (e.g., hemoglobin) that cause constriction of the vascular smooth muscle. Spasm, by reducing the cross-sectional area of the vessel, reduces flow.

In addition to the acute pathophysiology produced by hemorrhage and thrombosis, direct trauma can produce subacute, chronic, or occult injuries. The most common are arteriovenous fistula and pseudoaneurysm. An arteriovenous fistula typically occurs after penetrating trauma that causes injury to an artery and vein in close proximity. The high-pressure flow from the artery will follow the path of least vascular resistance into the vein, producing local, regional, and systemic signs and symptoms. These include local tenderness and edema, regional ischemia from steal, and congestive heart failure if the fistula enlarges.[7] A pseudoaneurysm is a result of a puncture or laceration of an artery that bleeds into and is controlled by the surrounding tissue. The artery remains patent; blood flows into and out of the pseudoaneurysm, much like flow from the ocean into a tide pool. These can enlarge and produce local compressive symptoms, erode adjacent structures or, rarely, be a source of distal emboli. Initially, they can be clinically occult, but with time become symptomatic.

Not all arterial injuries require operative management. During the past 2 decades, it has been convincingly demonstrated that patients with a normal vascular physical examination and asymptomatic nonocclusive intimal flaps, segmental arterial narrowing, small (<2-cm) false aneurysms, or small arteriovenous fistulas discovered on arterial imaging (i.e., duplex scanning or arteriography) have a benign clinical course.[8] Approximately 10% of these minimal injuries will progress to require a surgical or endovascular repair and most within the first week after injury. Thus, it is imperative that these patients have close follow-up with physical examination and duplex imaging, if needed. In rare cases, when a nonocclusive minimal injury increases in size or becomes symptomatic, requiring operative or endovascular repair, morbidity is not increased by the delay.

## Clinical Presentation

Vascular injuries can present with a broad spectrum of clinical manifestations, from profound hemorrhagic shock to subtle findings, such as an asymptomatic bruit. Patients who present in hemorrhagic shock must be assumed to have a major vascular injury until proven otherwise. There are five anatomic areas to consider, each with specific considerations. In the head and neck, external hemorrhage is required for vascular injuries to result in shock. Relatively small and tightly organized tissue planes preclude significant internal hemorrhage. In the chest, each hemithorax can accommodate lethal amounts of hemorrhage from cardiac, pulmonary, or great vessel arterial and venous injuries. Abdominal and pelvic vascular injuries can also result in lethal hemorrhage, particularly from the aorta and iliac arteries. Like the head and neck, extremity vascular injuries generally cause hemorrhagic shock only if there is significant external hemorrhage. The patient with hypotension and a lack of chest, abdominal, and pelvic findings may have what appears to be a trivial neck or extremity laceration, but which initially communicated with a major vessel injury. It is important to remember that hemorrhage sufficient to produce hypotension can be followed by thrombosis. It is therefore necessary to obtain a history from the prehospital personnel about the amount of blood at the scene or the initial presence of severe wound hemorrhage. It is also necessary to examine the patient thoroughly for additional wounds and to assess each of them carefully.

Extremity vascular trauma may be immediately apparent on presentation because of external hemorrhage, hematoma, or obvious limb ischemia. A history of penetrating trauma associated with hypotension, pulsatile bleeding, or a large quantity of blood at the scene suggest vascular injury. Blunt trauma is also capable of causing significant vascular injury that can be overlooked when serious head, chest, or abdominal injuries are present. Extremity fractures may result in vascular injury. Supracondylar humerus fractures can be associated with brachial artery injury and knee dislocation carries a significant risk of popliteal artery injury.[9] Crush injuries of the extremity without fracture may also result in vascular injury.

A relatively small number of vascular injuries present in a delayed fashion, without initial findings. These are limited to thrombosis of a previously partially disrupted but initially patent vessel, distal emboli from an intimal tear of the arterial wall with formation of platelet debris and, least commonly, rupture or expansion of a pseudoaneurysm that was initially small and contained by the outer arterial wall and local tissue.[9] Local signs of hematoma, diminished pulses, and the presence of patterns of associated injuries should indicate the presence of these vascular injuries. A thorough history and physical examination and appropriate adjunctive imaging studies will result in an effective initial diagnosis and result in a decrease in the frequency of these delayed presentations.

Because there is such a broad spectrum of clinical findings associated with vascular trauma, it is best to assume that vascular injury is present until proven otherwise in all patients with hemorrhagic shock and all patients with extremity fractures.

## Diagnosis

### Physical Examination

Vascular injury can produce systemic symptoms of hypotension, tachycardia, and altered mental status because of hypovolemic shock produced by hemorrhage. As a result, vascular injury can be life-threatening and attention must initially be directed to the primary survey using the principles of advanced trauma life support (ATLS).[10] The airway must be assessed, adequate oxygenation and ventilation ensured, and intravenous access achieved. Once this is completed and resuscitation is underway, the secondary survey is undertaken. A thorough history is obtained and careful physical examination is performed. This examination must include a careful inspection of the injured sites and wounds, complete sensory and motor assessment, and pulse examination of each extremity. The presence of a hematoma, bruit, or thrill must be noted. If distal pulses are diminished or absent, ankle or wrist systolic blood pressure should be determined with a continuous wave Doppler device and compared with the uninjured side. A significant difference in systolic blood pressure (>10 mm Hg) between extremities may be an indication of vascular injury. Patients with hard findings of vascular injury (Box 64-1) should be taken directly to the operating room.

In patients without hard findings, but with soft findings (see Box 64-1), vascular imaging can be used to rule out the need for operation. Additionally, patients with hard findings but with multilevel injuries in the same extremity may also need imaging. Catheter arteriography is sensitive and specific for the diagnosis of extremity vascular injuries (Fig. 64-1). Computed tomography angiography (CTA) with the latest generation scanners has proved to be an acceptable alternative to formal arteriography (Fig. 64-2).[11,12] Although this imaging technique requires a contrast infusion, it does not require arterial catheterization, is easily performed and is less costly and time-consuming than conventional angiography.

Some severely injured patients must be taken to the operating room to treat severe life-threatening associated injuries (e.g., subdural hematoma, ruptured spleen). In such cases, it is not prudent to delay operative therapy to obtain formal vascular imaging. An arteriogram can be obtained in the operating room by cannulating the artery proximal to the suspected vascular injury, injecting 20 to 25 mL of full-strength contrast, and

**BOX 64-1 Findings of Vascular Injury**

**Hard Findings**

These indicate need the for operative intervention for vascular injury:

- Pulsatile bleeding
- Expanding hematoma
- Palpable thrill or audible bruit
- Evidence of extremity ischemia
  - Pallor
  - Paresthesia
  - Paralysis
  - Pain
  - Pulselessness
  - Poikilothermia

**Soft Findings**

Consider further imaging and evaluation for vascular injury:

- History of moderate hemorrhage
- Injury (e.g., fracture, dislocation, penetrating wound)
- Diminished but palpable pulse
- Peripheral nerve deficit
- Wounds in proximity to extremity or neck vessels in patients with unexplained hemorrhagic shock

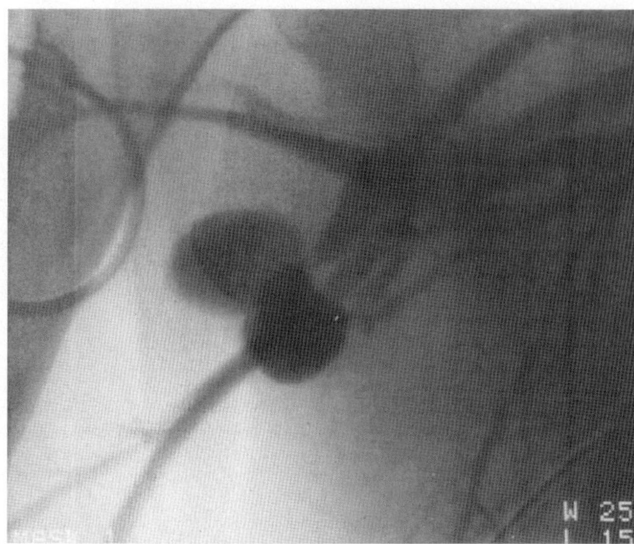

**FIGURE 64-1** Catheter arteriogram demonstrating an acute pseudoaneurysm and arteriovenous fistula of the right axillary artery and vein in a patient with a stab wound of the right anterolateral chest wall.

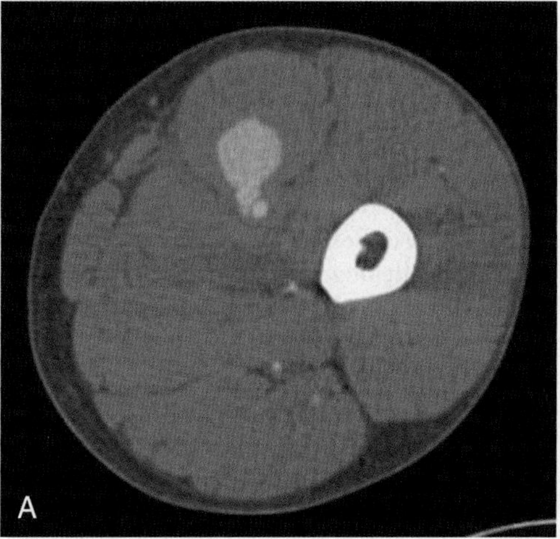


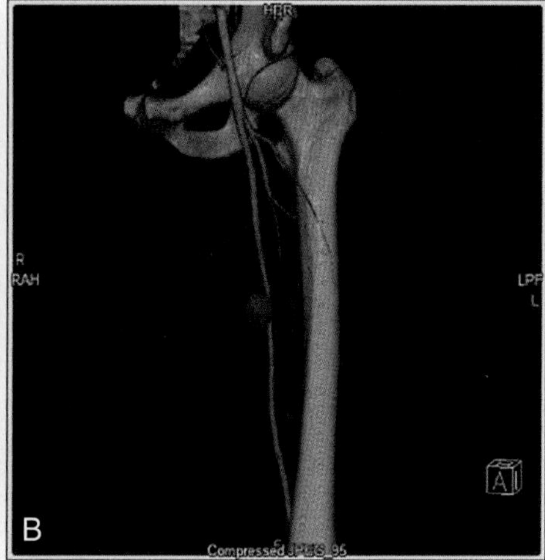


**FIGURE 64-2** CT angiogram. **A,** Cross-sectional view of the upper thigh. **B,** Volume rendering tomography view of femoral pseudoaneurysm in a patient with a metal fragment injury to the left superficial femoral artery.

taking an x-ray or using fluoroscopy (Fig. 64-3).[13,14] If doubt remains about the presence of a vascular injury and imaging studies and other diagnostic tests are inconclusive, there is a role for operative exploration and direct assessment of the artery. Routine operative exploration in the stable patient with soft signs, however, has a 5% to 30% incidence of morbidity, occasional mortality, and low diagnostic yield.[15] These patients are better served with formal vascular imaging.

Duplex color flow imaging is not used for the acute assessment of vascular injury. Wounds, swelling, presence of air in the tissue, and presence of dressings or splints impair the ability to obtain satisfactory images. Duplex imaging does have a role in the follow-up of treated lesions (e.g., to assess patency of bypass grafts or detect luminal stenosis at an anastomosis) or in the follow-up of nonoperative management of minimal vascular injury, such as small pseudoaneurysms or arteriovenous fistulas.

## Treatment

### Minimal Vascular Injury and Nonoperative Management

The widespread application of arteriography in the evaluation of injured extremities has resulted in the detection of clinically insignificant lesions. There is now an extensive body of experience with lesions that are not clinically significant. These minimal vascular injuries include intimal irregularity, focal spasm with minimal narrowing, and small pseudoaneurysms. They are often asymptomatic and usually do not progress.

A small, nonocclusive intimal flap is the most common clinically insignificant minimal vascular injury. The likelihood

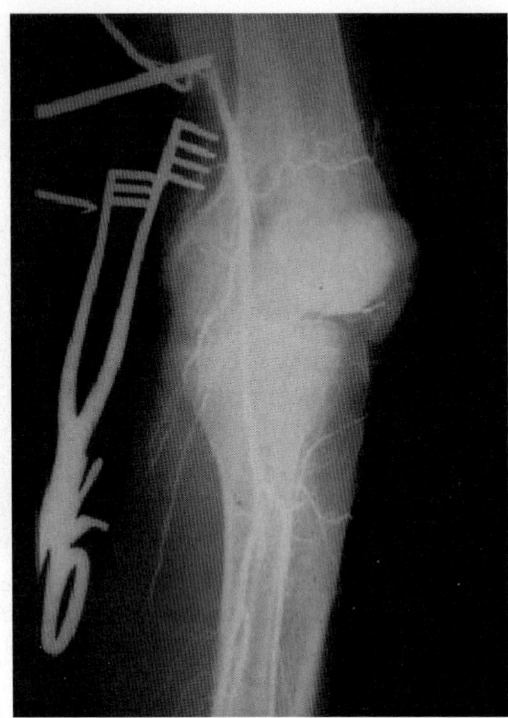

**FIGURE 64-3** Intraoperative plain film (direct injection arteriogram) in patient explored for penetrating left knee joint injury and determination of popliteal arterial injury.

that it will progress to cause occlusion or distal embolization is approximately 10% to 15%.[8,16] This progression, if it occurs, will be early in the postinjury course. Spasm is another common minimal vascular injury. This finding should resolve promptly after initial discovery. Failure of the return of normal extremity perfusion pressure indicates that a more serious vascular injury is present and intervention is needed. Small pseudoaneurysms are more likely to progress to the point of needing repair and must be actively followed with Duplex color flow imaging. Arteriovenous fistulas always enlarge over time and should be promptly repaired.

Considerable evidence suggests that nonoperative therapy of many asymptomatic lesions is safe and effective. However, successful nonoperative therapy requires continuous surveillance for subsequent progression, occlusion, or hemorrhage. Operative therapy is required for thrombosis, symptoms of chronic ischemia, and failure of small pseudoaneurysms to resolve.

### Endovascular Management

The use of endovascular therapy for the treatment of atherosclerotic arterial disease has become widespread. Endoluminal stent deployment for occlusive lesions and stent graft for aortic aneurysms have been used successively in select patients; there is now a strong tendency to generalize from this elective experience in older patients with atherosclerosis to the treatment of younger patients with acute vascular injuries. Most major trauma centers have some experience with endoluminal treatment of acute vascular lesions. However, the evidence to support these approaches is not well developed and there have been problems.[17-19] A review of available evidence combined with common sense should help identify the appropriate role of endovascular management of traumatic injuries.[9,18]

**Torso Injuries** Endovascular techniques offer various options for hemorrhage control in the torso. Intra-arterial catheter-directed embolization has become a mainstay of the management of solid organ hemorrhage in the abdomen.[20,21] Whether used as the sole treatment or in combination with open procedures, this approach has been effective for liver, spleen, and kidney injuries. Less commonly used intra-arterial balloon occlusion for proximal control is a promising adjunct to open repair.[22,23] These techniques are quick, accurate, and easily performed. The major obstacle to their widespread popularity has been the reluctance of surgeons to adopt catheter skills or partner with interventional radiologists to bring these techniques to the trauma operating room (OR). It does not require a dedicated endovascular suite to perform these techniques. A digital C arm and the proper catheters transforms any OR to an endovascular-capable room.

The early use of catheter-directed control of hemorrhage associated with pelvic fracture is an effective method of limiting blood loss and improving outcome.[24] This approach is well tolerated and has proven superior to open attempts at hemorrhage control by packing in most patients. Unstable patients benefit from an immediate trip to the operating room. If intraoperative endovascular capability is available, a combined approach may offer the best results.

Enthusiasm for stent graft management of great vessel injuries in the chest has steadily grown. The success of stent grafts for the treatment of aneurysm disease in the infrarenal aorta has led to the use of similar devices to treat contained thoracic aortic lacerations following blunt trauma. The initial results have been encouraging but are not without complications.[18] Lifelong CT imaging is necessary because of the possibility of delayed endoleak and possible loss of device fixation as the aorta enlarges over time. There is a promising role for covered stents in proximal branches of the aorta in the thorax and abdomen. In stable injuries at risk for delayed hemorrhage or thrombosis, carefully placed stents have the potential to lower morbidity compared with open procedures that require extensive operative dissection for exposure and control. Endoluminal management with stent grafts appears most effective in those torso injuries that are surgically inaccessible, with the potential for significant hemorrhage in stable patients (Fig. 64-4). These techniques should only be used in centers with an active elective endovascular practice that has experience in treating trauma patients.

**Cerebrovascular Injuries** Endovascular techniques offer advantages in anatomic regions in which direct operative control is difficult or impossible. For example, hemorrhage from a penetrating injury at the base of the skull is extremely difficult to control. Catheter-directed placement of coil, balloon, or hemostatic agent in the injured carotid or vertebral artery could be lifesaving. Initially, stent placement appeared to be less effective than anticoagulation in partially occluded injuries without associated hemorrhage.[17,25] However, the role of stents in cerebrovascular trauma has yet to be defined and may prove safe.[26] This use of endoluminal interventions, however, requires significant expertise and experience. If such experience does not exist at the receiving hospital, consideration should be given to transferring

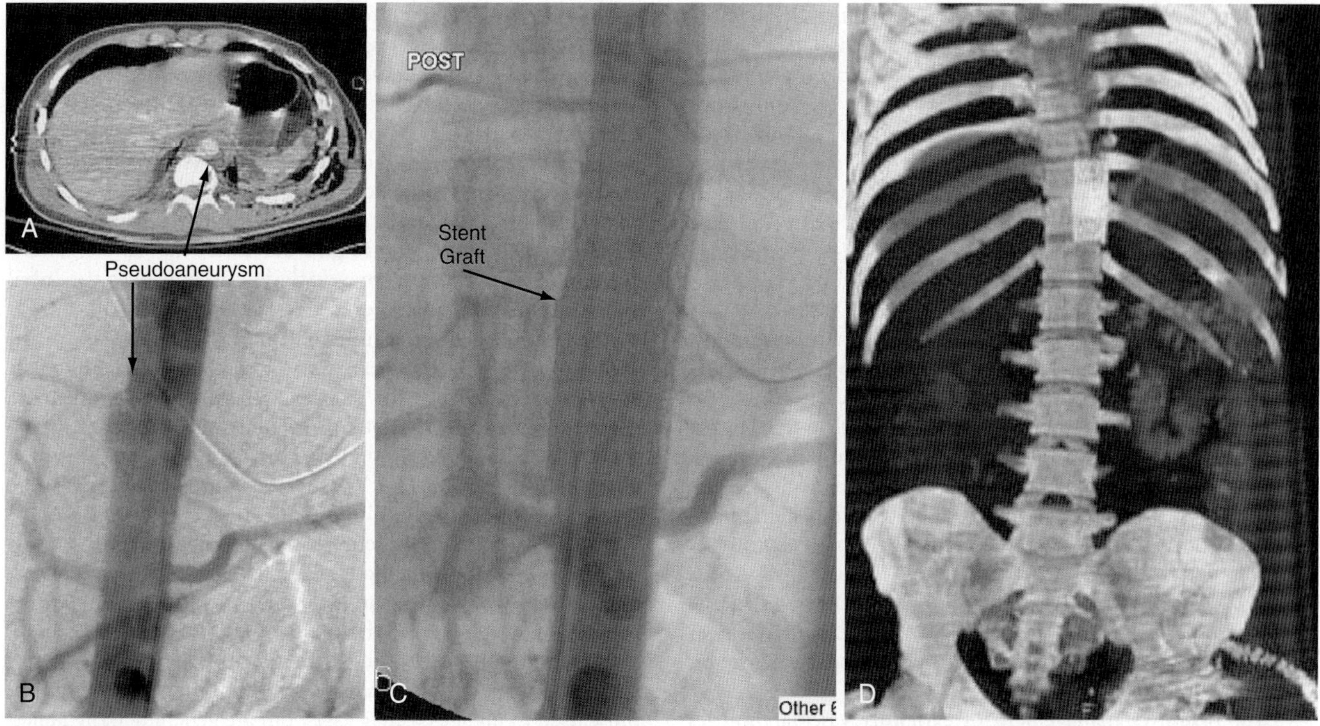


**FIGURE 64-4** Endovascular repair of difficult to expose aortic injury with pseudoaneurysm at the diaphragm from blunt force trauma. **A,** CT angiogram showing cross-sectional view of pseudoaneurysm and associated thoracic spine fracture, **B,** Catheter arteriogram demonstrating the pseudoaneurysm. **C,** Deployed stent graft. **D,** CT scan of level of aortic stent graft in midtorso (VTR view).

the patient to a medical center with experience in this mode of therapy.

**Extremity Vascular Injury** The use of stent grafts in the extremities is becoming more common [27,28] The long-term results, however, have not been documented and caution should be used when considering this type of treatment. Covered stents can be used to improve intraluminal diameter in partially occluded traumatized vessels with favorable early patency rates; however, they are prone to occlusion and long-term outcomes are as yet unknown. Autologous vein interposition grafts have excellent long-term patency rates and remain the gold standard for vascular repairs in the extremities.

Catheter-directed therapies for controlling hemorrhage from large branch vessels in the extremities are often effective and sufficient to manage these injuries.[29] Endoluminal treatment is not advocated for pseudoaneurysms of the extremity arteries. Small pseudoaneurysms are likely to resolve without any intervention and large pseudoaneurysms are best treated with open techniques because the risk of arterial thrombosis or distal embolization is high with this endovascular intervention.

**Who Should Perform Endovascular Repairs?** Successful management of vascular injuries requires that the most qualified person perform the indicated intervention in the appropriate patient, in the appropriate place, and at the appropriate time. Endovascular surgery is one of many approaches and, like all surgical procedures, should be performed by readily available trained clinicians who are cognizant of not only the technical aspects of a procedure, but who are also knowledgeable about the disease for which the procedure is being performed. In many centers, this person is the interventional radiologist. Other centers have catheter-trained vascular surgeons and others have trauma surgeons capable of performing endovascular procedures.

Endoluminal management of vascular trauma does not require a full endovascular suite. Rather, a modern digital C arm for fluoroscopy, appropriate radiation protection for the OR team, and access to a wide variety of catheters converts any OR into an endovascular-capable room. Planning and preparation are, however, essential for the success of such a conversion, which occasionally is done in the middle of the night. Preparing a team that can perform these techniques and organize the appropriate equipment with brief notice requires commitment, dedication, collaboration, and repeated training.

### Surgical Treatment

**Preparation for Operative Management** Operative procedures to manage vascular injuries should be limited to those surgeons who are capable, experienced, and qualified. Board certification in vascular surgery is not enough to qualify a surgeon as capable of handling these injuries, just as the lack of certification does not necessarily disqualify a surgeon. Many surgeons who perform elective vascular surgery are not sufficiently experienced in the management of vascular trauma. Conversely, there are many trauma surgeons who are skilled in vascular technique by virtue of their interest and experience.

Successful operative management of vascular injuries requires a systematic approach, with careful preparation. This begins with airway control, adequate intravenous access, and availability of blood products. However, these blood products should not be administered before obtaining control of hemorrhage unless the patient is profoundly hypotensive.[30-32] If the blood pressure (BP) is below approximately 80 to 90 mm Hg, the goal should be to provide adequate volume restoration with O-negative packed cells and type AB fresh-frozen plasma infusion to support transport to the operating room for definitive hemorrhage control without delay. Volume infusion that raises the blood pressure above a systolic pressure of 90 to 100 mm Hg may increase bleeding and negatively affect outcome, particularly if the infusion delays transport to the OR.

Broad-spectrum preoperative antibiotics (and tetanus toxoid, if it is a penetrating wound) should be administered; if there is an isolated extremity injury without significant hemorrhage, an IV bolus of 5000 U of heparin should also be given. Systemic heparinization should be avoided in patients with torso injuries, head injuries, or multiple extremity injuries.

The most commonly omitted step in preparation is a failure to document preoperative extremity neurologic status. The presence of a neurologic deficit after operative vascular repair without knowing the preoperative status presents a difficult management challenge. A new neurologic deficit after vascular repair merits investigation and, possibly, reoperation. Therefore, a thorough preoperative neurologic examination and careful documentation are essential to effective management.

The operative management of extremity vascular injuries must be carefully orchestrated with the overall care of the patient. The choice between definitive repair and damage control should be made as soon as possible in patients with life-threatening torso injuries or severe head injuries. This includes coordinating two surgical teams to work simultaneously to care for the torso injury and extremity vascular injury at the same time. Associated injuries to the soft tissue and bone require a coordinated assessment and treatment with orthopedic and plastic surgery consultants. These specialists should be involved as early as possible to facilitate any additional imaging or diagnostic procedures prior to proceeding to the OR. The conduct of the operation should also be discussed with these colleagues.[32] For example, the use of damage control procedures with shunt placement, followed by orthopedic stabilization, can remove the sense of urgency to restore blood flow. Extensive soft tissue injuries may compromise the proper coverage of vascular repairs and fracture fixation. The advice and assistance of a plastic and reconstructive surgeon can be helpful in obtaining coverage of exposed grafts and fractures.

**Vascular Exposure and Control** A generous sterile field should be prepared to allow for the adequate exposure of vessels to obtain proximal and distal control. In torso injuries, this includes prepping the chest and abdomen to the table laterally on both sides and both legs in case distal access or an autologous conduit is needed. For proximal vascular injuries of the extremities, at the groin crease or axilla, the chest or abdomen should be prepared to obtain proximal control out of the zone of injury. An uninjured leg should be also prepared for harvesting of autologous venous conduit.

Proximal control is the first priority in the exposure of vascular injuries.[33] In the torso, chest injuries with life-threatening hemorrhage are best approached through a fourth intercostal space anterolateral thoracotomy that can be extended across the sternum into the third intercostal space of the right chest to create a clamshell incision. Thoracic outlet and proximal neck vascular injuries may require median sternotomy, with extension above the clavicle, up along the ipsilateral sternocleidomastoid muscle. For abdominal vascular injuries, a generous xiphoid to pubis incision is needed for adequate exposure. Proximal control for aortic injuries can be obtained just below the aortic hiatus of the diaphragm or may require a left anterolateral thoracotomy to clamp the distal thoracic aorta.

In proximal extremity injuries with active hemorrhage, the first incision site is chosen to give the fastest exposure of inflow vessels for clamping; this may include incisions over the infraclavicular region of the chest to expose the axillary artery. For injuries in the groin, prepare to enter the lower quadrant of the abdomen for access to the external iliac vessels. In mid and distal extremity vascular injuries associated with active hemorrhage, tourniquets can rapidly obtain control in the trauma resuscitation room. In the operating room, have one team member compress the bleeding site precisely with a gloved hand and a sponge, remove the tourniquet, and prepare the extremity. A 5000-U heparin bolus is then given, if appropriate, the extremity is prepared and draped, and a sterile tourniquet is placed proximal to the wound and inflated. The injury site can then be explored in a controlled fashion and clamps or vessel loops placed above and below the vascular injury.

Incisions used to manage vascular injuries are the same as those used to mange elective cases, but are generally more generous. The use of smaller incisions may lead to errors in identifying the extent of vascular injury, adequately controlling branch vessel hemorrhage, and identifying associated venous lacerations. This is particularly true for popliteal artery and vein injuries. A limited approach with separate medial above- and below-knee incisions will not expose the site of injury adequately. A medial incision from the proximal popliteal space to the distal popliteal space, with division of the medial head of the gastrocnemius, semimembranosus, and semitendinosus muscles, with full exposure of the popliteal artery and vein and tibial nerve, provides adequate exposure. This ensures adequate vascular control and the opportunity for successful repair. Closure of the wound to include approximation of the divided muscles yields an excellent functional result. Dividing the inguinal ligament in the groin, dividing the pectoralis major in the axilla, and removing the midclavicle may rarely be necessary. In the presence of life-threatening hemorrhage that cannot be controlled by any other approach, these structures should not stand in the way of adequate exposure and control.

There are various adjunctive measures that can obtain temporary control. In the resuscitation bay, insertion and inflation of a Foley catheter in a wound in the neck or extremities with active hemorrhage can obtain temporary control and allow for safe transfer to the operating room.[30] In the OR, insertion of Fogarty balloon tip catheters under direct vision at sites in the artery above or below the injury also serves to gain control in difficult to reach anatomic areas.

**Vascular Damage Control** Damage control has gained wide acceptance in trauma surgery and is directed at rapid control of hemorrhage and closure of enteric wounds so that the patient can be warmed and resuscitated. The choice between definitive, time-consuming vascular repair and temporary measures that achieve control must be made early in the care of patients with vascular injury and hypovolemic shock. This is particularly important when an extremity vascular injury is associated with major torso injuries. The use of ligation or placement of intra-luminal shunts are the mainstays of vascular damage control.[32,34,35]

Ligation should be reserved for vessels with adequate distal collateral flow. In the torso, this includes the subclavian and innominate arteries, celiac artery, and inferior mesenteric artery. In the upper extremity, proximal injuries of the axillary artery and distal injuries to the radial or ulnar arteries may be ligated, provided there is evidence of adequate distal collateral flow assessed by physical examination or continuous wave Doppler interrogation. Similarly, in the lower extremity, ligation of a single tibial vessel or peroneal can be performed after a similar assessment. If distal perfusion is compromised, an intraluminal shunt should be inserted, rather than ligating the vessel. Superior mesenteric artery ligation is associated with a high risk of bowel necrosis and damage control is best accomplished with placement of an intraluminal shunt. In the extremities, ligation of the brachial, external iliac, superficial femoral, or popliteal artery has a high likelihood of producing limb-threatening ischemia and should be avoided, if possible.

There are various commercially available shunts that can be used for damage control. If these are not available, sterile IV tubing is of adequate size to shunt the artery and vein, if necessary. Venous shunt placement, instead of ligation, may improve extremity perfusion and lower the risk of compartment syndrome. Damage control shunt placement begins with obtaining adequate proximal and distal control. Thrombus should be cleared with a Fogarty embolectomy catheter, followed by the instillation of regional heparinized saline (10 U heparin/1 mL saline). The shunt should be placed in a straight line and long enough to remain safely held in place in the proximal and distal vessels with a tied umbilical tape or 2-0 silk tie at each end. Long looped shunts run the risk of becoming dislodged during subsequent dressing changes and should be avoided. The ties securing the shunt cause intimal damage, and those portions of the artery must be resected at the time of definitive vascular repair.

The condition of the patient determines the timing of definitive vascular repair following damage control. Hemorrhage must be controlled, coagulopathy and acidosis corrected, and temperature normalized.

**Choice of Repair and Graft Material** Vessel injuries that cannot be repaired by primary end-to-end technique will require an interposition graft. The most desirable graft is an autologous greater saphenous vein harvested from an uninjured leg.[9] Native vein graft is preferable for several reasons: it has elastic properties that make it compliant with the normal pulsatile flow of an artery; its diameter approximates that of an extremity artery, producing an adequately sized match for grafting in the arm and leg; it is not thrombogenic; and it has superior long-term patency in elective vascular surgery when compared with prosthetic material when used with smaller vessels (e.g., popliteal, tibial). The cephalic vein and lesser saphenous vein have been suggested as suitable second choices, but cephalic vein is less muscular than the greater saphenous vein and, like the lesser saphenous vein, may present problems with harvesting in a trauma patient.[36] Also, upper extremity venous access becomes compromised when the cephalic vein is used.

Saphenous vein may not be suitable in all cases because of inadequate size or because it has been traumatized or harvested previously.[37] In such cases, a prosthetic conduit may be needed. Initial experiences with the use of prosthetic material (Dacron) in traumatic vascular injuries were not good. Rich and Hughes[38] have reported a complication rate of 77%—infection and thrombosis were the most common—in 26 patients. However, experience with a newer graft material, polytetrafluoroethylene (PTFE), has shown improved patency (70% to 90% short term) and rare infection, even in contaminated wounds.[39,40] It is clear that patency with PTFE is equivalent to that of a vein for injuries proximal to the popliteal artery, but inferior to a vein for popliteal and more distal vessels, and that PTFE grafts smaller than 6 mm should not be used. PTFE and vein grafts must be covered or there is a significant risk of hemorrhage from desiccation of the vein, with subsequent autolysis or breakdown of the anastomosis.[41]

**Intraoperative Imaging and Noninvasive Evaluation** The successful management of vascular injury requires knowing the status of the blood flow in the area of the vessel injury precisely. Preoperative imaging with catheter angiography or CTA is not always possible. In addition, when a vascular repair has been completed, the presence of thrombus, kinking, or unexpected technical problems may cause early failure. Intraoperative imaging is, therefore, an important part of assessing the injured vessels and repair site.[36] A single injection of contrast with single shot radiography or fluoroscopy is effective in providing images in the operating room (see Fig. 64-3). Intraoperative duplex scanning is also effective but requires significant training and experience to perform it adequately. Hand-held continuous wave Doppler interrogation can be helpful, but requires considerable experience to be effective. Ankle or wrist pressure measurements may be misleading because of regional vasospasm in the proximal injured extremity, resulting in a reduced distal pressure compared with that of the uninjured leg. Intraoperative radiographic imaging remains the most accurate and useful method to detect technical problems with a vascular repair and determine the presence of thrombus in the runoff vessels distal to a repair. Routine completion arteriography following vascular repairs will yield findings of clinical importance in approximately 10% of patients.

### Role of Tissue Coverage

All vascular repairs must be covered to prevent desiccation and disruption. In crushed or badly mangled extremities, this can be a difficult challenge. Rotation of regional muscle or skin flaps may be required. The early involvement of a plastic and reconstructive surgeon is essential to obtain tissue coverage when there is extensive soft tissue injury or loss. Local muscle can be advanced into the wound at the initial operation. If there is a large contaminated wound and local muscle viability is questionable (e.g., which may occur following a shotgun wound or blast injury) temporary coverage can be obtained using a homograft (cadaver skin) or xenograft (pigskin).[42] The homograft or xenograft will be temporarily accepted by an immunocompromised trauma patient and often can stay in place for 5 to 7 days or longer. This will allow sufficient time for planning and carrying out definitive coverage.

Occasionally, tissue loss may be so extensive that an extra-anatomic course for an interposition graft may be required. Attention to coverage is also essential in damage control procedures to avoid shunt dislodgment during dressing changes.

### Fasciotomy

Failure to perform an adequate fasciotomy after revascularization of an acutely ischemic limb is the most common cause of preventable limb loss.[36] Calf compartment syndrome is the most common indication for fasciotomy. Forearm and thigh compartment syndromes are less common. Any muscle group can develop compartment syndrome, including those in the hands and feet.

Compartment syndrome may present 12 to 24 hours after reperfusion. If not promptly diagnosed and treated, the risk of limb loss or limb dysfunction is high. Calf compartment syndrome most commonly results from prolonged ischemia or a crush injury. Frequent physical examinations augmented with compartment pressure measurements are necessary to detect this complication in its early stage. The first clinical finding is loss of light touch sensation in the distribution of the nerve in the compartment (i.e., peroneal in the anterior compartment of the leg). The diagnosis of compartment syndrome should be suspected in any patient complaining of increasing pain following injury. The physical findings include a tense compartment, pain on passive range of motion, progressive loss of sensation, and weakness. The loss of arterial pulses is a late finding, which usually indicates a poor prognosis. Neurologic signs and symptoms, although helpful, are neither sensitive nor specific in the upper extremity following arterial injury because associated peripheral nerve injury often exists. Early diagnosis must be predicated on measurement of compartment pressures. The normal tissue compartment pressure ranges from 0 to 9 mm Hg. Much controversy exists about what constitutes a pathologic elevation. However, the safest approach is to perform fasciotomy when the compartment pressure exceeds 25 mm Hg.[43]

A compartment syndrome can also develop in the upper arm (triceps, deltoid, or along the axillary sheath) or forearm. The forearm compartment syndrome is more common. Increased tissue pressure can follow blunt or penetrating trauma because of hematoma, post-traumatic transudation of serum into the interstitial space, venous thrombosis, or reperfusion following ischemia.[36] The possibility of a compartment syndrome must always be a consideration in a patient who has been injured, particularly one with prolonged ischemia prior to reperfusion.

### Role of Immediate Amputation

A very limited role for primary amputation exists in the management of complex extremity vascular injuries. Patients with extensive soft tissue loss, neurologic deficit, extensive fractures, and vascular injuries should be evaluated collaboratively with orthopedic, neurosurgical, and plastic and reconstructive surgery colleagues to determine if primary amputation is the best initial management (Fig. 64-5). The use of scoring systems to predict the need for amputation have not been useful.[43] Damage control techniques with vascular shunt placement and temporary closure allow time for the extent of tissue destruction to become evident. Re-exploration at 24 to 36 hours will result in a more accurate assessment of viability. Documentation of operative findings with photographs placed in the chart is often helpful when explaining to patients and their families why amputation was necessary. This time interval allows communication with the patient and family and implementation of a more planned approach. Immediate amputation should also be considered for patients with extensive soft tissue, bone, and neurovascular disruption who have life-threatening torso injuries (see earlier discussion of damage control techniques). If immediate amputation is required, extensive documentation of the extremity injury with photographs placed in the chart will be helpful in explaining the decision to the patient and family later and will help with their acceptance of this drastic surgical procedure.

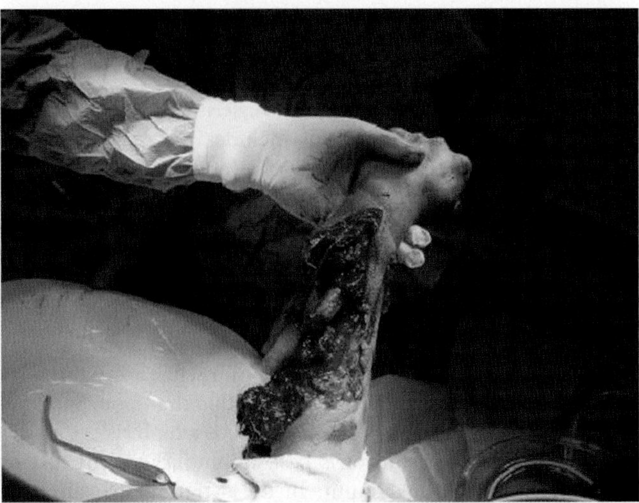

**FIGURE 64-5** Devastating left forearm injury with destruction of all three vessels and all major nerves with missing bone fragments. It was caused by a close-range shotgun blast and required immediate amputation. This is one of the digital photographs placed in the medical record.

### Common Errors and Pitfalls

The management of vascular injuries is challenging. An organized approach is necessary to avoid common errors and pitfalls. One of the most common errors is the lack of recognition of an extremity vascular injury in a patient with multiple torso injuries. Failure to recognize and adequately treat compartment syndrome is another error that is all too common and can have devastating consequences. In torso injuries to the great vessels, failure to expose and control the injured site adequately can lead to a rapid death from exsanguination. Finally, failure to recognize the need for damage control techniques and a rapid completion of the operation in an unstable patient can also be deadly. The three most common factors in generating errors when caring for the injured are fatigue, distraction, and familiarity.[44] Each of these factors is inherent in the process of care at busy trauma centers. An organized approach mitigates these factors and intercepts error in progress before they are completed and the patients suffer.

## SPECIFIC INJURIES

### Head, Neck, and Thoracic Outlet

Vascular injuries of the head, neck, and thoracic outlet can present significant problems. Penetrating trauma can injure large vessels, such as the innominate or subclavian, which can lead to exsanguination. Blunt trauma to the carotid or vertebral, collectively known as *blunt cerebrovascular injuries*, are often occult and, if not diagnosed and treated rapidly, can lead to cerebral ischemia, infarction, and death.

The principles of management of penetrating trauma to this region are based on the location of the injury relative to the three zones of the neck originally described by Monson:

- Zone 1: Inferior to the cricoid cartilage
- Zone 2: Cricoid cartilage to the angle of the mandible
- Zone 3: Cephalad from the angle of the mandible

In a stable patient with a suspected vascular injury in zone 1 or 3, vascular imaging is mandatory to confirm the suspicion of vascular injury and plan proximal and distal control.[45] Vascular imaging is also recommended for stable patients with penetrating trauma in zone 2, but exploration should be undertaken expeditiously for patients with an expanding hematoma or impending airway compromise, manifested by hoarseness and tracheal deviation.[46] In the unstable patient, a Fogarty thrombectomy catheter or Foley urinary catheter can be inserted into the wound to achieve temporary tamponade of injuries in these regions. Conventional angiography can have a dual role for injuries in zone 1 or 3. It not only provides the diagnosis, but also may provide a venue for endoluminal management—coiling of bleeding vessels or pseudoaneurysms in zone 3 or placement of covered stents in zone 1.

Blunt cerebrovascular injuries (BCVIs) are often occult and asymptomatic. Therefore, rapid diagnostic screening is essential and provides the underpinning of successful management. Initially, BCVIs were thought to be rare, occurring in approximately 0.1% of patients, but using the screening criteria developed by the group at Denver General Hospital, the incidence is actually 10 to 20 times that (Box 64-2).[47] Carotid and vertebral artery injuries occur from stretching or tearing of the intima of the vessels caused by rapid extreme extension or flexion of the neck or by direct blunt force injury. The carotid artery is particularly vulnerable where it lies in close proximity to the secondhand sixth cervical transverse processes. The vertebral artery is also vulnerable to stretch injuries and fractures of the transverse process of the cervical vertebrae that involve the foramen transversum.

Patients who fulfill the Denver criteria should undergo CTA of the neck.[48,49] The treatment of blunt carotid and vertebral artery injuries is anticoagulation in patients who do not have a contraindication.[47] Aspirin is the only alternative for patients who cannot be safely anticoagulated. The use of endovascular techniques has a limited role, as discussed earlier.

Vascular injuries of the thoracic outlet can be problematic because they can involve large-caliber vessels that can be difficult to expose and control. Unstable patients with vascular injury in the region of the thoracic outlet should be expeditiously taken to the operating room. Stable patients should have preoperative imaging to locate the injury and determine its extent. This will allow planning for endoluminal treatment or open exposure. Operative control may require a simple supraclavicular incision, sternotomy, or combination of the two, depending on the location and extent of the injury. Clamp application on the proximal subclavian and carotid arteries should be precise to avoid injury to the vagus, phrenic, or recurrent laryngeal nerves, all of which reside in this anatomic region. Sternotomy is frequently used for proximal innominate, proximal right subclavian, and proximal right carotid arterial injuries. Left subclavian artery proximal control is best obtained through a posterolateral thoracotomy for definitive repair. However, for supraclavicular injuries, a third intercostal space anterolateral thoracotomy provides exposure for proximal control. Distal control of the carotid arteries is obtained by extending the median sternotomy superiorly along the border of the ipsilateral sternocleidomastoid muscle. Distal subclavian arterial control is obtained through a supraclavicular incision. Resection of the clavicle has little or no morbidity and can be achieved quickly to control hemorrhage if needed. Suturing of the subclavian and axillary arteries must be done with extreme caution. Undue tension or traction will result in a tear of these vessels.

**BOX 64-2 Risk Factors for Blunt Cerebrovascular Injury**

High-energy transfer associated with the following:

- Displaced midface fracture (Le Fort fracture type II or III)
- Basilar skull fracture with carotid canal involvement
- Closed head injury consistent with diffuse axonal injury and Glascow coma scale <6
- Cervical vertebral body or transverse process fracture, subluxation, or ligamentous injury at any level; any fracture at C1-3
- Near-hanging, with anoxia
- Clothesline type of injury or seat belt abrasion with significant swelling, pain, or altered mental status

From Biffl WL, Cothren CC, Moore EE, et al: Western Trauma Association critical decisions in trauma: Screening for and treatment of blunt cerebrovascular injuries. J Trauma 67:1150–1153, 2009.

### Intrathoracic Great Vessel Injuries

Penetrating injuries of the great vessel injuries in the mediastinum are life-threatening and patients usually present in extremis, often necessitating a resuscitative thoracotomy. Access to the branches of the aortic arch and pulmonary vessels may require extending the resuscitative thoracotomy incision across the midline to create a clamshell incision.[50] This allows access to all but the most distal portions of the arch vessels. Injuries of the pulmonary hilum will occasionally require pneumonectomy for control of hemorrhage.

Great vessel injury following blunt injury is infrequent. The most common lesion is a pseudoaneurysm; the most common vessel involved is the thoracic aorta, The mechanism is rapid deceleration, such as that caused by high-speed, head-on ("T-bone" collision) motor vehicle accidents (MVAs) or falls from a height. The diagnosis can be suspected on an anteroposterior (AP) chest x-ray that shows a widened mediastinum, apical cap (extrapleural blood at the apex of the lung), widened paravertebral stripe (suggesting blood around the descending aorta, or depression of the left mainstem bronchus; Fig. 64-6).[51] Definitive diagnosis is made with multidetector row CT (MDCT) or catheter angiography, if the CT scan is indeterminate (Fig. 64-7).[52] Once diagnosed, treatment should occur expeditiously but not necessarily immediately, allowing time for complete resuscitation, evaluation for associated injuries, control of blood pressure with beta blockade, and management of comorbidities.[53] Treatment can be performed with an open procedure (e.g., posterolateral thoracotomy with graft insertion) (Fig. 64-8) or endovascular (e.g., insertion of a balloon-expandable stent graft) procedure (Fig. 64-9). Endovascular procedures are associated with a significantly lower risk-adjusted mortality, but device complications (e.g., endoleak, migration, collapse) remain as high as 20%.[54] In addition, there is almost no long-term follow-up, which is particularly important in the younger population because the aorta increases in diameter over time, which could result in migration or collapse of the graft. Stent grafts are likely to have the greatest impact in those older than 55 years, in which open procedures have significant morbidity and mortality.[55,56]

## Abdominal Vascular Injury

Major abdominal vascular injury should be suspected in any patient with a penetrating torso injury who remains hemodynamically unstable after initial fluid infusion. These patients should be taken expeditiously to the OR, where the diagnosis of vascular injury is made.[57] Exsanguinating hemorrhage from the retroperitoneum is the most common initial intraoperative finding.[58] Obtaining vascular control is the priority, first by tamponading the apparent site of bleeding with direct packs and manual pressure. This will limit bleeding and give the anesthesiologist time to gain additional intravenous access and infuse blood products to restore intravascular volume. Next, the proximal aorta is controlled at the diaphragmatic hiatus and the incision is extended, if necessary, from the xiphoid to pubis. Aortic control will not only slow bleeding from a distal arterial injury, but will also elevate the diastolic pressure and improve myocardial perfusion. This increased exposure will allow for an assistant to obtain distal control (out of the hematoma) and allow visualization while packs are temporarily released to determine the nature of the bleeding, venous or arterial, and plan further exposure. Left-sided medial visceral rotation is used for the management of proximal abdominal aortic injury and, on the right side, medial visceral rotation exposes the vena cava and portal vein (Fig. 64-10). This exposure can be extended medially along the root of the mesentery (Cattell-Braasch maneuver) to expose the inferior vena cava, renal arteries, infrarenal aorta, and iliac arteries. Median sternotomy with division of the central tendon of the diaphragm is required to expose injured hepatic veins.[59]

After the injury is exposed, repair should be kept as simple and rapid as possible. Direct suture, patch angioplasty, and graft interposition are used as needed.[57] Arterial and venous repair in the abdomen use the same general principles of vascular technique used elsewhere. The use of synthetic graft material is reserved for large defects not amenable to primary repair. Closure of the retroperitoneum over the vascular repair or coverage of the repair with a well-vascularized omental pedicle may protect the repair or graft from infection if there is associated bowel or pancreatic injury. Concomitant bowel, pancreas, and biliary tract injuries are common and should be promptly controlled

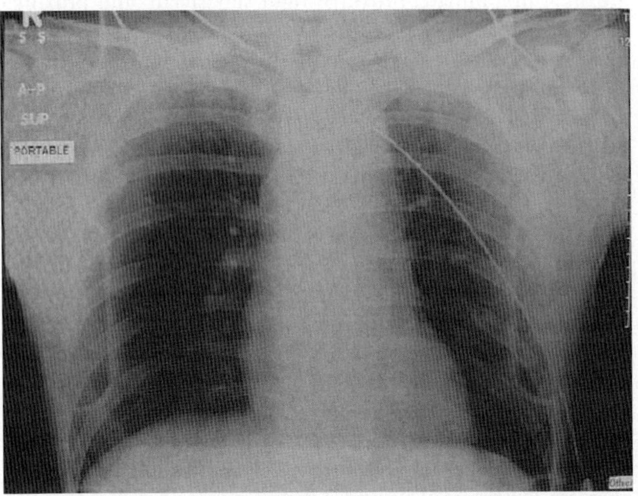


**FIGURE 64-6** Supine portable chest x-ray revealing widened mediastinum and loss of aortic contour in patient in high-speed MVA with restraints and air bag deployment. This patient was found to have a traumatic thoracic pseudoaneurysm. See CT angiographic views of this patient in Figure 64-7.

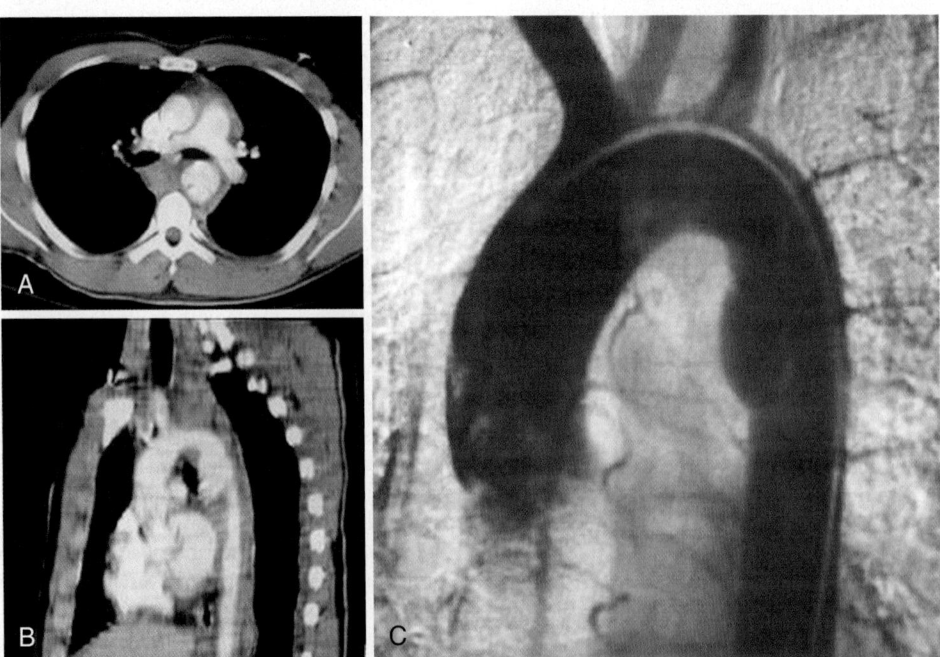


**FIGURE 64-7** CT angiogram demonstrating traumatic aortic pseudoaneurysm in patient shown in Figure 64-6, with widened mediastinum on portable chest x-ray. **A,** Cross-sectional view. **B,** Sagittal reconstruction. **C,** Catheter arteriogram of a similar injury.

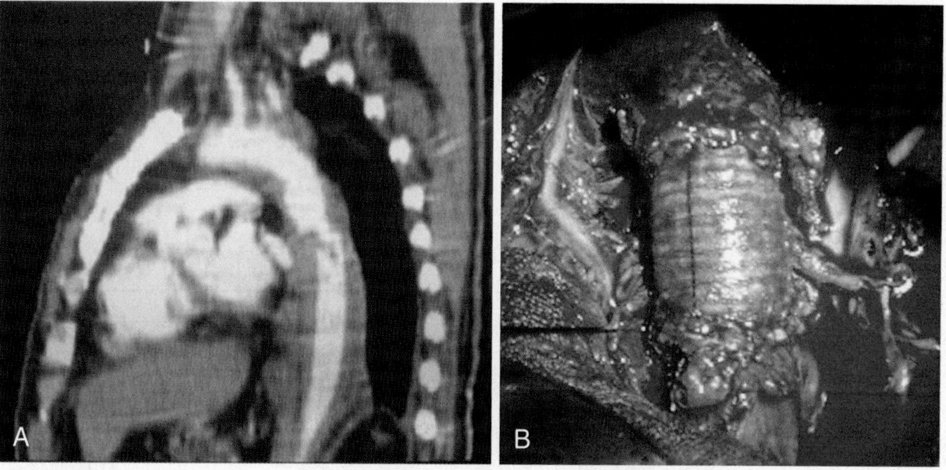


**FIGURE 64-8** Repair of traumatic aortic pseudoaneurysm with interposition graft placement through posterolateral left thoracotomy. **A,** Sagittal reconstruction view of CT angiogram. **B,** Dacron aortic interposition graft.

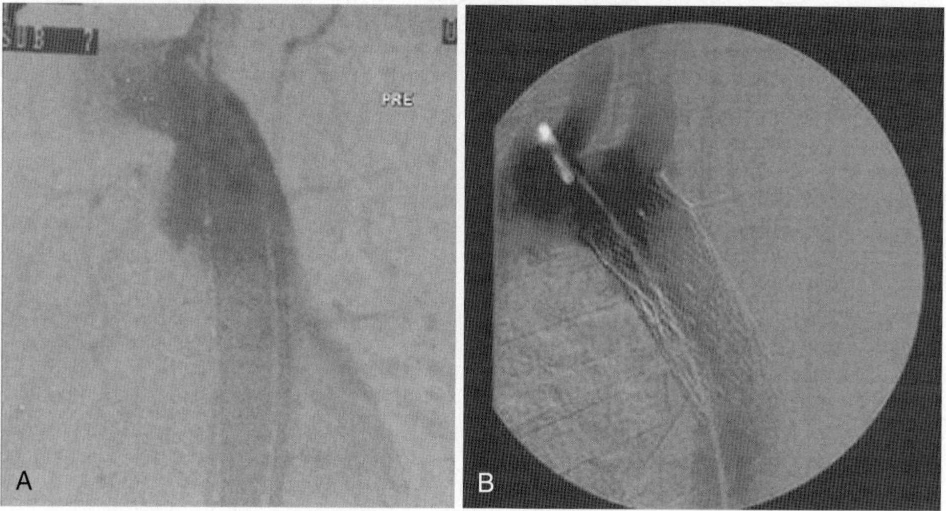


**FIGURE 64-9** Repair of traumatic aortic pseudoaneurysm with stent graft placement. **A,** Intraoperative digital subtraction arteriography. **B,** Deployed stent with proximal end just distal to the origin of the left subclavian artery.

or repaired to avoid spillage of the enteric contents. Because most of these patients are in shock on presentation, it is best to proceed with a damage control approach after the repair is covered and enteric injuries are stapled.

## Upper Extremity

Penetrating injury often presents with a history of arterial hemorrhage or ongoing bleeding. Blunt injury usually causes thrombosis and the signs of acute arterial occlusion, with resultant ischemia. Significant neurologic injury, usually involving the median nerve, is present in 60% of patients with upper extremity arterial injury.[60,61] Concomitant venous injury is common. In the setting of multisystem injury, arterial occlusion in the upper extremity is easily missed. Delay in diagnosis, resulting in prolonged ischemia, is an important contributing factor to preventable limb loss or long-term disability from irreversible ischemic nerve injury. All significant vascular injuries of the upper extremity result in clinical findings that are apparent on a thorough physical examination. Unfortunately, associate severe torso or lower extremity injuries distract the trauma team from the injured and ischemic upper extremity. Delays in diagnosis and treatment are common in collected series of patients with upper extremity arterial injury and are more common following blunt force trauma.

The diagnosis of upper extremity arterial injury is often made on the physical examination alone, particularly in penetrating injuries. Noninvasive evaluation of the injured upper extremity adds little to a thorough history and physical examination. Patients with obvious arterial or venous laceration from penetrating trauma or those with blunt trauma and hard findings (see Box 64-1) should be taken directly to the OR. The arterial bed of the upper extremity is extremely reactive to vasoconstriction produced by hypovolemic shock, pain, and drugs, including cocaine and methamphetamine. Absent pulses in the presence of complex fractures or crush injuries of the upper extremity need to be assessed with imaging (MDCT or conventional angiography) if normal perfusion does not return following resuscitation and administration of adequate pain medications.

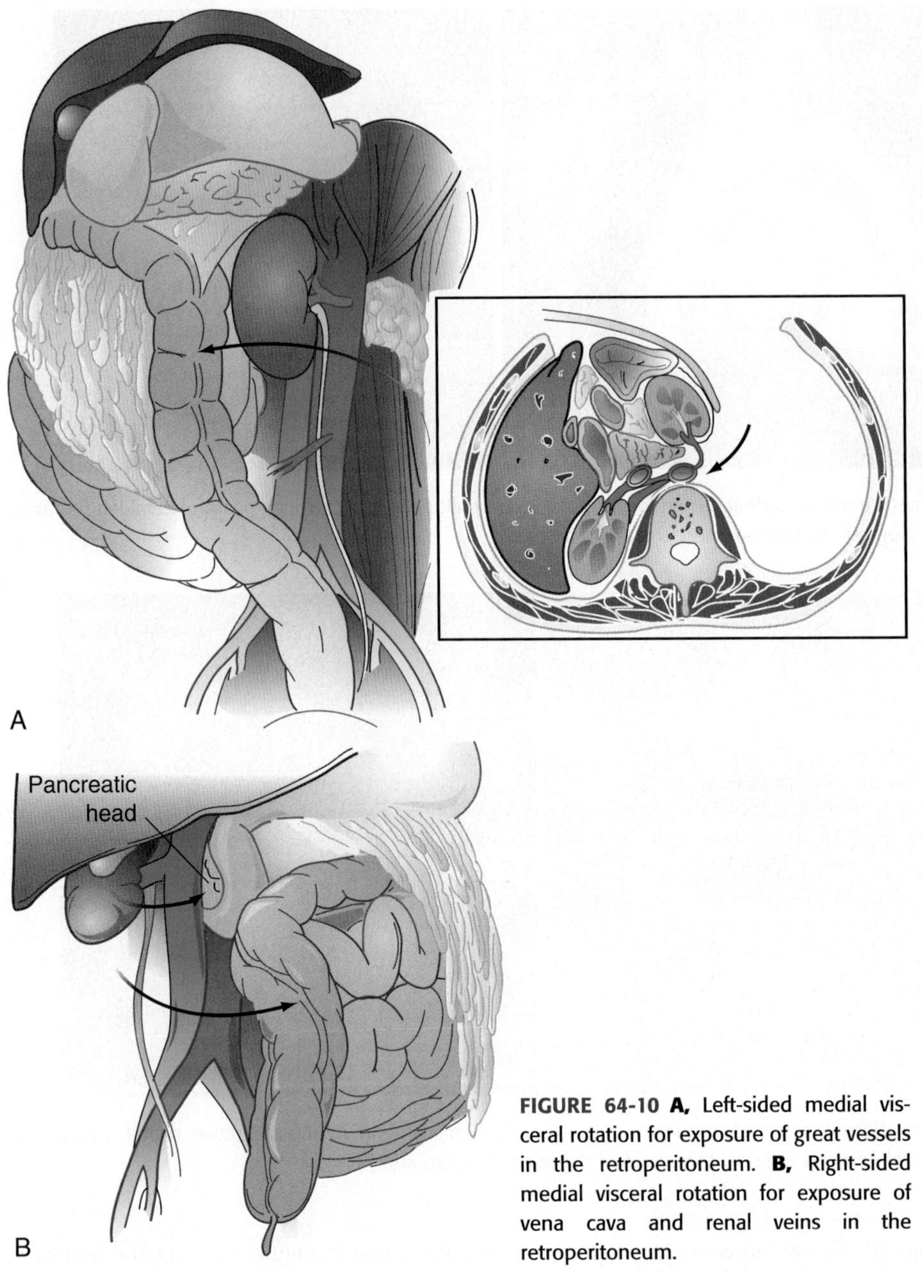


**FIGURE 64-10** **A,** Left-sided medial visceral rotation for exposure of great vessels in the retroperitoneum. **B,** Right-sided medial visceral rotation for exposure of vena cava and renal veins in the retroperitoneum.

There is currently no role for endovascular therapy in the brachial artery and forearm vessels. Traditional operative exposure, catheter thrombectomy, and repair represent the best approach to optimize results.[36]

Vascular injuries in the upper extremity are often associated with significant musculoskeletal, neurologic, and soft tissue injuries. When this occurs, a multidisciplinary approach is often required, with orthopedics, neurosurgery, and plastic surgery.

Venous injuries of the upper extremity can be ligated unless there is extensive soft tissue injury and loss of venous collaterals. In that setting, some form of venous reconstruction should be considered.

Occasionally, bleeding from a partially transected arm or forearm vessel can be significant. The senior surgeon should make certain that adequate control is obtained and maintained during resuscitation, transportation to the operating room, and surgical preparation and draping. Pneumatic tourniquets should be used sparingly and only placed and carefully monitored for adequacy of compression and duration of application by the senior surgeon.

The patient should be widely prepared and draped, with generous inclusion of the entire upper extremity, shoulder, and anterosuperior aspect of the chest to allow for incisions for proximal control. An uninjured leg should also be prepared and draped from the inguinal region to the toes to allow for saphenous vein harvest. Adjunctive measures such as bolus IV systemic heparinization, administration of a continuous infusion of low-molecular-weight Dextran, and administration of IV antibiotics should be considered and used when appropriate. In patients with multisystem injuries, especially a head injury, local or regional infusion of heparin should be used in place of systemic administration. Loupe magnification and coaxial lighting (headlight) are technical adjuncts that may be useful when suturing small blood vessels with fine sutures.

Surgical exposure requires generous incisions placed to maximize exposure and provide appropriate options for further exploration and repair. The brachial artery is best exposed through a longitudinal incision along the medial aspect of the upper arm, over the groove between the triceps and biceps muscles. The incision can be extended distally with an S-shaped extension across the antecubital fossa from the ulnar to radial aspect and onto the forearm to expose the origins of the forearm vessels. Proximal brachial artery injuries may require control of the infraclavicular axillary artery.

Vascular repair requires attention to detail in all phases. Balloon catheter thrombectomy and flushing with heparinized saline, followed by débridement of the damaged arterial wall, are essential to successful repair. Lacerated veins should be ligated unless there is extensive soft tissue injury and collateral venous flow is compromised. In these cases, the vein should be repaired. When repairing venous and arterial injuries, the vein should be repaired first. If the duration of arterial occlusion and ischemia is a concern, temporary intraluminal shunts may be placed in the artery. Primary arterial repair of undamaged ends of vessel (end-to-end anastomosis) should only be performed if the repair is tension-free. Saphenous vein interposition should be chosen whenever vessel injury is extensive or if primary tension-free repair is not possible. PTFE has no role in the management of injuries distal to the axillary artery.[36,39]

Forearm fasciotomy, particularly in the setting of prolonged ischemia, must always be considered prior to completion of the operation and compartment pressures should be measured at the completion of the procedure. If normal pressures are obtained, fasciotomy is not necessary, but pressure measurements should be repeated frequently because compartment syndrome can occur in the postoperative period as a consequence of reperfusion.

There is a limited but important role for primary or early amputation in the management of upper extremity vascular injuries. Patients with extensive soft tissue loss or with scapulothoracic dissociation, who have severe neurologic deficits, extensive fractures, and vascular injuries, should be evaluated collaboratively with orthopedic, neurosurgery, and plastic surgery colleagues to determine whether early amputation is appropriate. The best approach is intraoperative multidisciplinary assessment, damage control, and plan for reoperative assessment in 24 to 48 hours. This will allow discussions with the patient and family and enable a second look to take place.

A combined ulnar and radial artery injury in the forearm requires repair of at least one vessel. The ulnar artery is usually larger in the proximal forearm and is a better target for direct repair or saphenous vein bypass. Distally, the vessel repair should be performed in whichever vessel is largest or amenable to simple repair.

Isolated ulnar or radial artery injuries can be managed with simple ligation only if there is absolute certainty that flow through the remaining vessel is adequate. Close inspection of the forearm and hand with palpation of pulses augmented by continuous wave (hand-held) Doppler interrogation is essential.[36]

### Lower Extremity

Vascular injuries in the legs are more common in military series (30% to 40%) than in civilian practice (20%).[2,62] Although penetrating injuries are more common, blunt vascular trauma in the lower extremity remains a significant challenge. In the thigh and leg, fractures and dislocations can be associated with vascular injuries. The popliteal artery is at particularly high risk of injury following dislocation of the knee.[36]

Findings at presentation vary from significant hemorrhage from a wound (e.g., open fracture, knife or gunshot wound) to occult arterial occlusion from blunt injury. A systematic approach with a thorough extremity vascular examination is essential to avoid errors in recognition and delays in treatment.

Exposure is obtained with incisions used for elective surgical procedures. The common femoral artery is best exposed through a longitudinal incision overlying its course from the inguinal ligament inferiorly for 8 to 12 cm. Proximal control may require exposure of the external iliac artery, best accomplished through an oblique, muscle-splitting, lower quadrant abdominal incision carried into the retroperitoneum, where the artery and vein can be controlled. Superficial femoral artery (SFA) injuries are best exposed through a longitudinal groin incision, similar to that used for femoral bifurcation exposure for the proximal portion. The mid-SFA is approached through an oblique incision over the sartorius muscle. The junction of the SFA and popliteal can be exposed by extending this incision, dividing the adductor tendon.

Popliteal injuries are exposed through a generous medial incision. Exposure of the artery in the area at the knee joint requires division of the medial head of the gastrocnemius muscle and semimembranosus and semitendinosus muscles. The distal popliteal artery is exposed with an incision along the posterior margin of the tibia.

Repair of lower extremity vascular injuries usually requires an interposition graft. This is particularly true for the popliteal artery. A reverse saphenous vein from the contralateral extremity is the first choice for interposition grafts. In the common femoral artery, PTFE is an acceptable choice for interposition if the saphenous vein is not large enough, but should not be used in the below-knee popliteal arteries.[39]

Injuries below the popliteal artery at the level of the tibial vessels are best managed by ligation if two of the three calf vessels are patent and there is adequate collateral flow. In the presence of anterior and posterior tibial vessel occlusion, the peroneal artery is usually not sufficiently connected to the distal arterial bed by collaterals and one of the injured vessels should be repaired. The choice of which vessel to repair is based on the extent of associated soft tissue injury and on the patency of the distal segments of those vessels.

## OPERATIVE TECHNIQUES FOR EXTREMITY FASCIOTOMY

Fasciotomy of the forearm compartments requires release of individual muscle bundles. Generous incisions are required to release the dorsal and volar compartments and the mobile wad. Fasciotomy in the leg requires release of the anterior and lateral compartments on the anterior lateral aspect of the calf and of the deep and superficial posterior compartments through incisions on the lateral and medial aspects of the calf (Fig. 64-11). These incisions should be generous in their length to accommodate subsequent muscle swelling and avoid further compression.

Thigh compartment syndrome is uncommon. The most common cause is a thigh crush injury associated with femur fracture. Fasciotomy should release the three

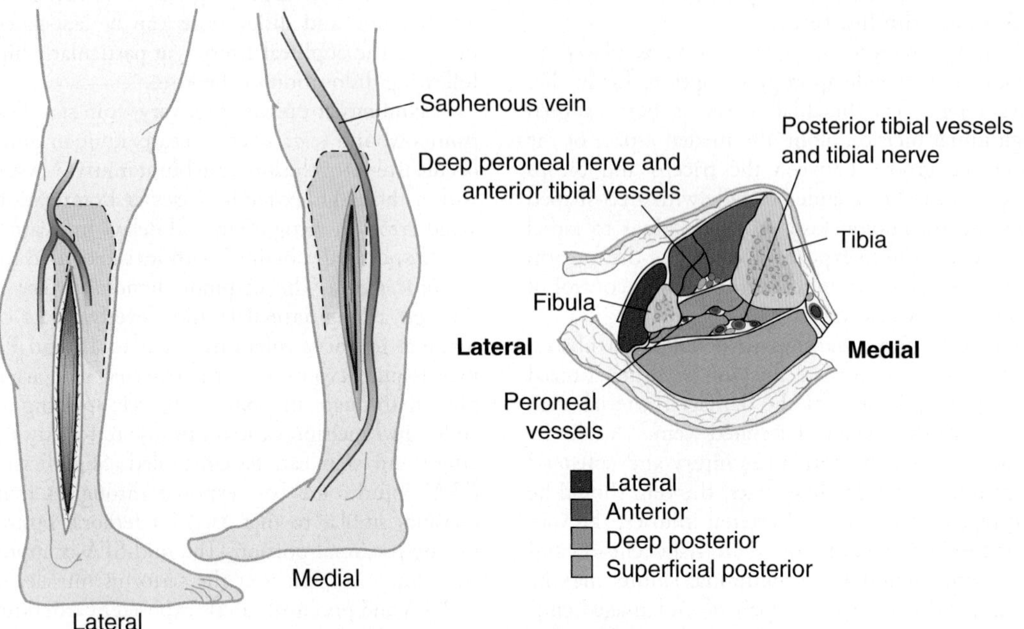


**FIGURE 64-11** Calf muscle compartments and incisions for fasciotomy.

compartments—lateral, medial, and posterior. Two incisions, one lateral for the lateral compartment and one medial for the other two compartments, are sufficient. These need to be generous in their length.

Compartment syndromes occur in the hands and feet. These are best managed by orthopedic or hand surgeons.

## POSTOPERATIVE MANAGEMENT

The cornerstone of postoperative management is diligent surveillance for a change in the vascular examination, which includes a frequent assessment of blood pressure, heart rate, distal pulse, continuous wave Doppler signal, capillary refill, and patient's temperature and overall condition (i.e., complaints of pain or increasing difficulty in feeling the extremity). If there is concern about any portion of the examination, a return to the operating room for reexploration can alleviate that concern and, more importantly, may avert a potentially limb-threatening problem. Because failure of a vascular repair caused by thrombosis can occur during the first 48 hours following repair, compulsive surveillance should continue for at least that long.

Reperfusion edema or intracompartmental hemorrhage can lead to delayed onset of a compartment syndrome.[36] The physical examination alone may not detect the presence of compartment syndrome. Frequent postoperative compartment pressure measurements are the only way to assess the injured extremity accurately in patients who are not conscious and cooperative. The presence of new postoperative extremity neurologic deficits is an important indicator of ongoing ischemia and should prompt assessment of the patency of the vascular repair and the pressure within muscle compartments.

## OUTCOMES AND FOLLOW-UP

The most common cause of amputation following vascular injury is caused by the neurologic insult, direct trauma to the nerve or ischemia. This should be remembered as one contemplates repairing a vascular injury in a flail extremity.[63] Functional outcome following vascular repair is related to the severity of the associated injuries—muscle, bone, and nerve. Regular follow-up of patients with vascular repairs is done to assess patency of the repair and determine the presence of late complications, such as aneurysmal dilation or segmental stenosis of vein grafts, venous insufficiency from venous ligation or thrombosis pseudoaneurysm, and arteriovenous fistula. Ideally, these patients should be followed up annually. Pulse examination and, if indicated, noninvasive imaging should be performed on a regular basis. Imaging with CTA or catheter angiography should be used if there is a suspicion of a complication.

Torso vascular injuries have relatively few late complications. Venous interposition grafts, when used, should be followed with periodic noninvasive imaging and, if indicated, CTA. Aortic and iliac arterial repairs should be followed similarly and surveillance for signs and symptoms of arterial occlusive disease, such as upper or lower extremity claudication, should be ongoing.

Patients with synthetic interposition grafts should be counseled on the need for antibiotic prophylaxis during subsequent dental work or invasive procedures. Although late infections are uncommon, patients should be made aware of this possibility and advised to notify all their health care providers about the presence of a vascular prosthesis.

## SELECTED REFERENCES

Bickell WH, Wall MJ, Jr, Pepe PE, et al: Immediate versus delayed fluid resuscitation for hypotensive patients with penetrating torso injuries. N Engl J Med 331:1105–1109, 1994.

This is the only prospective randomized study in the literature that examined delayed fluid resuscitation in penetrating torso trauma and showed that delayed fluid resuscitation favorably affects outcome. This reference is particularly relevant in light of modern damage control resuscitation strategies that use permissive hypotension, limiting crystalloid, and transfusing reconstituted whole blood.

Davis TP, Feliciano DV, Rozycki GS, et al: Results with abdominal vascular trauma in the modern era. Am Surg 67:565–570, 2001.

This report is an excellent series on abdominal vascular injury and sets a reasonable expectation of management challenges, practical approaches, and outcomes.

Demetriades D, Velmahos GC, Scalea TM, et al: Blunt traumatic thoracic aortic injuries: Early or delayed repair—results of an American Association for the Surgery of Trauma prospective study. J Trauma 66:967–973, 2009.

This report is a valuable guide to planning the appropriate timing for repair of thoracic aortic injuries. It focuses on the safety of temporizing until the patient is prepared for operation.

Mattox KL, Feliciano DV, Burch J, et al: Five thousand seven hundred sixty cardiovascular injuries in 4459 patients. Epidemiologic evolution 1958 to 1987. Ann Surg 209:698–705, 1989.

This is The largest epidemiologic study in the literature on civilian vascular injuries and it remains the best work on the subject.

Reuben BC, Whitten MG, Sarfati M, et al: Increasing use of endovascular therapy in acute arterial injuries: Analysis of the National Trauma Data Bank. J Vasc Surg 46:1222–1226, 2007.

This report from the NTDB demonstrates the growing use of endovascular therapy and raises the question of whether this is a practice based on evidence of efficacy or on convenience because of the growing availability of endovascular physicians.

Rich NM: Historic review of arteriovenous fistulas and traumatic false aneurysms. In Rich NM, Mattox KL, Hirshberg A, editors: Vascular trauma, ed 2, Philadelphia, 2004, Elsevier Saunders, pp 457–524.

The second edition of this classic textbook contains detailed discussions of every aspect of the modern management of major vascular injuries, operative and endovascular management options, techniques, and complications.

Subramanian A, Vercruysse G, Dente C, et al: A decade's experience with temporary intravascular shunts at a civilian level I trauma center. J Trauma 65:316–324, 2008.

This report gives a practical report a civilian center's use of damage control for vascular injuries and serves as a reference for other centers as they design their damage control strategies.

White PW, Gillespie DL, Feurstein I, et al: Sixty-four slice multidetector computed tomographic angiography in the evaluation of vascular trauma. J Trauma 68:96–102, 2010.

This work demonstrates the use and efficacy of high-resolution CT scanning in the workup of vascular injuries obviating catheter angiography in most patients and expediting care.

## REFERENCES


1. Davis TP, Feliciano DV, Rozycki GS, et al: Results with abdominal vascular trauma in the modern era. Am Surg 67:565–570, 2001.
2. Mattox KL, Feliciano DV, Burch J, et al: Five thousand seven hundred sixty cardiovascular injuries in 4459 patients. Epidemiologic evolution 1958 to 1987. Ann Surg 209:698–705, 1989.
3. Hirshberg A, Wall MJ, Jr, Allen MK, et al: Causes and patterns of missed injuries in trauma. Am J Surg 168:299–303, 1994.
4. Dimond FC, Jr, Rich NM: M-16 rifle wounds in Vietnam. J Trauma 7:619–625, 1967.
5. Rich NM, Manion WC, Hughes CW: Surgical and pathological evaluation of vascular injuries in Vietnam. J Trauma 9:279–291, 1969.
6. Amato JJ, Rich NM, Billy LJ, et al: High-velocity arterial injury: A study of the mechanism of injury. J Trauma 11:412–416, 1971.
7. Rich NM: Historic review of arteriovenous fistulas and traumatic false aneurysms. In Rich NM, Mattox KL, Hirshberg A, editors: Vascular trauma, ed 2, Philadelphia, 2004, Elsevier Saunders, pp 457–524.
8. Dennis JW, Frykberg ER, Veldenz HC, et al: Validation of nonoperative management of occult vascular injuries and accuracy of physical examination alone in penetrating extremity trauma: 5- to 10-year follow-up. J Trauma 44:243–252, 1998.
9. Sise MJ, Shackford SR: Extremity vascular trauma. In Rich NM, Mattox KL, Hirshberg A, editors: Vascular trauma, ed 2, Philadelphia, 2004, Elsevier Saunders, pp 353–389.
10. American College of Surgeons: Advanced trauma life support for doctors, 2008 (http://www.facs.org/trauma/atls/index.html).
11. Seamon MJ, Smoger D, Torres DM, et al: A prospective validation of a current practice: The detection of extremity vascular injury with CT angiography. J Trauma 67:238–243, 2009.
12. White PW, Gillespie DL, Feurstein I, et al: Sixty-four slice multidetector computed tomographic angiography in the evaluation of vascular trauma. J Trauma 68:96–102, 2010.
13. Callcut RA, Acher CW, Hoch J, et al: Impact of intraoperative arteriography on limb salvage for traumatic popliteal artery injury. J Trauma 67:252–257, 2009.
14. O'Gorman RB, Feliciano DV: Arteriography performed in the emergency center. Am J Surg 152:323–325, 1986.
15. Sirinek KR, Levine BA, Gaskill HV 3rd, et al: Reassessment of the role of routine operative exploration in vascular trauma. J Trauma 21:339–344, 1981.
16. Dennis JW: Minimal vascular injury. In Rich NM, Mattox KL, Hirshberg A, editors: Vascular trauma, ed 2, Philadelphia, 2004, Elsevier Saunders, pp 85–96.
17. Cothren CC, Moore EE, Ray CE, Jr, et al: Carotid artery stents for blunt cerebrovascular injury: risks exceed benefits. Arch Surg 140:480–485, 2005.
18. Mattox KL, Whigham C, Fisher RG, et al: Blunt trauma to the thoracic aorta: current challenges. In Lumsden AB, Lin PH, Chen C, et al, editors: Advanced endovascular therapy of aortic disease, Malden, Mass, 2007, Blackwell Futura, pp 127–134.
19. Xenos ES, Freeman M, Stevens S, et al: Covered stents for injuries of subclavian and axillary arteries. J Vasc Surg 38:451–454, 2003.
20. Dent D, Alsabrook G, Erickson BA, et al: Blunt splenic injuries: High nonoperative management rate can be achieved with selective embolization. J Trauma 56:1063–1067, 2004.
21. Richardson JD, Franklin GA, Lukan JK, et al: Evolution in the management of hepatic trauma: A 25-year perspective. Ann Surg 232:324–330, 2000.

22. Kayoko O, Yasuhiro K, Hideki T, et al: Intra-aortic balloon occlusion of the descending thoracic aorta for intra-abdominal hemorrhage. Jpn J Anesth 48:1323–1327, 1999.
23. Matsuda H, Tanaka Y, Hino Y, et al: Transbrachial arterial insertion of aortic occlusion balloon catheter in patients with shock from ruptured abdominal aortic aneurysm. J Vasc Surg 38:1293–1296, 2003.
24. Scalea TM, Stein DM, O'Toole RV: Pelvic fracture. In Feliciano DV, Mattox KL, Moore EE, editors: Trauma, ed 6, New York, 2008, McGraw-Hill, pp 759–788.
25. Eskandari MK: Commentary. Carotid artery stents for blunt cerebrovascular injury. Perspect Vasc Surg Endovasc Ther 18:73–74, 2006.
26. Inamasu J, Guiot BH: Vertebral artery injury after blunt cervical trauma: An update. Surg Neurol 65:238–245, 2006.
27. Brandt MM, Kazanjian S, Wahl WL: The utility of endovascular stents in the treatment of blunt arterial injuries. J Trauma 51:901–905, 2001.
28. Reuben BC, Whitten MG, Sarfati M, et al: Increasing use of endovascular therapy in acute arterial injuries: Analysis of the National Trauma Data Bank. J Vasc Surg 46:1222–1226, 2007.
29. Baum S, Pentecost MJ, editors: Abrams' angiography: Interventional radiology, ed 2, Philadelphia, 2006, Lippincott Williams & Wilkins.
30. Bickell WH, Wall MJ, Jr, Pepe PE, et al: Immediate versus delayed fluid resuscitation for hypotensive patients with penetrating torso injuries. N Engl J Med 331:1105–1109, 1994.
31. Harbrecht BG, Forsythe RM, Peitzman AB: Management of shock. In Feliciano DV, Mattox KL, Moore EE, editors: Trauma, ed 6, New York, 2008, McGraw-Hill, pp 213–233.
32. Hirschberg A, Scott BG: Vascular damage control. In Rich NM, Mattox KL, Hirshberg A, editors: Vascular trauma, ed 2, Philadelphia, 2004, Elsevier Saunders, pp 165–179.
33. Mattox KL, Hirschberg A: Access, control and repair techniques. In Rich NM, Mattox KL, Hirshberg A, editors: Vascular trauma, ed 2, Philadelphia, 2004, Elsevier Saunders, pp 137–164.
34. Gifford SM, Aidinian G, Clouse WD, et al: Effect of temporary shunting on extremity vascular injury: An outcome analysis from the Global War on Terror vascular injury initiative. J Vasc Surg 50:549–555, 2009.
35. Subramanian A, Vercruysse G, Dente C, et al: A decade's experience with temporary intravascular shunts at a civilian level I trauma center. J Trauma 65:316–324, 2008.
36. Frykberg ER, Schinco MA: Peripheral vascular injury. In Feliciano DV, Mattox KL, Moore EE, editors: Trauma, ed 6, New York, 2008, McGraw-Hill, pp 941–971.
37. Vertrees A, Fox CJ, Quan RW, et al: The use of prosthetic grafts in complex military vascular trauma: A limb salvage strategy for patients with severely limited autologous conduit. J Trauma 66:980–983, 2009.
38. Rich NM, Hughes CW: The fate of prosthetic material used to repair vascular injuries in contaminated wounds. J Trauma 12:459–467, 1972.
39. Feliciano DV, Mattox KL, Graham JM, et al: Five-year experience with PTFE grafts in vascular wounds. J Trauma 25:71–82, 1985.
40. Martin LC, McKenney MG, Sosa JL, et al: Management of lower extremity arterial trauma. J Trauma 37:591–598, 1994.
41. Lau JM, Mattox KL, Beall AC, Jr., et al: Use of substitute conduits in traumatic vascular injury. J Trauma 17:541–546, 1977.
42. Ledgerwood AM, Lucas CE: Biological dressings for exposed vascular grafts: A reasonable alternative. J Trauma 15:567–574, 1975.
43. Feliciano DV, Cruse PA, Spjut-Patrinely V, et al: Fasciotomy after trauma to the extremities. Am J Surg 156:533–536, 1988.
44. Dekker S: The field guide to understanding human error, Hampshire, England, 2006, Ashgate.
45. Monson DO, Saletta JD, Freeark RJ: Carotid vertebral trauma. J Trauma 9:987–999, 1969.
46. Tisherman SA, Bokhari F, Collier B, et al: Clinical practice guideline: Penetrating zone II neck trauma. J Trauma 64:1392–1405, 2008.
47. Cothren CC, Biffl WL, Moore EE, et al: Treatment for blunt cerebrovascular injuries: Equivalence of anticoagulation and antiplatelet agents. Arch Surg 144:685–690, 2009.
48. Biffl WL, Cothren CC, Moore EE, et al: Western Trauma Association critical decisions in trauma: Screening for and treatment of blunt cerebrovascular injuries. J Trauma 67:1150–1153, 2009.
49. Eastman AL, Muraliraj V, Sperry JL, et al: CTA-based screening reduces time to diagnosis and stroke rate in blunt cervical vascular injury. J Trauma 67:551–556, 2009.
50. Mattox KL, Wall MJ: Thoracic great vessel injury. In Feliciano DV, Mattox KL, Moore EE, editors: Trauma, ed 6, New York, 2008, McGraw-Hill, pp 588–606.
51. Cook AD, Klein JS, Rogers FB, et al: Chest radiographs of limited utility in the diagnosis of blunt traumatic aortic laceration. J Trauma 50:843–847, 2001.
52. Fabian TC, Davis KA, Gavant ML, et al: Prospective study of blunt aortic injury: Helical CT is diagnostic and antihypertensive therapy reduces rupture. Ann Surg 227:666–676, 1998.
53. Demetriades D, Velmahos GC, Scalea TM, et al: Blunt traumatic thoracic aortic injuries: Early or delayed repair—results of an American Association for the Surgery of Trauma prospective study. J Trauma 66:967–973, 2009.
54. Demetriades D, Velmahos GC, Scalea TM, et al: Operative repair or endovascular stent graft in blunt traumatic thoracic aortic injuries: Results of an American Association for the Surgery of Trauma Multicenter Study. J Trauma 64:561–570, 2008.
55. Camp PC, Shackford SR: Outcome after blunt traumatic thoracic aortic laceration: Identification of a high-risk cohort. Western Trauma Association Multicenter Study Group. J Trauma 43:413–422, 1997.
56. Camp PC Jr, Rogers FB, Shackford SR, et al: Blunt traumatic thoracic aortic lacerations in the elderly: An analysis of outcome. J Trauma 37:418–423, 1994.
57. Dente CJ, Feliciano DV: Abdominal vascular trauma. In Feliciano DV, Mattox KL, Moore EE, editors: Trauma, ed 6, New York, 2008, McGraw-Hill, pp 738–757.
58. Feliciano DV: Injuries to the great vessels of the abdomen. In Souba WW, Fink MP, Jurkovich GJ, et al, editors: ACS surgery: Principles and practice, ed 6, Philadelphia, 2007, BC Decker, pp 1341–1352.
59. Chen RJ, Fang JF, Lin BC, et al: Surgical management of juxtahepatic venous injuries in blunt hepatic trauma. J Trauma 38:886–890, 1995.
60. Fields CE, Latifi R, Ivatury RR: Brachial and forearm vessel injuries. Surg Clin North Am 82:105–114, 2002.
61. McCroskey BL, Moore EE, Pearce WH, et al: Traumatic injuries of the brachial artery. Am J Surg 156:553–555, 1988.
62. Rich NM, Baugh JH, Hughes CW: Acute arterial injuries in Vietnam: 1,000 cases. J Trauma 10:359–369, 1970.
63. Sampson LN, Britton JC, Eldrup-Jorgensen J, et al: The neurovascular outcome of scapulothoracic dissociation. J Vasc Surg 17:1083–1088, 1993.

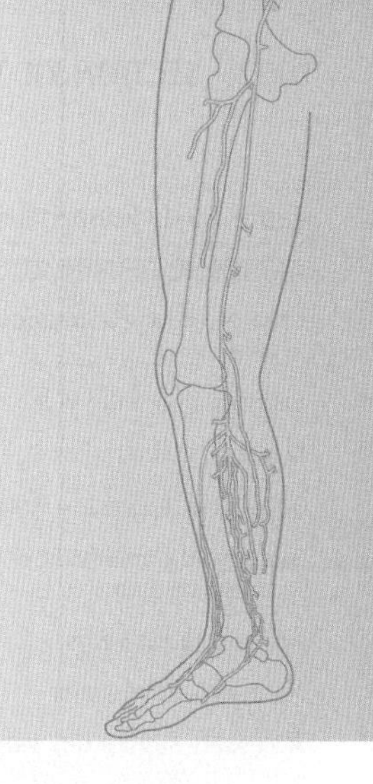

CHAPTER 65

# VENOUS DISEASE

Julie A. Freischlag and Jennifer A. Heller



An understanding of venous physiology provides the surgeon with valuable information with which to formulate a diagnostic and treatment plan. Technologic advances have broadened the therapeutic armamentarium. This chapter will provide the reader with a thorough overview of the physiology and pathophysiology of the venous system, followed by an evaluation of available diagnostic modalities and therapeutic interventions and then by a discussion of specific venous disorders.

## ANATOMY

To determine whether pathophysiology is present, precise knowledge of venous anatomy is essential. After the location and type of venous incompetence have been determined, a therapeutic plan can be constructed. Venous drainage of the legs is the function of two parallel and connected systems, the deep and superficial systems. The nomenclature of the venous system of the lower limb was revised in 2002 and the most relevant changes are addressed here.[1] The revised nomenclature is delineated in Tables 65-1 and 65-2.

### Superficial Venous System

The superficial veins of the lower extremity form a network that connects the superficial dorsal veins of the foot and deep plantar veins. The dorsal venous arch, into which empty the dorsal metatarsal veins, is continuous with the great saphenous vein medially and the small saphenous vein laterally (Fig. 65-1).

The great saphenous vein, in close proximity to the saphenous nerve, ascends anterior to the medial malleolus, crosses and then medial to the knee (Fig. 65-2). It ascends in the superficial compartment and empties into the common femoral vein after entering the fossa ovalis. Before its entry into the common femoral vein, it receives medial and lateral accessory saphenous veins, as well as small tributaries from the inguinal region, pudendal region, and anterior abdominal wall. The posterior arch vein drains the area around the medial malleolus and, as it ascends up the posterior medial aspect of the calf, it receives medial perforating veins, termed *Cockett's perforators,* before joining the great saphenous vein at or below the knee.

The small saphenous vein arises from the dorsal venous arch at the lateral aspect of the foot and ascends posterior to the lateral malleolus, rising cephalad in the midposterior calf. The small saphenous vein continues to ascend, penetrates the superficial fascia of the calf, and then terminates into the popliteal vein. The exact entry of the small saphenous vein into the popliteal vein is variable. The sural nerve lies parallel to the small saphenous vein.

### Deep Venous System

The plantar digital veins in the foot empty into a network of metatarsal veins that compose the deep plantar venous arch. This continues into the medial and lateral plantar veins, which then drain into the posterior tibial veins. The dorsalis pedis veins on the dorsum of the foot form the paired anterior tibial veins at the ankle.

The paired posterior tibial veins, adjacent to and flanking the posterior tibial artery, run under the fascia of the deep posterior compartment. These veins enter the soleus and join the popliteal vein, after joining with the paired peroneal and anterior tibial veins. There are large venous sinuses within the soleus muscle—soleal sinuses—that empty into the posterior tibial and peroneal veins. Bilateral gastrocnemius veins empty into the popliteal vein distal to the point of entry of the small saphenous vein into the popliteal vein.

The popliteal vein enters a window in the adductor magnus, at which point it is termed the *femoral vein,* previously known as the *superficial femoral vein.* The femoral vein ascends and receives venous drainage from the profunda femoris vein, or deep femoral vein and, after this confluence, it is the common femoral vein. As the common femoral vein crosses the inguinal ligament, it becomes the external iliac vein.

### Perforating Venous System

Perforating veins connect the superficial venous system to the deep venous system by penetrating the fascial layers of the lower extremity. These perforators run in a perpendicular fashion to the axial veins previously described. Although the total number of perforator veins is variable, up to 100 have been documented. The perforators enter at various points in the leg—the foot, medial and lateral calf, and mid and distal thigh (Fig. 65-3) Some have been named Cockett's perforators, which connect the posterior arch and posterior tibial veins, Boyd's perforators, which connect the great saphenous and gastrocnemius veins, and Hunterian and Dodd's perforators, which connect the great saphenous and superficial femoral veins. The perforator veins

**Table 65-1 Superficial Veins**

| ANATOMIC TERMINOLOGY | PROPOSED TERMINOLOGY |
|---|---|
| Greater or long saphenous vein | Great saphenous vein<br>Superficial inguinal veins |
| External pudendal vein | External pudendal vein |
| Superficial circumflex vein | Superficial circumflex iliac vein |
| Superficial epigastric vein | Superficial epigastric vein |
| Superficial dorsal vein of clitoris or penis | Superficial dorsal vein of clitoris or penis |
| Anterior labial veins | Anterior labial veins |
| Anterior scrotal veins | Anterior scrotal veins |
| Accessory saphenous vein | Anterior accessory great saphenous vein<br>Posterior accessory great saphenous vein<br>Superficial accessory great saphenous vein |
| Smaller or short saphenous vein | Small saphenous vein<br>Cranial extension of small saphenous vein<br>Superficial accessory small saphenous vein<br>Anterior thigh circumflex vein<br>Posterior thigh circumflex vein<br>Intersaphenous veins<br>Lateral venous system |
| Dorsal venous network of the foot | Dorsal venous network of the foot |
| Dorsal venous arch of the foot | Dorsal venous arch of the foot |
| Dorsal metatarsal veins | Superficial metatarsal veins (dorsal and plantar) |
| Plantar venous network<br>Plantar venous arch | Plantar venous subcutaneous network |
| Plantar metatarsal veins | Superficial digital veins (dorsal and plantar) |
| Lateral marginal vein | Lateral marginal vein |
| Medial marginal vein | Medial marginal vein |

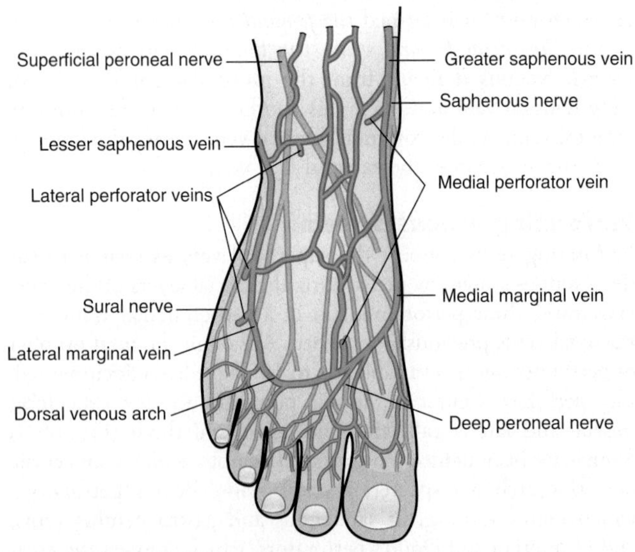


**FIGURE 65-1** Venous drainage of the foot.

**Table 65-2 Deep Veins**

| ANATOMIC TERMINOLOGY | PROPOSED TERMINOLOGY |
|---|---|
| Femoral vein | Common femoral vein<br>Femoral vein |
| Profunda femoris vein or deep vein of thigh | Profunda femoris vein or deep femoral vein |
| Medial circumflex femoral vein | Medial circumflex femoral vein |
| Lateral circumflex femoral vein | Lateral circumflex femoral vein |
| Perforating veins | Deep femoral communicating veins (accompanying veins of perforating arteries)<br>Sciatic vein |
| Popliteal vein | Popliteal vein<br>Sural veins<br>Soleal veins<br>Gastrocnemius veins<br>Medial gastrocnemius veins<br>Lateral gastrocnemius veins<br>Intergemellar vein |
| Genicular veins | Genicular venous plexus |
| Anterior tibial veins | Anterior tibial veins |
| Posterior tibial veins | Posterior tibial veins |
| Fibular or peroneal veins | Fibular or peroneal veins<br>Medial plantar veins<br>Lateral plantar veins<br>Deep plantar venous arch<br>Deep metatarsal veins (plantar and dorsal)<br>Deep digital veins (plantar and dorsal)<br>Pedal vein |

have an important function. Their valve system aids in preventing reflux from the deep to the superficial system, particularly during periods of standing and ambulation.

## Normal Venous Histology and Function

The venous wall is composed of three layers, the intima, media, and adventitia. Vein walls have less smooth muscle and elastin than their arterial counterparts. The venous intima has an endothelial cell layer resting on a basement membrane. The media is composed of smooth muscle cells and elastin connective tissue. The adventitia of the venous wall contains adrenergic fibers, particularly in the cutaneous veins. Central sympathetic discharge and brainstem thermoregulatory centers can alter venous tone, as can other stimuli, such as temperature changes, pain, emotional stimuli, and volume changes.

The histologic features of veins vary, depending on the caliber of the veins. The venules, the smallest veins, rangefrom 0.1 to 1 mm and contain mostly smooth muscle cells, whereas the larger extremity veins contain relatively few smooth muscle cells. These larger caliber veins have limited contractile capacity in comparison to the thicker walled great saphenous vein. The venous valves prevent retrograde flow; it is their failure or valvular incompetence that leads to reflux and its associated symptoms. Venous valves are most prevalent in the distal lower extremity, whereas as one proceeds proximally, the number of valves decreases to the point that no valves are present in the superior vena cava and inferior vena cava (IVC),.

Most of the capacitance of the vascular tree is in the venous system. Because veins do not have significant amounts of elastin,

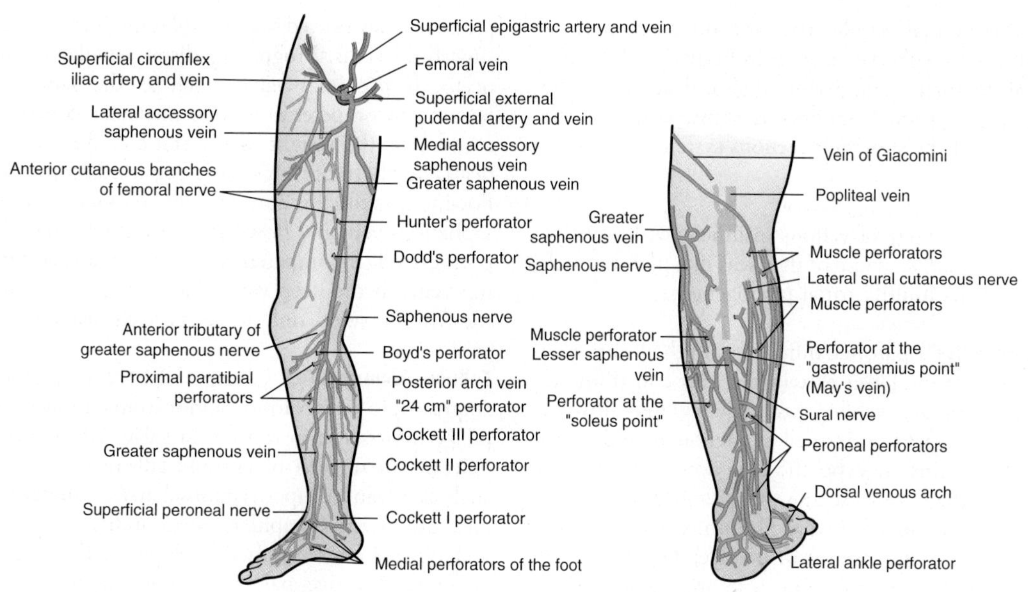


**FIGURE 65-2** Venous drainage of the lower limb.

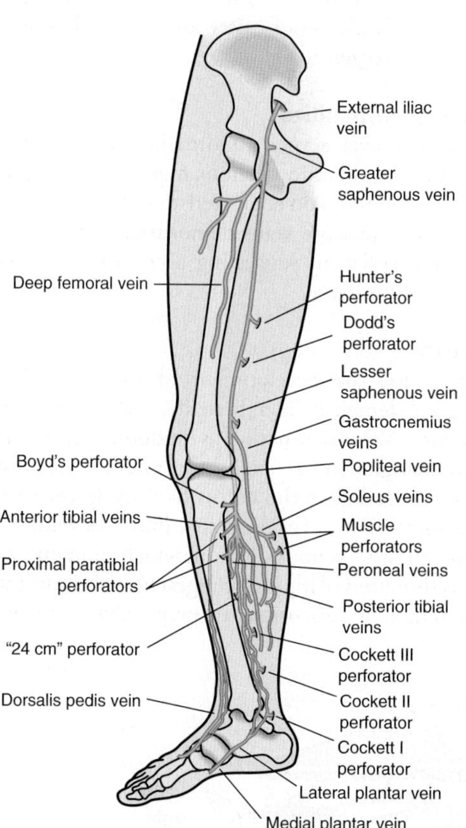


**FIGURE 65-3** Perforating veins of the lower limb.

veins can withstand large volume shifts with comparatively small changes in pressure. A vein has a normal elliptical configuration until the limit of its capacitance is reached, at which point the vein assumes a round configuration.

The calf muscles augment venous return by functioning as a pump. In the supine state, the resting venous pressure in the foot is the sum of the residual kinetic energy minus the resistance in the arterioles and precapillary sphincters. Thus, a pressure gradient is generated to the right atrium of approximately 10 to 12 mm Hg. In the upright position, the resting venous pressure of the foot is a reflection of the hydrostatic pressure from the upright column of blood extending from the right atrium to the foot.

The return of the blood to the heart from the lower extremity is facilitated by the muscle pump function of the calf, a mechanism whereby the calf muscle, functioning as a bellows during exercise, compresses the gastrocnemius and soleal sinuses and propels the blood toward the heart. The normally functioning valves in the venous system prevent retrograde flow; when one or more of these valves become incompetent, symptoms of venous insufficiency can develop. During calf muscle contraction, the venous pressure of the foot and ankle drop dramatically. The pressures developing in the muscle compartments during exercise range from 150 to 200 mm Hg and, when there is failure of perforating veins, these high pressures are transmitted to the superficial system.

## VENOUS INSUFFICIENCY

There are three categories of venous insufficiency—congenital, primary, and secondary. Congenital venous insufficiency is comprised of predominantly anatomic variants that are present at birth. Examples of congenital venous anomalies include venous ectasias, absence of venous valves, and syndromes such as Klippel-Trenaunay syndrome. Primary venous insufficiency is an acquired idiopathic entity. This is the largest clinical category and represents most of the superficial venous insufficiency encountered in the office. Secondary venous insufficiency arises from a post-thrombotic or obstructive state and is caused by a deep vein thrombus or primary chronic obstructive process.

### Primary Venous Insufficiency

There are three main anatomic categories of primary venous insufficiency—telangiectasias, reticular veins, and varicose veins. Telangiectasias, reticular varicosities, and varicose veins are similar but exhibit distinct variations in caliber. Telangiectasias are very small intradermal venules that are too diminutive to demonstrate reflux. Reticular veins are vein branches that enter the tributaries of the main axial, perforating, or deep veins. The axial veins, the great or small saphenous veins, represent the largest caliber veins of the superficial venous system.

### Pathology

The precise pathophysiology of venous insufficiency has yet to be elucidated. This describes some of the areas in which research has started to reveal its multifactorial pathogenesis.

**Mechanical Abnormalities** Anatomic differences in the location of the superficial veins of the lower extremities may contribute to the pathogenesis. Primary venous insufficiency may involve both the axial veins (great and small saphenouss), either, or neither. Perforating veins may be the sole source of venous pathophysiology, perhaps because the great saphenous vein is supported by a well-developed medial fibromuscular layer and fibrous connective tissue that bind it to the deep fascia. In contrast, tributaries to the small saphenous vein are less supported in the subcutaneous fat and are superficial to the membranous layer of superficial fascia (Fig. 65-4). These tributaries also contain less muscle mass in their walls. Thus, these veins, and not the main trunk, may become selectively varicose.

When these fundamental anatomic peculiarities are recognized, the intrinsic competence or incompetence of the valve system becomes important. For example, failure of a valve protecting a tributary vein from the pressures of the small saphenous vein allows a cluster of varicosities to develop. Furthermore, communicating veins connecting the deep with the superficial compartment may have valve failure. Pressure studies have shown that there are two sources of venous hypertension. The first is gravitational and is a result of venous blood coursing in a distal direction down linear axial venous segments. This is referred to as hydrostatic pressure and is the weight of the blood column from the right atrium. The highest pressure generated by this mechanism is evident at the ankle and foot, where measurements are expressed in centimeters of water or millimeters of mercury. The second source of venous hypertension is dynamic. It is the force of muscular contraction, usually contained within the compartments of the leg. If a perforating vein fails, high pressures (range, 150 to 200 mm Hg) developed within the muscular compartments during exercise are transmitted directly to the superficial venous system. Here, the sudden pressure transmitted causes dilation and lengthening of the superficial veins. Progressive distal valvular incompetence may occur. If proximal valves such as the saphenofemoral valve become incompetent, systolic muscular contraction is supplemented by the weight of the static column of blood from the heart. Furthermore, this static column becomes a barrier. Blood flowing proximally through the femoral vein spills into the saphenous vein and flows distally. As it refluxes distally through progressively incompetent valves, it is returned through perforating veins to the deep veins. Here, it is conveyed once again to the femoral veins, only to be recycled distally.

**Cellular Abnormalities** Changes also occur at the cellular level. Angioscopic observation demonstrates monocytic and macrophage infiltration in those vein valves affected by venous insufficiency. In regions of chronic advanced venous insufficiency, such as advanced lipodermatosclerosis, capillary proliferation is seen and extensive capillary permeability occurs as a result of the widening of interendothelial cell pores. Transcapillary leakage of osmotically active particles occurs, mainly of fibrinogen. In chronic venous insufficiency (CVI), venous fibrinolytic capacity is diminished and the extravascular fibrin remains to prevent the normal exchange of oxygen and nutrients in the surrounding cells.[2] However, little proof exists for an actual abnormality in the delivery of oxygen to the tissues.

### Molecular Abnormalities

On a molecular level, several abnormalities have been identified in extremities that manifest venous hypertension. Fundamental defects in the strength and characteristics of the venous wall have been identified. Varicose veins demonstrate decreased amounts of elastin and collagen, suggesting a contributing role toward venous pathophysiology.[3]

### Risk Factors

Risk factors for the development of varicose veins include advancing age, female gender, heredity, and history of trauma to the extremity. Venous function is undoubtedly influenced by hormonal changes. In particular, progesterone liberated by the corpus luteum stabilizes the uterus by causing the relaxation of smooth muscle fibers.[2] This directly influences venous function. The result is passive venous dilation, which in many cases causes valvular dysfunction. Although progesterone is implicated in the first appearance of varicosities in pregnancy, estrogen also has

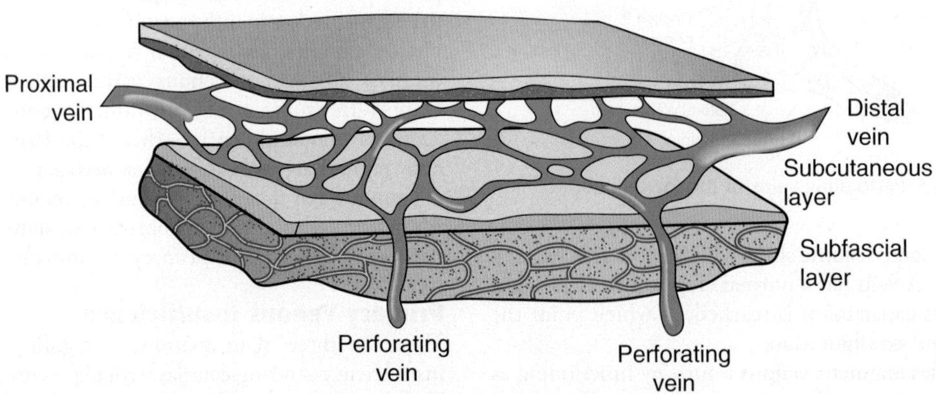


**FIGURE 65-4** Dilation of superficial venous tributaries caused by increased transmission of pressure by the perforating veins.

profound effects. It produces the relaxation of smooth muscle and a softening of collagen fibers. Furthermore, the estrogen-to-progesterone ratio influences venous distensibility. This ratio may explain the predominance of venous insufficiency symptoms on the first day of a menstrual period, when a profound shift occurs from the progesterone phase of the menstrual cycle to the estrogen phase. Although heredity is widely acknowledged as a risk factor for varicose vein development, the precise genetic mechanism has yet to be elucidated.

## Symptoms

Venous valvular dysfunction causes venous hypertension and, as such, patients' symptoms are attributed to excess venous pooling. The patient with symptomatic varicose veins commonly reports heaviness, discomfort, and extremity fatigue. The pain is characteristically dull, does not usually occur during recumbency or early in the morning, and is exacerbated in the afternoon, especially after periods of prolonged standing. Swelling is commonly described. The discomforts of aching, heaviness, and/or fatigue are usually relieved by leg elevation or elastic support. Cutaneous burning, termed *venous neuropathy,* can also occur in patients with advanced venous insufficiency. Pruritus occurs from excess hemosiderin deposition and tends to be located at the distal calf or in areas of phlebitic varicose branch segments.

## Physical Examination

A comprehensive examination includes assessment of the arterial circulation. Briefly, palpation of the femoral, popliteal, dorsalis pedis, and posterior tibialis pulses is performed. Nonpalpable pulses necessitate further evaluation. Auscultation of pulse flow is indicated when a thrill or widened pulse is appreciated. Demonstration of decreased hair, dependent rubor, pallor on elevation, and tissue loss are all indicative of advanced arterial ischemia.

The venous examination includes assessment of the patient in the standing and supine positions. Standing increases venous hypertension and dilates veins, thereby facilitating examination. Patients with superficial axial incompetence commonly exhibit palpable great saphenous veins (Fig. 65-5). Palpable cords may be present. Visual inspection is critical. Signs of advanced venous insufficiency include hyperpigmentation in the gaiter distribution, secondary to hemosiderin deposition, and lipodermatosclerosis. Lipodermatosclerosis develops over time, due to prolonged ambulatory venous hypertension and chronic inflammation. Physical examination findings that reflect lipodermatosclerosis are: brawny edema of the distal calf, "champagne bottle leg," fibrotic, hypertrophic skin, and hyperpigmentation. Advanced lipodermatosclerosis may involve fibrosis of the Achilles tendon, impairing motor function of the extremity. Atrophie blanche is an area of pale hue, visualized around the medial malleolus; it is commonly mistaken for a healed ulcer because of its lighter pigmentation (Fig. 65-6). *Corona phlebectica* is a term used to describe an accumulation of tiny telangiectasias or venous flare, usually located at the medial malleolus.

Venous stasis ulcers exhibit pathognomonic features that distinguish them from their arterial or neuropathic counterparts. Venous ulcers are not generally painful and appear at the medial malleolus, not in the mid to distal foot. Lack of arterial pulses in patients with a venous ulcer isunusual.

Venous stasis dermatitis is visualized at the distal ankle and can mimic eczema or dermatitis of another cause. It is this important attention to supporting features of the physical examination and history, as well as confirmation with duplex reflux examination, that will distinguish advanced venous stasis disease from dermatologic conditions.

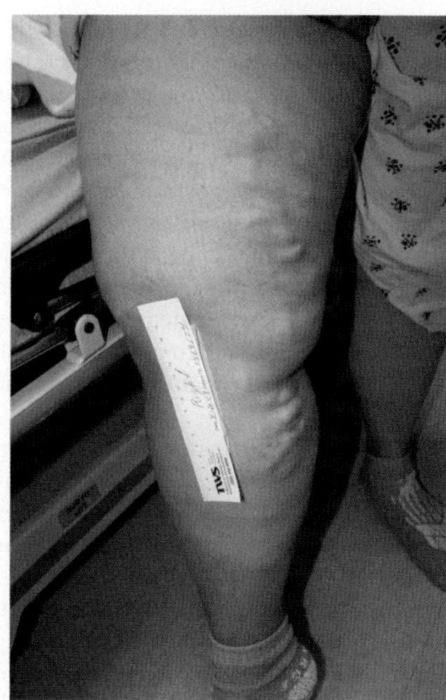


**FIGURE 65-5** Varicose veins.

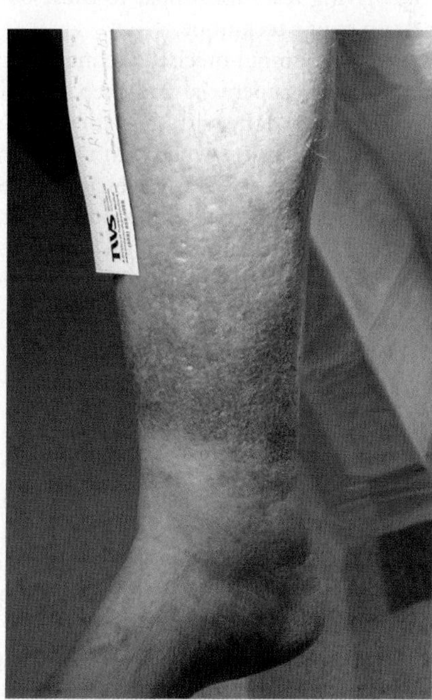


**FIGURE 65-6** Lipodermatosclerosis, atrophie blanche, and brawny edema.

## Diagnostic Evaluation of Venous Dysfunction

The Perthes test for deep venous occlusion and Brodie-Trendelenburg test of axial reflux have been replaced by in-office use of the continuous wave, hand-held Doppler instrument supplemented by duplex evaluation. The hand-held Doppler instrument can confirm an impression of saphenous reflux, which in turn dictates the operative procedure to be performed in a given patient. A common misconception is the belief that the Doppler instrument is used to locate perforating veins. Instead, it is used in specific locations to determine incompetent valves—for example, the hand-held, continuous wave, 8-MHz flow detector placed over the greater and lesser saphenous veins near their terminations. With distal augmentation of flow and release, normal deep breathing, and performance of a Valsalva maneuver, valve reflux is accurately identified. Formerly, the Doppler examination was supplemented by other objective studies, including photoplethysmography, mercury strain gauge plethysmography, and photorheography. These are no longer in common use.

Another instrument reintroduced to assess physiologic function of the muscle pump and venous valves is air displacement plethysmography.[4] Its use was discontinued after the 1960s because of its cumbersome nature. Computer technology has now allowed its reintroduction, as championed by Christopoulos and colleagues.[5] It consists of an air chamber that surrounds the leg from knee to ankle. During calibration, leg veins are emptied by leg elevation and the patient is then asked to stand so that leg venous volume can be quantitated and the time for filling recorded. The filling rate is then expressed in milliliters per second, thus giving readings similar to those obtained with the mercury strain gauge technique.

Duplex technology more precisely defines which veins are refluxing by imaging the superficial and deep veins. The duplex examination is commonly done with the patient supine, but this yields an erroneous evaluation of reflux. In the supine position, even when no flow is present, the valves remain open. Valve closure requires a reversal of flow with a pressure gradient that is higher proximally than distally. Thus, the duplex examination needs to be done with the patient standing or in the markedly trunk-elevated position.[6,7]

Imaging is obtained with a 7.5- or 10-MHz probe; the pulsed Doppler consists of a 3.0-MHz probe. The patient stands, with the probe placed longitudinally on the groin. After imaging, sample volumes can be obtained from the femoral and saphenous veins. This flow can be observed during quiet respiration or distal augmentation. Sudden release of augmentation allows the assessment of valvular competence. The small saphenous vein and popliteal veins are similarly examined. Reflux times of 3 seconds or longer is considered significant. Perforator veins can be visualized well with the duplex examination. Demonstration of duplex images of to and fro flow, with the presence of dilated segments, constitutes findings compatible with a refluxing perforator. Additionally, Doppler studies can provide the clinician with information about the deep system. Widespread use of duplex scanning has allowed a comparison of findings between standard clinical examinations and duplex Doppler studies.[8]

**Phlebography and Venography** In general, phlebography is unnecessary in the diagnosis and treatment of primary venous insufficiency. In cases of secondary chronic venous insufficiency, phlebography has specific usefulness. Ascending phlebography is performed via injection of contrast into a superficial pedal vein after a tourniquet is applied at the ankle to prevent flow into the superficial venous system. Observation of flow indicates defines anatomy and regions of thrombus or obstruction. Therefore, ascending phlebology differentiates primary from secondary venous insufficiency. Descending phlebography is performed with retrograde injection of contrast into the deep venous system at the groin or popliteal fossa (femoral vein or popliteal vein). This diagnostic modality identifies specific valvular incompetence suspected on B mode scanning and clinical examination. These studies are only performed as preoperative adjuncts when deep venous reconstruction is being planned.

**Magnetic Resonance Venous Imaging** Magnetic resonance venous imaging (MRVI) is a diagnostic imaging modality reserved for evaluation of the abdominal and pelvic venous vasculature. MRVI, unlike venography, is noninvasive and does not require IV contrast. Furthermore, studies have documented similar rates of specificity and sensitivity when compared with venography. MRVI is used for the evaluation of congenital malformations and identification of chronic and acute venous thrombi.

### Classification Systems

In 1994, the American Venous Forum devised the CEAP classification system, which is a scoring system that stratifies venous disease based on ***c***linical presentation, ***e***tiology, ***a***natomy, and ***p***athophysiology (Table 65-3). It is useful in helping the physician assess a limb afflicted with venous insufficiency and then arrive at an appropriate treatment plan. A revised CEAP was introduced that included a venous disability score (VDS) to document a patient's ability to perform activities of daily living.[9] Although the CEAP classification is a valuable tool to grade venous disease, assessment of outcomes following intervention cannot be realized. As a result, two additional scoring systems, the venous clinical severity scoring system (VCSS) and venous segmental disease score (VSDS), enhance the CEAP score with the increased ability to plot outcome. These three classification modalities now provide clinical researchers with invaluable tools to study treatment outcomes.[10]

### Treatment of Superficial Venous Insufficiency

**Nonoperative Management** As noted, symptoms of primary venous insufficiency are manifestations of valvular incompetence. Therefore, the objective of conservative management is to improve the symptoms caused by venous hypertension. The first measure is external compression using elastic hose, 20 to 30 mm Hg, to be worn during the daytime hours. Although the exact mechanism whereby compression is of benefit is not entirely known, a number of physiologic alterations have been observed with compression. These include reduction in ambulatory venous pressure, improvement in skin microcirculation, and increase in subcutaneous pressure, which counters transcapillary fluid leakage. Patients are instructed to wear the hose during the day only, but to put the stockings on as soon as the day begins; swelling with standing will make stocking placement difficult. Care must be taken with patients who have concomitant arterial insufficiency because the compression stockings may exacerbate arterial outflow to the foot. Therefore, these patients require less compression—in some cases no compression whatsoever—depending on the severity of the arterial disease.

The second part of conservative therapy is to practice lower extremity elevation for two brief periods during the day, instructing the patient that the feet must be above the level of the heart, or "toes above the nose." With good compliance, these measures may ameliorate symptoms so that patients may not require further intervention. Third, patients are encouraged to

**Table 65-3 Classification of Chronic Lower Extremity Venous Disease**

| | |
|---|---|
| C | Clinical signs (grade$_{0\text{-}6}$), supplemented by "A" for asymptomatic and "S" for symptomatic presentation |
| E | Classification by cause (etiology)—congenital, *p*rimary, *s*econdary |
| A | Anatomic distribution—*s*uperficial, *d*eep, or *p*erforator, alone or in combination |
| P | Pathophysiologic dysfunction—*r*eflux or *o*bstruction, alone or in combination |

**Clinical Classification ($C_{0\text{-}6}$)**

Any limb with possible chronic venous disease is first placed into one of seven clinical classes ($C_{0\text{-}6}$), according to the objective signs of disease.

***Clinical Classification of Chronic Lower Extremity Venous Disease****

| CLASS | FEATURES |
|---|---|
| 0 | No visible or palpable signs of venous disease |
| 1 | Telangiectasia, reticular veins, malleolar flare |
| 2 | Varicose veins |
| 3 | Edema without skin changes |
| 4 | Skin changes ascribed to venous disease (e.g., pigmentation, venous eczema, lipodermatosclerosis) |
| 5 | Skin changes as defined above with healed ulceration |
| 6 | Skin changes as defined above with active ulceration |

*Limbs in higher categories have more severe signs of chronic venous disease and may have some or all of the findings defining a less severe clinical category. Each limb is further characterized as asymptomatic (A)—for example, $C_{0\text{-}6,A}$—or symptomatic (S)—for example, $C_{0\text{-}6,S}$. Symptoms that may be associated with telangiectatic, reticular, or varicose veins include lower extremity aching, pain, and skin irritation. Therapy may alter the clinical category of chronic venous disease. Limbs should therefore be reclassified after any form of medical or surgical treatment.

**Classification by Cause ($E_C$, $E_P$, or $E_S$)**

Venous dysfunction may be congenital, primary, or secondary. These categories are mutually exclusive. Congenital venous disorders are present at birth but may not be recognized until later. The method of diagnosis of congenital abnormalities must be described. Primary venous dysfunction is defined as venous dysfunction of unknown cause but not of congenital origin. Secondary venous dysfunction denotes an acquired condition resulting in chronic venous disease—for example, deep venous thrombosis.

***Classification by Cause of Chronic Lower Extremity Venous Disease***

| | |
|---|---|
| Congenital ($E_C$) | Cause of the chronic venous disease present since birth |
| Primary ($E_P$) | Chronic venous disease of undetermined cause |
| Secondary ($E_S$) | Chronic venous disease with an associated known cause (e.g., post-thrombotic, post-traumatic, other) |

**Anatomic Classification ($A_S$, $A_D$, or $A_P$)**

The anatomic site(s) of the venous disease should be described as superficial ($A_S$), deep ($A_D$), or perforating ($A_P$) vein(s). One, two, or three systems may be involved in any combination. For reports requiring greater detail, the involvement of the superficial, deep, and perforating veins may be localized by use of the anatomic segments.

***Segmental Localization of Chronic Lower Extremity Venous Disease***

| SEGMENT NO. | VEIN(s) |
|---|---|
| *Superficial Veins ($A_{S1\text{-}5}$)* | |
| 1 | Telangiectasia/reticular veins<br>Greater (long) saphenous vein |
| 2 | Above knee |
| 3 | Below knee |
| 4 | Lesser (short) saphenous vein |
| 5 | Nonsaphenous |
| *Deep Veins ($A_{D6\text{-}16}$)* | |
| 6 | Inferior vena cava<br>ILIAC |
| 7 | Common |
| 8 | Internal |
| 9 | External |
| 10 | Pelvic: gonadal, broad ligament<br>FEMORAL |
| 11 | Common |

*Continued*

**Table 65-3 Classification of Chronic Lower Extremity Venous Disease—cont'd**

| SEGMENT NO. | VEIN(s) |
|---|---|
| 12 | Deep |
| 13 | Superficial |
| 14 | Popliteal |
| 15 | Tibial (anterior, posterior, or peroneal) |
| 16 | Muscular (gastrointestinal, soleal, other) |
| 17 | Thigh |
| 18 | Calf |
| **Pathophysiologic Classification ($P_{R,O}$)** | |
| Clinical signs or symptoms of chronic venous disease result from reflux ($P_R$), obstruction ($P_O$), or both ($P_{R,O}$). | |
| ***Pathophysiologic Classification of Chronic Lower Extremity Venous Disease*** | |
| Reflux ($P_R$) | |
| Obstruction ($P_O$) | |
| Reflux and obstruction ($P_{R,O}$) | |

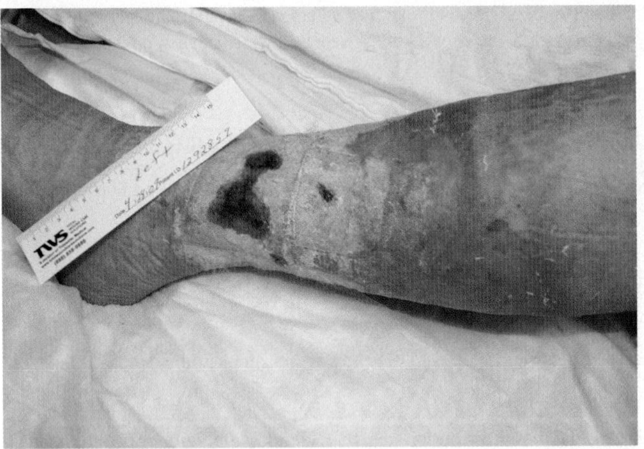

**FIGURE 65-7** Venous stasis ulcer.

participate in activities that activate the calf musculovenous pump, thereby decreasing ambulatory venous hypertension. These activities include frequent ambulation and exercise.

Patients who exhibit venous stasis ulceration will require local wound care (Fig. 65-7). A triple-layer compression dressing, with a zinc oxide paste gauze wrap in contact with the skin, is used most commonly, from the base of the toes to the anterior tibial tubercle with snug graded compression. This is an example of what is generally known as an *Unna boot*. A 15-year review of 998 patients with one or more venous ulcers treated with a similar compression bandage demonstrated that 73% of the ulcers healed in patients who returned for care (Fig. 65-8). The median time to healing for individual ulcers was 9 weeks. In general, snug, graded-pressure, triple-layer compression dressings result in more rapid healing than compression stockings alone.

For most patients, well-applied, sustained compression therapy offers the most cost-effective and efficacious therapy in the healing of venous ulcers. After healing, most cases of CVI are controlled with elastic compression stockings to be worn during waking hours. Occasionally, older patients and those

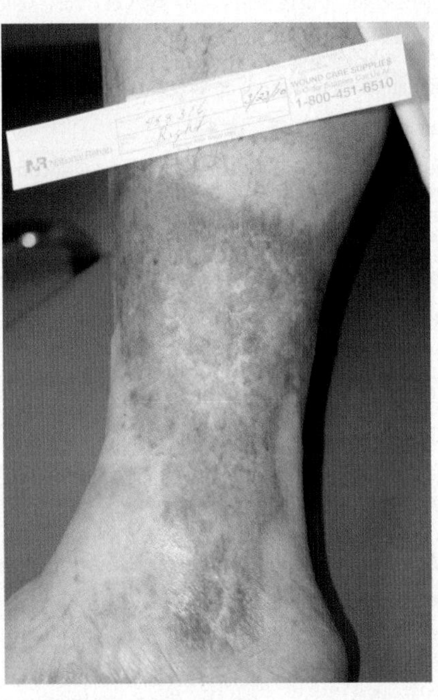

**FIGURE 65-8** Healed venous stasis ulcer.

with arthritic conditions cannot apply the compression stocking required, and control must be maintained by triple-layer zinc oxide compression dressings, which can usually be left in place and changed once a week.

Indications for interventional treatment are symptoms refractory to conservative therapy, recurrent superficial thrombophlebitis, variceal bleeding, and venous stasis ulceration. After clinical and objective criteria have established the presence of symptomatic varicose veins, the next step is to plan a course of therapy.[11]

***Venous Ablation of Telangiectasias*** Cutaneous venectasia with vessels smaller than 1 mm in diameter does not lend itself to surgical treatment (Fig. 65-9). However, all sources of spider

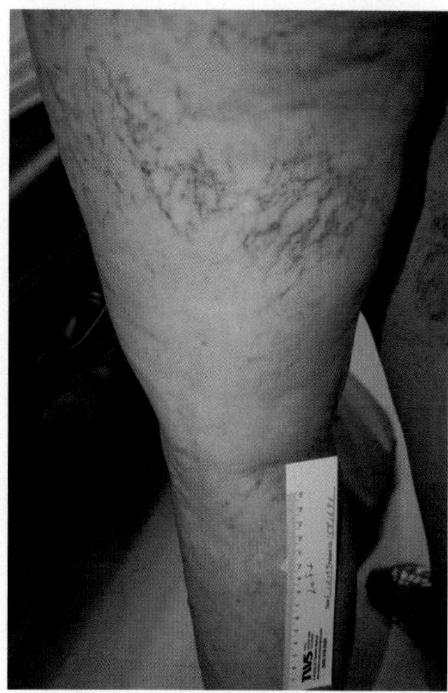

**FIGURE 65-9** Spider telangiectasias.

vein formation must be treated first; otherwise, unsatisfactory spider vein recurrence will take place. Axial venous incompetence is addressed and treated. Secondary branch varicosities are also addressed. Finally, treatment options for spider veins are considered. These include injection sclerotherapy, laser treatment, and radioablation.

**INJECTION SCLEROTHERAPY** The venectasia can be ablated successfully using the injection sclerotherapy technique. Dilute solutions of sclerosant (e.g., 1% to 3% sodium sotradecol solution) can be injected directly into the venules. Care must be taken to ensure that no single injection dose exceeds 0.1 mL but that multiple injections completely fill all feeding vessels. When the session is complete, a pressure dressing is applied, consisting of cotton balls at each injection site, and then covered with a pressure dressing of Coban wrap or low-grade compression stockings. Patients are advised to ambulate frequently over the first 24 hours and to abstain from direct sun exposure and airline travel for 2 weeks. Occasionally, entrapped blood may form, and patients report significant discomfort. Needle drainage is performed at the site, which facilitates healing, and cosmesis and rapidly improves discomfort. This liberation of entrapped blood is as important to success as the primary injection. This therapy is remarkably successful in achieving an excellent cosmetic result. In patients with a known allergy to sodium tetradecyl (Sotradecol), hypertonic saline can be used. Pain can occur with the use of pure hypertonic solutions, so lidocaine is added to the solution to decrease discomfort. Venules larger than 1 mm and smaller than 3 mm can also be injected with a sclerosant of slightly greater concentration, but the amount injected needs to be limited to less than 0.5 mL. Although injection sclerotherapy has met with significant success, complications do occur. They include hyperpigmentation, venous matting, postsclerotherapy necrosis, and an allergic reaction to the sclerosant. In addition, telangiectasia formation after injection sclerotherapy treatment tends to recur. Patients will commonly observe return of spider veins from 8 to 12 months after treatment. Although patients may report localized discomfort, sclerotherapy of telangiectasias is considered cosmetic and does not influence the venous circulation of the extremity.

**FOAM SCLEROTHERAPY** Foam sclerotherapy is a modality that has been introduced in Europe and has achieved great success, not only with spider veins, but also as a treatment option for perforator vein ablation. However, paradoxical embolism can occur, which is the main reason that foam sclerosant therapy has not been widely used in the United States. Standardization of technique and formal studies will likely demonstrate the appropriate safety of foam sclerotherapy for venous therapy.[12]

**LASER TREATMENT** Laser treatment of spider telangiectasias has been performed using a variety of wavelengths and varying techniques, such as high-intensity pulsed light (IPL), fiber-guided laser coagulation, and Nd:YAG laser with a wavelength of 1064 nm. Evaluation of all existing laser modalities has suggested that the Nd:YAG laser has the most success. However, to date, there have not been any prospective randomized trials to support this presumption. Laser treatment does tend to be more painful. Laser treatement in most centers will be used in conjunction with injection sclerotherapy—that is, injection treats the feeding venules; laser treatment will be used to treat the extremely small branches not adequately addressed with the injection technique. Most patients are satisfied with the injection-only method.

### Surgical Management

#### *Surgery for Axial Venous Incompetence*

**PHLEBECTOMY** There are two techniques to treat secondary branch varicosities, conventional stab phlebectomy and powered phlebectomy (TRIVEX, Inavein, Lexington, MA). Ambulatory phlebectomy is performed using the stab avulsion technique (Fig. 65-10). The patient's varicosities are marked after standing to allow for optimal dilation and visualization of affected veins. A variety of anesthetic methods are used successfully, including local anesthesia with tumescence and IV sedation. First, 1-mm incisions are made along Langer skin lines and the vein is retrieved with a hook. Continuous retraction of the vein segment affords maximal removal of the vein and direct pressure is applied over the site. Incisions are made at approximately 2-cm intervals. The extremity is wrapped with a layered compression dressing, and patients are instructed to ambulate on the day of surgery. The postoperative course is brief, and rarely do patients require more than acetaminophen or nonsteroidal anti-inflammatory drugs (NSAIDs) for discomfort. Compression stockings are worn for 2 weeks following the procedure. Complications are unusual, but include bleeding, infection, temporary or permanent paresthesias, and phlebitis from retained vein segments. There can be recurrence.

Powered phlebectomy (TriVex) is a modality that can be used to treat extensive secondary branch varicosities. The patient's varicosities are circumferentially marked preoperatively; in the operating room, 2-mm incisions are made at these boundary sites. These incisions permit placement of a transilluminator and resection device. The instruments are inserted through a subcutaneous plane, just deep to the varicosities. The transilluminator not only provides visualization of the veins, but also administers tumescent anesthesia. The resector is a rotating blade that transects the veins and then removes them via a

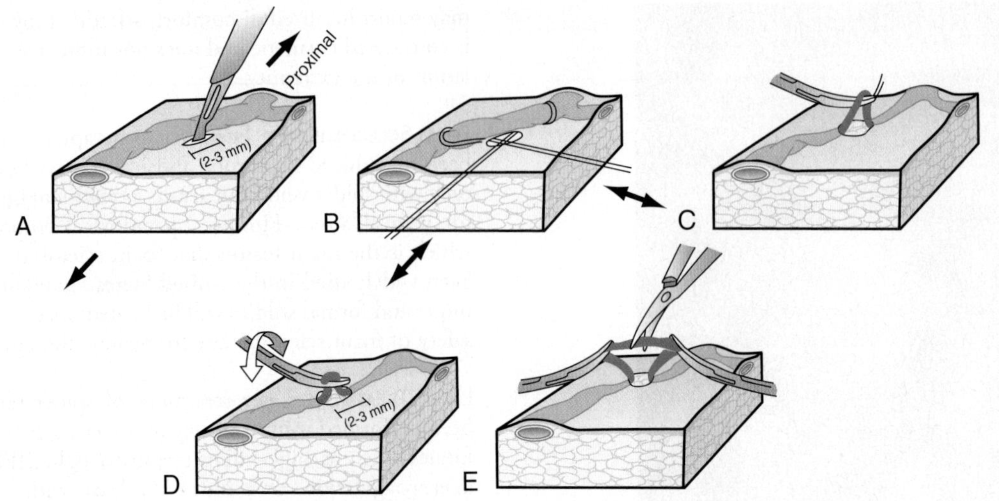


**FIGURE 65-10 A-E,** Technique of ambulatory phlebectomy (otherwise known as *stab avulsions* of varicosities).

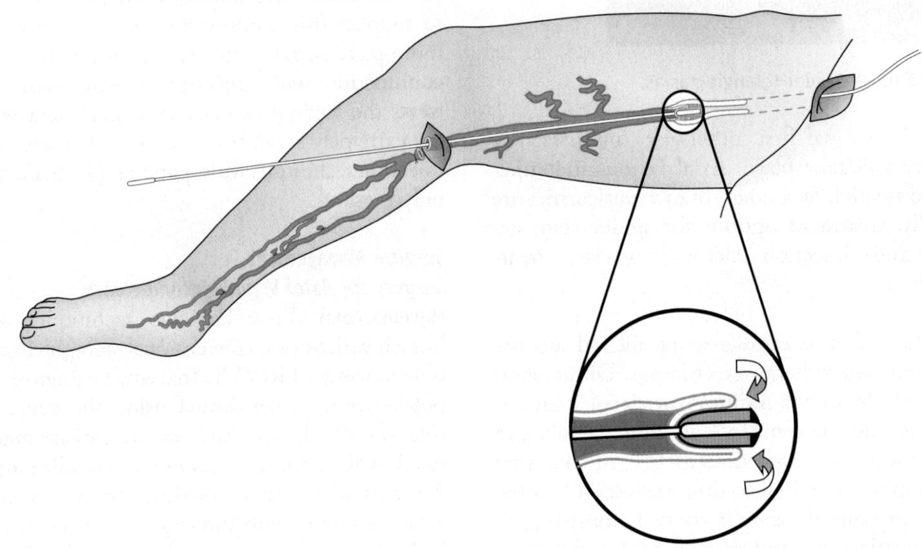

**FIGURE 65-11** Inversion stripping of the saphenous vein for superficial venous reflux caused by an incompetent saphenofemoral junction.

high-suction tubing system. The extremity is wrapped with a multilayer compression dressing and the patient is discharged, with instructions to ambulate hourly. The patient returns to the office for a dressing change within 48 hours and usually is changed to standard compression hose. Discomfort is minimal and over-the- counter analgesia is sufficient. A second-generation TriVex device has been developed; technical issues with the first-generation instrument were revised and studies now focus on methods to use the TriVex system in an outpatient setting. A steep learning curve occurs with this device but, once achieved, experienced physicians can perform most TriVex procedures within 30 minutes. Complications are unusual but can include contained hematoma, bleeding, temporary or permanent paresthesias, and phlebitis.[13]

**Stripping** When great or small saphenous incompetence is present, the removal of clusters is preceded by limited removal of the saphenous vein (stripping). Stripping techniques are best done from above downward to avoid lymphatic and cutaneous nerve damage (Fig. 65-11). A number of techniques have been described that adapt new instruments to minimally invasive removal of the saphenous vein.

The question of preservation or stripping of the saphenous vein is an important one; therefore, a 5-year clinical and duplex scan follow-up examination of a group of patients has been performed.[14] Patients were randomized to stripping of the small saphenous vein during varicose vein surgery versus saphenofemoral ligation with stab avulsion of varices. It was found that reoperation, done or awaited, was necessary for only 3 of 52 legs that underwent stripping, as compared with 12 of 58 limbs in which proximal ligation had been done. Neovascularization at the saphenofemoral junction was responsible for 10 of 12 recurrent varicose veins that underwent reoperation, and it was the cause of recurrence of saphenofemoral incompetence in 12 of the 52 limbs that were stripped versus 30 of the 58 limbs in which ligation was done. Clearly, the problem of neovascularization and recurrent varicose veins was not solved by the stripping operation, but stripping reduced the risk for reoperation by two

**BOX 65-1 Indications for Varicose Vein Intervention**

Cosmesis
Symptoms refractory to conservative therapy
Bleeding from a varix
Superficial thrombophlebitis
Lipodermatosclerosis
Venous stasis ulcer

thirds after 5 years of observation. It was the conclusion of the authors that stripping "should be routine for primary long saphenous varicose veins."[14]

Although axial venous stripping was considered the gold standard of therapy for several decades, several disadvantages to the technique have been realized. Patients required general anesthesia and a hospitalization. Additionally, once discharged, patients experienced a prolonged convalescence before resuming baseline activity. Also, the problems of nerve injury and neovascularization were frustrating to surgeons and patients.

In an effort to address and correct these limitations, endovenous techniques have been developed. They will be discussed in the next section. As a result of their efficacy, stripping is now considered in only select cases.

**ENDOVENOUS THERAPY** Recent advances in ablation of the incompetent great and small saphenous veins include radiofrequency closure and endovenous laser ablation. Both methods use a duplex-guided percutaneous access to the great or small saphenous vein. Tumescent anesthesia is administered along the course of the vein to be treated, which is then examined for complete administration with the duplex. Closure of the vein is accomplished with radiofrequency heat or laser. Confirmation of closure is obtained with postprocedure duplex at the conclusion of the intervention. Advantages of these procedures are that they are percutaneous and performed on an outpatient basis. General anesthesia is not used. Patients can return to baseline activities within 1 or 2 days. Risks of the procedures include development of a deep venous thrombosis (DVT), pulmonary embolism, skin burn, thrombophlebitis, paresthesias, and/or recurrence.[15] A 2-year follow-up study has compared endovenous radiofrequency closure with ligation and vein stripping. The findings revealed similar closure rates of the great saphenous vein. Interestingly, the authors did not find that ligation of the vein at the saphenofemoral junction improved long-term outcome. However, patients' quality of life index was superior in the endovenous radiofrequency group. Although initial findings are promising for radiofrequency and endovenous laser therapies, to date, there is no prospective randomized trial to compare these three modalities (Box 65-1).[15,16]

## Secondary Venous Insufficiency

Secondary venous insufficiency is usually caused by a deep venous thrombus. Clinical manifestations of secondary venous insufficiency usually present in a more advanced stage than their primary counterparts. Additionally, patients may describe venous claudication, or a bursting pain in the calf, that is classic for secondary venous insufficiency. Conservative treatment regimens are similar to those described in the previous section for primary insufficiency; however, these patients require a higher grade of compression for efficacy (30 to 40 mm Hg). Interventional treatment will focus on the superficial and deep systems. Diagnostic interrogation of the deep venous system must be more comprehensive in these patients to determine whether they are candidates for deep surgical or endovenous reconstruction.

### Treatment

**Surgery for Deep Venous Insufficiency** While conservative therapy is being pursued or ulcer healing is achieved, appropriate diagnostic studies generally reveal patterns of venous reflux or segments of venous occlusion so that specific therapy can be prescribed for the individual limb being evaluated. Imaging by duplex suffices for the detection of reflux if the examination is carried out in the patient while he or she is standing. Such noninvasive imaging may prove the only testing necessary beyond the hand-held, continuous wave Doppler instrument if superficial venous ablation is contemplated. If direct venous reconstruction by bypass or valvuloplasty techniques is planned, ascending and descending phlebography are required.[17]

Surprisingly, superficial reflux may be the only abnormality present in advanced chronic venous stasis. Correction goes a long way toward permanent relief of the chronic venous dysfunction and its cutaneous effects. Using duplex technology, Hanrahan and associates[18] found that in 95 extremities with current venous ulceration, 16.8% had only superficial incompetence and another 19% showed superficial incompetence combined with perforator incompetence. Another study has demonstrated ulcer healing and decreased ulcer recurrence with perforator reconstruction.[19]

A significant proportion of patients with venous ulceration have normal function in the deep veins and surgical treatment is a useful option that can definitively address the hemodynamic derangements. Maintaining that all venous ulcers are surgically incurable is not reasonable when data suggest that superficial vein surgery holds the potential for ameliorating the venous hypertension. A randomized controlled trial comparing compression therapy and surgery for superficial reflux versus conservative management alone has revealed significant improvement in patients who had been treated by the surgical component.[19] Early success in patients with CVI, superficial valvular incompetence, and venous ulceration has been obtained with endovenous radiofrequency and laser therapies.

In the 1938, Linton[20] emphasized the importance of perforating veins and their direct surgical interruption was advocated. This has fallen into disfavor because of a high incidence of postoperative wound healing complications. However, video techniques that allow direct visualization through small-diameter endoscopes have made endoscopic subfascial exploration and perforator vein interruption the desirable alternative to the Linton technique, minimizing morbidity and wound complications. The connective tissue between the fascia cruris and underlying flexor muscles is so loose that this potential space can be opened up easily and dissected with the endoscope. This operation, done with a vertical proximal incision, accomplishes the objective of perforator vein interruption on an outpatient basis.

The availability of subfascial endoscopic perforator vein surgery has had an impact on the care of venous ulcers in Western countries, albeit not as dramatic as its proponents had hoped. As patient limbs with severe CVI were studied accurately, the term *post-thrombotic syndrome* had to give way to the term *chronic venous insufficiency;* a link to platelet and monocyte aggregates in the circulation reflected the leukocytic infiltrate of the ankle skin, with its lipodermatosclerosis and healed and open ulcerations.[21]

Data regarding leukocytes in CVI accumulated and were consistent, showing that the activation of leukocytes sequestered in the cutaneous microcirculation during venous stasis was important to the development of the skin changes of CVI. This is reflected in the finding of adhesion markers between leukocytes and endothelial cells and increased production of leukocyte degranulation enzymes and oxygen free radicals. Nevertheless, experimental evidence was still required for decisive proof of the leukocyte hypothesis.

In the United States, several groups have performed perforating vein division using laparoscopic instrumentation. Initial data have suggested that perforator interruption produces rapid ulcer healing and a low rate of recurrence. The North American Registry, which voluntarily recorded the results of perforating venous surgery, has confirmed a low 2-year recurrence rate of ulcers and more rapid ulcer healing.[22]

A comparison of the three methods of perforator vein interruption, including the classic Linton procedure, laparoscopic instrumentation procedure, and single open-endoscope procedure, has revealed that the endoscopic techniques produces results comparable with those of the open Linton operation, with much less scarring and a greater tendency toward a fast recovery. More perforating veins were identified with the open technique. However, the mean hospital stay and period of convalescence were more favorable with the endoscope procedures.[23]

In general, registry reports and individual institution clinical experience have shown that patients with true post-thrombotic limbs are disadvantaged by the procedure, enough so that at Leicester (England), the students of the procedure said, "We conclude that perforating vein surgery is not indicated for the treatment of venous ulceration in limbs with primary deep venous incompetence."[23] Nevertheless, studies were reported in which previous superficial reflux was corrected with failures of such treatment. Rescue of these limbs with perforating vein division produced satisfactory results and verified that perforating veins are important in the genesis of venous ulceration, and that their division accelerates healing and may reduce recurrence of ulceration.

Part of the difficulty in understanding the need for perforating vein division is the disparity between venous hemodynamics and the severity of cutaneous changes. This is not surprising, because the cutaneous changes of CVI are dependent on leukocyte-endothelium interactions, which may not be directly related to venous hemodynamics. However, endoscopic perforator vein division has improved venous hemodynamics in some limbs, as would be expected, by removing superficial reflux and perforating vein outflow. In an effort to eliminate incompetent perforator veins without the associated morbidity described earlier, ultrasound-guided sclerotherapy has been developed as an alternative technique. Early study results are promising and have revealed improved wound healing rates compared with the subfascial endoscopic perforator surgery (SEPS). More data will be required before definitive recommendations can be made.[24]

**Direct Venous Reconstruction** Historically, the first successful procedures done to reconstruct major veins were the femorofemoral crossover graft of Eduardo Palma and the saphenopopliteal bypass he described, and also used by Richard Warren of Boston. These operations were elegant in their simplicity, use of autogenous tissue, and reconstruction by a single venovenous anastomosis.

With regard to femorofemoral crossover grafts, the only group to provide long-term physiologic data on a large number of patients has been Halliday and coworkers from Sydney, Australia. Although phlebography was used in selecting patients for surgery, no other details of preoperative indications were given. These investigators documented that 34 of 50 grafts remained patent in the long term, as assessed by postoperative phlebography. They believed that the best clinical results were achieved in relief of postexercise calf pain, but thought that a patent graft also slowed the progression of distal liposclerosis and controlled recurrent ulceration. No proof of this was given in their report. The history of application of bypass procedures for venous obstruction is a fascinating one. Nevertheless, the advent of endovascular techniques has made those operations almost obsolete.[25]

Perforator interruption, combined with superficial venous ablation, has been effective in controlling venous ulceration in 75% to 85% of patients. However, emphasis on failures of this technique led to Masuda and Kistner's[26] significant breakthrough in direct venous reconstruction with valvuloplasty in 1968 and the general recognition of this procedure after 1975. Late evaluations of direct valve reconstruction have indicated good to excellent long-term results in more than 80% of patients.[27] One cannot overestimate Kistner's contributions. The technique of directing the incompetent venous stream through a competent proximal valve by venous segment transfer was his next achievement. After Kistner's studies, surgeons were provided with an armamentarium that included Palma's venous bypass, direct valvuloplasty (of Kistner), and venous segment transfer (of Kistner). Moreover, external valvular reconstruction, as performed by various techniques, including monitoring by endoscopy, has led to renewed interest in this form of treatment of venous insufficiency. Axillary to popliteal autotransplantation of valve-containing venous segments has been considered since the early observations of Taheri and colleagues.[28] However, long-term verification of the preliminary excellent results has not been accomplished.

## DEEP VENOUS THROMBOSIS

### Lower Extremity Deep Venous Thrombosis

Acute DVT is a major cause of morbidity and mortality in the hospitalized patient, particularly in the surgical patient. The triad of venous stasis, endothelial injury, and hypercoagulable state, first posited by Virchow in 1856, has held true more than a century and a half later.

Acute DVT poses several risks and has significant morbid consequences. The thrombotic process initiated in a venous segment, in the absence of anticoagulation or in the presence of inadequate anticoagulation, can propagate to involve more proximal segments of the deep venous system, thus resulting in edema, pain, and immobility. The most dreaded sequel to acute DVT is that of pulmonary embolism, a condition of potentially lethal consequence. The late consequence of DVT, particularly of the iliofemoral veins, can be CVI and ultimately post-thrombotic syndrome as a result of valvular dysfunction in the presence of luminal obstruction.

Thus, understanding the pathophysiology, standardizing protocols to prevent or reduce DVT, and instituting optimal treatment promptly all are critical to reducing the incidence and morbidity of this unfortunately common condition.

### Causes

The triad of stasis, hypercoagulable state, and vessel injury is present in most surgical patients. It is also clear that increasing age places a patient at a greater risk, with those older than 65 years representing a higher risk population. In addition, many epidemiologic studies have reviewed additional factors that place patients at risk for the development of deep venous thrombus, including malignancy, increased body mass index (BMI), increasing age (especially >60 years), pregnancy, prolonged immobilization, tobacco use, and prior deep vein thrombus.[29]

**Stasis** Labeled fibrinogen studies in patients, as well as autopsy studies, have demonstrated convincingly that the soleal sinuses are the most common sites of initiation of venous thrombosis. The stasis may contribute to the endothelial cellular layer contacting activated platelets and procoagulant factors, thereby leading to DVT. Stasis, in and of itself, has never been shown to be a causative factor for DVT.

**Hypercoagulable State** Our knowledge of hypercoagulable conditions continues to improve, but it is still in its early stages. The standard array of conditions screened for when searching for a hypercoagulable state is listed in Box 65-2. If any of these conditions is identified, a treatment regimen of anticoagulation is instituted for life, unless specific contraindications exist. It is generally appreciated that the postoperative patient, following major surgery, is predisposed to the formation of DVT. After major operations, large amounts of tissue factor may be released into the bloodstream from damaged tissues. Tissue factor is a potent procoagulant expressed on the leukocyte cell surface as well as in a soluble form in the bloodstream. Increases in platelet count, adhesiveness, changes in coagulation cascade, and endogenous fibrinolytic activity result from physiologic stress, such as major operation or trauma, and have been associated with an increased risk for thrombosis.

**Venous Injury** It has been clearly established that venous thrombosis occurs in veins that are distant from the site of operation; for example, it is well known that patients undergoing total hip replacement frequently develop contralateral lower extremity DVT.

In a series of experiments, animal models of abdominal and total hip operations were used to study the possibility of venous endothelial damage distant from the operative site. In these studies, jugular veins were excised after the animals were perfusion-fixed. These experiments demonstrated that endothelial damage occurred after abdominal operations and were more severe after hip operations. There were multiple microtears noted within the valve cusps that resulted in exposure of the subendothelial matrix. The exact mechanisms whereby this injury at a distant site occurs, and which mediators, cellular or humoral, are responsible, are not clearly understood, but that the injury occurs is evident from these and other studies.

**BOX 65-2 Hypercoagulable States**

Factor V Leiden mutation
Prothrombin gene mutation
Protein C deficiency
Protein S deficiency
Antithrombin III deficiency
Homocysteinemia
Antiphospholipid syndrome
Lupus antibody
Anticardiolipin antibody

### Diagnostic Considerations

**Incidence** Venous thromboembolism occurs for the first time in approximately 100 persons/100,000 each year in the United States. This incidence increases with increasing age, with an incidence of 0.5%/100,000 at 80 years of age. More than two thirds of these patients have DVT alone, and the rest have evidence of pulmonary embolism. The recurrence rate with anticoagulation has been noted to be 6% to 7% in the ensuing 6 months.

In the United States, pulmonary embolism causes 50,000 to 200,000 deaths annually. A 28-day case-fatality rate of 9.4% after first-time DVT and of 15.1% after first-time pulmonary thromboembolism has been observed. Aside from pulmonary embolism, secondary CVI (resulting from DVT) is significant in terms of cost, morbidity, and lifestyle limitations.

If the consequences of DVT, in terms of pulmonary embolism and CVI, are to be prevented, the prevention, diagnosis, and treatment of DVT must be optimized.

**Clinical Diagnosis** The diagnosis of DVT requires a high index of suspicion. Most are familiar with *Homan's sign*, which refers to pain in the calf on dorsiflexion of the foot. Although the absence of this sign is not a reliable indicator of the absence of venous thrombus, the finding of a positive Homan's sign should prompt one to attempt to confirm the diagnosis. The extent of venous thrombosis in the lower extremity is an important factor in the manifestation of symptoms. For example, most calf thrombi may be asymptomatic unless there is proximal propagation. This is one reason why radiolabeled fibrinogen testing demonstrates a higher incidence of DVT than studies using imaging modalities. Only 40% of patients with venous thrombosis have any clinical manifestations of the condition.

Major venous thrombosis involving the iliofemoral venous system results in a massively swollen leg, with pitting edema (Fig. 65-12), pain, and blanching, a condition known as *phlegmasia alba dolens*. With further progression of disease, there may be such massive edema that arterial inflow can be compromised. This condition results in a painful blue leg, a condition called *phlegmasia cerulea dolens*. With this evolution of the condition, venous gangrene can develop unless flow is restored.

Post-thrombotic syndrome (PTS) is a common and unfortunate manifestation of deep venous thrombus. It occurs in 20% to 50% of patients after a documented episode of DVT. The clinical presentation includes chronic edema, pain, and venous claudication. Venous ulcerations occur. Risk factors for the development of PTS include persistent leg symptoms for months after the acute episode of DVT, an anatomically extensive DVT involving the iliofemoral system, recurrent ipsilateral DVTs, and a prolonged state of subtherapeutic anticoagulation for DVT. Unfortunately, treatment of PTS remains supportive and compression therapy remains the mainstay of treatment for

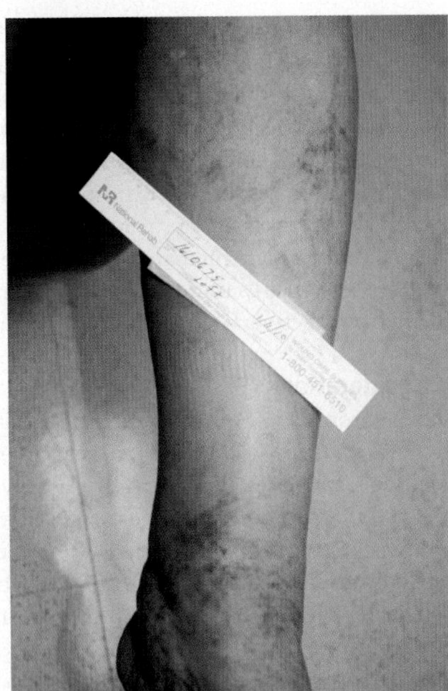

**FIGURE 65-12** Edema. Note the loss of ankle definition.

PTS. Some investigators have advocated the early use of thrombolysis to prevent PTS, but that has not been consistently proven.

### Imaging Studies and Laboratory Tests

***Venography*** Injection of contrast material into the venous system is the most accurate method of confirming DVT and its location. The superficial venous system has to be occluded with a tourniquet and the veins in the foot are injected for visualization of the deep venous system. Although this is a good test for finding occlusive and nonocclusive thrombus, it is also invasive, subject to risks of contrast, and requires interpretation, with a 5% to 10% error rate.

***Impedance Plethysmography*** Impedance plethysmography measures the change in venous capacitance and rate of emptying of the venous volume on temporary occlusion and release of the occlusion of the venous system. A cuff is inflated around the upper thigh until the electrical signal has plateaued. When the cuff is deflated, there is usually rapid outflow and reduction of volume. With a venous thrombosis, one notes a prolongation of the outflow wave. It is not useful clinically for the detection of calf venous thrombosis and of patients with prior venous thrombosis.

***Fibrin and Fibrinogen Assays*** Fibrin and fibrinogen levels can be determined by measuring the degradation of intravascular fibrin. The D-dimer test measures cross-linked degradation products, which is a surrogate of plasmin's activity on fibrin. In combination with clinical evaluation and assessment, the sensitivity exceeds 90% to 95%. The negative predictive value is 99.3% for proximal evaluation and 98.6% for distal evaluation. In the postoperative patient, D-dimer is causally elevated because of surgery and, as such, a positive D-dimer assay for evaluating for DVT is not useful. However, a negative D-dimer test in patients with suspected DVT has a high negative predictive value, ranging from 97% to 99%.[30]

***Duplex Ultrasound*** The current diagnostic test of choice for the diagnosis of DVT is duplex ultrasound, a modality that combines Doppler ultrasound and color flow imaging. The advantage of this test is that it is noninvasive, comprehensive, and without any risk of reaction to contrast angiography. This test is also highly operator-dependent, which is one of its potential drawbacks.

Doppler ultrasound is based on the principle of the impairment of an accelerated flow signal caused by an intraluminal thrombus. A detailed interrogation begins at the calf with imaging of the tibial veins and then proximally over the popliteal and femoral veins. A properly done examination evaluates flow with distal compression, which results in augmentation of flow, and with proximal compression, which should interrupt flow. If any segment of the venous system being examined fails to demonstrate augmentation on compression, venous thrombosis is suspected.

Real-time B mode ultrasonography with color flow imaging has improved the sensitivity and specificity of ultrasound scanning. With color flow duplex imaging, blood flow can be imaged in the presence of a partially occluding thrombus. The probe is also used to compress the vein. A normal vein is easily compressed, whereas in the presence of a thrombus, there is resistance to compression. In addition, the chronicity of the thrombus can be evaluated based on its imaging characteristics—namely, increased echogenicity and heterogeneity. Duplex imaging is significantly more sensitive than indirect physiologic testing.

***Magnetic Resonance Venous Imaging*** With major advances in imaging technology, MRVI has come to the forefront of imaging for proximal venous disease. The cost and issue of patient tolerance because of claustrophobia limit its widespread application, but this has been changing. It is a useful test for imaging the iliac veins and IVC, an area where the use of duplex ultrasound is limited.

### Prophylaxis

The patient who has undergone major abdominal or orthopedic surgery, has sustained major trauma, or has prolonged immobility (>3 days) represents an elevated risk for the development of venous thromboembolism. The specific risk factor analysis and epidemiologic studies detailing the causes of venous thromboembolism are beyond the scope of this chapter. The reader is referred to a more extensive analysis of this problem.[29]

The methods of prophylaxis can be mechanical or pharmacologic. The simplest method is for the patient to walk. Activation of the calf pump mechanism is an effective means of prophylaxis, as evidenced by the fact that few active people without underlying risk factors develop venous thrombosis. A patient who is expected to be up and walking within 24 to 48 hours is at low risk for developing venous thrombosis. The practice of having a patient out of bed into a chair is one of the most thrombogenic positions that could be ordered for a patient. Sitting in a chair, with the legs in a dependent position, causes venous pooling, which in the postoperative milieu could easily be a predisposing factor for the development of thromboembolism.

The most common method of surgical prophylaxis has traditionally revolved around sequential compression devices, which periodically compress the calves and essentially replicate the calf bellows mechanism. This has clearly reduced the incidence of venous thromboembolism in the surgical patient. The most likely mechanism for the efficacy of this device is prevention of venous stasis. Some studies have suggested that fibrinolytic activity systemically is enhanced by a sequential compression device. However, this has not been definitively established, because a considerable number of studies have demonstrated no enhancement of fibrinolytic activity.[31]

Another traditional method of thromboprophylaxis has been the use of low-dose unfractionated heparin. The dosage traditionally used was 5000 U of unfractionated heparin every 12 hours. However, analyses of trials comparing placebo versus fixed-dose heparin have shown that the stated dose of 5000 U SC every 12 hours is no more effective than placebo. When subcutaneous heparin is used on a dosing regimen every 8 hours, rather than every 12 hours, there is a reduction in the development of venous thromboembolism.

More recently, a number of studies have revealed the efficacy of fractionated low-molecular-weight heparin (LMWH) for the prophylaxis and treatment of venous thromboembolism. LMWH inhibits factor Xa and IIA activity, with the ratio of anti–factor Xa to anti–factor IIA activity ranging from 1 : 1 to 4 : 1. LMWH has a longer plasma half-life and significantly higher bioavailability. The consistent bioavailability and clearance of LMWH do not require monitoring of factor Xa levels, which facilitates patient use. Dosing is merely based on the patient's weight. There is a more predictable anticoagulant response than with unfractionated heparin. No laboratory monitoring is necessary because the partial thromboplastin time (PTT) is unaffected. Various analyses, including a major meta-analysis, have shown that LMWH results in equivalent, if not better, efficacy, with significantly less bleeding complications. It was first thought that LMWH results in less bleeding than unfractionated heparin, but no clinical observations have confirmed this. This property may be more a function of dose than an intrinsic drug action.

Comparison of LMWH with mechanical prophylaxis has demonstrated the superiority of LMWH for reduction of the development of venous thromboembolic disease.[32-34] Prospective trials evaluating LMWH in head-injured and trauma patients have also proved the safety of LMWH, with no increase in intracranial bleeding or major bleeding at other sites.[35] In addition, LMWH shows a significant reduction in the development of venous thromboembolism compared with other methods.

Thus, LMWH is considered the optimal method of prophylaxis for moderate- and high-risk patients. Even the traditional reluctance to use heparin in high-risk groups, such as the multiply injured trauma patient and head-injured patient, must be reexamined, given the efficacy and safety profile of LMWH in multiple prospective trials.

### Treatment

After a diagnosis of venous thrombosis has been made, a treatment plan must be instituted. Complications of calf DVT include proximal propagation of thrombus in up to one third of hospitalized patients and PTS. In addition, untreated lower extremity DVT carries a 30% recurrence rate.

Any venous thrombosis involving the femoropopliteal system is treated with full anticoagulation. Traditionally, the treatment of DVT has centered around heparin treatment to maintain the PTT at 60 to 80 seconds, followed by warfarin therapy to obtain an international normalized ratio (INR) of 2.5 to 3.0. If unfractionated heparin is used, it is important to use a nomogram-based dosing therapy. The incidence of recurrent venous thromboembolism increases if the time to therapeutic anticoagulation is prolonged. Therefore, it is important to reach therapeutic levels within 24 hours. An initial bolus of 80 U/kg or 5000 units IV bolus is administered, followed by 18 U/kg/hr. The rate is dependent on a target PTT corresponding to anti-factor Xa level of 0.3 to 0.7 unit/mL.[41] The PTT needs to be checked 6 hours after any change in heparin dosing. Warfarin is started on the same day. If warfarin is initiated without heparin, the risk for a transient hypercoagulable state exists because protein C and S levels fall before the other vitamin K–dependent factors are depleted. With the advent of LMWH, it is no longer necessary to admit the patient for IV heparin therapy. It is now accepted practice to administer LMWH on an outpatient basis, as a bridge to warfarin therapy, which is also monitored on an outpatient basis.

The recommended duration of anticoagulant therapy continues to evolve. A minimum treatment time of 3 months is advocated in most cases. The recurrence rate is the same with 3 versus 6 months of warfarin therapy. If the patient has a known hypercoagulable state or has experienced episodes of venous thrombosis, however, lifetime anticoagulation is required in the absence of contraindications. The accepted INR range is 2.0 to 3.0; a randomized double-blind study has confirmed that a goal INR of 2.0 to 3.0 is more effective in preventing recurrent venous thromboembolism than a low-intensity regimen with a goal INR of 1.0 to 1.9.[36] Additionally, the low-intensity regimen did not reduce the risk for clinically important bleeding.

Oral anticoagulants are teratogenic and thus cannot be used during pregnancy. In the case of the pregnant patient with venous thrombosis, LMWH is the treatment of choice; this is continued through delivery and can be continued postpartum, as indicated.

**Thrombolysis** The advent of thrombolysis has resulted in increased interest in thrombolysis for DVT. The purported benefit is preservation of valve function, with a subsequently lesser chance of developing CVI. However, there have been few definitive convincing studies to support the use of thrombolytic therapy for DVT.

One exception is the patient with phlegmasia, for whom thrombolysis is advocated for relief of significant venous obstruction. In this condition, thrombolytic therapy probably results in better relief of symptoms and less long-term sequelae than heparin anticoagulation alone. The alternative for this condition is surgical venous thrombectomy. No matter which treatment is chosen, long-term anticoagulation is indicated. The incidence of major bleeding is higher with lytic therapy.[25]

**Endovascular Reconstruction** Chronic proximal venous occlusion of the iliofemoral system is a challenging clinical problem. The presentation is variable, and there is no reliable diagnostic modality to measure proximal iliofemoral venous stenosis and assess outflow obstruction accurately. The pathophysiology is often a combination of primary and secondary venous insufficiency. Therefore, evaluation and treatment can be challenging. Endovascular reconstruction removes the need for surgical bypass, and has been used successfully. Recanalization of the occluded iliac vein is performed endovascularly. Balloon dilation of the lesion is then performed, and a stent is placed across the dilated segment. Excellent results have been achieved, thereby obviating an open surgical procedure. Endovascular iliac therapy has evolved to become first-line therapy for iliac occlusions.

## Upper Extremity Deep Venous Thrombosis

Upper extremity DVT is much less common than its lower extremity counterpart, constituting only approximately 5% of all documented DVTs. Although not as common, it is a serious problem; pulmonary embolism occurs in up to one third of all patients with an upper extremity DVT. *Upper extremity DVT* usually refers to thrombosis of the axillary or subclavian veins. The syndrome can be divided into two categories, primary idiopathic and secondary.

Primary causes include Paget-Schroetter syndrome and idiopathic upper extremity DVT. Patients with Paget-Schroetter syndrome develop effort thrombosis of the extremity caused by compression of the subclavian vein, the venous component of thoracic outlet syndrome. A classic presentation involves a young athlete who uses the upper extremity in a repetitive motion, such as swimming, which causes repetitive extrinsic compression of the subclavian vein. In these patients, anatomic anomalies such as a cervical rib or myofascial bands cause the venous compression. Plain films are one of the first diagnostic tests used to confirm thoracic outlet syndrome. Treatment with initial thrombolysis followed by first rib resection is the standard of care. Idiopathic upper extremity DVT is sometimes eventually attributed to an occult malignancy, and therefore a diagnosis of idiopathic upper extremity DVT warrants evaluation for an undetected malignancy.

Secondary causes of upper extremity DVT are more common. These include an indwelling central venous catheter, pacemaker, thrombophilia, or malignancy.

Classic findings on physical examination include unilateral swelling, pain, extremity discomfort, erythema, and a palpable cord. Diagnosis is confirmed by duplex ultrasonography. Because the clavicle obscures the midportion of the subclavian vein, venography or magnetic resonance venography may be required; these are second-line imaging modalities.

### Treatment

Treatment of upper extremity DVT involves anticoagulation therapy. Therapeutic dosing parameters are the same as for lower extremity DVT. Long-term complications of upper extremity DVT include recurrence and PTS. PTS is treated with extremity elevation and graduated elastic compression.[37,38]

**Vena Cava Filter** The most worrisome and potentially lethal complication of DVT is pulmonary embolism. The symptoms of pulmonary embolism, ranging from dyspnea, chest pain, and hypoxia to acute cor pulmonale, are nonspecific and require a high index of suspicion. The gold standard remains pulmonary angiography but, increasingly, this has been displaced by computed tomography angiography (CTA).

Adequate anticoagulation is usually effective for stabilizing venous thrombosis but, if a patient develops a pulmonary embolism in the presence of adequate anticoagulation, a vena cava filter is indicated. The general indications for a vena cava filter are listed in Box 65-3. Modern filters are placed percutaneously over a guidewire. The Greenfield filter, most extensively used and studied, has a 95% patency rate and a 4% recurrent embolism rate. This high patency rate allows for safe suprarenal placement if there is involvement of the IVC up to the renal veins or if it is placed in a woman in her childbearing years.

**BOX 65-3 Indications for a Vena Cava Filter**

- Recurrent thromboembolism despite adequate anticoagulation
- Deep venous thrombosis in a patient with contraindications to anticoagulation
- Chronic pulmonary embolism and resultant pulmonary hypertension
- Complications of anticoagulation
- Propagating iliofemoral venous thrombus in anticoagulation

Device-related complications are wound hematoma, migration of the device into the pulmonary artery, and caval occlusion caused by trapping of a large embolus. In the latter situation, the dramatic hypotension that accompanies acute caval occlusion can be mistaken for a massive pulmonary embolism. The distinction between the hypovolemia of caval occlusion and the right heart failure from pulmonary embolism can be made by measuring filling pressures of the right side of the heart. The treatment of caval occlusion is volume resuscitation.

**Retrievable Vena Cava Filters** Although generally safe, IVC filters are not without risk and significant morbidity. Therefore, permanent placement of a caval filter, particularly in a young patient who may only require short-term caval protection, is not generally accepted. Retrievable filters entered the field as a potential solution for the patient with temporary indications for pulmonary embolus prophylaxis. There are three retrievable IVC filters that have U.S. Food and Drug Administration (FDA) approval—the Recovery filter (Bard, Helsingborg, Sweden), OptEase filter (Cordis, Johnson & Johnson Gateway, Piscataway, NJ), and Gunther-Tulip filter (Cook Medical, Bloomington, Ind). These filters vary slightly with respect to shape and length. All can be deployed from the internal jugular vein or femoral vein and retrieved from the right jugular vein (Gunther-Tulip and Recovery) or right femoral vein (OptEase). Before retrieval, venography is performed to ensure that there is no nidus of IVC thrombus in the filter. These filters can be placed in an angiography suite or at the bedside using intravascular ultrasound. A major advantage to retrievable filters is that they may be removed when the patient no longer requires pulmonary embolism protection or can undergo anticoagulation. Patient groups that may benefit from retrievable filters include multiple-trauma patients and high-risk surgical patients. Insertion complications reported include vena cava perforation, filter migration, and venous thrombosis at the insertion site. Retrieval complications include failure to retrieve the filter, thrombus embolization from the filter, vein retrieval site thrombus, and groin hematoma. However, the role of retrievable filters continues to be a work in progress. Further investigation is required before definitive practice guidelines can be established (Box 65-4).[39,40]

## Superficial Thrombophlebitis

Superficial thrombophlebitis is a common disorder, diagnosed in the hospital and outpatient setting. In hospitalized patients, superficial thrombophlebitis is usually caused by an indwelling

**BOX 65-4 Indications for Placement of a Retrievable Inferior Vena Cava Filter**

Prophylactic placement in a high-risk trauma patient (orthopedic, spinal cord patients)
Short-term duration, contraindication of anticoagulation therapy
Protection during venous thrombolytic therapy
Extensive iliocaval thrombosis

catheter. In the clinic, patients with thrombophlebitis report common predisposing risk factors, such as recent surgery, recent childbirth, venous stasis, varicose veins, or IV drug use. Patients who deny any of these factors may be classified with idiopathic thrombophlebitis. In these cases, care must be taken to ensure that the patient does not harbor an occult hypercoagulable state or occult malignancy. In 1876, Trousseau identified the phenomenon of migratory thrombophlebitis and malignancy, particularly involving the tail of the pancreas. Mondor's disease involves superficial thrombophlebitis of the superficial veins of the breast. Diagnosis of superficial thrombophlebitis can be easily made by physical examination of an erythematous palpable cord coursing along a superficial vein, usually located along the lower extremities. Duplex ultrasonography is used if there is suspicion of proximal propagation into the deep venous system. With this diagnosis of DVT, anticoagulation is indicated. If, however, thrombus abuts the saphenofemoral junction, treatment of this more elusive condition is controversial. Some authors recommend serial ultrasound and others anticoagulation; another alternative is operative ligation at the junction.

The treatment of localized noncomplicated thrombophlebitis involves conservative therapy, which consists of anti-inflammatory medication and compression stockings. When the thrombophlebitis involves clusters of varicosities, particularly in the lower extremities, excision is indicated. Selective removal of the entire vein along its course is only indicated in the rare case of suppurative septic thrombophlebitis after all other sources of sepsis have been excluded.

## CONCLUSION

The spectrum of venous disease is widespread and diverse, providing surgeons who fully understand the unique physiology of veins a rewarding and rich arena for future investigation.

## SELECTED REFERENCES

Caggiati A, Bergan JJ, Gloviczki P, et al: Nomenclature of the veins of the lower limbs: An international interdisciplinary consensus statement. J Vasc Surg 36:416–422, 2002.

Outlines revised terminology for the venous anatomy of the lower extremity.

Bergan JJ, Pascarella L, Schmid-Schönbein GW: Pathogenesis of primary chronic venous disease: Insights from animal models of venous hypertension. J Vasc Surg 47:183–192, 2008.

Provides comprehensive review of the known aspects of venous hypertension pathophysiology.

Eklöf B, Rutherford RB, Bergan JJ, et al: American Venous Forum International Ad Hoc Committee for Revision of the CEAP Classification: Revision of the CEAP classification for chronic venous disorders: Consensus statement. J Vasc Surg 40:1248–1252, 2004.

Essential adjunct to the original CEAP document.

Leopardi D, Hoggan BL, Fitridge RA, et al: Systematic review of treatments for varicose veins. Ann Vasc Surg 23:264–276, 2009.

Systematic overview of current treatment modalities for superficial venous disease.

Meissner MH, Gloviczki P, Bergan J, et al: Primary chronic venous disorders. J Vasc Surg 46(Suppl):54S–67S, 2007.
Meissner MH, Eklof B, Smith PC, et al: Secondary chronic venous disorders. J Vasc Surg 46(Suppl):68S–83S, 2007.

These two supplements provide an extremely comprehensive evaluation of venous insufficiency, including pathophysiology, medical and surgical management, and outstanding references.

Wakefield TW, Caprini J, Comerota AJ: Thromboembolic diseases. Curr Probl Surg 45:844–899, 2008.

Excellent review of secondary venous disorders.

## REFERENCES

1. Caggiati A, Bergan JJ, Gloviczki P, et al: Nomenclature of the veins of the lower limbs: An international interdisciplinary consensus statement. J Vasc Surg 36:416–422, 2002.
2. Pascarella L, Schonbein GW, Bergan JJ: Microcirculation and venous ulcers: A review. Ann Vasc Surg 19:921–927, 2005.
3. Kowalewski R, Malkowski A, Sobolewski K, et al: Evaluation of transforming growth factor-beta signaling pathway in the wall of normal and varicose veins. Pathobiology 77:1–6, 2010.
4. Neglen P, Raju S: A rational approach to detection of significant reflux with duplex Doppler scanning and air plethysmography. J Vasc Surg 17:590–595, 1993.
5. Christopoulos D, Nicolaides AN, Szendro G: Venous reflux: quantification and correlation with the clinical severity of chronic venous disease. Br J Surg 75:352–356, 1988.
6. van Bemmelen PS, Bedford G, Beach K, et al: Quantitative segmental evaluation of venous valvular reflux with duplex ultrasound scanning. J Vasc Surg 10:425–431, 1989.
7. Vasdekis SN, Clarke GH, Nicolaides AN: Quantification of venous reflux by means of duplex scanning. J Vasc Surg 10:670–677, 1989.
8. Singh S, Lees TA, Donlon M, et al: Improving the preoperative assessment of varicose veins. Br J Surg 84:801–802, 1997.
9. Eklof B, Rutherford RB, Bergan JJ, et al: Revision of the CEAP classification for chronic venous disorders: Consensus statement. J Vasc Surg 40:1248–1252, 2004.
10. Rutherford RB, Padberg FT, Jr., Comerota AJ, et al: Venous severity scoring: An adjunct to venous outcome assessment. J Vasc Surg 31:1307–1312, 2000.
11. Raju S, Hollis K, Neglen P: Use of compression stockings in chronic venous disease: Patient compliance and efficacy. Ann Vasc Surg 21:790–795, 2007.
12. Bunke N, Brown K, Bergan J: Foam sclerotherapy: Techniques and uses. Perspect Vasc Surg Endovasc Ther 21:91–93, 2009.

13. Franz RW, Knapp ED: Transilluminated powered phlebectomy surgery for varicose veins: A review of 339 consecutive patients. Ann Vasc Surg 23:303–309, 2009.
14. Dwerryhouse S, Davies B, Harradine K, et al: Stripping the long saphenous vein reduces the rate of reoperation for recurrent varicose veins: five-year results of a randomized trial. J Vasc Surg 29:589–592, 1999.
15. van den Bos R, Arends L, Kockaert M, et al: Endovenous therapies of lower extremity varicosities: A meta-analysis. J Vasc Surg 49:230–239, 2009.
16. Marston WA, Owens LV, Davies S, et al: Endovenous saphenous ablation corrects the hemodynamic abnormality in patients with CEAP clinical class 3-6 CVI due to superficial reflux. Vasc Endovascular Surg 40:125–130, 2006.
17. Neglen P, Hollis KC, Olivier J, et al: Stenting of the venous outflow in chronic venous disease: Long-term stent-related outcome, clinical, and hemodynamic result. J Vasc Surg 46:979–990, 2007.
18. Hanrahan LM, Araki CT, Rodriguez AA, et al: Distribution of valvular incompetence in patients with venous stasis ulceration. J Vasc Surg 13:805–811, 1991.
19. O'Donnell TF, Jr.: The present status of surgery of the superficial venous system in the management of venous ulcer and the evidence for the role of perforator interruption. J Vasc Surg 48:1044–1052, 2008.
20. Linton RR: The communicating veins of the lower leg and the operative technic for their ligation. Ann Surg 107:582–593, 1938.
21. Powell CC, Rohrer MJ, Barnard MR, et al: Chronic venous insufficiency is associated with increased platelet and monocyte activation and aggregation. J Vasc Surg 30:844–851, 1999.
22. Gloviczki P, Bergan JJ, Rhodes JM, et al: Mid-term results of endoscopic perforator vein interruption for chronic venous insufficiency: Lessons learned from the North American subfascial endoscopic perforator surgery registry. The North American Study Group. J Vasc Surg 29:489–502, 1999.
23. Murray JD, Bergan JJ, Riffenburgh RH: Development of open-scope subfascial perforating vein surgery: Lessons learned from the first 67 cases. Ann Vasc Surg 13:372–377, 1999.
24. Masuda EM, Kessler DM, Lurie F, et al: The effect of ultrasound-guided sclerotherapy of incompetent perforator veins on venous clinical severity and disability scores. J Vasc Surg 43:551–556, 2006.
25. Sillesen H, Just S, Jorgensen M, et al: Catheter-directed thrombolysis for treatment of iliofemoral deep venous thrombosis is durable, preserves venous valve function and may prevent chronic venous insufficiency. Eur J Vasc Endovasc Surg 30:556–562, 2005.
26. Kistner RL: Surgical repair of the incompetent femoral vein valve. Arch Surg 110:1336–1342, 1975.
27. Masuda EM, Kistner RL: Long-term results of venous valve reconstruction: A four- to twenty-one-year follow-up. J Vasc Surg 19:391–403, 1994.
28. Taheri SA, Lazar L, Elias S, et al: Surgical treatment of post-phlebitic syndrome with vein valve transplant. Am J Surg 144: 221–224, 1982.
29. Anderson FA, Jr, Spencer FA: Risk factors for venous thromboembolism. Circulation 107(Suppl 1):9–16, 2003.
30. Kovacs MJ, MacKinnon KM, Anderson D, et al: A comparison of three rapid D-dimer methods for the diagnosis of venous thromboembolism. Br J Haematol 115:140–144, 2001.
31. Killewich LA, Cahan MA, Hanna DJ, et al: The effect of external pneumatic compression on regional fibrinolysis in a prospective randomized trial. J Vasc Surg 36:953–958, 2002.
32. Bernardi E, Prandoni P: Safety of low molecular weight heparins in the treatment of venous thromboembolism. Expert Opin Drug Saf 2:87–94, 2003.
33. Couturaud F, Julian JA, Kearon C: Low molecular weight heparin administered once versus twice daily in patients with venous thromboembolism: A meta-analysis. Thromb Haemost 86:980–984, 2001.
34. Mismetti P, Laporte S, Darmon JY, et al: Meta-analysis of low molecular weight heparin in the prevention of venous thromboembolism in general surgery. Br J Surg 88:913–930, 2001.
35. Norwood SH, McAuley CE, Berne JD, et al: Prospective evaluation of the safety of enoxaparin prophylaxis for venous thromboembolism in patients with intracranial hemorrhagic injuries. Arch Surg 137:696–701, 2002.
36. Kearon C, Ginsberg JS, Kovacs MJ, et al: Comparison of low-intensity warfarin therapy with conventional-intensity warfarin therapy for long-term prevention of recurrent venous thromboembolism. N Engl J Med 349:631–639, 2003.
37. Joffe HV, Goldhaber SZ: Upper-extremity deep vein thrombosis. Circulation 106:1874–1880, 2002.
38. Martinelli I, Battaglioli T, Bucciarelli P, et al: Risk factors and recurrence rate of primary deep vein thrombosis of the upper extremities. Circulation 110:566–570, 2004.
39. Offner PJ, Hawkes A, Madayag R, et al: The role of temporary inferior vena cava filters in critically ill surgical patients. Arch Surg 138:591–594; discussion 594-595, 2003.
40. Rosenthal D, Wellons ED, Lai KM, et al: Retrievable inferior vena cava filters: Initial clinical results. Ann Vasc Surg 20:157–165, 2006.
41. Kearon C, Kahn SR, Agnelli G, et al: Antithrombotic therapy for venous thromboembolic disease: American College of Chest Physicians evidence-based clinical practice guidelines, ed 8. Chest 133(6 Suppl):454S–545S, 2008.

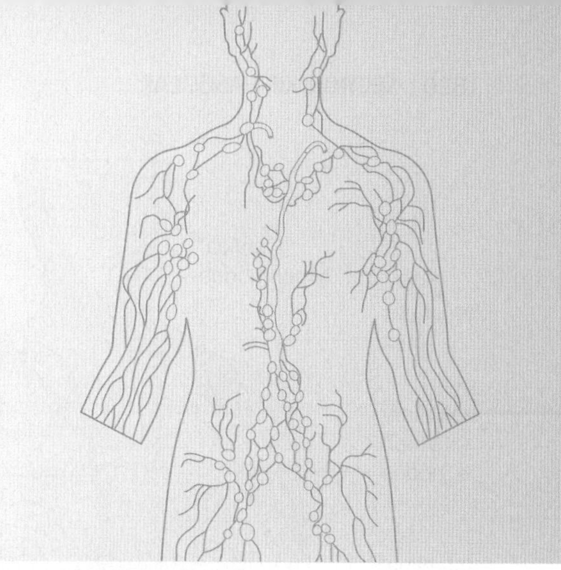

CHAPTER 66

# THE LYMPHATICS

Iraklis I. Pipinos and B. Timothy Baxter



## EMBRYOLOGY AND ANATOMY

The primordial lymphatic system is first seen during the sixth week of development in the form of lymph sacs located next to the jugular veins. During the eighth week, the cisterna chyli forms just dorsal to the aorta and, at the same time, two additional lymphatic sacs corresponding to the iliofemoral vascular pedicles begin forming. Communicating channels connecting the lymph sacs, which will become the thoracic duct, develop during the ninth week.

From this primordial lymphatic system sprout endothelial buds that grow with the venous system to form the peripheral lymphatic plexus (Fig. 66-1). Failure of one of the initial jugular lymphatic sacs to develop proper connections and drainage with the lymphatic and, subsequently, venous system may produce focal lymph cysts (cavernous lymphangiomas), also known as *cystic hygromas*.[1] Similarly, failure of embryologic remnants of lymphatic tissues to connect to efferent channels lead to the development of cystic lymphatic formations (simple capillary lymphangiomas) that, depending on their location, are classified as truncal, mesenteric, intestinal, and retroperitoneal lymphangiomas. Hypoplasia or failure of development of drainage channels connecting the lymphatic systems of extremities to the main primordial lymphatic system of the torso may result in primary lymphedema of the extremities.

Lymphangiogenesis appears to be regulated by vascular endothelial growth factors C and D (VEGF-C, VEGF-D), their receptor VEGFR-3, and their binding protein, neurophilin-2 (Nrp2). Consistent with these findings, Nrp2-deficient mice have lymphatic hypoplasia and the heterozygous inactivating mutation of VEGFR-3 is found in Chy mice, an animal model of primary lymphedema, which appears to be the underlying problem in patients with Milroy's disease (congenital familial lymphedema).[2]

## FUNCTION AND STRUCTURE

The lymphatic system is composed of three elements:

1. Initial or terminal lymphatic capillaries, which absorb lymph
2. Collecting vessels, which serve primarily as conduits for lymph transport
3. Lymph nodes, which are interposed in the pathway of the conducting vessels, filtering the lymph and serving a primary immunologic role

The terminal lymphatics have special structural characteristics that allow entry not only of large macromolecules, but even cells and microbes. Their most important structural feature is a high porosity resulting from a very small number of tight junctions between endothelial cells, a limited and incomplete basement membrane, and anchoring filaments (4 to 10 nm) tethering the interstitial matrix to the endothelial cells. These filaments, once the turgor of the tissue increases, are able to pull on the endothelial cells, and essentially introduce large gaps between them, which then allow for low-resistance influx of interstitial fluid and macromolecules into the lymphatic channels. The collecting vessels ascend alongside the primary blood vessels of the organ or limb, pass through the regional lymph nodes, and drain into the main lymph channels of the torso. These channels eventually empty into the venous system via the thoracic duct. There are additional communications between the lymphatic and venous systems. These smaller lymphovenous shunts mostly occur at the level of lymph nodes and around major venous structures, such as the jugular, subclavian, and iliac veins. Several structures in the body contain no lymphatics. Specifically, lymphatics have not been found in the epidermis, cornea, central nervous system, cartilage, tendon, and muscle.

The lymphatic system has three main functions. First, tissue fluid and macromolecules that undergo ultrafiltration at the level of the arterial capillaries are reabsorbed and returned to the circulation through the lymphatic system. Every day, 50% to 100% of the intravascular proteins are filtered this way in the interstitial space. Normally, they then enter the terminal lymphatics and are transported through the collecting lymphatics back into the venous circulation. Second, microbes arriving in the interstitial space enter the lymphatic system and are presented to the lymph nodes, which represent the first line of the immune system. Third, at the level of the gastrointestinal tract, lymph vessels are responsible for the uptake and transport of most of the fat absorbed from the bowel.

In contrast to what happens with venous forward flow, lymph's centripetal transport occurs mainly through intrinsic

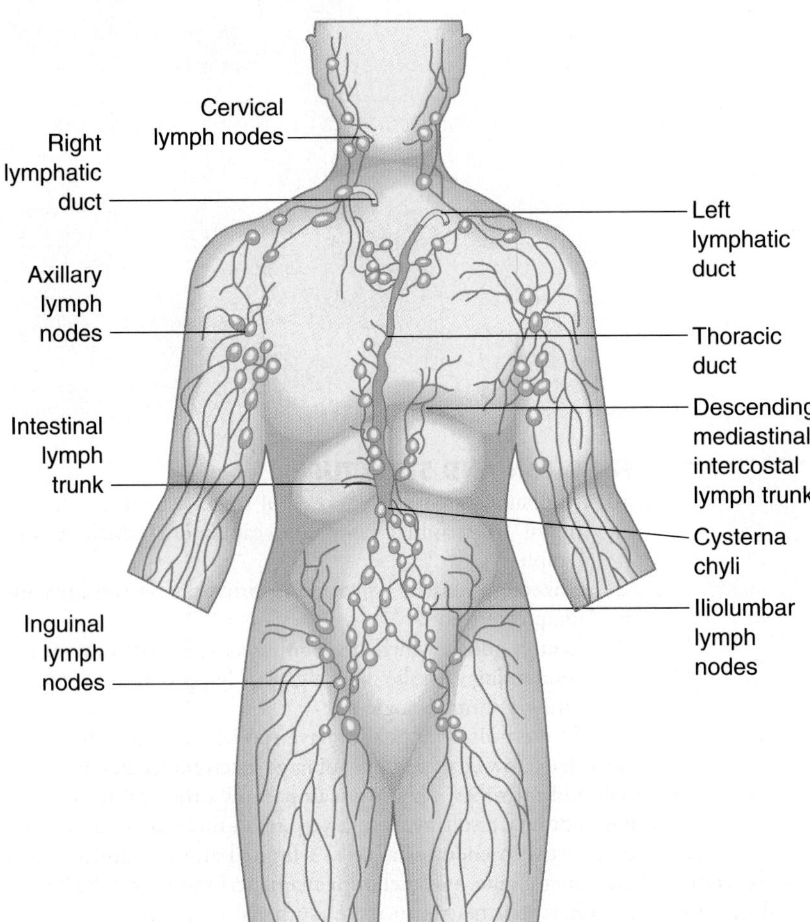


**FIGURE 66-1** Major anatomic pathways and lymph node groups of the lymphatic system.

contractility of the individual lymphatic vessels, which, in concert with competent valvular mechanisms, is effective in establishing constant forward flow of lymph. In addition to the intrinsic contractility, other factors, such as surrounding muscular activity, negative pressure secondary to breathing, and transmitted arterial pulsations, have a lesser role in the forward lymph flow. These secondary factors appear to become more important under conditions of lymph stasis and congestion of the lymphatic vessels.

## PATHOPHYSIOLOGY AND STAGING

Lymphedema is the result of an inability of the existing lymphatic system to accommodate the protein and fluid entering the interstitial compartment at the tissue level.[3] In the first stage of lymphedema, impaired lymphatic drainage results in protein-rich fluid accumulation in the interstitial compartment. Clinically, this manifests as soft pitting edema. In the second stage of lymphedema, the clinical condition is further exacerbated by the accumulation of fibroblasts, adipocytes and, perhaps most importantly, macrophages in the affected tissues, which culminate in a local inflammatory response. This results in important structural changes from the deposition of connective tissue and adipose elements at the skin and subcutaneous level. In the second stage of lymphedema, tissue edema is more pronounced, is nonpitting, and has a spongy consistency. In the third and most advanced stage of lymphedema, the affected tissues sustain further injury as a result of the local inflammatory response and recurrent infectious episodes that typically result from minimal subclinical skin breaks in the skin. Such repeated episodes injure the incompetent remaining lymphatic channels, progressively worsening the underlying insufficiency of the lymphatic system. This eventually results in excessive subcutaneous fibrosis and scarring, with associated severe skin changes characteristic of lymphostatic elephantiasis.

## DIFFERENTIAL DIAGNOSIS

In most patients with second- or third-stage lymphedema, the characteristic findings of the physical examination can usually establish the diagnosis. The edematous limb has a firm and hardened consistency. There is loss of the normal perimalleolar shape, resulting in a tree trunk pattern. The dorsum of the foot is characteristically swollen, resulting in the appearance of the so-called *buffalo hump*, and the toes become thick and squared (Fig. 66-2). In advanced lymphedema, the skin undergoes characteristic changes such as lichenification, development of peau d'orange, and hyperkeratosis.[3] Also, patients give a history of recurrent episodes of cellulitis and lymphangitis after trivial trauma, and frequently present with fungal infections affecting the forefoot and toes. Patients with isolated lymphedema usually do not have the hyperpigmentation or ulceration one typically sees in patients with chronic venous insufficiency. Lymphedema does not respond significantly to overnight elevation, whereas edema secondary to central organ failure or venous insufficiency does.

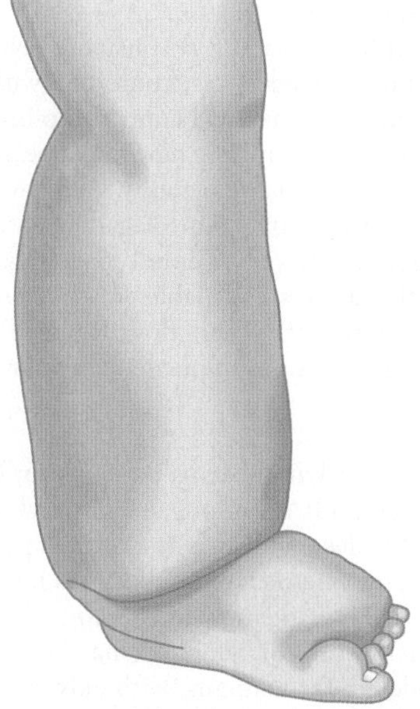

**FIGURE 66-2** Lymphedema with characteristic loss of the normal perimalleolar shape, resulting in a tree trunk pattern. The dorsum of the foot is characteristically swollen, resulting in the appearance of the so-called *buffalo hump*.

The evaluation of a swollen extremity should start with a detailed history and physical examination. The usual causes of bilateral extremity edema are of systemic origin; the most common is cardiac failure, followed by renal failure.[4] Hypoproteinemia secondary to cirrhosis, nephrotic syndrome, and malnutrition can also produce bilateral lower extremity edema. Another important cause to consider with bilateral leg enlargement is lipedema. Lipedema is not true edema but, rather, excessive subcutaneous fat typically found in obese women. It is bilateral, nonpitting, and greatest at the ankle and legs, with characteristic sparing of the feet. There are no skin changes and the enlargement is not affected by elevation. The history usually indicates that this has been a lifelong problem that runs in the family.

Once the systemic causes of edema are excluded, edema secondary to venous and lymphatic pathology should be considered in the patient with unilateral extremity involvement. Venous pathology is the most common cause of unilateral leg edema. Leg edema secondary to venous disease is usually pitting and is greatest at the legs and ankles, with a sparing of the feet. The edema responds promptly to overnight leg elevation. In the later stages, the skin is atrophic, with brawny pigmentation. Ulceration associated with venous insufficiency occurs above or posterior to and beneath the malleoli.

## CLASSIFICATION

Lymphedema is generally classified as primary when there is no known cause and as secondary when its cause is a known disease or disorder.[5] Primary lymphedema has generally been classified on the basis of the age of onset and presence of familial clustering. Primary lymphedema with onset before the first year of life is called *congenital*. The familial version of congenital lymphedema is known as *Milroy's disease* and is inherited as a dominant trait. Primary lymphedema with onset between the ages of 1 and 35 years is called *lymphedema praecox*. The familial version of lymphedema praecox is known as Meige's disease. Finally, primary lymphedema with onset after the age of 35 years is called *lymphedema tarda*.

The primary lymphedemas are relatively uncommon, occurring in 1/10,000 individuals. The most common form of primary lymphedema is praecox, which accounts for approximately 80% of patients. Congenital and tarda lymphedemas each account for the remaining 10%. Worldwide, the most common cause of secondary lymphedema is infestation of the lymph nodes by the parasite *Wuchereria bancrofti* in the disease state called *lymphatic filariasis*. In developed countries, the most common causes of secondary lymphedema involve resection or ablation of regional lymph nodes by surgery, radiation therapy, tumor invasion, direct trauma or, less commonly, an infectious process.

## DIAGNOSTIC TESTS

The diagnosis of lymphedema is relatively easy in the patient who presents in the second or third stage of the disease. It can, however, be a difficult diagnosis to make in the first stage, particularly when the edema is mild, pitting, and relieved with simple maneuvers such as elevation.[5,6] For patients with suspected secondary forms of lymphedema, computed tomography (CT) and magnetic resonance imaging (MRI) are valuable and essential for the exclusion of underlying oncologic disease states.[7] In patients with known lymph node excision and radiation treatment as the underlying problem of their lymphedema, additional diagnostic studies are rarely needed, except as they relate to follow-up of an underlying malignancy. For patients with edema of unknown cause and a suspicion for lymphedema, lymphoscintigraphy is the diagnostic test of choice. When lymphoscintigraphy confirms that lymphatic drainage is delayed, the diagnosis of primary lymphedema should never be made until neoplasia involving the regional and central lymphatic drainage of the limb has been excluded via CT or MRI. If a more detailed diagnostic interpretation of lymphatic channels is needed for operative planning, contrast lymphangiography may be considered.

Lymphoscintigraphy (or isotope lymphography) has emerged as the test of choice in patients with suspected lymphedema.[7,8] It cannot differentiate between primary and secondary lymphedemas, but it has a sensitivity of 70% to 90% and a specificity of almost 100% in differentiating lymphedema from other causes of limb swelling. The test assesses lymphatic function by quantitating the rate of clearance of a radiolabeled macromolecular tracer (Fig. 66-3). The advantages of the technique are that it is simple, safe, and reproducible, with low exposure to radioactivity (≈5 mCi). It involves the injection of a small amount (2-3 mCi injection in 0.2 mL of saline) of radioiodinated human albumin or $^{99}$Tc-labeled sulfide colloid into the first interdigital space of the foot or hand. Migration of the radiotracer within the skin and subcutaneous lymphatics is easily monitored with a whole-body gamma camera, thus producing clear images of the major lymphatic channels in the leg and amount of radioactivity at the inguinal nodes 30 and 60 minutes after injection of the radiolabeled substance in the feet. An uptake value less than 0.3% of the total injected dose at 30 minutes is diagnostic of lymphedema. The normal range of uptake is from 0.6% to 1.6%. In patients with edema secondary to venous disease, isotope clearance is usually abnormally rapid, resulting in more than 2% ilioinguinal uptake.

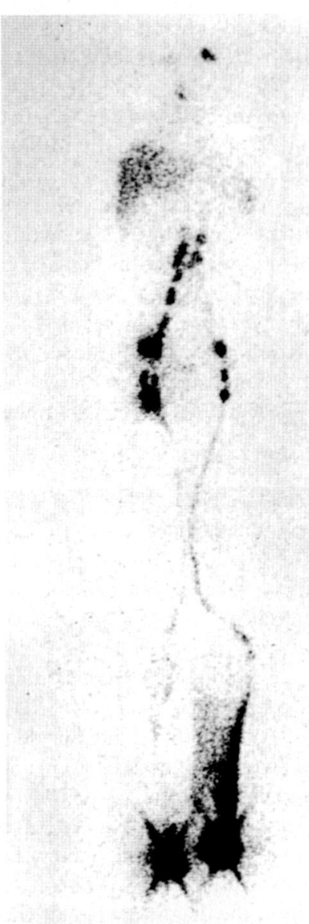

**FIGURE 66-3** Lymphoscintigraphic pattern in primary lymphedema. Note the area of dermal backflow on the left and diminished number of lymph nodes in the groin. (From Cambria RA, Gloviczki P, Naessens JM, Wahner HW: Noninvasive evaluation of the lymphatic system with lymphoscintigraphy: A prospective, semiquantitative analysis in 386 extremities. J Vasc Surg 18:773–782, 1993.)

Note that variations in the degree of edema involving the lower extremity do not appear to change the rate of isotope clearance significantly.

Direct contrast lymphangiography provides the finest details of the lymphatic anatomy.[9] However, it is an invasive study that involves exposure and cannulation of lymphatics at the dorsum of the forefoot, followed by slow injection of contrast medium (ethiodized oil). The procedure is tedious, the cannulation often necessitates the use of magnification optics (an operating microscope is often needed), and the dissection requires some form of anesthetic. After cannulation of a superficial lymph vessel, contrast material is slowly injected into the lymphatic system. A total of 7 to 10 mL of contrast is ideal for lower extremity and 4 to 5 mL for upper extremity evaluation. Potential complications include damage of the visualized lymphatics, allergic reactions, and pulmonary embolism if the oil-based contrast enters the venous system through lymphovenous anastomoses. At present, lymphangiography in the practice of vascular surgery is used infrequently and is reserved for the preoperative evaluation of select patients who are candidates for direct surgery on their lymphatic vessels.

### New Diagnostic Tests

The field of lymphatic imaging is constantly evolving. We can expect that technologic advances, combined with the development of new contrast agents, will continue to improve diagnostic accuracy.[7] The most promising new test appears to be contrast magnetic resonance lymphangiography.[10] This test is performed after the intracutaneous injection of gadobenate dimeglumine into the interdigital webs of the dorsal foot. Reported data have suggested that the new test is capable of visualizing the anatomy and functional status of lymph flow transport of lymphatic vessels and lymph nodes of lymphedematous limbs.

## TREATMENT

The large majority of lymphedema patients can be treated with a combination of limb elevation, a high quality compression garment, complex decongestive physical therapy, and compression pump therapy. The class of medications known as *benzopyrones* is still under investigation in the United States, but may find a place in the care of lymphedema. Operative treatment may be considered for patients with advanced complicated lymphedema who fail management with nonoperative means.

### General Therapeutic Measures

All patients with lymphedema should be educated in meticulous skin care and avoidance of injuries.[6,11,12] Patients should always be instructed to see their physician early for signs of infections because these may progress rapidly to serious systemic infections. Infections should be aggressively and promptly treated with appropriate antibiotics directed at gram-positive cocci. Eczema at the level of the forefoot and toes requires treatment; hydrocortisone-based creams may be considered. Additionally, basic range of motion exercises for the extremities have been shown to be of value in the management of lymphedema in the long term. Finally, patients should make every effort to maintain ideal body weight.

### Specific Treatment Measures

#### Elevation and Compression Garments

For lymphedema patients in all stages of disease, management with high-quality elastic garments is necessary at all times, except when the legs are elevated above the heart.[13,14] The ideal compression garment is custom-fitted and delivers pressures in the range of 30 to 60 mm Hg. These garments may have the additional benefit of protecting the extremity from injuries such as burns, lacerations, and insect bites. Patients should avoid standing for prolonged periods and should elevate their legs at night by supporting the foot of the bed on 15-cm blocks.

#### Complex Decongestive Physical Therapy

This specialized massage technique for patients with lymphedema is designed to stimulate the still-functioning lymph vessels, evacuate stagnant protein-rich fluid by breaking up subcutaneous deposits of fibrous tissue, and redirect lymph fluid to areas of the body where lymph flow is normal.[15] The technique is initiated on the normal contralateral side of the body, evacuating excessive fluid and preparing first the lymphatic zones of the nonaffected extremity, followed by the zones in the trunk quadrant adjacent to the affected limb, before attention is turned to the swollen extremity. The affected extremity is massaged in a segmental fashion, with the proximal zones being massaged first and then proceeding to the distal limb. The technique is time-consuming but effective in reducing the volume of the lymphedematous limbs. After the massage session is complete, the extremity is wrapped with a low-stretch wrap and the limb is placed in the custom-fitted garment to maintain the decreased girth obtained with the massage therapy. This type of therapy is appropriate for patients with all stages of lymphedema.

When the patient is first referred for complex decongestive physical therapy (CDP), the patient undergoes daily to weekly massage sessions for up to 8 to 12 weeks. Limb elevation and elastic stockings are a necessary adjunct in this phase. After maximal volume reduction is achieved, the patient returns for maintenance massage treatments every 2 to 3 months.

### Compression Pump Therapy

Pneumatic compression pump therapy is another effective method for reducing the volume of the lymphedematous limb, using a principle similar to that for massage therapy. The device consists of a sleeve containing several compartments. The lymphedematous limb is positioned inside the sleeve and the compartments are serially inflated to milk the stagnant fluid out of the extremity.[16]

When a patient with advanced lymphedema is first referred for therapy, an initial approach with hospitalization for 3 to 4 days, involving strict limb elevation, daily CDP, and compression pump treatments, may be necessary to achieve optimal control of the lymphedema. Patients with cardiac or renal dysfunction should be monitored for fluid overload. Following this initial period of intensive therapy, the patient is fitted with a high-quality compression garment to maintain the limb volume. Maintenance sessions are then prescribed for the patients on an as-needed basis.

## Drug Therapy

Benzopyrones can be effective agents in the treatment of lymphedema. This class of medications, including coumarin (1,2-benzopyrone), is thought to reduce lymphedema through stimulation of proteolysis by tissue macrophages and stimulation of the peristalsis and pumping action of the collecting lymphatics. Benzopyrones have no anticoagulant activity. The first randomized crossover trial of coumarin in patients with lymphedema of the arms and legs was reported in 1993.[17] The study concluded that coumarin was more effective than placebo in reducing not only volume; other important parameters, such as skin temperature, attacks of secondary acute inflammation, discomfort of the lymphedematous extremities, skin turgor, and suppleness were improved with coumarin. A second randomized crossover trial was reported in 1999.[18] This study focused on the effects of coumarin in women with secondary lymphedema after treatment for breast cancer, but the study found that coumarin was not effective therapy for this specific group of women. Because of the disagreement between these two major trials, the enthusiasm for the use of benzopyrones in the United States has been tempered. Additional trials should be undertaken to clarify the potential effects of the medications on primary and secondary lymphedemas in different extremities and stages.

Diuretics may temporarily improve the appearance of the lymphedematous extremity, with stage I disease leading patients to request continuous therapy. However, other than producing temporary intravascular volume depletion, there is no long-term benefit. Thus, diuretics have no role in the treatment of lymphedema at any stage.

### Molecular Lymphangiogenesis

Fundamental discoveries in lymphatic development have pointed to the potential of new treatments for lymphedema. These molecular treatments are based on the activation of the VEGFR-3 pathway by administration of cognate ligands VEGF-C and VEGF-D using a variety of methods.[19] At this point these treatments have only been tested in animal models with promising results. Formal clinical trials are now needed to evaluate the therapeutic potential and possible untoward effects (including the possibility of stimulation of dormant tumor cells as a consequence of increased angiogenesis) of therapeutic lymphangiogenesis.[20]

## Operative Treatment

Of patients with lymphedema, 95% can be managed nonoperatively. Surgical intervention may be considered for patients with stage II and III lymphedema who have severe functional impairment, recurrent episodes of lymphangitis, and severe pain, despite optimal medical therapy. Two main categories of operations are available for the care of patients with lymphedema, reconstructive and excisional.

Reconstructive surgery[21,22] should be considered for those patients with proximal (primary or secondary) obstruction of the extremity lymphatic circulation with preserved dilated lymphatics distal to the obstruction. In these patients, the residual dilated lymphatics can be anastomosed to nearby veins or to transposed healthy lymphatic channels, usually mobilized or harvested from the contralateral extremity, in an attempt to restore effective drainage of the lymphedematous extremity. Treatment of selected lymphedema patients with lymphovenous anastomoses has resulted in objective improvement in 30% to 60% of the patients, with an average initial reduction in the excess limb volume of 40% to 50%.[23,24]

For patients with primary lymphedema who have hypoplastic and fibrotic distal lymphatic vessels, such reconstructions are not an option. For these patients, surgical strategy involving the transfer of lymphatic-bearing tissue (portion of the greater omentum) into the affected limb has been attempted. This is intended to connect the residual hypoplastic lymphatic channels of the leg to competent lymphatics in the transferred tissue. Omental flap operations have been found to have poor results.[25] Alternatively, a segment of the ileum can be disconnected from the rest of the bowel, stripped of its mucosa, and mobilized to be sewn onto the cut surface of residual ilioinguinal nodes in an attempt to bridge the lower extremity with mesenteric lymphatics. When this enteromesenteric bridge procedure was applied to a group of eight carefully selected patients, the outcomes were promising, with six patients showing sustained clinical improvement over a long follow-up.[26]

Excisional operations are essentially the only viable option for patients without residual lymphatics of adequate size for reconstructive procedures. For patients with recalcitrant stage II and early stage III lymphedema, in whom the edema is moderate and the skin is relatively healthy, an excisional procedure that removes a large segment of the lymphedematous subcutaneous tissues and overlying skin is the procedure of choice. This palliative procedure was introduced by Kontoleon in 1918 and was

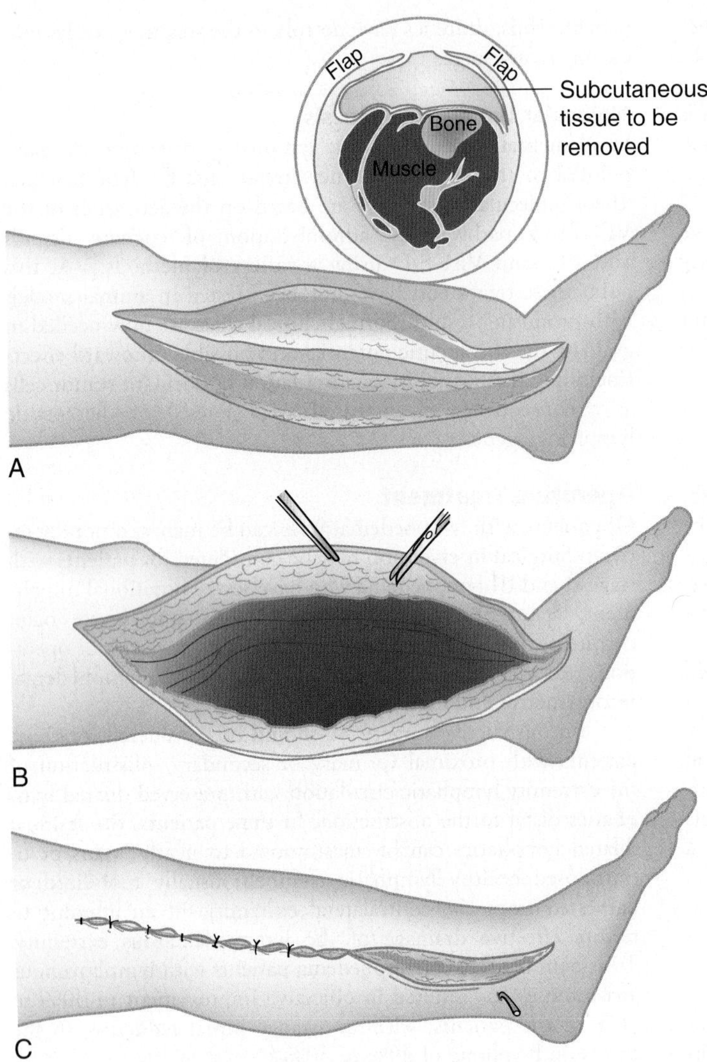


**FIGURE 66-4 A-C,** Schematic representation of Kontoleon's or Homan's procedure. Relatively thick skin flaps are raised anteriorly and posteriorly and all subcutaneous tissue beneath the flaps and underlying medial calf deep fascia is removed, along with the necessary redundant skin.

later popularized by Homan as "staged subcutaneous excision underneath flaps" (Fig. 66-4).

The operative approach starts with a medial incision extending from the level of the medial malleolus through the calf into the midthigh.[27,28] Flaps approximately 1 to 2 cm thick are elevated anteriorly and posteriorly and all subcutaneous tissue beneath the flaps, along with the underlying medial calf deep fascia, are removed with the redundant skin. The sural nerve is preserved. After the first-stage procedure is completed and if additional lymphedematous tissue removal is necessary, a second operation is performed, usually 3 to 6 months later. The second-stage operation is carried out using a similar technique through an incision on the lateral aspect of the limb. In a long-term follow-up study, 80% of patients undergoing staged subcutaneous excision underneath flaps had significant and long-lasting reduction in extremity size associated with improved function and contour of the treated extremity contour. Wound complications were encountered in 10% of patients.[27] A minimally invasive version of the Kontoleon procedure has been gaining increasing support among lymphedema experts.[29] Recent reports have demonstrated that the use of liposuction through small incisions is safe and is able to achieve control, at least over a short term, of clinically disabling conditions associated with advanced stages of lymphedema. Surgeons with experience in this technique recommend initial conservative treatment of pitting lymphedema to remove excess fluid, followed by liposuction to remove remaining excess volume bothersome to the patient.[30]

When the lymphedema is extremely pronounced and the skin is unhealthy and infected, the simple reducing operation of Kontoleon is not adequate. In this case, the classic excisional operation originally described by Charles in 1912 is performed (Fig. 66-5). The procedure involves complete and circumferential excision of the skin, subcutaneous tissue, and deep fascia of the involved leg and dorsum of the foot.[31] The excision is usually performed in one stage and coverage is provided preferably by full-thickness grafting from the excised skin. In a follow-up study, patients subjected to Charles' operation had immediate volume and circumference reduction. The skin graft take was 88%; complications consisted primarily of wound infections, hematomas, and necrosis of skin flaps. The hospital stay was 21 to 36 days.[32] Although this is a successful and radically reducing operation, the behavior in the healing skin graft is unpredictable. From 10% to 15% of the grafted segments do not take and can be difficult to manage because of frequent localized sloughing, excessive scarring, focal recurrent infections, and hyperkeratosis

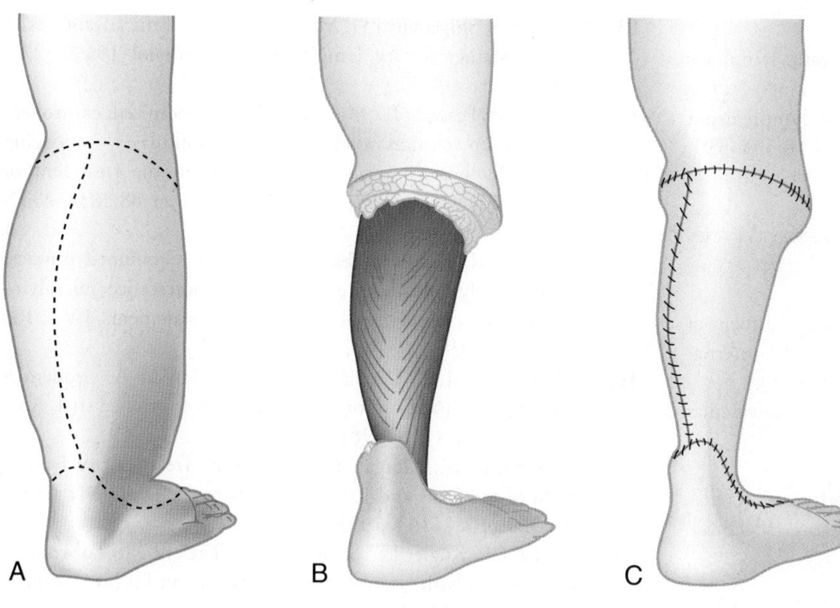


FIGURE 66-5 **A-C,** Schematic representation of Charles' procedure. This involves complete and circumferential excision of the skin, subcutaneous tissue, and deep fascia of the involved leg and dorsum of the foot. Coverage is provided preferably by full-thickness grafting from the excised skin.

or dermatitis. These complications seem to be worse in patients in whom leg resurfacing was performed using split-thickness grafts from the opposite extremity. In advanced cases, exophytic changes within the grafted skin, chronic cellulitis, and skin breakdown may eventually lead to leg amputation.[33]

## LYMPHATIC DISORDERS

### Chylothorax

Chylous pleural effusion is usually secondary to thoracic duct trauma—usually iatrogenic after chest surgery—and rarely a manifestation of advanced malignant disease with lymphatic metastasis.[34] The presence of chylomicrons on lipoprotein analysis and a triglyceride level higher than 110 mg/dL in the pleural fluid are diagnostic. Initially, patients can be treated nonoperatively with tube thoracostomy and a medium-chain triglyceride diet or total parenteral nutrition. For patients with thoracic duct injury and an effusion that persists after 1 week of drainage, video-assisted thoracoscopy or thoracotomy should be used to identify and ligate the thoracic duct above and below the leak. The site of the leak can be identified if cream is given to the patient a few hours before surgery. For patients with cancer-related chylothorax and persistent drainage, despite optimal chemotherapy and radiation therapy, pleurodesis is highly successful in preventing recurrence.[35]

### Chyloperitoneum

In contrast to chylothorax, the most common cause of chylous ascites is congenital lymphatic abnormalities in children and malignancy involving the abdominal lymph nodes in adults. Postoperative injury to abdominal lymphatics resulting in chylous ascites is rare.[36] The presence of chylomicrons on lipoprotein analysis and a triglyceride level higher than 110 mg/dL are, again diagnostic. Initial treatment includes paracentesis followed by a medium-chain triglyceride diet or total parenteral nutrition. In patients with postoperative chyloperitoneum, if ascites does not respond after 1 to 2 weeks of nonoperative management, exploration should be used to identify and ligate the leaking lymphatic duct. Congenital and malignant causes should be given longer periods (up to 4 to 6 weeks) of nonoperative management. If ascites persists in patients with congenital ascites, lymphoscintigraphy or lymphangiography is performed prior to attempting to control the leak with celiotomy. At the time of exploration, control of the leak can be achieved by ligation of leaking lymphatic vessels or resection of the bowel associated with the leak. Patients with malignancies should receive aggressive management for their underlying disease, which generally is effective at controlling the chyloperitoneum.

### Tumors of the Lymphatics

Lymphangiomas are the lymphatic analogue of the hemangiomas of blood vessels. They are generally divided into two types: (1) simple or capillary lymphangioma; and (2) cavernous lymphangioma, or cystic hygroma.[37] They are thought to represent isolated and sequestered segments of the lymphatic system that retain the ability to produce lymph. As the volume of lymph inside the cystic tumor increases, they grow larger within the surrounding tissues. Most of these benign tumors are present at birth and 90% of them can be identified by the end of the first year of life. Cavernous lymphangiomas almost invariably occur in the neck or the axilla, and very rarely in the retroperitoneum. The simple capillary lymphangiomas also tend to occur subcutaneously in the head and neck region, as well as the axilla. Rarely, however, they can be found in the trunk within the internal organs or connective tissue in and about the abdominal or thoracic cavities. The treatment of lymphangiomas should be surgical excision, taking care to preserve all normal surrounding infiltrated structures.

Lymphangiosarcoma is a rare tumor that develops as a complication of long-standing lymphedema (usually >10 years).[38] Clinically, patients present with acute worsening of the edema and appearance of subcutaneous nodules that have a propensity toward hemorrhage and ulceration. The tumor can be treated, like other sarcomas, with preoperative chemotherapy and radiation followed by surgical excision, which may take the form of radical amputation. Overall, the tumor has a very poor prognosis.[39]

## SELECTED REFERENCES

Gloviczki P: Principles of surgical treatment of chronic lymphoedema. Int Angiol 18:42–46, 1999.

Nagase T, Gonda K, Inoue K, et al: Treatment of lymphedema with lymphaticovenular anastomoses. Int J Clin Oncol 10:304–310, 2005.

These comprehensive reviews summarize the important elements in the management of patients with lymphedema.

International Society of Lymphology: The diagnosis and treatment of peripheral lymphedema. 2009 Consensus Document of the International Society of Lymphology. Lymphology 42:51–60, 2009.

Rockson SG: Diagnosis and management of lymphatic vascular disease. J Am Coll Cardiol 52:799–806, 2008.

These two current reviews illustrate the current knowledge and controversies in the pathophysiology, classification, natural history, differential diagnosis, and treatment of lymphedema

Wyatt LEMT: Lymphedema and tumors of the lymphatics. In Moore W, editor: Vascular surgery, a comprehensive review, Philadelphia, 1998, WB Saunders, pp 829–843.

This authoritative treatise provides a succinct summary of the diagnosis and treatment of lymphatic disorders.

## REFERENCES

1. Levine C: Primary disorders of the lymphatic vessels—a unified concept. J Pediatr Surg 24:233–240, 1989.
2. Alitalo K, Tammela T, Petrova TV: Lymphangiogenesis in development and human disease. Nature 438:946–953, 2005.
3. Browse NL, Stewart G: Lymphoedema: Pathophysiology and classification. J Cardiovasc Surg (Torino) 26:91–106, 1985.
4. Cho S, Atwood JE: Peripheral edema. Am J Med 113:580–586, 2002.
5. Radhakrishnan K, Rockson SG: The clinical spectrum of lymphatic disease. Ann N Y Acad Sci 1131:155–184, 2008.
6. Rockson SG: Diagnosis and management of lymphatic vascular disease. J Am Coll Cardiol 52:799–806, 2008.
7. Barrett T, Choyke PL, Kobayashi H: Imaging of the lymphatic system: New horizons. Contrast Media Mol Imaging 1:230–245, 2006.
8. Szuba A, Shin WS, Strauss HW, et al: The third circulation: Radionuclide lymphoscintigraphy in the evaluation of lymphedema. J Nucl Med 44:43–57, 2003.
9. Weissleder H, Weissleder R: Interstitial lymphangiography: initial clinical experience with a dimeric nonionic contrast agent. Radiology 170:371–374, 1989.
10. Liu NF, Lu Q, Jiang ZH, et al: Anatomic and functional evaluation of the lymphatics and lymph nodes in diagnosis of lymphatic circulation disorders with contrast magnetic resonance lymphangiography. J Vasc Surg 49:980–987, 2009.
11. International Society of Lymphology: The diagnosis and treatment of peripheral lymphedema. 2009 Consensus Document of the International Society of Lymphology. Lymphology 42:51–60, 2009.
12. Kerchner K, Fleischer A, Yosipovitch G: Lower extremity lymphedema update: Pathophysiology, diagnosis, and treatment guidelines. J Am Acad Dermatol 59:324–331, 2008.
13. Yasuhara H, Shigematsu H, Muto T: A study of the advantages of elastic stockings for leg lymphedema. Int Angiol 15:272–277, 1996.
14. Badger CM, Peacock JL, Mortimer PS: A randomized, controlled, parallel-group clinical trial comparing multilayer bandaging followed by hosiery versus hosiery alone in the treatment of patients with lymphedema of the limb. Cancer 88:2832–2837, 2000.
15. Franzeck UK, Spiegel I, Fischer M, et al: Combined physical therapy for lymphedema evaluated by fluorescence microlymphography and lymph capillary pressure measurements. J Vasc Res 34:306–311, 1997.
16. Richmand DM, O'Donnell TF, Jr., Zelikovski A: Sequential pneumatic compression for lymphedema. A controlled trial. Arch Surg 120:1116–1119, 1985.
17. Casley-Smith JR, Morgan RG, Piller NB: Treatment of lymphedema of the arms and legs with 5,6-benzo-α-pyrone. N Engl J Med 329:1158–1163, 1993.
18. Loprinzi CL, Kugler JW, Sloan JA, et al: Lack of effect of coumarin in women with lymphedema after treatment for breast cancer. N Engl J Med 340:346–350, 1999.
19. Nakamura K, Rockson SG: Molecular targets for therapeutic lymphangiogenesis in lymphatic dysfunction and disease. Lymphat Res Biol 6:181–189, 2008.
20. Tervala T, Suominen E, Saaristo A: Targeted treatment for lymphedema and lymphatic metastasis. Ann N Y Acad Sci 1131:215–224, 2008.
21. Campisi C, Boccardo F: Lymphedema and microsurgery. Microsurgery 22:74–80, 2002.
22. Gloviczki P: Principles of surgical treatment of chronic lymphoedema. Int Angiol 18:42–46, 1999.
23. Damstra RJ, Voesten HG, van Schelven WD, et al: Lymphatic venous anastomosis (LVA) for treatment of secondary arm lymphedema. A prospective study of 11 LVA procedures in 10 patients with breast cancer–related lymphedema and a critical review of the literature. Breast Cancer Res Treat 113:199–206, 2009.
24. Nagase T, Gonda K, Inoue K, et al: Treatment of lymphedema with lymphaticovenular anastomoses. Int J Clin Oncol 10:304–310, 2005.
25. Goldsmith HS: Long-term evaluation of omental transposition for chronic lymphedema. Ann Surg 180:847–849, 1974.
26. Hurst PA, Stewart G, Kinmonth JB, et al: Long-term results of the enteromesenteric bridge operation in the treatment of primary lymphoedema. Br J Surg 72:272–274, 1985.
27. Miller TA, Wyatt LE, Rudkin GH: Staged skin and subcutaneous excision for lymphedema: A favorable report of long-term results. Plast Reconstr Surg 102:1486–1498, 1998.
28. Wyatt LEMT: Lymphedema and tumors of the lymphatics. In Moore W, editor: Vascular Surgery, a comprehensive review, Philadelphia, 1998, WB Saunders, pp 829–843.
29. Espinosa-de-Los-Monteros A, Hinojosa CA, Abarca L, et al: Compression therapy and liposuction of lower legs for bilateral hereditary primary lymphedema praecox. J Vasc Surg 49:222–224, 2009.
30. Brorson H, Ohlin K, Olsson G, et al: Controlled compression and liposuction treatment for lower extremity lymphedema. Lymphology 41:52–63, 2008.
31. Dellon AL, Hoopes JE: The Charles procedure for primary lymphedema. Long-term clinical results. Plast Reconstr Surg 60:589–595, 1977.

**32.** Dandapat MC, Mohapatro SK, Mohanty SS: Filarial lymphoedema and elephantiasis of lower limb: A review of 44 cases. Br J Surg 73:451–453, 1986.

**33.** Miller TA: Charles procedure for lymphedema: A warning. Am J Surg 139:290–292, 1980.

**34.** Platis IE, Nwogu CE: Chylothorax. Thorac Surg Clin 16:209–214, 2006.

**35.** Romero S: Nontraumatic chylothorax. Curr Opin Pulm Med 6:287–291, 2000.

**36.** Aalami OO, Allen DB, Organ CH, Jr: Chylous ascites: A collective review. Surgery 128:761–778, 2000.

**37.** Fonkalsrud EW: Congenital malformations of the lymphatic system. Semin Pediatr Surg 3:62–69, 1994.

**38.** Nakazono T, Kudo S, Matsuo Y, et al: Angiosarcoma associated with chronic lymphedema (Stewart-Treves syndrome) of the leg: MR imaging. Skeletal Radiol 29:413–416, 2000.

**39.** Sordillo PP, Chapman R, Hajdu SI, et al: Lymphangiosarcoma. Cancer 48:1674–1679, 1981.

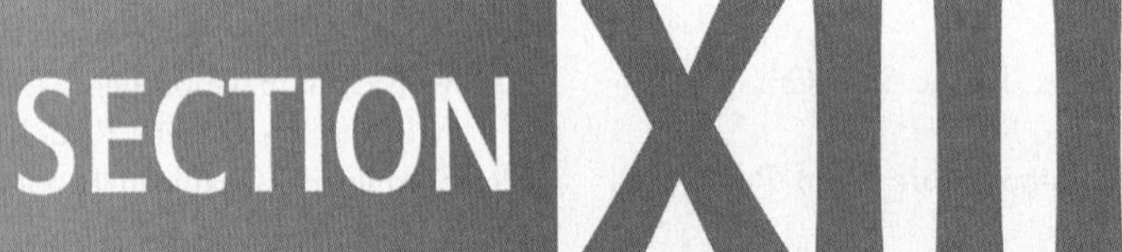


# SPECIALTIES IN GENERAL SURGERY

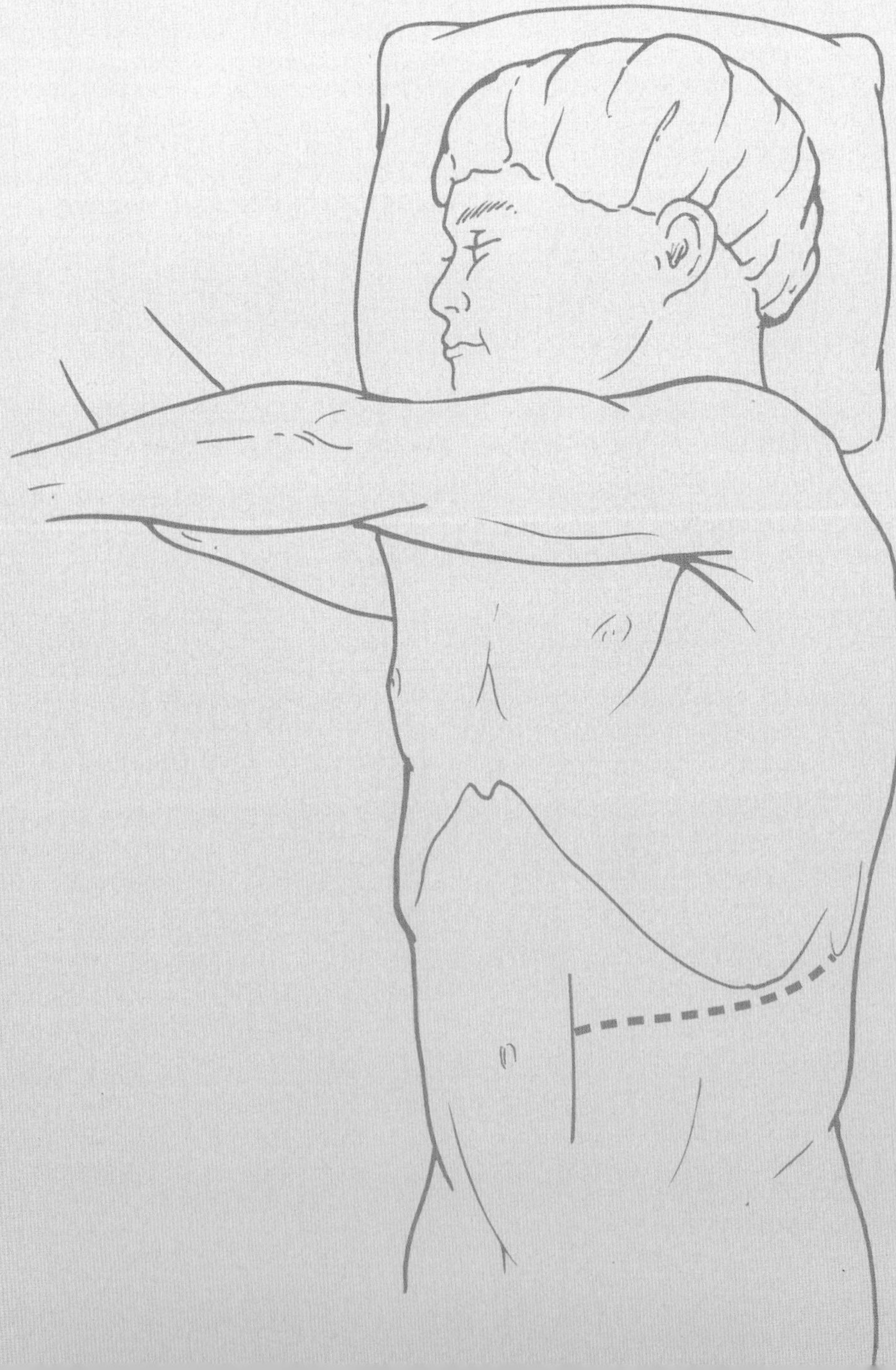

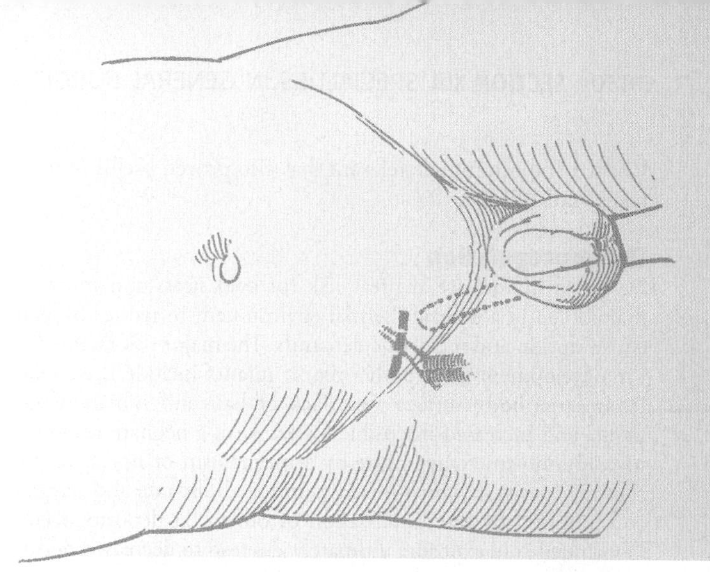

CHAPTER 67

# PEDIATRIC SURGERY

DAI H. CHUNG



Pediatric surgery remains as a true general surgical specialty, providing total care for infants and children of all ages. The range of clinical pathology is broad and not limited to specific anatomic organ systems. Pediatric surgeons are challenged by dealing with a wide spectrum of pathologies involving multiple organ systems from neonates to young adults. Although the pathogenesis of many pediatric surgical conditions remains unknown, there have been recent significant basic science and clinical advances in pediatric surgery, which have resulted in improvement in the management of complex pediatric surgical conditions. This chapter highlights common and unique pediatric surgical conditions.

## NEWBORN PHYSIOLOGY

The newborn infant is physiologically distinct from the adult patient in many respects. The smaller size, differing volume capacities, and functional immaturity of organ systems present unique challenges in the management of surgical conditions.

### Cardiovascular System

In the fetal circulation, arterial blood from the placenta bypasses the lungs through the patent foramen ovale and ductus arteriosus. After first breath, the foramen ovale closes, along with a precipitous drop in pulmonary arterial pressure caused by decreases in pulmonary vascular resistance, thereby promoting pulmonary blood flow. Decreased blood flow along with a higher oxygen content also promote closure of the ductus arteriosus. Many factors can contribute to persistent pulmonary hypertension (PPHN) with right-to-left shunt. Hypoxemia, acidosis, and sepsis all contribute to PPHN. Prematurity is also a significant risk factor for persistent ductus arteriosus. Nonsteroidal anti-inflammatory drugs (NSAIDs), such as indomethacin, have been used to close a patent ductus arteriosus in premature infants pharmacologically. If unsuccessful, surgical ligation may be necessary. An infant heart has a limited capacity to increase the stroke volume and, therefore, cardiac output is largely rate-dependent. Cardiac output is significantly affected by bradycardic episodes. Capillary refill is an ideal clinical indicator of adequate cardiac perfusion. A prolonged capillary refill longer than 1 to 2 seconds may represent significant shunting of blood from the peripheral tissues to the central organs, as may occur with cardiogenic and/or hypovolemic shock.

### Pulmonary System

The lungs are not fully matured at birth and continue to form new terminal bronchioles and alveoli until about 8 years of age. In premature infants, lung immaturity is one of the greatest contributors to morbidity and mortality. Immature lungs have fewer type II pneumocytes and a lower production of surfactant, which is critical for reducing alveolar surface tension and thereby increasing functional residual capacity. Hence, premature infants are at significant risks for alveolar collapse, hyaline membrane formation, and barotrauma. Surfactant is a lipoprotein mixture of phospholipid, protein, and neutral fats. Lecithin, the most predominant phospholipid, can be measured in amniotic fluid, and the lecithin-to-sphingomyelin ratio is used to determine fetal lung maturity. In addition to pulmonary parenchymal issues, the airway of the newborn is small (tracheal diameter = 2.5 to 4 mm) and easily plugged with secretions. The respiratory rate for a normal newborn may range from 40 to 60 breaths/min, with a tidal volume of 6 to 10 mL/kg. Nasal flaring, grunting, intercostal and substernal retractions, and cyanosis constitute symptoms of respiratory distress. Infants are obligate nasal and diaphragmatic breathers and any condition that obstructs the nasal passages (including the nasogastric tube) or interferes with diaphragmatic function may result in severe respiratory compromise. A major contributor to the treatment of premature infants, therefore, has been the ability to provide exogenous surfactant. This has resulted in improved survival and decreased incidence of bronchopulmonary dysplasia, a condition characterized by oxygen dependence, radiologic abnormality, and chronic respiratory symptoms beyond the first 28 days of life. The administration of inhaled nitric oxide, a potent inducer of vascular smooth muscle relaxant, has also proven useful in neonates with PPHN.

### Thermoregulation

Newborn infants are at great risk for cold stress and must be maintained in a neutral thermal environment to reduce oxygen consumption and metabolic demands. The major risk factors for the development of hypothermia in infants include their relatively large body surface area, lack of hair and subcutaneous tissue, and increased insensible losses. Also, a neonate responds to cold ambient temperature by a mechanism of nonshivering thermogenesis, in which increases in metabolic rate and oxygen consumption by the mobilization of brown fat deposits occur. Continued cold exposure ultimately can lead to decreased perfusion and metabolic acidosis. To avoid radiant and evaporative heat loss, the use of overhead radiant heaters and warming lights is a common practice, but a caution for significant insensible water losses should be made. All fluids should be warmed, especially when transfusing cold stored blood products.

### Immunologic Function

Neonates are immunodeficient with reduced levels of immunoglobulins (IgA, IgG, IgM) and of the C3b component of complement. As such, premature infants are at increased risk for severe infection. The evaluation of sepsis in neonates requires an extensive workup of surveillance cultures of blood, urine, and cerebrospinal fluid as well as a complete blood count with platelet count, differential smear, and plain radiography. Sepsis may result from various invasive devices that are essential to the care of premature infants, such as prolonged endotracheal intubation, umbilical catheters, and bladder catheterization. Based on subtle clinical changes (e.g., reduced tolerance of enteral feeding, temperature instability, reduced capillary refill, tachypnea, irritability), implementation of empirical antibiotic therapy targeted at common bacterial pathogens such as group B beta-hemolytic streptococci, methicillin-resistant *Staphylococcus aureus,* and *Escherichia coli* may be lifesaving.

## FLUIDS, ELECTROLYTES, AND NUTRITION

### Fluid Requirements

Fluid and electrolyte therapy in pediatrics requires careful assessment of fluid intake, fluid losses, and electrolyte abnormalities prior to initiating fluid management. It also requires frequent monitoring during the course of therapy to assess the adequacy of treatment. Accurate estimation of IV fluid and electrolytes is critical, especially in small infants with a narrow margin of error. Because of increased insensible water losses through thinner immature skin, fluid requirements for premature infants are substantial. Insensible water losses are directly related to gestational age, ranging from 45 to 60 mL/kg/day for premature infants weighing less than 1500 g to 30 to 35 mL/kg/day for term infants. Other factors, such as radiant heat warmers, phototherapy for hyperbilirubinemia, and respiratory distress, further increase losses. In the first 3 to 5 days of life, there is a physiologic water loss of up to 10% of the body weight of the infant. As such, fluid replacement volumes are less over the first several days of life. These fluid volumes are regarded as estimates and may change according to differing patient factors.

Fluid requirements are calculated according to body weight (Table 67-1). During the first few days of life, the fluid recommendations are conservative; however, most neonates require 100 to 130 mL/kg/day for maintenance fluids by the fourth day of life. Neonates with conditions that are associated with excessive fluid losses (e.g., gastroschisis) can require as much as 1.5 times maintenance volume. The two best indicators of sufficient fluid intake are urine output and osmolarity. The minimum urine output in a newborn and young child is 1 to 2 mL/kg/day. Although adults can concentrate urine in the range of 1200 mOsm/kg, an infant responding to water deprivation is only able to concentrate urine to a maximum of 700 mOsm/kg. Clinically, this indicates that greater fluid intake and urine output are necessary to excrete the solute load presented to the kidney during normal metabolism. In general, the daily requirements for sodium and potassium are 2 to 4 and 1 to 2 mEq/kg, respectively. These requirements are usually met with a solution of 5% dextrose in 0.45% normal saline with 20 mEq KCl/liter at the calculated maintenance rate. Fluid losses from gastric drainage, ostomy output, or diarrhea should also be carefully assessed and replaced with an appropriate solution. Gastric losses should be replaced in equal volumes with 0.45% NS with 20 mEq KCl/liter. Diarrheal, pancreatic, and biliary losses are replaced with isotonic lactated Ringer's solution. Acutely hypovolemic patients requiring rapid volume expansion should be treated with an IV bolus of 10 to 20 mL/kg body weight of whole blood, plasma, or 5% albumin. Transfusions of packed red blood cells are given in increments of 5 to 10 mL/kg.

**Table 67-1 Daily Fluid Requirements for Neonates and Infants**

| WEIGHT | VOLUME |
|---|---|
| Premature infants <2 kg | 140-150 mL/kg/day |
| Infants, 2-10 kg | 100 mL/kg/day for first 10 kg |
| Children, 10-20 kg | 1000 mL + 50 mL/kg/day for weight 10-20 kg |
| Children >20 kg | 1500 mL + 20 mL/kg/day for weight >20 kg |

### Nutrition

#### Total Parenteral Nutrition

Total parenteral nutrition (TPN) is reserved for neonates for whom gastrointestinal (GI) delivery of adequate calories is not feasible for various reasons. Deposition of body fat occurs in the later stages of fetal development, leaving premature infants poorly equipped to deal with periods of starvation as short as 2 to 3 days. Thus, a neonate's need for parenteral nutrition should be addressed early in the hospital stay. The key to prescribing pediatric TPN is that the maintenance IV rate remains constant whereas the concentration of nutrients is gradually increased each day until nutritional goals are met. This is unlike TPN orders for adults, for whom a standard solution is ordered and the rate is gradually adjusted. Surgical infants often become cholestatic during their recovery, usually caused by lengthy TPN therapy; however, other causes should be ruled out. Serum bile acid levels are usually elevated first, then direct bilirubin followed by liver enzyme levels. The best treatment for TPN-associated cholestasis is enteral feeding. A medium-chain triglyceride containing formula is used and, if an infant

**Table 67-2 Average Caloric and Protein Requirement by Age**

| AGE (yr) | CALORIES (kcal/kg/day) | PROTEIN (g/kg/day) |
|---|---|---|
| 0-1 | 90-124 | 2.0-3.5 |
| 1-7 | 75-90 | 2.0-2.5 |
| 7-12 | 60-75 | 2.0 |
| 12-18 | 30-60 | 1.5 |
| >18 | 25-30 | 1.0 |

is on total enteral nutrition, fat-soluble vitamins should be supplemented.

### Caloric Requirements

Energy requirements vary significantly from birth to childhood and also under different clinical conditions (Table 67-2). The parameter that is most indicative of sufficient delivery of calories in neonates is weight gain. Total daily caloric requirements and the expected daily weight gain decrease with age. Neonates have the highest energy requirements necessary to maintain growth. Almost 50% of the energy used in term infants younger than 2 weeks and 60% of energy intake in premature infants weighing less than 1200 g is devoted to growth. A general guideline for enteral caloric requirement for neonate is 120 calories/kg/day to achieve an ideal growth of 25 to 35 g/kg/day of weight gain (≈1% body weight gain/day). Most standard infant formulas, as well as breast milk, contain 20 calories/ounce. Formulas with higher caloric density are available for neonates who are unable to consume sufficient volumes to meet their caloric requirements and/or require fluid restriction. Breast milk or a protein hydrolysate formula (e.g., Pregestimil, Alimentum) should be used when beginning feedings in neonates with compromised gut functions (e.g., necrotizing enterocolitis [NEC]) or short gut caused by massive bowel resection. In general, continuous feedings are initiated for infants with a stressed gut and transition to bolus feedings is made later. Enteral feeding tolerance is carefully monitored by assessing for abdominal girth, gastric residuals, and stool or ostomy output.

### Protein

The average intake of protein comprises approximately 15% of the total daily calories and ranges from 2 to 3.5 g/kg/day in infants. This protein requirement is reduced in half by age 12 and approaches adult requirement levels (1 g/kg/day) by 18 years of age (see Table 67-2). The provision of greater amounts of protein relative to nonprotein calories will result in rising blood urea nitrogen levels. The nonprotein calorie (carbohydrate plus fat calories)-to-protein calorie ratio (when expressed in grams of nitrogen) is therefore not less than 150 : 1. For infants receiving parenteral nutrition, the amount of protein provided is usually begun at 0.5 g/kg/day and advanced in daily increments of 0.5 g/kg/day to the target goal.

### Carbohydrate

Carbohydrates are stored mainly as glycogen in the liver and muscles. Because neonatal liver and muscle masses are proportionately much smaller than those of the adult, neonates are susceptible to hypoglycemia with risks for seizures and neurologic impairment. The minimum glucose infusion rate (GIR) for neonates is 4 to 6 mg/kg/min. This rate needs to be calculated daily for every neonate receiving parenteral nutrition. For TPN, the amount of GIR is increased in daily increments of 2 mg/kg/min to a maximum of 10 to 12 mg/kg/min. Ultimately, the amount of weight gain should dictate the need to continue advancing glucose calories. Furthermore, hyperglycemia from too rapid advancement or underlying sepsis needs to be avoided because it can lead to rapid hyperosmolarity and dehydration.

### Fat

Fat comprises the other major source of nonprotein calories. Linoleic acid, an 18-carbon chain with two double bonds, is considered an essential fatty acid; its deficiency results in dryness, rash, and desquamation of skin. In pediatric patients, fat is provided as a major source of calories to prevent the development of essential fatty acid deficiency. The lipid requirements for growth are significant, and fat is a robust caloric source. Similar to protein, fat infusions are started at 0.5 g/kg/day and advanced up to 2.5 to 3.5 g/kg/day. In infants with unconjugated hyperbilirubinemia, fat is administered with caution because fatty acids may displace bilirubin from albumin. The free unconjugated bilirubin may then cross the blood-brain barrier and can lead to kernicterus, resulting in mental retardation.

## NECK LESIONS

### Cervical Lymphadenopathy

Enlarged lymph nodes is one of the most common pediatric conditions, resulting in frequent referral to a surgeon for biopsy and/or resection. They occur usually along the sternocleidomastoid muscle border, often presenting in clusters. The cause is multifocal but often thought to be infectious. A careful history and physical examination are typically sufficient to determine surgical indications; however, the use of diagnostic ultrasound has significantly increased in recent years. In most healthy children, cervical lymphadenopathy presents as a small, mobile, rubbery, palpable mass in the anterior cervical triangle. However, relatively fixed, nontender, progressively enlarging nodes in the supraclavicular region should raise suspicion for more serious underlying conditions. Other associated symptoms, such as night sweats and a history of weight loss, should also be thoroughly investigated. Chest radiography is often performed as a screening method to detect mediastinal adenopathy. If enlarged anterior mediastinal nodes are seen, a computed tomography (CT) scan of the chest is obtained to assess nodes better and identify potential airway compression. Patients with acute, bilateral cervical lymphadenitis are usually managed nonoperatively because respiratory viral infectious causes (e.g., adenovirus, influenza virus, respiratory syncytial virus) are common. *S. aureus* and group A streptococci are responsible for most cases of acute pyogenic lymphadenitis. When nodes become fluctuant because of a central area of liquefying necrosis, needle aspiration or incision and drainage should be performed.

Cat scratch disease is a self-limiting infectious condition characterized by painful regional lymphadenopathy. *Bartonella henselae,* a gram-negative bacillus, is responsible for most cases. A history of exposure to cats is helpful, but not always present. Indirect immunofluorescent antibody testing has only moderate specificity and, therefore, the use of the polymerase chain reaction assay from a lymph node biopsy is more useful for diagnosis. There is no specific treatment for cat scratch disease because it is usually self-limited. A less common infectious cause for cervical lymphadenitis is nontuberculous mycobacterial infection.[1] In general, the nodes are fluctuant, with a violaceous appearance of the overlying skin. The diagnosis is typically made by positive cultures for nontuberculous acid-fast bacilli, along with a tuberculin skin test. Surgical excision is usually indicated because most nontuberculous mycobacteria are resistant to conventional chemotherapy.

## Cystic Hygroma

Cystic hygromas are multiloculated cystic spaces lined by endothelial cells; they occur as a result of lymphatic malformation. Most cystic hygromas involve the lymphatic jugular sacs and present in the posterior neck region. The other common sites are the axillary, mediastinum, inguinal, and retroperitoneal regions, and approximately 50% of them present at birth. Cystic hygromas usually present as soft cystic masses that distort the surrounding anatomy, including the airway, which can result in acute airway obstruction. Prenatal recognition of a large cystic mass of the neck is associated with a significant risk to the airway, greater association with chromosomal abnormalities, and higher mortality rates. Advanced prenatal imaging modalities allow for careful coordination of surgical intervention at the time of delivery.

Aside from distorting adjacent normal structures, cystic hygromas are prone to infection and hemorrhage within the mass. Imaging studies, such as magnetic resonance imaging (MRI), can play a crucial role in preoperative planning. In general, complete surgical excision is the preferred treatment. However, this may be difficult because of the intimate involvement with surrounding vital structures. Resections are generally tedious, requiring careful isolation and ligation of lymphatic branches. Aggressive blunt and electrocautery dissections can lead to inadequate control of lymphatics, often resulting in recurrence and/or infection caused by accumulation of the lymphatic leak. Radical resection with sacrifice of vital structures is not advocated. Injection of sclerosing agents such as bleomycin or OK-432, derived from *Streptococcus pyogenes*, has been reported to be effective in the nonoperative management of cystic hygromas.[2]

## Thyroglossal Duct Cyst

A thyroglossal duct cyst is a midline neck lesion that originates at the base of the tongue at foramen cecum and descends through the central portion of the hyoid bone. It is one of the most common midline neck lesions presenting in preschool-aged children (Fig. 67-1*A*). Although thyroglossal duct cysts may occur anywhere from the base of the tongue to the thyroid gland, most are found at or just below the hyoid bone. The standard operation for thyroglossal duct cysts has remained unchanged since it was described by Sistrunk in 1928. It involves complete excision of the cyst in continuity with its tract, the central portion of the hyoid bone, and the tissue above the hyoid bone, extending to the base of the tongue (see Fig. 67-1*B*). Failure to remove these tissues will result in a high risk for recurrence because multiple sinuses have been histologically identified in these locations. Embryologically, a thyroid diverticulum develops as a median endodermal thickening at the foramen cecum. As the embryo develops, the thyroid diverticulum descends in the neck and remains attached to the base of tongue by the thyroglossal duct. Also, as the thyroid gland descends to its normal pretracheal position, the ventral cartilages of the second and third branchial arches form the hyoid bone—hence, the intimate anatomic relationship of the thyroglossal duct remnant with the central portion of the hyoid bone. Normally, the thyroglossal duct regresses by the time the thyroid gland reaches its final position. When the elements of the duct persist despite complete thyroid descent, a thyroglossal duct cyst may develop. Failure of normal caudal migration of thyroid gland results in a lingual thyroid, in which no other thyroid tissue is present in the neck. Ultrasound or radionuclide imaging may provide useful information to identify the presence of a normal thyroid gland within the neck.

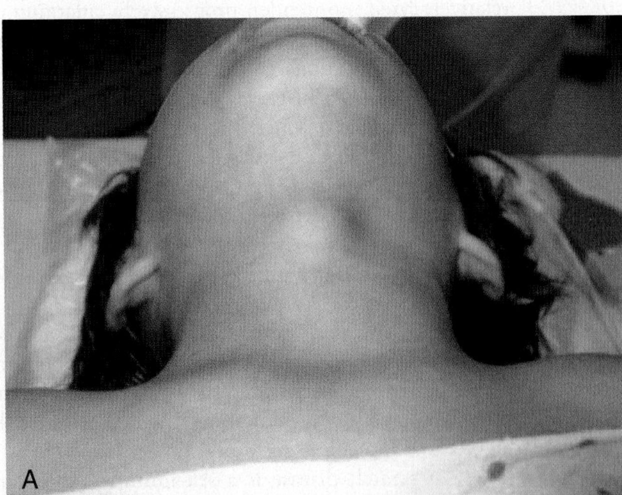


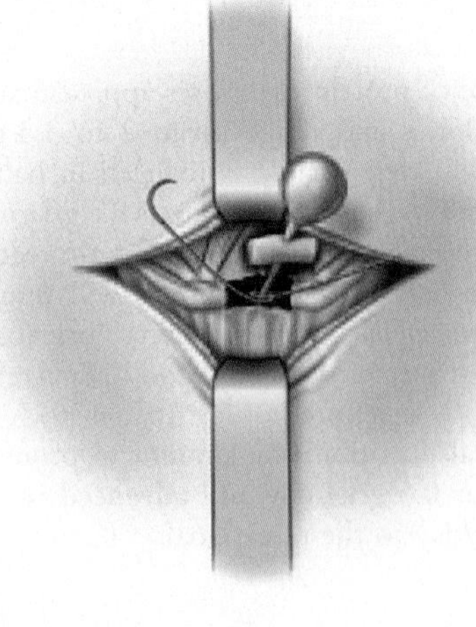


**FIGURE 67-1** **A,** Thyroglossal duct cyst presents as a midline neck mass. **B,** Sistrunk procedure consists of excision of the thyroglossal duct cyst up to its origin at the foramen cecum, including the central portion of hyoid bone. (From Josephs MD: Thyroglossal duct cyst. In Chung DH, Chen MK [eds]: Atlas of pediatric surgical techniques, Philadelphia, 2010, Elsevier Saunders, pp 28–33.)

## Branchial Cleft Remnants

The branchial cleft remnants typically present as a lateral neck mass on a toddler. The structures of the head and neck are derived from six pairs of branchial arches, their intervening clefts, and pouches. Congenital cysts, sinuses, or fistulas result from failure of these structures to regress, persisting in an aberrant location. The location of these remnants generally dictates their embryologic origin and guides the subsequent operative approach. Failure to understand the embryology may result in incomplete resection or injury to adjacent structures. All branchial remnants are present at the time of birth; however, they are often not recognized until later in life. These lesions may present as sinuses, fistulas, or cartilaginous rests in infants. However, they occur more commonly as cysts in older children and adolescents. The clinical presentation may range from a continuous mucoid drainage from a fistula or sinus to the development of a cystic mass that may become infected. Branchial remnants may also be palpable as cartilaginous lumps or cords corresponding with a fistulous tract. Dermal pits or skin tags may also be evident.

First branchial remnants are typically located in the front or back of the ear or in the upper neck near the mandible. Fistulas typically course through the parotid gland, deep or through branches of the facial nerve, and end in the external auditory canal. Remnants from the second branchial cleft are the most common. The external ostium of these remnants is located along the anterior border of the sternocleidomastoid muscle, usually in the vicinity of the upper half to lower third of the muscle. The course of the fistula must be anticipated preoperatively because stepladder counterincisions are often necessary to excise the fistula completely. Typically, the fistula penetrates the platysma, ascends along the carotid sheath to the level of the hyoid bone, and turns medially to extend between the carotid artery bifurcation. The fistula then courses behind the posterior belly of the digastric and stylohyoid muscles to end in the tonsillar fossa. Third branchial cleft remnants usually do not have associated sinuses or fistulas and are located in the suprasternal notch or clavicular region. These most often contain cartilage and present clinically as a firm mass or subcutaneous abscess.

## Torticollis

Torticollis is a state of abnormal muscle tone in the neck, resulting in the head to twist and turn to one side. It may be congenital or acquired and can occur at any age. In infants with congenital torticollis, the head is typically tilted toward the side of the affected muscle and rotated in the opposite direction. Although the true cause is unknown, birth trauma is most frequently considered. Congenital torticollis presents within a few weeks after birth as an isolated condition. However, acquired torticollis may be associated with a range of conditions, including acute myositis, brainstem tumors, atlantoaxial subluxation, and infectious causes, such as retropharyngeal abscess, cervical adenitis, or tonsillitis. The diagnosis is typically based solely on the clinical history and examination findings. Treatment of congenital torticollis is largely nonoperative, with passive range-of-motion stretching of the affected muscle for several months. Surgical resection or division of the involved muscle is rarely indicated.

# EXTRACORPOREAL LIFE SUPPORT

Extracorporeal life support (ECLS) is a form of cardiopulmonary bypass that provides temporary support for the critically ill patient with acute refractory respiratory and/or cardiac failure. In general, ECLS delivers sufficient gas exchange and maintains circulatory support, thus allowing for physiologic recovery. The largest experience with ECLS has been with respiratory failure in newborns; however, it is applicable for various clinical conditions resulting in respiratory and/or cardiovascular failure in pediatric and adult patients. Since its first reported neonatal case in 1976, the use of ECLS has now become the standard therapy option for refractory neonatal respiratory failure unresponsive to maximum conventional medical treatment. There are over 170 centers around the world contributing to the Extracorporeal Life Support Organization database.

## Indications

The major indications for neonatal ECLS include meconium aspiration, respiratory distress syndrome, PPHN, sepsis, and congenital diaphragmatic hernia (CDH). Neonates with complex congenital cardiac defects may be supported with ECLS perioperatively. Meconium aspiration is the most common indication for neonatal ECLS and is associated with the highest survival rate (>90%). Selection criteria for the initiation of neonatal ECLS vary slightly among institutions. Generally, an infant must have at least an 80% predicted mortality with continued conventional medical treatment to justify ECLS therapy. Two guidelines have been historically used as a means to predict survival without ECLS. The alveolar-arterial difference in the partial pressure of oxygen ($PAO_2 - PaO_2$ [also known as $AaDO_2$]) is calculated as follows:

$$AaDO_2 = (\text{atmospheric pressure} - 47) - (PaO_2 + PaCO_2)$$

$AaDO_2$ more than 610 for longer than 8 to 12 hours, and $AaDO_2$ more than 620 for 6 hours associated with extensive barotrauma and severe hypotension requiring inotropic support, are considered to be criteria for ECLS. The oxygen index (OI) is calculated as the fraction of inspired oxygen (usually 1.0) multiplied by the mean airway pressure ×100 divided by $PaO_2$. An 80% mortality is noted with an OI more than 40. Exclusion criteria include gestational age less than 34 weeks, birth weight less than 2 kg, and a nonreversible pulmonary pathology. Additional exclusion criteria include the presence of cyanotic congenital heart disease or another major congenital anomaly that precludes survival, intractable coagulopathy or hemorrhage, sonographic evidence of a significant intracranial hemorrhage (higher than a grade I intraventricular hemorrhage), and more than 10 to 14 days of high-pressure mechanical ventilatory support. Before the initiation of ECLS, all infants must undergo echocardiography to rule out congenital heart disease and cranial ultrasound to exclude the presence of significant intracranial hemorrhage.

## Physiologic Considerations

The basic concept of ECLS is to drain venous blood, remove carbon dioxide, add oxygen through the artificial membrane lung, and then return warmed blood back into the circulation. Venoarterial bypass provides cardiac and respiratory support, whereas venovenous bypass provides only respiratory support. Venoarterial bypass is used most commonly; the right internal jugular vein and common carotid artery are typically chosen for cannulation because of their vessel sizes, accessibility, and adequate collateral circulation. The ECLS circuit is composed of a silicone rubber bladder, which collapses when venous return is

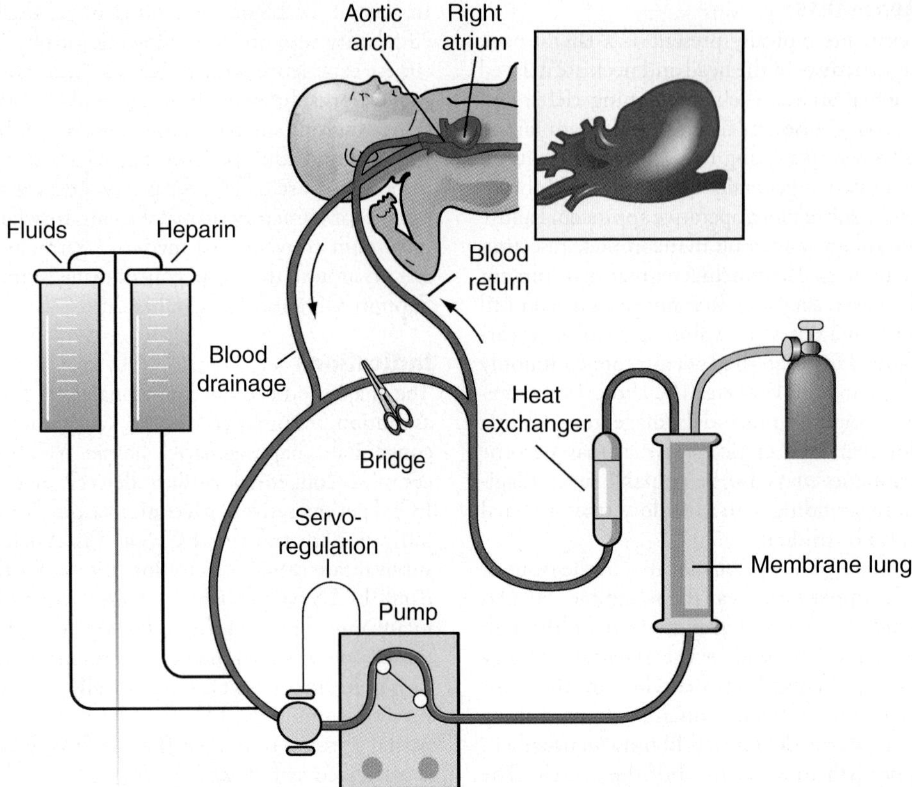


**FIGURE 67-2** Extracorporeal life support circuit. A venoarterial circuit is shown here . (From Shanley CJ, Bartlett RH: Extracorporeal life support: Techniques, indications, and results. In Cameron JL [ed]: Current surgical therapy, ed 4, St. Louis, 1992, Mosby Year Book, pp 1062–1066.)

diminished, roller pump, membrane oxygenator, heat exchanger, tubing, and connectors. Venous blood from the right atrium drains through the venous cannula to the bladder and is pumped to the membrane oxygenator, where carbon dioxide is removed and oxygen is added (Fig. 67-2). The oxygenated blood then passes through the heat exchanger and is returned to the patient through the arterial cannula. The patient is systemically anticoagulated to prevent clotting of the ECLS circuit; hence, patients are at risk for bleeding complications. As such, hematocrit values, platelet counts, and fibrinogen levels must be closely monitored and maintained at acceptable ranges. Cranial ultrasound is performed for the first few days of ECLS to monitor for hemorrhage and then done on an as-needed basis. Extracorporeal flow is gradually weaned as native cardiac or pulmonary function improves. Indicators of lung recovery include an increasing $PaO_2$, improved lung compliance, and clearing of the chest x-ray. Once the extracorporeal flow rate reaches minimal levels, the patient is trialed off bypass by temporarily clamping cannulas. If tolerated, the patient is taken off ECLS support on moderate conventional ventilatory settings.

### Complications

Bleeding is the most common complication of ECLS and may result in medical (e.g., intracranial) or surgical (e.g., neck cannulation site, intrathoracic, GI) problems. Birth weight and gestational age are the most significant correlates of intracranial hemorrhage on ECLS; infants weighing less than 2.2 kg and younger than 35 weeks gestational age are at highest risk. Other significant complications associated with ECLS include seizures, neurologic impairment, renal failure requiring hemofiltration or hemodialysis, hypertension, infection, and mechanical malfunction (e.g., failure of the membrane oxygenator, pump, and heat exchanger). Other potential complications include mechanical failure of the circuit.

## CONGENITAL DIAPHRAGMATIC HERNIA

Despite early prenatal detection of CDH, it remains one of the most challenging conditions to manage in pediatric surgery. CDH is a relatively common cause of neonatal respiratory distress, with an overall incidence of 1 in 2000 to 5000 live births. Most CDH defects occur on the left side (80%); bilateral condition is extremely rare. A hernia sac is present 20% of the time. Despite recent innovative treatment strategies, such as fetal hernia repair or tracheal occlusion, extracorporeal membrane oxygenation, inhaled nitric oxide, partial liquid ventilation, and respiratory management protocol of permissive hypercapnea, the overall survival rates have not changed significantly and remain in the range of 70% to 90%. Accurate determination of true survival is complicated by the fact that many infants with CDH are stillborn, and many reports tend to exclude infants with complex associated anomalies from survival calculations.

### Pathogenesis

The specific cause for CDH is unknown, but it is thought to result from failure of closure of the pleuroperitoneal canal in the developing fetus. Normally, the pleuroperitoneal cavities become separated by the developing membrane in weeks 8 to10 of gestation. When this process fails, closure of the pleuroperitoneal canal is incomplete and a posterolateral diaphragmatic defect results. The posterolateral location of this hernia is known as *Bochdalek's hernia*; it is distinguished from a CDH of the anteromedial location known as *Morgagni's hernia*. As a result of the defect, abdominal contents herniate through the resultant defect in the posterolateral aspect and compress the ipsilateral developing lung. These lungs have smaller bronchi, with less bronchial branching and less alveolar surface area than lungs in normal infants. The ipsilateral lung is affected more severely; however, lungs from both sides are affected by pulmonary hypoplasia. In addition to the abnormal airway development, the pulmonary vasculature is also significantly affected by increased thickness of arteriolar smooth muscle. Also, arteriolar vasculature is extremely sensitive to the multiple local and systemic vasoactive factors. Hence, the severity of pulmonary hypoplasia and pulmonary hypertension significantly affect the overall morbidity and mortality in CDH infants.

## Clinical Presentation

The most frequent clinical presentation of CDH is respiratory distress caused by severe hypoxemia. The initial symptoms and signs include grunting respiration, chest retractions, dyspnea, and cyanosis with scaphoid abdomen. Breath sounds are decreased and bowel sounds may be heard in the chest. The shifting of heart sounds to the right (for left CDH) is common. A significant differential between preductal and postductal pulse oximetry indicates the presence of right-to-left shunting as a result of PPHN. The diagnosis of CDH is frequently made prenatally as early as 15 weeks of gestation by ultrasonography during an otherwise unremarkable pregnancy. Infants who have a late onset of CDH (after 25 weeks of gestation) have been reported to have better overall survival rates. The herniation of the stomach and liver, along with polyhydramnios, has all been associated with poor outcome. The presence of associated anomalies also significantly decreases the overall survival. With prenatal diagnosis, delivery of a fetus with CDH should take place at an institution capable of providing advanced neonatal critical care, including extracorporeal membrane oxygenation (ECMO) support.

## Diagnosis

At birth, CDH infants demonstrate symptoms of respiratory distress with a classic chest radiographic appearance of multiple bowel loops in the thoracic cavity, along with mediastinal shift (Fig. 67-3). An orogastric tube may appear to coil in the chest. The differential diagnosis of CDH includes congenital cystic adenomatoid malformation, bronchogenic cyst, diaphragmatic eventration, and cystic teratoma. In Morgagni's hernia, the diagnosis is often delayed until childhood because most infants are asymptomatic. Chest radiographs may reveal an air-fluid level immediately posterior to the sternum. Usually, the infant does well for several hours after delivery during the so-called *honeymoon period* and then begins to demonstrate worsening respiratory function. Therapeutic interventions are targeted to reduce PPHN. In approximately 10% to 20% of cases, CDH is diagnosed beyond the first 24 hours of life, at which time infants present with various symptoms of feeding difficulties, respiratory distress, and pneumonia.

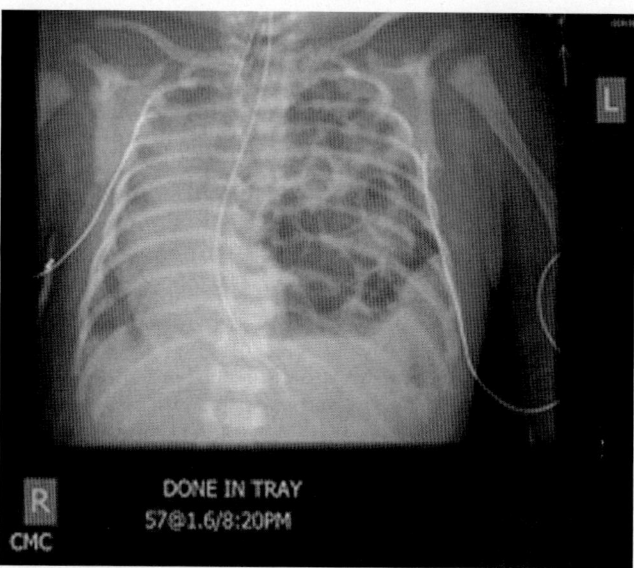


**FIGURE 67-3** Congenital diaphragmatic hernia. Multiple gas-filled bowel loops are located in the left hemithorax and the mediastinum is shifted to the right.

## Treatment

The open fetal surgery for CDH has failed to show significant overall survival advantage. Occlusion of the fetal trachea, resulting in accumulation of lung fluid to stimulate lung growth, has garnered significant recent interest. A laparoscopic approach has also been used to apply external clips or place balloons and sponges to occlude the fetal trachea. However, the fetal occlusion technique has not significantly influenced the overall survival rate with CDH, and fetal interventions for CDH remain limited to a few centers. The postnatal management of CDH is directed toward stabilization of the cardiorespiratory status while minimizing iatrogenic injury from therapeutic interventions. Immediate securing of the airway with endotracheal intubation is critical. Excessive mean airway pressure ventilation can result in pneumothorax and compromised venous blood return to the heart. An orogastric tube is placed to prevent gastric distention, which may worsen the lung compression, mediastinal shift, and ability to ventilate. The use of tolazoline, a nonselective $\alpha$-adrenergic blocking agent, as a pharmacologic pulmonary vasodilator has not produced clinically significant results. Inhaled nitric oxide is used by most centers as a pulmonary vasodilator. Surfactant administration and high-frequency ventilation have also resulted in variable overall outcome for CDH infants. However, the *recent use* of gentle ventilation with permissive hypercapnia and stable hypoxemia has resulted in a significantly higher survival rate (≈75%) for CDH infants.

### Surgical Repair

It has been well established that CDH repair should be delayed for 2 to 4 days until cardiopulmonary stabilization has occurred. The preferred operative approach for a posterolateral CDH is through a subcostal abdominal incision. The viscera are reduced into the abdominal cavity and the posterolateral defect in the diaphragm is closed using interrupted nonabsorbable sutures. When present (10% to 15% of cases), a hernia sac should be excised. Typically, the hernia defect is large, with only a small anteromedial leaflet of diaphragmatic tissue present. A number of reconstructive techniques and materials are available for the repair of large hernia defects. The surgical technique of abdominal or thoracic muscle flaps can be considered, but the use of prosthetic material (e.g., Gore-Tex, W.L. Gore, Elkton, Md) has become more widespread. The advantages of a prosthetic patch are shorter operative time and a tension-free repair. However, the major potential problems with prosthetic patches are the risks of infection and recurrence of the hernia. Recently, the use of regenerative extracellular matrix biomaterials has garnered significant interest as an ideal biodegradable patch to repair diaphragmatic hernia defects. At times, the abdominal cavity may be too small to accommodate the reduced viscera from the thoracic cavity. A temporary abdominal silo may be considered, but allowing for an incisional hernia with skin-only closure until the definitive fascia closure can be performed is an alternative surgical option. The timing of CDH repair relative to ECLS remains controversial. A recent CDH study group report has suggested that CDH repair after ECLS therapy is associated with improved survival when compared with repair while on ECLS.[3]

### Outcomes

Beyond the immediate postoperative period, many infants with CDH experience significant morbidity because of PPHN and respiratory dysfunction. Many children who survive aggressive management of severe respiratory failure manifest neurologic problems, such as abnormalities in motor and cognitive skills, developmental delay, seizures, and hearing loss. Other problems include a high incidence of gastroesophageal reflux (GER) and foregut dysmotility. Other morbidities associated with CDH survivors include chronic lung disease, scoliosis, growth retardation, and pectus excavatum deformities.

## BRONCHOPULMONARY MALFORMATIONS

Bronchopulmonary malformations are congenital abnormalities of the airway, such as bronchogenic cysts, intralobar and extralobar sequestrations (ELSs), congenital pulmonary airway malformations (CPAMs), and congenital lobar emphysema (CLE). Their natural histories vary widely. In the perinatal period, these lung lesions can result in pleural effusions, polyhydramnios, hydrops, and pulmonary hypoplasia with subsequent respiratory distress and airway obstruction. If severe enough, fetal demise can ensue. With increasing importance placed on prenatal care, many of these lesions are being diagnosed prenatally with serial imaging. Fetal surgery has been pursued when fetal viability is at risk. Although these congenital abnormalities are often asymptomatic and may even spontaneously regress, there is concern that these anomalies may cause recurrent infections and exhibit long-term malignant potential.

### Bronchogenic Cyst

Bronchogenic cyst is the most common cystic lesion of the mediastinum. The cyst wall consists of fibroelastic tissue, smooth muscle, and cartilage, whereas the cyst itself is lined with respiratory tract epithelia (ciliated columnar cells). It can also contain mucus-producing cuboidal cells, which contribute to enlargement of the cyst with mucus. They may occur anywhere along the tracheobronchial tree but are usually found around the carina and right hilum. Less frequently, they present in the neck, lung, pleura, pericardium, or below the diaphragm. When the cysts are large, they can compress surrounding vital structures, including the airway. Infants are particularly at risk because of their narrow, easily compressible airway. Bronchogenic cysts can also cause dysphagia, pneumothorax, cough, and hemoptysis or become infected, which is how older children present. Often picked up on postnatal chest x-ray, the diagnosis is confirmed by CT as a spherical nonenhancing mass. It is fluid- or mucus-filled, although an air-fluid level is apparent if the cyst communicates with the airway. Cysts within the pulmonary parenchyma typically communicate with a bronchus, whereas those in the mediastinum usually do not. Bronchogenic cysts are routinely resected even if asymptomatic, although recently there have been debates on observation alone for this condition.[4] Rare cases of malignant transformation have been reported. Resection is performed by video-assisted thoracic surgery (VATS) or thoracotomy.

### Congenital Pulmonary Airway Malformation

CPAMs have been controversially described as hamartomatous lesions in which a multicystic mass replaces normal lung tissue. They are connected to the tracheobronchial tree and its blood supply is pulmonary. Although they are usually unilateral and unilobar, they can present in the immediate perinatal period with life-threatening respiratory distress. If asymptomatic during this time, infants and older children can go on to present with fevers, persistent cough, and recurrent pneumonia. CPAMs can undergo malignant transformation; rhabdomyosarcoma has been reported. They are classified based on their appearance on imaging and confirmation is made by pathologic examination. According to the Stocker classification, type I lesions account for almost 75% of all cases and consist of a small number of large, 2- to 10-cm cysts that can compress normal lung parenchyma. Type II lesions have numerous cysts, usually measuring less than 1 cm in diameter. Type III lesions are rare and appear to be only a few millimeters in diameter.[5] However, they are associated with mediastinal shift, hydrops, and a poor prognosis.

Ultrasound and, less commonly, MRI, are used to locate the lesion, characterize its appearance, determine its blood supply and venous drainage, and evaluate whether there is any displacement of other thoracic structures. Also, when there is any uncertainty, prenatal MRI has been used to differentiate CPAM from other congenital thoracic abnormalities. Postnatally, a chest radiograph is usually diagnostic, revealing a mass with a possible mediastinal shift and air-fluid levels, but a chest CT is frequently obtained for confirmation. When fetal distress occurs in utero, options include fetal thoracotomy and thoracoamniotic shunting (if the fetus is <32 weeks). Most fetuses with a prenatally diagnosed CPAM experience partial regression in the third trimester and can be treated with expectant management. They can then undergo postnatal resection at 5 to 8 weeks of life.[4] Postnatal management of the symptomatic patient necessitates resection via a thoracotomy or VATS. The treatment of asymptomatic patients is more controversial but it is generally agreed that they should be resected, given the risk of infection and malignancy.

### Pulmonary Sequestration

Bronchopulmonary sequestrations (BPSs) are nonfunctional nests of microcystic pulmonary tissue that have no connection to the tracheobronchial tree but are fed by an aberrant systemic artery. There are two types, intralobar (IL) and extralobar (EL);

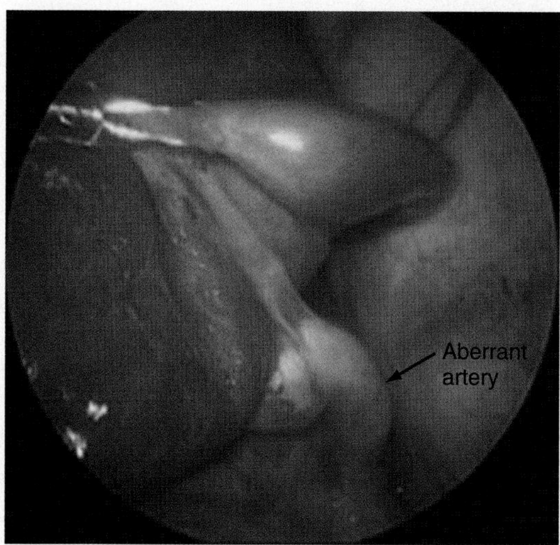


**FIGURE 67-4** Anomalous arterial vascular pedicle to extralobar pulmonary sequestration. The arterial branch comes directly off the thoracic aorta.

the former is contained within normal lung parenchyma and the latter is separate and encased by its own pleura.[4] ELSs occur predominantly in males and, in 40% of cases, other congenital anomalies, such as posterolateral diaphragmatic hernia, pectus excavatum and carinatum, and enteric duplication cysts, can be found.

Lacking a communication to the airway, sequestrations do not form enlarged cysts or cause spontaneous pneumothoraces. They can, however, infarct, become infected, and cause hemoptysis. It has been reported that ELSs can undergo torsion as well. Because of their aberrant systemic vascular supply (Fig. 67-4), BPSs can result in significant left-to-right shunting in infants, who are then susceptible to high-output cardiac failure.[6] For an initial evaluation, Doppler ultrasound may reveal a systemic arterial supply from the infradiaphragmatic or thoracic aorta. The lesion itself may appear solid, but can also be cystic. CT or MRI can aid in further defining the vascular anatomy. Accounting for 75% of all BPSs, intralobar sequestrations (ILSs) are found within the medial or posterior segments of the lower lobes, more on the left side. Most ELSs are found posteromedially in the left lower chest but can occur within or below the diaphragm. Air within an ILS usually signifies infection, whereas the same finding in an ELS suggests the presence of a fistulous connection with the esophagus.[4]

If a BPS is identified on prenatal ultrasound, the fetus is followed with serial ultrasound, looking for mass enlargement and the development of complications such as hydrops, pleural effusion, or polyhydramnios.[6] BPS has been reported to spontaneously regress. In fact, it is estimated that 68% of BPSs undergo spontaneous regression before birth as they become isodense with the surrounding lung. The involution may occur as the lesion outgrows its blood supply. Because of the risk for infection and bleeding, ILSs are usually resected by segmentectomy or lobectomy. ELSs are usually asymptomatic and, because there is generally no tracheobronchial communication, the risk of infection is low. As such, many of these lesions can be observed.

### Congenital Lobar Emphysema

CLE describes a progressively distended, hyperlucent lobe caused by abnormal bronchopulmonary development. Air trapping in the emphysematous lobes occurs with intrinsic or extrinsic obstruction, which includes endobronchial obstruction from mucosal proliferation and extrinsic compression from vascular anomalies. In over 90% of cases, it involves the left upper or right middle lobe. CLE is rarely diagnosed prenatally, but its prevalence is 1 in every 20,000 to 30,000 deliveries.[4] It tends to present in the first few days of life and as late as 6 months after birth. On ultrasound, CLE appears as an echogenic homogenous lung mass. When CLE is discovered in an asymptomatic patient, observation is recommended because these lesions have a tendency to regress. A chest radiograph is customarily diagnostic because it reveals overdistention of the involved lobe. Importantly, the lucency should not be mistaken for a pneumothorax, and positive-pressure ventilation should be used with caution because of the propensity of these patients to undergo auto-PEEP (positive end-expiratory pressure; auto-PEEP is defined as the end-expiratory intrapulmonary pressure that develops as a result of dynamic airflow resistance during mechanical ventilation). When the CLE progresses to the point that it causes mediastinal shift and worsening symptoms, an open thoracotomy with lobectomy is indicated.

## ALIMENTARY TRACT

### Esophageal Atresia and Tracheoesophageal Fistula

Esophageal atresia is a congenital condition of esophageal discontinuity that results in proximal esophageal obstruction. A tracheoesophageal fistula (TEF) is an abnormal fistula communication between the esophagus and trachea. Esophageal atresia and TEF can occur alone or in combination. The incidence of this anomaly is 1 in 1500 to 3000 live births, with a slight male predominance. Approximately one third of infants with esophageal atresia or TEF have a low birth weight, and 60% to 70% have associated anomalies. During the fourth week of gestation, the esophagotracheal diverticulum of the foregut fails to divide completely to form the esophagus and trachea. In 10% of patients, there is a nonrandom, nonhereditary association of anomalies referred to by the acronym VATER (***v***ertebral, ***a***norectal, ***t***racheal, ***e***sophageal, ***r***enal or ***r***adial limb); an alternative acronym is VACTERL (***v***ertebral, ***a***norectal, ***c***ardiac, ***t***racheal, ***e***sophageal, ***r***enal, and ***l***imb). Five anatomic variants of esophageal atresia are depicted in Figure 67-5. In the most common type (C lesion) of esophageal atresia with TEF, the proximal blind pouch ends approximately the distance of one to two vertebral bodies from the distal TEF. The distal TEF is typically located 1 cm above the carina in the membranous portion of the trachea.

#### Clinical Presentation and Diagnosis

The diagnosis of esophageal atresia is considered in an infant with excessive salivation along with coughing or choking during the first oral feeding. A maternal history of polyhydramnios is often present, more often in isolated proximal atresia (86%). In an infant with esophageal atresia and TEF, acute gastric distention may occur as a result of air entering the distal esophagus and stomach with each inspired breath. Reflux of gastric contents into the distal esophagus will traverse the TEF and spill

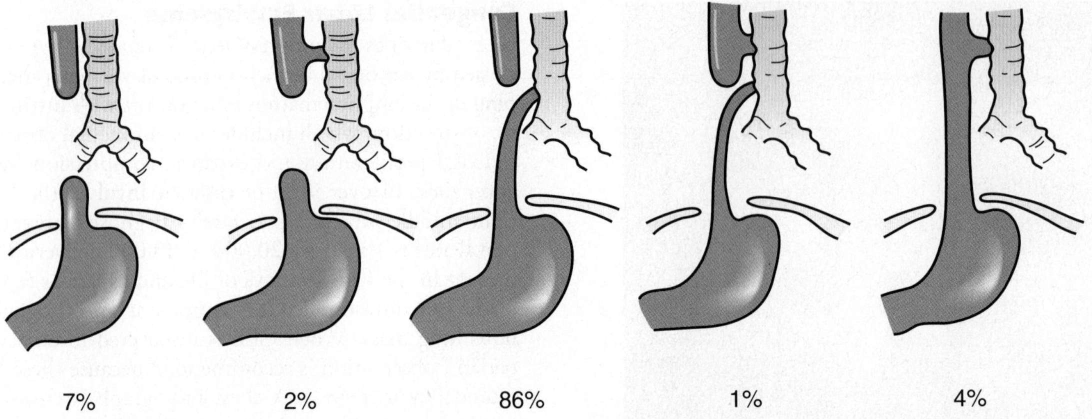


**FIGURE 67-5** Anatomic variants and incidence of esophageal atresia with tracheoesophageal fistula.

into the trachea, resulting in cough, tachypnea, apnea, and/or cyanosis. The presentation of isolated TEF without esophageal atresia may be more subtle, often beyond the newborn period. In general, these infants have choking and coughing associated with oral feeding. The inability to pass a nasogastric tube into the stomach of the neonate is a cardinal feature for the diagnosis of esophageal atresia. If gas is present in the GI tract below the diaphragm, an associated TEF is confirmed (Fig. 67-6*A*). Conversely, the inability to pass a nasogastric tube in an infant with absent radiographic evidence of GI gas is almost diagnostic of an isolated esophageal atresia. The use of isotonic contrast by mouth to demonstrate the presence and/or level of the proximal esophageal atresia is strongly discouraged because of risk for aspiration. The diagnostic evaluation includes screening for other associated anomalies. Echocardiography and renal ultrasound are performed to evaluate for congenital heart defects (including aortic arch anomaly) and genitourinary malformations.

## Treatment

**Preoperative Management** Initial treatment includes decompression of the proximal esophageal pouch with a sump tube (e.g., Replogle tube) placed on continuous suction. The infant is positioned in an upright prone position to minimize GER and prevent aspiration. Broad-spectrum IV antibiotic coverage should be started empirically. Routine endotracheal intubation is avoided because positive-pressure ventilation may be inadequate to inflate the lungs because air is directed into the TEF through the path of least resistance. Ventilation may be compounded further by the resultant gastric distention. Gastrostomy to decompress the distended stomach should be avoided because it may abruptly worsen the ability to ventilate the patient. In these circumstances, manipulation of the endotracheal tube to be positioned distal to the TEF (e.g., right mainstem intubation) may minimize the leak and permit adequate ventilation. Furthermore, placement of an occlusive balloon catheter (Fogarty) into the fistula through a bronchoscope may be useful, but this maneuver can be risky. As a last resort, emergent thoracotomy with ligation of the fistula alone may be required. A preoperative chest radiograph and echocardiogram provide sufficient information to determine the side of the aortic arch. A right thoracotomy is performed for the operative repair in patients with a normal left-sided aortic arch. However, for infants with a right-sided arch, a left thoracotomy would be preferred. A higher incidence of aortic arch anomalies (e.g., vascular rings) and postoperative complications has been reported with right-sided aortic arch.[7]

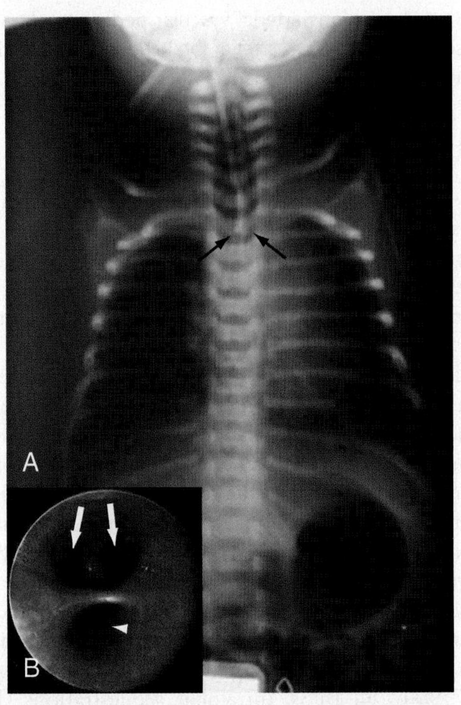


**FIGURE 67-6 A,** Plain chest radiograph of infant with proximal esophageal atresia with distal TEF. The distal tip of the orogastric tube is noted, with a surrounding gas-filled proximal esophagus *(arrows)*. The TEF is also indicated by the presence of gastric air. **B,** Rigid bronchoscopy inspection of distal tracheoesophageal fistula. The luminal size of the fistula *(arrowhead)* is equal to that of either main bronchus *(arrows)*.

**Surgical Management** The typical surgical approach for the most common esophageal atresia with TEF involves an open thoracotomy, with an extrapleural approach through the fourth intercostal space. Bronchoscopy is routinely performed to determine the relative site of the fistula and exclude the presence of a second

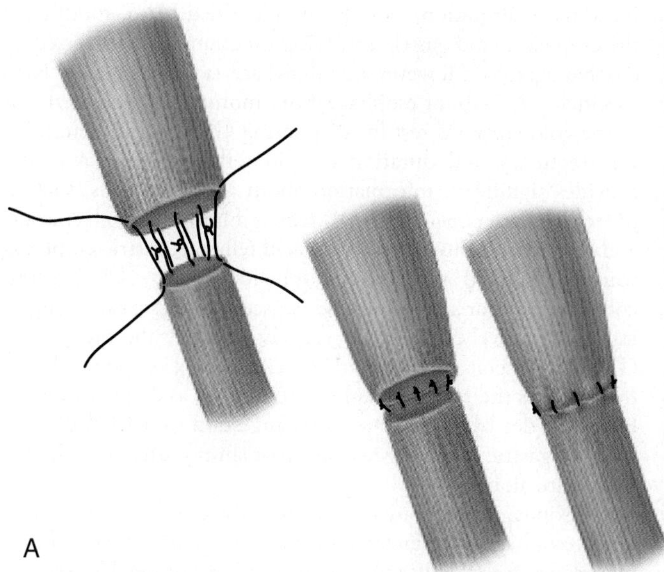


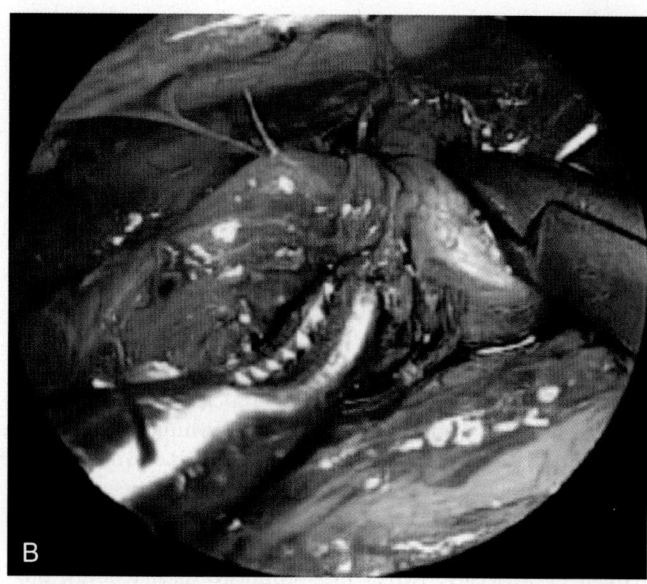


**FIGURE 67-7 A,** A single-layer end-to-end anastomosis is performed using nonabsorbable sutures. Two corner stitches are placed and a back row anastomosis is completed first. Just prior to completing the anterior row of the anastomosis, a nasogastric tube is placed across it. **B,** Thoracoscopic esophageal anastomosis. (**A** from Ricketts R: Esophageal atresia with tracheoesophageal fistula. In Chung DH, Chen MK [eds]: Atlas of pediatric surgical techniques, Philadelphia, 2010, Elsevier Saunders, pp 44–53; **B** from Wulkan ML: Thoracoscopic repair of esophageal atresia with tracheoesophageal fistula. In Chung DH, Chen MK [eds]: Atlas of pediatric surgical techniques, Philadelphia, 2010, Elsevier Saunders, pp 59–65.)

fistula (see Fig. 67-6*B*). After extrapleural dissection to expose the posterior mediastinum, the azygos vein is divided to reveal the underlying TEF. The TEF is dissected circumferentially and its attachment to the membranous portion of trachea is taken down. The tracheal opening is approximated using interrupted nonabsorbable sutures. The proximal esophageal pouch is then mobilized as high as possible to afford a tension-free esophageal anastomosis. The blood supply to the upper esophageal pouch is generally robust and is based on arteries derived from the thyrocervical trunk. However, the blood supply to the lower esophagus is more tenuous and segmental, originating from intercostal vessels. As such, significant mobilization of the lower esophagus is avoided to prevent ischemia at the esophageal anastomosis. The anastomosis is performed using a single- or double-layer technique (Fig. 67-7*A*). The rates of anastomotic leak are slightly higher with the single-layer anastomosis, whereas the rates of esophageal stricture are higher with the double-layer technique.

In case of a long gap between the two ends of the esophagus, there are several options. The first option is to suture the divided end of the distal esophagus to the prevertebral fascia, mark its location with a metal clip, and close the thoracotomy. Over a 2- to 3-month period, the proximal esophageal pouch may grow so that a subsequent primary esophageal anastomosis may be possible. Second, a circular or spiral esophagomyotomy of the upper pouch may be performed to gain esophageal length and facilitate a primary anastomosis. Another technique involves the placement of traction sutures through the proximal and distal ends of the esophagus, brought out through the chest. These sutures are then progressively tightened and a primary esophageal anastomosis is performed after several days.[8] Alternatively, a cervical esophagostomy may be constructed and a formal esophageal replacement performed at a later date.

In patients with pure esophageal atresia, primary anastomosis in the newborn period is not feasible because of a long gap between the two esophageal ends. Initially, a cervical esophagostomy for drainage of oral secretions and gastrostomy for enteral feeding access are performed. An esophageal replacement using the stomach, small intestine, or colon is then carried out at approximately 1 year of age. In some cases, the two ends of the esophagus may spontaneously grow so that a primary anastomosis may be accomplished by 4 months of age. The swallowing of saliva may actually promote elongation of the upper pouch, and an esophagostomy is therefore avoided. In patients with pure TEF, without esophageal atresia, the site of the TEF is usually in the region of the thoracic inlet. In this case, the surgical approach is through a cervical incision. At the time of surgical repair, it is often helpful to perform rigid bronchoscopy and cannulate the TEF with a guidewire to facilitate its identification. Recently, thoracoscopic repair has been described by several pediatric surgical centers (see Fig. 67-7*B*).[9]

The mortality rate of esophageal atresia or TEF is directly related to associated anomalies, particularly cardiac defects and chromosomal abnormalities. In the absence of these factors, survival of more than 95% of patients is expected. Postoperative complications unique to esophageal atresia or TEF include esophageal motility disorders, GER (25% to 50%), anastomotic stricture (15% to 30%), anastomotic leak (10% to 20%), and tracheomalacia (8% to 15%).

## Gastroesophageal Reflux

GER is a common problem in infants and children. During the first year of life, infants normally experience some degree of vomiting, thought to be the result of an incompetent lower esophageal sphincter mechanism. This physiologic vomiting usually resolves spontaneously after 6 to 12 months. Pathologic GER can present with a spectrum of clinical symptoms. Although diagnostic studies can determine the presence of significant reflux, the patient's symptoms remain as the most important factor in determining the surgical treatment of GER. Neurologically impaired children who are in need of enteral feeding access also have to be evaluated for concomitant reflux prior to gastrostomy placement. Today, a laparoscopic approach has become a standard for fundoplication with gastrostomy in pediatric patients.

### Clinical Presentation

Pathologic symptoms of GER vary considerably, depending on the age of the patient and underlying associated medical conditions. Although vomiting is a common symptom, failure to thrive (FTT) as a result of caloric deprivation is one of the most critical complications of persistent GER in infants and children. Aspiration of gastric contents can also result in recurrent bronchitis or pneumonia, presenting initially with a chronic cough or wheezing. Reflux may stimulate vagal reflexes, producing laryngospasm or bronchospasm and leading to an asthma-like clinical picture.[10] The significant airway spasm caused by reflux can result in apnea or choking spells, and may contribute to near-miss sudden infant death syndrome (SIDS). Irritability and crying in infants may also represent pain because of esophagitis induced by chronic reflux. Chronic acid insult to the lower esophagus can progress to the formation of stricture from chronic scarring and produce obstructive symptoms. Although rare in pediatric patients, chronic progressive esophagitis can lead to metaplastic replacement of normal lower esophageal squamous mucosa by columnar epithelium. This condition, known as *Barrett's esophagus*, requires close surveillance to detect the progression of premalignant dysplastic changes.

Many children referred for antireflux surgery are neurologically impaired, usually secondary to such factors as metabolic conditions, head trauma, or birth asphyxia. Thus, most of these patients require permanent feeding access in the form of a gastrostomy tube, so antireflux surgery is often considered at the time of the gastrostomy placement, especially in patients who are unable to protect their airway reliably or who already have significant vomiting associated with intragastric tube feeding. However, the concept of prophylactic fundoplication at the time of gastrostomy in neurologically impaired children remains controversial. These patients are also at high risk for delayed gastric emptying because of upper gastroduodenal dysmotility. However, fundoplication alone may result in enhanced gastric emptying function.[11]

### Evaluation

A detailed evaluation of the clinical history and associated symptoms will provide valuable guidance to determine the significance of GER. Clinical situations such as a near-miss SIDS episode or progressive neurologic disorders may indicate the desirability of performing an antireflux procedure, regardless of diagnostic study results. There are various diagnostic tools to objectively assess the presence of pathologic GER.

Barium esophagogram is used most frequently and provides anatomic and functional information about the esophagus and stomach. Esophageal stricture or mechanical evidence of gastric outlet obstruction, such as antral, duodenal web, or intestinal malrotation, can also be identified. Also, motility of the esophagus and gastric emptying function can be assessed by esophagography. However, one drawback is that this study lacks specificity. A 24-hour esophageal pH monitoring study remains as the gold standard test for diagnosing GER. It can determine the frequency and duration of acid reflux episodes and also provides significant information about reflux patterns, such as the total length of acid ($pH < 4$) reflux, duration of each episode, and longest continuous period of acid reflux. A gastric emptying scan is obtained when a radionuclide-labeled ($^{99m}Tc$ sulfur colloid) liquid or semisolid food is used to assess gastric emptying quantitatively. This study can also identify the presence of GER. In general, approximately 50% of the isotope meal normally leaves the stomach within 60 minutes and approximately 80% empties by 90 minutes after ingestion of a labeled meal. Delayed gastric emptying may improve simply after an antireflux procedure alone.

Esophageal manometry measures the esophageal body and lower esophageal sphincter pressures and helps identify abnormal esophageal motility. Although relatively simple to perform, manometry is infrequently used to evaluate GER disorders in children. The severity of GER in infants does not always correlate with an incompetent lower esophageal sphincter mechanism. There has also been considerably less experience with manometric studies in pediatric patients. However, identifying patients with esophageal dysmotility may be important for selecting the appropriate antireflux procedure. Children with poor esophageal motility are prone to develop refractory dysphagia after complete wrap fundoplication. Endoscopic evaluation of the esophageal mucosa provides a gross and microscopic assessment of mucosal injury secondary to GER. Patients who present with hematemesis or dysphagia may have significant underlying esophagitis. Esophagoscopy can determine the spectrum of esophagitis from inflammation to ulceration to stricture, and is also helpful in identifying Barrett's esophagus (columnar epithelium in the lower esophagus) via mucosal biopsy.

### Treatment

Conservative management of significant GER includes thickening of formula with cereal, reducing the volume of feeding, and postural maneuvers. In addition, pharmacologic acid suppression may be useful. Indications for surgical intervention include severe GER that is unresponsive to aggressive medical management. Surgery is generally warranted for patients with life-threatening near-miss SIDS episodes, FTT, or esophageal stricture. Other relative indications include those requiring complex surgical airway reconstruction, neurologic impairment requiring permanent feeding access, and a history of recurrent pneumonias or persistent asthma. In general, the gold standard surgical procedure for children with GER remains Nissen fundoplication (complete esophageal wrap). It is the most effective method to control the symptoms of GER; however, the undesirable side effect of gas bloat or dysphagia is more likely to occur after a complete wrap than after a partial wrap. A partial wrap ( e.g., Toupet, 270 degrees; Thal, 180 degrees) has been reported to produce less frequent complications, but is less effective in controlling the reflux symptoms as compared with a complete wrap. Regardless of which type of fundoplication is performed, a laparoscopic approach has become the standard technique.

## Hypertrophic Pyloric Stenosis

Hypertrophic pyloric stenosis (HPS) is a disease of newborns, with an incidence of 1 in 300 to 900 live births. It is one of the most common GI surgical disorders in early infancy; it is most common between the ages of 2 and 8 weeks. Boys are affected four times as often as girls, with first-born male infants being at highest risk. Hypertrophy of the circular muscle of the pylorus results in constriction and obstruction of the gastric outlet, leading to nonbilious, projectile emesis, loss of hydrochloric acid with the onset of hypokalemic hypochloremic metabolic alkalosis, and dehydration. Although the exact cause for HPS remains unknown, a lack of nitric oxide synthase in pyloric tissue has been implicated.

### Clinical Presentation

Infants with HPS generally present with progressively worsening nonbilious emesis. With time, the emesis becomes more frequent, forceful, and projectile in nature. Occasionally, visible gastric peristalsis may be observed as a wave of contractions from the left upper quadrant to the epigastrium. Shortly after emesis, infants usually crave additional feedings. A plain abdominal radiograph shows an upper abdominal gas bubble in the stomach. Palpation of the pyloric tumor (olive-shaped) in the epigastrium or right upper quadrant by an experienced examiner is pathognomonic for the diagnosis of HPS. If the olive is palpated, no additional diagnostic testing is necessary. When the olive is nonpalpable, the diagnosis of HPS can be made by ultrasound. A persistent pyloric muscle thickness more than 3 to 4 mm or a pyloric length more than 15 to 18 mm in the presence of functional gastric outlet obstruction is generally considered diagnostic. With equivocal clinical history, an upper GI contrast study is useful to evaluate for other causes of vomiting.

### Treatment: Surgical Management

The treatment of HPS is pyloromyotomy, consisting of incising through thickened pyloric musculature while preserving the underlying mucosa. This can be performed through a right upper quadrant or periumbilical incision. Recently, laparoscopic pyloromyotomy (Fig. 67-8) has gained popularity because of better cosmesis, with similar outcomes to those of the open technique.[12] Before surgery, it is important that the infant be fully rehydrated with IV fluids to establish an adequate urine output and correct electrolyte disturbances such as metabolic alkalosis. Because the infant with underlying metabolic alkalosis will compensate with respiratory acidosis, postoperative apnea may occur. Thus, the serum $HCO_3^-$ level needs to be normalized before surgery. Postoperatively, infants are usually allowed to resume enteral feedings. Vomiting after surgery occurs frequently but is generally self-limited. Potential complications include incomplete myotomy, mucosal perforation, and wound infection.

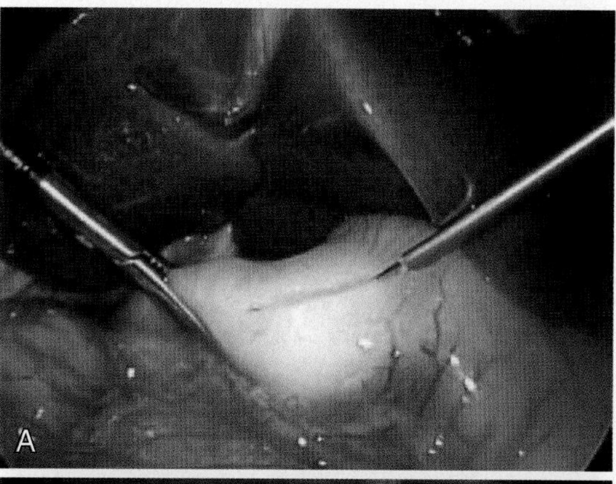


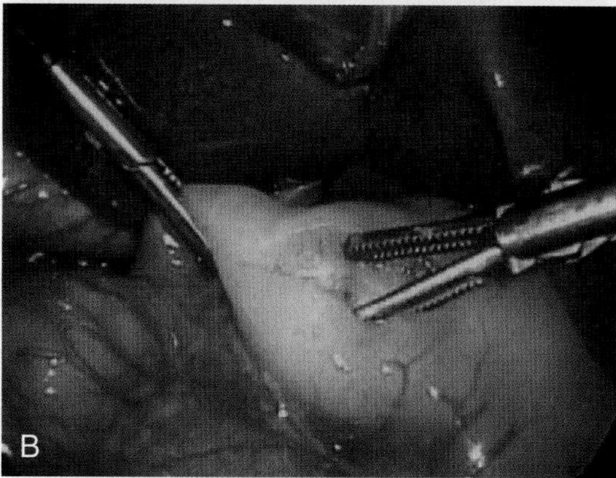


**FIGURE 67-8 A,** Laparoscopic pyloromyotomy is started using a retractable blade. **B,** A spreader with grooves on the outer surface is used to complete the pyloromyotomy. Intact mucosal bulging along with independent muscular wall motion is confirmed. (From St. Peter SD, Ostlie DJ: Laparoscopic and open pyloromyotomy. In Chung DH, Chen MK [eds]: Atlas of pediatric surgical techniques, Philadelphia, 2010, Elsevier Saunders, pp 253–265.)

## Duodenal Atresia

Duodenal atresia is thought to occur as a result of failure of vacuolization of the duodenum from its solid cord stage. The range of anatomic variants includes duodenal stenosis, mucosal web with intact muscular wall (so-called *windsock deformity*), two ends separated by a fibrous cord, and complete separation, with a gap within the duodenum. It is associated with several conditions, including prematurity, Down syndrome, maternal polyhydramnios, malrotation, annular pancreas, and biliary atresia (BA). Other anomalies, such as cardiac, renal, esophageal, and anorectal anomalies, are also common. In most cases, the duodenal obstruction is distal to the ampulla of Vater (85%), and therefore infants present with bilious emesis. In patients with a mucosal web, the symptoms of postprandial emesis may occur later in life.

### Clinical Presentation and Diagnosis

Infants with duodenal obstruction are generally first detected during a prenatal ultrasound evaluation. Immediately after birth, a plain abdominal radiograph shows a typical double-bubble sign, if obtained before orogastric tube decompression of swallowed gastric air (Fig. 67-9*A*). If distal air is present, an upper GI contrast study should be obtained rapidly, not only to confirm the diagnosis of duodenal stenosis or atresia but also to exclude midgut volvulus, which would constitute a surgical emergency.

### Treatment: Surgical Management

The management is by surgical bypass of the duodenal obstruction as a side-to-side or proximal transverse to distal longitudinal (diamond-shaped) duodenoduodenostomy (see Fig. 67-9*B*). At the time of anastomosis, a concomitant distal intestinal atresia

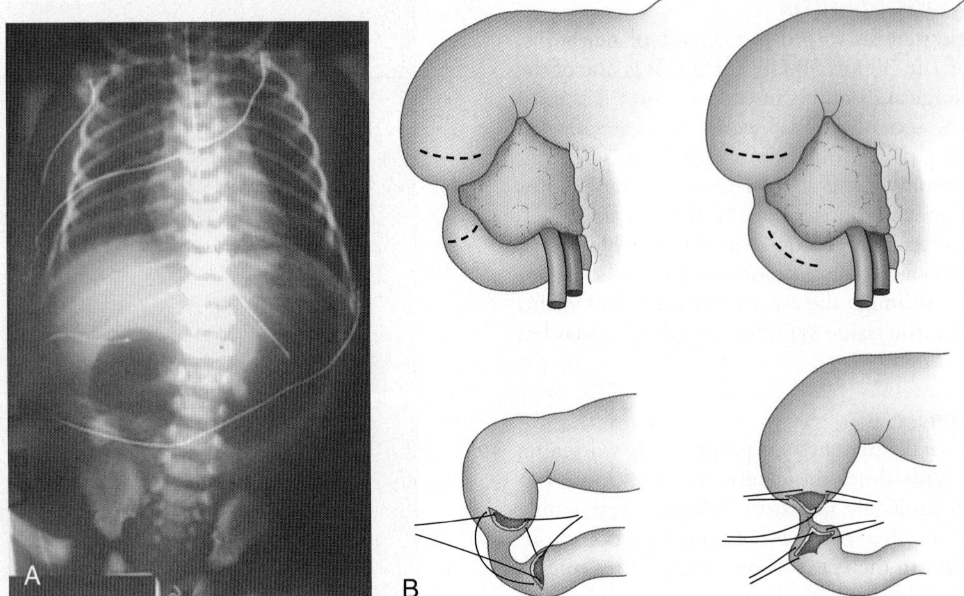


**FIGURE 67-9** **A,** Plain abdominal radiograph shows double-bubble appearance of duodenal atresia. **B,** Proximal transverse to distal longitudinal (diamond-shaped) or side-to-side duodenoduodenostomy is performed for congenital duodenal obstruction. (From Duodenal obstruction. In O'Neill JA Jr, Grosfeld JL, Fonkaksrud EW, et al [eds]: Principles of pediatric surgery, ed 2, St. Louis, 2003, Mosby, p 474.)

should be ruled out by injecting saline into a distal limb using a soft red rubber catheter. When the proximal duodenum is markedly dilated, a tapering duodenoplasty with staples or sutures should be considered to reduce the duodenal caliber, which may improve postoperative gastric emptying. In patients with a duodenal mucosal web, the web is excised transduodenally. Caution must be exercised to preserve the ampulla during the web excision.

## Jejunoileal Atresia

Jejunoileal atresia is the most common GI atresia; it occurs in approximately 1 in 2000 live births. It is thought to occur as a result of an intrauterine mesenteric vascular occlusion. Atresias occur slightly more frequently in the jejunum than in the ileum. Jejunoileal atresias are classified as type I, a mucosal web or diaphragm (Fig. 67-10*A*), type II, with an atretic cord between two blind ends of bowel with intact mesentery, type IIIa, a complete separation of the blind ends of the bowel by a V-shaped mesenteric gap, and type IIIb, an apple peel or Christmas tree deformity with a large mesenteric gap (see Fig. 67-10*B*), in which the distal bowel receives a retrograde blood supply from the ileocolic or right colic artery. This tenuous blood supply has implications for reanastomosis and the potential for ischemic necrosis caused by an antenatal volvulus. Thus, many of these infants with this type of atresia are born with reduced intestinal length. Finally, in type IV, there are multiple atresias, with a string of sausage appearance.

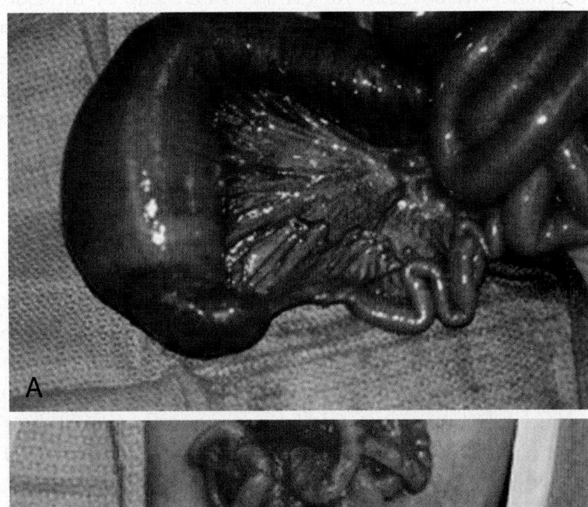


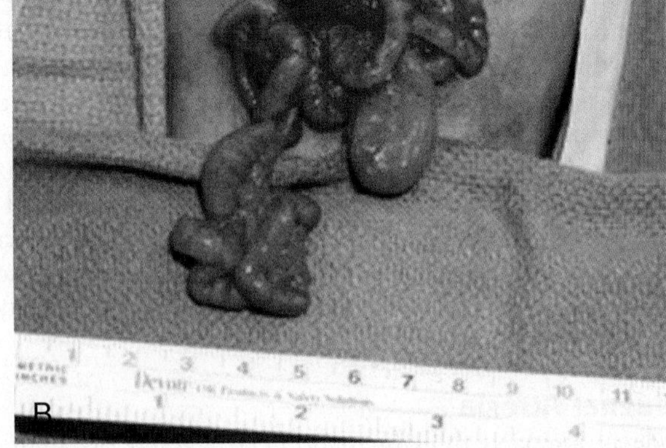


**FIGURE 67-10** Jejunoileal atresia. **A,** Massively dilated jejunum with narrow distal bowel segment. **B,** Apple peel type of atresia with a large mesenteric gap.

### Clinical Presentation

Infants present with bilious emesis, abdominal distention, and failure to pass meconium. Typically, the overall clinical presentation is dependent on the level of obstruction. In proximal atresia, abdominal distention is less, but significant bilious emesis is present. Plain abdominal radiographs show air-fluid levels with absent distal gas. With distal atresias, abdominal distention is present more frequently. A barium enema demonstrates a small unused colon and may also be useful to exclude multiple atresias, which may be present in 10% to 15% of cases. Jejunoileal atresia is typically not associated with other anomalies except cystic fibrosis (CF) in approximately 10% of patients.

### Treatment: Surgical Management

Infants are managed in a manner similar to that for other conditions of neonatal bowel obstruction. An orogastric tube is placed and appropriate IV fluid resuscitation is implemented. At operation, the main goal is to reestablish intestinal continuity while preserving as much intestinal length as possible. In multiple atresias, multiple anastomoses over an endoluminal stent may be necessary. If the proximal intestine is significantly dilated, prolonged dysmotility may persist and, therefore, a tapering enteroplasty of the dilated bowel should be considered. However, in cases of adequate bowel length, resection of the dilated bowel segment can result in faster recovery. The overall survival for infants with jejunoileal atresia is more than 90%.

## Intestinal Malrotation and Midgut Volvulus

The actual incidence of rotational anomalies of the midgut is difficult to determine, but is estimated to occur in 1 in 6000 live births. The midgut normally herniates out of the coelomic cavity through the umbilical ring at approximately the fourth week of fetal development. By week 10 of gestation, the intestine begins to migrate back into the abdominal cavity in a counterclockwise rotation around the axis of the superior mesenteric artery (SMA) for 270 degrees. The duodenojejunal segment returns first and rotates beneath and to the right of the SMA to fix in the left upper quadrant at the ligament of Treitz. The cecocolic segment also rotates counterclockwise around the SMA to rest in its final position in the right lower quadrant. By the week 12, this process of intestinal rotation is complete and the colon becomes fixed to the retroperitoneum. An interruption or reversal of any of these coordinated movements implies an embryologic explanation for the range of anomalies seen.

### Abnormal Intestinal Rotation

Complete nonrotation of the midgut is the most common anomaly and occurs when neither the duodenojejunal nor the cecocolic limb undergoes correct rotation. Consequently, duodenojejunal and ileocecal junctions lie close together and the midgut is suspended on a narrow SMA stalk, which can twist in a clockwise fashion to result in midgut volvulus. Nonrotation of the duodenojejunal limb, followed by normal rotation and fixation of the cecocolic limb, result in duodenal obstruction by abnormal mesenteric bands (Ladd's bands) that extend from the colon across the anterior duodenum. In this anomaly, although obstructive symptoms may be severe, the risk of midgut volvulus is low because there is a relatively broad mesenteric base between the duodenojejunal junction and cecum. Normal rotation of the duodenojejunal limb with nonrotation of the cecocolic segment carries the same risk for midgut volvulus as a complete nonrotation anomaly. In this case, the risks for volvulus are high because of a narrow mesenteric base.

**Clinical Presentation** The clinical presentation varies, depending on the specific mechanism of obstruction and whether it involves vascular compromised bowel. The major symptoms are related to the presence of midgut volvulus, duodenal obstruction, or intermittent or chronic abdominal pain, or as an incidental finding in an otherwise asymptomatic patient. Most patients develop symptoms during the first month of life. Midgut volvulus is a true surgical emergency because of evolving ischemic bowel loops. The acute onset of bilious emesis in a particularly somnolent or lethargic newborn is an ominous sign. Midgut volvulus may also be incomplete or intermittent. Patients may have chronic abdominal pain, intermittent episodes of emesis (which may be nonbilious), early satiety, weight loss, failure to thrive, and/or malabsorption and diarrhea. With partial volvulus, the resultant mesenteric venous and lymphatic obstruction may impair nutrient absorption and produce protein loss into the gut lumen, as well as mucosal ischemia and melena as a result of arterial insufficiency.

**Diagnosis** Abdominal radiographs may demonstrate upper intestinal obstruction or a gasless abdomen; however, these findings are nonspecific. The upper GI contrast series remains the diagnostic study of choice; it demonstrates an abnormal position of the ligament of Treitz along with the appearance of a bird's beak in the third portion of the duodenum, which indicates an obstruction. The ultrasound examination has proven to be a useful tool for the diagnosis of intestinal malrotation with midgut volvulus, in which the normal relationship of the superior mesenteric vessels (the vein is to the right of artery) is reversed or altered.[13] In the acutely ill child with midgut volvulus and obstruction, immediate operative correction is indicated, and little time is available for IV fluid resuscitation, catheterization, type and crossmatching, or administration of broad-spectrum antibiotics. Time is critical in terms of intestinal salvage.

**Treatment: Surgical Management** Midgut volvulus is a surgical emergency. Once the diagnosis is made, a child must be promptly explored. Ladd's procedure is the operation of choice for most rotational anomalies of the intestine (Fig. 67-11). On entering the peritoneal cavity, ascites (chyle from obstructive lymphatics) is frequently encountered. The volvulus is untwisted in a counterclockwise fashion. After detorsion, the intestine may be congested and edematous and some areas may appear necrotic. Placement of warm sponges and observation for a period of time may improve the appearance of the intestine when the vascular integrity has been compromised. Necrotic segment(s) are resected; however, marginally ischemic segments may be left in place and a second-look laparotomy performed after 24 to 36 hours. Ladd's bands are divided as they extend from the ascending colon across the duodenum to the posterior aspect of the right upper quadrant. In dividing the medial bands, the cecum is mobilized and the mesenteric base is broadened to prevent recurrent volvulus. There has been no demonstrated benefit to pexing the cecum or duodenum to the abdominal wall. In addition, an intraluminal duodenal obstruction may coexist, and therefore a catheter may be passed through the mouth and advanced beyond the pylorus into the distal duodenum to exclude any associated anomaly. An incidental appendectomy is performed because the cecum will ultimately lie on the left side of the abdomen after this procedure. The intestine is replaced into the abdominal cavity, with the small bowel lying entirely on the right side while the colon is positioned on the left.

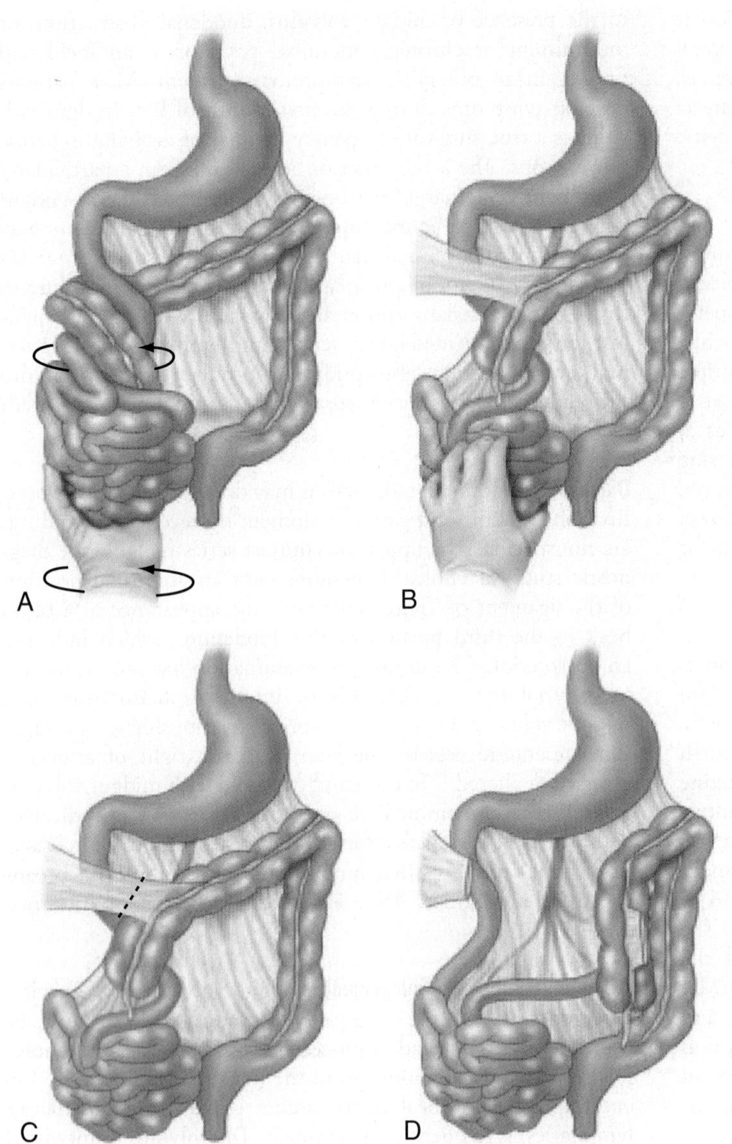


**FIGURE 67-11** Ladd procedure. **A,** The bowel is eviscerated. **B,** The intestine is derotated in a counterclockwise fashion. **C,** The peritoneal attachment between the cecum and retroperitoneum (Ladd's band) is divided. **D,** The base of the mesentery is widened and an appendectomy is performed. (From Warner BW: Imperforate anus. In Chung DH, Chen MK [eds]: Atlas of pediatric surgical techniques, Philadelphia, 2010, Elsevier Saunders, pp 138–142.)

### Outcomes

Recurrent volvulus is relatively infrequent but has been reported in up to 10% of children undergoing Ladd's procedure. The more common cause for postoperative obstruction is adhesive bands. Prolonged ileus is common, particularly if a volvulus has progressed to necrosis, requiring extensive resection. Midgut volvulus accounts for approximately 18% of cases of short gut syndrome in the pediatric population. Urgent recognition and treatment are the most important factors in preventing this complication.

## Necrotizing Enterocolitis

NEC is the most common GI emergency in the neonatal period. Although several contributing factors such as ischemia, bacteria, cytokines, and enteral feeding have been identified, prematurity is the single most important risk factor. Recent medical advances in the management of premature infants have led to improved overall survival, hence resulting in a greater number of premature infants at risk for developing NEC. Despite the tremendous impact of NEC on neonatal morbidity and mortality, progress in understanding this condition is hampered by the fact that a reliable animal study model for NEC does not exist.

### Clinical Presentation and Diagnosis

The clinical presentation for NEC can be variable and unpredictable. Acute abdominal distention, tenderness, and feeding intolerance with gross or occult blood in the stool are hallmark features for NEC. Other nonspecific clinical signs include irritability, temperature instability, and episodes of apnea or bradycardia. NEC typically occurs in the first few days of life with the initiation of enteral feedings. In approximately 80% of cases, however, it occurs within the first month of life. As NEC progresses, systemic sepsis develops, with hemodynamic deterioration and coagulopathy. The pathognomonic radiographic feature of NEC is pneumatosis intestinalis (see Fig. 67-12*A*). Pneumatosis is composed of hydrogen gas generated by the bacterial fermentation of luminal substrates. Other radiographic findings may include portal venous gas, ascites, fixed loops of small bowel, and free air (see Fig. 67-12*B*). The distal ileum and

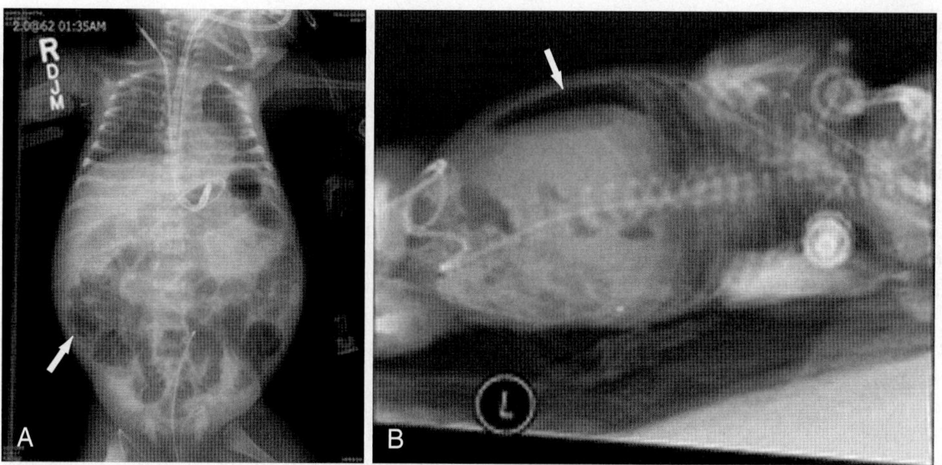


**FIGURE 67-12 A,** Pneumatosis intestinalis *(arrows)*, a pathognomonic radiographic sign for NEC. **B,** Pneumoperitoneum *(arrow)* on lateral decubitus radiograph.

ascending colon are the usual affected areas, although the entire GI tract (NEC totalis) may also be involved.

### Treatment

**Medical Treatment** Initial medical management consists of nasogastric tube decompression, fluid resuscitation, blood and platelet transfusion, and administration of broad-spectrum antibiotics. In general, NEC can be successfully treated medically in approximately 50% of cases with a 7- to 10-day course of antibiotics. Serial abdominal examinations are performed to closely monitor for any subtle signs that would indicate that surgery is required. The absolute indication for operative management of NEC is the presence of intestinal perforation, as revealed by free air on plain abdominal radiographs. Other relative indications for surgery include overall clinical deterioration, abdominal wall cellulitis, worsening acidosis, falling white blood cell or platelet count, a palpable abdominal mass, and a persistent fixed radiographic bowel loop.

**Surgical Management** The general principles of surgical management of NEC include resection of all nonviable segments of intestine with the creation of a stoma. All efforts need to be made to preserve as much intestinal length as possible. Thus, it may be necessary to resect multiple intervening necrotic segments of bowel, preserving all viable intestine. In cases in which the bowel is ischemic but not frankly necrotic, a second-look operation may be performed after 24 hours. Bowel resection with primary reanastomosis may be considered in the rare stable infant with focal involvement of NEC with minimal peritoneal contamination. However, the risks for anastomotic leak and stricture formation have tempered widespread enthusiasm for this approach.

Another operative approach to the management of the infant with perforated NEC is bedside placement of peritoneal drains. Drainage of the contaminated peritoneal fluid may improve ventilation and halt the progression of sepsis in select critically ill preterm infants. Surprisingly, drainage of the peritoneum may be the only necessary intervention in few select patients. However, in a multicenter cohort study, percutaneous drainage was found to be used commonly, but with poor outcomes in extremely low-birth-weight infants (<1000 g).[14] Evidence to support peritoneal drainage as an accepted mode of treatment for NEC has been recently established in a multicenter, randomized prospective clinical trial.[15] In this study, survival, need for parenteral nutrition, and length of hospital stay were similar for NEC infants weighing less than 1500 g treated by peritoneal drainage or laparotomy.

### Outcomes

The overall mortality rate for surgically managed NEC ranges from 10% to 50%. NEC is currently the single most common cause of short gut syndrome in children. Intestinal strictures may develop after medical or surgical management of NEC in approximately 10% of infants. The most common site of involvement is the splenic flexure of the colon. Because of this risk for post-NEC stricture, a radiographic contrast study of the distal intestine is carried out routinely prior to elective stoma reversal. Neurodevelopmental delay is also a frequent long-term problem in these infants.

## Short Bowel Syndrome

Short bowel syndrome (SBS) is a clinical condition in which there is inadequate length of functional intestine to sustain normal enteral nutrition, generally as a result of massive small bowel resection. Common conditions that could result in SBS are intestinal atresia, midgut volvulus, NEC, and gastroschisis. In patients with SBS, intestinal function depends on a number of factors, such as total bowel length, presence of the ileocecal valve, and residual segments of intestine. The jejunum is the site of absorption of most macronutrients and minerals. GI hormones that are critical for gut function, such as cholecystokinin and secretin, are produced in the jejunum. The ileum is essential for the absorption of carbohydrates, proteins, fluids, and electrolytes. Bile acids, vitamin $B_{12}$, and the fat-soluble vitamins (A, D, E, K) are primarily absorbed in the ileum. The presence or absence of an ileocecal valve is particularly critical in SBS, in which intestinal transit time can be significantly altered. The colon is particularly important in SBS patients to absorb water and electrolytes. After massive small bowel resection, a physiologic process known as *intestinal adaptation* occurs to compensate for the loss of intestinal length. Many factors are involved in this adaptive process to enhance the absorptive function of the residual intestine. Medical treatment of SBS patients includes the use of an elemental diet, glutamine and various growth factors, and careful delivery of TPN.[16] Many surgical techniques (excluding small bowel transplantation) aimed at slowing intestinal transit time and/or increasing the mucosal surface area for enhanced absorption have been described.[17] These include reversed intestinal segment, recirculating loop, artificial intestinal valve, colon interposition, and intestinal pacing. Two procedures that are generally used are the Bianchi procedure and serial transverse enteroplasty.

### Treatment: Surgical Management

**Bianchi Procedure** Bianchi originally described an intestinal lengthening procedure in which the mesenteric vascular bed is separated into two systems, the dilated small intestine is split into two parallel segments, each with its own blood supply, and the ends are approximated (Fig. 67-13*A*). This results in a 50% decreased diameter of the small intestine and increased length by 200%. The Bianchi procedure has shown to be an effective surgical option for treating patients with SBS.[18]

**Serial Transverse Enteroplasty** Since its first description in 2003, the STEP procedure (*s*erial *t*ransverse *e*ntero*p*lasty) has garnered significant interest by the pediatric surgical community. In contrast to the Bianchi procedure, dilated small intestine is serially stapled in a transverse fashion to create a narrower lumen and longer intestinal length (see Fig. 67-13*B*). In a report of early experience with 16 patients, the STEP procedure improved enteral feeding tolerance, resulting in significant catch-up growth, and was not associated with increased mortality.[19]

## Meconium Ileus

Meconium ileus is a unique form of neonatal obstruction that occurs in infants with CF. CF results from a mutation in the CF transmembrane regulator gene*(CFTR)* and is autosomal recessive. It is estimated that 3.3% of the Caucasian population in the United States are asymptomatic carriers of the mutated CF gene. The abnormal chloride transport in patients with CF results in tenacious viscous secretions with a protein concentration of almost 80 to 90%. It affects a wide variety of organs, including the intestine, pancreas, lungs, salivary glands, reproductive organs, and biliary tract. Meconium ileus is classified as simple or complicated.

### Clinical Presentation

Meconium ileus in the newborn represents the earliest clinical manifestation of CF; it affects approximately 10% to 15% of patients with this inherited disease. The incidence of CF ranges from 1 in 1000 to 2000 live births. Infants present with three cardinal signs in the first 24 to 48 hours of life: (1) generalized abdominal distention; (2) bilious emesis; and (3) failure to pass meconium. Maternal polyhydramnios occurs in approximately 20% of cases. In simple meconium ileus, the terminal ileum is dilated and filled with thick, tarlike, inspissated meconium. Smaller pellets of meconium are found in the more distal ileum, leading into a relatively small colon. In patients with simple meconium ileus, important plain abdominal radiographic findings include dilate, gas-filled loops of small bowel, absence of air-fluid levels, and a mass of meconium in the right side of the abdomen mixed with gas to give a ground glass or soap bubble appearance.

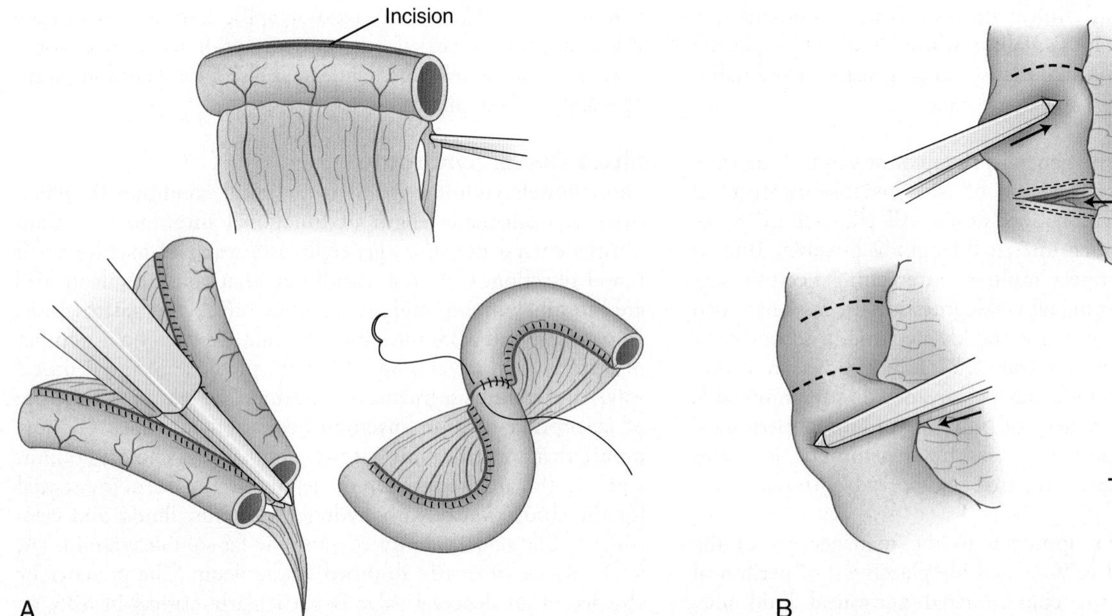


**FIGURE 67-13** Bowel-lengthening procedures. **A,** Bianchi technique separates two mesenteric planes. A dilated segment of bowel is stapled longitudinally to create two narrower segments for sequential anastomosis. **B,** STEP (serial transverse enteroplasty) involves stapling a dilated bowel into V shapes on alternating sides, decreasing width and increasing length. (**A** adapted from Abu-Elmagd KM, Bond G, Costa G, et al: Gut rehabilitation and intestinal transplantation. Therapy 2:853–864, 2005; **B** from Kim HB, Fauza D, Garza J, et al: Serial transverse enteroplasty (STEP): A novel bowel-lengthening procedure. J Pediatr Surg 38:425–429, 2003.)

### Simple Meconium Ileus

Plain abdominal radiographs show dilated bowel loops with relative absent air-fluid levels because of thick viscous meconium. A ground glass appearance is noted in the right lower quadrant corresponding to bowel loops filled with thick meconium mixed with air. The initial diagnostic study of choice is a contrast enema using a water-soluble ionic contrast solution. In simple meconium ileus, a Gastrografin contrast enema study can demonstrate a small unused colon and inspissated meconium pellets in the terminal ileum (Fig. 67-14*A*). Gastrografin is a hypertonic solution, which can aid in the evacuation of meconium. However, it is important that the infants are well hydrated and electrolytes and vital signs carefully monitored following the Gastrografin study. Contrast enema is successful in relieving the obstruction in up to 75% of cases, with a bowel perforation rate of less than 3%. The pilocarpine iontophoresis sweat test revealing a chloride concentration higher than 60 mEq/L is the most reliable and definitive method to confirm the diagnosis of CF. A more immediate test includes detection of the mutated *CFTR* gene.

**Treatment: Surgical Management** Operative management of simple meconium ileus is required when the obstruction cannot be relieved with Gastrografin contrast enema, along with 5 mL of 10% N-acetylcysteine (Mucomyst) solution administered every 6 hours through a nasogastric tube. Historically, the dilated terminal ileum was resected and various types of stomas were created, allowing for intestinal decompression and recovery. More recently, enterotomy, irrigation with warmed saline solution or 4% N-acetylcysteine, and simple evacuation of the luminal meconium without a stoma has been advocated (see Fig. 67-14*B*). N-acetylcysteine serves to break the disulfide bonds in the meconium and facilitate separation from the bowel mucosa. The meconium is manipulated into the distal colon or removed through the enterotomy. After the obstruction is relieved, the enterotomy is closed in standard fashion. If meconium evacuation is incomplete, a T tube may be left in place in the ileum to facilitate continued postoperative irrigation.

### Complicated Meconium Ileus

Meconium ileus is considered complicated when perforation of the intestine has taken place in utero or in the early neonatal period. Extravasated meconium can result in severe peritonitis, with a dense inflammatory response and calcification. The variable clinical presentation includes a meconium pseudocyst, adhesive peritonitis with or without secondary bacterial infection, and ascites. Plain abdominal radiographs can demonstrate calcifications, bowel dilation, mass effect, and ascites.

### Outcomes

The long-term outcomes of patients with CF, with or without meconium ileus, are not significantly variable. A meconium ileus equivalent (distal ileal obstructive syndrome) may develop as a consequence of noncompliance with oral enzyme replacement therapy or bouts of dehydration. This is managed nonoperatively in most patients with enemas or oral polyethylene glycol purging solutions. Other diagnoses must also be considered, including simple adhesive intestinal obstruction. Furthermore, with the introduction of enteric-coated, high-strength pancreatic enzyme replacement therapy, a fibrosing cholangiopathy has been described. Resection of the inflammatory colon stricture may be necessary.

## Colonic Atresia

Colonic atresia is uncommon, with an estimated incidence of 1 in 20,000 live births. It is the least common intestinal atresia, accounting for only 5% to 10% of cases. Infants with colonic atresia usually present with failure to pass meconium, abdominal distention, and bilious vomiting. Plain radiographs may demonstrate distal bowel obstruction pattern, but the diagnosis is confirmed by barium enema. The classification of colonic atresias is the same as that for the small intestine. At operation, depending on the location of the atretic point, primary anastomosis after partial resection or tapering of the proximal colon may be considered; however, a diverting end colostomy with delayed reversal is preferred.

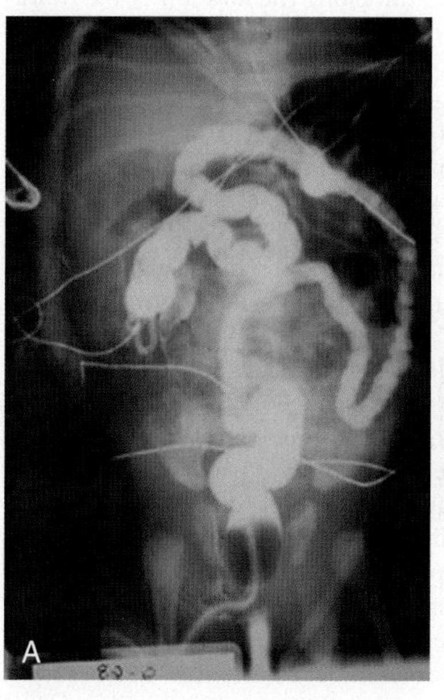


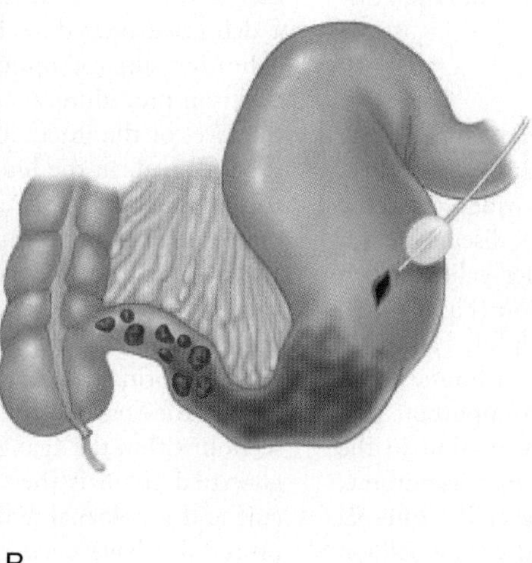


**FIGURE 67-14** Surgical management of simple meconium ileus. **A,** Contrast enema study shows microcolon with soap bubble appearance in the right lower quadrant. **B,** Removal of meconium can be facilitated by gentle use of a catheter along with a 2% to 4% N-acetylcysteine solution. (From Brandt, ML: Meconium disease. In Chung DH, Chen MK [eds]: Atlas of pediatric surgical techniques, Philadelphia, 2010, Elsevier Saunders, pp 44–53.)

### Meconium Plug Syndrome

Meconium plug syndrome is unrelated to meconium ileus and, in most cases is not a sequela of CF. However, it is a frequent cause of neonatal intestinal obstruction and is associated with a number of conditions, including Hirschsprung's disease, maternal diabetes, and hypothyroidism. In general, infants present with significant abdominal distention and failure to pass meconium in the first 24 hours of life. Barium enema shows a microcolon extending up to where the colon is dilated, filled with a thickened meconium plug. Often, a barium enema study is diagnostic and therapeutic. Although most children with meconium plug syndrome are normal, follow-up studies should be performed to rule out Hirschsprung's disease and CF.

### Hirschsprung's Disease

Hirschsprung's disease is a developmental disorder characterized by an absence of ganglion cells in the myenteric (Auerbach) and submucosal (Meissner) plexus. It occurs in 1 in 5000 live births, with boys being affected four times more frequently than girls. This neurogenic parasympathetic abnormality is associated with muscular spasm of the distal colon and internal anal sphincter, resulting in a functional obstruction. Hence, the abnormal bowel is the contracted distal segment, whereas the normal bowel is the proximal dilated portion. Aganglionosis begins at the anorectal line and the rectosigmoid is affected in approximately 80% of cases, splenic or transverse colon in 17%, and entire colon in 8%. The area between the dilated and contracted segments is referred to as the transition zone. In this area, ganglion cells begin to appear, but in reduced numbers. Of these patients, 3% to 5% have Down syndrome, and the risk for Hirschsprung's disease is greater if there is a family history. An abnormal locus on the chromosome 10 has been identified in some families and is associated with the *RET* oncogene.[20]

#### Clinical Presentation

Most infants (>90%) present with progressive abdominal distention and bilious emesis, with failure to pass meconium within the first 24 hours of life. In some cases, diarrhea may develop as a result of enterocolitis. For missed Hirschsprung's disease infants, they may present at an older age with a history of poor feeding, chronic abdominal distention, and significant constipation. Enterocolitis is the most common cause of death in patients with uncorrected Hirschsprung's disease and may manifest as diarrhea alternating with periods of obstipation, abdominal distention, fever, hematochezia, and peritonitis.

#### Diagnosis

The initial diagnostic step in a newborn with radiographic evidence of a distal bowel obstruction is a barium enema. In a normal barium enema study, the rectum is wider than the sigmoid colon. In patients with Hirschsprung's disease, spasm of the distal rectum usually results in a smaller caliber when compared with the more proximal sigmoid colon (Fig. 67-15). Identification of a transition zone may be helpful. Failure to evacuate the instilled contrast completely after 24 hours would also be indicative of Hirschsprung's disease. An important goal of the study is to exclude other causes of constipation in the newborn, such as meconium plug, small left colon syndrome, and atresia. The manometric finding of failure of the internal sphincter to relax when the rectum is distended with a balloon can also be useful information in older patients. A rectal biopsy is the gold standard for the diagnosis of Hirschsprung's disease. In the newborn period, this is performed at the bedside using a special suction rectal biopsy instrument. It is important to obtain the sample at least 2 cm above the dentate line to avoid sampling the normal transition from ganglionated bowel to the paucity or absence of ganglia in the region of the internal sphincter. In older children, a full-thickness biopsy is obtained under general anesthesia because the thicker rectal mucosa is not amenable to suction biopsy. Absent ganglia, hypertrophied nerve trunks, and robust immunostaining for acetylcholinesterase (AChE) are the histopathologic criteria. Recently, loss of calretinin immunostaining has been shown to be superior to AChE technique in the evaluation of suction rectal biopsies for Hirschsprung's disease.[21]

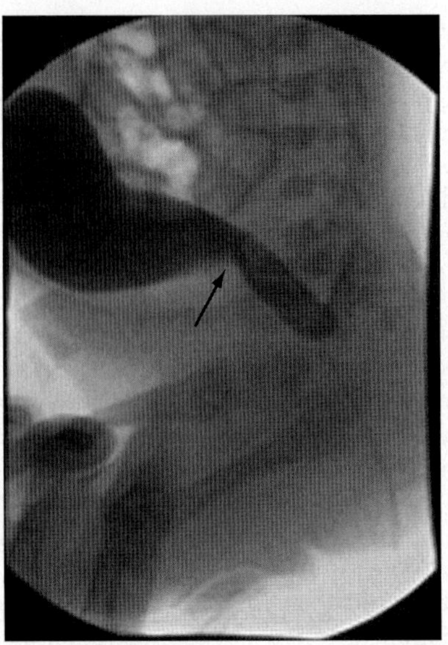

**FIGURE 67-15** Contrast enema demonstrating transition point *(arrow)* in Hirschsprung's disease.

#### Treatment: Surgical Management

Traditionally, a leveling colostomy was performed initially via a left lower quadrant surgical incision. The location of the transition zone is confirmed by frozen section evaluation of multiple seromuscular biopsies. A diverting colostomy (end or loop) is then performed in the region of normal ganglionated bowel and a definitive procedure is performed at a later age. There are definitive surgical options for Hirschsprung's disease. In the Swenson procedure, the aganglionic bowel is removed down to the level of the internal sphincters and a coloanal anastomosis is performed. In the Duhamel procedure, the aganglionic rectal stump is left in place and the ganglionated normal colon is pulled behind the stump. A stapler is then inserted through the anus, with one arm within the normal ganglionated bowel posteriorly and the other in the aganglionic rectum anteriorly. Firing of the stapler results in the formation of a neorectum that empties normally because of the posterior patch of ganglionated bowel. The Soave technique involves an endorectal mucosal dissection within the aganglionic distal rectum. The normally ganglionated colon is then pulled through the remnant muscular cuff and a coloanal anastomosis is performed. Recently, these procedures have been performed in the newborn period as a primary procedure without an initial colostomy.[22] Furthermore, the same procedures have been described in infants that are performed completely through a transanal approach, with or without laparoscopic guidance. The overall survival of patients with Hirschsprung's disease is excellent; however, long-term stooling problems are not infrequent. Constipation is the most frequent postoperative problem followed by soiling, incontinence, and enterocolitis.

## Anorectal Malformation

The incidence of imperforate anus is 1 in 5000 live births, and boys are more commonly affected (58%). The spectrum of anorectal malformations ranges from simple anal stenosis to the persistence of a cloaca. The most common defect is an imperforate anus with a fistula between the distal colon and urethra in boys or the vestibule of the vagina in girls.

### Embryology

By 6 weeks of gestation, the urorectal septum moves caudally to divide the cloaca into the anterior urogenital sinus and posterior anorectal canal. Failure of this septum to form results in a fistula between the bowel and urinary tract (in boys) or the vagina (in girls). Complete or partial failure of the anal membrane to resorb results in an anal membrane or stenosis. The perineum also contributes to the development of the external anal opening and genitalia by the formation of cloacal folds, which extend from the anterior genital tubercle to the anus. The perineal body is formed by fusion of the cloacal folds between the anal and urogenital membranes. Breakdown of the cloacal membrane anywhere along its course results in the external anal opening being anterior to the external sphincter (i.e., anteriorly displaced anus).

### Classification

An anatomic classification of anorectal anomalies is based on the level at which the blind-ending rectal pouch ends—low, intermediate, or high in relationship to the levator ani musculature. A more therapeutic and prognostically oriented classification is depicted in Box 67-1. An invertogram, a lateral pelvic radiograph taken after the infant is held upside-down for several minutes, was used often in the past to determine the level of the rectal pouch. In most cases, a careful inspection of the perineum alone can predict the pouch level. If an anocutaneous fistula is observed anywhere on the perineal skin of a boy or external to the hymen of a girl, a low lesion can be assumed. Most other types of lesions are high or intermediate. *Rectal atresia* refers to an unusual lesion in which the lumen of the rectum is completely or partially interrupted, with the upper rectum being dilated and the lower rectum consisting of a small anal canal. A persistent cloaca is defined as a defect in which the rectum, vagina, and urethra all fuse to form a single common channel. In girls, the type of defect may be indicated by the number of orifices at the perineum. A single orifice would be consistent with a cloaca. If two orifices are seen (i.e., urethra and vagina), the defect represents a high imperforate anus or, less commonly, a persistent urogenital sinus comprising one orifice and a normal anus as the other orifice. Anorectal malformation often coexists with other lesions and the VACTERL association must be considered during evaluation. Bony abnormalities of the sacrum and spine such as absent, accessory, or hemivertebrae or an asymmetrical or short sacrum can occur in approximately one third of patients. Absence of two or more vertebrae is associated with a poor prognosis for bowel and bladder continence. Occult dysraphism of the spinal cord may also be present; this consists of a tethered cord, lipomeningocele, or fat within the filum terminale.

**BOX 67-1 Classification of Congenital Anomalies of the Anorectum**

**Female**
Cutaneous (perineal fistula)
Vestibular fistula
Imperforate anus without fistula
Rectal atresia
Cloaca
Complex malformation

**Male**
Cutaneous (perineal fistula)
Recto-urethral fistula
Bulbar
Prostatic
Recto-bladder neck fistula
Imperforate anus without fistula
Rectal atresia

### Treatment

**Preoperative Evaluation** Aside from a detailed physical examination, plain radiography of the spine and ultrasound of the spinal cord are performed. Genitourinary abnormalities other than the rectourinary fistula occur in 25% to 60% of patients. Vesicoureteral reflux and hydronephrosis are the most common but other conditions, such as horseshoe, dysplastic, or absent kidney, as well as hypospadias or cryptorchidism, must be considered. In general, the higher the anorectal malformation, the greater the frequency of associated urologic abnormalities. In patients with a persistent cloaca or rectovesical fistula, the likelihood of a genitourinary abnormality is approximately 90%. In contrast, the frequency is only 10% with low defects (e.g., perineal fistula). Renal ultrasonography and voiding cystourethrography are frequently performed to evaluate the urinary tract. If a cardiac defect is suspected, echocardiography is performed before any surgical procedure. Esophageal atresia can also be ruled out with a nasogastric tube placement. The decision making algorithms for the management of male and female newborns with anorectal malformation are shown in Figures 67-16 and 67-17.

#### Surgical Management

***Low Lesions*** The newborn infant with a low lesion can undergo a primary single-stage repair without a colostomy. For anal stenosis in which the anal opening is in a normal location, serial dilation alone is usually curative. Dilations are performed daily with gradual dilator size increases over time. If the anal opening is anterior to the external sphincter (i.e., anteriorly displaced anus), with a small distance between the opening and the center of the external sphincter, and the perineal body is intact, a cutback anoplasty may be performed. This consists of an incision extending from the ectopic anal orifice to the central part of the anal sphincter, thus enlarging the anal opening. Alternatively, if there is a large distance between the anal opening and central portion of the external anal sphincter, a transposition anoplasty

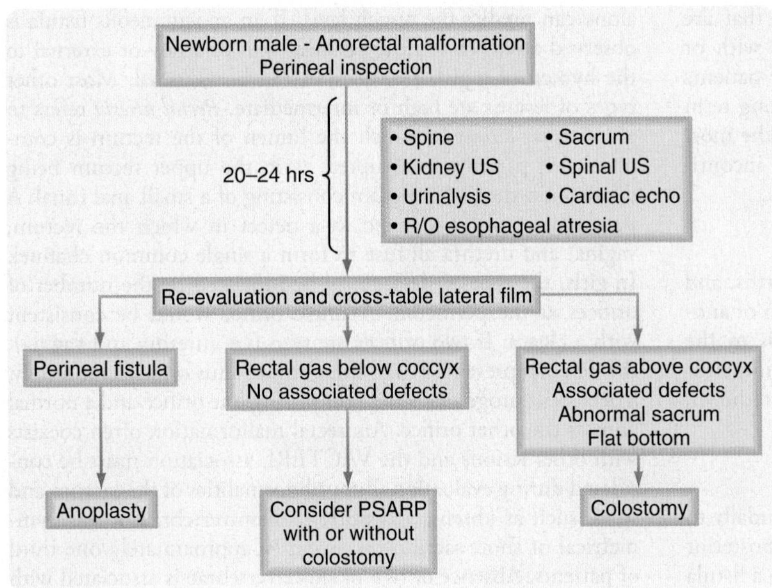


**FIGURE 67-16** Decision algorithm for the management of male patients with anorectal malformation. *PSARP,* Posterior sagittal anorectoplasty. (From Levitt M, Peña A: Imperforate anus. In Chung DH, Chen MK [eds]: Atlas of pediatric surgical techniques, Philadelphia, 2010, Elsevier Saunders, pp 185–205.)

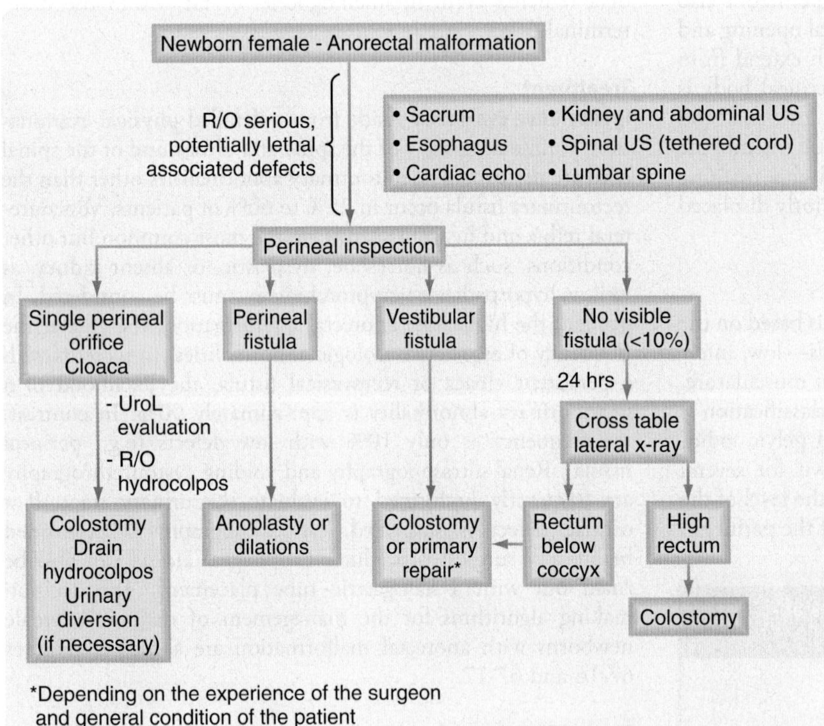


**FIGURE 67-17** Decision algorithm for the management of female patients with anorectal malformation. (From Levitt M, Peña A: Imperforate anus. In Chung DH, Chen MK [eds]: Atlas of pediatric surgical techniques, Philadelphia, 2010, Elsevier Saunders, pp 185–205.)

is performed in which the aberrant anal opening is transposed to the normal position within the center of the sphincter muscles and the perineal body is reconstructed.

***Intermediate or High Lesions*** Infants with intermediate or high lesions traditionally require a colostomy as the first part of a three-stage reconstruction. The colon is completely divided and an end sigmoid colostomy with a mucous fistula is constructed to minimize fecal contamination into the area of a rectourinary fistula. Furthermore, the distal mucous fistula limb can be evaluated radiographically to determine the location of the rectourinary fistula. The second-stage procedure usually is performed at 3 to 6 months of age. The operation consists of dividing the rectourinary or rectovaginal fistula with a pull-through of the terminal rectal pouch into the normal anal position. A posterior sagittal anorectoplasty, as first described by deVries and Pena, is the procedure of choice.[23] This consists of determining the location of the central position of the anal sphincter by electrical stimulation of the perineum. An incision is then made in the midline, extending from the coccyx to the anterior perineum and through the sphincter and levator musculature until the rectum is identified. The fistula from the rectum to the vagina or urinary tract is divided. The rectum is mobilized and the perineal musculature reconstructed. The third and final stage is closure of the colostomy, which is performed several weeks later. Anal dilations begin 2 weeks after the anorectoplasty and continue for several months after the colostomy closure.

Recently, a minimally invasive intra-abdominal approach to repair a high-type imperforate anus has gained significant interest, with some promising early results.[24] This technique offers the theoretical advantages of placing the neorectum within the central position of the sphincter and levator muscle complex under direct vision and avoids the need to cut across these structures. The long-term outcome of this new approach when compared with the standard posterior sagittal method is presently unknown.

### Outcomes

Most of the morbidity in patients with anorectal malformations is related to the presence of associated anomalies. Fecal continence is the major goal regarding correction of the defect. Prognostic factors for continence include the level of the pouch and whether the sacrum is normal. In general, 75% of patients have voluntary bowel movements. However, 50% of this group still soils their underwear occasionally while the other 50% is considered totally continent. Constipation is the most common sequela. A bowel management program consisting of daily enemas is an important postoperative plan to reduce the frequency of soilage and improve the quality of life for these patients.

## Intussusception

Intussusception is the telescoping of one portion of the intestine into the other; it is usually idiopathic, without an obvious anatomic lead point. It occurs predominantly at the ileocecal junction. Invariably, there is marked swelling of the lymphoid tissue in the region of the ileocecal valve. It is unknown whether this represents the cause or effect of the intussusception. The incidence of intussusception is associated with a history of recent episodes of viral gastroenteritis, upper respiratory infections, and even administration of rotavirus vaccine, implying lymphoid swelling in the pathogenesis of intussusception. In older children, the incidence of a pathologic lead point is up to 12%, where Meckel's diverticulum is found to be the most common lead point for intussusception. However, other causes such as intestinal polyps, inflamed appendix, submucosal hemorrhage associated with Henoch-Schönlein purpura, foreign body, ectopic pancreatic or gastric tissue, and intestinal duplication must also be considered. Postoperative small bowel intussusception in the absence of a lead point can also occur; this represents up to 5% of all pediatric cases of intussusception.

### Clinical Presentation and Diagnosis

Intussusception produces severe cramping abdominal pain in an otherwise healthy child from 3 months to 3 years. Two thirds of children presenting with intussusception are younger than 1 year. The child often draws the legs up during the pain episodes and is usually quiet during the intervening periods. Other symptoms include vomiting, passage of bloody mucous (currant jelly stool), and a palpable abdominal mass. In approximately 50% of cases, the diagnosis of intussusception can be suspected on plain abdominal radiographs based on the presence of a mass, sparse colonic gas, or complete distal small bowel obstruction. Currently, abdominal ultrasound is used as an initial diagnostic test. The characteristic sonographic findings of intussusception include the target sign of the intussuscepted layers of bowel on a transverse view or the pseudokidney sign when seen longitudinally.

### Treatment

**Nonoperative Management** Hydrostatic reduction by enema using contrast or air is the therapeutic procedure of choice. Contraindications to this approach include the presence of peritonitis or hemodynamic instability. Furthermore, an intussusception located entirely within the small intestine is unlikely to be reduced by an enema and more likely to have an associated lead point. Hydrostatic reduction using barium had been the mainstay of therapy; however, the use of air enema has become more widespread in recent years. Successful reduction is accomplished in more than 80% of cases and confirmed by resolution of the mass, along with reflux of air into the terminal ileum. The recurrence rate after hydrostatic reduction is approximately 11%, and it usually occurs within the 24 hours after the reduction. When it recurs, it is usually managed by another hydrostatic reduction. A third recurrence is an indication for operative management.

**Surgical Management** The operative indications with intussusception include the presence of peritonitis or complete small bowel obstruction at initial presentation, as well as failed hydrostatic reduction or multiple recurrences. The intussusceptum is delivered through a transverse incision in the right side of the abdomen and reduced in a retrograde fashion by pushing the mass proximally. Once reduced, warm lap pads may be placed over the bowel and a period of observation may be warranted in cases of questionable bowel viability. The lymphoid tissue in the ileocecal region is thickened and edematous and may be mistaken for a tumor within the small bowel; therefore, great caution should be exercised before committing to surgical resection. Recurrence rates are extremely low after surgical reduction. Bowel resection is required in cases in which the intussusception cannot be reduced, the viability of the bowel is uncertain, and/or a lead point is identified. An ileocolectomy with primary reanastomosis is usually performed. An appendectomy is an essential component, irrespective of bowel resection. Recently, the use of laparoscopy in the management of intussusception has gained popularity.

## Meckel's Diverticulum

Meckel's diverticulum is the most common congenital anomaly of the GI tract and occurs in approximately 2% of the population. More than 70% of symptomatic patients have heterotopic gastric mucosa and another 5% have pancreatic tissue. The rule of 2s is often cited in association with Meckel's diverticulum. Aside from its 2% incidence and two types of heterotopic mucosa, it is located within 2 feet of ileocecal valve, approximately 2 inches in length, and usually symptomatic by 2 years of age. Meckel's diverticulum is caused by a failure of normal regression of the vitelline duct that occurs during weeks 5 to 7 of gestation. Meckel's diverticulum is a true diverticulum containing all normal intestinal layers.

### Diagnosis

In general, clinical symptoms are related to hemorrhage, obstruction, or inflammation; the most common presenting symptom is a painless, massive, lower GI bleed in children younger than 5 years. Diagnosis of a persistent vitelline duct remnant may be established by umbilical ultrasound and/or lateral contrast radiography. The bleeding Meckel's diverticulum may be confirmed by a $^{99m}$Tc-pertechnetate isotope scan to detect gastric mucosa. Of note, ectopic gastric mucosa can also be present in patients with intestinal duplication.

#### Treatment: Surgical Management

Surgical treatment is the definitive therapy for Meckel's diverticulum. A simple V-shaped diverticulectomy with transverse closure of the ileum is the ideal surgical approach. In patients in whom there is ulceration or inflammation involving the ileum at the base of the diverticulum, resection of the involved ileum with a primary end-to-end anastomosis is preferred.

## HEPATOBILIARY CONDITIONS

### Extrahepatic Biliary Atresia

BA is a rare disease of neonates characterized by the inflammatory obliteration of intrahepatic and extrahepatic bile ducts. The incidence is estimated to be 1 in 5,000 to 12,000 infants, depending on region. It may be associated with other congenital malformations, particularly splenic abnormalities (e.g., asplenia, double spleen), absence of the inferior vena cava (IVC), and intestinal malformation. If BA is left untreated, progressive cirrhosis and death occur by 2 years of age.

#### Pathophysiology

The exact mechanism whereby BA develops is unknown, but several theories exist. The first is that the ductal injury is immune-mediated—inflammatory cells infiltrate and obliterate the bile ducts. Proinflammatory cytokines, such as interleukin-2, interferon-γ, and tumor necrosis factor, have been shown to be present. $CD4^+$, $CD8^+$ T cells, and natural killer cells are also prominent.[25] However, it remains unclear how the inflammatory process is initiated and progresses. Another hypothesis is that a viral insult, group C rotavirus infection, triggers the immune-mediated fibrosclerosis and obstruction of the extrahepatic bile ducts. Interestingly, animal studies have shown that infection of newborn mice with rotavirus leads to a similar presentation as infants, with the onset of hyperbilirubinemia, jaundice, and acholic stools. On histologic examination, inflammation and obstruction of the extrahepatic bile duct are observed. However, this theory has yet to be proven in human newborns, because many lack serologic evidence of viral infection. Another hypothesis is that there are genetic components that contribute to the development of BA. There may be an association with human leukocyte antigen (HLA) type. For example, patients with BA have a significantly high frequency of HLA-B12. It is unclear whether this is causal, but some have argued that abnormal expression of HLA makes biliary ductal epithelial cells a susceptible target for immunologic assault. Another putative gene, *CFC1,* encodes for a protein important in the embryonic differentiation of the left-right axis and, when mutated, is thought to predispose to the development of BA. Regardless of the mechanism, the end point is the same. Histopathologically, there is significant extrahepatic biliary obstruction with portal tract fibrosis, inflammatory cell infiltration, bile duct proliferation, and cholestasis with bile plugging.

#### Clinical Presentation and Diagnosis

The disease is classified according to the level of the most proximal biliary obstruction. For example, type 1 BA has patency to the level of the common bile duct. Type 2 has patency to the level of the common hepatic duct and type 3, which accounts for more than 90% of cases, occurs when the left and right hepatic ducts at the level of the porta hepatis are involved. This aids in the differentiation between correctable and noncorrectable BA. Correctable BA requires that patent hepatic ducts exist to the porta hepatis. Types 1 and 2 may be amenable to a direct extrahepatic biliary duct–intestinal anastomosis.

Infants present shortly after birth with jaundice, pale stools, and dark urine. Older infants may have failure to thrive and present with hepatomegaly and ascites suggestive of cirrhosis. If, in the postnatal period, the jaundice persists after 14 days in a term infant, a workup for liver disease should be initiated. This consists of measuring the direct, or conjugated, bilirubin level, which will be elevated (>2.0 mg/dL) in those with liver disease. Liver function tests should also be checked because derangements are typically seen. Coagulopathy is not generally encountered early because hepatic synthetic function is intact. Other exclusion studies include serologic testing for TORCH (***to***xoplasmosis, ***r***ubella, ***c***ytomegalovirus, and ***h***erpes) and hepatitis B and C infections, $\alpha_1$-antitrypsin, and CF. Metabolic disorders such as galactosemia and tyrosinemia and endocrine abnormalities must also be ruled out.

Evaluation of the biliary anatomy often begins with ultrasound. The gallbladder may be shrunken or absent and intrahepatic ducts may also be notably absent. The liver may appear echogenic. Other imaging modalities, such as hepatobiliary iminodiacetic acid (HIDA) scintigraphy, magnetic resonance cholangiopancreatography (MRCP), and endoscopic retrograde cholangiopancreatography (ERCP), have been used, with varying success. A HIDA scan would reveal uptake of the technetium isotope but an absence of emptying into the duodenum. MRCP or ERCP can better define the biliary anatomy, but because of the relative small size of the ducts, it is difficult from a technical and resolution standpoint. Although these are useful adjuncts, liver biopsy is the gold standard for the diagnosis of BA and can safely be done percutaneously under local anesthesia.

#### Treatment: Surgical Management

Once the diagnosis is strongly suspected, an exploratory laparotomy is warranted and intraoperative cholangiography is performed for confirmation. A Kasai hepatoportoenterostomy is the surgical procedure of choice. In this procedure, the extrahepatic biliary tree is dissected proximally to the level of the liver capsule, where the porta hepatis (portal plate) is transected. The reconstruction is performed via a Roux-en-Y hepaticojejunostomy (Fig. 67-18). Some have advocated the use of medications that augment biliary drainage, such as ursodeoxycholic acid and phenobarbital, but it is uncertain whether this actually improves outcomes. The use of perioperative steroids after the Kasai procedure remains controversial. The administration of perioperative steroids after the Kasai procedure has resulted in a shorter hospital stay.[26] The Biliary Atresia Clinical Research Consortium's randomized, double-blinded, placebo-controlled trial of steroid therapy following the Kasai procedure should shed some insight. Antibiotics are also continued postoperatively, because the risk of cholangitis is high (45% to 60%) due to the ease with

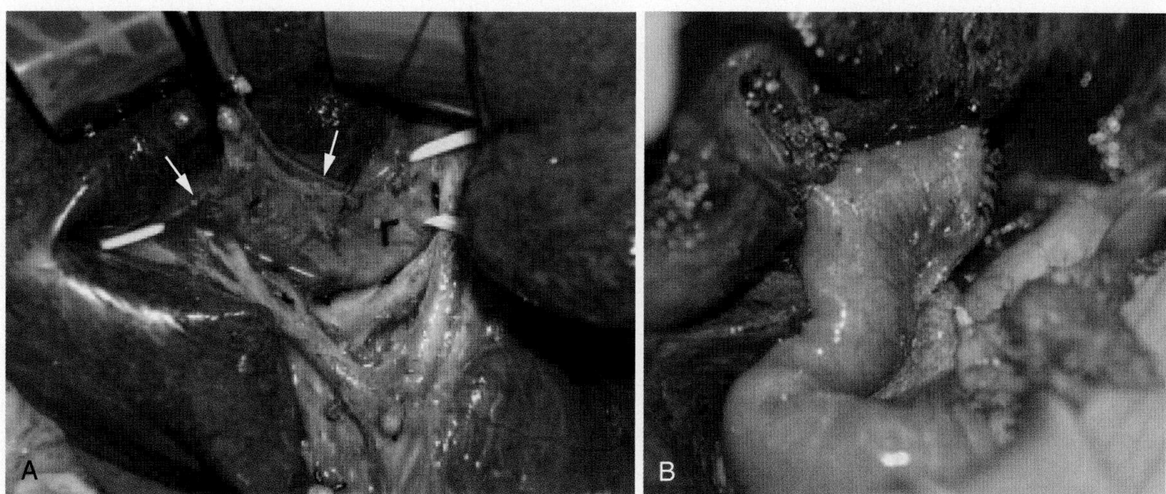


**FIGURE 67-18** Kasai portoenterostomy. **A,** The dissection of fibrous extrahepatic biliary remnant is continued up to the capsular surface of the liver within the bifurcation of the portal vein (*arrows* indicate fibrous portal plate; yellow vessel loops mark lateral dissection margins). **B,** Completed Roux-en-Y portoenterostomy. (From Nathan JD, Ryckman FC: Biliary atresia. In Chung DH, Chen MK [eds]: Atlas of pediatric surgical techniques, Philadelphia, 2010, Elsevier Saunders, pp 220–231.)

which intestinal bacteria can ascend and colonize the bile ducts. Unfortunately, if the Kasai procedure is unable to reestablish bile flow, and liver failure and/or cirrhosis ensue, liver transplantation is indicated.

### Outcomes

Kasai hepatoportoenterostomy does not cure BA, which will inevitably progress in more than 70% of infants who undergo this procedure. The rate with which the disease progresses, as evidenced by cirrhosis and portal hypertension, is variable, but may be expedited by recurrent cholangitis. It is estimated, however, that 80% of those who have successfully undergone a Kasai procedure can live up to 10 years before liver transplantation is needed. In those infants who undergo transplantation, outcomes are good, with 10-year graft survival and overall patient survival of 73% and 86%, respectively.[27]

## Choledochal Cysts

Choledochal cysts are cystic dilations of the common bile duct (CBD), and are rare. They have an incidence of 1 in 100,000 to 150,000 live births, with a 3:1 to 4:1 female-to-male preponderance. They are classified based on location and their frequency varies (Fig. 67-19). Type I (50% to 80%) is a simple cyst that can involve any portion of the CBD and type II (2%) describes a diverticulum arising off the CBD. Termed *choledochoceles,* type III cysts (1.4% to 4.5%) consist of dilation confined to the distal intrapancreatic portion of the CBD. Although type IV (15% to 35%) involves intrahepatic and extrahepatic bile ducts, type V (20%) is limited to the intrahepatic ducts only. Choledochal cysts can be associated with other congenital anomalies, including duodenal and colonic atresia, imperforate anus, pancreatic arteriovenous malformation, and pancreatic divisum.[28] Moreover, choledochal cysts are considered premalignant lesions.

### Pathogenesis

The pathogenesis of choledochal cysts remains unknown, but one well-established hypothesis is that pancreaticobiliary reflux allows for the activation of pancreatic enzymes within the duct. The subsequent inflammatory response compromises the integrity of the duct wall, which eventually results in dilation. In support of this theory, amylase and trypsinogen levels in the bile from patients with choledochal cysts are often elevated.[28] Another theory is that these cysts arise from CBD obstruction, which can occur with functional obstruction at the sphincter of Oddi.

### Clinical Presentation and Diagnosis

The classic triad of jaundice, a palpable right upper quadrant mass, and abdominal pain is seen in less than 20% of patients, but 85% of children have at least two of these symptoms on presentation. Patients younger than 12 months generally present with obstructive jaundice and abdominal masses, whereas older patients complain of pain, fever, nausea with vomiting, and jaundice. Common complications include cholangitis, pancreatitis, and bile peritonitis secondary to cyst rupture.[28] Abdominal ultrasound can reveal a cystic mass that is separate from the gallbladder and also allows for anatomic assessment of the biliary tree. When the diagnosis is unclear, a HIDA scan can be used because it will show absent filling of the cyst initially, followed by uptake in the cyst, and finally delayed emptying into the duodenum. CT is a useful modality for defining the intrahepatic biliary anatomy and evaluating the distal CBD and pancreatic head. Moreover, it has better resolution with regard to confirming continuity of the cyst with the CBD. Rarely, ERCP and/or MRCP is needed for preoperative confirmation of the diagnosis but, when necessary, MRCP is preferred, given the potential complications and invasiveness associated with ERCP.

### Treatment and Outcomes

Prompt excision of the cysts is recommended. Following cyst excision, a Roux-en-Y hepaticojejunostomy is performed for reconstruction. Complete excision is important because the risk of a primary malignancy is as high as 6% with a retained choledochal cyst. If the cyst cannot be completely excised because of scarring from chronic inflammation, the cyst should be

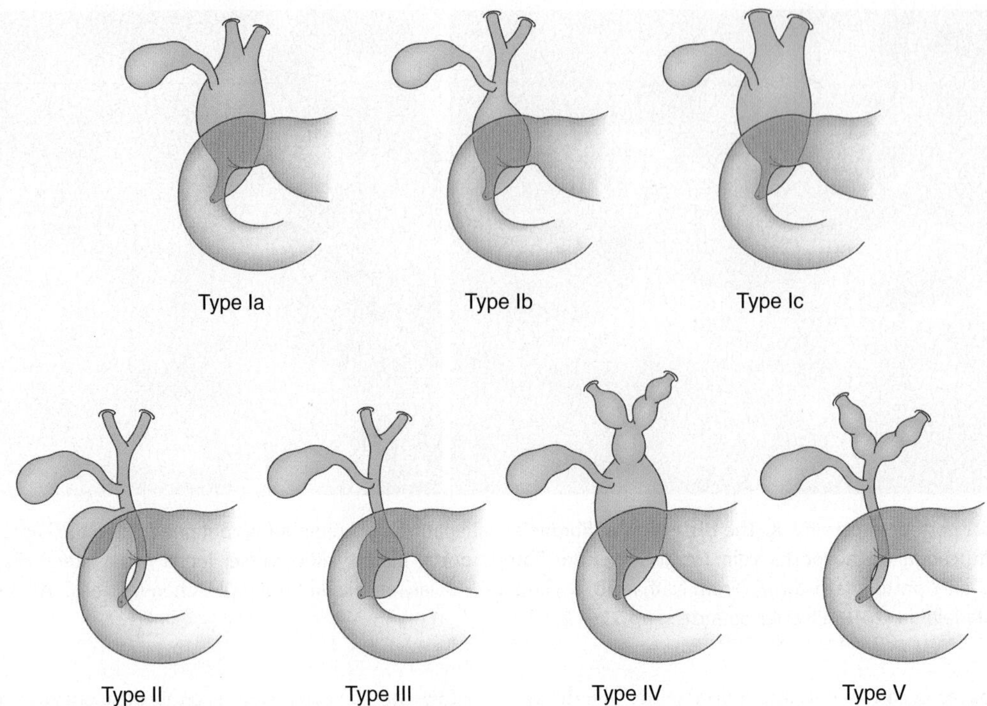


**FIGURE 67-19** Classification of choledochal cyst. (From O'Neill JA: Choledochal cyst. In Grosfeld JL, O'Neill JA, Fonkalsrud EW, et al [eds]: Pediatric surgery, ed 6, Philadelphia, 2006, Mosby Elsevier, pp 16–21.)

enucleated. These patients should be monitored via ultrasound. Postoperative anastomotic strictures are a common complication and probably arise from chronic intrahepatic cholelithiasis and recurrent cholangitis. Aside from this, outcomes are generally good.

### Hereditary Pancreatitis and Pancreas Divisum

Hereditary pancreatitis is an autosomal dominant disorder with a high degree of penetrance. It is rare, representing less than 1% of instances of chronic pancreatitis. The disease results from a mutation in the cationic trypsinogen gene *(PRSS1),* which leads to an increase in the autoactivation of trypsin and resistance to deactivation. The gene has been mapped to chromosome 7q35; the two most common allelic mutations are *R122H* and *N29I.*[29] Recurrent bouts of pancreatitis usually begin in childhood, between 5 to 10 years of age, with no identifiable cause. Aside from the age of onset, the presentation, natural history, diagnosis, and treatment of this disease are similar to those for other causes of pancreatitis.

Hereditary pancreatitis should be suspected in any patient who experiences at least two bouts of acute pancreatitis without obvious risk factors, such as trauma, hyperlipidemia, gallstones, or pancreas divisum. It should also be considered in any child with acute pancreatitis and a family history of this disease and in children with an unexplained episode of pancreatitis that requires admission. Making the correct diagnosis is important because there is an extremely high lifetime risk of malignancy. It is estimated that these patients have a 50- to 70-fold increase in the risk of developing pancreatic adenocarcinoma within 7 to 30 years of disease onset. The cumulative lifetime risk is estimated to be 40% by the age of 70 years.[29] Therefore, screening by endoscopic ultrasound is recommended, starting at 30 years of age.

Pancreas divisum is a congenital anatomical anomaly in which the ventral and dorsal pancreas fail to fuse. The resultant pancreas has dual drainage, with the dorsal pancreas draining through the duct of Santorini and the ventral pancreas (head and uncinate process) draining through the duct of Wirsung. The onset of symptoms is variable, ranging from early childhood to adulthood. Although ultrasound and CT are usually performed, ERCP is frequently used to confirm the diagnosis. However, MCRP has been touted as more advantageous because it can delineate the dorsal pancreatic duct in its entirety, as opposed to ERCP, which can only assess the ventral duct on cannulation of the major duodenal papilla. The significance of pancreas divisum and its predisposition to chronic pancreatitis remains controversial. Some have suggested that it may result in pancreatitis because all pancreatic output is forced to empty through the smaller lesser papilla. The result is an outflow obstruction that leads to ductal dilation. Treatment consists of transduodenal sphincteroplasty or a Puestow procedure (pancreaticojejunostomy); the latter is preferred if the dorsal pancreatic duct is dilated or obstructed.

## ABDOMINAL WALL

### Abdominal Wall Defects

Anterior abdominal wall defects are a relatively frequent neonatal surgical condition in pediatric surgery. During normal development of the human embryo, the midgut herniates outward through the umbilical ring and continues to grow. By the 11th week of gestation, the midgut returns to the coelomic cavity and undergoes proper rotation and fixation, along with closure of the umbilical ring. If the intestine fails to return, the infant is born with the abdominal contents protruding directly through the umbilical ring, with an intact sac covering the abdominal

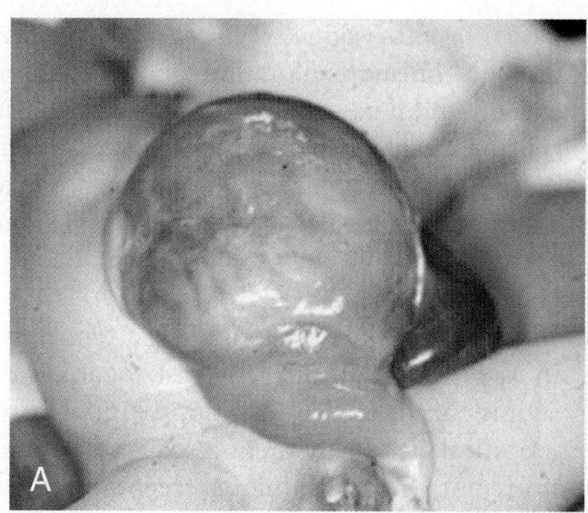


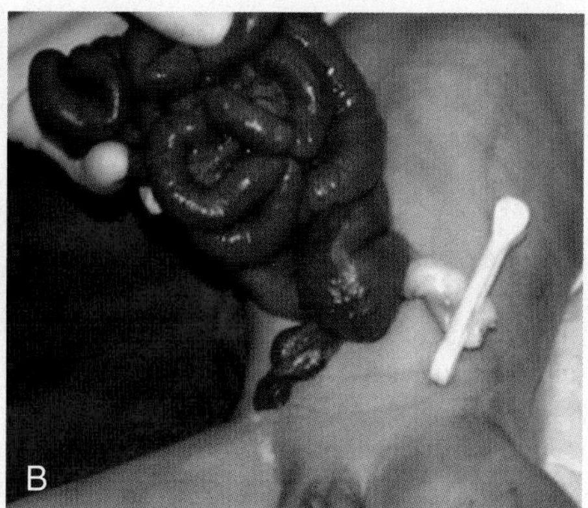


**FIGURE 67-20** Abdominal wall defects. **A,** Omphalocele with intact sac. **B,** Gastroschisis with eviscerated multiple bowel loops to the right of the umbilical cord.

viscera, termed an *omphalocele* (Fig. 67- 20*A*). In contrast, gastroschisis represents the abdominal wall defect, which is always to the right of an intact umbilical cord, and without sac covering the abdominal viscera (see Fig. 67-20*B*). No specific causes for abdominal wall defects have been identified.

### Omphalocele

At birth, omphalocele is recognized as a central defect of the abdominal wall. Its fascial defect is generally more than 4 cm in diameter with an intact membranous sac, which is composed of an outer layer of amnion and an inner layer of peritoneum. Defects less than 4 cm in diameter are arbitrarily designated as hernias of the cord. Infants with an omphalocele exhibit an approximately 50% incidence of associated anomalies. Beckwith-Wiedemann syndrome represents a combination of gigantism, macroglossia, and an umbilical defect, either hernia or omphalocele. Chromosomal abnormalities such as trisomy 13, 15, 18, and 21, have also been associated with omphalocele. Other major associated anomalies include exstrophy of the bladder or cloaca and the pentalogy of Cantrell—omphalocele, anterior diaphragmatic hernia, sternal cleft, ectopia cordis, and intracardiac defect, such as ventricular septal defect.

Neonatal treatment of omphalocele begins with the preservation of the intact sac with sterile, moistened, saline gauze or transparent bowel bag. IV fluid should be promptly started, along with gastric tube decompression and IV antibiotics. Great care should be taken to prevent hypothermia. A thorough diagnostic workup should be performed to identify associated anomalies. Primary surgical closure of the small to medium-sized defect is preferred. Alternative options to primary closure include prosthetic patch closure (e.g., Gore-Tex), porcine small intestinal submucosa-derived biomaterial (e.g., Surgisis, Cook Medical Bloomington, In), skin flap closure, or placement of a silo for sequential reduction and staged closure. Giant omphaloceles may be treated by topical application of escharotic agents such as povidone-iodine (Betadine) ointment, merbromin (Mercurochrome), or silver nitrate, allowing the sac to thicken and epithelialize gradually. The overall survival for infants with omphalocele depends on the size of the defect and severity of associated anomalies.

### Gastroschisis

The gastroschisis defect is usually just to the right of the umbilical cord, at the site of the obliterated right umbilical vein. The fascial defect is typically approximately 4 cm in diameter. Because of the absence of a sac and direct exposure of the intestine to amniotic fluid in utero, the intestine is often thickened, edematous, and foreshortened. Associated anomalies are rare but intestinal atresia is present in up to 15% of cases. Infants born with gastroschisis should be carefully handled to avoid injury to exposed bowel loops and minimize fluid losses. Typically, infants are placed in a warm, saline-filled plastic organ bag up to the nipple line. This allows for gross inspection of eviscerated bowel at all times and also lessens fluid losses. One should be cautious for potential volvulus of eviscerated malrotated intestine. IV fluids are started at 1.5 times maintenance along with IV antibiotics. In general, fluid requirements are greater than those required for omphalocele because of increased fluid losses. An orogastric tube is placed to decompress the stomach.

For primary closure, bowel loops are reduced and the fascia and skin are approximated. For defects requiring a prosthetic patch closure, a Gore-Tex patch can be used and the skin closed over it. Recently, other biomaterial substitutes (e.g., AlloDerm, LifeCell, Branchburg, NJ; Surgisis) have been used, with variable success.[30] If the viscera cannot be reduced into the abdomen, a silo is placed at the bedside and the eviscerated intestines are reduced serially over 5 to 7 days, followed by operative fascial closure. During the immediate postoperative period, if the abdominal wall closure is tight, patients may require paralysis along with frequent volume boluses to maintain adequate tissue perfusion and to prevent metabolic acidosis. Patients are often maintained on TPN until they gain bowel function. In cases of associated intestinal atresia or stenosis, inflammation of the bowel may preclude an immediate repair. Hence, the abdominal wall is repaired in a usual fashion and intestinal pathology is addressed in 6 to 8 weeks, when the inflammation resolves. Late occurrence of NEC has been reported in up to 20% of patients after gastroschisis repair.[31] Undescended testes are also present in 10% to 20% of infants born with gastroschisis. When found outside the coelomic cavity, the testes should be manually placed into the abdominal cavity at the time of abdominal wall closure or silo bag placement. They should be followed for a period of time to monitor potential spontaneous descent into the scrotum. If not, orchidopexy should be performed. Almost all infants have a prolonged postoperative ileus. Although TPN has been a lifesaving maneuver, it is associated with a high incidence of cholestasis and cirrhosis. One of the most difficult challenges in the management of gastroschisis remains dealing with dysfunctional intestine and/or short gut syndrome, which occurs despite adequate surgical closure of the abdominal wall defect.

## Hernias

### Inguinal Hernia

Inguinal hernia repair is one of the most common surgical procedures in pediatric surgery. The incidence of inguinal hernia, which is almost all indirect and congenital in nature, is approximately 3% to 5% in term infants and 9% to 11% in premature infants. It affects boys approximately six times more often than girls. Sixty percent of inguinal hernias occur on the right side, 30% are on the left side, and 10% are bilateral. The processes vaginalis is an elongated diverticulum of the peritoneum, which accompanies the testicle on its descent into the scrotum; it generally obliterates during the ninth month of gestation, or soon after birth. The variable persistence of the processes vaginalis results in a spectrum of clinical presentations, including a scrotal hernia with protrusion of intestine, ovaries, omentum, or communicating hydrocele, with intermittent accumulation of peritoneal fluid. All communicating hydroceles are repaired in the same manner as an indirect inguinal hernia.

**Diagnosis and Clinical Presentation** Diagnosis is established by clinical history and examination alone, especially when the contents of the hernia reduce into the peritoneal cavity. Communicating hydroceles can be difficult to reduce at times, and therefore can be misdiagnosed as simple hydroceles. Transillumination of the scrotum to distinguish a hydrocele from a hernia can also be misleading because a gas-filled herniated bowel loop can easily be transilluminated. Palpation of the cord may elicit a silk glove sign, which is produced by rubbing the opposing peritoneal membranes of the empty sac. At times, palpation of a thickened cord in comparison to the contralateral side, and a reliable history are sufficient to confirm a diagnosis. The acute development of hydrocele may also be associated with the onset of other conditions such as epididymitis, testicular torsion, and torsion of testicular appendage. In these clinical settings, ultrasound may be helpful to determine the diagnosis. The major risk factor of inguinal hernia is bowel incarceration, with potential strangulation. The incidence of incarceration is higher in premature infants in the first year of life.

**Treatment: Surgical Management** Although early hernia repair may be associated with a higher risk for injury to the cord structures, recurrence rate, and postoperative apneic episodes, most pediatric surgeons advocate operative repair prior to discharge from the hospital for premature infants because of their significant risks for incarceration. However, for those infants diagnosed after hospital discharge, elective hernia repair may be deferred until the infant is beyond 52 weeks postconceptional age, when postoperative apnea risk decreases. In patients presenting with incarcerated inguinal hernia, unless there is clinical evidence of peritonitis, attempts are made to reduce the hernia. Manual reduction is successful in up to 70% of cases. Once reduced, the patient is admitted for observation and hernia repair is performed at 24 to 48 hours, when local tissue edema resolves. A nonreducible incarcerated hernia should be promptly explored in the operating room. Routine contralateral inguinal exploration at the time of symptomatic hernia repair for infants is standard practice based on the high incidence of contralateral patent process vaginalis (4% to 65%). However, the issue regarding the routine exploration of the asymptomatic contralateral side in toddlers remains unresolved. Most pediatric surgeons routinely explore the asymptomatic contralateral side in children 2 years of age or younger; some surgeons extend the contralateral exploration criteria to those up to 5 years of age.

### Umbilical Hernia

In general, umbilical hernia has a tendency to close on its own in approximately 80% of cases, and therefore elective repair should be deferred until approximately 5 years of age. Also, umbilical hernia is rarely associated with significant complications but there are unique exceptions to this general rule, for which an earlier elective repair should be considered. Although rare, a history of incarceration clearly warrants prompt surgical repair, irrespective of age. Enlarging umbilical hernia over time, in particular with a large skin proboscis more than 3 cm, or a significantly large umbilical fascial defect (>2 cm) is unlikely to resolve spontaneously; therefore, surgical repair should be considered at an early age.

## CHEST WALL DEFORMITIES

The two major types of congenital chest wall deformities are pectus excavatum and pectus carinatum. Pectus excavatum is the most common type, five times more common than pectus carinatum (Fig. 67-21*A*). Its incidence is estimated at approximately 1 in 100 children, with a male-to-female ratio of 3 : 1 to 4 : 1. The deformity is usually present at birth and becomes more prominent during the first few years of life. It can become more pronounced between 8 and 10 years of age, and later again during puberty. It is also common to have associated kyphosis and scoliosis. Although the exact cause is unknown, abnormalities of costal cartilage development have been implicated most frequently. Pectus excavatum can be associated with congenital heart disease, including mitral valve prolapse, Ehlers-Danlos syndrome, and Marfan syndrome; therefore, thorough preoperative evaluation, such as ophthalmologic evaluation and echocardiography, must be considered. Asthma is also common, but it is unknown whether asthma contributes to the development of the defect or occurs as a result of it.

## Evaluation

To determine the severity of pectus excavatum and assess the indications for surgery, two or more of the following criteria should be met: (1) Haller index more than 3.2; (2) pulmonary function studies indicating restrictive or obstructive airway disease; (3) cardiology evaluation showing that the compression is causing mitral valve prolapse, murmurs, or conduction abnormalities; and (4) documentation of progression of deformity. Despite these objective criteria, the most common indication for surgery in patients with pectus deformities is cosmetic. This is a critical issue, particularly for adolescents with significant concerns regarding body image and development of self-esteem. A recent multicenter study has shown that surgical repair of pectus excavatum significantly improves body image and perceived ability for physical activity.[32]

### Preoperative Evaluation

A complete history and physical examination are obtained on all patients and they are encouraged to perform exercises to strengthen the chest and back muscles and maintain proper

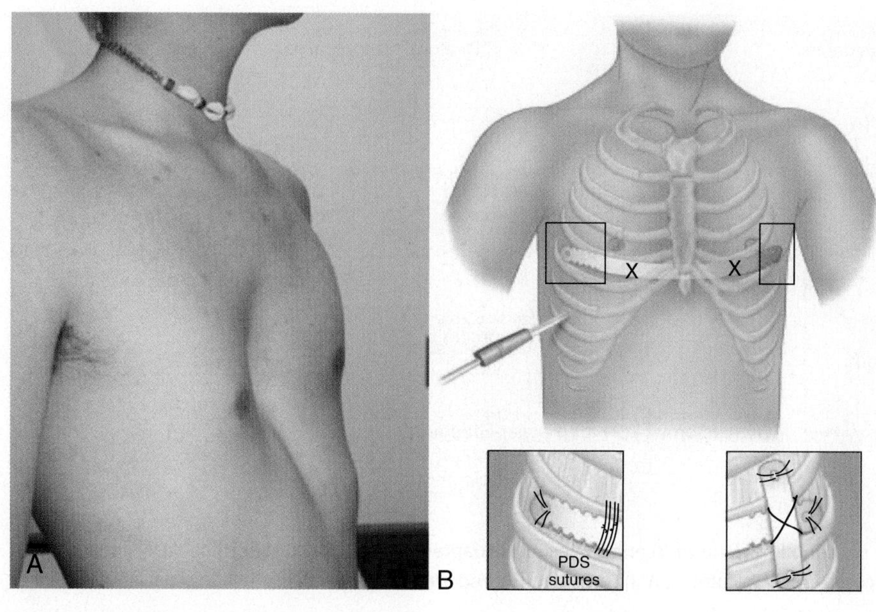


**FIGURE 67-21 A,** Pectus excavatum, **B,** A bar is placed beneath the sternum and secured onto the chest wall using stabilizers. (From Goretsky MJ, Nuss D: Surgical treatment of chest wall deformities: Nuss procedure. In Chung DH, Chen MK [eds]: Atlas of pediatric surgical techniques, Philadelphia, 2010, Elsevier Saunders, pp 97–103.)

posture. Standard anteroposterior and lateral chest radiographs are essential to serve as a baseline of the degree of deformity and detect the presence of thoracic scoliosis. Pulmonary function studies are important to document restrictive or obstructive abnormalities. If a heart murmur is detected on physical examination, echocardiography is indicated. A plain chest radiograph or CT scan allows for the calculation of a Haller index by dividing the measured transverse diameter of the chest by the anteroposterior diameter to document the severity of the defect more objectively.

### Treatment: Surgical Management

The optimal age for pectus excavatum repair is 10 to 14 years because the chest wall is still soft and malleable. Also, recovery seems faster in this age group. After puberty, the chest wall is more rigid, thus requiring a longer period of bar support, even with the insertion of two bars. Presently, there are two main methods for operative correction. The Ravitch technique was originally described in 1949 and remains as the standard against which other procedures are compared. This procedure is applied to patients with excavatum or carinatum deformities; it consists of a transverse skin incision overlying the deformity, bilateral subchondral resection of abnormal costal cartilages, sternal osteotomy, and anterior fixation of the sternum with a retrosternal stainless steel strut. The strut is removed as a secondary procedure in 6 to 12 months. The results are excellent.

As described by Nuss, a minimally invasive technique has been developed for pectus excavatum, in which a C-shaped bar is passed in a retrosternal plane from one hemithorax into the other through two lateral intercostal incisions (see Fig. 67-21*B*). The bar is then flipped so that the convexity is outward, and the chest wall defect is immediately corrected. The bar is left in place for approximately 2 years. This technique avoids the creation of pectoral flaps, cartilage resection, and sternal osteotomy, thus significantly lowering surgical morbidity. A multicenter prospective study has demonstrated that surgical repair for pectus excavatum can be performed safely with adequate pain management.[33] Pectus carinatum, or pigeon or chicken breast, occurs much less frequently than pectus excavatum. Preoperative considerations are similar to those for pectus excavatum. It is surgically repaired by open costal cartilage resection and sternal fixation, similar to that for pectus excavatum. Although moderate success can be achieved with external brace application for pectus carinatum,[34] there is compliance difficulty with teenage patients wearing an external brace for 16 to 18 hours daily.

## GENITOURINARY TRACT CONDITIONS

### Cryptorchidism

Cryptorchidism is a condition in which one or both testes fail to descend into the scrotum before birth. Up to 30% of preterm infants can present with an undescended testis, but it also occurs in approximately 3% of full-term infants. Some undescended testes eventually descend by 1 year of age, but are unlikely to descend after this time. The undescended testis is associated with histologic and morphologic changes as early as 6 months of age; atrophy of Leydig cells, decrease in tubular diameter, and spermatogenesis can also occur by 2 years of age. A true undescended testis has had its descent halted somewhere along the path of normal descent and can be found in the inguinal canal at exploration. A retractile testis is a normally descended testis that retracts into the inguinal canal, but can be brought down into the scrotal sac during the examination. It is thought to result from a hyperreflexive cremasteric muscle contraction and should be managed nonoperatively. Nonpalpable testes may include an intra-abdominal, absent, or vanishing testis. Ectopic testis have had an aberrant path of descent; these can be found in perineal, femoral canal, and suprapubic regions.

#### Diagnosis and Treatment

Although ultrasound has been used increasingly to evaluate for undescended testis, an examination by an experienced surgeon has a higher sensitivity for locating an undescended testis. For a unilateral palpable testis in the inguinal canal, standard dartos pouch orchidopexy is performed. The recommended timing for this procedure is at or near 1 year of age. A general management algorithm for nonpalpable testes is shown in Figure 67-22. For a nonpalpable unilateral testis, diagnostic laparoscopy is useful.

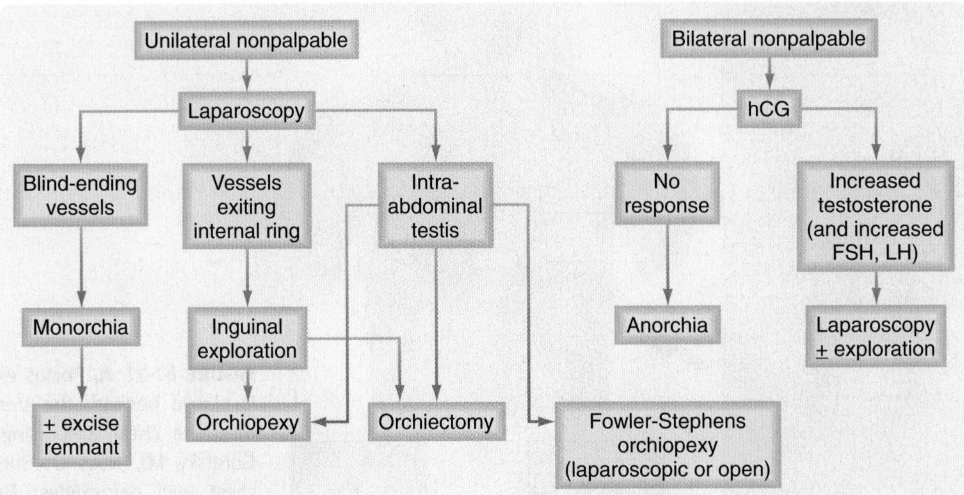


**FIGURE 67-22** Algorithm for the management of nonpalpable undescended testes. (Adapted from Lee KL, Shortliffe LD: Undescended testis and testicular tumors. In Ashcraft KW, Holcomb GW, Holcomb GW III, Murphy PJ: Pediatric surgery, ed 4, Philadelphia, 2005, Elsevier Saunders, pp 706–716.)

If the testicular vessels are seen exiting the internal ring, an open inguinal orchidopexy is performed. For an intra-abdominal testis, two-stage Fowler-Stephen orchidopexy can be considered, in which testicular vessels are ligated as a first stage to allow collateral circulation to develop for 6 months before performing orchidopexy as a second stage of the procedure. However, single-stage laparoscopic orchidopexy is being performed with increasing frequency for intra-abdominal testes. If both testes are nonpalpable, a human chorionic gonadotropin (hCG) stimulation test is carried out to confirm the presence of functioning testicular tissues. If present, diagnostic laparoscopy is performed to determine surgical therapy.

For nonpalpable testes, laparoscopy has proven to be useful, with 95% sensitivity. The risk of malignancy has been reported to be significantly greater for men with a history of undescended testes. Although orchidopexy does not decrease the malignancy risk associated with undescended testes, it allows for earlier detection. Nonseminomatous germ cell tumors are usually associated with undescended testes.

## Testicular Torsion

Torsion of the testis is the most common genitourinary tract emergency of childhood. The serious underlying pathogenesis is acute arterial ischemia; prompt surgical detorsion with testicular fixation is the mainstay of therapy. Extravaginal torsion is more common in neonates, in whom there can be torsion of the spermatic cord along its course outside the tunica vaginalis. Intravaginal torsion is associated with bell clapper deformity, in which the suspended testis can twist to torsion. Torsion of the testis occurs most frequently in late childhood and early adolescence, with a peak incidence at 14 years of age. Scrotal pain that is abrupt or gradual in nature is the primary symptom. On examination, the involved testis may be high-riding, edematous, and significantly tender. The presence of other urinary tract symptoms such as frequency, urgency, dysuria, and fever tend to occur more frequently with infectious or inflammatory conditions such as epididymitis; however, in no way does this it rule out testicular torsion. In most cases, a careful history and physical examination are sufficient to confirm the diagnosis of testicular torsion. However, if the diagnosis is unclear, prompt ultrasonography may be helpful to determine vascular flow to the testicles. Radioisotope scanning is the most specific diagnostic test but it can be more time-consuming to obtain. The time for diagnosis and surgical repair directly correlate with the testicular salvage rate. Immediate surgical detorsion via a scrotal medial raphe approach is the treatment of choice. The affected testis is detorsed, assessed for viability, and fixed to the scrotum. In all cases, the contralateral testis should also be fixed in the scrotum. For torsion of less than 6 hours, 90% of testes can be salvaged. However, this salvage rate significantly decreases to less than 10% with more than 24 hours of symptoms.

## Testicular Tumors

Testicular cancer accounts for less than 2% of all pediatric solid tumors. The peak incidence is 2 years of age, with a second peak during puberty. These tumors typically present as a painless scrotal mass, often discovered incidentally. An ultrasound examination is useful but CT is critical to evaluate for retroperitoneal lymphadenopathy and chest or abdominal metastatic disease. Serum tumor markers are useful for diagnosis and for follow-up. For example, α-fetoprotein (AFP) is a glycoprotein produced by the fetal yolk sac and its level is elevated in yolk sac tumors of the testes; β-hCG is produced by embryonal carcinomas and mixed teratomas. The most common prepubertal testicular cancer is of germ cell origin; yolk sac tumor, also known as *endodermal sinus* tumor, and embryonal carcinomas account for almost 40%. Children with yolk sac tumors present with elevated serum AFP levels and tumors are typically localized to the testis. The standard surgical approach is radical inguinal orchiectomy. The role of retroperitoneal lymph node dissection with yolk sac tumor is controversial. Tumors with microscopic node involvement or nodal disease require systemic chemotherapy, with modified retroperitoneal lymphadenectomy. The overall survival from yolk sac tumors is approximately 70% to 90%.

## SOLID TUMORS OF CHILDHOOD

### Neuroblastoma

Neuroblastoma is the most common extracranial solid tumor in infants and children, representing 8% to 10% of all childhood tumors and 15% of all cancer-related deaths in the pediatric population.[35] There are approximately 600 new diagnoses reported annually. Although 90% of cases are diagnosed before the age of 5 years, 30% of those are diagnosed in the first year of life. The median age at diagnosis is 22 months.

#### Involved Sites and Clinical Presentation

Arising from neural crest cells, neuroblastoma is a malignancy of the sympathetic nervous system and therefore occurs in sympathetic ganglia. Almost 65% of tumors are found in the abdomen, with 50% localized to the adrenal medulla. They can also occur in the neck (5%), chest (20%), or pelvis (5%), and 1% of patients have no detectable primary.[35] A patient's clinical presentation varies with tumor location, size, extent of invasion, metabolic activity, and presence of paraneoplastic syndromes. Many patients are asymptomatic, although it is not uncommon for some to present with constitutional symptoms (e.g., malaise, fevers, weight loss), an enlarging mass, pain, abdominal distention, lymphadenopathy, or respiratory distress. Pelvic masses may cause constipation or bladder dysfunction, whereas thoracic lesions can cause dysphagia or dyspnea. For cervical tumors, a patient may develop Horner's syndrome or stridor and, in up to 15% of patients, epidural involvement may result in neurologic deficits, which, when progressive, can lead to paralysis.

At diagnosis, 50% of patients have localized disease and 35% already have regional lymph node spread. Metastasis to distant organs (e.g., liver, bone, skin) occurs by hematogenous and lymphatic routes. For bone marrow invasion, patients may become anemic, bruise easily, and complain of weakness. Bony metastasis can result in pain, swelling, limp, and pathologic fractures. The orbits are frequently involved, which manifests as periorbital swelling and proptosis (raccoon eyes). When dissemination occurs to the skin, patients develop blue subcutaneous nodules associated with the blueberry muffin syndrome. With its neuroendocrine characteristics, neuroblastoma can secrete catecholamines, resulting in early-onset hypertension and tachycardia.[36] Patients may also experience paraneoplastic syndromes, which include intractable diarrhea caused by vasoactive intestinal peptide secretion, encephalomyelitis, and neuropathy. Opsoclonus-myoclonus syndrome—rapid, conjugate eye nystagmus with involuntary spasms of the limbs—although rare, occurs when antibodies cross-react with cerebellar tissue.

#### Genomics

Neuroblastoma occurs as whole chromosome gains, which result in hyperdiploidy and are associated with a favorable prognosis, or segmental chromosomal aberrations, which encompass *MYCN* amplification and gains or losses that tend to be associated with worse outcomes. The *MYCN* oncogene, which is amplified at chromosome 2p24 in 25% of cases, is overexpressed in 30% to 40% of stage 3 and 4 neuroblastomas, but only in 5% of localized or stage 4S tumors. Therefore, it is used as a biomarker for disease stratification. It has been shown that deletion of the 1p36 region occurs in 70% of tumors and is usually associated with *MYCN*-amplified, high-stage tumors that confer a poor prognosis.[37] Conversely, a whole chromosome 17 gain is associated with a good prognosis. Deletions of chromosome 11q have been identified in 15% to 22% of neuroblastomas and are also associated with unfavorable patient outcomes and a reduced time of progression-free survival.

#### Diagnosis

An initial workup includes basic serum tests, imaging studies, and determination of levels of urine catecholamine or their metabolites (e.g., dopamine, vanillylmandelic acid, homovanillic acid). Patients may have elevated levels of nonspecific biomarkers such as lactate dehydrogenase (>1500 U/mL), ferritin (>142 ng/mL), and neuron-specific enolase (>100 ng/mL), which have been associated with advanced stage and/or relapse. For confirmation, CT is the gold standard because it serves to localize the tumor and determine the degree of involvement (Fig. 67-23*A*). Ultrasonography may be used to initially

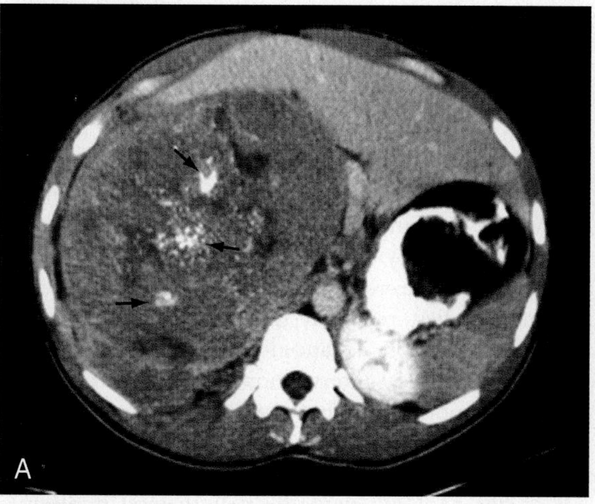


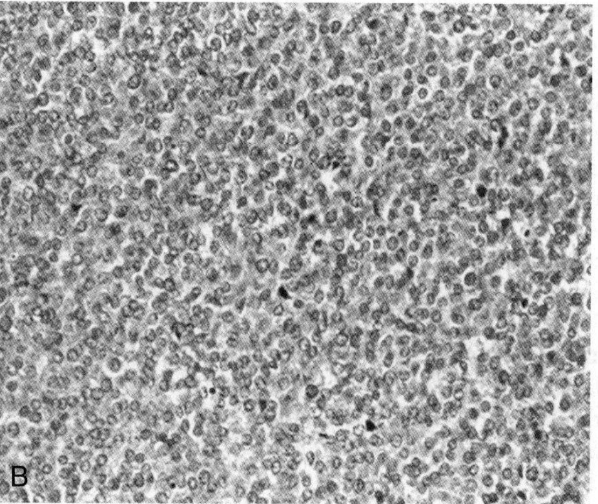


**FIGURE 67-23 A,** CT scan of neuroblastoma demonstrating areas of calcification *(arrows).* **B,** Classic small blue round cells of undifferentiated hyperchromatic neuroblasts. (**A** from Kim S, Chung DH: Pediatric solid malignancies: Neuroblastoma and Wilms' tumor. Surg Clin North Am 86:469–487, 2006.)

**Table 67-3 International Neuroblastoma Staging System**

| STAGE | DEFINITION |
|---|---|
| 1 | Localized tumor with complete gross excision, with or without microscopic residual disease; representative ipsilateral lymph nodes negative for tumor microscopically (nodes attached to and removed with the primary tumor may be positive). |
| 2A | Localized tumor with incomplete gross excision; representative ipsilateral nonadherent lymph nodes negative for tumor microscopically. |
| 2B | Localized tumor with or without complete gross excision, with ipsilateral nonadherent lymph nodes positive for tumor; enlarged contralateral lymph nodes must be negative microscopically. |
| 3 | Unresectable unilateral tumor with contralateral regional lymph node involvement or midline tumor with bilateral extension by infiltration (unresectable) or by lymph node involvement. |
| 4 | Any primary tumor with dissemination to distant lymph nodes, bone, bone marrow, liver, skin, and/or other organs (except as defined for stage 4S). |
| 4S | Localized primary tumor (as defined for stage 1, 2A, or 2B), with dissemination limited to skin, liver, and/or bone marrow (limited to infant <1 yr of age). |

characterize the mass. MRI may be useful if there is concern for spinal extension, and imaging of the brain is only needed in the setting of neurologic symptoms. Although not routinely used, a $^{131}$I- metaiodobenzylguanidine (MIBG) scan is valuable in the detection of primary tumor and metastases because a norepinephrine analogue is selectively concentrated in sympathetic tissue. The $^{131}$I-MIBG scan is also used for the surveillance of treatment response and recurrence. The diagnosis of neuroblastoma is made by demonstrating undifferentiated small round blue cells on histologic section (see Fig. 67-23*B*). Specimens can be obtained during resection of the primary tumor for stage 1 or 2 disease or as a biopsy from the unresectable disease and/or bone marrow. Molecular studies, such as fluorescent in situ hybridization, can be performed on tissue samples to note ploidy, *MYCN* amplification, and presence of other chromosomal abnormalities. This information is required to outline specific risk category–based therapy for individual patients.

### Staging

Neuroblastoma can be classified based on the degree of neuroblastic differentiation and mitosis-karyorrhexis index (MKI; low, intermediate, or high). Histologically, neuroblastoma has limited Schwann cell production, is stroma-poor, and has abundant neuroblasts.[36] The modified Shimada classification, on which the International Neuroblastoma Staging System (INSS; Table 67-3) is based, has been used to predict prognosis based on the histopathology of the tumor and age of the patient. This system takes into account the degree of cell differentiation, MKI, and presence of Schwann cells. The Children's Oncology Group currently stratifies patients into low-, intermediate-, or high-risk categories based on patient age at diagnosis, INSS stage, tumor histopathology, DNA index, and *MYCN* amplification status.[38] Thus, treatment recommendations depend on the patient's stage.

### Treatment

The standard multimodality therapy is based on disease risk classification and treatment stratification (Table 67-4). Induction chemotherapy consists of a multidrug regimen, including but not limited to cyclophosphamide, doxorubicin, cisplatin, carboplatin, etoposide, and vincristine. The goal of induction chemotherapy is to achieve remission and reduce the tumor burden, allowing for a more complete resection. However, many aggressive neuroblastomas acquire resistance to chemotherapeutic agents, thus resulting in a high relapse rate. This usually necessitates autologous hematopoietic stem cell transplantation. Surgery is recommended based on the ability to obtain a complete resection. Resection is correlated with a reduced risk of local recurrence, especially in combination with induction chemotherapy and local radiotherapy. Thus, some advocate that surgical resection should be considered only after adjuvant therapy because it increases the degree of complete excision and decreases morbidity. Based on results from outcomes studies, resection is recommended for stage 1 to 2B tumors. For more advanced-stage neuroblastoma (stages 3 and 4), initial surgical intervention is limited to an open or laparoscopic tumor biopsy. For stage 4S infants, surgical resection is not recommended because of the high rate of spontaneous differentiation and regression.

**Table 67-4 Patient Risk Group Categories for Neuroblastoma**

| RISK GROUP | STAGE | FACTORS |
|---|---|---|
| Low | 1 | |
| | 2 | <1 yr<br>>1 yr, low N-*myc*<br>>1 yr, amplified N-*myc;* favorable histology |
| | 4S | Favorable biology* |
| Intermediate | 3 | <1 yr, low N-*myc*<br>>1 yr, favorable biology* |
| | 4 | <1 yr, low N-*myc* |
| | 4S | Low N-*myc* |
| High | 2 | >1 yr, all unfavorable biology* |
| | 3 | <1 yr, amplified N-*myc*<br>>1 yr, any unfavorable biology* |
| | 4 | <1 yr, amplified N-*myc*<br>>1 yr |
| | 4S | Amplified N-*myc* |

*Favorable biology denotes low N-*myc,* favorable histology, and hyperdiploidy (infants).

For high-risk patients, radiotherapy is often needed for local and metastatic control. Radiation is contraindicated for intraspinal tumors because it can lead to vertebral damage, growth arrest, and scoliosis. However, it may be necessary for palliation in the setting of pain, hepatomegaly with respiratory compromise, or acute neurologic symptoms caused by tumor compression of the cord. It is further indicated when there is minimal residual disease post–induction chemotherapy and resection. The combination of chemotherapy, surgery, and radiation therapy has resulted in a local relapse rate lower than 10%.[39]

### Outcomes

The overall outcomes in patients with neuroblastoma have improved somewhat over the last 30 years, with 5-year survival rates rising from 52% to 74%.[38] The improvement is the result of improved cure rates in the low-risk group, which has survival rates of up to 92%. It is estimated that 50% to 60% of patients in the high-risk group experience relapse and, accordingly, have only seen a modest decrease in mortality.[38] Taken together, their overall survival rates remain dismal (~20% at 5 years), despite more aggressive therapies.

## Wilms' Tumor

Wilms' tumor (WT), also known as *nephroblastoma,* is an embryonal renal neoplasm consisting of metanephric blastema; it accounts for 85% of cases.[40] It represents 5.9% of all pediatric malignant tumors and has an annual incidence of 7.6 cases/million children younger than 15 years. There are 500 reported new cases annually and approximately 75% of WT cases are diagnosed in children younger than 5 years. The peak incidence occurs at 2 to 3 years. Of all patients, 13% can present with a bilateral tumor, which is usually synchronous in 60% of cases.

### Causes and Genomics

Divided into overgrowth and nonovergrowth disorders, a number of syndromes can predispose to the development of WT. These include Beckwith-Wiedemann (macroglossia, macrosomia, midline abdominal wall defects, and neonatal hypoglycemia), Li-Fraumeni (*p53* germline mutation with predisposition to various cancers), and Denys-Drash (gonadal dysgenesis, nephropathy, and WT) syndromes and neurofibromatosis. In 10% of patients, WT can be associated with other congenital anomalies, collectively known as *WAGR syndrome* (aniridia, hemihypertrophy, genitourinary malformations, and mental retardation).[41]

The WT suppressor gene *WT1* is located on chromosome 11p13, which contains genes responsible for the development of the kidney, genitourinary tract, and eyes. Mutations in *WT1* result in genitourinary abnormalities such as cryptorchidism and hypospadia but also increase the risk of developing WT. Aniridia is found in 1.1% of WT patients and, when *WT1* deletions are found in these patients, there is a 40% rate of WT development. Moreover, mutations in *WT2,* located at 11p15, have been linked to Beckwith-Wiedemann syndrome, and there is a 4% to 10% risk of developing WT in those who also have hemihypertrophy. A recent study has determined that the X-linked tumor suppressor gene *WTX* can be inactivated in up to one third of WT cases.[41] The exact significance of this finding remains unknown.

### Clinical Presentation

WT is typically discovered incidentally during a physical examination or because parents palpate an abdominal mass. Other presenting symptoms include abdominal pain and hematuria, which may signify tumor invasion into the collecting system or ureter. Another 25% develop hypertension, which is thought to occur secondary to disturbances in the renin-angiotensin feedback loop. Fewer than 10% of patients have atypical presentations; these include varicocele, hepatomegaly caused by hepatic vein obstruction, ascites, and congestive heart failure. WT may also be associated with predisposing syndromes and the index of suspicion in these cases should be high, with a low threshold to obtain a screening ultrasound study.

### Diagnosis

Ultrasonography is initially performed to determine whether the tumor is actually of renal origin, is cystic or solid, or extends into renal vein or IVC. An abdominopelvic CT scan can also achieve similar results while helping differentiate WT from neuroblastoma (Fig. 67-24). This study also evaluates for metastases, adenopathy, and adjacent structural involvement. Equally important, the contralateral kidney and/or bilaterality of disease can be assessed. MRI is also a useful adjunct for evaluating intravascular invasion; however, an ultrasound study may be preferred. Lung metastases, which are present in 8% at the time of diagnosis, can be identified on an initial chest radiograph. A chest CT could be used as well, although its use is controversial in those with normal chest x-rays.

### Pathology

The histology of WT is categorized as favorable or unfavorable. Favorable histology is more common, characterized by the presence of three elements—blastemal, stromal, and epithelial cells. Tumors with predominantly epithelial differentiation behave less aggressively and tend to be stage I when diagnosed early. Blastemal-predominant tumors tend to be clinically aggressive and are associated with advanced disease. Outcomes are correlated with histopathology and tumor stage. Unfavorable histology is defined by the presence of anaplasia, clear cell sarcoma, or rhabdoid tumor. Anaplastic WT can be focal or diffuse and is synonymous with unfavorable histology whenever it is encountered. It is associated with an increased risk of tumor recurrence and resistance to standard chemotherapy. Nephrogenic rests are

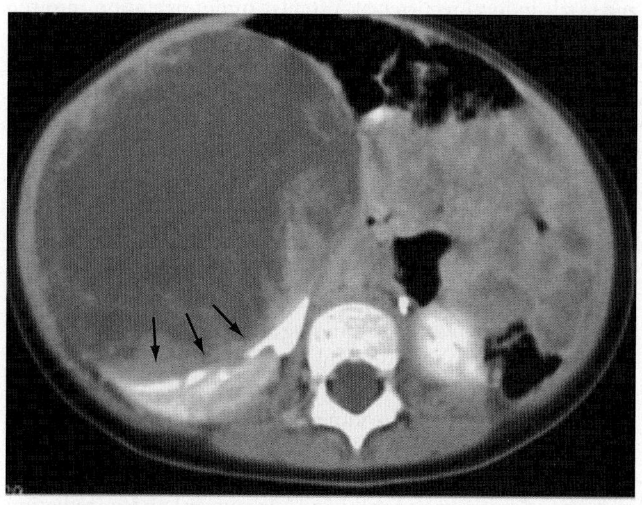

**FIGURE 67-24** CT image of Wilms' tumor with a claw sign *(arrows).* (From Kim S, Chung DH: Pediatric solid malignancies: Neuroblastoma and Wilms' tumor. Surg Clin North Am 86:469–487, 2006.)

**Table 67-5 National Wilms' Tumor Study Group Staging System**

| STAGE | DEFINITION |
|---|---|
| I | Tumor limited to the kidney and completely excised without rupture or biopsy. Surface of the renal capsule is intact. |
| II | Tumor extends through the renal capsule but is completely removed, with no microscopic involvement of the margins. Vessels outside the kidney contain tumor. Also placed in stage II are cases in which the kidney has undergone biopsy before removal or where there is local spillage of tumor (during resection) limited to the tumor bed. |
| III | Residual tumor is confined to the abdomen and of nonhematogenous spread. Includes tumors with involvement of the abdominal lymph nodes, diffuse peritoneal contamination by rupture of the tumor extending beyond the tumor bed, peritoneal implants, and microscopic or grossly positive resection margins. |
| IV | Hematogenous metastases at any site. |
| V | Bilateral renal involvement. |

precursor lesions found in 25% to 40% of kidneys with WT, but do not have oncologic potential. Instead, they can undergo differentiation and spontaneously regress through unclear mechanisms.

### Staging

Stage is one of the most important criteria in the therapeutic and prognostic consideration of WT. The International Society of Pediatric Oncology (SIOP) staging system is based on preoperative chemotherapy, but is applied postresection. The presence of metastases is evaluated at presentation, relying on imaging studies, and chemotherapy is instituted prior to operative intervention. The National Wilms' Tumor Study Group (NWTSG) has also developed a staging system that incorporates the clinical, surgical, and pathologic information that was obtained at the time of resection but stratifies patients prior to the initiation of chemotherapy (Table 67-5). The advantage of this system is that it favors stage-based therapy, thereby avoiding unnecessary chemotherapy in patients who might not otherwise benefit from it.[42]

### Treatment

The mainstay of therapy for WT is surgery and chemotherapy. Surgical exploration is necessary for formal staging and a radical nephrectomy is the standard. Utmost care must be taken to ensure en bloc resection because contamination and tumor spillage result in local recurrence. Vascular tumor extension into the IVC constitutes stage III disease and is managed accordingly. Sampling of the hilar, para-aortic, and paracaval lymph nodes is critical. Nephron-sparing surgery is usually reserved for children with a solitary kidney or bilateral WT. In these patients, preoperative chemotherapy may be used to induce tumor shrinkage to allow for a more complete resection. However, there is an increased risk of positive surgical margins and local tumor recurrence. Partial nephrectomy may be considered if the tumor involves only one pole of the kidney, there is no evidence of collecting system or vascular involvement, clear margins exist between the tumor and surrounding structures, and the involved kidney demonstrates appreciable function. Unfortunately, less than 5% of patients meet these criteria, and it is uncertain whether this approach provides any long-term benefit.[41] According to NWTSG recommendations (Box 67-2), the typical chemotherapy regimen consists of vincristine and dactinomycin, with the addition of doxorubicin (Adriamycin) and/or radiation therapy based on tumor stage and histologic favorability. The SIOP advocated the use of preoperative chemotherapy to improve cure and disease-free survival rates at 5 years.

**BOX 67-2 Treatment Regimens for Wilms' Tumor***

- Stage I (FH, focal anaplasia): Surgery, VA × 18 wk, no XRT
- Stage II (FH): Surgery, VA × 18 wk, no XRT
- Stage II (focal anaplasia): Surgery, VDA × 24 wk, XRT to tumor bed
- Stage III (FH, focal anaplasia): Surgery, VDA × 24 wk, XRT to tumor bed
- Stage III (focal anaplasia): Surgery; VDA × 24 wk, XRT to tumor bed
- Stage IV (FH; focal anaplasia): Surgery, VDA × 24 wk, XRT to tumor bed according to local tumor stage, and lung and/or other metastatic sites
- Stages II-IV (diffuse anaplasia): Surgery, VDEC × 24 wk, XRT to whole lung and abdomen
- Stages I-IV (clear cell sarcoma): Surgery, VDEC × 24 wk, XRT to abdomen; whole lung for stage IV only
- Stages I-IV (rhabdoid tumor): Surgery, ECCa × 24 wk, XRT

*A,* Dactinomycin; *C,* cyclophosphamide; *Ca,* carboplatin; *D,* doxorubicin; *E,* etoposide; *FH,* favorable histology; *I,* ifosfamide; *V,* vincristine; *XRT,* radiation therapy.

*National Wilms' Tumor Study. Infants <11 mo are given half the recommended dose of all drugs.

### Outcomes

The overall survival for children with WT has improved from 30% to almost 90% of patients now exhibiting a 5- to 7-year survival. Survival rates of patients with stage I or II favorable history or stage I unfavorable histology are approximately 95%. For patients with unfavorable histology, stages II, III, and IV are associated with 70%, 56%, and 17% 4-year survival rates, respectively. Similar to neuroblastoma, this improvement can be attributed to advances in diagnosis, imaging, improved staging, and appropriate risk-stratified treatment.

## Rhabdomyosarcoma

Derived from embryonic mesenchymal cells that can later differentiate into skeletal muscle, rhabdomyosarcoma is a soft tissue malignancy that accounts for approximately 4% of all pediatric malignancies. The incidence is 4.3 cases/million children, with approximately 350 new cases diagnosed annually.[43] With a bimodal peak incidence, children are affected between the ages of 2 and 5 years and again from 15 to 19 years of age. Almost 50% are diagnosed before the age of 5 years. Most cases occur sporadically, with no recognizable risk factors, although rhabdomyosarcoma is known to occur with increased frequency in patients with neurofibromatosis type I and Li-Fraumeni, and Beckwith-Wiedemann syndromes.

### Sites of Involvement

Rhabdomyosarcoma can appear at any site in the body, including those that do not typically contain skeletal muscle. The most common sites in children are the head and neck (35%), genitourinary tract (25%), and extremities (20%). Less common primary sites include the trunk, GI tract, intrathoracic, and perineal regions. Head and neck lesions tend to occur in the parameningeal region, orbits, and pharynx. Other specific sites include the bladder, prostate, vagina, uterus, liver, biliary tract, paraspinal region, and chest wall.

### Pathology

Rhabdomyosarcoma has been pathologically classified into three types. embryonal, alveolar, and pleomorphic. Embryonal rhabdomyosarcoma is the most common, accounting for more than two thirds of all rhabdomyosarcomas. Two subtypes of embryonal rhabdomyosarcoma—botryoides and spindle cell—appear to be associated with a better prognosis than others of similar histology. On examination of a sample, characteristic rhabdomyoblasts may be present; immunohistochemical staining for muscle-specific proteins, such as myosin and actin, desmin, and myoglobin, can bolster the diagnosis.

### Clinical Presentation

Manifestations of rhabdomyosarcoma depend on its size, location, age of the patient, and presence of metastatic disease. The mass is typically asymptomatic, although most symptoms are related to compressive effects and can result in pain. Orbital tumors can produce proptosis, decreased visual acuity, and ophthalmoplegia. Those arising from parameningeal sites frequently produce headaches and nasal or sinus obstruction that can be accompanied by a mucopurulent or bloody discharge. Moreover, these tumors can invade intracranially to produce cranial nerve palsies. For genitourinary rhabdomyosarcoma, paratesticular tumors may present as painless swelling in the scrotum, which may be confused with a hernia, hydrocele, or varicocele. Bladder tumors, commonly located at the base and trigone, result in hematuria and urinary obstruction. Prostate tumors can cause polyuria and constipation caused by compression of the bladder or bowel. Vaginal tumors in girls present with a protruding mass or vaginal bleeding and discharge.

In the case of extremity rhabdomyosarcoma, distal involvement is more common than proximal, and the lower extremities are more commonly involved than the upper extremities. These tumors present as a painless mass, and some children may develop a limp or disuse of the affected limb. At the time of diagnosis, almost 50% of patients have regional lymph node metastasis. Retroperitoneal tumors can grow large, making them difficult to resect. Symptoms arise secondary to invasion of adjacent structures and the associated pain and distention are typical late features of disease. Biliary tract tumors comprise 0.8% of all rhabdomyosarcomas and, like other signs of biliary obstruction, patients present with jaundice, abdominal swelling, fever, and loss of appetite.

### Diagnosis and Staging

The patient should be thoroughly examined and diagnostic imaging and basic laboratory studies performed. With concern for parameningeal involvement, cerebrospinal fluid should also be evaluated. There are no specific serum tumor markers for diagnosis. Depending on tumor location, MRI or CT should be used to characterize the mass better and evaluate for adjacent structural invasion, vessel encasement, metastasis, and adenopathy. One of the most critical aspects of the diagnostic process is obtaining tissue for histologic confirmation, which is usually accomplished by an incisional or core needle biopsy. On confirmation, surgical resection can be completed, although it may necessitate preoperative chemotherapy for tumor shrinkage. It should also be noted that during preoperative planning, the biopsy site should also be excised because there can be local recurrence. Based on histologic variances, rhabdomyosarcoma subtypes are associated with prognosis. For example, botryoid (cluster of grapes) and spindle cell sarcomas are noted to have a favorable prognosis, embryonal and pleomorphic histologies have an intermediate prognosis, and alveolar and undifferentiated histologies exhibit a poor prognosis.

Pretreatment staging serves to stratify patients, determine the most appropriate treatment regimen, and compare outcomes. Because it relies on preoperative imaging, this is technically clinical staging, although it is still based on TNM criteria (Box 67-3). It should be stressed that intraoperative or pathologic results from resected samples should have no bearing on patient stage. This is reserved for what is known as *clinical grouping*, which consists of selection into a group depending on operative findings, pathology, margins, and node status. Taken together, clinical grouping and pretreatment staging have been shown to correlate with outcomes. For example, low-risk patients have an estimated 3-year failure-free survival rate of 88%, intermediate-risk patients have an estimated 3-year failure-free survival rate of 55% to 76%, and high-risk patients have a 3-year failure-free survival rate less than 30%.

### Treatment

The main goal of therapy is to achieve cure or, if that is not feasible, at least to obtain local control. This requires a multimodality approach, with a combination of surgery, chemotherapy, and radiation therapy. Equally important is the need to minimize the short- and long-term effects of therapy. Currently,

**BOX 67-3 Staging for Rhabdomyosarcoma**

Group I: Localized disease that is completely resected, with no regional node involvement

Group II

- A: Localized, grossly resected tumor with microscopic residual disease but no regional nodal involvement
- B: Locoregional disease with tumor-involved lymph nodes with complete resection and no residual disease
- C: Locoregional disease with involved nodes, grossly resected, but with evidence of microscopic residual tumor at the primary site and/or histologic involvement of the most distal regional node (from the primary site)

Group III: Localized, gross residual disease including incomplete resection, or biopsy only of the primary site

Group IV: Distant metastatic disease present at time of diagnosis all patients with rhabdomyosarcoma receive some combination chemotherapy because it improves progression-free and overall survival. The recommended regimen depends on the risk stratification, with low-risk patients in subgroup A receiving vincristine and dactinomycin. For patients in the low-risk subgroup B and higher, cyclophosphamide is added to this therapy. Radiation therapy has been found to be effective for the local control of rhabdomyosarcoma, especially in patients who have microscopic disease after resection. It has also been successfully used in patients in whom surgery could result in significant disfigurement, such as with head and neck lesions. However, complications of radiation therapy are not negligible, including the potential development of secondary malignancies.

As is the case with most surgical approaches, a complete resection with negative margins and nodal sampling is the mainstay of treatment. The specific operative guidelines depend on the location of the tumor. For example, for head and neck tumors that are superficial and nonorbital, wide excision of the primary tumor with sampling of ipsilateral cervical lymph nodes is acceptable. Parameningeal lesions are particularly difficult to resect completely, given their degree of extension into critical structures. In these patients, and in patients with tumors that are considered unresectable, chemotherapy and radiation therapy are first-line treatment. For extremity lesions, it is important to achieve complete resection through wide local excision. Amputation is rarely necessary, except for distal tumors in the hand or foot that involve neurovascular structures. Given that trunk and extremity lesions have a high incidence of lymph node metastasis, sentinel lymph node mapping is being increasingly recommended. Reexcision may also be considered with evidence of minimal residual disease after initial resection. Patients with extremity tumors receive combination chemotherapy but, because of the high incidence of the alveolar histology, radiotherapy is also often used. Finally, the approach for patients with genitourinary tumors depends on which organ is affected. Preservation of bladder function is the key in resection of tumors involving the bladder or prostate. If this goal cannot be met, preoperative chemoradiation is usually recommended. If residual disease remains despite this, more aggressive measures can be considered, including a partial cystectomy, prostatectomy, or anterior (rectum-sparing) exenteration. Patients with paratesticular rhabdomyosarcoma should undergo a radical inguinal orchiectomy with a retroperitoneal lymph node dissection in boys younger than 10 years because of the frequent prevalence of metastasis. When the tumor is clearly fixed to scrotal skin, resection is required. Chemotherapy is standard, whereas radiation therapy is indicated only with positive nodes. For patients with vaginal or vulvar rhabdomyosarcoma, vaginectomy and wide local excision, respectively, and multiagent chemotherapy are recommended.

#### Outcomes

Approximately 15% of children present with metastatic disease and their prognosis remains poor. Approximately 30% of patients with rhabdomyosarcoma will relapse, and 50% to 95% of them will die as the disease progresses. Median survival from the first recurrence is 0.8 years, with an estimated 5-year survival rate of only 17%. Despite this harrowing data, however, rhabdomyosarcoma is a curable disease in most children, with more than 60% surviving 5 years after diagnosis. Survival for children with this malignancy has improved secondary to a number of factors, including better imaging and pathologic classification, use of multiagent chemotherapy, and appropriate use of radiotherapy.

### Liver Tumors

Primary tumors of the liver are rare in the pediatric population and are malignant in approximately 60% of cases. The two most common tumors are hepatoblastoma (HB) and hepatocellular carcinoma (HCC). HB represents approximately 80% of all malignant liver neoplasms and 1% of all pediatric malignancies. The peak incidence of HB occurs at 3 years of age; the median age for children with HCC is 10 to 11.2 years. This correlates with the observation that more than 90% of patients younger than 5 years with primary liver tumors are found to have HB, whereas 87% of those between 15 and 19 years have HCC.[44]

#### Causes and Risk Factors

Patients with familial adenomatous polyposis, Gardner's, and Beckwith-Wiedemann syndromes are at increased risk of developing HB. HCC is associated with acquired hepatitis B and C and has been observed in children with several types of congenital diseases, including tyrosinemia, glycogen storage disease type I, $\alpha_1$-antitrypsin deficiency, and cholestasis caused by BA.

#### Clinical Presentation

HB typically presents as a painless but palpable abdominal mass. Other symptoms are nonspecific and include anorexia, weight loss and failure to thrive, abdominal pain, anemia, and abdominal distention. Jaundice is not commonly encountered because liver function remains intact. Some patients present with fever and it is possible for the tumor to rupture, leading to intra-abdominal bleeding and peritonitis. HCC presents similarly, although stigmata of cirrhosis, such as jaundice, spider angiomas, ascites, and splenomegaly, may be encountered. Almost 25% of patients have metastatic spread to abdominal and mediastinal lymph nodes, lung, bone marrow, and brain.

#### Diagnosis and Staging

Basic laboratory blood tests usually reveal normal liver function in HB, whereas there will be abnormalities in HCC. There may be evidence of anemia; thrombocytopenia or pancytopenia can be found with splenomegaly caused by sequestration. AFP levels are elevated in more than 70% of patients and also correspond to HB and HCC disease activity. An elevated AFP level is not pathognomic and, depending on the age of the patient, other disease processes must be ruled out. For example, in infants younger than 6 months, elevated AFP levels may also be seen in sarcomas, yolk sac tumors, and hamartomas. Finally, all children who are being evaluated for HCC should be screened for exposure to and subsequently tested for hepatitis B and C.

Abdominal ultrasonography is an excellent initial diagnostic study. Doppler ultrasound can also detect the presence of tumor extension into or thrombosis of major vessels—namely, the hepatic veins, IVC, and portal vein. For better resolution, a helical CT is critical in assessing the relationship of the tumor to adjacent vital structures, such as bile ducts and vessels, and exclude intra-abdominal tumor extension beyond the liver. An MRI can similarly be used in this setting. Because HB frequently spreads hematologically to the lungs, chest CT should also be performed. Bone scintigraphy is recommended for staging in children with HCC because of the high incidence of bone

**Table 67-6 Liver Tumor Staging**

| STAGE | DEFINITION |
|---|---|
| I | Tumors confined to the liver and completely resectable |
| II | Tumor resection with microscopic residual disease (i.e., positive margins), tumor rupture, or tumor spillage at the time of operation |
| III | Unresectable or only partially resectable at the initial operation because of gross residual tumor or presence of regional lymph node involvement |
| IV | Distant organ metastases |

metastases. HB characteristically appears as a unifocal mass surrounded by a pseudocapsule; it may be a pure epithelial type that contains fetal or embryonal cells or a mixture of the two histologic subtypes, which contains mesenchymal tissue in addition to epithelial components. On the other hand, HCC is characterized by large, pleomorphic epithelial cells that appear much like mature hepatocytes. Grossly, HCC forms multifocal nodules that lack a fibrous tumor and often lead to diffuse intrahepatic involvement. Unlike adults, there has been no indisputable evidence that histopathology has any bearing on prognosis.

A standard TNM system (Table 67-6) has been used for staging purposes, but much effort has been placed into the development of a pretreatment staging system, known as the *pretreatment evaluation of tumor extension* (PRETEXT) *staging system*. Spearheaded by the SIOP group, the PRETEXT system divides the liver into four sections and the tumor is subsequently classified based on the number of tumor-free sections of liver. This system takes caudate lobe involvement, tumor rupture, ascites, extension into the stomach or diaphragm, tumor focality, lymph node involvement, presence of distant metastases, and vascular involvement into further consideration. Thus, patients are considered high risk if they meet the following criteria: serum AFP level higher than 100 ng/mL, extension beyond the liver, distant metastases, intraperitoneal hemorrhage, and invasion of the hepatic veins, IVC, or portal vein.

### Treatment

Unlike other pediatric solid tumors, liver transplantation is a surgical option for patients with unresectable disease. Neoadjuvant chemotherapy is used for tumor reduction in the hope that it can aid in a more complete resection. Interestingly, some advocate the use of preoperative chemotherapy to treat what would otherwise be residual microscopic disease left behind postresection. They argue that doing so eliminates tumor cells that could respond to hepatotrophic factors during liver regeneration, thereby decreasing the risk of recurrence.

There are two currently acceptable approaches to HB, tumor resection followed by chemotherapy and tumor biopsy followed by chemotherapy and delayed resection. Stage I patients with pure fetal histology usually do not receive postoperative chemotherapy. However, patients who are stage II or higher or who have any other type of histology do require this. The current chemotherapy regimen consists of cisplatin, 5-fluorouracil, and vincristine. For patients with residual tumor after resection, chemotherapy should be coupled with an evaluation for transplantation.[45] Criteria for transplantation include having no more than three tumors smaller than 3 cm in diameter, and no evidence of extrahepatic disease or vascular invasion. When relapses occur, doxorubicin, irinotecan, and ifosfamide have been used, often with some success. Another modality being used with variable success in children whose tumors are unresponsive to systemic chemotherapy is direct arterial chemotherapy and/or chemoembolization. Long-term outcomes have yet to be determined.

### Outcomes

Long-term disease-free survival of more than 85% to 90% can be achieved for resectable HB, although similar estimates have been seen noted for patients with unresectable HB treated by liver transplantation. The same cannot be said for HCC, in which survival rates with partial hepatectomy remain poor because of relapse. Nonetheless, in the past decade, early transplantation has been shown to result in better outcomes in experienced transplantation centers.

## Teratoma

Teratomas are typically benign neoplasms that contain elements derived from more than one of the three embryonic germ layers, endoderm, mesoderm, and ectoderm. By definition, they are comprised of tissue that is foreign to the anatomic site in which they are found. Although teratomas may occur anywhere along the midline, they are usually found in sacrococcygeal, mediastinal, retroperitoneal, and gonadal locations. Teratomas may be solid, cystic, or mixed and are classified as mature or immature. Although the latter can be potentially malignant, the incidence of malignant transformation in mature teratomas is low. There is a preponderance based on gender; almost 80% of all teratomas occur in females. Moreover, location has been associated with age, as evidenced by the fact that extragonadal tumors occur primarily in neonates and young children, whereas gonadal tumors are more commonly noted in adolescents.

### Sacrococcygeal Teratomas

Sacrococcygeal teratomas (SCTs) account for 60% of all teratomas and can present as large exophytic masses in utero. In such cases, they are detected on prenatal ultrasound. Complications include polyhydramnios and fetal hydrops, which can result in fetal demise caused by a tumor-induced vascular steal syndrome that leads to high-output heart failure. In infants and children, symptoms can include weakness, paralysis, bowel or bladder dysfunction, and other neurologic symptoms that may indicate intradural spinal extension. Because the mass is usually external and visible (Fig. 67-25*A*), the diagnosis is usually made by inspection. If the AFP or β-hCG level is elevated, yolk sac or choriocarcinoma components, respectively, make up the teratoma. Ultrasonography, CT, or MRI may be necessary to detect intra-abdominal lesions or determine whether there is pelvic or abdominal extension.

Surgical resection is the standard of care and should be performed promptly because of the risk of hemorrhage and tumor rupture. Operative planning must take into account the degree of intra-abdominal extension. Most tumors can be resected by a posterior approach, in which a Chevron incision allows for the division of the gluteal muscles, ligation of the blood supply, and en bloc resection of the tumor and coccyx (see Fig. 67-25*B*). It is important to preserve the anorectal complex to maintain long-term continence. External tumors

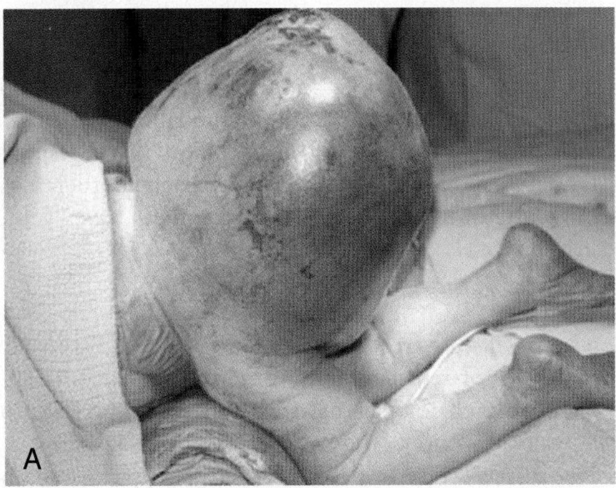

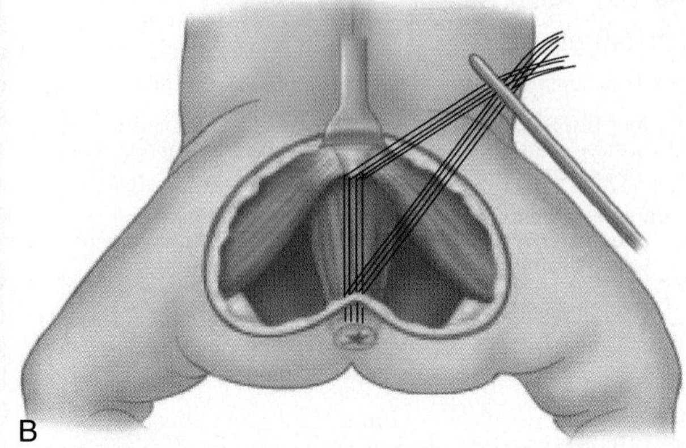

**FIGURE 67-25** **A,** Sacrococcygeal teratoma. **B,** Levator ani and gluteal muscles are reconstructed and a drain left in place. (**B** from Dicken BJ, Rescorla FJ: Sacrococcygeal teratoma. In Chung DH, Chen MK [eds]: Atlas of pediatric surgical techniques, Philadelphia, 2010, Elsevier Saunders, pp 364–373.)

with significant intra-abdominal extension require a combined abdominal and posterior approach, whereas teratomas that are entirely intra-abdominal may be approached via laparotomy or laparoscopy.

Outcomes have been favorable from survival and quality of life standpoints. The age of diagnosis is the most important factor; those diagnosed at less than 30 weeks' gestation or after 2 months postnatally tend to have a poor prognosis. The risk of malignancy associated with embryonal histology is 15% to 20%. Risk of local recurrence ranges from 4% to 11%, although failure to resect the coccyx is associated with a 37% risk of recurrence. Monitoring AFP levels at 3-month intervals for 3 to 4 years has been strongly recommended; if the mass recurs, reexcision is performed after a formal evaluation for staging purposes, given the high risk of malignancy.

## Ovarian Neoplasms

Approximately 50% of all ovarian lesions in children are neoplastic, but are rarely malignant. It is estimated that ovarian malignancies comprise 10% of all ovarian masses but only 1% of childhood cancers. Primary ovarian malignancies can be classified as germ cell, epithelial cell, and sex cord stromal tumors. Germ cell tumors include teratomas and choriocarcinoma; sex cord stromal tumors consist of granulosa (thecal) and Sertoli (Leydig) cells. Epithelial cell tumors encompass serous and mucinous cystadenomas and cystadenocarcinomas.[46] Symptoms are usually pain-related because of mass compression. The presence of ascites, omental masses, peritoneal or diaphragmatic implants, adherence to surrounding organs, aortoiliac adenopathy, size more than 8 cm, or contralateral ovarian mass should raise suspicion for malignancy.

### Types

**Germ Cell Tumors** An ovarian teratoma is the most common ovarian germ cell tumor. It also represents the most common pediatric ovarian neoplasm and accounts for 25% of all childhood teratomas. These tumors occur with equal frequency in either ovary and may even be bilateral in 10% of patients. They typically present with abdominal or pelvic pain and may involve ovarian torsion in approximately 25% of patients. Germ cell tumors account for 7% to 80% of all neoplastic ovarian masses. Dysgerminomas are the least differentiated of the germ cell tumors and are bilateral in 10% to 15% of cases. Although pure dysgerminomas are malignant, they tend to present while still localized and are highly responsive to chemoradiation. Survival is almost 90% with complete surgical resection.

**Sex Cord Tumors** Sex cord tumors arise from the stromal elements of the ovary, producing hormones that may result in precocious puberty. Interestingly, these tumors have been associated with Peutz-Jeghers syndrome. Abnormal menstruation, swelling, and pain are common chief complaints. Outcomes after resection are good in this group because most lesions are still limited to the ovary. Advanced-stage tumors are responsive to platinum-based chemotherapy. Granulosa cell tumors account for 1% to 10% of ovarian malignancies in females under the age of 20, whereas Sertoli-Leydig cell tumors account for 20% of ovarian sex cord stromal tumors. Because they are androgenic, serum testosterone metabolite levels can be elevated. With estrogen excess, patients develop early sexual characteristics, such as breast or labial enlargement, axillary and pubic hair growth, and/or galactorrhea.

**Epithelial Tumors** Less than 20% of ovarian tumors in childhood are epithelial in nature, given that they are rare before menarche. The two main histologic subtypes include serous and mucinous tumors, which can be further described as benign, malignant, or borderline malignant. It is possible to classify the subtypes as adenoma or adenocarcinoma; the latter is extremely rare but is associated with a poor prognosis.

### Diagnosis

Aside from a thorough physical examination and routine laboratory studies, AFP and β-HCG levels should be determined because they help provide information about tumor biology and can be used to measure treatment response. Although nonspecific, the lactate dehydrogenase level may also be elevated. Also, if there is any evidence of menstrual abnormalities or precocious puberty, luteinizing hormone (LH) and follicle-stimulating hormone (FSH) levels should also be checked. Abdominal ultrasound is performed to evaluate the tumor and contralateral ovary. It is not uncommon to obtain a CT scan, which will provide information regarding tumor extension, regional adenopathy, and metastasis.

### Treatment

Surgery is the mainstay of therapy and aims to ensure complete resection, with preservation of reproductive function when possible. Definitive treatment is oophorectomy or salpingo-oophorectomy. Care should be taken to resect the tumor without disrupting the capsule or spilling tumor contents, because this will result in upstaging of malignant lesions. Ascitic fluid, if present, should be tested for cytologic evidence of tumor. Intraoperatively, time should be taken to inspect the diaphragm, peritoneal surfaces, and omentum to look for ovarian implants, which, when present, should be biopsied for staging and treatment purposes. According to the staging system of the International Federation of Gynecology and Obstetrics, the liver, peritoneum, omentum, and contralateral ovary should be closely examined and suspicious lesions should be biopsied or resected. Bilateral retroperitoneal, iliac, para-aortic, and perirenal lymph nodes should be sampled for appropriate staging. Finally, ascites or peritoneal washings should be sent for cytology.[46] Chemotherapy is indicated for any ovarian tumor with extension beyond the affected ovary, which is often the case with germ cell and epithelial cell tumors. The combination of low-dose bleomycin, etoposide, and cisplatin treatment in patients with stage II disease has resulted in event-free and overall survival rates, of 87.5% and 93.8%, respectively.

### Summary

Solid tumors in children represent a challenging therapeutic problem but, with advances in diagnosis, staging, and treatment, outcomes are steadily improving. However, those with high-stage disease continue to be a subpopulation that requires increasingly aggressive approaches, only to see a modest improvement in outcomes. It is this patient population that stands to gain the most as energy is focused on a better understanding of the mechanisms that drive cancer cell proliferation and metastasis so that therapy can be designed more efficaciously.

## TRAUMA

Traumatic injury, intentional or unintentional, results in more deaths in children and adolescents than all other causes combined. Most pediatric trauma occurs as a result of blunt trauma, although penetrating injury accounts for 10% to 20% of all pediatric trauma admissions with the increase in violence among 13- to 18-year-olds. It must be stressed that the pediatric patient is different physiologically from an adult counterpart, but the basic principles remain the same.

## ABCs of Trauma

Evaluation of the pediatric patient's airway is of utmost importance. A child who is crying or able to verbalize is able to protect his or her airway. If a patient is drooling, gurgling, or wheezing, one must rule out correctable causes of airway obstruction, such as a retrievable foreign object in the oropharynx. The threshold for endotracheal intubation, especially with excessive sedation, should be low. The appropriate endotracheal tube size can be estimated as being equivalent to the diameter of the child's fifth digit. Alternatively, the endotracheal tube inner diameter can be calculated by 4 plus the patient's age in years divided by 4. It should also be noted that the trachea is shorter and narrower in children, which makes intubation more challenging.

After securing the airway, attention should be focused on the patient's respiratory status. A quick assessment should be made to determine the presence of flail chest, dyspnea, tachypnea, or unequal breath sounds. Caution should be exercised when using pulse oximetry because it does not reflect proper ventilation. Next, circulation should be assessed to ensure adequate oxygen delivery. The patient should be examined for general color, capillary refill, and presence of peripheral pulses. A weak and thready pulse, along with hypotension, indicates hypovolemic shock. Blood transfusion should be considered in those with hypovolemic shock unresponsive to two boluses of 20 mL/kg crystalloid. In children younger than 6 years, intraosseous access may be considered with peripheral IV difficulties.

Once the patient has been stabilized, a secondary survey should be performed. Hypothermia must be avoided to prevent complications of coagulopathy and acidosis. A Foley catheter should be placed to monitor adequate fluid resuscitation, ensuring urine output of more than 1 mL/kg/hr. Finally, if there is no contraindication to enteral feeding, nutrition should be established early, given that there is a significant increase in metabolic demand because of a stimulated inflammatory state associated with traumatic injuries. This blunts the catabolic breakdown of glycogen and fat, stimulates immune competency, decreases infections, and reduces the risk of bacterial translocation.[47]

## Types of Trauma

### Head and Spine Injuries

Central nervous system injury is the leading cause of death among injured children. In children 2 years or younger, physical abuse, such as that seen in shaken baby syndrome, is the most common cause of serious head injury. This may manifest as retinal, subdural, or subarachnoid hemorrhages. In children aged 3 years and older, falls and motor vehicle, bicycle, and pedestrian accidents are responsible for most traumatic brain injuries (TBIs). The response to head injury in children is diffuse edema, which may be difficult to identify on an initial noncontrasted CT scan of the head. However, with time, the injury may evolve, with evidence of diffuse axonal injury, hemorrhage, or parenchymal damage. Children with a mild head injury usually complain of headache and nausea or exhibit amnesia, impaired concentration, and behavior disturbances. Up to 20% of children who sustain mild TBIs (MTBIs) can have an intracranial hemorrhage, and approximately 3% will eventually require operative intervention. There is no consensus on how to approach the child with a MTBI; many advocate the use of a screening head CT with close clinical examination. When appropriate, cerebral perfusion pressure must be monitored. Because of its transient effect and propensity to induce vasospasm, prophylactic hyperventilation should be avoided unless there is imminent concern for herniation. Aside from diuretics and hypertonic saline, a barbiturate-induced coma and hypothermia are other maneuvers that can be used to lower the intracranial pressure (ICP). If increased ICP is refractory to medical treatment, a decompressive craniectomy may be required. Lesions that result in focal neurologic symptoms or mass effect should similarly be evacuated.

Although spinal cord injuries are relatively uncommon in the pediatric population, motor vehicle accidents (MVAs) account for most traumatic spinal cord injuries. Fractures of the C1 and C2 vertebrae are commonly seen in younger children, whereas compression and chance fractures, frequently associated with improper seat belt use, are seen in older children. Spinal cord injury without radiologic abnormality (SCIWORA) is a clinical condition in which a child (<8 years of age) can present with transient neurologic deficits. It is thought to occur because incomplete vertebral ossification and ligament laxity allow the cord and nerve roots to stretch or impact on the opposing bony surfaces of the spinal canal. The use of steroids in the setting of acute spinal injury remains controversial, because it is unclear whether it improves outcomes.

### Thoracic Trauma

Thoracic injury is the second leading cause of death in pediatric trauma cases and accounts for 5% of trauma-related hospital admissions. Blunt trauma, particularly from MVAs, is responsible for most thoracic injuries. However, it should be noted that the pediatric ribs are primarily cartilaginous and are therefore more pliable. Thus, a child may present with a significant intrathoracic injury (e.g., pulmonary contusion, pneumothorax, hemothorax) without obvious evidence of rib fractures. Pulmonary contusions result in an inflammatory response with edema, atelectasis, and subsequent consolidation. Hypoxemia, hypercarbia, and tachypnea can be significant and necessitate intubation. Radiographic findings are variable and unreliable. Nonetheless, most patients respond to conservative management without long-term sequelae. Traumatic asphyxia is a rare presentation after blunt trauma, but sudden compression or crushing of the thorax can result in airway obstruction and retrograde high-pressure flow in the superior vena cava. When this occurs, patients present dramatically with head and neck cyanosis, subconjunctival hemorrhaging, and petechiae. Rib fractures in children younger than 3 years should be approached with a high index of suspicion for child abuse. Surgical exploration of the chest may be indicated with a gross bloody chest tube output of more than 20% of the patient's blood volume or an output of 2 mL/kg/hr. Intercostal artery bleeding is a common cause.

Tracheobronchial injuries usually occur near the carina and are thought to result from anteroposterior compression of the pliable pediatric chest. The patient can present with pneumothorax, pneumomediastinum, and subcutaneous emphysema. Tracheobronchial disruption results in massive air leak with potential tension pneumothorax, compromising respiratory function and venous return. Aside from hemodynamic instability, primary repair is indicated if the injury involves more than one third of the diameter of the bronchus or if nonoperative management fails. A widened mediastinum on the chest radiograph is rare in children. Most of these injuries result from blunt trauma and are found at the ligamentum arteriosum. Traumatic diaphragmatic rupture with herniation of the stomach and bowel occurs in approximately 1% of children with blunt chest trauma. Left-sided rupture is more common because the liver protects against right-sided rupture.

### Abdominal Trauma

When a seat belt sign, a bruising of the midanterior abdominal wall after an MVA, is present on a child, the CT scan should be thoroughly reviewed for any subtle signs of bowel injury and/or presence of free peritoneal fluid. The presence of intra-abdominal fluid on a CT scan without a solid organ injury should raise the index of suspicion for a hollow viscous injury. Blunt injuries to the stomach occur more frequently in children than in adults and are generally seen in children who are struck by a vehicle or who fall across bicycle handlebars. The injury is usually a blowout or perforation of the greater curvature. Usually seen in restrained children involved in MVAs, intestinal injury secondary to blunt trauma is estimated to be less than 15%. Several mechanisms can explain the injury pattern, such as rapid deceleration causing the lap belt to compress the intestines against the spine. The increase in intraluminal pressure may predispose to perforation or rupture. Small intestinal injuries occur predominantly in areas of fixation, such as at the ligament of Treitz or ileocecal valve. A duodenal or mesenteric hematoma may ensue and cause obstruction, with subsequent nausea and bilious emesis. It is not uncommon to encounter retroperitoneal injuries as well. With abdominal pain and no objective source, conservative management with serial abdominal examinations is appropriate.

**Treatment of Solid Organ Injuries** The intra-abdominal solid organs are particularly vulnerable to blunt trauma in children. Nonoperative management is the standard of care for most hemodynamically stable children with blunt solid organ injury. Those who fail nonoperative management usually do so within the first 12 hours. The American Pediatric Surgical Association (APSA) has detailed guidelines regarding the management of isolated liver and spleen injuries based on initial CT findings; these have been shown to reduce the length of hospital stay significantly, without adverse outcomes (Table 67-7). Splenic injuries are relatively common in pediatric trauma. Because of the risk of overwhelming sepsis following splenectomy, splenic injuries are managed conservatively unless there is evidence of hemodynamic instability. An ultrasound, CT scan, or red blood cell–tagged scan can be used to isolate the source of a bleed. A blush or active extravasation may prompt splenectomy. The role of splenic artery embolization in the treatment of pediatric splenic injury has not yet been fully determined. An isolated hepatic injury without involvement of the hepatic vein, IVC, or portal vein can also be managed conservatively. Some have reported that 85% to 90% of patients can successfully be treated with nonoperative management. However, those who fail do so because of hemodynamic instability, changes in clinical examination, or transfusion requirements more than 25 to 40 mL/kg/day. Findings on the initial CT scan can provide clues regarding the potential for complications, such as hemobilia or delayed rupture. Delayed bleeding after liver injury has been reported as late as 6 weeks postinjury and may be seen in 1% to 3% of patients. As is the case with splenic lacerations, one should proceed with definitive surgical treatment with any indication of hemodynamic instability.

### Pancreatic Injury

Pancreatic injuries frequently occur from blunt trauma, such as falling into bicycle handlebars. A significantly elevated level of amylase or lipase may be seen. Moreover, a CT scan is a useful diagnostic modality for evaluating most pancreatic trauma, although it can miss ductal injuries. ERCP with possible stent placement is often indicated in this setting. Operative exploration may be required to evaluate the degree of pancreatic injury

**Table 67-7 Classification of Intra-Abdominal Solid Organ Injuries**

| GRADE | LIVER | SPLEEN | KIDNEY |
|---|---|---|---|
| I | Hematoma: <10% subcapsular surface area<br>Laceration: Capsular tear <1 cm | Hematoma: <10% subcapsular<br>Laceration: Capsular tear <1 cm | Contusion: Microscopic or gross hematuria<br>Hematoma: Subcapsular, nonexpanding, no parenchymal tear |
| II | Hematoma: 10%-50% subcapsular surface area, <10 cm intraparenchymal hemorrhage<br>Laceration: Capsular tear 1-3 cm deep, <10 cm length | Hematoma: 10%-50% subcapsular surface area, <5 cm intraparenchymal hemorrhage<br>Laceration: Capsular tear, 1-3 cm parenchymal depth not involving a trabecular vessel | Hematoma: Nonexpanding perirenal hematoma confined to retroperitoneum<br>Laceration: <1 cm parenchymal depth of renal cortex without collecting system rupture or urinary extravasation |
| III | Hematoma: >50% expanding subcapsular surface area, ruptured subcapsular with active bleeding, or intraparenchymal hematoma ≥2 cm or expanding<br>Laceration: >3 cm parenchymal depth | Hematoma: Ruptured subcapsular or parenchymal hematoma; intraparenchymal hematoma >5 cm or expanding<br>Laceration: >3 cm parenchymal depth involving trabecular vessels | Laceration: >1 cm parenchymal depth of renal cortex without collecting system rupture or urinary extravasation |
| IV | Hematoma: Ruptured parenchyma with active bleeding<br>Laceration: Parenchymal disruption involving 25%-75% of hepatic | Hematoma: Ruptured parenchyma with active bleeding<br>Laceration: Hilar vessels with major devascularization (>25% of spleen) | Laceration: Parenchymal laceration extending through the renal cortex, medulla, and collecting system<br>Vascular: Main renal artery or vein injury with contained hemorrhage |
| V | Laceration: Parenchymal disruption involving >50% of hepatic lobe<br>Vascular: Juxtahepatic venous injuries (retrohepatic vena cava, central major hepatic veins) | Laceration: Completely shattered spleen<br>Vascular: Hilar vascular injury with total devascularization | Laceration: Completely shattered kidney<br>Vascular: Avulsion of renal hilum with devascularization of kidney |
| VI | Vascular: Hepatic avulsion | | |

fully, especially with concern for pancreatic necrosis. With severe ductal injury or pancreatic transaction, a distal pancreatectomy may be indicated.

### Renal Injury

The concept of nonoperative treatment has been extended to include renal injuries. Retroperitoneal injuries are frequently seen with direct blows to the back or flank and the kidney is involved in 10% to 20% of cases. In children, there is a lack of perinephric fat, which makes the kidney a susceptible target. Contusion is the most common renal injury encountered in children, whereas fracture of the renal pelvis occurs in children who have congenital renal abnormalities. Interestingly, the presence of hematuria does not correlate with the severity of renal injury. Conservative management is standard for low-grade renal injuries (grades I to III), and there is no consensus on the controversial management of high-grade renal injuries (grades IV and V). An absolute indication for renal exploration is an expanding or pulsatile hematoma. Relative indications include urinary extravasation, necrosis, and arterial injury. In the case of urinary extravasation, ureteral stenting can be attempted. Grade V injuries usually require operative management, but the salvage rate is poor.

## FETAL SURGERY

With the advent of modern prenatal care, many congenital conditions are diagnosed before birth. Although these anomalies rarely progress in such a way that fetal survival is threatened, there are cases when an intervention is warranted. Fetal surgery is a progressive field that aims to alter the natural progression of congenital disease in utero. Many of these anomalies have severe complications associated with fetal demise if left untreated. However, given the high-risk nature of the procedures themselves, selection of which patients would benefit most and how best to manage them is the key. Indications for fetal surgery include hydrops caused by CPAM, steal syndrome and cardiac failure from SCTs, and oligohydramnios with renal failure from lower urinary tract obstruction. Although initial outcomes were disappointing, recent improvements have been made in selection criteria based on outcomes research, which aims to identify patients with malformations who would see reasonable benefit from prenatal intervention. Ultrasonography continues to be the primary method of diagnosis because it is noninvasive, nonirradiating, and inexpensive. However, ultrafast MRI has become a useful imaging adjunct, particularly when the diagnosis is unclear or needs further evaluation.

### Open Fetal Surgery

Open fetal surgery was attempted in the treatment of CDH to prevent pulmonary hypoplasia and hypertension. Unfortunately, studies have shown that it did little to decrease neonatal morbidity and mortality. In high-risk fetuses with CDH complicated by thoracic herniation of the liver, reduction of the liver back into the abdomen was associated with kinking of the umbilical vein and subsequent fetal demise. Therefore, the focus has shifted to reversible tracheal occlusion with clips or endoluminal balloons to induce lung growth. Outcomes have been controversial and not significantly improved survival, with premature rupture of membranes being a frequent complication of the procedure itself.[48]

Procedures involving tracheal occlusion have led to the development of the ex utero intrapartum treatment (EXIT) procedure, which is a delivery technique used for fetuses with airway compression that may be caused by the presence of a thoracic mass. To secure the fetus' airway during delivery, the mother is given tocolytics and anesthesia to induce maximal uterine relaxation while maintaining uteroplacental circulation. This allows for an airway to be established by endotracheal intubation before the umbilical cord is clamped. After delivery, the newborn can be stabilized for postnatal interventions, when indicated.

SCT is another condition for which fetal surgery may be indicated, but reports of in utero resection are rare. The development of hydrops in a fetus with SCT is caused by high-output cardiac failure from arteriovenous shunting through the tumor. To reduce blood flow to the tumor, coagulation of the arteriovenous shunt, laser photocoagulation, and radiofrequency ablation of the feeding vessels have been used with some success in small studies. Open fetal surgery for SCT is controversial. Because most fetuses with SCT undergo postnatal resection without complication, intrauterine intervention is advocated only for those patients with symptoms related to hydrops. It is unclear whether these interventions change overall survival, given the poor prognosis associated with the development of these symptoms.

CPAM can result in hydrops and pulmonary hypoplasia when large enough. One study has found a correlation between the volume of the CPAM and head circumference, which indicated that when the ratio is more than 1.6, the risk of developing hydrops was found to be 80%. It is this patient subset that benefits from in utero intervention. Typically, microcystic lesions can be resected with a lobectomy and macrocystic masses can be aspirated or shunted. Outcomes are good; these interventions reverse hydropic symptoms and result in a survival rate of more than 70%.[49]

### Fetoscopic Surgery

The application of minimally invasive techniques has been increasing and its role in fetal surgery is still being explored. It is used for lower urinary tract obstructions, in which oligohydramnios causes pulmonary insufficiency and compression deformities of the face and limbs. These patients may benefit from vesicoamniotic shunting and ablation of posterior valves. Fetoscopic surgery has also been successfully used in the laser ablation of the communicating placental blood vessels in twin-twin transfusion syndrome, characterized by hypovolemia, oliguria, and oligohydramnios in the donor twin and hypervolemia, polyuria, and polyhydramnios in the recipient twin. The procedure is associated with a 75% survival rate of at least one twin.

## SELECTED REFERENCES

Ashcraft KW, Holcomb GW III, Murphy JP, editors: Pediatric surgery, ed 5, Philadelphia, 2009, Elsevier Saunders.

This is an excellent reference source for most pediatric surgical conditions. This textbook is easy to read and serves as an outstanding practical resource, especially for young surgical residents and medical students.

Deprest JA, Flake AW, Gratacos E, et al: The making of fetal surgery. Prenat Diagn 30:653–667, 2010.

This is an excellent overview of progress that has been made in fetal surgery in the past 3 decades.

Grosfeld JL, O'Neill JA, Fonkalsrud EW, et al, editors: Pediatric surgery, ed 6, Philadelphia, 2006, Mosby Elsevier.

This two-volume set is a comprehensive textbook on pediatric surgery, considered to be the most authoritative textbook for pediatric surgeons.

Maris J: Recent advances in neuroblastoma. N Engl J Med 362: 2202–2211, 2010.

This is an excellent review of recent scientific as well as clinical advances made in neuroblastoma.

O'Neill JA, Grosfeld JL, Fonkaksrud EW, et al, editors: Principles of pediatric surgery, ed 2, St. Louis, 2004, Mosby.

This is an outstanding textbook for surgical residents and fellows in training. It is comprehensive, yet highlights essential core elements of pediatric surgical knowledge in a concise and clear fashion. Interestingly, five editors and 10 associate editors wrote this textbook without specific contributor(s) for each chapter.

## REFERENCES

1. Timmerman MK, Morley AD, Buwalda J: Treatment of non-tuberculous mycobacterial cervicofacial lymphadenitis in children: Critical appraisal of the literature. Clin Otolaryngol 33:546–552, 2008.
2. Perkins JA, Manning SC, Tempero RM, et al: Lymphatic malformations: Review of current treatment. Otolaryngol Head Neck Surg 142:795–803, 2010.
3. Bryner BS, West BT, Hirschl RB, et al: Congenital diaphragmatic hernia requiring extracorporeal membrane oxygenation: Does timing of repair matter? J Pediatr Surg 44:1165–1171, 2009.
4. Correia-Pinto J, Gonzaga S, Huang Y, et al: Congenital lung lesions—underlying molecular mechanisms. Semin Pediatr Surg 19:171–179, 2010.
5. Masters IB: Congenital airway lesions and lung disease. Pediatr Clin North Am 56:227–242, 2009.
6. Liechty KW, Flake AW: Pulmonary vascular malformations. Semin Pediatr Surg 17:9–16, 2008.
7. Allen SR, Ignacio R, Falcone RA, et al: The effect of a right-sided aortic arch on outcome in children with esophageal atresia and tracheoesophageal fistula. J Pediatr Surg 41:479–483, 2006.
8. Foker JE, Kendall Krosch TC, Catton K, et al: Long-gap esophageal atresia treated by growth induction: The biological potential and early follow-up results. Semin Pediatr Surg 18:23–29, 2009.
9. Patkowsk D, Rysiakiewicz K, Jaworski W, et al: Thoracoscopic repair of tracheoesophageal fistula and esophageal atresia. J Laparoendosc Adv Surg Tech A 19(Suppl 1):S19–S22, 2009.
10. Tannuri AC, Tannuri U, Mathias AL, et al: Gastroesophageal reflux disease in children: Efficacy of Nissen fundoplication in treating digestive and respiratory symptoms. Experience of a single center. Dis Esophagus 21:746–750, 2008.
11. Pacilli M, Pierro A, Lindley KJ, et al: Gastric emptying is accelerated following laparoscopic Nissen fundoplication. Eur J Pediatr Surg 18:395–397, 2008.

12. Sola JE, Neville HL: Laparoscopic vs open pyloromyotomy: A systematic review and meta-analysis. J Pediatr Surg 44:1631–1637, 2009.
13. Green P, Swischuk LE, Hernandez JA: Delayed presentation of malrotation and midgut volvulus: Imaging findings. Emerg Radiol 14:379–382, 2007.
14. Blakely ML, Tyson JE, Lally KP, et al: Laparotomy versus peritoneal drainage for necrotizing enterocolitis or isolated intestinal perforation in extremely low birth weight infants: Outcomes through 18 months adjusted age. Pediatrics 117:e680–687, 2006.
15. Moss RL, Dimmitt RA, Barnhart DC, et al: Laparotomy versus peritoneal drainage for necrotizing enterocolitis and perforation. N Engl J Med 354:2225–2234, 2006.
16. McMellen ME, Wakeman D, Longshore SW, et al: Growth factors: Possible roles for clinical management of the short bowel syndrome. Semin Pediatr Surg 19:35–43, 2010.
17. Jones BA, Hull MA, McGuire MM, et al: Autologous intestinal reconstruction surgery. Semin Pediatr Surg 19:59–67, 2010.
18. Walker SR, Nucci A, Yaworski JA, et al: The Bianchi procedure: A 20-year single institution experience. J Pediatr Surg 41:113–119, 2006.
19. Ching YA, Fitzgibbons S, Valim C, et al: Long-term nutritional and clinical outcomes after serial transverse enteroplasty at a single institution. J Pediatr Surg 44:939–943, 2009.
20. Sanchez-Mejias A, Fernandez RM, Lopez-Alonso M, et al: Contribution of RET, NTRK3 and EDN3 to the expression of Hirschsprung disease in a multiplex family. J Med Genet 46:862–864, 2009.
21. Kapur RP, Reed RC, Finn LS, et al: Calretinin immunohistochemistry versus acetylcholinesterase histochemistry in the evaluation of suction rectal biopsies for Hirschsprung disease. Pediatr Dev Pathol 12:6–15, 2009.
22. Keckler SJ, Yang JC, Fraser JD, et al: Contemporary practice patterns in the surgical management of Hirschsprung's disease. J Pediatr Surg 44:1257–1260, 2009.
23. deVries PA, Pena A: Posterior sagittal anorectoplasty. J Pediatr Surg 17:638–643, 1982.
24. Podevin G, Petit T, Mure PY, et al: Minimally invasive surgery for anorectal malformation in boys: A multicenter study. J Laparoendosc Adv Surg Tech A 19(Suppl 1):S233–S235, 2009.
25. Bassett MD, Murray KF: Biliary atresia: Recent progress. J Clin Gastroenterol 42:720–729, 2008.
26. Lao OB, Larison C, Garrison M, et al: Steroid use after the Kasai procedure for biliary atresia. Am J Surg 199:680–684, 2010.
27. Hartley JL, Davenport M, Kelly DA: Biliary atresia. Lancet 374:1704–1713, 2009.
28. Singham J, Yoshida EM, Scudamore CH: Choledochal cysts: Part 1 of 3: Classification and pathogenesis. Can J Surg 52:434–440, 2009.
29. Charnley RM: Hereditary pancreatitis. World J Gastroenterol 9:1–4, 2003.
30. Gabriel A, Gollin G: Management of complicated gastroschisis with porcine small intestinal submucosa and negative pressure wound therapy. J Pediatr Surg 41:1836–1840, 2006.
31. Lao OB, Larison C, Garrison MM, et al: Outcomes in neonates with gastroschisis in U.S. children's hospitals. Am J Perinatol 27:97–101, 2010.
32. Kelly RE, Jr, Cash TF, Shamberger RC, et al: Surgical repair of pectus excavatum markedly improves body image and perceived ability for physical activity: Multicenter study. Pediatrics 122:1218–1222, 2008.
33. Kelly RE, Jr, Shamberger RC, Mellins RB, et al: Prospective multicenter study of surgical correction of pectus excavatum: Design, perioperative complications, pain, and baseline pulmonary function facilitated by Internet-based data collection. J Am Coll Surg 205:205–216, 2007.
34. Martinez-Ferro M, Fraire C, Bernard S: Dynamic compression system for the correction of pectus carinatum. Semin Pediatr Surg 17:194–200, 2008.
35. Park JR, Eggert A, Caron H: Neuroblastoma: Biology, prognosis, and treatment. Hematol Oncol Clin North Am 24:65–86, 2010.
36. Ishola TA, Chung DH: Neuroblastoma. Surg Oncol 16:149–156, 2007.
37. Brodeur GM: Neuroblastoma: Biological insights into a clinical enigma. Nat Rev Cancer 3:203–216, 2003.
38. Maris JM: Recent advances in neuroblastoma. N Engl J Med 362:2202–2211, 2010.
39. Modak S, Cheung NK: Neuroblastoma: Therapeutic strategies for a clinical enigma. Cancer Treat Rev 36:307–317, 2010.
40. Vujanic GM, Sandstedt B: The pathology of Wilms' tumour (nephroblastoma): The International Society of Paediatric Oncology approach. J Clin Pathol 63:102–109, 2010.
41. Ko EY, Ritchey ML: Current management of Wilms' tumor in children. J Pediatr Urol 5:56–65, 2009.
42. Kaste SC, Dome JS, Babyn PS, et al: Wilms tumour: Prognostic factors, staging, therapy and late effects. Pediatr Radiol 38:2–17, 2008.
43. Paulino AC, Okcu MF: Rhabdomyosarcoma. Curr Probl Cancer 32:7–34, 2008.
44. Otte JB: Progress in the surgical treatment of malignant liver tumors in children. Cancer Treat Rev 36:360–371, 2010.
45. Barksdale EM, Jr, Obokhare I: Teratomas in infants and children. Curr Opin Pediatr 21:344–349, 2009.
46. von Allmen D: Malignant lesions of the ovary in childhood. Semin Pediatr Surg 14:100–105, 2005.
47. Cook RC, Blinman TA: Nutritional support of the pediatric trauma patient. Semin Pediatr Surg 19:242–251, 2010.
48. Rossi AC: Indications and outcomes of intrauterine surgery for fetal malformations. Curr Opin Obstet Gynecol 22:159–165, 2010.
49. Deprest JA, Flake AW, Gratacos E, et al: The making of fetal surgery. Prenat Diagn 30:653–667, 2010.

# CHAPTER 68

# NEUROSURGERY

Jaime Gasco, Aaron Mohanty, Fadi Hanbali, and Joel T. Patterson

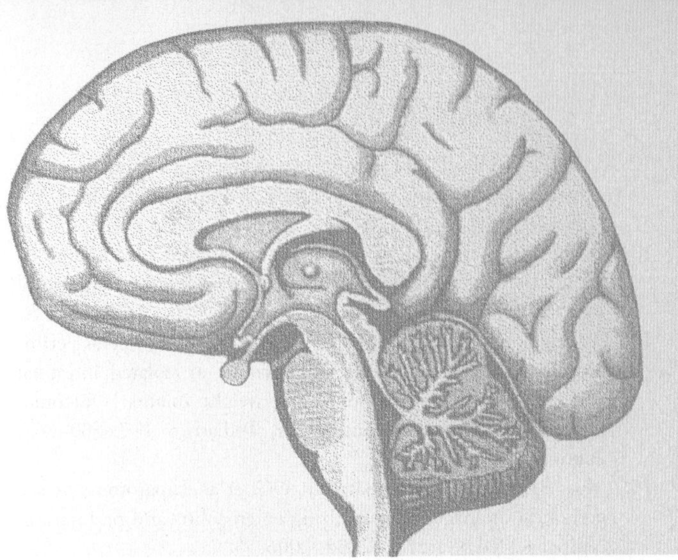



Neurosurgery is defined as surgery of the brain, spinal cord, peripheral nerves, and their supporting structures, including the blood supply, and protective elements, spinal fluid spaces, bony cranium, and spine. Although it may be intuitive to think of neurosurgery as mostly concerned with the neural tissue itself, it is common that the pathophysiology and opportunity for therapy involve its infrastructure. Thus, it is easy to understand that neurosurgeons are often focused on intracranial pressure (ICP), cerebrospinal fluid (CSF) dynamics, cerebral blood flow (CBF), and compression syndromes of the spinal cord, nerve roots, and peripheral nerves. Whatever may be happening to the neural tissue, whose complexity often defies direct intervention, its environment must be optimized for improvement or recovery to occur. The rigid closed space around the brain and spinal cord is often said to set neurosurgery apart from other branches of surgery. A prime example is the contrast between intra-abdominal and intracranial hemorrhage. Whereas bleeding in the abdomen may focus concern on blood loss and hypotension, bleeding within the closed space of the cranium causes problems with an increased ICP, with attendant decreased CBF, infarction, edema, and obstruction of spinal fluid absorption. These intracranial mechanisms can be lethal at volumes of intracranial bleeding that have no effect on systemic blood pressure through the mechanism of hypovolemia.

The chapter is intended for non-neurosurgeons who want to initiate a framework on which to add further knowledge and experience. It hopefully will also help personnel in a community hospital emergency room, or a medical student on the ward for the first time, communicate patient problems efficiently to neurosurgeons. The chapter first provides an overview of the underlying principles of neurosurgery, with a focus on intracranial dynamics. The remaining sections include a discussion of the following: cerebrovascular disorders, which include subarachnoid hemorrhage, intracerebral hemorrhage, aneurysm, and arteriovenous malformation (AVM); central nervous system (CNS) tumors, which include neoplasms of the brain, skull base, cranial nerves, spinal cord, meninges, and peripheral nerves; traumatic brain injury; degenerative diseases of the spine; functional neurosurgery, which includes stereotactic radiosurgery (SRS), epilepsy surgery, and surgery for the management of pain and movement disorders; hydrocephalus and pediatric neurosurgery; and neurosurgical management of CNS infections. The field of neurosurgery is simply too broad to make a detailed encyclopedic overview realistic, but some introduction to these issues will hopefully be useful to the reader.

## INTRACRANIAL DYNAMICS

A few basic principles concerning intracranial dynamics, CSF, CBF, and ICP are essential to grasp at the outset and are summarized here for quick review. Some of these principles are obvious whereas others might be considered counterintuitive.

The first principle is obvious. The cranial cavity has a fixed volume comprised of (1) brain tissue (parenchyma), (2) CSF, and (3) blood vessels and intravascular blood. According to the Monro-Kellie doctrine, the sum of these components within the fixed volume of the cranial cavity implies that an increase in one component must be accompanied by an equal and opposite decrease in one or both of the remaining components.[1] If this does not occur, the ICP will rise to levels close to the systemic blood pressure, producing a reverberating blood flow pattern with no net flow. The clinical implications are also straightforward. For each intracranial component, there is a family of pathologic conditions of excess volume and a means to improve that excess (Table 68-1). A consequence of this principle is that if there is an elevation in the volume of any one compartment, there is a stage of compensation in which the volume of one or more other compartments can be reduced to avoid elevations in the ICP.

The second principle is not obvious, and may seem counterintuitive. Spinal fluid is produced at a constant rate (≈15 to 20 mL/hr), by an energy-dependent, physicochemical process, mainly by the choroid plexus of the ventricles. It is essential to understand that production is little affected by any intracranial backpressure; thus, CSF production continues unabated, even to lethal elevations of intracranial pressure. Because production is almost always constant, it follows that derangement of CSF dynamics almost always involves some aspect of impeding CSF absorption through obstruction along the CSF pathways inside the brain, subarachnoid spaces at the basal cisterns or cerebral

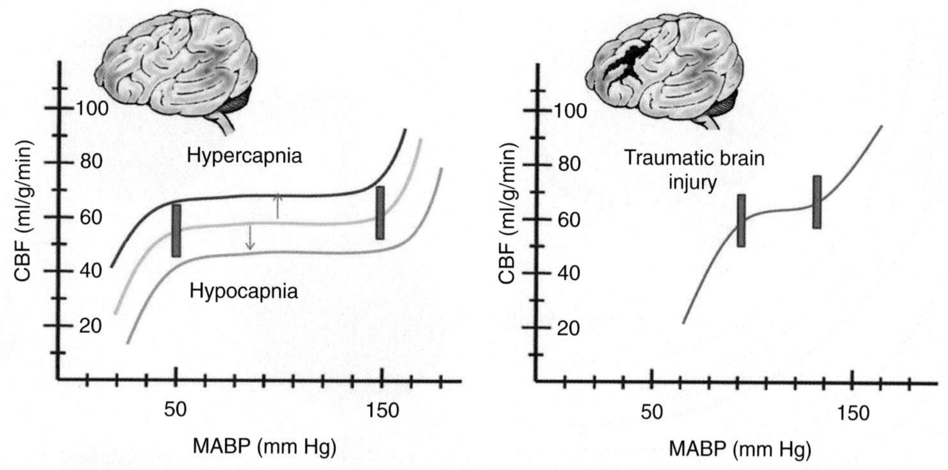


**FIGURE 68-1** CBF as a function of MAP. Note the upward and downward shifts with hypercapnia and hypocapnia, respectively. In traumatic brain injury, the curve is steeper, with large CBF changes occurring with small pressure changes. (Adapted from Rangel-Castilla L, Gasco J, Nauta HJ, et al: Cerebral pressure autoregulation in traumatic brain injury. Neurosurg Focus 25:E7, 2008.)

**Table 68-1 Intracranial Excess Volume Syndromes and Therapy**

| COMPONENT | EXCESS VOLUME SYNDROME | SPECIFIC TREATMENT |
|---|---|---|
| Brain tissue | Edema: Cytotoxic, vasogenic, perineoplastic, inflammatory | Diuretics: Mannitol, furosemide, hypertonic saline; steroids for perineoplastic and inflammatory vasogenic edema |
| Vascular | Elevated $PCO_2$: Hyperperfusion state with loss of autoregulation as in severe hypertension, after trauma or AVM removal; relative venous obstruction | Increased ventilation; diuretics (in hyperperfusion state, avoid mannitol), barbiturates; clear venous obstruction; elevate head of bed (to reduce venous volume) |
| Cerebrospinal fluid | Impaired absorption with congenital, posthemorrhagic, or postinfectious hydrocephalus, communicating or obstructive; loculations; arachnoid or periventricular cysts; rare increased production of CSF with choroid plexus papilloma | Ventricular external drainage (or lumbar drainage only if no threat of herniation) or shunt; with flocculation, or with some types of obstructive hydrocephalus, endoscopic fenestration or third ventriculostomy may be possible; acetazolamide and steroids may temporarily decrease CSF production |
| Mass lesion | Tumor, cyst, abscess, hematoma, radiation necrosis, or cerebral infarction necrosis | Remove, fenestrate, aspirate lesion (often with stereotactic guidance); less commonly, might be useful to enlarge intracranial volume by decompression |

convexity, or arachnoid granulations from which most absorption occurs. In the following discussions on tumors, infection, intracranial hemorrhage, and trauma, many examples will become apparent whereby impaired CSF absorption contributes to the pathologic condition. The only exceptions to the almost constant CSF production are the excess production associated with the rare choroid plexus papilloma tumor and the occasional decreased CSF production seen with some gram-negative bacterial meningitis with ventriculitis, usually in neonates.

The third basic principle is that the CBF normally varies over a wide range (30 to 100 mL/100 g brain tissue/min), depending on metabolic demand from neuronal activity within a particular area of the brain. The CBF may be considered in aggregate or of specific small regions, pathologic or normal.

The blood flow to any brain area is generally abundant, exceeding demand by a wide margin, so that $O_2$ extraction ratios are often low. The brain vasculature matches the blood flow to tissue metabolic demand and the CBF generally maintains what is needed, despite wide variations in systemic blood pressure, by a phenomenon known as *autoregulation*. Factors such as an elevated or decreased arterial $PCO_2$ shift the curve as indicated. In the setting of traumatic brain injury, the curve becomes more pronounced (i.e., smaller changes in blood pressure or $PCO_2$) and affects the CBF dramatically (Fig. 68-1). If tissue demand exceeds autoregulation, or if CBF declines for pathologic reasons, the first defense is that the $O_2$ extraction will increase (i.e., arteriovenous $O_2$ difference, $AVDO_2$). The tissue begins to dysfunction at levels below 0.25 mL per g of brain tissue per minute. With levels between 0.15 and 0.20 we may encounter reversible ischemia; however, infarction will occur when levels range between 0.10 and 0.15 (Fig. 68-2). The metabolic consumption of oxygen in the brain ($CMRO_2$) is decreased after traumatic brain injury to levels between 0.6 and 1.2 µmol/mg/min. Complete loss of blood flow to any brain area results in infarction (irreversible damage) within a few minutes. Swelling of the infarcted tissue takes days to peak and weeks to resolve.[2]

An important implication is that if brain dysfunction is occurring clinically because compensatory mechanisms (e.g., autoregulation changing the vascular resistance, capacity to elevate mean systemic arterial pressure, ability to increase $O_2$ extraction) have been exceeded, the tolerance for further decline in blood flow is low, and tissue damage is seriously threatened. Therapy to increase blood pressure or decrease ICP may be urgently needed. When time permits because the dysfunction

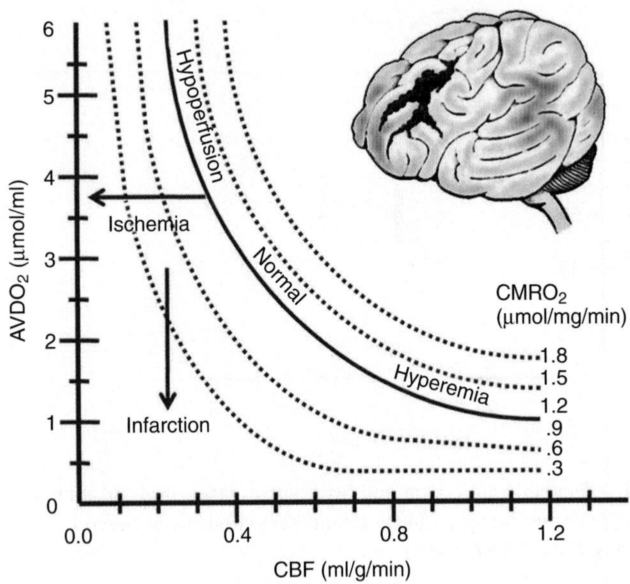


**FIGURE 68-2** Relationships among cerebral flow, metabolism, and oxygen extraction in normal and pathologic circumstances. (From Rangel-Castilla L, Gasco J, Nauta HJ, et al: Cerebral pressure autoregulation in traumatic brain injury. Neurosurg Focus 25:E7, 2008.)

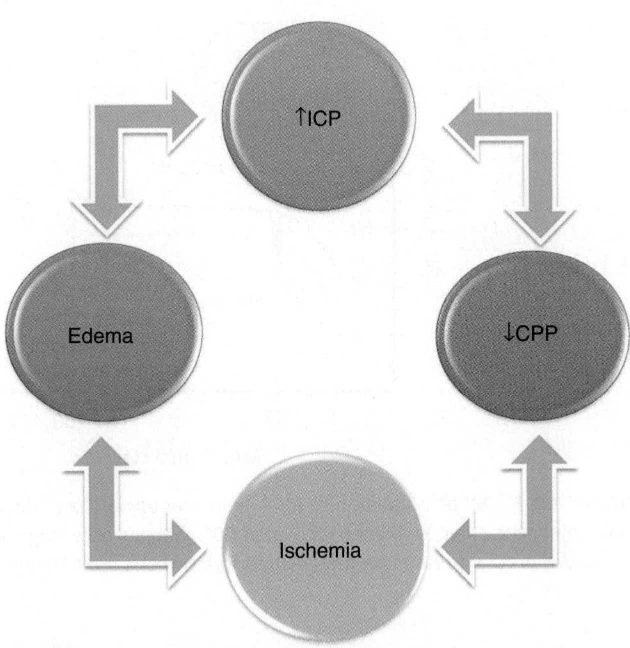


**FIGURE 68-3** Relationship among increased ICP, reduced CPP, development of ischemia and infarction, and cerebral edema.

fluctuates chronically, it may sometimes be appropriate to measure $O_2$ extraction ratios as one index of the overall adequacy of the CBF. At a low CBF, $O_2$ extraction is increased with a lower venous $Po_2$. It is interesting to note that the variations in CBF and extraction ratios related to neuronal activity are said to underlie the ability to image function by functional magnetic resonance imaging (MRI), a technique that is finding wider usage in the clinical neurosciences.

A fourth principle derives from the other three and the fact that injured tissue swells, making obvious the potential for a cascading injury by a vicious cycle mechanism (Fig. 68-3). If the stage of compensation (see earlier), even with therapy, is exceeded, and ICP is elevated high enough by some mechanism so that cerebral perfusion pressure (CPP) declines, CBF can decline to levels at which tissue injury occurs.

$$\text{CPP} = \text{mean arterial pressure (MAP)} - \text{ICP}$$

Brain edema swelling within the closed cranium will lead to further increases in ICP with even further decreases in CPP in a stage of decompensation. When the capacity for autoregulation is exceeded or damaged so that it can no longer play a role, CBF is linked directly to the CPP.

In the management of intracranial pathology, ICP and CPP are easy to measure continuously and thus serve as highly practical surrogates for the more fundamental, but much more difficult to measure, CBF. However, these are not equivalent, and the limitations of these parameters for guiding therapy need to be remembered. Regardless of causation, when concern arises about the possibility of cascading injury, every effort is made to keep the CPP in the realm of 60 mm Hg (range, 50 to 70 mm Hg) and ICP below 20 mm, Hg if possible. Routinely using pressors and volume expansion to maintain CPP higher than 70 mm Hg is not supported based on systemic complications.[3]

A fifth principle concerns focal mass effect and its progression in regard to the complex anatomy of the cranial cavity. The cranial cavity is not just a hollow spherical space but contains several almost knifelike projections of folded dura, the falx and tentorium, which divide the cavity into right and left supratentorial compartment and an infratentorial compartment, the posterior fossa. The sphenoid wing is a prominent, mostly bony ridge that separates the anterior fossa containing the frontal lobe from the middle fossa containing the temporal lobe. A narrow opening, the incisura, edged by the tentorium, surrounds the midbrain and is the only passage between the supratentorial and infratentorial compartments. Apart from the small openings for the cranial nerves and arteries, the foramen magnum is the only sizable opening from the cranial cavity as a whole.

The condition that classically illustrates the expanding mass lesion is the acute epidural hematoma, seen after trauma with skull fracture. Regardless of the source, however, the progression can be similar and has been termed *rostrocaudal decay* to reflect the early and late stages, as listed in order below:

- Focal distortion only
- Effacement of gyri and sulci
- Compression of the lateral (or other) ventricle
- Midline shift
- Subfalcial herniation
- Temporal lobe tentorial herniation
  - Third nerve compression (unilateral dilated pupil)
  - Obliteration of basal cisterns
  - Midbrain compression
  - Midbrain infarction, Duret's hemorrhages (both pupils dilate, with irreversible damage to midbrain)

- Further brainstem compression
  - Loss of brainstem reflexes: Progression from flexor posturing to extensor posturing; vestibulo-ocular and oculocephalic reflexes; corneal reflexes
  - Medullary compression syndrome: Respiratory reflexes; vasomotor reflexes, Cushing's reflex with elevation of the systolic blood pressure, widening of the pulse pressure, bradycardia.
- Foramen magnum herniation

At stages beyond tentorial herniation, it is unusual for focal mass effects not to be accompanied by an overall increase in ICP. The point at which focal mass effect evolves to include a rise in overall ICP depends largely on the compliance within the cranial cavity. Young patients with so-called *tight brains* can develop raised ICP, even with relatively small volumes of mass that produce only effacement of the cortical gyri. On the other hand, patients with advanced cerebral atrophy can, for example, tolerate large frontal intracerebral hematomas or chronic subdural hematomas with compression of the lateral ventricle and midline shift while maintaining a tolerable ICP and a surprising degree of intact neurologic function.

The Glasgow Coma Score (GCS; see later, "Traumatic Brain Injury") provides a clinical functional measure of the degree of mass effect and advanced raised ICP. Although it is a useful standardized functional measure of the more advanced stages of mass effect or raised ICP, it was never really intended to focus on more subtle functional changes. A recently introduced coma scale by Widjicks and colleagues[4] has delineated the FOUR score (***f***ull ***o***utline of ***u****n****r***esponsiveness) consisting of four components (eye, motor, brainstem, respiration). Each has a maximal score of 4 and takes into account the subtleties related to brainstem activity and breathing patterns occurring during the rostrocaudal decay described.

A sixth principle concerns the separateness of the phenomenology of the following: (1) focal mass effect (as described earlier); (2) diffuse raised ICP; and (3) ventriculomegaly (enlargement of the cerebral ventricles). Although these three processes often occur in combination, the notion that they are separable comes from the observation that there is a pure form of each. The ability to recognize these separate phenomena clinically is often useful in deciding priorities for diagnosis and treatment. This requires some explanation. The pure form of raised ICP—without focal mass lesion, trauma or enlargement of the ventricular system—is a condition known as *idiopathic intracranial hypertension* or *pseudotumor cerebri*. The pure form of ventriculomegaly is a condition known as *adult chronic idiopathic* or *normal-pressure hydrocephalus* (NPH). The pure form of the focal mass lesion without increased ICP or ventriculomegaly is common; it occurs with tumors too small to raise ICP on their own that are not in a location to interfere with CSF pathways. Instead, there focal mass lesions are typically discovered incidentally or because of symptoms from a focal neurologic deficit or seizure disorder.

Normal ICP varies over a wide range, with generally accepted values between 0 and 20 mm Hg. Diffuse raised ICP, in the fully evolved pure form, results in a clinical picture that may include symptoms of headache, nausea and vomiting, double vision, and obscuration of vision. The accompanying clinical signs may include papilledema and sixth cranial nerve palsy with lateral rectus weakness and side by side diplopia, initially worse on far vision or gaze directed toward the side of the palsy. The papilledema is a mostly chronic phenomenon and is not seen acutely. The sixth nerve palsy of raised ICP can occur regardless of its cause and does not imply direct involvement by a mass lesion, large or small, on the sixth nerve. In this situation, the sixth nerve palsy is a false localizing sign. With raised ICP, there may also be obscurations of vision, in which patients report that their vision temporarily fades or becomes gray, in combination with headache. Again, these obscurations are caused by the effect of diffusely increased ICP on the sensitive optic nerves. They do not imply the presence of a focal mass lesion directly affecting the optic nerves or pathways. Intuitively, it seems that if there is a slow increase in a process raising ICP, the pressure would also rise slowly and evenly, in pace with the evolving process. However, as first shown by Lundberg in 1960,[5] the intermediate stages of decompensation are characterized by transient pronounced elevations in ICP (to 60 mm Hg) that characteristically plateau for up to 45 minutes and then transiently cycle down again to a more normal range.

The original form of this condition of chronic, diffuse, raised ICP is known by the old term *pseudotumor cerebri* or the more descriptive *idiopathic intracranial hypertension.* Because it is often not benign, causing disabling chronic headache and visual loss, sometimes even to permanent blindness, the term *benign intracranial hypertension* is falling out of favor. The basis for the condition is not entirely understood. It usually occurs in obese young women. Treatment is with acetazolamide diuretics, steroids, and intermittent lumbar puncture. Severe cases with threatened permanent visual loss may require a lumboperitoneal or ventriculoperitoneal CSF shunt or optic nerve fenestration, in which the meninges around the optic nerves are opened to vent CSF in the orbit.

Pure ventriculomegaly—specifically, enlargement of the lateral ventricles—is characterized by gait disturbance and incontinence early in the clinical picture. As the process worsens, cognitive disturbances may be added on. The early appearance of gait disturbance and urinary incontinence is attributed to dysfunction of the medial cerebral hemispheres in which the leg area of the primary motor cortex and bladder control area reside. Nerve fiber pathways inside the brain must pass around the lateral ventricles to reach these areas on the medial hemisphere and therefore are especially vulnerable to pressure or distortion by the enlarged ventricle. This syndrome is called *NPH.* The usual diagnostic difficulty is in differentiating the condition from cerebral atrophy. Ventricular enlargement more prominent than enlargement of the CSF subarachnoid spaces over the cerebral convexity is typically seen in NPH. The clinical impression that gait disturbance and incontinence occur early and predominate over dementia is considered an important feature of NPH. Treatment is with CSF shunt, lumboperitoneal or ventriculoperitoneal. The differentiation between NPH and cerebral atrophy is important because of the increased risk for subdural hematoma with shunting in cerebral atrophy.

Table 68-2 summarizes the relationships among ICP, mass lesions, and ventriculomegaly.

## CEREBROVASCULAR DISORDERS

Cerebrovascular disorders encompass a host of disorders, congenital and acquired (Box 68-1).

**Table 68-2 Intracranial Hypertension Syndromes**

| RAISED ICP | SMALL MASS LESION | LARGE MASS LESION | VENTRICULOMEGALY | SYNDROME |
|---|---|---|---|---|
| ++++ | 0 | 0 | 0 | Pseudotumor cerebri |
| 0 | 0 | 0 | ++++ | Normal-pressure hydrocephalus |
| +++ | 0 | 0 | ++++ | Typical hydrocephalus, communicating or noncommunicating, requiring shunt or ventriculostomy |
| ++++ | + | 0 | ++++ | Small tumor such as colloid cyst obstructing the foramen of Monroe |
| +++ | + | 0 | 0 | Subdural empyema in which widespread inflammatory cerebral swelling dominates over the small mass of empyema itself |
| +++ | 0 | +++ | 0 | Frontal brain tumor reaching large size because local effects are on functionally silent brain |
| 0 | + | 0 | 0 | Typical small tumor, with only focal mass effect and focal dysfunction or seizure disorder |

**BOX 68-1 Cerebral Vascular Disease**

**Congenital**

Arteriovenous malformation and fistula
Cavernous malformation
Telangiectasis
Venous anomaly (angioma)

**Acquired**

- Traumatic

Some arteriovenous fistulas (type I carotid cavernous fistula)
Traumatic aneurysm

- Degenerative

Atherosclerotic, occlusive disease
Most cerebral (berry) aneurysms
Some arterial dissections
Spontaneous intracerebral hemorrhage

- Infectious

Mycotic aneurysms

**Idiopathic**

- Moyamoya

Some arteriovenous fistulas–dural AVM–like or type 2 carotid cavernous fistulas

## Arteriovenous Malformation and Fistula

In the early embryonic stage, the circulatory system does not yet have capillaries between the arterial and venous sides. Instead, there are vascular channels approximately 200 µm in diameter that must undergo further development and maturation to form the capillary bed. There is reason to believe that when this does not occur perfectly, a focal failure of maturation can lead to a nidus of persistent embryonic, low-resistance vessels connecting the arteries and veins. Over time, the high blood flow in these circuits leads to secondary changes that enlarge the nidus and the afferent arteries and efferent veins, often to impressive proportions. The high flow in the nidus, afferent, and efferent vessels predisposes to degenerative events, sometimes with aneurysm formation, causing hemorrhage, intracerebral, subarachnoid, or both. Brain tissue at the edge or intermixed with the abnormal vessels may develop dysfunction to become an epileptic focus or, less commonly, progressive ischemic deficits occur as the low-resistance AVM draws blood flow away from adjacent areas with normal vascular resistance.

It follows that AVMs can have a wide variety of configurations and sizes, depending on which part(s) of the vascular bed fail to mature and which consequences of the increased flow occur over time. If the venous outflow is restricted, the venous side of the complex may enlarge disproportionately and form a venous varix; so-called *vein of Galen* aneurysm is the prime example. Here, the vein of Galen, restricted by the downstream outflow limitations of the stiff dura–contained straight sinus, dilates, sometimes massively, and can cause obstructive hydrocephalus in the newborn, often together with high-output heart failure. Usually, the venous outflow channels enlarge to a moderate degree and become thickened in the vessel wall, or arterialized. They do not generally cause symptoms by mass effect.

Clinical presentation is usually that of a hemorrhagic stroke picture, typically an intracerebral or subarachnoid hemorrhage, or some combination. The patient complains of sudden-onset severe headache with or without focal neurologic deficit and meningismus. These symptoms can occur in all degrees of severity, but are less commonly fatal than after aneurysmal subarachnoid hemorrhage into the basal cisterns. Investigation usually begins in the emergency department with a computed tomography (CT) scan showing the hemorrhage. MRI or magnetic resonance angiography (MRA) studies typically follow, often showing enlarged afferent and efferent vessels. The role of CT angiography is evolving. Regardless of the mode of presentation, diagnosis is ultimately made by conventional catheter cerebral angiography (Fig. 68-4). It is based on demonstration of arteries and veins on the same conventional angiographic image, proving the high-flow shunting of blood through the nidus network or fistulous vessels. In an arteriovenous fistula, the shunting occurs through short, sparse, larger-diameter channels so that a cloudlike nidus of smaller vessels is not evident. Instead, the enlarged afferent arteries appear to connect directly with the enlarged efferent veins. In the typical AVM, there is a cloudlike nidus, or network of smaller vessels, seen well on angiography but not necessarily fully appreciated on MRI or MRA. The AVM can occur in all locations and with varying degrees of size, complexity, and compactness.

When the patient presents with a new-onset seizure, the next most common presentation, the investigation typically begins with brain MRI showing enlarged afferent and efferent

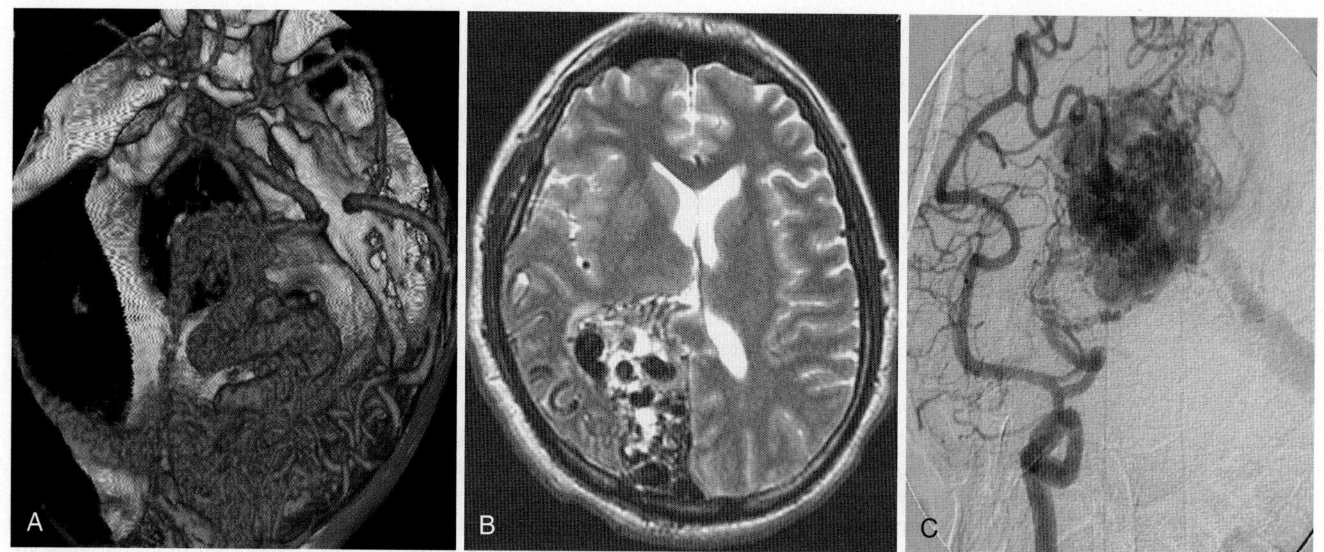


**FIGURE 68-4** CT angiography with three-dimensional reconstruction **(A)**, MRI **(B)**, and conventional angiogram **(C)** of a large AVM with supply from the middle and posterior cerebral arteries and ill-defined nidus. Complex deep and superficial venous drainage are present.

vessels. MRI, however, may not suggest the diagnosis if the afferent and efferent vessels are not grossly enlarged; however, this is rare in lesions presenting with seizure. Again, definitive diagnosis is with conventional catheter angiography, but this may sometimes be omitted if the diagnosis is sufficiently suggestive on MRI alone and there is reluctance to consider surgery, with only anticonvulsant treatment planned.

It is important to pay attention to the nidus or fistula as the prime mover of the process and realize that the secondary changes in the afferent and efferent vessels, however impressive they may seem, will generally revert to normal once the nidus or fistula has been resected or occluded. The assessment of AVM size refers to the size of the nidus and not the conglomeration of large feeding or draining vessels.

Therapy can include surgical excision, endovascular embolization of the nidus, and/or SRS. The decision to embark on any treatment depends on the assessment of the patient's treatment risk in comparison with the natural risk. The studies of Ondra and associates[6] have fairly well characterized the natural risk. Hemorrhage occurs with a frequency of approximately 4%/year, and because only approximately 25% of these are severe, with permanently severe disability or death, the catastrophe risk is only approximately1%/year. The treatment risk, therefore, must be favorably low to justify action in most situations, and delays in treatment to allow for patient acceptance and optimize the circumstances for therapy are understandable and reasonable. The main reason to recommend treatment is that the treatment may offer a lower risk over the long term. Younger patients have the most to gain by such an assessment. It may be possible to define features of individual AVMs that adjust the natural risk upward or downward, but so far these have been difficult to prove. For the purposes of clinical decision making, the hemorrhage risk is generally taken across the board for all AVMs as a starting point. An across-the-board assessment of treatment risk, however, is clearly not warranted because each AVM. Size, location relative to access by the treatment method considered, and location relative to proximity to deficit-prone brain structures are all important variables to consider. Another feature is the compactness of the AVM, with some forming a tightly clustered nidus, with little brain tissue in between, and others being diffuse and rambling, with scattered small clusters of nidus vessels encompassing large intervening areas of functional brain.

Obviously, the smaller, more compact AVMs located superficially in areas of silent brain function are the most attractive for open surgical resection. Diffuse large AVMs encompassing deficit-prone areas of brain are least attractive to open surgery and other methods. Spetzler and Martin[7] have devised a grading system for assessing risk with open operation. However, any decision is ultimately based on how an individual neurosurgeon assesses the risk for that AVM in a patient, with his or her limits of risk tolerance.

Surgical excision is carried out by craniotomy and microsurgical techniques. The lesions are evident at operation as a bright red blood–containing network of vessels. Feeding arteries are thicker walled than the generally larger, thinner walled draining veins. Nidus vessels are thin, bright red, and very thin walled, so that they resist coagulation. This feature makes it important to remain just at the edge of the lesion, if possible. Entry into the AVM nidus results in vigorous bleeding, which is time-consuming to control. Recent innovations in surgical therapy include the more common use of frameless stereotaxy or neuronavigation, which allows more accurate localization and definition of the margins, important feeders, and draining veins. Also, newer bipolar cautery instruments with advanced nonstick features have been helpful. A risk of open surgery is the unintended occlusion of vessels passing through the lesion to supply important functional areas of brain. Also, there is the potential to leave part of the nidus behind inadvertently, so the hemorrhage risk would be unpredictable. Postprocedure angiography is essential to perform at the end of the procedure, or as soon as possible thereafter. Any residual AVM is addressed as soon as practical. Another category of concern is hemorrhage resulting from a sudden increased blood flow at the periphery of the resected lesion, exceeding the limited autoregulatory capacity there. For the larger more complex AVM, intentionally staged surgery is sometimes an option and is probably reasonably safe as long as the remaining venous drainage of the AVM stays in balance with its residual afferent blood supply at each stage.

SRS is most attractive for small (<2.5 cm diameter) deep lesions that are difficult to access by open surgery. This method has the obvious attraction that hospitalization and craniotomy can be avoided, and patient acceptance is often high. The size of the nidus is the major limitation, however; that the smaller the nidus, the higher the dose of radiation that can be given safely and the more effective the treatment is likely to be. Negative considerations are that the radiation is not immediately effective and the risk for hemorrhage during the latent interval must be factored in. Approximately 60% of treated AVMs will be obliterated in 1 year (and ≈80% by 2 years). The obliteration rate is probably higher in younger patients and in those with nidus vessels of smaller diameter. The larger normal vessels generally escape obliteration by SRS, even when passing through the treatment volume to supply distant areas of the brain. However, this may also mean that the more fistulous type of AVMs, with sparse, large-diameter nidus channels, is less likely to be treated successfully. When an AVM reacts to SRS, there may be a period of edema in the surrounding or intervening brain. Usually, the edema evident by MRI is not symptomatic. However, the edema can be extensive and sometimes is temporarily disabling for up to several months. Steroids may be helpful in this setting. Seizures may also be more likely during a reactive interval and require upward adjustments of anticonvulsant medication, but the eventual seizure risk is not increased. Overall risk for permanent neurologic deficit with SRS is low, approximately 2% or 3%, when pooling large numbers of patients but, as with other treatment modalities, the risk for permanent deficit is dependent on proximity to deficit-prone structures. The optic nerves and chiasm and brainstem are of particular concern with radiation. It is safest not to target lesions within 5 mm of the optic pathways, which limits its application in treating parasellar or pituitary lesions.

Endovascular therapy is a rapidly evolving field, making it difficult to assess in terms of predicting actual patient outcomes with methods currently available. Whatever criticisms apply currently may be overcome with newer methods, but that remains to be proved. It is increasingly being carried out by neurosurgeons, although the familiarity with catheter angiography has made it largely the domain of the interventional neuroradiologist. Endovascular therapy has the allure of avoiding open surgery, but the likelihood of obliterating an entire AVM by this method alone is limited at present. To be effective in any permanent way, the embolic material must reach the nidus vessels but not pass readily through to the venous side. This can be more difficult than it seems because the diameter of the nidus vessels may not be uniform. Initially, the high blood flow to the nidus draws the embolic material to it but, as the nidus progressively occludes, the embolic material is progressively more likely to reflux into normal vessels and the risk for stroke increases. The method is safest in situations in which there is a long segment of feeding vessel dedicated to the AVM because then reflux to the normal circulation is less likely. As with any endovascular technique, some areas of the circulation are easier to access than others. The method can be effective alone for treating the smaller, more fistulous lesions with single feeding and draining vessels. These lesions are rare, however, and the method is generally used to reduce the size or complexity of an AVM just before open surgical resection. However, afferent vessel occlusion alone, without penetration of the nidus, is not effective in any other context. Over time, an occluded feeding vessel recruits a network of replacement channels that may make it even more difficult to treat definitively. When used in conjunction with radiosurgery, the embolic material must reach the nidus, reducing the nidus volume permanently in a dimension and making radiosurgery of the remainder more effective. Risks for permanent deficit with embolization have been described as high as 5% per embolization session, but this figure is based on older techniques. The problem with clinical decision making is that currently we do not know the risks of evolving techniques accurately.

### Cavernous Angioma: Cavernous Malformation

The cavernous angioma is a highly characteristic, usually almost spherical, discrete lesion, composed of a cluster of vascular sinusoids fed by small vessels in the arteriolar size range or smaller. Unlike the AVM, large feeding arteries and draining veins are not seen, and diagnosis by catheter angiography is not possible. The sinusoids are tightly compacted and there is no intervening brain tissue, a diagnostic feature. At surgery, they often appear as a discrete, mulberry-like collection of thin-walled vascular sinusoids with a greenish hemosiderin rim in the surrounding brain edge. When incised, bleeding from the lesion is minimal and easy to control, unlike the AVM, which bleeds vigorously if entered. The sinusoids often seem to be admixed with small chronic hematomas containing blood in various stages of decomposition. Many are older and contain birefringent yellow cholesterol crystals. Early autopsy studies[8] noted out that they should be more common than recognized clinically. However, the lesions were not usually evident on CT or conventional catheter angiography available at that time. The clinical entity was not fully appreciated until the more widespread availability of MRI in the 1980s. The lesions are easily seen on MRI, where their appearance is diagnostic. They show a center containing some small, high-intensity signal foci surrounded by a null signal corona, dark on T1- and T2-weighted images, that corresponds to hemosiderin deposition in the adjacent brain.

Like the true AVM, cavernous angiomas can present with symptomatic hemorrhage or new-onset seizures. Unlike AVM, they can also present as a slowly growing mass lesion. At least part of this growth appears to result from the accumulation of multiple small hemorrhagic foci in various stages of healing. The lesion can be particularly problematic in this manner when located in the brainstem. The hemorrhage frequency is not understood completely, partly because most hemorrhages are probably small and asymptomatic and not recorded as events. When located in the cerebral cortex or medial temporal lobe structures, they can be a focus of seizures and can be solitary or multiple, incidental or symptomatic. The multiple form is more common in women and in those of Hispanic descent and has been linked to the *KRIT-1/CCM1* gene locus on chromosome 7q21.2. Cavernous angioma can appear de novo in patients with earlier, completely negative MRI scans. Because of these features, cavernous angiomas occupy a position somewhere between congenital vascular malformations and vascular tumors. The term *angioma* probably reflects this tumor-like nature better than the term *malformation* and is preferred here for that reason.

Many lesions are followed conservatively with interval MRI scans for years, without signs of activity. At the other extreme, they can sometimes bleed to produce a large symptomatic or life-threatening intracerebral or brainstem hematoma, but this is relatively uncommon. The threat of such hemorrhage is generally not held out as a reason to operate, as it is for the true AVM. Surgical excision is usually reserved for lesions that are problematic because of hemorrhage, demonstrated growth, or seizures difficult to control with medication alone. Surgical excision is practical in most locations because of the distinct margins and minor bleeding encountered at operation. Lesions in the brainstem can pose major challenges but, even there, surgical resection is not ruled out as long as access can be achieved without the need to traverse crucial structures anticipated to produce a major new deficit. Intraoperative ultrasound and frame-based or frameless stereotaxy can be helpful in locating the lesions if they are small and in deep locations. Radiosurgery can be performed for these lesions but is not of demonstrated benefit. The hazards of radiosurgery in critical brainstem locations remain a concern.

## Capillary Telangiectasia

The telangiectasis is composed of vascular channels with extremely thin walls similar to those of dilated capillaries. These are usually grouped in small clusters, generally with prominent intervening brain tissue. They are often clinically silent and generally do not appear on imaging studies. They are not evident on conventional catheter angiography unless large, and then only in the capillary venous phase. They clearly differ from an AVM in that flow through the lesion is not fast enough to demonstrate arteries and veins in the same conventional angiographic image. These lesions are not treated surgically.

## Developmental Venous Anomaly: Venous Angioma

These lesions are composed of an abnormally configured venous drainage system converging on a single, enlarged venous outflow channel. The typical appearance is that of a hydra, with radially converging veins. A characteristic feature of this lesion appears to be that the abnormal venous bed is poorly collateralized. The abnormal venous drainage may or may not be fully adequate to the needs of the brain tissue supplied. Slowly evolving degenerative changes in the brain tissue supplied can occur as a result but, unfortunately, this is not helped by any known intervention. However inadequate, the venous anomaly represents the only venous drainage available to that area of brain, and therefore removal of the venous anomaly is not recommended. Doing so could lead to a venous infarction with swelling and hemorrhage, the consequences of which are particularly dangerous in the posterior fossa.

## Traumatic Arteriovenous Fistula

Both the internal carotid artery (ICA) and vertebral artery enter the cranial cavity immediately after passing through a venous network. The ICA passes through the cavernous sinus, which communicates with the superior ophthalmic vein, petrosal sinus, and sphenoparietal sinus. The vertebral artery passes through a venous plexus at the occipital-C1 epidural space, which communicates with the jugular vein, epidural venous plexus, and paraspinal venous plexus. Trauma leading to a tear in the carotid or vertebral artery at its tether point passing through the skull base can lead to fistula with the surrounding venous plexus. The consequences may vary in severity and suddenness but typically include periorbital swelling, with proptosis and scleral edema in the case of the carotid-cavernous fistula (CCF) and prominent pulsatile bruit in the case of the vertebral-jugular fistula. Intraocular pressure measurement by tonometry can guide the urgency in treating CCF. Radiologically, dilation of the superior ophthalmic vein is characteristic (Fig. 68-5). These lesions are usually treated by endovascular techniques. A catheter is advanced through the tear in the artery into the venous side of the fistula. The high-flow and large fistulous channel facilitate this process. Embolic material, a coil, or a detachable balloon is then used to occlude the venous side of the fistula. When conventional transvenous routes fail, a direct approach via transorbital puncture may be required to provide endovascular therapy.[9]

## Cerebral Saccular (Berry) Aneurysms

Saccular or berry cerebral aneurysms form as a degenerative change in the wall of the larger intracranial arteries in and around the circle of Willis. They are rare in children and occur with increased frequency in older age groups, sooner in patients with connective tissue defects, such as polycystic kidney disease, Marfan syndrome, and Ehlers-Danlos syndrome.

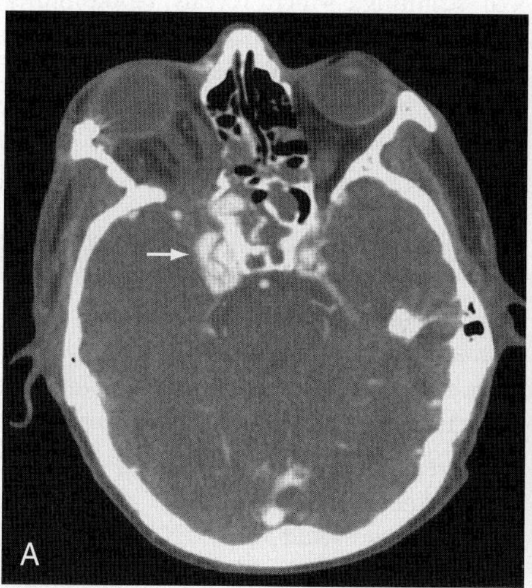


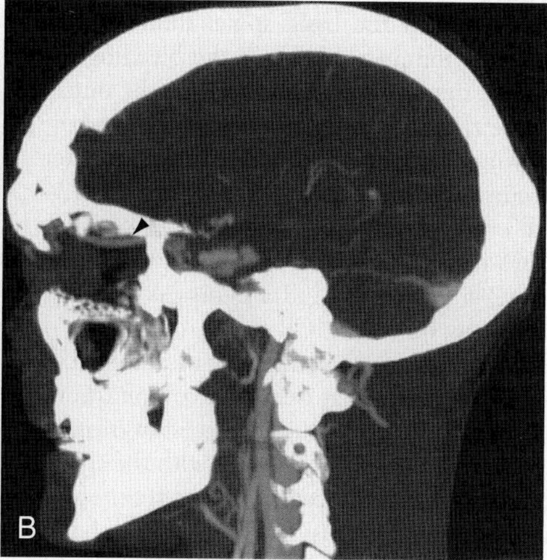


**FIGURE 68-5** Right internal carotid cavernous sinus fistula *(left arrow)* with dilation of the superior ophthalmic drain *(right arrow),* a typical imaging finding of this pathology.

Aneurysms form in relation to defects in the smooth muscle–containing media layer. Such defects are common at branch points in the arteries and can also occur in relation to shear forces at the edge of stiffened parts of the vessel wall containing atheroma. The defect in the media then allows the intima to stretch outward, fragmenting the internal elastic lamina in the process and carrying the connective tissue of the external adventitial layer outward with it. The connective tissue in the dilating intima and adventitia is capable of proliferation so that the aneurysm can reach a size considerably larger than stretching alone would allow. The Laplace equation predicts that at any given pressure, the stretching force on the wall of the aneurysm increases as the diameter increases. The process is therefore inherently not self-limited, but progressive. With robust connective tissue proliferation in the wall, a minority of aneurysms enlarge to surprising dimensions; hence, the blood flow within slows to allow thrombus formation, usually in concentric layers, to form a partly solid mass of much greater outer diameter than the lumen would suggest on angiography alone.

Distal embolization of clot material is a rare occurrence. Calcification can occur in the wall in advanced cases and the adjacent brain can become gliotic from chronic pressure, making seizures also a possible presentation. An enlarging aneurysm can also compress an adjacent cranial nerve; the optic and third nerves are usually affected by this mechanism. Generally, however, it is much more common for an aneurysm to present with subarachnoid hemorrhage. The proliferative ability of the connective tissue in the dome of the forming aneurysm can be exceeded by the stretching force, leading to rupture. The onset is unpredictable and appears to occur at a surprisingly low rate. Incidentally discovered unruptured aneurysms bleed at a rate depending on size. Those smaller than 1 cm bleed at a rate of 0.05% to 0.5%/year, whereas those larger than 1 cm bleed at a rate of 1% to 2%/year. Treatment recommendations for unruptured aneurysms smaller than 5 mm in diameter vary widely based on patient preference, aneurysm accessibility to treatment, and surgeon's assessment of risk. Once hemorrhage from an aneurysm occurs, the situation changes dramatically. Bleeding of highly oxygenated arterial blood occurs suddenly into the surrounding CSF-containing subarachnoid space, which initially offers little backpressure. Aneurysmal subarachnoid hemorrhage can occur in all gradations of severity. In most patients, accumulated blood in the basal spinal fluid cisterns leads to a coagulum that spontaneously stops the bleeding. In 10% to 15% of patients, the bleeding is so severe at the outset that death occurs before they even reach the hospital. Approximately 40% die following the initial hemorrhage but at a later stage. Rebleeding occurs with a peak incidence in the first 24 hours after the initial event. If the aneurysm is left unsecured, the rebleed rate is 20% in the first 2 weeks, 50% in the first 6 months, and thereafter 3% to 4%/year.[10] Rebleeding is the principal cause of death, usually by raised ICP.

Subarachnoid hemorrhage, with or without increased ICP, sets in motion a series of problems that can cause complications and poor outcomes, regardless of the technical success of treating the aneurysm itself. First, the blood can interfere with the spinal fluid circulation so that acute hydrocephalus can result in a raised ICP and reduced cerebral perfusion. The hydrocephalus is evident as ventricular enlargement on CT and can usually be readily treated with ventricular drainage. Second, the highly oxygenated blood coagulum surrounds the vessels traversing the subarachnoid space. Whereas these vessels are usually in an environment of clear colorless CSF, they now are in a milieu of decomposing blood, triggering the activation of lysosomal and proteolytic enzymes and generating chemically active free radicals. The smooth muscle coating of the otherwise intact vessels can become irritated to trigger vasospasm, at first reversible but, in severe cases evolving to a damaged and swollen arterial wall, with persistent luminal narrowing. The vessels eventually remodel over 3 to 6 weeks and return to a normal configuration but, all too often, ischemic deficits in the supplied brain occur in the interim. Unfortunately, these ischemic neurologic deficits are not rare and are the single major cause of serious morbidity after successful aneurysm treatment following subarachnoid hemorrhage. The blood coagulum eventually clears from the subarachnoid space but sometimes initiates a progressive slow fibrosis that results in delayed hydrocephalus, distinct from the early hydrocephalus caused by the coagulum itself. Cerebral vasospasm following subarachnoid hemorrhage starts on days 3 to 5 and peaks during days 5 to 14, resolving slowly over the weeks following the initial insult.

Treatment of the vasospasm includes elevating the blood pressure, blood volume, and cardiac output in an attempt to bring more blood flow past the narrowing in the vessels (Box 68-2). The calcium channel blocker nimodipine appears to reduce the incidence of delayed ischemic neurologic deficits and prevents vasospasm, probably through opening collaterals to the ischemic brain. Its direct effect on the vasospasm is still in question. Phase IIA trials with clazosentan, an endothelin A antagonist, have been promising in reducing the frequency and severity of cerebral vasospasm.[11] Attenuation of vasospasm by statins or magnesium sulfate is controversial according to recent literature.[12,13]

Investigation of patients with a suspected aneurysmal subarachnoid hemorrhage begins with an assessment of the history. Because the hemorrhage occurs into the subarachnoid space and not brain tissue, there is usually no focal neurologic deficit. Symptoms of sudden-onset headache with meningismus are classic and reflect a sudden rise in ICP and irritation of the basal meninges by the blood. In severe cases, the patient may be comatose or uncooperative. A report of a strokelike picture of sudden onset of neurologic signs and symptoms should prompt CT scanning, which reveals blood filling the subarachnoid cisterns (Fig. 68-6*A*). Because the hemorrhage can occur in all gradations of severity, the difficulty comes in recognizing the patient with the small sentinel hemorrhage who arrives in good condition with only the complaint of an alarmingly severe

**BOX 68-2 Treatment of Vasospasm**

**Prevention of Arterial Narrowing**
Subarachnoid blood removal
Prevention of dehydration and hypotension
Calcium channel blockers (nimodipine)

**Reversal of Arterial Narrowing**
Intra-arterial papaverine
Intra-arterial nimodipine
Transluminal balloon angioplasty

**Prevention and Reversal of Ischemic Neurologic Deficit**
Hypertension, hypervolemia, hemodilution

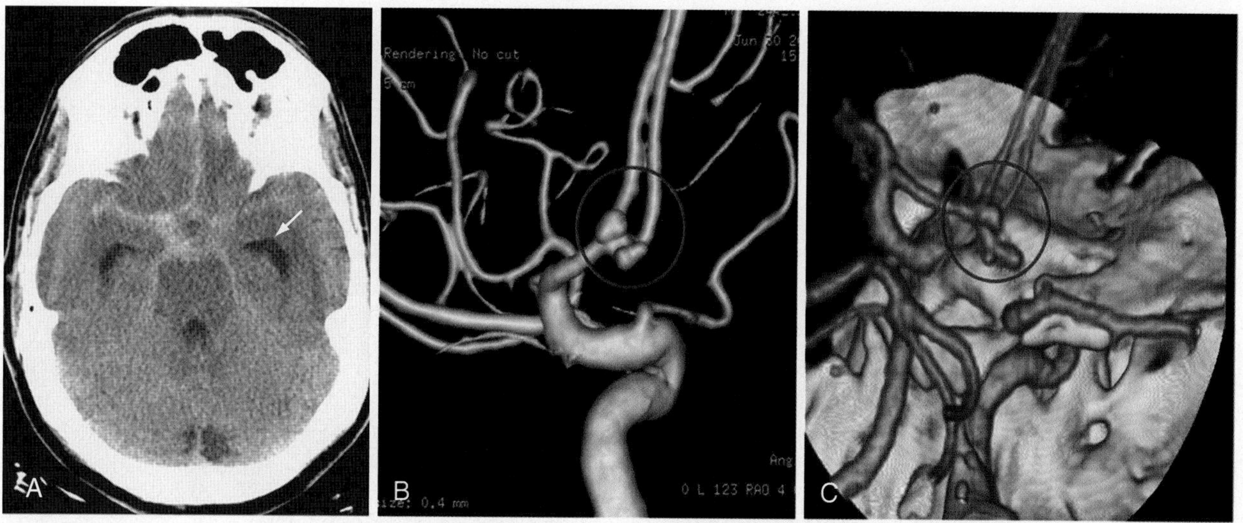

**FIGURE 68-6 A,** CT scan of brain showing subarachnoid blood in the basal cisterns. Dilated temporal horns *(yellow arrow)* indicate the presence of hydrocephalus. **B,** Cerebral angiogram shows two aneurysms located at the junction of the A1 and A2 segments of the anterior cerebral artery *(red circle)*. **C,** CT angiography with three-dimensional reconstruction showing the relationship of the aneurysms *(red circle)* with the skull base.

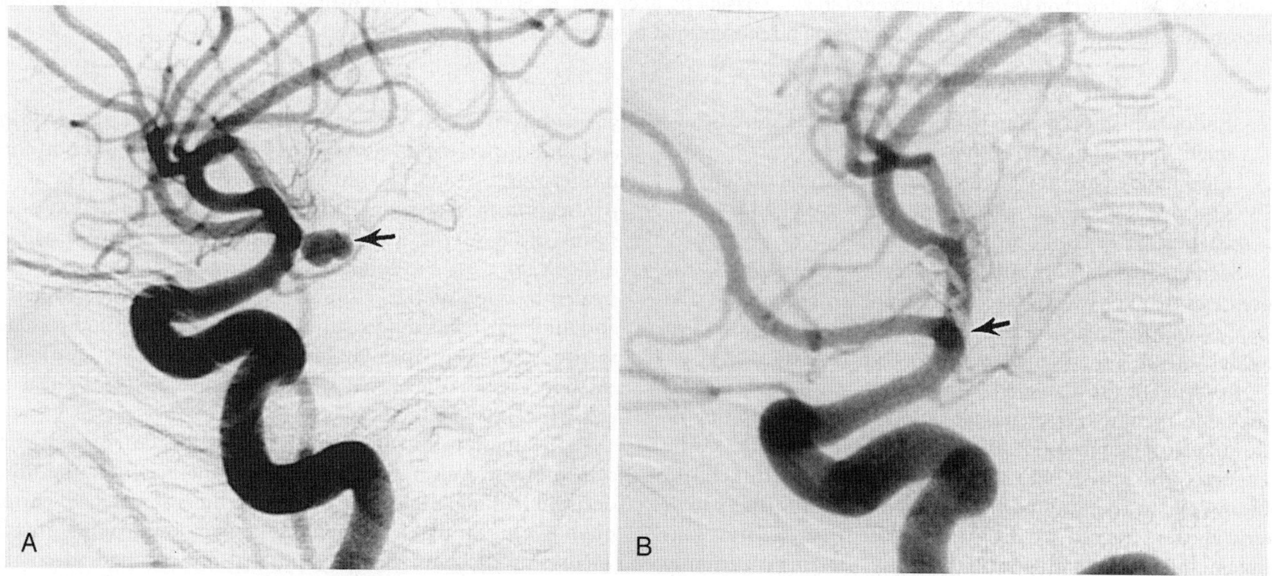

**FIGURE 68-7 A,** Subtraction carotid angiogram shows a 4- × 6-mm berry aneurysm *(arrow)* originating from the distal internal carotid artery. **B,** Postoperative carotid angiogram shows clip placement *(arrow)*, with total obliteration of the aneurysm.

sudden onset of headache. Headache from increased ICP may be only transient until compensatory mechanisms occur. Residual headache and neck stiffness from meningismus, although usually present, may not be impressive.

A high index of suspicion is required for these patients. It is important to focus on the suddenness of symptom onset rather than severity because reports of severity are more subjective or may be tainted by a strong psychological overlay of denial or exaggeration; also, the headache caused by a very small hemorrhage may be dissipating naturally to some extent by the time the patient is finally assessed. If the headache onset is truly or almost instantaneous, lumbar puncture is usually advised in cases in which the CT scan is negative. Blood in the CSF with xanthochromia in the supernatant is diagnostic.

If the CT scan or lumbar puncture is positive for subarachnoid blood, the next step is usually conventional catheter cerebral angiography (see Fig. 68-6*B*). CT angiography with bolus IV contrast has become increasingly convenient and accurate; thus, it is being used more frequently. Newer scanners are capable of large numbers of simultaneous slices so that three-dimensional reconstruction with good registration and surprising detail is possible (see Fig. 68-6*C*). With selections in density windowing, the relation of the aneurysm to any blood clot can also be visualized.

Treatment of a cerebral aneurysm can be performed in a variety of ways:

1. Open craniotomy with microdissection and clipping of the neck (Fig. 68-7)

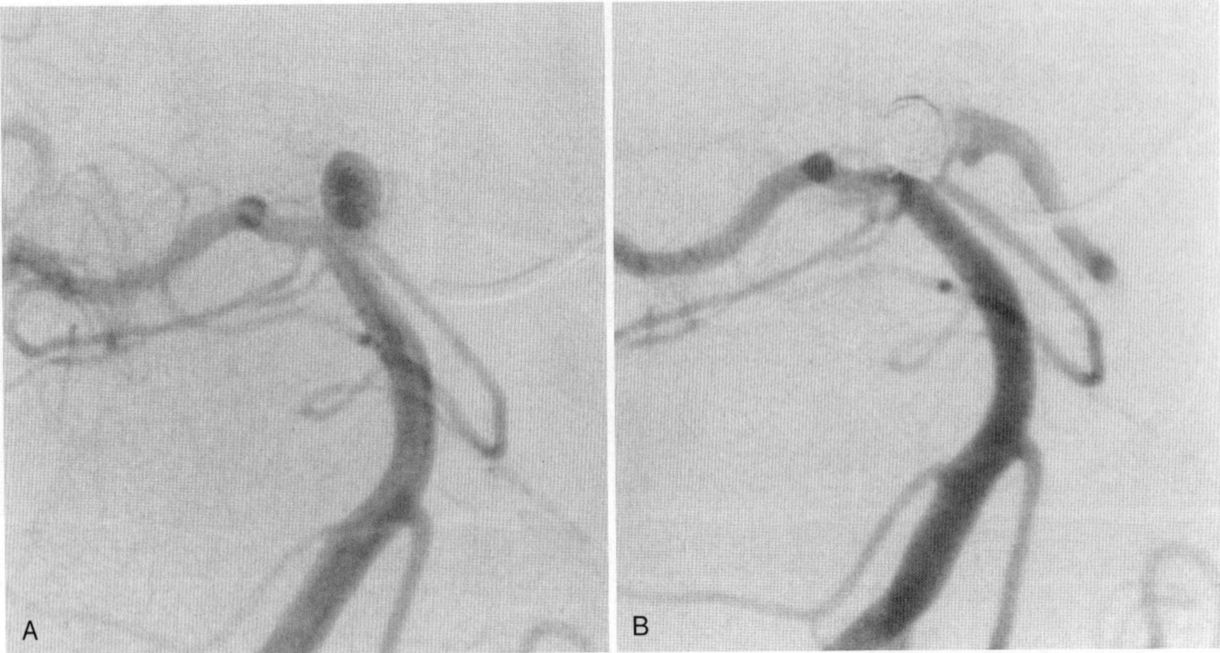


**FIGURE 68-8 A,** Subtraction vertebral angiogram shows a basilar tip aneurysm. **B,** Subtracted vertebral angiogram after the placement of coils demonstrates excellent obliteration of the aneurysm and preservation of adjacent vessels.

2. Endovascular occlusion with detachable coil placement in the fundus (Fig. 68-8)
3. Elimination from the circulation by segmental occlusion of the parent artery proximal and distal to the aneurysm neck, with or without bypass

Segmental occlusion and bypass are usually reserved for those cases that are awkward to treat by any other method. The choice of endovascular coil occlusion versus open surgical clipping has, on the other hand, become a complex issue.

In terms of the aneurysm configuration, a narrow neck is a favorable attribute for treatment by open surgical clipping or endovascular embolization methods. Wide-necked or sessile aneurysms with a high neck-to-fundus ratio make it difficult to contain coils in the fundus without protrusion into the parent artery. A stent placed in the parent artery may address this problem, but the technology is evolving and stenting is currently practical only in more proximal locations. Generally, wide-necked aneurysms gravitate toward open surgical treatment, although stent-assisted coiling can be also used in some cases. Particularly interesting is the recently introduced concept of functional reconstruction with the use of flow diverters. These stents induce reverse remodeling and delayed disappearance of the aneurysm via thrombosis. They are especially useful for very small, giant, wide-necked, or otherwise difficult to treat aneurysms and can be used with intramural coil placement.[14,15]

In regard to aneurysm location, the more proximal the aneurysm, the easier it is to reach by endovascular means, whereas the more distal the aneurysm, the more difficult it is to reach and treat effectively by that method. Aneurysms in the cavernous sinus are considered difficult to reach by any open surgical method and are generally only treated by endovascular means or by parent artery occlusion with bypass. Aneurysms of the ICA at the level of the ophthalmic artery origin can be treated by open surgery or endovascular methods, as can most aneurysms of the ICA, proximal middle cerebral artery (MCA), and anterior cerebral artery (ACA), as far as the anterior communicating artery. The more distal MCA aneurysms, at the trifurcation in the sylvian fissure and beyond, and ACA aneurysms distal to the anterior communicating artery are more difficult to treat by endovascular methods and generally are treated by open surgical clipping. The basilar artery termination and midbasilar area can usually be reached easily by endovascular methods, whereas open surgery is possible but not feasible in these locations. The vertebral artery aneurysms can be reached easily by either method.

In situations in which the aneurysm location or configuration presents a clear advantage of one method over the other, decision making is fairly easy, even at centers at which all current methods are available. Problems in decision making involve aneurysms that are favorably situated and configured so that they would be attractive to treat by open surgical clipping or endovascular coil occlusion. In the past, open surgical clipping was considered first,and the patient was referred for endovascular coil occlusion only if there were reasons to avoid open surgery. However, since the European prospective randomized trial of surgery versus open clipping, this paradigm is now open to question; it is becoming more common to consider endovascular treatment before open surgical clipping in aneurysms treatable by either method.[16]

Increasingly, the patient is treated by a team approach in which all treatment methods are available and considered in view of the patient's aneurysm location, configuration, general medical condition, and expressed personal or family preference(s). Endovascular treatment avoids craniotomy, but has an aneurysm recurrence rate of 15% or higher. The recurrence rate after open surgical clipping appears to be much lower.

Results of treatment of unruptured aneurysms are generally good by any method, but these usually involve a carefully selected group for whom treatment conditions are favorable and, most importantly, there is no aftermath of subarachnoid hemorrhage to overcome. These beneficial results in patients with unruptured aneurysms, without subarachnoid hemorrhage, contrast markedly with the overall disappointing outcomes in patients with aneurysmal subarachnoid hemorrhage. Regardless of the type of treatment, the risks for disabling ischemic complications from cerebral vasospasm and hydrocephalus are much higher in patients with subarachnoid hemorrhage. Patients with aneurysmal subarachnoid hemorrhage who present at the hospital in reasonable condition, at least awake and talking, still have only a 60% chance of returning home without functional deficit. The treatment contributes approximately 5% to the complications. Vasospasm and the comorbidities associated with prolonged treatment account for most of the rest. Infection from the ventriculostomy needed to treat hydrocephalus and control ICP is a minor component of the complication rate.

## Spontaneous Intracerebral Hemorrhage

Spontaneous intracerebral hemorrhages into the brain parenchyma are common, accounting for approximately 10% of all strokes. They generally occur in older patients, usually because of degenerative changes in the cerebral vessels that are often associated with chronic hypertension (Box 68-3). In younger patients, they are more likely related to drug abuse or vascular malformation. They can occur anywhere in the cerebral circulation or brainstem but are classically described in association with small degenerative aneurysms (microaneurysms; also known as *Charcot-Bouchard aneurysms*) at the junctions of the perforating vessels and larger vessels at the skull base. They are typically on the MCA junctions with the small perforating lenticulostriate vessels, leading to hemorrhage into the putamen. The clinical presentation is with a stroke pattern of sudden-onset neurologic signs and symptoms that depend on the area of brain affected. Symptoms are more likely to include headache than ischemic stroke. The diagnosis is with CT, usually done in an emergency department setting. The size and location of the acute hematoma are well visualized with CT, as well as any associated brain shift or hydrocephalus (Figs. 68-9*A* and 68-10). In older patients with a known history of hypertension and classic CT appearance of a hematoma in the putamen, thalamus, cerebellum, or pons, further diagnostic studies are generally not indicated. Rehemorrhage is unlikely in that setting. However, further investigation might be warranted with an atypical hematoma location or appearance, especially if there is any component of subarachnoid blood. Also, investigation is usually recommended for younger patients without known hypertension and those with a potential underlying cause for hemorrhage (e.g., history of neoplasm, blood dyscrasias, bacterial endocarditis).

Further investigation is generally done with contrast MRI or MRA. Any suggestion of aneurysm or AVM is followed by conventional catheter angiography. In older patients with a history of early dementia and multiple episodes of more peripherally located intracerebral hematomas, the diagnosis of amyloid angiopathy needs to be considered.

**BOX 68-3 Causes of Spontaneous Intracerebral Hemorrhage**

Hypertension
Vascular anomaly
Cerebral aneurysm
Arteriovenous malformation
Cavernous malformation
Cerebral infarction (stroke) transformation
Cerebral amyloid angiopathy
Coagulopathy
Tumors
Drug abuse
Other

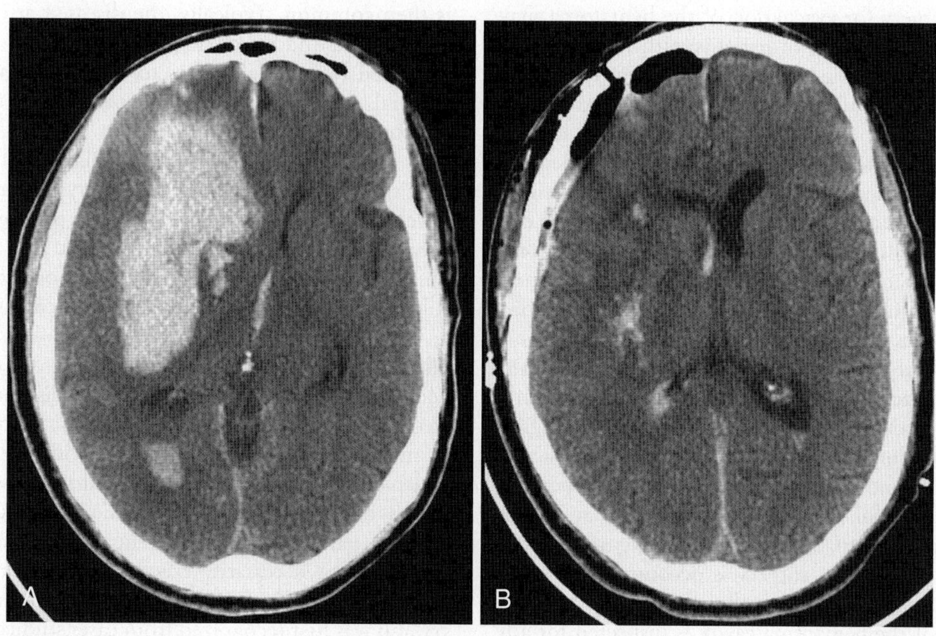


**FIGURE 68-9** Nonenhanced CT scan of the head. **A,** Spontaneous hypertensive intracerebral hematoma in the right basal ganglia, with extension to the frontal and temporal lobes. **B,** Immediate postoperative CT scan shows near-total removal of the intracerebral hematoma.

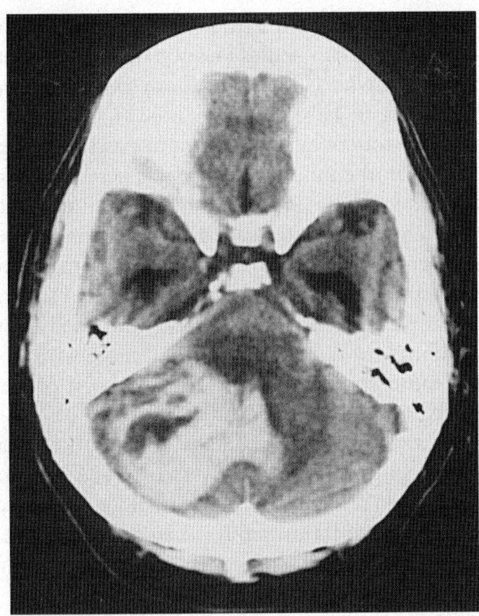

**FIGURE 68-10** Nonenhanced CT scan of the brain shows a large, hypertensive, intracerebellar hematoma with obstruction of the fourth ventricle and enlargement of the temporal horns, indicating obstructive hydrocephalus.

Most cases of spontaneous intracerebral hemorrhage do not require an operative procedure. Many hemorrhages are small enough to be well tolerated and do not require surgery. Others are so large at the outset that surgery is of little benefit. Relief of any obstructive hydrocephalus by ventricular drainage is usually offered, except in the most impossible cases. Patients who obey commands and can be monitored by changes in their neurologic examination can generally be managed conservatively with hospital observation for at least 5 to 7 days. Peak swelling and decompensation are probably most likely to occur within that time frame. Surgery for evacuation of the hematoma may be appropriate in a small group of patients with intermediate-sized hemorrhages in accessible locations who appear to tolerate the hematoma initially, but then deteriorate in a delayed fashion with edema, despite medical therapy. Steroids have not demonstrated benefit. Attempts to predict which patients will deteriorate based solely on hematoma volume have been frustrated by the broad spectrum of intracranial compliance exhibited by different patients. Generally, younger patients with smaller ventricles and small subarachnoid spaces have a lower compliance, with lower tolerance, than older patients with cerebral atrophy and generous ventricles and subarachnoid spaces.

The Surgical Trial in Intracerebral Hemorrhage has noted a lack of clinical outcome difference when comparing early surgery with conservative management.[17] If indicated, surgical evacuation is usually done by craniotomy over the most accessible part of the hematoma (see Fig. 68-9*B*). Intraoperative ultrasound is often helpful in finding hematomas that do not quite come to the cortical surface and in monitoring the progress of the evacuation. The goal of surgery is decompression more than complete removal, but is generally done as far as safely practical. The wall of the hematoma cavity is inspected for any underlying cause and a biopsy is taken, if indicated. Putamen hemorrhage can sometimes be evacuated with minimal surgical damage to the overlying brain by a trans-sylvian fissure–transinsular approach. Stereotactic aspiration and methods with fibrinolytic agents are being developed and may be a consideration for patients with hematomas in deep locations that are otherwise difficult to access.

A special situation to consider is the patient with cerebellar hemorrhage (see Fig. 68-10). Surgery is offered more readily in these cases because the danger of sudden deterioration from brainstem compression is more of a concern, and because even extensive damage to the cerebellum itself is generally survivable, with good functional outcome. Patients with fourth ventricular obstruction and hydrocephalus from cerebellar hemorrhage can sometimes be treated with ventricular drainage alone but are usually offered surgical evacuation of the hematoma by suboccipital craniotomy because of the risk for brainstem compression.

## Mycotic Aneurysms

These aneurysms are associated with a systemic infection capable of showering small particles of bacteria-infected material into the cerebral vascular bed. Subacute bacterial endocarditis and some pulmonary infections can do this. A distinguishing feature of these aneurysms is that they are generally found more distal in the cerebral vascular bed, as opposed to berry aneurysms, which are usually found on larger vessels near the circle of Willis. There can also be many of them. When the bacterial emboli lodge in distal cerebral arterial branches, they can erode through the wall of these smaller vessels, often creating a hemorrhage contained by the perivascular tissue. Maximal antibiotic treatment is essential at the outset. The presence of an intracerebral hematoma may force immediate craniotomy for evacuation. Operation on the aneurysm at this early stage often reveals a component of subarachnoid hemorrhage and an early inflammatory reaction in the subarachnoid space, with only a blood collection covering the erosion defect in the wall of the small artery. Attempts to dissect and define a neck are frustrated by a lack of developed fibrous tissues and intraoperative hemorrhage is then common. Typically, the diseased arterial segment must be occluded and resected when operated on in this early stage. The need for arterial bypass to maintain blood flow to critical cerebral areas should be anticipated, but this is not always possible.

If the mycotic aneurysms are discovered or treated at some later stage, a fibrous wall to the aneurysm may have had time to develop, and clipping can then be a possibility. However, the surgeon needs to be forewarned that it may be difficult to find the aneurysm in a distal location, often buried deep in a cerebral sulcus thickened with reactive fibrous scar tissue.

## Moyamoya Disease

Moyamoya disease is a cerebrovascular disorder that is characterized by an idiopathic nonatherosclerotic narrowing or occlusion of major intracranial blood vessels with the development of a conspicuous compensatory collateral rete vessel network, which allows continued cerebral perfusion around the occluded or severely narrowed segment. The disorder is usually bilateral, although not necessarily exactly symmetrical. Although generally rare, the disease is more common in persons of Asian ancestry and was first recognized from cases studied with angiography in Japan before the advent of CT and MRI. The term *moyamoya* comes from the Japanese word for "puff of smoke," or mist. The actual disease is sometimes confused with the less conspicuous collateral vascular networks seen around severe narrowing of common atherosclerotic origin in persons of Western origin. In the juvenile form, moyamoya typically presents as cognitive decline, with deteriorating school performance and evidence of multiple infarcts. Angiography reveals the ICA, proximal MCA, or proximal ACA with severe narrowing or occlusion and, generally, multiple clusters of fine collateral vessels. In the adult form of moyamoya disease, the rete vessels cause subarachnoid or basal ganglia hemorrhage, the most common presentations. The hemorrhage can usually be treated conservatively. Some form of extracranial to intracranial bypass is generally attempted to take the load off the collateral vascular network. In younger patients, the results are good, with an onlay interposition of the superficial temporal artery sewed into the dura after a strip craniotomy. A feature of the disorder is the vigor with which collaterals form from the onlay transposed vessel. In the adult form, a microvascular anastomosis with the superficial temporal artery or grafted vessel may be preferred.

### Dural Arteriovenous Malformations

Dural AVMs (type 2 CCF is a subtype) are not often seen in younger patients. The lesions seem to occur only in adults and are probably acquired lesions that follow a dural sinus thrombosis, usually of the cavernous sinus or sigmoid-transverse sinus junction area. With subsequent healing, the thrombosed segment triggers a neovascular response that evolves to an AVM configuration with fistulous channels that can gradually enlarge. Usually, there is associated stenosis of the affected dural segment, suggesting the earlier thrombosis. The lesions are generally not dangerous unless they cause retrograde venous drainage into the cerebral circulation. The risk for intracranial hemorrhage is then fairly high; it is important at least to separate the dural AVM drainage from the cerebral circulation when that occurs. In the case of transverse-sigmoid sinus dural AVM, the patient usually complains of a bruit and embolization or resection is optional, depending on symptom tolerance. In the case of type 2 CCF, the problem is usually intraocular and intraorbital venous hypertension, with proptosis, chemosis, and sometimes threatened vision. Ocular tonometry can help determine the extent of the threat to vision. Treatment of type 2 CCF involves endovascular embolization of prominent feeders, followed by occlusion of the affected venous dural sinus. As long as the dural AVM drainage is separated from the cerebral circulation, occlusion of the affected venous drainage is safe and curative. The affected stenotic transverse-sigmoid sinus segment can be reached by endovascular techniques through the jugular vein. The cavernous sinus can be reached by the petrosal sinus or, with neurosurgical assistance, through the superior orbital vein.

## CENTRAL NERVOUS SYSTEM TUMORS

### Intracranial Tumors

Intracranial tumors can be classified as primary versus secondary, pediatric versus adult, by cell of origin, or by location in the nervous system. Primary tumors arise from tissues in the nervous system, whereas secondary tumors originate from tissues outside the nervous system and metastasize secondarily to the brain. They may represent local extension of regional tumors such as chordoma or scalp cancer but usually reach the nervous system through the hematogenous route.

In general, the incidence of primary brain tumors is higher in whites than in blacks, and mortality is higher in males than in females. According to the Central Brain Tumor Registry of the United States (CBTUS), the overall incidence of primary brain tumors was 14.8/100,000 person-years between 1998 and 2002 (CBTUS statistical report, 2005-2006). On the other hand, secondary tumors outnumber primary brain tumors by 10 : 1 and occur in 20% to 40% of cancer patients.[18] Because no national cancer registry documents brain metastases, the exact incidence is unknown, but it has been estimated that 98,000 to 170,000 new cases are diagnosed in the United States each year.[19]

### Clinical Presentation

The clinical manifestations of various brain tumors can be divided into those caused by focal compression and irritation by the tumor itself and those attributed to secondary consequences—namely, increased ICP, peritumoral edema, and hydrocephalus. Usually, symptoms are caused by a combination of these factors.

The clinical presentation does not differ much by tumor histology but rather by rate of growth and location of the tumor. A meningioma peripherally located in a relatively silent area of the brain, with a slow rate of growth, may enlarge to a significant size in a neurologically intact patient because the brain can accommodate to a slowly growing lesion. On the other hand, a small metastatic lesion at the foramen of Monro or in the sensorimotor strip can cause acute hydrocephalus or seizures, respectively.

Headache occurs in 50% to 60% of primary brain tumors and in 35% to 50% of metastatic tumors. It is classically described as being worse in the morning, probably because of hypoventilation during sleep, with consequent elevation of the $P_{CO_2}$ and cerebrovascular dilation. The headache is associated with nausea and vomiting in 40% of patients and may be temporarily relieved by vomiting as a result of hyperventilation. Seizures may be the first symptom of a brain tumor. Patients older than 20 years presenting with a new-onset seizure are aggressively investigated for a brain tumor.

Infratentorial lesions may present with headache, nausea and vomiting, gait disturbance and ataxia, vertigo, cranial nerve deficits leading to diplopia (abducens nerve), facial numbness and pain (trigeminal nerve), unilateral hearing deficit and tinnitus (vestibulocochlear nerve), facial weakness (facial nerve), dysphagia (glossopharyngeal and vagus nerves), and CSF obstruction causing hydrocephalus and papilledema. Supratentorial lesions may present with different symptoms, depending on the location. Frontal lobe lesions manifest as personality changes, dementia, hemiparesis, or dysphasia. Temporal lobe lesions may present with memory changes, auditory or olfactory hallucinations, or contralateral quadrantanopsia. Patients with parietal lobe lesions may develop contralateral motor or sensory impairment, apraxias, and homonymous hemianopsias, whereas those with occipital lobe lesions may show contralateral visual field deficits and alexia.

### Imaging Studies

The initial workup generally involves a relatively inexpensive diagnostic tool, a CT scan of the brain. CT provides a rapid means of evaluating changes in brain density such as calcifications, hyperacute hemorrhages (<24 hours old), and skull lesions. MRI of the brain, however, is the gold standard modality for diagnosis, presurgical planning, and post-therapeutic monitoring of brain tumors. Gadolinium contrast enhancement with MRI is more sensitive in demonstrating defects in the blood-brain barrier and localizing small metastases (up to 5 mm). It can be used in patients allergic to iodine and those with renal failure. Advances in MRI techniques have evolved from strictly morphology-based imaging to a modality that encompasses function, physiology, and anatomy. Diffusion-weighted imaging can help distinguish between gliomas and abscesses, and perfusion-weighted imaging can predict response to radiotherapy in low-grade gliomas. Functional MRI can be used when planning surgery for tumors in eloquent areas of the brain to enable radical resection with less morbidity. Diffusion tensor imaging can demonstrate the effect of a tumor on white matter tracts. MRA is used more routinely as a noninvasive modality to evaluate the vascularity of a tumor or anatomic relationship of a tumor to normal cerebral vasculature.[20]

### Surgery

Dexamethasone is recommended for the management of brain tumors because of its propensity to reduce peritumoral edema by stabilizing the cell membrane. An antiepileptic drug is also recommended for tumors close to the sensorimotor strip. Mannitol administration prior to dural opening and operative resection is often used.

Technical advances have made tumor surgery safer and more effective. The intraoperative microscope provides superior illumination and magnification, thereby allowing the surgeon to resect tumors from critical areas through small cranial openings. The cavitational ultrasonic surgical aspirator (CUSA) simultaneously breaks up and sucks away firm tumors while protecting vital neural and vascular structures. Intraoperative ultrasonography provides real-time imaging of tumors and cysts in subcortical and deep areas of the brain. Intraoperative CT or MRI is standard practice in some centers, enabling on-table imaging of the extent of resection (Fig. 68-11*A*). CT and MRI also allow real-time visualization of a biopsy needle within a target. Image-guided (CT or MRI) frameless surgical navigation allows instant and accurate localization of the tip a probe during a craniotomy by displaying that point on a preoperative CT or MRI scan (see Fig. 68-11*B*).

The primary goals of surgery include histologic diagnosis and reduction of mass effect by removing as much tumor as is safely possible to preserve neurologic function. The decision between a needle biopsy and more radical surgical resection depends on the location and size of the tumor, its sensitivity to radiation or chemotherapy, preoperative Karnofsky performance score of the patient, and systemic status of the primary cancer in case of metastatic brain lesions.

## PRIMARY BRAIN TUMORS

Primary tumors of the brain are divided into intra-axial (those arising from within the brain parenchyma) and extra-axial (those arising from outside the brain parenchyma).

### Intra-Axial Brain Tumors

Intra-axial brain tumors develop from the glia, or supportive structures, of the neurons and are collectively called *gliomas*. Total surgical resection of gliomas is extremely rare because of their ability to infiltrate widely along the white matter tracts and

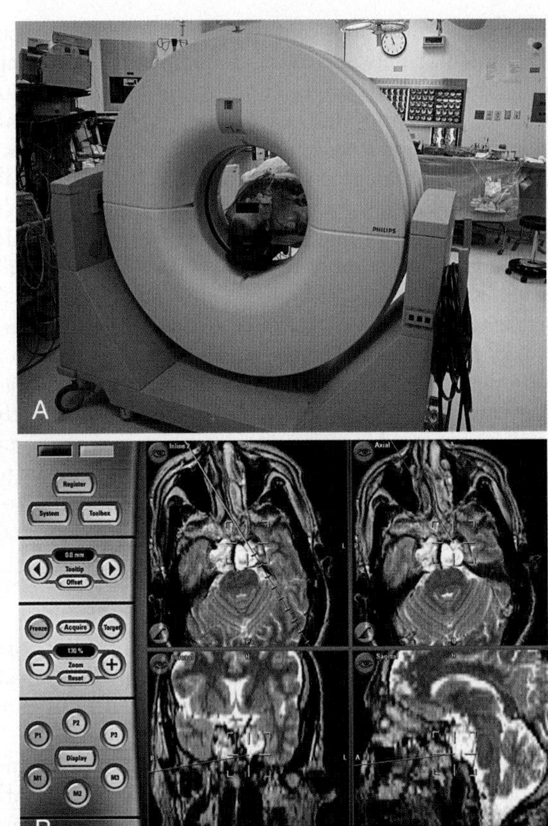


**FIGURE 68-11** Technologic advances in the operating room. **A,** Intraoperative CT scanner. **B,** Computer-guided surgical navigation showing real-time location of a surgical probe tip on the preoperative MRI study during resection of clival chordoma.

cross the corpus callosum into the contralateral hemisphere. Radiation therapy and chemotherapy options vary according to the histology of the brain tumor. Therapy involving surgically implanted carmustine-impregnated polymer combined with postoperative radiation therapy has a role in the treatment of de novo and recurrent high-grade gliomas. Biologic therapies being evaluated clinically for patients with brain tumors include dendritic cell vaccination, tyrosine kinase receptor inhibitors, farnesyl transferase inhibitors, viral-based gene therapy, and oncolytic viruses. An ideal therapy will target rapidly growing malignant glioma cells along with infiltrating tumor cells, with minimal toxicity to normal cells. This will require the therapeutic vehicle of choice to have access to all cells in the brain and be able to distinguish invasive or quiescent tumor cells from normal cells.[21]

The current histopathologic classification of brain tumors was recently updated by the World Health Organization (WHO).[22] WHO classifies intra-axial brain tumors by cell type and grades them on a scale of I to IV based on light microscopy characteristics that include the degree of cellularity, pleomorphism, mitotic figures, endothelial proliferation, and necrosis. The higher the grade, the more aggressive and malignant the tumor.

**Astrocytoma** Astrocytomas arise from astrocytes and account for 50% of all primary brain tumors. Grade I astrocytomas, also called *pilocytic astrocytomas*, are a special group of tumors that

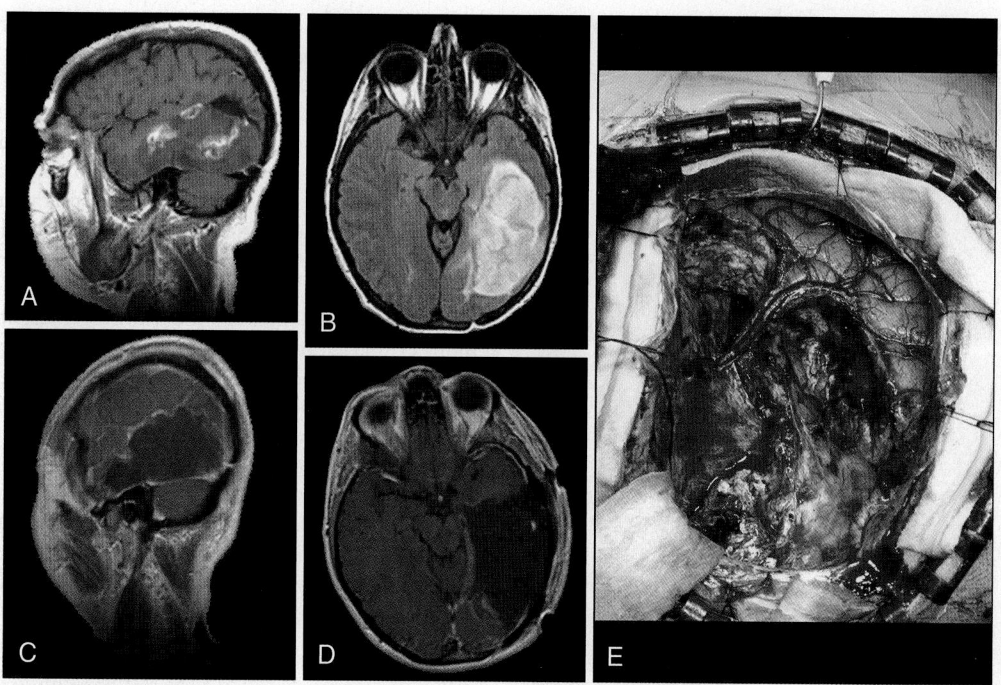


**FIGURE 68-12** Radiographic and intraoperative images of a patient with a left temporal anaplastic astrocytoma. **A,** A partially enhancing tumor is noted in the left temporal lobe on this gadolinium-enhanced sagittal MRI study. **B,** Fluid-attenuated inversion recovery (FLAIR) sequence axial MRI shows the extent of the tumor. The postoperative gadolinium-enhanced sagittal **(C)** and axial **(D)** MRI scans show near-total resection of the tumor. **E,** Intraoperative illustration of the surgical field after resection of the tumor.

are discrete appearing, contrast-enhancing, and often cystic, with a mural nodule. The mean age of occurrence is lower than for typical astrocytomas, generally in the first 2 decades of life. Patients have a median survival time of 8 to 10 years. Astrocytomas represent the most common glioma in children, representing 10% of cerebral and 85% of cerebellar astrocytomas. They tend to occur in the cerebellum, optic tract, and hypothalamus. These lesions are usually curable by radical resection. Radiation therapy and chemotherapy have no role in their treatment.[22]

Low-grade, or grade II, astrocytomas tend to occur in children and young adults. Most patients present with seizures. They typically demonstrate one histologic criterion, usually nuclear atypia, have a low degree of cellularity, and manifest preservation of normal brain elements. They appear hypointense on T1-weighted MRI sequences and hyperintense on T2, and fail to show contrast enhancement. The ultimate behavior of these tumors is usually not benign. Treatment is controversial and can include observant management and follow-up, radiation with or without chemotherapy, and surgery. Surgery is not curative because most of these tumors are infiltrative, with no clear margins. The median survival time is 7 to 8 years.

Grade III (anaplastic) and grade IV (glioblastoma multiforme [GBM]) astrocytomas are considered high-grade tumors. The presence of endothelial proliferation or necrosis on histology makes the tumor grade IV. Reports have suggested correlations between the presence of *p53* mutations on chromosome 17p and a number of findings, including an increased likelihood of anaplastic progression, longer survival time, correlation with the presence of aneuploidy, young age at diagnosis, and correlation with subsets of GBM.[23] These tumors are seen in older patients (>50 years). Malignant astrocytomas may develop from low-grade astrocytomas by dedifferentiation. GBM is the most common primary brain tumor. Anaplastic astrocytomas tend to have irregular enhancement on MRI (Fig. 68-12), whereas GBMs will have ring enhancement, with central necrosis (Fig. 68-13).

The optimal treatment includes a cytoreductive surgery followed by external beam radiation therapy (EBRT) to a dose of 60 Gy. The extent of tumor resection has a significant effect on time to tumor progression and median survival. All chemotherapeutic agents in use have no more than a 30% to 40% response rate, and most have a 10% to 20% response rate, primarily because of lack of adequate permeability through the blood-brain tumor barrier, with insufficient time to maintain therapeutic concentrations in individual tumor cells.[24] Carmustine (BCNU) and cisplatin have been the primary agents used against malignant gliomas. More recently, temozolomide, an oral alkylating agent that tags to guanine within the tumor cell, ultimately triggering apoptosis, has shown some promise in the management of newly diagnosed and recurrent GBM, with an overall survival time of 13.6 months.[25] Median survival time for anaplastic astrocytoma is 2 to 3 years and for GBM is less than 1 year.

**Oligodendroglioma** This tumor frequently presents with seizures, has a predilection for the cortex and white matter of the cerebral hemispheres (frontal lobe in 50% to 65% of patients), and has a classic histologic feature of so-called *fried egg cytoplasm*, chicken wire vasculature, and microscopic calcifications. The most frequent genetic alterations include loss of heterozygosity on chromosome 19q, followed by loss of heterozygosity on chromosome 1p. These alterations are usually associated with a better prognosis.[22] Brain CT may show tumoral calcifications

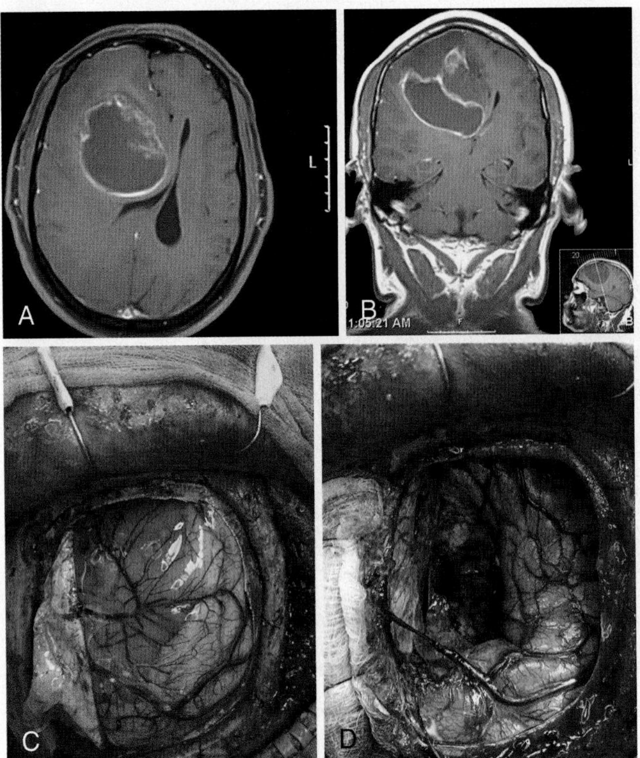


**FIGURE 68-13** MRI and intraoperative pictures of a patient with a glioblastoma multiforme. Gadolinium-enhanced axial **(A)** and coronal **(B)** MRI scans show a large tumor with ring enhancement causing a 1-cm subfalcine shift of midline structures. Intraoperative pictures show the yellowish tumor surrounded by normal brain gyri **(C)** and the surgical field after resection of the tumor **(D)**.

and MRI findings are similar to those with the astrocytomas. This tumor is classified as low or high grade. Chemotherapy is the primary modality of treatment after an appropriate surgical resection. Median survival times ranging from 3 to 5 years have been reported for patient with oligodendroglial tumors of all histologic grades. Benefits of radiation therapy are controversial.

**Ependymoma** These neoplasms arise from the ependymal lining of the cerebral hemispheres and from the remnants of the central canal of the spinal cord. They manifest predominantly in children (within the fourth ventricle) and young adults. MRI findings include a well-circumscribed lesion, with varying degrees of enhancement. Ventricular or brainstem displacement and hydrocephalus are frequent features. Optimal treatment includes maximal possible resection without causing neurologic deficits, followed by EBRT (45 to 56 Gy). Ependymomas have the potential to spread through the neuraxis by seeding of the CSF; craniospinal radiation is recommended in this case.

**Primitive Neuroectodermal Tumors** Primitive neuroectodermal tumors (PNETs) originate from primitive neuroectodermal cells (actual cell of origin is unknown) and encompass medulloblastoma, the most common PNET, retinoblastoma, pineoblastoma, neuroblastoma, esthesioneuroblastoma, and ependymoblastoma. These tumors also have a tendency to seed the CSF. Medulloblastoma is the most common pediatric brain malignancy, usually arises in the roof of the fourth ventricle (often producing hydrocephalus), and may invade the brainstem. The treatment of choice includes maximal surgical debulking, followed by craniospinal irradiation. BCNU and vincristine are primarily used for recurrences, in poor-risk patients, and in children younger than 3 years to avoid radiation therapy. Patients without a residual tumor on postoperative MRI and with negative CSF seeding have more than a 75% 5-year survival rate.

**Hemangioblastoma** Hemangioblastoma represents the most common primary intra-axial tumor in the adult posterior fossa, is histologically benign, and may be associated with erythrocytosis. Hemangioblastomas may be solid or cystic, with a mural nodule. They may occur sporadically and 20% of cases may be associated with von Hippel-Lindau disease (hemangioblastomas, retinal angiomas, renal cell carcinoma, pheochromocytoma, renal and pancreatic cysts). These lesions may also occur in the brainstem and spinal cord. Optimal surgical treatment involves resection of the mural nodule in a cystic lesion (cyst wall need not be removed). Solid lesions tend to be more difficult to remove.

**Primary Central Nervous System Lymphoma** The incidence of CNS lymphoma is rising relative to other brain lesions. This is partly because of the high frequency of CNS lymphoma in AIDS patients and transplant recipients. The median age at diagnosis is 52 years (younger in the immunocompromised population). It has a predilection for periventricular areas, deep nuclei, and the frontal lobes. It may also occur in the cerebellum. Primary CNS lymphoma is also known as a *ghost cell tumor* because of its tendency for partial to complete resolution on CT after the administration of steroids. A stereotactic needle biopsy is indicated when the index of suspicion for CNS lymphoma is high because these lesions are highly sensitive to radiation. In non-AIDS patients, chemotherapy combined with EBRT prolongs survival compared with EBRT alone. Without therapy, median survival time is 1.8 to 3.3 months. With radiation, median survival time is 10 months. In AIDS-related cases, the median survival time is only 3 to 5 months.

### Extra-Axial Brain Tumors

**Meningiomas** Meningiomas can occur wherever arachnoid cap cells are found (e.g., surface of brain and cord, ventricles). They are slow-growing, generally benign, tumors, usually located along the falx, convexity, or sphenoid bone, and can cause hyperostosis of adjacent bone. They tend to occur more in women, with a peak incidence at age 45 years. In one series, 32% of primary brain tumors seen on imaging were meningiomas, and 39% of these were asymptomatic.[26]

Meningiomas appear isointense on T1- and T2-weighted sequences on MRI but enhance strongly and homogeneously (Fig. 68-14*A*). A dural tail is a relatively common finding on MRI (Fig. 68-15*A* and *B*). Surgery is the treatment of choice for symptomatic meningiomas, with the extent of resection being the most important factor in the prevention of recurrence. Recurrence after gross total resection occurs in 11% to 15% of cases. Radiation therapy—conventional fractionated or, more commonly radiosurgery using a gamma knife or linear accelerator—may be of benefit in subtotally resected tumors located in critical areas (e.g., petroclival region, cavernous sinus),

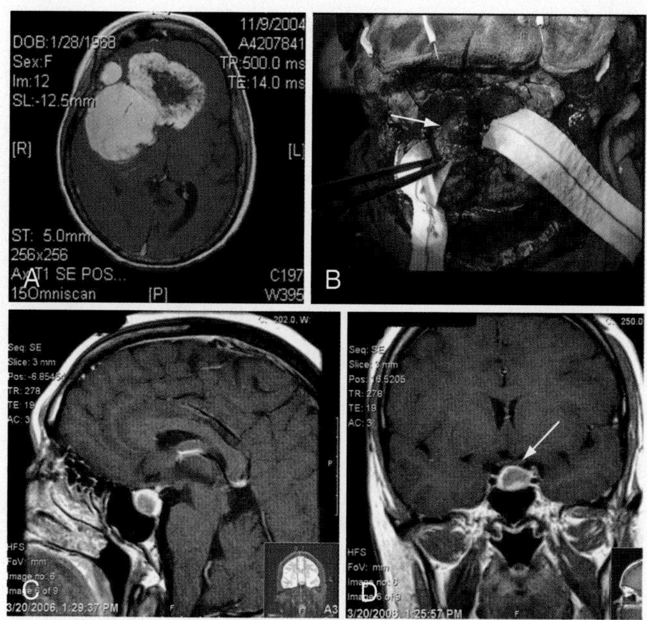


**FIGURE 68-14 A,** A large homogeneously enhancing meningioma can be seen in this gadolinium-enhanced axial MRI study. **B,** Intraoperative picture showing dissection of the meningioma *(arrow)* from the surrounding gyri. Gadolinium-enhanced sagittal **(C)** and coronal **(D)** MRI scans of a patient with a pituitary macroadenoma show impingement on the optic chiasm *(arrow)*.

in patients whose age or medical condition would prohibit surgery, and in those with tumor recurrence after previous surgery.[27]

**Schwannomas** Schwannomas are benign tumors that arise from Schwann cells of the myelin sheath around cranial and spinal nerves after they emerge from the brainstem and spinal cord. Vestibular schwannomas, the most common type, arise from the superior division of the vestibulocochlear nerve and manifest as unilateral sensorineural hearing loss, tinnitus, and disequilibrium. Characteristic findings on MRI include a round or oval enhancing tumor centered on the internal auditory canal (see Fig. 68-15*C* and *D*). Treatment options include expectant management with MRI and hearing audiometrics to detect tumor growth, surgical resection, and radiation therapy in the form of EBRT or radiosurgery (alone or in conjunction with surgery). A complete surgical resection may result in a cure; however, the primary risks of surgery include cranial nerve deficits, namely the facial nerve. In one series of 157 patients with tumors smaller than 3 cm treated with radiosurgery, with a median follow-up of 9.1 years, 73% of patients had a decrease in tumor size, 95% maintained normal facial function, and hearing remained at serviceable levels in 50%.[28] Vestibular schwannomas are at least 95% unilateral. Bilateral occurrence is associated with a neurocutaneous disorder, neurofibromatosis type 2, which is autosomal dominant (gene, 22q12.2). Other commonly affected cranial nerves include the facial, trigeminal, and glossopharyngeal and vagus.

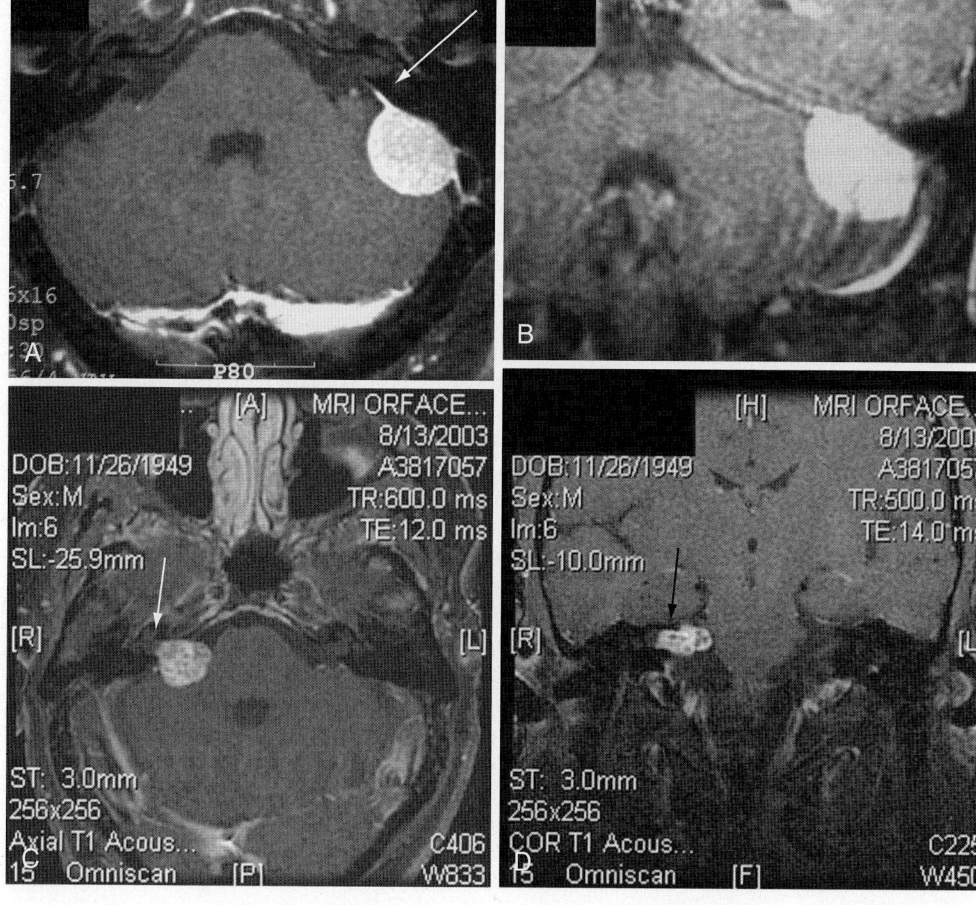


**FIGURE 68-15** MRI studies of two patients presenting with cerebellopontine angle tumors. Gadolinium-enhanced axial **(A)** and coronal **(B)** MRI studies show a well-circumscribed, homogeneously enhancing tumor with a dural tail *(arrow)* arising from the tentorium. Gadolinium-enhanced axial **(C)** and coronal **(D)** MRI studies show a vestibular schwannoma extending into the internal auditory meatus *(arrow)*.

**Pituitary Adenomas** Pituitary adenomas arise primarily from the anterior pituitary gland and are classified as functional (secreting) or nonfunctional (nonsecreting) tumors; the former presents earlier with symptoms caused by physiologic effects and the latter presents when large enough to cause neurologic deficits by mass effect on the chiasm, with consequent bitemporal hemianopsia. Tumors smaller than 1 cm in diameter are called *microadenomas* and larger than 1 cm are considered macroadenomas; 50% of pituitary tumors are smaller than 5 mm at the time of diagnosis. Their incidence is increased in multiple endocrine neoplasia. They usually occur in the third and fourth decades of life and affect both genders equally. The most common functional tumor is the prolactinoma, which causes amenorrhea and galactorrhea in women. Oversecretion of adrenocorticotropic hormone by the adenoma may lead to Cushing's disease, characterized by centripetal obesity, moon facies, hypertension, buffalo hump, hyperpigmentation, hyperglycemia, and psychiatric disturbances. Overproduction of growth hormone (GH) by the tumor manifests as acromegaly, with resultant skeletal overgrowth, deformities of the hands and feet, hypertension, cardiomyopathy, hyperglycemia, soft tissue swelling, and peripheral nerve entrapment syndromes. The latter two may be reversible with normalization of GH levels. Thyrotropin- and gonadotropin-secreting adenomas are rare.

MRI is the imaging test for pituitary tumors, providing information about location and invasion or compression of nearby structures, such as the optic chiasm and cavernous sinus (see Fig. 68-14*C* and *D*). Typically, the pituitary gland enhances rapidly because of a lack of the blood-brain barrier. As a result, the microadenoma may appear as a nonenhancing area within the gland. Diagnostic workup includes a full endocrinologic profile and formal visual fields test. Oral administration of a dopamine agonist (e.g., bromocriptine, cabergoline) can shrink prolactinomas in 75% of patients with macroadenomas in 6 to 8 weeks, but only while therapy is maintained. Bromocriptine may also work on GH-secreting tumors, with tumor shrinkage in less than 20%. Octreotide, a somatostatin analogue, can reduce GH levels in 71% of patients, with a significant reduction in tumor volume in 30% of cases.

Surgical treatment is indicated as initial treatment for most GH-secreting tumors, primary Cushing's disease, non–prolactin-secreting macroadenomas causing symptoms by mass effect, and any adenoma causing acute visual deterioration. Surgery is indicated for prolactinomas when mass effect occurs or there is failure of medical therapy. The surgical approach of choice is a sublabial or intranasal trans-sphenoidal approach, an extracranial procedure that requires no brain retraction. This procedure can be done using the microscope or via an endoscopic technique. It is a minimally invasive procedure that allows access to the sella through the sphenoid sinus. Care is taken to avoid injury to the carotid arteries located within the cavernous sinus, which constitutes the lateral margins of the sella turcica. A transcranial approach is sometimes chosen for surgery on a primarily suprasellar tumor or residual suprasellar component after a subtotal transsphenoidal resection.

The incidence of recurrence is approximately 12%, with most recurring 4 to 8 years after surgery. Consequently, patients are followed up with annual MRI. Radiosurgery can also be used as primary therapy, as adjuvant therapy after subtotal resection, or for recurrent disease. The main dose-limiting structure is proximity to the optic chiasm and optic nerves (within 3 to 5 mm). In this case, fractionated EBRT may be indicated as adjuvant therapy.

## Secondary Brain Tumors

### Metastatic Brain Tumors

Metastatic brain tumors are the most common brain tumors. They outnumber primary brain tumors by 10 : 1. In patients with no cancer history, a brain metastasis is the presenting symptom in 15%. The distribution of metastases in the brain is directly related to the amount of blood flow to each part of the brain; 80% percent of brain metastases occur in the cerebral hemispheres, mainly the frontal lobes, 15% occur in the cerebellum, and 5% occur in the brainstem. The most common primary sites are lung cancer (50%), breast cancer (15% to 20%), unknown primary cancer (10%-15%), melanoma (10%), and colon cancer (5%). Metastases to the brain are multiple in more than 70% of cases, but solitary metastases do occur. Dural metastases may constitute as much as 9% of total CNS metastases.[29]

MRI with gadolinium enhancement is the diagnostic study of choice for metastases (Fig. 68-16). It shows a lesion at the gray matter and white matter junction, well-circumscribed, surrounded by edema. Planning therapy depends on the number of lesions, their location in deep or eloquent areas of the brain, size, radiosensitivity of the primary cancer, systemic status of the primary cancer, and Karnofsky performance score. Surgery is recommended for accessible lesions (up to three) causing mass effect, followed by whole-brain radiation therapy to eradicate micrometastases. SRS followed by whole-brain radiation therapy has also been shown to be as effective as surgery in the management of metastatic brain tumors (<3 cm). The median survival time with optimal treatment remains 7 to 12 months. Chemotherapy is not useful for most brain metastases, except small cell lung cancer and seminomas.

### Regional Tumors

Brain involvement can occur with cancers of the nasopharyngeal region by direct extension along the cranial nerves or through the foramina at the base of the skull. Skull base tumors may cause symptoms of headache, diplopia, or other cranial nerve deficits. Clival chordoma, a remnant of the primitive notochord, is a skull base tumor that is locally invasive. Treatment consists of surgery followed by proton beam radiotherapy.

### Intraspinal Tumors

Intraspinal tumors are commonly divided into three groups—extradural, intradural extramedullary, and intramedullary.

**Extradural Tumors** These tumors originate in the vertebral body or, less commonly, the epidural space. Most tend to be malignant and represent metastatic tumors, particularly from the lung, breast, and prostate. Spinal epidural metastases occur in up to 10% of cancer patients. Other common extradural tumors include lymphomas and multiple myelomas. Pain is usually the first symptom and may be exacerbated by recumbency, especially at night, by movements, and by coughing or sneezing. Pathologic fractures are common. The pain may be mechanical or axial because of an inherent instability in the diseased spine, or may be radicular or referred because of epidural extension and compression of radicular nerves. As the tumor enlarges and

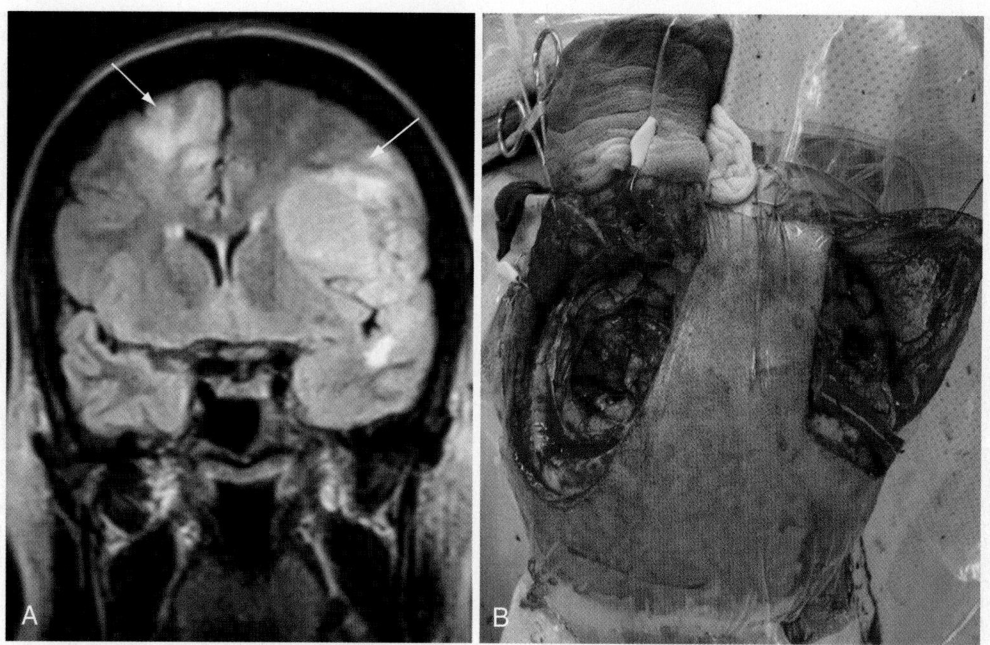


**FIGURE 68-16 A,** FLAIR sequence coronal MRI of a patient with two simultaneous metastatic tumors along the right and left frontal lobes *(arrows).* **B,** Simultaneous right and left frontal craniotomies for resection of both metastatic lesions.

compresses the spinal cord, myelopathic signs may be evident in the form of paraparesis or paraplegia, hyperreflexia, and spasticity. A sensory level deficit appropriate to the spinal level in question may also be found.

Diagnostic workup includes CT to visualize the extent of bony destruction and MRI with gadolinium to visualize the neural elements and soft tissue invasion. A CT-guided needle biopsy is also recommended to establish the diagnosis in case of an absent primary cancer. A metastatic workup includes chest x-ray, CT of the chest, abdomen, and pelvis, bone scan, serum prostate-specific antigen level determination, and mammography in women. Treatment consists of surgery with or without EBRT, depending on the radiosensitivity of the tumor. Surgery is indicated in patients with the following:

1. Progressive neurologic deficit
2. Pain refractory to medications
3. Progressive kyphotic deformity
4. Radioresistant tumor (e.g., melanoma, renal cell carcinoma)

The surgical approach is directed toward the tumor area whether it involves a simple laminectomy posteriorly or posterolateral thoracotomy or thoracoabdominal approach for a vertebrectomy. Stabilization in the form of instrumentation is always recommended in radical spinal oncology surgery (Fig. 68-17).

**Intradural Extramedullary Tumors** These tumors are located within the dura, but outside the substance of the spinal cord. Most are benign and arise from the meninges (meningioma) or nerve roots (schwannomas, neurofibromas). Metastatic tumors may also seed this area through subarachnoid spreading (lymphoma, ependymoma, medulloblastoma). Lymphomatous spread into the subarachnoid space may lead to meningeal carcinomatosis—leptomeningeal disease— typically diagnosed with CSF cytology through a lumbar puncture and MRI studies.

Spinal meningiomas (Fig. 68-18*A* and *B*) are more common in women and involve mainly the thoracic region (82%). They tend to occur lateral (68%), posterior (18%), and anterior (15%) to the spinal cord. Schwannomas and neurofibromas can originate wherever there is a nerve root. Schwannomas usually develop from the sensory portion of the nerve root (dorsal), thereby sparing the motor portion (anterior). They may extend through the nerve root foramen into the extraspinal space, giving the shape of a dumbbell appearance on MRI. These lesions are best evaluated by MRI with gadolinium, which shows the relationship of the tumor to the spinal cord and roots. They are frequently amenable to surgical resection with minimal morbidity. Sacrifice of the dorsal root during resection of a nerve sheath tumor is sometimes warranted, without any significant complications.

**Intramedullary Tumors** These tumors originate from the substance of the spinal cord. Patients usually experience myelopathy and sensory disturbances below the level of involvement. The two most common tumors are astrocytoma and ependymoma. MRI with gadolinium is the preferred imaging study. The treatment of intramedullary tumors is laminectomy followed by maximal tumor resection without causing significant neurologic deficits. The CUSA and operating microscope are indispensable tools in this type of surgery. Ependymomas are the most common glioma of the lower cord, conus, and filum (50%). The next most common location is the cervical cord (see Fig. 68-18*C* and *D*). They are generally slow-growing and benign and are typically encapsulated with a cleavage plane between the tumor and normal cord, which makes gross total resection feasible.[30] Astrocytomas, conversely, tend to be more infiltrative and less amenable to a total resection without significant neurologic deficits. If total resection was not possible, EBRT can be used for residual ependymomas and most astrocytomas. Other less

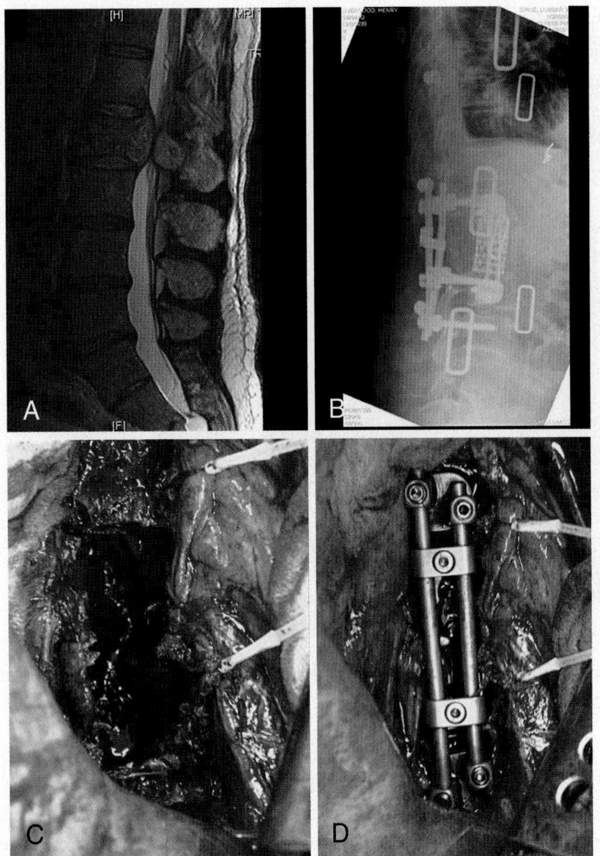

**FIGURE 68-17** Radiographic and intraoperative pictures of a patient presenting with metastatic renal cell carcinoma to L2. **A,** An expansile bony lesion with an epidural component at L2 causing obliteration of the spinal canal can be seen on this T2-weighted sagittal MRI study. **B,** A postoperative lateral radiograph shows the spinal instrumentation with a posterior L1, L3, and L4 pedicle screw-rod system and anterior L1 to L3 titanium cage with a lateral L1 to L3 vertebral body screw-rod system. Intraoperative pictures show the surgical field after L2 vertebrectomy **(C)** and the implanted cage at the vertebrectomy site covered by the lateral L1 to L3 screw-rod system **(D)**.

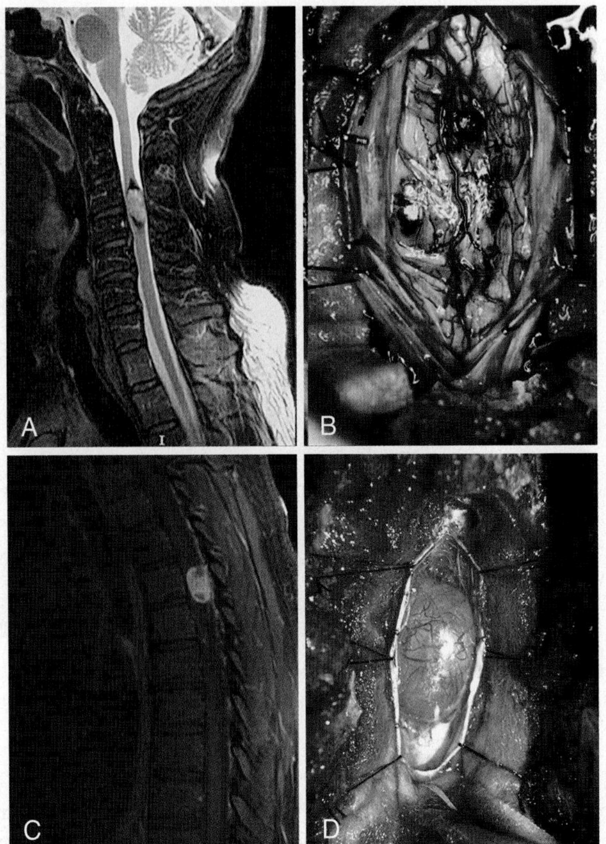

**FIGURE 68-18** Radiographic and intraoperative pictures of spinal intradural tumors. **A,** A gadolinium-enhanced sagittal MRI shows a T4 meningioma. **B,** An intraoperative picture shows the spinal cord and overlying meningioma. **C,** A T2-weighted sagittal MRI study shows an intramedullary cervical cord ependymoma at the C3-4 level with a small rostral and caudal syrinx. **D,** An intraoperative picture shows the dura splayed open, with the ependymoma showing in the cord.

common intramedullary tumors include dermoid and epidermoid neoplasms, lipomas, and hemangioblastomas.

## TRAUMATIC BRAIN INJURY

The goal of this section on traumatic brain injury is not to present a comprehensive review of the epidemiology, basic science research, and outcome studies on brain injury, but to give a practical, common sense approach to the management of injuries of the brain. There is bound to be overlap between this section and other parts of this text. Guidelines for the management of severe head injury were first published by the Brain Trauma Foundation in 1995 and last reviewed in 2007.[31] These evidence-based guidelines have been a tremendous aid to the physician caring for brain-injured patients. The following discussion on the management of severe traumatic brain injury is based largely on these guidelines. As with all practice guidelines, they can and need to be modified, as dictated by the experience of the treating physician and in accordance with the needs of the patient. This report and the protocols laid out in the advanced trauma life support guidelines, published by the American College of Surgeons Committee on Trauma, are also invaluable resources for the student and physician.

We first present the epidemiology, pathophysiology, prehospital and emergency management, and definitive treatment of severe traumatic brain injury. Concussion and mild to moderate brain injuries are then discussed.

### Epidemiology

Depending on the source of information, it is estimated that there are anywhere from 500,000 to well over 1 million cases of head injury every year. Most of these are classified as mild injuries, with approximately 20% classified as moderate to severe. Approximately 50% of the 150,000 trauma deaths every year are caused by head injury. It is estimated that 5.3 million people are living with brain injury–related disabilities, and the estimated cost to society exceeds $4 billion annually. The social, medical, and economic implications are profound. Fortunately, prevention programs appear to be decreasing the incidence of severe traumatic brain injury.

## PATHOPHYSIOLOGY

Traumatic brain injury can be classified into primary and secondary injuries. Primary injury occurs at impact and is considered first. It includes bone fracture, intracranial hemorrhage, and diffuse axonal injury (DAI). Fractures of the cranial vault and skull base are indicative of the forces applied to the skull at the time of impact. Fractures of the skull base may be associated with cranial nerve deficit, arterial dissection, and CSF fistula formation. Fractures of the cranial vault are classified as follows:

1. Open or closed
2. Depressed or nondepressed
3. Linear or comminuted

Any fracture of the cranial vault can cause disruption of the underlying meningeal arteries or dural venous sinuses, which can lead to intracranial bleeding. Intracranial hemorrhage can be classified as epidural, subdural, subarachnoid, and intraparenchymal or intracerebral. Epidural hemorrhage occurs between the dura and skull and is usually the result of a skull fracture causing the laceration of a meningeal artery.

Rarely, a fracture crossing a dural venous sinus can cause a venous epidural hematoma, especially in children. Subdural hemorrhage occurs in the potential space between the dura and arachnoid. This is often the result of shearing of the bridging veins between the brain and the dural venous sinuses. Sometimes, it comes from injury to cortical vessels, which then bleed into the subdural space. Subarachnoid hemorrhage (SAH) from trauma consists of bleeding into the spinal fluid spaces surrounding the blood vessels feeding the cerebral cortex. Trauma is the most common cause of subarachnoid hemorrhage. Rupture of an intracranial aneurysm is the second most common cause of subarachnoid hemorrhage and is generally distinguished from traumatic SAH by history and sometimes by the distribution of blood on a CT scan. Intraparenchymal or intracerebral hemorrhage is bleeding into the brain itself. This can run the spectrum from small contusions (bruises of the brain) to large intracerebral clots that require emergent surgical evacuation, which usually are the result of coup and contrecoup injuries. Although often small and nonsurgical at first, these can blossom and become life-threatening over a period of hours to days. DAI is a rotational acceleration-deceleration injury to the white matter pathways of the brain. This results in a functional or anatomic disruption of these pathways and is cited as the cause of loss of consciousness in patients without mass lesions. DAI can occur with or without other primary injuries, such as an epidural or subdural hematoma (Fig. 68-19). In addition to being one of the many primary injuries seen in severe traumatic brain injury, DAI can also be considered as a secondary injury.

Secondary injury to the brain occurs as a result of decreased oxygen delivery to the brain, which in turn sets off a cascade of events that causes even more damage than the initial injury. With severe traumatic brain injury, there can be an alteration in cerebral vessel autoregulation. Systemic hypotension in the presence of this altered autoregulation results in decreased CBF and decreased oxygen delivery. This ischemia is exacerbated even further by systemic hypoxemia; intracranial hypertension, which decreases CBF even further, and a cascade of events involving mediators of inflammation, excitotoxicity, calcium influx, and $Na^+$,$K^+$-ATPase dysfunction leads to neuronal cell dysfunction and death. The prevention of secondary injury is therefore thought to lead to increased cell survival and improved outcome. This is achieved by preventing hypotension and hypoxia while taking measures to control ICP and maintain CPP.

### Prehospital and Emergency Department Management

The prehospital and emergency department management of the traumatized patient is reviewed elsewhere in this and other texts. Here we will deal more specifically with issues critical to the patient with severe brain injury. The ABCs must always be addressed first, regardless of the severity of the patient's injury. Attention is first paid to securing a patent airway, establishing adequate ventilation and oxygenation, and maintaining adequate circulation. By doing this, one may avoid hypotension and hypoxia and, in so doing, avoid or minimize secondary brain injury. In patients with severe traumatic brain injury, a systolic blood pressure less than 90 mm Hg or a $PaO_2$ less than 60 mm Hg is a predictor of poor outcome. Appropriate spine precautions are observed in the initial resuscitation of the patient with a severe traumatic brain injury.

Once airway, breathing, and circulation have been addressed, neurologic evaluation may proceed. The Glasgow Coma Scale (GCS) is a simple and reproducible method of neurologic assessment. It is also used to grade traumatic brain injury as mild, moderate, or severe. The GCS consists of three components—intensity of stimulus required to cause eye opening, verbal response, and motor response (Table 68-3). Pupillary size and reactivity are also essential components of the initial neurologic examination. Hypoxia, hypotension, alcohol, and drugs may all contribute to an abnormal neurologic examination result. In the absence of hypotension and hypoxia, an abnormal examination is considered to be a primary brain injury until proven otherwise. Once all life-threatening injuries have been addressed and stabilized, the patient with a suspected traumatic brain injury undergoes CT. The CT scan is used to evaluate the presence or absence of fracture, epidural and subdural hematomas, intracerebral hematomas and contusions, shift of the midline structures, and appearance of the basal and perimesencephalic cisterns. In many centers with multislice scanners, routine scanning of the cervical spine is also performed to rule out acute fractures or traumatic dislocations. If life-threatening injuries elsewhere necessitate immediate transport of the patient to the operating room, and the patient has a suspected intracranial hematoma (e.g., unilateral fixed and dilated pupil on one side, with a contralateral hemiparesis), exploratory burr holes may be performed in the operating room concurrently with the laparotomy or thoracotomy.

Not infrequently, trauma patients with brain injury will require transfer to a hospital equipped to provide those patients with a higher level of care. In preparing these patients for transfer, the physician needs to follow the advanced trauma life support guidelines and secure the airway, ensure adequate ventilation, and maintain circulation. Anemia is treated with transfusion, as necessary. Hypoxia and hypotension need to be avoided. Adequate immobilization with a backboard and cervical collar are mandatory. In patients with obvious intracranial hypertension or mass lesions, treatment with mannitol may be considered after neurosurgical consultation. Vigilance and attention to detail, as well as communication between the transferring and accepting physicians, is key to the successful transfer and treatment of these patients.

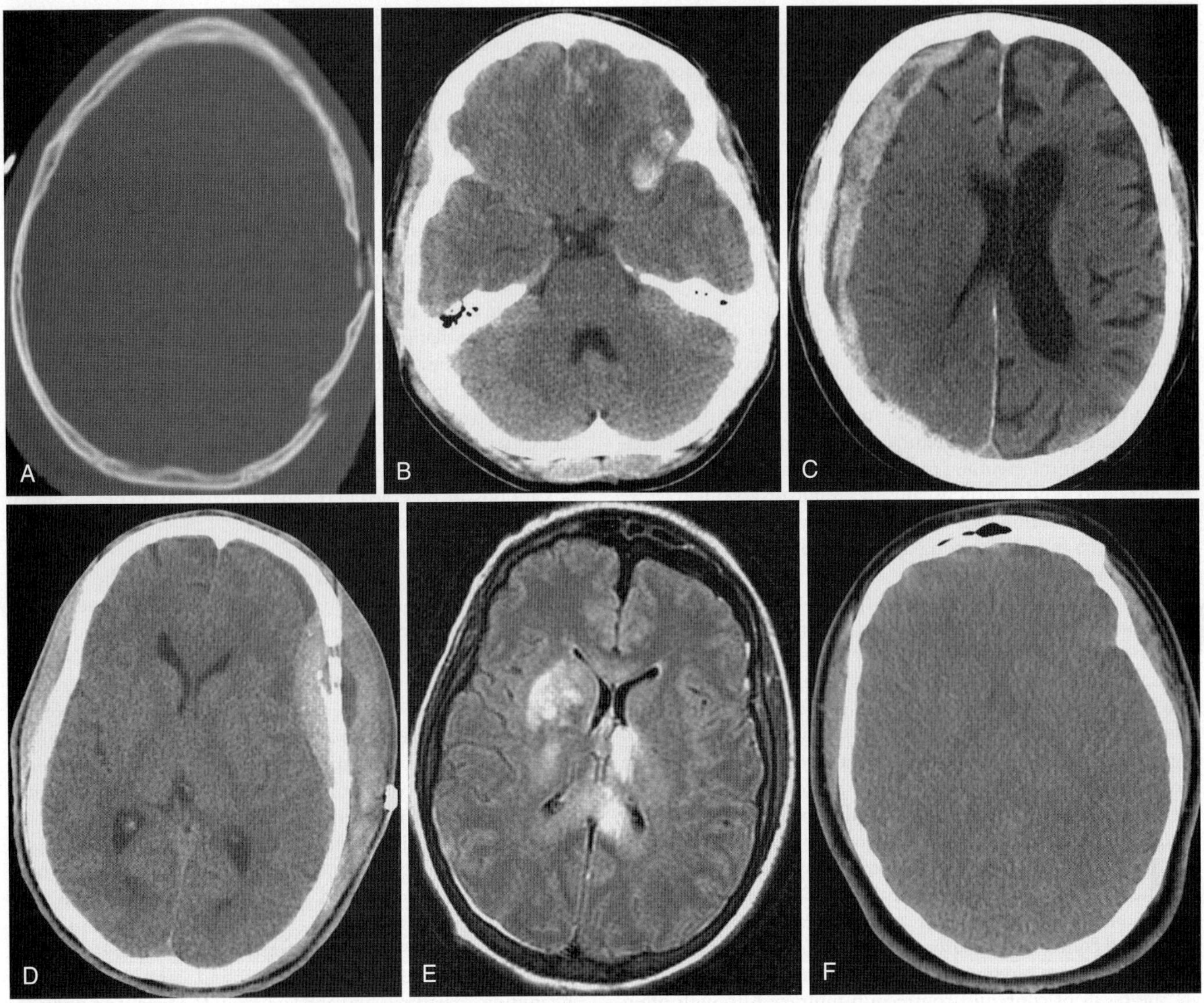

**FIGURE 68-19** Typical radiologic findings in traumatic brain injury. **A,** Skull fracture shown on CT. **B,** Intraparenchymal contusions. **C,** Subdural hematoma. **D,** Epidural hematoma. **E,** Diffuse axonal injury. **F,** Intracranial hypertension. Note the effacement of sulci and gray-white matter differentiation.

**Table 68-3 Neurologic Assessment Using the Glasgow Coma Scale**

| Eye-Opening Response | | Verbal Response | | Motor Response | |
|---|---|---|---|---|---|
| **SCORE** | **RESPONSE** | **SCORE** | **RESPONSE** | **SCORE** | **RESPONSE** |
| 4 | Spontaneous | 5 | Oriented | 6 | Obeys commands |
| 3 | To speech | 4 | Confused | 5 | Localizes to painful stimulus |
| 2 | To pain | 3 | Inappropriate responses | 4 | Withdraws to painful stimulus |
| 1 | No response | 2 | Incomprehensible responses | 3 | Flexion to painful stimulus |
| | | 1 | No response | 2 | Extension to painful stimulus |
| | | | | 1 | No response |

### Treatment

When the workup of a patient reveals an intracranial mass lesion and deficits thought to be related to that lesion, operative intervention is indicated. In general, any clot or contusion more than 30 mL is thought to be operable. Epidural and subdural hematomas (see Fig. 68-19) are addressed with similar approaches, with the craniotomy centered on the clot. Intracerebral hematomas are addressed through appropriately located craniotomies. ICP monitors are often placed at operation. These can be intraventricular drains, intraparenchymal monitors, or devices placed in the epidural or subdural spaces. The decision about when to place an ICP monitor depends on the patient's preoperative examination, appearance of the brain at operation, and potential risk for deterioration. In general, all patients with a GCS of 8 or less have ICP monitors placed. Some patients with moderate traumatic brain injury may also benefit from ICP monitoring. Postoperatively, the patient is managed similarly to those with nonoperable traumatic brain injury (see later).

The following is a simplified algorithm for the management of intracranial hypertension in the intensive care setting. The head of the bed is elevated to 30 degrees, with the head placed in a neutral position. Care is taken to ensure that any cervical spine immobilization device is not obstructing jugular venous flow because this can increase ICP. The goal of treatment is to try to keep the ICP less than 20 mm Hg and maintain CPP at or above 70 mm Hg. (Remember that CPP is MAP minus ICP.) If the ICP is persistently elevated above 20 mm Hg, it is treated. CSF drainage is now the first line of therapy in decreasing ICP. This is accomplished by an external ventricular drain, or ventriculostomy, which is a drain placed in the operating room or at bedside in the intensive care unit (ICU) in an appropriately monitored patient. If ICP remains persistently elevated despite CSF drainage, the patient can be sedated and even paralyzed pharmacologically to keep the ICP down. The physician is dependent on the pupillary examination and ICP reading in this situation. If the ICP changes rapidly, or the pupillary examination changes (i.e., blown pupil), emergent CT of the head is indicated. Sedation and paralysis can be occasionally discontinued to allow for an adequate neurologic evaluation in this situation.

If the ICP remains persistently elevated despite these interventions, mannitol and other diuretic agents may be used. Mannitol is administered as an IV bolus of 0.25 to 1 g/kg every 4 to 6 hours. Serum osmolality is followed closely when giving mannitol, and the drug is withheld if the serum osmolality exceeds 320 mOsm/kg. It is also important to maintain euvolemia in these patients. If ICP is still elevated, hyperventilation to a $\text{Paco}_2$ of 30 to 35 mm Hg may be used judiciously. At this point, second-tier therapeutic interventions (e.g., hypertonic saline, high-dose barbiturate therapy, decompressive craniectomy) may be considered.[32,33] Serial CT scans are critical throughout this treatment algorithm, and their use is tailored to the individual patient.

Several comments regarding nutrition, steroids, anticonvulsants and $\text{Paco}_2$ are appropriate here. Energy requirements after traumatic brain injury are increased. The nonparalyzed patient requires replacement of 140% of his or her resting metabolism expenditure and the paralyzed patient requires 100%. Of this, 15% is protein. Feeding begins within 7 days of injury. Steroids have no proven benefit in the management of traumatic brain injury and are not used. Prophylactic use of anticonvulsant drugs (e.g., phenytoin, carbamazepine phenobarbital) is not indicated for the prevention of late post-traumatic seizures. Anticonvulsants may, however, be used to prevent early post-traumatic seizures, primarily in patients at high risk for early seizures who may suffer adverse effects if they were to seize early in their hospital course. These can usually be tapered after 1 week of therapy. Hyperventilation causes a decrease in ICP by lowering $\text{Paco}_2$, which causes vasoconstriction and decreases intracranial blood volume. Unfortunately, it also causes decreased CBF. If hyperventilation to a $\text{Paco}_2$ of less than 30 mm Hg is required for the maintenance of an acceptable ICP and CPP, monitoring of CBF is strongly recommended by some. Jugular venous $O_2$ saturation and cerebral oxygen extraction may also be useful in this clinical scenario. Table 68-4 presents a summary of the recommendations of the 2007 guidelines provided by the Brain Trauma Foundation for traumatic brain injury.

## DEGENERATIVE DISORDERS OF THE SPINE

### Degenerative Disease of the Lumbar Spine

According to the National Institute of Neurological Disorders and Stroke, 25.9 million Americans complain of low back pain per year, with a cumulative expense of about $50 billion per year. Low back pain is the most common cause of job-related disability and a leading contributor to missed days at work. Back pain is the second most common neurologic ailment in the United States; only headache is more common.

A good understanding of the normal anatomy of the spine is of utmost importance for the appreciation of spinal disorders. The lumbar spine consists of five lumbar vertebrae with five intervening intervertebral discs (IVDs). Each vertebra is made up of an anterior vertebral body and posterior neural arch. Each neural arch is, in turn, composed of pedicles, facet joints, transverse processes, laminae, and a spinous process. The IVD consists of three components:

1. Cartilaginous end plates for nutrition and anchoring
2. Annulus fibrosus made of concentric sheets of collagen for containing the pressurized nucleus
3. Nucleus pulposus made of a soft semigelatinous collagen that can absorb axial compressive loads

The spinal cord ends at the L1 level, beyond which lumbar and sacral nerve roots, collectively called the *cauda equina*, continue distally and exit at their corresponding neural foramen. At each segmental level, a nerve root containing motor and sensory components exits the thecal sac, crosses the IVD space, travels a short distance within the lateral recess of the spinal canal, and passes underneath the pedicle on its way to exit the spine through the intervertebral foramen.

Biomechanically, as we age, the nucleus loses its ability to bear compressive loads. The load transfer then shifts to the anulus, a structure that is poorly suited to withstand compression, thereby causing fatigue failure, fissuring, and possibly rupture. A herniation of a fragment of the nucleus pulposus may follow. As the mechanical integrity of the nucleus deteriorates further, the load transfer is concentrated at the periphery of the vertebral end plates, leading to osteophyte formation, a process called *spondylosis*. Subsequently, as the degenerating disc becomes less able to resist rotations and shear, additional stresses are transferred to the posterior elements, with resultant facet arthrosis and hypertrophy and thickening and buckling of the ligamentum flavum.

**Table 68-4 Brain Trauma Foundation Recommendations for Traumatic Brain Injury (TBI)**

| PARAMETER | GUIDELINE |
|---|---|
| Hyperosmolar therapy | Mannitol effective for control of raised ICP (0.25-1 g/kg) |
| Prophylactic hypothermia | Mortality could be decreased when target temperatures are maintained >48 hr |
| Infection prophylaxis | Routine external ventricular catheter exchange not recommended; indicated if GCS = 3-8 on admission and abnormal CT; in severe TBI and normal CT, indicated with two or more of the following: age >40 yr, unilateral posturing, hypotension with SBP <90 mm Hg |
| ICP monitoring | Ventricular catheters are most reliable and cost-effective method; ICP should be kept <20 mm Hg |
| CPP threshold | CPP <50 mm Hg should be avoided; aggressive interventions to maintain it above 70 mm Hg have a considerable risk of ARDS |
| Brain oxygen monitoring and thresholds | Jugular venous saturation (50%) or brain tissue oxygen tension (15 mm Hg) are treatment thresholds |
| Blood pressure and oxygenation | Blood pressure should be monitored, hypotension (systolic blood pressure = 90 mm Hg) avoided; hypoxia (saturation <90% or $Po_2$ <60 mm Hg should be avoided |
| Nutrition | Should be initiated within 7 days of injury |
| Sedatives | High-dose barbiturates recommended to control refractory ICP in the hemodynamically stable patient; propofol recommended for ICP control but does not improve mortality |
| Seizure prophylaxis | Decreases early post traumatic seizures (<7 days postinjury) |
| Hyperventilation | Recommended as temporizing measure. $PCO_2$ below 25 mm Hg not recommended; avoid in first 24 hr after injury |
| Steroids | Not recommended, contraindicated |

*ARDS,* Acute respiratory distress syndrome.

**Table 68-5 Clinical Findings in Common Lumbar Disc Herniations**

| DISC | INCIDENCE (%) | ROOT | PAIN DISTRIBUTION | MUSCLE INVOLVED | SENSORY DEFICITS | REFLEX LOSS |
|---|---|---|---|---|---|---|
| L3-L4 | 3-10 | L4 | Anterior thigh | Quadriceps femoris | Medial malleolus and medial foot | Knee jerk |
| L4-L5 | 40-45 | L5 | Posterolateral thigh and leg | Tibialis anterior; extensor hallucis longus | Large toe web, dorsum of foot | None |
| L5-S1 | 45-50 | S1 | Posterolateral thigh and leg down to ankle | Gastrocnemius | Lateral malleolus, lateral foot | Ankle jerk |

### Lumbar Radiculopathy

Disc herniations can occur in any direction but usually follow a posterolateral direction at the site at which the posterior longitudinal ligament is thinnest. Disc material extruded in this location can compress a nerve root, leading to low back pain and radicular symptoms in a specific dermatomal distribution (Table 68-5). The back pain is usually a minor component. Large, more central disc herniations may compress the cauda equina, with resultant cauda equina syndrome consisting of saddle anesthesia, urinary retention with possible overflow incontinence, and significant motor weakness. In this case, it is advisable to decompress the thecal sac within 24 hours of onset of symptoms.

An initial period of nonsurgical management for at least 4 to 8 weeks is indicated unless the patient presents with cauda equina syndrome, progressive neurologic deficit, recurrent episodes of incapacitating pain, and/or profound motor weakness. Conservative therapy includes rest, activity modification, physical therapy, weight loss, analgesics, muscle relaxants, oral steroids, and epidural steroid injections. If conservative measures fail to control the pain, imaging of the spine is indicated. MRI is the diagnostic test of choice (Fig. 68-20); postmyelography CT may be indicated in patients who have pacemakers.

The standard treatment of these herniations involves a midline approach centered over the affected interspace, followed by a hemilaminectomy to expose the thecal sac and nerve root. The herniated fragment is usually located medial to the root along its shoulder. Removal of the herniated or extruded fragment is sufficient to relieve the symptoms. A minimally invasive procedure through a 1-cm paramedian incision with a muscle-splitting technique can also be used under microscopic or endoscopic visualization, with less postoperative morbidity. Most patients experience good results immediately after surgery. A recurrent herniated disc at the same level may occur in 3% to 19% of patients, with the higher rates usually in series with long-term follow-up.

### Lumbar Spinal Stenosis

Advanced degeneration of the lumbar spine may result in spondylosis, with arthrosis and hypertrophy of the facet joint as well as thickening and buckling of the ligamentum flavum. These changes lead to narrowing of the spinal canal, with resultant constriction of the thecal sac and development of neurologic deficits. Patients typically present with neurogenic claudication—unilateral or bilateral dermatomal discomfort precipitated by standing or walking or prolonged maintenance of the same posture, and characteristically relieved by a change in posture such as sitting, squatting, or recumbency. This discomfort may be in the form of pain, weakness, or paresthesias.

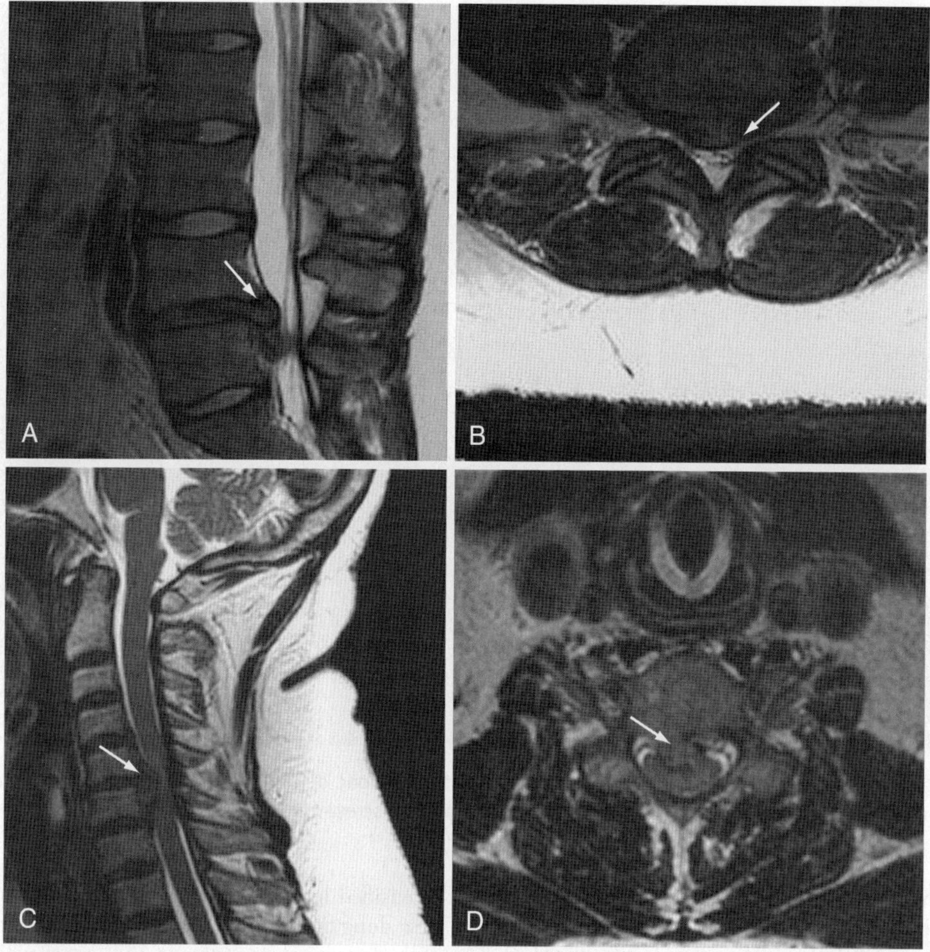


**FIGURE 68-20** **A,** T2-weighted sagittal MRI study showing a herniated lumbar disc fragment *(arrow)* at the L4-5 level. **B,** T2-weighted axial MRI showing the same fragment *(arrow)* compressing the thecal sac. **C,** T2 sagittal MRI of a patient with a large anterior disc prolapse at C5-6 level *(arrow)*. **D,** Axial images showing the disc compressing the spinal cord *(arrow)*.

Neurogenic claudication is thought to arise from ischemic root changes as a result of increased metabolic demands from exercise in the presence of vascular compromise of the root from the surrounding constriction. The clinical history is important if spinal stenosis is suspected because most of these patients have nonspecific neurologic findings such as absent or reduced reflexes. Again, MRI is the diagnostic test of choice for lumbar stenosis and typically shows an hourglass appearance on a T2-weighted sagittal sequence (see Fig. 68-20). Nonsteroidal anti-inflammatory drugs (NSAIDs), analgesics, and physical therapy are the mainstays of nonsurgical management. Surgical decompression is warranted for patients with recurrent and disabling pain that limits their daily activity. Laminotomies or laminectomies of the involved levels with undercutting of the superior articular facet are required to decompress the nerves in the foramina. Wide aggressive decompression of the spinal canal may result in lumbar instability.

### Lumbar Instrumentation and Fusion

The instrumentation is an adjunct to the fusion. It provides immediate rigid fixation while the spine completes the process of bony fusion that ensures long-term stabilization. The most common indication for fusion and instrumentation is spondylolisthesis (vertebral body subluxation). Lumbar fusion can be a potential adjunct to disc excision in cases of a herniated or recurrent herniated disc in patients with evidence of preoperative lumbar spinal deformity or instability or in patients with chronic mechanical and discogenic back pain.[34] Lumbar fusion is also recommended for carefully selected patients with disabling low back pain caused by one- or two-level degenerative disease without stenosis or spondylolisthesis.

Lumbar fusion and instrumentation can be performed through a number of approaches:

1. Posterolateral fusion (PLF), whereby the transverse processes of the involved segments are decorticated and covered with a mixture of bone autograft or allograft
2. Pedicle screw fixation (PSF), whereby screws are inserted into the pedicles of the involved segments and then attached to each other under compression with a rod (Fig. 68-21), alone or in conjunction with PLF
3. Posterior lumbar interbody fusion (PLIF), whereby an intervertebral body spacer, a bone allograft or cage packed with bone, is inserted in the disc space through a laminotomy on each side of the midline, together with PSF, alone or in conjunction with PLF

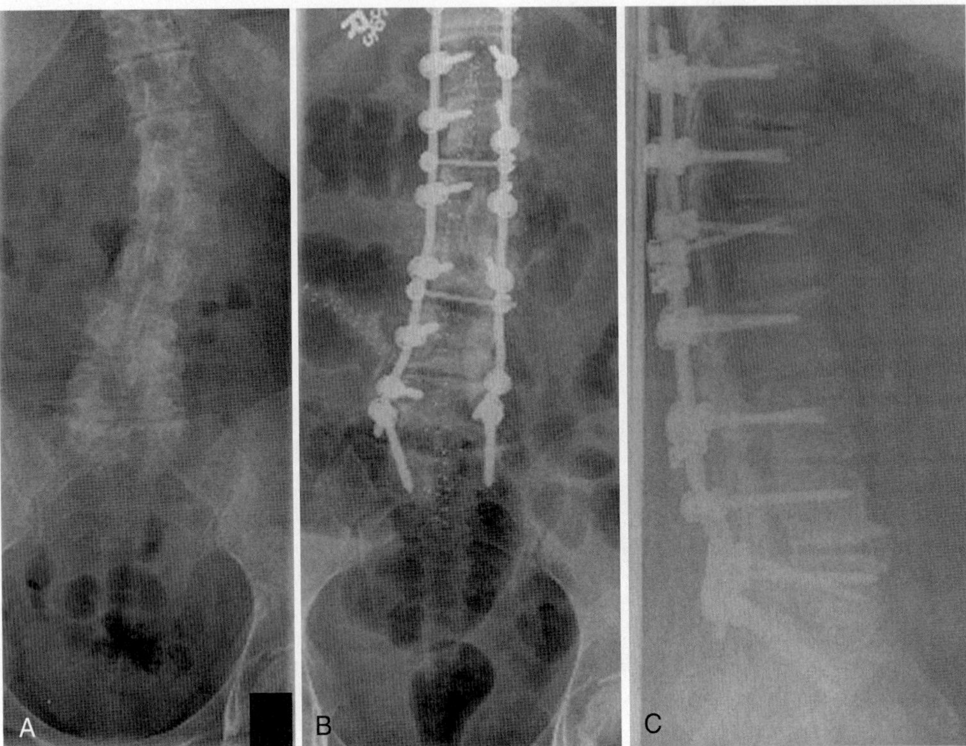

**FIGURE 68-21 A,** Posteroanterior (PA) x-ray of a patient with degenerative scoliotic deformity of the thoracolumbar spine. Postoperative PA **(B)** and lateral **(C)** x-rays show correction of the deformity using a long pedicle screw-rod construct from T11 to S1.

4. Transforaminal interbody fusion (TLIF), whereby the facet joint and the isthmus on one side are removed and a single bone graft or cage is introduced into the disc space in an oblique fashion, together with unilateral or bilateral PSF, alone or in conjunction with PLF
5. Anterior lumbar interbody fusion (ALIF), whereby the interbody space is fused using a bone graft or cage augmented by a metallic interbody plate through an anterior retroperitoneal approach

Bony fusion can also be augmented with bony extenders or substitutes such as demineralized bone matrix or recombinant human bone morphogenetic protein (rhBMP-2) in an attempt to avoid harvesting autologous bone grafts.

## Degenerative Diseases of the Cervical Spine

The pathophysiology of the degenerative changes of the cervical spine is essentially similar to that of the lumbar spine. An important distinction is that the spinal canal in the cervical spine contains the spinal cord, rather than the cauda equina and, consequently, a minor reduction in the canal space may lead to compression of the spinal cord, with devastating neurologic results. There are seven cervical vertebrae, but eight pairs of cervical nerves.

### Cervical Radiculopathy

The most common scenario for patients with herniated cervical disc is that the symptoms were present on awakening in the morning without identifiable trauma or stress. The pain usually radiates from the proximal arm distally, together with numbness and paresthesia, in a dermatomal distribution. The pain may be intensified by neck movements. In severe cases, a motor weakness along the same nerve may be noticed. On examination, pain with downward pressure on the vertex while tilting the head toward the symptomatic side (Spurling's sign) is a mechanical sign of disc herniation. Nerve root compression in the upper cervical spine is unusual. Compression of C2 root causes occipital neuralgia, whereas compression of C3 and C4 may lead to nonspecific neck and shoulder pain. Compression of the other cervical roots leads to the manifestations noted in Table 68-6.

### Cervical Myelopathy

Compression of the cervical cord, acutely by a large herniated disc fragment or chronically by osteophytic bony spurs as a result of advanced spondylosis or stenosis, causes cervical myelopathy. Myelopathy is manifested by spasticity, hyperreflexia, increased deep tendon reflexes, clonus, and the Babinski and Hoffman signs. Patients also complain of clumsiness in their hands as a result of poor muscle coordination. If left untreated, patients may become quadriparetic and wheelchair-bound (Fig. 68-22).

### Diagnosis and Treatment

MRI is the study of choice for the initial evaluation of a herniated cervical disc. CT myelography is indicated for patients who cannot undergo MRI or when anatomic bony details are required. MRI is less accurate than CT myelography for identifying foraminal fragments but is less invasive. A cervical spine x-ray is always recommended to evaluate the degree of spondylosis in the cervical spine before surgery. Electromyography and nerve conduction studies can be useful when other causes need to be excluded, such as plexopathies or peripheral nerve entrapment.

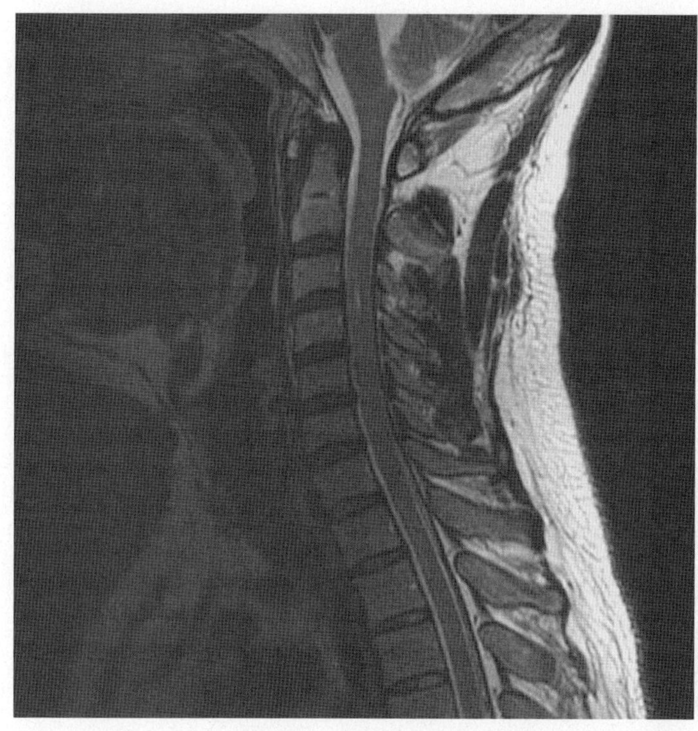

**FIGURE 68-22** T2-weighted sagittal MRI scan of a patient with significant cervical canal stenosis. Note the hyperintensity in the cervical spinal cord at the C3-4 level, suggesting myelomalacic changes. This may be indicative of permanent residual deficits.

**Table 68-6 Clinical Findings in Common Cervical Disc Herniations**

| DISC | INCIDENCE (%) | ROOT | PAIN DISTRIBUTION | MUSCLE INVOLVED | REFLEX LOSS |
|---|---|---|---|---|---|
| C4-5 | 2 | C5 | Shoulder | Deltoid | Deltoid |
| C5-6 | 19 | C6 | Upper arm, thumb, radial forearm | Biceps, extensor carpi radialis | Biceps, brachioradialis |
| C6-7 | 69 | C7 | Fingers 2 and 3, all fingertips | Triceps | Triceps |
| C7-T1 | 10 | C8 | Fingers 4 and 5 | Hand intrinsics | Finger jerk |

More than 90% of patients with acute cervical radiculopathy as a result of disc herniation can improve without surgery. Conservative therapy includes a combination of oral steroids, NSAIDs, analgesics, muscle relaxants, intermittent cervical traction, and physical therapy. Surgery is indicated for those who fail to improve and those with progressive neurologic deficit while undergoing conservative therapy. The aim of the surgery is to decompress the nerve root, which can be accomplished through an anterior or posterior approach. Both procedures carry an excellent outcome, approximately 90% to 96% improvement in preoperative symptoms.

With anterior pathology (paracentral herniation or large uncovertebral osteophyte), an anterior cervical discectomy, nerve root decompression, and fusion are indicated (Fig. 68-23). The approach is fairly simple, through the avascular plane between the carotid sheath and tracheoesophageal complex. The operative microscope is used to remove the IVD, decompress the thecal sac, and free the nerve roots. A bone graft, usually an allograft, is applied in the disc space. Next, a metallic plate can be applied between the two vertebral bodies, thereby accomplishing rigid fixation and minimizing the need for a postoperative cervical collar.

A posterior approach, also called *keyhole foraminotomy*, is indicated for patients with unilateral radiculopathy with soft disc herniation or small lateral osteophyte, professional speakers or singers who want to avoid the small risk for permanent injury to the recurrent laryngeal nerve (5%), and patients with a short thick neck. With the aid of an operating microscope, a small foraminotomy is performed with a high-speed drill to unroof the nerve root. The disc fragment can be removed, if accessible.

Patients with cervical spondylosis and myelopathy present a difficult problem. The approach is tailored to the patient's specific pathology. Patients who suffer from multiple discs or osteophytes with myelopathy and those with significant cervical stenosis in addition to a superimposed disc herniation can benefit from posterior cervical laminectomy. This, in turn, may need to be reinforced by lateral mass instrumentation and fusion, depending on the degree of spinal instability (Fig. 68-24). Patients with chronic spondylosis who manifest anterior and posterior compression may require complex surgery. In these cases, patients may undergo a staged surgical approach with an initial anterior exposure for multiple cervical discectomies or even cervical corpectomies with reconstruction with bone grafts

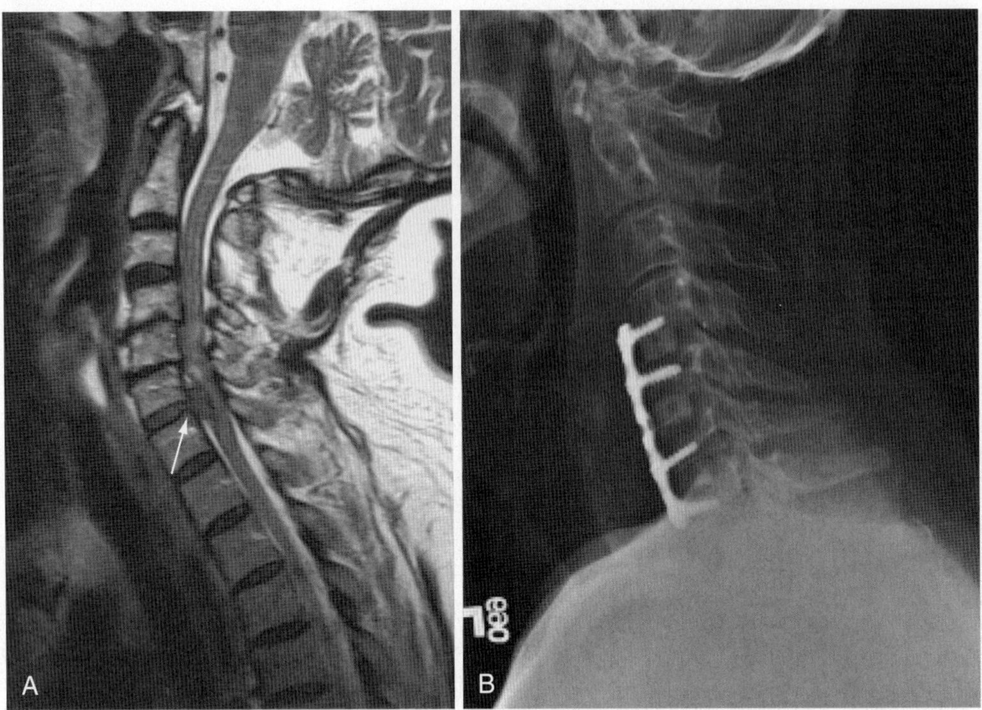

**FIGURE 68-23** **A,** T2-weighted sagittal MRI study of a patient with advanced cervical spondylosis and stenosis from C3-4 down to C6-7 with an acute herniated disc fragment at C6-7 *(arrow)* after cervical spine manipulation. **B,** Postoperative lateral x-ray showing C4-5, C5-6, and C6-7 anterior cervical discectomy and fusion using a bone allograft and titanium plate and screws.

or cages, followed by an anterior cervical plate. Next, the patient would undergo posterior cervical laminectomies reinforced with lateral mass plating. Unfortunately, the outcome from surgery for cervical spondylosis with myelopathy is often disappointing. The aim of the surgery is to arrest the progression of the myelopathy. In one series, 66% of patients had relief from radicular pain, whereas only 33% had improvement in sensory or motor complaints.[34]

## FUNCTIONAL AND STEREOTACTIC NEUROSURGERY

Functional neurosurgery is concerned with the anatomic or physiologic alteration of the nervous system to achieve a desired effect. This can be done with focal electrical stimulation procedures, ablative procedures, or implantation of pumps to deliver drugs, usually to the CSF but possibly also to the parenchyma. The field of functional neurosurgery deals primarily with the treatment of pain, movement disorders, epilepsy, and some psychiatric disorders when refractory to conventional treatments. These disorders all have in common hyperfunction or deranged function of some part(s) of the CNS. Sometimes, the hyperfunction results from a loss of function in some other part of the brain, such as in the output pathways of the globus pallidus (GPi) when the dopamine system in the brain degenerates, as in Parkinson's disease. The transmitter of the overactive GPi output system is inhibitory; the overall effect on the motor system is also inhibitory. The physiology of each functional disorder is often complex and only partly understood. It is not our focus here to detail what is known about the mechanism underlying each of these disorders; we focus on the surgery, especially the stereotactic techniques and possible interventions at the target site. This section also discusses SRS in general terms.

In considering brain stimulation, if the reader could image the consequences of placing two electrodes on the central processing unit of a computer and running a pulsatile stimulating current across it, not many would expect that the functioning of the computer would be enhanced. Rather, we would expect part of the computer not to work at all as a result. Although we talk about neuroaugmentation as if it were always adding something to the function of the nervous system, most of the interventions are actually effective because they stop certain unwanted activity in the brain. It may be a surprise to many but, in most situations, brain stimulation results in a temporary lesion of the stimulated structure. In almost all cases in the older neurosurgical literature in which a focal lesion was found to be effective, modern stimulation of that same structure is also effective. The difference is that a lesion is permanent and static in size and location. The advantage of stimulation is that it can be turned on or off, increased or decreased and, in the case of an implanted electrode array, changed in location, depending somewhat on which of the several contacts are activated. Thus, stimulation provides a reversible, scalable, and somewhat moveable functional lesion.

There are exceptions to the concept that stimulation is equivalent to a functional lesion. The frequency of stimulation can determine its overall effect and the neurotransmitters at the site of stimulation can also have an effect. The cerebral cortex, with its high concentrations of excitatory neurotransmitters, may actually be turned on with stimulation. Thus, certain crude visual prostheses may be effective on that basis.

Stereotaxis, as applied to neurosurgery, is concerned with the localization of a target in three-dimensional space. The target deep in the brain is not seen directly at surgery. This can be a

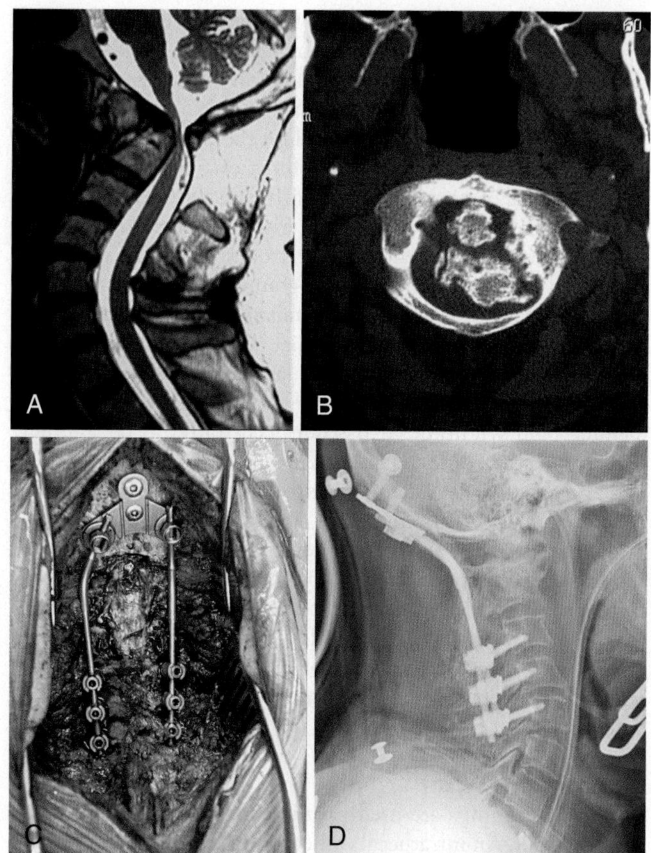


**FIGURE 68-24** Radiographic and intraoperative pictures of a patient presenting with a C2 odontoid fracture. A T2-weighted sagittal MRI study **(A)** and axial CT image at the level of C1 **(B)** show an odontoid fracture with anterior displacement of the odontoid fragment and settling of the C2 body into the C1 ring, resulting in significant compromise of the spinal canal and cord. Intraoperative picture **(C)** and lateral radiograph of the cervical spine **(D)** show an occipitocervical fusion after an anterior transoral approach for a C2 vertebrectomy.

tumor, white matter pathway, cranial nerve, vascular malformation, or nucleus deep within the brain. The field has evolved using frame-based and frameless systems but, in each case, a calculated inference is used to reach the target accurately.

Frame-based systems use a rigid frame attached to the skull by pins that penetrate the outer table of the skull (Fig. 68-25). This can easily be done under local anesthesia, with the patient wide awake. The patient is then taken for CT or MRI with a localizer on the frame. Using Cartesian coordinates, the x, y, and z coordinates of the target can then be determined. In other words, the position of the target in relation to the frame is known. Using an arc system, which is mounted on the frame, the target can be accessed by different trajectories. When the target is a vascular lesion, arteriography can be performed with a localizing frame and the position of the vascular lesion in three-dimensional space can be determined. Frame-based systems are used for brain biopsies, deep brain stimulation, ablative procedures, and SRS.

SRS involves the delivery of a concentrated dose of radiation to a defined volume in the brain. The dose of radiation delivered would be toxic if given in a broad field to the entire brain. When delivered in multiple collimated beams from numerous different angles, or in arcs at different angles, the effect on the surrounding brain is minimized. Two methods of frame-based SRS are currently used widely. The gamma knife uses cobalt-201 radiation sources focused on one point. Once the target is localized in three dimensions, it is placed at this point and different collimators are used to focus the radiation. Modified linear accelerators deliver the radiation dose in multiple arcs, thereby minimizing the effect on surrounding brain tissue. Both systems use multiple isocenters for the treatment of irregularly shaped lesions. SRS has been used in the treatment of almost every intracranial lesion but is commonly used in the treatment of metastatic tumors, benign lesions of the cranial nerves, AVMs and, trigeminal neuralgia.[35-37] The primary risks of SRS are radiation necrosis and radiation injury to surrounding structures.

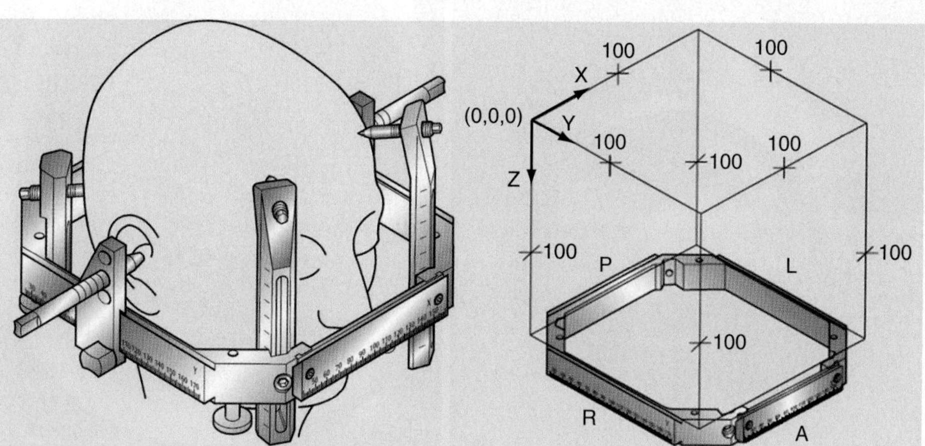


**FIGURE 68-25** The Leksell stereotactic coordinate frame is rigidly attached to the head by four threaded pins. The fiducial box is mounted on the frame during the imaging study (MRI or CT). The x, y, and z coordinates are determined directly from the imaging study. The center of the frame is arbitrarily given the coordinates 100, 100, 100. (Courtesy Elekta, Stockholm.)

Frameless stereotactic techniques use advanced imaging techniques, fiducials, and reference markers in place of a fixed frame. Robotic arms, infrared reflectors, and light-emitting diodes provide the surgeon with real-time information about the anatomy at hand. This technology can also be fused with a display from the operating microscope, aiding in the operative dissection. It is useful for the planning of incisions and craniotomies and, when combined with intraoperative ultrasound, may be of use in determining the extent of tumor resection. Frameless stereotactic radiosurgical devices are commercially available.[34,35,38,39]

## Brain Stimulation

Electrical stimulation of the nervous system is used in the treatment of movement disorders, pain, and epilepsy. Stimulation involves placement of an electrode, which is then connected to a subcutaneously placed generator. Here we discuss neurostimulation as it applies to the treatment of movement disorders, chronic pain states, and epilepsy.

Parkinson's disease is the most common movement disorder for which patients have surgery. Stereotactic techniques developed in the 1950s were used to create lesions in the pallidum and thalamus. These ablative procedures fell by the wayside for a time with the introduction and widespread use of L-dopa (L-3,4-dihydroxyphenylalanine). In the early 1990s, there was a renewed interest in the use of surgical techniques for Parkinson's patients who had become unresponsive to pharmacologic agents or intolerant of their side effects. Lesions of the internal segment of the GPi saw a tremendous resurgence. With improvements in imaging and intraoperative microelectrode recording, deep brain stimulation soon replaced ablative procedures in the surgical treatment of these patients. Stimulation induces a reversible inhibition of neuronal activity, which can be adjusted as the clinical situation demands. The subthalamic nucleus has replaced the GPi as the target of choice. Subthalamic nucleus stimulation is most effective for the treatment of rigidity and akinesia. Tremor is best addressed with stimulation of the ventralis intermedius nucleus of the thalamus (Fig. 68-26).

Spinal cord stimulation is used for the treatment of chronic pain, dystonia, and bladder dysfunction. Patients typically undergo a trial of stimulation in which wire electrodes are placed percutaneously and attached to an external generator. If symptoms improve, permanent wire electrodes or paddle electrodes are placed and connected to a programmable generator placed subcutaneously. The precise mechanism of action is unknown. The most common indication is that of the so-called *postlaminectomy syndrome*, especially when leg pain is worse than back pain. There is also some benefit for those patients with chronic regional pain syndrome. It has not been found to be routinely effective in the treatment of cancer pain.

Vagal nerve stimulation has been approved by the U.S. Food and Drug Administration (FDA) for the treatment of intractable seizures and severe depression. The mechanism of action is not clear but is thought to be the result of afferent stimulation of higher cortical centers in the hypothalamus, amygdala, insular cortex, and cerebral cortex through the nucleus of the solitary tract. Stimulation of the left vagus nerve decreases seizure frequency by approximately 50% but rarely makes patients seizure-free.[40]

## Implantable Pumps

Implantable pumps are used for the treatment of chronic pain and spasticity. An intrathecal catheter is inserted into the lumber spinal canal and a trial infusion used to gauge response. Many patients with cancer pain will respond favorably to intrathecal administration of narcotics through a programmable pump. Baclofen is the agent of choice for the treatment of spasticity with this modality.

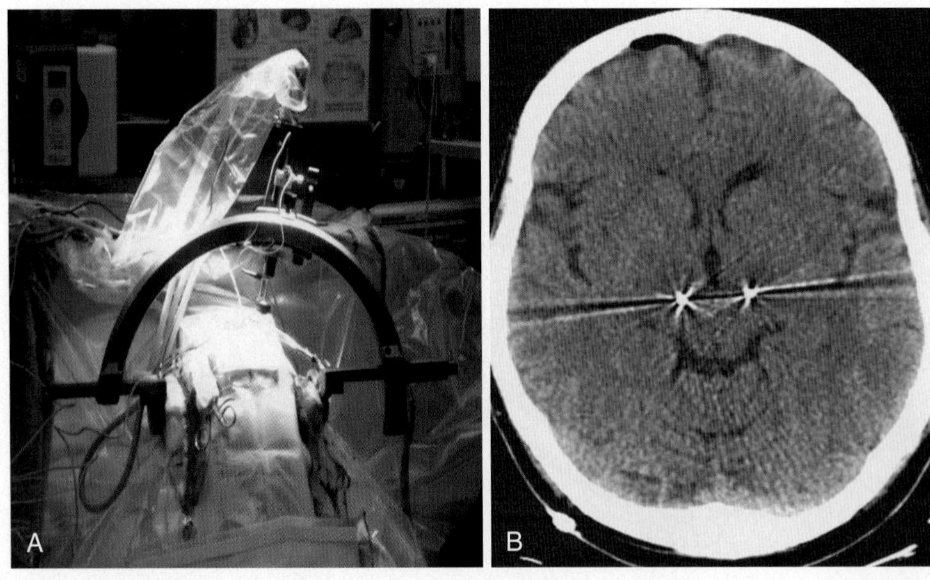


**FIGURE 68-26 A,** Intraoperative display in functional neurosurgery for deep brain stimulation. **B,** CT scan revealing deep brain stimulation electrodes at the ventral intermediate nucleus for the treatment of essential tremor. (**A** Courtesy Dr. Daniel Dilorenzo, University of Texas Medical Branch, Galveston, Tex.)

## Destructive Lesions

Ablative lesioning of the CNS for the treatment of pain, movement disorders, epilepsy, and psychiatric diseases has a long history. Before the advent of antipsychotic drugs, institutionalization and psychosurgery were thought to be the most efficient way of curing and controlling some patients with severe psychiatric disease. Before the development of the technologies described earlier, lesioning of different pathways in the brain and spinal cord was the only method for treating patients with chronic pain and movement disorders. Even though neuroaugmentative procedures and drug infusion technology have replaced many of the neuroablative procedures formerly in widespread use, a few ablative procedures still retain their clinical usefulness.

Dorsal root entry zone lesions are particularly useful for patients with deafferentation pain related to brachial plexus injury and, to a lesser extent, patients with spinal cord injury who have so-called *end zone pain*. In these conditions, deafferentation of the spinothalamic tract neurons results in spontaneous firing and the sensation of pain. The procedure creates lesions of the dorsal horn of the affected levels using a thermocouple probe. Extension of this concept has been applied to the caudal nucleus of the trigeminal nerve for the treatment of facial pain syndromes.

Myelotomy has traditionally been used in the treatment of bilateral cancer pain. It involves sectioning of the anterior commissure at and above the involved levels, which interrupts pain fibers on their way to the contralateral spinothalamic tract. A modified technique that only interrupts the median raphe of the dorsal columns has been described.[41] This presumably interrupts the second-order visceral pain pathway demonstrated to travel up the mammalian dorsal funiculus.[42]

Cordotomy involves lesioning the anterolateral quadrant of the spinal cord at cervical levels, thereby eliminating input from the spinothalamic tract on the contralateral side of the body. Historically, it was most useful in the treatment of unilateral cancer pain. Bilateral lesioning increases the risk for neurologically mediated sleep apnea (Ondine's curse). It can be performed percutaneously or as an open procedure.

Sympathectomy involves surgical interruption of the sympathetic chain at the high thoracic or lumbar level. A variety of endoscopic, thoracoscopic, radiofrequency, and open techniques are used. It is primarily used in patients with hyperhidrosis, sympathetically mediated pain, causalgia, chronic regional pain syndrome, and Raynaud's disease.

Nerve block or neurectomy uses local anesthetic, sometimes with corticosteroids, which can be injected into the tissues surrounding a peripheral nerve, blocking conductivity and relieving pain. This can result in a long-lasting effect but typically is short-lived. Neurolytic agents (phenol or absolute alcohol) can also be used. Nerves can also be surgically divided or interrupted using radiofrequency techniques. There is a significant risk for recurrence with ablative neurectomy. Local nerve blocks are generally used in diagnostic procedures but can be repeated as necessary for the relief of pain. Ablative neurectomy is usually reserved for short-term relief in patients with a poor prognosis and short life expectancy.

## Epilepsy

Epilepsy is not a distinct clinical entity with an identifiable cause, but rather is a complex collection of disorders of the brain that all share seizures as part of the complex. Seizures are classified as partial, generalized, or unclassified. Partial seizures are simple (consciousness not impaired) or complex (consciousness impaired). Generalized seizures are convulsive or nonconvulsive. Incidence rates in developed countries (40 to 70/100,000) are lower than those in developing countries (100 to 190/100,000). Approximately 20% to 40% of patients with seizures do not respond to anticonvulsant therapy. Failure to respond to three anticonvulsant medications prompts referral to a center specializing in epilepsy evaluation and treatment, and approximately 1.33% to 4.50% of those patients are candidates for surgical intervention.[43]

The goal of the workup of the patient who is a potential candidate for the surgical treatment of epilepsy is to identify the cortical area responsible for the onset of the seizure. When the radiographic workup (MRI, CT, or both) reveals an obvious lesion causing the seizure (e.g., tumor, vascular malformation), the treatment is relatively straightforward and involves removal of the lesion. In other cases, the offending lesion is not as obvious on imaging, and intensive and often invasive monitoring is necessary to determine the epileptogenic focus. It is also important to determine language dominance and areas of the brain that are functionally abnormal during the interictal period. Noninvasive techniques that have become more widely available and better characterized include magnetoencephalography, positron emission tomography, single-photon emission CT (SPECT), and functional MRI. Invasive modalities used in the evaluation of patients for seizure surgery include the Wada test for language dominance, stereotactically implanted depth electrodes, implanted strip electrodes, and implanted grid electrodes (Fig. 68-27). Any or all of these techniques may be useful in brain mapping. It has long been possible to map critical speech and limb movement areas in awake, locally anesthetized craniotomy patients at the time of seizure focus resection.

Based on the information obtained in a noninvasive workup, the patient may be taken to surgery. Dominant hemisphere lesions are often operated on with the patient awake to

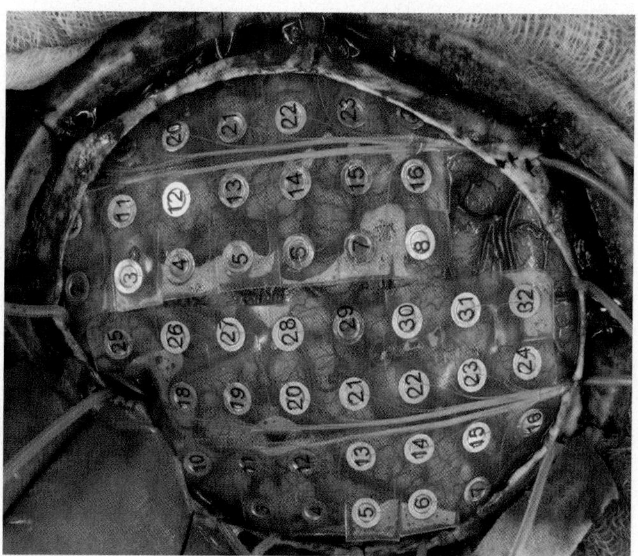

**FIGURE 68-27** Intraoperative view of grid electrode placement for epilepsy surgery. (Courtesy Dr. Nitin Tandon, University of Texas, Houston.)

allow for intraoperative confirmatory brain mapping. This is accomplished by stimulating the cortex and observing and monitoring the patient's response, looking for speech arrest, anomia, or limb weakness or numbness. The most common surgical procedures performed for epilepsy are anterior temporal lobectomy, focal cortical resection, multiple subpial transection, hemispherectomy, and corpus callosotomy.

Anterior temporal lobectomy is the most common operation for seizures. An entirely unilateral interictal focus is the ideal indication (Fig. 68-28). The anterior temporal lobe, anterior hippocampus, and amygdala are excised. If the epileptogenic focus is not completely excised, the patient may continue to experience intractable seizures. If too much temporal lobe is resected, it can result in a contralateral superior quadrantanopsia or, in dominant hemisphere lesions, speech and language dysfunction.

Focal cortical resection is usually performed in the frontal cortex. The results are more variable than those with temporal lobectomy.

Multiple subpial transection is used in more eloquent areas of the brain and involves making cortical incisions perpendicular to the surface of the gyrus in question. This presumably preserves descending fibers and function while interrupting spread of any epileptogenic activity within the cortical mantel itself.

Corpus callosotomy is used to prevent the rapid spread of seizures, rather than eliminate the focus. It is primarily useful in seizures that suddenly generalize, resulting in atonic drop attacks, as in Lennox-Gastaut syndrome.

Hemispherectomy is usually reserved for young children with seizures restricted to one hemisphere but threatening the good hemisphere by secondary effects of repeated seizures, as in Rasmussen's syndrome. There is usually some abnormality of cellular migration. In the past, the entire cortex was removed, leaving the basal ganglia intact. Even though there was a significant decrease in seizure activity, the procedure led to a high complication rate, with ex vacuo brain shifts. A newer technique now involves preservation of portions of the cortex and its blood supply while disconnecting them from the rest of the brain by extensive undercutting of the adjacent white matter.[44]

## Trigeminal Neuralgia

Trigeminal neuralgia affects approximately 4 in 100,000 individuals and is characterized by brief episodes of severe, lancinating pain in one or more of the three divisions of the trigeminal nerve, usually V2 and V3. Patients often describe that it is precipitated by touch or extremes of temperature. In extreme cases, a patient may refuse to eat or shave to avoid triggering the severe jolts of pain. Sensation usually remains intact, and significant numbness or jaw weakness leads to suspicion of a compressive mass lesion such as tumor. Often, patients are referred with an already established diagnosis. It is reassuring if the patient has responded at some point to carbamazepine or an appropriate medication. MRI is used to rule out posterior fossa tumors and multiple sclerosis, which can present with related symptoms. Most patients respond to the oral administration of carbamazepine. Baclofen and gabapentin also have some clinical usefulness in medical treatment. The most common mechanism is presumed to be related to vascular compression of the fifth cranial nerve as it enters the brainstem (Fig. 68-29). With aging, the arteries elongate and can then begin to loop against the cranial nerves. At its entry to the pons, the fifth nerve has lost its peripheral nerve supportive architecture, the reticulin and mesenchymal elements that toughen the nerve more peripherally. Focal pulsatile pressure of the artery against this vulnerable part of nerve results in ephaptic transmission from large myelinated fibers to small myelinated (A delta) and unmyelinated fibers.

Surgical therapy is usually reserved for patients who fail medical treatment. Microvascular decompression involves a small suboccipital craniotomy for microsurgical exploration of the dorsal root entry zone of the trigeminal nerve on the affected

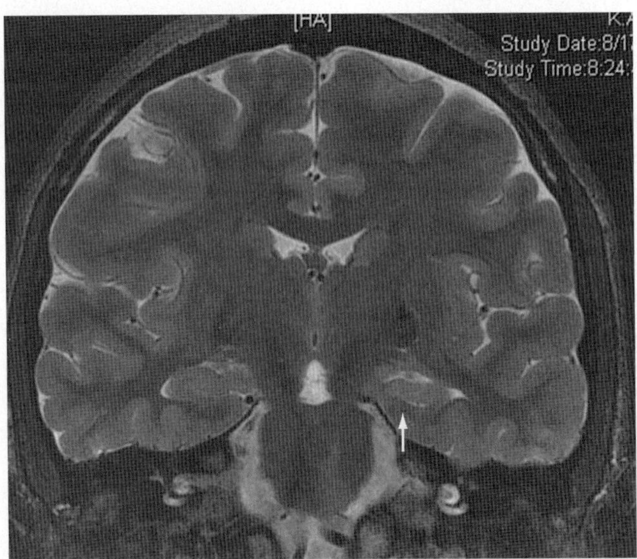


**FIGURE 68-28** T2-weighted coronal MRI study shows gliosis and atrophy of the left mesial temporal structure *(arrow).* (Courtesy Dr. James E. Baumgartner, University of Texas, Houston.)

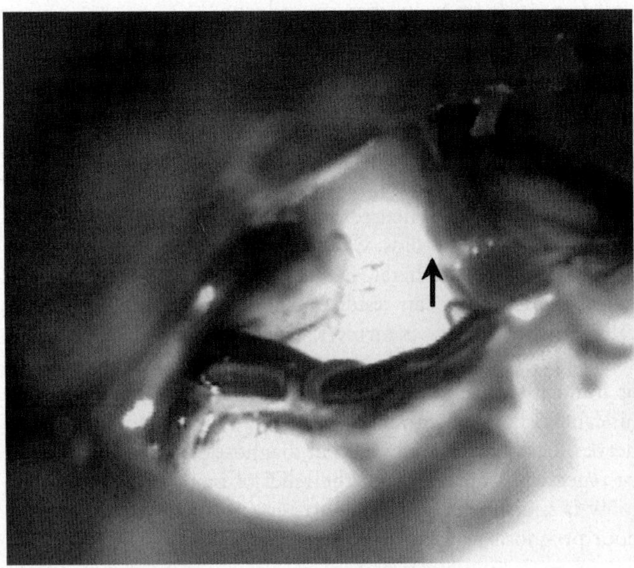

**FIGURE 68-29** Intraoperative photograph through of a patient with typical trigeminal neuralgia. The left trigeminal nerve is compressed superiorly by an arterial branch of the superior cerebellar artery *(arrow).*

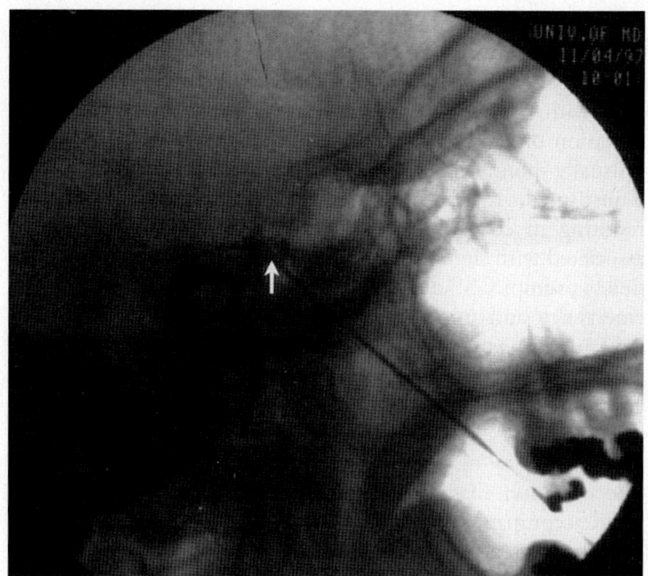


**FIGURE 68-30** Lateral skull film in a patient undergoing glycerol rhizotomy for typical trigeminal neuralgia. A 20-gauge spinal needle is directed to the foramen ovale and nonionic contrast agent is injected to outline the trigeminal ganglion *(arrow)*.

side. The offending vessel, usually the superior cerebellar artery, is then dissected off the nerve and a barrier (Teflon or PVA [polyvinyl alcohol] sponge) is placed between the vessel and nerve to prevent continued pulsatile focal compression. In especially favorable situations, the offending artery can be dissected free to loop away from the nerve, without the need for padding. A small sling of arterial patch graft material can also be sewn to hold the artery loop away from the nerve.

Percutaneous trigeminal rhizotomy techniques generally involve radiofrequency heat lesioning of the trigeminal ganglion, glycerol injection (Fig. 68-30) into the spinal fluid of Meckel's cave (which causes an osmotic damage preferentially to the smaller pain-carrying nerve fibers), or mechanical trauma to the nerve or ganglion by transient inflation of a no. 4 Fogarty catheter balloon. Each method has its own proponents along with advantages and disadvantages.

SRS has been described for the treatment of trigeminal neuralgia.[35] Although initial results have been encouraging, long-term efficacy has yet to be determined.

## HYDROCEPHALUS

Hydrocephalus denotes excessive accumulation of the CSF in the intracranial compartment. The accumulation of fluid can be in the intracerebral (ventricular) or extracerebral (subarachnoid spaces and cisterns) compartments.

Normally, there is a fine balance between CSF production by the choroid plexus and absorption at the arachnoid villi along the superior sagittal sinuses. CSF production has been found to be 0.33 mL/kg/hr (20 mL/hr). Almost all the fluid produced is absorbed within 8 hours. Any imbalance in this will lead to excessive accumulation of CSF, causing hydrocephalus. Thus, hydrocephalus can be caused by excessive production, decreased absorption, or obstruction anywhere in the pathways. Usually, the obstruction is never complete and there is some absorption from the ependyma.

### Types

#### Communicating and Obstructive Hydrocephalus

This distinction was made several decades ago to explain whether the obstructed ventricular CSF communicated with the subarachnoid CSF. In obstructive hydrocephalus, the obstruction is at or proximal to the fourth ventricular outlet foramina (foramen of Magendie, foramen of Luschka). However, if the obstruction is beyond the fourth ventricular outlet foramina (cisterns or arachnoid granulations), it is classified as communicating hydrocephalus. Common examples of obstructive hydrocephalus are aqueductal stenosis and hydrocephalus associated with tumors. When the term was initially coined, it took into account the findings of ventriculography and pneumoencephalography. However, with the arrival of CT and MRI, these investigations are no longer necessary in most cases and the terms *communicating* and *obstructive* were no longer clinically important. However, as will be discussed later, the advent of endoscopic third ventriculostomy has generated renewed interest in these terms.

#### Acute and Chronic Hydrocephalus

Hydrocephalus developing within days or few weeks (e.g., hydrocephalus caused by tumor) manifests with rapid progression of symptoms is known as *acute hydrocephalus*. It requires early attention and treatment. On the other hand, CSF accumulation over months (or even years) presents with subtle signs of memory impairment, walking difficulty, or urinary incontinence and is termed *chronic hydrocephalus*. A classic example is NPH, which is seen usually in older adults. At times, chronic hydrocephalus can present acutely because of changes in the pathophysiology of the CSF absorption or flow.

#### Congenital and Acquired Hydrocephalus

Hydrocephalus present at birth is known as *congenital hydrocephalus*. At times, congenital hydrocephalus is apparent a few weeks or months after birth; the process may even have started while the child was in utero. Although congenital hydrocephalus is commonly obstructive in nature, it can be communicating, as in intrauterine toxoplasmosis or cytomegalovirus infections. In acquired hydrocephalus, the pathologic process starts after birth and includes post-traumatic hydrocephalus, hydrocephalus associated with tumors, and NPH.

**Hydrocephalus Ex Vacuo (Compensatory Hydrocephalus)** Here, the ventricles enlarge in a compensatory manner because of overall shrinking of the brain tissue. This can mislead an inexperienced physician to diagnose hydrocephalus, whereas the enlargement of the ventricles is actually caused by the shrinkage of brain tissue. This is commonly seen in those of advanced age with brain atrophy, following diffuse head injury or stroke, and with various neurodegenerative conditions. The most important condition that is usually confused with hydrocephalus ex vacuo is NPH, unfortunately also seen in older adults.

#### Porencephaly

Porencephaly, or porencephalic cyst, commonly refers to a condition in which a focal brain substance has suffered some loss of volume (e.g., stroke, postsurgical change in volume) leading to the collection of CSF in the cavity. Porencephalic cyst is usually differentiated from hydrocephalus ex vacuo by its localized nature.

### Arrested Hydrocephalus

This represents a condition in which the ventricles are large, with the patient having no significant symptoms to require a surgical procedure. However, this term should be used with caution because it is well known that these patients may develop symptoms over a prolonged period or may manifest acutely following a precipitating event such as minor trauma or infection, which alters the CSF dynamics.

## Clinical Features

In hydrocephalus, CSF retained inside the cranial compartment results in increased ICP and dilation of ventricles, causing compression of the adjacent brain. The symptoms differ considerably in different age groups. In infants, a thin and relatively nonrigid skull allows for an overall cranial expansion, whereas in older children and adults the rigid fused skull prevents its enlargement. Considering this, in infantile hydrocephalus, either the infant is born with a large head or the head grows abnormally during the first few months of life. The anterior fontanel is usually full; it may or may not be bulging. In extreme cases, a relatively higher ICP allows the blood to be diverted from the intracranial to extracranial compartment, resulting in prominent and dilated scalp veins. A late feature is the classic sunset sign, manifested with downward deviation of the eyeballs, like a setting sun. This is caused by compression of the midbrain tectum by the posterior part of the dilated third ventricle. In later stages, the child will be irritable, fussy, and may not accept feeds. It may be associated with vomiting. Usually, there is no associated fever or diarrhea. Lethargy, drowsiness and, in extreme cases, lapsing into a comatose state will follow if the child remains untreated.

In older children and adults, fusion of the skull bones no longer permits the cranium to enlarge. The enlarging ventricles result in raised ICP and compression of the adjacent brain. There are two common modes of presentation, rapidly progressive hydrocephalus and chronic hydrocephalus. In rapidly progressive hydrocephalus, the increasing accumulation of CSF increases the ICP, causing new-onset headache and vomiting (commonly known as features of raised ICP). If untreated, these symptoms worsen and blurring of vision often occurs. In patients with long-standing raised pressure, papilledema can result in secondary optic atrophy. If still untreated, drowsiness and progression to coma follow. Focal neurologic deficits are not experienced, although walking difficulty or the sensation of giving way at the knees can occur.

In chronic hydrocephalus, the CSF accumulates more slowly, thus gradually compressing the brain. This type of presentation is predominantly seen in older adults, although it can occur at a younger age. The patient becomes progressively dull, apathetic, and uninvolved with her or his surroundings. Memory impairment for recent events is commonly seen, but usually the remote memory is well preserved. A short stepped gait with a wide stance and unsteadiness is evident. Urinary incontinence initially accompanies the form of urgency of micturition. Although it is uncertain why most of these patients do not have significant headache, it is assumed that slow dilation of the ventricles compresses the adjacent brain to accommodate for the CSF without causing raised ICP.

Seizures are uncommon because of hydrocephalus per se, but they may be caused by the process that initiates the hydrocephalus. It is worthwhile to note a phenomenon seen in late stages of untreated hydrocephalus known as *cerebellar fits* or *hydrocephalic attacks*. Preceded by progressively severe headache, the patient lapses into transient sudden unconsciousness associated with a decerebrate or decorticate response, downward deviation of the eyeballs, and respiratory distress. The recovery is usually spontaneous. These episodes recur until CSF diversion is instituted. This is caused by acute transtentorial herniation, resulting in compression of the brainstem. The condition is associated with significant morbidity and can be uniformly fatal unless prompt CSF drainage is instituted. This is a true medical emergency and under no circumstances should treatment be delayed. Survivors often develop permanent hemianopia caused by occipital infarcts from compression of the posterior cerebral arteries against the tentorial edge during the herniation.

## Diagnosis

The common diagnostic modality for hydrocephalus is CT, often accompanied by MRI. Cranial ultrasound evaluation has been used predominantly in the newborn and infants with an open fontanel. The CT scan shows dilated ventricles and often indicates the pathology and site of obstruction. The ventricular system dilates proximal to the obstruction, whereas the CSF pathways distal to the obstruction are not well visualized. One can infer the level of obstruction from by CT because all the ventricles are usually well visualized. Most of the tumorous pathology can also be well visualized by CT. However, it cannot delineate the exact site or nature of the obstruction. Probably the best use of CT for managing hydrocephalus has been in assessing patients with shunt malfunction. An obstructed shunt often, although not always, leads to dilation of the ventricles, which can easily be identified by CT. In addition, the radio-opaque shunt tube is well visualized by CT.

MRI has been the imaging choice for newly diagnosed hydrocephalus. The ability of MRI to obtain images in three different planes—coronal, sagittal and axial—has been of considerable value in diagnosing the exact cause of the hydrocephalus and site of obstruction. With a properly done MRI, the site of obstruction can be well visualized in most patients with obstructive hydrocephalus (Fig. 68-31). This is of considerable importance because small tumors or cysts causing the hydrocephalus can be visualized and, when removed, can relieve the hydrocephalus. Also, as discussed later, MRI is considered essential prior to considering endoscopic third ventriculostomy or aqueductoplasty; these are exciting alternatives for managing hydrocephalus and assessing the effectiveness of endoscopic third ventriculostomy during follow-up.

## Treatment

The ultimate goal in the treatment of hydrocephalus is to reverse the neurologic damage caused by the raised ICP. Reconstitution of the cerebral mantle to allow normal intellectual development and avoidance of shunt dependency should be considered as additional management goals. A cerebral mantle thickness of 2.8 cm or more has been found to be associated with a good outcome. However, cortical mantle reconstitution is not satisfactory if treatment is delayed for longer than 5 months.

Surgery for hydrocephalus involves diversion of the accumulated CSF by one of the following procedures: (1) by reopening the obstruction to allow the CSF to flow into its natural pathway; (2) by creating a diversion before the obstruction to allow the CSF to drain into the intracranial pathways distal to

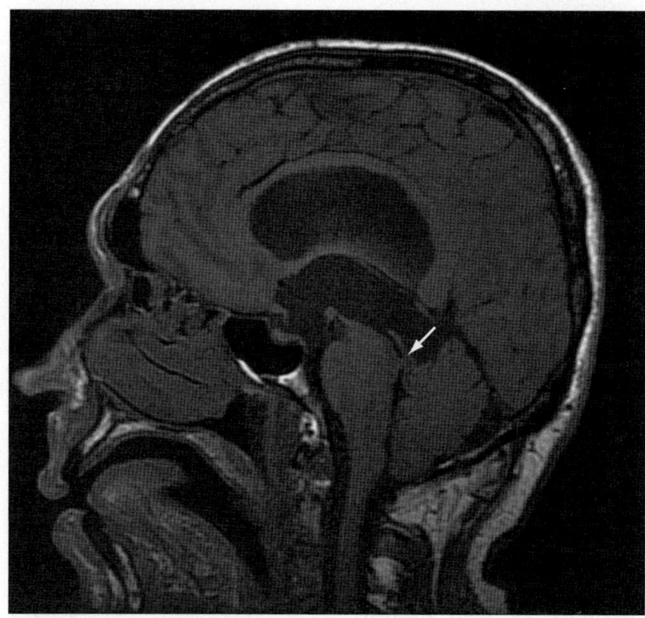

**FIGURE 68-31** T1-weighted sagittal MRI scan of patient with gross obstructive hydrocephalus caused by aqueductal stenosis *(arrow).*

the block; or (3) by diversion of the CSF into another cavity so it becomes absorbed into the bloodstream. Examples of reopening of the obstructed pathway include endoscopic aqueductoplasty and excision of the tumor causing hydrocephalus; endoscopic third ventriculostomy falls into the second category. Ventriculoperitoneal shunts, which have been the mainstay of treatment in hydrocephalus, belong in the third group.

Although shunts have been the mainstay of treatment for several decades, endoscopic procedures have now become more popular. These include endoscopic third ventriculostomy, endoscopic aqueductoplasty, and endoscopic aqueductal stenting. These alternative procedures appear exciting, but strict patient selection criteria are required.

It is often difficult for a pediatric neurosurgeon to decide whether the patient with ventriculomegaly needs a CSF diversion procedure. Imaging studies and invasive procedures such as ICP monitoring have not been able to predict which patients are likely to develop intellectual deterioration as a result of hydrocephalus reliably. Children younger than 5 years with moderate to severe hydrocephalus without any symptoms often are considered for a CSF diversion procedure because it is often difficult to assess intellectual development in this age group. It is also considered that mere attainment of developmental milestones is not indicative of adequate development of intellectual function. Insertion of shunt protects these children against the effects of persistent ventriculomegaly and ensures an optimal environment for future intellectual development. However, children older than 5 years and adults with asymptomatic ventriculomegaly often are closely watched, with frequent assessment of intellectual development, before considering a shunt insertion.

Medical treatment has not proved to be useful for hydrocephalus. It is often used as a temporary measure and in conjunction with surgical management. Acetazolamide has been commonly used because it has been found to reduce CSF production. However, benefits are minimal and high doses of the drug, which cause metabolic acidosis, are required to achieve the effect.

### Cerebrospinal Fluid Shunts

Although initially the concept of shunting appeared to be simple, it has proven to be more complex over the years. Being purely mechanical devices, shunts have not been able to manage the complexity of the CSF dynamics associated with hydrocephalus effectively. Basically, CSF shunts are tubes with valves that drain the CSF out from one compartment into another. The shunt contains three parts, the ventricular end, valve complex, and distal end. The distal end is usually named after the organ into which it is inserted; for example, in ventriculoperitoneal shunts, it is known as the *peritoneal end* and in ventriculoatrial shunts, it is known as the *atrial end.* Often, antisiphon devices that prevent the CSF siphoning effect, which can result in overdrainage when the person is in an upright position, are included in the valve complex.

Shunt malfunction, infection, overdrainage, brain injury, seizures, and distal complications are the major complications associated with shunts; shunt malfunction is the main complication of shunt procedures. Malfunction is so common that sometimes it is not considered as a complication but as part of the natural history of shunt surgery. Of the several predisposing factors for shunt malfunction, age has been found to be significant . In a multicenter study involving 38 neurosurgical centers and 773 patients, 29% of shunts failed in the first year, requiring reoperation. Approximately half of the shunts (47%) inserted in children younger than 6 months failed as compared with 14% of the shunts that failed in children older than 6 months. It was also found that shunts placed as an emergency procedure failed more often (34%) than shunts placed electively (29%).[45] Shunt components can also become disconnected at the junctions and migrate to either of the cavities. If the distal end of the tube migrates into the abdominal cavity, the tube is usually left behind. It generally floats freely in the abdominal cavity and does not precipitate bowel obstruction. Some neurosurgeons, however, would prefer to remove the abdominal catheter with a laparoscopic device. Similar to subcutaneous tissue, the catheter has to be removed if the shunt is infected or there is some other abdominal infection.

The incidence of shunt infection, the second significant complication, ranges from 4% to 7%. Common organisms include *Staphylococcus epidermidis* (50% to 60%), *Staphylococcus aureus* (20% to 30%), gram-negative bacilli, and *Propionibacterium* spp. Most shunt infections occur within 3 months of insertion, with a small percentage occurring as late as 6 months postinsertion. Most shunts are inoculated at the time of insertion although, uncommonly, it can be a hematogenous spread. *S. epidermidis* forms a biofilm and adheres to the shunt tube, which protects the bacteria against oral or IV antibiotics. The colonization permits the bacteria to remain quiescent for weeks or sometimes a few months before the infection manifests. The clinical picture depends on the severity of the infection, time of diagnosis, and site of infection. Shunt infections can be infection of the shunt tube in its subcutaneous tract or wound (wound infection or of the CSF spaces (meningitis), ventricles (ventriculitis), or abdominal space (peritonitis). Early subcutaneous infections manifest with low-grade fever, redness along the shunt tube, and purulent discharge from the incision. Wound breakage and exposure of the shunt tube can occur. Later, as the infection involves the CSF and ventricles, it may be associated with decreased sensorium, seizures, and neurologic deficits. If the infection involves the abdominal cavity, it can present with features of peritonitis. A high degree of suspicion for infection in the postoperative period is key for an early diagnosis. The possibility of a shunt infection should be considered in any patient with a shunt; however, only occasionally is the shunt related to the fever. The diagnosis is confirmed by shunt tap and CSF culture. Complete removal of the shunt tube is recommended, with reinsertion of a new shunt once the infection clears. The incidence of shunt infection is reduced by the use of catheters impregnated with rifampicin and clindamycin, which are effective against gram-positive bacteria.

It is imperative that the general surgeon be acquainted with the distal complications of ventriculoperitoneal shunts because they may be encountered with relative frequency in a general surgery practice. The two common distal complications are ascites and pseudoperitoneal cyst. Reduction in absorption of the CSF, causing generalized fluid accumulation in the peritoneal cavity, results in ascites. Common causes include a reduced absorbing surface (premature infants), high protein content of the CSF, peritoneal scarring from previous infections, or elevated venous pressure. Although usually sterile, ascites can be infected in as many as 15% of cases. Not uncommonly, ascites can present as shunt malfunction caused by backpressure and reduction in CSF drainage from intracranial compartment. In infected ascites, there will be associated signs of local and systemic infection. The shunt is usually removed and placed in another cavity, such as the atrium. In infected ascites, the shunt is externalized and replaced into an alternate site (e.g., atrium, pleura) after the infection is cleared. In premature infants with a reduced absorptive surface, it is not uncommon to find that the peritoneum often functions satisfactorily after few years.

In pseudoperitoneal cyst, there is a loculated pocket of CSF in the peritoneal cavity walled off by bowel and omental tissue. This results in a cystic fluid collection, which often presents as a mass in the abdomen. Generally, this is associated with a low-grade infection of the shunt tube or abdomen, a previous infection, or surgery of the abdominal cavity that has resulted in scarring and reduced absorption. This is usually easy to diagnose because the shunt tube can be seen lying inside a fluid-filled cavity in the abdomen. Pseudoperitoneal cyst often presents with shunt malfunction, with abdominal distention. Surgery involves exteriorizing the shunt tube, treating the infection, if present, and then reinserting the shunt into another compartment (i.e., converting it into ventriculoatrial shunt) or into another site in the abdominal cavity. Surprisingly, the second approach works for most patients.

The distinction between ascites and pseudoperitoneal cyst is significant because a pseudoperitoneal cyst is associated with a higher infection rate than ascites. Also, in ascites, the shunt needs to be removed from the peritoneal cavity because the entire peritoneal cavity cannot absorb fluid, whereas in the pseudoperitoneal cavity it is usually sufficient to remove the shunt and replace it into another region of the peritoneal cavity.

### Alternatives to Shunting

As noted, advances in endoscopic neurosurgery have created several alternative options to the placement of shunts. Endoscopic third ventriculostomy, endoscopic aqueductoplasty, endoscopic aqueductal stenting, and endoscopic septostomy are available as alternatives to shunt procedures. However, all these procedures are currently only effective for certain types of obstructive hydrocephalus, and not all procedures are effective for all types of obstructive hydrocephalus. In aqueductoplasty, the obstructed aqueduct is recanalized with the help of a 3 Fr Fogarty catheter under direct endoscopic vision; in aqueductal stenting, a stent is placed in the aqueduct to prevent further reclosure. The stent is usually attached to a subcutaneous reservoir to prevent its migration. Both these procedures are only indicated for obstructive hydrocephalus with short-segment aqueductal stenosis, for which an adequate reopening can be made without risking injury to the adjacent midbrain. Endoscopic third ventriculostomy involves the creation of a fenestration in the floor of the third ventricle to bypass the obstructed CSF into the basal cisterns (Fig. 68-32).[46,47] Endoscopic third

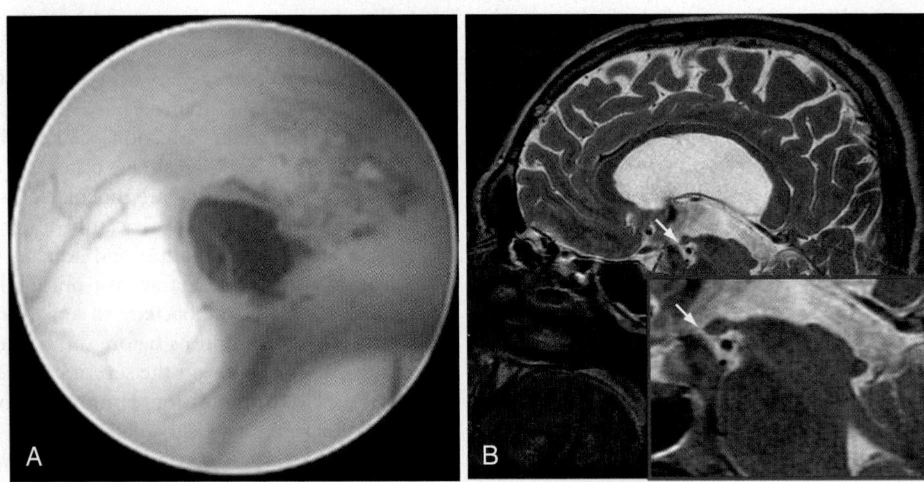


**FIGURE 68-32 A,** Endoscopic view of the third ventricular floor after the third ventriculostomy. **B,** Follow-up MRI scan 4 years later demonstrating good flow at the fenestration site *(arrow).*

ventriculostomy is effective for obstructive hydrocephalus associated with obstruction at or beyond the aqueduct (e.g., aqueductal stenosis, tumors of the fourth ventricle, fourth ventricular outlet obstruction). However, the effectiveness of these alternative procedures varies with age, with the procedure being least effective (20% to 40% success rate) in neonates and 80% effective in older children and adults. Although the cause for this is uncertain, failure of absorption of CSF by the normal absorptive process (arachnoid granulations) has been the most common explanation.

## Special Types of Hydrocephalus

Two common but distinct types of hydrocephalus seen in two different age groups need further mention. These are benign external hydrocephalus seen in infants and NPH seen in older adults.

### Benign External Hydrocephalus

This is seen exclusively in children and is often mistaken for subdural hematoma or hygroma in infants. A relative immaturity of the arachnoid villi, which fail to absorb the required amount of CSF into the bloodstream, has been postulated as the cause. With the obstruction at the level of the arachnoid villi, a communicating type of hydrocephalus develops. The child usually presents with a macrocrania, with mild delayed milestones. CT or MRI usually reveals evidence of a prominent ventricular system, with prominent subarachnoid spaces. Usually a self-limiting condition, this is corrected by 2 years of age and, uncommonly, may require a subduroperitoneal shunt.

### Normal-Pressure Hydrocephalus

This is another form of communicating hydrocephalus seen in older patients with excessive accumulation of the CSF in the intracranial compartment leading to dilation of the ventricles and subarachnoid spaces. The clinical picture is typically of an older patient who presents with the triad of gait ataxia, dementia, and urinary incontinence. Unfortunately, most patients with NPH are underdiagnosed or misdiagnosed in clinical practice. The exact cause is unknown, but reduction in absorption of CSF by the arachnoid granulations has been postulated. In these patients, the brain parenchyma is less stiff (more compliant) to allow it to be compressed by the developing ventriculomegaly and thus does not result in increased ICP. However, this is not always true, because intermittent increases in ICP have been detected by several investigators.

Hydrocephalus developing after several primary insults (e.g., trauma, infection, previous neurosurgical procedure) can present as NPH. The diagnosis is usually a combination of clinical features associated with prominent ventricles seen by CT and MRI, with no other abnormalities. A therapeutic trial of CSF drainage has been used for patients suspected of having NPH to predict response to treatment. Diversion of CSF, usually by a ventriculoperitoneal shunt or from the lumbar space by a lumboperitoneal shunt, has been the mainstay of treatment. Variable-pressure programmable shunt valves have been found to be extremely useful in regulating the flow to avoid complications of overdrainage while optimizing the overall outcome. Early diagnosis and treatment are associated with higher success rates, justifying an early recognition of this treatable form of dementia.

## Other Considerations

### Shunts and Intra-Abdominal Surgeries

Often, patients with ventriculoperitoneal shunts require other surgical procedures. It is not uncommon for the neurosurgeon to be asked about the safety of the procedure before it is contemplated. The circumstances can be broadly divided into two categories: (1) surgery when the shunt tube is not exposed and (2) surgery when the shunt tube will or may be exposed.

**Surgery When the Shunt Tube Is Not Exposed** These procedures should not cause any mechanical obstruction to the shunt. However, the risk of shunt infection is a potential concern and the risk is higher if the surgery is performed through a contaminated field with a predisposition for bacterial dissemination (e.g., lower gastrointestinal tract—colorectal biopsy).

**Surgery When the Shunt Tube Is or May Be Exposed** This group presents some concerns about functioning of the shunt in the postoperative period because the shunt tube is expected to be exposed during the procedure. Exposure of the shunt tube also increases the likelihood of shunt infection caused by direct contamination or dissemination during the surgery. These procedures include abdominal surgeries with an indwelling ventriculoperitoneal shunt and thoracic surgeries with a ventriculopleural shunt. Preoperative discussion with a neurosurgeon and his or her presence in the operating room is considered ideal under such circumstances.

### Shunts and Appendicitis

Appendicitis is a common condition in the general population and it is not uncommon to find patients with shunts in the emergency room being diagnosed with appendicitis. Diagnostic errors are common and can cause delay in initiating appropriate treatment. Uncomplicated appendicitis often can be effectively managed by conventional treatment protocols. If the shunt tube is seen during the appendicectomy, these often can be managed by replacing the catheter away from the operative site. These patients need to be followed up closely to assess for any chronic abdominal infection, which may present several weeks after the initial surgery. Patients with a ruptured appendix usually need the shunt to be externalized and broad spectrum antibiotic therapy initiated; once the peritoneal infection has cleared, another site in the peritoneal cavity may be chosen to insert the shunt. Alternatively, a ventriculoatrial or ventriculopleural shunt can be considered.

### Hernia, Hydrocele, and Shunts

It is not uncommon to see an infant with a shunt developing a hydrocele or hernia a few months after insertion of the shunt. One study has reported that 15% of shunted children developed inguinal hernias and hydroceles were seen in another 6% of boys.[48] Persistence of the peritoneovaginal canal causes the CSF to track from the peritoneal cavity into the scrotum, thus causing hydrocele. If the communication is large, bowel loops can migrate into the scrotal sac, which results in inguinal hernia. Usually, the collection is lax and supple. Uncommonly, the distal end of the shunt tube can migrate into the sac. In most cases, these spontaneously reduce in size and do not need any surgical intervention. However, tense or growing collections need a repositioning of the catheter with correction of the defect.

## Pediatric Neurosurgery

Neurosurgical conditions in infants and children are significantly different than those in adults. Congenital malformations, hydrocephalus, neoplasms, and pediatric trauma are the major neurosurgical disorders commonly encountered by a pediatric neurosurgeon. Hydrocephalus, pediatric brain tumors, and pediatric trauma have been discussed earlier. Here, we will discuss the following congenital malformations: spinal and cranial dysraphism, Chiari malformation, and craniosynostosis.

## Spinal Dysraphism

Of the three embryonic layers (ectoderm, mesoderm, and endoderm), the neural structures develop from the ectoderm. The neural tube forms from the neural placode at approximately 21 days of gestation. Failure to form the neural tube results in neural tube defects, such as spinal dysraphism. It is important to realize that neural tube defects have already formed by the time pregnancy is diagnosed; thus, prevention of these defects by the administration of folic acid has to commence prior to 21 days of gestation.

The spinal dysraphic state can be classified as spina bifida aperta (open defects, usually apparent) and spina bifida occulta (closed defects, commonly missed by an untrained observer; Fig. 68-33). The most common forms of spina bifida aperta are myelomeningocele and meningocele. The common forms of the spinal bifida occulta include simple spina bifida occulta, spinal dermal sinus, lipomyelomeningocele, diastematomyelia, and tethered spinal cord. Some of these may coexist with each other.

### Spina Bifida Aperta

**Myelomeningocele** Myelomeningocele, the most common type of spina bifida aperta, has an average incidence of 1/1000 live births. In this disorder, there is protrusion of a varying amount of spinal neural tissue outside the spinal canal confines. It has been associated with folate deficiency in the mother; intake of folate during pregnancy has reduced the incidence considerably. There is a deficiency of the skin, muscle, and bony elements, with the open neural placode exposed anywhere from the thoracic to sacral levels (Fig. 68-34). Varying degrees of motor and sensory deficits with autonomic (bladder and bowel) dysfunction accompany this defect. It is important to note that the degree of the deficit is directly related to the level of the defect, which often determines the child's capability to ambulate in the future. Hence, thoracic defects have the highest incidence of weakness and sacral defects often have only bladder involvement. Hydrocephalus is also present in 80% of patients and sometimes manifests after surgical closure of the defect. The incidence of hydrocephalus is also directly related to the level of the defect; thus, thoracic defects have the highest incidence and low sacral defects the lowest. The other significant association is the Chiari II malformation, which occurs in 90% to 95% of cases. Associated brain anomalies include corpus callosal anomalies, fused tectal plates, and thalamic fusion.

Surgical closure of the myelomeningocele is undertaken within 24 to 48 hours of birth to avoid CNS infection (e.g., meningitis, ventriculitis). Prior to the closure, the child is usually nursed prone, with the defect covered by moist sterile dressings, and given prophylactic antibiotics. All exposed neural tissue is considered as viable unless otherwise proven. During the closure, adequate care is taken to separate the neural tissue (placode) from the cutaneous element to prevent an inclusion dermoid. The dura is closed in a watertight fashion and is supplemented by myofascial closure. Skin grafts often are required for large defects. The child is usually also nursed in the prone position in the postoperative period. Ventricular shunts, if indicated, are placed concurrently with myelomeningocele closure or at a later date. Of children with myelomeningocele, 60% to 70% will ultimately require a shunt insertion, whereas only 15% to 30% of children will require a Chiari decompression.

Serum and amniotic fluid α-fetoprotein screening and prenatal ultrasound have been significantly helpful in diagnosing open neural tube defects in the prenatal period. Prenatal counseling should include a discussion of overall long-term mortality (24% over a 25-year period),[49] cognitive development (75% have an IQ higher than 80 if adequately treated for hydrocephalus), future ambulatory assistance, depending on the level of the defect, and the presence of incontinence. A 20% to 65% incidence of latex allergies in this population has led to universal latex allergy precautions for this group of children.

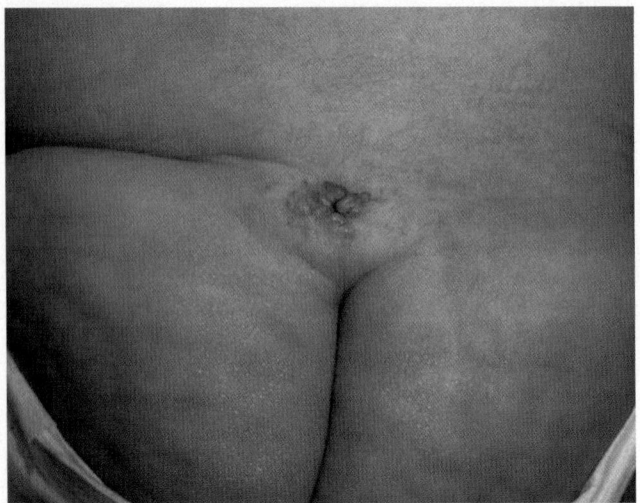

**FIGURE 68-33** Child with lumbar cutaneous hemangioma. This often accompanies an underlying spina bifida (spina bifida occulta) during the clinical evaluation.

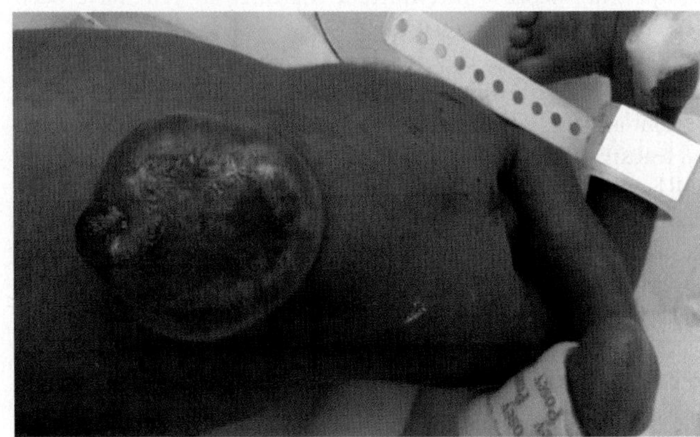

**FIGURE 68-34** Myelomeningocele in a neonate. Note the deformity of the lower limbs.

**Meningocele** Here, there is a protrusion of dura and arachnoid outside the confines of the spinal canal, with neural tissue remaining within the spinal canal confines. Because no neural elements are present, there are no associated neural deficits and repair is simpler. Meningoceles occur less commonly than myelomeningoceles and can be at any location in the spine, although they are most common in the lumbar region.

### Spinal Bifida Occulta

**Simple Spina Bifida Occulta** A posterior lumbar bony defect is often present in 5% to 10% of the normal population, without any symptoms or deficits. However, association of other markers such as a tuft of hair, cutaneous hemangioma, or sinus tract should be viewed with suspicion and warrants further investigation.

**Dermal Sinus** Occurrence of a dermal sinus tract from the cutaneous to spinal subarachnoid space is often associated with a cutaneous dimple or pit. These are most common in the lumbosacral region but can be seen in the cervical and thoracic regions. Although initially asymptomatic, it can cause ascending infection or be symptomatic, with tethering of the cord. It may be associated with intraspinal inclusion tumors such as dermoids. MRI is helpful for assessing the course of the tract and its termination. The tract usually is usually excised surgically, with care taken to untether the cord.

**Diastematomyelia** In diastematomyelia, the spinal cord is split into two hemicords, often by a bony or fibrous band that tethers the cord, preventing its free movement and ascent. It is often associated with a hairy patch on the back at the defect level. These need to be repaired surgically.

**Lipomyelomeningocele** In lipomyelomeningocele, there is a varying amount of fatty tissue in the spinal cord and in the spinal canal tethering the cord. Often associated with a large dural defect, these are complex congenital anomalies. Associated neurologic deficits, although uncommon at birth, usually develop later because of the tethering. Almost all lipomyelomeningoceles have a well-developed skin cover, which allows these children to be operated on electively at a later date. The relatively high incidence of postsurgical neurologic deficits (16% to 47%) in otherwise neurologically intact patients has triggered a controversy regarding the appropriate timing for the surgery; some favor early surgery and others consider surgery only when the child has developed deficits.

## Cranial Dysraphism

This includes encephalocele, meningocele, and a cranial dermal sinus. The encephalocele can be in the cranial vault or cranial base. The occipital encephalocele is the most common, followed by anterior encephalocele and then basal encephalocele. Encephaloceles may be associated with other developmental anomalies such as polydactyly, retinal dysplasia, micro-opthalmia, and orofacial clefts. Cranial vault encephaloceles present with an observable swelling at birth and have brain tissue and blood vessels contained in the sac. Although the brain tissue is thought to be dysplastic, large encephaloceles often contain functional brain. Excision and repair of the defect in the first few days of life is the usual surgical treatment. Cranial expansion may be required for patients with functional brain tissue in the sac. The outcome is generally directly proportional to the amount of neural tissue in the sac, with poorer outcomes seen in encephaloceles with a large amount of brain tissue. Basal encephaloceles present with a CSF leak from the nose or ear, or as a polyp.

## Chiari Malformation

Abnormal descent of the cerebellar tonsils below the level of the foramen magnum is known as a *Chiari malformation*. A descent of one tonsil of more than 5 mm or a 3-mm descent with associated syringohydromyelia is suggestive of Chiari malformation. Often, the tonsils are peg- shaped and associated with crowding of the craniocervical subarachnoid space. Usually, they are classified as Chiari I, II, and III malformations. These are grouped together, but there is a significant difference in cause among these three types. An isolated descent of the tonsils below the rim of the foramen magnum without any spina bifida is known as *Chiari I malformation*. Chiari II is invariably associated with open spina bifida and has several other diagnostic features, such as descent of the brainstem and fourth ventricle into the upper spinal canal. In the uncommon Chiari type III malformation, there is an associated high cervical encephalocele containing herniated cerebellar and brainstem tissue. We will limit the discussion here to the most common types, Chiari I and II malformations.

### Chiari I Malformation

As noted, descent of the cerebellar tonsils more than 5 mm below the rim of the foramen magnum is considered as Chiari malformation. The 5-mm classification is somewhat arbitrary because many have tonsillar descent and are asymptomatic. The descended tonsils are usually peg-shaped and the descent is associated with crowding of the soft tissue, obstructing CSF flow. There may or may not be associated syringomyelia (Fig. 68-35). Occipital headache, precipitated or aggravated by maneuvers that increase the intrathoracic pressure (e.g., cough, headaches) is typical. There may be associated tingling or numbness in the extremities and impairment of joint position. In patients with advanced compression, cavitation of the spinal cord (syringomyelia) can occur and can be associated with wasting and weakness of the extremities, scoliosis, and varying degrees of sensory impairment. Coexistent hydrocephalus is seen in 10% of cases.

The aim of surgery is to decompress the region of the foramen magnum and establish CSF flow. Removal of the rim of the foramen magnum, posterior arch of C1, and duraplasty are the most commonly performed procedures. Some also decompress the cerebellar tonsils. Associated hydrocephalus requires ventriculoperitoneal shunt placement or an endoscopic third ventriculostomy. Rescarring is a concern during follow-up and may require repeat surgery.

### Chiari II Malformation

Chiari II malformation is characterized by elongation and caudal displacement of the brainstem and cerebellar tonsils and by association with myelomeningocele. Hydrocephalus is common and syrinx occurs frequently. Although it is a common accompaniment of myelomeningocele, surgery is reserved for children who are symptomatic with lower cranial nerve paresis, weakness, respiratory distress, or syrinx.

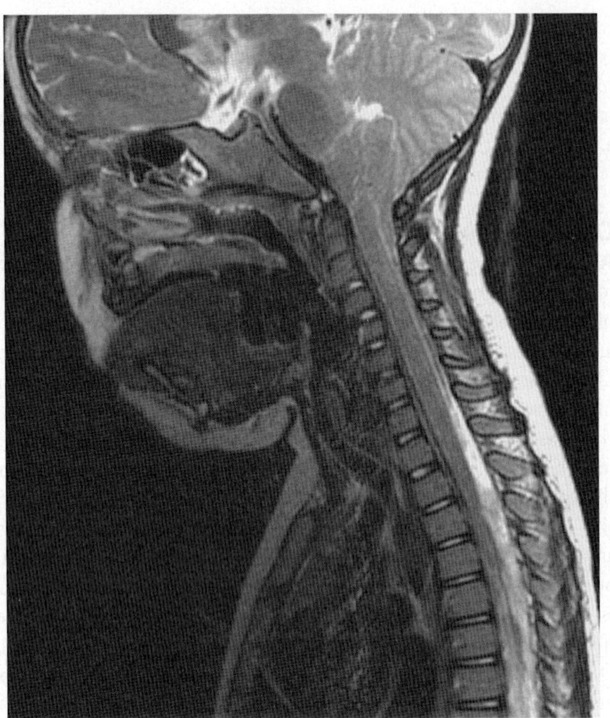

**FIGURE 68-35** T2-weighted sagittal MRI scan of a child with a significant type 1 Chiari malformation. Note the tonsillar descent below the rim of foramen of magnum.

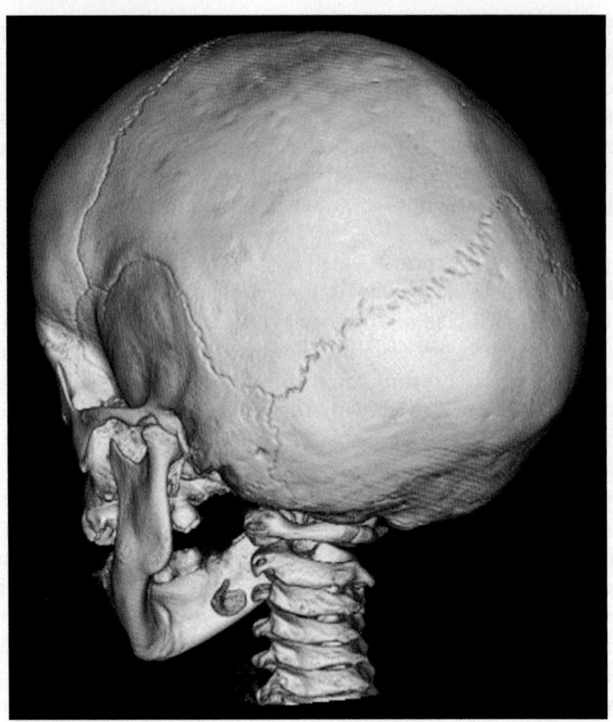

**FIGURE 68-36** Three-dimensional reconstruction CT scan of a child with sagittal synostosis. The coronal and lambdoid sutures are well visualized.

## Craniosynostosis

Craniosynostosis involves premature fusion of the cranial sutures. This results in restricted growth of the skull bones at the involved suture and compensatory growth at the adjacent patent sutures, causing disfigurement of the cranial shape. In multisutural synostosis, restriction of the cranial growth at various sutures can cause impairment of growth of the developing brain. The incidence of nonsyndromic craniosynostosis varies from 0.25 to 0.6/1000 live births. The most common suture involved is sagittal suture (50% to 60%), followed by coronal suture (30% to 35%), metopic suture (5%), and lambdoid suture (2%). Lambdoid suture synostosis has to be distinguished from positional plagiocephaly because the latter is common and does not require surgical intervention. Genetic patterns are found in 8% of patients with isolated coronal synostosis and 2% of those with sagittal synostosis. However, more complex disorders such as Crouzon, Apert, and Pfeiffer syndromes have a genetic predisposition. The clinical picture is recognized by the abnormal skull shape associated with each sutural fusion—sagittal, elongated skull, or scaphocephaly; coronal, brachycephaly; and metopic, trigonocephaly—and is confirmed by skull x-rays and CT scans. Three-dimensional reconstruction of the calvarium is often beneficial (Fig. 68-36). Surgical correction involves a wide suturectomy and placement in a cranial remodeling helmet in children younger than 4 months and a craniotomy and cranial vault reconstruction in older children. In recent years, simple suturectomies have been performed in children younger than 6 months of age under endoscopic guidance with a small incision.[50] Patients with coronal craniosynostosis will usually require advancement of the orbital rim in addition to the cranial remodeling.

# CENTRAL NERVOUS SYSTEM INFECTIONS

This section discusses infections of the CNS and its surrounding structures. Timely diagnosis and treatment of CNS infections are critical because failure to diagnose and appropriately treat these infections can have long-lasting and devastating consequences.

## Meningitis

Acute bacterial meningitis is an infection of the subarachnoid spaces and meninges. Symptoms and signs include fever, malaise, altered mental status, neck stiffness, and headache. These result from leptomeningeal irritation and increased ICP. The causative organism varies with patient age. Neonatal meningitis is caused by group B streptococcus, *Escherichia coli,* or *Listeria* spp. infection. Late neonatal meningitis can be caused by any of these organisms, as well as staphylococci or *Pseudomonas aeruginosa.* In children, *Streptococcus pneumoniae* (pneumococcus) and *Neisseria meningitidis* (meningococcus) are the most common causative organisms. In the past, *Haemophilus influenzae* was a common cause of meningitis in children, but its prevalence has decreased secondary to vaccination. Pneumococci and meningococci are the most common causative organisms in adults. Treatment consists of prompt CSF culture and immediate IV administration of antibiotics. Altered mental status secondary to communicating hydrocephalus may necessitate placement of an external ventricular drain and eventual placement of a ventriculoperitoneal shunt once the CSF is sterilized. Recurrent episodes of bacterial meningitis prompt investigation into abnormal communication between the CNS and the exterior environment (dermal sinus or CSF fistula).

## Postoperative Infections

Infections of the CNS occurring after neurosurgical procedures are typically caused by staphylococci. Enteric organisms and pseudomonal and streptococcal pathogens can also be problematic. As with any infection, treatment involves identification of the causative organism and appropriate antibiotic administration. Postoperative abscesses are addressed with drainage, surgery, or both, as dictated by the clinical situation.

## Post-Traumatic Meningitis

Meningeal infection after head injury is typically related to CSF fistula. Most post-traumatic fistulas stop spontaneously within days of injury. The incidence of meningitis increases if a leak persists for longer than 7 days. Clinically obvious leaks manifest as CSF rhinorrhea or otorrhea. The prophylactic antibiotic treatment of CSF fistula is controversial and needs to be tailored to the clinical situation. A persistent post-traumatic CSF fistula is addressed surgically to prevent the risks associated with recurrent bouts of meningitis.

## Brain Abscess

Cerebral abscesses present with signs and symptoms related to an expanding mass lesion. Patients can present with altered mental status, focal neurologic deficit, headache, nausea and vomiting, and/or seizures. Fever, elevated white blood cell count, and signs of meningeal irritation are often absent. Contrast-enhanced CT and MRI reveal a ring-enhancing lesion, usually at the gray-white interface, with surrounding edema. This can be confused with tumor. Acute deterioration of patients can occur when the abscess ruptures into the ventricle or subarachnoid space, with resultant ventriculitis or meningitis. Brain abscesses develop by contiguous spread from adjacent structures (paranasal sinuses, petrous bone) or hematogenous spread from a distant site. They can be solitary or multiple. Causative organisms are extremely varied and include aerobic and anaerobic organisms, fungi, and parasites. Principles of treatment revolve around accurate identification of the causative organism, relief of mass effect, administration of appropriate antibiotic therapy, and treatment of the underlying cause (e.g., paranasal sinus infection, dental caries, ear infection, bronchiectasis). Controversy exists as to whether surgical excision or aspiration of the abscess yields better results (Fig. 68-37).

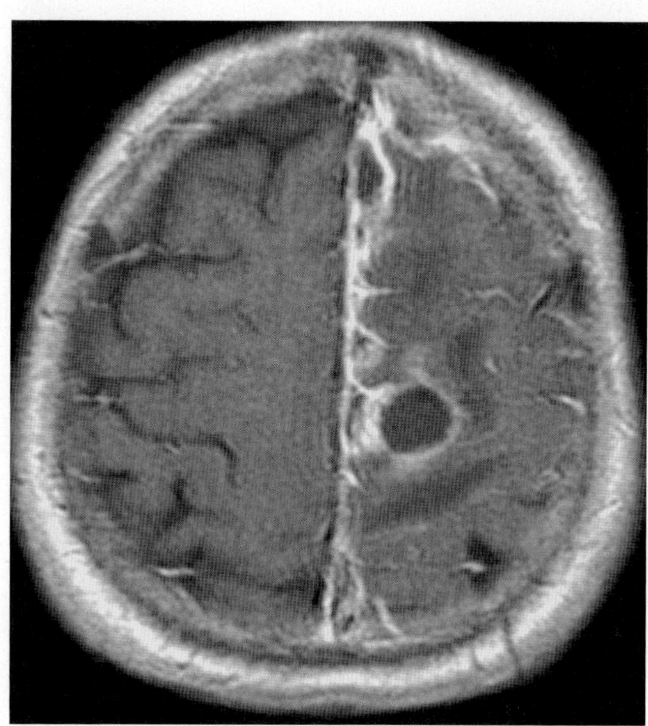

**FIGURE 68-37** Brain abscess *(arrow),* with an area of frontal subdural empyema in the convexity *(arrowheads).*

## Subdural Empyema

Subdural empyema is a collection of pus in the subdural space. It is typically related to contiguous spread from the paranasal sinuses or ear infection. Patients can present with fever, meningeal signs, headache, seizures, focal neurologic deficits, and altered mental status. It is often heralded by rapid clinical deterioration. Diagnosis is made based on index of suspicion and presence of a subdural fluid collection, sometimes adjacent to a known focus of sinus infection. Often, the collection is interhemispheric. Prompt institution of surgical (drainage and irrigation) and medical (antibiotics) therapy is critical in the treatment of this disease (see Fig. 68-37).

## Spinal Infections

Spinal infections can be divided into those affecting the bone (vertebral osteomyelitis), disc space (discitis), and epidural space (spinal epidural abscess). Occasionally, infectious processes can involve more than one, or even all three.

Osteomyelitis of the bone is generally seen in IV drug users, diabetic patients, hemodialysis patients, and older adults. The causative organism is usually *S. aureus* and spread is hematogenous, although postoperative infections are also seen. These infections can and do affect the integrity of the bone, resulting in collapse. This in turn can result in pain and neurologic compromise. Treatment consists of organism identification, appropriate long-term antibiotics, and maintenance of anatomic spinal alignment, with or without surgical intervention.

Discitis often occurs concomitantly with osteomyelitis and is seen in the same patient population. Fever, back pain, and an elevated sedimentation rate or C-reactive protein level are often seen. The white blood cell count may or may not be elevated. It may occur spontaneously or postoperatively. Treatment may or may not be surgical. Long-term antibiotic therapy is usually indicated (Fig. 68-38).

Spinal epidural abscess usually occurs in the setting of an infectious process elsewhere in the body. Spread occurs hematogenously or by direct extension. Patients present initially with localized back pain and possible radiculopathy. Spinal cord compromise can follow rapidly, with paraplegia or quadriplegia. Predisposing factors are the same as those for osteomyelitis and discitis. Diagnosis is made with contrast-enhanced MRI. When spinal cord compression is evident, surgery is usually performed for decompression and diagnosis. Spinal epidural abscess can sometimes be managed medically, with close neurologic observation and imaging studies. This is usually reserved for cases in which the causative organism is known, the abscess is small, and there is no neurologic compromise. As in all fields of medicine, treatment must be tailored to the individual patient.

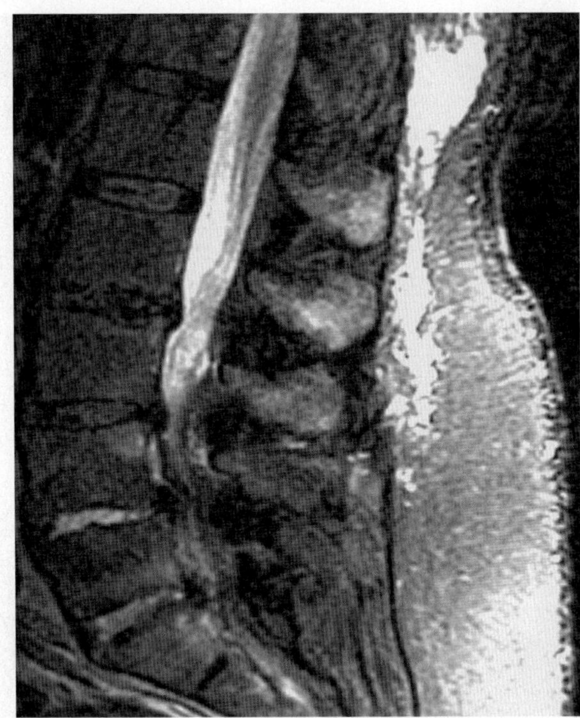

**FIGURE 68-38** MRI with gadolinium short T1 inversion recovery (STIR) sequence revealing disc osteomyelitis in the L4-5 and L5-S1 interspaces suggestive of an infectious process.

## Acquired Immunodeficiency Syndrome

The most common CNS opportunistic infection in patients with AIDS is toxoplasmosis caused by *Toxoplasma gondii*. The lesions usually present with ring enhancement on contrast-enhanced imaging studies and are usually in the basal ganglia. They may be solitary or multiple. Primary CNS lymphoma occurs in approximately 10% of AIDS patients and presents as an irregularly enhancing mass (target lesion). Progressive multifocal leukoencephalopathy presents with hypodense, nonenhancing white matter lesions. Fungal abscess and viral encephalopathy are not uncommon in this patient population. Even though the incidence of CNS opportunistic infections has decreased with the widespread use of highly active antiretroviral therapy (HAART), the treatment of these problems remains a challenge.

### SELECTED REFERENCES

Benzel EC: Spine surgery: Techniques, complication avoidance, and management, ed 2, Philadelphia, 2004, Churchill Livingstone.

A nice review of spine surgery and biomechanics in two volumes; thorough explanation and details from an authority in the field.

Fessler RG, Sekhar LN, editors: Atlas of neurosurgical techniques. Spine and peripheral nerves, New York, 2006, Thieme.

Compendium of a significant amount of the current neurosurgical approaches for the spine and peripheral nerves. The book covers trauma and degenerative pathology, and instrumented and noninstrumented surgery.

Sekhar LN, Fessler RG: Atlas of neurosurgical techniques. Brain, New York, 2006, Thieme.

Compendium of a significant amount of the current neurosurgical approaches for the cerebrum.

Winn HR, Youmans JR: Youmans neurological surgery, Philadelphia, 2004, Saunders.

The traditional source for neurosurgery residents and faculty as a core text.

### REFERENCES


1. Stern WE: Intracranial fluid dynamics: The relationship of intracranial pressure to the Monro-Kellie doctrine and the reliability of pressure assessment. J R Coll Surg Edinb 9:18–36, 1963.
2. Rangel-Castilla L, Gasco J, Nauta HJ, et al: Cerebral pressure autoregulation in traumatic brain injury. Neurosurg Focus 25:E7, 2008.
3. Bratton SL, Chestnut RM, Ghajar J, et al: Guidelines for the management of severe traumatic brain injury. IX. Cerebral perfusion thresholds. J Neurotrauma 24(Suppl 1):S59–S64, 2007.
4. Wijdicks EF, Bamlet WR, Maramattom BV, et al: Validation of a new coma scale: The FOUR score. Ann Neurol 58:585–593, 2005.
5. Lundberg N: Continuous recording and control of ventricular fluid pressure in neurosurgical practice. Acta Psychiatr Scand Suppl 36:1–193, 1960.
6. Ondra SL, Troupp H, George ED, et al: The natural history of symptomatic arteriovenous malformations of the brain: A 24-year follow-up assessment. J Neurosurg 73:387–391, 1990.
7. Spetzler RF, Martin NA: A proposed grading system for arteriovenous malformations. J Neurosurg 65:476–483, 1986.
8. McCormick WF, Hardman JM, Boulter TR: Vascular malformations ("angiomas") of the brain, with special reference to those occurring in the posterior fossa. J Neurosurg 28:241–251, 1968.
9. Ong CK, Wang LL, Parkinson RJ, et al: Onyx embolisation of cavernous sinus dural arteriovenous fistula via direct percutaneous transorbital puncture. J Med Imaging Radiat Oncol 53:291–295, 2009.
10. Winn HR, Richardson AE, Jane JA: The long-term prognosis in untreated cerebral aneurysms: I. The incidence of late hemorrhage in cerebral aneurysm: A 10-year evaluation of 364 patients. Ann Neurol 1:358–370, 1977.
11. Vajkoczy P, Meyer B, Weidauer S, et al: Clazosentan (AXV-034343), a selective endothelin A receptor antagonist, in the prevention of cerebral vasospasm following severe aneurysmal subarachnoid hemorrhage: Results of a randomized, double-blind, placebo-controlled, multicenter phase IIa study. J Neurosurg 103:9–17, 2005.
12. Kern M, Lam MM, Knuckey NW, et al: Statins may not protect against vasospasm in subarachnoid haemorrhage. J Clin Neurosci 16:527–530, 2009.
13. Wong GK, Poon WS, Chan MT, et al: Intravenous magnesium sulphate for aneurysmal subarachnoid hemorrhage (IMASH): A randomized, double-blinded, placebo-controlled, multicenter phase III trial. Stroke 41:921–926, 2010.
14. Kulcsar Z, Wetzel SG, Augsburger L, et al: Effect of flow diversion treatment on very small ruptured aneurysms. Neurosurgery 67:789–793, 2010.

15. Szikora I, Berentei Z, Kulcsar Z, et al: Treatment of intracranial aneurysms by functional reconstruction of the parent artery: The Budapest experience with the pipeline embolization device. AJNR Am J Neuroradiol 31:1139–1147, 2010.
16. Molyneux A, Kerr R, Stratton I, et al: International Subarachnoid Aneurysm Trial (ISAT) of neurosurgical clipping versus endovascular coiling in 2143 patients with ruptured intracranial aneurysms: A randomised trial. Lancet 360:1267–1274, 2002.
17. Mendelow AD, Gregson BA, Fernandes HM, et al: Early surgery versus initial conservative treatment in patients with spontaneous supratentorial intracerebral haematomas in the International Surgical Trial in Intracerebral Haemorrhage (STICH): A randomised trial. Lancet 365:387–397, 2005.
18. Patchell RA: The management of brain metastases. Cancer Treat Rev 29:533–540, 2003.
19. Levin VALS, Gutin PH: Neoplasms of the central nervous system. In De Vita VT, Jr, Hellman S, Rosenberg SA, editors: Cancer: Principles and practice of oncology, Philadelphia, 2001, Lippincott Williams & Wilkins, pp 2100–2160.
20. Gupta A, Shah A, Young RJ, et al: Imaging of brain tumors: Functional magnetic resonance imaging and diffusion tensor imaging. Neuroimaging Clin N Am 20:379–400, 2010.
21. Kew Y, Levin VA: Advances in gene therapy and immunotherapy for brain tumors. Curr Opin Neurol 16:665–670, 2003.
22. Louis DN, International Agency for Research on Cancer, World Health Organization: WHO classification of tumours of the central nervous system, ed 4, Lyon, France, 2007, International Agency for Research on Cancer.
23. Popko B, Pearl DK, Walker DM, et al: Molecular markers that identify human astrocytomas and oligodendrogliomas. J Neuropathol Exp Neurol 61:329–338, 2002.
24. Sarin H: Recent progress towards development of effective systemic chemotherapy for the treatment of malignant brain tumors. J Transl Med 7:77, 2009.
25. Galanis E, Buckner JC: Chemotherapy of brain tumors. Curr Opin Neurol 13:619–625, 2000.
26. Kuratsu J, Kochi M, Ushio Y: Incidence and clinical features of asymptomatic meningiomas. J Neurosurg 92:766–770, 2000.
27. Suh JH, Vogelbaum MA, Barnett GH: Update of stereotactic radiosurgery for brain tumors. Curr Opin Neurol 17:681–686, 2004.
28. Kondziolka D, Nathoo N, Flickinger JC, et al: Long-term results after radiosurgery for benign intracranial tumors. Neurosurgery 53:815–821, 2003.
29. Suki D: The epidemiology of brain metastases. In Sawaya R, editor: Intracranial metastases: Current management strategies, Malden, Mass, 2004, Blackwell, pp 20–35.
30. Hanbali F, Fourney DR, Marmor E, et al: Spinal cord ependymoma: Radical surgical resection and outcome. Neurosurgery 51:1162–1172, 2002.
31. Brain Trauma Foundation; American Association of Neurological Surgeons; Congress of Neurological Surgeons; Joint Section on Neurotrauma and Critical Care, AANS/CNS, Bratton SL, Chestnut RM, Ghajar J, et al: Guidelines for the management of severe traumatic brain injury. J Neurotrauma 24(Suppl 1):S1–S106, 2007.
32. Ogden AT, Mayer SA, Connolly ES, Jr: Hyperosmolar agents in neurosurgical practice: The evolving role of hypertonic saline. Neurosurgery 57:207–215; discussion 207–215, 2005.
33. Kakar V, Nagaria J, John Kirkpatrick P: The current status of decompressive craniectomy. Br J Neurosurg 23:147–157, 2009.
34. Lunsford LD, Bissonette DJ, Zorub DS: Anterior surgery for cervical disc disease. Part 2: Treatment of cervical spondylotic myelopathy in 32 cases. J Neurosurg 53:12–19, 1980.
35. Kondziolka D, Lunsford LD, Flickinger JC, et al: Emerging indications in stereotactic radiosurgery. Clin Neurosurg 52:229–233, 2005.
36. Chang SD, Adler JR, Jr: Current treatment of patients with multiple brain metastases. Neurosurg Focus 9:e5, 2000.
37. Flickinger JC, Barker FG, 2nd: Clinical results: Radiosurgery and radiotherapy of cranial nerve schwannomas. Neurosurg Clin N Am 17:121–128, vi, 2006.
38. Kuo JS, Yu C, Petrovich Z, et al: The CyberKnife stereotactic radiosurgery system: Description, installation, and an initial evaluation of use and functionality. Neurosurgery 62(Suppl 2): 785–789, 2008.
39. Romanelli P, Schaal DW, Adler JR: Image-guided radiosurgical ablation of intra- and extra-cranial lesions. Technol Cancer Res Treat 5:421–428, 2006.
40. Groves DA, Brown VJ: Vagal nerve stimulation: A review of its applications and potential mechanisms that mediate its clinical effects. Neurosci Biobehav Rev 29:493–500, 2005.
41. Nauta HJ, Soukup VM, Fabian RH, et al: Punctate midline myelotomy for the relief of visceral cancer pain. J Neurosurg 92:125–130, 2000.
42. Willis WD, Jr, Westlund KN: The role of the dorsal column pathway in visceral nociception. Curr Pain Headache Rep 5:20–26, 2001.
43. Zimmerman RS, Sirven JI: An overview of surgery for chronic seizures. Mayo Clin Proc 78:109–117, 2003.
44. Devlin AM, Cross JH, Harkness W, et al: Clinical outcomes of hemispherectomy for epilepsy in childhood and adolescence. Brain 126:556–566, 2003.
45. Di Rocco C, Marchese E, Velardi F: A survey of the first complication of newly implanted CSF shunt devices for the treatment of nontumoral hydrocephalus. Cooperative survey of the 1991-1992 Education Committee of the ISPN. Childs Nerv Syst 10:321–327, 1994.
46. Kulkarni AV, Drake JM, Mallucci CL, et al: Endoscopic third ventriculostomy in the treatment of childhood hydrocephalus. J Pediatr 155:254–259 e251, 2009.
47. Schroeder HW, Oertel J, Gaab MR: Endoscopic treatment of cerebrospinal fluid pathway obstructions. Neurosurgery 62:1084–1092, 2008.
48. Clarnette TD, Lam SK, Hutson JM: Ventriculo-peritoneal shunts in children reveal the natural history of closure of the processus vaginalis. J Pediatr Surg 33:413–416, 1998.
49. Bowman RM, McLone DG, Grant JA, et al: Spina bifida outcome: A 25-year prospective. Pediatr Neurosurg 34:114–120, 2001.
50. Jimenez DF, Barone CM: Multiple-suture nonsyndromic craniosynostosis: Early and effective management using endoscopic techniques. J Neurosurg Pediatr 5:223–231, 2010.

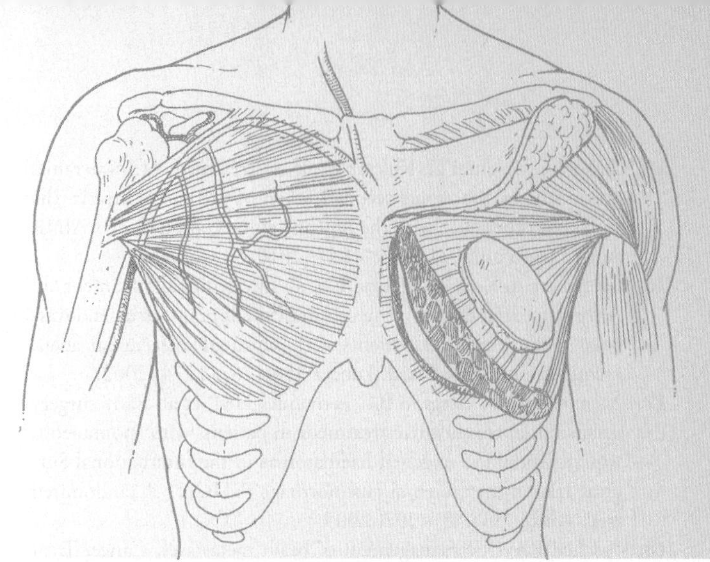

CHAPTER 69

# PLASTIC SURGERY

MARY H. MCGRATH AND JASON POMERANTZ



Challenged by complex clinical problems, the pace of innovation in plastic surgery has accelerated steadily over the past 30 years. The specialty benefits from the absence of anatomic or organ system boundaries, and from the collaboration with other surgical specialists who engage plastic surgeons, as new reconstructive and aesthetic challenges accompany surgical advances in all areas. With growing sophistication, plastic surgery has matured into areas of specialization, including congenital, maxillofacial, breast surgery, hand surgery, head and neck surgery, skin and soft tissue surgery, aesthetic surgery, body contouring, wound care, microsurgery, and burn care. As a relatively small specialty, plastic surgeons are abreast of innovations in each of these areas and are quick to use new ideas developed through the clinical and research experience of other plastic surgeons. With the breadth of exposure that this collaboration brings, it is not surprising that unique solutions for perplexing clinical problems sustain the momentum of innovation.

## RECONSTRUCTIVE TECHNIQUES

The concept of a reconstructive ladder is used to guide surgical reconstruction. Ascending the rungs of the ladder represents moving from simple to complex reconstructive techniques in a systemized way that considers the requirements of the defect to be repaired. Direct closure is the simplest and most straightforward technique. This may be precluded by the size of the wound or consequences of wound tension at the closure site, including distorting the surrounding tissue. In this case, a more complex closure technique, such as a skin graft that brings in additional tissue from a distant site, is required. A wound with exposed structures that do not accept a skin graft mandates a step up to a local flap for coverage. A local flap with no distant donor site may not be an option if the surrounding area is within the zone of injury, in which case a regional flap from an adjacent body region is needed. Microvascular free tissue transfer represents the most complex flap option and is usually the top rung on the reconstructive ladder.

When using the concept of the reconstructive ladder, the triad of form, function, and safety is the basis for setting the reconstructive goals for any given defect. For example, when reconstructing the face, awareness of form would suggest a more complex technique, such as tissue expansion, instead of the simpler technique of skin grafting because it is optimal to restore with skin and soft tissue of the same thickness, texture, and color. For any specific reconstructive situation, this matrix of going from simple to complex, considering form and function, and keeping safety paramount provides direction.

### Primary Wound Closure

Good suture technique starts with an incision with the scalpel at right angles to the skin and continues with careful handling of tissue to avoid devitalizing the skin margins, débridement of skin edges if needed, everting the wound margin, and precise approximation without tension. The skin edges need to be lined up at the same level and wound edges should just touch each other. Postoperative edema is predictable and will create additional tension.

Minimizing tension is essential to reduce scarring. This can be done by using buried deep dermal and subdermal sutures to lessen tension on the skin sutures. It is also accomplished by aligning skin incisions along relaxed skin tension lines. These lines of minimal tension, also called *natural skin lines*, wrinkle lines, or lines of facial expression, run at right angles to the long axis of the underlying muscles. When underlying muscles contract, the lines of facial expression deepen. For example, transverse forehead furrows appear when the eyebrows are raised by the frontalis muscle and, if an incision is placed in one of these furrows, it will be under minimal tension and will heal with minimal scarring.

### Skin Grafts

A skin graft is a segment of dermis and epidermis that is separated from its blood supply and donor site and transplanted to another recipient site on the body. Survival of the skin graft in the new site requires a vascularized wound recipient bed. Graftable beds with adequate blood supply include healthy soft tissues, periosteum, perichondrium, paratenon, and bone surface that is perforated to encourage granulation tissue growth. Poor graft surfaces with inadequate blood supply include exposed bone, cartilage, tendon, and fibrotic chronic granulation tissue.

The wound must be free of infection and debris interposed as a barrier between the graft and bed.

Skin grafts are classified in the following manner: autograft, self; allograft, other person; homograft, same species; heterograft, different species. Partial-thickness skin grafts consist of the epidermis and a portion of the dermis and are called *split-thickness skin grafts* (STSG). Full-thickness skin grafts (FTSG) include the epidermis and entire dermis, with portions of the sweat glands, sebaceous glands, and hair follicles. A STSG is harvested with a dermatome, which is an air- or electric-powered instrument that can be adjusted for width and depth to cut uniformly thick grafts, usually in strips from 0.006 to 0.024 inch in thickness. A STSG can be meshed by cutting slits into the sheet of graft and expanding it, usually in a 1 : 1.5 or 1 : 2 ratio. Meshed grafts are useful when there is a paucity of available donor skin, the recipient bed is bumpy or convoluted, or the recipient bed is suboptimal, as with exudate. A STSG can be taken from anywhere on the body; donor site considerations include color, texture, thickness, amount of skin required, and scar visibility. The STSG takes readily on the recipient site and the donor site reepithelializes quickly. Its disadvantages are contracture over time, abnormal pigmentation, and poor durability if subject to trauma. A FTSG is removed with a scalpel and is necessarily small in size because the donor site must be sutured closed. Containing skin appendages, a FTSG can grow hair and secrete sebum to lubricate the skin, has the color and texture of normal skin, and has the potential for growth. Generally, FTSGs are taken from areas at which the skin is thin and can be spared without deformity, such as the upper eyelids, postauricular crease, supraclavicular area, hairless groin, or elbow crease. The greater thickness makes a FTSG more durable than a STSG but this thickness also means that the graft take is not as predictable because more tissue must be revascularized from the recipient bed.

The take of either type of skin graft occurs in three phases:

- Plasmatic circulation, also called *serum imbibition*, during the first 48 hours nourishes the graft with plasma exudate from host bed capillaries.
- Revascularization starts after 48 hours with two processes. The primary is neovascularization, in which blood vessels grow from the recipient bed into the graft, and the secondary is inosculation, in which graft and host vessels form anastomoses.
- Organization begins immediately after grafting with a fibrin layer at the graft-bed interface holding the graft in place. This is replaced by postgraft day 7 with fibroblasts; generally, grafts are securely adherent to the bed by days 10 to 14.

Sensibility returns to the graft over time, with reinnervation beginning at approximately 4 to 5 weeks and completed by 12 to 24 months. Pain returns first, with light touch and temperature returning later.

The most common cause of skin graft failure is hematoma under the graft, where the blood clot is a barrier to contact of the graft and bed for revascularization. Similarly, shearing or movement of the graft on the bed will preclude revascularization and cause graft loss. Additional causes are infection, poor quality of the recipient bed, and characteristics of the graft itself, such as thickness or vascularity of the donor site. Dressings can prevent some impediments to graft take. A light pressure dressing minimizes the risk of fluid accumulation. A bolster or tie-over dressing left in place for 4 to 5 days improves survival by maintaining adherence of the graft to the bed, minimizing shearing, and preventing hematoma or seroma. A vacuum-assisted compression device can be placed on the grafted surface to stabilize the graft in place; this is especially useful for larger wounds with an irregular three-dimensional surface.

Skin grafts composed of tissue-cultured skin cells are used for the treatment of burns or other extensive skin wounds. Human epidermal cells in a single-cell suspension are grown in monolayers in vitro over a period of 3 to 6 weeks. Concerns with tissue-cultured skin are fragility, sensitivity to infection, length of time to cultivate, and potential risk of malignancy caused by mitogens present during culturing.

## Skin Flap Surgery

A surgical flap consists of tissue that is moved from one part of the body to another with a vascular pedicle to maintain blood supply. The vascular pedicle may be kept intact, or it can be transected for microvascular anastomosis of the flap vessels to vessels at another site. Flap defines the tongue of tissue; pedicle is used to describe the base or stem with the vascular supply.

Skin-bearing flaps are classified according to three basic characteristics—composition, method of movement, and blood supply. Composition refers to the tissue contained within the flap, such as cutaneous, musculocutaneous, fasciocutaneous, osseocutaneous, and sensory flaps. The method of movement is local transfer, as with advancement or rotation flaps, or distant transfer, as with pedicle flaps from the abdomen to the perineum or microvascular free flaps.

With regard to blood supply, arteries perfusing the surgical flap reach the skin component in two basic ways. Musculocutaneous arteries travel perpendicularly through muscle to the overlying skin. Septocutaneous arteries arising from segmental or musculocutaneous vessels travel with intermuscular fascial septae to supply the overlying skin. With either of these patterns, the flap can have a random pattern, which means that it derives its blood supply from the dermal and subdermal vascular plexus of vessels supplied by perforating arteries. Alternatively, it can be an axial flap designed to include a named musculocutaneous or septocutaneous vessel running longitudinally along the axis of the flap to penetrate the overlying cutaneous circulation at multiple points along the course of the flap's length to provide greater length and reliability.

### Skin Flaps

Local skin flaps contain tissue lying adjacent to the defect that usually matches the skin at the recipient site in color, texture, hair, and thickness. Flaps should be the same size and thickness as the defect and be designed to avoid distortion of local anatomic landmarks, such as the eyebrow or hairline. They can be planned so that the donor site can be closed directly and usually are elevated with incision lines placed in relaxed skin tension lines. Local flaps rely on the inherent elasticity of skin and are most useful in the older patient whose skin is looser. In some cases, the site from which the flap is raised is closed with a skin graft. Commonly used local skin flaps include the following:

- Rotation flaps are semicircular flaps of skin and subcutaneous tissue that revolve in an arc around a pivot point to shift tissue in a circle.
- Transposition flaps are rectangular or square and turn laterally to reach the defect.

- Advancement flaps move directly forward and rely on skin elasticity to stretch and fill a defect.
- V-Y advancement flaps advance skin on each side of a V-shaped incision to close the wound with a Y-shaped closure.
- Rhomboid flaps rely on the looseness of adjacent skin to transfer a rhomboid-shaped flap into a defect that has been converted into a similar rhomboid shape.
- Z-plasty transposes two interdigitating triangular flaps without tension to use lateral skin to produce a gain in length along the direction of the common limb of the Z.

Failure of a skin flap usually involves necrosis of the most distal portion of the transferred tissue. This could be caused by a flap design in which the size of the flap exceeds its inherent vascular supply, or could be a result of extrinsic mechanical compromise of the flap pedicle by pressure from a hematoma, compressive dressings, or twisting or kinking of the flap. Measures to optimize viability include proper flap design and avoiding extrinsic pedicle compression, undue tension with wound closure, and venous congestion caused by excessive flap dependency.

### Muscle and Musculocutaneous Flaps

Consideration of a muscle as a potential flap is possible because muscles have independent, intrinsic blood supply. The motor nerves of a muscle are accompanied by an arteriovenous system that often is the major source of blood supply to that muscle. This vascular pedicle may be a dominant one, capable of sustaining the entire muscle independently. A minor pedicle, regardless of the size of the vessel, is defined as one that maintains only a lesser portion of the muscle. Many muscles have multiple unrelated sources of blood supply so that each nourishes only a segment of the muscle, thus called *segmental pedicles*. Some muscles have both a dominant pedicle and segmental blood supply. One example is the latissimus dorsi muscle with a dominant pedicle, the thoracodorsal artery in the axilla, and additional segmental perforating branches from the intercostal and lumbar vessels posteriorly. In these muscles, the dominant pedicle can be ligated and the muscle moved on the secondary vessels as a reverse muscle flap.

Muscle flaps are classified according to their principal means of blood supply and the patterns of vascular anatomy (Fig. 69-1):

- Type I: Single pedicle (e.g., gastrocnemius, tensor fascia lata)
- Type II: Dominant pedicle with minor pedicles (e.g., gracilis, trapezius)
- Type III: Dual dominant pedicles (e.g., gluteus maximus, serratus anterior)
- Type IV: Segmental pedicles (e.g., sartorius, tibialis anterior)
- Type V: Dominant pedicle, with secondary segmental pedicles (e.g., latissimus dorsi)

In terms of reliability of the vascular anatomy and usefulness as a flap, large muscles with a recognized dominant pedicle supplying most of a flap (types I, III, and V) are most useful. The territory of the pedicles in type II muscles may vary, and type IV muscles are useful only when smaller flaps are needed. Connections between regions within a given muscle supplied by more than one pedicle are via small-caliber choke vessels with bidirectional flow. An example of a flap depending on these choke vessels is the transverse rectus abdominis musculocutaneous (TRAM) flap, in which the superior epigastric pedicle alone can support the lower half of the muscle normally supplied by the inferior epigastric vessels below the watershed level at the umbilicus. In muscle, venous territories are in parallel with arterial vessels. This means that venous outflow is adjacent to, and in a direction opposite from, flow in the major arterial pedicles. In a pattern analogous to that of the bidirectional choke vessels,

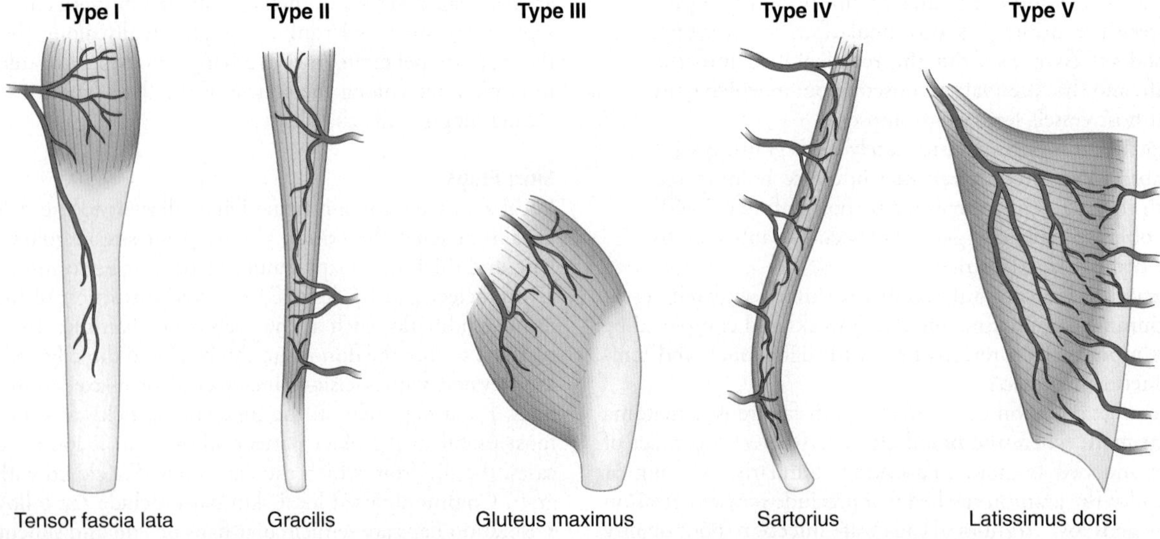


**FIGURE 69-1** Classification of muscle and musculocutaneous flaps according to their vascular supply: type I, one vascular pedicle; type II, dominant pedicle and minor pedicles; type III, two dominant pedicles; type IV, segmental vascular pedicles; type V, one dominant pedicle and secondary segmental pedicles. (From Mathes SJ, Nahai F: Classification of the vascular anatomy of muscles: experimental and clinical correlation. Plast Reconstr Surg 67:177–187, 1981.)

venous flow from one territory to another occurs through oscillating veins that are devoid of valves.

Compared with skin flaps, muscle flaps are less bulky, less stiff, and more malleable to conform to wounds with irregular three-dimensional contours. They have more robust blood supply and demonstrate superiority in wounds compromised by irradiation or infection. The vascular anatomy is predictable and easily identifiable, and the muscle can be put into use as a functional unit for a dynamic tissue transfer. A major consideration with muscle flaps is whether the loss of function is acceptable. In an effort to limit the functional loss associated with use of an entire muscle, methods of functional preservation have been devised. If some portion of the muscle chosen as the flap is left innervated and attached at its insertion and origin, function is preserved after transfer of the remainder of the muscle. This can be done by splitting the muscle into segments, provided that each is supplied by a different dominant pedicle. An example is the gluteus maximus, which extends and rotates the thigh laterally. This is not an expendable muscle, but the superior or inferior half of the muscle can be elevated as a flap, with function of the intact half of the muscle preserved.

A musculocutaneus flap, also called a *myocutaneous flap*, is a muscle flap designed with an attached skin paddle. Each superficial skeletal muscle carries blood supply to the skin lying directly over it through musculocutaneous perforators. The number and pattern of these musculocutaneous perforators varies with each specific muscle; this means that the extent of the skin territory is different for each muscle unit. Through dissection of injected cadaver specimens, the number, size, and location of musculocutaneous perforators have been described; this information, combined with clinical experience, is used to predict the cutaneous territories on the superficial muscles.

In addition to the musculocutaneous branches supplying the overlying skin, source vessels, also called *mother vessels*, branch within muscle into channels that perforate the deep fascia to anastomose within the subdermal plexus and nourish the skin. The source vessel and its perforating muscular branches can be dissected out of the muscle without jeopardizing skin perfusion. This requires intramuscular dissection to separate the perforators from the muscle and is the basis for the development of muscle perforator flaps. This makes the retention of muscle unnecessary for the survival of the skin paddle; thus, its inclusion serves a passive role, primarily to avoid tedious intramuscular dissection of the vascular tree. To spare the muscle unit, a growing number of muscle perforator flaps have been described, including the deep inferior epigastric perforator flap, which carries the same skin and subcutaneous tissue as the TRAM flap for breast reconstruction. By sparing the rectus muscle, abdominal wall bulging and other complications are less likely. The superior gluteal artery perforator flap (SGAP) carries the skin territory of the gluteus maximus musculocutaneous flap and preserves the muscle.

### Fascia and Fasciocutaneous Flaps

Growing knowledge about musculocutaneous skin circulation has led to the identification of vascular pedicles emerging between muscles, traveling in the intermuscular septum, and entering the deep fascia. Termed *septocutaneous perforators,* these vessels supply the fascial plexus, which gives off branches to an overlying cutaneous territory. Some state that a fasciocutaneous flap, by definition, should include a specific known septocutaneous perforator. Others accept a less strict definition of a fasciocutaneous flap as a skin flap including the deep fascia.

The anatomic features of a fasciocutaneous flap are the fascial feeder vessels, also called the *fascial perforators*, which are branches of source vessels to a given angiosome. An angiosome is the three-dimensional block of tissue supplied by a source artery; the entire surface of the body is comprised of a multitude of angiosome units. The fascial feeder vessels do not perforate the deep fascia, but terminate within the fascial plexus. The fascial plexus is not a structure but is a confluence of multiple adjacent vascular intercommunications that exist at the subfascial, fascial, suprafascial, subcutaneous, and subdermal levels (Fig. 69-2).

The concept of fasciocutaneous flaps arose from the observation that the size of a skin flap could be increased if it were oriented along a longitudinal axis on the extremity, and if the deep fascia were included. Subsequent anatomic studies have confirmed the presence of septocutaneous pedicles supplying a regional fascial vascular system. The larger septocutaneous pedicles tend to be fairly constant in location and a number of specific fasciocutaneous flaps have come into wide use (e.g., anterior lateral thigh flap, radial forearm flap, scapular flap).

The design of fasciocutaneous flaps has been learned by experience and the limits of these flaps still remain to be discovered. There are no set rules, because deep fascial perforators are frequently anomalous in caliber and location, not only among individuals but also on opposite sides of the same person. The expected range of flap size is learned through the experience of other surgeons.[1,2]

One of the most useful features of a fasciocutaneous flap is that it can be distally based. Unlike a muscle flap, in which the dominant pedicle is closest to the heart, blood flow in the fascial plexus is multidirectional. The flow to the corresponding

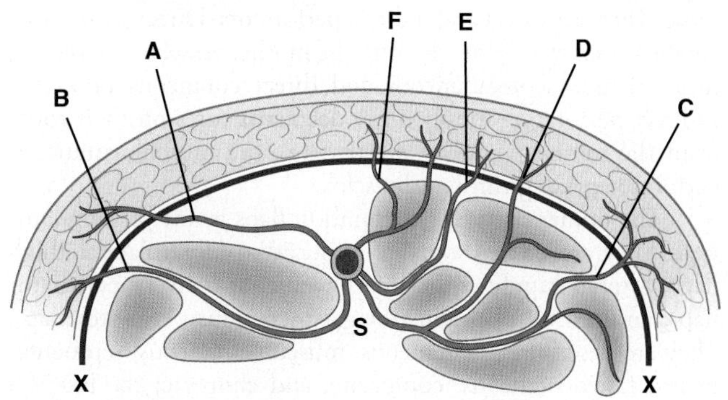


**FIGURE 69-2** Pathways of the various known cutaneous perforators that pierce the deep fascia to supply the fascial plexus. *S*, Source vessel; *X*, deep fascia. (From Hallock GG: Direct and indirect perforator flaps: the history and the controversy. Plast Reconstr Surg 111:855–865, 2003.)

angiosome is equivalent for a distal fascial perforator and proximal facial perforator. This means that a flap pedicle can be distally based with a reliable skin territory and transposed to cover a defect located at the end of an extremity. For example, the distal-based sural flap uses the skin of the calf, based on a distal perforator of the peroneal artery, for transfer to cover the foot and ankle. Obviating the need for a free microvascular transfer, this has become a standard for foot coverage.

In addition to the advantages provided by a distally based flap design, a fasciocutaneous flap can confer sensibility if a sensory nerve is included. Compared with musculocutaneous flaps, they are accessible on the surface of the body, and have the great advantage that no functioning muscle is expended. The comparative disadvantages are the anatomic anomalies in the fascial vascular system and the unanswered question as to whether they are as effective as muscle in the radiated or infected wound.

### Perforator Flaps

Perforator flaps evolved as an improvement over musculocutaneous and fasciocutaneous flaps. They rely on evidence that neither a passive muscle carrier nor the underlying fascial plexus of vessels is necessary for flap survival, provided that the musculocutaneous or fasciocutaneous vessel is carefully dissected out and preserved. Advantages of perforator flaps include preservation of functional muscle and fascia at the donor site and versatility of flap design with regard to including as little or as much bulk tissue as required. Disadvantages are the difficult dissection needed to isolate the perforator vessels, longer operating time associated with this dissection, anatomic variability of position and size of perforator vessels, short pedicle length available, and fragile nature of these small blood vessels.

A perforator is a blood vessel passing through the deep fascia and contributing blood supply to the fascial plexus. Perforators arise from a source, or mother, vessel to a given angiosome. There are direct and indirect perforators. Direct perforators are those that travel directly from the mother vessel to the plexus; these include septocutaneous and direct cutaneous branches. Indirect perforators supply other deep structures on their route from the mother vessel to plexus (e.g., the musculocutaneous perforator passing through muscle).

The nomenclature of perforation flaps is not yet standardized. They are named variably by location (anterolateral thigh flap), arterial supply (deep inferior epigastric artery perforator flap), and muscle of origin (the gastrocnemius perforator flap). They are described as cutaneous, musculocutaneous, septocutaneous, fasciocutaneous, composite, and chimeric; the last is a perforator flap with two separate muscular components with a common vascular source. Several suggestions for an ordering nomenclature have been made.

Because of the small size of the vessels and their anatomic variability, Doppler ultrasound is used routinely to locate the perforators before perforator flap elevation. This is not highly accurate and other technologies such as color flow duplex scanning and thermography may be useful in the future. Technical recommendations for harvesting a perforator flap include identification of at least one vessel with a diameter of 0.5 mm or more, inclusion of at least two or more perforators, sufficient pedicle length for the procedure, and preservation of a subcutaneous vein to use for venous outflow in situations in which the deep system of perforator veins proves anomalous.

The use of perforator flaps continues to evolve. Current work includes flap thinning, a technique for removing excess adipose tissue from the perforator flap as it is raised. This would provide a large delicate segment of vascularized skin for reconstruction in areas such as the ear, in which contour is important. Another innovation is the discovery of new flaps based on perforators smaller than 0.8 mm in diameter found superficial to the fascial plane. By eliminating the dissection needed to trace a perforator through the muscle, operating time is shortened and there is potential for developing a much larger number of suitable flaps. The challenge with these suprafascial free flaps is the supermicrosurgery needed for anastomoses in such small vessels.[3]

### Microvascular Free Tissue Transfer

A microvascular free tissue transfer, also called a free flap, brings distant tissue with a pedicled arterial and venous supply from another part of the body to be anastomosed to vessels at the recipient site to reestablish blood flow. The transferred tissue may be skin, fat, muscle, fascia, bone, nerves, small bowel, large bowel, or omentum as needed to reconstruct a given defect. Selection of tissue for transfer depends on the size, composition, and functional capabilities of the tissue needed, technical considerations such as vessel size and pedicle length, and donor site deformity that will be created with regard to function and aesthetic appearance.

Preoperative planning starts with patient selection and analysis of the defect. Environmental factors such as previous surgery or prior irradiation, which impair the quality of tissue and vessels, may be an indication for angiography to assess the available vasculature. Muscle does not tolerate warm ischemia for longer than 2 hours; skin and fasciocutaneous flaps can tolerate ischemia times from 4 to 6 hours. Planning is the most important factor to minimize the effects of ischemia and all structures at the recipient site should be ready for the tissue transfer when the donor pedicle is divided. Sound technique requires healthy vessels of reasonable size with good outflow for the anastomosis, which must be made without tension. This may require mobilization of the vessels to gain more length. Vein grafts have been shown to reduce the success rate and are not a primary choice, but may be needed if the pedicle is short or the vessels in the field are damaged. Vein grafts can be obtained from the saphenous vein, dorsum of the foot, volar forearm, or donor site. Adventitia is removed from the vessel ends to improve visualization of the vessel walls for accurate suture placement. Both end-to-end and end-to-side arterial anastomoses have similar patency rates, although end-to-side is preferred if there is vessel size or wall thickness discrepancy, or the continuity of the recipient vessel must be preserved. Dissection and manipulation of the microvessels frequently cause vasospasm. This can be relieved with topical lidocaine or papaverine, stripping the adventitia to remove sympathetic nerve fibers, or mechanical dilation of the vessels. Failure of reperfusion in an ischemic organ after reestablishment of blood supply is termed the *no-reflow phenomenon.* The causative mechanism is thought to be endothelial injury, platelet aggregation, and leakage of intravascular fluid. The severity of this effect correlates with ischemia time.

The use of postoperative anticoagulation is not a uniform practice for elective microvascular transfers. If pharmacologic agents are part of postoperative care, aspirin is generally used, followed by dextran and low-molecular-weight heparin (LMWH). Surveys of microsurgical centers have shown equal success rates for transplants with and without anticoagulation; the concern with the use of anticoagulants is an increased chance of hematoma at donor and recipient sites. Postoperative monitoring of free tissue transfers is critical because rapid identification of postoperative free flap ischemia permits intervention and flap salvage. Most free flap thromboses occur in the first 48 hours after surgery and salvage rates are high. Clinical evaluation includes observation of skin color, capillary refill, fullness, and color of capillary bleeding, which can be determined by pinprick testing of the flap. If a flap is buried, a temporary skin island can be added for monitoring purposes or an implantable monitoring device can be used. Many devices are available for flap monitoring, including temperature probes, pulse oximetry, photoplethysmography, hand-held pencil Doppler probes (low-frequency continuous ultrasonography), and implantable Doppler probes.

Tissue survival rates for free tissue transfers exceed 95%. Reexploration rates range from 6% to 25% and thrombosis of the arterial anastomosis is the most common finding at reoperation. This is termed *primary thrombosis* when technical faults lead to anastomotic failure. These faults include narrowing of the lumen, sutures tied too loosely so that media of the vessel is exposed in the gap and clot forms, sutures tied too tightly that tear through the vessel, too many sutures with subendothelial exposure and clot formation, and sutures that inadvertently take a bite of the back wall of the vessel, which obstructs the lumen. The term *secondary thrombosis* refers to kinking or compression of vessels by hematoma or edema, which leads to decreased inflow. With reexploration, salvage rates have been seen to vary from 54% to 100% in different series.[4]

The principles and techniques of microvascular surgery are under continual refinement. Areas of current emphasis include identification of tissue transfers that better suit the needs of the recipient site and minimize donor site sequelae. The latter has led to minimally invasive and endoscopic techniques for harvesting flap tissue through smaller incisions. It has also led to the development of tissue transfers, such as perforator flaps that preserve functional muscle and fascia at the donor site, and suprafascial free flaps, which require supermicrosurgery techniques.

### Supermicrosurgery

The introduction of supermicrosurgery, which allows the anastomosis of smaller caliber vessels and microvascular dissection of vessels ranging from 0.3 to 0.8 mm in diameter, has led to the development of new reconstructive techniques. Free perforator-to-perforator flaps using suprafascial vessels can be transferred more quickly and the tissue can be obtained from better concealed parts of the body.[5] If a discrete perforator can be identified anywhere on the body, a flap can be designed around it. This has been called a "freestyle flap." The constraints of using only described territories can be disregarded and the donor site selected solely on the basis of the best possible match for color, contour, and texture at the recipient site. Disadvantages are the anatomic variation of the perforators and the need for supermicrosurgical technique. The latter includes the use of 12-0 nylon sutures with 50- to 30-μm needles; the surgeons who pioneered "freestyle reconstruction" have noted that it is difficult to learn and can be tedious.[6]

### Tissue Expansion

Tissue expansion is a technique that uses a mechanical stimulus to induce tissue growth so as to generate soft tissue for reconstructive use. It involves placing a prosthesis that is gradually enlarged by the addition of saline, which causes an increase in the surface area of the overlying soft tissue. Initially, the expanded skin is the result of stretching as interstitial fluid is forced out of the tissue, elastic fibers are fragmented, viscoelastic changes (termed *creep*) occur in the collagen, and adjacent mobile soft tissue is recruited. Over time, it is not just stretching but actual growth of the skin flap that creates an increase in the surface area, with accompanying increases in collagen and ground substance. Histologic changes in the skin include dermal thinning, epidermal thickening, subcutaneous fat atrophy, and no effect on the skin appendages.

Tissue undergoing expansion must have the capacity for growth. Prior radiation or scar formation may slow the rate of expansion or make it impossible. Expanders perform poorly under skin grafts, under very tight tissue, and in the hands and feet. Contraindications include expansion near a malignancy, hemangioma, or open leg wound.

Expanders come in various styles, and sizes range from a few cubic centimeters to 1 liter or more. They can be round, square, rectangular, or horseshoe–shaped. The injection ports can be remote or integrated into the wall of the expander so that no dissection of a pocket for the remote port is required. The envelope can be smooth or textured for better stabilization at one location in the tissue pocket.

Expanders should be placed under tissue that best matches the lost tissue (Fig. 69-3). Normal landmarks such as the eyebrow or hairline should not be distorted. The incision to insert the expander can be placed at the edge of the defect that later will be excised, because a scar in this position will be removed at the time of the next surgery. The most common reason for expander failure is construction of a pocket that is too small for the device. An expander with a curled edge may later protrude through the incision or erode through the overlying tissue. Filling of the expander is initiated approximately 2 weeks after surgery and continued at weekly or biweekly intervals. The rate of expansion is limited by the relaxation and growth of the tissue overlying the expander. Pain and palpable tightness over the expander are clinical indicators that guide the rate of expansion. The patient is ready for the second surgical procedure when the expanded tissue is adequate to produce the desired effect. If the flap is to be advanced, it must be measured to ensure that it is large enough and has the correct geometry to cover the defect. At the second surgery, the skin is incised through the old scar, the capsule around the expander is opened, the expander is removed, and the expanded flap is advanced over the defect. It is important to confirm that the expanded tissue will replace the defect before excising the defect. If it is not sufficient, this is handled by subtotal resection of the defect and leaving the expander in place for a second round of expansion.[7]

Tissue expansion can be combined with other reconstructive techniques. Expander placement in the subcutaneous or submuscular plane can facilitate later repair of abdominal wall hernias. Preexpansion of transposition or rotation flaps increases the amount of tissue, enhances the flap's blood supply, and lessens donor site morbidity. Preexpansion of free flaps increases the surface area and augments the blood supply of the future flap, may make primary closure of the free flap donor

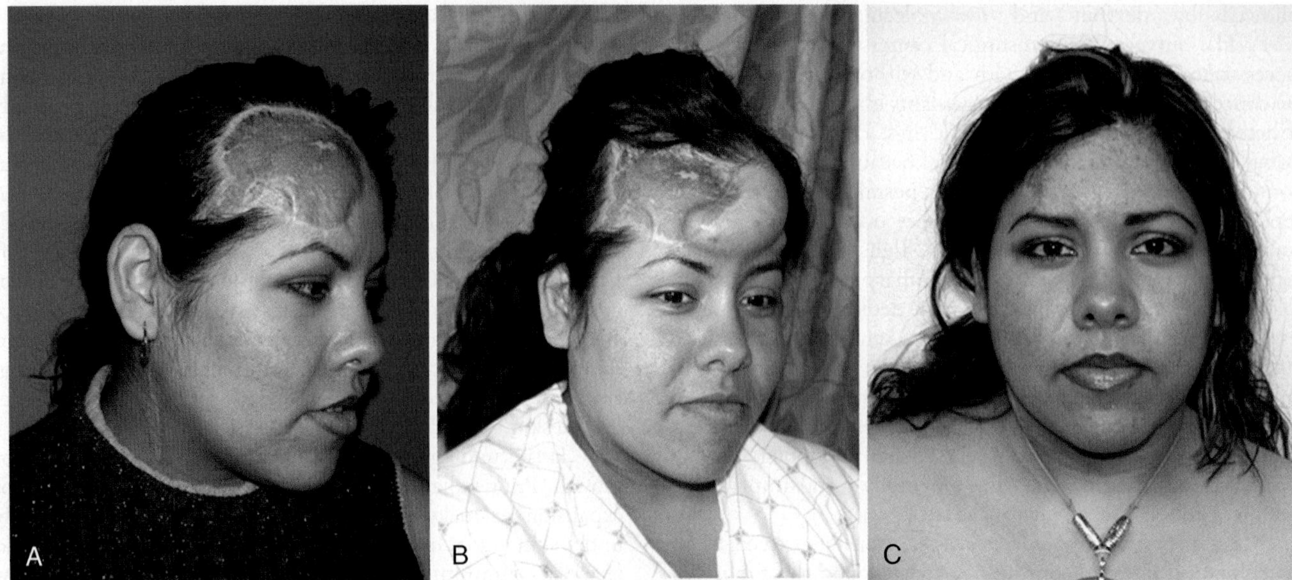


**FIGURE 69-3** The use of tissue expansion to generate new soft tissue to restore the forehead and hairline. The expanders are placed under tissue that best matches the lost tissue. **A,** Young woman with a STSG after a motor vehicle accident. **B,** Crescent-shaped expander in the forehead and two large rectangular expanders under the scalp. **C,** Postoperative result after the second procedure when the flaps were advanced and the split-thickness skin graft removed.

site possible, and thins the flap, which may be desirable for reconstructions calling for thinner and more pliable coverage. A disadvantage of the preexpansion of free flaps is the time needed for the expansion process, because delay may not be acceptable for oncologic defects and complex wounds. In addition, the preexpanded free flap procedure is technically more difficult because of distortion of the vascular pedicle.

The advantages of expansion are the provision of matching tissue for reconstruction, normal sensibility of the transferred tissue, negligible donor defect, and enhanced success of preexpanded traditional flaps because of enhanced vascularity.

## Alloplastic Materials

An alloplastic material is a synthetic substance implanted in living tissue. Its advantages are as follows: availability when autologous tissue is not; absence of donor site morbidity or scarring; nonbiodegradable alloplastic materials do not undergo resorption, as do bone or cartilage grafts; and it can be manufactured to meet special needs, such as implant systems for controlled-release drug delivery systems.

The tissue response to different implants varies with the chemical composition and the micro- and macrostructure of the synthetic material; these differences are used clinically. For example, the vigorous tissue ingrowth with polypropylene mesh in a hernia repair provides strong and lasting support, whereas the fibrous encapsulation around a silicone tendon prosthesis ensures free gliding of a tendon graft. However, certain properties and concerns are common to all implants—noncarcinogenic, nontoxic, nonallergenic, nonimmunogenic, mechanical reliability, and biocompatibility.

Categorization by chemical composition is the most useful framework for the description and comparison of surgical implants. This materials science approach recognizes that the commonality of different groups of materials arises more from their composition than for the organ systems in which they are used. Chemically, there are three major classes of biomaterials, metallic, ceramic, and polymeric. Although they are polymers, biologic materials such as collagen need to be classified separately because they introduce new considerations of protein antigenicity.

Metals in clinical use are stainless steel, Vitallium (cobalt-chromium-molybdenum alloy), and titanium. The general requirements for a metal device are mechanical strength, suitable elastic modulus, density and weight comparable to that of the surrounding tissue, and resistance to corrosion. Very few metals have sufficient corrosion resistance to be used in the hostile environment of the living organism. Corrosion results from the electrochemical activity of unstable metal ions and electrons in physiologic salt solutions; corrosion products can be cytotoxic, leading to pain, inflammation, allergic reactions, and loosening of the device.

Ceramic materials have high stability and resistance to chemical alteration and include carbon compounds such as hydroxyapatite, which is capable of bonding strongly to adjacent bone. Used to augment the facial skeleton or as a bone graft substitute, it is a permanent microporous implant that undergoes osteointegration by providing a matrix for the deposition of new bone from adjacent living bone.

Polymers are large, long-chain, high-molecular-weight macromolecules made up of repeat units, or mers. There are a vast number of these synthetic implants in surgical use. To a large extent, this is because of the ease and low cost of fabrication, and because they can be processed easily into tubes, fibers, fabrics, meshes, films, and foams. Polymers vary across an enormous range of chemical compositions, degree of polymerization, cross linking between chains, and presence of chemical additives such as plasticizers to increase flexibility or resins to catalyze polymerization. With the exception of resorbable polymers, most surgical polymers are relatively inert and stimulate fibrous encapsulation. The physical form of the implant, solid versus mesh, or smooth versus rough, will determine whether the entire structure is encapsulated as a whole or whether fibrous tissue will penetrate the interstices. Tissue reaction to the implant is influenced also by the chemical composition and factors such as hydrophilicity and ionic charge, as well as the chemical durability of the polymer. Silicone rubber, polytetrafluoroethylene, and polyethylene terephthalate polyester (Dacron) are among the most stable of polymers whereas polyamide (nylon) is vulnerable to hydrolytic reaction and undergoes substantial degradation.

## PEDIATRIC PLASTIC SURGERY

### Craniofacial Surgery

*Craniosynostosis* refers to the premature fusion of one or more of the cranial sutures, leading to characteristic deformities of the skull and face. It occurs at an overall frequency of approximately 1 in 2500 live births and is usually sporadic. Any suture may be involved in craniosynostosis and skull growth is restricted perpendicular to the affected suture. Treatment of craniosynostosis is indicated to correct the deformity and normalize the shape of the head, protect the eyes by restoring brow projection, and minimize the risk of developing increased intracranial pressure (ICP) and associated developmental and visual sequelae. The timing of treatment is based on which suture is fused and on the protocol at a given center, but correction during the first year of life is indicated.

Surgical treatment of craniosynostosis is generally done with a coronal approach; techniques differ, but all involve release or excision of the fused suture. The cranium then expands and remodels. Residual bony defects reossify secondarily, a process that is robust in the infant up to 2 years of age.

Other less common congenital abnormalities of the head include agenesis of one or a number of layers of scalp or cranium. *Aplasia cutis congenita* usually refers to a focal defect of skin on the vertex. The defect may include any proportion of skin, bone, or dura. Treatment depends on the size of the defect and layers involved and may involve local wound care or surgical reconstruction with flaps or grafts in infancy. The cause of this rare condition is unknown and likely varies from case to case. A classification system for aplasia cutis congenita has been developed and is related to the presence of other associated anomalies.

#### Congenital Ear Deformities

Congenital anomalies of the external ear may occur in isolation or as part of craniofacial microsomia. Common external ear deformities include prominent ears, constricted ears, cryptotia (failure of the upper pole of the ear to stand out from the head), and microtia (a small and/or abnormally formed outer ear). The most common type of microtia is a malformed vestigial cartilaginous structure associated with a soft tissue component of lobule. In cases of isolated microtia, there is often conductive hearing loss associated with absence of the external auditory canal. This is most important in bilateral cases in which a bone-anchored hearing aid is required.

Reconstruction of typical microtia can take two general approaches, autologous or nonautologous. Nonautologous reconstruction involves placement of a high-density polyethylene implant under the skin. This approach results in good form without the need to harvest tissue from another site or the requirement of shaping a framework. Disadvantages include the presence of a foreign body that may become exposed through the thin skin envelope, is susceptible to infection, and is difficult to salvage in case of complications. The second approach is preferred. This involves the use of autologous tissue (rib cartilage) to shape an ear framework, which is then buried in a subcutaneous pocket. The meticulous shaping of the framework, creation of a thin skin pocket, and use of drains allows the skin to contour around the intricate framework. The procedure requires multiple stages but results in a reconstructed ear that has good form and is capable of responding to trauma and infection like other parts of the body. The disadvantage is the need to harvest cartilage from the rib.

#### Craniofacial Microsomia

Craniofacial microsomia, also known as *hemifacial microsomia*, is a constellation of abnormalities involving deficient development of parts of the face related to the first and second branchial arches.[8] Deformity can be unilateral or bilateral and can involve the orbit, mandible, external ear, facial nerve, and facial soft tissue. Each or all of the structures may be involved and to varying degrees. The cause is unknown but is thought to be related to in utero vascular compromise of the stapedial artery. Treatment of craniofacial microsomia is complex and the approach has to be tailored for individual patients. Functional problems such as airway compromise or eye exposure are treated in childhood; reconstruction of other structural defects is delayed until the patient is almost full-grown.

For patients with craniofacial anomalies such as those described, as well as those with cleft lip and palate, the current standard is team care at an established craniofacial center. With referral to a craniofacial center at birth, the craniofacial team can make a diagnosis, carry out genetic testing, educate the family, and outline short- and long-term plans in a coordinated manner, bringing in multiple specialists (e.g., plastic surgeons, neurosurgeons, oral surgeons, orthodontists, speech pathologists, otolaryngologists, ophthalmologists, social workers, nurse practitioners, developmental psychologists, pediatricians).

#### Cleft Lip and Palate

Cleft lip and palate are relatively common congenital anomalies. They may be unilateral or bilateral. Most are isolated anomalies, but many syndromes have clefts as one of the features. The genetics of cleft lip and palate is complex and the condition is multifactorial. The pathophysiology of cleft lip and palate is incompletely understood, but the deformity and its variations are well described. A minimum of three operations, and usually four, will be required to correct the deformity. These are performed at specific times corresponding to the developmental stage of the patient:

- Cleft lip repair at 3 months
- Cleft palate repair before 1 year, or before speech development begins
- Alveolar bone graft when permanent dentition begins and after orthodontic preparation
- Possible septorhinoplasty in the late teenage years
- Possible lip and/or nose revision
- LeFort I maxillary advancement, if indicated
- Secondary procedures for speech improvement in 15% of cases

A cleft lip is characterized by a partial or complete lack of circumferential continuity of the lip. Most cleft lips occur at a typical location in the upper lip where one of the philtral columns normally lies, and they extend into the nose. The deformity involves the mucosa, orbicularis oris muscle, and skin. The nasal deformity is characterized by a slumped and widened ala (nostril) that is posteriorly misplaced at its base. The nasal floor is nonexistent in complete clefts and the nasal septum is deviated.

There are many techniques for repair of a cleft lip, but most are a variation of the rotation advancement repair. Millard introduced this technique of downward rotation of the medial portion of the lip and advancement of the lateral portion into the defect created by the rotation. The repair is based on the principle that existing elements need to be returned to their normal position to restore the normal anatomy while remaining cognizant of future growth and the effects of surgery on growth (Fig. 69-4).[9]

Cleft palate can also be complete or incomplete. The goals of palatal repair are the development of normal speech and prevention of regurgitation of food into the nose. Normal speech requires velopharyngeal competence to close the oral cavity off from the nasal cavity to produce pressure consonants. This requires static physical separation of the two cavities in the region of the hard palate and dynamic closure of the soft palate against the posterior pharyngeal wall with a functioning levator veli palatini muscle. In a cleft palate, the levator veli palatini muscle fibers are oriented abnormally along the cleft. Thus, all modern techniques of cleft palate repair involve repair of the nasal lining, oral mucosa, and reorientation and repair of the levator veli palatini muscle. The primary measure of outcome of cleft palate repair is normal speech. The third procedure necessary in most cases is alveolar bone grafting. Cancellous bone, usually from the ilium, is used to restore bony continuity along the dental arch as a foundation for dental implants for missing teeth associated with the cleft, close a nasolabial fistula, if present, and produce support for the nose.

Other procedures are indicated for some patients, but this generally cannot be predicted in infancy. Approximately 15% of patients will continue to demonstrate velopharyngeal insufficiency after initial palate repair and secondary palatal lengthening or other approaches to promote velopharyngeal closure are indicated, typically after 3 years of age.[10] Septorhinoplasty is usually necessary to correct residual nasal deformity in the teenage years after final dental restoration and orthodontics. A subset of unilateral cleft lip and palate patients will develop maxillary hypoplasia that is iatrogenic and related to scarring and growth retardation from lip and palate surgery. Depending on the degree of maxillary hypoplasia, LeFort I maxillary advancement in the teenage years may be indicated. In sum, treatment of a child born with a cleft lip and palate does not end after palate repair, but rather requires observation by a craniofacial team throughout development into adulthood and must be tailored for each individual.

## Vascular Anomalies

Vascular anomalies are divided into two major groups, tumors and malformations. Vascular tumors are characterized by increased abnormal proliferation of endothelium. Hemangioma is the most common vascular tumor; others include hemangioendotheliomas, tufted angiomas, hemangiopericytomas, and malignant tumors, such as angiosarcoma. Vascular malformations are the result of abnormal development of arterial, capillary, venous, or lymphatic components of the vascular system.

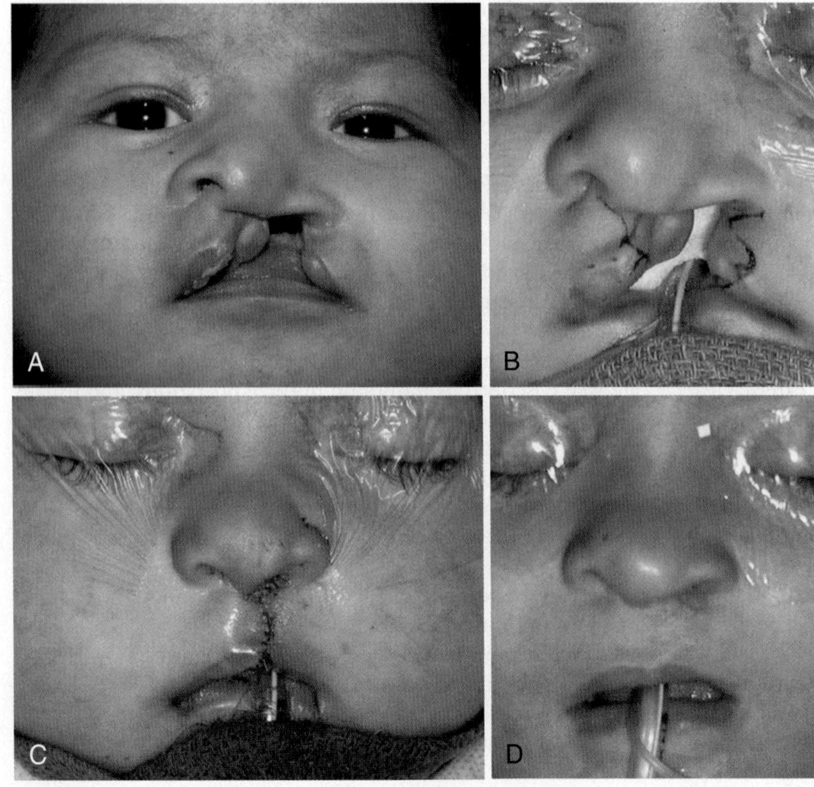


**FIGURE 69-4** Infant girl with a wide, left-sided, unilateral complete cleft lip and palate. **A,** Preoperative view shows the deformity—a wide cleft and absence of the nasal floor, malrotated central lip element, twisted premaxilla, and nasal deformity. **B,** Intraoperative markings for rotation-advancement cleft lip repair at age 3 months. **C,** Immediate postoperative views. **D,** Postoperative views at 11 months of age taken at the time of cleft palate repair.

They may involve only one component or may be mixed and are named for the component vessels. They can be high-flow, low-flow, or mixed. Correct diagnosis depends on the history (e.g., hemangiomas develop in infancy and are usually not visible at birth), physical examination (e.g., malformations with an arterial component may have a palpable pulse or thrill), and imaging to determine the extent of disease and assist with making the diagnosis.

The natural histories of the different anomalies are diverse. Hemangiomas typically involute spontaneously; 50% involute completely by the age of 5 years. This natural history reduces the indications for surgery to those lesions that are affecting vision or the airway, or are large enough that even after involution, the abnormal remaining skin will require surgical modification. In contrast, capillary malformations start as patches but, over time, they typically enlarge and become thick and verrucous; for these lesions, early treatment is indicated. Some vascular malformations or tumors have systemic effects, depending on their mass, status as high- or low-flow, and thrombosis and consumption of coagulation factors. Treatment of these lesions involves complete resection, when feasible, or debulking if complete resection is not possible. Sclerotherapy is the mainstay of treatment of venous malformations. For arteriovenous malformations, sclerotherapy is useful as an adjunct to surgery but insufficient alone because of the development of collaterals. For these malformations, sclerotherapy and embolization are followed immediately by surgical resection.

### Pediatric Neck Masses

Neck masses in the pediatric patient are most likely infectious or congenital noncancerous lesions. In addition to vascular malformations, other common pediatric neck masses include dermoid cysts, teratomas, branchial cleft anomalies, thyroglossal duct cysts, thymic cysts, ranulas, cartilaginous rests, heterotopic neurectodermal tissue, neurofibromas, ectopic salivary tissue, lymphadenopathy, and malignant tumors. Branchial cleft anomalies may be cysts, sinuses, or fistulas. Cysts and sinuses are located in the anterior cervical triangle and are derived from the first cleft (near the external auditory meatus) and second cleft (below the hyoid) 98% of the time. The treatment of these lesions is surgical excision. Thyroglossal duct cysts may arise anywhere along the course of the thyroglossal duct, from the foramen cecum at the base of the tongue to the thyroid gland. Thyroglossal duct cysts usually present in the first or second decade of life as painless anterior neck masses and there may be an associated sinus tract. Indications for surgery include recurrent infection, tissue diagnosis, and improved cosmesis. Thyroid scan is indicated prior to excision to rule out a functioning ectopic thyroid gland.

### Melanocytic Nevi

Congenital melanocytic nevi are hamartomas consisting of nevus cells. Nevi are classified by size—small (<1.5 cm), medium (1.5 to 19.9 cm), large (>20 cm), and giant (>50 cm). The classification dictates the prognosis and reconstructive approach. Risk of melanoma occurring in a melanocytic nevus varies by report, but is estimated to be less than 5% in small or medium lesions and typically presents after puberty. In large and giant nevi, the reported risk of melanoma development is up to 10%.[11] Unlike the case for small or medium nevi, malignancy in large and giant nevi typically occurs in the first 3 years of life. Large and giant nevi also have an increased incidence of leptomeningeal involvement that can be diagnosed by magnetic resonance imaging (MRI). In addition, psychosocial and developmental issues associated with larger nevi are significant, so early excision and reconstruction are recommended for large and giant nevi.

Options for removal of larger nevi include serial excision, excision and grafting, excision and closure with distant flaps, and tissue expansion. Replacement with like tissue is the goal and therefore tissue expansion is the mainstay approach.

## PLASTIC SURGERY OF THE HEAD AND NECK

### Maxillofacial Trauma

Facial trauma has decreased in frequency in the United States, and this is attributed in part to the advent of seat belt laws and improved collision safety. However, it remains part of multisystem trauma from motor vehicle accidents, assaults, and combat injuries. In the latter, improvements in body armor have resulted in better survival but proportionally more facial injuries.

#### Emergent Management

Surgical emergencies in the facial trauma patient include airway compromise, life-threatening hemorrhage, and reversible structural injury to the eye or optic nerve. Other injuries such as lacerations or extraocular muscle entrapment are treated within the first 24 hours. Fractures are treated within the first 2 weeks. Evaluation of the facial trauma patient follows advanced trauma life support (ATLS) protocol and includes looking for intracranial trauma and cervical spine injury. Acute airway compromise usually occurs in the setting of combined mandibular-maxillary trauma, with hemorrhage and soft tissue swelling. Endotracheal intubation should be attempted and need not be avoided because of concern about the facial injury. Nasotracheal intubation is contraindicated in the case of severe naso-orbitoethmoid and skull base fractures. Cricothyroidotomy is performed if oral or nasal endotracheal intubation is unsuccessful, and should be converted to tracheostomy after the patient has been stabilized. Maxillomandibular fixation by itself is not an indication for tracheostomy because endotracheal intubation may be maintained via the nasal or oral route using an armored tube that can be routed behind the molars without kinking. An alternative technique is to exit the endotracheal tube through a submental incision, which alleviates some of the practical difficulties of working around an oral tube.

Life-threatening hemorrhage, defined as 3 U of blood loss or hematocrit below 29%, occurs in a small percentage of facial trauma patients. In most cases, bleeding is effectively controlled with pressure, packing and, in the case of significant soft tissue avulsion, the rapid placement of temporary bolster sutures. Blind attempts to clamp and ligate vessels should be avoided because this is usually unnecessary and may result in injury to critical structures, such as the facial nerve. With penetrating trauma, hemorrhage is controlled in the operating room with vessel identification and ligation and, if unsuccessful, by angiographic selective embolization. With blunt trauma, severe hemorrhage is usually from the internal maxillary artery. The most effective way to control bleeding, especially when it is associated with midfacial fractures, is fracture reduction and stabilization. This can be accomplished quickly by temporary placement in maxillomandibular fixation using rapid techniques such as fixation screws. Severe hemorrhage from skull base and nasoethmoid fractures can often be controlled with anteroposterior nasal packing. Placement of Foley balloon catheters in each nasal airway serves to tamponade the bleeding and also stabilizes the packing. Current protocols for control of hemorrhage in blunt facial trauma settings involve selective angiography if these measures fail (Fig. 69-5).[12] Angiographic embolization is effective but is associated with significant morbidity, including the possibility of stroke or necrosis of midfacial structures such as the palate. In unstable patients, fracture reduction and nasal packing may be attempted on the angiography table to be followed immediately with embolization, if necessary.

Injuries to the orbit and contents can result in blindness; it is critical to recognize promptly and treat reversible injuries that are vision-threatening. Conditions that require emergent intervention include increased intraocular pressure, globe rupture, and optic nerve impingement. Acute increased ICP is manifested by pain and vision loss and can result from causes such as hematoma or decreased orbital volume because of fracture or a foreign body. Treatment involves rapid alleviation of intraocular hypertension by lateral canthotomy and administration of mannitol, acetazolamide (Diamox), and steroids. Urgent ophthalmology consultation is indicated. Vision loss may result from mechanical compression of the optic nerve. Computed tomography (CT) will diagnose the presence of a bone fragment or foreign body; such a finding should prompt emergent surgical decompression to preserve vision. Extraocular muscle entrapment presents as the inability to move the eye on the trajectory controlled by the entrapped muscle and is associated with pain on attempted motion. Especially in children, the pain may be severe and accompanied by nausea or vomiting. Muscle entrapment should be treated by surgical release of the entrapped contents. This should be done fairly soon after injury because delaying the treatment of entrapment for 1 week or longer after injury typically results in failure of the entrapped muscle to regain excursion.

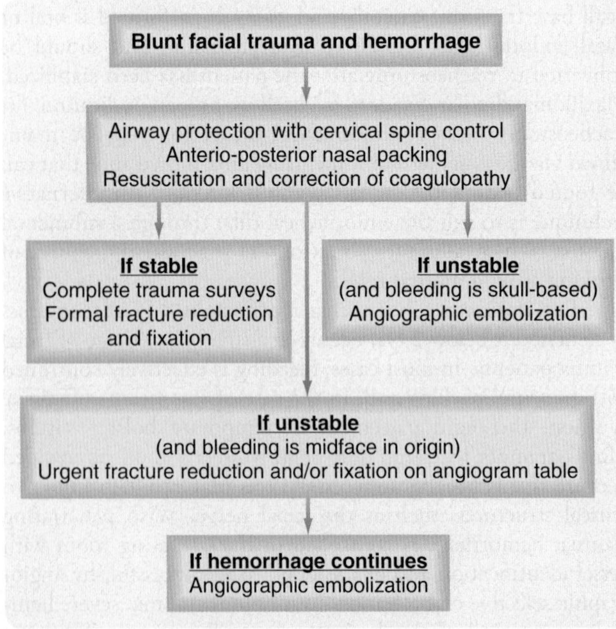


**FIGURE 69-5** Algorithm for the management of life-threatening hemorrhage in the setting of blunt facial trauma. (Adapted from Ho K, Hutter JJ, Eskridge J, et al: The management of life-threatening haemorrhage following blunt facial trauma. J Plast Reconstr Aesthet Surg 59:1257–1262, 2006.)

## Evaluation and Diagnosis

The primary diagnostic studies for facial injury are physical examination and CT. Systematic physical examination can detect deformity, soft tissue injury, cerebrospinal fluid (CSF) leak, and facial nerve injury. Palpation is used to identify bony stepoffs or midface instability. The eyes are examined for proptosis or enophthalmos, extraocular muscle function, and visual acuity. In patients who cannot cooperate with a physical examination and for whom there is reasonable suspicion of periorbital injury, a forced duction test should be performed. The occlusion is evaluated for subjective or objective malocclusion. Extraocular muscle entrapment, acute enophthalmos, and malocclusion are indications that surgical treatment of facial fractures will be required. Fine-cut CT of the face with direct or reformatted coronal and sagittal views is used to diagnose facial trauma and direct nonsurgical and surgical treatment (Fig. 69-6). With

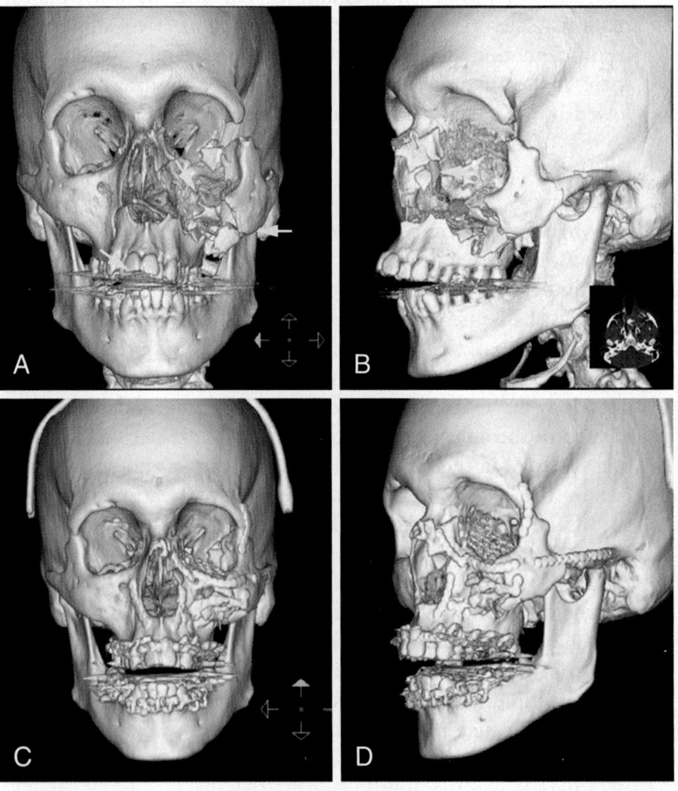


**FIGURE 69-6** Three-dimensional reconstruction of a fine-cut facial CT scan of a patient who sustained severe injuries in a sledding accident. **A,** *Arrows* clockwise from top show (1) massive orbital floor blowout fracture, (2) severely displaced zygoma, (3) displaced LeFort I fracture causing malocclusion. **B,** Lateral preoperative view showing the presence of a naso-orbitoethmoid fracture as well *(arrow)*. **C, D,** Postoperative CT scan shows reduction of the fractures and fixation with titanium plates and screws. Cranial bone grafts were used to reconstruct the left lateral maxillary buttress. The orbital floor was repaired using a Medpor implant (Stryker, Newnan, Ga) containing embedded titanium mesh.

current CT scanning technology, plain films are not necessary and provide less information. An exception is the Panorex, which is used by many physicians as an adjunct or primary study for mandible fractures and to assess teeth and their roots in particular.

### Soft Tissue Injuries

Because of its rich blood supply, even questionable tissue should be salvaged when treating facial lacerations and avulsions. The robust perfusion of facial tissue provides resistance to infection and repair can be done after a longer delay than would be safe elsewhere on the body. Although there is no strict cutoff, generally primary repair is done up to 24 hours after injury. Even grossly contaminated wounds or those from animal bites are irrigated extensively, débrided, and closed primarily. If there is the possibility of facial nerve injury, this is confirmed by the physical examination revealing weakness or absence of function of a portion of the muscles of facial expression. It is important to recognize a facial nerve laceration so that the distal cut ends can be identified with a nerve stimulator and tagged if they are not to be repaired immediately. Identification of distal stumps by nerve stimulation is not possible after a few days because conduction ceases. Parotid duct injuries should be identified and treated acutely to prevent the formation of sialocele or salivary fistula. In a sharp laceration or penetrating injury to the cheek, a parotid duct injury can be confirmed by direct visualization or injection of dye. This is done by cannulating Stensen's duct on the mucosal surface of the cheek and injecting a small amount of methylene blue dye. Extravasation of the dye into the wound indicates a parotid duct laceration and repair over a stent should be done in the operating room.

### Craniofacial Fractures

Current concepts in facial fracture treatment rest on craniofacial techniques to provide surgical exposure of the craniofacial skeleton, anatomic reduction of fractures, rigid bony fixation with low profile, titanium plates, and bone-grafting techniques. Failure to reconstruct the bony facial skeleton invariably results in shrinkage and tightening of the facial soft tissue envelope, a sequela that is almost impossible to correct secondarily.

Treatment of forehead fractures involves assessment of the frontal sinus and cranial base. The approach is dictated by injury to the anterior or posterior table of the frontal bone or skull base, and whether there is a dural injury or injury to the nasofrontal ducts that drain the frontal sinuses into the nose. Fractures of the upper midface include malar (zygoma) fractures, naso-orbitoethmoid fractures, and orbital fractures. There is considerable overlap in this region. For example, malar fractures occur in association with orbital fractures to a varying degree because the zygoma, in addition to producing cheek projection and determining facial width, is also part of the orbit. Treatment of fractures of the lower midface, the maxilla, focuses on the restoration of the preinjury dental occlusion. It is important to determine the patient's preoperative occlusion; the relationship of the upper and lower teeth is described by the Angle classification.

Maxillary fractures are classified using the LeFort system based on the level at which the midface is separated from the rest of the craniofacial skeleton. Repairs focus on the restoration of facial height and projection. With significant comminution or bone loss, bone grafting may be required to maintain the appropriate position of the maxilla in space. Rigid plate and screw fixation obviates the need for prolonged maxillomandibular fixation. Fractures of the mandible are treated by reduction and rigid fixation using restoration of occlusion as the principle intraoperative and postoperative goal. Many mandibular fractures are treated with open reduction and internal fixation, which may make maxillomandibular fixation unnecessary.[13] Certain fractures, however, are best treated closed, and the decision to pursue an open or closed approach depends on the fracture location and orientation.

The same principles of fracture repair apply in the pediatric patient, with some differences; early treatment within 1 week is necessary given the rapid healing in children, and fixation is complicated by the presence of permanent teeth embedded in the maxilla and mandible that are easily damaged by hardware. Resorbable hardware is frequently used for children but does not have the mechanical strength required for the most adult fractures.

## Scalp Reconstruction

The scalp is comprised of skin, subcutaneous tissue, an aponeurotic fascial layer continuous with the frontalis and occipital muscles, a loose areolar layer, and periosteum. Small defects up to a few centimeters in size may be closed primarily, depending on the defect location and mobility of the surrounding scalp. A skin graft can be placed on intact periosteum. If periosteum is absent, the outer calvarial table can be opened with a burr to expose the diploic space from which granulation tissue will develop to support a skin graft. In the irradiated scalp or in the case of an open wound with alloplastic material at the base, secondary healing or grafting will not provide stable, durable coverage and a flap will be needed.

Scalp flaps are elevated at the subgaleal level and many possible designs exist. In theory, defects as large as 30% of the scalp can be closed with scalp flaps elevated on major vessels. Incising, or scoring, the inelastic galea can extend the reach of a scalp flap. Tissue expansion also can be used for the reconstruction of larger defects with hair-bearing tissue.

For large scalp defects not amenable to closure by local remaining scalp, distant flaps may be used. Pedicled flaps with usefulness for scalp coverage include the trapezius, latissimus, and pectoralis major muscle flaps. Pedicled flaps are limited by their arc of rotation, so free microvascular tissue transfer offers more flexibility. The free latissimus dorsi muscle flap is preferred for coverage of near-total or total scalp defects because of its flat contour and ability to cover a large surface area. Traumatic scalp avulsions occur in the subgaleal plane and may be replanted based on a single dominant vessel, with good results.

## Facial Reconstruction

Defects of the face are usually the result of tumor resection or trauma. STSG coverage of facial defects has limited application because the tissue match is imperfect. FTSGs are taken from donor sites in the preauricular, postauricular, and supraclavicular areas for the best color match. Local flaps provide tissue of appropriate thickness and have the color and texture of the defect.

Nasal defects up to approximately 1.5 cm in size can be closed with local nasal flaps. For larger defects, the forehead flap is preferred. The forehead flap is based on the supratrochlear vessels and the reconstruction is performed in a staged fashion

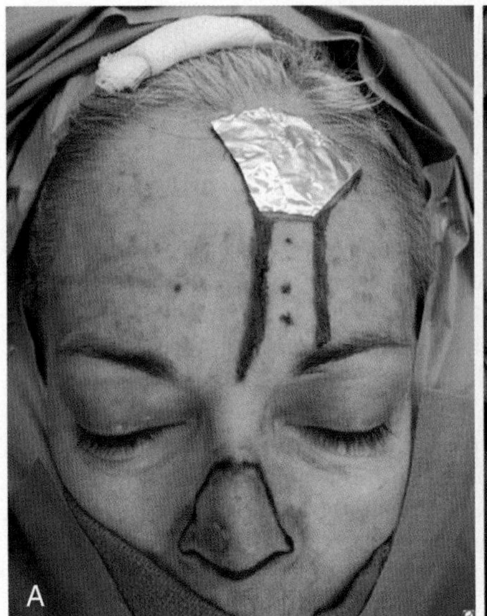


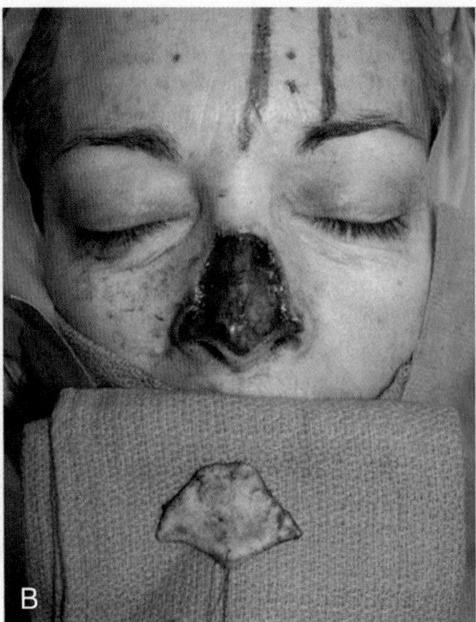


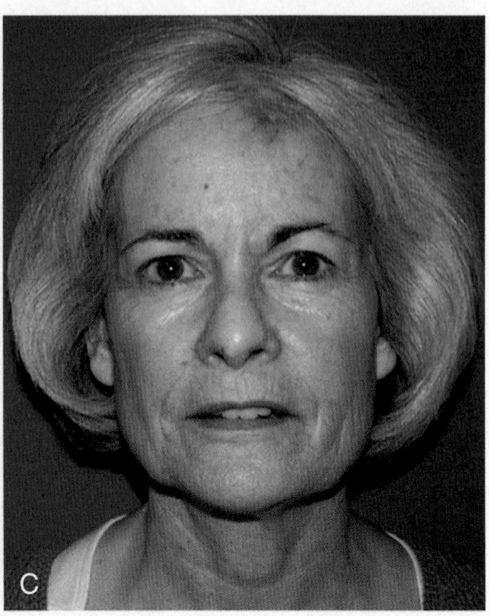


**FIGURE 69-7** A paramedian forehead flap is used for nasal reconstruction in a patient with melanoma on the right side of the nose. **A, B,** Although the tumor is on the right side, the entire nasal subunit is removed and the nasal cover flap designed so that there will be no scars on the anterior nose. **C,** Postoperative result at 4 months.

(Fig. 69-7). The forehead may be expanded prior to elevation for closure of larger defects and to assist with primary closure of the donor defect. With nasal defects, different components may be lost and restoration of skin, mucosal lining, and cartilage may be required. Composite grafts from the ear that contain skin and cartilage are useful for defects of the nasal ala. Reconstruction of total nasal defects is complex and may require bone grafting and free tissue transfer.

In the eyelid, FTSGs are a good option for skin loss alone. For a small, full-thickness lid defect, creating a V-shaped wedge can permit primary closure in layers. Adding a lateral canthotomy helps mobilize the lid margin for closure of larger defects and, in some cases, the incision can be carried out into the temporal skin to mobilize the lid further. Eyelid defects can be repaired with flaps rotated from the other lid; this is useful to provide similar tissue. Extensive eyelid defects require support, typically in the form of a chondromucosal graft obtained from the nasal septum or external ear. The graft is placed and covered with a regional skin flap.

For reconstruction of the cheek, a number of different, smaller local flaps can be designed. For larger defects, cervicofacial rotation flaps mobilize skin from the neck and side of the face for transposition to the more central areas of the face.

In the lip, precise alignment of the vermillion border is critical, as is repair of the orbicularis oris muscle to maintain lip competence. Defects are closed in layers and direct closure is possible for defects up to one third of the transverse width of the lip. Repair of larger defects requires mobilization of the surrounding tissue to reconstruct the oral sphincter. Central defects of the upper lip are best reconstructed using an Abbé flap, which is a mucosal musculocutaneous flap from the lower lip based on the labial artery. The flap is transferred in a staged fashion, with the donor pedicle divided 2 to 3 weeks after flap inset. Large defects of the lower lip are reconstructed with mucosal musculocutaneous flaps from the surrounding area. These reconstructions should preserve motor function of the orbicularis muscle, thus ensuring oral competence. Microstomia may be produced but is often temporary, because the tissues will stretch over time.

## Facial Transplantation

The first successful face transplantation was done in November 2005 in Amiens, France. Since then, there have been eight additional reports of successful facial composite tissue transplantation. All were done for devastating defects and were complex three-dimensional reconstructions, with variable amounts of skin, muscle, nerve, bone, and parts such as eyelids, noses, and lips. As of mid-2010, all the recipients had experienced at least one episode of acute graft rejection and two of the recipients have died, one from sepsis and the second after noncompliance with his immunosuppressive program. Functional recovery in the faces has been satisfactory in the long-term cases, with sensory function recovering at 3 to 6 months and acceptable motor recovery between 9 and 12 months. Aesthetic outcomes have been variable.[14]

The benefit of facial transplantation is that for a select number of severely disfigured individuals, it can provide a better functional and aesthetic outcome than conventional reconstructive methods and, in doing so, improve their quality of life. The immediate risks associated with surgery to transplant facial tissues are essentially the same as those for conventional reconstructive procedures. The important difference is the risk posed by the lifelong immunosuppression required to prevent rejection of the transplanted facial tissue. It is also assumed that there would be risks associated with the process of facial tissue rejection itself should that occur in any of these patients. At present, face transplantation is a technique of last resort after traditional facial reconstructive techniques have failed.

## Facial Aesthetic Surgery

Aesthetic surgery starts with an initial patient consultation for discussion and evaluation of the patient's perceptions and wishes, current health and past medical history, and realistic assessment of the benefits and risks of surgery to change appearance. The motivation to have aesthetic surgery is often psychological and involves body image, so the key to achieving success is selection of patients. The core value of the surgery lies not in the objective beauty of the visible result, but in the patient's opinion of and response to the change. Thus, being able to predict the likelihood that a patient will be satisfied with the surgical result is critical. Persons who consider their deformities greater than they actually are, who harbor unrealistic expectations, or who have substance abuse or mental health problems are not good candidates for aesthetic surgery because the surgery is unlikely to meet their needs.

### Forehead and Brow Lift

With aging, the eyebrow descends below its youthful location at or above the superior orbital rim. This ptosis is accompanied by a wrinkled brow, excess tissue hooding of the upper eyelids, especially in the temporal brow area, and creasing at the outer canthi (crow's feet) and over the dorsum of the upper nose. These changes can be corrected with a forehead or brow lift done as an open or endoscopic procedure. With an open lift, a bicoronal or modified anterior hairline incision is made. The forehead is elevated as a flap with the plane of dissection between the galea and pericranium, drawn taut, and the excess tissue in the frontal scalp excised. An endoscopic forehead lift is done through several small incisions within the hairline, extensive subperiosteal dissection to include the orbital rim and root of the nose, release and resection of the corrugator and procerus muscles, preservation of the supratrochlear and supraorbital nerves, and forehead elevation and fixation with percutaneous screws or other devices to reattach it in a higher position. The advantages of an endoscopic forehead lift are minimal scarring and no scalp resection; it is especially useful for patients with frontal baldness.

### Blepharoplasty

Blepharoplasty, derived from the Greek *blepharon,* meaning "eyelid," is done for dermatochalasis and corrects bagginess, fatty protrusions, and lax hanging skin around the eyes. If the eyelid itself is drooping, this is termed *blepharoptosis* and is corrected with a different procedure, a ptosis repair.

Upper eyelid blepharoplasty is done through an incision in the crease of the lid after marking the degree of excess skin to prevent overresection and resultant lagophthalmos (inability to close the eye completely). A strip of orbicularis oculus muscle can be taken and, if excess postseptal fat is present, this protruding orbital fat is resected. Lower eyelid blepharoplasty requires elevation of skin or skin–orbicularis oculi muscle flaps, with removal of skin, muscle, and fat. A transconjunctival approach to the lower eyelid is used for removal of lower lid fat or orbital septum tightening, with little or no skin resection. If the lower lid is lax and poorly adherent to the globe, a lateral canthopexy is done for mild laxity and a lateral canthoplasty is performed for significant laxity.

Complications after blepharoplasty include dry eye syndrome, scleral show, and ectropion. All patients should be tested preoperatively for preexisting dry eye and a Schirmer test may be predictive of this outcome in those who are prone to this. Scleral show is a complication after lower eyelid blepharoplasty in which the white sclera below the colored iris of the globe is exposed when the patient is in forward gaze. Scleral show is caused by lower eyelid retraction, with shortening of the middle lamella of the orbital septum; patients with preoperative laxity of the lower eyelids are predisposed to this complication if the laxity is not addressed at the time of surgery. Ectropion is eversion of the eyelid with exposure of the conjunctiva and is fairly common in the postoperative period, when the lower eyelid is edematous. Persistent ectropion requires surgery to increase lower lid support, possibly with the addition of skin grafts to augment the lower lid tissue.

### Facelift

A facelift, or rhytidectomy, derived from the Greek *rhytis,* meaning "wrinkle," is designed to correct the appearance of facial aging by removing lax, redundant facial and neck tissues. Facial aging is characterized by midface infraorbital flattening, prominent nasolabial folds, deepening of the labiomental crease, downturn of the lateral commissures of the mouth, deepening grooves at the outer corners of the mouth (marionette lines), jowl formation, vertical banding of the platysma muscles in the neck, and laxity of the neck skin. The traditional facelift is a subcutaneous dissection to elevate and redrape the skin of the face and neck. This has been eclipsed by procedures that also correct the effects of aging and gravity on the deeper tissues and structures of the face.

In addition to skin undermining and redraping, the superficial musculoaponeurotic system (SMAS) of the facial and neck fascia can be tightened by plication. With a lateral SMASectomy, a strip of SMAS is excised along the anterior border of the parotid and the mobile SMAS is brought up and sutured to the fixed SMAS at the malar prominence, which produces durable elevation of the superficial fascia and facial fat. It is effective for patients with a wide variety of anatomic differences and is reproducible and safe. With deep plane rhytidectomy, the facelift flap includes everything down to the fat over the zygomaticus muscles. This procedure corrects midface descent and ptosis, but is associated with prolonged facial edema and long recovery.

A number of ancillary procedures are available to enhance the outcome with facelift. Submental lipectomy removes the subcutaneous fat under the chin to improve the contour of the cervical portion of the facelift. Platysmaplasty corrects vertical banding by incising the platysma muscles at the level of the thyroid cartilage and suturing them together in the midline of the upper neck. Fat injection to selected areas under the facelift flaps before closure can fill hollows caused by subcutaneous fat atrophy in areas such as the temple.

Hematoma is the most common complication after facelift; other complications include scarring, alopecia, skin slough, and nerve injury. The most common nerve injury during facelift, occurring at a rate of 3% to 5%, involves the greater auricular nerve, which provides sensation to the lower ear.

### Rhinoplasty

Rhinoplasty is a difficult operation because it is a composite of procedures on a number of anatomic structures. When a patient describes a large nose or a long nose, this global description may encompass a dozen contributing structures. Laying the groundwork for a rhinoplasty starts with analysis of the facial proportions, followed by systematic analysis of the nasal components. Starting superiorly, the nasal frontal angle height and depth are noted. The bony pyramid, upper lateral cartilages and supratip are evaluated for their height, width, and symmetry. The nasal tip is analyzed in terms of its projection, rotation, symmetry, and position of the tip-defining points. The alae are inspected for increased width, collapse, or retraction. The columella is examined for increased or decreased show and the columellar-labial angle is measured. An internal nasal examination determines whether there is functional deformity by evaluating the septum, turbinates, and internal nasal valves. The soft tissue envelope and thickness of the skin are studied so the effect of underlying changes can be predicted.

Once thorough analysis is complete, this is converted into a surgical plan of action. The initial decision is whether to use an open or endonasal approach. The open rhinoplasty affords excellent exposure and makes it possible to manipulate the osteocartilaginous framework under direct vision. The closed rhinoplasty avoids a visible scar. After the surgical approach is decided on, the rest of the strategy involves choosing techniques based on location-specific criteria. These could include an osteotomy for changing the bony contour of the upper third of the nose, spreader grafts and dorsal resection of the upper lateral cartilages for internal valve collapse and dorsal contour in the middle third of the nose, resection and interdomal sutures for tip refinement and symmetry in the lower third of the nose, and columellar resection or a strut graft for overprojection or loss of tip support at the base of the nose.

The most common surgical complication with rhinoplasty is bleeding, which occurs in up to 3.6% of patients. A more challenging issue is that approximately 5% to 10% of patients require revision or a secondary rhinoplasty for aesthetic or functional reasons. The goal in rhinoplasty is to produce reliable, long-lasting, and natural-appearing results with consistency. It is thought that the key to achieving this goal is component analysis and management of the dorsal, tip, base, and internal nasal structures.[15]

### Skin Resurfacing

Several modalities are available to improve the texture, tone, and color of the skin. These include chemical peeling and dermabrasion, but the most rapidly growing technique for skin rejuvenation is laser technology. The use of light as a medical treatment was introduced in the 1960s with the development of the laser (***l****ight* ***a****mplification by* ***s****timulated* ***e****mission of* ***r****adiation*). Ablative lasers ($CO_2$ and erbium:YAG) have proved highly effective for skin treatment. Removing the epidermis and upper layers of the dermis, this ablation, combined with thermal coagulation of the dermis, heals with robust dermal remodeling that translates into clinical improvement. The problem was resultant scarring in some patients, prolonged edema and erythema, permanent pigmentation abnormalities, and increased risk of infection. Thus, a new concept of fractional photothermolysis was introduced in 2003, which has revolutionized laser surgery. Fractional $CO_2$ laser resurfacing represents a new class of therapy by delivering dermal coagulative injury without confluent epidermal damage. Distinct lesions of thermal damage are surrounded by larger zones of undisturbed normal skin; this combination allows complete reepithelialization within 24 to 48 hours while producing enough coagulation of the dermal collagen to stimulate connective tissue synthesis and produce skin tightening. With the fractional approach, results are comparable to those with full-surface ablative lasers without the associated side effects.[16]

The indications for laser resurfacing are facial rhytides, sun-damaged skin, and acne scarring. Benefits of treatment include softening or disappearance of mild to moderate wrinkles, improved skin texture and tone, decreased pore size, and reduction of skin laxity. The entire face, neck, and chest can be treated. Clinical improvement is seen with one or two treatments, scarring and hypopigmentation are rare, and the risk of infection in patients given prophylactic antiviral and antibiotic medications is low because the epidermal layer is restored promptly. When used to treat scars, fractional photothermolysis can flatten out and smooth hypertrophic scars and increases collagen production beneath depressed, atrophic scars, which summate in smoothing of the skin topography. For scarring, a series of treatments at 6- to 12-week intervals may be needed.

### Injectable Fillers

In the last few years, there has been more appreciation for the role that loss of volume plays in the contours of the aging face. Contrasting the youthful and aging face shows that areas such as the upper and lateral cheek, temple, nasojugal groove under the eye, and perioral area become atrophic, flat, and hollow in appearance. Restoring volume to reverse the atrophic changes in these areas produces a surprising rejuvenative change.

Volume restoration procedures can include lipotransfer of autologous fat or the use of an increasing number of materials, temporary or permanent, for soft tissue augmentation. Fat grafting is a technique-dependent procedure in which atraumatic handing and methodic layering of the autologous fat is emphasized for long-lasting results. An unexpected finding is that in addition to the volume restoration, fat grafting appears to have rejuvenative effects on the skin itself. The quality of the skin appears to be improved, with softening of wrinkles, decreased pore size, and more even pigmentation.[17] Similar observations are made when fat is injected beneath depressed scars; not only the indentation but the character of the skin itself appears to improve. With reports of the transformative power of fat grafted in areas of radiation damage, chronic ulcers, and other defects, there is much interest in documenting the extent and identifying the mechanism of these effects.[18]

In addition to autologous material, there are a number of biologic and synthetic products available for use as soft tissue fillers. Biologic materials derived from organic sources offer the benefits of ready off-the-shelf availability and ease of use, but introduce issues of sensitization to foreign animal or human proteins, transmission of disease, and immunogenicity. Also, as the tissue is processed to reduce these untoward side effects, the molecular structure is destabilized so that lack of persistence at the recipient site becomes the rule. The search over the last few years has been for new materials that are better tolerated and have greater longevity. The two major types of biologic tissue fillers are collagen products and hyaluronic acid products.[19]

Synthetic materials can offer permanence. Many injectable and surgically implantable synthetic products have been used over the years, and many have been condemned for complications such as granulomas, acute and delayed infections, migration or displacement, and deformity, which can result from complications or if the material is removed. Thus, only a limited number of synthetic materials are marketed in the United States for facial augmentation.

## PLASTIC SURGERY OF THE TRUNK

### Reconstruction of the Chest Wall

New techniques for repairing increasingly complex chest wall defects have accompanied advances in surgical and medical treatment of thoracic disease. Indications for chest wall reconstruction include defects arising from oncologic resection, irradiation ulceration, infection, or trauma and congenital defects. Considerations with reconstruction are the status of the pleural cavity, requirement for skeletal support, and provision of soft tissue coverage.

For management of the pleural cavity, principles include adequate débridement and the introduction of well-vascularized tissue to obliterate intrathoracic dead space. Extrathoracic muscles can be transposed to obliterate empyema spaces after pneumonectomy and to close bronchopleural or tracheoesophageal fistulas. Combined with adequate débridement and resection of poorly vascularized tissue, these muscle flaps can be passed through a thoracotomy incision with a two-rib resection and sutured into the defect, with thoracostomy drainage. The choice of muscle depends on the location of the defect; options include the latissimus dorsi, serratus anterior, and pectoralis major muscle flaps. Other muscle flaps with limited but specific uses are the trapezius and superiorly based rectus abdominis. The greater omentum can be transposed on the right gastroepiploic artery as a pedicle flap to provide well-vascularized tissue with the bulk and pliability to obliterate dead space, but it is a secondary choice because of the risks of intra-abdominal complications.

When evaluating a chest wall defect, a number of variables influence the decision about whether skeletal reconstruction or stabilization is required. These include the site of the chest wall defect, number of ribs resected, extent of resection of other bony structures of the chest wall, history of irradiation, and whether there is wound contamination or infection. The goals of skeletal reconstruction are protection of underlying vital structures, chest wall stability to preserve pulmonary function, and structural support for shoulder and upper limb function.

The number of resected ribs is accepted as the primary clinical determinant of the need for skeletal reconstruction. Stabilization is recommended when four or more consecutive ribs, or 5 cm or more of lateral chest wall, are resected because the resulting flail segment may impair respiratory mechanics. However, there are no conclusive data about the critical size for flail segment reconstruction and studies of pulmonary ventilation deficits from skeletal chest resection are controversial, particularly in the case of sternal resection.[20] Some of this lack of clarity may be caused by the presence of other factors that influence chest wall stability. Prior irradiation changes affect chest wall stability because soft tissues with radiation fibrosis have the rigidity and stiffness to limit chest wall motion. Location of the defect is relevant because lateral defects are more prone to flail chest deformity than those stabilized by proximity to the sternum or spine. Pancoast tumor resections are stabilized by scapular support and upper chest wall defects above the fourth rib generally can be closed with soft tissue only.

In the past, reconstruction of the chest skeleton with rib bone grafts or fascia lata was constrained by the limited availability of autologous tissue. One of the important advances in chest wall reconstruction has been the availability of suitable synthetic materials. The ideal characteristics of prosthetic material for chest wall reconstruction are semirigidity, flexibility, biocompatibility, and radiolucency. Several mesh materials are available, including polypropylene (Prolene), crystalline polypropylene and high-density polyethylene (Marlex), and polytetrafluoroethylene (Gore-Tex). Manufactured in a thick sheet, or doubled by folding, these materials provide support and malleability when sutured under tension. If additional rigidity is desired, methyl methacrylate glue can be sandwiched between sheets of mesh and allowed to harden into a rigid shell incorporated within the mesh. These synthetic materials provide good support and stability and perform well, provided they are covered with well-vascularized tissue to prevent infection. Chest wall infections in the presence of synthetic materials can be managed with drainage and antibiotic therapy; if removal of the foreign material can be delayed, a thickened fibrous layer will form to furnish some chest wall stability. In situations in which a chest defect is contaminated or infected at the outset, consideration can be given to the use of a temporary absorbable mesh, but this may have to be replaced when the infection has cleared.

Soft tissue coverage is the final stage of chest wall reconstruction. If a chest wall defect is limited to the skin and subcutaneous tissues, a skin graft is a reconstructive option. Its drawbacks are the eventual contraction that makes it a less attractive form of coverage than a flap and the poor success with graft healing on an irradiated bed. Thus, for chest wall defects with a radiation ulcer or osteoradionecrosis, there is little indication for a skin graft. The healing of skin grafts on the chest wall has been enhanced by the use of the vacuum-assisted closure device, which improves graft stabilization on a bed that is in motion with respiration.

In chest wall reconstruction, vascularized soft tissue flaps are used to close larger defects, control infection, obliterate dead space, cover synthetic materials, and close wounds with radiation necrosis. Although skin flaps or fasciocutaneous flaps are of some use, the muscle or musculocutaneous pedicle flap is preferred for its robust blood supply. The latissimus dorsi muscle is used frequently for its reliability, large area, and ability to reach almost any chest wall defect on the ipsilateral thorax. Other muscle flaps used for anterolateral soft tissue reconstruction include rectus abdominis, pectoralis major, external oblique, and serratus anterior. Trapezius muscle flaps are useful for defects of the upper third of the back, midback, and shoulders. Free flaps that transfer distant tissue with microvascular anastomoses are not often used and are reserved for situations in which regional flaps are unavailable or have failed, or for very large defects. In one series, in which aggressive resections of oncologic disease left chest wall defects as large as 300 to 400 $cm^2$, up to four muscle flaps and free flaps were required to achieve wound closure.[21]

One series of 200 chest wall reconstructions reported a mortality of 6%, with complete or partial flap loss in 5% of patients, and pneumonia, respiratory distress, infection, hematoma, and delayed wound healing in 27% of patients. Results were better in patients having immediate reconstruction at the time of resection than in those having delayed reconstruction.[22]

### Sternotomy Wounds: Treatment and Prevention

Sternal wound infection and mediastinitis after median sternotomy often require reoperation for débridement and reconstruction. Risk factors include diabetes, smoking, chronic obstructive pulmonary disease, immunosuppression, harvest of

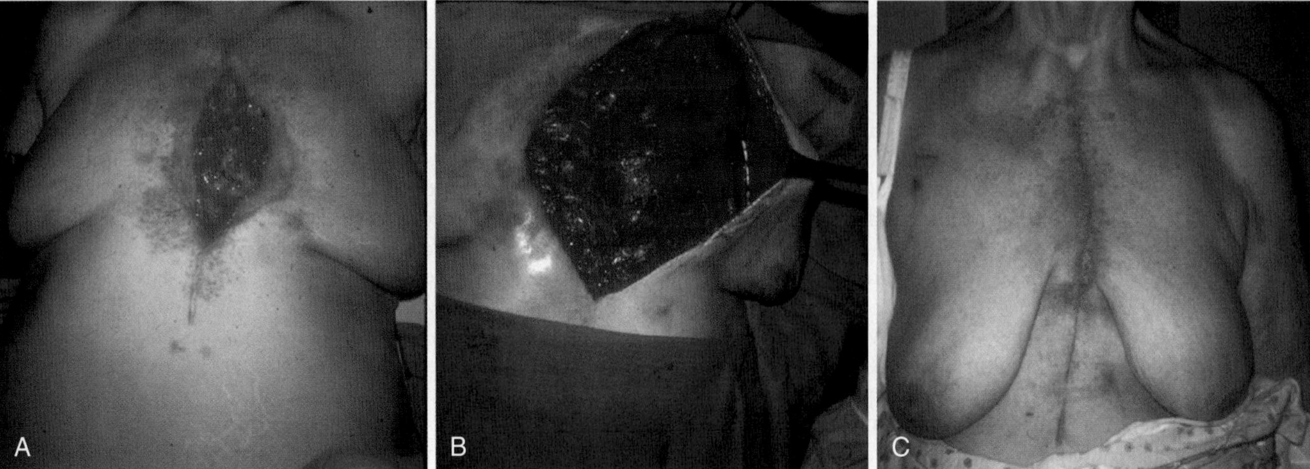


**FIGURE 69-8** **A,** 62-year-old woman 1 month after coronary artery bypass procedure with an open infected median sternotomy incision. **B,** The sternal wound was extensively débrided and covered with bilateral pectoralis major muscle flaps. Because the blood supply to the internal mammary perforators was damaged, each pectoralis major muscle was based on its thoracoacromial vascular pedicle after the insertion on the humerus and origin from the ribs was divided to permit muscle transposition. **C,** Postoperative result at 3 months.

internal mammary artery grafts, and use of assist devices. Primary rigid plate fixation of the sternum decreases the incidence of serious complications and there is current enthusiasm for introducing this surgical method for prevention in high-risk situations.[23]

For sternal instability or infection, débridement, use of wound vacuum-assisted closure devices, muscle and omental flaps, and fixation of the sternum have been described. Although minimal débridement may be needed in the wounds without costochondritis or osteomyelitis, single-stage or serial débridement bridged by vacuum-assisted closure as a sole or adjunct measure for definitive closure of the sternum may be required.[24] Fixation of the separated remaining sternal bone with plates before soft tissue coverage is advocated for earlier extubation, shorter length of stay, a more stable base for an overlying flap, and less long-term chest or shoulder pain. The pectoralis major muscle is the flap of choice for reconstruction of median sternotomy wounds. It is mobilized through the midline incision by detaching it from the sternum, ribs, clavicle, and humeral insertion while preserving the thoracoacromial pedicle (Fig. 69-8). It is advanced medially and, because of its size and arc of rotation, can cover almost the entire sternum. If an aortic vascular graft is exposed, the muscle is mobile enough to wrap around the graft and fill the mediastinum. Another option with the pectoralis major muscle is a turnover flap, in which one or both muscles are left attached on either side of the midline on the perforating branches of the internal mammary artery, dissected free from the remainder of the chest wall, and turned over like a book page to cover the sternum. If the pectoralis muscles are not sufficient, which is sometimes the case over the lower third of the sternum, the rectus abdominis muscle can mobilized. This is based on the superior epigastric artery and rotated 180 degrees to cover the sternum. If this is done in a patient in whom the ipsilateral internal mammary artery has been harvested for bypass grafting, the rectus abdominis muscle flap can be based on the eighth intercostal vessel, but with this as the pedicle the distal third may be poorly vascularized. With muscle flap reconstruction, the rates of successful sternal closure are approximately 85%.[25]

The greater omentum has been used for 40 years for the closure of sternal defects and provides reliable coverage. It has been claimed that omentum controls median sternotomy infection more successfully than pedicle muscle flaps, but is not used commonly because of exposure of the peritoneal cavity to infection, possibility of later intraperitoneal adhesions, and omentum's unavailability in some patients with previous abdominal surgery.

## Breast Surgery

### Reduction Mammoplasty

Hypertrophy or overgrowth of the breast is excessive development without any pathologic process. It can be familial, with a typical onset during puberty and pregnancy, when hormonal changes exert an abnormal influence on growth in some individuals. Reduction mammoplasty is the resection of excess fat, breast tissue, and skin to achieve a breast size proportional to the body. The principles guiding reduction mammoplasty for breast hypertrophy are to improve the patient's symptoms, decrease the volume of the breast, reshape the beast to correct ptosis, elevate the breast tissue to an anatomically correct position on the chest wall, reposition the nipple and areola on the reduced and reshaped breast, preserve the nerve supply to the skin and nipple-areolar complex, maintain blood supply to the breast tissue, and minimize scars. Surgical techniques are described by the location of the block of tissue to which the nipple and areola are left attached, and by the pattern of incisions and subsequent scars.

The pedicle is the portion of the breast tissue preserved with its blood and nerve supply while the surrounding breast tissue is removed. An inferior pedicle technique is used most often but there are central, superior, medial, lateral, and doubly attached vertical and horizontal pedicles. All variants are designed to maximize blood supply while allowing adequate tissue removal. Suction-assisted lipectomy is used with excision techniques to remove excess fat laterally and there are a small number of patients with mild to moderate hypertrophy, fatty breasts, good skin tone, no ptosis, and good breast shape for whom liposuction alone will reduce volume, with small scars. In the very large pendulous breast, in which the pedicle would be exceptionally long, the nipple-areolar complex is removed and transplanted as a graft. This technique is useful also for patients with vascular disorders or impaired wound healing.

Prior to reduction mammoplasty, breast cancer screening with examination and mammography usually is done in patients 35 years of age and older. A small number of breast cancers are discovered at the time of reduction by identifying a suspicious area or during routine pathologic study of the tissue; all breast tissue removed surgically should be sent for histopathologic study. There is no set lower age limit but, for the adolescent with breast hypertrophy, reduction is deferred until the breasts have stopped growing and are stable in size for at least 12 months before surgery. Secondary or repeat breast reduction has a higher complication rate because problems associated with a damaged blood supply, such as delayed wound healing, fat necrosis, and loss of the nipple and areola, are seen when a pedicle is developed again in a previously reduced breast. Wound healing is impaired in the previously irradiated breast because of radiation-induced vascular changes. Recommendations in these patients include the following: (1) delay between radiation and mammoplasty to allow some of the vascular changes to subside; and (2) technical modifications using pedicles that are broader and shorter than usual and minimizing adjustments to the breast tissue. Obese patients are poor candidates for breast reductions, with more local and systemic complications. Smoking is a contraindication to breast reduction.

Sequelae of reduction mammoplasty include changes in the sensibility of the nipple and areola in 20% to 25% of cases, usually a decrease but occasionally increased sensation. Lactation and breastfeeding are not always possible after breast reduction. Complications with reduction mammoplasty include wound dehiscence, skin slough, loss of tissue, hematoma, infection, and fat necrosis with palpable nodules of poorly vascularized fat. Fat necrosis may prompt later investigation or biopsy to distinguish these lumps from breast neoplasms.

Outcome studies after reduction mammoplasty have shown that patients gain relief from symptoms, can engage more in activities of daily life, and are happy with the results. In one study of 185 women, 97% reported improvement in back shoulder and neck pain, 95% said they were happy or very happy with the results of surgery, and 98% said they would recommend it to others.[26]

### Breast Augmentation

Augmentation mammoplasty is a cosmetic procedure done to resolve the dissatisfaction that some women feel with small breasts, either because their breasts never developed to a desired size or because their breasts lost volume after pregnancy or weight loss, or with aging. With the development of the sealed silicone gel breast implant in 1962, breast augmentation became widely accepted. All U.S. Food and Drug Administration (FDA)–approved breast implants, regardless of filling material, have an outer shell or envelope constructed of silicone elastomer. Silicone gel–filled implants are polymerized to a consistency similar to that of breast tissue. Newer gel implants have a thicker, more viscous gel than previous generations of these devices. Called *cohesive gel*, the material tends to stay in place, even if the shell of the implant is damaged. Gel implants are prefilled and sealed and cannot be adjusted in size in the operating room. Saline-filled implants are silicone rubber shells filled in the operating room. Advantages of the saline implants are the benign nature of saline, some flexibility in adjusting size by varying the amount of fluid put in the implant, and smaller incisions, because the implants are inserted while empty. The primary disadvantage is a higher incidence of visible rippling or wrinkling of the implant under the skin, particularly in thin patients.

Breast augmentation requires an incision in the skin and subcutaneous tissue, with creation of a pocket in which a breast implant is placed and positioned. There are a number of technical variations. One of three incisions can be used, each with advantages and drawbacks. The inframammary incision provides excellent access and does not require dissection within the breast parenchyma; the disadvantage is a scar that may be noticeable in the smaller breast. A periareolar incision is camouflaged in the areola and heals with little visible scarring but has the disadvantage of possible changes in sensation in the nipple-areolar area. An axillary incision leaves no scars on the breast but it is more difficult to create the pocket with this approach. The pocket into which the implant will be placed can be in one of two positions relative to the breast tissue and pectoralis major muscle. Subglandular placement superficial to the pectoralis muscle fascia provides more ability to control the shape of the breast and is associated with a more rapid postoperative recovery. With submuscular placement of the implant, the contour of the breast may be smoother because the edges of the implant are blunted by the muscle, there is less chance of developing capsular contracture (hardened scar around the implant), nipple sensation is protected, and mammogram interpretation may be more accurate when the breast tissue is lifted up and away from the implant by the muscle. Disadvantages include more postoperative discomfort and longer recovery, movement of the implant when the muscle is flexed, and less ability to lift the parenchyma in a breast with some degree of ptosis.

When considering potential problems that can develop after augmentation mammoplasty, it is useful to distinguish between operative complications and implant concerns. Perioperative complications are relatively low, with bleeding or hematoma in 1% to 3%, wound infections in 1% to 2%, and some degree of diminished sensibility of the nipple-areolar complex in approximately 15% of patients, depending on the incision used and position of the implant relative to the muscle. More numerous and more serious are the sequelae presenting weeks or years after the surgery. These include capsular contracture, implant deflation, implant rupture, and implant displacement.

**Capsular Contraction.** This occurs when the normal envelope of fibrous tissue around an implant becomes thicker or tighter so that the implant no longer feels soft and pliant. If the degree of capsular contracture is great, there can be pain, distortion, and palpability or distortion of the implant. Capsular contracture occurs in approximately 15% of patients, and it is not possible to predict who will develop it or take preventive measures. Treatment involves removing the fibrous capsule surgically and replacing the implant, but this often results in recurrence of the capsular contracture. The only permanent correction is removal of the implant.

**Implant Deflation.** Saline-filled implants can deflate when the fluid leaks out of the implant through the valve or implant shell. This occurs in approximately 7% of patients within the first 5 years after surgery. Causes include damage from handling at the time of surgery, pressure from capsular contracture, compression of the implant due to trauma, and other reasons that remain unknown.

**Implant Rupture.** Silicone gel implants can rupture, releasing the gel material; its frequency is similar to that of deflation of saline implants. However, there is an important difference in how the rupture is detected. When a gel implant ruptures, the breast volume will not change because the gel remains in the area; in many cases, the rupture remains undiagnosed—a silent rupture. Thus, it is recommended that gel implants be studied by MRI at intervals of 3 to 5 years so that silent ruptures can be detected and treated. Mammograms are not reliable diagnostic tools for rupture and surveillance with MRI is the standard.[27]

Two areas of extensive study have been the questions of whether breast implants are associated with breast cancer, and whether the silicone material in breast implants is associated with connective tissue disease. No study has ever suggested that the presence of a breast implant is a cause of breast cancer. The primary question has been whether the presence of an implant is responsible for delayed detection or poorer prognosis because of compromise of screening mammography. Standard mammograms in a woman with breast implants show only approximately 75% of the breast tissue because the remainder is obscured by the implant. Displacement techniques are used to address this, and additional views are needed. Studies have shown no significant difference between women with and without implants who develop breast cancer in terms of the size or stage of the tumor when it is diagnosed. One series of 3182 women followed for 18.7 years after breast augmentation has shown no increased risk, no delay in diagnosis, and no worse prognosis for these patients compared with a comparable group of women without implants.[28]

Concern about the association of breast implants with the development of autoimmune or connective tissue diseases, such as lupus, scleroderma, or rheumatoid arthritis, arose because of cases reported in the literature in the early 1980s. Since then, an increasing number of epidemiologic analyses have failed to support this association. A committee of the Institute of Medicine of the National Academies of Science reviewed over 2000 peer-reviewed studies and 1200 data sets. In 1999, they concluded that there was no definitive evidence linking breast implants to cancer, immunologic disease, or neurologic disease, and that women with breast implants were no more likely to develop these disorders than those in the rest of the population.

### Breast Ptosis and Mastopexy

Breast ptosis describes the downward displacement of the glandular tissue of the breast. Sagging and drooping develop when lax skin with poor elasticity cannot support and shape the underlying breast parenchyma and the fascial attachments, the suspensory ligaments of Cooper, lose elasticity and become attenuated. These changes are seen with significant weight loss, postpartum atrophy, postmenopausal involution, and the continual gravitational pull associated with aging. Breast ptosis is classified by the position of the nipple-areolar complex relative to the inframammary fold and breast mound; the degree of ptosis is considered when choosing the technique for surgical correction. There are numerous options for mastopexy and these draw on both breast reduction and breast augmentation techniques. The key elements are the removal and tightening of redundant skin and breast tissue and the possible addition of a breast implant. The primary intention when introducing a breast implant is not increased size; rather, the implant adds volume to the flattened upper pole of the breast and provides support and lift for a soft, involuted breast with thin, inelastic skin. The challenge with mastopexy is balancing tightening with restoration of volume. The effects of surgery are only temporary and ptosis recurs with the passage of time depending on the age of the patient, the cause of the ptosis, the size of the breast, and whether an implant was used.

### Fat Grafting to the Breast

Autologous fat injection into the breast is a controversial subject. It has been used successfully for breast enlargement, correction of breast deformities, additional coverage to disguise breast implants, and treatment of radiation damage to the chest. However, fat injections in the breast are associated with fat necrosis, oil cysts, and calcifications and there is concern that these abnormalities can hinder breast cancer screening. This prompted the American Society of Plastic Surgeons to issue a position paper in 1987 deploring the use of autologous fat injections for breast augmentation because of the scarring and calcification that would develop if the injected fat did not survive. Drawing on experience with fat grafting in the face, procedural modifications for harvesting fat with minimal trauma and injecting it into the breast in small aliquots were described 20 years later.[29] Taking care to avoid placing large amounts of fat at one site, the incidence of fat necrosis is lower and lipografting in the breast is being performed and studied actively. Adjunctive techniques include expanding the skin envelope and generating a recipient matrix prior to serial seeding with micrografts, placing the grafts outside the breast parenchyma itself, and layering the fat into different levels. With evidence that technical performance is critical, excellent long-lasting results are being reported. However, an accurate figure for the incidence of calcifications after fat grafting to the breast remains to be determined, as does the ability of breast screening studies to differentiate scattered microcalcifications and dispersed radiolucent oil cysts of fat injections from abnormalities suspicious for malignancy.[30] Another area of intense interest is the use of adipose stem cells when using fat grafting for breast enlargement. Still largely theoretical in clinical practice, the possibility of stimulating permanent fat survival in the breast is being weighed against the risk of introducing growing cell lines into tissue that will develop malignancy in some percentage of the treated population. Although it is clear that autologous fat transfer to the breast is effective, the safety of the procedure is unsettled at this time.

### Gynecomastia

Male breast enlargement occurs bilaterally in 50% to 55% of cases; most patients are asymptomatic or report some tenderness, soreness, or sensitivity. Caused by an increased estrogen-to-androgen ratio, the incidence is increased with generalized obesity because of increased conversion of testosterone to estradiol in adipose tissue. Histologically, variable degrees of ductal proliferation and stromal hyperplasia present in three patterns, described as florid, intermediate, or fibrous. The florid pattern shows ductal hyperplasia surrounded by loose cellular connective tissue. The fibrous pattern has extensive fibrosis of the stroma with little ductal proliferation and is seen with longer than 1 year duration of gynecomastia. The intermediate pattern represents a transition between the florid and fibrous types.

There are physiologic, pathologic, and pharmacologic causes. Physiologic or idiopathic gynecomastia, with no pathologic basis, develops transiently in more than 60% of newborns because of exposure to transplacental estrogens. During puberty, estrogen and testosterone shifts result in a prevalence of 50% to 60%, with presentation during midpuberty (14 years) and a self-limited average duration of 1 to 2 years. With increasing age, the prevalence gradually increases to more than 70% in the seventh decade. Pathologic gynecomastia is associated with cirrhosis, malnutrition, hypogonadism, Klinefelter's syndrome, renal disease, hyperthyroidism, hypothyroidism, and neoplastic disease. Tumors that may lead to gynecomastia are testicular tumors (e.g., Leydig cell and Sertoli cell tumors, choriocarcinomas), adrenal tumors, pituitary adenomas, and lung carcinoma. Gynecomastia is not associated with male breast cancer except in patients with Klinefelter's syndrome, in whom the incidence of mammary carcinoma is 20 to 60 times greater than in men without this chromosomal aberration. Pharmacologic gynecomastia is caused by drugs from a number of classes, including antiandrogens, antibiotics, chemotherapeutic agents, cardiovascular disease drugs, and drugs of abuse (e.g., alcohol, heroin, amphetamines, marijuana).[31]

For the patient presenting with gynecomastia, pertinent history includes duration, concomitant disease, and medication use. The breasts, thyroid, abdomen, testes and overall degree of virilization are examined. Laboratory studies include determinations of hormone levels and, as indicated, additional selected studies, such as checking karyotype, testicular ultrasound, hepatic or renal function tests, mammography, and imaging studies of the chest or adrenals. Treatment of an underlying disorder may lead to regression of gynecomastia, especially when an offending medication can be identified and withdrawn in drug-related cases, or when testosterone is administered for testicular failure. However, gynecomastia of long duration, with a fibrous pattern, is unlikely to resolve spontaneously.

Indications for surgery include symptomatic gynecomastia, adolescent males with enlargement persisting for more than 18 to 24 months, gynecomastia of long duration that has progressed to fibrosis, and patients at risk for breast cancer (e.g., those with Klinefelter's syndrome). Surgical approaches depend on the degree of enlargement and whether there is associated ptosis (drooping) of the breasts. For patients with mild to moderate gynecomastia with minimal drooping, there are several options, including suction-assisted liposuction, ultrasound-assisted liposuction, direct excision through a small incision confined to the areola, or a combination of these techniques. For the patient with moderate to large gynecomastia and associated laxity and descent of the breast, skin resection and transposition of the nipple-areolar complex superiorly to an appropriate position on the chest wall are required. This necessitates additional incisions, with resultant scarring; there are various techniques to minimize the appearance of these scars. For the patient with massive gynecomastia, an en bloc resection of excessive skin and breast tissue is needed, with free nipple grafting or repositioning of the nipple areolar complex on a pedicle flap.

The challenge with surgical excision of gynecomastia is achieving perfect symmetry of the two breasts and producing a smooth contour, without indentations or irregularities. Suction-assisted lipectomy is helpful to smooth the contours and taper the area of resection into the surrounding subcutaneous tissue on the chest wall to make it undetectable. Postoperative complications include hematoma or seroma caused by the extensive dissection and undermining of the skin through a small incision; these can be mitigated with good hemostasis and the use of drains and compression garments. Less common complications include infection or tissue loss, including loss of a portion of the nipple areolar complex.

### Congenital and Developmental Deformities

Breast and chest wall deformities range from hyperplastic anomalies, such as polymastia and polythelia, to hypoplastic deformational anomalies characterized by a paucity of breast tissue, as seen in Poland syndrome. Described by Alfred Poland in 1841, this syndrome is a severe form of chest wall and breast hypoplasia that occurs in approximately 1 in 25,000 live births. It occurs sporadically, is generally unilateral, and affects males more frequently than females (3 : 1). The syndrome includes a spectrum of deformities, the most consistent of which is absence of the sternocostal head of the pectoralis major muscle. Other features can include absence of the ipsilateral pectoralis major and minor muscles, absence of the anterior portions of ribs 2 to 5, loss of the latissimus dorsi and serratus anterior muscles, absence of axillary hair, limited subcutaneous chest wall fat, and brachysyndactyly of the ipsilateral hand. There can be absence of the breast or a varying degree of hypoplasia, and the nipple can be absent or displaced.

Treatment options for Poland syndrome include autologous tissue, alone or in combination with synthetic implant materials, to correct the contour deformity of the chest wall and reconstruct the breast. Because of its proximity, a pedicled latissimus dorsi muscle flap is preferred if it itself is not involved; as an alternative, the rectus abdominis muscle can be introduced as a pedicle or free flap. The timing of surgery requires careful consideration. In general, reconstruction is deferred until late adolescence to avoid the risk of growth inhibition with early operative trauma and minimize the need for multiple revisions to keep pace with chest wall and breast growth.

## Abdominal Wall Surgery

### Components Separation and Flap Coverage

Acquired abdominal wall defects are caused by incisional hernia, tumor resection, infection, irradiation, and trauma. The goals of abdominal wall reconstruction are protection of the abdominal contents, restoration of the integrity of the musculofascial wall, and provision of dynamic muscle support. Treatment is selected on the basis of a number of factors, including the medical status of the patient, wound bed preparedness, size of the defect, position of the defect, and whether there is loss of stable skin and subcutaneous tissue or loss of myofascial tissue. If skin coverage and myofascial continuity are absent, the defect is a complete, full-thickness loss and both layers will have to be restored using more complex approaches.

The timing of immediate versus delayed reconstruction depends on the clinical situation. Patient assessment includes body mass index (BMI) and pulmonary evaluation because postoperative loss of domain may decrease vital capacity, total lung capacity, and functional residual capacity.[32] Nutritional status, tobacco use, and fluid and electrolyte imbalance are corrected. Assessment of the wound bed includes identification of bacterial contamination, exposed viscera, adherent bowel, enterocutaneous fistulae, previous radiation, prosthetic material used in previous operations, and previous incisions or scars that interrupt the abdominal circulation. The presence of inflammation and edema, even in a clean wound, limits local tissue advancement; significant inflammation may be present after dehiscence, traumatic defects, fistulas, or recent infection.

Immediate and one-stage reconstruction of a wall defect is the approach of choice for a patient who is medically stable, with a clean wound bed and reliable reconstructive options. This approach is suitable for patients having ventral herniorrhaphy or tumor extirpation requiring concomitant reconstruction. Definitive repair is delayed if the patient is unstable, the wound is contaminated, further explorations are planned, or there is abdominal distention or inflammation. In these cases, the wound is managed with skin grafts, prosthetic mesh, or vacuum-assisted closure device as a temporary measure until reconstruction can be done.

STSGs have a high rate of success, even in colonized wounds, provide stable coverage to protect from infection, and prevent continued fluid and protein loss from granulation tissue. In addition, they aid in eventual closure by reducing the size the wound through contracture. The problem is that STSGs become fixed to the viscera on which they are placed; the consequences of skin grafting include hernia, abdominal wall bulge, and possible trauma to the viscera. Later reconstruction involving removal of the skin grafts should be delayed for a minimum of 6 months, until the wound has matured. This will decrease the density of the adhesions and scar tissue and help control the rate of inadvertent enterotomy, which converts a clean case in which prosthetic mesh could be used into a contaminated one.

If temporary fascial support of a contaminated wound is needed to prevent evisceration and maintain domain, an absorbable mesh can be used while the acute problems are addressed. Absorbable mesh made from polyglycolic acid can remain in place for 3 to 4 months, protecting the intra-abdominal contents and providing support while granulation tissue develops and is skin-grafted. This type of mesh undergoes hydrolytic degradation so its usefulness is temporally limited because of loss of structural strength, with ulceration and delayed hernia formation. If left in place, there will be eventual loss of support but there will be no difficulty removing the prosthetic material 6 to 12 months later in a patient undergoing definitive repair of the defect.

The vacuum-assisted closure device is effective for providing temporary closure of an abdominal wall defect by providing the support of an nondistensible dressing, limiting fascial retraction by applying constant medial tension, and stimulating granulation tissue growth. With modification of the standard vacuum pack dressing, visceral adherence to the abdominal wall can be limited whereas fascial closure is encouraged. Studies in a laboratory model have shown that the vacuum-assisted closure device results in a fourfold increase in vascularization to the wound, decreased bacterial colonization, increased formation of granulation tissue by 103%, and increased flap survival by 21% when compared with controls.[33]

When planning definitive repair, reconstructive options are considered in terms of the type of abdominal wall defect, which can be broadly classified into one of three categories:

- Loss of skin and subcutaneous tissue only. These partial defects are closed primarily if small, with skin grafting, random or local flaps, fasciocutaneous flaps, vacuum-assisted closure device, or tissue expander prior to primary closure.
- Loss of musculofascial tissue, with intact skin coverage. These partial defects are repaired with prosthetic mesh or with autologous tissue reconstruction. Autologous techniques include primary repair, open or endoscopic-assisted components separation, or local flap and distant flaps selected on the basis of the location of the fascial defect on the trunk.
- Loss of both the skin and fascial layers, with a full-thickness open defect. These complete defects can be approached with staged reconstruction to close the skin and return later to provide fascial replacement. Alternatively, a local or distant muscle flap, musculocutaneous flap, fasciocutaneous flap, or free tissue transfer can supply well-vascularized tissue with the use of prosthetic material for fascial support as needed.

Components separation is a technique in which a series of fascial incisions are used to separate the structural components of the abdominal wall and mobilize the musculofascial tissue for closure of a midline abdominal wall defect (Fig. 69-9). The anterior rectus sheath is separated from the external oblique aponeurosis by making a longitudinal relaxing incision along the linea semilunaris. This allows the anterior rectus sheath and muscle to move medially while maintaining its neurovascular supply, which comes from between the internal oblique and transversus abdominis in a segmental fashion. Posteriorly, the rectus muscle is released from its posterior sheath with medial advancement of 5 cm in the epigastric region, 10 cm at the umbilicus, and 3 cm in the suprapubic region. With the modification of also dividing the internal oblique component of the anterior rectus sheath, unilateral advancement increases to 8 to 10 cm in the epigastrium, 10 to 15 cm in the midabdomen, and 6 to 8 cm in the suprapubic region. With the components separation technique, the reported rate of hernia recurrence is variable, from below 5% to over 30%, presumably dependent on a number of factors, including the dimensions of the defect. To address this, techniques for augmenting, but not bridging, the fascial closure with prosthetic mesh have been described, with good results for larger, more complex hernias.[34] The components separation technique eliminates the need for prosthetic material in many patients, restores the dynamic abdominal wall function, and results in improvement in back pain and postural abnormalities. A common complication with this technique is wound breakdown caused by devascularized skin flaps consequent to the wide undermining required. Attention to preserving the periumbilical perforators can reduce the number of wound-healing complications; the use of endoscopic-assisted components separation has been described as a means to preserve midline perforators to the skin during release of the external oblique. In contrast to midline defects, components separation has limited use in lateral defects in which the achievable advancement decreases by 50%. In addition, use of components separation in lateral repairs

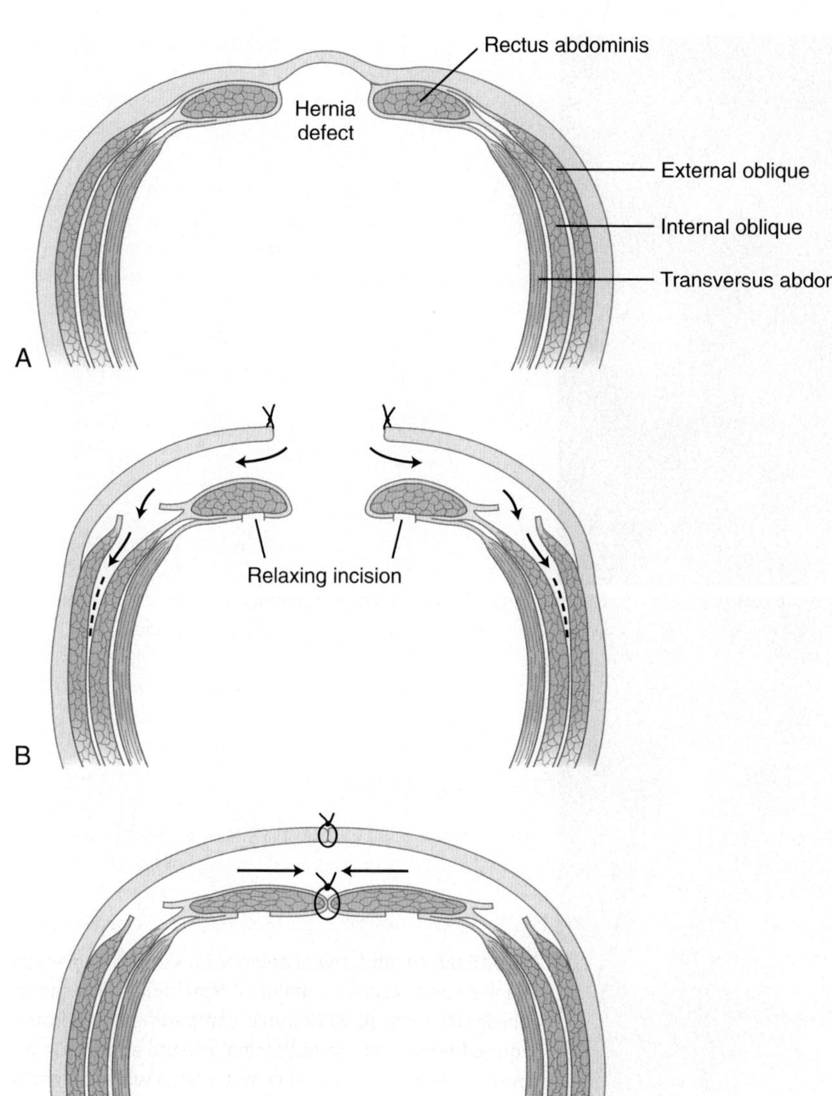


**FIGURE 69-9** Components separation to mobilize the musculofascial tissue for closure of a midline abdominal wall defect. **A,** Anterior midline abdominal wall defect. **B,** Anterior rectus sheath separated from the external oblique aponeurosis. Longitudinal relaxing incisions are made anteriorly along the linea semilunaris and posteriorly in the posterior rectus sheath. **C,** Relaxing incisions in anterior and posterior rectus sheath. These allow stretching of the rectus muscle as the anterior rectus wall is pulled medially to correct the defect. (From Nozaki M, Sasaki K, Huang TT: Reconstruction of the abdominal wall. In Mathes SJ, editor: Plastic surgery, ed 2, Philadelphia, 2006, Saunders Elsevier, p 1182.)

can result in loss of fascial congruity of the abdominal wall, with hernia formation at the donor site.

Various prosthetic materials are available for use as structural support of the abdominal wall. A number of trials have shown that the recurrence rate is halved after repair of incisional hernias more than 5 to 6 cm in size when the use of prosthetic mesh is compared with primary suture repair.[35] From this has come the consensus that prosthetic materials are useful in the presence of adequate skin and subcutaneous coverage and adequate wound bed. The incidence of infection is higher with the use of prosthetics than with primary repair; excessive wound tension, poor wound status, and a history of infection are associated with prosthetic material failure. The materials are classified as meshed or nonmeshed and absorbable or nonabsorbable. There is less fibrous ingrowth with a nonmeshed material such as Gore-Tex, which minimizes adhesions between the prosthesis and viscera; reopening of the abdominal cavity through nonmeshed material is easier. Alternatively, meshed material such as Marlex permits the effusion of fluid for a reduced incidence of seroma and promotes fibrous ingrowth, which enhances tissue strength. Although preferred, complications can include infection, extrusion of the prosthetic material, and bowel erosion when folds and wrinkles in the mesh exert pressure again the bowel wall. Softer, smoother mesh, made from Prolene, is more pliable and erosion into bowel is less common. In an effort to avoid these complications of infection, extrusion, abdominal wall stiffness, pain, and fistula formation that are associated with nonabsorbable materials, biomaterials derived from human and animal sources have been developed. These bioprostheses are absorbable; they include human acellular dermis (AlloDerm), porcine acellular dermis (Permacol), and porcine small intestinal submucosa (Surgisis). These materials have an acellular collagen matrix that promotes host tissue remodeling and replacement. Although resistant to infection, biocompatible, and mechanically stable over the short term, their disadvantages are high cost and few long-term studies establishing outcomes with regard to hernia recurrence.

Several techniques are used to place prosthetic material—mesh onlay, mesh inlay, retrorectus placement, and intraperitoneal underlay. For onlay grafts, the material is cut larger

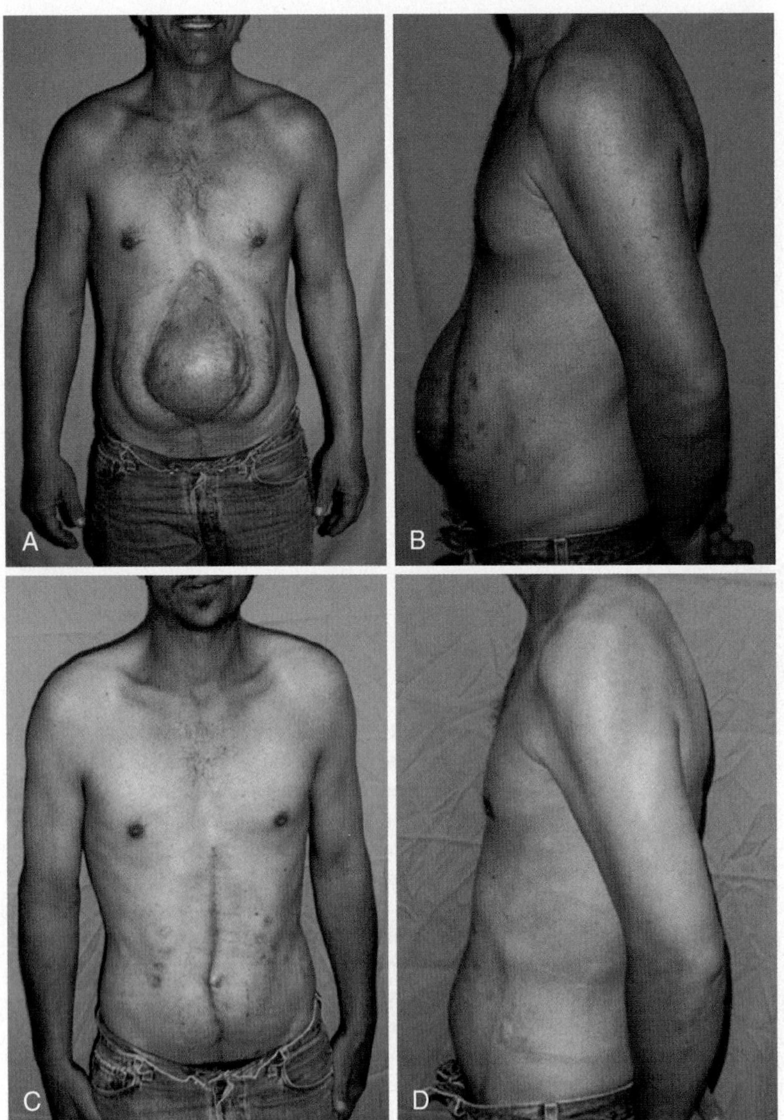


**FIGURE 69-10** Abdominal defect with skin graft coverage in a man who sustained major visceral injuries in a motor vehicle accident. **A,** Abdominal compartment syndrome required release of the abdominal closure and STSGs for coverage. **B,** Lateral view of ventral hernia with skin grafts on viscera. **C, D,** Postoperative view 1 year after peritoneal mesh reconstruction of abdominal wall.

than the fascial defect, placed superficially to the anterior rectus sheath, and anchored at its margins with sutures. With inlay grafts, the prosthetic material is cut to the same size as the fascial defect, placed in the defect, and anchored to the edges with sutures. With these techniques for mesh repair, recurrence is not uncommon. This is not caused by intrinsic failure of the prosthetic material, but by herniation at the suture line of the graft fascial interface. Therefore, underlay techniques are preferred. With the retrorectus approach, the material is placed in the preperitoneal space between the rectus muscle and posterior rectus sheath. Alternatively, the underlay graft can be placed intraperitoneally, using an endoscopic approach in selected cases, and secured with sutures, tacks, or staples (Fig. 69-10). In an underlay location, intra-abdominal pressure bolsters the repair by holding the graft in apposition to the fascia; at least 4 cm of contact at the margins between the mesh and fascia is desirable to increase the surface area for fibrous ingrowth at the material-fascial interface. When possible, the viscera are protected by interposing omentum between the mesh and abdominal contents. With use of these measures, secure and physiologic repairs with recurrence rates below 10% have been reported.

A number of autologous tissue flaps are available for defects with absent or unstable skin coverage. These include skin flaps, muscle flaps, fasciocutaneous flaps, musculocutaneous flaps, and free tissue transfers. Flap selection depends on the location and size of the defect and algorithms have been suggested for defect analysis and selecting the flap of choice.[36] For lower abdominal wall reconstruction, the tensor fascia lata musculofasciocutaneous flap based on the lateral circumflex femoral artery is the flap of choice. A dense strong sheet of vascularized fascia and its overlying skin can be transferred from the lateral thigh in a single stage to resurface the suprapubic region, lower abdominal quadrants, or as high as the upper quadrant on the ipsilateral abdomen. It is useful in irradiated and contaminated fields because it provides autologous fascia and conveys protective sensation when the lateral femoral cutaneous nerve is included. The rectus femoris musculocutaneous flap, based on the descending branch of the lateral circumflex femoral artery, is another choice for repair of the lower half of the abdomen or ipsilateral abdominal wall. Its drawback is the donor site morbidity of weakened quadriceps function in the leg associated loss of the muscle. This flap can be extended by incorporating adjacent fascia lata, and this "mutton chop" modification has been used to reconstruct into the epigastrium. Additional flaps for lower abdominal coverage include the anterior thigh flap, external oblique muscle, and rectus abdominis musculocutaneous flap, based inferiorly on the inferior epigastric vessels, which is also the flap of choice for lateral defects of the lower two thirds of the abdomen. In the upper half of the abdomen, the superiorly based vertical or transverse abdominis musculocutaneous flap, based on the superior epigastric artery, is useful for central defects, and the latissimus dorsi musculocutaneous flap, based on the thoracodorsal vessels, is suitable for reconstruction of the lateral parts of the upper abdomen. Free flaps are considered when local tissues are not available or when a pedicle flap cannot reach or is too small to cover a defect. In the case of a free tissue transfer to the abdomen, suitable recipient vessels are required. Usually, the inferior epigastric, deep circumflex iliac, superior epigastric, internal thoracic or saphenous vein graft may be used. Because it contains fascia, tensor fascia latae flaps are the most commonly used free flaps, but use of an innervated free latissimus dorsi flap has been described as a means to bring contractile function and strength to the lost abdominal wall.

## Abdominoplasty

Abdominoplasty removes fat and skin from the abdominal wall and repairs fascial laxity or dehiscence to produce an abdominal profile that is smoother and firmer. It is most effective in persons of normal weight who have loose sagging skin because of heredity, multiple pregnancies, fluctuations in weight, or significant weight loss. The basic technique includes a horizontal skin incision low on the abdominal wall between the umbilicus and pubic hairline, elevation of the skin and subcutaneous tissue from the deep fascia up to the level of the xiphoid and costal margins, incision around the umbilicus, leaving it attached to the underlying fascia as an isolated island, repairing a diastasis or plicating the muscle fascia, drawing the flap inferiorly under mild tension, excising excess skin and subcutaneous tissue, securing the flap inferiorly to scarpa or deep fascia, creating a new opening in the flap for exteriorization of the umbilicus, and placing multiple drains under the abdominal flap.

In addition to the traditional abdominoplasty, there are several variations. A miniabdominoplasty is a limited abdominoplasty, useful when the excess skin and fat are primarily below the umbilicus. *Fleur-de-lis abdominoplasty* refers to an inverted T type of abdominoplasty, which is useful for individuals with large amounts of excess skin. An umbilical float may be used in conjunction with a miniabdominoplasty to avoid the incision and scarring around the umbilicus. Here, the umbilicus is left attached to the skin, cut loose from the underlying abdominal fascia, and allowed to descend or float toward the pubic area as the skin is tightened. This shortens the distance between the umbilicus and pubic bone, so it is not suitable if the distance will be shortened greatly.

Complications occur in 12% to 32% of abdominoplasty patients, most frequently surgical site infection, hematoma, seroma, marginal skin loss, and minor wound separation.[37] Major complications are reported in 1.4% of cases and include major skin loss, deep vein thrombosis, and pulmonary embolus. Risk factors include diabetes, hypertension, and smoking. Complications are magnified dramatically in obese patients, with reports of complications in 80% of obese patients. Adherence to the guideline that a patient should be at or near his or her ideal BMI results in fewer serious complications and higher patient satisfaction. Preoperative smoking cessation is mandatory.

## Reconstruction of the Perineum

The indications for perineal wound reconstruction have escalated rapidly over the last few years. This is a consequence of more radical surgical resections, in which abdominoperineal resection (APR) may be combined with vaginectomy, sacrectomy, or exenteration of pelvic organs, and of the expanded role for adjuvant radiotherapy in the treatment of rectal cancer. When APR follows chemoradiotherapy, perineal wound complications, including nonhealing wounds, abscess, dehiscence, and fistula, have been reported in 41% of primary perineal wound closures.[38] These complications are caused by the presence of a wide cavity with dead space, poor vascularity of the surrounding tissue, use of irradiated skin in the closure, and bacterial contamination with bowel resection. Musculocutaneous flap reconstruction of a pelvic soft tissue defect introduces well-vascularized nonirradiated tissue with enough bulk to obliterate dead space, brings in a skin paddle for cutaneous wound closure, and provides functional restoration following vaginectomy.

Immediate flap reconstruction has been readily accepted for large perineal defects when the skin cannot be closed primarily or a massive dead space is present. More recently, there has been interest in extending the role of a flap into situations in which a skin paddle is not essential for cutaneous closure of the perineal wound or a large amount of tissue bulk is not needed to fill pelvic dead space. Early results using a musculocutaneous flap to reconstruct irradiated APR defects that could alternatively be closed primarily have shown a reduced incidence of major perineal wound complications. Comparing the outcomes of immediate vertical rectus abdominis musculocutaneous (VRAM) flap reconstruction to outcomes with primary closure in patients with similar irradiated APR defects has shown a fourfold reduction in major perineal wound dehiscence and a 10-fold reduction in perineal abscess formation associated with flap use.[39]

Flap reconstruction is preferably accomplished at the time of the original extirpative procedure, rather than in a delayed manner. Functional issues can be addressed at the same time and, in the pelvic area, typically involves vaginal or penile reconstruction, ideally using the same flap for reparative and functional purposes. Clinical indications for flap reconstruction of the perineum include the following:

- Repair after APR with extensive skin resection
- Repair after APR following chemoradiation of the pelvis to bring in well-vascularized tissue, even when skin is sufficient
- Repair after extended APR with wide tissue resection
- Repair after pelvic exenteration for urologic and gynecologic cancer
- Reconstruction after partial or complete vaginectomy
- Repair of a radical sacrectomy defect
- Repair of the perineum in severe, perianal Crohn's disease

- Neovaginal reconstruction in congenital absence of the vagina
- Repair of postirradiation ulcerated wounds of the perineum
- Pelvic excisions with intraoperative radiation therapy

Commonly used flaps for perineal reconstruction include the rectus abdominis musculocutaneous, gracilis musculocutaneous, posterior thigh fasciocutaneous, and gluteus maximus musculocutaneous flaps. An omental flap is an option in select cases. In the past, thigh-based flaps were regarded as most useful and unilateral or bilateral gracilis musculocutaneous flaps were preferred for many applications. Today, use of an abdominal musculocutaneous flap has become the technique of choice.

A pedicled rectus abdominis flap based inferiorly on the inferior epigastric vessels can be designed with a skin paddle oriented obliquely (Taylor's flap), horizontally (TRAM), or vertically along the muscle (VRAM). This last design, the VRAM, is particularly well suited for perineal reconstruction (Fig. 69-11). The VRAM flap has bulk for filling dead space, adequate length to reach to the perineum and sacrum, reliable blood supply, and consistent anatomy, and can be designed with a large, sturdy skin paddle from 5- to 10-cm wide for perineal skin reconstruction or vaginal reconstruction. In one study of surgical outcomes and complications in patients undergoing immediate reconstruction of the perineum, VRAM flaps performed well, with a 15% rate of major complications versus 42% with thigh flaps.[40] Although harvesting a VRAM flap results in greater tension on the abdominal wall fascial closure, higher rates of abdominal wound separation and incisional hernias have not been reported. Reinforcement of the donor site with synthetic mesh material is helpful, but other options include using a components separation technique to close the abdominal wall on the donor side and the development of perforator flaps to spare the muscle and fascia.[41]

Use of the VRAM requires careful planning, because taking one of the rectus abdominis muscles with the flap has implications for ostomy placement. If one rectus muscle is used, a colostomy can be brought out through the opposite rectus muscle. However, if a second ostomy is required for an ileal conduit for urinary diversion after pelvic exenteration or for colostomy relocation to treat a parastomal hernia, there will be no intact, untouched rectus muscle remaining through which the second ostomy can be placed. This can be addressed by placing the new ostomy through the abdominal wall on the flap donor side, lateral to the empty rectus sheath. This is successful in some series, but others have found it problematic, with localized wound infections, abdominal wound dehiscence, and malposition of the associated stoma.[42]

There may be situations encountered that limit the use of a VRAM flap. These include situations in which the rectus

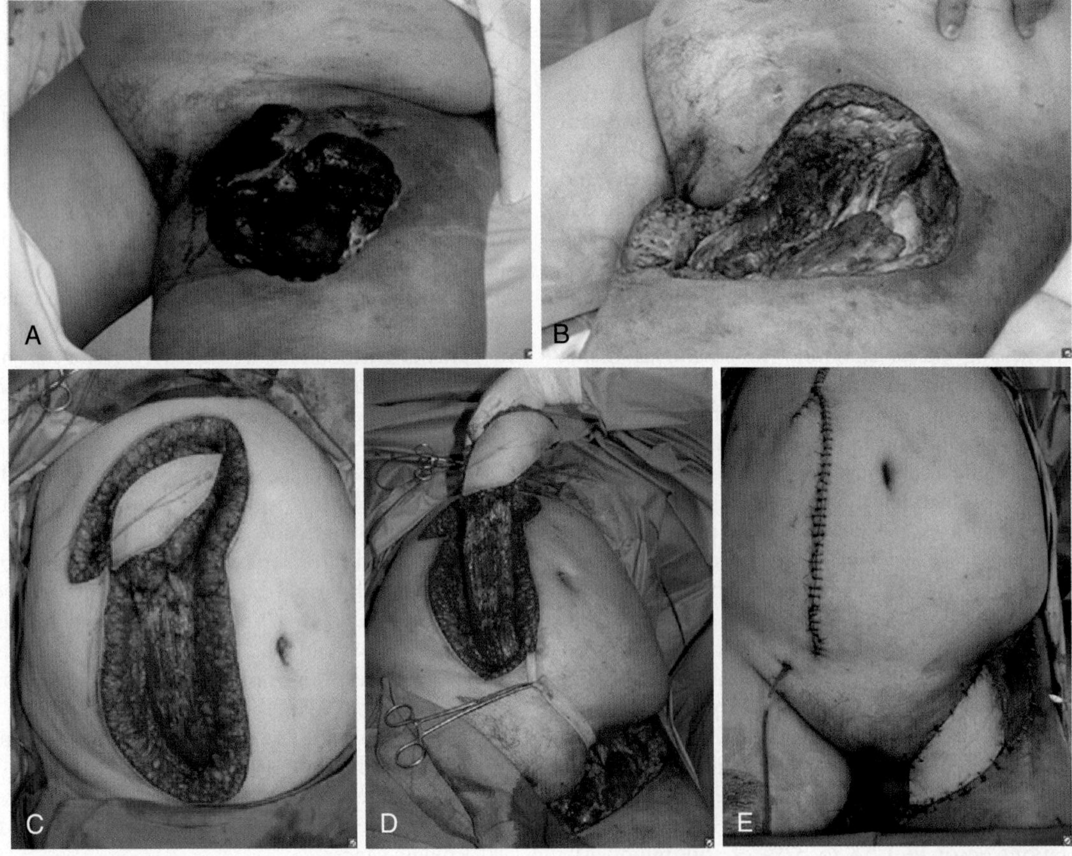


**FIGURE 69-11 A, B,** Extensive recurrent melanoma in the groin of a patient previously treated with surgery and irradiation. Resection of the tumor left a large defect with exposed femoral vessels. **C,** An obliquely oriented VRAM flap is elevated on the contralateral side of the abdomen. **D, E,** The flap is passed through a subcutaneous tunnel into the groin and used to cover the femoral triangle. A skin graft is placed on the lateral portion of the groin wound where the fascia lata was intact and there were no exposed neurovascular structures.

muscle or inferior epigastric pedicle has been divided by previous abdominal incisions and scarring, prior elevation of an abdominal flap, as with ventral hernia repair or cosmetic abdominoplasty, and preexisting stomas for fecal and urinary diversion exiting through the rectus muscles. In addition, transfer of the VRAM flap into the pelvis typically requires a laparotomy. Therefore, in cases that can be approached from the perineum alone, a thigh-based flap might be preferable to avoid a transabdominal procedure.

The pedicled gracilis muscle or musculocutaneous flap is a suitable alternative if the need to fill dead space is relatively small. The gracilis muscle originates from the pubis symphysis and inserts on the medial tibial condyle. Its blood supply is from the medial circumflex branch of the profunda femoris vessel and can be found 8 to 10 cm from its origin. This distal location of the dominant vascular pedicle, at the junction of the proximal and middle thirds of the thigh, means a restricted arc of rotation and limits how far the flap can reach onto the perineum and into the pelvis. When gracilis flaps are used for vaginal reconstruction, the depth of the reconstructed vault may be limited. In addition, the skin paddle is smaller and less reliable than the VRAM, and flap-specific complications, with wound healing and flap loss, are significantly higher with the gracilis flap.

Another alternative is the posterior thigh flap, a fasciocutaneous flap based on the descending branch of the inferior gluteal artery. This flap can provide an abundant and reliable amount of soft tissue for transfer from the posterior thigh and, because the vascular pedicle is proximal, the flap can easily reach high into the pelvis. The skin is innervated by the posterior femoral cutaneous nerve (S1-3) so the flap can provide sensate soft tissue for perineal or vaginal reconstruction, although this is dysesthetic in some patients. There is a relatively high rate of wound-healing complications with this flap but it is a suitable choice when other flaps are unavailable or unsuitable for an individual patient.

A pedicled gluteus maximus musculocutaneous flap based on the inferior gluteal artery has application for some anorectal wounds but will not reach deep into the pelvis. Similarly, flaps of the greater omentum can protect abdominal contents and reach the sacrum, but do not provide vascularized skin for tension-free perineal wound closure. However, both these flaps have been shown to improve perineal healing in certain settings. This highlights the importance of preoperative planning for flap selection in clinical practice. Flap choice depends on previous scars, where new incisions will be made, planned location of stomas, vascular patency, and availability of donor sites. Whichever flap is preferred, comparative studies have shown that immediate reconstruction can result in significant improvements in wound healing after radical perineal surgery.

## Surgery of Back Defects

Posterior trunk defects result from traumatic wounds, defects following oncologic resection, with or without radiation necrosis, wound breakdown or infection following spinal surgery, with or without exposed orthopedic hardware, and congenital deformities (e.g., spina bifida with myelomeningocele). Posterior trunk reconstruction must provide coverage for exposed major neurovascular structures, coverage for exposed bone and skeletal prostheses, and stable soft tissue to obliterate dead space, protect dura, control infection, and permit tension-free wound closure. To meet these needs, reconstruction generally involves muscle or musculocutaneous flaps to provide bulky, durable, well-vascularized tissue. Depth and location are the two wound parameters that determine flap selection. Deep wounds of the spine can be repaired with paraspinal muscle flaps, whereas more superficial wounds are treated with surface muscle flaps. The length of the back means that various regional muscle units can treat different areas of the posterior trunk.

Preparation for surgical coverage depends on the pathogenesis of the defect. Although exposed meninges must be covered promptly, necrotic or infected tissue may require débridement over time, treatment with antibiotic-impregnated materials for exposed hardware, and negative-pressure wound therapy to promote granulation tissue. As spine surgery has become more sophisticated, the need has grown for immediate, complex, soft tissue coverage and for strategies for salvage of postoperative complications. Techniques for covering the spine, exposed dura, and any exposed implants rely on mobilization, advancement, and midline closure of the bilateral paraspinous muscles that run the length of the vertebral column deep to the thoracolumbar fascia. This is done as a precautionary measure in patients with multiple previous operations, radiation, attenuated skin, or stiff, heavily scarred soft tissue.

Conceptually, the posterior trunk is divided into upper, middle, and lower thirds. Each has muscle flap options that are best suited for that part of the posterior trunk. Posterior cervical and upper back defects are reconstructed with the pedicled trapezius muscle or musculocutaneous flap, or with the dorsal scapular artery perforator flap (Fig. 69-12). The trapezius flap is reliable, versatile, and can include a large skin paddle. It is based on the transverse cervical artery, which has two major branches. The trapezius thus offers two separate muscular territories; the lower portion of the muscle can be elevated and transposed superiorly to cover the cervical spine. Alternatively, a trapezius turnover flap is an easily elevated, reliable solution for cervicothoracic wounds. For the midback, latissimus dorsi muscle and musculocutaneous flaps can be mobilized on the thoracodorsal branch of the subscapular vessels to be rotated for broad, reliable coverage. To extend coverage to the midline further inferiorly, the latissimus flap can be raised as a reverse turnover flap based on secondary segmental intercostal and lumbar artery perforators. The upper portion of the lower third of the back is the most difficult to cover. More inferiorly on the back, the gluteus maximus muscles provide excellent coverage for the sacrum (see later, "Pressure Sores"). However, in the lumbar area, where it is difficult for the more conventional muscle flaps to reach, perforator flaps, latissimus dorsi with a thoracolumbar fasciocutaneous extension, or vein grafting to the thoracodorsal vessels may be required. The pedicled omental flap also is used for the coverage of lumbar defects. The omentum can be transferred, based on the right or left gastroepiploic artery, by dividing attachments to the transverse colon, ligating one gastroepiploic artery, mobilizing the omentum off the greater curvature of the stomach, and passing it through the retroperitoneum and lumbar fascia to cover the spinal column while the back wound is closed with cutaneous advancement flaps.[43]

With partial or total sacrectomy, extensive soft tissue defects are created by oncologic ablation for chordoma, osteogenic sarcoma, or extension of pelvic carcinoma (Fig. 69-13). An anterior and posterior approach is generally used for resection of the tumor, which creates a large communication between the abdominal cavity and gluteal area. These ablations often

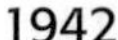



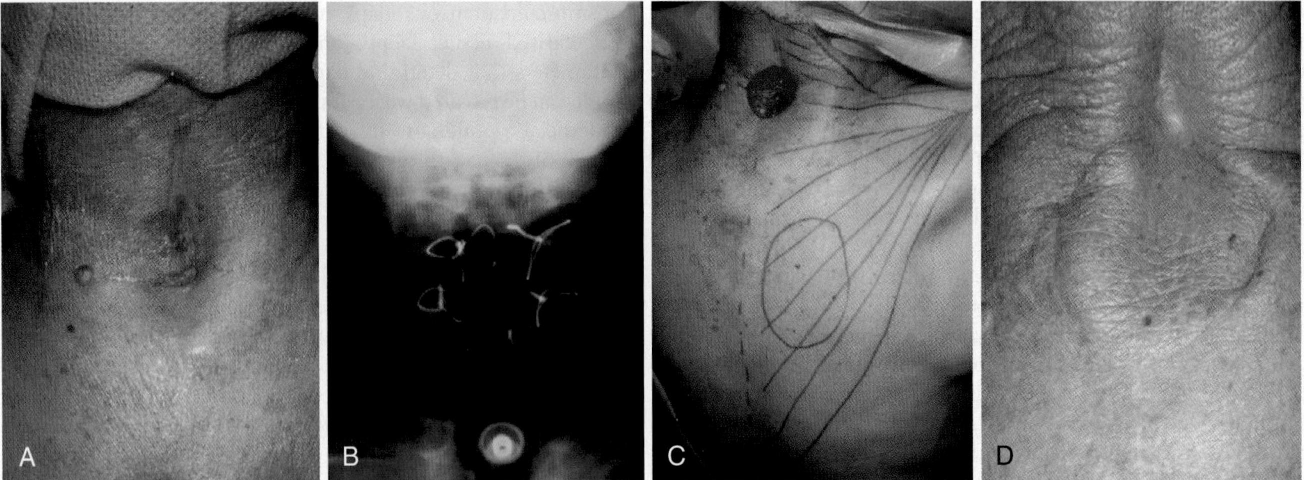

**FIGURE 69-12 A,** Posterior neck with a chronic open wound, with exposed bone and unstable surrounding soft tissue. **B,** Radiographs show surgical hardware in the cervical vertebrae. **C,** The defect is débrided back to healthy margins and the skin paddle on the posterior trapezius musculocutaneous flap is planned. **D,** Postoperative view at 6 months with the healed flap in place. The donor site for the flap was closed primarily.

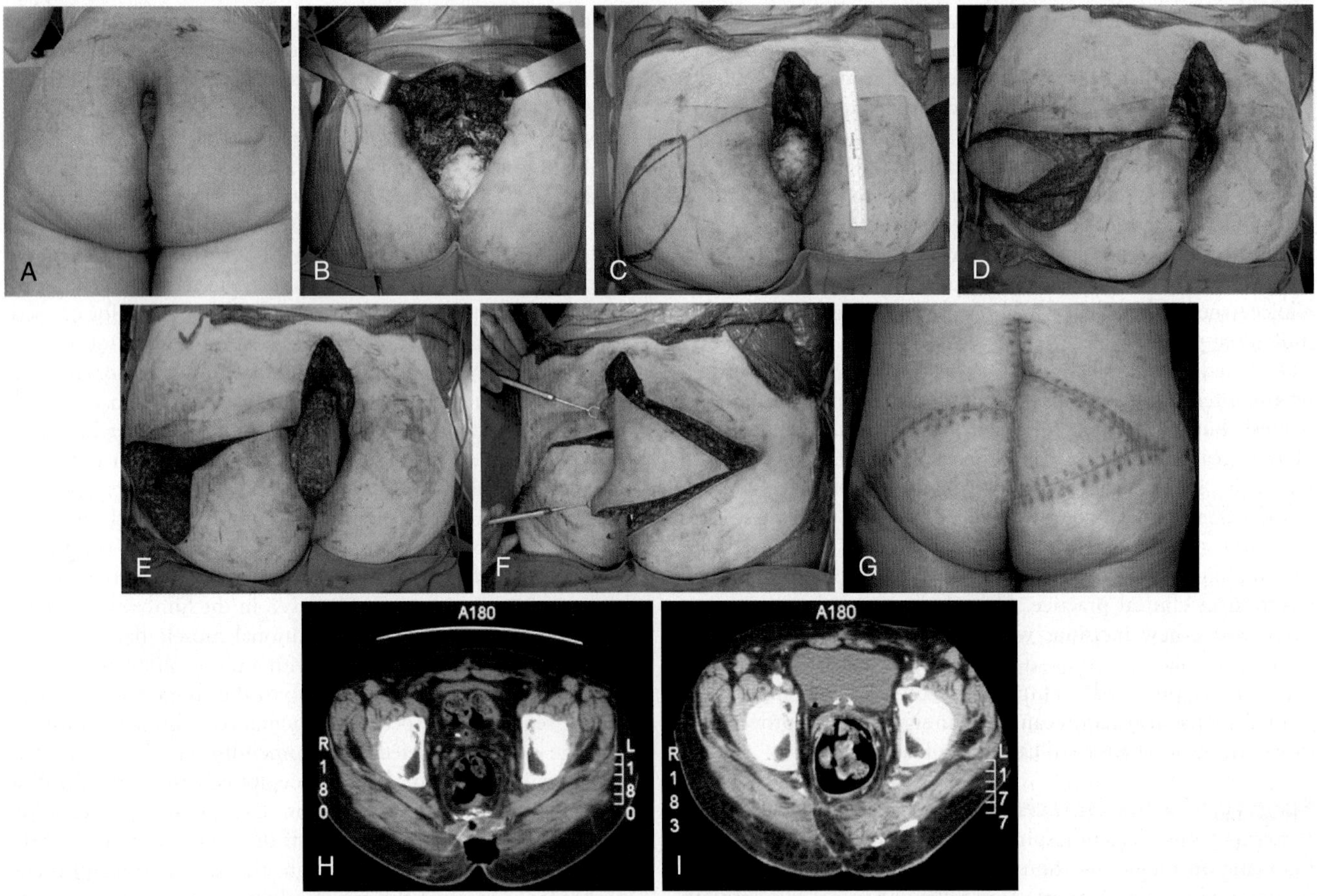

**FIGURE 69-13** Patient with metastatic tumor involving the sacrum. **A,** Preoperative view showing the tumor. **B,** Large soft tissue and bone defect after resection of the tumor and inferior portion of the sacrum. A sponge is present at the base of the wound. Reconstruction required obliteration of the large dead space created by the tumor resection and durable closure of the superficial wound. **C-E,** A musculocutaneous gluteal island flap is designed based on the inferior portion of the left gluteus maximus muscle. The skin is deepithelialized and the flap rotated into the defect to fill the resection cavity. **F,** V-Y fasciocutaneous flap is designed over the right buttock and advanced to close the wound. **G,** Postoperative views show a stable healed wound. **H,** Preoperative CT scan. **I,** Postoperative CT scan showing the buried gluteal island flap that is providing soft tissue bulk.

require large amounts of hardware for bony repair by the orthopedic surgeon; the hypogastric and gluteal vessels are divided during resection, which eliminates the use of potential local back flaps for repair. Successful reconstruction in these cases calls for well-vascularized tissue to fill the defect, cover the orthopedic appliances, close the abdominal cavity to prevent herniation, and close the skin on the posterior trunk. Initial efforts with gluteal flaps and omentum and the placement of synthetic mesh to prevent herniation had some usefulness. More recently, an inferiorly based, pedicled VRAM passed transabdominally has proven effective. With no need for mesh, the VRAM has a high success rate, with a low incidence of complications and low morbidity.[44]

### Meningomyelocele

Meningomyelocele is a congenital spinal malformation that results from failure of the neural tube to close during the first month of gestation. The most common of the four types of spina bifida, meningomyelocele is a cystic herniation of the meninges and neural tissue that presents as a defect on the surface of the lumbosacral skin. The open meningomyelocele defect should be closed soon after birth to prevent meningitis and protect the exposed neural structure from desiccation and further damage. Early closure has been shown to be a determinant in the neurosurgical outcome. Approximately 75% of meningomyelocele defects are small enough that soft tissue closure can be achieved by simple undermining of the skin edges and tension-free closure in the midline following dural repair. For defects larger than 5 to 8 cm in diameter, a number of techniques have been described.

The surgical options for closing a meningomyelocele defect include skin grafting, local flaps, musculocutaneous flaps, and fasciocutaneous flaps. Local skin flaps including advancement flaps, bipedicle flaps, transposition flaps, double Z-plasty, bilobed flaps, rhomboid flaps, and V-Y advancement flaps have all been used successfully. For larger defects, latissimus dorsi and gluteus maximus musculocutaneous flaps have been described.[45] For all of these, the first criterion is reliable wound healing so that the defect is closed securely and definitively to avoid CSF leakage and its accompanying morbidity. Also see Chapter 68, "Neurosurgery: Pediatric Neurosurgery."

## PRESSURE SORES

Prolonged weight bearing, as in an immobilized or paralyzed patient, can elevate tissue pressure above arterial capillary perfusion pressure (32 mm Hg) and result in compromised oxygenation, ischemia, and eventual tissue necrosis. In models of ischemia, external pressure higher than 60 mm Hg for 2 hours leads to irreversible tissue damage, and clinical studies have confirmed this. The clinical sequelae of this damage are pressure sores with ulceration, infection, and exposure of bone. In order of occurrence, the surfaces most commonly involved are those over the sacrum, calcaneus, ischium, and greater trochanter.

Extrinsic and intrinsic factors contribute to the pathogenesis of pressure ulcers. Extrinsic factors include unrelieved pressure seen in debilitated or spinal cord injury patients and factors that worsen the local wound environment, such as moisture in the perineal area, incontinence, and shearing forces from patient repositioning. Intrinsic factors include underlying conditions that lead to poor wound healing, such as advanced age, diabetes, malnutrition, and edema. The Braden Scale for Predicting Pressure Sore Risk is a widely used nursing assessment tool to help predict patients' risk of developing pressure sores. Although there is no clear evidence that using risk assessment scales decreases the incidence of pressure ulcers, the Braden scale has reasonable predictive capacity, with high interrater reliability. This scale accounts for several extrinsic and intrinsic causative factors by scoring six subscales—sensory perception, moisture, activity, mobility, nutrition, and friction and shear.

### Stages of Pressure Ulcers

The National Pressure Ulcer Advisory Panel has defined the stages of pressure ulcers, including an original four stages and adding two stages in 2007:

- Stage I: Skin intact but reddened for longer than 1 hour after relief of pressure: This stage represents intact skin with various degrees of erythema that does not blanch when compressed. This wound is potentially reversible if extrinsic forces and intrinsic wound-healing factors are optimized.
- Stage II: Blister or other break in the dermis with or without infection. Here, the skin has broken down, with a partial-thickness loss of dermis. By maintaining coverage over the wound, these wounds often can generate granulation tissue and undergo wound contraction to heal by secondary intention. Because there is violation of skin, the local environment must be monitored carefully for moisture and soiling to allow this stage to heal. Stages I and II pressure ulcers are the most prevalent.
- Stage III: Full-thickness tissue loss with visible subcutaneous fat but no exposed bone, tendon, or muscle: In the absence of bone exposure, these sores can heal and contract over a bony prominence. However, this is usually a temporally brief stage because muscle is the most oxygen-sensitive tissue and is most sensitive to ischemic necrosis, quickly reaching the final stage of exposed bone.
- Stage IV: Exposed bone, joint, muscle or tendon, with or without infection, often including undermining and tunneling: This is the most common stage that prompts a surgical consultation, because the ulcer is down to the causative bony prominence.

### Suspected Deep Tissue Injury

Purple or maroon localized area of discolored intact skin or blood-filled blister caused by damage of underlying soft tissue from pressure and/or shear: This stage identifies clinically suspicious deep tissue injury.

### Unstageable

Full-thickness tissue loss in which the base of the ulcer is covered by slough (yellow, tan, gray, green, or brown) and/or eschar (tan, brown, or black) in the wound bed: Until enough slough or eschar is removed to expose the base of the wound, the true depth and stage cannot be determined.

Swab cultures of the surface of a pressure sore invariably are positive because of local contamination, so cultures must be taken from biopsies of soft tissue and bone deep to the surface. Infections generally are polymicrobial with *Proteus, Bacteroides, Pseudomonas,* and *Escherichia coli* accompanying staphylococcal and streptococcal species. More than 50% of long-term care patients harbor methicillin-resistant *Staphylococcus aureus* (MRSA) organisms. In stage IV pressure ulcers with bone exposure, the desiccation and bacterial colonization of the surface of the bone is termed *osteitis.* If the deep bone has good blood supply and the patient is not immunocompromised, the bony inflammation of osteitis can be tolerated for protracted periods as long as wound care can contain the zone of injury. Osteomyelitis is infection of the bone requiring long-term systemic antibiotics; definitive diagnosis is made with bone biopsy and bacterial culture. Imaging modalities to diagnose osteomyelitis include radiography, tagged white blood cell scans, and MRI. Appropriate imaging is useful to evaluate the extent of bone involvement and to identify the source of infection in pressure sores associated with perianal fistulas or spinal hardware abscesses.

The management of a pressure sore starts with the correction of causative factors. Surgical interventions will not heal and the sores will recur unless the cause is addressed with pressure-relieving cushions and beds, relief of spasticity, correction of joint contractures, incontinence aids, nutritional support, and infection control.[46] Surgical treatment involves drainage of collections, wide débridement of devitalized and scarred soft tissue, excision of sinus tracts and the bursa-like lining of the chronic wound, ostectomy of involved bone, hemostasis with suction drainage, and obliteration of all residual dead space with well-vascularized tissue introduced to cover bone, provide padding, and close the open wound without tension.

Intraoperative débridement of superficial bone is carried out by visual assessment of avascular bone versus bleeding bone. Using rongeurs and rasps to smooth jutting prominences or excise heterotopic bone accomplishes the second purpose of bone resection, reducing the physical prominence of bone that causes pressure and predisposes to recurrence of the sore. After adequate bone débridement, a biopsy of the deeper, healthy-appearing bone is sent for bone culture. If positive, the remaining bone is still infected and the patient will need a long-term course of IV antibiotics to treat the osteomyelitis. Bone resection must be approached thoughtfully because resecting one of a paired set of pressure points, such as the ischia, shifts the patient's weight to the contralateral side, increasing the risk of a new pressure sore on the second side.

Reconstruction with a flap is necessary for most pressure sores because less complex options such as primary closure or skin grafting have limited usefulness. Primary closure places the surgical suture line directly over the area of pressure, whereas a flap shifts the closure and scar away from the pressure point. A skin graft is a thin and fragile coverage option, subject to the shearing forces that created the ulcer in the first place. In addition, a skin graft requires a clean, healthy recipient site, with good blood supply and no exposed bone. Only the most superficial of pressure sores meets these requirements for a base that can be covered successfully with a skin graft. Transferring healthy tissue with its own blood supply to fill the pressure sore can be accomplished with cutaneous, fasciocutaneous, musculocutaneous, muscle-only, and free microvascular flaps.

Sacral pressure sores develop in supine or semireclining patients and, because of the broad pointed shape of the sacrum and thinness of the overlying soft tissue, most ulcers have exposed bone. The soft tissues surrounding the sacrum receive their blood supply from perforators from the superior and inferior gluteal arteries, which are also the arteries supplying the gluteus maximus muscle. This muscle extends and rotates the thigh laterally and is required for ambulation, so the gluteus maximus is not considered expendable except in the spinal cord injury patient. However, the gluteus maximus can survive on either vascular pedicle alone and using only the superior or inferior half of the muscle will preserve function. Muscle or musculocutaneous flaps of the superior half of the muscle are constructed and moved in two primary ways, a rotational flap or V-Y advancement flap. A rotational flap can be an advancement or with a musculocutaneous skin island. The V-Y advancement technique involves creating a triangular-shaped skin island over the muscle, with one side being the defect and the other two sides forming a V. The central V is shifted into the open wound and the defect is closed in a Y configuration. To get extended coverage of the sacrum, bilateral V-Y advancement flaps can be used, one based on the right and one based on the left gluteal area.

The ischial tuberosities are under high pressure in a seated patient. Unilateral or bilateral ischial sores develop in individuals who are seated for protracted periods of time without adjusting their position and weight distribution. Ischial ulcers are challenging for several reasons. The pressure points are bilateral, which means that unweighting one side for pressure-reducing purposes shifts increased pressure onto the contralateral ischium. Resecting bone on both sides runs the risk of shifting weight bearing onto the perineal soft tissues, which can cause later scrotal or urethral sores. There can be fistulas involving the rectum or urethra; these may require diversion and control before addressing the ischial ulcers. Finally, because of the strong hip flexors, there can be flexion contractures with varying degrees of deformity, which reduce mobility and the capacity for normal weight distribution in the sitting or lying position. Because the ischium has a number of surrounding muscles, various flaps suitable for coverage have been described. These include the inferior gluteus maximus rotational, inferior gluteal fasciocutaneous thigh, V-Y hamstring advancement, gracilis muscle, tensor fascia lata rotational, and rectus abdominis rotational flaps.

Because of the mobility of the hip, pressure sores over the greater trochanter characteristically have extensive bursa formation with smaller areas of skin loss. After resection of the trochanter, flaps available for the repair of trochanteric pressure sores include local fasciocutaneous rotational, tensor fascia lata musculocutaneous, inferior gluteal thigh fasciocutaneous, and muscle flaps incorporating the vastus lateralis, rectus femoris, or rectus abdominis muscles.

On the feet, pressure sores can present over the heels, malleoli, and plantar surfaces. Unlike other pressure sores, foot ulcers lack a thick subcutaneous layer, are often modest in size and depth, and may respond favorably to conservative treatment. Stable (dry, adherent, intact, without erythema or fluctuance) eschar on the heels acts as a biologic dressing and need not be removed. In non–weight-bearing areas requiring a less durable surface, pressure sores may be treated conservatively because a scar left by wound contraction and epithelialization may suffice. For larger wounds, débridement and STSG may be useful. If the ulceration involves a large portion of the weight-bearing surface or if osteomyelitis of the calcaneus is present, débridement of devitalized bone with flap coverage is needed. Muscle flaps of the abductor digiti minimi, abductor hallucis, and flexor digitorum brevis have been described. Fasciocutaneous flaps based on the dorsalis pedis, medial plantar, and lateral plantar arteries can also provide coverage.

Postoperative protocols call for 2 to 6 weeks of strict pressure precautions because a newly transferred flap is vulnerable to pressure necrosis. When weight bearing is resumed in the area of the previous pressure sore, the transition is planned with progressive increases in time each day and frequent wound checks.

## RECONSTRUCTION OF THE LOWER EXTREMITY

The goal of lower extremity reconstruction is restoration or maintenance of function. For functionality, there must be a stable skeleton to support weight, muscle to power motion and joint movement, neural supply for proprioception and plantar sensibility, blood supply to sustain the underlying structures, and soft tissue to provide a stable skin envelope. Based on these needs, reconstruction may be needed for open fractures, defects from sarcoma resections, radiation wounds, chronic traumatic wounds of the distal third of the leg, diabetic ulcers, venous ulcers, osteomyelitis of the tibia, unstable scars, and infected vascular grafts. Many reconstructions are complex because they need to contribute more than one element, such as vascularized bone grafts or composite flaps with sensory potential, and many require a multidisciplinary surgical team.

### Soft Tissue Coverage of Traumatic Wounds

The loss of soft tissue cover over a fracture, particularly when interrupted endosteal blood supply is combined with periosteal damage, demands coverage of the exposed bone with vascularized tissue after thorough débridement of devitalized tissue. Determinants of outcome after open fractures are wound size, degree of soft tissue injury, and amount of contamination. The Gustilo classification system is used to categorize open fractures of the leg into subtypes predictive of prognosis:

- Gustilo I: Open fractures with wound <1 cm
- Gustilo II: Open fractures with wound 1-10 cm with moderate tissue damage
- Gustilo III: Open fractures with wound >10 cm and extensive tissue damage making it difficult to cover bone or hardware
  - Gustilo IIIA: Adequate soft tissue coverage of bone with extensive soft tissue laceration or flaps
  - Gustilo IIIB: Inadequate soft tissue with periosteal stripping and bone exposure
  - Gustilo IIIC: As above, with vascular injury and ischemia requiring repair

Gustilo grade I, and most grade II fractures, can be closed primarily after débridement and orthopedic fixation are applied. However, larger grade II and most grade III fractures require advanced reconstructive techniques. When flap coverage is required, it can be done at the time of fracture stabilization or as a secondary procedure. Early coverage of exposed bone, tendons, and neurovascular structures decreases the risk of infection, osteomyelitis, nonunion, and ongoing tissue loss. Although the advantages of radical débridement and early wound closure have been accepted, the definition of the duration of the early phase varies. Earlier bone healing and reduced infection rates have been demonstrated if coverage is completed within 72 hours of fracture stabilization; others have shown comparable results when the wounds are closed within the first 6 days after injury. Early reconstruction may be precluded by other patient injuries or when severely contaminated wounds require serial débridements before delayed reconstruction.[47]

For many years, muscle flaps have been the choice for traumatic lower limb defects. The gastrocnemius or soleus are accessible as local flaps to cover the upper and middle thirds of the leg, and smaller muscles such as the tibialis anterior, extensor digitorum longus, and peroneus brevis can be used for more distal small defects. For larger defects of the distal third of the leg, ankle, and foot, microvascular free tissue transfers of muscles such as the latissimus dorsi, gracilis, serratus anterior, or rectus abdominis are preferred. These free tissue transfers provide more bulk, have longer pedicles for greater flexibility in positioning, and are not dependent on blood supply within the injured area. Most series of lower extremity reconstructions have reported flap failure rates just below 10%. This is higher than at other sites on the body because of associated vascular injuries and preexisting vascular disease in these patients.

More recently, novel wound technologies, combined with growing experience with local fasciocutaneous flaps, are creating new options for reconstruction. Use of the vacuum-assisted closure device reduces edema, decreases wound area, and stimulates granulation tissue, making it possible in some cases to close previously large wounds with local or regional flaps. Fasciocutaneous flaps can cover small to moderate-sized defects, and use of the reverse sural, perforator, and bipedicle flaps is decreasing the need for free microvascular transfers. Clinical advantages of this shift from free flaps to a wider use of skin grafts and local flaps include shorter operations in the trauma patient and elimination of the need for anastomosis to a major leg artery, which may not be available in some traumatic cases.

In injuries with bone loss and a soft tissue defect, the options for skeletal reconstruction include autogenous bone grafts, vascularized bone transfer (pedicle or free), and the Iliazarov technique for osteosynthesis. Bone grafts generally are delayed for approximately 6 weeks after soft tissue reconstruction while orthopedic hardware holds the fracture fragments at length across the gap. The size and location of the bone defect will determine bone graft technique, with a vascularized procedure preferred for larger losses. An alternative to delayed bone grafting is immediate one-stage reconstruction of the bone and soft tissue with an osteocutaneous free tissue transfer.

There are contraindications to salvage of a Gustilo grade IIIC injury of the lower extremity. The most important element when considering primary amputation is disruption of the sciatic or posterior tibial nerve. With laceration of the posterior tibial nerve, the plantar surface is insensate, which results predictably in recurrent ulceration, infection, and osteomyelitis. Other elements include severe infection or contamination, tibial bone loss more than 8 cm, multilevel severe injury, ischemia time longer than 6 hours, and preexisting severe medical illness. There are several scoring systems to assist making a decision about limb salvage versus amputation but these tend to identify patients with good potential for salvage rather than those who will need eventual amputation. The Mangled Extremity Severity Score (MESS) is used widely but should not be the sole criterion on which an amputation decision is made.[48] Replantation of a severed lower limb is rarely done in the adult because of the inability to restore neurologic function to the foot. A nonfunctional or marginally functional lower extremity is a greater liability than a prosthetic limb capable of allowing high-level function. Absolute contraindications to replantation are older age, poor baseline health, multilevel injury that results in immobility of the knee or ankle, and warm ischemia time longer than 6 hours.

## Soft Tissue Reconstruction in the Groin and Thigh

The groin is the most common site of distal extremity prosthetic graft infections. Traditional treatment included removal of the graft material or a salvage attempt at graft preservation with secondary intention healing and its attendant risks of thrombosis, superinfection, and anastomotic disruption. Today, muscle flaps are the mainstay for managing vascular graft infections. Healthy muscle increases tissue oxygen tension in the wound, augments the delivery of antibiotics to the site, and eliminates dead space. Muscle flaps are useful to aid graft salvage in the presence of established infection, when there is increased dead space after drainage of a seroma or hematoma, or in situations in which the tissue bed is compromised by previous surgeries and scarring.

Several muscle flaps are useful for coverage of the femoral vessels. The sartorius muscle is used as first-line treatment because of its proximity, expendability, and relative ease of elevation. The muscle originates on the anterior superior iliac spine, inserts at the medial tibial condyle, and has a segmental blood supply with five to six direct branches from the superficial femoral artery. The muscle is mobilized by dividing the origin and two proximal vascular pedicles, which frees the proximal end of the muscle to be transposed medially and sutured to the inguinal ligament to provide vascularized muscle coverage of the femoral vessels. Disadvantages of the sartorius flap are that it is divided by some surgical incisions in the groin, and that division of more than two adjacent pedicles results in devascularization of the muscle. Another local flap option is the rectus femoris muscle; distant pedicled muscle flaps for groin coverage are the gracilis and rectus abdominis.

Defects after oncologic surgery in the thigh and groin are distinctive because extirpation of lower extremity tumors, typically sarcomas, often necessitates wide or radical margins combined with adjuvant radiation therapy. There is a higher incidence of infection and dehiscence after limb-sparing surgery in the thigh and groin than in more distal parts of the lower extremity because of greater dead space, exposure of neurovascular structures, difficulty keeping the wound clean and dry, and tension with ambulation and hip abduction. For these larger irradiated defects, flap reconstruction is necessary. There are a number of thigh muscles that can be used as a local flap, with or without skin grafts or a skin paddle; these include gracilis, tensor fascia lata, and vastus lateralis flaps. Fasciocutaneous flaps such as the medial thigh, lateral posterior thigh, and anterior lateral thigh are also available. In some cases, these local options are no longer useful because of inclusion in the field of radiation, so distant or free flaps are needed for coverage. Reported outcomes after reconstruction of these difficult wounds with a VRAM flap have been promising, with a 9.4% incidence of postoperative wound complications with immediate reconstruction but a significantly higher incidence of 47% in patients with delayed reconstruction.[49]

## Soft Tissue Coverage of the Knee, Leg, and Foot

Wounds around the knee can result from trauma, tumor extirpation, or exposure of an infected knee endoprosthesis after total knee replacement (Fig. 69-14). For each of these defects, durable soft tissue coverage is required; a pedicled medial gastrocnemius muscle or musculocutaneous flap based on the medial sural artery is preferred for genicular soft tissue reconstruction. The gastrocnemius muscle has a medial head and lateral head originating from the medial and lateral condyles of the femur, respectively; the two heads share a common insertion on the calcaneus via the Achilles tendon. As a result, one head can be detached from the Achilles tendon independently and transposed with its robust blood supply and vascular drainage without impairing foot dorsiflexion. Because the medial head is longer, it is preferred for knee wounds and can be transposed with or without a skin paddle. In situations in which a pedicled gastrocnemius flap has failed or is unavailable, free tissue transfer of a latissimus dorsi or rectus abdominis muscle flap has led to a high rate of salvage of limbs and knee prostheses.

Options for soft tissue coverage of the leg are determined by the position of the defect relative to the tibia:

- Proximal tibia: Medial gastrocnemius, lateral gastrocnemius, fasciocutaneous flap
- Middle tibia: Soleus, gastrocnemius, extensor digitorum longus, tibialis anterior, fasciocutaneous flap
- Distal tibia: Peroneus brevis, extensor brevis, distal-based soleus, reverse sural artery flap, lateral supramalleolar flap, dorsalis pedis fasciocutaneous flap, free flap
- Foot: Flexor digitorum brevis, abductor hallucis, abductor digiti minimi, reverse sural flap, medial plantar artery flap, lateral calcaneal artery flap, V-Y advancement, free flap

Muscle flaps are often unreliable in treating distal third leg wounds. Except for the soleus and gastrocnemius muscles, local muscles on the lower leg are only adequate to cover small defects. This, along with several other factors, means that treatment of the distal tibia, ankle, and foot is difficult. The area is vulnerable to injury because the distal portion of the leg has poor skin elasticity, bone lying in the subcutaneous space, and may be edematous. The distal third of the leg has little muscle but many tendinous structures, and they support skin grafts poorly. Finally, the foot and ankle require especially durable integument because they are exposed continually to friction and shear with walking and footwear. Any transferred flap may slip or slide at the interface with the underlying structures because the transferred tissue lacks the glabrous quality of the native plantar skin. If the transferred tissue is insensate, it will be at significant risk for eventual breakdown.

For larger defects, reconstruction in the distal third of the leg relies on free tissue transfer techniques. The vascular status of the extremity and recipient vessel selection are key factors for success. Guidelines for the use of free flaps in the lower extremity include making anastomoses to healthy recipient vessels outside the zone of injury and using end-to-side arterial anastomoses, whereas venous anastomoses can be end-to-side or end-to-end. Free tissue transfer remains the best option for large defects, wounds with trauma (e.g., crush injury to the surrounding vicinity that damages blood supply to all local tissues), and when the transfer of vascularized bone with the free flap is desirable. Free fibula flaps with skin paddles are preferred for lower extremity wounds with bony and soft tissue deficits.

More recently, the advent of local fasciocutaneous flaps has begun to change the treatment of difficult lower leg wounds. Recognition that the vascular plexus accompanying cutaneous sensory nerves can supply overlying skin and soft tissue has allowed the development of many useful, axial pattern fasciocutaneous flaps.[50] Currently, one of the most versatile of these is the distally based, or reverse, sural fasciocutaneous flap. One to three arteries accompany the sural nerve as it travels

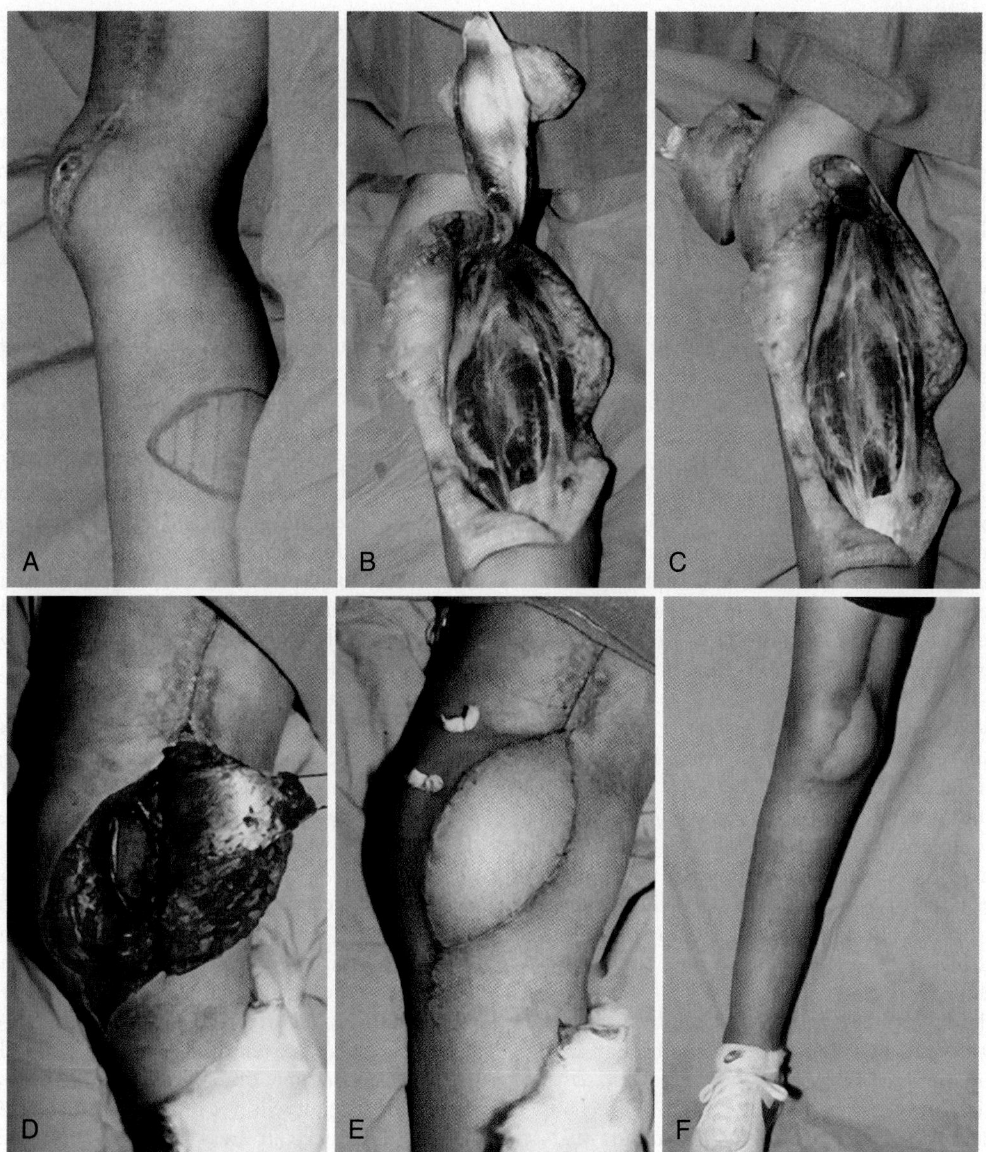


**FIGURE 69-14** Gastrocnemius musculocutaneous flap for repair of an open wound with an exposed prosthesis after total knee replacement. **A,** Soft tissue defect and planned incision of the skin paddle over the medial gastrocnemius muscle. **B,** The muscle with its attached skin paddle is elevated. **C,** The flap is tunneled under an intact bridge of skin into the defect anteriorly. **D,** The muscle flap is placed directly over the knee prosthesis after débridement. **E,** The skin paddle is sutured in place to close the wound without tension. **F,** Postoperative result. The flap provides stable wound coverage.

subcutaneously in the posterior calf. A skin paddle as large as 14 cm in diameter can be elevated on the proximal posterior calf as part of a distally based sural nerve flap; this tissue may be transposed to cover distal leg and foot wounds. Because the sural nerve flap is supported by perforators from the peroneal artery, the patency of this vessel must be ensured for flap success.

## BODY CONTOURING

### Following Bariatric Surgery

With the advent of bariatric surgery and successful treatment of severe obesity, a new deformity has emerged. After massive weight loss, the patient is left with excess skin and subcutaneous tissue that fails to retract and hangs from the torso, abdomen, and extremities. More than a cosmetic issue, this extreme skin redundancy can be painful, limits mobility, and is susceptible to recurrent infection in the intertriginous areas hooded by overhanging tissue. Patients seek body contouring surgery because many are deeply distressed by their appearance. These patients should be no less than 12 to 18 months post–bariatric surgery, stable in weight for 3 to 4 months, have a BMI less than 30, and be well-nourished, with no protein or vitamin deficiencies. Proceeding before these criteria are met can result in recurrent skin laxity and delayed wound healing, and may be inconsistent with the patient's health insurer's requirements.

Postbariatric body contouring is different from similar procedures in those who have not been obese. The postbariatric deformity is more severe because the skin damage and associated loss of tone and elasticity do not recover, and the laxity is global. A number of procedures may be required; some of these involve restoring volume to areas of deficiency, rather than removing tissue. When surgery is done in multiple stages, the procedures are separated by 4 to 6 months to optimize wound healing. The procedures are lengthy and deep vein thrombosis (DVT) prophylaxis is required. Abdominal wall hernias, particularly at surgical port sites, are found frequently and are repaired during the course of abdominal contouring. Except for large ventral hernias, these repairs are accomplished easily because the fascia can be approximated readily after massive weight loss. Various techniques are used for contouring:

- Panniculectomy is removal of excess skin and soft tissue from the abdominal wall without umbilical transposition. It is limited to removal of the overhanging pannus without mobilizing surrounding soft tissue.
- Abdominoplasty includes panniculectomy with wide undermining of the upper abdominal flap and umbilical transposition. Unlike a traditional abdominoplasty, a vertical ellipse, or fleur-de-lis, pattern of excision often is necessary to remove significant excess skin in the horizontal dimension superior to the umbilicus.
- Reverse abdominoplasty uses incisions in the inframammary crease to remove rolls of excess skin from the upper quadrants of the abdomen.
- Belt lipectomy is also termed a *lower body lift;* it corrects the circumferential roll of excess tissue found in most patients by extending the abdominal resection around the sides of the abdomen to include the lower back. In the course of resecting this circumferential ring of tissue, the lateral thighs and buttocks are also lifted.
- An upper body lift removes excess skin from the lateral sides of the chest and upper back through a horizontal incision across the back.
- A medial thigh lift is excision of a long ellipse of excess tissue parallel to the long axis of the thigh to remove hanging skin on the inner thigh.
- A mastopexy is a breast lift for ptosis. No breast tissue is removed because the volume of breast tissue may be small in the drooping, deflated, pancake breast after massive weight loss. The breast skin is resected as the breast is reshaped and the nipple-areolar complex is elevated and centralized. In some cases, augmentation with breast implants is done to restore volume. Alternatively, excess folds of skin under the arms can be deepithelialized and rotated anteriorly to augment the volume of the breast.
- Male mastopexy removes excess drooping skin to reduce fullness, with superior elevation of the nipple-areolar complex as a flap or with free nipple grafting.
- Brachioplasty is the excision of a long ellipse of excess tissue parallel to the long axis of the arm to correct the excess skin, or "bat wing," hanging from the proximal half of the arm.
- A minibrachioplasty excises an ellipse of tissue just distal to the axilla perpendicular to the long axis of the arm to remove a mild excess of tissue. The scar is placed in the axilla.

Postbariatric body contouring is a component in the treatment of the obese patient and is well accepted by patients, despite the extensive scarring with all of the surgical procedures. There is evidence that postbariatric surgery patients who have subsequent body contouring surgery maintain their weight loss. This could merely be a reflection of the motivation of this cohort of patients, but ongoing work is focused on better understanding of the psychological impact of extreme body contouring.

## Suction-Assisted Lipectomy

Suction-assisted lipectomy, also termed *liposuction, lipoplasty,* or *liposculpture,* was introduced in the late 1970s and early 1980s when plastic surgeons developed the concept of inserting a blunt-ended hollow cannula under the skin and connecting it to a vacuum pump, which generates negative pressure to aspirate the fatty tissue. Before making a small opening in the skin to introduce the cannula, the area to be treated is injected with a wetting solution, which is saline supplemented with local anesthetic and low concentrations of epinephrine. Terms used to describe variations in this fluid infiltrate are based on the amount of fluid used; these are *dry, wet, superwet,* and *tumescent.* Although the more generous use of saline, lidocaine, and epinephrine results in less blood loss, greater ease of fat removal, and decreased postoperative pain, it also raises concerns about fluid overload and drug toxicity, which call for close intraoperative monitoring of ventilation, circulation, and cardiac function.

The areas usually treated with liposuction are the neck, abdomen and waist, back, and hips and thighs. Good results can be obtained provided the volume of fat is not too great and there is good skin elasticity. Large-volume liposuction is associated with hemodynamic instability and a risk of damaging the blood supply to the overlying skin, causing skin necrosis. Elastic rebound of the skin after the underlying fat is removed is essential to the success of liposuction. In general, even when large amounts of fat are removed, skin has good elasticity and will conform to the new underlying volume. However, skin that is flaccid or sagging will not retract and therefore good results are harder to achieve in areas such as the face, arms, and inner thighs. The looseness of the skin and likelihood that it will exhibit poor adaptability means that liposuction will exacerbate the drooping and leave significant surface irregularities.

Suction-assisted lipectomy is a useful surgical treatment for several medical disorders. It is a treatment of choice for gynecomastia when combined, as needed, with resection of any glandular tissue. The skin of the chest wall tends to retract well and liposuction is particularly useful for tapering the boundaries of the treated area for a smooth contour. Liposuction alone is less often useful to reduce the size of the female breast because the large breast will become droopy if volume is removed without lifting and tightening the skin. The greater benefit of liposuction is in combination with surgical breast reduction techniques, in which it is used to smooth the contours under the arms and at the margins of the breast. For patients with a buffalo hump, liposuction makes it possible to reduce fat deposits on the upper back and lower neck that previously could not be removed without extensive surgery. For patients with HIV infection, lipodystrophy is a syndrome of abnormal fat distribution associated with the therapeutic use of protease inhibitors. The lipodystrophy may be in the form of a neck and upper back fat pad, fat deposition in the trunk and lower face, or increase in the adipose tissue of the breasts. All these respond well to treatment with liposuction.

The most common complications with suction-assisted lipectomy are contour deformity, excessive blood loss, hematoma, seroma, fluid overload, and asymmetry. Less commonly, overlying skin loss, skin burns, DVT, and pulmonary embolus are seen. There have been infrequent reports of fat embolus, cannula penetration of the abdominal cavity, lidocaine toxicity, and surgical shock. A national survey conducted in 2001 found that combining liposuction with other procedures such as abdominoplasty increased the mortality risk almost fivefold. This is presumably related to the longer length of the surgery, greater blood loss, and larger fluid shifts. Based on this information, subsequent technical and practice guidelines include limiting the performance of concomitant procedures at the time of liposuction, stricter criteria for patient selection with regard to obesity and general health factors, removing less fat in one operative session, placing limits on the length of the surgery, modifications in anesthetic techniques, and additional patient monitoring.

## CONCLUSIONS

Plastic surgery continues to evolve with the development of new approaches for the care of people with congenital and acquired deformities. With therapeutic advances in medicine and surgery, new problems have emerged that call for novel reconstructive techniques. Challenged by these difficult problems, plastic surgery continues to look for ways to treat life- and limb- threatening problems and, at the same time, restore form and function. Chest wall, abdominal wall, and perineal reconstruction are progressing rapidly, and defects that were incapacitating a decade ago are now correctable. Lower extremity salvage after devastating injury is now commonplace. With the advent of new specialties such as bariatric surgery, entirely new areas requiring plastic surgery have emerged. Old techniques, such as perforator flaps, continue to evolve and supply better ways to reconstruct defects. New techniques such as fat grafting, which may revolutionize clinical practice, have come from empirical observations. Developed from new research studies, tissue engineering, gene therapy, and stem cell work will change reconstruction in unforeseeable ways in the future. The search continues for the most reliable, durable, and aesthetic ways to "restore, repair, and make whole those parts . . . which fortune has taken away" (Gaspare Tagliacozzi [Italian surgeon who became famous for his skill in reconstructive surgery], *De Curtorum Chirurgia per Insitionem*, Venice, 1579).

## SELECTED REFERENCES

Siemionow MZ, Papay F, Djohan R, et al: First U.S. near-total human face transplantation: A paradigm shift for massive complex injuries. Plast Reconstr Surg 125:111–122, 2010.

This article describes the 5-year process of preparing for the first U.S. clinical case of face transplantation in humans. It includes the institutional review board protocol, informed consent, organ procurement organization approval process, and description of the technical aspects of the near-total face transplantation.

Coleman SR: Structural fat grafting: More than a permanent filler. Plast Reconstr Surg 118:108S–120S, 2006.

This is an early report about fat grafting that recognized an effect that is increasingly well-documented today. The transplanted fat survives and achieves a desired volume replacement at the recipient site. Unexpectedly, it also improves the quality of the soft tissue, producing significant improvement in conditions such as radiation damage and chronic ulceration. The mechanism and role of adipose-derived stem cells and preadipocytes are under investigation.

Koshima I, Yamamoto T, Narushima M, et al: Perforator flaps and supermicrosurgery. Clin Plast Surg 37:683–689, 2010.

The introduction of supermicrosurgery, the microvascular anastomosis of vessels ranging from 0.3 to 0.8 mm in diameter, opens up a wide array of new reconstructive options. Free perforator flaps can be obtained from anywhere on the body and provide thinner, more pliant tissue for repair of extremity and facial defects. This paper reviews these new options as well as the technical challenges of supermicrosurgery.

Rohrich RJ, Lowe JB, Hackney FL, et al: An algorithm for abdominal wall reconstruction. Plast Reconstr Surg 105:202–216, 2000.

This paper reviews the anatomy of the abdominal wall with the goals, components, timing, and techniques of abdominal wall reconstruction. Based on the depth, size, and position of an abdominal wall defect, an algorithm is provided for the use of tissue expansion, vacuum-assisted closure device, abdominal components separation, prosthetic materials, local and distant muscle flaps, and free tissue transfer.

Ko JH, Wang EC, Salvay DM, et al: Abdominal wall reconstruction: Lessons learned from 200 "components separation" procedures. Arch Surg 144:1047–1055, 2009.

Recurrence and complication rates were compared with variations in the components separation procedure for the repair of ventral hernias. The study groups included primary components separation and the use of biologic and permanent meshes to augment the repair; the results support the use of permanent mesh.

Nelson RA, Butler CE: Surgical outcomes of VRAM versus thigh flaps for immediate reconstruction of pelvic and perineal cancer resection defects. Plast Reconstr Surg 123:175–183, 2009.

Results in this series of 133 patients support the move away from thigh-based flaps for reconstruction following APR or pelvic exenteration. Complication rates decreased from 42% to 15% with use of an anterior abdominal wall flap.

## REFERENCES

1. Saint-Cyr M, Schaverien M, Wong C, et al: The extended anterolateral thigh flap: anatomical basis and clinical experience. Plast Reconstr Surg 123:1245–1255, 2009.
2. Avery CM: Review of the radial free flap: Is it still evolving, or is it facing extinction? Part one: Soft-tissue radial flap. Br J Oral Maxillofac Surg 48:245–252, 2010.
3. Hong JP, Koshima I: Using perforators as recipient vessels (supermicrosurgery) for free flap reconstruction of the knee region. Ann Plast Surg 64:291–293, 2010.
4. Wei F, Suominen S: Principles and techniques of microvascular surgery. In Mathes SJ, editor: Plastic surgery, ed 2, Philadelphia, 2006, Saunders Elsevier, pp 507–538.

5. Koshima I, Yamamoto T, Narushima M, et al: Perforator flaps and supermicrosurgery. Clin Plast Surg 37:683–689, 2010.
6. Hong JP: The use of supermicrosurgery in lower extremity reconstruction: The next step in evolution. Plast Reconstr Surg 123: 230–235, 2009.
7. Argenta LC, Marks MW: Principles of tissue expansion. In Mathes SJ, editor: Plastic surgery, ed 2, Philadelphia, 2006, Saunders Elsevier, pp 539–567.
8. Gougoutas AJ, Singh DJ, Low DW, et al: Hemifacial microsomia: Clinical features and pictographic representations of the OMENS classification system. Plast Reconstr Surg 120:112e–120e, 2007.
9. Stal S, Brown RH, Higuera S, et al: Fifty years of the Millard rotation-advancement: Looking back and moving forward. Plast Reconstr Surg 123:1364–1377, 2009.
10. Sullivan SR, Marrinan EM, LaBrie RA, et al: Palatoplasty outcomes in nonsyndromic patients with cleft palate: a 29-year assessment of one surgeon's experience. J Craniofac Surg 20 (Suppl 1):612–616, 2009.
11. Tromberg J, Bauer B, Benvenuto-Andrade C, et al: Congenital melanocytic nevi needing treatment. Dermatol Ther 18:136–150, 2005.
12. Ho K, Hutter JJ, Eskridge J, et al: The management of life-threatening haemorrhage following blunt facial trauma. J Plast Reconstr Aesthet Surg 59:1257–1262, 2006.
13. Ellis E, 3rd, Miles BA: Fractures of the mandible: A technical perspective. Plast Reconstr Surg 120:76S–89S, 2007.
14. Siemionow MZ, Papay F, Djohan R, et al: First U.S. near-total human face transplantation: A paradigm shift for massive complex injuries. Plast Reconstr Surg 125:111–122, 2010.
15. Janis JE, Rohrich RJ: Clinical decision-making in rhinoplasty. In Nahai F, editor: The art of aesthetic surgery: Principles and techniques, St. Louis, 2005, Quality Medical, pp 1515–1533.
16. Cohen SR, Henssler C, Johnston J: Fractional photothermolysis for skin rejuvenation. Plast Reconstr Surg 124:281–290, 2009.
17. Coleman SR: Structural fat grafting: More than a permanent filler. Plast Reconstr Surg 118:108S–120S, 2006.
18. Rigotti G, Marchi A, Galie M, et al: Clinical treatment of radiotherapy tissue damage by lipoaspirate transplant: A healing process mediated by adipose-derived adult stem cells. Plast Reconstr Surg 119:1409–1422, 2007.
19. Carruthers JD, Glogau RG, Blitzer A: Advances in facial rejuvenation: Botulinum toxin type a, hyaluronic acid dermal fillers, and combination therapies—consensus recommendations. Plast Reconstr Surg 121:5S–30S, 2008.
20. Netscher DT, Baumholtz MA: Chest reconstruction: I. Anterior and anterolateral chest wall and wounds affecting respiratory function. Plast Reconstr Surg 124:240e–252e, 2009.
21. Chang RR, Mehrara BJ, Hu QY, et al: Reconstruction of complex oncologic chest wall defects: A 10-year experience. Ann Plast Surg 52:471–479, 2004.
22. Losken A, Thourani VH, Carlson GW, et al: A reconstructive algorithm for plastic surgery following extensive chest wall resection. Br J Plast Surg 57:295–302, 2004.
23. Lee JC, Raman J, Song DH: Primary sternal closure with titanium plate fixation: Plastic surgery effecting a paradigm shift. Plast Reconstr Surg 125:1720–1724, 2010.
24. Agarwal JP, Ogilvie M, Wu LC, et al: Vacuum-assisted closure for sternal wounds: A first-line therapeutic management approach. Plast Reconstr Surg 116:1035–1040, 2005.
25. Davison SP, Clemens MW, Armstrong D, et al: Sternotomy wounds: Rectus flap versus modified pectoral reconstruction. Plast Reconstr Surg 120:929–934, 2007.
26. Dabbah A, Lehman JA, Jr, Parker MG, et al: Reduction mammoplasty: An outcome analysis. Ann Plast Surg 35:337–341, 1995.
27. Gorczyca DP, Gorczyca SM, Gorczyca KL: The diagnosis of silicone breast implant rupture. Plast Reconstr Surg 120:49S–61S, 2007.
28. Deapen D, Hamilton A, Bernstein L, et al: Breast cancer stage at diagnosis and survival among patients with prior breast implants. Plast Reconstr Surg 105:535–540, 2000.
29. Coleman SR, Saboeiro AP: Fat grafting to the breast revisited: Safety and efficacy. Plast Reconstr Surg 119:775–785, 2007.
30. Hyakusoku H, Ogawa R, Ono S, et al: Complications after autologous fat injection to the breast. Plast Reconstr Surg 123: 360–370, 2009.
31. Johnson RE, Murad MH: Gynecomastia: Pathophysiology, evaluation, and management. Mayo Clin Proc 84:1010–1015, 2009.
32. Agnew SP, Small W, Jr, Wang E, et al: Prospective measurements of intra-abdominal volume and pulmonary function after repair of massive ventral hernias with the components separation technique. Ann Surg 251:981–988, 2010.
33. Morykwas MJ, Argenta LC, Shelton-Brown EI, et al: Vacuum-assisted closure: A new method for wound control and treatment:Animal studies and basic foundation. Ann Plast Surg 38:553–562, 1997.
34. Ko JH, Wang EC, Salvay DM, et al: Abdominal wall reconstruction: lessons learned from 200 "components separation" procedures. Arch Surg 144:1047–1055, 2009.
35. den Hartog D, Dur AH, Tuinebreijer WE, et al: Open surgical procedures for incisional hernias. Cochrane Database Syst Rev (3):CD006438, 2008.
36. Rohrich RJ, Lowe JB, Hackney FL, et al: An algorithm for abdominal wall reconstruction. Plast Reconstr Surg 105:202–216, 2000.
37. Hensel JM, Lehman JA, Jr, Tantri MP, et al: An outcomes analysis and satisfaction survey of 199 consecutive abdominoplasties. Ann Plast Surg 46:357–363, 2001.
38. Bullard KM, Trudel JL, Baxter NN, et al: Primary perineal wound closure after preoperative radiotherapy and abdominoperineal resection has a high incidence of wound failure. Dis Colon Rectum 48:438–443, 2005.
39. Butler CE, Gundeslioglu AO, Rodriguez-Bigas MA: Outcomes of immediate vertical rectus abdominis myocutaneous flap reconstruction for irradiated abdominoperineal resection defects. J Am Coll Surg 206:694–703, 2008.
40. Nelson RA, Butler CE: Surgical outcomes of VRAM versus thigh flaps for immediate reconstruction of pelvic and perineal cancer resection defects. Plast Reconstr Surg 123:175–183, 2009.
41. Sinna R, Qassemyar Q, Benhaim T, et al: Perforator flaps: A new option in perineal reconstruction. J Plast Reconstr Aesthet Surg 63:e766–e774, 2010.
42. Friedman JD, Reece GR, Eldor L: The utility of the posterior thigh flap for complex pelvic and perineal reconstruction. Plast Reconstr Surg 126:146–155, 2010.
43. O'Shaughnessy BA, Dumanian GA, Liu JC, et al: Pedicled omental flaps as an adjunct in the closure of complex spinal wounds. Spine (Phila Pa 1976) 32:3074–3080, 2007.
44. Glatt BS, Disa JJ, Mehrara BJ, et al: Reconstruction of extensive partial or total sacrectomy defects with a transabdominal vertical

rectus abdominis myocutaneous flap. Ann Plast Surg 56:526–530; discussion 530–521, 2006.

**45.** Zakaria Y, Hasan EA: Reversed turnover latissimus dorsi muscle flap for closure of large myelomeningocele defects. J Plast Reconstr Aesthet Surg 63:1513–1518, 2010.

**46.** Bass MJ, Phillips LG: Pressure sores. Curr Probl Surg 44:101–143, 2007.

**47.** Ong YS, Levin LS: Lower limb salvage in trauma. Plast Reconstr Surg 125:582–588, 2010.

**48.** Shawen SB, Keeling JJ, Branstetter J, et al: The mangled foot and leg: salvage versus amputation. Foot Ankle Clin 15:63–75, 2010.

**49.** Parrett BM, Winograd JM, Garfein ES, et al: The vertical and extended rectus abdominis myocutaneous flap for irradiated thigh and groin defects. Plast Reconstr Surg 122:171–177, 2008.

**50.** Parrett BM, Talbot SG, Pribaz JJ, et al: A review of local and regional flaps for distal leg reconstruction. J Reconstr Microsurg 25:445–455, 2009.

CHAPTER 70

# HAND SURGERY

David Netscher, Kevin Murphy,
and Nicholas A. Fiore, II

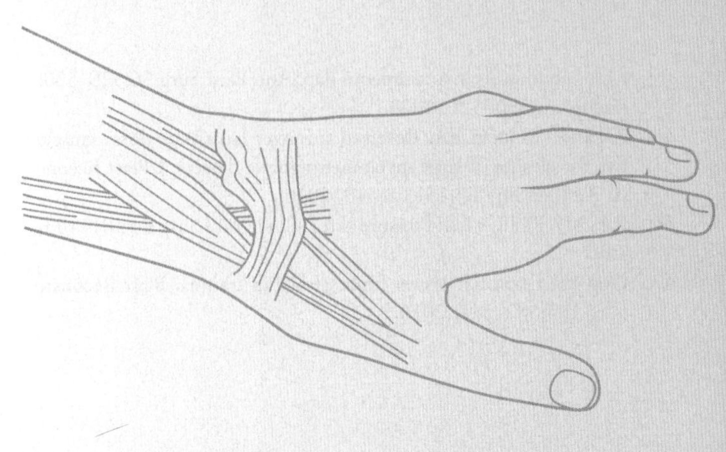

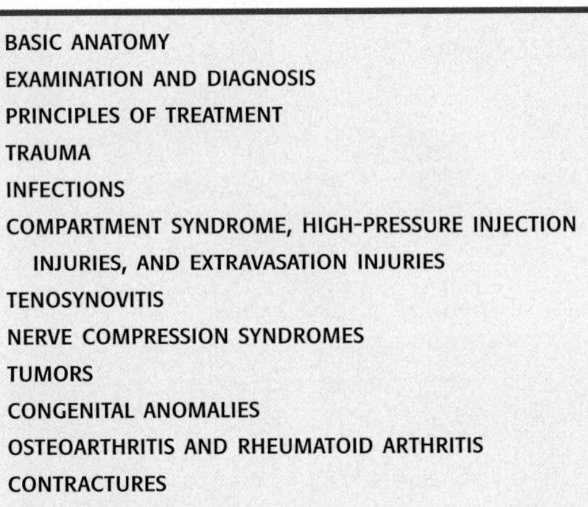


Although hand surgery fellowships traditionally receive trainees primarily with backgrounds in orthopedic surgery or plastic surgery, fellowship training in hand surgery may also be undertaken by those having completed a residency in general surgery. Basic tenets of hand surgery must be acquired by all general surgeons. Depending on the practice locale (rural or urban), type of hospital, and residency rotations (e.g., surgical intern covering the emergency department), or even for the purposes of board examinations, the ability to evaluate and manage hand injuries and problems is a necessary skill for the general surgeon. The purpose of this chapter is not to provide the general surgeon with an exhaustive study of hand surgery, because specialty texts are more appropriate, but to provide an overview of hand pathology encountered more commonly by the general surgeon, and especially to emphasize basics in anatomy, physical examination, and treatment of common hand and upper extremity emergencies.

## BASIC ANATOMY

The arm and hand are divided into volar or palmar, and also dorsal, aspects. Distal to the elbow, structures are termed *radial* or *ulnar* to the middle finger axis rather than lateral and medial, respectively, because with forearm pronation and supination, the latter terms become confusing. The nomenclature of digits has become standardized. The hand has five digits, namely the thumb and four fingers (the thumb is not called a finger). The four fingers are respectively termed the *index, long (middle), ring,* and *small (little) fingers.* The use of numbers to designate digits is no longer accepted (Fig. 70-1). Within the hand, those structures close to the fingertips are termed *distal,* whereas those further up toward the wrist are termed *proximal.* Motion in a palmar direction is flexion, whereas dorsal motion is termed *extension.* Finger motion away from the long finger axis is termed *abduction,* whereas motion toward the axis of the long finger is termed *adduction.* The description of the motion of the thumb is sometimes confusing. Extension of the thumb is in the plane of the palm of the hand, whereas palmar abduction of the thumb is the motion that occurs at 90 degrees away from the plane of the palm. Finally, side to side motion of the wrist is termed *radial* and *ulnar deviation.*

Intrinsic muscles of the hand are those that have their origins and insertions in the hand, whereas the extrinsic muscles have their muscle bellies in the forearm and their tendon insertions in the hand. The intrinsic muscles that make up the thenar eminence are the abductor pollicis brevis (APB), flexor pollicis brevis (FPB), opponens pollicis (OP), and adductor pollicis (AP). There are four dorsal interossei that arise from adjacent sides of each metacarpal and provide abduction of the metacarpophalangeal (MP) joints of the index, middle, and ring fingers. There are three palmar interossei that adduct the index, ring, and little fingers toward the middle finger. Four lumbricals originate on the flexor digitorum profundus (FDP) tendons in the palm and insert on the radial sides of the extensor mechanisms of the four fingers. Together with the interossei, these bring about flexion of the MP joints and extension of the interphalangeal (IP) joints of the fingers (Fig. 70-2). The FPB flexes the thumb at the MP joint, in contrast with the extrinsic flexor pollicis longus (FPL), which flexes the thumb IP joint.

The hypothenar muscles consist of the flexor digiti minimi (FDM), which flexes the little finger at the MP joint, as well as the abductor digiti minimi (ADM) and opponens digiti minimi (ODM). A small muscle called the *palmaris brevis* is located transversally in the subcutaneous tissue at the base of the hypothenar imminence. It is innervated by the ulnar nerve, puckers the skin, and helps in cupping the skin of the palm during grip (Table 70-1).

The extrinsic muscles originate proximal to the wrist and comprise the long flexors and extensors of the wrist and digits. The extensors are located dorsally and are divided into three subgroups. The radialmost subgroup is termed the *mobile wad* and comprises the brachioradialis (BR), extensor carpi radialis longus (ECRL), and extensor carpi radialis brevis (ECRB). The ECRL and ECRB extend the wrist and deviate it radially.

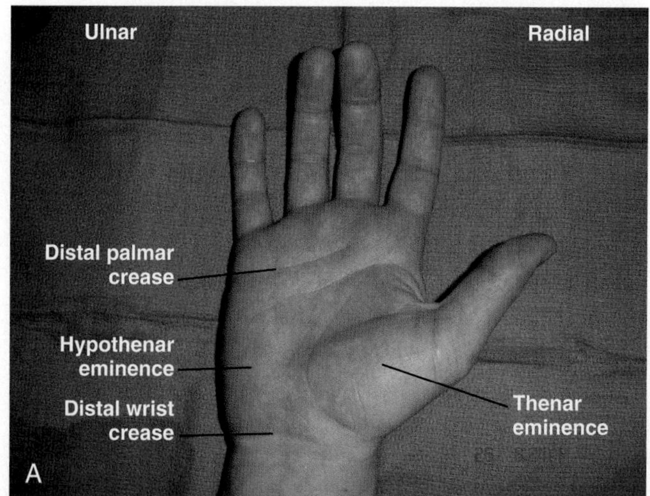


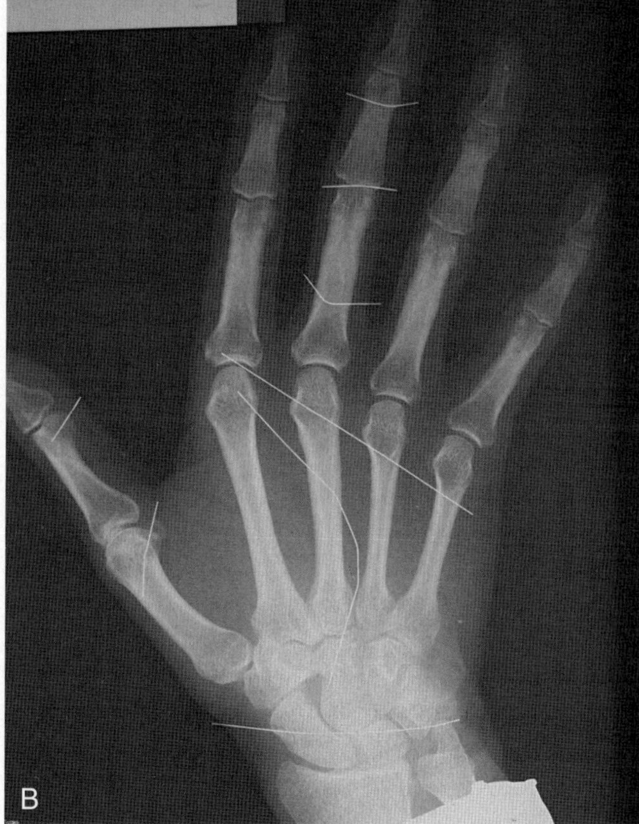


**FIGURE 70-1** Surface anatomy of the hand. **A,** Hand surfaces and nomenclature. **B,** Skin creases of the hand superimposed on the skeletal structures.

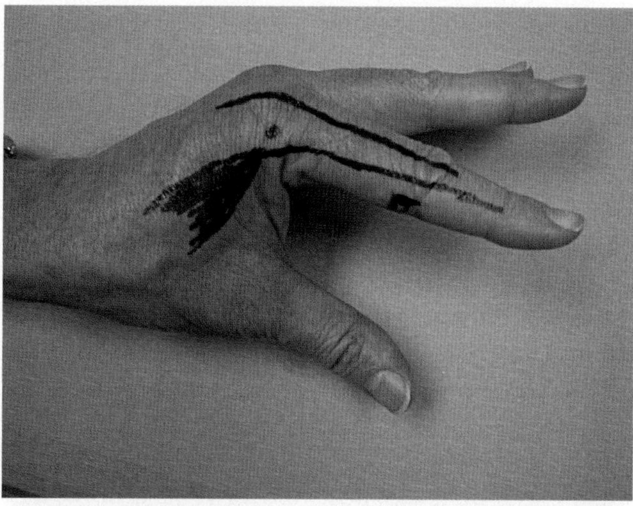

**FIGURE 70-2** Outline of first dorsal interosseous muscle on the index finger shows how it passes volar to the fulcrum of flexion of the metacarpophalangeal joint (MP) and dorsal to the IP joints. Interossei flex MP joints and extend proximal and distal IP joints. The long extrinsic extensor tendon passes dorsal to all joints.

The second group is located in a more superficial layer and comprises three muscles—namely, the extensor carpi ulnaris (ECU), extensor digiti minimi-quinti (EDM-Q), and extensor digitorum communis (EDC). The ECU deviates the wrist in an ulnar direction and extends the wrist, whereas the EDM and EDC extend the MP joints of the fingers. The third and deeper subgroup comprises four muscles, three of which act on the thumb; the remaining muscle influences the index finger. The abductor pollicis longus (APL), extensor pollicis longus (EPL), and extensor pollicis brevis (EPB) provide function to the

**Table 70-1 Intrinsic Muscles of the Hand**

| MUSCLE | INNERVATION* | FUNCTION |
|---|---|---|
| Abductor pollicis brevis (APB) | Median | Abducts the thumb |
| Flexor pollicis brevis (FPB) | Median | Flexes the thumb |
| Opponens pollicis (OP) | Median | Opposes the thumb |
| Lumbricals | Median and ulnar | Flexes metacarpal phalangeal (MCP) joints and extends interphalangeal (IP) joints |
| Palmaris brevis | Ulnar | Wrinkles the skin on the medial (ulnar) side of the palm |
| Adductor pollicis (AdP) | Ulnar | Adducts the thumb |
| Abductor digiti minimi (ADM) | Ulnar | Abducts the small finger |
| Flexor digiti minimi (FDM) | Ulnar | Flexes the small digit |
| Opponens digiti minimi (ODM) | Ulnar | Opposes the small finger |
| Dorsal interossei | Ulnar | Abducts the fingers; flexes MCP joints and extends the IP joints |
| Palmar interossei | Ulnar | Adducts the fingers; flexes MCP joints and extends the IP joints |

*All the thenar intrinsic muscles are supplied by the median nerve except the AdP; all the remaining intrinsic muscles are supplied by the ulnar nerve except the two radial lumbricals.

thumb, and the extensor indicis proprius (EIP) extends the MP joint to the index finger. Last of the deep muscles is the supinator, which is located proximally in the forearm (Table 70-2).

The extensor tendons pass through six compartments deep to the extensor retinaculum at the dorsum of the wrist. From radial to ulnar side, these tendons and compartments are arranged as follows. The first compartment contains the APL and EPB, which also forms the radial boundary of the so-called *anatomic snuffbox*. The second compartment consists of the ECRL and ECRB, and the third compartment (which also forms the ulnar boundary of the anatomic snuffbox) contains the EPL. The EIP and EDC pass through the fourth compartment and the EDM through the fifth compartment, where they overlie the distal radioulnar joint. The sixth compartment contains the ECU (Fig. 70-3).

At the level of the MP joints, the long extrinsic extensor tendons broaden out to form the extensor hood. The proximal part of the hood at this level is called the *sagittal band*. It loops around the MP joint and blends into the volar plate, thus forming a lasso around the base of the proximal phalanx, through which it extends the MP joint. The insertions of the interossei and lumbricals enter into the extensor hood as the lateral bands. These lateral bands insert distally and dorsally to the axis of the PIP joint, and it is through this distal insertion that the intrinsic muscles (the interossei and lumbricals) are flexors of the MP joints and yet extensors of the IP joints. The extensor hood inserts to the base of the middle phalanx, which is termed the *central slip*, and finally proceeds on to the base of the distal phalanx, where it inserts through the terminal slip, thus extending the distal interphalangeal (DIP) joint (Fig. 70-4).

The extrinsic flexor muscles are located on the volar aspect of the forearm and are arranged in three layers. The superficial layer comprises four muscles—pronator teres (PT), flexor carpi radialis (FCR), flexor carpi ulnaris (FCU), and palmaris longus (PL). The PL muscle may be absent in as many as 10% to 12% of individuals. These muscles originate from the medial humeral epicondyle in the proximal forearm and function to flex the wrist and pronate the forearm. The intermediate layer consists of the flexor digitorum superficialis (FDS), which allows independent flexion of the proximal interphalangeal (PIP) joints of the fingers. In the deep layer, there are three muscles: the FPL, which flexes the IP joint to the thumb; the FDP, which flexes the DIP joints of the fingers; and a distal quadrangular muscle that spans between the radius and ulna termed the *pronator quadratus*, which helps in pronation of the forearm (Table 70-3).

**Table 70-2 Extrinsic Muscles of the Dorsal Forearm**

| MUSCLE | INNERVATION* | FUNCTION |
|---|---|---|
| Extensor pollicis brevis (EPB) | Radial | Abducts the hand and extends the thumb at the proximal phalanx |
| Abductor pollicis longus (APL) | Radial | Abducts the hand and thumb |
| Extensor carpi radialis longus (ECRL) | Radial | Extends and radially deviates the hand |
| Extensor carpi radialis brevis (ECRB) | Radial | Extends and radially deviates the hand |
| Extensor pollicis longus (EPL) | Radial | Extends the distal phalanx of the thumb |
| Extensor digitorum communis (EDC) | Radial | Extends the fingers and the hand |
| Extensor indicis proprius (EIP) | Radial | Extends the index finger |
| Extensor digiti minimi/quinti (EDM/Q) | Radial | Extends the small finger |
| Extensor carpi ulnaris (ECU) | Radial | Extends and ulnarly deviates the wrist |
| Supinator | Radial | Supination |
| Brachioradialis | Radial | Flexes the forearm |

*All muscles of the dorsal forearm are innervated by the radial nerve and its respective branches.

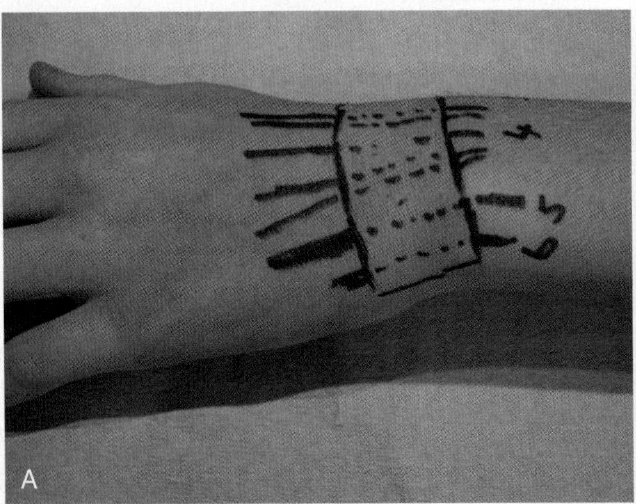


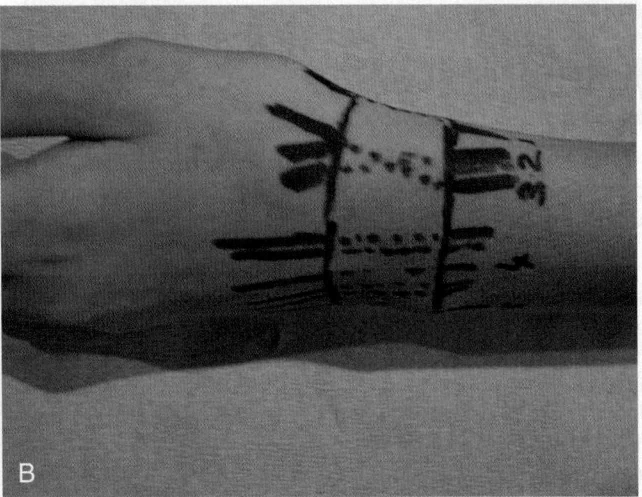


**FIGURE 70-3 A, B,** Surface anatomy of the six dorsal extensor compartments at the wrist. Note that the first (APL and EPB) and third (EPL) compartments form the radial and ulnar boundaries, respectively, of the anatomic snuffbox.

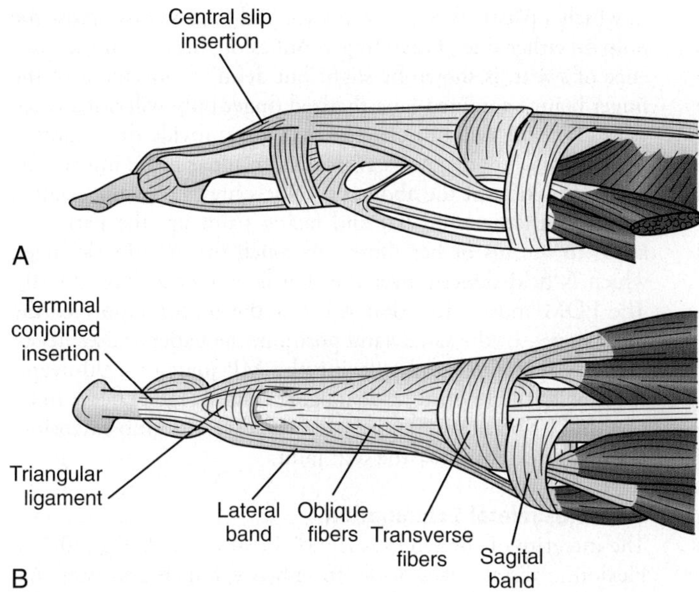


**FIGURE 70-4** Extensor mechanism of the fingers. **A,** Lateral view. **B,** Dorsal view.

**Table 70-3 Extrinsic Muscles of the Volar Forearm**

| MUSCLE | INNERVATION* | FUNCTION |
|---|---|---|
| Pronator teres (PT) | Median | Pronation |
| Flexor carpi radialis (FCR) | Median | Flexion and radial deviation of the wrist |
| Palmaris longus (PL) | Median | Flexion of the wrist |
| Flexor carpi ulnaris (FCU) | Ulnar | Flexion and ulnar deviation of the wrist |
| Flexor digitorum superficialis (FDS) | Median | Flexion of the proximal interphalangeal (PIP) joint |
| Flexor digitorum profundus (FDP) | Median and ulnar | Flexion of the distal interphalangeal (DIP) joint |
| Pronator quadratus | Median | Pronation |
| Flexor pollicis longus (FPL) | Median | Flexion of the thumb |

*All muscles of the volar forearm are innervated by the median nerve and its branches except the two ulnar digits of the FDP and FCU, which are innervated by the ulnar nerve.

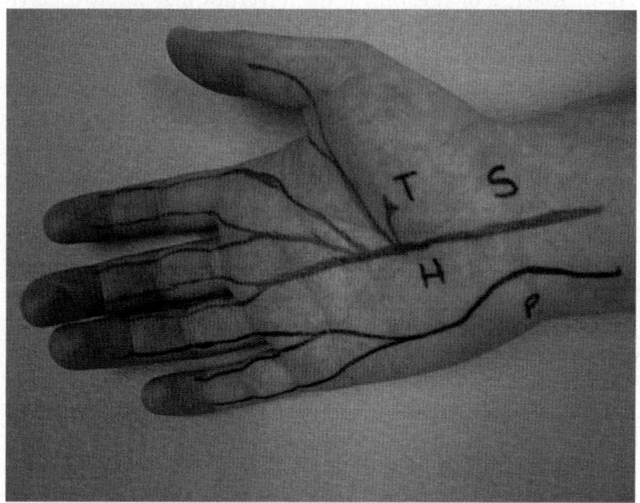


**FIGURE 70-5** Surface anatomy of median *(red)* and ulnar *(black)* nerves. *H,* Hook of hamate; *P,* pisiform; *S,* scaphoid; *T,* trapezium.

Nerve supply to the hand is by three nerves, the median, ulnar, and radial nerves. A knowledge of the surface anatomy of nerves helps when evaluating specific lacerating injuries (Fig. 70-5). The ulnar attachment to the flexor retinaculum is to the pisiform and hook of the hamate, and the radial attachment is to the scaphoid and ridge of the trapezium. The median nerve passes through the carpal tunnel between these landmarks. It gives sensation to the thumb, index finger, middle finger, and radial half of the ring finger. The palmar cutaneous branch of the median nerve originates from its radial side 5 to 6 cm proximal to the wrist, providing sensation to the palmar triangle. The ulnar nerve travels to the radial side of the pisiform and passes to the ulnar side of the hook of the hamate in its passage through Guyon's canal. It gives sensation to the little finger and ulnar half of the ring finger; the dorsal branch of the ulnar nerve (arising proximal to the wrist and curving dorsally around the head of the ulna) supplies the same digits on their dorsal aspects. The superficial radial sensory nerve emerges from under the brachioradialis in the distal forearm, dividing into two or three branches proximal to the radial styloid, which then proceed in a subcutaneous course across the anatomic snuffbox, innervating the skin of the dorsum of the first web space. The number of fingers served by each nerve is variable. However, as an absolute rule, the palmar surfaces of the index and little fingers are always served by the median and ulnar nerves, respectively.

With regard to the motor supply of these nerves, the ulnar nerve supplies the hypothenar muscles, interossei, ulnar two lumbricals, adductor pollicis, and deep head of the flexor pollicis brevis. The median nerve supplies the abductor pollicis brevis, opponens pollicis, radial two lumbricals, and superficial head of the flexor pollicis brevis. In summary, the median nerve thus supplies all the extrinsic digit flexors and wrist flexors (except the FDP to the ring and little fingers and the FCU, which are supplied by the ulnar nerve) and all the thumb intrinsic muscles (except the AP, innervated by the ulnar nerve). The ulnar nerve supplies all the interossei, all the lumbricals (except the radial two, supplied by the median nerve), and the adductor of the thumb. The radial nerve innervates all of the wrist, finger, and thumb extrinsic long extensors.

## EXAMINATION AND DIAGNOSIS

### Evaluation

Basic instruments used in hand examination are shown in Figure 70-6. Examination of the resting posture of the hand can provide valuable information; for example, if a finger flexor tendon is severed, that affected finger does not assume its normal resting position in line with the natural flexion cascade of the adjacent digits (Fig. 70-7). Extensor tendon injuries may be indicated by a droop at the affected joint. A clawed posture of the little and ring fingers may be characteristic of an ulnar nerve injury (Fig. 70-8). Absence of sweating at the fingertips may imply a nerve injury in that particular distribution. Swelling and erythema may indicate a hand infection, and a purulent flexor tenosynovitis always results in a flexed posture of the digits. Rotational and angular digital deformities may occur when there are underlying fractures.

#### Neurovascular Examination

The Allen test confirms patency of the ulnar and radial arteries. Two-point sensory discrimination is the most sensitive method for testing for sensory loss and is easily done by using a bent paperclip (Fig. 70-9). The paperclip ends are set to a distance of approximately 5 mm apart for fingertip pulp sensory testing. The points are aligned along the axis of the finger. If this test is not reproducible because of an uncooperative patient, suspicion of a nerve injury can be confirmed by the tactile adherence test, in which a plastic pen is passed back and forth gently across the pulp on either side of each finger. Adhesion, because of the presence of sweat, is shown by slight but definite movement of the finger being examined (anesthetized finger pulp will not sweat).

There are two muscle tests that may provide the examiner with an absolute diagnosis of median or ulnar nerve injury. The motor function of the abductor pollicis brevis tests the median nerve. With the hand flat and facing palm up, the patient is asked to use his or her thumb to touch the examiner's finger, which is held directly over the thenar eminence (Fig. 70-10). The FDM muscle function will test the motor supply of the ulnar nerve. In the same hand position, the patient raises her or his little finger vertically, flexing the MP joint to a 90-degree angle, with the IP joint held straight. Tests for radial nerve function and its branches require wrist extension, thumb extension, and finger extension at the MP joint.

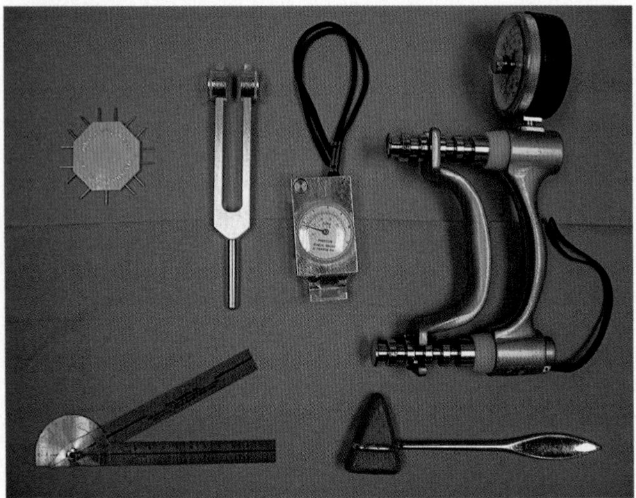

**FIGURE 70-6** Basic instruments used in hand examination include a tuning fork, pinch meter, grip dynamometer, two-point discriminator (paperclip also suffices), goniometer, and patella hammer.

#### Musculoskeletal Examination

The integrity of the tendons is individually tested (Fig. 70-11). Flexion at distal joints of the thumb and fingers confirms that the FPL and FDP, respectively, are intact. Testing of FDS tendons is more complex. It is not possible to flex the DIP joints independently of one another because of a common origin of the FDP tendons. Thus, the other fingers are fixed in extension by the examiner and the patient is asked to flex the remaining digits. Movement is produced by the FDS and occurs at the PIP joint. In approximately one third of patients, the FDS cannot produce little finger flexion. In 50% of these, in turn, there is a common origin with the ring finger, so flexion will occur if the ring finger is permitted to flex simultaneously. More uncommonly, there is no profundus tendon to the little finger and the superficialis inserts into the middle and distal phalanges. The long and short extensors (EPL and EPB) and long abductor of the thumb are tested by asking the patient to extend his or her thumb against resistance, whereas these tendons are individually palpated. Long extensors of the fingers are tested by asking the patient to extend them against resistance applied to the dorsum of the proximal phalanx.

#### Special Investigations

Radiographs are necessary in almost every case. These help in the diagnosis and evaluation of fractures and also in the investigation of foreign bodies. Multiple radiographic views of the affected part are required to define the precise pathology or fracture pattern. Glass is often seen on plain radiographs and, if not seen but suspected, may be visualized by computed tomography (CT) or magnetic resonance imaging (MRI). If plastic is painted, it may be seen on routine radiographs; it is generally poorly visualized with CT but can be clearly seen with MRI. Wooden foreign bodies may be seen by CT or MRI, but not by routine radiography.

Various stress radiographic views and cineradiography may be useful for demonstrating dynamic wrist instability patterns, especially scapholunate separation. Arthrography may detect ligamentous tears by extravasation of contrast material between the radiocarpal, distal radioulnar, and midcarpal joints. This is best combined with MRI, especially for the detection of triangular fibrocartilage tears at the ulnocarpal joint. Radionuclide bone scanning may help diagnose osteomyelitis but, in the hand, a false-positive result may occur because of the close proximity of soft tissue infections to the bones. Occult wrist fractures may

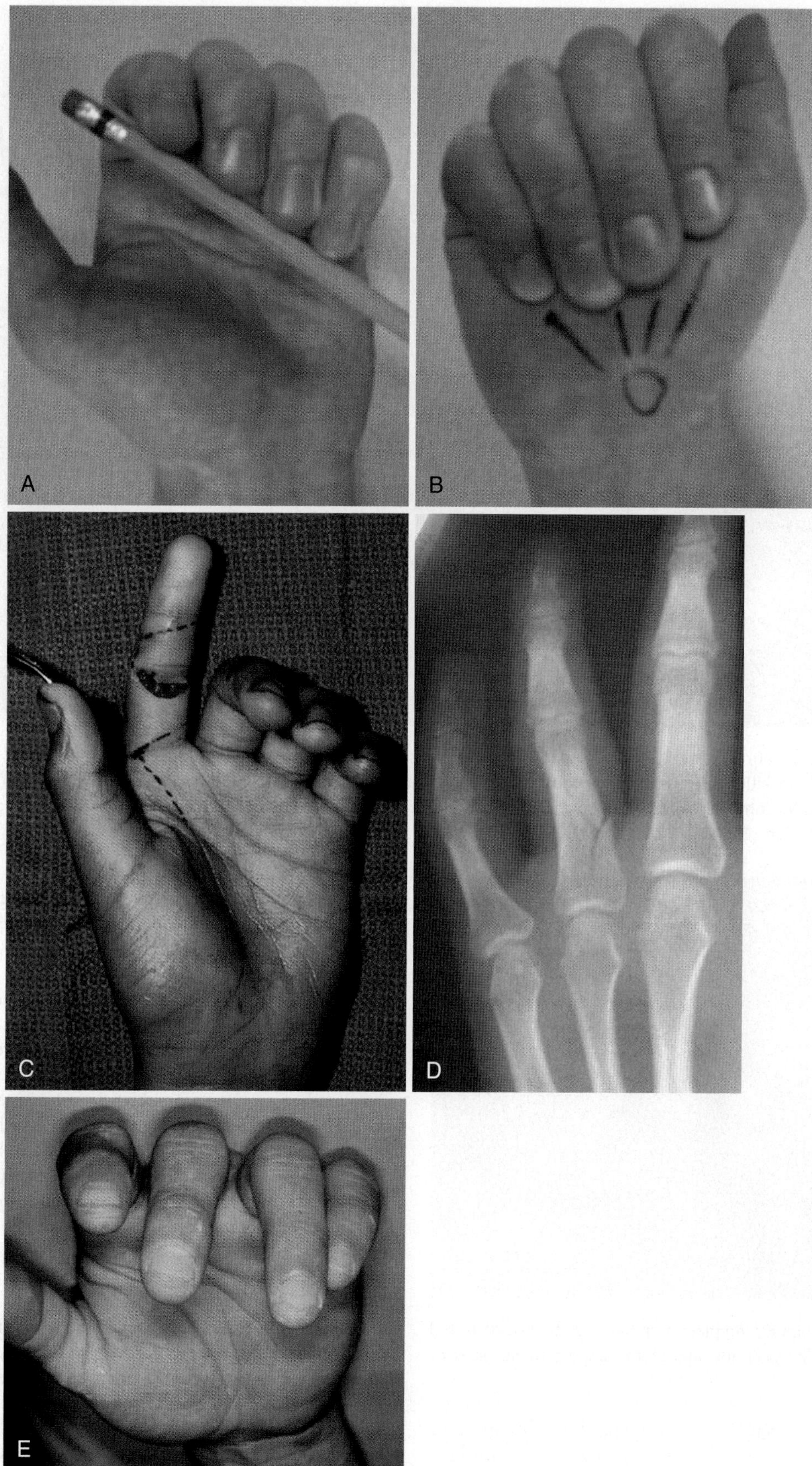


**FIGURE 70-7 A, B,** Natural finger flexion cascade of the hand in repose. Note the fingertips pointing to the distal pole of the scaphoid. **C,** With flexor tendon injury, the affected digit does not adopt this resting flexed posture. **D, E,** Spiral finger fractures produce a rotational deformity, which is also noted as an interruption in the finger flexion cascade.

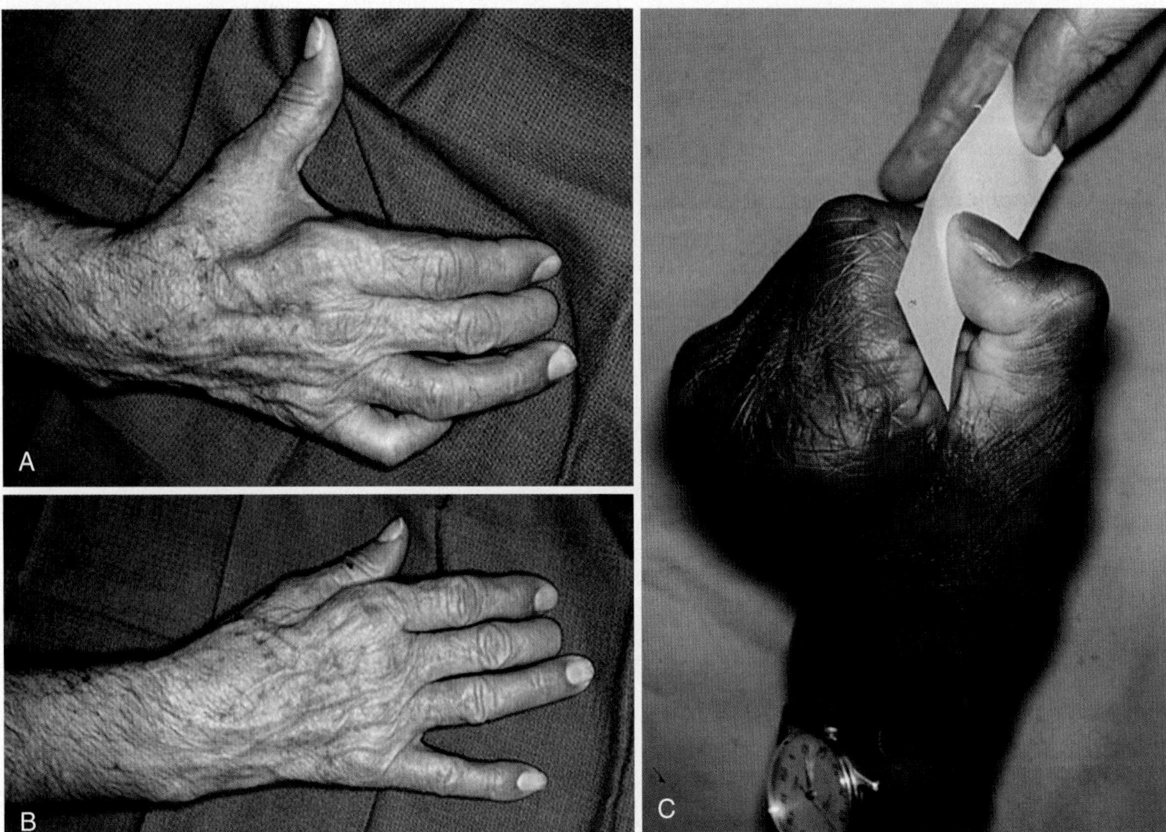


**FIGURE 70-8** **A,** Marked atrophy in the first web space dorsal interosseous muscle is noted with ulnar nerve palsy, with clawing of the little and ring fingers. **B,** The little finger assumes an abducted position and cannot be adducted to the adjacent fingers (Wartenberg's sign). **C,** Because thumb adduction is weak, attempts to grasp a piece of paper between the adducted thumb and index finger produce compensatory thumb IP joint flexion (Froment's sign).

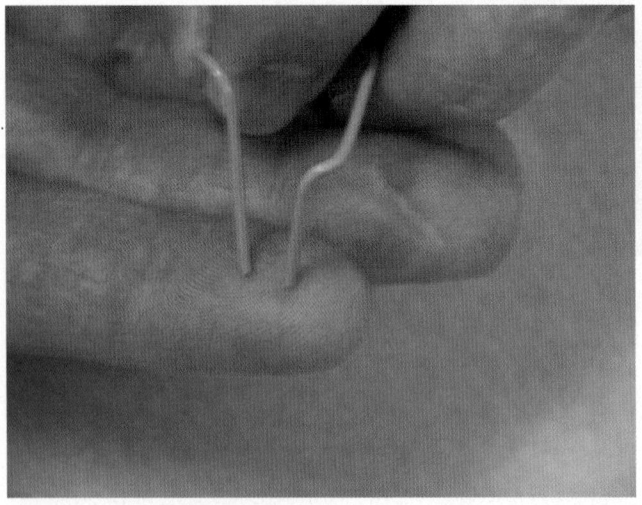

**FIGURE 70-9** Two-point discrimination on the fingertip can be tested with a bent paperclip, with the tips of the paperclips set specific distances apart.

be localized by increased radionuclide uptake, but a false-positive result when evaluating for a fracture may also occur with ligamentous injuries. CT is a helpful modality for diagnosing suspected carpal fractures, (e.g., a scaphoid fracture that may not be seen on a routine x-ray), although most prefer MRI.

Wrist arthroscopy is useful as a diagnostic and therapeutic modality for a number of wrist problems, especially for disorders of the triangular fibrocartilage. Minimally invasive surgery with arthroscopic guidance has added a new dimension to the treatment of acute wrist disorders such as scaphoid and distal radius intra-articular fractures.

Patients with ischemic problems often require noninvasive vascular studies. Doppler pressure measurements help localize the site of a vascular lesion. Angiography in the upper extremity is always carried out in the presence of a vasodilator (e.g., tolazoline [Priscoline], nitroglycerin) or an axillary block to differentiate apparent vessel occlusion from vasospasm. Subtraction radiographs with magnification help improve the detail and definition of the vascular study, especially in the distal forearm and hand.

## PRINCIPLES OF TREATMENT

In the case of injuries, treatment is directed at the specific structures damaged—skeletal, tendon, nerve, vessel, integument.[1,2] In emergency situations, the goals of treatment are to maintain or restore distal circulation, obtain a healed wound, preserve motion, and retain distal sensation. Stable skeletal architecture is established in the primary phase of care because skeletal stability is essential for effective motion and function of the extremity. This also reestablishes skeletal length, straightens deformities, and corrects the compression or kinking of nerves and vessels.

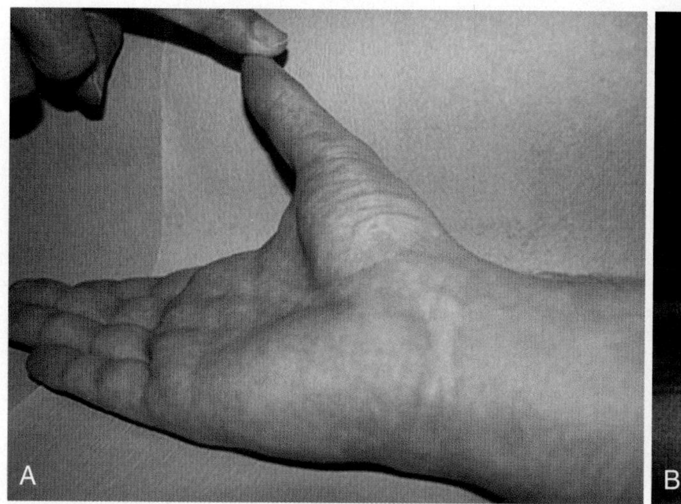


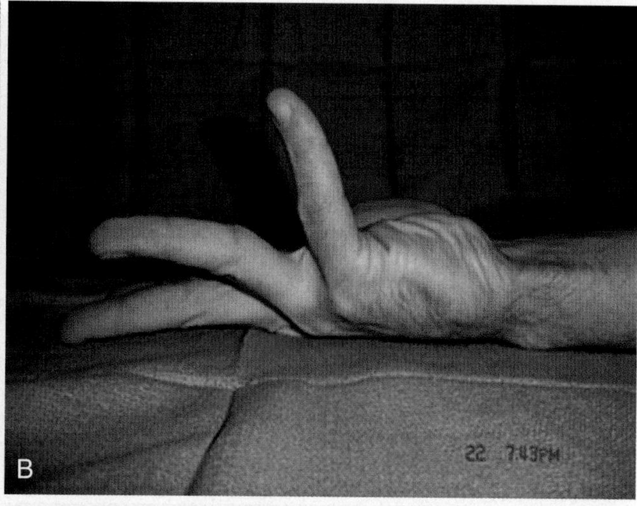


**FIGURE 70-10** Motor innervation of muscles of the hand. **A,** Thumb abduction tests median motor nerve function. **B,** Little finger flexion at the metacarpophalangeal joint with simultaneous IP joint extension tests ulnar motor nerve function.

Arteries are also repaired in the acute phase of treatment to maintain distal tissue viability. Also, extrinsic compression on arteries must be released emergently, such as with compartment pressure problems. In clean-cut injuries, tendons can be repaired primarily. In situations in which there is a chance that tendon adhesions may form, such as when there are associated fractures, it is nonetheless better to repair tendons primarily with preservation of their length and, if necessary at a later date, to perform tenolysis. However, when there are open and contaminated wounds or a severe crushing injury, it is best to delay repair of tendon and nerve injuries.

In clean-cut sharp wounds, primary nerve repair lessens the possibility of nerve end retraction and therefore the need for later nerve grafting. However, primary nerve repair must not be performed in situations in which there is contusion of the nerve (e.g., gunshot wounds, power saw injuries, blunt crushing trauma) because the extent of proximal axonal injury may not be immediately evident. If nerve repair is performed before this is apparent, it may result in abnormal nerve ends being reattached, negating the chance for functional return.

In severe soft tissue injuries, wound closure may not be possible immediately. Initial open treatment of the wound is directed to prevent an infection and protect critical deep structures by proper dressing and wound management (Fig. 70-12). Adequate débridement is essential, but appropriate soft tissue coverage must be achieved as soon as possible thereafter. The sooner the soft tissue coverage can be achieved, the less likely there will be a secondary deformity caused by fibrosis and joint contractures. The more rapidly hand therapy can be started, the better the chance for maximizing functional return. The treatment regimen must consist of débridement, rigid skeletal fixation, and early soft tissue resurfacing, possibly even requiring microvascular soft tissue reconstruction, followed by protected range-of-motion exercises as soon as possible. It has been shown that early soft tissue reconstruction results in improved function, decreased morbidity, and shortened hospital stay.

Appropriate treatment of upper extremity problems requires a thorough knowledge of local and regional anesthesia, use of a tourniquet to provide a bloodless field, correct placement of incisions to minimize later scar contracture, and appropriate use of dressings and splints to reduce edema and maintain a functional position. Above all, a clear knowledge of the unique anatomy of the hand and upper extremity not only aids in obtaining an accurate clinical diagnosis, but also enables the safe performance of surgery.

## Anesthesia

The choice of general, regional (e.g., IV Bier block, brachial plexus block that might be a supraclavicular or axillary block), or local anesthesia is governed by the extent and length of the operation. An upper arm or forearm tourniquet can be used in the unanesthetized extremity with only local anesthetic field infiltration or digital block for 30 to 45 minutes in a relaxed, cooperative patient provided that the arm is well exsanguinated. After this time, tourniquet pain will not permit more extensive local anesthetic procedures. If one has to operate in other areas, such as for harvesting of bone, nerve, tendon, or skin graft, or if more extensive surgical procedures are planned, general anesthesia will be required.

A digital block or median, ulnar, or radial wrist nerve block may be useful, especially for more limited emergency room procedures (Fig. 70-13). Digital nerve blocks usually do not include epinephrine, which could lead to vasospasm, but evidence has indicated the safety of distal blocks using an epinephrine solution. A maximum safe dose of lidocaine is 4 mg/kg.

## Tourniquet Application

The tourniquet is used to provide a bloodless field so that clear visualization of all structures in the operative field is obtained. Penrose drains, rolled rubber glove fingers, or commercially available tourniquets can be used on digits. Great care must be taken when using any constrictive device on digits because narrow bands cause direct injury to underlying nerves and digital vessels. With the use of an arm tourniquet, the skin beneath the cuff must be protected with several wraps of cast padding. During skin preparation, this area must be kept dry to prevent blistering of the skin under an inflated cuff over moist padding. The cuff selected needs to be as wide as the diameter of the arm. Standard pressures used are 100 to 150 mm Hg higher than systolic blood pressure. The cuff is deflated every 2

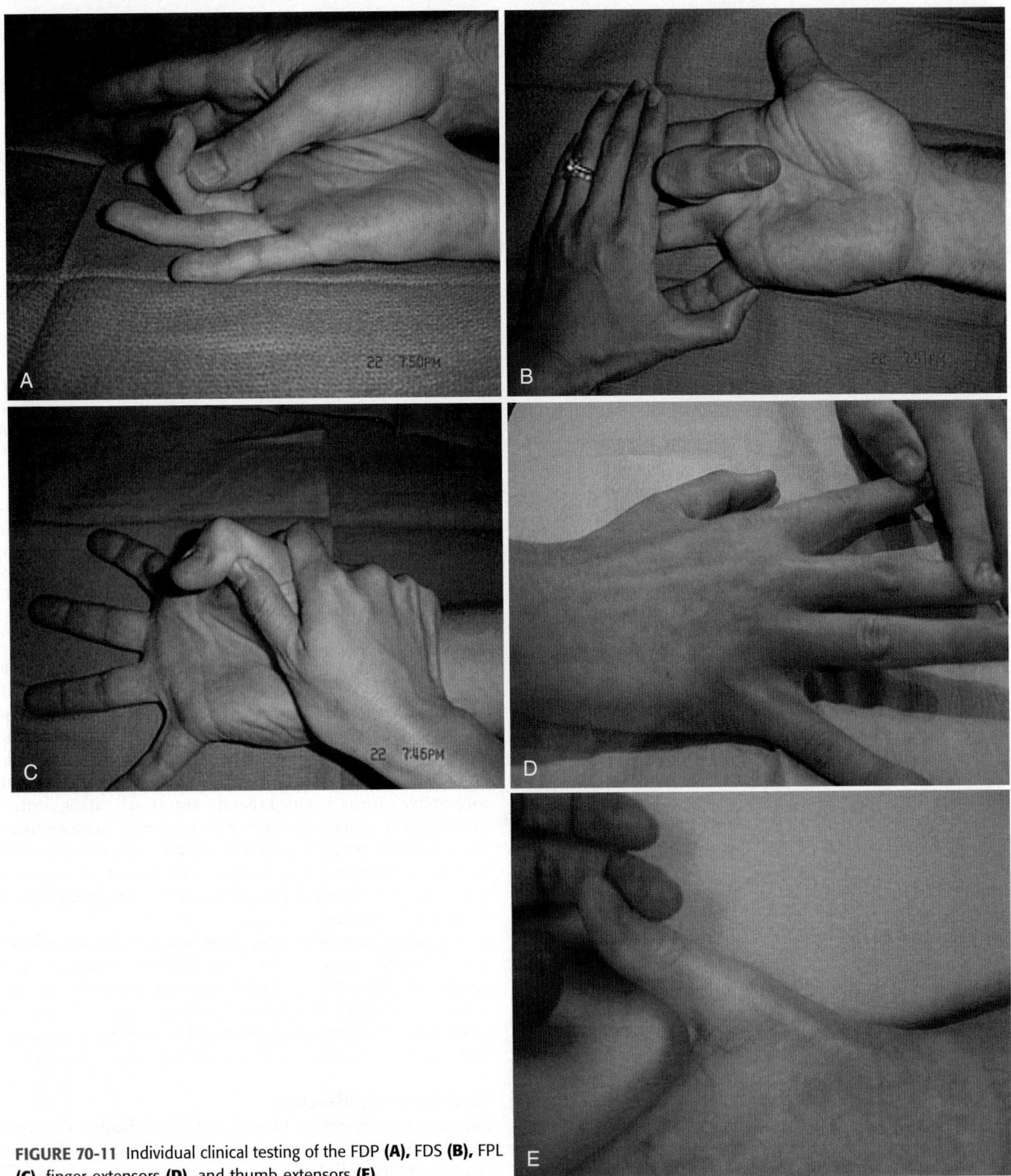

**FIGURE 70-11** Individual clinical testing of the FDP **(A)**, FDS **(B)**, FPL **(C)**, finger extensors **(D)**, and thumb extensors **(E)**.

hours for 15 to 20 minutes (5 minutes of reperfusion for every 30 minutes of tourniquet time) to revascularize distal tissues and relieve pressure on nerves locally before reinflating the cuff for more extensive procedures.[3] Exsanguination of the extremities is performed by wrapping the extremity with a Martin's bandage in all cases, except those involving infection or tumors. In these latter cases, because of the possibility of embolization by mechanical pressure, exsanguination by bandage wrapping needs to be avoided. Simple elevation of the extremity for a few minutes before tourniquet inflation suffices.[1]

## Incisions

Incisions are of the Bruner zigzag or midaxial type, or combinations of these, to avoid longitudinal motion-restricting scars that cross palmar flexion creases (Fig. 70-14). The marginal edge of a skin graft with healthy skin is also a potential scar line, so the

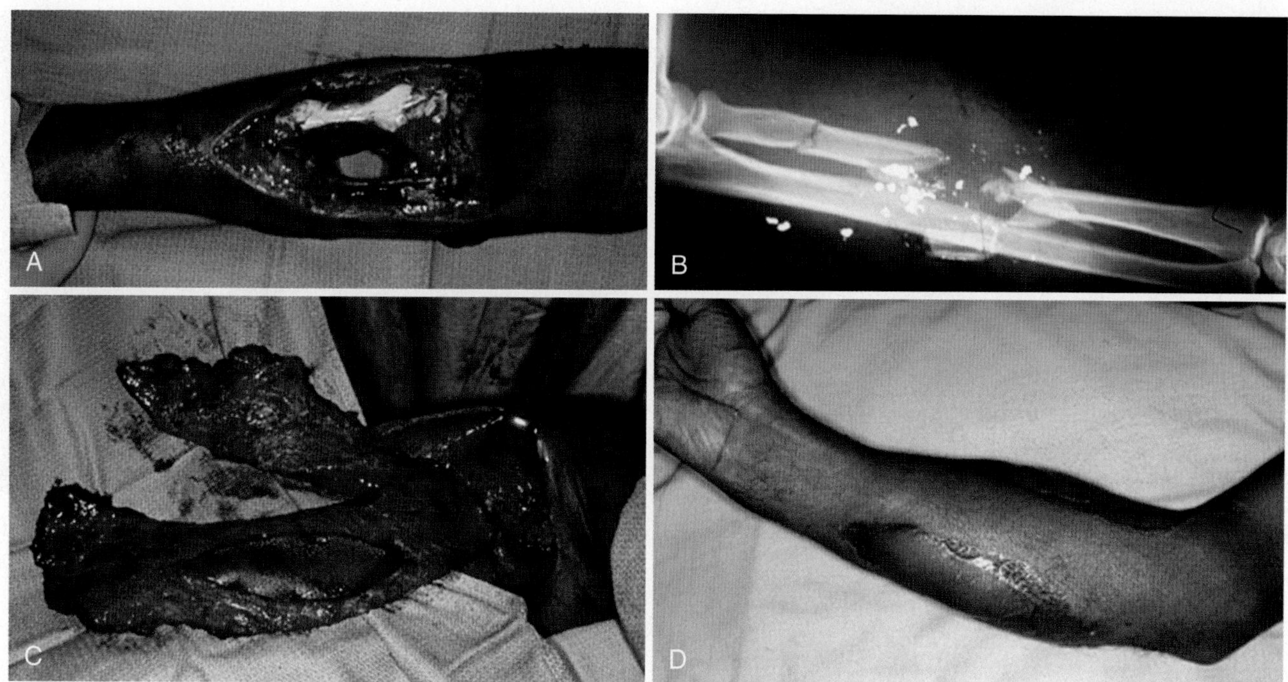

**FIGURE 70-12 A,** Gunshot wound of forearm showing extensive soft tissue injury. **B,** Initial radiograph. **C,** Microvascular reconstruction using a bilobed latissimus dorsi musculocutaneous flap was done in association with fracture fixation. **D,** Long-term follow-up of reconstructed forearm that also required sural nerve grafting to a segmental injury of the median nerve.

margin of the skin graft is designed to be in these same lines to prevent contractures across flexion creases. Palmar incisions follow the pattern of skin creases. Dorsal incisions on the fingers and wrist and incisions on the forearm may follow longitudinal straight lines.

### Dressings and Splints

The purposes of dressings are to protect wounds, absorb drainage, and help splint repaired structures. The first layer consists of a nonadherent dressing and may contain an antibiotic. The next layer is soft and bulky and is usually followed by a firmer, more conforming external wrap. Conforming compression is useful, but constriction is harmful. Splints are made to protect only the part necessary to be immobilized and must not prevent motion in the remainder of the extremity. Often, patients keep the injured, operated, or infected hand in a flexed wrist position, which automatically causes the MP joints to extend, thereby placing the collateral ligaments in their shortest lengths. Edema fluid collects dorsally and the resulting dorsal hand swelling causes stiff joints. Thus, a splint that keeps the hand in the protected position extends the wrist 40 to 50 degrees, maintaining the MP joints at 70 degrees of flexion and the IP joints in a neutral position (Fig. 70-15). Postoperative hand elevation is essential to reduce edema.

## TRAUMA

### Emergency Control of Bleeding

Bleeding in the extremity can often be profuse when first encountered. A reasoned and controlled assessment of the situation almost invariably results in the control of bleeding and minimization of further blood loss, and facilitates necessary stabilization of the patient and appropriate assessment of the upper limb injury. Bleeding in the upper extremity often results when vessels lie in a superficial location, such as at the wrist. Bleeding can originate from superficial veins that bleed more profusely when poorly applied dressings result in venous engorgement. The thicker media of transected arterial walls contract strongly, resulting in hemostasis. Partially lacerated arteries continue to bleed profusely.

Elevation and accurately placed point pressure over bleeding points result in hemostatic control in almost all cases. Brief use of tourniquets may be a useful adjunct to allow temporary control of blood loss in the emergency room (ER). Poorly applied dressings may be removed, bleeding points identified, point pressure dressings applied, and the hand elevated. This should take no more than 5 to 10 minutes. Extended tourniquet application results in hyperemic bleeding on deflation and subsequently hinders the surgeon. Tourniquets should not be applied for any significant period of time before definitive repair in the operating room (OR), except for control of torrential hemorrhage caused by major amputation in the field. Misguided attempts to control upper extremity bleeding with clamps, ligatures, and cauterization in the ER frequently result in additional avoidable injury to adjacent uninjured structures and to vessels that may need to be repaired for adequate limb perfusion. Fracture reduction and stabilization will improve distal perfusion and facilitate hemorrhage control by restoring the limb to its correct anatomic alignment.

### Lacerations, Fingertip, and Complex Soft Tissue Injuries

Although it is tempting to look within a wound to determine whether any tendon or nerve injuries exist, the same information can be obtained by careful physical examination without further violating a potential operative field and causing the patient

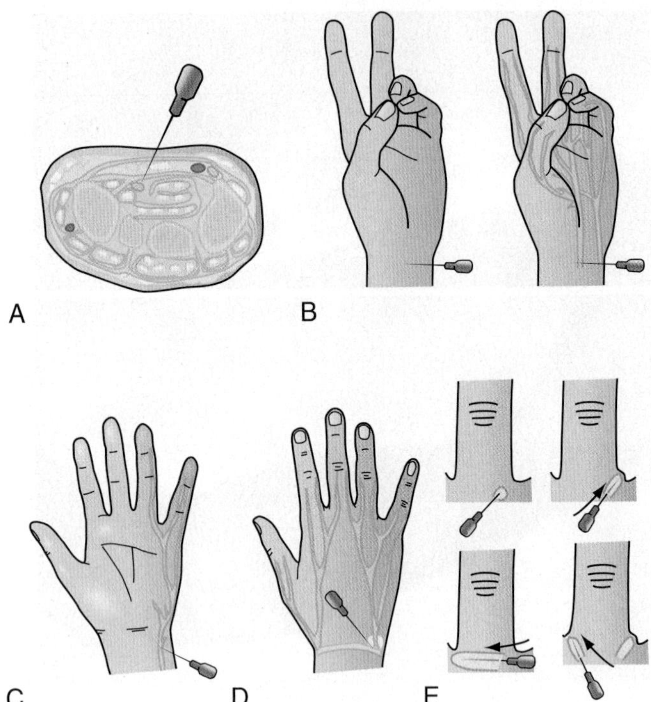


**FIGURE 70-13** **A,** Median nerve block is done at the wrist, where the median nerve is superficial to all the flexor tendons in the carpal tunnel. **B,** At the wrist, when a median nerve block is performed, the needle is directed between the PL and FCR tendons. **C,** Ulnar nerve block at the wrist is done by passing the injecting needle around the ulnar deep aspect of the FCU tendon just proximal to the pisiform. Intravascular injection into the immediately adjacent ulnar artery is avoided by first aspirating before injection. **D,** Dorsal branches of the ulnar nerve and superficial sensory radial nerve are anesthetized by raising a broad weal of local anesthetic across the dorsum of the wrist. **E,** A dorsal approach to the finger can be used for digital nerve block.

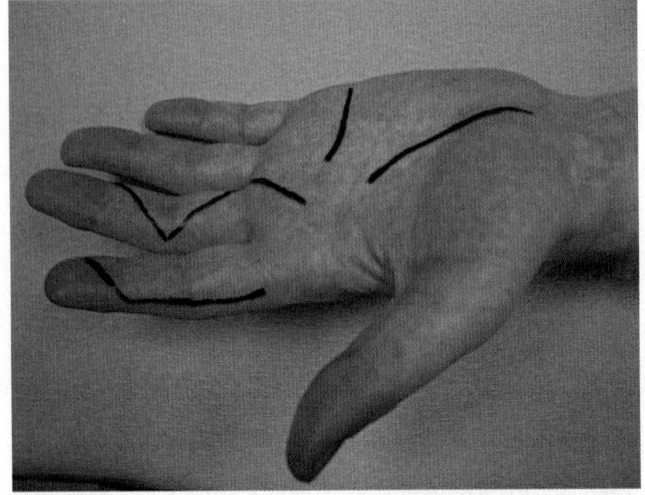

**FIGURE 70-14** Incisions used on the palmar surface of the hand must respect the creases. These may be zigzag Brunner incisions or midaxial incisions of the digits.

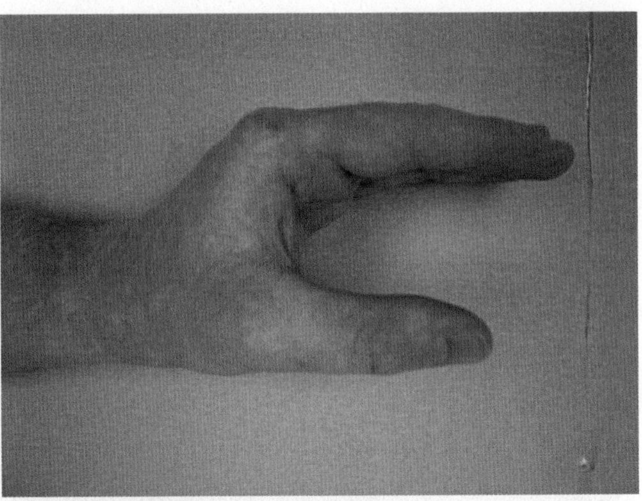

**FIGURE 70-15** Application of a splint and dressings to demonstrate the safe or protected position of the wrist, hand, and digits. The thumb is palmar-abducted.

extreme discomfort. A combination of knowledge of anatomy, presence of sensory or motor deficits, and presence or absence of radial or ulnar pulses can narrow the differential diagnosis of injured structures to a minimum. Control of bleeding is attempted by direct pressure with dressings and not by blind clamping of vessels because vital structures may be inadvertently injured in the depths of the wound. However, a tourniquet may be used if the initial pressure measures fail. Tourniquets are generally not used initially because the entire limb will be ischemic during patient transport. If the trauma has caused complete obliteration of anatomy, incisions can be extended into nonviolated areas in which control of bleeding vessels and delineation of injured tendons and nerves may be easier, using the guidelines presented earlier for extremity incisions.

All patients who present with extremity injuries undergo radiography. Fractures of the distal phalanx are among the more commonly encountered hand fractures.[4] A distal phalangeal fracture is appropriately splinted, reduced to improve alignment, or occasionally fixated internally if the fracture is unstable. Internal fixation is usually provided by simply placing a longitudinal 0.028-inch Kirschner wire. Appropriate antibiotics are administered because, technically, these are open fractures.

The least severe injury of the dorsum of the fingertip is a nail bed hematoma. When seen early, the hematoma can be decompressed by perforating the nail plate after the administration of a digital local anesthetic block. Fingertip and nail bed injuries can be managed with digital block anesthesia and a Penrose drain at the base of the finger as a tourniquet. After the nail plate has been stripped, simple gentle removal of the nail to examine the underlying nail bed is done and suture repair of the nail bed is performed using loupe magnification and a 6-0 catgut suture. Once the nail bed has been repaired, it is best to place the thoroughly cleansed nail back under the nailfold, where it serves as a rigid splint for an underlying distal phalangeal fracture and prevents adhesions from forming between the adjacent surfaces of the nailfold, which might lead to an unsightly split nail deformity. If there is a piece of nail bed missing, the undersurface of the avulsed nail plate is examined. Frequently, the missing piece may still be adherent to the nail, and it can be

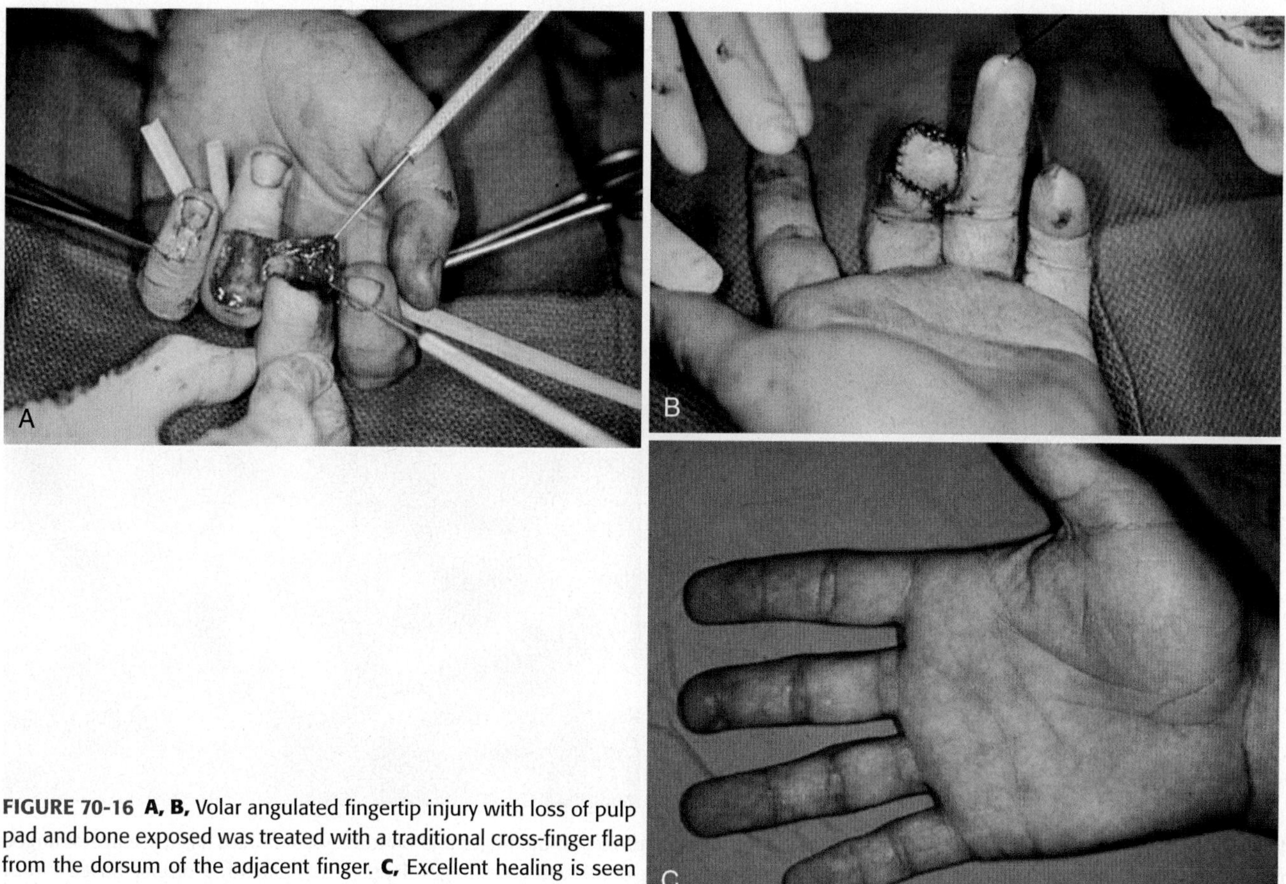

**FIGURE 70-16** **A, B,** Volar angulated fingertip injury with loss of pulp pad and bone exposed was treated with a traditional cross-finger flap from the dorsum of the adjacent finger. **C,** Excellent healing is seen in the long term after flap division.

gently removed and replaced as a nail bed graft. Some fingertip injuries may be so severe that amputation revision may be the most sensible and functional solution.

Volar fingertip injuries range from simple to more complex. Multiple digits may be involved, such as with lawnmower injuries. If bone is not exposed and a soft tissue defect of the finger pulp is smaller than 1 cm, the wound is best left open and managed with dressings. Such an injury will heal with excellent functional and cosmetic results. Larger soft tissue defects of the fingertip pulp are more appropriately treated with a small, full-thickness skin graft. However, if bone is exposed and the soft tissue wound is larger, flap coverage or revision of amputation by trimming back exposed bone to obtain soft tissue coverage should be considered. In a dorsally angulated fingertip amputation, soft tissue coverage can be achieved by a neurovascular V-Y advancement flap. If the soft tissue loss is angulated in a more volar direction, a cross-finger flap, adjacent finger digital island flap, or homodigital flap may be performed (Figs. 70-16 to 70-18).

## Tendon Injuries

### Flexor Tendons

Flexor tendon injuries usually result from lacerations or puncture wounds on the palmar surface of the hand, although flexor tendons can be avulsed from their distal bony insertions by sudden violent contractions. These are best treated by a surgeon experienced in the treatment of such injuries. Flexor tendon injuries are divided into five zones (Fig. 70-19). In zones 1, 2, and 4, each tendon is surrounded by a synovial sheath and contained within a semirigid fibro-osseous canal, either within the flexor tendon sheath of the digit or carpal tunnel. In the other zones, the flexor tendons are surrounded by loose areolar (paratenon) tissue. Those parts devoid of a fibrous sheath usually heal very well because of the good blood supply from the paratenon. Tendons in the carpal tunnel (zone 4) have their rich blood supply provided by the mesotenon; however, zones 1 and 2 have a precarious blood supply through the vincula; complementary nutritional support is provided by the synovial fluid in these latter two zones. For tendon gliding to occur, the mesotenon has disappeared in the digital flexor sheath except at the sites of the vincula that carry the vessels from the periosteum to the tendons (Fig. 70-20). Tendon zones to the thumb are T1 through T3.

Primary tendon repair undertaken within a few hours of injury is generally reserved for cleanly cut tendons. Delayed primary repair is performed from several hours up to 10 days after injury and is indicated for tidy, but potentially contaminated, wounds to allow for prophylaxis against infection before the tendon repair. Relative contraindications to immediate tendon repair include the following:

1. Injuries more than 12 hours old
2. Crush wounds with poor skin coverage
3. Contaminated wounds, especially human bites
4. Tendon loss more than 1 cm
5. Injury at multiple sites along the tendon
6. Destruction of the pulley system

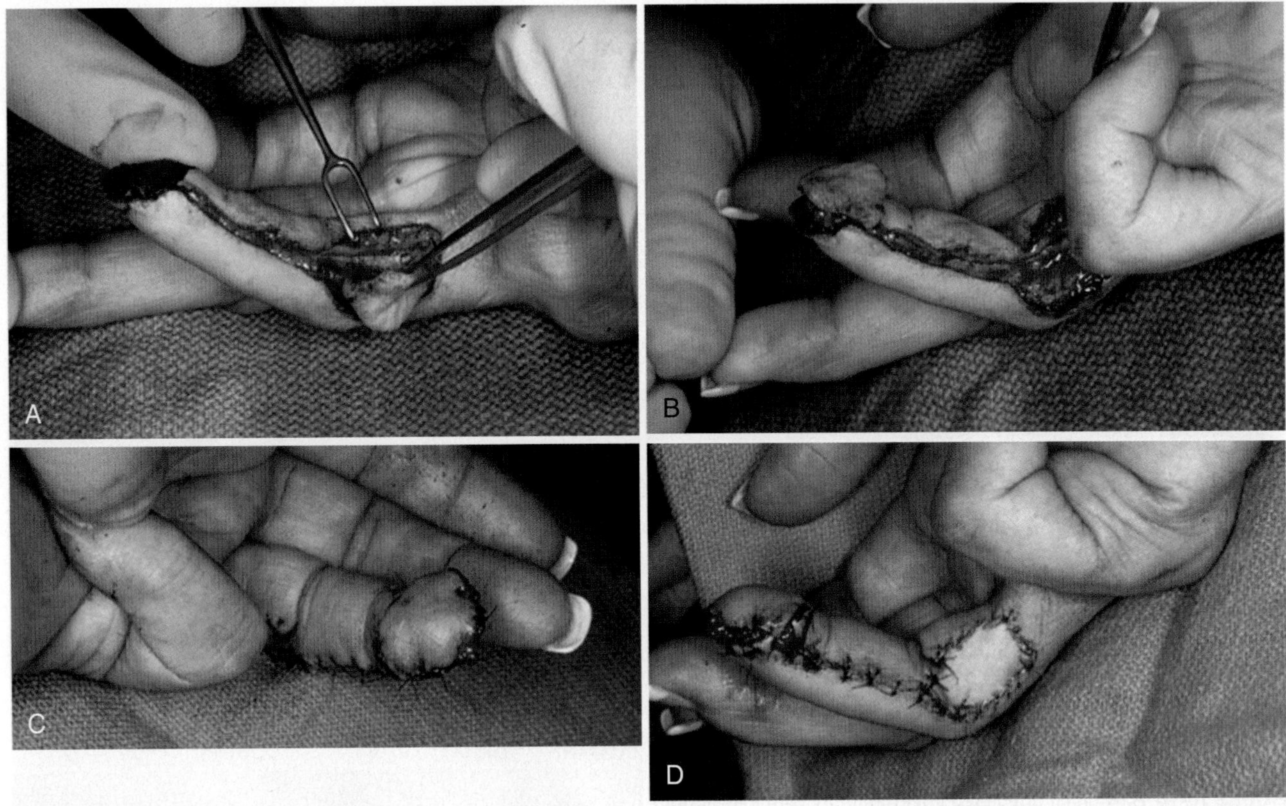

**FIGURE 70-17 A-D,** More recent understanding of the vascular skin territories of the finger and hand enable intrinsic flap coverage of fingertip injuries and avoid the cumbersome tethering of adjacent fingers, as is done with cross-finger flaps. In this patient, a distally based turnover vascular island flap reconstructs an avulsed fingertip. The reverse-flow perforating vessels at the proximal IP joint cross from the opposite side to nourish this flap.

After 4 weeks, a later secondary repair is generally not possible because of retraction of the musculotendinous unit so that reapproximation of the tendon ends produces undesirable joint flexion. In this situation, tendon graft repair may be required. The surgeon's endeavors are directed at avoiding the four major complications that interfere with smooth gliding and the integrated action of tendons—adhesions, attenuation of the repair, repair rupture, and joint and soft tissue contractures. Prerequisites for tendon repair are aseptic conditions in the OR, with good lighting, good instruments, adequate anesthesia, and loupe magnification. A well-performed technical operation can be futile without proper postoperative hand therapy, splinting, and excellent patient compliance.[5]

Appropriate treatment of partial flexor tendon injuries is necessary to produce a smooth juncture at the injury site. Prevention of complications requires exploration of all wounds likely to cause partial flexor tendon lacerations. A partial tendon injury of 50% or less is treated by simple trimming of the lacerated portion. Those injuries greater than 50% are repaired. Failure to diagnose a partial flexor tendon laceration at the time of primary repair may lead to delayed tendon rupture, entrapment between the tendon laceration and the laceration in the flexor sheath, or trigger finger.

Zone 2 flexor tendon injuries require special attention. This zone is also called *Bunnell's no man's land.* There are three tendons—the profundus and two slips of superficialis—that traverse zone 2 and they constantly interchange their mutual spatial relationships. Tendon injury in this region requires opening the existing laceration in the flexor tendon sheath by making a longitudinal trap door so that a flap of tendon sheath can be elevated. Care must be taken to avoid excising excessive portions of the flexor tendon sheath because bowstringing may result in ineffective finger flexion, although portions can be vented or excised to facilitate repair or prevent postoperative triggering. Total preservation of the A2 and A4 pulleys, previously thought to be essential, is no longer believed to be critical to success. One can excise up to 50% of the A2 and A4 pulleys without creating unnecessary tendon bowstringing if this is thought to be prudent to avoid the tendon repair impinging under the pulley.[6] It has also been shown that one can incise the full length of the A4 pulley (but not excise it), without any biomechanical consequences.[7] This is especially helpful when the zone 2 repair occurs proximate to the A4 pulley, the narrowest part of the flexor tendon sheath. Finally, wide awake anesthesia, which is local anesthetic infiltration using a solution of xylocaine with epinephrine, enables flexor tendon repair without the use of a tourniquet and ensures full patient cooperation during the procedure.[8] This was previously thought to be unwise, but this has been proven to be unsubstantiated. Thus, one can determine intraoperatively that there is full flexor tendon excursion at the repair site without impingement under the pulleys as the patient flexes and extends his or her fingers before the skin incision is finally closed. All these novel and revolutionary concepts challenge previously accepted dogma with regard to zone 2 flexor

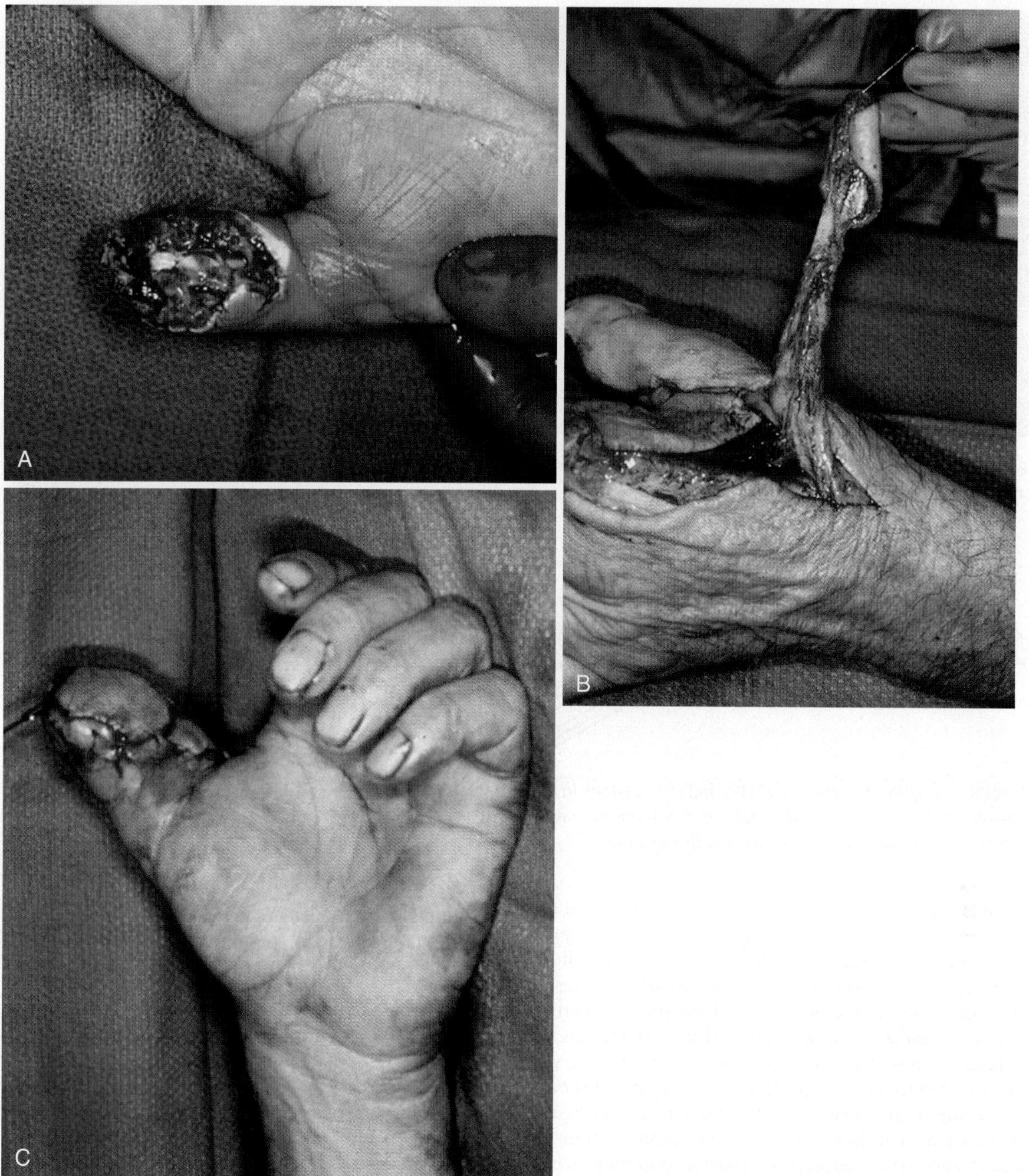


**FIGURE 70-18 A-C,** The first dorsal metacarpal artery flap is a vascularized island flap that is transposed from the dorsoradial aspect of the index finger to the distal pulp of the thumb following a crushing injury.

tendon repairs and the significance of the various annular pulleys. It is often difficult to repair profundus and superficialis tendons if they are injured in zone 2. Nonetheless, both can be repaired because resection of the superficialis reduces overall grip strength, predisposes to a recurvatum and swan neck deformity at the PIP joint, and damages the vincula supply to the profundus.

Usually, skin wounds have to be extended proximally and distally in a zigzag fashion to display the retracted divided tendon ends. Tendon ends are handled with a fine-toothed forceps and the tendon surface is never touched. The wrist is flexed and a small Keith needle is passed transversely through the proximal tendon, approximately 2 cm from the end, transfixing it to the skin and tendon sheath. In this way, immobilization of the tendon end facilitates a tension-free repair. Ragged tendon ends may be squared off sharply, but no more than 1 cm is resected or permanent finger contracture will result. The tendon ends are brought together by a single tension-holding, locking, core suture. Various locking core suture techniques have been described, but usually a modified Kessler-type suture is placed. A specifically placed locking loop increases the ultimate tensile strength of the tendon repair by 10% to 50% compared

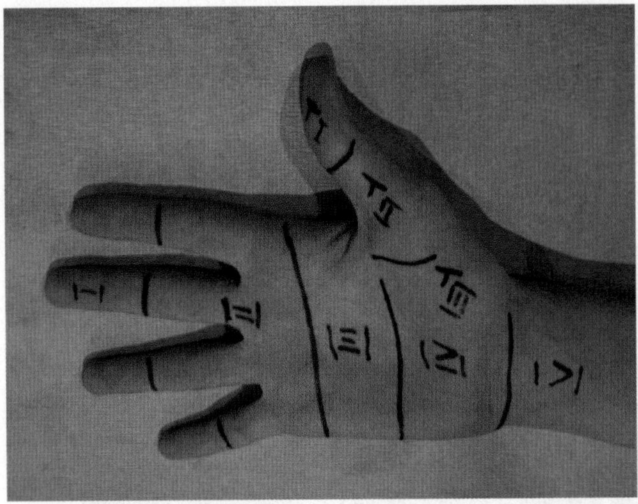

**FIGURE 70-19** Zones of flexor tendon injuries on the fingers, thumb, and hand.

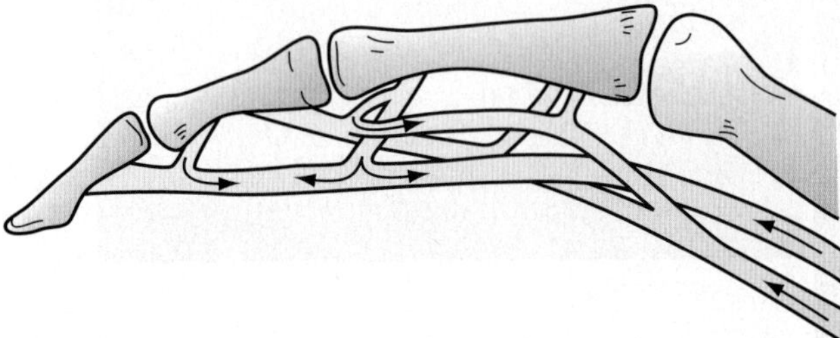

**FIGURE 70-20** Complex arrangement of FDS and FDP tendons in the flexor sheath of the fingers. Blood supply to the tendons travels through the vincula from the dorsal aspects of the tendons.

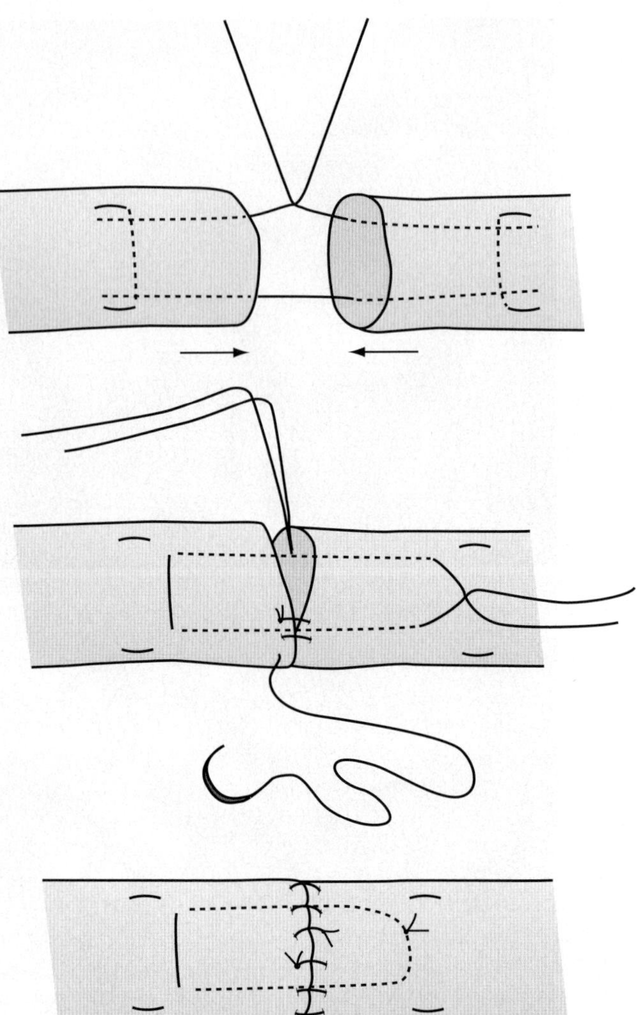

**FIGURE 70-21** Technique of performing a four-strand flexor tendon core suture repair is demonstrated in association with a peripheral running suture.

with a simple mattress suture. If this is not done, tension on the suture line can open up the repair, increasing the propensity for tendon gapping at the repair site. The ideal suture material for tendon repairs has not been found. A 4-0 coated polyester or braided nylon suture is the best material for the core suture. Increasing the number of suture strands that cross the tendon repair site and obtaining suture bites of at least 0.7 cm will increase the overall tensile strength of the actual repair.[9] However, the more suture strands that are added, the greater will be the friction and edema within the flexor tendon sheath. A four- or six-stranded core repair appears to provide optimum repair strength and does not increases stiffness and friction at the repair site excessively. Some perform a four-stranded core repair by simply using a double-stranded type of suture material, whereas others place a second core suture with a single-stranded material. A four-stranded core repair permits a light, protected, composite grip for the duration of postoperative healing. Also, a running circumferential epitenon suture repair is also placed (Fig. 70-21). This not only helps smooth the repair but also adds to the ultimate tensile strength at the repair site and reduces gap formation. A peripheral 6-0 nylon suture serves this purpose.

The forces generated on FDP flexor tendons during passive finger flexion are 600 g and during active finger flexion are 2000 g; with strong active finger flexion, they are 8000 g. However, after tendon repair, the effects of wound healing, changes in elasticity, and added friction between the flexor tendons and their surrounding tissues will affect the overall work of flexion. There will be added frictional forces caused by edema, the presence of suture material, and the pulley system. The estimated work of flexion (resistance) increases by a factor of 50% after tendon repair. Thus, the estimated forces on repaired tendons, with 50% added for the work of flexion, are 900 g for passive finger flexion, 3000 g for active finger flexion, and 12,000 g for strong active flexion. The ultimate tensile strengths of various repairs are 2600 g for two-stranded and simple epitendinous repair, 4600 g for four-stranded and simple epitendinous repair, and 6800 g for six-stranded and simple epitendinous repair. The strength of the initial tendon repair decreases by approximately 25% during the first 3 weeks and then steadily increased thereafter to 6 weeks. Hence, if one is to undertake a postoperative active finger flexion protocol, then at least a four- or six-stranded core suture tendon repair is needed.[10]

Zone 1 flexor tendon injury may be caused by a penetrating injury. However, closed-traction injury may also cause profundus tendon avulsion, which most frequently involves the ring or middle finger. In the repair of a zone 1 injury, a pullout suture is necessary if the distal tendon length is insufficient to repair

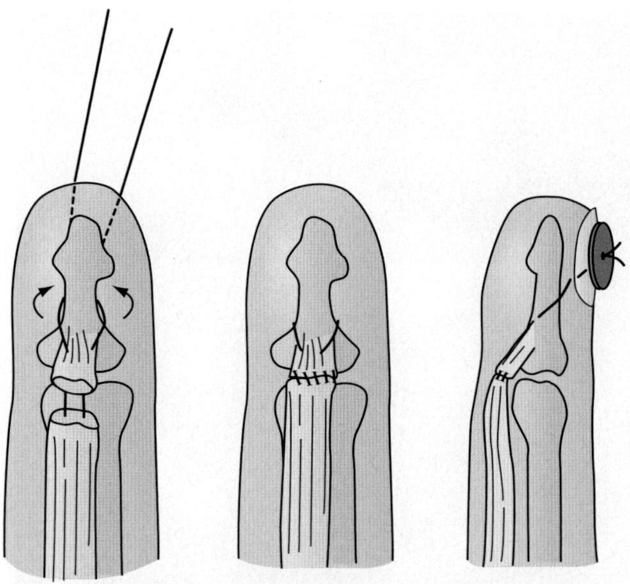

**FIGURE 70-22** Zone 1 flexor tendon repair to reattach tendon to bone.

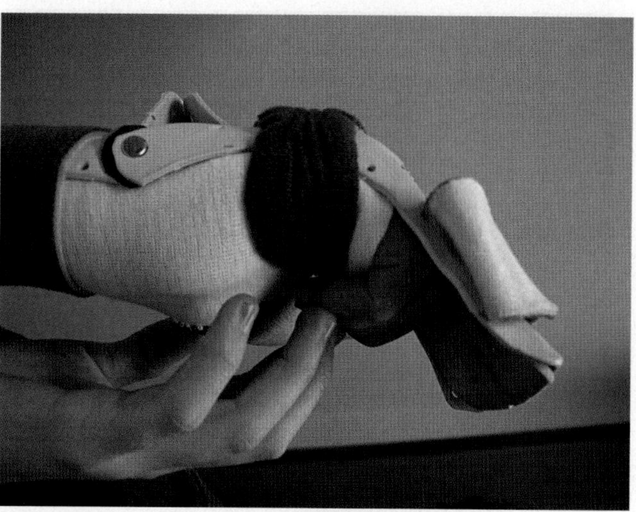

**FIGURE 70-23** Flexor hinge brace with place-and-hold technique of finger mobilization is one of the preferred methods for postoperative rehabilitation after flexor tendon repair.

the tendon securely (Fig. 70-22), although suture bone anchors have facilitated this mode of tendon repair into bone at the base of the distal phalanx.

Postoperatively, hand elevation is important to reduce edema. The wrist is placed in approximately 20 degrees of flexion and the MP joint at approximately 60 to 70 degrees of flexion. The splint is molded against the fingers, with the IP joints fully extended. A system of rubber band dynamic traction may be used following the repair of flexor tendons in zone 2, with good results obtained in more than 80% of cases. Differential excursion between the two digital flexors is dramatically increased by a synergistic splint that allows for wrist extension and finger flexion. This position of wrist extension and MP joint flexion produces the least tension on a repaired flexor tendon during active digital flexion; thus, we have come to use the flexor hinge brace technique and the so-called *place-and-hold protocol* (Fig. 70-23). Of all the postoperative flexor tendon protocols, this enables the greatest overall tendon excursion of each of the FDS and FDP tendons and the most significant differential tendon gliding between the FDS and FDP repair sites, which theoretically would then reduce the risk of adhesion formation between the two tendons. A tenodesis brace with a wrist hinge is fabricated to allow for full wrist flexion, wrist extension of 30 degrees, and maintenance of MP joint flexion of at least 60 degrees. After composite passive digital flexion, the wrist is extended and passive finger flexion is maintained. The patient actively maintains digital flexion and holds that position for approximately 5 seconds. The patient is instructed to use the lightest muscle power necessary to maintain digital flexion. Wrist flexion and finger extension follow. This protected motion postoperative protocol is continued for 6 weeks.

### Extensor Tendons

Proper diagnosis of extensor tendon injuries requires full knowledge of the relatively complex anatomy of the extensor mechanism of the dorsum of the finger. The subcutaneous location of extensor tendons makes them susceptible to crush, laceration, and avulsion injuries. The presence of juncturae tendinum prevents proximal retraction of the EDC tendons. Extensor tendon injuries have been divided into nine zones, which ascend numerically from the dorsum of the DIP joints to the forearm. The odd-numbered zones begin at the DIP joint and are located over the joints; the even-numbered zones are located between the joints.

Extensor tendons are thinner than flexor tendons and, over the dorsum of the digits, are spread out to form the extensor hood. It may occasionally be possible to use conventional tendon repair techniques in the proximal parts of the tendons, but this is usually not the case in the extensor hood region. Here, horizontal mattress sutures or figure-of-eight mattress sutures may be needed. All lacerations are repaired if 50% or more of the tendon is divided.

Extensor tendon avulsions are most likely to occur at the DIP joint from a jamming type of injury that results in a mallet finger deformity (Fig. 70-24). If a bone fragment representing 50% or more of the articular surface is involved, or if there is volar subluxation of the DIP joint, an open reduction with internal fixation is performed. If there is a tendon rupture only or a small piece of bone is avulsed with the tendon, good results can be obtained by 6 weeks of continuous splinting with the DIP joint in extension (Fig. 70-25). After this period of splinting, the DIP joint is further protected during sleep for 2 more weeks.

Closed tears through the triangular ligament may be caused by PIP joint subluxation or a jamming type of injury that results in a boutonniere deformity. The central slip attachment at the base of the middle phalanx is disrupted, so that extension of that joint is altered. The lateral bands lose their support dorsal to the PIP joint axis and slip volar and become flexors at the PIP joint and extensors of the DIP joint. The consequent deformity is one of flexion at the PIP joint and hyperextension at the DIP joint. Within 6 weeks of injury, these can be treated satisfactorily by extension splinting at the PIP joint, maintaining the DIP joint free for active flexion and extension (see Fig. 70-25). If there is an open laceration to the central slip mechanism and adjacent triangular ligament, direct suture repair or reinsertion into bone

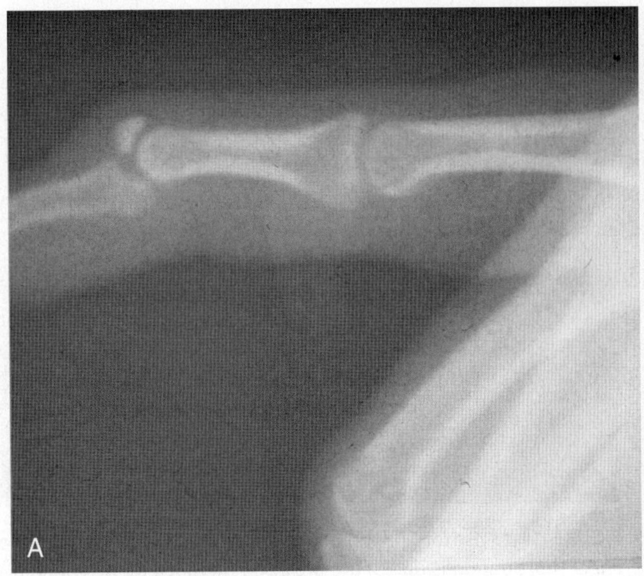

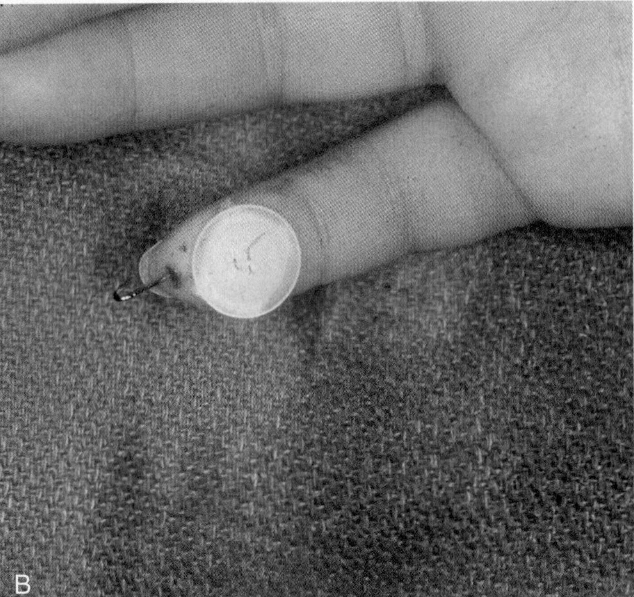

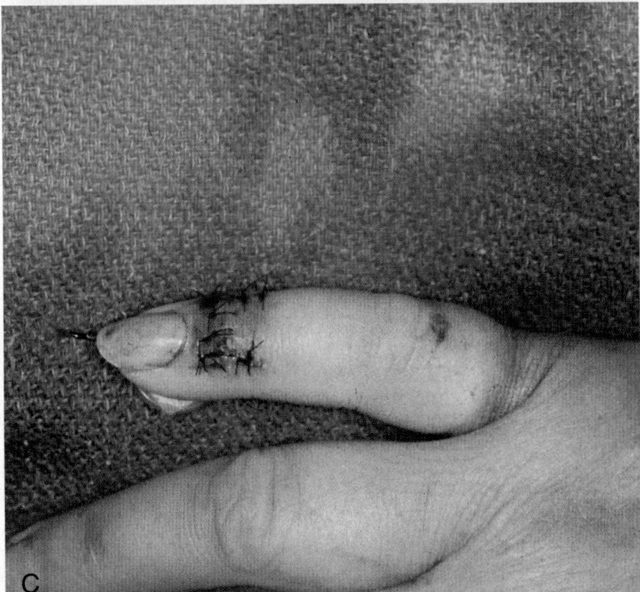

**FIGURE 70-24 A-C,** Mallet fracture with avulsed bony fragment involving more than 50% of the articular surface with volar subluxation of the distal phalanx. The bony fragment is reapproximated with a tie-over volar suture and a longitudinal pin traversing the DIP joint.

by means of bone anchor minisutures is performed, followed by the same postoperative protocol.

Extensor tendon injuries proximal to the PIP joint result in a drop finger (Fig. 70-26). These are repaired and splinted for 4 weeks. Common extensor tendon injuries over the dorsum of the hand and at the wrist must be repaired and then treated postoperatively by various different controlled motion protocols. One is a dynamic rubber band extension outrigger brace or use of a relative motion splint, in which the affected digit is kept at a more dorsal pitch to the adjacent fingers, thus relaxing the repaired tendon. This latter splint causes minimal interference with daily activities during rehabilitation (Fig. 70-27).[11]

## Nerve Injuries

Sunderland's classification, the most widely used classification, describes five types of nerve injury: neuropraxia (grade I), axonotmesis (grades II to IV), and neurotmesis (grade V). Neuropraxia is a physiologic block of impulse conduction without anatomic destruction of nerve fibers. This might occur with a closed injury, such as a radial nerve injury in the spiral groove associated with a midshaft humerus fracture. Neuropraxia may occur because of prolonged pressure in a tight anatomic location (e.g., carpal tunnel) or prolonged application of a tourniquet. Provided the offending cause is promptly removed, spontaneous recovery is generally the rule but can take as long as 3 months. In axonotmesis, axonal fibers are completely ruptured, generally from traction on the nerve (II). With higher energy injuries, the endoneurial (III) and perineurial (IV) nerve sheaths that support and nourish the axons and fascicles are progressively injured, leading to poorer nerve recovery, with increasing damage to intraneural architecture. *Neurotmesis* refers to complete transection of a nerve and is the most severe degree of nerve injury. It may result from direct sharp trauma or a violent traction injury. Accurate approximation of the cut

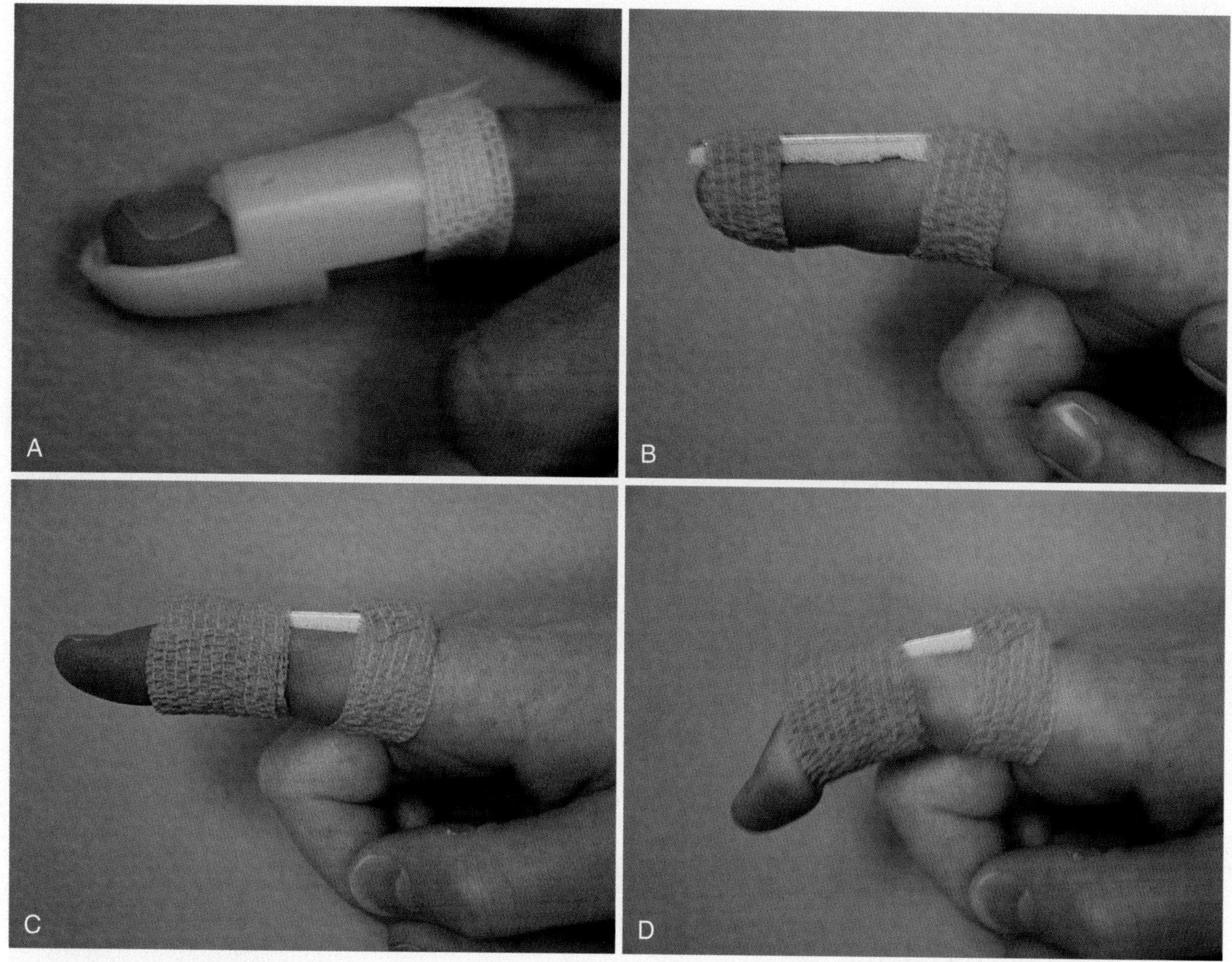


**FIGURE 70-25 A,** Prefabricated stack splint may be used for the closed treatment of a mallet finger. **B,** A simple dorsal aluminum splint may serve equally well for mallet finger treatment. **C, D,** Dorsal splinting across the PIP joint enables closed treatment of a boutonniere injury. The DIP is left free for flexion and extension.

nerve ends and meticulous repair are required for the best possible recovery. Axonal regeneration following axonotmesis or successful nerve repair following neurotmesis occurs at a rate of 1 mm/day. Traction injuries may result in a combination of all grades of nerve injury but, with intact external nerve sheaths, grades II to IV may be difficult to distinguish from one another clinically.

Severance of a peripheral nerve involves an acute loss of sensory, motor, and sympathetic functions. Knowledge of the motor and sensory distribution of the nerve is essential for clinical evaluation. However, associated injuries, such as fractures and muscle and tendon lacerations, may complicate the evaluation. Loss of pseudomotor activity occurs within 30 minutes of the nerve injury. Clinically, loss of sweating can sometimes be observed and denervated skin will not wrinkle if placed in water. Sensory denervation can also be demonstrated with a ninhydrin test. Nerve conduction studies are not immediately helpful but become valuable 3 weeks after injury, when fibrillation and denervation potentials can be measured in completely denervated muscles. In a closed injury, they may differentiate between a neuropraxia and neurotmesis. Later, nerve conduction studies may help monitor nerve regeneration following repair.

Primary nerve repair is done within 72 hours of injury, delayed primary repair from 72 hours to 14 days, and secondary nerve repairs 14 days or longer after injury. Primary neurorrhaphy is recommended in the following situations:

1. The nerve is sharply incised.
2. There is minimal wound contamination.
3. There are no injuries that preclude obtaining skeletal stability or adequate skin cover.
4. The patient is medically stable to undergo an operation.
5. Appropriate facilities and instrumentation are available.

In a completely severed nerve, wallerian degeneration occurs in the entire segment distal to the injury and 1 to 2 cm proximal to it. In closed injuries, when the severity of the nerve injury is unknown, repeat clinical evaluation and electrical studies every 3 to 6 weeks help distinguish between neuropraxia and axonal injury. In most cases, surgical exploration with repair is indicated after 3 months if no clinical recovery is detected.

The nerve repair must be tensionless. Stretching a nerve more than 10% compromises epineurial blood flow and thus its recovery. With sharp nerve lacerations, an epineurial repair

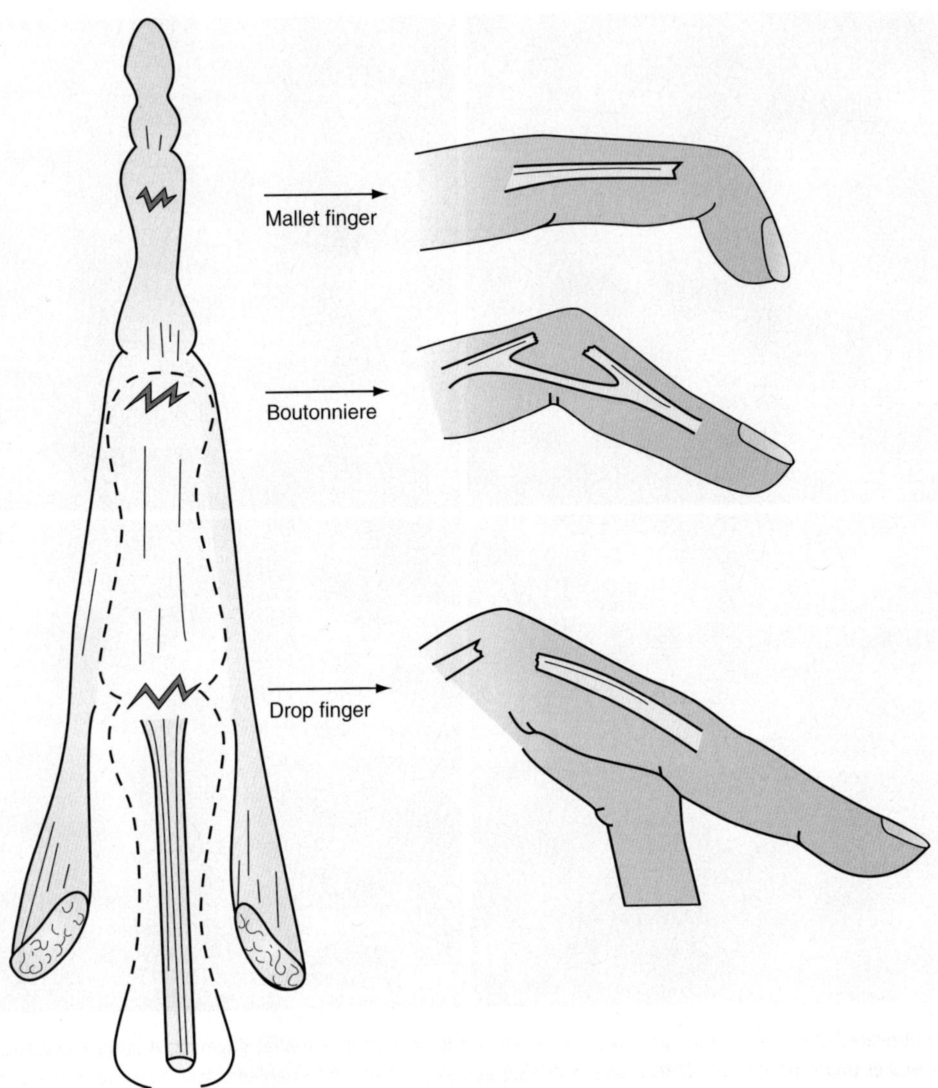


**FIGURE 70-26** Extensor tendon injuries on the dorsum of the finger. Injury at the distal insertion causes a mallet finger and, at the central slip over the PIP joint, causes a boutonniere deformity. Proximal to the PIP joint, over the proximal phalanx, injury results in a drop finger.

provides as good a functional recovery as fascicular (perineurial) repair, provided that anatomic landmarks such as the vasa nervorum are accurately realigned to provide precise matching of fascicles at the severed nerve ends.

A nerve gap may exist because of segmental nerve loss or when a crushed nerve segment is unsuitable for repair and must be resected. This may be overcome by proximal and distal mobilization of the nerve ends or, in the case of the ulnar nerve, by transposition of the nerve to the front of the elbow. If there is too much tension on the repair (cannot be held with an 8-0 nylon suture), a nerve conduit or nerve graft must be used.

It has been suggested that optimal nerve regeneration and appropriate matching of axons in proximal and distal nerve segments result from a combination of paracrine-mediated neurotropism and contact guidance of sprouting proximal axons. Experimental evidence has suggested that the neurotropic chemical gradient can effectively guide regenerating axons at least 14 mm through a hollow nerve conduit in the rat model. The conduit allows diffusion of the neurotropic signal while preventing a mechanical fibrous block between the proximal and distal nerve segments. However, large-gap animal models (30 mm) have shown poor or no recovery using nerve conduits, suggesting that a finite limit exists for this technique. Although the gap length that can be bridged successfully in humans is still uncertain, many surgeons consider the use of bioresorbable nerve conduits for gap lengths up to 2 cm to be appropriate for small peripheral nerves. Nerve grafting remains the gold standard for large or mixed nerves and the brachial plexus. Appropriate conduits are polyglycolic acid tubes and semipermeable collagen tubes, which have shown similar experimental outcomes (Fig. 70-28).[12]

With nerve grafting, fascicular matching, when chosen by the surgeon, may not always be appropriate. However, the additional contact guidance provided to regenerating axons makes successful nerve regeneration possible over longer distances than with conduits. Donor sources for nerve grafting usually include the terminal sensory portion of the posterior interosseous nerve and the medial antebrachial cutaneous nerve for small digital nerves. The sural nerve(s) are used for nerve gaps involving larger nerves.

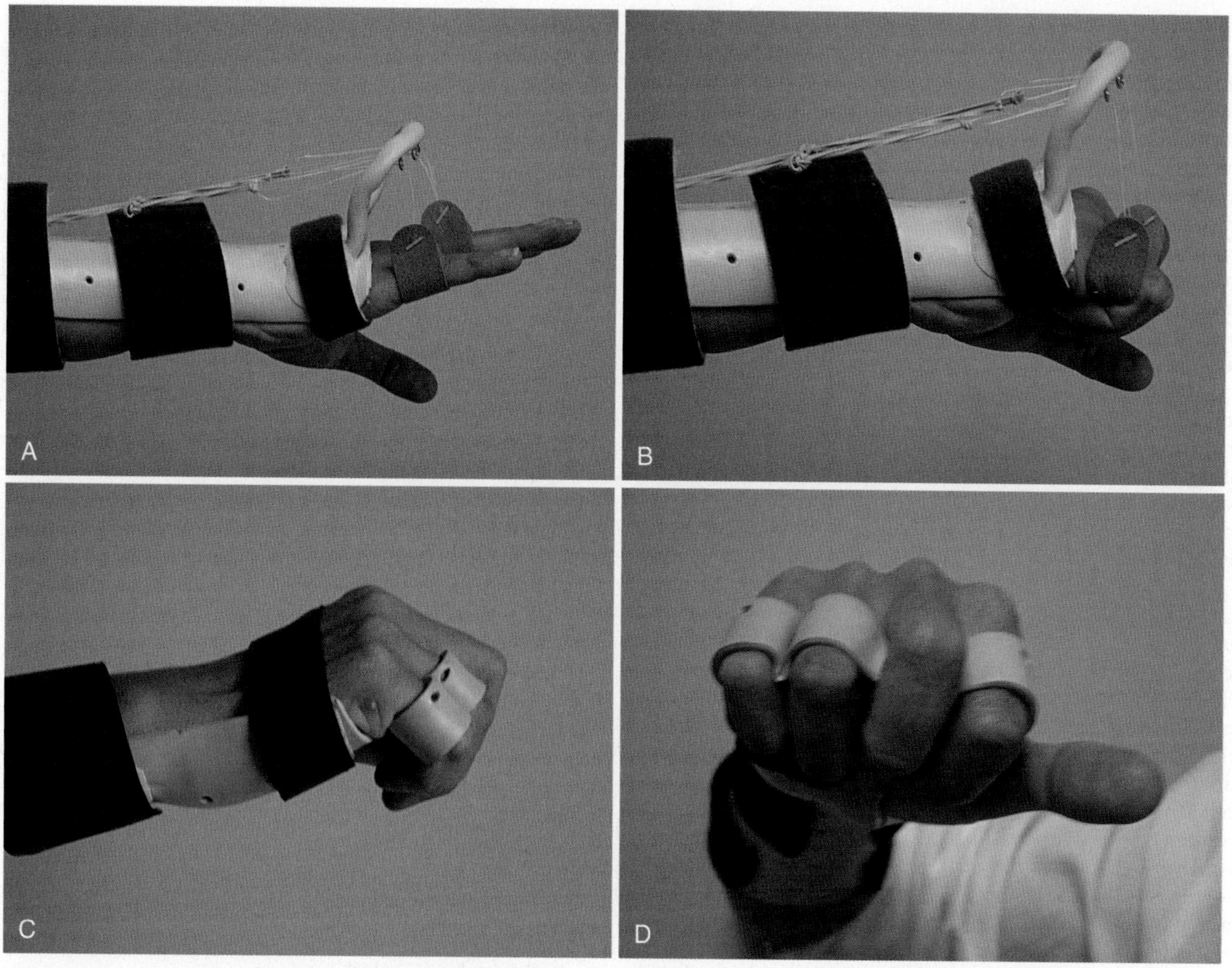

**FIGURE 70-27 A, B,** Extension outrigger dynamic splint commonly used for extensor tendon injuries postoperatively (extension and flexion views). **C, D,** Relative motion splint has the advantage of being low profile and causes minimal interference with daily activities and yet provides protection to the freshly repaired extensor tendon.

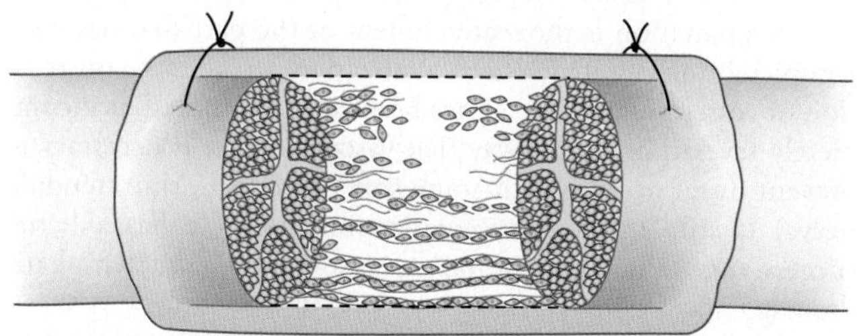

**FIGURE 70-28** Nerve conduits may be an appropriate treatment for short nerve gaps in the hand.

After nerve repair, the affected part is splinted for 3 weeks to protect the repair site in the position of least tension. Tinel's sign indicates the position of axonal regrowth; advancing distal progression of Tinel's sign with time indicates successful repair and nerve regeneration.

## Nerve Transfers

If there may be a long distance between the site of nerve injury and distal muscle target, primary nerve repair may be fruitless, because muscle degeneration would have occurred by the time distal neural growth occurs. Muscle recovery is unlikely after an 18-month lapse. Thus, if nerve growth occurs at the rate of approximately 1 mm/day, a proximal motor nerve lesion more than 540 mm proximal to the hand will be doomed to failure. Hence, for proximal arm nerve and brachial plexus injuries, nerve transfers may result in a nerve repair that is closer to the muscle target. The donor nerve must be chosen so as to minimize morbidity from loss of the donor nerve. The donor nerve must be closely related to the denervated muscle so that the repair is performed much closer to the muscle target. Nerve transfers have revolutionized the repair of proximal nerve injuries so that distal muscle atrophy is minimized. For example, the classic Oberlin transfer uses part of the ulnar nerve (usually a single fascicle) for transfer to the musculocutaneous nerve and to the brachialis in the upper arm to restore elbow flexion.[13] It is technically easy, quick, and effective. No significant motor or sensory deficits result in the territory of the ulnar nerve. This technique has become popular and is indicated for C5-6 brachial plexus lesions when C8-T1 is intact. It can also be used to neurotize a functioning free muscle transfer that may be required if the native muscles have already sustained atrophy because of prolonged denervation.

## Vascular Injuries

Acute vascular injuries may follow closed or penetrating trauma or iatrogenic injury. Fractures or dislocations may cause vascular injury. Indirect vascular trauma may be caused by traction injuries, which can avulse vessels, or by intimal damage or repetitive microtrauma from vibratory tools, which can lead to thrombosis. The latter usually affects the ulnar artery in Guyon's canal at the wrist and is called the *hypothenar hammer syndrome*. Regardless of the cause, vascular injuries may lead to a critical compromise of circulation in the extremity. With a closed injury, the onset of symptoms may be delayed, because swelling, hypotension, and intimal injury combine and result in late thrombosis and vascular insufficiency.

Following an acute arterial injury, symptoms result from a combination of the adequacy of collateral circulation, post-traumatic sympathetic tone, and vasomotor control mechanisms. Patients with an upper extremity arterial injury who have adequate collateral circulation and normal vasomotor control may have minimal symptoms, so reconstruction is not necessarily mandatory and the injury can be treated with simple arterial ligation. If there is a noncritical arterial injury, such as to the radial artery alone, reconstruction may be advocated to restore parallel flow in case of future arterial injury, enhance nerve recovery, facilitate healing, and prevent cold intolerance. However, the reported patency rate, even with microvascular techniques for single vessel repairs, varies from 47% to 82%. The following injuries are optimally managed by vascular repair and reconstruction: axillary or brachial artery injury; combined radial and ulnar artery injury; and radial or ulnar artery injury associated with poor collateral circulation. Relative indications for repair of a noncritical vascular injury are extensive distal soft tissue injury, technical ability to achieve repair without compromising the patient's well-being, and a combined vascular and neural injury. The need for arterial reconstruction necessitates assessing the adequacy of collateral circulation; this is based primarily on initial clinical judgment. However, the final decision regarding arterial reconstruction is often made in the OR after exploration. Once the injured structures have been isolated, potential bleeding sites controlled, and hematoma evacuated, the distal extremity can be assessed more adequately. At this time, lacerated vessel ends are controlled by atraumatic vascular clamps and a tourniquet can be released. Capillary refill and perfusion of the distal extremity can then be assessed, as can backflow from the distal lacerated vessel ends. Digital blood pressure can be quantified with a sterile Doppler probe and cuff; a digital brachial index of 0.7 or greater suggests adequate perfusion. If there is poor collateral flow, arterial reconstruction is performed. At this time, standard of care does not require arterial repair of isolated noncritical vessels. In combined radial and ulnar artery injuries, one or both vessels are reconstructed. If possible, both vessels are repaired.[14]

Muscles often swell after prolonged periods of ischemia. This can lead to an increase of pressure within the closed compartment of the forearm, resulting in a compartment syndrome. It is thus the practice of most surgeons to perform a routine fasciotomy to decompress the forearm compartment after a true revascularization procedure has been performed. During the period of ischemia to the muscles, there may be a buildup of lactic acid. Furthermore, myonecrosis might occur. Restoration of circulation to such a limb can cause a sudden flooding of the circulation with myoglobin, lactic acid, and other toxic substances. This is called *reperfusion syndrome* and can lead to multiorgan failure, especially affecting the renal and cardiac systems.

## Replantation and Amputations

It can often be frustrating for the novice general surgeon being told by a replantation surgeon in the middle of the night that a consultation was obtained inappropriately or not soon enough. There are general indications for the replantation of amputated parts, but the overriding decision is still to save life before limb. Although patients and family members may desire—and in some cases have even been promised by members of the primary team—replantation, it is not performed in patients with severe associated medical problems or injuries. Replantation is also generally not considered under the following circumstances[2,15]:

1. Severe crush or multilevel injury of the amputated part
2. A psychotic patient who has willfully self-amputated the part
3. Amputation of a single digit proximal to the FDS distal insertion (zone 2), except for single-digit amputations in children or those with a demanding profession (e.g., a musician)
4. Amputation in patients with severely atherosclerotic arteries (sometimes this can only be determined when exploring the vessels in the OR)

Indications for replantation of amputated parts are as follows:

1. Whenever possible for a thumb amputation (it provides >40% of the overall hand function)[15]
2. Single digits that have been amputated distal to the FDS insertion (e.g., a manual worker may likely desire revision of amputation and desires to return to work quickly)
3. Multiple injured digits
4. Most amputations in children, including single-digit amputations
5. Guillotine-sharp clean amputations at the hand, wrist, or distal forearm

Replantation is the reattachment of the part that has been completely amputated. Revascularization requires reconstruction of vessels in a limb that has been severely injured or incompletely severed in such a way that vascular repair is necessary to prevent distal necrosis, but some soft tissue (e.g., skin, tendon, nerve) is still intact. Revascularization generally has a better success rate than replantation because venous and lymphatic drainage may be intact.

Minor replantation is a reattachment at the wrist, hand, or digital level, whereas major replantation is performed proximal to the wrist. This clinical distinction exists because in the case of a major replantation, ischemic time is crucial to the viability of muscle and to functional outcome. Ischemic muscle may result in myonecrosis, myoglobinemia, and infection, which may threaten the patient's life (as well as limb). There are three types of amputations:

1. Guillotine amputation, whereby the tissue is cut with a sharp object and is minimally damaged
2. Crush amputation, in which a local crushing injury can be converted into a guillotine injury simply by débriding back the edges, although this may not be possible in a diffusely crushing amputation

3. Avulsion amputation, which is the most unfavorable type for replanting because structures are injured at different levels

Avulsion amputation may occur, for example, with a so-called *ring avulsion injury*. The extensor tendons are shredded, flexor tendons are often avulsed at the musculotendinous junctions, and nerves are stretched and may be ripped from end organs.

Ischemia time is also an important consideration when evaluating a patient for replantation. For amputated digits, more than 12 hours of warm ischemia is a relative contraindication. Promptly cooling the part to 4° C dramatically alters the ischemia factor, but even ischemia exceeding 24 hours does not necessarily preclude successful digital replantation. Ischemia time is more crucial for replantation above the proximal forearm, and reimplantation is not considered after more than 6 to 10 hours of warm ischemia time. Single digits in adults, other than the thumb in zone 2, are generally not reattached because of the consequent adverse overall functional result on the hand, with a single stiff finger.[15]

Amputation is not an outmoded operation; rather, it is necessary in a patient in whom replantation might not be indicated. When primary amputation is performed, the stump is preserved with as much length as possible. An exception might be made if there is only a very short segment of proximal phalanx. A short proximal phalangeal remnant at the index finger position may serve as an impediment for thumb to middle finger prehension, and one might consider a formal ray amputation in this case to improve overall hand function. The ends of the cut nerve are cut sharply and allowed to retract to minimize the occurrence of painful neuromas at the amputation tip. Tendons are also divided sharply and allowed to retract. The practice of suturing flexor and extensor tendons over the ends of the middle, ring, or small finger stump seriously impairs the motion of the uninjured fingers because of the common origin of the flexors. There will be an active flexion deficit in the uninjured digits, the quadriga syndrome; this is corrected simply by release of the flexor tendon remnant at the injured amputated digit.

If it is anticipated that the amputated part will be considered for replantation, it is critical to transport the patient and the part in an appropriate manner. The amputated part is placed in a clean, dry, plastic bag, which is sealed and placed on top of ice in a Styrofoam container. This keeps the part sufficiently cool at 4° to 10° C without freezing. The amputated part is wrapped in a lightly moistened saline gauze to prevent tissue drying.

With only a few minor variations, the sequence of replantation has been standardized. Preliminary exploration of the distal amputated part under a microscope by an initial surgical team not only determines whether a replantation is technically feasible, but also can be started while the patient is being prepared for the operating room. Bone shortening allows skin to be débrided back to where it is free of contusion and direct tension-free closure can be achieved. In the thumb, bone shortening is minimized to less than 10 mm. The order of repair is usually bone, tendons, muscle units, arteries, nerves, and finally veins. Establishment of arterial flow before venous flow clears lactic acid from the replanted part. The functional veins can now also be detected by spurting bleeding. However, blood loss must be closely monitored.

For major replantations, reestablishing arterial circulation as rapidly as possible is crucial to limiting ischemia time. A dialysis shunt or carotid shunt may be placed between the arterial ends. Intermittent clamping of the shunt may be necessary to restrict blood loss. In the upper extremity, bone shortening can be aggressive to achieve primary skin closure and primary nerve repair. Judicious use of anticoagulants may enhance the success of replantation. Topical application of 2% lidocaine or papaverine may help relieve vasospasm. Postoperative dressings consist of nonadherent mesh gauze, loose flap gauze, and a plaster splint, with postoperative elevation to minimize edema and venous congestion. The patient's room must be kept warm, and smoking is forbidden postoperatively. Aside from antibiotics and analgesics, one aspirin tablet daily for its retarding effect on platelet aggregation is suggested. Postoperative monitoring is done hourly to assess color, pulp turgor, capillary refill, and digital temperature.

## Fractures and Dislocations

Pain, swelling, limited motion, and deformities suggest the presence of a fracture or dislocation. Standard anteroposterior and lateral x-rays may miss some fractures and dislocations and multiple views may be necessary to establish the exact diagnosis. Fractures may be rotated, angulated, telescoped, or displaced. Angulation is described by the direction in which the apex of the fracture is pointing, and displacement is described by the direction of the distal fragment. Fractures may be open or closed, depending on whether a wound is involved. They may also be complete, incomplete, or comminuted (more than two pieces). Fractures are also described by their pattern; they may be transverse, longitudinal, oblique, or spiral. Open fractures need to be thoroughly irrigated and débrided urgently. Displaced fractures or dislocations are repositioned as soon as possible. A dislocation is described according to the direction of displacement of the distal bone in the involved joint. The separation of joints may be complete or incomplete (subluxed), depending on the severity of the capsular injury.[4,16,17]

Displaced fractures or dislocations are repositioned as soon as possible to decrease soft tissue injury, decompress nerves that might be stretched, and relieve kinking of blood vessels. Good bony contact and stability are necessary for fractures to heal. Some fractures are stable and require only external support in a splint or cast, whereas others are unstable and require internal support, which can be provided by Kirschner wires, internal wire sutures through drill holes in the fracture fragments, screws, plates, or even external fixation devices (Table 70-4). The more complicated the fixation, the more dissection is required to apply that fixation and therefore the greater the potential for scarring around adjacent tendons and consequential stiffness. Plates and screws, however, can nonetheless establish a degree of rigid fixation that allows early motion of the part and thus potentially reduces the risk for cicatricial stiffness. Intra-articular fractures require accurate reduction to preserve motion and minimize the risk for later development of arthrosis. Persistent rotational and significant lateral angular deformities generally do not remodel with time; these can be avoided by observing the alignment of the injured fingers as compared with adjacent digits while passively and gently flexing them into a fist after reduction is attained. If they do not fit comfortably adjacent to each other and do not point toward the distal pole of the scaphoid, a fresh attempt at reduction must be performed. A thorough

**Table 70-4 Comparison of Methods of Skeletal Fixation**

| METHOD OF FIXATION | ADVANTAGES | DISADVANTAGES |
|---|---|---|
| Kirschner wires | Come in varying diameters | Pins can loosen |
| | Can be applied percutaneously or open | Cannot provide rigid fixation |
| | Second surgery not required for removal | Soft tissue may be transfixed (but can be avoided by careful placement) |
| | Require less soft tissue dissection than plates and screws | Infection can occur along pin tracks |
| Screws | Have high stability | Frequently require open approach (although not always) |
| | Allow for early finger mobilization | |
| Plates | Can be used when fracture line is not oblique enough for screws | Require open approach<br>Require extensive soft tissue dissection |
| | Allow for early finger mobilization | Have relatively high profile and may be palpable through the dorsum of fingers and hand |
| | | May promote extensor tendon adhesions by their relative bulk and dissection required for placement |

neurovascular examination is always performed before and after fracture reduction has been completed.

### Distal Phalangeal Fractures

Fractures of the distal phalanx are the most frequent hand fractures, representing 50% of all hand fractures. Most result from crush injuries with associated nail bed injuries. Precise reduction is generally not required and treatment typically consists of splinting alone. However, unstable shaft fractures with overriding fragments are indications for reduction and longitudinal Kirschner wire fixation.

Most closed mallet fractures can be managed by splinting the DIP joint in extension, provided that the fracture involves less than 50% of the joint surface and is not associated with DIP joint subluxation. If fixation is required, the fracture fragment is held in place with a monofilament wire or nonabsorbable suture passed through to the palmar aspect of the finger through the distal phalanx. A transarticular longitudinal Kirschner wire is used to keep the joint in neutral position. A so-called *jersey finger* is an avulsion fracture of the insertion of the FDP tendon into the distal phalanx. It occurs after a pull of the FDP against resistance, as can occur when a footballer catches onto the jersey of an opponent. Occasionally, the avulsed fragment may lie as far proximally as the palm. This fracture fragment generally requires open reduction and internal fixation.[4]

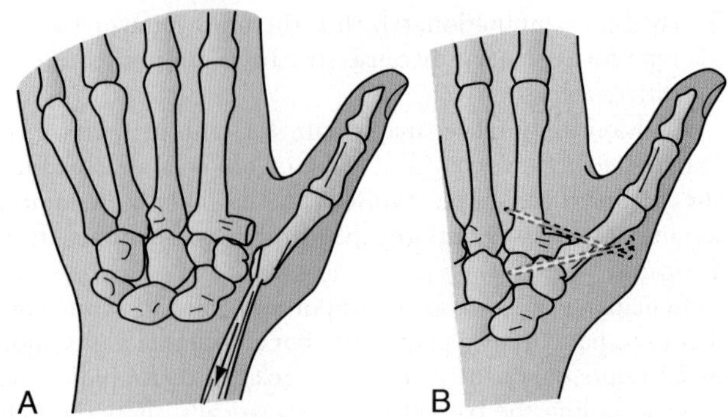


**FIGURE 70-29 A,** Fracture-dislocation at the base of the thumb metacarpal is called *Bennett's fracture*. The deforming force is produced by the pull of the APL muscle. **B,** Open reduction and pinning of the fracture are frequently required.

### Middle Phalanx and Proximal Phalanx Fractures

Fractures may involve the head, neck, shaft, or base of the respective bone. Head and base fractures may be intra-articular. A middle phalangeal shaft fracture is displaced according to the forces exerted by the insertions of the FDS and central slip mechanism. If the fracture lies distal to the FDS insertion, the proximal fragment is flexed by this muscle, resulting in a volar angulation. In contrast, if the fracture is proximal to the FDS insertion, the proximal fragment is extended by the central slip, whereas the distal part is flexed by the FDS. This results in a dorsal angulation. Most shaft fractures of the proximal phalanx tend to angulate volarward because the interossei reflect the proximal fragment and the central slip, through the PIP joint, extends the distal fragment. Displaced and unstable shaft fractures require open reduction followed by fixation with Kirschner wires, plates, and/or screws.

### Metacarpal Fractures

Stable metacarpal fractures may be treated with splinting alone. Fractures with dorsal or volar angulation can be stabilized by percutaneous insertion of intramedullary fixation pins. If they are displaced or unstable, such as oblique, spiral, or multiple metacarpal fractures, open reduction and internal fixation of these metacarpal fractures are performed. The internal fixation can be achieved with Kirschner wires, lag screws, or plate and screws, depending on the fracture pattern configuration. Dorsally angulated fractures at the neck of the little finger metacarpal, the so-called *boxer's fracture*, do not require reduction if the dorsal angulation is less than 30 degrees. The mobility of the carpometacarpal joint will compensate for this degree of angulation. The index and middle finger metacarpals are less mobile than the ring and little finger metacarpals. Therefore, a maximum of 15 degrees of angular deformity can be tolerated in the index and middle finger metacarpals.

Oblique fractures at the base of the thumb metacarpal (Bennett's fracture) result in the small proximal fragment being held in position by the volar oblique ligament to the trapezium. The remaining portion of the thumb metacarpal is displaced dorsally and radially because of the pull of the APL tendon (Fig. 70-29). These fracture fragments must be properly reduced and secured with internal fixation with Kirschner wires or a screw.

Comminuted fractures at the base of the thumb metacarpal (Rolando's fracture) are infrequently treated by closed reduction. If the fragments are large and badly displaced, an open reduction is indicated to ensure accurate restoration of the joint surface at the base of the thumb metacarpal. Fractures of the shaft of the thumb metacarpal tend to become displaced by the opposing muscle forces of the abductor and adductor on the proximal and distal fragments, respectively. Even undisplaced fractures may become progressively more displaced and angulated over time, necessitating an internal fixation. If initial splint immobilization is chosen for an undisplaced thumb metacarpal fracture, close follow-up is required to detect the earliest signs of displacement and instability. Fracture at the base of the little finger metacarpal is analogous to Bennett's fracture of the thumb and is sometimes called a *reverse Bennett's fracture*. This results in a fracture dislocation, with the deforming force being the insertion of the extensor carpi ulnaris tendon.

### Scaphoid Fractures

The scaphoid is the most common carpal bone fracture and accounts for approximately 60% of all carpal injuries. Clinical examination shows tenderness over the anatomic snuffbox and over the scaphoid tubercle. If a scaphoid fracture is suspected, the initial radiographic examination includes not only the standard three views of the wrist but also a scaphoid view, which is a posteroanterior image with the wrist in full ulnar deviation (Fig 70-30). Frequently, immediate postinjury radiographs may not reveal a fracture. CT or MRI may help in these cases or one may elect to apply a splint and repeat the radiographs in 2 weeks.[18]

Treatment of a nondisplaced scaphoid fracture is with a long arm cast that includes the thumb. The thumb spica cast is maintained for 6 weeks, followed by a short arm cast until radiographic healing has occurred. There has been a trend toward percutaneous screw fixation of even, undisplaced scaphoid fractures.

Displaced scaphoid fractures require open reduction with internal fixation, generally using a compression screw. Complications with inadequately treated scaphoid fractures are notorious. The blood vessels enter the scaphoid mainly through its distal half and fractures through the waist of the scaphoid may deprive the proximal half of its blood supply, leading to avascular necrosis of the proximal pole of the scaphoid. Nonunion also occurs with relative frequency, and these cases need to be treated with cancellous bone grafting or even a pedicle vascularized bone graft. Early diagnosis of scaphoid fractures is essential so that appropriate treatment can be instituted to reduce the risks for these complications. Modern cannulated compression screws, intraoperative fluoroscopy, and arthroscopy have allowed minimally invasive percutaneous fixation of some of these scaphoid fractures, resulting in a trend toward more aggressive surgical treatment of these fractures.

### Fractures in Children

The Salter-Harris classification describes five types of epiphyseal injuries (Fig. 70-31). Pediatric bones are still growing and thus permit a greater degree of remodeling. Hence, moderate angular and translational displacement of fractures tend to correct with age. However, rotational deformities never correct in the hand and are totally unacceptable, even in children. Implants that cross the epiphysis must have minimal potential for damage. Hence, smooth Kirschner wires are generally used for the fixation of pediatric skeletal injuries and threaded screws are usually avoided.

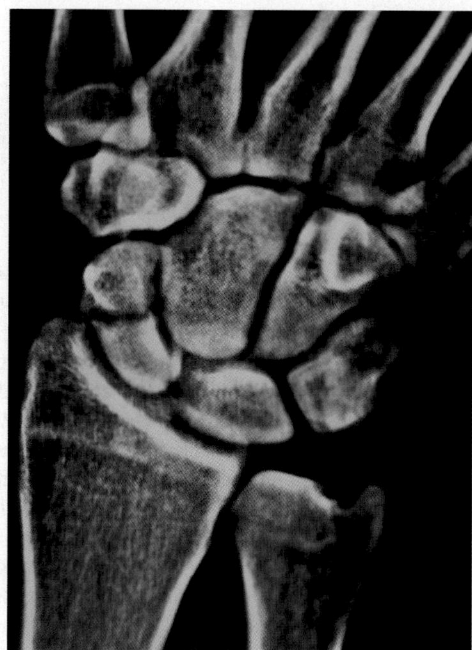

**FIGURE 70-30** Anteroposterior (AP) radiograph of the wrist demonstrating a fracture of the waist of the scaphoid, the bone in the hand that is usually fractured.

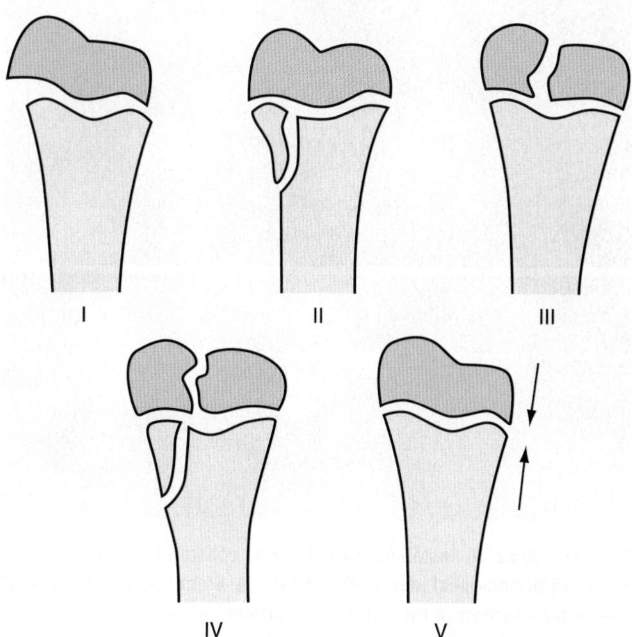


**FIGURE 70-31** Salter-Harris fracture patterns involving the epiphysis in children.

### Dislocations

Dislocations are more frequently seen at the PIP joint. A closed dislocation of the PIP joint can frequently be managed by closed reduction and splinting. If the joint is unstable after reduction, it needs exploration for collateral ligament repair. The most common type of PIP joint dislocation is a dorsal dislocation. A PIP joint volar dislocation is often associated with a tear in the triangular ligament of the extensor mechanism through which the head of the proximal phalanx protrudes and becomes trapped. Attempts at closed reduction fail because they tighten the fibers of the lateral bands and central slip around each side of the protruding proximal phalangeal neck; these injuries often require open reduction with repair of the extensor tear.

Palmar dislocations of the head of the index finger metacarpal often require open reduction. The head of the metacarpal becomes trapped between the superficial transverse metacarpal ligament, flexor tendons, and lumbrical muscles, whereas the volar plate becomes trapped between the metacarpal head and base of the proximal phalanx. Attempts at closed reduction are fruitless because of the entrapment resulting from this arrangement.

MP joint dislocation of the thumb often results from jamming it in a radial direction, thus tearing the ulnar collateral ligament. The ulnar collateral ligament may pull proximally and come to rest dorsal to the extensor hood (Stener's lesion; Fig. 70-32). It cannot heal spontaneously because the ulnar collateral ligament is prevented from reattaching to bone. This so-called *ski pole injury* may then require operative repair. Stress radiography, sometimes able to be performed only after anesthetizing the digit with a metacarpal block, may be required to facilitate diagnosis of a complete ulnar collateral ligament injury of the thumb metacarpal joint.

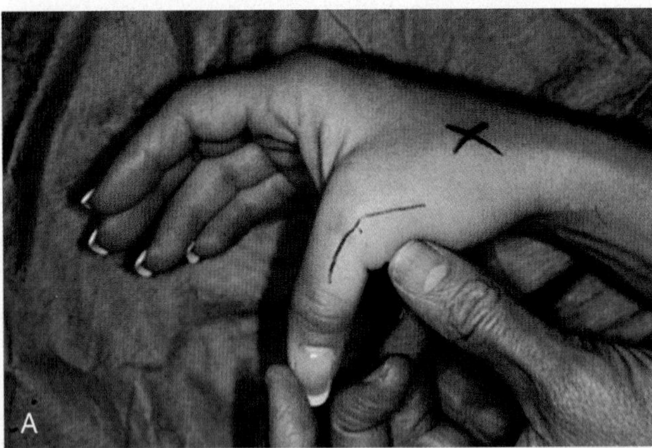

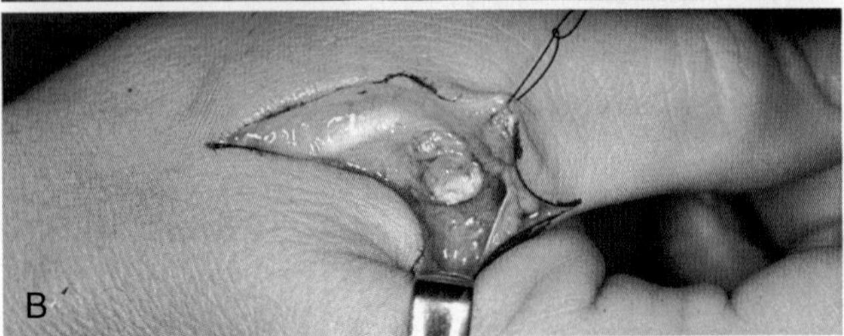

**FIGURE 70-32 A,** Instability of the ulnar collateral ligament of the metacarpophalangeal joint of the thumb. **B,** Stener lesion shows that the distal insertion of the collateral ligament has avulsed proximal to the extensor hood and is thus blocked from spontaneous reattachment. Open operation is required to reanchor the collateral ligament insertion to the base of the proximal phalanx.

## INFECTIONS

Hand infections commonly present to the surgical resident covering the emergency room. When diagnosed and treated properly initially, most patients do well. The extent of deep palmar infections may often be underestimated during the early phases because the volar aspect of the hand does not show edema as readily as the dorsal aspect of the hand. Thus, if infections in the hand are not diagnosed at an early stage, infections may spread from one anatomic compartment to another along natural tissue planes. Hand infections can then result in significant morbidity and severe functional compromise if not appropriately diagnosed and treated (Fig. 70-33). Some of the more common types of infections are discussed here.

### Superficial Paronychial Infections

Paronychia is the most common infection of the hand; it usually results from trauma to the eponychial or paronychial region. The infection localizes around the nail base, advances around the nail fold, and burrows beneath the base of the nail. If pus is trapped beneath the nail, pressure on the nail evokes exquisite pain. The most common causative organism is *Staphylococcus aureus*. Early treatment is with antibiotics, preferably penicillin in combination with a β-lactamase inhibitor such as sulbactam or clavulanic acid. However, there has now been an increasing incidence of methicillin-resistant *S. aureus* (MRSA) in community-acquired infections. After an abscess develops, surgical drainage is required. The surgical approach to an acute paronychia depends on the extent of the infection. Incisions may not be necessary. A Freer elevator is used to lift approximately 25% of the nail adjacent

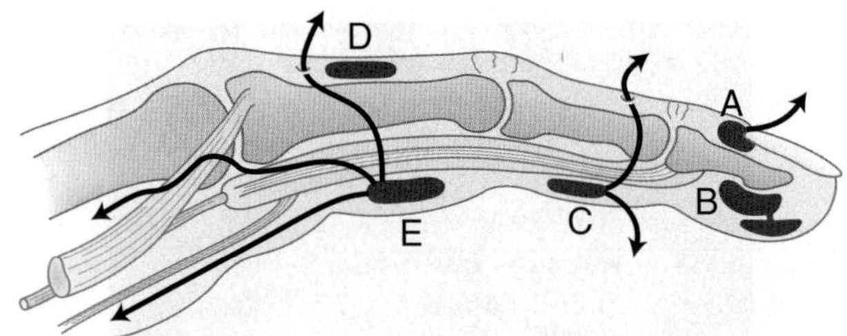


**FIGURE 70-33** Spread of soft tissue infections in the hand occurs through loss of containment from the original site and erosion into and spread through contiguous anatomic compartments. **A,** Paronychium. Infecting organisms access periungal tissues through fissures in the epinychial or paronychial tissues and often discharge spontaneously in these areas. **B,** Infection of pulp tissues (felon). Fibrous septae within the pulp create collar stud abscesses within the pulp. **C,** Volar subcutaneous infections in the digit may discharge percutaneously on either surface of the digit, or penetrate dorsally and spread along the sheaths of the flexor or extensor tendons. **D,** Subcutaneous infections on the dorsum of the digit usually discharge percutaneously because of the thin and areolar nature of the soft tissues. **E,** Proximally located digital infections or web space infections may rupture into the palmar spaces by tracking along tendon sheaths, palmar fascia, or lumbrical canal. The continuous sheaths of the thumb and little fingers (radial and ulnar bursae) are continuous with the carpal tunnel and space of Parona at the wrist.

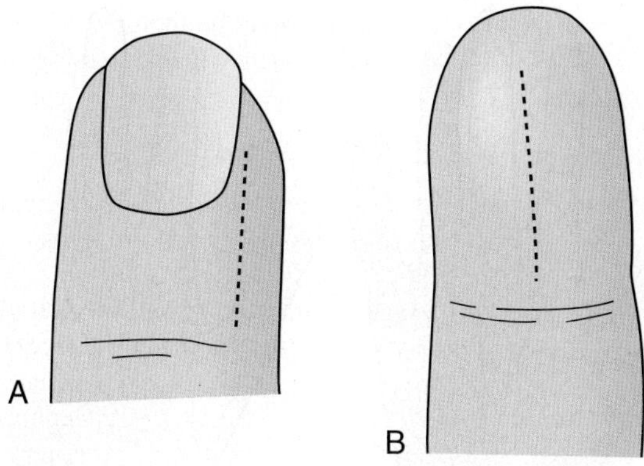


**FIGURE 70-34** Incisions for paronychia **(A)** and felon **(B)**.

to the infected perionychium, extending proximally to the edge of the nail. This portion of the nail is transected and gauze packing is inserted beneath the nail fold. A single incision to drain the affected perionychium also allows elevation of the eponychial fold when both eponychium and paronychium are involved (Fig. 70-34).[19-21]

## Infections of Intermediate-Depth Spaces

Infections of intermediate-depth spaces are pulp space infections (felons) and also deep web space infections. The former may involve the terminal or middle or proximal volar pulp spaces and may result from direct implantation with a penetrating injury, or may represent spread from a more superficial subcutaneous infection. The volar pulp of the distal digital segment is a fascial space closed proximally by a septum joining the distal flexion crease to the periosteum, where the long flexor tendon is inserted. This space is also partitioned by fibrous septa. Tension in the distal digital segment can become so great that the arteries to the bone are compressed, resulting in gangrene of the fingertip and necrosis of the distal 75% of the terminal phalanx. With infection of the digital pulp space, one must not wait for fluctuance before making the decision for surgery because of the danger of ischemic necrosis of the skin and bone. Clinical diagnosis is made by the rapid onset of throbbing pain, swelling, and exquisite tenderness of the affected pulp space. Surgical drainage is required. A single volar or unilateral longitudinal incision may be used (see Fig. 70-34). Postoperative care includes packing of the wound and elevation of the extremity. Use of antibiotics is guided by the results of Gram staining. Similar to a paronychia, *S. aureus* is the most common causative agent. Spread from a pulp space infection may move into a joint space or underlying bone, or burst through the septum proximally to involve the rest of the finger. More proximally, a pulp space infection at the base of the finger can travel through the lumbrical canal into the palm to create a deep palmar space infection.[21]

Web space abscesses result from direct implantation or spread from a pulp space. An inflamed and tender mass in the web space separates the fingers. There is loss of the normal palmar concavity, with a widened space between the fingers. Dorsal swelling is present and must not be mistaken for the infection site. A surgical incision is placed transversely across the web space, and a counter longitudinal incision may be placed dorsally between the bases of the proximal phalanges; a generous communication is established between these two incisions (Fig. 70-35).

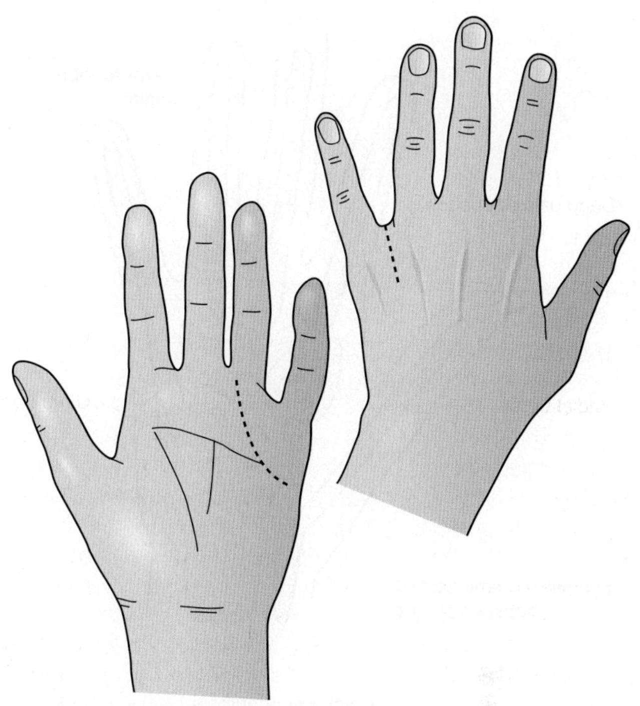

**FIGURE 70-35** Incisions for web space abscess between the little and ring fingers.

## Deep Infections

### Palmar Space Infections

These infections are localized to the deep space of the hand between the metacarpals and palmar aponeurosis. A transverse septum to the metacarpal of the middle finger divides the deep space into an ulnar midpalmar and radial thenar space. The transverse head of the adductor pollicis partitions the thenar space from the retroadductor space. There may be ballooning of the palm, thenar eminence, or posterior aspect of the first web space, depending on which of the affected spaces is involved with an abscess. The dorsal subaponeurotic space of the hand deep to the extensor tendons may also be affected by an isolated infection, generally as the result of direct implantation (Fig. 70-36*A*). For a thenar space infection, the preferred approach to surgical drainage is a dual volar and dorsal incision (see Fig. 70-36*B*). On the volar side, an incision is made adjacent and parallel to the thenar crease. Great care is taken to avoid injury to the palmar cutaneous branch of the median nerve in the proximal part of the incision and motor branch of the median nerve in a deeper plane. A second, slightly curved longitudinal incision is made on the dorsum of the first web space. Dissection is continued more deeply into this area between the first dorsal interosseous muscle and adductor pollicis. A drain is placed in the incision after thorough exploration of the respective spaces. With midpalmar space infections, dorsal swelling of the hand will be present, as is the case with all palmar infections, and must not be mistaken for the infection site. Motion of the middle and ring fingers is limited and painful. A longitudinal curvilinear incision is the preferred approach for drainage of this space.

Infection of Parona's space occurs in the potential space deep to the flexor tendons in the distal forearm and superficial to the pronator quadratus muscle. It is usually the result of

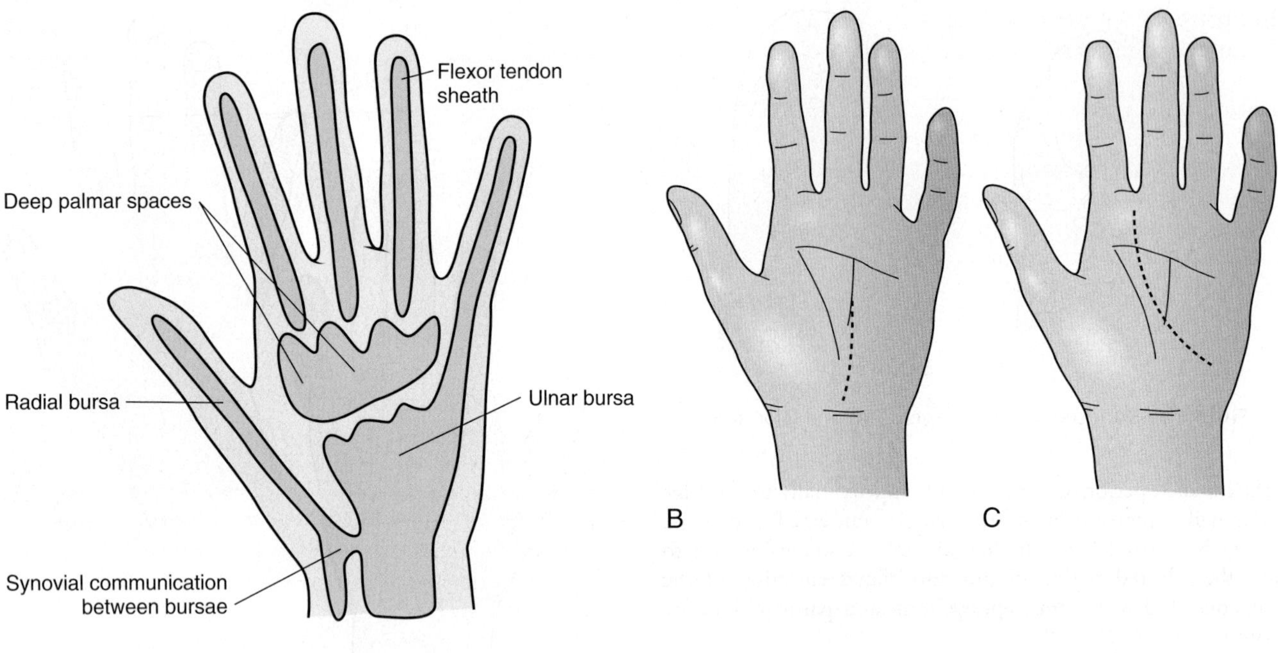


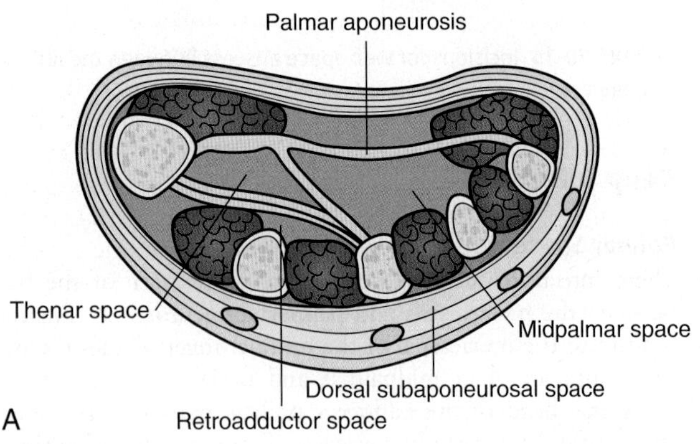


**FIGURE 70-36** **A,** Deep spaces of the hand and synovial bursae. Infections may be bound by these spaces or may track along anatomic dissection planes between these spaces. **B,** Incision for thenar space infection. A dorsal first web space incision is also often required. **C,** Incision for midpalmar space abscess.

spread from the adjacent contiguous midpalmar space or from the radial or ulnar bursa. Swelling, tenderness, and fluctuation will be present in the distal volar forearm. A midpalmar infection may be associated. Active digital flexion is painful, as is passive finger extension. A surgical incision must be planned so as to leave the median nerve adequately covered with soft tissue.

### Pyogenic Flexor Tenosynovitis

Kanavel's four cardinal signs include the following: (1) the finger is held flexed because this position allows the synovial sheath its maximum volume and eases pain; (2) symmetrical fusiform swelling of the entire finger is present, with edema of the back of the hand; (3) the slightest attempt at passive extension of the affected digit produces exquisite pain; and (4) the site of maximum tenderness is at the proximal cul-de-sac of the index, middle, and ring finger synovial sheaths in the distal palm or, in the case of infection of the sheaths of the thumb and little finger, more proximally in the palm (see Fig. 70-36). The radial and ulnar bursae communicate in approximately 80% of cases and may be simultaneously infected. Bursal infections may spread into the forearm space of Parona, deep to the flexor tendons in the distal part of the forearm, creating a horseshoe abscess.

Pyogenic flexor tenosynovitis may be aborted with parenteral antibiotics, extremity elevation, and hand immobilization if the patient is seen within the first 24 hours of onset of infection. If this course is unsuccessful, or if the patient is seen more than 48 hours after onset of infection, surgical drainage is undertaken. The preferred surgical approach is through two separate incisions, with the first being a midaxial incision made on the finger, usually on the ulnar side of the digit (on the radial side of the thumb or little finger); the digital artery and nerve remain in the volar flap, with the dissection proceeding directly to the tendon sheath. The synovium between the A3 and A4 pulleys is incised and cloudy fluid is encountered. A second incision is made in the palm over the tendon to drain the cul-de-sac. A 16-gauge polyethylene catheter is inserted beneath the A1 pulley into the sheath and the sheath is flushed manually with sterile saline every 2 hours after surgery. A bulky hand dressing absorbs the drainage. Studies have found that postoperative catheter drainage may not always be necessary.[22,23]

## Chronic and Atypical Infections

Chronic paronychia are generally the result of *Candida albicans* (>95%) infection and are not bacterial. When bacteria are involved, they are more commonly atypical mycobacteria or gram-negative organisms. These chronic paronychia generally respond to treatment with topical antifungal agents, although oral antifungal agents are sometimes used. Occasionally, surgical treatment by means of marsupialization of the eponychial fold is required. If the lesion is refractory to treatment, the possibility of a malignancy is entertained.

Chronic tenosynovitis can occur in the flexor tendons or in the dorsum of the wrist and extensor tendons. It is usually of a granulomatous type and is caused by mycobacteria or fungi. Treatment includes surgical excision of the involved synovium and prolonged treatment with the appropriate antimicrobial agents. Chronic infected tenosynovitis must be differentiated from other causes of chronic granulomatous synovitis, such as sarcoidosis, amyloidosis, gout, and rheumatoid arthritis.

## Herpetic Whitlow

Herpetic whitlow is caused by type 1 or 2 herpes simplex virus and may be confused with a paronychia. Infection begins with the appearance of small clear vesicles with localized swelling, erythema, and intense pain. The vesicles may subsequently appear turbid and coalesce over the next few days before ulcerating. Diagnosis is confirmed by culturing the virus from the vesicular fluid, assessing immunofluorescent serum antibody titers, or performing a Tzanck smear. However, these measures are rarely required because clinical diagnosis is usually sufficient. Infection can occur from autoinoculation from an oral or genital lesion or exposure as a health care worker. Pain is often out of proportion to the physical findings. Treatment is generally nonoperative because this infection is usually self-limited. Antivirals such as acyclovir or famciclovir may be of some benefit if started within the first 48 hours of symptom onset. Surgical incision and drainage can lead to systemic involvement and possible viral encephalitis.

## Animal and Human Bites

The most striking difference in the microbial flora of human and animal bite wounds is the higher number of bacterial isolates per wound in human bites, the difference being mostly caused by the presence of anaerobic bacteria. Human bites can occasionally transmit other infectious diseases, such as hepatitis B, tuberculosis, syphilis, or actinomycosis. The incidence of *Eikenella corrodens* in human bite infections of the hand has been reported to vary between 7% and 29%. Usually, isolated organisms from infected human bite wounds are, as in animal bites, alpha-hemolytic streptococci and *S. aureus,* β-lactamase–producing strains of *S. aureus,* and *Bacteroides* spp. Anaerobic bacteria are more prevalent in human bite infections than previously recognized, including *Bacteroides, Clostridium, Peptococcus,* and *Veillonella.* Most studies of animal bite wounds have focused on the isolation of *Pasteurella multocida,* disregarding the role of anaerobes. However, more recent studies have shown that dog bite wounds indicate multiple organisms, with *P. multocida* being isolated from only 26% of dog bite wounds in adults. Most animal bites cause mixed infections of aerobic and anaerobic bacteria.

Pyogenic joint infections usually result from trauma, such as a bite wound from a tooth when the assailant's hand strikes the jaw. A tooth struck by the clenched fist of an attacker penetrates the skin, tendon, joint capsule, and metacarpal head. Once the finger is extended, the four puncture wounds separate from each other to create a closed space within the joint. All these so-called *fight bite wounds* of the MP joint need to be explored surgically, débrided, and thoroughly lavaged. Human bite wounds are not closed primarily and are treated with appropriate antibiotics.

# COMPARTMENT SYNDROME, HIGH-PRESSURE INJECTION INJURIES, AND EXTRAVASATION INJURIES

## High-Pressure Injection Injuries

High-pressure injection injuries to the hand are relatively uncommon, but consequences of a misdiagnosis are serious. Urgent treatment is required. High-pressure injection guns are used for painting, lubricating, cleaning, and farm animal vaccinations. Materials that may be injected with these devices include paint, paint thinners, oil, grease, water, plastic, vaccines, and cement. These high-pressure injection guns may generate pressures ranging between 3000 and 12,000 psi. Injection injuries can also be caused by other sources, such as defective lines and valves, pneumatic hoses, and hydraulic lines. The type of material injected is the most important prognostic factor. Oil-based paints and paint thinners can generate significant early inflammation leading to severe fibrosis. Because tendon sheaths at the index, middle, and ring fingers end at the level of the MP joints, material injected at the DIP or PIP flexion creases will remain within these digits. However, tendon sheaths at the thumb and little finger extend all the way into the radial and ulnar bursae. Thus, material injected at the little finger or at the IP flexion crease of the thumb may potentially extend all the way into the forearm, and even cause a compartment syndrome.

Initial presentation of a patient with a high-pressure injection may be benign and subtle. This may result in mismanagement by minimizing the patient's complaints. The break in the skin may be a benign-looking, pinhole-sized puncture site. However, within several hours, the digit becomes increasingly more painful, swollen, and pale. Prompt recognition and realization of the severity of injury are paramount. Radiographs may help determine the extent and dispersion of the injected material, either in the form of subcutaneous emphysema or, with lead-based paints, appearing as radiopaque soft tissue densities. The entire digit must be surgically decompressed and all foreign material and necrotic tissue débrided (Fig 70-37). Wounds are closed loosely over Penrose drains or in a delayed manner. Appropriate antibiotics must be administered. Despite prompt recognition and treatment, many such injuries ultimately result in surgical amputation of the digits.

## Extravasation Injuries

In the past, extravasation injuries of chemotherapeutic agents frequently affected the upper extremity. However, subcutaneously tunneled central lines have now reduced the incidence of these injuries. If extravasation is suspected, infusion must be stopped immediately. Cold packs are applied for 15 minutes four times a day and the extremity elevated over the next 48 hours. This treatment is generally effective for most extravasation injuries. However, if blistering, ulceration, and pain occur in the

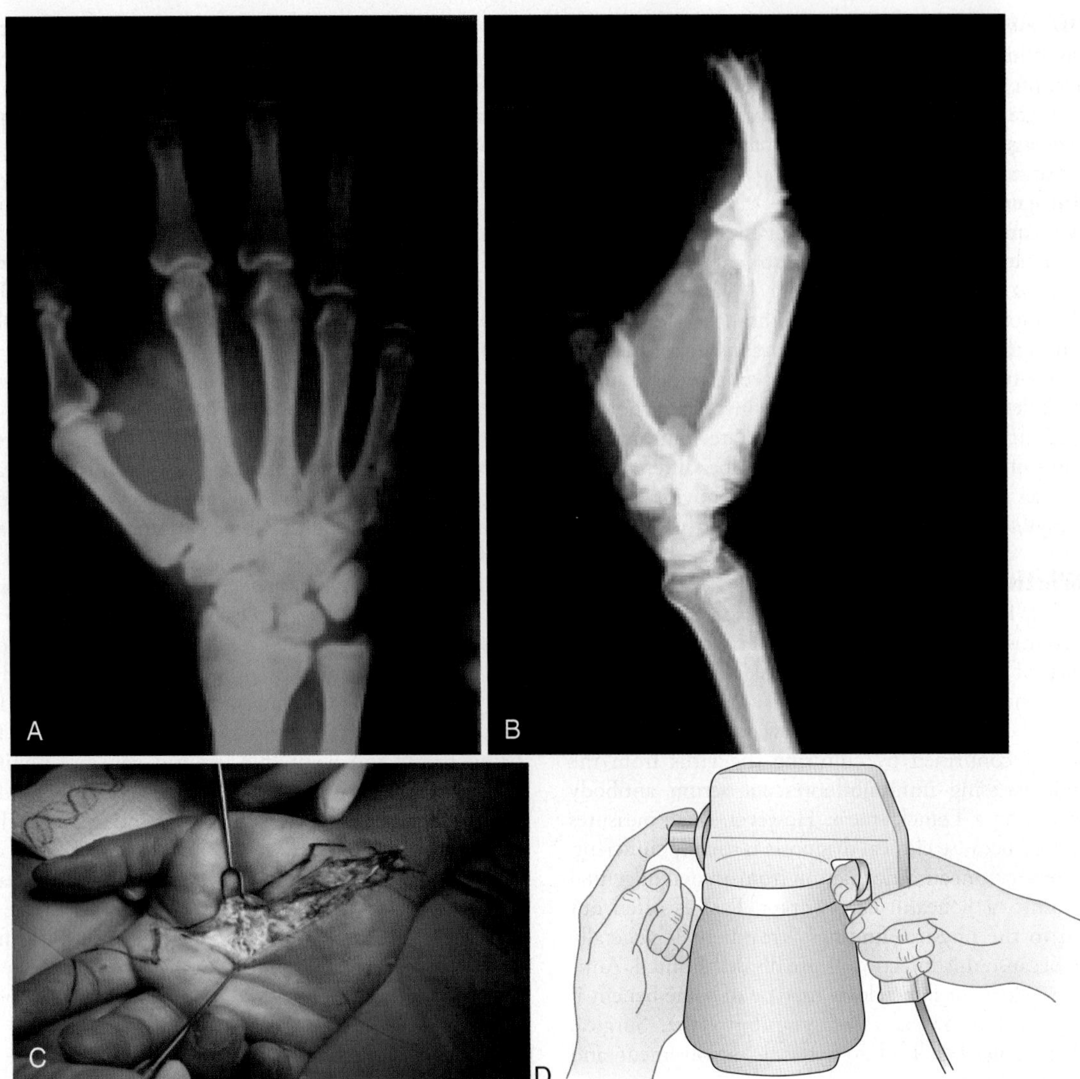


**FIGURE 70-37** High-pressure injection injury from paint gun appears completely innocuous, with tiny puncture wound on presentation. **A, B,** AP and lateral radiographs of the right hand show widely disseminated radio-opaque foreign material in soft tissues of the palm and thenar eminence. **C,** Introperative photo of left-handed man with palmar high-pressure injection injury from a paint gun on the nondominant palm. The tissues are extensively infiltrated by paint from the base of the finger to the wrist and require urgent débridement and decompression. **D,** Removal of the guard allows the nozzle to come into close contact, exponentially increasing the pressure delivered to soft tissues.

damaged tissue, progressive necrosis to the limits of the extravasation will follow, and surgical excision of all damaged tissue is necessary. Most subsequent wounds can generally be treated with delayed split-thickness skin grafting, although the options for wound coverage after débridement depend on the extent of the débridement that was required.

### Compartment Syndrome

Compartment syndrome results in symptoms and signs caused by increased pressure within a limited space that compromises circulation and function of the tissues in that space. Volkmann's ischemic contracture is the sequel of untreated compartment syndrome; it results in muscle that is fibrosed, contracted, and functionless and nerves that are insensible. Various injuries are known to cause compartment syndrome:

1. Decreased compartment volume (e.g., from externally applied tight dressings or casts, lying on a limb in a comatose state)
2. Increased compartment content (e.g., from bleeding or trauma with fractures or finger injuries, increased capillary permeability such as reperfusion after ischemic injury, electrical burn injuries)
3. Other injuries (e.g., snakebites, high-pressure injection injuries)[24]

The diagnosis of compartment syndrome is based primarily on clinical evaluation. Although it is possible to measure intracompartment pressure, the decision to perform fasciotomy is based on a high degree of clinical suspicion. Compartment ischemia may be severe and still not affect the color or temperature of the distal fingers, and the distal pulses are rarely obliterated by compartment swelling. However, circulation in the muscle and nerve may be greatly reduced. Muscle ischemia that lasts for more than 4 hours leads to muscle death and may also cause significant myoglobinuria. After 8 hours of total ischemia, irreversible nerve changes are complete. The hallmark of muscle and nerve ischemia is pain, which is progressive and persistent. The pain is accentuated by passive muscle stretching; this is the most reliable clinical test for diagnosing compartment syndrome. The next most important clinical finding is diminished sensation, which indicates nerve ischemia. The closed compartments of the forearm and hand are also palpated and found to be tense and tender, confirming the diagnosis of compartment syndrome. A passive muscle stretch test elicits severe pain in the presence of compartment syndrome. An arterial injury and nerve injury need to be distinguished in the differential diagnosis of compartment syndrome. All three of these injuries produce paresthesias and paresis, pain with passive stretch is present in compartment syndrome and arterial occlusion, but not in neuropraxia, and pulses are intact in compartment syndrome and neuropraxia, but not with arterial occlusion.

In situations in which the clinical diagnosis is difficult because the patient cannot cooperate because of inebriation or unconsciousness, compartment pressure can be measured.

Release of a forearm compartment syndrome always requires carpal tunnel release (Fig. 70-38). The palmar incision starts in the valley between the thenar and hypothenar muscles and the incision then curves transversely across the flexion crease of the wrist at the ulnar border. This incision must avoid the palmar cutaneous branch of the median nerve and prevent flexion contracture across the wrist crease. It also provides an opportunity to release Guyon's canal. The incision then extends proximally up the forearm before curving back in a radial direction so as to have a large skin flap that will cover the median nerve and distal forearm tendons. At the elbow, the incision for the flap then curves again across the antecubital fossa, providing cover for the brachial artery and median nerve and preventing linear contracture across the antecubital fossa. The dorsal and so-called *mobile wad compartments* of the forearm are readily released through a straight incision, as needed. Appropriate release of the various intrinsic compartments of the hand may

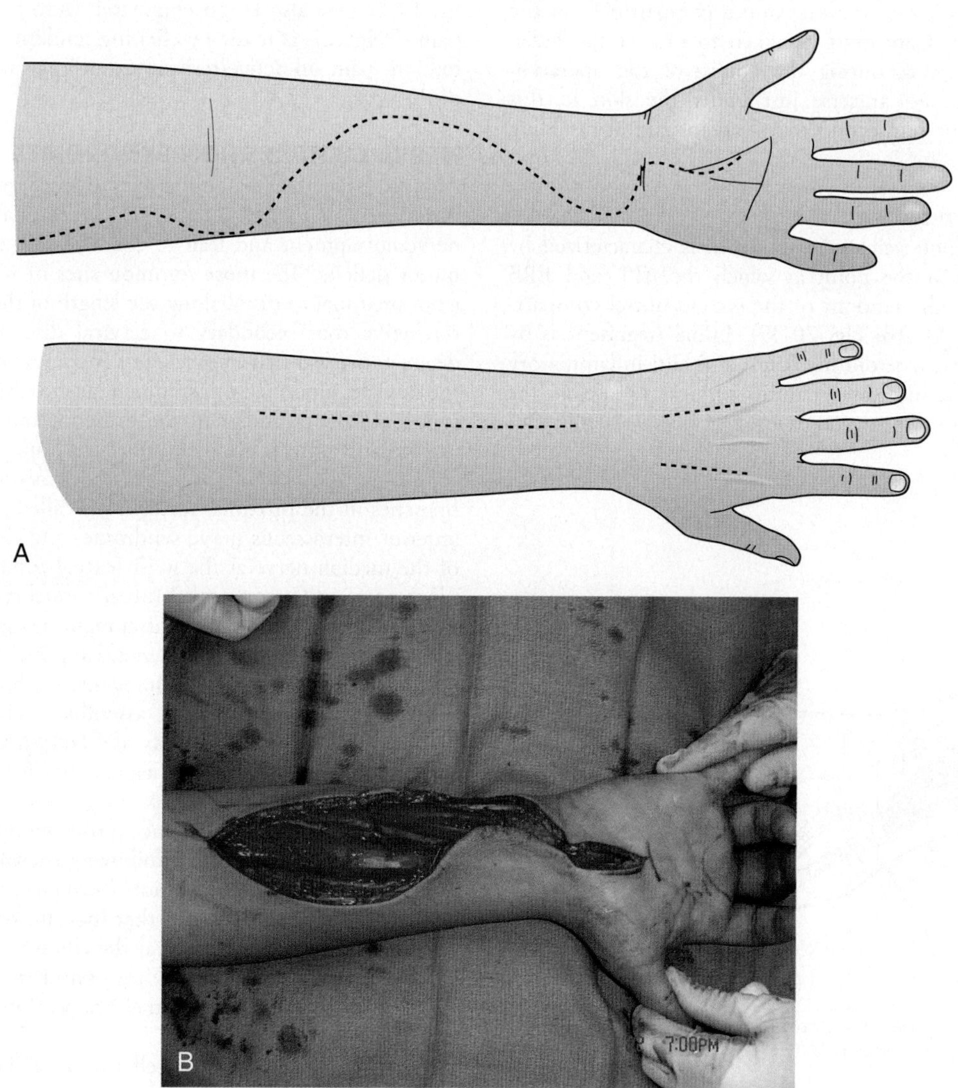


**FIGURE 70-38 A,** Incisions for forearm fasciotomy. **B,** Fasciotomy in a child for compartment syndrome following a snakebite.

also be required. Most wounds can be partially closed at 5 days. If the skin cannot be closed secondarily within 10 days, a split-thickness skin graft can be applied.

## TENOSYNOVITIS

### De Quervain's Disease

De Quervain's disease is a stenosing tenosynovitis of the first dorsal compartment of the wrist and is a common cause of pain and disability. Diagnosis is easily made from a history of pain localized to the radial side of the wrist and aggravated by movement of the thumb. There is frequently a history of chronic overuse of the wrist and hand. Other features are local tenderness and swelling over the first dorsal compartment of the wrist and a positive Finkelstein's test—the patient clasps the thumb and brisk ulnar deviation to the hand elicits extreme pain. Crepitus may be palpable. This condition must be differentiated by radiographic and physical examination from arthritis of the thumb carpometacarpal joint.

Nonoperative treatment includes local steroid injection, thumb and wrist immobilization, local heat, and systemic anti-inflammatory medications. If these nonoperative measures fail, surgical decompression of the first dorsal compartment at the wrist is performed. Care must be taken to protect the radial sensory nerve branches during the course of the operation because these branches traverse just under the skin in this area, and trauma or transection may lead to painful disabling neuromas.

### Intersection Syndrome

This condition is not well understood but is characterized by pain and crepitus at the point at which the APL and EPB tendons cross over the tendons of the second dorsal compartment (ECRL and ECRB; Fig. 70-39). Initial treatment is by splinting, local corticosteroid injection, and anti-inflammatory medications. Refractory cases require surgical release at the second dorsal compartment and excision of involved tenosynovial membranes.

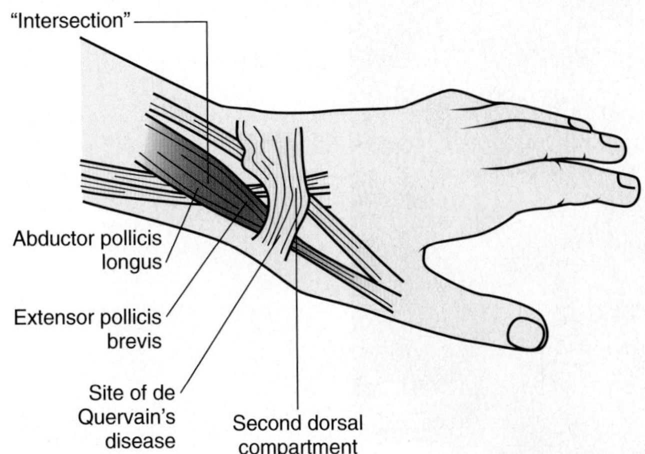


**FIGURE 70-39** Anatomic locations for de Quervain's stenosing tenosynovitis and intersection syndrome.

### Trigger Thumb and Fingers

Trigger finger is a constricting tenosynovitis of the flexor tendons. generally at the level of the A1 pulley. The patient can flex the digit, but an apparent nodule catches at the proximal edge of the A1 pulley, locking the PIP joint (or the IP joint of the thumb) in this flexed position. Attempts at extending the digit cause it to snap back suddenly, much like the trigger of a gun. Often, the patient needs to use the opposite hand to unlock and extend the digit. In its most severe form, the constriction is so tight that the patient cannot flex the digit or it gets fixed in a flexed position and can no longer be fully extended. A congenital form of trigger thumb or finger presents in infants, but most cases resolve by the time the patient reaches 1 year of age; if not, an operation is indicated.

Nonoperative treatment in adults includes local injection of corticosteroids. If this regimen fails, the A1 pulley is longitudinally divided by surgery.[25]

### Other Sites of Tenosynovitis

Other sites include the FCR and FCU tendons. They can frequently be treated by splinting and local corticosteroid injection, although surgery occasionally may be required. Inflammation of the ECU may also be an enigmatic cause of ulnar-sided wrist pain. Diagnosis is made by eliciting tenderness along the ECU tendon, pain on active-resisted extension, and ulnar deviation of the wrist.

## NERVE COMPRESSION SYNDROMES

Along the length of the upper extremity, nerves pass through a number of anatomic bottlenecks. These are all possible sites of nerve entrapment and lead to characteristic distal sensory and motor deficits. The most common sites of nerve compression, from proximal to distal along the length of the extremity, are at the nerve root secondary to cervical disc disease or cervical degenerative arthritis, thoracic outlet compression at the level of the clavicle, ulnar nerve entrapment at the elbow (cubital tunnel syndrome), entrapment of the posterior interosseous nerve in the proximal forearm (radial tunnel syndrome, posterior interosseous syndrome), entrapment of the median nerve and its branches in the proximal forearm (so-called *pronator syndrome*, anterior interosseous nerve syndrome) and, finally, entrapment of the median nerve at the wrist (carpal tunnel syndrome) and ulnar nerve in Guyon's canal (ulnar tunnel syndrome).

In most cases of nerve entrapment, no specific aggravating causative factor is found. An increasing incidence of compression neuropathy is reported in patients whose works involves chronic repetitive stress (e.g., assemblers, chicken cutters). In some, there may be a clearly defined extrinsic compressive problem on the nerve or an aggravating factor. These include the following:

- Trauma that can produce bony compression—for example, carpal tunnel following carpal dislocations or a distal radius malunion (median) and supracondylar humerus fractures that increase the elbow carrying angle (ulnar nerve at the elbow)
- Synovial thickening of the bursa in rheumatoid arthritis in the carpal tunnel (median) or at the elbow (posterior interosseous)
- Tumors such as giant cell tumor in Guyon's canal (ulnar) or a lipoma in the radial tunnel (posterior interosseous)

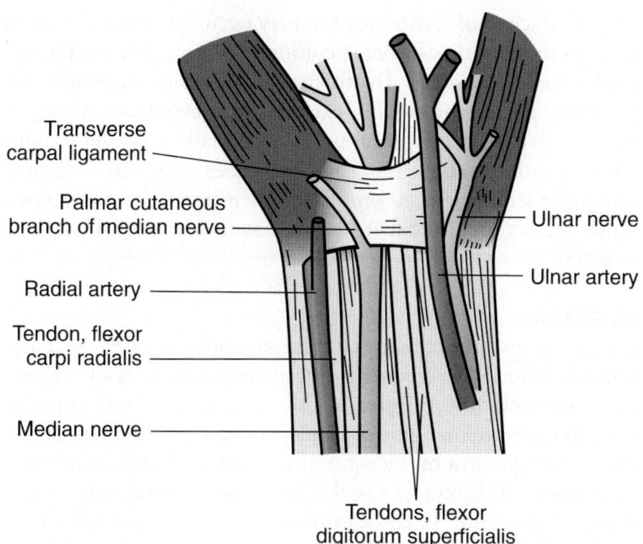


**FIGURE 70-40** Anatomy of the carpal tunnel. The transverse carpal ligament (flexor retinaculum) is divided longitudinally during a carpal tunnel release.

- Developmental, with anomalous muscles present in the carpal tunnel (median), Guyon's canal (ulnar), or the forearm (median)
- Metabolic, in which disturbances of fluid balance cause increased pressure on the nerve, particularly at the carpal tunnel (e.g., myxedema, pregnancy)

Carpal tunnel syndrome is the most common peripheral nerve entrapment syndrome, followed by ulnar nerve entrapment at the elbow.[26] The other entrapment syndromes are less common.

## Carpal Tunnel Syndrome

The carpal tunnel is a packed fibro-osseous tunnel at the wrist that is traversed by the median nerve and nine long extrinsic digital flexor tendons (Fig. 70-40). Its floor is formed by the carpal bones and roofed by the flexor retinaculum (transverse carpal ligament). Normal pressures in this tunnel are 20 to 30 mm Hg. A rise in pressure above this causes a chronic compressive ischemic injury to the nerve segment, resulting first in demyelination and eventually in axonal death. There is progressive conduction block in the nerve, with subsequent sensory and motor dysfunction. The earliest symptoms are pain and paresthesias, which are characteristically more obvious at night, after prolonged activity, and with positional postural changes at the wrist, such as when driving, using a hand-held hair dryer, or reading a book. The patient may complain of clumsiness and a tendency to drop objects. The paresthesias characteristically follow the distribution of the median nerve, including the thumb and index and middle fingers. Physical examination consists of compressing the carpal canal, percussing the median nerve, and hyperflexing the wrist to produce paresthesias (Durkin's sign, Tinel's sign, and Phalen's test, respectively). Sensory evaluation reveals hypoesthesia in the distribution of the median nerve and may reveal a widened two-point sensory discrimination. Thenar weakness or muscle wasting is a late finding. Nerve conduction studies and electromyography are useful adjuncts to the clinical examination.

Initial treatment of carpal tunnel syndrome includes use of wrist splints (especially at night), occasional local corticosteroid injections, and modification in work patterns. If symptoms persist, or if the initial presentation shows severe carpal tunnel syndrome, surgical decompression is required. This is performed by longitudinally dividing the flexor retinaculum by open or endoscopic means. Both the Agee (single-portal) and Chow (two-portal) procedures have shown similar efficacy to the open approach.[27] Synovectomy and removal of any mass lesion may also be required if that is the cause of the problem.[28]

## Pronator Syndrome

In the proximal forearm, the median nerve may be compressed at the fibrous arch between the two heads of the FDS, two heads of the pronator teres, lacertus fibrosis (bicipital aponeurosis at the elbow), and ligament of Struthers. Compression at any or all of these sites is loosely grouped under the pronator syndrome. The symptoms produced are similar to those of carpal tunnel, although nocturnal symptoms are uncommon. The palm may also feel numb because the palmar cutaneous branch is involved, but is specifically spared in carpal tunnel syndrome because that nerve branch passes superficial to the flexor retinaculum and arises proximal to the retinaculum. Symptoms may be reproduced or worsened by attempting pronation against resistance and by resisted flexion of the middle finger. However, it may be difficult to locate the compressive cause in the pronator syndrome precisely, and surgical decompression often involves release of all four potential sites of compression.

The anterior interosseus nerve branch of the median nerve may occasionally be compressed in isolation. This does not produce any sensory symptoms, but specifically targets the three muscles innervated by the anterior interosseous nerve—FPL, FDP to the index and middle fingers, and pronator quadratus.

## Ulnar Nerve Compression

The ulnar nerve may be compressed in Guyon's canal at the wrist or in the so-called *cubital tunnel* at the elbow and distal upper arm.

### Guyon's Canal Compression

This canal is bounded by the hook of the hamate, pisiform, pisohamate ligament, and palmar carpal ligament. Compression by mass lesions may occur at this site, including a ganglion, giant cell tumor, ulnar artery thrombosis, and ulnar artery aneurysm, as in the hypothenar hammer syndrome. Compression at this site may also be idiopathic. Distal ulnar deficits may be in the motor or sensory distribution or both, depending on where in the canal the compression occurs relative to the takeoff of the deep motor branch of the ulnar nerve. There may be a positive Tinel's sign and worsening of symptoms by direct compression over Guyon's canal. Treatment is surgical; it consists of dividing the palmaris brevis muscle and palmar carpal ligament, as well as removing any offending mass in this region.

### Cubital Tunnel Syndrome

The cubital tunnel is a long tunnel starting in the distal upper arm and extending into the proximal forearm. As the ulnar nerve passes into the forearm, it curves tightly around the grooved posterior and inferior surfaces of the medial epicondyle of the humerus. This groove is bridged by the aponeurosis between the two heads of the FCU, the leading edge of which may be thickened and fibrosed, called *Osborne's ligament.* More proximally, the ulnar nerve passes from the anterior compartment of the arm into the posterior compartment, which may be bridged by a long tunnel called the *arcade of Struthers.* The medial intermuscular septum in the upper arm may also cause ulnar nerve compression. The most distal fibro-osseous tunnel is more accurately termed the *cubital tunnel.* However, compression on the ulnar nerve can occur at any of these sites, proximal to distal, starting in the upper arm and extending into the forearm. Motor and sensory symptoms develop in the distribution of the ulnar nerve and are worsened by adopting a flexed position at the elbow. Examination reveals a positive Tinel's sign over the tunnel. Paresthesias are described in the distribution of the ulnar nerve to the little and ring fingers and ulnar border of the hand. A differential diagnosis includes thoracic outlet syndrome, compression of the ulnar nerve in Guyon's canal, and nerve root compression in the neck.

Initial treatment consists of splinting the elbow in extension at night. Use of soft extension elbow pads prevents elbow flexion and direct pressure on the nerve. Failure of nonoperative measures, together with significant changes in electrodiagnostic studies, are indications for surgical decompression. Usually, all the fibrous restraints on the ulnar nerve around the elbow are released and the nerve is transposed anteriorly to the medial epicondyle into a subcutaneous or submuscular position. There have been preliminary reports of success with endoscopic in situ decompression of the ulnar nerve at the elbow.

### Radial Nerve Compression

The radial nerve may be compressed proximally in the triangular space in the axilla (specifically involving the axillary branch), spiral groove posterior to the humerus in the arm, and lateral intermuscular septum proximal to the elbow. More distally in the forearm, the posterior interosseous nerve. The principle motor division of the radial nerve can be compressed in the so-called *radial tunnel,* starting at the leading fibrous edge of the supinator (ligament of Frohse). There may be a variable degree of interosseous nerve paresis or there may be pain radiating down the dorsoradial aspect of the forearm (the latter is called *radial tunnel syndrome*). Initial treatment is nonoperative with splinting but, if this fails, surgical decompression may occasionally be required.

### Thoracic Outlet Compression

The thoracic outlet is a narrow space at the base of the neck bounded by the first rib medially, scalenus anterior muscle and clavicle anteriorly, and scalenus medius muscle posteriorly. All elements of the brachial plexus, as well as the subclavian artery and vein, pass through this narrow space and can be potentially compressed at this site. A positive Tinel's sign can often be elicited at the supraclavicular and infraclavicular regions. A Roos test is performed by asking the patient to hold both arms overhead in a surrender position while opening and closing the fists. This reproduces symptoms within 1 minute and, if continued, the arm collapses at the side. Adson's test involves palpating the radial pulse while the patient turns the chin toward the same side, inhales deeply, and holds his or her breath. The radial pulse disappears or diminishes. The costoclavicular compression test involves sustained downward pressure on the clavicle, and the symptoms are reproduced. Radiographic evaluation may reveal a cervical rib. Nerve conduction studies are often normal.

Thoracic outlet compression may occur in association with other peripheral sites of nerve compression, a condition termed *double-crush syndrome.* Treatment is primarily nonoperative, involving posture-improving exercises and avoidance of aggravating activities. If symptoms persist, especially if associated with vascular compression, the thoracic outlet may be surgically decompressed. This is accomplished by a transcervical or transaxillary resection of the first rib, often with release of the scalene muscles.

## TUMORS

Ganglions and mucous cysts represent 60% to 70% of hand tumors, followed in frequency by inclusion cysts, warts (verrucae), giant cell tumors in tendon sheaths, foreign body granulomas, lipomas, hemangiomas, and pyogenic granulomas (Table 70-5). Benign tumors account for 95% of hand neoplasms. Squamous cell carcinoma is the most frequent primary malignancy of the hand, basal cell carcinoma is rare, and melanoma is relatively uncommon in the upper extremity. Acral lentiginous melanoma (e.g., in the palm, sole, nail bed) has a tendency for early metastasis. Primary bone tumors of the hand are generally benign; the most common are enchondromas and osteochondromas. Giant cell tumors of bone are rare in the hand, occurring usually in the distal radius. They are locally aggressive and may occasionally metastasize. Of malignant bone tumors, only 1.2% affect the hand. Although bone metastases in other parts of the body are relatively common, bones of the hand are rarely affected by metastases from other sites.[29,30]

Soft tissue sarcomas are rare, representing 1% of all malignancies of the body, excluding skin tumors. Although uncommon, certain types predominate in the hand. Epithelioid, synovial, and clear cell sarcomas are relatively rare in other sites but, by comparison are more common in the hand.

Within the spectrum of benign and malignant tumors, there is a group with intermediate malignancy. Giant cell and desmoid tumors (of soft tissue) have a propensity for local recurrence after surgical excision. Their histologic patterns may belie their behavior. Juvenile aponeurotic fibroma and nodular fasciitis may appear histologically more aggressive than desmoid tumors, but are self-limiting. The tiny glomus tumor is uncommon but has a propensity for the fingertips and subungual regions. It may be an enigmatic cause of severe and exquisite pain at the fingertips and can be recognized by a pinpoint site of extreme local tenderness and a violaceous hue deep to the nail plate. MRI may occasionally detect these tiny lesions at the fingertip.

If a lesion is thought to be benign, excision without further workup, except perhaps for routine radiographs, is appropriate. However, if a primary malignancy of bone or soft tissue is suspected, additional studies must be undertaken before biopsy. CT may help delineate tumor boundaries. Desmoid tumors have radiographic density identical to that of muscle and are better demonstrated by MRI.

### Soft Tissue Tumors

#### Ganglion Cysts

Ganglions are formed by an outpouching of the synovial membrane from a joint or tendon sheath and contain thick, jelly-like, mucinous material similar in composition to synovial fluid (Fig. 70-41). Of ganglions, 60% occur on the dorsal aspect of the wrist, arising in the region of the scapholunate ligament. Other

**Table 70-5 Benign Connective Tissue Tumors of the Hand**

| SOFT TISSUE TUMORS | PRESENTATION | MOST COMMON LOCATIONS | TISSUE OF ORIGIN AND APPEARANCE | TREATMENT | RADIOGRAPHIC APPEARANCE |
|---|---|---|---|---|---|
| Ganglion | Swelling, sometimes painful; DIP mucous cyst may spontaneously drain clear gelatinous fluid; 70% of hand swellings | Volar and dorsal wrist, flexor tendon sheath, dorsum of DIP joint | Synovial cyst containing thick gelatinous fluid | No treatment versus aspiration versus excision | No radiographic alterations; mucous cyst at DIP joint may have osteophytes associated with osteoarthritis |
| Giant cell tumor of tendon sheath | Progressive enlargement, painless, deeply adherent; potential recurrence after excision; second most common hand tumor | Any synovial site, including tendon sheath, joint, palmar plate, usually in a digit | Synovium and histiocytes; bosselated and yellow-brown color from hemosiderin pigmentation | Excision | Pressure resorption of bone |
| Lipoma | Painless enlarging mass, usually on volar surface of hand or finger; may reach very large size; seldom nerve compression symptoms | Volar hand and finger | Mature fat cells | Excision (shell out) | Characteristic water-clear appearance on x-ray |
| Inclusion cyst (implantation dermoid) | Painless, enlarging lesion, adherent to overlying dermis; more common in laborers and those subject to minor hand trauma; may become infected | Palm and fingertips | Implanted epidermis cyst containing keratinous debris | Excision of entire epithelium-lined sac | May cause pressure resorption of bone |
| Neurofibroma | May be localized, diffuse, or plexiform; may be associated with von Recklinghausen disease; painless enlargement, but pain arouses suspicion of malignant change | Less common on hand than elsewhere; seen more frequently on palm | Perineurial fibroblasts | Excision if noncritical nerve; biopsy if malignancy suspected; possible nerve grafting | Characteristic MRI lobulated appearance |
| Schwannoma | Painless small mass in a peripheral nerve that is laterally mobile; may be an incidental finding at time of carpal tunnel surgery; occasional distal dysesthesias | Median and digital nerves | Schwann cells | Microneural surgery can shell the tumor out of the nerve without leaving neurologic deficit | No changes on plain x-ray |
| Pyogenic granuloma | Often at site of previous trivial skin injury on the fingers; friable and bleeds easily; grows rapidly | Fingers | Granulation tissue | Small lesions—can be cauterized; excise larger lesions | No x-ray changes |
| Glomus tumor | Very small lesions; exquisitely painful, localized tenderness, cold-sensitive; patients sometimes labeled as malingering | Subungual or volar fingertip; may be multiple | Neuromyoarterial apparatus | Excision; repair nail bed if subungual | May show indentation of distal phalanx |

sites for ganglions in the hand are at the volar wrist arising from one of the scaphoid articulations, the flexor tendon sheath at the area of the A1 pulley, and at the dorsum of the DIP joint, called a *mucous cyst*, where they are often associated with osteoarthritis of that DIP joint. In the latter location, the ganglion cyst can exert pressure on the germinal matrix of the nail bed, resulting in a deformed or grooved nail.

Ganglions are most common in women in the third decade of life. They are innocuous and can often be left alone. However, treatment may be required for cosmetic purposes or to relieve pressure effects on adjacent structures (Fig. 70-42). The dorsal wrist ganglion can sometimes be painful as a result of pressure on the posterior interosseous nerve at that location. A very small impalpable dorsal wrist ganglion can become quite painful, the so-called *occult ganglion* and, on occasion may best be diagnosed by MRI. Treatment of a dorsal wrist ganglion may be performed by aspiration of the mucinous substance with a large-bore needle. If this fails, the ganglion can then be surgically excised. Care must be taken to trace and resect the pedicle of the ganglion all the way down to the joint or tendon sheath from which it arises.[31] A volar wrist ganglion may often be closely related to the radial artery. Aspiration of volar wrist ganglions is seldom advised because of the potential risk of injury to the radial artery. At the level of the DIP joint, optimal treatment

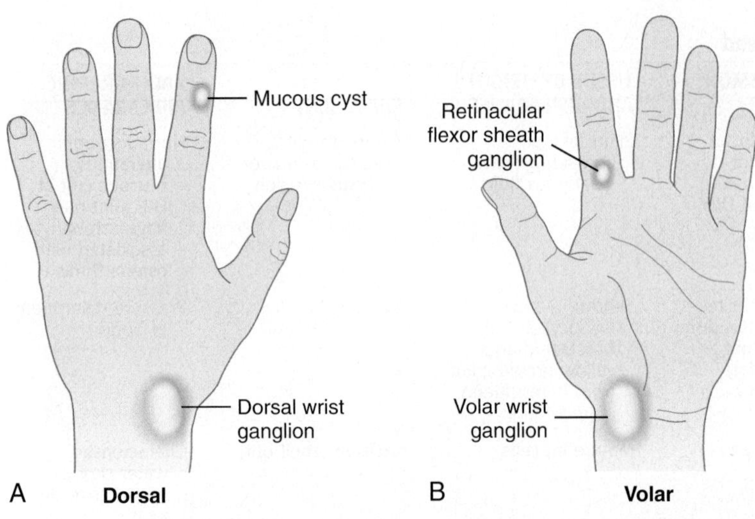


**FIGURE 70-41** Dorsal **(A)** and volar **(B)** aspects of the hand and wrist showing common types of ganglions, including the dorsal wrist ganglion, volar wrist ganglion, flexor sheath ganglion (volar retinacular cyst), and mucous cyst.

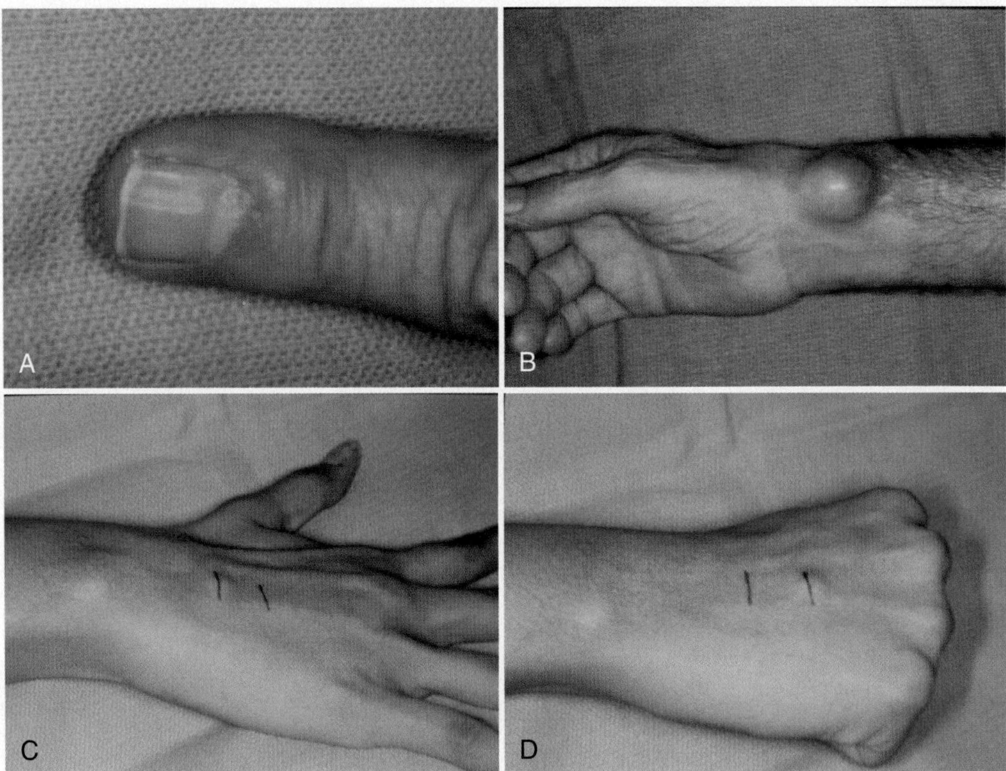


**FIGURE 70-42** Ganglions in the hand. **A,** Ganglion associated with osteoarthritis of the DIP joint (mucous cyst), causing longitudinal linear groove in the nail plate from pressure on the germinal matrix. **B,** Volar wrist ganglion on the radial side of the FCR tendon is closely related to the radial artery and should not be aspirated. **C,** Ganglion arising from the EDC tendon of the ring finger located at the level of the proximal skin marking with fingers extended. **D,** Movement of ganglion 2 cm to the level of the more distal skin marking when the fist is clenched. Distal movement of the swelling with the gliding extensor tendon confirms its attachment to the tendon.

includes not only meticulous excision of the ganglion but also the removal of associated osteophytes from the joint. Arthroscopic decompression of dorsal wrist ganglions has been described.

## Giant Cell Tumor

Giant cell tumor (GCT), also called *pigmented villonodular synovitis* (PVNS), is the second most common hand tumor. It occurs in soft tissues (e.g., synovial membrane of joints, tendon sheaths) and, less commonly, in bone. This yellow-brown multilobular tumor is composed of multinucleated giant cells. Although usually benign, the tumor pushes deeply into the soft tissues of the digits and extends along tendon sheaths and around neurovascular structures. It is frequently asymptomatic and is often larger than suspected clinically. Radiologic notching of bone may be evident in larger, soft tissue GCTs. Complete surgical excision is the treatment of choice. Failure to discern

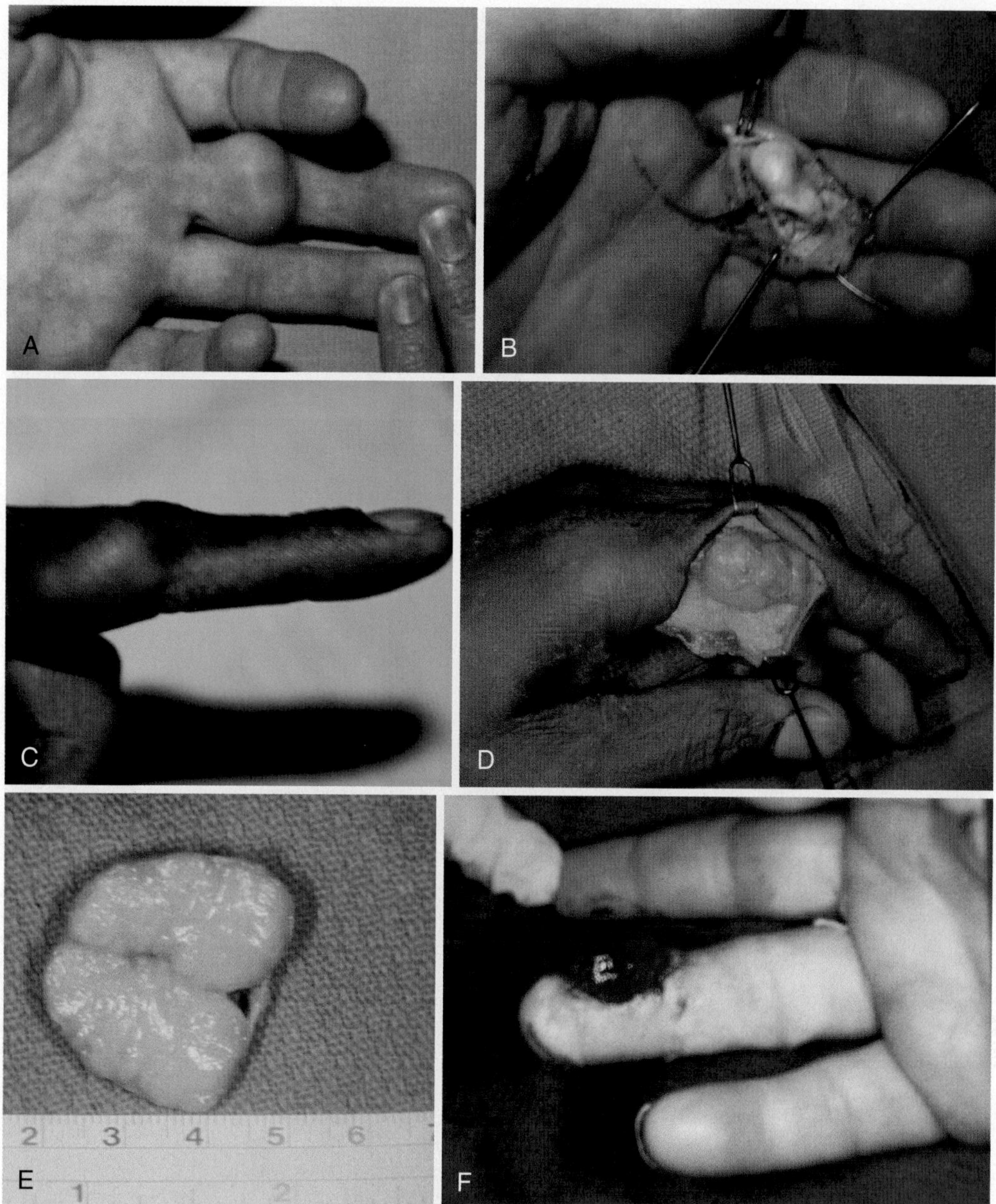

**FIGURE 70-43** Soft tissue tumors of the hand. **A,** Traumatically induced inclusion cyst on the palmar aspect of the middle finger in a manual worker. **B,** Intraoperative photograph demonstrates cyst filled with toothpaste-like gel derived from keratin. **C,** Firm, progressively enlarging swelling on the radial side of the left index finger. **D,** Firm, lobulated, yellow-brown giant cell tumor insinuating onto the dorsal and volar aspects of the finger is noted intraoperatively. **E,** Giant cell tumor is the most common solid soft tissue tumor encountered in the hand. **F,** Fleshy friable pyogenic granuloma bleeds easily on contact.

and remove each lobule substantially increases the reported local recurrence rate of almost 10%. Synovectomy of the joint of origin may be necessary (Fig. 70-43; see Fig. 70-45*B*).

### Epidermal Inclusion Cysts

Epidermal inclusion cysts, also called *implantation dermoids*, frequently occur after trauma as keratin-producing epidermal cells become lodged in the subcutaneous tissues (Fig. 70-43). The resulting cystic mass contains a thick toothpaste-like material. They occur more commonly in men, especially in manual laborers, and most frequently involve the palm of the hand and fingertips. They may also occur in previous surgical scars. Treatment is surgical excision and recurrence is rare.

### Lipoma

Lipomas are small, benign, soft, fluctuant, fatty tumors (Fig. 70-44). In the hand, they usually occur on the thenar eminence. Although generally painless, they may enlarge significantly, insinuating into deep palmar spaces and causing pain by compression on adjacent nerves. Intracarpal lipoma is a rarer cause of carpal tunnel syndrome. Resection of symptomatic lipomas is curative, although 1% to 2% may recur.

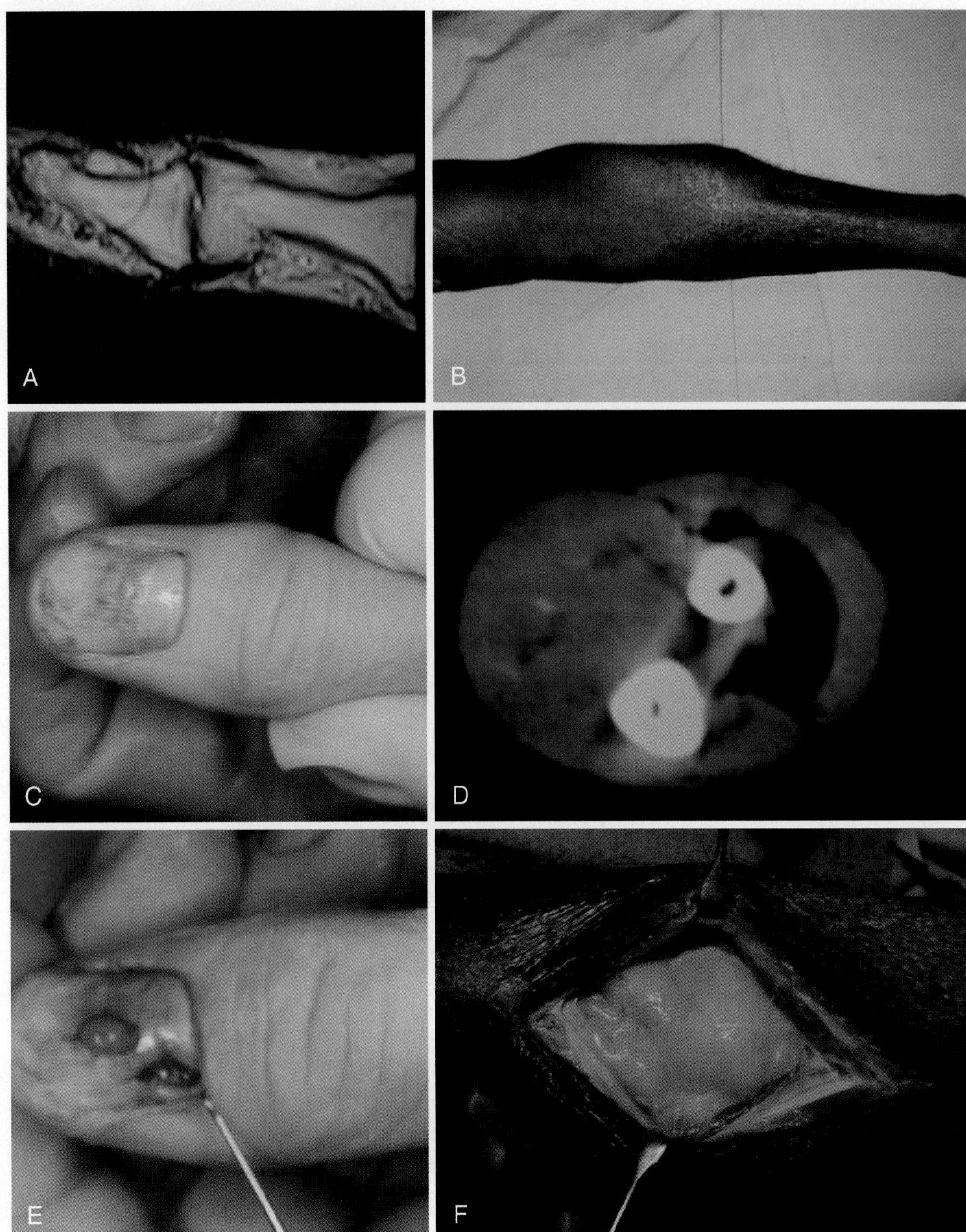

**FIGURE 70-44** Soft tissue tumors of the hand. **A,** Patient presenting with pain in tip of thumb, exacerbated in cold weather. Exquisite pain on palpation of the thumb nail plate is typical of a subungal glomus tumor that can be demonstrated by MRI. **B,** Occult subungal glomus tumor may be difficult to appreciate, even after removal of the nail plate, but can often be identified by a surface bulge of the nail bed. **C,** Excised glomus tumor sitting on nail bed. A nail bed defect requires repair with fine absorbable sutures. **D,** Man with swelling of left dorsoradial forearm and weakness of finger and thumb extension. **E,** MRI reveals a dorsal forearm mass compressing the posterior interosseous nerve. **F,** Dorsal approach over the mass reveals intramuscular benign lipoma when extensor muscles are split.

### Pyogenic Granuloma

Pyogenic granuloma is a misnomer for an exuberant outburst of highly vascular granulation tissue at the site of previous relatively trivial trauma. These lesions are very friable, bleed easily, and may grow rapidly. They respond to curettage or simple excision. They usually occur on the fingertips. Histologic confirmation of the diagnosis is necessary because of occasional confusion with aggressive malignant lesions, such as ulcerated, amelanotic, malignant melanomas.

### Verruca Vulgaris

Verrucae vulgaris are common contagious warts associated with human papilloma virus type 1 (HPV-1). They occur usually as hyperkeratotic filiform lesions on the digits or about the nail bed. The most effective topical treatments are salicylates, liquid nitrogen cryotherapy, and especially currettage. Recalcitrant lesions respond to oral cimetidine given for 6 to 8 weeks and to imiquimod, an immunomodulator that increases interferon production.[32] Like squamous cell carcinomas, their incidence is increased in immunocompromised patients, such as in those after transplantations. Recurrence is relatively common.[33]

### Seborrheic Keratoses

Seborrheic keratoses are benign, hyperkeratotic, scaly lesions. They are frequently pigmented, and common on the dorsum of the hand in older adults. Occasional confusion occurs with pigmented basal cell carcinomas. When necessary, these superficial scaly lesions are best treated by shave excision, and sutures are unnecessary. Rapid reepithelialization occurs.

### Keratoacanthoma

Keratoacanthoma occurs on exposed body parts such as the dorsum of the hand. It grows rapidly over approximately 3 weeks into a nodule with a central umbilicated keratotic plug, often followed by spontaneous resolution over many weeks or months. The resulting scar is often worse than if the lesion had been excised initially.[34] There may be diagnostic uncertainty in regard to well-differentiated squamous cell carcinomas. Hence, most authors recommend surgical excision.

### Dermatofibroma

A dermatofibroma arises from fibrous dermal tissue as a firm erythematous plaque, sometimes having central umbilication. It is often adherent to the overlying epidermis. Surgery is required primarily for diagnosis.

### Vascular Malformations and Hemangiomas

Hemangiomas are hamartomas that are rarely visible at birth and are usually noticed weeks to months later. Rapid proliferation occurs in the first year of life. Histologically, proliferation of endothelial cells with increased mitotic activity is seen in conjunction with pericytes and dendritic and mast cells. Hemangiomas occur 10 times more commonly than vascular malformations and approximately 70% involute by the age of 7 years, leaving a fibrofatty scar with redundant skin. Excision is seldom required and, after involution, is usually cosmetic. Occasionally, oral or injectable steroids may be necessary to control rapidly proliferating lesions that cause pain or interfering with function. Propranolol, which reduces basic fibroblast growth factor (bFGF) and vascular endothelial growth factor (VEGF) expression, is sometimes added in conjunction with steroids for problematic hemangiomas.[35]

By contrast, vascular malformations show normal endothelial growth characteristics and normal mast cell counts. They are often noted at birth and growth is usually commensurate with the child for low-flow lesions. They do not undergo spontaneous involution.

Vascular malformations are subclassified into low-flow lesions; capillary, venous, and lymphatic lesions predominate. Arterial and arteriovenous fistulas predominate in high-flow lesions and accelerated growth may occur relative to the patient. Pressure effects, ulceration, bleeding and high-output cardiac failure can occur in severe cases. Enlarging lesions hinder hand function. Compression garments can provide symptomatic relief in some cases. Pain is often caused by vascular engorgement, phlebitis, or intralesional coagulation. D-dimer levels may be elevated and some patients obtain relief from aspirin. Combined surgical excision[36] and radiologic embolization[37] are most effective in preventing recurrence caused by dilation of collateral vascular channels after simple excision.

Lymphaticovenous malformations may also be associated with generalized hypertrophy of an extremity. Vascular malformations and isolated macrodactyly are seen in Klippel-Trenaunay syndrome.

## Malignant Skin Tumors

### Basal Cell Carcinoma

Basal cell carcinoma is rare on the hand and is generally located on the dorsum. It is usually an ulcer with raised pearly edges. Treatment consists of excision with a margin of normal adjacent tissue. Nail bed lesions can be mistaken for paronychial infection and amputation at the distal interphalangeal joint may be required.[38]

### Squamous Cell Carcinoma

Squamous cell carcinoma (SCC) may arise de novo from ultraviolet (UV) light exposure because of occupation or climate, usually on the sun-exposed dorsum of the hand. Approximately 16% of actinic keratoses may progress to SCC. Arsenical keratoses may develop secondary to exposure to inorganic arsenic compounds but have a predilection for the palm.

Bowen's disease is an intraepidermal squamous cell carcinoma (carcinoma in situ).[39] It is a plaquelike lesion with crusting. Complete surgical excision with a margin of normal tissue is curative. When the nail matrix is involved, amputation at the distal interphalangeal joint may be necessary.

For squamous cell carcinoma lesions smaller than 2.5 cm in diameter, wide excision with approximately a 6-mm clear margin is recommended. However, for larger lesions, more radical excision may be required, which may even include ray or segmental amputation for deeply adherent and invasive lesions. Mohs micrographic surgery and three-dimensional histologic reconstruction with a pathologist at the time of radical resection help ensure complete excision. Routine prophylactic lymphadenectomy is not beneficial.[40] However, lymphadenectomy may be advised for recurrent tumors, even though lymph nodes may not be clinically palpable. Malignant degeneration may occur in cicatricial tissue and chronic ulcers (e.g., Marjolin's ulcer) and, in particular, occurs in burn scars. Prognosis tends to be poorer.[41]

### Malignant Melanomas

Melanoma of the hand is cutaneous or subungual. There is an almost equal distribution of cases between the two types.[42] Frequently, there is a delay in treatment, particularly with subungual melanomas. Suspicious lesions should be biopsied.

Any subungual pigmented lesions should generally be biopsied. Under tourniquet control and with loupe magnification, the nail plate is atraumatically removed and a longitudinal, elliptical, full-thickness excision of the lesion is performed. Careful nail bed repair is done following biopsy by the advancement of adjacent tissues and using fine absorbable sutures. The nail plate is then reapplied to act as a splint.

Benign melanocytic hyperplasia, without evidence of atypia, is completely treated by this form of biopsy. If there is any evidence of melanocytic atypia, absolute confirmation of complete excision is required. In the absence of a clear margin, or recurrence of such a lesion, total nail bed excision and reconstruction with a full-thickness skin graft is required. Melanoma in situ is similarly treated. Invasive melanoma of the nail bed is

**Table 70-6 Bone Tumors of the Hand**

| TUMOR | PRESENTATION | MOST COMMON LOCATIONS | TISSUE OF ORIGIN AND APPEARANCE | TREATMENT | RADIOGRAPHIC APPEARANCE |
|---|---|---|---|---|---|
| Enchondroma | Often incidental finding on routine hand x-ray; presents as pain secondary to pathologic fracture; most common bone tumor of hand | Proximal and middle phalanges and metacarpals | Fragments of cartilage nests; multiple (Ollier's disease); when associated with hemangiomas (Mafucci syndrome), may undergo malignant change | Curettage, filling of defect with cancellous bone if structural bone integrity is compromised | Lesion eccentric in bone shaft with calcific stippling |
| Osteochondroma | Benign bony prominence (capped with cartilage); rare in hand; may cause angular growth and interfere with joint motion | Fingers and wrist; growth stops after skeletal maturity reached | Aberrant focus of cartilage; multiple osteochondromatosis is autosomal dominant*; malignant change may occur | Surgery may be necessary, generally after epiphyseal closure | Exostosis, often at base of proximal phalanx; often shortening of parent bone |
| Osteoid osteoma | Aching pain, greatest at night, sometimes responding specifically to aspirin; patient may be labeled as malingerer | Phalanges, metacarpals, carpals | Nidus composed of loose fibrovascular connective tissue between bars of osteoid and bony trabeculae | Surgical excision to include the nidus | Very small lesion; some not seen on plain x-rays and require CT scan; cortical sclerosis surrounding a radiolucent area of nidus |
| Giant cell tumor of bone | Expansile bony swelling at distal radius or in phalanx | Distal radius most common site | May be locally aggressive and even metastasize | Curettage for low-grade lesions, but en bloc resection for high-grade lesions; do not irradiate because could induce sarcomatous change | Expansile soap bubble lesion in bone; high-grade lesions break through cortex |

treated by amputation at the next most proximal joint. Acral lentiginous melanoma of the palm may sometimes be mistaken for a wart, which may also delay diagnosis. These tumors are aggressively treated with wide local excision and potential sentinel node biopsy, as might be treated anywhere else on the body.

## Bone Tumors

### Osteoid Osteoma

This may occur in the hand and classically causes pain that is worse at night and unrelated to use or motion of the hand (Table 70-6). Osteoid osteomas produce prostaglandins; symptoms are relieved by nonsteroidal anti-inflammatory drugs (NSAIDs). Radiologically, a round lucent tumor with sclerotic edges is seen (Fig. 70-45*A*). Conservative treatments with NSAIDs may be considered, but definitive treatment is surgical.

### Aneurysmal Bone Cyst

This is an expansile osteolytic bony lesion with a thin wall. It is usually derived from a preexisting bony tumor, usually a GCT (20% to 40% of cases). Of these, 25% occur in the upper extremity, causing pain that peaks over 2 to 3 months. A bony swelling may be detectable, with increased overlying skin temperature.

### Enchondroma

Enchondromas usually occur in the hand and are the most common bony tumor of the hand. Peak incidence is in the second decade, with equal gender distribution. They are frequently asymptomatic and noted incidentally as lytic lesions on plain radiology. Pain, bony swelling, or pathologic fracture may occur as these cartilaginous intraosseous cysts compromise bony structural integrity (see Fig. 70-45*D*). Treatment is by curettage and bone grafting of the osseous defect. Multiple enchondromatosis occurs in Ollier's disease and is associated with angiomas in Maffucci syndrome.

### Primary Bone Sarcomas

These malignant tumors are rare in the hand.

### Secondary (Metastatic) Bone Tumors

Metastatic tumors, even those with a tendency to metastasize to bone, usually occur in the axial skeleton and long bones. They are very rare in the hand.

## CONGENITAL ANOMALIES

The causes of congenital hand anomalies may be genetic, teratogenic, or idiopathic and may also have a syndromic association with anomalies elsewhere in the body. Knowledge of these associations is important because the more life-threatening associated problems frequently need to be treated first, before the hand and upper extremity reconstruction can be performed. Such an association is found in a constellation of problems that occur in the VACTERL association of congenital defects (***v***ertebral anomalies, ***a***nal atresia, ***c***ardiac abnormalities, ***t***racheo***e***sophageal fistula, ***r***enal agenesis, and ***l***imb anomalies). A number of factors must be considered in optimizing the timing of each surgical procedure to the upper extremity, including the psychosocial development of the child, presence of other illnesses, size of the structures to be operated on, and normal growth and

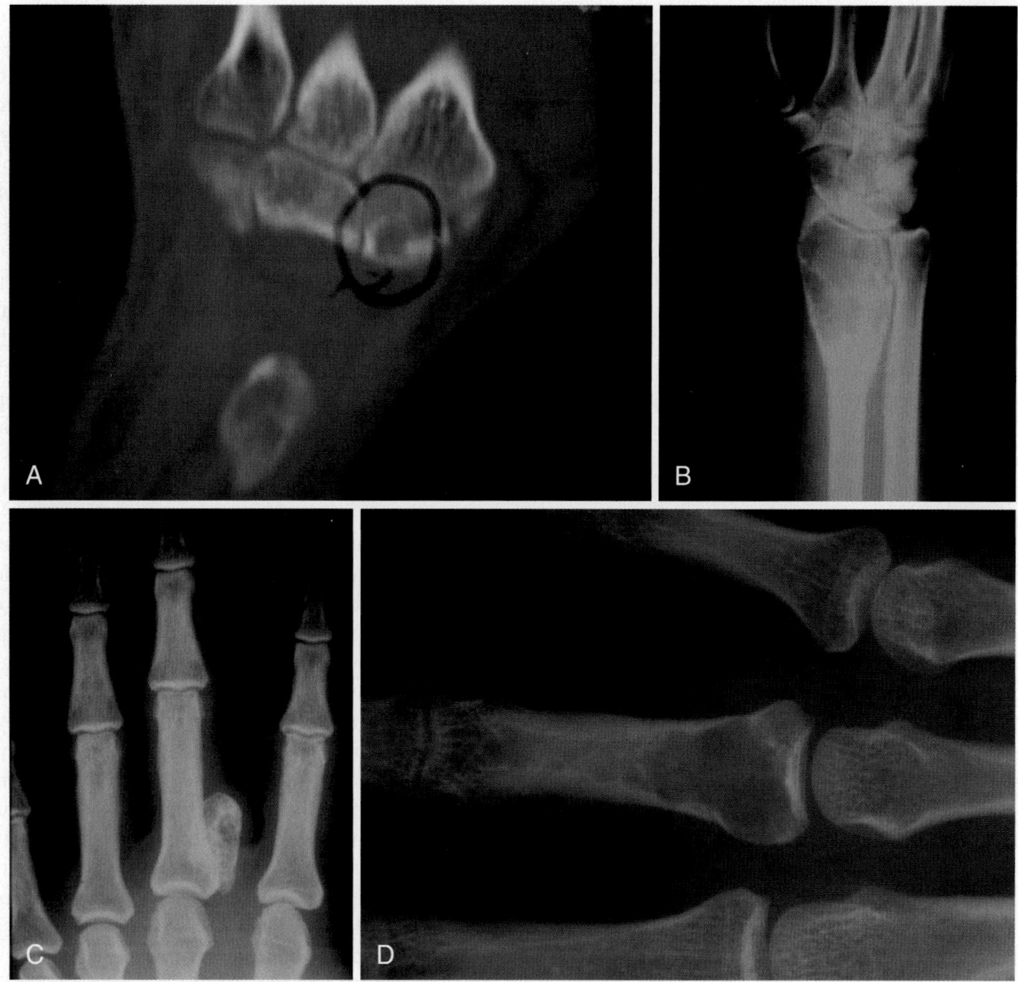


**FIGURE 70-45** Plain radiographs of the upper extremity. **A,** Osteoid osteoma of carpus. **B,** Soap bubble appearance of giant cell tumor expanding the metaphysis of the distal radius. **C,** Osteochondroma of proximal phalanx of middle (long) finger. **D,** Patient with finger pain after trivial injury. This is a pathologic fracture of the base of the proximal phalanx through an enchondroma that has replaced most of proximal metaphysis and medulla.

development of the hand. Modern technologic advances have allowed us to operate on smaller structures; the timing of the procedure can now be guided by knowledge of the anatomy and development of the growing hand. Optimal function is the primary goal of surgery. Principles of treatment of congenital hand anomalies recognize that infant immunity to infection develops over time, early surgery prevents the emotional scarring associated with a child's awareness of the deformity, and some congenital problems may not be apparent in the neonate. The hand surgeon must work closely with the pediatrician to identify general conditions that may affect the child's health. Some congenital anomalies of the extremities, especially those with the radial ray, may be associated with bone marrow failure (Fanconi's syndrome) or heart defects that may not be immediately apparent in the neonate. Children with congenital anomalies will attempt to keep up with their peers and often develop successful hand substitution techniques. However, once a child experiences the cruel ridicule of playmates or the unintentional but sometimes overly solicitous supervision of a teacher, his or her deformity becomes important. Generally plans for surgical reconstruction are designed to be completed by school age, so that the child may adapt to and fully use the reconstructed limb.[43]

The rationale for early surgery includes the avoidance of deformity and malfunction and optimal use of infantile tissue plasticity. Because hand length almost doubles during the first 2 years of life, a digit tethered to another digit that fails to grow can produce a major deformity during the early growth spurt. For example, with separation of syndactyly that involves the border digits of the hand, because of adjacent tethering to a digit of unequal length, surgical separation of the syndactyly is required at an early age, as early as 6 months, to avoid secondary angular deformity of the digits.

In rare circumstances, urgent treatment in the neonate is required. The distal lymphedema of a severe constriction band syndrome may be so marked as to inhibit function totally or even threaten distal viability. This may require urgent release. The unusual clinical entity of aplasia cutis may result in exposure of vital structures, requiring urgent soft tissue coverage, even in the neonatal period.

Early operation, although not urgent, may be required, not only because of the rapid growth that occurs in the first 2 years of life but also because of functional consequences. Surgery at a young age is considered mandatory in children with malformations in which hand function may be altered by surgery or in those who are at risk for developing certain grasping habits that would have to be unlearned after corrective surgery. An older child, 12 to 14 years of age, has developed grasp patterns that would have to be altered by prolonged periods of physical therapy after corrective surgery.[43,44]

The ability to place the upper limbs in space (a cortical function) and development of a strong grasp are established by 1 year of age, as are grasp and pinch maneuvers between the thumb and fingers. Accuracy of prehension and refinement of coordination continue until 3 years of age. Surgery must be performed early to allow the affected parts to develop differently when the function of the parts of the hand is altered by transposition (e.g., pollicization of an index finger for thumb aplasia). Duplicated thumb correction is carried out before 1 year of age, well in advance of the development of integrated thumb grasp patterns.

Finally, the physical ability of infant bone and soft tissues to adapt to change produced by surgery is also a key factor in deciding when to operate. In the early pollicization of the index finger, the first dorsal interosseous muscle hypertrophies to form a thenar eminence and the first metacarpal (formerly known as the *proximal phalanx* of the index finger) broadens. If centralization of the wrist for radial dysplasia (formerly known as *radial club hand*) has been undertaken early, the head of the ulna broadens to resemble the distal end of the radius.

Thus, a number of issues are taken into consideration when deciding on the optimum time for surgical reconstruction of congenital hand and upper extremity anomalies. The more common hand anomalies include syndactyly, polydactyly, constriction band syndrome, and absent or hypoplastic thumb.

Syndactyly results from the failure of programmed cell death (apoptosis) between the individual finger rays. Consequently, there is a resulting fusion of adjacent digits. It can involve part or all of the length of the digits (incomplete or complete) and may be limited to skin and soft tissue only (simple syndactyly), or can also involve skeletal fusion (complex syndactyly). Apert's syndrome also involves craniofacial anomalies and is a severe form of bilaterally symmetrical complex syndactyly. Surgical treatment involves digit separation using a local flap to reconstruct the depths of the commissure between the fingers and release of the finger borders with zigzag incisions and the use of full-thickness skin grafts (Fig. 70-46*A*).

Polydactyly is the presence of extranumerary digits on the hand. Preaxial (radial) polydactyly involves the thumb. It is not as common as postaxial (ulnar) polydactyly, which is the most frequent congenital hand anomaly in African Americans. Polydactyly can be as simple as the presence of a skin tag–like structure or may have a complex arrangement of shared vessels, nerves, and bones. Thumb polydactyly is not merely a duplication but a splitting of a single digit, with variable degrees of development in each of the separate parts. It is typically classified into seven subtypes using the Wassel classification, which is based on the specific duplication, progressing from distal to proximal. Type IV is the most common type, with total duplication of proximal and distal phalanges and a shared metacarpophalangeal joint. *Type VII* refers to associated triphalangia with a duplication. Reconstructive goals include stabilization without sacrificing mobility, proper alignment of joints along the longitudinal axis of the thumb, balanced motor units, and a cosmetically acceptable nail plate (see Fig. 70-46*B* and *C*).

The Blauth classification categorizes thumb hypoplasia from type I, which represents minor hypoplasia, to type V, which is a total thumb absence. Surgical correction ranges from reconstruction of the existing hypoplastic thumb to pollicization (creating a thumb from the index finger) for complete absence or for the more severe types of hypoplasia (Fig. 70-47).

Clinodactyly is a curving of the digits in a radial or ulnar direction. It is common, particularly involving the little finger in many individuals, but a curvature of more than 10 degrees is considered abnormal. The distal phalanx is usually affected and a delta phalanx may be associated. A delta phalanx occurs when the epiphysis forms a C shape around the metaphyseal core in the middle phalanx. Most patients present with little or no functional or cosmetic deformity, and operative intervention is seldom required. If there is a functionally impairing deviation of the finger, corrective osteotomy can be done.

Camptodactyly is a congenital flexion deformity of digits. It usually occurs in the little finger PIP joint. The exact cause is unclear, but has been attributed to a variety of different structures around the PIP joint, including a skin pterygium, collateral ligaments, volar plate, flexor tendon, abnormal insertions of lumbrical or interosseous muscles, and size and shape of the head of the proximal phalanx. Treatment is generally nonoperative and may involve serial splinting. If no improvement occurs and the flexion deformity is sufficient to cause a functional problem, surgical intervention may be required; this includes correction of the deformity with Z-plasty and possibly grafts. One author has reported that all his patients who had reconstructive surgery on one hand did not ask for corrective surgery on the opposite affected hand.

Constriction band syndrome is secondary to intrauterine amniotic bands (see Fig. 70-46*D*). These can act like tourniquets and threaten the viability of digits and even limbs, resulting in congenital amputation. Infants may suffer from a similar problem from the external ligature effect of cotton strands coming off protective booties and even from a human hair, termed the *hair-thread-tourniquet syndrome.*

## OSTEOARTHRITIS AND RHEUMATOID ARTHRITIS

Osteoarthritis may be primary or post-traumatic (secondary). Primary osteoarthritis is a degenerative joint disease occurring in later life. An injury that leaves articular surfaces of a joint incongruous can precipitate secondary osteoarthritis. Osteoarthritis begins with biochemical alteration of the water content of articular cartilage. The cartilage weakens and develops cracks, called *fibrillation.* Progressive erosion and thinning of the cartilage results and the subchondral bone becomes sclerotic, termed *eburnation.* New bone forms around the edges of the articular cartilage and these outcroppings are call osteophytes (Fig. 70-48).

The joints usually affected in the hand are the DIP and PIP joints of the fingers and carpometacarpal joint at the base of the thumb. Osteophytes at the DIP joint are called *Heberden's nodes* and those at the PIP joint are known as *Bouchard's nodes.* The involved joints may be painful, stiff, deformed, or subluxated. Radiographs reveal narrowing of the joint space, sclerosis of subchondral bone, and presence of osteophytes.

Initial treatment may be symptomatic and may include splinting and even local corticosteroid injections. NSAIDs may

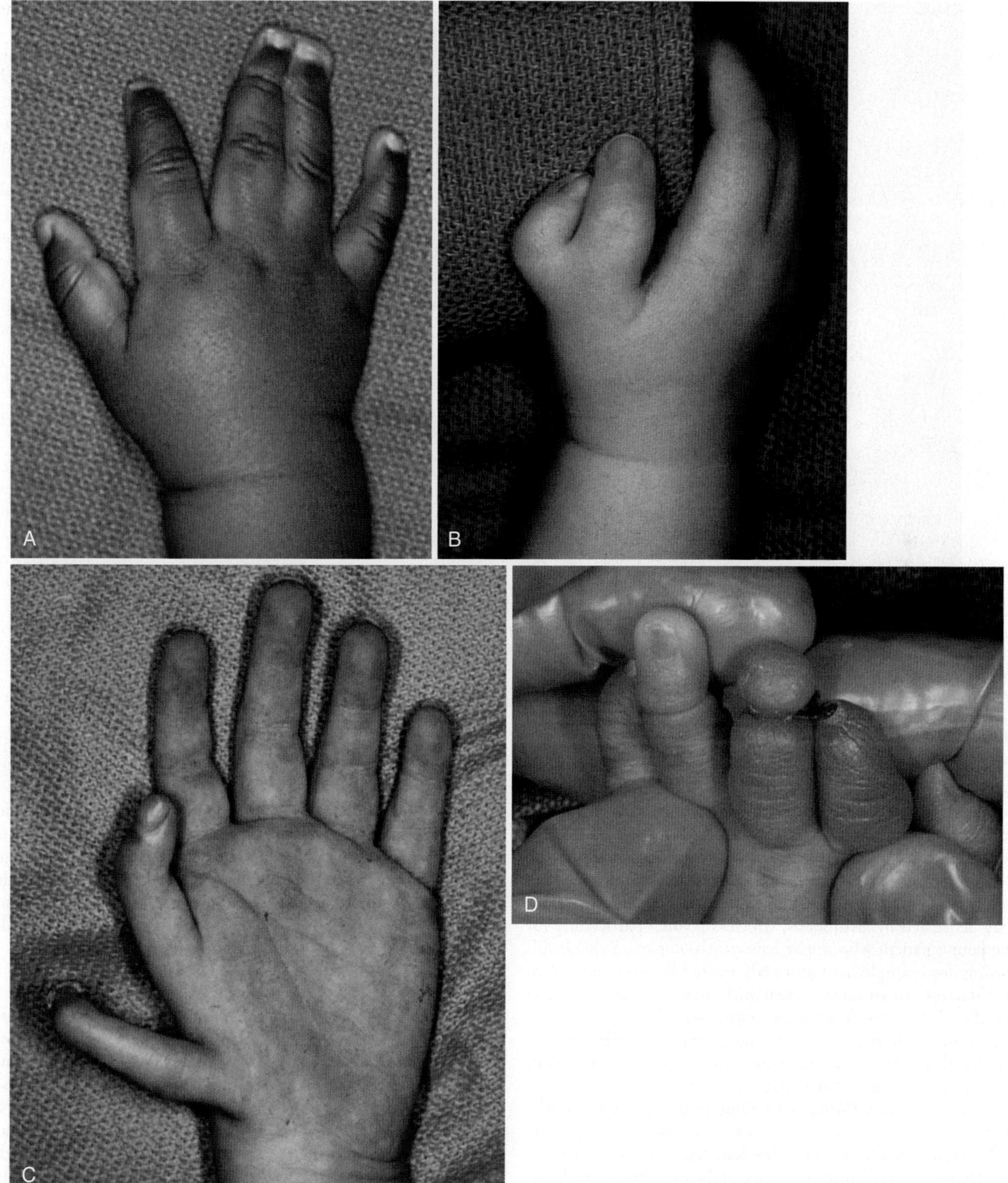


**FIGURE 70-46** Congenital hand anomalies include syndactyly **(A)**, Wassel type IV thumb polydactyly **(B)**, Wassel type VI polydactyly **(C)**, and constriction band **(D)**.

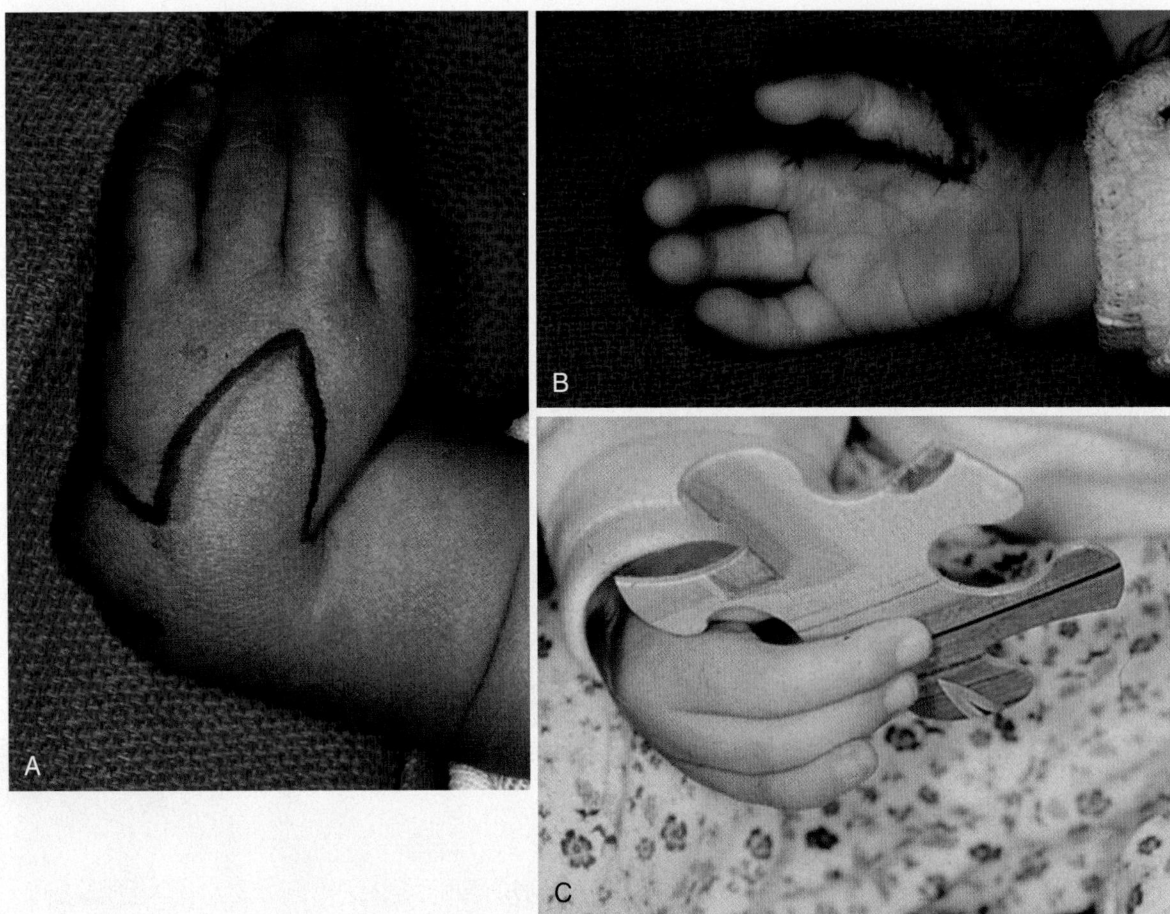

**FIGURE 70-47 A,** Patient with radial dysplasia and absent thumb. **B,** After centralization of the wrist on the distal ulna, pollicization of the index finger is performed. **C,** Natural prehension has been restored to this three-finger hand with a reconstructed wrist and thumb.

be helpful and chondroprotective medications such as glucosamine and chondroitin sulfate can reduce symptoms. In advanced cases, the DIP joints respond best to arthrodesis. The PIP joints may be surgically treated by replacement arthroplasty or by arthrodesis (Fig. 70-49). The thumb carpometacarpal joint may be treated by arthrodesis, which is favored particularly for the young patient who might have post-traumatic arthritis following, for example, an improperly treated Bennett's or Orlando's fracture. In an older patient with primary osteoarthritis at the thumb base, excision of the trapezium followed by tendon suspension (interposition) arthroplasty may be preferred. This uses local tendons for construction of a sling arthroplasty, with interposition of tendon material.

Rheumatoid arthritis is an autoimmune process whereby destruction of the musculoskeletal system may occur. Synovial inflammation results in pain, joint destruction, tendon ruptures, and characteristic deformities. Some of the more common deformities associated with rheumatoid arthritis include a swan neck deformity (hyperextension of the PIP joint with concurrent flexion at the DIP joint), boutonniere deformity (flexion at the PIP joint, with concurrent hyperextension at the DIP joint), joint subluxation, radial deviation of the wrist, and ulnar deviation and flexion of the fingers (Fig. 70-50). Rheumatoid arthritis is primarily a medical illness for which a number of medications are currently available. Thus, there must be excellent lines of communication between the rheumatologist and surgeon. NSAIDs are used, as well as disease-modifying antirheumatoid drugs. Rheumatoid arthritis is a progressive disorder and ongoing slow destruction may be anticipated, despite surgery (Fig. 70-51). Some of the more common surgical procedures include joint synovectomy, tenosynovectomy, tendon transfers, joint replacements (especially at the MP and PIP joints), and arthrodesis (more commonly at the wrist and thumb MP joint).[45]

## CONTRACTURES

Volkmann's ischemic contracture develops as a result of myofascial contractures in response to prolonged ischemia. This most common contracture results from untreated compartment syndrome of the forearm and hand. The muscles necrose and become replaced by fibrous scar tissue. The FDP and FPL muscles are usually affected, being in the deepest forearm volar compartment, and digits are characteristically flexed, with passive extension of the wrist worsening the flexion deformity of the digits. Intrinsic contractures can occur in the hand; these can be investigated using Bunnell's test, in which passive extension of the MP joint makes passive flexion of the PIP joint more difficult.

In the milder forms of Volkmann's ischemic contracture, serial splinting and passive stretching exercises may resolve the problem. In more severe contractures, Z-type lengthening of tendons may be required. A flexor pronator muscle slide, in which subperiosteal elevation of the common flexor origin from

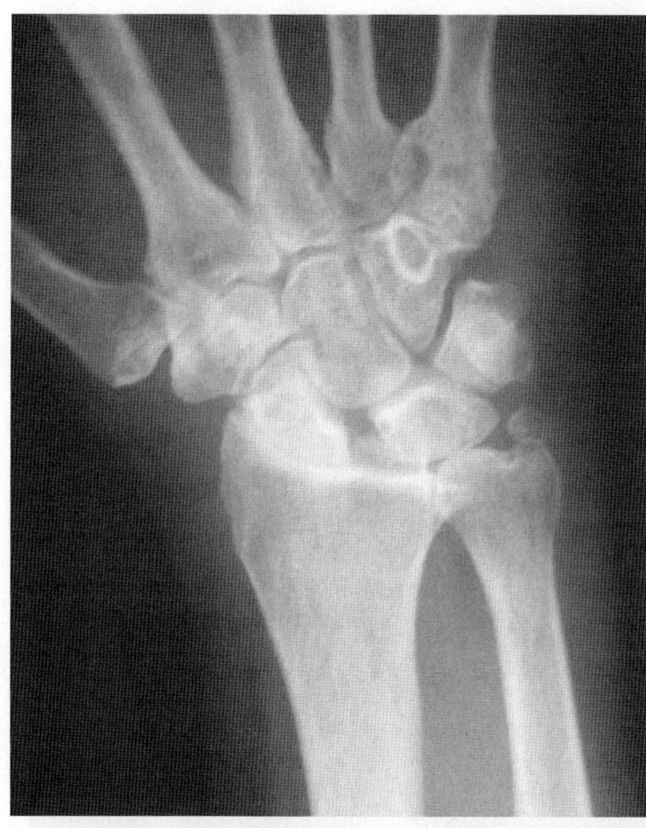

**FIGURE 70-48** Radiograph of a hand with a scapholunate advanced collapse wrist showing post-traumatic osteoarthritis at the radioscaphoid junction. This is many years after a wrist sprain in which the scapholunate ligament was torn; there is a wide scapholunate gap visible on radiograph.

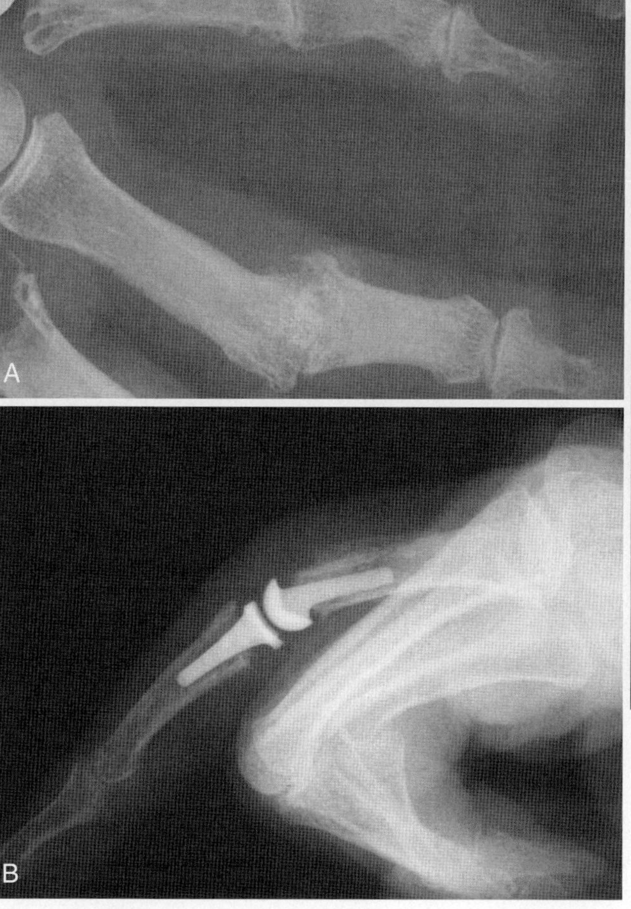



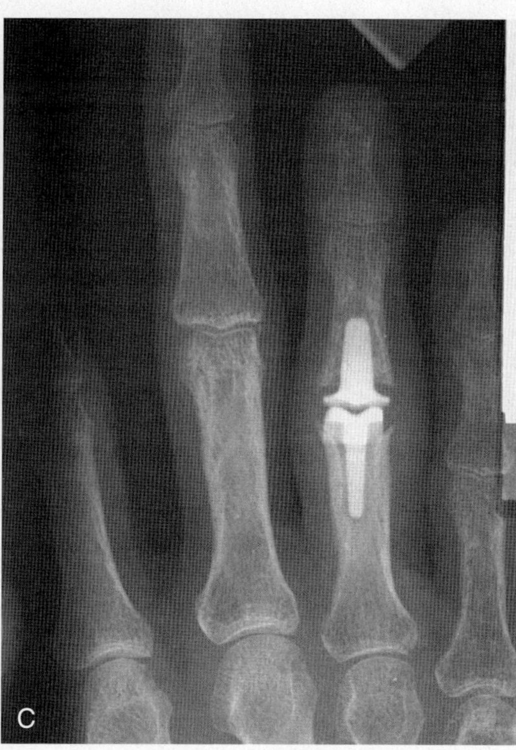



**FIGURE 70-49 A,** Patient with painful and unstable PIP joint from osteoarthritis. **B, C,** Reconstruction is performed by implant arthroplasty. An advantage over arthrodesis is that motion is retained, although there remains the potential for future recurrent joint instability and wear of the artificial joint.

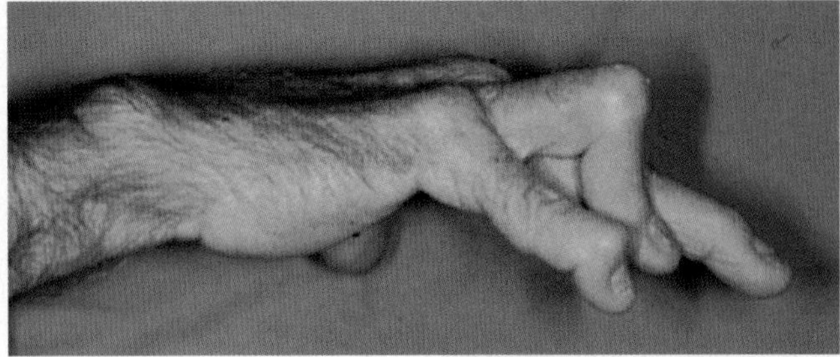

**FIGURE 70-50** Patient with inflammatory arthritis has both boutonniere deformity and swan neck deformity on the same hand.

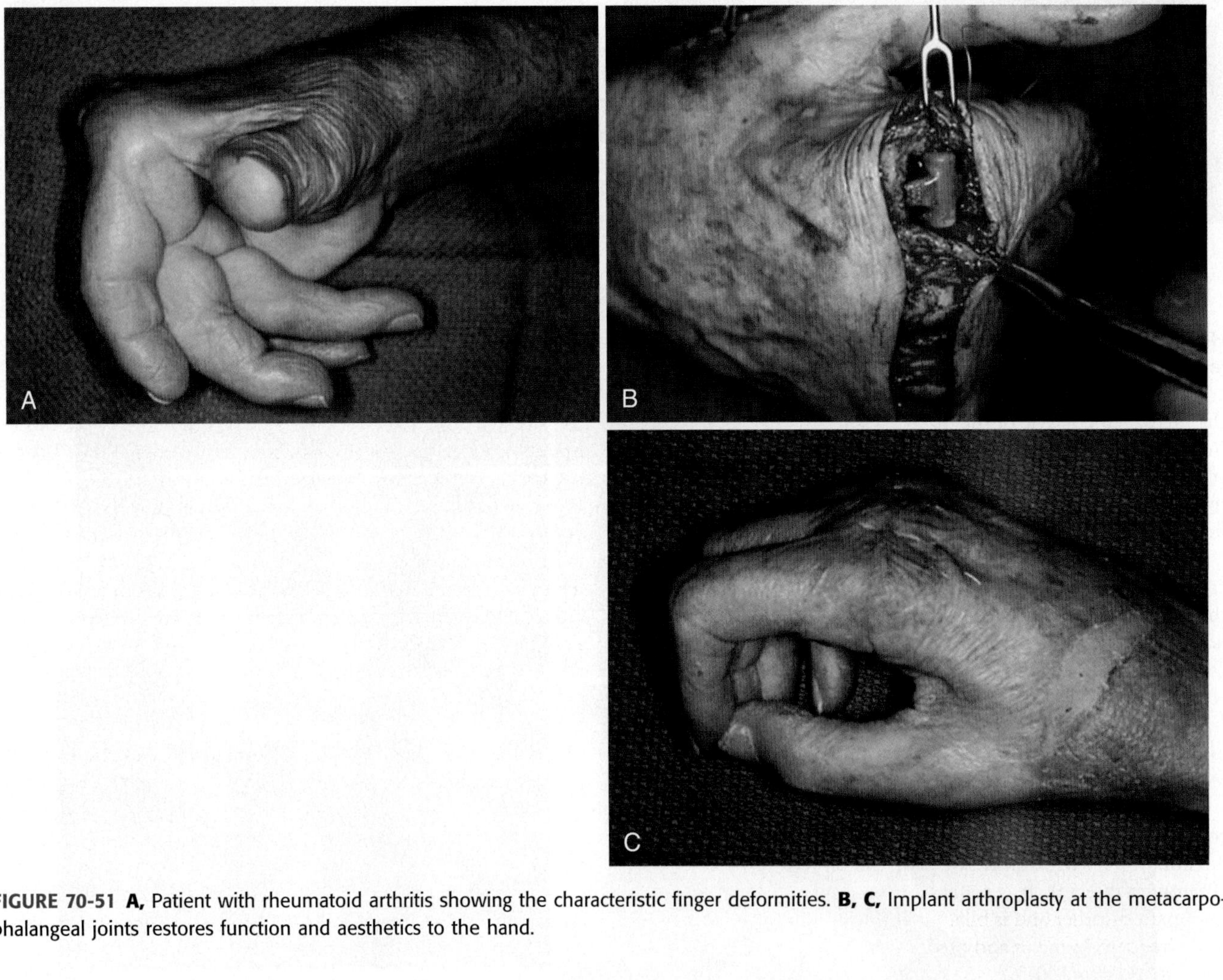

**FIGURE 70-51 A,** Patient with rheumatoid arthritis showing the characteristic finger deformities. **B, C,** Implant arthroplasty at the metacarpophalangeal joints restores function and aesthetics to the hand.

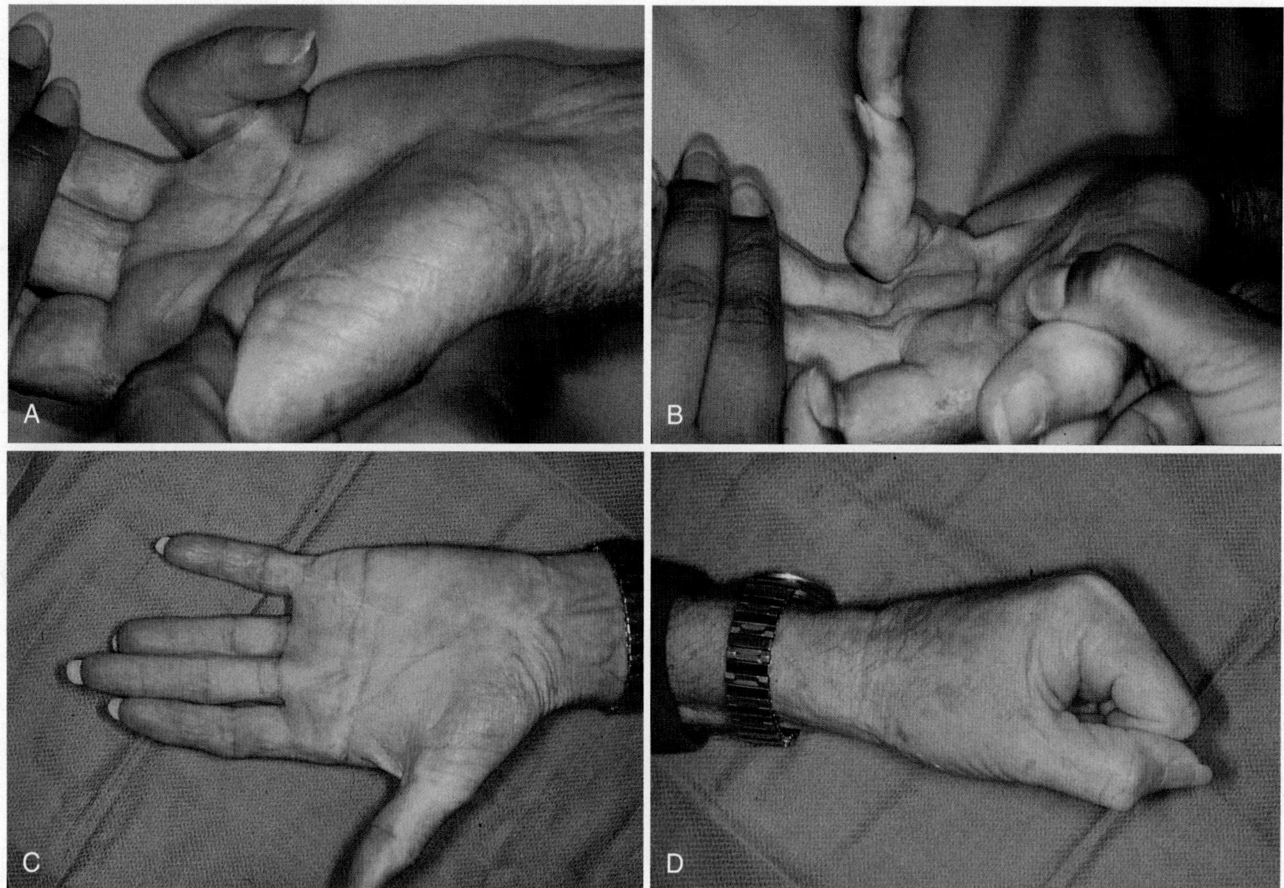


**FIGURE 70-52 A-D,** Patient with Dupuytren's contracture is treated by regional palmar and digital fasciectomy, and good hand function is restored.

the medial epicondyle of the humerus and from the ulna, allows the muscles to slide distally until the contracture is corrected. In the most severe form, all the muscles of the volar forearm may be affected, requiring tendon transfers, even microvascular functional muscle transfers to provide some functional return.

Post-traumatic contractures are the most common type of contracture. These can be prevented by appropriate treatment of the primary injury, especially with attention to detail in how the hand and upper extremity are splinted and immobilized. Once contractures have developed, if they are mild, they may be able to be stretched out by exercises and hand therapy. If these contractures are severe and functionally deforming, surgical release of joint contractures and release of tendon adhesions may be required.

Dupuytren's contracture is a disease process of contracting collagen affecting the palmar fascia, which can also affect the dorsum of the fingers (knuckle pads), soles of the feet, and penis (Peyronie's disease). It is thought to be a hereditary mendelian dominant disorder and is bilateral in 65% of cases. It is six times more frequent in males and predominantly involves the ring and little fingers (Fig. 70-52).

The process of Dupuytren's contracture occurs in the normal bands of collagen tissue that form the palmar fascia, natatory ligaments, and digital sheaths. Nodules containing myofibroblasts and immature collagen (type III) develop in these tissues or in the dermis. The nodules progressively increase in size, leading to thickened contractures and shortened fascial bands that develop into cords extending up the digits. Treatment is surgical excision; it is indicated in metacarpophalangeal contractures of 30 degrees or more, when the patient fails the so-called *tabletop test* and cannot place the palm of the hand flat on a surface, and whenever there is a PIP joint contracture. Careful surgical technique is necessary to avoid complications such as skin necrosis, hematoma, and digital nerve injuries. Collagenase injections using enzyme derived from *Clostridium histolyticum* have been attempted and have shown some promise in the treatment of Dupuytren's contracture. However, long-term follow-up in patients who had these injections is still necessary.[46-48]

## CONCLUSION

The specialty of hand surgery is exhaustive and a number of specialty textbooks are available. Although general surgeons may be responsible for the basic tenets of hand surgery, knowledge of minute details is often not necessary; thus, most details have been omitted from this chapter because the its purpose has been to see the big picture in regard to hand surgery. Those topics of hand surgery that the general surgeon is most likely to encounter have been emphasized, particularly with regard to principles of anatomy, physical examination, and emergency treatments. Taking this into consideration, Table 70-7 includes some high-yield facts relevant to hand surgery that have been compiled from various general surgery review books, as well as topics discussed in the American Board of Surgery (ABS) In-Training Examination (ABSITE).[49,50] This list is provided for the convenience of general surgeons preparing for ABSITE or board examinations.

**Table 70-7 American Board of Surgery Review Topics**

| TOPIC | ANSWER |
|---|---|
| Fracture of the distal radius | Injury to the median nerve |
| Innervation of FDP to the ring and small fingers | Ulnar nerve |
| Injury to the ulnar nerve at the elbow | Weakness in abduction and adduction of the index finger through small digits |
| Midshaft humeral fracture | Associated with radial nerve injury |
| Distal phalanx fractures | >50% of all hand fractures |
| Joint involved in Bennett's fracture | Carpometacarpal (CMC) joint of the thumb |
| Common name for metacarpal fracture of the small finger | Boxer's fracture |
| Most frequently fractured carpal bone | Scaphoid |
| Complications associated with displaced fractures | Avascular necrosis and nonunion of the scaphoid |
| Axonal nerve growth rate | 1 mm/day |
| Common maximum intraoperative tourniquet time in hand surgery | 2 hr |
| Single digits that are primarily replanted | Thumbs in adults and children, all digits whenever possible in children |
| Maximal period of anoxia compatible with replantation | Finger—8 hr (warm ischemia), but longer times have been anecdotally reported; upper and lower extremity—6 hr |
| Proper method for transportation of an amputated body part to maximize replantation success | Cleaned of debris, wrapped in sterile towel or gauze, moistened with sterile lactated Ringer's solution, placed in sterile plastic bag, transported in insulated cooler with ice water (ideal temperature, 4° C) |
| Complications if nerve repair is delayed >2 wk | Retraction of nerve's ends resulting in need for nerve grafting |
| Zone 2, no man's land | Area of flexor tendon injury between metacarpal phalangeal (MCP) and FDS insertion |
| Mallet finger | Injury to extensor mechanism at level of DIP joint |
| Gamekeeper's thumb | Rupture of ulnar collateral ligament of thumb MCP joint, with resultant instability of the joint to radial-directed force |
| Most common organism causing hand infections | *Staphylococcus aureus* |
| Classic symptoms of carpal tunnel syndrome | Paresthesias in median nerve distribution, often waking the patient at night |
| Most effective therapy for full-thickness burns of the hand | Early excision and grafting |
| Most common location of ganglion cysts | Scapholunate interosseous ligament at the dorsal wrist |
| Treatment of de Quervain's stenosing tenosynovitis after failed nonoperative management | Surgical release of first extensor compartment |
| Cause of trigger finger | Stenosing tenosynovitis in the region of the MCP joint, A1 pulley |
| Late findings of rheumatoid arthritis | Subluxation of involved joints resulting in deformity |
| Swan neck deformity | Hyperextension of PIP joint with flexion of DIP joint |
| Boutonnière deformity | Flexion of PIP joint with hyperextension of DIP joint |
| Nonoperative measures of Dupuytren's contracture | Exercise, local steroid injections, collagenase injections, radiotherapy |
| Digits usually affected in Dupuytren's contracture | Ring and small fingers |
| Cause of Dupuytren's contracture | Proliferation and fibrosis of the palmar fascia |
| Fractures likely to cause compartment syndrome, Volkmann's ischemic contracture | Supracondylar fracture of the humerus |
| Artery and nerve compromised in Volkmann's ischemic contracture | Median nerve and anterior interosseous artery |
| Complication of cast placement for supracondylar fractures of the humerus | Volkmann's ischemic contracture |

## SELECTED REFERENCES

### General

Patel MM, Catalano LW: Bone graft substitutes: Current uses in hand surgery. J Hand Surg Am 34:555–556, 2009.

Bone grafts are used for structural support and biologic properties. The use of bone graft substitutes limits donor morbidity and also shortens operative time.

Slutsky DJ, Nagle DJ: Wrist arthroscopy: Current Concepts. J Hand Surg Am 33:1228–1244, 2008.

Wrist arthroscopy has grown from a diagnostic procedure to a valuable treatment modality for a variety of wrist disorders such as degenerative arthritis, acute carpal and metacarpal fractures, wrist instability, and ganglions.

Cordill LL, Schubkegel T, Light TR, Ahmad F: Lipid infusion rescue for bupivacaine-induced cardiac arrest after axillary block. J Hand Surg Am 35:144–146, 2010.

Successful resuscitation of a hand surgery patient after inadvertent intravascular injection of bupivacaine during administration of an axillary block is discussed.

Harness NG: Digital block anesthesia. J Hand Surg Am 34:142–145, 2009.

The optimum techniques for providing digital block anesthesia are discussed.

Bruen KJ, Gowski WF: Treatment of digital frostbite: Current concepts. J Hand Surg Am 34:553–554, 2009.

Experience with tissue plasminogen activator is reported. It shows promise in decreasing rates of digital amputation.

Omer, GE: Development of hand surgery: Education of hand surgeons. J Hand Surg Am 25:616–628, 2000.

This article traces the development of hand surgery from the publication, in 1916, of Kanavel's classic book on infections of the hand, through the recognition of the specialty of hand surgery, to the training of modern-day hand surgeons and their educational requirements. The article contains historical vignettes and mentions many giants in hand surgery.

### Soft Tissue

Foucher G, Khouri RK: Digital reconstruction with island flaps. Clin Plast Surg 24:1–32, 1997.

New information of the intrinsic flaps of the hand enables ingenious soft tissue reconstructions using local tissues from the hand and fingers as pedicled, vascularized, island flaps. A thorough knowledge of the vasculature of the hand is required in addition to that in standard anatomy texts.

Godina M: Early microsurgical reconstruction of complex trauma of the extremities. Plast Reconstr Surg 78:285–292, 1986.

This paper emphasizes the concept of primary repair and reconstruction of all damaged tissues (including microvascular soft tissue coverage) acutely following major trauma.

Martin D, Bakhach J, Casoli V, et al: Reconstruction of the hand with forearm island flaps. Clin Plast Surg 24:33–48, 1997.

Knowledge of the vascular anatomy of the forearm enables an array of pedicled flaps to be used for soft tissue reconstruction of the hand, thus avoiding the need to use microvascular anastomoses.

### Flexor Tendons

Hunter JM, Salisbury RE: Flexor tendon reconstruction in severely damaged hands: A two-stage procedure using a silicone-dacron reinforced gliding prosthesis prior to tendon grafting. J Bone Joint Surg 53:829–858, 1971.

This paper introduces the concept of two-stage flexor tendon repair in patients in whom the flexor tendon sheath is scarred in a late repair. A tendon spacer is placed as a preliminary procedure to later tendon grafting. This remains a time-honored way of dealing with late flexor tendon reconstructions.

Kim HM, Nelson G, Thomopoulos S, et al: Technical and biological modifications for enhanced flexor tendon repair. J Hand Surg Am 35:1031–1037, 2010.

An up-to-date current concept on technical essentials to enhance outcome and the potential for future biologic manipulation of the tendon repair site.

Kleinert H, Kutz JE, Atasoy E, Stormo A: Primary repair of flexor tendons. Orthop Clin North Am 4:865–876, 1973.

This article was the first substantive evidence that flexor tendons could be safely and effectively repaired in no man's land, emphasizing the importance of postoperative controlled mobilization of the fingers.

Strickland JW: Development of flexor tendon surgery: Twenty-five years of progress. J Hand Surg Am 25:214–235, 2000.

This excellent review article describes the current state of the art for treatment of flexor tendon injuries.

### Nerve Injuries

Isaacs T: Treatment of acute peripheral nerve injures: Current Concepts. J Hand Surg Am 35: 491–497, 2010.

Although outcomes following nerve repair are not always excellent, this article assesses well-established basic principles and also includes a number of strategies for repair techniques for small and large traumatic nerve gaps.

Millesi H, Meissel G, Berger A: The interfascicular nerve-grafting of the median and ulnar nerves. J Bone Joint Surg 54:727–750, 1972.

This landmark article emphasizes the importance of tension-free nerve repair, matching of proximal and distal fascicular groups, and use of nerve grafts in cases of a large nerve gap injury.

Lundborg G: A 25-year perspective of peripheral nerve surgery: Evolving neuroscientific concepts and classical significance. J Hand Surg Am 25:391–414, 2000.

This excellent article establishes the experimental basis and neuroscience behind nerve repair and nerve regeneration. The rationale for nerve conduits is discussed.

Weber RV, Mackinnon S: Nerve transfers in the upper extremity. J Am Soc Surg Hand 4:200–213, 2004.

The innovative use of nerve transfers is described to bypass and overcome long nerve gaps following nerve injury to hasten and improve functional recovery.

### Replantation

Buncke HJ: Microvascular hand surgery—transplants and replants—over the past 25 years. J Hand Surg Am 25:415–428, 2000.

This article traces the history of microvascular surgery as it applies to the upper extremities and of the milestones achieved. It discusses the many microvascular reconstructive options available for free tissue transfer and microvascular toe to hand transfers and also evaluates anticipated survival and functional outcomes for replantation surgery.

### Fractures

Kawamura K, Chung KC: Treatment of scaphoid fractures and nonunions. J Hand Surg Am 33:938–997, 2008.

Scaphoid fractures are a common injury presenting with unique challenges because of a tenuous scaphoid blood supply. This article updates the reader about diagnostic imaging and current treatment strategies for displaced and nondisplaced acute scaphoid fractures, scaphoid nonunions, and avascular necrosis.

Carlsen BT, Moran SL: Thumb trauma: Bennett fractures, Rolando fractures and ulnar collateral ligament injuries. J Hand Surg Am 34:945–952, 2009.

Recent advancements for the treatment of these common injuries are discussed.

Stern PJ: Management of fractures of the hand over the last 25 years. J Hand Surg Am 25:817–823, 2000.

Fluoroscopic imaging has greatly facilitated the operative management of hand fractures. The evolution from Kirschner wires to plates and screws is discussed. Innovations included self-tapping screws, low-profile plates, and cannulated screws, with the goal of achieving rigid bone fixation to enable restoration of early digital motion to minimize the risk for tendon adhesions and joint contractures.

Russe O: Fracture of the carpal navicular: Diagnosis, non-operative, and operative treatment. J Bone Joint Surg Am 42:759–768, 1960.

Although new innovations of cannulated compression screw and minimally invasive surgery have changed the management of scaphoid fractures, this article is still relevant in regard to understanding and treating of scaphoid fractures and their complications.

### Infections

Kanavel AB: An anatomical, experimental, and clinical study of acute phlegmons of the hand. Surg Gynecol Obstet 1:221–259, 1905.

This is classic paper described the anatomic spaces of the hand. It changed the course of infection treatment and also saw the origins of hand surgery. The clinical outcome was changed from amputation to surgical management, which preserved the function of structures, emphasizing that hand surgery is founded in a sound knowledge of anatomy. The basic principles of this article, written in the preantibiotic era, still remain true.

### Compartment Syndrome

Mubarak SJ, Hargens AR: Acute compartment syndromes. Surg Clin North Am 63:539–565, 1983.

This excellent article describes the pathogenesis of acute compartment syndrome, including the diagnosis and surgical management in the upper extremity.

### Entrapment Neuropathy

Bickel KD: Carpal tunnel syndrome. J Hand Surg Am 35:147–152, 2010.

This is the most common compressive neuropathy in the upper extremity. Evidence-based guidelines for diagnosis and treatment are provided.

Palmer BA, Hughes TB: Cubital tunnel syndrome. J Hand Surg Am 35:153–163, 2010.

This up to date article provides current concepts in diagnosis and treatment strategies for cubital tunnel syndrome.

Koo JT, Szabo RM: Compression neuropathies of the median nerve. J Am Soc Surg Hand 4:156–175, 2004.

This comprehensive article gives excellent anatomic descriptions of all the anatomic sites in the upper extremity in which chronic compression of the median nerve can occur. Nonsurgical and surgical management guidelines are outlined for each.

Phalen GS: The carpal-tunnel syndrome: Seventeen years' experience in diagnosis and treatment of six hundred fifty-four hands. J Bone Joint Surg 48:211–228, 1966.

This is a classic paper written by a founder and past president of the American Society for Surgery of the Hand. It presents an understanding of median nerve compression at the wrist that is surgically treated by decompression and release of the transverse carpal ligament. The most common procedure performed by hand surgeons today is median nerve decompression.

### Vascular Tumors

Mulliken JB, Glowacki J: Hemangioma and vascular malformations in infants and children: A classification based on endothelial characteristics. Plast Reconstr Surg 69:412–422, 1982.

The authors attempted to unify the classification of hemangiomas and vascular malformations. Suggested classifications fall into six broad categories—embryology, histology, clinical features, dynamics of growth, hemodynamic patterns, and cell biology. A classification is useful only if it has diagnostic applicability and aids in planning therapy and understanding pathogenesis.

### Congenital Anomalies

McCarroll HR: Congenital anomalies: A 25-year overview. J Hand Surg Am 25:1007–1037, 2000.

This excellent review discusses the more commonly treated congenital hand anomalies. It also identifies some of the newer (at that time) developments in surgical treatment, which include distraction lengthening, pollicization, microvascular surgery, and potential for in utero interventions. Useful classifications for treatment management are provided.

Netscher DT, Scheker LR: Timing and decision making in the treatment of congenital upper extremity deformities. Clin Plast Surg 17:113–131, 1990.

This review describes commonly treated congenital hand anomalies and provides a rational basis for timing surgical interventions to meet critical hand functional milestones.

### Osteoarthritis

Burton RI, Pellegrini VD: Surgical management of basal joint arthritis of the thumb. Part II. Ligament reconstruction with tendon interposition arthroplasty. J Hand Surg Am 11:324–332, 1986.

An excellent description of the pathogenesis and surgical management of basilar joint osteoarthritis of the thumb. This is the usually performed surgical procedure for carpometacarpal joint osteoarthritis of the thumb.

Eaton RG, Littler JW: Ligament reconstruction for the painful thumb carpometacarpal joint. J Bone Joint Surg Am 55:1655–1666, 1973.

One of the most common joints affected by osteoarthritis is at the base of the thumb. This operation, originally described by these authors for surgical management, still forms the basis of surgical treatment today, with few modifications in technique.

### Rheumatoid Arthritis

Brasington R: TNF-α antagonists and other recombinant proteins for treatment of rheumatoid arthritis. J Hand Surg Am 34:349–350, 2009.

Disease modifying antirheumatic drugs are discussed that specifically target individual molecules. Medical treatment of rheumatoid conditions has changed dramatically in recent years.

Swanson AB: Flexible implant arthroplasty for arthritic finger joints: Rationale, technique, and results of treatment. J Bone Joint Surg Am 54:435–455, 1972.

A landmark article that changed the course of treatment for rheumatoid arthritis. In this paper, Swanson introduced small joint arthroplasty.

### Contractures

Curtis RM: Capsulectomy of the interphalangeal joints of the fingers. J Bone Joint Surg Am 36:1219–1232, 1954.

This classic article changed the course of treatment of the stiff hand and promoted interest in the complex anatomy of the proximal interphalangeal joint. The author was meticulous in technique and insisted on rigid postoperative therapy.

McFarlane RM: Patterns of the diseased fascia in the fingers in Dupuytren's contracture: Displacement of the neurovascular bundle. Plast Reconstr Surg 54:31–44, 1974.

This article clearly outlines the pathology, anatomy, and proposed surgical treatment for Dupuytren's contracture. The author describes the patterns of diseased fascia in the palm and fingers and how displacement of the digital neurovascular bundle may occur.

## REFERENCES


1. Green DP: General principles. In Hotchkiss RN, Pederson WC, Wolfe SW, et al, editors: Green's operative hand surgery, ed 5, Philadelphia, 2005, Elsevier, pp 3–24.
2. Idler RS, Manktelow RT: The hand: Primary care of common problems, ed 2, Philadelphia, 1990, Churchill Livingstone.
3. Klenerman L: Tourniquet time—how long? Hand 12:231–234, 1980.
4. Netscher DT, Cohen V: Phalangeal fractures. In Evans GRD, editor: Operative plastic surgery, New York, 2000, McGraw-Hill, pp 979–991.
5. Hunter JM, Salisbury RE: Flexor-tendon reconstruction in severely damaged hands. A two-stage procedure using a silicone-dacron reinforced gliding prosthesis prior to tendon grafting. J Bone Joint Surg Am 53:829–858, 1971.
6. Tomaino M, Mitsionis G, Basitidas J, et al: The effect of partial excision of the A2 and A4 pulleys on the biomechanics of finger flexion. J Hand Surg Br 23:50–52, 1998.
7. Tang JB: Indications, methods, postoperative motion and outcome evaluation of primary flexor tendon repairs in zone 2. J Hand Surg Eur 32:118–129, 2007.
8. Lalonde DH: Wide-awake flexor tendon repair. Plast Reconstr Surg 123:623–625, 2009.
9. Tang JB, Zhang Y, Cao Y, et al: Core suture purchase affects strength of tendon repairs. J Hand Surg Am 30:1262–1266, 2005.
10. Williamson DT, Richards RS: Flexor tendon injuries and reconstruction. In Mathes SJ, Hentz VR, editors: Plastic surgery, ed 2, Philadelphia, 2006, Elsevier, pp 351–391.
11. Netscher DT: Extensor tendon injuries. In Goldwyn RM, Cohen MN, editors: The unfavorable result in plastic surgery, Philadelphia, 2001, Lippincott Williams and Wilkins, pp 751–770.
12. Cheng CJ: Synthetic nerve conduits for digital nerve reconstruction. J Hand Surg Am 34:1718–1721, 2009.
13. Oberlin C, Beal D, Leechavengvongs S, et al: Nerve transfer to biceps muscle using a part of ulnar nerve for C5-C6 avulsion of the brachial plexus: Anatomical study and report of four cases. J Hand Surg Am 19:232–237, 1994.
14. McClinton MA, Wilgis EFS: Ischemic conditions of the hand. In Mathes SJ, Hentz VR, editors: Plastic surgery, ed 2, Philadelphia, 2006, Elsevier, pp 791–822.
15. Soucacos PN: Indications and selection for digital amputation and replantation. J Hand Surg Br 26:572–581, 2001.

16. Netscher DT, Cohen MN: Metacarpals and phalanges. In Evans GRD, editor: Operative plastic surgery, New York, 2000, McGraw-Hill, pp 959–978.
17. Stern PJ: Fractures of the metacarpals and phalanges. In Hotchkiss RN, Pederson WC, Wolfe SW, et al, editors: Green's operative hand surgery, ed 5, Philadelphia, 2005, Elsevier, pp 277–342.
18. Kumar S, O'Connor A, Despois M, et al: Use of early magnetic resonance imaging in the diagnosis of occult scaphoid fractures: the CAST Study (Canberra Area Scaphoid Trial). N Z Med J 118:U1296, 2005.
19. Clark DC: Common acute hand infections. Am Fam Physician 68:2167–2176, 2003.
20. Rockwell PG: Acute and chronic paronychia. Am Fam Physician 63:1113–1116, 2001.
21. Stevanovic MV, Sharpe F: Acute infections in the hand. In Hotchkiss RN, Pederson WC, Wolfe SW, et al, editors: Green's operative hand surgery, ed 5, Philadelphia, 2005, Elsevier, pp 55–93.
22. Lille S, Hayakawa T, Neumeister MW, et al: Continuous post-operative catheter irrigation is not necessary for the treatment of suppurative flexor tenosynovitis. J Hand Surg Br 25:304–307, 2000.
23. Mollitt DL: Infection control: Avoiding the inevitable. Surg Clin North Am 82:365–378, 2002.
24. Kare JA: Volkmann contracture, 2010 (http://emedicine.medscape.com/article/1270462-overview).
25. Patel MR, Bassini L: Trigger fingers and thumb: When to splint, inject, or operate. J Hand Surg Am 17:110–113, 1992.
26. Trumble TE: Compressive neuropathies. In Trumble TE, editor: Principles of hand surgery and therapy, Philadelphia, 2000, WB Saunders, pp 324–342.
27. Trumble TE, Diao E, Abrams RA, et al: Single-portal endoscopic carpal tunnel release compared with open release: A prospective, randomized trial. J Bone Joint Surg Am 84-A:1107–1115, 2002.
28. Mackinnon SE, Novak CB: Compression neuropathies. In Hotchkiss RN, Pederson WC, Wolfe SW, et al, editors: Green's operative hand surgery, ed 5, Philadelphia, 2005, Elsevier, pp 999–1046.
29. Athanasian EA: Bone and soft tissue tumors. In Hotchkiss RN, Pederson WC, Wolfe SW, et al, editors: Green's operative hand surgery, ed 5, Philadelphia, 2005, Elsevier, pp 2211–2265.
30. Netscher DT, Hildreth DH, Kleinert HE: Tumors of the hand. In Georgiade GS, Riefkohl R, Levin LS, editors: Plastic, maxillofacial, and reconstructive surgery, Baltimore, 1997, Williams and Wilkins, pp 1046–1070.
31. Cohen V, Netscher DT: Excision of ganglion cysts. In Evans GRD, editor: Operative plastic surgery, New York, 2000, McGraw-Hill, pp 924–935.
32. Glass AT, Solomon BA: Cimetidine therapy for recalcitrant warts in adults. Arch Dermatol 132:680–682, 1996.
33. Shenefelt PD: Warts, nongenital, 2010 (http://emedicine.medscape.com/article/1133317-overview).
34. Kopf AW: Keratoacanthoma: Clinical aspects. In Andrade R, Gumport SL, Popkin GL, et al, editors: Cancer of the skin, Philadelphia, 1976, WB Saunders, pp 755–781.
35. Buckmiller LM, Munson PD, Dyamenahalli U, et al: Propranolol for infantile hemangiomas: Early experience at a tertiary vascular anomalies center. Laryngoscope 120:676–681, 2010.
36. Sofocleous CT, Rosen RJ, Raskin K, et al: Congenital vascular malformations in the hand and forearm. J Endovasc Ther 8:484–494, 2001.
37. Koman LA, Ruch DS, Paterson SB: Vascular disorders. In Hotchkiss RN, Pederson WC, Wolfe SW, et al, editors: Green's operative hand surgery, ed 5, Philadelphia, 2005, Elsevier, pp 2265–2313.
38. Butler ED, Hamill JP, Seipel RS, et al: Tumors of the hand. A ten-year survey and report of 437 cases. Am J Surg 100:293–302, 1960.
39. Bowen JT: Pre-cancerous dermatosis. J Cutan Dis 33:787–802, 1915.
40. Johnson RE, Ackerman LV: Epidermoid carcinoma of the hand. Cancer 3:657–666, 1950.
41. Novick M, Gard DA, Hardy SB, et al: Burn scar carcinoma: A review and analysis of 46 cases. J Trauma 17:809–817, 1977.
42. Glat PM, Shapiro RL, Roses DF, et al: Management considerations for melanonychia striata and melanoma of the hand. Hand Clin 11:183–189, 1995.
43. Netscher DT: Congenital hand problems. Terminology, cause, and management. Clin Plast Surg 25:537–552, 1998.
44. McCarroll HR: Congenital anomalies: A 25-year overview. J Hand Surg Am 25:1007–1037, 2000.
45. Feldon P, Terrono AL, Nalebluff EA: Rheumatoid arthritis and other connective tissue diseases. In Hotchkiss RN, Pederson WC, Wolfe SW, et al, editors: Green's operative hand surgery, ed 5, Philadelphia, 2005, Elsevier, pp 2049–2136.
46. Hurst LC, Badalamente MA: Nonoperative treatment of Dupuytren's disease. Hand Clin 15:97–107, vii, 1999.
47. Reilly RM, Stern PJ, Goldfarb CA: A retrospective review of the management of Dupuytren's nodules. J Hand Surg Am 30:1014–1018, 2005.
48. Saar JD, Grothaus PC: Dupuytren's disease: An overview. Plast Reconstr Surg 106:125–134, 2000.
49. Blecha M, Brown A: Orthopedic and hand surgery pearls. In Blecha M, Brown A: General surgery: Pearls of wisdom, Lincoln, Mass, 2004, Boston Medical, pp 217–224.
50. Deziel DJ, Witt TR, Bines SD: Hand surgery. In Deziel DJ, Witt TR, Bines SD, et al, editors: Rush University review of surgery, ed 3, Philadelphia, 2000, WB Saunders, pp 579–589.

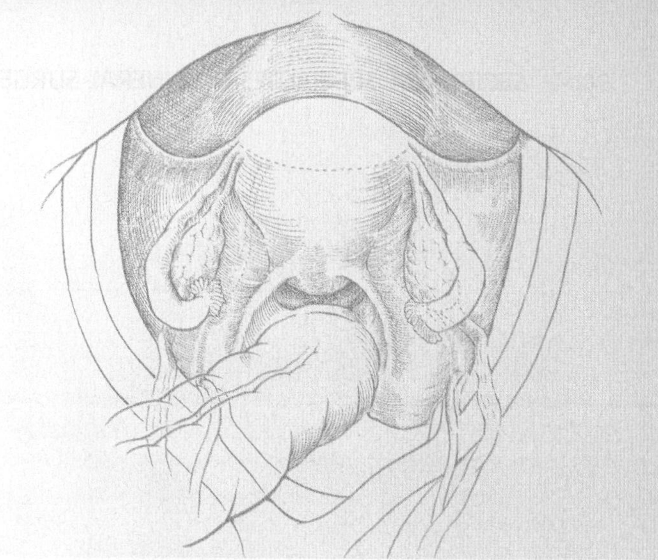

## CHAPTER 71

# GYNECOLOGIC SURGERY

Howard W. Jones, III

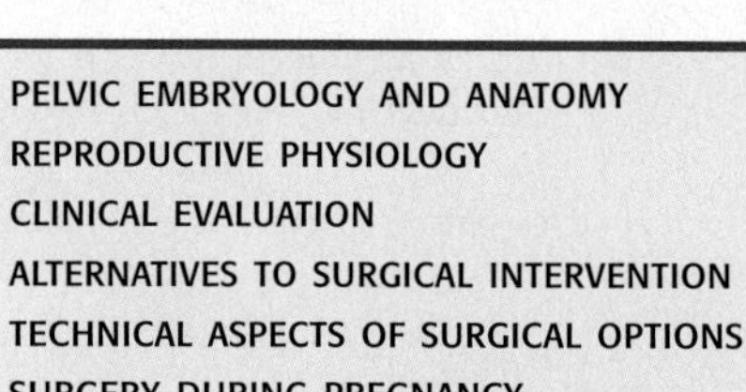



Gynecologic surgery involves the operative treatment of benign and malignant conditions of the female genital tract. Because of the hormonal responsiveness of these tissues and organs during the menstrual cycle and during the premenarchal, reproductive, and postmenopausal periods of life, the diagnosis, management, and even surgical approach may differ because of the hormonal milieu and the patient's desire for future fertility. All these factors may be even further complicated in pregnant women in whom the surgical and anesthetic approach must consider the pregnant uterus and fetus. The surgeon who understands and is able to consider the physiology, endocrinology, and anatomy of the female pelvis is most prepared to select the most appropriate and successful operative procedure. In addition, by knowing the alternatives to surgery and risks and advantages of several possible management approaches, a treatment most likely to correct the problem and be consistent with the patient's desires for fertility preservation, minimally invasive surgical approach, or even no surgery at all can be accomplished with the best opportunity for a good outcome.

The general surgeon may be called on to assist the gynecologic surgeon when endometriosis or ovarian cancer involves the sigmoid colon, when a diverticular abscess or carcinoma of the colon involves the ovary, in the pregnant women with acute appendicitis or cholecystitis, or in smaller communities in which there is no gynecologist at all.

Although a full discussion of gynecologic surgery is beyond the scope of a single chapter, I will attempt to address the basics of pelvic anatomy, reproductive physiology, clinical evaluation of common gynecologic symptoms, surgical technique for several common operations, and surgical approach to the pregnant patient.

## PELVIC EMBRYOLOGY AND ANATOMY

### Embryology

The female external genitalia are derived embryologically from the genital tubercle, which, in the absence of testosterone, fails to undergo fusion and devolves to the vulvar structures. The labial structures are of ectodermal origin. The urethra, vaginal introitus, and vulvar vestibule are derived from uroepithelial entoderm. The lower third of the vagina develops from the invagination of the urogenital sinus.

The internal genitalia are derived from the genital ridge. The ovaries develop from the incorporation of primordial germ cells into coelomic epithelium of the mesonephric (wolffian) duct and the tubes, uterus, cervix, and upper two thirds of the vagina develop from the paramesonephric (mullerian) duct. The embryologic ovaries migrate caudad to the true pelvis. Primordial ovarian follicles develop but remain dormant until stimulation in adolescence by gonadotropins. The paired mullerian ducts migrate caudad and medially to form the fallopian tubes and fuse in the midline to form the uterus, cervix, and upper vagina. The wolffian ducts regress. Failure or partial failure of these processes can result in distortions of anatomy and potential diagnostic dilemmas (Table 71-1).

### Anatomy

#### External Genitalia

The external genitalia consist of the mons veneris, labia majora, labia minora, clitoris, vulvar vestibule, urethral meatus, and ostia of the accessory glandular structures (Fig. 71-1). These structures overlie the fascial and muscle layers of the perineum. The perineum is the most caudal region of the trunk; it includes the pelvic floor and those structures occupying the pelvic outlet. It is bounded superiorly by the funnel-shaped pelvic diaphragm and inferiorly by the skin covering the external genitalia, anus, and adjacent structures. Laterally, the perineum is bounded by the medial surface of the inferior pubic rami, obturator internus muscle below the origin of the levator ani muscle, coccygeus muscle, medial surface of the sacrotuberous ligaments, and overlapping margins of the gluteus maximus muscles (Fig. 71-2).

The pelvic outlet can be divided into two triangles separated by a line drawn between the ischial tuberosities. The anterior or urogenital triangle has its apex anteriorly at the symphysis pubis and the posterior or anal triangle has its apex at the coccyx.

The urogenital triangle contains the urogenital diaphragm, a muscular shelf extending between the pubic rami and penetrated by the urethra and vagina, and the external genitalia, consisting of the mons pubis, labia majora and minora, clitoris, and vestibule. The mons pubis is a suprapubic fat pad covered by dense skin appendages. The labia majora extend posteriorly from the mons, forming the lateral borders of the vulva. They

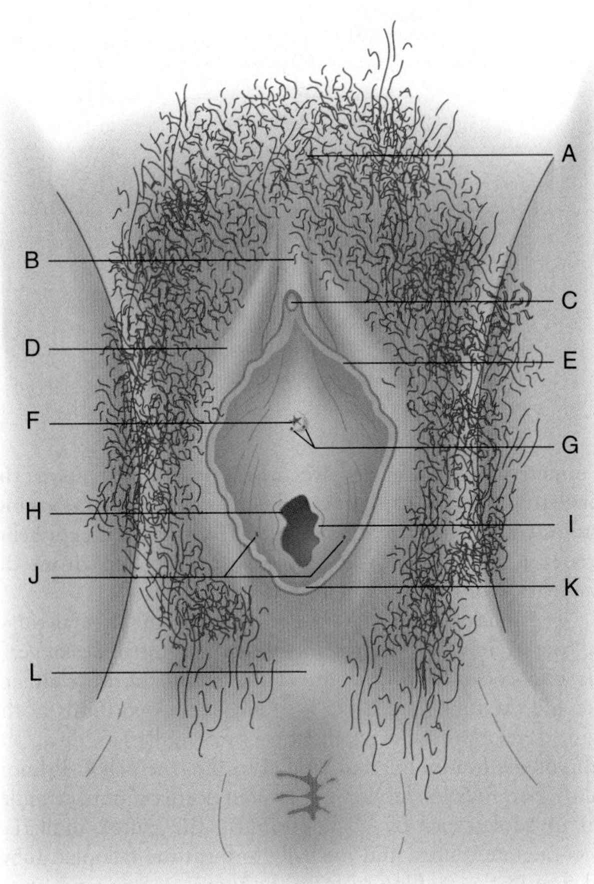


FIGURE 71-1 The external genitalia. A, Mons pubis; B, prepuce; C, clitoris; D, labia majora; E, labia minora; F, urethral meatus; G, Skene's ducts; H, vagina; I, hymen; J, Bartholin's glands; K, posterior fourchette; L, perineal body.

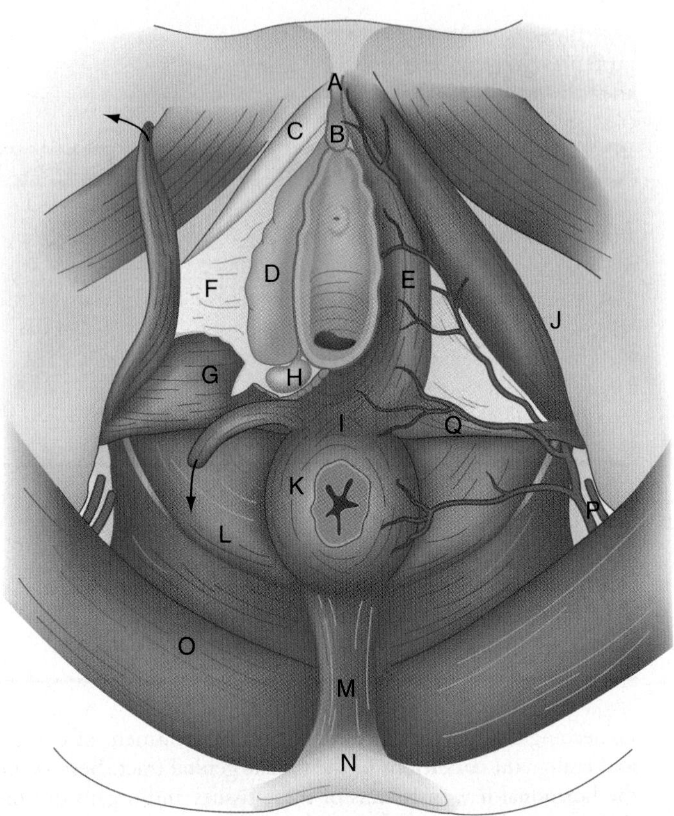


FIGURE 71-2 The muscles and fascia of the perineum: A, Suspensory ligament of clitoris; B, clitoris; C, crus of clitoris; D, vestibular bulb; E, bulbocavernosus muscle; F, inferior fascia of urogenital diaphragm; G, deep transverse perineal muscle; H, Bartholin's gland; I, perineal body; J, ischiocavernosus muscle; K, external anal sphincter; L, levator ani muscle; M, anococcygeal body; N, coccyx; O, gluteus maximus muscle; P, pudendal artery and vein; Q, superficial transverse perineal muscle.

**Table 71-1 Selected Anatomic Abnormalities as a Result of Disrupted Embryogenesis**

| ORGAN | ABNORMALITY |
|---|---|
| Ovary | Duplication of ovary; secondary ovarian rests; paraovarian cysts (wolffian remnants) |
| Tube | Congenital absence; paratubal cyst (hydatid of Morgagni) |
| Uterus | Agenesis; complete or partial duplication of the uterine fundus |
| Cervix | Agenesis; complete or partial duplication of the cervix |
| Vagina | Agenesis; transverse or longitudinal septum; paravaginal (Gartner's duct) cyst |
| Vulva | Fusion; hermaphroditism; cyst of the canal of Nuck (round ligament cyst) |

have a keratinized, stratified squamous epithelium with all the normal skin appendages and extend posteriorly to the lateral perineum. Within the confines of the labium are fat and the insertion of the round ligament. Medial to the labia majora are interlabial grooves and the labia minora, of similar cutaneous origin, but devoid of hair follicles. The labia minora are richly vascularized, with an erectile venous plexus. The bilateral roots of the clitoris fuse in the midline to form the glans at the lower edge of the pubic symphysis. The labia minora fuse over the clitoris to form the hood and, to a variable degree, below to create the clitoral frenulum.

Contiguous to the medial aspect of the labia minora, demarcated by Hart's line, is the vulvar vestibule, extending to the hymeneal sulcus. The vestibular surface is a stratified, squamous mucous membrane that shares embryology and has similar characteristics to the distal urethra and urethral meatus. Bartholin's glands, at 5 and 7 o'clock, the paraurethral Skene's glands, and minor vestibular glands positioned around the lateral vestibule are all under the vestibular bulb, subjacent to the bulbocavernosus muscle. The ostia of these glands pass through the vestibular mucosa, directly adjacent to the hymeneal ring.

The muscles of the external genitalia consist of the deep and superficial transverse perineal muscles, paired ischiocavernosus muscles that cover the crura of the clitoris, and bulbocavernosus muscles lying on either side of the vagina, covering the vestibular bulbs.

The anal triangle contains the anal canal, with surrounding internal and external sphincters, ischiorectal fossa, filled with fatty tissue, median raphe, and overlying skin.

Blood supply to the perineum is predominantly from a posterior direction from the internal pudendal artery, which, after arising from the internal iliac artery, passes through Alcock's canal, a fascial tunnel along the obturator internus muscle below the origin of the levator ani muscle. On emerging from Alcock's canal, the internal pudendal artery sends branches to the urogenital triangle anteriorly and to the anal triangle posteriorly. Anteriorly, there is blood supply to the mons pubis from the inferior epigastric artery, a branch of the femoral artery. Laterally, the external pudendal artery arises from the femoral artery and supplies the lateral aspect of the vulva. Venous return from the perineum accompanies the arterial supply and therefore drains into the internal iliac and femoral veins. It is important for the surgeon dissecting the external genitalia to be cognizant of the variability of direction from which the blood supply of the operative field is derived.

The major nerve supply to the perineum comes from the internal pudendal nerve, which originates from the S2 to S4 anterior rami of the sacral plexus and travels through Alcock's canal, along with the internal pudendal artery and vein. Anterior branches supply the urogenital diaphragm and external genitalia, whereas posterior branches, the inferior rectal nerve, supply the anus, anal canal, ischiorectal fossa, and adjacent skin. Branches of the posterior femoral cutaneous nerve from the sacral plexus innervate the lateral aspects of the ischiorectal fossa and adjacent structures. The mons pubis and anterior labia are supplied by the ilioinguinal and genitofemoral nerves from the lumbar plexus; they travel through the inguinal canal and exit through the superficial inguinal ring. All these paired nerves routinely cross the midline for partial innervation of the contralateral side. The visceral efferent nerves responsible for clitoral erection are derived from the pelvic splanchnic nerves and reach the external genitalia along with the urethra and vagina as they pass through the urogenital diaphragm.

Surgical injury to the pelvic nerve plexus can result in neuropathic pain and diminished sexual, voiding, and excretory function.

The lymphatic drainage of the perineum, including the urogenital and anogenital triangles, travels for the most part with the external pudendal vessels to the superficial inguinal nodes. The deep parts of the perineum, including the urethra, vagina, and anal canal, drain in part through the lymphatics that accompany the internal pudendal vessels and into the internal iliac lymph nodes.

The fascia and fascial spaces of the perineum are important regarding the spread of extravasated fluids and superficial and deep infections. Fascia covers each of the muscles bounding the perineum, including the deep surface of the levator ani, obturator internus, and coccygeus, as well as other perineal muscles, such as the urogenital diaphragm. The fascia of the levator ani muscles fuses with the obturator internus fascia and pubic rami, creating well-defined fascial spaces, the ischiorectal fosse. Beneath the skin of the external genitalia is a layer of fat; deep to this is Colles' fascia, which is attached to the ischiopubic rami laterally and the posterior edge of the urogenital diaphragm. Anteriorly, Colles' fascia of the vulva is continuous with Colles' fascia of the anterior abdominal wall.

Infections or collections of extravasated urine deep to the urogenital diaphragm are usually confined to the ischiorectal fossa, including the anterior recess, which is superior to the urogenital diaphragm. Collections of fluid or infections superficial to the urogenital diaphragm may pass to the abdominal wall deep to Colles' fascia. Because of various fascial fusions, infections spreading from the vulva to the anterior abdominal wall do not spread into the inguinal regions or the thigh.

### Internal Genitalia

The internal genitalia consist of the ovaries, fallopian tubes, uterus, cervix, and vagina, with associated blood supply and lymphatic drainage (Figs. 71-3 to 71-5).

**Ovary** The oblong ovaries, glistening white in color, vary in size, which is dependent on age and status of the ovulatory cycle. In the prepubescent girl, the ovary will appear as a white sliver of tissue smaller than 1 cm in any dimension. The ovary of a woman during her reproductive years will vary in size and shape. The size of the nonovulating ovary will typically be in the range of $3 \times 2 \times 1$ cm. When a follicular or corpus luteum cyst is present, the size may extend up to 5 to 6 cm. A follicular cyst is an asymmetrical, translucent, clear structure. A corpus luteum cyst will generally be characterized by areas of golden yellow and, occasionally, by hematoma. The ovaries are suspended from the lateral side wall of the pelvis below the pelvic brim by the infundibulopelvic ligament and attach to the superolateral aspect of the uterine fundus by the utero-ovarian ligament.

The primary blood supply to the ovary is the ovarian artery. It arises directly from the aorta and courses with the vein through the infundibulopelvic ligament into the medulla on the lateral aspect of the ovary. The right ovarian vein generally drains to the inferior vena cava and the left ovarian vein drains to the common iliac vein; however, variations commonly occur. There is a rich anastomotic arterial complex arising from the uterine artery that spreads across the broad ligament and mesosalpinx. The venous return accompanies that arterial supply. There is no somatic innervation to the ovary, but the autonomic fibers arise from the lumbar sympathetic and sacral parasympathetic plexuses. Lymphatic drainage parallels the iliac and aortic arteries.

There are three important relationships to be considered when carrying out surgical dissection. The infundibulopelvic ligament, with the ovarian blood supply, crosses over the ureter as it descends into the pelvis. As the surgeon divides and ligates the ovarian vessels, it is critical that this relationship be identified to avoid transecting, ligating, or kinking the ureter. The risk for ureteral injury is greater with a more proximal dissection of the ligament. Also, in its natural position, the suspended ovary drops along the pelvic sidewall along the course of the midureter. If there are adhesions between the ovary and peritoneum of the pelvic sidewall, careful dissection is necessary to avoid tenting the peritoneum with the attached ureter and causing injury. The third surgical relationship is the complex of external iliac vessels and femoral nerve, which course along the iliopsoas muscle, directly below the course of the ovarian vessels; with anterior adhesions of an ovary, these structures may be subjacent to the malpositioned ovary.

**Fallopian Tubes** The fallopian tubes are cylindrical structures approximately 8 cm in length. They originate at the uterine cavity in the uterine cornua, with an intramural segment of 1 to 2 cm and a narrow isthmic segment of 4 to 5 cm, flaring over 2 to 3 cm to the funnel of the infundibular segment and terminating in the fimbriated end of the tube. The fimbria are fine, delicate mucosal projections that are positioned to allow for

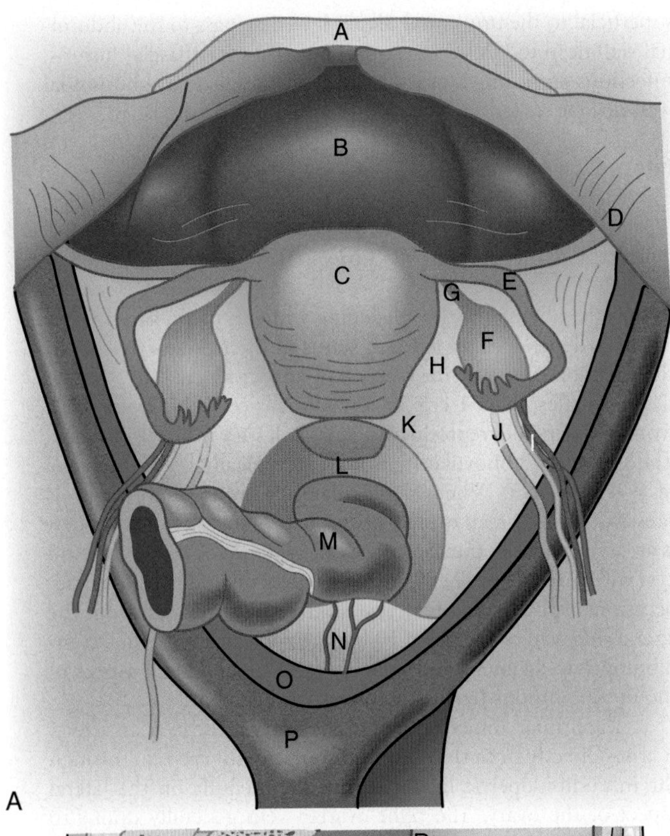


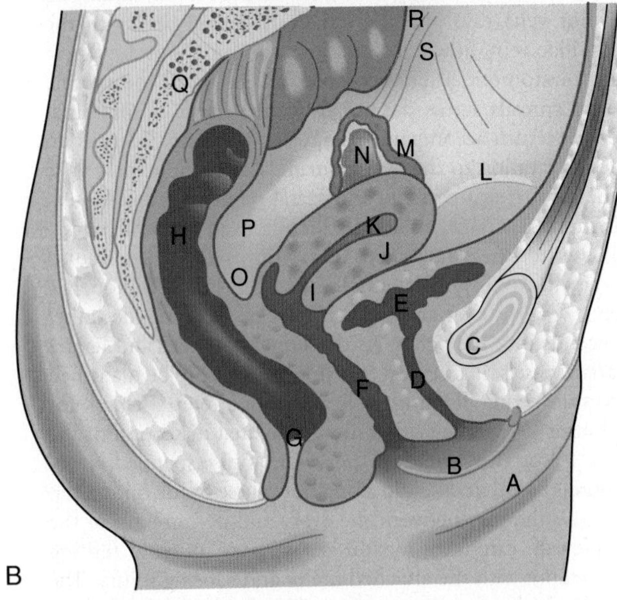


**FIGURE 71-3** The internal genitalia. **A,** A, Symphysis pubis; B, bladder; C, corpus uteri; D, round ligament; E, fallopian tube; F, ovary; G, utero-ovarian ligament; H, broad ligament; I, ovarian artery and vein; J, ureter; K, uterosacral ligament; L, cul-de-sac; M, rectum; N, middle sacral artery and vein; O, vena cava; P, aorta. **B,** A, Labium majus; B, labium minus; C, symphysis pubis, D, urethra; E, bladder; F, vagina; G, anus; H, rectum; I, cervix uteri; J, corpus uteri; K, endometrial cavity; L, round ligament; M, fallopian tube; N, ovary; O, cul-de-sac; P, uterosacral ligament; Q, sacrum; R, ureter; S, ovarian artery and vein.

capture of the extruded oocyte to promote the potential for fertilization. The blood supply to the tube is derived primarily from branches of the uterine artery, with a delicate cascade of vessels in the mesosalpinx. There is a secondary supply from the anastomosis with the ovarian vessels.

The surgeon must be aware of the fragility of the fallopian tube and handle this structure delicately, especially in women wishing to preserve their fertility. The mucosa lining the tubal lumen, especially at the fimbriated end, is highly specialized to facilitate transport of the oocyte and fertilized zygote. Traumatic manipulation of the tube can induce tubal infertility or predispose to later tubal pregnancy through damage to the mucosa or distortion of the tubal position by adhesions, thereby interfering with the access or transport mechanisms.

**Uterus and Cervix** The uterus, with the cervix, is a midline, pear-shaped organ suspended in the midplane of the pelvis by the cardinal and uterosacral ligaments. The cardinal ligaments are dense fibrous condensations arising from the fascial covering of the levator ani muscles of the pelvic floor and inserting into the lateral portions of the uterocervical junction. The uterosacral ligaments arise posterolaterally from the uterocervical junction and course obliquely in a posterolateral direction to insert into the parietal fascia of the pelvic floor at the sacroiliac joint. The round ligaments of the uterus arise from the anterolateral superior aspect of the uterine fundus, course anterolaterally to the internal inguinal ring, and insert into the labia majora. The round ligaments are highly stretchable and serve no function in pelvic organ support. The broad ligaments are composed of a visceral peritoneal surface containing loose adventitious tissue. These ligaments also provide no pelvic organ support, but do allow access to an avascular plane of the pelvis through which the retroperitoneal vasculature and ureter can be exposed.

The size of the uterus is influenced by age, hormonal status, prior pregnancy, and common benign neoplasms. The normal uterus during the reproductive years is approximately $8 \times 6 \times 4$ cm and weighs approximately 100 g. The prepubertal or postmenopausal uterus is substantially smaller. The mass of the uterus is almost exclusively made up of myometrium, a complex of interlacing bundles of smooth muscle. The uterine cavity is 4 to 6 cm from the internal cervical os to the uterine fundus, shaped as an inverted triangle, 2 to 3 mm wide at the cervix, and 3 to 4 cm across the fundus, extending from cornua to cornua. It is only a few millimeters deep between the anterior and posterior walls, with no defined lateral walls in the nonpregnant state. The most common reason for variation in size is current pregnancy followed by uterine fibroids.

If, during a surgical procedure, the surgeon encounters an enlarged uterus, undiagnosed pregnancy must be considered. The morphologic differences between a uterus enlarged by a pregnancy and one enlarged by fibroid include symmetrical enlargement in pregnancy with generally asymmetrical enlargement with fibroids. If symmetrical, consider the origin of the round ligaments. With pregnancy, the round ligaments stretch as the uterus grows and continue to originate from the normal site; even with an apparently symmetrical fibroid uterus, the origin of the round ligaments is frequently displaced from the top of the uterine fundus or asymmetrical course through the pelvis. Finally, the pregnant uterus is usually dusky and soft, whereas fibroids are generally firm and nodular masses can be palpated in the myometrial wall.

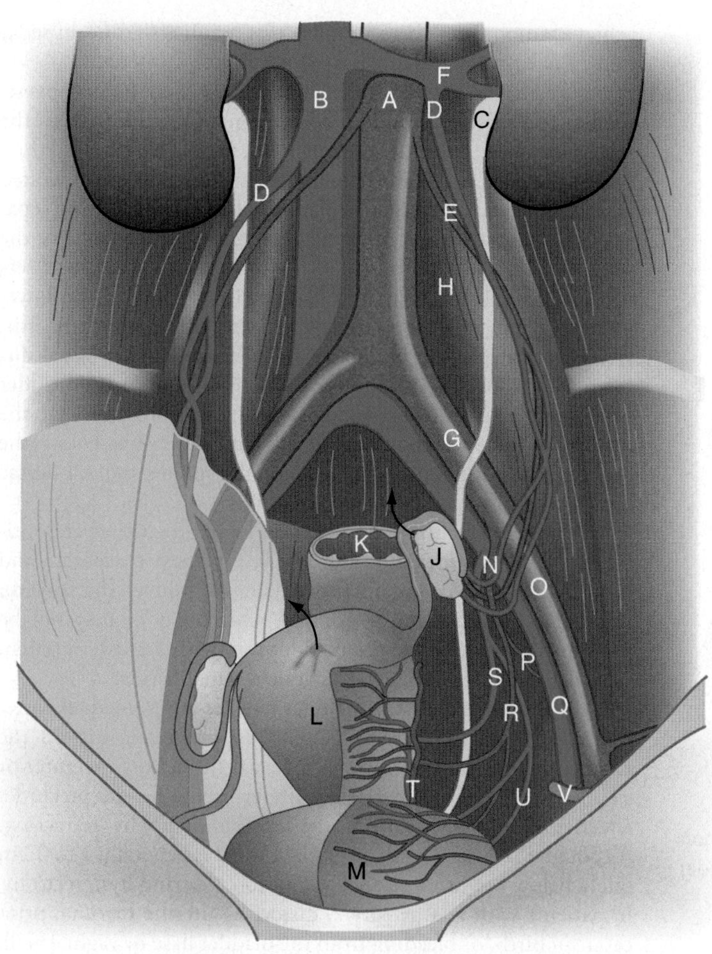


**FIGURE 71-4** Blood supply of the pelvis. A, Aorta; B, inferior vena cava; C, ureter; D, ovarian vein; E, ovarian artery; F, renal vein; G, common iliac artery; H, psoas muscle; J, ovary; K, rectum; L, corpus uteri; M, bladder; N, internal iliac (hypogastric) artery, anterior branch; O, external iliac artery; P, obturator artery; Q, external iliac vein; R, uterine artery; S, uterine vein; T, vaginal artery; U, superior vesicle artery; V, inferior epigastric artery.

The uterine cavity is lined by the endometrium, a complex epithelial-stromal-vascular secretory tissue. The arterial supply to the endometrium is derived from branches of the uterine artery that perforate the myometrium to the inactive basalis layer. There, they form the arcuate vessels, which produce radial branches extending through the functional layer toward the compacted surface layer. There will be further description of the menstrual cycle here but, during the postovulatory phase, these vessels differentiate into spiral arteries, uniquely suited to allow menstruation and subsequent hemostasis.

The uterine cervix is histologically dynamic, with changes in cervical mucus production during the ovarian cycle. In the follicular phase, under estrogen stimulation, copious clear mucus is produced that facilitates the transport of sperm through the cervical canal to ascend through the uterine cavity to the fallopian tubes. During progesterone-dominant states, either luteal phase, or with exogenous hormones, the mucus becomes viscous and plugs the cervix. The secretory epithelium of the endocervical canal has a dynamic metaplastic interaction with the stratified squamous epithelium of the portio vaginalis of the ectocervix under hormonal stimulation. Because the cervical canal is continuous with the vagina, surgical procedures involving the uterus and tubes are considered to be clean-contaminated cases.

The major sources of blood supply for the uterus and cervix are the uterine arteries, which are branches of the anterior division of the internal iliac (hypogastric) arteries. Although the origin of the uterine artery is usually a single identifiable vessel, it divides into multiple ascending and descending branches as it courses medially to the lateral margins of the cervicouterine junction. The distance from the uterus at which this division occurs is highly variable. Venous return from the uterus flows into the companion internal iliac vein. Lymphatics from the cervix and upper vagina drain primarily through the internal iliac nodes but, from the uterine fundus, drainage occurs primarily along a presacral path directly to the para-aortic nodes.

The primary surgical consideration for managing the uterine vessels is the close proximity of the ureter, which courses approximately 1 cm below the artery and 1 cm lateral to the cervix. If the surgeon loses control of one of the branches of the vessel, it is important to use techniques that avoid clamping or kinking the ureter. Often, the most prudent way to secure the uterine artery is to expose its origin and place hemostatic clips on the vessel.

Innervation of the uterus and cervix is derived from the autonomic plexus. Autonomic pain fibers are activated with dysmenorrhea, in labor, and with instrumentation of the cervix and uterus.

In the retroperitoneal space lateral to the uterus is the obturator nerve, which arises from the lumbosacral plexus and passes through the pelvic floor by way of the obturator canal to innervate the medial thigh. With relatively normal pelvic anatomy, it is unlikely to be subjected to injury; however, under circumstances in which the surgeon must dissect the

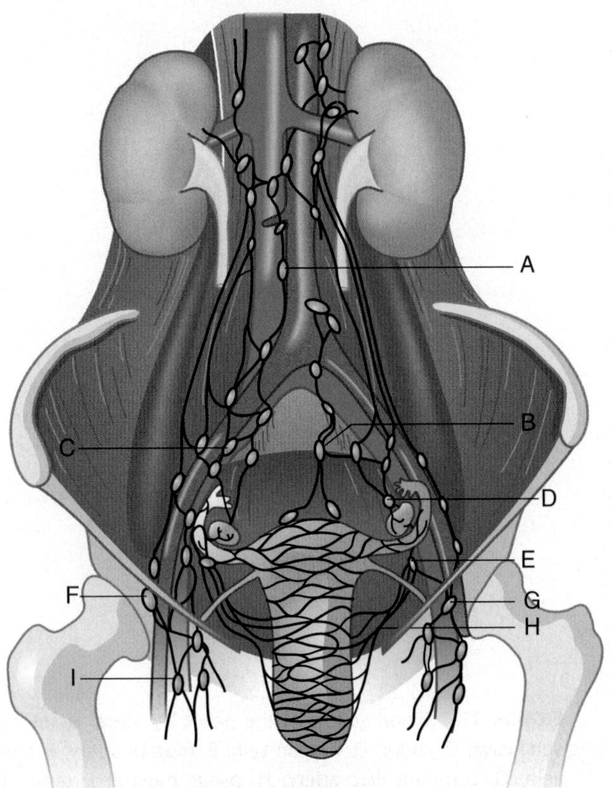


**FIGURE 71-5** Lymphatics of the pelvis. A, Aortic; B, sacral; C, common iliac; D, hypogastric; E, obturator; F, deep inguinal; G, Cloquet's node; H, parametrial; I, superficial inguinal.

retroperitoneal or paravaginal spaces, this relatively subtle structure can be injured, with significant neuropathic residual.

**Vagina** The vagina originates at the cervix and terminates at the hymeneal ring. The anatomic axis of the upper vagina is posterior to anterior in a caudad direction. The anterior and posterior walls of the upper two thirds of the vagina are normally opposed to each other to create a transverse potential space, distensible through pliability of the lateral sulci. The lower third of the vagina has a relatively vertically oriented caudad lumen. The mucosa of the vagina is nonkeratinized, stratified, squamous epithelium that responds to estrogen stimulation.

The blood supply to the vagina is provided by descending branches of the uterine artery and vein and ascending branches of the internal pudendal artery and its companion vein. These vessels course along the lateral walls of the vagina. Innervation is derived from the autonomic plexus and pudendal nerve, which track with the vessels.

Traumatic lacerations of the vagina are usually located along the lateral sidewalls, and the degree to which there is major injury to the vessels can be associated not only with significant evident hemorrhage, but also with concealed hemorrhage. Spaces in which a hematoma can be concealed are the retroperitoneum of the broad ligaments, paravesical and pararectal spaces, and ischiorectal fossa. Because of the proximity of the pudendal nerve, attempts to ligate the vessels require maintaining orientation to the location of Alcock's canal to avoid creating neuropathic injury. In the absence of an accumulating hematoma, the best approach to management is often a bulk vaginal pack to achieve tamponade. To accomplish this requires significant sedation or anesthesia and an indwelling urinary catheter.

The uterus, cervix, and vagina, with their fascial investments, comprise the middle compartment of the pelvis. The structures of the anterior compartment, the bladder and urethra, and of the posterior compartment, the rectum, are each invested with a fascial layer. Avascular planes of loose areolar tissue separate the posterior fascia of the bladder and anterior fascia of the vagina and the anterior fascia of the rectum and posterior fascia of the vagina. Anteriorly, the bladder is attached to the lower uterine segment by the continuous visceral peritoneum. This vesicouterine fold can be incised transversely with minimal difficulty to expose the plane and allow dissection of the bladder from the cervix and vagina. Posteriorly, the proximity of the rectum to the posterior vagina is significant only below the peritoneum of the cul-de-sac of Douglas, unless the cul-de-sac anatomy is distorted by dense adhesions.

Operative techniques for gynecologic procedures are optimized by careful identification of these planes to separate and protect the adjacent organs from operative injury. The surgeon can create an incidental cystotomy, which may or may not be recognized, or devitalize the bladder wall with a crush or stitch, with delayed development of a vesicovaginal fistula.

In the lower pelvis, the ureter courses anteromedially after it passes under the uterine vessels and progresses toward the trigone of the bladder through a fascial tunnel on the anterior vaginal wall. The fixation of the ureter by the tunnel precludes effective displacement from the operative site by retracting. Although the location of the fascial tunnel is generally 1 to 2 cm safely below the usual site for vaginotomy during hysterectomy, in patients with a large cervix, distorting uterine myoma, prior cesarean birth, or bleeding from the bladder base or vaginal wall, the ureter can be transected, crushed, or kinked with a stitch.

The rectovaginal septum is surgically relevant during the repair of an episiotomy or obstetric laceration, repair of rectovaginal fistula, or pelvic support procedures. Identification of the fascial layers investing the subjacent structures and using the tissue strength is critical to an optimal repair.

## REPRODUCTIVE PHYSIOLOGY

The development of a differential diagnosis of gynecologic complaints is facilitated by an understanding of the reproductive cycle and eliciting a careful menstrual history. Many conditions are a direct consequence of aberrations in the hypothalamic-pituitary-ovarian cycle and the effects of the hormonal milieu on the endometrium. Others tend to be mere variations in the presentation of different phases of the cycle. A detailed description of the cycle is beyond our scope here, but the surgeon needs to have a basic understanding of the relationships in this complex process to elicit an adequate history, interpret the findings on physical examination, use ancillary tests appropriately, and formulate the differential diagnosis (Fig. 71-6).

### Ovarian Cycle

Under the stimulus of hypothalamic secretion of gonadotropin-releasing hormone (GnRH) to the pituitary gland, follicle-stimulating hormone (FSH) is released into the systemic circulation. During this secretory phase of the ovarian cycle, the primordial follicles of the ovary are targeted and stimulated toward growth and maturity. Multiple follicles are recruited each cycle, but generally only one follicle becomes dominant,

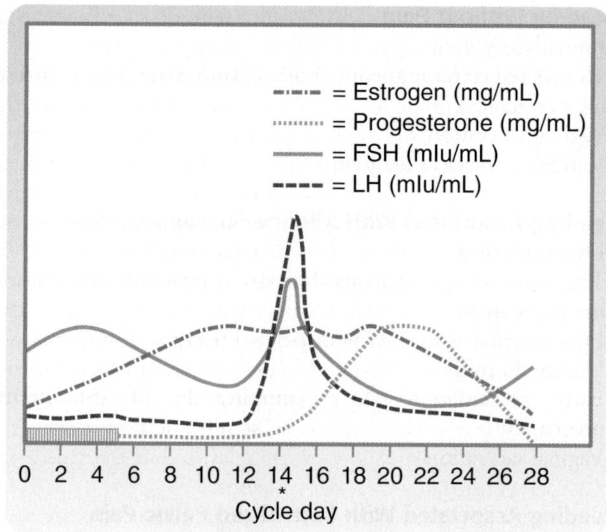


**FIGURE 71-6** Hormonal changes during the menstrual cycle. Menses, days 0 to 5; ovulation, day 14.

destined to reach maturity and extrusion at ovulation. The effects of the maturation process include not only the completion of meiotic germ cell development but also the stimulation of the granulosa cells that surround the follicle to secrete estradiol, other estrogenic compounds, and inhibin. As the estradiol level increases in the circulation, it has a positive regulatory effect on GnRH, which in turn stimulates the pituitary gland to release a surge of luteinizing hormone (LH). The LH surge stimulates the release of the oocyte from the follicle. After release, the follicle site converts to the corpus luteum; the dominant hormone secreted during this luteal phase is progesterone. This sequence of hormonal events prepares the cervix, uterus, and tubes for sperm transport into the upper genital tract, fertilization, implantation, and support of the early gestation. In the absence of conception, the corpus luteum undergoes atresia and the next ovarian cycle begins.

## Endometrial Cycle

The hormonal sequence of the ovarian cycle controls the physiologic changes in the endometrium. By convention, each endometrial cycle begins on day 1, defined as the onset of menses. In an idealized cycle, the LH surge and ovulation occur on day 14. Atresia of the corpus luteum occurs on day 28 and menses begin the next day, day 1 of the new cycle.

During the follicular phase of the ovarian cycle, estrogen exerts a stimulatory effect on the endometrium, producing the proliferative phase of the endometrial cycle. The endometrial tissues that are affected include the surface and glandular epithelium, stromal matrix, and vascular bed. The stromal layer thickens, the glandular elements elongate, and the terminal arterioles of the endometrial circulation extend from the basalis toward the endometrial surface. The mucous secretions of the glands of the endometrium, and the endocervix, become profuse and watery, facilitating the ascent of spermatozoa for potential fertilization.

During the luteal phase of the ovarian cycle, corresponding to the secretory phase of the endometrial cycle, progesterone domination converts the endometrium toward receptivity for implantation of the fertilized oocyte. Several endometrial changes occur under progesterone stimulation. The growth of the endometrial stroma is terminated, the surface layer of the endometrium becomes compacted, the glandular secretions become more viscous, and the terminal arterioles become coiled, creating the spiral arterioles. Cervical mucus similarly becomes more viscous and tenacious, creating a relative barrier between the vagina and uterine cavity.

In the absence of fertilization, and with the withdrawal of progesterone because of atresia of the corpus luteum, there is a complex sequence of arteriolar spasm, leading to ischemic necrosis of the endometrial surface and endometrial shedding, or menses. Normal menses, in the absence of structural pathology, is an orderly process because these arteriolar changes occur in the entire mucosa simultaneously and universally, with vasospasm and coagulation occluding the terminal vessels. Bleeding associated with normal menses is notable for the absence of clotting because of fibrinolysis within the uterine cavity before flow. With fertilization and implantation, menses are absent (amenorrhea). Alternatively, a disordered ovarian cycle leads to a disordered endometrial cycle and abnormal uterine bleeding patterns.

## Early Pregnancy

A brief description of the events leading to pregnancy is useful for understanding the possible complications of early pregnancy. Coitus during the 48 hours before ovulation or during the periovulatory period establishes the conditions for fertilization. As noted, sperm transport is facilitated by the estrogenic environment; the spermatozoa ascend through the cervix and uterine cavity to the fallopian tube. When a mature oocyte and spermatozoa come into contact in the distal fallopian tube, fertilization can occur, usually 3 to 5 days after ovulation. During tubal transport, the zygote undergoes multiple divisions to reach the stage of the morula by the time it reaches the cavity. Implantation generally occurs approximately 5 to 7 days after fertilization.

There are two significant clinical implications to delay in the fertilization-transport sequence. If the zygote has not matured adequately before reaching the endometrial cavity, implantation will not occur and a preclinical unrecognized pregnancy will be lost. If there is delay in the fertilization-transport sequence, either because of the randomness of coital timing or because of altered tubal structure or function, the zygote can reach the stage at which it is programmed to adhere to genital mucosa while still in the fallopian tube, resulting in an ectopic pregnancy.

## Amenorrhea and Abnormal Menses

A disrupted sequence of the hypothalamic-pituitary-ovarian interaction has a profound effect on the endometrium and menses. There are two broad classes of amenorrheic disorders, hypogonadotropic and anovulatory. Although the details of the pathology and evaluation are beyond our scope of this text, hypogonadotropic conditions result from central disruption of the hypothalamic-pituitary axis. Common causes for this condition include stress, hyperprolactinemia, and low body mass (e.g., those with anorexia nervosa, athletes [distance runners, gymnasts, ballerinas]). Because of the hypogonadotropic state, follicles are not stimulated, estrogen is not secreted, and endometrial proliferation does not occur. The result is an atrophic endometrium.

An atrophic endometrium can be identified with ultrasound, measuring the endometrial bilayer. Although local equipment and operator experience will vary, an endometrial bilayer less than 5 mm in a young amenorrheic woman is highly supportive of the diagnosis. This must be followed by a thorough investigation of the entire axis.

Anovulation results from a disrupted sequence of the axis from failure of the feedback loop to trigger the LH surge. The patient may have normal or elevated FSH levels, but FSH continues to stimulate the continuous production of estrogen from the granulosa cells. The chronic unopposed estrogen promotes continuous proliferation of the endometrium, without the maturing sequence induced by progesterone. The proliferation of the endometrium results in excessive thickness. This becomes clinically manifest by prolonged amenorrhea, often followed by prolonged and profuse uterine bleeding (hypermenorrhea, menorrhagia). The most common cause for this presentation is polycystic ovarian disease, but physiologic or social stress can produce a similar clinical scenario.

Ultrasound measurement of the endometrial bilayer can exceed 20 mm. Patients with chronic anovulation with chronic unopposed estrogen are at risk for endometrial hyperplasia and even endometrial cancer. The evaluation of the patient must address the cause for the chronic anovulation and the endometrial consequences. Histologic diagnosis requires an endometrial biopsy or curettage.

After prolonged amenorrhea with excessive proliferation of the endometrial lining, hypermenorrhea and menorrhagia may occur as a result of four parallel mechanisms. The growth of tissue from the basalis to the surface extends beyond the terminal branches of the arterioles, resulting in surface ischemia and necrosis. The volume of endometrial tissue is obviously increased. The normal hemostatic mechanisms of the spiral arterioles in the menstrual cycle are absent. Finally, the shedding of the endometrial surface is not a universal event, but is random and leads to multiple foci of bleeding that are dyssynchronous and occur over a prolonged time. Frequently, the rate of bleeding exceeds the capacity of the normal intracavitary fibrinolytic processes, and blood clots are common in the flow.

## CLINICAL EVALUATION

Acute life-threatening conditions frequently involve pregnancy, such as a ruptured ectopic pregnancy and heavy vaginal bleeding associated with miscarriage. Therefore, in the acute setting, the possibility of pregnancy must be considered and history focused on this area. It is immediately apparent that many questions in a gynecologic or obstetric history are personal and sensitive, so it may be helpful to conduct the interview or at least part of it in private, without the presence of family members and after attempting to gain the patient's trust and understanding.

Patients will typically present with aberrant bleeding patterns, pelvic-abdominal pain or ill-defined discomfort, or a combination of these symptoms. With a focused history, the differential diagnosis can be constructed with further refinement from physical findings and ancillary tests. The key elements to be elicited are age, pregnancy history, recent and past menstrual history, sexual history, contraception, prior gynecologic disease and procedures, and evolution of the current complaints.

### Diagnostic Considerations

Although there are always atypical crossover presentations for any of the possible diagnoses, the most common considerations for the differential diagnosis of symptom complexes are as presented here.

#### Bleeding Without Pain

- Anovulatory cycle
- Threatened or spontaneous abortion (miscarriage of intrauterine pregnancy)
- Vaginal laceration
- Vaginal or cervical neoplasm

#### Bleeding Associated With Midline Suprapubic Pain

- Dysmenorrhea
- Threatened or spontaneous abortion (miscarriage of intrauterine pregnancy)
- Endometritis associated with pelvic infection
- Uterine fibroids
- Early presentation of a complication of extrauterine pregnancy
- Vaginal laceration

#### Bleeding Associated With Lateralized Pelvic Pain

- Extrauterine pregnancy, prerupture
- Functional ovarian cyst
- Ruptured functional ovarian cyst
- Ruptured corpus luteum, with or without an intrauterine pregnancy
- Vaginal trauma

#### Bleeding Associated With Generalized Pelvic Pain

- Ruptured extrauterine pregnancy
- Ruptured corpus luteum, with or without an intrauterine pregnancy
- Septic spontaneous or induced abortion
- Vaginal trauma

#### Midline Pelvic Pain Without Bleeding

- Endometritis or pelvic inflammatory disease (PID)
- Endometriosis
- Pelvic neoplasm
- Urinary tract infection
- Constipation

#### Lateralized Pelvic Pain Without Bleeding

- Extrauterine pregnancy
- Functional ovarian cyst, with or without intraparenchymal hemorrhage
- Functional ovarian cyst with rupture
- Functional or neoplastic ovarian cyst with intermittent torsion
- Pedunculated paratubal or paraovarian cyst with intermittent torsion
- Endometriosis
- Ovarian remnant syndrome
- Ureteritis
- Constipation

#### Generalized Abdominal Pain Without Bleeding

- Ruptured extrauterine pregnancy
- Ruptured ovarian cyst
- PID with pelvic peritonitis
- Endometriosis

#### Obstipation

- Cul-de-sac hematoma
- Cul-de-sac adnexal mass

- Posterior uterine fibroid
- Pelvic abscess
- Endometriosis

#### Flank Pain

- Pyelonephritis
- Ureteral obstruction
- Ovarian remnant syndrome, with or without ureteral obstruction

### Other Acute Clinical Presentations

#### Acute Vulvovaginitis

Acute vulvovaginitis is a common presenting emergency complaint. Presenting symptoms are intense pruritus or cutaneous pain with discharge. The most frequent pathogens are mycotic or herpetic infections. Mycotic infections are generally characterized by a thick, white, cottage cheese–like discharge. Primary herpetic infections often present with profuse watery discharge, inguinal adenopathy, and signs of a viremia. In contrast, other common vaginal infections, such as bacterial vaginosis and trichomoniasis, may cause irritative symptoms and malodorous discharge, but rarely cause pain.

Common acute vulvar complaints include infection of skin appendages—folliculitis, furunculosis, and cellulitis. The ostium of the Bartholin's gland may become occluded, with or without infection. Sterile cysts are only minimally uncomfortable, but a Bartholin's cyst abscess is exquisitely painful.

#### Necrotizing Fasciitis

Necrotizing fasciitis is a life-threatening infection that can occur in the vulva. It can begin as a cellulitis, from infected skin appendages, or following biopsy or episiotomy. Once established, it can quickly extend through the fascial planes. Women at risk are patients with obesity, diabetes, and steroid or other immunosuppressive drug use. Treatment is immediate surgical débridement. Patients may require several débridements to determine the extent of the fascial involvement. Skin grafts are often needed to repair large defects. It is important that women with risk factors for necrotizing fasciitis who present with a vulvar cellulitis be admitted for treatment with IV antibiotics and possible surgery.

#### Pelvic Masses

Masses identified in the pelvis can be functional, congenital, neoplastic, hemorrhagic, or inflammatory and can arise from the ovary or the uterus. Also, the anatomy of the cul-de-sac of Douglas in its dependent position in the pelvis facilitates restriction of pelvic infection as collections or abscesses to that location.

Common ovarian masses include functional cysts, hemorrhagic cysts, paraovarian or paratubal wolffian remnants, endometrioma, and benign or malignant tumors (e.g., epithelial, germ cell, stromal). The most common neoplastic mass in young women is the benign cystic teratoma. Because of the sebaceous content of these lesions, they frequently float to the anterior cul-de-sac between the uterus and bladder. Diagnostic considerations for differentiating among ovarian masses of various causes are discussed in detail in the later section on ovarian cancer.

Common uterine masses include leiomyoma, adenomyoma, and bicornuate uterus. Common inflammatory masses are tubo-ovarian abscesses (TOAs), pelvic collection, and appendiceal or diverticular abscesses.

Inflammatory masses in the anterior cul-de-sac most commonly originate from sigmoid diverticular disease.

## History

#### Age

Patient age is relevant primarily because of the phases of the reproductive life cycle—menarche at adolescence, perimenopause in middle age, and menopause.

At the time of menarche, the synchrony of the hypothalamic-pituitary-ovarian axis is immature and the sequence of hypergonadotropic, anovulatory, amenorrhea-hypermenorrhea is common. Similarly, this is the age group in which emotional stress, anorexia nervosa, and excessive athleticism commonly occur, and the amenorrheic patient may have hypogonadotropic amenorrhea. Finally, however, the young patient may be fertile and sexually active, so pregnancy with complications must always be considered.

In the perimenopausal years, the ovary is less responsive to the gonadotropic stimulus and anovulation with the amenorrhea-hypermenorrhea sequence is common. In this age group, however, anatomic abnormalities such as uterine leiomyomas or endometrial polyps may confound the presentation.

Menopause is defined as cessation of menses for 1 year or more. Any postmenopausal woman who presents with uterine bleeding must be presumed to have uterine pathology and needs to undergo an appropriate evaluation for possible hyperplastic or neoplastic endometrial pathology.

#### Pregnancy History

The commonly used notation for describing pregnancy history is G, T, P, A, L—***g***ravidity (number of pregnancies), ***t***erm births, ***p***reterm births, ***a***bortions (spontaneous, induced, or ectopic), and ***l***iving children. Additional comment is made if there have been recurring spontaneous abortions, ectopic pregnancies, or multiple gestations.

Although any pregnancy can develop complications, the patient with a history of poor outcomes in prior pregnancies will be at higher risk for another adverse outcome. In the acute setting, with pain or bleeding, pregnancy complications must be considered.

#### Menstrual History

The date of the last menstrual period (LMP) and the prior menstrual period (PMP) must be determined as accurately as possible. It is often necessary to elicit menstrual events over several prior months to establish a pattern. Additionally, it is important to obtain a description of any variation from the patient's normal pattern of quantity and duration of menstrual flow. One can place the current complaints of bleeding and pain in perspective in the context of this menstrual history.

The amenorrhea-hypermenorrhea sequence has been described earlier. The patient who describes "two periods this month" may merely be describing a normal 28-day cycle beginning early and then late in the same calendar month. Alternating episodes of light bleeding with normal flow may suggest breakthrough bleeding at the time of ovulation or when the patient is on oral contraceptives. Excessive flow (menorrhagia) associated with regular cycles at normal intervals suggests structural abnormalities of the endometrial cavity, usually submucous leiomyomas or endometrial polyps. Random or intermittent bleeding episodes during the cycle prompt consideration of a lesion of the cervix, endometrial hyperplasia or, occasionally, adenocarcinoma of the endometrium.

Dysmenorrhea (menstrual cramps) is generally considered to occur only with ovulatory cycles. The patient who typically has dysmenorrhea but who currently denies cramps, even with a current episode of heavy flow, may be having an anovulatory bleeding episode, regardless of the interval between periods. Patients with high-volume flow, with insufficient intracavitary fibrinolysis, may experience cramps as the uterus contracts to expel the clot. Bleeding associated with threatened pregnancy loss or from an extrauterine pregnancy must be considered, whether heavy or light flow, continuous or episodic, anteceded by reported normal cycles, or occurring after amenorrhea. Bleeding after menopause demands consideration of endometrial pathology and appropriate workup to rule out hyperplasia or carcinoma. Postcoital bleeding suggests cervical lesions, including cervicitis, polyps, and neoplasia.

### Sexual History

Sexual activity, a sensitive and personal subject that is often difficult to elicit reliably in the acute setting, may significantly influence the formulation of the differential diagnosis. Beyond the possibility of pregnancy, the patient who will acknowledge unprotected coitus with casual sexual partners is considered to be at high risk for sexually transmitted infections (STIs). Reliable reports of the use of barrier contraception reduce, but do not eliminate, the possibility of an STI.

Pregnancy must be ruled out in any circumstance in which there is a clinical presentation that is not inconsistent with complications of pregnancy.

### Contraception

Reliable use of contraception does not totally preclude the possibility of pregnancy but raises other possible diagnoses to a higher level in the differential diagnosis. Breakthrough bleeding on hormonal contraception is typically low volume and is rarely associated with cramps or pain. In the presence of other symptoms, however, pregnancy complications and genital tract infections need to be considered. Patients with an intrauterine contraceptive device (IUD) may have spotting and cramping but, because use of an IUD increases the risk for endometrial infection, and because a disproportionate percentage of pregnancies that are conceived with an IUD are extrauterine, these patients need careful evaluation.

Patients with previous tubal sterilization have a 1% to 3% lifetime risk for pregnancy, with a disproportionate number of extrauterine pregnancies. Irregular bleeding associated with pain mandates careful evaluation.

### Prior Gynecologic Diseases and Procedures

The past gynecologic history may indicate recurring conditions suggesting lifestyle issues that create risk for recurrence or raise consideration for complications of previous interventions. Tubal ligation, prior tubal injury from an ectopic pregnancy, endometriosis, and PID all increase the risk for extrauterine pregnancy. Endometriosis with an intraperitoneal inflammatory response may cause significant pain. Patients with a history of functional ovarian cysts, with or without intraparenchymal hemorrhage, have a higher risk for recurrence. Previous pelvic surgery with periovarian adhesions can cause significant pain, even with benign, self-limited ovarian cyst accidents, but also may predispose to ovarian torsion.

The ovarian remnant syndrome is an interesting and confusing entity. It can cause pelvic pain in ill-defined patterns. The cause of the syndrome is a retained fragment of ovarian capsule after previous ovarian surgery. The fragment is adherent to the peritoneum and remains viable through a parasitic blood supply. Active follicles can be recruited through gonadotropin stimulation and the dynamics of peritoneal inflammation can be severely symptomatic. These remnants are usually found after resection of a densely adherent ovary with endometriosis or purulent infection of the pelvis. They are frequently located along the course of the ureter and may present with flank pain from urinary obstruction.

### History of Present Illness

The surgeon elicits the elements of the history, as described, to determine the evolution of the presenting complaint and formulate a plan for further evaluation and treatment. This section will focus on the most common emergency presentations, bleeding and pain.

#### Bleeding

- When did bleeding begin?
- How does the current flow compare with normal? Are there clots in the menstrual flow normally? Currently?
- How did the timing of onset relate to previous menses? Was there any prolongation of the interval between the last period and the onset of the current bleeding event?
- Were recent menses normal? Expected timing, flow, duration?
- Are menstrual periods normally associated with menstrual cramps? Is the current episode associated with similar cramps? No cramps, more intense discomfort?

#### Pain

- When did the pain begin? Relationship to last menses, ovulatory?
- What is the character of the pain—cramping, sharp, pressure, stabbing, colicky?
- What is the pattern of the pain—constant, intermittent, episodic?
- Where is the pain located—generalized, midline suprapubic, lateralized?
- Does the pain radiate—vagina, rectum, legs, back, upper abdomen, shoulder?
- Were there changes in the character, pattern, or location of the pain over time? For example, did cramping midline pain become acute sharp lateralized pain, followed by relief, evolving to generalized abdominal pain radiating to the shoulder? Did lateralized constant intense pressure evolve to acute sharp pain or intermittent colicky pain?
- Is there exacerbation of the pain with movement, intercourse, coughing?
- Are there any urinary tract symptoms, dysuria?
- Are there any intestinal symptoms, constipation, obstipation, diarrhea?

## Physical Examination

The approach to the physical examination of the gynecologic patient must account for the threat to dignity and modesty that a genital examination poses. In the emergency setting, against a background of fear or pain, and especially in young and older patients, the patient must be afforded maximum comfort. This includes an adequate sense of physical privacy, continuous presence of a chaperone, comfortable examination table on which to assume the lithotomy position, and patience by the examiner.

Although the chief complaint might suggest that only a focused pelvic examination is necessary, the examiner will enhance comfort and trust by a more general examination before the pelvic examination. The examiner must remember that the patient cannot see and cannot anticipate what she will experience next; the examiner or assistant informs the patient at every step in the process what the next sensation will be.

At the beginning of the pelvic examination, the examiner encourages relaxation and exposure by having the patient relax her medial thighs to allow the knees to drop out toward laterally placed hands. The knees must never be pushed apart by the examiner. Before contacting the genitalia, gentle touch of the gloved hand on the medial thigh, with gentle pressure and movement toward the vulva, will orient the patient to the progress of the examination. The external genitalia are inspected for lesions and evidence of trauma. This is followed by the insertion of a properly sized, lubricated vaginal speculum. The patient needs to be prepared for the speculum by the examiner placing a finger on the perineum and exerting gentle pressure with encouragement to relax the introital muscles. The speculum is placed at the hymeneal ring at a 30-degree angle from the vertical to minimize lateral or urethral pressure. After the leading edge is through the introitus, the speculum is rotated to the horizontal plane as it is advanced toward the apex of the vagina. The blades are gently separated as the midvagina is approached so that the cervix can be visualized and the blades are spread to surround the cervix. During the advancement and subsequent withdrawal, the walls of the vagina are visualized for lesions or trauma. The cervix is inspected for lesions, lacerations, dilation, products of conception, and/or purulent discharge. Support of the pelvic structures in the anterior, posterior, and superior compartments is evaluated. Vaginal swabs for microscopic wet mount examination of the vaginal environment, for gonorrhea and chlamydia, and for a Papanicolaou (Pap) test are obtained as indicated.

After the speculum examination, the index and middle fingers of the examiner's dominant hand are inserted into the vagina. Before placing his or her abdominal hand, the examiner's fingers gently palpate the vaginal walls to elicit tenderness or detect fullness or mass. The cervix is palpated for size and consistency. The examiner's fingers are placed sequentially along the side in all four quadrants of the cervix and gentle pressure is exerted to move the cervix in the opposite direction to elicit cervical motion tenderness.

Because the major supporting structures for the uterus are the cardinal and uterosacral ligaments that insert at the cervicouterine junction, the junction serves as the fulcrum for leverage. As the cervix is moved in one direction, it is likely that the uterine fundus is being displaced in the opposite direction. Tenderness with cervical motion may be related to traction on the ligamentous attachments, collision of the cervix against a structure in the direction to which the cervix is being displaced, or collision of the fundus against a structure on the opposite side.

The bimanual examination is performed with gentle pressure from the examiner's nondominant hand systematically mobilizing pelvic contents against the vaginal fingers. Except for large masses that are palpable on abdominal examination, the primary information gathered is detected by the examiner's vaginal fingers. The examiner should specifically note lateralized tenderness and masses. The rectovaginal examination provides additional perspective, especially for the cul-de-sac and adnexal structures.

Very young women and some older women will not tolerate the insertion of two fingers, or occasionally even one. Under these circumstances, a rectal finger along with the abdominal placement of the other hand can simulate a bimanual examination.

## Ancillary Tests

### Imaging

The single most effective and efficient modality for assessing pelvic anatomy and pathology is real-time ultrasound, especially with a transvaginal transducer. This technique not only allows assessment of the size and relationship of the pelvic structures but also, by clear delineation of echogenicity, can provide strong suspicion of the nature of pathology. With real-time Doppler flow assessment, blood flow to an organ or mass and fetal heart motion are readily apparent.

Axial tomography and magnetic resonance imaging (MRI) rarely provide additional information for benign pelvic pathology but are valuable techniques for assessing malignancies. IV pyelography may be useful if ultrasound assessment of the urinary tract is inadequate to delineate obstruction or anatomic distortion.

### Pregnancy Tests

There are two useful endocrine tests for determining the presence and health of a pregnancy, the β subunit of human chorionic gonadotropin (β-hCG) and progesterone.

Pregnancy tests measure the β-hCG level; the value obtained by the qualitative urine assay can be as low as 20 mIU/mL. This is sufficiently low as almost to exclude all but the earliest of gestations. Unless a viable fetus can be detected clinically or by ultrasound, a positive urine test in the clinical setting that might suggest an ectopic pregnancy must be followed with a quantitative serum radioimmunoassay. A result lower than 5 mIU/mL is a negative test. In most laboratories and, depending on the quality of the ultrasound equipment and experience of the sonographer, a healthy intrauterine pregnancy that has produced 2000 mIU/mL of β-hCG is generally visualized. In the absence of that threshold, serial β-hCG tests are scheduled at 2-day intervals.[1]

In the so-called typical healthy intrauterine pregnancy, serum β-hCG levels double every 48 hours. However, this description is based on pooled aggregated data; within data sets, there are many patients with successful pregnancies who will have intervals with a lower slope of increase followed by an interval with a steep increase. A decline in value over a 2-day period is always ominous and therefore demands a clinical decision about an intrauterine versus extrauterine failed pregnancy. The greater challenge occurs when the rate of increase is less than

60% over 48 hours. This is ambiguous; if the β-hCG level is below the discriminatory value of 2000 mIU/mL, clinical presentation and clinical judgment are vital to determine whether continued observation or intervention is the appropriate course.[2]

Note that there are three commonly used reference standards for β-hCG, as well as significant interlaboratory variation in test results. It is critical to understand the standard used and to be certain that sequential tests are performed in the same laboratory. If a change in laboratories is necessary, repeated parallel testing in the new laboratory using the residual serum from the original sample will resolve the question. Significantly elevated β-hCG levels raise suspicion of a hydatidiform mole or germ cell tumor.

Determining the serum progesterone level can be a useful adjunct in assessing the viability of a pregnancy. The quantitative relationship with pregnancy status is not as discrete, and cutoff values must be established in each laboratory. Progesterone levels lower than 5 ng/mL are rarely associated with successful pregnancies. Studies have demonstrated 100% sensitivity for ectopic pregnancy and 100% negative predictive value for a progesterone level cutoff of 22 ng/mL, but specificity and positive predictive value were poor. The role of the progesterone assay results in the clinical management of the acute patient is not yet clear.

#### Serum Hormone Assays

Other than the assessment of pregnancy, there is relatively little value to ordering the determination of reproductive hormone levels in the acute setting. These tests are relatively expensive, and the sequence of ordering them is determined by the clinical findings. The laboratory turn-around time is rarely less than 1 day.

#### Cervicovaginal Cultures, Gram Staining, and Vaginal Wet Mount

Because the healthy vagina is a polymicrobial environment, there are only four organisms for which cervicovaginal cultures are clinically useful—gonococcus, *Chlamydia trachomatis,* herpes simplex and, in pregnancy, group B beta-hemolytic streptococci. The tests for gonococcus and chlamydia can be combined in a single-swab medium kit for their molecular analysis.

Gram staining of purulent cervical discharge is useful in the emergency setting for identification of the gram-negative intracellular diplococci, diagnostic of gonococcus. The test may also be useful in helping identify *Trichomonas vaginalis.* Culture and Gram staining of purulent material from an abscess of Bartholin's gland may allow the physician to select a narrow-spectrum antibiotic as an adjunct to drainage.

The vaginal wet mount (wet prep) is useful for diagnosis of the offending organism in acute vaginitis. A sample of discharge is taken from the vaginal pool and by rubbing the vaginal walls with a cotton swab. The swab is placed in 1 to 2 mm of saline in a tube to create a slurry. One drop of the slurry is placed on a slide with a cover slip and examined by low- and high-power light microscopy for polymorphonuclear leukocytes, clue cells, trichomonads, hyphae, and budding yeast forms. If hyphae and budding yeast forms are not identified, a second slide is prepared by mixing one drop of the slurry with one drop of potassium hydroxide, which will lyse the epithelial cells and highlight the fungal organisms.

The clue cell is an epithelial cell with densely adherent bacteria, creating a stippled effect. To make this diagnosis, the density of bacteria must obscure cell margins in a substantial percentage of the cells. These, along with a strong amine ("fishy") odor, are diagnostic of bacterial vaginosis. There is rarely a significant white cell response to this condition because it is not an infection per se, but a shift in the normal vaginal ecosystem.

Trichomonads are often obvious as flagellated motile organisms similar in size to white blood cells. The organism is fragile, however, and motility can be inhibited by severe infection or cooling of the specimen during a delay before inspecting.

#### Lower Genital Cytology

The Pap cytology technique has had significant public health impact, reducing the incidence of invasive cervical cancer. Although the processing time for the smear limits usefulness in the acute setting, there are two important reasons to consider obtaining the sample. The first is to take the opportunity of the visit to test a previously noncompliant patient. The second is to satisfy any significant concern about a high-grade cervical lesion before surgical manipulation of the cervix.

There are two fundamental approaches for obtaining and preparing the specimen. In the older technique, a cervical spatula is placed in the cervical os and rotated circumferentially against the cervical epithelium. This is followed by a cotton swab placed in the cervical canal and rotated on its long axis. As each step is completed, the instrument is wiped across a glass slide and spray fixative is applied. In the more recent technique, the specimen from the instrument is swirled in a fluid-based preservative, which is processed to provide a more homogeneous slide for Pap staining. Although the cost of the fluid-based technique is higher, the improved accuracy and reduction of false-positive and false-negative results makes this more cost-effective.

### ALTERNATIVES TO SURGICAL INTERVENTION

There are valid indications for medical or observational management of many acute gynecologic conditions, even if there is also a surgical option available. Because acute pelvic pathology is often accompanied by severe pain or bleeding to a degree that the general surgeon would consider it as a surgical emergency in the upper abdomen, some guidance is provided here about the clinical judgment to allow the surgeon to avoid, or defer, surgery. Also provided is an overview approach to medical treatment and the points to observe during follow-up observation.

#### Dysfunctional Uterine Bleeding

Dysfunctional uterine bleeding is uterine bleeding that occurs as a result of abnormal or dyssynchronous pituitary hormonal stimulation of the ovary, abnormal ovarian hormone production, or abnormal response of the endometrium to normal hormonal stimulation.[1-3] If a pregnancy related-condition has been ruled out and the bleeding is not too severe, medical treatment does not require a tissue or even ultrasound diagnosis. Emergency implementation of dilation and curettage (D&C) is not necessary. The episode can be truncated by inducing acute proliferation and regeneration of the endometrium with high-dose estrogens, followed by induction of a secretory endometrium with a progestin.

An oral or IV bolus of estrogens (e.g., conjugated estrogens, 5 mg orally every 6 hours for 4 to 6 doses, or 25 mg IV in two doses 6 hours apart) with simultaneous administration of an active progestin (micronized progesterone, 100 mg orally twice daily, or medroxyprogesterone, 10 mg four times daily) will stabilize the endometrium. The progestin must be continued for at least 7 days and then withdrawn to simulate atresia of the corpus luteum. This will mimic the orderly menses of an ovulatory cycle, although perhaps with heavy bleeding. The patient receives oral contraceptives for several months to stabilize iron stores, allow for orderly evaluation of structural pathology, and initiate a plan to assess underlying hypothalamic-pituitary-ovarian cycle pathology.

### Spontaneous Abortion

First-trimester pregnancies fail 10% to 15% of the time, often with minimal symptoms. For the patient who presents with pain or bleeding, confirm that this is an early gestation. On inspection of the cervix, observe whether there is placental tissue in the dilated cervical os; if so, it can often be removed with a sponge forceps, which will often resolve the event. The need for acute surgical intervention with curettage is wholly dependent on the amount of blood loss and intensity of pain. The patient who is hemodynamically stable and has pain control may spontaneously complete her miscarriage without any procedural intervention.

### Ectopic Pregnancy

Ruptured ectopic pregnancy is a surgical emergency, but there are two other tubal pregnancy scenarios that are amenable to less aggressive treatment for the patient who is hemodynamically stable and has limited intraperitoneal blood loss, tubal abortion and unruptured ectopic pregnancy. A tubal abortion results when the pregnancy is extruded from the fimbriated end of the tube. Pain is often described as lateralized cramping, and the volume of blood identified in the cul-de-sac is approximately 100 mL. These events may be self-limited and, if pain and hemodynamic status are under control during observation, surgery may be avoided.

A patient may present with pain and vaginal bleeding; an intact tubal pregnancy is identified by ultrasound. There are varying sets of criteria for medical management of the unruptured tubal pregnancy, based on gestational size (<3 to 5 cm) and the presence of fetal cardiac activity, but the physician must actively consider medical rather than surgical management.[4]

Surgical procedures for managing an ectopic pregnancy include salpingectomy, salpingostomy, and segmental resection.[5] For the patient desiring to maintain maximal future fertility, preservation of the tube is preferable.

The medical treatment of tubal pregnancy relies on the cytotoxic effect of methotrexate. There are several protocols for dosage (e.g., 1 mg/kg) and follow-up. Consultation with an experienced gynecologist before initiation is advisable.

### Pelvic Infection

The diagnosis of PID can be challenging. Usually, the differential diagnosis includes appendicitis, urinary tract infection, ruptured ovarian cyst, and ectopic pregnancy, all of which share some of the signs and symptoms of PID. The diagnosis of PID is made only when the patient has fever, leukocytosis, purulent discharge from the cervix, bilateral adnexal tenderness on gentle palpation, and peritoneal signs limited to the pelvis. Appendicitis is differentiated by anteceding gastrointestinal symptoms, evolving pain pattern, absence of cervical discharge, and generalized peritonitis. Lower urinary tract infection is distinguished by dysuria and obvious pyuria. Rarely do ovarian cysts or ectopic pregnancy present with significant fever or leukocytosis. In a classic study, Wølner-Hanssen and associates[6] concluded that the sensitivity and specificity of clinical assessment for PID was so poor that laparoscopic inspection of the pelvis is necessary to make a firm diagnosis. Although that may be unduly aggressive in many cases, this diagnosis must be applied cautiously because it is stigmatizing and labels the patient, disproportionately a woman of color, from lower socioeconomic status, or with a counterculture lifestyle.

Acute PID, as a polymicrobial infection, is a medical, not a surgical, disease. The major acute complication of this disease is a TOA. In contrast to abscesses related to the intestine, however, initial management of a TOA is with broad-spectrum IV antibiotics. Indications for surgical intervention are a ruptured TOA with generalized peritonitis or failure to respond to medical therapy.

A pelvic inflammatory collection is a clinical variant of a TOA. Whereas an abscess is an infectious process bounded by an inflammatory response across natural tissue planes, the collection, which may be indistinguishable on ultrasound or CT scan, is bounded by anatomic surfaces of the posterior cul-de-sac, rectum, uterus, and intestine. Pelvic collections are more common than true abscesses and are much more likely to respond to medical therapy than abscesses.

### Functional Ovarian Cysts

Rupture of a follicle or corpus luteum cyst, or intraparenchymal hemorrhage in the corpus luteum, can result in extreme pain, with signs of localized peritoneal irritation. If ultrasound evaluation reveals a simple cyst and does not demonstrate significant intraperitoneal bleeding, and if Doppler flow rules out an ovarian torsion, this acute condition will resolve in 12 to 24 hours. Fluids and analgesic support are all that is necessary.

If the right ovary is affected, the acuity clearly will force the consideration of appendicitis, but prior gastrointestinal symptoms, fever, and leukocytosis are rarely present.

Ovarian torsion is a surgical emergency and sometimes mandates oophorectomy. However, unless the ovary is obviously necrotic at the time of laparoscopic inspection, the surgeon needs to untwist the ovarian pedicle and directly observe for return of blood flow before considering removal.

### Uterine Leiomyomas

Uterine leiomyomas are benign myometrial tumors present in up to 40% of women, more prevalent in African American women. With clinical or ultrasound confirmation of the diagnosis, observation for stability over time is indicated. Surgical intervention is warranted if the patient has unresponsive menorrhagia, intolerable pressure symptoms, rapid growth, or change in consistency of palpable masses. Leiomyosarcoma is sufficiently rare that hysterectomy or myomectomy to rule out malignancy carries a greater statistical risk than the lesion itself.

Observational management is especially valid in women who are approaching menopause because leiomyomas are estrogen-dependent and, with the decline in estrogen production, typically the lesions will decrease in size. Continued observation is important after menopause because progressive growth during this period may reflect malignant transformation.

### Endometriosis and Endometriomas

Endometriosis is a complex disease created by the presence of ectopic endometrial tissue in the peritoneal cavity or adnexa. The endometrial tissue transforms and bleeds with the ovarian cycle. This process induces a sterile inflammatory response, resulting in pain, pelvic adhesions and, when located in the ovary, a complex hemorrhagic mass, known as an *endometrioma.* First-line therapy for this disease is medical induction of temporary menopause and suppression of ovarian estrogen. Surgical treatment for younger women is conservative, with local destruction of lesions and maximum conservation of reproductive organs. Women who have completed their reproductive plans will benefit from hysterectomy and oophorectomy.

## TECHNICAL ASPECTS OF SURGICAL OPTIONS

### Surgical Approaches

Similar to all the surgical specialties, minimally invasive surgical approaches have become increasingly adopted in gynecologic surgery over the past decade. Laparoscopy and, more recently, robotically-assisted surgery has become more widely used for benign and malignant gynecologic conditions.[7-9] These minimally invasive techniques offer fewer postoperative complications and a shorter postoperative recovery. Postoperative adhesions are markedly reduced in many studies; this translates to a lower risk of infertility, which can be an important consideration following pelvic surgery. Shorter hospitalization and rapid recovery to full function are also major advantages to many patients. Today, most patients are discharged the morning following their hysterectomy if laparoscopy or robotic surgery is used; a 5-day hospitalization with slow return of bowel function is typical for patients managed by a traditional open abdominal hysterectomy.

Although these minimally invasive approaches are popular with patients and surgeons, they often require a longer operative time and definitely require advanced surgical training and skills. They also require significant specialized instrumentation and a well-trained and experienced surgical team. Because of their complexity and special instrumentation required for these approaches, they will not be discussed in detail in this chapter. The transvaginal approach is commonly used by gynecologic surgeons and is also highly effective for pelvic pathology, especially for the correction of pelvic organ prolapse and various urogynecologic conditions. These techniques also require special training and experience and will not be discussed in this chapter, although they are commonly used by gynecologic surgeons.

### Surgery for Menorrhagia or Abnormal Uterine Bleeding

D&C is the classic gynecologic procedure for the evaluation and possible therapeutic treatment of menorrhagia, menometrorrhagia, and abnormal uterine bleeding. It is now understood that its therapeutic success is 25% or less and is usually temporary. Because it is a blind procedure, it is difficult to ensure that the entire endometrium is curetted uniformly, much like attempting to scoop cake batter out of a bowl with a spoon. Therefore, more commonly now, hysteroscopy is used in conjunction with D&C so that the cavity can be visualized and any pathology seen can be directly resected or removed. The combination of the two adds to the evaluation and therapeutic success.

In addition, ablative techniques are being used for improved therapy for nonstructural bleeding abnormalities. These ablative techniques (e.g., rollerball, thermal balloon, hydrotherapy, cryotherapy, microwave) are advanced techniques best reserved for a surgeon with extensive experience in hysteroscopy and the evaluation and manipulation of the endometrial cavity.

#### Technique: Dilation and Curettage

A weighted speculum and anterior retracting blade or a bivalve Graves speculum are used in the vagina to visualize the cervix. The cervix is grasped transversely on the anterior lip with a single-toothed tenaculum. A Kevorkian curette is used to curette the endocervix for a specimen. A sound is placed through the cervix and into the uterus and gently tapped on the fundus of the uterus to measure the depth of the cavity. This step is important to help prevent or recognize uterine perforation for the remainder of the procedure. The cervix is dilated with graduated dilators of increasing diameter. At this time, if hysteroscopy is going to be performed, the hysteroscope is introduced through the cervix and into the uterus for visualization of the endometrial cavity; glycine or saline is commonly used as a distention medium. The curettage phase is performed. A sharp curette, the largest diameter that will easily fit through the cervix, is introduced gently into the cervix and endometrial cavity. This is done without excessive pressure or undue force. The fundus is found and a firm withdrawal stroke is applied until the curette reaches the cervicouterine junction. This is repeated while moving circumferentially around the uterine cavity, attempting to curette as much of the endometrial cavity as possible. The procedure is then terminated; the instruments are removed with careful attention to the cervix, which may bleed when the tenaculum is removed. The bleeding usually stops with pressure, silver nitrate, or Monsel's solution.

**Potential Complications** As with any surgical procedure, infection from instrumenting the cavity or bleeding from the denuded endometrial lining can occur. In addition, perforation of the uterine cavity is possible and can occur during any phase of the procedure. However, it usually occurs during the sounding of the uterus, and bleeding from the perforated area can result. The perforation is usually midline and self-limited. Generally, observation for 24 hours is all that is required. If there is continued bleeding, as evidenced by a decreasing hemoglobin level or increased abdominal pain, or if other symptoms are present, exploration by laparoscopy or laparotomy may be required. Injury to the bowel is possible, although rare, with perforation.

### Treatment of Bartholin's Gland Cyst or Abscess

Large, symptomatic Bartholin's gland cysts or painful abscesses may not respond to conservative treatment. Surgical treatment options are as follows:

1. Incision and drainage with Word catheter placement
2. Marsupialization
3. Excision of the gland itself

Excision of the gland is rarely indicated. Typically, incision and drainage with appropriate follow-up, with or without marsupialization, is all that is needed to treat this condition.

Incision and drainage are generally done on the vestibular side at the hymeneal ring in a lower dependent portion of the cyst or abscess using a sharp knife. The cyst is stabilized

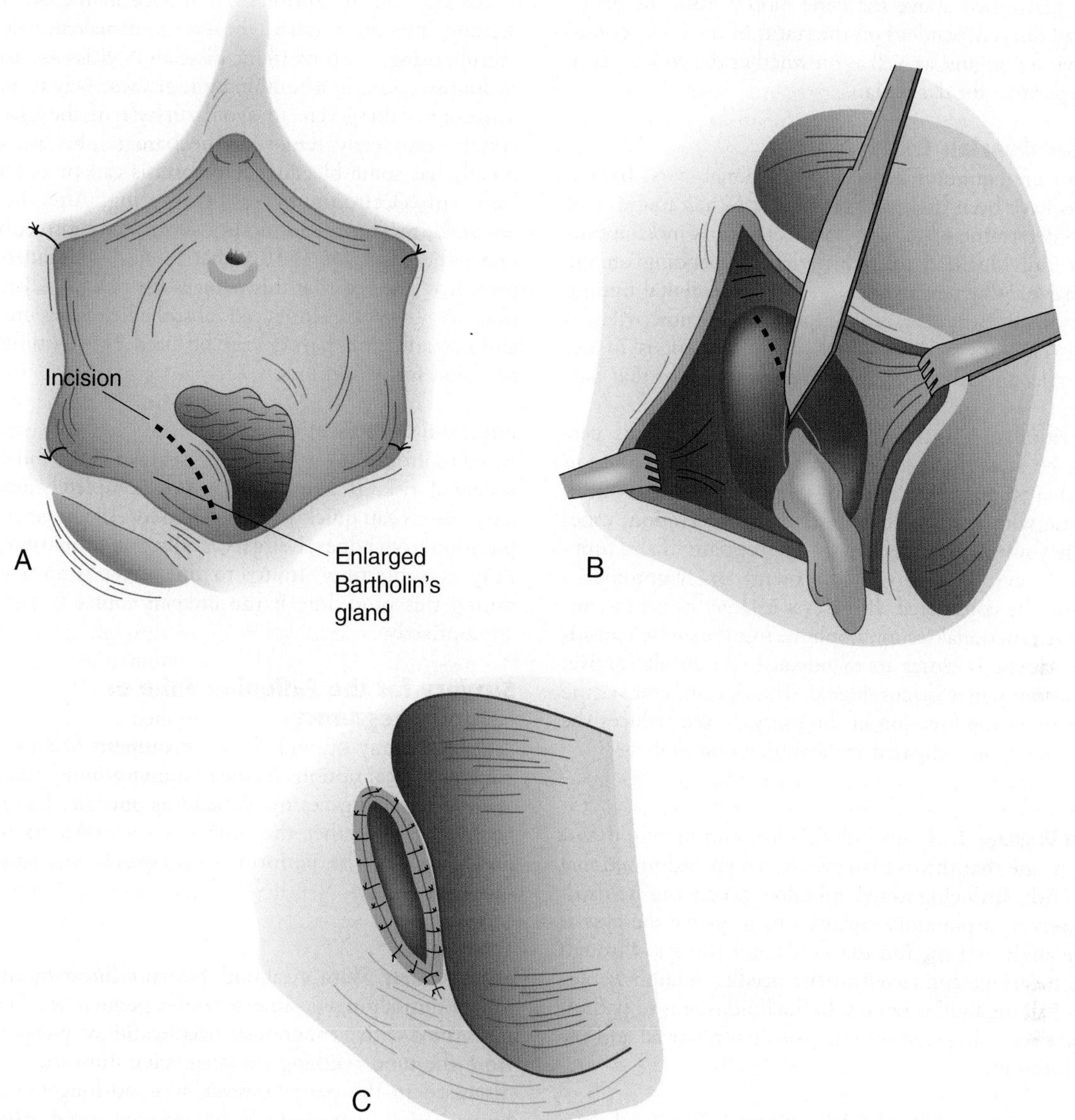


**FIGURE 71-7** Bartholin's gland marsupialization. **A,** Retraction of the labia and incision over the mucosa of the vagina. **B,** Wall of the gland is excised. **C,** Completed marsupialization. (Adapted from Mitchell CW, Wheeless CR: Atlas of pelvic surgery, ed 3, Philadelphia, 1997, Lippincott Williams & Wilkins.)

and an incision is made into the cyst itself. A small Word catheter is placed into the cyst for drainage and is reevaluated on a weekly basis. Patients with abscesses are pretreated with antibiotics.

To perform a marsupialization, an elliptical incision is made in the vestibular mucosa down to the wall of the gland. The wall of the gland is incised along the entire length of the ellipse. The contents are evacuated and the wall of the cyst is sutured to the vestibular mucosa with 3-0 synthetic absorbable sutures in an interrupted fashion or using a baseball stitch (Fig. 71-7). The patient is placed on a regimen of hot sitz baths. If the lesion is an abscess, the patient is given antibiotics. Whether marsupialization or incision and drainage have been performed, sexual intercourse is avoided until the area has completely healed.

## Cone Procedure

Conization can be performed with a cold knife, or a LEEP. A LEEP (loop electrosurgical excision procedure) conization entails removal of the transformation zone with an ectocervical loop followed by removal of an endocervical specimen with an endocervical loop. This is called a top hat procedure and allows for sampling of the canal. If a cold knife conization is done in the operating room, a single-toothed tenaculum is placed on the anterior lip of the cervix. Figure-of-eight retention sutures of 0-0 Vicryl are placed at 3 and 9 o'clock. A circumferential incision is made around the transformation zone and lesion. The specimen is grasped with Allis clamps to maintain orientation and a deeper circumferential incision is made in the cervix. The specimen is removed with a scalpel or Mayo scissors. A marking stitch is placed at 12 o'clock on the specimen and an endocervical curetting is performed above the cone biopsy. Risk for recurrence of dysplasia is dependent on the status of the endocervical and ectocervical margins, as well as on whether the endocervical curetting is positive for dysplasia.

## Surgery for Ovarian Cysts

Ovarian cysts are common, especially functional cysts. Benign ovarian cysts have been discussed previously. When found, it is necessary to determine which type of treatment is most appropriate. It is individualized to each patient, depending on the clinical scenario. When an ovarian cyst is an incidental finding at the time of other surgery, it is important to know what, if any, are the patient's symptoms, where the patient is in her menstrual cycle, and what size of follicle is normal for that part of the cycle.

It is critical to remember that whenever surgery is performed on the adnexal structures, there is a risk for adhesion formation that might inhibit fertility. If the patient has been asymptomatic with a small functional cyst, observation, especially for the younger patient, is most appropriate. If the functional ovarian cyst is large (>5 to 6 cm) or symptomatic, aspiration may be considered. If the cyst is larger or is not consistent with a functional lesion, oophorectomy may be considered if the patient is closer to menopause. As an alternative, ovarian cystectomy may be considered. This option removes the cyst but preserves the function of the ovary. It also reduces the risk for recurrence as compared with ovarian cyst drainage.

### Technique

**Ovarian Cyst Drainage** It is imperative, before considering drainage, to determine that the ovarian cyst is benign and functional in nature. With this being noted, a hollow needle can be used, by laparoscopy or exploratory laparotomy, to pierce the cyst at a 90-degree angle and suction the fluid from the cyst through tubing and a syringe connected to the needle. Suction is performed until all the fluid is removed. The fluid is sent to pathology to ensure accurate diagnosis. The needle is removed and the procedure is terminated.

**Oophorectomy With or Without Salpingectomy** When oophorectomy is desired, the infundibulopelvic (IP) ligament is identified and isolated. The ipsilateral ureter must be identified and noted to be remote from the area of the IP ligament to be ligated. With the IP ligament isolated, the following strategies can be followed:

1. Clamp, cut, and suture-ligate the IP ligament.
2. Ligate the IP ligament with one or two Endoloops and then surgically dissect it.
3. Cauterize the IP ligament with bipolar cautery and sharply dissect it.

If the ipsilateral tube is to be removed, dissection across the mesosalpinx is performed with clamp, sharp dissection, and suture ligation or with bipolar coagulation and sharp dissection. If the uterus is present, attention is directed to the utero-ovarian ligament. This ligament is dissected in a similar fashion, as described, through bipolar cautery or the clamping technique. The ovary, completely dissected, possibly in conjunction with the fallopian tube, can be removed.

**Ovarian Cystectomy** To begin an ovarian cystectomy, a surgical line into the ovarian capsule is developed sharply over the area of the cyst, on the antimesovarian side of the ovary. After the incision into the capsule, the cyst is dissected away from the capsule using sharp or blunt dissection. Scissors, knife, kitner, hydrodissection, or a combination of these may be used for this dissection, taking care to avoid rupture of the cyst. After the cyst is completely removed, the base of the ovarian capsule usually has some bleeding. Hemostasis can be obtained at the base with electrocautery or by suturing. After hemostasis is obtained, most surgeons do not suture the capsule, but approximate the edges loosely together to heal spontaneously on its own. It is believed that this reduces the risk for adhesion formation. A Gynecare Interceed absorbable adhesion barrier or another adhesion barrier can be used at this time to reduce adhesion formation.

### Potential Complications

Bleeding from the large vascular pedicles is the most dangerous potential risk. If hemostasis is not completely obtained, the large vessels can quickly bleed profusely. The more chronic complication from adnexal surgery is adhesion formation, with infertility or subfertility. Injury to the ureter is always a concern during this procedure if the ureteral course is not monitored appropriately.

## Surgery for the Fallopian Tube or Ectopic Pregnancy

There are many options for the treatment of an ectopic pregnancy. Surgical options include salpingostomy, segmental resection, and salpingectomy, depending on the desire for future fertility and whether the tube is salvageable. As noted, these procedures can be performed by laparoscopy, laparotomy, or minilaparotomy.

### Technique

**Salpingostomy** With a salpingostomy, a linear incision is made in the antisalpingetic line over the pregnancy. This is usually performed with a monopolar needle. The pregnancy is removed from the tube. Milking the pregnancy from the tube has been discussed in the past; however, it is no longer recommended because of an increased risk for retained tissue. After the pregnancy is completely removed, hemostasis is achieved with monopolar or bipolar cautery. The tube is not sutured, but rather left open to heal spontaneously. This has been shown to improve patency rates and fertility (Fig. 71-8).

**Segmental Resection** In segmental resection, the portion of the tube encompassing the products of conception is resected and the proximal and distal ends are left in situ. This gives the option of reanastomosis at a later date if the patient chooses. The mesosalpinx is perforated in an avascular space. Ligatures are placed on each side of the pregnancy. The segment is sharply resected within the ligatures; the vessels of the mesosalpinx are inspected for injury, and secured if necessary.

**Salpingectomy** In salpingectomy, the tube is grasped and the mesosalpinx is secured using bipolar cautery, an Endoloop, or clamps with a suture ligation. The tube is sharply excised. The area is examined closely for hemostasis (Fig. 71-9).

In rare cases, the ectopic pregnancy is in the abdomen and not in the fallopian tube. In these situations, the fetus is removed with ligation of the umbilical cord near its insertion

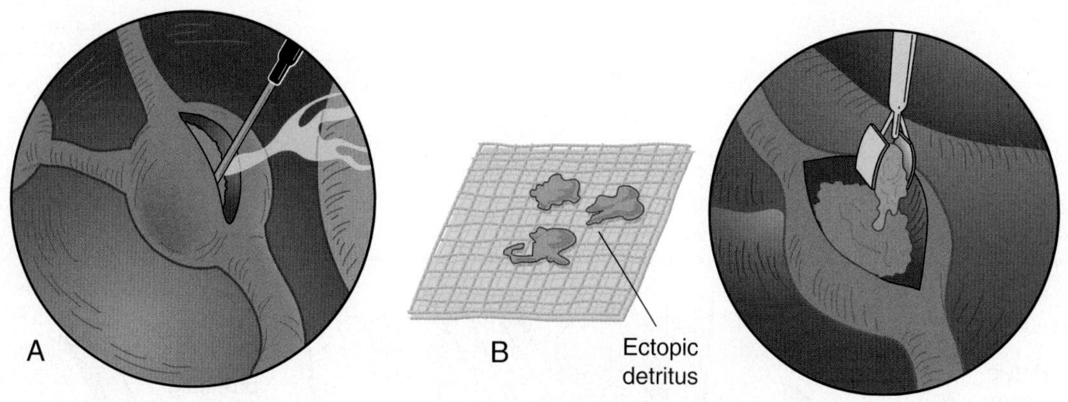


**FIGURE 71-8** Salpingostomy. **A,** Fallopian tube is opened in a longitudinal manner. **B,** Trophoblastic tissue is removed in pieces. (Adapted from Mitchell CW, Wheeless CR: Atlas of pelvic surgery, ed 3, Philadelphia,1997, Lippincott Williams & Wilkins.)

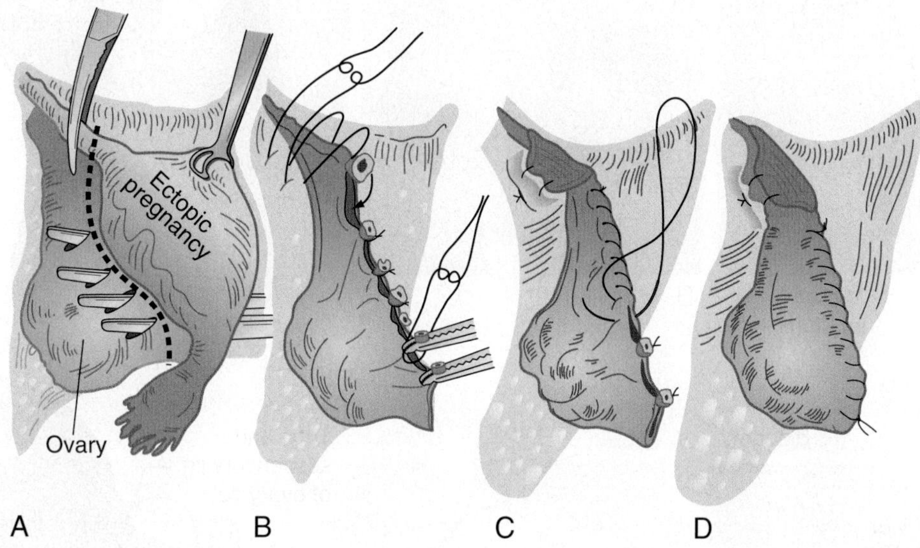


**FIGURE 71-9** Salpingectomy. **A,** Tube is excised from the cornual portion across the mesosalpinx to the fimbria. **B,** Pedicles are tied, peritoneal lining is reestablished, and cornual portion of the tube is buried into the posterior segment of the uterine cornu. **C,** Mesosalpinx is reperitonealized. **D,** Mesosalpinx is closed and the procedure completed. (Adapted from Mitchell CW, Wheeless CR: Atlas of pelvic surgery, ed 3, Philadelphia,1997, Lippincott Williams & Wilkins.)

into the placenta. Because of the vascularity of the placenta, the placenta is left in situ, with subsequent medical therapy with methotrexate.

### Potential Complications

The vascular supply of the tube in pregnancy is markedly increased; therefore, bleeding is a risk during and after the surgery is completed. If the tube is preserved, there is a risk for subsequent recurrent ectopic pregnancy. Also, there is a risk for retained placental tissue in the tube and persistent ectopic pregnancy. Adhesions of the affected adnexa are also a significant risk, whether the tube is preserved or removed.

## Hysterectomy

Hysterectomy is one of the most common gynecologic procedures performed. The route of hysterectomy depends on the indication for surgery, size of the uterus, descent of the cervix and uterus, shape of the vagina, size of the patient, and skill and preference of the surgeon. Surgical routes for hysterectomy include total abdominal hysterectomy (TAH), total vaginal hysterectomy (TVH), laparoscopically assisted vaginal hysterectomy (LAVH), and two more recent techniques—total laparoscopic hysterectomy (TLH) and laparoscopic supracervical hysterectomy (LSH). Robotically assisted total laparoscopic hysterectomy is a popular variation of total laparoscopic hysterectomy.

Because of the significant impact of the transvaginal approach on appreciating anatomic relationships, vaginal hysterectomy and laparoscopically assisted hysterectomy must only be performed by an experienced vaginal surgeon.

### Technique

Any lower abdominal incision (vertical, Pfannenstiel, Maylard, Cherney) can be used. The bowel is packed from the pelvis and the patient placed in the Trendelenburg position. The ureters are identified and the following steps are performed bilaterally (Fig. 71-10).

The round ligament is identified, incised between clamps, and ligated with 0-0 absorbable suture. The leaves of the broad ligament are sharply opened anteriorly and posteriorly, with the

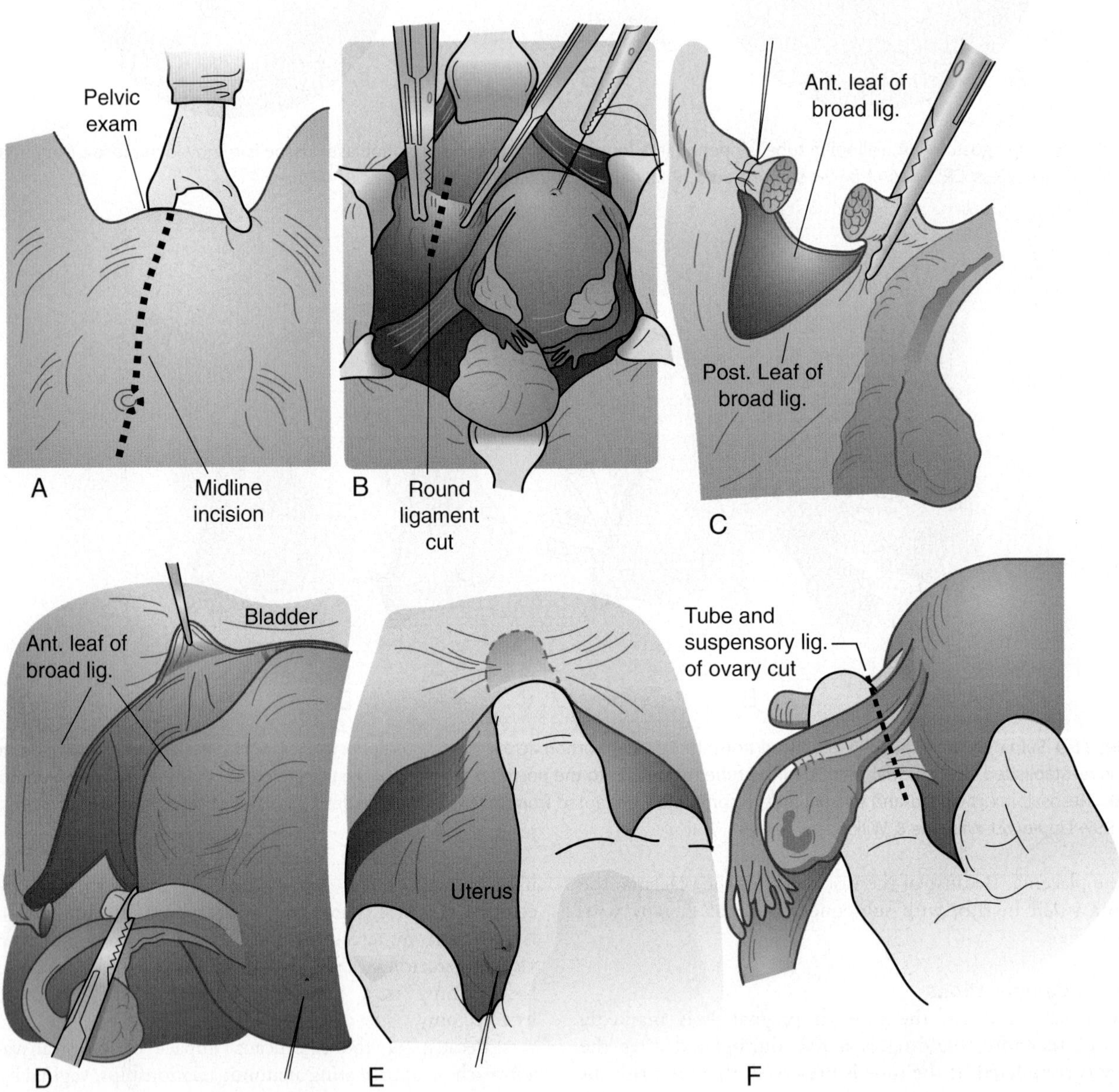


**FIGURE 71-10 A–N,** Hysterectomy. (Adapted from Mitchell CW, Wheeless CR: Atlas of pelvic surgery, ed 3, Philadelphia, 1997, Lippincott Williams & Wilkins.)

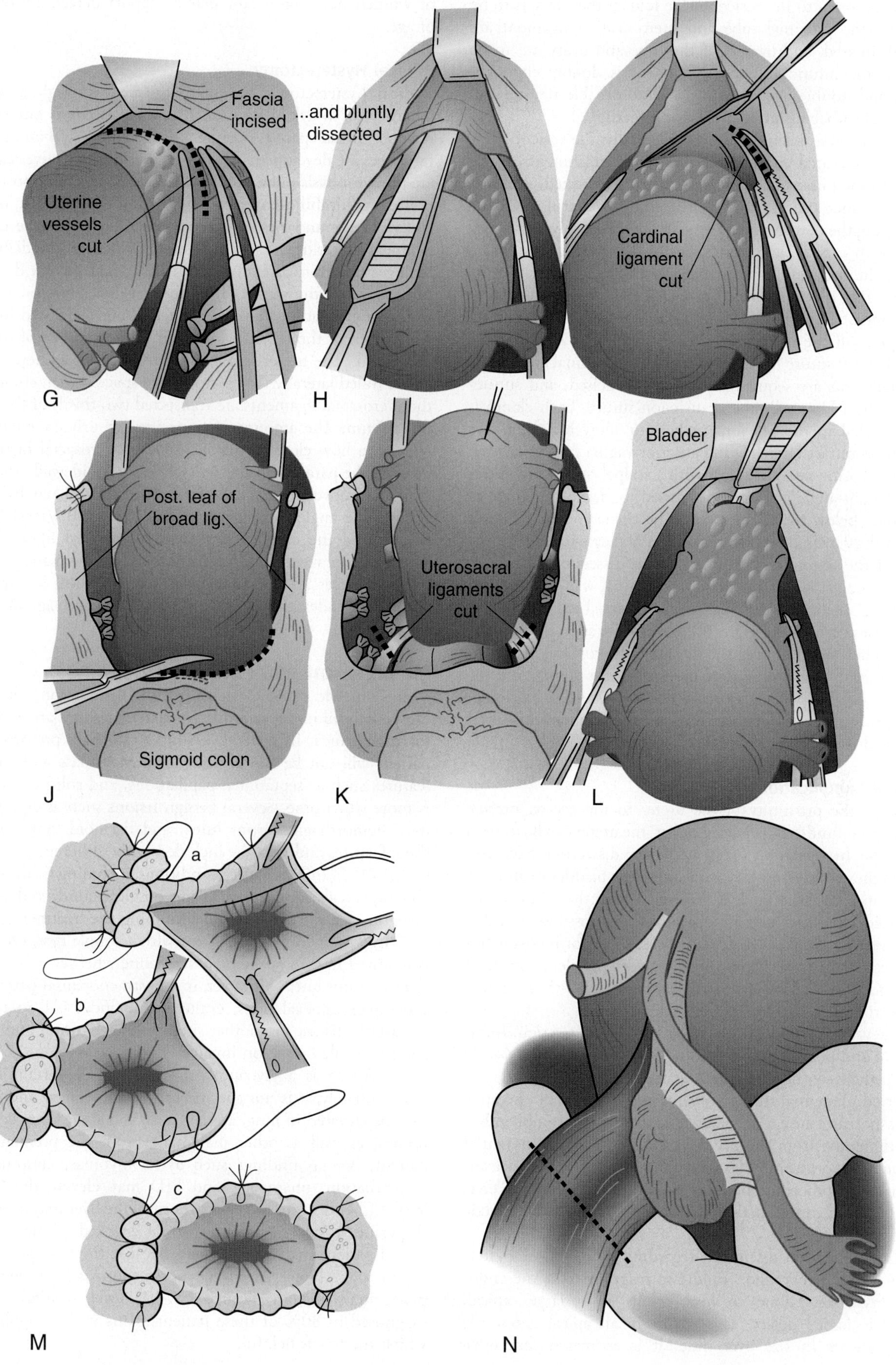


**FIGURE 71-10, Cont'd**

anterior leaf open to the vesicouterine fold. If the ovary is to be preserved, the proximal tube and utero-ovarian ligament are clamped, incised, and ligated. If the tube and ovary are to be removed, the infundibulopelvic ligament is doubly clamped, incised, and double-ligated with a 0-0 absorbable tie and 0-0 synthetic absorbable suture, as described earlier.

After this has been performed bilaterally, the vesicoperitoneal fold is elevated and incised. The filmy attachments of the bladder to the pubovesical fascia are sharply dissected, mobilizing the bladder off the cervix. The filmy adventitious tissue surrounding the uterine vessels is skeletonized sharply, dissecting the tissue to expose the uterine vessels. The uterine vessels are clamped, incised, and ligated at the level of the lower uterine segment. This is accomplished by placing the tip of the clamp on the uterus at a right angle to the axis of the cervix and sliding or stepping off the uterus. The pedicle is incised and a simple absorbable 0-0 suture ligature is placed. The cardinal and uterosacral ligaments are sequentially clamped, incised, and suture-ligated with a Haney double transfixion suture. Each clamp is placed medial to the previous pedicle to allow for the ureter passively to retract laterally. The anterior vagina can be entered by a stab incision and cut across with a scalpel or scissors. Alternatively, right-angle clamps can be used to clamp the angle of the vagina, below the distal cervix. The tissue above this angle clamp is then incised and ligated with a Haney stitch. With the lumen of the vagina now exposed, sharp dissection is used to complete the vaginal transection. The vaginal wall, incorporating perivaginal fascia, muscularis, and mucosal edge, is closed with a series of figure-of-eight 0-0 absorbable sutures, with the angle stitches incorporating the ipsilateral uterosacral ligament. Ligatures need to be snug, but they must not strangulate the vaginal edges. The pelvic peritoneum does not need to be closed. The pelvis is irrigated, hemostasis ensured, and abdominal incision closed routinely.

### Potential Complications

Because of the proximity of the ureter to the cervix, uterine vessels, and infundibulopelvic ligament, the ureter can be injured during the hysterectomy and, with the dissection necessary between the bladder and cervix, injury to the bladder is similarly a common complication. It is imperative that these injuries be recognized and repaired intraoperatively, if possible. Fistulas, such as vesicovaginal or ureterovaginal, can also form postoperatively secondary to ischemic injury caused by denudation of the bladder muscularis or partial entrapment with a vaginal closure stitch.

The vascular supply to the uterus and ovaries is rich. Intraoperative and postoperative bleeding is a concern. A previously secure pedicle can begin to bleed acutely during the postoperative period. A vaginal stump vessel, missed because of operative vasospasm, can cause a pelvic cuff hematoma. Thromboembolism originating from the pelvic vasculature is also a potential postoperative problem. Hysterectomy is considered a clean-contaminated procedure because of entering the vagina. Pelvic cuff infection is common, despite the routine use of prophylactic antibiotics.

There has been discussion regarding the effect of hysterectomy on the pelvic floor. Failure to reapproximate the endopelvic fascia or failure to heal results in a large, apical, endopelvic fascial defect. This results in an apical enterocele that progresses in size over time. It is estimated that 60% of women have significant pelvic support defects by 60 years of age.

### Radical Hysterectomy

Radical hysterectomy can be performed through a vertical, Cherney, or Maylard incision. After the pelvis is entered, the retroperitoneal space is opened and the paravesical and pararectal spaces are developed. The boundaries of the paravesical space are the symphysis pubis anteriorly, cardinal ligament posteriorly, obliterated umbilical artery medially, and external iliac vein laterally. The boundaries of the pararectal space are the cardinal ligament anteriorly, sacrum posteriorly, ureter medially, and hypogastric artery laterally. The bladder flap is then developed to the level of the vagina. The uterine arteries are isolated back to the origin and ligated. The ureter is then separated from the medial leaf of the broad ligament and the parametrial tunnel is developed. The ureter is separated from the parametrial tissue and is rolled laterally. The rectovaginal space is then entered and the uterosacral ligaments are transected two thirds of the way to the sacrum. The amount of postoperative urinary retention is related to how close to the sacrum the uterosacral ligament is ligated. The parametria are then taken at the sidewall. The specimen is removed when the vagina is entered 1 cm below the cervix. The angle sutures are secured with 0-0 Vicryl Heaney sutures and the cuff is closed with 0-0 Vicryl figure-of-eight sutures. More recent surgical techniques for the management of cervical cancer include total laparoscopic radical hysterectomy with lymphadenectomy and fertility-sparing vaginal radical trachelectomy.

## Management of a Pelvic Mass

When a pelvic mass is discovered on examination, ultrasound can be helpful in determining characteristics that are worrisome for malignancy. In general, a simple cyst in a premenopausal patient will not be cancerous. However, a mass with complex features such as septations, papillations, and solid components is more worrisome. Several benign lesions such as endometriomas, hemorrhagic corpus lutea, and dermoid cysts can have these features and must be included in the differential diagnosis (Table 71-2). Inflammatory conditions, including a tubo-ovarian abscess, can also appear worrisome on ultrasound, so the clinical scenario is important when determining the treatment plan.

In a premenopausal patient with a simple cyst, ultrasound is repeated in 6 to 8 weeks to determine whether it is a hemorrhagic corpus lutea. However, in a postmenopausal patient with a complex adnexal mass, evaluation includes CT to rule out metastatic disease or another site of primary tumor and barium enema to rule out colon involvement or primary.[10]

CA-125 is a glycoprotein produced by certain tumors. Unfortunately, it is not specific for ovarian cancer and its level may be elevated in lung, appendiceal, and signet ring cell carcinomas, as well as other malignancies. In the premenopausal patient, benign findings such as leiomyomas, endometriosis, menstruation, pregnancy, and PID may elevate the CA-125 level. Other diseases such as cirrhosis of the liver may also elevate the value. CA-125, therefore, is not checked in the premenopausal patient with a pelvic mass because the false-positive rate is too high. However, in the postmenopausal patient with a pelvic mass and an elevated CA-125 level, ovarian cancer is diagnosed in 80% of these patients. This is the population in which the test is helpful.

**Table 71-2 Differential Diagnosis of Ovarian Masses**

| MASS | DIFFERENTIAL DIAGNOSIS |
|---|---|
| Benign disease | Hemorrhagic corpus luteum, endometrioma, tubo-ovarian abscess, ectopic pregnancy, serous or mucinous cystadenoma, cystadenofibroma, fibroma, Brenner's tumor, dermoid |
| Malignant disease | Serous borderline tumor, mucinous epithelial borderline tumor, invasive cancer (papillary serous, endometrioid, transitional cell, clear cell, neuroendocrine or small cell, malignant mixed mullerian tumor) |
| Germ cell | Dysgerminoma, endodermal sinus tumor, choriocarcinoma, immature teratoma, embryonal carcinoma, polyembryoma |
| Stromal | Sertoli-Leydig cell tumor, granulosa cell tumor |
| Metastasis | Colon cancer, stomach cancer, breast cancer, lymphoma |

Definitive diagnosis of a pelvic mass requires visual inspection and histologic diagnosis. Laparoscopy or laparotomy can be done, depending on the clinical suspicion of malignancy. In patients with potential for carcinomatosis, laparoscopy is not done because of port site metastasis that occurs quickly and can make debulking difficult. At the time of surgery, pelvic washings are done, and the mass is visually inspected to augment prior information from ultrasound. If all indications are that the lesion is benign, ovarian cystectomy or drainage (see earlier, "Technical Aspects of Surgical Options") are indicated, with evaluation of cyst cytology or gross or microscopic evaluation of the tissue to confirm a benign lesion. If there is a higher level of suspicion or the patient is menopausal, oophorectomy is performed and frozen section histologic diagnosis is carried out.[11-13]

Serous and mucinous cystadenomas are common benign tumors of the ovary that can occur in any age group. Treatment can be cystectomy or oophorectomy, depending on the amount of ovary involved. Brenner's tumors are benign transitional cell tumors of the ovary that can also be managed in a similar fashion.

If the lesion is an invasive, epithelial ovarian cancer, treatment includes hysterectomy, bilateral salpingo-oophorectomy, omentectomy, peritoneal biopsies of the diaphragm, bilateral paracolic gutters, bilateral pelvis, and cul-de-sac and lymph node sampling. If the cell type is mucinous, an appendectomy is also performed to rule out metastasis from the appendix. Attention has turned toward minimally invasive (laparoscopic) and fertility-sparing surgical approaches. Interval laparoscopic staging of newly diagnosed ovarian tumors, with no suspicion of carcinomatosis, may be performed in selected patients.[8]

Extensive disease mandates tumor debulking to remove all possible tumor. Patients who undergo optimal tumor reductive surgery (<2 cm of visible disease) have a survival advantage over patients who cannot be or are not optimally debulked. Complete staging is important because patients who have a grade 1 or 2 stage 1A ovarian cancer do not require chemotherapy. With other stages, surgery is followed by chemotherapy.

Borderline tumors do not behave like invasive ovarian cancers. Typically, they are treated with surgery alone and do not require chemotherapy. They tend to occur in younger women. If found at frozen section and the patient is finished with childbearing, pelvic washings, hysterectomy, bilateral salpingo-oophorectomy, omentectomy, peritoneal biopsies, and lymph node biopsies are performed. If the patient desires future fertility, a unilateral oophorectomy, omentectomy, peritoneal biopsies, and lymph node biopsies on the side of the tumor can be performed. The other ovary can then be monitored with ultrasound. Staging is done in case an invasive ovarian cancer is found at the time of final pathology. Mucinous borderline tumors have also been associated with abnormalities in the appendix. Therefore, an appendectomy is performed in conjunction with other staging.

Other types of ovarian tumors include sex cord stromal tumors, such as granulosa cell and Sertoli-Leydig cell tumors. These typically appear solid but occasionally have a cystic appearance. Hysterectomy, bilateral salpingo-oophorectomy, and staging are performed. For stage I tumors of the adult type, no further therapy is needed. For patients with a higher stage, postoperative chemotherapy or radiation therapy is added.

Germ cell tumors must be considered in girls and young women,. The most common cell type is a dysgerminoma; 90% of these are diagnosed at stage I. Conservative surgery with unilateral oophorectomy and staging can be performed, leaving the uterus and other tube and ovary in place. No further treatment is needed.[14] Other germ cell tumors include endodermal sinus tumor, choriocarcinoma, immature teratoma, and embryonal carcinoma. A mixture of these cancers can be present. Tumor markers such as β-hCG, α-fetoprotein, and lactate dehydrogenase (LDH) may be detected in certain germ cell tumors. Patients who have a gonadoblastoma must be tested by chromosome evaluation. If XY chromosomes are discovered, the gonads are removed to prevent the development of dysgerminoma. This may occur in 20% of patients with gonadoblastoma.

Because these are potentially aggressive tumors, postoperative chemotherapy is implemented with the diagnoses of teratoma (stage IA, grade 2 or 3 immature teratoma, or any higher stage), dysgerminoma (stage II and above), any endodermal sinus tumor, or choriocarcinoma.

## SURGERY DURING PREGNANCY

Approximately 0.1% to 2.2% of pregnant women require surgery during pregnancy. Changes in maternal-fetal physiology, enlarging gestation, and changes in maternal organ placement can make diagnosis and treatment challenging. This section addresses important issues for the surgeon to consider before proceeding to the operating room.

### Physiologic Changes

During pregnancy, multisystem adaptions result in altered physiology.

#### Cardiovascular System

Blood volume increases by 45% to 50% at term. Placental hormone production stimulates maternal erythropoiesis, which increases red cell mass by approximately 20%. This results in a functional hemodilution manifested by a physiologic anemia. Therefore, pregnancy needs to be considered as a hypervolemic state.

The maternal heart rate increases as early as 7 weeks' gestation. In late pregnancy, the maternal heart rate is increased by approximately 20% over antepartum values. Systemic vascular

**Table 71-3 Physiologic Changes of Pregnancy**

| SYSTEM | CHANGES | RESULT |
|---|---|---|
| Cardiovascular, hemodynamic | Blood volume increased by 50%; red cell mass increased by 20%; cardiac output increased by 50%; heart rate increased by 20%; systemic vascular resistance decreased by 20% | High-output cardiac state with a hemodilutional anemia |
| Respiratory | Minute volume increased by 20%; functional residual capacity decreased by 15%; tidal volume increased by 20% to 30%; oxygen consumption increased by 20% | Compensated respiratory alkalosis |
| Gastrointestinal | Smooth muscle relaxation; delayed gastrointestinal emptying | Full stomach; constipation |
| Coagulation | Fibrinogen increased by 30%; protein S decreased by 30% to 40% | Hypercoagulable state regardless of risk factors |
| Renal | Glomerular filtration rate increased by 50%; serum creatinine decreased 40%; physiologic hydronephrosis | Increased urination; increased risk for upper tract infection |

resistance decreases by 20%, but gradually increases near term. This results in a decrease in systolic and diastolic blood pressure during pregnancy, with a gradual recovery to nonpregnant values by term. Because there is increased pressure in the venous system, there is decreased return from the lower extremities, resulting in dependent edema.

### Respiratory System

In pregnancy, minute volume is increased, whereas functional residual volume is decreased (Table 71-3). Although it seems intuitive that lung volume would decrease during pregnancy, an increase in minute volume in association with an expansion of the anterior and posterior diameter of the chest results in increased tidal volume, thereby also increasing minute ventilation. These changes result in a compensated respiratory alkalosis. Normal $Pco_2$ values in pregnancy ranges from 28 to 35 mm Hg. The $Po_2$ value is usually 100 mm Hg or higher. Oxygen consumption and basal metabolic rate are also increased during pregnancy by approximately 20%.

These physiologic changes result in less pulmonary reserve for the acutely ill pregnant patient, reducing the time needed for the deterioration of respiratory distress to respiratory failure. Early intervention is mandatory.

### Gastrointestinal Tract

During pregnancy, there is a decrease in gastrointestinal motility caused by mechanical changes in the abdomen, with the enlarging uterus and smooth muscle relaxation resulting from the increased production of progesterone in pregnancy. Gastric emptying may be delayed for up to 8 hours. Pregnant women are considered to have a functionally full stomach at all times. In addition, a decrease in large intestine motility may result in constipation severe enough to cause significant abdominal pain.

### Coagulation Changes

Pregnancy is a hypercoagulable state. Fibrinogen is increased approximately 30% over baseline values. The hypercoagulable state of pregnancy is associated with an increased risk for deep venous thrombosis and pulmonary embolus. This is particularly compounded when bed rest or immobilization occurs during the gestational period.

### Renal Changes

Pregnancy increases blood flow to the renal pelvis by approximately 50%. This results in an increased glomerular filtration rate. Frequent urination is common. The serum creatinine level is approximately 40% less than in a nonpregnant state. Therefore, a creatinine level of 1 mg/dL during gestation is considered abnormal.

Ureteral diameter increases in pregnancy secondary to compression and smooth muscle relaxation. Peristalsis is delayed and reflux occurs freely from the bladder into the lower ureteral segment. This results in an increased incidence of pyelonephritis during pregnancy. Therefore, asymptomatic bacteruria must be aggressively treated.

## Diagnostic Considerations and Evaluation

### Imaging Techniques

The most common imaging technique used during pregnancy is ultrasound, which is considered the safest modality and is used for fetal assessment. In patients with abdominal pain, an ultrasound is considered the first-line diagnostic test. During ultrasound, the presence of an intrauterine pregnancy needs to be documented, if possible. In addition, evaluation of the cul-de-sac for fluid, the ureter for dilation or stones, the gallbladder for the presence of gallstones, and the placenta for abnormalities can be carried out.

MRI also can be used during pregnancy. To date, no evidence has suggested an increased risk from this modality; in fact, MRI is used to diagnose fetal abnormalities, especially abnormalities of the central nervous system.

Although there are theoretical risks associated with ionizing radiation, most diagnostic x-ray procedures are associated with minimal or no risk to the fetus. Evidence suggests that there is no increased risk to the fetus with regard to congenital malformations, growth restriction, or abortion from x-ray procedures that expose the fetus to doses of 5 cGy or less. In 1995, the American College of Obstetrics and Gynecology published guidelines regarding diagnostic imaging during pregnancy. Women need to be reassured that concern about radiation exposure must not prevent medically indicated diagnostic procedures. It cannot be stressed enough that maternal well-being is of the utmost importance, and appropriate diagnostic procedures need to be performed to facilitate a rapid diagnosis.

### Clinical Evaluation

Abdominal pain during pregnancy can be confusing to the clinician. It is natural for the clinician to attribute most abdominal pain to the pregnancy; however, other organ systems are affected during pregnancy at the rate of the general population. In addition to these diagnoses, diagnosis specific to pregnancy also needs to be considered.

## Common Surgical Complications of Pregnancy

### Appendicitis

Appendicitis is one of the most common surgical complications of pregnancy, with an incidence of approximately 2/1000 pregnant women. This incidence is no higher than that of the general population; however, appendiceal location during pregnancy changes with the upward displacement of the appendix with advancing gestation (Fig. 71-11). Nevertheless, the most common presenting symptom is pain in the right lower quadrant, which presents regardless of gestational age. The diagnosis of appendicitis in pregnancy may be difficult because many of the symptoms of appendicitis are seen during pregnancy. Pain in the right lower quadrant may be mistaken for round ligament pain, and nausea, vomiting, and abdominal discomfort may be mistaken for hyperemesis gravidarum. Because mild leukocytosis is commonly seen in pregnancy, it may confound the diagnosis. However, other symptoms, such as fever and anorexia, can help the clinician establish the diagnosis. Ultrasonography may be used but is of limited value if bowel loops are distended. CT without contrast can be used, if needed, to assist in the diagnosis.

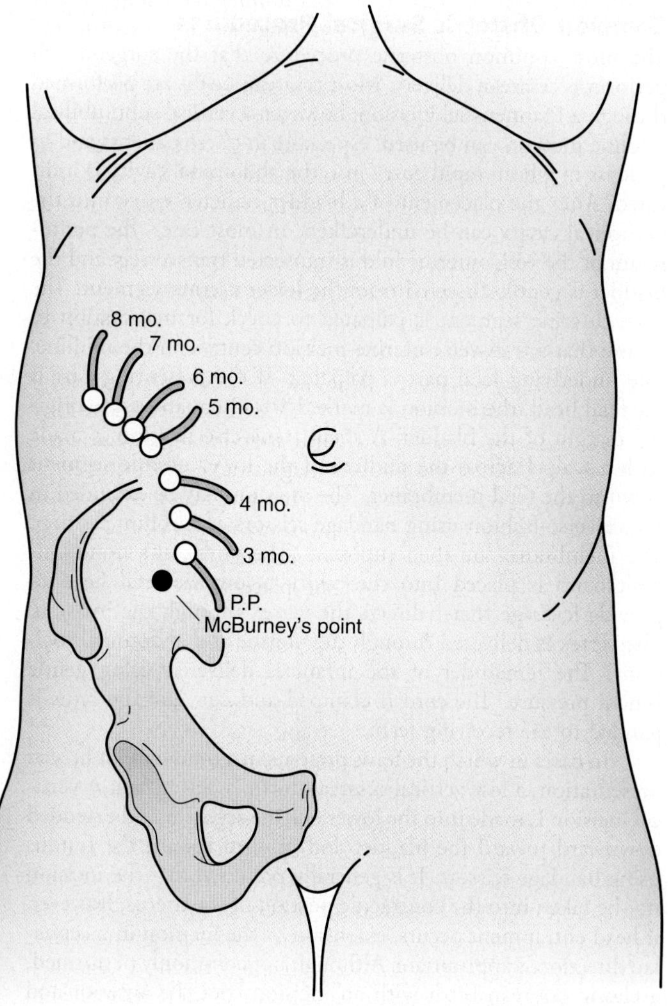


**FIGURE 71-11** The approximate location of the appendix during succeeding months of pregnancy is illustrated. In planning an operation, it is better to make the abdominal incision over the point of maximum tenderness unless there is a great disparity between that point and the theoretical location of the appendix. (From Ludmir J, Stubblefield PG: Surgical procedures in pregnancy. In Gabbe S, Neibyl JR, Simpson JL [eds]: Obstetrics: Normal and problem pregnancies, ed 4, Philadelphia, 2002, Churchill Livingstone, p 617.)

Rupture of the appendix during pregnancy increases perinatal morbidity and mortality. This is particularly true when rupture occurs after 20 weeks' gestation. Peritonitis increases the risk for preterm labor and preterm delivery. Therefore, it is prudent that the clinician make an early diagnosis and proceed immediately with surgical intervention.

### Cholelithiasis

After appendicitis, biliary tract disease is the second most common general surgical condition encountered during pregnancy. Cholelithiasis of pregnancy usually develops from obstruction of the cystic duct. The clinical presentation ranges from intermittent attacks of biliary colic to persistent pain radiating into the subcapsular area in patients in whom the common bile duct is obstructed by a stone. Ultrasound is helpful for detecting the presence of stones. The differential diagnosis of acute cholelithiasis includes acute pain in the liver of pregnancy, the HELLP (***h***emolysis, ***e***levated ***l***iver enzymes, ***l***ow ***p***latelets) syndrome, and severe preeclampsia. Initial attacks may be treated conservatively with IV fluids, antibiotics, and antispasmodics; however, without prompt resolution of symptoms, surgery needs to be considered. Delay of surgery in a patient with cholecystitis may increase perinatal morbidity. Despite the potential difficulty of operating on a pregnant woman, lower morbidity has been shown in patients managed surgically, particularly in cases involving obstruction. In early gestation, laparoscopic cholecystectomy can be considered.

Although rare, pancreatitis may present during pregnancy. The most common cause of pancreatitis in pregnant women is cholelithiasis. However, pancreatitis can be a complication of severe preeclampsia or HELLP syndrome. Pancreatitis caused by milk-alkali toxicity may be seen in patients with an excessive intake of antacids.[15]

### Intestinal Obstruction

The incidence of intestinal obstruction in pregnant women is similar to that of the general population. Patients present with classic symptoms of the abdominal colicky pain associated with hyperactive peristalsis. Nausea and vomiting are present in approximately 80% of cases. Bowel distention is marked. Laparotomy needs to be performed before bowel necrosis and perforation occur. If perforation occurs during pregnancy, there is a significant increase in maternal and perinatal morbidity and mortality.

### Ovarian Masses

With the frequent use of ultrasound in early pregnancy, the corpus luteum cyst of pregnancy is frequently identified. This is physiologic and, in the absence of symptoms of torsion, requires only follow-up to ensure the diagnosis. The progesterone produced in the first 14 weeks of gestation is necessary to support the pregnancy until placental production of progesterone replaces it. Therefore, if surgery is required for symptoms of torsion or bleeding, every effort must be made to preserve the corpus luteum in the first trimester.[16]

## Obstetric Complications Resulting in Abdominal Pain

### Placental Abruption

Placental abruption usually occurs in the third trimester and may be associated with excruciating abdominal pain. Contrary to popular belief, overt vaginal bleeding does not need to be present in order for the diagnosis to be made. Ultrasonography is of little use because only 5% to 10% of abruptions can be seen. Therefore, the diagnosis of abruption is clinical. Abruptions are usually associated with uterine hypertonicity, resulting in fetal heart rate abnormalities. It is important for the clinician to diagnose abruption rapidly.

Trauma may increase the risk for abruption. There are three distinct mechanisms for post-traumatic placental abruption:

1. Blunt trauma to the uterus—for example, assault or seat belt placement can cause a direct injury to the placental implantation site.
2. The sudden acceleration-deceleration cycle that occurs in motor vehicle crashes can cause a contrecoup shearing injury.
3. Even in the absence of any overt physical injury, the acute adrenergic reaction to stress can result in sufficient uterine vasospasm to create ischemic necrosis at the implantation site; with reperfusion, a subplacental hematoma can dissect the plane of the implantation site.

The pregnant patient and her fetus who experience trauma need to be monitored for at least 4 hours, with the possibility of prolonged monitoring for 24 hours. Abruption may quickly become a surgical emergency, requiring immediate delivery of the fetus. Laboratory studies that may be helpful in the diagnosis of abruption include a platelet count and measurement of the fibrinogen level. As the retroplacental hematoma expands, clotting factors, especially fibrinogen and platelets, are consumed. This may assist the clinician in the diagnosis in occult cases.

### Pregnancy-Related Hepatic Complications

HELLP syndrome and acute fatty liver of pregnancy can present as right upper quadrant pain and nausea and vomiting. HELLP is a form of severe preeclampsia. It is important that the clinician not mistake this for cholelithiasis or some other gastrointestinal pathology. Progression of this disease can result in rupture of the hepatic capsule and maternal death if the diagnosis is missed.

Acute fatty liver of pregnancy, which also carries a serious risk for maternal and fetal morbidity and mortality, can present in a similar fashion. Laboratory studies useful in the diagnosis include platelet count and determination of LDH, serum glutamic-oxaloacetic transaminase (SGOT), creatinine, uric acid, and hematocrit levels. SGOT and LDH levels will be elevated, platelets will be decreased, and the hematocrit value may be increased, especially when seen in association with intravascular volume depletion. In patients with acute fatty liver, the glucose level may also be decreased. It is important that the clinician remember the physiologic changes when interpreting values discussed at the beginning of this chapter.

### Trauma

Trauma from accidental injuries occurs in 6% to 7% of all pregnancies. In addition to the risk for placental abruption noted, blunt trauma may increase the risk for preterm labor and preterm rupture of the membranes. It is important that pregnant trauma patients be assessed for the same spectrum of injuries as nonpregnant patients. A number of studies have established that fetal-maternal hemorrhage is increased in women who have suffered trauma. Women who are RhD-negative need to have a quantitative assessment of the volume of fetal cells in maternal circulation and an appropriate dose of anti-D immune globulin administered. Peritoneal lavage is not contraindicated in pregnancy and can be performed safely in those patients in whom the possibility of a ruptured viscus is suspected.

## Common Obstetric Surgical Procedures

The most common obstetric procedure that the surgeon will perform is cesarean delivery. Most cesarean births are performed through a Pfannenstiel incision; however, a vertical subumbilical midline incision can be used, especially in obese patients and in patients in whom rapid entry into the abdominal cavity is indicated. After the placement of a bladder catheter, entry into the peritoneal cavity can be undertaken. In most cases, the peritoneum of the vesicouterine fold is transected transversely and the bladder is gently dissected from the lower uterine segment. The lower uterine segment is palpated to check for malrotation to ensure that a transverse uterine incision centers on the midline. The underlying fetal part is palpated. If the presenting part is the fetal head, the incision is marked 1 to 2 cm above the original margin of the bladder. A small transverse incision is made with a scalpel across the midline of the lower uterine segment down to the fetal membranes. The incision may be extended in a transverse fashion using bandage scissors or in blunt fashion. The membranes are then ruptured. The physician's nondominant hand is placed into the cavity below the fetal head to provide leverage that redirects the vertex through the incision. The vertex is delivered through the uterine and abdominal incisions. The remainder of the infant is delivered using gentle fundal pressure. The cord is clamped and cut, and the fetus is handed to the receiving team.

In cases in which the fetus presents in a transverse or breech presentation, a low vertical cesarean birth is performed. A vertical incision is made into the lower uterine segment and extended downward toward the bladder and upward toward the fundus using bandage scissors. It is generally preferred that the incision not be taken into the contractile portion of the uterus; however, if head entrapment occurs, extension of the incision in a cephalad direction is appropriate. Although not commonly performed, a classic cesarean birth with an incision over the anterior and superior uterine fundus can be used in patients in whom obstruction of the lower uterine segment occurs secondary to uterine fibroids or in very early gestation.

After the infant is delivered through the incision of choice, closure of the uterine incision may be aided by removing the uterine fundus through the abdominal incision. Delivery of the fundus also facilitates uterine massage. Oxytocin is administered via an IV line. It is recommended that 20 U of oxytocin be placed into a 1-liter bag of IV fluid, with care taken not to run the fluids at a rate of more than 200 mL/hr in most cases. The uterine incision is closed using an interlocking suture of 1-0 Vicryl or a chromic suture. A second imbricating layer may be used to achieve hemostasis. After the uterus incision is reapproximated and completed, care is taken to investigate for bleeding. The abdomen may be irrigated if there is spillage of meconium or vernix outside the operative field. There is no need to reapproximate the peritoneum or rectus muscles. The abdominal wall is closed in the usual fashion with absorbable suture.

It is possible that the surgeon may be called to assist a patient with postpartum hemorrhage. Therefore, it is important to recognize factors that may be unique to pregnancy. As noted at the beginning of the chapter, blood volume is increased during pregnancy. Hemorrhage in pregnancy is defined as blood loss in excess of 1000 mL. Because of the increase in blood volume by term, however, the patient may lose 1500 to 2000 mL of blood before symptoms are manifest. The most common cause of postpartum hemorrhage is uterine atony. Risk factors for uterine atony include prolonged labor, uterine infection, cesarean birth, and overdistention of the uterus. Hemorrhage can also be seen in abruption of the placenta and in patients with placenta previa, before or after delivery. It is recommended that therapy be initiated after the loss of 600 mL.[15,17]

The first step is to assess for vaginal, cervical, or uterine lacerations. If negative, and uterine atony is the mechanism, manual exploration of the uterus is initiated to ensure complete removal of the placenta and aggressive fundal massage begun. If this is unsuccessful, the administration of a solution of oxytocin, 20 U/liter of physiologic saline solution at a rate of 200 mL/hr, may assist with uterine contractility. A rate of as high as 500 mL in 10 minutes can be administered without significant cardiovascular complications; however, maternal hypotension may occur with an IV bolus injection of as low as 5 U.

When oxytocin fails to provide an adequate response, a synthetic 15-methyl-$F_{2\alpha}$ prostaglandin (carboprost) is administered IM or in the uterine wall. In addition, methylergonovine maleate (Methergine), 0.2 mg given IM, may be administered. Methergine is contraindicated in patients with hypertension. Prostaglandin $F_{2\alpha}$ is contraindicated in patients with asthma. Misoprostol (Cytotec) also has uterotonic properties and can be used at a dose of 1000 μg per rectum.

When pharmacologic measures fail to control hemorrhage, surgical measures are undertaken. If the hemorrhage is secondary to uterine atony, ligation of the uterine vessels may be successful. The first step in ligating the uterine arteries is at the anastomosis of the uterine and ovarian artery high on the fundus, just below the utero-ovarian ligament. A large suture on the atraumatic needle can be passed from the uterus around the vessel and tied. If bilateral utero-ovarian vessel ligation does not stop the bleeding, temporary atraumatic occlusion of the ovarian arteries in the infundibulopelvic ligaments may be attempted. By decreasing perfusion pressure, thrombosis in the vascular bed may produce hemostasis.

If conservative measures are unsuccessful, a cesarean hysterectomy may need to be performed before sequelae of coagulopathy and hemorrhagic shock occur. In the case of postpartum hemorrhage, supracervical hysterectomy is often the procedure of choice. As for the gynecologic hysterectomy described earlier, the superior attachments of the uterus are separated but, following ligation of the uterine arteries, the fundus of the uterus is amputated from the cervix, which is closed with figure-of-eight sutures. This procedure also maintains the integrity of the uterosacral ligaments.

It is difficult to remove the cervix, especially after a vaginal delivery secondary to dilation of the lower uterine segment. Only surgeons who are skilled in this procedure can proceed without consultation.

### Other Procedures

On rare occasions, the surgeon may be consulted to assist with the repair of an episiotomy and extension. Episiotomy is an incision into the perineal body made to help facilitate delivery. Most episiotomies are cut in the midline from the posterior fourchette toward the rectum. Although more comfortable for the patient, these incisions may extend through the anal sphincter (third degree) or through the rectal wall (fourth degree). An inappropriate repair may result in a rectovaginal fistula. These fistulas present with the same symptoms as those seen in other rectal fistulas associated with Crohn's disease but are much easier to repair and have a lower rate of recurrence.

Repair of an episiotomy requires reapproximation of the vaginal tissue and perineal body. Repair of the anal sphincter requires that the fascial capsule that usually retracts posteriorly be identified and reapproximated. If the rectal wall has been compromised, a multilayer closure of mucosa, muscularis, rectovaginal fascia, anal sphincter, vaginal muscularis, and vaginal mucosa using 2-0 or 3-0 absorbable sutures will provide the best opportunity to avoid a fistula. Because of the increased vascularity associated with pregnancy, with an adequate closure without stitch-induced tissue necrosis, healing is not usually a problem.

## ACKNOWLEDGMENT

This chapter is a revision of the chapter written by Stephen S. Entman, Cornelia R. Graves, Barry K. Jarnagin, and Gautam G. Rao for the 18th edition of *Sabiston Textbook of Surgery*. I gratefully acknowledge their contribution and am honored to build on their work.

## SELECTED REFERENCES

Baggish MS, Karram MM, editors: Atlas of pelvic anatomy and gynecologic surgery, ed 3, Philadelphia, 2011, WB Saunders.

Detailed pelvic anatomy and comprehensive coverage of gynecologic procedures with excellent illustrations are presented.

Edge SB, Byrd DR, Compton CC, et al: AJCC cancer staging handbook, ed 7, Philadelphia, 2010, Springer.

Comprehensive staging handbook for gynecologic and other cancers.

Fritz MA, Speroff L: Clinical gynecologic endocrinology and infertility, ed 8, Philadelphia, 2011, Lippincott Williams & Wilkins.

This is the classic text that explains the pathophysiology and endocrinology of menstrual abnormalities in practical clinical terms.

Hacker NF, Gambone JC, Hobel CJ, editors: Hacker and Moore's essential of obstetrics and gynecology, ed 5, Philadelphia, 2010, WB Saunders.

Excellent coverage of obstetrics and gynecology, with color illustrations and photographs.

Rock JA, Jones HWJ, III, editors: TeLinde's operative gynecology, ed 10, Philadephia, 2003, Lippincott Williams & Wilkins.

Encyclopedic coverage addresses all areas of gynecologic surgery, with an expanded oncology section.

## REFERENCES

1. Espindola D, Kennedy KA, Fischer EG: Management of abnormal uterine bleeding and the pathology of endometrial hyperplasia. Obstet Gynecol Clin North Am 34:717–737, 2007.
2. Goldstein SR: Abnormal uterine bleeding: The role of ultrasound. Radiol Clin North Am 44:901–910, 2006.
3. Dimitraki M, Tsikouras P, Bouchlariotou S, et al: Clinical evaluation of women with PMB. Is it always necessary an endometrial biopsy to be performed? A review of the literature. Arch Gynecol Obstet 283:261–266, 2011.
4. Barnhart KT: Clinical practice. Ectopic pregnancy. N Engl J Med 361:379–387, 2009.
5. Ehrenberg-Buchner S, Sandadi S, Moawad NS, et al: Ectopic pregnancy: Role of laparoscopic treatment. Clin Obstet Gynecol 52:372–379, 2009.
6. Wølner-Hanssen P, Mårdh PA, Svensson L, Weström L: Laparoscopy in women with chlamydial infection and pelvic pain: A comparison of patients with and without salpingitis. Obstet Gynecol 61:299–303, 1983.
7. Jonsdottir GM, Jorgensen S, Cohen SL, et al: Increasing minimally invasive hysterectomy: Effect on cost and complications. Obstet Gynecol 117:1142–1149, 2011.
8. Subramaniam A, Kim KH, Bryant SA, et al: A cohort study evaluating robotic versus laparotomy surgical outcomes of obese women with endometrial carcinoma. Gynecol Oncol 122:604–607, 2011.
9. Paley PJ, Veljovich DS, Shah CA, et al: Surgical outcomes in gynecologic oncology in the era of robotics: Analysis of first 1000 cases. Am J Obstet Gynecol 204:551, e1-e9, 2011.
10. Guzel AI, Kuyumcuoglu U, Erdemoglu M: Adnexal masses in postmenopausal and reproductive age women. J Exp Ther Oncol 9:167–169, 2011.
11. Liu JH, Zanotti KM: Management of the adnexal mass. Obstet Gynecol 117:1413–1428, 2011.
12. Gad MS, El Khouly NI, Soto E, et al: Differences in perioperative outcomes after laparoscopic management of benign and malignant adnexal masses. J Gynecol Oncol 22:18–24, 2011.
13. Perutelli A, Garibaldi S, Basile S, et al: Laparoscopic adnexectomy of suspect ovarian masses: Surgical technique used to avert spillage. J Minim Invasive Gynecol 18:372–377, 2011.
14. 13. Eskander RN, Bristow RE, Saenz NC, et al: A retrospective review of the effect of surgeon specialty on the management of 190 benign and malignant pediatric and adolescent adnexal masses. J Pediatr Adolesc Gynecol 24:282–285, 2011.
15. Hull AD, Resnik R: Placenta accreta and postpartum hemorrhage. Clin Obstet Gynecol 53:228–236, 2010.
16. Hoover K, Jenkins TR: Evaluation and management of adnexal mass in pregnancy. Am J Obstet Gynecol 2011.
17. Gonsalves M, Belli A: The role of interventional radiology in obstetric hemorrhage. Cardiovasc Intervent Radiol 33:887–895, 2010.

CHAPTER 72

# SURGERY IN THE PREGNANT PATIENT

Dean J. Mikami, Paul R. Beery, and E. Christopher Ellison

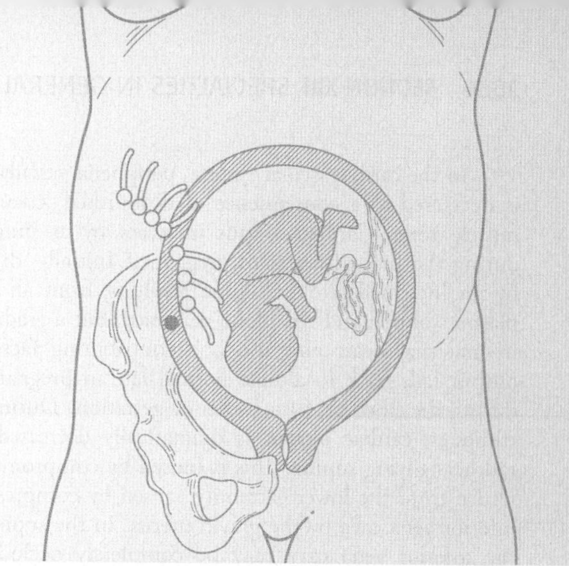



The pregnant patient presents a unique clinical challenge. An estimated 1% to 2% of pregnant women require surgical procedures, with nonobstetric surgery necessary in up to 1% of pregnancies in the United States each year. In a review of 44 papers and 12,452 patients, the effects of nonobstetric surgical procedures on maternal and fetal outcomes were studied; a maternal death rate of 0.006% and a miscarriage rate of 5.8% were reported. Most indications for surgical intervention are common for the patient's age group and unrelated to pregnancy, such as acute appendicitis, symptomatic cholelithiasis, breast masses, or trauma. Changes in maternal anatomy and physiology and safety of the fetus are among the issues of which the surgeon must be cognizant. The presentation of surgical diseases in the pregnant patient may be atypical or may mimic signs and symptoms associated with a normal pregnancy, and a standard evaluation may be unreliable because of pregnancy-associated changes in diagnostic tests or laboratory test results. Finally, many physicians may be more conservative in regard to diagnostic evaluation and treatment. Any of these factors may result in a delay in diagnosis and treatment, adversely affecting maternal and fetal outcome. Although consultation with an obstetrician is ideal when caring for a pregnant patient, the surgeon needs to be aware of certain fundamental principles when this resource is unavailable. This chapter discusses key points when caring for the pregnant patient who presents with nonobstetric surgical disorders.

## PHYSIOLOGIC CHANGES OF PREGNANCY

Progesterone and estrogen, two of the principal hormones of pregnancy, mediate many of the maternal physiologic changes in pregnancy. Normal laboratory values differ in the gravid compared with the nonpregnant patient. The diaphragm can be elevated in pregnancy up to 4 cm and the lower chest wall can widen up to 7 cm.[1] These changes may also mimic similar pathophysiology that occurs in nonpregnant women who have cardiac or liver disease. Elevated progesterone levels, as well as decreased serum motilin, result in smooth muscle relaxation, producing multiple effects on several organ systems. In the stomach, this decreased smooth muscle tone results in diminished gastric tone and motility. The lower esophageal sphincter tone is also decreased and, when combined with increased intra-abdominal pressure, results in an increase in the incidence of gastroesophageal reflux. Small bowel motility is reduced, increasing small bowel transit time. Absorption of nutrients, however, remains unchanged, with the exception of iron absorption, which is increased because of increased iron requirements. In the colon, pregnancy-related changes usually manifest as constipation. This is caused by a combination of increased colonic sodium and water absorption, decreased motility, and mechanical obstruction by the gravid uterus. An increase in portal venous pressure, and therefore an increase in the pressure in the collateral venous circulation, results in dilation of the veins at the gastroesophageal junction. This is of importance only if the patient had esophageal varices before becoming pregnant. The most common result of the increased portal venous pressure is dilation of the hemorrhoidal veins, leading to the well-known complaint of hemorrhoids.

In addition to alterations in smooth muscle tone and motility, other notable changes occur in the gastrointestinal tract. The function of the gallbladder is altered, as is the chemical composition of bile. During the second and third trimesters, the volume of the gallbladder may be twice that found in the nonpregnant state, and gallbladder emptying is markedly slower. Up to 4% of pregnant patients have gallstones on routine obstetric ultrasound.[2] Still, only 1 of every 1000 pregnant patients develops symptoms. It is unknown whether the increased biliary stasis, changes in bile composition, or combination of these two factors results in an increased risk for gallstone formation, but the risk for developing gallstones increases with multiparity. However, the incidence of symptomatic cholelithiasis during pregnancy is similar to the incidence in age-related nonpregnant women.

Some of the changes of pregnancy closely resemble those of liver disease. These include spider angiomas and palmar erythema from elevated serum estrogen levels. Hypoalbuminemia is also seen, along with elevated serum cholesterol, alkaline phosphatase, and fibrinogen levels. Serum bilirubin and hepatic transaminase levels remain unchanged during pregnancy.

In the cardiovascular system, peripheral vascular resistance is decreased as a consequence of diminished vascular smooth muscle tone. Cardiac output increases by as much as 50% during the first trimester of pregnancy. Initially, this is caused by an increased stroke volume resulting from an increase in plasma volume and red blood cell mass, but a gradual increase in maternal heart rate also is a contributing factor. Cardiac output falls back to almost normal late in pregnancy, usually during the 36th to 40th weeks of gestation. During the third trimester, cardiac output is dramatically decreased when the mother is lying supine. This is caused by compromised venous return from the lower extremity caused by compression of the inferior vena cava by the gravid uterus. In the supine position, the inferior vena cava may be completely occluded; venous drainage of the lower extremities is through collateral channels. With this drop in preload, an increase in sympathetic tone usually maintains peripheral vascular resistance and blood pressure. However, up to 10% of patients may experience supine hypotensive syndrome, in which the sympathetic response is not adequate to maintain blood pressure. During anesthesia induction in the operating room, anesthetic agents may inhibit the compensatory sympathetic response, causing a more precipitous fall in blood pressure. From a surgeon's perspective, it may be necessary to place the patient in the left lateral decubitus position during procedures performed during the third trimester, relieving caval compression by the enlarged uterus.

Inguinal swelling secondary to varicosities of the round ligament is also a phenomenon that occurs during pregnancy. The increase in swelling is a result of hormonal and mechanical changes. It is often mistaken for an inguinal or femoral hernia. Appropriate treatment includes careful physical examination and ultrasound if needed. The varicosities generally resolve postpartum.

Oxygen consumption increases during pregnancy. Minute ventilation increases by 50% because of an increase in tidal volume, which appears to be a result of an elevated serum progesterone level.[1] Progesterone not only increases the sensitivity of the respiratory centers to $CO_2$ but also acts as a direct stimulant to the respiratory centers. As a consequence of the increased minute ventilation, the maternal $PaO_2$ level during late pregnancy ranges from 104 to 108 mm Hg and the maternal $PaCO_2$ level ranges from 27 to 32 mm Hg. Renal compensation maintains a normal maternal pH. The decreased $PaCO_2$ level increases the $CO_2$ gradient from the fetus to the mother, facilitating $CO_2$ transfer from the fetus to the mother. The oxygen-hemoglobin dissociation curve of maternal blood is shifted to the right; this, coupled with the increased affinity of fetal hemoglobin for oxygen, results in increased oxygen transfer to the fetus. Elevation of the diaphragm by as much as 4 cm results in a decrease in total lung volume by 5%. Diminished expiratory reserve volume and residual volume result in a functional residual capacity that is 20% lower than that in the nonpregnant woman. Vital capacity and inspiratory reserve volume remain stable.

In the kidney, there is an increase in the glomerular filtration rate by 50% that accompanies a 75% increase in renal plasma flow. Urinary glucose excretion increases as a direct consequence of the increased glomerular filtration rate. The blood urea nitrogen level decreases by 25% during the first trimester and is maintained at that level for the remainder of the pregnancy. The serum creatinine level also decreases by the end of the first trimester from a nonpregnant value of 0.8 to 0.7 mg/dL and may be as low as 0.5 mg/dL by term. A five- to tenfold increase in the serum renin level occurs, with a subsequent four- to fivefold increase in the angiotensin level. Although the pregnant patient is apparently less sensitive to the hypertensive effects of the increased angiotensin, elevated aldosterone levels result in an increase in sodium reabsorption, overcoming the natriuresis produced by elevated progesterone levels. Serum sodium levels are decreased, however, because the increase in sodium reabsorption is less than the increase in plasma volume. Serum osmolality is decreased to 270 to 280 mOsm/kg.[1]

The increase in plasma volume and red blood cell mass is accompanied by a progressive rise in the leukocyte count during pregnancy. During the first trimester, the white blood cell count ranges from 3,000 to 15,000 cells/$mm^3$, increasing to a range of 6,000 to 16,000 cells/$mm^3$ during the second and third trimesters.[1] The platelet count progressively declines throughout pregnancy, whereas the mean platelet volume tends to increase after 28 weeks' gestation. As noted, fibrinogen levels are elevated to a range of 400 to 500 mg/dL. Plasma levels of factors VII, VIII, IX, and X also rise progressively, whereas levels of factors XI and XIII decline, and levels of factors II, V, and XII remain unchanged. Despite these alterations in the coagulation cascade and platelet count, bleeding and clotting times are unchanged.

## SAFETY CONCERNS IN PREGNANCY

### Radiologic Concerns

Radiographic studies remain useful diagnostic tools for the pregnant patient. Of greatest concern with radiation exposure is the risk to the fetus from the exposure. The accepted maximum dose of ionizing radiation during the entire pregnancy is 5 cGy. The fetus is at the highest risk from radiation exposure from the preimplantation period to approximately 15 weeks' gestation. Primary organogenesis occurs during this time and the teratogenic effects of radiation, particularly to the developing central nervous system, are at their highest. Perinatal radiation exposure has also been associated with childhood leukemia and certain childhood malignancies. The radiation dose that has been associated with congenital malformation is higher than 10 cGy. As shown in Table 72-1, radiation exposure to the fetus with the doses from the more common radiology procedures is well below that threshold. Nonetheless, prudence on the part of the clinician is required to avoid unnecessary fetal exposure to ionizing

**Table 72-1 Fetal Radiation Exposure With Radiographic Imaging**

| EXAMINATION TYPE | ESTIMATED FETAL RADIATION EXPOSURE (cGy) |
|---|---|
| Two-view chest radiography | 0.00007 |
| Cervical spine radiography | 0.002 |
| Pelvis radiography | 0.04 |
| Head CT | <0.050 |
| Abdomen CT | 2.60 |
| Upper GI series | 0.056 |
| Barium enema | 3.986 |
| Hepatobiliary (HIDA) scanning | 0.150 |

*GI,* Gastrointestinal; *HIDA,* hepatobiliary iminodiacetic acid.

radiation, especially during the first and early second trimesters, when the risk from exposure is greatest.

Magnetic resonance imaging (MRI) avoids exposure to ionizing radiation but poses an unknown risk to the fetus. Animal studies have shown no teratogenic effect or increased incidence of fetal death or congenital malformations from the electromagnetic radiation, static magnetic field, radiofrequency magnetic fields, or IV contrast agents used during MRI. Theoretically, the gradient magnetic fields may produce electric currents in the patient and the high-frequency currents induced by radiofrequency fields may cause local generation of heat. The long-term effect of exposure is not known.[3] The National Radiological Protection Board has advised against the use of MRI during the first trimester of pregnancy.

Contrast media may be administered with various techniques of body imaging. If computed tomography (CT) has been performed during pregnancy with iodide contrast, neonatal thyroid function should be checked during the first week after delivery. No effect on the fetus has been observed after the use of gadolinium contrast medium with MRI.

Ultrasonography is routinely used by obstetricians during pregnancy. Although tissue heating and cavitation are theoretical effects of ultrasound exposure, such effects have never been reported. Ultrasound may be a helpful alternative diagnostic tool when trying to avoid exposure to ionizing radiation, but does have some limitations. Deeper structures are difficult to visualize and may be obscured by superficial structures that are more echodense. Ultrasound imaging has a limited field of view and is highly operator-dependent. Despite these limitations, certain disease processes, such as a palpable breast mass or suspected appendicitis, may be evaluated effectively and safely.

## Medication Concerns

The surgeon will on occasion need to prescribe medications to treat the pregnant patient with surgical disease. In this section, we provide an overview of medications that the surgeon may commonly prescribe. The list is by no means comprehensive and, prior to using any medication, consultation with the patient's obstetrician is necessary.

The U.S. Food and Drug Administration (FDA) ranks the following as the least harmful classes of drugs during pregnancy:

Category A: These drugs have been tested and found to be safe during pregnancy. Category A includes drugs such as folic acid, vitamin B6, and some thyroid medicines in prescribed doses.

Category B: These drugs are frequently used during pregnancy and do not appear to cause major birth defects or other problems. Category B includes some antibiotics, prednisone, insulin, acetaminophen (Tylenol), aspartame (Equal, NutraSweet), famotidine (Pepcid), and ibuprofen (Advil, Motrin) before the third trimester. Pregnant women should not take ibuprofen during the last 3 months of pregnancy.

The FDA offers the following classifications for prescription drugs that should not be taken during pregnancy:

Category C: These are drugs that are more likely to cause problems for the mother or fetus, and drugs for which safety studies have not been finished. Most of these drugs do not have safety studies in progress. These drugs often come with a warning that they should be used only if the benefits of taking them outweigh the risks. This is something the surgeon would need to discuss with the patient's obstetrician. These drugs include prochlorperazine (Compazine), pseudoephedrine (Sudafed), fluconazole (Diflucan), and ciprofloxacin (Cipro). Some antidepressants are also included in this group.

Category D: These include drugs that have clear health risks for the fetus and include alcohol, lithium, phenytoin (Dilantin), and most forms of chemotherapy. In some cases, chemotherapy is given during pregnancy.

Category X: These drugs have been shown to cause birth defects and should never be taken during pregnancy. These include drugs to treat skin conditions such as cystic acne (isotretinoin [Accutane]) and psoriasis (etretinate [Tegison], acitretin [Soriatane]), thalidomide (sedative), and diethylstilbestrol (DES; prevents miscarriage) that was used up until 1971 in the United States and until 1983 in Europe.

### Analgesics

**Over-the-Counter Medications** Acetaminophen, the active ingredient in Tylenol, is considered safe during pregnancy. Well researched by scientists, acetaminophen is used primarily for headaches, fever, aches, pains, and sore throat. It can be used during all three trimesters of pregnancy.

Nonsteroidal anti-inflammatory drugs (NSAIDs) include aspirin and ibuprofen (Advil, Motrin) and naproxen (Aleve). Aspirin, which contains salicylic acid as its active ingredient, should not be taken by expectant mothers because it can cause problems for the mother and fetus. Also, if aspirin is taken 1 or 2 days before delivery, it can lead to heavy bleeding during labor. There are occasions when aspirin may be prescribed for women who have certain other medical problems (e.g., preeclampsia, for risk of blood clots). Ibuprofen and naproxen are safer options, but both should be used with caution during pregnancy. They are considered safe in the first two trimesters but are ill-advised in the final 3 months because they can also increase bleeding during delivery.

**Prescription Drugs** Prescription analgesics are available in several different forms and brand names, including codeine, oxycodone (OxyContin), oxycodone and acetaminophen (Percocet), morphine (Roxanol), meperidine (Demerol), fentanyl (Duragesic) and hydrocodone and acetaminophen (Vicodin). These drugs may be used occasionally in pregnant patients when the benefits of the drug outweigh the potential risks.

However, there is no known safe level of narcotic use during pregnancy. Risks to the fetus include miscarriage, stillbirth, and premature delivery. At birth, the baby is also at increased risk of low birth weight (i.e., <5.5 pounds), breathing difficulties, and extreme drowsiness, which can lead to feeding problems.

### Antibiotics

Antibiotics may be necessary to treat various surgery-related illnesses in pregnancy. These are listed by class.

#### Aminoglycosides

***Gentamicin*** No epidemiologic studies of congenital anomalies have been conducted in infants whose mothers were treated with gentamicin during pregnancy. However, nephrotoxicity has been observed in many patients receiving gentamicin, which raises the concern of whether fetal kidney damage may occur with maternal treatment. Although fetal renal damage after maternal gentamicin treatment has not been documented, there have been cases of severe neonatal nephropathy after therapy with this drug. Furthermore, because gentamicin is an aminoglycoside, maternal treatment with this drug may be associated with an increased risk for fetal auditory nerve damage, similar to the possible risks associated with streptomycin exposure. It is important to note, however, that although these theoretical risks cannot be excluded, no studies to date have demonstrated these findings with gentamicin treatment in humans.

***Neomycin*** No increased frequency of malformations was found on investigation of pregnant patients treated with this antibiotic. Although neomycin is similar to related antibiotics such as gentamicin in that ototoxicity is a clearly defined side effect, no reports have been noted that demonstrate neomycin ototoxicity in infants who were exposed in utero.

**Polymyxins: Polymyxin B** No epidemiologic studies of infants who were exposed in utero to polymyxin B have been reported. One retrospective study found no adverse effects associated with the use of polymyxin B during pregnancy. However, these data are not sufficient to estimate the safety of using this compound during pregnancy, and therefore this drug has an undetermined risk for use during pregnancy.

**Tetracyclines** Administration of tetracyclines, including doxycycline, tetracycline, and minocycline, during the second or third trimester of pregnancy can cause staining of the teeth of the childhood. Up to a 40% depression of bone growth (especially of the fibula in preterm pregnancies) can occur following in utero exposure to doxycycline.

No epidemiologic studies have been reported of infants exposed in utero to doxycycline. Therefore, a small risk cannot be excluded, but there is no indication that there is an increased risk of malformations in the children of women treated with this agent during pregnancy. Although data on the specific safety of the use of doxycycline during pregnancy are limited, it is assumed that the risks of the dental staining and depression of bone growth that pertain to tetracyclines in general also pertain to doxycycline use during the second and third trimesters.

**5-Nitromidazoles: Metronidazole** Rare reports and studies have shown no consistent pattern of congenital malformations in infants exposed to metronidazole in utero. Given the limited information available, and no conclusive human studies, there is probably no increased risk of birth defects caused by exposure to metronidazole during pregnancy.

**Penicillins** Penicillins are a widely used group of antibiotics that include ampicillin, amoxicillin, azlocillin, mezlocillin, penicillin G, penicillin V, piperacillin, and ticarcillin. Although penicillins accumulate in amniotic fluid in large amounts during maternal ingestion, no adverse fetal effects have been associated with this group of medications. It must be noted that all penicillins may produce anaphylaxis during pregnancy or immediately after delivery. If anaphylaxis is severe and uncontrolled, it could result in compromising placental circulation and cause fetal damage or death. However, in general, the penicillins have not been shown to be teratogenic in humans, and there have been no recognized adverse effects caused by exposure to these drugs.

**Cephalosporins** Cephalosporins are the most widely used class of antibiotics. Based on their spectrum of activity against gram-negative bacteria, they are classified into three generations. Many of the first- and second-generation cephalosporins have been studied extensively in pregnant patients. Although there are limited data available at this time, it is thought that most of them are not associated with any known or suspected teratogenic effects and are assumed safe for use during pregnancy The third-generation cephalosporins, however, have not been used extensively during pregnancy and therefore there is little information known about their effects.

**Macrolides**

***Erythromycin*** No increase in the frequency of congenital anomalies was observed among children of women treated with erythromycin at any time during pregnancy. The estolate ester of erythromycin has been associated with a relatively high incidence of subclinical reversible hepatotoxicity when used during pregnancy.

***Clarithromycin*** Clarithromycin is structurally similar to erythromycin. Currently, there have been no epidemiologic studies of congenital anomalies conducted on infants who were exposed to this antibiotic in utero. Animal studies have reported adverse effects such as cardiovascular abnormalities, cleft palate, fetal growth retardation, and embryonic loss. Although these findings occurred when the animal was given doses much higher than the typical therapeutic dose for humans, these reports stand in sharp contrast to the minimal effects reported in animal studies in which erythromycin was given during pregnancy. Therefore, these data suggest that clarithromycin may be more toxic during development than its parent compound, erythromycin.

**Sulfonamides** A recent study found an association between sulfonamides and rare birth defects. Although there is no direct proof that these antibiotics cause birth defects, additional research is needed. In the meantime, physicians should be cautious about prescribing these medications during pregnancy.

**Quinolones**

***Ciprofloxacin*** The use of ciprofloxacin during human gestation does not appear to be associated with an increased risk of major congenital malformations. Although a number of birth defects have occurred in the offspring of women who had taken this drug during pregnancy, the lack of a pattern among the anomalies is reassuring. In addition, a meta-analysis has shown that the use of quinolones during the first trimester of pregnancy does not appear to represent an increased risk for major malformations after birth, stillbirths, preterm births, or low birth weight.[4]

However, a causal relationship with some of the birth defects cannot be fully excluded. Because of this and available animal data, the use of ciprofloxacin during pregnancy, especially during the first trimester. should be avoided if an acceptable alternative is available. A review on the safety of quinolones has concluded that these antibacterials should be avoided during pregnancy because of the difficulty in extrapolating animal mutagenicity results to humans and because interpretation of this toxicity is still controversial. Others have also concluded that fluoroquinolones should be considered contraindicated in pregnancy because safer alternatives are usually available

**Summary of Antibiotic Use** Although antibiotics are commonly prescribed to pregnant women, details relating to the effects of many of these drugs remains poorly understood. If an antibiotic must be prescribed, it is important to be aware of the effects these drugs can have on pregnancies and to prescribe the most suitable agent with the least risk to the pregnancy.

### Sedatives

#### Benzodiazepines

***Diazepam*** The use of benzodiazepines, specifically diazepam, was previously thought to be associated with an increased frequency of cleft lip and/or palate; this finding has not been supported by most recent studies. Although the balance of evidence from human studies of the benzodiazepines (chiefly diazepam) does not show first-trimester usage to be teratogenic, the surgeon should check with the patient's obstetrician before administering this class of drugs.

***Midazolam*** Midazolam is generally considered unsafe for use during pregnancy. Midazolam was given a pregnancy category D rating by the FDA because it is a benzodiazepine and other benzodiazepines have been shown to cause birth defects and other problems. However, studies of midazolam in pregnant rabbits and rats did not show any problems.

## Anesthesia Concerns

Anesthesia concerns during pregnancy include the safety of the mother and fetus. The fetus may be affected by exposure to teratogenic effects of anesthetic agents, risk for preterm labor, and risk from changes in maternal physiology as a consequence of anesthesia. Changes in uterine blood flow and maternal acid-base status may cause hypoxemia or asphyxia in the fetus. These can be a result of maternal hypotension or hypoxia, maternal hyperventilation, or placental passage of anesthetic agents that affect the fetal central nervous or cardiovascular system.

The effects of anesthesia during pregnancy can be divided into direct, or active, and indirect, or passive, effects. The direct effects relate to the possible teratogenic or embryotoxic properties of the drugs used for anesthesia, some of which cross the placenta. The indirect effects are those mechanisms whereby an anesthetic agent or surgical procedure may interfere with maternal or fetal physiology and, in doing so, harm the fetus. For the most part, the fetus experiences indirect effects as a consequence of anesthetic agents administered to the mother and hemodynamic changes in the mother from blood loss or anesthetic agents. The most profound effects on the fetus are related to decreased uterine blood flow or decreased oxygen content of uterine blood. Unlike circulation to other vital organs, most notably the brain, the uterine circulation is not autoregulated. During the third trimester, uterine circulation represents almost 10% of cardiac output. When treating maternal hypotension, vasopressors such as dopamine and epinephrine, although increasing the maternal systemic pressure, have little or no effect on uterine circulation. Phenylephrine and metaraminol are alpha agonists that are effective in maintaining maternal blood pressure and preventing fetal acidosis.[5] Other maneuvers, such as fluid bolus, Trendelenburg position, compression stockings, and leg elevation, have a larger impact on increasing uterine blood flow.

In addition to the risks related to maternal hypoxia or hypotension, the risk for spontaneous abortion and teratogenesis related to anesthetic agents is of major concern. Many nonhuman studies have demonstrated different teratogenic effects with similar agents but have not led to definitive conclusions regarding their teratogenic potential in humans. For a congenital defect to result, exposure to the teratogen must occur during the vulnerable differentiation stage of the affected organ system. As noted, differentiation of the major organ systems occurs during the first trimester of human embryonic development. Therefore, delaying semielective surgical procedures until after the first trimester may reduce the risk for teratogenicity. However, large survey studies have demonstrated an increased risk for spontaneous abortions, intrauterine growth retardation, and low-birth-weight neonates in women who require surgery during pregnancy. These studies lacked information on the indications for nonobstetric surgical procedures.

Elective surgical procedures are delayed until at least 6 weeks after delivery, when maternal physiology has returned to the nonpregnant state and when the impact on the fetus is no longer a concern. When emergent procedures are required, obviously the life of the mother takes priority, although an experienced anesthesiologist will be able to modify the anesthesia used according to maternal physiology and fetal well-being. For semielective surgical procedures, attempts are made to delay surgery until after the first trimester, whenever possible. This needs to be determined on an individual basis because continued exposure to the underlying disease process may be more harmful than the operative risk to the mother and fetus. During the second trimester, after organ system differentiation has occurred, there is almost no risk for anesthetic-induced malformation or spontaneous abortion. Later in pregnancy, during the third trimester, the risk for preterm delivery is at its highest.

When the pregnant patient requires surgical intervention, consultation with the obstetrician and possibly a perinatologist is essential. The specialist is helpful in determining the optimum technique to monitor fetal status and can assist with perioperative management and diagnose and manage preterm labor. Typically, when emergent surgery occurs during the first or early second trimester, fetal heart tones are monitored before and after anesthesia exposure. During the late second and third trimesters, when the fetus is of viable age, continuous intraoperative monitoring is performed when possible. Transvaginal ultrasound can be used when the surgical field involves the abdomen. Continuous monitoring is used if significant blood loss is possible or anticipated to assess fetal well-being. Checking the fetal heart rate for fetal status and tocometer monitoring for uterine activity are done before and after the procedure, even if intraoperative monitoring is not believed necessary or is unavailable.

Postoperative pain control in the pregnant patient needs to be monitored closely. NSAIDs are not used in pregnancy because of the risk for premature closure of the ductus arteriosis.[6] Morphine and fentanyl are both good IV choices postoperatively. Morphine has a higher associated incidence of nausea and vomiting, but most surgeons have extensive experience with it. A patient-controlled analgesia pump after surgery may be the best choice because of the associated low incidence of maternal respiratory depression and drug transfer to the fetus.

Postoperative oral narcotic use is generally considered safe in pregnancy. Narcotic analgesics have not been found to cause birth defects in humans in normal dosages. Oxycodone, hydrocodone, and codeine are commonly used narcotics and can be safely used in moderation. Chronic use of narcotics during pregnancy may cause fetal dependency. It is recommended that the pregnant postsurgical patient be weaned off narcotic use as soon as possible.

## PREVENTION OF PRETERM LABOR

The incidence of preterm labor associated with nonobstetric surgery is related to gestational age and the indication for surgery. Studies have suggested that the rate of premature labor induced by nonobstetric surgical intervention is 3.5%. Gestational age at treatment and severity of the underlying disease are the most predictive indicators of patients at risk for preterm labor. The later in gestation is the patient, the higher the risk for preterm contractions or preterm labor. Intraperitoneal surgeries and disease processes with intraperitoneal inflammation are the most likely to have a postoperative course complicated by preterm contractions and preterm labor. In a number of studies, a significant difference was found in the number of patients with preterm contractions based on the average time from onset of symptoms to operative intervention. A delay in treatment appears to increase the chance of preterm labor, likely related to the primary disease process. Laparoscopic and open techniques have an equal associated incidence of preterm labor.

There is no general consensus on the use of prophylactic tocolytics after nonobstetric surgery during pregnancy. Tocolytic use varies widely among centers and physicians. Most studies have suggested that tocolytics only be used if contractions are noted during postoperative monitoring or are appreciated by the patient. Tocolytics used as needed are generally successful at preventing preterm labor and preterm delivery when postoperative contractions are detected. Terbutaline, magnesium, and indomethacin (Indocin) have been used in different studies, with equivalent results. Almost 100% of patients with postoperative contractions were successfully given tocolytics and delivered at term. In general, for patients with postoperative contractions before 32 weeks, indomethacin would be a reasonable treatment, whereas terbutaline could be used as first-line treatment for patients at more than 32 weeks' gestation. The use of prophylactic tocolysis is individualized, depending on the patient's gestational age and underlying disease process.

## ABDOMINAL PAIN AND THE ACUTE ABDOMEN IN PREGNANCY

When the pregnant patient presents with abdominal pain, it may be difficult to distinguish a pathophysiologic cause from normal pregnancy-associated symptoms. Changes in the position and orientation of abdominal viscera from the enlarging uterus, and the alterations in physiology already described, may modify the perception or manifestation of an intra-abdominal process. If it is early in the pregnancy, the woman may not know that she is pregnant. Also, some intra-abdominal processes are exclusive to pregnancy, such as ectopic pregnancy, HELLP (***h****emolysis,* ***e****levated* ***l****iver enzymes,* ***l****ow* ***p****latelets*) syndrome, or acute fatty liver of pregnancy. Both patient and physician may attribute the patient's complaints to normal pregnancy, resulting in a delay in evaluation and treatment. These delays in diagnosis and definitive intervention are the most serious adverse events affecting maternal and fetal outcome. It is usually not the treatment but the delay in diagnosis and severity of the primary disease process that affects outcomes poorly. Box 72-1 lists the more common causes of abdominal pain in the pregnant patient, classified according to location.

**BOX 72-1 Common Causes of Abdominal Pain in the Pregnant Patient**

**Right Upper Quadrant**
Gastroesophageal reflux
Peptic ulcer disease
Acute cholecystitis
Biliary colic
Acute pancreatitis
Hepatitis
Acute fatty liver of pregnancy
HELLP syndrome
Preeclampsia
Pneumothorax
Pneumonia
Acute appendicitis
Hepatic adenoma
Hemangioma

**Right Lower Quadrant**
Acute appendicitis
Ectopic pregnancy
Renal or ureteral colic
Pelvic inflammatory disease
Tubo-ovarian abscess
Endometriosis
Adnexal torsion
Ruptured ovarian cyst
Ruptured corpus luteum

**Lower Abdomen**
Threatened, incomplete, or complete abortion
Abruptio placentae
Preterm labor
Pelvic inflammatory disease
Tubo-ovarian abscess
Inflammatory bowel disease
Irritable bowel syndrome
Pyelonephritis

**Flank**
Pyelonephritis
Hydronephrosis of pregnancy
Acute appendicitis (retrocecal appendix)

**Diffuse Abdominal Pain**
Early acute appendicitis
Small bowel obstruction
Acute intermittent porphyria
Sickle cell crisis

## MINIMALLY INVASIVE SURGERY IN PREGNANCY

When laparoscopic techniques were initially described, pregnancy was considered to be a contraindication to laparoscopy. Effects of $CO_2$ pneumoperitoneum on venous return and cardiac output, uterine perfusion, and fetal acid-base status were

**BOX 72-2 Advantages and Disadvantages of Laparoscopy Instead of Laparotomy During Pregnancy**

**Advantages**

Decreased fetal depression secondary to decreased narcotic requirement
Lower rates of wound infections and incisional hernias
Diminished postoperative maternal hypoventilation
Decreased manipulation of the uterus
Faster recovery with early return to normal function
Decreased risk for ileus

**Disadvantages**

Possible uterine injury during trocar placement
Decreased uterine blood flow
Preterm labor risk secondary to increased intra-abdominal pressure
Increased risk of fetal acidosis and unknown effects of $CO_2$ pneumoperitoneum
Decreased visualization with gravid uterus

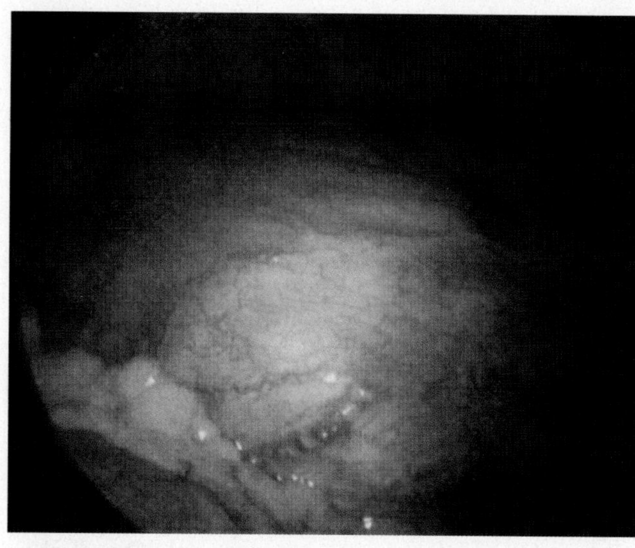

**FIGURE 72-1** Intraoperative image of a 24-week gravid uterus taken with a 5-mm, 30-degree, high-definition camera.

unknown. Laparoscopy was safely used in several series to evaluate pregnant patients for ectopic pregnancy. Patients with an intrauterine pregnancy had no increase in fetal loss or observed negative effect on long-term outcome.[7,8] When comparing laparoscopic and open techniques in nonpregnant patients, patients who underwent laparoscopic procedures had decreased pain, shorter hospital stays, and a quicker return to normal activity.

Major concerns of laparoscopy during pregnancy include injury to the uterus, decreased uterine blood flow, fetal acidosis, and preterm labor from increased intra-abdominal pressure. During the second trimester, the uterus is no longer contained within the pelvis. The open technique for abdominal access can reduce the risk for injury. Using a Veress needle for insufflation or optical trocar can be done safely if the site of initial abdominal access is adjusted according to fundal height and the abdominal wall is elevated. Decreased uterine blood flow from pneumoperitoneum remains a theoretical concern because significant changes in intra-abdominal pressure occur normally during pregnancy with maternal Valsalva maneuvers. The risk for pneumoperitoneum may also be less than the risk for direct uterine manipulation that occurs with laparotomy. Fetal respiratory acidosis with subsequent fetal hypertension and tachycardia have been observed in a pregnant ewe model but were reversed by maintaining maternal respiratory alkalosis.[9] Also, in the largest series comparing laparoscopy and open techniques, no significant differences in preterm labor or delivery-related side effects were observed.[7] Box 72-2 illustrates the general comparison between laparoscopic and open technique.

The Society of American Gastrointestinal Endoscopic Surgeons recommends the following guidelines for laparoscopic surgery during pregnancy[10]:

1. Obstetric consultation is obtained preoperatively.
2. When possible, operative intervention is deferred until the second trimester, when fetal risk is lowest.
3. Pneumoperitoneum enhances lower extremity venous stasis already present in the gravid patient, and pregnancy induces a hypercoagulable state. Therefore, pneumatic compression devices are used whenever possible.
4. Fetal and uterine status, as well as maternal end-tidal $CO_2$ and arterial blood gas levels, need to be monitored.
5. The uterus needs to be protected with a lead shield if intraoperative cholangiography is a possibility. Fluoroscopy is used selectively.
6. Given the enlarged gravid uterus, abdominal access is attained using an open technique.
7. Dependent positioning is used to shift the uterus off the inferior vena cava.
8. Pneumoperitoneum pressures are minimized to 8 to 12 mm Hg and not allowed to exceed 15 mm Hg.

Trocar placement in the pregnant patient does not differ radically from placement in the nonpregnant patient early in pregnancy. Later in pregnancy, the camera port must be placed in a supraumbilical location and the remaining ports are placed under direct camera visualization. The gravid uterus enlarges superiorly (Fig. 72-1); adjustments in trocar placement must be made to avoid uterine injury and improve visualization. An angled endoscope may aid in viewing over or around the uterus. The uterus should be manipulated as little as possible.

## BREAST MASSES IN PREGNANCY

Pregnancy-associated breast cancer is defined as breast cancer diagnosed during pregnancy or within 1 year after pregnancy. It has become increasingly more prominent as more women delay childbearing until they are in their 30s and 40s; the incidence of breast cancer is higher in women in those age groups. Overall, pregnancy-associated breast cancer has been reported to occur in 1 in 3000 pregnancies.[11,12]

Breast cancer is the most common nongynecologic malignancy associated with pregnancy. It usually presents as a painless palpable mass, with or without nipple discharge. Studies have demonstrated that pregnancy-associated breast cancer may be more common in women with a genetic predisposition to breast cancer. In a group of 292 women diagnosed with breast cancer before age 40 years, those with a known *BRCA1* or *BRCA2* gene mutation were more likely to develop cancer during pregnancy.[13] As is true for nonpregnant patients, ductal carcinoma is the most common pathologic type of tumor, accounting for 75% to 90% of breast cancers in pregnant patients.[14]

Delays in diagnosis and treatment are common, although this has improved. Previous studies demonstrated delays in diagnosis of almost 6 months, but more recent data have shown a mean delay of 1 to 2 months. Given a tumor doubling size of 130 days, a delay in diagnosis and treatment of 1 month increases the risk for nodal metastasis by 0.9%, whereas a delay of 6 months increases the risk by 5.1%.[12] Although the initial reports of pregnancy-associated breast cancer more than 100 years ago proposed a dismal prognosis, more recent literature has suggested that this is because of a more advanced stage at the time of diagnosis.[15] When compared with age-matched nonpregnant controls, women with pregnancy-associated breast cancer present with a larger primary tumor and higher risk for positive axillary lymph nodes. However, women with pregnancy-associated breast cancer have a similar stage-related prognosis compared with nonpregnant controls. Overall, these women bear a worse prognosis because of the more advanced disease at presentation. Pregnancy is a hyperestrogenic state and may correlate with rapid tumor proliferation and axillary lymph node metastases,[16] although pregnant women and nonpregnant young women have a higher percentage of estrogen receptor–negative cancers than older women. In a series comparing 75 patients with pregnancy-associated breast cancer and 182 nonpregnant patients with breast cancer, 42% of cancers were estrogen receptor–negative in the pregnant group and 21% were estrogen receptor–negative in the nonpregnant control group.[17] This higher incidence of estrogen receptor–negative cancer is likely caused by a downregulation of estrogen receptors during pregnancy. Physiologic changes of breast engorgement, rapid cellular proliferation, and increased vascularity make a reliable physical examination difficult; masses of similar size that would be easily palpable in the nonpregnant state may be obscured, or palpable masses may be attributed to normal pregnancy-related changes. Benign breast lesions such as galactoceles, mastitis, abscesses, lipomas, fibroadenomas, lobular hyperplasia, and lactational adenomas account for 80% of breast masses that occur during pregnancy or lactation. However, any palpable mass that persists for 4 weeks or longer needs to be evaluated.

Because of the changes in the breast tissue with pregnancy, imaging modality findings may be difficult to interpret. If used with appropriate shielding, mammography carries a limited risk to the fetus. Mammography has a high false-negative rate because of the increased density of the fibroglandular breast tissue, however, so it has limited usefulness in evaluation of the pregnant patient. Ultrasonography can safely be performed as an initial evaluation or in conjunction with mammography. Ultrasound is able to distinguish solid from cystic lesions in 97% of patients and is helpful in guiding fine-needle aspiration (FNA) or biopsy. MRI of the breast is highly sensitive but only moderately specific and has been used more frequently in the nonpregnant patient. Its usefulness in the pregnant patient is yet to be determined. Although MRI does not use ionizing radiation, the two main risks to the fetus from the magnetic field and electromagnetic radiation are heating and cavitation. Gadolinium contrast is listed as a pregnancy category C drug, to be used only if the potential benefit outweighs the potential risk. Gadolinium crosses the placenta and has been associated with fetal abnormalities in rats. With other reliable imaging modalities available, MRI is not currently recommended for breast imaging in the pregnant patient.[2]

Tissue diagnosis is essential. Core needle biopsy, with or without ultrasound guidance, is a safe and reliable method for obtaining tissue. The major risks are hematoma formation and milk fistula development. A pressure dressing is applied following the biopsy to minimize the risk for hematoma from the hypervascularity of the breasts. The risk for milk fistula may be reduced by stopping lactation for several days before biopsy and by emptying the breast of milk just before the procedure. If the biopsy is done postpartum, a 1-week course of bromocriptine may also be given before biopsy. FNA may be a reliable alternative to core needle or open biopsy. It can be performed safely with ultrasound guidance under local anesthesia without exposing the patient and fetus to the risks involved with general anesthesia, but its accuracy is dependent on the pathologist's experience in distinguishing the proliferative changes of pregnancy from those of cancer.

The mainstay of therapy for pregnancy-associated breast cancer is surgical resection. Modified radical mastectomy has long been considered the appropriate choice for local control. It eliminates the need for adjuvant radiation and its risk to the fetus. More recent data have suggested that the combination of local control and adjuvant therapy may be tailored to the patient according to the stage of pregnancy, as well as the stage of the cancer.[15] In stages I and II cancer, mastectomy with axillary dissection is preferred. Axillary dissection is necessary because of the aggressive nature of pregnancy-associated breast cancer and the higher incidence of nodal metastasis. Sentinel node biopsy poses an unknown risk to the fetus and is avoided until the safety of the radioisotope has been determined.

In patients diagnosed during the late second trimester or later, immediate breast-conserving lumpectomy and axillary dissection, followed with radiation postpartum, is a treatment option. If the diagnosis of breast cancer is made in the first or early second trimester of pregnancy, lumpectomy and axillary dissection can be followed by chemotherapy after the first trimester and by radiation after delivery. Chemotherapy is indicated for node-positive cancers or node-negative tumors larger than 1 cm. Current chemotherapeutic regimens are relatively safe after the first trimester, when the teratogenic risk is greatest. The increased plasma volume, hypoalbuminemia, and the fact that almost all chemotherapeutic agents cross the placenta change drug pharmacokinetics and make accurate dosing difficult. Antimetabolites such as methotrexate are avoided because of the high risk for spontaneous abortion, even after the first trimester. Other agents have been associated with congenital malformations and complications such as preterm delivery, low birth weight, hyaline membrane disease, transient leukopenia, transient tachypnea of the newborn, and intrauterine growth retardation, but most of these effects occurred when the chemotherapeutic agent was administered during the first trimester. In one study, 24 patients with pregnancy-associated breast cancer were given a chemotherapeutic regimen during the second and third trimesters that included fluorouracil, cyclophosphamide, and doxorubicin. None of the infants had congenital malformations; the median age at delivery was 38 weeks.[18] Long-term effects of the chemotherapeutic agents used for pregnancy-associated breast cancer on growth and development of children are still not known. Cyclophosphamide and doxorubicin

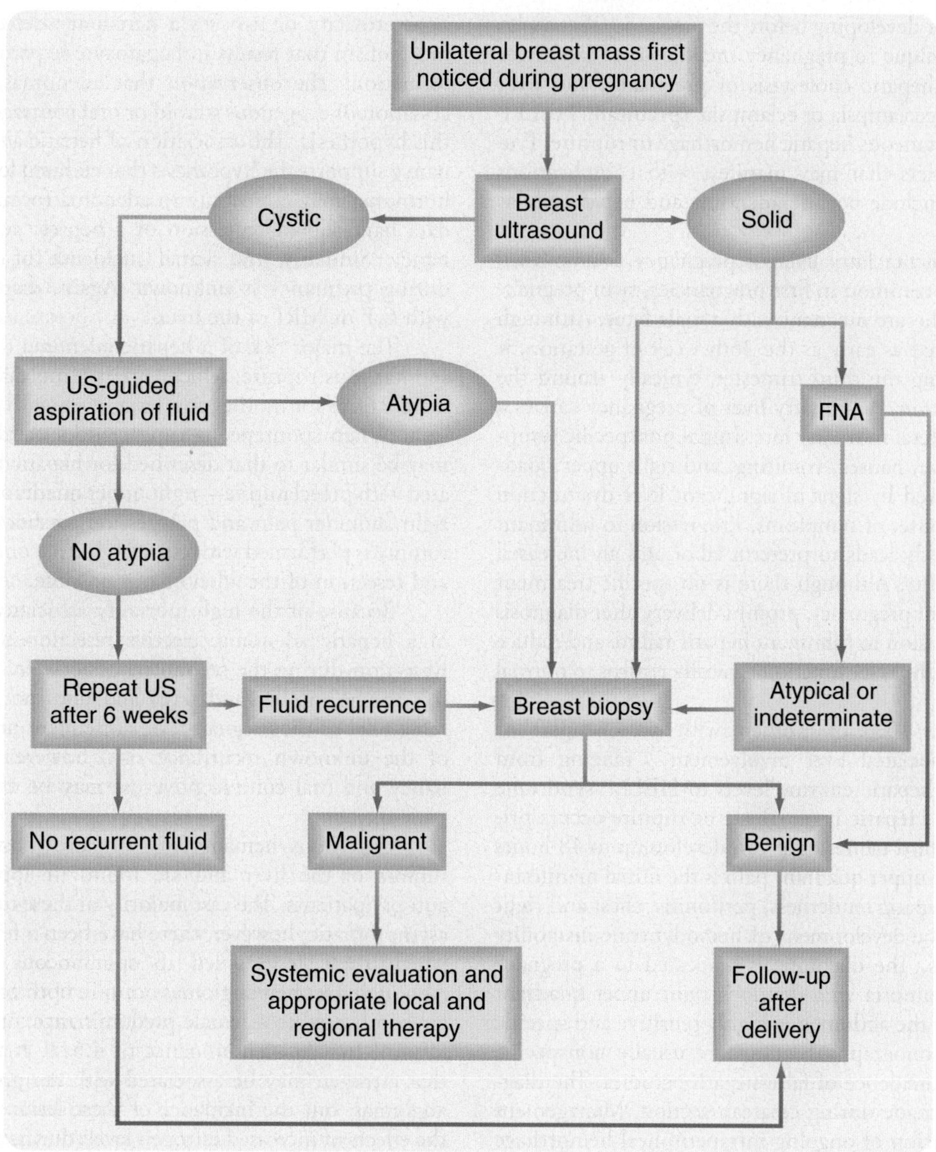


**FIGURE 72-2** Algorithm for the management of a breast mass during pregnancy. *US,* Ultrasound.

can enter breast milk; breastfeeding is contraindicated during chemotherapy.

Radiation is typically not offered during pregnancy because of its teratogenic risk and risk for induction of childhood malignancies. The risk is directly related to dose and developmental stage. During the preimplantation stage and continuing to 15 weeks after conception, during organogenesis, the rapidly proliferating cells of the fetus are most sensitive to radiation, and exposure greater than 1 Gy during this period has a high likelihood of causing fetal death. The standard therapeutic course of 50 Gy results in varying exposure to the fetus, depending on the gestational age and proximity of the gravid uterus to the radiation bed. Even with abdominal shielding, the greatest fetal exposure is caused by scatter. Although there have been several case reports of healthy infants born after maternal radiation exposure, radiation is not recommended during pregnancy because of the risks to the fetus.

Elective termination of the pregnancy to receive appropriate therapy without the risk for fetal malformation is no longer routinely recommended because no improvement in survival has been demonstrated. With the treatment options available to the pregnant patient with breast cancer, a combined approach among the patient, surgeon, oncologist, and maternal-fetal medicine specialist ensures optimal treatment of the disease while minimizing risk to the patient and fetus. A suggested algorithm for the treatment of breast masses in pregnancy is shown in Figure 72-2.

## SURGERY FOR DISEASES IN PREGNANCY

### Hepatobiliary Disease

Liver abnormalities during pregnancy can be classified as occurring exclusively during pregnancy as a direct result of conditions during pregnancy, occurring simultaneously but not exclusively during pregnancy, or developing before the pregnancy. Examples of liver disorders unique to pregnancy include acute fatty liver of pregnancy, intrahepatic cholestasis of pregnancy, and liver disease related to preeclampsia or eclampsia, specifically HELLP syndrome and spontaneous hepatic hemorrhage or rupture. Preexisting liver disorders that may manifest with complications during pregnancy include hepatic adenoma and hepatocellular carcinoma.

The cause of acute fatty liver of pregnancy is unknown, although it is more common in first pregnancies, twin pregnancies, and women who are pregnant with a male fetus. Although it has been diagnosed as early as the 26th week of gestation, it usually occurs during the third trimester, typically around the 35th week of gestation. Acute fatty liver of pregnancy carries a 20% maternal and fetal mortality rate. Initial nonspecific symptoms such as malaise, nausea, vomiting, and right upper quadrant pain are followed by signs of significant liver dysfunction within 2 weeks of onset of symptoms. Progression to fulminant hepatic failure quickly leads to preterm labor and an increased risk for fetal mortality. Although there is no specific treatment for acute fatty liver of pregnancy, prompt delivery after diagnosis may prevent progression to fulminant hepatic failure and reduce the risk for fetal death. Liver function typically returns to normal after delivery.

Approximately 10% of women with preeclampsia or eclampsia have associated liver involvement,[19] ranging from severe elevation of hepatic enzyme levels to HELLP syndrome to hepatic rupture. Hepatic hemorrhage or rupture occurs primarily during the third trimester or can develop up to 48 hours after delivery. Right upper quadrant pain is the initial manifestation, followed by hepatic tenderness, peritonitis, chest and right shoulder pain, or the development of hemodynamic instability within a few hours. The diagnosis is suspected in a pregnant patient with preeclampsia who develops right upper quadrant pain. A CT scan of the abdomen is highly sensitive and specific in diagnosis; ultrasonography findings are usually nonspecific and have a higher incidence of false-negative studies. The diagnosis may also be made during cesarean section. Management depends on a suspicion of ongoing intraperitoneal hemorrhage or vascular instability. Hepatic hematomas without evidence of ongoing bleeding in hemodynamically stable patients may be managed nonoperatively with serial imaging and close monitoring, and these lesions typically heal without intervention. If there is evidence or suspicion of rupture, immediate intervention is required because maternal and fetal mortality rates from hepatic hemorrhage are 60% and 85%; respectively. Immediate laparotomy with abdominal packing or hepatic artery ligation reduces maternal and fetal mortality. Coagulopathy must be corrected aggressively. If the patient is relatively stable or abdominal packing has been unsuccessful in controlling hemorrhage, angiography with selective embolization may be performed. Angiography is most useful when the diagnosis is made postpartum.

Hepatic adenomas are uncommon benign lesions usually associated with oral contraceptive use in young women.[20] Hepatic adenomas are also associated with glycogen storage disease, diabetes, exogenous steroids, and pregnancy. They are usually solitary lesions but may be multifocal, and have a low potential for malignant transformation. Although the specific cause is unknown, it has been hypothesized that a change in hormone levels, specifically of the sex steroids, leads to hepatotoxicity or exposes a hereditary defect in carbohydrate metabolism that results in hepatocyte hyperplasia and adenoma formation. The observation that adenomas may resolve after cessation of exogenous steroid or oral contraceptive use supports this hypothesis. The association of hepatic adenomas with pregnancy supports the hypothesis that elevated levels of endogenous hormones may contribute to adenoma formation, although no data have shown regression of a hepatic adenoma after pregnancy. Similarly, the actual incidence of hepatic adenomas during pregnancy is unknown. Again, diagnosis is best done with CT or MRI of the liver.

The major risk of a hepatic adenoma during pregnancy is spontaneous rupture, which carries a mortality rate of approximately 60% for mother and fetus, even with operative intervention. When spontaneous rupture does occur, the presentation may be similar to that described for hepatic hemorrhage associated with preeclampsia—right upper quadrant pain with referred right shoulder pain and progression to shock. Immediate laparotomy is performed with cesarean birth, control of hemorrhage, and resection of the adenoma, if possible.

Because of the high mortality associated with the rupture of a hepatic adenoma, elective resection may be performed. Resection during the second trimester minimizes the operative risk to the mother and fetus and does not interfere with the remainder of the pregnancy or subsequent pregnancies. Because of the unknown recurrence risk, however, subsequent pregnancy and oral contraceptive use may be discouraged in these patients.

Cavernous hemangiomas are the most common benign tumors of the liver and are found in approximately 2% of autopsy patients. The vast majority of these tumors are small and asymptomatic; however, there have been a few reported cases in which these lesions led to spontaneous fatal hemorrhage. Although liver hemangiomas occur in both genders, most studies have indicated to a female predominance; one study reported a ratio of female predominance of 4.5 : 1. It has been suggested that estrogen may be associated with the growth of liver hemangiomas, but the incidence of these lesions in pregnancy and the effects of increased estrogen levels during pregnancy on them are unknown. Symptomatic liver hemangiomas have been treated by steroids, radiation therapy, surgical resection and, recently embolization, but surgeons may sometimes be confronted with intra-abdominal hemorrhage originating from the rupture of asymptomatic liver hemangiomas. A case of an incidental intra-abdominal hemorrhage originating from a liver hemangioma in a 36-week twin pregnancy being delivered emergently by cesarean section because of fetal distress has been reported.

Cholecystectomy for symptomatic cholelithiasis is second to appendectomy as the most common nonobstetric surgical procedure performed during pregnancy. As noted, pregnancy is associated with an increased incidence of cholelithiasis. Most pregnant women are asymptomatic. Although an estimated 2% to 4% of pregnant women may be found to have gallstones by ultrasound, only 0.05% to 0.1% of them will be symptomatic. The symptoms of biliary colic are the same in pregnant and nonpregnant patients. In patients with symptoms consistent with cholelithiasis, ultrasound is the diagnostic examination of choice. In pregnant patients, ultrasound is as accurate in identifying gallstones and signs of inflammation as in nonpregnant patients.

Historically, pregnant patients with a clear operative indication, such as obstructive jaundice, gallstone pancreatitis, and choledocholithiasis, underwent cholecystectomy regardless of gestational age. Patients with recurrent biliary colic or acute cholecystitis that responded to medical management were treated expectantly until after delivery, at which time they underwent cholecystectomy. As it became understood that adverse maternal and fetal outcomes are related more to the disease process and not the surgical intervention, management patterns have changed.[21] Also, complications from nonoperative management of gallstone disease result in an increase in maternal and fetal mortality. With gallstone pancreatitis during pregnancy, a maternal mortality rate of 15% and a fetal mortality rate of 60% have been reported. In a study of 63 patients who were admitted with symptomatic cholelithiasis, surgical management reduced the need for labor induction, rate of preterm deliveries, and fetal mortality.[22] Therefore, surgical intervention is considered as primary treatment of gallstones in pregnancy.

The timing of cholecystectomy for biliary colic depends on the gestational age and severity of symptoms. A spontaneous abortion rate of 12% with open cholecystectomy during the first trimester falls to 5.6% and 0% during the second and third trimesters, respectively. The risk for preterm labor is almost 0% during the second trimester and 40% during the third trimester.[2] The optimum time for cholecystectomy is the second trimester, when the risks for spontaneous abortion and preterm labor are the lowest, unless the patient develops a complication of cholelithiasis. In a study of 122 patients who were admitted with biliary colic, 69 (56.5%) underwent minimally invasive intervention. Eight patients were treated during the first, 54 during the second, and 7 during the last trimester. There was no fetal morbidity or mortality and only minor maternal morbidity, with no mortality.[23]

Laparoscopic cholecystectomy is relatively safe during the second trimester. The gravid uterus is not usually large enough at this gestational age to interfere with visualization; the uterus also is less likely to be inadvertently instrumented at this size. The open technique using the Hasson trocar is recommended for obtaining access to the abdomen. If intraoperative cholangiography or endoscopic retrograde cholangiopancreatography is indicated for choledocholithiasis, the uterus needs to be protected with appropriate shielding. If the severity of symptoms prevents delaying surgical intervention until after delivery, laparoscopic cholecystectomy can be safely performed during the third trimester, although the risk for preterm labor is substantially increased. In several small series of patients, preterm labor was successfully managed with tocolytics and the patients delivered healthy term infants.[24]

## Endocrine Disease

### Adrenal Disease

Pheochromocytomas originate from chromaffin cells in the adrenal medulla or from extramedullary paraganglion cells. They are hormonally active tumors, secreting the catecholamines norepinephrine, epinephrine and, less commonly, dopamine. Pheochromocytomas are usually described by the rule of 10, which states that 10% of pheochromocytomas are extra-adrenal, 10% are bilateral, 10% are malignant, and 10% are familial. These tumors can occur sporadically or as part of a syndrome, such as multiple endocrine neoplasia (MEN) type 2A, MEN 2B, or von Hippel-Lindau disease.

Although pheochromocytomas are uncommon in pregnancy, they have devastating effects on the mother and fetus. Pheochromocytomas that remain undiagnosed during pregnancy have a postpartum maternal mortality as high as 55%, with fetal mortality also exceeding 50%. The greatest risk occurs from the onset of labor to 48 hours after delivery. The index of suspicion must be high in any patient with preeclampsia, paroxysmal hypertension, or unexplained fever after delivery. With diagnosis and appropriate treatment, the maternal mortality rate is reduced to almost 0% and the fetal mortality rate is decreased to 15%. Diagnosis is made by elevated urine catecholamine levels; urinary catecholamine levels in the pregnant patient without a pheochromocytoma are the same as in the nonpregnant patient. Lack of proteinuria also helps eliminate preeclampsia as a cause of hypertension. Metaiodobenzylguanidine (MIBG) imaging is not recommended during pregnancy because the small molecule may cross the placenta; however, the use of MIBG imaging has not been evaluated in pregnancy.

Surgical resection needs to be performed before 20 weeks' gestation, when spontaneous abortion is less likely and the size of the gravid uterus does not interfere with the procedure. If the diagnosis is made late in the second trimester or during the third trimester, medical management followed by combined cesarean birth and resection of the pheochromocytoma may be an option. It is unknown whether the standard preoperative management with alpha blockade or calcium channel blockade followed by perioperative beta blockade in nonpregnant patients is safe during pregnancy. The long-term effects of the alpha blocker phenoxybenzamine on the fetus have not been determined, although calcium channel blockers are safe to use during pregnancy. Beta blockers are frequently used during pregnancy with close monitoring for intrauterine growth retardation. Consultation with a maternal-fetal medicine specialist is essential to determine the preoperative management that will ensure the optimal postoperative result for the patient and fetus. In nonpregnant patients, the method of approach depends on suspected malignancy, unilateral versus bilateral tumors, extra-adrenal location, size of the tumor, and surgeon's preference and experience. In all series comparing the different approaches, including open versus laparoscopic technique, pregnant patients were not included. Recent studies have indicated the safety of the laparoscopic approach in pregnancy.

### Thyroid Disease

Thyroid disease during pregnancy can be categorized into three groups—hypothyroidism, hyperthyroidism, and thyroid cancer. Hypothyroidism is found in 2.5% of pregnancies. Of these, only 20% to 30% of patients develop symptoms. The first step is to obtain a serum thyroid-stimulating hormone (TSH) concentration. This will help categorize primary hypothyroidism versus hypothyroidism resulting from pituitary or hypothalamic causes.

Current guidelines from LeBeau and Mandel[25] for the treatment of hypothyroidism during pregnancy are as follows:

1. Check serum TSH level.
2. Initial levothyroxine dosage is based on severity of symptoms. Levothyroxine is started at 2 μg/kg/day. If TSH is less than 10 mU/L, dose is adjusted to 0.1 mg/day.

3. For previously diagnosed hypothyroidism, monitor TSH level every 3 to 4 weeks.
4. Goal TSH level is less than 2.5 mU/L.
5. Monitor serum TSH and total TSH every 3 to 4 weeks with each dose change.

Hyperthyroidism during pregnancy has an incidence of 0.1% to 0.4%.[26] Gestational thyrotoxicosis is a multifactorial phenomenon. High serum concentrations of human chorionic gonadotropin (hCG) during pregnancy activate the TSH receptors. Elevated serum-free thyroxine ($T_4$) and low-serum TSH levels are seen with this form of thyrotoxicosis. Gestational thyrotoxicosis is usually self-limited and spontaneously resolves by 20 weeks' gestation, when the hCG level declines. Repeat evaluation is warranted if thyrotoxicosis persists. Most cases of hyperthyroidism are a result of Graves' disease. After the diagnosis is made, medical treatment with thionamides (e.g., propylthiouracil, methimazole) is the mainstay of treatment. Iodides are avoided, except in patients preparing for thyroidectomy during pregnancy. Subtotal thyroidectomy for Graves' disease is reserved for patients who are taking high-dose propylthiouracil (>600 mg/day) or methimazole (>40 mg/day), are allergic to thionamides, are noncompliant, or have compressive symptoms because of goiter size. Surgery is performed during the second trimester before 24 weeks' gestation to minimize the risk for miscarriage. A 2-week course of a β-adrenergic agent, along with potassium iodide, is implemented before surgery to minimize perioperative complications. Radioactive iodine therapy is contraindicated during pregnancy.

Because of hormonal changes, thyroid nodules may have a higher prevalence during pregnancy, but thyroid cancers do not. Thyroid cancers are worked up in the traditional fashion during pregnancy. FNA, along with ultrasonic evaluation, remain the cornerstone of diagnosis. If cytology shows thyroid cancer, surgery is recommended during the second trimester, before 24 weeks' gestation. If thyroid cancer is found after the second half of pregnancy, surgery can be performed after delivery. This statement is supported by a recent study in which 201 pregnant women underwent thyroid ($n$ = 165) and parathyroid ($n$ = 36) procedures. Of these patients, 46% had thyroid cancer. When compared with nonpregnant women ($n$ = 31), the pregnant patients had a higher rate of endocrine (15.9% versus 8.1%; $P < .001$) and general complications (11.4% versus 3.6%; $P < .001$) and longer unadjusted lengths of stay (2 days versus 1 day; $P < .001$). The fetal and maternal complication rates were 5.5% and 4.5%, respectively.[27] Postoperative radioactive iodine therapy also needs to be delayed until after delivery.

## Small Bowel Disease

Intestinal obstruction is the third most common nonobstetric surgical issue in pregnancy, after acute appendicitis and acute cholecystitis. The incidence of small bowel obstruction during pregnancy has been reported to be between 1 in 1,500 to 17,000 pregnancies. Small bowel obstructions usually occur during the second and third trimesters. Adhesions resulting from prior abdominal and pelvic surgeries are the most frequent causes of intestinal obstruction in pregnancy, accounting for 53% to 59% of cases. Other causes of small bowel obstruction in the pregnant patient include volvulus, intussusception, malignancy, and hernia, although the displacement of the small bowel out of the pelvis by the enlarging uterus makes this a rare cause.

The symptoms of an obstruction are identical to those in the nonpregnant patient and consist of the triad of abdominal pain, vomiting, and obstipation. Pain, present in 85% to 98% of cases, is usually colicky in nature and located in the midabdomen, although the character and duration are highly variable. Nausea and vomiting are seen in 80% of pregnant patients with small bowel obstruction; however, nausea and vomiting are not uncommon during the first trimester of normal pregnancy. Nausea and vomiting that persist or begin later in pregnancy should arouse suspicion and be evaluated. Bowel distention may be marked but difficult to assess because of the gravid uterus. Diagnosis is made by serial examination and plain abdominal radiography.

Treatment for small bowel obstruction in pregnancy is identical to that in the nonpregnant patient. Therapy consists of nasogastric decompression and IV fluids. However, a lower threshold for operative management is necessary. If, after 6 to 8 hours of nonoperative treatment, there is no satisfactory patient response, a laparotomy is performed before perforation or bowel necrosis occurs. Maternal mortality ranges from 6% to 20% because of sepsis and multisystem organ failure, and fetal loss is as high as 26% to 50%. To avoid the risk to the mother and fetus, a more aggressive approach is used.

Midgut volvulus remains a dreaded diagnosis during the postpartum period. It is usually more common in the pregnant patient if she has undergone previous abdominal surgery; however, spontaneous midgut volvulus may occur. A case report of maternal death caused by midgut volvulus after bariatric surgery has been reported.[28] The key is increased vigilance for all those involved in the patient's care. Early exploration is warranted if the diagnosis is unclear.

## Colon and Rectal Disease

Acute appendicitis is the most common nonobstetric surgical problem in the pregnant patient, occurring in 1 in 1500 pregnancies. The incidence of acute appendicitis is fairly evenly distributed among the trimesters of pregnancy, with a slight predominance during the second trimester. Timely and accurate diagnosis is challenging because the typical clinical findings of nausea, vomiting, abdominal pain, and mild leukocytosis may be seen in a normal pregnancy. Delay in diagnosis results in an increased perforation rate of 10%, which has significant consequences for the patient and fetus. Fetal mortality increases from 1.5% in acute appendicitis to 35% in perforated appendicitis; preterm labor and premature delivery rates are as high as 40% in perforated appendicitis[29] compared with a 13% rate of preterm labor and 4% rate of premature delivery in acute appendicitis.[30]

In 1932, Baer studied 78 normal pregnant women with radiographic studies at regular intervals from the second month of pregnancy to 10 days postpartum. As the uterus enlarges, the appendix is driven upward with a counterclockwise rotation. Baer concluded that early in pregnancy, pain is low and that as the gestation progresses, pain is located higher in the abdomen.[31] A review of 45 pregnant patients with acute appendicitis demonstrated that pain in the right lower quadrant is the most common symptom, regardless of gestational age (first trimester, 86%; second trimester, 83%; third trimester, 85%).[29] Despite the inconsistency, acute appendicitis needs to be included in the differential diagnosis of every pregnant woman who presents with right-sided abdominal pain. Treatment of suspected acute appendicitis in the pregnant patient is emergent appendectomy. Although helical CT scans have demonstrated higher than 90% sensitivity and specificity in the diagnosis of acute appendicitis, few data are available in pregnant patients. In nonpregnant patients, a 10% to 15% negative laparotomy rate is considered acceptable. Because of the increased risk to mother and fetus with appendiceal perforation, a negative rate of 30% to 33% has been widely accepted until recently, when it was reported that even negative appendectomy may be associated with an increased risk of fetal loss. In a series of 3133 patients, the rates of fetal loss and preterm delivery in complicated appendicitis were 6% and 11%, respectively, in comparison to the rates of fetal loss and preterm delivery of 4% and 10%, respectively, in patients who underwent negative appendectomy.[32] It was concluded that improvement in fetal outcomes would result from improvement in diagnostic accuracy and reduction of the rate of negative appendectomy. In a small series of 47 patients, a positive ultrasound was considered to be diagnostic for appendicitis, with MRI without gadolinium or CT being used to confirm or exclude the diagnosis in a negative or nondiagnostic ultrasound diagnosis of appendicitis in pregnancy.[33] The debate is then for an open or laparoscopic technique. The argument for open appendectomy is that the laparoscopic approach exposes the fetus to risks for pneumoperitoneum and trocar placement without the benefit of a significantly smaller incision. The laparoscopic technique enables examination of a larger portion of the abdomen with less uterine manipulation and allows locating the appendix as it is pushed into the right upper quadrant by the enlarging uterus.

Colonic pseudo-obstruction, or Ogilvie's syndrome, is a functional obstruction, or adynamic ileus, without a mechanical cause. Of all cases of Ogilvie's syndrome, 10% occur in postpartum patients. It is characterized by massive abdominal distention with cecal dilation. Although neostigmine is effective first-line therapy in nonpregnant patients, its safety in pregnancy is unknown. It can be used safely in the postpartum period. Colonoscopic decompression has been described in postpartum patients, with laparotomy indicated only in suspected perforation.

### Vascular Disease

Of more than 400 cases of ruptured splenic artery aneurysms in the literature, approximately 100 cases of ruptured splenic artery aneurysm during pregnancy have been reported, with only 12 cases of maternal and fetal survival.[34] Rupture occurred during the third trimester in two thirds of cases and was typically misdiagnosed as splenic rupture or uterine rupture. The maternal mortality rate was 75%, with a fetal mortality rate of 95%. Increased portal pressures, high splenic artery flow caused by distal aortic compression, and progressive arterial wall weakening are contributing factors. Multiparity may increase the risk; 78% of patients with ruptured splenic artery aneurysms have been in their third pregnancy. Survival is most likely related to a two-stage rupture, in which the lesser sac temporarily tamponades the bleeding aneurysm.

When treated electively in nonpregnant patients, the mortality rate is only 0.5% to 1.3%. When the diagnosis is made in a woman of childbearing age or in a pregnant patient, a splenic artery aneurysm of 2 cm or larger is treated electively because of the increased risk for rupture during pregnancy.[34]

Acute iliofemoral venous thrombosis is six times more frequent in pregnant than nonpregnant patients. Pregnancy may increase the risk for thrombosis via a number of factors, including mechanical obstruction of venous drainage by the enlarging uterus, decreased activity in late pregnancy and at time of delivery, intimal injury from vascular distention or surgical manipulation during cesarean section, and abnormal levels of coagulation factors (see earlier). Also, a wide spectrum of pathologic abnormalities, such as the presence of lupus anticoagulant antibodies and deficiencies of proteins C and S, may further increase the risk for thrombotic disease. Protein S serves as a cofactor for activated protein C, which has anticoagulant activity. Therefore, a deficiency of protein S leads to spontaneous, recurrent thromboembolic complications in nonpregnant adults. Even in normal individuals, protein S levels are substantially reduced during pregnancy.

The management of acute iliofemoral venous thrombosis during pregnancy is controversial because thrombolytic therapy poses hazards to the fetus. The risk for pulmonary thromboembolism with manipulation of the clot during thrombectomy would have catastrophic effects on both the patient and fetus. Techniques that have been described include interruption of the inferior vena cava through a right retroperitoneal approach or interruption of the inferior vena cava by passage of a Fogarty catheter through the unaffected contralateral femoral vein. The disadvantage of the retroperitoneal approach is that an extensive dissection is required. The disadvantages of the Fogarty catheter are that the catheter may still dislodge clots that have extended into the vena cava and that once the catheter is removed, an inferior vena cava filter must still be placed. However, the most effective technique is filter placement in the inferior vena cava through the internal jugular vein using ultrasound guidance, followed by thrombectomy.

## TRAUMA IN PREGNANCY

Trauma is the leading nonobstetric cause of maternal mortality and occurs in approximately 5% of pregnancies.[35] The most common mechanisms of injury are from falls or from motor vehicle accidents.[36] When compared with age-matched pregnant controls, pregnant women who sustained trauma had a higher incidence of spontaneous abortion, preterm labor, fetomaternal hemorrhage, abruptio placentae, and uterine rupture.[37] A number of studies have attempted to identify risk factors that predict morbidity and mortality in the pregnant trauma patient. The maternal Injury Severity Score, mechanism of injury, and physical findings are unable to predict adverse outcomes adequately, such as abruptio placentae and fetal loss. Pregnant patients with severe head, abdominal, thoracic, or lower extremity injuries are at high risk for pregnancy loss.[38] Early involvement of an available obstetrician is important to evaluate maternal and fetal well-being.

In the treatment of the pregnant trauma patient, the critical point is that resuscitation of the fetus is accomplished by resuscitation of the mother. Therefore, the initial evaluation and treatment of the pregnant injured patient is identical to that of the nonpregnant injured patient. Rapid assessment of the maternal airway, breathing, and circulation, as well as ensuring an adequate airway, avoids maternal and fetal hypoxia. In the later stages of pregnancy, as described earlier, uterine compression of the vena cava may result in hypotension from diminished venous return; thus, the pregnant trauma patient needs to be placed in a left lateral decubitus position. If spinal cord injury is suspected, the patient may be secured to a backboard and then tilted to the left.

The increased blood volume associated with pregnancy has important implications in the trauma patient. Signs of blood loss such as tachycardia and hypotension may be delayed until the patient loses almost 30% of her blood volume. As a result, the fetus may be experiencing hypoperfusion long before the mother manifests any signs. Early and rapid fluid resuscitation should be initiated, even in the pregnant patient who is normotensive.

As with the primary survey, the secondary survey proceeds in a fashion similar to that in the nonpregnant patient. Special attention is given to the abdominal examination. The uterus remains protected by the pelvis until approximately 12 weeks' gestation and is relatively well sheltered from the abdominal injury until then. As the uterus grows, it becomes more prominent and more vulnerable to injury. Measurement of fundal height provides a rapid approximation of gestational age. At 20 weeks' gestation, it is at the level of the umbilicus and is approximately 1 cm per week of gestation. Intrauterine hemorrhage or uterine rupture may result in a discrepancy in measurement. A pelvic examination is performed, by an obstetrician if possible, to evaluate for vaginal bleeding, ruptured membranes, or a bulging perineum. Vaginal bleeding may indicate abruptio placentae, placenta previa, or preterm labor. Rupture of the amniotic membrane may result in umbilical cord prolapse, which compresses the umbilical vessels and compromises fetal blood flow. This requires immediate cesarean delivery. If cloudy white or greenish fluid is seen from the cervical os or perineum, the presence of amniotic fluid is confirmed by testing with Nitrazine paper, which indicates pH and changes from green to blue.

The Kleihauer-Betke (KB) test for the assessment of fetomaternal transfusion is useful after maternal trauma and is ordered with the initial laboratory studies, which include typing and crossmatching. Because of the sensitivity of the KB test, a small amount of fetomaternal transfusion may be undetected. Therefore, all Rh-negative pregnant trauma patients are considered for Rh immunoglobulin (RhoGAM) therapy.

The most common cause of fetal death after blunt injury is abruptio placentae. Deceleration of the fetal heart rate may be the earliest sign of abruption. The uterus needs to be evaluated for contractions, rupture, and abruptio placentae. Early initiation of cardiotocographic fetal monitoring adequately warns of deterioration in the condition of the fetus.

Penetrating trauma results in maternal death in fewer than 5% of cases. Penetrating trauma is primarily from gunshot wounds and knife wounds. The incidence of visceral injury with penetrating trauma during pregnancy is 16% to 38% in comparison to 80% to 90% in nonpregnant patients.[39] Fetal injury occurs in up to 70% of cases, with a 40% to 70% rate of fetal death as a result of direct fetal injury or preterm labor.[35] A number of factors contribute to the nature of the injuries. Bullets produce a transient shock wave and cavitation as they transmit kinetic energy to body tissues. The density of the tissue, such as the thick density of the uterus during early pregnancy, may rapidly dissipate the lower amount of kinetic energy from a low-velocity projectile, protecting the fetus from significant injury. Higher velocity projectiles may produce more serious injuries to mother and fetus. As pregnancy progresses and the growing uterus displaces the abdominal viscera, location of the injury becomes crucial in determining which of the maternal viscera are injured and whether the fetus has sustained a direct injury. Management of penetrating injuries during pregnancy is similar to that for nonpregnant patients. It should be individualized, with early involvement by an obstetrician. Diagnostic and treatment options include surgical exploration, supraumbilical diagnostic peritoneal lavage, diagnostic laparoscopy, CT, local wound exploration, and observation.[40] Emergency cesarean delivery may be indicated in maternal arrest after 4 minutes of unsuccessful resuscitation, fetal compromise with a stable mother if the fetus is of viable gestational age, obvious impending maternal death, or when the gravid uterus interferes with trauma-related surgical intervention.[41] Also, emergent cesarean delivery may also improve chances of maternal survival by removing aortocaval compression and increasing cardiac output. Maternal and fetal survival rates as high as 72% and 45%, respectively, have been reported following emergency cesarean delivery at more than 25 weeks/ gestational age. No fetal survival has been documented when fetal heart tones were absent before emergent delivery, but a 75% chance of fetal survival has been reported when fetal heart tones were present and gestational age was at least 26 weeks.[42] The best chance for fetal survival with an intact infant is when cesarean delivery occurs within 5 minutes of maternal death. Four minutes of resuscitation followed by a 1-minute cesarean delivery offers the best chance for infant survival. In a review of 61 infants born by perimortem cesarean delivery between 1900 and 1985, 70% of the infants survived who were delivered within 5 minutes of maternal death, and all of the survivors were neurologically intact.[43]

## PREGNANCY AFTER MAJOR ABDOMINAL SURGERY

Not infrequently, the surgeon will be asked about pregnancy following treatment of surgical disease. Each case should be individualized. The conditions can be divided into those involving benign and malignant disease.

### Benign Disease

After most abdominal procedures for benign disease, there is no contraindication for pregnancy. Special circumstances include bariatric surgery and total colectomy with ileal pouch–anal anastomosis.

#### Bariatric Surgery

Bariatric surgery is rapidly becoming one of the most common procedures done in the United States. With approximately 160,000 women undergoing weight loss surgery in 2009, pregnancy after bariatric surgery is a common occurrence. There is an improvement in infertility and pregnancy outcomes after weight loss surgery.[44] There is also a decreased incidence in patients who have undergone bariatric surgery in regard to maternal complications, such as diabetes mellitus, hypertensive disorders, and fetal macrosomia as compared with their morbidly obese counterparts.[45] Currently, the consensus of studies has supported that pregnancy should be delayed for up to 2 years following bariatric surgery. Outcomes in maternal or fetal health do not differ whether a patient has had a Roux-en Y gastric bypass or restrictive procedure (e.g., vertical-banded gastroplasty [VBG]; laparoscopic adjustable gastric banding [LAGB]).[46] Current recommendations for women who become pregnant after bariatric surgery are to continue with a prenatal multivitamin, vitamin $B_{12}$, iron, and folate supplement. Protein supplementation may also be necessary for patients who have undergone malabsorptive operations. For patients who have undergone adjustable gastric band placement, deflation of the band is recommended to aid in optimal nutrition.

### Ileal Pouch–Anal Anastomosis

Ulcerative colitis can be a debilitating disease that might eventually require a total colectomy with an ileal pouch–anal anastomosis. Long-term outcomes of pregnancy after this procedure have been generally positive.[47] In a study of 37 women who became pregnant before and after ileal pouch–anal anastomosis, there were no differences in birth weight, duration of labor, complications, and unplanned cesarean sections.[48] Another study comparing patients who underwent cesarean section versus vaginal delivery after ileal pouch–anal anastomosis has demonstrated that the vaginal delivery patients have a significant higher incidence of anterior sphincter defect (13% versus 50%) and worse quality of life evaluated by the time trade-off method.[49]

### Malignant Disease

This discussion will be limited to breast cancer because this occurs more often in women of reproductive age in comparison to most oncologic disease treated by the general surgeon or surgical oncologist. The issues that patients will need advice on are the following: (1) maintenance of fertility; (2) the impact of pregnancy on disease progression and survival; (3) the timing of pregnancy relative to the diagnosis of breast cancer; and (4) pregnancy outcome.

Breast cancer often affects women of reproductive age. Although treatment is effective, cytotoxic chemotherapy causes ovarian reserve depletion, whereas hormonal therapy necessitates a delay in pregnancy, resulting in potential infertility in some patients, but some patients retain normal fertility. On diagnosis of breast cancer in patients of reproductive age who are interested in having children after treatment, the surgeon or medical oncologist may consider referral to a fertility specialist to explore methods of fertility preservation. The best established method of fertility preservation is embryo cryopreservation. This involves ovarian stimulation to retrieve oocytes for in vitro fertilization prior to freezing; this remains the best known option for fertility preservation in women with early-stage breast cancer whose risk of fertility may be compromised by adjuvant chemotherapy. However, little is known about the impact, if any, of ovarian stimulation on disease progression.

Studies have shown that pregnancy is more likely to occur in patients with prolonged survival and no evidence of disease recurrence. In addition, there is no evidence of a negative effect of pregnancy on recurrence rate and survival in patients treated for breast cancer. This includes those who have had a mastectomy as well as breast-conserving therapy. Survival was based on initial stage and not affected by hormonal receptor status or pregnancy.[50,51]

The timing of pregnancy varies with the treatment protocol and reassessment for recurrent disease. Some recommend that women wait 2 years from the time of diagnosis, but this is controversial. The population-based study of Ives and colleagues[51] did not support the current medical advice given to premenopausal women with a diagnosis of with breast cancer to wait 2 years before attempting to conceive. It was concluded that although this recommendation may be valid for women who are receiving treatment or have systemic disease at diagnosis, and for women with localized disease, early conception, 6 months after completing their treatment, is unlikely to reduce survival. The occurrence of preterm labor or miscarriage is similar in patients with a previous diagnosis of breast cancer compared with those with no history of breast cancer.

## SUMMARY

Pregnant patients are susceptible to the same surgical diseases as nonpregnant patients of similar age. Maternal physiologic changes, as well as the enlarging uterus, may result in atypical presentation of surgical disease or symptoms may be attributed to normal pregnancy. A delay in diagnosis and treatment of surgical illnesses in pregnancy poses a greater risk to maternal and fetal well-being than the risks of anesthesia or surgical intervention. Early consultation with an obstetrician, maternal-fetal medicine specialist, and perinatologist can ensure optimal outcomes and avoid pitfalls. Laparoscopy is becoming increasingly accepted in the pregnant patient and future advances should make it even safer for these women. Preterm labor prevention needs to be individualized, given the patient's gestational age and underlying disease process.

## SELECTED REFERENCES

Baer JL, Reis RA, Arens RA: Appendicitis in pregnancy: with changes in position and axis of the normal appendix in pregnancy. JAMA 98:1359–1364, 1932.

Landmark article illustrating the changes in appendiceal location during pregnancy.

Freeland M, King E, Safcsak K, et al: Diagnosis of appendicitis in pregnancy. Am J Surg 198:753–758, 2009.

This study shows that when ultrasound is read as positive for appendicitis, no further confirmatory test other than surgery is required. However, if the ultrasound is nondiagnostic, further imaging with MRI or CT may avoid a negative appendectomy.

Jackson H, Granger S, Price R, et al: Diagnosis and laparoscopic treatment of surgical diseases during pregnancy: An evidence-based review. Surg Endosc 22:1917–1927, 2008.

The literature supporting the safety and efficacy of laparoscopy in cholecystectomy, appendectomy, solid organ resection, and oophorectomy in the gravid patient is outlined. Based on the level of evidence, the authors review recommendations specific to surgical approach, trimester of pregnancy, patient positioning, port placement, insufflation pressure, monitoring, venous thromboembolic prophylaxis, obstetric consultation, and use of tocolytics in the pregnant patient.

Kuy S, Roman SA, Desai R, et al: Outcomes following thyroid and parathyroid surgery in pregnant women. Arch Surg 144:399–406, 2009.

The authors review in a retrospective study 201 pregnant women who underwent thyroid ($n$ = 165) and parathyroid ($n$ = 36) procedures and compared with nonpregnant women ($n$ = 31). On multivariate regression analysis, pregnancy was an independent predictor of higher combined surgical complications (odds ratio, 2; $P < .001$), longer adjusted length of stay (0.3 days longer; $P < .001$), and higher adjusted hospital costs ($300; $P < .001$). Other independent predictors of outcome were surgeon volume, patient race or ethnicity, and insurance status. The authors conclude that pregnant women have worse clinical and economic outcomes following thyroid and parathyroid surgery than nonpregnant women. In addition, they found disparities in outcomes based on race, insurance, and access to high-volume surgeons.

LeBeau SO, Mandel SJ: Thyroid disorders during pregnancy. Endocrinol Metab Clin North Am 35:117–136, 2006.

Comprehensive review of all the major thyroid abnormalities that occur during pregnancy.

Mourad J, Elliott JP, Erickson L, et al: Appendicitis in pregnancy: New information that contradicts long-held clinical beliefs. Am J Obstet Gynecol 182:1027–1029, 2000.

This paper, which retrospectively reviewed more than 66,000 deliveries and found 45 pregnant patients with appendicitis, challenged the original landmark paper by Baer regarding the presentation of acute appendicitis in pregnant patients.

Sadot E, Telem DA, Arora M, et al: Laparoscopy: A safe approach to appendicitis during pregnancy. Surg Endosc 24:383–389, 2010.

This article is the largest hospital-based series evaluating the laparoscopic versus open approach for pregnant patients with presumed acute appendicitis. Based on their findings, the authors conclude that laparoscopy appears to be a safe, feasible, and efficacious approach for pregnant patients with presumed acute appendicitis. They concluded that it is likely not the surgical approach but the underlying diagnosis combined with maternal factors that determine the risk for pregnancy complications.

Soper NJ: SAGES' guidelines for diagnosis, treatment, and use of laparoscopy for surgical problems during pregnancy, Surg Endosc 25:3477–3478, 2011.

These are current guidelines for laparoscopy in pregnancy.

Tang SJ, Mayo MJ, Rodriguez-Frias E, et al: Safety and utility of ERCP during pregnancy. Gastrointest Endosc 69:453–461, 2009.

Endoscopic retrograde cholangiopancreatography (ERCP) is an important diagnostic and therapeutic tool in patients with biliary and pancreatic disease. Its usefulness and safety during pregnancy are largely unknown because it is not often required and because its use has been only infrequently reported in the published literature. This is a retrospective review, from a single academic center, from 2000 to 2006. During the study period, 68 ERCPs were performed on 65 pregnant women. There were no perforations, sedation-related adverse event, postsphincterotomy bleeding, cholangitis, or procedure-related maternal or fetal deaths. Post-ERCP pancreatitis was diagnosed in 11 patients (16%); 59 patients had complete follow-up. Endoscopic therapy at the time of ERCP was undertaken in all patients. Term pregnancy was achieved in 53 patients (89.8%). Patients having ERCP in the first trimester had the lowest percentage of term pregnancy (73.3%) and the highest risk of preterm delivery (20.0%) and low-birth-weight newborns (21.4%). The authors reported that none of the 59 patients with long-term follow-up had spontaneous fetal loss, perinatal death, stillbirth, or fetal malformation.

Vinatier E, Merlot B, Poncelet E, et al: Breast cancer during pregnancy. Eur J Obstet Gynecol Reprod Biol 147:9–14, 2009.

Breast cancer in pregnancy is an uncommon situation but poses dilemmas for patients and physicians. There is a paucity of prospective studies regarding the diagnosis and treatment of breast cancer during pregnancy. Women diagnosed with breast cancer during pregnancy have similar disease characteristics to age-matched controls. Current evidence suggests that diagnosis may be carried out with limitations regarding staging. Surgical treatment may be performed as for nonpregnant women. Radiotherapy and endocrine or antibody treatment should be postponed until after delivery. Chemotherapy is allowed after the first trimester. Physicians should be aggressive in the workup of breast symptoms in the pregnant population to expedite diagnosis and allow multidisciplinary treatment without delay.

## REFERENCES


1. Chesnutt AN: Physiology of normal pregnancy. Crit Care Clin 20:609–615, 2004.
2. Melnick DM, Wahl WL, Dalton VK: Management of general surgical problems in the pregnant patient. Am J Surg 187:170–180, 2004.
3. Harrison BP, Crystal CS: Imaging modalities in obstetrics and gynecology. Emerg Med Clin North Am 21:711–735, 2003.
4. Bar-Oz B, Moretti ME, Boskovic R, et al: The safety of quinolones—a meta-analysis of pregnancy outcomes. Eur J Obstet Gynecol Reprod Biol 143:75–78, 2009.
5. Ni Mhuireachtaigh R, O'Gorman DA: Anesthesia in pregnant patients for nonobstetric surgery. J Clin Anesth 18:60–66, 2006.
6. Schecter WP, Farmer D, Horn JK, et al: Special considerations in perioperative pain management: Audiovisual distraction, geriatrics, pediatrics, and pregnancy. J Am Coll Surg 201:612–618, 2005.
7. Jackson H, Granger S, Price R, et al: Diagnosis and laparoscopic treatment of surgical diseases during pregnancy: An evidence-based review. Surg Endosc 22:1917–1927, 2008.
8. Sadot E, Telem DA, Arora M, et al: Laparoscopy: A safe approach to appendicitis during pregnancy. Surg Endosc 24:383–389, 2010.
9. Hunter JG, Swanstrom L, Thornburg K: Carbon dioxide pneumoperitoneum induces fetal acidosis in a pregnant ewe model. Surg Endosc 9:272–277, 1995.
10. Society of American Gastrointestinal Endoscopic Surgeons (SAGES): Guidelines for laparoscopic surgery during pregnancy. Surg Endosc 12:189–190, 1998.
11. Keleher AJ, Theriault RL, Gwyn KM, et al: Multidisciplinary management of breast cancer concurrent with pregnancy. J Am Coll Surg 194:54–64, 2002.
12. Falkenberry SS: Breast cancer in pregnancy. Obstet Gynecol Clin North Am 29:225–232, 2002.
13. Johannsson O, Loman N, Borg A, et al: Pregnancy-associated breast cancer in BRCA1 and BRCA2 germline mutation carriers. Lancet 352:1359–1360, 1998.
14. Woo JC, Yu T, Hurd TC: Breast cancer in pregnancy: A literature review. Arch Surg 138:91–98, 2003.
15. Vinatier E, Merlot B, Poncelet E, et al: Breast cancer during pregnancy. Eur J Obstet Gynecol Reprod Biol 147:9–14, 2009.
16. Leslie KK, Lange CA: Breast cancer and pregnancy. Obstet Gynecol Clin North Am 32:547–558, 2005.

17. Bonnier P, Romain S, Dilhuydy JM, et al: Influence of pregnancy on the outcome of breast cancer: a case-control study. Societe Francaise de Senologie et de Pathologie Mammaire Study Group. Int J Cancer 72:720–727, 1997.
18. Berry DL, Theriault RL, Holmes FA, et al: Management of breast cancer during pregnancy using a standardized protocol. J Clin Oncol 17:855–861, 1999.
19. Doshi S, Zucker SD: Liver emergencies during pregnancy. Gastroenterol Clin North Am 32:1213–1227, 2003.
20. Cobey FC, Salem RR: A review of liver masses in pregnancy and a proposed algorithm for their diagnosis and management. Am J Surg 187:181–191, 2004.
21. Tang SJ, Mayo MJ, Rodriguez-Frias E, et al: Safety and utility of ERCP during pregnancy. Gastrointest Endosc 69:453–461, 2009.
22. Lu EJ, Curet MJ, El-Sayed YY, et al: Medical versus surgical management of biliary tract disease in pregnancy. Am J Surg 188:755–759, 2004.
23. Eichenberg BJ, Vanderlinden J, Miguel C, et al: Laparoscopic cholecystectomy in the third trimester of pregnancy. Am Surg 62:874–877, 1996.
24. Chiappetta Porras LT, Napoli ED, Canullan CM, et al: Minimally invasive management of acute biliary tract disease during pregnancy, 2009 (http://www.hindawi.com/journals/hpb/2009/829020.html).
25. LeBeau SO, Mandel SJ: Thyroid disorders during pregnancy. Endocrinol Metab Clin North Am 35:117–136, 2006.
26. Mandel SJ: Thyroid disease and pregnancy. In Copper DS, editor: Medical management of thyroid disease, New York, 2001, Marcel Dekker, pp 380–418.
27. Kuy S, Roman SA, Desai R, et al: Outcomes following thyroid and parathyroid surgery in pregnant women. Arch Surg 144:399–406, 2009.
28. Loar PV, 3rd, Sanchez-Ramos L, Kaunitz AM, et al: Maternal death caused by midgut volvulus after bariatric surgery. Am J Obstet Gynecol 193:1748–1749, 2005.
29. Rollins MD, Chan KJ, Price RR: Laparoscopy for appendicitis and cholelithiasis during pregnancy: A new standard of care. Surg Endosc 18:237–241, 2004.
30. Mourad J, Elliott JP, Erickson L, et al: Appendicitis in pregnancy: New information that contradicts long-held clinical beliefs. Am J Obstet Gynecol 182:1027–1029, 2000.
31. Baer JL, Reis RA, Arens RA: Appendicitis in pregnancy: With changes in position and axis of the normal appendix in pregnancy. JAMA 98:1359–1364, 1932.
32. McGory ML, Zingmond DS, Tillou A, et al: Negative appendectomy in pregnant women is associated with a substantial risk of fetal loss. J Am Coll Surg 205:534–540, 2007.
33. Freeland M, King E, Safcsak K, et al: Diagnosis of appendicitis in pregnancy. Am J Surg 198:753–758, 2009.
34. Herbeck M, Horbach T, Putzenlechner C, et al: Ruptured splenic artery aneurysm during pregnancy: A rare case with both maternal and fetal survival. Am J Obstet Gynecol 181:763–764, 1999.
35. Mattox KL, Goetzl L: Trauma in pregnancy. Crit Care Med 33:S385–S389, 2005.
36. Schiff MA, Holt VL, Daling JR: Maternal and infant outcomes after injury during pregnancy in Washington State from 1989 to 1997. J Trauma 53:939–945, 2002.
37. Pak LL, Reece EA, Chan L: Is adverse pregnancy outcome predictable after blunt abdominal trauma? Am J Obstet Gynecol 179:1140–1144, 1998.
38. Ikossi DG, Lazar AA, Morabito D, et al: Profile of mothers at risk: An analysis of injury and pregnancy loss in 1,195 trauma patients. J Am Coll Surg 200:49–56, 2005.
39. Shah AJ, Kilcline BA: Trauma in pregnancy. Emerg Med Clin North Am 21:615–629, 2003.
40. Muench MV, Canterino JC: Trauma in pregnancy. Obstet Gynecol Clin North Am 34:555–583, 2007.
41. Hill CC, Pickinpaugh J: Trauma and surgical emergencies in the obstetric patient. Surg Clin North Am 88:421–440, 2008.
42. Morris JA, Jr, Rosenbower TJ, Jurkovich GJ, et al: Infant survival after cesarean section for trauma. Ann Surg 223:481–488, 1996.
43. Katz VL, Dotters DJ, Droegemueller W: Perimortem cesarean delivery. Obstet Gynecol 68:571–576, 1986.
44. Patel JA, Colella JJ, Esaka E, et al: Improvement in infertility and pregnancy outcomes after weight loss surgery. Med Clin North Am 91:515–528, 2007.
45. Weintraub AY, Levy A, Levi I, et al: Effect of bariatric surgery on pregnancy outcome. Int J Gynaecol Obstet 103:246–251, 2008.
46. Sheiner E, Balaban E, Dreiher J, et al: Pregnancy outcome in patients following different types of bariatric surgeries. Obes Surg 19:1286–1292, 2009.
47. Ravid A, Richard CS, Spencer LM, et al: Pregnancy, delivery, and pouch function after ileal pouch-anal anastomosis for ulcerative colitis. Dis Colon Rectum 45:1283–1288, 2002.
48. Hahnloser D, Pemberton JH, Wolff BG, et al: Pregnancy and delivery before and after ileal pouch-anal anastomosis for inflammatory bowel disease: Immediate and long-term consequences and outcomes. Dis Colon Rectum 47:1127–1135, 2004.
49. Remzi FH, Gorgun E, Bast J, et al: Vaginal delivery after ileal pouch-anal anastomosis: A word of caution. Dis Colon Rectum 48:1691–1699, 2005.
50. Velentgas P, Daling JR, Malone KE, et al: Pregnancy after breast carcinoma: Outcomes and influence on mortality. Cancer 85:2424–2432, 1999.
51. Ives A, Saunders C, Bulsara M, et al: Pregnancy after breast cancer: Population based study, 2007 (http://www.bmj.com/cgi/reprint/334/7586/194).

# CHAPTER 73

# UROLOGIC SURGERY

Michael Coburn

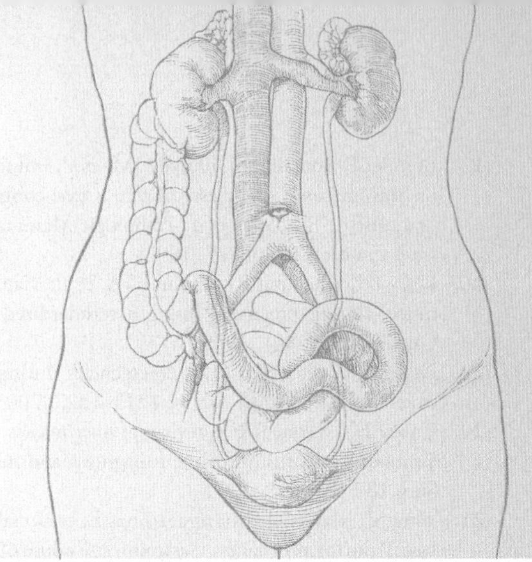



Urology as a specialty discipline has much in common with general surgery. Our focus on abdominal and retroperitoneal anatomy, surgical approach, combined use of endoscopic, laparoscopic, robotic, and open surgical technologies, and remarkable diversity of disease processes connects us in the surgical sciences. Urologists work closely with general surgeons regularly, and can profit greatly from each other's skills and knowledge.

During my experience as Chief of Urology at Ben Taub General Hospital in Houston over the past 20 years, I have had the great privilege of enjoying an outstanding collaborative relationship with the superb general, vascular, and trauma surgeons at our institution. We have worked closely under the stress of major trauma surgery, complexity of exenterative surgery for advanced pelvic malignancies, management of iatrogenic urologic and surgical injury, and challenges of necrotizing infections of the genitalia and perineum.

The surgical resident in training, while moving along the path to becoming a competent general surgeon, must acquire a thorough understanding of urologic disease and urologic surgery. This is equally important for those who practice in settings in which a urologist is likely unavailable, as well as in the setting in which appropriate consultation, surgical planning, and regular operative collaboration are routine.

The following discussion is intended to provide a fundamental overview of urologic surgery for the general surgery resident. As your colleagues in the house of surgery, I welcome and encourage your in-depth pursuit of the fascinating history and practice of urology as your career unfolds.

## UROLOGIC ANATOMY FOR THE GENERAL SURGEON

It is essential for the general abdominal surgeon to be intimately familiar with genitourinary anatomy to complete standard general surgical procedures, avoid iatrogenic injury, and deal with abnormal anatomy.[1] Examples of particular areas of risk or challenge include the renal vasculature in major vascular and retroperitoneal tumor surgery, ureteral mobilization and injury avoidance in complex colonic procedures, urethral and prostatic relationship to the rectum, and spermatic cord and scrotal contents in complex inguinal hernia surgery.

### Upper Abdomen and Retroperitoneum

The kidneys are located anterior to the psoas and quadratus lumborum muscles; adjacent to the left kidney are the body and tail of the pancreas, spleen, splenic flexure of the colon, and colonic mesentery. On the right, the kidney is adjacent to the liver, duodenum, and head of the pancreas. In the setting of neoplastic or inflammatory processes involving any of these structures, or the kidney, complex adhesions can form that create challenging dissection planes and increase the risk of organ injury with surgical exploration or mobilization. Although the perirenal fascia (Gerota's fascia) separates the kidney capsule and parenchyma from these adjacent organs and reduces the risk of renal injury with local dissection, renal parenchymal injury is possible with abnormal anatomy. In the setting of inflammatory disease, the Gerota's fascia may be densely adherent and inseparable from the kidney, requiring an additional approach to renal mobilization to avoid capsular or parenchymal injury. In the setting of retroperitoneal trauma, it is easy to strip the renal capsule from the parenchyma inadvertently when the kidney is rapidly dissected digitally; this maneuver is therefore best done with care and under direct vision whenever possible, because preserving the capsule enhances renal reconstructive efforts.

The renal pedicle has a predictable anatomic orientation, although anomalies of the venous system and the renal collecting system are not uncommon and can confuse the operating surgeon. The renal vein is typically most anterior, the renal artery just posterior to the vein, and the renal pelvis and ureter most posterior. On the left side, the renal vein typically passes anterior to the aorta and inferior to the superior mesenteric vein as it courses toward the vena cava. On the right, the renal vein can be short and enters the vena cava laterally. The major branches of the renal vein are the gonadal vein on the left (the right gonadal vein enters the vena cava directly), the adrenal vein, which joins the left renal vein superiorly on the left, and enters the vena cava directly and at times posteriorly on the right, and variable lumbar veins, which may be found entering the renal veins posteriorly, coursing directly posterior just lateral to the aorta on the left, or near the vena cava on the right. These major branches are particularly prone to injury with dissection of the renal pedicle and can result in troublesome bleeding. It is the presence of these predictable renal vein branches that allows ligation of the left renal vein near the vena cava in the trauma setting, with preservation of renal venous drainage in most cases. On the right, ligation of the renal vein will typically result in renal vein thrombosis and renal infarction. Renal vascular anomalies for which the surgeon must beware include the circumaortic or retroaortic renal vein on the left and multiple renal veins or arteries on either side. Congenital anomalies involving the kidneys and upper urinary tract may result in unintended injury if not appreciated preoperatively. Renal malrotation, duplication, and fusion anomalies are of particular concern. A pelvic kidney could be removed if thought to represent a pelvic mass of neoplastic origin and the isthmus of a horseshoe kidney might be injured if not appreciated prior to exposure to the great vessels in retroperitoneal surgery, because it invariably crosses anterior to the aorta, just inferior to the inferior mesenteric artery. Renal ectopia is accompanied by markedly variable and unpredictable renal vasculature, with multiple branches, possibly arising from the iliac arteries or aortic bifurcation. Duplication of the renal collecting system with a supernumerary renal pelvis and ureter is notorious for precipitating iatrogenic injury; the unsuspecting surgeon might be caught unaware after identifying a single ureter on either side.

### Ureter

The ureter travels from the renal pedicle to the bladder hiatus in a predictable manner, but can be difficult to identify when the region is anatomically hostile because of prior surgery, hematoma, fibrosis, inflammation, or neoplasm. The ureter is found lateral to the aorta or vena cava in the upper abdomen, typically just anterior to the psoas muscle. It then courses laterally, passing over the iliac vessels at the level of the bifurcation of the common iliac into the external and internal iliac branches. The ureter then follows the lateral pelvis, extending deep into the pelvis and passing posterior to the vas deferens in the male and behind the uterine vessels in the female pelvis, before penetrating the detrusor muscle of the bladder posterolaterally. The ureter is best identified in an area of normal anatomy and then followed to the area of concern. This is readily accomplished medial to the lower pole of the kidney or at the iliac bifurcation. When mobilizing the ureter, it is important to avoid undue traction, which could tear or avulse the ureter when it is friable or fixed by surrounding fibrosis, and to achieve the proper dissection plane to avoid devascularization, which is outside the adventitial sheath. The primary longitudinal blood supply to the ureter is found between the muscularis and the adventitia; it is important to preserve this vascular network. The blood supply to the upper third of the ureter arises mainly from branches of the renal artery and small direct branches of the aorta. The middle third of the ureter draws its blood supply from small iliac branches and, at times, branches from the gonadal vessels. The lower third of the ureter has blood supply from gonadal, hemorrhoidal, internal iliac, and superior and inferior vesical branches. In the female, uterine and cervical vessel branches support the ureter, as do vasal branches in the male. Following prior surgery or retroperitoneal disease processes, any of these rich collateral blood supply sources may not be contributory; thus, it is critical to avoid unnecessary extensive circumferential dissection of the ureter and be cognizant of the potential to cause ischemic injury with injudicious dissection, particularly if the longitudinal vessels are disrupted and the branches from the deep pelvis are unreliable following prior insults to the ureteral feeding vessels.

### Pelvic Anatomy: Bladder, Prostate, and Seminal Vesicles

The bladder has a rich adventitial layer covered by the pelvic peritoneum along the dome and upper posterior wall, under which lies the detrusor muscle, with the submucosa and mucosa internally. The blood supply to the bladder comes from the superior and inferior vesical arteries, which are branches of the internal iliac artery. The prostate lies just caudal to the bladder neck and gains blood supply from the inferior vesical artery branches. Anterior to the lower bladder segment and the prostate lies the dorsal venous plexus (Santorini's plexus), which runs behind the pubic symphysis and is contiguous with the dorsal venous system of the penis or the clitoris in the female. The anterior and lateral bladder walls do not have a peritoneal surface but reside within pelvic fat or may abut the musculature of the pelvic sidewall and pubis anteriorly. The bladder can be injured when entering the abdomen through a midline incision if care is not taken to enter the superior retropubic space (of Retzius) and displace the bladder posteriorly with simple blunt dissection when extending the midline rectus fascial incision to the pubis. By transperitoneal palpation, the balloon of a Foley catheter can be palpated within the bladder, ensuring its correct position and confirming that the bladder is well-drained.

When performing complex pelvic surgery in which the bladder is adherent to a pathologic process, such as diverticulitis or sigmoid colon or rectal cancer, I recommend having full sterile access to the urinary tract, with the genitalia prepped into the operative field and any urinary catheters inserted in a sterile fashion. This allows easy intraoperative filling and drainage of the bladder to aid in its identification and also supports the efforts of a consulting urologist if the bladder needs to be entered, repaired, or partially excised. This may be followed by changing to a larger bore catheter to encourage drainage postoperatively.

When ureteral catheters are placed prior to abdominal surgery to aid in ureteral identification, these catheters are typically tied to the exiting Foley catheter with sutures, allowing all catheters to drain during the operative procedure and enabling ready manipulation of all the tubes intraoperatively. In pelvic trauma, particularly from penetrating injuries, when gross hematuria is present, it is sometimes most expeditious to open the bladder via a longitudinal anterior cystotomy incision to perform inspection and repair. The efflux from the ureteral orifices can be observed through this approach, the entire surface can be evaluated, and the entire bladder is accessible through this exposure, which is easily closed, with minimal morbidity. The prostate and seminal vesicles are typically encountered by the general surgeon during pelvic exploration for trauma or during abdominoperineal resection for rectal cancer. Following pelvic radiotherapy and/or chemotherapy, the dissection plane between the Denonvilliers' fascia, which is just posterior to the prostate, may become fibrotic or obliterated, causing the surgeon to be at risk to enter the prostatic parenchyma or bulbomembranous urethra while trying to separate the perirectal tissues from the urinary tract. When recognized early, the correct dissection plane can be reestablished, although prostatic and urethral repair may be challenging if tissues from the genitourinary side of this dissection are excised or extensively damaged before recognition of the errant plane of dissection. The presence of the Foley catheter is most helpful in guiding the proper dissection, but does not eliminate the potential for iatrogenic injury. The seminal vesicles extend superolaterally from the base (cephalad extent) of the prostate and are prone to injury in the same situations as noted; if entered, they can be sutured or excised with little concern, unless fertility is an issue for the patient.

### Groin, Genitalia, and Perineum

Inguinal anatomy is well known to all general surgeons. The relevant urologic issues in this anatomic region relate to the spermatic cord and male genitalia. The detailed anatomy of the scrotal contents is beyond the scope of this discussion; suffice it to say that the testis lies within a mesothelial envelope, the tunica vaginalis. The vascular and genital ductal structures leave the testis from the mediastinum in the posterosuperior portion and travel via the scrotal neck into the inguinal canal. The spermatic cord is invested by the internal spermatic fascia, derived from the transversalis fascia. The cremaster muscle is derived from the internal oblique. The external spermatic fascia, derived from the external oblique aponeurosis, joins the cord below the external ring. The cord is susceptible to injury during inguinal dissection for hernia repair, especially in redo cases, when it may be encased in fibrosis and injured without recognition. Significant injury to the cord may put the viability of the testis at risk, even though the testis is supported by three collateral blood supply sources—external spermatic artery from the external iliac, internal spermatic or gonadal artery from the aorta, and vasal artery from the internal iliac branches. The vas deferens itself may also be injured anywhere along its course, from the midscrotal level to the inguinal canal to its intrapelvic portion. When inguinal herniorrhaphy is performed, care must be taken to avoid excessive tightening at the internal ring level, because compression of the cord at this level can result in venous, lymphatic, or arterial obstruction. In addition, the common use of nonabsorbable mesh materials in hernia repair, whether performed through an open inguinal or laparoscopic approach, may result in fibrotic and inflammatory changes involving the vas deferens, which can cause late occlusion and potentially azoospermia and infertility. This phenomenon has been well-documented in the literature; patients in their reproductive years should be counseled about this risk of groin surgery.[2]

At times, exploration for inguinal hernia may reveal other forms of scrotal pathology that were misdiagnosed preoperatively, including hydrocele and spermatocele. Urologic consultation may be helpful when atypical groin or scrotal anatomy is anticipated preoperatively or encountered at the time of surgery.

The evaluation of the acute scrotum requires a sophisticated knowledge of genital structure and normal anatomy, as well as extensive clinical experience, for accurate diagnosis. The epididymis is located posteriorly and slightly lateral position to the testis; distinguishing acute epididymitis or epididymo-orchitis from testicular torsion or trauma is a commonly encountered clinical challenge. Scrotal ultrasound may be a helpful adjunct to history and physical examination in the rapid assessment of patients,[3] because it is critical to rule out testicular torsion promptly to avoid permanent ischemic injury.

Penile anatomy is seldom relevant to the general surgeon, aside from issues related to urethral catheterization. Urologists are well versed in penile and urethral surgery in the elective and emergency settings and can be helpful to the general surgeon when urethral catheterization is challenging, in the trauma setting, and in the setting of neoplastic and inflammatory disease when anatomy is obscure.

In perineal surgical approaches, urology consultation may be helpful to the general surgeon, as noted, when performing abdominoperineal resection for rectal cancer and when performing incision and drainage or débridement for a perirectal abscess, perineal gangrene, or local neoplasms. The male and female urethras are palpable throughout their length, from the tip of the penis to the prostate in the male or from the urethral meatus to the bladder neck in the female. In the male, the bulbomembranous and prostatic urethra are immediately adjacent to the sites of dissection for these entities. The presence of a urethral catheter is helpful in palpating the location of the urethra, but the corpus spongiosum surrounding the bulbar urethra and the prostatic urethra and parenchyma are still vulnerable to injury with dissection in an errant or obliterated anatomic plane. At the level of the membranous urethra, within the external sphincter of the pelvic floor, the corpus spongiosum essentially disappears, leaving only the relatively thin-walled urethra, which must be approached with great care to avoid inadvertent laceration, transection, or excision.

## ENDOSCOPIC UROLOGIC SURGERY

Urology was the first surgical specialty to embrace diagnostic and therapeutic endoscopic surgery. The history of the development of the cystoscope and the modern evolution of ureteroscopy, percutaneous nephroscopy, and urologic laparoscopy represent fascinating stories in the book of surgical history. Urology as a discipline has the good fortune of being able, in most situations, to assess the urinary tract fully with endourologic techniques and high-resolution imaging; thus, in urology, exploration of the various components of this organ system, without a reasonably well-formulated preoperative diagnosis, is uncommon. The general surgeon should have a basic working knowledge of urologic endoscopy because it affects what we can provide as consultants and how we can support surgical interventions to enhance safety and contend with complex anatomy, trauma, and surgical complications.

Cystoscopy (or, technically, cystourethroscopy) may be performed with rigid or flexible fiberoptic instrumentation. In the pediatric setting, endoscopes range from approximately 7 to 14 Fr sizes; in the adult, rigid cystoscopes or resectoscopes generally range from 15 Fr flexible and17 French diagnostic rigid scopes to 26 to 28 Fr operating resectoscopes.

Extensive training in lower tract endoscopy is an important part of a urology residency program because injudicious use of lower tract scopes can result in significant iatrogenic injury. Flexible cystoscopy may readily be performed under local anesthesia alone, using 2% lidocaine jelly instilled into the urethra as a topical anesthetic. Rigid lower tract endoscopy is more difficult to perform in the awake patient, although it is much better tolerated in the female than in the male because of the short, straight female urethra. In general, male rigid cystoscopy is performed under conscious sedation or regional or general anesthesia in most modern practice settings. The flexible cystoscope is fully deflectable, allowing complete examination of the bladder and also allowing retroflexion to look back at the bladder neck or prostate without difficulty. To observe the entire bladder lumen with a rigid scope, I generally use interchangeable lenses with a standard metal sheath and connecting bridge; commonly available telescopes include 0- or 5-degree lenses for urethral surgery and 30- and 70-degree telescopes to view the entire bladder surface. Various biopsy and grasping instruments are compatible with flexible and rigid scopes.

Via a standard cystoscope, upper tract anatomy may be demonstrated by performing retrograde ureterography or retrograde pyelography. Cone-tipped or straight injectable ureteral catheters may be used to inject water-soluble iodinated contrast into the upper urinary tract under fluoroscopic or plain film guidance to obtain high-quality images of the ureters and renal collecting systems. Even in patients with a history of allergy to iodinated contrast, retrograde pyelography may be safely performed as long as unduly forceful injection with resultant contrast extravasation is avoided. It is wise to provide medical suppression of a possible allergic reaction (e.g., antihistamine, corticosteroid) in such cases, when it is imperative to perform these studies in a patient with a history of contrast allergy.

Cystoscopically, ureteral catheters can be inserted and left in position during a general surgery procedure to aid in identifying the ureters in an abnormal anatomic field. I generally use open-ended 5 or 6 Fr catheters for this purpose and tie the catheter to a Foley catheter for retention.

More advanced lower tract endoscopy may involve dilation, incision, or ablation of urethral lesions or stricture, lithotripsy for lower tract calculi, removal of foreign bodies from the urinary tract, and biopsy or resection of bladder tumors or obstructing prostatic or bladder neck tissue, benign or malignant. Urethral stricture incision, which is usually palliative and not curative, may be performed using a specialized cystoscope called an *internal* or *optical urethrotome* to which a variety of types of cutting blades or laser fibers may be applied. For resection of prostate tissue or bladder lesions of tumors, a cold cup biopsy forceps may be passed through a standard cystoscope to obtain small tissue biopsies, which can then be cauterized by a cautery electrode. For extensive tissue resection tasks in the prostate or bladder, an electroresectoscope is typically used. Traditional resection procedures use a cutting loop that can remove tissue in chips using the cutting current of the electroresection unit, with the coagulation current then used to obtain hemostasis. Newer technologies have now come into common use as well, including the GreenLight laser (American Medical Systems, Minnetonka, Minn) for ablating benign prostatic tissue, Holmium laser (Boston Scientific, Natick, Mass) for treating some bladder tumors, and the normal saline bipolar resection system, which uses cutting loop or button electrodes for the ablation of tissue without the hemolysis or hyponatremia risk of the use of sterile water or 1.5% glycine, which is generally used for lower tract endoscopic surgery. After resection of prostatic or bladder tumor tissue, the fragments must be removed from the bladder by irrigating them out through the scope using commonly available instruments, such as the Ellik evacuator (C.R. Bard, Madison, Ga). When resecting lesions near the ureteral orifices, I always take care to avoid applying coagulating current to the orifice circumferentially because this may result in scarring and obstruction.

Following lower tract endoscopic surgery, I routinely consider whether an indwelling drainage catheter is necessary. This depends on the adequacy of hemostasis, thinness of the bladder wall following resection of a tumor, and desire to have a catheter across the prostate and to allow the prostatic fossa to clot and be defunctionalized temporarily following transurethral resection of the prostate (TURP). Depending on the specific situation, I may often choose to implement continuous bladder irrigation (CBI) with normal saline following lower tract endoscopic surgery. This is most commonly performed using a three-way catheter, a Foley catheter with an additional infusion port that allows saline to be dripped into the bladder and efflux to be drained continuously to a drainage bag. After TURP, CBI is particularly helpful to avoid clot formation in the bladder, which could occlude the catheter and require manual irrigation. One pitfall with this approach is that if the outflow lumen of the catheter becomes occluded with a clot and the inflow continues, significant bladder distention can occur unrecognized, putting the bladder at risk for perforation or encouraging more bleeding by distending the recently operated bladder wall or prostatic fossa. The nursing staff responsible for monitoring CBI must be aware of this potential, must turn off the inflow, and have instructions on whether and how to irrigate the outflow port of the catheter if this situation arises.

Surgeons caring for urologic surgery patients in a postoperative or intensive care unit (ICU) setting should have close communication with their urologic colleagues regarding catheter management—whether a catheter can be safely irrigated or exchanged, what degree of hematuria is expected or acceptable, how to treat bladder spasms, when the catheter can be safely removed, and whether imaging studies will be necessary prior to doing this.

## UROLOGIC INFECTIOUS DISEASE

Genitourinary infection encompasses a wide range of disorders that cross paths with the clinical experience of the general surgeon. These include uncomplicated urinary infections, which may affect whether to proceed with elective surgery, complex necrotizing genital infections, for which the surgeon's expertise may be needed for judicious and complete débridement, and chronic renal infection, which may fistulize to the colon or flank. Urinary tract obstruction with concomitant closed space infection may result in urosepsis and septic shock, challenging the skills of the urologist and surgical critical care specialist.

### Uncomplicated Urinary Tract Infection

Urinary infection is considered uncomplicated when it occurs in the immunocompetent host, without underlying anatomic or physiologic abnormalities of the urinary tract. Risk factors include prior infections, sexual activity in the premenopausal female and, in some settings, an uncircumcised penis. Patients may present with asymptomatic bacteriuria prior to elective surgery or with typical irritative symptoms, such as frequency, dysuria, hematuria, and/or suprapubic or perineal pain or discomfort. Significant infection is diagnosed on culture, based on the presence of more than 100,000 colony forming units (CFU)/mL and, typically, by the presence of pyuria and nitrite positivity on urinalysis. Common organisms include *Escherichia coli,* other Enterobacteriacae, and *Enterococcus* spp.

As a general principle, it is desirable to eradicate asymptomatic bacteriuria or symptomatic infection prior to urologic or neurologic surgery to minimize the risk of the development of febrile infection in the perioperative period, because manipulation of the urinary tract in the presence of infection, even as limited as Foley catheter placement or bladder distention following anesthesia, may promote the development of a significant clinical infection. Deciding whether elective surgery should be cancelled if urinary infection or colonization is noted soon before surgery must be based on the urgency of the planned procedure and anticipated risk of promoting clinical infection by the planned manipulation. In the higher risk patient (e.g., older or infirm patients, or when urinary tract manipulation is anticipated), postponement of elective surgery until treatment has been provided is the most cautious approach. Treatment is best based on specific culture data whenever possible in the setting of surgical preparation, but the empirical use of fluoroquinolones, trimethoprim-sulfamethoxazole, cephalosporins, or broad-spectrum penicillin derivatives is common, preferably with confirmation that the urine chemical dipstick and microscopic findings have normalized and the culture has become negative.

Recurrent uncomplicated infections may occur in the absence of any significant urinary tract pathology. Typically caused by changing flora, common clinical settings include young, sexually active females and older patients. Although recurrent asymptomatic bacteriuria may be observed without treatment in some settings, in most cases it is treated with oral antibiotics.

Uncomplicated infection also is common postoperatively following urologic or nonurologic surgery; technically, however, this may be more appropriately viewed as a complicated infection when the patient has been hospitalized, catheterized, or has had urologic manipulation during surgery. Patients may commonly complain of urinary irritation following urethral catheterization but, if such complaints are persistent or substantial, or are accompanied by hematuria or progressively worsening symptoms, urinalysis and culture should be carried out and empirical therapy commenced while awaiting the culture results if the urinalysis suggests infection.

It is important for the surgeon to remember that in specific clinical settings, the urine may not show signs of infection while the patient is, in fact, seriously infected. For example, this can occur with complete unilateral upper tract obstruction from stone, stricture, or iatrogenic occlusion. If no urine is reaching the bladder from the obstructed upper tract, the bladder urine may be negative microscopically and on culture. Failure to appreciate this possibility can result in failure to diagnose a dangerous obstruction with infection and may lead to preventable morbidity or mortality.

## Complicated Urinary Tract Infection

Complicated urinary infection occurs in the setting of underlying abnormalities of the physiology or anatomy of the genitourinary system or in the presence of an immunocompromised host.[4] Patients who recently have been catheterized or have undergone hospitalization and/or urologic or nonurologic surgery also fall into the category of patients with complicated urinary infection, because they may be experiencing transient functional or anatomic problems or may have acquired a nosocomial infection by resistant or atypical organism. Certain specific infections of the genitourinary system may require the surgeon's involvement in the operative or critical care support setting. Patients with relapsing infection— that is, recurrent infection with the same organism following standard treatment for which eradication should be expected—should undergo urologic evaluation to determine whether there is a complicating factor preventing the infection from fully responding to standard treatment (e.g., unrecognized obstructed kidney or ureter, chronic abscess, impaired bladder emptying, foreign body in the urinary tract, ischemic state, urinary fistula).

Patients for whom a complicated infection is suspected should have culture data obtained and be aggressively treated with antibacterial therapy based on culture-specific antibiotic selection. Investigations to rule out an occult source of persistent infection should be pursued. These should include a careful urologic history and physical examination with urologic consultation, urologic imaging with ultrasound or CT, and measurement of postvoid residual (PVR) urine volume using an ultrasound-based bladder scan device or catheter drainage.

A patient who is sick enough to warrant hospitalization for a febrile urinary infection, particularly if there are lateralizing signs potentially indicative of an upper tract inflammatory process (e.g., flank pain, tenderness, swelling, erythema), should have upper tract imaging performed urgently (ultrasound or CT). This should be done to ensure there is no undrained infection in an obstructed upper tract. I teach our residents that "the sun should never set on the obstructed, infected urinary tract"; these patients may deteriorate rapidly, despite antibiotic therapy, hydration, and supportive care, if prompt drainage is not instituted.[5] I have witnessed deaths that might have been preventable when a patient was hospitalized for presumed pyelonephritis, but without upper tract imaging, which would have demonstrated an obstructing ureteral calculus with proximal pyonephrosis.

When urinary tract obstruction with infection is diagnosed, drainage may be achieved by Foley catheter or suprapubic cystostomy placement for lower tract. For upper tract obstruction, cystoscopic insertion of a ureteral stent or percutaneous nephrostomy placement is necessary. The selection of drainage approach is a judgment call in every case, based on the technical resources and expertise available, promptness of access to such resources, condition of the patient, and specific tasks to be achieved and challenges anticipated in achieving them. If, for example, a patient is floridly septic, with hydronephrosis and an obstructing ureteral calculus, the urologist must consider the potentially adverse impact of an anesthetic procedure with lower tract manipulation, which might allow a ureteral stent to pass a tightly obstructing ureteral occlusion, versus the risk of renal bleeding and passage of infected urine into the bloodstream with an attempt at a percutaneous drainage approach. With the latter option, the coagulation status of the patient is also a critical consideration, because percutaneous nephrostomy placement in a coagulopathic or anticoagulated patient could introduce a significant bleeding risk.

In achieving retrograde ureteral stent insertion, the urologist may choose a double-J internalized stent or an externally draining open-ended catheter, which is typically tied to a Foley catheter with sutures, similar to the approach used when a ureteral catheter is placed prior to pelvic or retroperitoneal surgery to aid in ureteral identification. Internal stents have the advantage of being less prone to dislodgment, and may be more comfortable for longer indwelling times, but the externally draining catheter has the advantage of being available for continuous monitoring of urine output and irrigation if it becomes clogged with pus, debris, or blood clots. Externally draining ureteral catheters generally are not left in place for more than a few days at a time. With internal stents, it is important to document their presence and discuss with the patient and family, when they could be reasonably expected to comprehend and recall the discussion, the temporary nature of the stent and importance of follow-up and removal to avoid late encrustation, occlusion, infection, obstruction, and potential loss of kidney function.[6] This is an important medicolegal issue in the critical care and trauma settings that has been the source of litigation.

With the drainage approach, aspirated material from the kidney or ureter should be sent for Gram staining and culture including, in the appropriate clinical setting, aerobes, anaerobes, fungi, and acid-fast bacilli. For patients already on antibiotics prior to obtaining specimens for culture, Gram staining may be of particular value because an organism may not grow in the presence of high urinary concentrations of antibiotics and Gram staining might indicate the type of organism present.

The presence of polymicrobial flora with a complicated urinary infection could indicate a contaminated specimen or may be meaningful, as in the presence of an enterourinary fistula. A number of organisms may be observed in the presence of indwelling catheters, neurogenic bladder dysfunction, or foreign body. Initial empirical therapy for presumed complicated urinary infection should cover resistant gram-negative bacilli, gram-positive cocci, including enterococcal and resistant staphylococcal organisms and, at times, anaerobes. Antibiotic selection for the wide variety of surgical infections is covered in detail elsewhere in this text.

## Specific Complicated Genitourinary Infectious States

### Emphysematous Infection and Infections in the Diabetic Patient

Gas-forming or emphysematous infection of the urinary tract is usually seen in the poorly controlled diabetic patient. Emphysematous pyelonephritis typically presents as a fulminant infection involving the renal parenchyma, which may progress to involve the perinephric space[7] (Fig. 73-1). A lesser form of this process, emphysematous pyelitis, results in gas within the renal collecting system but not within the parenchyma. The causative agent most commonly is *E. coli*, which produces gas through a facultative anaerobic or fermentative process. Significant soft tissue destruction may result and a picture consistent with urosepsis is common. Control of the metabolic abnormalities and aggressive antibiotic and supportive therapy in a critical care setting are essential. If there is upper tract obstruction present, it should be relieved promptly with retrograde or antegrade tube drainage. If discrete purulent collections are present based on computed tomography (CT) imaging, percutaneous drainage may be attempted while the sepsis is being controlled medically. These patients often require urgent nephrectomy, although if the

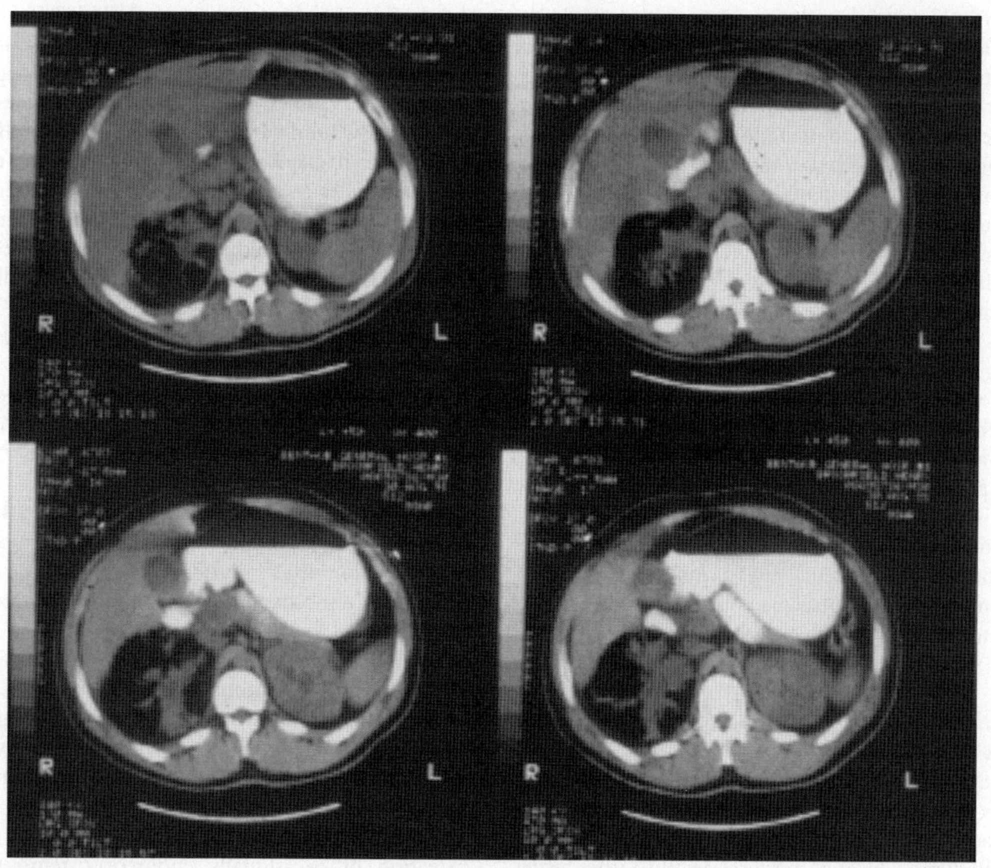


**FIGURE 73-1** Emphysematous pyelonephritis. This CT scan demonstrates extensive destruction of the right kidney with intraparenchymal gas on the right, obliterating the renal architecture. The left kidney is normal.

overall clinical status is improving with medical treatment, there may be an advantage to delaying surgical intervention until the patient is more stable. At times, the process may be focal or segmental and may respond solely to medical therapy and indicated drainage procedures.

Emphysematous cystitis is a gas-forming infection involving the bladder wall, with gas evident in the submucosa and/or detrusor level, also best demonstrated on a CT scan. Therapy consists of urinary catheter drainage, aggressive antibiotic therapy, and supportive care.

Acute papillary necrosis is also most commonly seen in the diabetic patient.[8] Often, there is an underlying ischemic state involving the renal papillae, which progresses to frank necrosis and passage of the sloughed papilla into the collecting system and ureter, causing obstruction and, if concomitant infection is present, often progresses to urosepsis. These patients require urgent drainage of the obstructed upper tract and, after their infection is resolved, endoscopic evacuation of the necrotic tissue. This process may present as a fulminant infectious illness or as a chronically progressive process.

Gas may be present in the urinary tract from anaerobic urinary infection in the absence of these emphysematous processes. Gas may also be present because of instrumentation or catheterization or the presence of urinary tract fistulae; the most common is the colovesical fistula secondary to complications of diverticulitis or colonic neoplasms.

### Xanthogranulomatous Pyelonephritis

Xanthogranulomatous pyelonephritis (XGP) is a specific clinical and histologic entity that involves the presence of a foamy, lipid-laden, macrophage infiltrate in the renal parenchyma, with extensive inflammation, fibrosis, and loss of function. It is thought to result from chronic bacterial infection, usually in the presence of stones and chronic obstruction.[9] The kidney is typically nonfunctional or poorly functioning and may be a source of chronic disease, pain, persistent infection, and sometimes fistulization to the flank or adjacent organs. Nephrectomy is usually indicated. Radiographically, by CT, there may be an apparent collecting system dilation; however, drainage attempts often are unproductive because the material is often solid or too viscous to drain. Patients may present with active infection and require a cooling off period with antibiotics and supportive care to be readied for surgery. The general surgeon may become involved in such cases because of this lesion's propensity to become densely adherent to surrounding structures, particularly the diaphragm, pancreas, duodenum, great vessels, iliac vessels, and flank wall. The risk of iatrogenic adjacent organ injury is high in these nephrectomies. Often, the renal hilum is so inflamed and fibrotic that the renal vessels cannot be individually dissected; in these cases, placement of a vascular pedicle clamp with renal excision and oversewing the pedicle is necessary.

### Epididymitis, Epididymo-Orchitis, Without and With abscess

The topic of the acute scrotum is important to urologists and general surgeons because the differential diagnosis can be challenging and an accurate diagnosis may only be achievable surgically.[10] The epididymis, located posterolateral to the testis, becomes infected through ascending infection from the urinary tract down the vas deferens into the scrotum. When infection is advanced, the entire scrotal contents ipsilaterally become involved, with overlying skin fixation and edema. It may be difficult to distinguish this entity from late torsion, incarcerated inguinal hernia, or testicular tumor with necrosis and inflammation. Scrotal ultrasound is useful diagnostically, especially to rule out associated abscess. Cultures should be obtained and patients should be treated with broad-spectrum antibiotics. If abscess is present, surgical drainage and often orchiectomy is indicated. If improvement is seen with medical therapy, rest, and scrotal elevation, continued observation may result in eventual, although often slow, resolution with medical therapy alone. If there is persistent pain and mass, or signs of testicular ischemia are noted by repeat Doppler imaging, exploration and orchiectomy may still be necessary to resolve the process.

### Fournier's Gangrene

Gas-forming and necrotizing soft tissue infections are covered in detail elsewhere in this text. When the genitalia are involved, patients typically present with significant pain and tenderness, scrotal and genital swelling, discoloration or frank necrosis, crepitus and, at times, foul-smelling discharge (Fig. 73-2). Bacteriologically, these infections are usually polymicrobial, with aerobes, anaerobes, gram-positive, and gram-negative organisms. Necrotizing soft tissue infections of the genitalia, as in other anatomic regions, require aggressive broad-spectrum antibiotic treatment, supportive care, and urgent surgical drainage with aggressive débridement of the necrotic tissue.[11] The magnitude of the débridement depends entirely on the degree of progression of the process. It is rare for the process to involve the testicles or deep tissues of the penis, so these structures should be preserved, if possible. I prefer to separate the parietal tunica vaginalis of the testes from the overlying necrotic dartos and skin and preserve the tunical compartment intact, which helps with wound care and patient comfort. If the penile skin is necrotic, it can be débrided down to but not through the Buck's fascial layer. It is uncommon for the urethra to be involved although, occasionally, a defined urinary tract source may be evident, such as a urethral stricture with perforation and local infection. Suprapubic tube diversion is generally not necessary; urethral catheter drainage is generally sufficient. Wound vacuum-assisted closure (VAC) device placement after purulence has resolved results in rapid wound size reduction and fluid evacuation. Grafting large defects with meshed split-thickness grafts for the scrotum and nonmeshed thick split-thickness grafts for the penile shaft yields favorable results.

### Genitourinary Fungal and Tuberculous Infections

Fungal infections of the urinary tract are most often seen in diabetics, immunocompromised patients, and those who have had extensive nosocomial and antibiotic exposure. These infections vary markedly, from superficial candidal infections of the groins and genitalia, treatable with standard topical agents, to invasive fungal infections of the bladder or kidneys that may cause urosepsis and be life-threatening.[12] Fungal infections are addressed in general terms elsewhere in this text. Specific issues related to the urinary tract include the occasional need for antifungal bladder irrigation, potential for fungal deposits (fungus balls) forming in the renal colleting system requiring direct irrigation or occasionally endoscopic removal, and complex cutaneous involvement of the genitalia. Infectious disease consultation and support are valuable in such cases because the

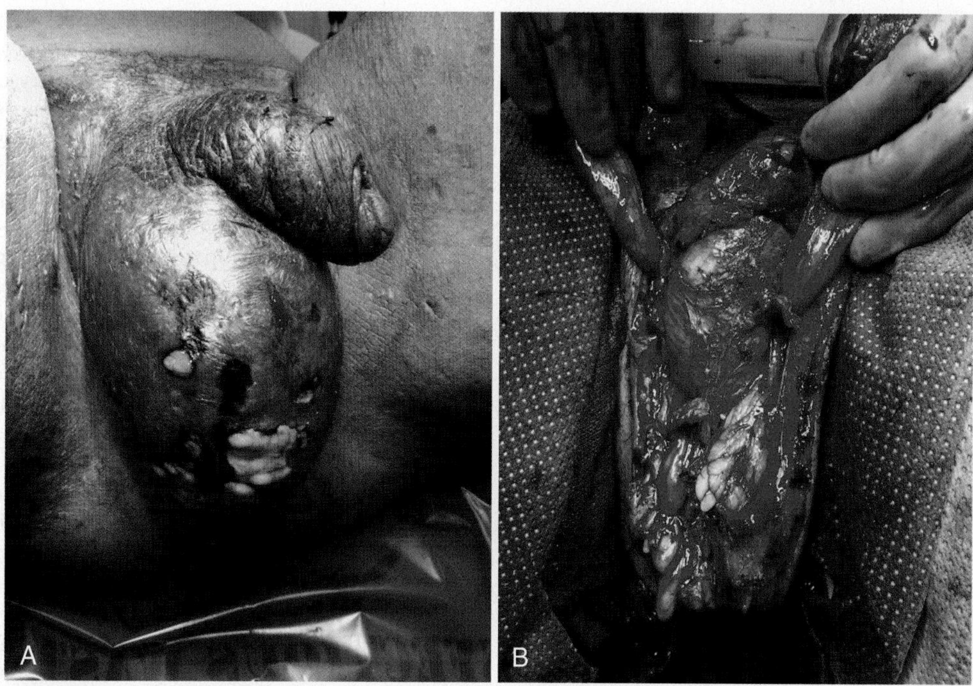


**FIGURE 73-2** Fournier's gangrene. **A,** Skin necrosis, purulence, and edema of the scrotum. The skin can also be normal-appearing, with much more subtle physical findings in some cases. **B,** Appearance following extensive débridement of scrotal skin and underlying tissues. The base of the penis is visible centrally; the testes are elevated out of the field and the spermatic cords are visible anteriorly.

organisms may be resistant and atypical, and selection of treatment agents may not be straightforward.

Genitourinary (GU) tuberculosis may be manifested as an isolated GU infection (e.g., tuberculous cystitis, epididymitis) or as part of a systemic infection.[13] Urine cultures from the first morning void are most effective in detecting infection. Current references should be consulted to address specific anti-infective therapy agent selection. Upper urinary tract tuberculosis infection may cause ureteral strictures, which may progress even with therapy and result in silent obstruction and renal loss if not promptly detected. These patients should be regularly monitored by ultrasound to assure adequate upper tract drainage. Tuberculous epididymitis should be suspected if chronic epididymitis results in cutaneous fistula formation; following adequate medical therapy, epididymectomy or orchiectomy may be indicated for residual mass, pain, or fistula. Renal nonfunction following diagnosis and treatment may occasionally require partial or total nephrectomy. As a general principle, atypical infections of the genitourinary system should prompt testing for an immunocompromised state, including testing for HIV status, because varied urologic manifestations of such viral infections may be observed.[14]

## VOIDING DYSFUNCTION, BLADDER OUTLET OBSTRUCTION, BENIGN PROSTATIC HYPERPLASIA, AND INCONTINENCE

The accurate diagnosis and tailored management of voiding dysfunction is an important aspect of general urologic care. From simple postoperative urinary retention caused by immobility, local pain, and medication side effects, to female or male stress incontinence following pelvic surgery, to the complex neurourologic disorders of the spinal cord injury patient, voiding dysfunction is one of the most common reasons to consult an urologist. To focus on the most important and common entities in this broad range of pathology, I will discuss four examples, as well as male voiding dysfunction caused by benign prostatic hyperplasia (BPH).

### Postoperative Acute Urinary Retention

This problem can have many causes. Common contributing factors are immobility, narcosis, anticholinergic side effects of anesthetic agents, underlying subclinical bladder outlet obstruction, and local pain and spasm (typical after hemorrhoid or groin hernia surgery). If a patient requires straight catheterization once, it is reasonable to allow a voiding trial but, if a second catheterization is required, it may be best to leave an indwelling Foley catheter for 1 or more days, depending on the volume of distention. Short-term treatment with $\alpha$-adrenergic blocking agents (e.g., tamsulosin) and adequate analgesics may be beneficial in bringing about prompt resolution. If the patient fails another voiding trial after a short period of catheter drainage, further investigation, including urodynamic studies and cystoscopy, may be necessary to determine the cause of the retention and appropriate management. Following coronary bypass surgery or other procedures requiring cardiopulmonary bypass, it appears that postoperative retention is particularly common, possibly because of transient prostatic swelling, among other factors. Similar management principles apply.

### Urinary Incontinence

Incontinence, or the inability to exercise full volitional control of urine passage, is often classified symptomatically. Urgency incontinence is loss of urine associated with an urge to void. Stress incontinence is loss of urine with movement, straining, or increase in abdominal pressure. Overflow incontinence is loss of urine when the bladder becomes full and there is an inability to empty volitionally. Mixed incontinence combines these.

Urge incontinence is most commonly caused by overactive bladder or detrusor instability. This may be age-related, caused by a specific anatomic bladder irritative focus, or be neurologic in origin. Urologic consultation may be necessary to determine the cause; anticholinergic or antimuscarinic medication therapy is the mainstay of treatment once critical underlying issues (e.g., bladder tumor, carcinoma in situ, obstruction) are excluded. There is a burgeoning variety of overactive bladder medications on the market. They generally have predictable side effects, including dry mouth, constipation, and often confusion in older adults, and should be avoided in patients with a history of narrow-angle glaucoma; an ophthalmologist's approval should be sought for these patients. These drugs will decrease urgency and episodes of urge incontinence in most patients and are typically safe for long-term use. Refractory cases may require more complex interventions, including nerve stimulator devices, intravesical botulinum toxin injections and, rarely, surgical bladder augmentation.[15]

Stress incontinence results from anatomic changes in the pelvic floor or sphincteric apparatus that lead to excessive bladder hypermobility or sphincteric incompetence, so that with an increase in abdominal pressure, urine is involuntarily lost. Common clinical settings would be following multiple vaginal deliveries, with stretching of the pelvic floor supports and bladder prolapse, and male incontinence after radical prostatectomy. The treatment may be behavioral (e.g., biofeedback training, pelvic floor exercises), involve injectable bulking agents (injected into the sphincteric region) or surgical (e.g., female pelvic floor reconstruction, female or male sling device implants, artificial urinary sphincter device implant). This is a specialized area of urologic care and surgery. Urodynamics testing may be useful in assessing the sphincter anatomy and function prior to initiating therapy.

Overflow incontinence is involuntary loss of urine caused by excessive bladder fullness. It is often missed as a diagnosis; careful history, physical examination to palpate or percuss the full bladder, and/or measurement of postvoid residual by ultrasound or catheter drainage are essential. Treatment is based on determining the cause of the bladder distention (obstructive versus detrusor dysfunction) and managing that issue accordingly—for example, by corrective surgery for bladder outlet obstruction or self-intermittent catheterization for refractory detrusor failure.

It is common for incontinence to be mixed—that is, to have elements of stress and urgency. Urodynamic testing is important in such cases to distinguish obstruction from detrusor dysfunction and to plan therapy.[16] In general, the medical component (e.g., bladder control medicine for urgency) is treated first, with surgical intervention reserved for patients in whom medical management is not effective or does not address a critical underlying problem, such as high-grade outlet obstruction.

## Neurourology and Voiding Dysfunction of the Neurologically Impaired

This complex area of specialization in urology requires a working knowledge of the neurologic basis of voiding function and understanding how lesions of the central and peripheral nervous systems affect bladder and outlet function. Briefly, patients with cerebral dysfunction (e.g., dementia) may develop uninhibited detrusor function with challenges to urinary control; they may respond to bladder control medicines. Patients with cervical cord lesions often develop detrusor-sphincter dyssynergia, in which the outlet paradoxically closes against high bladder contraction pressures. This entity can cause serious damage to the lower and upper urinary tracts and must be managed by a neurourologist expert in caring for such patients; anticholinergic therapy, intermittent catheterization, and other surgical interventions may be necessary, with close upper tract anatomy monitoring. These patients may be prone to autonomic dysreflexia, which can result in severe episodic hypertension. Patients with lower lumbar or sacral lesions typically develop bladder flaccidity and impaired emptying, requiring mechanical assistance to aid in bladder drainage.

## Benign Prostatic Hyperplasia and Bladder Outlet and Urethral Obstruction

BPH is generally considered to be the most common benign internal neoplasm of the adult male. It is an almost ubiquitous process in men, although varying greatly in degree, bothersomeness, and complications.

BPH may result in LUTS (lower urinary tract symptoms) and BOO (bladder outlet obstruction). The process involves hypertrophy and hyperplasia, with increased glandular and stromal elements of the prostate in varying amounts. There is little correlation between the measured volume of the prostate and degree of symptomatology that results. In addition, the degree of BOO does not necessarily correlate with the severity of LUTS. Symptoms may be mild and manageable just with watchful waiting, or may be more significant, requiring long-term medical therapy and, at times, surgical intervention. Complications of BPH may include bladder damage and loss of function from chronic distention, upper tract deterioration, troublesome hematuria, bladder stone formation, and recurrent urinary infection. Practice guidelines for BPH have been produced by the American Urologic Association to guide providers in the diagnosis and management of BPH.[17] The basic evaluation involves history and physical examination, digital rectal examination, urinalysis, prostate-specific antigen (PSA) level testing (in select patients), other interventions to rule out prostate cancer and, at times, other tests to rule out other significant urologic pathology (e.g., urine cytology, upper tract imaging, cystoscopy). A quantitative symptom score may be useful. Checking PVR urine volume may be valuable as well. After the basic assessment, patients are directed toward some therapeutic approach, such as watchful waiting, medical therapy, or minimally invasive or standard surgical intervention. The management selection reflects patient preferences and the presence of complicating factors.

Medical therapy options consist of $\alpha$-adrenergic blocking agents and/or 5-alpha-reductase inhibitors. The former work on the $\alpha$ or $\alpha_{1a}$ receptors (e.g., tamsulosin) of the bladder outlet, relaxing smooth muscle in the prostatic stroma and bladder neck region. They may cause some orthostatic side effects, which are usually mild. 5-Alpha-reductase inhibitors (e.g., finasteride, dutasteride) block the conversion of testosterone to dihydrotestosterone, the active agent that causes and maintains BPH. These agents will reduce the actual volume of the prostate, with maximal effects seen by 6 months, and maintain that volume

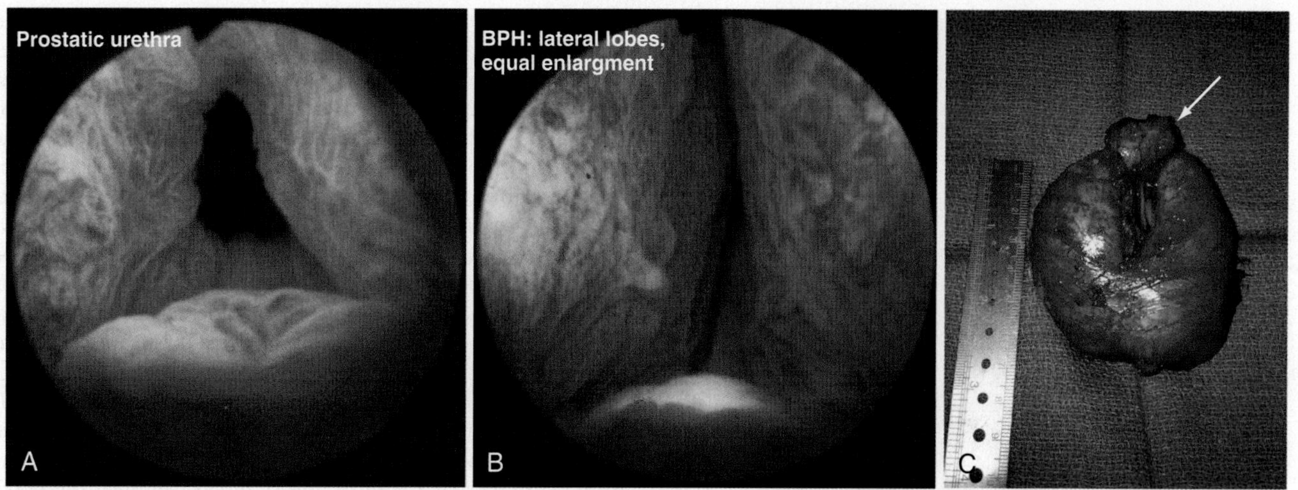


**FIGURE 73-3** BPH. **A,** Normal cystoscopic appearance of the prostate in a young man. **B,** Moderate BPH, viewed cystoscopically. The size of the prostate correlates poorly with the magnitude of voiding symptoms. **C,** Prostatic adenoma following simple open prostatectomy. Note the small medial lobe *(arrow, top center),* with large lateral lobes (130-g specimen).

reduction during continued use. This class of drugs also alters the serum PSA level (reduces it ≈50%), which must be kept in mind with regard to prostate cancer screening.

When medical therapy is ineffective and symptoms remain bothersome, or when there is an objective surgical indication (e.g., severe obstruction based on urodynamic data, recurrent hematuria or infection, urinary tract anatomic deterioration from obstruction), surgical intervention is considered. The standard approaches include minimally invasive options (e.g., laser procedures, thermotherapy, microwave procedure), TURP or, when the adenomatous growth is particularly large, open simple prostatectomy to enucleate the adenoma surgically (Fig. 73-3). Complications of these surgical procedures include persistent bleeding, prostatic capsular perforation, or perforation into periprostatic venous sinuses, with fluid absorption, which may result in hyponatremia because of the glycine irrigation typically used (newer electroresection systems use normal saline with a bipolar electrode, eliminating the hyponatremia risk) and, rarely, injury of an adjacent structure (e.g., rectal injury with TURP or open prostatectomy).

Because BOO and LUTS from BPH are so common in today's aging population, the general surgeon will deal with many patients with this diagnosis. If any difficulty is encountered when catheterizing a patient with BPH, a coude-tipped catheter should be used, with the angulated tip oriented cephalad; this will allow atraumatic catheterization for many BPH patients. If this is not successful, a urologist should be consulted to assess the patient and determine whether there is another cause of obstruction, such as a urethral stricture or bladder neck contracture, which may be present in up to 10% of patients post-TURP; this may require a more specialized technique for urethral passage.

## MALE REPRODUCTIVE AND SEXUAL DYSFUNCTION

An area of practice to which urologists devote significant attention is male infertility and sexual dysfunction.[18] Diagnostic evaluation, medical treatment, and surgical therapy represent sophisticated aspects of urologic care; general surgeons should have a basic familiarity with the management of these disorders. They may at times be called on to participate in the treatment of surgical complications of genital surgery and prosthetic implant surgery; the patient's history of having undergone these procedures may affect the precautions and challenges of nonurologic pelvic and groin procedures.

### Male Infertility: Evaluation and Treatment

Infertility affects approximately 15% to 20% of couples; the male factor is primary or sole factor in 50% of these cases. Couples are often referred to the urologist following a period of infertility, and referrals are generally from a primary care physician and often from the evaluating gynecologist. It is not uncommon in my experience as a urologist to receive a patient following an exhaustive workup and extensive treatment for female reproductive dysfunction only to discover late in the process that there is a significant male factor, typically identified by semen analysis.

The standard male factor evaluation involves a detailed history, physical examination, and basic laboratory and imaging evaluation. The history should include a discussion regarding sexual and reproductive history, including potential gonadotoxic exposure, urologic and sexually transmitted infections, trauma and prior surgery involving the pelvis, groin, and genitalia, and family history of infertility. Physical assessment should include a general evaluation of masculinization, genital findings, including normal meatal location, testicular size and, consistently, presence and normalcy of the epididymis and vas deferens, and possible presence of a varicocele (Fig. 73-4). Perineal and rectal examinations are routine parts of this assessment.

#### Basic Laboratory Assessment

Laboratory evaluation includes a semen analysis and serum hormone studies. Semen analysis parameters of importance include semen volume and consistency, sperm concentration and total count, percentage motility and quality of sperm movement, sperm morphology, and presence of red and white blood cells or bacteria. The World Health Organization has defined parameters of normal for routine semen analyses.

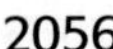

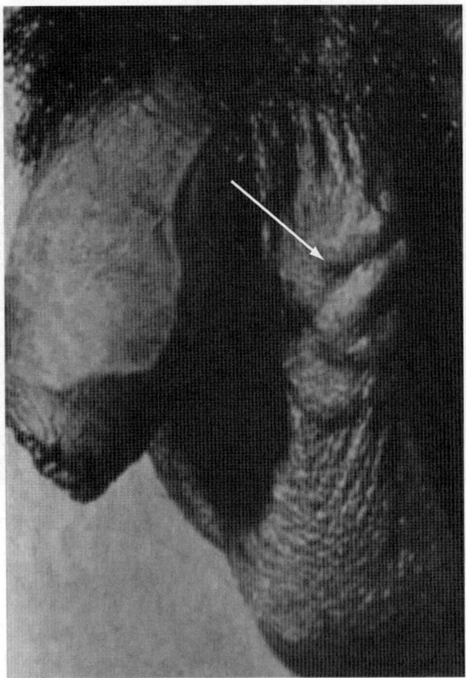

**FIGURE 73-4** Varicocele. The bag of worms appearance is visible and palpable through the scrotal skin, representing the dilated branches of the internal spermatic venous system.

Semen analysis abnormalities fall into two main categories—azoospermia (the complete absence of sperm from the semen), and abnormal bulk semen parameters (e.g., reduced concentration, motility, morphology [in isolation or in combination], and abnormal sperm function). Azoospermia results from ablative pathology of the germinal epithelium of the testis with absence of the production of mature sperm or from defects in sperm transport or ejaculation, often caused by ductal obstruction or ejaculatory dysfunction. When azoospermia is caused by lack of sperm production, this is often accompanied by normal semen volume and by a markedly elevated serum follicle-stimulating hormone (FSH) level. There are exceptions to this rule; however, because certain forms of maturational arrest of intratesticular sperm development, as well as other sperm production defects, can be seen with normal serum hormone parameters. Abnormalities of sperm transport are commonly caused by epididymal obstruction or obstruction at the level of the ejaculatory duct within the prostate, or may be caused by remote iatrogenic injury (e.g., vasal occlusion in the groin from pediatric inguinal hernia repair, and adult hernia repair with vasal entrapment from permanent polypropylene mesh). Abnormal bulk semen parameters may be indicative of a wide range of disorders that go beyond the scope of this discussion; important entities that may cause reduced sperm numbers, motility, or morphology include varicocele, antisperm antibodies causing immunologic infertility, genital duct infection with pyospermia causing sperm dysfunction, and prior or current gonadotoxic exposure. Reduced semen volume may be artifactual, indicating incomplete ejaculation or specimen collection, or may represent true pathology, including, for example, congenital absence of the seminal vesical, ejaculatory duct obstruction, or retrograde ejaculation caused by diabetes or neurologic injury or prior bladder neck surgery or medications.

Serum hormone testing includes determining levels of FSH, luteinizing hormone (LH), testosterone, free testosterone (measured or calculated based on binding protein levels), and prolactin. It may be possible to diagnose hypogonadotropic hypogonadism on the basis of serum hormone studies or note significant elevation in the FSH level, which is often indicative of significant ablative intratesticular pathology. In any situation in which the serum testosterone level is below normal, the serum prolactin level should be measured to rule out a prolactinoma, a benign but potentially clinically significant neoplasm of the pituitary gland.

Additional testing of value in the evaluation of the infertile male may include ultrasound imaging and additional sperm function or genetic testing. Ultrasound of the scrotum is useful to measure testicular volume and symmetry, exclude the possibility of testicular neoplasm, identify epididymal anatomy, and define or confirm the presence of a varicocele, which is an abnormal dilation of the pampiniform venous plexus of the internal spermatic venous system. This may cause testicular overheating, reduction in the level and quality of sperm production, testicular atrophy, and discomfort or pain. Transrectal ultrasound of the prostate may provide evidence of ejaculatory duct obstruction with seminal vesical dilation or congenital absence of the seminal vesicle, which may accompany congenital absence of the vas deferens.

Additional laboratory testing may include ultrastructural studies of sperm for motility analysis, semen leukocyte assay, antisperm antibody assay, and biologic tests of sperm-egg interaction; these more advanced tests have value in pursute of a diagnosis in cases of unexplained infertility. Patients with severe oligospermia or azoospermia should have genetic testing performed to rule out a significant genetic cause of the infertility; this information may affect a couple's decision about whether and how to proceed with fertility treatment attempts. Screening for cystic fibrosis mutations, Y chromosome microdeletion assays, sperm chromatin damage assays, and basic karyotype analysis are typically included in this genetic evaluation.

Treatment of male infertility depends on the identified cause and on the availability and affordability of assisted reproductive technologies support options for specific or empirical treatment of failure to conceive. Commonly used medical therapies include hormonal stimulation of spermatogenesis, which has had mixed success, and anti-inflammatory or antibiotic therapy for pyospermia or genital duct infection. Surgical therapies may include microsurgical reconstruction for vasal or epididymal occlusion (including vasectomy reversal), transurethral resection of the ejaculatory duct for obstructive lesions, and varicocele repair, which may be performed by open groin surgery approach, laparoscopically, or through interventional radiology internal spermatic vein embolization.

Surgeons must be aware of the potential for groin and pelvic surgical procedures to cause male infertility via damage to the spermatic cord vasculature, vas deferens, or ejaculatory duct region, or from vasal entrapment from mesh used for inguinal hernia repair. The vas and testicular blood supply is vulnerable to injury, particularly when the groin is explored in a reoperative setting for recurrent inguinal hernia or when the anatomy is obscure because of trauma, because the specific identification of these structures may be challenging. If the vas is injured during a general surgical procedure and the patient is in his reproductive years, intraoperative urologic consultation may be appropriate.

## Male Sexual Dysfunction and Treatment

Sexual dysfunction refers to a range of disorders, including erectile dysfunction, diminished libido, hypogonadism, and ejaculatory dysfunction. The general surgeon should be aware of certain basic aspects of sexual dysfunction as they relate to the possible presence of undiagnosed neuropathy, endocrinopathy, vasculopathy, and psychological abnormalities and how these may affect planned nonurologic surgery.

Male sexual dysfunction is a common condition, being discernible in approximately 40% of men at age 40 and 70% of men at age 70 years. Although mild dysfunction of psychogenic cause is more common in younger age groups, more severe or complete absence of erectile function, often caused by vascular insufficiency, is more typical in those in older age groups. Several studies have demonstrated that erectile dysfunction can be an early indication of significant atherosclerotic vascular disease because the endothelial deterioration that results in loss of penile tumescence is often a systemic process, also manifested in other critical vascular tissue beds.[19] Urologists will pursue any other signs of systemic vascular disease in patients with vasculogenic erectile dysfunction, and have a low threshold to pursue cardiologic or vascular surgical referral if lower extremity pulses are diminished or other signs or symptoms of vasculopathy are noted.

Based on the patient's history, much can be determined regarding cause when discussing sexual dysfunction with patients. Often, psychogenic dysfunction is situational and connected with relationship stress or performance anxiety. Neurogenic dysfunction is typically secondary to identifiable disorders, such as neural injury following radical prostatectomy or other diagnosed neurologic disease. Vasculogenic dysfunction can be documented by various types of testing; it is most often studied with duplex Doppler ultrasound of the penis and related arteries, with intracavernosal injection of arterial vasodilating substances. Endocrine assessment is routinely obtained in sexual dysfunction evaluation and is especially relevant when patients also complain of diminished libido. In diabetic patients, erectile dysfunction is particularly common; this often has multifactorial causes, with small vessel disease and neuropathic components.

Treatment for erectile dysfunction may involve psychotherapy, noninvasive vacuum erection support devices, oral medications (e.g., phosphodiesterase-5 inhibitors), intraurethral suppository therapy with prostaglandin compounds, intracavernosal self-injection programs, and surgical intervention. Surgery for erectile dysfunction includes vascular reconstruction, most relevant in younger patients and particularly effective after traumatic vascular injury, and prosthetic implantation and other forms of penile reconstructive surgery. Rearterialization of the penis to restore erectile function, following arteriography for anatomic documentation, is usually achieved using an inferior epigastric artery pedicle flap, whereby new arterial inflow is brought to the corpora cavernosa. In older patients with diabetes or vascular disease, rearterialization has not been successful.

Penile implant surgery may involve malleable implants, which have a flexible wire core inside a silicone sleeve, implanted bilaterally in the corpora or, more commonly, inflatable penile implants. These are fluid-containing, completely internalized systems that may include paired corporal cylinders, a scrotal pumping device, and a fluid reservoir, which is typically positioned in the retropubic space or extraperitoneal lower abdominal quadrant. Intraperitoneal positioning may also occur, intentionally or through erosion through the peritoneal membrane, so that the reservoir and/or system tubing may be encountered during nonurologic abdominopelvic surgery. Care should be taken not to contaminate any of the implant components with enteric material or inadvertently injure the tubing or device components. If it is known that an implant is in place and surgery in the relevant anatomic area(s) is planned, urologic consultation may be helpful in handling any issues that arise with the implant (Fig. 73-5). Other forms of penile reconstructive surgery commonly performed include repairs of injuries for trauma and penile surgery for congenital or acquired curvature or angulation, common in Peyronie's disease.

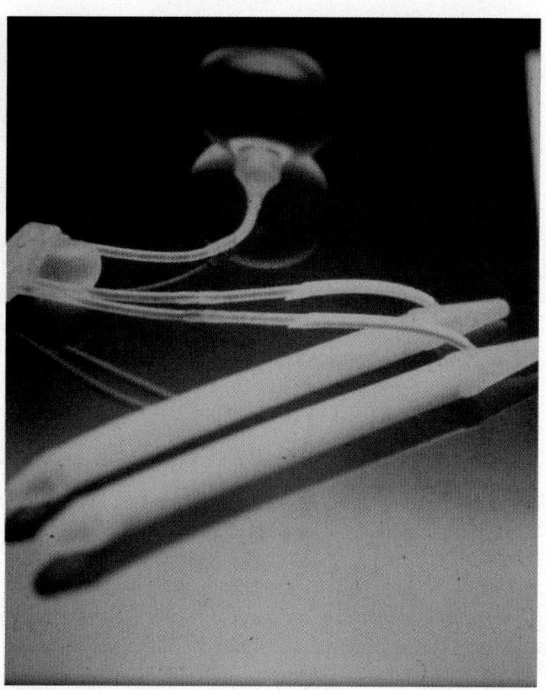

**FIGURE 73-5** Inflatable penile prosthesis. A three-component device is shown. The reservoir *(top)* is placed retropubically in an extraperitoneal position. The paired cylinders *(right)* are placed within the corpora cavernosa. The pump *(left)* is placed in the scrotum, adjacent to the testes.

# UROLITHIASIS

Urinary tract stones are a common cause of visits to the emergency room (ER). General surgeons in training will encounter many such patients and must have a working knowledge of basic evaluation and management.[20]

Urolithiasis presentations vary depending on the size and location of the stone, degree of obstruction caused, and other anatomic and host factors. Nonobstructing renal calyceal stones are typically found incidentally or during a hematuria evaluation. Stones that are obstructing the renal pelvic outlet or ureter typically present acutely, with pain, hematuria, and possibly nausea, vomiting, and ileus. These patients typically present to the ER and their findings prompt abdominal imaging. Ultrasound of the kidneys may show hydronephrosis;

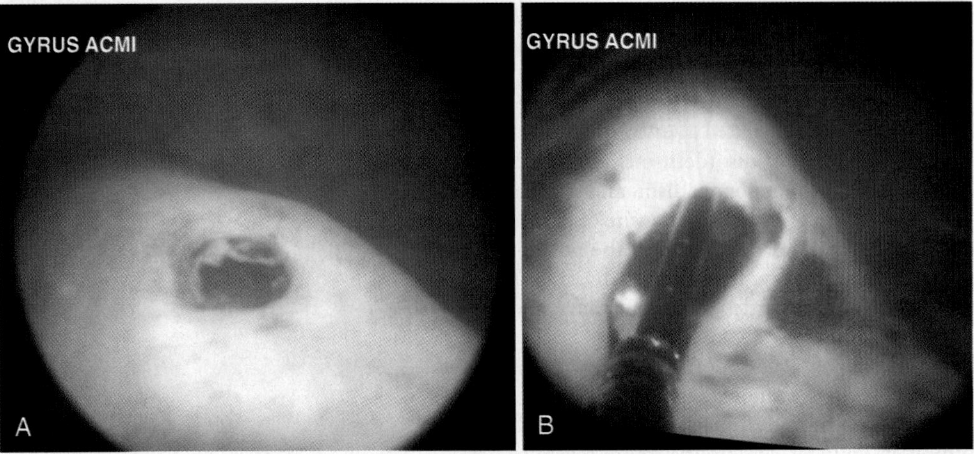


**FIGURE 73-6** Ureteral stone. **A,** An obstructing calculus is shown crowning within the right ureteral orifice. **B,** Cystoscopic extraction performed with a grasping forceps.

the now-standard stone protocol CT scan (without contrast) demonstrates the stone and the dilated collecting system proximal to it. On plain radiographs (of the kidney, ureter, and bladder), 90% of stones are visible as a radio-opacity. In the United States and other industrialized nations, the most common stone chemistry is calcium oxalate. For most patients, if a careful search is made, a metabolic risk factor for stone formation can be determined.

Stones may be classified by their chemistry, location, and clinical impact. Calcium oxalate stones are the most common variety. The most common metabolic cause found in calcium stone formers is absorptive hypercalciuria. These are opaque on plain radiography. Magnesium ammonium phosphate (struvite) stones, commonly combined with calcium phosphate, are related to chronic urinary infection with urease-producing bacteria (e.g., *Proteus* spp., *Klebsiella*). They form in the alkaline urine environment created by these chronically infecting bacteria and often form branched calculi in the collecting system (staghorn stones). Uric acid calculi are often lucent on a plain radiograph and form in acidic urine. Although they are common in patients with a history of gout and elevated serum uric acid levels, most patients with uric acid stones are not found to be hyperuricosemic. These stones are soluble in alkaline urine; they can be dissolved clinically in situ using urinary alkalinizing agents. Cystine stones are caused by an inborn error of metabolism (homocystinuria, usually homozygous). They form in acid urine and also can be dissolved medically. Other less common stones include those caused by indinavir (Crixivan, a protease inhibitor used in AIDS patients), matrix stones (radiolucent, composed of proteinaceous material), and ammonium acid urate stones.

Clinical evaluation involves urinalysis, culture, imaging (usually by CT, ultrasound, or retrograde pyelography), and possibly metabolic assessment, with a 24-hour urine collection for various urinary constituents that affect stone risk factors.

Various underlying disease states can affect stone formation. Chronic urinary infection was noted. Sarcoidosis, renal tubular acidosis, hyperoxaluria, cystinuria, inflammatory bowel disease, short gut syndrome, and medullary sponge kidney are some of the important stone risk factors. Relative dehydration (living and working in a hot environment) is also a risk factor.

Acute episodes related to urolithiasis usually reflect obstruction, infection, or both. When the ureter is obstructed by a stone, the pressure in the proximal collecting system rises and, with progressive distention, the patient experiences significant pain and visceral symptoms, including nausea, vomiting, and ileus. If the patient is free of signs of infection (based on urinalysis and absence of chills, fever, and leukocytosis), many patients can be managed on an ambulatory basis, as long as they can hydrate orally, their pain is adequately controlled by oral analgesics, they are not having persistent nausea or vomiting, and their stone is potentially passable, based on x-ray findings. If these factors are not relevant, patients should be admitted for hydration, pain control, and possible surgical intervention. If they show signs of infection on the obstructed side, this is a surgical emergency and the patient needs aggressive antibiotic administration. The upper tract must be decompressed urgently by cystoscopy and retrograde ureteral stent insertion or by percutaneous nephrostomy insertion to avoid progressive deterioration and potentially sepsis and septic shock. In the setting of upper tract infection, the goal is simply to decompress and drain the infected and obstructed upper tract, not to treat the stone definitively. It is contraindicated to perform a ureteroscopic lithotripsy at this juncture; this should be done electively, in another setting, when the patient is stable and the infection is fully resolved. It is important to remember that if one upper tract is totally obstructed by stone, the patient could have a serious infection with pyonephrosis, and the voided urine would be deceptively normal. The whole clinical picture needs to be considered; I believe that if a patient is deemed sick enough to be admitted to the hospital for a febrile urinary infection, he or she should have upper tract imaging on admission to ensure that there is no upper tract obstruction requiring urgent intervention (Fig. 73-6).

If a patient is discharged for outpatient management, she or he should be followed closely to determine whether the stone has passed. It should not be assumed that because their pain has resolved, they must have passed the stone. With persistent upper tract obstruction, the pressure in the collecting system eventually declines as renal blood flow diminishes and urine output drops; the pain can disappear and the kidney can remain obstructed, undergoing silent destruction in the weeks and months that follow. Reimaging is necessary if there is no definitive evidence that the stone has been passed (e.g., the patient brings it in for analysis).

If the trial of stone passage is not successful, the patient will require intervention to eliminate the stone. This can be performed by extracorporeal shock wave lithotripsy (ESWL), ureteroscopic stone manipulation or laser ablation, or percutaneous lithotripsy. Open stone surgery has become rare with the current, less invasive technologies available.

When presenting on a more elective basis, stones are handled in an elective surgical manner, when indicated. Not every small nonobstructing calyceal stone requires treatment; monitoring is reasonable in many cases, with treatment being pursued if symptoms develop or growth is noted on serial imaging. Often, patients who have experienced the misery of ureteral colic or those who just prefer to be stone-free (e.g., pilots, those living in remote areas) prefer to have their stones treated, even when small and asymptomatic, which is certainly appropriate.

Occasionally, complications of stone management will involve the general surgeon. Percutaneous lithotripsy may result in hydrothorax or pneumothorax from transpleural or peripleural access tracts and require evacuation. Injuries to adjacent organs (spleen, colon) and, rarely, vascular injuries have also occurred with percutaneous renal access procedures, requiring surgical intervention.

Stones can also form in the bladder, requiring removal, usually via a cystoscopic lithotripsy approach (Fig. 73-7). Stones can lodge in the urethra, causing urinary outlet obstruction, which also requires intervention. In industrialized nations, most bladder stones result from long-term Foley catheter use or bladder outlet obstruction and urinary stasis, as opposed to the nutritionally based bladder stone formation problems seen in developing nations.

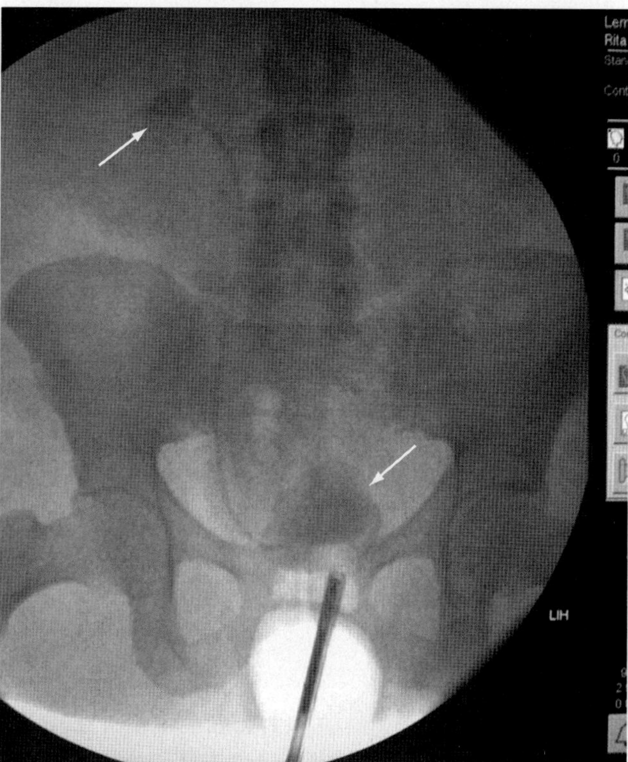


**FIGURE 73-7** Retained calcified ureteral stent. A large bladder stone and a moderate-sized right renal stone have formed on the distal and proximal coils of the stent, which was forgotten by the patient and was in place for 3 years. Endoscopic management involved laser lithotripsy and evacuation of the bladder stone fragments, followed by ureteroscopic lithotripsy of the upper calcifications, after which the stent was removed. Such cases raise challenging clinical management and medicolegal concerns.

## UROLOGIC TRAUMA

Urologic injury is present in approximately 10% of penetrating abdominal trauma cases and in a markedly variable percentage of blunt abdominal trauma cases, depending on the setting (e.g., urban, rural, athletic, military). Renal injuries, for example, are reported to occur in 1.4% to 3.25% of all trauma patients and in 4% to 8% of penetrating trauma patients. In many centers, injuries are typically initially assessed by an emergency physician or general surgeon and may be addressed by a nonurologist, whereas in other centers, and for many types of injuries, the input of an experienced urologist is essential. The urologist may therefore be called on to deal with a wide variety of types of urologic injuries, often consulted on an urgent basis and with little advanced notice; these consultations often occur years after residency training and possibly years after the last such consultation. Although the general surgeon is capable of performing an expeditious nephrectomy for a high-grade, nonreconstructible renal injury, he or she may be less comfortable performing a complex renorrhaphy for a renal injury with an extensive parenchymal and collecting system laceration. The repair of a straightforward intraperitoneal bladder rupture can be competently performed by a nonurologist surgeon, extensive injury of the trigonal region involving the intramural ureter, or in continuity with a significant penetrating rectal injury, may challenge urologists and nonurologists. Overall, urologic expertise can enhance the quality of care provided for all urologic injuries, whether managed operatively or nonoperatively; this collaboration should be a standard approach in trauma centers.

The focus of the following discussion on urologic trauma will be the practical acute management of a variety of urologic injuries.[21,22] The optimal interaction between the urologist and general trauma surgeon in such cases will be addressed. I will discuss specific, common injuries throughout the urinary tract, as well as the optimal timing of such interventions. The role of damage control techniques—the decision to delay immediate management of injuries because of concern for patient stability—in the management of urologic trauma has been an area of interest at our center for many years, and our experience with and perspective on these management strategies will also be presented as part of a unified approach to patient management.[23]

### Injury Staging and Evidence-Based Management Consensus

The Organ Injury Scaling System of the American Association for the Surgery of Trauma (AAST) describes an objective approach to the description of urologic injuries. The staging system for renal trauma has become well established in the urologic literature (Fig. 73-8; Table 73-1). Staging criteria also exist for the other primary organ injury sites (e.g., ureter, bladder, urethra), but these are not in common use, partly because of the

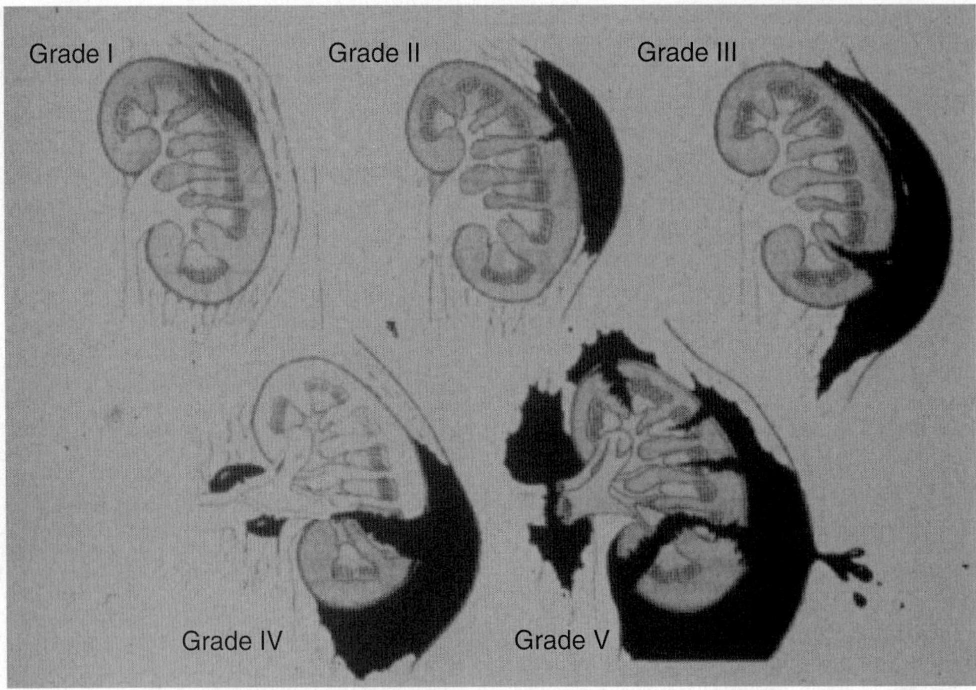


**FIGURE 73-8** AAST Organ Injury Scaling System for renal injuries.

**Table 73-1 Organ Injury Scaling System: Kidney**

| GRADE | INJURY DESCRIPTION | AIS-90 |
|---|---|---|
| I | Contusion: Microscopic or gross hematuria, urologic studies normal | 2 |
| | Hematoma: Subcapsular, nonexpanding, without parenchymal laceration | 2 |
| II | Hematoma: Nonexpanding perirenal haematoma confined to renal retroperitoneum | 2 |
| | Laceration: <1-cm parenchymal depth of renal cortex without urinary extravasation | 2 |
| III | Laceration: >1-cm depth of renal cortex, without collecting system rupture or urinary extravasation | 3 |
| IV | Laceration: Parenchymal laceration extending through the renal cortex, medulla, and collecting system | 4 |
| | Vascular: Main renal artery or vein injury, with contained hemorrhage | 5 |
| V | Laceration: Completely shattered kidney | 5 |
| | Vascular: Avulsion of renal hilum, which devascularizes kidney | 5 |

From trauma.org: Organ injury scaling: Kidney, 2011 (http://www.trauma.org/archive/scores/ois-renal.html).

difficulty in assigning an injury stage for these organ sites in the nonoperative setting.

In 2002, a consensus conference for the diagnosis and treatment of urologic injuries was convened by the World Health Organization and the Societé Internationale d'Urologie. The conference brought together international participants and focused on performing a comprehensive literature review and analysis, divided into five subcommittees, organized by organ site—kidney, ureter, bladder, urethra, and external genitalia. The reports of the subcommittees, based on available literature and consensus on management approaches, were published in the *British Journal of Urology* in 2004 to 2005.[24-28]

## Renal Injuries

### Imaging

The relevance of imaging to detect and stage urinary tract injury prior to abdominal trauma surgery has been debated in the general surgical and urologic literature. Extensive literature supports limiting imaging for blunt renal trauma to those patients with hypotension or gross hematuria. Other patients who may profit from imaging, even in the absence of these two criteria, may include those who have suffered significant deceleration injury, those with altered mental status for whom physical examination data is unreliable, and those for whom bony injury noted on plain film assessment may suggest an increased risk of urologic injury (e.g., transverse process spinal, long bone, or lower rib fractures). When selecting patients for nonoperative management of renal injuries, contrast-enhanced CT imaging is clearly useful for initial patient selection and as a baseline for subsequent reassessment. CT has the advantage of detailed assessment of the renal vasculature and of parenchymal lacerations, detection of displaced or nonperfused parenchymal fragments and urinary extravasation, and evaluation of nonurologic injuries (Fig. 73-9). The "shock room" IV pyelogram (IVP) has limited usefulness in the trauma setting, but may demonstrate gross anatomic abnormalities and indicate that the contralateral uninjured kidney is functional, which may be reassuring prior to exploring the injured kidney. Recent general surgery trauma literature has held a rather negative view of the usefulness of the preexploration IVP and there is disagreement in the urologic trauma community regarding its value. In our center, I generally

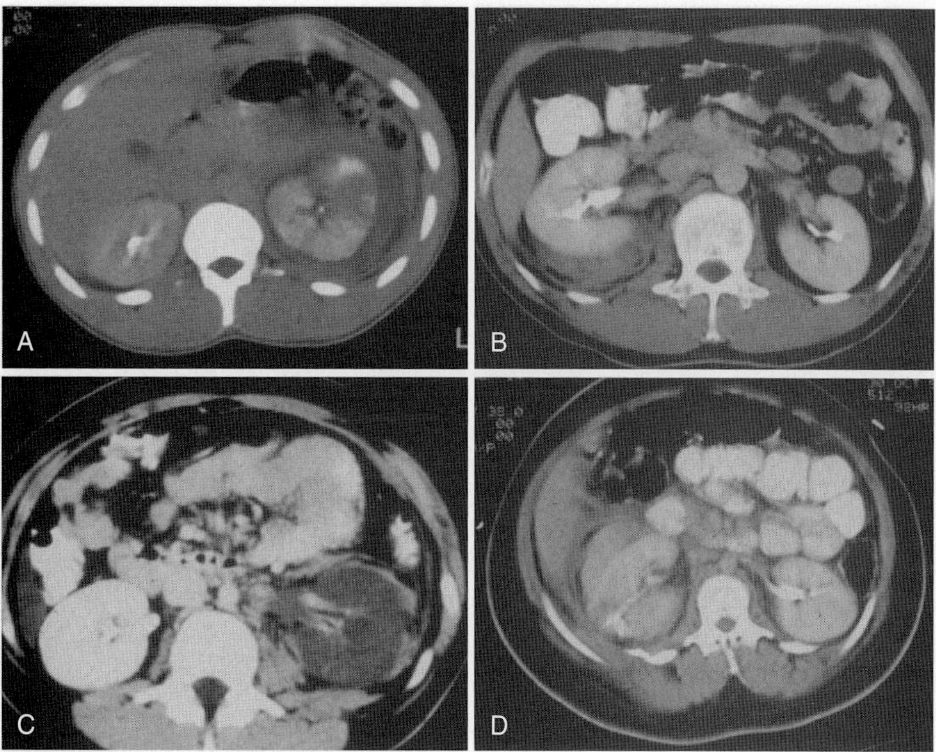


**FIGURE 73-9** CT scans depicting renal trauma. **A,** Left renal contusion with heterogeneous contrast enhancement. **B,** Small right posterior pericapsular renal hematoma. **C,** Nonperfused left kidney following deceleration trauma and intimal disruption, with thrombosis of the renal artery. Vessel cutoff sign and some pericapsular enhancement are demonstrated. **D,** Grade 4 laceration to the posterolateral right kidney, with posterolateral contrast extravasation.

do not perform this study, using clinical and intraoperative assessment to decide whether to explore a retroperitoneal hematoma. For patients on track for early laparotomy following blunt or penetrating trauma, preoperative CT may be used to stage a renal injury potentially to avoid exploration, which would otherwise add time and morbidity. Alternatively, this imaging may provide anatomic information useful for understanding the injury and assessing function of the contralateral uninjured kidney. Although often impractical and inappropriately time-consuming in the emergency setting, such imaging is often useful when clinically and logistically appropriate. When intraoperative imaging is of value, a one-shot IVP may be obtained 10 minutes after the injection of iodinated contrast.

## Treatment

**Selection of Operative Versus Nonoperative Management** When selecting operative versus nonoperative management for renal injuries, one needs to consider several variables, such as whether the patient requires laparotomy for nonurologic injuries, hemodynamic stability of the patient, findings on imaging studies, when available, and intraoperative observations and course. For the fully staged injury in a patient not requiring emergent laparotomy for other indications, imaging data play a pivotal role in management selection. Low grade injuries (grades 1 to 3) are routinely managed nonoperatively, whereas grade 5 injuries fare better with operative intervention. Grade 4 injuries are more controversial, with some experts suggesting lower complication and nephrectomy rates with aggressive operative management and others reserving such interventions for patients with clear hemodynamic indications for surgery. Interventional radiology options should also be considered in decision making for such injuries. Selected penetrating injuries to the kidney may be managed nonoperatively using similar criteria as for blunt trauma, although with abdominal gunshot wounds, laparotomy can be avoided only occasionally, such as when CT reveals a tangential course without peritoneal penetration. Renal stab wounds that are shown to exist in the absence of any other abdominal injuries (again, usually by CT findings) are also amenable to nonoperative management in select cases (Fig. 73-10).

When urgent laparotomy occurs, if one has had the luxury of obtaining optimal preoperative renal images, a preoperative judgment can be made as to whether the renal injury is amenable to nonoperative management with a reasonable likelihood of success. If the kidney's appearance on CT and grade of injury support the impression that nonoperative management is appropriate, exploration is not performed and the renal fossa is not violated. In the absence of imaging, several criteria may be used to select patients for renal exploration when the urologist is consulted intraoperatively to assess an apparent retroperitoneal hematoma. Active significant bleeding from the renal fossa into the peritoneal cavity, or a visibly expanding or pulsatile hematoma, will typically prompt exploration because of the concern for significant vascular injury requiring urgent control. In the absence of such findings, or in patients in whom a damage control approach is to be implemented, exploration may be avoided if the surgeon is uncomfortable with the potential requirements for reconstructive renal surgery. The question of

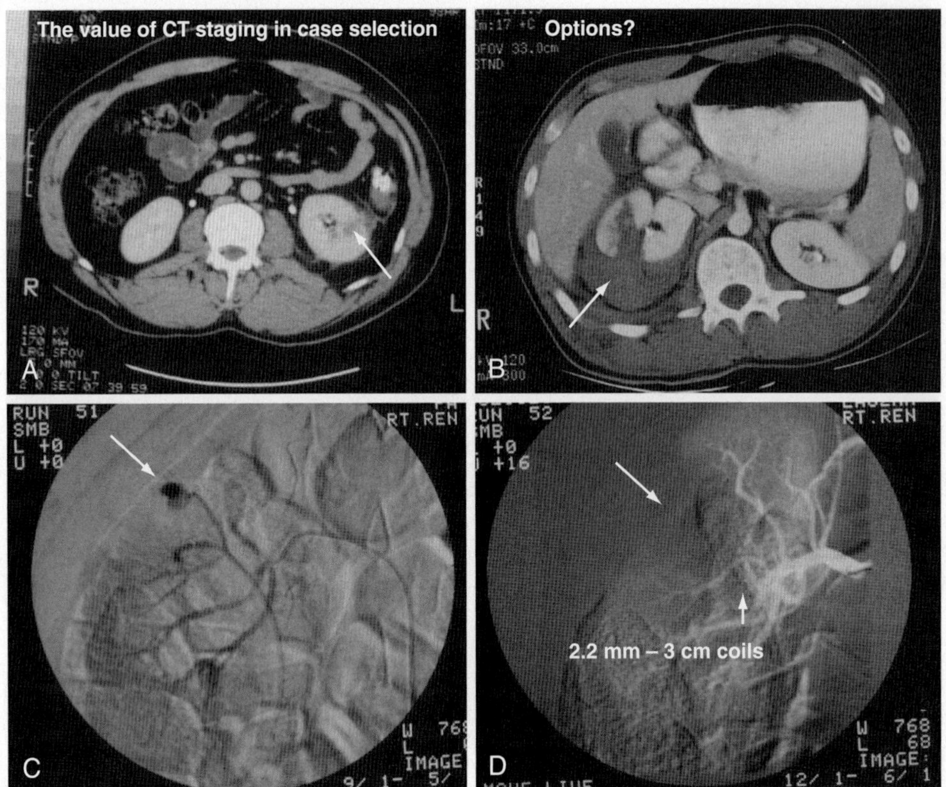


**FIGURE 73-10** CT scans depicting penetrating renal injury. **A,** Superficial laceration to the lateral left kidney from a stab wound. Note minimal hematoma and proximity of the posterior descending colon to the track of injury. Nonoperative management was selected and was successful. **B,** Deep laceration to the right kidney following a stab wound. Note the proximity to renal hilar structures and moderate-sized hematoma. **C,** Renal angiography performed for a significant postinjury hematuria with hemodynamic instability, demonstrating pseudoaneurysm. **D,** Postembolization appearance of the right kidney showing a wedge-shaped defect following coil placement, which was successful.

whether nephrectomy rates are higher when one adopts a more conservative versus a more aggressive approach to exploration for renal trauma is difficult to determine from the published literature. However, overall, it seems that if exploration is performed by a surgeon not highly skilled in reconstructive renal surgery in the trauma setting, the nephrectomy rate will be lower if a relatively conservative approach to selecting patients for renal exploration is adopted. One should keep in mind that as long as the patient can be determined to be at low risk for exsanguinating hemorrhage in the perioperative period, reoperating for the renal injury is always an option, based on clinical developments or postoperative imaging findings.

For renal pedicle injuries resulting from blunt trauma, a high index of suspicion is essential for injury detection, because hematuria is frequently absent in such cases. The mechanism of injury with rapid deceleration should raise suspicion of these injuries, which result from stretching of the vascular pedicle and intimal disruption, with subsequent thrombosis of the renal artery. When detected early after the injury, and in patients for whom revascularization is appropriate in terms of the prioritization of multiple injuries, good results may be obtained. The time frame for predicting success is difficult to anticipate because there is a continuum of evolution of these injuries, with warm ischemia developing at variable intervals postinjury, depending on the specific features of the arterial disruption. Interventional radiologic treatment of these injuries with endovascular stenting may be applicable in certain cases, especially those in which there is still distal perfusion noted on initial angiography. These injuries are best managed, in my experience, by an expeditious multidisciplinary discussion among urology, trauma, and vascular surgeons and interventional radiologists to select a treatment and implement the decision quickly.

**Intraoperative Approach** Urologists are typically trained to approach the injured kidney anteriorly through a midline incision and to obtain vascular control of the renal vessels prior to opening Gerota's fascia and exposing the kidney. The purpose of this traditional approach is to avoid a situation in which severe renal bleeding is encountered, which may necessitate an urgent nephrectomy that might have otherwise been preventable. In my experience, an abbreviated approach to the control of the renal pedicle can produce excellent results. This pedicle access maneuver, which I routinely use prior to renal trauma exploration, involves bluntly creating a window medial to the lower pole of the kidney and lateral to the aorta (left) or vena cava (right), spreading digitally down to the psoas muscle fascia, and creating a space using cephalad blunt dissection, which allows a vascular pedicle clamp to be placed if bleeding is encountered on renal exposure. This maneuver avoids the somewhat tedious, technically difficult, and potentially morbid individual dissection of the renal vessels in the setting of surrounding hematoma while still providing access for rapid, atraumatic pedicle occlusion when necessary. For cases in which active bleeding is emanating directly from the renal pedicle or vessels, direct dissection and control of the vessels are initiated in the traditional manner. For renal reconstruction in the trauma setting, pedicle clamping with a warm ischemia time less than 30 minutes generally will not have a permanent adverse impact on renal function.

Once vascular access is achieved, the kidney is exposed through an anterior vertical incision in Gerota's fascia, which extends from the upper to the lower pole of the kidney. If there is parenchymal injury, care must be taken to identify the plane external to the renal capsule when exposing and mobilizing the kidney to avoid stripping the entire capsule from the renal parenchyma, which attempts at reconstruction. The entire kidney should be exposed to reveal any lacerations, evacuate hematoma, and facilitate full mobility for repair.

The selection of reconstruction or nephrectomy depends on the details of the injury. If half the kidney can be preserved, renal reconstruction has benefit. If there is extensive destruction of the hilar region, successful reconstruction is unlikely. If the injury is polar or lateral in the parenchyma, and if the depth of the injury is limited, reconstruction is typically straightforward and carries a high likelihood of favorable anatomic and functional outcomes. Renorrhaphy with suture of bleeding vessels, collecting system closure, and parenchymal and preferably capsular approximation is a relatively straightforward task. For destructive polar injuries, a polar nephrectomy can be performed, controlling the collecting system and adjacent vessels with direct suturing. Absorbable sutures should be used for parenchymal and collecting system repair to prevent subsequent calcification, which would result if nonabsorbable sutures were exposed to the urinary tract lumen postoperatively. The use of hemostatic agents and tissue sealants may aid in the reconstructive effort and have been shown, at least in animal studies, to decrease postoperative bleeding and urinary extravasation. Institution of closed suction drainage is of benefit when a collecting system injury has been noted and for drainage of blood in the perioperative period. Prophylactic antibiotic coverage should be provided and continued until urinary extravasation is resolved or an established drainage tract is established.

It should be kept in mind that interventional radiologic techniques (e.g., angiography with selective embolization, percutaneous collecting system drainage) may constitute highly effective means of dealing with renal bleeding or urinary extravasation, and can be integrated into the treatment algorithm, especially when a urologist experienced in dealing with renal reconstruction is not immediately available at the time of surgery or when a postoperative complication occurs.

## Ureteral Injuries

### Imaging

Contrast-enhanced CT or a complete IVP is accurate for the detection of ureteral trauma, although CT provides significantly more information regarding additional injuries and therefore is favored in the trauma setting. With modern spiral CT systems, the imaging sequences are obtained rapidly and it is necessary to have a protocol in place, or specifically request a delayed excretory phase, so as not to miss collecting system or ureteral contrast extravasation, which would not be appreciated with only a renal parenchymal enhancement phase. Ureteral injuries are among the most common missed injuries in the trauma setting, and may result in significant preventable morbidity. When CT imaging raises concern for an extrarenal collecting system, renal pelvic, or ureteral injury, but provides incomplete staging, cystoscopy with retrograde pyelography is an option to gain more definitive information.

In the setting of penetrating abdominal trauma, ureteral injury may occur in 5% to 10% of patients. Ureteral injury from blunt trauma is uncommon, but may occasionally be seen in the setting of an underlying anatomic abnormality (e.g., prior retroperitoneal or urologic surgery, congenital anomalies) or with sudden stretch or compressive forces causing pelvic rupture or ureteropelvic or ureteral avulsion. A high index of suspicion is necessary to detect such injuries, because gross hematuria may be absent (i.e., no urine may be conducted to the bladder from the injured side in these cases).

### Treatment

**Selection of Operative Versus Nonoperative Management** As a general principle, penetrating injuries to the ureter or blunt avulsion injuries are best managed by surgical repair. Cystoscopically or radiologically guided ureteral stenting or diversion as definitive therapy is generally reserved for missed injuries and for patients for whom reoperation is prohibitively morbid, or the timing would make a successful repair unlikely. Ureteral contusions from adjacent penetrating trauma may benefit from prophylactic stenting to reduce progressive edema, occlusion, and ischemia and potentially diminish the risk of postinjury extravasation, according to limited published reports.

There are exceptions to these principles that dictate an aggressive operative approach to ureteral trauma. For example, minimal puncture defects in the ureter (e.g., from small-gauge shotgun pellets) may be effectively managed by stenting alone after determining by contrast-enhanced CT or retrograde pyelography that there is minimal tissue injury. These injuries would be analogous to minimal endoscopic perforations during stone procedures, which urologists routinely manage with stent insertion alone.

**Intraoperative Approach** The ureter can be approached surgically at any level by finding an area of normal anatomy and proceeding expeditiously to the area(s) in question. While dissecting around the ureter and mobilizing it from surrounding tissues, it is important to avoid devascularization. The longitudinal blood supply to the ureter runs between the muscularis and adventitial sheath. It is important to avoid dissecting in a subadventitial plane to prevent ischemic injury.

For penetrating injuries to the distal ureter, the necessary extensive dissection can be difficult and potentially morbid because visualization in this region is limited following trauma caused by infiltrating hematoma, and the potential for creating further vascular or other iatrogenic injury is a realistic concern. In my practice, I sometimes open the bladder and perform intraoperative contrast retrograde pyelography with a catheter inserted into the ureteral orifice when dealing with penetrating trauma to the pelvis and when the status of the lower ureter is in question. Exposing the most distal ureter by direct dissection may require taking down the bladder pedicle on the ipsilateral side and is better avoided if not essential.

If a ureteral injury is encountered, repair usually involves minimal débridement to viable tissue with a spatulated, tension-free anastomosis (for injuries to the middle and upper thirds), or reimplantation into the bladder (for injuries below the internal iliac vessels). For gunshot wounds to the proximal ureter and midureter, resection of the injured segment with primary anastomosis is superior to simple closure of the defect. In the penetrating trauma setting, it should be assumed that the viability of the distal ureteral stump may be compromised because of local tissue injury; reimplantation is more reliable for very distal injuries. Fine absorbable suture is used in a running or interrupted fashion. Stent placement (an internal double-J or single-J externalized through the anterolateral bladder wall) is desirable to allow low-pressure drainage, minimize postoperative urinary extravasation, and prevent angulation. As noted later, ureteral injuries are highly amenable to damage control approaches when repair acutely is not appropriate because of the patient's condition or the need to prioritize the management of other, more critical injuries. If a general surgeon is responsible for the initial operative management, a ureteral injury is recognized intraoperatively, and urologic expertise is not immediately available, temporizing maneuvers with a plan for delayed definitive repair may be preferable to a suboptimal repair in the acute setting.

## Bladder Injuries

### Imaging

Bladder injury, in the setting of penetrating or blunt pelvic trauma, is generally suspected because of the presence of gross hematuria, which is almost invariably present. In penetrating injuries to the pelvis for which laparotomy is planned, no preoperative bladder imaging is needed in most cases. Direct inspection of the injury site intraoperatively will allow full assessment of the injury. For blunt trauma, a stress cystogram is of value in distinguishing intraperitoneal from extraperitoneal injury, which directly affects selection of treatment. Regardless of whether a standard radiographic, fluoroscopic, or CT cystographic technique is used, the bladder must be adequately distended to its expected capacity, or until the patient describes a sense of fullness, to demonstrate extravasation through any defect present and avoid false-negative results (Figs. 73-11 to 73-13). Blunt extraperitoneal rupture typically involves the lower bladder segment, usually in the anterolateral retropubic portion. These injuries usually accompany pelvic fracture and result from tearing and shear forces related to injury to the pelvic ring. Intraperitoneal rupture generally results from sudden compression of the bladder by impact to the lower anterior abdominal wall, resulting in a large laceration of the bladder dome. The classic radiographic findings of each type of bladder rupture have been well described and indicate whether the contrast extravasation pattern is intraperitoneal or extraperitoneal.

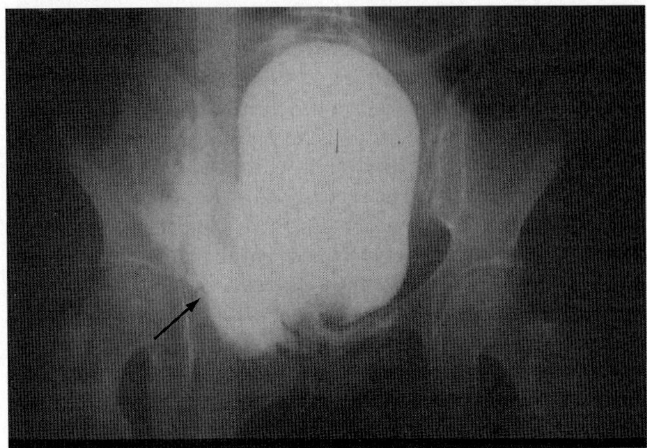

**FIGURE 73-11** Static cystogram in patient with pelvic fracture and gross hematuria showing extraperitoneal contrast extravasation on the right side.

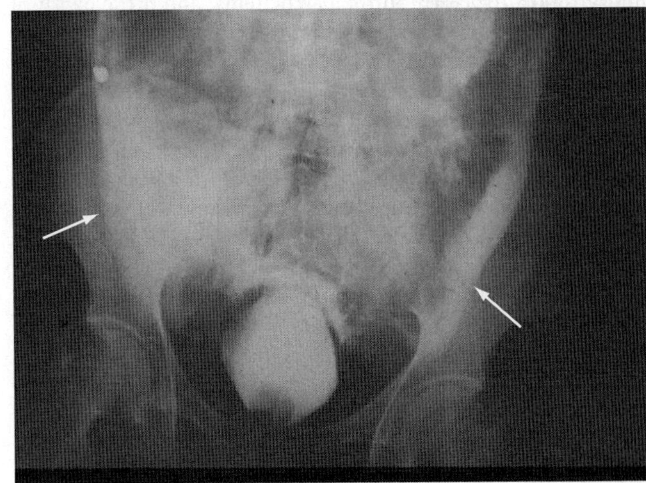

**FIGURE 73-12** Static cystogram in patient following blunt injury to the lower abdomen showing the typical contrast extravasation pattern of intraperitoneal bladder rupture. Note contrast outlining the left and right colic gutters and present within the peritoneal cavity.

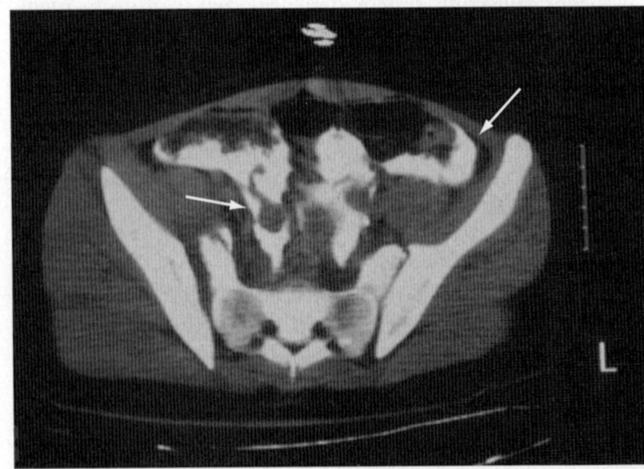


**FIGURE 73-13** CT cystogram demonstrating intraperitoneal contrast extravasation pattern of intraperitoneal bladder rupture. Note contrast in the colic gutters, within the deep pelvis, and outlining the ovaries.

### Treatment

**Selection of Operative Versus Nonoperative Management** Penetrating injuries to the bladder are generally managed with operative exploration and repair. In select cases of penetrating bladder trauma, nonoperative management is appropriate—when the injury to the bladder wall is minimal and extraperitoneal, hematuria not problematic, and no other indication for laparotomy is present (i.e., no rectal vascular or intraperitoneal trauma). Selecting such cases can be difficult and may require cystoscopic assessment. For most patients, the standard approach for penetrating bladder injury is exploration and repair.

For blunt injury to the bladder resulting in intraperitoneal rupture, operative exploration and repair should be performed. Such an approach prevents ongoing leakage of urine into the peritoneal cavity and avoids the delayed abdominal sepsis that often results from uncontrolled intraperitoneal extravasation. Blunt injuries to the bladder with extraperitoneal rupture, typically occurring in the setting of pelvic fracture, are usually manageable with catheter drainage alone. Operative repair for these injuries may still be necessary for cases in which there is failure of catheter management (e.g., persistent hematuria with catheter occlusion). In addition, certain types of complex bladder injuries, such as bladder neck avulsion injuries (mainly seen in women and children), extensive lacerations of the bladder neck in women, or concomitant injury to the lower bladder segment and rectum or vagina, will require operative repair, although the definitive reconstructive procedure may be best accomplished subacutely (1 to 3 days postinjury; see later, "Damage Control Techniques for Urologic Injuries").

**Intraoperative Approach** Surgical exploration of the bladder is performed through a generous midline anterior cystotomy. The interior of the bladder is examined, the clot evacuated, and critical structures (intramural ureters, ureteral orifices, bladder neck) assessed. Passing feeding tubes up the ureters to assess efflux or performing intraoperative retrograde pyelography through the cystotomy may be useful in completing this assessment. Defects in the bladder wall are closed with strong, absorbable 2-0 sutures, preferably in two layers to enhance watertightness. Care should be taken when suturing the bladder near the ureteral orifices or intramural ureter to avoid occluding the ureter; intraoperative stenting may be of benefit in these cases. Injuries in continuity with rectal or vaginal injuries may benefit from viable tissue interposition (e.g., omental flap) to prevent fistula formation, depending on whether the defects directly overlap and whether there is extensive tissue loss. Diversion with a large-bore Foley catheter (at least 20 Fr, usually 22 to 24 Fr in the adult) allows bloody urine to drain and allows careful irrigation, if necessary. Suprapubic cystostomy tubes are used for cases of tenuous bladder closure, extensive injuries requiring complex repairs, or if prolonged bladder drainage is anticipated (e.g., concomitant rectal or vaginal injury, significant head injury).

## Urethral Injuries

### Imaging

When suspicion of urethral injury exists, retrograde urethrography should be performed prior to Foley catheter insertion. The classic indication of urethral injury is blood per the urethra or blood at the urethral meatus following blunt trauma (e.g., pelvic fracture, straddle injury with perineal impact) or penetrating trauma, although mechanism and pattern of injury (e.g., severe pubic diastasis, marked vertical shear pelvic fracture), regardless of physical findings, may prompt urethrography as well. Proper performance of retrograde urethrography involves adequate filling of the entire urethra, with passage of contrast into the bladder, when such continuity has not been lost because of the injury (Fig. 73-14).

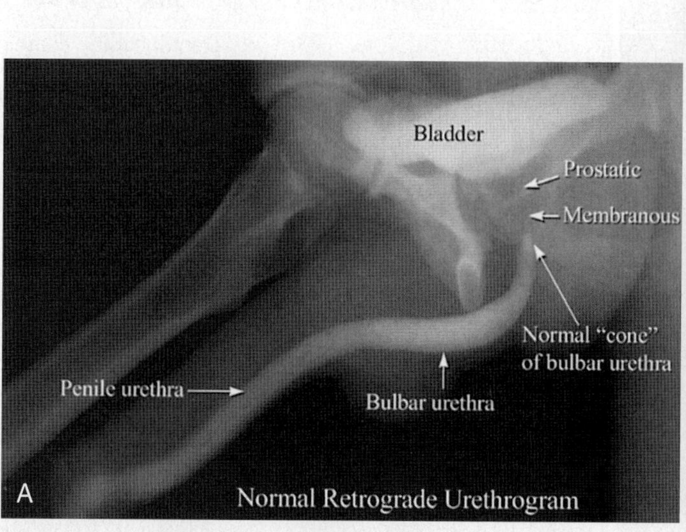


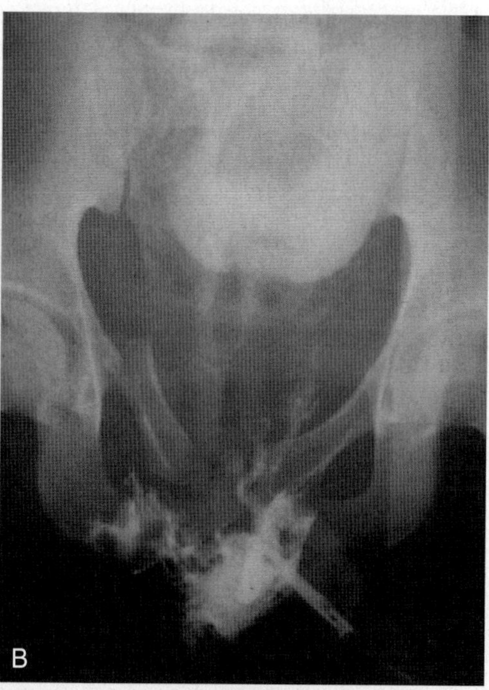


**FIGURE 73-14** Retrograde urethrograms. **A,** Standard technique with patient in an oblique position and complete contrast filling of the anterior and posterior urethra. **B,** Posterior urethral disruption in patient with displaced pelvic fracture. Note the deformity of the right superior pubic ramus and extensive contrast extravasation, extending above and below the urogenital diaphragm, on retrograde contrast injection into the urethra. The bladder, which is greatly displaced cephalad, is filling with contrast administered IV. The photograph demonstrates the so-called *pie in the sky bladder* resulting from dramatic displacement by a large pelvic hematoma following the prostatomembranous disruption Injury. (**A** from Older RA, Hertz M: Cystourethrography. In Pollack HM, McClennan BL, Dyer R, Kenney PJ [eds]: Clinical urography, ed 2, Philadelphia, 2000, WB Saunders.)

### Treatment

**Operative Versus Nonoperative Management** The primary immediate goal in managing urethral injury is to provide urinary bladder drainage and avoid further injury. Few urethral injuries, barring those resulting in significant ongoing external bleeding, such as with penetrating perineal trauma, require acute operative reconstruction. A delayed approach can almost always be implemented and, based on available literature, often produces better outcomes than acute repair, so the surgeon with limited experience with these injuries should liberally use temporizing maneuvers for these cases. Urethral reconstruction is a highly specialized area of urology; definitive reconstructive surgery can be performed in a subacute or delayed fashion, with good results.

For injuries to the posterior or anterior urethra, if extravasation is present on retrograde urethrography and adequate urologic expertise is not immediately available, a suprapubic catheter should be inserted rather than instrumenting the traumatized urethra and risking further injury. If the bladder is palpably distended and there is no evidence of prior lower abdominal surgery, or the bladder can be clearly localized with ultrasound, percutaneous tube placement in the ER is appropriate. Prepackaged kits may be safely used for this purpose. If these criteria are not met, open surgical cystostomy tube placement is safer and can be accomplished through a small anterior cystotomy (Fig. 73-15). A 24 Fr Foley or Malecot catheter works well for this purpose. It should be anchored at the anterior bladder wall with absorbable sutures and at the skin exit site. When the procedure is performed acutely following pelvic fracture, one should try to avoid violating the retropubic hematoma by entering the bladder cephalad. It is important to assess the bladder if gross hematuria is noted because a concomitant bladder injury may be present. This can be accomplished by direct inspection or cystographically if a percutaneous suprapubic (SP) tube is placed.

If surgical exploration of the urethra is necessary because of ongoing external bleeding and limited urologic expertise is available, interventions should be limited to gaining hemostasis meticulously by focused suturing of bleeding tissues, again leaving reconstructive maneuvers for another occasion. If there is an opportunity to place a catheter across a penetrating trauma defect, this is reasonable and, if simple suturing can reapproximate the injured urethral edges, doing so with absorbable sutures (3-0 or 4-0) is also reasonable.

In recent years, there has been increased interest in early catheter realignment for posterior urethral disruption in the setting of pelvic fracture; the results of these strategies have been reported. This technique requires substantial expertise in urologic endoscopic procedures and the risk of creating further injury is substantial. If one lacks experience with these techniques, it is best to treat such injuries with suprapubic tube insertion alone. Catheter realignment can be performed at any time soon after injury, often using the suprapubic access that has been established acutely, so there is no need to feel a sense of urgency in doing this on the day of injury. Controversy exists in the urologic literature regarding the benefit of catheter realignment for these injuries, with most reports indicating that 30% to 50% of patients can avoid ultimate urethroplasty, although strictures typically develop and require at least endoscopic management, often involving multiple procedures.

## Genital Injuries

Penetrating injuries to the external genitalia warrant surgical exploration in the vast majority of cases. Functional and structural outcomes are greatly improved by early exploration and

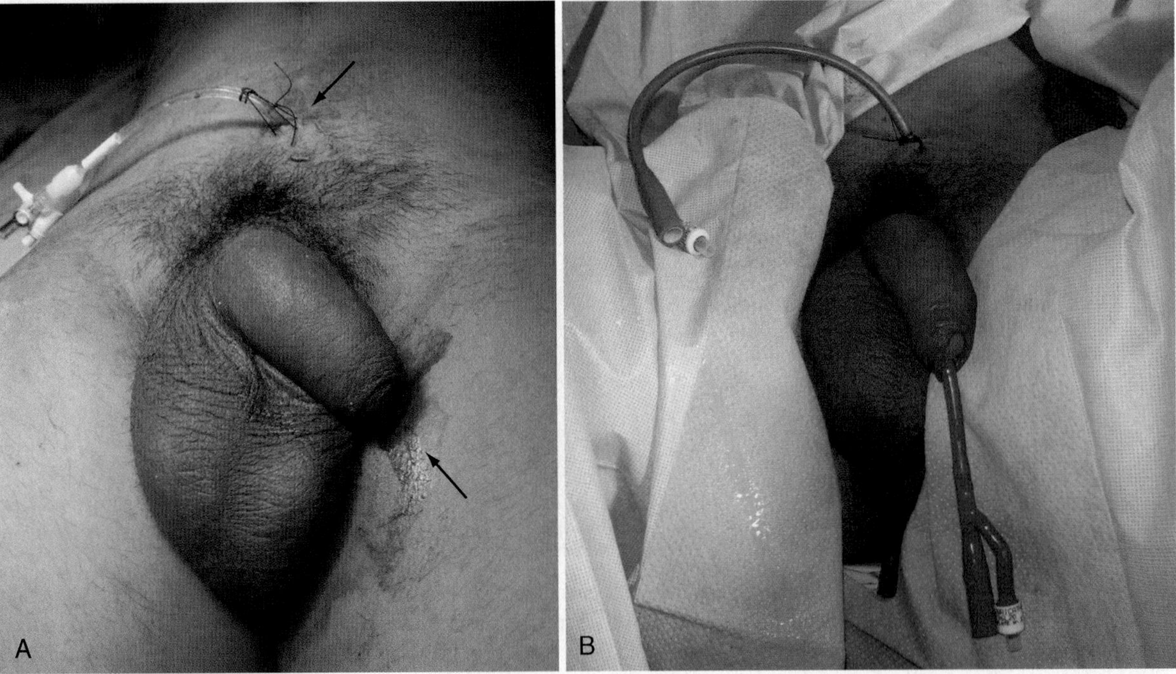


**FIGURE 73-15** Posterior urethral disruption injury. **A,** Patient with blood visible at penile meatus, managed with percutaneously placed suprapubic cystostomy tube. **B,** Patient initially managed similarly has undergone an endoscopic, fluoroscopically guided realignment procedure, with placement of urethral and suprapubic Foley catheters.

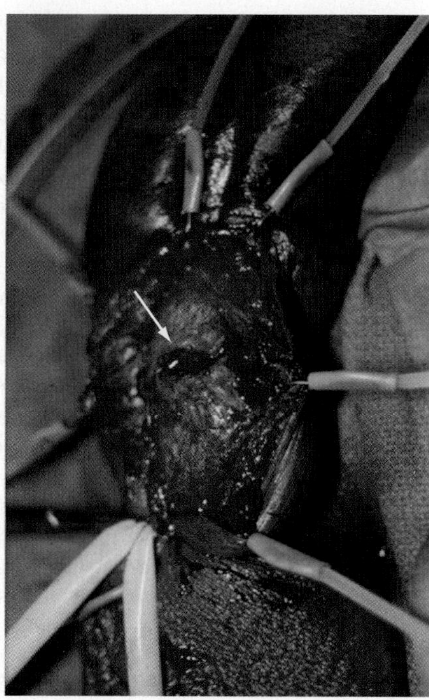

**FIGURE 73-16** Penile fracture. This patient was undergoing surgical exploration for a suspected penile fracture injury sustained during sexual activity. A ventral midline penoscrotal incision is used to expose the transverse laceration in the ventral right tunica albuginea of the corpus cavernosum, shown centrally. The Penrose drain at the bottom was used briefly as a tourniquet to control bleeding during suture repair of the injury. The hook and ring retractor system shown is useful for genital surgery.

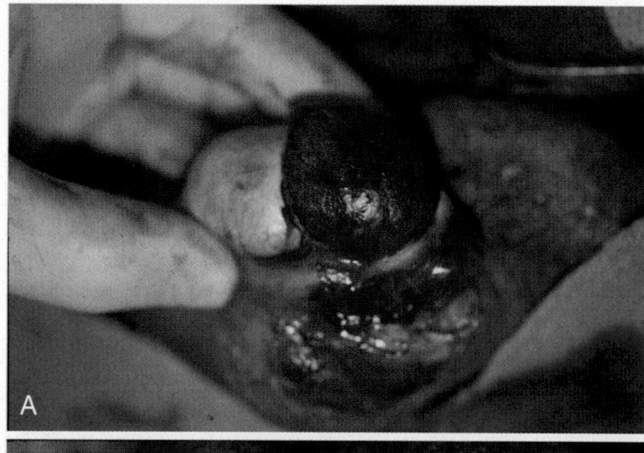



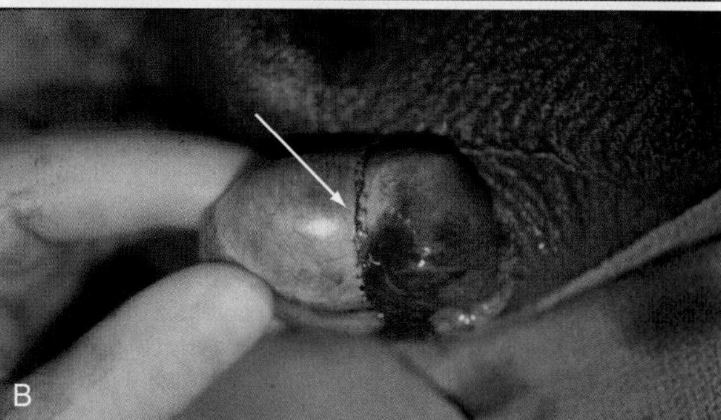



**FIGURE 73-17** Testicular rupture from blunt trauma. **A,** Intact tunica albuginea with a large transverse laceration *(left);* the extruded testicular parenchyma from the upper portion of the testis is also shown *(right).* **B,** Appearance following repair with running absorbable sutures.

repair for penetrating penile, scrotal, and testicular injuries. For penile injuries, the goal is to remove foreign material, cleanse the wound, obtain hemostasis, identify any defects in the tunica albuginea or urethra, and proceed with appropriate repair, while exercising caution not to be excessively aggressive with débridement of tissues of uncertain viability. For testicular injuries, débridement of devitalized parenchyma, closure of the capsule (tunica albuginea of the testis), and repair of the scrotum are key tasks.

For blunt penile and scrotal injuries, whether to operate depends on whether the tunica albuginea structures are ruptured. For the penis, this determination is made. In the typical suspected penile fracture type of injury that results from sudden flexion of the erect penis during sexual activity, if there is significant swelling and hematoma, these injuries are usually explored and the tunical defect is repaired (Fig. 73-16). For blunt scrotal injuries, scrotal ultrasound may be helpful in determining whether the testis is ruptured. If ultrasound shows gross disruption of the capsule, or shows marked heterogeneity of the testicular parenchyma, there is a high risk of testicular rupture and exploration, and repair should be pursued (Fig. 73-17). Orchiectomy is reserved for those injuries that thoroughly destroy the blood supply to the testis or those parenchymal injuries in which there is no viable parenchyma available to salvage.

## Damage Control Techniques for Urologic Injuries

Many urologic injuries are amenable to initial management by applying damage control strategies.[23] As noted briefly, damage control surgery refers to the concept of limiting the initial operative interventions, in the unstable trauma patient, to those maneuvers that are immediately lifesaving (e.g., control of surgical hemorrhage, control of continued fecal contamination). More time-consuming, definitive reconstructive efforts are delayed until later, following resuscitation, when the patient is more stable and can tolerate such reconstructive efforts.

The physiologic rationale for damage control surgery relates to the metabolic consequences of extensive blood loss and blood and fluid replacement. These patients develop progressive hypothermia, acidosis, and coagulopathy (the so-called *lethal triad*), which can only be corrected, following the essential interventions noted, when the patient can be brought to the intensive care unit, with appropriate warming and other critical care interventions provided.

Initially described in the military trauma literature, and then applied to civilian penetrating abdominal trauma, these principles have now been successfully applied to a wide range of penetrating and blunt injuries. Extensive studies now support the view that appropriately selected patients managed by damage control strategies demonstrate improved survival compared with patients who undergo prolonged reconstructive efforts during the initial postinjury operative period. With the exception of patients with severe renal or bladder bleeding, urinary tract injuries do not directly result in early mortality. In the surgeon's judgment, when the patient would not tolerate the magnitude of the reconstructive effort needed to deal definitively with a urologic injury at initial laparotomy— because of pattern of injury, hypothermia, acidosis, coagulopathy, or other parameters that mandate a damage control approach—certain temporary solutions may be desirable. I have gained substantial experience with these in my center and have achieved an effective working relationship with the trauma surgeons in regard to patient selection and technical approaches. The complexity of patient selection for damage control surgery requires a multidisciplinary interaction with the trauma surgeon and surgical specialists involved in the case to determine which injuries must be addressed initially and which can be definitively handled in a delayed manner. Earlier selection of damage control surgery candidates, based on patterns of injury and initial presentation factors, represents an emerging trend in the trauma surgery community, with improved survival being observed when the initial operative procedure can be concluded before significant metabolic deterioration occurs.

Renal injuries that are incompletely staged or unstaged may be approached with delayed assessment and exploration, as long as a determination has been made that early exsanguinating bleeding from the injury is unlikely. In the absence of significant bleeding from the renal fossa into the peritoneal cavity, a large midline hematoma, or an expanding or pulsatile renal hematoma, one can elect to leave the perinephric hematoma undisturbed and perform postoperative imaging during the resuscitation phase following initial laparotomy, or explore at the time of a second-look procedure. If the kidney is exposed, hemostasis for major bleeding from the parenchyma or branch renal vessels can be rapidly obtained. If a major reconstructive effort is still needed in the unstable patient, packing the kidney and returning for reconstructive interventions later is also an option.

Ureteral injuries may be managed initially with externalized stenting, ligation, or simple local drainage. Of these options, I favor externalized stenting, because it allows control of the urinary output, minimizes ongoing urinary extravasation, and can be maintained for several days until the patient is stable enough to return to surgery for definitive reconstruction. A 7 or 8.5 Fr single-J urinary diversion stent can be placed into the ureter through the injury site, advanced proximally into the kidney, and then externalized through the abdominal wall. The catheter should be tied to the very end of the injured ureter at the injury site so as not to lose ureteral length by ligating it more proximally and making later reconstruction more challenging. The distal ureteral limb is best left undisturbed; ligating it requires subsequent débridement and causes further tissue loss.

A similar approach can be used for extensive bladder injuries; the ureteral orifices can be catheterized, the catheters externalized, and the pelvis packed, leaving bladder reconstruction to be performed at a more suitable time, following appropriate resuscitation. Urethral and genital injuries are also amenable to damage control approaches, generally involving tube diversion, placement of moistened dressings, and tissue preservation until definitive reconstruction following appropriate resuscitation.

### Relationship With the Trauma Surgeon

The urologist involved in the care of the trauma patient has the privilege of sharing the injured abdomen with the trauma surgeon. Usually, the trauma surgeon has more training and experience in critical care and response to injury than the urologist. In academic centers and training settings, exposure to abdominal trauma is of critical importance to urology residents. There is a valuable, mutual learning opportunity for the urologist and surgeon to collaborate in decision making and in the technical aspects of trauma care. The ability of the urologist to play a meaningful role in acute trauma is enhanced by the creation of standardized protocols for factors such as the timing of consultation and implementation of damage control maneuvers. Consultation of the urologist from the shock room in any patient with obvious signs of urologic injury (e.g., gross hematuria, blood at the urethral meatus, genital injury) will allow early mobilization of specialty expertise and allow active participation at all phases of injury management. I have had the good fortune of having an excellent, collaborative working relationship with the trauma surgeons at my institution and I believe that such interaction can greatly benefit the patient.

## NONTRAUMATIC UROLOGIC EMERGENCIES

Although mentioned in other contexts within this chapter, several nontraumatic urologic emergencies warrant additional discussion.

### Testicular Torsion

Testicular torsion is a time-sensitive ischemic process for which rapid diagnosis and intervention are necessary to enhance the likelihood of testicular salvage. In theory, torsion occurs in the setting of a congenital deformity (e.g., bell clapper deformity) in which the testis is not attached normally within the scrotal compartment, so that it is able to rotate freely on its spermatic cord pedicle. When this type of twisting occurs, if spontaneous detorsion does not occur promptly, there is progressive edema and venous and arterial occlusion, which will result in testicular infarction without intervention. The best results are obtained if detorsion occurs within 4 hours of the onset of pain. After 8 to 12 hours, the likelihood of maintaining testicular viability and function decreases significantly. From a management standpoint, it is essential to have a high index of suspicion for torsion. Although occurring usually in the pediatric, adolescent, and young adult groups, torsion can occur at any age. Differential diagnosis includes trauma, epididymitis, incarcerated hernia, and torsion of the appendix testis or appendix epididymis. Diagnosis can be confirmed by Doppler ultrasound, which shows absence of arterial flow to the testis. If there is a high suspicion of torsion, and ultrasound is not available in a reasonable time frame (≈1 hour after presentation), it is appropriate to proceed with surgical exploration because an inordinate delay in definitive intervention can adversely affect the outcome. Surgery consists of a scrotal incision, inspection of the testis with detorsion, and suture fixation to the interior scrotal wall, followed by also performing orchiopexy on the contralateral side at the same setting (Fig. 73-18). Even in patients in whom a late torsion is suspected (e.g., several days of fixed swelling, firmness), urgent exploration is still indicated, because it is difficult to know definitively how long complete ischemia has been present and whether there is salvageability. Medicolegal considerations are also relevant in these cases.

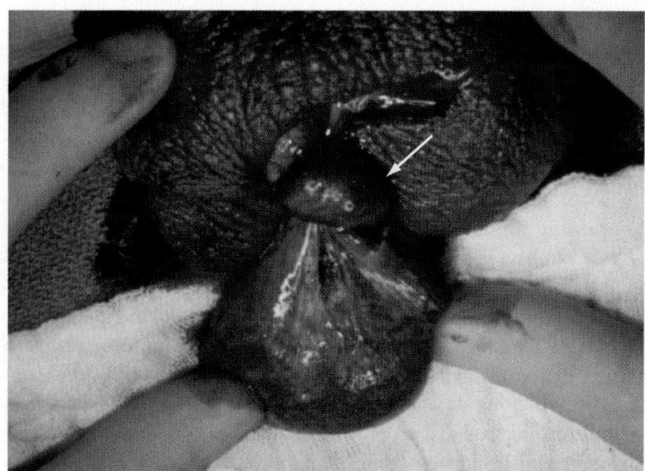

**FIGURE 73-18** Testicular torsion. Exploration through a transverse scrotal incision demonstrates the torsed cord *(top).* Note the degree of edema, erythema, and ecchymosis present following several hours of torsion.

## Gross Hematuria With Clot Retention

Asymptomatic gross hematuria without significant blood loss is not an emergency and can be evaluated electively with urine testing, upper tract imaging, and lower tract endoscopy. Severe gross hematuria with a hazardous degree of blood loss and/or urinary clot retention is potentially a surgical emergency. In certain conditions (e.g., postoperative bleeding after TURP or transurethral resection of bladder tumor [TURBT], radiation cystitis, pelvic trauma, arteriocalyceal fistula), urinary tract bleeding can be voluminous and a risk to a patient's life. If bleeding does not respond to catheter irrigation and is heavy enough to require transfusion, consideration should be given to operative intervention. This generally starts with cystoscopy and possible fulguration, which also allows one to determine the site of bleeding and pathologic process. If a patient has a significant amount of blood clot in the bladder, it will be necessary to place a large-bore irrigation catheter (in the adult, often 20 to 26 Fr) and adequately irrigate the clots from the bladder using normal saline irrigation (Figs. 73-19 and 73-20). Three-way catheters may also be useful in instituting continuous bladder irrigation, as noted. In some cases, complete evacuation of clots from the bladder is best accomplished in the operating room under anesthesia so that a rigid cystoscopy or resectoscope sheath can be placed and irrigation pursued with a piston syringe and irrigation process. It is difficult to judge the amount of blood that is being lost from the urinary tract with gross hematuria, because only a small amount of blood mixed with urine will darken the bladder efflux. If, however, copious amounts of clot are evacuated from the bladder, one should suspect at least moderate blood loss and monitor the patient with vital signs and hemoglobin measurements. Upper tract clot formation may produce a so-called *clot colic,* with renal pain similar to that experienced from passage of a stone. Supportive care and, in some cases, stent insertion may be helpful in addition to addressing the underlying problem. If unexplained, significant, gross hematuria occurs following minor trauma, one should suspect an underlying abnormality of the urinary tract, such as a neoplasm or congenital anomaly.

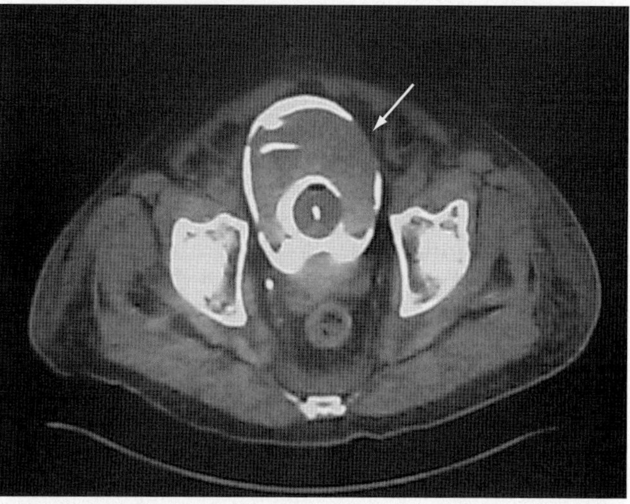

**FIGURE 73-19** CT scan of the pelvis with cystography in a patient with urinary clot retention caused by chronic hemorrhagic cystitis following radiation therapy for prostate cancer. A clot may be seen surrounding the Foley catheter balloon, with instilled contrast outlining the balloon and intact bladder wall.

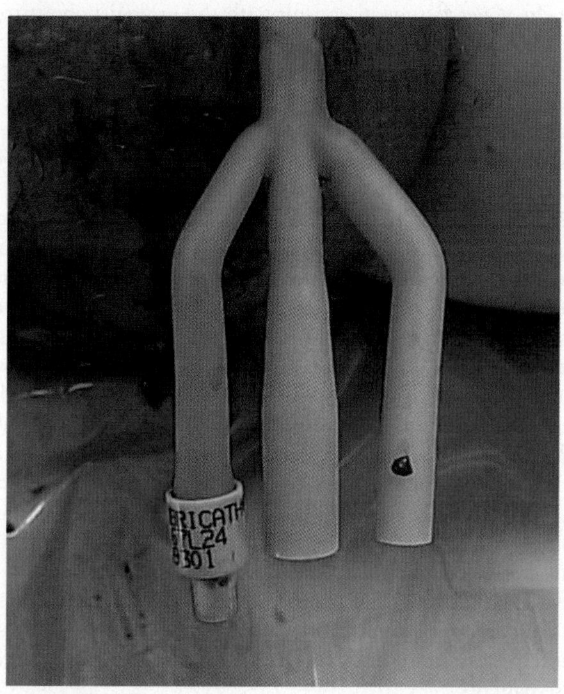

**FIGURE 73-20** Use of large-bore (24 Fr), three-way Foley catheter for initial treatment of a patient with gross hematuria following the removal of all clots from the bladder by catheter irrigation. Care must be taken to avoid overdistention of the bladder when using continuous bladder irrigation for gross hematuria because the outflow lumen can become occluded with clot material.

## Priapism

Priapism is a prolonged, unwanted, often painful penile disturbance that occurs in the absence of sexual arousal. Important causes of priapism include sickle cell disease, certain types of drug or medication use, pelvic or genital trauma, and hematologic malignancy. Priapism may resolve spontaneously but, if it persists longer than 2 to 3 hours, measures should be taken to reverse the process in most cases. Urologists classify priapism as low-flow or high-flow priapism. Low-flow priapism is typical of sickle cell patients; the sludging of blood in the corpora cavernosa results in the accumulation of dark thick material that is noted on needle aspiration when performing a percutaneous shunt. High-flow priapism is typical of that seen after penile or perineal trauma, in which a fistula develops between a central corporal artery and the vascular space within the corpus cavernosum. Aspirated blood has an arterial appearance and arterial blood gas parameters. Urologic consultation is almost always needed if priapism does not respond easily to needle aspiration with the injection of small doses of a vasoconstrictive substance such as dilute phenylephrine. For priapism related to sickle cell disease, medical treatment of the sickle crisis (e.g., hydration, oxygenation, pain management, addressing hemoglobin and transfusion status) with hematology support is a mainstay of therapy to resolve priapism. The urologist may continue irrigation and aspiration with further vasoactive injections or may proceed to a shunting procedure between the corpus cavernosum and corpus spongiosum. There are several commonly performed shunting procedures, but the technical details are beyond the scope of this discussion. It is important that the general surgeon consult with the urologist about treatment, because corporal fibrosis and loss of erectile function are risks that increase with significant delays in therapy.

## UROLOGIC ONCOLOGY

In addition to urologic trauma and related reconstructive surgery, urologic oncology is probably the specialty area of urology for which the general, plastic, vascular, or cardiothoracic surgeon is most likely to become involved as a consultant, in the planned scheduled setting or on an emergent basis. Urologic cancers may involve adjacent viscera, vasculature, and soft tissue and body wall structures so that additional surgical expertise is necessary to complete the exenterative task at hand and support reconstructive efforts. The multidisciplinary approach to modern cancer care often involves surgeons of multiple specialties when addressing complex urologic decision making. Postoperative and critical care support provided by the surgical critical care specialist are essential in ensuring favorable outcomes from complex urologic cancer surgery. The major anatomic types of urologic cancers will be discussed in this section, with a focus on the essential basic background knowledge important for the surgeon, the fundamental therapeutic approaches for various stages of cancer presentation, and the role of the surgeon in support of these patients.[29]

### Renal Tumors

With the current use of ultrasound and CT for a number of indications, most renal tumors are discovered incidentally, with the patient being asymptomatic. When signs and symptoms are present, the most typical of these are hematuria, pain, flank mass, weight loss, or constitutional symptoms stemming from metastatic disease, which is present approximately 25% of newly presenting renal cell cancers. Currently, the classic triad—flank pain, flank mass, and hematuria—is actually present in less than 10% of renal cell cancers. Underlying risk factors for renal cell carcinoma include tobacco smoking, von Hippel-Lindau syndrome (VHL), tuberous sclerosis, acquired renal cystic disease from chronic renal failure, and a number of specific genetic and familial factors. Because most (≈65% to 75%) of solid renal tumors larger than 3 cm represent renal cell carcinomas, biopsy of renal lesions prior to surgical extirpation is reserved for specific indications, such as suspicion that the lesion represents a metastasis from a nonrenal primary, or that one is dealing with an atypical renal neoplasm, such as lymphoma, minimally fat-containing angiomyolipoma, sarcoma, or pseudotumor. Renal cell carcinoma is one of the malignancies for which paraneoplastic syndromes have been well described, including hypercalcemia, anemia, Stauffer's syndrome, and erythrocyte sedimentation rate (ESR) elevation. Variants of renal cell carcinoma include clear cell, papillary, collecting duct type, medullary, and sarcomatoid. Although these histologic variants have different prognostic implications, the technical considerations relevant to the surgeon are similar.

Cystic renal masses present diagnostic challenges. Depending on specific aspects of renal cystic lesions, their risk of representing cystic malignancies must be considered.[30] The Bosniak classification system describes cystic renal masses according to their malignant risk, ranging from category I (simple cysts) to category IV (cysts associated with enhancing or solid elements). Category III and IV cysts are usually treated as representing cystic renal cell carcinomas. Various benign renal masses are also described, with the most common and important being renal adenomas, angiomyolipomas, and oncocytomas.

Evaluation for renal masses includes imaging of the primary tumor, usually with a multiphase contrast-enhanced CT scan or MRI study, and a metastatic evaluation that includes abdominal, retroperitoneal, and chest imaging. Also, based on clinical suspicion or abnormal laboratory studies, bone and brain imaging are performed.

Staging for the more common and important urologic malignancies, including renal cell carcinoma, is described in Box 73-1. The grading system for renal cell carcinoma is the Fuhrman grading system, on a scale from I to IV.

Renal cell carcinoma is primarily a surgical disease. For renal tumors that are diagnosed in the absence of metastases, or for those with a solitary metastasis, extirpative surgery is the standard approach, with resection of solitary synchronous metastases when technically feasible. With the advent of modern immunotherapy protocols and chemotherapeutic drugs such as sunitinib (a small-molecule, protein receptor tyrosine kinase inhibitor) for the treatment of metastatic renal cell carcinoma, many cancerous kidneys are currently removed (cytoreductive nephrectomy). This is done even for widely metastatic disease, assuming that the performance status of the patient justifies surgery, as part of an adjuvant treatment program.

#### Surgery for Renal Cell Carcinoma

The primary lesion of renal cell carcinoma may be treated with radical or partial nephrectomy. Recent studies comparing the achievement of a negative surgical margin and long-term local recurrence rates for partial nephrectomy (nephron-sparing surgery) versus radical nephrectomy have supported an aggressive approach to renal preservation for many cases of renal cell carcinoma. Evidence has shown that a complete tumor resection can be achieved while leaving a meaningful amount of perfused functional parenchyma with adequate collecting system drainage. Partial nephrectomy surgery may be straightforward when dealing with a small, well-encapsulated, superficial, exophytic,

**BOX 73-1 Staging of Urologic Malignancies**

**Staging of Kidney Cancer: Primary Tumor (T)**

TX: Primary tumor cannot be assessed
T0: No evidence of primary tumor
T1: Tumor ≤7 cm, limited to kidney
T2: Tumor >7 cm, limited to kidney
T3: Tumor extends into major veins, adrenal, perinephric tissue, but not beyond Gerota's fascia
T3a: Tumors with direct adrenal involvement, perinephric fat, but not beyond Gerota's fascia
T3b: Tumor extends into renal vein(s) or IVC below the diaphragm
T3c: IVC involvement above diaphragm
T4: Tumor invades beyond Gerota's fascia

**Staging of Bladder Cancer**

- Stage 0: Cancer cells are found only on the inner lining of the bladder (this stage also often called *stage Ta*).
- Stage I: Cancer cells have proliferated to the layer beyond the inner lining of the urinary bladder but not to the muscles of the urinary bladder.
- Stage II: Cancer cells have proliferated to the muscles in the bladder wall but not to the fatty tissue that surrounds the urinary bladder.
- Stage III: Cancer cells have proliferated to the fatty tissue surrounding the urinary bladder and to the prostate gland, vagina, or uterus, but not to the lymph nodes or other organs.
- Stage IV: Cancer cells have proliferated to the lymph nodes, pelvic or abdominal wall, and/or other organs.

**Staging of Prostate Cancer**

The 2002 tumor node metastases (TNM) staging system is used to stage prostate cancer, as follows:

- T: Primary tumor
- TX: Primary tumor cannot be assessed
- T0: No evidence of primary tumor
- T1: Clinically inapparent tumor not palpable or visible by imaging
- T1a: Tumor incidental histologic finding in ≤5% of tissue resected
- T1b: Tumor incidental histologic finding in >5% of tissue resected
- T1c: Tumor identified by needle biopsy (because of elevated PSA level); tumors found in one or both lobes by needle biopsy but not palpable or reliably visible by imaging
- T2: Tumor confined within prostate
- T2a: Tumor involving less than half a lobe
- T2b: Tumor involving less than or equal to one lobe
- T2c: Tumor involving both lobes
- T3: Tumor extending through the prostatic capsule; no invasion into the prostatic apex or into, but not beyond, the prostatic capsule
- T3a: Extracapsular extension (unilateral or bilateral)
- T3b: Tumor invading seminal vesicle(s)
- T4: Tumor fixed or invading adjacent structures other than seminal vesicles (e.g., bladder neck, external sphincter, rectum, levator muscles, pelvic wall)

**Staging of Testicular Cancer***

- Stage I: Cancer is found only in the testicle. Removing the testicle alone should cure the patient, although many will choose some form of additional treatment just to be sure.
- Stage II: Cancer has spread to the lymph nodes in the abdomen. Removing the testicle alone will not cure the patient, and more treatment is necessary.
- Stage III: Cancer has spread to areas above the diaphragm such as the lungs, neck, or brain. There may be also be cancer in some parts of the body such as the bones or liver. In this situation, chemotherapy is absolutely required. Surgery may also be needed.
- Stage IV: To the best of my knowledge, there is no such entity as stage IV testicular cancer. However, it is possible that the term *stage IV testicular cancer* may still be used in some places in Europe. Stage IV is probably very similar to stage III.
- Recurrent: Recurrent disease means that the cancer has come back after it has been treated. It may recur in the same place or in another part of the body.

**TNM Definitions**

Primary tumor (T): The extent of primary tumor is classified after radical orchiectomy.

- pTX: Primary tumor cannot be assessed (if no radical orchiectomy has been performed, TX is used).
- pT0: No evidence of primary tumor (e.g., histologic scar in testis)
- pTis: Intratubular germ cell neoplasia (carcinoma in situ)
- pT1: Tumor limited to testis and epididymis without lymphatic or vascular invasion
- pT2: Tumor limited to testis and epididymis with vascular or lymphatic invasion, or tumor extending through the tunica albuginea with involvement of the tunica vaginalis
- pT3: Tumor invades spermatic cord, with or without vascular or lymphatic invasion
- pT4: Tumor invades scrotum, with or without vascular or lymphatic invasion

Regional lymph nodes (N)

- NX: Regional lymph nodes cannot be assessed.
- N0: No regional lymph node metastasis
- N1: Metastasis in a single lymph node, ≤2 cm in greatest dimension
- N2: Metastasis in a single lymph node, >2 cm but not >5 cm in greatest dimension, or multiple lymph nodes, none >5 cm in greatest dimension
- N3: Metastasis in a lymph node >5 cm in greatest dimension

Distant metastasis (M)

- MX: Presence of distant metastasis cannot be assessed.
- M0: No distant metastasis
- M1: Distant metastasis
- M1a: Nonregional nodal or pulmonary metastasis
- M1b: Distant metastasis other than to nonregional nodes and lungs

*IVC,* Inferior vena cava.

*In reality, however, there are many subclasses as well, so it can become complicated. The complete TNM Staging Protocol is used by most physicians worldwide today, as defined by the American Joint Committee on Cancer (AJCC).

polar lesion, or complex when dealing with larger central lesions that involve the renal hilar structures. When a kidney contains multiple tumors or a large central tumor not amenable to partial nephrectomy, or when a partial nephrectomy presents an unreasonable level of risk with regard to postoperative hemorrhage, necrosis, or loss of collecting system integrity, radical nephrectomy is appropriate. All urologists who manage renal cell carcinoma surgically should be comfortable with radical nephrectomy and varying levels of complexity of partial nephrectomy. In many centers, many renal surgery procedures are performed laparoscopically or robotically, including complex partial nephrectomy procedures and radical nephrectomies for large tumors, when the requisite specialty expertise and technology support capabilities are available.

Whether performed through a standard open surgical approach or laparoscopic or robotic technique, the anatomic principles of radical nephrectomy are the same. Selecting an incision requires a thorough knowledge of abdominal and flank anatomy and an appreciation for the relational anatomy of the kidney when distorted by tumor. Although a midline incision is workable for renal surgery, transverse anterior abdominal, flank, or thoracoabdominal incisions may have advantages in certain situations, especially when dealing with a large upper pole mass that may be adherent to upper abdominal viscera. When working with a renal vein or inferior vena caval thrombus, additional considerations come into play, with extensive exposure to the great vessels in the uppermost abdomen or, potentially, exposure to the chest, heart, or atrium becoming necessary.

Dissection of the renal pedicle with ligation of a renal artery must precede vein ligation to prevent massive swelling, rupture, and dangerous bleeding from the kidney. The renal artery may be approached on the left side by identifying and following the aorta to the point at which the left renal vein crosses it anteriorly; the arterial pulse can often be palpated at that level and, with cautious mobilization of the vein, the artery, which typically lies posterior to the vein, can be ligated. Alternatively, the kidney, encased in Gerota's fascia, may be rotated anteriorly and the artery may be approached and ligated from a posterior approach. After determination that no accessory arteries are present (by reviewing the preoperative imaging studies and direct assessment in the operating room), the renal vein may be ligated and divided. For renal cell carcinoma, an extra-Gerotal nephrectomy is performed. That is, the entire perinephric fascial envelope containing the perinephric fat as a margin around the kidney parenchyma and tumor are excised intact. The ureter is ligated and divided where convenient. If a negative surgical margin around the tumor can be achieved and the adjacent tissues appear benign, the ipsilateral adrenal gland is generally spared whenever possible. This is certainly feasible in most cases of lower pole and midkidney lesions.

Bulky tumors may be adherent to or invade other local nonurologic structures. In these cases, adequate radical nephrectomy may require splenectomy (on the left side), distal pancreatectomy, partial resection of the colon and/or mesentery, and resection of flank musculature. On the right side, segmental or wedge resection of the liver, duodenum, colon, or other adjacent structures may be necessary. Although the need for surgical support for such adjacent organ resection efforts may be suspected on the basis of physical examination findings or preoperative imaging, loss of fat planes between adjacent organs does not necessarily predict direct adhesion or invasion. Only on operative assessment may it be possible to determine what else needs to be excised along with the kidney and Gerota's fascia. A regional lymph node dissection is often performed with a radical nephrectomy although, based on most evidence, it is more helpful as a staging and prognostic endeavor than a therapeutic one,.

If a renal vein or vena caval tumor thrombus is present, the surgical approach will vary, depending on the level of the thrombus and features of the primary tumor. The specific details of the approach to the renal vein and vena cava when a tumor thrombus is present basically relate to obtaining complete proximal and distal control of the vena cava and all major collaterals and being prepared, possibly, to deal with massive transfusion requirements, Cell Saver blood recirculation capability and, if the thrombus extends above the diaphragm or into the right atrium, cardiopulmonary bypass. Excellent descriptions of the medical challenges and surgical extirpative approaches for renal vein and vena caval thrombus resection are available in the urologic literature.[31]

In most cases, in the setting of macroscopic lymph node involvement, distant metastases, and/or cytoreductive nephrectomy, the primary goal is just to remove the involved kidney. When dealing with bilateral renal cell carcinomas, both kidneys may be addressed at the same initial operative setting, or the surgery may be staged, with a decision being made as to whether a partial nephrectomy (versus a radical nephrectomy) is feasible on one or both sides and a decision made as to which kidney to approach first. Many urologic oncologists will deal with the larger and more challenging kidney initially and then proceed with the contralateral resection if the procedure is progressing well and the patient can tolerate the additional surgery at the same setting.

For partial nephrectomy, a negative margin should be obtained with the parenchymal resection, although the trend has moved toward more emphasis on preservation of parenchyma and only a few millimeters of normal parenchyma around the tumor is often considered necessary. Various techniques for safe partial nephrectomy using laparoscopic or robotic instrumentation have been described, with the a high success rate for renal salvage and the positive margin and local recurrence rate reported as being in the acceptable range of less than 5%. The general principles for partial nephrectomy include achieving a negative surgical margin, identification and suturing of significant segmental renal vessel branches, and collecting system repair when the collecting system is entered and/or partially resected. To complete a meticulous partial nephrectomy without undue blood loss, regional hypothermia with atraumatic vascular clamping of the renal artery and surface cooling of the kidney with iced saline slush are effective. When the tumor is in a polar or peripheral lateral location, direct parenchymal compression may be adequate to provide reasonable hemostasis during partial nephrectomy without renal hypothermia. When laparoscopic or robotic approaches are used for partial nephrectomy, the same options exist (direct parenchymal compression versus renal artery clamping with a laparoscopic bulldog clamp); local hypothermia is more cumbersome to use laparoscopically and, with rapid tumor resection and clamp times of less than 30 minutes, the risk of irreversible loss of renal function with this approach is minimal. Tissue sealants, hemostatic agents, and absorbable mesh reconstruction of the kidney are all useful techniques to aid in the completion of a partial nephrectomy in the open surgical, laparoscopic, or robotic setting.

## Urothelial Cancer: Upper and Lower Tract

Urothelial carcinoma may affect any part of the urinary tract, from the renal calyces to the external urethral meatus. Cancer of the urinary bladder is the most common malignancy involving the urinary tract and represents one of the most common causes of cancer-related death in adult male patients. Most cases are diagnosed in the aging population.

The causes of many bladder and other urothelial cancers haves been well-described. Tobacco smoking is the most common identifiable cause in the Western Hemisphere. Other important contributing causative factors include chronic inflammation from indwelling catheters, stones, foreign bodies, or recurrent infection. There is a well-known association between bladder cancer and schistosomiasis, with *Schistosoma hematobium* infection being most frequently described. Certain types of industrial exposure history are also well known to cause bladder cancer; aniline dyes and various aromatic amine compounds are important culprits, as are other common chemical exposures, such as among rubber, leather, dye and petroleum workers. Cyclophosphamide (Cytoxan) exposure also is a risk factor for bladder cancer.

The most common presenting finding for bladder cancer is gross painless hematuria, which is present in over 75% of patients. Other signs or symptoms that should raise suspicion of urothelial neoplasm include chronic irritative voiding symptoms, pelvic mass and, for upper tract urothelial cancers, signs related to upper tract obstruction, such as flank pain or flank mass.

Staging of bladder cancers and upper tract urothelial malignancies relates to the depth of invasion and involvement of adjacent or remote structures. Ta disease refers to papillary tumors, with involvement of only the mucosa. T1 tumors involve the lamina propria, and T2 disease involves the detrusor muscle. Higher stages of the local tumor reflect involvement of perivesical fat or adjacent organs. The standard TNM staging system describes lymph node and distant metastatic disease. Tumors are graded (1 to 4) based on histologic and cytologic indications of aggressiveness.

Urine cytology or bladder wash cytology is highly sensitive for the diagnosis of high-grade urothelial malignancies but insensitive for low-grade papillary disease, so a negative cytology result should never dissuade one from pursuing a hematuria evaluation or other suspicious signs of potential urothelial malignancy.

The most common histology for bladder cancer is transitional cell carcinoma (TCC), comprising over 90% of cases in most populations. Squamous cell carcinoma (5% to 10%) is related to schistosomal infection, chronic inflammatory states, and smoking. It often presents with a high stage and is typically muscle-invasive at presentation. Adenocarcinoma (1% to 2% in the United States) may be urachal in origin, is typically seen at the upper bladder dome, and is also related to a history of bladder exstrophy. Any patient determined to have an adenocarcinoma of the bladder should have a complete evaluation of the gastrointestinal (GI) and other systems to ensure that the tumor has not arisen from another organ system. Adenocarcinoma of the bladder also typically presents with high grade and stage and is usually muscle-invasive on presentation. Some adenocarcinomas of the urothelium may be mucin-producing.

Most TCCs present as low-grade, noninvasive, papillary lesions, which are amenable to control with transurethral resection (TUR). A small percentage of patients with low-grade papillary bladder TCC may develop a simultaneous or metachronous upper tract tumor, so upper tract imaging should be considered at diagnosis or follow-up. Patients with low-grade papillary TCC of the bladder, after having definitive TUR, should be followed periodically with office cystoscopy and cytology because the long-term recurrence rate is approximately 50%.

Carcinoma in situ of the bladder (Tis) is a flat, high-grade neoplasm involving the mucosa. Urinary cytology is usually positive, and patients may describe irritative voiding symptoms. Cystoscopically, patients may be noted to have reddish patches or irregularity of the mucosa; it is difficult to distinguish such lesions visually from inflammatory processes so, when suspicious, bladder biopsies for histology should be obtained in addition to bladder washes for cytology. In addition to fulguration for focal lesions, standard therapy for carcinoma in situ of the bladder consists of serial Bacille Calmette-Guérin (BCG) intravesical instillations. Intravesical BCG significantly decreases the invasion and progression rate for carcinoma in situ of the bladder, compared with transurethral fulguration alone. Optimized regimens of BCG plus interferon have also been described, particularly for initial BCG unresponsiveness. Many urologists also will pursue maintenance BCG instillations over the following 2 years after an initial response.

In addition to BCG intravesical immunotherapy, various intravesical chemotherapeutic agents are available, such as mitomycin C. Mitomycin C is often instilled into the bladder immediately following standard TUR of papillary low-grade tumors (with 1-hour indwelling time), because it has been shown to decrease the risk of tumor recurrence.

For muscle-invasive bladder cancer, for select cases of problematic recurrences of high-volume noninvasive disease, and for carcinoma in situ of the bladder that has failed or recurred following intravesical therapy, radical cystectomy is the standard approach. Although the standard approach is through a midline laparotomy incision, laparoscopic cystectomy with urinary diversion subsequently being performed through a smaller incision is gaining popularity in some referral centers. Staging prior to cystectomy should involve CT of the abdomen and pelvis, preferably contrast-enhanced, chest imaging and, depending on laboratory findings or clinical suspicion, occasionally bone or brain imaging. In the male, radical cystectomy involves the removal of the entire urinary bladder en bloc with the perivesical fat, prostate, seminal vesicles, and pelvic lymph nodes. In the female, radical cystectomy typically involves en bloc removal of the female pelvic viscera, although salvage of these structures may at times be considered, depending on the details of the case. The level of aggressiveness of the nodal dissection varies among urologists, but may include internal, external iliac, and obturator nodes and may extend up to the aortic bifurcation. Bulky disease may require involvement of the general surgeon for resection of mesentery or rectosigmoid tissue. If a lesion is fixed to the pelvic sidewall and is immobile on preoperative bimanual examination, neoadjuvant chemotherapy is generally provided and, at times, radiation therapy, rather than entrance into the pelvis with the attendant morbidity and high risk of obtaining a grossly positive tumor margin.

In certain situations, a urethrectomy is also performed along with a radical cystectomy, particularly if there is extension of urothelial disease into the urethra or the presence of certain types of prostatic or prostate urothelial involvement, or bladder neck involvement in the female. If the urethra is left in situ, one must consider the possibility of delayed urethral recurrence (approximately 10% risk), and the urethra should undergo appropriate surveillance with washings and endoscopy.

There are various approaches to urinary diversion available to the urologist, including a simple ileal conduit, more complex forms of cutaneous catheterizable reservoirs with continence mechanisms, and orthotopic bladder substitution or neobladder creation, which involves anastomosis to the urethra and allows relatively normal voiding. There is an extensive and complex history involving the use of intestinal segments in the urinary tract for urinary diversion following cystectomy and in other reconstructive settings. The surgeon should be familiar with the metabolic, mechanical, and other risk factors associated with the use of intestinal segments in the reconstructed urinary tract, including electrolyte abnormalities, bone demineralization, mucus production, stone formation, chronic infection, diarrhea, vitamin $B_{12}$ deficiency, and increased cancer risk.[32]

The selection of the type of urinary diversion following cystectomy must take into account any history of pelvic radiation, the presence of renal insufficiency, liver function abnormalities, and the mechanical tasks for which the patient will be responsible.

For advanced bladder cancer, typical chemotherapy regimens are combination platinum-based, the most commonly used is MVAC (***m***ethotrexate, ***v***inblastine, ***A***driamycin [doxorubicin], ***c***isplatin) or GC (***g***emcitabine, ***c***isplatin). For patients who cannot tolerate full platinum-based regimens, modified regimens of lower potential toxicity (e.g., carboplatin) are available. The complete response and long-term disease-free survival rates for metastatic bladder cancer are low.

For upper tract TCC, the standard treatment is surgical resection. For low-grade papillary lesions of the ureter or renal pelvis, endoscopic ablation may be attempted using a ureteroscopic or percutaneous nephroscopic approach and electroresection or laser ablation procedures. For bulkier or more invasive lesions of the upper urinary tract, the standard approach is complete nephroureterectomy, including the entire ipsilateral ureter with the ureteral orifice. For lesions involving the lower ureter only, distal ureterectomy with ureteral reimplantation into the bladder is appropriate therapy, as long as more proximal disease has been definitively excluded through imaging and endoscopic assessment. Laparoscopic approaches have been developed for the surgical management of upper tract TCC, including laparoscopic nephroureterectomy, along with cystoscopically guided and electroresection-based mobilization of the ureteral orifice and intramural ureter. For high-grade, aggressive, upper tract TCC, especially if there is a high suspicion of extrarenal or extraurethral disease, neoadjuvant chemotherapy is typically offered prior to any surgical extirpative procedure.

## Prostate Cancer

Cancer of the prostate is the most common noncutaneous malignancy and the second most common cause of cancer-related deaths in men in the United States. Nevertheless, many prostate cancers are never diagnosed and are likely to be clinically insignificant. The challenge facing the urologist is in diagnosing clinically significant cancers accurately and treating them effectively while avoiding the unnecessary morbidity of treating clinically insignificant cancers. Much contemporary clinical and basic research has gone into distinguishing among these entities.

Most prostate cancers present in men older than 60 years. The vast majority of newly diagnosed cancers found on prostate-specific antigen (PSA) screening or digital rectal examination (DRE) and are asymptomatic at the time of diagnosis. Factors that are thought to increase prostate cancer risk include a family history of prostate cancer, particularly when present in an individual's father or brothers, advancing age, and African American heritage.

Prostate cancer may be discovered incidentally during radical cystectomy for bladder cancer or at the time of prostate resection procedures for benign prostatic hyperplasia. Most prostate cancers are adenocarcinomas (≈95%). Other malignant neoplasms include TCC invading the prostate, sarcomas, lymphomas, and neuroendocrine tumors. Most prostate cancers arise in the peripheral zone of the gland.

Screening for prostate cancer is recommended by the American Cancer Society and American Urologic Association. Studies are ongoing that will further address the value of screening programs and policies. Much of the available evidence supports the contention that PSA and DRE screening improve survival, although there is some controversy. Standard screening should be considered in all men older than 50 years. For men with elevated risk factors (e.g., African American, family history, worrisome symptoms), screening should commence at age 40 or 45 years. PSA screening in contemporary practice uses an age-specific, normal-range approach. Men younger than 50 years should have a PSA level less than 2.5 ng/mL and younger than 60, less than 3.5 ng/mL, with corresponding increases per decade. Serum PSA level testing is also often ordered to obtain the total and percentage of free PSA, because the percentage of free PSA has important predictive value for gauging the risk of having or developing prostate cancer. A percentage of free PSA exceeding 25% suggests less than a 10% risk of having prostate cancer, whereas a percentage of free PSA less than 10% may predict as high as a 50% risk of cancer.

The concept of PSA velocity is also useful for gauging the risk of prostate cancer. If the total PSA increases more than 0.75 U/year, the patient should be assessed for a possible increased risk of prostate cancer. These findings also assist the urologist in determining when and whether to rebiopsy patients with a negative biopsy, and how suspicious they should be of occult disease. Most urologists cease annual PSA screening at an advanced age (typically, by 80 years), although an individualized approach is appropriate based on medical comorbidities. Prostate biopsy is generally done in the office using a transrectal ultrasound (TRUS)–guided procedure, performed under local or regional anesthesia, and usually with a transrectal approach. In certain cases, a transperineal approach is used. The standard biopsy template involves 12 cores with a spring-loaded biopsy instrument, obtaining tissue from the base, mid, and apex regions, medially and laterally, and from the left and right sides. Prophylactic antibiotics are routinely administered, cleansing enemas are often advised, and ceasing anticoagulants is desirable when feasible. Common adverse events following TRUS biopsy include rectal bleeding and gross hematuria, both usually self-limiting. Fever and urinary infection and retention occur in less than 5% of patients; urosepsis occurs, but is rare (<1%). Occasionally, rectal bleeding may be troublesome and require proctoscopy, fulguration, and suturing of the bleeding sites in the rectal wall. Approximately two thirds of prostate cancers are hypoechoic on TRUS, but approximately one third have the ultrasound appearance of normal prostatic parenchyma.

Important findings that may be noted on histologic examination of biopsy specimens include cancer (graded using the Gleason grading system, on a scale of 1 to 5), prostatic intraepithelial neoplasia (PIN, which has premalignant potential in some patients), atrophy, and inflammation. The Gleason score is the sum of the two highest and most prominent grades observed (e.g., Gleason 3 + 4, score = 7). If a positive biopsy for cancer is obtained, staging may be appropriate, particularly if the cancer has any high-grade foci (Gleason grade 4 or 5), the PSA level is markedly elevated (>10 ng/mL), there is suspicion by DRE or TRUS of extracapsular extension, or there is any clinical suspicion of metastatic disease. Staging typically includes CT of the abdomen and pelvis and a nuclear medicine bone scan, because the local lymph nodes and bone are important early metastatic sites for prostate cancer.

Treatment decision making is largely based on whether the disease is thought to be localized to the prostate (and therefore locally curable) and whether the patient's age and medical status justify an aggressive treatment approach, considering the anticipated natural history of the disease. For localized disease, standard forms of therapy include watchful waiting, radical prostatectomy (open, laparoscopic, or more commonly today in the United States, robotic-assisted laparoscopic prostatectomy [RALP]), or local radiotherapy via external beam conformal therapy or interstitial radiotherapy using one of several available isotopes. For advanced disease, androgen ablation therapy is often used, generally via luteinizing hormone-releasing hormone (LHRH) agonists or, less commonly done today, via a bilateral simple orchiectomy.

The ideal candidate for watchful waiting has a low PSA level, a low-grade, low-volume tumor, and little chance of progressing based on age and medical status. Such patients should have regular examinations and periodic serum PSA level measurements; they may be advised to undergo rebiopsy to determine if their cancer is evolving to a higher grade or volume status over time.

Radical prostatectomy (RP), regardless of the approach, involves the complete removal of the prostate and seminal vesicles through an anterior surgical approach. When technically feasible and oncologically appropriate, a nerve-sparing approach is used, which avoids injury to the cavernous nerves that run posterolaterally along the prostate in the neurovascular bundle and mediate penile erection. Important landmarks for RP are the dorsal venous plexus anteriorly, bladder neck cephalad, prostatomembranous urethral junction distally, and rectal wall posteriorly. The correct plane of posterior dissection in RP is just posterior to the Denonvilliers' fascia. Rectal injury is an uncommon but known risk during RP and may prompt intraoperative general surgical consultation if it occurs. In most cases, these injuries can be successfully managed with primary closure and without colostomy diversion unless there has been prior radiation to the region. Laparoscopic prostatectomy and RALP may be performed through a transperitoneal or extraperitoneal approach, although the transperitoneal approach is most commonly used in the United States. RALP seems to involve a somewhat more rapid postoperative recovery and often results in less blood loss and decreased transfusion requirements compared with traditional open surgery. The anastomotic technique in RALP is usually a running, monofilament suture, as opposed to the interrupted anastomotic technique commonly used in the open RP.

Patients with localized prostate cancer may select radiation therapy—external beam therapy (XRT) or permanent or temporary brachytherapy. Other forms of treatment that can be considered for local treatment of prostate cancer include cryotherapy and proton beam therapy, although long-term results for these modalities are still being reported.

Following prostate cancer therapy, patients are monitored for post-treatment morbidities (e.g., continence, erectile function, voiding adequacy) and possible cancer recurrence. The latter involves PSA testing and potentially repeat metastatic evaluation, when indicated. If a patient has a positive surgical margin after RP, he may be referred for postoperative XRT or, at times, observed for signs of a PSA recurrence. If postoperative XRT is planned, it is usually delayed for approximately 6 weeks until initial recovery of continence is observed. Long-term follow-up for prostate cancer patients should continue at least 10 years, if not permanently, because very late recurrences can occur. If the PSA level becomes significantly detectable or is rising after definitive treatment, it may be appropriate to consider repeat TRUS of the anastomotic region, possibly with rebiopsy, and repeat metastatic evaluation to decide whether to proceed with local XRT, androgen ablation therapy, or observation. In advanced prostate cancer, androgen deprivation therapy may become ineffective, with clinical and/or PSA progression observed in spite of appropriate hormonal therapy. In these cases, second-line treatment includes antiandrogens, chemotherapy, and investigational agents.

## Testicular Cancer

Curative treatment for testicular cancer is one of the great success stories of modern oncology. The vast majority of testicular tumors represent germ cell tumors (>90%); interstitial cell (Leydig, Sertoli cell) tumors, other malignant lesions (lymphoma, metastatic lesions) and benign lesions represent less than 10% of lesions. Any solid intratesticular mass is likely to represent a malignant germ cell tumor and is typically treated as such unless there is a strong suspicion to the contrary.

Malignant germ cell tumors are categorized as seminomas or nonseminomatous tumors. Seminomas are mostly of the classic or typical variety (85%); less common are anaplastic seminomas (10%) and spermatocytic (5%) varieties. Spermatocytic seminomas typically present in older men. Nonseminomatous tumor types include embryonal carcinoma, yolk sac tumor (presenting in infants and children), choriocarcinoma, and teratoma; each of these may manifest in pure form or as a mixed tumor type. The non–germ cell tumors are usually nonmalignant; less than 10% of Leydig or Sertoli cell tumors are considered malignant. Intratubular germ cell neoplasia (ICGN, or carcinoma in situ of the testis) is an important entity to delineate by histology. It often accompanies malignant tumors and may also be found in the palpably normal, contralateral testis on biopsy, in which case it often prompts the initiation of radiotherapy to prevent a gross tumor from forming contralaterally in the future.

Risk factors for the development of germ cell tumors include an undescended testis and cryptorchidism. The risk is greatest with the intra-abdominal undescended testis; there is a lower risk, but still elevated, in testes located in a groin position. Various intersex abnormalities are also risk factors for germ cell tumor. HIV infection is thought to be a risk factor for testicular cancer. It is controversial whether testicular atrophy of a benign cause elevates germ cell tumor risk.

Patients typically present with a painless enlargement, heaviness, or mass involving the testis. On examination, a nontender mass is usually appreciable. Any scrotal mass lesion that cannot be definitively determined to be benign on physical examination should undergo scrotal ultrasound. Patients who have a hydrocele or other cystic lesion of the scrotal contents should also undergo ultrasound if the testis cannot be definitively palpated and determined to be entirely normal. Other lesions of the scrotal contents that may at times be difficult to distinguish from a testis tumor include epididymo-orchitis, epididymal tumors (usually benign), torsion, and trauma. Patients may also manifest constitutional symptoms related to metastatic disease, such as back pain, pulmonary symptoms, weight loss, or abdominal mass.

Patients with seminoma are 30 to 40 years old; nonseminomatous tumor patients often present at younger ages (25 to 35 years). Yolk sac tumors manifest in infants or children younger than 10 years. Lymphomas of the testis usually are seen in men older than 50 years.

Metastatic disease from testicular cancer typically follows a predictable retroperitoneal lymphatic path, although choriocarcinoma is notorious for hematogenous spread early to distant sites. From the right testis, initial lymph node metastasis is to the pericaval, and interaortocaval nodes; on the left, to left para-aortic nodes, and then on to other retroperitoneal nodal levels on either side. If the patient has had prior groin or pelvic surgery, the natural lymphatic distributions may be altered and the metastatic pattern may be unpredictable, potentially leading to involvement of the inguinal or pelvic nodes. Distant metastases are typically seen to the lung, liver, brain, bone, kidney, and adrenal gland. The likelihood of a man's presenting with metastatic disease is approximately 20% for seminoma and higher (30% to 60%) with nonseminomatous tumors.

Testis tumor patients should undergo complete metastatic evaluation. This includes complete laboratory studies with serum tumor markers (β-human chorionic gonadotropin [hCG], alpha-fetoprotein [AFP], lactate dehydrogenase [LDH]), and CT scanning of the chest, abdomen, and pelvis, preferably prior to orchiectomy to avoid postsurgical artifacts. Bone and/or brain imaging would be included based on suspicion in individual cases, although brain imaging should be performed for all choriocarcinomas. The staging approach uses the standard TNM system.

The standard tumor markers noted are particularly useful in managing testicular cancer. On the basis of their predictable half-lives, one can gain information regarding metastatic disease and also follow patients with precision after definitive treatment. The half-life of β-hCG is 24 to 36 hours; for AFP, it is 5 to 7 days. Patients are categorized into risk categories based on their histology, staging, and sites of disease.

The standard initial treatment for testicular tumors is a radical inguinal orchiectomy (Fig. 73-21). This is performed through a groin incision, with mobilization of the spermatic cord from within the inguinal canal and mobilization of the testis from the scrotum within the intact parietal tunica vaginalis sac. It is important not to enter the tunica vaginalis inadvertently during the mobilization, because there is a small risk of tumor spillage or contamination of the wound with malignant cells from a surrounding hydrocele. The spermatic cord is ligated high at the level of the internal inguinal ring; a permanent marking suture should be left at that level as a landmark in case further

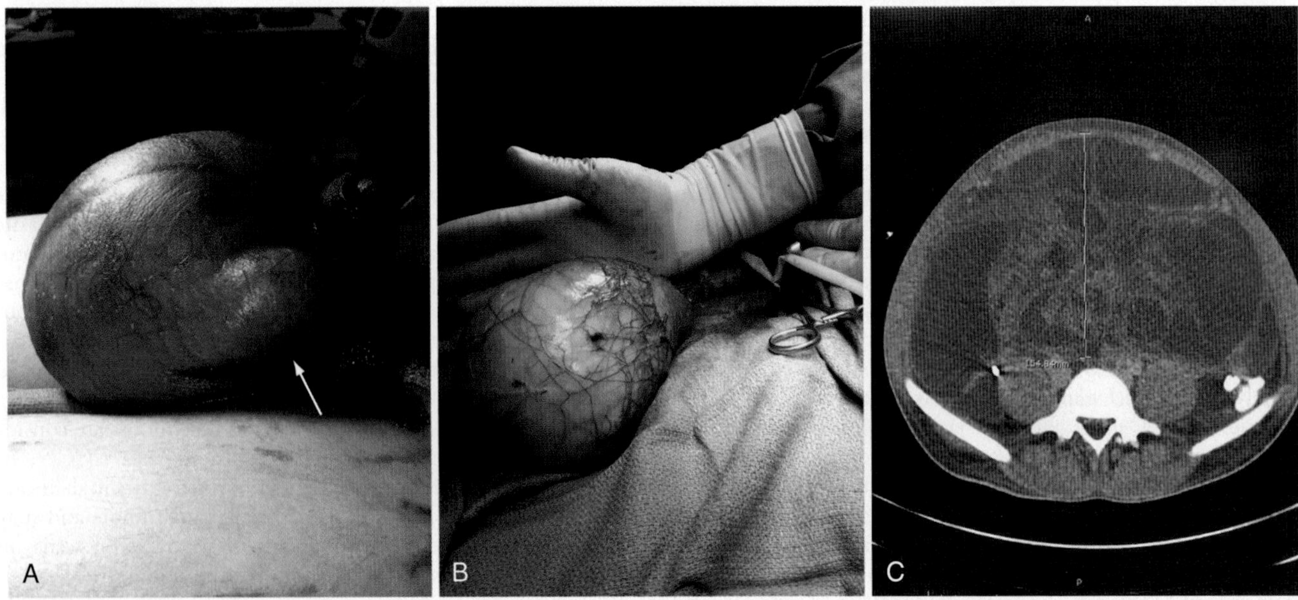


**FIGURE 73-21** Advanced testicular carcinoma. **A,** Preoperative appearance of the scrotum in a patient with a large right testis tumor. The normal left testis is seen pushed cephalad by the right-sided mass. **B,** Surgical exploration through right inguinal incision, showing the right testis that has been dissected from the scrotum in an extravaginal plane, still attached by the spermatic cord pedicle to the right. **C,** Massive retroperitoneal lymphadenopathy in the same patient. Note that the descending colon is opacified with contrast, but all other viscera are pushed cephalad so that no small intestine is seen in this image. The patient was managed with primary chemotherapy following by retroperitoneal lymphadenectomy for the residual mass.

surgery with cord stump removal is indicated. Trans-scrotal biopsy of the contralateral testis may be considered in certain cases, particularly if the patient is known to be azoospermic or severely oligospermic, the other testis is atrophic or has a history of corrected cryptorchidism, or compliance with regular follow-up is unlikely.

Following orchiectomy, further treatment depends on the histology, risk category, stage of disease, and patient preferences. Further treatment may consist of regular surveillance, retroperitoneal radiation therapy, retroperitoneal lymphadenectomy (RPLND), systemic chemotherapy, or a multimodal therapy approach. The decision making is complex, is still evolving, and is beyond the scope of this discussion, but several general principles apply:

- For seminoma stage I disease, one must decide among surveillance, radiation to regional lymph nodes (25 to 30 Gy), or limited prophylactic chemotherapy. Seminoma is a radiosensitive tumor but the radiation has potential morbidity, with a risk of delayed secondary malignancy as high as 15% within 25 years of treatment.
- For nonseminoma stage I disease, the options include RPLND, surveillance, and chemotherapy.
- For seminoma stage II, abdominal radiation therapy is typically favored; for stage IIC or III, platinum-based chemotherapy is offered.
- For nonseminoma stage IIA or IIB, RPLND is most often recommended; chemotherapy is recommended for stage IIC or III disease.

Standard, commonly used chemotherapy regimens for metastatic testicular cancer include BEP (***b***leomycin, ***e***toposide, cis***p***latin). If one elects to proceed with RPLND, this can be accomplished through an open surgical or laparoscopic approach (requiring advanced skill) using a standard dissection template and, when possible, a nerve-sparing approach to preserve ejaculatory function. The general surgeon may become involved in these procedures based on the need to deal with involved viscera or severe adhesions to major abdominal vasculature; this is particularly relevant in the post-XRT or postchemotherapy setting, in which severe desmoplastic reaction may be encountered. Dense adhesions between a residual nodal mass and the wall of the aorta are frequently encountered following chemotherapy, at times requiring great vessel excision and replacement. Liver mesenteric involvement and other complexities of the abnormal retroperitoneal anatomy may require general surgical or vascular surgical expertise and should be preplanned whenever possible. Many patients undergoing RPLND will have been exposed to bleomycin chemotherapy, which requires meticulous intraoperative anesthetic management because of the exquisite sensitivity of these patients to elevated oxygen exposure; often, the anesthetic is run essentially on room air ventilation in these cases.

Following orchiectomy and prior to any additional therapy for testicular cancer, consideration should be given to preservation of fertility. Patients should be made aware of the potential impact of radiation, chemotherapy, or RPLND on the ability to ejaculate and on spermatogenesis. It is essential that patients be offered sperm cryopreservation prior to therapies that could adversely affect their reproductive potential.

Overall, long-term survival for testicular cancer ranges from 98% to 99% for stage I seminoma or nonseminoma to 40% to 80% for stage II or III seminoma or nonseminoma.

## Penile, Urethral, and Other Genital Malignancies

Other less common genitourinary neoplasms will occasionally require the involvement of the general surgeon. Penile cancer is an uncommon malignancy, generally squamous cell histologically, and often associated with the uncircumcised state, chronic phimosis, and local infection. Chronic infection with human papillomavirus (HPV) has been implicated in many cases. The mainstay of therapy is local excisional control of the primary lesion by circumcision, if isolated to the prepuce, distal penectomy, or radical penectomy. For invasive lesions, inguinal lymphadenectomy may be advised. This dissection may expose the femoral vessels, which requires local flap coverage, typically using the medially rotated sartorius muscle. The surgeon may need to assist with vascular repair or dissection.

Urethral cancer is more common in women than in men, but is often seen in association with chronic inflammatory states or with urethral stricture disease in men. Transitional cell carcinoma may be seen in the most proximal urethra; most bulbar and distal male urethral cancers are squamous cell. Local control may involve partial or total urethrectomy and sometimes an aggressive en bloc resection of the external genitalia, with cystoprostatectomy and partial pubectomy.

Squamous cell cancers of the scrotum were first described in chimney sweeps because of the carcinogenic effects of inspissated soot. Local excision is the mainstay of therapy.

## REFERENCES


1. Wein AJ, Kavoussi LR, Novick AC, et al, editors: Campbell-Walsh urology, ed 9, New York, 2007, Elsevier.
2. Shin D, Lipshultz LI, Goldstein M, et al: Herniorrhaphy with polypropylene mesh causing inguinal vasal obstruction: A preventable cause of obstructive azoospermia. Ann Surg 241:553–558, 2005.
3. Dudea SM, Ciurea A, Chiorean A, Botar-Jid C: Doppler applications in testicular and scrotal disease. Med Ultrason 12:43–51, 2010.
4. Bader MS, Hawboldt J, Brooks A: Management of complicated urinary tract infections in the era of antimicrobial resistance. Postgrad Med 122:7–15, 2010.
5. Coburn M, Zimmerman JL: Sepsis and septic shock in the urology patient. AUA Update Series 21:Lesson 14, 2002.
6. Weedin JW, Coburn M, Link RE: The impact of proximal stone burden on the management of encrusted and retained ureteral stents. J Urol 185:542–547, 2011.
7. Mokabberi R, Ravakhah K: Emphysematous urinary tract infections: Diagnosis, treatment and survival (case review series). Am J Med Sci 333:111–116, 2007.
8. Brix AE: Renal papillary necrosis. Toxicol Pathol 30:672–674, 2002.
9. Korkes F, Favoretto RL, Bróglio M, et al: Xanthogranulomatous pyelonephritis: Clinical experience with 41 cases. Urology 71:178–180, 2008.
10. Raynor MC, Carson CC, 3rd: Urinary infections in men. Med Clin North Am 95:43–54, 2011.
11. Koukouras D, Kallidonis P, Panagopoulos C, et al: Fournier's gangrene, a urologic and surgical emergency: Presentation of a multi-institutional experience with 45 cases. Urol Int 86:167–172, 2011.
12. Hollenbach E: To treat or not to treat—critically ill patients with candiduria. Mycoses 51:(Suppl 2):12–24, 2008.

13. Wise GJ, Marella VK: Genitourinary manifestations of tuberculosis. Urol Clin North Am 30:111–121, 2003.
14. Coburn M: Urologic manifestations of HIV infection. AIDS Res Hum Retroviruses 14:S23–S25, 1998.
15. Gomelsky A, Dmochowski RR: Treatment of mixed urinary incontinence in women. Curr Opin Obstet Gynecol 23:371–375, 2011.
16. McGuire EJ: Urodynamics of the neurogenic bladder. Urol Clin North Am 37:507–516, 2010.
17. McVary KT, Roehrborn CG, Avins AL, et al: Update on AUA guideline on the management of benign prostatic hyperplasia. J Urol 185(5):1793–1803, 2011.
18. Lipshultz LI, Howards SS, Niederberger CS, editors: Infertility in the male, ed 4, Cambridge, England, 2009, Cambridge University Press.
19. Albersen M, Orabi H, Lue TF: Evaluation and treatment of erectile dysfunction in the aging male: A mini-review. Gerontology 2011 (Epub ahead of print).
20. Eisner BH, McQuaid JW, Hyams E, Matlaga BR: Nephrolithiasis: What surgeons need to know. AJR Am J Roentgenol 196:1274–1278, 2011.
21. Coburn M: Genitourinary trauma. In Feliciano D, Mattox K, Moore E, editors: Trauma, ed 7, New York, 2011, McGraw Hill, in press.
22. Coburn M, Guerriero WG: Complications of genitourinary trauma. In Mattox KL, editor: Complications of trauma, New York, 1994, Churchill Livingstone.
23. Coburn M: Damage control for urologic injuries. Surg Clin North Am 77:821–834, 1977.
24. Santucci RA, Wessels H, Bartsch G, et al: Consensus on genitourinary trauma. Evaluation and management of renal injuries: Consensus statement of the renal trauma subcommittee. Br J Urol 93:937, 2004.
25. Chapple C, Barbagli G, Jordan G, et al: Consensus on genitourinary trauma. Consensus statement on urethral trauma. Br J Urol 93:1195, 2004.
26. Gomez RG, Ceballos L, Coburn M, et al: Consensus on genitourinary trauma. Consensus statement on bladder injuries. Br J Urol 94:27, 2004.
27. Brandes S, Coburn M, Armenakas N, et al: Consensus on genitourinary trauma. Diagnosis and management of ureteric injury: An evidence-based analysis. Br J Urol 94:277, 2004.
28. Morey AF, Metro MJ, Carney KJ, et al: Consensus on genitourinary trauma. Consensus on genitourinary trauma: External genitalia. Br J Urol 94:507, 2004.
29. Vogelzang NJ, Scardino PT, Shipley WU, et al, editors: Comprehensive textbook of genitourinary oncology, ed 3, Philadelphia, 2005, Lippincott Williams & Wilkins.
30. McGuire BB, Fitzpatrick JM: The diagnosis and management of complex renal cysts. Curr Opin Urol 20:349–354, 2010.
31. Pouliot F, Shuch B, Larochelle JC, et al: Contemporary management of renal tumors with venous tumor thrombus. J Urol 184:833–841, 2010.
32. Gerharz EW, Turner WH, Kälble T, Woodhouse CR: Metabolic and functional consequences of urinary reconstruction with bowel. BJU Int 91:143–149, 2003.

# INDEX



Note: Page numbers followed by "f" refer to illustrations; page numbers followed by "t" refer to tables; page numbers followed by "b" refer to boxes.

## C

## E

## F

## G

## H

## M

## Q



## R

## V

## X



## Y



## Z